EXPERT

D1384634

# 2018

# ICD-10-CM Expert for Hospitals

The complete official code set

Codes valid October 1, 2017 through September 30, 2018

## Publisher's Notice

The *ICD-10-CM Expert for Hospitals: The Complete Official Code Set* is designed to be an accurate and authoritative source regarding coding and every reasonable effort has been made to ensure accuracy and completeness of the content. However, Optum360 makes no guarantee, warranty, or representation that this publication is accurate, complete, or without errors. It is understood that Optum360 is not rendering any legal or other professional services or advice in this publication and that Optum360 bears no liability for any results or consequences that may arise from the use of this book.

## Acknowledgments

Lauri Gray, RHIT, CPC, AHIMA-approved ICD-10-CM/PCS Trainer, *Product Manager*
Karen Schmidt, BSN, *Technical Director*
Anita Schmidt, BS, RHIT, AHIMA-approved ICD-10-CM/PCS Trainer, *Clinical Technical Editor*
Anne Kenney, BA, MBA, CCA, CCS, *Clinical Technical Editor*
Karen Krawzik, RHIT, CCS, AHIMA-approved ICD-10-CM/PCS Trainer, *Clinical Technical Editor*
Peggy Willard, CCS, AHIMA-approved ICD-10-CM/PCS Trainer, *Clinical Technical Editor*
Leanne Patterson, CPC, *Clinical Technical Editor*
Stacy Perry, *Manager, Desktop Publishing*
Lisa Singley, *Project Manager*
Tracy Betzler, *Senior Desktop Publishing Specialist*
Hope M. Dunn, *Senior Desktop Publishing Specialist*
Katie Russell, *Desktop Publishing Specialist*
Kate Holden, *Editor*

## Our Commitment to Accuracy

Optum360 is committed to producing accurate and reliable materials.

To report corrections, please visit www.optum360coding.com/accuracy or email accuracy@optum.com. You can also reach customer service by calling 1.800.464.3649, option 1.

## Anita Schmidt, BS, RHIT, AHIMA-approved ICD-10-CM/PCS Trainer

Ms. Schmidt has expertise in Level I Adult and Pediatric Trauma hospital coding, specializing in ICD-9-CM, ICD-10-CM/PCS, DRG, and CPT coding. Her experience includes analysis of medical record documentation, assignment of ICD-10-CM and PCS codes, DRG validation, as well as CPT code assignments for same-day surgery cases. She has conducted coding training and auditing, including DRG validation, conducted electronic health record training, and worked with clinical documentation specialists to identify documentation needs and potential areas for physician education. Most recently she has been developing content for resource and educational products related to ICD-10-CM and ICD-10-PCS. Ms. Schmidt is an AHIMA-approved ICD-10-CM/PCS trainer, and is an active member of the American Health Information Management Association (AHIMA) and the Minnesota Health Information Management Association (MHIMA).

## Anne Kenney, BA, MBA, CCA, CCS

Ms. Kenney has expertise in ICD-10-CM/PCS, ICD-9-CM, DRG, and CPT coding. Most recently she has been developing content for ICD-10-CM and ICD-10-PCS applications. Her prior experience in a major teaching hospital includes assignment of ICD-9-CM codes and DRGs, CPT code assignments, and determining physician evaluation and management levels for inpatient, emergency department, and observation cases. Ms. Kenney is an active member of the American Health Information Management Association (AHIMA) and the Minnesota Health Information Management Association (MHIMA).

## Peggy Willard, CCS, AHIMA-approved ICD-10-CM/PCS Trainer

Ms. Willard's expertise is ICD-10-CM and PCS including in-depth analysis of medical record documentation, ICD-10-CM/PCS code and DRG assignment. In recent years she has been responsible for the creation and development of several print products and e-books designed to assist with appropriate application of ICD-10-CM and PCS coding system. Ms. Willard has several years of prior experience in Level I Adult and Pediatric Trauma hospital coding, specializing in ICD-9-CM, DRG, and CPT coding with emphasis in conducting coding audits, and conducting coding training for coding staff and clinical documentation specialists. Ms. Willard is an active member of the American Health Information Management Association (AHIMA) and the Minnesota Health Information Management Association (MHIMA).

> Let Optum360 help you find the best product for your needs.

Together with you, Optum360® can help drive financial results across your organization with industry-leading resources that cut through the complexity of medical coding challenges.

**Let us help you find the best coding solution, at the best price.**

Contact your Medallion representative directly or call Customer Service at 1-800-464-3649, option 1.

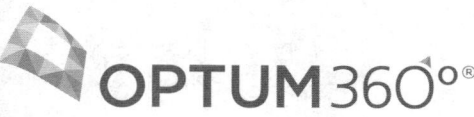

# Optum360 Learning

## Earn your CEUs with US

You've worked hard for your coding credentials, and now you need an easy way to maintain your certification.

Optum360® offers the most complete training in the marketplace, designed to address exactly what you and your organization need. We offer eLearning courses you can take online at your desk; you can invite a specialist to your office for on-the-job preparation; or ask our consulting professionals to create a tailor-made program specific for your organization.

Our strategy is simple — education must be concise, relevant and accurate. Choose the delivery method that works best for you:

- **eLearning:** Web-based courses offered at the most convenient times for your learners. eLearning courses are interactive, task-focused and developed around practical scenarios. These self-paced courses include "try-it" functionality, knowledge checks and downloadable resources.

- **Instructor-led training (ILT):** On-site or remote courses, built specifically for your organization.

- **Webinars:** Online courses, geared toward a broad market of learners, delivered in a live or recorded setting.

- **Podcasts and videos:** Physician-focused online courses available when and where convenient.

## NO MATTER HOW YOU CHOOSE TO EARN YOUR CEUs, OPTUM360 IS HERE TO HELP YOU.

 VISIT

**optum360coding.com/learning**

 CALL

**1-800-464-3649, option 1**

# OPTUM360°®

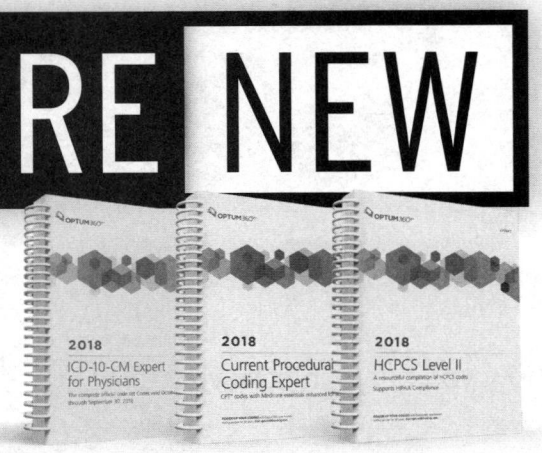

RE NEW

It's time to renew your Optum360 coding tools.

## SAVE UP TO 25%*

when you renew your 2018 coding essentials.

| ITEM # | TITLE<br>INDICATE THE ITEMS YOU WISH TO PURCHASE | QUANTITY | PRICE<br>PER PRODUCT | TOTAL |
|---|---|---|---|---|
| | | | | |
| | | | | |
| | | | | |
| | | | | |
| | | | | |
| | | Subtotal | | |
| | (AK, DE, HI, MT, NH & OR are exempt) | Sales Tax | | |
| | 1 item $10.95 • 2–4 items $12.95 • 5+ CALL | Shipping & Handling | | |
| | | TOTAL AMOUNT ENCLOSED | | |

## Save up to 25% when you renew.

**PROMO CODE: RENEW18B**

Visit **optum360coding.com** and enter the promo code above.

Call **1-800-464-3649, option 1,** and mention the promo code above.

Fax this order form with purchase order to **1-801-982-4033.** *Optum360 no longer accepts credit cards by fax.*

Mail this order form with payment and/or purchase order to: **Optum360, PO Box 88050, Chicago, IL 60680-9920.** *Optum360 no longer accepts credit cards by mail.*

Name _____

Address _____

_____

Customer Number _____  Contact Number _____

○ CHECK ENCLOSED (PAYABLE TO OPTUM360)

○ BILL ME  ○ P.O.# _____

( ___ ) _____
Telephone
( ___ ) _____
Fax
_____ @ _____
E-mail

Optum360 respects your right to privacy. We will not sell or rent your email address or fax number to anyone outside Optum360 and its business partners. If you would like to remove your name from Optum360 promotions, please call 1-800-464-3649, option 1.

*Save 20% when you order by phone, fax or mail; save 25% when you order online. Save 15% on AMA and custom fee products. Offer excludes digital coding tools, workers' comp and bookstore products.

# Contents

# Preface

## ICD-10-CM Official Preface

This FY 2018 update of the International Statistical Classification of Diseases and Related Health Problems, 10th revision, Clinical Modification (ICD-10-CM) is being published by the United States government in recognition of its responsibility to promulgate this classification throughout the United States for morbidity coding. The International Statistical Classification of Diseases and Related Health Problems, 10th Revision (ICD-10), published by the World Health Organization (WHO), is the foundation of ICD-10-CM. ICD-10 continues to be the classification used in cause-of-death coding in the United States. The ICD-10-CM is comparable with the ICD-10. The WHO Collaborating Center for the Family of International Classifications in North America, housed at the Centers of Disease Control and Prevention's National Center for Health Statistics (NCHS), has responsibility for the implementation of ICD and other WHO-FIC classifications and serves as a liaison with the WHO, fulfilling international obligations for comparable classifications and the national health data needs of the United States. The historical background of ICD and ICD-10 can be found in the Introduction to the International Classification of Diseases and Related Health Problems (ICD-10), 2010, World Health Organization, Geneva, Switzerland.

ICD-10-CM is the United States' clinical modification of the World Health Organization's ICD-10. The term "clinical" is used to emphasize the modification's intent: to serve as a useful tool in the area of classification of morbidity data for indexing of health records, medical care review, and ambulatory and other health care programs, as well as for basic health statistics. To describe the clinical picture of the patient the codes must be more precise than those needed only for statistical groupings and trend analysis.

## Characteristics of ICD-10-CM

ICD-10-CM far exceeds its predecessors in the number of concepts and codes provided. The disease classification has been expanded to include health-related conditions and to provide greater specificity at the 6th and 7th character level. The 6th and 7th characters are not optional and are intended for use in recording the information documented in the clinical record.

ICD-10-CM extensions, interpretations, modifications, addenda, or errata other than those approved by the Centers for Disease Control and Prevention are not to be considered official and should not be utilized. Continuous maintenance of the ICD-10- CM is the responsibility of the aforementioned agencies. However, because the ICD-10-CM represents the best in contemporary thinking of clinicians, nosologists, epidemiologists, and statisticians from both public and private sectors, when future modifications are considered, advice will be sought from all stakeholders.

All official authorized addenda since the last complete update (October 1, 2017) have been included in this revision. For more detailed information please see the complete official authorized addenda to ICD-10-CM, including the "ICD-10-CM Official Guidelines for Coding and Reporting," and a description of the ICD-10-CM updating and maintenance process.

## Official Updates

The National Center for Health Statistics (NCHS), a section of the Centers for Disease Control and Prevention (CDC), is the agency charged with maintaining and updating ICD-10-CM. The 2018 official addendum was posted to the Centers for Medicare and Medicaid Services (CMS) website on June 13, 2017, identifying the changes to the ICD-10-CM code set for fiscal 2018. A summary of changes is provided below:

- 360 new codes added
- 226 code descriptions revised
- 34 codes changed from valid to invalid

**Note:** Validity changes are the result of new codes being added to the classification, changing a previously valid code to an invalid code, creating a new subcategory

| | |
|---|---|
| A04.7 | Enterocolitis due to Clostridium difficile |
| C96.2 | Malignant mast cell tumor |
| D47.0 | Histiocytic and mast cell tumors of uncertain behavior |
| E85.8 | Other amyloidosis |
| H54.0 | Blindness, both eyes |
| H54.11 | Blindness, right eye, low vision left eye |
| H54.12 | Blindness, left eye, low vision right eye |
| H54.2 | Low vision, both eyes |
| H54.41 | Blindness, right eye, normal vision left eye |
| H54.42 | Blindness, left eye, normal vision right eye |
| H54.51 | Low vision, right eye, normal vision left eye |
| H54.52 | Low vision, left eye, normal vision right eye |
| I27.2 | Other secondary pulmonary hypertension |
| K06.0 | Gingival recession |
| K56.5 | Intestinal adhesions [bands] with obstruction (postprocedural) (postinfection) |
| K56.60 | Unspecified intestinal obstruction |
| K56.69 | Other intestinal obstruction |
| K91.3 | Postprocedural intestinal obstruction |
| M48.06 | Spinal stenosis, lumbar region |
| N63 | Unspecified lump in breast |
| O00.10 | Tubal pregnancy without intrauterine pregnancy |
| O00.11 | Tubal pregnancy with intrauterine pregnancy |
| O00.20 | Ovarian pregnancy without intrauterine pregnancy |
| O00.21 | Ovarian pregnancy with intrauterine pregnancy |
| P29.3 | Persistent fetal circulation |
| P83.8 | Other specified conditions of integument specific to newborn |
| P91.8 | Other specified disturbances of cerebral status of newborn |
| Q53.11 | Abdominal testis, unilateral |
| Q53.21 | Abdominal testis, bilateral |
| T07 | Unspecified multiple injuries |
| T14.8 | Other injury of unspecified body region |
| T14.90 | Injury, unspecified |
| T14.91 | Suicide attempt |
| Z36 | Encounter for antenatal screening of mother |

- 122 codes deleted from the classification

| | |
|---|---|
| S06.1X7D | Traumatic cerebral edema with loss of consciousness of any duration with death due to brain injury prior to regaining consciousness, subsequent encounter |
| S06.1X7S | Traumatic cerebral edema with loss of consciousness of any duration with death due to brain injury prior to regaining consciousness, sequela |
| S06.1X8D | Traumatic cerebral edema with loss of consciousness of any duration with death due to other cause prior to regaining consciousness, subsequent encounter |
| S06.1X8S | Traumatic cerebral edema with loss of consciousness of any duration with death due to other cause prior to regaining consciousness, sequela |
| S06.2X7D | Diffuse traumatic brain injury with loss of consciousness of any duration with death due to brain injury prior to regaining consciousness, subsequent encounter |
| S06.2X7S | Diffuse traumatic brain injury with loss of consciousness of any duration with death due to brain injury prior to regaining consciousness, sequela |
| S06.2X8D | Diffuse traumatic brain injury with loss of consciousness of any duration with death due to other cause prior to regaining consciousness, subsequent encounter |
| S06.2X8S | Diffuse traumatic brain injury with loss of consciousness of any duration with death due to other cause prior to regaining consciousness, sequela |
| S06.307D | Unspecified focal traumatic brain injury with loss of consciousness of any duration with death due to brain injury prior to regaining consciousness, subsequent encounter |
| S06.307S | Unspecified focal traumatic brain injury with loss of consciousness of any duration with death due to brain injury prior to regaining consciousness, sequela |
| S06.308D | Unspecified focal traumatic brain injury with loss of consciousness of any duration with death due to other cause prior to regaining consciousness, subsequent encounter |
| S06.308S | Unspecified focal traumatic brain injury with loss of consciousness of any duration with death due to other cause prior to regaining consciousness, sequela |
| S06.317D | Contusion and laceration of right cerebrum with loss of consciousness of any duration with death due to brain injury prior to regaining consciousness, subsequent encounter |
| S06.317S | Contusion and laceration of right cerebrum with loss of consciousness of any duration with death due to brain injury prior to regaining consciousness, sequela |
| S06.318D | Contusion and laceration of right cerebrum with loss of consciousness of any duration with death due to other cause prior to regaining consciousness, subsequent encounter |
| S06.318S | Contusion and laceration of right cerebrum with loss of consciousness of any duration with death due to other cause prior to regaining consciousness, sequela |
| S06.327D | Contusion and laceration of left cerebrum with loss of consciousness of any duration with death due to brain injury prior to regaining consciousness, subsequent encounter |

S06.327S   Contusion and laceration of left cerebrum with loss of consciousness of any duration with death due to brain injury prior to regaining consciousness, sequela

S06.328D   Contusion and laceration of left cerebrum with loss of consciousness of any duration with death due to other cause prior to regaining consciousness, subsequent encounter

S06.328S   Contusion and laceration of left cerebrum with loss of consciousness of any duration with death due to other cause prior to regaining consciousness, sequela

S06.337D   Contusion and laceration of cerebrum, unspecified, with loss of consciousness of any duration with death due to brain injury prior to regaining consciousness, subsequent encounter

S06.337S   Contusion and laceration of cerebrum, unspecified, with loss of consciousness of any duration with death due to brain injury prior to regaining consciousness, sequela

S06.338D   Contusion and laceration of cerebrum, unspecified, with loss of consciousness of any duration with death due to other cause prior to regaining consciousness, subsequent encounter

S06.338S Contusion and laceration of cerebrum, unspecified, with loss of consciousness of any duration with death due to other cause prior to regaining consciousness, sequela

S06.347D   Traumatic hemorrhage of right cerebrum with loss of consciousness of any duration with death due to brain injury prior to regaining consciousness, subsequent encounter

S06.347S   Traumatic hemorrhage of right cerebrum with loss of consciousness of any duration with death due to brain injury prior to regaining consciousness, sequela

S06.348D   Traumatic hemorrhage of right cerebrum with loss of consciousness of any duration with death due to other cause prior to regaining consciousness, subsequent encounter

S06.348S   Traumatic hemorrhage of right cerebrum with loss of consciousness of any duration with death due to other cause prior to regaining consciousness, sequela

S06.357D   Traumatic hemorrhage of left cerebrum with loss of consciousness of any duration with death due to brain injury prior to regaining consciousness, subsequent encounter

S06.357S   Traumatic hemorrhage of left cerebrum with loss of consciousness of any duration with death due to brain injury prior to regaining consciousness, sequela

S06.358D   Traumatic hemorrhage of left cerebrum with loss of consciousness of any duration with death due to other cause prior to regaining consciousness, subsequent encounter

S06.358S   Traumatic hemorrhage of left cerebrum with loss of consciousness of any duration with death due to other cause prior to regaining consciousness, sequela

S06.367D   Traumatic hemorrhage of cerebrum, unspecified, with loss of consciousness of any duration with death due to brain injury prior to regaining consciousness, subsequent encounter

S06.367S   Traumatic hemorrhage of cerebrum, unspecified, with loss of consciousness of any duration with death due to brain injury prior to regaining consciousness, sequela

S06.368D   Traumatic hemorrhage of cerebrum, unspecified, with loss of consciousness of any duration with death due to

other cause prior to regaining consciousness, subsequent encounter

S06.368S   Traumatic hemorrhage of cerebrum, unspecified, with loss of consciousness of any duration with death due to other cause prior to regaining consciousness, sequela

S06.377D   Contusion, laceration, and hemorrhage of cerebellum with loss of consciousness of any duration with death due to brain injury prior to regaining consciousness, subsequent encounter

S06.377S   Contusion, laceration, and hemorrhage of cerebellum with loss of consciousness of any duration with death due to brain injury prior to regaining consciousness, sequela

S06.378D   Contusion, laceration, and hemorrhage of cerebellum with loss of consciousness of any duration with death due to other cause prior to regaining consciousness, subsequent encounter

S06.378S   Contusion, laceration, and hemorrhage of cerebellum with loss of consciousness of any duration with death due to other cause prior to regaining consciousness, sequela

S06.387D   Contusion, laceration, and hemorrhage of brainstem with loss of consciousness of any duration with death due to brain injury prior to regaining consciousness, subsequent encounter

S06.387S   Contusion, laceration, and hemorrhage of brainstem with loss of consciousness of any duration with death due to brain injury prior to regaining consciousness, sequela

S06.388D   Contusion, laceration, and hemorrhage of brainstem with loss of consciousness of any duration with death due to other cause prior to regaining consciousness, subsequent encounter

S06.388S   Contusion, laceration, and hemorrhage of brainstem with loss of consciousness of any duration with death due to other cause prior to regaining consciousness, sequela

S06.4X7D   Epidural hemorrhage with loss of consciousness of any duration with death due to brain injury prior to regaining consciousness, subsequent encounter

S06.4X7S   Epidural hemorrhage with loss of consciousness of any duration with death due to brain injury prior to regaining consciousness, sequela

S06.4X8D   Epidural hemorrhage with loss of consciousness of any duration with death due to other causes prior to regaining consciousness, subsequent encounter

S06.4X8S   Epidural hemorrhage with loss of consciousness of any duration with death due to other causes prior to regaining consciousness, sequela

S06.5X7D   Traumatic subdural hemorrhage with loss of consciousness of any duration with death due to brain injury before regaining consciousness, subsequent encounter

S06.5X7S   Traumatic subdural hemorrhage with loss of consciousness of any duration with death due to brain injury before regaining consciousness, sequela

S06.5X8D   Traumatic subdural hemorrhage with loss of consciousness of any duration with death due to other cause before regaining consciousness, subsequent encounter

| | |
|---|---|
| S06.5X8S | Traumatic subdural hemorrhage with loss of consciousness of any duration with death due to other cause before regaining consciousness, sequela |
| S06.6X7D | Traumatic subarachnoid hemorrhage with loss of consciousness of any duration with death due to brain injury prior to regaining consciousness, subsequent encounter |
| S06.6X7S | Traumatic subarachnoid hemorrhage with loss of consciousness of any duration with death due to brain injury prior to regaining consciousness, sequela |
| S06.6X8D | Traumatic subarachnoid hemorrhage with loss of consciousness of any duration with death due to other cause prior to regaining consciousness, subsequent encounter |
| S06.6X8S | Traumatic subarachnoid hemorrhage with loss of consciousness of any duration with death due to other cause prior to regaining consciousness, sequela |
| S06.817D | Injury of right internal carotid artery, intracranial portion, not elsewhere classified with loss of consciousness of any duration with death due to brain injury prior to regaining consciousness, subsequent encounter |
| S06.817S | Injury of right internal carotid artery, intracranial portion, not elsewhere classified with loss of consciousness of any duration with death due to brain injury prior to regaining consciousness, sequela |
| S06.818D | Injury of right internal carotid artery, intracranial portion, not elsewhere classified with loss of consciousness of any duration with death due to other cause prior to regaining consciousness, subsequent encounter |
| S06.818S | Injury of right internal carotid artery, intracranial portion, not elsewhere classified with loss of consciousness of any duration with death due to other cause prior to regaining consciousness, sequela |
| S06.827D | Injury of left internal carotid artery, intracranial portion, not elsewhere classified with loss of consciousness of any duration with death due to brain injury prior to regaining consciousness, subsequent encounter |
| S06.827S | Injury of left internal carotid artery, intracranial portion, not elsewhere classified with loss of consciousness of any duration with death due to brain injury prior to regaining consciousness, sequela |
| S06.828D | Injury of left internal carotid artery, intracranial portion, not elsewhere classified with loss of consciousness of any duration with death due to other cause prior to regaining consciousness, subsequent encounter |
| S06.828S | Injury of left internal carotid artery, intracranial portion, not elsewhere classified with loss of consciousness of any duration with death due to other cause prior to regaining consciousness, sequela |
| S06.897D | Other specified intracranial injury with loss of consciousness of any duration with death due to brain injury prior to regaining consciousness, subsequent encounter |
| S06.897S | Other specified intracranial injury with loss of consciousness of any duration with death due to brain injury prior to regaining consciousness, sequela |
| S06.898D | Other specified intracranial injury with loss of consciousness of any duration with death due to other cause prior to regaining consciousness, subsequent encounter |
| S06.898S | Other specified intracranial injury with loss of consciousness of any duration with death due to other cause prior to regaining consciousness, sequela |
| S06.9X7D | Unspecified intracranial injury with loss of consciousness of any duration with death due to brain injury prior to regaining consciousness, subsequent encounter |
| S06.9X7S | Unspecified intracranial injury with loss of consciousness of any duration with death due to brain injury prior to regaining consciousness, sequela |
| S06.9X8D | Unspecified intracranial injury with loss of consciousness of any duration with death due to other cause prior to regaining consciousness, subsequent encounter |
| S06.9X8S | Unspecified intracranial injury with loss of consciousness of any duration with death due to other cause prior to regaining consciousness, sequela |
| S63.13 | Subluxation and dislocation of proximal interphalangeal joint of thumb |
| S63.131 | Subluxation of proximal interphalangeal joint of right thumb |
| S63.131A | Subluxation of proximal interphalangeal joint of right thumb, initial encounter |
| S63.131D | Subluxation of proximal interphalangeal joint of right thumb, subsequent encounter |
| S63.131S | Subluxation of proximal interphalangeal joint of right thumb, sequela |
| S63.132 | Subluxation of proximal interphalangeal joint of left thumb |
| S63.132A | Subluxation of proximal interphalangeal joint of left thumb, initial encounter |
| S63.132D | Subluxation of proximal interphalangeal joint of left thumb, subsequent encounter |
| S63.132S | Subluxation of proximal interphalangeal joint of left thumb, sequela |
| S63.133 | Subluxation of proximal interphalangeal joint of unspecified thumb |
| S63.133A | Subluxation of proximal interphalangeal joint of unspecified thumb, initial encounter |
| S63.133D | Subluxation of proximal interphalangeal joint of unspecified thumb, subsequent encounter |
| S63.133S | Subluxation of proximal interphalangeal joint of unspecified thumb, sequela |
| S63.134 | Dislocation of proximal interphalangeal joint of right thumb |
| S63.134A | Dislocation of proximal interphalangeal joint of right thumb, initial encounter |
| S63.134D | Dislocation of proximal interphalangeal joint of right thumb, subsequent encounter |
| S63.134S | Dislocation of proximal interphalangeal joint of right thumb, sequela |
| S63.135 | Dislocation of proximal interphalangeal joint of left thumb |
| S63.135A | Dislocation of proximal interphalangeal joint of left thumb, initial encounter |
| S63.135D | Dislocation of proximal interphalangeal joint of left thumb, subsequent encounter |
| S63.135S | Dislocation of proximal interphalangeal joint of left thumb, sequela |
| S63.136 | Dislocation of proximal interphalangeal joint of unspecified thumb |

| | |
|---|---|
| S63.136A | Dislocation of proximal interphalangeal joint of unspecified thumb, initial encounter |
| S63.136D | Dislocation of proximal interphalangeal joint of unspecified thumb, subsequent encounter |
| S63.136S | Dislocation of proximal interphalangeal joint of unspecified thumb, sequela |
| S63.14 | Subluxation and dislocation of distal interphalangeal joint of thumb |
| S63.141 | Subluxation of distal interphalangeal joint of right thumb |
| S63.141A | Subluxation of distal interphalangeal joint of right thumb, initial encounter |
| S63.141D | Subluxation of distal interphalangeal joint of right thumb, subsequent encounter |
| S63.141S | Subluxation of distal interphalangeal joint of right thumb, sequela |
| S63.142 | Subluxation of distal interphalangeal joint of left thumb |
| S63.142A | Subluxation of distal interphalangeal joint of left thumb, initial encounter |
| S63.142D | Subluxation of distal interphalangeal joint of left thumb, subsequent encounter |
| S63.142S | Subluxation of distal interphalangeal joint of left thumb, sequela |
| S63.143 | Subluxation of distal interphalangeal joint of unspecified thumb |
| S63.143A | Subluxation of distal interphalangeal joint of unspecified thumb, initial encounter |
| S63.143D | Subluxation of distal interphalangeal joint of unspecified thumb, subsequent encounter |
| S63.143S | Subluxation of distal interphalangeal joint of unspecified thumb, sequela |
| S63.144 | Dislocation of distal interphalangeal joint of right thumb |
| S63.144A | Dislocation of distal interphalangeal joint of right thumb, initial encounter |
| S63.144D | Dislocation of distal interphalangeal joint of right thumb, subsequent encounter |
| S63.144S | Dislocation of distal interphalangeal joint of right thumb, sequela |
| S63.145 | Dislocation of distal interphalangeal joint of left thumb |
| S63.145A | Dislocation of distal interphalangeal joint of left thumb, initial encounter |

| | |
|---|---|
| S63.145D | Dislocation of distal interphalangeal joint of left thumb, subsequent encounter |
| S63.145S | Dislocation of distal interphalangeal joint of left thumb, sequela |
| S63.146 | Dislocation of distal interphalangeal joint of unspecified thumb |
| S63.146A | Dislocation of distal interphalangeal joint of unspecified thumb, initial encounter |
| S63.146D | Dislocation of distal interphalangeal joint of unspecified thumb, subsequent encounter |
| S63.146S | Dislocation of distal interphalangeal joint of unspecified thumb, sequela |

## Proprietary Updates

The following proprietary features have also been added:

- 150+ new definitions that describe, in lay terms, a specific condition or disease process

- 50+ new illustrations

- Updated *AHA Coding Clinic* references through second quarter 2017

- Updated pharmacology list

- New HCC icon identifying CMS hierarchical condition category (CMS-HCC) codes

- New appendix outlining the Medicare Advantage risk-adjustment model

- Updated coding examples in the chapter-specific guideline sections, specific to the inpatient setting

- New POA Exempt list, provided as a searchable data file, available at Optum360coding.com

# Introduction

## History of ICD-10-CM

The ICD-10-CM classification system was developed by the National Center for Health Statistics (NCHS) as a clinical modification to the ICD-10 system developed by the World Health Organization (WHO), primarily as a unique system for use in the United States for morbidity and mortality reporting. Although ICD-10 replaced ICD-9 for use in coding and classifying of mortality data from death certificates beginning January 1, 1999, ICD-10-CM implementation was postponed many years until legislation to replace ICD-9-CM, volumes 1 and 2, with ICD-10-CM was approved.

ICD-10 is the copyrighted product of the World Health Organization (WHO), which has authorized the development of a clinical modification (CM) of ICD-10 for use in the United States. However, all modifications to the ICD-10 must conform to WHO conventions for ICD. The development of ICD-10-CM included comprehensive evaluation by a Technical Advisory Panel and extensive consultation with physician groups, clinical coders, and other industry experts.

The ICD-10-CM draft and crosswalk between ICD-9-CM and ICD-10-CM were made available on the Centers for Medicare and Medicaid Services (CMS) website for public comment. The initial public comment period extended from December 1997 through February 1998. A field test for ICD-10-CM was conducted in the summer of 2003 jointly by the American Hospital Association (AMA) and the American Health Information Management Association (AHIMA). Public comments and suggestions were reviewed and additional modifications to ICD-10-CM were made. Revisions were made to ICD-10-CM based on the established update process for ICD-10-CM (the ICD-10-CM Coordination and Maintenance Committee) and the World Health Organization's ICD-10 (the Update and Revision Committee).

These revisions to ICD-10-CM have included:

- Information relevant to ambulatory and managed care encounters
- Expanded injury codes
- Creation of combination diagnosis/symptom codes to reduce the number of codes needed to fully describe a condition
- The addition of 6th and 7th character classifications
- Incorporation of common 4th and 5th character classifications
- Classifications specific to laterality
- Classification refinement for increased data granularity

This new structure allows for further expansion than was possible with the ICD-9-CM classification system.

The Department of Health and Human Services (HHS) published the final rule regarding the adoption of both ICD-10-CM and ICD-10-PCS in the January 16, 2009, *Federal Register* (45 CFR part 162 [CMS—0013—F]). The initial compliance date for implementation of ICD-10-CM and ICD-10-PCS as a replacement for ICD-9-CM was set at October 1, 2013. On April 17, 2012, the Department of Health and Human Services (HHS) released a notice to postpone the date by which certain health care entities have to comply with International Classification of Diseases, 10th Revision diagnosis and procedure codes (ICD-10). The compliance date for implementation of ICD-10-CM and ICD-10-PCS as a replacement for ICD-9-CM was changed to October 1, 2014. On April 1, 2014, Congress enacted the Protecting Access to Medicare Act of 2014, which contained a provision to delay the implementation of ICD-10-CM/PCS by at least one year, prohibiting the Department of Health and Human Services (HHS) from adopting the ICD-10-CM/PCS code sets as the mandatory standard until October 1, 2015. Eventually, the ICD-10-CM/PCS code sets were implemented in their entirety on October 1, 2015, and ICD-9-CM, volumes 1 and 2, were retired.

## ICD-10-CM for Hospitals: The Complete Official Code Set

*ICD-10-CM for Hospitals: The Complete Official Code Set 2018* includes many of the enhancements described below in direct response to requests from our subscribers.

As you review the content, you will find the following:

- Optum360 Exclusive feature — Check Placeholder Alert symbol, indicating the need for one or more "filler" X character assignments in the 5th and/or 6th character position to appropriately assign a required character in the 7th character position
- Optum360 Exclusive feature — Key word differentiation by the use of a green font that highlights the differentiating terms in similar code descriptions in a given category
- Optum360 Exclusive feature — Exclusive *following* references and Check Additional Character symbol in the indexes. The *following* references (designed and used exclusively by Optum360) help coders locate those alphanumeric codes that are out of sequence in the tabular section.
- Optum360 Exclusive feature — Exclusive shaded guides in the index that help users easily follow the indent levels for the subterms under a main term
- Illustrations throughout the tabular list and at the back of the book that feature anatomy and terminology included in the ICD-10-CM classification system
- Optum360 Exclusive feature — Detailed muscle/tendon tables that correspond with codes in chapters 13 and 19
- The complete ICD-10-CM Official Guidelines for Coding and Reporting, published by the U.S. Department of Health and Human Services and approved by the cooperating parties (American Health Information Management Association, National Center for Health Statistics, Centers for Medicare and Medicaid Services, American Hospital Association)
- Optum360 Exclusive feature — Official chapter-specific guidelines with coding examples specific to the hospital setting at the beginning of each chapter
- Exclusive color coding, symbols, and footnotes that alert coders to coding and reimbursement issues, including the majority of the Medicare code edits and identification of conditions that significantly affect DRG assignment
- A searchable data file for complication and comorbidity (CC) exclusions with a reference beneath applicable codes to make it easier to determine complications and comorbidities excluded from a particular principal diagnosis
- All official ICD-10-CM codes, indexes, notes, footnotes, and symbols
- Icons and definitions to differentiate between the two types of Excludes notes
- Check 4th, 5th, 6th, and 7th character symbols that identify codes that require the addition of a 4th, 5th, 6th, or 7th character for code specificity and validity
- Color coding and symbol legend at the bottom of each page

Please review "How to Use *ICD-10-CM Expert for Hospitals*" in this manual to learn about the features that will help you assign and report correct codes, ensuring appropriate reimbursement.

# How to Use ICD-10-CM Expert for Hospitals 2018

This International Classification of Diseases, 10th Revision, Clinical Modification (ICD-10-CM) is being published by the United States Government in recognition of its responsibility to promulgate this classification throughout the United States for morbidity coding. This code book represents an adaptation of ICD-10 that was created specifically for use in the United States. Revisions to ICD-10-CM will be made based on the established update process for ICD-10-CM (the ICD-10-CM Coordination and Maintenance Committee) and the World Health Organization's ICD-10 (the Update and Revision Committee).

## Use of Official Sources

The *ICD-10-CM Expert for Hospitals* contains the official U.S. Department of Health and Human Services, Tenth Revision, Clinical Modification (ICD-10-CM) codes, effective for the current year.

Much of the color coding and many of the symbols and footnotes that identify coding and reimbursement issues are derived from official federal government sources, including Medicare Code Editor (MCE), version 34, ICD-10 MS-DRG Definitions Manual Files, version 34, and the *Federal Register,* volume 82, number 81, April 28, 2017 ("Hospital Inpatient Prospective Payment Systems for Acute Care Hospitals and the Long-Term Care Hospital Prospective Payment System and Proposed Policy Changes and Fiscal Year 2018 Rates; Proposed Rule").

For the most current files related to IPPS please refer to the following:

https://www.cms.gov/Medicare/Medicare-Fee-for-Service-Payment/AcuteInpatientPPS/IPPS-Regulations-and-Notices.html.

## Steps to Correct Coding

1. Before beginning to use this code book, review section I.A., "Conventions for the ICD-10-CM," and section I.B., "General Coding Guidelines," of the ICD-10-CM Official Guidelines for Coding and Reporting.

2. Look up the main term in the alphabetic index and scan the subterm entries as appropriate. Review continued lines and additional subterms that may appear in the next column or on the next page.

3. Note all parenthetical terms (nonessential modifiers) that help in code selection but do not affect code assignment. Shaded vertical guidelines in the index are provided to help determine the indentation level for each subterm in relation to the main terms.

4. Pay close attention to the following instructions in the index:
   - "See," "see also," and "see category" cross-references
   - "With"/"without" notes
   - "Omit code" notes
   - "Due to" subterms
   - Other instructions found in note boxes, such as "code by site"
   - *Following* references and Check Additional Character symbol in the indexes. The *following* references (designed and used exclusively by Optum360) help coders locate those alphanumeric codes that are out of sequence in the tabular section.

5. Do not code from the alphabetic index without verifying the accuracy of the code in the Tabular List. Locate the code in the alphanumerically arranged Tabular List.

6. To determine the appropriateness of the code selection and proper coding, read all instructional material:
   - "Includes" and both types of "Excludes" notes
   - "Use additional code" and "code first underlying disease" instructions
   - "Code also"
   - 4th, 5th, and 6th character requirements and 7th character extension requirements
   - CC Exclusions
   - Age and sex symbols

7. Consult the official ICD-10-CM guidelines, which govern the use of specific codes. These guidelines provide both general and chapter-specific coding guidance.

8. Confirm and assign the correct code.

## Organization

This book is organized in the following manner:

### Introduction

The introductory material in this book includes the ICD-10-CM Official Preface, the history of ICD-10-CM as well as an overview of the classification system.

### Official ICD-10-CM Conventions and Guidelines

This section provides an explanation of the conventions and guidelines regulating the appropriate assignment and reporting of ICD-10-CM codes. This coding guidance is presented by the National Center for Health Statistics (NCHS), a governmental agency of the Centers for Disease Control and Prevention (CDC), within the United States Department of Health and Human Services (DHHS). **Note: The 2018 *ICD-10-CM Official Guidelines for Coding and Reporting* were not available at the time this book went to print. Updated guidelines will be posted on our website at https://www.optum360coding.com/ProductUpdates/ as soon as they are available.**

### Alphabetic Index to Diseases

The Alphabetic Index to Diseases is arranged in alphabetic order by disease — by specific illness, injury, eponym, abbreviation, or other descriptive diagnostic term. The index also lists diagnostic terms for other reasons for encounters with health care professionals.

### Neoplasm Table

The Neoplasm Table provides the proper code based upon histology of the neoplasm and site.

### Table of Drugs and Chemicals

The Table of Drugs and Chemicals lists the drug and the specific codes that identify the drug and the intent. No additional external cause of injury and poisoning code is assigned in ICD-10-CM.

### Index to External Causes

The Alphabetic Index to External Causes of injuries is arranged in alphabetic order by main term indicating the event.

# Tabular List of Diseases

ICD-10-CM codes and descriptors are arranged numerically within the Tabular List of diseases within 21 separate chapters according to body system or nature of injury and disease. Classifications which were previously considered supplemental to ICD-9-CM (e.g., V codes and E codes) are incorporated into the Tabular Listing of ICD-10-CM as individual chapters. Chapters 20, "External Causes of Morbidity," and 21, "Factors Influencing Health Status and Contact with Health Services," include chapter-specific guidelines.

# Appendixes

The resources described below have been included as appendixes for the *ICD-10-CM Expert for Hospitals: The Complete Official Code Set*. These resources further instruct the inpatient coder on the appropriate application of the ICD-10-CM code set.

## Appendix A: 10 Steps to Correct Coding

This step-by-step tutorial walks the coder through the process of locating the correct code in the alphabetic index and verifying it in the tabular section while following applicable conventions and guidelines. Detailed examples are provided and explained along with advice for proper sequencing.

## Appendix B: Valid 3-character ICD-10-CM Codes

The user may consult this table to confirm that no further specificity, such as the use of 4th, 5th, 6th, or 7th characters or placeholders (X), is necessary. All ICD-10-CM codes that are valid at the three-character level are listed.

## Appendix C: Pharmacology List 2018

This reference is a comprehensive but not all-inclusive list of pharmacological agents used to treat acute and/or chronic conditions. Drugs are listed in alphabetical order by their brand and/or generic names along with their drug action and indications for which they may commonly be prescribed. Some drugs have also been mapped to their appropriate long-term drug use Z code.

## Appendix D: Z Codes for Long-Term Drug Use with Associated Drugs

This resource correlates Z codes that are used to identify current long-term drug use with a list of drugs that are typically categorized to that class of drug.

**Note:** These tables are not all-inclusive but list some of the more commonly used drugs.

## Appendix E: Major Complication and Comorbidity (MCC) Code List

This is a full listing of conditions considered to be major complications and/or comorbidities that when present as a secondary diagnosis may affect DRG assignment under the Medicare Severity DRG (MS-DRG) system.

## Appendix F: Complication and Comorbidity (CC) Code List

This is a full listing of conditions considered to be complications and/or comorbidities that when present as a secondary diagnosis may affect DRG assignment under the MS-DRG system.

## Appendix G: Lists of Principal Diagnoses That Are Their Own CC and Their Own MCC

This listing displays those ICD-10-CM combination codes that may function as their own CC or MCC when sequenced as a principal diagnosis based on the MS-DRG system.

## Appendix H: Present on Admission (POA) Tutorial

This tutorial walks the coder through the process of assigning the appropriate present-on-admission (POA) indicator for inpatient codes based on the POA reporting guidelines. Detailed scenarios for a variety of situations are provided and discussed.

## Appendix I: Hospital Acquired Conditions

This comprehensive table displays codes that identify conditions that are considered reasonably preventable when occurring during the hospital admission and may prevent the case from grouping to a higher-paying MS-DRG. Many of these HACs are conditional and are based on reporting the specific diagnosis code(s) in combination with certain procedure codes, which are also noted in this table.

## Appendix J: Centers for Medicare & Medicaid Services (CMS) Hierarchical Condition Categories (HCC) (CMS-HCC)

This resource provides the framework behind CMS's Medicare Advantage (MA) program, a risk-adjustment model developed as a means of compensating health care plans with large numbers of Medicare Part C beneficiaries. It includes a brief synopsis of the evolution of the program from its inception; insight into the various elements needed to predict risk, including the principles used to develop the hierarchical condition categories (HCCs), one of the fundamental components of the risk adjustment model; and a description of the audit process used to ensure the accuracy of payments made to MA plans.

# Illustrations

This section includes illustrations of normal anatomy with ICD-10-CM specific terminology.

# ICD-10-CM Hospital Data Files

To save space in this coding manual and provide more comprehensive references for the user, Optum360 has provided searchable data files for certain features in this manual. These data files can be accessed at the following:

http://www.optum360coding.com/ProdcutUpdates/

Two data files are available for FY 2018; the titles and passwords to each of these are provided below:

- CC Exclusions Data File

  Title: "2018 ICD-10-CM for Hospitals CC Excludes Data File"

  Password: OptumCCExcl18

- POA Exempt Data File

  Title: "2018 ICD-10-CM for Hospitals POA Exemption Data File"

  Password: OptumPOAExempt18

# Overview of ICD-10-CM Official Conventions

This is an overview of the ICD-10-CM official conventions, which are general rules for the use of the classification system, independent of the guidelines. The official conventions and instructions of the classification, which take precedence over the guidelines, are incorporated within the alphabetic index and tabular list as instructional notes and are applicable regardless of the health care setting. For the full version of the official conventions, see the ICD-10-CM Official Guidelines for Coding and Reporting, section I.A., which is included in this book.

## Format

ICD-10-CM is divided into two main parts: the index, an alphabetical list of terms and their corresponding code, and the Tabular List, a sequential, alphanumeric list of codes divided into chapters based on body system or condition. The index contains the Index to Diseases and Injuries (main index) and the Index to External Causes of Injury. Also included in the main Index is the Neoplasm Table and a Table of Drugs and Chemicals.

The Tabular List contains categories, subcategories, and valid codes. ICD-10-CM is an alphanumeric classification system. The 1st character of a three-character category is a letter. The 2nd and 3rd characters may be numbers or alpha characters. A three-character category without further subclassification is equivalent to a valid three-character code. Subcategories are either four or five characters. Subcategory characters include either letters or numbers. Codes may be three, four, five, six, or seven characters in length, in which each level of subdivision after a category is a subcategory. The final level of subdivision is a valid code. The final character in a code may be either a letter or a number.

The ICD-10-CM uses the letter "X" as a placeholder. A placeholder "X" is used as a 5th character placeholder at certain six character codes to allow for future expansion, without disturbing the 6th character structure. For instance, an initial encounter for accidental poisoning by penicillin is coded to T36.0X1A. The "X" in the 5th character position is a placeholder, or filler character.

Similarly, certain categories have applicable 7th character extensions. In these cases, the 7th character extension is required for all codes within the category, or as otherwise instructed in the tabular list notations. 7th character extensions must always be the last character in the data field. If a code is not a full six characters in length, a dummy placeholder "X" must be used to fill in the empty characters when a 7th character extension is required.

## Punctuation

[ ]   In the Tabular List, brackets are used to enclose synonyms, alternative wording, or explanatory phrases. In the index, brackets are used to identify manifestation codes.

( )   Parentheses are used in both the index and tabular list to enclose nonessential modifiers; supplementary words that may be present or absent in the statement of a disease or procedure without affecting the code number to which it is assigned.

:   Colons are used in the tabular list after an incomplete term that needs one or more of the modifiers following the colon to make it assignable to a given category.

## Abbreviations

### NEC

The abbreviation NEC, "Not elsewhere classifiable" represents "other specified" in the ICD-10-CM. An Index entry that states NEC directs the coder to an "other specified" code in the Tabular List. Codes titled "Other" or "Other specified" in the Tabular List (usually a code with a 4th or 6th character 8 and 5th character 9) are for use when the information in the medical record provides detail for which a specific code does not exist.

### NOS

The abbreviation NOS, "Not otherwise specified," in the Tabular List may be interpreted as "unspecified." Codes in the Tabular List with "Unspecified" in the title (usually a code with a 4th or 6th character 9 and 5th character Ø) are for use when the information in the medical record is insufficient to assign a more specific code.

## Typeface

### Boldface

Boldface type is used for main term entries in the alphabetic index, and all codes and descriptions in the Tabular List.

## General Notes

The following conventions and notes appear only in the Tabular List of Diseases:

### Includes Notes

The word INCLUDES appears immediately under certain categories to further define, clarify, or give examples of the content of a code category.

### Inclusion Terms

Lists of inclusion terms are included under certain codes. These terms indicate some of the conditions for which that code number may be used. Inclusion terms may be synonyms with the code title, or, in the case of "other specified" codes, the terms may also provide a list of various conditions included within a classification code. The inclusion terms are not exhaustive. The index may provide additional terms that may also be assigned to a given code.

### Excludes Notes

ICD-10-CM has two types of excludes notes. Each note has a different definition for use. However, they are similar in that they both indicate that codes excluded from each other are independent of each other.

#### Excludes 1

An EXCLUDES 1 note is a "pure" excludes. It means "NOT CODED HERE!" An Excludes 1 note indicates mutually exclusive codes: two conditions that cannot be reported together. For example, a congenital form of a disease may not be reported with the acquired form of the same condition. The code excluded should never be reported with the applicable codes listed above the excludes notation.

An exception to the Excludes1 definition is the circumstance when the two conditions are unrelated to each other. If it is not clear whether the two conditions involving an Excludes1 note are related or not, query the provider. For example, code F45.8, Other somatoform disorders, has an Excludes1 note for "sleep related teeth grinding (G47.63)," because "teeth grinding" is an inclusion term under F45.8. Only one of these two codes should be assigned for teeth grinding. However psychogenic dysmenorrhea is also an inclusion term under F45.8, and a patient could have both this condition and sleep related teeth grinding. In this case, the two conditions are clearly unrelated to each other, and so it would be appropriate to report F45.8 and G47.63 together.

## Excludes 2

An EXCLUDES 2 note means "NOT INCLUDED HERE." An Excludes 2 note indicates that although the excluded condition is not part of the condition it is excluded from, a patient may have both conditions at the same time. Therefore, when an Excludes 2 note appears under a code, it may be acceptable to use both the code and the excluded code together if supported by the medical documentation.

## Note

NOTE The term "NOTE" appears as an icon and precedes the instructional information. These notes function as alerts to highlight coding instructions within the text.

## Default Codes

In the Index, the default code is the code listed next to the main term. The default code represents the condition most commonly associated with the main term. This code may be assigned when documentation does not facilitate reporting a more specific code. Alternatively, it may provide an unspecified code for the condition.

## Syndromes

Follow the Alphabetic Index guidance when coding syndromes. In the absence of index guidance, assign codes for the documented manifestations of the syndrome.

## And

When the term "and" is used in a narrative statement or code title, it may be interpreted as "and/or."

## With

The word "with" should be interpreted to mean "associated with" or "due to" when it appears in a code title, the Alphabetic Index, or an instructional note in the Tabular List. The classification presumes a causal relationship between the two conditions linked by these terms in the Alphabetic Index and Tabular List. These conditions should be coded as related even in the absence of provider documentation linking them unless the documentation clearly states that they are not related. Conditions not linked by these terms in the index or tabular section need provider documentation of a link in order to code them as related.

## See and See Also

The instruction "See" following a main term in the alphabetic index indicates that another term must be referenced in order to locate the correct code. The instructional note "See also" simply provides alternative terms that may be useful in determining the correct code but are not necessary to look up if the main term supplies the appropriate code.

## Instructional Notes Used in the Tabular List

In the tabular section, the following instructional notes appear in red type for emphasis:

### Code First/Use additional/In diseases classified elsewhere code:

These instructional notes provide sequencing instruction. They may appear independently of each other or to designate certain etiology/manifestation paired codes. These instructions signal the coder that an additional code should be reported to provide a more complete picture of that diagnosis.

In etiology/manifestation coding, ICD-10-CM requires the underlying condition to be sequenced first, followed by the manifestation. In these situations, codes with "In diseases classified elsewhere" in the code description are never permitted as a first-listed or principal diagnosis code and must be sequenced following the underlying condition code.

### Code Also:

A "code also" note alerts the coder that more than one code may be required to fully describe the condition. Code sequencing is discretionary. Factors that may determine sequencing include severity and reason for the encounter.

## Code Assignment and Clinical Criteria

Diagnosis code assignment must be based on the provider's diagnostic statement that the condition exists and is not based on clinical criteria used by the provider to establish the diagnosis. Conflicting documentation must be queried.

# Additional Annotations

## Code-Level Notations

The tabular section of ICD-10-CM has various colors, symbol, and other tabular annotations that may help in code selection, provide clinical or coding information, or alert the coder to reimbursement issues affected by the diagnosis code assignment. Some codes may have more than one annotation. For quick reference to the meanings of the colors and symbols, look at the color/symbol legend at the bottom of each page in the tabular list.

## Italics

Italicized type is used for all exclusion notes and to identify manifestation codes, those codes that should not be reported as first-listed (principal) diagnoses.

## Color Coding/Symbols

### New Code
This ● icon identifies the codes that are new to the classification system for the current year. The new code icon is to the left of the code.

### Revised Code Title
This ▲ icon to the left of a code alerts the user to a change in that code's title. This change may be as simple as adding or removing punctuation, which may or may not change the intent of the code, to adding or removing specific terms from a code description that completely alter the circumstances in which the code would be used.

### Revised Text
The revised text ►◄ "bow ties" alert the user to changes in parenthetical notes for the current year. Revised text may include the following:

- A change in a current parenthetical description
- A change in the code(s) associated with a current parenthetical note
- A change in how a current parenthetical note is classified (e.g., an Excludes 1 note that changed to an Excludes 2 note)
- Addition of a new parenthetical note(s) to a code

### Deleted Text
Strikethrough on code description(s) and/or code note(s) indicates a deletion from the classification for the current year. For example:

√4ᵗʰ **N25 Disorders resulting from impaired renal tubular function**
    *EXCLUDES 1* ~~metabolic disorders classifiable to E70-E88~~

The strikethrough over the Excludes 1 note indicates that this note was deleted from the classification and is no longer applicable to codes in category N25.

    √7ᵗʰ ~~**S63.131 Subluxation of proximal interphalangeal joint of right thumb**~~

The strikethrough over the code and the code description indicates that all codes in subcategory S63.131 (S63.131A, S63.131D, and S63.131S) have been deleted from the classification.

### Additional Characters Required
√4ᵗʰ This symbol indicates that the code requires a 4th character.

√5ᵗʰ This symbol indicates that the code requires a 5th character.

√6ᵗʰ This symbol indicates that the code requires a 6th character.

√7ᵗʰ This symbol indicates that the code requires a 7th character.

√x7ᵗʰ This symbol indicates that the code requires a 7th character following the placeholder "X". Codes with fewer than six characters that require a 7th character must contain placeholder "X" to fill in the empty character(s).

## Key Word
Green font is used throughout the Tabular List of Diseases to differentiate the key words that appear in similar code descriptions in a given category or subcategory.

For example, refer to the list of codes below from category C7A:

C7A.020    Malignant carcinoid tumor of the **appendix**

C7A.021    Malignant carcinoid tumor of the **cecum**

C7A.022    Malignant carcinoid tumor of the **ascending colon**

C7A.023    Malignant carcinoid tumor of the **transverse colon**

C7A.024    Malignant carcinoid tumor of the **descending colon**

C7A.025    Malignant carcinoid tumor of the **sigmoid colon**

C7A.026    Malignant carcinoid tumor of the **rectum**

C7A.029    Malignant carcinoid tumor of the large intestine, **unspecified portion**

The portion of the code description that appears in **green font** in the tabular list helps the coder quickly identify the key terms and the correct code. This convention is especially useful when the codes describe laterality, such as the following codes from subcategory H40.22:

H40.221    Chronic angle-closure glaucoma, **right** eye

H40.222    Chronic angle-closure glaucoma, **left** eye

H40.223    Chronic angle-closure glaucoma, **bilateral**

H40.229    Chronic angle-closure glaucoma, **unspecified** eye

The key word convention is used only in those categories in which there are multiple codes with very similar descriptions with only a few words that differentiate them.

## Medicare Code Edits
Medicare Administrative Contractors (MACs) and many payers use Medicare code edits to check the coding accuracy on claims. The coding edit information in this manual is used for acute care hospital inpatient admissions and has been updated to reflect v34 changes to the Medicare Code Editor (MCE) and ICD-10 MS-DRG Definitions Manual as well as changes identified in *Federal Register,* volume 82, number 81, April 28, 2017 ("Hospital Inpatient Prospective Payment Systems for Acute Care Hospitals and the Long-Term Care Hospital Prospective Payment System and Proposed Policy Changes and Fiscal Year 2018 Rates; Proposed Rule").

The Medicare code edits for diagnoses are listed below:

- Invalid diagnosis or procedure code
- External causes of morbidity codes as principal diagnosis
- Duplicate of PDx
- *Age conflict
- *Sex conflict
- *Manifestation code as principal diagnosis
- *Questionable principal diagnosis
- *Unacceptable principal diagnosis
- Invalid age
- Invalid sex
- *Wrong procedure performed

Starred edits above are identified in this manual by color bars, symbols, or footnotes as described below.

## Age and Sex Edit

The age and sex edits below are used to detect inconsistencies between the patient's age and/or sex and the patient's diagnosis. The following edit symbols appear in the tabular list to the right of the code description.

### Newborn Age: 0                                                      N

These diagnoses are intended for newborns and neonates and the patient's age must be 0 years.

### Pediatric Age: 0-17                                                 P

These diagnoses are intended for children and the patient's age must between 0 and 17 years.

### Maternity Age: 12-55                                                M

These diagnoses are intended for childbearing patients between the age of 12 and 55 years.

### Adult Age: 15-124                                                   A

These diagnoses are intended for patients between the age of 15 and 124 years.

### Male diagnosis only                                                 ♂

### Female diagnosis only                                               ♀

## Manifestation Code

These codes appear in italic type, with a **_blue color bar_** over the title. A manifestation code cannot be reported as a first-listed or principal diagnosis. By definition, a manifestation code represents a demonstration of some aspect of an underlying disease, which is separately classifiable. In the alphabetic index, these codes are listed as the secondary code in brackets. The underlying disease code is listed first.

## Unacceptable PDx/Questionable Admission Dx

Unacceptable principal diagnoses will appear with a gray color bar over the code title. These codes do not describe a current illness or injury, but a circumstance which influences a patient's health status. They are considered an unacceptable principal diagnosis for *inpatient* admission.

Questionable admission diagnoses will also appear with a gray color bar over the code title along with a reference to footnote 4. These codes, although not unacceptable as a PDx, may be considered a "questionable admission" when used as PDx in an acute care hospital.

## Wrong Procedure Performed Edit

The Wrong Procedure Performed edit was created to identify cases in which wrong surgeries occurred. Any claim with a code from the Y65.51-Y65.53 will be denied and returned to the provider. A surgical or other invasive procedure is considered to be a wrong procedure if:

- The procedure was performed on the wrong site
- The procedure was performed on the wrong patient, or
- The incorrect procedure was performed on a patient.

# ICD-10 MS-DRG Definitions Manual Edits

An MS-DRG is assigned based on specific patient attributes, such as principal diagnosis, secondary diagnoses, procedures, and discharge status. The attributes (edits) provided in this manual are only those directly related to ICD-10-CM diagnoses and are used for acute care hospital inpatient admissions.

## Hospital Acquired Condition (HAC)                           H1 — H14

These codes identify conditions that are high cost or high volume or both, are either a complication or comorbidity (CC) or major complication or comorbidity (MCC) that as a secondary diagnosis results in assignment of a case to a higher-paying MS-DRG. These conditions are reasonably preventable through the application of evidence-based guidelines. If the condition is not present on admission (meaning it developed during the hospital admission), the case will not group to the higher-paying MS-DRG

based solely upon the reporting of the HAC code. Many of these HACs are conditional, and are based on reporting the specific diagnosis code(s) in combination with certain procedure codes, notated in footnotes.

The HAC icon with the specific HAC table number in which this code is classified appears to the right of the code description. The comprehensive list of HAC tables that coincide with these icon numbers appears in appendix I of this book.

## CC Condition                                                        CC

This symbol designates a complication or comorbidity diagnosis that may affect DRG assignment. A complication or comorbidity diagnosis, CC condition, is defined as a significant acute disease, a significant acute manifestation of a chronic disease, an advanced or end-stage chronic disease, or a chronic disease associated with systemic physiological decompensation and debility that have consistently greater impact on hospital resources.

A CC icon appears to the right of the code description.

## MCC Condition                                                       MCC

This symbol designates a major complication or comorbidity diagnosis that may affect DRG assignment. An MCC condition meets the same criteria as a CC condition but is associated with a higher acuity level and hospital resource consumption is expected to be higher than that for a CC condition. There are fewer conditions that meet the criteria as an MCC than those for a CC condition.

An MCC icon appears to the right of the code description.

## CC Excludes Notations

The assignment of an MS-DRG often depends on the presence or absence of a secondary diagnosis code that is designated as an MCC or CC. However, in some instances the MCC or CC designation for that secondary diagnosis code is negated due to its relationship with the principal diagnosis.

To save space in this coding manual and provide a more comprehensive reference for the user, the CC Exclusion notations have been restructured. Instead of the individual codes being listed in the reference, which can in many cases be extensive, only the principal diagnosis collection (PDX collection) number is provided. A PDX collection contains a specific list of ICD-10-CM codes and their official descriptions that when used as principal diagnosis would render the MCC/CC designation ineffective. Each PDX collection is provided in an easily searchable data file which can be accessed at the following:

https://www.optum360coding.com/ProductUpdates/

Title: "2018 ICD-10-CM for Hospitals CC Excludes Data File"

Password: OptumCCExcl18

Similar to the parenthetical notes, the CC Exclusion notations are provided at the category, subcategory, and/or code level. If a CC Exclusion notation is found at the category or subcategory level, all the CC and/or MCC codes in that category or subcategory share the same PDX collection listed in that notation. For example:

**G43.6       Persistent migraine aura with cerebral infarction**

> **CC Excl: For CC codes in subcategory G43.6, unless otherwise noted:** PDX collection 584

There are four codes with a CC designation in subcategory G43.6; the CC Excludes notation applies to all four codes.

Often a CC exclusion reference is specific to laterality for CC/MCC codes in a category or subcategory. Where possible, a CC exclusion reference is placed at the category or subcategory level with the PDX collection identified for the right, left, or unspecified side. For example:

**S58**     **Traumatic amputation of elbow and forearm**

> **CC Excl: For CC codes in category S58:**
> **Right side:** PDX collection 1266
> **Left side:** PDX collection 1267
> **Unspecified side:** PDX collection 1268

All CC codes that are specific to the right side in category S58 are excluded from being a CC for any principal diagnosis found in PDX collection 1266.

Where possible a "see" reference may also be used, referring the user to a previously designated CC excludes notation. For example:

**S72.0**     **Fracture of head and neck of femur**

> **CC Excl: For CC/MCC codes in subcategory S72.0:**
> **Right side:** See code S72.001
> **Left side:** See code S72.002
> **Unspecified side:** See code S72.009

If users want to know the principal diagnoses to which code S72.022 Displaced fracture of epiphysis (separation) (upper) of left femur, may not function as a CC or MCC, they would be referred to the CC excludes notation under code S72.002.

Certain codes may also have no principal diagnosis codes to which they would be excluded from functioning as a CC or MCC. These are identified as follows:

**A17.83**     **Tuberculosis neuritis**
> **CC Excl:** No Excl

By definition of being a condition that acts as its own CC or MCC, the CC exclusion concept (two conditions being too interrelated) does not apply to PDxCC or PDxMCC (see "PDxCC or PDxMCC Condition"). However, if a condition carries separate PDxCC/PDxMCC and MCC/CC designations, a CC Excludes notation does appear for the CC and/or MCC designations.

### *PDxCC or PDxMCC Condition*                          `PDxCC` `PDxMCC`

Many ICD-10-CM codes identify multiple clinical concepts, typically describing an underlying condition and its associated acute manifestation; these are often referred to as combination codes. To continue to appropriately capture the complication/comorbidity (CC) or major complication/comorbidity (MCC) included in these combination codes, CMS introduced the concept of a diagnosis combination code acting as its own CC or MCC. For example, code I26.09 Other pulmonary embolism with acute cor pulmonale, is designated as a principal diagnosis that can act as its own MCC to capture the severity and resource consumption related to a pulmonary embolism that is exacerbated by acute cor pulmonale but is represented by one ICD-10-CM code.

The PDxCC and PDxMCC icons appear to the right of the code description.

### *HIV*                                                    `HIV`

This symbol indicates that the condition is considered a major HIV-related diagnosis. When the condition is coded in combination with a diagnosis of human immunodeficiency virus (HIV), code B20, the case will move from MS-DRG 977 to MS-DRGs 974-976.

The HIV icon appears to the right of the code description.

## Medicare Advantage Risk Adjustment Edits

Medicare Advantage plans provided as part of the Medicare Part C program uses a risk-adjustment model to plan for future healthcare costs to Medicare Part C participants. The risk-adjustment model measures disease burden by designating certain ICD-10-CM diagnosis codes as falling into hierarchical condition categories (HCC). The HCC information in this manual has been updated to reflect the CMS-HCC model category for v22 of the CMS-HCC risk-adjustment software.

### *HCC*                                                    `HCC`

This symbol indicates that the condition is considered a CMS-HCC diagnosis. All HCC conditions that are appropriately documented are used in the risk-adjustment model for Medicare Advantage to provide a means of comparing quality of care across Medicare Part C participants as well as predict future healthcare costs.

The HCC icon appears to the right of the code description.

## Other Code-Level Notations

### AHA:

This symbol precedes official citations from AHA's *Coding Clinic for ICD-10-CM/PCS*. Similar to the parenthetical notes, AHA references are placed in a hierarchical pattern at the chapter, code block, category, subcategory, or valid code level. This means that the information found in the reference applies to one or more codes depending on where the citation is placed.

The citations appear in purple type and are listed with the most current citation first. *Coding Clinic* citations included in this edition have been updated through second quarter 2017.

### DEF:

This symbol precedes a definition of a condition or disease.

The definition appears in purple type directly under the code.

### TIP:

This symbol precedes coding advice that is not readily available within the ICD-10-CM classification. It may relate official coding guidelines, indexing nuances, or advice from *AHA's Coding Clinic for ICD-10-CM/PCS*.

The tip appears in purple type directly under the code.

## Footnotes

All footnotes are identified by a numerical superscript that appears to the upper left of the code. For example:

[1] **I49.01**     **Ventricular fibrillation**                    `MCC`

The footnote 1 indicates "MCC = Only if patient is discharged alive." This means that ventricular fibrillation is considered a major complication or comorbidity that may affect DRG assignment only if the patient is discharged alive. Otherwise ventricular fibrillation is assigned as a non-MCC condition.

The following list identifies the meaning of each footnote number in the Tabular List of diseases:

1     These codes are considered major complication/comorbidity (MCC) conditions and may affect MS-DRG assignment only if the patient is discharged alive.

2     These codes indicate that the wrong procedure was performed on the patient and reimbursement may be affected.

3     This condition represents an unacceptable PDx for all encounters – initial, subsequent, and sequela (7th character A, D or S).

4     These codes, although not unacceptable as PDx, would be considered questionable as a PDx for acute care hospital admissions.

5     This code is considered an unacceptable PDx unless a relevant secondary diagnosis is also reported.

6     This condition is considered an MCC only when reported as an initial encounter for an open fracture (7th character B or C specific to category).

7     This condition is considered a CC only when reported as an initial encounter for a fracture (7th character A, B, or C specific to category) or a subsequent encounter for nonunion or malunion fracture (7th character K, M, N, P, Q, or R specific to category).

8   This condition is considered a CC only when reported as a subsequent encounter for a nonunion or malunion fracture (7th character K, M, N, P, Q, or R specific to category).

9   This condition is considered a CC only when reported as an initial encounter or subsequent encounter (7th character A or D).

10  This condition is considered an HCC when reported as initial encounter (7th character A, B, or C specific to category).

11  This condition is considered an HCC when reported as initial encounter (7th character A or B specific to category) or as a sequela.

12  This condition is considered an HCC when reported as a sequela.

## Chapter-Level Notations

### Chapter-Specific Guidelines with Coding Examples

Each chapter begins with the Official Guidelines for Coding and Reporting specific to that chapter, where provided. Coding examples specific to inpatient care settings have been provided to illustrate the coding and/or sequencing guidance in these guidelines.

### Muscle and Tendon Table

ICD-10-CM categorizes certain muscles and tendons in the upper and lower extremities by their action (e.g., extension or flexion) as well as their anatomical location. The Muscle/Tendon table is provided at the beginning of chapter 13 and chapter 19 to help users when code selection depends on the action of the muscle and/or tendon.

**Note:** This table is not all-inclusive, and proper code assignment should be based on the provider's documentation.

## Index Notations

▽   Subterms under main terms may continue to next column or page. This warning statement is a reminder to always check for additional subterms and information that may continue onto the next page or column before making a final selection.

### *Following* References

The Index includes following references to assist in locating "out-of-sequence" codes in the tabular list. "Out-of-sequence" codes contain an alphabetic character (letter) in the 3rd or 4th character position. These codes are placed according to the classification rules — the placement of the codes according to condition — not according to alphabetic or numeric sequencing rules.

*Examples:*

**Carcinoma (malignant)** (*see also* Neoplasm, by site, malignant)
neuroendocrine (*see also* Tumor, neuroendocrine)
    high grade, any site C7A.1 (*following* C75)
    poorly differentiated, any site C7A.1 (*following* C75)

In the tabular rubric, C7A is included after rubric C75 and before C76.

**Gout, chronic** (*see also* Gout, gouty) M1A.9
    drug-induced M1A.2Ø (*following* MØ8)
        ankle M1A.27-(*following* MØ8)
        elbow M1A.22-(*following* MØ8)

In the tabular rubric, M1A is included after rubric MØ8 and before M1Ø.

# ICD-10-CM Official Guidelines for Coding and Reporting

Note: The 2017 *ICD-10-CM Official Guidelines for Coding and Reporting* have been included as the 2018 guidelines were not available at the time of printing. As soon as the 2018 guidelines become available a downloadable PDF version will be posted to our website. You will also receive a booklet containing the updated 2018 ICD-10-CM guidelines in a separate shipment.

Narrative changes appear in **bold** text

Items underlined have been moved within the guidelines since the FY 2017 version

*Italics* are used to indicate revisions to heading changes

The Centers for Medicare and Medicaid Services (CMS) and the National Center for Health Statistics (NCHS), two departments within the U.S. Federal Government's Department of Health and Human Services (DHHS) provide the following guidelines for coding and reporting using the International Classification of Diseases, 10th Revision, Clinical Modification (ICD-10-CM). These guidelines should be used as a companion document to the official version of the ICD-10-CM as published on the NCHS website. The ICD-10-CM is a morbidity classification published by the United States for classifying diagnoses and reason for visits in all health care settings. The ICD-10-CM is based on the ICD-10, the statistical classification of disease published by the World Health Organization (WHO).

These guidelines have been approved by the four organizations that make up the Cooperating Parties for the ICD-10-CM: the American Hospital Association (AHA), the American Health Information Management Association (AHIMA), CMS, and NCHS.

These guidelines are a set of rules that have been developed to accompany and complement the official conventions and instructions provided within the ICD-10-CM itself. The instructions and conventions of the classification take precedence over guidelines. These guidelines are based on the coding and sequencing instructions in the Tabular List and Alphabetic Index of ICD-10-CM, but provide additional instruction. Adherence to these guidelines when assigning ICD-10-CM diagnosis codes is required under the Health Insurance Portability and Accountability Act (HIPAA). The diagnosis codes (Tabular List and Alphabetic Index) have been adopted under HIPAA for all healthcare settings. A joint effort between the healthcare provider and the coder is essential to achieve complete and accurate documentation, code assignment, and reporting of diagnoses and procedures. These guidelines have been developed to assist both the healthcare provider and the coder in identifying those diagnoses that are to be reported. The importance of consistent, complete documentation in the medical record cannot be overemphasized. Without such documentation accurate coding cannot be achieved. The entire record should be reviewed to determine the specific reason for the encounter and the conditions treated.

The term encounter is used for all settings, including hospital admissions. In the context of these guidelines, the term provider is used throughout the guidelines to mean physician or any qualified health care practitioner who is legally accountable for establishing the patient's diagnosis. Only this set of guidelines, approved by the Cooperating Parties, is official.

The guidelines are organized into sections. Section I includes the structure and conventions of the classification and general guidelines that apply to the entire classification, and chapter-specific guidelines that correspond to the chapters as they are arranged in the classification. Section II includes guidelines for selection of principal diagnosis for non-outpatient settings. Section III includes guidelines for reporting additional diagnoses in non-outpatient settings. Section IV is for outpatient coding and reporting. It is necessary to review all sections of the guidelines to fully understand all of the rules and instructions needed to code properly.

# Section I. Conventions, general coding guidelines and chapter specific guidelines

The conventions, general guidelines and chapter-specific guidelines are applicable to all health care settings unless otherwise indicated. The conventions and instructions of the classification take precedence over guidelines.

## A. Conventions for the ICD-10-CM

The conventions for the ICD-10-CM are the general rules for use of the classification independent of the guidelines. These conventions are incorporated within the Alphabetic Index and Tabular List of the ICD-10-CM as instructional notes.

1.  **The Alphabetic Index and Tabular List**
    The ICD-10-CM is divided into the Alphabetic Index, an alphabetical list of terms and their corresponding code, and the Tabular List, a structured list of codes divided into chapters based on body system or condition. The Alphabetic Index consists of the following parts: the Index of Diseases and Injury, the Index of External Causes of Injury, the Table of Neoplasms and the Table of Drugs and Chemicals.

    *See Section I.C2. General guidelines*

    *See Section I.C.19. Adverse effects, poisoning, underdosing and toxic effects*

2.  **Format and Structure:**
    The ICD-10-CM Tabular List contains categories, subcategories and codes. Characters for categories, subcategories and codes may be either a letter or a number. All categories are 3 characters. A three-character category that has no further subdivision is equivalent to a code. Subcategories are either 4 or 5 characters. Codes may be 3, 4, 5, 6 or 7 characters. That is, each level of subdivision after a category is a subcategory. The final level of subdivision is a code. Codes that have applicable 7th characters are still referred to as codes, not subcategories. A code that has an applicable 7th character is considered invalid without the 7th character.

    The ICD-10-CM uses an indented format for ease in reference.

3.  **Use of codes for reporting purposes**
    For reporting purposes only codes are permissible, not categories or subcategories, and any applicable 7th character is required.

4.  **Placeholder character**
    The ICD-10-CM utilizes a placeholder character "X". The "X" is used as a placeholder at certain codes to allow for future expansion. An example of this is at the poisoning, adverse effect and underdosing codes, categories T36-T50.

    Where a placeholder exists, the X must be used in order for the code to be considered a valid code.

5.  **7th Characters**
    Certain ICD-10-CM categories have applicable 7th characters. The applicable 7th character is required for all codes within the category, or as the notes in the Tabular List instruct. The 7th character must always be the 7th character in the data field. If a code that requires a 7th character is not 6 characters, a placeholder X must be used to fill in the empty characters.

6.  **Abbreviations**
    a. **Alphabetic Index abbreviations**
       NEC     "Not elsewhere classifiable"

This abbreviation in the Alphabetic Index represents "other specified." When a specific code is not available for a condition, the Alphabetic Index directs the coder to the "other specified" code in the Tabular List.
   NOS    "Not otherwise specified"
        This abbreviation is the equivalent of unspecified.

   b. **Tabular List abbreviations**
     NEC    "Not elsewhere classifiable"
         This abbreviation in the Tabular List represents "other specified". When a specific code is not available for a condition, the Tabular List includes an NEC entry under a code to identify the code as the "other specified" code.
     NOS    "Not otherwise specified"
         This abbreviation is the equivalent of unspecified.

7.  **Punctuation**
    [ ]   Brackets are used in the Tabular List to enclose synonyms, alternative wording or explanatory phrases. Brackets are used in the Alphabetic Index to identify manifestation codes.

    ( )   Parentheses are used in both the Alphabetic Index and Tabular List to enclose supplementary words that may be present or absent in the statement of a disease or procedure without affecting the code number to which it is assigned. The terms within the parentheses are referred to as nonessential modifiers. The nonessential modifiers in the Alphabetic Index to Diseases apply to subterms following a main term except when a nonessential modifier and a subentry are mutually exclusive, the subentry takes precedence. For example, in the ICD-10-CM Alphabetic Index under the main term Enteritis, "acute" is a nonessential modifier and "chronic" is a subentry. In this case, the nonessential modifier "acute" does not apply to the subentry "chronic".

    :    Colons are used in the Tabular List after an incomplete term which needs one or more of the modifiers following the colon to make it assignable to a given category.

8.  **Use of "and".**
    *See Section I.A.14. Use of the term "And"*

9.  **Other and Unspecified codes**
    a. **"Other" codes**
    Codes titled "other" or "other specified" are for use when the information in the medical record provides detail for which a specific code does not exist. Alphabetic Index entries with NEC in the line designate "other" codes in the Tabular List. These Alphabetic Index entries represent specific disease entities for which no specific code exists so the term is included within an "other" code.

    b. **"Unspecified" codes**
    Codes titled "unspecified" are for use when the information in the medical record is insufficient to assign a more specific code. For those categories for which an unspecified code is not provided, the "other specified" code may represent both other and unspecified.

    *See Section I.B.18 Use of Signs/Symptom/Unspecified Codes*

10. **Includes Notes**
    This note appears immediately under a three character code title to further define, or give examples of, the content of the category.

11. **Inclusion terms**
    List of terms is included under some codes. These terms are the conditions for which that code is to be used. The terms may be synonyms of the code title, or, in the case of "other specified" codes, the terms are a list of the various conditions assigned to that code. The inclusion terms are not necessarily exhaustive. Additional terms found only in the Alphabetic Index may also be assigned to a code.

12. **Excludes Notes**
    The ICD-10-CM has two types of excludes notes. Each type of note has a different definition for use but they are all similar in that they indicate that codes excluded from each other are independent of each other.

    a. **Excludes1**
    A type 1 Excludes note is a pure excludes note. It means "NOT CODED HERE!" An Excludes1 note indicates that the code excluded should never be used at the same time as the code above the Excludes1 note. An Excludes1 is used when two conditions cannot occur together, such as a congenital form versus an acquired form of the same condition.

An exception to the Excludes1 definition is the circumstance when the two conditions are unrelated to each other. If it is not clear whether the two conditions involving an Excludes1 note are related or not, query the provider. For example, code F45.8, Other somatoform disorders, has an Excludes1 note for "sleep related teeth grinding (G47.63)," because "teeth grinding" is an inclusion term under F45.8. Only one of these two codes should be assigned for teeth grinding. However psychogenic dysmenorrhea is also an inclusion term under F45.8, and a patient could have both this condition and sleep related teeth grinding. In this case, the two conditions are clearly unrelated to each other, and so it would be appropriate to report F45.8 and G47.63 together.

**b. Excludes2**

A type 2 Excludes note represents "Not included here." An excludes2 note indicates that the condition excluded is not part of the condition represented by the code, but a patient may have both conditions at the same time. When an Excludes2 note appears under a code, it is acceptable to use both the code and the excluded code together, when appropriate.

**13. Etiology/manifestation convention ("code first", "use additional code" and "in diseases classified elsewhere" notes)**

Certain conditions have both an underlying etiology and multiple body system manifestations due to the underlying etiology. For such conditions, the ICD-10-CM has a coding convention that requires the underlying condition be sequenced first, if applicable, followed by the manifestation. Wherever such a combination exists, there is a "use additional code" note at the etiology code, and a "code first" note at the manifestation code. These instructional notes indicate the proper sequencing order of the codes, etiology followed by manifestation.

In most cases the manifestation codes will have in the code title, "in diseases classified elsewhere." Codes with this title are a component of the etiology/ manifestation convention. The code title indicates that it is a manifestation code. "In diseases classified elsewhere" codes are never permitted to be used as first-listed or principal diagnosis codes. They must be used in conjunction with an underlying condition code and they must be listed following the underlying condition. See category F02, Dementia in other diseases classified elsewhere, for an example of this convention.

There are manifestation codes that do not have "in diseases classified elsewhere" in the title. For such codes, there is a "use additional code" note at the etiology code and a "code first" note at the manifestation code, and the rules for sequencing apply.

In addition to the notes in the Tabular List, these conditions also have a specific Alphabetic Index entry structure. In the Alphabetic Index both conditions are listed together with the etiology code first followed by the manifestation codes in brackets. The code in brackets is always to be sequenced second.

An example of the etiology/manifestation convention is dementia in Parkinson's disease. In the Alphabetic Index, code G20 is listed first, followed by code F02.80 or F02.81 in brackets. Code G20 represents the underlying etiology, Parkinson's disease, and must be sequenced first, whereas codes F02.80 and F02.81 represent the manifestation of dementia in diseases classified elsewhere, with or without behavioral disturbance.

"Code first" and "Use additional code" notes are also used as sequencing rules in the classification for certain codes that are not part of an etiology/ manifestation combination.

*See Section I.B.7. Multiple coding for a single condition.*

**14. "And"**

The word "and" should be interpreted to mean either "and" or "or" when it appears in a title.

For example, cases of "tuberculosis of bones", "tuberculosis of joints" and "tuberculosis of bones and joints" are classified to subcategory A18.0, Tuberculosis of bones and joints.

**15. "With"**

The word "with" should be interpreted to mean "associated with" or "due to" when it appears in a code title, the Alphabetic Index, or an instructional note in the Tabular List. The classification presumes a causal relationship between the two conditions linked by these terms in the Alphabetic Index or Tabular List. These conditions should be coded as related even in the absence of provider documentation explicitly linking

them, unless the documentation clearly states the conditions are unrelated. For conditions not specifically linked by these relational terms in the classification, provider documentation must link the conditions in order to code them as related. The word "with" in the Alphabetic Index is sequenced immediately following the main term, not in alphabetical order.

**16. "See" and "See Also"**

The "see" instruction following a main term in the Alphabetic Index indicates that another term should be referenced. It is necessary to go to the main term referenced with the "see" note to locate the correct code.

A "see also" instruction following a main term in the Alphabetic Index instructs that there is another main term that may also be referenced that may provide additional Alphabetic Index entries that may be useful. It is not necessary to follow the "see also" note when the original main term provides the necessary code.

**17. "Code also" note**

A "code also" note instructs that two codes may be required to fully describe a condition, but this note does not provide sequencing direction.

**18. Default codes**

A code listed next to a main term in the ICD-10-CM Alphabetic Index is referred to as a default code. The default code represents that condition that is most commonly associated with the main term, or is the unspecified code for the condition. If a condition is documented in a medical record (for example, appendicitis) without any additional information, such as acute or chronic, the default code should be assigned.

**19. Code assignment and Clinical Criteria**

The assignment of a diagnosis code is based on the provider's diagnostic statement that the condition exists. The provider's statement that the patient has a particular condition is sufficient. Code assignment is not based on clinical criteria used by the provider to establish the diagnosis.

# B. General Coding Guidelines

**1. Locating a code in the ICD-10-CM**

To select a code in the classification that corresponds to a diagnosis or reason for visit documented in a medical record, first locate the term in the Alphabetic Index, and then verify the code in the Tabular List. Read and be guided by instructional notations that appear in both the Alphabetic Index and the Tabular List.

It is essential to use both the Alphabetic Index and Tabular List when locating and assigning a code. The Alphabetic Index does not always provide the full code. Selection of the full code, including laterality and any applicable 7th character can only be done in the Tabular List. A dash (-) at the end of an Alphabetic Index entry indicates that additional characters are required. Even if a dash is not included at the Alphabetic Index entry, it is necessary to refer to the Tabular List to verify that no 7th character is required.

**2. Level of Detail in Coding**

Diagnosis codes are to be used and reported at their highest number of characters available.

ICD-10-CM diagnosis codes are composed of codes with 3, 4, 5, 6 or 7 characters. Codes with three characters are included in ICD-10-CM as the heading of a category of codes that may be further subdivided by the use of fourth and/or fifth characters and/or sixth characters, which provide greater detail.

A three-character code is to be used only if it is not further subdivided. A code is invalid if it has not been coded to the full number of characters required for that code, including the 7th character, if applicable.

**3. Code or codes from A00.0 through T88.9, Z00-Z99.8**

The appropriate code or codes from A00.0 through T88.9, Z00-Z99.8 must be used to identify diagnoses, symptoms, conditions, problems, complaints or other reason(s) for the encounter/visit.

**4. Signs and symptoms**

Codes that describe symptoms and signs, as opposed to diagnoses, are acceptable for reporting purposes when a related definitive diagnosis has not been established (confirmed) by the provider. Chapter 18 of ICD-10-CM, Symptoms, Signs, and Abnormal Clinical and Laboratory Findings, Not Elsewhere Classified (codes R00.0 - R99) contains many, but not all, codes for symptoms.

*See Section I.B.18 Use of Signs/Symptom/Unspecified Codes*

**5. Conditions that are an integral part of a disease process**
Signs and symptoms that are associated routinely with a disease process should not be assigned as additional codes, unless otherwise instructed by the classification.

**6. Conditions that are not an integral part of a disease process**
Additional signs and symptoms that may not be associated routinely with a disease process should be coded when present.

**7. Multiple coding for a single condition**
In addition to the etiology/manifestation convention that requires two codes to fully describe a single condition that affects multiple body systems, there are other single conditions that also require more than one code. "Use additional code" notes are found in the Tabular List at codes that are not part of an etiology/manifestation pair where a secondary code is useful to fully describe a condition. The sequencing rule is the same as the etiology/manifestation pair, "use additional code" indicates that a secondary code should be added.

For example, for bacterial infections that are not included in chapter 1, a secondary code from category B95, Streptococcus, Staphylococcus, and Enterococcus, as the cause of diseases classified elsewhere, or B96, Other bacterial agents as the cause of diseases classified elsewhere, may be required to identify the bacterial organism causing the infection. A "use additional code" note will normally be found at the infectious disease code, indicating a need for the organism code to be added as a secondary code.

"Code first" notes are also under certain codes that are not specifically manifestation codes but may be due to an underlying cause. When there is a "code first" note and an underlying condition is present, the underlying condition should be sequenced first.

"Code, if applicable, any causal condition first" notes indicate that this code may be assigned as a principal diagnosis when the causal condition is unknown or not applicable. If a causal condition is known, then the code for that condition should be sequenced as the principal or first-listed diagnosis.

Multiple codes may be needed for sequela, complication codes and obstetric codes to more fully describe a condition. See the specific guidelines for these conditions for further instruction.

**8. Acute and Chronic Conditions**
If the same condition is described as both acute (subacute) and chronic, and separate subentries exist in the Alphabetic Index at the same indentation level, code both and sequence the acute (subacute) code first.

**9. Combination Code**
A combination code is a single code used to classify:
Two diagnoses, or
A diagnosis with an associated secondary process (manifestation)
A diagnosis with an associated complication

Combination codes are identified by referring to subterm entries in the Alphabetic Index and by reading the inclusion and exclusion notes in the Tabular List.

Assign only the combination code when that code fully identifies the diagnostic conditions involved or when the Alphabetic Index so directs. Multiple coding should not be used when the classification provides a combination code that clearly identifies all of the elements documented in the diagnosis. When the combination code lacks necessary specificity in describing the manifestation or complication, an additional code should be used as a secondary code.

**10. Sequela (Late Effects)**
A sequela is the residual effect (condition produced) after the acute phase of an illness or injury has terminated. There is no time limit on when a sequela code can be used. The residual may be apparent early, such as in cerebral infarction, or it may occur months or years later, such as that due to a previous injury. Examples of sequela include: scar formation resulting from a burn, deviated septum due to a nasal fracture, and infertility due to tubal occlusion from old tuberculosis. Coding of sequela generally requires two codes sequenced in the following order: the condition or nature of the sequela is sequenced first. The sequela code is sequenced second.

An exception to the above guidelines are those instances where the code for the sequela is followed by a manifestation code identified in the Tabular List and title, or the sequela code has been expanded (at the fourth, fifth or sixth character levels) to include the manifestation(s). The code for the acute phase of an illness or injury that led to the sequela is never used with a code for the late effect.

*See Section I.C.9. Sequelae of cerebrovascular disease*

*See Section I.C.15. Sequelae of complication of pregnancy, childbirth and the puerperium*

*See Section I.C.19. Application of 7th characters for Chapter 19*

**11. Impending or Threatened Condition**
Code any condition described at the time of discharge as "impending" or "threatened" as follows:

If it did occur, code as confirmed diagnosis.
If it did not occur, reference the Alphabetic Index to determine if the condition has a subentry term for "impending" or "threatened" and also reference main term entries for "Impending" and for "Threatened."
If the subterms are listed, assign the given code.
If the subterms are not listed, code the existing underlying condition(s) and not the condition described as impending or threatened.

**12. Reporting Same Diagnosis Code More than Once**
Each unique ICD-10-CM diagnosis code may be reported only once for an encounter. This applies to bilateral conditions when there are no distinct codes identifying laterality or two different conditions classified to the same ICD-10-CM diagnosis code.

**13. Laterality**
Some ICD-10-CM codes indicate laterality, specifying whether the condition occurs on the left, right or is bilateral. If no bilateral code is provided and the condition is bilateral, assign separate codes for both the left and right side. If the side is not identified in the medical record, assign the code for the unspecified side.

When a patient has a bilateral condition and each side is treated during separate encounters, assign the "bilateral" code (as the condition still exists on both sides), including for the encounter to treat the first side. For the second encounter for treatment after one side has previously been treated and the condition no longer exists on that side, assign the appropriate unilateral code for the side where the condition still exists (e.g., cataract surgery performed on each eye in separate encounters). The bilateral code would not be assigned for the subsequent encounter, as the patient no longer has the condition in the previously-treated site. If the treatment on the first side did not completely resolve the condition, then the bilateral code would still be appropriate.

**14. Documentation for BMI, Depth of Non-pressure ulcers, Pressure Ulcer Stages, Coma Scale, and NIH Stroke Scale**
For the Body Mass Index (BMI), depth of non-pressure chronic ulcers, pressure ulcer stage, coma scale, and NIH stroke scale (NIHSS) codes, code assignment may be based on medical record documentation from clinicians who are not the patient's provider (i.e., physician or other qualified healthcare practitioner legally accountable for establishing the patient's diagnosis), since this information is typically documented by other clinicians involved in the care of the patient (e.g., a dietitian often documents the BMI, a nurse often documents the pressure ulcer stages, and an emergency medical technician often documents the coma scale). However, the associated diagnosis (such as overweight, obesity, acute stroke, or pressure ulcer) must be documented by the patient's provider. If there is conflicting medical record documentation, either from the same clinician or different clinicians, the patient's attending provider should be queried for clarification.

The BMI, coma scale, and NIHSS codes should only be reported as secondary diagnoses.

**15. Syndromes**
Follow the Alphabetic Index guidance when coding syndromes. In the absence of Alphabetic Index guidance, assign codes for the documented manifestations of the syndrome. Additional codes for manifestations that are not an integral part of the disease process may also be assigned when the condition does not have a unique code.

**16. Documentation of Complications of Care**
Code assignment is based on the provider's documentation of the relationship between the condition and the care or procedure, unless otherwise instructed by the classification. The guideline extends to any complications of care, regardless of the chapter the code is located in. It is important to note that not all conditions that occur during or following medical care or surgery are classified as complications. There must be a cause-and-effect relationship between the care provided and

the condition, and an indication in the documentation that it is a complication. Query the provider for clarification, if the complication is not clearly documented.

### 17. Borderline Diagnosis

If the provider documents a "borderline" diagnosis at the time of discharge, the diagnosis is coded as confirmed, unless the classification provides a specific entry (e.g., borderline diabetes). If a borderline condition has a specific index entry in ICD-10-CM, it should be coded as such. Since borderline conditions are not uncertain diagnoses, no distinction is made between the care setting (inpatient versus outpatient). Whenever the documentation is unclear regarding a borderline condition, coders are encouraged to query for clarification.

### 18. Use of Sign/Symptom/Unspecified Codes

Sign/symptom and "unspecified" codes have acceptable, even necessary, uses. While specific diagnosis codes should be reported when they are supported by the available medical record documentation and clinical knowledge of the patient's health condition, there are instances when signs/symptoms or unspecified codes are the best choices for accurately reflecting the healthcare encounter. Each healthcare encounter should be coded to the level of certainty known for that encounter.

If a definitive diagnosis has not been established by the end of the encounter, it is appropriate to report codes for sign(s) and/or symptom(s) in lieu of a definitive diagnosis. When sufficient clinical information isn't known or available about a particular health condition to assign a more specific code, it is acceptable to report the appropriate "unspecified" code (e.g., a diagnosis of pneumonia has been determined, but not the specific type). Unspecified codes should be reported when they are the codes that most accurately reflect what is known about the patient's condition at the time of that particular encounter. It would be inappropriate to select a specific code that is not supported by the medical record documentation or conduct medically unnecessary diagnostic testing in order to determine a more specific code.

## C. Chapter-Specific Coding Guidelines

In addition to general coding guidelines, there are guidelines for specific diagnoses and/or conditions in the classification. Unless otherwise indicated, these guidelines apply to all health care settings. Please refer to Section II for guidelines on the selection of principal diagnosis.

### 1. Chapter 1: Certain Infectious and Parasitic Diseases (A00-B99)

#### a. Human Immunodeficiency Virus (HIV) Infections

##### 1) Code only confirmed cases

Code only confirmed cases of HIV infection/illness. This is an exception to the hospital inpatient guideline Section II, H.

In this context, "confirmation" does not require documentation of positive serology or culture for HIV; the provider's diagnostic statement that the patient is HIV positive, or has an HIV-related illness is sufficient.

##### 2) Selection and sequencing of HIV codes

###### (a) Patient admitted for HIV-related condition

If a patient is admitted for an HIV-related condition, the principal diagnosis should be B20, Human immunodeficiency virus [HIV] disease followed by additional diagnosis codes for all reported HIV-related conditions.

###### (b) Patient with HIV disease admitted for unrelated condition

If a patient with HIV disease is admitted for an unrelated condition (such as a traumatic injury), the code for the unrelated condition (e.g., the nature of injury code) should be the principal diagnosis. Other diagnoses would be B20 followed by additional diagnosis codes for all reported HIV-related conditions.

###### (c) Whether the patient is newly diagnosed

Whether the patient is newly diagnosed or has had previous admissions/encounters for HIV conditions is irrelevant to the sequencing decision.

###### (d) Asymptomatic human immunodeficiency virus

Z21, Asymptomatic human immunodeficiency virus [HIV] infection status, is to be applied when the patient without any documentation of symptoms is listed as being "HIV positive," "known HIV," "HIV test positive," or similar terminology. Do not use this code if the term "AIDS" is used or if the patient is treated for any HIV-related illness or is described as having any condition(s) resulting from his/her HIV positive status; use B20 in these cases.

###### (e) Patients with inconclusive HIV serology

Patients with inconclusive HIV serology, but no definitive diagnosis or manifestations of the illness, may be assigned code R75, Inconclusive laboratory evidence of human immunodeficiency virus [HIV].

###### (f) Previously diagnosed HIV-related illness

Patients with any known prior diagnosis of an HIV-related illness should be coded to B20. Once a patient has developed an HIV-related illness, the patient should always be assigned code B20 on every subsequent admission/encounter. Patients previously diagnosed with any HIV illness (B20) should never be assigned to R75 or Z21, Asymptomatic human immunodeficiency virus [HIV] infection status.

###### (g) HIV Infection in Pregnancy, Childbirth and the Puerperium

During pregnancy, childbirth or the puerperium, a patient admitted (or presenting for a health care encounter) because of an HIV-related illness should receive a principal diagnosis code of O98.7-, Human immunodeficiency [HIV] disease complicating pregnancy, childbirth and the puerperium, followed by B20 and the code(s) for the HIV-related illness(es). Codes from Chapter 15 always take sequencing priority.

Patients with asymptomatic HIV infection status admitted (or presenting for a health care encounter) during pregnancy, childbirth, or the puerperium should receive codes of O98.7- and Z21.

###### (h) Encounters for testing for HIV

If a patient is being seen to determine his/her HIV status, use code Z11.4, Encounter for screening for human immunodeficiency virus [HIV]. Use additional codes for any associated high risk behavior.

If a patient with signs or symptoms is being seen for HIV testing, code the signs and symptoms. An additional counseling code Z71.7, Human immunodeficiency virus [HIV] counseling, may be used if counseling is provided during the encounter for the test.

When a patient returns to be informed of his/her HIV test results and the test result is negative, use code Z71.7, Human immunodeficiency virus [HIV] counseling.

If the results are positive, see previous guidelines and assign codes as appropriate.

#### b. Infectious agents as the cause of diseases classified to other chapters

Certain infections are classified in chapters other than Chapter 1 and no organism is identified as part of the infection code. In these instances, it is necessary to use an additional code from Chapter 1 to identify the organism. A code from category B95, Streptococcus, Staphylococcus, and Enterococcus as the cause of diseases classified to other chapters, B96, Other bacterial agents as the cause of diseases classified to other chapters, or B97, Viral agents as the cause of diseases classified to other chapters, is to be used as an additional code to identify the organism. An instructional note will be found at the infection code advising that an additional organism code is required.

#### c. Infections resistant to antibiotics

Many bacterial infections are resistant to current antibiotics. It is necessary to identify all infections documented as antibiotic resistant. Assign a code from category Z16, Resistance to antimicrobial drugs, following the infection code only if the infection code does not identify drug resistance.

**d. Sepsis, Severe Sepsis, and Septic Shock**

**1) Coding of Sepsis and Severe Sepsis**

**(a) Sepsis**

For a diagnosis of sepsis, assign the appropriate code for the underlying systemic infection. If the type of infection or causal organism is not further specified, assign code A41.9, Sepsis, unspecified organism.

A code from subcategory R65.2, Severe sepsis, should not be assigned unless severe sepsis or an associated acute organ dysfunction is documented.

**(i) Negative or inconclusive blood cultures and sepsis**

Negative or inconclusive blood cultures do not preclude a diagnosis of sepsis in patients with clinical evidence of the condition; however, the provider should be queried.

**(ii) Urosepsis**

The term urosepsis is a nonspecific term. It is not to be considered synonymous with sepsis. It has no default code in the Alphabetic Index. Should a provider use this term, he/she must be queried for clarification.

**(iii) Sepsis with organ dysfunction**

If a patient has sepsis and associated acute organ dysfunction or multiple organ dysfunction (MOD), follow the instructions for coding severe sepsis.

**(iv) Acute organ dysfunction that is not clearly associated with the sepsis**

If a patient has sepsis and an acute organ dysfunction, but the medical record documentation indicates that the acute organ dysfunction is related to a medical condition other than the sepsis, do not assign a code from subcategory R65.2, Severe sepsis. An acute organ dysfunction must be associated with the sepsis in order to assign the severe sepsis code. If the documentation is not clear as to whether an acute organ dysfunction is related to the sepsis or another medical condition, query the provider.

**(b) Severe sepsis**

The coding of severe sepsis requires a minimum of 2 codes: first a code for the underlying systemic infection, followed by a code from subcategory R65.2, Severe sepsis. If the causal organism is not documented, assign code A41.9, Sepsis, unspecified organism, for the infection. Additional code(s) for the associated acute organ dysfunction are also required.

Due to the complex nature of severe sepsis, some cases may require querying the provider prior to assignment of the codes.

**2) Septic shock**

**(a)** Septic shock generally refers to circulatory failure associated with severe sepsis, and therefore, it represents a type of acute organ dysfunction.

For cases of septic shock, the code for the systemic infection should be sequenced first, followed by code R65.21, Severe sepsis with septic shock or code T81.12, Postprocedural septic shock. Any additional codes for the other acute organ dysfunctions should also be assigned. As noted in the sequencing instructions in the Tabular List, the code for septic shock cannot be assigned as a principal diagnosis.

**3) Sequencing of severe sepsis**

If severe sepsis is present on admission, and meets the definition of principal diagnosis, the underlying systemic infection should be assigned as principal diagnosis followed by the appropriate code from subcategory R65.2 as required by the sequencing rules in the Tabular List. A code from subcategory R65.2 can never be assigned as a principal diagnosis.

When severe sepsis develops during an encounter (it was not present on admission), the underlying systemic infection and

the appropriate code from subcategory R65.2 should be assigned as secondary diagnoses.

Severe sepsis may be present on admission, but the diagnosis may not be confirmed until sometime after admission. If the documentation is not clear whether severe sepsis was present on admission, the provider should be queried.

**4) Sepsis and severe sepsis with a localized infection**

If the reason for admission is both sepsis or severe sepsis and a localized infection, such as pneumonia or cellulitis, a code(s) for the underlying systemic infection should be assigned first and the code for the localized infection should be assigned as a secondary diagnosis. If the patient has severe sepsis, a code from subcategory R65.2 should also be assigned as a secondary diagnosis. If the patient is admitted with a localized infection, such as pneumonia, and sepsis/severe sepsis doesn't develop until after admission, the localized infection should be assigned first, followed by the appropriate sepsis/severe sepsis codes.

**5) Sepsis due to a postprocedural infection**

**(a) Documentation of causal relationship**

As with all postprocedural complications, code assignment is based on the provider's documentation of the relationship between the infection and the procedure.

**(b) Sepsis due to a postprocedural infection**

For such cases, the postprocedural infection code, such as T80.2, Infections following infusion, transfusion, and therapeutic injection, T81.4, Infection following a procedure, T88.0, Infection following immunization, or O86.0, Infection of obstetric surgical wound, should be coded first, followed by the code for the specific infection. If the patient has severe sepsis, the appropriate code from subcategory R65.2 should also be assigned with the additional code(s) for any acute organ dysfunction.

**(c) Postprocedural infection and postprocedural septic shock**

In cases where a postprocedural infection has occurred and has resulted in severe sepsis the code for the precipitating complication such as code T81.4, Infection following a procedure, or O86.0, Infection of obstetrical surgical wound should be coded first followed by code R65.20, Severe sepsis without septic shock. A code for the systemic infection should also be assigned.

If a postprocedural infection has resulted in postprocedural septic shock, the code for the precipitating complication such as code T81.4, Infection following a procedure, or O86.0, Infection of obstetrical surgical wound should be coded first followed by code T81.12-, Postprocedural septic shock. A code for the systemic infection should also be assigned.

**6) Sepsis and severe sepsis associated with a noninfectious process (condition)**

In some cases a noninfectious process (condition), such as trauma, may lead to an infection which can result in sepsis or severe sepsis. If sepsis or severe sepsis is documented as associated with a noninfectious condition, such as a burn or serious injury, and this condition meets the definition for principal diagnosis, the code for the noninfectious condition should be sequenced first, followed by the code for the resulting infection. If severe sepsis is present, a code from subcategory R65.2 should also be assigned with any associated organ dysfunction(s) codes. It is not necessary to assign a code from subcategory R65.1, Systemic inflammatory response syndrome (SIRS) of non-infectious origin, for these cases.

If the infection meets the definition of principal diagnosis, it should be sequenced before the non-infectious condition. When both the associated non-infectious condition and the infection meet the definition of principal diagnosis, either may be assigned as principal diagnosis.

Only one code from category R65, Symptoms and signs specifically associated with systemic inflammation and infection, should be assigned. Therefore, when a non-infectious condition leads to an infection resulting in severe sepsis, assign the appropriate code from subcategory R65.2, Severe sepsis. Do not additionally assign a code from subcategory R65.1, Systemic inflammatory response syndrome (SIRS) of non-infectious origin.

*See Section I.C.18. SIRS due to non-infectious process*

**7) Sepsis and septic shock complicating abortion, pregnancy, childbirth, and the puerperium**
*See Section I.C.15. Sepsis and septic shock complicating abortion, pregnancy, childbirth and the puerperium*

**8) Newborn sepsis**
*See Section I.C.16. f. Bacterial sepsis of Newborn*

**e. Methicillin Resistant *Staphylococcus aureus* (MRSA) Conditions**
**1) Selection and sequencing of MRSA codes**
**(a) Combination codes for MRSA infection**
When a patient is diagnosed with an infection that is due to methicillin resistant *Staphylococcus aureus* (MRSA), and that infection has a combination code that includes the causal organism (e.g., sepsis, pneumonia) assign the appropriate combination code for the condition (e.g., code A41.02, Sepsis due to Methicillin resistant Staphylococcus aureus or code J15.212, Pneumonia due to Methicillin resistant Staphylococcus aureus). Do not assign code B95.62, Methicillin resistant Staphylococcus aureus infection as the cause of diseases classified elsewhere, as an additional code, because the combination code includes the type of infection and the MRSA organism. Do not assign a code from subcategory Z16.11, Resistance to penicillins, as an additional diagnosis.

*See Section C.1. for instructions on coding and sequencing of sepsis and severe sepsis.*

**(b) Other codes for MRSA infection**
When there is documentation of a current infection (e.g., wound infection, stitch abscess, urinary tract infection) due to MRSA, and that infection does not have a combination code that includes the causal organism, assign the appropriate code to identify the condition along with code B95.62, Methicillin resistant Staphylococcus aureus infection as the cause of diseases classified elsewhere for the MRSA infection. Do not assign a code from subcategory Z16.11, Resistance to penicillins.

**(c) Methicillin susceptible Staphylococcus aureus (MSSA) and MRSA colonization**
The condition or state of being colonized or carrying MSSA or MRSA is called colonization or carriage, while an individual person is described as being colonized or being a carrier. Colonization means that MSSA or MSRA is present on or in the body without necessarily causing illness. A positive MRSA colonization test might be documented by the provider as "MRSA screen positive" or "MRSA nasal swab positive".

Assign code Z22.322, Carrier or suspected carrier of Methicillin resistant Staphylococcus aureus, for patients documented as having MRSA colonization. Assign code Z22.321, Carrier or suspected carrier of Methicillin susceptible Staphylococcus aureus, for patient documented as having MSSA colonization. Colonization is not necessarily indicative of a disease process or as the cause of a specific condition the patient may have unless documented as such by the provider.

**(d) MRSA colonization and infection**
If a patient is documented as having both MRSA colonization and infection during a hospital admission, code Z22.322, Carrier or suspected carrier of Methicillin resistant Staphylococcus aureus, and a code for the MRSA infection may both be assigned.

**f. Zika virus infections**
**1) Code only confirmed cases**
Code only a confirmed diagnosis of Zika virus (A92.5, Zika virus disease) as documented by the provider. This is an exception to the hospital inpatient guideline Section II, H.

In this context, "confirmation" does not require documentation of the type of test performed; the physician's diagnostic statement that the condition is confirmed is sufficient. This code should be assigned regardless of the stated mode of transmission.

If the provider documents "suspected", "possible" or "probable" Zika, do not assign code A92.5. Assign a code(s) explaining the reason for encounter (such as fever, rash, or joint pain) or Z20.828, Contact with and (suspected) exposure to other viral communicable diseases.

**2. Chapter 2: Neoplasms (C00-D49)**
**General guidelines**
Chapter 2 of the ICD-10-CM contains the codes for most benign and all malignant neoplasms. Certain benign neoplasms, such as prostatic adenomas, may be found in the specific body system chapters. To properly code a neoplasm it is necessary to determine from the record if the neoplasm is benign, in-situ, malignant, or of uncertain histologic behavior. If malignant, any secondary (metastatic) sites should also be determined.

Primary malignant neoplasms overlapping site boundaries

A primary malignant neoplasm that overlaps two or more contiguous (next to each other) sites should be classified to the subcategory/code .8 ('overlapping lesion'), unless the combination is specifically indexed elsewhere. For multiple neoplasms of the same site that are not contiguous such as tumors in different quadrants of the same breast, codes for each site should be assigned.

Malignant neoplasm of ectopic tissue

Malignant neoplasms of ectopic tissue are to be coded to the site of origin mentioned, e.g., ectopic pancreatic malignant neoplasms involving the stomach are coded to pancreas, unspecified (C25.9).

The neoplasm table in the Alphabetic Index should be referenced first. However, if the histological term is documented, that term should be referenced first, rather than going immediately to the Neoplasm Table, in order to determine which column in the Neoplasm Table is appropriate. For example, if the documentation indicates "adenoma," refer to the term in the Alphabetic Index to review the entries under this term and the instructional note to "see also neoplasm, by site, benign." The table provides the proper code based on the type of neoplasm and the site. It is important to select the proper column in the table that corresponds to the type of neoplasm. The Tabular List should then be referenced to verify that the correct code has been selected from the table and that a more specific site code does not exist.

*See Section I.C.21. Factors influencing health status and contact with health services, Status, for information regarding Z15.0, codes for genetic susceptibility to cancer.*

**a. Treatment directed at the malignancy**
If the treatment is directed at the malignancy, designate the malignancy as the principal diagnosis.

The only exception to this guideline is if a patient admission/encounter is solely for the administration of chemotherapy, immunotherapy or radiation therapy, assign the appropriate Z51.-- code as the first-listed or principal diagnosis, and the diagnosis or problem for which the service is being performed as a secondary diagnosis.

**b. Treatment of secondary site**
When a patient is admitted because of a primary neoplasm with metastasis and treatment is directed toward the secondary site only, the secondary neoplasm is designated as the principal diagnosis even though the primary malignancy is still present.

**c. Coding and sequencing of complications**
Coding and sequencing of complications associated with the malignancies or with the therapy thereof are subject to the following guidelines:

**1) Anemia associated with malignancy**
When admission/encounter is for management of an anemia associated with the malignancy, and the treatment is only for anemia, the appropriate code for the malignancy is sequenced as the principal or first-listed diagnosis followed by the appropriate code for the anemia (such as code D63.0, Anemia in neoplastic disease).

**2)** **Anemia associated with chemotherapy, immunotherapy and radiation therapy**

When the admission/encounter is for management of an anemia associated with an adverse effect of the administration of chemotherapy or immunotherapy and the only treatment is for the anemia, the anemia code is sequenced first followed by the appropriate codes for the neoplasm and the adverse effect (T45.1X5, Adverse effect of antineoplastic and immunosuppressive drugs).

When the admission/encounter is for management of an anemia associated with an adverse effect of radiotherapy, the anemia code should be sequenced first, followed by the appropriate neoplasm code and code Y84.2, Radiological procedure and radiotherapy as the cause of abnormal reaction of the patient, or of later complication, without mention of misadventure at the time of the procedure.

**3)** **Management of dehydration due to the malignancy**

When the admission/encounter is for management of dehydration due to the malignancy and only the dehydration is being treated (intravenous rehydration), the dehydration is sequenced first, followed by the code(s) for the malignancy.

**4)** **Treatment of a complication resulting from a surgical procedure**

When the admission/encounter is for treatment of a complication resulting from a surgical procedure, designate the complication as the principal or first-listed diagnosis if treatment is directed at resolving the complication.

**d. Primary malignancy previously excised**

When a primary malignancy has been previously excised or eradicated from its site and there is no further treatment directed to that site and there is no evidence of any existing primary malignancy, a code from category Z85, Personal history of malignant neoplasm, should be used to indicate the former site of the malignancy. Any mention of extension, invasion, or metastasis to another site is coded as a secondary malignant neoplasm to that site. The secondary site may be the principal or first-listed with the Z85 code used as a secondary code.

**e. Admissions/Encounters involving chemotherapy, immunotherapy and radiation therapy**

**1)** **Episode of care involves surgical removal of neoplasm**

When an episode of care involves the surgical removal of a neoplasm, primary or secondary site, followed by adjunct chemotherapy or radiation treatment during the same episode of care, the code for the neoplasm should be assigned as principal or first-listed diagnosis.

**2)** **Patient admission/encounter solely for administration of chemotherapy, immunotherapy and radiation therapy**

If a patient admission/encounter is solely for the administration of chemotherapy, immunotherapy or radiation therapy assign code Z51.0, Encounter for antineoplastic radiation therapy, or Z51.11, Encounter for antineoplastic chemotherapy, or Z51.12, Encounter for antineoplastic immunotherapy as the first-listed or principal diagnosis. If a patient receives more than one of these therapies during the same admission more than one of these codes may be assigned, in any sequence.

The malignancy for which the therapy is being administered should be assigned as a secondary diagnosis.

**3)** **Patient admitted for radiation therapy, chemotherapy or immunotherapy and develops complications**

When a patient is admitted for the purpose of radiotherapy, immunotherapy or chemotherapy and develops complications such as uncontrolled nausea and vomiting or dehydration, the principal or first-listed diagnosis is Z51.0, Encounter for antineoplastic radiation therapy, or Z51.11, Encounter for antineoplastic chemotherapy, or Z51.12, Encounter for antineoplastic immunotherapy followed by any codes for the complications.

**f. Admission/encounter to determine extent of malignancy**

When the reason for admission/encounter is to determine the extent of the malignancy, or for a procedure such as paracentesis or thoracentesis, the primary malignancy or appropriate metastatic site is designated as the principal or first-listed diagnosis, even though chemotherapy or radiotherapy is administered.

**g. Symptoms, signs, and abnormal findings listed in Chapter 18 associated with neoplasms**

Symptoms, signs, and ill-defined conditions listed in Chapter 18 characteristic of, or associated with, an existing primary or secondary site malignancy cannot be used to replace the malignancy as principal or first-listed diagnosis, regardless of the number of admissions or encounters for treatment and care of the neoplasm.

*See section I.C.21. Factors influencing health status and contact with health services, Encounter for prophylactic organ removal.*

**h. Admission/encounter for pain control/management**

*See Section I.C.6. for information on coding admission/encounter for pain control/management.*

**i. Malignancy in two or more noncontiguous sites**

A patient may have more than one malignant tumor in the same organ. These tumors may represent different primaries or metastatic disease, depending on the site. Should the documentation be unclear, the provider should be queried as to the status of each tumor so that the correct codes can be assigned.

**j. Disseminated malignant neoplasm, unspecified**

Code C80.0, Disseminated malignant neoplasm, unspecified, is for use only in those cases where the patient has advanced metastatic disease and no known primary or secondary sites are specified. It should not be used in place of assigning codes for the primary site and all known secondary sites.

**k. Malignant neoplasm without specification of site**

Code C80.1, Malignant (primary) neoplasm, unspecified, equates to Cancer, unspecified. This code should only be used when no determination can be made as to the primary site of a malignancy. This code should rarely be used in the inpatient setting.

**l. Sequencing of neoplasm codes**

**1)** **Encounter for treatment of primary malignancy**

If the reason for the encounter is for treatment of a primary malignancy, assign the malignancy as the principal/first-listed diagnosis. The primary site is to be sequenced first, followed by any metastatic sites.

**2)** **Encounter for treatment of secondary malignancy**

When an encounter is for a primary malignancy with metastasis and treatment is directed toward the metastatic (secondary) site(s) only, the metastatic site(s) is designated as the principal/first-listed diagnosis. The primary malignancy is coded as an additional code.

**3)** **Malignant neoplasm in a pregnant patient**

When a pregnant woman has a malignant neoplasm, a code from subcategory O9A.1-, Malignant neoplasm complicating pregnancy, childbirth, and the puerperium, should be sequenced first, followed by the appropriate code from Chapter 2 to indicate the type of neoplasm.

**4)** **Encounter for complication associated with a neoplasm**

When an encounter is for management of a complication associated with a neoplasm, such as dehydration, and the treatment is only for the complication, the complication is coded first, followed by the appropriate code(s) for the neoplasm.

The exception to this guideline is anemia. When the admission/encounter is for management of an anemia associated with the malignancy, and the treatment is only for anemia, the appropriate code for the malignancy is sequenced as the principal or first-listed diagnosis followed by code D63.0, Anemia in neoplastic disease.

**5)** **Complication from surgical procedure for treatment of a neoplasm**

When an encounter is for treatment of a complication resulting from a surgical procedure performed for the treatment of the neoplasm, designate the complication as the principal/first-listed diagnosis. See guideline regarding the coding of a current malignancy versus personal history to determine if the code for the neoplasm should also be assigned.

6) **Pathologic fracture due to a neoplasm**
When an encounter is for a pathological fracture due to a neoplasm, and the focus of treatment is the fracture, a code from subcategory M84.5, Pathological fracture in neoplastic disease, should be sequenced first, followed by the code for the neoplasm.

If the focus of treatment is the neoplasm with an associated pathological fracture, the neoplasm code should be sequenced first, followed by a code from M84.5 for the pathological fracture.

m. **Current malignancy versus personal history of malignancy**
When a primary malignancy has been excised but further treatment, such as an additional surgery for the malignancy, radiation therapy or chemotherapy is directed to that site, the primary malignancy code should be used until treatment is completed.

When a primary malignancy has been previously excised or eradicated from its site, there is no further treatment (of the malignancy) directed to that site, and there is no evidence of any existing primary malignancy, a code from category Z85, Personal history of malignant neoplasm, should be used to indicate the former site of the malignancy.

*See Section I.C.21. Factors influencing health status and contact with health services, History (of)*

n. **Leukemia, Multiple Myeloma, and Malignant Plasma Cell Neoplasms in remission versus personal history**
The categories for leukemia, and category C90, Multiple myeloma and malignant plasma cell neoplasms, have codes indicating whether or not the leukemia has achieved remission. There are also codes Z85.6, Personal history of leukemia, and Z85.79, Personal history of other malignant neoplasms of lymphoid, hematopoietic and related tissues. If the documentation is unclear as to whether the leukemia has achieved remission, the provider should be queried.

*See Section I.C.21. Factors influencing health status and contact with health services, History (of)*

o. **Aftercare following surgery for neoplasm**
*See Section I.C.21. Factors influencing health status and contact with health services, Aftercare*

p. **Follow-up care for completed treatment of a malignancy**
*See Section I.C.21. Factors influencing health status and contact with health services, Follow-up*

q. **Prophylactic organ removal for prevention of malignancy**
*See Section I.C. 21, Factors influencing health status and contact with health services, Prophylactic organ removal*

r. **Malignant neoplasm associated with transplanted organ**
A malignant neoplasm of a transplanted organ should be coded as a transplant complication. Assign first the appropriate code from category T86.-, Complications of transplanted organs and tissue, followed by code C80.2, Malignant neoplasm associated with transplanted organ. Use an additional code for the specific malignancy.

3. **Chapter 3: Disease of the blood and blood-forming organs and certain disorders involving the immune mechanism (D50-D89)**
Reserved for future guideline expansion

4. **Chapter 4: Endocrine, Nutritional, and Metabolic Diseases (E00-E89)**
a. **Diabetes mellitus**
The diabetes mellitus codes are combination codes that include the type of diabetes mellitus, the body system affected, and the complications affecting that body system. As many codes within a particular category as are necessary to describe all of the complications of the disease may be used. They should be sequenced based on the reason for a particular encounter. Assign as many codes from categories E08 – E13 as needed to identify all of the associated conditions that the patient has.

1) **Type of diabetes**
The age of a patient is not the sole determining factor, though most type 1 diabetics develop the condition before reaching puberty. For this reason type 1 diabetes mellitus is also referred to as juvenile diabetes.

2) **Type of diabetes mellitus not documented**
If the type of diabetes mellitus is not documented in the medical record the default is E11.-, Type 2 diabetes mellitus.

3) **Diabetes mellitus and the use of insulin and oral hypoglycemics**
If the documentation in a medical record does not indicate the type of diabetes but does indicate that the patient uses insulin, code E11, Type 2 diabetes mellitus, should be assigned. Code Z79.4, Long-term (current) use of insulin, or Z79.84, Long term (current) use of oral hypoglycemic drugs, should also be assigned to indicate that the patient uses insulin or hypoglycemic drugs. Code Z79.4 should not be assigned if insulin is given temporarily to bring a type 2 patient's blood sugar under control during an encounter.

4) **Diabetes mellitus in pregnancy and gestational diabetes**
*See Section I.C.15. Diabetes mellitus in pregnancy.*

*See Section I.C.15. Gestational (pregnancy induced) diabetes*

5) **Complications due to insulin pump malfunction**
(a) **Underdose of insulin due to insulin pump failure**
An underdose of insulin due to an insulin pump failure should be assigned to a code from subcategory T85.6, Mechanical complication of other specified internal and external prosthetic devices, implants and grafts, that specifies the type of pump malfunction, as the principal or first-listed code, followed by code T38.3X6-, Underdosing of insulin and oral hypoglycemic [antidiabetic] drugs. Additional codes for the type of diabetes mellitus and any associated complications due to the underdosing should also be assigned.

(b) **Overdose of insulin due to insulin pump failure**
The principal or first-listed code for an encounter due to an insulin pump malfunction resulting in an overdose of insulin, should also be T85.6-, Mechanical complication of other specified internal and external prosthetic devices, implants and grafts, followed by code T38.3X1-, Poisoning by insulin and oral hypoglycemic [antidiabetic] drugs, accidental (unintentional).

6) **Secondary diabetes mellitus**
Codes under categories E08, Diabetes mellitus due to underlying condition, E09, Drug or chemical induced diabetes mellitus, and E13, Other specified diabetes mellitus, identify complications/manifestations associated with secondary diabetes mellitus. Secondary diabetes is always caused by another condition or event (e.g., cystic fibrosis, malignant neoplasm of pancreas, pancreatectomy, adverse effect of drug, or poisoning).

(a) **Secondary diabetes mellitus and the use of insulin or hypoglycemic drugs**
For patients who routinely use insulin or hypoglycemic drugs, code Z79.4, Long-term (current) use of insulin, or Z79.84, Long term (current) use of oral hypoglycemic drugs should also be assigned. Code Z79.4 should not be assigned if insulin is given temporarily to bring a patient's blood sugar under control during an encounter.

(b) **Assigning and sequencing secondary diabetes codes and its causes**
The sequencing of the secondary diabetes codes in relationship to codes for the cause of the diabetes is based on the Tabular List instructions for categories E08, E09 and E13.

(i) **Secondary diabetes mellitus due to pancreatectomy**
For postpancreatectomy diabetes mellitus (lack of insulin due to the surgical removal of all or part of the pancreas), assign code E89.1, Postprocedural hypoinsulinemia. Assign a code from category E13 and a code from subcategory Z90.41-, Acquired absence of pancreas, as additional codes.

**(ii) Secondary diabetes due to drugs**

Secondary diabetes may be caused by an adverse effect of correctly administered medications, poisoning or sequela of poisoning.

*See section I.C.19.e for coding of adverse effects and poisoning, and section I.C.20 for external cause code reporting.*

5. **Chapter 5: Mental, Behavioral and Neurodevelopmental disorders (F01-F99)**

a. **Pain disorders related to psychological factors**

Assign code F45.41, for pain that is exclusively related to psychological disorders. As indicated by the Excludes 1 note under category G89, a code from category G89 should not be assigned with code F45.41.

Code F45.42, Pain disorders with related psychological factors, should be used with a code from category G89, Pain, not elsewhere classified, if there is documentation of a psychological component for a patient with acute or chronic pain.

*See Section I.C.6. Pain*

b. **Mental and behavioral disorders due to psychoactive substance use**

1) **In Remission**

Selection of codes for "in remission" for categories F10-F19, Mental and behavioral disorders due to psychoactive substance use (categories F10-F19 with -.21) requires the provider's clinical judgment. The appropriate codes for "in remission" are assigned only on the basis of provider documentation (as defined in the Official Guidelines for Coding and Reporting).

2) **Psychoactive Substance Use, Abuse And Dependence**

When the provider documentation refers to use, abuse and dependence of the same substance (e.g. alcohol, opioid, cannabis, etc.), only one code should be assigned to identify the pattern of use based on the following hierarchy:

- If both use and abuse are documented, assign only the code for abuse
- If both abuse and dependence are documented, assign only the code for dependence
- If use, abuse and dependence are all documented, assign only the code for dependence
- If both use and dependence are documented, assign only the code for dependence.

3) **Psychoactive Substance Use**

As with all other diagnoses, the codes for psychoactive substance use (F10.9-, F11.9-, F12.9-, F13.9-, F14.9-, F15.9-, F16.9-) should only be assigned based on provider documentation and when they meet the definition of a reportable diagnosis (see Section III, Reporting Additional Diagnoses). The codes are to be used only when the psychoactive substance use is associated with a mental or behavioral disorder, and such a relationship is documented by the provider.

6. **Chapter 6: Diseases of the Nervous System (G00-G99)**

a. **Dominant/nondominant side**

Codes from category G81, Hemiplegia and hemiparesis, and subcategories G83.1, Monoplegia of lower limb, G83.2, Monoplegia of upper limb, and G83.3, Monoplegia, unspecified, identify whether the dominant or nondominant side is affected. Should the affected side be documented, but not specified as dominant or nondominant, and the classification system does not indicate a default, code selection is as follows:

- For ambidextrous patients, the default should be dominant.
- If the left side is affected, the default is non-dominant.
- If the right side is affected, the default is dominant.

b. **Pain - Category G89**

1) **General coding information**

Codes in category G89, Pain, not elsewhere classified, may be used in conjunction with codes from other categories and chapters to provide more detail about acute or chronic pain and neoplasm-related pain, unless otherwise indicated below.

If the pain is not specified as acute or chronic, post-thoracotomy, postprocedural, or neoplasm-related, do not assign codes from category G89.

A code from category G89 should not be assigned if the underlying (definitive) diagnosis is known, unless the reason for the encounter is pain control/ management and not management of the underlying condition.

When an admission or encounter is for a procedure aimed at treating the underlying condition (e.g., spinal fusion, kyphoplasty), a code for the underlying condition (e.g., vertebral fracture, spinal stenosis) should be assigned as the principal diagnosis. No code from category G89 should be assigned.

(a) **Category G89 Codes as Principal or First-Listed Diagnosis**

Category G89 codes are acceptable as principal diagnosis or the first-listed code:

- When pain control or pain management is the reason for the admission/encounter (e.g., a patient with displaced intervertebral disc, nerve impingement and severe back pain presents for injection of steroid into the spinal canal). The underlying cause of the pain should be reported as an additional diagnosis, if known.

- When a patient is admitted for the insertion of a neurostimulator for pain control, assign the appropriate pain code as the principal or first-listed diagnosis. When an admission or encounter is for a procedure aimed at treating the underlying condition and a neurostimulator is inserted for pain control during the same admission/encounter, a code for the underlying condition should be assigned as the principal diagnosis and the appropriate pain code should be assigned as a secondary diagnosis.

(b) **Use of Category G89 Codes in Conjunction with Site Specific Pain Codes**

(i) **Assigning Category G89 and Site-Specific Pain Codes**

Codes from category G89 may be used in conjunction with codes that identify the site of pain (including codes from chapter 18) if the category G89 code provides additional information. For example, if the code describes the site of the pain, but does not fully describe whether the pain is acute or chronic, then both codes should be assigned.

(ii) **Sequencing of Category G89 Codes with Site-Specific Pain Codes**

The sequencing of category G89 codes with site-specific pain codes (including chapter 18 codes), is dependent on the circumstances of the encounter/admission as follows:

- If the encounter is for pain control or pain management, assign the code from category G89 followed by the code identifying the specific site of pain (e.g., encounter for pain management for acute neck pain from trauma is assigned code G89.11, Acute pain due to trauma, followed by code M54.2, Cervicalgia, to identify the site of pain).

- If the encounter is for any other reason except pain control or pain management, and a related definitive diagnosis has not been established (confirmed) by the provider, assign the code for the specific site of pain first, followed by the appropriate code from category G89.

2) **Pain due to devices, implants and grafts**

*See Section I.C.19. Pain due to medical devices*

3) **Postoperative Pain**

The provider's documentation should be used to guide the coding of postoperative pain, as well as *Section III. Reporting Additional Diagnoses* and *Section IV. Diagnostic Coding and Reporting in the Outpatient Setting.*

The default for post-thoracotomy and other postoperative pain not specified as acute or chronic is the code for the acute form.

Routine or expected postoperative pain immediately after surgery should not be coded.

(a) **Postoperative pain not associated with specific postoperative complication**
Postoperative pain not associated with a specific postoperative complication is assigned to the appropriate postoperative pain code in category G89.

(b) **Postoperative pain associated with specific postoperative complication**
Postoperative pain associated with a specific postoperative complication (such as painful wire sutures) is assigned to the appropriate code(s) found in Chapter 19, Injury, poisoning, and certain other consequences of external causes. If appropriate, use additional code(s) from category G89 to identify acute or chronic pain (G89.18 or G89.28).

4) **Chronic pain**
Chronic pain is classified to subcategory G89.2. There is no time frame defining when pain becomes chronic pain. The provider's documentation should be used to guide use of these codes.

5) **Neoplasm Related Pain**
Code G89.3 is assigned to pain documented as being related, associated or due to cancer, primary or secondary malignancy, or tumor. This code is assigned regardless of whether the pain is acute or chronic.

This code may be assigned as the principal or first-listed code when the stated reason for the admission/encounter is documented as pain control/pain management. The underlying neoplasm should be reported as an additional diagnosis.

When the reason for the admission/encounter is management of the neoplasm and the pain associated with the neoplasm is also documented, code G89.3 may be assigned as an additional diagnosis. It is not necessary to assign an additional code for the site of the pain.

*See Section I.C.2 for instructions on the sequencing of neoplasms for all other stated reasons for the admission/encounter (except for pain control/pain management).*

6) **Chronic pain syndrome**
Central pain syndrome (G89.0) and chronic pain syndrome (G89.4) are different than the term "chronic pain," and therefore codes should only be used when the provider has specifically documented this condition.

*See Section I.C.5. Pain disorders related to psychological factors*

7. **Chapter 7: Diseases of the Eye and Adnexa (H00-H59)**
a. **Glaucoma**
1) **Assigning Glaucoma Codes**
Assign as many codes from category H40, Glaucoma, as needed to identify the type of glaucoma, the affected eye, and the glaucoma stage.

2) **Bilateral glaucoma with same type and stage**
When a patient has bilateral glaucoma and both eyes are documented as being the same type and stage, and there is a code for bilateral glaucoma, report only the code for the type of glaucoma, bilateral, with the seventh character for the stage.

When a patient has bilateral glaucoma and both eyes are documented as being the same type and stage, and the classification does not provide a code for bilateral glaucoma (i.e. subcategories H40.10, H40.11 and H40.20) report only one code for the type of glaucoma with the appropriate seventh character for the stage.

3) **Bilateral glaucoma stage with different types or stages**
When a patient has bilateral glaucoma and each eye is documented as having a different type or stage, and the classification distinguishes laterality, assign the appropriate code for each eye rather than the code for bilateral glaucoma.

When a patient has bilateral glaucoma and each eye is documented as having a different type, and the classification does not distinguish laterality (i.e. subcategories H40.10, H40.11 and H40.20), assign one code for each type of glaucoma with the appropriate seventh character for the stage.

When a patient has bilateral glaucoma and each eye is documented as having the same type, but different stage, and the classification does not distinguish laterality (i.e. subcategories H40.10, H40.11 and H40.20), assign a code for the type of glaucoma for each eye with the seventh character for the specific glaucoma stage documented for each eye.

4) **Patient admitted with glaucoma and stage evolves during the admission**
If a patient is admitted with glaucoma and the stage progresses during the admission, assign the code for highest stage documented.

5) **Indeterminate stage glaucoma**
Assignment of the seventh character "4" for "indeterminate stage" should be based on the clinical documentation. The seventh character "4" is used for glaucomas whose stage cannot be clinically determined. This seventh character should not be confused with the seventh character "0", unspecified, which should be assigned when there is no documentation regarding the stage of the glaucoma.

8. **Chapter 8: Diseases of the Ear and Mastoid Process (H60-H95)**
Reserved for future guideline expansion

9. **Chapter 9: Diseases of the Circulatory System (I00-I99)**
a. **Hypertension**
The classification presumes a causal relationship between hypertension and heart involvement and between hypertension and kidney involvement, as the two conditions are linked by the term "with" in the Alphabetic Index. These conditions should be coded as related even in the absence of provider documentation explicitly linking them, unless the documentation clearly states the conditions are unrelated.

For hypertension and conditions not specifically linked by relational terms such as "with," "associated with" or "due to" in the classification, provider documentation must link the conditions in order to code them as related.

1) **Hypertension with Heart Disease**
Hypertension with heart conditions classified to I50.- or I51.4-I51.9, are assigned to a code from category I11, Hypertensive heart disease. Use an additional code from category I50, Heart failure, to identify the type of heart failure in those patients with heart failure.

The same heart conditions (I50.-, I51.4-I51.9) with hypertension are coded separately if the provider has specifically documented a different cause. Sequence according to the circumstances of the admission/encounter.

2) **Hypertensive Chronic Kidney Disease**
Assign codes from category I12, Hypertensive chronic kidney disease, when both hypertension and a condition classifiable to category N18, Chronic kidney disease (CKD), are present. CKD should not be coded as hypertensive if the physician has specifically documented a different cause.

The appropriate code from category N18 should be used as a secondary code with a code from category I12 to identify the stage of chronic kidney disease.

*See Section I.C.14. Chronic kidney disease.*

If a patient has hypertensive chronic kidney disease and acute renal failure, an additional code for the acute renal failure is required.

3) **Hypertensive Heart and Chronic Kidney Disease**
Assign codes from combination category I13, Hypertensive heart and chronic kidney disease, when there is hypertension with both heart and kidney involvement. If heart failure is present, assign an additional code from category I50 to identify the type of heart failure.

The appropriate code from category N18, Chronic kidney disease, should be used as a secondary code with a code from category I13 to identify the stage of chronic kidney disease.

*See Section I.C.14. Chronic kidney disease.*

The codes in category I13, Hypertensive heart and chronic kidney disease, are combination codes that include hypertension, heart disease and chronic kidney disease. The

Includes note at I13 specifies that the conditions included at I11 and I12 are included together in I13. If a patient has hypertension, heart disease and chronic kidney disease, then a code from I13 should be used, not individual codes for hypertension, heart disease and chronic kidney disease, or codes from I11 or I12.

For patients with both acute renal failure and chronic kidney disease, an additional code for acute renal failure is required.

### 4) Hypertensive Cerebrovascular Disease
For hypertensive cerebrovascular disease, first assign the appropriate code from categories I60-I69, followed by the appropriate hypertension code.

### 5) Hypertensive Retinopathy
Subcategory H35.0, Background retinopathy and retinal vascular changes, should be used with a code from category I10 – I15, Hypertensive disease to include the systemic hypertension. The sequencing is based on the reason for the encounter.

### 6) Hypertension, Secondary
Secondary hypertension is due to an underlying condition. Two codes are required: one to identify the underlying etiology and one from category I15 to identify the hypertension. Sequencing of codes is determined by the reason for admission/encounter.

### 7) Hypertension, Transient
Assign code R03.0, Elevated blood pressure reading without diagnosis of hypertension, unless patient has an established diagnosis of hypertension. Assign code O13.-, Gestational [pregnancy-induced] hypertension without significant proteinuria, or O14.-, Pre-eclampsia, for transient hypertension of pregnancy.

### 8) Hypertension, Controlled
This diagnostic statement usually refers to an existing state of hypertension under control by therapy. Assign the appropriate code from categories I10-I15, Hypertensive diseases.

### 9) Hypertension, Uncontrolled
Uncontrolled hypertension may refer to untreated hypertension or hypertension not responding to current therapeutic regimen. In either case, assign the appropriate code from categories I10-I15, Hypertensive diseases.

### 10) Hypertensive Crisis
Assign a code from category I16, Hypertensive crisis, for documented hypertensive urgency, hypertensive emergency or unspecified hypertensive crisis. Code also any identified hypertensive disease (I10-I15). The sequencing is based on the reason for the encounter.

## b. Atherosclerotic Coronary Artery Disease and Angina
ICD-10-CM has combination codes for atherosclerotic heart disease with angina pectoris. The subcategories for these codes are I25.11, Atherosclerotic heart disease of native coronary artery with angina pectoris and I25.7, Atherosclerosis of coronary artery bypass graft(s) and coronary artery of transplanted heart with angina pectoris.

When using one of these combination codes it is not necessary to use an additional code for angina pectoris. A causal relationship can be assumed in a patient with both atherosclerosis and angina pectoris, unless the documentation indicates the angina is due to something other than the atherosclerosis.

If a patient with coronary artery disease is admitted due to an acute myocardial infarction (AMI), the AMI should be sequenced before the coronary artery disease.

*See Section I.C.9. Acute myocardial infarction (AMI)*

## c. Intraoperative and Postprocedural Cerebrovascular Accident
Medical record documentation should clearly specify the cause-and-effect relationship between the medical intervention and the cerebrovascular accident in order to assign a code for intraoperative or postprocedural cerebrovascular accident.

Proper code assignment depends on whether it was an infarction or hemorrhage and whether it occurred intraoperatively or postoperatively. If it was a cerebral hemorrhage, code assignment depends on the type of procedure performed.

## d. Sequelae of Cerebrovascular Disease
### 1) Category I69, Sequelae of Cerebrovascular disease
Category I69 is used to indicate conditions classifiable to categories I60-I67 as the causes of sequela (neurologic deficits), themselves classified elsewhere. These "late effects" include neurologic deficits that persist after initial onset of conditions classifiable to categories I60-I67. The neurologic deficits caused by cerebrovascular disease may be present from the onset or may arise at any time after the onset of the condition classifiable to categories I60-I67.

Codes from category I69, Sequelae of cerebrovascular disease, that specify hemiplegia, hemiparesis and monoplegia identify whether the dominant or nondominant side is affected. Should the affected side be documented, but not specified as dominant or nondominant, and the classification system does not indicate a default, code selection is as follows:

- For ambidextrous patients, the default should be dominant.
- If the left side is affected, the default is non-dominant.
- If the right side is affected, the default is dominant.

### 2) Codes from category I69 with codes from I60-I67
Codes from category I69 may be assigned on a health care record with codes from I60-I67, if the patient has a current cerebrovascular disease and deficits from an old cerebrovascular disease.

### 3) Codes from category I69 and Personal history of transient ischemic attack (TIA) and cerebral infarction (Z86.73)
Codes from category I69 should not be assigned if the patient does not have neurologic deficits.

*See Section I.C.21. 4. History (of) for use of personal history codes*

## e. Acute myocardial infarction (AMI)
### 1) ST elevation myocardial infarction (STEMI) and non ST elevation myocardial infarction (NSTEMI)
The ICD-10-CM codes for acute myocardial infarction (AMI) identify the site, such as anterolateral wall or true posterior wall. Subcategories I21.0-I21.2 and code I21.3 are used for ST elevation myocardial infarction (STEMI). Code I21.4, Non-ST elevation (NSTEMI) myocardial infarction, is used for non ST elevation myocardial infarction (NSTEMI) and nontransmural MIs.

If NSTEMI evolves to STEMI, assign the STEMI code. If STEMI converts to NSTEMI due to thrombolytic therapy, it is still coded as STEMI.

For encounters occurring while the myocardial infarction is equal to, or less than, four weeks old, including transfers to another acute setting or a postacute setting, and the myocardial infarction meets the definition for "other diagnoses" (see Section III, Reporting Additional Diagnoses), codes from category I21 may continue to be reported. For encounters after the 4 week time frame and the patient is still receiving care related to the myocardial infarction, the appropriate aftercare code should be assigned, rather than a code from category I21. For old or healed myocardial infarctions not requiring further care, code I25.2, Old myocardial infarction, may be assigned.

### 2) Acute myocardial infarction, unspecified
Code I21.3, ST elevation (STEMI) myocardial infarction of unspecified site, is the default for unspecified acute myocardial infarction. If only STEMI or transmural MI without the site is documented, assign code I21.3.

### 3) AMI documented as nontransmural or subendocardial but site provided
If an AMI is documented as nontransmural or subendocardial, but the site is provided, it is still coded as a subendocardial AMI.

*See Section I.C.21.3 for information on coding status post administration of tPA in a different facility within the last 24 hours.*

### 4) Subsequent acute myocardial infarction
A code from category I22, Subsequent ST elevation (STEMI) and non ST elevation (NSTEMI) myocardial infarction, is to be used when a patient who has suffered an AMI has a new AMI within the 4 week time frame of the initial AMI. A code from category I22 must be used in conjunction with a code from category I21.

The sequencing of the I22 and I21 codes depends on the circumstances of the encounter.

10. **Chapter 10: Diseases of the Respiratory System (J00-J99)**
   a. **Chronic Obstructive Pulmonary Disease [COPD] and Asthma**
      1) **Acute exacerbation of chronic obstructive bronchitis and asthma**
      The codes in categories J44 and J45 distinguish between uncomplicated cases and those in acute exacerbation. An acute exacerbation is a worsening or a decompensation of a chronic condition. An acute exacerbation is not equivalent to an infection superimposed on a chronic condition, though an exacerbation may be triggered by an infection.

   b. **Acute Respiratory Failure**
      1) **Acute respiratory failure as principal diagnosis**
      A code from subcategory J96.0, Acute respiratory failure, or subcategory J96.2, Acute and chronic respiratory failure, may be assigned as a principal diagnosis when it is the condition established after study to be chiefly responsible for occasioning the admission to the hospital, and the selection is supported by the Alphabetic Index and Tabular List. However, chapter-specific coding guidelines (such as obstetrics, poisoning, HIV, newborn) that provide sequencing direction take precedence.

      2) **Acute respiratory failure as secondary diagnosis**
      Respiratory failure may be listed as a secondary diagnosis if it occurs after admission, or if it is present on admission, but does not meet the definition of principal diagnosis.

      3) **Sequencing of acute respiratory failure and another acute condition**
      When a patient is admitted with respiratory failure and another acute condition, (e.g., myocardial infarction, cerebrovascular accident, aspiration pneumonia), the principal diagnosis will not be the same in every situation. This applies whether the other acute condition is a respiratory or nonrespiratory condition. Selection of the principal diagnosis will be dependent on the circumstances of admission. If both the respiratory failure and the other acute condition are equally responsible for occasioning the admission to the hospital, and there are no chapter-specific sequencing rules, the guideline regarding two or more diagnoses that equally meet the definition for principal diagnosis *(Section II, C.)* may be applied in these situations.

      If the documentation is not clear as to whether acute respiratory failure and another condition are equally responsible for occasioning the admission, query the provider for clarification.

   c. **Influenza due to certain identified influenza viruses**
   Code only confirmed cases of influenza due to certain identified influenza viruses (category J09), and due to other identified influenza virus (category J10). This is an exception to the hospital inpatient guideline Section II, H. (Uncertain Diagnosis).

   In this context, "confirmation" does not require documentation of positive laboratory testing specific for avian or other novel influenza A or other identified influenza virus. However, coding should be based on the provider's diagnostic statement that the patient has avian influenza, or other novel influenza A, for category J09, or has another particular identified strain of influenza, such as H1N1 or H3N2, but not identified as novel or variant, for category J10.

   If the provider records "suspected" or "possible" or "probable" avian influenza, or novel influenza, or other identified influenza, then the appropriate influenza code from category J11, Influenza due to unidentified influenza virus, should be assigned. A code from category J09, Influenza due to certain identified influenza viruses, should not be assigned nor should a code from category J10, Influenza due to other identified influenza virus.

   d. **Ventilator associated Pneumonia**
      1) **Documentation of Ventilator associated Pneumonia**
      As with all procedural or postprocedural complications, code assignment is based on the provider's documentation of the relationship between the condition and the procedure.

      Code J95.851, Ventilator associated pneumonia, should be assigned only when the provider has documented ventilator

associated pneumonia (VAP). An additional code to identify the organism (e.g., Pseudomonas aeruginosa, code B96.5) should also be assigned. Do not assign an additional code from categories J12-J18 to identify the type of pneumonia.

Code J95.851 should not be assigned for cases where the patient has pneumonia and is on a mechanical ventilator and the provider has not specifically stated that the pneumonia is ventilator-associated pneumonia. If the documentation is unclear as to whether the patient has a pneumonia that is a complication attributable to the mechanical ventilator, query the provider.

   2) **Ventilator associated Pneumonia Develops after Admission**
   A patient may be admitted with one type of pneumonia (e.g., code J13, Pneumonia due to Streptococcus pneumonia) and subsequently develop VAP. In this instance, the principal diagnosis would be the appropriate code from categories J12-J18 for the pneumonia diagnosed at the time of admission. Code J95.851, Ventilator associated pneumonia, would be assigned as an additional diagnosis when the provider has also documented the presence of ventilator associated pneumonia.

11. **Chapter 11: Diseases of the Digestive System (K00-K95)**
   Reserved for future guideline expansion

12. **Chapter 12: Diseases of the Skin and Subcutaneous Tissue (L00-L99)**
   a. **Pressure ulcer stage codes**
      1) **Pressure ulcer stages**
      Codes from category L89, Pressure ulcer, identify the site of the pressure ulcer as well as the stage of the ulcer.

      The ICD-10-CM classifies pressure ulcer stages based on severity, which is designated by stages 1-4, unspecified stage and unstageable.

      Assign as many codes from category L89 as needed to identify all the pressure ulcers the patient has, if applicable.

      2) **Unstageable pressure ulcers**
      Assignment of the code for unstageable pressure ulcer (L89.--0) should be based on the clinical documentation. These codes are used for pressure ulcers whose stage cannot be clinically determined (e.g., the ulcer is covered by eschar or has been treated with a skin or muscle graft) and pressure ulcers that are documented as deep tissue injury but not documented as due to trauma. This code should not be confused with the codes for unspecified stage (L89.--9). When there is no documentation regarding the stage of the pressure ulcer, assign the appropriate code for unspecified stage (L89.--9).

      3) **Documented pressure ulcer stage**
      Assignment of the pressure ulcer stage code should be guided by clinical documentation of the stage or documentation of the terms found in the Alphabetic Index. For clinical terms describing the stage that are not found in the Alphabetic Index, and there is no documentation of the stage, the provider should be queried.

      4) **Patients admitted with pressure ulcers documented as healed**
      No code is assigned if the documentation states that the pressure ulcer is completely healed.

      5) **Patients admitted with pressure ulcers documented as healing**
      Pressure ulcers described as healing should be assigned the appropriate pressure ulcer stage code based on the documentation in the medical record. If the documentation does not provide information about the stage of the healing pressure ulcer, assign the appropriate code for unspecified stage.

      If the documentation is unclear as to whether the patient has a current (new) pressure ulcer or if the patient is being treated for a healing pressure ulcer, query the provider.

      For ulcers that were present on admission but healed at the time of discharge, assign the code for the site and stage of the pressure ulcer at the time of admission.

**6) Patient admitted with pressure ulcer evolving into another stage during the admission**

If a patient is admitted with a pressure ulcer at one stage and it progresses to a higher stage, two separate codes should be assigned: one code for the site and stage of the ulcer on admission and a second code for the same ulcer site and the highest stage reported during the stay.

## 13. Chapter 13: Diseases of the Musculoskeletal System and Connective Tissue (M00-M99)

### a. Site and laterality

Most of the codes within Chapter 13 have site and laterality designations. The site represents the bone, joint or the muscle involved. For some conditions where more than one bone, joint or muscle is usually involved, such as osteoarthritis, there is a "multiple sites" code available. For categories where no multiple site code is provided and more than one bone, joint or muscle is involved, multiple codes should be used to indicate the different sites involved.

#### 1) Bone versus joint

For certain conditions, the bone may be affected at the upper or lower end, (e.g., avascular necrosis of bone, M87, Osteoporosis, M80, M81). Though the portion of the bone affected may be at the joint, the site designation will be the bone, not the joint.

### b. Acute traumatic versus chronic or recurrent musculoskeletal conditions

Many musculoskeletal conditions are a result of previous injury or trauma to a site, or are recurrent conditions. Bone, joint or muscle conditions that are the result of a healed injury are usually found in chapter 13. Recurrent bone, joint or muscle conditions are also usually found in chapter 13. Any current, acute injury should be coded to the appropriate injury code from chapter 19. Chronic or recurrent conditions should generally be coded with a code from chapter 13. If it is difficult to determine from the documentation in the record which code is best to describe a condition, query the provider.

### c. Coding of Pathologic Fractures

7th character A is for use as long as the patient is receiving active treatment for the fracture. While the patient may be seen by a new or different provider over the course of treatment for a pathological fracture, assignment of the 7th character is based on whether the patient is undergoing active treatment and not whether the provider is seeing the patient for the first time.

7th character D is to be used for encounters after the patient has completed active treatment. The other 7th characters, listed under each subcategory in the Tabular List, are to be used for subsequent encounters for routine care of fractures during the healing and recovery phase as well as treatment of problems associated with the healing, such as malunions, nonunions, and sequelae.

Care for complications of surgical treatment for fracture repairs during the healing or recovery phase should be coded with the appropriate complication codes.

*See Section I.C.19. Coding of traumatic fractures.*

### d. Osteoporosis

Osteoporosis is a systemic condition, meaning that all bones of the musculoskeletal system are affected. Therefore, site is not a component of the codes under category M81, Osteoporosis without current pathological fracture. The site codes under category M80, Osteoporosis with current pathological fracture, identify the site of the fracture, not the osteoporosis.

#### 1) Osteoporosis without pathological fracture

Category M81, Osteoporosis without current pathological fracture, is for use for patients with osteoporosis who do not currently have a pathologic fracture due to the osteoporosis, even if they have had a fracture in the past. For patients with a history of osteoporosis fractures, status code Z87.310, Personal history of (healed) osteoporosis fracture, should follow the code from M81.

#### 2) Osteoporosis with current pathological fracture

Category M80, Osteoporosis with current pathological fracture, is for patients who have a current pathologic fracture at the time of an encounter. The codes under M80 identify the site of the fracture. A code from category M80, not a traumatic fracture

code, should be used for any patient with known osteoporosis who suffers a fracture, even if the patient had a minor fall or trauma, if that fall or trauma would not usually break a normal, healthy bone.

## 14. Chapter 14: Diseases of Genitourinary System (N00-N99)

### a. Chronic kidney disease

#### 1) Stages of chronic kidney disease (CKD)

The ICD-10-CM classifies CKD based on severity. The severity of CKD is designated by stages 1-5. Stage 2, code N18.2, equates to mild CKD; stage 3, code N18.3, equates to moderate CKD; and stage 4, code N18.4, equates to severe CKD. Code N18.6, End stage renal disease (ESRD), is assigned when the provider has documented end-stage-renal disease (ESRD).

If both a stage of CKD and ESRD are documented, assign code N18.6 only.

#### 2) Chronic kidney disease and kidney transplant status

Patients who have undergone kidney transplant may still have some form of chronic kidney disease (CKD) because the kidney transplant may not fully restore kidney function. Therefore, the presence of CKD alone does not constitute a transplant complication. Assign the appropriate N18 code for the patient's stage of CKD and code Z94.0, Kidney transplant status. If a transplant complication such as failure or rejection or other transplant complication is documented, see section I.C.19.g for information on coding complications of a kidney transplant. If the documentation is unclear as to whether the patient has a complication of the transplant, query the provider.

#### 3) Chronic kidney disease with other conditions

Patients with CKD may also suffer from other serious conditions, most commonly diabetes mellitus and hypertension. The sequencing of the CKD code in relationship to codes for other contributing conditions is based on the conventions in the Tabular List.

*See I.C.9. Hypertensive chronic kidney disease.*

*See I.C.19. Chronic kidney disease and kidney transplant complications.*

## 15. Chapter 15: Pregnancy, Childbirth, and the Puerperium (O00-O9A)

### a. General Rules for Obstetric Cases

#### 1) Codes from chapter 15 and sequencing priority

Obstetric cases require codes from chapter 15, codes in the range O00-O9A, Pregnancy, Childbirth, and the Puerperium. Chapter 15 codes have sequencing priority over codes from other chapters. Additional codes from other chapters may be used in conjunction with chapter 15 codes to further specify conditions. Should the provider document that the pregnancy is incidental to the encounter, then code Z33.1, Pregnant state, incidental, should be used in place of any chapter 15 codes. It is the provider's responsibility to state that the condition being treated is not affecting the pregnancy.

#### 2) Chapter 15 codes used only on the maternal record

Chapter 15 codes are to be used only on the maternal record, never on the record of the newborn.

#### 3) Final character for trimester

The majority of codes in Chapter 15 have a final character indicating the trimester of pregnancy. The timeframes for the trimesters are indicated at the beginning of the chapter. If trimester is not a component of a code, it is because the condition always occurs in a specific trimester, or the concept of trimester of pregnancy is not applicable. Certain codes have characters for only certain trimesters because the condition does not occur in all trimesters, but it may occur in more than just one. Assignment of the final character for trimester should be based on the provider's documentation of the trimester (or number of weeks) for the current admission/encounter. This applies to the assignment of trimester for pre-existing conditions as well as those that develop during or are due to the pregnancy. The provider's documentation of the number of weeks may be used to assign the appropriate code identifying the trimester.

Whenever delivery occurs during the current admission, and there is an "in childbirth" option for the obstetric complication being coded, the "in childbirth" code should be assigned.

**4) Selection of trimester for inpatient admissions that encompass more than one trimester**

In instances when a patient is admitted to a hospital for complications of pregnancy during one trimester and remains in the hospital into a subsequent trimester, the trimester character for the antepartum complication code should be assigned on the basis of the trimester when the complication developed, not the trimester of the discharge. If the condition developed prior to the current admission/encounter or represents a pre-existing condition, the trimester character for the trimester at the time of the admission/encounter should be assigned.

**5) Unspecified trimester**

Each category that includes codes for trimester has a code for "unspecified trimester." The "unspecified trimester" code should rarely be used, such as when the documentation in the record is insufficient to determine the trimester and it is not possible to obtain clarification.

**6) 7th character for Fetus Identification**

Where applicable, a 7th character is to be assigned for certain categories (O31, O32, O33.3 - O33.6, O35, O36, O40, O41, O60.1, O60.2, O64, and O69) to identify the fetus for which the complication code applies.

Assign 7th character "0":

- For single gestations
- When the documentation in the record is insufficient to determine the fetus affected and it is not possible to obtain clarification.
- When it is not possible to clinically determine which fetus is affected.

**b. Selection of OB Principal or First-listed Diagnosis**

**1) Routine outpatient prenatal visits**

For routine outpatient prenatal visits when no complications are present, a code from category Z34, Encounter for supervision of normal pregnancy, should be used as the first-listed diagnosis. These codes should not be used in conjunction with chapter 15 codes.

**2) Supervision of High-Risk Pregnancy**

Codes from category O09, Supervision of high-risk pregnancy, are intended for use only during the prenatal period. For complications during the labor or delivery episode as a result of a high-risk pregnancy, assign the applicable complication codes from Chapter 15. If there are no complications during the labor or delivery episode, assign code O80, Encounter for full-term uncomplicated delivery.

For routine prenatal outpatient visits for patients with high-risk pregnancies, a code from category O09, Supervision of high-risk pregnancy, should be used as the first-listed diagnosis. Secondary chapter 15 codes may be used in conjunction with these codes if appropriate.

**3) Episodes when no delivery occurs**

In episodes when no delivery occurs, the principal diagnosis should correspond to the principal complication of the pregnancy which necessitated the encounter. Should more than one complication exist, all of which are treated or monitored, any of the complications codes may be sequenced first.

**4) When a delivery occurs**

When an obstetric patient is admitted and delivers during that admission, the condition that prompted the admission should be sequenced as the principal diagnosis. If multiple conditions prompted the admission, sequence the one most related to the delivery as the principal diagnosis. A code for any complication of the delivery should be assigned as an additional diagnosis. In cases of cesarean delivery, if the patient was admitted with a condition that resulted in the performance of a cesarean procedure, that condition should be selected as the principal diagnosis. If the reason for the admission was unrelated to the condition resulting in the cesarean delivery, the condition related to the reason for the admission should be selected as the principal diagnosis.

**5) Outcome of delivery**

A code from category Z37, Outcome of delivery, should be included on every maternal record when a delivery has occurred. These codes are not to be used on subsequent records or on the newborn record.

**c. Pre-existing conditions versus conditions due to the pregnancy**

Certain categories in Chapter 15 distinguish between conditions of the mother that existed prior to pregnancy (pre-existing) and those that are a direct result of pregnancy. When assigning codes from Chapter 15, it is important to assess if a condition was pre-existing prior to pregnancy or developed during or due to the pregnancy in order to assign the correct code.

Categories that do not distinguish between pre-existing and pregnancy-related conditions may be used for either. It is acceptable to use codes specifically for the puerperium with codes complicating pregnancy and childbirth if a condition arises postpartum during the delivery encounter.

**d. Pre-existing hypertension in pregnancy**

Category O10, Pre-existing hypertension complicating pregnancy, childbirth and the puerperium, includes codes for hypertensive heart and hypertensive chronic kidney disease. When assigning one of the O10 codes that includes hypertensive heart disease or hypertensive chronic kidney disease, it is necessary to add a secondary code from the appropriate hypertension category to specify the type of heart failure or chronic kidney disease.

*See Section I.C.9. Hypertension.*

**e. Fetal Conditions Affecting the Management of the Mother**

**1) Codes from categories O35 and O36**

Codes from categories O35, Maternal care for known or suspected fetal abnormality and damage, and O36, Maternal care for other fetal problems, are assigned only when the fetal condition is actually responsible for modifying the management of the mother, i.e., by requiring diagnostic studies, additional observation, special care, or termination of pregnancy. The fact that the fetal condition exists does not justify assigning a code from this series to the mother's record.

**2) In utero surgery**

In cases when surgery is performed on the fetus, a diagnosis code from category O35, Maternal care for known or suspected fetal abnormality and damage, should be assigned identifying the fetal condition. Assign the appropriate procedure code for the procedure performed.

No code from Chapter 16, the perinatal codes, should be used on the mother's record to identify fetal conditions. Surgery performed in utero on a fetus is still to be coded as an obstetric encounter.

**f. HIV Infection in Pregnancy, Childbirth and the Puerperium**

During pregnancy, childbirth or the puerperium, a patient admitted because of an HIV-related illness should receive a principal diagnosis from subcategory O98.7-, Human immunodeficiency [HIV] disease complicating pregnancy, childbirth and the puerperium, followed by the code(s) for the HIV-related illness(es).

Patients with asymptomatic HIV infection status admitted during pregnancy, childbirth, or the puerperium should receive codes of O98.7- and Z21, Asymptomatic human immunodeficiency virus [HIV] infection status.

**g. Diabetes mellitus in pregnancy**

Diabetes mellitus is a significant complicating factor in pregnancy. Pregnant women who are diabetic should be assigned a code from category O24, Diabetes mellitus in pregnancy, childbirth, and the puerperium, first, followed by the appropriate diabetes code(s) (E08-E13) from Chapter 4.

**h. Long term use of insulin and oral hypoglycemics**

Code Z79.4, Long-term (current) use of insulin, or code Z79.84, Long-term (current) use of oral hypoglycemic drugs, should also be assigned if the diabetes mellitus is being treated with insulin or oral medications. If the patient is treated with both oral medications and insulin, only the code for insulin-controlled should be assigned.

i. **Gestational (pregnancy induced) diabetes**
Gestational (pregnancy induced) diabetes can occur during the second and third trimester of pregnancy in women who were not diabetic prior to pregnancy. Gestational diabetes can cause complications in the pregnancy similar to those of pre-existing diabetes mellitus. It also puts the woman at greater risk of developing diabetes after the pregnancy. Codes for gestational diabetes are in subcategory O24.4, Gestational diabetes mellitus. No other code from category O24, Diabetes mellitus in pregnancy, childbirth, and the puerperium, should be used with a code from O24.4.

The codes under subcategory O24.4 include diet controlled, insulin controlled, and controlled by oral hypoglycemic drugs. If a patient with gestational diabetes is treated with both diet and insulin, only the code for insulin-controlled is required. If a patient with gestational diabetes is treated with both diet and oral hypoglycemic medications, only the code for "controlled by oral hypoglycemic drugs" is required. Code Z79.4, Long-term (current) use of insulin or code Z79.84, Long-term (current) use of oral hypoglycemic drugs, should not be assigned with codes from subcategory O24.4.

An abnormal glucose tolerance in pregnancy is assigned a code from subcategory O99.81, Abnormal glucose complicating pregnancy, childbirth, and the puerperium.

j. **Sepsis and septic shock complicating abortion, pregnancy, childbirth and the puerperium**
When assigning a chapter 15 code for sepsis complicating abortion, pregnancy, childbirth, and the puerperium, a code for the specific type of infection should be assigned as an additional diagnosis. If severe sepsis is present, a code from subcategory R65.2, Severe sepsis, and code(s) for associated organ dysfunction(s) should also be assigned as additional diagnoses.

k. **Puerperal sepsis**
Code O85, Puerperal sepsis, should be assigned with a secondary code to identify the causal organism (e.g., for a bacterial infection, assign a code from category B95-B96, Bacterial infections in conditions classified elsewhere). A code from category A40, Streptococcal sepsis, or A41, Other sepsis, should not be used for puerperal sepsis. If applicable, use additional codes to identify severe sepsis (R65.2-) and any associated acute organ dysfunction.

l. **Alcohol and tobacco use during pregnancy, childbirth and the puerperium**
   1) **Alcohol use during pregnancy, childbirth and the puerperium**
   Codes under subcategory O99.31, Alcohol use complicating pregnancy, childbirth, and the puerperium, should be assigned for any pregnancy case when a mother uses alcohol during the pregnancy or postpartum. A secondary code from category F10, Alcohol related disorders, should also be assigned to identify manifestations of the alcohol use.

   2) **Tobacco use during pregnancy, childbirth and the puerperium**
   Codes under subcategory O99.33, Smoking (tobacco) complicating pregnancy, childbirth, and the puerperium, should be assigned for any pregnancy case when a mother uses any type of tobacco product during the pregnancy or postpartum. A secondary code from category F17, Nicotine dependence, should also be assigned to identify the type of nicotine dependence.

m. **Poisoning, toxic effects, adverse effects and underdosing in a pregnant patient**
A code from subcategory O9A.2, Injury, poisoning and certain other consequences of external causes complicating pregnancy, childbirth, and the puerperium, should be sequenced first, followed by the appropriate injury, poisoning, toxic effect, adverse effect or underdosing code, and then the additional code(s) that specifies the condition caused by the poisoning, toxic effect, adverse effect or underdosing.

*See Section I.C.19. Adverse effects, poisoning, underdosing and toxic effects.*

n. **Normal Delivery, Code O80**
   1) **Encounter for full term uncomplicated delivery**
   Code O80 should be assigned when a woman is admitted for a full-term normal delivery and delivers a single, healthy infant without any complications antepartum, during the delivery, or postpartum during the delivery episode. Code O80 is always a principal diagnosis. It is not to be used if any other code from chapter 15 is needed to describe a current complication of the antenatal, delivery, or perinatal period. Additional codes from other chapters may be used with code O80 if they are not related to or are in any way complicating the pregnancy.

   2) **Uncomplicated delivery with resolved antepartum complication**
   Code O80 may be used if the patient had a complication at some point during the pregnancy, but the complication is not present at the time of the admission for delivery.

   3) **Outcome of delivery for O80**
   Z37.0, Single live birth, is the only outcome of delivery code appropriate for use with O80.

o. **The Peripartum and Postpartum Periods**
   1) **Peripartum and Postpartum periods**
   The postpartum period begins immediately after delivery and continues for six weeks following delivery. The peripartum period is defined as the last month of pregnancy to five months postpartum.

   2) **Peripartum and postpartum complication**
   A postpartum complication is any complication occurring within the six-week period.

   3) **Pregnancy-related complications after 6 week period**
   Chapter 15 codes may also be used to describe pregnancy-related complications after the peripartum or postpartum period if the provider documents that a condition is pregnancy related.

   4) **Admission for routine postpartum care following delivery outside hospital**
   When the mother delivers outside the hospital prior to admission and is admitted for routine postpartum care and no complications are noted, code Z39.0, Encounter for care and examination of mother immediately after delivery, should be assigned as the principal diagnosis.

   5) **Pregnancy associated cardiomyopathy**
   Pregnancy associated cardiomyopathy, code O90.3, is unique in that it may be diagnosed in the third trimester of pregnancy but may continue to progress months after delivery. For this reason, it is referred to as peripartum cardiomyopathy. Code O90.3 is only for use when the cardiomyopathy develops as a result of pregnancy in a woman who did not have pre-existing heart disease.

p. **Code O94, Sequelae of complication of pregnancy, childbirth, and the puerperium**
   1) **Code O94**
   Code O94, Sequelae of complication of pregnancy, childbirth, and the puerperium, is for use in those cases when an initial complication of a pregnancy develops a sequelae requiring care or treatment at a future date.

   2) **After the initial postpartum period**
   This code may be used at any time after the initial postpartum period.

   3) **Sequencing of Code O94**
   This code, like all sequela codes, is to be sequenced following the code describing the sequelae of the complication.

q. **Termination of Pregnancy and Spontaneous abortions**
   1) **Abortion with Liveborn Fetus**
   When an attempted termination of pregnancy results in a liveborn fetus, assign code Z33.2, Encounter for elective termination of pregnancy and a code from category Z37, Outcome of Delivery.

   2) **Retained Products of Conception following an abortion**
   Subsequent encounters for retained products of conception following a spontaneous abortion or elective termination of pregnancy are assigned the appropriate code from category

O03, Spontaneous abortion, or codes O07.4, Failed attempted termination of pregnancy without complication and Z33.2, Encounter for elective termination of pregnancy. This advice is appropriate even when the patient was discharged previously with a discharge diagnosis of complete abortion.

### 3) Complications leading to abortion
Codes from Chapter 15 may be used as additional codes to identify any documented complications of the pregnancy in conjunction with codes in categories in O07 and O08.

### r. Abuse in a pregnant patient
For suspected or confirmed cases of abuse of a pregnant patient, a code(s) from subcategories O9A.3, Physical abuse complicating pregnancy, childbirth, and the puerperium, O9A.4, Sexual abuse complicating pregnancy, childbirth, and the puerperium, and O9A.5, Psychological abuse complicating pregnancy, childbirth, and the puerperium, should be sequenced first, followed by the appropriate codes (if applicable) to identify any associated current injury due to physical abuse, sexual abuse, and the perpetrator of abuse.

*See Section I.C.19. Adult and child abuse, neglect and other maltreatment.*

## 16. Chapter 16: Certain Conditions Originating in the Perinatal Period (P00-P96)
For coding and reporting purposes the perinatal period is defined as before birth through the 28th day following birth. The following guidelines are provided for reporting purposes.

### a. General Perinatal Rules

#### 1) Use of Chapter 16 Codes
Codes in this chapter are never for use on the maternal record. Codes from Chapter 15, the obstetric chapter, are never permitted on the newborn record. Chapter 16 codes may be used throughout the life of the patient if the condition is still present.

#### 2) Principal Diagnosis for Birth Record
When coding the birth episode in a newborn record, assign a code from category Z38, Liveborn infants according to place of birth and type of delivery, as the principal diagnosis. A code from category Z38 is assigned only once, to a newborn at the time of birth. If a newborn is transferred to another institution, a code from category Z38 should not be used at the receiving hospital.

A code from category Z38 is used only on the newborn record, not on the mother's record.

#### 3) Use of Codes from other Chapters with Codes from Chapter 16
Codes from other chapters may be used with codes from chapter 16 if the codes from the other chapters provide more specific detail. Codes for signs and symptoms may be assigned when a definitive diagnosis has not been established. If the reason for the encounter is a perinatal condition, the code from chapter 16 should be sequenced first.

#### 4) Use of Chapter 16 Codes after the Perinatal Period
Should a condition originate in the perinatal period, and continue throughout the life of the patient, the perinatal code should continue to be used regardless of the patient's age.

#### 5) Birth process or community acquired conditions
If a newborn has a condition that may be either due to the birth process or community acquired and the documentation does not indicate which it is, the default is due to the birth process and the code from Chapter 16 should be used. If the condition is community-acquired, a code from Chapter 16 should not be assigned.

#### 6) Code all clinically significant conditions
All clinically significant conditions noted on routine newborn examination should be coded. A condition is clinically significant if it requires:

- clinical evaluation; or
- therapeutic treatment; or
- diagnostic procedures; or
- extended length of hospital stay; or

- increased nursing care and/or monitoring; or
- has implications for future health care needs

**Note:** The perinatal guidelines listed above are the same as the general coding guidelines for "additional diagnoses", except for the final point regarding implications for future health care needs. Codes should be assigned for conditions that have been specified by the provider as having implications for future health care needs.

### b. Observation and Evaluation of Newborns for Suspected Conditions not Found

#### 1)
Assign a code from category Z05, Observation and evaluation of newborns and infants for suspected conditions ruled out, to identify those instances when a healthy newborn is evaluated for a suspected condition that is determined after study not to be present. Do not use a code from category Z05 when the patient has identified signs or symptoms of a suspected problem; in such cases code the sign or symptom.

#### 2)
A code from category Z05 may also be assigned as a principal or first-listed code for readmissions or encounters when the code from category Z38 code no longer applies. Codes from category Z05 are for use only for healthy newborns and infants for which no condition after study is found to be present.

#### 3) Z05 on a birth record
A code from category Z05 is to be used as a secondary code after the code from category Z38, Liveborn infants according to place of birth and type of delivery.

### c. Coding Additional Perinatal Diagnoses

#### 1) Assigning codes for conditions that require treatment
Assign codes for conditions that require treatment or further investigation, prolong the length of stay, or require resource utilization.

#### 2) Codes for conditions specified as having implications for future health care needs
Assign codes for conditions that have been specified by the provider as having implications for future health care needs.

**Note:** This guideline should not be used for adult patients.

### d. Prematurity and Fetal Growth Retardation
Providers utilize different criteria in determining prematurity. A code for prematurity should not be assigned unless it is documented. Assignment of codes in categories P05, Disorders of newborn related to slow fetal growth and fetal malnutrition, and P07, Disorders of newborn related to short gestation and low birth weight, not elsewhere classified, should be based on the recorded birth weight and estimated gestational age. Codes from category P05 should not be assigned with codes from category P07.

When both birth weight and gestational age are available, two codes from category P07 should be assigned, with the code for birth weight sequenced before the code for gestational age.

### e. Low birth weight and immaturity status
Codes from category P07, Disorders of newborn related to short gestation and low birth weight, not elsewhere classified, are for use for a child or adult who was premature or had a low birth weight as a newborn and this is affecting the patient's current health status.

*See Section I.C.21. Factors influencing health status and contact with health services, Status.*

### f. Bacterial Sepsis of Newborn
Category P36, Bacterial sepsis of newborn, includes congenital sepsis. If a perinate is documented as having sepsis without documentation of congenital or community acquired, the default is congenital and a code from category P36 should be assigned. If the P36 code includes the causal organism, an additional code from category B95, Streptococcus, Staphylococcus, and Enterococcus as the cause of diseases classified elsewhere, or B96, Other bacterial agents as the cause of diseases classified elsewhere, should not be assigned. If the P36 code does not include the causal organism, assign an additional code from category B96. If applicable, use additional codes to identify severe sepsis (R65.2-) and any associated acute organ dysfunction.

g. **Stillbirth**
Code P95, Stillbirth, is only for use in institutions that maintain separate records for stillbirths. No other code should be used with P95. Code P95 should not be used on the mother's record.

17. **Chapter 17: Congenital malformations, deformations, and chromosomal abnormalities (Q00-Q99)**
Assign an appropriate code(s) from categories Q00-Q99, Congenital malformations, deformations, and chromosomal abnormalities when a malformation/deformation or chromosomal abnormality is documented. A malformation/deformation/or chromosomal abnormality may be the principal/first-listed diagnosis on a record or a secondary diagnosis.

When a malformation/deformation or chromosomal abnormality does not have a unique code assignment, assign additional code(s) for any manifestations that may be present.

When the code assignment specifically identifies the malformation/deformation or chromosomal abnormality, manifestations that are an inherent component of the anomaly should not be coded separately. Additional codes should be assigned for manifestations that are not an inherent component.

Codes from Chapter 17 may be used throughout the life of the patient. If a congenital malformation or deformity has been corrected, a personal history code should be used to identify the history of the malformation or deformity. Although present at birth, malformation/deformation/or chromosomal abnormality may not be identified until later in life. Whenever the condition is diagnosed by the physician, it is appropriate to assign a code from codes Q00-Q99.For the birth admission, the appropriate code from category Z38, Liveborn infants, according to place of birth and type of delivery, should be sequenced as the principal diagnosis, followed by any congenital anomaly codes, Q00- Q99.

18. **Chapter 18: Symptoms, signs, and abnormal clinical and laboratory findings, not elsewhere classified (R00-R99)**
Chapter 18 includes symptoms, signs, abnormal results of clinical or other investigative procedures, and ill-defined conditions regarding which no diagnosis classifiable elsewhere is recorded. Signs and symptoms that point to a specific diagnosis have been assigned to a category in other chapters of the classification.

a. **Use of symptom codes**
Codes that describe symptoms and signs are acceptable for reporting purposes when a related definitive diagnosis has not been established (confirmed) by the provider.

b. **Use of a symptom code with a definitive diagnosis code**
Codes for signs and symptoms may be reported in addition to a related definitive diagnosis when the sign or symptom is not routinely associated with that diagnosis, such as the various signs and symptoms associated with complex syndromes. The definitive diagnosis code should be sequenced before the symptom code.

Signs or symptoms that are associated routinely with a disease process should not be assigned as additional codes, unless otherwise instructed by the classification.

c. **Combination codes that include symptoms**
ICD-10-CM contains a number of combination codes that identify both the definitive diagnosis and common symptoms of that diagnosis. When using one of these combination codes, an additional code should not be assigned for the symptom.

d. **Repeated falls**
Code R29.6, Repeated falls, is for use for encounters when a patient has recently fallen and the reason for the fall is being investigated.

Code Z91.81, History of falling, is for use when a patient has fallen in the past and is at risk for future falls. When appropriate, both codes R29.6 and Z91.81 may be assigned together.

e. **Coma scale**
The coma scale codes (R40.2-) can be used in conjunction with traumatic brain injury codes, acute cerebrovascular disease or sequelae of cerebrovascular disease codes. These codes are primarily for use by trauma registries, but they may be used in any setting where this information is collected. The coma scale may also be used to assess the status of the central nervous system for other non-trauma conditions, such as monitoring patients in the intensive care unit regardless of medical condition. The coma scale codes should be sequenced after the diagnosis code(s).

These codes, one from each subcategory, are needed to complete the scale. The 7th character indicates when the scale was recorded. The 7th character should match for all three codes.

At a minimum, report the initial score documented on presentation at your facility. This may be a score from the emergency medicine technician (EMT) or in the emergency department. If desired, a facility may choose to capture multiple coma scale scores.

Assign code R40.24, Glasgow coma scale, total score, when only the total score is documented in the medical record and not the individual score(s).

f. **Functional quadriplegia**
Functional quadriplegia (code R53.2) is the lack of ability to use one's limbs or to ambulate due to extreme debility. It is not associated with neurologic deficit or injury, and code R53.2 should not be used for cases of neurologic quadriplegia. It should only be assigned if functional quadriplegia is specifically documented in the medical record.

g. **SIRS due to Non-Infectious Process**
The systemic inflammatory response syndrome (SIRS) can develop as a result of certain non-infectious disease processes, such as trauma, malignant neoplasm, or pancreatitis. When SIRS is documented with a noninfectious condition, and no subsequent infection is documented, the code for the underlying condition, such as an injury, should be assigned, followed by code R65.10, Systemic inflammatory response syndrome (SIRS) of non-infectious origin without acute organ dysfunction, or code R65.11, Systemic inflammatory response syndrome (SIRS) of non-infectious origin with acute organ dysfunction. If an associated acute organ dysfunction is documented, the appropriate code(s) for the specific type of organ dysfunction(s) should be assigned in addition to code R65.11. If acute organ dysfunction is documented, but it cannot be determined if the acute organ dysfunction is associated with SIRS or due to another condition (e.g., directly due to the trauma), the provider should be queried.

h. **Death NOS**
Code R99, Ill-defined and unknown cause of mortality, is only for use in the very limited circumstance when a patient who has already died is brought into an emergency department or other healthcare facility and is pronounced dead upon arrival. It does not represent the discharge disposition of death.

i. **NIHSS Stroke Scale**
The NIH stroke scale (NIHSS) codes (R29.7- -) can be used in conjunction with acute stroke codes (I63) to identify the patient's neurological status and the severity of the stroke. The stroke scale codes should be sequenced after the acute stroke diagnosis code(s).

At a minimum, report the initial score documented. If desired, a facility may choose to capture multiple stroke scale scores.

*See Section I.B.14. for information concerning the medical record documentation that may be used for assignment of the NIHSS codes.*

19. **Chapter 19: Injury, poisoning, and certain other consequences of external causes (S00-T88)**
a. **Application of 7th Characters in Chapter 19**
Most categories in chapter 19 have a 7th character requirement for each applicable code. Most categories in this chapter have three 7th character values (with the exception of fractures): A, initial encounter, D, subsequent encounter and S, sequela. Categories for traumatic fractures have additional 7th character values. While the patient may be seen by a new or different provider over the course of treatment for an injury, assignment of the 7th character is based on whether the patient is undergoing active treatment and not whether the provider is seeing the patient for the first time.

For complication codes, active treatment refers to treatment for the condition described by the code, even though it may be related to an earlier precipitating problem. For example, code T84.50XA, Infection and inflammatory reaction due to unspecified internal joint prosthesis, initial encounter, is used when active treatment is provided for the infection, even though the condition relates to the prosthetic device, implant or graft that was placed at a previous encounter.

7th character "A", initial encounter is used for each encounter where the patient is receiving active treatment for the condition.

7th character "D" subsequent encounter is used for encounters after the patient has completed active treatment of the condition and is receiving routine care for the condition during the healing or recovery phase.

The aftercare Z codes should not be used for aftercare for conditions such as injuries or poisonings, where 7th characters are provided to identify subsequent care. For example, for aftercare of an injury, assign the acute injury code with the 7th character "D" (subsequent encounter).

7th character "S", sequela, is for use for complications or conditions that arise as a direct result of a condition, such as scar formation after a burn. The scars are sequelae of the burn. When using 7th character "S", it is necessary to use both the injury code that precipitated the sequela and the code for the sequela itself. The "S" is added only to the injury code, not the sequela code. The 7th character "S" identifies the injury responsible for the sequela. The specific type of sequela (e.g. scar) is sequenced first, followed by the injury code.

*See Section I.B.10 Sequelae, (Late Effects)*

b.  **Coding of Injuries**
When coding injuries, assign separate codes for each injury unless a combination code is provided, in which case the combination code is assigned. Code T07, Unspecified multiple injuries should not be assigned in the inpatient setting unless information for a more specific code is not available. Traumatic injury codes (S00-T14.9) are not to be used for normal, healing surgical wounds or to identify complications of surgical wounds.

The code for the most serious injury, as determined by the provider and the focus of treatment, is sequenced first.

1)  **Superficial injuries**
Superficial injuries such as abrasions or contusions are not coded when associated with more severe injuries of the same site.

2)  **Primary injury with damage to nerves/blood vessels**
When a primary injury results in minor damage to peripheral nerves or blood vessels, the primary injury is sequenced first with additional code(s) for injuries to nerves and spinal cord (such as category S04), and/or injury to blood vessels (such as category S15). When the primary injury is to the blood vessels or nerves, that injury should be sequenced first.

c.  **Coding of Traumatic Fractures**
The principles of multiple coding of injuries should be followed in coding fractures. Fractures of specified sites are coded individually by site in accordance with both the provisions within categories S02, S12, S22, S32, S42, S49, S52, S59, S62, S72, S79, S82, S89, S92 and the level of detail furnished by medical record content.

A fracture not indicated as open or closed should be coded to closed. A fracture not indicated whether displaced or not displaced should be coded to displaced.

More specific guidelines are as follows:

1)  **Initial vs. Subsequent Encounter for Fractures**
Traumatic fractures are coded using the appropriate 7th character for initial encounter (A, B, C) for each encounter where the patient is receiving active treatment for the fracture. The appropriate 7th character for initial encounter should also be assigned for a patient who delayed seeking treatment for the fracture or nonunion.

Fractures are coded using the appropriate 7th character for subsequent care for encounters after the patient has completed active treatment of the fracture and is receiving routine care for the fracture during the healing or recovery phase.

Care for complications of surgical treatment for fracture repairs during the healing or recovery phase should be coded with the appropriate complication codes.

Care of complications of fractures, such as malunion and nonunion, should be reported with the appropriate 7th character for subsequent care with nonunion (K, M, N,) or subsequent care with malunion (P, Q, R).

Malunion/nonunion: The appropriate 7th character for initial encounter should also be assigned for a patient who delayed seeking treatment for the fracture or nonunion.

The open fracture designations in the assignment of the 7th character for fractures of the forearm, femur and lower leg, including ankle are based on the Gustilo open fracture classification. When the Gustilo classification type is not specified for an open fracture, the 7th character for open fracture type I or II should be assigned (B, E, H, M, Q).

A code from category M80, not a traumatic fracture code, should be used for any patient with known osteoporosis who suffers a fracture, even if the patient had a minor fall or trauma, if that fall or trauma would not usually break a normal, healthy bone.

*See Section I.C.13. Osteoporosis.*

The aftercare Z codes should not be used for aftercare for traumatic fractures. For aftercare of a traumatic fracture, assign the acute fracture code with the appropriate 7th character.

2)  **Multiple fractures sequencing**
Multiple fractures are sequenced in accordance with the severity of the fracture.

d.  **Coding of Burns and Corrosions**
The ICD-10-CM makes a distinction between burns and corrosions. The burn codes are for thermal burns, except sunburns, that come from a heat source, such as a fire or hot appliance. The burn codes are also for burns resulting from electricity and radiation. Corrosions are burns due to chemicals. The guidelines are the same for burns and corrosions.

Current burns (T20-T25) are classified by depth, extent and by agent (X code). Burns are classified by depth as first degree (erythema), second degree (blistering), and third degree (full-thickness involvement). Burns of the eye and internal organs (T26-T28) are classified by site, but not by degree.

1)  **Sequencing of burn and related condition codes**
Sequence first the code that reflects the highest degree of burn when more than one burn is present.

a.  When the reason for the admission or encounter is for treatment of external multiple burns, sequence first the code that reflects the burn of the highest degree.

b.  When a patient has both internal and external burns, the circumstances of admission govern the selection of the principal diagnosis or first-listed diagnosis.

c.  When a patient is admitted for burn injuries and other related conditions such as smoke inhalation and/or respiratory failure, the circumstances of admission govern the selection of the principal or first-listed diagnosis.

2)  **Burns of the same local site**
Classify burns of the same local site (three-character category level, T20-T28) but of different degrees to the subcategory identifying the highest degree recorded in the diagnosis.

3)  **Non-healing burns**
Non-healing burns are coded as acute burns.

Necrosis of burned skin should be coded as a non-healed burn.

4)  **Infected Burn**
For any documented infected burn site, use an additional code for the infection.

5)  **Assign separate codes for each burn site**
When coding burns, assign separate codes for each burn site. Category T30, Burn and corrosion, body region unspecified is extremely vague and should rarely be used.

6)  **Burns and Corrosions Classified According to Extent of Body Surface Involved**
Assign codes from category T31, Burns classified according to extent of body surface involved, or T32, Corrosions classified according to extent of body surface involved, when the site of the burn is not specified or when there is a need for additional data. It is advisable to use category T31 as additional coding when needed to provide data for evaluating burn mortality,

such as that needed by burn units. It is also advisable to use category T31 as an additional code for reporting purposes when there is mention of a third-degree burn involving 2Ø percent or more of the body surface.

Categories T31 and T32 are based on the classic "rule of nines" in estimating body surface involved: head and neck are assigned nine percent, each arm nine percent, each leg 18 percent, the anterior trunk 18 percent, posterior trunk 18 percent, and genitalia one percent. Providers may change these percentage assignments where necessary to accommodate infants and children who have proportionally larger heads than adults, and patients who have large buttocks, thighs, or abdomen that involve burns.

**7)   Encounters for treatment of sequela of burns**
Encounters for the treatment of the late effects of burns or corrosions (i.e., scars or joint contractures) should be coded with a burn or corrosion code with the 7th character "S" for sequela.

**8)   Sequelae with a late effect code and current burn**
When appropriate, both a code for a current burn or corrosion with 7th character "A" or "D" and a burn or corrosion code with 7th character "S" may be assigned on the same record (when both a current burn and sequelae of an old burn exist). Burns and corrosions do not heal at the same rate and a current healing wound may still exist with sequela of a healed burn or corrosion.

*See Section I.B.10 Sequela (Late Effects)*

**9)   Use of an external cause code with burns and corrosions**
An external cause code should be used with burns and corrosions to identify the source and intent of the burn, as well as the place where it occurred.

**e.   Adverse Effects, Poisoning, Underdosing and Toxic Effects**
Codes in categories T36-T65 are combination codes that include the substance that was taken as well as the intent. No additional external cause code is required for poisonings, toxic effects, adverse effects and underdosing codes.

**1)   Do not code directly from the Table of Drugs**
Do not code directly from the Table of Drugs and Chemicals. Always refer back to the Tabular List.

**2)   Use as many codes as necessary to describe**
Use as many codes as necessary to describe completely all drugs, medicinal or biological substances.

**3)   If the same code would describe the causative agent**
If the same code would describe the causative agent for more than one adverse reaction, poisoning, toxic effect or underdosing, assign the code only once.

**4)   If two or more drugs, medicinal or biological substances**
If two or more drugs, medicinal or biological substances are reported, code each individually unless a combination code is listed in the Table of Drugs and Chemicals.

**5)   The occurrence of drug toxicity is classified in ICD-10-CM as follows:**
**(a)   Adverse Effect**
When coding an adverse effect of a drug that has been correctly prescribed and properly administered, assign the appropriate code for the nature of the adverse effect followed by the appropriate code for the adverse effect of the drug (T36-T5Ø). The code for the drug should have a 5th or 6th character "5" (for example T36.ØX5-) Examples of the nature of an adverse effect are tachycardia, delirium, gastrointestinal hemorrhaging, vomiting, hypokalemia, hepatitis, renal failure, or respiratory failure.

**(b)   Poisoning**
When coding a poisoning or reaction to the improper use of a medication (e.g., overdose, wrong substance given or taken in error, wrong route of administration), first assign the appropriate code from categories T36-T5Ø. The poisoning codes have an associated intent as their 5th or 6th character (accidental, intentional self-harm, assault and undetermined. If the intent of the poisoning is unknown or unspecified, code the intent as accidental intent. The

undetermined intent is only for use if the documentation in the record specifies that the intent cannot be determined. Use additional code(s) for all manifestations of poisonings.

If there is also a diagnosis of abuse or dependence of the substance, the abuse or dependence is assigned as an additional code.

Examples of poisoning include:

(i)   Error was made in drug prescription

Errors made in drug prescription or in the administration of the drug by provider, nurse, patient, or other person.

(ii)   Overdose of a drug intentionally taken

If an overdose of a drug was intentionally taken or administered and resulted in drug toxicity, it would be coded as a poisoning.

(iii)   Nonprescribed drug taken with correctly prescribed and properly administered drug

If a nonprescribed drug or medicinal agent was taken in combination with a correctly prescribed and properly administered drug, any drug toxicity or other reaction resulting from the interaction of the two drugs would be classified as a poisoning.

(iv)   Interaction of drug(s) and alcohol

When a reaction results from the interaction of a drug(s) and alcohol, this would be classified as poisoning.

*See Section I.C.4. if poisoning is the result of insulin pump malfunctions.*

**(c)   Underdosing**
Underdosing refers to taking less of a medication than is prescribed by a provider or a manufacturer's instruction. For underdosing, assign the code from categories T36-T5Ø (fifth or sixth character "6").

Codes for underdosing should never be assigned as principal or first-listed codes. If a patient has a relapse or exacerbation of the medical condition for which the drug is prescribed because of the reduction in dose, then the medical condition itself should be coded.

Noncompliance (Z91.12-, Z91.13-) or complication of care (Y63.6-Y63.9) codes are to be used with an underdosing code to indicate intent, if known.

**(d)   Toxic Effects**
When a harmful substance is ingested or comes in contact with a person, this is classified as a toxic effect. The toxic effect codes are in categories T51-T65.

Toxic effect codes have an associated intent: accidental, intentional self-harm, assault and undetermined.

**f.   Adult and child abuse, neglect and other maltreatment**
Sequence first the appropriate code from categories T74.- (Adult and child abuse, neglect and other maltreatment, confirmed) or T76.- (Adult and child abuse, neglect and other maltreatment, suspected) for abuse, neglect and other maltreatment, followed by any accompanying mental health or injury code(s).

If the documentation in the medical record states abuse or neglect it is coded as confirmed (T74.-). It is coded as suspected if it is documented as suspected (T76.-).

For cases of confirmed abuse or neglect an external cause code from the assault section (X92-YØ9) should be added to identify the cause of any physical injuries. A perpetrator code (YØ7) should be added when the perpetrator of the abuse is known. For suspected cases of abuse or neglect, do not report external cause or perpetrator code.

If a suspected case of abuse, neglect or mistreatment is ruled out during an encounter code ZØ4.71, Encounter for examination and observation following alleged physical adult abuse, ruled out, or code ZØ4.72, Encounter for examination and observation following alleged child physical abuse, ruled out, should be used, not a code from T76.

If a suspected case of alleged rape or sexual abuse is ruled out during an encounter code Z04.41, Encounter for examination and observation following alleged adult rape or code Z04.42, Encounter for examination and observation following alleged child rape, should be used, not a code from T76.

*See Section I.C.15. Abuse in a pregnant patient.*

### g. Complications of care

#### 1) General guidelines for complications of care

##### (a) Documentation of complications of care
*See Section I.B.16. for information on documentation of complications of care.*

#### 2) Pain due to medical devices
Pain associated with devices, implants or grafts left in a surgical site (for example painful hip prosthesis) is assigned to the appropriate code(s) found in Chapter 19, Injury, poisoning, and certain other consequences of external causes. Specific codes for pain due to medical devices are found in the T code section of the ICD-10-CM. Use additional code(s) from category G89 to identify acute or chronic pain due to presence of the device, implant or graft (G89.18 or G89.28).

#### 3) Transplant complications

##### (a) Transplant complications other than kidney
Codes under category T86, Complications of transplanted organs and tissues, are for use for both complications and rejection of transplanted organs. A transplant complication code is only assigned if the complication affects the function of the transplanted organ. Two codes are required to fully describe a transplant complication: the appropriate code from category T86 and a secondary code that identifies the complication.

Pre-existing conditions or conditions that develop after the transplant are not coded as complications unless they affect the function of the transplanted organs.

*See I.C.21. for transplant organ removal status*

*See I.C.2. for malignant neoplasm associated with transplanted organ.*

##### (b) Kidney transplant complications
Patients who have undergone kidney transplant may still have some form of chronic kidney disease (CKD) because the kidney transplant may not fully restore kidney function. Code T86.1- should be assigned for documented complications of a kidney transplant, such as transplant failure or rejection or other transplant complication. Code T86.1- should not be assigned for post kidney transplant patients who have chronic kidney (CKD) unless a transplant complication such as transplant failure or rejection is documented. If the documentation is unclear as to whether the patient has a complication of the transplant, query the provider.

Conditions that affect the function of the transplanted kidney, other than CKD, should be assigned a code from subcategory T86.1, Complications of transplanted organ, Kidney, and a secondary code that identifies the complication.

For patients with CKD following a kidney transplant, but who do not have a complication such as failure or rejection, *see section I.C.14. Chronic kidney disease and kidney transplant status.*

#### 4) Complication codes that include the external cause
As with certain other T codes, some of the complications of care codes have the external cause included in the code. The code includes the nature of the complication as well as the type of procedure that caused the complication. No external cause code indicating the type of procedure is necessary for these codes.

#### 5) Complications of care codes within the body system chapters
Intraoperative and postprocedural complication codes are found within the body system chapters with codes specific to the organs and structures of that body system. These codes

should be sequenced first, followed by a code(s) for the specific complication, if applicable.

## 20. Chapter 20: External Causes of Morbidity (V00-Y99)
The external causes of morbidity codes should never be sequenced as the first-listed or principal diagnosis.

External cause codes are intended to provide data for injury research and evaluation of injury prevention strategies. These codes capture how the injury or health condition happened (cause), the intent (unintentional or accidental; or intentional, such as suicide or assault), the place where the event occurred the activity of the patient at the time of the event, and the person's status (e.g., civilian, military).

There is no national requirement for mandatory ICD-10-CM external cause code reporting. Unless a provider is subject to a state-based external cause code reporting mandate or these codes are required by a particular payer, reporting of ICD-10-CM codes in Chapter 20, External Causes of Morbidity, is not required. In the absence of a mandatory reporting requirement, providers are encouraged to voluntarily report external cause codes, as they provide valuable data for injury research and evaluation of injury prevention strategies.

### a. General External Cause Coding Guidelines

#### 1) Used with any code in the range of A00.0-T88.9, Z00-Z99
An external cause code may be used with any code in the range of A00.0-T88.9, Z00-Z99, classification that is a health condition due to an external cause. Though they are most applicable to injuries, they are also valid for use with such things as infections or diseases due to an external source, and other health conditions, such as a heart attack that occurs during strenuous physical activity.

#### 2) External cause code used for length of treatment
Assign the external cause code, with the appropriate 7th character (initial encounter, subsequent encounter or sequela) for each encounter for which the injury or condition is being treated.

Most categories in chapter 20 have a 7th character requirement for each applicable code. Most categories in this chapter have three 7th character values: A, initial encounter, D, subsequent encounter and S, sequela. While the patient may be seen by a new or different provider over the course of treatment for an injury or condition, assignment of the 7th character for external cause should match the 7th character of the code assigned for the associated injury or condition for the encounter.

#### 3) Use the full range of external cause codes
Use the full range of external cause codes to completely describe the cause, the intent, the place of occurrence, and if applicable, the activity of the patient at the time of the event, and the patient's status, for all injuries, and other health conditions due to an external cause.

#### 4) Assign as many external cause codes as necessary
Assign as many external cause codes as necessary to fully explain each cause. If only one external code can be recorded, assign the code most related to the principal diagnosis.

#### 5) The selection of the appropriate external cause code
The selection of the appropriate external cause code is guided by the Alphabetic Index of External Causes and by Inclusion and Exclusion notes in the Tabular List.

#### 6) External cause code can never be a principal diagnosis
An external cause code can never be a principal (first-listed) diagnosis.

#### 7) Combination external cause codes
Certain of the external cause codes are combination codes that identify sequential events that result in an injury, such as a fall which results in striking against an object. The injury may be due to either event or both. The combination external cause code used should correspond to the sequence of events regardless of which caused the most serious injury.

#### 8) No external cause code needed in certain circumstances
No external cause code from Chapter 20 is needed if the external cause and intent are included in a code from another chapter (e.g. T36.0X1- Poisoning by penicillins, accidental (unintentional)).

**b. Place of Occurrence Guideline**

Codes from category Y92, Place of occurrence of the external cause, are secondary codes for use after other external cause codes to identify the location of the patient at the time of injury or other condition.

Generally, a place of occurrence code is assigned only once, at the initial encounter for treatment. However, in the rare instance that a new injury occurs during hospitalization, an additional place of occurrence code may be assigned. No 7th characters are used for Y92.

Do not use place of occurrence code Y92.9 if the place is not stated or is not applicable.

**c. Activity Code**

Assign a code from category Y93, Activity code, to describe the activity of the patient at the time the injury or other health condition occurred.

An activity code is used only once, at the initial encounter for treatment. Only one code from Y93 should be recorded on a medical record.

The activity codes are not applicable to poisonings, adverse effects, misadventures or sequela.

Do not assign Y93.9, Unspecified activity, if the activity is not stated.

A code from category Y93 is appropriate for use with external cause and intent codes if identifying the activity provides additional information about the event.

**d. Place of Occurrence, Activity, and Status Codes Used with other External Cause Code**

When applicable, place of occurrence, activity, and external cause status codes are sequenced after the main external cause code(s). Regardless of the number of external cause codes assigned, generally there should be only one place of occurrence code, one activity code, and one external cause status code assigned to an encounter. However, in the rare instance that a new injury occurs during hospitalization, an additional place of occurrence code may be assigned.

**e. If the Reporting Format Limits the Number of External Cause Codes**

If the reporting format limits the number of external cause codes that can be used in reporting clinical data, report the code for the cause/intent most related to the principal diagnosis. If the format permits capture of additional external cause codes, the cause/intent, including medical misadventures, of the additional events should be reported rather than the codes for place, activity, or external status.

**f. Multiple External Cause Coding Guidelines**

More than one external cause code is required to fully describe the external cause of an illness or injury. The assignment of external cause codes should be sequenced in the following priority:

If two or more events cause separate injuries, an external cause code should be assigned for each cause. The first-listed external cause code will be selected in the following order:

External codes for child and adult abuse take priority over all other external cause codes.

*See Section I.C.19., Child and Adult abuse guidelines.*

External cause codes for terrorism events take priority over all other external cause codes except child and adult abuse.

External cause codes for cataclysmic events take priority over all other external cause codes except child and adult abuse and terrorism.

External cause codes for transport accidents take priority over all other external cause codes except cataclysmic events, child and adult abuse and terrorism.

Activity and external cause status codes are assigned following all causal (intent) external cause codes.

The first-listed external cause code should correspond to the cause of the most serious diagnosis due to an assault, accident, or self-harm, following the order of hierarchy listed above.

**g. Child and Adult Abuse Guideline**

Adult and child abuse, neglect and maltreatment are classified as assault. Any of the assault codes may be used to indicate the external cause of any injury resulting from the confirmed abuse.

For confirmed cases of abuse, neglect and maltreatment, when the perpetrator is known, a code from Y07, Perpetrator of maltreatment and neglect, should accompany any other assault codes.

*See Section I.C.19. Adult and child abuse, neglect and other maltreatment*

**h. Unknown or Undetermined Intent Guideline**

If the intent (accident, self-harm, assault) of the cause of an injury or other condition is unknown or unspecified, code the intent as accidental intent. All transport accident categories assume accidental intent.

**1) Use of undetermined intent**

External cause codes for events of undetermined intent are only for use if the documentation in the record specifies that the intent cannot be determined.

**i. Sequelae (Late Effects) of External Cause Guidelines**

**1) Sequelae external cause codes**

Sequela are reported using the external cause code with the 7th character "S" for sequela. These codes should be used with any report of a late effect or sequela resulting from a previous injury.

*See Section I.B.10 Sequela (Late Effects)*

**2) Sequela external cause code with a related current injury**

A sequela external cause code should never be used with a related current nature of injury code.

**3) Use of sequela external cause codes for subsequent visits**

Use a late effect external cause code for subsequent visits when a late effect of the initial injury is being treated. Do not use a late effect external cause code for subsequent visits for follow-up care (e.g., to assess healing, to receive rehabilitative therapy) of the injury when no late effect of the injury has been documented.

**j. Terrorism Guidelines**

**1) Cause of injury identified by the Federal Government (FBI) as terrorism**

When the cause of an injury is identified by the Federal Government (FBI) as terrorism, the first-listed external cause code should be a code from category Y38, Terrorism. The definition of terrorism employed by the FBI is found at the inclusion note at the beginning of category Y38. Use additional code for place of occurrence (Y92.-). More than one Y38 code may be assigned if the injury is the result of more than one mechanism of terrorism.

**2) Cause of an injury is suspected to be the result of terrorism**

When the cause of an injury is suspected to be the result of terrorism a code from category Y38 should not be assigned. Suspected cases should be classified as assault.

**3) Code Y38.9, Terrorism, secondary effects**

Assign code Y38.9, Terrorism, secondary effects, for conditions occurring subsequent to the terrorist event. This code should not be assigned for conditions that are due to the initial terrorist act.

It is acceptable to assign code Y38.9 with another code from Y38 if there is an injury due to the initial terrorist event and an injury that is a subsequent result of the terrorist event.

**k. External cause status**

A code from category Y99, External cause status, should be assigned whenever any other external cause code is assigned for an encounter, including an Activity code, except for the events noted below. Assign a code from category Y99, External cause status, to indicate the work status of the person at the time the event occurred. The status code indicates whether the event occurred during military activity, whether a non-military person was at work, whether an individual including a student or volunteer was involved in a non-work activity at the time of the causal event.

A code from Y99, External cause status, should be assigned, when applicable, with other external cause codes, such as transport accidents and falls. The external cause status codes are not applicable to poisonings, adverse effects, misadventures or late effects.

Do not assign a code from category Y99 if no other external cause codes (cause, activity) are applicable for the encounter.

An external cause status code is used only once, at the initial encounter for treatment. Only one code from Y99 should be recorded on a medical record.

Do not assign code Y99.9, Unspecified external cause status, if the status is not stated.

21. **Chapter 21: Factors influencing health status and contact with health services (Z00-Z99)**
**Note:** The chapter specific guidelines provide additional information about the use of Z codes for specified encounters.

   a. **Use of Z codes in any healthcare setting**
   Z codes are for use in any healthcare setting. Z codes may be used as either a first-listed (principal diagnosis code in the inpatient setting) or secondary code, depending on the circumstances of the encounter. Certain Z codes may only be used as first-listed or principal diagnosis.

   b. **Z Codes indicate a reason for an encounter**
   Z codes are not procedure codes. A corresponding procedure code must accompany a Z code to describe any procedure performed.

   c. **Categories of Z Codes**
   1) **Contact/Exposure**
   Category Z20 indicates contact with, and suspected exposure to, communicable diseases. These codes are for patients who do not show any sign or symptom of a disease but are suspected to have been exposed to it by close personal contact with an infected individual or are in an area where a disease is epidemic.

   Category Z77, Other contact with and (suspected) exposures hazardous to health, indicates contact with and suspected exposures hazardous to health.

   Contact/exposure codes may be used as a first-listed code to explain an encounter for testing, or, more commonly, as a secondary code to identify a potential risk.

   2) **Inoculations and vaccinations**
   Code Z23 is for encounters for inoculations and vaccinations. It indicates that a patient is being seen to receive a prophylactic inoculation against a disease. Procedure codes are required to identify the actual administration of the injection and the type(s) of immunizations given. Code Z23 may be used as a secondary code if the inoculation is given as a routine part of preventive health care, such as a well-baby visit.

   3) **Status**
   Status codes indicate that a patient is either a carrier of a disease or has the sequelae or residual of a past disease or condition. This includes such things as the presence of prosthetic or mechanical devices resulting from past treatment. A status code is informative, because the status may affect the course of treatment and its outcome. A status code is distinct from a history code. The history code indicates that the patient no longer has the condition.

   A status code should not be used with a diagnosis code from one of the body system chapters, if the diagnosis code includes the information provided by the status code. For example, code Z94.1, Heart transplant status, should not be used with a code from subcategory T86.2, Complications of heart transplant. The status code does not provide additional information. The complication code indicates that the patient is a heart transplant patient.

   For encounters for weaning from a mechanical ventilator, assign a code from subcategory J96.1, Chronic respiratory failure, followed by code Z99.11, Dependence on respirator [ventilator] status.

The status Z codes/categories are:

Z14   Genetic carrier

Genetic carrier status indicates that a person carries a gene, associated with a particular disease, which may be passed to offspring who may develop that disease. The person does not have the disease and is not at risk of developing the disease.

Z15   Genetic susceptibility to disease

Genetic susceptibility indicates that a person has a gene that increases the risk of that person developing the disease.

Codes from category Z15 should not be used as principal or first-listed codes. If the patient has the condition to which he/she is susceptible, and that condition is the reason for the encounter, the code for the current condition should be sequenced first. If the patient is being seen for follow-up after completed treatment for this condition, and the condition no longer exists, a follow-up code should be sequenced first, followed by the appropriate personal history and genetic susceptibility codes. If the purpose of the encounter is genetic counseling associated with procreative management, code Z31.5, Encounter for genetic counseling, should be assigned as the first-listed code, followed by a code from category Z15. Additional codes should be assigned for any applicable family or personal history.

Z16   Resistance to antimicrobial drugs

This code indicates that a patient has a condition that is resistant to antimicrobial drug treatment. Sequence the infection code first.

Z17   Estrogen receptor status

Z18   Retained foreign body fragments

Z19   Hormone sensitivity malignancy status

Z21   Asymptomatic HIV infection status

This code indicates that a patient has tested positive for HIV but has manifested no signs or symptoms of the disease.

Z22   Carrier of infectious disease

Carrier status indicates that a person harbors the specific organisms of a disease without manifest symptoms and is capable of transmitting the infection.

Z28.3   Underimmunization status

Z33.1   Pregnant state, incidental

This code is a secondary code only for use when the pregnancy is in no way complicating the reason for visit. Otherwise, a code from the obstetric chapter is required.

Z66   Do not resuscitate

This code may be used when it is documented by the provider that a patient is on do not resuscitate status at any time during the stay.

Z67   Blood type

Z68   Body mass index (BMI)

As with all other secondary diagnosis codes, the BMI codes should only be assigned when they meet the definition of a reportable diagnosis (see Section III, Reporting Additional Diagnoses).

Z74.01   Bed confinement status

Z76.82   Awaiting organ transplant status

Z78   Other specified health status

Code Z78.1, Physical restraint status, may be used when it is documented by the provider that a patient has been put in restraints during the current encounter. Please note that this code should not be reported when it is documented by the provider that a patient is temporarily restrained during a procedure.

**Z79**    Long-term (current) drug therapy

Codes from this category indicate a patient's continuous use of a prescribed drug (including such things as aspirin therapy) for the long-term treatment of a condition or for prophylactic use. It is not for use for patients who have addictions to drugs. This subcategory is not for use of medications for detoxification or maintenance programs to prevent withdrawal symptoms in patients with drug dependence (e.g., methadone maintenance for opiate dependence). Assign the appropriate code for the drug dependence instead.

Assign a code from Z79 if the patient is receiving a medication for an extended period as a prophylactic measure (such as for the prevention of deep vein thrombosis) or as treatment of a chronic condition (such as arthritis) or a disease requiring a lengthy course of treatment (such as cancer). Do not assign a code from category Z79 for medication being administered for a brief period of time to treat an acute illness or injury (such as a course of antibiotics to treat acute bronchitis).

**Z88**    Allergy status to drugs, medicaments and biological substances

Except: Z88.9, Allergy status to unspecified drugs, medicaments and biological substances status

**Z89**    Acquired absence of limb

**Z90**    Acquired absence of organs, not elsewhere classified

**Z91.0-**   Allergy status, other than to drugs and biological substances

**Z92.82** Status post administration of tPA (rtPA) in a different facility within the last 24 hours prior to admission to a current facility

Assign code Z92.82, Status post administration of tPA (rtPA) within the last 24 hours prior to admission to current facility, as a secondary diagnosis when a patient is received by transfer into a facility and documentation indicates they were administered tissue plasminogen activator (tPA) within the last 24 hours prior to admission to the current facility.

This guideline applies even if the patient is still receiving the tPA at the time they are received into the current facility.

The appropriate code for the condition for which the tPA was administered (such as cerebrovascular disease or myocardial infarction) should be assigned first.

Code Z92.82 is only applicable to the receiving facility record and not to the transferring facility record.

**Z93**    Artificial opening status

**Z94**    Transplanted organ and tissue status

**Z95**    Presence of cardiac and vascular implants and grafts

**Z96**    Presence of other functional implants

**Z97**    Presence of other devices

**Z98**    Other postprocedural states

Assign code Z98.85, Transplanted organ removal status, to indicate that a transplanted organ has been previously removed. This code should not be assigned for the encounter in which the transplanted organ is removed. The complication necessitating removal of the transplant organ should be assigned for that encounter.

*See section I.C19. for information on the coding of organ transplant complications.*

**Z99**    Dependence on enabling machines and devices, not elsewhere classified

**Note:** Categories Z89-Z90 and Z93-Z99 are for use only if there are no complications or malfunctions of the organ or tissue replaced, the amputation site or the equipment on which the patient is dependent.

**4)  History (of)**

There are two types of history Z codes, personal and family. Personal history codes explain a patient's past medical condition that no longer exists and is not receiving any treatment, but that has the potential for recurrence, and therefore may require continued monitoring.

Family history codes are for use when a patient has a family member(s) who has had a particular disease that causes the patient to be at higher risk of also contracting the disease.

Personal history codes may be used in conjunction with follow-up codes and family history codes may be used in conjunction with screening codes to explain the need for a test or procedure. History codes are also acceptable on any medical record regardless of the reason for visit. A history of an illness, even if no longer present, is important information that may alter the type of treatment ordered.

The history Z code categories are:

**Z80**    Family history of primary malignant neoplasm

**Z81**    Family history of mental and behavioral disorders

**Z82**    Family history of certain disabilities and chronic diseases (leading to disablement)

**Z83**    Family history of other specific disorders

**Z84**    Family history of other conditions

**Z85**    Personal history of malignant neoplasm

**Z86**    Personal history of certain other diseases

**Z87**    Personal history of other diseases and conditions

**Z91.4-**   Personal history of psychological trauma, not elsewhere classified

**Z91.5**   Personal history of self-harm

**Z91.8-**   Other specified personal risk factors, not elsewhere classified

Exception: Z91.83, Wandering in diseases classified elsewhere

**Z92**    Personal history of medical treatment

Except: Z92.0, Personal history of contraception

Except: Z92.82, Status post administration of tPA (rtPA) in a different facility within the last 24 hours prior to admission to a current facility

**5)  Screening**

Screening is the testing for disease or disease precursors in seemingly well individuals so that early detection and treatment can be provided for those who test positive for the disease (e.g., screening mammogram).

The testing of a person to rule out or confirm a suspected diagnosis because the patient has some sign or symptom is a diagnostic examination, not a screening. In these cases, the sign or symptom is used to explain the reason for the test.

A screening code may be a first-listed code if the reason for the visit is specifically the screening exam. It may also be used as an additional code if the screening is done during an office visit for other health problems. A screening code is not necessary if the screening is inherent to a routine examination, such as a pap smear done during a routine pelvic examination.

Should a condition be discovered during the screening then the code for the condition may be assigned as an additional diagnosis.

The Z code indicates that a screening exam is planned. A procedure code is required to confirm that the screening was performed.

The screening Z codes/categories:

**Z11**    Encounter for screening for infectious and parasitic diseases

**Z12**    Encounter for screening for malignant neoplasms

**Z13**    Encounter for screening for other diseases and disorders

Except: Z13.9, Encounter for screening, unspecified

Z36    Encounter for antenatal screening for mother

### 6) Observation

There are three observation Z code categories. They are for use in very limited circumstances when a person is being observed for a suspected condition that is ruled out. The observation codes are not for use if an injury or illness or any signs or symptoms related to the suspected condition are present. In such cases the diagnosis/symptom code is used with the corresponding external cause code.

The observation codes are to be used as principal diagnosis only. The only exception to this is when the principal diagnosis is required to be a code from category Z38, Liveborn infants according to place of birth and type of delivery. Then a code from category Z05, Encounter for observation and evaluation of newborn for suspected diseases and conditions ruled out, is sequenced after the Z38 code. Additional codes may be used in addition to the observation code, but only if they are unrelated to the suspected condition being observed.

Codes from subcategory Z03.7, Encounter for suspected maternal and fetal conditions ruled out, may either be used as a first-listed or as an additional code assignment depending on the case. They are for use in very limited circumstances on a maternal record when an encounter is for a suspected maternal or fetal condition that is ruled out during that encounter (for example, a maternal or fetal condition may be suspected due to an abnormal test result). These codes should not be used when the condition is confirmed. In those cases, the confirmed condition should be coded. In addition, these codes are not for use if an illness or any signs or symptoms related to the suspected condition or problem are present. In such cases the diagnosis/symptom code is used.

Additional codes may be used in addition to the code from subcategory Z03.7, but only if they are unrelated to the suspected condition being evaluated.

Codes from subcategory Z03.7 may not be used for encounters for antenatal screening of mother. *See Section I.C.21. Screening.*

For encounters for suspected fetal condition that are inconclusive following testing and evaluation, assign the appropriate code from category O35, O36, O40 or O41.

The observation Z code categories:

Z03    Encounter for medical observation for suspected diseases and conditions ruled out

Z04    Encounter for examination and observation for other reasons

       Except: Z04.9, Encounter for examination and observation for unspecified reason

Z05    Encounter for observation and evaluation of newborn for suspected diseases and conditions ruled out

### 7) Aftercare

Aftercare visit codes cover situations when the initial treatment of a disease has been performed and the patient requires continued care during the healing or recovery phase, or for the long-term consequences of the disease. The aftercare Z code should not be used if treatment is directed at a current, acute disease. The diagnosis code is to be used in these cases. Exceptions to this rule are codes Z51.0, Encounter for antineoplastic radiation therapy, and codes from subcategory Z51.1, Encounter for antineoplastic chemotherapy and immunotherapy. These codes are to be first-listed, followed by the diagnosis code when a patient's encounter is solely to receive radiation therapy, chemotherapy, or immunotherapy for the treatment of a neoplasm. If the reason for the encounter is more than one type of antineoplastic therapy, code Z51.0 and a code from subcategory Z51.1 may be assigned together, in which case one of these codes would be reported as a secondary diagnosis.

The aftercare Z codes should also not be used for aftercare for injuries. For aftercare of an injury, assign the acute injury code with the appropriate 7th character (for subsequent encounter).

The aftercare codes are generally first-listed to explain the specific reason for the encounter. An aftercare code may be used as an additional code when some type of aftercare is provided in addition to the reason for admission and no diagnosis code is applicable. An example of this would be the closure of a colostomy during an encounter for treatment of another condition.

Aftercare codes should be used in conjunction with other aftercare codes or diagnosis codes to provide better detail on the specifics of an aftercare encounter visit, unless otherwise directed by the classification. Should a patient receive multiple types of antineoplastic therapy during the same encounter, code Z51.0, Encounter for antineoplastic radiation therapy, and codes from subcategory Z51.1, Encounter for antineoplastic chemotherapy and immunotherapy, may be used together on a record. The sequencing of multiple aftercare codes depends on the circumstances of the encounter.

Certain aftercare Z code categories need a secondary diagnosis code to describe the resolving condition or sequelae**.** For others, the condition is included in the code title.

Additional Z code aftercare category terms include fitting and adjustment, and attention to artificial openings.

Status Z codes may be used with aftercare Z codes to indicate the nature of the aftercare. For example code Z95.1, Presence of aortocoronary bypass graft, may be used with code Z48.812, Encounter for surgical aftercare following surgery on the circulatory system, to indicate the surgery for which the aftercare is being performed. A status code should not be used when the aftercare code indicates the type of status, such as using Z43.0, Encounter for attention to tracheostomy, with Z93.0, Tracheostomy status.

The aftercare Z category/codes:

Z42    Encounter for plastic and reconstructive surgery following medical procedure or healed injury

Z43    Encounter for attention to artificial openings

Z44    Encounter for fitting and adjustment of external prosthetic device

Z45    Encounter for adjustment and management of implanted device

Z46    Encounter for fitting and adjustment of other devices

Z47    Orthopedic aftercare

Z48    Encounter for other postprocedural aftercare

Z49    Encounter for care involving renal dialysis

Z51    Encounter for other aftercare and medical care

### 8) Follow-up

The follow-up codes are used to explain continuing surveillance following completed treatment of a disease, condition, or injury. They imply that the condition has been fully treated and no longer exists. They should not be confused with aftercare codes, or injury codes with a 7th character for subsequent encounter, that explain ongoing care of a healing condition or its sequelae. Follow-up codes may be used in conjunction with history codes to provide the full picture of the healed condition and its treatment. The follow-up code is sequenced first, followed by the history code.

A follow-up code may be used to explain multiple visits. Should a condition be found to have recurred on the follow-up visit, then the diagnosis code for the condition should be assigned in place of the follow-up code.

The follow-up Z code categories:

Z08    Encounter for follow-up examination after completed treatment for malignant neoplasm

Z09    Encounter for follow-up examination after completed treatment for conditions other than malignant neoplasm

Z39    Encounter for maternal postpartum care and examination

### 9) Donor

Codes in category Z52, Donors of organs and tissues, are used for living individuals who are donating blood or other body tissue. These codes are only for individuals donating for others, not for self-donations. They are not used to identify cadaveric donations.

### 10) Counseling

Counseling Z codes are used when a patient or family member receives assistance in the aftermath of an illness or injury, or when support is required in coping with family or social problems. They are not used in conjunction with a diagnosis code when the counseling component of care is considered integral to standard treatment.

The counseling Z codes/categories:

Z30.0-  Encounter for general counseling and advice on contraception

Z31.5  Encounter for genetic counseling

Z31.6-  Encounter for general counseling and advice on procreation

Z32.2  Encounter for childbirth instruction

Z32.3  Encounter for childcare instruction

Z69  Encounter for mental health services for victim and perpetrator of abuse

Z70  Counseling related to sexual attitude, behavior and orientation

Z71  Persons encountering health services for other counseling and medical advice, not elsewhere classified

Z76.81  Expectant mother prebirth pediatrician visit

### 11) Encounters for Obstetrical and Reproductive Services

*See Section I.C.15. Pregnancy, Childbirth, and the Puerperium, for further instruction on the use of these codes.*

Z codes for pregnancy are for use in those circumstances when none of the problems or complications included in the codes from the Obstetrics chapter exist (a routine prenatal visit or postpartum care). Codes in category Z34, Encounter for supervision of normal pregnancy, are always first-listed and are not to be used with any other code from the OB chapter.

Codes in category Z3A, Weeks of gestation, may be assigned to provide additional information about the pregnancy. Category Z3A codes should not be assigned for pregnancies with abortive outcomes (categories O00-O08), elective termination of pregnancy (code Z33.32), nor for postpartum conditions, as category Z3A is not applicable to these conditions. The date of the admission should be used to determine weeks of gestation for inpatient admissions that encompass more than one gestational week.

The outcome of delivery, category Z37, should be included on all maternal delivery records. It is always a secondary code. Codes in category Z37 should not be used on the newborn record.

Z codes for family planning (contraceptive) or procreative management and counseling should be included on an obstetric record either during the pregnancy or the postpartum stage, if applicable.

Z codes/categories for obstetrical and reproductive services:

Z30  Encounter for contraceptive management

Z31  Encounter for procreative management

Z32.2  Encounter for childbirth instruction

Z32.3  Encounter for childcare instruction

Z33  Pregnant state

Z34  Encounter for supervision of normal pregnancy

Z36  Encounter for antenatal screening of mother

Z3A  Weeks of gestation

Z37  Outcome of delivery

Z39  Encounter for maternal postpartum care and examination

Z76.81  Expectant mother prebirth pediatrician visit

### 12) Newborns and Infants

*See Section I.C.16. Newborn (Perinatal) Guidelines, for further instruction on the use of these codes.*

Newborn Z codes/categories:

Z76.1  Encounter for health supervision and care of foundling

Z00.1-  Encounter for routine child health examination

Z38  Liveborn infants according to place of birth and type of delivery

### 13) Routine and administrative examinations

The Z codes allow for the description of encounters for routine examinations, such as, a general check-up, or, examinations for administrative purposes, such as, a pre-employment physical. The codes are not to be used if the examination is for diagnosis of a suspected condition or for treatment purposes. In such cases the diagnosis code is used. During a routine exam, should a diagnosis or condition be discovered, it should be coded as an additional code. Pre-existing and chronic conditions and history codes may also be included as additional codes as long as the examination is for administrative purposes and not focused on any particular condition.

Some of the codes for routine health examinations distinguish between "with" and "without" abnormal findings. Code assignment depends on the information that is known at the time the encounter is being coded. For example, if no abnormal findings were found during the examination, but the encounter is being coded before test results are back, it is acceptable to assign the code for "without abnormal findings." When assigning a code for "with abnormal findings," additional code(s) should be assigned to identify the specific abnormal finding(s).

Pre-operative examination and pre-procedural laboratory examination Z codes are for use only in those situations when a patient is being cleared for a procedure or surgery and no treatment is given.

The Z codes/categories for routine and administrative examinations:

Z00  Encounter for general examination without complaint, suspected or reported diagnosis

Z01  Encounter for other special examination without complaint, suspected or reported diagnosis

Z02  Encounter for administrative examination

Except: Z02.9, Encounter for administrative examinations, unspecified

Z32.0-  Encounter for pregnancy test

### 14) Miscellaneous Z codes

The miscellaneous Z codes capture a number of other health care encounters that do not fall into one of the other categories. Certain of these codes identify the reason for the encounter; others are for use as additional codes that provide useful information on circumstances that may affect a patient's care and treatment.

**Prophylactic Organ Removal**

For encounters specifically for prophylactic removal of an organ (such as prophylactic removal of breasts due to a genetic susceptibility to cancer or a family history of cancer), the principal or first-listed code should be a code from category Z40, Encounter for prophylactic surgery, followed by the appropriate codes to identify the associated risk factor (such as genetic susceptibility or family history).

If the patient has a malignancy of one site and is having prophylactic removal at another site to prevent either a new primary malignancy or metastatic disease, a code for the malignancy should also be assigned in addition to a code from subcategory Z40.0, Encounter for prophylactic surgery for risk factors related to malignant neoplasms. A Z40.0 code should not be assigned if the patient is having organ removal for treatment of a malignancy, such as the removal of the testes for the treatment of prostate cancer.

Miscellaneous Z codes/categories:

Z28    Immunization not carried out

Except: Z28.3, Underimmunization status

Z29    Encounter for other prophylactic measures

Z40    Encounter for prophylactic surgery

Z41    Encounter for procedures for purposes other than remedying health state

Except: Z41.9, Encounter for procedure for purposes other than remedying health state, unspecified

Z53    Persons encountering health services for specific procedures and treatment, not carried out

Z55    Problems related to education and literacy

Z56    Problems related to employment and unemployment

Z57    Occupational exposure to risk factors

Z58    Problems related to physical environment

Z59    Problems related to housing and economic circumstances

Z60    Problems related to social environment

Z62    Problems related to upbringing

Z63    Other problems related to primary support group, including family circumstances

Z64    Problems related to certain psychosocial circumstances

Z65    Problems related to other psychosocial circumstances

Z72    Problems related to lifestyle

**Note:** These codes should be assigned only when the documentation specifies that the patient has an associated problem

Z73    Problems related to life management difficulty

Z74    Problems related to care provider dependency

Except: Z74.01, Bed confinement status

Z75    Problems related to medical facilities and other health care

Z76.0    Encounter for issue of repeat prescription

Z76.3    Healthy person accompanying sick person

Z76.4    Other boarder to healthcare facility

Z76.5    Malingerer [conscious simulation]

Z91.1-   Patient's noncompliance with medical treatment and regimen

Z91.83    Wandering in diseases classified elsewhere

Z91.89    Other specified personal risk factors, not elsewhere classified

15) **Nonspecific Z codes**

Certain Z codes are so non-specific, or potentially redundant with other codes in the classification, that there can be little justification for their use in the inpatient setting. Their use in the outpatient setting should be limited to those instances when there is no further documentation to permit more precise coding. Otherwise, any sign or symptom or any other reason for visit that is captured in another code should be used.

Nonspecific Z codes/categories:

Z02.9    Encounter for administrative examinations, unspecified

Z04.9    Encounter for examination and observation for unspecified reason

Z13.9    Encounter for screening, unspecified

Z41.9    Encounter for procedure for purposes other than remedying health state, unspecified

Z52.9    Donor of unspecified organ or tissue

Z86.59    Personal history of other mental and behavioral disorders

Z88.9    Allergy status to unspecified drugs, medicaments and biological substances status

Z92.0    Personal history of contraception

16) **Z Codes That May Only be Principal/First-Listed Diagnosis**

The following Z codes/categories may only be reported as the principal/first-listed diagnosis, except when there are multiple encounters on the same day and the medical records for the encounters are combined:

Z00    Encounter for general examination without complaint, suspected or reported diagnosis

Except: Z00.6

Z01    Encounter for other special examination without complaint, suspected or reported diagnosis

Z02    Encounter for administrative examination

Z03    Encounter for medical observation for suspected diseases and conditions ruled out

Z04    Encounter for examination and observation for other reasons

Z33.2    Encounter for elective termination of pregnancy

Z31.81    Encounter for male factor infertility in female patient

Z31.83    Encounter for assisted reproductive fertility procedure cycle

Z31.84    Encounter for fertility preservation procedure

Z34    Encounter for supervision of normal pregnancy

Z39    Encounter for maternal postpartum care and examination

Z38    Liveborn infants according to place of birth and type of delivery

Z42    Encounter for plastic and reconstructive surgery following medical procedure or healed injury

Z51.0    Encounter for antineoplastic radiation therapy

Z51.1-   Encounter for antineoplastic chemotherapy and immunotherapy

Z52    Donors of organs and tissues

Except: Z52.9, Donor of unspecified organ or tissue

Z76.1    Encounter for health supervision and care of foundling

Z76.2    Encounter for health supervision and care of other healthy infant and child

Z99.12    Encounter for respirator [ventilator] dependence during power failure

# Section II. Selection of Principal Diagnosis

The circumstances of inpatient admission always govern the selection of principal diagnosis. The principal diagnosis is defined in the Uniform Hospital Discharge Data Set (UHDDS) as "that condition established after study to be chiefly responsible for occasioning the admission of the patient to the hospital for care."

The UHDDS definitions are used by hospitals to report inpatient data elements in a standardized manner. These data elements and their definitions can be found in the July 31, 1985, Federal Register (Vol. 50, No, 147), pp. 31038-40.

Since that time the application of the UHDDS definitions has been expanded to include all non-outpatient settings (acute care, short term, long term care and psychiatric hospitals; home health agencies; rehab facilities; nursing homes, etc). The UHDDS definitions also apply to hospice services (all levels of care).

In determining principal diagnosis, coding conventions in the ICD-10-CM, the Tabular List and Alphabetic Index take precedence over these official coding guidelines.

*(See Section I.A., Conventions for the ICD-10-CM)*

The importance of consistent, complete documentation in the medical record cannot be overemphasized. Without such documentation the application of all coding guidelines is a difficult, if not impossible, task.

A. **Codes for symptoms, signs, and ill-defined conditions**

Codes for symptoms, signs, and ill-defined conditions from Chapter 18 are not to be used as principal diagnosis when a related definitive diagnosis has been established.

**B. Two or more interrelated conditions, each potentially meeting the definition for principal diagnosis.**

When there are two or more interrelated conditions (such as diseases in the same ICD-10-CM chapter or manifestations characteristically associated with a certain disease) potentially meeting the definition of principal diagnosis, either condition may be sequenced first, unless the circumstances of the admission, the therapy provided, the Tabular List, or the Alphabetic Index indicate otherwise.

**C. Two or more diagnoses that equally meet the definition for principal diagnosis**

In the unusual instance when two or more diagnoses equally meet the criteria for principal diagnosis as determined by the circumstances of admission, diagnostic workup and/or therapy provided, and the Alphabetic Index, Tabular List, or another coding guidelines does not provide sequencing direction, any one of the diagnoses may be sequenced first.

**D. Two or more comparative or contrasting conditions**

In those rare instances when two or more contrasting or comparative diagnoses are documented as "either/or" (or similar terminology), they are coded as if the diagnoses were confirmed and the diagnoses are sequenced according to the circumstances of the admission. If no further determination can be made as to which diagnosis should be principal, either diagnosis may be sequenced first.

**E. A symptom(s) followed by contrasting/comparative diagnoses**

GUIDELINE HAS BEEN DELETED EFFECTIVE OCTOBER 1, 2014

**F. Original treatment plan not carried out**

Sequence as the principal diagnosis the condition, which after study occasioned the admission to the hospital, even though treatment may not have been carried out due to unforeseen circumstances.

**G. Complications of surgery and other medical care**

When the admission is for treatment of a complication resulting from surgery or other medical care, the complication code is sequenced as the principal diagnosis. If the complication is classified to the T80-T88 series and the code lacks the necessary specificity in describing the complication, an additional code for the specific complication should be assigned.

**H. Uncertain Diagnosis**

If the diagnosis documented at the time of discharge is qualified as "probable", "suspected", "likely", "questionable", "possible", or "still to be ruled out", or other similar terms indicating uncertainty, code the condition as if it existed or was established. The bases for these guidelines are the diagnostic workup, arrangements for further workup or observation, and initial therapeutic approach that correspond most closely with the established diagnosis.

**Note:** This guideline is applicable only to inpatient admissions to short-term, acute, long-term care and psychiatric hospitals.

**I. Admission from Observation Unit**

**1. Admission Following Medical Observation**

When a patient is admitted to an observation unit for a medical condition, which either worsens or does not improve, and is subsequently admitted as an inpatient of the same hospital for this same medical condition, the principal diagnosis would be the medical condition which led to the hospital admission.

**2. Admission Following Post-Operative Observation**

When a patient is admitted to an observation unit to monitor a condition (or complication) that develops following outpatient surgery, and then is subsequently admitted as an inpatient of the same hospital, hospitals should apply the Uniform Hospital Discharge Data Set (UHDDS) definition of principal diagnosis as "that condition established after study to be chiefly responsible for occasioning the admission of the patient to the hospital for care."

**J. Admission from Outpatient Surgery**

When a patient receives surgery in the hospital's outpatient surgery department and is subsequently admitted for continuing inpatient care at the same hospital, the following guidelines should be followed in selecting the principal diagnosis for the inpatient admission:

- If the reason for the inpatient admission is a complication, assign the complication as the principal diagnosis.

- If no complication, or other condition, is documented as the reason for the inpatient admission, assign the reason for the outpatient surgery as the principal diagnosis.

- If the reason for the inpatient admission is another condition unrelated to the surgery, assign the unrelated condition as the principal diagnosis.

**K. Admissions/Encounters for Rehabilitation**

When the purpose for the admission/encounter is rehabilitation, sequence first the code for the condition for which the service is being performed. For example, for an admission/encounter for rehabilitation for right-sided dominant hemiplegia following a cerebrovascular infarction, report code I69.351, Hemiplegia and hemiparesis following cerebral infarction affecting right dominant side, as the first-listed or principal diagnosis. If the condition for which the rehabilitation service is no longer present, report the appropriate aftercare code as the first-listed or principal diagnosis. For example, if a patient with severe degenerative osteoarthritis of the hip, underwent hip replacement and the current encounter/admission is for rehabilitation, report code Z47.1, Aftercare following joint replacement surgery, as the first-listed or principal diagnosis.

*See Section I.C.21.c.7, Factors influencing health states and contact with health services, Aftercare.*

# Section III. Reporting Additional Diagnoses

GENERAL RULES FOR OTHER (ADDITIONAL) DIAGNOSES

For reporting purposes the definition for "other diagnoses" is interpreted as additional conditions that affect patient care in terms of requiring:

clinical evaluation; or

therapeutic treatment; or

diagnostic procedures; or

extended length of hospital stay; or

increased nursing care and/or monitoring.

The UHDDS item #11-b defines Other Diagnoses as "all conditions that coexist at the time of admission, that develop subsequently, or that affect the treatment received and/or the length of stay. Diagnoses that relate to an earlier episode which have no bearing on the current hospital stay are to be excluded." UHDDS definitions apply to inpatients in acute care, short-term, long term care and psychiatric hospital setting. The UHDDS definitions are used by acute care short-term hospitals to report inpatient data elements in a standardized manner. These data elements and their definitions can be found in the July 31, 1985, Federal Register (Vol. 50, No, 147), pp. 31038-40.

Since that time the application of the UHDDS definitions has been expanded to include all non-outpatient settings (acute care, short term, long term care and psychiatric hospitals; home health agencies; rehab facilities; nursing homes, etc). The UHDDS definitions also apply to hospice services (all levels of care).

The following guidelines are to be applied in designating "other diagnoses" when neither the Alphabetic Index nor the Tabular List in ICD-10-CM provide direction. The listing of the diagnoses in the patient record is the responsibility of the attending provider.

**A. Previous conditions**

If the provider has included a diagnosis in the final diagnostic statement, such as the discharge summary or the face sheet, it should ordinarily be coded. Some providers include in the diagnostic statement resolved conditions or diagnoses and status-post procedures from previous admission that have no bearing on the current stay. Such conditions are not to be reported and are coded only if required by hospital policy.

However, history codes (categories Z80-Z87) may be used as secondary codes if the historical condition or family history has an impact on current care or influences treatment.

**B. Abnormal findings**

Abnormal findings (laboratory, x-ray, pathologic, and other diagnostic results) are not coded and reported unless the provider indicates their clinical significance. If the findings are outside the normal range and the attending provider has ordered other tests to evaluate the condition or prescribed treatment, it is appropriate to ask the provider whether the abnormal finding should be added.

**Please note:** This differs from the coding practices in the outpatient setting for coding encounters for diagnostic tests that have been interpreted by a provider.

**C. Uncertain Diagnosis**

If the diagnosis documented at the time of discharge is qualified as "probable", "suspected", "likely", "questionable", "possible", or "still to be ruled out" or other similar terms indicating uncertainty, code the condition as if it existed or was established. The bases for these guidelines are the diagnostic workup, arrangements for further workup or observation, and initial therapeutic approach that correspond most closely with the established diagnosis.

**Note:** This guideline is applicable only to inpatient admissions to short-term, acute, long-term care and psychiatric hospitals.

# Section IV. Diagnostic Coding and Reporting Guidelines for Outpatient Services

These coding guidelines for outpatient diagnoses have been approved for use by hospitals/ providers in coding and reporting hospital-based outpatient services and provider-based office visits. Guidelines in Section I, Conventions, general coding guidelines and chapter-specific guidelines, should also be applied for outpatient services and office visits.

Information about the use of certain abbreviations, punctuation, symbols, and other conventions used in the ICD-10-CM Tabular List (code numbers and titles), can be found in Section IA of these guidelines, under "Conventions Used in the Tabular List." Section I.B. contains general guidelines that apply to the entire classification. Section I.C. contains chapter-specific guidelines that correspond to the chapters as they are arranged in the classification. Information about the correct sequence to use in finding a code is also described in Section I.

The terms encounter and visit are often used interchangeably in describing outpatient service contacts and, therefore, appear together in these guidelines without distinguishing one from the other.

Though the conventions and general guidelines apply to all settings, coding guidelines for outpatient and provider reporting of diagnoses will vary in a number of instances from those for inpatient diagnoses, recognizing that:

> The Uniform Hospital Discharge Data Set (UHDDS) definition of principal diagnosis does not apply to hospital-based outpatient services and provider-based office visits.
>
> Coding guidelines for inconclusive diagnoses (probable, suspected, rule out, etc.) were developed for inpatient reporting and do not apply to outpatients.

**A. Selection of first-listed condition**

In the outpatient setting, the term first-listed diagnosis is used in lieu of principal diagnosis.

In determining the first-listed diagnosis the coding conventions of ICD-10-CM, as well as the general and disease specific guidelines take precedence over the outpatient guidelines.

Diagnoses often are not established at the time of the initial encounter/visit. It may take two or more visits before the diagnosis is confirmed.

The most critical rule involves beginning the search for the correct code assignment through the Alphabetic Index. Never begin searching initially in the Tabular List as this will lead to coding errors.

**1. Outpatient Surgery**

When a patient presents for outpatient surgery (same day surgery), code the reason for the surgery as the first-listed diagnosis (reason for the encounter), even if the surgery is not performed due to a contraindication.

**2. Observation Stay**

When a patient is admitted for observation for a medical condition, assign a code for the medical condition as the first-listed diagnosis.

When a patient presents for outpatient surgery and develops complications requiring admission to observation, code the reason for the surgery as the first reported diagnosis (reason for the encounter), followed by codes for the complications as secondary diagnoses.

**B. Codes from A00.0 through T88.9, Z00-Z99**

The appropriate code(s) from A00.0 through T88.9, Z00-Z99 must be used to identify diagnoses, symptoms, conditions, problems, complaints, or other reason(s) for the encounter/visit.

**C. Accurate reporting of ICD-10-CM diagnosis codes**

For accurate reporting of ICD-10-CM diagnosis codes, the documentation should describe the patient's condition, using terminology which includes specific diagnoses as well as symptoms, problems, or reasons for the encounter. There are ICD-10-CM codes to describe all of these.

**D. Codes that describe symptoms and signs**

Codes that describe symptoms and signs, as opposed to diagnoses, are acceptable for reporting purposes when a diagnosis has not been established (confirmed) by the provider. Chapter 18 of ICD-10-CM, Symptoms, Signs, and Abnormal Clinical and Laboratory Findings Not Elsewhere Classified (codes R00-R99) contain many, but not all codes for symptoms.

**E. Encounters for circumstances other than a disease or injury**

ICD-10-CM provides codes to deal with encounters for circumstances other than a disease or injury. The Factors Influencing Health Status and Contact with Health Services codes (Z00-Z99) are provided to deal with occasions when circumstances other than a disease or injury are recorded as diagnosis or problems.

*See Section I.C.21. Factors influencing health status and contact with health services.*

**F. Level of Detail in Coding**

**1. ICD-10-CM codes with 3, 4, 5, 6 or 7 characters**

ICD-10-CM is composed of codes with 3, 4, 5, 6 or 7 characters. Codes with three characters are included in ICD-10-CM as the heading of a category of codes that may be further subdivided by the use of fourth, fifth, sixth or seventh characters to provide greater specificity.

**2. Use of full number of characters required for a code**

A three-character code is to be used only if it is not further subdivided. A code is invalid if it has not been coded to the full number of characters required for that code, including the 7th character, if applicable.

**G. ICD-10-CM code for the diagnosis, condition, problem, or other reason for encounter/visit**

List first the ICD-10-CM code for the diagnosis, condition, problem, or other reason for encounter/visit shown in the medical record to be chiefly responsible for the services provided. List additional codes that describe any coexisting conditions. In some cases the first-listed diagnosis may be a symptom when a diagnosis has not been established (confirmed) by the physician.

**H. Uncertain diagnosis**

Do not code diagnoses documented as "probable", "suspected," "questionable," "rule out," or "working diagnosis" or other similar terms indicating uncertainty. Rather, code the condition(s) to the highest degree of certainty for that encounter/visit, such as symptoms, signs, abnormal test results, or other reason for the visit.

**Please note:** This differs from the coding practices used by short-term, acute care, long-term care and psychiatric hospitals.

**I. Chronic diseases**

Chronic diseases treated on an ongoing basis may be coded and reported as many times as the patient receives treatment and care for the condition(s)

**J. Code all documented conditions that coexist**

Code all documented conditions that coexist at the time of the encounter/visit, and require or affect patient care treatment or management. Do not code conditions that were previously treated and no longer exist. However, history codes (categories Z80-Z87) may be used as secondary codes if the historical condition or family history has an impact on current care or influences treatment.

**K. Patients receiving diagnostic services only**

For patients receiving diagnostic services only during an encounter/visit, sequence first the diagnosis, condition, problem, or other reason for encounter/visit shown in the medical record to be chiefly responsible for the outpatient services provided during the encounter/visit. Codes for other diagnoses (e.g., chronic conditions) may be sequenced as additional diagnoses.

For encounters for routine laboratory/radiology testing in the absence of any signs, symptoms, or associated diagnosis, assign Z01.89, Encounter for other specified special examinations. If routine testing is performed during the same encounter as a test to evaluate a sign, symptom, or diagnosis, it is appropriate to assign both the Z code and the code describing the reason for the non-routine test.

For outpatient encounters for diagnostic tests that have been interpreted by a physician, and the final report is available at the time of coding, code any confirmed or definitive diagnosis(es) documented in the interpretation. Do not code related signs and symptoms as additional diagnoses.

**Please note:** This differs from the coding practice in the hospital inpatient setting regarding abnormal findings on test results.

**L. Patients receiving therapeutic services only**
For patients receiving therapeutic services only during an encounter/visit, sequence first the diagnosis, condition, problem, or other reason for encounter/visit shown in the medical record to be chiefly responsible for the outpatient services provided during the encounter/visit. Codes for other diagnoses (e.g., chronic conditions) may be sequenced as additional diagnoses.

The only exception to this rule is that when the primary reason for the admission/encounter is chemotherapy or radiation therapy, the appropriate Z code for the service is listed first, and the diagnosis or problem for which the service is being performed listed second.

**M. Patients receiving preoperative evaluations only**
For patients receiving preoperative evaluations only, sequence first a code from subcategory Z01.81, Encounter for pre-procedural examinations, to describe the pre-op consultations. Assign a code for the condition to describe the reason for the surgery as an additional diagnosis. Code also any findings related to the pre-op evaluation.

**N. Ambulatory surgery**
For ambulatory surgery, code the diagnosis for which the surgery was performed. If the postoperative diagnosis is known to be different from the preoperative diagnosis at the time the diagnosis is confirmed, select the postoperative diagnosis for coding, since it is the most definitive.

**O. Routine outpatient prenatal visits**
See Section I.C.15. Routine outpatient prenatal visits.

**P. Encounters for general medical examinations with abnormal findings**
The subcategories for encounters for general medical examinations, Z00.0-, provide codes for with and without abnormal findings. Should a general medical examination result in an abnormal finding, the code for general medical examination with abnormal finding should be assigned as the first-listed diagnosis. An examination with abnormal findings refers to a condition/diagnosis that is newly identified or a change in severity of a chronic condition (such as uncontrolled hypertension, or an acute exacerbation of chronic obstructive pulmonary disease) during a routine physical examination. A secondary code for the abnormal finding should also be coded.

**Q. Encounters for routine health screenings**
See Section I.C.21. Factors influencing health status and contact with health services, Screening

# Appendix I. Present on Admission Reporting Guidelines

## Introduction
These guidelines are to be used as a supplement to the *ICD-10-CM Official Guidelines for Coding and Reporting* to facilitate the assignment of the Present on Admission (POA) indicator for each diagnosis and external cause of injury code reported on claim forms (UB-04 and 837 Institutional).

These guidelines are not intended to replace any guidelines in the main body of the *ICD-10-CM Official Guidelines for Coding and Reporting*. The POA guidelines are not intended to provide guidance on when a condition should be coded, but rather, how to apply the POA indicator to the final set of diagnosis codes that have been assigned in accordance with Sections I, II, and III of the official coding guidelines. Subsequent to the assignment of the ICD-10-CM codes, the POA indicator should then be assigned to those conditions that have been coded.

As stated in the Introduction to the ICD-10-CM Official Guidelines for Coding and Reporting, a joint effort between the healthcare provider and the coder is essential to achieve complete and accurate documentation, code assignment, and reporting of diagnoses and procedures. The importance of consistent, complete documentation in the medical record cannot be overemphasized.

Medical record documentation from any provider involved in the care and treatment of the patient may be used to support the determination of whether a condition was present on admission or not. In the context of the official coding guidelines, the term "provider" means a physician or any qualified healthcare practitioner who is legally accountable for establishing the patient's diagnosis.

These guidelines are not a substitute for the provider's clinical judgment as to the determination of whether a condition was/was not present on admission. The provider should be queried regarding issues related to the linking of signs/symptoms, timing of test results, and the timing of findings.

Please see the CDC website for the detailed list of ICD-10-CM codes that do not require the use of a POA indicator (ftp://ftp.cdc.gov/pub/Health_Statistics/NCHS/Publications/ICD10CM/2017/). The conditions on this exempt list represent categories and/or codes for circumstances regarding the healthcare encounter or factors influencing health status that do not represent a current disease or injury or are always present on admission.

## General Reporting Requirements
All claims involving inpatient admissions to general acute care hospitals or other facilities that are subject to a law or regulation mandating collection of present on admission information.

Present on admission is defined as present at the time the order for inpatient admission occurs -- conditions that develop during an outpatient encounter, including emergency department, observation, or outpatient surgery, are considered as present on admission.

POA indicator is assigned to principal and secondary diagnoses (as defined in Section II of the Official Guidelines for Coding and Reporting) and the external cause of injury codes.

Issues related to inconsistent, missing, conflicting or unclear documentation must still be resolved by the provider.

If a condition would not be coded and reported based on UHDDS definitions and current official coding guidelines, then the POA indicator would not be reported.

Reporting Options

Y - Yes

N - No

U - Unknown

W – Clinically undetermined

Unreported/Not used – (Exempt from POA reporting)

Reporting Definitions

Y = present at the time of inpatient admission

N = not present at the time of inpatient admission

U = documentation is insufficient to determine if condition is present on admission

W = provider is unable to clinically determine whether condition was present on admission or not

## Timeframe for POA Identification and Documentation
There is no required timeframe as to when a provider (per the definition of "provider" used in these guidelines) must identify or document a condition to be present on admission. In some clinical situations, it may not be possible for a provider to make a definitive diagnosis (or a condition may not be recognized or reported by the patient) for a period of time after admission. In some cases it may be several days before the provider arrives at a definitive diagnosis. This does not mean that the condition was not present on admission. Determination of whether the condition was present on admission or not will be based on the applicable POA guideline as identified in this document, or on the provider's best clinical judgment.

If at the time of code assignment the documentation is unclear as to whether a condition was present on admission or not, it is appropriate to query the provider for clarification.

## Assigning the POA Indicator

**Condition is on the "Exempt from Reporting" list**

Leave the "present on admission" field blank if the condition is on the list of ICD-10-CM codes for which this field is not applicable. This is the only circumstance in which the field may be left blank.

**POA Explicitly Documented**

Assign Y for any condition the provider explicitly documents as being present on admission.

Assign N for any condition the provider explicitly documents as not present at the time of admission.

**Conditions diagnosed prior to inpatient admission**

Assign "Y" for conditions that were diagnosed prior to admission (example: hypertension, diabetes mellitus, asthma)

**Conditions diagnosed during the admission but clearly present before admission**

Assign "Y" for conditions diagnosed during the admission that were clearly present but not diagnosed until after admission occurred.

Diagnoses subsequently confirmed after admission are considered present on admission if at the time of admission they are documented as suspected, possible, rule out, differential diagnosis, or constitute an underlying cause of a symptom that is present at the time of admission.

**Condition develops during outpatient encounter prior to inpatient admission**

Assign Y for any condition that develops during an outpatient encounter prior to a written order for inpatient admission.

**Documentation does not indicate whether condition was present on admission**

Assign "U" when the medical record documentation is unclear as to whether the condition was present on admission. "U" should not be routinely assigned and used only in very limited circumstances. Coders are encouraged to query the providers when the documentation is unclear.

**Documentation states that it cannot be determined whether the condition was or was not present on admission**

Assign "W" when the medical record documentation indicates that it cannot be clinically determined whether or not the condition was present on admission.

**Chronic condition with acute exacerbation during the admission**

If a single code identifies both the chronic condition and the acute exacerbation, see POA guidelines pertaining to codes that contain multiple clinical concepts.

If a single code only identifies the chronic condition and not the acute exacerbation (e.g., acute exacerbation of chronic leukemia), assign "Y."

**Conditions documented as possible, probable, suspected, or rule out at the time of discharge**

If the final diagnosis contains a possible, probable, suspected, or rule out diagnosis, and this diagnosis was based on signs, symptoms or clinical findings suspected at the time of inpatient admission, assign "Y."

If the final diagnosis contains a possible, probable, suspected, or rule out diagnosis, and this diagnosis was based on signs, symptoms or clinical findings that were not present on admission, assign "N".

**Conditions documented as impending or threatened at the time of discharge**

If the final diagnosis contains an impending or threatened diagnosis, and this diagnosis is based on symptoms or clinical findings that were present on admission, assign "Y".

If the final diagnosis contains an impending or threatened diagnosis, and this diagnosis is based on symptoms or clinical findings that were not present on admission, assign "N".

**Acute and Chronic Conditions**

Assign "Y" for acute conditions that are present at time of admission and N for acute conditions that are not present at time of admission.

Assign "Y" for chronic conditions, even though the condition may not be diagnosed until after admission.

If a single code identifies both an acute and chronic condition, see the POA guidelines for codes that contain multiple clinical concepts.

**Codes That Contain Multiple Clinical Concepts**

Assign "N" if at least one of the clinical concepts included in the code was not present on admission (e.g., COPD with acute exacerbation and the exacerbation was not present on admission; gastric ulcer that does not start bleeding until after admission; asthma patient develops status asthmaticus after admission).

Assign "Y" if all of the clinical concepts included in the code were present on admission (e.g., duodenal ulcer that perforates prior to admission).

For infection codes that include the causal organism, assign "Y" if the infection (or signs of the infection) were present on admission, even though the culture results may not be known until after admission (e.g., patient is admitted with pneumonia and the provider documents Pseudomonas as the causal organism a few days later).

**Same Diagnosis Code for Two or More Conditions**

When the same ICD-10-CM diagnosis code applies to two or more conditions during the same encounter (e.g. two separate conditions classified to the same ICD-10-CM diagnosis code):

Assign "Y" if all conditions represented by the single ICD-10-CM code were present on admission (e.g. bilateral unspecified age-related cataracts).

Assign "N" if any of the conditions represented by the single ICD-10-CM code was not present on admission (e.g. traumatic secondary and recurrent hemorrhage and seroma is assigned to a single code T79.2, but only one of the conditions was present on admission).

**Obstetrical conditions**

Whether or not the patient delivers during the current hospitalization does not affect assignment of the POA indicator. The determining factor for POA assignment is whether the pregnancy complication or obstetrical condition described by the code was present at the time of admission or not.

If the pregnancy complication or obstetrical condition was present on admission (e.g., patient admitted in preterm labor), assign "Y".

If the pregnancy complication or obstetrical condition was not present on admission (e.g., 2nd degree laceration during delivery, postpartum hemorrhage that occurred during current hospitalization, fetal distress develops after admission), assign "N".

If the obstetrical code includes more than one diagnosis and any of the diagnoses identified by the code were not present on admission assign "N".

(e.g., Category O11, Pre-existing hypertension with pre-eclampsia)

**Perinatal conditions**

Newborns are not considered to be admitted until after birth. Therefore, any condition present at birth or that developed in utero is considered present at admission and should be assigned "Y". This includes conditions that occur during delivery (e.g., injury during delivery, meconium aspiration, exposure to streptococcus B in the vaginal canal).

**Congenital conditions and anomalies**

Assign "Y" for congenital conditions and anomalies except for categories Q00-Q99, Congenital anomalies, which are on the exempt list. Congenital conditions are always considered present on admission.

**External cause of injury codes**

Assign "Y" for any external cause code representing an external cause of morbidity that occurred prior to inpatient admission (e.g., patient fell out of bed at home, patient fell out of bed in emergency room prior to admission)

Assign "N" for any external cause code representing an external cause of morbidity that occurred during inpatient hospitalization (e.g., patient fell out of hospital bed during hospital stay, patient experienced an adverse reaction to a medication administered after inpatient admission)

# ICD-10-CM Index to Diseases and Injuries

## A

**Aarskog's syndrome** Q87.1
**Abandonment** — *see* Maltreatment
**Abasia** (-astasia) (hysterical) F44.4
**Abderhalden-Kaufmann-Lignac syndrome** (cystinosis) E72.04
**Abdomen, abdominal** (*see also* condition)
  acute R10.0
  angina K55.1
  muscle deficiency syndrome Q79.4
**Abdominalgia** — *see* Pain, abdominal
**Abduction contracture, hip or other joint** — *see* Contraction, joint
**Aberrant** (congenital) (*see also* Malposition, congenital)
  adrenal gland Q89.1
  artery (peripheral) Q27.8
    basilar NEC Q28.1
    cerebral Q28.3
    coronary Q24.5
    digestive system Q27.8
    eye Q15.8
    lower limb Q27.8
    precerebral Q28.1
    pulmonary Q25.79
    renal Q27.2
    retina Q14.1
    specified site NEC Q27.8
    subclavian Q27.8
    upper limb Q27.8
    vertebral Q28.1
  breast Q83.8
  endocrine gland NEC Q89.2
  hepatic duct Q44.5
  pancreas Q45.3
  parathyroid gland Q89.2
  pituitary gland Q89.2
  sebaceous glands, mucous membrane, mouth, congenital Q38.6
  spleen Q89.09
  subclavian artery Q27.8
  thymus (gland) Q89.2
  thyroid gland Q89.2
  vein (peripheral) NEC Q27.8
    cerebral Q28.3
    digestive system Q27.8
    lower limb Q27.8
    precerebral Q28.1
    specified site NEC Q27.8
    upper limb Q27.8
**Aberration**
  distantial — *see* Disturbance, visual
  mental F99
**Abetalipoproteinemia** E78.6
**Abiotrophy** R68.89
**Ablatio, ablation**
  retinae — *see* Detachment, retina
**Ablepharia, ablepharon** Q10.3
**Abnormal, abnormality, abnormalities** (*see also* Anomaly)
  acid-base balance (mixed) E87.4
  albumin R77.0
  alphafetoprotein R77.2
  alveolar ridge K08.9
  anatomical relationship Q89.9
  apertures, congenital, diaphragm Q79.1
  auditory perception H93.29- ☑
    diplacusis — *see* Diplacusis
    hyperacusis — *see* Hyperacusis
    recruitment — *see* Recruitment, auditory
    threshold shift — *see* Shift, auditory threshold
  autosomes Q99.9
    fragile site Q95.5
  basal metabolic rate R94.8
  biosynthesis, testicular androgen E29.1
  bleeding time R79.1
  blood level (of)
    cobalt R79.0
    copper R79.0
    iron R79.0
    lithium R78.89
    magnesium R79.0

**Abnormal, abnormality, abnormalities** — *continued*
  blood level — *continued*
    mineral NEC R79.0
    zinc R79.0
  blood pressure
    elevated R03.0
    low reading (nonspecific) R03.1
  blood sugar R73.09
  blood-gas level R79.81
  bowel sounds R19.15
    absent R19.11
    hyperactive R19.12
  brain scan R94.02
  breathing R06.9
  caloric test R94.138
  cerebrospinal fluid R83.9
    cytology R83.6
    drug level R83.2
    enzyme level R83.0
    hormones R83.1
    immunology R83.4
    microbiology R83.5
    nonmedicinal level R83.3
    specified type NEC R83.8
  chemistry, blood R79.9
    C-reactive protein R79.82
    drugs — *see* Findings, abnormal, in blood
    gas level R79.81
    minerals R79.0
    pancytopenia D61.818
    PTT R79.1
    specified NEC R79.89
    toxins — *see* Findings, abnormal, in blood
  chest sounds (friction) (rales) R09.89
  chromosome, chromosomal Q99.9
    with more than three X chromosomes, female Q97.1
    analysis result R89.8
      bronchial washings R84.8
      cerebrospinal fluid R83.8
      cervix uteri NEC R87.89
      nasal secretions R84.8
      nipple discharge R89.8
      peritoneal fluid R85.89
      pleural fluid R84.8
      prostatic secretions R86.8
      saliva R85.89
      seminal fluid R86.8
      sputum R84.8
      synovial fluid R89.8
      throat scrapings R84.8
      vagina R87.89
      vulva R87.89
      wound secretions R89.8
    dicentric replacement Q93.2
    ring replacement Q93.2
    sex Q99.8
      female phenotype Q97.9
        specified NEC Q97.8
      male phenotype Q98.9
        specified NEC Q98.8
      structural male Q98.6
    specified NEC Q99.8
  clinical findings NEC R68.89
  coagulation D68.9
    newborn, transient P61.6
    profile R79.1
    time R79.1
  communication — *see* Fistula
  conjunctiva, vascular H11.41- ☑
  coronary artery Q24.5
  cortisol-binding globulin E27.8
  course, eustachian tube Q17.8
  creatinine clearance R94.4
  cytology
    anus R85.619
      atypical squamous cells cannot exclude high grade squamous intraepithelial lesion (ASC-H) R85.611
      atypical squamous cells of undetermined significance (ASC-US) R85.610
      cytologic evidence of malignancy R85.614

**Abnormal, abnormality, abnormalities** — *continued*
  cytology — *continued*
    anus — *continued*
      high grade squamous intraepithelial lesion (HGSIL) R85.613
      human papillomavirus (HPV) DNA test
        high risk positive R85.81
        low risk postive R85.82
      inadequate smear R85.615
      low grade squamous intraepithelial lesion (LGSIL) R85.612
      satisfactory anal smear but lacking transformation zone R85.616
      specified NEC R85.618
      unsatisfactory smear R85.615
    female genital organs — *see* Abnormal, Papanicolaou (smear)
  dark adaptation curve H53.61
  dentofacial NEC — *see* Anomaly, dentofacial
  development, developmental Q89.9
    central nervous system Q07.9
  diagnostic imaging
    abdomen, abdominal region NEC R93.5
    biliary tract R93.2
    bladder R93.41
    breast R92.8
    central nervous system NEC R90.89
    cerebrovascular NEC R90.89
    coronary circulation R93.1
    digestive tract NEC R93.3
    gastrointestinal (tract) R93.3
    genitourinary organs R93.8
    head R93.0
    heart R93.1
    intrathoracic organ NEC R93.8
    kidney R93.42- ☑
    limbs R93.6
    liver R93.2
    lung (field) R91.8
    musculoskeletal system NEC R93.7
    renal pelvis R93.41
    retroperitoneum R93.5
    site specified NEC R93.8
    skin and subcutaneous tissue R93.8
    skull R93.0
    ureter R93.41
    urinary organs specified NEC R93.49
  direction, teeth, fully erupted M26.30
  ear ossicles, acquired NEC H74.39- ☑
    ankylosis — *see* Ankylosis, ear ossicles
    discontinuity — *see* Discontinuity, ossicles, ear
    partial loss — *see* Loss, ossicles, ear (partial)
  Ebstein Q22.5
  echocardiogram R93.1
  echoencephalogram R90.81
  echogram — *see* Abnormal, diagnostic imaging
  electrocardiogram [ECG] [EKG] R94.31
  electroencephalogram [EEG] R94.01
  electrolyte — *see* Imbalance, electrolyte
  electromyogram [EMG] R94.131
  electro-oculogram [EOG] R94.110
  electrophysiological intracardiac studies R94.39
  electroretinogram [ERG] R94.111
  erythrocytes
    congenital, with perinatal jaundice D58.9
  feces (color) (contents) (mucus) R19.5
  finding — *see* Findings, abnormal, without diagnosis
  fluid
    amniotic — *see* Abnormal, specimen, specified
    cerebrospinal — *see* Abnormal, cerebrospinal fluid
    peritoneal — *see* Abnormal, specimen, digestive organs
    pleural — *see* Abnormal, specimen, respiratory organs
    synovial — *see* Abnormal, specimen, specified
    thorax (bronchial washings) (pleural fluid) — *see* Abnormal, specimen, respiratory organs
    vaginal — *see* Abnormal, specimen, female genital organs
  form
    teeth K00.2
    uterus — *see* Anomaly, uterus

**Abnormal, abnormality, abnormalities** —
    *continued*
function studies
    auditory R94.120
    bladder R94.8
    brain R94.09
    cardiovascular R94.30
    ear R94.128
    endocrine NEC R94.7
    eye NEC R94.118
    kidney R94.4
    liver R94.5
    nervous system
        central NEC R94.09
        peripheral NEC R94.138
    pancreas R94.8
    placenta R94.8
    pulmonary R94.2
    special senses NEC R94.128
    spleen R94.8
    thyroid R94.6
    vestibular R94.121
gait — *see* Gait
    hysterical F44.4
gastrin secretion E16.4
globulin R77.1
    cortisol-binding E27.8
    thyroid-binding E07.89
glomerular, minor (*see also* N00-N07 with fourth
        character .0) N05.0
glucagon secretion E16.3
glucose tolerance (test) (non-fasting) R73.09
gravitational (G) forces or states (effect of) T75.81 ☑
hair (color) (shaft) L67.9
    specified NEC L67.8
hard tissue formation in pulp (dental) K04.3
head movement R25.0
heart
    rate R00.9
        specified NEC R00.8
    shadow R93.1
    sounds NEC R01.2
hemoglobin (disease) (*see also* Disease, hemoglobin)
        D58.2
    trait — *see* Trait, hemoglobin, abnormal
histology NEC R89.7
immunological findings R89.4
    in serum R76.9
        specified NEC R76.8
increase in appetite R63.2
involuntary movement — *see* Abnormal, movement,
        involuntary
jaw closure M26.51
karyotype R89.8
kidney function test R94.4
knee jerk R29.2
leukocyte (cell) (differential) NEC D72.9
liver function test R94.5
loss of
    height R29.890
    weight R63.4
mammogram NEC R92.8
    calcification (calculus) R92.1
    microcalcification R92.0
Mantoux test R76.11
movement (disorder) (*see also* Disorder, movement)
    head R25.0
    involuntary R25.9
        fasciculation R25.3
        of head R25.0
        spasm R25.2
        specified type NEC R25.8
        tremor R25.1
myoglobin (Aberdeen) (Annapolis) R89.7
neonatal screening P09
oculomotor study R94.113
palmar creases Q82.8
Papanicolaou (smear)
    anus R85.619
        atypical squamous cells cannot exclude high
                grade squamous intraepithelial lesion
                (ASC-H) R85.611
        atypical squamous cells of undetermined signif-
                icance (ASC-US) R85.610
        cytologic evidence of malignancy R85.614
        high grade squamous intraepithelial lesion
                (HGSIL) R85.613
        human papillomavirus (HPV) DNA test
            high risk positive R85.81

**Abnormal, abnormality, abnormalities** —
    *continued*
Papanicolaou — *continued*
    anus — *continued*
        human papillomavirus DNA test — *contin-
                ued*
            low risk postive R85.82
        inadequate smear R85.615
        low grade squamous intraepithelial lesion
                (LGSIL) R85.612
        satisfactory anal smear but lacking transforma-
                tion zone R85.616
        specified NEC R85.618
        unsatisfactory smear R85.615
    bronchial washings R84.6
    cerebrospinal fluid R83.6
    cervix R87.619
        atypical squamous cells cannot exclude high
                grade squamous intraepithelial lesion
                (ASC-H) R87.611
        atypical squamous cells of undetermined signif-
                icance (ASC-US) R87.610
        cytologic evidence of malignancy R87.614
        high grade squamous intraepithelial lesion
                (HGSIL) R87.613
        inadequate smear R87.615
        low grade squamous intraepithelial lesion
                (LGSIL) R87.612
        non-atypical endometrial cells R87.618
        satisfactory cervical smear but lacking transfor-
                mation zone R87.616
        specified NEC R87.618
        thin preparaton R87.619
        unsatisfactory smear R87.615
    nasal secretions R84.6
    nipple discharge R89.6
    peritoneal fluid R85.69
    pleural fluid R84.6
    prostatic secretions R86.6
    saliva R85.69
    seminal fluid R86.6
    sites NEC R89.6
    sputum R84.6
    synovial fluid R89.6
    throat scrapings R84.6
    vagina R87.629
        atypical squamous cells cannot exclude high
                grade squamous intraepithelial lesion
                (ASC-H) R87.621
        atypical squamous cells of undetermined signif-
                icance (ASC-US) R87.620
        cytologic evidence of malignancy R87.624
        high grade squamous intraepithelial lesion
                (HGSIL) R87.623
        inadequate smear R87.625
        low grade squamous intraepithelial lesion
                (LGSIL) R87.622
        specified NEC R87.628
        thin preparation R87.629
        unsatisfactory smear R87.625
    vulva R87.69
    wound secretions R89.6
partial thromboplastin time (PTT) R79.1
pelvis (bony) — *see* Deformity, pelvis
percussion, chest (tympany) R09.89
periods (grossly) — *see* Menstruation
phonocardiogram R94.39
plantar reflex R29.2
plasma
    protein R77.9
        specified NEC R77.8
    viscosity R70.1
pleural (folds) Q34.0
posture R29.3
product of conception O02.9
    specified type NEC O02.89
prothrombin time (PT) R79.1
pulmonary
    artery, congenital Q25.79
    function, newborn P28.89
    test results R94.2
pulsations in neck R00.2
pupillary H21.56- ☑
    function (reaction) (reflex) — *see* Anomaly, pupil,
            function
radiological examination — *see* Abnormal, diagnostic
        imaging
red blood cell(s) (morphology) (volume) R71.8
reflex — *see* Reflex

**Abnormal, abnormality, abnormalities** —
    *continued*
renal function test R94.4
response to nerve stimulation R94.130
retinal correspondence H53.31
retinal function study R94.111
rhythm, heart (*see also* Arrhythmia)
saliva — *see* Abnormal, specimen, digestive organs
scan
    kidney R94.4
    liver R93.2
    thyroid R94.6
secretion
    gastrin E16.4
    glucagon E16.3
semen, seminal fluid — *see* Abnormal, specimen, male
        genital organs
serum level (of)
    acid phosphatase R74.8
    alkaline phosphatase R74.8
    amylase R74.8
    enzymes R74.9
        specified NEC R74.8
    lipase R74.8
    triacylglycerol lipase R74.8
shape
    gravid uterus — *see* Anomaly, uterus
sinus venosus Q21.1
size, tooth, teeth K00.2
spacing, tooth, teeth, fully erupted M26.30
specimen
    digestive organs (peritoneal fluid) (saliva) R85.9
        cytology R85.69
        drug level R85.2
        enzyme level R85.0
        histology R85.7
        hormones R85.1
        immunology R85.4
        microbiology R85.5
        nonmedicinal level R85.3
        specified type NEC R85.89
    female genital organs (secretions) (smears) R87.9
        cytology R87.69
            cervix R87.619
                human papillomavirus (HPV) DNA test
                    high risk positive R87.810
                    low risk positive R87.820
                inadequate (unsatisfactory) smear
                    R87.615
                non-atypical endometrial cells R87.618
                specified NEC R87.618
            vagina R87.629
                human papillomavirus (HPV) DNA test
                    high risk positive R87.811
                    low risk positive R87.821
                inadequate (unsatisfactory) smear
                    R87.625
            vulva R87.69
        drug level R87.2
        enzyme level R87.0
        histological R87.7
        hormones R87.1
        immunology R87.4
        microbiology R87.5
        nonmedicinal level R87.3
        specified type NEC R87.89
    male genital organs (prostatic secretions) (semen)
            R86.9
        cytology R86.6
        drug level R86.2
        enzyme level R86.0
        histological R86.7
        hormones R86.1
        immunology R86.4
        microbiology R86.5
        nonmedicinal level R86.3
        specified type NEC R86.8
    nipple discharge — *see* Abnormal, specimen,
            specified
    respiratory organs (bronchial washings) (nasal se-
            cretions) (pleural fluid) (sputum) R84.9
        cytology R84.6
        drug level R84.2
        enzyme level R84.0
        histology R84.7
        hormones R84.1
        immunology R84.4
        microbiology R84.5
        nonmedicinal level R84.3

**Abnormal, abnormality, abnormalities** —
*continued*
specimen — *continued*
respiratory organs — *continued*
specified type NEC R84.8
specified organ, system and tissue NOS R89.9
cytology R89.6
drug level R89.2
enzyme level R89.0
histology R89.7
hormones R89.1
immunology R89.4
microbiology R89.5
nonmedicinal level R89.3
specified type NEC R89.8
synovial fluid — *see* Abnormal, specimen, specified
thorax (bronchial washings) (pleural fluids) — *see* Abnormal, specimen, respiratory organs
vagina (secretion) (smear) R87.629
vulva (secretion) (smear) R87.69
wound secretion — *see* Abnormal, specimen, specified
spermatozoa — *see* Abnormal, specimen, male genital organs
sputum (amount) (color) (odor) R09.3
stool (color) (contents) (mucus) R19.5
bloody K92.1
guaiac positive R19.5
synchondrosis Q78.8
thermography (*see also* Abnormal, diagnostic imaging) R93.8
thyroid-binding globulin E07.89
tooth, teeth (form) (size) K00.2
toxicology (findings) R78.9
transport protein E88.09
tumor marker NEC R97.8
ultrasound results — *see* Abnormal, diagnostic imaging
umbilical cord complicating delivery O69.9 ☑
urination NEC R39.198
urine (constituents) R82.90
bile R82.2
cytological examination R82.8
drugs R82.5
fat R82.0
glucose R81
heavy metals R82.6
hemoglobin R82.3
histological examination R82.8
ketones R82.4
microbiological examination (culture) R82.79
myoglobin R82.1
positive culture R82.79
protein — *see* Proteinuria
specified substance NEC R82.99
chromoabnormality NEC R82.91
substances nonmedical R82.6
uterine hemorrhage — *see* Hemorrhage, uterus
vectorcardiogram R94.39
visually evoked potential (VEP) R94.112
white blood cells D72.9
specified NEC D72.89
X-ray examination — *see* Abnormal, diagnostic imaging
**Abnormity** (any organ or part) — *see* Anomaly
**Abocclusion** M26.29
hemolytic disease (newborn) P55.1
incompatibility reaction ABO — *see* Complication(s), transfusion, incompatibility reaction, ABO
**Abolition, language** R48.8
**Aborter, habitual or recurrent** — *see* Loss (of), pregnancy, recurrent
**Abortion** (complete) (spontaneous) O03.9
with
retained products of conception — *see* Abortion, incomplete
attempted (elective) (failed) O07.4
complicated by O07.30
afibrinogenemia O07.1
cardiac arrest O07.36
chemical damage of pelvic organ(s) O07.34
circulatory collapse O07.31
cystitis O07.38
defibrination syndrome O07.1
electrolyte imbalance O07.33
embolism (air) (amniotic fluid) (blood clot) (fat) (pulmonary) (septic) (soap) O07.2
endometritis O07.0

**Abortion** — *continued*
attempted — *continued*
complicated by — *continued*
genital tract and pelvic infection O07.0
hemolysis O07.1
hemorrhage (delayed) (excessive) O07.1
infection
genital tract or pelvic O07.0
urinary tract tract O07.38
intravascular coagulation O07.1
laceration of pelvic organ(s) O07.34
metabolic disorder O07.33
oliguria O07.32
oophoritis O07.0
parametritis O07.0
pelvic peritonitis O07.0
perforation of pelvic organ(s) O07.34
renal failure or shutdown O07.32
salpingitis or salpingo-oophoritis O07.0
sepsis O07.37
shock O07.31
specified condition NEC O07.39
tubular necrosis (renal) O07.32
uremia O07.32
urinary tract infection O07.38
venous complication NEC O07.35
embolism (air) (amniotic fluid) (blood clot) (fat) (pulmonary) (septic) (soap) O07.2
complicated (by) (following) O03.80
afibrinogenemia O03.6
cardiac arrest O03.86
chemical damage of pelvic organ(s) O03.84
circulatory collapse O03.81
cystitis O03.88
defibrination syndrome O03.6
electrolyte imbalance O03.83
embolism (air) (amniotic fluid) (blood clot) (fat) (pulmonary) (septic) (soap) O03.7
endometritis O03.5
genital tract and pelvic infection O03.5
hemolysis O03.6
hemorrhage (delayed) (excessive) O03.6
infection
genital tract or pelvic O03.5
urinary tract O03.88
intravascular coagulation O03.6
laceration of pelvic organ(s) O03.84
metabolic disorder O03.83
oliguria O03.82
oophoritis O03.5
parametritis O03.5
pelvic peritonitis O03.5
perforation of pelvic organ(s) O03.84
renal failure or shutdown O03.82
salpingitis or salpingo-oophoritis O03.5
sepsis O03.87
shock O03.81
specified condition NEC O03.89
tubular necrosis (renal) O03.82
uremia O03.82
urinary tract infection O03.88
venous complication NEC O03.85
embolism (air) (amniotic fluid) (blood clot) (fat) (pulmonary) (septic) (soap) O03.7
failed — *see* Abortion, attempted
habitual or recurrent N96
with current abortion — *see* categories O03-O04
without current pregnancy N96
care in current pregnancy O26.2- ☑
incomplete (spontaneous) O03.4
complicated (by) (following) O03.30
afibrinogenemia O03.1
cardiac arrest O03.36
chemical damage of pelvic organ(s) O03.34
circulatory collapse O03.31
cystitis O03.38
defibrination syndrome O03.1
electrolyte imbalance O03.33
embolism (air) (amniotic fluid) (blood clot) (fat) (pulmonary) (septic) (soap) O03.2
endometritis O03.0
genital tract and pelvic infection O03.0
hemolysis O03.1
hemorrhage (delayed) (excessive) O03.1
infection
genital tract or pelvic O03.0
urinary tract O03.38
intravascular coagulation O03.1
laceration of pelvic organ(s) O03.34

**Abortion** — *continued*
incomplete — *continued*
complicated — *continued*
metabolic disorder O03.33
oliguria O03.32
oophoritis O03.0
parametritis O03.0
pelvic peritonitis O03.0
perforation of pelvic organ(s) O03.34
renal failure or shutdown O03.32
salpingitis or salpingo-oophoritis O03.0
sepsis O03.37
shock O03.37
specified condition NEC O03.39
tubular necrosis (renal) O03.32
uremia O03.32
urinary infection O03.38
venous complication NEC O03.35
embolism (air) (amniotic fluid) (blood clot) (fat) (pulmonary) (septic) (soap) O03.2
induced (encounter for) Z33.2
complicated by O04.80
afibrinogenemia O04.6
cardiac arrest O04.86
chemical damage of pelvic organ(s) O04.84
circulatory collapse O04.81
cystitis O04.88
defibrination syndrome O04.6
electrolyte imbalance O04.83
embolism (air) (amniotic fluid) (blood clot) (fat) (pulmonary) (septic) (soap) O04.7
endometritis O04.5
genital tract and pelvic infection O04.5
hemolysis O04.6
hemorrhage (delayed) (excessive) O04.6
infection
genital tract or pelvic O04.5
urinary tract O04.88
intravascular coagulation O04.6
laceration of pelvic organ(s) O04.84
metabolic disorder O04.83
oliguria O04.82
oophoritis O04.5
parametritis O04.5
pelvic peritonitis O04.5
perforation of pelvic organ(s) O04.84
renal failure or shutdown O04.82
salpingitis or salpingo-oophoritis O04.5
sepsis O04.87
shock O04.81
specified condition NEC O04.89
tubular necrosis (renal) O04.82
uremia O04.82
urinary tract infection O04.88
venous complication NEC O04.85
embolism (air) (amniotic fluid) (blood clot) (fat) (pulmonary) (septic) (soap) O04.7
missed O02.1
spontaneous — *see* Abortion (complete) (spontaneous)
threatened O20.0
threatened (spontaneous) O20.0
tubal O00.10- ☑
with intrauterine pregnancy O00.11- ☑
**Abortus fever** A23.1
**Aboulomania** F60.7
**Abrami's disease** D59.8
**Abramov-Fiedler myocarditis** (acute isolated myocarditis) I40.1
**Abrasion** T14.8 ☑
abdomen, abdominal (wall) S30.811 ☑
alveolar process S00.512 ☑
ankle S90.51- ☑
antecubital space — *see* Abrasion, elbow
anus S30.817 ☑
arm (upper) S40.81- ☑
auditory canal — *see* Abrasion, ear
auricle — *see* Abrasion, ear
axilla — *see* Abrasion, arm
back, lower S30.810 ☑
breast S20.11- ☑
brow S00.81 ☑
buttock S30.810 ☑
calf — *see* Abrasion, leg
canthus — *see* Abrasion, eyelid
cheek S00.81 ☑
internal S00.512 ☑
chest wall — *see* Abrasion, thorax

**Index**

**Abrasion — Abscess**

**Abrasion** — *continued*
chin S00.81 ☑
clitoris S30.814- ☑
cornea S05.0- ☑
costal region — *see* Abrasion, thorax
dental K03.1
digit(s)
    foot — *see* Abrasion, toe
    hand — *see* Abrasion, finger
ear S00.41- ☑
elbow S50.31- ☑
epididymis S30.813 ☑
epigastric region S30.811 ☑
epiglottis S10.11 ☑
esophagus (thoracic) S27.818 ☑
    cervical S10.11 ☑
eyebrow — *see* Abrasion, eyelid
eyelid S00.21- ☑
face S00.81 ☑
finger(s) S60.41- ☑
    index S60.41- ☑
    little S60.41- ☑
    middle S60.41- ☑
    ring S60.41- ☑
flank S30.811 ☑
foot (except toe(s) alone) S90.81- ☑
    toe — *see* Abrasion, toe
forearm S50.81- ☑
    elbow only — *see* Abrasion, elbow
forehead S00.81 ☑
genital organs, external
    female S30.816 ☑
    male S30.815 ☑
groin S30.811 ☑
gum S00.512 ☑
hand S60.51- ☑
head S00.91 ☑
    ear — *see* Abrasion, ear
    eyelid — *see* Abrasion, eyelid
    lip S00.511 ☑
    nose S00.31 ☑
    oral cavity S00.512 ☑
    scalp S00.01 ☑
    specified site NEC S00.81 ☑
heel — *see* Abrasion, foot
hip S70.21- ☑
inguinal region S30.811 ☑
interscapular region S20.419 ☑
jaw S00.81 ☑
knee S80.21- ☑
labium (majus) (minus) S30.814 ☑
larynx S10.11 ☑
leg (lower) S80.81- ☑
    knee — *see* Abrasion, knee
    upper — *see* Abrasion, thigh
lip S00.511 ☑
lower back S30.810 ☑
lumbar region S30.810 ☑
malar region S00.81 ☑
mammary — *see* Abrasion, breast
mastoid region S00.81 ☑
mouth S00.512 ☑
nail
    finger — *see* Abrasion, finger
    toe — *see* Abrasion, toe
nape S10.81 ☑
nasal S00.31 ☑
neck S10.91 ☑
    specified site NEC S10.81 ☑
    throat S10.11 ☑
nose S00.31 ☑
occipital region S00.01 ☑
oral cavity S00.512 ☑
orbital region — *see* Abrasion, eyelid
palate S00.512 ☑
palm — *see* Abrasion, hand
parietal region S00.01 ☑
pelvis S30.810 ☑
penis S30.812 ☑
perineum
    female S30.814 ☑
    male S30.810 ☑
periocular area — *see* Abrasion, eyelid
phalanges
    finger — *see* Abrasion, finger
    toe — *see* Abrasion, toe

**Abrasion** — *continued*
pharynx S10.11 ☑
pinna — *see* Abrasion, ear
popliteal space — *see* Abrasion, knee
prepuce S30.812 ☑
pubic region S30.810 ☑
pudendum
    female S30.816 ☑
    male S30.815 ☑
sacral region S30.810 ☑
scalp S00.01 ☑
scapular region — *see* Abrasion, shoulder
scrotum S30.813 ☑
shin — *see* Abrasion, leg
shoulder S40.21- ☑
skin NEC T14.8 ☑
sternal region S20.319 ☑
submaxillary region S00.81 ☑
submental region S00.81 ☑
subungual
    finger(s) — *see* Abrasion, finger
    toe(s) — *see* Abrasion, toe
supraclavicular fossa S10.81 ☑
supraorbital S00.81 ☑
temple S00.81 ☑
temporal region S00.81 ☑
testis S30.813 ☑
thigh S70.31- ☑
thorax, thoracic (wall) S20.91 ☑
    back S20.41- ☑
    front S20.31- ☑
throat S10.11 ☑
thumb S60.31- ☑
toe(s) (lesser) S90.416 ☑
    great S90.41- ☑
tongue S00.512 ☑
tooth, teeth (dentifrice) (habitual) (hard tissues) (occupational) (ritual) (traditional) K03.1
trachea S10.11 ☑
tunica vaginalis S30.813 ☑
tympanum, tympanic membrane — *see* Abrasion, ear
uvula S00.512 ☑
vagina S30.814 ☑
vocal cords S10.11 ☑
vulva S30.814 ☑
wrist S60.81- ☑
**Abrism** — *see* Poisoning, food, noxious, plant
**Abruptio placentae** O45.9- ☑
    with
        afibrinogenemia O45.01- ☑
        coagulation defect O45.00- ☑
            specified NEC O45.09- ☑
        disseminated intravascular coagulation O45.02- ☑
        hypofibrinogenemia O45.01- ☑
    specified NEC O45.8- ☑
**Abruption, placenta** — *see* Abruptio placentae
**Abscess** (connective tissue) (embolic) (fistulous) (infective) (metastatic) (multiple) (pernicious) (pyogenic) (septic) L02.91
    with
        diverticular disease (intestine) K57.80
            with bleeding K57.81
            large intestine K57.20
                with
                    bleeding K57.21
                    small intestine K57.40
                        with bleeding K57.41
                small intestine K57.00
                    with
                        bleeding K57.01
                        large intestine K57.40
                            with bleeding K57.41
        lymphangitis — *code by* site under Abscess
    abdomen, abdominal
        cavity K65.1
        wall L02.211
    abdominopelvic K65.1
    accessory sinus — *see* Sinusitis
    adrenal (capsule) (gland) E27.8
    alveolar K04.7
        with sinus K04.6
    ambic A06.4
        brain (and liver or lung abscess) A06.6
        genitourinary tract A06.82
        liver (without mention of brain or lung abscess) A06.4

**Abscess** — *continued*
    amebic — *continued*
        lung (and liver) (without mention of brain abscess) A06.5
        specified site NEC A06.89
        spleen A06.89
    anerobic A48.0
    ankle — *see* Abscess, lower limb
    anorectal K61.2
    antecubital space — *see* Abscess, upper limb
    antrum (chronic) (Highmore) — *see* Sinusitis, maxillary
    anus K61.0
    apical (tooth) K04.7
        with sinus (alveolar) K04.6
    appendix K35.3
    areola (acute) (chronic) (nonpuerperal) N61.1
        puerperal, postpartum or gestational — *see* Infection, nipple
    arm (any part) — *see* Abscess, upper limb
    artery (wall) I77.89
    atheromatous I77.2
    auricle, ear — *see* Abscess, ear, external
    axilla (region) L02.41- ☑
        lymph gland or node L04.2
    back (any part, except buttock) L02.212
    Bartholin's gland N75.1
        with
            abortion — *see* Abortion, by type complicated by, sepsis
            ectopic or molar pregnancy O08.0
        following ectopic or molar pregnancy O08.0
    Bezold's — *see* Mastoiditis, acute
    bilharziasis B65.1
    bladder (wall) — *see* Cystitis, specified type NEC
    bone (subperiosteal) (*see also* Osteomyelitis, specified type NEC)
        accessory sinus (chronic) — *see* Sinusitis
        chronic or old — *see* Osteomyelitis, chronic
        jaw (lower) (upper) M27.2
        mastoid — *see* Mastoiditis, acute, subperiosteal
        petrous — *see* Petrositis
        spinal (tuberculous) A18.01
            nontuberculous — *see* Osteomyelitis, vertebra
    bowel K63.0
    brain (any part) (cystic) (otogenic) G06.0
        amebic (with abscess of any other site) A06.6
        gonococcal A54.82
        pheomycotic (chromomycotic) B43.1
        tuberculous A17.81
    breast (acute) (chronic) (nonpuerperal) N61.1
        newborn P39.0
        puerperal, postpartum, gestational — *see* Mastitis, obstetric, purulent
    broad ligament N73.2
        acute N73.0
        chronic N73.1
    Brodie's (localized) (chronic) M86.8X- ☑
    bronchi J98.09
    buccal cavity K12.2
    bulbourethral gland N34.0
    bursa M71.00
        ankle M71.07- ☑
        elbow M71.02- ☑
        foot M71.07- ☑
        hand M71.04- ☑
        hip M71.05- ☑
        knee M71.06- ☑
        multiple sites M71.09
        pharyngeal J39.1
        shoulder M71.01- ☑
        specified site NEC M71.08
        wrist M71.03- ☑
    buttock L02.31
    canthus — *see* Blepharoconjunctivitis
    cartilage — *see* Disorder, cartilage, specified type NEC
    cecum K35.3
    cerebellum, cerebellar G06.0
        sequelae G09
    cerebral (embolic) G06.0
        sequelae G09
    cervical (meaning neck) L02.11
        lymph gland or node L04.0
    cervix (stump) (uteri) — *see* Cervicitis
    cheek (external) L02.01
        inner K12.2
    chest J86.9
        with fistula J86.0
        wall L02.213

**Abscess** — *continued*
- chin L02.01
- choroid — *see* Inflammation, chorioretinal
- circumtonsillar J36
- cold (lung) (tuberculous) (*see also* Tuberculosis, abscess, lung)
  - articular — *see* Tuberculosis, joint
- colon (wall) K63.0
- colostomy K94.02
- conjunctiva — *see* Conjunctivitis, acute
- cornea H16.31- ☑
- corpus
  - cavernosum N48.21
  - luteum — *see* Oophoritis
- Cowper's gland N34.0
- cranium G06.0
- cul-de-sac (Douglas') (posterior) — *see* Peritonitis, pelvic, female
- cutaneous — *see* Abscess, by site
- dental K04.7
  - with sinus (alveolar) K04.6
- dentoalveolar K04.7
  - with sinus K04.6
- diaphragm, diaphragmatic K65.1
- Douglas' cul-de-sac or pouch — *see* Peritonitis, pelvic, female
- Dubois A50.59
- ear (middle) (*see also* Otitis, media, suppurative)
  - acute — *see* Otitis, media, suppurative, acute
  - external H60.0- ☑
- entamebic — *see* Abscess, amebic
- enterostomy K94.12
- epididymis N45.4
- epidural G06.2
  - brain G06.0
  - spinal cord G06.1
- epiglottis J38.7
- epiploon, epiploic K65.1
- erysipelatous — *see* Erysipelas
- esophagus K20.8
- ethmoid (bone) (chronic) (sinus) J32.2
- external auditory canal — *see* Abscess, ear, external
- extradural G06.2
  - brain G06.0
    - sequelae G09
  - spinal cord G06.1
- extraperitoneal K68.19
- eye — *see* Endophthalmitis, purulent
- eyelid H00.03- ☑
- face (any part, except ear, eye and nose) L02.01
- fallopian tube — *see* Salpingitis
- fascia M72.8
- fauces J39.1
- fecal K63.0
- femoral (region) — *see* Abscess, lower limb
- filaria, filarial — *see* Infestation, filarial
- finger (any) (*see also* Abscess, hand)
  - nail — *see* Cellulitis, finger
- foot L02.61- ☑
- forehead L02.01
- frontal sinus (chronic) J32.1
- gallbladder K81.0
- genital organ or tract
  - female (external) N76.4
  - male N49.9
    - multiple sites N49.8
    - specified NEC N49.8
- gestational mammary O91.11- ☑
- gestational subareolar O91.11- ☑
- gingival — *see* Peridontitis, aggressive, localized
- gland, glandular (lymph) (acute) — *see* Lymphadenitis, acute
- gluteal (region) L02.31
- gonorrheal — *see* Gonococcus
- groin L02.214
- gum — *see* Peridontitis, aggressive, localized
- hand L02.51- ☑
- head NEC L02.811
  - face (any part, except ear, eye and nose) L02.01
- heart — *see* Carditis
- heel — *see* Abscess, foot
- helminthic — *see* Infestation, helminth
- hepatic (cholangitic) (hematogenic) (lymphogenic) (pylephlebitic) K75.0
  - amebic A06.4
- hip (region) — *see* Abscess, lower limb
- ileocecal K35.3
- ileostomy (bud) K94.12

**Abscess** — *continued*
- iliac (region) L02.214
  - fossa K35.3
- infraclavicular (fossa) — *see* Abscess, upper limb
- inguinal (region) L02.214
  - lymph gland or node L04.1
- intestine, intestinal NEC K63.0
  - rectal K61.1
- intra-abdominal (*see also* Abscess, peritoneum) K65.1
  - postprocedural T81.4 ☑
    - retroperitoneal K68.11
- intracranial G06.0
- intramammary — *see* Abscess, breast
- intraorbital — *see* Abscess, orbit
- intraperitoneal K65.1
- intrasphincteric (anus) K61.4
- intraspinal G06.1
- intratonsillar J36
- ischiorectal (fossa) K61.3
- jaw (bone) (lower) (upper) M27.2
- joint — *see* Arthritis, pyogenic or pyemic
  - spine (tuberculous) A18.01
    - nontuberculous — *see* Spondylopathy, infective
- kidney N15.1
  - with calculus N20.0
    - with hydronephrosis N13.6
  - puerperal (postpartum) O86.21
- knee (*see also* Abscess, lower limb)
  - joint M00.9
- labium (majus) (minus) N76.4
- lacrimal
  - caruncle — *see* Inflammation, lacrimal, passages, acute
  - gland — *see* Dacryoadenitis
  - passages (duct) (sac) — *see* Inflammation, lacrimal, passages, acute
- lacunar N34.0
- larynx J38.7
- lateral (alveolar) K04.7
  - with sinus K04.6
- leg (any part) — *see* Abscess, lower limb
- lens H27.8
- lingual K14.0
  - tonsil J36
- lip K13.0
- Littre's gland N34.0
- liver (cholangitic) (hematogenic) (lymphogenic) (pylephlebitic) (pyogenic) K75.0
  - amebic (due to Entamoeba histolytica) (dysenteric) (tropical) A06.4
    - with
      - brain abscess (and liver or lung abscess) A06.6
      - lung abscess A06.5
- loin (region) L02.211
- lower limb L02.41- ☑
- lumbar (tuberculous) A18.01
  - nontuberculous L02.212
- lung (miliary) (putrid) J85.2
  - with pneumonia J85.1
    - due to specified organism (see Pneumonia, in (due to))
  - amebic (with liver abscess) A06.5
    - with
      - brain abscess A06.6
      - pneumonia A06.5
- lymph, lymphatic, gland or node (acute) (*see also* Lymphadenitis, acute)
  - mesentery I88.0
- malar M27.2
- mammary gland — *see* Abscess, breast
- marginal, anus K61.0
- mastoid — *see* Mastoiditis, acute
- maxilla, maxillary M27.2
  - molar (tooth) K04.7
    - with sinus K04.6
  - premolar K04.7
  - sinus (chronic) J32.0
- mediastinum J85.3
- meibomian gland — *see* Hordeolum
- meninges G06.2
- mesentery, mesenteric K65.1
- mesosalpinx — *see* Salpingitis
- mons pubis L02.215
- mouth (floor) K12.2
- muscle — *see* Myositis, infective
- myocardium I40.0

**Abscess** — *continued*
- nabothian (follicle) — *see* Cervicitis
- nasal J32.9
- nasopharyngeal J39.1
- navel L02.216
  - newborn P38.9
    - with mild hemorrhage P38.1
    - without hemorrhage P38.9
- neck (region) L02.11
  - lymph gland or node L04.0
- nephritic — *see* Abscess, kidney
- nipple N61.1
  - associated with
    - lactation — *see* Pregnancy, complicated by
    - pregnancy — *see* Pregnancy, complicated by
- nose (external) (fossa) (septum) J34.0
  - sinus (chronic) — *see* Sinusitis
- omentum K65.1
- operative wound T81.4 ☑
- orbit, orbital — *see* Cellulitis, orbit
- otogenic G06.0
- ovary, ovarian (corpus luteum) — *see* Oophoritis
- oviduct — *see* Oophoritis
- palate (soft) K12.2
  - hard M27.2
- palmar (space) — *see* Abscess, hand
- pancreas (duct) — *see* Pancreatitis, acute
- parafrenal N48.21
- parametric, parametrium N73.2
  - acute N73.0
  - chronic N73.1
- paranephric N15.1
- parapancreatic — *see* Pancreatitis, acute
- parapharyngeal J39.0
- pararectal K61.1
- parasinus — *see* Sinusitis
- parauterine (*see also* Disease, pelvis, inflammatory) N73.2
- paravaginal — *see* Vaginitis
- parietal region (scalp) L02.811
- parodontal — *see* Peridontitis, aggressive, localized
- parotid (duct) (gland) K11.3
  - region K12.2
- pectoral (region) L02.213
- pelvis, pelvic
  - female — *see* Disease, pelvis, inflammatory
  - male, peritoneal K65.1
- penis N48.21
  - gonococcal (accessory gland) (periurethral) A54.1
- perianal K61.0
- periapical K04.7
  - with sinus (alveolar) K04.6
- periappendicular K35.3
- pericardial I30.1
- pericecal K35.3
- pericemental — *see* Peridontitis, aggressive, localized
- pericholecystic — *see* Cholecystitis, acute
- pericoronal — *see* Peridontitis, aggressive, localized
- peridental — *see* Peridontitis, aggressive, localized
- perimetric (*see also* Disease, pelvis, inflammatory) N73.2
- perinephric, perinephritic — *see* Abscess, kidney
- perineum, perineal (superficial) L02.215
  - urethra N34.0
- periodontal (parietal) — *see* Peridontitis, aggressive, localized
  - apical K04.7
- periosteum, periosteal (*see also* Osteomyelitis, specified type NEC)
  - with osteomyelitis (*see also* Osteomyelitis, specified type NEC)
    - acute — *see* Osteomyelitis, acute
    - chronic — *see* Osteomyelitis, chronic
- peripharyngeal J39.0
- peripleuritic J86.9
  - with fistula J86.0
- periprostatic N41.2
- perirectal K61.1
- perirenal (tissue) — *see* Abscess, kidney
- perisinuous (nose) — *see* Sinusitis
- peritoneum, peritoneal (perforated) (ruptured) K65.1
  - with appendicitis K35.3
  - pelvic
    - female — *see* Peritonitis, pelvic, female
    - male K65.1
  - postoperative T81.4 ☑
  - puerperal, postpartum, childbirth O85
  - tuberculous A18.31

**Abscess** — *continued*
  peritonsillar J36
  perityphlic K35.3
  periureteral N28.89
  periurethral N34.0
    gonococcal (accessory gland) (periurethral) A54.1
  periuterine (*see also* Disease, pelvis, inflammatory)
    N73.2
  perivesical — *see* Cystitis, specified type NEC
  petrous bone — *see* Petrositis
  phagedenic NOS L02.91
    chancroid A57
  pharynx, pharyngeal (lateral) J39.1
  pilonidal L05.01
  pituitary (gland) E23.6
  pleura J86.9
    with fistula J86.0
  popliteal — *see* Abscess, lower limb
  postcecal K35.3
  postlaryngeal J38.7
  postnasal J34.0
  postoperative (any site) T81.4 ☑
    retroperitoneal K68.11
  postpharyngeal J39.0
  posttonsillar J36
  post-typhoid A01.09
  pouch of Douglas — *see* Peritonitis, pelvic, female
  premammary — *see* Abscess, breast
  prepatellar — *see* Abscess, lower limb
  prostate N41.2
    gonococcal (acute) (chronic) A54.22
  psoas muscle K68.12
  puerperal — *code by* site under Puerperal, abscess
  pulmonary — *see* Abscess, lung
  pulp, pulpal (dental) K04.01
    irreversible K04.02
    reversible K04.01
  rectovaginal septum K63.0
  rectovesical — *see* Cystitis, specified type NEC
  rectum K61.1
  renal — *see* Abscess, kidney
  retina — *see* Inflammation, chorioretinal
  retrobulbar — *see* Abscess, orbit
  retrocecal K65.1
  retrolaryngeal J38.7
  retromammary — *see* Abscess, breast
  retroperitoneal NEC K68.19
    postprocedural K68.11
  retropharyngeal J39.0
  retrouterine — *see* Peritonitis, pelvic, female
  retrovesical — *see* Cystitis, specified type NEC
  root, tooth K04.7
    with sinus (alveolar) K04.6
  round ligament (*see also* Disease, pelvis, inflammatory)
    N73.2
  rupture (spontaneous) NOS L02.91
  sacrum (tuberculous) A18.01
    nontuberculous M46.28
  salivary (duct) (gland) K11.3
  scalp (any part) L02.811
  scapular — *see* Osteomyelitis, specified type NEC
  sclera — *see* Scleritis
  scrofulous (tuberculous) A18.2
  scrotum N49.2
  seminal vesicle N49.0
  septal, dental K04.7
    with sinus (alveolar) K04.6
  serous — *see* Periostitis
  shoulder (region) — *see* Abscess, upper limb
  sigmoid K63.0
  sinus (accessory) (chronic) (nasal) (*see also* Sinusitis)
    intracranial venous (any) G06.0
  Skene's duct or gland N34.0
  skin — *see* Abscess, by site
  specified site NEC L02.818
  spermatic cord N49.1
  sphenoidal (sinus) (chronic) J32.3
  spinal cord (any part) (staphylococcal) G06.1
    tuberculous A17.81
  spine (column) (tuberculous) A18.01
    epidural G06.1
    nontuberculous — *see* Osteomyelitis, vertebra
  spleen D73.3
    amebic A06.89
  stitch T81.4 ☑
  subarachnoid G06.2
    brain G06.0
    spinal cord G06.1

**Abscess** — *continued*
  subareolar — *see* Abscess, breast
  subcecal K35.3
  subcutaneous (*see also* Abscess, by site)
    pheomycotic (chromomycotic) B43.2
  subdiaphragmatic K65.1
  subdural G06.2
    brain G06.0
      sequelae G09
    spinal cord G06.1
  subgaleal L02.811
  subhepatic K65.1
  sublingual K12.2
    gland K11.3
  submammary — *see* Abscess, breast
  submandibular (region) (space) (triangle) K12.2
    gland K11.3
  submaxillary (region) L02.01
    gland K11.3
  submental L02.01
    gland K11.3
  subperiosteal — *see* Osteomyelitis, specified type NEC
  subphrenic K65.1
    postoperative T81.4 ☑
  suburethral N34.0
  sudoriparous L75.8
  supraclavicular (fossa) — *see* Abscess, upper limb
  suprapelvic, acute N73.0
  suprarenal (capsule) (gland) E27.8
  sweat gland L74.8
  tear duct — *see* Inflammation, lacrimal, passages,
    acute
  temple L02.01
  temporal region L02.01
  temporosphenoidal G06.0
  tendon (sheath) M65.00
    ankle M65.07- ☑
    foot M65.07- ☑
    forearm M65.03- ☑
    hand M65.04- ☑
    lower leg M65.06- ☑
    pelvic region M65.05- ☑
    shoulder region M65.01- ☑
    specified site NEC M65.08
    thigh M65.05- ☑
    upper arm M65.02- ☑
  testis N45.4
  thigh — *see* Abscess, lower limb
  thorax J86.9
    with fistula J86.0
  throat J39.1
  thumb (*see also* Abscess, hand)
    nail — *see* Cellulitis, finger
  thymus (gland) E32.1
  thyroid (gland) E06.0
  toe (any) (*see also* Abscess, foot)
    nail — *see* Cellulitis, toe
  tongue (staphylococcal) K14.0
  tonsil(s) (lingual) J36
  tonsillopharyngeal J36
  tooth, teeth (root) K04.7
    with sinus (alveolar) K04.6
    supporting structures NEC — *see* Peridontitis, ag-
      gressive, localized
  trachea J39.8
  trunk L02.219
    abdominal wall L02.211
    back L02.212
    chest wall L02.213
    groin L02.214
    perineum L02.215
    umbilicus L02.216
  tubal — *see* Salpingitis
  tuberculous — *see* Tuberculosis, abscess
  tubo-ovarian — *see* Salpingo-oophoritis
  tunica vaginalis N49.1
  umbilicus L02.216
  upper
    limb L02.41- ☑
    respiratory J39.8
  urethral (gland) N34.0
  urinary N34.0
  uterus, uterine (wall) (*see also* Endometritis)
    ligament (*see also* Disease, pelvis, inflammatory)
      N73.2
    neck — *see* Cervicitis
  uvula K12.2
  vagina (wall) — *see* Vaginitis

**Abscess** — *continued*
  vaginorectal — *see* Vaginitis
  vas deferens N49.1
  vermiform appendix K35.3
  vertebra (column) (tuberculous) A18.01
    nontuberculous — *see* Osteomyelitis, vertebra
  vesical — *see* Cystitis, specified type NEC
  vesico-uterine pouch — *see* Peritonitis, pelvic, female
  vitreous (humor) — *see* Endophthalmitis, purulent
  vocal cord J38.3
  von Bezold's — *see* Mastoiditis, acute
  vulva N76.4
  vulvovaginal gland N75.1
  web space — *see* Abscess, hand
  wound T81.4 ☑
  wrist — *see* Abscess, upper limb
**Absence** (of) (organ or part) (complete or partial)
  adrenal (gland) (congenital) Q89.1
    acquired E89.6
  albumin in blood E88.09
  alimentary tract (congenital) Q45.8
    upper Q40.8
  alveolar process (acquired) — *see* Anomaly, alveolar
  ankle (acquired) Z89.44- ☑
  anus (congenital) Q42.3
    with fistula Q42.2
  aorta (congenital) Q25.41
  appendix, congenital Q42.8
  arm (acquired) Z89.20- ☑
    above elbow Z89.22- ☑
      congenital (with hand present) — *see* Agenesis,
        arm, with hand present
        and hand — *see* Agenesis, forearm, and
          hand
      below elbow Z89.21- ☑
        congenital (with hand present) — *see* Agenesis,
          arm, with hand present
        and hand — *see* Agenesis, forearm, and
          hand
    congenital — *see* Defect, reduction, upper limb
    shoulder (following explantation of shoulder joint
      prosthesis) (joint) (with or without presence
      of antibiotic-impregnated cement spacer)
      Z89.23- ☑
      congenital (with hand present) — *see* Agenesis,
        arm, with hand present
  artery (congenital) (peripheral) Q27.8
    brain Q28.3
    coronary Q24.5
    pulmonary Q25.79
    specified NEC Q27.8
    umbilical Q27.0
  atrial septum (congenital) Q21.1
  auditory canal (congenital) (external) Q16.1
  auricle (ear), congenital Q16.0
  bile, biliary duct, congenital Q44.5
  bladder (acquired) Z90.6
    congenital Q64.5
  bowel sounds R19.11
  brain Q00.0
    part of Q04.3
  breast(s) (and nipple(s)) (acquired) Z90.1- ☑
    congenital Q83.8
  broad ligament Q50.6
  bronchus (congenital) Q32.4
  canaliculus lacrimalis, congenital Q10.4
  cerebellum (vermis) Q04.3
  cervix (acquired) (with uterus) Z90.710
    with remaining uterus Z90.712
    congenital Q51.5
  chin, congenital Q18.8
  cilia (congenital) Q10.3
    acquired — *see* Madarosis
  clitoris (congenital) Q52.6
  coccyx, congenital Q76.49
  cold sense R20.8
  congenital
    lumen — *see* Atresia
    organ or site NEC — *see* Agenesis
    septum — *see* Imperfect, closure
  corpus callosum Q04.0
  cricoid cartilage, congenital Q31.8
  diaphragm (with hernia), congenital Q79.1
  digestive organ(s) or tract, congenital Q45.8
    acquired NEC Z90.49
    upper Q40.8
  ductus arteriosus Q28.8
  duodenum (acquired) Z90.49

☑ Additional Character Required — Refer to the Tabular List for Character Selection

△ Subterms under main terms may continue to next column or page

**Absence** — *continued*
  duodenum — *continued*
    congenital Q41.0
  ear, congenital Q16.9
    acquired H93.8- ☑
    auricle Q16.0
    external Q16.0
    inner Q16.5
    lobe, lobule Q17.8
    middle, except ossicles Q16.4
      ossicles Q16.3
    ossicles Q16.3
  ejaculatory duct (congenital) Q55.4
  endocrine gland (congenital) NEC Q89.2
    acquired E89.89
  epididymis (congenital) Q55.4
    acquired Z90.79
  epiglottis, congenital Q31.8
  esophagus (congenital) Q39.8
    acquired (partial) Z90.49
  eustachian tube (congenital) Q16.2
  extremity (acquired) Z89.9
    congenital Q73.0
    knee (following explantation of knee joint prosthesis) (joint) (with or without presence of antibiotic-impregnated cement spacer) Z89.52- ☑
    lower (above knee) Z89.619
      below knee Z89.51- ☑
    upper — *see* Absence, arm
  eye (acquired) Z90.01
    congenital Q11.1
    muscle (congenital) Q10.3
  eyeball (acquired) Z90.01
  eyelid (fold) (congenital) Q10.3
    acquired Z90.01
  face, specified part NEC Q18.8
  fallopian tube(s) (acquired) Z90.79
    congenital Q50.6
  family member (causing problem in home) NEC (*see also* Disruption, family) Z63.32
  femur, congenital — *see* Defect, reduction, lower limb, longitudinal, femur
  fibrinogen (congenital) D68.2
    acquired D65
  finger(s) (acquired) Z89.02- ☑
    congenital — *see* Agenesis, hand
  foot (acquired) Z89.43- ☑
    congenital — *see* Agenesis, foot
  forearm (acquired) — *see* Absence, arm, below elbow
  gallbladder (acquired) Z90.49
    congenital Q44.0
  gamma globulin in blood D80.1
    hereditary D80.0
  genital organs
    acquired (female) (male) Z90.79
    female, congenital Q52.8
      external Q52.71
      internal NEC Q52.8
    male, congenital Q55.8
  genitourinary organs, congenital NEC
    female Q52.8
    male Q55.8
  globe (acquired) Z90.01
    congenital Q11.1
  glottis, congenital Q31.8
  hand and wrist (acquired) Z89.11- ☑
    congenital — *see* Agenesis, hand
  head, part (acquired) NEC Z90.09
  heat sense R20.8
  hip (following explantation of hip joint prosthesis) (joint) (with or without presence of antibiotic-impregnated cement spacer) Z89.62- ☑
  hymen (congenital) Q52.4
  ileum (acquired) Z90.49
    congenital Q41.2
  immunoglobulin, isolated NEC D80.3
    IgA D80.2
    IgG D80.3
    IgM D80.4
  incus (acquired) — *see* Loss, ossicles, ear
    congenital Q16.3
  inner ear, congenital Q16.5
  intestine (acquired) (small) Z90.49
    congenital Q41.9
      specified NEC Q41.8
    large Z90.49
      congenital Q42.9

**Absence** — *continued*
  intestine — *continued*
    large — *continued*
      congenital — *continued*
        specified NEC Q42.8
  iris, congenital Q13.1
  jejunum (acquired) Z90.49
    congenital Q41.1
  joint
    acquired
      hip (following explantation of hip joint prosthesis) (with or without presence of antibiotic-impregnated cement spacer) Z89.62- ☑
      knee (following explantation of knee joint prosthesis) (with or without presence of antibiotic-impregnated cement spacer) Z89.52- ☑
      shoulder (following explantation of shoulder joint prosthesis) (with or without presence of antibiotic-impregnated cement spacer) Z89.23- ☑
    congenital NEC Q74.8
  kidney(s) (acquired) Z90.5
    congenital Q60.2
      bilateral Q60.1
      unilateral Q60.0
  knee (following explantation of knee joint prosthesis) (joint) (with or without presence of antibiotic-impregnated cement spacer) Z89.52- ☑
  labyrinth, membranous Q16.5
  larynx (congenital) Q31.8
    acquired Z90.02
  leg (acquired) (above knee) Z89.61- ☑
    below knee (acquired) Z89.51- ☑
    congenital — *see* Defect, reduction, lower limb
  lens (acquired) (*see also* Aphakia)
    congenital Q12.3
    post cataract extraction Z98.4- ☑
  limb (acquired) — *see* Absence, extremity
  lip Q38.6
  liver (congenital) Q44.7
  lung (fissure) (lobe) (bilateral) (unilateral) (congenital) Q33.3
    acquired (any part) Z90.2
  menstruation — *see* Amenorrhea
  muscle (congenital) (pectoral) Q79.8
    ocular Q10.3
  neck, part Q18.8
  neutrophil — *see* Agranulocytosis
  nipple(s) (with breast(s)) (acquired) Z90.1- ☑
    congenital Q83.2
  nose (congenital) Q30.1
    acquired Z90.09
  organ
    of Corti, congenital Q16.5
    or site, congenital NEC Q89.8
      acquired NEC Z90.89
  osseous meatus (ear) Q16.4
  ovary (acquired)
    bilateral Z90.722
    congenital
      bilateral Q50.02
      unilateral Q50.01
    unilateral Z90.721
  oviduct (acquired)
    bilateral Z90.722
    congenital Q50.6
    unilateral Z90.721
  pancreas (congenital) Q45.0
    acquired Z90.410
      complete Z90.410
      partial Z90.411
      total Z90.410
  parathyroid gland (acquired) E89.2
    congenital Q89.2
  patella, congenital Q74.1
  penis (congenital) Q55.5
    acquired Z90.79
  pericardium (congenital) Q24.8
  pituitary gland (congenital) Q89.2
    acquired E89.3
  prostate (acquired) Z90.79
    congenital Q55.4
  pulmonary valve Q22.0
  punctum lacrimale (congenital) Q10.4
  radius, congenital — *see* Defect, reduction, upper limb, longitudinal, radius

**Absence** — *continued*
  rectum (congenital) Q42.1
    with fistula Q42.0
    acquired Z90.49
  respiratory organ NOS Q34.9
  rib (acquired) Z90.89
    congenital Q76.6
  sacrum, congenital Q76.49
  salivary gland(s), congenital Q38.4
  scrotum, congenital Q55.29
  seminal vesicles (congenital) Q55.4
    acquired Z90.79
  septum
    atrial (congenital) Q21.1
    between aorta and pulmonary artery Q21.4
    ventricular (congenital) Q20.4
  sex chromosome
    female phenotype Q97.8
    male phenotype Q98.8
  skull bone (congenital) Q75.8
    with
      anencephaly Q00.0
      encephalocele — *see* Encephalocele
      hydrocephalus Q03.9
        with spina bifida — *see* Spina bifida, by site, with hydrocephalus
      microcephaly Q02
  spermatic cord, congenital Q55.4
  spine, congenital Q76.49
  spleen (congenital) Q89.01
    acquired Z90.81
  sternum, congenital Q76.7
  stomach (acquired) (partial) Z90.3
    congenital Q40.2
  superior vena cava, congenital Q26.8
  teeth, tooth (congenital) K00.0
    acquired (complete) K08.109
      class I K08.101
      class II K08.102
      class III K08.103
      class IV K08.104
      due to
        caries K08.139
          class I K08.131
          class II K08.132
          class III K08.133
          class IV K08.134
        periodontal disease K08.129
          class I K08.121
          class II K08.122
          class III K08.123
          class IV K08.124
        specified NEC K08.199
          class I K08.191
          class II K08.192
          class III K08.193
          class IV K08.194
        trauma K08.119
          class I K08.111
          class II K08.112
          class III K08.113
          class IV K08.114
      partial K08.409
        class I K08.401
        class II K08.402
        class III K08.403
        class IV K08.404
        due to
          caries K08.439
            class I K08.431
            class II K08.432
            class III K08.433
            class IV K08.434
          periodontal disease K08.429
            class I K08.421
            class II K08.422
            class III K08.423
            class IV K08.424
          specified NEC K08.499
            class I K08.491
            class II K08.492
            class III K08.493
            class IV K08.494
          trauma K08.419
            class I K08.411
            class II K08.412
            class III K08.413
            class IV K08.414
  tendon (congenital) Q79.8

**Index**

**Absence — Abuse**

**Absence** — *continued*
  testis (congenital) Q55.0
    acquired Z90.79
  thumb (acquired) Z89.01- ☑
    congenital — *see* Agenesis, hand
  thymus gland Q89.2
  thyroid (gland) (acquired) E89.0
    cartilage, congenital Q31.8
    congenital E03.1
  toe(s) (acquired) Z89.42- ☑
    with foot — *see* Absence, foot and ankle
    congenital — *see* Agenesis, foot
    great Z89.41- ☑
  tongue, congenital Q38.3
  trachea (cartilage), congenital Q32.1
  transverse aortic arch, congenital Q25.49
  tricuspid valve Q22.4
  umbilical artery, congenital Q27.0
  upper arm and forearm with hand present, congenital
    — *see* Agenesis, arm, with hand present
  ureter (congenital) Q62.4
    acquired Z90.6
  urethra, congenital Q64.5
  uterus (acquired) Z90.710
    with cervix Z90.710
    with remaining cervical stump Z90.711
    congenital Q51.0
  uvula, congenital Q38.5
  vagina, congenital Q52.0
  vas deferens (congenital) Q55.4
    acquired Z90.79
  vein (peripheral) congenital NEC Q27.8
    cerebral Q28.3
    digestive system Q27.8
    great Q26.8
    lower limb Q27.8
    portal Q26.5
    precerebral Q28.1
    specified site NEC Q27.8
    upper limb Q27.8
  vena cava (inferior) (superior), congenital Q26.8
  ventricular septum Q20.4
  vertebra, congenital Q76.49
  vulva, congenital Q52.71
  wrist (acquired) Z89.12- ☑
**Absorbent system disease** I87.8
**Absorption**
  carbohydrate, disturbance K90.49
  chemical — *see* Table of Drugs and Chemicals
    through placenta (newborn) P04.9
      environmental substance P04.6
      nutritional substance P04.5
      obstetric anesthetic or analgesic drug P04.0
  drug NEC — *see* Table of Drugs and Chemicals
    addictive
      through placenta (newborn) P04.49
        cocaine P04.41
    medicinal
      through placenta (newborn) P04.1
    through placenta (newborn) P04.1
      obstetric anesthetic or analgesic drug P04.0
  fat, disturbance K90.49
    pancreatic K90.3
  noxious substance — *see* Table of Drugs and Chemicals
  protein, disturbance K90.49
  starch, disturbance K90.49
  toxic substance — *see* Table of Drugs and Chemicals
  uremic — *see* Uremia
**Abstinence symptoms, syndrome**
  alcohol F10.239
    with delirium F10.231
  cocaine F14.23
  neonatal P96.1
  nicotine — *see* Dependence, drug, nicotine, with, withdrawal
  opioid F11.93
    with dependence F11.23
  psychoactive NEC F19.939
    with
      delirium F19.931
      dependence F19.239
        with
          delirium F19.231
          perceptual disturbance F19.232
        uncomplicated F19.230
      perceptual disturbance F19.932
    uncomplicated F19.930

**Abstinence symptoms, syndrome** — *continued*
  sedative F13.939
    with
      delirium F13.931
      dependence F13.239
        with
          delirium F13.231
          perceptual disturbance F13.232
        uncomplicated F13.230
      perceptual disturbance F13.932
    uncomplicated F13.930
  stimulant NEC F15.93
    with dependence F15.23
**Abulia** R68.89
**Abulomania** F60.7
**Abuse**
  adult — *see* Maltreatment, adult
    as reason for
      couple seeking advice (including offender) Z63.0
  alcohol (non-dependent) F10.10
    with
      anxiety disorder F10.180
      intoxication F10.129
        with delirium F10.121
        uncomplicated F10.120
      mood disorder F10.14
      other specified disorder F10.188
      psychosis F10.159
        delusions F10.150
        hallucinations F10.151
      sexual dysfunction F10.181
      sleep disorder F10.182
      unspecified disorder F10.19
    counseling and surveillance Z71.41
    in remission (early) (sustained) F10.11
  amphetamine (or related substance) — *see* Abuse, drug, stimulant NEC
  analgesics (non-prescribed) (over the counter) F55.8
  antacids F55.0
  antidepressants — *see* Abuse, drug, psychoactive NEC
  anxiolytic — *see* Abuse, drug, sedative
  barbiturates — *see* Abuse, drug, sedative
  caffeine — *see* Abuse, drug, stimulant NEC
  cannabis, cannabinoids — *see* Abuse, drug, cannabis
  child — *see* Maltreatment, child
  cocaine — *see* Abuse, drug, cocaine
  drug NEC (non-dependent) F19.10
    with sleep disorder F19.182
    amphetamine type — *see* Abuse, drug, stimulant NEC
    analgesics (non-prescribed) (over the counter) F55.8
    antacids F55.0
    antidepressants — *see* Abuse, drug, psychoactive NEC
    anxiolytics — *see* Abuse, drug, sedative
    barbiturates — *see* Abuse, drug, sedative
    caffeine — *see* Abuse, drug, stimulant NEC
    cannabis F12.10
      with
        anxiety disorder F12.180
        intoxication F12.129
          with
            delirium F12.121
            perceptual disturbance F12.122
          uncomplicated F12.120
        other specified disorder F12.188
        psychosis F12.159
          delusions F12.150
          hallucinations F12.151
        unspecified disorder F12.19
      in remission (early) (sustained) F12.11
    cocaine F14.10
      with
        anxiety disorder F14.180
        intoxication F14.129
          with
            delirium F14.121
            perceptual disturbance F14.122
          uncomplicated F14.120
        mood disorder F14.14
        other specified disorder F14.188
        psychosis F14.159
          delusions F14.150
          hallucinations F14.151
        sexual dysfunction F14.181
        sleep disorder F14.182

**Abuse** — *continued*
  drug — *continued*
    cocaine — *continued*
      with — *continued*
        unspecified disorder F14.19
      in remission (early) (sustained) F14.11
    counseling and surveillance Z71.51
    hallucinogen F16.10
      with
        anxiety disorder F16.180
        flashbacks F16.183
        intoxication F16.129
          with
            delirium F16.121
            perceptual disturbance F16.122
          uncomplicated F16.120
        mood disorder F16.14
        other specified disorder F16.188
        perception disorder, persisting F16.183
        psychosis F16.159
          delusions F16.150
          hallucinations F16.151
        unspecified disorder F16.19
      in remission (early) (sustained) F16.11
    hashish — *see* Abuse, drug, cannabis
    herbal or folk remedies F55.1
    hormones F55.3
    hypnotics — *see* Abuse, drug, sedative
    in remission (early) (sustained) F19.11
    inhalant F18.10
      with
        anxiety disorder F18.180
        dementia, persisting F18.17
        intoxication F18.129
          with delirium F18.121
          uncomplicated F18.120
        mood disorder F18.14
        other specified disorder F18.188
        psychosis F18.159
          delusions F18.150
          hallucinations F18.151
        unspecified disorder F18.19
      in remission (early) (sustained) F18.11
    laxatives F55.2
    LSD — *see* Abuse, drug, hallucinogen
    marihuana — *see* Abuse, drug, cannabis
    morphine type (opioids) — *see* Abuse, drug, opioid
    opioid F11.10
      with
        intoxication F11.129
          with
            delirium F11.121
            perceptual disturbance F11.122
          uncomplicated F11.120
        mood disorder F11.14
        other specified disorder F11.188
        psychosis F11.159
          delusions F11.150
          hallucinations F11.151
        sexual dysfunction F11.181
        sleep disorder F11.182
        unspecified disorder F11.19
      in remission (early) (sustained) F11.11
    PCP (phencyclidine) (or related substance) — *see* Abuse, drug, hallucinogen
    psychoactive NEC F19.10
      with
        amnestic disorder F19.16
        anxiety disorder F19.180
        dementia F19.17
        intoxication F19.129
          with
            delirium F19.121
            perceptual disturbance F19.122
          uncomplicated F19.120
        mood disorder F19.14
        other specified disorder F19.188
        psychosis F19.159
          delusions F19.150
          hallucinations F19.151
        sexual dysfunction F19.181
        sleep disorder F19.182
        unspecified disorder F19.19
    sedative, hypnotic or anxiolytic F13.10
      with
        anxiety disorder F13.180
        intoxication F13.129
          with delirium F13.121
          uncomplicated F13.120

**Abuse** — *continued*
  drug — *continued*
    sedative, hypnotic or anxiolytic — *continued*
      with — *continued*
        mood disorder F13.14
        other specified disorder F13.188
        psychosis F13.159
          delusions F13.150
          hallucinations F13.151
        sexual dysfunction F13.181
        sleep disorder F13.182
        unspecified disorder F13.19
      in remission (early) (sustained) F13.11
    solvent — *see* Abuse, drug, inhalant
    steroids F55.3
    stimulant NEC F15.10
      with
        anxiety disorder F15.180
        intoxication F15.129
          with
            delirium F15.121
            perceptual disturbance F15.122
          uncomplicated F15.120
        mood disorder F15.14
        other specified disorder F15.188
        psychosis F15.159
          delusions F15.150
          hallucinations F15.151
        sexual dysfunction F15.181
        sleep disorder F15.182
        unspecified disorder F15.19
      in remission (early) (sustained) F15.11
    tranquilizers — *see* Abuse, drug, sedative
    vitamins F55.4
  hallucinogens — *see* Abuse, drug, hallucinogen
  hashish — *see* Abuse, drug, cannabis
  herbal or folk remedies F55.1
  hormones F55.3
  hypnotic — *see* Abuse, drug, sedative
  inhalant — *see* Abuse, drug, inhalant
  laxatives F55.2
  LSD — *see* Abuse, drug, hallucinogen
  marihuana — *see* Abuse, drug, cannabis
  morphine type (opioids) — *see* Abuse, drug, opioid
  non-psychoactive substance NEC F55.8
    antacids F55.0
    folk remedies F55.1
    herbal remedies F55.1
    hormones F55.3
    laxatives F55.2
    steroids F55.3
    vitamins F55.4
  opioids — *see* Abuse, drug, opioid
  PCP (phencyclidine) (or related substance) — *see* Abuse, drug, hallucinogen
  physical (adult) (child) — *see* Maltreatment
  psychoactive substance — *see* Abuse, drug, psychoactive NEC
  psychological (adult) (child) — *see* Maltreatment
  sedative — *see* Abuse, drug, sedative
  sexual — *see* Maltreatment
  solvent — *see* Abuse, drug, inhalant
  steroids F55.3
  vitamins F55.4
**Acalculia** R48.8
  developmental F81.2
**Acanthamebiasis** (with) B60.10
  conjunctiva B60.12
  keratoconjunctivitis B60.13
  meningoencephalitis B60.11
  other specified B60.19
**Acanthocephaliasis** B83.8
**Acanthocheilonemiasis** B74.4
**Acanthocytosis** E78.6
**Acantholysis** L11.9
**Acanthosis** (acquired) (nigricans) L83
  benign Q82.8
  congenital Q82.8
  seborrheic L82.1
    inflamed L82.0
  tongue K14.3
**Acapnia** E87.3
**Acarbia** E87.2
**Acardia, acardius** Q89.8
**Acardiacus amorphus** Q89.8
**Acardiotrophia** I51.4
**Acariasis** B88.0
  scabies B86

**Acarodermatitis** (urticarioides) B88.0
**Acarophobia** F40.218
**Acatalasemia, acatalasia** E80.3
**Acathisia** (drug induced) G25.71
**Accelerated atrioventricular conduction** I45.6
**Accentuation of personality traits** (type A) Z73.1
**Accessory** (congenital)
  adrenal gland Q89.1
  anus Q43.4
  appendix Q43.4
  atrioventricular conduction I45.6
  auditory ossicles Q16.3
  auricle (ear) Q17.0
  biliary duct or passage Q44.5
  bladder Q64.79
  blood vessels NEC Q27.9
    coronary Q24.5
  bone NEC Q79.8
  breast tissue, axilla Q83.1
  carpal bones Q74.0
  cecum Q43.4
  chromosome(s) NEC (nonsex) Q92.9
    with complex rearrangements NEC Q92.5
      seen only at prometaphase Q92.8
    13 — *see* Trisomy, 13
    18 — *see* Trisomy, 18
    21 — *see* Trisomy, 21
    partial Q92.9
    sex
      female phenotype Q97.8
  coronary artery Q24.5
  cusp(s), heart valve NEC Q24.8
    pulmonary Q22.3
  cystic duct Q44.5
  digit(s) Q69.9
  ear (auricle) (lobe) Q17.0
  endocrine gland NEC Q89.2
  eye muscle Q10.3
  eyelid Q10.3
  face bone(s) Q75.8
  fallopian tube (fimbria) (ostium) Q50.6
  finger(s) Q69.0
  foreskin N47.8
  frontonasal process Q75.8
  gallbladder Q44.1
  genital organ(s)
    female Q52.8
      external Q52.79
      internal NEC Q52.8
    male Q55.8
  genitourinary organs NEC Q89.8
    female Q52.8
    male Q55.8
  hallux Q69.2
  heart Q24.8
    valve NEC Q24.8
      pulmonary Q22.3
  hepatic ducts Q44.5
  hymen Q52.4
  intestine (large) (small) Q43.4
  kidney Q63.0
  lacrimal canal Q10.6
  leaflet, heart valve NEC Q24.8
  ligament, broad Q50.6
  liver Q44.7
    duct Q44.5
  lobule (ear) Q17.0
  lung (lobe) Q33.1
  muscle Q79.8
  navicular of carpus Q74.0
  nervous system, part NEC Q07.8
  nipple Q83.3
  nose Q30.8
  organ or site not listed — *see* Anomaly, by site
  ovary Q50.31
  oviduct Q50.6
  pancreas Q45.3
  parathyroid gland Q89.2
  parotid gland (and duct) Q38.4
  pituitary gland Q89.2
  preauricular appendage Q17.0
  prepuce N47.8
  renal arteries (multiple) Q27.2
  rib Q76.6
    cervical Q76.5
  roots (teeth) K00.2
  salivary gland Q38.4
  sesamoid bones Q74.8

**Accessory** — *continued*
  sesamoid bones — *continued*
    foot Q74.2
    hand Q74.0
  skin tags Q82.8
  spleen Q89.09
  sternum Q76.7
  submaxillary gland Q38.4
  tarsal bones Q74.2
  teeth, tooth K00.1
  tendon Q79.8
  thumb Q69.1
  thymus gland Q89.2
  thyroid gland Q89.2
  toes Q69.2
  tongue Q38.3
  tooth, teeth K00.1
  tragus Q17.0
  ureter Q62.5
  urethra Q64.79
  urinary organ or tract NEC Q64.8
  uterus Q51.2
  vagina Q52.10
  valve, heart NEC Q24.8
    pulmonary Q22.3
  vertebra Q76.49
  vocal cords Q31.8
  vulva Q52.79
**Accident**
  birth — *see* Birth, injury
  cardiac — *see* Infarct, myocardium
  cerebral I63.9
  cerebrovascular (embolic) (ischemic) (thrombotic) I63.9
    aborted I63.9
    hemorrhagic — *see* Hemorrhage, intracranial, intracerebral
    old (without sequelae) Z86.73
      with sequelae (of) — *see* Sequelae, infarction, cerebral
  coronary — *see* Infarct, myocardium
  craniovascular I63.9
  vascular, brain I63.9
**Accidental** — *see* condition
**Accommodation** (disorder) (*see also* condition)
  hysterical paralysis of F44.89
  insufficiency of H52.4
  paresis — *see* Paresis, of accommodation
  spasm — *see* Spasm, of accommodation
**Accouchement** — *see* Delivery
**Accreta placenta** O43.21- ☑
**Accretio cordis** (nonrheumatic) I31.0
**Accretions, tooth, teeth** K03.6
**Acculturation difficulty** Z60.3
**Accumulation secretion, prostate** N42.89
**Acephalia, acephalism, acephalus, acephaly** Q00.0
**Acephalobrachia monster** Q89.8
**Acephalochirus monster** Q89.8
**Acephalogaster** Q89.8
**Acephalostomus monster** Q89.8
**Acephalothorax** Q89.8
**Acerophobia** F40.298
**Acetonemia** R79.89
  in Type 1 diabetes E10.10
    with coma E10.11
**Acetonuria** R82.4
**Achalasia** (cardia) (esophagus) K22.0
  congenital Q39.5
  pylorus Q40.0
  sphincteral NEC K59.8
**Ache**(s) — *see* Pain
**Acheilia** Q38.6
**Achillobursitis** — *see* Tendinitis, Achilles
**Achillodynia** — *see* Tendinitis, Achilles
**Achlorhydria, achlorhydric** (neurogenic) K31.83
  anemia D50.8
  diarrhea K31.83
  psychogenic F45.8
  secondary to vagotomy K91.1
**Achluophobia** F40.228
**Acholia** K82.8
**Acholuric jaundice** (familial) (splenomegalic) (*see also* Spherocytosis)
  acquired D59.8
**Achondrogenesis** Q77.0
**Achondroplasia** (osteosclerosis congenita) Q77.4
**Achroma, cutis** L80

---

**Achromat** (ism), achromatopsia (acquired) (congenital) H53.51
**Achromia, congenital** — see Albinism
**Achromia parasitica** B36.0
**Achylia gastrica** K31.89
  psychogenic F45.8
**Acid**
  burn — see Corrosion
  deficiency
    amide nicotinic E52
    ascorbic E54
    folic E53.8
    nicotinic E52
    pantothenic E53.8
  intoxication E87.2
  peptic disease K30
  phosphatase deficiency E83.39
  stomach K30
    psychogenic F45.8
**Acidemia** E87.2
  argininosuccinic E72.22
  isovaleric E71.110
  metabolic (newborn) P19.9
    first noted before onset of labor P19.0
    first noted during labor P19.1
    noted at birth P19.2
  methylmalonic E71.120
  pipecolic E72.3
  propionic E71.121
**Acidity, gastric** (high) K30
  psychogenic F45.8
**Acidocytopenia** — see Agranulocytosis
**Acidocytosis** D72.1
**Acidopenia** — see Agranulocytosis
**Acidosis** (lactic) (respiratory) E87.2
  in Type 1 diabetes E10.10
    with coma E10.11
  kidney, tubular N25.89
  lactic E87.2
  metabolic NEC E87.2
    with respiratory acidosis E87.4
    late, of newborn P74.0
  mixed metabolic and respiratory, newborn P84
  newborn P84
  renal (hyperchloremic) (tubular) N25.89
  respiratory E87.2
    complicated by
      metabolic
        acidosis E87.4
        alkalosis E87.4
**Aciduria**
  argininosuccinic E72.22
  glutaric (type I) E72.3
    type II E71.313
    type III E71.5- ☑
  orotic (congenital) (hereditary) (pyrimidine deficiency) E79.8
    anemia D53.0
**Acladiosis** (skin) B36.0
**Aclasis, diaphyseal** Q78.6
**Acleistocardia** Q21.1
**Aclusion** — see Anomaly, dentofacial, malocclusion
**Acne** L70.9
  artificialis L70.8
  atrophica L70.2
  cachecticorum (Hebra) L70.8
  conglobata L70.1
  cystic L70.0
  decalvans L66.2
  excoriée (des jeunes filles) L70.5
  frontalis L70.2
  indurata L70.0
  infantile L70.4
  keloid L73.0
  lupoid L70.2
  necrotic, necrotica (miliaris) L70.2
  neonatal L70.4
  nodular L70.0
  occupational L70.8
  picker's L70.5
  pustular L70.0
  rodens L70.2
  rosacea L71.9
  specified NEC L70.8
  tropica L70.3
  varioliformis L70.2
  vulgaris L70.0
**Acnitis** (primary) A18.4

**Acosta's disease** T70.29 ☑
**Acoustic** — see condition
**Acousticophobia** F40.298
**Acquired** (see also condition)
  immunodeficiency syndrome (AIDS) B20
**Acrania** Q00.0
**Acroangiodermatitis** I78.9
**Acroasphyxia, chronic** I73.89
**Acrobystitis** N47.7
**Acrocephalopolysyndactyly** Q87.0
**Acrocephalosyndactyly** Q87.0
**Acrocephaly** Q75.0
**Acrochondrohyperplasia** — see Syndrome, Marfan's
**Acrocyanosis** I73.8 ☑
  newborn P28.2
    meaning transient blue hands and feet — omit code
**Acrodermatitis** L30.8
  atrophicans (chronica) L90.4
  continua (Hallopeau) L40.2
  enteropathica (hereditary) E83.2
  Hallopeau's L40.2
  infantile papular L44.4
  perstans L40.2
  pustulosa continua L40.2
  recalcitrant pustular L40.2
**Acrodynia** — see Poisoning, mercury
**Acromegaly, acromegalia** E22.0
**Acromelalgia** I73.81
**Acromicria, acromikria** Q79.8
**Acronyx** L60.0
**Acropachy, thyroid** — see Thyrotoxicosis
**Acroparesthesia** (simple) (vasomotor) I73.89
**Acropathy, thyroid** — see Thyrotoxicosis
**Acrophobia** F40.241
**Acroposthitis** N47.7
**Acroscleriasis, acroscleroderma, acrosclerosis** — see Sclerosis, systemic
**Acrosphacelus** I96
**Acrospiroma, eccrine** — see Neoplasm, skin, benign
**Acrostealgia** — see Osteochondropathy
**Acrotrophodynia** — see Immersion
**ACTH ectopic syndrome** E24.3
**Actinic** — see condition
**Actinobacillosis, actinobacillus** A28.8
  mallei A24.0
  muris A25.1
**Actinomyces israelii** (infection) — see Actinomycosis
**Actinomycetoma** (foot) B47.1
**Actinomycosis, actinomycotic** A42.9
  with pneumonia A42.0
  abdominal A42.1
  cervicofacial A42.2
  cutaneous A42.89
  gastrointestinal A42.1
  pulmonary A42.0
  sepsis A42.7
  specified site NEC A42.89
**Actinoneuritis** G62.82
**Action, heart**
  disorder I49.9
  irregular I49.9
    psychogenic F45.8
**Activated protein C resistance** D68.51
**Activation**
  mast cell (disorder) (syndrome) D89.40
    idiopathic D89.42
    monoclonal D89.41
    secondary D89.43
    specified type NEC D89.49
**Active** — see condition
**Acute** (see also condition)
  abdomen R10.0
  gallbladder — see Cholecystitis, acute
**Acyanotic heart disease** (congenital) Q24.9
**Acystia** Q64.5
**Adair-Dighton syndrome** (brittle bones and blue sclera, deafness) Q78.0
**Adamantinoblastoma** — see Ameloblastoma
**Adamantinoma** (see also Cyst, calcifying odontogenic)
  long bones C40.90
    lower limb C40.2- ☑
    upper limb C40.0- ☑
  malignant C41.1
    jaw (bone) (lower) C41.1
      upper C41.0
  tibial C40.2- ☑

**Adamantoblastoma** — see Ameloblastoma
**Adams-Stokes** (-Morgagni) disease or syndrome I45.9
**Adaption reaction** — see Disorder, adjustment
**Addiction** (see also Dependence) F19.20
  alcohol, alcoholic (ethyl) (methyl) (wood) (without remission) F10.20
    with remission F10.21
  drug — see Dependence, drug
  ethyl alcohol (without remission) F10.20
    with remission F10.21
  heroin — see Dependence, drug, opioid
  methyl alcohol (without remission) F10.20
    with remission F10.21
  methylated spirit (without remission) F10.20
    with remission F10.21
  morphine (-like substances) — see Dependence, drug, opioid
  nicotine — see Dependence, drug, nicotine
  opium and opioids — see Dependence, drug, opioid
  tobacco — see Dependence, drug, nicotine
**Addison-Biermer anemia** (pernicious) D51.0
**Addisonian crisis** E27.2
**Addison's**
  anemia (pernicious) D51.0
  disease (bronze) or syndrome E27.1
    tuberculous A18.7
  keloid L94.0
**Addison-Schilder complex** E71.528
**Additional** (see also Accessory)
  chromosome(s) Q99.8
    21 — see Trisomy, 21
    sex — see Abnormal, chromosome, sex
**Adduction contracture, hip or other joint** — see Contraction, joint
**Adenitis** (see also Lymphadenitis)
  acute, unspecified site L04.9
  axillary I88.9
    acute L04.2
    chronic or subacute I88.1
  Bartholin's gland N75.8
  bulbourethral gland — see Urethritis
  cervical I88.9
    acute L04.0
    chronic or subacute I88.1
  chancroid (Hemophilus ducreyi) A57
  chronic, unspecified site I88.1
  Cowper's gland — see Urethritis
  due to Pasteurella multocida (P. septica) A28.0
  epidemic, acute B27.09
  gangrenous L04.9
  gonorrheal NEC A54.89
  groin I88.9
    acute L04.1
    chronic or subacute I88.1
  infectious (acute) (epidemic) B27.09
  inguinal I88.9
    acute L04.1
    chronic or subacute I88.1
  lymph gland or node, except mesenteric I88.9
    acute — see Lymphadenitis, acute
    chronic or subacute I88.1
  mesenteric (acute) (chronic) (nonspecific) (subacute) I88.0
  parotid gland (suppurative) — see Sialoadenitis
  salivary gland (any) (suppurative) — see Sialoadenitis
  scrofulous (tuberculous) A18.2
  Skene's duct or gland — see Urethritis
  strumous, tuberculous A18.2
  subacute, unspecified site I88.1
  sublingual gland (suppurative) — see Sialoadenitis
  submandibular gland (suppurative) — see Sialoadenitis
  submaxillary gland (suppurative) — see Sialoadenitis
  tuberculous — see Tuberculosis, lymph gland
  urethral gland — see Urethritis
  Wharton's duct (suppurative) — see Sialoadenitis
**Adenoacanthoma** — see Neoplasm, malignant, by site
**Adenoameloblastoma** — see Cyst, calcifying odontogenic
**Adenocarcinoid** (tumor) — see Neoplasm, malignant, by site
**Adenocarcinoma** (see also Neoplasm, malignant, by site)
  acidophil
    specified site — see Neoplasm, malignant, by site
    unspecified site C75.1
  adrenal cortical C74.0- ☑
  alveolar — see Neoplasm, lung, malignant

**Adenocarcinoma** — *continued*
  apocrine
    breast — *see* Neoplasm, breast, malignant
    in situ
      breast D05.8- ☑
      specified site NEC — *see* Neoplasm, skin, in situ
      unspecified site D04.9
    specified site NEC — *see* Neoplasm, skin, malignant
    unspecified site C44.99
  basal cell
    specified site — *see* Neoplasm, skin, malignant
    unspecified site C08.9
  basophil
    specified site — *see* Neoplasm, malignant, by site
    unspecified site C75.1
  bile duct type C22.1
    liver C22.1
    specified site NEC — *see* Neoplasm, malignant, by site
    unspecified site C22.1
  bronchiolar — *see* Neoplasm, lung, malignant
  bronchioloalveolar — *see* Neoplasm, lung, malignant
  ceruminous C44.29- ☑
  cervix, in situ (*see also* Carcinoma, cervix uteri, in situ) D06.9
  chromophobe
    specified site — *see* Neoplasm, malignant, by site
    unspecified site C75.1
  diffuse type
    specified site — *see* Neoplasm, malignant, by site
    unspecified site C16.9
  duct
    infiltrating
      with Paget's disease — *see* Neoplasm, breast, malignant
      specified site — *see* Neoplasm, malignant, by site
      unspecified site (female) C50.91- ☑
        male C50.92- ☑
    specified site — *see* Neoplasm, malignant, by site
    unspecified site
      female C56.9
      male C61
  eosinophil
    specified site — *see* Neoplasm, malignant, by site
    unspecified site C75.1
  follicular
    with papillary C73
    moderately differentiated C73
    specified site — *see* Neoplasm, malignant, by site
    trabecular C73
    unspecified site C73
    well differentiated C73
  Hurthle cell C73
  in
    adenomatous
      polyposis coli C18.9
  infiltrating duct
    with Paget's disease — *see* Neoplasm, breast, malignant
    specified site — *see* Neoplasm, by site, malignant
    unspecified site (female) C50.91- ☑
      male C50.92- ☑
  inflammatory
    specified site — *see* Neoplasm, by site, malignant
    unspecified site (female) C50.91- ☑
      male C50.92- ☑
  intestinal type
    specified site — *see* Neoplasm, by site, malignant
    unspecified site C16.9
  intracystic papillary
  intraductal
    breast D05.1- ☑
    noninfiltrating
      breast D05.1- ☑
      papillary
        with invasion
          specified site — *see* Neoplasm, by site, malignant
          unspecified site (female) C50.91- ☑
            male C50.92- ☑
        breast D05.1- ☑
        specified site NEC — *see* Neoplasm, in situ, by site
        unspecified site D05.1- ☑
      specified site NEC — *see* Neoplasm, in situ, by site

**Adenocarcinoma** — *continued*
  intraductal — *continued*
    noninfiltrating — *continued*
      unspecified site D05.1- ☑
    papillary
      with invasion
        specified site — *see* Neoplasm, malignant, by site
        unspecified site (female) C50.91- ☑
          male C50.92- ☑
      breast D05.1- ☑
      specified site — *see* Neoplasm, in situ, by site
      unspecified site D05.1- ☑
    specified site NEC — *see* Neoplasm, in situ, by site
    unspecified site D05.1- ☑
  islet cell
    with exocrine, mixed
      specified site — *see* Neoplasm, malignant, by site
      unspecified site C25.9
    pancreas C25.4
    specified site NEC — *see* Neoplasm, malignant, by site
    unspecified site C25.4
  lobular
    in situ
      breast D05.0- ☑
      specified site NEC — *see* Neoplasm, in situ, by site
      unspecified site D05.0- ☑
    specified site — *see* Neoplasm, malignant, by site
    unspecified site (female) C50.91- ☑
      male C50.92- ☑
  mucoid (*see also* Neoplasm, malignant, by site)
    cell
      specified site — *see* Neoplasm, malignant, by site
      unspecified site C75.1
  nonencapsulated sclerosing C73
  papillary
    with follicular C73
    follicular variant C73
    intraductal (noninfiltrating)
      with invasion
        specified site — *see* Neoplasm, malignant, by site
        unspecified site (female) C50.91- ☑
          male C50.92- ☑
      breast D05.1- ☑
      specified site NEC — *see* Neoplasm, in situ, by site
      unspecified site D05.1- ☑
    serous
      specified site — *see* Neoplasm, malignant, by site
      unspecified site C56.9
  papillocystic
    specified site — *see* Neoplasm, malignant, by site
    unspecified site C56.9
  pseudomucinous
    specified site — *see* Neoplasm, malignant, by site
    unspecified site C56.9
  renal cell C64- ☑
  sebaceous — *see* Neoplasm, skin, malignant
  serous (*see also* Neoplasm, malignant, by site)
    papillary
      specified site — *see* Neoplasm, malignant, by site
      unspecified site C56.9
  sweat gland — *see* Neoplasm, skin, malignant
  water-clear cell C75.0
**Adenocarcinoma-in-situ** (*see also* Neoplasm, in situ, by site)
  breast D05.9- ☑
**Adenofibroma**
  clear cell — *see* Neoplasm, benign, by site
  endometrioid D27.9
    borderline malignancy D39.10
    malignant C56- ☑
  mucinous
    specified site — *see* Neoplasm, benign, by site
    unspecified site D27.9
  papillary
    specified site — *see* Neoplasm, benign, by site
    unspecified site D27.9
  prostate — *see* Enlargement, enlarged, prostate

**Adenofibroma** — *continued*
  serous
    specified site — *see* Neoplasm, benign, by site
    unspecified site D27.9
  specified site — *see* Neoplasm, benign, by site
  unspecified site D27.9
**Adenofibrosis**
  breast — *see* Fibroadenosis, breast
  endometrioid N80.0
**Adenoiditis** (chronic) J35.02
  with tonsillitis J35.03
  acute J03.90
    recurrent J03.91
    specified organism NEC J03.80
      recurrent J03.81
    staphylococcal J03.80
      recurrent J03.81
    streptococcal J03.00
      recurrent J03.01
**Adenoids** — *see* condition
**Adenolipoma** — *see* Neoplasm, benign, by site
**Adenolipomatosis, Launois-Bensaude** E88.89
**Adenolymphoma**
  specified site — *see* Neoplasm, benign, by site
  unspecified site D11.9
**Adenoma** (*see also* Neoplasm, benign, by site)
  acidophil
    specified site — *see* Neoplasm, benign, by site
    unspecified site D35.2
  acidophil-basophil, mixed
    specified site — *see* Neoplasm, benign, by site
    unspecified site D35.2
  adrenal (cortical) D35.00
    clear cell D35.00
    compact cell D35.00
    glomerulosa cell D35.00
    heavily pigmented variant D35.00
    mixed cell D35.00
  alpha-cell
    pancreas D13.7
    specified site NEC — *see* Neoplasm, benign, by site
    unspecified site D13.7
  alveolar D14.30
  apocrine
    breast D24- ☑
    specified site NEC — *see* Neoplasm, skin, benign, by site
    unspecified site D23.9
  basal cell D11.9
  basophil
    specified site — *see* Neoplasm, benign, by site
    unspecified site D35.2
  basophil-acidophil, mixed
    specified site — *see* Neoplasm, benign, by site
    unspecified site D35.2
  beta-cell
    pancreas D13.7
    specified site NEC — *see* Neoplasm, benign, by site
    unspecified site D13.7
  bile duct D13.4
    common D13.5
    extrahepatic D13.5
    intrahepatic D13.4
    specified site NEC — *see* Neoplasm, benign, by site
    unspecified site D13.4
  black D35.00
  bronchial D38.1
    cylindroid type — *see* Neoplasm, lung, malignant
  ceruminous D23.2- ☑
  chief cell D35.1
  chromophobe
    specified site — *see* Neoplasm, benign, by site
    unspecified site D35.2
  colloid
    specified site — *see* Neoplasm, benign, by site
    unspecified site D34
  duct
  eccrine, papillary — *see* Neoplasm, skin, benign
  endocrine, multiple
    single specified site — *see* Neoplasm, uncertain behavior, by site
    two or more specified sites D44- ☑
    unspecified site D44.9
  endometrioid (*see also* Neoplasm, benign)
    borderline malignancy — *see* Neoplasm, uncertain behavior, by site
  eosinophil
    specified site — *see* Neoplasm, benign, by site

**Adenoma** — *continued*
  eosinophil — *continued*
    unspecified site D35.2
  fetal
    specified site — *see* Neoplasm, benign, by site
    unspecified site D34
  follicular
    specified site — *see* Neoplasm, benign, by site
    unspecified site D34
  hepatocellular D13.4
  Hurthle cell D34
  islet cell
    pancreas D13.7
    specified site NEC — *see* Neoplasm, benign, by site
    unspecified site D13.7
  liver cell D13.4
  macrofollicular
    specified site — *see* Neoplasm, benign, by site
    unspecified site D34
  malignant, malignum — *see* Neoplasm, malignant, by site
  microcystic
    pancreas D13.6
    specified site NEC — *see* Neoplasm, benign, by site
    unspecified site D13.6
  microfollicular
    specified site — *see* Neoplasm, benign, by site
    unspecified site D34
  mucoid cell
    specified site — *see* Neoplasm, benign, by site
    unspecified site D35.2
  multiple endocrine
    single specified site — *see* Neoplasm, uncertain behavior, by site
    two or more specified sites D44- ☑
    unspecified site D44.9
  nipple D24- ☑
  papillary (*see also* Neoplasm, benign, by site)
    eccrine — *see* Neoplasm, skin, benign, by site
  Pick's tubular
    specified site — *see* Neoplasm, benign, by site
    unspecified site
      female D27.9
      male D29.20
  pleomorphic
    carcinoma in — *see* Neoplasm, salivary gland, malignant
      specified site — *see* Neoplasm, malignant, by site
      unspecified site C08.9
  polypoid (*see also* Neoplasm, benign)
    adenocarcinoma in — *see* Neoplasm, malignant, by site
    adenocarcinoma in situ — *see* Neoplasm, in situ, by site
  prostate — *see* Neoplasm, benign, prostate
  rete cell D29.20
  sebaceous — *see* Neoplasm, skin, benign
  Sertoli cell
    specified site — *see* Neoplasm, benign, by site
    unspecified site
      female D27.9
      male D29.20
  skin appendage — *see* Neoplasm, skin, benign
  sudoriferous gland — *see* Neoplasm, skin, benign
  sweat gland — *see* Neoplasm, skin, benign
  testicular
    specified site — *see* Neoplasm, benign, by site
    unspecified site
      female D27.9
      male D29.20
  tubular (*see also* Neoplasm, benign, by site)
    adenocarcinoma in — *see* Neoplasm, malignant, by site
    adenocarcinoma in situ — *see* Neoplasm, in situ, by site
    Pick's
      specified site — *see* Neoplasm, benign, by site
      unspecified site
        female D27.9
        male D29.20
  tubulovillous (*see also* Neoplasm, benign, by site)
    adenocarcinoma in — *see* Neoplasm, malignant, by site
    adenocarcinoma in situ — *see* Neoplasm, in situ, by site
  villous — *see* Neoplasm, uncertain behavior, by site

**Adenoma** — *continued*
  villous — *see* Neoplasm, uncertain behavior, by site — *continued*
    adenocarcinoma in — *see* Neoplasm, malignant, by site
    adenocarcinoma in situ — *see* Neoplasm, in situ, by site
  water-clear cell D35.1
**Adenomatosis**
  endocrine (multiple) E31.20
    single specified site — *see* Neoplasm, uncertain behavior, by site
  erosive of nipple D24- ☑
  pluriendocrine — *see* Adenomatosis, endocrine
  pulmonary D38.1
    malignant — *see* Neoplasm, lung, malignant
  specified site — *see* Neoplasm, benign, by site
  unspecified site D12.6
**Adenomatous**
  goiter (nontoxic) E04.9
    with hyperthyroidism — *see* Hyperthyroidism, with, goiter, nodular
    toxic — *see* Hyperthyroidism, with, goiter, nodular
**Adenomyoma** (*see also* Neoplasm, benign, by site)
  prostate — *see* Enlarged, prostate
**Adenomyometritis** N80.0
**Adenomyosis** N80.0
**Adenopathy** (lymph gland) R59.9
  generalized R59.1
  inguinal R59.0
  localized R59.0
  mediastinal R59.0
  mesentery R59.0
  syphilitic (secondary) A51.49
  tracheobronchial R59.0
    tuberculous A15.4
      primary (progressive) A15.7
  tuberculous (*see also* Tuberculosis, lymph gland)
    tracheobronchial A15.4
      primary (progressive) A15.7
**Adenosalpingitis** — *see* Salpingitis
**Adenosarcoma** — *see* Neoplasm, malignant, by site
**Adenosclerosis** I88.8
**Adenosis** (sclerosing) breast — *see* Fibroadenosis, breast
**Adenovirus, as cause of disease classified elsewhere** B97.0
**Adentia** (complete) (partial) — *see* Absence, teeth
**Adherent** (*see also* Adhesions)
  labia (minora) N90.89
  pericardium (nonrheumatic) I31.0
    rheumatic I09.2
  placenta (with hemorrhage) O72.0
    without hemorrhage O73.0
  prepuce, newborn N47.0
  scar (skin) L90.5
  tendon in scar L90.5
**Adhesions, adhesive** (postinfective) K66.0
  with intestinal obstruction K56.50
    complete K56.52
    incomplete K56.51
    partial K56.51
  abdominal (wall) — *see* Adhesions, peritoneum
  appendix K38.8
  bile duct (common) (hepatic) K83.8
  bladder (sphincter) N32.89
  bowel — *see* Adhesions, peritoneum
  cardiac I31.0
    rheumatic I09.2
  cecum — *see* Adhesions, peritoneum
  cervicovaginal N88.1
    congenital Q52.8
    postpartal O90.89
      old N88.1
  cervix N88.1
  ciliary body NEC — *see* Adhesions, iris
  clitoris N90.89
  colon — *see* Adhesions, peritoneum
  common duct K83.8
  congenital (*see also* Anomaly, by site)
    fingers — *see* Syndactylism, complex, fingers
    omental, anomalous Q43.3
    peritoneal Q43.3
    tongue (to gum or roof of mouth) Q38.3
  conjunctiva (acquired) H11.21- ☑
    congenital Q15.8
  cystic duct K82.8
  diaphragm — *see* Adhesions, peritoneum
  due to foreign body — *see* Foreign body

**Adhesions, adhesive** — *continued*
  duodenum — *see* Adhesions, peritoneum
  ear
    middle H74.1- ☑
  epididymis N50.89
  epidural — *see* Adhesions, meninges
  epiglottis J38.7
  eyelid H02.59
  female pelvis N73.6
  gallbladder K82.8
  globe H44.89
  heart I31.0
    rheumatic I09.2
  ileocecal (coil) — *see* Adhesions, peritoneum
  ileum — *see* Adhesions, peritoneum
  intestine (*see also* Adhesions, peritoneum)
    with obstruction K56.50
      complete K56.52
      incomplete K56.51
      partial K56.51
  intra-abdominal — *see* Adhesions, peritoneum
  iris H21.50- ☑
    anterior H21.51- ☑
    goniosynechiae H21.52- ☑
    posterior H21.54- ☑
    to corneal graft T85.898 ☑
  joint — *see* Ankylosis
    knee M23.8X ☑
    temporomandibular M26.61- ☑
  labium (majus) (minus), congenital Q52.5
  liver — *see* Adhesions, peritoneum
  lung J98.4
  mediastinum J98.59
  meninges (cerebral) (spinal) G96.12
    congenital Q07.8
    tuberculous (cerebral) (spinal) A17.0
  mesenteric — *see* Adhesions, peritoneum
  nasal (septum) (to turbinates) J34.89
  ocular muscle — *see* Strabismus, mechanical
  omentum — *see* Adhesions, peritoneum
  ovary N73.6
    congenital (to cecum, kidney or omentum) Q50.39
  paraovarian N73.6
  pelvic (peritoneal)
    female N73.6
      postprocedural N99.4
    male — *see* Adhesions, peritoneum
    postpartal (old) N73.6
    tuberculous A18.17
  penis to scrotum (congenital) Q55.8
  periappendiceal (*see also* Adhesions, peritoneum)
  pericardium (nonrheumatic) I31.0
    focal I31.8
    rheumatic I09.2
    tuberculous A18.84
  pericholecystic K82.8
  perigastric — *see* Adhesions, peritoneum
  periovarian N73.6
  periprostatic N42.89
  perirectal — *see* Adhesions, peritoneum
  perirenal N28.89
  peritoneum, peritoneal (postinfective)
    with obstruction (intestinal) K56.50
      complete K56.52
      incomplete K56.51
      partial K56.51
    congenital Q43.3
    pelvic, female N73.6
      postprocedural N99.4
    postpartal, pelvic N73.6
    postprocedural K66.0
    to uterus N73.6
  peritubal N73.6
  periureteral N28.89
  periuterine N73.6
  perivesical N32.89
  perivesicular (seminal vesicle) N50.89
  pleura, pleuritic J94.8
    tuberculous NEC A15.6
  pleuropericardial J94.8
  postoperative (gastrointestinal tract) K66.0
    with obstruction (*see also* Obstruction, intestine, postoperative) K91.30
    due to foreign body accidentally left in wound — *see* Foreign body, accidentally left during a procedure
    pelvic peritoneal N99.4
  urethra — *see* Stricture, urethra, postprocedural

**Adhesions, adhesive** — *continued*
  postoperative — *continued*
    vagina N99.2
  postpartal, old (vulva or perineum) N90.89
  preputial, prepuce N47.5
  pulmonary J98.4
  pylorus — *see* Adhesions, peritoneum
  sciatic nerve — *see* Lesion, nerve, sciatic
  seminal vesicle N50.89
  shoulder (joint) — *see* Capsulitis, adhesive
  sigmoid flexure — *see* Adhesions, peritoneum
  spermatic cord (acquired) N50.89
    congenital Q55.4
  spinal canal G96.12
  stomach — *see* Adhesions, peritoneum
  subscapular — *see* Capsulitis, adhesive
  temporomandibular M26.61- ☑
  tendinitis (*see also* Tenosynovitis, specified type NEC)
    shoulder — *see* Capsulitis, adhesive
  testis N44.8
  tongue, congenital (to gum or roof of mouth) Q38.3
    acquired K14.8
  trachea J39.8
  tubo-ovarian N73.6
  tunica vaginalis N44.8
  uterus N73.6
    internal N85.6
    to abdominal wall N73.6
  vagina (chronic) N89.5
    postoperative N99.2
  vitreomacular H43.82- ☑
  vitreous H43.89
  vulva N90.89

**Adiaspiromycosis** B48.8

**Adie** (-Holmes) **pupil or syndrome** — *see* Anomaly, pupil, function, tonic pupil

**Adiponecrosis neonatorum** P83.88

**Adiposis** (*see also* Obesity)
  cerebralis E23.6
  dolorosa E88.2

**Adiposity** (*see also* Obesity)
  heart — *see* Degeneration, myocardial
  localized E65

**Adiposogenital dystrophy** E23.6

**Adjustment**
  disorder — *see* Disorder, adjustment
  implanted device — *see* Encounter (for), adjustment (of)
  prosthesis, external — *see* Fitting
  reaction — *see* Disorder, adjustment

**Administration of tPA** (rtPA) in a different facility within the last 24 hours prior to admission to current facility Z92.82

**Admission** (for) (*see also* Encounter (for))
  adjustment (of)
    artificial
      arm Z44.00- ☑
        complete Z44.01- ☑
        partial Z44.02- ☑
      eye Z44.2 ☑
      leg Z44.10- ☑
        complete Z44.11- ☑
        partial Z44.12- ☑
    brain neuropacemaker Z46.2
      implanted Z45.42
    breast
      implant Z45.81 ☑
      prosthesis (external) Z44.3 ☑
    colostomy belt Z46.89
    contact lenses Z46.0
    cystostomy device Z46.6
    dental prosthesis Z46.3
    device NEC
      abdominal Z46.89
      implanted Z45.89
        cardiac Z45.09
          defibrillator (with synchronous cardiace pacemaker) Z45.02
          pacemaker (cardiac resynchronization therapy (CRT-P)) Z45.018
            pulse generator Z45.010
          resynchronization therapy defibrillator (CRT-D) Z45.02
        hearing device Z45.328
          bone conduction Z45.320
          cochlear Z45.321
        infusion pump Z45.1
        nervous system Z45.49

**Admission** — *continued*
  adjustment — *continued*
    device — *continued*
      implanted — *continued*
        nervous system — *continued*
          CSF drainage Z45.41
          hearing device — *see* Admission, adjustment, device, implanted, hearing device
          neuropacemaker Z45.42
          visual substitution Z45.31
        specified NEC Z45.89
        vascular access Z45.2
        visual substitution Z45.31
      nervous system Z46.2
        implanted — *see* Admission, adjustment, device, implanted, nervous system
      orthodontic Z46.4
      prosthetic Z44.9
        arm — *see* Admission, adjustment, artificial, arm
        breast Z44.3 ☑
        dental Z46.3
        eye Z44.2 ☑
        leg — *see* Admission, adjustment, artificial, leg
        specified type NEC Z44.8
      substitution
        auditory Z46.2
          implanted — *see* Admission, adjustment, device, implanted, hearing device
        nervous system Z46.2
          implanted — *see* Admission, adjustment, device, implanted, nervous system
        visual Z46.2
          implanted Z45.31
      urinary Z46.6
    hearing aid Z46.1
      implanted — *see* Admission, adjustment, device, implanted, hearing device
    ileostomy device Z46.89
    intestinal appliance or device NEC Z46.89
    neuropacemaker (brain) (peripheral nerve) (spinal cord) Z46.2
      implanted Z45.42
    orthodontic device Z46.4
    orthopedic (brace) (cast) (device) (shoes) Z46.89
    pacemaker (cardiac resynchronization therapy (CRT-P)
      cardiac Z45.018
        pulse generator Z45.010
      nervous system Z46.2
        implanted Z45.42
    portacath (port-a-cath) Z45.2
    prosthesis Z44.9
      arm — *see* Admission, adjustment, artificial, arm
      breast Z44.3 ☑
      dental Z46.3
      eye Z44.2 ☑
      leg — *see* Admission, adjustment, artificial, leg
      specified NEC Z44.8
    spectacles Z46.0
  aftercare (*see also* Aftercare) Z51.89
    postpartum
      immediately after delivery Z39.0
      routine follow-up Z39.2
    radiation therapy (antineoplastic) Z51.0
  attention to artificial opening (of) Z43.9
    artificial vagina Z43.7
    colostomy Z43.3
    cystostomy Z43.5
    enterostomy Z43.4
    gastrostomy Z43.1
    ileostomy Z43.2
    jejunostomy Z43.4
    nephrostomy Z43.6
    specified site NEC Z43.8
      intestinal tract Z43.4
      urinary tract Z43.6
    tracheostomy Z43.0
    ureterostomy Z43.6
    urethrostomy Z43.6
  breast augmentation or reduction Z41.1
  breast reconstruction following mastectomy Z42.1

**Admission** — *continued*
  change of
    dressing (nonsurgical) Z48.00
    neuropacemaker device (brain) (peripheral nerve) (spinal cord) Z46.2
      implanted Z45.42
    surgical dressing Z48.01
  circumcision, ritual or routine (in absence of diagnosis) Z41.2
  clinical research investigation (control) (normal comparison) (participant) Z00.6
  contraceptive management Z30.9
  cosmetic surgery NEC Z41.1
  counseling (*see also* Counseling)
    dietary Z71.3
    gestational carrier Z31.7
    HIV Z71.7
    human immunodeficiency virus Z71.7
    nonattending third party Z71.0
    procreative management NEC Z31.69
  delivery, full-term, uncomplicated O80
    cesarean, without indication O82
  desensitization to allergens Z51.6
  dietary surveillance and counseling Z71.3
  ear piercing Z41.3
  examination at health care facility (adult) (*see also* Examination) Z00.00
    with abnormal findings Z00.01
    clinical research investigation (control) (normal comparison) (participant) Z00.6
    dental Z01.20
      with abnormal findings Z01.21
    donor (potential) Z00.5
    ear Z01.10
      with abnormal findings NEC Z01.118
    eye Z01.00
      with abnormal findings Z01.01
    general, specified reason NEC Z00.8
    hearing Z01.10
      with abnormal findings NEC Z01.118
    postpartum checkup Z39.2
    psychiatric (general) Z00.8
      requested by authority Z04.6
    vision Z01.00
      with abnormal findings Z01.01
  fitting (of)
    artificial
      arm — *see* Admission, adjustment, artificial, arm
      eye Z44.2 ☑
      leg — *see* Admission, adjustment, artificial, leg
    brain neuropacemaker Z46.2
      implanted Z45.42
    breast prosthesis (external) Z44.3 ☑
    colostomy belt Z46.89
    contact lenses Z46.0
    cystostomy device Z46.6
    dental prosthesis Z46.3
    dentures Z46.3
    device NEC
      abdominal Z46.89
      nervous system Z46.2
        implanted — *see* Admission, adjustment, device, implanted, nervous system
      orthodontic Z46.4
      prosthetic Z44.9
        breast Z44.3 ☑
        dental Z46.3
        eye Z44.2 ☑
      substitution
        auditory Z46.2
          implanted — *see* Admission, adjustment, device, implanted, hearing device
        nervous system Z46.2
          implanted — *see* Admission, adjustment, device, implanted, nervous system
        visual Z46.2
          implanted Z45.31
    hearing aid Z46.1
    ileostomy device Z46.89
    intestinal appliance or device NEC Z46.89
    neuropacemaker (brain) (peripheral nerve) (spinal cord) Z46.2
      implanted Z45.42
    orthodontic device Z46.4
    orthopedic device (brace) (cast) (shoes) Z46.89

☞ Subterms under main terms may continue to next column or page     ☑ **Additional Character Required** — Refer to the Tabular List for Character Selection     **13**

**Index**

**Adhesions, adhesive — Admission**

**Admission** — *continued*
  fitting — *continued*
    prosthesis Z44.9
      arm — *see* Admission, adjustment, artificial,
          arm
      breast Z44.3 ☑
      dental Z46.3
      eye Z44.2 ☑
      leg — *see* Admission, adjustment, artificial, leg
      specified type NEC Z44.8
    spectacles Z46.0
  follow-up examination Z09
  intrauterine device management Z30.431
    initial prescription Z30.014
  mental health evaluation Z00.8
    requested by authority Z04.6
  observation — *see* Observation
  Papanicolaou smear, cervix Z12.4
    for suspected malignant neoplasm Z12.4
  plastic and reconstructive surgery following medical
      procedure or healed injury NEC Z42.8
  plastic surgery, cosmetic NEC Z41.1
  postpartum observation
    immediately after delivery Z39.0
    routine follow-up Z39.2
  poststerilization (for restoration) Z31.0
    aftercare Z31.42
  procreative management Z31.9
  prophylactic (measure) — (*see also* Encounter, prophy-
      lactic measures)
    organ removal Z40.00
      breast Z40.01
      fallopian tube(s) Z40.03
        with ovary(s) Z40.02
      ovary(s) Z40.02
      specified organ NEC Z40.09
      testes Z40.09
    vaccination Z23
  psychiatric examination (general) Z00.8
    requested by authority Z04.6
  radiation therapy (antineoplastic) Z51.0
  reconstructive surgery following medical procedure
      or healed injury NEC Z42.8
  removal of
    cystostomy catheter Z43.5
    drains Z48.03
    dressing (nonsurgical) Z48.00
    implantable subdermal contraceptive Z30.46
    intrauterine contraceptive device Z30.432
    neuropacemaker (brain) (peripheral nerve) (spinal
        cord) Z46.2
      implanted Z45.42
    staples Z48.02
    surgical dressing Z48.01
    sutures Z48.02
    ureteral stent Z46.6
  respirator [ventilator] use during power failure Z99.12
  restoration of organ continuity (poststerilization) Z31.0
    aftercare Z31.42
  sensitivity test (*see also* Test, skin)
    allergy NEC Z01.82
    Mantoux Z11.1
  tuboplasty following previous sterilization Z31.0
    aftercare Z31.42
  vasoplasty following previous sterilization Z31.0
    aftercare Z31.42
  vision examination Z01.00
    with abnormal findings Z01.01
  waiting period for admission to other facility Z75.1
**Adnexitis** (suppurative) — *see* Salpingo-oophoritis
**Adolescent X-linked adrenoleukodystrophy** E71.521
**Adrenal** (gland) — *see* condition
**Adrenalism, tuberculous** A18.7
**Adrenalitis, adrenitis** E27.8
  autoimmune E27.1
  meningococcal, hemorrhagic A39.1
**Adrenarche, premature** E27.0
**Adrenocortical syndrome** — *see* Cushing's, syndrome
**Adrenogenital syndrome** E25.9
  acquired E25.8
  congenital E25.0
  salt loss E25.0
**Adrenogenitalism, congenital** E25.0
**Adrenoleukodystrophy** E71.529
  neonatal E71.511
  X-linked E71.529
    Addison only phenotype E71.528
    Addison-Schilder E71.528

**Adrenoleukodystrophy** — *continued*
  X-linked — *continued*
    adolescent E71.521
    adrenomyeloneuropathy E71.522
    childhood cerebral E71.520
    other specified E71.528
**Adrenomyeloneuropathy** E71.522
**Adventitious bursa** — *see* Bursopathy, specified type
    NEC
**Adverse effect** — *see* Table of Drugs and Chemicals,
    categories T36-T50, with 6th character 5
**Advice** — *see* Counseling
**Adynamia** (episodica) (hereditary) (periodic) G72.3
**Aeration lung imperfect, newborn** — *see* Atelectasis
**Aerobullosis** T70.3 ☑
**Aerocele** — *see* Embolism, air
**Aerodermectasia**
  subcutaneous (traumatic) T79.7 ☑
**Aerodontalgia** T70.29 ☑
**Aeroembolism** T70.3 ☑
**Aerogenes capsulatus infection** A48.0
**Aero-otitis media** T70.0 ☑
**Aerophagy, aerophagia** (psychogenic) F45.8
**Aerophobia** F40.228
**Aerosinusitis** T70.1 ☑
**Aerotitis** T70.0 ☑
**Affection** — *see* Disease
**Afibrinogenemia** (*see also* Defect, coagulation) D68.8
  acquired D65
  congenital D68.2
  following ectopic or molar pregnancy O08.1
  in abortion — *see* Abortion, by type, complicated by,
      afibrinogenemia
  puerperal O72.3
**African**
  sleeping sickness B56.9
  tick fever A68.1
  trypanosomiasis B56.9
    gambian B56.0
    rhodesian B56.1
**Aftercare** (*see also* Care) Z51.89
  following surgery (for) (on)
    amputation Z47.81
    attention to
      drains Z48.03
      dressings (nonsurgical) Z48.00
        surgical Z48.01
      sutures Z48.02
    circulatory system Z48.812
    delayed (planned) wound closure Z48.1
    digestive system Z48.815
    explantation of joint prosthesis (staged procedure)
      hip Z47.32
      knee Z47.33
      shoulder Z47.31
    genitourinary system Z48.816
    joint replacement Z47.1
    neoplasm Z48.3
    nervous system Z48.811
    oral cavity Z48.814
    organ transplant
      bone marrow Z48.290
      heart Z48.21
      heart-lung Z48.280
      kidney Z48.22
      liver Z48.23
      lung Z48.24
      multiple organs NEC Z48.288
      specified NEC Z48.298
    orthopedic NEC Z47.89
    planned wound closure Z48.1
    removal of internal fixation device Z47.2
    respiratory system Z48.813
    scoliosis Z47.82
    sense organs Z48.810
    skin and subcutaneous tissue Z48.817
    specified body system
      circulatory Z48.812
      digestive Z48.815
      genitourinary Z48.816
      nervous Z48.811
      oral cavity Z48.814
      respiratory Z48.813
      sense organs Z48.810
      skin and subcutaneous tissue Z48.817
      teeth Z48.814
    specified NEC Z48.89
    spinal Z47.89

**Aftercare** — *continued*
  following surgery — *continued*
    teeth Z48.814
  fracture — *code to* fracture with seventh character D
  involving
    removal of
      drains Z48.03
      dressings (nonsurgical) Z48.00
      staples Z48.02
      surgical dressings Z48.01
      sutures Z48.02
    neuropacemaker (brain) (peripheral nerve) (spinal
        cord) Z46.2
      implanted Z45.42
    orthopedic NEC Z47.89
    postprocedural — *see* Aftercare, following surgery
**After-cataract** — *see* Cataract, secondary
**Agalactia** (primary) O92.3
  elective, secondary or therapeutic O92.5
**Agammaglobulinemia** (acquired (secondary) (nonfamil-
    ial) D80.1
  with
    immunoglobulin-bearing B-lymphocytes D80.1
    lymphopenia D81.9
  autosomal recessive (Swiss type) D80.0
  Bruton's X-linked D80.0
  common variable (CVAgamma) D80.1
  congenital sex-linked D80.0
  hereditary D80.0
  lymphopenic D81.9
  Swiss type (autosomal recessive) D80.0
  X-linked (with growth hormone deficiency) (Bruton)
      D80.0
**Aganglionosis** (bowel) (colon) Q43.1
**Age** (old) — *see* Senility
**Agenesis**
  adrenal (gland) Q89.1
  alimentary tract (complete) (partial) NEC Q45.8
    upper Q40.8
  anus, anal (canal) Q42.3
    with fistula Q42.2
  aorta Q25.41
  appendix Q42.8
  arm (complete) Q71.0- ☑
    with hand present Q71.1- ☑
  artery (peripheral) Q27.9
    brain Q28.3
    coronary Q24.5
    pulmonary Q25.79
    specified NEC Q27.8
    umbilical Q27.0
  auditory (canal) (external) Q16.1
  auricle (ear) Q16.0
  bile duct or passage Q44.5
  bladder Q64.5
  bone Q79.9
  brain Q00.0
    part of Q04.3
  breast (with nipple present) Q83.8
    with absent nipple Q83.0
  bronchus Q32.4
  canaliculus lacrimalis Q10.4
  carpus — *see* Agenesis, hand
  cartilage Q79.9
  cecum Q42.8
  cerebellum Q04.3
  cervix Q51.5
  chin Q18.8
  cilia Q10.3
  circulatory system, part NOS Q28.9
  clavicle Q74.0
  clitoris Q52.6
  coccyx Q76.49
  colon Q42.9
    specified NEC Q42.8
  corpus callosum Q04.0
  cricoid cartilage Q31.8
  diaphragm (with hernia) Q79.1
  digestive organ(s) or tract (complete) (partial) NEC
      Q45.8
    upper Q40.8
  ductus arteriosus Q28.8
  duodenum Q41.0
  ear Q16.9
    auricle Q16.0
    lobe Q17.8
  ejaculatory duct Q55.4
  endocrine (gland) NEC Q89.2

**Agenesis** — *continued*
  epiglottis Q31.8
  esophagus Q39.8
  eustachian tube Q16.2
  eye Q11.1
    adnexa Q15.8
  eyelid (fold) Q10.3
  face
    bones NEC Q75.8
    specified part NEC Q18.8
  fallopian tube Q50.6
  femur — *see* Defect, reduction, lower limb, longitudinal, femur
  fibula — *see* Defect, reduction, lower limb, longitudinal, fibula
  finger (complete) (partial) — *see* Agenesis, hand
  foot (and toes) (complete) (partial) Q72.3- ☑
  forearm (with hand present) — *see* Agenesis, arm, with hand present
    and hand Q71.2- ☑
  gallbladder Q44.0
  gastric Q40.2
  genitalia, genital (organ(s))
    female Q52.8
      external Q52.71
      internal NEC Q52.8
    male Q55.8
  glottis Q31.8
  hair Q84.0
  hand (and fingers) (complete) (partial) Q71.3- ☑
  heart Q24.8
    valve NEC Q24.8
      pulmonary Q22.0
  hepatic Q44.7
  humerus — *see* Defect, reduction, upper limb
  hymen Q52.4
  ileum Q41.2
  incus Q16.3
  intestine (small) Q41.9
    large Q42.9
      specified NEC Q42.8
  iris (dilator fibers) Q13.1
  jaw M26.09
  jejunum Q41.1
  kidney(s) (partial) Q60.2
    bilateral Q60.1
    unilateral Q60.0
  labium (majus) (minus) Q52.71
  labyrinth, membranous Q16.5
  lacrimal apparatus Q10.4
  larynx Q31.8
  leg (complete) Q72.0- ☑
    with foot present Q72.1- ☑
    lower leg (with foot present) — *see* Agenesis, leg, with foot present
      and foot Q72.2- ☑
  lens Q12.3
  limb (complete) Q73.0
    lower — *see* Agenesis, leg
    upper — *see* Agenesis, arm
  lip Q38.0
  liver Q44.7
  lung (fissure) (lobe) (bilateral) (unilateral) Q33.3
  mandible, maxilla M26.09
  metacarpus — *see* Agenesis, hand
  metatarsus — *see* Agenesis, foot
  muscle Q79.8
    eyelid Q10.3
    ocular Q15.8
  musculoskeletal system NEC Q79.8
  nail(s) Q84.3
  neck, part Q18.8
  nerve Q07.8
  nervous system, part NEC Q07.8
  nipple Q83.2
  nose Q30.1
  nuclear Q07.8
  organ
    of Corti Q16.5
    or site not listed — *see* Anomaly, by site
  osseous meatus (ear) Q16.1
  ovary
    bilateral Q50.02
    unilateral Q50.01
  oviduct Q50.6
  pancreas Q45.0
  parathyroid (gland) Q89.2
  parotid gland(s) Q38.4

**Agenesis** — *continued*
  patella Q74.1
  pelvic girdle (complete) (partial) Q74.2
  penis Q55.5
  pericardium Q24.8
  pituitary (gland) Q89.2
  prostate Q55.4
  punctum lacrimale Q10.4
  radioulnar — *see* Defect, reduction, upper limb
  radius — *see* Defect, reduction, upper limb, longitudinal, radius
  rectum Q42.1
    with fistula Q42.0
  renal Q60.2
    bilateral Q60.1
    unilateral Q60.0
  respiratory organ NEC Q34.8
  rib Q76.6
  roof of orbit Q75.8
  round ligament Q52.8
  sacrum Q76.49
  salivary gland Q38.4
  scapula Q74.0
  scrotum Q55.29
  seminal vesicles Q55.4
  septum
    atrial Q21.1
    between aorta and pulmonary artery Q21.4
    ventricular Q20.4
  shoulder girdle (complete) (partial) Q74.0
  skull (bone) Q75.8
    with
      anencephaly Q00.0
      encephalocele — *see* Encephalocele
      hydrocephalus Q03.9
        with spina bifida — *see* Spina bifida, by site, with hydrocephalus
      microcephaly Q02
  spermatic cord Q55.4
  spinal cord Q06.0
  spine Q76.49
  spleen Q89.01
  sternum Q76.7
  stomach Q40.2
  submaxillary gland(s) (congenital) Q38.4
  tarsus — *see* Agenesis, foot
  tendon Q79.8
  testicle Q55.0
  thymus (gland) Q89.2
  thyroid (gland) E03.1
    cartilage Q31.8
  tibia — *see* Defect, reduction, lower limb, longitudinal, tibia
  tibiofibular — *see* Defect, reduction, lower limb, specified type NEC
  toe (and foot) (complete) (partial) — *see* Agenesis, foot
  tongue Q38.3
  trachea (cartilage) Q32.1
  ulna — *see* Defect, reduction, upper limb, longitudinal, ulna
  upper limb — *see* Agenesis, arm
  ureter Q62.4
  urethra Q64.5
  urinary tract NEC Q64.8
  uterus Q51.0
  uvula Q38.5
  vagina Q52.0
  vas deferens Q55.4
  vein(s) (peripheral) Q27.9
    brain Q28.3
    great NEC Q26.8
    portal Q26.5
  vena cava (inferior) (superior) Q26.8
  vermis of cerebellum Q04.3
  vertebra Q76.49
  vulva Q52.71
**Ageusia** R43.2
**Agitated** — *see* condition
**Agitation** R45.1
**Aglossia** (congenital) Q38.3
**Aglossia-adactylia syndrome** Q87.0
**Aglycogenosis** E74.00
**Agnosia** (body image) (other senses) (tactile) R48.1
  developmental F88
  verbal R48.1
    auditory R48.1
      developmental F80.2

**Agnosia** — *continued*
  verbal — *continued*
    developmental F80.2
  visual (object) R48.3
**Agoraphobia** F40.00
  with panic disorder F40.01
  without panic disorder F40.02
**Agrammatism** R48.8
**Agranulocytopenia** — *see* Agranulocytosis
**Agranulocytosis** (chronic) (cyclical) (genetic) (infantile) (periodic) (pernicious) (*see also* Neutropenia) D70.9
  congenital D70.0
  cytoreductive cancer chemotherapy sequela D70.1
  drug-induced D70.2
    due to cytoreductive cancer chemotherapy D70.1
  due to infection D70.3
  secondary D70.4
    drug-induced D70.2
      due to cytoreductive cancer chemotherapy D70.1
**Agraphia** (absolute) R48.8
  with alexia R48.0
  developmental F81.81
**Ague** (dumb) — *see* Malaria
**Agyria** Q04.3
**Ahumada-del Castillo syndrome** E23.0
**Aichomophobia** F40.298
**AIDS** (related complex) B20
**Ailment heart** — *see* Disease, heart
**Ailurophobia** F40.218
**AIN** — *see* Neoplasia, intraepithelial, anal
**Ainhum** (disease) L94.6
**AIPHI** (acute idiopathic pulmonary hemorrhage in infants (over 28 days old)) R04.81
**Air**
  anterior mediastinum J98.2
  compressed, disease T70.3 ☑
  conditioner lung or pneumonitis J67.7
  embolism (artery) (cerebral) (any site) T79.0 ☑
    with ectopic or molar pregnancy O08.2
    due to implanted device NEC — *see* Complications, by site and type, specified NEC
    following
      abortion — *see* Abortion by type, complicated by, embolism
      ectopic or molar pregnancy O08.2
    infusion, therapeutic injection or transfusion T80.0 ☑
    in pregnancy, childbirth or puerperium — *see* Embolism, obstetric
    traumatic T79.0 ☑
  hunger, psychogenic F45.8
  rarefied, effects of — *see* Effect, adverse, high altitude
  sickness T75.3 ☑
**Airplane sickness** T75.3 ☑
**Akathisia** (drug-induced) (treatment-induced) G25.71
  neuroleptic induced (acute) G25.71
  tardive G25.71
**Akinesia** R29.898
**Akinetic mutism** R41.89
**Akureyri's disease** G93.3
**Alactasia, congenital** E73.0
**Alagille's syndrome** Q44.7
**Alastrim** B03
**Albers-Schönberg syndrome** Q78.2
**Albert's syndrome** — *see* Tendinitis, Achilles
**Albinism, albino** E70.30
  with hematologic abnormality E70.339
    Chédiak-Higashi syndrome E70.330
    Hermansky-Pudlak syndrome E70.331
    other specified E70.338
  I E70.320
  II E70.321
  ocular E70.319
    autosomal recessive E70.311
    other specified E70.318
    X-linked E70.310
  oculocutaneous E70.329
    other specified E70.328
    tyrosinase (ty) negative E70.320
    tyrosinase (ty) positive E70.321
  other specified E70.39
**Albinismus** E70.30
**Albright** (-McCune)(-Sternberg) syndrome Q78.1
**Albuminous** — *see* condition
**Albuminuria, albuminuric** (acute) (chronic) (subacute) (*see also* Proteinuria) R80.9

**Albuminuria, albuminuric** — *continued*
  complicating pregnancy — *see* Proteinuria, gestational
    with
      gestational hypertension — *see* Pre-eclampsia
      pre-existing hypertension — *see* Hypertension,
        complicating pregnancy, pre-existing,
        with, pre-eclampsia
  gestational — *see* Proteinuria, gestational
    with
      gestational hypertension — *see* Pre-eclampsia
      pre-existing hypertension — *see* Hypertension,
        complicating pregnancy, pre-existing,
        with, pre-eclampsia
  orthostatic R80.2
  postural R80.2
  pre-eclamptic — *see* Pre-eclampsia
  scarlatinal A38.8
**Albuminurophobia** F40.298
**Alcaptonuria** E70.29
**Alcohol, alcoholic, alcohol-induced**
  addiction (without remission) F10.20
    with remission F10.21
  amnestic disorder, persisting F10.96
    with dependence F10.26
  anxiety disorder F10.980
  bipolar and related disorder F10.94
  brain syndrome, chronic F10.97
    with dependence F10.27
  cardiopathy I42.6
  counseling and surveillance Z71.41
    family member Z71.42
  delirium (acute) (tremens) (withdrawal) F10.231
    with intoxication F10.921
      in
        abuse F10.121
        dependence F10.221
  dementia F10.97
    with dependence F10.27
  depressive disorder F10.94
  deterioration F10.97
    with dependence F10.27
  hallucinosis (acute) F10.951
    in
      abuse F10.151
      dependence F10.251
  insanity F10.959
  intoxication (acute) (without dependence) F10.129
    with
      delirium F10.121
      dependence F10.229
        with delirium F10.221
        uncomplicated F10.220
      uncomplicated F10.120
  jealousy F10.988
  Korsakoff's, Korsakov's, Korsakow's F10.26
  liver K70.9
    acute — *see* Disease, liver, alcoholic, hepatitis
  major neurocognitive disorder, amnestic-confabulato-
    ry type F10.96
  major neurocognitive disorder, nonamnestic-confab-
    ulatory type F10.97
  mania (acute) (chronic) F10.959
  mild neurocognitive disorder F10.988
  paranoia, paranoid (type) psychosis F10.950
  pellagra E52
  poisoning, accidental (acute) NEC — *see* Table of Drugs
    and Chemicals, alcohol, poisoning
  psychosis — *see* Psychosis, alcoholic
  psychotic disorder F10.959
  sexual dysfunction F10.981
  sleep disorder F10.982
  withdrawal (without convulsions) F10.239
    with delirium F10.231
**Alcoholism** (chronic) (without remission) F10.20
  with
    psychosis — *see* Psychosis, alcoholic
    remission F10.21
  Korsakov's F10.96
    with dependence F10.26
**Alder** (-Reilly) **anomaly or syndrome** (leukocyte granulation) D72.0
**Aldosteronism** E26.9
  familial (type I) E26.02
  glucocorticoid-remediable E26.02
  primary (due to (bilateral) adrenal hyperplasia) E26.09
  primary NEC E26.09
  secondary E26.1
  specified NEC E26.89

**Aldosteronoma** D44.10
**Aldrich** (-Wiskott) **syndrome** (eczema-thrombocytopenia) D82.0
**Alektorophobia** F40.218
**Aleppo boil** B55.1
**Aleukemic** — *see* condition
**Aleukia**
  congenital D70.0
  hemorrhagica D61.9
    congenital D61.09
  splenica D73.1
**Alexia** R48.0
  developmental F81.0
  secondary to organic lesion R48.0
**Algoneurodystrophy** M89.00
  ankle M89.07- ☑
  foot M89.07- ☑
  forearm M89.03- ☑
  hand M89.04- ☑
  lower leg M89.06- ☑
  multiple sites M89.0- ☑
  shoulder M89.01- ☑
  specified site NEC M89.08
  thigh M89.05- ☑
  upper arm M89.02- ☑
**Algophobia** F40.298
**Alienation, mental** — *see* Psychosis
**Alkalemia** E87.3
**Alkalosis** E87.3
  metabolic E87.3
    with respiratory acidosis E87.4
  respiratory E87.3
**Alkaptonuria** E70.29
**Allen-Masters syndrome** N83.8
**Allergy, allergic** (reaction) (to) T78.40 ☑
  air-borne substance NEC (rhinitis) J30.89
  alveolitis (extrinsic) J67.9
    due to
      Aspergillus clavatus J67.4
      Cryptostroma corticale J67.6
      organisms (fungal, thermophilic actinomycete)
        growing in ventilation (air conditioning)
        systems J67.7
    specified type NEC J67.8
  anaphylactic reaction or shock T78.2 ☑
  angioneurotic edema T78.3
  animal (dander) (epidermal) (hair) (rhinitis) J30.81
  bee sting (anaphylactic shock) — *see* Toxicity, venom,
    arthropod, bee
  biological — *see* Allergy, drug
  colitis (*see also* Colitis, allergic) K52.29
  dander (animal) (rhinitis) J30.81
  dandruff (rhinitis) J30.81
  dental restorative material (existing) K08.55
  dermatitis — *see* Dermatitis, contact, allergic
  diathesis — *see* History, allergy
  drug, medicament & biological (any) (external) (inter-
    nal) T78.40 ☑
    correct substance properly administered — *see*
      Table of Drugs and Chemicals, by drug, ad-
      verse effect
    wrong substance given or taken NEC (by accident)
      — *see* Table of Drugs and Chemicals, by
      drug, poisoning
  due to pollen J30.1
  dust (house) (stock) (rhinitis) J30.89
    with asthma — *see* Asthma, allergic extrinsic
  eczema — *see* Dermatitis, contact, allergic
  epidermal (animal) (rhinitis) J30.81
  feathers (rhinitis) J30.89
  food (any) (ingested) NEC T78.1 ☑
    anaphylactic shock — *see* Shock, anaphylactic, due
      to food
    dermatitis — *see* Dermatitis, due to, food
    dietary counseling and surveillance Z71.3
    in contact with skin L23.6
    rhinitis J30.5
    status (without reaction) Z91.018
      eggs Z91.012
      milk products Z91.011
      peanuts Z91.010
      seafood Z91.013
      specified NEC Z91.018
  gastrointestinal — *see also* specific type of allergic
    reaction
    meaning colitis (*see also* Colitis, allergic) K52.29

**Allergy, allergic** — *continued*
  gastrointestinal — *see also* specific type of allergic re-
    action — *continued*
    meaning gastroenteritis (*see also* Gastroenteritis,
      allergic) K52.29
    meaning other adverse food reaction not else-
      where classified T78.1 ☑
  grain J30.1
  grass (hay fever) (pollen) J30.1
    asthma — *see* Asthma, allergic extrinsic
  hair (animal) (rhinitis) J30.81
  history (of) — *see* History, allergy
  horse serum — *see* Allergy, serum
  inhalant (rhinitis) J30.89
    pollen J30.1
  kapok (rhinitis) J30.89
  medicine — *see* Allergy, drug
  milk protein (*see also* Allergy, food) Z91.011
    anaphylactic reaction T78.07 ☑
    dermatitis L27.2
    enterocolitis syndrome K52.21
    enteropathy K52.22
    gastroenteritis K52.29
    gastroesophageal reflux (*see also* Reaction, adverse,
      food) K21.9
      with esophagitis K21.0
    proctocolitis K52.82
  nasal, seasonal due to pollen J30.1
  pneumonia J82
  pollen (any) (hay fever) J30.1
    asthma — *see* Asthma, allergic extrinsic
  primrose J30.1
  primula J30.1
  proctocolitis K52.82
  purpura D69.0
  ragweed (hay fever) (pollen) J30.1
    asthma — *see* Asthma, allergic extrinsic
  rose (pollen) J30.1
  seasonal NEC J30.2
  Senecio jacobae (pollen) J30.1
  serum (*see also* Reaction, serum) T80.69 ☑
    anaphylactic shock T80.59 ☑
  shock (anaphylactic) T78.2 ☑
    due to
      administration of blood and blood products
        T80.51 ☑
      adverse effect of correct medicinal substance
        properly administered T88.6 ☑
      immunization T80.52 ☑
      serum NEC T80.59 ☑
      vaccination T80.52 ☑
  specific NEC T78.49 ☑
  tree (any) (hay fever) (pollen) J30.1
    asthma — *see* Asthma, allergic extrinsic
  upper respiratory J30.9
  urticaria L50.0
  vaccine — *see* Allergy, serum
  wheat — *see* Allergy, food
**Allescheriasis** B48.2
**Alligator skin disease** Q80.9
**Allocheiria, allochiria** R20.8
**Almeida's disease** — *see* Paracoccidioidomycosis
**Alopecia** (hereditaria) (seborrheica) L65.9
  androgenic L64.9
    drug-induced L64.0
    specified NEC L64.8
  areata L63.9
    ophiasis L63.2
    specified NEC L63.8
    totalis L63.0
    universalis L63.1
  cicatricial L66.9
    specified NEC L66.8
  circumscripta L63.9
  congenital, congenitalis Q84.0
  due to cytotoxic drugs NEC L65.8
  mucinosa L65.2
  postinfective NEC L65.8
  postpartum L65.0
  premature L64.8
  specific (syphilitic) A51.32
  specified NEC L65.8
  syphilitic (secondary) A51.32
  totalis (capitis) L63.0
  universalis (entire body) L63.1
  X-ray L58.1
**Alpers' disease** G31.81
**Alpine sickness** T70.29 ☑

☑ **Additional Character Required** — Refer to the Tabular List for Character Selection    ▽ **Subterms under main terms may continue to next column or page**

**Alport syndrome** Q87.81
**ALTE** (apparent life threatening event) **in newborn and infant** R68.13
**Alteration** (of), **Altered**
  awareness
    transient R40.4
      unintended under general anesthesia, during procedure T88.53 ☑
  mental status R41.82
  pattern of family relationships affecting child Z62.898
  sensation
    following
      cerebrovascular disease I69.998
        cerebral infarction I69.398
        intracerebral hemorrhage I69.198
        nontraumatic intracranial hemorrhage NEC I69.298
        specified disease NEC I69.898
        subarachnoid hemorrhage I69.098
**Alternating** — *see* condition
**Altitude, high** (effects) — *see* Effect, adverse, high altitude
**Aluminosis** (of lung) J63.0
**Alveolitis**
  allergic (extrinsic) — *see* Pneumonitis, hypersensitivity
  due to
    Aspergillus clavatus J67.4
    Cryptostroma corticale J67.6
  fibrosing (cryptogenic) (idiopathic) J84.112
  jaw M27.3
  sicca dolorosa M27.3
**Alveolus, alveolar** — *see* condition
**Alymphocytosis** D72.810
  thymic (with immunodeficiency) D82.1
**Alymphoplasia, thymic** D82.1
**Alzheimer's disease or sclerosis** — *see* Disease, Alzheimer's
**Amastia** (with nipple present) Q83.8
  with absent nipple Q83.0
**Amathophobia** F40.228
**Amaurosis** (acquired) (congenital) (*see also* Blindness)
  fugax G45.3
  hysterical F44.6
  Leber's congenital H35.50
  uremic — *see* Uremia
**Amaurotic idiocy** (infantile) (juvenile) (late) E75.4
**Amaxophobia** F40.248
**Ambiguous genitalia** Q56.4
**Amblyopia** (congenital) (ex anopsia) (partial) (suppression) H53.00- ☑
  anisometropic — *see* Amblyopia, refractive
  deprivation H53.01- ☑
  hysterical F44.6
  nocturnal (*see also* Blindness, night)
    vitamin A deficiency E50.5
  refractive H53.02- ☑
  strabismic H53.03- ☑
  suspect H53.04- ☑
  tobacco H53.8
  toxic NEC H53.8
  uremic — *see* Uremia
**Ameba, amebic** (histolytica) (*see also* Amebiasis)
  abscess (liver) A06.4
**Amebiasis** A06.9
  with abscess — *see* Abscess, amebic
  acute A06.0
  chronic (intestine) A06.1
    with abscess — *see* Abscess, amebic
  cutaneous A06.7
  cutis A06.7
  cystitis A06.81
  genitourinary tract NEC A06.82
  hepatic — *see* Abscess, liver, amebic
  intestine A06.0
  nondysenteric colitis A06.2
  skin A06.7
  specified site NEC A06.89
**Ameboma** (of intestine) A06.3
**Amelia** Q73.0
  lower limb — *see* Agenesis, leg
  upper limb — *see* Agenesis, arm
**Ameloblastoma** (*see also* Cyst, calcifying odontogenic)
  long bones C40.9- ☑
    lower limb C40.2- ☑
    upper limb C40.0- ☑
  malignant C41.1
    jaw (bone) (lower) C41.1

**Ameloblastoma** — *continued*
  malignant — *continued*
    jaw — *continued*
      upper C41.0
    tibial C40.2- ☑
**Amelogenesis imperfecta** K00.5
  nonhereditaria (segmentalis) K00.4
**Amenorrhea** N91.2
  hyperhormonal E28.8
  primary N91.0
  secondary N91.1
**Amentia** — *see* Disability, intellectual
  Meynert's (nonalcoholic) F04
**American**
  leishmaniasis B55.2
  mountain tick fever A93.2
**Ametropia** — *see* Disorder, refraction
**AMH** (asymptomatic microscopic hematuria) R31.21
**Amianthosis** J61
**Amimia** R48.8
**Amino-acid disorder** E72.9
  anemia D53.0
**Aminoacidopathy** E72.9
**Aminoaciduria** E72.9
**Amnesia** R41.3
  anterograde R41.1
  auditory R48.8
  dissociative F44.0
    with dissociative fugue F44.1
  hysterical F44.0
  postictal in epilepsy — *see* Epilepsy
  psychogenic F44.0
  retrograde R41.2
  transient global G45.4
**Amnes(t)ic syndrome** (post-traumatic) F04
  induced by
    alcohol F10.96
      with dependence F10.26
    psychoactive NEC F19.96
      with
        abuse F19.16
        dependence F19.26
    sedative F13.96
      with dependence F13.26
**Amnion, amniotic** — *see* condition
**Amnionitis** — *see* Pregnancy, complicated by
**Amok** F68.8
**Amoral traits** F60.89
**Amphetamine** (or other stimulant) **-induced**
  anxiety disorder F15.980
  bipolar and related disorder F15.94
  delirium F15.921
  depressive disorder F15.94
  obsessive-compulsive and related disorder F15.988
  psychotic disorder F15.959
  sexual dysfunction F15.981
  sleep disorder F15.982
  stimulant withdrawal F15.23
**Ampulla**
  lower esophagus K22.8
  phrenic K22.8
**Amputation** (*see also* Absence, by site, acquired)
  neuroma (postoperative) (traumatic) — *see* Complications, amputation stump, neuroma
  stump (surgical)
    abnormal, painful, or with complication (late) — *see* Complications, amputation stump
    healed or old NOS Z89.9
  traumatic (complete) (partial)
    arm (upper) (complete) S48.91- ☑
      at
        elbow S58.01- ☑
          partial S58.02- ☑
        shoulder joint (complete) S48.01- ☑
          partial S48.02- ☑
      between
        elbow and wrist (complete) S58.11- ☑
          partial S58.12- ☑
        shoulder and elbow (complete) S48.11- ☑
          partial S48.12- ☑
      partial S48.92- ☑
    breast (complete) S28.21- ☑
      partial S28.22- ☑
    clitoris (complete) S38.211
      partial S38.212
    ear (complete) S08.11- ☑
      partial S08.12- ☑

**Amputation** — *continued*
  traumatic — *continued*
    finger (complete) (metacarpophalangeal)
      S68.11- ☑
      index S68.11- ☑
      little S68.11- ☑
      middle S68.11- ☑
      partial S68.12- ☑
        index S68.12- ☑
        little S68.12- ☑
        middle S68.12- ☑
        ring S68.12- ☑
      ring S68.11- ☑
      thumb — *see* Amputation, traumatic, thumb
      transphalangeal (complete) S68.61- ☑
        index S68.61- ☑
        little S68.61- ☑
        middle S68.61- ☑
        partial S68.62- ☑
          index S68.62- ☑
          little S68.62- ☑
          middle S68.62- ☑
          ring S68.62- ☑
        ring S68.61- ☑
    foot (complete) S98.91- ☑
      at ankle level S98.01- ☑
        partial S98.02- ☑
      midfoot S98.31- ☑
        partial S98.32- ☑
      partial S98.92- ☑
    forearm (complete) S58.91- ☑
      at elbow level (complete) S58.01- ☑
        partial S58.02- ☑
      between elbow and wrist (complete) S58.11- ☑
        partial S58.12- ☑
      partial S58.92- ☑
    genital organ(s) (external)
      female (complete) S38.211 ☑
        partial S38.212 ☑
      male
        penis (complete) S38.221 ☑
          partial S38.222 ☑
        scrotum (complete) S38.231 ☑
          partial S38.232 ☑
        testes (complete) S38.231 ☑
          partial S38.232 ☑
    hand (complete) (wrist level) S68.41- ☑
      finger(s) alone — *see* Amputation, traumatic, finger
      partial S68.42- ☑
      thumb alone — *see* Amputation, traumatic, thumb
      transmetacarpal (complete) S68.71- ☑
        partial S68.72- ☑
    head
      ear — *see* Amputation, traumatic, ear
      nose (partial) S08.812 ☑
        complete S08.811 ☑
      part S08.89 ☑
        scalp S08.0 ☑
    hip (and thigh) (complete) S78.91- ☑
      at hip joint (complete) S78.01- ☑
        partial S78.02- ☑
      between hip and knee (complete) S78.11- ☑
        partial S78.12- ☑
      partial S78.92- ☑
    labium (majus) (minus) (complete) S38.21- ☑
      partial S38.21- ☑
    leg (lower) S88.91- ☑
      at knee level S88.01- ☑
        partial S88.02- ☑
      between knee and ankle S88.11- ☑
        partial S88.12- ☑
      partial S88.92- ☑
    nose (partial) S08.812 ☑
      complete S08.811 ☑
    penis (complete) S38.221 ☑
      partial S38.222 ☑
    scrotum (complete) S38.231 ☑
      partial S38.232 ☑
    shoulder — *see* Amputation, traumatic, arm
      at shoulder joint — *see* Amputation, traumatic, arm, at shoulder joint
    testes (complete) S38.231 ☑
      partial S38.232 ☑
    thigh — *see* Amputation, traumatic, hip

**Index** *(side tab)*

**Amputation** — *continued*
  traumatic — *continued*
    thorax, part of S28.1 ☑
      breast — *see* Amputation, traumatic, breast
    thumb (complete) (metacarpophalangeal)
        S68.01- ☑
      partial S68.02- ☑
      transphalangeal (complete) S68.51- ☑
        partial S68.52- ☑
    toe (lesser) S98.13- ☑
      great S98.11- ☑
        partial S98.12- ☑
      more than one S98.21- ☑
        partial S98.22- ☑
      partial S98.14- ☑
    vulva (complete) S38.211 ☑
      partial S38.212 ☑
**Amputee** (bilateral) (old) Z89.9
**Amsterdam dwarfism** Q87.1
**Amusia** R48.8
  developmental F80.89
**Amyelencephalus, amyelencephaly** Q00.0
**Amyelia** Q06.0
**Amygdalitis** — *see* Tonsillitis
**Amygdalolith** J35.8
**Amyloid heart** (disease) E85.4 [I43]
**Amyloidosis** (generalized) (primary) E85.9
  with lung involvement E85.4 [J99]
  familial E85.2
  genetic E85.2
  heart E85.4 [I43]
  hemodialysis-associated E85.3
  light chain (AL) E85.81
  liver E85.4 [K77]
  localized E85.4
  neuropathic heredofamilial E85.1
  non-neuropathic heredofamilial E85.0
  organ limited E85.4
  Portuguese E85.1
  pulmonary E85.4 [J99]
  secondary systemic E85.3
  senile systemic (SSA) E85.82
  skin (lichen) (macular) E85.4 [L99]
  specified NEC E85.89
  subglottic E85.4 [J99]
  wild-type transthyretin-related (ATTR) E85.82
**Amylopectinosis** (brancher enzyme deficiency) E74.03
**Amylophagia** — *see* Pica
**Amyoplasia congenita** Q79.8
**Amyotonia** M62.89
  congenita G70.2
**Amyotrophia, amyotrophy, amyotrophic** G71.8
  congenita Q79.8
  diabetic — *see* Diabetes, amyotrophy
  lateral sclerosis G12.21
  neuralgic G54.5
  spinal progressive G12.25
**Anacidity, gastric** K31.83
  psychogenic F45.8
**Anaerosis of newborn** P28.89
**Analbuminemia** E88.09
**Analgesia** — *see* Anesthesia
**Analphalipoproteinemia** E78.6
**Anaphylactic**
  purpura D69.0
  shock or reaction — *see* Shock, anaphylactic
**Anaphylactoid shock or reaction** — *see* Shock, anaphylactic
**Anaphylactoid syndrome of pregnancy** O88.01- ☑
**Anaphylaxis** — *see* Shock, anaphylactic
**Anaplasia cervix** (see also Dysplasia, cervix) N87.9
**Anaplasmosis, human** A77.49
**Anarthria** R47.1
**Anasarca** R60.1
  cardiac — *see* Failure, heart, congestive
  lung J18.2
  newborn P83.2
  nutritional E43
  pulmonary J18.2
  renal N04.9
**Anastomosis**
  aneurysmal — *see* Aneurysm
  arteriovenous ruptured brain I60.8
  intestinal K63.89
    complicated NEC K91.89
      involving urinary tract N99.89
  retinal and choroidal vessels (congenital) Q14.8

**Anatomical narrow angle** H40.03- ☑
**Ancylostoma, ancylostomiasis** (braziliense) (caninum)
    (ceylanicum) (duodenale) B76.0
  Necator americanus B76.1
**Andersen's disease** (glycogen storage) E74.09
**Anderson-Fabry disease** E75.21
**Andes disease** T70.29 ☑
**Andrews' disease** (bacterid) L08.89
**Androblastoma**
  benign
    specified site — *see* Neoplasm, benign, by site
    unspecified site
      female D27.9
      male D29.20
  malignant
    specified site — *see* Neoplasm, malignant, by site
    unspecified site
      female C56.9
      male C62.90
  specified site — *see* Neoplasm, uncertain behavior,
    by site
  tubular
    with lipid storage
      specified site — *see* Neoplasm, benign, by site
      unspecified site
        female D27.9
        male D29.20
    specified site — *see* Neoplasm, benign, by site
    unspecified site
      female D27.9
      male D29.20
  unspecified site
    female D39.10
    male D40.10
**Androgen insensitivity syndrome** (see also Syndrome,
    androgen insensitivity) E34.50
**Androgen resistance syndrome** (see also Syndrome,
    androgen insensitivity) E34.50
**Android pelvis** Q74.2
  with disproportion (fetopelvic) O33.3 ☑
    causing obstructed labor O65.3
**Androphobia** F40.290
**Anectasis, pulmonary** (newborn) — *see* Atelectasis
**Anemia** (essential) (general) (hemoglobin deficiency)
    (infantile) (primary) (profound) D64.9
  with (due to) (in)
    disorder of
      anaerobic glycolysis D55.2
      pentose phosphate pathway D55.1
    koilonychia D50.9
  achlorhydric D50.8
  achrestic D53.1
  Addison (-Biermer) (pernicious) D51.0
  agranulocytic — *see* Agranulocytosis
  amino-acid-deficiency D53.0
  aplastic D61.9
    congenital D61.09
    drug-induced D61.1
    due to
      drugs D61.1
      external agents NEC D61.2
      infection D61.2
      radiation D61.2
    idiopathic D61.3
    red cell (pure) D60.9
      chronic D60.0
      congenital D61.01
      specified type NEC D60.8
      transient D60.1
    specified type NEC D61.89
    toxic D61.2
  aregenerative
    congenital D61.09
  asiderotic D50.9
  atypical (primary) D64.9
  Baghdad spring D55.0
  Balantidium coli A07.0
  Biermer's (pernicious) D51.0
  blood loss (chronic) D50.0
    acute D62
  bothriocephalus B70.0 [D63.8]
  brickmaker's B76.9 [D63.8]
  cerebral I67.89
  childhood D58.9
  chlorotic D50.8
  chronic
    blood loss D50.0
    hemolytic D58.9

**Anemia** — *continued*
  chronic — *continued*
    hemolytic — *continued*
      idiopathic D59.9
    simple D53.9
  chronica congenita aregenerativa D61.09
  combined system disease NEC D51.0 [G32.0]
    due to dietary vitamin B12 deficiency D51.3 [G32.0]
  complicating pregnancy, childbirth or puerperium —
    *see* Pregnancy, complicated by (management
    affected by), anemia
  congenital P61.4
    aplastic D61.09
    due to isoimmunization NOS P55.9
    dyserythropoietic, dyshematopoietic D64.4
    following fetal blood loss P61.3
    Heinz body D58.2
    hereditary hemolytic NOS D58.9
    pernicious D51.0
    spherocytic D58.0
  Cooley's (erythroblastic) D56.1
  cytogenic D51.0
  deficiency D53.9
    6-PGD D55.1
    2, 3 diphosphoglycurate mutase D55.2
    2, 3 PG D55.2
    6 phosphogluconate dehydrogenase D55.1
    amino-acid D53.0
    combined B12 and folate D53.1
    enzyme D55.9
      drug-induced (hemolytic) D59.2
      glucose-6-phosphate dehydrogenase (G6PD)
        D55.0
      glycolytic D55.2
      nucleotide metabolism D55.3
      related to hexose monophosphate (HMP) shunt
        pathway NEC D55.1
      specified type NEC D55.8
    erythrocytic glutathione D55.1
    folate D52.9
      dietary D52.0
      drug-induced D52.1
    folic acid D52.9
      dietary D52.0
      drug-induced D52.1
    G SH D55.1
    G6PD D55.0
    GGS-R D55.1
    glucose-6-phosphate dehydrogenase D55.0
    glutathione reductase D55.1
    glyceraldehyde phosphate dehydrogenase D55.2
    hexokinase D55.2
    iron D50.9
      secondary to blood loss (chronic) D50.0
    nutritional D53.9
      with
        poor iron absorption D50.8
        specified deficiency NEC D53.8
    phosphofructo-aldolase D55.2
    phosphoglycerate kinase D55.2
    PK D55.2
    protein D53.0
    pyruvate kinase D55.2
    transcobalamin II D51.2
    triose-phosphate isomerase D55.2
    vitamin B12 NOS D51.9
      dietary D51.3
      due to
        intrinsic factor deficiency D51.0
        selective vitamin B12 malabsorption with
          proteinuria D51.1
      pernicious D51.0
      specified type NEC D51.8
  Diamond-Blackfan (congenital hypoplastic) D61.01
  dibothriocephalus B70.0 [D63.8]
  dimorphic D53.1
  diphasic D53.1
  Diphyllobothrium (Dibothriocephalus) B70.0 [D63.8]
  due to (in) (with)
    antineoplastic chemotherapy D64.81
    blood loss (chronic) D50.0
      acute D62
    chemotherapy, antineoplastic D64.81
    chronic disease classified elsewhere NEC D63.8
    chronic kidney disease D63.1
    deficiency
      amino-acid D53.0
      copper D53.8
      folate (folic acid) D52.9

☑ **Additional Character Required** — Refer to the Tabular List for Character Selection    ▽ Subterms under main terms may continue to next column or page

**Amputation — Anemia** *(side tab)*

**Anemia** — *continued*
  due to — *continued*
    deficiency — *continued*
      folate — *continued*
        dietary D52.0
        drug-induced D52.1
      molybdenum D53.8
      protein D53.0
      zinc D53.8
    dietary vitamin B12 deficiency D51.3
    disorder of
      glutathione metabolism D55.1
      nucleotide metabolism D55.3
    drug — *see* Anemia, by type (*see also* Table of Drugs and Chemicals)
    end stage renal disease D63.1
    enzyme disorder D55.9
    fetal blood loss P61.3
    fish tapeworm (D.latum) infestation B70.0 [D63.8]
    hemorrhage (chronic) D50.0
      acute D62
    impaired absorption D50.9
    loss of blood (chronic) D50.0
      acute D62
    myxedema E03.9 [D63.8]
    Necator americanus B76.1 [D63.8]
    prematurity P61.2
    selective vitamin B12 malabsorption with proteinuria D51.1
    transcobalamin II deficiency D51.2
  Dyke-Young type (secondary) (symptomatic) D59.1
  dyserythropoietic (congenital) D64.4
  dyshematopoietic (congenital) D64.4
  Egyptian B76.9 [D63.8]
  elliptocytosis — *see* Elliptocytosis
  enzyme-deficiency, drug-induced D59.2
  epidemic (*see also* Ancylostomiasis) B76.9 [D63.8]
  erythroblastic
    familial D56.1
    newborn (*see also* Disease, hemolytic) P55.9
    of childhood D56.1
  erythrocytic glutathione deficiency D55.1
  erythropoietin-resistant anemia (EPO resistant anemia) D63.1
  Faber's (achlorhydric anemia) D50.9
  factitious (self-induced blood letting) D50.0
  familial erythroblastic D56.1
  Fanconi's (congenital pancytopenia) D61.09
  favism D55.0
  fish tapeworm (D. latum) infestation B70.0 [D63.8]
  folate (folic acid) deficiency D52.9
  glucose-6-phosphate dehydrogenase (G6PD) deficiency D55.0
  glutathione-reductase deficiency D55.1
  goat's milk D52.0
  granulocytic — *see* Agranulocytosis
  Heinz body, congenital D58.2
  hemolytic D58.9
    acquired D59.9
      with hemoglobinuria NEC D59.6
      autoimmune NEC D59.1
      infectious D59.4
      specified type NEC D59.8
      toxic D59.4
    acute D59.9
      due to enzyme deficiency specified type NEC D55.8
      Lederer's D59.1
    autoimmune D59.1
      drug-induced D59.0
    chronic D58.9
      idiopathic D59.9
    cold type (secondary) (symptomatic) D59.1
    congenital (spherocytic) — *see* Spherocytosis
    due to
      cardiac conditions D59.4
      drugs (nonautoimmune) D59.2
        autoimmune D59.1
      enzyme disorder D55.9
        drug-induced D59.2
      presence of shunt or other internal prosthetic device D59.4
    familial D58.9
    hereditary D58.9
      due to enzyme disorder D55.9
        specified type NEC D55.8
      specified type NEC D58.8
    idiopathic (chronic) D59.9
    mechanical D59.4

**Anemia** — *continued*
  hemolytic — *continued*
    microangiopathic D59.4
    nonautoimmune D59.4
      drug-induced D59.2
    nonspherocytic
      congenital or hereditary NEC D55.8
        glucose-6-phosphate dehydrogenase deficiency D55.0
        pyruvate kinase deficiency D55.2
        type
          I D55.1
          II D55.2
      type
        I D55.1
        II D55.2
    secondary D59.4
      autoimmune D59.1
    specified (hereditary) type NEC D58.8
    Stransky-Regala type (*see also* Hemoglobinopathy) D58.8
    symptomatic D59.4
      autoimmune D59.1
    toxic D59.4
    warm type (secondary) (symptomatic) D59.1
  hemorrhagic (chronic) D50.0
    acute D62
  Herrick's D57.1
  hexokinase deficiency D55.2
  hookworm B76.9 [D63.8]
  hypochromic (idiopathic) (microcytic) (normoblastic) D50.9
    due to blood loss (chronic) D50.0
      acute D62
    familial sex-linked D64.0
    pyridoxine-responsive D64.3
    sideroblastic, sex-linked D64.0
  hypoplasia, red blood cells D61.9
    congenital or familial D61.01
  hypoplastic (idiopathic) D61.9
    congenital or familial (of childhood) D61.01
  hypoproliferative (refractive) D61.9
  idiopathic D64.9
    aplastic D61.3
    hemolytic, chronic D59.9
  in (due to) (with)
    chronic kidney disease D63.1
    end stage renal disease D63.1
    failure, kidney (renal) D63.1
    neoplastic disease (*see also* Neoplasm) D63.0
  intertropical (*see also* Ancylostomiasis) D63.8
  iron deficiency D50.9
    secondary to blood loss (chronic) D50.0
      acute D62
    specified type NEC D50.8
  Joseph-Diamond-Blackfan (congenital hypoplastic) D61.01
  Lederer's (hemolytic) D59.1
  leukoerythroblastic D61.82
  macrocytic D53.9
    nutritional D52.0
    tropical D52.8
  malarial (*see also* Malaria) B54 [D63.8]
  malignant (progressive) D51.0
  malnutrition D53.9
  marsh (*see also* Malaria) B54 [D63.8]
  Mediterranean (with other hemoglobinopathy) D56.9
  megaloblastic D53.1
    combined B12 and folate deficiency D53.1
    hereditary D51.1
    nutritional D52.0
    orotic aciduria D53.0
    refractory D53.1
    specified type NEC D53.1
  megalocytic D53.1
  microcytic (hypochromic) D50.9
    due to blood loss (chronic) D50.0
      acute D62
    familial D56.8
  microdrepanocytosis D57.40
  microelliptopoikilocytic (Rietti-Greppi- Micheli) D56.9
  miner's B76.9 [D63.8]
  myelodysplastic D46.9
  myelofibrosis D75.81
  myelogenous D64.89
  myelopathic D64.89
  myelophthisic D61.82
  myeloproliferative D47.Z9 (*following* D47.4)
  newborn P61.4

**Anemia** — *continued*
  newborn — *continued*
    due to
      ABO (antibodies, isoimmunization, maternal/fetal incompatibility) P55.1
      Rh (antibodies, isoimmunization, maternal/fetal incompatibility) P55.0
    following fetal blood loss P61.3
    posthemorrhagic (fetal) P61.3
    nonspherocytic hemolytic — *see* Anemia, hemolytic, nonspherocytic
  normocytic (infectional) D64.9
    due to blood loss (chronic) D50.0
      acute D62
    myelophthisic D61.82
  nutritional (deficiency) D53.9
    with
      poor iron absorption D50.8
      specified deficiency NEC D53.8
    megaloblastic D52.0
  of prematurity P61.2
  orotaciduric (congenital) (hereditary) D53.0
  osteosclerotic D64.89
  ovalocytosis (hereditary) — *see* Elliptocytosis
  paludal (*see also* Malaria) B54 [D63.8]
  pernicious (congenital) (malignant) (progressive) D51.0
  pleochromic D64.89
    of sprue D52.8
  posthemorrhagic (chronic) D50.0
    acute D62
    newborn P61.3
  postoperative (postprocedural)
    due to (acute) blood loss D62
      chronic blood loss D50.0
    specified NEC D64.9
  postpartum O90.81
  pressure D64.89
  progressive D64.9
    malignant D51.0
    pernicious D51.0
  protein-deficiency D53.0
  pseudoleukemica infantum D64.89
  pure red cell D60.9
    congenital D61.01
  pyridoxine-responsive D64.3
  pyruvate kinase deficiency D55.2
  refractory D46.4
    with
      excess of blasts D46.20
        1 (RAEB 1) D46.21
        2 (RAEB 2) D46.22
        in transformation (RAEB T) — *see* Leukemia, acute myeloblastic
      hemochromatosis D46.1
      sideroblasts (ring) (RARS) D46.1
    without ring sideroblasts, so stated D46.0
    without sideroblasts without excess of blasts D46.0
    megaloblastic D53.1
    sideroblastic D46.1
    sideropenic D50.9
  Rietti-Greppi-Micheli D56.9
  scorbutic D53.2
  secondary to
    blood loss (chronic) D50.0
      acute D62
    hemorrhage (chronic) D50.0
      acute D62
  semiplastic D61.89
  sickle-cell — *see* Disease, sickle-cell
  sideroblastic D64.3
    hereditary D64.0
    hypochromic, sex-linked D64.0
    pyridoxine-responsive NEC D64.3
    refractory D46.1
    secondary (due to)
      disease D64.1
      drugs and toxins D64.2
    specified type NEC D64.3
  sideropenic (refractory) D50.9
    due to blood loss (chronic) D50.0
      acute D62
  simple chronic D53.9
  specified type NEC D64.89
  spherocytic (hereditary) — *see* Spherocytosis
  splenic D64.89
  splenomegalic D64.89
  stomatocytosis D58.8
  syphilitic (acquired) (late) A52.79 [D63.8]
  target cell D64.89

**Anemia** — *continued*
  thalassemia D56.9
  thrombocytopenic — *see* Thrombocytopenia
  toxic D61.2
  tropical B76.9 [D63.8]
    macrocytic D52.8
  tuberculous A18.89 [D63.8]
  vegan D51.3
  vitamin
    B6-responsive D64.3
    B12 deficiency (dietary) pernicious D51.0
  von Jaksch's D64.89
  Witts' (achlorhydric anemia) D50.8
**Anemophobia** F40.228
**Anencephalus, anencephaly** Q00.0
**Anergasia** — *see* Psychosis, organic
**Anesthesia, anesthetic** R20.0
  complication or reaction NEC (*see also* Complications, anesthesia) T88.59 ☑
    due to
      correct substance properly administered — *see* Table of Drugs and Chemicals, by drug, adverse effect
      overdose or wrong substance given — *see* Table of Drugs and Chemicals, by drug, poisoning
    unintended awareness under general anesthesia during procedure T88.53 ☑
      personal history of Z92.84
  cornea H18.81- ☑
  dissociative F44.6
  functional (hysterical) F44.6
  hyperesthetic, thalamic G89.0
  hysterical F44.6
  local skin lesion R20.0
  sexual (psychogenic) F52.1
  shock (due to) T88.2 ☑
  skin R20.0
  testicular N50.9
**Anetoderma** (maculosum) (of) L90.8
  Jadassohn-Pellizzari L90.2
  Schweniger-Buzzi L90.1
**Aneurin deficiency** E51.9
**Aneurysm** (anastomotic) (artery) (cirsoid) (diffuse) (false) (fusiform) (multiple) (saccular) I72.9
  abdominal (aorta) I71.4
    ruptured I71.3
    syphilitic A52.01
  aorta, aortic (nonsyphilitic) I71.9
    abdominal I71.4
      ruptured I71.3
    arch I71.2
      ruptured I71.1
    arteriosclerotic I71.9
      ruptured I71.8
    ascending I71.2
      ruptured I71.1
    congenital Q25.43
    descending I71.9
      abdominal I71.4
        ruptured I71.3
      ruptured I71.8
      thoracic I71.2
        ruptured I71.1
    root Q25.43
    ruptured I71.8
    sinus, congenital Q25.43
    syphilitic A52.01
    thoracic I71.2
      ruptured I71.1
    thoracoabdominal I71.6
      ruptured I71.5
    thorax, thoracic (arch) I71.2
      ruptured I71.1
    transverse I71.2
      ruptured I71.1
    valve (heart) (*see also* Endocarditis, aortic) I35.8
  arteriosclerotic I72.9
    cerebral I67.1
      ruptured — *see* Hemorrhage, intracranial, subarachnoid
  arteriovenous (congenital) (*see also* Malformation, arteriovenous)
    acquired I77.0
      brain I67.1
      coronary I25.41
      pulmonary I28.0
    brain Q28.2

**Aneurysm** — *continued*
  arteriovenous (*see also* Malformation, arteriovenous) — *continued*
    brain — *continued*
      ruptured I60.8
    peripheral — *see* Malformation, arteriovenous, peripheral
    precerebral vessels Q28.0
    specified site NEC (*see also* Malformation, arteriovenous)
      acquired I77.0
  basal — *see* Aneurysm, brain
  basilar (trunk) I72.5
  berry (congenital) (nonruptured) I67.1
    ruptured I60.7
  brain I67.1
    arteriosclerotic I67.1
      ruptured — *see* Hemorrhage, intracranial, subarachnoid
    arteriovenous (congenital) (nonruptured) Q28.2
      acquired I67.1
        ruptured I60.8
      ruptured I60.8
    berry (congenital) (nonruptured) I67.1
      ruptured (*see also* Hemorrhage, intracranial, subarachnoid) I60.7
    congenital Q28.3
      ruptured I60.7
    meninges I67.1
      ruptured I60.8
    miliary (congenital) (nonruptured) I67.1
      ruptured (*see also* Hemorrhage, intracranial, subarachnoid) I60.7
    mycotic I33.0
    ruptured — *see* Hemorrhage, intracranial, subarachnoid
    syphilitic (hemorrhage) A52.05
  cardiac (false) (*see also* Aneurysm, heart) I25.3
  carotid artery (common) (external) I72.0
    internal (intracranial) I67.1
      extracranial portion I72.0
    ruptured into brain I60.0- ☑
    syphilitic A52.09
      intracranial A52.05
  cavernous sinus I67.1
    arteriovenous (congenital) (nonruptured) Q28.3
      ruptured I60.8
  celiac I72.8
  central nervous system, syphilitic A52.05
  cerebral — *see* Aneurysm, brain
  chest — *see* Aneurysm, thorax
  circle of Willis I67.1
    congenital Q28.3
      ruptured I60.6
    ruptured I60.6
  common iliac artery I72.3
  congenital (peripheral) Q27.8
    aorta (root) (sinus) Q25.43
    brain Q28.3
      ruptured I60.7
    coronary Q24.5
    digestive system Q27.8
    lower limb Q27.8
    pulmonary Q25.79
    retina Q14.1
    specified site NEC Q27.8
    upper limb Q27.8
  conjunctiva — *see* Abnormality, conjunctiva, vascular
  conus arteriosus — *see* Aneurysm, heart
  coronary (arteriosclerotic) (artery) I25.41
    arteriovenous, congenital Q24.5
    congenital Q24.5
    ruptured — *see* Infarct, myocardium
    syphilitic A52.06
    vein I25.89
  cylindroid (aorta) I71.9
    ruptured I71.8
    syphilitic A52.01
  ductus arteriosus Q25.0
  endocardial, infective (any valve) I33.0
  femoral (artery) (ruptured) I72.4
  gastroduodenal I72.8
  gastroepiploic I72.8
  heart (wall) (chronic or with a stated duration of over 4 weeks) I25.3
    valve — *see* Endocarditis
  hepatic I72.8
  iliac (common) (artery) (ruptured) I72.3

**Aneurysm** — *continued*
  infective I72.9
    endocardial (any valve) I33.0
  innominate (nonsyphilitic) I72.8
    syphilitic A52.09
  interauricular septum — *see* Aneurysm, heart
  interventricular septum — *see* Aneurysm, heart
  intrathoracic (nonsyphilitic) I71.2
    ruptured I71.1
    syphilitic A52.01
  lower limb I72.4
  lung (pulmonary artery) I28.1
  mediastinal (nonsyphilitic) I72.8
    syphilitic A52.09
  miliary (congenital) I67.1
    ruptured — *see* Hemorrhage, intracerebral, subarachnoid, intracranial
  mitral (heart) (valve) I34.8
  mural — *see* Aneurysm, heart
  mycotic I72.9
    endocardial (any valve) I33.0
    ruptured, brain — *see* Hemorrhage, intracerebral, subarachnoid
  myocardium — *see* Aneurysm, heart
  neck I72.0
  pancreaticoduodenal I72.8
  patent ductus arteriosus Q25.0
  peripheral NEC I72.8
    congenital Q27.8
      digestive system Q27.8
      lower limb Q27.8
      specified site NEC Q27.8
      upper limb Q27.8
  popliteal (artery) (ruptured) I72.4
  precerebral
    congenital (nonruptured) Q28.1
    specified site, NEC I72.5
  pulmonary I28.1
    arteriovenous Q25.72
      acquired I28.0
    syphilitic A52.09
    valve (heart) — *see* Endocarditis, pulmonary
  racemose (peripheral) I72.9
    congenital — *see* Aneurysm, congenital
  radial I72.1
  Rasmussen NEC A15.0
  renal (artery) I72.2
  retina (*see also* Disorder, retina, microaneurysms)
    congenital Q14.1
    diabetic — *see* Diabetes, microaneurysms, retinal
  sinus of Valsalva Q25.49
  specified NEC I72.8
  spinal (cord) I72.8
    syphilitic (hemorrhage) A52.09
  splenic I72.8
  subclavian (artery) (ruptured) I72.8
    syphilitic A52.09
  superior mesenteric I72.8
  syphilitic (aorta) A52.01
    central nervous system A52.05
    congenital (late) A50.54 [I79.0]
    spine, spinal A52.09
  thoracoabdominal (aorta) I71.6
    ruptured I71.5
    syphilitic A52.01
  thorax, thoracic (aorta) (arch) (nonsyphilitic) I71.2
    ruptured I71.1
    syphilitic A52.01
  traumatic (complication) (early), specified site — *see* Injury, blood vessel
  tricuspid (heart) (valve) I07.8
  ulnar I72.1
  upper limb (ruptured) I72.1
  valve, valvular — *see* Endocarditis
  venous (*see also* Varix) I86.8
    congenital Q27.8
      digestive system Q27.8
      lower limb Q27.8
      specified site NEC Q27.8
      upper limb Q27.8
  ventricle — *see* Aneurysm, heart
  vertebral artery I72.6
  visceral NEC I72.8
**Angelman syndrome** Q93.5
**Anger** R45.4
**Angiectasis, angiectopia** I99.8
**Angiitis** I77.6
  allergic granulomatous M30.1

| | |
|---|---|

**Angiitis** — *continued*
  hypersensitivity M31.0
  necrotizing M31.9
    specified NEC M31.8
  nervous system, granulomatous I67.7
**Angina** (attack) (cardiac) (chest) (heart) (pectoris) (syn-
    drome) (vasomotor) I20.9
  with
    atherosclerotic heart disease — *see* Arteriosclerosis,
      coronary (artery),
      documented spasm I20.1
  abdominal K55.1
  accelerated — *see* Angina, unstable
  agranulocytic — *see* Agranulocytosis
  angiospastic — *see* Angina, with documented spasm
  aphthous B08.5
  crescendo — *see* Angina, unstable
  croupous J05.0
  cruris I73.9
  de novo effort — *see* Angina, unstable
  diphtheritic, membranous A36.0
  equivalent I20.8
  exudative, chronic J37.0
  following acute myocardial infarction I23.7
  gangrenous diphtheritic A36.0
  intestinal K55.1
  Ludovici K12.2
  Ludwig's K12.2
  malignant diphtheritic A36.0
  membranous J05.0
    diphtheritic A36.0
    Vincent's A69.1
  mesenteric K55.1
  monocytic — *see* Mononucleosis, infectious
  of effort — *see* Angina, specified NEC
  phlegmonous J36
    diphtheritic A36.0
  post-infarctional I23.7
  pre-infarctional I23.7
  Prinzmetal — *see* Angina, with documented spasm
  progressive — *see* Angina, unstable
  pseudomembranous A69.1
  pultaceous, diphtheritic A36.0
  spasm-induced — *see* Angina, with documented
      spasm
  specified NEC I20.8
  stable I20.8
  stenocardia — *see* Angina, specified NEC
  stridulous, diphtheritic A36.2
  tonsil J36
  trachealis J05.0
  unstable I20.0
  variant — *see* Angina, with documented spasm
  Vincent's A69.1
  worsening effort — *see* Angina, unstable
**Angioblastoma** — *see* Neoplasm, connective tissue,
    uncertain behavior
**Angiocholecystitis** — *see* Cholecystitis, acute
**Angiocholitis** (*see also* Cholecystitis, acute) K83.0
**Angiodysgenesis spinalis** G95.19
**Angiodysplasia** (cecum) (colon) K55.20
  with bleeding K55.21
  duodenum (and stomach) K31.819
    with bleeding K31.811
  stomach (and duodenum) K31.819
    with bleeding K31.811
**Angioedema** (allergic) (any site) (with urticaria) T78.3 ☑
  hereditary D84.1
**Angioendothelioma** — *see* Neoplasm, uncertain behav-
    ior, by site
  benign D18.00
    intra-abdominal D18.03
    intracranial D18.02
    skin D18.01
    specified site NEC D18.09
  bone — *see* Neoplasm, bone, malignant
  Ewing's — *see* Neoplasm, bone, malignant
**Angioendotheliomatosis** C85.8-
**Angiofibroma** (*see also* Neoplasm, benign, by site)
  juvenile
    specified site — *see* Neoplasm, benign, by site
    unspecified site D10.6
**Angiohemophilia** (A) (B) D68.0
**Angioid streaks** (choroid) (macula) (retina) H35.33
**Angiokeratoma** — *see* Neoplasm, skin, benign
  corporis diffusum E75.21
**Angioleiomyoma** — *see* Neoplasm, connective tissue,
    benign

**Angiolipoma** (*see also* Lipoma)
  infiltrating — *see* Lipoma
**Angioma** (*see also* Hemangioma, by site)
  capillary I78.1
  hemorrhagicum hereditaria I78.0
  intra-abdominal D18.03
  intracranial D18.02
  malignant — *see* Neoplasm, connective tissue, malig-
    nant
  plexiform D18.00
    intra-abdominal D18.03
    intracranial D18.02
    skin D18.01
    specified site NEC D18.09
  senile I78.1
  serpiginosum L81.7
  skin D18.01
  specified site NEC D18.09
  spider I78.1
  stellate I78.1
  venous Q28.3
**Angiomatosis** Q82.8
  bacillary A79.89
  encephalotrigeminal Q85.8
  hemorrhagic familial I78.0
  hereditary familial I78.0
  liver K76.4
**Angiomyolipoma** — *see* Lipoma
**Angiomyoliposarcoma** — *see* Neoplasm, connective
    tissue, malignant
**Angiomyoma** — *see* Neoplasm, connective tissue, be-
    nign
**Angiomyosarcoma** — *see* Neoplasm, connective tissue,
    malignant
**Angiomyxoma** — *see* Neoplasm, connective tissue, un-
    certain behavior
**Angioneurosis** F45.8
**Angioneurotic edema** (allergic) (any site) (with urticaria)
    T78.3 ☑
  hereditary D84.1
**Angiopathia, angiopathy** I99.9
  cerebral I67.9
    amyloid E85.4 [I68.0]
  diabetic (peripheral) — *see* Diabetes, angiopathy
  peripheral I73.9
    diabetic — *see* Diabetes, angiopathy
    specified type NEC I73.89
  retinae syphilitica A52.05
  retinalis (juvenilis)
    diabetic — *see* Diabetes, retinopathy
    proliferative — *see* Retinopathy, proliferative
**Angiosarcoma** (*see also* Neoplasm, connective tissue,
    malignant)
  liver C22.3
**Angiosclerosis** — *see* Arteriosclerosis
**Angiospasm** (peripheral) (traumatic) (vessel) I73.9
  brachial plexus G54.0
  cerebral G45.9
  cervical plexus G54.2
  nerve
    arm — *see* Mononeuropathy, upper limb
      axillary G54.0
      median — *see* Lesion, nerve, median
      ulnar — *see* Lesion, nerve, ulnar
    axillary G54.0
    leg — *see* Mononeuropathy, lower limb
    median — *see* Lesion, nerve, median
    plantar — *see* Lesion, nerve, plantar
    ulnar — *see* Lesion, nerve, ulnar
**Angiospastic disease or edema** I73.9
**Angiostrongyliasis**
  due to
    Parastrongylus
      cantonensis B83.2
      costaricensis B81.3
    intestinal B81.3
**Anguillulosis** — *see* Strongyloidiasis
**Angulation**
  cecum — *see* Obstruction, intestine
  coccyx (acquired) (*see also* subcategory) M43.8 ☑
    congenital NEC Q76.49
  femur (acquired) (*see also* Deformity, limb, specified
    type NEC, thigh)
    congenital Q74.2
  intestine (large) (small) — *see* Obstruction, intestine
  sacrum (acquired) (*see also* subcategory) M43.8 ☑
    congenital NEC Q76.49
  sigmoid (flexure) — *see* Obstruction, intestine

**Angulation** — *continued*
  spine — *see* Dorsopathy, deforming, specified NEC
  tibia (acquired) (*see also* Deformity, limb, specified
      type NEC, lower leg)
    congenital Q74.2
  ureter N13.5
    with infection N13.6
  wrist (acquired) (*see also* Deformity, limb, specified
      type NEC, forearm)
    congenital Q74.2
**Angulus infectiosus** (lips) K13.0
**Anhedonia** R45.84
  sexual F52.0
**Anhidrosis** L74.4
**Anhydration** E86.0
**Anhydremia** E86.0
**Anidrosis** L74.4
**Aniridia** (congenital) Q13.1
**Anisakiasis** (infection) (infestation) B81.0
**Anisakis larvae infestation** B81.0
**Aniseikonia** H52.32
**Anisocoria** (pupil) H57.02
  congenital Q13.2
**Anisocytosis** R71.8
**Anisometropia** (congenital) H52.31
**Ankle** — *see* condition
**Ankyloblepharon** (eyelid) (acquired) (*see also* Ble-
    pharophimosis)
  filiforme (adnatum) (congenital) Q10.3
  total Q10.3
**Ankyloglossia** Q38.1
**Ankylosis** (fibrous) (osseous) (joint) M24.60
  ankle M24.67- ☑
  arthrodesis status Z98.1
  cricoarytenoid (cartilage) (joint) (larynx) J38.7
  dental K03.5
  ear ossicles H74.31- ☑
  elbow M24.62- ☑
  foot M24.67- ☑
  hand M24.64- ☑
  hip M24.65- ☑
  incostapedial joint (infectional) — *see* Ankylosis, ear
    ossicles
  jaw (temporomandibular) M26.61- ☑
  knee M24.66- ☑
  lumbosacral (joint) M43.27
  postoperative (status) Z98.1
  produced by surgical fusion, status Z98.1
  sacro-iliac (joint) M43.28
  shoulder M24.61- ☑
  spine (joint) (*see also* Fusion, spine)
    spondylitic — *see* Spondylitis, ankylosing
  surgical Z98.1
  temporomandibular M26.61- ☑
  tooth, teeth (hard tissues) K03.5
  wrist M24.63- ☑
**Ankylostoma** — *see* Ancylostoma
**Ankylostomiasis** — *see* Ancylostomiasis
**Ankylurethria** — *see* Stricture, urethra
**Annular** (*see also* condition)
  detachment, cervix N88.8
  organ or site, congenital NEC — *see* Distortion
  pancreas (congenital) Q45.1
**Anodontia** (complete) (partial) (vera) K00.0
  acquired K08.10 ☑
**Anomaly, anomalous** (congenital) (unspecified type)
    Q89.9
  abdominal wall NEC Q79.59
  acoustic nerve Q07.8
  adrenal (gland) Q89.1
  Alder (-Reilly) (leukocyte granulation) D72.0
  alimentary tract Q45.9
    upper Q40.9
  alveolar M26.70
    hyperplasia M26.79
      mandibular M26.72
      maxillary M26.71
    hypoplasia M26.79
      mandibular M26.74
      maxillary M26.73
    ridge (process) M26.79
    specified NEC M26.79
  ankle (joint) Q74.2
  anus Q43.9
  aorta (arch) NEC Q25.40
    coarctation (preductal) (postductal) Q25.1
  aortic cusp or valve Q23.9

**Anomaly, anomalous** — *continued*
  appendix Q43.8
  apple peel syndrome Q41.1
  aqueduct of Sylvius Q03.0
    with spina bifida — *see* Spina bifida, with hydrocephalus
  arm Q74.0
  arteriovenous NEC
    coronary Q24.5
    gastrointestinal Q27.33
      acquired — *see* Angiodysplasia
  artery (peripheral) Q27.9
    basilar NEC Q28.1
    cerebral Q28.3
    coronary Q24.5
    digestive system Q27.8
    eye Q15.8
    great Q25.9
      specified NEC Q25.8
    lower limb Q27.8
    peripheral Q27.9
      specified NEC Q27.8
    pulmonary NEC Q25.79
    renal Q27.2
    retina Q14.1
    specified site NEC Q27.8
    subclavian Q27.8
      origin Q25.48
    umbilical Q27.0
    upper limb Q27.8
    vertebral NEC Q28.1
  aryteno-epiglottic folds Q31.8
  atrial
    bands or folds Q20.8
    septa Q21.1
  atrioventricular
    excitation I45.6
    septum Q21.0
  auditory canal Q17.8
  auricle
    ear Q17.8
      causing impairment of hearing Q16.9
    heart Q20.8
  Axenfeld's Q15.0
  back Q89.9
  band
    atrial Q20.8
    heart Q24.8
    ventricular Q24.8
  Bartholin's duct Q38.4
  biliary duct or passage Q44.5
  bladder Q64.70
    absence Q64.5
    diverticulum Q64.6
    exstrophy Q64.10
      cloacal Q64.12
      extroversion Q64.19
      specified type NEC Q64.19
      supravesical fissure Q64.11
    neck obstruction Q64.31
    specified type NEC Q64.79
  bone Q79.9
    arm Q74.0
    face Q75.9
    leg Q74.2
    pelvic girdle Q74.2
    shoulder girdle Q74.0
    skull Q75.9
      with
        anencephaly Q00.0
        encephalocele — *see* Encephalocele
        hydrocephalus Q03.9
          with spina bifida — *see* Spina bifida, by site, with hydrocephalus
        microcephaly Q02
  brain (multiple) Q04.9
    vessel Q28.3
  breast Q83.9
  broad ligament Q50.6
  bronchus Q32.4
  bulbus cordis Q21.9
  bursa Q79.9
  canal of Nuck Q52.4
  canthus Q10.3
  capillary Q27.9
  cardiac Q24.9
    chambers Q20.9
      specified NEC Q20.8
    septal closure Q21.9

**Anomaly, anomalous** — *continued*
  cardiac — *continued*
    septal closure — *continued*
      specified NEC Q21.8
    valve NEC Q24.8
      pulmonary Q22.3
  cardiovascular system Q28.8
  carpus Q74.0
  caruncle, lacrimal Q10.6
  cascade stomach Q40.2
  cauda equina Q06.3
  cecum Q43.9
  cerebral Q04.9
    vessels Q28.3
  cervix Q51.9
  Chédiak-Higashi (-Steinbrinck) (congenital gigantism of peroxidase granules) E70.330
  cheek Q18.9
  chest wall Q67.8
    bones Q76.9
  chin Q18.9
  chordae tendineae Q24.8
  choroid Q14.3
    plexus Q07.8
  chromosomes, chromosomal Q99.9
    D (1) — *see* condition, chromosome 13
    E (3) — *see* condition, chromosome 18
    G — *see* condition, chromosome 21
    sex
      female phenotype Q97.8
      gonadal dysgenesis (pure) Q99.1
      Klinefelter's Q98.4
      male phenotype Q98.9
      Turner's Q96.9
    specified NEC Q99.8
  cilia Q10.3
  circulatory system Q28.9
  clavicle Q74.0
  clitoris Q52.6
  coccyx Q76.49
  colon Q43.9
  common duct Q44.5
  communication
    coronary artery Q24.5
    left ventricle with right atrium Q21.0
  concha (ear) Q17.3
  connection
    portal vein Q26.5
    pulmonary venous Q26.4
      partial Q26.3
      total Q26.2
    renal artery with kidney Q27.2
  cornea (shape) Q13.4
  coronary artery or vein Q24.5
  cranium — *see* Anomaly, skull
  cricoid cartilage Q31.8
  cystic duct Q44.5
  dental
    alveolar — *see* Anomaly, alveolar
    arch relationship M26.20
      specified NEC M26.29
  dentofacial M26.9
    alveolar — *see* Anomaly, alveolar
    dental arch relationship M26.20
      specified NEC M26.29
    functional M26.50
      specified NEC M26.59
    jaw size M26.00
      macrogenia M26.05
      mandibular
        hyperplasia M26.03
        hypoplasia M26.04
      maxillary
        hyperplasia M26.01
        hypoplasia M26.02
      microgenia M26.06
      specified type NEC M26.09
    jaw-cranial base relationship M26.10
      asymmetry M26.12
        maxillary M26.11
      specified type NEC M26.19
    malocclusion M26.4
      dental arch relationship NEC M26.29
      jaw size — *see* Anomaly, dentofacial, jaw size
      jaw-cranial base relationship — *see* Anomaly, dentofacial, jaw-cranial base relationship
    specified type NEC M26.89
    temporomandibular joint M26.60- ☑

**Anomaly, anomalous** — *continued*
  dentofacial — *continued*
    temporomandibular joint — *continued*
      adhesions M26.61- ☑
      ankylosis M26.61- ☑
      arthralgia M26.62- ☑
      articular disc M26.63- ☑
      specified type NEC M26.69
    tooth position, fully erupted M26.30
    specified NEC M26.39
  dermatoglyphic Q82.8
  diaphragm (apertures) NEC Q79.1
  digestive organ(s) or tract Q45.9
    lower Q43.9
    upper Q40.9
  distance, interarch (excessive) (inadequate) M26.25
  distribution, coronary artery Q24.5
  ductus
    arteriosus Q25.0
    botalli Q25.0
  duodenum Q43.9
  dura (brain) Q04.9
    spinal cord Q06.9
  ear (external) Q17.9
    causing impairment of hearing Q16.9
    inner Q16.5
    middle (causing impairment of hearing) Q16.4
      ossicles Q16.3
  Ebstein's (heart) (tricuspid valve) Q22.5
  ectodermal Q82.9
  Eisenmenger's (ventricular septal defect) Q21.8
  ejaculatory duct Q55.4
  elbow Q74.0
  endocrine gland NEC Q89.2
  epididymis Q55.4
  epiglottis Q31.8
  esophagus Q39.9
  eustachian tube Q17.8
  eye Q15.9
    anterior segment Q13.9
      specified NEC Q13.89
    posterior segment Q14.9
      specified NEC Q14.8
    ptosis (eyelid) Q10.0
    specified NEC Q15.8
  eyebrow Q18.8
  eyelid Q10.3
    ptosis Q10.0
  face Q18.9
    bone(s) Q75.9
  fallopian tube Q50.6
  fascia Q79.9
  femur NEC Q74.2
  fibula NEC Q74.2
  finger Q74.0
  fixation, intestine Q43.3
  flexion (joint) NOS Q74.9
    hip or thigh Q65.89
  foot NEC Q74.2
    varus (congenital) Q66.3
  foramen
    Botalli Q21.1
    ovale Q21.1
  forearm Q74.0
  forehead Q75.8
  form, teeth K00.2
  fovea centralis Q14.1
  frontal bone — *see* Anomaly, skull
  gallbladder (position) (shape) (size) Q44.1
  Gartner's duct Q52.4
  gastrointestinal tract Q45.9
  genitalia, genital organ(s) or system
    female Q52.9
      external Q52.70
      internal NOS Q52.9
    male Q55.9
      hydrocele P83.5
      specified NEC Q55.8
  genitourinary NEC
    female Q52.9
    male Q55.9
  Gerbode Q21.0
  glottis Q31.8
  granulation or granulocyte, genetic (constitutional) (leukocyte) D72.0
  gum Q38.6
  gyri Q07.9
  hair Q84.2
  hand Q74.0

22

☑ Additional Character Required — Refer to the Tabular List for Character Selection    ▽ Subterms under main terms may continue to next column or page

**Anomaly, anomalous** — *continued*
 hard tissue formation in pulp K04.3
 head — *see* Anomaly, skull
 heart Q24.9
  auricle Q20.8
  bands or folds Q24.8
  fibroelastosis cordis I42.4
  obstructive NEC Q22.6
  patent ductus arteriosus (Botalli) Q25.0
  septum Q21.9
   auricular Q21.1
   interatrial Q21.1
   interventricular Q21.0
    with pulmonary stenosis or atresia, dextra-
     position of aorta and hypertrophy of
     right ventricle Q21.3
   specified NEC Q21.8
   ventricular Q21.0
    with pulmonary stenosis or atresia, dextra-
     position of aorta and hypertrophy of
     right ventricle Q21.3
  tetralogy of Fallot Q21.3
  valve NEC Q24.8
   aortic
    bicuspid valve Q23.1
    insufficiency Q23.1
    stenosis Q23.0
     subaortic Q24.4
   mitral
    insufficiency Q23.3
    stenosis Q23.2
   pulmonary Q22.3
    atresia Q22.0
    insufficiency Q22.2
    stenosis Q22.1
     infundibular Q24.3
     subvalvular Q24.3
   tricuspid
    atresia Q22.4
    stenosis Q22.4
  ventricle Q20.8
 heel NEC Q74.2
 Hegglin's D72.0
 hemianencephaly Q00.0
 hemicephaly Q00.0
 hemicrania Q00.0
 hepatic duct Q44.5
 hip NEC Q74.2
 hourglass stomach Q40.2
 humerus Q74.0
 hydatid of Morgagni
  female Q50.5
  male (epididymal) Q55.4
   testicular Q55.29
 hymen Q52.4
 hypersegmentation of neutrophils, hereditary D72.0
 hypophyseal Q89.2
 ileocecal (coil) (valve) Q43.9
 ileum Q43.9
 ilium NEC Q74.2
 integument Q84.9
  specified NEC Q84.8
 interarch distance (excessive) (inadequate) M26.25
 intervertebral cartilage or disc Q76.49
 intestine (large) (small) Q43.9
  with anomalous adhesions, fixation or malrotation
   Q43.3
 iris Q13.2
 ischium NEC Q74.2
 jaw — *see* Anomaly, dentofacial
  alveolar — *see* Anomaly, alveolar
 jaw-cranial base relationship — *see* Anomaly, dentofacial, jaw-cranial base relationship
 jejunum Q43.8
 joint Q74.9
  specified NEC Q74.8
 Jordan's D72.0
 kidney(s) (calyx) (pelvis) Q63.9
  artery Q27.2
  specified NEC Q63.8
 Klippel-Feil (brevicollis) Q76.1
 knee Q74.1
 labium (majus) (minus) Q52.70
 labyrinth, membranous Q16.5
 lacrimal apparatus or duct Q10.6
 larynx, laryngeal (muscle) Q31.9
  web (bed) Q31.0
 lens Q12.9
 leukocytes, genetic D72.0

**Anomaly, anomalous** — *continued*
 leukocytes, genetic — *continued*
  granulation (constitutional) D72.0
 lid (fold) Q10.3
 ligament Q79.9
  broad Q50.6
  round Q52.8
 limb Q74.9
  lower NEC Q74.2
   reduction deformity — *see* Defect, reduction,
    lower limb
  upper Q74.0
 lip Q38.0
 liver Q44.7
  duct Q44.5
 lower limb NEC Q74.2
 lumbosacral (joint) (region) Q76.49
  kyphosis — *see* Kyphosis, congenital
  lordosis — *see* Lordosis, congenital
 lung (fissure) (lobe) Q33.9
 mandible — *see* Anomaly, dentofacial
 maxilla — *see* Anomaly, dentofacial
 May (-Hegglin) D72.0
 meatus urinarius NEC Q64.79
 meningeal bands or folds Q07.9
  constriction of Q07.8
  spinal Q06.9
 meninges Q07.9
  cerebral Q04.8
  spinal Q06.9
 meningocele Q05.9
 mesentery Q45.9
 metacarpus Q74.0
 metatarsus NEC Q74.2
 middle ear Q16.4
  ossicles Q16.3
 mitral (leaflets) (valve) Q23.9
  insufficiency Q23.3
  specified NEC Q23.8
  stenosis Q23.2
 mouth Q38.6
 Müllerian (*see also* Anomaly, by site)
  uterus NEC Q51.818
 multiple NEC Q89.7
 muscle Q79.9
  eyelid Q10.3
 musculoskeletal system, except limbs Q79.9
 myocardium Q24.8
 nail Q84.6
 narrowness, eyelid Q10.3
 nasal sinus (wall) Q30.8
 neck (any part) Q18.9
 nerve Q07.9
  acoustic Q07.8
  optic Q07.8
 nervous system (central) Q07.9
 nipple Q83.9
 nose, nasal (bones) (cartilage) (septum) (sinus) Q30.9
  specified NEC Q30.8
 ocular muscle Q15.8
 omphalomesenteric duct Q43.0
 opening, pulmonary veins Q26.4
 optic
  disc Q14.2
  nerve Q07.8
 opticociliary vessels Q13.2
 orbit (eye) Q10.7
 organ Q89.9
  of Corti Q16.5
 origin
  artery
   innominate Q25.8
   pulmonary Q25.79
   renal Q27.2
   subclavian Q25.48
 osseous meatus (ear) Q16.1
 ovary Q50.39
 oviduct Q50.6
 palate (hard) (soft) NEC Q38.5
 pancreas or pancreatic duct Q45.3
 papillary muscles Q24.8
 parathyroid gland Q89.2
 paraurethral ducts Q64.79
 parotid (gland) Q38.4
 patella Q74.1
 Pelger-Huët (hereditary hyposegmentation) D72.0
 pelvic girdle NEC Q74.2
 pelvis (bony) NEC Q74.2
  rachitic E64.3

**Anomaly, anomalous** — *continued*
 penis (glans) Q55.69
 pericardium Q24.8
 peripheral vascular system Q27.9
 Peter's Q13.4
 pharynx Q38.8
 pigmentation L81.9
  congenital Q82.8
 pituitary (gland) Q89.2
 pleural (folds) Q34.0
 portal vein Q26.5
  connection Q26.5
 position, tooth, teeth, fully erupted M26.30
  specified NEC M26.39
 precerebral vessel Q28.1
 prepuce Q55.69
 prostate Q55.4
 pulmonary Q33.9
  artery NEC Q25.79
  valve Q22.3
   atresia Q22.0
   insufficiency Q22.2
   specified type NEC Q22.3
   stenosis Q22.1
    infundibular Q24.3
    subvalvular Q24.3
  venous connection Q26.4
   partial Q26.3
   total Q26.2
 pupil Q13.2
  function H57.00
   anisocoria H57.02
   Argyll Robertson pupil H57.01
   miosis H57.03
   mydriasis H57.04
   specified type NEC H57.09
   tonic pupil H57.05- ☑
 pylorus Q40.3
 radius Q74.0
 rectum Q43.9
 reduction (extremity) (limb)
  femur (longitudinal) — *see* Defect, reduction,
   lower limb, longitudinal, femur
  fibula (longitudinal) — *see* Defect, reduction, lower
   limb, longitudinal, fibula
  lower limb — *see* Defect, reduction, lower limb
  radius (longitudinal) — *see* Defect, reduction, upper limb, longitudinal, radius
  tibia (longitudinal) — *see* Defect, reduction, lower
   limb, longitudinal, tibia
  ulna (longitudinal) — *see* Defect, reduction, upper
   limb, longitudinal, ulna
  upper limb — *see* Defect, reduction, upper limb
 refraction — *see* Disorder, refraction
 renal Q63.9
  artery Q27.2
  pelvis Q63.9
   specified NEC Q63.8
 respiratory system Q34.9
  specified NEC Q34.8
 retina Q14.1
 rib Q76.6
  cervical Q76.5
 Rieger's Q13.81
 rotation — *see* Malrotation
  hip or thigh Q65.89
 round ligament Q52.8
 sacroiliac (joint) NEC Q74.2
 sacrum NEC Q76.49
  kyphosis — *see* Kyphosis, congenital
  lordosis — *see* Lordosis, congenital
 saddle nose, syphilitic A50.57
 salivary duct or gland Q38.4
 scapula Q74.0
 scrotum — *see* Malformation, testis and scrotum
 sebaceous gland Q82.9
 seminal vesicles Q55.4
 sense organs NEC Q07.8
 sex chromosomes NEC (*see also* Anomaly, chromosomes)
  female phenotype Q97.8
  male phenotype Q98.9
 shoulder (girdle) (joint) Q74.0
 sigmoid (flexure) Q43.9
 simian crease Q82.8
 sinus of Valsalva Q25.49
 skeleton generalized Q78.9
 skin (appendage) Q82.9

**Anomaly, anomalous** — *continued*
  skull Q75.9
    with
      anencephaly Q00.0
      encephalocele — *see* Encephalocele
      hydrocephalus Q03.9
        with spina bifida — *see* Spina bifida, by site, with hydrocephalus
      microcephaly Q02
  specified organ or site NEC Q89.8
  spermatic cord Q55.4
  spine, spinal NEC Q76.49
    column NEC Q76.49
      kyphosis — *see* Kyphosis, congenital
      lordosis — *see* Lordosis, congenital
    cord Q06.9
    nerve root Q07.8
  spleen Q89.09
    agenesis Q89.01
  stenonian duct Q38.4
  sternum NEC Q76.7
  stomach Q40.3
  submaxillary gland Q38.4
  tarsus NEC Q74.2
  tendon Q79.9
  testis — *see* Malformation, testis and scrotum
  thigh NEC Q74.2
  thorax (wall) Q67.8
    bony Q76.9
  throat Q38.8
  thumb Q74.0
  thymus gland Q89.2
  thyroid (gland) Q89.2
    cartilage Q31.8
  tibia NEC Q74.2
    saber A50.56
  toe Q74.2
  tongue Q38.3
  tooth, teeth K00.9
    eruption K00.6
    position, fully erupted M26.30
    spacing, fully erupted M26.30
  trachea (cartilage) Q32.1
  tragus Q17.9
  tricuspid (leaflet) (valve) Q22.9
    atresia or stenosis Q22.4
    Ebstein's Q22.5
  Uhl's (hypoplasia of myocardium, right ventricle) Q24.8
  ulna Q74.0
  umbilical artery Q27.0
  union
    cricoid cartilage and thyroid cartilage Q31.8
    thyroid cartilage and hyoid bone Q31.8
    trachea with larynx Q31.8
  upper limb Q74.0
  urachus Q64.4
  ureter Q62.8
    obstructive NEC Q62.39
      cecoureterocele Q62.32
      orthotopic ureterocele Q62.31
  urethra Q64.70
    absence Q64.5
    double Q64.74
    fistula to rectum Q64.73
    obstructive Q64.39
      stricture Q64.32
    prolapse Q64.71
    specified type NEC Q64.79
  urinary tract Q64.9
  uterus Q51.9
    with only one functioning horn Q51.4
  uvula Q38.5
  vagina Q52.4
  valleculae Q31.8
  valve (heart) NEC Q24.8
    coronary sinus Q24.5
    inferior vena cava Q24.8
    pulmonary Q22.3
    sinus coronario Q24.5
    venae cavae inferioris Q24.8
  vas deferens Q55.4
  vascular Q27.9
    brain Q28.3
    ring Q25.45
  vein(s) (peripheral) Q27.9
    brain Q28.3
    cerebral Q28.3
    coronary Q24.5
    developmental Q28.3

**Anomaly, anomalous** — *continued*
  vein(s) — *continued*
    great Q26.9
      specified NEC Q26.8
  vena cava (inferior) (superior) Q26.9
  venous — *see* Anomaly, vein(s)
  venous return Q26.8
  ventricular
    bands or folds Q24.8
    septa Q21.0
  vertebra Q76.49
    kyphosis — *see* Kyphosis, congenital
    lordosis — *see* Lordosis, congenital
  vesicourethral orifice Q64.79
  vessel(s) Q27.9
    optic papilla Q14.2
    precerebral Q28.1
  vitelline duct Q43.0
  vitreous body or humor Q14.0
  vulva Q52.70
  wrist (joint) Q74.0
**Anomia** R48.8
**Anonychia** (congenital) Q84.3
  acquired L60.8
**Anophthalmos, anophthalmus** (congenital) (globe) Q11.1
  acquired Z90.01
**Anopia, anopsia** H53.46- ☑
  quadrant H53.46- ☑
**Anorchia, anorchism, anorchidism** Q55.0
**Anorexia** R63.0
  hysterical F44.89
  nervosa F50.00
    atypical F50.9
    binge-eating type F50.2
      with purging F50.02
    restricting type F50.01
**Anorgasmy, psychogenic** (female) F52.31
  male F52.32
**Anosmia** R43.0
  hysterical F44.6
  postinfectional J39.8
**Anosognosia** R41.89
**Anosteoplasia** Q78.9
**Anovulatory cycle** N97.0
**Anoxemia** R09.02
  newborn P84
**Anoxia** (pathological) R09.02
  altitude T70.29 ☑
  cerebral G93.1
    complicating
      anesthesia (general) (local) or other sedation T88.59 ☑
        in labor and delivery O74.3
        in pregnancy O29.21- ☑
        postpartum, puerperal O89.2
      delivery (cesarean) (instrumental) O75.4
    during a procedure G97.81
    newborn P84
    resulting from a procedure G97.82
  due to
    drowning T75.1 ☑
    high altitude T70.29 ☑
  heart — *see* Insufficiency, coronary
  intrauterine P84
  myocardial — *see* Insufficiency, coronary
  newborn P84
  spinal cord G95.11
  systemic (by suffocation) (low content in atmosphere) — *see* Asphyxia, traumatic
**Anteflexion** — *see* Anteversion
**Antenatal**
  care (normal pregnancy) Z34.90
  screening (encounter for) of mother (*see also* Encounter, antenatal screening) Z36.9
**Antepartum** — *see* condition
**Anterior** — *see* condition
**Antero-occlusion** M26.220
**Anteversion**
  cervix — *see* Anteversion, uterus
  femur (neck), congenital Q65.89
  uterus, uterine (cervix) (postinfectional) (postpartal) (old) N85.4
    congenital Q51.818
    in pregnancy or childbirth — *see* Pregnancy, complicated by
**Anthophobia** F40.228
**Anthracosilicosis** J60

**Anthracosis** (lung) (occupational) J60
  lingua K14.3
**Anthrax** A22.9
  with pneumonia A22.1
  cerebral A22.8
  colitis A22.2
  cutaneous A22.0
  gastrointestinal A22.2
  inhalation A22.1
  intestinal A22.2
  meningitis A22.8
  pulmonary A22.1
  respiratory A22.1
  sepsis A22.7
  specified manifestation NEC A22.8
**Anthropoid pelvis** Q74.2
  with disproportion (fetopelvic) O33.0
**Anthropophobia** F40.10
  generalized F40.11
**Antibodies, maternal** (blood group) — *see* Isoimmunization, affecting management of pregnancy
  anti-D — *see* Isoimmunization, affecting management of pregnancy, Rh
  newborn P55.0
**Antibody**
  anticardiolipin R76.0
    with
      hemorrhagic disorder D68.312
      hypercoagulable state D68.61
  antiphosphatidylglycerol R76.0
    with
      hemorrhagic disorder D68.312
      hypercoagulable state D68.61
  antiphosphatidylinositol R76.0
    with
      hemorrhagic disorder D68.312
      hypercoagulable state D68.61
  antiphosphatidylserine R76.0
    with
      hemorrhagic disorder D68.312
      hypercoagulable state D68.61
  antiphospholipid R76.0
    with
      hemorrhagic disorder D68.312
      hypercoagulable state D68.61
**Anticardiolipin syndrome** D68.61
**Anticoagulant, circulating** (intrinsic) (*see also* Disorder, hemorrhagic) D68.318
  drug-induced (extrinsic) (*see also* Disorder, hemorrhagic) D68.32
  iatrogenic D68.32
**Antidiuretic hormone syndrome** E22.2
**Antimonial cholera** — *see* Poisoning, antimony
**Antiphospholipid**
  antibody
    with hemorrhagic disorder D68.312
    syndrome D68.61
**Antisocial personality** F60.2
**Antithrombinemia** — *see* Circulating anticoagulants
**Antithromboplastinemia** D68.318
**Antithromboplastinogenemia** D68.318
**Antitoxin complication or reaction** — *see* Complications, vaccination
**Antlophobia** F40.228
**Antritis** J32.0
  maxilla J32.0
    acute J01.00
      recurrent J01.01
  stomach K29.60
    with bleeding K29.61
**Antrum, antral** — *see* condition
**Anuria** R34
  calculous (impacted) (recurrent) (*see also* Calculus, urinary) N20.9
  following
    abortion — *see* Abortion by type complicated by, renal failure
    ectopic or molar pregnancy O08.4
  newborn P96.0
  postprocedural N99.0
  postrenal N13.8
  traumatic (following crushing) T79.5 ☑
**Anus, anal** — *see* condition
**Anusitis** K62.89
**Anxiety** F41.9
  depression F41.8
  episodic paroxysmal F41.0
  generalized F41.1

**Anxiety** — *continued*
　hysteria F41.8
　neurosis F41.1
　panic type F41.0
　reaction F41.1
　separation, abnormal (of childhood) F93.0
　specified NEC F41.8
　state F41.1
**Aorta, aortic** — *see* condition
**Aortectasia** — *see* Ectasia, aorta
　with aneurysm — *see* Aneurysm, aorta
**Aortitis** (nonsyphilitic) (calcific) I77.6
　arteriosclerotic I70.0
　Doehle-Heller A52.02
　luetic A52.02
　rheumatic — *see* Endocarditis, acute, rheumatic
　specific (syphilitic) A52.02
　syphilitic A52.02
　　congenital A50.54 [I79.1]
**Apathetic thyroid storm** — *see* Thyrotoxicosis
**Apathy** R45.3
**Apeirophobia** F40.228
**Apepsia** K30
　psychogenic F45.8
**Aperistalsis, esophagus** K22.0
**Apertognathia** M26.29
**Apert's syndrome** Q87.0
**Aphagia** R13.0
　psychogenic F50.9
**Aphakia** (acquired) (postoperative) H27.0- ☑
　congenital Q12.3
**Aphasia** (amnestic) (global) (nominal) (semantic) (syntactic) R47.01
　acquired, with epilepsy (Landau-Kleffner syndrome)
　　— *see* Epilepsy, specified NEC
　auditory (developmental) F80.2
　developmental (receptive type) F80.2
　　expressive type F80.1
　　Wernicke's F80.2
　following
　　cerebrovascular disease I69.920
　　　cerebral infarction I69.320
　　　intracerebral hemorrhage I69.120
　　　nontraumatic intracranial hemorrhage NEC
　　　　I69.220
　　　specified disease NEC I69.820
　　　subarachnoid hemorrhage I69.020
　primary progressive G31.01 [F02.80]
　　with behavioral disturbance G31.01 [F02.81]
　progressive isolated G31.01 [F02.80]
　　with behavioral disturbance G31.01 [F02.81]
　sensory F80.2
　syphilis, tertiary A52.19
　Wernicke's (developmental) F80.2
**Aphonia** (organic) R49.1
　hysterical F44.4
　psychogenic F44.4
**Aphthae, aphthous** (*see also* condition)
　Bednar's K12.0
　cachectic K14.0
　epizootic B08.8
　fever B08.8
　oral (recurrent) K12.0
　stomatitis (major) (minor) K12.0
　thrush B37.0
　ulcer (oral) (recurrent) K12.0
　　genital organ(s) NEC
　　　female N76.6
　　　male N50.89
　　larynx J38.7
**Apical** — *see* condition
**Apiphobia** F40.218
**Aplasia** (*see also* Agenesis)
　abdominal muscle syndrome Q79.4
　alveolar process (acquired) — *see* Anomaly, alveolar
　　congenital Q38.6
　aorta (congenital) Q25.41
　axialis extracorticalis (congenita) E75.29
　bone marrow (myeloid) D61.9
　　congenital D61.01
　brain Q00.0
　　part of Q04.3
　bronchus Q32.4
　cementum K00.4
　cerebellum Q04.3
　cervix (congenital) Q51.5
　congenital pure red cell D61.01
　corpus callosum Q04.0

**Aplasia** — *continued*
　cutis congenita Q84.8
　erythrocyte congenital D61.01
　extracortical axial E75.29
　eye Q11.1
　fovea centralis (congenital) Q14.1
　gallbladder, congenital Q44.0
　iris Q13.1
　labyrinth, membranous Q16.5
　limb (congenital) Q73.8
　　lower — *see* Defect, reduction, lower limb
　　upper — *see* Agenesis, arm
　lung, congenital (bilateral) (unilateral) Q33.3
　pancreas Q45.0
　parathyroid-thymic D82.1
　Pelizaeus-Merzbacher E75.29
　penis Q55.5
　prostate Q55.4
　red cell (with thymoma) D60.9
　　acquired D60.9
　　　due to drugs D60.9
　　adult D60.9
　　chronic D60.0
　　congenital D61.01
　　constitutional D61.01
　　due to drugs D60.9
　　hereditary D61.01
　　of infants D61.01
　　primary D61.01
　　pure D61.01
　　　due to drugs D60.9
　　specified type NEC D60.8
　　transient D60.1
　round ligament Q52.8
　skin Q84.8
　spermatic cord Q55.4
　spleen Q89.01
　testicle Q55.0
　thymic, with immunodeficiency D82.1
　thyroid (congenital) (with myxedema) E03.1
　uterus Q51.0
　ventral horn cell Q06.1
**Apnea, apneic** (of) (spells) R06.81
　newborn NEC P28.4
　　obstructive P28.4
　　sleep (central) (obstructive) (primary) P28.3
　prematurity P28.4
　sleep G47.30
　　central (primary) G47.31
　　　idiopathic G47.31
　　　in conditions classified elsewhere G47.37
　　obstructive (adult) (pediatric) G47.33
　　　hypopnea G47.33
　　primary central G47.31
　　specified NEC G47.39
**Apneumatosis, newborn** P28.0
**Apocrine metaplasia** (breast) — *see* Dysplasia, mammary, specified type NEC
**Apophysitis** (bone) (*see also* Osteochondropathy)
　calcaneus M92.8
　juvenile M92.9
**Apoplectiform convulsions** (cerebral ischemia) I67.82
**Apoplexia, apoplexy, apoplectic**
　adrenal A39.1
　heart (auricle) (ventricle) — *see* Infarct, myocardium
　heat T67.0 ☑
　hemorrhagic (stroke) — *see* Hemorrhage, intracranial
　meninges, hemorrhagic — *see* Hemorrhage, intracranial, subarachnoid
　uremic N18.9 [I68.8]
**Appearance**
　bizarre R46.1
　specified NEC R46.89
　very low level of personal hygiene R46.0
**Appendage**
　epididymal (organ of Morgagni) Q55.4
　intestine (epiploic) Q43.8
　preauricular Q17.0
　testicular (organ of Morgagni) Q55.29
**Appendicitis** (pneumococcal) (retrocecal) K37
　with
　　perforation or rupture K35.2
　　peritoneal abscess K35.3
　　peritonitis NEC K35.3
　　　generalized (with perforation or rupture) K35.2
　　　localized (with perforation or rupture) K35.3
　acute (catarrhal) (fulminating) (gangrenous) (obstructive) (retrocecal) (suppurative) K35.80

**Appendicitis** — *continued*
　acute — *continued*
　　with
　　　peritoneal abscess K35.3
　　　peritonitis NEC K35.3
　　　　generalized (with perforation or rupture)
　　　　　K35.2
　　　　localized (with perforation or rupture) K35.3
　　　specified NEC K35.89
　　amebic A06.89
　　chronic (recurrent) K36
　　exacerbation — *see* Appendicitis, acute
　　gangrenous — *see* Appendicitis, acute
　　healed (obliterative) K36
　　interval K36
　　neurogenic K36
　　obstructive K36
　　recurrent K36
　　relapsing K36
　　subacute (adhesive) K36
　　subsiding K36
　　suppurative — *see* Appendicitis, acute
　　tuberculous A18.32
**Appendicopathia oxyurica** B80
**Appendix, appendicular** (*see also* condition)
　epididymis Q55.4
　Morgagni
　　female Q50.5
　　male (epididymal) Q55.4
　　　testicular Q55.29
　testis Q55.29
**Appetite**
　depraved — *see* Pica
　excessive R63.2
　lack or loss (*see also* Anorexia) R63.0
　　nonorganic origin F50.89
　　psychogenic F50.89
　perverted (hysterical) — *see* Pica
**Apple peel syndrome** Q41.1
**Apprehension state** F41.1
**Apprehensiveness, abnormal** F41.9
**Approximal wear** K03.0
**Apraxia** (classic) (ideational) (ideokinetic) (ideomotor) (motor) (verbal) R48.2
　following
　　cerebrovascular disease I69.990
　　　cerebral infarction I69.390
　　　intracerebral hemorrhage I69.190
　　　nontraumatic intracranial hemorrhage NEC
　　　　I69.290
　　　specified disease NEC I69.890
　　　subarachnoid hemorrhage I69.090
　oculomotor, congenital H51.8
**Aptyalism** K11.7
**Apudoma** — *see* Neoplasm, uncertain behavior, by site
**Aqueous misdirection** H40.83- ☑
**Arabicum elephantiasis** — *see* Infestation, filarial
**Arachnitis** — *see* Meningitis
**Arachnodactyly** — *see* Syndrome, Marfan's
**Arachnoiditis** (acute) (adhesive) (basal) (brain) (cerebrospinal) — *see* Meningitis
**Arachnophobia** F40.210
**Arboencephalitis, Australian** A83.4
**Arborization block** (heart) I45.5
**ARC** (AIDS-related complex) B20
**Arch**
　aortic Q25.49
　bovine Q25.49
**Arches** — *see* condition
**Arcuate uterus** Q51.810
**Arcuatus uterus** Q51.810
**Arcus** (cornea) senilis — *see* Degeneration, cornea, senile
**Arc-welder's lung** J63.4
**Areflexia** R29.2
**Areola** — *see* condition
**Argentaffinoma** (*see also* Neoplasm, uncertain behavior, by site)
　malignant — *see* Neoplasm, malignant, by site
　syndrome E34.0
**Argininemia** E72.21
**Arginosuccinic aciduria** E72.22
**Argyll Robertson phenomenon, pupil or syndrome** (syphilitic) A52.19
　atypical H57.09
　nonsyphilitic H57.09
**Argyria, argyriasis**
　conjunctival H11.13- ☑

**Argyria, argyriasis** — *continued*
  from drug or medicament — *see* Table of Drugs and Chemicals, by substance
**Argyrosis, conjunctival** H11.13- ☑
**Arhinencephaly** Q04.1
**Ariboflavinosis** E53.0
**Arm** — *see* condition
**Arnold-Chiari disease, obstruction or syndrome** (type II) Q07.00
  with
    hydrocephalus Q07.02
      with spina bifida Q07.03
    spina bifida Q07.01
      with hydrocephalus Q07.03
  type III — *see* Encephalocele
  type IV Q04.8
**Aromatic amino-acid metabolism disorder** E70.9
  specified NEC E70.8
**Arousals, confusional** G47.51
**Arrest, arrested**
  cardiac I46.9
    complicating
      abortion — *see* Abortion, by type, complicated by, cardiac arrest
      anesthesia (general) (local) or other sedation — *see* Table of Drugs and Chemicals, by drug
        in labor and delivery O74.2
        in pregnancy O29.11- ☑
        postpartum, puerperal O89.1
      delivery (cesarean) (instrumental) O75.4
    due to
      cardiac condition I46.2
      specified condition NEC I46.8
    intraoperative I97.71- ☑
    newborn P29.31
    personal history, successfully resuscitated Z86.74
    postprocedural I97.12- ☑
      obstetric procedure O75.4
  cardiorespiratory — *see* Arrest, cardiac
  circulatory — *see* Arrest, cardiac
  deep transverse O64.0 ☑
  development or growth
    bone — *see* Disorder, bone, development or growth
    child R62.50
    tracheal rings Q32.1
  epiphyseal
    complete
      femur M89.15- ☑
      humerus M89.12- ☑
      tibia M89.16- ☑
      ulna M89.13- ☑
      forearm M89.13- ☑
        specified NEC M89.13- ☑
        ulna — *see* Arrest, epiphyseal, by type, ulna
      lower leg M89.16- ☑
        specified NEC M89.168
        tibia — *see* Arrest, epiphyseal, by type, tibia
    partial
      femur M89.15- ☑
      humerus M89.12- ☑
      tibia M89.16- ☑
      ulna M89.13- ☑
    specified NEC M89.18
  granulopoiesis — *see* Agranulocytosis
  growth plate — *see* Arrest, epiphyseal
  heart — *see* Arrest, cardiac
  legal, anxiety concerning Z65.3
  physeal — *see* Arrest, epiphyseal
  respiratory R09.2
    newborn P28.81
  sinus I45.5
  spermatogenesis (complete) — *see* Azoospermia
    incomplete — *see* Oligospermia
  transverse (deep) O64.0 ☑
**Arrhenoblastoma**
  benign
    specified site — *see* Neoplasm, benign, by site
    unspecified site
      female D27.9
      male D29.20
  malignant
    specified site — *see* Neoplasm, malignant, by site
    unspecified site
      female C56.9
      male C62.90

**Arrhenoblastoma** — *continued*
  specified site — *see* Neoplasm, uncertain behavior, by site
  unspecified site
    female D39.10
    male D40.10
**Arrhythmia** (auricle) (cardiac) (juvenile) (nodal) (reflex) (sinus) (supraventricular) (transitory) (ventricle) I49.9
  block I45.9
  extrasystolic I49.49
  newborn
    bradycardia P29.12
    occurring before birth P03.819
      before onset of labor P03.810
      during labor P03.811
    tachycardia P29.11
  psychogenic F45.8
  specified NEC I49.8
  vagal R55
  ventricular re-entry I47.0
**Arrillaga-Ayerza syndrome** (pulmonary sclerosis with pulmonary hypertension) I27.0
**Arsenical pigmentation** L81.8
  from drug or medicament — *see* Table of Drugs and Chemicals
**Arsenism** — *see* Poisoning, arsenic
**Arterial** — *see* condition
**Arteriofibrosis** — *see* Arteriosclerosis
**Arteriolar sclerosis** — *see* Arteriosclerosis
**Arteriolith** — *see* Arteriosclerosis
**Arteriolitis** I77.6
  necrotizing, kidney I77.5
  renal — *see* Hypertension, kidney
**Arteriolosclerosis** — *see* Arteriosclerosis
**Arterionephrosclerosis** — *see* Hypertension, kidney
**Arteriopathy** I77.9
**Arteriosclerosis, arteriosclerotic** (diffuse) (obliterans) (of) (senile) (with calcification) I70.90
  aorta I70.0
  arteries of extremities — *see* Arteriosclerosis, extremities
  brain I67.2
  bypass graft
    coronary — *see* Arteriosclerosis, coronary, bypass graft
    extremities — *see* Arteriosclerosis, extremities, bypass graft
  cardiac — *see* Disease, heart, ischemic, atherosclerotic
  cardiopathy — *see* Disease, heart, ischemic, atherosclerotic
  cardiorenal — *see* Hypertension, cardiorenal
  cardiovascular — *see* Disease, heart, ischemic, atherosclerotic
  carotid (see also Occlusion, artery, carotid) I65.2- ☑
  central nervous system I67.2
  cerebral I67.2
  cerebrovascular I67.2
  coronary (artery) I25.10
    bypass graft I25.810
      with
        angina pectoris I25.709
          with documented spasm I25.701
          specified type NEC I25.708
          unstable I25.700
        ischemic chest pain I25.709
      autologous artery I25.810
        with
          angina pectoris I25.729
            with documented spasm I25.721
            specified type I25.728
            unstable I25.720
          ischemic chest pain I25.729
      autologous vein I25.810
        with
          angina pectoris I25.719
            with documented spasm I25.711
            specified type I25.718
            unstable I25.710
          ischemic chest pain I25.719
      nonautologous biological I25.810
        with
          angina pectoris I25.739
            with documented spasm I25.731
            specified type I25.738
            unstable I25.730
          ischemic chest pain I25.739
      specified type NEC I25.810

**Arteriosclerosis, arteriosclerotic** — *continued*
  coronary — *continued*
    bypass graft — *continued*
      specified type — *continued*
        with
          angina pectoris I25.799
            with documented spasm I25.791
            specified type I25.798
            unstable I25.790
          ischemic chest pain I25.799
    due to
      calcified coronary lesion (severely) I25.84
      lipid rich plaque I25.83
    native vessel
      with
        angina pectoris I25.119
          with documented spasm I25.111
          specified type NEC I25.118
          unstable I25.110
        ischemic chest pain I25.119
    transplanted heart I25.811
      bypass graft I25.812
        with
          angina pectoris I25.769
           with documented spasm I25.761
           specified type I25.768
           unstable I25.760
         ischemic chest pain I25.769
      native coronary artery I25.811
        with
          angina pectoris I25.759
           with documented spasm I25.751
           specified type I25.758
           unstable I25.750
         ischemic chest pain I25.759
  extremities (native arteries) I70.209
    bypass graft I70.309
      autologous vein graft I70.409
        leg I70.409
          with
            gangrene (and intermittent claudication, rest pain and ulcer) I70.469
            intermittent claudication I70.419
            rest pain (and intermittent claudication) I70.429
          bilateral I70.403
            with
              gangrene (and intermittent claudication, rest pain and ulcer) I70.463
             intermittent claudication I70.463
             rest pain (and intermittent claudication) I70.423
            specified type NEC I70.493
          left I70.402
            with
              gangrene (and intermittent claudication, rest pain and ulcer) I70.462
             intermittent claudication I70.412
             rest pain (and intermittent claudication) I70.422
             ulceration (and intermittent claudication and rest pain) I70.449
              ankle I70.443
              calf I70.442
              foot site NEC I70.445
              heel I70.444
              lower leg NEC I70.448
              midfoot I70.444
              thigh I70.441
            specified type NEC I70.492
          right I70.401
            with
              gangrene (and intermittent claudication, rest pain and ulcer) I70.461
             intermittent claudication I70.411
             rest pain (and intermittent claudication) I70.421
             ulceration (and intermittent claudication and rest pain) I70.439
              ankle I70.433
              calf I70.432
              foot site NEC I70.435
              heel I70.434

☑ **Additional Character Required** — **Refer to the Tabular List for Character Selection**   ▽ **Subterms under main terms may continue to next column or page**

**Arteriosclerosis, arteriosclerotic** — *continued*
 extremities — *continued*
  bypass graft — *continued*
   autologous vein graft — *continued*
    leg — *continued*
     right — *continued*
      with — *continued*
       ulceration — *continued*
        lower leg NEC I70.438
        midfoot I70.434
        thigh I70.431
       specified type NEC I70.491
      specified type NEC I70.499
     specified NEC I70.408
      with
       gangrene (and intermittent claudication, rest pain and ulcer) I70.468
       intermittent claudication I70.418
       rest pain (and intermittent claudication) I70.428
       ulceration (and intermittent claudication and rest pain) I70.45
      specified type NEC I70.498
    leg I70.309
     with
      gangrene (and intermittent claudication, rest pain and ulcer) I70.369
      intermittent claudication I70.319
      rest pain (and intermittent claudication) I70.329
     bilateral I70.303
      with
       gangrene (and intermittent claudication, rest pain and ulcer) I70.363
       intermittent claudication I70.313
       rest pain (and intermittent claudication) I70.323
      specified type NEC I70.393
     left I70.302
      with
       gangrene (and intermittent claudication, rest pain and ulcer) I70.362
       intermittent claudication I70.312
       rest pain (and intermittent claudication) I70.322
       ulceration (and intermittent claudication and rest pain) I70.349
        ankle I70.343
        calf I70.342
        foot site NEC I70.345
        heel I70.344
        lower leg NEC I70.348
        midfoot I70.344
        thigh I70.341
      specified type NEC I70.392
     right I70.301
      with
       gangrene (and intermittent claudication, rest pain and ulcer) I70.361
       intermittent claudication I70.311
       rest pain (and intermittent claudication) I70.321
       ulceration (and intermittent claudication and rest pain I70.339
        ankle I70.333
        calf I70.332
        foot site NEC I70.335
        heel I70.334
        lower leg NEC I70.338
        midfoot I70.334
        thigh I70.331
      specified type NEC I70.391
     specified type NEC I70.399
   nonautologous biological graft I70.509
    leg I70.509
     with
      gangrene (and intermittent claudication, rest pain and ulcer) I70.569
      intermittent claudication I70.519
      rest pain (and intermittent claudication) I70.529
     bilateral I70.503

**Arteriosclerosis, arteriosclerotic** — *continued*
 extremities — *continued*
  bypass graft — *continued*
   nonautologous biological graft — *continued*
    leg — *continued*
     bilateral — *continued*
      with
       gangrene (and intermittent claudication, rest pain and ulcer) I70.563
       intermittent claudication I70.513
       rest pain (and intermittent claudication) I70.523
      specified type NEC I70.593
     left I70.502
      with
       gangrene (and intermittent claudication, rest pain and ulcer) I70.562
       intermittent claudication I70.512
       rest pain (and intermittent claudication) I70.522
       ulceration (and intermittent claudication and rest pain) I70.549
        ankle I70.543
        calf I70.542
        foot site NEC I70.545
        heel I70.544
        lower leg NEC I70.548
        midfoot I70.544
        thigh I70.541
      specified type NEC I70.592
     right I70.501
      with
       gangrene (and intermittent claudication, rest pain and ulcer) I70.561
       intermittent claudication I70.511
       rest pain (and intermittent claudication) I70.521
       ulceration (and intermittent claudication and rest pain) I70.539
        ankle I70.533
        calf I70.532
        foot site NEC I70.535
        heel I70.534
        lower leg NEC I70.538
        midfoot I70.534
        thigh I70.531
      specified type NEC I70.591
     specified type NEC I70.599
    specified NEC I70.508
     with
      gangrene (and intermittent claudication, rest pain and ulcer) I70.568
      intermittent claudication I70.518
      rest pain (and intermittent claudication) I70.528
      ulceration (and intermittent claudication and rest pain) I70.55
     specified type NEC I70.598
   nonbiological graft I70.609
    leg I70.609
     with
      gangrene (and intermittent claudication, rest pain and ulcer) I70.669
      intermittent claudication I70.619
      rest pain (and intermittent claudication) I70.629
     bilateral I70.603
      with
       gangrene (and intermittent claudication, rest pain and ulcer) I70.663
       intermittent claudication I70.613
       rest pain (and intermittent claudication) I70.623
      specified type NEC I70.693
     left I70.602
      with
       gangrene (and intermittent claudication, rest pain and ulcer) I70.662
       intermittent claudication I70.612

**Arteriosclerosis, arteriosclerotic** — *continued*
 extremities — *continued*
  bypass graft — *continued*
   nonbiological graft — *continued*
    leg — *continued*
     left — *continued*
      with — *continued*
       rest pain (and intermittent claudication) I70.622
       ulceration (and intermittent claudication and rest pain) I70.649
        ankle I70.643
        calf I70.642
        foot site NEC I70.645
        heel I70.644
        lower leg NEC I70.648
        midfoot I70.644
        thigh I70.641
      specified type NEC I70.692
     right I70.601
      with
       gangrene (and intermittent claudication, rest pain and ulcer) I70.661
       intermittent claudication I70.611
       rest pain (and intermittent claudication) I70.621
       ulceration (and intermittent claudication and rest pain) I70.639
        ankle I70.633
        calf I70.632
        foot site NEC I70.635
        heel I70.634
        lower leg NEC I70.638
        midfoot I70.634
        thigh I70.631
      specified type NEC I70.691
     specified type NEC I70.699
    specified NEC I70.608
     with
      gangrene (and intermittent claudication, rest pain and ulcer) I70.668
      intermittent claudication I70.618
      rest pain (and intermittent claudication) I70.628
      ulceration (and intermittent claudication and rest pain) I70.65
     specified type NEC I70.698
   specified graft NEC I70.709
    leg I70.709
     with
      gangrene (and intermittent claudication, rest pain and ulcer) I70.769
      intermittent claudication I70.719
      rest pain (and intermittent claudication) I70.729
     bilateral I70.703
      with
       gangrene (and intermittent claudication, rest pain and ulcer) I70.763
       intermittent claudication I70.713
       rest pain (and intermittent claudication) I70.723
      specified type NEC I70.793
     left I70.702
      with
       gangrene (and intermittent claudication, rest pain and ulcer) I70.762
       intermittent claudication I70.712
       rest pain (and intermittent claudication) I70.722
       ulceration (and intermittent claudication and rest pain) I70.749
        ankle I70.743
        calf I70.742
        foot site NEC I70.745
        heel I70.744
        lower leg NEC I70.748
        midfoot I70.744
        thigh I70.741
      specified type NEC I70.792
     right I70.701

**Arteriosclerosis, arteriosclerotic** — *continued*
  extremities — *continued*
    bypass graft — *continued*
      specified graft — *continued*
        leg — *continued*
          right — *continued*
            with
              gangrene (and intermittent claudication, rest pain and ulcer) I70.761
              intermittent claudication I70.711
              rest pain (and intermittent claudication) I70.721
              ulceration (and intermittent claudication and rest pain) I70.739
                ankle I70.733
                calf I70.732
                foot site NEC I70.735
                heel I70.734
                lower leg NEC I70.738
                midfoot I70.734
                thigh I70.731
              specified type NEC I70.791
        specified type NEC I70.799
      specified NEC I70.708
        with
          gangrene (and intermittent claudication, rest pain and ulcer) I70.768
          intermittent claudication I70.718
          rest pain (and intermittent claudication) I70.728
          ulceration (and intermittent claudication and rest pain) I70.75
          specified type NEC I70.798
    specified NEC I70.308
      with
        gangrene (and intermittent claudication, rest pain and ulcer) I70.368
        intermittent claudication I70.318
        rest pain (and intermittent claudication) I70.328
        ulceration (and intermittent claudication and rest pain) I70.35
        specifiec type NEC I70.398
  leg I70.209
    with
      gangrene (and intermittent claudication, rest pain and ulcer) I70.269
      intermittent claudication I70.219
      rest pain (and intermittent claudication) I70.229
    bilateral I70.203
      with
        gangrene (and intermittent claudication, rest pain and ulcer) I70.263
        intermittent claudication I70.213
        rest pain (and intermittent claudication) I70.223
        specified type NEC I70.293
    left I70.202
      with
        gangrene (and intermittent claudication, rest pain and ulcer) I70.262
        intermittent claudication I70.212
        rest pain (and intermittent claudication) I70.222
        ulceration (and intermittent claudication and rest pain) I70.249
          ankle I70.243
          calf I70.242
          foot site NEC I70.245
          heel I70.244
          lower leg NEC I70.248
          midfoot I70.244
          thigh I70.241
        specified type NEC I70.292
    right I70.201
      with
        gangrene (and intermittent claudication, rest pain and ulcer) I70.261
        intermittent claudication I70.211
        rest pain (and intermittent claudication) I70.221
        ulceration (and intermittent claudication and rest pain) I70.239
          ankle I70.233
          calf I70.232

**Arteriosclerosis, arteriosclerotic** — *continued*
  extremities — *continued*
    leg — *continued*
      right — *continued*
        with — *continued*
          ulceration — *continued*
            foot site NEC I70.235
            heel I70.234
            lower leg NEC I70.238
            midfoot I70.234
            thigh I70.231
          specified type NEC I70.291
        specified type NEC I70.299
      specified site NEC I70.208
        with
          gangrene (and intermittent claudication, rest pain and ulcer) I70.268
          intermittent claudication I70.218
          rest pain (and intermittent claudication) I70.228
          ulceration (and intermittent claudication and rest pain) I70.25
          specified type NEC I70.298
  generalized I70.91
  heart (disease) — *see* Arteriosclerosis, coronary (artery),
  kidney — *see* Hypertension, kidney
  medial — *see* Arteriosclerosis, extremities
  mesenteric (artery) K55.1
  Mönckeberg's — *see* Arteriosclerosis, extremities
  myocarditis I51.4
  peripheral (of extremities) — *see* Arteriosclerosis, extremities
  pulmonary (idiopathic) I27.0
  renal (arterioles) (*see also* Hypertension, kidney)
    artery I70.1
  retina (vascular) I70.8 [H35.0-] ☑
  specified artery NEC I70.8
  spinal (cord) G95.19
  vertebral (artery) I67.2
**Arteriospasm** I73.9
**Arteriovenous** — *see* condition
**Arteritis** I77.6
  allergic M31.0
  aorta (nonsyphilitic) I77.6
    syphilitic A52.02
  aortic arch M31.4
  brachiocephalic M31.4
  brain I67.7
    syphilitic A52.04
  cerebral I67.7
    in systemic lupus erythematosus M32.19
    listerial A32.89
    syphilitic A52.04
    tuberculous A18.89
  coronary (artery) I25.89
    rheumatic I01.8
      chronic I09.89
    syphilitic A52.06
  cranial (left) (right), giant cell M31.6
  deformans — *see* Arteriosclerosis
  giant cell NEC M31.6
    with polymyalgia rheumatica M31.5
  necrosing or necrotizing M31.9
    specified NEC M31.8
  nodosa M30.0
  obliterans — *see* Arteriosclerosis
  pulmonary I28.8
  rheumatic — *see* Fever, rheumatic
  senile — *see* Arteriosclerosis
  suppurative I77.2
  syphilitic (general) A52.09
    brain A52.04
    coronary A52.06
    spinal A52.09
  temporal, giant cell M31.6
  young female aortic arch syndrome M31.4
**Artery, arterial** (*see also* condition)
  abscess I77.89
  single umbilical Q27.0
**Arthralgia** (allergic) (*see also* Pain, joint)
  in caisson disease T70.3 ☑
  temporomandibular M26.62- ☑
**Arthritis, arthritic** (acute) (chronic) (nonpyogenic) (subacute) M19.90
  allergic — *see* Arthritis, specified form NEC
  ankylosing (crippling) (spine) (*see also* Spondylitis, ankylosing)

  ankylosing (*see also* Spondylitis, ankylosing) — *continued*
    sites other than spine — *see* Arthritis, specified form NEC
  atrophic — *see* Osteoarthritis
    spine — *see* Spondylitis, ankylosing
  back — *see* Spondylopathy, inflammatory
  blennorrhagic (gonococcal) A54.42
  Charcot's — *see* Arthropathy, neuropathic
    diabetic — *see* Diabetes, arthropathy, neuropathic
    syringomyelic G95.0
  chylous (filarial) (*see also* category M01) B74.9
  climacteric (any site) NEC — *see* Arthritis, specified form NEC
  crystal (-induced) — *see* Arthritis, in, crystals
  deformans — *see* Osteoarthritis
  degenerative — *see* Osteoarthritis
  due to or associated with
    acromegaly E22.0
    brucellosis — *see* Brucellosis
    caisson disease T70.3 ☑
    diabetes — *see* Diabetes, arthropathy
    dracontiasis (*see also* category M01) B72
    enteritis NEC
      regional — *see* Enteritis, regional
    erysipelas (*see also* category M01) A46
    erythema
      epidemic A25.1
      nodosum L52
    filariasis NOS B74.9
    glanders A24.0
    helminthiasis (*see also* category M01) B83.9
    hemophilia D66 [M36.2]
    Henoch- (Schönlein) purpura D69.0 [M36.4]
    human parvovirus (*see also* category M01) B97.6
    infectious disease NEC M01 ☑
    leprosy (see also category M01) (*see also* Leprosy) A30.9
    Lyme disease A69.23
    mycobacteria (*see also* category M01) A31.8
    parasitic disease NEC (*see also* category M01) B89
    paratyphoid fever (see also category M01) (*see also* Fever, paratyphoid) A01.4
    rat bite fever (*see also* category M01) A25.1
    regional enteritis — *see* Enteritis, regional
    respiratory disorder NOS J98.9
    serum sickness (*see also* Reaction, serum) T80.69 ☑
    syringomyelia G95.0
    typhoid fever A01.04
  epidemic erythema A25.1
  febrile — *see* Fever, rheumatic
  gonococcal A54.42
  gouty (acute) — *see* Gout
  in (due to)
    acromegaly (*see also* subcategory M14.8-) E22.0
    amyloidosis (*see also* subcategory M14.8-) E85.4
    bacterial disease (*see also* subcategory M01) A49.9
    Behçet's syndrome M35.2
    caisson disease (*see also* subcategory M14.8-) T70.3 ☑
    coliform bacilli (Escherichia coli) — *see* Arthritis, in, pyogenic organism NEC
    crystals M11.9
      dicalcium phosphate — *see* Arthritis, in, crystals, specified type NEC
      hydroxyapatite M11.0- ☑
      pyrophosphate — *see* Arthritis, in, crystals, specified type NEC
      specified type NEC M11.80
        ankle M11.87- ☑
        elbow M11.82- ☑
        foot joint M11.87- ☑
        hand joint M11.84- ☑
        hip M11.85- ☑
        knee M11.86- ☑
        multiple sites M11.8- ☑
        shoulder M11.81- ☑
        vertebrae M11.88
        wrist M11.83- ☑
    dermatoarthritis, lipoid E78.81
    dracontiasis (dracunculiasis) (*see also* category M01) B72
    endocrine disorder NEC (*see also* subcategory M14.8-) E34.9
    enteritis, infectious NEC (*see also* category M01) A09

28

☑ **Additional Character Required** — Refer to the Tabular List for Character Selection
   Subterms under main terms may continue to next column or page

**Arthritis, arthritic** — *continued*
  in — *continued*
    enteritis, infectious (*see also* category M01) —
      *continued*
      specified organism NEC (*see also* category M01)
        A08.8
    erythema
      multiforme (*see also* subcategory M14.8-) L51.9
      nodosum (*see also* subcategory M14.8-) L52
    gout — *see* Gout
    helminthiasis NEC (*see also* category M01) B83.9
    hemochromatosis (*see also* subcategory M14.8-)
      E83.118
    hemoglobinopathy NEC D58.2 [M36.3]
    hemophilia NEC D66 [M36.2]
    Hemophilus influenzae M00.8- ☑ [B96.3]
    Henoch (-Schönlein) purpura D69.0 [M36.4]
    hyperparathyroidism NEC (*see also* subcategory
      M14.8-) E21.3
    hypersensitivity reaction NEC T78.49 ☑ [M36.4]
    hypogammaglobulinemia (*see also* subcategory
      M14.8-) D80.1
    hypothyroidism NEC (*see also* subcategory M14.8-)
      E03.9
    infection — *see* Arthritis, pyogenic or pyemic
      spine — *see* Spondylopathy, infective
    infectious disease NEC M01 ☑
    leprosy (*see also* category M01) A30.9
    leukemia NEC C95.9- ☑ [M36.1]
    lipoid dermatoarthritis E78.81
    Lyme disease A69.23
    Mediterranean fever, familial (*see also* subcategory
      M14.8-) M04.1
    Meningococcus A39.83
    metabolic disorder NEC (*see also* subcategory
      M14.8-) E88.9
    multiple myelomatosis C90.0- ☑ [M36.1]
    mumps B26.85
    mycosis NEC (*see also* category M01) B49
    myelomatosis (multiple) C90.0- ☑ [M36.1]
    neurological disorder NEC G98.0
    ochronosis (*see also* subcategory M14.8-) E70.29
    O'nyong-nyong (*see also* category M01) A92.1
    parasitic disease NEC (*see also* category M01) B89
    paratyphoid fever (*see also* category M01) A01.4
    Pseudomonas — *see* Arthritis, pyogenic, bacterial
      NEC
    psoriasis L40.50
    pyogenic organism NEC — *see* Arthritis, pyogenic,
      bacterial NEC
    Reiter's disease — *see* Reiter's disease
    respiratory disorder NEC (*see also* subcategory
      M14.8-) J98.9
    reticulosis, malignant (*see also* subcategory M14.8-
      ) C86.0
    rubella B06.82
    Salmonella (arizonae) (cholerae-suis) (enteritidis)
      (typhimurium) A02.23
    sarcoidosis D86.86
    specified bacteria NEC — *see* Arthritis, pyogenic,
      bacterial NEC
    sporotrichosis B42.82
    syringomyelia G95.0
    thalassemia NEC D56.9 [M36.3]
    tuberculosis — *see* Tuberculosis, arthritis
    typhoid fever A01.04
    urethritis, Reiter's — *see* Reiter's disease
    viral disease NEC (*see also* category M01) B34.9
  infectious or infective (*see also* Arthritis, pyogenic or
    pyemic)
    spine — *see* Spondylopathy, infective
  juvenile M08.90
    with systemic onset — *see* Still's disease
    ankle M08.97- ☑
    elbow M08.92- ☑
    foot joint M08.97- ☑
    hand joint M08.94- ☑
    hip M08.95- ☑
    knee M08.96- ☑
    multiple site M08.99
    pauciarticular M08.40
      ankle M08.47- ☑
      elbow M08.42- ☑
      foot joint M08.47- ☑
      hand joint M08.44- ☑
      hip M08.45- ☑
      knee M08.46- ☑

**Arthritis, arthritic** — *continued*
  juvenile — *continued*
    pauciarticular — *continued*
      shoulder M08.41- ☑
      vertebrae M08.48
      wrist M08.43- ☑
    psoriatic L40.54
    rheumatoid — *see* Arthritis, rheumatoid, juvenile
    shoulder M08.91- ☑
    specified type NEC M08.80
      ankle M08.87- ☑
      elbow M08.82- ☑
      foot joint M08.87- ☑
      hand joint M08.84- ☑
      hip M08.85- ☑
      knee M08.86- ☑
      multiple site M08.89
      shoulder M08.81- ☑
      specified joint NEC M08.88
      vertebrae M08.88
      wrist M08.83- ☑
    wrist M08.93- ☑
  meaning osteoarthritis — *see* Osteoarthritis
  meningococcal A39.83
  menopausal (any site) NEC — *see* Arthritis, specified
    form NEC
  mutilans (psoriatic) L40.52
  mycotic NEC (*see also* category M01) B49
  neuropathic (Charcot) — *see* Arthropathy, neuropathic
    diabetic — *see* Diabetes, arthropathy, neuropathic
    nonsyphilitic NEC G98.0
    syringomyelic G95.0
  ochronotic (*see also* subcategory M14.8-) E70.29
  palindromic (any site) — *see* Rheumatism, palindromic
  pneumococcal M00.10
    ankle M00.17- ☑
    elbow M00.12- ☑
    foot joint — *see* Arthritis, pneumococcal, ankle
    hand joint M00.14- ☑
    hip M00.15- ☑
    knee M00.16- ☑
    multiple site M00.19
    shoulder M00.11- ☑
    vertebra M00.18
    wrist M00.13- ☑
  postdysenteric — *see* Arthropathy, postdysenteric
  postmeningococcal A39.84
  postrheumatic, chronic — *see* Arthropathy,
    postrheumatic, chronic
  primary progressive (*see also* Arthritis, specified form
    NEC)
    spine — *see* Spondylitis, ankylosing
  psoriatic L40.50
  purulent (any site except spine) — *see* Arthritis, pyo-
    genic or pyemic
    spine — *see* Spondylopathy, infective
  pyogenic or pyemic (any site except spine) M00.9
    bacterial NEC M00.80
      ankle M00.87- ☑
      elbow M00.82- ☑
      foot joint — *see* Arthritis, pyogenic, bacterial
        NEC, ankle
      hand joint M00.84- ☑
      hip M00.85- ☑
      knee M00.86- ☑
      multiple site M00.89
      shoulder M00.81- ☑
      vertebra M00.88
      wrist M00.83- ☑
    pneumococcal — *see* Arthritis, pneumococcal
    spine — *see* Spondylopathy, infective
    staphylococcal — *see* Arthritis, staphylococcal
    streptococcal — *see* Arthritis, streptococcal NEC
      pneumococcal — *see* Arthritis, pneumococcal
  reactive — *see* Reiter's disease
  rheumatic (*see also* Arthritis, rheumatoid)
    acute or subacute — *see* Fever, rheumatic
  rheumatoid M06.9
    with
      carditis — *see* Rheumatoid, carditis
      endocarditis — *see* Rheumatoid, carditis
      heart involvement NEC — *see* Rheumatoid,
        carditis
      lung involvement — *see* Rheumatoid, lung
      myocarditis — *see* Rheumatoid, carditis
      myopathy — *see* Rheumatoid, myopathy
      pericarditis — *see* Rheumatoid, carditis

**Arthritis, arthritic** — *continued*
  rheumatoid — *continued*
    with — *continued*
      polyneuropathy — *see* Rheumatoid, polyneu-
        ropathy
      rheumatoid factor — *see* Arthritis, rheumatoid,
        seropositive
      splenoadenomegaly and leukopenia — *see*
        Felty's syndrome
      vasculitis — *see* Rheumatoid, vasculitis
      visceral involvement NEC — *see* Rheumatoid,
        arthritis, with involvement of organs NEC
    juvenile (with or without rheumatoid factor)
      M08.00
      ankle M08.07- ☑
      elbow M08.02- ☑
      foot joint M08.07- ☑
      hand joint M08.04- ☑
      hip M08.05- ☑
      knee M08.06- ☑
      multiple site M08.09
      shoulder M08.01- ☑
      vertebra M08.08
      wrist M08.03- ☑
    seronegative M06.00
      ankle M06.07- ☑
      elbow M06.02- ☑
      foot joint M06.07- ☑
      hand joint M06.04- ☑
      hip M06.05- ☑
      knee M06.06- ☑
      multiple site M06.09
      shoulder M06.01- ☑
      vertebra M06.08
      wrist M06.03- ☑
    seropositive M05.9
      without organ involvement M05.70
        ankle M05.77- ☑
        elbow M05.72- ☑
        foot joint M05.77- ☑
        hand joint M05.74- ☑
        hip M05.75- ☑
        knee M05.76- ☑
        multiple sites M05.79
        shoulder M05.71- ☑
        vertebra — *see* Spondylitis, ankylosing
        wrist M05.73- ☑
      specified NEC M05.80
        ankle M05.87- ☑
        elbow M05.82- ☑
        foot joint M05.87- ☑
        hand joint M05.84- ☑
        hip M05.85- ☑
        knee M05.86- ☑
        multiple sites M05.89
        shoulder M05.81- ☑
        vertebra — *see* Spondylitis, ankylosing
        wrist M05.83- ☑
    specified type NEC M06.80
      ankle M06.87- ☑
      elbow M06.82- ☑
      foot joint M06.87- ☑
      hand joint M06.84- ☑
      hip M06.85- ☑
      knee M06.86- ☑
      multiple site M06.89
      shoulder M06.81- ☑
      vertebra M06.88
      wrist M06.83- ☑
    spine — *see* Spondylitis, ankylosing
  rubella B06.82
  scorbutic (*see also* subcategory M14.8-) E54
  senile or senescent — *see* Osteoarthritis
  septic (any site except spine) — *see* Arthritis, pyogenic
    or pyemic
    spine — *see* Spondylopathy, infective
  serum (nontherapeutic) (therapeutic) — *see*
    Arthropathy, postimmunization
  specified form NEC M13.80
    ankle M13.87- ☑
    elbow M13.82- ☑
    foot joint M13.87- ☑
    hand joint M13.84- ☑
    hip M13.85- ☑
    knee M13.86- ☑
    multiple site M13.89

**Arthritis, arthritic** — *continued*
　specified form — *continued*
　　shoulder M13.81- ☑
　　specified joint NEC M13.88
　　wrist M13.83- ☑
　spine (*see also* Spondylopathy, inflammatory)
　　infectious or infective NEC — *see* Spondylopathy,
　　　infective
　　Marie-Strümpell — *see* Spondylitis, ankylosing
　　pyogenic — *see* Spondylopathy, infective
　　rheumatoid — *see* Spondylitis, ankylosing
　　traumatic (old) — *see* Spondylopathy, traumatic
　　tuberculous A18.01
　staphylococcal M00.00
　　ankle M00.07- ☑
　　elbow M00.02- ☑
　　foot joint — *see* Arthritis, staphylococcal, ankle
　　hand joint M00.04- ☑
　　hip M00.05- ☑
　　knee M00.06- ☑
　　multiple site M00.09
　　shoulder M00.01- ☑
　　vertebra M00.08
　　wrist M00.03- ☑
　streptococcal NEC M00.20
　　ankle M00.27- ☑
　　elbow M00.22- ☑
　　foot joint — *see* Arthritis, streptococcal, ankle
　　hand joint M00.24- ☑
　　hip M00.25- ☑
　　knee M00.26- ☑
　　multiple site M00.29
　　shoulder M00.21- ☑
　　vertebra M00.28
　　wrist M00.23- ☑
　suppurative — *see* Arthritis, pyogenic or pyemic
　syphilitic (late) A52.16
　　congenital A50.55 [M12.80]
　syphilitica deformans (Charcot) A52.16
　temporomandibular M26.69
　toxic of menopause (any site) — *see* Arthritis, specified
　　form NEC
　transient — *see* Arthropathy, specified form NEC
　traumatic (chronic) — *see* Arthropathy, traumatic
　tuberculous A18.02
　　spine A18.01
　uratic — *see* Gout
　urethritica (Reiter's) — *see* Reiter's disease
　vertebral — *see* Spondylopathy, inflammatory
　villous (any site) — *see* Arthropathy, specified form
　　NEC
**Arthrocele** — *see* Effusion, joint
**Arthrodesis status** Z98.1
**Arthrodynia** (*see also* Pain, joint)
**Arthrodysplasia** Q74.9
**Arthrofibrosis, joint** — *see* Ankylosis
**Arthrogryposis** (congenital) Q68.8
　multiplex congenita Q74.3
**Arthrokatadysis** M24.7
**Arthropathy** (*see also* Arthritis) M12.9
　Charcot's — *see* Arthropathy, neuropathic
　　diabetic — *see* Diabetes, arthropathy, neuropathic
　　syringomyelic G95.0
　cricoarytenoid J38.7
　crystal (-induced) — *see* Arthritis, in, crystals
　diabetic NEC — *see* Diabetes, arthropathy
　distal interphalangeal, psoriatic L40.51
　enteropathic M07.60
　　ankle M07.67- ☑
　　elbow M07.62- ☑
　　foot joint M07.67- ☑
　　hand joint M07.64- ☑
　　hip M07.65- ☑
　　knee M07.66- ☑
　　multiple site M07.69
　　shoulder M07.61- ☑
　　vertebra M07.68
　　wrist M07.63- ☑
　following intestinal bypass M02.00
　　ankle M02.07- ☑
　　elbow M02.02- ☑
　　foot joint M02.07- ☑
　　hand joint M02.04- ☑
　　hip M02.05- ☑
　　knee M02.06- ☑
　　multiple site M02.09
　　shoulder M02.01- ☑

**Arthropathy** — *continued*
　following intestinal bypass — *continued*
　　vertebra M02.08
　　wrist M02.03- ☑
　gouty (*see also* Gout)
　　in (due to)
　　　Lesch-Nyhan syndrome E79.1 [M14.8-] ☑
　　　sickle-cell disorders D57- ☑ [M14.8-] ☑
　hemophilic NEC D66 [M36.2]
　　in (due to)
　　　hyperparathyroidism NEC E21.3 [M14.8-] ☑
　　　metabolic disease NOS E88.9 [M14.8-] ☑
　in (due to)
　　acromegaly E22.0 [M14.8-] ☑
　　amyloidosis E85.4 [M14.8-] ☑
　　blood disorder NOS D75.9 [M36.3]
　　diabetes — *see* Diabetes, arthropathy
　　endocrine disease NOS E34.9 [M14.8-] ☑
　　erythema
　　　multiforme L51.9 [M14.8-] ☑
　　　nodosum L52 [M14.8-] ☑
　　hemochromatosis E83.118 [M14.8-] ☑
　　hemoglobinopathy NEC D58.2 [M36.3]
　　hemophilia NEC D66 [M36.2]
　　Henoch-Schönlein purpura D69.0 [M36.4]
　　hyperthyroidism E05.90 [M14.8-] ☑
　　hypothyroidism E03.9 [M14.8-] ☑
　　infective endocarditis I33.0 [M12.80]
　　leukemia NEC C95.9- ☑ [M36.1]
　　malignant histiocytosis C96.A [M36.1]
　　metabolic disease NOS E88.9 [M14.8-] ☑
　　multiple myeloma C90.0- ☑ [M36.1]
　　neoplastic disease NOS (*see also* Neoplasm)
　　　D49.9 [M36.1]
　　nutritional deficiency (*see also* subcategory
　　　M14.8-) E63.9
　　psoriasis NOS L40.50
　　sarcoidosis D86.86
　　syphilis (late) A52.77
　　　congenital A50.55 [M12.80]
　　thyrotoxicosis (*see also* subcategory M14.8-) E05.90
　　ulcerative colitis K51.90 [M07.60]
　　viral hepatitis (postinfectious) NEC B19.9 [M12.80]
　　Whipple's disease (*see also* subcategory M14.8-)
　　　K90.81
　Jaccoud — *see* Arthropathy, postrheumatic, chronic
　juvenile — *see* Arthritis, juvenile
　　psoriatic L40.54
　mutilans (psoriatic) L40.52
　neuropathic (Charcot) M14.60
　　ankle M14.67- ☑
　　diabetic — *see* Diabetes, arthropathy, neuropathic
　　elbow M14.62- ☑
　　foot joint M14.67- ☑
　　hand joint M14.64- ☑
　　hip M14.65- ☑
　　knee M14.66- ☑
　　multiple site M14.69
　　nonsyphilitic NEC G98.0
　　shoulder M14.61- ☑
　　syringomyelic G95.0
　　vertebra M14.68
　　wrist M14.63- ☑
　osteopulmonary — *see* Osteoarthropathy, hyper-
　　trophic, specified NEC
　postdysenteric M02.10
　　ankle M02.17- ☑
　　elbow M02.12- ☑
　　foot joint M02.17- ☑
　　hand joint M02.14- ☑
　　hip M02.15- ☑
　　knee M02.16- ☑
　　multiple site M02.19
　　shoulder M02.11- ☑
　　vertebra M02.18
　　wrist M02.13- ☑
　postimmunization M02.20
　　ankle M02.27- ☑
　　elbow M02.22- ☑
　　foot joint M02.27- ☑
　　hand joint M02.24- ☑
　　hip M02.25- ☑
　　knee M02.26- ☑
　　multiple site M02.29
　　shoulder M02.21- ☑
　　vertebra M02.28
　　wrist M02.23- ☑

**Arthropathy** — *continued*
　postinfectious NEC B99 ☑ [M12.80]
　　in (due to)
　　　enteritis due to Yersinia enterocolitica
　　　　A04.6 [M12.80]
　　　syphilis A52.77
　　　viral hepatitis NEC B19.9 [M12.80]
　postrheumatic, chronic (Jaccoud) M12.00
　　ankle M12.07- ☑
　　elbow M12.02- ☑
　　foot joint M12.07- ☑
　　hand joint M12.04- ☑
　　hip M12.05- ☑
　　knee M12.06- ☑
　　multiple site M12.09
　　shoulder M12.01- ☑
　　specified joint NEC M12.08
　　vertebrae M12.08
　　wrist M12.03- ☑
　psoriatic NEC L40.59
　　interphalangeal, distal L40.51
　reactive M02.9
　　in (due to)
　　　infective endocarditis I33.0 [M02.9]
　　specified type NEC M02.80
　　　ankle M02.87- ☑
　　　elbow M02.82- ☑
　　　foot joint M02.87- ☑
　　　hand joint M02.84- ☑
　　　hip M02.85- ☑
　　　knee M02.86- ☑
　　　multiple site M02.89
　　　shoulder M02.81- ☑
　　　vertebra M02.88
　　　wrist M02.83- ☑
　specified form NEC M12.80
　　ankle M12.87- ☑
　　elbow M12.82- ☑
　　foot joint M12.87- ☑
　　hand joint M12.84- ☑
　　hip M12.85- ☑
　　knee M12.86- ☑
　　multiple site M12.89
　　shoulder M12.81- ☑
　　specified joint NEC M12.88
　　vertebrae M12.88
　　wrist M12.83- ☑
　syringomyelic G95.0
　tabes dorsalis A52.16
　tabetic A52.16
　transient — *see* Arthropathy, specified form NEC
　traumatic M12.50
　　ankle M12.57- ☑
　　elbow M12.52- ☑
　　foot joint M12.57- ☑
　　hand joint M12.54- ☑
　　hip M12.55- ☑
　　knee M12.56- ☑
　　multiple site M12.59
　　shoulder M12.51- ☑
　　specified joint NEC M12.58
　　vertebrae M12.58
　　wrist M12.53- ☑
**Arthropyosis** — *see* Arthritis, pyogenic or pyemic
**Arthrosis** (deformans) (degenerative) (localized) (*see also*
　Osteoarthritis) M19.90
　spine — *see* Spondylosis
**Arthus' phenomenon or reaction** T78.41 ☑
　due to
　　drug — *see* Table of Drugs and Chemicals, by drug
**Articular** — *see* condition
**Articulation, reverse** (teeth) M26.24
**Artificial**
　insemination complication — *see* Complications, arti-
　　ficial, fertilization
　opening status (functioning) (without complication)
　　Z93.9
　　anus (colostomy) Z93.3
　　colostomy Z93.3
　　cystostomy Z93.50
　　　appendico-vesicostomy Z93.52
　　　cutaneous Z93.51
　　　specified NEC Z93.59
　　enterostomy Z93.4
　　gastrostomy Z93.1
　　ileostomy Z93.2
　　intestinal tract NEC Z93.4

☑ Additional Character Required — Refer to the Tabular List for Character Selection　　　▽ Subterms under main terms may continue to next column or page

**Artificial** — *continued*
  opening status — *continued*
    jejunostomy Z93.4
    nephrostomy Z93.6
    specified site NEC Z93.8
    tracheostomy Z93.0
    ureterostomy Z93.6
    urethrostomy Z93.6
    urinary tract NEC Z93.6
    vagina Z93.8
  vagina status Z93.8
**Arytenoid** — *see* condition
**Asbestosis** (occupational) J61
**Ascariasis** B77.9
  with
    complications NEC B77.89
    intestinal complications B77.0
    pneumonia, pneumonitis B77.81
**Ascaridosis, ascariasis** — *see* Ascariasis
**Ascaris** (infection) (infestation) (lumbricoides) — *see* Ascariasis
**Ascending** — *see* condition
**ASC-H** (atypical squamous cells cannot exclude high grade squamous intraepithelial lesion on cytologic smear)
  anus R85.611
  cervix R87.611
  vagina R87.621
**Aschoff's bodies** — *see* Myocarditis, rheumatic
**Ascites** (abdominal) R18.8
  cardiac (*see also* Failure, heart, right) I50.810
  chylous (nonfilarial) I89.8
    filarial — *see* Infestation, filarial
  due to
    cirrhosis, alcoholic K70.31
    hepatitis
      alcoholic K70.11
      chronic active K71.51
    S. japonicum B65.2
  heart (*see also* Failure, heart, right) I50.810
  malignant R18.0
  pseudochylous R18.8
  syphilitic A52.74
  tuberculous A18.31
**ASC-US** (atypical squamous cells of undetermined significance on cytologic smear)
  anus R85.610
  cervix R87.610
  vagina R87.620
**Aseptic** — *see* condition
**Asherman's syndrome** N85.6
**Asialia** K11.7
**Asiatic cholera** — *see* Cholera
**Asimultagnosia** (simultanagnosia) R48.3
**Askin's tumor** — *see* Neoplasm, connective tissue, malignant
**Asocial personality** F60.2
**Asomatognosia** R41.4
**Aspartylglucosaminuria** E77.1
**Asperger's disease or syndrome** F84.5
**Aspergilloma** — *see* Aspergillosis
**Aspergillosis** (with pneumonia) B44.9
  bronchopulmonary, allergic B44.81
  disseminated B44.7
  generalized B44.7
  pulmonary NEC B44.1
    allergic B44.81
    invasive B44.0
  specified NEC B44.89
  tonsillar B44.2
**Aspergillus** (flavus) (fumigatus) (infection) (terreus) — *see* Aspergillosis
**Aspermatogenesis** — *see* Azoospermia
**Aspermia** (testis) — *see* Azoospermia
**Asphyxia, asphyxiation** (by) R09.01
  antenatal P84
  birth P84
  bunny bag — *see* Asphyxia, due to, mechanical threat to breathing, trapped in bed clothes
  crushing S28.0 ☑
  drowning T75.1 ☑
  gas, fumes, or vapor — *see* Table of Drugs and Chemicals
  inhalation — *see* Inhalation
  intrauterine P84
  local I73.00
    with gangrene I73.01

**Asphyxia, asphyxiation** — *continued*
  mucus (*see also* Foreign body, respiratory tract, causing asphyxia)
  newborn P84
  pathological R09.01
  postnatal P84
    mechanical — *see* Asphyxia, due to, mechanical threat to breathing
  prenatal P84
  reticularis R23.1
  strangulation — *see* Asphyxia, due to, mechanical threat to breathing
  submersion T75.1 ☑
  traumatic T71.9 ☑
    due to
      crushed chest S28.0 ☑
      foreign body (in) — *see* Foreign body, respiratory tract, causing asphyxia
      low oxygen content of ambient air T71.20 ☑
        due to
          being trapped in
            low oxygen environment T71.29 ☑
            in car trunk T71.221 ☑
              circumstances undetermined T71.224 ☑
              done with intent to harm by another person T71.223 ☑
              self T71.222 ☑
            in refrigerator T71.231 ☑
              circumstances undetermined T71.234 ☑
              done with intent to harm by another person T71.233 ☑
              self T71.232 ☑
        cave-in T71.21 ☑
      mechanical threat to breathing (accidental) T71.191 ☑
        circumstances undetermined T71.194 ☑
        done with intent to harm by another person T71.193 ☑
        self T71.192 ☑
        hanging T71.161 ☑
          circumstances undetermined T71.164 ☑
          done with intent to harm by another person T71.163 ☑
          self T71.162 ☑
        plastic bag T71.121 ☑
          circumstances undetermined T71.124 ☑
          done with intent to harm by another person T71.123 ☑
          self T71.122 ☑
        smothering
          in furniture T71.151 ☑
            circumstances undetermined T71.154 ☑
            done with intent to harm by another person T71.153 ☑
            self T71.152 ☑
          under
            another person's body T71.141 ☑
              circumstances undetermined T71.144 ☑
              done with intent to harm T71.143 ☑
            pillow T71.111 ☑
              circumstances undetermined T71.114 ☑
              done with intent to harm by another person T71.113 ☑
              self T71.112 ☑
        trapped in bed clothes T71.131 ☑
          circumstances undetermined T71.134 ☑
          done with intent to harm by another person T71.133 ☑
          self T71.132 ☑
  vomiting, vomitus — *see* Foreign body, respiratory tract, causing asphyxia
**Aspiration**
  amniotic (clear) fluid (newborn) P24.10
    with
      pneumonia (pneumonitis) P24.11
      respiratory symptoms P24.11
  blood
    newborn (without respiratory symptoms) P24.20
      with
        pneumonia (pneumonitis) P24.21
        respiratory symptoms P24.21

**Aspiration** — *continued*
  blood — *continued*
    specified age NEC — *see* Foreign body, respiratory tract
  bronchitis J69.0
  food or foreign body (with asphyxiation) — *see* Asphyxia, food
  liquor (amnii) (newborn) P24.10
    with
      pneumonia (pneumonitis) P24.11
      respiratory symptoms P24.11
  meconium (newborn) (without respiratory symptoms) P24.00
    with
      pneumonitis (pneumonitis) P24.01
      respiratory symptoms P24.01
  milk (newborn) (without respiratory symptoms) P24.30
    with
      pneumonia (pneumonitis) P24.31
      respiratory symptoms P24.31
    specified age NEC — *see* Foreign body, respiratory tract
  mucus (*see also* Foreign body, by site, causing asphyxia)
    newborn P24.10
      with
        pneumonia (pneumonitis) P24.11
        respiratory symptoms P24.11
  neonatal P24.9
    specific NEC (without respiratory symptoms) P24.80
      with
        pneumonia (pneumonitis) P24.81
        respiratory symptoms P24.81
  newborn P24.9
    specific NEC (without respiratory symptoms) P24.80
      with
        pneumonia (pneumonitis) P24.81
        respiratory symptoms P24.81
  pneumonia J69.0
  pneumonitis J69.0
  syndrome of newborn — *see* Aspiration, by substance, with pneumonia
  vernix caseosa (newborn) P24.80
    with
      pneumonia (pneumonitis) P24.81
      respiratory symptoms P24.81
  vomitus (*see also* Foreign body, respiratory tract)
    newborn (without respiratory symptoms) P24.30
      with
        pneumonia (pneumonitis) P24.31
        respiratory symptoms P24.31
**Asplenia** (congenital) Q89.01
  postsurgical Z90.81
**Assam fever** B55.0
**Assault, sexual** — *see* Maltreatment
**Assmann's focus NEC** A15.0
**Astasia** (-abasia) (hysterical) F44.4
**Asteatosis cutis** L85.3
**Astereognosia, astereognosis** R48.1
**Asterixis** R27.8
  in liver disease K71.3
**Asteroid hyalitis** — *see* Deposit, crystalline
**Asthenia, asthenic** R53.1
  cardiac (*see also* Failure, heart) I50.9
    psychogenic F45.8
  cardiovascular (*see also* Failure, heart) I50.9
    psychogenic F45.8
  heart (*see also* Failure, heart) I50.9
    psychogenic F45.8
  hysterical F44.4
  myocardial (*see also* Failure, heart) I50.9
    psychogenic F45.8
  nervous F48.8
  neurocirculatory F45.8
  neurotic F48.8
  psychogenic F48.8
  psychoneurotic F48.8
  psychophysiologic F48.8
  reaction (psychophysiologic) F48.8
  senile R54
**Asthenopia** (*see also* Discomfort, visual)
  hysterical F44.6
  psychogenic F44.6
**Asthenospermia** — *see* Abnormal, specimen, male genital organs
**Asthma, asthmatic** (bronchial) (catarrh) (spasmodic) J45.909

**Asthma, asthmatic** — *continued*
  with
    chronic obstructive bronchitis J44.9
      with
        acute lower respiratory infection J44.0
        exacerbation (acute) J44.1
    chronic obstructive pulmonary disease J44.9
      with
        acute lower respiratory infection J44.0
        exacerbation (acute) J44.1
    exacerbation (acute) J45.901
    hay fever — *see* Asthma, allergic extrinsic
    rhinitis, allergic — *see* Asthma, allergic extrinsic
    status asthmaticus J45.902
  allergic extrinsic J45.909
    with
      exacerbation (acute) J45.901
      status asthmaticus J45.902
  atopic — *see* Asthma, allergic extrinsic
  cardiac — *see* Failure, ventricular, left
  cardiobronchial I50.1
  childhood J45.909
    with
      exacerbation (acute) J45.901
      status asthmaticus J45.902
  chronic obstructive J44.9
    with
      acute lower respiratory infection J44.0
      exacerbation (acute) J44.1
  collier's J60
  cough variant J45.991
  detergent J69.8
  due to
    detergent J69.8
    inhalation of fumes J68.3
  eosinophilic J82
  extrinsic, allergic — *see* Asthma, allergic extrinsic
  grinder's J62.8
  hay — *see* Asthma, allergic extrinsic
  heart I50.1
  idiosyncratic — *see* Asthma, nonallergic
  intermittent (mild) J45.20
    with
      exacerbation (acute) J45.21
      status asthmaticus J45.22
  intrinsic, nonallergic — *see* Asthma, nonallergic
  Kopp's E32.8
  late-onset J45.909
    with
      exacerbation (acute) J45.901
      status asthmaticus J45.902
  mild intermittent J45.20
    with
      exacerbation (acute) J45.21
      status asthmaticus J45.22
  mild persistent J45.30
    with
      exacerbation (acute) J45.31
      status asthmaticus J45.32
  Millar's (laryngismus stridulus) J38.5
  miner's J60
  mixed J45.909
    with
      exacerbation (acute) J45.901
      status asthmaticus J45.902
  moderate persistent J45.40
    with
      exacerbation (acute) J45.41
      status asthmaticus J45.42
  nervous — *see* Asthma, nonallergic
  nonallergic (intrinsic) J45.909
    with
      exacerbation (acute) J45.901
      status asthmaticus J45.902
  persistent
    mild J45.30
      with
        exacerbation (acute) J45.31
        status asthmaticus J45.32
    moderate J45.40
      with
        exacerbation (acute) J45.41
        status asthmaticus J45.42
    severe J45.50
      with
        exacerbation (acute) J45.51
        status asthmaticus J45.52
  platinum J45.998

**Asthma, asthmatic** — *continued*
  pneumoconiotic NEC J64
  potter's J62.8
  predominantly allergic J45.909
  psychogenic F54
  pulmonary eosinophilic J82
  red cedar J67.8
  Rostan's I50.1
  sandblaster's J62.8
  sequoiosis J67.8
  severe persistent J45.50
    with
      exacerbation (acute) J45.51
      status asthmaticus J45.52
  specified NEC J45.998
  stonemason's J62.8
  thymic E32.8
  tuberculous — *see* Tuberculosis, pulmonary
  Wichmann's (laryngismus stridulus) J38.5
  wood J67.8
**Astigmatism** (compound) (congenital) H52.20- ☑
  irregular H52.21- ☑
  regular H52.22- ☑
**Astraphobia** F40.220
**Astroblastoma**
  specified site — *see* Neoplasm, malignant, by site
  unspecified site C71.9
**Astrocytoma** (cystic)
  anaplastic
    specified site — *see* Neoplasm, malignant, by site
    unspecified site C71.9
  fibrillary
    specified site — *see* Neoplasm, malignant, by site
    unspecified site C71.9
  fibrous
    specified site — *see* Neoplasm, malignant, by site
    unspecified site C71.9
  gemistocytic
    specified site — *see* Neoplasm, malignant, by site
    unspecified site C71.9
  juvenile
    specified site — *see* Neoplasm, malignant, by site
    unspecified site C71.9
  pilocytic
    specified site — *see* Neoplasm, malignant, by site
    unspecified site C71.9
  piloid
    specified site — *see* Neoplasm, malignant, by site
    unspecified site C71.9
  protoplasmic
    specified site — *see* Neoplasm, malignant, by site
    unspecified site C71.9
  specified site NEC — *see* Neoplasm, malignant, by site
  subependymal D43.2
    giant cell
      specified site — *see* Neoplasm, uncertain behavior, by site
      unspecified site D43.2
    specified site — *see* Neoplasm, uncertain behavior, by site
    unspecified site D43.2
  unspecified site C71.9
**Astroglioma**
  specified site — *see* Neoplasm, malignant, by site
  unspecified site C71.9
**Asymbolia** R48.8
**Asymmetry** (*see also* Distortion)
  between native and reconstructed breast N65.1
  face Q67.0
  jaw (lower) — *see* Anomaly, dentofacial, jaw-cranial base relationship, asymmetry
**Asynergia, asynergy** R27.8
  ventricular I51.89
**Asystole** (heart) — *see* Arrest, cardiac
**At risk**
  for
    dental caries Z91.849
      high Z91.843
      low Z91.841
      moderate Z91.842
    falling Z91.81
**Ataxia, ataxy, ataxic** R27.0
  acute R27.8
  brain (hereditary) G11.9
  cerebellar (hereditary) G11.9
    with defective DNA repair G11.3
    alcoholic G31.2
    early-onset G11.1

**Ataxia, ataxy, ataxic** — *continued*
  cerebellar — *continued*
    in
      alcoholism G31.2
      myxedema E03.9 [G13.2]
      neoplastic disease (*see also* Neoplasm) D49.9 [G32.81]
      specified disease NEC G32.81
    late-onset (Marie's) G11.2
  cerebral (hereditary) G11.9
  congenital nonprogressive G11.0
  family, familial — *see* Ataxia, hereditary
  following
    cerebrovascular disease I69.993
      cerebral infarction I69.393
      intracerebral hemorrhage I69.193
      nontraumatic intracranial hemorrhage NEC I69.293
      specified disease NEC I69.893
      subarachnoid hemorrhage I69.093
  Friedreich's (heredofamilial) (cerebellar) (spinal) G11.1
  gait R26.0
    hysterical F44.4
  general R27.8
  gluten M35.9 [G32.81]
    with celiac disease K90.0 [G32.81]
  hereditary G11.9
    with neuropathy G60.2
    cerebellar — *see* Ataxia, cerebellar
    spastic G11.4
    specified NEC G11.8
    spinal (Friedreich's) G11.1
  heredofamilial — *see* Ataxia, hereditary
  Hunt's G11.1
  hysterical F44.4
  locomotor (progressive) (syphilitic) (partial) (spastic) A52.11
    diabetic — *see* Diabetes, ataxia
  Marie's (cerebellar) (heredofamilial) (late-onset) G11.2
  nonorganic origin F44.4
  nonprogressive, congenital G11.0
  psychogenic F44.4
  Roussy-Lévy G60.0
  Sanger-Brown's (hereditary) G11.2
  spastic hereditary G11.4
  spinal
    hereditary (Friedreich's) G11.1
    progressive (syphilitic) A52.11
  spinocerebellar, X-linked recessive G11.1
  telangiectasia (Louis-Bar) G11.3
**Ataxia-telangiectasia** (Louis-Bar) G11.3
**Atelectasis** (massive) (partial) (pressure) (pulmonary) J98.11
  newborn P28.10
    due to resorption P28.11
    partial P28.19
    primary P28.0
    secondary P28.19
  primary (newborn) P28.0
  tuberculous — *see* Tuberculosis, pulmonary
**Atelocardia** Q24.9
**Atelomyelia** Q06.1
**Atheroembolism**
  of
    extremities
      lower I75.02- ☑
      upper I75.01- ☑
    kidney I75.81
    specified NEC I75.89
**Atheroma, atheromatous** (*see also* Arteriosclerosis) I70.90
  aorta, aortic I70.0
    valve (*see also* Endocarditis, aortic) I35.8
  aorto-iliac I70.0
  artery — *see* Arteriosclerosis
  basilar (artery) I67.2
  carotid (artery) (common) (internal) I67.2
  cerebral (arteries) I67.2
  coronary (artery) I25.10
    with angina pectoris — *see* Arteriosclerosis, coronary (artery)
  degeneration — *see* Arteriosclerosis
  heart, cardiac — *see* Disease, heart, ischemic, atherosclerotic
  mitral (valve) I34.8
  myocardium, myocardial — *see* Disease, heart, ischemic, atherosclerotic

**Atheroma, atheromatous** — *continued*
  pulmonary valve (heart) (valve) (*see also* Endocarditis, pulmonary) I37.8
  tricuspid (heart) (valve) I36.8
  valve, valvular — *see* Endocarditis
  vertebral (artery) I67.2
**Atheromatosis** — *see* Arteriosclerosis
**Atherosclerosis** (*see also* Arteriosclerosis)
  coronary
    artery I25.1Ø
      with angina pectoris — *see* Arteriosclerosis, coronary (artery),
      due to
        calcified coronary lesion (severely) I25.84
        lipid rich plaque I25.83
    transplanted heart I25.811
      bypass graft I25.812
        with angina pectoris — *see* Arteriosclerosis, coronary (artery),
      native coronary artery I25.811
        with angina pectoris — *see* Arteriosclerosis, coronary (artery),
**Athetosis** (acquired) R25.8
  bilateral (congenital) G8Ø.3
  congenital (bilateral) (double) G8Ø.3
  double (congenital) G8Ø.3
  unilateral R25.8
**Athlete's**
  foot B35.3
  heart I51.7
**Athrepsia** E41
**Athyrea** (acquired) (*see also* Hypothyroidism)
  congenital EØ3.1
**Atonia, atony, atonic**
  bladder (sphincter) (neurogenic) N31.2
  capillary I78.8
  cecum K59.8
    psychogenic F45.8
  colon — *see* Atony, intestine
  congenital P94.2
  esophagus K22.8
  intestine K59.8
    psychogenic F45.8
  stomach K31.89
    neurotic or psychogenic F45.8
  uterus (during labor) O62.2
    with hemorrhage (postpartum) O72.1
    postpartum (with hemorrhage) O72.1
      without hemorrhage O75.89
**Atopy** — *see* History, allergy
**Atransferrinemia, congenital** E88.Ø9
**Atresia, atretic**
  alimentary organ or tract NEC Q45.8
    upper Q4Ø.8
  ani, anus, anal (canal) Q42.3
    with fistula Q42.2
  aorta (ring) Q25.29
  aortic (orifice) (valve) Q23.Ø
    arch Q25.21
    congenital with hypoplasia of ascending aorta and defective development of left ventricle (with mitral stenosis) Q23.4
    in hypoplastic left heart syndrome Q23.4
  aqueduct of Sylvius QØ3.Ø
    with spina bifida — *see* Spina bifida, with hydrocephalus
  artery NEC Q27.8
    cerebral Q28.3
    coronary Q24.5
    digestive system Q27.8
    eye Q15.8
    lower limb Q27.8
    pulmonary Q25.5
    specified site NEC Q27.8
    umbilical Q27.Ø
    upper limb Q27.8
  auditory canal (external) Q16.1
  bile duct (common) (congenital) (hepatic) Q44.2
    acquired — *see* Obstruction, bile duct
  bladder (neck) Q64.39
    obstruction Q64.31
  bronchus Q32.4
  cecum Q42.8
  cervix (acquired) N88.2
    congenital Q51.828
    in pregnancy or childbirth — *see* Anomaly, cervix, in pregnancy or childbirth
      causing obstructed labor O65.5

**Atresia, atretic** — *continued*
  choana Q3Ø.Ø
  colon Q42.9
    specified NEC Q42.8
  common duct Q44.2
  cricoid cartilage Q31.8
  cystic duct Q44.2
    acquired K82.8
      with obstruction K82.Ø
  digestive organs NEC Q45.8
  duodenum Q41.Ø
  ear canal Q16.1
  ejaculatory duct Q55.4
  epiglottis Q31.8
  esophagus Q39.Ø
    with tracheoesophageal fistula Q39.1
  eustachian tube Q17.8
  fallopian tube (congenital) Q5Ø.6
    acquired N97.1
  follicular cyst N83.Ø- ☑
  foramen of
    Luschka QØ3.1
      with spina bifida — *see* Spina bifida, with hydrocephalus
    Magendie QØ3.1
      with spina bifida — *see* Spina bifida, with hydrocephalus
  gallbladder Q44.1
  genital organ
    external
      female Q52.79
      male Q55.8
    internal
      female Q52.8
      male Q55.8
  glottis Q31.8
  gullet Q39.Ø
    with tracheoesophageal fistula Q39.1
  heart valve NEC Q24.8
    pulmonary Q22.Ø
    tricuspid Q22.4
  hymen Q52.3
    acquired (postinfective) N89.6
  ileum Q41.2
  intestine (small) Q41.9
    large Q42.9
      specified NEC Q42.8
  iris, filtration angle Q15.Ø
  jejunum Q41.1
  lacrimal apparatus Q1Ø.4
  larynx Q31.8
  meatus urinarius Q64.33
  mitral valve Q23.2
    in hypoplastic left heart syndrome Q23.4
  nares (anterior) (posterior) Q3Ø.Ø
  nasopharynx Q34.8
  nose, nostril Q3Ø.Ø
    acquired J34.89
  organ or site NEC Q89.8
  osseous meatus (ear) Q16.1
  oviduct (congenital) Q5Ø.6
    acquired N97.1
  parotid duct Q38.4
    acquired K11.8
  pulmonary (artery) Q25.5
    valve Q22.Ø
  pulmonic Q22.Ø
  pupil Q13.2
  rectum Q42.1
    with fistula Q42.Ø
  salivary duct Q38.4
    acquired K11.8
  sublingual duct Q38.4
    acquired K11.8
  submandibular duct Q38.4
    acquired K11.8
  submaxillary duct Q38.4
    acquired K11.8
  thyroid cartilage Q31.8
  trachea Q32.1
  tricuspid valve Q22.4
  ureter Q62.1Ø
    pelvic junction Q62.11
    vesical orifice Q62.12
  ureteropelvic junction Q62.11
  ureterovesical orifice Q62.12
  urethra (valvular) Q64.39
    stricture Q64.32
  urinary tract NEC Q64.8

**Atresia, atretic** — *continued*
  uterus Q51.818
    acquired N85.8
  vagina (congenital) Q52.4
    acquired (postinfectional) (senile) N89.5
  vas deferens Q55.3
  vascular NEC Q27.8
    cerebral Q28.3
    digestive system Q27.8
    lower limb Q27.8
    specified site NEC Q27.8
    upper limb Q27.8
  vein NEC Q27.8
    digestive system Q27.8
    great Q26.8
    lower limb Q27.8
    portal Q26.5
    pulmonary Q26.4
      partial Q26.3
      total Q26.2
    specified site NEC Q27.8
    upper limb Q27.8
  vena cava (inferior) (superior) Q26.8
  vesicourethral orifice Q64.31
  vulva Q52.79
    acquired N9Ø.5
**Atrichia, atrichosis** — *see* Alopecia
**Atrophia** (*see also* Atrophy)
  cutis senilis L9Ø.8
    due to radiation L57.8
  gyrata of choroid and retina H31.23
  senilis R54
    dermatological L9Ø.8
      due to radiation (nonionizing) (solar) L57.8
  unguium L6Ø.3
    congenita Q84.6
**Atrophie blanche** (en plaque) (de Milian) L95.Ø
**Atrophoderma, atrophodermia** (of) L9Ø.9
  diffusum (idiopathic) L9Ø.4
  maculatum L9Ø.8
    et striatum L9Ø.8
      due to syphilis A52.79
    syphilitic A51.39
  neuriticum L9Ø.8
  Pasini and Pierini L9Ø.3
  pigmentosum Q82.1
  reticulatum symmetricum faciei L66.4
  senile L9Ø.8
    due to radiation (nonionizing) (solar) L57.8
  vermiculata (cheeks) L66.4
**Atrophy, atrophic** (of)
  adrenal (capsule) (gland) E27.49
    primary (autoimmune) E27.1
  alveolar process or ridge (edentulous) KØ8.2Ø
  anal sphincter (disuse) N81.84
  appendix K38.8
  arteriosclerotic — *see* Arteriosclerosis
  bile duct (common) (hepatic) K83.8
  bladder N32.89
    neurogenic N31.8
  blanche (en plaque) (of Milian) L95.Ø
  bone (senile) NEC (*see also* Disorder, bone, specified type NEC)
    due to
      tabes dorsalis (neurogenic) A52.11
  brain (cortex) (progressive) G31.9
    frontotemporal circumscribed G31.Ø1 [FØ2.8Ø]
      with behavioral disturbance G31.Ø1 [FØ2.81]
    senile NEC G31.1
  breast N64.2
    obstetric — *see* Disorder, breast, specified type NEC
  buccal cavity K13.79
  cardiac — *see* Degeneration, myocardial
  cartilage (infectional) (joint) — *see* Disorder, cartilage, specified NEC
  cerebellar — *see* Atrophy, brain
  cerebral — *see* Atrophy, brain
  cervix (mucosa) (senile) (uteri) N88.8
    menopausal N95.8
  Charcot-Marie-Tooth G6Ø.Ø
  choroid (central) (macular) (myopic) (retina) H31.1Ø- ☑
    diffuse secondary H31.12- ☑
    gyrate H31.23
    senile H31.11- ☑
  ciliary body — *see* Atrophy, iris
  conjunctiva (senile) H11.89
  corpus cavernosum N48.89

**Atrophy, atrophic** — *continued*
- cortical — *see* Atrophy, brain
- cystic duct K82.8
- Déjérine-Thomas G23.8
- disuse NEC — *see* Atrophy, muscle
- Duchenne-Aran G12.21
- ear H93.8- ☑
- edentulous alveolar ridge K08.20
- endometrium (senile) N85.8
  - cervix N88.8
- enteric K63.89
- epididymis N50.89
- eyeball — *see* Disorder, globe, degenerated condition, atrophy
- eyelid (senile) — *see* Disorder, eyelid, degenerative
- facial (skin) L90.9
- fallopian tube (senile) N83.32- ☑
  - with ovary N83.33- ☑
- fascioscapulohumeral (Landouzy- Déjérine) G71.0
- fatty, thymus (gland) E32.8
- gallbladder K82.8
- gastric K29.40
  - with bleeding K29.41
- gastrointestinal K63.89
- glandular I89.8
- globe H44.52- ☑
- gum — *see* Recession, gingival
- hair L67.8
- heart (brown) — *see* Degeneration, myocardial
- hemifacial Q67.4
  - Romberg G51.8
- infantile E41
  - paralysis, acute — *see* Poliomyelitis, paralytic
- intestine K63.89
- iris (essential) (progressive) H21.26- ☑
  - specified NEC H21.29
- kidney (senile) (terminal) (*see also* Sclerosis, renal) N26.1
  - congenital or infantile Q60.5
    - bilateral Q60.4
    - unilateral Q60.3
  - hydronephrotic — *see* Hydronephrosis
- lacrimal gland (primary) H04.14- ☑
  - secondary H04.15- ☑
- Landouzy-Déjérine G71.0
- laryngitis, infective J37.0
- larynx J38.7
- Leber's optic (hereditary) H47.22
- lip K13.0
- liver (yellow) K72.90
  - with coma K72.91
  - acute, subacute K72.00
    - with coma K72.01
  - chronic K72.10
    - with coma K72.11
- lung (senile) J98.4
- macular (dermatological) L90.8
  - syphilitic, skin A51.39
    - striated A52.79
- mandible (edentulous) K08.20
  - minimal K08.21
  - moderate K08.22
  - severe K08.23
- maxilla K08.20
  - minimal K08.24
  - moderate K08.25
  - severe K08.26
- muscle, muscular (diffuse) (general) (idiopathic) (primary) M62.50
  - ankle M62.57- ☑
  - Duchenne-Aran G12.21
  - foot M62.57- ☑
  - forearm M62.53- ☑
  - hand M62.54- ☑
  - infantile spinal G12.0
  - lower leg M62.56- ☑
  - multiple sites M62.59
  - myelopathic — *see* Atrophy, muscle, spinal
  - myotonic G71.11
  - neuritic G58.9
  - neuropathic (peroneal) (progressive) G60.0
  - pelvic (disuse) N81.84
  - peroneal G60.0
  - progressive (bulbar) G12.21
    - adult G12.1
    - infantile (spinal) G12.0
    - spinal G12.25
      - adult G12.1

**Atrophy, atrophic** — *continued*
- muscle, muscular — *continued*
  - progressive — *continued*
    - spinal — *continued*
      - infantile G12.0
  - pseudohypertrophic G71.0
  - shoulder region M62.51- ☑
  - specified site NEC M62.58
  - spinal G12.9
    - adult form G12.1
    - Aran-Duchenne G12.21
    - childhood form, type II G12.1
    - distal G12.1
    - hereditary NEC G12.1
    - infantile, type I (Werdnig-Hoffmann) G12.0
    - juvenile form, type III (Kugelberg- Welander) G12.1
    - progressive G12.25
    - scapuloperoneal form G12.1
    - specified NEC G12.8
  - syphilitic A52.78
  - thigh M62.55- ☑
  - upper arm M62.52- ☑
- myocardium — *see* Degeneration, myocardial
- myometrium (senile) N85.8
  - cervix N88.8
- myopathic NEC — *see* Atrophy, muscle
- myotonia G71.11
- nail L60.3
- nasopharynx J31.1
- nerve (*see also* Disorder, nerve)
  - abducens — *see* Strabismus, paralytic, sixth nerve
  - accessory G52.8
  - acoustic or auditory H93.3 ☑
  - cranial G52.9
    - eighth (auditory) H93.3 ☑
    - eleventh (accessory) G52.8
    - fifth (trigeminal) G50.8
    - first (olfactory) G52.0
    - fourth (trochlear) — *see* Strabismus, paralytic, fourth nerve
    - second (optic) H47.20
    - sixth (abducens) — *see* Strabismus, paralytic, sixth nerve
    - tenth (pneumogastric) (vagus) G52.2
    - third (oculomotor) — *see* Strabismus, paralytic, third nerve
    - twelfth (hypoglossal) G52.3
  - hypoglossal G52.3
  - oculomotor — *see* Strabismus, paralytic, third nerve
  - olfactory G52.0
  - optic (papillomacular bundle)
    - syphilitic (late) A52.15
      - congenital A50.44
  - pneumogastric G52.2
  - trigeminal G50.8
  - trochlear — *see* Strabismus, paralytic, fourth nerve
  - vagus (pneumogastric) G52.2
- neurogenic, bone, tabetic A52.11
- nutritional E41
- old age R54
- olivopontocerebellar G23.8
- optic (nerve) H47.20
  - glaucomatous H47.23- ☑
  - hereditary H47.22
  - primary H47.21- ☑
  - specified type NEC H47.29- ☑
  - syphilitic (late) A52.15
    - congenital A50.44
- orbit H05.31- ☑
- ovary (senile) N83.31- ☑
  - with fallopian tube N83.33- ☑
- oviduct (senile) — *see* Atrophy, fallopian tube
- palsy, diffuse (progressive) G12.22
- pancreas (duct) (senile) K86.89
- parotid gland K11.0
- pelvic muscle N81.84
- penis N48.89
- pharynx J39.2
- pluriglandular E31.8
  - autoimmune E31.0
- polyarthritis M15.9
- prostate N42.89
- pseudohypertrophic (muscle) G71.0
- renal (*see also* Sclerosis, renal) N26.1
- retina, retinal (postinfectional) H35.89
- rhinitis J31.0

**Atrophy, atrophic** — *continued*
- salivary gland K11.0
- scar L90.5
- sclerosis, lobar (of brain) G31.09 [F02.80]
  - with behavioral disturbance G31.09 [F02.81]
- scrotum N50.89
- seminal vesicle N50.89
- senile R54
  - due to radiation (nonionizing) (solar) L57.8
- skin (patches) (spots) L90.9
  - degenerative (senile) L90.8
  - due to radiation (nonionizing) (solar) L57.8
  - senile L90.8
- spermatic cord N50.89
- spinal (acute) (cord) G95.89
  - muscular — *see* Atrophy, muscle, spinal
  - paralysis G12.20
    - acute — *see* Poliomyelitis, paralytic
    - meaning progressive muscular atrophy G12.21
- spine (column) — *see* Spondylopathy, specified NEC
- spleen (senile) D73.0
- stomach K29.40
  - with bleeding K29.41
- striate (skin) L90.6
  - syphilitic A52.79
- subcutaneous L90.9
- sublingual gland K11.0
- submandibular gland K11.0
- submaxillary gland K11.0
- Sudeck's — *see* Algoneurodystrophy
- suprarenal (capsule) (gland) E27.49
  - primary E27.1
- systemic affecting central nervous system in
  - myxedema E03.9 [G13.2]
  - neoplastic disease (*see also* Neoplasm) D49.9 [G13.1]
  - specified disease NEC G13.8
- tarso-orbital fascia, congenital Q10.3
- testis N50.0
- thenar, partial — *see* Syndrome, carpal tunnel
- thymus (fatty) E32.8
- thyroid (gland) (acquired) E03.4
  - with cretinism E03.1
  - congenital (with myxedema) E03.1
- tongue (senile) K14.8
  - papillae K14.4
- trachea J39.8
- tunica vaginalis N50.89
- turbinate J34.89
- tympanic membrane (nonflaccid) H73.82- ☑
  - flaccid H73.81- ☑
- upper respiratory tract J39.8
- uterus, uterine (senile) N85.8
  - cervix N88.8
  - due to radiation (intended effect) N85.8
    - adverse effect or misadventure N99.89
- vagina (senile) N95.2
- vas deferens N50.89
- vascular I99.8
- vertebra (senile) — *see* Spondylopathy, specified NEC
- vulva (senile) N90.5
- Werdnig-Hoffmann G12.0
- yellow — *see* Failure, hepatic

**Attack, attacks**
- with alteration of consciousness (with automatisms) — *see* Epilepsy, localization-related, symptomatic, with complex partial seizures
- without alteration of consciousness — *see* Epilepsy, localization-related, symptomatic, with simple partial seizures
- Adams-Stokes I45.9
- akinetic — *see* Epilepsy, generalized, specified NEC
- angina — *see* Angina
- atonic — *see* Epilepsy, generalized, specified NEC
- benign shuddering G25.83
- cataleptic — *see* Catalepsy
- coronary — *see* Infarct, myocardium
- cyanotic, newborn P28.2
- drop NEC R55
- epileptic — *see* Epilepsy
- heart — *see* infarct, myocardium
- hysterical F44.9
- jacksonian — *see* Epilepsy, localization-related, symptomatic, with simple partial seizures
- myocardium, myocardial — *see* Infarct, myocardium
- myoclonic — *see* Epilepsy, generalized, specified NEC
- panic F41.0

☑ **Additional Character Required** — **Refer to the Tabular List for Character Selection**     ▽ **Subterms under main terms may continue to next column or page**

**Attack, attacks** — *continued*
- psychomotor — *see* Epilepsy, localization-related, symptomatic, with complex partial seizures
- salaam — *see* Epilepsy, spasms
- schizophreniform, brief F23
- shuddering, benign G25.83
- Stokes-Adams I45.9
- syncope R55
- transient ischemic (TIA) G45.9
  - specified NEC G45.8
- unconsciousness R55
  - hysterical F44.89
- vasomotor R55
- vasovagal (paroxysmal) (idiopathic) R55

**Attention** (to)
- artificial
  - opening (of) Z43.9
    - digestive tract NEC Z43.4
      - colon Z43.3
      - ilium Z43.2
      - stomach Z43.1
    - specified NEC Z43.8
    - trachea Z43.0
    - urinary tract NEC Z43.6
      - cystostomy Z43.5
      - nephrostomy Z43.6
      - ureterostomy Z43.6
      - urethrostomy Z43.6
    - vagina Z43.7
- colostomy Z43.3
- cystostomy Z43.5
- deficit disorder or syndrome F98.8
  - with hyperactivity — *see* Disorder, attention-deficit hyperactivity
- gastrostomy Z43.1
- ileostomy Z43.2
- jejunostomy Z43.4
- nephrostomy Z43.6
- surgical dressings Z48.01
- sutures Z48.02
- tracheostomy Z43.0
- ureterostomy Z43.6
- urethrostomy Z43.6

**Attrition**
- gum — *see* Recession, gingival
- tooth, teeth (excessive) (hard tissues) K03.0

**Atypical, atypism** (*see also* condition)
- cells (on cytolgocial smear) (endocervical) (endometrial) (glandular)
  - cervix R87.619
  - vagina R87.629
- cervical N87.9
- endometrium N85.9
  - hyperplasia N85.00
- parenting situation Z62.9

**Auditory** — *see* condition
**Aujeszky's disease** B33.8
**Aurantiasis, cutis** E67.1
**Auricle, auricular** (*see also* condition)
- cervical Q18.2

**Auriculotemporal syndrome** G50.8
**Austin Flint murmur** (aortic insufficiency) I35.1
**Australian**
- Q fever A78
- X disease A83.4

**Autism, autistic** (childhood) (infantile) F84.0
- atypical F84.9
- spectrum disorder F84.0

**Autodigestion** R68.89
**Autoerythrocyte sensitization** (syndrome) D69.2
**Autographism** L50.3
**Autoimmune**
- disease (systemic) M35.9
- inhibitors to clotting factors D68.311
- lymphoproliferative syndrome [ALPS] D89.82
- thyroiditis E06.3

**Autointoxication** R68.89
**Automatism** G93.89
- with temporal sclerosis G93.81
- epileptic — *see* Epilepsy, localization-related, symptomatic, with complex partial seizures
- paroxysmal, idiopathic — *see* Epilepsy, localization-related, symptomatic, with complex partial seizures

**Autonomic, autonomous**
- bladder (neurogenic) N31.2
- hysteria seizure F44.5

**Autosensitivity, erythrocyte** D69.2

**Autosensitization, cutaneous** L30.2
**Autosome** — *see* condition by chromosome involved
**Autotopagnosia** R48.1
**Autotoxemia** R68.89
**Autumn** — *see* condition
**Avellis' syndrome** G46.8
**Aversion**
- oral R63.3
  - newborn P92.- ☑
  - nonorganic origin F98.2 ☑
- sexual F52.1

**Aviator's**
- disease or sickness — *see* Effect, adverse, high altitude
- ear T70.0 ☑

**Avitaminosis** (multiple) (*see also* Deficiency, vitamin) E56.9
- B E53.9
  - with
    - beriberi E51.11
    - pellagra E52
  - B2 E53.0
  - B6 E53.1
  - B12 E53.8
- D E55.9
  - with rickets E55.0
- G E53.0
- K E56.1
- nicotinic acid E52

**AVNRT** (atrioventricular nodal re-entrant tachycardia) I47.1
**AVRT** (atrioventricular nodal re-entrant tachycardia) I47.1
**Avulsion** (traumatic)
- blood vessel — *see* Injury, blood vessel
- bone — *see* Fracture, by site
- cartilage (*see also* Dislocation, by site)
  - symphyseal (inner), complicating delivery O71.6
- external site other than limb — *see* Wound, open, by site
- eye S05.7- ☑
- head (intracranial)
  - external site NEC S08.89 ☑
  - scalp S08.0 ☑
- internal organ or site — *see* Injury, by site
- joint (*see also* Dislocation, by site)
  - capsule — *see* Sprain, by site
- kidney S37.06- ☑
- ligament — *see* Sprain, by site
- limb (*see also* Amputation, traumatic, by site)
  - skin and subcutaneous tissue — *see* Wound, open, by site
- muscle — *see* Injury, muscle
- nerve (root) — *see* Injury, nerve
- scalp S08.0 ☑
- skin and subcutaneous tissue — *see* Wound, open, by site
- spleen S36.032 ☑
- symphyseal cartilage (inner), complicating delivery O71.6
- tendon — *see* Injury, muscle
- tooth S03.2 ☑

**Awareness of heart beat** R00.2
**Axenfeld's**
- anomaly or syndrome Q15.0
- degeneration (calcareous) Q13.4

**Axilla, axillary** (*see also* condition)
- breast Q83.1

**Axonotmesis** — *see* Injury, nerve
**Ayerza's disease or syndrome** (pulmonary artery sclerosis with pulmonary hypertension) I27.0
**Azoospermia** (organic) N46.01
- due to
  - drug therapy N46.021
  - efferent duct obstruction N46.023
  - infection N46.022
  - radiation N46.024
  - specified cause NEC N46.029
  - systemic disease N46.025

**Azotemia** R79.89
- meaning uremia N19

**Aztec ear** Q17.3
**Azygos**
- continuation inferior vena cava Q26.8
- lobe (lung) Q33.1

# B

**Baastrup's disease** — *see* Kissing spine

**Babesiosis** B60.0
**Babington's disease** (familial hemorrhagic telangiectasia) I78.0
**Babinski's syndrome** A52.79
**Baby**
- crying constantly R68.11
- floppy (syndrome) P94.2

**Bacillary** — *see* condition
**Bacilluria** R82.71
**Bacillus** (*see also* Infection, bacillus)
- abortus infection A23.1
- anthracis infection A22.9
- coli infection (*see also* Escherichia coli) B96.20
- Flexner's A03.1
- mallei infection A24.0
- Shiga's A03.0
- suipestifer infection — *see* Infection, salmonella

**Back** — *see* condition
**Backache** (postural) M54.9
- sacroiliac M53.3
- specified NEC M54.89

**Backflow** — *see* Reflux
**Backward reading** (dyslexia) F81.0
**Bacteremia** R78.81
- with sepsis — *see* Sepsis

**Bactericholia** — *see* Cholecystitis, acute
**Bacterid, bacteride** (pustular) L40.3
**Bacterium, bacteria, bacterial**
- agent NEC, as cause of disease classified elsewhere B96.89
- in blood — *see* Bacteremia
- in urine — *see* Bacteriuria

**Bacteriuria, bacteruria** R82.71
- asymptomatic R82.71

**Bacteroides**
- fragilis, as cause of disease classified elsewhere B96.6

**Bad**
- heart — *see* Disease, heart
- trip
  - due to drug abuse — *see* Abuse, drug, hallucinogen
  - due to drug dependence — *see* Dependence, drug, hallucinogen

**Baelz's disease** (cheilitis glandularis apostematosa) K13.0
**Baerensprung's disease** (eczema marginatum) B35.6
**Bagasse disease or pneumonitis** J67.1
**Bagassosis** J67.1
**Baker's cyst** — *see* Cyst, Baker's
**Bakwin-Krida syndrome** (metaphyseal dysplasia) Q78.5
**Balancing side interference** M26.56
**Balanitis** (circinata) (erosiva) (gangrenosa) (phagedenic) (vulgaris) N48.1
- amebic A06.82
- candidal B37.42
- due to Haemophilus ducreyi A57
- gonococcal (acute) (chronic) A54.09
- xerotica obliterans N48.0

**Balanoposthitis** N47.6
- gonococcal (acute) (chronic) A54.09
- ulcerative (specific) A63.8

**Balanorrhagia** — *see* Balanitis
**Balantidiasis, balantidiosis** A07.0
**Bald tongue** K14.4
**Baldness** (*see also* Alopecia)
- male-pattern — *see* Alopecia, androgenic

**Balkan grippe** A78
**Balloon disease** — *see* Effect, adverse, high altitude
**Balo's disease** (concentric sclerosis) G37.5
**Bamberger-Marie disease** — *see* Osteoarthropathy, hypertrophic, specified type NEC
**Bancroft's filariasis** B74.0
**Band**(s)
- adhesive — *see* Adhesions, peritoneum
- anomalous or congenital (*see also* Anomaly, by site)
  - heart (atrial) (ventricular) Q24.8
  - intestine Q43.3
  - omentum Q43.3
- cervix N88.1
- constricting, congenital Q79.8
- gallbladder (congenital) Q44.1
- intestinal (adhesive) — *see* Adhesions, peritoneum
- obstructive
  - intestine K56.50
    - complete K56.52
    - incomplete K56.51
    - partial K56.51
  - peritoneum K56.50

**Band**(s) — *continued*
> obstructive — *continued*
>> peritoneum — *continued*
>>> complete K56.52
>>> incomplete K56.51
>>> partial K56.51
>> periappendiceal, congenital Q43.3
>> peritoneal (adhesive) — *see* Adhesions, peritoneum
>> uterus N73.6
>>> internal N85.6
>> vagina N89.5

**Bandemia** D72.825
**Bandl's ring** (contraction), complicating delivery O62.4
**Bangkok hemorrhagic fever** A91
**Bang's disease** (brucella abortus) A23.1
**Bankruptcy, anxiety concerning** Z59.8
**Bannister's disease** T78.3 ☑
> hereditary D84.1

**Banti's disease or syndrome** (with cirrhosis) (with portal hypertension) K76.6
**Bar, median, prostate** — *see* Enlargement, enlarged, prostate
**Barcoo disease or rot** — *see* Ulcer, skin
**Barlow's disease** E54
**Barodontalgia** T70.29 ☑
**Baron Münchausen syndrome** — *see* Disorder, factitious
**Barosinusitis** T70.1 ☑
**Barotitis** T70.0 ☑
**Barotrauma** T70.29 ☑
> odontalgia T70.29 ☑
> otitic T70.0 ☑
> sinus T70.1 ☑

**Barraquer** (-Simons) **disease or syndrome** (progressive lipodystrophy) E88.1
**Barré-Guillain disease or syndrome** G61.0
**Barrel chest** M95.4
**Barré-Liéou syndrome** (posterior cervical sympathetic) M53.0
**Barrett's**
> disease — *see* Barrett's, esophagus
> esophagus K22.70
>> with dysplasia K22.719
>>> high grade K22.711
>>> low grade K22.710
>> without dysplasia K22.70
> syndrome — *see* Barrett's, esophagus
> ulcer K22.10
>> with bleeding K22.11
>> without bleeding K22.10

**Bársony** (-Polgár) (-Teschendorf) **syndrome** (corkscrew esophagus) K22.4
**Barth syndrome** E78.71
**Bartholinitis** (suppurating) N75.8
> gonococcal (acute) (chronic) (with abscess) A54.1

**Bartonellosis** A44.9
> cutaneous A44.1
> mucocutaneous A44.1
> specified NEC A44.8
> systemic A44.0

**Barton's fracture** S52.56- ☑
**Bartter's syndrome** E26.81
**Basal** — *see* condition
**Basan's** (hidrotic) ectodermal dysplasia Q82.4
**Baseball finger** — *see* Dislocation, finger
**Basedow's disease** (exophthalmic goiter) — *see* Hyperthyroidism, with, goiter
**Basic** — *see* condition
**Basilar** — *see* condition
**Bason's** (hidrotic) ectodermal dysplasia Q82.4
**Basopenia** — *see* Agranulocytosis
**Basophilia** D72.824
**Basophilism** (cortico-adrenal) (Cushing's) (pituitary) E24.0
**Bassen-Kornzweig disease or syndrome** E78.6
**Bat ear** Q17.5
**Bateman's**
> disease B08.1
> purpura (senile) D69.2

**Bathing cramp** T75.1 ☑
**Bathophobia** F40.248
**Batten** (-Mayou) **disease** E75.4
> retina E75.4 [H36]

**Batten-Steinert syndrome** G71.11
**Battered** — *see* Maltreatment
**Battey Mycobacterium infection** A31.0
**Battle exhaustion** F43.0

**Battledore placenta** O43.19- ☑
**Baumgarten-Cruveilhier cirrhosis, disease or syndrome** K74.69
**Bauxite fibrosis** (of lung) J63.1
**Bayle's disease** (general paresis) A52.17
**Bazin's disease** (primary) (tuberculous) A18.4
**Beach ear** — *see* Swimmer's, ear
**Beaded hair** (congenital) Q84.1
**Béal conjunctivitis or syndrome** B30.2
**Beard's disease** (neurasthenia) F48.8
**Beat**(s)
> atrial, premature I49.1
> ectopic I49.49
> elbow — *see* Bursitis, elbow
> escaped, heart I49.49
> hand — *see* Bursitis, hand
> knee — *see* Bursitis, knee
> premature I49.40
>> atrial I49.1
>> auricular I49.1
>> supraventricular I49.1

**Beau's**
> disease or syndrome — *see* Degeneration, myocardial
> lines (transverse furrows on fingernails) L60.4

**Bechterev's syndrome** — *see* Spondylitis, ankylosing
**Becker's**
> cardiomyopathy I42.8
> disease
>> idiopathic mural endomyocardial disease I42.3
>> myotonia congenita, recessive form G71.12
> dystrophy G71.0
> pigmented hairy nevus D22.5

**Beck's syndrome** (anterior spinal artery occlusion) I65.8
**Beckwith-Wiedemann syndrome** Q87.3
**Bed confinement status** Z74.01
**Bed sore** — *see* Ulcer, pressure, by site
**Bedbug bite**(s) — *see* Bite(s), by site, superficial, insect
**Bedclothes, asphyxiation or suffocation by** — *see* Asphyxia, traumatic, due to, mechanical, trapped
**Bednar's**
> aphthae K12.0
> tumor — *see* Neoplasm, malignant, by site

**Bedridden** Z74.01
**Bedsore** — *see* Ulcer, pressure, by site
**Bedwetting** — *see* Enuresis
**Bee sting** (with allergic or anaphylactic shock) — *see* Toxicity, venom, arthropod, bee
**Beer drinker's heart** (disease) I42.6
**Begbie's disease** (exophthalmic goiter) — *see* Hyperthyroidism, with, goiter
**Behavior**
> antisocial
>> adult Z72.811
>> child or adolescent Z72.810
> disorder, disturbance — *see* Disorder, conduct
> disruptive — *see* Disorder, conduct
> drug seeking Z76.5
> inexplicable R46.2
> marked evasiveness R46.5
> obsessive-compulsive R46.81
> overactivity R46.3
> poor responsiveness R46.4
> self-damaging (life-style) Z72.89
> sleep-incompatible Z72.821
> slowness R46.4
> specified NEC R46.89
> strange (and inexplicable) R46.2
> suspiciousness R46.5
> type A pattern Z73.1
> undue concern or preoccupation with stressful events R46.6
> verbosity and circumstantial detail obscuring reason for contact R46.7

**Behçet's disease or syndrome** M35.2
**Behr's disease** — *see* Degeneration, macula
**Beigel's disease or morbus** (white piedra) B36.2
**Bejel** A65
**Bekhterev's syndrome** — *see* Spondylitis, ankylosing
**Belching** — *see* Eructation
**Bell's**
> mania F30.8
> palsy, paralysis G51.0
>> infant or newborn P11.3
> spasm G51.3

**Bence Jones albuminuria or proteinuria NEC** R80.3
**Bends** T70.3 ☑
**Benedikt's paralysis or syndrome** G46.3

**Benign** (*see also* condition)
> prostatic hyperplasia — *see* Hyperplasia, prostate

**Bennett's fracture** (displaced) S62.21- ☑
**Benson's disease** — *see* Deposit, crystalline
**Bent**
> back (hysterical) F44.4
> nose M95.0
>> congenital Q67.4

**Bereavement** (uncomplicated) Z63.4
**Bergeron's disease** (hysterical chorea) F44.4
**Berger's disease** — *see* Nephropathy, IgA
**Beriberi** (dry) E51.11
> heart (disease) E51.12
> polyneuropathy E51.11
> wet E51.12
>> involving circulatory system E51.11

**Berlin's disease or edema** (traumatic) S05.8X- ☑
**Berlock** (berloque) **dermatitis** L56.2
**Bernard-Horner syndrome** G90.2
**Bernard-Soulier disease or thrombopathia** D69.1
**Bernhardt** (-Roth) **disease** — *see* Mononeuropathy, lower limb, meralgia paresthetica
**Bernheim's syndrome** — *see* Failure, heart, right
**Bertielliasis** B71.8
**Berylliosis** (lung) J63.2
**Besnier-Boeck** (-Schaumann) **disease** — *see* Sarcoidosis
**Besnier's**
> lupus pernio D86.3
> prurigo L20.0

**Bestiality** F65.89
**Best's disease** H35.50
**Betalipoproteinemia, broad or floating** E78.2
**Beta-mercaptolactate-cysteine disulfiduria** E72.09
**Betting and gambling** Z72.6
> pathological (compulsive) F63.0

**Bezoar** T18.9 ☑
> intestine T18.3 ☑
> stomach T18.2 ☑

**Bezold's abscess** — *see* Mastoiditis, acute
**Bianchi's syndrome** R48.8
**Bicornate or bicornis uterus** Q51.3
> in pregnancy or childbirth O34.00
>> causing obstructed labor O65.5

**Bicuspid aortic valve** Q23.1
**Biedl-Bardet syndrome** Q87.89
**Bielschowsky** (-Jansky) disease E75.4
**Biermer's** (pernicious) anemia or disease D51.0
**Biett's disease** L93.0
**Bifid** (congenital)
> apex, heart Q24.8
> clitoris Q52.6
> kidney Q63.8
> nose Q30.2
> patella Q74.1
> scrotum Q55.29
> toe NEC Q74.2
> tongue Q38.3
> ureter Q62.8
> uterus Q51.3
> uvula Q35.7

**Biforis uterus** (suprasimplex) Q51.3
**Bifurcation** (congenital)
> gallbladder Q44.1
> kidney pelvis Q63.8
> renal pelvis Q63.8
> rib Q76.6
> tongue, congenital Q38.3
> trachea Q32.1
> ureter Q62.8
> urethra Q64.74
> vertebra Q76.49

**Big spleen syndrome** D73.1
**Bigeminal pulse** R00.8
**Bilateral** — *see* condition
**Bile**
> duct — *see* condition
> pigments in urine R82.2

**Bilharziasis** (*see also* Schistosomiasis)
> chyluria B65.0
> cutaneous B65.3
> galacturia B65.0
> hematochyluria B65.0
> intestinal B65.1
> lipemia B65.9
> lipuria B65.0
> oriental B65.2
> piarhemia B65.9

**Band — Bilharziasis**

36     ☑ **Additional Character Required** — Refer to the Tabular List for Character Selection     ▽ Subterms under main terms may continue to next column or page

**Bite**(s) — *continued*
  genital organs, external — *continued*
    male — *continued*
      testes — *see* Bite, testis
    groin — *see* Bite, abdomen, wall
    gum — *see* Bite, oral cavity
    hand S61.45- ☑
      finger — *see* Bite, finger
      superficial NEC S60.57- ☑
        insect S60.56- ☑
      thumb — *see* Bite, thumb
    head S01.95 ☑
      cheek — *see* Bite, cheek
      ear — *see* Bite, ear
      eyelid — *see* Bite, eyelid
      lip — *see* Bite, lip
      nose — *see* Bite, nose
      oral cavity — *see* Bite, oral cavity
      scalp — *see* Bite, scalp
      specified site NEC S01.85 ☑
        superficial NEC S00.87 ☑
          insect S00.86 ☑
      superficial NEC S00.97 ☑
        insect S00.96 ☑
      temporomandibular area — *see* Bite, cheek
    heel — *see* Bite, foot
    hip S71.05- ☑
      superficial NEC S70.27- ☑
        insect S70.26- ☑
    hymen S31.45 ☑
    hypochondrium — *see* Bite, abdomen, wall
    hypogastric region — *see* Bite, abdomen, wall
    inguinal region — *see* Bite, abdomen, wall
    insect — *see* Bite, by site, superficial, insect
    instep — *see* Bite, foot
    interscapular region — *see* Bite, thorax, back
    jaw — *see* Bite, head, specified site NEC
    knee S81.05- ☑
      superficial NEC S80.27- ☑
        insect S80.26- ☑
    labium (majus) (minus) — *see* Bite, vulva
    lacrimal duct — *see* Bite, eyelid
    larynx S11.015 ☑
      superficial NEC S10.17 ☑
        insect S10.16 ☑
    leg (lower) S81.85- ☑
      ankle — *see* Bite, ankle
      foot — *see* Bite, foot
      knee — *see* Bite, knee
      superficial NEC S80.87- ☑
        insect S80.86- ☑
      toe — *see* Bite, toe
      upper — *see* Bite, thigh
    lip S01.551 ☑
      superficial NEC S00.571 ☑
        insect S00.561 ☑
    lizard (venomous) — *see* Venom, bite, reptile
    loin — *see* Bite, abdomen, wall
    lower back — *see* Bite, back, lower
    lumbar region — *see* Bite, back, lower
    malar region — *see* Bite, head, specified site NEC
    mammary — *see* Bite, breast
    marine animals (venomous) — *see* Toxicity, venom, marine animal
    mastoid region — *see* Bite, head, specified site NEC
    mouth — *see* Bite, oral cavity
    nail
      finger — *see* Bite, finger
      toe — *see* Bite, toe
    nape — *see* Bite, neck, specified site NEC
    nasal (septum) (sinus) — *see* Bite, nose
    nasopharynx — *see* Bite, head, specified site NEC
    neck S11.95 ☑
      involving
        cervical esophagus — *see* Bite, esophagus, cervical
        larynx — *see* Bite, larynx
        pharynx — *see* Bite, pharynx
        thyroid gland S11.15 ☑
        trachea — *see* Bite, trachea
      specified site NEC S11.85 ☑
        superficial NEC S10.87 ☑
          insect S10.86 ☑
      superficial NEC S10.97 ☑
        insect S10.96 ☑
      throat S11.85 ☑

**Bite**(s) — *continued*
  neck — *continued*
    throat — *continued*
      superficial NEC S10.17 ☑
      pelvis S10.16 ☑
    nose (septum) (sinus) S01.25 ☑
      superficial NEC S00.37 ☑
        insect S00.36 ☑
    occipital region — *see* Bite, scalp
    oral cavity S01.552 ☑
      superficial NEC S00.572 ☑
        insect S00.562 ☑
    orbital region — *see* Bite, eyelid
    palate — *see* Bite, oral cavity
    palm — *see* Bite, hand
    parietal region — *see* Bite, scalp
    pelvis S31.050 ☑
      with penetration into retroperitoneal space S31.051 ☑
      superficial NEC S30.870 ☑
        insect S30.860 ☑
    penis S31.25 ☑
      superficial NEC S30.872 ☑
        insect S30.862 ☑
    perineum
      female — *see* Bite, vulva
      male — *see* Bite, pelvis
    periocular area (with or without lacrimal passages) — *see* Bite, eyelid
    phalanges
      finger — *see* Bite, finger
      toe — *see* Bite, toe
    pharynx S11.25 ☑
      superficial NEC S10.17 ☑
        insect S10.16 ☑
    pinna — *see* Bite, ear
    poisonous — *see* Venom
    popliteal space — *see* Bite, knee
    prepuce — *see* Bite, penis
    pubic region — *see* Bite, abdomen, wall
    rectovaginal septum — *see* Bite, vulva
    red bug B88.0
    reptile NEC (*see also* Venom, bite, reptile)
      nonvenomous — *see* Bite, by site
      snake — *see* Venom, bite, snake
    sacral region — *see* Bite, back, lower
    sacroiliac region — *see* Bite, back, lower
    salivary gland — *see* Bite, oral cavity
    scalp S01.05 ☑
      superficial NEC S00.07 ☑
        insect S00.06 ☑
    scapular region — *see* Bite, shoulder
    scrotum S31.35 ☑
      superficial NEC S30.873 ☑
        insect S30.863 ☑
    sea-snake (venomous) — *see* Toxicity, venom, snake, sea snake
    shin — *see* Bite, leg
    shoulder S41.05- ☑
      superficial NEC S40.27- ☑
        insect S40.26- ☑
    snake (*see also* Venom, bite, snake)
      nonvenomous — *see* Bite, by site
    spermatic cord — *see* Bite, testis
    spider (venomous) — *see* Toxicity, venom, spider
      nonvenomous — *see* Bite, by site, superficial, insect
    sternal region — *see* Bite, thorax, front
    submaxillary region — *see* Bite, head, specified site NEC
    submental region — *see* Bite, head, specified site NEC
    subungual
      finger(s) — *see* Bite, finger
      toe — *see* Bite, toe
    superficial — *see* Bite, by site, superficial
    supraclavicular fossa S11.85 ☑
    supraorbital — *see* Bite, head, specified site NEC
    temple, temporal region — *see* Bite, head, specified site NEC
    temporomandibular area — *see* Bite, cheek
    testis S31.35 ☑
      superficial NEC S30.873 ☑
        insect S30.863 ☑
    thigh S71.15- ☑
      superficial NEC S70.37- ☑
        insect S70.36- ☑
    thorax, thoracic (wall) S21.95 ☑

**Bite**(s) — *continued*
  thorax, thoracic — *continued*
    back S21.25- ☑
      with penetration into thoracic cavity S21.45- ☑
    breast — *see* Bite, breast
    front S21.15- ☑
      with penetration into thoracic cavity S21.35- ☑
    superficial NEC S20.97 ☑
      back S20.47- ☑
      front S20.37- ☑
      insect S20.96 ☑
        back S20.46- ☑
        front S20.36- ☑
  throat — *see* Bite, neck, throat
  thumb S61.05- ☑
    with
      damage to nail S61.15- ☑
    superficial NEC S60.37- ☑
      insect S60.36- ☑
  thyroid S11.15 ☑
    superficial NEC S10.87 ☑
      insect S10.86 ☑
  toe(s) S91.15- ☑
    with
      damage to nail S91.25- ☑
    great S91.15- ☑
      with
        damage to nail S91.25- ☑
    lesser S91.15- ☑
      with
        damage to nail S91.25- ☑
    superficial NEC S90.47- ☑
      great S90.47- ☑
      insect S90.46- ☑
        great S90.46- ☑
  tongue S01.552 ☑
  trachea S11.025 ☑
    superficial NEC S10.17 ☑
      insect S10.16 ☑
  tunica vaginalis — *see* Bite, testis
  tympanum, tympanic membrane — *see* Bite, ear
  umbilical region S31.155 ☑
  uvula — *see* Bite, oral cavity
  vagina — *see* Bite, vulva
  venomous — *see* Venom
  vocal cords S11.035 ☑
    superficial NEC S10.17 ☑
      insect S10.16 ☑
  vulva S31.45 ☑
    superficial NEC S30.874 ☑
      insect S30.864 ☑
  wrist S61.55- ☑
    superficial NEC S60.87- ☑
      insect S60.86- ☑
**Biting, cheek or lip** K13.1
**Biventricular failure** (heart) I50.82
**Björck** (-Thorson) **syndrome** (malignant carcinoid) E34.0
**Black**
  death A20.9
  eye S00.1- ☑
  hairy tongue K14.3
  heel (foot) S90.3- ☑
  lung (disease) J60
  palm (hand) S60.22- ☑
**Blackfan-Diamond anemia or syndrome** (congenital hypoplastic anemia) D61.01
**Blackhead** L70.0
**Blackout** R55
**Bladder** — *see* condition
**Blast** (air) (hydraulic) (immersion) (underwater)
  blindness S05.8X- ☑
  injury
    abdomen or thorax — *see* Injury, by site
    ear (acoustic nerve trauma) — *see* Injury, nerve, acoustic, specified type NEC
  syndrome NEC T70.8 ☑
**Blastoma** — *see* Neoplasm, malignant, by site
  pulmonary — *see* Neoplasm, lung, malignant
**Blastomycosis, blastomycotic** B40.9
  Brazilian — *see* Paracoccidioidomycosis
  cutaneous B40.3
  disseminated B40.7
  European — *see* Cryptococcosis
  generalized B40.7
  keloidal B48.0
  North American B40.9

☑ Additional Character Required — Refer to the Tabular List for Character Selection    ▽ Subterms under main terms may continue to next column or page

**Blastomycosis, blastomycotic** — *continued*
  primary pulmonary B40.0
  pulmonary B40.2
    acute B40.0
    chronic B40.1
  skin B40.3
  South American — *see* Paracoccidioidomycosis
  specified NEC B40.89
**Bleb**(s) R23.8
  emphysematous (lung) (solitary) J43.9
  endophthalmitis H59.43
  filtering (vitreous), after glaucoma surgery Z98.83
  inflamed (infected), postprocedural H59.40
    stage 1 H59.41
    stage 2 H59.42
    stage 3 H59.43
  lung (ruptured) J43.9
    congenital — *see* Atelectasis
    newborn P25.8
  subpleural (emphysematous) J43.9
**Blebitis, postprocedural** H59.40
  stage 1 H59.41
  stage 2 H59.42
  stage 3 H59.43
**Bleeder** (familial) (hereditary) — *see* Hemophilia
**Bleeding** (*see also* Hemorrhage)
  anal K62.5
  anovulatory N97.0
  atonic, following delivery O72.1
  capillary I78.8
    puerperal O72.2
  contact (postcoital) N93.0
  due to uterine subinvolution N85.3
  ear — *see* Otorrhagia
  excessive, associated with menopausal onset N92.4
  familial — *see* Defect, coagulation
  following intercourse N93.0
  gastrointestinal K92.2
  hemorrhoids — *see* Hemorrhoids
  intermenstrual (regular) N92.3
    irregular N92.1
  intraoperative — *see* Complication, intraoperative, hemorrhage
  irregular N92.6
  menopausal N92.4
  newborn, intraventricular — *see* Newborn, affected by, hemorrhage, intraventricular
  nipple N64.59
  nose R04.0
  ovulation N92.3
  postclimacteric N95.0
  postcoital N93.0
  postmenopausal N95.0
  postoperative — *see* Complication, postprocedural, hemorrhage
  preclimacteric N92.4
  pre-pubertal vaginal N93.1
  puberty (excessive, with onset of menstrual periods) N92.2
  rectum, rectal K62.5
    newborn P54.2
  tendencies — *see* Defect, coagulation
  throat R04.1
  tooth socket (post-extraction) K91.840
  umbilical stump P51.9
  uterus, uterine NEC N93.9
    climacteric N92.4
    dysfunctional or functional N93.8
    menopausal N92.4
    preclimacteric or premenopausal N92.4
    unrelated to menstrual cycle N93.9
  vagina, vaginal (abnormal) N93.9
    dysfunctional or functional N93.8
    newborn P54.6
    pre-pubertal N93.1
  vicarious N94.89
**Blennorrhagia, blennorrhagic** — *see* Gonorrhea
**Blennorrhea** (acute) (chronic) (*see also* Gonorrhea)
  inclusion (neonatal) (newborn) P39.1
  lower genitourinary tract (gonococcal) A54.00
  neonatorum (gonococcal ophthalmia) A54.31
**Blepharelosis** — *see* Entropion
**Blepharitis** (angularis) (ciliaris) (eyelid) (marginal) (nonulcerative) H01.009
  herpes zoster B02.39
  left H01.006
    lower H01.005
    upper H01.004

**Blepharitis** — *continued*
  right H01.003
    lower H01.002
    upper H01.001
  squamous H01.029
    left H01.026
      lower H01.025
      upper H01.024
    right H01.023
      lower H01.022
      upper H01.021
  ulcerative H01.019
    left H01.016
      lower H01.015
      upper H01.014
    right H01.013
      lower H01.012
      upper H01.011
**Blepharochalasis** H02.30
  congenital Q10.0
  left H02.36
    lower H02.35
    upper H02.34
  right H02.33
    lower H02.32
    upper H02.31
**Blepharoclonus** H02.59
**Blepharoconjunctivitis** H10.50- ☑
  angular H10.52- ☑
  contact H10.53- ☑
  ligneous H10.51- ☑
**Blepharophimosis** (eyelid) H02.529
  congenital Q10.3
  left H02.526
    lower H02.525
    upper H02.524
  right H02.523
    lower H02.522
    upper H02.521
**Blepharoptosis** H02.40- ☑
  congenital Q10.0
  mechanical H02.41- ☑
  myogenic H02.42- ☑
  neurogenic H02.43- ☑
  paralytic H02.43- ☑
**Blepharopyorrhea, gonococcal** A54.39
**Blepharospasm** G24.5
  drug induced G24.01
**Blighted ovum** O02.0
**Blind** (*see also* Blindness)
  bronchus (congenital) Q32.4
  loop syndrome K90.2
    congenital Q43.8
  sac, fallopian tube (congenital) Q50.6
  spot, enlarged — *see* Defect, visual field, localized, scotoma, blind spot area
  tract or tube, congenital NEC — *see* Atresia, by site
**Blindness** (acquired) (congenital) (both eyes) H54.0X- ☑
  blast S05.8X- ☑
  color — *see* Deficiency, color vision
  concussion S05.8X- ☑
  cortical H47.619
    left brain H47.612
    right brain H47.611
  day H53.11
  due to injury (current episode) S05.9- ☑
    sequelae — *code to* injury with seventh character S
  eclipse (total) — *see* Retinopathy, solar
  emotional (hysterical) F44.6
  face H53.16
  hysterical F44.6
  legal (both eyes) (USA definition) H54.8
  mind R48.8
  night H53.60
    abnormal dark adaptation curve H53.61
    acquired H53.62
    congenital H53.63
    specified type NEC H53.69
    vitamin A deficiency E50.5
  one eye (other eye normal) H54.40
    left (normal vision on right) H54.42- ☑
      low vision on right H54.12- ☑
      low vision, other eye H54.10
    right (normal vision on left) H54.41- ☑
      low vision on left H54.11- ☑
  psychic R48.8
  river B73.01

**Blindness** — *continued*
  snow — *see* Photokeratitis
  sun, solar — *see* Retinopathy, solar
  transient — *see* Disturbance, vision, subjective, loss, transient
  traumatic (current episode) S05.9- ☑
  word (developmental) F81.0
    acquired R48.0
    secondary to organic lesion R48.0
**Blister** (nonthermal)
  abdominal wall S30.821 ☑
  alveolar process S00.522 ☑
  ankle S90.52- ☑
  antecubital space — *see* Blister, elbow
  anus S30.827 ☑
  arm (upper) S40.82- ☑
  auditory canal — *see* Blister, ear
  auricle — *see* Blister, ear
  axilla — *see* Blister, arm
  back, lower S30.820 ☑
  beetle dermatitis L24.89
  breast S20.12- ☑
  brow S00.82 ☑
  calf — *see* Blister, leg
  canthus — *see* Blister, eyelid
  cheek S00.82 ☑
    internal S00.522 ☑
  chest wall — *see* Blister, thorax
  chin S00.82 ☑
  costal region — *see* Blister, thorax
  digit(s)
    foot — *see* Blister, toe
    hand — *see* Blister, finger
  due to burn — *see* Burn, by site, second degree
  ear S00.42- ☑
  elbow S50.32- ☑
  epiglottis S10.12 ☑
  esophagus, cervical S10.12 ☑
  eyebrow — *see* Blister, eyelid
  eyelid S00.22- ☑
  face S00.82 ☑
  fever B00.1
  finger(s) S60.429 ☑
    index S60.42- ☑
    little S60.42- ☑
    middle S60.42- ☑
    ring S60.42- ☑
  foot (except toe(s) alone) S90.82- ☑
    toe — *see* Blister, toe
  forearm S50.82- ☑
    elbow only — *see* Blister, elbow
  forehead S00.82 ☑
  fracture — *omit code*
  genital organ
    female S30.826 ☑
    male S30.825 ☑
  gum S00.522 ☑
  hand S60.52- ☑
  head S00.92 ☑
    ear — *see* Blister, ear
    eyelid — *see* Blister, eyelid
    lip S00.521 ☑
    nose S00.32 ☑
    oral cavity S00.522 ☑
    scalp S00.02 ☑
    specified site NEC S00.82 ☑
  heel — *see* Blister, foot
  hip S70.22- ☑
  interscapular region S20.429 ☑
  jaw S00.82 ☑
  knee S80.22- ☑
  larynx S10.12 ☑
  leg (lower) S80.82- ☑
    knee — *see* Blister, knee
    upper — *see* Blister, thigh
  lip S00.521 ☑
  malar region S00.82 ☑
  mammary — *see* Blister, breast
  mastoid region S00.82 ☑
  mouth S00.522 ☑
  multiple, skin, nontraumatic R23.8
  nail
    finger — *see* Blister, finger
    toe — *see* Blister, toe
  nasal S00.32 ☑
  neck S10.92 ☑

**Blister** — *continued*
  neck — *continued*
    specified site NEC S10.82 ☑
      throat S10.12 ☑
  nose S00.32 ☑
  occipital region S00.02 ☑
  oral cavity S00.522 ☑
  orbital region — *see* Blister, eyelid
  palate S00.522 ☑
  palm — *see* Blister, hand
  parietal region S00.02 ☑
  pelvis S30.820 ☑
  penis S30.822 ☑
  periocular area — *see* Blister, eyelid
  phalanges
    finger — *see* Blister, finger
    toe — *see* Blister, toe
  pharynx S10.12 ☑
  pinna — *see* Blister, ear
  popliteal space — *see* Blister, knee
  scalp S00.02 ☑
  scapular region — *see* Blister, shoulder
  scrotum S30.823 ☑
  shin — *see* Blister, leg
  shoulder S40.22- ☑
  sternal region S20.329 ☑
  submaxillary region S00.82 ☑
  submental region S00.82 ☑
  subungual
    finger(s) — *see* Blister, finger
    toe(s) — *see* Blister, toe
  supraclavicular fossa S10.82 ☑
  supraorbital S00.82 ☑
  temple S00.82 ☑
  temporal region S00.82 ☑
  testis S30.823 ☑
  thermal — *see* Burn, second degree, by site
  thigh S70.32- ☑
  thorax, thoracic (wall) S20.92 ☑
    back S20.42- ☑
    front S20.32- ☑
  throat S10.12 ☑
  thumb S60.32- ☑
  toe(s) S90.42- ☑
    great S90.42- ☑
  tongue S00.522 ☑
  trachea S10.12 ☑
  tympanum, tympanic membrane — *see* Blister, ear
  upper arm — *see* Blister, arm (upper)
  uvula S00.522 ☑
  vagina S30.824 ☑
  vocal cords S10.12 ☑
  vulva S30.824 ☑
  wrist S60.82- ☑
**Bloating** R14.0
**Bloch-Sulzberger disease or syndrome** Q82.3
**Block, blocked**
  alveolocapillary J84.10
  arborization (heart) I45.5
  arrhythmic I45.9
  atrioventricular (incomplete) (partial) I44.30
    with atrioventricular dissociation I44.2
    complete I44.2
      congenital Q24.6
    congenital Q24.6
    first degree I44.0
    second degree (types I and II) I44.1
    specified NEC I44.39
    third degree I44.2
    types I and II I44.1
  auriculoventricular — *see* Block, atrioventricular
  bifascicular (cardiac) I45.2
  bundle-branch (complete) (false) (incomplete) I45.4
    bilateral I45.2
    left I44.7
      with right bundle branch block I45.2
      hemiblock I44.60
        anterior I44.4
        posterior I44.5
      incomplete I44.7
        with right bundle branch block I45.2
    right I45.10
      with
        left bundle branch block I45.2
        left fascicular block I45.2
      specified NEC I45.19
    Wilson's type I45.19

**Block, blocked** — *continued*
  cardiac I45.9
  conduction I45.9
    complete I44.2
  fascicular (left) I44.60
    anterior I44.4
    posterior I44.5
    right I45.0
    specified NEC I44.69
  foramen Magendie (acquired) G91.1
    congenital Q03.1
      with spina bifida — *see* Spina bifida, by site, with hydrocephalus
  heart I45.9
    bundle branch I45.4
      bilateral I45.2
    complete (atrioventricular) I44.2
    congenital Q24.6
    first degree (atrioventricular) I44.0
    second degree (atrioventricular) I44.1
    specified type NEC I45.5
    third degree (atrioventricular) I44.2
  hepatic vein I82.0
  intraventricular (nonspecific) I45.4
    bundle branch
      bilateral I45.2
  kidney N28.9
    postcystoscopic or postprocedural N99.0
  Mobitz (types I and II) I44.1
  myocardial — *see* Block, heart
  nodal I45.5
  organ or site, congenital NEC — *see* Atresia, by site
  portal (vein) I81
  second degree (types I and II) I44.1
  sinoatrial I45.5
  sinoauricular I45.5
  third degree I44.2
  trifascicular I45.3
  tubal N97.1
  vein NOS I82.90
  Wenckebach (types I and II) I44.1
**Blockage** — *see* Obstruction
**Blocq's disease** F44.4
**Blood**
  constituents, abnormal R78.9
  disease D75.9
  donor — *see* Donor, blood
  dyscrasia D75.9
    with
      abortion — *see* Abortion, by type, complicated by, hemorrhage
      ectopic pregnancy O08.1
      molar pregnancy O08.1
      following ectopic or molar pregnancy O08.1
    newborn P61.9
    puerperal, postpartum O72.3
  flukes NEC — *see* Schistosomiasis
  in
    feces K92.1
      occult R19.5
    urine — *see* Hematuria
  mole O02.0
  occult in feces R19.5
  pressure
    decreased, due to shock following injury T79.4 ☑
    examination only Z01.30
    fluctuating I99.8
    high — *see* Hypertension
      borderline R03.0
      incidental reading, without diagnosis of hypertension R03.0
    low (*see also* Hypotension)
      incidental reading, without diagnosis of hypotension R03.1
  spitting — *see* Hemoptysis
  staining cornea — *see* Pigmentation, cornea, stromal
  transfusion
    reaction or complication — *see* Complications, transfusion
  type
    A (Rh positive) Z67.10
      Rh negative Z67.11
    AB (Rh positive) Z67.30
      Rh negative Z67.31
    B (Rh positive) Z67.20
      Rh negative Z67.21
    O (Rh positive) Z67.40
      Rh negative Z67.41

**Blood** — *continued*
  type — *continued*
    Rh (positive) Z67.90
      negative Z67.91
  vessel rupture — *see* Hemorrhage
  vomiting — *see* Hematemesis
**Blood-forming organs, disease** D75.9
**Bloodgood's disease** — *see* Mastopathy, cystic
**Bloom** (-Machacek)(-Torre) **syndrome** Q82.8
**Blount's disease or osteochondrosis** — *see* Osteochondrosis, juvenile, tibia
**Blue**
  baby Q24.9
  diaper syndrome E72.09
  dome cyst (breast) — *see* Cyst, breast
  dot cataract Q12.0
  nevus D22.9
  sclera Q13.5
    with fragility of bone and deafness Q78.0
  toe syndrome I75.02- ☑
**Blueness** — *see* Cyanosis
**Blues, postpartal** O90.6
  baby O90.6
**Blurring, visual** H53.8
**Blushing** (abnormal) (excessive) R23.2
**BMI** — *see* Body, mass index
**Boarder, hospital NEC** Z76.4
  accompanying sick person Z76.3
  healthy infant or child Z76.2
    foundling Z76.1
**Bockhart's impetigo** L01.02
**Bodechtel-Guttman disease** (subacute sclerosing panencephalitis) A81.1
**Boder-Sedgwick syndrome** (ataxia-telangiectasia) G11.3
**Body, bodies**
  Aschoff's — *see* Myocarditis, rheumatic
  asteroid, vitreous — *see* Deposit, crystalline
  cytoid (retina) — *see* Occlusion, artery, retina
  drusen (degenerative) (macula) (retinal) (*see also* Degeneration, macula, drusen)
    optic disc — *see* Drusen, optic disc
  foreign — *see* Foreign body
  loose
    joint, except knee — *see* Loose, body, joint
      knee M23.4- ☑
    sheath, tendon — *see* Disorder, tendon, specified type NEC
  mass index (BMI)
    adult
      19.9 or less Z68.1
      20.0-20.9 Z68.20
      21.0-21.9 Z68.21
      22.0-22.9 Z68.22
      23.0-23.9 Z68.23
      24.0-24.9 Z68.24
      25.0-25.9 Z68.25
      26.0-26.9 Z68.26
      27.0-27.9 Z68.27
      28.0-28.9 Z68.28
      29.0-29.9 Z68.29
      30.0-30.9 Z68.30
      31.0-31.9 Z68.31
      32.0-32.9 Z68.32
      33.0-33.9 Z68.33
      34.0-34.9 Z68.34
      35.0-35.9 Z68.35
      36.0-36.9 Z68.36
      37.0-37.9 Z68.37
      38.0-38.9 Z68.38
      39.0-39.9 Z68.39
      40.0-44.9 Z68.41
      45.0-49.9 Z68.42
      50.0-59.9 Z68.43
      60.0-69.9 Z68.44
      70 and over Z68.45
    pediatric
      5th percentile to less than 85th percentile for age Z68.52
      85th percentile to less than 95th percentile for age Z68.53
      less than fifth percentile for age Z68.51
      greater than or equal to ninety-fifth percentile for age Z68.54
  Mooser's A75.2
  rice (*see also* Loose, body, joint)
    knee M23.4- ☑
  rocking F98.4

☑ Additional Character Required — Refer to the Tabular List for Character Selection    Subterms under main terms may continue to next column or page

**Boeck's**
- disease or sarcoid — *see* Sarcoidosis
- lupoid (miliary) D86.3

**Boerhaave's syndrome** (spontaneous esophageal rupture) K22.3

**Boggy**
- cervix N88.8
- uterus N85.8

**Boil** (*see also* Furuncle, by site)
- Aleppo B55.1
- Baghdad B55.1
- Delhi B55.1
- lacrimal
  - gland — *see* Dacryoadenitis
  - passages (duct) (sac) — *see* Inflammation, lacrimal, passages, acute
- Natal B55.1
- orbit, orbital — *see* Abscess, orbit
- tropical B55.1

**Bold hives** — *see* Urticaria

**Bombé, iris** — *see* Membrane, pupillary

**Bone** — *see* condition

**Bonnevie-Ullrich syndrome** (*see also* Turner's syndrome) Q87.1

**Bonnier's syndrome** H81.8

**Bonvale dam fever** T73.3 ☑

**Bony block of joint** — *see* Ankylosis

**BOOP** (bronchiolitis obliterans organized pneumonia) J84.89

**Borderline**
- diabetes mellitus R73.03
- hypertension R03.0
- osteopenia M85.8- ☑
- pelvis, with obstruction during labor O65.1
- personality F60.3

**Borna disease** A83.9

**Bornholm disease** B33.0

**Boston exanthem** A88.0

**Botalli, ductus** (patent) (persistent) Q25.0

**Bothriocephalus latus infestation** B70.0

**Botulism** (foodborne intoxication) A05.1
- infant A48.51
- non-foodborne A48.52
- wound A48.52

**Bouba** — *see* Yaws

**Bouchard's nodes** (with arthropathy) M15.2

**Bouffée délirante** F23

**Bouillaud's disease or syndrome** (rheumatic heart disease) I01.9

**Bourneville's disease** Q85.1

**Boutonniere deformity** (finger) — *see* Deformity, finger, boutonniere

**Bouveret** (-Hoffmann) **syndrome** (paroxysmal tachycardia) I47.9

**Bovine heart** — *see* Hypertrophy, cardiac

**Bowel** — *see* condition

**Bowen's**
- dermatosis (precancerous) — *see* Neoplasm, skin, in situ
- disease — *see* Neoplasm, skin, in situ
- epithelioma — *see* Neoplasm, skin, in situ
- type
  - epidermoid carcinoma-in-situ — *see* Neoplasm, skin, in situ
  - intraepidermal squamous cell carcinoma — *see* Neoplasm, skin, in situ

**Bowing**
- femur (*see also* Deformity, limb, specified type NEC, thigh)
  - congenital Q68.3
- fibula (*see also* Deformity, limb, specified type NEC, lower leg)
  - congenital Q68.4
- forearm — *see* Deformity, limb, specified type NEC, forearm
- leg(s), long bones, congenital Q68.5
- radius — *see* Deformity, limb, specified type NEC, forearm
- tibia (*see also* Deformity, limb, specified type NEC, lower leg)
  - congenital Q68.4

**Bowleg**(s) (acquired) M21.16- ☑
- congenital Q68.5
- rachitic E64.3

**Boyd's dysentery** A03.2

**Brachial** — *see* condition

**Brachycardia** R00.1

**Brachycephaly** Q75.0

**Bradley's disease** A08.19

**Bradyarrhythmia, cardiac** I49.8

**Bradycardia** (sinoatrial) (sinus) (vagal) R00.1
- neonatal P29.12
- reflex G90.09
- tachycardia syndrome I49.5

**Bradykinesia** R25.8

**Bradypnea** R06.89

**Bradytachycardia** I49.5

**Brailsford's disease or osteochondrosis** — *see* Osteochondrosis, juvenile, radius

**Brain** (*see also* condition)
- death G93.82
- syndrome — *see* Syndrome, brain

**Branched-chain amino-acid disorder** E71.2

**Branchial** — *see* condition
- cartilage, congenital Q18.2

**Branchiogenic remnant** (in neck) Q18.0

**Brandt's syndrome** (acrodermatitis enteropathica) E83.2

**Brash** (water) R12

**Bravais-jacksonian epilepsy** — *see* Epilepsy, localization-related, symptomatic, with simple partial seizures

**Braxton Hicks contractions** — *see* False, labor

**Brazilian leishmaniasis** B55.2

**BRBPR** K62.5

**Break, retina** (without detachment) H33.30- ☑
- with retinal detachment — *see* Detachment, retina
  - horseshoe tear H33.31- ☑
  - multiple H33.33- ☑
  - round hole H33.32- ☑

**Breakdown**
- device, graft or implant (*see also* Complications, by site and type, mechanical) T85.618 ☑
  - arterial graft NEC — *see* Complication, cardiovascular device, mechanical, vascular
  - breast (implant) T85.41 ☑
  - catheter NEC T85.618 ☑
    - cystostomy T83.010 ☑
    - dialysis (renal) T82.41 ☑
      - intraperitoneal T85.611 ☑
    - Hopkins T83.018 ☑
    - ileostomy T83.018 ☑
    - infusion NEC T82.514 ☑
      - cranial T85.610- ☑
      - epidural T85.610 ☑
      - intrathecal T85.610 ☑
      - spinal T85.610 ☑
      - subarachnoid T85.610 ☑
      - subdural T85.610 ☑
    - nephrostomy T83.012 ☑
    - urethral indwelling T83.011 ☑
    - urinary NEC T83.018 ☑
    - urostomy T83.018 ☑
  - electronic (electrode) (pulse generator) (stimulator)
    - bone T84.310 ☑
    - cardiac T82.119 ☑
      - electrode T82.110 ☑
      - pulse generator T82.111 ☑
      - specified type NEC T82.118 ☑
    - nervous system — *see* Complication, prosthetic device, mechanical, electronic nervous system stimulator
    - urinary — *see* Complication, genitourinary, device, urinary, mechanical
  - fixation, internal (orthopedic) NEC — *see* Complication, fixation device, mechanical
  - gastrointestinal — *see* Complications, prosthetic device, mechanical, gastrointestinal device
  - genital NEC T83.418 ☑
    - intrauterine contraceptive device T83.31 ☑
    - penile prosthesis (cylinder) (implanted) (pump) (resevoir) T83.410 ☑
    - testicular prosthesis T83.411 ☑
  - heart NEC — *see* Complication, cardiovascular device, mechanical
  - intrathecal infusion pump T85.615 ☑
  - joint prosthesis — *see* Complications..., joint prosthesis,internal, mechanical, by site
  - nervous system, specified device NEC T85.615 ☑
  - ocular NEC — *see* Complications, prosthetic device, mechanical, ocular device
  - orthopedic NEC — *see* Complication, orthopedic, device, mechanical
  - specified NEC T85.618 ☑

**Breakdown** — *continued*
- device, graft or implant (*see also* Complications, by site and type, mechanical) — *continued*
  - subcutaneous device pocket
    - nervous system prosthetic device, implant, or graft T85.890 ☑
    - other internal prosthetic device, implant, or graft T85.898 ☑
  - sutures, permanent T85.612 ☑
    - used in bone repair — *see* Complications, fixation device, internal (orthopedic), mechanical
  - urinary NEC T83.118 ☑
    - graft T83.21 ☑
    - sphincter, implanted T83.111 ☑
    - stent (ileal conduit) (nephroureteral) T83.113 ☑
    - ureteral indwelling T83.112 ☑
  - vascular NEC — *see* Complication, cardiovascular device, mechanical
  - ventricular intracranial shunt T85.01 ☑
- nervous F48.8
- perineum O90.1
- respirator J95.850
  - specified NEC J95.859
- ventilator J95.850
  - specified NEC J95.859

**Breast** (*see also* condition)
- buds E30.1
  - in newborn P96.89
- dense R92.2
- nodule (*see also* Lump, breast) N63.0

**Breath**
- foul R19.6
- holder, child R06.89
- holding spell R06.89
- shortness R06.02

**Breathing**
- labored — *see* Hyperventilation
- mouth R06.5
  - causing malocclusion M26.5 ☑
- periodic R06.3
  - high altitude G47.32

**Breathlessness** R06.81

**Breda's disease** — *see* Yaws

**Breech presentation** (mother) O32.1 ☑
- causing obstructed labor O64.1 ☑
- footling O32.8 ☑
  - causing obstructed labor O64.8 ☑
- incomplete O32.8 ☑
  - causing obstructed labor O64.8 ☑

**Breisky's disease** N90.4

**Brennemann's syndrome** I88.0

**Brenner**
- tumor (benign) D27.9
  - borderline malignancy D39.1- ☑
  - malignant C56 ☑
  - proliferating D39.1- ☑

**Bretonneau's disease or angina** A36.0

**Breus' mole** O02.0

**Brevicollis** Q76.49

**Brickmakers' anemia** B76.9 [D63.8]

**Bridge, myocardial** Q24.5

**Bright red blood per rectum** (BRBPR) K62.5

**Bright's disease** (*see also* Nephritis)
- arteriosclerotic — *see* Hypertension, kidney

**Brill** (-Zinsser) **disease** (recrudescent typhus) A75.1
- flea-borne A75.2
- louse-borne A75.1

**Brill-Symmers' disease** C82.90

**Brion-Kayser disease** — *see* Fever, parathyroid

**Briquet's disorder or syndrome** F45.0

**Brissaud's**
- infantilism or dwarfism E23.0
- motor-verbal tic F95.2

**Brittle**
- bones disease Q78.0
- nails L60.3
  - congenital Q84.6

**Broad** (*see also* condition)
- beta disease E78.2
- ligament laceration syndrome N83.8

**Broad- or floating-betalipoproteinemia** E78.2

**Brock's syndrome** (atelectasis due to enlarged lymph nodes) J98.19

**Brocq-Duhring disease** (dermatitis herpetiformis) L13.0

**Brodie's abscess or disease** M86.8X- ☑

**Broken**
arches (see also Deformity, limb, flat foot)
arm (meaning upper limb) — see Fracture, arm
back — see Fracture, vertebra
bone — see Fracture
implant or internal device — see Complications, by site and type, mechanical
leg (meaning lower limb) — see Fracture, leg
nose S02.2 ☑
tooth, teeth — see Fracture, tooth
**Bromhidrosis, bromidrosis** L75.0
**Bromidism, bromism** G92
chronic (dependence) F13.20
due to
correct substance properly administered — see Table of Drugs and Chemicals, by drug, adverse effect
overdose or wrong substance given or taken — see Table of Drugs and Chemicals, by drug, poisoning
**Bromidrosiphobia** F40.298
**Bronchi, bronchial** — see condition
**Bronchiectasis** (cylindrical) (diffuse) (fusiform) (localized) (saccular) J47.9
with
acute
bronchitis J47.0
lower respiratory infection J47.0
exacerbation (acute) J47.1
congenital Q33.4
tuberculous NEC — see Tuberculosis, pulmonary
**Bronchiolectasis** — see Bronchiectasis
**Bronchiolitis** (acute) (infective) (subacute) J21.9
with
bronchospasm or obstruction J21.9
influenza, flu or grippe — see Influenza, with, respiratory manifestations NEC
chemical (chronic) J68.4
acute J68.0
chronic (fibrosing) (obliterative) J44.9
due to
external agent — see Bronchitis, acute, due to
human metapneumovirus J21.1
respiratory syncytial virus J21.0
specified organism NEC J21.8
fibrosa obliterans J44.9
influenzal — see Influenza, with, respiratory manifestations NEC
obliterans J42
with organizing pneumonia (BOOP) J84.89
obliterative (chronic) (subacute) J44.9
due to chemicals, gases, fumes or vapors (inhalation) J68.4
due to fumes or vapors J68.4
respiratory, interstitial lung disease J84.115
**Bronchitis** (diffuse) (fibrinous) (hypostatic) (infective) (membranous) J40
with
influenza, flu or grippe — see Influenza, with, respiratory manifestations NEC
obstruction (airway) (lung) J44.9
tracheitis (15 years of age and above) J40
acute or subacute J20.9
chronic J42
under 15 years of age J20.9
acute or subacute (with bronchospasm or obstruction) J20.9
with
bronchiectasis J47.0
chronic obstructive pulmonary disease J44.0
chemical (due to gases, fumes or vapors) J68.0
due to
fumes or vapors J68.0
Haemophilus influenzae J20.1
Mycoplasma pneumoniae J20.0
radiation J70.0
specified organism NEC J20.8
Streptococcus J20.2
virus
coxsackie J20.3
echovirus J20.7
parainfluenzae J20.4
respiratory syncytial J20.5
rhinovirus J20.6
viral NEC J20.8
allergic (acute) J45.909
with
exacerbation (acute) J45.901

**Bronchitis** — continued
allergic — continued
with — continued
status asthmaticus J45.902
arachidic T17.528 ☑
aspiration (due to fumes or vapors) J68.0
asthmatic J45.9 ☑
chronic J44.9
with
acute lower respiratory infection J44.0
exacerbation (acute) J44.1
capillary — see Pneumonia, broncho
caseous (tuberculous) A15.5
Castellani's A69.8
catarrhal (15 years of age and above) J40
acute — see Bronchitis, acute
chronic J41.0
under 15 years of age J20.9
chemical (acute) (subacute) J68.0
chronic J68.4
due to fumes or vapors J68.0
chronic J68.4
chronic J42
with
airways obstruction J44.9
tracheitis (chronic) J42
asthmatic (obstructive) J44.9
catarrhal J41.0
chemical (due to fumes or vapors) J68.4
due to
chemicals, gases, fumes or vapors (inhalation) J68.4
radiation J70.1
tobacco smoking J41.0
emphysematous J44.9
mucopurulent J41.1
non-obstructive J41.0
obliterans J44.9
obstructive J44.9
purulent J41.1
simple J41.0
croupous — see Bronchitis, acute
due to gases, fumes or vapors (chemical) J68.0
emphysematous (obstructive) J44.9
exudative — see Bronchitis, acute
fetid J41.1
grippal — see Influenza, with, respiratory manifestations NEC
in those under 15 years age — see Bronchitis, acute
chronic — see Bronchitis, chronic
influenzal — see Influenza, with, respiratory manifestations NEC
mixed simple and mucopurulent J41.8
moulder's J62.8
mucopurulent (chronic) (recurrent) J41.1
acute or subacute J20.9
simple (mixed) J41.8
obliterans (chronic) J44.9
obstructive (chronic) (diffuse) J44.9
pituitous J41.1
pneumococcal, acute or subacute J20.2
pseudomembranous, acute or subacute — see Bronchitis, acute
purulent (chronic) (recurrent) J41.1
acute or subacute — see Bronchitis, acute
putrid J41.1
senile (chronic) J42
simple and mucopurulent (mixed) J41.8
smokers' J41.0
spirochetal NEC A69.8
subacute — see Bronchitis, acute
suppurative (chronic) J41.1
acute or subacute — see Bronchitis, acute
tuberculous A15.5
under 15 years of age — see Bronchitis, acute
chronic — see Bronchitis, chronic
viral NEC, acute or subacute (see also Bronchitis, acute) J20.8
**Bronchoalveolitis** J18.0
**Bronchoaspergillosis** B44.1
**Bronchocele meaning goiter** E04.0
**Broncholithiasis** J98.09
tuberculous NEC A15.5
**Bronchomalacia** J98.09
congenital Q32.2
**Bronchomycosis NOS** B49 [J99]
candidal B37.1
**Bronchopleuropneumonia** — see Pneumonia, broncho

**Bronchopneumonia** — see Pneumonia, broncho
**Bronchopneumonitis** — see Pneumonia, broncho
**Bronchopulmonary** — see condition
**Bronchopulmonitis** — see Pneumonia, broncho
**Bronchorrhagia** (see Hemoptysis)
**Bronchorrhea** J98.09
acute J20.9
chronic (infective) (purulent) J42
**Bronchospasm** (acute) J98.01
with
bronchiolitis, acute J21.9
bronchitis, acute (conditions in J20) — see Bronchitis, acute
due to external agent — see condition, respiratory, acute, due to
exercise induced J45.990
**Bronchospirochetosis** A69.8
Castellani A69.8
**Bronchostenosis** J98.09
**Bronchus** — see condition
**Brontophobia** F40.220
**Bronze baby syndrome** P83.88
**Brooke's tumor** — see Neoplasm, skin, benign
**Brown enamel of teeth** (hereditary) K00.5
**Brown's sheath syndrome** H50.61- ☑
**Brown-Séquard disease, paralysis or syndrome** G83.81
**Bruce sepsis** A23.0
**Brucellosis** (infection) A23.9
abortus A23.1
canis A23.3
dermatitis A23.9
melitensis A23.0
mixed A23.8
sepsis A23.9
melitensis A23.0
specified NEC A23.8
suis A23.2
**Bruck-de Lange disease** Q87.1
**Bruck's disease** — see Deformity, limb
**BRUE** (brief resolved unexplained event) R68.13
**Brugsch's syndrome** Q82.8
**Bruise** (skin surface intact) (see also Contusion)
with
open wound — see Wound, open
internal organ — see Injury, by site
newborn P54.5
scalp, due to birth injury, newborn P12.3
umbilical cord O69.5 ☑
**Bruit** (arterial) R09.89
cardiac R01.1
**Brush burn** — see Abrasion, by site
**Bruton's X-linked agammaglobulinemia** D80.0
**Bruxism**
psychogenic F45.8
sleep related G47.63
**Bubbly lung syndrome** P27.0
**Bubo** I88.8
blennorrhagic (gonococcal) A54.89
chancroidal A57
climatic A55
due to Haemophilus ducreyi A57
gonococcal A54.89
indolent (nonspecific) I88.8
inguinal (nonspecific) I88.8
chancroidal A57
climatic A55
due to H. ducreyi A57
infective I88.8
scrofulous (tuberculous) A18.2
soft chancre A57
suppurating — see Lymphadenitis, acute
syphilitic (primary) A51.0
congenital A50.07
tropical A55
virulent (chancroidal) A57
**Bubonic plague** A20.0
**Bubonocele** — see Hernia, inguinal
**Buccal** — see condition
**Buchanan's disease or osteochondrosis** M91.0
**Buchem's syndrome** (hyperostosis corticalis) M85.2
**Bucket-handle fracture or tear** (semilunar cartilage) — see Tear, meniscus
**Budd-Chiari syndrome** (hepatic vein thrombosis) I82.0
**Budgerigar fancier's disease or lung** J67.2
**Buds**
breast E30.1

☑ **Additional Character Required** — Refer to the Tabular List for Character Selection ▽ Subterms under main terms may continue to next column or page

**Buds** — *continued*
  breast — *continued*
    in newborn P96.89
**Buerger's disease** (thromboangiitis obliterans) I73.1
**Bulbar** — *see* condition
**Bulbus cordis** (left ventricle) (persistent) Q21.8
**Bulimia** (nervosa) F50.2
  atypical F50.9
  normal weight F50.9
**Bulky**
  stools R19.5
  uterus N85.2
**Bulla** (e) R23.8
  lung (emphysematous) (solitary) J43.9
    newborn P25.8
**Bullet wound** (*see also* Wound, open)
  fracture — *code as* Fracture, by site
  internal organ — *see* Injury, by site
**Bundle**
  branch block (complete) (false) (incomplete) — *see* Block, bundle-branch
  of His — *see* condition
**Bunion** M21.61- ☑
  tailor's M21.62- ☑
**Bunionette** M21.62- ☑
**Buphthalmia, buphthalmos** (congenital) Q15.0
**Burdwan fever** B55.0
**Bürger-Grütz disease or syndrome** E78.3
**Buried**
  penis (congenital) Q55.64
    acquired N48.83
  roots K08.3
**Burke's syndrome** K86.89
**Burkitt**
  cell leukemia C91.0- ☑
  lymphoma (malignant) C83.7- ☑
    small noncleaved, diffuse C83.7- ☑
    spleen C83.77
    undifferentiated C83.7- ☑
  tumor C83.7- ☑
  type
    acute lymphoblastic leukemia C91.0- ☑
    undifferentiated C83.7- ☑
**Burn** (electricity) (flame) (hot gas, liquid or hot object) (radiation) (steam) (thermal) T30.0
  abdomen, abdominal (muscle) (wall) T21.02 ☑
    first degree T21.12 ☑
    second degree T21.22 ☑
    third degree T21.32 ☑
  above elbow T22.039 ☑
    first degree T22.139 ☑
    left T22.032 ☑
      first degree T22.132 ☑
      second degree T22.232 ☑
      third degree T22.332 ☑
    right T22.031 ☑
      first degree T22.131 ☑
      second degree T22.231 ☑
      third degree T22.331 ☑
    second degree T22.239 ☑
    third degree T22.339 ☑
  acid (caustic) (external) (internal) — *see* Corrosion, by site
  alimentary tract NEC T28.2 ☑
    esophagus T28.1 ☑
    mouth T28.0 ☑
    pharynx T28.0 ☑
  alkaline (caustic) (external) (internal) — *see* Corrosion, by site
  ankle T25.019 ☑
    first degree T25.119 ☑
    left T25.012 ☑
      first degree T25.112 ☑
      second degree T25.212 ☑
      third degree T25.312 ☑
    multiple with foot — *see* Burn, lower, limb, multiple, ankle and foot
    right T25.011 ☑
      first degree T25.111 ☑
      second degree T25.211 ☑
      third degree T25.311 ☑
    second degree T25.219 ☑
    third degree T25.319 ☑
  anus — *see* Burn, buttock
  arm (lower) (upper) — *see* Burn, upper, limb
  axilla T22.049 ☑

**Burn** — *continued*
  axilla — *continued*
    first degree T22.149 ☑
    left T22.042 ☑
      first degree T22.142 ☑
      second degree T22.242 ☑
      third degree T22.342 ☑
    right T22.041 ☑
      first degree T22.141 ☑
      second degree T22.241 ☑
      third degree T22.341 ☑
    second degree T22.249 ☑
    third degree T22.349 ☑
  back (lower) T21.04 ☑
    first degree T21.14 ☑
    second degree T21.24 ☑
    third degree T21.34 ☑
    upper T21.03 ☑
      first degree T21.13 ☑
      second degree T21.23 ☑
      third degree T21.33 ☑
  blisters — *code as* Burn, second degree, by site
  breast(s) — *see* Burn, chest wall
  buttock(s) T21.05 ☑
    first degree T21.15 ☑
    second degree T21.25 ☑
    third degree T21.35 ☑
  calf T24.039 ☑
    first degree T24.139 ☑
    left T24.032 ☑
      first degree T24.132 ☑
      second degree T24.232 ☑
      third degree T24.332 ☑
    right T24.031 ☑
      first degree T24.131 ☑
      second degree T24.231 ☑
      third degree T24.331 ☑
    second degree T24.239 ☑
    third degree T24.339 ☑
  canthus (eye) — *see* Burn, eyelid
  caustic acid or alkaline — *see* Corrosion, by site
  cervix T28.3 ☑
  cheek T20.06 ☑
    first degree T20.16 ☑
    second degree T20.26 ☑
    third degree T20.36 ☑
  chemical (acids) (alkalines) (caustics) (external) (internal) — *see* Corrosion, by site
  chest wall T21.01 ☑
    first degree T21.11 ☑
    second degree T21.21 ☑
    third degree T21.31 ☑
  chin T20.03 ☑
    first degree T20.13 ☑
    second degree T20.23 ☑
    third degree T20.33 ☑
  colon T28.2 ☑
  conjunctiva (and cornea) — *see* Burn, cornea
  cornea (and conjunctiva) T26.1- ☑
    chemical — *see* Corrosion, cornea
  corrosion (external) (internal) — *see* Corrosion, by site
  deep necrosis of underlying tissue — *code as* Burn, third degree, by site
  dorsum of hand T23.069 ☑
    first degree T23.169 ☑
    left T23.062 ☑
      first degree T23.162 ☑
      second degree T23.262 ☑
      third degree T23.362 ☑
    right T23.061 ☑
      first degree T23.161 ☑
      second degree T23.261 ☑
      third degree T23.361 ☑
    second degree T23.269 ☑
    third degree T23.369 ☑
  due to ingested chemical agent — *see* Corrosion, by site
  ear (auricle) (external) (canal) T20.01 ☑
    first degree T20.11 ☑
    second degree T20.21 ☑
    third degree T20.31 ☑
  elbow T22.029 ☑
    first degree T22.129 ☑
    left T22.022 ☑
      first degree T22.122 ☑
      second degree T22.222 ☑

**Burn** — *continued*
  elbow — *continued*
    left — *continued*
      third degree T22.322 ☑
    right T22.021 ☑
      first degree T22.121 ☑
      second degree T22.221 ☑
      third degree T22.321 ☑
    second degree T22.229 ☑
    third degree T22.329 ☑
  epidermal loss — *code as* Burn, second degree, by site
  erythema, erythematous — *code as* Burn, first degree, by site
  esophagus T28.1 ☑
  extent (percentage of body surface)
    less than 10 percent T31.0
    10-19 percent T31.10
      with 0-9 percent third degree burns T31.10
      with 10-19 percent third degree burns T31.11
    20-29 percent T31.20
      with 0-9 percent third degree burns T31.20
      with 10-19 percent third degree burns T31.21
      with 20-29 percent third degree burns T31.22
    30-39 percent T31.30
      with 0-9 percent third degree burns T31.30
      with 10-19 percent third degree burns T31.31
      with 20-29 percent third degree burns T31.32
      with 30-39 percent third degree burns T31.33
    40-49 percent T31.40
      with 0-9 percent third degree burns T31.40
      with 10-19 percent third degree burns T31.41
      with 20-29 percent third degree burns T31.42
      with 30-39 percent third degree burns T31.43
      with 40-49 percent third degree burns T31.44
    50-59 percent T31.50
      with 0-9 percent third degree burns T31.50
      with 10-19 percent third degree burns T31.51
      with 20-29 percent third degree burns T31.52
      with 30-39 percent third degree burns T31.53
      with 40-49 percent third degree burns T31.54
      with 50-59 percent third degree burns T31.55
    60-69 percent T31.60
      with 0-9 percent third degree burns T31.60
      with 10-19 percent third degree burns T31.61
      with 20-29 percent third degree burns T31.62
      with 30-39 percent third degree burns T31.63
      with 40-49 percent third degree burns T31.64
      with 50-59 percent third degree burns T31.65
      with 60-69 percent third degree burns T31.66
    70-79 percent T31.70
      with 0-9 percent third degree burns T31.70
      with 10-19 percent third degree burns T31.71
      with 20-29 percent third degree burns T31.72
      with 30-39 percent third degree burns T31.73
      with 40-49 percent third degree burns T31.74
      with 50-59 percent third degree burns T31.75
      with 60-69 percent third degree burns T31.76
      with 70-79 percent third degree burns T31.77
    80-89 percent T31.80
      with 0-9 percent third degree burns T31.80
      with 10-19 percent third degree burns T31.81
      with 20-29 percent third degree burns T31.82
      with 30-39 percent third degree burns T31.83
      with 40-49 percent third degree burns T31.84
      with 50-59 percent third degree burns T31.85
      with 60-69 percent third degree burns T31.86
      with 70-79 percent third degree burns T31.87
      with 80-89 percent third degree burns T31.88
    90 percent or more T31.90
      with 0-9 percent third degree burns T31.90
      with 10-19 percent third degree burns T31.91
      with 20-29 percent third degree burns T31.92
      with 30-39 percent third degree burns T31.93
      with 40-49 percent third degree burns T31.94
      with 50-59 percent third degree burns T31.95
      with 60-69 percent third degree burns T31.96
      with 70-79 percent third degree burns T31.97
      with 80-89 percent third degree burns T31.98
      with 90 percent or more third degree burns T31.99
  extremity — *see* Burn, limb
  eye(s) and adnexa T26.4- ☑
    with resulting rupture and destruction of eyeball T26.2- ☑
    conjunctival sac — *see* Burn, cornea
    cornea — *see* Burn, cornea
    lid — *see* Burn, eyelid
    periocular area — *see* Burn, eyelid

▽ Subterms under main terms may continue to next column or page      ☑ Additional Character Required — Refer to the Tabular List for Character Selection      **43**

Buds — Burn

Index

**Burn** — *continued*
  eye(s) and adnexa — *continued*
    specified site NEC T26.3- ✔
  eyeball — *see* Burn, eye
  eyelid(s) T26.0- ✔
    chemical — *see* Corrosion, eyelid
  face — *see* Burn, head
  finger T23.029 ✔
    first degree T23.129 ✔
    left T23.022 ✔
      first degree T23.122 ✔
      second degree T23.222 ✔
      third degree T23.322 ✔
    multiple sites (without thumb) T23.039 ✔
      with thumb T23.049 ✔
        first degree T23.149 ✔
        left T23.042 ✔
          first degree T23.142 ✔
          second degree T23.242 ✔
          third degree T23.342 ✔
        right T23.041 ✔
          first degree T23.141 ✔
          second degree T23.241 ✔
          third degree T23.341 ✔
      second degree T23.249 ✔
      third degree T23.349 ✔
    first degree T23.139 ✔
    left T23.032 ✔
      first degree T23.132 ✔
      second degree T23.232 ✔
      third degree T23.332 ✔
    right T23.031 ✔
      first degree T23.131 ✔
      second degree T23.231 ✔
      third degree T23.331 ✔
    second degree T23.239 ✔
    third degree T23.339 ✔
    right T23.021 ✔
      first degree T23.121 ✔
      second degree T23.221 ✔
      third degree T23.321 ✔
    second degree T23.229 ✔
    third degree T23.329 ✔
  flank — *see* Burn, abdominal wall
  foot T25.029 ✔
    first degree T25.129 ✔
    left T25.022 ✔
      first degree T25.122 ✔
      second degree T25.222 ✔
      third degree T25.322 ✔
    multiple with ankle — *see* Burn, lower, limb, mul-
      tiple, ankle and foot
    right T25.021 ✔
      first degree T25.121 ✔
      second degree T25.221 ✔
      third degree T25.321 ✔
    second degree T25.229 ✔
    third degree T25.329 ✔
  forearm T22.019 ✔
    first degree T22.119 ✔
    left T22.012 ✔
      first degree T22.112 ✔
      second degree T22.212 ✔
      third degree T22.312 ✔
    right T22.011 ✔
      first degree T22.111 ✔
      second degree T22.211 ✔
      third degree T22.311 ✔
    second degree T22.219 ✔
    third degree T22.319 ✔
  forehead T20.06 ✔
    first degree T20.16 ✔
    second degree T20.26 ✔
    third degree T20.36 ✔
  fourth degree — *code as* Burn, third degree, by site
  friction — *see* Burn, by site
  from swallowing caustic or corrosive substance NEC
    — *see* Corrosion, by site
  full thickness skin loss — *code as* Burn, third degree,
    by site
  gastrointestinal tract NEC T28.2 ✔
    from swallowing caustic or corrosive substance
      T28.7 ✔
  genital organs
    external
      female T21.07 ✔

**Burn** — *continued*
  genital organs — *continued*
    external — *continued*
      female — *continued*
        first degree T21.17 ✔
        second degree T21.27 ✔
        third degree T21.37 ✔
      male T21.06 ✔
        first degree T21.16 ✔
        second degree T21.26 ✔
        third degree T21.36 ✔
    internal T28.3 ✔
      from caustic or corrosive substance T28.8 ✔
  groin — *see* Burn, abdominal wall
  hand(s) T23.009 ✔
    back — *see* Burn, dorsum of hand
    finger — *see* Burn, finger
    first degree T23.109 ✔
    left T23.002 ✔
      first degree T23.102 ✔
      second degree T23.202 ✔
      third degree T23.302 ✔
    multiple sites with wrist T23.099 ✔
      first degree T23.199 ✔
      left T23.092 ✔
        first degree T23.192 ✔
        second degree T23.292 ✔
        third degree T23.392 ✔
      right T23.091 ✔
        first degree T23.191 ✔
        second degree T23.291 ✔
        third degree T23.391 ✔
      second degree T23.299 ✔
      third degree T23.399 ✔
    palm — *see* Burn, palm
    right T23.001 ✔
      first degree T23.101 ✔
      second degree T23.201 ✔
      third degree T23.301 ✔
    second degree T23.209 ✔
    third degree T23.309 ✔
    thumb — *see* Burn, thumb
  head (and face) (and neck) T20.00 ✔
    cheek — *see* Burn, cheek
    chin — *see* Burn, chin
    ear — *see* Burn, ear
    eye(s) only — *see* Burn, eye
    first degree T20.10 ✔
    forehead — *see* Burn, forehead
    lip — *see* Burn, lip
    multiple sites T20.09 ✔
      first degree T20.19 ✔
      second degree T20.29 ✔
      third degree T20.39 ✔
    neck — *see* Burn, neck
    nose — *see* Burn, nose
    scalp — *see* Burn, scalp
    second degree T20.20 ✔
    third degree T20.30 ✔
  hip(s) — *see* Burn, thigh
  inhalation — *see* Burn, respiratory tract
    caustic or corrosive substance (fumes) — *see* Cor-
      rosion, respiratory tract
  internal organ(s) T28.40 ✔
    alimentary tract T28.2 ✔
      esophagus T28.1 ✔
    eardrum T28.41 ✔
    esophagus T28.1 ✔
    from caustic or corrosive substance (swallowing)
      NEC — *see* Corrosion, by site
    genitourinary T28.3 ✔
    mouth T28.0 ✔
    pharynx T28.0 ✔
    respiratory tract — *see* Burn, respiratory tract
    specified organ NEC T28.49 ✔
  interscapular region — *see* Burn, back, upper
  intestine (large) (small) T28.2 ✔
  knee T24.029 ✔
    first degree T24.129 ✔
    left T24.022 ✔
      first degree T24.122 ✔
      second degree T24.222 ✔
      third degree T24.322 ✔
    right T24.021 ✔
      first degree T24.121 ✔
      second degree T24.221 ✔

**Burn** — *continued*
  knee — *continued*
    right — *continued*
      third degree T24.321 ✔
    second degree T24.229 ✔
    third degree T24.329 ✔
  labium (majus) (minus) — *see* Burn, genital organs,
    external, female
  lacrimal apparatus, duct, gland or sac — *see* Burn, eye,
    specified site NEC
  larynx T27.0 ✔
    with lung T27.1 ✔
  leg(s) (lower) (upper) — *see* Burn, lower, limb
  lightning — *see* Burn, by site
  limb(s)
    lower (except ankle or foot alone) — *see* Burn,
      lower, limb
    upper — *see* Burn, upper limb
  lip(s) T20.02 ✔
    first degree T20.12 ✔
    second degree T20.22 ✔
    third degree T20.32 ✔
  lower
    back — *see* Burn, back
    limb T24.009 ✔
      ankle — *see* Burn, ankle
      calf — *see* Burn, calf
      first degree T24.109 ✔
      foot — *see* Burn, foot
      hip — *see* Burn, thigh
      knee — *see* Burn, knee
      left T24.002 ✔
        first degree T24.102 ✔
        second degree T24.202 ✔
        third degree T24.302 ✔
      multiple sites, except ankle and foot T24.099 ✔
        ankle and foot T25.099 ✔
          first degree T25.199 ✔
          left T25.092 ✔
            first degree T25.192 ✔
            second degree T25.292 ✔
            third degree T25.392 ✔
          right T25.091 ✔
            first degree T25.191 ✔
            second degree T25.291 ✔
            third degree T25.391 ✔
          second degree T25.299 ✔
          third degree T25.399 ✔
        first degree T24.199 ✔
        left T24.092 ✔
          first degree T24.192 ✔
          second degree T24.292 ✔
          third degree T24.392 ✔
        right T24.091 ✔
          first degree T24.191 ✔
          second degree T24.291 ✔
          third degree T24.391 ✔
        second degree T24.299 ✔
        third degree T24.399 ✔
      right T24.001 ✔
        first degree T24.101 ✔
        second degree T24.201 ✔
        third degree T24.301 ✔
      second degree T24.209 ✔
      thigh — *see* Burn, thigh
      third degree T24.309 ✔
      toe — *see* Burn, toe
  lung (with larynx and trachea) T27.1 ✔
  mouth T28.0 ✔
  neck T20.07 ✔
    first degree T20.17 ✔
    second degree T20.27 ✔
    third degree T20.37 ✔
  nose (septum) T20.04 ✔
    first degree T20.14 ✔
    second degree T20.24 ✔
    third degree T20.34 ✔
  ocular adnexa — *see* Burn, eye
  orbit region — *see* Burn, eyelid
  palm T23.059 ✔
    first degree T23.159 ✔
    left T23.052 ✔
      first degree T23.152 ✔
      second degree T23.252 ✔
      third degree T23.352 ✔
    right T23.051 ✔

✔ Additional Character Required — Refer to the Tabular List for Character Selection    ▽ Subterms under main terms may continue to next column or page

**Burn** — *continued*
palm — *continued*
　right — *continued*
　　first degree T23.151 ☑
　　second degree T23.251 ☑
　　third degree T23.351 ☑
　　second degree T23.259 ☑
　　third degree T23.359 ☑
　partial thickness — *code as* Burn, unspecified degree, by site
　pelvis — *see* Burn, trunk
　penis — *see* Burn, genital organs, external, male
　perineum
　　female — *see* Burn, genital organs, external, female
　　male — *see* Burn, genital organs, external, male
　periocular area — *see* Burn, eyelid
　pharynx T28.0 ☑
　rectum T28.2 ☑
　respiratory tract T27.3 ☑
　　larynx — *see* Burn, larynx
　　specified part NEC T27.2 ☑
　　trachea — *see* Burn, trachea
　sac, lacrimal — *see* Burn, eye, specified site NEC
　scalp T20.05 ☑
　　first degree T20.15 ☑
　　second degree T20.25 ☑
　　third degree T20.35 ☑
　scapular region T22.069 ☑
　　first degree T22.169 ☑
　　left T22.062 ☑
　　　first degree T22.162 ☑
　　　second degree T22.262 ☑
　　　third degree T22.362 ☑
　　right T22.061 ☑
　　　first degree T22.161 ☑
　　　second degree T22.261 ☑
　　　third degree T22.361 ☑
　　second degree T22.269 ☑
　　third degree T22.369 ☑
　sclera — *see* Burn, eye, specified site NEC
　scrotum — *see* Burn, genital organs, external, male
　shoulder T22.059 ☑
　　first degree T22.159 ☑
　　left T22.052 ☑
　　　first degree T22.152 ☑
　　　second degree T22.252 ☑
　　　third degree T22.352 ☑
　　right T22.051 ☑
　　　first degree T22.151 ☑
　　　second degree T22.251 ☑
　　　third degree T22.351 ☑
　　second degree T22.259 ☑
　　third degree T22.359 ☑
　stomach T28.2 ☑
　temple — *see* Burn, head
　testis — *see* Burn, genital organs, external, male
　thigh T24.019 ☑
　　first degree T24.119 ☑
　　left T24.012 ☑
　　　first degree T24.112 ☑
　　　second degree T24.212 ☑
　　　third degree T24.312 ☑
　　right T24.011 ☑
　　　first degree T24.111 ☑
　　　second degree T24.211 ☑
　　　third degree T24.311 ☑
　　second degree T24.219 ☑
　　third degree T24.319 ☑
　thorax (external) — *see* Burn, trunk
　throat (meaning pharynx) T28.0 ☑
　thumb(s) T23.019 ☑
　　first degree T23.119 ☑
　　left T23.012 ☑
　　　first degree T23.112 ☑
　　　second degree T23.212 ☑
　　　third degree T23.312 ☑
　　multiple sites with fingers T23.049 ☑
　　　first degree T23.149 ☑
　　　left T23.042 ☑
　　　　first degree T23.142 ☑
　　　　second degree T23.242 ☑
　　　　third degree T23.342 ☑
　　　right T23.041 ☑
　　　　first degree T23.141 ☑
　　　　second degree T23.241 ☑
　　　　third degree T23.341 ☑

**Burn** — *continued*
thumb(s) — *continued*
　multiple sites with fingers — *continued*
　　second degree T23.249 ☑
　　third degree T23.349 ☑
　　right T23.011 ☑
　　　first degree T23.111 ☑
　　　second degree T23.211 ☑
　　　third degree T23.311 ☑
　　second degree T23.219 ☑
　　third degree T23.319 ☑
　toe T25.039 ☑
　　first degree T25.139 ☑
　　left T25.032 ☑
　　　first degree T25.132 ☑
　　　second degree T25.232 ☑
　　　third degree T25.332 ☑
　　right T25.031 ☑
　　　first degree T25.131 ☑
　　　second degree T25.231 ☑
　　　third degree T25.331 ☑
　　second degree T25.239 ☑
　　third degree T25.339 ☑
　tongue T28.0 ☑
　tonsil(s) T28.0 ☑
　trachea T27.0 ☑
　　with lung T27.1 ☑
　trunk T21.00 ☑
　　abdominal wall — *see* Burn, abdominal wall
　　anus — *see* Burn, buttock
　　axilla — *see* Burn, upper limb
　　back — *see* Burn, back
　　breast — *see* Burn, chest wall
　　buttock — *see* Burn, buttock
　　chest wall — *see* Burn, chest wall
　　first degree T21.10 ☑
　　flank — *see* Burn, abdominal wall
　　genital
　　　female — *see* Burn, genital organs, external, female
　　　male — *see* Burn, genital organs, external, male
　　groin — *see* Burn, abdominal wall
　　interscapular region — *see* Burn, back, upper
　　labia — *see* Burn, genital organs, external, female
　　lower back — *see* Burn, back
　　penis — *see* Burn, genital organs, external, male
　　perineum
　　　female — *see* Burn, genital organs, external, female
　　　male — *see* Burn, genital organs, external, male
　　scapula region — *see* Burn, scapular region
　　scrotum — *see* Burn, genital organs, external, male
　　second degree T21.20 ☑
　　specified site NEC T21.09 ☑
　　　first degree T21.19 ☑
　　　second degree T21.29 ☑
　　　third degree T21.39 ☑
　　testes — *see* Burn, genital organs, external, male
　　third degree T21.30 ☑
　　upper back — *see* Burn, back, upper
　　vulva — *see* Burn, genital organs, external, female
　unspecified site with extent of body surface involved specified
　　less than 10 percent T31.0
　　10-19 percent (0-9 percent third degree) T31.10
　　　with 10-19 percent third degree T31.11
　　20-29 percent (0-9 percent third degree) T31.20
　　　with
　　　　10-19 percent third degree T31.21
　　　　20-29 percent third degree T31.22
　　30-39 percent (0-9 percent third degree) T31.30
　　　with
　　　　10-19 percent third degree T31.31
　　　　20-29 percent third degree T31.32
　　　　30-39 percent third degree T31.33
　　40-49 percent (0-9 percent third degree) T31.40
　　　with
　　　　10-19 percent third degree T31.41
　　　　20-29 percent third degree T31.42
　　　　30-39 percent third degree T31.43
　　　　40-49 percent third degree T31.44
　　50-59 percent (0-9 percent third degree) T31.50
　　　with
　　　　10-19 percent third degree T31.51
　　　　20-29 percent third degree T31.52
　　　　30-39 percent third degree T31.53
　　　　40-49 percent third degree T31.54

**Burn** — *continued*
unspecified site with extent of body surface involved specified — *continued*
　50-59 percent — *continued*
　　with — *continued*
　　　50-59 percent third degree T31.55
　　60-69 percent (0-9 percent third degree) T31.60
　　　with
　　　　10-19 percent third degree T31.61
　　　　20-29 percent third degree T31.62
　　　　30-39 percent third degree T31.63
　　　　40-49 percent third degree T31.64
　　　　50-59 percent third degree T31.65
　　　　60-69 percent third degree T31.66
　　70-79 percent (0-9 percent third degree) T31.70
　　　with
　　　　10-19 percent third degree T31.71
　　　　20-29 percent third degree T31.72
　　　　30-39 percent third degree T31.73
　　　　40-49 percent third degree T31.74
　　　　50-59 percent third degree T31.75
　　　　60-69 percent third degree T31.76
　　　　70-79 percent third degree T31.77
　　80-89 percent (0-9 percent third degree) T31.80
　　　with
　　　　10-19 percent third degree T31.81
　　　　20-29 percent third degree T31.82
　　　　30-39 percent third degree T31.83
　　　　40-49 percent third degree T31.84
　　　　50-59 percent third degree T31.85
　　　　60-69 percent third degree T31.86
　　　　70-79 percent third degree T31.87
　　　　80-89 percent third degree T31.88
　　90 percent or more (0-9 percent third degree) T31.90
　　　with
　　　　10-19 percent third degree T31.91
　　　　20-29 percent third degree T31.92
　　　　30-39 percent third degree T31.93
　　　　40-49 percent third degree T31.94
　　　　50-59 percent third degree T31.95
　　　　60-69 percent third degree T31.96
　　　　70-79 percent third degree T31.97
　　　　80-89 percent third degree T31.98
　　　　90-99 percent third degree T31.99
upper limb T22.00 ☑
　above elbow — *see* Burn, above elbow
　axilla — *see* Burn, axilla
　elbow — *see* Burn, elbow
　first degree T22.10 ☑
　forearm — *see* Burn, forearm
　hand — *see* Burn, hand
　interscapular region — *see* Burn, back, upper
　multiple sites T22.099 ☑
　　first degree T22.199 ☑
　　left T22.092 ☑
　　　first degree T22.192 ☑
　　　second degree T22.292 ☑
　　　third degree T22.392 ☑
　　right T22.091 ☑
　　　first degree T22.191 ☑
　　　second degree T22.291 ☑
　　　third degree T22.391 ☑
　　second degree T22.299 ☑
　　third degree T22.399 ☑
　scapular region — *see* Burn, scapular region
　second degree T22.20 ☑
　shoulder — *see* Burn, shoulder
　third degree T22.30 ☑
　wrist — *see* Burn, wrist
uterus T28.3 ☑
vagina T28.3 ☑
vulva — *see* Burn, genital organs, external, female
wrist T23.079 ☑
　first degree T23.179 ☑
　left T23.072 ☑
　　first degree T23.172 ☑
　　second degree T23.272 ☑
　　third degree T23.372 ☑
　multiple sites with hand T23.099 ☑
　　first degree T23.199 ☑
　　left T23.092 ☑
　　　first degree T23.192 ☑
　　　second degree T23.292 ☑
　　　third degree T23.392 ☑
　　right T23.091 ☑
　　　first degree T23.191 ☑

**Burn** — *continued*
 wrist — *continued*
  multiple sites with hand — *continued*
   right — *continued*
    second degree T23.291 ☑
    third degree T23.391 ☑
   second degree T23.299 ☑
   third degree T23.399 ☑
  right T23.071 ☑
   first degree T23.171 ☑
   second degree T23.271 ☑
   third degree T23.371 ☑
  second degree T23.279 ☑
  third degree T23.379 ☑
**Burnett's syndrome** E83.52
**Burning**
 feet syndrome E53.9
 sensation R20.8
 tongue K14.6
**Burn-out** (state) Z73.0
**Burns' disease or osteochondrosis** — *see* Osteochondrosis, juvenile, ulna
**Bursa** — *see* condition
**Bursitis** M71.9
 Achilles — *see* Tendinitis, Achilles
 adhesive — *see* Bursitis, specified NEC
 ankle — *see* Enthesopathy, lower limb, ankle, specified type NEC
 calcaneal — *see* Enthesopathy, foot, specified type NEC
 collateral ligament, tibial — *see* Bursitis, tibial collateral
 due to use, overuse, pressure (*see also* Disorder, soft tissue, due to use, specified type NEC)
  specified NEC — *see* Disorder, soft tissue, due to use, specified NEC
 Duplay's M75.0 ☑
 elbow NEC M70.3- ☑
  olecranon M70.2- ☑
 finger — *see* Disorder, soft tissue, due to use, specified type NEC, hand
 foot — *see* Enthesopathy, foot, specified type NEC
 gonococcal A54.49
 gouty — *see* Gout
 hand M70.1- ☑
 hip NEC M70.7- ☑
  trochanteric M70.6- ☑
 infective NEC M71.10
  abscess — *see* Abscess, bursa
  ankle M71.17- ☑
  elbow M71.12- ☑
  foot M71.17- ☑
  hand M71.14- ☑
  hip M71.15- ☑
  knee M71.16- ☑
  multiple sites M71.19
  shoulder M71.11- ☑
  specified site NEC M71.18
  wrist M71.13- ☑
 ischial — *see* Bursitis, hip
 knee NEC M70.5- ☑
  prepatellar M70.4- ☑
 occupational NEC (*see also* Disorder, soft tissue, due to, use)
 olecranon — *see* Bursitis, elbow, olecranon
 pharyngeal J39.1
 popliteal — *see* Bursitis, knee
 prepatellar M70.4- ☑
 radiohumeral M77.8
 rheumatoid M06.20
  ankle M06.27- ☑
  elbow M06.22- ☑
  foot joint M06.27- ☑
  hand joint M06.24- ☑
  hip M06.25- ☑
  knee M06.26- ☑
  multiple site M06.29
  shoulder M06.21- ☑
  vertebra M06.28
  wrist M06.23- ☑
 scapulohumeral — *see* Bursitis, shoulder
 semimembranous muscle (knee) — *see* Bursitis, knee
 shoulder M75.5- ☑
  adhesive — *see* Capsulitis, adhesive
 specified NEC M71.50
  ankle M71.57- ☑

**Bursitis** — *continued*
 specified — *continued*
  due to use, overuse or pressure — *see* Disorder, soft tissue, due to, use
  elbow M71.52- ☑
  foot M71.57- ☑
  hand M71.54- ☑
  hip M71.55- ☑
  knee M71.56- ☑
  shoulder — *see* Bursitis, shoulder
  specified site NEC M71.58
  tibial collateral M76.4- ☑
  wrist M71.53- ☑
 subacromial — *see* Bursitis, shoulder
 subcoracoid — *see* Bursitis, shoulder
 subdeltoid — *see* Bursitis, shoulder
 syphilitic A52.78
 Thornwaldt, Tornwaldt J39.2
 tibial collateral M76.4- ☑
 toe — *see* Enthesopathy, foot, specified type NEC
 trochanteric (area) — *see* Bursitis, hip, trochanteric
 wrist — *see* Bursitis, hand
**Bursopathy** M71.9
 specified type NEC M71.80
  ankle M71.87- ☑
  elbow M71.82- ☑
  foot M71.87- ☑
  hand M71.84- ☑
  hip M71.85- ☑
  knee M71.86- ☑
  multiple sites M71.89
  shoulder M71.81- ☑
  specified site NEC M71.88
  wrist M71.83- ☑
**Burst stitches or sutures** (complication of surgery) T81.31 ☑
 external operation wound T81.31 ☑
 internal operation wound T81.32 ☑
**Buruli ulcer** A31.1
**Bury's disease** L95.1
**Buschke's**
 disease B45.3
 scleredema — *see* Sclerosis, systemic
**Busse-Buschke disease** B45.3
**Buttock** — *see* condition
**Button**
 Biskra B55.1
 Delhi B55.1
 oriental B55.1
**Buttonhole deformity** (finger) — *see* Deformity, finger, boutonniere
**Bwamba fever** A92.8
**Byssinosis** J66.0
**Bywaters' syndrome** T79.5 ☑

# C

**Cachexia** R64
 cancerous R64
 cardiac — *see* Disease, heart
 dehydration E86.0
 due to malnutrition R64
 exophthalmic — *see* Hyperthyroidism
 heart — *see* Disease, heart
 hypophyseal E23.0
 hypopituitary E23.0
 lead — *see* Poisoning, lead
 malignant R64
 marsh — *see* Malaria
 nervous F48.8
 old age R54
 paludal — *see* Malaria
 pituitary E23.0
 renal N28.9
 saturnine — *see* Poisoning, lead
 senile R54
 Simmonds' E23.0
 splenica D73.0
 strumipriva E03.4
 tuberculous NEC — *see* Tuberculosis
**Café, au lait spots** L81.3
**Caffeine-induced**
 anxiety disorder F15.980
 sleep disorder F15.982
**Caffey's syndrome** Q78.8
**Caisson disease** T70.3 ☑
**Cake kidney** Q63.1

**Caked breast** (puerperal, postpartum) O92.79
**Calabar swelling** B74.3
**Calcaneal spur** — *see* Spur, bone, calcaneal
**Calcaneo-apophysitis** M92.8
**Calcareous** — *see* condition
**Calcicosis** J62.8
**Calciferol** (vitamin D) deficiency E55.9
 with rickets E55.0
**Calcification**
 adrenal (capsule) (gland) E27.49
  tuberculous E35 [B90.8]
 aorta I70.0
 artery (annular) — *see* Arteriosclerosis
 auricle (ear) — *see* Disorder, pinna, specified type NEC
 basal ganglia G23.8
 bladder N32.89
  due to Schistosoma hematobium B65.0
 brain (cortex) — *see* Calcification, cerebral
 bronchus J98.09
 bursa M71.40
  ankle M71.47- ☑
  elbow M71.42- ☑
  foot M71.47- ☑
  hand M71.44- ☑
  hip M71.45- ☑
  knee M71.46- ☑
  multiple sites M71.49
  shoulder M75.3- ☑
  specified site NEC M71.48
  wrist M71.43- ☑
 cardiac — *see* Degeneration, myocardial
 cerebral (cortex) G93.89
  artery I67.2
 cervix (uteri) N88.8
 choroid plexus G93.89
 conjunctiva — *see* Concretion, conjunctiva
 corpora cavernosa (penis) N48.89
 cortex (brain) — *see* Calcification, cerebral
 dental pulp (nodular) K04.2
 dentinal papilla K00.4
 fallopian tube N83.8
 falx cerebri G96.19
 gallbladder K82.8
 general E83.59
 heart (*see also* Degeneration, myocardial)
  valve — *see* Endocarditis
 idiopathic infantile arterial (IIAC) Q28.8
 intervertebral cartilage or disc (postinfective) — *see* Disorder, disc, specified NEC
 intracranial — *see* Calcification, cerebral
 joint — *see* Disorder, joint, specified type NEC
 kidney N28.89
  tuberculous N29 [B90.1]
 larynx (senile) J38.7
 lens — *see* Cataract, specified NEC
 lung (active) (postinfectional) J98.4
  tuberculous B90.9
 lymph gland or node (postinfectional) I89.8
  tuberculous (*see also* Tuberculosis, lymph gland) B90.8
 mammographic R92.1
 massive (paraplegic) — *see* Myositis, ossificans, in, quadriplegia
 medial — *see* Arteriosclerosis, extremities
 meninges (cerebral) (spinal) G96.19
 metastatic E83.59
 Mönckeberg's — *see* Arteriosclerosis, extremities
 muscle M61.9
  due to burns — *see* Myositis, ossificans, in, burns
  paralytic — *see* Myositis, ossificans, in, quadriplegia
  specified type NEC M61.40
   ankle M61.47- ☑
   foot M61.47- ☑
   forearm M61.43- ☑
   hand M61.44- ☑
   lower leg M61.46- ☑
   multiple sites M61.49
   pelvic region M61.45- ☑
   shoulder region M61.41- ☑
   specified site NEC M61.48
   thigh M61.45- ☑
   upper arm M61.42- ☑
 myocardium, myocardial — *see* Degeneration, myocardial
 ovary N83.8
 pancreas K86.89
 penis N48.89

**Calcification** — *continued*
- periarticular — *see* Disorder, joint, specified type NEC
- pericardium (*see also* Pericarditis) I31.1
- pineal gland E34.8
- pleura J94.8
  - postinfectional J94.8
  - tuberculous NEC B90.9
- pulpal (dental) (nodular) K04.2
- sclera H15.89
- spleen D73.89
- subcutaneous L94.2
- suprarenal (capsule) (gland) E27.49
- tendon (sheath) (*see also* Tenosynovitis, specified type NEC)
  - with bursitis, synovitis or tenosynovitis — *see* Tendinitis, calcific
- trachea J39.8
- ureter N28.89
- uterus N85.8
- vitreous — *see* Deposit, crystalline

**Calcified** — *see* Calcification

**Calcinosis** (interstitial) (tumoral) (universalis) E83.59
- with Raynaud's phenomenon, esophageal dysfunction, sclerodactyly, telangiectasia (CREST syndrome) M34.1
- circumscripta (skin) L94.2
- cutis L94.2

**Calciphylaxis** (*see also* Calcification, by site) E83.59

**Calcium**
- deposits — *see* Calcification, by site
- metabolism disorder E83.50
- salts or soaps in vitreous — *see* Deposit, crystalline

**Calciuria** R82.99

**Calculi** — *see* Calculus

**Calculosis, intrahepatic** — *see* Calculus, bile duct

**Calculus, calculi, calculous**
- ampulla of Vater — *see* Calculus, bile duct
- anuria (impacted) (recurrent) (*see also* Calculus, urinary) N20.9
- appendix K38.1
- bile duct (common) (hepatic) K80.50
  - with
    - calculus of gallbladder — *see* Calculus, gallbladder and bile duct
    - cholangitis K80.30
      - with
        - cholecystitis — *see* Calculus, bile duct, with cholecystitis
        - obstruction K80.31
      - acute K80.32
        - with
          - chronic cholangitis K80.36
            - with obstruction K80.37
          - obstruction K80.33
      - chronic K80.34
        - with
          - acute cholangitis K80.36
            - with obstruction K80.37
          - obstruction K80.35
    - cholecystitis (with cholangitis) K80.40
      - with obstruction K80.41
      - acute K80.42
        - with
          - chronic cholecystitis K80.46
            - with obstruction K80.47
          - obstruction K80.43
      - chronic K80.44
        - with
          - acute cholecystitis K80.46
            - with obstruction K80.47
          - obstruction K80.45
  - biliary (*see also* Calculus, gallbladder)
    - specified NEC K80.80
      - with obstruction K80.81
- bilirubin, multiple — *see* Calculus, gallbladder
- bladder (encysted) (impacted) (urinary) (diverticulum) N21.0
- bronchus J98.09
- calyx (kidney) (renal) — *see* Calculus, kidney
- cholesterol (pure) (solitary) — *see* Calculus, gallbladder
- common duct (bile) — *see* Calculus, bile duct
- conjunctiva — *see* Concretion, conjunctiva
- cystic N21.0
  - duct — *see* Calculus, gallbladder
- dental (subgingival) (supragingival) K03.6
- diverticulum
  - bladder N21.0
  - kidney N20.0

**Calculus, calculi, calculous** — *continued*
- epididymis N50.89
- gallbladder K80.20
  - with
    - bile duct calculus — *see* Calculus, gallbladder and bile duct
    - cholecystitis K80.10
      - with obstruction K80.11
      - acute K80.00
        - with
          - chronic cholecystitis K80.12
            - with obstruction K80.13
          - obstruction K80.01
      - chronic K80.10
        - with
          - acute cholecystitis K80.12
            - with obstruction K80.13
          - obstruction K80.11
    - specified NEC K80.18
      - with obstruction K80.19
    - obstruction K80.21
  - gallbladder and bile duct K80.70
    - with
      - cholecystitis K80.60
        - with obstruction K80.61
        - acute K80.62
          - with
            - chronic cholecystitis K80.66
              - with obstruction K80.67
            - obstruction K80.63
        - chronic K80.64
          - with
            - acute cholecystitis K80.66
              - with obstruction K80.67
            - obstruction K80.65
      - obstruction K80.71
- hepatic (duct) — *see* Calculus, bile duct
- ileal conduit N21.8
- intestinal (impaction) (obstruction) K56.49
- kidney (impacted) (multiple) (pelvis) (recurrent) (staghorn) N20.0
  - with calculus, ureter N20.2
  - congenital Q63.8
- lacrimal passages — *see* Dacryolith
- liver (impacted) — *see* Calculus, bile duct
- lung J98.4
- mammographic R92.1
- nephritic (impacted) (recurrent) — *see* Calculus, kidney
- nose J34.89
- pancreas (duct) K86.89
- parotid duct or gland K11.5
- pelvis, encysted — *see* Calculus, kidney
- prostate N42.0
- pulmonary J98.4
- pyelitis (impacted) (recurrent) N20.0
  - with hydronephrosis N13.2
- pyelonephritis (impacted) (recurrent) N20 ☑
  - with hydronephrosis N13.2
- renal (impacted) (recurrent) — *see* Calculus, kidney
- salivary (duct) (gland) K11.5
- seminal vesicle N50.89
- staghorn — *see* Calculus, kidney
- Stensen's duct K11.5
- stomach K31.89
- sublingual duct or gland K11.5
  - congenital Q38.4
- submandibular duct, gland or region K11.5
- submaxillary duct, gland or region K11.5
- suburethral N21.8
- tonsil J35.8
- tooth, teeth (subgingival) (supragingival) K03.6
- tunica vaginalis N50.89
- ureter (impacted) (recurrent) N20.1
  - with calculus, kidney N20.2
    - with hydronephrosis N13.2
      - with infection N13.6
- urethra (impacted) N21.1
- urinary (duct) (impacted) (passage) (tract) N20.9
  - with hydronephrosis N13.2
    - with infection N13.6
  - in (due to)
  - lower N21.9
    - specified NEC N21.8
- vagina N89.8
- vesical (impacted) N21.0
- Wharton's duct K11.5
- xanthine E79.8 [N22]

**Calicectasis** N28.89

**Caliectasis** N28.89

**California**
- disease B38.9
- encephalitis A83.5

**Caligo cornea** — *see* Opacity, cornea, central

**Callositas, callosity** (infected) L84

**Callus** (infected) L84
- bone — *see* Osteophyte
  - excessive, following fracture — *code as* Sequelae of fracture

**CALME** (childhood asymmetric labium majus enlargement) N90.61

**Calorie deficiency or malnutrition** (*see also* Malnutrition) E46

**Calvé-Perthes disease** — *see* Legg-Calvé-Perthes disease

**Calvé's disease** — *see* Osteochondrosis, juvenile, spine

**Calvities** — *see* Alopecia, androgenic

**Cameroon fever** — *see* Malaria

**Camptocormia** (hysterical) F44.4

**Camurati-Engelmann syndrome** Q78.3

**Canal** (*see also* condition)
- atrioventricular common Q21.2

**Canaliculitis** (lacrimal) (acute) (subacute) H04.33- ☑
- Actinomyces A42.89
- chronic H04.42- ☑

**Canavan's disease** E75.29

**Canceled procedure** (surgical) Z53.9
- because of
  - contraindication Z53.09
    - smoking Z53.01
  - left against medical advice (AMA) Z53.21
  - patient's decision Z53.20
    - for reasons of belief or group pressure Z53.1
    - specified reason NEC Z53.29
  - specified reason NEC Z53.8

**Cancer** (*see also* Neoplasm, by site, malignant)
- bile duct type liver C22.1
- blood — *see* Leukemia
- breast (*see also* Neoplasm, breast, malignant) C50.91- ☑
- hepatocellular C22.0
- lung (*see also* Neoplasm, lung, malignant) C34.90
- ovarian (*see also* Neoplasm ovary, malignant) C56.9
- unspecified site (primary) C80.1

**Cancer (o)phobia** F45.29

**Cancerous** — *see* Neoplasm, malignant, by site

**Cancrum oris** A69.0

**Candidiasis, candidal** B37.9
- balanitis B37.42
- bronchitis B37.1
- cheilitis B37.83
- congenital P37.5
- cystitis B37.41
- disseminated B37.7
- endocarditis B37.6
- enteritis B37.82
- esophagitis B37.81
- intertrigo B37.2
- lung B37.1
- meningitis B37.5
- mouth B37.0
- nails B37.2
- neonatal P37.5
- onychia B37.2
- oral B37.0
- osteomyelitis B37.89
- otitis externa B37.84
- paronychia B37.2
- perionyxis B37.2
- pneumonia B37.1
- proctitis B37.82
- pulmonary B37.1
- pyelonephritis B37.49
- sepsis B37.7
- skin B37.2
- specified site NEC B37.89
- stomatitis B37.0
- systemic B37.7
- urethritis B37.41
- urogenital site NEC B37.49
- vagina B37.3
- vulva B37.3
- vulvovaginitis B37.3

**Candidid** L30.2

**Candidosis** — *see* Candidiasis

**Candiru infection or infestation** B88.8

**Canities** (premature) L67.1

**Carcinoma** — *continued*
  intracystic
    noninfiltrating — *see* Neoplasm, in situ, by site
  intraductal (noninfiltrating)
    with Paget's disease — *see* Neoplasm, breast, malignant
    breast D05.1- ☑
    papillary
      with invasion
        specified site — *see* Neoplasm, malignant, by site
        unspecified site (female) C50.91- ☑
          male C50.92- ☑
      breast D05.1- ☑
      specified site NEC — *see* Neoplasm, in situ, by site
      unspecified site (female) D05.1- ☑
    specified site NEC — *see* Neoplasm, in situ, by site
    unspecified site (female) D05.1- ☑
  intraepidermal — *see* Neoplasm, in situ
    squamous cell, Bowen's type — *see* Neoplasm, skin, in situ
  intraepithelial — *see* Neoplasm, in situ, by site
    squamous cell — *see* Neoplasm, in situ, by site
  intraosseous C41.1
    upper jaw (bone) C41.0
  islet cell
    with exocrine, mixed
      specified site — *see* Neoplasm, malignant, by site
      unspecified site C25.9
    pancreas C25.4
    specified site NEC — *see* Neoplasm, malignant, by site
    unspecified site C25.4
  juvenile, breast — *see* Neoplasm, breast, malignant
  large cell
    small cell
      specified site — *see* Neoplasm, malignant, by site
      unspecified site C34.90
  Leydig cell (testis)
    specified site — *see* Neoplasm, malignant, by site
    unspecified site
      female C56.9
      male C62.90
  lipid-rich (female) C50.91- ☑
    male C50.92- ☑
  liver cell C22.0
  liver NEC C22.7
  lobular (infiltrating)
    with intraductal
      specified site — *see* Neoplasm, malignant, by site
      unspecified site (female) C50.91- ☑
        male C50.92- ☑
    noninfiltrating
      breast D05.0- ☑
      specified site NEC — *see* Neoplasm, in situ, by site
      unspecified site D05.0- ☑
    specified site — *see* Neoplasm, malignant, by site
    unspecified site (female) C50.91- ☑
      male C50.92- ☑
  medullary
    with
      amyloid stroma
        specified site — *see* Neoplasm, malignant, by site
        unspecified site C73
      lymphoid stroma
        specified site — *see* Neoplasm, malignant, by site
        unspecified site (female) C50.91- ☑
          male C50.92- ☑
  Merkel cell C4A.9 (*following* C43)
    anal margin C4A.51 (*following* C43)
    anal skin C4A.51 (*following* C43)
    canthus C4A.1- ☑ (*following* C43)
    ear and external auricular canal C4A.2- ☑ (*following* C43)
    external auricular canal C4A.2- ☑ (*following* C43)
    eyelid, including canthus C4A.1- ☑ (*following* C43)
    face C4A.30 (*following* C43)
      specified NEC C4A.39 (*following* C43)
    hip C4A.7- ☑ (*following* C43)
    lip C4A.0 (*following* C43)

**Carcinoma** — *continued*
  Merkel cell — *continued*
    lower limb, including hip C4A.7- ☑ (*following* C43)
    neck C4A.4 (*following* C43)
    nodal presentation C7B.1 (*following* C75)
    nose C4A.31 (*following* C43)
    overlapping sites C4A.8 (*following* C43)
    perianal skin C4A.51 (*following* C43)
    scalp C4A.4 (*following* C43)
    secondary C7B.1 (*following* C75)
    shoulder C4A.6- ☑ (*following* C43)
    skin of breast C4A.52 (*following* C43)
    trunk NEC C4A.59 (*following* C43)
    upper limb, including shoulder C4A.6- ☑ (*following* C43)
    visceral metastatic C7B.1 (*following* C75)
  metastatic — *see* Neoplasm, secondary, by site
  metatypical — *see* Neoplasm, skin, malignant
  morphea, basal cell — *see* Neoplasm, skin, malignant
  mucoid
    cell
      specified site — *see* Neoplasm, malignant, by site
      unspecified site C75.1
  neuroendocrine (*see also* Tumor, neuroendocrine)
    high grade, any site C7A.1 (*following* C75)
    poorly differentiated, any site C7A.1 (*following* C75)
  nonencapsulated sclerosing C73
  noninfiltrating
    intracystic — *see* Neoplasm, in situ, by site
    intraductal
      breast D05.1- ☑
      papillary
        breast D05.1- ☑
        specified site NEC — *see* Neoplasm, in situ, by site
        unspecified site D05.1- ☑
      specified site — *see* Neoplasm, in situ, by site
      unspecified site D05.1- ☑
    lobular
      breast D05.0- ☑
      specified site NEC — *see* Neoplasm, in situ, by site
      unspecified site (female) D05.0- ☑
  oat cell
    specified site — *see* Neoplasm, malignant, by site
    unspecified site C34.90
  odontogenic C41.1
    upper jaw (bone) C41.0
  papillary
    with follicular (mixed) C73
    follicular variant C73
    intraductal (noninfiltrating)
      with invasion
        specified site — *see* Neoplasm, malignant, by site
        unspecified site (female) C50.91- ☑
          male C50.92- ☑
      breast D05.1- ☑
      specified site NEC — *see* Neoplasm, in situ, by site
      unspecified site D05.1- ☑
    serous
      specified site — *see* Neoplasm, malignant, by site
    surface
      specified site — *see* Neoplasm, malignant, by site
      unspecified site C56.9
    unspecified site C56.9
  papillocystic
    specified site — *see* Neoplasm, malignant, by site
    unspecified site C56.9
  parafollicular cell
    specified site — *see* Neoplasm, malignant, by site
    unspecified site C73
  pilomatrix — *see* Neoplasm, skin, malignant
  pseudomucinous
    specified site — *see* Neoplasm, malignant, by site
    unspecified site C56.9
  renal cell C64- ☑
  Schmincke — *see* Neoplasm, nasopharynx, malignant
  Schneiderian
    specified site — *see* Neoplasm, malignant, by site
    unspecified site C30.0
  sebaceous — *see* Neoplasm, skin, malignant

**Carcinoma** — *continued*
  secondary (*see also* Neoplasm, secondary, by site)
    Merkel cell C7B.1 (*following* C75)
  secretory, breast — *see* Neoplasm, breast, malignant
  serous
    papillary
      specified site — *see* Neoplasm, malignant, by site
      unspecified site C56.9
    surface, papillary
      specified site — *see* Neoplasm, malignant, by site
      unspecified site C56.9
  Sertoli cell
    specified site — *see* Neoplasm, malignant, by site
    unspecified site C62.90
      female C56.9
      male C62.90
  skin appendage — *see* Neoplasm, skin, malignant
  small cell
    fusiform cell
      specified site — *see* Neoplasm, malignant, by site
      unspecified site C34.90
    intermediate cell
      specified site — *see* Neoplasm, malignant, by site
      unspecified site C34.90
    large cell
      specified site — *see* Neoplasm, malignant, by site
      unspecified site C34.90
  solid
    with amyloid stroma
      specified site — *see* Neoplasm, malignant, by site
      unspecified site C73
    microinvasive
      specified site — *see* Neoplasm, malignant, by site
      unspecified site C53.9
  sweat gland — *see* Neoplasm, skin, malignant
  theca cell C56.- ☑
  thymic C37
  unspecified site (primary) C80.1
  water-clear cell C75.0
**Carcinoma-in-situ** (*see also* Neoplasm, in situ, by site)
  breast NOS D05.9- ☑
    specified type NEC D05.8- ☑
  epidermoid (*see also* Neoplasm, in situ, by site)
    with questionable stromal invasion
      cervix D06.9
      specified site NEC — *see* Neoplasm, in situ, by site
      unspecified site D06.9
    Bowen's type — *see* Neoplasm, skin, in situ
  intraductal
    breast D05.1- ☑
    specified site NEC — *see* Neoplasm, in situ, by site
    unspecified site D05.1- ☑
  lobular
    with
      infiltrating duct
        breast (female) C50.91- ☑
          male C50.92- ☑
        specified site NEC — *see* Neoplasm, malignant
        unspecified site (female) C50.91- ☑
          male C50.92- ☑
      intraductal
        breast D05.8- ☑
        specified site NEC — *see* Neoplasm, in situ, by site
        unspecified site (female) D05.8- ☑
    breast D05.0- ☑
    specified site NEC — *see* Neoplasm, in situ, by site
    unspecified site D05.0- ☑
  squamous cell (*see also* Neoplasm, in situ, by site)
    with questionable stromal invasion
      cervix D06.9
      specified site NEC — *see* Neoplasm, in situ, by site
      unspecified site D06.9
**Carcinomaphobia** F45.29
**Carcinomatosis** C80.0
  peritonei C78.6

⚐ Subterms under main terms may continue to next column or page    ☑ Additional Character Required — Refer to the Tabular List for Character Selection    49

Carcinoma — Carcinomatosis

**Carcinomatosis** — *continued*
    unspecified site (primary) (secondary) C80.0
**Carcinosarcoma** — *see* Neoplasm, malignant, by site
    embryonal — *see* Neoplasm, malignant, by site
**Cardia, cardial** — *see* condition
**Cardiac** (*see also* condition)
    death, sudden — *see* Arrest, cardiac
    pacemaker
        in situ Z95.0
        management or adjustment Z45.018
    tamponade I31.4
**Cardialgia** — *see* Pain, precordial
**Cardiectasis** — *see* Hypertrophy, cardiac
**Cardiochalasia** K21.9
**Cardiomalacia** I51.5
**Cardiomegalia glycogenica diffusa** E74.02 [I43]
**Cardiomegaly** (*see also* Hypertrophy, cardiac)
    congenital Q24.8
    glycogen E74.02 [I43]
    idiopathic I51.7
**Cardiomyoliposis** I51.5
**Cardiomyopathy** (familial) (idiopathic) I42.9
    alcoholic I42.6
    amyloid E85.4 [I43]
        transthyretin-related (ATTR) familial E85.4
    arteriosclerotic — *see* Disease, heart, ischemic,
        atherosclerotic
    beriberi E51.12
    cobalt-beer I42.6
    congenital I42.4
    congestive I42.0
    constrictive NOS I42.5
    dilated I42.0
    due to
        alcohol I42.6
        beriberi E51.12
        cardiac glycogenosis E74.02 [I43]
        drugs I42.7
        external agents NEC I42.7
        Friedreich's ataxia G11.11
        myotonia atrophica G71.11 [I43]
        progressive muscular dystrophy G71.0 [I43]
    glycogen storage E74.02 [I43]
    hypertensive — *see* Hypertension, heart
    hypertrophic (nonobstructive) I42.2
        obstructive I42.1
            congenital Q24.8
    in
        Chagas' disease (chronic) B57.2
            acute B57.0
        sarcoidosis D86.85
    ischemic I25.5
    metabolic E88.9 [I43]
        thyrotoxic E05.90 [I43]
            with thyroid storm E05.91 [I43]
    newborn I42.8
        congenital I42.4
    nutritional E63.9 [I43]
        beriberi E51.12
    obscure of Africa I42.8
    peripartum O90.3
    postpartum O90.3
    restrictive NEC I42.5
    rheumatic I09.0
    secondary I42.9
    stress induced I51.81
    takotsubo I51.81
    thyrotoxic E05.90 [I43]
        with thyroid storm E05.91 [I43]
    toxic NEC I42.7
    transthyretin-related (ATTR) familial amyloid E85.4
    tuberculous A18.84
    viral B33.24
**Cardionephritis** — *see* Hypertension, cardiorenal
**Cardionephropathy** — *see* Hypertension, cardiorenal
**Cardionephrosis** — *see* Hypertension, cardiorenal
**Cardiopathia nigra** I27.0
**Cardiopathy** (*see also* Disease, heart) I51.9
    idiopathic I42.9
    mucopolysaccharidosis E76.3 [I52]
**Cardiopericarditis** — *see* Pericarditis
**Cardiophobia** F45.29
**Cardiorenal** — *see* condition
**Cardiorrhexis** — *see* Infarct, myocardium
**Cardiosclerosis** — *see* Disease, heart, ischemic,
    atherosclerotic
**Cardiosis** — *see* Disease, heart
**Cardiospasm** (esophagus) (reflex) (stomach) K22.0

**Cardiospasm** — *continued*
    congenital Q39.5
        with megaesophagus Q39.5
**Cardiostenosis** — *see* Disease, heart
**Cardiosymphysis** I31.0
**Cardiovascular** — *see* condition
**Carditis** (acute) (bacterial) (chronic) (subacute) I51.89
    meningococcal A39.50
    rheumatic — *see* Disease, heart, rheumatic
    rheumatoid — *see* Rheumatoid, carditis
    viral B33.20
**Care** (of) (for) (following)
    child (routine) Z76.2
    family member (handicapped) (sick)
        creating problem for family Z63.6
        provided away from home for holiday relief Z75.5
        unavailable, due to
            absence (person rendering care) (sufferer) Z74.2
            inability (any reason) of person rendering care
                Z74.2
    foundling Z76.1
    holiday relief Z75.5
    improper — *see* Maltreatment
    lack of (at or after birth) (infant) — *see* Maltreatment,
        child, neglect
    lactating mother Z39.1
    palliative Z51.5
    postpartum
        immediately after delivery Z39.0
        routine follow-up Z39.2
    respite Z75.5
    unavailable, due to
        absence of person rendering care Z74.2
        inability (any reason) of person rendering care
            Z74.2
    well-baby Z76.2
**Caries**
    bone NEC A18.03
    dental (dentino enamel junction) (early childhood) (of
        dentine) (pre-eruptive) (recurrent) (to the pulp)
        K02.9
        arrested (coronal) (root) K02.3
        chewing surface
            limited to enamel K02.51
            penetrating into dentin K02.52
            penetrating into pulp K02.53
        coronal surface
            chewing surface
                limited to enamel K02.51
                penetrating into dentin K02.52
                penetrating into pulp K02.53
            pit and fissure surface
                limited to enamel K02.51
                penetrating into dentin K02.52
                penetrating into pulp K02.53
            smooth surface
                limited to enamel K02.61
                penetrating into dentin K02.62
                penetrating into pulp K02.63
        pit and fissure surface
            limited to enamel K02.51
            penetrating into dentin K02.52
            penetrating into pulp K02.53
        primary, cervical origin K02.52
        root K02.7
        smooth surface
            limited to enamel K02.61
            penetrating into dentin K02.62
            penetrating into pulp K02.63
    external meatus — *see* Disorder, ear, external, speci-
        fied type NEC
    hip (tuberculous) A18.02
    initial (tooth)
        chewing surface K02.51
        pit and fissure surface K02.51
        smooth surface K02.61
    knee (tuberculous) A18.02
    labyrinth H83.8 ☑
    limb NEC (tuberculous) A18.03
    mastoid process (chronic) — *see* Mastoiditis, chronic
        tuberculous A18.03
    middle ear H74.8 ☑
    nose (tuberculous) A18.03
    orbit (tuberculous) A18.03
    ossicles, ear — *see* Abnormal, ear ossicles
    petrous bone — *see* Petrositis
    root (dental) (tooth) K02.7
    sacrum (tuberculous) A18.01

**Caries** — *continued*
    spine, spinal (column) (tuberculous) A18.01
    syphilitic A52.77
        congenital (early) A50.02 [M90.80]
    tooth, teeth — *see* Caries, dental
    tuberculous A18.03
    vertebra (column) (tuberculous) A18.01
**Carious teeth** — *see* Caries, dental
**Carneous mole** O02.0
**Carnitine insufficiency** E71.40
**Carotid body or sinus syndrome** G90.01
**Carotidynia** G90.01
**Carotinemia** (dietary) E67.1
**Carotinosis** (cutis) (skin) E67.1
**Carpal tunnel syndrome** — *see* Syndrome, carpal tunnel
**Carpenter's syndrome** Q87.0
**Carpopedal spasm** — *see* Tetany
**Carr-Barr-Plunkett syndrome** Q97.1
**Carrier** (suspected) of
    amebiasis Z22.1
    bacterial disease NEC Z22.39
        diphtheria Z22.2
        intestinal infectious NEC Z22.1
            typhoid Z22.0
        meningococcal Z22.31
        sexually transmitted Z22.4
        specified NEC Z22.39
        staphylococcal (Methicillin susceptible) Z22.321
            Methicillin resistant Z22.322
        streptococcal Z22.338
            group B Z22.330
                complicating pregnancy or delivery
                    O99.82- ☑
        typhoid Z22.0
    cholera Z22.1
    diphtheria Z22.2
    gastrointestinal pathogens NEC Z22.1
    genetic Z14.8
        cystic fibrosis Z14.1
        hemophilia A (asymptomatic) Z14.01
            symptomatic Z14.02
    gestational, pregnant Z33.1
    gonorrhea Z22.4
    HAA (hepatitis Australian-antigen) B18.8
    HB (c)(s)-AG B18.1
    hepatitis (viral) B18.9
        Australia-antigen (HAA) B18.8
        B surface antigen (HBsAg) B18.1
            with acute delta- (super)infection B17.0
            C B18.2
        specified NEC B18.8
    human T-cell lymphotropic virus type-1 (HTLV-1) infec-
        tion Z22.6
    infectious organism Z22.9
        specified NEC Z22.8
    meningococci Z22.31
    Salmonella typhosa Z22.0
    serum hepatitis — *see* Carrier, hepatitis
    staphylococci (Methicillin susceptible) Z22.321
        Methicillin resistant Z22.322
    streptococci Z22.338
        group B Z22.330
            complicating pregnancy or delivery O99.82- ☑
    syphilis Z22.4
    typhoid Z22.0
    venereal disease NEC Z22.4
**Carrion's disease** A44.0
**Carter's relapsing fever** (Asiatic) A68.1
**Cartilage** — *see* condition
**Caruncle** (inflamed)
    conjunctiva (acute) — *see* Conjunctivitis, acute
    labium (majus) (minus) N90.89
    lacrimal — *see* Inflammation, lacrimal, passages
    myrtiform N89.8
    urethral (benign) N36.2
**Cascade stomach** K31.2
**Caseation lymphatic gland** (tuberculous) A18.2
**Cassidy** (-Scholte) syndrome (malignant carcinoid) E34.0
**Castellani's disease** A69.8
**Castration, traumatic, male** S38.231 ☑
**Casts in urine** R82.99
**Cat**
    cry syndrome Q93.4
    ear Q17.3
    eye syndrome Q92.8
**Catabolism, senile** R54
**Catalepsy** (hysterical) F44.2
    schizophrenic F20.2

☑ **Additional Character Required** — Refer to the Tabular List for Character Selection        ▽ **Subterms under main terms may continue to next column or page**

**Cataplexy** (idiopathic) — *see* Narcolepsy
**Cataract** (cortical) (immature) (incipient) H26.9
    with
        neovascularization — *see* Cataract, complicated
    age-related — *see* Cataract, senile
    anterior
        and posterior axial embryonal Q12.0
        pyramidal Q12.0
    associated with
        galactosemia E74.21 [H28]
        myotonic disorders G71.19 [H28]
    blue Q12.0
    central Q12.0
    cerulean Q12.0
    complicated H26.20
        with
            neovascularization H26.21- ☑
            ocular disorder H26.22- ☑
        glaucomatous flecks H26.23- ☑
    congenital Q12.0
    coraliform Q12.0
    coronary Q12.0
    crystalline Q12.0
    diabetic — *see* Diabetes, cataract
    drug-induced H26.3- ☑
    due to
        ocular disorder — *see* Cataract, complicated
        radiation H26.8
    electric H26.8
    extraction status Z98.4- ☑
    glass-blower's H26.8
    heat ray H26.8
    heterochromic — *see* Cataract, complicated
    hypermature — *see* Cataract, senile, morgagnian type
    in (due to)
        chronic iridocyclitis — *see* Cataract, complicated
        diabetes — *see* Diabetes, cataract
        endocrine disease E34.9 [H28]
        eye disease — *see* Cataract, complicated
        hypoparathyroidism E20.9 [H28]
        malnutrition-dehydration E46 [H28]
        metabolic disease E88.9 [H28]
        myotonic disorders G71.19 [H28]
        nutritional disease E63.9 [H28]
    infantile — *see* Cataract, presenile
    irradiational — *see* Cataract, specified NEC
    juvenile — *see* Cataract, presenile
    malnutrition-dehydration E46 [H28]
    morgagnian — *see* Cataract, senile, morgagnian type
    myotonic G71.19 [H28]
    myxedema E03.9 [H28]
    nuclear
        embryonal Q12.0
        sclerosis — *see* Cataract, senile, nuclear
    presenile H26.00- ☑
        combined forms H26.06- ☑
        cortical H26.01- ☑
        lamellar — *see* Cataract, presenile, cortical
        nuclear H26.03- ☑
        specified NEC H26.09
        subcapsular polar (anterior) H26.04- ☑
            posterior H26.05- ☑
        zonular — *see* Cataract, presenile, cortical
    secondary H26.40
        Soemmering's ring H26.41- ☑
        specified NEC H26.49- ☑
        to eye disease — *see* Cataract, complicated
    senile H25.9
        brunescens — *see* Cataract, senile, nuclear
        combined forms H25.81- ☑
        coronary — *see* Cataract, senile, incipient
        cortical H25.01- ☑
        hypermature — *see* Cataract, senile, morgagnian type
        incipient (mature) (total) H25.09- ☑
            cortical — *see* Cataract, senile, cortical
            subcapsular — *see* Cataract, senile, subcapsular
        morgagnian type (hypermature) H25.2- ☑
        nuclear (sclerosis) H25.1- ☑
        polar subcapsular (anterior) (posterior) — *see* Cataract, senile, incipient
        punctate — *see* Cataract, senile, incipient
        specified NEC H25.89
        subcapsular polar (anterior) H25.03- ☑
            posterior H25.04- ☑
    snowflake — *see* Diabetes, cataract
    specified NEC H26.8

**Cataract** — *continued*
    toxic — *see* Cataract, drug-induced
    traumatic H26.10- ☑
        localized H26.11- ☑
        partially resolved H26.12- ☑
        total H26.13- ☑
    zonular (perinuclear) Q12.0
**Cataracta** (*see also* Cataract)
    brunescens — *see* Cataract, senile, nuclear
    centralis pulverulenta Q12.0
    cerulea Q12.0
    complicata — *see* Cataract, complicated
    congenita Q12.0
    coralliformis Q12.0
    coronaria Q12.0
    diabetic — *see* Diabetes, cataract
    membranacea
        accreta — *see* Cataract, secondary
        congenita Q12.0
    nigra — *see* Cataract, senile, nuclear
    sunflower — *see* Cataract, complicated
**Catarrh, catarrhal** (acute) (febrile) (infectious) (inflammation) (*see also* condition) J00
    bronchial — *see* Bronchitis
    chest — *see* Bronchitis
    chronic J31.0
    due to congenital syphilis A50.03
    enteric — *see* Enteritis
    eustachian H68.009
    fauces — *see* Pharyngitis
    gastrointestinal — *see* Enteritis
    gingivitis K05.00
        nonplaque induced K05.01
        plaque induced K05.00
    hay — *see* Fever, hay
    intestinal — *see* Enteritis
    larynx, chronic J37.0
    liver B15.9
        with hepatic coma B15.0
    lung — *see* Bronchitis
    middle ear, chronic — *see* Otitis, media, nonsuppurative, chronic, serous
    mouth K12.1
    nasal (chronic) — *see* Rhinitis
    nasobronchial J31.1
    nasopharyngeal (chronic) J31.1
        acute J00
    pulmonary — *see* Bronchitis
    spring (eye) (vernal) — *see* Conjunctivitis, acute, atopic
    summer (hay) — *see* Fever, hay
    throat J31.2
    tubotympanal (*see also* Otitis, media, nonsuppurative)
        chronic — *see* Otitis, media, nonsuppurative, chronic, serous
**Catatonia** (schizophrenic) F20.2
**Catatonic**
    disorder due to known physiologic condition F06.1
    schizophrenia F20.2
    stupor R40.1
**Cat-scratch** (*see also* Abrasion)
    disease or fever A28.1
**Cauda equina** — *see* condition
**Cauliflower ear** M95.1- ☑
**Causalgia** (upper limb) G56.4- ☑
    lower limb G57.7- ☑
**Cause**
    external, general effects T75.89 ☑
**Caustic burn** — *see* Corrosion, by site
**Cavare's disease** (familial periodic paralysis) G72.3
**Cave-in, injury**
    crushing (severe) — *see* Crush
    suffocation — *see* Asphyxia, traumatic, due to low oxygen, due to cave-in
**Cavernitis** (penis) N48.29
**Cavernositis** N48.29
**Cavernous** — *see* condition
**Cavitation of lung** (*see also* Tuberculosis, pulmonary)
    nontuberculous J98.4
**Cavities, dental** — *see* Caries, dental
**Cavity**
    lung — *see* Cavitation of lung
    optic papilla Q14.2
    pulmonary — *see* Cavitation of lung
**Cavovarus foot, congenital** Q66.1
**Cavus foot** (congenital) Q66.7
    acquired — *see* Deformity, limb, foot, specified NEC
**Cazenave's disease** L10.2

**Cecitis** K52.9
    with perforation, peritonitis, or rupture K65.8
**Cecum** — *see* condition
**Celiac**
    artery compression syndrome I77.4
    disease (with steatorrhea) K90.0
    infantilism K90.0
**Cell**(s), **cellular** (*see also* condition)
    in urine R82.99
**Cellulitis** (diffuse) (phlegmonous) (septic) (suppurative) L03.90
    abdominal wall L03.311
    anaerobic A48.0
    ankle — *see* Cellulitis, lower limb
    anus K61.0
    arm — *see* Cellulitis, upper limb
    auricle (ear) — *see* Cellulitis, ear
    axilla L03.11- ☑
    back (any part) L03.312
    breast (acute) (nonpuerperal) (subacute) N61.0
        nipple N61.0
    broad ligament
        acute N73.0
    buttock L03.317
    cervical (meaning neck) L03.221
    cervix (uteri) — *see* Cervicitis
    cheek (external) L03.211
        internal K12.2
    chest wall L03.313
    chronic L03.90
    clostridial A48.0
    corpus cavernosum N48.22
    digit
        finger — *see* Cellulitis, finger
        toe — *see* Cellulitis, toe
    Douglas' cul-de-sac or pouch
        acute N73.0
    drainage site (following operation) T81.4 ☑
    ear (external) H60.1- ☑
    eosinophilic (granulomatous) L98.3
    erysipelatous — *see* Erysipelas
    external auditory canal — *see* Cellulitis, ear
    eyelid — *see* Abscess, eyelid
    face NEC L03.211
    finger (intrathecal) (periosteal) (subcutaneous) (subcuticular) L03.01- ☑
    foot — *see* Cellulitis, lower limb
    gangrenous — *see* Gangrene
    genital organ NEC
        female (external) N76.4
        male N49.9
            multiple sites N49.8
            specified NEC N49.8
    gluteal (region) L03.317
    gonococcal A54.89
    groin L03.314
    hand — *see* Cellulitis, upper limb
    head NEC L03.811
        face (any part, except ear, eye and nose) L03.211
    heel — *see* Cellulitis, lower limb
    hip — *see* Cellulitis, lower limb
    jaw (region) L03.211
    knee — *see* Cellulitis, lower limb
    labium (majus) (minus) — *see* Vulvitis
    lacrimal passages — *see* Inflammation, lacrimal, passages
    larynx J38.7
    leg — *see* Cellulitis, lower limb
    lip K13.0
    lower limb L03.11- ☑
        toe — *see* Cellulitis, toe
    mouth (floor) K12.2
    multiple sites, so stated L03.90
    nasopharynx J39.1
    navel L03.316
        newborn P38.9
            with mild hemorrhage P38.1
            without hemorrhage P38.9
    neck (region) L03.221
    nipple (acute) (nonpuerperal) (subacute) N61.0
    nose (septum) (external) J34.0
    orbit, orbital H05.01- ☑
    palate (soft) K12.2
    pectoral (region) L03.313
    pelvis, pelvic (chronic)
        female (*see also* Disease, pelvis, inflammatory) N73.2
            acute N73.0

⬇ Subterms under main terms may continue to next column or page      ☑ Additional Character Required — Refer to the Tabular List for Character Selection      51

Cataplexy — Cellulitis

**Cellulitis** — continued
  pelvis, pelvic — continued
    following ectopic or molar pregnancy O08.0
      male K65.0
  penis N48.22
  perineal, perineum L03.315
  periorbital L03.213
  perirectal K61.1
  peritonsillar J36
  periurethral N34.0
  periuterine (see also Disease, pelvis, inflammatory) N73.2
    acute N73.0
  pharynx J39.1
  preseptal L03.213
  rectum K61.1
  retroperitoneal K68.9
  round ligament
    acute N73.0
  scalp (any part) L03.811
  scrotum N49.2
  seminal vesicle N49.0
  shoulder — see Cellulitis, upper limb
  specified site NEC L03.818
  submandibular (region) (space) (triangle) K12.2
    gland K11.3
  submaxillary (region) K12.2
    gland K11.3
  thigh — see Cellulitis, lower limb
  thumb (intrathecal) (periosteal) (subcutaneous) (subcuticular) — see Cellulitis, finger
  toe (intrathecal) (periosteal) (subcutaneous) (subcuticular) L03.03- ☑
  tonsil J36
  trunk L03.319
    abdominal wall L03.311
    back (any part) L03.312
    buttock L03.317
    chest wall L03.313
    groin L03.314
    perineal, perineum L03.315
    umbilicus L03.316
  tuberculous (primary) A18.4
  umbilicus L03.316
  upper limb L03.11- ☑
    axilla — see Cellulitis, axilla
    finger — see Cellulitis, finger
    thumb — see Cellulitis, finger
  vaccinal T88.0 ☑
  vocal cord J38.3
  vulva — see Vulvitis
  wrist — see Cellulitis, upper limb
**Cementoblastoma, benign** — see Cyst, calcifying odontogenic
**Cementoma** — see Cyst, calcifying odontogenic
**Cementoperiostitis** — see Periodontitis
**Cementosis** K03.4
**Central auditory processing disorder** H93.25
**Central pain syndrome** G89.0
**Cephalematocele, cephal** (o)hematocele
  newborn P52.8
    birth injury P10.8
  traumatic — see Hematoma, brain
**Cephalematoma, cephalhematoma** (calcified)
  newborn (birth injury) P12.0
  traumatic — see Hematoma, brain
**Cephalgia, cephalalgia** (see also Headache)
  histamine G44.009
    intractable G44.001
    not intractable G44.009
  trigeminal autonomic (TAC) NEC G44.099
    intractable G44.091
    not intractable G44.099
**Cephalic** — see condition
**Cephalitis** — see Encephalitis
**Cephalocele** — see Encephalocele
**Cephalomenia** N94.89
**Cephalopelvic** — see condition
**Cerclage** (with cervical incompetence) in pregnancy — see Incompetence, cervix, in pregnancy
**Cerebellitis** — see Encephalitis
**Cerebellum, cerebellar** — see condition
**Cerebral** — see condition
**Cerebritis** — see Encephalitis
**Cerebro-hepato-renal syndrome** Q87.89
**Cerebromalacia** — see Softening, brain
  sequelae of cerebrovascular disease I69.398
**Cerebroside lipidosis** E75.22

**Cerebrospasticity** (congenital) G80.1
**Cerebrospinal** — see condition
**Cerebrum** — see condition
**Ceroid-lipofuscinosis, neuronal** E75.4
**Cerumen** (accumulation) (impacted) H61.2- ☑
**Cervical** (see also condition)
  auricle Q18.2
  dysplasia in pregnancy — see Abnormal, cervix, in pregnancy or childbirth
  erosion in pregnancy — see Abnormal, cervix, in pregnancy or childbirth
  fibrosis in pregnancy — see Abnormal, cervix, in pregnancy or childbirth
  fusion syndrome Q76.1
  rib Q76.5
  shortening (complicating pregnancy) O26.87- ☑
**Cervicalgia** M54.2
**Cervicitis** (acute) (chronic) (nonvenereal) (senile (atrophic)) (subacute) (with ulceration) N72
  with
    abortion — see Abortion, by type complicated by genital tract and pelvic infection
    ectopic pregnancy O08.0
    molar pregnancy O08.0
  chlamydial A56.09
  gonococcal A54.03
  herpesviral A60.03
  puerperal (postpartum) O86.11
  syphilitic A52.76
  trichomonal A59.09
  tuberculous A18.16
**Cervicocolpitis** (emphysematosa) (see also Cervicitis) N72
**Cervix** — see condition
**Cesarean delivery, previous, affecting management of pregnancy** O34.219
  classical (vertical) scar O34.212
  low transverse scar O34.211
**Céstan** (-Chenais) paralysis or syndrome G46.3
**Céstan-Raymond syndrome** I65.8
**Cestode infestation** B71.9
  specified type NEC B71.8
**Cestodiasis** B71.9
**Chabert's disease** A22.9
**Chacaleh** E53.8
**Chafing** L30.4
**Chagas'** (-Mazza) disease (chronic) B57.2
  with
    cardiovascular involvement NEC B57.2
    digestive system involvement B57.30
      megacolon B57.32
      megaesophagus B57.31
      other specified B57.39
    megacolon B57.32
    megaesophagus B57.31
    myocarditis B57.2
    nervous system involvement B57.40
      meningitis B57.41
      meningoencephalitis B57.42
      other specified B57.49
    specified organ involvement NEC B57.5
  acute (with) B57.1
    cardiovascular NEC B57.0
    myocarditis B57.0
**Chagres fever** B50.9
**Chairridden** Z74.09
**Chalasia** (cardiac sphincter) K21.9
**Chalazion** H00.19
  left H00.16
    lower H00.15
    upper H00.14
  right H00.13
    lower H00.12
    upper H00.11
**Chalcosis** (see also Disorder, globe, degenerative, chalcosis)
  cornea — see Deposit, cornea
  crystalline lens — see Cataract, complicated
  retina H35.89
**Chalicosis** (pulmonum) J62.8
**Chancre** (any genital site) (hard) (hunterian) (mixed) (primary) (seronegative) (seropositive) (syphilitic) A51.0
  congenital A50.07
  conjunctiva NEC A51.2
  Ducrey's A57
  extragenital A51.2
  eyelid A51.2

**Chancre** — continued
  lip A51.2
  nipple A51.2
  Nisbet's A57
  of
    carate A67.0
    pinta A67.0
    yaws A66.0
  palate, soft A51.2
  phagedenic A57
  simple A57
  soft A57
    bubo A57
    palate A51.2
  urethra A51.0
  yaws A66.0
**Chancroid** (anus) (genital) (penis) (perineum) (rectum) (urethra) (vulva) A57
**Chandler's disease** (osteochondritis dissecans, hip) — see Osteochondritis, dissecans, hip
**Change(s)** (in) (of) (see also Removal)
  arteriosclerotic — see Arteriosclerosis
  bone (see also Disorder, bone)
    diabetic — see Diabetes, bone change
  bowel habit R19.4
  cardiorenal (vascular) — see Hypertension, cardiorenal
  cardiovascular — see Disease, cardiovascular
  circulatory I99.9
  cognitive (mild) (organic) R41.89
  color, tooth, teeth
    during formation K00.8
    posteruptive K03.7
  contraceptive device Z30.433
  corneal membrane H18.30
    Bowman's membrane fold or rupture H18.31- ☑
    Descemet's membrane
      fold H18.32- ☑
      rupture H18.33- ☑
  coronary — see Disease, heart, ischemic
  degenerative, spine or vertebra — see Spondylosis
  dental pulp, regressive K04.2
  dressing (nonsurgical) Z48.00
    surgical Z48.01
  heart — see Disease, heart
  hip joint — see Derangement, joint, hip
  hyperplastic larynx J38.7
  hypertrophic
    nasal sinus J34.89
    turbinate, nasal J34.3
    upper respiratory tract J39.8
  indwelling catheter Z46.6
  inflammatory (see also Inflammation)
    sacroiliac M46.1
  job, anxiety concerning Z56.1
  joint — see Derangement, joint
  life — see Menopause
  mental status R41.82
  minimal (glomerular) (see also N00-N07 with fourth character .0) N05.0
  myocardium, myocardial — see Degeneration, myocardial
  of life — see Menopause
  pacemaker Z45.018
    pulse generator Z45.010
  personality (enduring) F68.8
    due to (secondary to)
      general medical condition F07.0
    secondary (nonspecific) F60.89
  regressive, dental pulp K04.2
  renal — see Disease, renal
  retina H35.9
    myopic (see also Myopia, degenerative) H44.2- ☑
  sacroiliac joint M53.3
  senile (see also condition) R54
  sensory R20.8
  skin R23.9
    acute, due to ultraviolet radiation L56.9
      specified NEC L56.8
    chronic, due to nonionizing radiation L57.9
      specified NEC L57.8
    cyanosis R23.0
    flushing R23.2
    pallor R23.1
    petechiae R23.3
    specified change NEC R23.8
    swelling — see Mass, localized
    texture R23.4

☑ **Additional Character Required — Refer to the Tabular List for Character Selection**      ▽ **Subterms under main terms may continue to next column or page**

**Change(s)** — *continued*
  trophic
    arm — *see* Mononeuropathy, upper limb
    leg — *see* Mononeuropathy, lower limb
  vascular I99.9
  vasomotor I73.9
  voice R49.9
    psychogenic F44.4
    specified NEC R49.8
**Changing sleep-work schedule, affecting sleep**
  G47.26
**Changuinola fever** A93.1
**Chapping skin** T69.8 ☑
**Charcot-Marie-Tooth disease, paralysis or syndrome**
  G60.0
**Charcot's**
  arthropathy — *see* Arthropathy, neuropathic
  cirrhosis K74.3
  disease (tabetic arthropathy) A52.16
  joint (disease) (tabetic) A52.16
    diabetic — *see* Diabetes, with, arthropathy
    syringomyelic G95.0
  syndrome (intermittent claudication) I73.9
**CHARGE association** Q89.8
**Charley-horse** (quadriceps) M62.831
  traumatic (quadriceps) S76.11- ☑
**Charlouis' disease** — *see* Yaws
**Cheadle's disease** E54
**Checking** (of)
  cardiac pacemaker (battery) (electrode(s)) Z45.018
    pulse generator Z45.010
  implantable subdermal contraceptive Z30.46
  intrauterine contraceptive device Z30.431
  wound Z48.0- ☑
    due to injury — code to Injury, by site, using appropriate seventh character for subsequent encounter
**Check-up** — *see* Examination
**Chédiak-Higashi** (-Steinbrinck) **syndrome** (congenital gigantism of peroxidase granules) E70.330
**Cheek** — *see* condition
**Cheese itch** B88.0
**Cheese-washer's lung** J67.8
**Cheese-worker's lung** J67.8
**Cheilitis** (acute) (angular) (catarrhal) (chronic) (exfoliative) (gangrenous) (glandular) (infectional) (suppurative) (ulcerative) (vesicular) K13.0
  actinic (due to sun) L56.8
    other than from sun L59.8
  candidal B37.83
**Cheilodynia** K13.0
**Cheiloschisis** — *see* Cleft, lip
**Cheilosis** (angular) K13.0
  with pellagra E52
  due to
    vitamin B2 (riboflavin) deficiency E53.0
**Cheiromegaly** M79.89
**Cheiropompholyx** L30.1
**Cheloid** — *see* Keloid
**Chemical burn** — *see* Corrosion, by site
**Chemodectoma** — *see* Paraganglioma, nonchromaffin
**Chemosis, conjunctiva** — *see* Edema, conjunctiva
**Chemotherapy** (session) (for)
  cancer Z51.11
  neoplasm Z51.11
**Cherubism** M27.8
**Chest** — *see* condition
**Cheyne-Stokes breathing** (respiration) R06.3
**Chiari's**
  disease or syndrome (hepatic vein thrombosis) I82.0
  malformation
    type I G93.5
    type II — *see* Spina bifida
    net Q24.8
**Chicago disease** B40.9
**Chickenpox** — *see* Varicella
**Chiclero ulcer or sore** B55.1
**Chigger** (infestation) B88.0
**Chignon** (disease) B36.8
  newborn (from vacuum extraction) (birth injury) P12.1
**Chilaiditi's syndrome** (subphrenic displacement, colon)
  Q43.3
**Chilblain**(s) (lupus) T69.1 ☑
**Child**
  custody dispute Z65.3
**Childbirth** — *see* Delivery

**Childhood**
  cerebral X-linked adrenoleukodystrophy E71.520
  period of rapid growth Z00.2
**Chill**(s) R68.83
  with fever R50.9
  without fever R68.83
  congestive in malarial regions B54
**Chilomastigiasis** A07.8
**Chimera 46,XX/46,XY** Q99.0
**Chin** — *see* condition
**Chinese dysentery** A03.9
**Chionophobia** F40.228
**Chitral fever** A93.1
**Chlamydia, chlamydial** A74.9
  cervicitis A56.09
  conjunctivitis A74.0
  cystitis A56.01
  endometritis A56.11
  epididymitis A56.19
  female
    pelvic inflammatory disease A56.11
    pelviperitonitis A56.11
  orchitis A56.19
  peritonitis A74.81
  pharyngitis A56.4
  proctitis A56.3
  psittaci (infection) A70
  salpingitis A56.11
  sexually-transmitted infection NEC A56.8
  specified NEC A74.89
  urethritis A56.01
  vulvovaginitis A56.02
**Chlamydiosis** — *see* Chlamydia
**Chloasma** (skin) (idiopathic) (symptomatic) L81.1
  eyelid H02.719
    hyperthyroid E05.90 [H02.719]
      with thyroid storm E05.91 [H02.719]
    left H02.716
      lower H02.715
      upper H02.714
    right H02.713
      lower H02.712
      upper H02.711
**Chloroma** C92.3- ☑
**Chlorosis** D50.9
  Egyptian B76.9 [D63.8]
  miner's B76.9 [D63.8]
**Chlorotic anemia** D50.8
**Chocolate cyst** (ovary) N80.1
**Choked**
  disc or disk — *see* Papilledema
  on food, phlegm, or vomitus NOS — *see* Foreign body, by site
  while vomiting NOS — *see* Foreign body, by site
**Chokes** (resulting from bends) T70.3 ☑
**Choking sensation** R09.89
**Cholangiectasis** K83.8
**Cholangiocarcinoma**
  with hepatocellular carcinoma, combined C22.0
  liver C22.1
  specified site NEC — *see* Neoplasm, malignant, by site
  unspecified site C22.1
**Cholangiohepatitis** K83.8
  due to fluke infestation B66.1
**Cholangiohepatoma** C22.0
**Cholangiolitis** (acute) (chronic) (extrahepatic) (gangrenous) (intrahepatic) K83.0
  paratyphoidal — *see* Fever, paratyphoid
  typhoidal A01.09
**Cholangioma** D13.4
  malignant — *see* Cholangiocarcinoma
**Cholangitis** (ascending) (primary) (recurrent) (sclerosing) (secondary) (stenosing) (suppurative) K83.0
  with calculus, bile duct — *see* Calculus, bile duct, with cholangitis
  chronic nonsuppurative destructive K74.3
**Cholecystectasia** K82.8
**Cholecystitis** K81.9
  with
    calculus, stones in
      bile duct (common) (hepatic) — *see* Calculus, bile duct, with cholecystitis
      cystic duct — *see* Calculus, gallbladder, with cholecystitis
      gallbladder — *see* Calculus, gallbladder, with cholecystitis
      choledocholithiasis — *see* Calculus, bile duct, with cholecystitis

**Cholecystitis** — *continued*
  with — *continued*
    cholelithiasis — *see* Calculus, gallbladder, with cholecystitis
  acute (emphysematous) (gangrenous) (suppurative) K81.0
    with
      calculus, stones in
        cystic duct — *see* Calculus, gallbladder, with cholecystitis, acute
        gallbladder — *see* Calculus, gallbladder, with cholecystitis, acute
      choledocholithiasis — *see* Calculus, bile duct, with cholecystitis, acute
      cholelithiasis — *see* Calculus, gallbladder, with cholecystitis, acute
    chronic cholecystitis K81.2
      with gallbladder calculus K80.12
        with obstruction K80.13
  chronic K81.1
    with acute cholecystitis K81.2
      with gallbladder calculus K80.12
        with obstruction K80.13
  emphysematous (acute) — *see* Cholecystitis, acute
  gangrenous — *see* Cholecystitis, acute
  paratyphoidal, current A01.4
  suppurative — *see* Cholecystitis, acute
  typhoidal A01.09
**Cholecystolithiasis** — *see* Calculus, gallbladder
**Choledochitis** (suppurative) K83.0
**Choledocholith** — *see* Calculus, bile duct
**Choledocholithiasis** (common duct) (hepatic duct) —
  *see* Calculus, bile duct
  cystic — *see* Calculus, gallbladder
  typhoidal A01.09
**Cholelithiasis** (cystic duct) (gallbladder) (impacted) (multiple) — *see* Calculus, gallbladder
  bile duct (common) (hepatic) — *see* Calculus, bile duct
  hepatic duct — *see* Calculus, bile duct
  specified NEC K80.80
    with obstruction K80.81
**Cholemia** (*see also* Jaundice)
  familial (simple) (congenital) E80.4
  Gilbert's E80.4
**Choleperitoneum, choleperitonitis** K65.3
**Cholera** (Asiatic) (epidemic) (malignant) A00.9
  antimonial — *see* Poisoning, antimony
  classical A00.0
  due to Vibrio cholerae 01 A00.9
    biovar cholerae A00.0
    biovar eltor A00.1
    el tor A00.1
  el tor A00.1
**Cholerine** — *see* Cholera
**Cholestasis NEC** K83.1
  with hepatocyte injury K71.0
  due to total parenteral nutrition (TPN) K76.89
  pure K71.0
**Cholesteatoma** (ear) (middle) (with reaction) H71.9- ☑
  attic H71.0- ☑
  external ear (canal) H60.4- ☑
  mastoid H71.2- ☑
  postmastoidectomy cavity (recurrent) — *see* Complications, postmastoidectomy, recurrent cholesteatoma
  recurrent (postmastoidectomy) — *see* Complications, postmastoidectomy, recurrent cholesteatoma
  tympanum H71.1- ☑
**Cholesteatosis, diffuse** H71.3- ☑
**Cholesteremia** E78.00
**Cholesterin in vitreous** — *see* Deposit, crystalline
**Cholesterol**
  deposit
    retina H35.89
    vitreous — *see* Deposit, crystalline
  elevated (high) E78.00
    with elevated (high) triglycerides E78.2
    screening for Z13.220
  imbibition of gallbladder K82.4
**Cholesterolemia** (essential) (pure) E78.00
  familial E78.01
  hereditary E78.01
**Cholesterolosis, cholesterosis** (gallbladder) K82.4
  cerebrotendinous E75.5
**Cholocolic fistula** K82.3
**Choluria** R82.2
**Chondritis** M94.8X9

---

**Chondritis** — *continued*
  aurical H61.03- ☑
  costal (Tietze's) M94.0
  external ear H61.03- ☑
  patella, posttraumatic — *see* Chondromalacia, patella
  pinna H61.03- ☑
  purulent M94.8X- ☑
  tuberculous NEC A18.02
    intervertebral A18.01
**Chondroblastoma** (*see also* Neoplasm, bone, benign)
  malignant — *see* Neoplasm, bone, malignant
**Chondrocalcinosis** M11.20
  ankle M11.27- ☑
  elbow M11.22- ☑
  familial M11.10
    ankle M11.17- ☑
    elbow M11.12- ☑
    foot joint M11.17- ☑
    hand joint M11.14- ☑
    hip M11.15- ☑
    knee M11.16- ☑
    multiple site M11.19
    shoulder M11.11- ☑
    vertebrae M11.18
    wrist M11.13- ☑
  foot joint M11.27- ☑
  hand joint M11.24- ☑
  hip M11.25- ☑
  knee M11.26- ☑
  multiple site M11.29
  shoulder M11.21- ☑
  specified type NEC M11.20
    ankle M11.27- ☑
    elbow M11.22- ☑
    foot joint M11.27- ☑
    hand joint M11.24- ☑
    hip M11.25- ☑
    knee M11.26- ☑
    multiple site M11.29
    shoulder M11.21- ☑
    vertebrae M11.28
    wrist M11.23- ☑
  vertebrae M11.28
  wrist M11.23- ☑
**Chondrodermatitis nodularis helicis or anthelicis**
  — *see* Perichondritis, ear
**Chondrodysplasia** Q78.9
  with hemangioma Q78.4
  calcificans congenita Q77.3
  fetalis Q77.4
  metaphyseal (Jansen's) (McKusick's) (Schmid's) Q78.8
  punctata Q77.3
**Chondrodystrophy, chondrodystrophia** (familial)
  (fetalis) (hypoplastic) Q78.9
  calcificans congenita Q77.3
  myotonic (congenital) G71.13
  punctata Q77.3
**Chondroectodermal dysplasia** Q77.6
**Chondrogenesis imperfecta** Q77.4
**Chondrolysis** M94.35- ☑
**Chondroma** (*see also* Neoplasm, cartilage, benign)
  juxtacortical — *see* Neoplasm, bone, benign
  periosteal — *see* Neoplasm, bone, benign
**Chondromalacia** (systemic) M94.20
  acromioclavicular joint M94.21- ☑
  ankle M94.27- ☑
  elbow M94.22- ☑
  foot joint M94.27- ☑
  glenohumeral joint M94.21- ☑
  hand joint M94.24- ☑
  hip M94.25- ☑
  knee M94.26- ☑
    patella M22.4- ☑
  multiple sites M94.29
  patella M22.4- ☑
  rib M94.28
  sacroiliac joint M94.259
  shoulder M94.21- ☑
  sternoclavicular joint M94.21- ☑
  vertebral joint M94.28
  wrist M94.23- ☑
**Chondromatosis** (*see also* Neoplasm, cartilage, uncertain
  behavior)
  internal Q78.4
**Chondromyxosarcoma** — *see* Neoplasm, cartilage,
  malignant

**Chondro-osteodysplasia** (Morquio-Brailsford type)
  E76.219
**Chondro-osteodystrophy** E76.29
**Chondro-osteoma** — *see* Neoplasm, bone, benign
**Chondropathia tuberosa** M94.0
**Chondrosarcoma** — *see* Neoplasm, cartilage, malignant
  juxtacortical — *see* Neoplasm, bone, malignant
  mesenchymal — *see* Neoplasm, connective tissue,
    malignant
  myxoid — *see* Neoplasm, cartilage, malignant
**Chordee** (nonvenereal) N48.89
  congenital Q54.4
  gonococcal A54.09
**Chorditis** (fibrinous) (nodosa) (tuberosa) J38.2
**Chordoma** — *see* Neoplasm, vertebral (column), malignant
**Chorea** (chronic) (gravis) (posthemiplegic) (senile)
  (spasmodic) G25.5
  with
    heart involvement I02.0
      active or acute (conditions in I01-) I02.0
      rheumatic I02.9
        with valvular disorder I02.0
      rheumatic heart disease (chronic) (inactive)(quies-
        cent) — *code to* rheumatic heart condition
        involved
  drug-induced G25.4
  habit F95.8
  hereditary G10
  Huntington's G10
  hysterical F44.4
  minor I02.9
    with heart involvement I02.0
  progressive G25.5
    hereditary G10
  rheumatic (chronic) I02.9
    with heart involvement I02.0
  Sydenham's I02.9
    with heart involvement — *see* Chorea, with
      rheumatic heart disease
    nonrheumatic G25.5
**Choreoathetosis** (paroxysmal) G25.5
**Chorioadenoma** (destruens) D39.2
**Chorioamnionitis** O41.12- ☑
**Chorioangioma** D26.7
**Choriocarcinoma** — *see* Neoplasm, malignant, by site
  combined with
    embryonal carcinoma — *see* Neoplasm, malignant,
      by site
    other germ cell elements — *see* Neoplasm, malig-
      nant, by site
    teratoma — *see* Neoplasm, malignant, by site
  specified site — *see* Neoplasm, malignant, by site
  unspecified site
    female C58
    male C62.90
**Chorioencephalitis** (acute) (lymphocytic) (serous) A87.2
**Chorioepithelioma** — *see* Choriocarcinoma
**Choriomeningitis** (acute) (lymphocytic) (serous) A87.2
**Chorionepithelioma** — *see* Choriocarcinoma
**Chorioretinitis** (*see also* Inflammation, chorioretinal)
  disseminated (*see also* Inflammation, chorioretinal,
    disseminated)
    in neurosyphilis A52.19
  Egyptian B76.9 [D63.8]
  focal (*see also* Inflammation, chorioretinal, focal)
  histoplasmic B39.9 [H32]
  in (due to)
    histoplasmosis B39.9 [H32]
    syphilis (secondary) A51.43
      late A52.71
    toxoplasmosis (acquired) B58.01
      congenital (active) P37.1 [H32]
    tuberculosis A18.53
  juxtapapillary, juxtapapillaris — *see* Inflammation,
    chorioretinal, focal, juxtapapillary
  leprous A30.9 [H32]
  miner's B76.9 [D63.8]
  progressive myopia (degeneration) (*see also* Myopia,
    degenerative) H44.2- ☑
  syphilitic (secondary) A51.43
    congenital (early) A50.01 [H32]
      late A50.32
    late A52.71
  tuberculous A18.53
**Chorioretinopathy, central serous** H35.71- ☑
**Choroid** — *see* condition
**Choroideremia** H31.21

**Choroiditis** — *see* Chorioretinitis
**Choroidopathy** — *see* Disorder, choroid
**Choroidoretinitis** — *see* Chorioretinitis
**Choroidoretinopathy, central serous** — *see* Chori-
  oretinopathy, central serous
**Christian-Weber disease** M35.6
**Christmas disease** D67
**Chromaffinoma** (*see also* Neoplasm, benign, by site)
  malignant — *see* Neoplasm, malignant, by site
**Chromatopsia** — *see* Deficiency, color vision
**Chromhidrosis, chromidrosis** L75.1
**Chromoblastomycosis** — *see* Chromomycosis
**Chromoconversion** R82.91
**Chromomycosis** B43.9
  brain abscess B43.1
  cerebral B43.1
  cutaneous B43.0
  skin B43.0
  specified NEC B43.8
  subcutaneous abscess or cyst B43.2
**Chromophytosis** B36.0
**Chromosome** — *see* Anomaly, by chromosome involved
  D (1) — *see* Anomaly, chromosome 13
  E (3) — *see* Anomaly, chromosome 18
  G — *see* Anomaly, chromosome 21
**Chromotrichomycosis** B36.8
**Chronic** — *see* condition
  fracture — *see* Fracture, pathological
**Churg-Strauss syndrome** M30.1
**Chyle cyst, mesentery** I89.8
**Chylocele** (nonfilarial) I89.8
  filarial (*see also* Infestation, filarial) B74.9 [N51]
  tunica vaginalis N50.89
    filarial (*see also* Infestation, filarial) B74.9 [N51]
**Chylomicronemia** (fasting) (with hyperprebetalipopro-
  teinemia) E78.3
**Chylopericardium** I31.3
  acute I30.9
**Chylothorax** (nonfilarial) I89.8
  filarial (*see also* Infestation, filarial) B74.9 [J91.8]
**Chylous** — *see* condition
**Chyluria** (nonfilarial) R82.0
  due to
    bilharziasis B65.0
    Brugia (malayi) B74.1
      timori B74.2
    schistosomiasis (bilharziasis) B65.0
    Wuchereria (bancrofti) B74.0
  filarial — *see* Infestation, filarial
**Cicatricial** (deformity) — *see* Cicatrix
**Cicatrix** (adherent) (contracted) (painful) (vicious) (*see
  also* Scar) L90.5
  adenoid (and tonsil) J35.8
  alveolar process M26.79
  anus K62.89
  auricle — *see* Disorder, pinna, specified type NEC
  bile duct (common) (hepatic) K83.8
  bladder N32.89
  bone — *see* Disorder, bone, specified type NEC
  brain G93.89
  cervix (postoperative) (postpartal) N88.1
  common duct K83.8
  cornea H17.9
    tuberculous A18.59
  duodenum (bulb), obstructive K31.5
  esophagus K22.2
  eyelid — *see* Disorder, eyelid function
  hypopharynx J39.2
  lacrimal passages — *see* Obstruction, lacrimal
  larynx J38.7
  lung J98.4
  middle ear H74.8 ☑
  mouth K13.79
  muscle M62.89
    with contracture — *see* Contraction, muscle NEC
  nasopharynx J39.2
  palate (soft) K13.79
  penis N48.89
  pharynx J39.2
  prostate N42.89
  rectum K62.89
  retina — *see* Scar, chorioretinal
  semilunar cartilage — *see* Derangement, meniscus
  seminal vesicle N50.89
  skin L90.5
    infected L08.89
    postinfective L90.5

☑ **Additional Character Required** — Refer to the Tabular List for Character Selection    ▽ Subterms under main terms may continue to next column or page

**Cicatrix** — *continued*
  skin — *continued*
    tuberculous B90.8
    specified site NEC L90.5
  throat J39.2
  tongue K14.8
  tonsil (and adenoid) J35.8
  trachea J39.8
  tuberculous NEC B90.9
  urethra N36.8
  uterus N85.8
  vagina N89.8
    postoperative N99.2
  vocal cord J38.3
  wrist, constricting (annular) L90.5
**CIDP** (chronic inflammatory demyelinating polyneuropathy ) G61.81
**CIN** — *see* Neoplasia, intraepithelial, cervix
**CINCA** (chronic infantile neurological, cutaneous and articular syndrome) M04.2
**Cinchonism** — *see* Deafness, ototoxic
  correct substance properly administered — *see* Table of Drugs and Chemicals, by drug, adverse effect
  overdose or wrong substance given or taken — *see* Table of Drugs and Chemicals, by drug, poisoning
**Circle of Willis** — *see* condition
**Circular** — *see* condition
**Circulating anticoagulants** (*see also* Disorder, hemorrhagic) D68.318
  due to drugs (*see also* Disorder, hemorrhagic) D68.32
  following childbirth O72.3
**Circulation**
  collateral, any site I99.8
  defective (lower extremity) I99.9
    congenital Q28.9
  embryonic Q28.9
  failure (peripheral) R57.9
    newborn P29.89
  fetal, persistent P29.38
  heart, incomplete Q28.9
**Circulatory system** — *see* condition
**Circulus senilis** (cornea) — *see* Degeneration, cornea, senile
**Circumcision** (in absence of medical indication) (ritual) (routine) Z41.2
**Circumscribed** — *see* condition
**Circumvallate placenta** O43.11- ☑
**Cirrhosis, cirrhotic** (hepatic) (liver) K74.60
  alcoholic K70.30
    with ascites K70.31
  atrophic — *see* Cirrhosis, liver
  Baumgarten-Cruveilhier K74.69
  biliary (cholangiolitic) (cholangitic) (hypertrophic) (obstructive) (pericholangiolitic) K74.5
    due to
      Clonorchiasis B66.1
      flukes B66.3
    primary K74.3
    secondary K74.4
  cardiac (of liver) K76.1
  Charcot's K74.3
  cholangiolitic, cholangitic, cholostatic (primary) K74.3
  congestive K76.1
  Cruveilhier-Baumgarten K74.69
  cryptogenic (liver) K74.69
  due to
    hepatolenticular degeneration E83.01
    Wilson's disease E83.01
    xanthomatosis E78.2
  fatty K76.0
    alcoholic K70.0
  Hanot's (hypertrophic) K74.3
  hepatic — *see* Cirrhosis, liver
  hypertrophic K74.3
  Indian childhood K74.69
  kidney — *see* Sclerosis, renal
  Laennec's K70.30
    with ascites K70.31
    alcoholic K70.30
      with ascites K70.31
    nonalcoholic K74.69
  liver K74.60
    alcoholic K70.30
      with ascites K70.31
      fatty K70.0
    congenital P78.81
    syphilitic A52.74

**Cirrhosis, cirrhotic** — *continued*
  lung (chronic) J84.10
  macronodular K74.69
    alcoholic K70.30
      with ascites K70.31
  micronodular K74.69
    alcoholic K70.30
      with ascites K70.31
  mixed type K74.69
  monolobular K74.3
  nephritis — *see* Sclerosis, renal
  nutritional K74.69
    alcoholic K70.30
      with ascites K70.31
  obstructive — *see* Cirrhosis, biliary
  ovarian N83.8
  pancreas (duct) K86.89
  pigmentary E83.110
  portal K74.69
    alcoholic K70.30
      with ascites K70.31
  postnecrotic K74.69
    alcoholic K70.30
      with ascites K70.31
  pulmonary J84.10
  renal — *see* Sclerosis, renal
  spleen D73.2
  stasis K76.1
  Todd's K74.3
  unilobar K74.3
  xanthomatous (biliary) K74.5
    due to xanthomatosis (familial) (metabolic) (primary) E78.2
**Cistern, subarachnoid** R93.0
**Citrullinemia** E72.23
**Citrullinuria** E72.23
**Civatte's disease or poikiloderma** L57.3
**Clam digger's itch** B65.3
**Clammy skin** R23.1
**Clap** — *see* Gonorrhea
**Clarke-Hadfield syndrome** (pancreatic infantilism) K86.89
**Clark's paralysis** G80.9
**Clastothrix** L67.8
**Claude Bernard-Horner syndrome** G90.2
  traumatic — *see* Injury, nerve, cervical sympathetic
**Claude's disease or syndrome** G46.3
**Claudicatio venosa intermittens** I87.8
**Claudication** (intermittent) I73.9
  cerebral (artery) G45.9
  spinal cord (arteriosclerotic) G95.19
    syphilitic A52.09
  venous (axillary) I87.8
**Claustrophobia** F40.240
**Clavus** (infected) L84
**Clawfoot** (congenital) Q66.89
  acquired — *see* Deformity, limb, clawfoot
**Clawhand** (acquired) (*see also* Deformity, limb, clawhand)
  congenital Q68.1
**Clawtoe** (congenital) Q66.89
  acquired — *see* Deformity, toe, specified NEC
**Clay eating** — *see* Pica
**Cleansing of artificial opening** — *see* Attention to, artificial, opening
**Cleft** (congenital) — *see also* Imperfect, closure
  alveolar process M26.79
  branchial (persistent) Q18.2
    cyst Q18.0
      fistula Q18.0
      sinus Q18.0
  cricoid cartilage, posterior Q31.8
  cyst Q18.0
    fistula Q18.0
    sinus Q18.0
  foot Q72.7 ☑
  hand Q71.6 ☑
  lip (unilateral) Q36.9
    with cleft palate Q37.9
      hard Q37.1
        with soft Q37.5
      soft Q37.3
        with hard Q37.5
    bilateral Q36.0
      with cleft palate Q37.8
        hard Q37.0
          with soft Q37.4
        soft Q37.2
          with hard Q37.4

**Cleft** — *continued*
  lip — *continued*
    median Q36.1
  nose Q30.2
  palate Q35.9
    with cleft lip (unilateral) Q37.9
      bilateral Q37.8
    hard Q35.1
      with
        cleft lip (unilateral) Q37.1
          bilateral Q37.0
        soft Q35.5
          with cleft lip (unilateral) Q37.5
            bilateral Q37.4
    medial Q35.5
    soft Q35.3
      with
        cleft lip (unilateral) Q37.3
          bilateral Q37.2
        hard Q35.5
          with cleft lip (unilateral) Q37.5
            bilateral Q37.4
  penis Q55.69
  scrotum Q55.29
  thyroid cartilage Q31.8
  uvula Q35.7
**Cleidocranial dysostosis** Q74.0
**Cleptomania** F63.2
**Clicking hip** (newborn) R29.4
**Climacteric** (female) (*see also* Menopause)
  arthritis (any site) NEC — *see* Arthritis, specified form NEC
  depression (single episode) F32.89
    recurrent episode F33.8
  male (symptoms) (syndrome) NEC N50.89
  melancholia (single episode) F32.89
    recurrent episode F33.8
  paranoid state F22
  polyarthritis NEC — *see* Arthritis, specified form NEC
  symptoms (female) N95.1
**Clinical research investigation** (clinical trial) (control subject) (normal comparison) (participant) Z00.6
**Clitoris** — *see* condition
**Cloaca** (persistent) Q43.7
**Clonorchiasis, clonorchis infection** (liver) B66.1
**Clonus** R25.8
**Closed bite** M26.29
**Clostridium** (C.) **perfringens, as cause of disease classified elsewhere** B96.7
**Closure**
  congenital, nose Q30.0
  cranial sutures, premature Q75.0
  defective or imperfect NEC — *see* Imperfect, closure
  fistula, delayed — *see* Fistula
  foramen ovale, imperfect Q21.1
  hymen N89.6
  interauricular septum, defective Q21.1
  interventricular septum, defective Q21.0
  lacrimal duct (*see also* Stenosis, lacrimal, duct)
    congenital Q10.5
  nose (congenital) Q30.0
    acquired M95.0
  of artificial opening — *see* Attention to, artificial, opening
  vagina N89.5
  valve — *see* Endocarditis
  vulva N90.5
**Clot** (blood) (*see also* Embolism)
  artery (obstruction) (occlusion) — *see* Embolism
  bladder N32.89
  brain (intradural or extradural) — *see* Occlusion, artery, cerebral
  circulation I74.9
  heart (*see also* Infarct, myocardium)
    not resulting in infarction I51.3
  vein — *see* Thrombosis
**Clouded state** R40.1
  epileptic — *see* Epilepsy, specified NEC
  paroxysmal — *see* Epilepsy, specified NEC
**Cloudy antrum, antra** J32.0
**Clouston's** (hidrotic) **ectodermal dysplasia** Q82.4
**Clubbed nail pachydermoperiostosis** M89.40 [L62]
**Clubbing of finger**(s) (nails) R68.3
**Clubfinger** R68.3
  congenital Q68.1
**Clubfoot** (congenital) Q66.89
  acquired — *see* Deformity, limb, clubfoot
  equinovarus Q66.0

**Clubfoot** — *continued*
paralytic — *see* Deformity, limb, clubfoot
**Clubhand** (congenital) (radial) Q71.4- ☑
acquired — *see* Deformity, limb, clubhand
**Clubnail** R68.3
congenital Q84.6
**Clump, kidney** Q63.1
**Clumsiness, clumsy child syndrome** F82
**Cluttering** F80.81
**Clutton's joints** A50.51 [M12.80]
**Coagulation, intravascular** (diffuse) (disseminated)
(*see also* Defibrination syndrome)
complicating abortion — *see* Abortion, by type, complicated by, intravascular coagulation
following ectopic or molar pregnancy O08.1
**Coagulopathy** (*see also* Defect, coagulation)
consumption D65
intravascular D65
newborn P60
**Coalition**
calcaneo-scaphoid Q66.89
tarsal Q66.89
**Coalminer's**
elbow — *see* Bursitis, elbow, olecranon
lung or pneumoconiosis J60
**Coalworker's lung or pneumoconiosis** J60
**Coarctation**
aorta (preductal) (postductal) Q25.1
pulmonary artery Q25.71
**Coated tongue** K14.3
**Coats' disease** (exudative retinopathy) — *see*
Retinopathy, exudative
**Cocaine-induced**
anxiety disorder F14.980
bipolar and related disorder F14.94
depressive disorder F14.94
obsessive-compulsive and related disorder F14.988
psychotic disorder F14.959
sexual dysfunction F14.981
sleep disorder F14.982
**Cocainism** — *see* Disorder, cocaine use
**Coccidioidomycosis** B38.9
cutaneous B38.3
disseminated B38.7
generalized B38.7
meninges B38.4
prostate B38.81
pulmonary B38.2
acute B38.0
chronic B38.1
skin B38.3
specified NEC B38.89
**Coccidioidosis** — *see* Coccidioidomycosis
**Coccidiosis** (intestinal) A07.3
**Coccydynia, coccygodynia** M53.3
**Coccyx** — *see* condition
**Cochin-China diarrhea** K90.1
**Cockayne's syndrome** Q87.1
**Cocked up toe** — *see* Deformity, toe, specified NEC
**Cock's peculiar tumor** L72.3
**Codman's tumor** — *see* Neoplasm, bone, benign
**Coenurosis** B71.8
**Coffee-worker's lung** J67.8
**Cogan's syndrome** H16.32- ☑
oculomotor apraxia H51.8
**Coitus, painful** (female) N94.10
male N53.12
psychogenic F52.6
**Cold** J00
with influenza, flu, or grippe — *see* Influenza, with,
respiratory manifestations NEC
agglutinin disease or hemoglobinuria (chronic) D59.1
bronchial — *see* Bronchitis
chest — *see* Bronchitis
common (head) J00
effects of T69.9 ☑
specified effect NEC T69.8 ☑
excessive, effects of T69.9 ☑
specified effect NEC T69.8 ☑
exhaustion from T69.8 ☑
exposure to T69.9 ☑
specified effect NEC T69.8 ☑
head J00
injury syndrome (newborn) P80.0
on lung — *see* Bronchitis
rose J30.1
sensitivity, auto-immune D59.1

**Cold** — *continued*
symptoms J00
virus J00
**Coldsore** B00.1
**Colibacillosis** A49.8
as the cause of other disease (*see also* Escherichia coli)
B96.20
generalized A41.50
**Colic** (bilious) (infantile) (intestinal) (recurrent) (spasmodic) R10.83
abdomen R10.83
psychogenic F45.8
appendix, appendicular K38.8
bile duct — *see* Calculus, bile duct
biliary — *see* Calculus, bile duct
common duct — *see* Calculus, bile duct
cystic duct — *see* Calculus, gallbladder
Devonshire NEC — *see* Poisoning, lead
gallbladder — *see* Calculus, gallbladder
gallstone — *see* Calculus, gallbladder
gallbladder or cystic duct — *see* Calculus, gallbladder
hepatic (duct) — *see* Calculus, bile duct
hysterical F45.8
kidney N23
lead NEC — *see* Poisoning, lead
mucous K58.9
with diarrhea K58.0
psychogenic F54
nephritic N23
painter's NEC — *see* Poisoning, lead
pancreas K86.89
psychogenic F45.8
renal N23
saturnine NEC — *see* Poisoning, lead
ureter N23
urethral N36.8
due to calculus N21.1
uterus NEC N94.89
menstrual — *see* Dysmenorrhea
worm NOS B83.9
**Colicystitis** — *see* Cystitis
**Colitis** (acute) (catarrhal) (chronic) (noninfective) (hemorrhagic) (*see also* Enteritis) K52.9
allergic K52.29
with
food protein-induced enterocolitis syndrome
K52.21
proctocolitis K52.82
amebic (acute) (*see also* Amebiasis) A06.0
nondysenteric A06.2
anthrax A22.2
bacillary — *see* Infection, Shigella
balantidial A07.0
Clostridium difficile
not specified as recurrent A04.72
recurrent A04.71
coccidial A07.3
collagenous K52.831
cystica superficialis K52.89
dietary counseling and surveillance (for) Z71.3
dietetic (*see also* Colitis, allergic) K52.29
drug-induced K52.1
due to radiation K52.0
eosinophilic K52.82
food hypersensitivity (*see also* Colitis, allergic) K52.29
giardial A07.1
granulomatous — *see* Enteritis, regional, large intestine
indeterminate, so stated K52.3
infectious — *see* Enteritis, infectious
ischemic K55.9
acute (subacute) (*see also* Ischemia, intestine,
acute) K55.039
chronic K55.1
due to mesenteric artery insufficiency K55.1
fulminant (acute) (*see also* Ischemia, intestine,
acute) K55.039
left sided K51.50
with
abscess K51.514
complication K51.519
specified NEC K51.518
fistula K51.513
obstruction K51.512
rectal bleeding K51.511
lymphocytic K52.832

**Colitis** — *continued*
membranous
psychogenic F54
microscopic K52.839
specified NEC K52.838
mucous — *see* Syndrome, irritable, bowel
psychogenic F54
noninfective K52.9
specified NEC K52.89
polyposa — *see* Polyp, colon, inflammatory
protozoal A07.9
pseudomembranous
not specified as recurrent A04.72
recurrent A04.71
pseudomucinous — *see* Syndrome, irritable, bowel
regional — *see* Enteritis, regional, large intestine
infectious A09
segmental — *see* Enteritis, regional, large intestine
septic — *see* Enteritis, infectious
spastic K58.9
with diarrhea K58.0
psychogenic F54
staphylococcal A04.8
foodborne A05.0
subacute ischemic (*see also* Ischemia, intestine, acute)
K55.039
thromboulcerative (*see also* Ischemia, intestine, acute)
K55.039
toxic NEC K52.1
due to Clostridium difficile
not specified as recurrent A04.72
recurrent A04.71
transmural — *see* Enteritis, regional, large intestine
trichomonal A07.8
tuberculous (ulcerative) A18.32
ulcerative (chronic) K51.90
with
complication K51.919
abscess K51.914
fistula K51.913
obstruction K51.912
rectal bleeding K51.911
specified complication NEC K51.918
enterocolitis — *see* Enterocolitis, ulcerative
ileocolitis — *see* Ileocolitis, ulcerative
mucosal proctocolitis — *see* Proctocolitis, mucosal
proctitis — *see* Proctitis, ulcerative
pseudopolyposis — *see* Polyp, colon, inflammatory
psychogenic F54
rectosigmoiditis — *see* Rectosigmoiditis, ulcerative
specified type NEC K51.80
with
complication K51.819
abscess K51.814
fistula K51.813
obstruction K51.812
rectal bleeding K51.811
specified complication NEC K51.818
**Collagenosis, collagen disease** (nonvascular) (vascular)
M35.9
cardiovascular I42.8
reactive perforating L87.1
specified NEC M35.8
**Collapse** R55
adrenal E27.2
cardiorespiratory R57.0
cardiovascular R57.0
newborn P29.89
circulatory (peripheral) R57.9
during or after labor and delivery O75.1
following ectopic or molar pregnancy O08.3
newborn P29.89
during or
after labor and delivery O75.1
resulting from a procedure, not elsewhere classified
T81.10 ☑
external ear canal — *see* Stenosis, external ear canal
general R55
heart — *see* Disease, heart
heat T67.1 ☑
hysterical F44.89
labyrinth, membranous (congenital) Q16.5
lung (massive) (*see also* Atelectasis) J98.19
pressure due to anesthesia (general) (local) or
other sedation T88.2 ☑
during labor and delivery O74.1
in pregnancy O29.02- ☑
postpartum, puerperal O89.09

☑ **Additional Character Required — Refer to the Tabular List for Character Selection**    ▽ **Subterms under main terms may continue to next column or page**

**Collapse** — *continued*
- myocardial — *see* Disease, heart
- nervous F48.8
- neurocirculatory F45.8
- nose M95.0
- postoperative T81.10 ☑
- pulmonary (*see also* Atelectasis) J98.19
  - newborn — *see* Atelectasis
- trachea J39.8
- tracheobronchial J98.09
- valvular — *see* Endocarditis
- vascular (peripheral) R57.9
  - during or after labor and delivery O75.1
  - following ectopic or molar pregnancy O08.3
  - newborn P29.89
- vertebra M48.50- ☑
  - cervical region M48.52- ☑
  - cervicothoracic region M48.53- ☑
  - in (due to)
    - metastasis — *see* Collapse, vertebra, in, specified disease NEC
    - osteoporosis (*see also* Osteoporosis) M80.88 ☑
      - cervical region M80.88 ☑
      - cervicothoracic region M80.88 ☑
      - lumbar region M80.88 ☑
      - lumbosacral region M80.88 ☑
      - multiple sites M80.88 ☑
      - occipito-atlanto-axial region M80.88 ☑
      - sacrococcygeal region M80.88 ☑
      - thoracic region M80.88 ☑
      - thoracolumbar region M80.88 ☑
    - specified disease NEC M48.50- ☑
      - cervical region M48.52- ☑
      - cervicothoracic region M48.53- ☑
      - lumbar region M48.56- ☑
      - lumbosacral region M48.57- ☑
      - occipito-atlanto-axial region M48.51- ☑
      - sacrococcygeal region M48.58- ☑
      - thoracic region M48.54- ☑
      - thoracolumbar region M48.55- ☑
  - lumbar region M48.56- ☑
  - lumbosacral region M48.57- ☑
  - occipito-atlanto-axial region M48.51- ☑
  - sacrococcygeal region M48.58- ☑
  - thoracic region M48.54- ☑
  - thoracolumbar region M48.55- ☑

**Collateral** (*see also* condition)
- circulation (venous) I87.8
- dilation, veins I87.8

**Colles' fracture** S52.53- ☑

**Collet** (-Sicard) syndrome G52.7

**Collier's asthma or lung** J60

**Collodion baby** Q80.2

**Colloid nodule** (of thyroid) (cystic) E04.1

**Coloboma** (iris) Q13.0
- eyelid Q10.3
- fundus Q14.8
- lens Q12.2
- optic disc (congenital) Q14.2
  - acquired H47.31- ☑

**Coloenteritis** — *see* Enteritis

**Colon** — *see* condition

**Colonization**
- MRSA (Methicillin resistant Staphylococcus aureus) Z22.322
- MSSA (Methicillin susceptible Staphylococcus aureus) Z22.321
- status — *see* Carrier (suspected) of

**Coloptosis** K63.4

**Color blindness** — *see* Deficiency, color vision

**Colostomy**
- attention to Z43.3
- fitting or adjustment Z46.89
- malfunctioning K94.03
- status Z93.3

**Colpitis** (acute) — *see* Vaginitis

**Colpocele** N81.5

**Colpocystitis** — *see* Vaginitis

**Colpospasm** N94.2

**Column, spinal, vertebral** — *see* condition

**Coma** R40.20
- with
  - motor response (none) R40.231 ☑
    - abnormal extensor posturing to pain or noxious stimuli (< 2 years of age) R40.232 ☑
    - abnormal flexure posturing to pain or noxious stimuli (0-5 years of age) R40.233 ☑

**Coma** — *continued*
- with — *continued*
  - motor response — *continued*
    - extensor posturing to pain or noxious stimuli (2-5 years of age) R40.232 ☑
    - flexion/decorticate posturing (< 2 years of age) R40.233 ☑
    - localizes pain (2-5 years of age) R40.235 ☑
    - normal or spontaneous movement (< 2 years of age) R40.236 ☑
    - obeys commands (2-5 years of age) R40.236 ☑
    - withdraws from pain or noxious stimuli (0-5 years of age) R40.234 ☑
    - withdraws to touch (< 2 years of age) R40.235 ☑
  - opening of eyes (never) R40.211 ☑
    - in response to
      - pain R40.212 ☑
      - sound R40.213 ☑
    - spontaneous R40.214 ☑
  - verbal response (none) R40.221 ☑
    - confused conversation R40.224 ☑
    - cooing or babbling or crying appropriately (< 2 years of age) R40.225 ☑
    - inappropriate crying or screaming (< 2 years of age) R40.223 ☑
    - inappropriate words (2-5 years of age) R40.224 ☑
    - incomprehensible sounds (2-5 years of age) R40.222 ☑
    - incomprehensible words R40.222 ☑
    - irritable cries (< 2 years of age) R40.224 ☑
    - moans/grunts to pain; restless (< 2 years old) R40.222 ☑
    - oriented R40.225 ☑
    - screaming (2-5 years of age) R40.223 ☑
    - uses appropriate words (2-5 years of age) R40.225 ☑
- eclamptic — *see* Eclampsia
- epileptic — *see* Epilepsy
- Glasgow, scale score — *see* Glasgow coma scale
- hepatic — *see* Failure, hepatic, by type, with coma
- hyperglycemic (diabetic) — *see* Diabetes, by type, with hyperosmolarity, with coma
- hyperosmolar (diabetic) — *see* Diabetes, by type, with hyperosmolarity, with coma
- hypoglycemic (diabetic) — *see* Diabetes, by type, with hypoglycemia, with coma
  - nondiabetic E15
- in diabetes — *see* Diabetes, coma
- insulin-induced — *see* Coma, hypoglycemic
- ketoacidotic (diabetic) — *see* Diabetes, by type, with ketoacidosis, with coma
- myxedematous E03.5
- newborn P91.5
- persistent vegetative state R40.3
- specified NEC, without documented Glasgow coma scale score, or with partial Glasgow coma scale score reported R40.244 ☑

**Comatose** — *see* Coma

**Combat fatigue** F43.0

**Combined** — *see* condition

**Comedo, comedones** (giant) L70.0

**Comedocarcinoma** (*see also* Neoplasm, breast, malignant)
- noninfiltrating
  - breast D05.8- ☑
  - specified site — *see* Neoplasm, in situ, by site
  - unspecified site D05.8- ☑

**Comedomastitis** — *see* Ectasia, mammary duct

**Comminuted fracture** — *code as* Fracture, closed

**Common**
- arterial trunk Q20.0
- atrioventricular canal Q21.2
- atrium Q21.1
- cold (head) J00
- truncus (arteriosus) Q20.0
- variable immunodeficiency — *see* Immunodeficiency, common variable
- ventricle Q20.4

**Commotio, commotion** (current)
- brain — *see* Injury, intracranial, concussion
- cerebri — *see* Injury, intracranial, concussion
- retinae S05.8X- ☑
- spinal cord — *see* Injury, spinal cord, by region
- spinalis — *see* Injury, spinal cord, by region

**Communication**
- between
  - base of aorta and pulmonary artery Q21.4
  - left ventricle and right atrium Q20.5
  - pericardial sac and pleural sac Q34.8
  - pulmonary artery and pulmonary vein, congenital Q25.72
  - congenital between uterus and digestive or urinary tract Q51.7

**Compartment syndrome** (deep) (posterior) (traumatic) T79.A0 ☑ (*following* T79.7)
- abdomen T79.A3 ☑ (*following* T79.7)
- lower extremity (hip, buttock, thigh, leg, foot, toes) T79.A2 ☑ (*following* T79.7)
- nontraumatic
  - abdomen M79.A3 (*following* M79.7)
  - lower extremity (hip, buttock, thigh, leg, foot, toes) M79.A2- ☑ (*following* M79.7)
  - specified site NEC M79.A9 (*following* M79.7)
  - upper extremity (shoulder, arm, forearm, wrist, hand, fingers) M79.A1- ☑ (*following* M79.7)
- specified site NEC T79.A9 ☑ (*following* T79.7)
- upper extremity (shoulder, arm, forearm, wrist, hand, fingers) T79.A1- ☑ (*following* T79.7)

**Compensation**
- failure — *see* Disease, heart
- neurosis, psychoneurosis — *see* Disorder, factitious

**Complaint** (*see also* Disease)
- bowel, functional K59.9
  - psychogenic F45.8
- intestine, functional K59.9
  - psychogenic F45.8
- kidney — *see* Disease, renal
- miners' J60

**Complete** — *see* condition

**Complex**
- Addison-Schilder E71.528
- cardiorenal — *see* Hypertension, cardiorenal
- Costen's M26.69
- disseminated mycobacterium avium- intracellulare (DMAC) A31.2
- Eisenmenger's (ventricular septal defect) I27.83
- hypersexual F52.8
- jumped process, spine — *see* Dislocation, vertebra
- primary, tuberculous A15.7
- Schilder-Addison E71.528
- subluxation (vertebral) M99.19
  - abdomen M99.19
  - acromioclavicular M99.17
  - cervical region M99.11
  - cervicothoracic M99.11
  - costochondral M99.18
  - costovertebral M99.18
  - head region M99.10
  - hip M99.15
  - lower extremity M99.16
  - lumbar region M99.13
  - lumbosacral M99.13
  - occipitocervical M99.10
  - pelvic region M99.15
  - pubic M99.15
  - rib cage M99.18
  - sacral region M99.14
  - sacrococcygeal M99.14
  - sacroiliac M99.14
  - specified NEC M99.19
  - sternochondral M99.18
  - sternoclavicular M99.17
  - thoracic region M99.12
  - thoracolumbar M99.12
  - upper extremity M99.17
- Taussig-Bing (transposition, aorta and overriding pulmonary artery) Q20.1

**Complication**(s) (from) (of)
- accidental puncture or laceration during a procedure (of) — *see* Complications, intraoperative (intraprocedural), puncture or laceration
- amputation stump (surgical) (late) NEC T87.9
  - dehiscence T87.81
  - infection or inflammation T87.40
    - lower limb T87.4- ☑
    - upper limb T87.4- ☑
  - necrosis T87.50
    - lower limb T87.5- ☑
    - upper limb T87.5- ☑
  - neuroma T87.30
    - lower limb T87.3- ☑
    - upper limb T87.3- ☑

**Complication**(s) — *continued*
  amputation stump — *continued*
    specified type NEC T87.89
  anastomosis (and bypass) (*see also* Complications, prosthetic device or implant)
    intestinal (internal) NEC K91.89
      involving urinary tract N99.89
    urinary tract (involving intestinal tract) N99.89
    vascular — *see* Complications, cardiovascular device or implant
  anesthesia, anesthetic (*see also* Anesthesia, complication) T88.59 ☑
    brain, postpartum, puerperal O89.2
    cardiac
      in
        labor and delivery O74.2
        pregnancy O29.19-
      postpartum, puerperal O89.1
    central nervous system
      in
        labor and delivery O74.3
        pregnancy O29.29- ☑
      postpartum, puerperal O89.2
    difficult or failed intubation T88.4 ☑
      in pregnancy O29.6- ☑
    failed sedation (conscious) (moderate) during procedure T88.52 ☑
    general, unintended awareness during procedure T88.53 ☑
    hyperthermia, malignant T88.3 ☑
    hypothermia T88.51 ☑
    intubation failure T88.4 ☑
    malignant hyperthermia T88.3 ☑
    pulmonary
      in
        labor and delivery O74.1
        pregnancy NEC O29.09- ☑
      postpartum, puerperal O89.09
    shock T88.2 ☑
    spinal and epidural
      in
        labor and delivery NEC O74.6
          headache O74.5
        pregnancy NEC O29.5X- ☑
      postpartum, puerperal NEC O89.5
        headache O89.4
    unintended awareness under general anesthesia during procedure T88.53 ☑
  anti-reflux device — *see* Complications, esophageal anti-reflux device
  aortic (bifurcation) graft — *see* Complications, graft, vascular
  aortocoronary (bypass) graft — *see* Complications, coronary artery (bypass) graft
  aortofemoral (bypass) graft — *see* Complications, extremity artery (bypass) graft
  arteriovenous
    fistula, surgically created T82.9 ☑
      embolism T82.818 ☑
      fibrosis T82.828 ☑
      hemorrhage T82.838 ☑
      infection or inflammation T82.7 ☑
      mechanical
        breakdown T82.510 ☑
        displacement T82.520 ☑
        leakage T82.530 ☑
        malposition T82.520 ☑
        obstruction T82.590 ☑
        perforation T82.590 ☑
        protrusion T82.590 ☑
      pain T82.848 ☑
      specified type NEC T82.898 ☑
      stenosis T82.858 ☑
      thrombosis T82.868 ☑
    shunt, surgically created T82.9 ☑
      embolism T82.818 ☑
      fibrosis T82.828 ☑
      hemorrhage T82.838 ☑
      infection or inflammation T82.7 ☑
      mechanical
        breakdown T82.511 ☑
        displacement T82.521 ☑
        leakage T82.531 ☑
        malposition T82.521 ☑
        obstruction T82.591 ☑
        perforation T82.591 ☑
        protrusion T82.591 ☑

**Complication**(s) — *continued*
  arteriovenous — *continued*
    shunt, surgically created — *continued*
      pain T82.848 ☑
      specified type NEC T82.898 ☑
      stenosis T82.858 ☑
      thrombosis T82.868 ☑
  arthroplasty — *see* Complications, joint prosthesis
  artificial
    fertilization or insemination N98.9
      attempted introduction (of)
        embryo in embryo transfer N98.3
        ovum following in vitro fertilization N98.2
      hyperstimulation of ovaries N98.1
      infection N98.0
      specified NEC N98.8
    heart T82.9 ☑
      embolism T82.817 ☑
      fibrosis T82.827 ☑
      hemorrhage T82.837 ☑
      infection or inflammation T82.7 ☑
      mechanical
        breakdown T82.512 ☑
        displacement T82.522 ☑
        leakage T82.532 ☑
        malposition T82.522 ☑
        obstruction T82.592 ☑
        perforation T82.592 ☑
        protrusion T82.592 ☑
      pain T82.847 ☑
      specified type NEC T82.897 ☑
      stenosis T82.857 ☑
      thrombosis T82.867 ☑
    opening
      cecostomy — *see* Complications, colostomy
      colostomy — *see* Complications, colostomy
      cystostomy — *see* Complications, cystostomy
      enterostomy — *see* Complications, enterostomy
      gastrostomy — *see* Complications, gastrostomy
      ileostomy — *see* Complications, enterostomy
      jejunostomy — *see* Complications, enterostomy
      nephrostomy — *see* Complications, stoma, urinary tract
      tracheostomy — *see* Complications, tracheostomy
      ureterostomy — *see* Complications, stoma, urinary tract
      urethrostomy — *see* Complications, stoma, urinary tract
  balloon implant or device
    gastrointestinal T85.9 ☑
      embolism T85.818 ☑
      fibrosis T85.828 ☑
      hemorrhage T85.838 ☑
      infection and inflammation T85.79 ☑
      pain T85.848 ☑
      specified type NEC T85.898 ☑
      stenosis T85.858 ☑
      thrombosis T85.868 ☑
    vascular (counterpulsation) T82.9 ☑
      embolism T82.818 ☑
      fibrosis T82.828 ☑
      hemorrhage T82.838 ☑
      infection or inflammation T82.7 ☑
      mechanical
        breakdown T82.513 ☑
        displacement T82.523 ☑
        leakage T82.533 ☑
        malposition T82.523 ☑
        obstruction T82.593 ☑
        perforation T82.593 ☑
        protrusion T82.593 ☑
      pain T82.848 ☑
      specified type NEC T82.898 ☑
      stenosis T82.858 ☑
      thrombosis T82.868 ☑
  bariatric procedure
    gastric band procedure K95.09
      infection K95.01
    specified procedure NEC K95.89
      infection K95.81
  bile duct implant (prosthetic) T85.9 ☑
    embolism T85.818 ☑
    fibrosis T85.828 ☑
    hemorrhage T85.838 ☑

**Complication**(s) — *continued*
  bile duct implant — *continued*
    infection and inflammation T85.79 ☑
    mechanical
      breakdown T85.510 ☑
      displacement T85.520 ☑
      malfunction T85.510 ☑
      malposition T85.520 ☑
      obstruction T85.590 ☑
      perforation T85.590 ☑
      protrusion T85.590 ☑
      specified NEC T85.590 ☑
    pain T85.848 ☑
    specified type NEC T85.898 ☑
    stenosis T85.858 ☑
    thrombosis T85.868 ☑
  bladder device (auxiliary) — *see* Complications, genitourinary, device or implant, urinary system
  bleeding (postoperative) — *see* Complication, postoperative, hemorrhage
    intraoperative — *see* Complication, intraoperative, hemorrhage
  blood vessel graft — *see* Complications, graft, vascular
  bone
    device NEC T84.9 ☑
      embolism T84.81 ☑
      fibrosis T84.82 ☑
      hemorrhage T84.83 ☑
      infection or inflammation T84.7 ☑
      mechanical
        breakdown T84.318 ☑
        displacement T84.328 ☑
        malposition T84.328 ☑
        obstruction T84.398 ☑
        perforation T84.398 ☑
        protrusion T84.398 ☑
      pain T84.84 ☑
      specified type NEC T84.89 ☑
      stenosis T84.85 ☑
      thrombosis T84.86 ☑
    graft — *see* Complications, graft, bone
    growth stimulator (electrode) — *see* Complications, electronic stimulator device, bone
    marrow transplant — *see* Complications, transplant, bone, marrow
  brain neurostimulator (electrode) — *see* Complications, electronic stimulator device, brain
  breast implant (prosthetic) T85.9 ☑
    capsular contracture T85.44 ☑
    embolism T85.818 ☑
    fibrosis T85.828 ☑
    hemorrhage T85.838 ☑
    infection and inflammation T85.79 ☑
    mechanical
      breakdown T85.41 ☑
      displacement T85.42 ☑
      leakage T85.43 ☑
      malposition T85.42 ☑
      obstruction T85.49 ☑
      perforation T85.49 ☑
      protrusion T85.49 ☑
      specified NEC T85.49 ☑
    pain T85.848 ☑
    specified type NEC T85.898 ☑
    stenosis T85.858 ☑
    thrombosis T85.868 ☑
  bypass (*see also* Complications, prosthetic device or implant)
    aortocoronary — *see* Complications, coronary artery (bypass) graft
    arterial (*see also* Complications, graft, vascular)
      extremity — *see* Complications, extremity artery (bypass) graft
  cardiac (*see also* Disease, heart)
    device, implant or graft T82.9 ☑
      embolism T82.817 ☑
      fibrosis T82.827 ☑
      hemorrhage T82.837 ☑
      infection or inflammation T82.7 ☑
        valve prosthesis T82.6 ☑
      mechanical
        breakdown T82.519 ☑
          specified device NEC T82.518 ☑
        displacement T82.529 ☑
          specified device NEC T82.528 ☑
        leakage T82.539 ☑

58    ☑ **Additional Character Required** — **Refer to the Tabular List for Character Selection**    ▽ **Subterms under main terms may continue to next column or page**

Complication — Complication

**Complication**(s) — *continued*
  cardiac (*see also* Disease, heart) — *continued*
    device, implant or graft — *continued*
      mechanical — *continued*
        leakage — *continued*
          specified device NEC T82.538 ☑
        malposition T82.529 ☑
          specified device NEC T82.528 ☑
        obstruction T82.599 ☑
          specified device NEC T82.598 ☑
        perforation T82.599 ☑
          specified device NEC T82.598 ☑
        protrusion T82.599 ☑
          specified device NEC T82.598 ☑
      pain T82.847 ☑
      specified type NEC T82.897 ☑
      stenosis T82.857 ☑
      thrombosis T82.867 ☑
  cardiovascular device, graft or implant T82.9 ☑
    aortic graft — *see* Complications, graft, vascular
    arteriovenous
      fistula, artificial — *see* Complication, arteriovenous, fistula, surgically created
      shunt — *see* Complication, arteriovenous, shunt, surgically created
    artificial heart — *see* Complication, artificial, heart
    balloon (counterpulsation) device — *see* Complication, balloon implant, vascular
    carotid artery graft — *see* Complications, graft, vascular
    coronary bypass graft — *see* Complication, coronary artery (bypass) graft
    dialysis catheter (vascular) — *see* Complication, catheter, dialysis
    electronic T82.9 ☑
      electrode T82.9 ☑
        embolism T82.817 ☑
        fibrosis T82.827 ☑
        hemorrhage T82.837 ☑
        infection T82.7 ☑
        mechanical
          breakdown T82.110 ☑
          displacement T82.120 ☑
          leakage T82.190 ☑
          obstruction T82.190 ☑
          perforation T82.190 ☑
          protrusion T82.190 ☑
          specified type NEC T82.190 ☑
        pain T82.847 ☑
        specified NEC T82.897 ☑
        stenosis T82.857 ☑
        thrombosis T82.867 ☑
      embolism T82.817 ☑
      fibrosis T82.827 ☑
      hemorrhage T82.837 ☑
      infection T82.7 ☑
      mechanical
        breakdown T82.119 ☑
        displacement T82.129 ☑
        leakage T82.199 ☑
        obstruction T82.199 ☑
        perforation T82.199 ☑
        protrusion T82.199 ☑
        specified type NEC T82.199 ☑
      pain T82.847 ☑
      pulse generator T82.9 ☑
        embolism T82.817 ☑
        fibrosis T82.827 ☑
        hemorrhage T82.837 ☑
        infection T82.7 ☑
        mechanical
          breakdown T82.111 ☑
          displacement T82.121 ☑
          leakage T82.191 ☑
          obstruction T82.191 ☑
          perforation T82.191 ☑
          protrusion T82.191 ☑
          specified type NEC T82.191 ☑
        pain T82.847 ☑
        specified NEC T82.897 ☑
        stenosis T82.857 ☑
        thrombosis T82.867 ☑
      specified condition NEC T82.897 ☑
      specified device NEC T82.9 ☑
        embolism T82.817 ☑
        fibrosis T82.827 ☑

**Complication**(s) — *continued*
  cardiovascular device, graft or implant — *continued*
    electronic — *continued*
      specified device — *continued*
        hemorrhage T82.837 ☑
        infection T82.7 ☑
        mechanical
          breakdown T82.118 ☑
          displacement T82.128 ☑
          leakage T82.198 ☑
          obstruction T82.198 ☑
          perforation T82.198 ☑
          protrusion T82.198 ☑
          specified type NEC T82.198 ☑
        pain T82.847 ☑
        specified NEC T82.897 ☑
        stenosis T82.857 ☑
        thrombosis T82.867 ☑
      stenosis T82.857 ☑
      thrombosis T82.867 ☑
    extremity artery graft — *see* Complication, extremity artery (bypass) graft
    femoral artery graft — *see* Complication, extremity artery (bypass) graft
    heart
      transplant — *see* Complication, transplant, heart
      valve — *see* Complication, prosthetic device, heart valve
        graft — *see* Complication, heart, valve, graft
    heart-lung transplant — *see* Complication, transplant, heart, with lung
    infection or inflammation T82.7 ☑
    umbrella device — *see* Complication, umbrella device, vascular
    vascular graft (or anastomosis) — *see* Complication, graft, vascular
  carotid artery (bypass) graft — *see* Complications, graft, vascular
  catheter (device) NEC (*see also* Complications, prosthetic device or implant)
    cranial infusion
      infection and inflammation T85.735 ☑
      mechanical
        breakdown T85.610 ☑
        displacement T85.620 ☑
        leakage T85.630 ☑
        malfunction T85.690 ☑
        malposition T85.620 ☑
        obstruction T85.690 ☑
        perforation T85.690 ☑
        protrusion T85.690 ☑
        specified NEC T85.690 ☑
    cystostomy T83.9 ☑
      embolism T83.81 ☑
      fibrosis T83.82 ☑
      hemorrhage T83.83 ☑
      infection and inflammation T83.510 ☑
      mechanical
        breakdown T83.010 ☑
        displacement T83.020 ☑
        leakage T83.030 ☑
        malposition T83.020 ☑
        obstruction T83.090 ☑
        perforation T83.090 ☑
        protrusion T83.090 ☑
        specified NEC T83.090 ☑
      pain T83.84 ☑
      specified type NEC T83.89 ☑
      stenosis T83.85 ☑
      thrombosis T83.86 ☑
    dialysis (vascular) T82.9 ☑
      embolism T82.818 ☑
      fibrosis T82.828 ☑
      hemorrhage T82.838 ☑
      infection and inflammation T82.7 ☑
      intraperitoneal — *see* Complications, catheter, intraperitoneal
      mechanical
        breakdown T82.41 ☑
        displacement T82.42 ☑
        leakage T82.43 ☑
        malposition T82.42 ☑
        obstruction T82.49 ☑
        perforation T82.49 ☑

**Complication**(s) — *continued*
  catheter (*see also* Complications, prosthetic device or implant) — *continued*
    dialysis — *continued*
      mechanical — *continued*
        protrusion T82.49 ☑
      pain T82.848 ☑
      specified type NEC T82.898 ☑
      stenosis T82.858 ☑
      thrombosis T82.868 ☑
    epidural infusion T85.9 ☑
      embolism T85.810 ☑
      fibrosis T85.820 ☑
      hemorrhage T85.830 ☑
      infection and inflammation T85.735 ☑
      mechanical
        breakdown T85.610 ☑
        displacement T85.620 ☑
        leakage T85.630 ☑
        malfunction T85.610 ☑
        malposition T85.620 ☑
        obstruction T85.690 ☑
        perforation T85.690 ☑
        protrusion T85.690 ☑
        specified NEC T85.690 ☑
      pain T85.840 ☑
      specified type NEC T85.890 ☑
      stenosis T85.850 ☑
      thrombosis T85.860 ☑
    intraperitoneal dialysis T85.9 ☑
      embolism T85.818 ☑
      fibrosis T85.828 ☑
      hemorrhage T85.838 ☑
      infection and inflammation T85.71 ☑
      mechanical
        breakdown T85.611 ☑
        displacement T85.621 ☑
        leakage T85.631 ☑
        malfunction T85.611 ☑
        malposition T85.621 ☑
        obstruction T85.691 ☑
        perforation T85.691 ☑
        protrusion T85.691 ☑
        specified NEC T85.691 ☑
      pain T85.848 ☑
      specified type NEC T85.898 ☑
      stenosis T85.858 ☑
      thrombosis T85.868 ☑
    intrathecal infusion
      infection and inflammation T85.735 ☑
      mechanical
        breakdown T85.610 ☑
        displacement T85.620 ☑
        leakage T85.630 ☑
        malfunction T85.690 ☑
        malposition T85.620 ☑
        obstruction T85.690 ☑
        perforation T85.690 ☑
        protrusion T85.690 ☑
        specified NEC T85.690 ☑
    intravenous infusion T82.9 ☑
      embolism T82.818 ☑
      fibrosis T82.828 ☑
      hemorrhage T82.838 ☑
      infection or inflammation T82.7 ☑
      mechanical
        breakdown T82.514 ☑
        displacement T82.524 ☑
        leakage T82.534 ☑
        malposition T82.524 ☑
        obstruction T82.594 ☑
        perforation T82.594 ☑
        protrusion T82.594 ☑
      pain T82.848 ☑
      specified type NEC T82.898 ☑
      stenosis T82.858 ☑
      thrombosis T82.868 ☑
    spinal infusion
      infection and inflammation T85.735 ☑
      mechanical
        breakdown T85.610 ☑
        displacement T85.620 ☑
        leakage T85.630 ☑
        malfunction T85.690 ☑
        malposition T85.620 ☑
        obstruction T85.690 ☑

**Complication**(s) — *continued*
catheter (*see also* Complications, prosthetic device or implant) — *continued*
  spinal infusion — *continued*
    mechanical — *continued*
      perforation T85.690 ☑
      protrusion T85.690 ☑
      specified NEC T85.690 ☑
    subarachnoid infusion
      infection and inflammation T85.735 ☑
      mechanical
        breakdown T85.610 ☑
        displacement T85.620 ☑
        leakage T85.630 ☑
        malfunction T85.690 ☑
        malposition T85.620 ☑
        obstruction T85.690 ☑
        perforation T85.690 ☑
        protrusion T85.690 ☑
        specified NEC T85.690 ☑
    subdural infusion T85.9 ☑
      embolism T85.810 ☑
      fibrosis T85.820 ☑
      hemorrhage T85.830 ☑
      infection and inflammation T85.735 ☑
      mechanical
        breakdown T85.610 ☑
        displacement T85.620 ☑
        leakage T85.630 ☑
        malfunction T85.610 ☑
        malposition T85.620 ☑
        obstruction T85.690 ☑
        perforation T85.690 ☑
        protrusion T85.690 ☑
        specified NEC T85.690 ☑
      pain T85.840 ☑
      specified type NEC T85.890 ☑
      stenosis T85.850 ☑
      thrombosis T85.860 ☑
  urethral T83.9 ☑
    displacement T83.028 ☑
    embolism T83.81 ☑
    fibrosis T83.82 ☑
    hemorrhage T83.83 ☑
    indwelling
      breakdown T83.011 ☑
      displacement T83.021 ☑
      infection and inflammation T83.511 ☑
      leakage T83.031 ☑
      specified complication NEC T83.091 ☑
    infection and inflammation T83.511 ☑
    leakage T83.038 ☑
    malposition T83.028 ☑
    mechanical
      breakdown T83.011 ☑
    obstruction (mechanical) T83.091 ☑
    pain T83.84 ☑
    perforation T83.091 ☑
    protrusion T83.091 ☑
    specified type NEC T83.091 ☑
    stenosis T83.85 ☑
    thrombosis T83.86 ☑
  urinary NEC
    breakdown T83.018 ☑
    displacement T83.028 ☑
    infection and inflammation T83.518 ☑
    leakage T83.038 ☑
    specified complication NEC T83.098 ☑
cecostomy (stoma) — *see* Complications, colostomy
cesarean delivery wound NEC O90.89
  disruption O90.0
  hematoma O90.2
  infection (following delivery) O86.0
chemotherapy (antineoplastic) NEC T88.7 ☑
chin implant (prosthetic) — *see* Complication, prosthetic device or implant, specified NEC
circulatory system I99.8
  intraoperative I97.88
  postprocedural I97.89
    following cardiac surgery (*see also* Infarct, myocardium, associated with revascularization procedure) I97.19- ☑
      postcardiotomy syndrome I97.0
    hypertension I97.3
    lymphedema after mastectomy I97.2
    postcardiotomy syndrome I97.0

**Complication**(s) — *continued*
circulatory system — *continued*
  postprocedural — *continued*
    specified NEC I97.89
colostomy (stoma) K94.00
  hemorrhage K94.01
  infection K94.02
  malfunction K94.03
  mechanical K94.03
  specified complication NEC K94.09
contraceptive device, intrauterine — *see* Complications, intrauterine, contraceptive device
cord (umbilical) — *see* Complications, umbilical cord
corneal graft — *see* Complications, graft, cornea
coronary artery (bypass) graft T82.9 ☑
  atherosclerosis — *see* Arteriosclerosis, coronary (artery),
  embolism T82.818 ☑
  fibrosis T82.828 ☑
  hemorrhage T82.838 ☑
  infection and inflammation T82.7 ☑
  mechanical
    breakdown T82.211 ☑
    displacement T82.212 ☑
    leakage T82.213 ☑
    malposition T82.212 ☑
    obstruction T82.218 ☑
    perforation T82.218 ☑
    protrusion T82.218 ☑
    specified NEC T82.218 ☑
  pain T82.848 ☑
  specified type NEC T82.898 ☑
  stenosis T82.858 ☑
  thrombosis T82.868 ☑
counterpulsation device (balloon), intra-aortic — *see* Complications, balloon implant, vascular
cystostomy (stoma) N99.518
  catheter — *see* Complications, catheter, cystostomy
  hemorrhage N99.510
  infection N99.511
  malfunction N99.512
  specified type NEC N99.518
delivery (*see also* Complications, obstetric) O75.9
  procedure (instrumental) (manual) (surgical) O75.4
  specified NEC O75.89
dialysis (peritoneal) (renal) (*see also* Complications, infusion)
  catheter (vascular) — *see* Complication, catheter, dialysis
  peritoneal, intraperitoneal — *see* Complications, catheter, intraperitoneal
dorsal column (spinal) neurostimulator — *see* Complications, electronic stimulator device, spinal cord
drug NEC T88.7 ☑
ear procedure (*see also* Disorder, ear)
  intraoperative H95.88
    hematoma — *see* Complications, intraoperative, hemorrhage (hematoma) (of), ear
    hemorrhage — *see* Complications, intraoperative, hemorrhage (hematoma) (of), ear
    laceration — *see* Complications, intraoperative, puncture or laceration..., ear
    specified NEC H95.88
  postoperative H95.89
    external ear canal stenosis H95.81- ☑
    hematoma — *see* Complications, postprocedural, hematoma (of), ear
    hemorrhage — *see* Complications, postprocedural, hemorrhage (of), ear
    postmastoidectomy — *see* Complications, postmastoidectomy
    seroma — *see* Complications, postprocedural, seroma (of), mastoid process
    specified NEC H95.89
ectopic pregnancy O08.9
  damage to pelvic organs O08.6
  embolism O08.2
  genital infection O08.0
  hemorrhage (delayed) (excessive) O08.1
  metabolic disorder O08.5
  renal failure O08.4
  shock O08.3
  specified type NEC O08.0
  venous complication NEC O08.7

**Complication**(s) — *continued*
electronic stimulator device
  bladder (urinary) — *see* Complications, electronic stimulator device, urinary
  bone T84.9 ☑
    breakdown T84.310 ☑
    displacement T84.320 ☑
    embolism T84.81 ☑
    fibrosis T84.82 ☑
    hemorrhage T84.83 ☑
    infection or inflammation T84.7 ☑
    malfunction T84.310 ☑
    malposition T84.320 ☑
    mechanical NEC T84.390 ☑
    obstruction T84.390 ☑
    pain T84.84 ☑
    perforation T84.390 ☑
    protrusion T84.390 ☑
    specified type NEC T84.89 ☑
    stenosis T84.85 ☑
    thrombosis T84.86 ☑
  brain T85.9 ☑
    embolism T85.810 ☑
    fibrosis T85.820 ☑
    hemorrhage T85.830 ☑
    infection and inflammation T85.731 ☑
    mechanical
      breakdown T85.110 ☑
      displacement T85.120 ☑
      leakage T85.190 ☑
      malposition T85.120 ☑
      obstruction T85.190 ☑
      perforation T85.190 ☑
      protrusion T85.190 ☑
      specified NEC T85.190 ☑
    pain T85.840 ☑
    specified type NEC T85.890 ☑
    stenosis T85.850 ☑
    thrombosis T85.860 ☑
  cardiac (defibrillator) (pacemaker) — *see* Complications, cardiovascular device or implant, electronic
  generator (brain) (gastric) (peripheral) (sacral) (spinal)
    breakdown T85.113 ☑
    displacement T85.123 ☑
    leakage T85.193 ☑
    malposition T85.123 ☑
    obstruction T85.193 ☑
    perforation T85.193 ☑
    protrusion T85.193 ☑
    specified type NEC T85.193 ☑
  muscle T84.9 ☑
    breakdown T84.418 ☑
    displacement T84.428 ☑
    embolism T84.81 ☑
    fibrosis T84.82 ☑
    hemorrhage T84.83 ☑
    infection or inflammation T84.7 ☑
    mechanical NEC T84.498 ☑
    pain T84.84 ☑
    specified type NEC T84.89 ☑
    stenosis T84.85 ☑
    thrombosis T84.86 ☑
  nervous system T85.9 ☑
    brain — *see* Complications, electronic stimulator device, brain
    cranial nerve — *see* Complications, electronic stimulator device, peripheral nerve
    embolism T85.810 ☑
    fibrosis T85.820 ☑
    gastric nerve — *see* Complications, electronic stimulator device, peripheral nerve
    hemorrhage T85.830 ☑
    infection and inflammation T85.738 ☑
    mechanical
      breakdown T85.118 ☑
      displacement T85.128 ☑
      leakage T85.199 ☑
      malposition T85.128 ☑
      obstruction T85.199 ☑
      perforation T85.199 ☑
      protrusion T85.199 ☑
      specified NEC T85.199 ☑
    pain T85.840 ☑

Complication(s) — *continued*
  electronic stimulator device — *continued*
    nervous system — *continued*
      peripheral nerve — *see* Complications, electronic stimulator device, peripheral nerve
      sacral nerve — *see* Complications, electronic stimulator device, peripheral nerve
      specified type NEC T85.890 ☑
      spinal cord — *see* Complications, electronic stimulator device, spinal cord
      stenosis T85.850 ☑
      thrombosis T85.860 ☑
      vagal nerve — *see* Complications, electronic stimulator device, peripheral nerve
    peripheral nerve T85.9 ☑
      embolism T85.810 ☑
      fibrosis T85.820 ☑
      hemorrhage T85.830 ☑
      infection and inflammation T85.732 ☑
      mechanical
        breakdown T85.111 ☑
        displacement T85.121 ☑
        leakage T85.191 ☑
        malposition T85.121 ☑
        obstruction T85.191 ☑
        perforation T85.191 ☑
        protrusion T85.191 ☑
        specified NEC T85.191 ☑
      pain T85.840 ☑
      specified type NEC T85.890 ☑
      stenosis T85.850 ☑
      thrombosis T85.860 ☑
    spinal cord T85.9 ☑
      embolism T85.810 ☑
      fibrosis T85.820 ☑
      hemorrhage T85.830 ☑
      infection and inflammation T85.733 ☑
      mechanical
        breakdown T85.112 ☑
        displacement T85.122 ☑
        leakage T85.192 ☑
        malposition T85.122 ☑
        obstruction T85.192 ☑
        perforation T85.192 ☑
        protrusion T85.192 ☑
        specified NEC T85.192 ☑
      pain T85.840 ☑
      specified type NEC T85.890 ☑
      stenosis T85.850 ☑
      thrombosis T85.860 ☑
  urinary T83.9 ☑
    embolism T83.81 ☑
    fibrosis T83.82 ☑
    hemorrhage T83.83 ☑
    infection and inflammation T83.598 ☑
    mechanical
      breakdown T83.110 ☑
      displacement T83.120 ☑
      malposition T83.120 ☑
      perforation T83.190 ☑
      protrusion T83.190 ☑
      specified NEC T83.190 ☑
    pain T83.84 ☑
    specified type NEC T83.89 ☑
    stenosis T83.85 ☑
    thrombosis T83.86 ☑
  electroshock therapy T88.9 ☑
    specified NEC T88.8 ☑
  endocrine E34.9
    postprocedural
      adrenal hypofunction E89.6
      hypoinsulinemia E89.1
      hypoparathyroidism E89.2
      hypopituitarism E89.3
      hypothyroidism E89.0
      ovarian failure E89.40
        asymptomatic E89.40
        symptomatic E89.41
      specified NEC E89.89
      testicular hypofunction E89.5
  endodontic treatment NEC M27.59
  enterostomy (stoma) K94.10
    hemorrhage K94.11
    infection K94.12
    malfunction K94.13
    mechanical K94.13

Complication(s) — *continued*
  enterostomy — *continued*
    specified complication NEC K94.19
  episiotomy, disruption O90.1
  esophageal anti-reflux device T85.9 ☑
    embolism T85.818 ☑
    fibrosis T85.828 ☑
    hemorrhage T85.838 ☑
    infection and inflammation T85.79 ☑
    mechanical
      breakdown T85.511 ☑
      displacement T85.521 ☑
      malfunction T85.511 ☑
      malposition T85.521 ☑
      obstruction T85.591 ☑
      perforation T85.591 ☑
      protrusion T85.591 ☑
      specified NEC T85.591 ☑
    pain T85.848 ☑
    specified type NEC T85.898 ☑
    stenosis T85.858 ☑
    thrombosis T85.868 ☑
  esophagostomy K94.30
    hemorrhage K94.31
    infection K94.32
    malfunction K94.33
    mechanical K94.33
    specified complication NEC K94.39
  extracorporeal circulation T80.90 ☑
  extremity artery (bypass) graft T82.9 ☑
    arteriosclerosis — *see* Arteriosclerosis, extremities, bypass graft
    embolism T82.818 ☑
    fibrosis T82.828 ☑
    hemorrhage T82.838 ☑
    infection and inflammation T82.7 ☑
    mechanical
      breakdown T82.318 ☑
        femoral artery T82.312 ☑
      displacement T82.328 ☑
        femoral artery T82.322 ☑
      leakage T82.338 ☑
        femoral artery T82.332 ☑
      malposition T82.328 ☑
        femoral artery T82.322 ☑
      obstruction T82.398 ☑
        femoral artery T82.392 ☑
      perforation T82.398 ☑
        femoral artery T82.392 ☑
      protrusion T82.398 ☑
        femoral artery T82.392 ☑
    pain T82.848 ☑
    specified type NEC T82.898 ☑
    stenosis T82.858 ☑
    thrombosis T82.868 ☑
  eye H57.9
    corneal graft — *see* Complications, graft, cornea
    implant (prosthetic) T85.9 ☑
      embolism T85.818 ☑
      fibrosis T85.828 ☑
      hemorrhage T85.838 ☑
      infection and inflammation T85.79 ☑
      mechanical
        breakdown T85.318 ☑
        displacement T85.328 ☑
        leakage T85.398 ☑
        malposition T85.328 ☑
        obstruction T85.398 ☑
        perforation T85.398 ☑
        protrusion T85.398 ☑
        specified NEC T85.398 ☑
      pain T85.848 ☑
      specified type NEC T85.898 ☑
      stenosis T85.858 ☑
      thrombosis T85.868 ☑
    intraocular lens — *see* Complications, intraocular lens
    orbital prosthesis — *see* Complications, orbital prosthesis
  female genital N94.9
    device, implant or graft NEC — *see* Complications, genitourinary, device or implant, genital tract
  femoral artery (bypass) graft — *see* Complication, extremity artery (bypass) graft
  fixation device, internal (orthopedic) T84.9 ☑
    infection and inflammation T84.60 ☑

Complication(s) — *continued*
  fixation device, internal — *continued*
    infection and inflammation — *continued*
      arm T84.61- ☑
        humerus T84.61- ☑
        radius T84.61- ☑
        ulna T84.61- ☑
      leg T84.629 ☑
        femur T84.62- ☑
        fibula T84.62- ☑
        tibia T84.62- ☑
      specified site NEC T84.89 ☑
      spine T84.63 ☑
    mechanical
      breakdown
        limb T84.119 ☑
          carpal T84.210 ☑
          femur T84.11- ☑
          fibula T84.11- ☑
          humerus T84.11- ☑
          metacarpal T84.210 ☑
          metatarsal T84.213 ☑
          phalanx
            foot T84.213 ☑
            hand T84.210 ☑
          radius T84.11- ☑
          tarsal T84.213 ☑
          tibia T84.11- ☑
          ulna T84.11- ☑
        specified bone NEC T84.218 ☑
        spine T84.216 ☑
      displacement
        limb T84.129 ☑
          carpal T84.220 ☑
          femur T84.12- ☑
          fibula T84.12- ☑
          humerus T84.12- ☑
          metacarpal T84.220 ☑
          metatarsal T84.223 ☑
          phalanx
            foot T84.223 ☑
            hand T84.220 ☑
          radius T84.12- ☑
          tarsal T84.223 ☑
          tibia T84.12- ☑
          ulna T84.12- ☑
        specified bone NEC T84.228 ☑
        spine T84.226 ☑
      malposition — *see* Complications, fixation device, internal, mechanical, displacement
      obstruction — *see* Complications, fixation device, internal, mechanical, specified type NEC
      perforation — *see* Complications, fixation device, internal, mechanical, specified type NEC
      protrusion — *see* Complications, fixation device, internal, mechanical, specified type NEC
      specified type NEC
        limb T84.199 ☑
          carpal T84.290 ☑
          femur T84.19- ☑
          fibula T84.19- ☑
          humerus T84.19- ☑
          metacarpal T84.290 ☑
          metatarsal T84.293 ☑
          phalanx
            foot T84.293 ☑
            hand T84.290 ☑
          radius T84.19- ☑
          tarsal T84.293 ☑
          tibia T84.19- ☑
          ulna T84.19- ☑
        specified bone NEC T84.298 ☑
        vertebra T84.296 ☑
    specified type NEC T84.89 ☑
      embolism T84.81 ☑
      fibrosis T84.82 ☑
      hemorrhage T84.83 ☑
      pain T84.84 ☑
      specified complication NEC T84.89 ☑
      stenosis T84.85 ☑
      thrombosis T84.86 ☑
  following
    acute myocardial infarction NEC I23.8

Complication(s) — *continued*
  following — *continued*
    acute myocardial infarction — *continued*
      aneurysm (false) (of cardiac wall) (of heart wall) (ruptured) I23.3
      angina I23.7
      atrial
        septal defect I23.1
        thrombosis I23.6
      cardiac wall rupture I23.3
      chordae tendinae rupture I23.4
      defect
        septal
          atrial (heart) I23.1
          ventricular (heart) I23.2
      hemopericardium I23.Ø
      papillary muscle rupture I23.5
      rupture
        cardiac wall I23.3
          with hemopericardium I23.Ø
        chordae tendineae I23.4
        papillary muscle I23.5
      specified NEC I23.8
      thrombosis
        atrium I23.6
        auricular appendage I23.6
        ventricle (heart) I23.6
      ventricular
        septal defect I23.2
        thrombosis I23.6
    ectopic or molar pregnancy OØ8.9
      cardiac arrest OØ8.81
      sepsis OØ8.82
      specified type NEC OØ8.89
      urinary tract infection OØ8.83
    termination of pregnancy — *see* Abortion
  gastrointestinal K92.9
    bile duct prosthesis — *see* Complications, bile duct implant
    esophageal anti-reflux device — *see* Complications, esophageal anti-reflux device
    postoperative
      colostomy — *see* Complications, colostomy
      dumping syndrome K91.1
      enterostomy — *see* Complications, enterostomy
      gastrostomy — *see* Complications, gastrostomy
      malabsorption NEC K91.2
      obstruction (*see also* Obstruction, intestine, postoperative) K91.3Ø
      postcholecystectomy syndrome K91.5
      specified NEC K91.89
      vomiting after GI surgery K91.Ø
    prosthetic device or implant
      bile duct prosthesis — *see* Complications, bile duct implant
      esophageal anti-reflux device — *see* Complications, esophageal anti-reflux device
      specified type NEC
        embolism T85.818 ☑
        fibrosis T85.828 ☑
        hemorrhage T85.838 ☑
        mechanical
          breakdown T85.518 ☑
          displacement T85.528 ☑
          malfunction T85.518 ☑
          malposition T85.528 ☑
          obstruction T85.598 ☑
          perforation T85.598 ☑
          protrusion T85.598 ☑
          specified NEC T85.598 ☑
        pain T85.848 ☑
        specified complication NEC T85.898 ☑
        stenosis T85.858 ☑
        thrombosis T85.868 ☑
  gastrostomy (stoma) K94.2Ø
    hemorrhage K94.21
    infection K94.22
    malfunction K94.23
    mechanical K94.23
    specified complication NEC K94.29
  genitourinary
    device or implant T83.9 ☑
      genital tract T83.9 ☑
        infection or inflammation T83.69 ☑
        intrauterine contraceptive device — *see* Complications, intrauterine, contraceptive device

Complication(s) — *continued*
  genitourinary — *continued*
    device or implant — *continued*
      genital tract — *continued*
        mechanical — *see* Complications, by device, mechanical
        mesh — *see* Complications, mesh
        penile prosthesis — *see* Complications, prosthetic device, penile
        specified type NEC T83.89 ☑
          embolism T83.81 ☑
          fibrosis T83.82 ☑
          hemorrhage T83.83 ☑
          pain T83.84 ☑
          specified complication NEC T83.89 ☑
          stenosis T83.85 ☑
          thrombosis T83.86 ☑
        vaginal mesh — *see* Complications, mesh
      urinary system T83.9
        cystostomy catheter — *see* Complication, catheter, cystostomy
        electronic stimulator — *see* Complications, electronic stimulator device, urinary
        indwelling urethral catheter — *see* Complications, catheter, urethral, indwelling
        infection or inflammation T83.598 ☑
          indwelling urethral catheter T83.511 ☑
        kidney transplant — *see* Complication, transplant, kidney
        organ graft — *see* Complication, graft, urinary organ
        specified type NEC T83.89 ☑
          embolism T83.81 ☑
          fibrosis T83.82 ☑
          hemorrhage T83.83 ☑
          mechanical T83.198 ☑
            breakdown T83.118 ☑
            displacement T83.128 ☑
            malfunction T83.118 ☑
            malposition T83.128 ☑
            obstruction T83.198 ☑
            perforation T83.198 ☑
            protrusion T83.198 ☑
            specified NEC T83.198 ☑
        sphincter implant — *see* Complications, implant, urinary sphincter
        sphincter, implanted T83.191 ☑
        stent (ileal conduit) (nephroureteral) T83.193 ☑
          pain T83.84 ☑
          specified complication NEC T83.89 ☑
          stenosis T83.85 ☑
          thrombosis T83.86 ☑
          ureteral indwelling T83.192 ☑
    postprocedural
      pelvic peritoneal adhesions N99.4
      renal failure N99.Ø
      specified NEC N99.89
      stoma — *see* Complications, stoma, urinary tract
      urethral stricture — *see* Stricture, urethra, postprocedural
      vaginal
        adhesions N99.2
        vault prolapse N99.3
  graft (bypass) (patch) (*see also* Complications, prosthetic device or implant)
    aorta — *see* Complications, graft, vascular
    arterial — *see* Complication, graft, vascular
    bone T86.839
      failure T86.831
      infection T86.832
      mechanical T84.318 ☑
        breakdown T84.318 ☑
        displacement T84.328 ☑
        protrusion T84.398 ☑
        specified type NEC T84.398 ☑
      rejection T86.83Ø
      specified type NEC T86.838
    carotid artery — *see* Complications, graft, vascular
    cornea T86.849
      failure T86.841
      infection T86.842
      mechanical T85.398 ☑
        breakdown T85.318 ☑
        displacement T85.328 ☑
        protrusion T85.398 ☑

Complication(s) — *continued*
  graft (*see also* Complications, prosthetic device or implant) — *continued*
    cornea — *continued*
      mechanical — *continued*
        specified type NEC T85.398 ☑
      rejection T86.84Ø
      retroprosthetic membrane T85.398 ☑
      specified type NEC T86.848
    femoral artery (bypass) — *see* Complication, extremity artery (bypass) graft
    genital organ or tract — *see* Complications, genitourinary, device or implant, genital tract
    muscle T84.9 ☑
      breakdown T84.41Ø ☑
      displacement T84.42Ø ☑
      embolism T84.81 ☑
      fibrosis T84.82 ☑
      hemorrhage T84.83 ☑
      infection and inflammation T84.7 ☑
      mechanical NEC T84.49Ø ☑
      pain T84.84 ☑
      specified type NEC T84.89 ☑
      stenosis T84.85 ☑
      thrombosis T84.86 ☑
    nerve — *see* Complication, prosthetic device or implant, specified NEC
    skin — *see* Complications, prosthetic device or implant, skin graft
    tendon T84.9 ☑
      breakdown T84.41Ø ☑
      displacement T84.42Ø ☑
      embolism T84.81 ☑
      fibrosis T84.82 ☑
      hemorrhage T84.83 ☑
      infection and inflammation T84.7 ☑
      mechanical NEC T84.49Ø ☑
      pain T84.84 ☑
      specified type NEC T84.89 ☑
      stenosis T84.85 ☑
      thrombosis T84.86 ☑
    urinary organ T83.9 ☑
      embolism T83.81 ☑
      fibrosis T83.82 ☑
      hemorrhage T83.83 ☑
      infection and inflammation T83.598 ☑
        indwelling urethral catheter T83.511 ☑
      mechanical
        breakdown T83.21 ☑
        displacement T83.22 ☑
        erosion T83.24 ☑
        exposure T83.25 ☑
        leakage T83.23 ☑
        malposition T83.22 ☑
        obstruction T83.29 ☑
        perforation T83.29 ☑
        protrusion T83.29 ☑
        specified NEC T83.29 ☑
      pain T83.84 ☑
      specified type NEC T83.89 ☑
      stenosis T83.85 ☑
      thrombosis T83.86 ☑
    vascular T82.9 ☑
      embolism T82.818 ☑
      femoral artery — *see* Complication, extremity artery (bypass) graft
      fibrosis T82.828 ☑
      hemorrhage T82.838 ☑
      mechanical
        breakdown T82.319 ☑
          aorta (bifurcation) T82.31Ø ☑
          carotid artery T82.311 ☑
          specified vessel NEC T82.318 ☑
        displacement T82.329 ☑
          aorta (bifurcation) T82.32Ø ☑
          carotid artery T82.321 ☑
          specified vessel NEC T82.328 ☑
        leakage T82.339 ☑
          aorta (bifurcation) T82.33Ø ☑
          carotid artery T82.331 ☑
          specified vessel NEC T82.338 ☑
        malposition T82.329 ☑
          aorta (bifurcation) T82.32Ø ☑
          carotid artery T82.321 ☑
          specified vessel NEC T82.328 ☑
        obstruction T82.399 ☑

**Complication**(s) — *continued*
  graft (*see also* Complications, prosthetic device or implant) — *continued*
    vascular — *continued*
      mechanical — *continued*
        obstruction — *continued*
          aorta (bifurcation) T82.390 ☑
          carotid artery T82.391 ☑
          specified vessel NEC T82.398 ☑
        perforation T82.399 ☑
          aorta (bifurcation) T82.390 ☑
          carotid artery T82.391 ☑
          specified vessel NEC T82.398 ☑
        protrusion T82.399 ☑
          aorta (bifurcation) T82.390 ☑
          carotid artery T82.391 ☑
          specified vessel NEC T82.398 ☑
      pain T82.848 ☑
      specified complication NEC T82.898 ☑
      stenosis T82.858 ☑
      thrombosis T82.868 ☑
  heart I51.9
    assist device
      infection and inflammation T82.7 ☑
    following acute myocardial infarction — *see*
        Complications, following, acute myocardial
        infarction
    postoperative — *see* Complications, circulatory
        system
    transplant — *see* Complication, transplant, heart
        and lung(s) — *see* Complications, transplant,
        heart, with lung
    valve
      graft (biological) T82.9 ☑
        embolism T82.817 ☑
        fibrosis T82.827 ☑
        hemorrhage T82.837 ☑
        infection and inflammation T82.7 ☑
        mechanical T82.228 ☑
          breakdown T82.221 ☑
          displacement T82.222 ☑
          leakage T82.223 ☑
          malposition T82.222 ☑
          obstruction T82.228 ☑
          perforation T82.228 ☑
          protrusion T82.228 ☑
        pain T82.847 ☑
        specified type NEC T82.897 ☑
        stenosis T82.857 ☑
        thrombosis T82.867 ☑
      prosthesis T82.9 ☑
        embolism T82.817 ☑
        fibrosis T82.827 ☑
        hemorrhage T82.837 ☑
        infection or inflammation T82.6 ☑
        mechanical T82.09 ☑
          breakdown T82.01 ☑
          displacement T82.02 ☑
          leakage T82.03 ☑
          malposition T82.02 ☑
          obstruction T82.09 ☑
          perforation T82.09 ☑
          protrusion T82.09 ☑
        pain T82.847 ☑
        specified type NEC T82.897 ☑
          mechanical T82.09 ☑
        stenosis T82.857 ☑
        thrombosis T82.867 ☑
  hematoma
    intraoperative — *see* Complication, intraoperative,
        hemorrhage
    postprocedural — *see* Complication, postprocedural, hematoma
  hemodialysis — *see* Complications, dialysis
  hemorrhage
    intraoperative — *see* Complication, intraoperative,
        hemorrhage
    postprocedural — *see* Complication, postprocedural, hemorrhage
  ileostomy (stoma) — *see* Complications, enterostomy
  immunization (procedure) — *see* Complications, vaccination
  implant (*see also* Complications, by site and type)
    urinary sphincter T83.9 ☑
      embolism T83.81 ☑
      fibrosis T83.82 ☑

**Complication**(s) — *continued*
  implant (*see also* Complications, by site and type) —
      *continued*
    urinary sphincter — *continued*
      hemorrhage T83.83 ☑
      infection and inflammation T83.591 ☑
      mechanical
        breakdown T83.111 ☑
        displacement T83.121 ☑
        leakage T83.191 ☑
        malposition T83.121 ☑
        obstruction T83.191 ☑
        perforation T83.191 ☑
        protrusion T83.191 ☑
        specified NEC T83.191 ☑
      pain T83.84 ☑
      specified type NEC T83.89 ☑
      stenosis T83.85 ☑
      thrombosis T83.86 ☑
  infusion (procedure) T80.90 ☑
    air embolism T80.0 ☑
    blood — *see* Complications, transfusion
    catheter — *see* Complications, catheter
    infection T80.29 ☑
    pump — *see* Complications, cardiovascular, device
        or implant
    sepsis T80.29 ☑
    serum reaction (*see also* Reaction, serum) T80.69 ☑
      anaphylactic shock (*see also* Shock, anaphylactic) T80.59 ☑
    specified type NEC T80.89 ☑
  inhalation therapy NEC T81.81 ☑
  injection (procedure) T80.90 ☑
    drug reaction — *see* Reaction, drug
    infection T80.29 ☑
    sepsis T80.29 ☑
    serum (prophylactic) (therapeutic) — *see* Complications, vaccination
    specified type NEC T80.89 ☑
    vaccine (any) — *see* Complications, vaccination
  inoculation (any) — *see* Complications, vaccination
  insulin pump
    infection and inflammation T85.72 ☑
    mechanical
      breakdown T85.614 ☑
      displacement T85.624 ☑
      leakage T85.633 ☑
      malposition T85.624 ☑
      obstruction T85.694 ☑
      perforation T85.694 ☑
      protrusion T85.694 ☑
      specified NEC T85.694 ☑
  intestinal pouch NEC K91.858
  intraocular lens (prosthetic) T85.9 ☑
    embolism T85.818 ☑
    fibrosis T85.828 ☑
    hemorrhage T85.838 ☑
    infection and inflammation T85.79 ☑
    mechanical
      breakdown T85.21 ☑
      displacement T85.22 ☑
      malposition T85.22 ☑
      obstruction T85.29 ☑
      perforation T85.29 ☑
      protrusion T85.29 ☑
      specified NEC T85.29 ☑
    pain T85.848 ☑
    specified type NEC T85.898 ☑
    stenosis T85.858 ☑
    thrombosis T85.868 ☑
  intraoperative (intraprocedural)
    cardiac arrest (*see also* Infarct, myocardium, associated with revascularization procedure)
      during cardiac surgery I97.710
      during other surgery I97.711
    cardiac functional disturbance NEC (*see also* Infarct, myocardium, associated with revascularization procedure)
      during cardiac surgery I97.790
      during other surgery I97.791
    hemorrhage (hematoma) (of)
      circulatory system organ or structure
        during cardiac bypass I97.411
        during cardiac catheterization I97.410
        during other circulatory system procedure
            I97.418

**Complication**(s) — *continued*
  intraoperative — *continued*
    hemorrhage — *continued*
      circulatory system organ or structure — *continued*
        during other procedure I97.42
      digestive system organ
        during procedure on digestive system
            K91.61
        during procedure on other organ K91.62
      ear
        during procedure on ear and mastoid process H95.21
        during procedure on other organ H95.22
      endocrine system organ or structure
        during procedure on endocrine system organ or structure E36.01
        during procedure on other organ E36.02
      eye and adnexa
        during ophthalmic procedure H59.11- ☑
        during other procedure H59.12- ☑
      genitourinary organ or structure
        during procedure on genitourinary organ or structure N99.61
        during procedure on other organ N99.62
      mastoid process
        during procedure on ear and mastoid process H95.21
        during procedure on other organ H95.22
      musculoskeletal structure
        during musculoskeletal surgery M96.810
        during non-orthopedic surgery M96.811
        during orthopedic surgery M96.810
      nervous system
        during a nervous system procedure G97.31
        during other procedure G97.32
      respiratory system
        during other procedure J95.62
        during procedure on respiratory system organ or structure J95.61
      skin and subcutaneous tissue
        during a dermatologic procedure L76.01
        during a procedure on other organ L76.02
      spleen
        during a procedure on other organ D78.02
        during a procedure on the spleen D78.01
    puncture or laceration (accidental) (unintentional)
        (of)
      brain
        during a nervous system procedure G97.48
        during other procedure G97.49
      circulatory system organ or structure
        during circulatory system procedure I97.51
        during other procedure I97.52
      digestive system
        during procedure on digestive system
            K91.71
        during procedure on other organ K91.72
      ear
        during procedure on ear and mastoid process H95.31
        during procedure on other organ H95.32
      endocrine system organ or structure
        during procedure on endocrine system organ or structure E36.11
        during procedure on other organ E36.12
      eye and adnexa
        during ophthalmic procedure H59.21- ☑
        during other procedure H59.22- ☑
      genitourinary organ or structure
        during procedure on genitourinary organ or structure N99.71
        during procedure on other organ N99.72
      mastoid process
        during procedure on ear and mastoid process H95.31
        during procedure on other organ H95.32
      musculoskeletal structure
        during musculoskeletal surgery M96.820
        during non-orthopedic surgery M96.821
        during orthopedic surgery M96.820
      nervous system
        during a nervous system procedure G97.48
        during other procedure G97.49
      respiratory system
        during other procedure J95.72
        during procedure on respiratory system organ or structure J95.71

**Complication**(s) — *continued*
  intraoperative — *continued*
    puncture or laceration — *continued*
      skin and subcutaneous tissue
        during a dermatologic procedure L76.11
        during a procedure on other organ L76.12
      spleen
        during a procedure on other organ D78.12
        during a procedure on the spleen D78.11
    specified NEC
      circulatory system I97.88
      digestive system K91.81
      ear H95.88
      endocrine system E36.8
      eye and adnexa H59.88
      genitourinary system N99.81
      mastoid process H95.88
      musculoskeletal structure M96.89
      nervous system G97.81
      respiratory system J95.88
      skin and subcutaneous tissue L76.81
      spleen D78.81
  intraperitoneal catheter (dialysis) (infusion) — *see* Complications, catheter, intraperitoneal
  intrathecal infusion pump
    infection and inflammation T85.738 ☑
    mechanical
      breakdown T85.615 ☑
      displacement T85.625 ☑
      leakage T85.635 ☑
      malfunction T85.695 ☑
      malposition T85.625 ☑
      obstruction T85.695 ☑
      perforation T85.695 ☑
      protrusion T85.695 ☑
      specified NEC T85.695 ☑
  intrauterine
    contraceptive device
      embolism T83.81 ☑
      fibrosis T83.82 ☑
      hemorrhage T83.83 ☑
      infection and inflammation T83.69 ☑
      mechanical
        breakdown T83.31 ☑
        displacement T83.32 ☑
        malposition T83.32 ☑
        obstruction T83.39 ☑
        perforation T83.39 ☑
        protrusion T83.39 ☑
        specified NEC T83.39 ☑
      pain T83.84 ☑
      specified type NEC T83.89 ☑
      stenosis T83.85 ☑
      thrombosis T83.86 ☑
    procedure (fetal), to newborn P96.5
  jejunostomy (stoma) — *see* Complications, enterostomy
  joint prosthesis, internal T84.9 ☑
    breakage (fracture) T84.01- ☑
    dislocation T84.02- ☑
    fracture T84.01- ☑
    infection or inflammation T84.50 ☑
      hip T84.5- ☑
      knee T84.5- ☑
      specified joint NEC T84.59 ☑
    instability T84.02- ☑
    malposition — *see* Complications, joint prosthesis, mechanical, displacement
    mechanical
      breakage, broken T84.01- ☑
      dislocation T84.02- ☑
      fracture T84.01- ☑
      instability T84.02- ☑
      leakage — *see* Complications, joint prosthesis, mechanical, specified NEC
      loosening T84.039 ☑
        hip T84.03- ☑
        knee T84.03- ☑
        specified joint NEC T84.038 ☑
      obstruction — *see* Complications, joint prosthesis, mechanical, specified NEC
      perforation — *see* Complications, joint prosthesis, mechanical, specified NEC
      osteolysis T84.059 ☑
        hip T84.05- ☑
        knee T84.05- ☑
        other specified joint T84.058 ☑

**Complication**(s) — *continued*
  joint prosthesis, internal — *continued*
    mechanical — *continued*
      protrusion — *see* Complications, joint prosthesis, mechanical, specified NEC
      specified complication NEC T84.099 ☑
        hip T84.09- ☑
        knee T84.09- ☑
        other specified joint T84.098 ☑
      subluxation T84.02- ☑
      wear of articular bearing surface T84.069 ☑
        hip T84.06- ☑
        knee T84.06- ☑
        other specified joint T84.068 ☑
    specified joint NEC T84.89 ☑
      embolism T84.81 ☑
      fibrosis T84.82 ☑
      hemorrhage T84.83 ☑
      pain T84.84 ☑
      specified complication NEC T84.89 ☑
      stenosis T84.85 ☑
      thrombosis T84.86 ☑
    subluxation T84.02- ☑
  kidney transplant — *see* Complications, transplant, kidney
  labor O75.9
    specified NEC O75.89
  liver transplant (immune or nonimmune) — *see* Complications, transplant, liver
  lumbar puncture G97.1
    cerebrospinal fluid leak G97.0
    headache or reaction G97.1
  lung transplant — *see* Complications, transplant, lung
    and heart — *see* Complications, transplant, lung, with heart
  male genital N50.9
    device, implant or graft — *see* Complications, genitourinary, device or implant, genital tract
    postprocedural or postoperative — *see* Complications, genitourinary, postprocedural
    specified NEC N99.89
  mastoid (process) procedure
    intraoperative H95.88
      hematoma — *see* Complications, intraoperative, hemorrhage (hematoma) (of), mastoid process
      hemorrhage — *see* Complications, intraoperative, hemorrhage (hematoma) (of), mastoid process
      laceration — *see* Complications, intraoperative, puncture or laceration, mastoid process
      specified NEC H95.88
    postmastoidectomy — *see* Complications, postmastoidectomy
    postoperative H95.89
      external ear canal stenosis H95.81 ☑
      hematoma — *see* Complications, postprocedural, hematoma (of), mastoid process
      hemorrhage — *see* Complications, postprocedural, hemorrhage (of), mastoid process
      postmastoidectomy — *see* Complications, postmastoidectomy
      seroma — *see* Complications, postprocedural, seroma (of), mastoid process
      specified NEC H95.89
  mastoidectomy cavity — *see* Complications, postmastoidectomy
  mechanical — *see* Complications, by site and type, mechanical
  medical procedures (*see also* Complication(s), intraoperative) T88.9 ☑
  metabolic E88.9
    postoperative E89.89
    specified NEC E89.89
  molar pregnancy NOS O08.9
    damage to pelvic organs O08.6
    embolism O08.2
    genital infection O08.0
    hemorrhage (delayed) (excessive) O08.1
    metabolic disorder O08.5
    renal failure O08.4
    shock O08.3
    specified type NEC O08.0
    venous complication NEC O08.7

**Complication**(s) — *continued*
  musculoskeletal system (*see also* Complication, intraoperative (intraprocedural), by site)
    device, implant or graft NEC — *see* Complications, orthopedic, device or implant
    internal fixation (nail) (plate) (rod) — *see* Complications, fixation device, internal
    joint prosthesis — *see* Complications, joint prosthesis
    post radiation M96.89
      kyphosis M96.2
      scoliosis M96.5
      specified complication NEC M96.89
    postoperative (postprocedural) M96.89
      with osteoporosis — *see* Osteoporosis
      fracture following insertion of device — *see* Fracture, following insertion of orthopedic implant, joint prosthesis or bone plate
      joint instability after prosthesis removal M96.89
      lordosis M96.4
      postlaminectomy syndrome NEC M96.1
        kyphosis M96.3
      pseudarthrosis M96.0
      specified complication NEC M96.89
  nephrostomy (stoma) — *see* Complications, stoma, urinary tract, external NEC
  nervous system G98.8
    central G96.9
    device, implant or graft (*see also* Complication, prosthetic device or implant, specified NEC)
      electronic stimulator (electrode(s)) — *see* Complications, electronic stimulator device
      specified NEC
        infection and inflammation T85.738 ☑
        mechanical T85.695 ☑
          breakdown T85.615 ☑
          displacement T85.625 ☑
          leakage T85.635 ☑
          malfunction T85.695 ☑
          malposition T85.625 ☑
          obstruction T85.695 ☑
          perforation T85.695 ☑
          protrusion T85.695 ☑
          specified NEC T85.695 ☑
      ventricular shunt — *see* Complications, ventricular shunt
    electronic stimulator (electrode(s)) — *see* Complications, electronic stimulator device
    postprocedural G97.82
      intracranial hypotension G97.2
      specified NEC G97.82
      spinal fluid leak G97.0
  newborn, due to intrauterine (fetal) procedure P96.5
  nonabsorbable (permanent) sutures — *see* Complication, sutures, permanent
  obstetric O75.9
    procedure (instrumental) (manual) (surgical) specified NEC O75.4
    specified NEC O75.89
    surgical wound NEC O90.89
      hematoma O90.2
      infection O86.0
  ocular lens implant — *see* Complications, intraocular lens
  ophthalmologic
    postprocedural bleb — *see* Blebitis
  orbital prosthesis T85.9 ☑
    embolism T85.818 ☑
    fibrosis T85.828 ☑
    hemorrhage T85.838 ☑
    infection and inflammation T85.79 ☑
    mechanical
      breakdown T85.31- ☑
      displacement T85.32- ☑
      malposition T85.32- ☑
      obstruction T85.39- ☑
      perforation T85.39- ☑
      protrusion T85.39- ☑
      specified NEC T85.39- ☑
    pain T85.848 ☑
    specified type NEC T85.898 ☑
    stenosis T85.858 ☑
    thrombosis T85.868 ☑
  organ or tissue transplant (partial) (total) — *see* Complications, transplant

☑ **Additional Character Required** — **Refer to the Tabular List for Character Selection**  ▽ **Subterms under main terms may continue to next column or page**

**Complication**(s) — *continued*
  orthopedic (*see also* Disorder, soft tissue)
    device or implant T84.9 ☑
      bone
        device or implant — *see* Complication,
          bone, device NEC
        graft — *see* Complication, graft, bone
      breakdown T84.418 ☑
      displacement T84.428 ☑
      electronic bone stimulator — *see* Complica-
        tions, electronic stimulator device, bone
      embolism T84.81 ☑
      fibrosis T84.82 ☑
      fixation device — *see* Complication, fixation
        device, internal
      hemorrhage T84.83 ☑
      infection or inflammation T84.7 ☑
      joint prosthesis — *see* Complication, joint
        prosthesis, internal
      malfunction T84.418 ☑
      malposition T84.428 ☑
      mechanical NEC T84.498 ☑
      muscle graft — *see* Complications, graft, muscle
      obstruction T84.498 ☑
      pain T84.84 ☑
      perforation T84.498 ☑
      protrusion T84.498 ☑
      specified complication NEC T84.89 ☑
      stenosis T84.85 ☑
      tendon graft — *see* Complications, graft, ten-
        don
      thrombosis T84.86 ☑
    fracture (following insertion of device) — *see*
      Fracture, following insertion of orthopedic
      implant, joint prosthesis or bone plate
    postprocedural M96.89
      fracture — *see* Fracture, following insertion of
        orthopedic implant, joint prosthesis or
        bone plate
      postlaminectomy syndrome NEC M96.1
        kyphosis M96.3
        lordosis M96.4
      postradiation
        kyphosis M96.2
        scoliosis M96.5
      pseudarthrosis post-fusion M96.0
      specified type NEC M96.89
  pacemaker (cardiac) — *see* Complications, cardiovas-
    cular device or implant, electronic
  pancreas transplant — *see* Complications, transplant,
    pancreas
  penile prosthesis (implant) — *see* Complications,
    prosthetic device, penile
  perfusion NEC T80.90 ☑
  perineal repair (obstetrical) NEC O90.89
    disruption O90.1
    hematoma O90.2
    infection (following delivery) O86.0
  phototherapy T88.9 ☑
    specified NEC T88.8 ☑
  postmastoidectomy NEC H95.19- ☑
    cyst, mucosal H95.13- ☑
    granulation H95.12- ☑
    inflammation, chronic H95.11- ☑
    recurrent cholesteatoma H95.0- ☑
  postoperative — *see* Complications, postprocedural
    circulatory — *see* Complications, circulatory system
    ear — *see* Complications, ear
    endocrine — *see* Complications, endocrine
    eye — *see* Complications, eye
    lumbar puncture G97.1
      cerebrospinal fluid leak G97.0
    nervous system (central) (peripheral) — *see* Com-
      plications, nervous system
    respiratory system — *see* Complications, respirato-
      ry system
  postprocedural (*see also* Complications, surgical pro-
    cedure)
    cardiac arrest (*see also* Infarct, myocardium, associ-
      ated with revascularization procedure)
      following cardiac surgery I97.120
      following other surgery I97.121
    cardiac functional disturbance NEC (*see also* Infarct,
      myocardium, associated with revascularia-
      tion procedure)
      following cardiac surgery I97.190

**Complication**(s) — *continued*
  postprocedural (*see also* Complications, surgical pro-
    cedure) — *continued*
    cardiac functional disturbance (*see also* Infarct,
      myocardium, associated with revasculariza-
      tion procedure) — *continued*
      following other surgery I97.191
    cardiac insufficiency
      following cardiac surgery I97.110
      following other surgery I97.111
    chorioretinal scars following retinal surgery
      H59.81- ☑
    following cataract surgery
      cataract (lens) fragments H59.02- ☑
      cystoid macular edema H59.03- ☑
      specified NEC H59.09- ☑
      vitreous (touch) syndrome H59.01- ☑
    heart failure
      following cardiac surgery I97.130
      following other surgery I97.131
    hematoma (of)
      circulatory system organ or structure
        following cardiac bypass I97.631
        following cardiac catheterization I97.630
        following other circulatory system proce-
          dure I97.638
        following other procedure I97.621
      digestive system
        following procedure on digestive system
          K91.870
        following procedure on other organ K91.871
      ear
        following other procedure H95.52
        following procedure on ear and mastoid
          process H95.51
      endocrine system
        following endocrine system procedure
          E89.820
        following other procedure E89.821
      eye and adnexa
        following ophthalmic procedure H59.33- ☑
        following other procedure H59.34- ☑
      genitourinary organ or structure
        following procedure on genitourinary organ
          or structure N99.840
        following procedure on other organ
          N99.841
      mastoid process
        following other procedure H95.52
        following procedure on ear and mastoid
          process H95.51
      musculoskeletal structure
        following musculoskeletal surgery M96.840
        following non-orthopedic surgery M96.841
        following orthopedic surgery M96.840
      nervous system
        following nervous system procedure G97.61
        following other procedure G97.62
      respiratory system
        following other procedure J95.861
        following procedure on respiratory system
          organ or structure J95.860
      skin and subcutaneous tissue
        following dermatologic procedure L76.31
        following procedure on other organ L76.32
      spleen
        following procedure on other organ D78.32
        following procedure on the spleen D78.31
    hemorrhage (of)
      circulatory system organ or structure
        following cardiac bypass I97.611
        following cardiac catheterization I97.610
        following other circulatory system proce-
          dure I97.618
        following other procedure I97.620
      digestive system
        following procedure on digestive system
          K91.840
        following procedure on other organ K91.841
      ear
        following other procedure H95.42
        following procedure on ear and mastoid
          process H95.41
      endocrine system
        following endocrine system procedure
          E89.810
        following other procedure E89.811

**Complication**(s) — *continued*
  postprocedural (*see also* Complications, surgical pro-
    cedure) — *continued*
    hemorrhage — *continued*
      eye and adnexa
        following ophthalmic procedure H59.31- ☑
        following other procedure H59.32- ☑
      genitourinary organ or structure
        following procedure on genitourinary organ
          or structure N99.820
        following procedure on other organ
          N99.821
      mastoid process
        following other procedure H95.42
        following procedure on ear and mastoid
          process H95.41
      musculoskeletal structure
        following musculoskeletal surgery M96.830
        following non-orthopedic surgery M96.831
        following orthopedic surgery M96.830
      nervous system
        following nervous system procedure G97.51
        following other procedure G97.52
      respiratory system
        following a respiratory system procedure
          J95.830
        following other procedure J95.831
      skin and subcutaneous tissue
        following a procedure on other organ
          L76.22
        following dermatologic procedure L76.21
      spleen
        following procedure on other organ D78.22
        following procedure on the spleen D78.21
    seroma (of)
      circulatory system organ or structure
        following cardiac bypass I97.641
        following cardiac catheterization I97.640
        following other circulatory system proce-
          dure I97.648
        following other procedure I97.622
      digestive system
        following procedure on digestive system
          K91.872
        following procedure on other organ K91.873
      ear
        following other procedure H95.54
        following procedure on ear and mastoid
          process H95.53
      endocrine system
        following endocrine system procedure
          E89.822
        following other procedure E89.823
      eye and adnexa
        following ophthalmic procedure H59.35- ☑
        following other procedure H59.36- ☑
      genitourinary organ or structure
        following procedure on genitourinary organ
          or structure N99.842
        following procedure on other organ
          N99.843
      mastoid process
        following other procedure H95.54
        following procedure on ear and mastoid
          process H95.53
      musculoskeletal structure
        following musculoskeletal surgery M96.842
        following non-orthopedic surgery M96.843
        following orthopedic surgery M96.842
      nervous system
        following nervous system procedure G97.63
        following other procedure G97.64
      respiratory system
        following other procedure J95.863
        following procedure on respiratory system
          organ or structure J95.862
      skin and subcutaneous tissue
        following dermatologic procedure L76.33
        following procedure on other organ L76.34
      spleen
        following procedure on other organ D78.34
        following procedure on the spleen D78.33
    specified NEC
      circulatory system I97.89
      digestive K91.89
      ear H95.89
      endocrine E89.89
      eye and adnexa H59.89
      genitourinary N99.89

**Complication**(s) — *continued*
  postprocedural (*see also* Complications, surgical procedure) — *continued*
    specified — *continued*
      mastoid process H95.89
      metabolic E89.89
      musculoskeletal structure M96.89
      nervous system G97.82
      respiratory system J95.89
      skin and subcutaneous tissue L76.82
      spleen D78.89
  pregnancy NEC — *see* Pregnancy, complicated by
  prosthetic device or implant T85.9 ☑
    bile duct — *see* Complications, bile duct implant
    breast — *see* Complications, breast implant
    bulking agent
      ureteral
        erosion T83.714 ☑
        exposure T83.724 ☑
      urethral
        erosion T83.713 ☑
        exposure T83.723 ☑
    cardiac and vascular NEC — *see* Complications, cardiovascular device or implant
    corneal transplant — *see* Complications, graft, cornea
    electronic nervous system stimulator — *see* Complications, electronic stimulator device
    epidural infusion catheter — *see* Complications, catheter, epidural
    esophageal anti-reflux device — *see* Complications, esophageal anti-reflux device
    genital organ or tract — *see* Complications, genitourinary, device or implant, genital tract
      specified NEC T83.79- ☑
    heart valve — *see* Complications, heart, valve, prosthesis
    infection or inflammation T85.79 ☑
      intestine transplant T86.892
      liver transplant T86.43
      lung transplant T86.812
      pancreas transplant T86.892
      skin graft T86.822
    intraocular lens — *see* Complications, intraocular lens
    intraperitoneal (dialysis) catheter — *see* Complications, catheter, intraperitoneal
    joint — *see* Complications, joint prosthesis, internal
    mechanical NEC T85.698 ☑
      dialysis catheter (vascular) (*see also* Complication, catheter, dialysis, mechanical)
        peritoneal — *see* Complication, catheter, intraperitoneal, mechanical
      gastrointestinal device T85.598 ☑
      ocular device T85.398 ☑
      subdural (infusion) catheter T85.690 ☑
      suture, permanent T85.692 ☑
        that for bone repair — *see* Complications, fixation device, internal (orthopedic), mechanical
      ventricular shunt
        breakdown T85.01 ☑
        displacement T85.02 ☑
        leakage T85.03 ☑
        malposition T85.02 ☑
        obstruction T85.09 ☑
        perforation T85.09 ☑
        protrusion T85.09 ☑
        specified NEC T85.09 ☑
    mesh
      erosion (to surrounding organ or tissue) T83.718 ☑
        urethral (into pelvic floor muscles) T83.712 ☑
        vaginal (into pelvic floor muscles) T83.711 ☑
      exposure (into surrounding organ or tissue) T83.728 ☑
        urethral (through urethral wall) T83.722 ☑
        vaginal (into vagina) (through vaginal wall) T83.721 ☑
    orbital — *see* Complications, orbital prosthesis
    penile T83.9 ☑
      embolism T83.81 ☑
      fibrosis T83.82 ☑
      hemorrhage T83.83 ☑
      infection and inflammation T83.61 ☑

**Complication**(s) — *continued*
  prosthetic device or implant — *continued*
    penile — *continued*
      mechanical
        breakdown T83.410 ☑
        displacement T83.420 ☑
        leakage T83.490 ☑
        malposition T83.420 ☑
        obstruction T83.490 ☑
        perforation T83.490 ☑
        protrusion T83.490 ☑
        specified NEC T83.490 ☑
      pain T83.84 ☑
      specified type NEC T83.89 ☑
      stenosis T83.85 ☑
      thrombosis T83.86 ☑
    prosthetic materials NEC
      erosion (to surrounding organ or tissue) T83.718 ☑
      exposure (into surrounding organ or tissue) T83.728 ☑
    skin graft T86.829
      artificial skin or decellularized allodermis
        embolism T85.818 ☑
        fibrosis T85.828 ☑
        hemorrhage T85.838 ☑
        infection and inflammation T85.79 ☑
        mechanical
          breakdown T85.613 ☑
          displacement T85.623 ☑
          malfunction T85.613 ☑
          malposition T85.623 ☑
          obstruction T85.693 ☑
          perforation T85.693 ☑
          protrusion T85.693 ☑
          specified NEC T85.693 ☑
        pain T85.848 ☑
        specified type NEC T85.898 ☑
        stenosis T85.858 ☑
        thrombosis T85.868 ☑
      failure T86.821
      infection T86.822
      rejection T86.820
      specified NEC T86.828
    sling
      urethral (female) (male)
        erosion T83.712 ☑
        exposure T83.722 ☑
    specified NEC T85.9 ☑
      embolism T85.818 ☑
      fibrosis T85.828 ☑
      hemorrhage T85.838 ☑
      infection and inflammation T85.79 ☑
      mechanical
        breakdown T85.618 ☑
        displacement T85.628 ☑
        leakage T85.638 ☑
        malfunction T85.618 ☑
        malposition T85.628 ☑
        obstruction T85.698 ☑
        perforation T85.698 ☑
        protrusion T85.698 ☑
        specified NEC T85.698 ☑
      pain T85.848 ☑
      specified type NEC T85.898 ☑
      stenosis T85.858 ☑
      thrombosis T85.868 ☑
    subdural infusion catheter — *see* Complications, catheter, subdural
    sutures — *see* Complications, sutures
    urinary organ or tract NEC — *see* Complications, genitourinary, device or implant, urinary system
    vascular — *see* Complications, cardiovascular device or implant
    ventricular shunt — *see* Complications, ventricular shunt (device)
  puerperium — *see* Puerperal
  puncture, spinal G97.1
    cerebrospinal fluid leak G97.0
    headache or reaction G97.1
  pyelogram N99.89
  radiation
    kyphosis M96.2
    scoliosis M96.5

**Complication**(s) — *continued*
  reattached
    extremity (infection) (rejection)
      lower T87.1X- ☑
      upper T87.0X- ☑
    specified body part NEC T87.2
  reconstructed breast
    asymmetry between native and reconstructed breast N65.1
    deformity N65.0
    disproportion between native and reconstructed breast N65.1
    excess tissue N65.0
    misshappen N65.0
  reimplant NEC (*see also* Complications, prosthetic device or implant)
    limb (infection) (rejection) — *see* Complications, reattached, extremity
    organ (partial) (total) — *see* Complications, transplant
    prosthetic device NEC — *see* Complications, prosthetic device
  renal N28.9
    allograft — *see* Complications, transplant, kidney
    dialysis — *see* Complications, dialysis
  respirator
    mechanical J95.850
      specified NEC J95.859
  respiratory system J98.9
    device, implant or graft — *see* Complication, prosthetic device or implant, specified NEC
    lung transplant — *see* Complications, prosthetic device or implant, lung transplant
    postoperative J95.89
      air leak J95.812
      Mendelson's syndrome (chemical pneumonitis) J95.4
      pneumothorax J95.811
      pulmonary insufficiency (acute) (after nonthoracic surgery) J95.2
        chronic J95.3
        following thoracic surgery J95.1
      respiratory failure (acute) J95.821
        acute and chronic J95.822
      specified NEC J95.89
      subglottic stenosis J95.5
      tracheostomy complication — *see* Complications, tracheostomy
    therapy T81.89 ☑
  sedation during labor and delivery O74.9
    cardiac O74.2
    central nervous system O74.3
    pulmonary NEC O74.1
  shunt (*see also* Complications, prosthetic device or implant)
    arteriovenous — *see* Complications, arteriovenous, shunt
    ventricular (communicating) — *see* Complications, ventricular shunt
  skin
    graft T86.829
      failure T86.821
      infection T86.822
      rejection T86.820
      specified type NEC T86.828
  spinal
    anesthesia — *see* Complications, anesthesia, spinal
    catheter (epidural) (subdural) — *see* Complications, catheter
    puncture or tap G97.1
      cerebrospinal fluid leak G97.0
      headache or reaction G97.1
  stent
    bile duct — *see* Complications, bile duct prosthesis
    ureteral indwelling
      breakdown T83.112 ☑
      displacement T83.122 ☑
      leakage T83.192 ☑
      malposition T83.122 ☑
      obstruction T83.192 ☑
      perforation T83.192 ☑
      protrusion T83.192 ☑
      specified NEC T83.192 ☑
    urinary NEC (ileal conduit) (nephroureteral) T83.193 ☑
      embolism T83.81 ☑
      fibrosis T83.82 ☑
      hemorrhage T83.83 ☑

**Complication**(s) — *continued*
  stent — *continued*
    urinary — *continued*
      infection and inflammation T83.593 ☑
      mechanical
        breakdown T83.113 ☑
        displacement T83.123 ☑
        leakage T83.193 ☑
        malposition T83.123 ☑
        obstruction T83.193 ☑
        perforation T83.193 ☑
        protrusion T83.193 ☑
        specified NEC T83.193 ☑
      pain T83.84 ☑
      specified type NEC T83.89 ☑
      stenosis T83.85 ☑
      thrombosis T83.86 ☑
    vascular
      end stent stenosis — *see* Restenosis, stent
      in stent stenosis — *see* Restenosis, stent
  stoma
    digestive tract
      colostomy — *see* Complications, colostomy
      enterostomy — *see* Complications, enterosto-
        my
      esophagostomy — *see* Complications,
        esophagostomy
      gastrostomy — *see* Complications, gastrostomy
    urinary tract N99.528
      continent N99.538
        hemorrhage N99.530
        herniation N99.533
        infection N99.531
        malfunction N99.532
        specified type NEC N99.538
        stenosis N99.534
      cystostomy — *see* Complications, cystostomy
      external NOS N99.528
      hemorrhage N99.520
      herniation N99.523
      incontinent N99.528
        hemorrhage N99.520
        herniation N99.523
        infection N99.521
        malfunction N99.522
        specified type NEC N99.528
        stenosis N99.524
      infection N99.521
      malfunction N99.522
      specified type NEC N99.528
      stenosis N99.524
  stomach banding — *see* Complication(s), bariatric
    procedure
  stomach stapling — *see* Complication(s), bariatric
    procedure
  surgical material, nonabsorbable — *see* Complication,
    suture, permanent
  surgical procedure (on) T81.9 ☑
    amputation stump (late) — *see* Complications,
      amputation stump
    cardiac — *see* Complications, circulatory system
    cholesteatoma, recurrent — *see* Complications,
      postmastoidectomy, recurrent
      cholesteatoma
    circulatory (early) — *see* Complications, circulatory
      system
    digestive system — *see* Complications, gastroin-
      testinal
    dumping syndrome (postgastrectomy) K91.1
    ear — *see* Complications, ear
    elephantiasis or lymphedema I97.89
      postmastectomy I97.2
    emphysema (surgical) T81.82 ☑
    endocrine — *see* Complications, endocrine
    eye — *see* Complications, eye
    fistula (persistent postoperative) T81.83 ☑
    foreign body inadvertently left in wound (sponge)
      (suture) (swab) — *see* Foreign body, acciden-
      tally left during a procedure
    gastrointestinal — *see* Complications, gastrointesti-
      nal
    genitourinary NEC N99.89
    hematoma
      intraoperative — *see* Complication, intraopera-
        tive, hemorrhage
      postprocedural — *see* Complication, postpro-
        cedural, hematoma

**Complication**(s) — *continued*
  surgical procedure — *continued*
    hemorrhage
      intraoperative — *see* Complication, intraopera-
        tive, hemorrhage
      postprocedural — *see* Complication, postpro-
        cedural, hemorrhage
    hepatic failure K91.82
    hyperglycemia (postpancreatectomy) E89.1
    hypoinsulinemia (postpancreatectomy) E89.1
    hypoparathyroidism (postparathyroidectomy)
      E89.2
    hypopituitarism (posthypophysectomy) E89.3
    hypothyroidism (post-thyroidectomy) E89.0
    intestinal obstruction (*see also* Obstruction, intes-
      tine, postoperative) K91.30
    intracranial hypotension following ventricular
      shunting (ventriculostomy) G97.2
    lymphedema I97.89
      postmastectomy I97.2
    malabsorption (postsurgical) NEC K91.2
      osteoporosis — *see* Osteoporosis, postsurgical
      malabsorption
    mastoidectomy cavity NEC — *see* Complications,
      postmastoidectomy
    metabolic E89.89
      specified NEC E89.89
    musculoskeletal — *see* Complications, muscu-
      loskeletal system
    nervous system (central) (peripheral) — *see* Com-
      plications, nervous system
    ovarian failure E89.40
      asymptomatic E89.40
      symptomatic E89.41
    peripheral vascular — *see* Complications, surgical
      procedure, vascular
    postcardiotomy syndrome I97.0
    postcholecystectomy syndrome K91.5
    postcommissurotomy syndrome I97.0
    postgastrectomy dumping syndrome K91.1
    postlaminectomy syndrome NEC M96.1
      kyphosis M96.3
    postmastectomy lymphedema syndrome I97.2
    postmastoidectomy cholesteatoma — *see* Compli-
      cations, postmastoidectomy, recurrent
      cholesteatoma
    postvagotomy syndrome K91.1
    postvalvulotomy syndrome I97.0
    pulmonary insufficiency (acute) J95.2
      chronic J95.3
      following thoracic surgery J95.1
    reattached body part — *see* Complications, reat-
      tached
    respiratory — *see* Complications, respiratory sys-
      tem
    shock (hypovolemic) T81.19 ☑
    spleen (postoperative) D78.89
      intraoperative D78.81
    stitch abscess T81.4 ☑
    subglottic stenosis (postsurgical) J95.5
    testicular hypofunction E89.5
    transplant — *see* Complications, organ or tissue
      transplant
    urinary NEC N99.89
    vaginal vault prolapse (posthysterectomy) N99.3
    vascular (peripheral)
      artery T81.719 ☑
        mesenteric T81.710 ☑
        renal T81.711 ☑
        specified NEC T81.718 ☑
      vein T81.72 ☑
    wound infection T81.4 ☑
  suture, permanent (wire) NEC T85.9 ☑
    with repair of bone — *see* Complications, fixation
      device, internal
    embolism T85.818 ☑
    fibrosis T85.828 ☑
    hemorrhage T85.838 ☑
    infection and inflammation T85.79 ☑
    mechanical
      breakdown T85.612 ☑
      displacement T85.622 ☑
      malfunction T85.612 ☑
      malposition T85.622 ☑
      obstruction T85.692 ☑
      perforation T85.692 ☑
      protrusion T85.692 ☑

**Complication**(s) — *continued*
  suture, permanent — *continued*
    mechanical — *continued*
      specified NEC T85.692 ☑
    pain T85.848 ☑
    specified type NEC T85.898 ☑
    stenosis T85.858 ☑
    thrombosis T85.868 ☑
  tracheostomy J95.00
    granuloma J95.09
    hemorrhage J95.01
    infection J95.02
    malfunction J95.03
    mechanical J95.03
    obstruction J95.03
    specified type NEC J95.09
    tracheo-esophageal fistula J95.04
  transfusion (blood) (lymphocytes) (plasma) T80.92 ☑
    air emblism T80.0 ☑
    circulatory overload E87.71
    febrile nonhemolytic transfusion reaction R50.84
    hemochromatosis E83.111
    hemolysis T80.89 ☑
    hemolytic reaction (antigen unspecified)
      T80.919 ☑
    incompatibility reaction (antigen unspecified)
      T80.919 ☑
      ABO T80.30 ☑
        delayed serologic (DSTR) T80.39 ☑
        hemolytic transfusion reaction (HTR) (un-
          specified time after transfusion)
          T80.319 ☑
          acute (AHTR) (less than 24 hours after
            transfusion) T80.310 ☑
          delayed (DHTR) (24 hours or more after
            transfusion) T80.311 ☑
        specified NEC T80.39 ☑
      acute (antigen unspecified) T80.910 ☑
      delayed (antigen unspecified) T80.911 ☑
      delayed serologic (DSTR) T80.89 ☑
      non-ABO (minor antigens (Duffy) (Kell) (Kidd)
        (Lewis) (M) (N) (P) (S)) T80.A0 ☑ (*follow-*
        *ing* T80.4)
        delayed serologic (DSTR) T80.A9 ☑ (*follow-*
          *ing* T80.4)
        hemolytic transfusion reaction (HTR) (un-
          specified time after transfusion)
          T80.A19 ☑ (*following* T80.4)
          acute (AHTR) (less than 24 hours after
            transfusion) T80.A10 ☑ (*following*
            T80.4)
          delayed (DHTR) (24 hours or more after
            transfusion) T80.A11 ☑ (*following*
            T80.4)
        specified NEC T80.A9 ☑ (*following* T80.4)
      Rh (antigens (C) (c) (D) (E) (e)) (factor) T80.40 ☑
        delayed serologic (DSTR) T80.49 ☑
        hemolytic transfusion reaction (HTR) (un-
          specified time after transfusion)
          T80.419 ☑
          acute (AHTR) (less than 24 hours after
            transfusion) T80.410 ☑
          delayed (DHTR) (24 hours or more after
            transfusion) T80.411 ☑
        specified NEC T80.49 ☑
    infection T80.29 ☑
      acute T80.22- ☑
    reaction NEC T80.89 ☑
    sepsis T80.29 ☑
    shock T80.89 ☑
  transplant T86.90
    bone T86.839
      failure T86.831
      infection T86.832
      rejection T86.830
      specified type NEC T86.838
    bone marrow T86.00
      failure T86.02
      infection T86.03
      rejection T86.01
      specified type NEC T86.09
    cornea T86.849
      failure T86.841
      infection T86.842
      rejection T86.840
      specified type NEC T86.848
    failure T86.92

**Complication**(s) — *continued*
transplant — *continued*
heart T86.20
with lung T86.30
cardiac allograft vasculopathy T86.290
failure T86.32
infection T86.33
rejection T86.31
specified type NEC T86.39
failure T86.22
infection T86.23
rejection T86.21
specified type NEC T86.298
infection T86.93
intestine T86.859
failure T86.851
infection T86.852
rejection T86.850
specified type NEC T86.858
kidney T86.10
failure T86.12
infection T86.13
rejection T86.11
specified type NEC T86.19
liver T86.40
failure T86.42
infection T86.43
rejection T86.41
specified type NEC T86.49
lung T86.819
with heart T86.30
failure T86.32
infection T86.33
rejection T86.31
specified type NEC T86.39
failure T86.811
infection T86.812
rejection T86.810
specified type NEC T86.818
malignant neoplasm C80.2
pancreas T86.899
failure T86.891
infection T86.892
rejection T86.890
specified type NEC T86.898
peripheral blood stem cells T86.5
post-transplant lymphoproliferative disorder (PTLD) D47.Z1 (*following* D47.4)
rejection T86.91
skin T86.829
failure T86.821
infection T86.822
rejection T86.820
specified type NEC T86.828
specified
tissue T86.899
failure T86.891
infection T86.892
rejection T86.890
specified type NEC T86.898
type NEC T86.99
stem cell (from peripheral blood) (from umbilical cord) T86.5
umbilical cord stem cells T86.5
trauma (early) T79.9 ☑
specified NEC T79.8 ☑
ultrasound therapy NEC T88.9 ☑
umbilical cord NEC
complicating delivery O69.9 ☑
specified NEC O69.89 ☑
umbrella device, vascular T82.9 ☑
embolism T82.818 ☑
fibrosis T82.828 ☑
hemorrhage T82.838 ☑
infection or inflammation T82.7 ☑
mechanical
breakdown T82.515 ☑
displacement T82.525 ☑
leakage T82.535 ☑
malposition T82.525 ☑
obstruction T82.595 ☑
perforation T82.595 ☑
protrusion T82.595 ☑
pain T82.848 ☑
specified type NEC T82.898 ☑
stenosis T82.858 ☑
thrombosis T82.868 ☑

**Complication**(s) — *continued*
urethral catheter — *see* Complications, catheter, urethral, indwelling
vaccination T88.1 ☑
anaphylaxis NEC T80.52 ☑
arthropathy — *see* Arthropathy, postimmunization
cellulitis T88.0 ☑
encephalitis or encephalomyelitis G04.02
infection (general) (local) NEC T88.0 ☑
meningitis G03.8
myelitis G04.02
protein sickness T80.62 ☑
rash T88.1 ☑
reaction (allergic) T88.1 ☑
serum T80.62 ☑
sepsis T88.0 ☑
serum intoxication, sickness, rash, or other serum reaction NEC T80.62 ☑
anaphylactic shock T80.52 ☑
shock (allergic) (anaphylactic) T80.52 ☑
vaccinia (generalized) (localized) T88.1 ☑
vas deferens device or implant — *see* Complications, genitourinary, device or implant, genital tract
vascular I99.9
device or implant T82.9 ☑
embolism T82.818 ☑
fibrosis T82.828 ☑
hemorrhage T82.838 ☑
infection or inflammation T82.7 ☑
mechanical
breakdown T82.519 ☑
specified device NEC T82.518 ☑
displacement T82.529 ☑
specified device NEC T82.528 ☑
leakage T82.539 ☑
specified device NEC T82.538 ☑
malposition T82.529 ☑
specified device NEC T82.528 ☑
obstruction T82.599 ☑
specified device NEC T82.598 ☑
perforation T82.599 ☑
specified device NEC T82.598 ☑
protrusion T82.599 ☑
specified device NEC T82.598 ☑
pain T82.848 ☑
specified type NEC T82.898 ☑
stenosis T82.858 ☑
thrombosis T82.868 ☑
dialysis catheter — *see* Complication, catheter, dialysis
following infusion, therapeutic injection or transfusion T80.1 ☑
graft T82.9 ☑
embolism T82.818 ☑
fibrosis T82.828 ☑
hemorrhage T82.838 ☑
mechanical
breakdown T82.319 ☑
aorta (bifurcation) T82.310 ☑
carotid artery T82.311 ☑
specified vessel NEC T82.318 ☑
displacement T82.329 ☑
aorta (bifurcation) T82.320 ☑
carotid artery T82.321 ☑
specified vessel NEC T82.328 ☑
leakage T82.339 ☑
aorta (bifurcation) T82.330 ☑
carotid artery T82.331 ☑
specified vessel NEC T82.338 ☑
malposition T82.329 ☑
aorta (bifurcation) T82.320 ☑
carotid artery T82.321 ☑
specified vessel NEC T82.328 ☑
obstruction T82.399 ☑
aorta (bifurcation) T82.390 ☑
carotid artery T82.391 ☑
specified vessel NEC T82.398 ☑
perforation T82.399 ☑
aorta (bifurcation) T82.390 ☑
carotid artery T82.391 ☑
specified vessel NEC T82.398 ☑
protrusion T82.399 ☑
aorta (bifurcation) T82.390 ☑
carotid artery T82.391 ☑
specified vessel NEC T82.398 ☑
pain T82.848 ☑

**Complication**(s) — *continued*
vascular — *continued*
graft — *continued*
specified complication NEC T82.898 ☑
stenosis T82.858 ☑
thrombosis T82.868 ☑
postoperative — *see* Complications, postoperative, circulatory
vena cava device (filter) (sieve) (umbrella) — *see* Complications, umbrella device, vascular
ventilation therapy NEC T81.81 ☑
ventilator
mechanical J95.850
specified NEC J95.859
ventricular (communicating) shunt (device) T85.9 ☑
embolism T85.810 ☑
fibrosis T85.820 ☑
hemorrhage T85.830 ☑
infection and inflammation T85.730 ☑
mechanical
breakdown T85.01 ☑
displacement T85.02 ☑
leakage T85.03 ☑
malposition T85.02 ☑
obstruction T85.09 ☑
perforation T85.09 ☑
protrusion T85.09 ☑
specified NEC T85.09 ☑
pain T85.840 ☑
specified type NEC T85.890 ☑
stenosis T85.850 ☑
thrombosis T85.860 ☑
wire suture, permanent (implanted) — *see* Complications, suture, permanent
**Compressed air disease** T70.3 ☑
**Compression**
with injury — *code by* Nature of injury
artery I77.1
celiac, syndrome I77.4
brachial plexus G54.0
brain (stem) G93.5
due to
contusion (diffuse) — *see* Injury, intracranial, diffuse
focal — *see* Injury, intracranial, focal
injury NEC — *see* Injury, intracranial, diffuse
traumatic — *see* Injury, intracranial, diffuse
bronchus J98.09
cauda equina G83.4
celiac (artery) (axis) I77.4
cerebral — *see* Compression, brain
cervical plexus G54.2
cord
spinal — *see* Compression, spinal
umbilical — *see* Compression, umbilical cord
cranial nerve G52.9
eighth H93.3 ☑
eleventh G52.8
fifth G50.8
first G52.0
fourth — *see* Strabismus, paralytic, fourth nerve
ninth G52.1
second — *see* Disorder, nerve, optic
seventh G51.8
sixth — *see* Strabismus, paralytic, sixth nerve
tenth G52.2
third — *see* Strabismus, paralytic, third nerve
twelfth G52.3
diver's squeeze T70.3 ☑
during birth (newborn) P15.9
esophagus K22.2
eustachian tube — *see* Obstruction, eustachian tube, cartilaginous
facies Q67.1
fracture
nontraumatic NOS — *see* Collapse, vertebra
pathological — *see* Fracture, pathological
traumatic — *see* Fracture, traumatic
heart — *see* Disease, heart
intestine — *see* Obstruction, intestine
laryngeal nerve, recurrent G52.2
with paralysis of vocal cords and larynx J38.00
bilateral J38.02
unilateral J38.01
lumbosacral plexus G54.1
lung J98.4
lymphatic vessel I89.0

☑ **Additional Character Required** — Refer to the Tabular List for Character Selection ▽ Subterms under main terms may continue to next column or page

**Compression** — *continued*
　medulla — *see* Compression, brain
　nerve (*see also* Disorder, nerve) G58.9
　　arm NEC — *see* Mononeuropathy, upper limb
　　axillary G54.0
　　cranial — *see* Compression, cranial nerve
　　leg NEC — *see* Mononeuropathy, lower limb
　　median (in carpal tunnel) — *see* Syndrome, carpal tunnel
　　optic — *see* Disorder, nerve, optic
　　plantar — *see* Lesion, nerve, plantar
　　posterior tibial (in tarsal tunnel) — *see* Syndrome, tarsal tunnel
　　root or plexus NOS (in) G54.9
　　　intervertebral disc disorder NEC — *see* Disorder, disc, with, radiculopathy
　　　　with myelopathy — *see* Disorder, disc, with, myelopathy
　　　neoplastic disease (*see also* Neoplasm) D49.9 [G55]
　　　spondylosis — *see* Spondylosis, with radiculopathy
　　sciatic (acute) — *see* Lesion, nerve, sciatic
　　sympathetic G90.8
　　traumatic — *see* Injury, nerve
　　ulnar — *see* Lesion, nerve, ulnar
　　upper extremity NEC — *see* Mononeuropathy, upper limb
　spinal (cord) G95.20
　　by displacement of intervertebral disc NEC (*see also* Disorder, disc, with, myelopathy)
　　nerve root NOS G54.9
　　　due to displacement of intervertebral disc NEC — *see* Disorder, disc, with, radiculopathy
　　　　with myelopathy — *see* Disorder, disc, with, myelopathy
　　specified NEC G95.29
　　spondylogenic (cervical) (lumbar, lumbosacral) (thoracic) — *see* Spondylosis, with myelopathy NEC
　　anterior — *see* Syndrome, anterior, spinal artery, compression
　　traumatic — *see* Injury, spinal cord, by region
　subcostal nerve (syndrome) — *see* Mononeuropathy, upper limb, specified NEC
　sympathetic nerve NEC G90.8
　syndrome T79.5 ☑
　trachea J39.8
　ulnar nerve (by scar tissue) — *see* Lesion, nerve, ulnar
　umbilical cord
　　complicating delivery O69.2 ☑
　　　cord around neck O69.1 ☑
　　　prolapse O69.0 ☑
　　　specified NEC O69.2 ☑
　ureter N13.5
　vein I87.1
　vena cava (inferior) (superior) I87.1
**Compulsion, compulsive**
　gambling F63.0
　neurosis F42.8
　personality F60.5
　states F42.8
　swearing F42.8
　　in Gilles de la Tourette's syndrome F95.2
　tics and spasms F95.9
**Concato's disease** (pericardial polyserositis) A19.9
　nontubercular I31.1
　pleural — *see* Pleurisy, with effusion
**Concavity chest wall** M95.4
**Concealed penis** Q55.69
**Concern** (normal) **about sick person in family** Z63.6
**Concrescence** (teeth) K00.2
**Concretio cordis** I31.1
　rheumatic I09.2
**Concretion** (*see also* Calculus)
　appendicular K38.1
　canaliculus — *see* Dacryolith
　clitoris N90.89
　conjunctiva H11.12- ☑
　eyelid — *see* Disorder, eyelid, specified type NEC
　lacrimal passages — *see* Dacryolith
　prepuce (male) N47.8
　salivary gland (any) K11.5
　seminal vesicle N50.89
　tonsil J35.8
**Concussion** (brain) (cerebral) (current) S06.0X9 ☑

**Concussion** — *continued*
　with
　　loss of consciousness of 30 minutes or less S06.0X1 ☑
　　loss of consciousness of unspecified duration S06.0X9 ☑
　　without loss of consciousness S06.0X0 ☑
　blast (air) (hydraulic) (immersion) (underwater)
　　abdomen or thorax — *see* Injury, blast, by site
　　ear with acoustic nerve injury — *see* Injury, nerve, acoustic, specified type NEC
　cauda equina S34.3 ☑
　conus medullaris S34.02 ☑
　ocular S05.8X- ☑
　spinal (cord)
　　cervical S14.0 ☑
　　lumbar S34.01 ☑
　　sacral S34.02 ☑
　　thoracic S24.0 ☑
　syndrome F07.81
**Condition** — *see* Disease
**Conditions arising in the perinatal period** — *see* Newborn, affected by
**Conduct disorder** — *see* Disorder, conduct
**Condyloma** A63.0
　acuminatum A63.0
　gonorrheal A54.09
　latum A51.31
　syphilitic A51.31
　　congenital A50.07
　venereal, syphilitic A51.31
**Conflagration** (*see also* Burn)
　asphyxia (by inhalation of gases, fumes or vapors) (*see also* Table of Drugs and Chemicals) T59.9- ☑
**Conflict** (with) (*see also* Discord)
　family Z73.9
　marital Z63.0
　　involving divorce or estrangement Z63.5
　parent-child Z62.820
　　parent-adopted child Z62.821
　　parent-biological child Z62.820
　　parent-foster child Z62.822
　social role NEC Z73.5
**Confluent** — *see* condition
**Confusion, confused** R41.0
　epileptic F05
　mental state (psychogenic) F44.89
　psychogenic F44.89
　reactive (from emotional stress, psychological trauma) F44.89
**Confusional arousals** G47.51
**Congelation** T69.9 ☑
**Congenital** (*see also* condition)
　aortic septum Q25.49
　intrinsic factor deficiency D51.0
　malformation — *see* Anomaly
**Congestion, congestive**
　bladder N32.89
　bowel K63.89
　brain G93.89
　breast N64.59
　bronchial J98.09
　catarrhal J31.0
　chest R09.89
　chill, malarial — *see* Malaria
　circulatory NEC I99.8
　duodenum K31.89
　eye — *see* Hyperemia, conjunctiva
　facial, due to birth injury P15.4
　general R68.89
　glottis J37.0
　heart — *see* Failure, heart, congestive
　hepatic K76.1
　hypostatic (lung) — *see* Edema, lung
　intestine K63.89
　kidney N28.89
　labyrinth H83.8 ☑
　larynx J37.0
　liver K76.1
　lung R09.89
　　active or acute — *see* Pneumonia
　malaria, malarial — *see* Malaria
　nasal R09.81
　nose R09.81
　orbit, orbital (*see also* Exophthalmos)
　　inflammatory (chronic) — *see* Inflammation, orbit
　ovary N83.8

**Congestion, congestive** — *continued*
　pancreas K86.89
　pelvic, female N94.89
　pleural J94.8
　prostate (active) N42.1
　pulmonary — *see* Congestion, lung
　renal N28.89
　retina H35.81
　seminal vesicle N50.1
　spinal cord G95.19
　spleen (chronic) D73.2
　stomach K31.89
　trachea — *see* Tracheitis
　urethra N36.8
　uterus N85.8
　　with subinvolution N85.3
　venous (passive) I87.8
　viscera R68.89
**Congestive** — *see* Congestion
**Conical**
　cervix (hypertrophic elongation) N88.4
　cornea — *see* Keratoconus
　teeth K00.2
**Conjoined twins** Q89.4
**Conjugal maladjustment** Z63.0
　involving divorce or estrangement Z63.5
**Conjunctiva** — *see* condition
**Conjunctivitis** (staphylococcal) (streptococcal) NOS H10.9
　Acanthamoeba B60.12
　acute H10.3- ☑
　　atopic H10.1- ☑
　　chemical (*see also* Corrosion, cornea) H10.21- ☑
　　mucopurulent H10.02- ☑
　　　follicular H10.01- ☑
　　pseudomembranous H10.22- ☑
　　serous except viral H10.23- ☑
　　viral — *see* Conjunctivitis, viral
　　toxic H10.21- ☑
　adenoviral (acute) (follicular) B30.1
　allergic (acute) — *see* Conjunctivitis, acute, atopic
　　chronic H10.45
　　　vernal H10.44
　anaphylactic — *see* Conjunctivitis, acute, atopic
　Apollo B30.3
　atopic (acute) — *see* Conjunctivitis, acute, atopic
　Béal's B30.2
　blennorrhagic (gonococcal) (neonatorum) A54.31
　chemical (acute) (*see also* Corrosion, cornea) H10.21- ☑
　chlamydial A74.0
　　due to trachoma A71.1
　　neonatal P39.1
　chronic (nodosa) (petrificans) (phlyctenular) H10.40- ☑
　　allergic H10.45
　　　vernal H10.44
　　follicular H10.43- ☑
　　giant papillary H10.41- ☑
　　simple H10.42- ☑
　　vernal H10.44
　coxsackievirus 24 B30.3
　diphtheritic A36.86
　due to
　　dust — *see* Conjunctivitis, acute, atopic
　　filariasis B74.9
　　mucocutaneous leishmaniasis B55.2
　enterovirus type 70 (hemorrhagic) B30.3
　epidemic (viral) B30.9
　　hemorrhagic B30.3
　gonococcal (neonatorum) A54.31
　granular (trachomatous) A71.1
　　sequelae (late effect) B94.0
　hemorrhagic (acute) (epidemic) B30.3
　herpes zoster B02.31
　in (due to)
　　Acanthamoeba B60.12
　　adenovirus (acute) (follicular) B30.1
　　Chlamydia A74.0
　　coxsackievirus 24 B30.3
　　diphtheria A36.86
　　enterovirus type 70 (hemorrhagic) B30.3
　　filariasis B74.9
　　gonococci A54.31
　　herpes (simplex) virus B00.53
　　　zoster B02.31
　　infectious disease NEC B99 ☑
　　meningococci A39.89
　　mucocutaneous leishmaniasis B55.2

**Conjunctivitis** — continued
- in — continued
  - rosacea L71.9
  - syphilis (late) A52.71
  - zoster B02.31
- inclusion A74.0
- infantile P39.1
  - gonococcal A54.31
- Koch-Weeks' — see Conjunctivitis, acute, mucopurulent
- light — see Conjunctivitis, acute, atopic
- ligneous — see Blepharoconjunctivitis, ligneous
- meningococcal A39.89
- mucopurulent — see Conjunctivitis, acute, mucopurulent
- neonatal P39.1
  - gonococcal A54.31
- Newcastle B30.8
- of Béal B30.2
- parasitic
  - filariasis B74.9
  - mucocutaneous leishmaniasis B55.2
- Parinaud's H10.89
- petrificans H10.89
- rosacea L71.9
- specified NEC H10.89
- swimming-pool B30.1
- trachomatous A71.1
  - acute A71.0
  - sequelae (late effect) B94.0
- traumatic NEC H10.89
- tuberculous A18.59
- tularemic A21.1
- tularensis A21.1
- viral B30.9
  - due to
    - adenovirus B30.1
    - enterovirus B30.3
  - specified NEC B30.8

**Conjunctivochalasis** H11.82- ☑

**Connective tissue** — see condition

**Conn's syndrome** E26.01

**Conradi** (-Hunermann) **disease** Q77.3

**Consanguinity** Z84.3
- counseling Z71.89

**Conscious simulation** (of illness) Z76.5

**Consecutive** — see condition

**Consolidation lung** (base) — see Pneumonia, lobar

**Constipation** (atonic) (neurogenic) (simple) (spastic) K59.00
- chronic K59.09
  - idiopathic K59.04
- drug-induced K59.03
- functional K59.04
- outlet dysfunction K59.02
- psychogenic F45.8
- slow transit K59.01
- specified NEC K59.09

**Constitutional** (see also condition)
- substandard F60.7

**Constitutionally substandard** F60.7

**Constriction** (see also Stricture)
- auditory canal — see Stenosis, external ear canal
- bronchial J98.09
- duodenum K31.5
- esophagus K22.2
- external
  - abdomen, abdominal (wall) S30.841 ☑
  - alveolar process S00.542 ☑
  - ankle S90.54- ☑
  - antecubital space — see Constriction, external, forearm
  - arm (upper) S40.84- ☑
  - auricle — see Constriction, external, ear
  - axilla — see Constriction, external, arm
  - back, lower S30.840 ☑
  - breast S20.14- ☑
  - brow S00.84 ☑
  - buttock S30.840 ☑
  - calf — see Constriction, external, leg
  - canthus — see Constriction, external, eyelid
  - cheek S00.84 ☑
    - internal S00.542 ☑
  - chest wall — see Constriction, external, thorax
  - chin S00.84 ☑
  - clitoris S30.844 ☑
  - costal region — see Constriction, external, thorax

**Constriction** — continued
- external — continued
  - digit(s)
    - foot — see Constriction, external, toe
    - hand — see Constriction, external, finger
  - ear S00.44- ☑
  - elbow S50.34- ☑
  - epididymis S30.843 ☑
  - epigastric region S30.841 ☑
  - esophagus, cervical S10.14 ☑
  - eyebrow — see Constriction, external, eyelid
  - eyelid S00.24- ☑
  - face S00.84 ☑
  - finger(s) S60.44- ☑
    - index S60.44- ☑
    - little S60.44- ☑
    - middle S60.44- ☑
    - ring S60.44- ☑
  - flank S30.841 ☑
  - foot (except toe(s) alone) S90.84- ☑
    - toe — see Constriction, external, toe
  - forearm S50.84- ☑
    - elbow only — see Constriction, external, elbow
  - forehead S00.84 ☑
  - genital organs, external
    - female S30.846 ☑
    - male S30.845 ☑
  - groin S30.841 ☑
  - gum S00.542 ☑
  - hand S60.54- ☑
  - head S00.94 ☑
    - ear — see Constriction, external, ear
    - eyelid — see Constriction, external, eyelid
    - lip S00.541 ☑
    - nose S00.34 ☑
    - oral cavity S00.542 ☑
    - scalp S00.04 ☑
    - specified site NEC S00.84 ☑
  - heel — see Constriction, external, foot
  - hip S70.24- ☑
  - inguinal region S30.841 ☑
  - interscapular region S20.449 ☑
  - jaw S00.84 ☑
  - knee S80.24- ☑
  - labium (majus) (minus) S30.844 ☑
  - larynx S10.14 ☑
  - leg (lower) S80.84- ☑
    - knee — see Constriction, external, knee
    - upper — see Constriction, external, thigh
  - lip S00.541 ☑
  - lower back S30.840 ☑
  - lumbar region S30.840 ☑
  - malar region S00.84 ☑
  - mammary — see Constriction, external, breast
  - mastoid region S00.84 ☑
  - mouth S00.542 ☑
  - nail
    - finger — see Constriction, external, finger
    - toe — see Constriction, external, toe
  - nasal S00.34 ☑
  - neck S10.94 ☑
    - specified site NEC S10.84 ☑
    - throat S10.14 ☑
  - nose S00.34 ☑
  - occipital region S00.04 ☑
  - oral cavity S00.542 ☑
  - orbital region — see Constriction, external, eyelid
  - palate S00.542 ☑
  - palm — see Constriction, external, hand
  - parietal region S00.04 ☑
  - pelvis S30.840 ☑
  - penis S30.842 ☑
  - perineum
    - female S30.844 ☑
    - male S30.840 ☑
  - periocular area — see Constriction, external, eyelid
  - phalanges
    - finger — see Constriction, external, finger
    - toe — see Constriction, external, toe
  - pharynx S10.14 ☑
  - pinna — see Constriction, external, ear
  - popliteal space — see Constriction, external, knee
  - prepuce S30.842 ☑
  - pubic region S30.840 ☑
  - pudendum
    - female S30.846 ☑

**Constriction** — continued
- external — continued
  - pudendum — continued
    - male S30.845 ☑
  - sacral region S30.840 ☑
  - scalp S00.04 ☑
  - scapular region — see Constriction, external, shoulder
  - scrotum S30.843 ☑
  - shin — see Constriction, external, leg
  - shoulder S40.24- ☑
  - sternal region S20.349 ☑
  - submaxillary region S00.84 ☑
  - submental region S00.84 ☑
  - subungual
    - finger(s) — see Constriction, external, finger
    - toe(s) — see Constriction, external, toe
  - supraclavicular fossa S10.84 ☑
  - supraorbital S00.84 ☑
  - temple S00.84 ☑
  - temporal region S00.84 ☑
  - testis S30.843 ☑
  - thigh S70.34- ☑
  - thorax, thoracic (wall) S20.94 ☑
    - back S20.44- ☑
    - front S20.34- ☑
  - throat S10.14 ☑
  - thumb S60.34- ☑
  - toe(s) (lesser) S90.44- ☑
    - great S90.44- ☑
  - tongue S00.542 ☑
  - trachea S10.14 ☑
  - tunica vaginalis S30.843 ☑
  - uvula S00.542 ☑
  - vagina S30.844 ☑
  - vulva S30.844 ☑
  - wrist S60.84- ☑
- gallbladder — see Obstruction, gallbladder
- intestine — see Obstruction, intestine
- larynx J38.6
  - congenital Q31.8
    - specified NEC Q31.8
    - subglottic Q31.1
- organ or site, congenital NEC — see Atresia, by site
- prepuce (acquired) (congenital) N47.1
- pylorus (adult hypertrophic) K31.1
  - congenital or infantile Q40.0
    - newborn Q40.0
- ring dystocia (uterus) O62.4
- spastic (see also Spasm)
  - ureter N13.5
- ureter N13.5
  - with infection N13.6
- urethra — see Stricture, urethra
- visual field (peripheral) (functional) — see Defect, visual field

**Constrictive** — see condition

**Consultation**
- without complaint or sickness Z71.9
  - feared complaint unfounded Z71.1
    - specified reason NEC Z71.89
- medical — see Counseling, medical
- religious Z71.81
- specified reason NEC Z71.89
- spiritual Z71.81

**Consumption** — see Tuberculosis

**Contact** (with) (see also Exposure (to))
- acariasis Z20.7
- AIDS virus Z20.6
- air pollution Z77.110
- algae and algae toxins Z77.121
- algae bloom Z77.121
- anthrax Z20.810
- aromatic amines Z77.020
- aromatic (hazardous) compounds NEC Z77.028
- aromatic dyes NOS Z77.028
- arsenic Z77.010
- asbestos Z77.090
- bacterial disease NEC Z20.818
- benzene Z77.021
- blue-green algae bloom Z77.121
- body fluids (potentially hazardous) Z77.21
- brown tide Z77.121
- chemicals (chiefly nonmedicinal) (hazardous) NEC Z77.098
- cholera Z20.09
- chromium compounds Z77.018

☑ Additional Character Required — Refer to the Tabular List for Character Selection ⓦ Subterms under main terms may continue to next column or page

**Contact** — *continued*
  communicable disease Z20.9
    bacterial NEC Z20.818
    specified NEC Z20.89
    viral NEC Z20.828
  cyanobacteria bloom Z77.121
  dyes Z77.098
  Escherichia coli (E. coli) Z20.01
  fiberglass — *see* Table of Drugs and Chemicals, fiberglass
  German measles Z20.4
  gonorrhea Z20.2
  hazardous metals NEC Z77.018
  hazardous substances NEC Z77.29
  hazards in the physical environment NEC Z77.128
  hazards to health NEC Z77.9
  HIV Z20.6
  HTLV-III/LAV Z20.6
  human immunodeficiency virus (HIV) Z20.6
  infection Z20.9
    specified NEC Z20.89
  infestation (parasitic) NEC Z20.7
  intestinal infectious disease NEC Z20.09
    Escherichia coli (E. coli) Z20.01
  lead Z77.011
  meningococcus Z20.811
  mold (toxic) Z77.120
  nickel dust Z77.018
  noise Z77.122
  parasitic disease Z20.7
  pediculosis Z20.7
  pfiesteria piscicida Z77.121
  poliomyelitis Z20.89
  pollution
    air Z77.110
    environmental NEC Z77.118
    soil Z77.112
    water Z77.111
  polycyclic aromatic hydrocarbons Z77.028
  rabies Z20.3
  radiation, naturally occurring NEC Z77.123
  radon Z77.123
  red tide (Florida) Z77.121
  rubella Z20.4
  sexually-transmitted disease Z20.2
  smallpox (laboratory) Z20.89
  syphilis Z20.2
  tuberculosis Z20.1
  uranium Z77.012
  varicella Z20.820
  venereal disease Z20.2
  viral disease NEC Z20.828
  viral hepatitis Z20.5
  water pollution Z77.111
**Contamination, food** — *see* Intoxication, foodborne
**Contraception, contraceptive**
  advice Z30.09
  counseling Z30.09
  device (intrauterine) (in situ) Z97.5
    causing menorrhagia T83.83 ☑
    checking Z30.431
    complications — *see* Complications, intrauterine, contraceptive device
    in place Z97.5
    initial prescription Z30.014
    reinsertion Z30.433
    removal Z30.432
    replacement Z30.433
  emergency (postcoital) Z30.012
  initial prescription Z30.019
    barrier Z30.018
    diaphragm Z30.018
    injectable Z30.013
    intrauterine device Z30.014
    pills Z30.011
    postcoital (emergency) Z30.012
    specified type NEC Z30.018
    subdermal implantable Z30.017
    transdermal patch hormonal Z30.016
    vaginal ring hormonal Z30.015
  maintenance Z30.40
    barrier Z30.49
    diaphragm Z30.49
    examination Z30.8
    injectable Z30.42
    intrauterine device Z30.431
    pills Z30.41
    specified type NEC Z30.49
    subdermal implantable Z30.46

**Contraception, contraceptive** — *continued*
  maintenance — *continued*
    transdermal patch hormonal Z30.45
    vaginal ring hormonal Z30.44
  management Z30.9
    specified NEC Z30.8
  postcoital (emergency) Z30.012
  prescription Z30.019
    repeat Z30.40
  sterilization Z30.2
  surveillance (drug) — *see* Contraception, maintenance
**Contraction(s), contracture, contracted**
  Achilles tendon (*see also* Short, tendon, Achilles)
    congenital Q66.89
  amputation stump (surgical) (flexion) (late) (next proximal joint) T87.89
  anus K59.8
  bile duct (common) (hepatic) K83.8
  bladder N32.89
    neck or sphincter N32.0
  bowel, cecum, colon or intestine, any part — *see* Obstruction, intestine
  Braxton Hicks — *see* False, labor
  breast implant, capsular T85.44 ☑
  bronchial J98.09
  burn (old) — *see* Cicatrix
  cervix — *see* Stricture, cervix
  cicatricial — *see* Cicatrix
  conjunctiva, trachomatous, active A71.1
    sequelae (late effect) B94.0
  Dupuytren's M72.0
  eyelid — *see* Disorder, eyelid function
  fascia (lata) (postural) M72.8
    Dupuytren's M72.0
    palmar M72.0
    plantar M72.2
  finger NEC (*see also* Deformity, finger)
    congenital Q68.1
    joint — *see* Contraction, joint, hand
  flaccid — *see* Contraction, paralytic
  gallbladder K82.0
  heart valve — *see* Endocarditis
  hip — *see* Contraction, joint, hip
  hourglass
    bladder N32.89
      congenital Q64.79
    gallbladder K82.0
      congenital Q44.1
    stomach K31.89
      congenital Q40.2
      psychogenic F45.8
    uterus (complicating delivery) O62.4
  hysterical F44.4
  internal os — *see* Stricture, cervix
  joint (abduction) (acquired) (adduction) (flexion) (rotation) M24.50
    ankle M24.57- ☑
    congenital NEC Q68.8
      hip Q65.89
    elbow M24.52- ☑
    foot joint M24.57- ☑
    hand joint M24.54- ☑
    hip M24.55- ☑
      congenital Q65.89
    hysterical F44.4
    knee M24.56- ☑
    shoulder M24.51- ☑
    wrist M24.53- ☑
  kidney (granular) (secondary) N26.9
    congenital Q63.8
    hydronephritic — *see* Hydronephrosis Page N26.2
    pyelonephritic — *see* Pyelitis, chronic
    tuberculous A18.11
  ligament (*see also* Disorder, ligament)
    congenital Q79.8
  muscle (postinfective) (postural) NEC M62.40
    with contracture of joint — *see* Contraction, joint
    ankle M62.47- ☑
    congenital Q79.8
      sternocleidomastoid Q68.0
    extraocular — *see* Strabismus
    eye (extrinsic) — *see* Strabismus
    foot M62.47- ☑
    forearm M62.43- ☑
    hand M62.44- ☑
    hysterical F44.4

**Contraction(s), contracture, contracted** — *continued*
  muscle — *continued*
    ischemic (Volkmann's) T79.6 ☑
    lower leg M62.46- ☑
    multiple sites M62.49
    pelvic region M62.45- ☑
    posttraumatic — *see* Strabismus, paralytic
    psychogenic F45.8
      conversion reaction F44.4
    shoulder region M62.41- ☑
    specified site NEC M62.48
    thigh M62.45- ☑
    upper arm M62.42- ☑
  neck — *see* Torticollis
  ocular muscle — *see* Strabismus
  organ or site, congenital NEC — *see* Atresia, by site
  outlet (pelvis) — *see* Contraction, pelvis
  palmar fascia M72.0
  paralytic
    joint — *see* Contraction, joint
    muscle (*see also* Contraction, muscle NEC)
      ocular — *see* Strabismus, paralytic
  pelvis (acquired) (general) M95.5
    with disproportion (fetopelvic) O33.1
      causing obstructed labor O65.1
      inlet O33.2
      mid-cavity O33.3 ☑
      outlet O33.3 ☑
  plantar fascia M72.2
  premature
    atrium I49.1
    auriculoventricular I49.49
    heart I49.49
    junctional I49.2
    supraventricular I49.1
    ventricular I49.3
  prostate N42.89
  pylorus NEC (*see also* Pylorospasm)
    psychogenic F45.8
  rectum, rectal (sphincter) K59.8
  ring (Bandl's) (complicating delivery) O62.4
  scar — *see* Cicatrix
  spine — *see* Dorsopathy, deforming
  sternocleidomastoid (muscle), congenital Q68.0
  stomach K31.89
    hourglass K31.89
      congenital Q40.2
      psychogenic F45.8
    psychogenic F45.8
  tendon (sheath) M62.40
    with contracture of joint — *see* Contraction, joint
    Achilles — *see* Short, tendon, Achilles
    ankle M62.47- ☑
      Achilles — *see* Short, tendon, Achilles
    foot M62.47- ☑
    forearm M62.43- ☑
    hand M62.44- ☑
    lower leg M62.46- ☑
    multiple sites M62.49
    neck M62.48
    pelvic region M62.45- ☑
    shoulder region M62.41- ☑
    specified site NEC M62.48
    thigh M62.45- ☑
    thorax M62.48
    trunk M62.48
    upper arm M62.42- ☑
  toe — *see* Deformity, toe, specified NEC
  ureterovesical orifice (postinfectional) N13.5
    with infection N13.6
  urethra (*see also* Stricture, urethra)
    orifice N32.0
  uterus N85.8
    abnormal NEC O62.9
    clonic (complicating delivery) O62.4
    dyscoordinate (complicating delivery) O62.4
    hourglass (complicating delivery) O62.4
    hypertonic O62.4
    hypotonic NEC O62.2
    inadequate
      primary O62.0
      secondary O62.1
    incoordinate (complicating delivery) O62.4
    poor O62.2
    tetanic (complicating delivery) O62.4
  vagina (outlet) N89.5
  vesical N32.89

**Contusion** — *continued*
  throat S10.0 ☑
  thumb S60.01- ☑
    with damage to nail S60.11- ☑
  toe(s) (lesser) S90.12- ☑
    with damage to nail S90.22- ☑
    great S90.11- ☑
      with damage to nail S90.21- ☑
  tongue S00.532 ☑
  trachea (cervical) S10.0 ☑
    thoracic S27.52 ☑
  tunica vaginalis S30.22 ☑
  tympanum, tympanic membrane — *see* Contusion,
    ear
  ureter S37.12 ☑
  urethra S37.32 ☑
  urinary organ NEC S37.892 ☑
  uterus S37.62 ☑
  uvula S00.532 ☑
  vagina S30.23 ☑
  vas deferens S37.892 ☑
  vesical S37.22 ☑
  vocal cord(s) S10.0 ☑
  vulva S30.23 ☑
  wrist S60.21- ☑
**Conus** (congenital) (any type) Q14.8
  cornea — *see* Keratoconus
  medullaris syndrome G95.81
**Conversion hysteria, neurosis or reaction** F44.9
**Converter, tuberculosis** (test reaction) R76.11
**Conviction** (legal), **anxiety concerning** Z65.0
  with imprisonment Z65.1
**Convulsions** (idiopathic) (*see also* Seizure(s)) R56.9
  apoplectiform (cerebral ischemia) I67.82
  dissociative F44.5
  epileptic — *see* Epilepsy
  epileptiform, epileptoid — *see* Seizure, epileptiform
  ether (anesthetic) — *see* Table of Drugs and Chemicals,
    by drug
  febrile R56.00
    with status epilepticus G40.901
    complex R56.01
      with status epilepticus G40.901
    simple R56.00
  hysterical F44.5
  infantile P90
    epilepsy — *see* Epilepsy
  jacksonian — *see* Epilepsy, localization-related,
    symptomatic, with simple partial seizures
  myoclonic G25.3
  newborn P90
  obstetrical (nephritic) (uremic) — *see* Eclampsia
  paretic A52.17
  post traumatic R56.1
  psychomotor — *see* Epilepsy, localization-related,
    symptomatic, with complex partial seizures
  recurrent R56.9
  reflex R25.8
  scarlatinal A38.8
  tetanus, tetanic — *see* Tetanus
  thymic E32.8
**Convulsive** (*see also* Convulsions)
**Cooley's anemia** D56.1
**Coolie itch** B76.9
**Cooper's**
  disease — *see* Mastopathy, cystic
  hernia — *see* Hernia, abdomen, specified site NEC
**Copra itch** B88.0
**Coprophagy** F50.89
**Coprophobia** F40.298
**Coproporphyria, hereditary** E80.29
**Cor**
  biloculare Q20.8
  bovis, bovinum — *see* Hypertrophy, cardiac
  pulmonale (chronic) I27.81
    acute I26.09
  triatriatum, triatrium Q24.2
  triloculare Q20.8
    biatrium Q20.4
    biventriculare Q21.1
**Corbus' disease** (gangrenous balanitis) N48.1
**Cord** (*see also* condition)
  around neck
    complicating delivery O69.81 ☑
      with compression O69.1 ☑
  bladder G95.89
    tabetic A52.19

**Cordis ectopia** Q24.8
**Corditis** (spermatic) N49.1
**Corectopia** Q13.2
**Cori's disease** (glycogen storage) E74.03
**Corkhandler's disease or lung** J67.3
**Corkscrew esophagus** K22.4
**Corkworker's disease or lung** J67.3
**Corn** (infected) L84
**Cornea** (*see also* condition)
  donor Z52.5
  plana Q13.4
**Cornelia de Lange syndrome** Q87.1
**Cornu cutaneum** L85.8
**Cornual gestation or pregnancy** O00.80
  with intrauterine pregnancy O00.81
**Coronary** (artery) — *see* condition
**Coronavirus, as cause of disease classified elsewhere**
  B97.29
  SARS-associated B97.21
**Corpora** (*see also* condition)
  amylacea, prostate N42.89
  cavernosa — *see* condition
**Corpulence** — *see* Obesity
**Corpus** — *see* condition
**Corrected transposition** Q20.5
**Corrosion** (injury) (acid) (caustic) (chemical) (lime) (exter-
  nal) (internal) T30.4
  abdomen, abdominal (muscle) (wall) T21.42 ☑
    first degree T21.52 ☑
    second degree T21.62 ☑
    third degree T21.72 ☑
  above elbow T22.439 ☑
    first degree T22.539 ☑
    left T22.432 ☑
      first degree T22.532 ☑
      second degree T22.632 ☑
      third degree T22.732 ☑
    right T22.431 ☑
      first degree T22.531 ☑
      second degree T22.631 ☑
      third degree T22.731 ☑
    second degree T22.639 ☑
    third degree T22.739 ☑
  alimentary tract NEC T28.7 ☑
  ankle T25.419 ☑
    first degree T25.519 ☑
    left T25.412 ☑
      first degree T25.512 ☑
      second degree T25.612 ☑
      third degree T25.712 ☑
    multiple with foot — *see* Corrosion, lower, limb,
      multiple, ankle and foot
    right T25.411 ☑
      first degree T25.511 ☑
      second degree T25.611 ☑
      third degree T25.711 ☑
    second degree T25.619 ☑
    third degree T25.719 ☑
  anus — *see* Corrosion, buttock
  arm(s) (meaning upper limb(s)) — *see* Corrosion, upper
    limb
  axilla T22.449 ☑
    first degree T22.549 ☑
    left T22.442 ☑
      first degree T22.542 ☑
      second degree T22.642 ☑
      third degree T22.742 ☑
    right T22.441 ☑
      first degree T22.541 ☑
      second degree T22.641 ☑
      third degree T22.741 ☑
    second degree T22.649 ☑
    third degree T22.749 ☑
  back (lower) T21.44 ☑
    first degree T21.54 ☑
    second degree T21.64 ☑
    third degree T21.74 ☑
    upper T21.43 ☑
      first degree T21.53 ☑
      second degree T21.63 ☑
      third degree T21.73 ☑
  blisters — *code as* Corrosion, second degree, by site
  breast(s) — *see* Corrosion, chest wall
  buttock(s) T21.45 ☑
    first degree T21.55 ☑
    second degree T21.65 ☑

**Corrosion** — *continued*
  buttock(s) — *continued*
    third degree T21.75 ☑
  calf T24.439 ☑
    first degree T24.539 ☑
    left T24.432 ☑
      first degree T24.532 ☑
      second degree T24.632 ☑
      third degree T24.732 ☑
    right T24.431 ☑
      first degree T24.531 ☑
      second degree T24.631 ☑
      third degree T24.731 ☑
    second degree T24.639 ☑
    third degree T24.739 ☑
  canthus (eye) — *see* Corrosion, eyelid
  cervix T28.8 ☑
  cheek T20.46 ☑
    first degree T20.56 ☑
    second degree T20.66 ☑
    third degree T20.76 ☑
  chest wall T21.41 ☑
    first degree T21.51 ☑
    second degree T21.61 ☑
    third degree T21.71 ☑
  chin T20.43 ☑
    first degree T20.53 ☑
    second degree T20.63 ☑
    third degree T20.73 ☑
  colon T28.7 ☑
  conjunctiva (and cornea) — *see* Corrosion, cornea
  cornea (and conjunctiva) T26.6- ☑
  deep necrosis of underlying tissue — *code as* Corro-
    sion, third degree, by site
  dorsum of hand T23.469 ☑
    first degree T23.569 ☑
    left T23.462 ☑
      first degree T23.562 ☑
      second degree T23.662 ☑
      third degree T23.762 ☑
    right T23.461 ☑
      first degree T23.561 ☑
      second degree T23.661 ☑
      third degree T23.761 ☑
    second degree T23.669 ☑
    third degree T23.769 ☑
  ear (auricle) (external) (canal) T20.41 ☑
    drum T28.91 ☑
    first degree T20.51 ☑
    second degree T20.61 ☑
    third degree T20.71 ☑
  elbow T22.429 ☑
    first degree T22.529 ☑
    left T22.422 ☑
      first degree T22.522 ☑
      second degree T22.622 ☑
      third degree T22.722 ☑
    right T22.421 ☑
      first degree T22.521 ☑
      second degree T22.621 ☑
      third degree T22.721 ☑
    second degree T22.629 ☑
    third degree T22.729 ☑
  entire body — *see* Corrosion, multiple body regions
  epidermal loss — *code as* Corrosion, second degree,
    by site
  epiglottis T27.4 ☑
  erythema, erythematous — *code as* Corrosion, first
    degree, by site
  esophagus T28.6 ☑
  extent (percentage of body surface)
    less than 10 percent T32.0
    10-19 percent (0-9 percent third degree) T32.10
      with 10-19 percent third degree T32.11
    20-29 percent (0-9 percent third degree) T32.20
      with
        10-19 percent third degree T32.21
        20-29 percent third degree T32.22
    30-39 percent (0-9 percent third degree) T32.30
      with
        10-19 percent third degree T32.31
        20-29 percent third degree T32.32
        30-39 percent third degree T32.33
    40-49 percent (0-9 percent third degree) T32.40
      with
        10-19 percent third degree T32.41

**Corrosion** — *continued*
extent — *continued*
40-49 percent — *continued*
with — *continued*
20-29 percent third degree T32.42
30-39 percent third degree T32.43
40-49 percent third degree T32.44
50-59 percent (0-9 percent third degree) T32.50
with
10-19 percent third degree T32.51
20-29 percent third degree T32.52
30-39 percent third degree T32.53
40-49 percent third degree T32.54
50-59 percent third degree T32.55
60-69 percent (0-9 percent third degree) T32.60
with
10-19 percent third degree T32.61
20-29 percent third degree T32.62
30-39 percent third degree T32.63
40-49 percent third degree T32.64
50-59 percent third degree T32.65
60-69 percent third degree T32.66
70-79 percent (0-9 percent third degree) T32.70
with
10-19 percent third degree T32.71
20-29 percent third degree T32.72
30-39 percent third degree T32.73
40-49 percent third degree T32.74
50-59 percent third degree T32.75
60-69 percent third degree T32.76
70-79 percent third degree T32.77
80-89 percent (0-9 percent third degree) T32.80
with
10-19 percent third degree T32.81
20-29 percent third degree T32.82
30-39 percent third degree T32.83
40-49 percent third degree T32.84
50-59 percent third degree T32.85
60-69 percent third degree T32.86
70-79 percent third degree T32.87
80-89 percent third degree T32.88
90 percent or more (0-9 percent third degree) T32.90
with
10-19 percent third degree T32.91
20-29 percent third degree T32.92
30-39 percent third degree T32.93
40-49 percent third degree T32.94
50-59 percent third degree T32.95
60-69 percent third degree T32.96
70-79 percent third degree T32.97
80-89 percent third degree T32.98
90-99 percent third degree T32.99
extremity — *see* Corrosion, limb
eye(s) and adnexa T26.9-
with resulting rupture and destruction of eyeball T26.7- ✓
conjunctival sac — *see* Corrosion, cornea
cornea — *see* Corrosion, cornea
lid — *see* Corrosion, eyelid
periocular area — *see* Corrosion eyelid
specified site NEC T26.8- ✓
eyeball — *see* Corrosion, eye
eyelid(s) T26.5- ✓
face — *see* Corrosion, head
finger T23.429 ✓
first degree T23.529 ✓
left T23.422 ✓
first degree T23.522 ✓
second degree T23.622 ✓
third degree T23.722 ✓
multiple sites (without thumb) T23.439 ✓
with thumb T23.449 ✓
first degree T23.549 ✓
left T23.442 ✓
first degree T23.542 ✓
second degree T23.642 ✓
third degree T23.742 ✓
right T23.441 ✓
first degree T23.541 ✓
second degree T23.641 ✓
third degree T23.741 ✓
second degree T23.649 ✓
third degree T23.749 ✓
first degree T23.539 ✓
left T23.432 ✓
first degree T23.532 ✓

**Corrosion** — *continued*
finger — *continued*
multiple sites — *continued*
left — *continued*
second degree T23.632 ✓
third degree T23.732 ✓
right T23.431 ✓
first degree T23.531 ✓
second degree T23.631 ✓
third degree T23.731 ✓
second degree T23.639 ✓
third degree T23.739 ✓
right T23.421 ✓
first degree T23.521 ✓
second degree T23.621 ✓
third degree T23.721 ✓
second degree T23.629 ✓
third degree T23.729 ✓
flank — *see* Corrosion, abdomen
foot T25.429 ✓
first degree T25.529 ✓
left T25.422 ✓
first degree T25.522 ✓
second degree T25.622 ✓
third degree T25.722 ✓
multiple with ankle — *see* Corrosion, lower, limb, multiple, ankle and foot
right T25.421 ✓
first degree T25.521 ✓
second degree T25.621 ✓
third degree T25.721 ✓
second degree T25.629 ✓
third degree T25.729 ✓
forearm T22.419 ✓
first degree T22.519 ✓
left T22.412 ✓
first degree T22.512 ✓
second degree T22.612 ✓
third degree T22.712 ✓
right T22.411 ✓
first degree T22.511 ✓
second degree T22.611 ✓
third degree T22.711 ✓
second degree T22.619 ✓
third degree T22.719 ✓
forehead T20.46 ✓
first degree T20.56 ✓
second degree T20.66 ✓
third degree T20.76 ✓
fourth degree — *code as* Corrosion, third degree, by site
full thickness skin loss — *code as* Corrosion, third degree, by site
gastrointestinal tract NEC T28.7 ✓
genital organs
external
female T21.47 ✓
first degree T21.57 ✓
second degree T21.67 ✓
third degree T21.77 ✓
male T21.46 ✓
first degree T21.56 ✓
second degree T21.66 ✓
third degree T21.76 ✓
internal T28.8 ✓
groin — *see* Corrosion, abdominal wall
hand(s) T23.409 ✓
back — *see* Corrosion, dorsum of hand
finger — *see* Corrosion, finger
first degree T23.509 ✓
left T23.402 ✓
first degree T23.502 ✓
second degree T23.602 ✓
third degree T23.702 ✓
multiple sites with wrist T23.499 ✓
first degree T23.599 ✓
left T23.492 ✓
first degree T23.592 ✓
second degree T23.692 ✓
third degree T23.792 ✓
right T23.491 ✓
first degree T23.591 ✓
second degree T23.691 ✓
third degree T23.791 ✓
second degree T23.699 ✓
third degree T23.799 ✓

**Corrosion** — *continued*
hand(s) — *continued*
palm — *see* Corrosion, palm
right T23.401 ✓
first degree T23.501 ✓
second degree T23.601 ✓
third degree T23.701 ✓
second degree T23.609 ✓
third degree T23.709 ✓
thumb — *see* Corrosion, thumb
head (and face) (and neck) T20.40 ✓
cheek — *see* Corrosion, cheek
chin — *see* Corrosion, chin
ear — *see* Corrosion, ear
eye(s) only — *see* Corrosion, eye
first degree T20.50 ✓
forehead — *see* Corrosion, forehead
lip — *see* Corrosion, lip
multiple sites T20.49 ✓
first degree T20.59 ✓
second degree T20.69 ✓
third degree T20.79 ✓
neck — *see* Corrosion, neck
nose — *see* Corrosion, nose
scalp — *see* Corrosion, scalp
second degree T20.60 ✓
third degree T20.70 ✓
hip(s) — *see* Corrosion, lower, limb
inhalation — *see* Corrosion, respiratory tract
internal organ(s) (*see also* Corrosion, by site) T28.90 ✓
alimentary tract T28.7 ✓
esophagus T28.6 ✓
esophagus T28.6 ✓
genitourinary T28.8 ✓
mouth T28.5 ✓
pharynx T28.5 ✓
specified organ NEC T28.99 ✓
interscapular region — *see* Corrosion, back, upper
intestine (large) (small) T28.7 ✓
knee T24.429 ✓
first degree T24.529 ✓
left T24.422 ✓
first degree T24.522 ✓
second degree T24.622 ✓
third degree T24.722 ✓
right T24.421 ✓
first degree T24.521 ✓
second degree T24.621 ✓
third degree T24.721 ✓
second degree T24.629 ✓
third degree T24.729 ✓
labium (majus) (minus) — *see* Corrosion, genital organs, external, female
lacrimal apparatus, duct, gland or sac — *see* Corrosion, eye, specified site NEC
larynx T27.4 ✓
with lung T27.5 ✓
leg(s) (meaning lower limb(s)) — *see* Corrosion, lower limb
limb(s)
lower — *see* Corrosion, lower, limb
upper — *see* Corrosion, upper limb
lip(s) T20.42 ✓
first degree T20.52 ✓
second degree T20.62 ✓
third degree T20.72 ✓
lower
back — *see* Corrosion, back
limb T24.409 ✓
ankle — *see* Corrosion, ankle
calf — *see* Corrosion, calf
first degree T24.509 ✓
foot — *see* Corrosion, foot
knee — *see* Corrosion, knee
left T24.402 ✓
first degree T24.502 ✓
second degree T24.602 ✓
third degree T24.702 ✓
multiple sites, except ankle and foot T24.499 ✓
ankle and foot T25.499 ✓
first degree T25.599 ✓
left T25.492 ✓
first degree T25.592 ✓
second degree T25.692 ✓
third degree T25.792 ✓
right T25.491 ✓

✓ **Additional Character Required** — **Refer to the Tabular List for Character Selection**    ⬇ Subterms under main terms may continue to next column or page

**Corrosion** — *continued*
  lower — *continued*
    limb — *continued*
      multiple sites, except ankle and foot — *continued*
        ankle and foot — *continued*
          right — *continued*
            first degree T25.591 ☑
            second degree T25.691 ☑
            third degree T25.791 ☑
          second degree T25.699 ☑
          third degree T25.799 ☑
        first degree T24.599 ☑
        left T24.492 ☑
          first degree T24.592 ☑
          second degree T24.692 ☑
          third degree T24.792 ☑
        right T24.491 ☑
          first degree T24.591 ☑
          second degree T24.691 ☑
          third degree T24.791 ☑
        second degree T24.699 ☑
        third degree T24.799 ☑
      right T24.401 ☑
        first degree T24.501 ☑
        second degree T24.601 ☑
        third degree T24.701 ☑
      second degree T24.609 ☑
      thigh — *see* Corrosion, thigh
      third degree T24.709 ☑
  lung (with larynx and trachea) T27.5 ☑
  mouth T28.5 ☑
  neck T20.47 ☑
    first degree T20.57 ☑
    second degree T20.67 ☑
    third degree T20.77 ☑
  nose (septum) T20.44 ☑
    first degree T20.54 ☑
    second degree T20.64 ☑
    third degree T20.74 ☑
  ocular adnexa — *see* Corrosion, eye
  orbit region — *see* Corrosion, eyelid
  palm T23.459 ☑
    first degree T23.559 ☑
    left T23.452 ☑
      first degree T23.552 ☑
      second degree T23.652 ☑
      third degree T23.752 ☑
    right T23.451 ☑
      first degree T23.551 ☑
      second degree T23.651 ☑
      third degree T23.751 ☑
    second degree T23.659 ☑
    third degree T23.759 ☑
  partial thickness — *code as* Corrosion, unspecified degree, by site
  pelvis — *see* Corrosion, trunk
  penis — *see* Corrosion, genital organs, external, male
  perineum
    female — *see* Corrosion, genital organs, external, female
    male — *see* Corrosion, genital organs, external, male
  periocular area — *see* Corrosion, eyelid
  pharynx T28.5 ☑
  rectum T28.7 ☑
  respiratory tract T27.7 ☑
    larynx — *see* Corrosion, larynx
    specified part NEC T27.6 ☑
    trachea — *see* Corrosion, larynx
  sac, lacrimal — *see* Corrosion, eye, specified site NEC
  scalp T20.45 ☑
    first degree T20.55 ☑
    second degree T20.65 ☑
    third degree T20.75 ☑
  scapular region T22.469 ☑
    first degree T22.569 ☑
    left T22.462 ☑
      first degree T22.562 ☑
      second degree T22.662 ☑
      third degree T22.762 ☑
    right T22.461 ☑
      first degree T22.561 ☑
      second degree T22.661 ☑
      third degree T22.761 ☑
    second degree T22.669 ☑

**Corrosion** — *continued*
  scapular region — *continued*
    third degree T22.769 ☑
  sclera — *see* Corrosion, eye, specified site NEC
  scrotum — *see* Corrosion, genital organs, external, male
  shoulder T22.459 ☑
    first degree T22.559 ☑
    left T22.452 ☑
      first degree T22.552 ☑
      second degree T22.652 ☑
      third degree T22.752 ☑
    right T22.451 ☑
      first degree T22.551 ☑
      second degree T22.651 ☑
      third degree T22.751 ☑
    second degree T22.659 ☑
    third degree T22.759 ☑
  stomach T28.7 ☑
  temple — *see* Corrosion, head
  testis — *see* Corrosion, genital organs, external, male
  thigh T24.419 ☑
    first degree T24.519 ☑
    left T24.412 ☑
      first degree T24.512 ☑
      second degree T24.612 ☑
      third degree T24.712 ☑
    right T24.411 ☑
      first degree T24.511 ☑
      second degree T24.611 ☑
      third degree T24.711 ☑
    second degree T24.619 ☑
    third degree T24.719 ☑
  thorax (external) — *see* Corrosion, trunk
  throat (meaning pharynx) T28.5 ☑
  thumb(s) T23.419 ☑
    first degree T23.519 ☑
    left T23.412 ☑
      first degree T23.512 ☑
      second degree T23.612 ☑
      third degree T23.712 ☑
    multiple sites with fingers T23.449 ☑
      first degree T23.549 ☑
      left T23.442 ☑
        first degree T23.542 ☑
        second degree T23.642 ☑
        third degree T23.742 ☑
      right T23.441 ☑
        first degree T23.541 ☑
        second degree T23.641 ☑
        third degree T23.741 ☑
      second degree T23.649 ☑
      third degree T23.749 ☑
    right T23.411 ☑
      first degree T23.511 ☑
      second degree T23.611 ☑
      third degree T23.711 ☑
    second degree T23.619 ☑
    third degree T23.719 ☑
  toe T25.439 ☑
    first degree T25.539 ☑
    left T25.432 ☑
      first degree T25.532 ☑
      second degree T25.632 ☑
      third degree T25.732 ☑
    right T25.431 ☑
      first degree T25.531 ☑
      second degree T25.631 ☑
      third degree T25.731 ☑
    second degree T25.639 ☑
    third degree T25.739 ☑
  tongue T28.5 ☑
  tonsil(s) T28.5 ☑
  total body — *see* Corrosion, multiple body regions
  trachea T27.4 ☑
    with lung T27.5 ☑
  trunk T21.40 ☑
    abdominal wall — *see* Corrosion, abdominal wall
    anus — *see* Corrosion, buttock
    axilla — *see* Corrosion, upper limb
    back — *see* Corrosion, back
    breast — *see* Corrosion, chest wall
    buttock — *see* Corrosion, buttock
    chest wall — *see* Corrosion, chest wall
    first degree T21.50 ☑
    flank — *see* Corrosion, abdominal wall

**Corrosion** — *continued*
  trunk — *continued*
    genital
      female — *see* Corrosion, genital organs, external, female
      male — *see* Corrosion, genital organs, external, male
    groin — *see* Corrosion, abdominal wall
    interscapular region — *see* Corrosion, back, upper
    labia — *see* Corrosion, genital organs, external, female
    lower back — *see* Corrosion, back
    penis — *see* Corrosion, genital organs, external, male
    perineum
      female — *see* Corrosion, genital organs, external, female
      male — *see* Corrosion, genital organs, external, male
    scapular region — *see* Corrosion, upper limb
    scrotum — *see* Corrosion, genital organs, external, male
    second degree T21.60 ☑
    shoulder — *see* Corrosion, upper limb
    specified site NEC T21.49 ☑
      first degree T21.59 ☑
      second degree T21.69 ☑
      third degree T21.79 ☑
    testes — *see* Corrosion, genital organs, external, male
    third degree T21.70 ☑
    upper back — *see* Corrosion, back, upper
    vagina T28.8 ☑
    vulva — *see* Corrosion, genital organs, external, female
  unspecified site with extent of body surface involved specified
    less than 10 percent T32.0
    10-19 percent (0-9 percent third degree) T32.10
      with 10-19 percent third degree T32.11
    20-29 percent (0-9 percent third degree) T32.20
      with
        10-19 percent third degree T32.21
        20-29 percent third degree T32.22
    30-39 percent (0-9 percent third degree) T32.30
      with
        10-19 percent third degree T32.31
        20-29 percent third degree T32.32
        30-39 percent third degree T32.33
    40-49 percent (0-9 percent third degree) T32.40
      with
        10-19 percent third degree T32.41
        20-29 percent third degree T32.42
        30-39 percent third degree T32.43
        40-49 percent third degree T32.44
    50-59 percent (0-9 percent third degree) T32.50
      with
        10-19 percent third degree T32.51
        20-29 percent third degree T32.52
        30-39 percent third degree T32.53
        40-49 percent third degree T32.54
        50-59 percent third degree T32.55
    60-69 percent (0-9 percent third degree) T32.60
      with
        10-19 percent third degree T32.61
        20-29 percent third degree T32.62
        30-39 percent third degree T32.63
        40-49 percent third degree T32.64
        50-59 percent third degree T32.65
        60-69 percent third degree T32.66
    70-79 percent (0-9 percent third degree) T32.70
      with
        10-19 percent third degree T32.71
        20-29 percent third degree T32.72
        30-39 percent third degree T32.73
        40-49 percent third degree T32.74
        50-59 percent third degree T32.75
        60-69 percent third degree T32.76
        70-79 percent third degree T32.77
    80-89 percent (0-9 percent third degree) T32.80
      with
        10-19 percent third degree T32.81
        20-29 percent third degree T32.82
        30-39 percent third degree T32.83
        40-49 percent third degree T32.84
        50-59 percent third degree T32.85
        60-69 percent third degree T32.86
        70-79 percent third degree T32.87

**Corrosion** — *continued*

unspecified site with extent of body surface involved
specified — *continued*
80-89 percent — *continued*
with — *continued*
80-89 percent third degree T32.88
90 percent or more (0-9 percent third degree)
T32.90
with
10-19 percent third degree T32.91
20-29 percent third degree T32.92
30-39 percent third degree T32.93
40-49 percent third degree T32.94
50-59 percent third degree T32.95
60-69 percent third degree T32.96
70-79 percent third degree T32.97
80-89 percent third degree T32.98
90-99 percent third degree T32.99
upper limb (axilla) (scapular region) T22.40 ☑
above elbow — *see* Corrosion, above elbow
axilla — *see* Corrosion, axilla
elbow — *see* Corrosion, elbow
first degree T22.50 ☑
forearm — *see* Corrosion, forearm
hand — *see* Corrosion, hand
interscapular region — *see* Corrosion, back, upper
multiple sites T22.499 ☑
first degree T22.599 ☑
left T22.492 ☑
first degree T22.592 ☑
second degree T22.692 ☑
third degree T22.792 ☑
right T22.491 ☑
first degree T22.591 ☑
second degree T22.691 ☑
third degree T22.791 ☑
second degree T22.699 ☑
third degree T22.799 ☑
scapular region — *see* Corrosion, scapular region
second degree T22.60 ☑
shoulder — *see* Corrosion, shoulder
third degree T22.70 ☑
wrist — *see* Corrosion, hand
uterus T28.8 ☑
vagina T28.8 ☑
vulva — *see* Corrosion, genital organs, external, female
wrist T23.479 ☑
first degree T23.579 ☑
left T23.472 ☑
first degree T23.572 ☑
second degree T23.672 ☑
third degree T23.772 ☑
multiple sites with hand T23.499 ☑
first degree T23.599 ☑
left T23.492 ☑
first degree T23.592 ☑
second degree T23.692 ☑
third degree T23.792 ☑
right T23.491 ☑
first degree T23.591 ☑
second degree T23.691 ☑
third degree T23.791 ☑
second degree T23.699 ☑
third degree T23.799 ☑
right T23.471 ☑
first degree T23.571 ☑
second degree T23.671 ☑
third degree T23.771 ☑
second degree T23.679 ☑
third degree T23.779 ☑

**Corrosive burn** — *see* Corrosion
**Corsican fever** — *see* Malaria
**Cortical** — *see* condition
**Cortico-adrenal** — *see* condition
**Coryza** (acute) J00
with grippe or influenza — *see* Influenza, with, respiratory manifestations NEC
syphilitic
congenital (chronic) A50.05
**Costen's syndrome or complex** M26.69
**Costiveness** — *see* Constipation
**Costochondritis** M94.0
**Cot death** R99
**Cotard's syndrome** F22
**Cotia virus** B08.8
**Cotton wool spots** (retinal) H35.81

**Cotungo's disease** — *see* Sciatica
**Cough** (affected) (chronic) (epidemic) (nervous) R05
with hemorrhage — *see* Hemoptysis
bronchial R05
with grippe or influenza — *see* Influenza, with, respiratory manifestations NEC
functional F45.8
hysterical F45.8
laryngeal, spasmodic R05
psychogenic F45.8
smokers' J41.0
tea taster's B49
**Counseling** (for) Z71.9
abuse NEC
perpetrator Z69.82
victim Z69.81
alcohol abuser Z71.41
family Z71.42
child abuse
nonparental
perpetrator Z69.021
victim Z69.020
parental
perpetrator Z69.011
victim Z69.010
consanguinity Z71.89
contraceptive Z30.09
dietary Z71.3
drug abuser Z71.51
family member Z71.52
exercise Z71.82
family Z71.89
fertility preservation (prior to cancer therapy) (prior to removal of gonads) Z31.62
for non-attending third party Z71.0
related to sexual behavior or orientation Z70.2
genetic
nonprocreative Z71.83
procreative NEC Z31.5
gestational carrier Z31.7
health (advice) (education) (instruction) — *see* Counseling, medical
human immunodeficiency virus (HIV) Z71.7
impotence Z70.1
insulin pump use Z46.81
medical (for) Z71.9
boarding school resident Z59.3
consanguinity Z71.89
feared complaint and no disease found Z71.1
human immunodeficiency virus (HIV) Z71.7
institutional resident Z59.3
on behalf of another Z71.0
related to sexual behavior or orientation Z70.2
person living alone Z60.2
specified reason NEC Z71.89
natural family planning
procreative Z31.61
to avoid pregnancy Z30.02
perpetrator (of)
abuse NEC Z69.82
child abuse
non-parental Z69.021
parental Z69.011
rape NEC Z69.82
spousal abuse Z69.12
procreative NEC Z31.69
fertility preservation (prior to cancer therapy) (prior to removal of gonads) Z31.62
using natural family planning Z31.61
promiscuity Z70.1
rape victim Z69.81
religious Z71.81
sex, sexual (related to) Z70.9
attitude(s) Z70.0
behavior or orientation Z70.1
combined concerns Z70.3
non-responsiveness Z70.1
on behalf of third party Z70.2
specified reason NEC Z70.8
specified reason NEC Z71.89
spiritual Z71.81
spousal abuse (perpetrator) Z69.12
victim Z69.11
substance abuse Z71.89
alcohol Z71.41
drug Z71.51
tobacco Z71.6
tobacco use Z71.6

**Counseling** — *continued*
use (of)
insulin pump Z46.81
victim (of)
abuse Z69.81
child abuse
by parent Z69.010
non-parental Z69.020
rape NEC Z69.81
**Coupled rhythm** R00.8
**Couvelaire syndrome or uterus** (complicating delivery) O45.8X- ☑
**Cowperitis** — *see* Urethritis
**Cowper's gland** — *see* condition
**Cowpox** B08.010
due to vaccination T88.1 ☑
**Coxa**
magna M91.4- ☑
plana M91.2- ☑
valga (acquired) (*see also* Deformity, limb, specified type NEC, thigh)
congenital Q65.81
sequelae (late effect) of rickets E64.3
vara (acquired) (*see also* Deformity, limb, specified type NEC, thigh)
congenital Q65.82
sequelae (late effect) of rickets E64.3
**Coxalgia, coxalgic** (nontuberculous) (*see also* Pain, joint, hip)
tuberculous A18.02
**Coxitis** — *see* Monoarthritis, hip
**Coxsackie** (virus) (infection) B34.1
as cause of disease classified elsewhere B97.11
carditis B33.20
central nervous system NEC A88.8
endocarditis B33.21
enteritis A08.39
meningitis (aseptic) A87.0
myocarditis B33.22
pericarditis B33.23
pharyngitis B08.5
pleurodynia B33.0
specific disease NEC B33.8
**Crabs, meaning pubic lice** B85.3
**Crack baby** P04.41
**Cracked nipple** N64.0
associated with
lactation O92.13
pregnancy O92.11- ☑
puerperium O92.12
**Cracked tooth** K03.81
**Cradle cap** L21.0
**Craft neurosis** F48.8
**Cramp**(s) R25.2
abdominal — *see* Pain, abdominal
bathing T75.1 ☑
colic R10.83
psychogenic F45.8
due to immersion T75.1 ☑
fireman T67.2 ☑
heat T67.2 ☑
immersion T75.1 ☑
intestinal — *see* Pain, abdominal
psychogenic F45.8
leg, sleep related G47.62
limb (lower) (upper) NEC R25.2
sleep related G47.62
linotypist's F48.8
organic G25.89
muscle (limb) (general) R25.2
due to immersion T75.1 ☑
psychogenic F45.8
occupational (hand) F48.8
organic G25.89
salt-depletion E87.1
sleep related, leg G47.62
stoker's T67.2 ☑
swimmer's T75.1 ☑
telegrapher's F48.8
organic G25.89
typist's F48.8
organic G25.89
uterus N94.89
menstrual — *see* Dysmenorrhea
writer's F48.8
organic G25.89
**Cranial** — *see* condition

☑ Additional Character Required — Refer to the Tabular List for Character Selection    Subterms under main terms may continue to next column or page

**Craniocleidodysostosis** Q74.0
**Craniofenestria** (skull) Q75.8
**Craniolacunia** (skull) Q75.8
**Craniopagus** Q89.4
**Craniopathy, metabolic** M85.2
**Craniopharyngeal** — *see* condition
**Craniopharyngioma** D44.4
**Craniorachischisis** (totalis) Q00.1
**Cranioschisis** Q75.8
**Craniostenosis** Q75.0
**Craniosynostosis** Q75.0
**Craniotabes** (cause unknown) M83.8
  neonatal P96.3
  rachitic E64.3
  syphilitic A50.56
**Cranium** — *see* condition
**Craw-craw** — *see* Onchocerciasis
**Creaking joint** — *see* Derangement, joint, specified type
  NEC
**Creeping**
  eruption B76.9
  palsy or paralysis G12.22
**Crenated tongue** K14.8
**Creotoxism** A05.9
**Crepitus**
  caput Q75.8
  joint — *see* Derangement, joint, specified type NEC
**Crescent or conus choroid, congenital** Q14.3
**CREST syndrome** M34.1
**Cretin, cretinism** (congenital) (endemic) (nongoitrous)
  (sporadic) E00.9
  pelvis
    with disproportion (fetopelvic) O33.0
      causing obstructed labor O65.0
  type
    hypothyroid E00.1
    mixed E00.2
    myxedematous E00.1
    neurological E00.0
**Creutzfeldt-Jakob disease or syndrome** (with dementia) A81.00
  familial A81.09
  iatrogenic A81.09
  specified NEC A81.09
  sporadic A81.09
  variant (vCJD) A81.01
**Crib death** R99
**Cribriform hymen** Q52.3
**Cri-du-chat syndrome** Q93.4
**Crigler-Najjar disease or syndrome** E80.5
**Crime, victim of** Z65.4
**Crimean hemorrhagic fever** A98.0
**Criminalism** F60.2
**Crisis**
  abdomen R10.0
  acute reaction F43.0
  addisonian E27.2
  adrenal (cortical) E27.2
  celiac K90.0
  Dietl's N13.8
  emotional (*see also* Disorder, adjustment)
    acute reaction to stress F43.0
    specific to childhood and adolescence F93.8
  glaucomatocyclitic — *see* Glaucoma, secondary, in-
    flammation
  heart — *see* Failure, heart
  nitritoid I95.2
    correct substance properly administered — *see*
      Table of Drugs and Chemicals, by drug, ad-
      verse effect
    overdose or wrong substance given or taken —
      *see* Table of Drugs and Chemicals, by drug,
      poisoning
  oculogyric H51.8
    psychogenic F45.8
  Pel's (tabetic) A52.11
  psychosexual identity F64.2
  renal N28.0
  sickle-cell D57.00
    with
      acute chest syndrome D57.01
      splenic sequestration D57.02
  state (acute reaction) F43.0
  tabetic A52.11
  thyroid — *see* Thyrotoxicosis with thyroid storm
  thyrotoxic — *see* Thyrotoxicosis with thyroid storm
**Crocq's disease** (acrocyanosis) I73.89

**Crohn's disease** — *see* Enteritis, regional
**Crooked septum, nasal** J34.2
**Cross syndrome** E70.328
**Crossbite** (anterior) (posterior) M26.24
**Cross-eye** — *see* Strabismus, convergent concomitant
**Croup, croupous** (catarrhal) (infectious) (inflammatory)
  (nondiphtheritic) J05.0
  bronchial J20.9
  diphtheritic A36.2
  false J38.5
  spasmodic J38.5
    diphtheritic A36.2
  stridulous J38.5
    diphtheritic A36.2
**Crouzon's disease** Q75.1
**Crowding, tooth, teeth, fully erupted** M26.31
**CRST syndrome** M34.1
**Cruchet's disease** A85.8
**Cruelty in children** (*see also* Disorder, conduct)
**Crural ulcer** — *see* Ulcer, lower limb
**Crush, crushed, crushing** T14.8 ☑
  abdomen S38.1 ☑
  ankle S97.0- ☑
  arm (upper) (and shoulder) S47.- ☑
  axilla — *see* Crush, arm
  back, lower S38.1 ☑
  buttock S38.1 ☑
  cheek S07.0 ☑
  chest S28.0 ☑
  cranium S07.1 ☑
  ear S07.0 ☑
  elbow S57.0- ☑
  extremity
    lower
      ankle — *see* Crush, ankle
      below knee — *see* Crush, leg
      foot — *see* Crush, foot
      hip — *see* Crush, hip
      knee — *see* Crush, knee
      thigh — *see* Crush, thigh
      toe — *see* Crush, toe
    upper
      below elbow S67.9- ☑
      elbow — *see* Crush, elbow
      finger — *see* Crush, finger
      forearm — *see* Crush, forearm
      hand — *see* Crush, hand
      thumb — *see* Crush, thumb
      upper arm — *see* Crush, arm
      wrist — *see* Crush, wrist
  face S07.0 ☑
  finger(s) S67.1- ☑
    with hand (and wrist) — *see* Crush, hand, specified
      site NEC
    index S67.19- ☑
    little S67.19- ☑
    middle S67.19- ☑
    ring S67.19- ☑
    thumb — *see* Crush, thumb
  foot S97.8- ☑
    toe — *see* Crush, toe
  forearm S57.8- ☑
  genitalia, external
    female S38.002 ☑
      vagina S38.03 ☑
      vulva S38.03 ☑
    male S38.001 ☑
      penis S38.01 ☑
      scrotum S38.02 ☑
      testis S38.02 ☑
  hand (except fingers alone) S67.2- ☑
    with wrist S67.4- ☑
  head S07.9 ☑
    specified NEC S07.8 ☑
  heel — *see* Crush, foot
  hip S77.0- ☑
    with thigh S77.2- ☑
  internal organ (abdomen, chest, or pelvis) NEC
    T14.8 ☑
  knee S87.0- ☑
  labium (majus) (minus) S38.03 ☑
  larynx S17.0 ☑
  leg (lower) S87.8- ☑
    knee — *see* Crush, knee
  lip S07.0 ☑

**Crush, crushed, crushing** — *continued*
  lower
    back S38.1 ☑
    leg — *see* Crush, leg
  neck S17.9 ☑
  nerve — *see* Injury, nerve
  nose S07.0 ☑
  pelvis S38.1 ☑
  penis S38.01 ☑
  scalp S07.8 ☑
  scapular region — *see* Crush, arm
  scrotum S38.02 ☑
  severe, unspecified site T14.8 ☑
  shoulder (and upper arm) — *see* Crush, arm
  skull S07.1 ☑
  syndrome (complication of trauma) T79.5 ☑
  testis S38.02 ☑
  thigh S77.1- ☑
    with hip S77.2- ☑
  throat S17.8 ☑
  thumb S67.0- ☑
    with hand (and wrist) — *see* Crush, hand, specified
      site NEC
  toe(s) S97.10- ☑
    great S97.11- ☑
    lesser S97.12- ☑
  trachea S17.0 ☑
  vagina S38.03 ☑
  vulva S38.03 ☑
  wrist S67.3- ☑
    with hand S67.4- ☑
**Crusta lactea** L21.0
**Crusts** R23.4
**Crutch paralysis** — *see* Injury, brachial plexus
**Cruveilhier-Baumgarten cirrhosis, disease or syn-
  drome** K74.69
**Cruveilhier's atrophy or disease** G12.8
**Crying** (constant) (continuous) (excessive)
  child, adolescent, or adult R45.83
  infant (baby) (newborn) R68.11
**Cryofibrinogenemia** D89.2
**Cryoglobulinemia** (essential) (idiopathic) (mixed) (primary) (purpura) (secondary) (vasculitis) D89.1
  with lung involvement D89.1 [J99]
**Cryptitis** (anal) (rectal) K62.89
**Cryptococcosis, cryptococcus** (infection) (neoformans)
  B45.9
  bone B45.3
  cerebral B45.1
  cutaneous B45.2
  disseminated B45.7
  generalized B45.7
  meningitis B45.1
  meningocerebralis B45.1
  osseous B45.3
  pulmonary B45.0
  skin B45.2
  specified NEC B45.8
**Cryptopapillitis** (anus) K62.89
**Cryptophthalmos** Q11.2
  syndrome Q87.0
**Cryptorchid, cryptorchism, cryptorchidism** Q53.9
  bilateral Q53.20
    abdominal Q53.211
    perineal Q53.22
  unilateral Q53.10
    abdominal Q53.111
    perineal Q53.12
**Cryptosporidiosis** A07.2
  hepatobiliary B88.8
  respiratory B88.8
**Cryptostromosis** J67.6
**Crystalluria** R82.99
**Cubitus**
  congenital Q68.8
  valgus (acquired) M21.0- ☑
    congenital Q68.8
    sequelae (late effect) of rickets E64.3
  varus (acquired) M21.1- ☑
    congenital Q68.8
    sequelae (late effect) of rickets E64.3
**Cultural deprivation or shock** Z60.3
**Curling esophagus** K22.4
**Curling's ulcer** — *see* Ulcer, peptic, acute
**Curschmann** (-Batten) (-Steinert) **disease or syndrome**
  G71.11
**Curse, Ondine's** — *see* Apnea, sleep

**Curvature**
- organ or site, congenital NEC — *see* Distortion
- penis (lateral) Q55.61
- Pott's (spinal) A18.01
- radius, idiopathic, progressive (congenital) Q74.0
- spine (acquired) (angular) (idiopathic) (incorrect) (postural) — *see* Dorsopathy, deforming
  - congenital Q67.5
  - due to or associated with
    - Charcot-Marie-Tooth disease (*see also* subcategory M49.8) G60.0
    - osteitis
      - deformans M88.88
      - fibrosa cystica (*see also* subcategory M49.8) E21.0
    - tuberculosis (Pott's curvature) A18.01
  - sequelae (late effect) of rickets E64.3
  - tuberculous A18.01

**Cushingoid due to steroid therapy** E24.2
- correct substance properly administered — *see* Table of Drugs and Chemicals, by drug, adverse effect
- overdose or wrong substance given or taken — *see* Table of Drugs and Chemicals, by drug, poisoning

**Cushing's**
- syndrome or disease E24.9
  - drug-induced E24.2
  - iatrogenic E24.2
  - pituitary-dependent E24.0
  - specified NEC E24.8
- ulcer — *see* Ulcer, peptic, acute

**Cusp, Carabelli** — *omit code*
**Cut** (external) (*see also* Laceration)
- muscle — *see* Injury, muscle

**Cutaneous** (*see also* condition)
- hemorrhage R23.3
- larva migrans B76.9

**Cutis** (*see also* condition)
- hyperelastica Q82.8
  - acquired L57.4
- laxa (hyperelastica) — *see* Dermatolysis
- marmorata R23.8
- osteosis L94.2
- pendula — *see* Dermatolysis
- rhomboidalis nuchae L57.2
- verticis gyrata Q82.8
  - acquired L91.8

**Cyanosis** R23.0
- due to
  - patent foramen botalli Q21.1
  - persistent foramen ovale Q21.1
- enterogenous D74.8
- paroxysmal digital — *see* Raynaud's disease
  - with gangrene I73.01
- retina, retinal H35.89

**Cyanotic heart disease** I24.9
- congenital Q24.9

**Cycle**
- anovulatory N97.0
- menstrual, irregular N92.6

**Cyclencephaly** Q04.9
**Cyclical vomiting** (*see also* Vomiting, cyclical) G43.A0
- (*following* G43.7)
- psychogenic F50.89

**Cyclitis** (*see also* Iridocyclitis) H20.9
- chronic — *see* Iridocyclitis, chronic
- Fuchs' heterochromic H20.81- ☑
- granulomatous — *see* Iridocyclitis, chronic
- lens-induced — *see* Iridocyclitis, lens-induced
- posterior H30.2- ☑

**Cycloid personality** F34.0
**Cyclophoria** H50.54
**Cyclopia, cyclops** Q87.0
**Cyclopism** Q87.0
**Cyclosporiasis** A07.4
**Cyclothymia** F34.0
**Cyclothymic personality** F34.0
**Cyclotropia** H50.41- ☑
**Cylindroma** (*see also* Neoplasm, malignant, by site)
- eccrine dermal — *see* Neoplasm, skin, benign
- skin — *see* Neoplasm, skin, benign

**Cylindruria** R82.99
**Cynanche**
- diphtheritic A36.2
- tonsillaris J36

**Cynophobia** F40.218
**Cynorexia** R63.2

**Cyphosis** — *see* Kyphosis
**Cyprus fever** — *see* Brucellosis
**Cyst** (colloid) (mucous) (simple) (retention)
- adenoid (infected) J35.8
- adrenal gland E27.8
  - congenital Q89.1
- air, lung J98.4
- allantoic Q64.4
- alveolar process (jaw bone) M27.40
- amnion, amniotic O41.8X- ☑
- aneurysmal M27.49
- anterior
  - chamber (eye) — *see* Cyst, iris
  - nasopalatine K09.1
- antrum J34.1
- anus K62.89
- apical (tooth) (periodontal) K04.8
- appendix K38.8
- arachnoid, brain (acquired) G93.0
  - congenital Q04.6
- arytenoid J38.7
- Baker's M71.2- ☑
  - ruptured M66.0
  - tuberculous A18.02
- Bartholin's gland N75.0
- bile duct (common) (hepatic) K83.5
- bladder (multiple) (trigone) N32.89
- blue dome (breast) — *see* Cyst, breast
- bone (local) NEC M85.60
  - aneurysmal M85.50
    - ankle M85.57- ☑
    - foot M85.57- ☑
    - forearm M85.53- ☑
    - hand M85.54- ☑
    - jaw M27.49
    - lower leg M85.56- ☑
    - multiple site M85.59
    - neck M85.58
    - rib M85.58
    - shoulder M85.51- ☑
    - skull M85.58
    - specified site NEC M85.58
    - thigh M85.55- ☑
    - toe M85.57- ☑
    - upper arm M85.52- ☑
    - vertebra M85.58
  - solitary M85.40
    - ankle M85.47- ☑
    - fibula M85.46- ☑
    - foot M85.47- ☑
    - hand M85.44- ☑
    - humerus M85.42- ☑
    - jaw M27.49
    - neck M85.48
    - pelvis M85.45- ☑
    - radius M85.43- ☑
    - rib M85.48
    - shoulder M85.41- ☑
    - skull M85.48
    - specified site NEC M85.48
    - tibia M85.46- ☑
    - toe M85.47- ☑
    - ulna M85.43- ☑
    - vertebra M85.48
  - specified type NEC M85.60
    - ankle M85.67- ☑
    - foot M85.67- ☑
    - forearm M85.63- ☑
    - hand M85.64- ☑
    - jaw M27.40
      - developmental (nonodontogenic) K09.1
      - odontogenic K09.0
      - latent M27.10
    - lower leg M85.66- ☑
    - multiple site M85.69
    - neck M85.68
    - rib M85.68
    - shoulder M85.61- ☑
    - skull M85.68
    - specified site NEC M85.68
    - thigh M85.65- ☑
    - toe M85.67- ☑
    - upper arm M85.62- ☑
    - vertebra M85.68
- brain (acquired) G93.0
  - congenital Q04.6
  - hydatid B67.99 [G94]

**Cyst** — *continued*
- brain — *continued*
  - third ventricle (colloid), congenital Q04.6
- branchial (cleft) Q18.0
- branchiogenic Q18.0
- breast (benign) (blue dome) (pedunculated) (solitary) N60.0- ☑
  - involution — *see* Dysplasia, mammary, specified type NEC
  - sebaceous — *see* Dysplasia, mammary, specified type NEC
- broad ligament (benign) N83.8
- bronchogenic (mediastinal) (sequestration) J98.4
  - congenital Q33.0
- buccal K09.8
- bulbourethral gland N36.8
- bursa, bursal NEC M71.30
  - with rupture — *see* Rupture, synovium
  - ankle M71.37- ☑
  - elbow M71.32- ☑
  - foot M71.37- ☑
  - hand M71.34- ☑
  - hip M71.35- ☑
  - multiple sites M71.39
  - pharyngeal J39.2
  - popliteal space — *see* Cyst, Baker's
  - shoulder M71.31- ☑
  - specified site NEC M71.38
  - wrist M71.33- ☑
- calcifying odontogenic D16.5
  - upper jaw (bone) (maxilla) D16.4
- canal of Nuck (female) N94.89
  - congenital Q52.4
- canthus — *see* Cyst, conjunctiva
- carcinomatous — *see* Neoplasm, malignant, by site
- cauda equina G95.89
- cavum septi pellucidi — *see* Cyst, brain
- celomic (pericardium) Q24.8
- cerebellopontine (angle) — *see* Cyst, brain
- cerebellum — *see* Cyst, brain
- cerebral — *see* Cyst, brain
- cervical lateral Q18.0
- cervix NEC N88.8
  - embryonic Q51.6
  - nabothian N88.8
- chiasmal optic NEC — *see* Disorder, optic, chiasm
- chocolate (ovary) N80.1
- choledochus, congenital Q44.4
- chorion O41.8X- ☑
- choroid plexus G93.0
- ciliary body — *see* Cyst, iris
- clitoris N90.7
- colon K63.89
- common (bile) duct K83.5
- congenital NEC Q89.8
  - adrenal gland Q89.1
  - epiglottis Q31.8
  - esophagus Q39.8
  - fallopian tube Q50.4
  - kidney Q61.00
    - more than one (multiple) Q61.02
      - specified as polycystic Q61.3
        - adult type Q61.2
        - infantile type NEC Q61.19
          - collecting duct dilation Q61.11
    - solitary Q61.01
  - larynx Q31.8
  - liver Q44.6
  - lung Q33.0
  - mediastinum Q34.1
  - ovary Q50.1
  - oviduct Q50.4
  - periurethral (tissue) Q64.79
  - prepuce Q55.69
  - salivary gland (any) Q38.4
  - sublingual Q38.6
  - submaxillary gland Q38.6
  - thymus (gland) Q89.2
  - tongue Q38.3
  - ureterovesical orifice Q62.8
  - vulva Q52.79
- conjunctiva H11.44- ☑
- cornea H18.89- ☑
- corpora quadrigemina G93.0
- corpus
  - albicans N83.29- ☑
  - luteum (hemorrhagic) (ruptured) N83.1- ☑
- Cowper's gland (benign) (infected) N36.8

☑ **Additional Character Required** — Refer to the Tabular List for Character Selection   ▽ Subterms under main terms may continue to next column or page

**Cyst** — *continued*
  paralabral — *continued*
    shoulder S43.43- ☑
  paramesonephric duct Q50.4
    female Q50.4
    male Q55.29
  paranephric N28.1
  paraphysis, cerebri, congenital Q04.6
  parasitic B89
  parathyroid (gland) E21.4
  paratubal N83.8
  paraurethral duct N36.8
  paroophoron Q50.5
  parotid gland K11.6
  parovarian Q50.5
  pelvis, female N94.89
    in pregnancy or childbirth O34.8- ☑
      causing obstructed labor O65.5
  penis (sebaceous) N48.89
  periapical K04.8
  pericardial (congenital) Q24.8
    acquired (secondary) I31.8
  pericoronal K09.0
  periodontal K04.8
    lateral K09.0
  peripelvic (lymphatic) N28.1
  peritoneum K66.8
    chylous I89.8
  periventricular, acquired, newborn P91.1
  pharynx (wall) J39.2
  pilar L72.11
  pilonidal (infected) (rectum) L05.91
    with abscess L05.01
    malignant C44.59- ☑
  pituitary (duct) (gland) E23.6
  placenta O43.19- ☑
  pleura J94.8
  popliteal — *see* Cyst, Baker's
  porencephalic Q04.6
    acquired G93.0
  postanal (infected) — *see* Cyst, pilonidal
  postmastoidectomy cavity (mucosal) — *see* Complications, postmastoidectomy, cyst
  preauricular Q18.1
  prepuce N47.4
    congenital Q55.69
  primordial (jaw) K09.0
  prostate N42.83
  pseudomucinous (ovary) D27.9
  pupillary, miotic H21.27- ☑
  radicular (residual) K04.8
  radiculodental K04.8
  ranular K11.8
  Rathke's pouch E23.6
  rectum (epithelium) (mucous) K62.89
  renal — *see* Cyst, kidney
  residual (radicular) K04.8
  retention (ovary) N83.29- ☑
    salivary gland K11.6
  retina H33.19- ☑
    ora serrata H33.11- ☑
    parasitic H33.12- ☑
  retroperitoneal K68.9
  sacrococcygeal (dermoid) — *see* Cyst, pilonidal
  salivary gland or duct (mucous extravasation or retention) K11.6
  Sampson's N80.1
  sclera H15.89
  scrotum L72.9
    sebaceous L72.3
  sebaceous (duct) (gland) L72.3
    breast — *see* Dysplasia, mammary, specified type NEC
    eyelid — *see* Cyst, eyelid
    genital organ NEC
      female N94.89
      male N50.89
    scrotum L72.3
  semilunar cartilage (knee) (multiple) — *see* Derangement, knee, meniscus, cystic
  seminal vesicle N50.89
  serous (ovary) N83.20- ☑
  sinus (accessory) (nasal) J34.1
  Skene's gland N36.8
  skin L72.9
    breast — *see* Dysplasia, mammary, specified type NEC
    epidermal, epidermoid L72.0

**Cyst** — *continued*
  skin — *continued*
    epithelial L72.0
    eyelid — *see* Cyst, eyelid
    genital organ NEC
      female N90.7
      male N50.89
    inclusion L72.0
    scrotum L72.9
    sebaceous L72.3
    sweat gland or duct L74.8
  solitary
    bone — *see* Cyst, bone, solitary
    jaw M27.40
    kidney N28.1
  spermatic cord N50.89
  sphenoid sinus J34.1
  spinal meninges G96.19
  spleen NEC D73.4
    congenital Q89.09
    hydatid (*see also* Echinococcus) B67.99 [D77]
  Stafne's M27.0
  subarachnoid intrasellar R93.0
  subcutaneous, pheomycotic (chromomycotic) B43.2
  subdural (cerebral) G93.0
    spinal cord G96.19
  sublingual gland K11.6
  submandibular gland K11.6
  submaxillary gland K11.6
  suburethral N36.8
  suprarenal gland E27.8
  suprasellar — *see* Cyst, brain
  sweat gland or duct L74.8
  synovial (*see also* Cyst, bursa)
    ruptured — *see* Rupture, synovium
  tarsal — *see* Chalazion
  tendon (sheath) — *see* Disorder, tendon, specified type NEC
  testis N44.2
    tunica albuginea N44.1
  theca lutein (ovary) N83.1- ☑
  Thornwaldt's J39.2
  thymus (gland) E32.8
  thyroglossal duct (infected) (persistent) Q89.2
  thyroid (gland) E04.1
  thyrolingual duct (infected) (persistent) Q89.2
  tongue K14.8
  tonsil J35.8
  tooth — *see* Cyst, dental
  Tornwaldt's J39.2
  trichilemmal (proliferating) L72.12
  trichodermal L72.12
  tubal (fallopian) N83.8
    inflammatory — *see* Salpingitis, chronic
  tubo-ovarian N83.8
    inflammatory N70.13
  tunica
    albuginea testis N44.1
    vaginalis N50.89
  turbinate (nose) J34.1
  Tyson's gland N48.89
  urachus, congenital Q64.4
  ureter N28.89
  ureterovesical orifice N28.89
  urethra, urethral (gland) N36.8
  uterine ligament N83.8
  uterus (body) (corpus) (recurrent) N85.8
    embryonic Q51.818
      cervix Q51.6
  vagina, vaginal (implantation) (inclusion) (squamous cell) (wall) N89.8
    embryonic Q52.4
  vallecula, vallecular (epiglottis) J38.7
  vesical (orifice) N32.89
  vitreous body H43.89
  vulva (implantation) (inclusion) N90.7
    congenital Q52.79
    sebaceous gland N90.7
  vulvovaginal gland N90.7
  wolffian
    female Q50.5
    male Q55.4

**Cystadenocarcinoma** — *see* Neoplasm, malignant, by site
  bile duct C22.1
  endometrioid — *see* Neoplasm, malignant, by site
    specified site — *see* Neoplasm, malignant, by site

**Cystadenocarcinoma** — *continued*
  endometrioid — *see* Neoplasm, malignant, by site — *continued*
    unspecified site
      female C56.9
      male C61
  mucinous
    papillary
      specified site — *see* Neoplasm, malignant, by site
      unspecified site C56.9
    specified site — *see* Neoplasm, malignant, by site
    unspecified site C56.9
  papillary
    mucinous
      specified site — *see* Neoplasm, malignant, by site
      unspecified site C56.9
    pseudomucinous
      specified site — *see* Neoplasm, malignant, by site
      unspecified site C56.9
    serous
      specified site — *see* Neoplasm, malignant, by site
      unspecified site C56.9
    specified site — *see* Neoplasm, malignant, by site
    unspecified site C56.9
  pseudomucinous
    papillary
      specified site — *see* Neoplasm, malignant, by site
      unspecified site C56.9
    specified site — *see* Neoplasm, malignant, by site
    unspecified site C56.9
  serous
    papillary
      specified site — *see* Neoplasm, malignant, by site
      unspecified site C56.9
    specified site — *see* Neoplasm, malignant, by site
    unspecified site C56.9

**Cystadenofibroma**
  clear cell — *see* Neoplasm, benign, by site
  endometrioid D27.9
    borderline malignancy D39.1- ☑
    malignant C56.- ☑
  mucinous
    specified site — *see* Neoplasm, benign, by site
    unspecified site D27.9
  serous
    specified site — *see* Neoplasm, benign, by site
    unspecified site D27.9
  specified site — *see* Neoplasm, benign, by site
  unspecified site D27.9

**Cystadenoma** (*see also* Neoplasm, benign, by site)
  bile duct D13.4
  endometrioid — *see* Neoplasm, benign, by site
    borderline malignancy — *see* Neoplasm, uncertain behavior, by site
  malignant — *see* Neoplasm, malignant, by site
  mucinous
    borderline malignancy
      ovary C56.- ☑
      specified site NEC — *see* Neoplasm, uncertain behavior, by site
      unspecified site C56.9
    papillary
      borderline malignancy
        ovary C56.- ☑
        specified site NEC — *see* Neoplasm, uncertain behavior, by site
        unspecified site C56.9
      specified site — *see* Neoplasm, benign, by site
      unspecified site D27.9
    specified site — *see* Neoplasm, benign, by site
    unspecified site D27.9
  papillary
    borderline malignancy
      ovary C56.- ☑
      specified site NEC — *see* Neoplasm, uncertain behavior, by site
      unspecified site C56.9
    lymphomatosum
      specified site — *see* Neoplasm, benign, by site
      unspecified site D11.9

☑ **Additional Character Required** — **Refer to the Tabular List for Character Selection**    Subterms under main terms may continue to next column or page

**Cystadenoma** — *continued*
  papillary — *continued*
    mucinous
      borderline malignancy
        ovary C56.- ☑
        specified site NEC — *see* Neoplasm, uncertain behavior, by site
        unspecified site C56.9
      specified site — *see* Neoplasm, benign, by site
      unspecified site D27.9
    pseudomucinous
      borderline malignancy
        ovary C56.- ☑
        specified site NEC — *see* Neoplasm, uncertain behavior, by site
        unspecified site C56.9
      specified site — *see* Neoplasm, benign, by site
      unspecified site D27.9
    serous
      borderline malignancy
        ovary C56.- ☑
        specified site NEC — *see* Neoplasm, uncertain behavior, by site
        unspecified site C56.9
      specified site — *see* Neoplasm, benign, by site
      unspecified site D27.9
  specified site — *see* Neoplasm, benign, by site
  unspecified site D27.9
  pseudomucinous
    borderline malignancy
      ovary C56.- ☑
      specified site NEC — *see* Neoplasm, uncertain behavior, by site
      unspecified site C56.9
    papillary
      borderline malignancy
        ovary C56.- ☑
        specified site NEC — *see* Neoplasm, uncertain behavior, by site
        unspecified site C56.9
      specified site — *see* Neoplasm, benign, by site
      unspecified site D27.9
    specified site — *see* Neoplasm, benign, by site
    unspecified site D27.9
  serous
    borderline malignancy
      ovary C56.- ☑
      specified site NEC — *see* Neoplasm, uncertain behavior, by site
      unspecified site C56.9
    papillary
      borderline malignancy
        ovary C56.- ☑
        specified site NEC — *see* Neoplasm, uncertain behavior, by site
        unspecified site C56.9
      specified site — *see* Neoplasm, benign, by site
      unspecified site D27.9
    specified site — *see* Neoplasm, benign, by site
    unspecified site D27.9
**Cystathionine synthase deficiency** E72.11
**Cystathioninemia** E72.19
**Cystathioninuria** E72.19
**Cystic** (*see also* condition)
  breast (chronic) — *see* Mastopathy, cystic
  corpora lutea (hemorrhagic) N83.1- ☑
  duct — *see* condition
  eyeball (congenital) Q11.0
  fibrosis — *see* Fibrosis, cystic
  kidney (congenital) Q61.9

**Cystic** — *continued*
  kidney — *continued*
    adult type Q61.2
    infantile type NEC Q61.19
      collecting duct dilatation Q61.11
    medullary Q61.5
  liver, congenital Q44.6
  lung disease J98.4
    congenital Q33.0
  mastitis, chronic — *see* Mastopathy, cystic
  medullary, kidney Q61.5
  meniscus — *see* Derangement, knee, meniscus, cystic
  ovary N83.20- ☑
**Cysticercosis, cysticerciasis** B69.9
  with
    epileptiform fits B69.0
    myositis B69.81
  brain B69.0
  central nervous system B69.0
  cerebral B69.0
  ocular B69.1
  specified NEC B69.89
**Cysticercus cellulose infestation** — *see* Cysticercosis
**Cystinosis** (malignant) E72.04
**Cystinuria** E72.01
**Cystitis** (exudative) (hemorrhagic) (septic) (suppurative) N30.90
  with
    fibrosis — *see* Cystitis, chronic, interstitial
    hematuria N30.91
    leukoplakia — *see* Cystitis, chronic, interstitial
    malakoplakia — *see* Cystitis, chronic, interstitial
    metaplasia — *see* Cystitis, chronic, interstitial
    prostatitis N41.3
  acute N30.00
    with hematuria N30.01
    of trigone N30.30
      with hematuria N30.31
  allergic — *see* Cystitis, specified type NEC
  amebic A06.81
  bilharzial B65.9 [N33]
  blennorrhagic (gonococcal) A54.01
  bullous — *see* Cystitis, specified type NEC
  calculous N21.0
  chlamydial A56.01
  chronic N30.20
    with hematuria N30.21
    interstitial N30.10
      with hematuria N30.11
    of trigone N30.30
      with hematuria N30.31
    specified NEC N30.20
      with hematuria N30.21
  cystic (a) — *see* Cystitis, specified type NEC
  diphtheritic A36.85
  echinococcal
    granulosus B67.39
    multilocularis B67.69
  emphysematous — *see* Cystitis, specified type NEC
  encysted — *see* Cystitis, specified type NEC
  eosinophilic — *see* Cystitis, specified type NEC
  follicular — *see* Cystitis, of trigone
  gangrenous — *see* Cystitis, specified type NEC
  glandularis — *see* Cystitis, specified type NEC
  gonococcal A54.01
  incrusted — *see* Cystitis, specified type NEC
  interstitial (chronic) — *see* Cystitis, chronic, interstitial
  irradiation N30.40
    with hematuria N30.41
  irritation — *see* Cystitis, specified type NEC

**Cystitis** — *continued*
  malignant — *see* Cystitis, specified type NEC
  of trigone N30.30
    with hematuria N30.31
  panmural — *see* Cystitis, chronic, interstitial
  polyposa — *see* Cystitis, specified type NEC
  prostatic N41.3
  puerperal (postpartum) O86.22
  radiation — *see* Cystitis, irradiation
  specified type NEC N30.80
    with hematuria N30.81
  subacute — *see* Cystitis, chronic
  submucous — *see* Cystitis, chronic, interstitial
  syphilitic (late) A52.76
  trichomonal A59.03
  tuberculous A18.12
  ulcerative — *see* Cystitis, chronic, interstitial
**Cystocele** (-urethrocele)
  female N81.10
    with prolapse of uterus — *see* Prolapse, uterus
    lateral N81.12
    midline N81.11
    paravaginal N81.12
  in pregnancy or childbirth O34.8- ☑
    causing obstructed labor O65.5
  male N32.89
**Cystolithiasis** N21.0
**Cystoma** (*see also* Neoplasm, benign, by site)
  endometrial, ovary N80.1
  mucinous
    specified site — *see* Neoplasm, benign, by site
    unspecified site D27.9
  serous
    specified site — *see* Neoplasm, benign, by site
    unspecified site D27.9
  simple (ovary) N83.29- ☑
**Cystoplegia** N31.2
**Cystoptosis** N32.89
**Cystopyelitis** — *see* Pyelonephritis
**Cystorrhagia** N32.89
**Cystosarcoma phyllodes** D48.6- ☑
  benign D24- ☑
  malignant — *see* Neoplasm, breast, malignant
**Cystostomy**
  attention to Z43.5
  complication — *see* Complications, cystostomy
  status Z93.50
    appendico-vesicostomy Z93.52
    cutaneous Z93.51
    specified NEC Z93.59
**Cystourethritis** — *see* Urethritis
**Cystourethrocele** (*see also* Cystocele)
  female N81.10
    with uterine prolapse — *see* Prolapse, uterus
    lateral N81.12
    midline N81.11
    paravaginal N81.12
  male N32.89
**Cytomegalic inclusion disease**
  congenital P35.1
**Cytomegalovirus infection** B25.9
**Cytomycosis** (reticuloendothelial) B39.4
**Cytopenia** D75.9
  refractory
    with multilineage dysplasia D46.A (*following* D46.2)
    and ring sideroblasts (RCMD RS) D46.B (*following* D46.2)
**Czerny's disease** (periodic hydrarthrosis of the knee) — *see* Effusion, joint, knee

# D

**Da Costa's syndrome** F45.8
**Daae** (-Finsen) **disease** (epidemic pleurodynia) B33.0
**Dabney's grip** B33.0
**Dacryoadenitis, dacryadenitis** H04.00- ☑
   acute H04.01- ☑
   chronic H04.02- ☑
**Dacryocystitis** H04.30- ☑
   acute H04.32- ☑
   chronic H04.41- ☑
   neonatal P39.1
   phlegmonous H04.31- ☑
   syphilitic A52.71
      congenital (early) A50.01
   trachomatous, active A71.1
      sequelae (late effect) B94.0
**Dacryocystoblenorrhea** — *see* Inflammation, lacrimal,
   passages, chronic
**Dacryocystocele** — *see* Disorder, lacrimal system,
   changes
**Dacryolith, dacryolithiasis** H04.51- ☑
**Dacryoma** — *see* Disorder, lacrimal system, changes
**Dacryopericystitis** — *see* Dacryocystitis
**Dacryops** H04.11- ☑
**Dacryostenosis** (*see also* Stenosis, lacrimal)
   congenital Q10.5
**Dactylitis**
   bone — *see* Osteomyelitis
   sickle-cell D57.00
      Hb C D57.219
      Hb SS D57.00
      specified NEC D57.819
   skin L08.9
   syphilitic A52.77
   tuberculous A18.03
**Dactylolysis spontanea** (ainhum) L94.6
**Dactylosymphysis** Q70.9
   fingers — *see* Syndactylism, complex, fingers
   toes — *see* Syndactylism, complex, toes
**Damage**
   arteriosclerotic — *see* Arteriosclerosis
   brain (nontraumatic) G93.9
      anoxic, hypoxic G93.1
         resulting from a procedure G97.82
      child NEC G80.9
      due to birth injury P11.2
   cardiorenal (vascular) — *see* Hypertension, cardiorenal
   cerebral NEC — *see* Damage, brain
   coccyx, complicating delivery O71.6
   coronary — *see* Disease, heart, ischemic
   eye, birth injury P15.3
   liver (nontraumatic) K76.9
      alcoholic K70.9
      due to drugs — *see* Disease, liver, toxic
      toxic — *see* Disease, liver, toxic
   medication T88.7 ☑
   pelvic
      joint or ligament, during delivery O71.6
      organ NEC
         during delivery O71.5
         following ectopic or molar pregnancy O08.6
   renal — *see* Disease, renal
   subendocardium, subendocardial — *see* Degeneration,
      myocardial
   vascular I99.9
**Dana-Putnam syndrome** (subacute combined sclerosis
   with pernicious anemia) — *see* Degeneration,
   combined
**Danbolt** (-Cross) **syndrome** (acrodermatitis enteropathica) E83.2
**Dandruff** L21.0
**Dandy-Walker syndrome** Q03.1
   with spina bifida — *see* Spina bifida
**Danlos' syndrome** Q79.6
**Darier** (-White) **disease** (congenital) Q82.8
   meaning erythema annulare centrifugum L53.1
**Darier-Roussy sarcoid** D86.3
**Darling's disease or histoplasmosis** B39.4
**Darwin's tubercle** Q17.8
**Dawson's** (inclusion body) **encephalitis** A81.1

**De Beurmann** (-Gougerot) **disease** B42.1
**De la Tourette's syndrome** F95.2
**De Lange's syndrome** Q87.1
**De Morgan's spots** (senile angiomas) I78.1
**De Quervain's**
   disease (tendon sheath) M65.4
   syndrome E34.51
   thyroiditis (subacute granulomatous thyroiditis) E06.1
**De Toni-Fanconi** (-Debré) **syndrome** E72.09
   with cystinosis E72.04
**Dead**
   fetus, retained (mother) O36.4 ☑
      early pregnancy O02.1
   labyrinth H83.2 ☑
   ovum, retained O02.0
**Deaf nonspeaking NEC** H91.3
**Deafmutism** (acquired) (congenital) NEC H91.3
   hysterical F44.6
   syphilitic, congenital (*see also* subcategory) H94.8
      A50.09
**Deafness** (acquired) (complete) (hereditary) (partial)
   H91.9- ☑
   with blue sclera and fragility of bone Q78.0
   auditory fatigue — *see* Deafness, specified type NEC
   aviation T70.0 ☑
      nerve injury — *see* Injury, nerve, acoustic, specified
         type NEC
   boilermaker's H83.3 ☑
   central — *see* Deafness, sensorineural
   conductive H90.2
      and sensorineural
         mixed H90.8
            bilateral H90.6
      bilateral H90.0
      unilateral H90.1- ☑
         with restricted hearing on the contralateral side
            H90.A- ☑
   congenital H90.5
      with blue sclera and fragility of bone Q78.0
   due to toxic agents — *see* Deafness, ototoxic
   emotional (hysterical) F44.6
   functional (hysterical) F44.6
   high frequency H91.9- ☑
   hysterical F44.6
   low frequency H91.9- ☑
   mental R48.8
   mixed conductive and sensorineural H90.8
      bilateral H90.6
      unilateral H90.7- ☑
   nerve — *see* Deafness, sensorineural
   neural — *see* Deafness, sensorineural
   noise-induced (*see also* subcategory) H83.3 ☑
      nerve injury — *see* Injury, nerve, acoustic, specified
         type NEC
   nonspeaking H91.3
   ototoxic H91.0 ☑
   perceptive — *see* Deafness, sensorineural
   psychogenic (hysterical) F44.6
   sensorineural H90.5
      and conductive
         bilateral H90.6
         mixed H90.8
            bilateral H90.6
      bilateral H90.3
      unilateral H90.4- ☑
         with restricted hearing on the contralateral side
            H90.A- ☑
   sensory — *see* Deafness, sensorineural
   specified type NEC H91.8
   sudden (idiopathic) H91.2- ☑
   syphilitic A52.15
   transient ischemic H93.01- ☑
   traumatic — *see* Injury, nerve, acoustic, specified type
      NEC
   word (developmental) H93.25
**Death** (cause unknown) (of) (unexplained) (unspecified
   cause) R99
   brain G93.82
   cardiac (sudden) (with successful resuscitation) —
      *code to* underlying disease
      family history of Z82.41
      personal history of Z86.74

**Death** — *continued*
   family member (assumed) Z63.4
**Debility** (chronic) (general) (nervous) R53.81
   congenital or neonatal NOS P96.9
   nervous R53.81
   old age R54
   senile R54
**Débove's disease** (splenomegaly) R16.1
**Decalcification**
   bone — *see* Osteoporosis
   teeth K03.89
**Decapsulation, kidney** N28.89
**Decay**
   dental — *see* Caries, dental
   senile R54
   tooth, teeth — *see* Caries, dental
**Deciduitis** (acute)
   following ectopic or molar pregnancy O08.0
**Decline** (general) — *see* Debility
   cognitive, age-associated R41.81
**Decompensation**
   cardiac (acute) (chronic) — *see* Disease, heart
   cardiovascular — *see* Disease, cardiovascular
   heart — *see* Disease, heart
   hepatic — *see* Failure, hepatic
   myocardial (acute) (chronic) — *see* Disease, heart
   respiratory J98.8
**Decompression sickness** T70.3 ☑
**Decrease** (d)
   absolute neutrophile count — *see* Neutropenia
   blood
      platelets — *see* Thrombocytopenia
      pressure R03.1
         due to shock following
            injury T79.4 ☑
            operation T81.19 ☑
   estrogen E28.39
      postablative E89.40
         asymptomatic E89.40
         symptomatic E89.41
   fragility of erythrocytes D58.8
   function
      lipase (pancreatic) K90.3
      ovary in hypopituitarism E23.0
      parenchyma of pancreas K86.89
      pituitary (gland) (anterior) (lobe) E23.0
         posterior (lobe) E23.0
   functional activity R68.89
   glucose R73.09
   hematocrit R71.0
   hemoglobin R71.0
   leukocytes D72.819
      specified NEC D72.818
   libido R68.82
   lymphocytes D72.810
   platelets D69.6
   respiration, due to shock following injury T79.4 ☑
   sexual desire R68.82
   tear secretion NEC — *see* Syndrome, dry eye
   tolerance
      fat K90.49
      glucose R73.09
      pancreatic K90.3
      salt and water E87.8
   vision NEC H54.7
   white blood cell count D72.819
      specified NEC D72.818
**Decubitus** (ulcer) — *see* Ulcer, pressure, by site
   cervix N86
**Deepening acetabulum** — *see* Derangement, joint,
   specified type NEC, hip
**Defect, defective** Q89.9
   3-beta-hydroxysteroid dehydrogenase E25.0
   11-hydroxylase E25.0
   21-hydroxylase E25.0
   abdominal wall, congenital Q79.59
   antibody immunodeficiency D80.9
   aorticopulmonary septum Q21.4
   atrial septal (ostium secundum type) Q21.1
      following acute myocardial infarction (current
         complication) I23.1
      ostium primum type Q21.2

**Defect, defective** — *continued*
  atrioventricular
    canal Q21.2
    septum Q21.2
  auricular septal Q21.1
  bilirubin excretion NEC E80.6
  biosynthesis, androgen (testicular) E29.1
  bulbar septum Q21.0
  catalase E80.3
  cell membrane receptor complex (CR3) D71
  circulation I99.9
    congenital Q28.9
    newborn Q28.9
  coagulation (factor) (*see also* Deficiency, factor) D68.9
    with
      ectopic pregnancy O08.1
      molar pregnancy O08.1
    acquired D68.4
    antepartum with hemorrhage — *see* Hemorrhage, antepartum, with coagulation defect
    due to
      liver disease D68.4
      vitamin K deficiency D68.4
    hereditary NEC D68.2
    intrapartum O67.0
    newborn, transient P61.6
    postpartum O99.13
      with hemorrhage O72.3
    specified type NEC D68.8
  complement system D84.1
  conduction (heart) I45.9
    bone — *see* Deafness, conductive
  congenital, organ or site not listed — *see* Anomaly, by site
  coronary sinus Q21.1
  cushion, endocardial Q21.2
  degradation, glycoprotein E77.1
  dental bridge, crown, fillings — *see* Defect, dental restoration
  dental restoration K08.50
    specified NEC K08.59
  dentin (hereditary) K00.5
  Descemet's membrane, congenital Q13.89
  developmental (*see also* Anomaly)
    cauda equina Q06.3
  diaphragm
    with elevation, eventration or hernia — *see* Hernia, diaphragm
    congenital Q79.1
      with hernia Q79.0
      gross (with hernia) Q79.0
  ectodermal, congenital Q82.9
  Eisenmenger's Q21.8
  enzyme
    catalase E80.3
    peroxidase E80.3
  esophagus, congenital Q39.9
  extensor retinaculum M62.89
  fibrin polymerization D68.2
  filling
    bladder R93.41
    kidney R93.42- ☑
    renal pelvis R93.41
    stomach R93.3
    ureter R93.41
    urinary organs, specified NEC R93.49
  Gerbode Q21.0
  glycoprotein degradation E77.1
  Hageman (factor) D68.2
  hearing — *see* Deafness
  high grade F70
  interatrial septal Q21.1
  interauricular septal Q21.1
  interventricular septal Q21.0
    with dextroposition of aorta, pulmonary stenosis and hypertrophy of right ventricle Q21.3
    in tetralogy of Fallot Q21.3
  learning (specific) — *see* Disorder, learning
  lymphocyte function antigen-1 (LFA-1) D84.0
  lysosomal enzyme, post-translational modification E77.0
  major osseous M89.70
    ankle M89.77- ☑
    carpus M89.74- ☑
    clavicle M89.71- ☑
    femur M89.75- ☑
    fibula M89.76- ☑
    fingers M89.74- ☑

**Defect, defective** — *continued*
  major osseous — *continued*
    foot M89.77- ☑
    forearm M89.73- ☑
    hand M89.74- ☑
    humerus M89.72- ☑
    lower leg M89.76- ☑
    metacarpus M89.74- ☑
    metatarsus M89.77- ☑
    multiple sites M89.79
    pelvic region M89.75- ☑
    pelvis M89.75- ☑
    radius M89.73- ☑
    scapula M89.71- ☑
    shoulder region M89.71- ☑
    specified NEC M89.78
    tarsus M89.77- ☑
    thigh M89.75- ☑
    tibia M89.76- ☑
    toes M89.77- ☑
    ulna M89.73- ☑
  mental — *see* Disability, intellectual
  modification, lysosomal enzymes, post-translational E77.0
  obstructive, congenital
    renal pelvis Q62.39
    ureter Q62.39
      atresia — *see* Atresia, ureter
      cecoureterocele Q62.32
      megaureter Q62.2
      orthotopic ureterocele Q62.31
  osseous, major M89.70
    ankle M89.77- ☑
    carpus M89.74- ☑
    clavicle M89.71- ☑
    femur M89.75- ☑
    fibula M89.76- ☑
    fingers M89.74- ☑
    foot M89.77- ☑
    forearm M89.73- ☑
    hand M89.74- ☑
    humerus M89.72- ☑
    lower leg M89.76- ☑
    metacarpus M89.74- ☑
    metatarsus M89.77- ☑
    multiple sites M89.9
    pelvic region M89.75- ☑
    pelvis M89.75- ☑
    radius M89.73- ☑
    scapula M89.71- ☑
    shoulder region M89.71- ☑
    specified NEC M89.78
    tarsus M89.77- ☑
    thigh M89.75- ☑
    tibia M89.76- ☑
    toes M89.77- ☑
    ulna M89.73- ☑
  osteochondral NEC (*see also* Deformity) M95.8
  ostium
    primum Q21.2
    secundum Q21.1
  peroxidase E80.3
  placental blood supply — *see* Insufficiency, placental
  platelets, qualitative D69.1
    constitutional D68.0
  postural NEC, spine — *see* Dorsopathy, deforming
  reduction
    limb Q73.8
      lower Q72.9- ☑
        absence — *see* Agenesis, leg
          foot — *see* Agenesis, foot
        longitudinal
          femur Q72.4- ☑
          fibula Q72.6- ☑
          tibia Q72.5- ☑
        specified type NEC Q72.89- ☑
        split foot Q72.7- ☑
      specified type NEC Q73.8
      upper Q71.9- ☑
        absence — *see* Agenesis, arm
          forearm — *see* Agenesis, forearm
          hand — *see* Agenesis, hand
        lobster-claw hand Q71.6- ☑
        longitudinal
          radius Q71.4- ☑
          ulna Q71.5- ☑

**Defect, defective** — *continued*
  reduction — *continued*
    limb — *continued*
      upper — *continued*
        specified type NEC Q71.89- ☑
  renal pelvis Q63.8
    obstructive Q62.39
  respiratory system, congenital Q34.9
  restoration, dental K08.50
    specified NEC K08.59
  retinal nerve bundle fibers H35.89
  septal (heart) NOS Q21.9
    acquired (atrial) (auricular) (ventricular) (old) I51.0
    atrial Q21.1
      concurrent with acute myocardial infarction — *see* Infarct, myocardium
      following acute myocardial infarction (current complication) I23.1
    ventricular (*see also* Defect, ventricular septal) Q21.0
  sinus venosus Q21.1
  speech R47.9
    developmental F80.9
    specified NEC R47.89
  Taussig-Bing (aortic transposition and overriding pulmonary artery) Q20.1
  teeth, wedge K03.1
  vascular (local) I99.9
    congenital Q27.9
  ventricular septal Q21.0
    concurrent with acute myocardial infarction — *see* Infarct, myocardium
    following acute myocardial infarction (current complication) I23.2
    in tetralogy of Fallot Q21.3
  vision NEC H54.7
  visual field H53.40
    bilateral
      heteronymous H53.47
      homonymous H53.46- ☑
    generalized contraction H53.48- ☑
    localized
      arcuate H53.43- ☑
      scotoma (central area) H53.41- ☑
        blind spot area H53.42- ☑
      sector H53.43- ☑
      specified type NEC H53.45- ☑
  voice R49.9
    specified NEC R49.8
  wedge, tooth, teeth (abrasion) K03.1
**Deferentitis** N49.1
  gonorrheal (acute) (chronic) A54.23
**Defibrination** (syndrome) D65
  antepartum — *see* Hemorrhage, antepartum, with coagulation defect, disseminated intravascular coagulation
  following ectopic or molar pregnancy O08.1
  intrapartum O67.0
  newborn P60
  postpartum O72.3
**Deficiency, deficient**
  3-beta hydroxysteroid dehydrogenase E25.0
  5-alpha reductase (with male pseudo-hermaphroditism) E29.1
  11-hydroxylase E25.0
  21-hydroxylase E25.0
  abdominal muscle syndrome Q79.4
  AC globulin (congenital) (hereditary) D68.2
    acquired D68.4
  accelerator globulin (Ac G) (blood) D68.2
  acid phosphatase E83.39
  activating factor (blood) D68.2
  adenosine deaminase (ADA) D81.3
  aldolase (hereditary) E74.19
  alpha-1-antitrypsin E88.01
  amino-acids E72.9
  anemia — *see* Anemia
  aneurin E51.9
  antibody with
    hyperimmunoglobulinemia D80.6
    near-normal immunoglobins D80.6
  antidiuretic hormone E23.2
  anti-hemophilic
    factor (A) D66
      B D67
      C D68.1
    globulin (AHG) NEC D66
  antithrombin (antithrombin III) D68.59

▼ Subterms under main terms may continue to next column or page    ☑ Additional Character Required — Refer to the Tabular List for Character Selection    83

Defect, defective — Deficiency, deficient

**Deficiency, deficient** — *continued*
  ascorbic acid E54
  attention (disorder) (syndrome) F98.8
    with hyperactivity — *see* Disorder, attention-deficit
        hyperactivity
  autoprothrombin
    C D68.2
    I D68.2
    II D67
  beta-glucuronidase E76.29
  biotin E53.8
  biotin-dependent carboxylase D81.819
  biotinidase D81.810
  brancher enzyme (amylopectinosis) E74.03
  C1 esterase inhibitor (C1-INH) D84.1
  calciferol E55.9
    with
        adult osteomalacia M83.8
        rickets — *see* Rickets
  calcium (dietary) E58
  calorie, severe E43
    with marasmus E41
        and kwashiorkor E42
  cardiac — *see* Insufficiency, myocardial
  carnitine E71.40
    due to
        hemodialysis E71.43
        inborn errors of metabolism E71.42
        Valproic acid therapy E71.43
    iatrogenic E71.43
    muscle palmityltransferase E71.314
    primary E71.41
    secondary E71.448
  carotene E50.9
  central nervous system G96.8
  ceruloplasmin (Wilson) E83.01
  choline E53.8
  Christmas factor D67
  chromium E61.4
  clotting (blood) (*see also* Deficiency, coagulation factor) D68.9
  clotting factor NEC (hereditary) (*see also* Deficiency, factor) D68.2
  coagulation NOS D68.9
    with
        ectopic pregnancy O08.1
        molar pregnancy O08.1
    acquired (any) D68.4
    antepartum hemorrhage — *see* Hemorrhage, antepartum, with coagulation defect
    clotting factor NEC (*see also* Deficiency, factor) D68.2
    due to
        hyperprothrombinemia D68.4
        liver disease D68.4
        vitamin K deficiency D68.4
    newborn, transient P61.6
    postpartum O72.3
    specified NEC D68.8
  cognitive F09
  color vision H53.50
    achromatopsia H53.51
    acquired H53.52
    deuteranomaly H53.53
    protanomaly H53.54
    specified type NEC H53.59
    tritanomaly H53.55
  combined glucocorticoid and mineralocorticoid E27.49
  contact factor D68.2
  copper (nutritional) E61.0
  corticoadrenal E27.40
    primary E27.1
  craniofacial axis Q75.0
  cyanocobalamin E53.8
  debrancher enzyme (limit dextrinosis) E74.03
  dehydrogenase
    long chain/very long chain acyl CoA E71.310
    medium chain acyl CoA E71.311
    short chain acyl CoA E71.312
  diet E63.9
  dihydropyrimidine dehydrogenase (DPD) E88.89
  disaccharidase E73.9
  edema — *see* Malnutrition, severe
  endocrine E34.9
  energy-supply — *see* Malnutrition
  enzymes, circulating NEC E88.09
  ergosterol E55.9

**Deficiency, deficient** — *continued*
  ergosterol — *continued*
    with
        adult osteomalacia M83.8
        rickets — *see* Rickets
  essential fatty acid (EFA) E63.0
  factor (*see also* Deficiency, coagulation)
    Hageman D68.2
    I (congenital) (hereditary) D68.2
    II (congenital) (hereditary) D68.2
    IX (congenital) (functional) (hereditary) (with functional defect) D67
    multiple (congenital) D68.8
        acquired D68.4
    V (congenital) (hereditary) D68.2
    VII (congenital) (hereditary) D68.2
    VIII (congenital) (functional) (hereditary) (with functional defect) D66
        with vascular defect D68.0
    X (congenital) (hereditary) D68.2
    XI (congenital) (hereditary) D68.1
    XII (congenital) (hereditary) D68.2
    XIII (congenital) (hereditary) D68.2
  femoral, proximal focal (congenital) — *see* Defect, reduction, lower limb, longitudinal, femur
  fibrinase D68.2
  fibrinogen (congenital) (hereditary) D68.2
    acquired D65
  fibrin-stabilizing factor (congenital) (hereditary) D68.2
    acquired D68.4
  folate E53.8
  folic acid E53.8
  foreskin N47.3
  fructokinase E74.11
  fructose 1,6-diphosphatase E74.19
  fructose-1-phosphate aldolase E74.19
  galactokinase E74.29
  galactose-1-phosphate uridyl transferase E74.29
  gammaglobulin in blood D80.1
    hereditary D80.0
  glass factor D68.2
  glucocorticoid E27.49
    mineralocorticoid E27.49
  glucose-6-phosphatase E74.01
  glucose-6-phosphate dehydrogenase anemia D55.0
  glucuronyl transferase E80.5
  glycogen synthetase E74.09
  gonadotropin (isolated) E23.0
  growth hormone (idiopathic) (isolated) E23.0
  Hageman factor D68.2
  hemoglobin D64.9
  hepatophosphorylase E74.09
  homogentisate 1,2-dioxygenase E70.29
  hormone
    anterior pituitary (partial) NEC E23.0
        growth E23.0
    growth (isolated) E23.0
    pituitary E23.0
    testicular E29.1
  hypoxanthine- (guanine)-phosphoribosyltransferase (HG- PRT) (total H-PRT) E79.1
  immunity D84.9
    cell-mediated D84.8
        with thrombocytopenia and eczema D82.0
    combined D81.9
    humoral D80.9
    IgA (secretory) D80.2
    IgG D80.3
    IgM D80.4
  immuno — *see* Immunodeficiency
  immunoglobulin, selective
    A (IgA) D80.2
    G (IgG) (subclasses) D80.3
    M (IgM) D80.4
  inositol (B complex) E53.8
  intrinsic
    factor (congenital) D51.0
    sphincter N36.42
        with urethral hypermobility N36.43
  iodine E61.8
    congenital syndrome — *see* Syndrome, iodine-deficiency, congenital
  iron E61.1
    anemia D50.9
  kalium E87.6
  kappa-light chain D80.8
  labile factor (congenital) (hereditary) D68.2
    acquired D68.4

**Deficiency, deficient** — *continued*
  lacrimal fluid (acquired) (*see also* Syndrome, dry eye)
    congenital Q10.6
  lactase
    congenital E73.0
    secondary E73.1
  Laki-Lorand factor D68.2
  lecithin cholesterol acyltransferase E78.6
  lipocaic K86.89
  lipoprotein (familial) (high density) E78.6
  liver phosphorylase E74.09
  lysosomal alpha-1, 4 glucosidase E74.02
  magnesium E61.2
  major histocompatibility complex
    class I D81.6
    class II D81.7
  manganese E61.3
  menadione (vitamin K) E56.1
    newborn P53
  mental (familial) (hereditary) — *see* Disability, intellectual
  methylenetetrahydrofolate reductase (MTHFR) E72.12
  mevalonate kinase M04.1
  mineralocorticoid E27.49
    with glucocorticoid E27.49
  mineral NEC E61.8
  molybdenum (nutritional) E61.5
  moral F60.2
  multiple nutrient elements E61.7
  muscle
    carnitine (palmityltransferase) E71.314
    phosphofructokinase E74.09
  myoadenylate deaminase E79.2
  myocardial — *see* Insufficiency, myocardial
  myophosphorylase E74.04
  NADH diaphorase or reductase (congenital) D74.0
  NADH-methemoglobin reductase (congenital) D74.0
  natrium E87.1
  niacin (amide) (-tryptophan) E52
  nicotinamide E52
  nicotinic acid E52
  number of teeth — *see* Anodontia
  nutrient element E61.9
    multiple E61.7
    specified NEC E61.8
  nutrition, nutritional E63.9
    sequelae — *see* Sequelae, nutritional deficiency
    specified NEC E63.8
  of interleukin 1 receptor antagonist [DIRA] M04.8
  ornithine transcarbamylase E72.4
  ovarian E28.39
  oxygen — *see* Anoxia
  pantothenic acid E53.8
  parathyroid (gland) E20.9
  perineum (female) N81.89
  phenylalanine hydroxylase E70.1
  phosphoenolpyruvate carboxykinase E74.4
  phosphofructokinase E74.19
  phosphomannomutase E74.8
  phosphomannose isomerase E74.8
  phosphomannosyl mutase E74.8
  phosphorylase kinase, liver E74.09
  pituitary hormone (isolated) E23.0
  plasma thromboplastin
    antecedent (PTA) D68.1
    component (PTC) D67
  platelet NEC D69.1
    constitutional D68.0
  polyglandular E31.8
    autoimmune E31.0
  potassium (K) E87.6
  prepuce N47.3
  proaccelerin (congenital) (hereditary) D68.2
    acquired D68.4
  proconvertin factor (congenital) (hereditary) D68.2
    acquired D68.4
  protein (*see also* Malnutrition) E46
    anemia D53.0
    C D68.59
    S D68.59
  prothrombin (congenital) (hereditary) D68.2
    acquired D68.4
  Prower factor D68.2
  pseudocholinesterase E88.09
  PTA (plasma thromboplastin antecedent) D68.1
  PTC (plasma thromboplastin component) D67
  purine nucleoside phosphorylase (PNP) D81.5

**Deficiency, deficient** — *continued*
pyracin (alpha) (beta) E53.1
pyridoxal E53.1
pyridoxamine E53.1
pyridoxine (derivatives) E53.1
pyruvate
  carboxylase E74.4
  dehydrogenase E74.4
riboflavin (vitamin B2) E53.0
salt E87.1
secretion
  ovary E28.39
  salivary gland (any) K11.7
  urine R34
selenium (dietary) E59
serum antitrypsin, familial E88.01
short stature homeobox gene (SHOX)
  with
    dyschondrosteosis Q78.8
    short stature (idiopathic) E34.3
    Turner's syndrome Q96.9
sodium (Na) E87.1
SPCA (factor VII) D68.2
sphincter, intrinsic N36.42
  with urethral hypermobility N36.43
stable factor (congenital) (hereditary) D68.2
  acquired D68.4
Stuart-Prower (factor X) D68.2
sucrase E74.39
sulfatase E75.29
sulfite oxidase E72.19
thiamin, thiaminic (chloride) E51.9
  beriberi (dry) E51.11
    wet E51.12
thrombokinase D68.2
  newborn P53
thyroid (gland) — *see* Hypothyroidism
tocopherol E56.0
tooth bud K00.0
transcobalamine II (anemia) D51.2
vanadium E61.6
vascular I99.9
vasopressin E23.2
vertical ridge K06.8
viosterol — *see* Deficiency, calciferol
vitamin (multiple) NOS E56.9
  A E50.9
    with
      Bitot's spot (corneal) E50.1
      follicular keratosis E50.8
      keratomalacia E50.4
      manifestations NEC E50.8
      night blindness E50.5
      scar of cornea, xerophthalmic E50.6
      xeroderma E50.8
      xerophthalmia E50.7
      xerosis
        conjunctival E50.0
          and Bitot's spot E50.1
        cornea E50.2
          and ulceration E50.3
    sequelae E64.1
  B (complex) NOS E53.9
    with
      beriberi (dry) E51.11
        wet E51.12
      pellagra E52
  B1 NOS E51.9
    beriberi (dry) E51.11
      with circulatory system manifestations
        E51.11
      wet E51.12
  B2 (riboflavin) E53.0
  B6 E53.1
  B12 E53.8
  C E54
    sequelae E64.2
  D E55.9
    with
      adult osteomalacia M83.8
      rickets — *see* Rickets
    25-hydroxylase E83.32
  E E56.0
  folic acid E53.8
  G E53.0
  group B E53.9
    specified NEC E53.8
  H (biotin) E53.8
  K E56.1

**Deficiency, deficient** — *continued*
vitamin — *continued*
  K — *continued*
    of newborn P53
  nicotinic E52
  P E56.8
  PP (pellagra-preventing) E52
  specified NEC E56.8
  thiamin E51.9
    beriberi — *see* Beriberi
zinc, dietary E60
**Deficit** (*see also* Deficiency)
attention and concentration R41.840
  disorder — *see* Attention, deficit
  following
    cerebral infarction I69.310
    cerebrovascular disease I69.910
      specified disease NEC I69.810
      nontraumatic
        intracerebral hemorrhage I69.110
        specified intracranial hemorrhage NEC
          I69.210
        subarachnoid hemorrhage I69.010
cognitive
  communication R41.841
  emotional
    following
      cerebral infarction I69.315
      cerebrovascular disease I69.915
        specified disease NEC I69.815
      nontraumatic
        intracerebral hemorrhage I69.115
        specified intracranial hemorrhage NEC
          I69.215
        subarachnoid hemorrhage I69.015
  following
    cerebral infarction I69.319
    cerebrovascular disease I69.919
      specified disease NEC I69.819
    nontraumatic
      intracerebral hemorrhage I69.119
      specified intracranial hemorrhage NEC
        I69.219
      subarachnoid hemorrhage I69.019
  social
    following
      cerebral infarction I69.315
      cerebrovascular disease I69.915
        specified disease NEC I69.815
      nontraumatic
        intracerebral hemorrhage I69.115
        specified intracranial hemorrhage NEC
          I69.215
        subarachnoid hemorrhage I69.015
cognitive NEC R41.89
  following
    cerebral infarction I69.318
    cerebrovascular disease I69.918
      specified disease NEC I69.818
    nontraumatic
      intracerebral hemorrhage I69.118
      specified intracranial hemorrhage NEC
        I69.218
      subarachnoid hemorrhage I69.018
concentration R41.840
executive function R41.844
  following
    cerebral infarction I69.314
    cerebrovascular disease I69.914
      specified disease NEC I69.814
    nontraumatic
      intracerebral hemorrhage I69.114
      specified intracranial hemorrhage NEC
        I69.214
      subarachnoid hemorrhage I69.014
frontal lobe R41.844
  following
    cerebral infarction I69.314
    cerebrovascular disease I69.914
      specified disease NEC I69.814
    nontraumatic
      intracerebral hemorrhage I69.114
      specified intracranial hemorrhage NEC
        I69.214
      subarachnoid hemorrhage I69.014
memory
  following
    cerebral infarction I69.311
    cerebrovascular disease I69.911

**Deficit** — *continued*
memory — *continued*
  following — *continued*
    cerebrovascular disease — *continued*
      specified disease NEC I69.811
    nontraumatic
      intracerebral hemorrhage I69.111
      specified intracranial hemorrhage NEC
        I69.211
      subarachnoid hemorrhage I69.011
neurologic NEC R29.818
  ischemic
    reversible (RIND) I63.9
      prolonged (PRIND) I63.9
oxygen R09.02
prolonged reversible ischemic neurologic (PRIND) I63.9
psychomotor R41.843
  following
    cerebral infarction I69.313
    cerebrovascular disease I69.913
      specified disease NEC I69.813
    nontraumatic
      intracerebral hemorrhage I69.113
      specified intracranial hemorrhage NEC
        I69.213
      subarachnoid hemorrhage I69.013
visuospatial R41.842
  following
    cerebral infarction I69.312
    cerebrovascular disease I69.912
      specified disease NEC I69.812
    nontraumatic
      intracerebral hemorrhage I69.112
      specified intracranial hemorrhage NEC
        I69.212
      subarachnoid hemorrhage I69.012
**Deflection**
radius — *see* Deformity, limb, specified type NEC,
  forearm
septum (acquired) (nasal) (nose) J34.2
spine — *see* Curvature, spine
turbinate (nose) J34.2
**Defluvium**
capillorum — *see* Alopecia
ciliorum — *see* Madarosis
unguium L60.8
**Deformity** Q89.9
abdomen, congenital Q89.9
abdominal wall
  acquired M95.8
  congenital Q79.59
acquired (unspecified site) M95.9
adrenal gland Q89.1
alimentary tract, congenital Q45.9
  upper Q40.9
ankle (joint) (acquired) (*see also* Deformity, limb, lower
  leg)
  abduction — *see* Contraction, joint, ankle
  congenital Q68.8
  contraction — *see* Contraction, joint, ankle
  specified type NEC — *see* Deformity, limb, foot,
    specified NEC
anus (acquired) K62.89
  congenital Q43.9
aorta (arch) (congenital) Q25.40
  acquired I77.89
aortic
  arch, acquired I77.89
  cusp or valve (congenital) Q23.8
    acquired (*see also* Endocarditis, aortic) I35.8
arm (acquired) (upper) (*see also* Deformity, limb, upper
  arm)
  congenital Q68.8
  forearm — *see* Deformity, limb, forearm
artery (congenital) (peripheral) NOS Q27.9
  acquired I77.89
  coronary (acquired) I25.9
    congenital Q24.5
  umbilical Q27.0
atrial septal Q21.1
auditory canal (external) (congenital) (*see also* Malformation, ear, external)
  acquired — *see* Disorder, ear, external, specified
    type NEC
auricle
  ear (congenital) (*see also* Malformation, ear, exter-
    nal)
    acquired — *see* Disorder, pinna, deformity

**Deformity** — *continued*

back — *see* Dorsopathy, deforming
bile duct (common) (congenital) (hepatic) Q44.5
    acquired K83.8
biliary duct or passage (congenital) Q44.5
    acquired K83.8
bladder (neck) (trigone) (sphincter) (acquired) N32.89
    congenital Q64.79
bone (acquired) NOS M95.9
    congenital Q79.9
    turbinate M95.0
brain (congenital) Q04.9
    acquired G93.89
    reduction Q04.3
breast (acquired) N64.89
    congenital Q83.9
    reconstructed N65.0
bronchus (congenital) Q32.4
    acquired NEC J98.09
bursa, congenital Q79.9
canaliculi (lacrimalis) (acquired) (*see also* Disorder, lacrimal system, changes)
    congenital Q10.6
canthus, acquired — *see* Disorder, eyelid, specified type NEC
capillary (acquired) I78.8
cardiovascular system, congenital Q28.9
caruncle, lacrimal (acquired) (*see also* Disorder, lacrimal system, changes)
    congenital Q10.6
cascade, stomach K31.2
cecum (congenital) Q43.9
    acquired K63.89
cerebral, acquired G93.89
    congenital Q04.9
cervix (uterus) (acquired) NEC N88.8
    congenital Q51.9
cheek (acquired) M95.2
    congenital Q18.9
chest (acquired) (wall) M95.4
    congenital Q67.8
    sequelae (late effect) of rickets E64.3
chin (acquired) M95.2
    congenital Q18.9
choroid (congenital) Q14.3
    acquired H31.8
    plexus Q07.8
        acquired G96.19
cicatricial — *see* Cicatrix
cilia, acquired — *see* Disorder, eyelid, specified type NEC
clavicle (acquired) M95.8
    congenital Q68.8
clitoris (congenital) Q52.6
    acquired N90.89
clubfoot — *see* Clubfoot
coccyx (acquired) — *see* subcategory M43.8 ☑
colon (congenital) Q43.9
    acquired K63.89
concha (ear), congenital (*see also* Malformation, ear, external)
    acquired — *see* Disorder, pinna, deformity
cornea (acquired) H18.70
    congenital Q13.4
    descemetocele — *see* Descemetocele
    ectasia — *see* Ectasia, cornea
    specified NEC H18.79- ☑
    staphyloma — *see* Staphyloma, cornea
coronary artery (acquired) I25.9
    congenital Q24.5
cranium (acquired) — *see* Deformity, skull
cricoid cartilage (congenital) Q31.8
    acquired J38.7
cystic duct (congenital) Q44.5
    acquired K82.8
Dandy-Walker Q03.1
    with spina bifida — *see* Spina bifida
diaphragm (congenital) Q79.1
    acquired J98.6
digestive organ NOS Q45.9
ductus arteriosus Q25.0
duodenal bulb K31.89
duodenum (congenital) Q43.9
    acquired K31.89
dura — *see* Deformity, meninges
ear (acquired) (*see also* Disorder, pinna, deformity)
    congenital (external) Q17.9
        internal Q16.5

**Deformity** — *continued*

ear (*see also* Disorder, pinna, deformity) — *continued*
    congenital — *continued*
        middle Q16.4
            ossicles Q16.3
        ossicles Q16.3
ectodermal (congenital) NEC Q84.9
ejaculatory duct (congenital) Q55.4
    acquired N50.89
elbow (joint) (acquired) (*see also* Deformity, limb, upper arm)
    congenital Q68.8
    contraction — *see* Contraction, joint, elbow
endocrine gland NEC Q89.2
epididymis (congenital) Q55.4
    acquired N50.89
epiglottis (congenital) Q31.8
    acquired J38.7
esophagus (congenital) Q39.9
    acquired K22.8
eustachian tube (congenital) NEC Q17.8
eye, congenital Q15.9
eyebrow (congenital) Q18.8
eyelid (acquired) (*see also* Disorder, eyelid, specified type NEC)
    congenital Q10.3
face (acquired) M95.2
    congenital Q18.9
fallopian tube, acquired N83.8
femur (acquired) — *see* Deformity, limb, specified type NEC, thigh
fetal
    with fetopelvic disproportion O33.7 ☑
    causing obstructed labor O66.3
finger (acquired) M20.00- ☑
    boutonniere M20.02- ☑
    congenital Q68.1
    flexion contracture — *see* Contraction, joint, hand
    mallet finger M20.01- ☑
    specified NEC M20.09- ☑
    swan-neck M20.03- ☑
flexion (joint) (acquired) (*see also* Deformity, limb, flexion) M21.20
    congenital NOS Q74.9
        hip Q65.89
foot (acquired) (*see also* Deformity, limb, lower leg)
    cavovarus (congenital) Q66.1
    congenital NOS Q66.9
        specified type NEC Q66.89
    specified type NEC — *see* Deformity, limb, foot, specified NEC
    valgus (congenital) Q66.6
        acquired — *see* Deformity, valgus, ankle
    varus (congenital) NEC Q66.3
        acquired — *see* Deformity, varus, ankle
forearm (acquired) (*see also* Deformity, limb, forearm)
    congenital Q68.8
forehead (acquired) M95.2
    congenital Q75.8
frontal bone (acquired) M95.2
    congenital Q75.8
gallbladder (congenital) Q44.1
    acquired K82.8
gastrointestinal tract (congenital) NOS Q45.9
    acquired K63.89
genitalia, genital organ(s) or system NEC
    female (congenital) Q52.9
        acquired N94.89
        external Q52.70
    male (congenital) Q55.9
        acquired N50.89
globe (eye) (congenital) Q15.8
    acquired H44.89
gum, acquired NEC K06.8
hand (acquired) — *see* Deformity, limb, hand
    congenital Q68.1
head (acquired) M95.2
    congenital Q75.8
heart (congenital) Q24.9
    septum Q21.9
        auricular Q21.1
        ventricular Q21.0
    valve (congenital) NEC Q24.8
        acquired — *see* Endocarditis
heel (acquired) — *see* Deformity, foot
hepatic duct (congenital) Q44.5
    acquired K83.8

**Deformity** — *continued*

hip (joint) (acquired) (*see also* Deformity, limb, thigh)
    congenital Q65.9
    due to (previous) juvenile osteochondrosis — *see* Coxa, plana
    flexion — *see* Contraction, joint, hip
hourglass — *see* Contraction, hourglass
humerus (acquired) M21.82- ☑
    congenital Q74.0
hypophyseal (congenital) Q89.2
ileocecal (coil) (valve) (acquired) K63.89
    congenital Q43.9
ileum (congenital) Q43.9
    acquired K63.89
ilium (acquired) M95.5
    congenital Q74.2
integument (congenital) Q84.9
intervertebral cartilage or disc (acquired) — *see* Disorder, disc, specified NEC
intestine (large) (small) (congenital) NOS Q43.9
    acquired K63.89
intrinsic minus or plus (hand) — *see* Deformity, limb, specified type NEC, forearm
iris (acquired) H21.89
    congenital Q13.2
ischium (acquired) M95.5
    congenital Q74.2
jaw (acquired) (congenital) M26.9
joint (acquired) NEC M21.90
    congenital Q68.8
    elbow M21.92- ☑
    hand M21.94- ☑
    hip M21.95- ☑
    knee M21.96- ☑
    shoulder M21.92- ☑
    wrist M21.93- ☑
kidney(s) (calyx) (pelvis) (congenital) Q63.9
    acquired N28.89
    artery (congenital) Q27.2
        acquired I77.89
Klippel-Feil (brevicollis) Q76.1
knee (acquired) NEC (*see also* Deformity, limb, lower leg)
    congenital Q68.2
labium (majus) (minus) (congenital) Q52.79
    acquired N90.89
lacrimal passages or duct (congenital) NEC Q10.6
    acquired — *see* Disorder, lacrimal system, changes
larynx (muscle) (congenital) Q31.8
    acquired J38.7
    web (glottic) Q31.0
leg (upper) (acquired) NEC (*see also* Deformity, limb, thigh)
    congenital Q68.8
    lower leg — *see* Deformity, limb, lower leg
lens (acquired) H27.8
    congenital Q12.9
lid (fold) (acquired) (*see also* Disorder, eyelid, specified type NEC)
    congenital Q10.3
ligament (acquired) — *see* Disorder, ligament
    congenital Q79.9
limb (acquired) M21.90
    clawfoot M21.53- ☑
    clawhand M21.51- ☑
    clubfoot M21.54- ☑
    clubhand M21.52- ☑
    congenital, except reduction deformity Q74.9
    flat foot M21.4- ☑
    flexion M21.20
        ankle M21.27- ☑
        elbow M21.22- ☑
        finger M21.24- ☑
        hip M21.25- ☑
        knee M21.26- ☑
        shoulder M21.21- ☑
        toe M21.27- ☑
        wrist M21.23- ☑
    foot
        claw — *see* Deformity, limb, clawfoot
        club — *see* Deformity, limb, clubfoot
        drop M21.37- ☑
        flat — *see* Deformity, limb, flat foot
        specified NEC M21.6X- ☑
    forearm M21.93- ☑
    hand M21.94- ☑
    lower leg M21.96- ☑

☑ **Additional Character Required — Refer to the Tabular List for Character Selection**  ▽ **Subterms under main terms may continue to next column or page**

**Deformity** — *continued*
  limb — *continued*
    specified type NEC M21.80
      forearm M21.83- ☑
        lower leg M21.86- ☑
        thigh M21.85- ☑
        upper arm M21.82- ☑
      thigh M21.95- ☑
    unequal length M21.70
      short site is
        femur M21.75- ☑
        fibula M21.76- ☑
        humerus M21.72- ☑
        radius M21.73- ☑
        tibia M21.76- ☑
        ulna M21.73- ☑
      upper arm M21.92- ☑
    valgus — *see* Deformity, valgus
    varus — *see* Deformity, varus
    wrist drop M21.33- ☑
  lip (acquired) NEC K13.0
    congenital Q38.0
  liver (congenital) Q44.7
    acquired K76.89
  lumbosacral (congenital) (joint) (region) Q76.49
    acquired — *see* subcategory M43.8 ☑
    kyphosis — *see* Kyphosis, congenital
    lordosis — *see* Lordosis, congenital
  lung (congenital) Q33.9
    acquired J98.4
  lymphatic system, congenital Q89.9
  Madelung's (radius) Q74.0
  mandible (acquired) (congenital) M26.9
  maxilla (acquired) (congenital) M26.9
  meninges or membrane (congenital) Q07.9
    cerebral Q04.8
      acquired G96.19
    spinal cord (congenital) G96.19
      acquired G96.19
  metacarpus (acquired) — *see* Deformity, limb, forearm
    congenital Q74.0
  metatarsus (acquired) — *see* Deformity, foot
    congenital Q66.9
  middle ear (congenital) Q16.4
    ossicles Q16.3
  mitral (leaflets) (valve) I05.8
    parachute Q23.2
    stenosis, congenital Q23.2
  mouth (acquired) K13.79
    congenital Q38.6
  multiple, congenital NEC Q89.7
  muscle (acquired) M62.89
    congenital Q79.9
      sternocleidomastoid Q68.0
  musculoskeletal system (acquired) M95.9
    congenital Q79.9
    specified NEC M95.8
  nail (acquired) L60.8
    congenital Q84.6
  nasal — *see* Deformity, nose
  neck (acquired) M95.3
    congenital Q18.9
      sternocleidomastoid Q68.0
  nervous system (congenital) Q07.9
  nipple (congenital) Q83.9
    acquired N64.89
  nose (acquired) (cartilage) M95.0
    bone (turbinate) M95.0
    congenital Q30.9
      bent or squashed Q67.4
    saddle M95.0
      syphilitic A50.57
    septum (acquired) J34.2
      congenital Q30.8
    sinus (wall) (congenital) Q30.8
      acquired M95.0
    syphilitic (congenital) A50.57
      late A52.73
  ocular muscle (congenital) Q10.3
    acquired — *see* Strabismus, mechanical
  opticociliary vessels (congenital) Q13.2
  orbit (eye) (acquired) H05.30
    atrophy — *see* Atrophy, orbit
    congenital Q10.7
    due to
      bone disease NEC H05.32- ☑
      trauma or surgery H05.33- ☑
    enlargement — *see* Enlargement, orbit

**Deformity** — *continued*
  orbit — *continued*
    exostosis — *see* Exostosis, orbit
  organ of Corti (congenital) Q16.5
  ovary (congenital) Q50.39
    acquired N83.8
  oviduct, acquired N83.8
  palate (congenital) Q38.5
    acquired M27.8
    cleft (congenital) — *see* Cleft, palate
  pancreas (congenital) Q45.3
    acquired K86.89
  parathyroid (gland) Q89.2
  parotid (gland) (congenital) Q38.4
    acquired K11.8
  patella (acquired) — *see* Disorder, patella, specified NEC
  pelvis, pelvic (acquired) (bony) M95.5
    with disproportion (fetopelvic) O33.0
      causing obstructed labor O65.0
    congenital Q74.2
    rachitic sequelae (late effect) E64.3
  penis (glans) (congenital) Q55.69
    acquired N48.89
  pericardium (congenital) Q24.8
    acquired — *see* Pericarditis
  pharynx (congenital) Q38.8
    acquired J39.2
  pinna, acquired (*see also* Disorder, pinna, deformity)
    congenital Q17.9
  pituitary (congenital) Q89.2
  posture — *see* Dorsopathy, deforming
  prepuce (congenital) Q55.69
    acquired N47.8
  prostate (congenital) Q55.4
    acquired N42.89
  pupil (congenital) Q13.2
    acquired — *see* Abnormality, pupillary
  pylorus (congenital) Q40.3
    acquired K31.89
  rachitic (acquired), old or healed E64.3
  radius (acquired) (*see also* Deformity, limb, forearm)
    congenital Q68.8
  rectum (congenital) Q43.9
    acquired K62.89
  reduction (extremity) (limb), congenital (*see also* condition and site) Q73.8
    brain Q04.3
    lower — *see* Defect, reduction, lower limb
    upper — *see* Defect, reduction, upper limb
  renal — *see* Deformity, kidney
  respiratory system (congenital) Q34.9
  rib (acquired) M95.4
    congenital Q76.6
    cervical Q76.5
  rotation (joint) (acquired) — *see* Deformity, limb, specified site NEC
    congenital Q74.9
    hip — *see* Deformity, limb, specified type NEC, thigh
      congenital Q65.89
  sacroiliac joint (congenital) — *see* subcategory Q74.2
    acquired — *see* subcategory M43.8 ☑
  sacrum (acquired) — *see* subcategory M43.8 ☑
  saddle
    back — *see* Lordosis
    nose M95.0
      syphilitic A50.57
  salivary gland or duct (congenital) Q38.4
    acquired K11.8
  scapula (acquired) M95.8
    congenital Q68.8
  scrotum (congenital) (*see also* Malformation, testis and scrotum)
    acquired N50.89
  seminal vesicles (congenital) Q55.4
    acquired N50.89
  septum, nasal (acquired) J34.2
  shoulder (joint) (acquired) — *see* Deformity, limb, upper arm
    congenital Q74.0
    contraction — *see* Contraction, joint, shoulder
  sigmoid (flexure) (congenital) Q43.9
    acquired K63.89
  skin (congenital) Q82.9
  skull (acquired) M95.2
    congenital Q75.8

**Deformity** — *continued*
  skull — *continued*
    congenital — *continued*
      with
        anencephaly Q00.0
        encephalocele — *see* Encephalocele
        hydrocephalus Q03.9
          with spina bifida — *see* Spina bifida, by site, with hydrocephalus
        microcephaly Q02
    soft parts, organs or tissues (of pelvis)
      in pregnancy or childbirth NEC O34.8- ☑
        causing obstructed labor O65.5
  spermatic cord (congenital) Q55.4
    acquired N50.89
    torsion — *see* Torsion, spermatic cord
  spinal — *see* Dorsopathy, deforming
    column (acquired) — *see* Dorsopathy, deforming
    congenital Q67.5
    cord (congenital) Q06.9
      acquired G95.89
    nerve root (congenital) Q07.9
  spine (acquired) (*see also* Dorsopathy, deforming)
    congenital Q67.5
    rachitic E64.3
    specified NEC — *see* Dorsopathy, deforming, specified NEC
  spleen
    acquired D73.89
    congenital Q89.09
  Sprengel's (congenital) Q74.0
  sternocleidomastoid (muscle), congenital Q68.0
  sternum (acquired) M95.4
    congenital NEC Q76.7
  stomach (congenital) Q40.3
    acquired K31.89
  submandibular gland (congenital) Q38.4
  submaxillary gland (congenital) Q38.4
    acquired K11.8
  talipes — *see* Talipes
  testis (congenital) (*see also* Malformation, testis and scrotum)
    acquired N44.8
    torsion — *see* Torsion, testis
  thigh (acquired) (*see also* Deformity, limb, thigh)
    congenital NEC Q68.8
  thorax (acquired) (wall) M95.4
    congenital Q67.8
    sequelae of rickets E64.3
  thumb (acquired) (*see also* Deformity, finger)
    congenital NEC Q68.1
  thymus (tissue) (congenital) Q89.2
  thyroid (gland) (congenital) Q89.2
    cartilage Q31.8
    acquired J38.7
  tibia (acquired) (*see also* Deformity, limb, specified type NEC, lower leg)
    congenital NEC Q68.8
    saber (syphilitic) A50.56
  toe (acquired) M20.6- ☑
    congenital Q66.9
    hallux rigidus M20.2- ☑
    hallux valgus M20.1- ☑
    hallux varus M20.3- ☑
    hammer toe M20.4- ☑
    specified NEC M20.5X- ☑
  tongue (congenital) Q38.3
    acquired K14.8
  tooth, teeth K00.2
  trachea (rings) (congenital) Q32.1
    acquired J39.8
  transverse aortic arch (congenital) Q25.49
  tricuspid (leaflets) (valve) I07.8
    atresia or stenosis Q22.4
    Ebstein's Q22.5
  trunk (acquired) M95.8
    congenital Q89.9
  ulna (acquired) (*see also* Deformity, limb, forearm)
    congenital NEC Q68.8
  urachus, congenital Q64.4
  ureter (opening) (congenital) Q62.8
    acquired N28.89
  urethra (congenital) Q64.79
    acquired N36.8
  urinary tract (congenital) Q64.9
    urachus Q64.4
  uterus (congenital) Q51.9
    acquired N85.8

**Deformity** — *continued*
uvula (congenital) Q38.5
vagina (acquired) N89.8
congenital Q52.4
valgus NEC M21.00
ankle M21.07- ☑
elbow M21.02- ☑
hip M21.05- ☑
knee M21.06- ☑
valve, valvular (congenital) (heart) Q24.8
acquired — *see* Endocarditis
varus NEC M21.10
ankle M21.17- ☑
elbow M21.12- ☑
hip M21.15 ☑
knee M21.16- ☑
tibia — *see* Osteochondrosis, juvenile, tibia
vas deferens (congenital) Q55.4
acquired N50.89
vein (congenital) Q27.9
great Q26.9
vertebra — *see* Dorsopathy, deforming
vertical talus (congenital) Q66.80
left foot Q66.82
right foot Q66.81
vesicourethral orifice (acquired) N32.89
congenital NEC Q64.79
vessels of optic papilla (congenital) Q14.2
visual field (contraction) — *see* Defect, visual field
vitreous body, acquired H43.89
vulva (congenital) Q52.79
acquired N90.89
wrist (joint) (acquired) (*see also* Deformity, limb, forearm)
congenital Q68.8
contraction — *see* Contraction, joint, wrist

**Degeneration, degenerative**
adrenal (capsule) (fatty) (gland) (hyaline) (infectional) E27.8
amyloid (*see also* Amyloidosis) E85.9
anterior cornua, spinal cord G12.29
anterior labral S43.49- ☑
aorta, aortic I70.0
fatty I77.89
aortic valve (heart) — *see* Endocarditis, aortic
arteriovascular — *see* Arteriosclerosis
artery, arterial (atheromatous) (calcareous) (*see also* Arteriosclerosis)
cerebral, amyloid E85.4 [I68.0]
medial — *see* Arteriosclerosis, extremities
articular cartilage NEC — *see* Derangement, joint, articular cartilage, by site
atheromatous — *see* Arteriosclerosis
basal nuclei or ganglia G23.9
specified NEC G23.8
bone NEC — *see* Disorder, bone, specified type NEC
brachial plexus G54.0
brain (cortical) (progressive) G31.9
alcoholic G31.2
arteriosclerotic I67.2
childhood G31.9
specified NEC G31.89
cystic G31.89
congenital Q04.6
in
alcoholism G31.2
beriberi E51.2
cerebrovascular disease I67.9
congenital hydrocephalus Q03.9
with spina bifida (*see also* Spina bifida)
Fabry-Anderson disease E75.21
Gaucher's disease E75.22
Hunter's syndrome E76.1
lipidosis
cerebral E75.4
generalized E75.6
mucopolysaccharidosis — *see* Mucopolysaccharidosis
myxedema E03.9 [G32.89]
neoplastic disease (*see also* Neoplasm) D49.6 [G32.89]
Niemann-Pick disease E75.249 [G32.89]
sphingolipidosis E75.3 [G32.89]
vitamin B12 deficiency E53.8 [G32.89]
senile NEC G31.1
breast N64.89
Bruch's membrane — *see* Degeneration, choroid
capillaries (fatty) I78.8

**Degeneration, degenerative** — *continued*
capillaries — *continued*
amyloid E85.89 [I79.8]
cardiac (*see also* Degeneration, myocardial)
valve, valvular — *see* Endocarditis
cardiorenal — *see* Hypertension, cardiorenal
cardiovascular (*see also* Disease, cardiovascular)
renal — *see* Hypertension, cardiorenal
cerebellar NOS G31.9
alcoholic G31.2
primary (hereditary) (sporadic) G11.9
cerebral — *see* Degeneration, brain
cerebrovascular I67.9
due to hypertension I67.4
cervical plexus G54.2
cervix N88.8
due to radiation (intended effect) N88.8
adverse effect or misadventure N99.89
chamber angle H21.21- ☑
changes, spine or vertebra — *see* Spondylosis
chorioretinal (*see also* Degeneration, choroid)
hereditary H31.20
choroid (colloid) (drusen) H31.10- ☑
atrophy — *see* Atrophy, choroidal
hereditary — *see* Dystrophy, choroidal, hereditary
ciliary body H21.22- ☑
cochlear — *see* subcategory H83.8 ☑
combined (spinal cord) (subacute) E53.8 [G32.0]
with anemia (pernicious) D51.0 [G32.0]
due to dietary vitamin B12 deficiency D51.3 [G32.0]
in (due to)
vitamin B12 deficiency E53.8 [G32.0]
anemia D51.9 [G32.0]
conjunctiva H11.10
concretions — *see* Concretion, conjunctiva
deposits — *see* Deposit, conjunctiva
pigmentations — *see* Pigmentation, conjunctiva
pinguecula — *see* Pinguecula
xerosis — *see* Xerosis, conjunctiva
cornea H18.40
calcerous H18.43
band keratopathy H18.42- ☑
familial, hereditary — *see* Dystrophy, cornea
hyaline (of old scars) H18.49
keratomalacia — *see* Keratomalacia
nodular H18.45- ☑
peripheral H18.46- ☑
senile H18.41- ☑
specified type NEC H18.49
cortical (cerebellar) (parenchymatous) G31.89
alcoholic G31.2
diffuse, due to arteriopathy I67.2
corticobasal G31.85
cutis L98.8
amyloid E85.4 [L99]
dental pulp K04.2
disc disease — *see* Degeneration, intervertebral disc NEC
dorsolateral (spinal cord) — *see* Degeneration, combined
extrapyramidal G25.9
eye, macular (*see also* Degeneration, macula)
congenital or hereditary — *see* Dystrophy, retina
facet joints — *see* Spondylosis
fatty
liver NEC K76.0
alcoholic K70.0
grey matter (brain) (Alpers') G31.81
heart (*see also* Degeneration, myocardial)
amyloid E85.4 [I43]
atheromatous — *see* Disease, heart, ischemic, atherosclerotic
ischemic — *see* Disease, heart, ischemic
hepatolenticular (Wilson's) E83.01
hepatorenal K76.7
hyaline (diffuse) (generalized)
localized — *see* Degeneration, by site
infrapatellar fat pad M79.4
intervertebral disc NOS
with
myelopathy — *see* Disorder, disc, with, myelopathy
radiculitis or radiculopathy — *see* Disorder, disc, with, radiculopathy
cervical, cervicothoracic — *see* Disorder, disc, cervical, degeneration

**Degeneration, degenerative** — *continued*
intervertebral disc — *continued*
cervical, cervicothoracic — *see* Disorder, disc, cervical, degeneration — *continued*
with
myelopathy — *see* Disorder, disc, cervical, with myelopathy
neuritis, radiculitis or radiculopathy — *see* Disorder, disc, cervical, with neuritis
lumbar region M51.36
with
myelopathy M51.06
neuritis, radiculitis, radiculopathy or sciatica M51.16
lumbosacral region M51.37
with
neuritis, radiculitis, radiculopathy or sciatica M51.17
sacrococcygeal region M53.3
thoracic region M51.34
with
myelopathy M51.04
neuritis, radiculitis, radiculopathy M51.14
thoracolumbar region M51.35
with
myelopathy M51.05
neuritis, radiculitis, radiculopathy M51.15
intestine, amyloid E85.4
iris (pigmentary) H21.23- ☑
ischemic — *see* Ischemia
joint disease — *see* Osteoarthritis
kidney N28.89
amyloid E85.4 [N29]
cystic, congenital Q61.9
fatty N28.89
polycystic Q61.3
adult type (autosomal dominant) Q61.2
infantile type (autosomal recessive) NEC Q61.19
collecting duct dilatation Q61.11
Kuhnt-Junius (*see also* Degeneration, macula) H35.32- ☑
lens — *see* Cataract
lenticular (familial) (progressive) (Wilson's) (with cirrhosis of liver) E83.01
liver (diffuse) NEC K76.89
amyloid E85.4 [K77]
cystic K76.89
congenital Q44.6
fatty NEC K76.0
alcoholic K70.0
hypertrophic K76.89
parenchymatous, acute or subacute K72.00
with coma K72.01
pigmentary K76.89
toxic (acute) K71.9
lung J98.4
lymph gland I89.8
hyaline I89.8
macula, macular (acquired) (age-related) (senile) H35.30
angioid streaks H35.33
atrophic age-related H35.31- ☑
congenital or hereditary — *see* Dystrophy, retina
cystoid H35.35- ☑
drusen H35.36- ☑
dry age-related H35.31- ☑
exudative H35.32- ☑
hole H35.34- ☑
nonexudative H35.31- ☑
puckering H35.37- ☑
toxic H35.38- ☑
wet age-related H35.32- ☑
membranous labyrinth, congenital (causing impairment of hearing) Q16.5
meniscus — *see* Derangement, meniscus
mitral — *see* Insufficiency, mitral
Mönckeberg's — *see* Arteriosclerosis, extremities
motor centers, senile G31.1
multi-system G90.3
mural — *see* Degeneration, myocardial
muscle (fatty) (fibrous) (hyaline) (progressive) M62.89
heart — *see* Degeneration, myocardial
myelin, central nervous system G37.9
myocardial, myocardium (fatty) (hyaline) (senile) I51.5
with rheumatic fever (conditions in I00) I09.9
active, acute or subacute I01.2
with chorea I02.0
inactive or quiescent (with chorea) I09.0

**Degeneration, degenerative** — *continued*
  myocardial, myocardium — *continued*
    hypertensive — *see* Hypertension, heart
    rheumatic — *see* Degeneration, myocardial, with rheumatic fever
    syphilitic A52.06
  nasal sinus (mucosa) J32.9
    frontal J32.1
    maxillary J32.0
  nerve — *see* Disorder, nerve
  nervous system G31.9
    alcoholic G31.2
    amyloid E85.4 [G99.8]
    autonomic G90.9
    fatty G31.89
    specified NEC G31.89
  nipple N64.89
  olivopontocerebellar (hereditary) (familial) G23.8
  osseous labyrinth — *see* subcategory H83.8 ☑
  ovary N83.8
    cystic N83.20- ☑
    microcystic N83.20- ☑
  pallidal pigmentary (progressive) G23.0
  pancreas K86.89
    tuberculous A18.83
  penis N48.89
  pigmentary (diffuse) (general)
    localized — *see* Degeneration, by site
    pallidal (progressive) G23.0
  pineal gland E34.8
  pituitary (gland) E23.6
  popliteal fat pad M79.4
  posterolateral (spinal cord) — *see* Degeneration, combined
  pulmonary valve (heart) I37.8
  pulp (tooth) K04.2
  pupillary margin H21.24- ☑
  renal — *see* Degeneration, kidney
  retina H35.9
    hereditary (cerebroretinal) (congenital) (juvenile) (macula) (peripheral) (pigmentary) — *see* Dystrophy, retina
    Kuhnt-Junius (*see also* Degeneration, macula) H35.32- ☑
    macula (cystic) (exudative) (hole) (nonexudative) (pseudohole) (senile) (toxic) — *see* Degeneration, macula
    peripheral H35.40
      lattice H35.41- ☑
      microcystoid H35.42- ☑
      paving stone H35.43- ☑
      secondary
        pigmentary H35.45- ☑
        vitreoretinal H35.46- ☑
      senile reticular H35.44- ☑
    pigmentary (primary) (*see also* Dystrophy, retina)
      secondary — *see* Degeneration, retina, peripheral, secondary
    posterior pole — *see* Degeneration, macula
  saccule, congenital (causing impairment of hearing) Q16.5
  senile R54
    brain G31.1
    cardiac, heart or myocardium — *see* Degeneration, myocardial
    motor centers G31.1
    vascular — *see* Arteriosclerosis
  sinus (cystic) (*see also* Sinusitis)
    polypoid J33.1
  skin L98.8
    amyloid E85.4 [L99]
    colloid L98.8
  spinal (cord) G31.89
    amyloid E85.4 [G32.89]
    combined (subacute) — *see* Degeneration, combined
    dorsolateral — *see* Degeneration, combined
    familial NEC G31.89
    fatty G31.89
    funicular — *see* Degeneration, combined
    posterolateral — *see* Degeneration, combined
    subacute combined — *see* Degeneration, combined
    tuberculous A17.81
  spleen D73.0
    amyloid E85.4 [D77]
  stomach K31.89
  striatonigral G23.2

**Degeneration, degenerative** — *continued*
  suprarenal (capsule) (gland) E27.8
  synovial membrane (pulpy) — *see* Disorder, synovium, specified type NEC
  tapetoretinal — *see* Dystrophy, retina
  thymus (gland) E32.8
    fatty E32.8
  thyroid (gland) E07.89
  tricuspid (heart) (valve) I07.9
  tuberculous NEC — *see* Tuberculosis
  turbinate J34.89
  uterus (cystic) N85.8
  vascular (senile) — *see* Arteriosclerosis
    hypertensive — *see* Hypertension
  vitreoretinal, secondary — *see* Degeneration, retina, peripheral, secondary, vitreoretinal
  vitreous (body) H43.81- ☑
  Wallerian — *see* Disorder, nerve
  Wilson's hepatolenticular E83.01
**Deglutition**
  paralysis R13.0
    hysterical F44.4
  pneumonia J69.0
**Degos' disease** I77.89
**Dehiscence** (of)
  amputation stump T87.81
  cesarean wound O90.0
  closure of
    cornea T81.31 ☑
    craniotomy T81.32 ☑
    fascia (muscular) (superficial) T81.32 ☑
    internal organ or tissue T81.32 ☑
    laceration (external) (internal) T81.33 ☑
    ligament T81.32 ☑
    mucosa T81.31 ☑
    muscle or muscle flap T81.32 ☑
    ribs or rib cage T81.32 ☑
    skin and subcutaneous tissue (full-thickness) (superficial) T81.31 ☑
    skull T81.32 ☑
    sternum (sternotomy) T81.32 ☑
    tendon T81.32 ☑
    traumatic laceration (external) (internal) T81.33 ☑
  episiotomy O90.1
  operation wound NEC T81.31 ☑
    external operation wound (superficial) T81.31 ☑
    internal operation wound (deep) T81.32 ☑
  perineal wound (postpartum) O90.1
  traumatic injury wound repair T81.33 ☑
  wound T81.30 ☑
    traumatic repair T81.33 ☑
**Dehydration** E86.0
  newborn P74.1
**Déjérine-Roussy syndrome** G89.0
**Déjérine-Sottas disease or neuropathy** (hypertrophic) G60.0
**Déjérine-Thomas atrophy** G23.8
**Delay, delayed**
  any plane in pelvis
    complicating delivery O66.9
  birth or delivery NOS O63.9
  closure, ductus arteriosus (Botalli) P29.38
  coagulation — *see* Defect, coagulation
  conduction (cardiac) (ventricular) I45.9
  delivery, second twin, triplet, etc O63.2
  development R62.50
    global F88
    intellectual (specific) F81.9
    language F80.9
      due to hearing loss F80.4
    learning F81.9
    pervasive F84.9
    physiological R62.50
      specified stage NEC R62.0
    reading F81.0
    sexual E30.0
    speech F80.9
      due to hearing loss F80.4
    spelling F81.81
  ejaculation F52.32
  gastric emptying K30
  menarche E30.0
  menstruation (cause unknown) N91.0
  milestone R62.0
  passage of meconium (newborn) P76.0
  primary respiration P28.9
  puberty (constitutional) E30.0

**Delay, delayed** — *continued*
  separation of umbilical cord P96.82
  sexual maturation, female E30.0
  sleep phase syndrome G47.21
  union, fracture — *see* Fracture, by site
  vaccination Z28.9
**Deletion**(s)
  autosome Q93.9
    identified by fluorescence in situ hybridization (FISH) Q93.89
    identified by in situ hybridization (ISH) Q93.89
  chromosome
    with complex rearrangements NEC Q93.7
    part of NEC Q93.5
    seen only at prometaphase Q93.89
    short arm
      22q11.2 Q93.81
      4 Q93.3
      5p Q93.4
    specified NEC Q93.89
  long arm chromosome 18 or 21 Q93.89
    with complex rearrangements NEC Q93.7
  microdeletions NEC Q93.88
**Delhi boil or button** B55.1
**Delinquency** (juvenile) (neurotic) F91.8
  group Z72.810
**Delinquent immunization status** Z28.3
**Delirium, delirious** (acute or subacute) (not alcohol- or drug-induced) (with dementia) R41.0
  alcoholic (acute) (tremens) (withdrawal) F10.921
    with intoxication F10.921
      in
        abuse F10.121
        dependence F10.221
    due to (secondary to)
      alcohol
        intoxication F10.921
          in
            abuse F10.121
            dependence F10.221
        withdrawal F10.231
      amphetamine intoxication F15.921
        in
          abuse F15.121
          dependence F15.221
      anxiolytic
        intoxication F13.921
          in
            abuse F13.121
            dependence F13.221
        withdrawal F13.231
      cannabis intoxication (acute) F12.921
        in
          abuse F12.121
          dependence F12.221
      cocaine intoxication (acute) F14.921
        in
          abuse F14.121
          dependence F14.221
      general medical condition F05
      hallucinogen intoxication F16.921
        in
          abuse F16.121
          dependence F16.221
      hypnotic
        intoxication F13.921
          in
            abuse F13.121
            dependence F13.221
        withdrawal F13.231
      inhalant intoxication (acute) F18.921
        in
          abuse F18.121
          dependence F18.221
      multiple etiologies F05
      opioid intoxication (acute) F11.921
        in
          abuse F11.121
          dependence F11.221
      other (or unknown) substance F19.921
      phencyclidine intoxication (acute) F16.921
        in
          abuse F16.121
          dependence F16.221
      psychoactive substance NEC intoxication (acute) F19.921
        in
          abuse F19.121
          dependence F19.221

**Delivery** — *continued*
  complicated — *continued*
    by — *continued*
      fetal — *continued*
        stress — *continued*
          specified NEC O77.8
          ultrasound evidence of O77.8
      fever during labor O75.2
      gastric banding status O99.844
      gastric bypass status O99.844
      gastrointestinal disease NEC O99.62
      gestational
        diabetes O24.429
          diet controlled O24.420
          insulin (and diet) controlled O24.424
          oral drug controlled (antidiabetic) (hypo-
            glycemic) O24.425
        edema O12.04
          with proteinuria O12.24
        proteinuria O12.14
      gonorrhea O98.22
      hematoma O71.7
        ischial spine O71.7
        pelvic O71.7
        vagina O71.7
        vulva or perineum O71.7
      hemorrhage (uterine) O67.9
        associated with
          afibrinogenemia O67.0
          coagulation defect O67.0
          hyperfibrinolysis O67.0
          hypofibrinogenemia O67.0
        due to
          low implantation of placenta O44.5- ☑
          low-lying placenta O44.5- ☑
          placenta previa O44.1- ☑
            marginal O44.3- ☑
            partial O44.3- ☑
          premature separation of placenta (nor-
            mally implanted) (*see also* Abrup-
            tio placentae) O45.9- ☑
          retained placenta O72.0
          uterine leiomyoma O67.8
        placenta NEC O67.8
        postpartum NEC (atonic) (immediate) O72.1
          with retained or trapped placenta O72.0
          delayed O72.2
          secondary O72.2
          third stage O72.0
      hourglass contraction, uterus O62.4
      hypertension, hypertensive (pre-existing) —
        *see* Hypertension, complicated by, child-
        birth (labor)
      hypotension O26.5- ☑
      incomplete dilatation (cervix) O62.0
      incoordinate uterus contractions O62.4
      inertia, uterus O62.2
        during latent phase of labor O62.0
        primary O62.0
        secondary O62.1
      infection (maternal) O98.92
        carrier state NEC O99.834
        gonorrhea O98.22
        human immunodeficiency virus (HIV)
          O98.72
        sexually transmitted NEC O98.32
        specified NEC O98.82
        syphilis O98.12
        tuberculosis O98.02
        viral hepatitis O98.42
        viral NEC O98.52
      injury (to mother) (*see also* Delivery, complicat-
        ed, by, damage to) O71.9
      nonobstetric O9A.22 (*following* O99)
        caused by abuse — *see* Delivery, compli-
          cated by, abuse
      intrauterine fetal death, early O02.1
      inversion, uterus O71.2
      laceration (perineal) O70.9
        anus (sphincter) O70.4
          with third degree laceration (*see also*
            Delivery, complicated, by, lacera-
            tion, perineum, third degree)
            O70.20
            with mucosa O70.3
          without third degree laceration O70.2 ☑
        bladder (urinary) O71.5
        bowel O71.5

**Delivery** — *continued*
  complicated — *continued*
    by — *continued*
      laceration — *continued*
        cervix (uteri) O71.3
        fourchette O70.0
        hymen O70.0
        labia O70.0
        pelvic
          floor O70.1
          organ NEC O71.5
        perineum, perineal O70.9
          first degree O70.0
          fourth degree O70.3
          muscles O70.1
          second degree O70.1
          skin O70.0
          slight O70.0
          third degree O70.20
            with
              less than 50% of external anal
                sphincter (EAS) thickness
                torn (IIIa) O70.21
              both external anal sphincter (EAS)
                and internal anal sphincter
                (IAS) torn (IIIc) O70.23
              more than 50% external anal
                sphincter (EAS) thickness
                torn (IIIb) O70.22
            IIIa O70.21
            IIIb O70.22
            IIIc O70.23
        peritoneum (pelvic) O71.5
        rectovaginal (septum) (without perineal
          laceration) O71.4
          with perineum (*see also* Delivery, compli-
            cated, by, laceration, perineum,
            third degree) O70.20
            with anal or rectal mucosa O70.3
        specified NEC O71.89
        sphincter ani — *see* Delivery, complicated,
          by, laceration, anus (sphincter)
        urethra O71.5
        uterus O71.81
          before labor O71.81
        vagina, vaginal (deep) (high) (without per-
          ineal laceration) O71.4
          with perineum O70.0
          muscles, with perineum O70.1
        vulva O70.0
      liver disorder O26.62
      malignancy O9A.12 (*following* O99)
      malnutrition O25.2
      malposition, malpresentation
        without obstruction (*see also* Delivery,
          complicated by, obstruction) O32.9 ☑
          breech O32.1 ☑
          compound O32.6 ☑
          face (brow) (chin) O32.3 ☑
          footling O32.8 ☑
          high head O32.4 ☑
          oblique O32.2 ☑
          specified NEC O32.8 ☑
          transverse O32.2 ☑
          unstable lie O32.0 ☑
        placenta O44.0- ☑
          with hemorrhage O44.1- ☑
        uterus or cervix O65.5
      meconium in amniotic fluid O77.0
      mental disorder NEC O99.344
      metrorrhexis — *see* Delivery, complicated by,
        rupture, uterus
      nervous system disorder O99.354
      obesity (pre-existing) O99.214
      obesity surgery status O99.844
      obstetric trauma O71.9
        specified NEC O71.89
      obstructed labor
        due to
          breech (complete) (frank) presentation
            O64.1 ☑
            incomplete O64.8 ☑
          brow presentation O64.3 ☑
          buttock presentation O64.1 ☑
          chin presentation O64.2 ☑
          compound presentation O64.5 ☑
          contracted pelvis O65.1
          deep transverse arrest O64.0 ☑

**Delivery** — *continued*
  complicated — *continued*
    by — *continued*
      obstructed labor — *continued*
        due to — *continued*
          deformed pelvis O65.0
          dystocia (fetal) O66.9
            due to
              conjoined twins O66.3
              fetal
                abnormality NEC O66.3
                ascites O66.3
                hydrops O66.3
                meningomyelocele O66.3
                sacral teratoma O66.3
                tumor O66.3
              hydrocephalic fetus O66.3
            shoulder O66.0
          face presentation O64.2 ☑
          fetopelvic disproportion O65.4
          footling presentation O64.8 ☑
          impacted shoulders O66.0
          incomplete rotation of fetal head
            O64.0 ☑
          large fetus O66.2
          locked twins O66.1
          malposition O64.9 ☑
            specified NEC O64.8 ☑
          malpresentation O64.9 ☑
            specified NEC O64.8 ☑
          multiple fetuses NEC O66.6
          pelvic
            abnormality (maternal) O65.9
              organ O65.5
              specified NEC O65.8
            contraction
              inlet O65.2
              mid-cavity O65.3
              outlet O65.3
          persistent (position)
            occipitoiliac O64.0 ☑
            occipitoposterior O64.0 ☑
            occipitosacral O64.0 ☑
            occipitotransverse O64.0 ☑
          prolapsed arm O64.4 ☑
          shoulder presentation O64.4 ☑
        specified NEC O66.8
      pathological retraction ring, uterus O62.4
      penetration, pregnant uterus by instrument
        O71.1
      perforation — *see* Delivery, complicated by,
        laceration
      placenta, placental
        ablatio (*see also* Abruptio placentae)
          O45.9- ☑
        abnormality O43.9- ☑
          specified NEC O43.89- ☑
        abruptio (*see also* Abruptio placentae)
          O45.9- ☑
        accreta O43.21- ☑
        adherent (with hemorrhage) O72.0
          without hemorrhage O73.0
        detachment (premature) (*see also* Abruptio
          placentae) O45.9- ☑
        disorder O43.9- ☑
          specified NEC O43.89- ☑
        hemorrhage NEC O67.8
        increta O43.22- ☑
        low (implantation) (lying) O44.4- ☑
          with hemorrhage O44.5- ☑
        malformation O43.10- ☑
        malposition O44.0- ☑
          without hemorrhage O44.1- ☑
        percreta O43.23- ☑
        previa (central) (complete) (lateral) (total)
          O44.0- ☑
          with hemorrhage O44.1- ☑
          marginal O44.2- ☑
            with hemorrhage O44.3- ☑
          partial O44.2- ☑
            with hemorrhage O44.3- ☑
        retained (with hemorrhage) O72.0
          without hemorrhage O73.0
        separation (premature) O45.9- ☑
          specified NEC O45.8X- ☑
        vicious insertion O44.1- ☑
      precipitate labor O62.3

Index

Delivery — Delivery

**Delivery** — *continued*
  complicated — *continued*
    by — *continued*
      premature rupture, membranes (*see also* Pregnancy, complicated by, premature rupture of membranes) O42.90
      prolapse
        arm or hand O32.2 ☑
        cord (umbilical) O69.0 ☑
        foot or leg O32.8 ☑
        uterus O34.52- ☑
      prolonged labor O63.9
        first stage O63.0
        second stage O63.1
      protozoal disease (maternal) O98.62
      respiratory disease NEC O99.52
      retained membranes or portions of placenta O72.2
        without hemorrhage O73.1
      retarded birth O63.9
      retention of secundines (with hemorrhage) O72.0
        without hemorrhage O73.0
        partial O72.2
          without hemorrhage O73.1
      rupture
        bladder (urinary) O71.5
        cervix O71.3
        pelvic organ NEC O71.5
        urethra O71.5
        uterus (during or after labor) O71.1
          before labor O71.0- ☑
      separation, pubic bone (symphysis pubis) O71.6
      shock O75.1
      shoulder presentation O64.4 ☑
      skin disorder NEC O99.72
      spasm, cervix O62.4
      stenosis or stricture, cervix O65.5
      streptococcus group B (GBS) carrier state O99.824
      subluxation of symphysis (pubis) O26.72
      syphilis (maternal) O98.12
      tear — *see* Delivery, complicated by, laceration
      tetanic uterus O62.4
      trauma (obstetrical) (*see also* Delivery, complicated, by, damage to) O71.9
        non-obstetric O9A.22 (*following* O99)
        periurethral O71.82
        specified NEC O71.89
      tuberculosis (maternal) O98.02
      tumor, pelvic organs or tissues NEC O65.5
      umbilical cord around neck
        with compression O69.1 ☑
        without compression O69.81 ☑
      uterine inertia O62.2
        during latent phase of labor O62.0
        primary O62.0
        secondary O62.1
      vasa previa O69.4 ☑
      velamentous insertion of cord O43.12- ☑
    specified complication NEC O75.89
  delayed NOS O63.9
    following rupture of membranes
      artificial O75.5
    second twin, triplet, etc. O63.2
  forceps, low following failed vacuum extraction O66.5
  missed (at or near term) O36.4 ☑
  normal O80
  obstructed — *see* Delivery, complicated by, obstructed labor
  precipitate O62.3
  preterm (*see also* Pregnancy, complicated by, preterm labor) O60.10 ☑
  spontaneous O80
  term pregnancy NOS O80
  uncomplicated O80
  vaginal, following previous cesarean delivery O34.219
    classical (vertical) scar O34.212
    low transverse scar O34.211
**Delusions** (paranoid) — *see* Disorder, delusional
**Dementia** (degenerative (primary)) (old age) (persisting) F03.90
  with
    aggressive behavior F03.91
    behavioral disturbance F03.91
    combative behavior F03.91
    Lewy bodies G31.83 [F02.80]
      with behavioral disturbance G31.83 [F02.81]

**Dementia** — *continued*
  with — *continued*
    Parkinsonism G31.83 [F02.80]
      with behavioral disturbance G31.83 [F02.81]
    Parkinson's disease G20 [F02.80]
      with behavioral disturbance G20 [F02.81]
    violent behavior F03.91
  alcoholic F10.97
    with dependence F10.27
  Alzheimer's type — *see* Disease, Alzheimer's
  arteriosclerotic — *see* Dementia, vascular
  atypical, Alzheimer's type — *see* Disease, Alzheimer's, specified NEC
  congenital — *see* Disability, intellectual
  frontal (lobe) G31.09 [F02.80]
    with behavioral disturbance G31.09 [F02.81]
  frontotemporal G31.09 [F02.80]
    with behavioral disturbance G31.09 [F02.81]
    specified NEC G31.09 [F02.80]
      with behavioral disturbance G31.09 [F02.81]
  Huntington's disease or chorea G10
    with dementia G10 [F02.80]
  in (due to)
    with behavioral disturbance G31.83 [F02.81]
    alcohol F10.97
      with dependence F10.27
    Alzheimer's disease — *see* Disease, Alzheimer's
    arteriosclerotic brain disease — *see* Dementia, vascular
    cerebral lipidoses E75.- ☑ [F02.80]
      with behavioral disturbance E75.- ☑ [F02.81]
    Creutzfeldt-Jakob disease (*see also* Creutzfeldt-Jakob disease or syndrome (with dementia)) A81.00
    epilepsy G40.- ☑ [F02.80]
      with behavioral disturbance G40.- ☑ [F02.81]
    hepatolenticular degeneration E83.01 [F02.80]
      with behavioral disturbance E83.01 [F02.81]
    human immunodeficiency virus (HIV) disease B20 [F02.80]
      with behavioral disturbance B20 [F02.81]
    Huntington's disease or chorea G10 [F02.80]
      with behavioral disturbance G10 [F02.81]
    hypercalcemia E83.52 [F02.80]
      with behavioral disturbance E83.52 [F02.81]
    hypothyroidism, acquired E03.9 [F02.80]
      with behavioral disturbance E03.9 [F02.81]
      due to iodine deficiency E01.8 [F02.80]
        with behavioral disturbance E01.8 [F02.81]
    inhalants F18.97
      with dependence F18.27
    multiple
      etiologies F03 ☑
      sclerosis G35 [F02.80]
        with behavioral disturbance G35 [F02.81]
    neurosyphilis A52.17 [F02.80]
      with behavioral disturbance A52.17 [F02.81]
      juvenile A50.49 [F02.80]
        with behavioral disturbance A50.49 [F02.81]
    niacin deficiency E52 [F02.80]
      with behavioral disturbance E52 [F02.81]
    paralysis agitans G20 [F02.80]
      with behavioral disturbance G20 [F02.81]
    Parkinson's disease G20 [F02.80]
      with behavioral disturbance G20 [F02.81]
    pellagra E52 [F02.80]
      with behavioral disturbance E52 [F02.81]
    Pick's G31.01 [F02.80]
      with behavioral disturbance G31.01 [F02.81]
    polyarteritis nodosa M30.0 [F02.80]
      with behavioral disturbance M30.0 [F02.81]
    psychoactive drug F19.97
      with dependence F19.27
      inhalants F18.97
        with dependence F18.27
      sedatives, hypnotics or anxiolytics F13.97
        with dependence F13.27
    sedatives, hypnotics or anxiolytics F13.97
      with dependence F13.27
    systemic lupus erythematosus M32.- ☑ [F02.80]
      with behavioral disturbance M32.- ☑ [F02.81]
    trypanosomiasis
      African B56.9 [F02.80]
        with behavioral disturbance B56.9 [F02.81]
    unknown etiology F03 ☑
    vitamin B12 deficiency E53.8 [F02.80]
      with behavioral disturbance E53.8 [F02.81]
    volatile solvents F18.97
      with dependence F18.27

**Dementia** — *continued*
  infantile, infantilis F84.3
  Lewy body G31.83 [F02.80]
    with behavioral disturbance G31.83 [F02.81]
  multi-infarct — *see* Dementia, vascular
  paralytica, paralytic (syphilitic) A52.17 [F02.80]
    with behavioral disturbance A52.17 [F02.81]
    juvenilis A50.45
  paretic A52.17
  praecox — *see* Schizophrenia
  presenile F03 ☑
    Alzheimer's type — *see* Disease, Alzheimer's, early onset
  primary degenerative F03 ☑
  progressive, syphilitic A52.17
  senile F03 ☑
    with acute confusional state F05
    Alzheimer's type — *see* Disease, Alzheimer's, late onset
    depressed or paranoid type F03 ☑
  vascular (acute onset) (mixed) (multi-infarct) (subcortical) F01.50
    with behavioral disturbance F01.51
**Demineralization, bone** — *see* Osteoporosis
**Demodex folliculorum** (infestation) B88.0
**Demophobia** F40.248
**Demoralization** R45.3
**Demyelination, demyelinization**
  central nervous system G37.9
    specified NEC G37.8
  corpus callosum (central) G37.1
  disseminated, acute G36.9
    specified NEC G36.8
  global G35
  in optic neuritis G36.0
**Dengue** (classical) (fever) A90
  hemorrhagic A91
  sandfly A93.1
**Dennie-Marfan syphilitic syndrome** A50.45
**Dens evaginatus, in dente or invaginatus** K00.2
**Dense breasts** R92.2
**Density**
  increased, bone (disseminated) (generalized) (spotted) — *see* Disorder, bone, density and structure, specified type NEC
  lung (nodular) J98.4
**Dental** (*see also* condition)
  examination Z01.20
    with abnormal findings Z01.21
  restoration
    aesthetically inadequate or displeasing K08.56
    defective K08.50
      specified NEC K08.59
    failure of marginal integrity K08.51
    failure of periodontal anatomical integrity K08.54
**Dentia praecox** K00.6
**Denticles** (pulp) K04.2
**Dentigerous cyst** K09.0
**Dentin**
  irregular (in pulp) K04.3
  opalescent K00.5
  secondary (in pulp) K04.3
  sensitive K03.89
**Dentinogenesis imperfecta** K00.5
**Dentinoma** — *see* Cyst, calcifying odontogenic
**Dentition** (syndrome) K00.7
  delayed K00.6
  difficult K00.7
  precocious K00.6
  premature K00.6
  retarded K00.6
**Dependence** (on) (syndrome) F19.20
  with remission F19.21
  alcohol (ethyl) (methyl) (without remission) F10.20
    with
      amnestic disorder, persisting F10.26
      anxiety disorder F10.280
      dementia, persisting F10.27
      intoxication F10.229
        with delirium F10.221
        uncomplicated F10.220
      mood disorder F10.24
      psychotic disorder F10.259
        with
          delusions F10.250
          hallucinations F10.251
      remission F10.21
      sexual dysfunction F10.281

**Dependence** — continued
  alcohol — continued
    with — continued
      sleep disorder F10.282
      specified disorder NEC F10.288
      withdrawal F10.239
        with
          delirium F10.231
          perceptual disturbance F10.232
        uncomplicated F10.230
    counseling and surveillance Z71.41
  amobarbital — see Dependence, drug, sedative
  amphetamine(s) (type) — see Dependence, drug, stimulant NEC
  amytal (sodium) — see Dependence, drug, sedative
  analgesic NEC F55.8
  anesthetic (agent) (gas) (general) (local) NEC — see Dependence, drug, psychoactive NEC
  anxiolytic NEC — see Dependence, drug, sedative
  barbital(s) — see Dependence, drug, sedative
  barbiturate(s) (compounds) (drugs classifiable to T42) — see Dependence, drug, sedative
  benzedrine — see Dependence, drug, stimulant NEC
  bhang — see Dependence, drug, cannabis
  bromide(s) NEC — see Dependence, drug, sedative
  caffeine — see Dependence, drug, stimulant NEC
  cannabis (sativa) (indica) (resin) (derivatives) (type) — see Dependence, drug, cannabis
  chloral (betaine) (hydrate) — see Dependence, drug, sedative
  chlordiazepoxide — see Dependence, drug, sedative
  coca (leaf) (derivatives) — see Dependence, drug, cocaine
  cocaine — see Dependence, drug, cocaine
  codeine — see Dependence, drug, opioid
  combinations of drugs F19.20
  dagga — see Dependence, drug, cannabis
  demerol — see Dependence, drug, opioid
  dexamphetamine — see Dependence, drug, stimulant NEC
  dexedrine — see Dependence, drug, stimulant NEC
  dextromethorphan — see Dependence, drug, opioid
  dextromoramide — see Dependence, drug, opioid
  dextro-nor-pseudo-ephedrine — see Dependence, drug, stimulant NEC
  dextrorphan — see Dependence, drug, opioid
  diazepam — see Dependence, drug, sedative
  dilaudid — see Dependence, drug, opioid
  D-lysergic acid diethylamide — see Dependence, drug, hallucinogen
  drug NEC F19.20
    with sleep disorder F19.282
    cannabis F12.20
      with
        anxiety disorder F12.280
        intoxication F12.229
          with
            delirium F12.221
            perceptual disturbance F12.222
          uncomplicated F12.220
        other specified disorder F12.288
        psychosis F12.259
          delusions F12.250
          hallucinations F12.251
        unspecified disorder F12.29
      in remission F12.21
    cocaine F14.20
      with
        anxiety disorder F14.280
        intoxication F14.229
          with
            delirium F14.221
            perceptual disturbance F14.222
          uncomplicated F14.220
        mood disorder F14.24
        other specified disorder F14.288
        psychosis F14.259
          delusions F14.250
          hallucinations F14.251
        sexual dysfunction F14.281
        sleep disorder F14.282
        unspecified disorder F14.29
        withdrawal F14.23
      in remission F14.21
      withdrawal symptoms in newborn P96.1
    counseling and surveillance Z71.51
    hallucinogen F16.20

**Dependence** — continued
  drug — continued
    hallucinogen — continued
      with
        anxiety disorder F16.280
        flashbacks F16.283
        intoxication F16.229
          with delirium F16.221
          uncomplicated F16.220
        mood disorder F16.24
        other specified disorder F16.288
        perception disorder, persisting F16.283
        psychosis F16.259
          delusions F16.250
          hallucinations F16.251
        unspecified disorder F16.29
      in remission F16.21
    in remission F19.21
    inhalant F18.20
      with
        anxiety disorder F18.280
        dementia, persisting F18.27
        intoxication F18.229
          with delirium F18.221
          uncomplicated F18.220
        mood disorder F18.24
        other specified disorder F18.288
        psychosis F18.259
          delusions F18.250
          hallucinations F18.251
        unspecified disorder F18.29
      in remission F18.21
    nicotine F17.200
      with disorder F17.209
        in remission F17.201
        specified disorder NEC F17.208
        withdrawal F17.203
      chewing tobacco F17.220
        with disorder F17.229
          in remission F17.221
          specified disorder NEC F17.228
          withdrawal F17.223
      cigarettes F17.210
        with disorder F17.219
          in remission F17.211
          specified disorder NEC F17.218
          withdrawal F17.213
      specified product NEC F17.290
        with disorder F17.299
          remission F17.291
          specified disorder NEC F17.298
          withdrawal F17.293
    opioid F11.20
      with
        intoxication F11.229
          with
            delirium F11.221
            perceptual disturbance F11.222
          uncomplicated F11.220
        mood disorder F11.24
        other specified disorder F11.288
        psychosis F11.259
          delusions F11.250
          hallucinations F11.251
        sexual dysfunction F11.281
        sleep disorder F11.282
        unspecified disorder F11.29
        withdrawal F11.23
      in remission F11.21
    psychoactive NEC F19.20
      with
        amnestic disorder F19.26
        anxiety disorder F19.280
        dementia F19.27
        intoxication F19.229
          with
            delirium F19.221
            perceptual disturbance F19.222
          uncomplicated F19.220
        mood disorder F19.24
        other specified disorder F19.288
        psychosis F19.259
          delusions F19.250
          hallucinations F19.251
        sexual dysfunction F19.281
        sleep disorder F19.282
        unspecified disorder F19.29
        withdrawal F19.239

**Dependence** — continued
  drug — continued
    psychoactive — continued
      with — continued
        withdrawal — continued
          with
            delirium F19.231
            perceptual disturbance F19.232
          uncomplicated F19.230
    sedative, hypnotic or anxiolytic F13.20
      with
        amnestic disorder F13.26
        anxiety disorder F13.280
        dementia, persisting F13.27
        intoxication F13.229
          with delirium F13.221
          uncomplicated F13.220
        mood disorder F13.24
        other specified disorder F13.288
        psychosis F13.259
          delusions F13.250
          hallucinations F13.251
        sexual dysfunction F13.281
        sleep disorder F13.282
        unspecified disorder F13.29
        withdrawal F13.239
          with
            delirium F13.231
            perceptual disturbance F13.232
          uncomplicated F13.230
      in remission F13.21
    stimulant NEC F15.20
      with
        anxiety disorder F15.280
        intoxication F15.229
          with
            delirium F15.221
            perceptual disturbance F15.222
          uncomplicated F15.220
        mood disorder F15.24
        other specified disorder F15.288
        psychosis F15.259
          delusions F15.250
          hallucinations F15.251
        sexual dysfunction F15.281
        sleep disorder F15.282
        unspecified disorder F15.29
        withdrawal F15.23
      in remission F15.21
  ethyl
    alcohol (without remission) F10.20
      with remission F10.21
    bromide — see Dependence, drug, sedative
    carbamate F19.20
    chloride F19.20
    morphine — see Dependence, drug, opioid
  ganja — see Dependence, drug, cannabis
  glue (airplane) (sniffing) — see Dependence, drug, inhalant
  glutethimide — see Dependence, drug, sedative
  hallucinogenics — see Dependence, drug, hallucinogen
  hashish — see Dependence, drug, cannabis
  hemp — see Dependence, drug, cannabis
  heroin (salt) (any) — see Dependence, drug, opioid
  hypnotic NEC — see Dependence, drug, sedative
  Indian hemp — see Dependence, drug, cannabis
  inhalants — see Dependence, drug, inhalant
  khat — see Dependence, drug, stimulant NEC
  laudanum — see Dependence, drug, opioid
  LSD (-25) (derivatives) — see Dependence, drug, hallucinogen
  luminal — see Dependence, drug, sedative
  lysergic acid — see Dependence, drug, hallucinogen
  maconha — see Dependence, drug, cannabis
  marihuana — see Dependence, drug, cannabis
  meprobamate — see Dependence, drug, sedative
  mescaline — see Dependence, drug, hallucinogen
  methadone — see Dependence, drug, opioid
  methamphetamine(s) — see Dependence, drug, stimulant NEC
  methaqualone — see Dependence, drug, sedative
  methyl
    alcohol (without remission) F10.20
      with remission F10.21
    bromide — see Dependence, drug, sedative
    morphine — see Dependence, drug, opioid

**Dependence** — *continued*
  methyl — *continued*
    phenidate — *see* Dependence, drug, stimulant
        NEC
    sulfonal — *see* Dependence, drug, sedative
  morphine (sulfate) (sulfite) (type) — *see* Dependence,
        drug, opioid
  narcotic (drug) NEC — *see* Dependence, drug, opioid
  nembutal — *see* Dependence, drug, sedative
  neraval — *see* Dependence, drug, sedative
  neravan — *see* Dependence, drug, sedative
  neurobarb — *see* Dependence, drug, sedative
  nicotine — *see* Dependence, drug, nicotine
  nitrous oxide F19.20
  nonbarbiturate sedatives and tranquilizers with similar
        effect — *see* Dependence, drug, sedative
  on
    artificial heart (fully implantable) (mechanical)
        Z95.812
    aspirator Z99.0
    care provider (because of) Z74.9
        impaired mobility Z74.09
        need for
            assistance with personal care Z74.1
            continuous supervision Z74.3
            no other household member able to render
                care Z74.2
            specified reason NEC Z74.8
    machine Z99.89
        enabling NEC Z99.89
        specified type NEC Z99.89
    renal dialysis (hemodialysis) (peritoneal) Z99.2
    respirator Z99.11
    ventilator Z99.11
    wheelchair Z99.3
  opiate — *see* Dependence, drug, opioid
  opioids — *see* Dependence, drug, opioid
  opium (alkaloids) (derivatives) (tincture) — *see* Depen-
        dence, drug, opioid
  oxygen (long-term) (supplemental) Z99.81
  paraldehyde — *see* Dependence, drug, sedative
  paregoric — *see* Dependence, drug, opioid
  PCP (phencyclidine) (or related substance) — *see* De-
        pendence, drug, hallucinogen
  pentobarbital — *see* Dependence, drug, sedative
  pentobarbitone (sodium) — *see* Dependence, drug,
        sedative
  pentothal — *see* Dependence, drug, sedative
  peyote — *see* Dependence, drug, hallucinogen
  phencyclidine (PCP) (or related substance) — *see* De-
        pendence, drug, hallucinogen
  phenmetrazine — *see* Dependence, drug, stimulant
        NEC
  phenobarbital — *see* Dependence, drug, sedative
  polysubstance F19.20
  psilocibin, psilocin, psilocyn, psilocyline — *see* Depen-
        dence, drug, hallucinogen
  psychostimulant NEC — *see* Dependence, drug, stim-
        ulant NEC
  secobarbital — *see* Dependence, drug, sedative
  seconal — *see* Dependence, drug, sedative
  sedative NEC — *see* Dependence, drug, sedative
  specified drug NEC — *see* Dependence, drug
  stimulant NEC — *see* Dependence, drug, stimulant
        NEC
  substance NEC — *see* Dependence, drug
  supplemental oxygen Z99.81
  tobacco — *see* Dependence, drug, nicotine
        counseling and surveillance Z71.6
  tranquilizer NEC — *see* Dependence, drug, sedative
  vitamin B6 E53.1
  volatile solvents — *see* Dependence, drug, inhalant
**Dependency**
  care-provider Z74.9
  passive F60.7
  reactions (persistent) F60.7
**Depersonalization** (in neurotic state) (neurotic) (syn-
        drome) F48.1
**Depletion**
  extracellular fluid E86.9
  plasma E86.1
  potassium E87.6
    nephropathy N25.89
  salt or sodium E87.1
    causing heat exhaustion or prostration T67.4 ☑
    nephropathy N28.9
  volume NOS E86.9

**Deployment** (current) (military) status Z56.82
  in theater or in support of military war, peacekeeping
        and humanitarian operations Z56.82
  personal history of Z91.82
    military war, peacekeeping and humanitarian de-
        ployment (current or past conflict) Z91.82
  returned from Z91.82
**Depolarization, premature** I49.40
  atrial I49.1
  junctional I49.2
  specified NEC I49.49
  ventricular I49.3
**Deposit**
  bone in Boeck's sarcoid D86.89
  calcareous, calcium — *see* Calcification
  cholesterol
    retina H35.89
    vitreous (body) (humor) — *see* Deposit, crystalline
  conjunctiva H11.11- ☑
  cornea H18.00- ☑
    argentous H18.02- ☑
    due to metabolic disorder H18.03- ☑
    Kayser-Fleischer ring H18.04- ☑
    pigmentation — *see* Pigmentation, cornea
  crystalline, vitreous (body) (humor) H43.2- ☑
  hemosiderin in old scars of cornea — *see* Pigmenta-
        tion, cornea, stromal
  metallic in lens — *see* Cataract, specified NEC
  skin R23.8
  tooth, teeth (betel) (black) (green) (materia alba) (or-
        ange) (tobacco) K03.6
  urate, kidney — *see* Calculus, kidney
**Depraved appetite** — *see* Pica
**Depressed**
  HDL cholesterol E78.6
**Depression** (acute) (mental) F32.9
  agitated (single episode) F32.2
  anaclitic — *see* Disorder, adjustment
  anxiety F41.8
    persistent F34.1
  arches (*see also* Deformity, limb, flat foot)
  atypical (single episode) F32.89
    recurrent episode F33.8
  basal metabolic rate R94.8
  bone marrow D75.89
  central nervous system R09.2
  cerebral R29.818
    newborn P91.4
  cerebrovascular I67.9
  chest wall M95.4
  climacteric (single episode) F32.89
    recurrent episode F33.8
  endogenous (without psychotic symptoms) F33.2
    with psychotic symptoms F33.3
  functional activity R68.89
  hysterical F44.89
  involutional (single episode) F32.89
    recurrent episode F33.8
  major F32.9
    with psychotic symptoms F32.3
    recurrent — *see* Disorder, depressive, recurrent
  manic-depressive — *see* Disorder, depressive, recur-
        rent
  masked (single episode) F32.89
  medullary G93.89
  menopausal (single episode) F32.89
    recurrent episode F33.8
  metatarsus — *see* Depression, arches
  monopolar F33.9
  nervous F34.1
  neurotic F34.1
  nose M95.0
  postnatal F53
  postpartum F53
  post-psychotic of schizophrenia F32.89
  post-schizophrenic F32.89
  psychogenic (reactive) (single episode) F32.9
  psychoneurotic F34.1
  psychotic (single episode) F32.3
    recurrent F33.3
  reactive (psychogenic) (single episode) F32.9
    psychotic (single episode) F32.3
  recurrent — *see* Disorder, depressive, recurrent
  respiratory center G93.89
  seasonal — *see* Disorder, depressive, recurrent
  senile F03 ☑
  severe, single episode F32.2
  situational F43.21

**Depression** — *continued*
  skull Q67.4
  specified NEC (single episode) F32.89
  sternum M95.4
  visual field — *see* Defect, visual field
  vital (recurrent) (without psychotic symptoms) F33.2
    with psychotic symptoms F33.3
    single episode F32.2
**Deprivation**
  cultural Z60.3
  effects NOS T73.9 ☑
    specified NEC T73.8 ☑
  emotional NEC Z65.8
    affecting infant or child — *see* Maltreatment, child,
        psychological
  food T73.0 ☑
  protein — *see* Malnutrition
  sleep Z72.820
  social Z60.4
    affecting infant or child — *see* Maltreatment, child,
        psychological
  specified NEC T73.8 ☑
  vitamins — *see* Deficiency, vitamin
  water T73.1 ☑
**Derangement**
  ankle (internal) — *see* Derangement, joint, ankle
  cartilage (articular) NEC — *see* Derangement, joint,
        articular cartilage, by site
  recurrent — *see* Dislocation, recurrent
  cruciate ligament, anterior, current injury — *see*
        Sprain, knee, cruciate, anterior
  elbow (internal) — *see* Derangement, joint, elbow
  hip (joint) (internal) (old) — *see* Derangement, joint,
        hip
  joint (internal) M24.9
    ankylosis — *see* Ankylosis
    articular cartilage M24.10
        ankle M24.17- ☑
        elbow M24.12- ☑
        foot M24.17- ☑
        hand M24.14- ☑
        hip M24.15- ☑
        knee NEC M23.9- ☑
        loose body — *see* Loose, body
        shoulder M24.11- ☑
        wrist M24.13- ☑
    contracture — *see* Contraction, joint
    current injury (*see also* Dislocation)
        knee, meniscus or cartilage — *see* Tear, menis-
            cus
    dislocation
        pathological — *see* Dislocation, pathological
        recurrent — *see* Dislocation, recurrent
    knee — *see* Derangement, knee
    ligament — *see* Disorder, ligament
    loose body — *see* Loose, body
    recurrent — *see* Dislocation, recurrent
    specified type NEC M24.80
        ankle M24.87- ☑
        elbow M24.82- ☑
        foot joint M24.87- ☑
        hand joint M24.84- ☑
        hip M24.85- ☑
        shoulder M24.81- ☑
        wrist M24.83- ☑
    temporomandibular M26.69
  knee (recurrent) M23.9- ☑
    ligament disruption, spontaneous M23.60- ☑
        anterior cruciate M23.61- ☑
        capsular M23.67- ☑
        instability, chronic M23.5- ☑
        lateral collateral M23.64- ☑
        medial collateral M23.63- ☑
        posterior cruciate M23.62- ☑
    loose body M23.4- ☑
    meniscus M23.30- ☑
        cystic M23.00- ☑
            lateral M23.002
                anterior horn M23.04- ☑
                posterior horn M23.05- ☑
                specified NEC M23.06- ☑
            medial M23.005
                anterior horn M23.01- ☑
                posterior horn M23.02- ☑
                specified NEC M23.03- ☑

**Derangement** — continued
  knee — continued
    meniscus — continued
      degenerate — see Derangement, knee, menis-
        cus, specified NEC
      detached — see Derangement, knee, meniscus,
        specified NEC
      due to old tear or injury M23.20- ☑
        lateral M23.20- ☑
          anterior horn M23.24- ☑
          posterior horn M23.25- ☑
          specified NEC M23.26- ☑
        medial M23.20- ☑
          anterior horn M23.21- ☑
          posterior horn M23.22- ☑
          specified NEC M23.23- ☑
      retained — see Derangement, knee, meniscus,
        specified NEC
      specified NEC M23.30- ☑
        lateral M23.30- ☑
          anterior horn M23.34- ☑
          posterior horn M23.35- ☑
          specified NEC M23.36- ☑
        medial M23.30- ☑
          anterior horn M23.31- ☑
          posterior horn M23.32- ☑
          specified NEC M23.33- ☑
      old M23.8X- ☑
      specified NEC — see subcategory M23.8 ☑
    low back NEC — see Dorsopathy, specified NEC
    meniscus — see Derangement, knee, meniscus
    mental — see Psychosis
    patella, specified NEC — see Disorder, patella, derange-
      ment NEC
    semilunar cartilage (knee) — see Derangement, knee,
      meniscus, specified NEC
    shoulder (internal) — see Derangement, joint, shoul-
      der
**Dercum's disease** E88.2
**Derealization** (neurotic) F48.1
**Dermal** — see condition
**Dermaphytid** — see Dermatophytosis
**Dermatitis** (eczematous) L30.9
  ab igne L59.0
  acarine B88.0
  actinic (due to sun) L57.8
    other than from sun L59.8
  allergic — see Dermatitis, contact, allergic
  ambustionis, due to burn or scald — see Burn
  amebic A06.7
  ammonia L22
  arsenical (ingested) L27.8
  artefacta L98.1
    psychogenic F54
  atopic L20.9
    psychogenic F54
    specified NEC L20.89
  autoimmune progesterone L30.8
  berlock, berloque L56.2
  blastomycotic B40.3
  blister beetle L24.89
  bullous, bullosa L13.9
    mucosynechial, atrophic L12.1
    seasonal L30.8
    specified NEC L13.8
  calorica L59.0
    due to burn or scald — see Burn
  caterpillar L24.89
  cercarial B65.3
  combustionis L59.0
    due to burn or scald — see Burn
  congelationis T69.1 ☑
  contact (occupational) L25.9
    allergic L23.9
      due to
        adhesives L23.1
        cement L23.5
        chemical products NEC L23.5
        chromium L23.0
        cosmetics L23.2
        dander (cat) (dog) L23.81
        drugs in contact with skin L23.3
        dyes L23.4
        food in contact with skin L23.6
        hair (cat) (dog) L23.81
        insecticide L23.5
        metals L23.0

**Dermatitis** — continued
  contact — continued
    allergic — continued
      due to — continued
        nickel L23.0
        plants, non-food L23.7
        plastic L23.5
        rubber L23.5
        specified agent NEC L23.89
      due to
        cement L25.3
        chemical products NEC L25.3
        cosmetics L25.0
        dander (cat) (dog) L23.81
        drugs in contact with skin L25.1
        dyes L25.2
        food in contact with skin L25.4
        hair (cat) (dog) L23.81
        plants, non-food L25.5
        specified agent NEC L25.8
    irritant L24.9
      due to
        cement L24.5
        chemical products NEC L24.5
        cosmetics L24.3
        detergents L24.0
        drugs in contact with skin L24.4
        food in contact with skin L24.6
        oils and greases L24.1
        plants, non-food L24.7
        solvents L24.2
        specified agent NEC L24.89
  contusiformis L52
  diabetic — see E08-E13 with .620
  diaper L22
  diphtheritica A36.3
  dry skin L85.3
  due to
    acetone (contact) (irritant) L24.2
    acids (contact) (irritant) L24.5
    adhesive(s) (allergic) (contact) (plaster) L23.1
      irritant L24.5
    alcohol (irritant) (skin contact) (substances in cate-
      gory T51) L24.2
      taken internally L27.8
    alkalis (contact) (irritant) L24.5
    arsenic (ingested) L27.8
    carbon disulfide (contact) (irritant) L24.2
    caustics (contact) (irritant) L24.5
    cement (contact) L25.3
    cereal (ingested) L27.2
    chemical(s) NEC L25.3
      taken internally L27.8
    chlorocompounds L24.2
    chromium (contact) (irritant) L24.81
    coffee (ingested) L27.2
    cold weather L30.8
    cosmetics (contact) L25.0
      allergic L23.2
      irritant L24.3
    cyclohexanes L24.2
    dander (cat) (dog) L23.81
    Demodex species B88.0
    Dermanyssus gallinae B88.0
    detergents (contact) (irritant) L24.0
    dichromate L24.81
    drugs and medicaments (generalized) (internal
      use) L27.0
      external — see Dermatitis, due to, drugs, in
        contact with skin
      in contact with skin L25.1
        allergic L23.3
        irritant L24.4
      localized skin eruption L27.1
      specified substance — see Table of Drugs and
        Chemicals
    dyes (contact) L25.2
      allergic L23.4
      irritant L24.89
    epidermophytosis — see Dermatophytosis
    esters L24.2
    external irritant NEC L24.9
    fish (ingested) L27.2
    flour (ingested) L27.2
    food (ingested) L27.2
      in contact with skin L25.4
    fruit (ingested) L27.2
    furs (allergic) (contact) L23.81
    glues — see Dermatitis, due to, adhesives

**Dermatitis** — continued
  due to — continued
    glycols L24.2
    greases NEC (contact) (irritant) L24.1
    hair (cat) (dog) L23.81
    hot
      objects and materials — see Burn
      weather or places L59.0
    hydrocarbons L24.2
    infrared rays L59.8
    ingestion, ingested substance L27.9
      chemical NEC L27.8
      drugs and medicaments — see Dermatitis, due
        to, drugs
      food L27.2
      specified NEC L27.8
    insecticide in contact with skin L24.5
    internal agent L27.9
      drugs and medicaments (generalized) — see
        Dermatitis, due to, drugs
      food L27.2
    irradiation — see Dermatitis, due to, radioactive
      substance
    ketones L24.2
    lacquer tree (allergic) (contact) L23.7
    light (sun) NEC L57.8
      acute L56.8
      other L59.8
    Liponyssoides sanguineus B88.0
    low temperature L30.8
    meat (ingested) L27.2
    metals, metal salts (contact) (irritant) L24.81
    milk (ingested) L27.2
    nickel (contact) (irritant) L24.81
    nylon (contact) (irritant) L24.5
    oils NEC (contact) (irritant) L24.1
    paint solvent (contact) (irritant) L24.2
    petroleum products (contact) (irritant) (substances
      in T52.0) L24.2
    plants NEC (contact) L25.5
      allergic L23.7
      irritant L24.7
    plasters (adhesive) (any) (allergic) (contact) L23.1
      irritant L24.5
    plastic (contact) L25.3
    preservatives (contact) — see Dermatitis, due to,
      chemical, in contact with skin
    primrose (allergic) (contact) L23.7
    primula (allergic) (contact) L23.7
    radiation L59.8
      nonionizing (chronic exposure) L57.8
      sun NEC L57.8
        acute L56.8
    radioactive substance L58.9
      acute L58.0
      chronic L58.1
    radium L58.9
      acute L58.0
      chronic L58.1
    ragweed (allergic) (contact) L23.7
    Rhus (allergic) (contact) (diversiloba) (radicans)
      (toxicodendron) (venenata) (verniciflua)
      L23.7
    rubber (contact) L24.5
    Senecio jacobaea (allergic) (contact) L23.7
    solvents (contact) (irritant) (substances in category
      T52) L24.2
    specified agent NEC (contact) L25.8
      allergic L23.89
      irritant L24.89
    sunshine NEC L57.8
      acute L56.8
    tetrachlorethylene (contact) (irritant) L24.2
    toluene (contact) (irritant) L24.2
    turpentine (contact) L24.2
    ultraviolet rays (sun NEC) (chronic exposure) L57.8
      acute L56.8
    vaccine or vaccination L27.0
      specified substance — see Table of Drugs and
        Chemicals
    varicose veins — see Varix, leg, with, inflammation
    X-rays L58.9
      acute L58.0
      chronic L58.1
  dyshydrotic L30.1
  dysmenorrheica N94.6
  escharotica — see Burn
  exfoliative, exfoliativa (generalized) L26

**Dermatitis** — *continued*
exfoliative, exfoliativa — *continued*
neonatorum L00
eyelid (*see also* Dermatosis, eyelid)
allergic H01.119
left H01.116
lower H01.115
upper H01.114
right H01.113
lower H01.112
upper H01.111
contact — *see* Dermatitis, eyelid, allergic
due to
Demodex species B88.0
herpes (zoster) B02.39
simplex B00.59
eczematous H01.139
left H01.136
lower H01.135
upper H01.134
right H01.133
lower H01.132
upper H01.131
facta, factitia, factitial L98.1
psychogenic F54
flexural NEC L20.82
friction L30.4
fungus B36.9
specified type NEC B36.8
gangrenosa, gangrenous infantum L08.0
harvest mite B88.0
heat L59.0
herpesviral, vesicular (ear) (lip) B00.1
herpetiformis (bullous) (erythematous) (pustular)
(vesicular) L13.0
juvenile L12.2
senile L12.0
hiemalis L30.8
hypostatic, hypostatica — *see* Varix, leg, with, inflammation
infectious eczematoid L30.3
infective L30.3
irritant — *see* Dermatitis, contact, irritant
Jacquet's (diaper dermatitis) L22
Leptus B88.0
lichenified NEC L28.0
medicamentosa (generalized) (internal use) — *see*
Dermatitis, due to drugs
mite B88.0
multiformis L13.0
juvenile L12.2
napkin L22
neurotica L13.0
nummular L30.0
papillaris capillitii L73.0
pellagrous E52
perioral L71.0
photocontact L56.2
polymorpha dolorosa L13.0
pruriginosa L13.0
pruritic NEC L30.8
psychogenic F54
purulent L08.0
pustular
contagious B08.02
subcorneal L13.1
pyococcal L08.0
pyogenica L08.0
repens L40.2
Ritter's (exfoliativa) L00
Schamberg's L81.7
schistosome B65.3
seasonal bullous L30.8
seborrheic L21.9
infantile L21.1
specified NEC L21.8
sensitization NOS L23.9
septic L08.0
solare L57.8
specified NEC L30.8
stasis I87.2
with
varicose ulcer — *see* Varix, leg, with ulcer, with
inflammation
varicose veins — *see* Varix, leg, with, inflammation
due to postthrombotic syndrome — *see* Syndrome,
postthrombotic

**Dermatitis** — *continued*
suppurative L08.0
traumatic NEC L30.4
trophoneurotica L13.0
ultraviolet (sun) (chronic exposure) L57.8
acute L56.8
varicose — *see* Varix, leg, with, inflammation
vegetans L10.1
verrucosa B43.0
vesicular, herpesviral B00.1
**Dermatoarthritis, lipoid** E78.81
**Dermatochalasis, eyelid** H02.839
left H02.836
lower H02.835
upper H02.834
right H02.833
lower H02.832
upper H02.831
**Dermatofibroma** (lenticulare) — *see* Neoplasm, skin,
benign
protuberans — *see* Neoplasm, skin, uncertain behavior
**Dermatofibrosarcoma** (pigmented) (protuberans) —
*see* Neoplasm, skin, malignant
**Dermatographia** L50.3
**Dermatolysis** (exfoliativa) (congenital) Q82.8
acquired L57.4
eyelids — *see* Blepharochalasis
palpebrarum — *see* Blepharochalasis
senile L57.4
**Dermatomegaly NEC** Q82.8
**Dermatomucosomyositis** M33.10
with
myopathy M33.12
respiratory involvement M33.11
specified organ involvement NEC M33.19
**Dermatomycosis** B36.9
furfuracea B36.0
specified type NEC B36.8
**Dermatomyositis** (acute) (chronic) (*see also* Dermatopolymyositis)
adult (*see also* Dermatomyositis, specified NEC) M33.10
in (due to) neoplastic disease (*see also* Neoplasm)
D49.9 [M36.0]
juvenile M33.00
with
myopathy M33.02
respiratory involvement M33.01
specified organ involvement NEC M33.09
without myopathy M33.03
specified NEC M33.10
with
myopathy M33.12
respiratory involvement M33.11
specified organ involvement NEC M33.19
without myopathy M33.13
**Dermatoneuritis of children** — *see* Poisoning, mercury
**Dermatophilosis** A48.8
**Dermatophytid** L30.2
**Dermatophytide** — *see* Dermatophytosis
**Dermatophytosis** (epidermophyton) (infection) (Microsporum) (tinea) (Trichophyton) B35.9
beard B35.0
body B35.4
capitis B35.0
corporis B35.4
deep-seated B35.8
disseminated B35.8
foot B35.3
granulomatous B35.8
groin B35.6
hand B35.2
nail B35.1
perianal (area) B35.6
scalp B35.0
specified NEC B35.8
**Dermatopolymyositis** M33.90
with
myopathy M33.92
respiratory involvement M33.91
specified organ involvement NEC M33.99
without myopathy M33.93
in neoplastic disease (*see also* Neoplasm)
D49.9 [M36.0]
juvenile M33.00
with
myopathy M33.02
respiratory involvement M33.01
specified organ involvement NEC M33.09

**Dermatopolymyositis** — *continued*
specified NEC M33.10
myopathy M33.12
respiratory involvement M33.11
specified organ involvement NEC M33.19
**Dermatopolyneuritis** — *see* Poisoning, mercury
**Dermatorrhexis** Q79.6
acquired L57.4
**Dermatosclerosis** (*see also* Scleroderma)
localized L94.0
**Dermatosis** L98.9
Andrews' L08.89
Bowen's — *see* Neoplasm, skin, in situ
bullous L13.9
specified NEC L13.8
exfoliativa L26
eyelid (noninfectious)
dermatitis — *see* Dermatitis, eyelid
discoid lupus erythematosus — *see* Lupus, erythematosus, eyelid
xeroderma — *see* Xeroderma, acquired, eyelid
factitial L98.1
febrile neutrophilic L98.2
gonococcal A54.89
herpetiformis L13.0
juvenile L12.2
linear IgA L13.8
menstrual NEC L98.8
neutrophilic, febrile L98.2
occupational — *see* Dermatitis, contact
papulosa nigra L82.1
pigmentary L81.9
progressive L81.7
Schamberg's L81.7
psychogenic F54
purpuric, pigmented L81.7
pustular, subcorneal L13.1
transient acantholytic L11.1
**Dermographia, dermographism** L50.3
**Dermoid** (cyst) (*see also* Neoplasm, benign, by site)
with malignant transformation C56- ☑
due to radiation (nonionizing) L57.8
**Dermopathy**
infiltrative with thyrotoxicosis — *see* Thyrotoxicosis
nephrogenic fibrosing L90.8
**Dermophytosis** — *see* Dermatophytosis
**Descemetocele** H18.73- ☑
**Descemet's membrane** — *see* condition
**Descending** — *see* condition
**Descensus uteri** — *see* Prolapse, uterus
**Desert**
rheumatism B38.0
sore — *see* Ulcer, skin
**Desertion** (newborn) — *see* Maltreatment
**Desmoid** (extra-abdominal) (tumor) — *see* Neoplasm,
connective tissue, uncertain behavior
abdominal D48.1
**Despondency** F32.9
**Desquamation, skin** R23.4
**Destruction, destructive** (*see also* Damage)
articular facet (*see also* Derangement, joint, specified
type NEC)
knee M23.8X- ☑
vertebra — *see* Spondylosis
bone (*see also* Disorder, bone, specified type NEC)
syphilitic A52.77
joint (*see also* Derangement, joint, specified type NEC)
sacroiliac M53.3
rectal sphincter K62.89
septum (nasal) J34.89
tuberculous NEC — *see* Tuberculosis
tympanum, tympanic membrane (nontraumatic) —
*see* Disorder, tympanic membrane, specified
NEC
vertebral disc — *see* Degeneration, intervertebral disc
**Destructiveness** (*see also* Disorder, conduct)
adjustment reaction — *see* Disorder, adjustment
**Desultory labor** O62.2
**Detachment**
cartilage — *see* Sprain
cervix, annular N88.8
complicating delivery O71.3
choroid (old) (postinfectional) (simple) (spontaneous)
H31.40- ☑
hemorrhagic H31.41- ☑
serous H31.42- ☑
ligament — *see* Sprain

☑ **Additional Character Required** — **Refer to the Tabular List for Character Selection**
▽ Subterms under main terms may continue to next column or page

**Detachment** — *continued*
　meniscus (knee) (*see also* Derangement, knee, meniscus, specified NEC)
　　current injury — *see* Tear, meniscus
　　due to old tear or injury — *see* Derangement, knee, meniscus, due to old tear
　retina (without retinal break) (serous) H33.2- ☑
　　with retinal:
　　　break H33.00- ☑
　　　　giant H33.03- ☑
　　　　multiple H33.02- ☑
　　　　single H33.01- ☑
　　　dialysis H33.04- ☑
　　pigment epithelium — *see* Degeneration, retina, separation of layers, pigment epithelium detachment
　　rhegmatogenous — *see* Detachment, retina, with retinal, break
　　specified NEC H33.8
　　total H33.05- ☑
　　traction H33.4- ☑
　vitreous (body) H43.81 ☑
**Detergent asthma** J69.8
**Deterioration**
　epileptic F06.8
　general physical R53.81
　heart, cardiac — *see* Degeneration, myocardial
　mental — *see* Psychosis
　myocardial, myocardium — *see* Degeneration, myocardial
　senile (simple) R54
**Deuteranomaly** (anomalous trichromat) H53.53
**Deuteranopia** (complete) (incomplete) H53.53
**Development**
　abnormal, bone Q79.9
　arrested R62.50
　　bone — *see* Arrest, development or growth, bone
　　child R62.50
　　due to malnutrition E45
　defective, congenital (*see also* Anomaly, by site)
　　cauda equina Q06.3
　　left ventricle Q24.8
　　　in hypoplastic left heart syndrome Q23.4
　　valve Q24.8
　　　pulmonary Q22.3
　delayed (*see also* Delay, development) R62.50
　　arithmetical skills F81.2
　　language (skills) (expressive) F80.1
　　learning skill F81.9
　　mixed skills F88
　　motor coordination F82
　　reading F81.0
　　specified learning skill NEC F81.89
　　speech F80.9
　　spelling F81.81
　　written expression F81.81
　imperfect, congenital (*see also* Anomaly, by site)
　　heart Q24.9
　　lungs Q33.6
　incomplete
　　bronchial tree Q32.4
　　organ or site not listed — *see* Hypoplasia, by site
　　respiratory system Q34.9
　sexual, precocious NEC E30.1
　tardy, mental (*see also* Disability, intellectual) F79
**Developmental** — *see* condition
　testing, infant or child — *see* Examination, child
**Devergie's disease** (pityriasis rubra pilaris) L44.0
**Deviation** (in)
　conjugate palsy (eye) (spastic) H51.0
　esophagus (acquired) K22.8
　eye, skew H51.8
　midline (jaw) (teeth) (dental arch) M26.29
　　specified site NEC — *see* Malposition
　nasal septum J34.2
　　congenital Q67.4
　opening and closing of the mandible M26.53
　organ or site, congenital NEC — *see* Malposition, congenital
　septum (nasal) (acquired) J34.2
　　congenital Q67.4
　sexual F65.9
　　bestiality F65.89
　　erotomania F52.8
　　exhibitionism F65.2
　　fetishism, fetishistic F65.0
　　　transvestism F65.1
　　frotteurism F65.81

**Deviation** — *continued*
　sexual — *continued*
　　masochism F65.51
　　multiple F65.89
　　necrophilia F65.89
　　nymphomania F52.8
　　pederosis F65.4
　　pedophilia F65.4
　　sadism, sadomasochism F65.52
　　satyriasis F52.8
　　specified type NEC F65.89
　　transvestism F64.1
　　voyeurism F65.3
　teeth, midline M26.29
　trachea J39.8
　ureter, congenital Q62.61
**Device**
　cerebral ventricle (communicating) in situ Z98.2
　contraceptive — *see* Contraceptive, device
　drainage, cerebrospinal fluid, in situ Z98.2
**Devic's disease** G36.0
**Devil's**
　grip B33.0
　pinches (purpura simplex) D69.2
**Devitalized tooth** K04.99
**Devonshire colic** — *see* Poisoning, lead
**Dextraposition, aorta** Q20.3
　in tetralogy of Fallot Q21.3
**Dextrinosis, limit** (debrancher enzyme deficiency) E74.03
**Dextrocardia** (true) Q24.0
　with
　　complete transposition of viscera Q89.3
　　situs inversus Q89.3
**Dextrotransposition, aorta** Q20.3
**d-glycericacidemia** E72.59
**Dhat syndrome** F48.8
**Dhobi itch** B35.6
**Di George's syndrome** D82.1
**Di Guglielmo's disease** C94.0- ☑
**Diabetes, diabetic** (mellitus) (sugar) E11.9
　with
　　amyotrophy E11.44
　　arthropathy NEC E11.618
　　autonomic (poly)neuropathy E11.43
　　cataract E11.36
　　Charcot's joints E11.610
　　chronic kidney disease E11.22
　　circulatory complication NEC E11.59
　　complication E11.8
　　　specified NEC E11.69
　　dermatitis E11.620
　　foot ulcer E11.621
　　gangrene E11.52
　　gastroparalysis E11.43
　　gastroparesis E11.43
　　glomerulonephrosis, intracapillary E11.21
　　glomerulosclerosis, intercapillary E11.21
　　hyperglycemia E11.65
　　hyperosmolarity E11.00
　　　with coma E11.01
　　hypoglycemia E11.649
　　　with coma E11.641
　　ketoacidosis E11.10
　　　with coma E11.11
　　kidney complications NEC E11.29
　　Kimmelstiel-Wilson disease E11.21
　　loss of protective sensation (LOPS) — *see* Diabetes, by type, with neuropathy
　　mononeuropathy E11.41
　　myasthenia E11.44
　　necrobiosis lipoidica E11.620
　　nephropathy E11.21
　　neuralgia E11.42
　　neurologic complication NEC E11.49
　　neuropathic arthropathy E11.610
　　neuropathy E11.40
　　ophthalmic complication NEC E11.39
　　oral complication NEC E11.638
　　osteomyelitis E11.69
　　periodontal disease E11.630
　　peripheral angiopathy E11.51
　　　with gangrene E11.52
　　polyneuropathy E11.42
　　renal complication NEC E11.29
　　renal tubular degeneration E11.29
　　retinopathy E11.319
　　　with macular edema E11.311

**Diabetes, diabetic** — *continued*
　with — *continued*
　　retinopathy — *continued*
　　　with macular edema — *continued*
　　　　resolved following treatment E11.37 ☑
　　　nonproliferative E11.329 ☑
　　　　with macular edema E11.321 ☑
　　　　mild E11.329 ☑
　　　　　with macular edema E11.321 ☑
　　　　moderate E11.339 ☑
　　　　　with macular edema E11.331 ☑
　　　　severe E11.349 ☑
　　　　　with macular edema E11.341 ☑
　　　proliferative E11.359 ☑
　　　　with
　　　　　combined traction retinal detachment and rhegmatogenous retinal detachment E11.354 ☑
　　　　　macular edema E11.351 ☑
　　　　　stable proliferative diabetic retinopathy E11.355 ☑
　　　　　traction retinal detachment involving the macula E11.352 ☑
　　　　　traction retinal detachment not involving the macula E11.353 ☑
　　skin complication NEC E11.628
　　skin ulcer NEC E11.622
　brittle — *see* Diabetes, type 1
　bronzed E83.110
　complicating pregnancy — *see* Pregnancy, complicated by, diabetes
　dietary counseling and surveillance Z71.3
　due to
　　autoimmune process — *see* Diabetes, type 1
　　immune mediated pancreatic islet beta-cell destruction — *see* Diabetes, type 1
　due to drug or chemical E09.9
　　with
　　　amyotrophy E09.44
　　　arthropathy NEC E09.618
　　　autonomic (poly)neuropathy E09.43
　　　cataract E09.36
　　　Charcot's joints E09.610
　　　chronic kidney disease E09.22
　　　circulatory complication NEC E09.59
　　　complication E09.8
　　　　specified NEC E09.69
　　　dermatitis E09.620
　　　foot ulcer E09.621
　　　gangrene E09.52
　　　gastroparalysis E09.43
　　　gastroparesis E09.43
　　　glomerulonephrosis, intracapillary E09.21
　　　glomerulosclerosis, intercapillary E09.21
　　　hyperglycemia E09.65
　　　hyperosmolarity E09.00
　　　　with coma E09.01
　　　hypoglycemia E09.649
　　　　with coma E09.641
　　　ketoacidosis E09.10
　　　　with coma E09.11
　　　kidney complications NEC E09.29
　　　Kimmelsteil-Wilson disease E09.21
　　　mononeuropathy E09.41
　　　myasthenia E09.44
　　　necrobiosis lipoidica E09.620
　　　nephropathy E09.21
　　　neuralgia E09.42
　　　neurologic complication NEC E09.49
　　　neuropathic arthropathy E09.610
　　　neuropathy E09.40
　　　ophthalmic complication NEC E09.39
　　　oral complication NEC E09.638
　　　periodontal disease E09.630
　　　peripheral angiopathy E09.51
　　　　with gangrene E09.52
　　　polyneuropathy E09.42
　　　renal complication NEC E09.29
　　　renal tubular degeneration E09.29
　　　retinopathy E09.319
　　　　with macular edema E09.311
　　　　nonproliferative E09.329 ☑
　　　　　with macular edema E09.321 ☑
　　　　　mild E09.329 ☑
　　　　　　with macular edema E09.321 ☑
　　　　　moderate E09.339 ☑
　　　　　　with macular edema E09.331 ☑
　　　　　severe E09.349 ☑

Index

Diabetes, diabetic — Diabetes, diabetic

**Diabetes, diabetic** — *continued*
  due to drug or chemical — *continued*
    with — *continued*
      retinopathy — *continued*
        nonproliferative — *continued*
          severe — *continued*
            with macular edema E09.341 ☑
          proliferative E09.359 ☑
            with
              combined traction retinal detachment and rhegmatogenous retinal detachment E09.354 ☑
              macular edema E09.351 ☑
              stable proliferative diabetic retinopathy E09.355 ☑
              traction retinal detachment involving the macula E09.352 ☑
              traction retinal detachment not involving the macula E09.353 ☑
        resolved following treatment E09.37 ☑
      skin complication NEC E09.628
      skin ulcer NEC E09.622
  due to underlying condition E08.9
    with
      amyotrophy E08.44
      arthropathy NEC E08.618
      autonomic (poly)neuropathy E08.43
      cataract E08.36
      Charcot's joints E08.610
      chronic kidney disease E08.22
      circulatory complication NEC E08.59
      complication E08.8
        specified NEC E08.69
      dermatitis E08.620
      foot ulcer E08.621
      gangrene E08.52
      gastroparalysis E08.43
      gastroparesis E08.43
      glomerulonephrosis, intracapillary E08.21
      glomerulosclerosis, intercapillary E08.21
      hyperglycemia E08.65
      hyperosmolarity E08.00
        with coma E08.01
      hypoglycemia E08.649
        with coma E08.641
      ketoacidosis E08.10
        with coma E08.11
      kidney complications NEC E08.29
      Kimmelstein-WIlson disease E08.21
      mononeuropathy E08.41
      myasthenia E08.44
      necrobiosis lipoidica E08.620
      nephropathy E08.21
      neuralgia E08.42
      neurologic complication NEC E08.49
      neuropathic arthropathy E08.610
      neuropathy E08.40
      ophthalmic complication NEC E08.39
      oral complication NEC E08.638
      periodontal disease E08.630
      peripheral angiopathy E08.51
        with gangrene E08.52
      polyneuropathy E08.42
      renal complication NEC E08.29
      renal tubular degeneration E08.29
      retinopathy E08.319
        with macular edema E08.311
        nonproliferative E08.329 ☑
          with macular edema E08.321 ☑
          mild E08.329 ☑
            with macular edema E08.321 ☑
          moderate E08.339 ☑
            with macular edema E08.331 ☑
          severe E08.349 ☑
            with macular edema E08.341 ☑
        proliferative E08.359 ☑
          with
            combined traction retinal detachment and rhegmatogenous retinal detachment E08.354 ☑
            macular edema E08.351 ☑
            stable proliferative diabetic retinopathy E08.355 ☑
            traction retinal detachment involving the macula E08.352 ☑
            traction retinal detachment not involving the macula E08.353 ☑
        resolved following treatment E08.37 ☑

**Diabetes, diabetic** — *continued*
  due to underlying condition — *continued*
    with — *continued*
      skin complication NEC E08.628
      skin ulcer NEC E08.622
  gestational (in pregnancy) O24.419
    affecting newborn P70.0
    diet controlled O24.410
    in childbirth O24.429
      diet controlled O24.420
      insulin (and diet) controlled O24.424
      oral drug controlled (antidiabetic) (hypoglycemic) O24.425
    insulin (and diet) controlled O24.414
    oral drug controlled (antidiabetic) (hypoglycemic) O24.415
    puerperal O24.439
      diet controlled O24.430
      insulin (and diet) controlled O24.434
      oral drug controlled (antidiabetic) (hypoglycemic) O24.435
  hepatogenous E13.9
  idiopathic — *see* Diabetes, type 1
  inadequately controlled — *code to* Diabetes, by type, with hyperglycemia
  insipidus E23.2
    nephrogenic N25.1
    pituitary E23.2
    vasopressin resistant N25.1
  insulin dependent — *code to* type of diabetes
  juvenile-onset — *see* Diabetes, type 1
  ketosis-prone — *see* Diabetes, type 1
  latent R73.03
  neonatal (transient) P70.2
  non-insulin dependent — *code to* type of diabetes
  out of control — *code to* Diabetes, by type, with hyperglycemia
  phosphate E83.39
  poorly controlled — *code to* Diabetes, by type, with hyperglycemia
  postpancreatectomy — *see* Diabetes, specified type NEC
  postprocedural — *see* Diabetes, specified type NEC
  secondary diabetes mellitus NEC — *see* Diabetes, specified type NEC
  specified type NEC E13.9
    with
      amyotrophy E13.44
      arthropathy NEC E13.618
      autonomic (poly)neuropathy E13.43
      cataract E13.36
      Charcot's joints E13.610
      chronic kidney disease E13.22
      circulatory complication NEC E13.59
      complication E13.8
        specified NEC E13.69
      dermatitis E13.620
      foot ulcer E13.621
      gangrene E13.52
      gastroparalysis E13.43
      gastroparesis E13.43
      glomerulonephrosis, intracapillary E13.21
      glomerulosclerosis, intercapillary E13.21
      hyperglycemia E13.65
      hyperosmolarity E13.00
        with coma E13.01
      hypoglycemia E13.649
        with coma E13.641
      ketoacidosis E13.10
        with coma E13.11
      kidney complications NEC E13.29
      Kimmelstein-Wilson disease E13.21
      mononeuropathy E13.41
      myasthenia E13.44
      necrobiosis lipoidica E13.620
      nephropathy E13.21
      neuralgia E13.42
      neurologic complication NEC E13.49
      neuropathic arthropathy E13.610
      neuropathy E13.40
      ophthalmic complication NEC E13.39
      oral complication NEC E13.638
      periodontal disease E13.630
      peripheral angiopathy E13.51
        with gangrene E13.52
      polyneuropathy E13.42
      renal complication NEC E13.29
      renal tubular degeneration E13.29

**Diabetes, diabetic** — *continued*
  specified type — *continued*
    with — *continued*
      retinopathy E13.319
        with macular edema E13.311
        nonproliferative E13.329 ☑
          with macular edema E13.321 ☑
          mild E13.329 ☑
            with macular edema E13.321 ☑
          moderate E13.339 ☑
            with macular edema E13.331 ☑
          severe E13.349 ☑
            with macular edema E13.341 ☑
        proliferative E13.359 ☑
          with
            combined traction retinal detachment and rhegmatogenous retinal detachment E13.354 ☑
            macular edema E13.351 ☑
            stable proliferative diabetic retinopathy E13.355 ☑
            traction retinal detachment involving the macula E13.352 ☑
            traction retinal detachment not involving the macula E13.353 ☑
        resolved following treatment E13.37 ☑
      skin complication NEC E13.628
      skin ulcer NEC E13.622
  steroid-induced — *see* Diabetes, due to, drug or chemical
  type 1 E10.9
    with
      amyotrophy E10.44
      arthropathy NEC E10.618
      autonomic (poly)neuropathy E10.43
      cataract E10.36
      Charcot's joints E10.610
      chronic kidney disease E10.22
      circulatory complication NEC E10.59
      complication E10.8
        specified NEC E10.69
      dermatitis E10.620
      foot ulcer E10.621
      gangrene E10.52
      gastroparalysis E10.43
      gastroparesis E10.43
      glomerulonephrosis, intracapillary E10.21
      glomerulosclerosis, intercapillary E10.21
      hyperglycemia E10.65
      hypoglycemia E10.649
        with coma E10.641
      ketoacidosis E10.10
        with coma E10.11
      kidney complications NEC E10.29
      Kimmelstein-Wilson disease E10.21
      mononeuropathy E10.41
      myasthenia E10.44
      necrobiosis lipoidica E10.620
      nephropathy E10.21
      neuralgia E10.42
      neurologic complication NEC E10.49
      neuropathic arthropathy E10.610
      neuropathy E10.40
      ophthalmic complication NEC E10.39
      oral complication NEC E10.638
      osteomyelitis E10.69
      periodontal disease E10.630
      peripheral angiopathy E10.51
        with gangrene E10.52
      polyneuropathy E10.42
      renal complication NEC E10.29
      renal tubular degeneration E10.29
      retinopathy E10.319
        with macular edema E10.311
        nonproliferative E10.329 ☑
          with macular edema E10.321 ☑
          mild E10.329 ☑
            with macular edema E10.321 ☑
          moderate E10.339 ☑
            with macular edema E10.331 ☑
          severe E10.349 ☑
            with macular edema E10.341 ☑
        proliferative E10.359 ☑
          with
            combined traction retinal detachment and rhegmatogenous retinal detachment E10.354 ☑
            macular edema E10.351 ☑

☑ **Additional Character Required** — **Refer to the Tabular List for Character Selection**

▽ **Subterms under main terms may continue to next column or page**

**Diabetes, diabetic** — *continued*
  type 1 — *continued*
    with — *continued*
      retinopathy — *continued*
        proliferative — *continued*
          with — *continued*
            stable proliferative diabetic
              retinopathy E10.355 ☑
            traction retinal detachment involving
              the macula E10.352 ☑
            traction retinal detachment not in-
              volving the macula E10.353 ☑
        resolved following treatment E10.37 ☑
      skin complication NEC E10.628
      skin ulcer NEC E10.622
  type 2 E11.9
    with
      amyotrophy E11.44
      arthropathy NEC E11.618
      autonomic (poly)neuropathy E11.43
      cataract E11.36
      Charcot's joints E11.610
      chronic kidney disease E11.22
      circulatory complication NEC E11.59
      complication E11.8
        specified NEC E11.69
      dermatitis E11.620
      foot ulcer E11.621
      gangrene E11.52
      gastroparalysis E11.43
      gastroparesis E11.43
      glomerulonephrosis, intracapillary E11.21
      glomerulosclerosis, intercapillary E11.21
      hyperglycemia E11.65
      hyperosmolarity E11.00
        with coma E11.01
      hypoglycemia E11.649
        with coma E11.641
      ketoacidosis E11.10
        with coma E11.11
      kidney complications NEC E11.29
      Kimmelstiel-Wilson disease E11.21
      mononeuropathy E11.41
      myasthenia E11.44
      necrobiosis lipoidica E11.620
      nephropathy E11.21
      neuralgia E11.42
      neurologic complication NEC E11.49
      neuropathic arthropathy E11.610
      neuropathy E11.40
      ophthalmic complication NEC E11.39
      oral complication NEC E11.638
      osteomyelitis E11.69
      periodontal disease E11.630
      peripheral angiopathy E11.51
        with gangrene E11.52
      polyneuropathy E11.42
      renal complication NEC E11.29
      renal tubular degeneration E11.29
      retinopathy E11.319
        with macular edema E11.311
        nonproliferative E11.329 ☑
          with macular edema E11.321 ☑
          mild E11.329 ☑
            with macular edema E11.321 ☑
          moderate E11.339 ☑
            with macular edema E11.331 ☑
          severe E11.349 ☑
            with macular edema E11.341 ☑
        proliferative E11.359 ☑
          with
            combined traction retinal detach-
              ment and rhegmatogenous
              retinal detachment E11.354 ☑
            macular edema E11.351 ☑
            stable proliferative diabetic
              retinopathy E11.355 ☑
            traction retinal detachment involving
              the macula E11.352 ☑
            traction retinal detachment not in-
              volving the macula E11.353 ☑
        resolved following treatment E11.37 ☑
      skin complication NEC E11.628
      skin ulcer NEC E11.622
  uncontrolled
    meaning
      hyperglycemia — *see* Diabetes, by type, with,
        hyperglycemia

**Diabetes, diabetic** — *continued*
  uncontrolled — *continued*
    meaning — *continued*
      hypoglycemia — *see* Diabetes, by type, with,
        hypoglycemia
**Diacyclothrombopathia** D69.1
**Diagnosis deferred** R69
**Dialysis** (intermittent) (treatment)
  noncompliance (with) Z91.15
  renal (hemodialysis) (peritoneal), status Z99.2
  retina, retinal — *see* Detachment, retina, with retinal,
    dialysis
**Diamond-Blackfan anemia** (congenital hypoplastic)
  D61.01
**Diamond-Gardener syndrome** (autoerythrocyte sensi-
  tization) D69.2
**Diaper rash** L22
**Diaphoresis** (excessive) R61
**Diaphragm** — *see* condition
**Diaphragmalgia** R07.1
**Diaphragmatitis, diaphragmitis** J98.6
**Diaphysial aclasis** Q78.6
**Diaphysitis** — *see* Osteomyelitis, specified type NEC
**Diarrhea, diarrheal** (disease) (infantile) (inflammatory)
  R19.7
  achlorhydric K31.83
  allergic K52.29
    due to
      colitis — *see* Colitis, allergic
      enteritis — *see* Enteritis, allergic
  ambic (*see also* Amebiasis) A06.0
    with abscess — *see* Abscess, amebic
    acute A06.0
    chronic A06.1
    nondysenteric A06.2
  bacillary — *see* Dysentery, bacillary
  balantidial A07.0
  cachectic NEC K52.89
  Chilomastix A07.8
  choleriformis A00.1
  chronic (noninfectious) K52.9
  coccidial A07.3
  Cochin-China K90.1
    strongyloidiasis B78.0
  Dientamoeba A07.8
  dietetic (*see also* Diarrhea, allergic) K52.29
  drug-induced K52.1
  due to
    bacteria A04.9
      specified NEC A04.8
    Campylobacter A04.5
    Capillaria philippinensis B81.1
    Clostridium difficile
      not specified as recurrent A04.72
      recurrent A04.71
    Clostridium perfringens (C) (F) A04.8
    Cryptosporidium A07.2
    drugs K52.1
    Escherichia coli A04.4
      enteroaggregative A04.4
      enterohemorrhagic A04.3
      enteroinvasive A04.2
      enteropathogenic A04.0
      enterotoxigenic A04.1
      specified NEC A04.4
    food hypersensitivity (*see also* Diarrhea, allergic)
      K52.29
    Necator americanus B76.1
    S. japonicum B65.2
    specified organism NEC A08.8
      bacterial A04.8
      viral A08.39
    Staphylococcus A04.8
    Trichuris trichiuria B79
    virus — *see* Enteritis, viral
    Yersinia enterocolitica A04.6
  dysenteric A09
  endemic A09
  epidemic A09
  flagellate A07.9
  Flexner's (ulcerative) A03.1
  functional K59.1
    following gastrointestinal surgery K91.89
    psychogenic F45.8
  Giardia lamblia A07.1
  giardial A07.1
  hill K90.1
  infectious A09

**Diarrhea, diarrheal** — *continued*
  malarial — *see* Malaria
  mite B88.0
  mycotic NEC B49
  neonatal (noninfectious) P78.3
  nervous F45.8
  neurogenic K59.1
  noninfectious K52.9
  postgastrectomy K91.1
  postvagotomy K91.1
  protozoal A07.9
    specified NEC A07.8
  psychogenic F45.8
  specified
    bacterium NEC A04.8
    virus NEC A08.39
  strongyloidiasis B78.0
  toxic K52.1
  trichomonal A07.8
  tropical K90.1
  tuberculous A18.32
  viral — *see* Enteritis, viral
**Diastasis**
  cranial bones M84.88
    congenital NEC Q75.8
  joint (traumatic) — *see* Dislocation
  muscle M62.00
    ankle M62.07- ☑
    congenital Q79.8
    foot M62.07- ☑
    forearm M62.03- ☑
    hand M62.04- ☑
    lower leg M62.06- ☑
    pelvic region M62.05- ☑
    shoulder region M62.01- ☑
    specified site NEC M62.08
    thigh M62.05- ☑
    upper arm M62.02- ☑
  recti (abdomen)
    complicating delivery O71.89
    congenital Q79.59
**Diastema, tooth, teeth, fully erupted** M26.32
**Diastematomyelia** Q06.2
**Diataxia, cerebral** G80.4
**Diathesis**
  allergic — *see* History, allergy
  bleeding (familial) D69.9
  cystine (familial) E72.00
  gouty — *see* Gout
  hemorrhagic (familial) D69.9
    newborn NEC P53
  spasmophilic R29.0
**Diaz's disease or osteochondrosis** (juvenile) (talus) —
  *see* Osteochondrosis, juvenile, tarsus
**Dibothriocephalus, dibothriocephaliasis** (latus) (infection) (infestation) B70.0
  larval B70.1
**Dicephalus, dicephaly** Q89.4
**Dichotomy, teeth** K00.2
**Dichromat, dichromatopsia** (congenital) — *see* Deficiency, color vision
**Dichuchwa** A65
**Dicroceliasis** B66.2
**Didelphia, didelphys** — *see* Double uterus
**Didymytis** N45.1
  with orchitis N45.3
**Dietary**
  inadequacy or deficiency E63.9
  surveillance and counseling Z71.3
**Dietl's crisis** N13.8
**Dieulafoy lesion** (hemorrhagic)
  duodenum K31.82
  esophagus K22.8
  intestine (colon) K63.81
  stomach K31.82
**Difficult, difficulty** (in)
  acculturation Z60.3
  feeding R63.3
    newborn P92.9
      breast P92.5
      specified NEC P92.8
    nonorganic (infant or child) F98.29
  intubation, in anesthesia T88.4
  mechanical, gastroduodenal stoma K91.89
    causing obstruction (*see also* Obstruction, intestine,
      postoperative) K91.30
  micturition
    need to immediately re-void R39.191

**Difficult, difficulty** — *continued*
  micturition — *continued*
    position dependent R39.192
    specified NEC R39.198
  reading (developmental) F81.Ø
    secondary to emotional disorders F93.9
  spelling (specific) F81.81
    with reading disorder F81.89
    due to inadequate teaching Z55.8
  swallowing — *see* Dysphagia
  walking R26.2
  work
    conditions NEC Z56.5
    schedule Z56.3
**Diffuse** — *see* condition
**Digestive** — *see* condition
**Dihydropyrimidine dehydrogenase disease** (DPD)
  E88.89
**Diktyoma** — *see* Neoplasm, malignant, by site
**Dilaceration, tooth** KØØ.4
**Dilatation**
  anus K59.8
    venule — *see* Hemorrhoids
  aorta (focal) (general) — *see* Ectasia, aorta
    with aneuysm — *see* Aneurysm, aorta
    congenital Q25.44
  artery — *see* Aneurysm
  bladder (sphincter) N32.89
    congenital Q64.79
  blood vessel I99.8
  bronchial J47.9
    with
      exacerbation (acute) J47.1
      lower respiratory infection J47.Ø
  calyx (due to obstruction) — *see* Hydronephrosis
  capillaries I78.8
  cardiac (acute) (chronic) (*see also* Hypertrophy, cardiac)
    congenital Q24.8
      valve NEC Q24.8
        pulmonary Q22.3
    valve — *see* Endocarditis
  cavum septi pellucidi QØ6.8
  cervix (uteri) (*see also* Incompetency, cervix)
    incomplete, poor, slow complicating delivery O62.Ø
  colon K59.39
    congenital Q43.1
    psychogenic F45.8
    toxic K59.31
  common duct (acquired) K83.8
    congenital Q44.5
  cystic duct (acquired) K82.8
    congenital Q44.5
  duct, mammary — *see* Ectasia, mammary duct
  duodenum K59.8
  esophagus K22.8
    congenital Q39.5
    due to achalasia K22.Ø
  eustachian tube, congenital Q17.8
  gallbladder K82.8
  gastric — *see* Dilatation, stomach
  heart (acute) (chronic) (*see also* Hypertrophy, cardiac)
    congenital Q24.8
    valve — *see* Endocarditis
  ileum K59.8
    psychogenic F45.8
  jejunum K59.8
    psychogenic F45.8
  kidney (calyx) (collecting structures) (cystic)
    (parenchyma) (pelvis) (idiopathic) N28.89
  lacrimal passages or duct — *see* Disorder, lacrimal
    system, changes
  lymphatic vessel I89.Ø
  mammary duct — *see* Ectasia, mammary duct
  Meckel's diverticulum (congenital) Q43.Ø
    malignant — *see* Table of Neoplasms, small intes-
      tine, malignant
  myocardium (acute) (chronic) — *see* Hypertrophy,
    cardiac
  organ or site, congenital NEC — *see* Distortion
  pancreatic duct K86.89
  pericardium — *see* Pericarditis
  pharynx J39.2
  prostate N42.89
  pulmonary
    artery (idiopathic) I28.8
    valve, congenital Q22.3
  pupil H57.Ø4
  rectum K59.39

**Dilatation** — *continued*
  saccule, congenital Q16.5
  salivary gland (duct) K11.8
  sphincter ani K62.89
  stomach K31.89
    acute K31.Ø
    psychogenic F45.8
  submaxillary duct K11.8
  trachea, congenital Q32.1
  ureter (idiopathic) N28.82
    congenital Q62.2
    due to obstruction N13.4
  urethra (acquired) N36.8
  vasomotor I73.9
  vein I86.8
  ventricular, ventricle (acute) (chronic) (*see also* Hyper-
    trophy, cardiac)
    cerebral, congenital QØ4.8
  venule NEC I86.8
  vesical orifice N32.89
**Dilated, dilation** — *see* Dilatation
**Diminished, diminution**
  hearing (acuity) — *see* Deafness
  sense or sensation (cold) (heat) (tactile) (vibratory)
    R2Ø.8
  vision NEC H54.7
  vital capacity R94.2
**Diminuta taenia** B71.Ø
**Dimitri-Sturge-Weber disease** Q85.8
**Dimple**
  congenital sacral Q82.6
  parasacral Q82.6
  pilonidal or postanal — *see* Cyst, pilonidal
**Dioctophyme renalis** (infection) (infestation) B83.8
**Dipetalonemiasis** B74.4
**Diphallus** Q55.69
**Diphtheria, diphtheritic** (gangrenous) (hemorrhagic)
  A36.9
  carrier (suspected) Z22.2
  cutaneous A36.3
  faucial A36.Ø
  infection of wound A36.3
  laryngeal A36.2
  myocarditis A36.81
  nasal, anterior A36.89
  nasopharyngeal A36.1
  neurological complication A36.89
  pharyngeal A36.Ø
  specified site NEC A36.89
  tonsillar A36.Ø
**Diphyllobothriasis** (intestine) B7Ø.Ø
  larval B7Ø.1
**Diplacusis** H93.22- ☑
**Diplegia** (upper limbs) G83.Ø
  congenital (cerebral) G8Ø.8
  facial G51.Ø
  lower limbs G82.2Ø
  spastic G8Ø.1
**Diplococcus, diplococcal** — *see* condition
**Diplopia** H53.2
**Dipsomania** F1Ø.2Ø
  with
    psychosis — *see* Psychosis, alcoholic
    remission F1Ø.21
**Dipylidiasis** B71.1
**DIRA** (deficiency of interleukin 1 receptor antagonist)
  MØ4.8
**Direction, teeth, abnormal, fully erupted** M26.3Ø
**Dirofilariasis** B74.8
**Dirt-eating child** F98.3
**Disability, disabilities**
  heart — *see* Disease, heart
  intellectual F79
    with
      autistic features F84.9
    mild (I.Q. 5Ø-69) F7Ø
    moderate (I.Q. 35-49) F71
    profound (I.Q. under 2Ø) F73
    severe (I.Q. 2Ø-34) F72
    specified level NEC F78
  knowledge acquisition F81.9
  learning F81.9
  limiting activities Z73.6
  spelling, specific F81.81
**Disappearance of family member** Z63.4
**Disarticulation** — *see* Amputation
  meaning traumatic amputation — *see* Amputation,
    traumatic

**Discharge** (from)
  abnormal finding in — *see* Abnormal, specimen
  breast (female) (male) N64.52
  diencephalic autonomic idiopathic — *see* Epilepsy,
    specified NEC
  ear (*see also* Otorrhea)
    blood — *see* Otorrhagia
  excessive urine R35.8
  nipple N64.52
  penile R36.9
  postnasal RØ9.82
  prison, anxiety concerning Z65.2
  urethral R36.9
    without blood R36.Ø
    hematospermia R36.1
  vaginal N89.8
**Discitis, diskitis** M46.4Ø
  cervical region M46.42
  cervicothoracic region M46.43
  lumbar region M46.46
  lumbosacral region M46.47
  multiple sites M46.49
  occipito-atlanto-axial region M46.41
  pyogenic — *see* Infection, intervertebral disc, pyogenic
  sacrococcygeal region M46.48
  thoracic region M46.44
  thoracolumbar region M46.45
**Discoid**
  meniscus (congenital) Q68.6
  semilunar cartilage (congenital) — *see* Derangement,
    knee, meniscus, specified NEC
**Discoloration**
  nails L6Ø.8
  teeth (posteruptive) KØ3.7
    during formation KØØ.8
**Discomfort**
  chest RØ7.89
  visual H53.14- ☑
**Discontinuity, ossicles, ear** H74.2- ☑
**Discord** (with)
  boss Z56.4
  classmates Z55.4
  counselor Z64.4
  employer Z56.4
  family Z63.8
  fellow employees Z56.4
  in-laws Z63.1
  landlord Z59.2
  lodgers Z59.2
  neighbors Z59.2
  probation officer Z64.4
  social worker Z64.4
  teachers Z55.4
  workmates Z56.4
**Discordant connection**
  atrioventricular (congenital) Q2Ø.5
  ventriculoarterial Q2Ø.3
**Discrepancy**
  centric occlusion maximum intercuspation M26.55
  leg length (acquired) — *see* Deformity, limb, unequal
    length
    congenital — *see* Defect, reduction, lower limb
  uterine size date O26.84- ☑
**Discrimination**
  ethnic Z6Ø.5
  political Z6Ø.5
  racial Z6Ø.5
  religious Z6Ø.5
  sex Z6Ø.5
**Disease, diseased** (*see also* Syndrome)
  absorbent system I87.8
  acid-peptic K3Ø
  Acosta's T7Ø.29 ☑
  Adams-Stokes (-Morgagni) (syncope with heart block)
    I45.9
  Addison's anemia (pernicious) D51.Ø
  adenoids (and tonsils) J35.9
  adrenal (capsule) (cortex) (gland) (medullary) E27.9
    hyperfunction E27.Ø
    specified NEC E27.8
  ainhum L94.6
  airway
    obstructive, chronic J44.9
      due to
        cotton dust J66.Ø
        specific organic dusts NEC J66.8
    reactive — *see* Asthma
  akamushi (scrub typhus) A75.3

**Disease, diseased** — *continued*
Albers-Schönberg (marble bones) Q78.2
Albert's — *see* Tendinitis, Achilles
alimentary canal K63.9
alligator-skin Q80.9
   acquired L85.0
alpha heavy chain C88.3
alpine T70.29 ☑
altitude T70.20 ☑
alveolar ridge
   edentulous K06.9
      specified NEC K06.8
alveoli, teeth K08.9
Alzheimer's G30.9 [F02.80]
   with behavioral disturbance G30.9 [F02.81]
   early onset G30.0 [F02.80]
      with behavioral disturbance G30.0 [F02.81]
   late onset G30.1 [F02.80]
      with behavioral disturbance G30.1 [F02.81]
   specified NEC G30.8 [F02.80]
      with behavioral disturbance G30.8 [F02.81]
amyloid — *see* Amyloidosis
Andersen's (glycogenosis IV) E74.09
Andes T70.29 ☑
Andrews' (bacterid) L08.89
angiospastic I73.9
   cerebral G45.9
   vein I87.8
anterior
   chamber H21.9
   horn cell G12.29
antiglomerular basement membrane (anti- GBM) anti-
    body M31.0
   tubulo-interstitial nephritis N12
antral — *see* Sinusitis, maxillary
anus K62.9
   specified NEC K62.89
aorta (nonsyphilitic) I77.9
   syphilitic NEC A52.02
aortic (heart) (valve) I35.9
   rheumatic I06.9
Apollo B30.3
aponeuroses — *see* Enthesopathy
appendix K38.9
   specified NEC K38.8
aqueous (chamber) H21.9
Arnold-Chiari — *see* Arnold-Chiari disease
arterial I77.9
   occlusive — *see* Occlusion, by site
      due to stricture or stenosis I77.1
arteriocardiorenal — *see* Hypertension, cardiorenal
arteriolar (generalized) (obliterative) I77.9
arteriorenal — *see* Hypertension, kidney
arteriosclerotic (*see also* Arteriosclerosis)
   cardiovascular — *see* Disease, heart, ischemic,
      atherosclerotic
   coronary (artery) — *see* Disease, heart, ischemic,
      atherosclerotic
   heart — *see* Disease, heart, ischemic, atherosclerot-
      ic
artery I77.9
   cerebral I67.9
   coronary I25.10
      with angina pectoris — *see* Arteriosclerosis,
         coronary (artery)
arthropod-borne NOS (viral) A94
   specified type NEC A93.8
atticoantral, chronic H66.20
   left H66.22
      with right H66.23
   right H66.21
      with left H66.23
auditory canal — *see* Disorder, ear, external
auricle, ear NEC — *see* Disorder, pinna
Australian X A83.4
autoimmune (systemic) NOS M35.9
   hemolytic (cold type) (warm type) D59.1
      drug-induced D59.0
   thyroid E06.3
aviator's — *see* Effect, adverse, high altitude
Ayerza's (pulmonary artery sclerosis with pulmonary
    hypertension) I27.0
Babington's (familial hemorrhagic telangiectasia) I78.0
bacterial A49.9
   specified NEC A48.8
   zoonotic A28.9
      specified type NEC A28.8
Baelz's (cheilitis glandularis apostematosa) K13.0

**Disease, diseased** — *continued*
bagasse J67.1
balloon — *see* Effect, adverse, high altitude
Bang's (brucella abortus) A23.1
Bannister's T78.3 ☑
barometer makers' — *see* Poisoning, mercury
Barraquer (-Simons') (progressive lipodystrophy) E88.1
Barrett's — *see* Barrett's, esophagus
Bartholin's gland N75.9
basal ganglia G25.9
   degenerative G23.9
      specified NEC G23.8
   specified NEC G25.89
Basedow's (exophthalmic goiter) — *see* Hyperthy-
    roidism, with, goiter (diffuse)
Bateman's B08.1
Batten-Steinert G71.11
Battey A31.0
Beard's (neurasthenia) F48.8
Becker
   idiopathic mural endomyocardial I42.3
   myotonia congenita G71.12
Begbie's (exophthalmic goiter) — *see* Hyperthy-
    roidism, with, goiter (diffuse)
behavioral, organic F07.9
Beigel's (white piedra) B36.2
Benson's — *see* Deposit, crystalline
Bernard-Soulier (thrombopathy) D69.1
Bernhardt (-Roth) — *see* Mononeuropathy, lower limb,
    meralgia paresthetica
Biermer's (pernicious anemia) D51.0
bile duct (common) (hepatic) K83.9
   with calculus, stones — *see* Calculus, bile duct
   specified NEC K83.8
biliary (tract) K83.9
   specified NEC K83.8
Billroth's — *see* Spina bifida
bird fancier's J67.2
black lung J60
bladder N32.9
   in (due to)
      schistosomiasis (bilharziasis) B65.0 [N33]
   specified NEC N32.89
bleeder's D66
blood D75.9
   forming organs D75.9
   vessel I99.9
Bloodgood's — *see* Mastopathy, cystic
Bodechtel-Guttmann (subacute sclerosing panen-
    cephalitis) A81.1
bone (*see also* Disorder, bone)
   aluminum M83.4
   fibrocystic NEC
      jaw M27.49
bone-marrow D75.9
Borna A83.9
Bornholm (epidemic pleurodynia) B33.0
Bouchard's (myopathic dilatation of the stomach)
    K31.0
Bouillaud's (rheumatic heart disease) I01.9
Bourneville (-Brissaud) (tuberous sclerosis) Q85.1
Bouveret (-Hoffmann) (paroxysmal tachycardia) I47.9
bowel K63.9
   functional K59.9
      psychogenic F45.8
brain G93.9
   arterial, artery I67.9
   arteriosclerotic I67.2
   congenital Q04.9
   degenerative — *see* Degeneration, brain
   inflammatory — *see* Encephalitis
   organic G93.9
      arteriosclerotic I67.2
   parasitic NEC B71.9 [G94]
   senile NEC G31.1
   specified NEC G93.89
breast (*see also* Disorder, breast) N64.9
   cystic (chronic) — *see* Mastopathy, cystic
   fibrocystic — *see* Mastopathy, cystic
   Paget's
      female, unspecified side C50.91- ☑
      male, unspecified side C50.92- ☑
   specified NEC N64.89
Breda's — *see* Yaws
Bretonneau's (diphtheritic malignant angina) A36.0
Bright's — *see* Nephritis
   arteriosclerotic — *see* Hypertension, kidney
Brill's (recrudescent typhus) A75.1

**Disease, diseased** — *continued*
Brill-Zinsser (recrudescent typhus) A75.1
Brion-Kayser — *see* Fever, paratyphoid
broad
   beta E78.2
   ligament (noninflammatory) N83.9
      inflammatory — *see* Disease, pelvis, inflamma-
        tory
      specified NEC N83.8
Brocq-Duhring (dermatitis herpetiformis) L13.0
Brocq's
   meaning
      dermatitis herpetiformis L13.0
      prurigo L28.2
bronchopulmonary J98.4
bronchus NEC J98.09
bronze Addison's E27.1
   tuberculous A18.7
budgerigar fancier's J67.2
Buerger's (thromboangiitis obliterans) I73.1
bullous L13.9
   chronic of childhood L12.2
   specified NEC L13.8
Bürger-Grütz (essential familial hyperlipemia) E78.3
bursa — *see* Bursopathy
caisson T70.3 ☑
California — *see* Coccidioidomycosis
capillaries I78.9
   specified NEC I78.8
Carapata A68.0
cardiac — *see* Disease, heart
cardiopulmonary, chronic I27.9
cardiorenal (hepatic) (hypertensive) (vascular) — *see*
    Hypertension, cardiorenal
cardiovascular (atherosclerotic) I25.10
   with angina pectoris — *see* Arteriosclerosis, coro-
      nary (artery),
   congenital Q28.9
   hypertensive — *see* Hypertension, heart
   newborn P29.9
      specified NEC P29.89
   renal (hypertensive) — *see* Hypertension, cardiore-
      nal
   syphilitic (asymptomatic) A52.00
cartilage — *see* Disorder, cartilage
Castellani's A69.8
Castleman (unicentric) (multicentric) D47.Z2
   HHV-8-associated (*see also* Herpesvirus, human, 8)
      D47.Z2
cat-scratch A28.1
Cavare's (familial periodic paralysis) G72.3
cecum K63.9
celiac (adult) (infantile) (with steatorrhea) K90.0
cellular tissue L98.9
central core G71.2
cerebellar, cerebellum — *see* Disease, brain
cerebral (*see also* Disease, brain)
   degenerative — *see* Degeneration, brain
cerebrospinal G96.9
cerebrovascular I67.9
   acute I67.89
      embolic I63.4- ☑
      thrombotic I63.3- ☑
   arteriosclerotic I67.2
   specified NEC I67.89
cervix (uteri) (noninflammatory) N88.9
   inflammatory — *see* Cervicitis
   specified NEC N88.8
Chabert's A22.9
Chandler's (osteochondritis dissecans, hip) — *see* Os-
    teochondritis, dissecans, hip
Charlouis — *see* Yaws
Chédiak-Steinbrinck (-Higashi) (congenital gigantism
    of peroxidase granules) E70.330
chest J98.9
Chiari's (hepatic vein thrombosis) I82.0
Chicago B40.9
Chignon B36.8
chigo, chigoe B88.1
childhood granulomatous D71
Chinese liver fluke B66.1
chlamydial A74.9
   specified NEC A74.89
cholecystic K82.9
choroid H31.9
   specified NEC H31.8
Christmas D67
chronic bullous of childhood L12.2

**Disease, diseased** — *continued*
- chylomicron retention E78.3
- ciliary body H21.9
  - specified NEC H21.89
- circulatory (system) NEC I99.8
  - newborn P29.9
  - syphilitic A52.00
    - congenital A50.54
- coagulation factor deficiency (congenital) — *see* Defect, coagulation
- coccidioidal — *see* Coccidioidomycosis
- cold
  - agglutinin or hemoglobinuria D59.1
    - paroxysmal D59.6
  - hemagglutinin (chronic) D59.1
- collagen NOS (nonvascular) (vascular) M35.9
  - specified NEC M35.8
- colon K63.9
  - functional K59.9
    - congenital Q43.2
  - ischemic (*see also* Ischemia, intestine, acute) K55.039
- colonic inflammatory bowel, unclassified (IBDU) K52.3
- combined system — *see* Degeneration, combined
- compressed air T70.3 ☑
- Concato's (pericardial polyserositis) A19.9
  - nontubercular I31.1
  - pleural — *see* Pleurisy, with effusion
- conjunctiva H11.9
  - chlamydial A74.0
  - specified NEC H11.89
  - viral B30.9
    - specified NEC B30.8
- connective tissue, systemic (diffuse) M35.9
  - in (due to)
    - hypogammaglobulinemia D80.1 [M36.8]
    - ochronosis E70.29 [M36.8]
  - specified NEC M35.8
- Conor and Bruch's (boutonneuse fever) A77.1
- Cooper's — *see* Mastopathy, cystic
- Cori's (glycogenosis III) E74.03
- corkhandler's or corkworker's J67.3
- cornea H18.9
  - specified NEC H18.89- ☑
- coronary (artery) — *see* Disease, heart, ischemic, atherosclerotic
  - congenital Q24.5
  - ostial, syphilitic (aortic) (mitral) (pulmonary) A52.03
- corpus cavernosum N48.9
  - specified NEC N48.89
- Cotugno's — *see* Sciatica
- coxsackie (virus) NEC B34.1
- cranial nerve NOS G52.9
- Creutzfeldt-Jakob — *see* Creutzfeldt-Jakob disease or syndrome
- Crocq's (acrocyanosis) I73.89
- Crohn's — *see* Enteritis, regional
- Curschmann G71.11
- cystic
  - breast (chronic) — *see* Mastopathy, cystic
  - kidney, congenital Q61.9
  - liver, congenital Q44.6
  - lung J98.4
    - congenital Q33.0
- cytomegalic inclusion (generalized) B25.9
  - with pneumonia B25.0
  - congenital P35.1
- cytomegaloviral B25.9
  - specified NEC B25.8
- Czerny's (periodic hydrarthrosis of the knee) — *see* Effusion, joint, knee
- Daae (-Finsen) (epidemic pleurodynia) B33.0
- Darling's — *see* Histoplasmosis capsulati
- de Quervain's (tendon sheath) M65.4
  - thyroid (subacute granulomatous thyroiditis) E06.1
- Débove's (splenomegaly) R16.1
- deer fly — *see* Tularemia
- Degos' I77.89
- demyelinating, demyelinizating (nervous system) G37.9
  - multiple sclerosis G35
  - specified NEC G37.8
- dense deposit (*see also* N00-N07 with fourth character .6) N05.6
- deposition, hydroxyapatite — *see* Disease, hydroxyapatite deposition
- Devergie's (pityriasis rubra pilaris) L44.0
- Devic's G36.0

**Disease, diseased** — *continued*
- diaphorase deficiency D74.0
- diaphragm J98.6
- diarrheal, infectious NEC A09
- digestive system K92.9
  - specified NEC K92.89
- disc, degenerative — *see* Degeneration, intervertebral disc
- discogenic (*see also* Displacement, intervertebral disc NEC)
  - with myelopathy — *see* Disorder, disc, with, myelopathy
- diverticular — *see* Diverticula
- Dubois (thymus) A50.59 [E35]
- Duchenne-Griesinger G71.0
- Duchenne's
  - muscular dystrophy G71.0
  - pseudohypertrophy, muscles G71.0
- ductless glands E34.9
- Duhring's (dermatitis herpetiformis) L13.0
- duodenum K31.9
  - specified NEC K31.89
- Dupré's (meningism) R29.1
- Dupuytren's (muscle contracture) M72.0
- Durand-Nicholas-Favre (climatic bubo) A55
- Duroziez's (congenital mitral stenosis) Q23.2
- ear — *see* Disorder, ear
- Eberth's — *see* Fever, typhoid
- Ebola (virus) A98.4
- Ebstein's heart Q22.5
- Echinococcus — *see* Echinococcus
- echovirus NEC B34.1
- Eddowes' (brittle bones and blue sclera) Q78.0
- edentulous (alveolar) ridge K06.9
  - specified NEC K06.8
- Edsall's T67.2 ☑
- Eichstedt's (pityriasis versicolor) B36.0
- Eisenmenger's (irreversible) I27.83
- Ellis-van Creveld (chondroectodermal dysplasia) Q77.6
- end stage renal (ESRD) N18.6
  - due to hypertension I12.0
- endocrine glands or system NEC E34.9
- endomyocardial (eosinophilic) I42.3
- English (rickets) E55.0
- enteroviral, enterovirus NEC B34.1
  - central nervous system NEC A88.8
- epidemic B99.9
  - specified NEC B99.8
- epididymis N50.9
- Erb (-Landouzy) G71.0
- Erdheim-Chester (ECD) E88.89
- esophagus K22.9
  - functional K22.4
  - psychogenic F45.8
  - specified NEC K22.8
- Eulenburg's (congenital paramyotonia) G71.19
- eustachian tube — *see* Disorder, eustachian tube
- external
  - auditory canal — *see* Disorder, ear, external
  - ear — *see* Disorder, ear, external
- extrapyramidal G25.9
  - specified NEC G25.89
- eye H57.9
  - anterior chamber H21.9
  - inflammatory NEC H57.8
  - muscle (external) — *see* Strabismus
  - specified NEC H57.8
  - syphilitic — *see* Oculopathy, syphilitic
- eyeball H44.9
  - specified NEC H44.89
- eyelid — *see* Disorder, eyelid
  - specified NEC — *see* Disorder, eyelid, specified type NEC
- eyeworm of Africa B74.3
- facial nerve (seventh) G51.9
  - newborn (birth injury) P11.3
- Fahr (of brain) G23.8
- Fahr Volhard (of kidney) I12.- ☑
- fallopian tube (noninflammatory) N83.9
  - inflammatory — *see* Salpingo-oophoritis
  - specified NEC N83.8
- familial periodic paralysis G72.3
- Fanconi's (congenital pancytopenia) D61.09
- fascia NEC (*see also* Disorder, muscle)
  - inflammatory — *see* Myositis
  - specified NEC M62.89
- Fauchard's (periodontitis) — *see* Periodontitis
- Favre-Durand-Nicolas (climatic bubo) A55

**Disease, diseased** — *continued*
- Fede's K14.0
- Feer's — *see* Poisoning, mercury
- female pelvic inflammatory (*see also* Disease, pelvis, inflammatory) N73.9
  - syphilitic (secondary) A51.42
  - tuberculous A18.17
- Fernels' (aortic aneurysm) I71.9
- fibrocaseous of lung — *see* Tuberculosis, pulmonary
- fibrocystic — *see* Fibrocystic disease
- Fiedler's (leptospiral jaundice) A27.0
- fifth B08.3
- file-cutter's — *see* Poisoning, lead
- fish-skin Q80.9
  - acquired L85.0
- Flajani (-Basedow) (exophthalmic goiter) — *see* Hyperthyroidism, with, goiter (diffuse)
- flax-dresser's J66.1
- fluke — *see* Infestation, fluke
- foot and mouth B08.8
- foot process N04.9
- Forbes' (glycogenosis III) E74.03
- Fordyce-Fox (apocrine miliaria) L75.2
- Fordyce's (ectopic sebaceous glands) (mouth) Q38.6
- Forestier's (rhizomelic pseudopolyarthritis) M35.3
  - meaning ankylosing hyperostosis — *see* Hyperostosis, ankylosing
- Fothergill's
  - neuralgia — *see* Neuralgia, trigeminal
  - scarlatina anginosa A38.9
- Fournier (gangrene) N49.3
  - female N76.89
- fourth B08.8
- Fox (-Fordyce) (apocrine miliaria) L75.2
- Francis' — *see* Tularemia
- Franklin C88.2
- Frei's (climatic bubo) A55
- Friedreich's
  - combined systemic or ataxia G11.1
  - myoclonia G25.3
- frontal sinus — *see* Sinusitis, frontal
- fungus NEC B49
- Gaisböck's (polycythemia hypertonica) D75.1
- gallbladder K82.9
  - calculus — *see* Calculus, gallbladder
  - cholecystitis — *see* Cholecystitis
  - cholesterolosis K82.4
  - fistula — *see* Fistula, gallbladder
  - hydrops K82.1
  - obstruction — *see* Obstruction, gallbladder
  - perforation K82.2
  - specified NEC K82.8
- gamma heavy chain C88.2
- Gamna's (siderotic splenomegaly) D73.2
- Gamstorp's (adynamia episodica hereditaria) G72.3
- Gandy-Nanta (siderotic splenomegaly) D73.2
- ganister J62.8
- gastric — *see* Disease, stomach
- gastroesophageal reflux (GERD) K21.9
  - with esophagitis K21.0
- gastrointestinal (tract) K92.9
  - amyloid E85.4
  - functional K59.9
    - psychogenic F45.8
  - specified NEC K92.89
- Gee (-Herter) (-Heubner) (-Thaysen) (nontropical sprue) K90.0
- genital organs
  - female N94.9
  - male N50.9
- Gerhardt's (erythromelalgia) I73.81
- Gibert's (pityriasis rosea) L42
- Gierke's (glycogenosis I) E74.01
- Gilles de la Tourette's (motor-verbal tic) F95.2
- gingiva K06.9
  - plaque induced K05.00
  - specified NEC K06.8
- gland (lymph) I89.9
- Glanzmann's (hereditary hemorrhagic thrombasthenia) D69.1
- glass-blower's (cataract) — *see* Cataract, specified NEC
  - salivary gland hypertrophy K11.1
- Glisson's — *see* Rickets
- globe H44.9
  - specified NEC H44.89
- glomerular (*see also* Glomerulonephritis)
  - with edema — *see* Nephrosis
  - acute — *see* Nephritis, acute

**Disease, diseased** — *continued*
  glomerular (*see also* Glomerulonephritis) — *continued*
    chronic — *see* Nephritis, chronic
    minimal change N05.0
    rapidly progressive N01.9
  glycogen storage E74.00
    Andersen's E74.09
    Cori's E74.03
    Forbes' E74.03
    generalized E74.00
    glucose-6-phosphatase deficiency E74.01
    heart E74.02 [I43]
    hepatorenal E74.09
    Hers' E74.09
    liver and kidney E74.09
    McArdle's E74.04
    muscle phosphofructokinase E74.09
    myocardium E74.02 [I43]
    Pompe's E74.02
    Tauri's E74.09
    type 0 E74.09
    type I E74.01
    type II E74.02
    type III E74.03
    type IV E74.09
    type V E74.04
    type VI-XI E74.09
    Von Gierke's E74.01
  Goldstein's (familial hemorrhagic telangiectasia) I78.0
  gonococcal NOS A54.9
  graft-versus-host (GVH) D89.813
    acute D89.810
    acute on chronic D89.812
    chronic D89.811
  grainhandler's J67.8
  granulomatous (childhood) (chronic) D71
  Graves' (exophthalmic goiter) — *see* Hyperthyroidism, with, goiter (diffuse)
  Griesinger's — *see* Ancylostomiasis
  Grisel's M43.6
  Gruby's (tinea tonsurans) B35.0
  Guillain-Barré G61.0
  Guinon's (motor-verbal tic) F95.2
  gum K06.9
  gynecological N94.9
  H (Hartnup's) E72.02
  Haff — *see* Poisoning, mercury
  Hageman (congenital factor XII deficiency) D68.2
  hair (color) (shaft) L67.9
    follicles L73.9
      specified NEC L73.8
  Hamman's (spontaneous mediastinal emphysema) J98.2
  hand, foot and mouth B08.4
  Hansen's — *see* Leprosy
  Hantavirus, with pulmonary manifestations B33.4
    with renal manifestations A98.5
  Harada's H30.81- ☑
  Hartnup (pellagra-cerebellar ataxia-renal aminoaciduria) E72.02
  Hart's (pellagra-cerebellar ataxia-renal aminoaciduria) E72.02
  Hashimoto's (struma lymphomatosa) E06.3
  Hb — *see* Disease, hemoglobin
  heart (organic) I51.9
    with
      pulmonary edema (acute) (*see also* Failure, ventricular, left) I50.1
      rheumatic fever (conditions in I00)
        active I01.9
          with chorea I02.0
          specified NEC I01.8
        inactive or quiescent (with chorea) I09.9
          specified NEC I09.89
    amyloid E85.4 [I43]
    aortic (valve) I35.9
    arteriosclerotic or sclerotic (senile) — *see* Disease, heart, ischemic, atherosclerotic
    artery, arterial — *see* Disease, heart, ischemic, atherosclerotic
    beer drinkers' I42.6
    beriberi (wet) E51.12
    black I27.0
    congenital Q24.9
      cyanotic Q24.9
      specified NEC Q24.8
    coronary — *see* Disease, heart, ischemic

**Disease, diseased** — *continued*
  heart — *continued*
    cryptogenic I51.9
    fibroid — *see* Myocarditis
    functional I51.89
      psychogenic F45.8
    glycogen storage E74.02 [I43]
    gonococcal A54.83
    hypertensive — *see* Hypertension, heart
    hyperthyroid (*see also* Hyperthyroidism) E05.90 [I43]
      with thyroid storm E05.91 [I43]
    ischemic (chronic or with a stated duration of over 4 weeks) I25.9
      atherosclerotic (of) I25.10
        with angina pectoris — *see* Arteriosclerosis, coronary (artery)
        coronary artery bypass graft — *see* Arteriosclerosis, coronary (artery), cardiomyopathy I25.5
        diagnosed on ECG or other special investigation, but currently presenting no symptoms I25.6
        silent I25.6
        specified form NEC I25.89
    kyphoscoliotic I27.1
    meningococcal A39.50
      endocarditis A39.51
      myocarditis A39.52
      pericarditis A39.53
    mitral I05.9
      specified NEC I05.8
    muscular — *see* Degeneration, myocardial
    psychogenic (functional) F45.8
    pulmonary (chronic) I27.9
      in schistosomiasis B65.9 [I52]
      specified NEC I27.89
    rheumatic (chronic) (inactive) (old) (quiescent) (with chorea) I09.9
      active or acute I01.9
        with chorea (acute) (rheumatic) (Sydenham's) I02.0
      specified NEC I09.89
    senile — *see* Myocarditis
    syphilitic A52.06
      aortic A52.03
        aneurysm A52.01
      congenital A50.54 [I52]
    thyrotoxic (*see also* Thyrotoxicosis) E05.90 [I43]
      with thyroid storm E05.91 [I43]
    valve, valvular (obstructive) (regurgitant) (*see also* Endocarditis)
      congenital NEC Q24.8
      pulmonary Q22.3
    vascular — *see* Disease, cardiovascular
  heavy chain NEC C88.2
    alpha C88.3
    gamma C88.2
    mu C88.2
  Hebra's
    pityriasis
      maculata et circinata L42
      rubra pilaris L44.0
    prurigo L28.2
  hematopoietic organs D75.9
  hemoglobin or Hb
    abnormal (mixed) NEC D58.2
      with thalassemia D56.9
    AS genotype D57.3
    Bart's D56.0
    C (Hb-C) D58.2
      with other abnormal hemoglobin NEC D58.2
      elliptocytosis D58.1
      Hb-S D57.2- ☑
      sickle-cell D57.2- ☑
      thalassemia D56.8
    Constant Spring D58.2
    D (Hb-D) D58.2
    E (Hb-E) D58.2
    E-beta thalassemia D56.5
    elliptocytosis D58.1
    H (Hb-H) (thalassemia) D56.0
      with other abnormal hemoglobin NEC D56.9
      Constant Spring D56.0
    I thalassemia D56.9
    M D74.0
    S or SS D57.1
    SC D57.2- ☑

**Disease, diseased** — *continued*
  hemoglobin or Hb — *continued*
    SD D57.8- ☑
    SE D57.8- ☑
    spherocytosis D58.0
    unstable, hemolytic D58.2
  hemolytic (newborn) P55.9
    autoimmune (cold type) (warm type) D59.1
    drug-induced D59.0
    due to or with
      incompatibility
        ABO (blood group) P55.1
        blood (group) (Duffy) (K(ell)) (Kidd) (Lewis) (M) (S) NEC P55.8
        Rh (blood group) (factor) P55.0
    Rh negative mother P55.0
    specified type NEC P55.8
    unstable hemoglobin D58.2
  hemorrhagic D69.9
    newborn P53
  Henoch (-Schönlein) (purpura nervosa) D69.0
  hepatic — *see* Disease, liver
  hepatolenticular E83.01
  heredodegenerative NEC
    spinal cord G95.89
  herpesviral, disseminated B00.7
  Hers' (glycogenosis VI) E74.09
  Herter (-Gee) (-Heubner) (nontropical sprue) K90.0
  Heubner-Herter (nontropical sprue) K90.0
  high fetal gene or hemoglobin thalassemia D56.9
  Hildenbrand's — *see* Typhus
  hip (joint) M25.9
    congenital Q65.89
    suppurative M00.9
    tuberculous A18.02
  His (-Werner) (trench fever) A79.0
  Hodgson's I71.2
    ruptured I71.1
  Holla — *see* Spherocytosis
  hookworm B76.9
    specified NEC B76.8
  host-versus-graft D89.813
    acute D89.810
    acute on chronic D89.812
    chronic D89.811
  human immunodeficiency virus (HIV) B20
  Huntington's G10
    with dementia G10 [F02.80]
  Hutchinson's (cheiropompholyx) — *see* Hutchinson's disease
  hyaline (diffuse) (generalized)
    membrane (lung) (newborn) P22.0
    adult J80
  hydatid — *see* Echinococcus
  hydroxyapatite deposition M11.00
    ankle M11.07- ☑
    elbow M11.02- ☑
    foot joint M11.07- ☑
    hand joint M11.04- ☑
    hip M11.05- ☑
    knee M11.06- ☑
    multiple site M11.09
    shoulder M11.01- ☑
    vertebra M11.08
    wrist M11.03- ☑
  hyperkinetic — *see* Hyperkinesia
  hypertensive — *see* Hypertension
  hypophysis E23.7
  Iceland G93.3
  I-cell E77.0
  immune D89.9
  immunoproliferative (malignant) C88.9
    small intestinal C88.3
    specified NEC C88.8
  inclusion B25.9
    salivary gland B25.9
  infectious, infective B99.9
    congenital P37.9
      specified NEC P37.8
      viral P35.9
        specified type NEC P35.8
    specified NEC B99.8
  inflammatory
    penis N48.29
      abscess N48.21
      cellulitis N48.22
    prepuce N47.7
      balanoposthitis N47.6

**Disease, diseased** — *continued*
- inflammatory — *continued*
  - tubo-ovarian — *see* Salpingo-oophoritis
  - intervertebral disc (*see also* Disorder, disc)
    - with myelopathy — *see* Disorder, disc, with, myelopathy
      - cervical, cervicothoracic — *see* Disorder, disc, cervical
        - with
          - myelopathy — *see* Disorder, disc, cervical, with myelopathy
          - neuritis, radiculitis or radiculopathy — *see* Disorder, disc, cervical, with neuritis
          - specified NEC — *see* Disorder, disc, cervical, specified type NEC
      - lumbar (with)
        - myelopathy M51.06
        - neuritis, radiculitis, radiculopathy or sciatica M51.16
        - specified NEC M51.86
      - lumbosacral (with)
        - neuritis, radiculitis, radiculopathy or sciatica M51.17
        - specified NEC M51.87
      - specified NEC — *see* Disorder, disc, specified NEC
      - thoracic (with)
        - myelopathy M51.04
        - neuritis, radiculitis or radiculopathy M51.14
        - specified NEC M51.84
      - thoracolumbar (with)
        - myelopathy M51.05
        - neuritis, radiculitis or radiculopathy M51.15
        - specified NEC M51.85
- intestine K63.9
  - functional K59.9
    - psychogenic F45.8
    - specified NEC K59.8
  - organic K63.9
  - protozoal A07.9
  - specified NEC K63.89
- iris H21.9
  - specified NEC H21.89
- iron metabolism or storage E83.10
- island (scrub typhus) A75.3
- itai-itai — *see* Poisoning, cadmium
- Jakob-Creutzfeldt — *see* Creutzfeldt-Jakob disease or syndrome
- jaw M27.9
  - fibrocystic M27.49
  - specified NEC M27.8
- jigger B88.1
- joint (*see also* Disorder, joint)
  - Charcot's — *see* Arthropathy, neuropathic (Charcot)
  - degenerative — *see* Osteoarthritis
    - multiple M15.9
    - spine — *see* Spondylosis
  - hypertrophic — *see* Osteoarthritis
  - sacroiliac M53.3
  - specified NEC — *see* Disorder, joint, specified type NEC
  - spine NEC — *see* Dorsopathy
  - suppurative — *see* Arthritis, pyogenic or pyemic
- Jourdain's (acute gingivitis) K05.00
  - nonplaque induced K05.01
  - plaque induced K05.00
- Kaschin-Beck (endemic polyarthritis) M12.10
  - ankle M12.17- ☑
  - elbow M12.12- ☑
  - foot joint M12.17- ☑
  - hand joint M12.14- ☑
  - hip M12.15- ☑
  - knee M12.16- ☑
  - multiple site M12.19
  - shoulder M12.11- ☑
  - vertebra M12.18
  - wrist M12.13- ☑
- Katayama B65.2
- Kedani (scrub typhus) A75.3
- Keshan E59
- kidney (functional) (pelvis) N28.9
  - chronic N18.9
    - hypertensive — *see* Hypertension, kidney
    - stage 1 N18.1
    - stage 2 (mild) N18.2
    - stage 3 (moderate) N18.3
    - stage 4 (severe) N18.4
    - stage 5 N18.5

**Disease, diseased** — *continued*
- kidney — *continued*
  - complicating pregnancy — *see* Pregnancy, complicated by, renal disease
  - cystic (congenital) Q61.9
  - fibrocystic (congenital) Q61.8
  - hypertensive — *see* Hypertension, kidney
  - in (due to)
    - schistosomiasis (bilharziasis) B65.9 [N29]
  - multicystic Q61.4
  - polycystic Q61.3
    - adult type Q61.2
    - childhood type NEC Q61.19
      - collecting duct dilatation Q61.11
- Kimmelstiel (-Wilson) (intercapillary polycystic (congenital) glomerulosclerosis) — *see* E08-E13 with .21
- Kinnier Wilson's (hepatolenticular degeneration) E83.01
- kissing — *see* Mononucleosis, infectious
- Klebs' (*see also* Glomerulonephritis) N05- ☑
- Klippel-Feil (brevicollis) Q76.1
- Köhler-Pellegrini-Stieda (calcification, knee joint) — *see* Bursitis, tibial collateral
- Kok Q89.8
- König's (osteochondritis dissecans) — *see* Osteochondritis, dissecans
- Korsakoff's (nonalcoholic) F04
  - alcoholic F10.96
    - with dependence F10.26
- Kostmann's (infantile genetic agranulocytosis) D70.0
- kuru A81.81
- Kyasanur Forest A98.2
- labyrinth, ear — *see* Disorder, ear, inner
- lacrimal system — *see* Disorder, lacrimal system
- Lafora's — *see* Epilepsy, generalized, idiopathic
- Lancereaux-Mathieu (leptospiral jaundice) A27.0
- Landry's G61.0
- Larrey-Weil (leptospiral jaundice) A27.0
- larynx J38.7
- legionnaires' A48.1
  - nonpneumonic A48.2
- Lenegre's I44.2
- lens H27.9
  - specified NEC H27.8
- Lev's (acquired complete heart block) I44.2
- Lewy body (dementia) G31.83 [F02.80]
  - with behavioral disturbance G31.83 [F02.81]
- Lichtheim's (subacute combined sclerosis with pernicious anemia) D51.0
- Lightwood's (renal tubular acidosis) N25.89
- Lignac's (cystinosis) E72.04
- lip K13.0
- lipid-storage E75.6
  - specified NEC E75.5
- Lipschütz's N76.6
- liver (chronic) (organic) K76.9
  - alcoholic (chronic) K70.9
    - acute — *see* Disease, liver, alcoholic, hepatitis
    - cirrhosis K70.30
      - with ascites K70.31
    - failure K70.40
      - with coma K70.41
    - fatty liver K70.0
    - fibrosis K70.2
    - hepatitis K70.10
      - with ascites K70.11
    - sclerosis K70.2
  - cystic, congenital Q44.6
  - drug-induced (idiosyncratic) (toxic) (predictable) (unpredictable) — *see* Disease, liver, toxic
  - end stage K72.90
    - due to hepatitis — *see* Hepatitis
  - fatty, nonalcoholic (NAFLD) K76.0
    - alcoholic K70.0
  - fibrocystic (congenital) Q44.6
  - fluke
    - Chinese B66.1
    - oriental B66.1
    - sheep B66.3
  - gestational alloimmune (GALD) P78.84
  - glycogen storage E74.09 [K77]
  - in (due to)
    - schistosomiasis (bilharziasis) B65.9 [K77]
  - inflammatory K75.9
    - alcoholic K70.1 ☑
    - specified NEC K75.89
  - polycystic (congenital) Q44.6

**Disease, diseased** — *continued*
- liver — *continued*
  - toxic K71.9
    - with
      - cholestasis K71.0
      - cirrhosis (liver) K71.7
      - fibrosis (liver) K71.7
      - focal nodular hyperplasia K71.8
      - hepatic granuloma K71.8
      - hepatic necrosis K71.10
        - with coma K71.11
      - hepatitis NEC K71.6
        - acute K71.2
        - chronic
          - active K71.50
            - with ascites K71.51
          - lobular K71.4
          - persistent K71.3
        - lupoid K71.50
          - with ascites K71.51
      - peliosis hepatis K71.8
      - veno-occlusive disease (VOD) of liver K71.8
  - veno-occlusive K76.5
- Lobo's (keloid blastomycosis) B48.0
- Lobstein's (brittle bones and blue sclera) Q78.0
- Ludwig's (submaxillary cellulitis) K12.2
- lumbosacral region M53.87
- lung J98.4
  - black J60
  - congenital Q33.9
  - cystic J98.4
    - congenital Q33.0
  - fibroid (chronic) — *see* Fibrosis, lung
  - fluke B66.4
    - oriental B66.4
  - in
    - amyloidosis E85.4 [J99]
    - sarcoidosis D86.0
    - Sjögren's syndrome M35.02
    - systemic
      - lupus erythematosus M32.13
      - sclerosis M34.81
  - interstitial J84.9
    - of childhood, specified NEC J84.848
    - respiratory bronchiolitis J84.115
    - specified NEC J84.89
  - obstructive (chronic) J44.9
    - with
      - acute
        - bronchitis J44.0
        - exacerbation NEC J44.1
        - lower respiratory infection J44.0
      - alveolitis, allergic J67.9
      - asthma J44.9
      - bronchiectasis J47.9
        - with
          - exacerbation (acute) J47.1
          - lower respiratory infection J47.0
      - bronchitis J44.9
        - with
          - exacerbation (acute) J44.1
          - lower respiratory infection J44.0
      - emphysema J43.9
      - hypersensitivity pneumonitis J67.9
    - decompensated J44.1
      - with
        - exacerbation (acute) J44.1
  - polycystic J98.4
    - congenital Q33.0
  - rheumatoid (diffuse) (interstitial) — *see* Rheumatoid, lung
- Lutembacher's (atrial septal defect with mitral stenosis) Q21.1
- Lyme A69.20
- lymphatic (gland) (system) (channel) (vessel) I89.9
- lymphoproliferative D47.9
  - specified NEC D47.Z9 (*following* D47.4)
  - T-gamma D47.Z9 (*following* D47.4)
  - X-linked D82.3
- Magitot's M27.2
- malarial — *see* Malaria
- malignant (*see also* Neoplasm, malignant, by site)
- Manson's B65.1
- maple bark J67.6
- maple-syrup-urine E71.0
- Marburg (virus) A98.3
- Marion's (bladder neck obstruction) N32.0
- Marsh's (exophthalmic goiter) — *see* Hyperthyroidism, with, goiter (diffuse)

☑ Additional Character Required — Refer to the Tabular List for Character Selection    ▽ Subterms under main terms may continue to next column or page

**Disease, diseased** — *continued*

mastoid (process) — *see* Disorder, ear, middle
Mathieu's (leptospiral jaundice) A27.Ø
Maxcy's A75.2
McArdle (-Schmid-Pearson) (glycogenosis V) E74.Ø4
mediastinum J98.59
medullary center (idiopathic) (respiratory) G93.89
Meige's (chronic hereditary edema) Q82.Ø
meningococcal — *see* Infection, meningococcal
mental F99
  organic FØ9
mesenchymal M35.9
mesenteric embolic (*see also* Ischemia, intestine, acute)
    K55.Ø39
metabolic, metabolism E88.9
  bilirubin E8Ø.7
metal-polisher's J62.8
metastatic (*see also* Neoplasm, secondary, by site)
    C79.9
microvascular - code to condition
microvillus
  atrophy Q43.8
  inclusion (MVD) Q43.8
middle ear — *see* Disorder, ear, middle
Mikulicz' (dryness of mouth, absent or decreased
    lacrimation) K11.8
Milroy's (chronic hereditary edema) Q82.Ø
Minamata — *see* Poisoning, mercury
minicore G71.2
Minor's G95.19
Minot's (hemorrhagic disease, newborn) P53
Minot-von Willebrand-Jürgens (angiohemophilia)
    D68.Ø
Mitchell's (erythromelalgia) I73.81
mitral (valve) IØ5.9
  nonrheumatic I34.9
mixed connective tissue M35.1
moldy hay J67.Ø
Monge's T7Ø.29 ☑
Morgagni-Adams-Stokes (syncope with heart block)
    I45.9
Morgagni's (syndrome) (hyperostosis frontalis interna)
    M85.2
Morton's (with metatarsalgia) — *see* Lesion, nerve,
    plantar
Morvan's G6Ø.8
motor neuron (bulbar) (mixed type) (spinal) G12.2Ø
  amyotrophic lateral sclerosis G12.21
  familial G12.24
  progressive bulbar palsy G12.22
  specified NEC G12.29
moyamoya I67.5
mu heavy chain disease C88.2
multicore G71.2
muscle (*see also* Disorder, muscle)
  inflammatory — *see* Myositis
  ocular (external) — *see* Strabismus
musculoskeletal system, soft tissue — *see also* Disor-
    der, soft tissue
  specified NEC — *see* Disorder, soft tissue, specified
      type NEC
mushroom workers' J67.5
mycotic B49
myelodysplastic, not classified C94.6
myeloproliferative, not classified C94.6
  chronic D47.1
myocardium, myocardial (*see also* Degeneration, my-
    ocardial) I51.5
  primary (idiopathic) I42.9
myoneural G7Ø.9
Naegeli's D69.1
nails L6Ø.9
  specified NEC L6Ø.8
Nairobi (sheep virus) A93.8
nasal J34.9
nemaline body G71.2
nerve — *see* Disorder, nerve
nervous system G98.8
  autonomic G9Ø.9
  central G96.9
    specified NEC G96.8
  congenital QØ7.9
  parasympathetic G9Ø.9
  specified NEC G98.8
  sympathetic G9Ø.9
  vegetative G9Ø.9
neuromuscular system G7Ø.9
Newcastle B3Ø.8

**Disease, diseased** — *continued*

Nicolas (-Durand)-Favre (climatic bubo) A55
nipple N64.9
  Paget's C5Ø.Ø1- ☑
    female C5Ø.Ø1- ☑
    male C5Ø.Ø2- ☑
Nishimoto (-Takeuchi) I67.5
nonarthropod-borne NOS (viral) B34.9
  enterovirus NEC B34.1
nonautoimmune hemolytic D59.4
  drug-induced D59.2
Nonne-Milroy-Meige (chronic hereditary edema) Q82.Ø
nose J34.9
nucleus pulposus — *see* Disorder, disc
nutritional E63.9
oast-house-urine E72.19
  ocular
    herpesviral BØØ.5Ø
    zoster BØ2.3Ø
obliterative vascular I77.1
Ohara's — *see* Tularemia
Opitz's (congestive splenomegaly) D73.2
Oppenheim-Urbach (necrobiosis lipoidica diabetico-
    rum) — *see* EØ8-E13 with .62Ø
optic nerve NEC — *see* Disorder, nerve, optic
orbit — *see* Disorder, orbit
Oriental liver fluke B66.1
Oriental lung fluke B66.4
Ormond's N13.5
Oropouche virus A93.Ø
Osler-Rendu (familial hemorrhagic telangiectasia) I78.Ø
osteofibrocystic E21.Ø
Otto's M24.7
outer ear — *see* Disorder, ear, external
ovary (noninflammatory) N83.9
  cystic N83.2Ø- ☑
  inflammatory — *see* Salpingo-oophoritis
  polycystic E28.2
  specified NEC N83.8
Owren's (congenital) — *see* Defect, coagulation
pancreas K86.9
  cystic K86.2
  fibrocystic E84.9
  specified NEC K86.89
panvalvular IØ8.9
  specified NEC IØ8.8
parametrium (noninflammatory) N83.9
parasitic B89
  cerebral NEC B71.9 [G94]
  intestinal NOS B82.9
  mouth B37.Ø
  skin NOS B88.9
  specified type — *see* Infestation
  tongue B37.Ø
parathyroid (gland) E21.5
  specified NEC E21.4
Parkinson's G2Ø
parodontal KØ5.6
Parrot's (syphilitic osteochondritis) A5Ø.Ø2
Parry's (exophthalmic goiter) — *see* Hyperthyroidism,
    with, goiter (diffuse)
Parson's (exophthalmic goiter) — *see* Hyperthyroidism,
    with, goiter (diffuse)
Paxton's (white piedra) B36.2
pearl-worker's — *see* Osteomyelitis, specified type
    NEC
Pellegrini-Stieda (calcification, knee joint) — *see* Bur-
    sitis, tibial collateral
pelvis, pelvic
  female NOS N94.9
    specified NEC N94.89
  gonococcal (acute) (chronic) A54.24
  inflammatory (female) N73.9
    acute N73.Ø
    chlamydial A56.11
    chronic N73.1
    specified NEC N73.8
    syphilitic (secondary) A51.42
      late A52.76
    tuberculous A18.17
  organ, female N94.9
  peritoneum, female NEC N94.89
penis N48.9
  inflammatory N48.29
    abscess N48.21
    cellulitis N48.22
  specified NEC N48.89
periapical tissues NOS KØ4.9Ø

**Disease, diseased** — *continued*

periodontal KØ5.6
  specified NEC KØ5.5
periosteum — *see* Disorder, bone, specified type NEC
peripheral
  arterial I73.9
  autonomic nervous system G9Ø.9
  nerves — *see* Polyneuropathy
  vascular NOS I73.9
peritoneum K66.9
  pelvic, female NEC N94.89
  specified NEC K66.8
persistent mucosal (middle ear) H66.2Ø
  left H66.22
    with right H66.23
  right H66.21
    with left H66.23
Petit's — *see* Hernia, abdomen, specified site NEC
pharynx J39.2
  specified NEC J39.8
Phocas' — *see* Mastopathy, cystic
photochromogenic (acid-fast bacilli) (pulmonary)
    A31.Ø
  nonpulmonary A31.9
Pick's G31.Ø1 [FØ2.8Ø]
  with behavioral disturbance G31.Ø1 [FØ2.81]
    brain G31.Ø1 [FØ2.8Ø]
      with behavioral disturbance G31.Ø1 [FØ2.81]
  of pericardium (pericardial pseudocirrhosis of liver)
      I31.1
pigeon fancier's J67.2
pineal gland E34.8
pink — *see* Poisoning, mercury
Pinkus' (lichen nitidus) L44.1
pinworm B8Ø
Piry virus A93.8
pituitary (gland) E23.7
pituitary-snuff-taker's J67.8
pleura (cavity) J94.9
  specified NEC J94.8
pneumatic drill (hammer) T75.21 ☑
Pollitzer's (hidradenitis suppurativa) L73.2
polycystic
  kidney or renal Q61.3
    adult type Q61.2
    childhood type NEC Q61.19
      collecting duct dilatation Q61.11
  liver or hepatic Q44.6
  lung or pulmonary J98.4
    congenital Q33.Ø
  ovary, ovaries E28.2
  spleen Q89.Ø9
polyethylene T84.Ø5- ☑
Pompe's (glycogenosis II) E74.Ø2
Posadas-Wernicke B38.9
Potain's (pulmonary edema) — *see* Edema, lung
prepuce N47.8
  inflammatory N47.7
    balanoposthitis N47.6
Pringle's (tuberous sclerosis) Q85.1
prion, central nervous system A81.9
  specified NEC A81.89
prostate N42.9
  specified NEC N42.89
protozoal B64
  acanthamebiasis — *see* Acanthamebiasis
  African trypanosomiasis — *see* African trypanoso-
      miasis
  babesiosis B6Ø.Ø
  Chagas disease — *see* Chagas disease
  intestine, intestinal AØ7.9
  leishmaniasis — *see* Leishmaniasis
  malaria — *see* Malaria
  naegleriasis B6Ø.2
  pneumocystosis B59
  specified organism NEC B6Ø.8
  toxoplasmosis — *see* Toxoplasmosis
pseudo-Hurler's E77.Ø
psychiatric F99
psychotic — *see* Psychosis
Puente's (simple glandular cheilitis) K13.Ø
puerperal (*see also* Puerperal) O9Ø.89
pulmonary (*see also* Disease, lung)
  artery I28.9
  chronic obstructive J44.9
    with
      acute bronchitis J44.Ø
      exacerbation (acute) J44.1

**Disease, diseased** — *continued*
pulmonary (*see also* Disease, lung) — *continued*
  chronic obstructive — *continued*
    with — *continued*
      lower respiratory infection (acute) J44.0
    decompensated J44.1
      with
        exacerbation (acute) J44.1
  heart I27.9
    specified NEC I27.89
  hypertensive (vascular) (*see also* Hypertension, pulmonary) I27.20
    primary (idiopathic) I27.0
    NEC I27.2 ☑
  valve I37.9
    rheumatic I09.89
pulp (dental) K04.90
pulseless M31.4
Putnam's (subacute combined sclerosis with pernicious anemia) D51.0
Pyle (-Cohn) (metaphyseal dysplasia) Q78.5
ragpicker's or ragsorter's A22.1
Raynaud's — *see* Raynaud's disease
reactive airway — *see* Asthma
Reclus' (cystic) — *see* Mastopathy, cystic
rectum K62.9
  specified NEC K62.89
Refsum's (heredopathia atactica polyneuritiformis) G60.1
renal (functional) (pelvis) (*see also* Disease, kidney) N28.9
  with
    edema — *see* Nephrosis
    glomerular lesion — *see* Glomerulonephritis
      with edema — *see* Nephrosis
    interstitial nephritis N12
  acute N28.9
  chronic (*see also* Disease, kidney, chronic) N18.9
  cystic, congenital Q61.9
  diabetic — *see* E08-E13 with .22
  end-stage (failure) N18.6
    due to hypertension I12.0
  fibrocystic (congenital) Q61.8
  hypertensive — *see* Hypertension, kidney
  lupus M32.14
  phosphate-losing (tubular) N25.0
  polycystic (congenital) Q61.3
    adult type Q61.2
    childhood type NEC Q61.19
      collecting duct dilatation Q61.11
  rapidly progressive N01.9
  subacute N01.9
Rendu-Osler-Weber (familial hemorrhagic telangiectasia) I78.0
renovascular (arteriosclerotic) — *see* Hypertension, kidney
respiratory (tract) J98.9
  acute or subacute NOS J06.9
    due to
      chemicals, gases, fumes or vapors (inhalation) J68.3
      external agent J70.9
        specified NEC J70.8
      radiation J70.0
      smoke inhalation J70.5
    noninfectious J39.8
  chronic NOS J98.9
    due to
      chemicals, gases, fumes or vapors J68.4
      external agent J70.9
        specified NEC J70.8
      radiation J70.1
    newborn P27.9
      specified NEC P27.8
  due to
    chemicals, gases, fumes or vapors J68.9
      acute or subacute NEC J68.3
      chronic J68.4
    external agent J70.9
      specified NEC J70.8
  newborn P28.9
    specified type NEC P28.89
  upper J39.9
    acute or subacute J06.9
    noninfectious NEC J39.8
    specified NEC J39.8
    streptococcal J06.9
retina, retinal H35.9

**Disease, diseased** — *continued*
retina, retinal — *continued*
  Batten's or Batten-Mayou E75.4 [H36]
    specified NEC H35.89
  rheumatoid — *see* Arthritis, rheumatoid
  rickettsial NOS A79.9
    specified type NEC A79.89
  Riga (-Fede) (cachectic aphthae) K14.0
  Riggs' (compound periodontitis) — *see* Periodontitis
  Ritter's L00
  Rivalta's (cervicofacial actinomycosis) A42.2
  Robles' (onchocerciasis) B73.01
  Roger's (congenital interventricular septal defect) Q21.0
  Rosenthal's (factor XI deficiency) D68.1
  Ross River B33.1
  Rossbach's (hyperchlorhydria) K30
  Rotes Quérol — *see* Hyperostosis, ankylosing
  Roth (-Bernhardt) — *see* Mononeuropathy, lower limb, meralgia paresthetica
  Runeberg's (progressive pernicious anemia) D51.0
sacroiliac NEC M53.3
salivary gland or duct K11.9
  inclusion B25.9
  specified NEC K11.8
  virus B25.9
sandworm B76.9
Schimmelbusch's — *see* Mastopathy, cystic
Schmorl's — *see* Schmorl's disease or nodes
Schönlein (-Henoch) (purpura rheumatica) D69.0
Schottmüller's — *see* Fever, paratyphoid
Schultz's (agranulocytosis) — *see* Agranulocytosis
Schwalbe-Ziehen-Oppenheim G24.1
Schwartz-Jampel G71.13
sclera H15.9
  specified NEC H15.89
scrofulous (tuberculous) A18.2
scrotum N50.9
sebaceous glands L73.9
semilunar cartilage, cystic (*see also* Derangement, knee, meniscus, cystic)
seminal vesicle N50.9
serum NEC (*see also* Reaction, serum) T80.69 ☑
sexually transmitted A64
  anogenital
    herpesviral infection — *see* Herpes, anogenital
    warts A63.0
  chancroid A57
  chlamydial infection — *see* Chlamydia
  gonorrhea — *see* Gonorrhea
  granuloma inguinale A58
  specified organism NEC A63.8
  syphilis — *see* Syphilis
  trichomoniasis — *see* Trichomoniasis
Sézary C84.1- ☑
shimamushi (scrub typhus) A75.3
shipyard B30.0
sickle-cell D57.1
  with crisis (vasoocclusive pain) D57.00
    with
      acute chest syndrome D57.01
      splenic sequestration D57.02
  elliptocytosis D57.8- ☑
  Hb-C D57.20
    with crisis (vasoocclusive pain) D57.219
      with
        acute chest syndrome D57.211
        splenic sequestration D57.212
    without crisis D57.20
  Hb-SD D57.80
    with crisis D57.819
      with
        acute chest syndrome D57.811
        splenic sequestration D57.812
  Hb-SE D57.80
    with crisis D57.819
      with
        acute chest syndrome D57.811
        splenic sequestration D57.812
  specified NEC D57.80
    with crisis D57.819
      with
        acute chest syndrome D57.811
        splenic sequestration D57.812
  spherocytosis D57.80
    with crisis D57.819
      with
        acute chest syndrome D57.811

**Disease, diseased** — *continued*
sickle-cell — *continued*
  spherocytosis — *continued*
    with crisis — *continued*
      with — *continued*
        splenic sequestration D57.812
  thalassemia D57.40
    with crisis (vasoocclusive pain) D57.419
      with
        acute chest syndrome D57.411
        splenic sequestration D57.412
    without crisis D57.40
silo-filler's J68.8
  bronchitis J68.0
  pneumonitis J68.0
  pulmonary edema J68.1
simian B B00.4
Simons' (progressive lipodystrophy) E88.1
sin nombre virus B33.4
sinus — *see* Sinusitis
Sirkari's B55.0
sixth B08.20
  due to human herpesvirus 6 B08.21
  due to human herpesvirus 7 B08.22
skin L98.9
  due to metabolic disorder NEC E88.9 [L99]
  specified NEC L98.8
slim (HIV) B20
small vessel I73.9
Sneddon-Wilkinson (subcorneal pustular dermatosis) L13.1
South African creeping B88.0
spinal (cord) G95.9
  congenital Q06.9
  specified NEC G95.89
spine (*see also* Spondylopathy)
  joint — *see* Dorsopathy
  tuberculous A18.01
spinocerebellar (hereditary) G11.9
  specified NEC G11.8
spleen D73.9
  amyloid E85.4 [D77]
  organic D73.9
  polycystic Q89.09
  postinfectional D73.89
sponge-diver's — *see* Toxicity, venom, marine animal, sea anemone
Startle Q89.8
Steinert's G71.11
Sticker's (erythema infectiosum) B08.3
Stieda's (calcification, knee joint) — *see* Bursitis, tibial collateral
Stokes' (exophthalmic goiter) — *see* Hyperthyroidism, with, goiter (diffuse)
Stokes-Adams (syncope with heart block) I45.9
stomach K31.9
  functional, psychogenic F45.8
  specified NEC K31.89
stonemason's J62.8
storage
  glycogen — *see* Disease, glycogen storage
  mucopolysaccharide — *see* Mucopolysaccharidosis
striatopallidal system NEC G25.89
Stuart-Prower (congenital factor X deficiency) D68.2
Stuart's (congenital factor X deficiency) D68.2
subcutaneous tissue — *see* Disease, skin
supporting structures of teeth K08.9
  specified NEC K08.89
suprarenal (capsule) (gland) E27.9
  hyperfunction E27.0
  specified NEC E27.8
sweat glands L74.9
  specified NEC L74.8
Sweeley-Klionsky E75.21
Swift (-Feer) — *see* Poisoning, mercury
swimming-pool granuloma A31.1
Sylvest's (epidemic pleurodynia) B33.0
sympathetic nervous system G90.9
synovium — *see* Disorder, synovium
syphilitic — *see* Syphilis
systemic tissue mast cell C96.20
tanapox (virus) B08.71
Tangier E78.6
Tarral-Besnier (pityriasis rubra pilaris) L44.0
Tauri's E74.09
tear duct — *see* Disorder, lacrimal system
tendon, tendinous (*see also* Disorder, tendon)
  nodular — *see* Trigger finger

☑ **Additional Character Required — Refer to the Tabular List for Character Selection**

▼ **Subterms under main terms may continue to next column or page**

**Disease, diseased** — *continued*
terminal vessel I73.9
testis N50.9
thalassemia Hb-S — *see* Disease, sickle-cell, tha-
    lassemia
Thaysen-Gee (nontropical sprue) K90.0
Thomsen G71.12
throat J39.2
    septic J02.0
thromboembolic — *see* Embolism
thymus (gland) E32.9
    specified NEC E32.8
thyroid (gland) E07.9
    heart (*see also* Hyperthyroidism) E05.90 [I43]
        with thyroid storm E05.91 [I43]
    specified NEC E07.89
Tietze's M94.0
tongue K14.9
    specified NEC K14.8
tonsils, tonsillar (and adenoids) J35.9
tooth, teeth K08.9
    hard tissues K03.9
        specified NEC K03.89
    pulp NEC K04.99
    specified NEC K08.89
Tourette's F95.2
trachea NEC J39.8
tricuspid I07.9
    nonrheumatic I36.9
triglyceride-storage E75.5
trophoblastic — *see* Mole, hydatidiform
tsutsugamushi A75.3
tube (fallopian) (noninflammatory) N83.9
    inflammatory — *see* Salpingitis
    specified NEC N83.8
tuberculous NEC — *see* Tuberculosis
tubo-ovarian (noninflammatory) N83.9
    inflammatory — *see* Salpingo-oophoritis
    specified NEC N83.8
tubotympanic, chronic — *see* Otitis, media, suppura-
    tive, chronic, tubotympanic
tubulo-interstitial N15.9
    specified NEC N15.8
tympanum — *see* Disorder, tympanic membrane
Uhl's Q24.8
Underwood's (sclerema neonatorum) P83.0
Unverricht (-Lundborg) — *see* Epilepsy, generalized,
    idiopathic
Urbach-Oppenheim (necrobiosis lipoidica diabetico-
    rum) — *see* E08-E13 with .620
ureter N28.9
    in (due to)
        schistosomiasis (bilharziasis) B65.0 [N29]
urethra N36.9
    specified NEC N36.8
urinary (tract) N39.9
    bladder N32.9
        specified NEC N32.89
    specified NEC N39.8
uterus (noninflammatory) N85.9
    infective — *see* Endometritis
    inflammatory — *see* Endometritis
    specified NEC N85.8
uveal tract (anterior) H21.9
    posterior H31.9
vagabond's B85.1
vagina, vaginal (noninflammatory) N89.9
    inflammatory NEC N76.89
    specified NEC N89.8
valve, valvular I38
    multiple I08.9
        specified NEC I08.8
van Creveld-von Gierke (glycogenosis I) E74.01
vas deferens N50.9
vascular I99.9
    arteriosclerotic — *see* Arteriosclerosis
    ciliary body NEC — *see* Disorder, iris, vascular
    hypertensive — *see* Hypertension
    iris NEC — *see* Disorder, iris, vascular
    obliterative I77.1
        peripheral I73.9
    occlusive I99.8
    peripheral (occlusive) I73.9
        in diabetes mellitus — *see* E08-E13 with .51
vasomotor I73.9
vasospastic I73.9
vein I87.9
venereal (*see also* Disease, sexually transmitted) A64

**Disease, diseased** — *continued*
venereal (*see also* Disease, sexually transmitted) —
    *continued*
    chlamydial NEC A56.8
        anus A56.3
        genitourinary NOS A56.2
        pharynx A56.4
        rectum A56.3
    fifth A55
    sixth A55
    specified nature or type NEC A63.8
vertebra, vertebral (*see also* Spondylopathy)
    disc — *see* Disorder, disc
vibration — *see* Vibration, adverse effects
viral, virus (*see also* Disease, by type of virus) B34.9
    arbovirus NOS A94
    arthropod-borne NOS A94
    congenital P35.9
        specified NEC P35.8
    Hanta (with renal manifestations) (Dobrava) (Pu-
        umala) (Seoul) A98.5
        with pulmonary manifestations (Andes) (Bayou)
            (Bermejo) (Black Creek Canal) (Choclo)
            (Juquitiba) (Laguna negra) (Lechiguanas)
            (New York) (Oran) (Sin nombre) B33.4
    Hantaan (Korean hemorrhagic fever) A98.5
    human immunodeficiency (HIV) B20
    Kunjin A83.4
    nonarthropod-borne NOS B34.9
    Powassan A84.8
    Rocio (encephalitis) A83.6
    Sin nombre (Hantavirus) (cardio)-pulmonary syn-
        drome) B33.4
    Tahyna B33.8
    vesicular stomatitis A93.8
vitreous H43.9
    specified NEC H43.89
vocal cord J38.3
Volkmann's, acquired T79.6 ☑
von Eulenburg's (congenital paramyotonia) G71.19
von Gierke's (glycogenosis I) E74.01
von Graefe's — *see* Strabismus, paralytic, ophthalmo-
    plegia, progressive
von Willebrand (-Jürgens) (angiohemophilia) D68.0
Vrolik's (osteogenesis imperfecta) Q78.0
vulva (noninflammatory) N90.9
    inflammatory NEC N76.89
    specified NEC N90.89
Wallgren's (obstruction of splenic vein with collateral
    circulation) I87.8
Wassilieff's (leptospiral jaundice) A27.0
wasting NEC R64
    due to malnutrition E41
Waterhouse-Friderichsen A39.1
Wegner's (syphilitic osteochondritis) A50.02
Weil's (leptospiral jaundice of lung) A27.0
Weir Mitchell's (erythromelalgia) I73.81
Werdnig-Hoffmann G12.0
Wermer's E31.21
Werner-His (trench fever) A79.0
Werner-Schultz (neutropenic splenomegaly) D73.81
Wernicke-Posadas B38.9
whipworm B79
white blood cells D72.9
    specified NEC D72.89
white matter R90.82
white-spot, meaning lichen sclerosus et atrophicus
    L90.0
    penis N48.0
    vulva N90.4
Wilkie's K55.1
Wilkinson-Sneddon (subcorneal pustular dermatosis)
    L13.1
Willis' — *see* Diabetes
Wilson's (hepatolenticular degeneration) E83.01
woolsorter's A22.1
yaba monkey tumor B08.72
yaba pox (virus) B08.72
Zika virus A92.5
zoonotic, bacterial A28.9
    specified type NEC A28.8
**Disfigurement** (due to scar) L90.5
**Disgerminoma** — *see* Dysgerminoma
**DISH** (diffuse idiopathic skeletal hyperostosis) — *see*
    Hyperostosis, ankylosing
**Disinsertion, retina** — *see* Detachment, retina
**Dislocatable hip, congenital** Q65.6

**Dislocation** (articular)
with fracture — *see* Fracture
acromioclavicular (joint) S43.10- ☑
    with displacement
        100%-200% S43.12- ☑
        more than 200% S43.13- ☑
    inferior S43.14- ☑
    posterior S43.15- ☑
ankle S93.0- ☑
astragalus — *see* Dislocation, ankle
atlantoaxial S13.121 ☑
atlantooccipital S13.111 ☑
atloidooccipital S13.111 ☑
breast bone S23.29 ☑
capsule, joint — *code by* site under Dislocation
carpal (bone) — *see* Dislocation, wrist
carpometacarpal (joint) NEC S63.05- ☑
    thumb S63.04- ☑
cartilage (joint) — *code by* site under Dislocation
cervical spine (vertebra) — *see* Dislocation, vertebra,
    cervical
chronic — *see* Dislocation, recurrent
clavicle — *see* Dislocation, acromioclavicular joint
coccyx S33.2 ☑
congenital NEC Q68.8
coracoid — *see* Dislocation, shoulder
costal cartilage S23.29 ☑
costochondral S23.29 ☑
cricoarytenoid articulation S13.29 ☑
cricothyroid articulation S13.29 ☑
dorsal vertebra — *see* Dislocation, vertebra, thoracic
ear ossicle — *see* Discontinuity, ossicles, ear
elbow S53.10- ☑
    congenital Q68.8
    pathological — *see* Dislocation, pathological NEC,
        elbow
    radial head alone — *see* Dislocation, radial head
    recurrent — *see* Dislocation, recurrent, elbow
    traumatic S53.10- ☑
        anterior S53.11- ☑
        lateral S53.14- ☑
        medial S53.13- ☑
        posterior S53.12- ☑
        specified type NEC S53.19- ☑
eye, nontraumatic — *see* Luxation, globe
eyeball, nontraumatic — *see* Luxation, globe
femur
    distal end — *see* Dislocation, knee
    proximal end — *see* Dislocation, hip
fibula
    distal end — *see* Dislocation, ankle
    proximal end — *see* Dislocation, knee
finger S63.25- ☑
    index S63.25- ☑
    interphalangeal S63.27- ☑
        distal S63.29- ☑
            index S63.29- ☑
            little S63.29- ☑
            middle S63.29- ☑
            ring S63.29- ☑
        index S63.27- ☑
        little S63.27- ☑
        middle S63.27- ☑
        proximal S63.28- ☑
            index S63.28- ☑
            little S63.28- ☑
            middle S63.28- ☑
            breast S63.28- ☑
        ring S63.27- ☑
    little S63.25- ☑
    metacarpophalangeal S63.26- ☑
        index S63.26- ☑
        little S63.26- ☑
        middle S63.26- ☑
        ring S63.26- ☑
    middle S63.25- ☑
    recurrent — *see* Dislocation, recurrent, finger
    ring S63.25- ☑
    thumb — *see* Dislocation, thumb
foot S93.30- ☑
    recurrent — *see* Dislocation, recurrent, foot
    specified site NEC S93.33- ☑
    tarsal joint S93.31- ☑
    tarsometatarsal joint S93.32- ☑
    toe — *see* Dislocation, toe
fracture — *see* Fracture

☑ Subterms under main terms may continue to next column or page          ☑ Additional Character Required — Refer to the Tabular List for Character Selection          107

Disease, diseased — Dislocation

**Dislocation** — *continued*
  glenohumeral (joint) — *see* Dislocation, shoulder
  glenoid — *see* Dislocation, shoulder
  habitual — *see* Dislocation, recurrent
  hip S73.00- ☑
    anterior S73.03- ☑
      obturator S73.02- ☑
    central S73.04- ☑
    congenital (total) Q65.2
      bilateral Q65.1
      partial Q65.5
        bilateral Q65.4
        unilateral Q65.3- ☑
      unilateral Q65.0- ☑
    developmental M24.85- ☑
    pathological — *see* Dislocation, pathological NEC, hip
    posterior S73.01- ☑
    recurrent — *see* Dislocation, recurrent, hip
  humerus, proximal end — *see* Dislocation, shoulder
  incomplete — *see* Subluxation, by site
  incus — *see* Discontinuity, ossicles, ear
  infracoracoid — *see* Dislocation, shoulder
  innominate (pubic junction) (sacral junction) S33.39 ☑
    acetabulum — *see* Dislocation, hip
  interphalangeal (joint(s))
    finger S63.279 ☑
      distal S63.29- ☑
        index S63.29- ☑
        little S63.29- ☑
        middle S63.29- ☑
        ring S63.29- ☑
      index S63.27- ☑
      little S63.27- ☑
      middle S63.27- ☑
      proximal S63.28- ☑
        index S63.28- ☑
        little S63.28- ☑
        middle S63.28- ☑
        ring S63.28- ☑
      ring S63.27- ☑
    foot or toe — *see* Dislocation, toe
    thumb S63.12- ☑
      distal joint S63.14- ☑
      proximal joint S63.13- ☑
  jaw (cartilage) (meniscus) S03.0- ☑
  joint prosthesis — *see* Complications, joint prosthesis, mechanical, displacement, by site
  knee S83.106 ☑
    cap — *see* Dislocation, patella
    congenital Q68.2
    old M23.8X- ☑
    patella — *see* Dislocation, patella
    pathological — *see* Dislocation, pathological NEC, knee
    proximal tibia
      anteriorly S83.11- ☑
      laterally S83.14- ☑
      medially S83.13- ☑
      posteriorly S83.12- ☑
    recurrent (*see also* Derangement, knee, specified NEC)
    specified type NEC S83.19- ☑
  lacrimal gland H04.16- ☑
  lens (complete) H27.10
    anterior H27.12- ☑
    congenital Q12.1
    ocular implant — *see* Complications, intraocular lens
    partial H27.11- ☑
    posterior H27.13- ☑
    traumatic S05.8X- ☑
  ligament — *code by* site under Dislocation
  lumbar (vertebra) — *see* Dislocation, vertebra, lumbar
  lumbosacral (vertebra) (*see also* Dislocation, vertebra, lumbar)
    congenital Q76.49
  mandible S03.0- ☑
  meniscus (knee) — *see* Tear, meniscus
    other sites - code by site under Dislocation
  metacarpal (bone)
    distal end — *see* Dislocation, finger
    proximal end S63.06- ☑
  metacarpophalangeal (joint)
    finger S63.26- ☑
      index S63.26- ☑

**Dislocation** — *continued*
  metacarpophalangeal — *continued*
    finger — *continued*
      little S63.26- ☑
      middle S63.26- ☑
      ring S63.26- ☑
      thumb S63.11- ☑
  metatarsal (bone) — *see* Dislocation, foot
  metatarsophalangeal (joint(s)) — *see* Dislocation, toe
  midcarpal (joint) S63.03- ☑
  midtarsal (joint) — *see* Dislocation, foot
  neck S13.20 ☑
    specified site NEC S13.29 ☑
    vertebra — *see* Dislocation, vertebra, cervical
  nose (septal cartilage) S03.1 ☑
  occipitoatloid S13.111 ☑
  old — *see* Derangement, joint, specified type NEC
  ossicles, ear — *see* Discontinuity, ossicles, ear
  partial — *see* Subluxation, by site
  patella S83.006 ☑
    congenital Q74.1
    lateral S83.01- ☑
    recurrent (nontraumatic) M22.0- ☑
      incomplete M22.1- ☑
    specified type NEC S83.09- ☑
  pathological NEC M24.30
    ankle M24.37- ☑
    elbow M24.32- ☑
    foot joint M24.37- ☑
    hand joint M24.34- ☑
    hip M24.35- ☑
    knee M24.36- ☑
    lumbosacral joint — *see* subcategory M53.2
    pelvic region — *see* Dislocation, pathological, hip
    sacroiliac — *see* subcategory M53.2
    shoulder M24.31- ☑
    wrist M24.33- ☑
  pelvis NEC S33.30 ☑
    specified NEC S33.39 ☑
  phalanx
    finger or hand — *see* Dislocation, finger
    foot or toe — *see* Dislocation, toe
  prosthesis, internal — *see* Complications, prosthetic device, by site, mechanical
  radial head S53.006 ☑
    anterior S53.01- ☑
    posterior S53.02- ☑
    specified type NEC S53.09- ☑
  radiocarpal (joint) S63.02- ☑
  radiohumeral (joint) — *see* Dislocation, radial head
  radioulnar (joint)
    distal S63.01- ☑
    proximal — *see* Dislocation, elbow
  radius
    distal end — *see* Dislocation, wrist
    proximal end — *see* Dislocation, radial head
  recurrent M24.40
    ankle M24.47- ☑
    elbow M24.42- ☑
    finger M24.44- ☑
    foot joint M24.47- ☑
    hand joint M24.44- ☑
    hip M24.45- ☑
    knee M24.46- ☑
      patella — *see* Dislocation, patella, recurrent
    patella — *see* Dislocation, patella, recurrent
    sacroiliac — *see* subcategory M53.2
    shoulder M24.41- ☑
    toe M24.47- ☑
    vertebra (*see also* subcategory) M43.5 ☑
      atlantoaxial M43.4
        with myelopathy M43.3
    wrist M24.43- ☑
  rib (cartilage) S23.29 ☑
  sacrococcygeal S33.2 ☑
  sacroiliac (joint) (ligament) S33.2 ☑
    congenital Q74.2
    recurrent — *see* subcategory M53.2
  sacrum S33.2 ☑
  scaphoid (bone) (hand) (wrist) — *see* Dislocation, wrist
    foot — *see* Dislocation, foot
  scapula — *see* Dislocation, shoulder, girdle, scapula
  semilunar cartilage, knee — *see* Tear, meniscus
  septal cartilage (nose) S03.1 ☑
  septum (nasal) (old) J34.2

**Dislocation** — *continued*
  sesamoid bone — *code by* site under Dislocation
  shoulder (blade) (ligament) (joint) (traumatic) S43.006 ☑
    acromioclavicular — *see* Dislocation, acromioclavicular
    chronic — *see* Dislocation, recurrent, shoulder
    congenital Q68.8
    girdle S43.30- ☑
      scapula S43.31- ☑
      specified site NEC S43.39- ☑
    humerus S43.00- ☑
      anterior S43.01- ☑
      inferior S43.03- ☑
      posterior S43.02- ☑
    pathological — *see* Dislocation, pathological NEC, shoulder
    recurrent — *see* Dislocation, recurrent, shoulder
    specified type NEC S43.08- ☑
  spine
    cervical — *see* Dislocation, vertebra, cervical
    congenital Q76.49
    due to birth trauma P11.5
    lumbar — *see* Dislocation, vertebra, lumbar
    thoracic — *see* Dislocation, vertebra, thoracic
  spontaneous — *see* Dislocation, pathological
  sternoclavicular (joint) S43.206 ☑
    anterior S43.21- ☑
    posterior S43.22- ☑
  sternum S23.29 ☑
  subglenoid — *see* Dislocation, shoulder
  symphysis pubis S33.4 ☑
  talus — *see* Dislocation, ankle
  tarsal (bone(s)) (joint(s)) — *see* Dislocation, foot
  tarsometatarsal (joint(s)) — *see* Dislocation, foot
  temporomandibular (joint) S03.0- ☑
  thigh, proximal end — *see* Dislocation, hip
  thorax S23.20 ☑
    specified site NEC S23.29 ☑
    vertebra — *see* Dislocation, vertebra
  thumb S63.10- ☑
    interphalangeal joint — *see* Dislocation, interphalangeal (joint), thumb
    metacarpophalangeal joint — *see* Dislocation, metacarpophalangeal (joint), thumb
  thyroid cartilage S13.29 ☑
  tibia
    distal end — *see* Dislocation, ankle
    proximal end — *see* Dislocation, knee
  tibiofibular (joint)
    distal — *see* Dislocation, ankle
    superior — *see* Dislocation, knee
  toe(s) S93.106 ☑
    great S93.10- ☑
      interphalangeal joint S93.11- ☑
      metatarsophalangeal joint S93.12- ☑
    interphalangeal joint S93.119 ☑
    lesser S93.106 ☑
      interphalangeal joint S93.11- ☑
      metatarsophalangeal joint S93.12- ☑
    metatarsophalangeal joint S93.12- ☑
  tooth S03.2 ☑
  trachea S23.29 ☑
  ulna
    distal end S63.07- ☑
    proximal end — *see* Dislocation, elbow
  ulnohumeral (joint) — *see* Dislocation, elbow
  vertebra (articular process) (body) (traumatic)
    cervical S13.101 ☑
      atlantoaxial joint S13.121 ☑
      atlantooccipital joint S13.111 ☑
      atloidooccipital joint S13.111 ☑
      joint between
        C0 and C1 S13.111 ☑
        C1 and C2 S13.121 ☑
        C2 and C3 S13.131 ☑
        C3 and C4 S13.141 ☑
        C4 and C5 S13.151 ☑
        C5 and C6 S13.161 ☑
        C6 and C7 S13.171 ☑
        C7 and T1 S13.181 ☑
      occipitoatloid joint S13.111 ☑
    congenital Q76.49
    lumbar S33.101 ☑
      joint between
        L1 and L2 S33.111 ☑

☑ **Additional Character Required** — **Refer to the Tabular List for Character Selection**      ▽ Subterms under main terms may continue to next column or page

**Dislocation** — continued
  vertebra — continued
    lumbar — continued
      joint between — continued
        L2 and L3 S33.121 ☑
        L3 and L4 S33.131 ☑
        L4 and L5 S33.141 ☑
      nontraumatic — see Displacement, intervertebral disc
      partial — see Subluxation, by site
      recurrent NEC — see subcategory M43.5 ☑
    thoracic S23.101 ☑
      joint between
        T1 and T2 S23.111 ☑
        T2 and T3 S23.121 ☑
        T3 and T4 S23.123 ☑
        T4 and T5 S23.131 ☑
        T5 and T6 S23.133 ☑
        T6 and T7 S23.141 ☑
        T7 and T8 S23.143 ☑
        T8 and T9 S23.151 ☑
        T9 and T10 S23.153 ☑
        T10 and T11 S23.161 ☑
        T11 and T12 S23.163 ☑
        T12 and L1 S23.171 ☑
  wrist (carpal bone) S63.006 ☑
    carpometacarpal joint — see Dislocation, carpometacarpal (joint)
    distal radioulnar joint — see Dislocation, radioulnar (joint), distal
    metacarpal bone, proximal — see Dislocation, metacarpal (bone), proximal end
    midcarpal — see Dislocation, midcarpal (joint)
    radiocarpal joint — see Dislocation, radiocarpal (joint)
    recurrent — see Dislocation, recurrent, wrist
    specified site NEC S63.09- ☑
    ulna — see Dislocation, ulna, distal end
  xiphoid cartilage S23.29 ☑
**Disorder** (of) (see also Disease)
  acantholytic L11.9
    specified NEC L11.8
  acute
    psychotic — see Psychosis, acute
    stress F43.0
  adjustment (grief) F43.20
    with
      anxiety F43.22
        with depressed mood F43.23
      conduct disturbance F43.24
        with emotional disturbance F43.25
      depressed mood F43.21
        with anxiety F43.23
      other specified symptom F43.29
  adrenal (capsule) (gland) (medullary) E27.9
    specified NEC E27.8
  adrenogenital E25.9
    drug-induced E25.8
    iatrogenic E25.8
    idiopathic E25.8
  adult personality (and behavior) F69
    specified NEC F68.8
  affective (mood) — see Disorder, mood
  aggressive, unsocialized F91.1
  alcohol use
    mild F10.10
      with
        alcohol intoxication F10.129
          delirium F10.121
        alcohol-induced
          anxiety disorder F10.180
          bipolar and related disorder F10.14
          depressive disorder F10.14
          psychotic disorder F10.159
          sexual dysfunction F10.181
          sleep disorder F10.182
      in remission (early) (sustained) F10.11
    moderate or severe F10.20
      with
        alcohol intoxication F10.229
          delirium F10.221
        alcohol-induced
          anxiety disorder F10.280
          bipolar and related disorder F10.24
          depressive disorder F10.24
          major neurocognitive disorder, amnestic-confabulatory type F10.26

**Disorder** — continued
  alcohol use — continued
    moderate or severe — continued
      with — continued
        alcohol-induced — continued
          major neurocognitive disorder, non-amnestic-confabulatory type F10.27
          mild neurocognitive disorder F10.288
          psychotic disorder F10.259
          sexual dysfunction F10.281
          sleep disorder F10.282
      in remission (early) (sustained) F10.21
  alcohol-related F10.99
    with
      amnestic disorder, persisting F10.96
      anxiety disorder F10.980
      dementia, persisting F10.97
      intoxication F10.929
        with delirium F10.921
        uncomplicated F10.920
      mood disorder F10.94
      other specified F10.988
      psychotic disorder F10.959
        with
          delusions F10.950
          hallucinations F10.951
      sexual dysfunction F10.981
      sleep disorder F10.982
  allergic — see Allergy
  alveolar NEC J84.09
  amino-acid
    cystathioninuria E72.19
    cystinosis E72.04
    cystinuria E72.01
    glycinuria E72.09
    homocystinuria E72.11
    metabolism — see Disturbance, metabolism, amino-acid
      specified NEC E72.8
    neonatal, transitory P74.8
    renal transport NEC E72.09
    transport NEC E72.09
  amnesic, amnestic
    alcohol-induced F10.96
      with dependence F10.26
    due to (secondary to) general medical condition F04
    psychoactive NEC-induced F19.96
      with
        abuse F19.16
        dependence F19.26
    sedative, hypnotic or anxiolytic-induced F13.96
      with dependence F13.26
  amphetamine (or other stimulant) use
    mild
      with
        amphetamine, cocaine, or other stimulant intoxication
          with perceptual disturbances F15.122
          without perceptual disturbances F15.129
        amphetamine (or other stimulant) -induced
          anxiety disorder F15.180
          bipolar and related disorder F15.14
          depressive disorder F15.14
          obsessive-compulsive and related disorder F15.188
          psychotic disorder F15.159
          sexual dysfunction F15.181
        intoxication delirium F15.121
    moderate or severe
      with
        amphetamine, cocaine, or other stimulant intoxication
          with perceptual disturbances F15.222
          without perceptual disturbances F15.229
        amphetamine (or other stimulant) -induced
          anxiety disorder F15.280
          bipolar and related disorder F15.24
          depressive disorder F15.24
          obsessive-compulsive and related disorder F15.288
          psychotic disorder F15.259
          sexual dysfunction F15.281
        intoxication delirium F15.221
  amphetamine-type substance use
    mild F15.10
      in remission (early) (sustained) F15.11
    moderate F15.20

**Disorder** — continued
  amphetamine-type substance use — continued
    moderate — continued
      in remission (early) (sustained) F15.21
    severe F15.20
      in remission (early) (sustained) F15.21
  anaerobic glycolysis with anemia D55.2
  anxiety F41.9
    due to (secondary to)
      alcohol F10.980
        in
          abuse F10.180
          dependence F10.280
      amphetamine F15.980
        in
          abuse F15.180
          dependence F15.280
      anxiolytic F13.980
        in
          abuse F13.180
          dependence F13.280
      caffeine F15.980
        in
          abuse F15.180
          dependence F15.280
      cannabis F12.980
        in
          abuse F12.180
          dependence F12.280
      cocaine F14.980
        in
          abuse F14.180
          dependence F14.180
      general medical condition F06.4
      hallucinogen F16.980
        in
          abuse F16.180
          dependence F16.280
      hypnotic F13.980
        in
          abuse F13.180
          dependence F13.280
      inhalant F18.980
        in
          abuse F18.180
          dependence F18.280
      phencyclidine F16.980
        in
          abuse F16.180
          dependence F16.280
      psychoactive substance NEC F19.980
        in
          abuse F19.180
          dependence F19.280
      sedative F13.980
        in
          abuse F13.180
          dependence F13.280
      volatile solvents F18.980
        in
          abuse F18.180
          dependence F18.280
    generalized F41.1
    illness F45.21
    mixed
      with depression (mild) F41.8
      specified NEC F41.3
    organic F06.4
    phobic F40.9
      of childhood F40.8
    specified NEC F41.8
  aortic valve — see Endocarditis, aortic
  aromatic amino-acid metabolism E70.9
    specified NEC E70.8
  arteriole NEC I77.89
  artery NEC I77.89
  articulation — see Disorder, joint
  attachment (childhood)
    disinhibited F94.2
    reactive F94.1
  attention-deficit hyperactivity (adolescent) (adult) (child) F90.9
    combined
      presentation F90.2
      type F90.2
    hyperactive
      impulsive presentation F90.1
      type F90.1

☑ **Additional Character Required** — Refer to the Tabular List for Character Selection    ▽ **Subterms under main terms may continue to next column or page**

**Disorder** — *continued*
  choroid — *continued*
    rupture — *see* Rupture, choroid
    scar — *see* Scar, chorioretinal
    solar retinopathy — *see* Retinopathy, solar
    specified type NEC H31.8
  ciliary body — *see* Disorder, iris
    degeneration — *see* Degeneration, ciliary body
  coagulation (factor) (*see also* Defect, coagulation)
    D68.9
    newborn, transient P61.6
  cocaine use
    mild F14.10
      with
        amphetamine, cocaine, or other stimulant
          intoxication
            with perceptual disturbances F14.122
            without perceptual disturbances F14.129
        cocaine intoxication delirium F14.121
        cocaine-induced
          anxiety disorder F14.180
          bipolar and related disorder F14.14
          depressive disorder F14.14
          obsessive-compulsive and related disor-
           der F14.188
          psychotic disorder F14.159
          sexual dysfunction F14.181
          sleep disorder F14.182
      in remission (early) (sustained) F14.11
    moderate or severe F14.20
      with
        amphetamine, cocaine, or other stimulant
          intoxication
            with perceptual disturbances F14.222
            without perceptual disturbances F14.229
        cocaine intoxication delirium F14.221
        cocaine-induced
          anxiety disorder F14.280
          bipolar and related disorder F14.24
          depressive disorder F14.24
          obsessive-compulsive and related disor-
           der F14.288
          psychotic disorder F14.259
          sexual dysfunction F14.281
          sleep disorder F14.282
      in remission (early) (sustained) F14.21
  coccyx NEC M53.3
  cognitive F09
    due to (secondary to) general medical condition
      F09
    persisting R41.89
      due to
        alcohol F10.97
          with dependence F10.27
        anxiolytics F13.97
          with dependence F13.27
        hypnotics F13.97
          with dependence F13.27
        sedatives F13.97
          with dependence F13.27
        specified substance NEC F19.97
          with
            abuse F19.17
            dependence F19.27
  communication F80.9
    social pragmatic F80.82
  conduct (childhood) F91.9
    adjustment reaction — *see* Disorder, adjustment
    adolescent onset type F91.2
    childhood onset type F91.1
    compulsive F63.9
    confined to family context F91.0
    depressive F91.8
    group type F91.2
    hyperkinetic — *see* Disorder, attention-deficit hy-
      peractivity
    oppositional defiance F91.3
    socialized F91.2
    solitary aggressive type F91.1
    specified NEC F91.8
    unsocialized (aggressive) F91.1
  conduction, heart I45.9
  congenital glycosylation (CDG) E74.8
  conjunctiva H11.9
    infection — *see* Conjunctivitis
  connective tissue, localized L94.9
    specified NEC L94.8

**Disorder** — *continued*
  conversion (functional neurological symptom disorder)
    with
      abnormal movement F44.4
      anesthesia or sensory loss F44.6
      attacks or seizures F44.5
      mixed symptoms F44.7
      special sensory symptoms F44.6
      speech symptoms F44.4
      swallowing symptoms F44.4
      weakness or paralysis F44.4
  convulsive (secondary) — *see* Convulsions
  cornea H18.9
    deformity — *see* Deformity, cornea
    degeneration — *see* Degeneration, cornea
    deposits — *see* Deposit, cornea
    due to contact lens H18.82- ☑
      specified as edema — *see* Edema, cornea
    edema — *see* Edema, cornea
    keratitis — *see* Keratitis
    keratoconjunctivitis — *see* Keratoconjunctivitis
    membrane change — *see* Change, corneal mem-
      brane
    neovascularization — *see* Neovascularization,
      cornea
    scar — *see* Opacity, cornea
    specified type NEC H18.89- ☑
    ulcer — *see* Ulcer, cornea
  corpus cavernosum N48.9
  cranial nerve — *see* Disorder, nerve, cranial
  cyclothymic F34.0
  defiant oppositional F91.3
  delusional (persistent) (systematized) F22
    induced F24
  depersonalization F48.1
  depressive F32.9
    due to known physiological condition
      with
        depressive features F06.31
        major depressive-like episode F06.32
        mixed features F06.34
    major F32.9
      with psychotic symptoms F32.3
      in remission (full) F32.5
        partial F32.4
      recurrent F33.9
        with psychotic features F33.3
      single episode F32.9
        mild F32.0
        moderate F32.1
        severe (without psychotic symptoms) F32.2
          with psychotic symptoms F32.3
    organic F06.31
    persistent F34.1
    recurrent F33.9
      current episode
        mild F33.0
        moderate F33.1
        severe (without psychotic symptoms) F33.2
          with psychotic symptoms F33.3
      in remission F33.40
        full F33.42
        partial F33.41
      specified NEC F33.8
    single episode — *see* Episode, depressive
    specified NEC F32.89
  developmental F89
    arithmetical skills F81.2
    coordination (motor) F82
    expressive writing F81.81
    language F80.9
      expressive F80.1
      mixed receptive and expressive F80.2
      receptive type F80.2
      specified NEC F80.89
    learning F81.9
      arithmetical F81.2
      reading F81.0
    mixed F88
    motor coordination or function F82
    pervasive F84.9
      specified NEC F84.8
    phonological F80.0
    reading F81.0
    scholastic skills (*see also* Disorder, learning)
      mixed F81.89
    specified NEC F88
    speech F80.9

**Disorder** — *continued*
  developmental — *continued*
    speech — *continued*
      articulation F80.0
      specified NEC F80.89
    written expression F81.81
  diaphragm J98.6
  digestive (system) K92.9
    newborn P78.9
      specified NEC P78.89
    postprocedural — *see* Complication, gastrointesti-
      nal
    psychogenic F45.8
  disc (intervertebral) M51.9
    with
      myelopathy
        cervical region M50.00
        cervicothoracic region M50.03
        high cervical region M50.01
        lumbar region M51.06
        mid-cervical region M50.020
        sacrococcygeal region M53.3
        thoracic region M51.04
        thoracolumbar region M51.05
      radiculopathy
        cervical region M50.10
        cervicothoracic region M50.13
        high cervical region M50.11
        lumbar region M51.16
        lumbosacral region M51.17
        mid-cervical region M50.120
        sacrococcygeal region M53.3
        thoracic region M51.14
        thoracolumbar region M51.15
    cervical M50.90
      with
        myelopathy M50.00
          C2-C3 M50.01
          C3-C4 M50.01
          C4-C5 M50.021
          C5-C6 M50.022
          C6-C7 M50.023
          C7-T1 M50.03
          cervicothoracic region M50.03
          high cervical region M50.01
          mid-cervical region M50.020
        neuritis, radiculitis or radiculopathy M50.10
          C2-C3 M50.11
          C3-C4 M50.11
          C4-C5 M50.121
          C5-C6 M50.122
          C6-C7 M50.123
          C7-T1 M50.13
          cervicothoracic region M50.13
          high cervical region M50.11
          mid-cervical region M50.120
      C2-C3 M50.91
      C3-C4 M50.91
      C4-C5 M50.921
      C5-C6 M50.922
      C6-C7 M50.923
      C7-T1 M50.93
      cervicothoracic region M50.93
      degeneration M50.30
        C2-C3 M50.31
        C3-C4 M50.31
        C4-C5 M50.321
        C5-C6 M50.322
        C6-C7 M50.323
        C7-T1 M50.33
        cervicothoracic region M50.33
        high cervical region M50.31
        mid-cervical region M50.320
      displacement M50.20
        C2-C3 M50.21
        C3-C4 M50.21
        C4-C5 M50.221
        C5-C6 M50.222
        C6-C7 M50.223
        C7-T1 M50.23
        cervicothoracic region M50.23
        high cervical region M50.21
        mid-cervical region M50.220
      high cervical region M50.91
      mid-cervical region M50.920
      specified type NEC M50.80
        C2-C3 M50.81
        C3-C4 M50.81
        C4-C5 M50.821

**Disorder** — *continued*
  disc — *continued*
    cervical — *continued*
      specified type — *continued*
        C5-C6 M50.822
        C6-C7 M50.823
        C7-T1 M50.83
        cervicothoracic region M50.83
        high cervical region M50.81
        mid-cervical region M50.820
      specified NEC
        lumbar region M51.86
        lumbosacral region M51.87
        sacrococcygeal region M53.3
        thoracic region M51.84
        thoracolumbar region M51.85
  disinhibited attachment (childhood) F94.2
  disintegrative, childhood NEC F84.3
  disruptive F91.9
    mood dysregulation F34.81
    specified NEC F91.8
  disruptive behavior — *see* Disorder, conduct
  dissocial personality F60.2
  dissociative F44.9
    affecting
      motor function F44.4
        and sensation F44.7
      sensation F44.6
        and motor function F44.7
    brief reactive F43.0
    due to (secondary to) general medical condition F06.8
    mixed F44.7
    organic F06.8
    other specified NEC F44.89
  double heterozygous sickling — *see* Disease, sickle-cell
  dream anxiety F51.5
  drug induced hemorrhagic D68.32
  drug related F19.99
    abuse — *see* Abuse, drug
    dependence — *see* Dependence, drug
  dysmorphic body F45.22
  dysthymic F34.1
  ear H93.9- ☑
    bleeding — *see* Otorrhagia
    deafness — *see* Deafness
    degenerative H93.09- ☑
    discharge — *see* Otorrhea
    external H61.9- ☑
      auditory canal stenosis — *see* Stenosis, external ear canal
      exostosis — *see* Exostosis, external ear canal
      impacted cerumen — *see* Impaction, cerumen
      otitis — *see* Otitis, externa
      perichondritis — *see* Perichondritis, ear
      pinna — *see* Disorder, pinna
      specified type NEC H61.89- ☑
    inner H83.9- ☑
      vestibular dysfunction — *see* Disorder, vestibular function
    middle H74.9- ☑
      adhesive H74.1- ☑
      ossicle — *see* Abnormal, ear ossicles
      polyp — *see* Polyp, ear (middle)
      specified NEC, in diseases classified elsewhere H75.8- ☑
    postprocedural — *see* Complications, ear, procedure
    specified NEC, in diseases classified elsewhere H94.8- ☑
  eating (adult) (psychogenic) F50.9
    anorexia — *see* Anorexia
    binge F50.81
    bulimia F50.2
    child F98.29
      pica F98.3
      rumination disorder F98.21
    pica F50.89
      childhood F98.3
  electrolyte (balance) NEC E87.8
    with
      abortion — *see* Abortion by type complicated by specified condition NEC
      ectopic pregnancy O08.5
      molar pregnancy O08.5
    acidosis (metabolic) (respiratory) E87.2
    alkalosis (metabolic) (respiratory) E87.3

**Disorder** — *continued*
  elimination, transepidermal L87.9
    specified NEC L87.8
  emotional (persistent) F34.9
    of childhood F93.9
      specified NEC F93.8
  endocrine E34.9
    postprocedural E89.89
    specified NEC E89.89
  erectile (male) (organic) (*see also* Dysfunction, sexual, male, erectile) N52.9
    nonorganic F52.21
  erythematous — *see* Erythema
  esophagus K22.9
    functional K22.4
    psychogenic F45.8
  eustachian tube H69.9- ☑
    infection — *see* Salpingitis, eustachian
    obstruction — *see* Obstruction, eustachian tube
    patulous — *see* Patulous, eustachian tube
    specified NEC H69.8- ☑
  exhibitionistic F65.2
  extrapyramidal G25.9
    in deseases classified elsewhere — *see* category G26
    specified type NEC G25.89
  eye H57.9
    postprocedural — *see* Complication, postprocedural, eye
  eyelid H02.9
    cyst — *see* Cyst, eyelid
    degenerative H02.70
      chloasma — *see* Chloasma, eyelid
      madarosis — *see* Madarosis
      specified type NEC H02.79
      vitiligo — *see* Vitiligo, eyelid
      xanthelasma — *see* Xanthelasma
    dermatochalasis — *see* Dermatochalasis
    edema — *see* Edema, eyelid
    elephantiasis — *see* Elephantiasis, eyelid
    foreign body, retained — *see* Foreign body, retained, eyelid
    function H02.59
      abnormal innervation syndrome — *see* Syndrome, abnormal innervation
      blepharochalasis — *see* Blepharochalasis
      blepharoclonus — *see* Blepharoclonus
      blepharophimosis — *see* Blepharophimosis
      blepharoptosis — *see* Blepharoptosis
      lagophthalmos — *see* Lagophthalmos
      lid retraction — *see* Retraction, lid
    hypertrichosis — *see* Hypertrichosis, eyelid
    specified type NEC H02.89
    vascular H02.879
      left H02.876
        lower H02.875
        upper H02.874
      right H02.873
        lower H02.872
        upper H02.871
  factitious F68.10
    with predominantly
      physical symptoms F68.12
        with psychological symptoms F68.13
      psychological symptoms F68.11
        with physical symptoms F68.13
  factor, coagulation — *see* Defect, coagulation
  fatty acid
    metabolism E71.30
      specified NEC E71.39
    oxidation
      LCAD E71.310
      MCAD E71.311
      SCAD E71.312
      specified deficiency NEC E71.318
  feeding (infant or child) (*see also* Disorder, eating) R63.3
    or eating disorder F50.9
    specified NEC F50.9
  feigned (with obvious motivation) Z76.5
    without obvious motivation — *see* Disorder, factitious
  female
    hypoactive sexual desire F52.0
    orgasmic F52.31
    sexual interest/arousal F52.22
  fetishistic F65.0
  fibroblastic M72.9

**Disorder** — *continued*
  fibroblastic — *continued*
    specified NEC M72.8
  fluency
    adult onset F98.5
    childhood onset F80.81
    following
      cerebral infarction I69.323
      cerebrovascular disease I69.923
        specified disease NEC I69.823
      intracerebral hemorrhage I69.123
      nontraumatic intracranial hemorrhage NEC I69.223
      subarachnoid hemorrhage I69.023
    in conditions classified elsewhere R47.82
  fluid balance E87.8
  follicular (skin) L73.9
    specified NEC L73.8
  frotteuristic F65.81
  fructose metabolism E74.10
    essential fructosuria E74.11
    fructokinase deficiency E74.11
    fructose-1, 6-diphosphatase deficiency E74.19
    hereditary fructose intolerance E74.12
    other specified E74.19
  functional polymorphonuclear neutrophils D71
  gallbladder, biliary tract and pancreas in diseases classified elsewhere K87
  gambling F63.0
  gamma-glutamyl cycle E72.8
  gastric (functional) K31.9
    motility K30
    psychogenic F45.8
    secretion K30
  gastrointestinal (functional) NOS K92.9
    newborn P78.9
    psychogenic F45.8
  gender-identity or -role F64.9
    childhood F64.2
    effect on relationship F66
    of adolescence or adulthood F64.0
      nontranssexual F64.8
    specified NEC F64.8
    uncertainty F66
  genito-pelvic pain penetration F52.6
  genitourinary system
    female N94.9
    male N50.9
    psychogenic F45.8
  globe H44.9
    degenerated condition H44.50
      absolute glaucoma H44.51- ☑
      atrophy H44.52- ☑
      leucocoria H44.53- ☑
    degenerative H44.30
      chalcosis H44.31- ☑
      myopia (*see also* Myopia, degenerative) H44.2- ☑
      siderosis H44.32- ☑
      specified type NEC H44.39- ☑
    endophthalmitis — *see* Endophthalmitis
    foreign body, retained — *see* Foreign body, intraocular, old, retained
    hemophthalmos — *see* Hemophthalmos
    hypotony H44.40
      due to
        ocular fistula H44.42- ☑
        specified disorder NEC H44.43- ☑
      flat anterior chamber H44.41- ☑
      primary H44.44- ☑
    luxation — *see* Luxation, globe
    specified type NEC H44.89
  glomerular (in) N05.9
    amyloidosis E85.4 [N08]
    cryoglobulinemia D89.1 [N08]
    disseminated intravascular coagulation D65 [N08]
    Fabry's disease E75.21 [N08]
    familial lecithin cholesterol acyltransferase deficiency E78.6 [N08]
    Goodpasture's syndrome M31.0
    hemolytic-uremic syndrome D59.3
    Henoch (-Schönlein) purpura D69.0 [N08]
    malariae malaria B52.0
    microscopic polyangiitis M31.7 [N08]
    multiple myeloma C90.0- ☑ [N08]
    mumps B26.83
    schistosomiasis B65.9 [N08]
    sepsis NEC A41.- ☑ [N08]

☑ **Additional Character Required — Refer to the Tabular List for Character Selection**    ▽ **Subterms under main terms may continue to next column or page**

**Disorder** — *continued*
  glomerular — *continued*
    sepsis — *continued*
      streptococcal A40.- ☑ [N08]
      sickle-cell disorders D57.- ☑ [N08]
      strongyloidiasis B78.9 [N08]
      subacute bacterial endocarditis I33.0 [N08]
      syphilis A52.75
      systemic lupus erythematosus M32.14
      thrombotic thrombocytopenic purpura
        M31.1 [N08]
      Waldenström macroglobulinemia C88.0 [N08]
      Wegener's granulomatosis M31.31
  gluconeogenesis E74.4
  glucosaminoglycan metabolism — *see* Disorder,
    metabolism, glucosaminoglycan
  glycine metabolism E72.50
    d-glycericacidemia E72.59
    hyperhydroxyprolinemia E72.59
    hyperoxaluria E72.53
    hyperprolinemia E72.59
    non-ketotic hyperglycinemia E72.51
    oxalosis E72.53
    oxaluria E72.53
    sarcosinemia E72.59
    trimethylaminuria E72.52
  glycoprotein metabolism E77.9
    specified NEC E77.8
  habit (and impulse) F63.9
    involving sexual behavior NEC F65.9
    specified NEC F63.89
  hallucinogen use
    mild F16.10
      with
        hallucinogen intoxication delirium F16.121
        hallucinogen-induced
          anxiety disorder F16.180
          bipolar and related disorder F16.14
          depressive disorder F16.14
          psychotic disorder F16.159
        other hallucinogen intoxication F16.129
      in remission (early) (sustained) F16.11
    moderate or severe F16.20
      with
        hallucinogen intoxication delirium F16.221
        hallucinogen-induced
          anxiety disorder F16.280
          bipolar and related disorder F16.24
          depressive disorder F16.24
          psychotic disorder F16.259
        other hallucinogen intoxication F16.229
      in remission (early) (sustained) F16.21
  heart action I49.9
  hematological D75.9
    newborn (transient) P61.9
      specified NEC P61.8
  hematopoietic organs D75.9
  hemorrhagic NEC D69.9
    drug-induced D68.32
    due to
      extrinsic circulating anticoagulants D68.32
      increase in
        anti-IIa D68.32
        anti-Xa D68.32
      intrinsic
        circulating anticoagulants D68.318
        increase in
          anti-IXa D68.318
          antithrombin D68.318
          anti-VIIIa D68.318
          anti-XIa D68.318
    following childbirth O72.3
  hemostasis — *see* Defect, coagulation
  histidine metabolism E70.40
    histidinemia E70.41
    other specified E70.49
  hoarding F42.3
  hyperkinetic — *see* Disorder, attention-deficit hyper-
    activity
  hyperleucine-isoleucinemia E71.19
  hypervalinemia E71.19
  hypoactive sexual desire F52.0
  hypochondriacal F45.20
    body dysmorphic F45.22
    neurosis F45.21
    other specified F45.29
  identity
    dissociative F44.81
    illness anxiety F45.21

**Disorder** — *continued*
  identity — *continued*
    of childhood F93.8
  immune mechanism (immunity) D89.9
    specified type NEC D89.89
  impaired renal tubular function N25.9
    specified NEC N25.89
  impulse (control) F63.9
  inflammatory
    pelvic, in diseases classified elsewhere — *see* cate-
      gory N74
    penis N48.29
      abscess N48.21
      cellulitis N48.22
  inhalant use
    mild F18.10
      with
        inhalant intoxication F18.129
        inhalant intoxication delirium F18.121
        inhalant-induced
          anxiety disorder F18.180
          depressive disorder F18.14
          major neurocognitive disorder F18.17
          mild neurocognitive disorder F18.188
          psychotic disorder F18.159
      in remission (early) (sustained) F18.11
    moderate or severe F18.20
      with
        inhalant intoxication F18.229
        inhalant intoxication delirium F18.221
        inhalant-induced
          anxiety disorder F18.280
          depressive disorder F18.24
          major neurocognitive disorder F18.27
          mild neurocognitive disorder F18.288
          psychotic disorder F18.259
      in remission (early) (sustained) F18.21
  integument, newborn P83.9
    specified NEC P83.88
  intermittent explosive F63.81
  internal secretion pancreas — *see* Increased, secretion,
    pancreas, endocrine
  intestine, intestinal
    carbohydrate absorption NEC E74.39
      postoperative K91.2
    functional NEC K59.9
      postoperative K91.89
    psychogenic F45.8
    vascular K55.9
      chronic K55.1
      specified NEC K55.8
  intraoperative (intraprocedural) — *see* Complications,
    intraoperative
  involuntary emotional expression (IEED) F07.89
  iris H21.9
    adhesions — *see* Adhesions, iris
    atrophy — *see* Atrophy, iris
    chamber angle recession — *see* Recession, cham-
      ber angle
    cyst — *see* Cyst, iris
    degeneration — *see* Degeneration, iris
    in diseases classified elsewhere H22
    iridodialysis — *see* Iridodialysis
    iridoschisis — *see* Iridoschisis
    miotic pupillary cyst — *see* Cyst, pupillary
    pupillary
      abnormality — *see* Abnormality, pupillary
      membrane — *see* Membrane, pupillary
    specified type NEC H21.89
    vascular NEC H21.1X- ☑
  iron metabolism E83.10
    specified NEC E83.19
  isovaleric acidemia E71.110
  jaw, developmental M27.0
    temporomandibular (*see also* Anomaly, dentofacial,
      temporomandibular joint) M26.60- ☑
  joint M25.9
    derangement — *see* Derangement, joint
    effusion — *see* Effusion, joint
    fistula — *see* Fistula, joint
    hemarthrosis — *see* Hemarthrosis
    instability — *see* Instability, joint
    osteophyte — *see* Osteophyte
    pain — *see* Pain, joint
    psychogenic F45.8
    specified type NEC M25.80
      ankle M25.87- ☑
      elbow M25.82- ☑

**Disorder** — *continued*
  joint — *continued*
    specified type — *continued*
      foot joint M25.87- ☑
      hand joint M25.84- ☑
      hip M25.85- ☑
      knee M25.86- ☑
      shoulder M25.81- ☑
      wrist M25.83- ☑
    stiffness — *see* Stiffness, joint
  ketone metabolism E71.32
  kidney N28.9
    functional (tubular) N25.9
    in
      schistosomiasis B65.9 [N29]
    tubular function N25.9
      specified NEC N25.89
  lacrimal system H04.9
    changes H04.69
      fistula — *see* Fistula, lacrimal
    gland H04.19
      atrophy — *see* Atrophy, lacrimal gland
      cyst — *see* Cyst, lacrimal, gland
      dacryops — *see* Dacryops
      dislocation — *see* Dislocation, lacrimal gland
      dry eye syndrome — *see* Syndrome, dry eye
      infection — *see* Dacryoadenitis
      granuloma — *see* Granuloma, lacrimal
      inflammation — *see* Inflammation, lacrimal
      obstruction — *see* Obstruction, lacrimal
    specified NEC H04.89
  lactation NEC O92.79
  language (developmental) F80.9
    expressive F80.1
    mixed receptive and expressive F80.2
    receptive F80.2
  late luteal phase dysphoric N94.89
  learning (specific) F81.9
    acalculia R48.8
    alexia R48.0
    mathematics F81.2
    reading F81.0
    specified
      with impairment in
        mathematics F81.2
        reading F81.0
        written expression F81.81
    specified NEC F81.89
    spelling F81.81
    written expression F81.81
  lens H27.9
    aphakia — *see* Aphakia
    cataract — *see* Cataract
    dislocation — *see* Dislocation, lens
    specified type NEC H27.8
  ligament M24.20
    ankle M24.27- ☑
    attachment, spine — *see* Enthesopathy, spinal
    elbow M24.22- ☑
    foot joint M24.27- ☑
    hand joint M24.24- ☑
    hip M24.25- ☑
    knee — *see* Derangement, knee, specified NEC
    shoulder M24.21- ☑
    vertebra M24.28
    wrist M24.23- ☑
  ligamentous attachments (*see also* Enthesopathy)
    spine — *see* Enthesopathy, spinal
  lipid
    metabolism, congenital E78.9
    storage E75.6
      specified NEC E75.5
  lipoprotein
    deficiency (familial) E78.6
    metabolism E78.9
      specified NEC E78.89
  liver K76.9
    malarial B54 [K77]
  low back (*see also* Dorsopathy, specified NEC)
  lumbosacral
    plexus G54.1
    root (nerve) NEC G54.4
  lung, interstitial, drug-induced J70.4
    acute J70.2
    chronic J70.3
  lymphoproliferative, post-transplant (PTLD) D47.Z1
    (*following* D47.4)
  lysine and hydroxylysine metabolism E72.3

**Disorder** — *continued*
major neurocognitive — *see* Dementia, in (due to)
male
  erectile (organic) (*see also* Dysfunction, sexual,
    male, erectile) N52.9
    nonorganic F52.21
  hypoactive sexual desire F52.0
  orgasmic F52.32
manic F30.9
  organic F06.33
mast cell activation — *see* Activation, mast cell
mastoid (*see also* Disorder, ear, middle)
  postprocedural — *see* Complications, ear, proce-
    dure
meniscus — *see* Derangement, knee, meniscus
menopausal N95.9
  specified NEC N95.8
menstrual N92.6
  psychogenic F45.8
  specified NEC N92.5
mental (or behavioral) (nonpsychotic) F99
  due to (secondary to)
    amphetamine
      due to drug abuse — *see* Abuse, drug,
        stimulant
      due to drug dependence — *see* Depen-
        dence, drug, stimulant
    brain disease, damage and dysfunction F09
    caffeine use
      due to drug abuse — *see* Abuse, drug,
        stimulant
      due to drug dependence — *see* Depen-
        dence, drug, stimulant
    cannabis use
      due to drug abuse — *see* Abuse, drug,
        cannabis
      due to drug dependence — *see* Depen-
        dence, drug, cannabis
    general medical condition F09
    sedative or hypnotic use
      due to drug abuse — *see* Abuse, drug,
        sedative
      due to drug dependence — *see* Depen-
        dence, drug, sedative
    tobacco (nicotine) use — *see* Dependence,
      drug, nicotine
  following organic brain damage F07.9
    frontal lobe syndrome F07.0
    personality change F07.0
    postconcussional syndrome F07.81
    specified NEC F07.89
  infancy, childhood or adolescence F98.9
  neurotic — *see* Neurosis
  organic or symptomatic F09
  presenile, psychotic F03 ☑
  problem NEC
  psychoneurotic — *see* Neurosis
  psychotic — *see* Psychosis
  puerperal F53
  senile, psychotic NEC F03 ☑
metabolic, amino acid, transitory, newborn P74.8
metabolism NOS E88.9
  amino-acid E72.9
    aromatic E70.9
      albinism — *see* Albinism
      histidine E70.40
        histidinemia E70.41
        other specified E70.49
      hyperphenylalaninemia E70.1
        classical phenylketonuria E70.0
      other specified E70.8
      tryptophan E70.5
      tyrosine E70.20
        hypertyrosinemia E70.21
        other specified E70.29
    branched chain E71.2
      3-methylglutaconic aciduria E71.111
      hyperleucine-isoleucinemia E71.19
      hypervalinemia E71.19
      isovaleric acidemia E71.110
      maple syrup urine disease E71.0
      methylmalonic acidemia E71.120
      organic aciduria NEC E71.118
      other specified E71.19
      proprionate NEC E71.128
      proprionic acidemia E71.121
    glycine E72.50
      d-glycericacidemia E72.59

**Disorder** — *continued*
metabolism — *continued*
  amino-acid — *continued*
    glycine — *continued*
      hyperhydroxyprolinemia E72.59
      hyperoxaluria E72.53
      hyperprolinemia E72.59
      non-ketotic hyperglycinemia E72.51
      other specified E72.59
      sarcosinemia E72.59
      trimethylaminuria E72.52
    hydroxylysine E72.3
    lysine E72.3
    ornithine E72.4
    other specified E72.8
      beta-amino acid E72.8
      gamma-glutamyl cycle E72.8
    straight-chain E72.8
    sulfur-bearing E72.10
      homocystinuria E72.11
      methylenetetrahydrofolate reductase defi-
        ciency E72.12
      other specified E72.19
  bile acid and cholesterol metabolism E78.70
  bilirubin E80.7
    specified NEC E80.6
  calcium E83.50
    hypercalcemia E83.52
    hypocalcemia E83.51
    other specified E83.59
  carbohydrate E74.9
    specified NEC E74.8
  cholesterol and bile acid metabolism E78.70
  congenital E88.9
  copper E83.00
    specified type NEC E83.09
    Wilson's disease E83.01
  cystinuria E72.01
  fructose E74.10
  galactose E74.20
  glucosaminoglycan E76.9
    mucopolysaccharidosis — *see* Mucopolysaccha-
      ridosis
    specified NEC E76.8
  glutamine E72.8
  glycine E72.50
  glycogen storage (hepatorenal) E74.09
  glycoprotein E77.9
    specified NEC E77.8
  glycosaminoglycan E76.9
    specified NEC E76.8
  in labor and delivery O75.89
  iron E83.10
  isoleucine E71.19
  leucine E71.19
  lipoid E78.9
  lipoprotein E78.9
    specified NEC E78.89
  magnesium E83.40
    hypermagnesemia E83.41
    hypomagnesemia E83.42
    other specified E83.49
  mineral E83.9
    specified NEC E83.89
  mitochondrial E88.40
    MELAS syndrome E88.41
    MERRF syndrome (myoclonic epilepsy associat-
      ed with ragged-red fibers) E88.42
    other specified E88.49
  ornithine E72.4
  phosphatases E83.30
  phosphorus E83.30
    acid phosphatase deficiency E83.39
    hypophosphatasia E83.39
    hypophosphatemia E83.39
      familial E83.31
    other specified E83.39
    pseudovitamin D deficiency E83.32
  plasma protein NEC E88.09
  porphyrin — *see* Porphyria
  postprocedural E89.89
    specified NEC E89.89
  purine E79.9
    specified NEC E79.8
  pyrimidine E79.9
    specified NEC E79.8
  pyruvate E74.4
  serine E72.8
  sodium E87.8

**Disorder** — *continued*
metabolism — *continued*
  specified NEC E88.89
  threonine E72.8
  valine E71.19
  zinc E83.2
methylmalonic acidemia E71.120
micturition NEC (*see also* Difficulty, micturition)
  R39.198
  feeling of incomplete emptying R39.14
  hesitancy R39.11
  poor stream R39.12
  psychogenic F45.8
  split stream R39.13
  straining R39.16
  urgency R39.15
mild neurocognitive G31.84
mitochondrial metabolism E88.40
mitral (valve) — *see* Endocarditis, mitral
mixed
  anxiety and depressive F41.8
  of scholastic skills (developmental) F81.89
  receptive expressive language F80.2
mood F39
  bipolar — *see* Disorder, bipolar
  depressive — *see* Disorder, depressive
  due to (secondary to)
    alcohol F10.94
    amphetamine F15.94
      in
        abuse F15.14
        dependence F15.24
    anxiolytic F13.94
      in
        abuse F13.14
        dependence F13.24
    cocaine F14.94
      in
        abuse F14.14
        dependence F14.24
    general medical condition F06.30
    hallucinogen F16.94
      in
        abuse F16.14
        dependence F16.24
    hypnotic F13.94
      in
        abuse F13.14
        dependence F13.24
    inhalant F18.94
      in
        abuse F18.14
        dependence F18.24
    opioid F11.94
      in
        abuse F11.14
        dependence F11.24
    phencyclidine (PCP) F16.94
      in
        abuse F16.14
        dependence F16.24
    physiological condition F06.30
      with
        depressive features F06.31
        major depressive-like episode F06.32
        manic features F06.33
        mixed features F06.34
    psychoactive substance NEC F19.94
      in
        abuse F19.14
        dependence F19.24
    sedative F13.94
      in
        abuse F13.14
        dependence F13.24
    volatile solvents F18.94
      in
        abuse F18.14
        dependence F18.24
  manic episode F30.9
    with psychotic symptoms F30.2
    without psychotic symptoms F30.10
      mild F30.11
      moderate F30.12
      severe F30.13
    in remission (full) F30.4
      partial F30.3
    specified type NEC F30.8
  organic F06.30

☑ **Additional Character Required** — **Refer to the Tabular List for Character Selection**      ▽ **Subterms under main terms may continue to next column or page**

**Disorder** — *continued*
  mood — *continued*
    organic — *continued*
      right hemisphere F07.89
    persistent F34.9
      cyclothymia F34.0
      dysthymia F34.1
      specified type NEC F34.89
    recurrent F39
    right hemisphere organic F07.89
  movement G25.9
    drug-induced G25.70
      akathisia G25.71
      specified NEC G25.79
    hysterical F44.4
    in diseases classified elsewhere — *see* category
      G26
    periodic limb G47.61
      sleep related G47.61
    sleep related NEC G47.69
    specified NEC G25.89
    stereotyped F98.4
    treatment-induced G25.9
  multiple personality F44.81
  muscle M62.9
    attachment, spine — *see* Enthesopathy, spinal
    in trichinellosis — *see* Trichinellosis, with muscle
      disorder
    psychogenic F45.8
    specified type NEC M62.89
    tone, newborn P94.9
      specified NEC P94.8
  muscular
    attachments (*see also* Enthesopathy)
      spine — *see* Enthesopathy, spinal
    urethra N36.44
  musculoskeletal system, soft tissue — *see* Disorder,
    soft tissue
    postprocedural M96.89
    psychogenic F45.8
  myoneural G70.9
    due to lead G70.1
    specified NEC G70.89
    toxic G70.1
  myotonic NEC G71.19
  nail, in diseases classified elsewhere L62
  neck region NEC — *see* Dorsopathy, specified NEC
  neonatal onset multisystemic inflammatory (NOMID)
    M04.2
  nerve G58.9
    abducent NEC — *see* Strabismus, paralytic, sixth
      nerve
    accessory G52.8
    acoustic — *see* subcategory H93.3 ☑
    auditory — *see* subcategory H93.3 ☑
    auriculotemporal G50.8
    axillary G54.0
    cerebral — *see* Disorder, nerve, cranial
    cranial G52.9
      eighth — *see* subcategory H93.3 ☑
      eleventh G52.8
      fifth G50.9
      first G52.0
      fourth NEC — *see* Strabismus, paralytic, fourth
        nerve
      multiple G52.7
      ninth G52.1
      second NEC — *see* Disorder, nerve, optic
      seventh NEC G51.8
      sixth NEC — *see* Strabismus, paralytic, sixth
        nerve
      specified NEC G52.8
      tenth G52.2
      third NEC — *see* Strabismus, paralytic, third
        nerve
      twelfth G52.3
    entrapment — *see* Neuropathy, entrapment
    facial G51.9
      specified NEC G51.8
    femoral — *see* Lesion, nerve, femoral
    glossopharyngeal NEC G52.1
    hypoglossal G52.3
    intercostal G58.0
    lateral
      cutaneous of thigh — *see* Mononeuropathy,
        lower limb, meralgia paresthetica
      popliteal — *see* Lesion, nerve, popliteal
    lower limb — *see* Mononeuropathy, lower limb

  nerve — *continued*
    medial popliteal — *see* Lesion, nerve, popliteal,
      medial
    median NEC — *see* Lesion, nerve, median
    multiple G58.7
    oculomotor NEC — *see* Strabismus, paralytic, third
      nerve
    olfactory G52.0
    optic NEC H47.09- ☑
      hemorrhage into sheath — *see* Hemorrhage,
        optic nerve
      ischemic H47.01- ☑
    peroneal — *see* Lesion, nerve, popliteal
    phrenic G58.8
    plantar — *see* Lesion, nerve, plantar
    pneumogastric G52.2
    posterior tibial — *see* Syndrome, tarsal tunnel
    radial — *see* Lesion, nerve, radial
    recurrent laryngeal G52.2
    root G54.9
      cervical G54.2
      lumbosacral G54.1
      specified NEC G54.8
      thoracic G54.3
    sciatic NEC — *see* Lesion, nerve, sciatic
    specified NEC G58.8
      lower limb — *see* Mononeuropathy, lower limb,
        specified NEC
      upper limb — *see* Mononeuropathy, upper
        limb, specified NEC
    sympathetic G90.9
    tibial — *see* Lesion, nerve, popliteal, medial
    trigeminal G50.9
      specified NEC G50.8
    trochlear NEC — *see* Strabismus, paralytic, fourth
      nerve
    ulnar — *see* Lesion, nerve, ulnar
    upper limb — *see* Mononeuropathy, upper limb
    vagus G52.2
  nervous system G98.8
    autonomic (peripheral) G90.9
      specified NEC G90.8
    central G96.9
      specified NEC G96.8
    parasympathetic G90.9
    specified NEC G98.8
    sympathetic G90.9
    vegetative G90.9
  neurocognitive R41.9
    major
      with
        aggressive behavior F01.51
        combative behavior F01.51
        violent behavior F01.51
      without behavioral disturbance F01.50
      due to vascular disease, with behavioral distur-
        bance F01.51
      in (due to) (other diseases classified elsewhere)
        (*see also* Dementia, in (due to)) F02.80
        with
          aggressive behavior F02.81
          combative behavior F02.81
          violent behavior F02.81
    mild G31.84
  neurodevelopmental F89
    specified NEC F88
  neurohypophysis NEC E23.3
  neurological NEC R29.818
  neuromuscular G70.9
    hereditary NEC G71.9
    specified NEC G70.89
    toxic G70.1
  neurotic F48.9
    specified NEC F48.8
  neutrophil, polymorphonuclear D71
  nicotine use — *see* Dependence, drug, nicotine
  nightmare F51.5
  non-rapid eye movement sleep arousal
    sleep terror type F51.4
    sleepwalking type F51.3
  nose J34.9
    specified NEC J34.89
  obsessive-compulsive F42.9
    and related disorder due to a known physiological
      condition F06.8
  odontogenesis NOS K00.9

  opioid use
    with
      opioid-induced psychotic disorder F11.959
        with
          delusions F11.950
          hallucinations F11.951
    due to drug abuse — *see* Abuse, drug, opioid
    due to drug dependence — *see* Dependence, drug,
      opioid
    mild F11.10
      with
        opioid intoxication
          with perceptual disturbances F11.122
          without perceptual disturbances F11.129
          delirium F11.121
        opioid-induced
          anxiety disorder F11.188
          depressive disorder F11.14
          sexual dysfunction F11.181
      in remission (early) (sustained) F11.11
    moderate or severe F11.20
      with
        opioid intoxication
          with perceptual disturbances F11.222
          without perceptual disturbances F11.229
          delirium F11.221
        opioid-induced
          anxiety disorder F11.288
          anxiety disorder F11.988
          depressive disorder F11.24
          depressive disorder F11.94
          sexual dysfunction F11.281
          sexual dysfunction F11.981
      in remission (early) (sustained) F11.21
  oppositional defiant F91.3
  optic
    chiasm H47.49
      due to
        inflammatory disorder H47.41
        neoplasm H47.42
        vascular disorder H47.43
    disc H47.39- ☑
      coloboma — *see* Coloboma, optic disc
      drusen — *see* Drusen, optic disc
      pseudopapilledema — *see* Pseudopapilledema
      radiations — *see* Disorder, visual, pathway
      tracts — *see* Disorder, visual, pathway
  orbit H05.9
    cyst — *see* Cyst, orbit
    deformity — *see* Deformity, orbit
    edema — *see* Edema, orbit
    enophthalmos — *see* Enophthalmos
    exophthalmos — *see* Exophthalmos
    hemorrhage — *see* Hemorrhage, orbit
    inflammation — *see* Inflammation, orbit
    myopathy — *see* Myopathy, extraocular muscles
    retained foreign body — *see* Foreign body, orbit,
      old
    specified type NEC H05.89
  organic
    anxiety F06.4
    catatonic F06.1
    delusional F06.2
    dissociative F06.8
    emotionally labile (asthenic) F06.8
    mood (affective) F06.30
    schizophrenia-like F06.2
  orgasmic (female) F52.31
    male F52.32
  ornithine metabolism E72.4
  overanxious F41.1
    of childhood F93.8
  pain
    with related psychological factors F45.42
    exclusively related to psychological factors F45.41
    genito-pelvic penetration disorder F52.6
  pancreatic internal secretion E16.9
    specified NEC E16.8
  panic F41.0
    with agoraphobia F40.01
  papulosquamous L44.9
    in diseases classified elsewhere L45
    specified NEC L44.8
  paranoid F22
    induced F24
    shared F24
  paraphilic F65.9

**Disorder** — *continued*

paraphilic — *continued*
   specified NEC F65.89
parathyroid (gland) E21.5
  specified NEC E21.4
parietoalveolar NEC J84.09
paroxysmal, mixed R56.9
patella M22.9- ☑
  chondromalacia — *see* Chondromalacia, patella
  derangement NEC M22.3X- ☑
  recurrent
     dislocation — *see* Dislocation, patella, recurrent
     subluxation — *see* Dislocation, patella, recurrent, incomplete
  specified NEC M22.8X- ☑
patellofemoral M22.2X- ☑
pedophilic F65.4
pentose phosphate pathway with anemia D55.1
perception, due to hallucinogens F16.983
  in
    abuse F16.183
    dependence F16.283
peripheral nervous system NEC G64
peroxisomal E71.50
  biogenesis
    neonatal adrenoleukodystrophy E71.511
    specified disorder NEC E71.518
    Zellweger syndrome E71.510
  rhizomelic chondrodysplasia punctata E71.540
  specified form NEC E71.548
    group 1 E71.518
    group 2 E71.53
    group 3 E71.542
  X-linked adrenoleukodystrophy E71.529
    adolescent E71.521
    adrenomyeloneuropathy E71.522
    childhood E71.520
    specified form NEC E71.528
  Zellweger-like syndrome E71.541
persistent
  (somatoform) pain F45.41
  affective (mood) F34.9
personality (*see also* Personality) F60.9
  affective F34.0
  aggressive F60.3
  amoral F60.2
  anankastic F60.5
  antisocial F60.2
  anxious F60.6
  asocial F60.2
  asthenic F60.7
  avoidant F60.6
  borderline F60.3
  change (secondary) due to general medical condition F07.0
  compulsive F60.5
  cyclothymic F34.0
  dependent (passive) F60.7
  depressive F34.1
  dissocial F60.2
  emotional instability F60.3
  expansive paranoid F60.0
  explosive F60.3
  following organic brain damage F07.9
  histrionic F60.4
  hyperthymic F34.0
  hypothymic F34.1
  hysterical F60.4
  immature F60.89
  inadequate F60.7
  labile F60.3
  mixed (nonspecific) F60.89
  moral deficiency F60.2
  narcissistic F60.81
  negativistic F60.89
  obsessional F60.5
  obsessive (-compulsive) F60.5
  organic F07.9
  overconscientious F60.5
  paranoid F60.0
  passive (-dependent) F60.7
  passive-aggressive F60.89
  pathological NEC F60.9
  pseudosocial F60.2
  psychopathic F60.2
  schizoid F60.1
  schizotypal F21
  self-defeating F60.7

**Disorder** — *continued*

personality (*see also* Personality) — *continued*
  specified NEC F60.89
  type A F60.5
  unstable (emotional) F60.3
pervasive, developmental F84.9
phencyclidine use
  mild F16.10
    with
      phencyclidine intoxication F16.129
      phencyclidine intoxication delirium F16.121
      phencyclidine-induced
        anxiety disorder F16.180
        bipolar and related disorder F16.14
        depressive disorder F16.14
        psychotic disorder F16.159
    in remission (early) (sustained) F16.11
  moderate or severe F16.20
    with
      phencyclidine intoxication F16.229
      phencyclidine intoxication delirium F16.221
      phencyclidine-induced
        anxiety disorder F16.280
        bipolar and related disorder F16.14
        depressive disorder F16.24
        psychotic disorder F16.259
    in remission (early) (sustained) F16.21
phobic anxiety, childhood F40.8
phosphate-losing tubular N25.0
pigmentation L81.9
  choroid, congenital Q14.3
  diminished melanin formation L81.6
  iron L81.8
  specified NEC L81.8
pinna (noninfective) H61.10- ☑
  deformity, acquired H61.11- ☑
  hematoma H61.12- ☑
  perichondritis — *see* Perichondritis, ear
  specified type NEC H61.19- ☑
pituitary gland E23.7
  iatrogenic (postprocedural) E89.3
  specified NEC E23.6
platelets D69.1
plexus G54.9
  specified NEC G54.8
polymorphonuclear neutrophils D71
porphyrin metabolism — *see* Porphyria
postconcussional F07.81
posthallucinogen perception F16.983
  in
    abuse F16.183
    dependence F16.283
postmenopausal N95.9
  specified NEC N95.8
postprocedural (postoperative) — *see* Complications, postprocedural
post-transplant lymphoproliferative D47.Z1 (*following* D47.4)
post-traumatic stress (PTSD) F43.10
  acute F43.11
  chronic F43.12
premenstrual dysphoric (PMDD) F32.81
prepuce N47.8
propionic acidemia E71.121
prostate N42.9
  specified NEC N42.89
psychogenic NOS (*see also* condition) F45.9
  anxiety F41.8
  appetite F50.9
  asthenic F48.8
  cardiovascular (system) F45.8
  compulsive F42.8
  cutaneous F54
  depressive F32.9
  digestive (system) F45.8
  dysmenorrheic F45.8
  dyspneic F45.8
  endocrine (system) F54
  eye NEC F45.8
  feeding — *see* Disorder, eating
  functional NEC F45.8
  gastric F45.8
  gastrointestinal (system) F45.8
  genitourinary (system) F45.8
  heart (function) (rhythm) F45.8
  hyperventilatory F45.8
  hypochondriacal — *see* Disorder, hypochondriacal
  intestinal F45.8

**Disorder** — *continued*

psychogenic (*see also* condition) — *continued*
  joint F45.8
  learning F81.9
  limb F45.8
  lymphatic (system) F45.8
  menstrual F45.8
  micturition F45.8
  monoplegic NEC F44.4
  motor F44.4
  muscle F45.8
  musculoskeletal F45.8
  neurocirculatory F45.8
  obsessive F42.8
  occupational F48.8
  organ or part of body NEC F45.8
  paralytic NEC F44.4
  phobic F40.9
  physical NEC F45.8
  rectal F45.8
  respiratory (system) F45.8
  rheumatic F45.8
  sexual (function) F52.9
  skin (allergic) (eczematous) F54
  sleep F51.9
  specified part of body NEC F45.8
  stomach F45.8
psychological F99
  associated with
    disease classified elsewhere F54
    sexual
      development F66
      relationship F66
    uncertainty about gender identity F64.9
psychomotor NEC F44.4
  hysterical F44.4
psychoneurotic (*see also* Neurosis)
  mixed NEC F48.8
psychophysiologic — *see* Disorder, somatoform
psychosexual F65.9
  development F66
  identity of childhood F64.2
psychosomatic NOS — *see* Disorder, somatoform
  multiple F45.0
  undifferentiated F45.1
psychotic — *see* Psychosis
  transient (acute) F23
puberty E30.9
  specified NEC E30.8
pulmonary (valve) — *see* Endocarditis, pulmonary
purine metabolism E79.9
pyrimidine metabolism E79.9
pyruvate metabolism E74.4
reactive attachment (childhood) F94.1
reading R48.0
  developmental (specific) F81.0
receptive language F80.2
receptor, hormonal, peripheral (*see also* Syndrome, androgen insensitivity) E34.50
recurrent brief depressive F33.8
reflex R29.2
refraction H52.7
  aniseikonia H52.32
  anisometropia H52.31
  astigmatism — *see* Astigmatism
  hypermetropia — *see* Hypermetropia
  myopia — *see* Myopia
  presbyopia H52.4
  specified NEC H52.6
relationship F68.8
  due to sexual orientation F66
REM sleep behavior G47.52
renal function, impaired (tubular) N25.9
resonance R49.9
  specified NEC R49.8
respiratory function, impaired (*see also* Failure, respiration)
  postprocedural — *see* Complication, postoperative, respiratory system
  psychogenic F45.8
retina H35.9
  angioid streaks H35.33
  changes in vascular appearance H35.01- ☑
  degeneration — *see* Degeneration, retina
  dystrophy (hereditary) — *see* Dystrophy, retina
  edema H35.81
  hemorrhage — *see* Hemorrhage, retina
  ischemia H35.82

☑ **Additional Character Required** — Refer to the Tabular List for Character Selection    ▽ Subterms under main terms may continue to next column or page

**Disorder** — *continued*
  retina — *continued*
    macular degeneration — *see* Degeneration, macula
    microaneurysms H35.04- ☑
    microvascular abnormality NEC H35.09
    neovascularization — *see* Neovascularization, retina
    retinopathy — *see* Retinopathy
    separation of layers H35.70
      central serous chorioretinopathy H35.71- ☑
      pigment epithelium detachment (serous) H35.72- ☑
      hemorrhagic H35.73- ☑
    specified type NEC H35.89
    telangiectasis — *see* Telangiectasis, retina
    vasculitis — *see* Vasculitis, retina
  retroperitoneal K68.9
  right hemisphere organic affective F07.89
  rumination (infant or child) F98.21
  sacrum, sacrococcygeal NEC M53.3
  schizoaffective F25.9
    bipolar type F25.0
    depressive type F25.1
    manic type F25.0
    mixed type F25.0
    specified NEC F25.8
  schizoid of childhood F84.5
  schizophrenia spectrum and other psychotic disorder F29
    specified NEC F28
  schizophreniform F20.81
    brief F23
  schizotypal (personality) F21
  secretion, thyrocalcitonin E07.0
  sedative, hypnotic, or anxiolytic use
    mild F13.10
      with
        sedative, hypnotic, or anxiolytic intoxication F13.129
        sedative, hypnotic, or anxiolytic intoxication delirium F13.121
        sedative, hypnotic, or anxiolytic-induced
          anxiety disorder F13.180
          bipolar and related disorder F13.14
          depressive disorder F13.14
          psychotic disorder F13.159
          sexual dysfunction F13.181
      in remission (early) (sustained) F13.11
    moderate or severe F13.20
      with
        sedative, hypnotic, or anxiolytic intoxication F13.229
        sedative, hypnotic, or anxiolytic intoxication delirium F13.221
        sedative, hypnotic, or anxiolytic-induced
          anxiety disorder F13.280
          bipolar and related disorder F13.24
          depressive disorder F13.24
          major neurocognitive disorder F13.27
          mild neurocognitive disorder F13.288
          psychotic disorder F13.259
          sexual dysfunction F13.281
      in remission (early) (sustained) F13.21
  seizure (*see also* Epilepsy) G40.909
    intractable G40.919
      with status epilepticus G40.911
  semantic pragmatic F80.89
    with autism F84.0
  sense of smell R43.1
    psychogenic F45.8
  separation anxiety, of childhood F93.0
  sexual
    aversion F52.1
    function, psychogenic F52.9
    interest/arousal, female F52.22
    masochism F65.51
    maturation F66
    nonorganic F52.9
    preference (*see also* Deviation, sexual) F65.9
      fetishistic transvestism F65.1
    relationship F66
    sadism F65.52
  shyness, of childhood and adolescence F40.10
  sibling rivalry F93.8
  sickle-cell (sickling) (homozygous) — *see* Disease, sickle-cell
    heterozygous D57.3
    specified type NEC D57.8- ☑

**Disorder** — *continued*
  sickle-cell — *see* Disease, sickle-cell — *continued*
    trait D57.3
  sinus (nasal) J34.9
    specified NEC J34.89
  skin L98.9
    atrophic L90.9
      specified NEC L90.8
    granulomatous L92.9
      specified NEC L92.8
    hypertrophic L91.9
      specified NEC L91.8
    infiltrative NEC L98.6
    newborn P83.9
      specified NEC P83.88
    picking F42.4
    psychogenic (allergic) (eczematous) F54
  sleep G47.9
    breathing-related — *see* Apnea, sleep
    circadian rhythm G47.20
      advance sleep phase type G47.22
      delayed sleep phase type G47.21
      due to
        alcohol
          abuse F10.182
          dependence F10.282
          use F10.982
        amphetamines
          abuse F15.182
          dependence F15.282
          use F15.982
        caffeine
          abuse F15.182
          dependence F15.282
          use F15.982
        cocaine
          abuse F14.182
          dependence F14.282
          use F14.982
        drug NEC
          abuse F19.182
          dependence F19.282
          use F19.982
        opioid
          abuse F11.182
          dependence F11.282
          use F11.982
        psychoactive substance NEC
          abuse F19.182
          dependence F19.282
          use F19.982
        sedative, hypnotic, or anxiolytic
          abuse F13.182
          dependence F13.282
          use F13.982
        stimulant NEC
          abuse F15.182
          dependence F15.282
          use F15.982
      free running type G47.24
      in conditions classified elsewhere G47.27
      irregular sleep wake type G47.23
      jet lag type G47.25
      non-24-hour sleep-wake type G47.24
      shift work type G47.26
      specified NEC G47.29
    due to
      alcohol
        abuse F10.182
        dependence F10.282
        use F10.982
      amphetamine
        abuse F15.182
        dependence F15.282
        use F15.982
      anxiolytic
        abuse F13.182
        dependence F13.282
        use F13.982
      caffeine
        abuse F15.182
        dependence F15.282
        use F15.982
      cocaine
        abuse F14.182
        dependence F14.282
        use F14.982
      drug NEC
        abuse F19.182

**Disorder** — *continued*
  sleep — *continued*
    due to — *continued*
      drug — *continued*
        dependence F19.282
        use F19.982
      hypnotic
        abuse F13.182
        dependence F13.282
        use F13.982
      opioid
        abuse F11.182
        dependence F11.282
        use F11.982
      psychoactive substance NEC
        abuse F19.182
        dependence F19.282
        use F19.982
      sedative
        abuse F13.182
        dependence F13.282
        use F13.982
      stimulant NEC
        abuse F15.182
        dependence F15.282
        use F15.982
    emotional F51.9
    excessive somnolence — *see* Hypersomnia
    hypersomnia type — *see* Hypersomnia
    initiating or maintaining — *see* Insomnia
    nightmares F51.5
    nonorganic F51.9
      specified NEC F51.8
    parasomnia type G47.50
    specified NEC G47.8
    terrors F51.4
    walking F51.3
  sleep-wake pattern or schedule (*see also* Disorder, sleep, circadian rhythm) G47.9
    specified NEC G47.8
  social
    anxiety (of childhood) F40.10
      generalized F40.11
    functioning in childhood F94.9
      specified NEC F94.8
    pragmatic F80.82
  soft tissue M79.9
    ankle M79.9
    due to use, overuse and pressure M70.90
      ankle M70.97- ☑
      bursitis — *see* Bursitis
      foot M70.97- ☑
      forearm M70.93- ☑
      hand M70.94- ☑
      lower leg M70.96- ☑
      multiple sites M70.99
      pelvic region M70.95- ☑
      shoulder region M70.91- ☑
      specified site NEC M70.98
      specified type NEC M70.80
        ankle M70.87- ☑
        foot M70.87- ☑
        forearm M70.83- ☑
        hand M70.84- ☑
        lower leg M70.86- ☑
        multiple sites M70.89
        pelvic region M70.85- ☑
        shoulder region M70.81- ☑
        specified site NEC M70.88
        thigh M70.85- ☑
        upper arm M70.82- ☑
      thigh M70.95- ☑
      upper arm M70.92- ☑
    foot M79.9
    forearm M79.9
    hand M79.9
    lower leg M79.9
    multiple sites M79.9
    occupational — *see* Disorder, soft tissue, due to use, overuse and pressure
    pelvic region M79.9
    shoulder region M79.9
    specified type NEC M79.89
    thigh M79.9
    upper arm M79.9
  somatic symptom F45.1
  somatization F45.0
  somatoform F45.9

**Disorder** — *continued*
somatoform — *continued*
  pain (persistent) F45.41
  somatization (multiple) (long-lasting) F45.0
  specified NEC F45.8
  undifferentiated F45.1
somnolence, excessive — *see* Hypersomnia
specific
  arithmetical F81.2
  developmental, of motor F82
  reading F81.0
  speech and language F80.9
  spelling F81.81
  written expression F81.81
speech R47.9
  articulation (functional) (specific) F80.0
  developmental F80.9
  specified NEC R47.89
speech-sound F80.0
spelling (specific) F81.81
spine (*see also* Dorsopathy)
  ligamentous or muscular attachments, peripheral — *see* Enthesopathy, spinal
  specified NEC — *see* Dorsopathy, specified NEC
stereotyped, habit or movement F98.4
stimulant use (other) (unspecified)
  mild F15.10
    in remission (early) (sustained) F15.11
  moderate or severe F15.20
    in remission (early) (sustained) F15.21
stomach (functional) — *see* Disorder, gastric
stress F43.9
  acute F43.0
  post-traumatic F43.10
    acute F43.11
    chronic F43.12
substance use (other) (unknown)
  mild F19.10
    with substance-induced
      anxiety disorder F19.180
      bipolar and related disorder F19.14
      depressive disorder F19.14
      major neurocognitive disorder F19.17
      mild neurocognitive disorder F19.188
      obsessive-compulsive and related disorder F19.188
      sexual dysfunction F19.181
      substance intoxication F19.129
      substance intoxication delirium F19.121
  moderate or severe F19.20
    with substance-induced
      anxiety disorder F19.280
      bipolar and related disorder F19.24
      depressive disorder F19.24
      major neurocognitive disorder F19.27
      mild neurocognitive disorder F19.288
      obsessive-compulsive and related disorder F19.288
      sexual dysfunction F19.281
    in remission (early) (sustained) F19.21
    substance intoxication F19.229
    substance intoxication delirium F19.221
sulfur-bearing amino-acid metabolism E72.10
sweat gland (eccrine) L74.9
  apocrine L75.9
    specified NEC L75.8
  specified NEC L74.8
synovium M67.90
  acromioclavicular M67.91- ☑
  ankle M67.97- ☑
  elbow M67.92- ☑
  foot M67.97- ☑
  forearm M67.93- ☑
  hand M67.94- ☑
  hip M67.95- ☑
  knee M67.96- ☑
  multiple sites M67.99
  rupture — *see* Rupture, synovium
  shoulder M67.91- ☑
  specified type NEC M67.80- ☑
    acromioclavicular M67.81- ☑
    ankle M67.87- ☑
    elbow M67.82- ☑
    foot M67.87- ☑
    hand M67.84- ☑
    hip M67.85- ☑
    knee M67.86- ☑
    multiple sites M67.89

**Disorder** — *continued*
synovium — *continued*
  specified type — *continued*
    wrist M67.83- ☑
  synovitis — *see* Synovitis
  upper arm M67.92- ☑
  wrist M67.93- ☑
temperature regulation, newborn P81.9
  specified NEC P81.8
temporomandibular joint M26.60- ☑
tendon M67.90
  acromioclavicular M67.91- ☑
  ankle M67.97- ☑
  contracture — *see* Contracture, tendon
  elbow M67.92- ☑
  foot M67.97- ☑
  forearm M67.93- ☑
  hand M67.94- ☑
  hip M67.95- ☑
  knee M67.96- ☑
  multiple sites M67.99
  rupture — *see* Rupture, tendon
  shoulder M67.91- ☑
  specified type NEC M67.80
    acromioclavicular M67.81- ☑
    ankle M67.87- ☑
    elbow M67.82- ☑
    foot M67.87- ☑
    hand M67.84- ☑
    hip M67.85- ☑
    knee M67.86- ☑
    multiple sites M67.89
    trunk M67.88
    wrist M67.83- ☑
  synovitis — *see* Synovitis
  tendinitis — *see* Tendinitis
  tenosynovitis — *see* Tenosynovitis
  trunk M67.98
  upper arm M67.92- ☑
  wrist M67.93- ☑
thoracic root (nerve) NEC G54.3
thyrocalcitonin hypersecretion E07.0
thyroid (gland) E07.9
  function NEC, neonatal, transitory P72.2
  iodine-deficiency related E01.8
  specified NEC E07.89
tic — *see* Tic
tobacco use
  chewing tobacco (mild) (moderate) (severe) Z72.0
    in remission (early) (sustained) F17.221
  cigarettes (mild) (moderate) (severe)
    in remission (early) (sustained) F17.211
  mild Z72.0
    in remission (early) (sustained) F17.201
  moderate F17.200
    in remission (early) (sustained) F17.201
  severe F17.200
    in remission (early) (sustained) F17.201
  specified product NEC (mild) (moderate) (severe)
    in remission (early) (sustained) F17.291
tooth K08.9
  development K00.9
    specified NEC K00.8
  eruption K00.6
Tourette's F95.2
trance and possession F44.89
transvestic F65.1
trauma and stressor-related F43.9
  other specified F43.8
tricuspid (valve) — *see* Endocarditis, tricuspid
tryptophan metabolism E70.5
tubular, phosphate-losing N25.0
tubulo-interstitial (in)
  brucellosis A23.9 [N16]
  cystinosis E72.04
  diphtheria A36.84
  glycogen storage disease E74.00 [N16]
  leukemia NEC C95.9- ☑ [N16]
  lymphoma NEC C85.9- ☑ [N16]
  mixed cryoglobulinemia D89.1 [N16]
  multiple myeloma C90.0- ☑ [N16]
  Salmonella infection A02.25
  sarcoidosis D86.84
  sepsis A41.9 [N16]
    streptococcal A40.9 [N16]
  systemic lupus erythematosus M32.15
  toxoplasmosis B58.83

**Disorder** — *continued*
tubulo-interstitial — *continued*
  transplant rejection T86.91 [N16]
  Wilson's disease E83.01 [N16]
tubulo-renal function, impaired N25.9
  specified NEC N25.89
tympanic membrane H73.9- ☑
  atrophy — *see* Atrophy, tympanic membrane
  infection — *see* Myringitis
  perforation — *see* Perforation, tympanum
  specified NEC H73.89- ☑
unsocialized aggressive F91.1
urea cycle metabolism E72.20
  argininemia E72.21
  argininosuccinic aciduria E72.22
  citrullinemia E72.23
  ornithine transcarbamylase deficiency E72.4
  other specified E72.29
ureter (in) N28.9
  schistosomiasis B65.0 [N29]
  tuberculosis A18.11
urethra N36.9
  specified NEC N36.8
urinary system N39.9
  specified NEC N39.8
valve, heart
  aortic — *see* Endocarditis, aortic
  mitral — *see* Endocarditis, mitral
  pulmonary — *see* Endocarditis, pulmonary
  rheumatic
    aortic — *see* Endocarditis, aortic, rheumatic
    mitral — *see* Endocarditis, mitral
    pulmonary — *see* Endocarditis, pulmonary, rheumatic
    tricuspid — *see* Endocarditis, tricuspid
  tricuspid — *see* Endocarditis, tricuspid
vestibular function H81.9- ☑
  specified NEC — *see* subcategory H81.8 ☑
    in diseases classified elsewhere H82.- ☑
  vertigo — *see* Vertigo
vision, binocular H53.30
  abnormal retinal correspondence H53.31
  diplopia H53.2
  fusion with defective stereopsis H53.32
  simultaneous perception H53.33
  suppression H53.34
visual
  cortex
    blindness H47.619
      left brain H47.612
      right brain H47.611
    due to
      inflammatory disorder H47.629
        left brain H47.622
        right brain H47.621
      neoplasm H47.639
        left brain H47.632
        right brain H47.631
      vascular disorder H47.649
        left brain H47.642
        right brain H47.641
  pathway H47.9
    due to
      inflammatory disorder H47.51- ☑
      neoplasm H47.52- ☑
      vascular disorder H47.53- ☑
    optic chiasm — *see* Disorder, optic, chiasm
vitreous body H43.9
  crystalline deposits — *see* Deposit, crystalline
  degeneration — *see* Degeneration, vitreous
  hemorrhage — *see* Hemorrhage, vitreous
  opacities — *see* Opacity, vitreous
  prolapse — *see* Prolapse, vitreous
  specified type NEC H43.89
voice R49.9
  specified type NEC R49.8
volatile solvent use
  due to drug abuse — *see* Abuse, drug, inhalant
  due to drug dependence — *see* Dependence, drug, inhalant
voyeuristic F65.3
white blood cells D72.9
  specified NEC D72.89
withdrawing, child or adolescent F40.10
**Disorientation** R41.0
**Displacement, displaced**
  acquired traumatic of bone, cartilage, joint, tendon NEC — *see* Dislocation

☑ **Additional Character Required** — Refer to the Tabular List for Character Selection

▽ **Subterms under main terms may continue to next column or page**

**Displacement, displaced** — *continued*
adrenal gland (congenital) Q89.1
appendix, retrocecal (congenital) Q43.8
auricle (congenital) Q17.4
bladder (acquired) N32.89
congenital Q64.19
brachial plexus (congenital) Q07.8
brain stem, caudal (congenital) Q04.8
canaliculus (lacrimalis), congenital Q10.6
cardia through esophageal hiatus (congenital) Q40.1
cerebellum, caudal (congenital) Q04.8
cervix — *see* Malposition, uterus
colon (congenital) Q43.3
device, implant or graft (*see also* Complications, by
site and type, mechanical) T85.628 ☑
arterial graft NEC — *see* Complication, cardiovascular device, mechanical, vascular
breast (implant) T85.42 ☑
catheter NEC T85.628 ☑
dialysis (renal) T82.42 ☑
intraperitoneal T85.621 ☑
infusion NEC T82.524 ☑
spinal (epidural) (subdural) T85.620 ☑
urinary
cystostomy T83.020 ☑
Hopkins T83.028 ☑
ileostomy T83.028 ☑
indwelling T83.021 ☑
nephrostomy T83.022 ☑
specified NEC T83.028 ☑
urostomy T83.028 ☑
electronic (electrode) (pulse generator) (stimulator)
— *see* Complication, electronic stimulator
fixation, internal (orthopedic) NEC — *see* Complication, fixation device, mechanical
gastrointestinal — *see* Complications, prosthetic
device, mechanical, gastrointestinal device
genital NEC T83.428 ☑
intrauterine contraceptive device (string)
T83.32 ☑
penile prosthesis (cylinder) (implanted) (pump)
(reservoir) T83.420 ☑
testicular prosthesis T83.421 ☑
heart NEC — *see* Complication, cardiovascular device, mechanical
joint prosthesis — *see* Complications, joint prosthesis, mechanical
ocular — *see* Complications, prosthetic device,
mechanical, ocular device
orthopedic NEC — *see* Complication, orthopedic,
device or graft, mechanical
specified NEC T85.628 ☑
urinary NEC T83.128 ☑
graft T83.22 ☑
sphincter, implanted T83.121 ☑
stent (ileal conduit) (nephroureteral) T83.123 ☑
ureteral indwelling T83.122 ☑
vascular NEC — *see* Complication, cardiovascular
device, mechanical
ventricular intracranial shunt T85.02 ☑
electronic stimulator
bone T84.320 ☑
cardiac — *see* Complications, cardiac device, electronic
nervous system — *see* Complication, prosthetic
device, mechanical, electronic nervous system stimulator
urinary — *see* Complications, electronic stimulator,
urinary
esophageal mucosa into cardia of stomach, congenital
Q39.8
esophagus (acquired) K22.8
congenital Q39.8
eyeball (acquired) (lateral) (old) — *see* Displacement,
globe
congenital Q15.8
current — *see* Avulsion, eye
fallopian tube (acquired) N83.4- ☑
congenital Q50.6
opening (congenital) Q50.6
gallbladder (congenital) Q44.1
gastric mucosa (congenital) Q40.2
globe (acquired) (old) (lateral) H05.21- ☑
current — *see* Avulsion, eye
heart (congenital) Q24.8
acquired I51.89
hymen (upward) (congenital) Q52.4

**Displacement, displaced** — *continued*
intervertebral disc NEC
with myelopathy — *see* Disorder, disc, with,
myelopathy
cervical, cervicothoracic (with) M50.20
myelopathy — *see* Disorder, disc, cervical, with
myelopathy
neuritis, radiculitis or radiculopathy — *see* Disorder, disc, cervical, with neuritis
due to trauma — *see* Dislocation, vertebra
lumbar region M51.26
with
myelopathy M51.06
neuritis, radiculitis, radiculopathy or sciatica
M51.16
lumbosacral region M51.27
with
neuritis, radiculitis, radiculopathy or sciatica
M51.17
sacrococcygeal region M53.3
thoracic region M51.24
with
myelopathy M51.04
neuritis, radiculitis, radiculopathy M51.14
thoracolumbar region M51.25
with
myelopathy M51.05
neuritis, radiculitis, radiculopathy M51.15
intrauterine device (string) T83.32 ☑
kidney (acquired) N28.83
congenital Q63.2
lachrymal, lacrimal apparatus or duct (congenital)
Q10.6
lens, congenital Q12.1
macula (congenital) Q14.1
Meckel's diverticulum Q43.0
malignant — *see* Table of Neoplasms, small intestine, malignant
nail (congenital) Q84.6
acquired L60.8
opening of Wharton's duct in mouth Q38.4
organ or site, congenital NEC — *see* Malposition,
congenital
ovary (acquired) N83.4- ☑
congenital Q50.39
free in peritoneal cavity (congenital) Q50.39
into hernial sac N83.4- ☑
oviduct (acquired) N83.4- ☑
congenital Q50.6
parathyroid (gland) E21.4
parotid gland (congenital) Q38.4
punctum lacrimale (congenital) Q10.6
sacro-iliac (joint) (congenital) Q74.2
current injury S33.2 ☑
old — *see* subcategory M53.2 ☑
salivary gland (any) (congenital) Q38.4
spleen (congenital) Q89.09
stomach, congenital Q40.2
sublingual duct Q38.4
tongue (downward) (congenital) Q38.3
tooth, teeth, fully erupted M26.30
horizontal M26.33
vertical M26.34
trachea (congenital) Q32.1
ureter or ureteric opening or orifice (congenital)
Q62.62
uterine opening of oviducts or fallopian tubes Q50.6
uterus, uterine — *see* Malposition, uterus
ventricular septum Q21.0
with rudimentary ventricle Q20.4
**Disproportion**
between native and reconstructed breast N65.1
fiber-type G71.2
**Disruptio uteri** — *see* Rupture, uterus
**Disruption** (of)
ciliary body NEC H21.89
closure of
cornea T81.31 ☑
craniotomy T81.32 ☑
fascia (muscular) (superficial) T81.32 ☑
internal organ or tissue T81.32 ☑
laceration (external) (internal) T81.33 ☑
ligament T81.32 ☑
mucosa T81.31 ☑
muscle or muscle flap T81.32 ☑
ribs or rib cage T81.32 ☑
skin and subcutaneous tissue (full-thickness) (superficial) T81.31 ☑

**Disruption** — *continued*
closure of — *continued*
skull T81.32 ☑
sternum (sternotomy) T81.32 ☑
tendon T81.32 ☑
traumatic laceration (external) (internal) T81.33 ☑
family Z63.8
due to
absence of family member due to military deployment Z63.31
absence of family member NEC Z63.32
alcoholism and drug addiction in family Z63.72
bereavement Z63.4
death (assumed) or disappearance of family
member Z63.4
divorce or separation Z63.5
drug addiction in family Z63.72
return of family member from military deployment (current or past conflict) Z63.71
stressful life events NEC Z63.79
iris NEC H21.89
ligament(s) (*see also* Sprain)
knee
current injury — *see* Dislocation, knee
old (chronic) — *see* Derangement, knee, instability
spontaneous NEC — *see* Derangement, knee,
disruption ligament
ossicular chain — *see* Discontinuity, ossicles, ear
pelvic ring (stable) S32.810 ☑
unstable S32.811 ☑
traumatic injury wound repair T81.33 ☑
wound T81.30 ☑
episiotomy O90.1
operation T81.31 ☑
cesarean O90.0
external operation wound (superficial)
T81.31 ☑
internal operation wound (deep) T81.32 ☑
perineal (obstetric) O90.1
traumatic injury repair T81.33 ☑
**Dissatisfaction with**
employment Z56.9
school environment Z55.4
**Dissecting** — *see* condition
**Dissection**
aorta I71.00
abdominal I71.02
thoracic I71.01
thoracoabdominal I71.03
artery I77.70
basilar (trunk) I77.75
carotid I77.71
cerebral (nonruptured) I67.0
ruptured — *see* Hemorrhage, intracranial,
subarachnoid
coronary I25.42
extremity
lower I77.77
upper I77.76
iliac I77.72
precerebral
congenital (nonruptured) Q28.1
specified site NEC I77.75
renal I77.73
specified NEC I77.79
vertebral I77.74
precerebral artery, congenital (nonruptured) Q28.1
Heartland A93.8
traumatic — *see* Wound, open, by site
vascular I99.8
wound — *see* Wound, open
**Disseminated** — *see* condition
**Dissociation**
auriculoventricular or atrioventricular (AV) (any degree) (isorhythmic) I45.89
with heart block I44.2
interference I45.89
**Dissociative reaction, state** F44.9
**Dissolution, vertebra** — *see* Osteoporosis
**Distension, distention**
abdomen R14.0
bladder N32.89
cecum K63.89
colon K63.89
gallbladder K82.8
intestine K63.89
kidney N28.89

**Distension, distention** — *continued*
- liver K76.89
- seminal vesicle N50.89
- stomach K31.89
  - acute K31.0
  - psychogenic F45.8
- ureter — *see* Dilatation, ureter
- uterus N85.8

**Distoma hepaticum infestation** B66.3

**Distomiasis** B66.9
- bile passages B66.3
- hemic B65.9
- hepatic B66.3
  - due to Clonorchis sinensis B66.1
- intestinal B66.5
- liver B66.3
  - due to Clonorchis sinensis B66.1
- lung B66.4
- pulmonary B66.4

**Distomolar** (fourth molar) K00.1

**Disto-occlusion** (Division I) (Division II) M26.212

**Distortion**(s) (congenital)
- adrenal (gland) Q89.1
- arm NEC Q68.8
- bile duct or passage Q44.5
- bladder Q64.79
- brain Q04.9
- cervix (uteri) Q51.9
- chest (wall) Q67.8
  - bones Q76.8
- clavicle Q74.0
- clitoris Q52.6
- coccyx Q76.49
- common duct Q44.5
- coronary Q24.5
- cystic duct Q44.5
- ear (auricle) (external) Q17.3
  - inner Q16.5
  - middle Q16.4
    - ossicles Q16.3
- endocrine NEC Q89.2
- eustachian tube Q17.8
- eye (adnexa) Q15.8
- face bone(s) NEC Q75.8
- fallopian tube Q50.6
- femur NEC Q68.8
- fibula NEC Q68.8
- finger(s) Q68.1
- foot Q66.9
- genitalia, genital organ(s)
  - female Q52.8
    - external Q52.79
    - internal NEC Q52.8
- gyri Q04.8
- hand bone(s) Q68.1
- heart (auricle) (ventricle) Q24.8
  - valve (cusp) Q24.8
- hepatic duct Q44.5
- humerus NEC Q68.8
- hymen Q52.4
- intrafamilial communications Z63.8
- jaw NEC M26.89
- labium (majus) (minus) Q52.79
- leg NEC Q68.8
- lens Q12.8
- liver Q44.7
- lumbar spine Q76.49
  - with disproportion O33.8
    - causing obstructed labor O65.0
- lumbosacral (joint) (region) Q76.49
  - kyphosis — *see* Kyphosis, congenital
  - lordosis — *see* Lordosis, congenital
- nerve Q07.8
- nose Q30.8
- organ
  - of Corti Q16.5
  - or site not listed — *see* Anomaly, by site
- ossicles, ear Q16.3
- oviduct Q50.6
- pancreas Q45.3
- parathyroid (gland) Q89.2
- pituitary (gland) Q89.2
- radius NEC Q68.8
- sacroiliac joint Q74.2
- sacrum Q76.49
- scapula Q74.0
- shoulder girdle Q74.0
- skull bone(s) NEC Q75.8

**Distortion**(s) — *continued*
- skull bone(s) — *continued*
  - with
    - anencephalus Q00.0
    - encephalocele — *see* Encephalocele
    - hydrocephalus Q03.9
      - with spina bifida — *see* Spina bifida, with hydrocephalus
    - microcephaly Q02
- spinal cord Q06.8
- spine Q76.49
  - kyphosis — *see* Kyphosis, congenital
  - lordosis — *see* Lordosis, congenital
- spleen Q89.09
- sternum NEC Q76.7
- thorax (wall) Q67.8
  - bony Q76.8
- thymus (gland) Q89.2
- thyroid (gland) Q89.2
- tibia NEC Q68.8
- toe(s) Q66.9
- tongue Q38.3
- trachea (cartilage) Q32.1
- ulna NEC Q68.8
- ureter Q62.8
- urethra Q64.79
  - causing obstruction Q64.39
- uterus Q51.9
- vagina Q52.4
- vertebra Q76.49
  - kyphosis — *see* Kyphosis, congenital
  - lordosis — *see* Lordosis, congenital
- visual (*see also* Disturbance, vision)
  - shape and size H53.15
- vulva Q52.79
- wrist (bones) (joint) Q68.8

**Distress**
- abdomen — *see* Pain, abdominal
- acute respiratory R06.03
  - syndrome (adult) (child) J80
- epigastric R10.13
- fetal P84
  - complicating pregnancy — *see* Stress, fetal
- gastrointestinal (functional) K30
  - psychogenic F45.8
- intestinal (functional) NOS K59.9
  - psychogenic F45.8
- maternal, during labor and delivery O75.0
- relationship, with spouse or intimate partner Z63.0
- respiratory (adult) (child) R06.03
  - newborn P22.9
    - specified NEC P22.8
  - orthopnea R06.01
  - psychogenic F45.8
  - shortness of breath R06.02
  - specified type NEC R06.09

**Distribution vessel, atypical** Q27.9
- coronary artery Q24.5
- precerebral Q28.1

**Districhiasis** L68.8

**Disturbance**(s) (*see also* Disease)
- absorption K90.9
  - calcium E58
  - carbohydrate K90.49
  - fat K90.49
    - pancreatic K90.3
  - protein K90.49
  - starch K90.49
  - vitamin — *see* Deficiency, vitamin
- acid-base equilibrium E87.8
  - mixed E87.4
- activity and attention (with hyperkinesis) — *see* Disorder, attention-deficit hyperactivity
- amino acid transport E72.00
- assimilation, food K90.9
- auditory nerve, except deafness — *see* subcategory H93.3 ☑
- behavior — *see* Disorder, conduct
- blood clotting (mechanism) (*see also* Defect, coagulation) D68.9
- cerebral
  - nerve — *see* Disorder, nerve, cranial
  - status, newborn P91.9
    - specified NEC P91.88
- circulatory I99.9
- conduct (*see also* Disorder, conduct) F91.9
  - adjustment reaction — *see* Disorder, adjustment
  - compulsive F63.9

**Disturbance**(s) — *continued*
- conduct (*see also* Disorder, conduct) — *continued*
  - disruptive F91.9
  - hyperkinetic — *see* Disorder, attention-deficit hyperactivity
  - socialized F91.2
  - specified NEC F91.8
  - unsocialized F91.1
- coordination R27.8
- cranial nerve — *see* Disorder, nerve, cranial
- deep sensibility — *see* Disturbance, sensation
- digestive K30
  - psychogenic F45.8
- electrolyte (*see also* Imbalance, electrolyte)
  - newborn, transitory P74.4
    - hyperammonemia P74.6
    - potassium balance P74.3
    - sodium balance P74.2
    - specified type NEC P74.4
- emotions specific to childhood and adolescence F93.9
  - with
    - anxiety and fearfulness NEC F93.8
    - elective mutism F94.0
    - oppositional disorder F91.3
    - sensitivity (withdrawal) F40.10
    - shyness F40.10
    - social withdrawal F40.10
  - involving relationship problems F93.8
  - mixed F93.8
  - specified NEC F93.8
- endocrine (gland) E34.9
  - neonatal, transitory P72.9
    - specified NEC P72.8
- equilibrium R42
- fructose metabolism E74.10
- gait — *see* Gait
  - hysterical F44.4
  - psychogenic F44.4
- gastrointestinal (functional) K30
  - psychogenic F45.8
- habit, child F98.9
- hearing, except deafness and tinnitus — *see* Abnormal, auditory perception
- heart, functional (conditions in I44-I50)
  - due to presence of (cardiac) prosthesis I97.19- ☑
  - postoperative I97.89
    - cardiac surgery (*see also* Infarct, myocardium, associated with revascularization procedure) I97.19- ☑
- hormones E34.9
- innervation uterus (parasympathetic) (sympathetic) N85.8
- keratinization NEC
  - gingiva K05.10
    - nonplaque induced K05.11
    - plaque induced K05.10
  - lip K13.0
  - oral (mucosa) (soft tissue) K13.29
  - tongue K13.29
- learning (specific) — *see* Disorder, learning
- memory — *see* Amnesia
  - mild, following organic brain damage F06.8
- mental F99
  - associated with diseases classified elsewhere F54
- metabolism E88.9
  - with
    - abortion — *see* Abortion, by type with other specified complication
    - ectopic pregnancy O08.5
    - molar pregnancy O08.5
  - amino-acid E72.9
    - aromatic E70.9
    - branched-chain E71.2
    - straight-chain E72.8
    - sulfur-bearing E72.10
  - ammonia E72.20
  - arginine E72.21
  - arginosuccinic acid E72.22
  - carbohydrate E74.9
  - cholesterol E78.9
  - citrulline E72.23
  - cystathionine E72.19
  - general E88.9
  - glutamine E72.8
  - histidine E70.40
  - homocystine E72.19
  - hydroxylysine E72.3
  - in labor or delivery O75.89

☑ Additional Character Required — Refer to the Tabular List for Character Selection    ▽ Subterms under main terms may continue to next column or page

**Disturbance(s)** — *continued*
metabolism — *continued*
iron E83.10
lipoid E78.9
lysine E72.3
methionine E72.19
neonatal, transitory P74.9
calcium and magnesium P71.9
specified type NEC P71.8
carbohydrate metabolism P70.9
specified type NEC P70.8
specified NEC P74.8
ornithine E72.4
phosphate E83.39
sodium NEC E87.8
threonine E72.8
tryptophan E70.5
tyrosine E70.20
urea cycle E72.20
motor R29.2
nervous, functional R45.0
neuromuscular mechanism (eye), due to syphilis A52.15
nutritional E63.9
nail L60.3
ocular motion H51.9
psychogenic F45.8
oculogyric H51.8
psychogenic F45.8
oculomotor H51.9
psychogenic F45.8
olfactory nerve R43.1
optic nerve NEC — *see* Disorder, nerve, optic
oral epithelium, including tongue NEC K13.29
perceptual due to
alcohol withdrawal F10.232
amphetamine intoxication F15.922
in
abuse F15.122
dependence F15.222
anxiolytic withdrawal F13.232
cannabis intoxication (acute) F12.922
in
abuse F12.122
dependence F12.222
cocaine intoxication (acute) F14.922
in
abuse F14.122
dependence F14.222
hypnotic withdrawal F13.232
opioid intoxication (acute) F11.922
in
abuse F11.122
dependence F11.222
phencyclidine intoxication (acute) F16.122
sedative withdrawal F13.232
personality (pattern) (trait) (*see also* Disorder, personality) F60.9
following organic brain damage F07.9
polyglandular E31.9
specified NEC E31.8
potassium balance, newborn P74.3
psychogenic F45.9
psychomotor F44.4
psychophysical visual H53.16
pupillary — *see* Anomaly, pupil, function
reflex R29.2
rhythm, heart I49.9
salivary secretion K11.7
sensation (cold) (heat) (localization) (tactile discrimination) (texture) (vibratory) NEC R20.9
hysterical F44.6
skin R20.9
anesthesia R20.0
hyperesthesia R20.3
hypoesthesia R20.1
paresthesia R20.2
specified type NEC R20.8
smell R43.9
and taste (mixed) R43.8
anosmia R43.0
parosmia R43.1
specified NEC R43.8
taste R43.9
and smell (mixed) R43.8
parageusia R43.2
specified NEC R43.8
sensory — *see* Disturbance, sensation

**Disturbance(s)** — *continued*
situational (transient) (*see also* Disorder, adjustment)
acute F43.0
sleep G47.9
nonorganic origin F51.9
smell — *see* Disturbance, sensation, smell
sociopathic F60.2
sodium balance, newborn P74.2
speech R47.9
developmental F80.9
specified NEC R47.89
stomach (functional) K31.9
sympathetic (nerve) G90.9
taste — *see* Disturbance, sensation, taste
temperature
regulation, newborn P81.9
specified NEC P81.8
sense R20.8
hysterical F44.6
tooth
eruption K00.6
formation K00.4
structure, hereditary NEC K00.5
touch — *see* Disturbance, sensation
vascular I99.9
arteriosclerotic — *see* Arteriosclerosis
vasomotor I73.9
vasospastic I73.9
vision, visual H53.9
following
cerebral infarction I69.398
cerebrovascular disease I69.998
specified NEC I69.898
intracerebral hemorrhage I69.198
nontraumatic intracranial hemorrhage NEC I69.298
specified disease NEC I69.898
subarachnoid hemorrhage I69.098
psychophysical H53.16
specified NEC H53.8
subjective H53.10
day blindness H53.11
discomfort H53.14- ☑
distortions of shape and size H53.15
loss
sudden H53.13- ☑
transient H53.12- ☑
specified type NEC H53.19
voice R49.9
psychogenic F44.4
specified NEC R49.8
**Diuresis** R35.8
**Diver's palsy, paralysis or squeeze** T70.3 ☑
**Diverticulitis** (acute) K57.92
bladder — *see* Cystitis
ileum — *see* Diverticulitis, intestine, small
intestine K57.92
with
abscess, perforation or peritonitis K57.80
with bleeding K57.81
bleeding K57.93
congenital Q43.8
large K57.32
with
abscess, perforation or peritonitis K57.20
with bleeding K57.21
bleeding K57.33
small intestine K57.52
with
abscess, perforation or peritonitis K57.40
with bleeding K57.41
bleeding K57.53
small K57.12
with
abscess, perforation or peritonitis K57.00
with bleeding K57.01
bleeding K57.13
large intestine K57.52
with
abscess, perforation or peritonitis K57.40
with bleeding K57.41
bleeding K57.53
**Diverticulosis** K57.90
with bleeding K57.91
large intestine K57.30

**Diverticulosis** — *continued*
large intestine — *continued*
with
bleeding K57.31
small intestine K57.50
with bleeding K57.51
small intestine K57.10
with
bleeding K57.11
large intestine K57.50
with bleeding K57.51
**Diverticulum, diverticula** (multiple) K57.90
appendix (noninflammatory) K38.2
bladder (sphincter) N32.3
congenital Q64.6
bronchus (congenital) Q32.4
acquired J98.09
calyx, calyceal (kidney) N28.89
cardia (stomach) K31.4
cecum — *see* Diverticulosis, intestine, large
congenital Q43.8
colon — *see* Diverticulosis, intestine, large
congenital Q43.8
duodenum — *see* Diverticulosis, intestine, small
congenital Q43.8
epiphrenic (esophagus) K22.5
esophagus (congenital) Q39.6
acquired (epiphrenic) (pulsion) (traction) K22.5
eustachian tube — *see* Disorder, eustachian tube, specified NEC
fallopian tube N83.8
gastric K31.4
heart (congenital) Q24.8
ileum — *see* Diverticulosis, intestine, small
jejunum — *see* Diverticulosis, intestine, small
kidney (pelvis) (calyces) N28.89
with calculus — *see* Calculus, kidney
Meckel's (displaced) (hypertrophic) Q43.0
malignant — *see* Table of Neoplasms, small intestine, malignant
midthoracic K22.5
organ or site, congenital NEC — *see* Distortion
pericardium (congenital) (cyst) Q24.8
acquired I31.8
pharyngoesophageal (congenital) Q39.6
acquired K22.5
pharynx (congenital) Q38.7
rectosigmoid — *see* Diverticulosis, intestine, large
congenital Q43.8
rectum — *see* Diverticulosis, intestine, large
Rokitansky's K22.5
seminal vesicle N50.89
sigmoid — *see* Diverticulosis, intestine, large
congenital Q43.8
stomach (acquired) K31.4
congenital Q40.2
trachea (acquired) J39.8
ureter (acquired) N28.89
congenital Q62.8
ureterovesical orifice N28.89
urethra (acquired) N36.1
congenital Q64.79
ventricle, left (congenital) Q24.8
vesical N32.3
congenital Q64.6
Zenker's (esophagus) K22.5
**Division**
cervix uteri (acquired) N88.8
glans penis Q55.69
labia minora (congenital) Q52.79
ligament (partial or complete) (current) (*see also* Sprain)
with open wound — *see* Wound, open
muscle (partial or complete) (current) (*see also* Injury, muscle)
with open wound — *see* Wound, open
nerve (traumatic) — *see* Injury, nerve
spinal cord — *see* Injury, spinal cord, by region
vein I87.8
**Divorce, causing family disruption** Z63.5
**Dix-Hallpike neurolabyrinthitis** — *see* Neuronitis, vestibular
**Dizziness** R42
hysterical F44.89
psychogenic F45.8
**DMAC** (disseminated mycobacterium avium- intracellulare complex) A31.2
**DNR** (do not resuscitate) Z66

**Doan-Wiseman syndrome** (primary splenic neutropenia) — *see* Agranulocytosis
**Doehle-Heller aortitis** A52.02
**Dog bite** — *see* Bite
**Dohle body panmyelopathic syndrome** D72.0
**Dolichocephaly** Q67.2
**Dolichocolon** Q43.8
**Dolichostenomelia** — *see* Syndrome, Marfan's
**Donohue's syndrome** E34.8
**Donor** (organ or tissue) Z52.9
  blood (whole) Z52.000
    autologous Z52.010
      specified component (lymphocytes) (platelets) NEC Z52.008
        autologous Z52.018
        specified donor NEC Z52.098
      specified donor NEC Z52.090
    stem cells Z52.001
      autologous Z52.011
      specified donor NEC Z52.091
  bone Z52.20
    autologous Z52.21
    marrow Z52.3
    specified type NEC Z52.29
  cornea Z52.5
  egg (Oocyte) Z52.819
    age 35 and over Z52.812
      anonymous recipient Z52.812
      designated recipient Z52.813
    under age 35 Z52.810
      anonymous recipient Z52.810
      designated recipient Z52.811
  kidney Z52.4
  liver Z52.6
  lung Z52.89
  lymphocyte — *see* Donor, blood, specified components NEC
  Oocyte — *see* Donor, egg
  platelets Z52.008
  potential, examination of Z00.5
  semen Z52.89
  skin Z52.10
    autologous Z52.11
    specified type NEC Z52.19
  specified organ or tissue NEC Z52.89
  sperm Z52.89
**Donovanosis** A58
**Dorsalgia** M54.9
  psychogenic F45.41
  specified NEC M54.89
**Dorsopathy** M53.9
  deforming M43.9
    specified NEC — *see* subcategory M43.8 ☑
  specified NEC M53.80
    cervical region M53.82
    cervicothoracic region M53.83
    lumbar region M53.86
    lumbosacral region M53.87
    occipito-atlanto-axial region M53.81
    sacrococcygeal region M53.88
    thoracic region M53.84
    thoracolumbar region M53.85
**Double**
  albumin E88.09
  aortic arch Q25.45
  auditory canal Q17.8
  auricle (heart) Q20.8
  bladder Q64.79
  cervix Q51.820
    with doubling of uterus (and vagina) Q51.10
      with obstruction Q51.11
  inlet ventricle Q20.4
  kidney with double pelvis (renal) Q63.0
  meatus urinarius Q64.75
  monster Q89.4
  outlet
    left ventricle Q20.2
    right ventricle Q20.1
  pelvis (renal) with double ureter Q62.5
  tongue Q38.3
  ureter (one or both sides) Q62.5
    with double pelvis (renal) Q62.5
  urethra Q64.74
  urinary meatus Q64.75
  uterus Q51.2
    with
      doubling of cervix (and vagina) Q51.10
        with obstruction Q51.11

**Double** — *continued*
  uterus — *continued*
    in pregnancy or childbirth O34.59- ☑
      causing obstructed labor O65.5
    vagina Q52.10
      with doubling of uterus (and cervix) Q51.10
        with obstruction Q51.11
    vision H53.2
    vulva Q52.79
**Douglas' pouch, cul-de-sac** — *see* condition
**Down syndrome** Q90.9
  meiotic nondisjunction Q90.0
  mitotic nondisjunction Q90.1
  mosaicism Q90.1
  translocation Q90.2
**DPD** (dihydropyrimidine dehydrogenase deficiency) E88.89
**Dracontiasis** B72
**Dracunculiasis, dracunculosis** B72
**Dream state, hysterical** F44.89
**Drepanocytic anemia** — *see* Disease, sickle-cell
**Dresbach's syndrome** (elliptocytosis) D58.1
**Dreschlera** (hawaiiensis) (infection) B43.8
**Dressler's syndrome** I24.1
**Drift, ulnar** — *see* Deformity, limb, specified type NEC, forearm
**Drinking** (alcohol)
  excessive, to excess NEC (without dependence) F10.10
    habitual (continual) (without remission) F10.20
      with remission F10.21
**Drip, postnasal** (chronic) R09.82
  due to
    allergic rhinitis — *see* Rhinitis, allergic
    common cold J00
    gastroesophageal reflux — *see* Reflux, gastroesophageal
    nasopharyngitis — *see* Nasopharyngitis
    other known condition — *code to* condition
    sinusitis — *see* Sinusitis
**Droop**
  facial R29.810
    cerebrovascular disease I69.992
      cerebral infarction I69.392
      intracerebral hemorrhage I69.192
      nontraumatic intracranial hemorrhage NEC I69.292
      specified disease NEC I69.892
      subarachnoid hemorrhage I69.092
**Drop** (in)
  attack NEC R55
  finger — *see* Deformity, finger
  foot — *see* Deformity, limb, foot, drop
  hematocrit (precipitous) R71.0
  hemoglobin R71.0
  toe — *see* Deformity, toe, specified NEC
  wrist — *see* Deformity, limb, wrist drop
**Dropped heart beats** I45.9
**Dropsy, dropsical** (*see also* Hydrops)
  abdomen R18.8
  brain — *see* Hydrocephalus
  cardiac, heart — *see* Failure, heart, congestive
  gangrenous — *see* Gangrene
  heart — *see* Failure, heart, congestive
  kidney — *see* Nephrosis
  lung — *see* Edema, lung
  newborn due to isoimmunization P56.0
  pericardium — *see* Pericarditis
**Drowned, drowning** (near) T75.1 ☑
**Drowsiness** R40.0
**Drug**
  abuse counseling and surveillance Z71.51
  addiction — *see* Dependence
  dependence — *see* Dependence
  habit — *see* Dependence
  harmful use — *see* Abuse, drug
  induced fever R50.2
  overdose — *see* Table of Drugs and Chemicals, by drug, poisoning
  poisoning — *see* Table of Drugs and Chemicals, by drug, poisoning
  resistant organism infection (*see also* Resistant, organism, to, drug) Z16.30
  therapy
    long term (current) (prophylactic) — *see* Therapy, drug long-term (current) (prophylactic)

**Drug** — *continued*
  therapy — *continued*
    short term — *omit code*
    wrong substance given or taken in error — *see* Table of Drugs and Chemicals, by drug, poisoning
**Drunkenness** (without dependence) F10.129
  acute in alcoholism F10.229
  chronic (without remission) F10.20
    with remission F10.21
  pathological (without dependence) F10.129
    with dependence F10.229
  sleep F51.9
**Drusen**
  macula (degenerative) (retina) — *see* Degeneration, macula, drusen
  optic disc H47.32- ☑
**Dry, dryness** (*see also* condition)
  larynx J38.7
  mouth R68.2
    due to dehydration E86.0
  nose J34.89
  socket (teeth) M27.3
  throat J39.2
**DSAP** L56.5
**Duane's syndrome** H50.81- ☑
**Dubin-Johnson disease or syndrome** E80.6
**Dubois' disease** (thymus gland) A50.59 [E35]
**Dubowitz' syndrome** Q87.1
**Duchenne-Aran muscular atrophy** G12.21
**Duchenne-Griesinger disease** G71.0
**Duchenne's**
  disease or syndrome
    motor neuron disease G12.22
    muscular dystrophy G71.0
  locomotor ataxia (syphilitic) A52.11
  paralysis
    birth injury P14.0
    due to or associated with
      motor neuron disease G12.22
      muscular dystrophy G71.0
**Ducrey's chancre** A57
**Duct, ductus** — *see* condition
**Duhring's disease** (dermatitis herpetiformis) L13.0
**Dullness, cardiac** (decreased) (increased) R01.2
**Dumb ague** — *see* Malaria
**Dumbness** — *see* Aphasia
**Dumdum fever** B55.0
**Dumping syndrome** (postgastrectomy) K91.1
**Duodenitis** (nonspecific) (peptic) K29.80
  with bleeding K29.81
**Duodenocholangitis** — *see* Cholangitis
**Duodenum, duodenal** — *see* condition
**Duplay's bursitis or periarthritis** — *see* Tendinitis, calcific, shoulder
**Duplication, duplex** (*see also* Accessory)
  alimentary tract Q45.8
  anus Q43.4
  appendix (and cecum) Q43.4
  biliary duct (any) Q44.5
  bladder Q64.79
  cecum (and appendix) Q43.4
  cervix Q51.820
  chromosome NEC
    with complex rearrangements NEC Q92.5
    seen only at prometaphase Q92.8
  cystic duct Q44.5
  digestive organs Q45.8
  esophagus Q39.8
  frontonasal process Q75.8
  intestine (large) (small) Q43.4
  kidney Q63.0
  liver Q44.7
  pancreas Q45.3
  penis Q55.69
  respiratory organs NEC Q34.8
  salivary duct Q38.4
  spinal cord (incomplete) Q06.2
  stomach Q40.2
**Dupré's disease** (meningism) R29.1
**Dupuytren's contraction or disease** M72.0
**Durand-Nicolas-Favre disease** A55
**Durotomy** (inadvertent) (incidental) G97.41
**Duroziez's disease** (congenital mitral stenosis) Q23.2
**Dutton's relapsing fever** (West African) A68.1
**Dwarfism** E34.3
  achondroplastic Q77.4
  congenital E34.3
  constitutional E34.3

**Dwarfism** — *continued*
 hypochondroplastic Q77.4
 hypophyseal E23.0
 infantile E34.3
 Laron-type E34.3
 Lorain (-Levi) type E23.0
 metatropic Q77.8
 nephrotic-glycosuric (with hypophosphatemic rickets) E72.09
 nutritional E45
 pancreatic K86.89
 pituitary E23.0
 renal N25.0
 thanatophoric Q77.1
**Dyke-Young anemia** (secondary) (symptomatic) D59.1
**Dysacusis** — *see* Abnormal, auditory perception
**Dysadrenocortism** E27.9
 hyperfunction E27.0
**Dysarthria** R47.1
 following
  cerebral infarction I69.322
  cerebrovascular disease I69.922
   specified disease NEC I69.822
  intracerebral hemorrhage I69.122
  nontraumatic intracranial hemorrhage NEC I69.222
  subarachnoid hemorrhage I69.022
**Dysautonomia** (familial) G90.1
**Dysbarism** T70.3 ☑
**Dysbasia** R26.2
 angiosclerotica intermittens I73.9
 hysterical F44.4
 lordotica (progressiva) G24.1
 nonorganic origin F44.4
 psychogenic F44.4
**Dysbetalipoproteinemia** (familial) E78.2
**Dyscalculia** R48.8
 developmental F81.2
**Dyschezia** K59.00
**Dyschondroplasia** (with hemangiomata) Q78.4
**Dyschromia** (skin) L81.9
**Dyscollagenosis** M35.9
**Dyscranio-pygo-phalangy** Q87.0
**Dyscrasia**
 blood (with) D75.9
  antepartum hemorrhage — *see* Hemorrhage, antepartum, with coagulation defect
  intrapartum hemorrhage O67.0
  newborn P61.9
   specified type NEC P61.8
  puerperal, postpartum O72.3
 polyglandular, pluriglandular E31.9
**Dysendocrinism** E34.9
**Dysentery, dysenteric** (catarrhal) (diarrhea) (epidemic) (hemorrhagic) (infectious) (sporadic) (tropical) A09
 abscess, liver A06.4
 amebic (*see also* Amebiasis) A06.0
  with abscess — *see* Abscess, amebic
  acute A06.0
  chronic A06.1
 arthritis (*see also* category M01) A09
  bacillary (*see also* category M01) A03.9
 bacillary A03.9
  arthritis (*see also* category M01) A03.9
  Boyd A03.2
  Flexner A03.1
  Schmitz (-Stutzer) A03.0
  Shiga (-Kruse) A03.0
  Shigella A03.9
   boydii A03.2
   dysenteriae A03.0
   flexneri A03.1
   group A A03.0
   group B A03.1
   group C A03.2
   group D A03.3
   sonnei A03.3
   specified type NEC A03.8
  Sonne A03.3
  specified type NEC A03.8
 balantidial A07.0
 Balantidium coli A07.0
 Boyd's A03.2
 candidal B37.82
 Chilomastix A07.8
 Chinese A03.9
 coccidial A07.3
 Dientamoeba (fragilis) A07.8
 Embadomonas A07.8

**Dysentery, dysenteric** — *continued*
 Entamoeba, entamebic — *see* Dysentery, amebic
 Flexner-Boyd A03.2
 Flexner's A03.1
 Giardia lamblia A07.1
 Hiss-Russell A03.1
 Lamblia A07.1
 leishmanial B55.0
 malarial — *see* Malaria
 metazoal B82.0
 monilial B37.82
 protozoal A07.9
 Salmonella A02.0
 schistosomal B65.1
 Schmitz (-Stutzer) A03.0
 Shiga (-Kruse) A03.0
 Shigella NOS — *see* Dysentery, bacillary
 Sonne A03.3
 strongyloidiasis B78.0
 trichomonal A07.8
 viral (*see also* Enteritis, viral) A08.4
**Dysequilibrium** R42
**Dysesthesia** R20.8
 hysterical F44.6
**Dysfibrinogenemia** (congenital) D68.2
**Dysfunction**
 adrenal E27.9
  hyperfunction E27.0
 autonomic
  due to alcohol G31.2
  somatoform F45.8
 bladder N31.9
  neurogenic NOS — *see* Dysfunction, bladder, neuromuscular
  neuromuscular NOS N31.9
   atonic (motor) (sensory) N31.2
   autonomous N31.2
   flaccid N31.2
   nonreflex N31.2
   reflex N31.1
   specified NEC N31.8
   uninhibited N31.0
 bleeding, uterus N93.8
 cerebral G93.89
 colon K59.9
  psychogenic F45.8
 colostomy K94.03
 cystic duct K82.8
 cystostomy (stoma) — *see* Complications, cystostomy
 ejaculatory N53.19
  anejaculatory orgasm N53.13
  painful N53.12
  premature F52.4
  retarded N53.11
 endocrine NOS E34.9
 endometrium N85.8
 enterostomy K94.13
 erectile — *see* Dysfunction, sexual, male, erectile
 gallbladder K82.8
 gastrostomy (stoma) K94.23
 gland, glandular NOS E34.9
 heart I51.89
 hemoglobin D75.89
 hepatic K76.89
 hypophysis E23.7
 hypothalamic NEC E23.3
 ileostomy (stoma) K94.13
 jejunostomy (stoma) K94.13
 kidney — *see* Disease, renal
 labyrinthine — *see* subcategory H83.2 ☑
 left ventricular, following sudden emotional stress I51.81
 liver K76.89
 male — *see* Dysfunction, sexual, male
 orgasmic (female) F52.31
  male F52.32
 ovary E28.9
  specified NEC E28.8
 papillary muscle I51.89
 parathyroid E21.4
 physiological NEC R68.89
  psychogenic F59
 pineal gland E34.8
 pituitary (gland) E23.3
 platelets D69.1
 polyglandular E31.9
  specified NEC E31.8
 psychophysiologic F59

**Dysfunction** — *continued*
 psychosexual F52.9
  with
   dyspareunia F52.6
   premature ejaculation F52.4
   vaginismus F52.5
 pylorus K31.9
 rectum K59.9
  psychogenic F45.8
 reflex (sympathetic) — *see* Syndrome, pain, complex regional I
 segmental — *see* Dysfunction, somatic
 senile R54
 sexual (due to) R37
  alcohol F10.981
  amphetamine F15.981
   in
    abuse F15.181
    dependence F15.281
  anxiolytic F13.981
   in
    abuse F13.181
    dependence F13.281
  cocaine F14.981
   in
    abuse F14.181
    dependence F14.281
  excessive sexual drive F52.8
  failure of genital response (male) F52.21
   female F52.22
  female N94.9
   aversion F52.1
   dyspareunia N94.10
    psychogenic F52.6
   frigidity F52.22
   nymphomania F52.8
   orgasmic F52.31
   psychogenic F52.9
    aversion F52.1
    dyspareunia F52.6
    frigidity F52.22
    nymphomania F52.8
    orgasmic F52.31
    vaginismus F52.5
   vaginismus N94.2
    psychogenic F52.5
  hypnotic F13.981
   in
    abuse F13.181
    dependence F13.281
  inhibited orgasm (female) F52.31
   male F52.32
  lack
   of sexual enjoyment F52.1
   or loss of sexual desire F52.0
  male N53.9
   anejaculatory orgasm N53.13
   ejaculatory N53.19
    painful N53.12
    premature F52.4
    retarded N53.11
   erectile N52.9
    drug induced N52.2
    due to
     disease classified elsewhere N52.1
     drug N52.2
    postoperative (postprocedural) N52.39
     following
      cryotherapy N52.37
      interstitial seed therapy N52.36
      prostate ablative therapy N52.37
      prostatectomy N52.34
       radical N52.31
      radiation therapy N52.35
      radical cystectomy N52.32
      ultrasound ablative therapy N52.37
      urethral surgery N52.33
    psychogenic F52.21
    specified cause NEC N52.8
    vasculogenic
     arterial insufficiency N52.01
      with corporo-venous occlusive N52.03
     corporo-venous occlusive N52.02
      with arterial insufficiency N52.03
   impotence — *see* Dysfunction, sexual, male, erectile
   psychogenic F52.9
    aversion F52.1

**Dysfunction** — *continued*
  sexual — *continued*
    male — *continued*
      psychogenic — *continued*
        erectile F52.21
        orgasmic F52.32
        premature ejaculation F52.4
        satyriasis F52.8
        specified type NEC F52.8
      specified type NEC N53.8
      nonorganic F52.9
        specified NEC F52.8
      opioid F11.981
        in
          abuse F11.181
          dependence F11.281
      orgasmic dysfunction (female) F52.31
        male F52.32
      premature ejaculation F52.4
      psychoactive substances NEC F19.981
        in
          abuse F19.181
          dependence F19.281
      psychogenic F52.9
      sedative F13.981
        in
          abuse F13.181
          dependence F13.281
      sexual aversion F52.1
      vaginismus (nonorganic) (psychogenic) F52.5
  sinoatrial node I49.5
  somatic M99.09
    abdomen M99.09
    acromioclavicular M99.07
    cervical region M99.01
    cervicothoracic M99.01
    costochondral M99.08
    costovertebral M99.08
    head region M99.00
    hip M99.05
    lower extremity M99.06
    lumbar region M99.03
    lumbosacral M99.03
    occipitocervical M99.00
    pelvic region M99.05
    pubic M99.05
    rib cage M99.08
    sacral region M99.04
    sacrococcygeal M99.04
    sacroiliac M99.04
    specified NEC M99.09
    sternochondral M99.08
    sternoclavicular M99.07
    thoracic region M99.02
    thoracolumbar M99.02
    upper extremity M99.07
  somatoform autonomic F45.8
  stomach K31.89
    psychogenic F45.8
  suprarenal E27.9
    hyperfunction E27.0
  symbolic R48.9
    specified type NEC R48.8
  temporomandibular (joint) M26.69
    joint-pain syndrome M26.62- ☑
  testicular (endocrine) E29.9
    specified NEC E29.8
  thymus E32.9
  thyroid E07.9
  ureterostomy (stoma) — *see* Complications, stoma, urinary tract
  urethrostomy (stoma) — *see* Complications, stoma, urinary tract
  uterus, complicating delivery O62.9
    hypertonic O62.4
    hypotonic O62.2
      primary O62.0
      secondary O62.1
  ventricular I51.9
    with congestive heart failure (*see also* Failure, heart) I50.9
    left, reversible, following sudden emotional stress I51.81

**Dysgenesis**
  gonadal (due to chromosomal anomaly) Q96.9
    pure Q99.1
  renal Q60.5
    bilateral Q60.4
    unilateral Q60.3

**Dysgenesis** — *continued*
  reticular D72.0
  tidal platelet D69.3
**Dysgerminoma**
  specified site — *see* Neoplasm, malignant, by site
  unspecified site
    female C56.9
    male C62.90
**Dysgeusia** R43.2
**Dysgraphia** R27.8
**Dyshidrosis, dysidrosis** L30.1
**Dyskaryotic cervical smear** R87.619
**Dyskeratosis** L85.8
  cervix — *see* Dysplasia, cervix
  congenital Q82.8
  uterus NEC N85.8
**Dyskinesia** G24.9
  biliary (cystic duct or gallbladder) K82.8
  drug induced
    orofacial G24.01
  esophagus K22.4
  hysterical F44.4
  intestinal K59.8
  nonorganic origin F44.4
  orofacial (idiopathic) G24.4
    drug induced G24.01
  psychogenic F44.4
  subacute, drug induced G24.01
  tardive G24.01
    neuroleptic induced G24.01
  trachea J39.8
  tracheobronchial J98.09
**Dyslalia** (developmental) F80.0
**Dyslexia** R48.0
  developmental F81.0
**Dyslipidemia** E78.5
  depressed HDL cholesterol E78.6
  elevated fasting triglycerides E78.1
**Dysmaturity** (*see also* Light for dates)
  pulmonary (newborn) (Wilson-Mikity) P27.0
**Dysmenorrhea** (essential) (exfoliative) N94.6
  congestive (syndrome) N94.6
  primary N94.4
  psychogenic F45.8
  secondary N94.5
**Dysmetabolic syndrome X** E88.81
**Dysmetria** R27.8
**Dysmorphism** (due to)
  alcohol Q86.0
  exogenous cause NEC Q86.8
  hydantoin Q86.1
  warfarin Q86.2
**Dysmorphophobia** (nondelusional) F45.22
  delusional F22
**Dysnomia** R47.01
**Dysorexia** R63.0
  psychogenic F50.89
**Dysostosis**
  cleidocranial, cleidocranialis Q74.0
  craniofacial Q75.1
  Fairbank's (idiopathic familial generalized osteophytosis) Q78.9
  mandibulofacial (incomplete) Q75.4
  multiplex E76.01
  oculomandibular Q75.5
**Dyspareunia** (female) N94.10
  deep N94.12
  male N53.12
  nonorganic F52.6
  psychogenic F52.6
  secondary N94.19
  specified NEC N94.19
  superficial (introital) N94.11
**Dyspepsia** R10.13
  atonic K30
  functional (allergic) (congenital) (gastrointestinal) (occupational) (reflex) K30
  intestinal K59.8
  nervous F45.8
  neurotic F45.8
  psychogenic F45.8
**Dysphagia** R13.10
  cervical R13.19
  following
    cerebral infarction I69.391
    cerebrovascular disease I69.991
      specified NEC I69.891
    intracerebral hemorrhage I69.191

**Dysphagia** — *continued*
  following — *continued*
    nontraumatic intracranial hemorrhage NEC I69.291
    specified disease NEC I69.891
    subarachnoid hemorrhage I69.091
  functional (hysterical) F45.8
  hysterical F45.8
  nervous (hysterical) F45.8
  neurogenic R13.19
  oral phase R13.11
  oropharyngeal phase R13.12
  pharyngeal phase R13.13
  pharyngoesophageal phase R13.14
  psychogenic F45.8
  sideropenic D50.1
  spastica K22.4
  specified NEC R13.19
**Dysphagocytosis, congenital** D71
**Dysphasia** R47.02
  developmental
    expressive type F80.1
    receptive type F80.2
  following
    cerebrovascular disease I69.921
      cerebral infarction I69.321
      intracerebral hemorrhage I69.121
      nontraumatic intracranial hemorrhage NEC I69.221
      specified disease NEC I69.821
      subarachnoid hemorrhage I69.021
**Dysphonia** R49.0
  functional F44.4
  hysterical F44.4
  psychogenic F44.4
  spastica J38.3
**Dysphoria**
  gender F64.9
    in
      adolescence and adulthood F64.0
      children F64.2
    specified NEC F64.8
  postpartal O90.6
**Dyspituitarism** E23.3
**Dysplasia** (*see also* Anomaly)
  acetabular, congenital Q65.89
  alveolar capillary, with vein misalignment J84.843
  anus (histologically confirmed) (mild) (moderate) K62.82
    severe D01.3
  arrhythmogenic right ventricular I42.8
  arterial, fibromuscular I77.3
  asphyxiating thoracic (congenital) Q77.2
  brain Q07.9
  bronchopulmonary, perinatal P27.1
  cervix (uteri) N87.9
    mild N87.0
    moderate N87.1
    severe D06.9
  chondroectodermal Q77.6
  colon D12.6
  craniometaphyseal Q78.8
  dentinal K00.5
  diaphyseal, progressive Q78.3
  dystrophic Q77.5
  ectodermal (anhidrotic) (congenital) (hereditary) Q82.4
    hydrotic Q82.8
  epithelial, uterine cervix — *see* Dysplasia, cervix
  eye (congenital) Q11.2
  fibrous
    bone NEC (monostotic) M85.00
      ankle M85.07- ☑
      foot M85.07- ☑
      forearm M85.03- ☑
      hand M85.04- ☑
      lower leg M85.06- ☑
      multiple site M85.09
      neck M85.08
      rib M85.08
      shoulder M85.01- ☑
      skull M85.08
      specified site NEC M85.08
      thigh M85.05- ☑
      toe M85.07- ☑
      upper arm M85.02- ☑
      vertebra M85.08
  diaphyseal, progressive Q78.3
  jaw M27.8
  polyostotic Q78.1

124

☑ **Additional Character Required** — Refer to the Tabular List for Character Selection    ▽ **Subterms under main terms may continue to next column or page**

**Dysplasia** — continued
- florid osseous (see also Cyst, calcifying odontogenic)
- high grade, focal D12.6
- hip, congenital Q65.89
- joint, congenital Q74.8
- kidney Q61.4
  - multicystic Q61.4
- leg Q74.2
- lung, congenital (not associated with short gestation) Q33.6
- mammary (gland) (benign) N60.9- ☑
  - cyst (solitary) — see Cyst, breast
  - cystic — see Mastopathy, cystic
  - duct ectasia — see Ectasia, mammary duct
  - fibroadenosis — see Fibroadenosis, breast
  - fibrosclerosis — see Fibrosclerosis, breast
  - specified type NEC N60.8- ☑
- metaphyseal Q78.5
- muscle Q79.8
- oculodentodigital Q87.0
- periapical (cemental) (cemento-osseous) — see Cyst, calcifying odontogenic
- periosteum — see Disorder, bone, specified type NEC
- polyostotic fibrous Q78.1
- prostate (see also Neoplasia, intraepithelial, prostate) N42.30
  - severe D07.5
  - specified NEC N42.39
- renal Q61.4
  - multicystic Q61.4
- retinal, congenital Q14.1
- right ventricular, arrhythmogenic I42.8
- septo-optic Q04.4
- skin L98.8
- spinal cord Q06.1
- spondyloepiphyseal Q77.7
- thymic, with immunodeficiency D82.1
- vagina N89.3
  - mild N89.0
  - moderate N89.1
  - severe NEC D07.2
- vulva N90.3
  - mild N90.0
  - moderate N90.1
  - severe NEC D07.1

**Dyspnea** (nocturnal) (paroxysmal) R06.00
- asthmatic (bronchial) J45.909
  - with
    - bronchitis J45.909
      - with
        - exacerbation (acute) J45.901
        - status asthmaticus J45.902
      - chronic J44.9
    - exacerbation (acute) J45.901
    - status asthmaticus J45.902
  - cardiac — see Failure, ventricular, left
- cardiac — see Failure, ventricular, left
- functional F45.8
- hyperventilation R06.4
- hysterical F45.8
- newborn P28.89
- orthopnea R06.01
- psychogenic F45.8
- shortness of breath R06.02
- specified type NEC R06.09

**Dyspraxia** R27.8
- developmental (syndrome) F82

**Dysproteinemia** E88.09
**Dysreflexia, autonomic** G90.4
**Dysrhythmia**
- cardiac I49.9
- newborn
  - bradycardia P29.12
  - occurring before birth P03.819
    - before onset of labor P03.810
    - during labor P03.811
  - tachycardia P29.11
- postoperative I97.89
- cerebral or cortical — see Epilepsy

**Dyssomnia** — see Disorder, sleep
**Dyssynergia**
- biliary K83.8
- bladder sphincter N36.44
- cerebellaris myoclonica (Hunt's ataxia) G11.1

**Dysthymia** F34.1
**Dysthyroidism** E07.9
**Dystocia** O66.9
- affecting newborn P03.1

**Dystocia** — continued
- cervical (hypotonic) O62.2
  - affecting newborn P03.6
  - primary O62.0
  - secondary O62.1
- contraction ring O62.4
- fetal O66.9
  - abnormality NEC O66.3
  - conjoined twins O66.3
  - oversize O66.2
- maternal O66.9
- positional O64.9 ☑
- shoulder (girdle) O66.0
  - causing obstructed labor O66.0
- uterine NEC O62.4

**Dystonia** G24.9
- deformans progressiva G24.1
- drug induced NEC G24.09
  - acute G24.02
  - specified NEC G24.09
- familial G24.1
- idiopathic G24.1
  - familial G24.1
  - nonfamilial G24.2
  - orofacial G24.4
- lenticularis G24.8
- musculorum deformans G24.1
- neuroleptic induced (acute) G24.02
- orofacial (idiopathic) G24.4
- oromandibular G24.4
  - due to drug G24.01
- specified NEC G24.8
- torsion (familial) (idiopathic) G24.1
  - acquired G24.8
  - genetic G24.1
  - symptomatic (nonfamilial) G24.2

**Dystonic movements** R25.8
**Dystrophy, dystrophia**
- adiposogenital E23.6
- Becker's type G71.0
- cervical sympathetic G90.2
- choroid (hereditary) H31.20
  - central areolar H31.22
  - choroideremia H31.21
  - gyrate atrophy H31.23
  - specified type NEC H31.29
- cornea (hereditary) H18.50
  - endothelial H18.51
  - epithelial H18.52
  - granular H18.53
  - lattice H18.54
  - macular H18.55
  - specified type NEC H18.59
- Duchenne's type G71.0
- due to malnutrition E45
- Erb's G71.0
- Fuchs' H18.51
- Gower's muscular G71.0
- hair L67.8
- infantile neuraxonal G31.89
- Landouzy-Déjérine G71.0
- Leyden-Möbius G71.0
- muscular G71.0
  - benign (Becker type) G71.0
  - congenital (hereditary) (progressive) (with specific morphological abnormalities of the muscle fiber) G71.0
    - myotonic G71.11
  - distal G71.0
  - Duchenne type G71.0
  - Emery-Dreifuss G71.0
  - Erb type G71.0
  - facioscapulohumeral G71.0
  - Gower's G71.0
  - hereditary (progressive) G71.0
  - Landouzy-Déjérine type G71.0
  - limb-girdle G71.0
  - myotonic G71.11
  - progressive (hereditary) G71.0
    - Charcot-Marie (-Tooth) type G60.0
  - pseudohypertrophic (infantile) G71.0
  - severe (Duchenne type) G71.0
- myocardium, myocardial — see Degeneration, myocardial
- nail L60.3
  - congenital Q84.6
- nutritional E45
- ocular G71.0
- oculocerebrorenal E72.03

**Dystrophy, dystrophia** — continued
- oculopharyngeal G71.0
- ovarian N83.8
- polyglandular E31.8
- reflex (neuromuscular) (sympathetic) — see Syndrome, pain, complex regional I
- retinal (hereditary) H35.50
  - in
    - lipid storage disorders E75.6 [H36]
    - systemic lipidoses E75.6 [H36]
  - involving
    - pigment epithelium H35.54
    - sensory area H35.53
  - pigmentary H35.52
  - vitreoretinal H35.51
- Salzmann's nodular — see Degeneration, cornea, nodular
- scapuloperoneal G71.0
- skin NEC L98.8
- sympathetic (reflex) — see Syndrome, pain, complex regional I
  - cervical G90.2
- tapetoretinal H35.54
- thoracic, asphyxiating Q77.2
- unguium L60.3
  - congenital Q84.6
- vitreoretinal H35.51
- vulva N90.4
- yellow (liver) — see Failure, hepatic

**Dysuria** R30.0
- psychogenic F45.8

# E

**Eales' disease** H35.06- ☑
**Ear** (see also condition)
- piercing Z41.3
- tropical NEC B36.9 [H62.40]
  - in
    - aspergillosis B44.89
    - candidiasis B37.84
    - moniliasis B37.84
- wax (impacted) H61.20
  - left H61.22
    - with right H61.23
  - right H61.21
    - with left H61.23

**Earache** — see subcategory H92.0 ☑
**Early satiety** R68.81
**Eaton-Lambert syndrome** — see Syndrome, Lambert-Eaton
**Eberth's disease** (typhoid fever) A01.00
**Ebola virus disease** A98.4
**Ebstein's anomaly or syndrome** (heart) Q22.5
**Eccentro-osteochondrodysplasia** E76.29
**Ecchondroma** — see Neoplasm, bone, benign
**Ecchondrosis** D48.0
**Ecchymosis** R58
- conjunctiva — see Hemorrhage, conjunctiva
- eye (traumatic) — see Contusion, eyeball
- eyelid (traumatic) — see Contusion, eyelid
- newborn P54.5
- spontaneous R23.3
- traumatic — see Contusion

**Echinococciasis** — see Echinococcus
**Echinococcosis** — see Echinococcus
**Echinococcus** (infection) B67.90
- granulosus B67.4
  - bone B67.2
  - liver B67.0
  - lung B67.1
  - multiple sites B67.32
  - specified site NEC B67.39
  - thyroid B67.31
- liver NOS B67.8
  - granulosus B67.0
  - multilocularis B67.5
- lung NEC B67.99
  - granulosus B67.1
  - multilocularis B67.69
- multilocularis B67.7
  - liver B67.5
  - multiple sites B67.61
  - specified site NEC B67.69
- specified site NEC B67.99
  - granulosus B67.39
  - multilocularis B67.69
- thyroid NEC B67.99

**Echinococcus** — continued
  thyroid — continued
    granulosus B67.31
    multilocularis B67.69 [E35]
**Echinorhynchiasis** B83.8
**Echinostomiasis** B66.8
**Echolalia** R48.8
**Echovirus, as cause of disease classified elsewhere**
  B97.12
**Eclampsia, eclamptic** (coma) (convulsions) (delirium)
  (with hypertension) NEC O15.9
  complicating
    labor and delivery O15.1
    postpartum O15.2
    pregnancy O15.0- ☑
    puerperium O15.2
**Economic circumstances affecting care** Z59.9
**Economo's disease** A85.8
**Ectasia, ectasis**
  annuloaortic I35.8
  aorta I77.819
    with aneurysm — see Aneurysm, aorta
    abdominal I77.811
    thoracic I77.810
    thoracoabdominal I77.812
  breast — see Ectasia, mammary duct
  capillary I78.8
  cornea H18.71- ☑
  gastric antral vascular (GAVE) K31.819
    with hemorrhage K31.811
    without hemorrhage K31.819
  mammary duct N60.4- ☑
  salivary gland (duct) K11.8
  sclera — see Sclerectasia
**Ecthyma** L08.0
  contagiosum B08.02
  gangrenosum L08.0
  infectiosum B08.02
**Ectocardia** Q24.8
**Ectodermal dysplasia** (anhidrotic) Q82.4
**Ectodermosis erosiva pluriorificialis** L51.1
**Ectopic, ectopia** (congenital)
  abdominal viscera Q45.8
    due to defect in anterior abdominal wall Q79.59
  ACTH syndrome E24.3
  adrenal gland Q89.1
  anus Q43.5
  atrial beats I49.1
  beats I49.49
    atrial I49.1
    ventricular I49.3
  bladder Q64.10
  bone and cartilage in lung Q33.5
  brain Q04.8
  breast tissue Q83.8
  cardiac Q24.8
  cerebral Q04.8
  cordis Q24.8
  endometrium — see Endometriosis
  gastric mucosa Q40.2
  gestation — see Pregnancy, by site
  heart Q24.8
  hormone secretion NEC E34.2
  kidney (crossed) (pelvis) Q63.2
  lens, lentis Q12.1
  mole — see Pregnancy, by site
  organ or site NEC — see Malposition, congenital
  pancreas Q45.3
  pregnancy — see Pregnancy, ectopic
  pupil — see Abnormality, pupillary
  renal Q63.2
  sebaceous glands of mouth Q38.6
  spleen Q89.09
  testis Q53.00
    bilateral Q53.02
    unilateral Q53.01
  thyroid Q89.2
  tissue in lung Q33.5
  ureter Q62.63
  ventricular beats I49.3
  vesicae Q64.10
**Ectromelia** Q73.8
  lower limb — see Defect, reduction, limb, lower,
    specified type NEC
  upper limb — see Defect, reduction, limb, upper,
    specified type NEC
**Ectropion** H02.109
  cervix N86

**Ectropion** — continued
  cervix — continued
    with cervicitis N72
  congenital Q10.1
  eyelid (paralytic) H02.109
    cicatricial H02.119
      left H02.116
        lower H02.115
        upper H02.114
      right H02.113
        lower H02.112
        upper H02.111
    congenital Q10.1
    left H02.106
      lower H02.105
      upper H02.104
    mechanical H02.129
      left H02.126
        lower H02.125
        upper H02.124
      right H02.123
        lower H02.122
        upper H02.121
    right H02.103
      lower H02.102
      upper H02.101
    senile H02.139
      left H02.136
        lower H02.135
        upper H02.134
      right H02.133
        lower H02.132
        upper H02.131
    spastic H02.149
      left H02.146
        lower H02.145
        upper H02.144
      right H02.143
        lower H02.142
        upper H02.141
  iris H21.89
  lip (acquired) K13.0
    congenital Q38.0
  urethra N36.8
  uvea H21.89
**Eczema** (acute) (chronic) (erythematous) (fissum)
  (rubrum) (squamous) (see also Dermatitis) L30.9
  contact — see Dermatitis, contact
  dyshydrotic L30.1
  external ear — see Otitis, externa, acute, eczematoid
  flexural L20.82
  herpeticum B00.0
  hypertrophicum L28.0
  hypostatic — see Varix, leg, with, inflammation
  impetiginous L01.1
  infantile (due to any substance) L20.83
    intertriginous L21.1
    seborrheic L21.1
  intertriginous NEC L30.4
    infantile L21.1
  intrinsic (allergic) L20.84
  lichenified NEC L28.0
  marginatum (hebrae) B35.6
  pustular L30.3
  stasis I87.2
    with varicose veins — see Varix, leg, with, inflam-
      mation
  vaccination, vaccinatum T88.1 ☑
  varicose — see Varix, leg, with, inflammation
**Eczematid** L30.2
**Eddowes** (-Spurway) **syndrome** Q78.0
**Edema, edematous** (infectious) (pitting) (toxic) R60.9
  with nephritis — see Nephrosis
  allergic T78.3 ☑
  amputation stump (surgical) (sequelae (late effect))
    T87.89
  angioneurotic (allergic) (any site) (with urticaria)
    T78.3 ☑
    hereditary D84.1
  angiospastic I73.9
  Berlin's (traumatic) S05.8X- ☑
  brain (cytotoxic) (vasogenic) G93.6
    due to birth injury P11.0
    newborn (anoxia or hypoxia) P52.4
      birth injury P11.0
    traumatic — see Injury, intracranial, cerebral edema
  cardiac — see Failure, heart, congestive
  cardiovascular — see Failure, heart, congestive

**Edema, edematous** — continued
  cerebral — see Edema, brain
  cerebrospinal — see Edema, brain
  cervix (uteri) (acute) N88.8
    puerperal, postpartum O90.89
  chronic hereditary Q82.0
  circumscribed, acute T78.3 ☑
    hereditary D84.1
  conjunctiva H11.42- ☑
  cornea H18.2- ☑
    idiopathic H18.22- ☑
    secondary H18.23- ☑
      due to contact lens H18.21- ☑
  due to
    lymphatic obstruction I89.0
    salt retention E87.0
  epiglottis — see Edema, glottis
  essential, acute T78.3 ☑
    hereditary D84.1
  extremities, lower — see Edema, legs
  eyelid NEC H02.849
    left H02.846
      lower H02.845
      upper H02.844
    right H02.843
      lower H02.842
      upper H02.841
  familial, hereditary Q82.0
  famine — see Malnutrition, severe
  generalized R60.1
  glottis, glottic, glottidis (obstructive) (passive) J38.4
    allergic T78.3 ☑
      hereditary D84.1
  heart — see Failure, heart, congestive
  heat T67.7 ☑
  hereditary Q82.0
  inanition — see Malnutrition, severe
  intracranial G93.6
  iris H21.89
  joint — see Effusion, joint
  larynx — see Edema, glottis
  legs R60.0
    due to venous obstruction I87.1
    hereditary Q82.0
  localized R60.0
    due to venous obstruction I87.1
  lower limbs — see Edema, legs
  lung J81.1
    with heart condition or failure — see Failure, ven-
      tricular, left
    acute J81.0
    chemical (acute) J68.1
      chronic J68.1
    chronic J81.1
      due to
        chemicals, gases, fumes or vapors (inhala-
          tion) J68.1
        external agent J70.9
          specified NEC J70.8
        radiation J70.1
    due to
      chemicals, fumes or vapors (inhalation) J68.1
      external agent J70.9
        specified NEC J70.8
      high altitude T70.29 ☑
      near drowning T75.1 ☑
      radiation J70.0
    meaning failure, left ventricle I50.1
  lymphatic I89.0
    due to mastectomy I97.2
  macula H35.81
    cystoid, following cataract surgery — see Compli-
      cations, postprocedural, following cataract
      surgery
    diabetic — see Diabetes, by type, with, retinopathy,
      with macular edema
  malignant — see Gangrene, gas
  Milroy's Q82.0
  nasopharynx J39.2
  newborn P83.30
    hydrops fetalis — see Hydrops, fetalis
    specified NEC P83.39
  nutritional (see also Malnutrition, severe)
    with dyspigmentation, skin and hair E40
  optic disc or nerve — see Papilledema
  orbit H05.22- ☑
  pancreas K86.89
  papilla, optic — see Papilledema

☑ **Additional Character Required** — Refer to the Tabular List for Character Selection      ▽ **Subterms under main terms may continue to next column or page**

**Edema, edematous** — *continued*
penis N48.89
periodic T78.3 ☑
hereditary D84.1
pharynx J39.2
pulmonary — *see* Edema, lung
Quincke's T78.3 ☑
hereditary D84.1
renal — *see* Nephrosis
retina H35.81
diabetic — *see* Diabetes, by type, with, retinopathy, with macular edema
salt E87.0
scrotum N50.89
seminal vesicle N50.89
spermatic cord N50.89
spinal (cord) (vascular) (nontraumatic) G95.19
starvation — *see* Malnutrition, severe
stasis — *see* Hypertension, venous, (chronic)
subglottic — *see* Edema, glottis
supraglottic — *see* Edema, glottis
testis N44.8
tunica vaginalis N50.89
vas deferens N50.89
vulva (acute) N90.89
**Edentulism** — *see* Absence, teeth, acquired
**Edsall's disease** T67.2 ☑
**Educational handicap** Z55.9
specified NEC Z55.8
**Edward's syndrome** — *see* Trisomy, 18
**Effect**(s) (of) (from) — *see* Effect, adverse NEC
**Effect, adverse**
abnormal gravitational (G) forces or states T75.81 ☑
abuse — *see* Maltreatment
air pressure T70.9 ☑
specified NEC T70.8 ☑
altitude (high) — *see* Effect, adverse, high altitude
anesthesia (*see also* Anesthesia) T88.59 ☑
in labor and delivery O74.9
local, toxic
in labor and delivery O74.4
in pregnancy NEC O29.3- ☑
postpartum, puerperal O89.3
postpartum, puerperal O89.9
specified NEC T88.59 ☑
in labor and delivery O74.8
postpartum, puerperal O89.8
spinal and epidural T88.59 ☑
headache T88.59 ☑
in labor and delivery O74.5
postpartum, puerperal O89.4
specified NEC
in labor and delivery O74.6
postpartum, puerperal O89.5
antitoxin — *see* Complications, vaccination
atmospheric pressure T70.9 ☑
due to explosion T70.8 ☑
high T70.3 ☑
low — *see* Effect, adverse, high altitude
specified effect NEC T70.8 ☑
biological, correct substance properly administered — *see* Effect, adverse, drug
blood (derivatives) (serum) (transfusion) — *see* Complications, transfusion
chemical substance — *see* Table of Drugs and Chemicals
cold (temperature) (weather) T69.9 ☑
chilblains T69.1 ☑
frostbite — *see* Frostbite
specified effect NEC T69.8 ☑
drugs and medicaments T88.7 ☑
specified drug — *see* Table of Drugs and Chemicals, by drug, adverse effect
specified effect — *code to* condition
electric current, electricity (shock) T75.4 ☑
burn — *see* Burn
exertion (excessive) T73.3 ☑
exposure — *see* Exposure
external cause NEC T75.89 ☑
foodstuffs T78.1 ☑
allergic reaction — *see* Allergy, food
causing anaphylaxis — *see* Shock, anaphylactic, due to food
noxious — *see* Poisoning, food, noxious
gases, fumes, or vapors T59.9- ☑
specified agent — *see* Table of Drugs and Chemicals

**Effect, adverse** — *continued*
glue (airplane) sniffing
due to drug abuse — *see* Abuse, drug, inhalant
due to drug dependence — *see* Dependence, drug, inhalant
heat — *see* Heat
high altitude NEC T70.29 ☑
anoxia T70.29 ☑
on
ears T70.0 ☑
sinuses T70.1 ☑
polycythemia D75.1
high pressure fluids T70.4 ☑
hot weather — *see* Heat
hunger T73.0 ☑
immersion, foot — *see* Immersion
immunization — *see* Complications, vaccination
immunological agents — *see* Complications, vaccination
infrared (radiation) (rays) NOS T66 ☑
dermatitis or eczema L59.8
infusion — *see* Complications, infusion
lack of care of infants — *see* Maltreatment, child
lightning — *see* Lightning
medical care T88.9 ☑
specified NEC T88.8 ☑
medicinal substance, correct, properly administered — *see* Effect, adverse, drug
motion T75.3 ☑
noise, on inner ear — *see* subcategory H83.3 ☑
overheated places — *see* Heat
psychosocial, of work environment Z56.5
radiation (diagnostic) (infrared) (natural source) (therapeutic) (ultraviolet) (X-ray) NOS T66 ☑
dermatitis or eczema — *see* Dermatitis, due to, radiation
fibrosis of lung J70.1
pneumonitis J70.0
pulmonary manifestations
acute J70.0
chronic J70.1
skin L59.9
radioactive substance NOS
dermatitis or eczema — *see* Radiodermatitis
reduced temperature T69.9 ☑
immersion foot or hand — *see* Immersion
specified effect NEC T69.8 ☑
serum NEC (*see also* Reaction, serum) T80.69 ☑
specified NEC T78.8 ☑
external cause NEC T75.89 ☑
strangulation — *see* Asphyxia, traumatic
submersion T75.1 ☑
thirst T73.1 ☑
toxic — *see* Toxicity
transfusion — *see* Complications, transfusion
ultraviolet (radiation) (rays) NOS T66 ☑
burn — *see* Burn
dermatitis or eczema — *see* Dermatitis, due to, ultraviolet rays
acute L56.8
vaccine (any) — *see* Complications, vaccination
vibration — *see* Vibration, adverse effects
water pressure NEC T70.9 ☑
specified NEC T70.8 ☑
weightlessness T75.82 ☑
whole blood — *see* Complications, transfusion
work environment Z56.5
**Effects, late** — *see* Sequelae
**Effluvium**
anagen L65.1
telogen L65.0
**Effort syndrome** (psychogenic) F45.8
**Effusion**
amniotic fluid — *see* Pregnancy, complicated by, premature rupture of membranes
brain (serous) G93.6
bronchial — *see* Bronchitis
cerebral G93.6
cerebrospinal (*see also* Meningitis)
vessel G93.6
chest — *see* Effusion, pleura
chylous, chyliform (pleura) J94.0
intracranial G93.6
joint M25.40
ankle M25.47- ☑
elbow M25.42- ☑
foot joint M25.47- ☑

**Effusion** — *continued*
joint — *continued*
hand joint M25.44- ☑
hip M25.45- ☑
knee M25.46- ☑
shoulder M25.41- ☑
specified joint NEC M25.48
wrist M25.43- ☑
malignant pleural J91.0
meninges — *see* Meningitis
pericardium, pericardial (noninflammatory) I31.3
acute — *see* Pericarditis, acute
peritoneal (chronic) R18.8
pleura, pleurisy, pleuritic, pleuropericardial J90
chylous, chyliform J94.0
due to systemic lupus erythematosis M32.13
in conditions classified elsewhere J91.8
influenzal — *see* Influenza, with, respiratory manifestations NEC
malignant J91.0
newborn P28.89
tuberculous NEC A15.6
primary (progressive) A15.7
spinal — *see* Meningitis
thorax, thoracic — *see* Effusion, pleura
**Egg shell nails** L60.3
congenital Q84.6
**Egyptian splenomegaly** B65.1
**Ehlers-Danlos syndrome** Q79.6
**Ehrlichiosis** A77.40
due to
E. chafeensis A77.41
E. sennetsu A79.81
specified organism NEC A77.49
**Eichstedt's disease** B36.0
**Eisenmenger's**
complex or syndrome I27.83
defect Q21.8
**Ejaculation**
delayed F52.32
painful N53.12
premature F52.4
retarded N53.11
retrograde N53.14
semen, painful N53.12
psychogenic F52.6
**Ekbom's syndrome** (restless legs) G25.81
**Ekman's syndrome** (brittle bones and blue sclera) Q78.0
**Elastic skin** Q82.8
acquired L57.4
**Elastofibroma** — *see* Neoplasm, connective tissue, benign
**Elastoma** (juvenile) Q82.8
Miescher's L87.2
**Elastomyofibrosis** I42.4
**Elastosis**
actinic, solar L57.8
atrophicans (senile) L57.4
perforans serpiginosa L87.2
senilis L57.4
**Elbow** — *see* condition
**Electric current, electricity, effects** (concussion) (fatal) (nonfatal) (shock) T75.4 ☑
burn — *see* Burn
**Electric feet syndrome** E53.8
**Electrocution** T75.4 ☑
from electroshock gun (taser) T75.4 ☑
**Electrolyte imbalance** E87.8
with
abortion — *see* Abortion by type, complicated by, electrolyte imbalance
ectopic pregnancy O08.5
molar pregnancy O08.5
**Elephantiasis** (nonfilarial) I89.0
arabicum — *see* Infestation, filarial
bancroftian B74.0
congenital (any site) (hereditary) Q82.0
due to
Brugia (malayi) B74.1
timori B74.2
mastectomy I97.2
Wuchereria (bancrofti) B74.0
eyelid H02.859
left H02.856
lower H02.855
upper H02.854
right H02.853
lower H02.852

**Elephantiasis** — *continued*
  eyelid — *continued*
    right — *continued*
      upper H02.851
  filarial, filariensis — *see* Infestation, filarial
  glandular I89.0
  graecorum A30.9
  lymphangiectatic I89.0
  lymphatic vessel I89.0
    due to mastectomy I97.2
  scrotum (nonfilarial) I89.0
  streptococcal I89.0
  surgical I97.89
    postmastectomy I97.2
  telangiectodes I89.0
  vulva (nonfilarial) N90.89
**Elevated, elevation**
  antibody titer R76.0
  basal metabolic rate R94.8
  blood pressure (*see also* Hypertension)
    reading (incidental) (isolated) (nonspecific), no di-
      agnosis of hypertension R03.0
  blood sugar R73.9
  body temperature (of unknown origin) R50.9
  cancer antigen 125 [CA 125] R97.1
  carcinoembryonic antigen [CEA] R97.0
  cholesterol E78.00
    with high triglycerides E78.2
  conjugate, eye H51.0
  C-reactive protein (CRP) R79.82
  diaphragm, congenital Q79.1
  erythrocyte sedimentation rate R70.0
  fasting glucose R73.01
  fasting triglycerides E78.1
  finding on laboratory examination — *see* Findings,
    abnormal, inconclusive, without diagnosis, by
    type of exam
  GFR (glomerular filtration rate) — *see* Findings, abnor-
    mal, inconclusive, without diagnosis, by type of
    exam
  glucose tolerance (oral) R73.02
  immunoglobulin level R76.8
  indoleacetic acid R82.5
  lactic acid dehydrogenase (LDH) level R74.0
  leukocytes D72.829
  lipoprotein a level E78.8 ☑
  liver function
    study R94.5
    test R79.89
      alkaline phosphatase R74.8
      aminotransferase R74.0
      bilirubin R17
      hepatic enzyme R74.8
      lactate dehydrogenase R74.0
  lymphocytes D72.820
  prostate specific antigen [PSA] R97.20
  Rh titer — *see* Complication(s), transfusion, incompat-
    ibility reaction, Rh (factor)
  scapula, congenital Q74.0
  sedimentation rate R70.0
  SGOT R74.0
  SGPT R74.0
  transaminase level R74.0
  triglycerides E78.1
    with high cholesterol E78.2
  tumor associated antigens [TAA] NEC R97.8
  tumor specific antigens [TSA] NEC R97.8
  urine level of
    17-ketosteroids R82.5
    catecholamine R82.5
    indoleacetic acid R82.5
    steroids R82.5
    vanillylmandelic acid (VMA) R82.5
  venous pressure I87.8
  white blood cell count D72.829
    specified NEC D72.828
**Elliptocytosis** (congenital) (hereditary) D58.1
  Hb C (disease) D58.1
  hemoglobin disease D58.1
  sickle-cell (disease) D57.8- ☑
    trait D57.3
**Ellison-Zollinger syndrome** E16.4
**Ellis-van Creveld syndrome** (chondroectodermal dysplasia) Q77.6
**Elongated, elongation** (congenital) (*see also* Distortion)
  bone Q79.9
  cervix (uteri) Q51.828
    acquired N88.4

**Elongated, elongation** — *continued*
  cervix — *continued*
    hypertrophic N88.4
  colon Q43.8
  common bile duct Q44.5
  cystic duct Q44.5
  frenulum, penis Q55.69
  labia minora (acquired) N90.69
  ligamentum patellae Q74.1
  petiolus (epiglottidis) Q31.8
  tooth, teeth K00.2
  uvula Q38.6
**Eltor cholera** A00.1
**Emaciation** (due to malnutrition) E41
**Embadomoniasis** A07.8
**Embedded tooth, teeth** K01.0
  root only K08.3
**Embolic** — *see* condition
**Embolism** (multiple) (paradoxical) I74.9
  air (any site) (traumatic) T79.0 ☑
    following
      abortion — *see* Abortion by type complicated
        by embolism
      ectopic pregnancy O08.2
      infusion, therapeutic injection or transfusion
        T80.0 ☑
      molar pregnancy O08.2
      procedure NEC
        artery T81.719 ☑
          mesenteric T81.710 ☑
          renal T81.711 ☑
          specified NEC T81.718 ☑
        vein T81.72 ☑
    in pregnancy, childbirth or puerperium — *see*
      Embolism, obstetric
  amniotic fluid (pulmonary) (*see also* Embolism, obstet-
    ric)
    following
      abortion — *see* Abortion by type complicated
        by embolism
      ectopic pregnancy O08.2
      molar pregnancy O08.2
  aorta, aortic I74.10
    abdominal I74.09
      saddle I74.01
    bifurcation I74.09
    saddle I74.01
    thoracic I74.11
  artery I74.9
    auditory, internal I65.8
    basilar — *see* Occlusion, artery, basilar
    carotid (common) (internal) — *see* Occlusion,
      artery, carotid
    cerebellar (anterior inferior) (posterior inferior)
      (superior) I66.3
    cerebral — *see* Occlusion, artery, cerebral
    choroidal (anterior) I65.8
    communicating posterior I65.8
    coronary (*see also* Infarct, myocardium)
      not resulting in infarction I24.0
    extremity I74.4
      lower I74.3
      upper I74.2
    hypophyseal I65.8
    iliac I74.5
    limb I74.4
      lower I74.3
      upper I74.2
    mesenteric (with gangrene) (*see also* Ischemia, in-
      testine, acute) K55.059
    ophthalmic — *see* Occlusion, artery, retina
    peripheral I74.4
    pontine I65.8
    precerebral — *see* Occlusion, artery, precerebral
    pulmonary — *see* Embolism, pulmonary
    renal N28.0
    retinal — *see* Occlusion, artery, retina
    septic I76
    specified NEC I74.8
    vertebral — *see* Occlusion, artery, vertebral
  basilar (artery) I65.1
  blood clot
    following
      abortion — *see* Abortion by type complicated
        by embolism
      ectopic or molar pregnancy O08.2
    in pregnancy, childbirth or puerperium — *see*
      Embolism, obstetric

**Embolism** — *continued*
  brain (*see also* Occlusion, artery, cerebral)
    following
      abortion — *see* Abortion by type complicated
        by embolism
      ectopic or molar pregnancy O08.2
    puerperal, postpartum, childbirth — *see* Embolism,
      obstetric
  capillary I78.8
  cardiac (*see also* Infarct, myocardium)
    not resulting in infarction I51.3
  carotid (artery) (common) (internal) — *see* Occlusion,
    artery, carotid
  cavernous sinus (venous) — *see* Embolism, intracranial
    venous sinus
  cerebral — *see* Occlusion, artery, cerebral
  cholesterol — *see* Atheroembolism
  coronary (artery or vein) (systemic) — *see* Occlusion,
    coronary
  due to device, implant or graft (*see also* Complications,
    by site and type, specified NEC)
    arterial graft NEC T82.818 ☑
    breast (implant) T85.818 ☑
    catheter NEC T85.818 ☑
      dialysis (renal) T82.818 ☑
        intraperitoneal T85.818 ☑
      infusion NEC T82.818 ☑
        spinal (epidural) (subdural) T85.810 ☑
      urinary (indwelling) T83.81 ☑
    electronic (electrode) (pulse generator) (stimulator)
      bone T84.81 ☑
      cardiac T82.817 ☑
      nervous system (brain) (peripheral nerve)
        (spinal) T85.810 ☑
      urinary T83.81 ☑
    fixation, internal (orthopedic) NEC T84.81 ☑
    gastrointestinal (bile duct) (esophagus) T85.818 ☑
    genital NEC T83.81 ☑
    heart (graft) (valve) T82.817 ☑
    joint prosthesis T84.81 ☑
    ocular (corneal graft) (orbital implant) T85.818 ☑
    orthopedic (bone graft) NEC T86.838
    specified NEC T85.818 ☑
    urinary (graft) NEC T83.81 ☑
    vascular NEC T82.818 ☑
    ventricular intracranial shunt T85.810 ☑
  extremities
    lower — *see* Embolism, vein, lower extremity
      arterial I74.3
    upper I74.2
  eye H34.9
  fat (cerebral) (pulmonary) (systemic) T79.1 ☑
    complicating delivery — *see* Embolism, obstetric
    following
      abortion — *see* Abortion by type complicated
        by embolism
      ectopic or molar pregnancy O08.2
  following
    abortion — *see* Abortion by type complicated by
      embolism
    ectopic or molar pregnancy O08.2
    infusion, therapeutic injection or transfusion
      air T80.0 ☑
  heart (fatty) (*see also* Infarct, myocardium)
    not resulting in infarction I51.3
  hepatic (vein) I82.0
  in pregnancy, childbirth or puerperium — *see* Em-
    bolism, obstetric
  intestine (artery) (vein) (with gangrene) (*see also* Is-
    chemia, intestine, acute) K55.039
  intracranial (*see also* Occlusion, artery, cerebral)
    venous sinus (any) G08
      nonpyogenic I67.6
  intraspinal venous sinuses or veins G08
    nonpyogenic G95.19
  kidney (artery) N28.0
  lateral sinus (venous) — *see* Embolism, intracranial,
    venous sinus
  leg — *see* Embolism, vein, lower extremity
    arterial I74.3
  longitudinal sinus (venous) — *see* Embolism, intracra-
    nial, venous sinus
  lung (massive) — *see* Embolism, pulmonary
  meninges I66.8
  mesenteric (artery) (vein) (with gangrene) (*see also*
    Ischemia, intestine, acute) K55.059

**Embolism** — *continued*
  obstetric (in) (pulmonary)
    childbirth O88.22
      air O88.02
      amniotic fluid O88.12
      blood clot O88.22
      fat O88.82
      pyemic O88.32
      septic O88.32
      specified type NEC O88.82
    pregnancy O88.21- ☑
      air O88.01- ☑
      amniotic fluid O88.11- ☑
      blood clot O88.21- ☑
      fat O88.81- ☑
      pyemic O88.31- ☑
      septic O88.31- ☑
      specified type NEC O88.81- ☑
    puerperal O88.23
      air O88.03
      amniotic fluid O88.13
      blood clot O88.23
      fat O88.83
      pyemic O88.33
      septic O88.33
      specified type NEC O88.83
  ophthalmic — *see* Occlusion, artery, retina
  penis N48.81
  peripheral artery NOS I74.4
  pituitary E23.6
  popliteal (artery) I74.3
  portal (vein) I81
  postoperative, postprocedural
    artery T81.719 ☑
      mesenteric T81.710 ☑
      renal T81.711 ☑
      specified NEC T81.718 ☑
    vein T81.72 ☑
  precerebral artery — *see* Occlusion, artery, precerebral
  puerperal — *see* Embolism, obstetric
  pulmonary (acute) (artery) (vein) I26.99
    with acute cor pulmonale I26.09
    chronic I27.82
    following
      abortion — *see* Abortion by type complicated
        by embolism
      ectopic or molar pregnancy O08.2
    healed or old Z86.711
    in pregnancy, childbirth or puerperium — *see*
      Embolism, obstetric
    personal history of Z86.711
    saddle I26.92
      with acute cor pulmonale I26.02
    septic I26.90
      with acute cor pulmonale I26.01
  pyemic (multiple) I76
    following
      abortion — *see* Abortion by type complicated
        by embolism
      ectopic or molar pregnancy O08.2
    Hemophilus influenzae A41.3
    pneumococcal A40.3
      with pneumonia J13
    puerperal, postpartum, childbirth (any organism)
      — *see* Embolism, obstetric
    specified organism NEC A41.89
    staphylococcal A41.2
    streptococcal A40.9
  renal (artery) N28.0
    vein I82.3
  retina, retinal — *see* Occlusion, artery, retina
  saddle
    abdominal aorta I74.01
    pulmonary artery I26.92
      with acute cor pulmonale I26.02
  septic (arterial) I76
    complicating abortion — *see* Abortion, by type,
      complicated by, embolism
  sinus — *see* Embolism, intracranial, venous sinus
  soap complicating abortion — *see* Abortion, by type,
    complicated by, embolism
  spinal cord G95.19
    pyogenic origin G06.1
  spleen, splenic (artery) I74.8
  upper extremity I74.2
  vein (acute) I82.90
    antecubital I82.61- ☑
      chronic I82.71- ☑

**Embolism** — *continued*
  vein — *continued*
    axillary I82.A1- ☑ (*following* I82.7)
      chronic I82.A2- ☑ (*following* I82.7)
    basilic I82.61- ☑
      chronic I82.71- ☑
    brachial I82.62- ☑
      chronic I82.72- ☑
    brachiocephalic (innominate) I82.290
      chronic I82.291
    cephalic I82.61- ☑
      chronic I82.71- ☑
    chronic I82.91
    deep (DVT) I82.40- ☑
      calf I82.4Z- ☑
        chronic I82.5Z- ☑
      lower leg I82.4Z- ☑
        chronic I82.5Z- ☑
      thigh I82.4Y- ☑
        chronic I82.5Y- ☑
      upper leg I82.4Y ☑
        chronic I82.5Y-
    femoral I82.41- ☑
      chronic I82.51- ☑
    iliac (iliofemoral) I82.42- ☑
      chronic I82.52- ☑
    innominate I82.290
      chronic I82.291
    internal jugular I82.C1- ☑ (*following* I82.7)
      chronic I82.C2- ☑ (*following* I82.7)
    lower extremity
      deep I82.40- ☑
        chronic I82.50- ☑
        specified NEC I82.49- ☑
          chronic NEC I82.59- ☑
      distal
        deep I82.4Z- ☑
      proximal
        deep I82.4Y- ☑
          chronic I82.5Y- ☑
      superficial I82.81- ☑
    popliteal I82.43- ☑
      chronic I82.53- ☑
    radial I82.62- ☑
      chronic I82.72- ☑
    renal I82.3
    saphenous (greater) (lesser) I82.81- ☑
    specified NEC I82.890
      chronic NEC I82.891
    subclavian I82.B1- ☑ (*following* I82.7)
      chronic I82.B2- ☑ (*following* I82.7)
    thoracic NEC I82.290
      chronic I82.291
    tibial I82.44- ☑
      chronic I82.54- ☑
    ulnar I82.62- ☑
      chronic I82.72- ☑
    upper extremity I82.60- ☑
      chronic I82.70- ☑
      deep I82.62- ☑
        chronic I82.72- ☑
      superficial I82.61- ☑
        chronic I82.71- ☑
  vena cava
    inferior (acute) I82.220
      chronic I82.221
    superior (acute) I82.210
      chronic I82.211
  venous sinus G08
  vessels of brain — *see* Occlusion, artery, cerebral
**Embolus** — *see* Embolism
**Embryoma** (*see also* Neoplasm, uncertain behavior, by
  site)
  benign — *see* Neoplasm, benign, by site
  kidney C64.- ☑
  liver C22.0
  malignant (*see also* Neoplasm, malignant, by site)
    kidney C64.- ☑
    liver C22.0
    testis C62.9- ☑
      descended (scrotal) C62.1- ☑
      undescended C62.0- ☑
  testis C62.9- ☑
    descended (scrotal) C62.1- ☑
    undescended C62.0- ☑

**Embryonic**
  circulation Q28.9
  heart Q28.9
  vas deferens Q55.4
**Embryopathia NOS** Q89.9
**Embryotoxon** Q13.4
**Emesis** — *see* Vomiting
**Emotional lability** R45.86
**Emotionality, pathological** F60.3
**Emotogenic disease** — *see* Disorder, psychogenic
**Emphysema** (atrophic) (bullous) (chronic) (interlobular)
  (lung) (obstructive) (pulmonary) (senile) (vesicular)
  J43.9
  cellular tissue (traumatic) T79.7 ☑
    surgical T81.82 ☑
  centrilobular J43.2
  compensatory J98.3
  congenital (interstitial) P25.0
  conjunctiva H11.89
  connective tissue (traumatic) T79.7 ☑
    surgical T81.82 ☑
  due to chemicals, gases, fumes or vapors J68.4
  eyelid(s) — *see* Disorder, eyelid, specified type NEC
    surgical T81.82 ☑
    traumatic T79.7 ☑
  interstitial J98.2
    congenital P25.0
    perinatal period P25.0
  laminated tissue T79.7 ☑
    surgical T81.82 ☑
  mediastinal J98.2
    newborn P25.2
  orbit, orbital — *see* Disorder, orbit, specified type NEC
  panacinar J43.1
  panlobular J43.1
  specified NEC J43.8
  subcutaneous (traumatic) T79.7 ☑
    nontraumatic J98.2
    postprocedural T81.82 ☑
    surgical T81.82 ☑
  surgical T81.82 ☑
  thymus (gland) (congenital) E32.8
  traumatic (subcutaneous) T79.7 ☑
  unilateral J43.0
**Empty nest syndrome** Z60.0
**Empyema** (acute) (chest) (double) (pleura) (supradi-
  aphragmatic) (thorax) J86.9
  with fistula J86.0
  accessory sinus (chronic) — *see* Sinusitis
  antrum (chronic) — *see* Sinusitis, maxillary
  brain (any part) — *see* Abscess, brain
  ethmoidal (chronic) (sinus) — *see* Sinusitis, ethmoidal
  extradural — *see* Abscess, extradural
  frontal (chronic) (sinus) — *see* Sinusitis, frontal
  gallbladder K81.0
  mastoid (process) (acute) — *see* Mastoiditis, acute
  maxilla, maxillary M27.2
    sinus (chronic) — *see* Sinusitis, maxillary
  nasal sinus (chronic) — *see* Sinusitis
  sinus (accessory) (chronic) (nasal) — *see* Sinusitis
  sphenoidal (sinus) (chronic) — *see* Sinusitis, sphe-
    noidal
  subarachnoid — *see* Abscess, extradural
  subdural — *see* Abscess, subdural
  tuberculous A15.6
  ureter — *see* Ureteritis
  ventricular — *see* Abscess, brain
**En coup de sabre lesion** L94.1
**Enamel pearls** K00.2
**Enameloma** K00.2
**Enanthema, viral** B09
**Encephalitis** (chronic) (hemorrhagic) (idiopathic)
  (nonepidemic) (spurious) (subacute) G04.90
  acute (*see also* Encephalitis, viral) A86
    disseminated G04.00
      infectious G04.01
      noninfectious G04.81
      postimmunization (postvaccination) G04.02
      postinfectious G04.01
    inclusion body A85.8
    necrotizing hemorrhagic G04.30
      postimmunization G04.32
      postinfectious G04.31
      specified NEC G04.39
  arboviral, arbovirus NEC A85.2
  arthropod-borne NEC (viral) A85.2
  Australian A83.4

---

**Encephalitis** — continued
  California (virus) A83.5
  Central European (tick-borne) A84.1
  Czechoslovakian A84.1
  Dawson's (inclusion body) A81.1
  diffuse sclerosing A81.1
  disseminated, acute G04.00
  due to
    cat scratch disease A28.1
    human immunodeficiency virus (HIV) disease
      B20 [G05.3]
    malaria — see Malaria
    rickettsiosis — see Rickettsiosis
    smallpox inoculation G04.02
    typhus — see Typhus
  Eastern equine A83.2
  endemic (viral) A86
  epidemic NEC (viral) A86
  equine (acute) (infectious) (viral) A83.9
    Eastern A83.2
    Venezuelan A92.2
    Western A83.1
  Far Eastern (tick-borne) A84.0
  following vaccination or other immunization proce-
    dure G04.02
  herpes zoster B02.0
  herpesviral B00.4
    due to herpesvirus 6 B10.01
    due to herpesvirus 7 B10.09
    specified NEC B10.09
  Ilheus (virus) A83.8
  in (due to)
    actinomycosis A42.82
    adenovirus A85.1
    African trypanosomiasis B56.9 [G05.3]
    Chagas' disease (chronic) B57.42
    cytomegalovirus B25.8
    enterovirus A85.0
    herpes (simplex) virus B00.4
      due to herpesvirus 6 B10.01
      due to herpesvirus 7 B10.09
      specified NEC B10.09
    infectious disease NEC B99 ☑ [G05.3]
    influenza — see Influenza, with, encephalopathy
    listeriosis A32.12
    measles B05.0
    mumps B26.2
    naegleriasis B60.2
    parasitic disease NEC B89 [G05.3]
    poliovirus A80.9 [G05.3]
    rubella B06.01
    syphilis
      congenital A50.42
      late A52.14
    systemic lupus erythematosus M32.19
    toxoplasmosis (acquired) B58.2
      congenital P37.1
    tuberculosis A17.82
    zoster B02.0
  inclusion body A81.1
  infectious (acute) (virus) NEC A86
  Japanese (B type) A83.0
  La Crosse A83.5
  lead — see Poisoning, lead
  lethargica (acute) (infectious) A85.8
  louping ill A84.8
  lupus erythematosus, systemic M32.19
  lymphatica A87.2
  Mengo A85.8
  meningococcal A39.81
  Murray Valley A83.4
  otitic NEC H66.40 [G05.3]
  parasitic NOS B71.9
  periaxial G37.0
  periaxialis (concentrica) (diffuse) G37.5
  postchickenpox B01.11
  postexanthematous NEC B09
  postimmunization G04.02
  postinfectious NEC G04.01
  postmeasles B05.0
  postvaccinal G04.02
  postvaricella B01.11
  postviral NEC A86
  Powassan A84.8
  Rasmussen G04.81
  Rio Bravo A85.8
  Russian
    autumnal A83.0
    spring-summer (taiga) A84.0

**Encephalitis** — continued
  saturnine — see Poisoning, lead
  specified NEC G04.81
  St. Louis A83.3
  subacute sclerosing A81.1
  summer A83.0
  suppurative G04.81
  tick-borne A84.9
  Torula, torular (cryptococcal) B45.1
  toxic NEC G92
  trichinosis B75 [G05.3]
  type
    B A83.0
    C A83.3
  van Bogaert's A81.1
  Venezuelan equine A92.2
  Vienna A85.8
  viral, virus A86
    arthropod-borne NEC A85.2
      mosquito-borne A83.9
        Australian X disease A83.4
        California virus A83.5
        Eastern equine A83.2
        Japanese (B type) A83.0
        Murray Valley A83.4
        specified NEC A83.8
        St. Louis A83.3
        type B A83.0
        type C A83.3
        Western equine A83.1
      tick-borne A84.9
        biundulant A84.1
        central European A84.1
        Czechoslovakian A84.1
        diphasic meningoencephalitis A84.1
        Far Eastern A84.0
        Russian spring-summer (taiga) A84.0
        specified NEC A84.8
    specified type NEC A85.8
  Western equine A83.1
**Encephalocele** Q01.9
  frontal Q01.0
  nasofrontal Q01.1
  occipital Q01.2
  specified NEC Q01.8
**Encephalocystocele** — see Encephalocele
**Encephaloduroarteriomyosynangiosis** (EDAMS) I67.5
**Encephalomalacia** (brain) (cerebellar) (cerebral) — see
  Softening, brain
**Encephalomeningitis** — see Meningoencephalitis
**Encephalomeningocele** — see Encephalocele
**Encephalomeningomyelitis** — see Meningoencephalitis
**Encephalomyelitis** (see also Encephalitis) G04.90
  acute disseminated G04.00
    infectious G04.01
    noninfectious G04.81
    postimmunization G04.02
    postinfectious G04.01
  acute necrotizing hemorrhagic G04.30
    postimmunization G04.32
    postinfectious G04.31
    specified NEC G04.39
  benign myalgic G93.3
  equine A83.9
    Eastern A83.2
    Venezuelan A92.2
    Western A83.1
  in diseases classified elsewhere G05.3
  myalgic, benign G93.3
  postchickenpox B01.11
  postinfectious NEC G04.01
  postmeasles B05.0
  postvaccinal G04.02
  postvaricella B01.11
  rubella B06.01
  specified NEC G04.81
  Venezuelan equine A92.2
**Encephalomyelocele** — see Encephalocele
**Encephalomyelomeningitis** — see Meningoencephalitis
**Encephalomyelopathy** G96.9
**Encephalomyeloradiculitis** (acute) G61.0
**Encephalomyeloradiculoneuritis** (acute) (Guillain-
  Barré) G61.0
**Encephalomyeloradiculopathy** G96.9
**Encephalopathia hyperbilirubinemica, newborn**
  P57.9

**Encephalopathia hyperbilirubinemica, newborn** —
  continued
  due to isoimmunization (conditions in P55) P57.0
**Encephalopathy** (acute) G93.40
  acute necrotizing hemorrhagic G04.30
    postimmunization G04.32
    postinfectious G04.31
    specified NEC G04.39
  alcoholic G31.2
  anoxic — see Damage, brain, anoxic
  arteriosclerotic I67.2
  centrolobar progressive (Schilder) G37.0
  congenital Q07.9
  degenerative, in specified disease NEC G32.89
  demyelinating callosal G37.1
  due to
    drugs (see also Table of Drugs and Chemicals) G92
  hepatic — see Failure, hepatic
  hyperbilirubinemic, newborn P57.9
    due to isoimmunization (conditions in P55) P57.0
  hypertensive I67.4
  hypoglycemic E16.2
  hypoxic — see Damage, brain, anoxic
  hypoxic ischemic P91.60
    mild P91.61
    moderate P91.62
    severe P91.63
  in (due to) (with)
    birth injury P11.1
    hyperinsulinism E16.1 [G94]
    influenza — see Influenza, with, encephalopathy
    lack of vitamin (see also Deficiency, vitamin)
      E56.9 [G32.89]
    neoplastic disease (see also Neoplasm)
      D49.9 [G13.1]
    serum (see also Reaction, serum) T80.69 ☑
    syphilis A52.17
    trauma (postconcussional) F07.81
      current injury — see Injury, intracranial
    vaccination G04.02
  lead — see Poisoning, lead
  metabolic G93.41
    drug induced G92
    toxic G92
  myoclonic, early, symptomatic — see Epilepsy, gener-
    alized, specified NEC
  necrotizing, subacute (Leigh) G31.82
  neonatal P91.819
    in diseases classified elsewhere P91.811
  pellagrous E52 [G32.89]
  portosystemic — see Failure, hepatic
  postcontusional F07.81
    current injury — see Injury, intracranial, diffuse
  posthypoglycemic (coma) E16.1 [G94]
  postradiation G93.89
  saturnine — see Poisoning, lead
  septic G93.41
  specified NEC G93.49
  spongioform, subacute (viral) A81.09
  toxic G92
    metabolic G92
  traumatic (postconcussional) F07.81
    current injury — see Injury, intracranial
  vitamin B deficiency NEC E53.9 [G32.89]
    vitamin B1 E51.2
  Wernicke's E51.2
**Encephalorrhagia** — see Hemorrhage, intracranial, intracerebral
**Encephalosis, posttraumatic** F07.81
**Enchondroma** (see also Neoplasm, bone, benign)
**Enchondromatosis** (cartilaginous) (multiple) Q78.4
**Encopresis** R15.9
  functional F98.1
  nonorganic origin F98.1
  psychogenic F98.1
**Encounter** (with health service) (for) Z76.89
  adjustment and management (of)
    breast implant Z45.81 ☑
    implanted device NEC Z45.89
    myringotomy device (stent) (tube) Z45.82
  administrative purpose only Z02.9
    examination for
      adoption Z02.82
      armed forces Z02.3
      disability determination Z02.71
      driving license Z02.4
      employment Z02.1
      insurance Z02.6

**Encounter** — *continued*
  administrative purpose only — *continued*
    examination for — *continued*
      medical certificate NEC Z02.79
      paternity testing Z02.81
      residential institution admission Z02.2
      school admission Z02.0
      sports Z02.5
      specified reason NEC Z02.89
  aftercare — *see* Aftercare
  antenatal screening Z36.9
    cervical length Z36.86
    chromosomal anomalies Z36.0
    congenital cardiac abnormalities Z36.83
    elevated maternal serum alphafetoprotein Z36.1
    fetal growth retardation Z36.4
    fetal lung maturity Z36.84
    fetal macrosomia Z36.88
    hydrops fetalis Z36.81
    intrauterine growth restriction (IUGR) /small-for-dates Z36.4
    isoimmunization Z36.5
    large-for-dates Z36.88
    malformations Z36.3
    non-visualized anatomy on a previous scan Z36.2
    nuchal translucency Z36.82
    raised alphafetoprotein level Z36.1
    risk of pre-term labor Z36.86
    specified follow-up NEC Z36.2
    specified genetic defects NEC Z36.8A
    specified type NEC Z36.89
    Streptococcus B Z36.85
    suspected anomaly Z36.3
    uncertain dates Z36.87
  assisted reproductive fertility procedure cycle Z31.83
  blood typing Z01.83
    Rh typing Z01.83
  breast augmentation or reduction Z41.1
  breast implant exchange (different material) (different size) Z45.81 ☑
  breast reconstruction following mastectomy Z42.1
  check-up — *see* Examination
  chemotherapy for neoplasm Z51.11
  colonoscopy, screening Z12.11
  counseling — *see* Counseling
  delivery, full-term, uncomplicated O80
    cesarean, without indication O82
  desensitization to allergens Z51.6
  ear piercing Z41.3
  examination — *see* Examination
  expectant parent(s) (adoptive) pre-birth pediatrician visit Z76.81
  fertility preservation procedure (prior to cancer therapy) (prior to removal of gonads) Z31.84
  fitting (of) — *see* Fitting (and adjustment) (of)
  genetic
    counseling
      nonprocreative Z71.83
      procreative Z31.5
    testing — *see* Test, genetic
  hearing conservation and treatment Z01.12
  immunotherapy for neoplasm Z51.12
  in vitro fertilization cycle Z31.83
  instruction (in)
    child care (postpartal) (prenatal) Z32.3
    childbirth Z32.2
    natural family planning
      procreative Z31.61
      to avoid pregnancy Z30.02
  insulin pump titration Z46.81
  joint prosthesis insertion following prior explantation of joint prosthesis (staged procedure)
    hip Z47.32
    knee Z47.33
    shoulder Z47.31
  laboratory (as part of a general medical examination) Z00.00
    with abnormal findings Z00.01
  mental health services (for)
    abuse NEC
      perpetrator Z69.82
      victim Z69.81
    child abuse
      nonparental
        perpetrator Z69.021
        victim Z69.020
      parental
        perpetrator Z69.011

**Encounter** — *continued*
  mental health services — *continued*
    child abuse — *continued*
      parental — *continued*
        victim Z69.010
    child neglect
      nonparental
        perpetrator Z69.021
        victim Z69.020
      parental
        perpetrator Z69.011
        victim Z69.010
    child psychological abuse
      nonparental
        perpetrator Z69.021
        victim Z69.020
      parental
        perpetrator Z69.011
        victim Z69.010
    child sexual abuse
      nonparental
        perpetrator Z69.021
        victim Z69.020
      parental
        perpetrator Z69.011
        victim Z69.010
    non-spousal adult abuse (perpetrator) (victim) Z69.81
    spousal or partner
      abuse
        perpetrator Z69.12
        victim Z69.11
      neglect
        perpetrator Z69.12
        victim Z69.11
      psychological abuse
        perpetrator Z69.12
        victim Z69.11
      violence
        perpetrator (physical) (sexual) Z69.12
        victim (physical) Z69.11
        sexual Z69.81
  observation (for) (ruled out)
    exposure to (suspected)
      anthrax Z03.810
      biological agent NEC Z03.818
  pediatrician visit, by expectant parent(s) (adoptive) Z76.81
  placental sample (taken vaginally) (*see also* Encounter, antenatal screening) Z36.9
  plastic and reconstructive surgery following medical procedure or healed injury NEC Z42.8
  pregnancy
    supervision of — *see* Pregnancy, supervision of
    test Z32.00
      result negative Z32.02
      result positive Z32.01
  procreative management and counseling for gestational carrier Z31.7
  prophylactic measures Z29.9
    antivenin Z29.12
    fluoride administration Z29.3
    immunotherapy for respiratory syncytial virus (RSV) Z29.11
    rabies immune globin Z29.14
    Rho (D) immune globulin Z29.13
    specified NEC Z29.8
  radiation therapy (antineoplastic) Z51.0
  radiological (as part of a general medical examination) Z00.00
    with abnormal findings Z00.01
  reconstructive surgery following medical procedure or healed injury NEC Z42.8
  removal (of) (*see also* Removal)
    artificial
      arm Z44.00- ☑
        complete Z44.01- ☑
        partial Z44.02- ☑
      eye Z44.2- ☑
      leg Z44.10- ☑
        complete Z44.11- ☑
        partial Z44.12- ☑
    breast implant Z45.81 ☑
      tissue expander (without synchronous insertion of permanent implant) Z45.81 ☑
    device Z46.9
      specified NEC Z46.89

**Encounter** — *continued*
  removal (*see also* Removal) — *continued*
    external
      fixation device — *code to* fracture with seventh character D
      prosthesis, prosthetic device Z44.9
        breast Z44.3- ☑
        specified NEC Z44.8
    implanted device NEC Z45.89
    insulin pump Z46.81
    internal fixation device Z47.2
    myringotomy device (stent) (tube) Z45.82
    nervous system device NEC Z46.2
      brain neuropacemaker Z46.2
      visual substitution device Z46.2
        implanted Z45.31
    non-vascular catheter Z46.82
    orthodontic device Z46.4
    stent
      ureteral Z46.6
    urinary device Z46.6
  repeat cervical smear to confirm findings of recent normal smear following initial abnormal smear Z01.42
  respirator [ventilator] use during power failure Z99.12
  Rh typing Z01.83
  screening — *see* Screening
  specified NEC Z76.89
  sterilization Z30.2
  suspected condition, ruled out
    amniotic cavity and membrane Z03.71
    cervical shortening Z03.75
    fetal anomaly Z03.73
    fetal growth Z03.74
    maternal and fetal conditions NEC Z03.79
    oligohydramnios Z03.71
    placental problem Z03.72
    polyhydramnios Z03.71
  suspected exposure (to), ruled out
    anthrax Z03.810
    biological agents NEC Z03.818
  termination of pregnancy, elective Z33.2
  testing — *see* Test
  therapeutic drug level monitoring Z51.81
  titration, insulin pump Z46.81
  to determine fetal viability of pregnancy O36.80 ☑
  training
    insulin pump Z46.81
  X-ray of chest (as part of a general medical examination) Z00.00
    with abnormal findings Z00.01
**Encystment** — *see* Cyst
**Endarteritis** (bacterial, subacute) (infective) I77.6
  brain I67.7
  cerebral or cerebrospinal I67.7
  deformans — *see* Arteriosclerosis
  embolic — *see* Embolism
  obliterans (*see also* Arteriosclerosis)
    pulmonary I28.8
  pulmonary I28.8
  retina — *see* Vasculitis, retina
  senile — *see* Arteriosclerosis
  syphilitic A52.09
    brain or cerebral A52.04
    congenital A50.54 [I79.8]
  tuberculous A18.89
**Endemic** — *see* condition
**Endocarditis** (chronic) (marantic) (nonbacterial) (thrombotic) (valvular) I38
  with rheumatic fever (conditions in I00)
    active — *see* Endocarditis, acute, rheumatic
    inactive or quiescent (with chorea) I09.1
  acute or subacute I33.9
    infective I33.0
    rheumatic (aortic) (mitral) (pulmonary) (tricuspid) I01.1
      with chorea (acute) (rheumatic) (Sydenham's) I02.0
  aortic (heart) (nonrheumatic) (valve) I35.8
    with
      mitral disease I08.0
        with tricuspid (valve) disease I08.3
        active or acute I01.1
          with chorea (acute) (rheumatic) (Sydenham's) I02.0
      rheumatic fever (conditions in I00)
        active — *see* Endocarditis, acute, rheumatic
        inactive or quiescent (with chorea) I06.9

Index

Endocarditis — Enlargement, enlarged

**Endocarditis** — continued
aortic — continued
with — continued
tricuspid (valve) disease I08.2
with mitral (valve) disease I08.3
acute or subacute I33.9
arteriosclerotic I35.8
rheumatic I06.9
with mitral disease I08.0
with tricuspid (valve) disease I08.3
active or acute I01.1
with chorea (acute) (rheumatic) (Sydenham's) I02.0
active or acute I01.1
with chorea (acute) (rheumatic) (Sydenham's) I02.0
specified NEC I06.8
specified cause NEC I35.8
syphilitic A52.03
arteriosclerotic I38
atypical verrucous (Libman-Sacks) M32.11
bacterial (acute) (any valve) (subacute) I33.0
candidal B37.6
congenital Q24.8
constrictive I33.0
Coxiella burnetii A78 [I39]
Coxsackie B33.21
due to
prosthetic cardiac valve T82.6 ☑
Q fever A78 [I39]
Serratia marcescens I33.0
typhoid (fever) A01.02
gonococcal A54.83
infectious or infective (acute) (any valve) (subacute) I33.0
lenta (acute) (any valve) (subacute) I33.0
Libman-Sacks M32.11
listerial A32.82
Löffler's I42.3
malignant (acute) (any valve) (subacute) I33.0
meningococcal A39.51
mitral (chronic) (double) (fibroid) (heart) (inactive) (valve) (with chorea) I05.9
with
aortic (valve) disease I08.0
with tricuspid (valve) disease I08.3
active or acute I01.1
with chorea (acute) (rheumatic) (Sydenham's) I02.0
rheumatic fever (conditions in I00)
active — see Endocarditis, acute, rheumatic
inactive or quiescent (with chorea) I05.9
tricuspid (valve) disease I08.1
with aortic (valve) disease I08.3
active or acute I01.1
with chorea (acute) (rheumatic) (Sydenham's) I02.0
bacterial I33.0
arteriosclerotic I34.8
nonrheumatic I34.8
acute or subacute I33.9
specified NEC I05.8
monilial B37.6
multiple valves I08.9
specified disorders I08.8
mycotic (acute) (any valve) (subacute) I33.0
pneumococcal (acute) (any valve) (subacute) I33.0
pulmonary (chronic) (heart) (valve) I37.8
with rheumatic fever (conditions in I00)
active — see Endocarditis, acute, rheumatic
inactive or quiescent (with chorea) I09.89
with aortic, mitral or tricuspid disease I08.8
acute or subacute I33.9
rheumatic I01.1
with chorea (acute) (rheumatic) (Sydenham's) I02.0
arteriosclerotic I37.8
congenital Q22.2
rheumatic (chronic) (inactive) (with chorea) I09.89
active or acute I01.1
with chorea (acute) (rheumatic) (Sydenham's) I02.0
syphilitic A52.03
purulent (acute) (any valve) (subacute) I33.0
Q fever A78 [I39]
rheumatic (chronic) (inactive) (with chorea) I09.1
active or acute (aortic) (mitral) (pulmonary) (tricuspid) I01.1

**Endocarditis** — continued
rheumatic — continued
active or acute — continued
with chorea (acute) (rheumatic) (Sydenham's) I02.0
rheumatoid — see Rheumatoid, carditis
septic (acute) (any valve) (subacute) I33.0
streptococcal (acute) (any valve) (subacute) I33.0
subacute — see Endocarditis, acute
suppurative (acute) (any valve) (subacute) I33.0
syphilitic A52.03
toxic I33.9
tricuspid (chronic) (heart) (inactive) (rheumatic) (valve) (with chorea) I07.9
with
aortic (valve) disease I08.2
mitral (valve) disease I08.3
mitral (valve) disease I08.1
aortic (valve) disease I08.3
rheumatic fever (conditions in I00)
active — see Endocarditis, acute, rheumatic
inactive or quiescent (with chorea) I07.8
active or acute I01.1
with chorea (acute) (rheumatic) (Sydenham's) I02.0
arteriosclerotic I36.8
nonrheumatic I36.8
acute or subacute I33.9
specified cause, except rheumatic I36.8
tuberculous — see Tuberculosis, endocarditis
typhoid A01.02
ulcerative (acute) (any valve) (subacute) I33.0
vegetative (acute) (any valve) (subacute) I33.0
verrucous (atypical) (nonbacterial) (nonrheumatic) M32.11
**Endocardium, endocardial** (see also condition)
cushion defect Q21.2
**Endocervicitis** (see also Cervicitis)
due to intrauterine (contraceptive) device T83.69 ☑
hyperplastic N72
**Endocrine** — see condition
**Endocrinopathy, pluriglandular** E31.9
**Endodontic**
overfill M27.52
underfill M27.53
**Endodontitis** K04.01
irreversible K04.02
reversible K04.01
**Endomastoiditis** — see Mastoiditis
**Endometrioma** N80.9
**Endometriosis** N80.9
appendix N80.5
bladder N80.8
bowel N80.5
broad ligament N80.3
cervix N80.0
colon N80.5
cul-de-sac (Douglas') N80.3
exocervix N80.0
fallopian tube N80.2
female genital organ NEC N80.8
gallbladder N80.8
in scar of skin N80.6
internal N80.0
intestine N80.5
lung N80.8
myometrium N80.0
ovary N80.1
parametrium N80.3
pelvic peritoneum N80.3
peritoneal (pelvic) N80.3
rectovaginal septum N80.4
rectum N80.5
round ligament N80.3
skin (scar) N80.6
specified site NEC N80.8
stromal D39.0
thorax N80.8
umbilicus N80.8
uterus (internal) N80.0
vagina N80.4
vulva N80.8
**Endometritis** (decidual) (nonspecific) (purulent) (senile) (atrophic) (suppurative) N71.9
with ectopic pregnancy O08.0
acute N71.0
blenorrhagic (gonococcal) (acute) (chronic) A54.24

**Endometritis** — continued
cervix, cervical (with erosion or ectropion) (see also Cervicitis)
hyperplastic N72
chlamydial A56.11
chronic N71.1
following
abortion — see Abortion by type complicated by genital infection
ectopic or molar pregnancy O08.0
gonococcal, gonorrheal (acute) (chronic) A54.24
hyperplastic (see also Hyperplasia, endometrial) N85.00
cervix N72
puerperal, postpartum, childbirth O86.12
subacute N71.0
tuberculous A18.17
**Endometrium** — see condition
**Endomyocardiopathy, South African** I42.3
**Endomyocarditis** — see Endocarditis
**Endomyofibrosis** I42.3
**Endomyometritis** — see Endometritis
**Endopericarditis** — see Endocarditis
**Endoperineuritis** — see Disorder, nerve
**Endophlebitis** — see Phlebitis
**Endophthalmia** — see Endophthalmitis, purulent
**Endophthalmitis** (acute) (infective) (metastatic) (subacute) H44.009
bleb associated (see also Bleb, inflammed (infected), postprocedural H59.4 ☑
gonorrheal A54.39
in (due to)
cysticercosis B69.1
onchocerciasis B73.01
toxocariasis B83.0
panuveitis — see Panuveitis
parasitic H44.12- ☑
purulent H44.00- ☑
panophthalmitis — see Panophthalmitis
vitreous abscess H44.02- ☑
specified NEC H44.19
sympathetic — see Uveitis, sympathetic
**Endosalpingioma** D28.2
**Endosalpingiosis** N94.89
**Endosteitis** — see Osteomyelitis
**Endothelioma, bone** — see Neoplasm, bone, malignant
**Endotheliosis** (hemorrhagic infectional) D69.8
**Endotoxemia** — code to condition
**Endotrachelitis** — see Cervicitis
**Engelmann** (-Camurati) **syndrome** Q78.3
**English disease** — see Rickets
**Engman's disease** L30.3
**Engorgement**
breast N64.59
newborn P83.4
puerperal, postpartum O92.79
lung (passive) — see Edema, lung
pulmonary (passive) — see Edema, lung
stomach K31.89
venous, retina — see Occlusion, retina, vein, engorgement
**Enlargement, enlarged** (see also Hypertrophy)
adenoids J35.2
with tonsils J35.3
alveolar ridge K08.89
congenital — see Anomaly, alveolar
apertures of diaphragm (congenital) Q79.1
gingival K06.1
heart, cardiac — see Hypertrophy, cardiac
labium majus, childhood asymmetric (CALME) N90.61
lacrimal gland, chronic H04.03- ☑
liver — see Hypertrophy, liver
lymph gland or node R59.9
generalized R59.1
localized R59.0
orbit H05.34- ☑
organ or site, congenital NEC — see Anomaly, by site
parathyroid (gland) E21.0
pituitary fossa R93.0
prostate N40.0
with lower urinary tract symptoms (LUTS) N40.1
without lower urinary tract symtpoms (LUTS) N40.0
sella turcica R93.0
spleen — see Splenomegaly
thymus (gland) (congenital) E32.0
thyroid (gland) — see Goiter
tongue K14.8
tonsils J35.1

**Enlargement, enlarged** — *continued*
  tonsils — *continued*
    with adenoids J35.3
  uterus N85.2
  vestibular aqueduct Q16.5
**Enophthalmos** H05.40- ☑
  due to
    orbital tissue atrophy H05.41- ☑
    trauma or surgery H05.42- ☑
**Enostosis** M27.8
**Entamebic, entamebiasis** — *see* Amebiasis
**Entanglement**
  umbilical cord(s) O69.82 ☑
    with compression O69.2 ☑
    without compression O69.82 ☑
    around neck (with compression) O69.81 ☑
      with compression O69.1 ☑
      without compression O69.81 ☑
    of twins in monoamniotic sac O69.2 ☑
**Enteralgia** — *see* Pain, abdominal
**Enteric** — *see* condition
**Enteritis** (acute) (diarrheal) (hemorrhagic) (noninfective) K52.9
  adenovirus A08.2
  aertrycke infection A02.0
  allergic K52.29
    with
      eosinophilic gastritis or gastroenteritis K52.81
      food protein-induced enterocolitis syndrome K52.21
      food protein-induced enteropathy K52.22
  amebic (acute) A06.0
    with abscess — *see* Abscess, amebic
    chronic A06.1
      with abscess — *see* Abscess, amebic
      nondysenteric A06.2
    nondysenteric A06.2
  astrovirus A08.32
  bacillary NOS A03.9
  bacterial A04.9
    specified NEC A04.8
  calicivirus A08.31
  candidal B37.82
  Chilomastix A07.8
  choleriformis A00.1
  chronic (noninfectious) K52.9
    ulcerative — *see* Colitis, ulcerative
  cicatrizing (chronic) — *see* Enteritis, regional, small intestine
  Clostridium
    botulinum (food poisoning) A05.1
    difficile
      not specified as recurrent A04.72
      recurrent A04.71
  coccidial A07.3
  coxsackie virus A08.39
  dietetic (*see also* Enteritis, allergic) K52.29
  drug-induced K52.1
  due to
    astrovirus A08.32
    calicivirus A08.31
    coxsackie virus A08.39
    drugs K52.1
    echovirus A08.39
    enterovirus NEC A08.39
    food hypersensitivity (*see also* Enteritis, allergic) K52.29
    infectious organism (bacterial) (viral) — *see* Enteritis, infectious
    torovirus A08.39
    Yersinia enterocolitica A04.6
  echovirus A08.39
  eltor A00.1
  enterovirus NEC A08.39
  eosinophilic K52.81
  epidemic (infectious) A09
  fulminant (*see also* Ischemia, intestine, acute) K55.019
  gangrenous — *see* Enteritis, infectious
  giardial A07.1
  infectious NOS A09
    due to
      adenovirus A08.2
      Aerobacter aerogenes A04.8
      Arizona (bacillus) A02.0
      bacteria NOS A04.9
        specified NEC A04.8
      Campylobacter A04.5

**Enteritis** — *continued*
  infectious — *continued*
    due to — *continued*
      Clostridium difficile
        not specified as recurrent A04.72
        recurrent A04.71
      Clostridium perfringens A04.8
      Enterobacter aerogenes A04.8
      enterovirus A08.39
      Escherichia coli A04.4
        enteroaggregative A04.4
        enterohemorrhagic A04.3
        enteroinvasive A04.2
        enteropathogenic A04.0
        enterotoxigenic A04.1
        specified NEC A04.4
      specified
        bacteria NEC A04.8
        virus NEC A08.39
      Staphylococcus A04.8
      virus NEC A08.4
        specified type NEC A08.39
      Yersinia enterocolitica A04.6
    specified organism NEC A08.8
  influenzal — *see* Influenza, with, digestive manifestations
  ischemic K55.9
    acute (*see also* Ischemia, intestine, acute) K55.019
    chronic K55.1
  microsporidial A07.8
  mucomembranous, myxomembranous — *see* Syndrome, irritable bowel
  mucous — *see* Syndrome, irritable bowel
  necroticans A05.2
  necrotizing of newborn — *see* Enterocolitis, necrotizing, in newborn
  neurogenic — *see* Syndrome, irritable bowel
  newborn necrotizing — *see* Enterocolitis, necrotizing, in newborn
  noninfectious K52.9
  norovirus A08.11
  parasitic NEC B82.9
  paratyphoid (fever) — *see* Fever, paratyphoid
  protozoal A07.9
    specified NEC A07.8
  radiation K52.0
  regional (of) K50.90
    with
      complication K50.919
        abscess K50.914
        fistula K50.913
        intestinal obstruction K50.912
        rectal bleeding K50.911
        specified complication NEC K50.918
    colon — *see* Enteritis, regional, large intestine
    duodenum — *see* Enteritis, regional, small intestine
    ileum — *see* Enteritis, regional, small intestine
    jejunum — *see* Enteritis, regional, small intestine
    large bowel — *see* Enteritis, regional, large intestine
    large intestine (colon) (rectum) K50.10
      with
        complication K50.119
          abscess K50.114
          fistula K50.113
          intestinal obstruction K50.112
          rectal bleeding K50.111
          small intestine (duodenum) (ileum) (jejunum) involvement K50.80
          with
            complication K50.819
              abscess K50.814
              fistula K50.813
              intestinal obstruction K50.812
              rectal bleeding K50.811
              specified complication NEC K50.818
        specified complication NEC K50.118
    rectum — *see* Enteritis, regional, large intestine
    small intestine (duodenum) (ileum) (jejunum) K50.00
      with
        complication K50.019
          abscess K50.014
          fistula K50.013
          intestinal obstruction K50.012
          large intestine (colon) (rectum) involvement K50.80

**Enteritis** — *continued*
  regional — *continued*
    small intestine — *continued*
      with — *continued*
        complication — *continued*
          large intestine involvement — *continued*
            with
              complication K50.819
                abscess K50.814
                fistula K50.813
                intestinal obstruction K50.812
                rectal bleeding K50.811
                specified complication NEC K50.818
            rectal bleeding K50.011
            specified complication NEC K50.018
  rotaviral A08.0
  Salmonella, salmonellosis (arizonae) (cholerae-suis) (enteritidis) (typhimurium) A02.0
  segmental — *see* Enteritis, regional
  septic A09
  Shigella — *see* Infection, Shigella
  small round structured NEC A08.19
  spasmodic, spastic — *see* Syndrome, irritable bowel
  staphylococcal A04.8
    due to food A05.0
  torovirus A08.39
  toxic NEC K52.1
    due to Clostridium difficile
      not specified as recurrent A04.72
      recurrent A04.71
  trichomonal A07.8
  tuberculous A18.32
  typhosa A01.00
  ulcerative (chronic) — *see* Colitis, ulcerative
  viral A08.4
    adenovirus A08.2
    enterovirus A08.39
    Rotavirus A08.0
    small round structured NEC A08.19
    specified NEC A08.39
    virus specified NEC A08.39
**Enterobiasis** B80
**Enterobius vermicularis** (infection) (infestation) B80
**Enterocele** (*see also* Hernia, abdomen)
  pelvic, pelvis (acquired) (congenital) N81.5
  vagina, vaginal (acquired) (congenital) NEC N81.5
**Enterocolitis** (*see also* Enteritis) K52.9
  due to Clostridium difficile
    not specified as recurrent A04.72
    recurrent A04.71
  fulminant ischemic (*see also* Ischemia, intestine, acute) K55.059
  granulomatous — *see* Enteritis, regional
  hemorrhagic (acute) (*see also* Ischemia, intestine, acute) K55.059
    chronic K55.1
  infectious NEC A09
  ischemic K55.9
  necrotizing K55.30
    with
      perforation K55.33
      pneumatosis K55.32
        and perforation K55.33
    without pneumatosis or perforation K55.31
    due to Clostridium difficile
      not specified as recurrent A04.72
      recurrent A04.71
    in newborn P77.9
      stage 1 (without pneumatosis, without perforation) P77.1
      stage 2 (with pneumatosis, without perforation) P77.2
      stage 3 (with pneumatosis, with perforation) P77.3
    in non-newborn K55.30
      stage 1 (without pneumatosis, without perforation) K55.31
      stage 2 (with pneumatosis, without perforation) K55.32
      stage 3 (with pneumatosis, with perforation) K55.33
  noninfectious K52.9
    newborn — *see* Enterocolitis, necrotizing, in newborn
  pseudomembranous (newborn)
    not specified as recurrent A04.72

**Enterocolitis** — continued
  pseudomembranous — continued
    recurrent A04.71
  radiation K52.0
    newborn — see Enterocolitis, necrotizing, in new-born
  ulcerative (chronic) — see Pancolitis, ulcerative (chronic)
**Enterogastritis** — see Enteritis
**Enteropathy** K63.9
  celiac-gluten-sensitive K90.0
    non-celiac K90.41
  food protein-induced enterocolitis K52.22
  hemorrhagic, terminal (see also Ischemia, intestine, acute) K55.059
  protein-losing K90.49
**Enteroperitonitis** — see Peritonitis
**Enteroptosis** K63.4
**Enterorrhagia** K92.2
**Enterospasm** (see also Syndrome, irritable, bowel)
  psychogenic F45.8
**Enterostenosis** (see also Obstruction, intestine, specified NEC) K56.699
**Enterostomy**
  complication — see Complication, enterostomy
  status Z93.4
**Enterovirus, as cause of disease classified elsewhere**
    B97.10
  coxsackievirus B97.11
  echovirus B97.12
  other specified B97.19
**Enthesopathy** (peripheral) M77.9
  Achilles tendinitis — see Tendinitis, Achilles
  ankle and tarsus M77.9
    specified type NEC — see Enthesopathy, foot, specified type NEC
  anterior tibial syndrome M76.81- ☑
  calcaneal spur — see Spur, bone, calcaneal
  elbow region M77.8
    lateral epicondylitis — see Epicondylitis, lateral
    medial epicondylitis — see Epicondylitis, medial
  foot NEC M77.9
    metatarsalgia — see Metatarsalgia
    specified type NEC M77.5- ☑
  forearm M77.9
  gluteal tendinitis — see Tendinitis, gluteal
  hand M77.9
  hip — see Enthesopathy, lower limb, specified type NEC
  iliac crest spur — see Spur, bone, iliac crest
  iliotibial band syndrome — see Syndrome, iliotibial band
  knee — see Enthesopathy, lower limb, lower leg, specified type NEC
  lateral epicondylitis — see Epicondylitis, lateral
  lower limb (excluding foot) M76.9
    Achilles tendinitis — see Tendinitis, Achilles
    anterior tibial syndrome M76.81- ☑
    gluteal tendinitis — see Tendinitis, gluteal
    iliac crest spur — see Spur, bone, iliac crest
    iliotibial band syndrome — see Syndrome, iliotibial band
    patellar tendinitis — see Tendinitis, patellar
    pelvic region — see Enthesopathy, lower limb, specified type NEC
    peroneal tendinitis — see Tendinitis, peroneal
    posterior tibial syndrome M76.82- ☑
    psoas tendinitis — see Tendinitis, psoas
    shoulder M77.9
    specified type NEC M76.89- ☑
    tibial collateral bursitis — see Bursitis, tibial collateral
  medial epicondylitis — see Epicondylitis, medial
  metatarsalgia — see Metatarsalgia
  multiple sites M77.9
  patellar tendinitis — see Tendinitis, patellar
  pelvis M77.9
  periarthritis of wrist — see Periarthritis, wrist
  peroneal tendinitis — see Tendinitis, peroneal
  posterior tibial syndrome M76.82- ☑
  psoas tendinitis — see Tendinitis, psoas
  shoulder region — see Lesion, shoulder
  specified site NEC M77.9
  specified type NEC M77.8
  spinal M46.00
    cervical region M46.02
    cervicothoracic region M46.03

**Enthesopathy** — continued
  spinal — continued
    lumbar region M46.06
    lumbosacral region M46.07
    multiple sites M46.09
    occipito-atlanto-axial region M46.01
    sacrococcygeal region M46.08
    thoracic region M46.04
    thoracolumbar region M46.05
  tibial collateral bursitis — see Bursitis, tibial collateral
  upper arm M77.9
  wrist and carpus NEC M77.8
    calcaneal spur — see Spur, bone, calcaneal
    periarthritis of wrist — see Periarthritis, wrist
**Entomophobia** F40.218
**Entomophthoromycosis** B46.8
**Entrance, air into vein** — see Embolism, air
**Entrapment, nerve** — see Neuropathy, entrapment
**Entropion** (eyelid) (paralytic) H02.009
  cicatricial H02.019
    left H02.016
      lower H02.015
      upper H02.014
    right H02.013
      lower H02.012
      upper H02.011
  congenital Q10.2
  left H02.006
    lower H02.005
    upper H02.004
  mechanical H02.029
    left H02.026
      lower H02.025
      upper H02.024
    right H02.023
      lower H02.022
      upper H02.021
  right H02.003
    lower H02.002
    upper H02.001
  senile H02.039
    left H02.036
      lower H02.035
      upper H02.034
    right H02.033
      lower H02.032
      upper H02.031
  spastic H02.049
    left H02.046
      lower H02.045
      upper H02.044
    right H02.043
      lower H02.042
      upper H02.041
**Enucleated eye** (traumatic, current) S05.7- ☑
**Enuresis** R32
  functional F98.0
  habit disturbance F98.0
  nocturnal N39.44
    psychogenic F98.0
  nonorganic origin F98.0
  psychogenic F98.0
**Eosinopenia** — see Agranulocytosis
**Eosinophilia** (allergic) (hereditary) (idiopathic) (secondary) D72.1
  with
    angiolymphoid hyperplasia (ALHE) D18.01
  infiltrative J82
  Löffler's J82
  peritoneal — see Peritonitis, eosinophilic
  pulmonary NEC J82
  tropical (pulmonary) J82
**Eosinophilia-myalgia syndrome** M35.8
**Ependymitis** (acute) (cerebral) (chronic) (granular) — see Encephalomyelitis
**Ependymoblastoma**
  specified site — see Neoplasm, malignant, by site
  unspecified site C71.9
**Ependymoma** (epithelial) (malignant)
  anaplastic
    specified site — see Neoplasm, malignant, by site
    unspecified site C71.9
  benign
    specified site — see Neoplasm, benign, by site
    unspecified site D33.2
  myxopapillary D43.2
    specified site — see Neoplasm, uncertain behavior, by site

**Ependymoma** — continued
  myxopapillary — continued
    unspecified site D43.2
  papillary D43.2
    specified site — see Neoplasm, uncertain behavior, by site
    unspecified site D43.2
  specified site — see Neoplasm, malignant, by site
  unspecified site C71.9
**Ependymopathy** G93.89
**Ephelis, ephelides** L81.2
**Epiblepharon** (congenital) Q10.3
**Epicanthus, epicanthic fold** (eyelid) (congenital) Q10.3
**Epicondylitis** (elbow)
  lateral M77.1- ☑
  medial M77.0- ☑
**Epicystitis** — see Cystitis
**Epidemic** — see condition
**Epidermidalization, cervix** — see Dysplasia, cervix
**Epidermis, epidermal** — see condition
**Epidermodysplasia verruciformis** B07.8
**Epidermolysis**
  bullosa (congenital) Q81.9
    acquired L12.30
      drug-induced L12.31
      specified cause NEC L12.35
    dystrophica Q81.2
    letalis Q81.1
    simplex Q81.0
    specified NEC Q81.8
  necroticans combustiformis L51.2
    due to drug — see Table of Drugs and Chemicals, by drug
**Epidermophytid** — see Dermatophytosis
**Epidermophytosis** (infected) — see Dermatophytosis
**Epididymis** — see condition
**Epididymitis** (acute) (nonvenereal) (recurrent) (residual) N45.1
  with orchitis N45.3
  blennorrhagic (gonococcal) A54.23
  caseous (tuberculous) A18.15
  chlamydial A56.19
  filarial (see also Infestation, filarial) B74.9 [N51]
  gonococcal A54.23
  syphilitic A52.76
  tuberculous A18.15
**Epididymo-orchitis** (see also Epididymitis) N45.3
**Epidural** — see condition
**Epigastrium, epigastric** — see condition
**Epigastrocele** — see Hernia, ventral
**Epiglottis** — see condition
**Epiglottitis, epiglottiditis** (acute) J05.10
  with obstruction J05.11
  chronic J37.0
**Epignathus** Q89.4
**Epilepsia partialis continua** (see also Kozhevnikof's epilepsy) G40.1- ☑
**Epilepsy, epileptic, epilepsia** (attack) (cerebral) (convulsion) (fit) (seizure) G40.909

> Note: the following terms are to be considered equivalent to intractable: pharmacoresistant (pharmacologically resistant), treatment resistant, refractory (medically) and poorly controlled

  with
    complex partial seizures — see Epilepsy, localization-related, symptomatic, with complex partial seizures
    grand mal seizures on awakening — see Epilepsy, generalized, specified NEC
    myoclonic absences — see Epilepsy, generalized, specified NEC
    myoclonic-astatic seizures — see Epilepsy, generalized, specified NEC
    simple partial seizures — see Epilepsy, localization-related, symptomatic, with simple partial seizures
  akinetic — see Epilepsy, generalized, specified NEC
  benign childhood with centrotemporal EEG spikes — see Epilepsy, localization-related, idiopathic
  benign myoclonic in infancy G40.80- ☑
  Bravais-jacksonian — see Epilepsy, localization-related, symptomatic, with simple partial seizures
  childhood
    with occipital EEG paroxysms — see Epilepsy, localization-related, idiopathic
    absence G40.A09 (following G40.3)

☑ Additional Character Required — Refer to the Tabular List for Character Selection     ▽ Subterms under main terms may continue to next column or page

**Epilepsy, epileptic, epilepsia** — *continued*
  childhood — *continued*
    absence — *continued*
      intractable G40.A19 (*following* G40.3)
        with status epilepticus G40.A11 (*following* G40.3)
        without status epilepticus G40.A19 (*following* G40.3)
      not intractable G40.A09 (*following* G40.3)
        with status epilepticus G40.A01 (*following* G40.3)
        without status epilepticus G40.A09 (*following* G40.3)
  climacteric — *see* Epilepsy, specified NEC
  cysticercosis B69.0
  deterioration (mental) F06.8
  due to syphilis A52.19
  focal — *see* Epilepsy, localization-related, symptomatic, with simple partial seizures
  generalized
    idiopathic G40.309
      intractable G40.319
        with status epilepticus G40.311
        without status epilepticus G40.319
      not intractable G40.309
        with status epilepticus G40.301
        without status epilepticus G40.309
    specified NEC G40.409
      intractable G40.419
        with status epilepticus G40.411
        without status epilepticus G40.419
      not intractable G40.409
        with status epilepticus G40.401
        without status epilepticus G40.409
  impulsive petit mal — *see* Epilepsy, juvenile myoclonic
  intractable G40.919
    with status epilepticus G40.911
    without status epilepticus G40.919
  juvenile absence G40.A09 (*following* G40.3)
    intractable G40.A19 (*following* G40.3)
      with status epilepticus G40.A11 (*following* G40.3)
      without status epilepticus G40.A19 (*following* G40.3)
    not intractable G40.A09 (*following* G40.3)
      with status epilepticus G40.A01 (*following* G40.3)
      without status epilepticus G40.A09 (*following* G40.3)
  juvenile myoclonic G40.B09 (*following* G40.3)
    intractable G40.B19 (*following* G40.3)
      with status epilepticus G40.B11 (*following* G40.3)
      without status epilepticus G40.B19 (*following* G40.3)
    not intractable G40.B09 (*following* G40.3)
      with status epilepticus G40.B01 (*following* G40.3)
      without status epilepticus G40.B09 (*following* G40.3)
  localization-related (focal) (partial)
    idiopathic G40.009
      with seizures of localized onset G40.009
        intractable G40.019
          with status epilepticus G40.011
          without status epilepticus G40.019
        not intractable G40.009
          with status epilepticus G40.001
          without status epilepticus G40.009
    symptomatic
      with complex partial seizures G40.209
        intractable G40.219
          with status epilepticus G40.211
          without status epilepticus G40.219
        not intractable G40.209
          with status epilepticus G40.201
          without status epilepticus G40.209
      with simple partial seizures G40.109
        intractable G40.119
          with status epilepticus G40.111
          without status epilepticus G40.119
        not intractable G40.109
          with status epilepticus G40.101
          without status epilepticus G40.109
  myoclonus, myoclonic — *see* Epilepsy, generalized, specified NEC
    progressive — *see* Epilepsy, generalized, idiopathic
  not intractable G40.909
    with status epilepticus G40.901

**Epilepsy, epileptic, epilepsia** — *continued*
  not intractable — *continued*
    without status epilepticus G40.909
  on awakening — *see* Epilepsy, generalized, specified NEC
  parasitic NOS B71.9 [G94]
  partialis continua (*see also* Kozhevnikof's epilepsy) G40.1- ☑
  peripheral — *see* Epilepsy, specified NEC
  procursiva — *see* Epilepsy, localization-related, symptomatic, with simple partial seizures
  progressive (familial) myoclonic — *see* Epilepsy, generalized, idiopathic
  reflex — *see* Epilepsy, specified NEC
  related to
    alcohol G40.509
      not intractable G40.509
        with status epilepticus G40.501
        without status eplliepticus G40.509
    drugs G40.509
      not intractable G40.509
        with status epilepticus G40.501
        without status eplliepticus G40.509
    external causes G40.509
      not intractable G40.509
        with status epilepticus G40.501
        without status eplliepticus G40.509
    hormonal changes G40.509
      not intractable G40.509
        with status epilepticus G40.501
        without status eplliepticus G40.509
    sleep deprivation G40.509
      not intractable G40.509
        with status epilepticus G40.501
        without status eplliepticus G40.509
    stress G40.509
      not intractable G40.509
        with status epilepticus G40.501
        without status eplliepticus G40.509
  somatomotor — *see* Epilepsy, localization-related, symptomatic, with simple partial seizures
  somatosensory — *see* Epilepsy, localization-related, symptomatic, with simple partial seizures
  spasms G40.822
    intractable G40.824
      with status epilepticus G40.823
      without status epilepticus G40.824
    not intractable G40.822
      with status epilepticus G40.821
      without status epilepticus G40.822
  specified NEC G40.802
    intractable G40.804
      with status epilepticus G40.803
      without status epilepticus G40.804
    not intractable G40.802
      with status epilepticus G40.801
      without status epilepticus G40.802
  syndromes
    generalized
      idiopathic G40.309
        intractable G40.319
          with status epilepticus G40.311
          without status epilepticus G40.319
        not intractable G40.309
          with status epilepticus G40.301
          without status epilepticus G40.309
      specified NEC G40.409
        intractable G40.419
          with status epilepticus G40.411
          without status epilepticus G40.419
        not intractable G40.409
          with status epilepticus G40.401
          without status epilepticus G40.409
    localization-related (focal) (partial)
      idiopathic G40.009
        with seizures of localized onset G40.009
          intractable G40.019
            with status epilepticus G40.011
            without status epilepticus G40.019
          not intractable G40.009
            with status epilepticus G40.001
            without status epilepticus G40.009
      symptomatic
        with complex partial seizures G40.209
          intractable G40.219
            with status epilepticus G40.211
            without status epilepticus G40.219
          not intractable G40.209

**Epilepsy, epileptic, epilepsia** — *continued*
  syndromes — *continued*
    localization-related — *continued*
      symptomatic — *continued*
        with complex partial seizures — *continued*
          not intractable — *continued*
            with status epilepticus G40.201
            without status epilepticus G40.209
        with simple partial seizures G40.109
          intractable G40.119
            with status epilepticus G40.111
            without status epilepticus G40.119
          not intractable G40.109
            with status epilepticus G40.101
            without status epilepticus G40.109
      specified NEC G40.802
        intractable G40.804
          with status epilepticus G40.803
          without status epilepticus G40.804
        not intractable G40.802
          with status epilepticus G40.801
          without status epilepticus G40.802
  tonic (-clonic) — *see* Epilepsy, generalized, specified NEC
  twilight F05
  uncinate (gyrus) — *see* Epilepsy, localization-related, symptomatic, with complex partial seizures
  Unverricht (-Lundborg) (familial myoclonic) — *see* Epilepsy, generalized, idiopathic
  visceral — *see* Epilepsy, specified NEC
  visual — *see* Epilepsy, specified NEC
**Epiloia** Q85.1
**Epimenorrhea** N92.0
**Epipharyngitis** — *see* Nasopharyngitis
**Epiphora** H04.20- ☑
  due to
    excess lacrimation H04.21- ☑
    insufficient drainage H04.22- ☑
**Epiphyseal arrest** — *see* Arrest, epiphyseal
**Epiphyseolysis, epiphysiolysis** — *see* Osteochondropathy
**Epiphysitis** (*see also* Osteochondropathy)
  juvenile M92.9
  syphilitic (congenital) A50.02
**Epiplocele** — *see* Hernia, abdomen
**Epiploitis** — *see* Peritonitis
**Epiplosarcomphalocele** — *see* Hernia, umbilicus
**Episcleritis** (suppurative) H15.10- ☑
  in (due to)
    syphilis A52.71
    tuberculosis A18.51
  nodular H15.12- ☑
  periodica fugax H15.11- ☑
    angioneurotic — *see* Edema, angioneurotic
  syphilitic (late) A52.71
  tuberculous A18.51
**Episode**
  affective, mixed F39
  depersonalization (in neurotic state) F48.1
  depressive F32.9
    major F32.9
      mild F32.0
      moderate F32.1
      severe (without psychotic symptoms) F32.2
        with psychotic symptoms F32.3
    recurrent F33.9
      brief F33.8
    specified NEC F32.89
  hypomanic F30.8
  manic F30.9
    with
      psychotic symptoms F30.2
      remission (full) F30.4
        partial F30.3
    without psychotic symptoms F30.10
      mild F30.11
      moderate F30.12
      severe (without psychotic symptoms) F30.13
        with psychotic symptoms F30.2
    other specified F30.8
    recurrent F31.89
  psychotic F23
    organic F06.8
  schizophrenic (acute) NEC, brief F23
**Epispadias** (female) (male) Q64.0
**Episplenitis** D73.89
**Epistaxis** (multiple) R04.0

**Epistaxis** — *continued*
  hereditary I78.0
  vicarious menstruation N94.89
**Epithelioma** (malignant) (*see also* Neoplasm, malignant, by site)
  adenoides cysticum — *see* Neoplasm, skin, benign
  basal cell — *see* Neoplasm, skin, malignant
  benign — *see* Neoplasm, benign, by site
  Bowen's — *see* Neoplasm, skin, in situ
  calcifying, of Malherbe — *see* Neoplasm, skin, benign
  external site — *see* Neoplasm, skin, malignant
  intraepidermal, Jadassohn — *see* Neoplasm, skin, benign
  squamous cell — *see* Neoplasm, malignant, by site
**Epitheliomatosis pigmented** Q82.1
**Epitheliopathy, multifocal placoid pigment** H30.14- ☑
**Epithelium, epithelial** — *see* condition
**Epituberculosis** (with atelectasis) (allergic) A15.7
**Eponychia** Q84.6
**Epstein's**
  nephrosis or syndrome — *see* Nephrosis
  pearl K09.8
**Epulis** (gingiva) (fibrous) (giant cell) K06.8
**Equinia** A24.0
**Equinovarus** (congenital) (talipes) Q66.0
  acquired — *see* Deformity, limb, clubfoot
**Equivalent**
  convulsive (abdominal) — *see* Epilepsy, specified NEC
  epileptic (psychic) — *see* Epilepsy, localization-related, symptomatic, with complex partial seizures
**Erb** (-Duchenne) **paralysis** (birth injury) (newborn) P14.0
**Erb-Goldflam disease or syndrome** G70.00
  with exacerbation (acute) G70.01
  in crisis G70.01
**Erb's**
  disease G71.0
  palsy, paralysis (brachial) (birth) (newborn) P14.0
    spinal (spastic) syphilitic A52.17
  pseudohypertrophic muscular dystrophy G71.0
**Erdheim's syndrome** (acromegalic macrospondylitis) E22.0
**Erection, painful** (persistent) — *see* Priapism
**Ergosterol deficiency** (vitamin D) E55.9
  with
    adult osteomalacia M83.8
    rickets — *see* Rickets
**Ergotism** (*see also* Poisoning, food, noxious, plant)
  from ergot used as drug (migraine therapy) — *see* Table of Drugs and Chemicals
**Erosio interdigitalis blastomycetica** B37.2
**Erosion**
  artery I77.2
    without rupture I77.89
  bone — *see* Disorder, bone, density and structure, specified NEC
  bronchus J98.09
  cartilage (joint) — *see* Disorder, cartilage, specified type NEC
  cervix (uteri) (acquired) (chronic) (congenital) N86
    with cervicitis N72
  cornea (nontraumatic) — *see* Ulcer, cornea
    recurrent H18.83- ☑
    traumatic — *see* Abrasion, cornea
  dental (idiopathic) (occupational) (due to diet, drugs or vomiting) K03.2
  duodenum, postpyloric — *see* Ulcer, duodenum
  esophagus K22.10
    with bleeding K22.11
  gastric — *see* Ulcer, stomach
  gastrojejunal — *see* Ulcer, gastrojejunal
  implanted mesh — *see* Complications, mesh
  intestine K63.3
  lymphatic vessel I89.8
  pylorus, pyloric (ulcer) — *see* Ulcer, stomach
  spine, aneurysmal A52.09
  stomach — *see* Ulcer, stomach
  subcutaneous device pocket
    nervous system prosthetic device, implant, or graft T85.890 ☑
    other internal prosthetic device, implant, or graft T85.898 ☑
  teeth (idiopathic) (occupational) (due to diet, drugs or vomiting) K03.2
  urethra N36.8
  uterus N85.8
**Erotomania** F52.8

**Error**
  metabolism, inborn — *see* Disorder, metabolism
  refractive — *see* Disorder, refraction
**Eructation** R14.2
  nervous or psychogenic F45.8
**Eruption**
  creeping B76.9
  drug (generalized) (taken internally) L27.0
    fixed L27.1
    in contact with skin — *see* Dermatitis, due to drugs
    localized L27.1
  Hutchinson, summer L56.4
  Kaposi's varicelliform B00.0
  napkin L22
  polymorphous light (sun) L56.4
  recalcitrant pustular L13.8
  ringed R23.8
  skin (nonspecific) R21
    creeping (meaning hookworm) B76.9
    due to inoculation/vaccination (generalized) (*see also* Dermatitis, due to, vaccine) L27.0
      localized L27.1
    erysipeloid A26.0
    feigned L98.1
    Kaposi's varicelliform B00.0
    lichenoid L28.0
    meaning dermatitis — *see* Dermatitis
    toxic NEC L53.0
  tooth, teeth, abnormal (incomplete) (late) (premature) (sequence) K00.6
  vesicular R23.8
**Erysipelas** (gangrenous) (infantile) (newborn) (phlegmonous) (suppurative) A46
  external ear A46 [H62.40]
  puerperal, postpartum O86.89
**Erysipeloid** A26.9
  cutaneous (Rosenbach's) A26.0
  disseminated A26.8
  sepsis A26.7
  specified NEC A26.8
**Erythema, erythematous** (infectional) (inflammation) L53.9
  ab igne L59.0
  annulare (centrifugum) (rheumaticum) L53.1
  arthriticum epidemicum A25.1
  brucellum — *see* Brucellosis
  chronic figurate NEC L53.3
  chronicum migrans (Borrelia burgdorferi) A69.20
  diaper L22
  due to
    chemical NEC L53.0
      in contact with skin L24.5
    drug (internal use) — *see* Dermatitis, due to, drugs
  elevatum diutinum L95.1
  endemic E52
  epidemic, arthritic A25.1
  figuratum perstans L53.3
  gluteal L22
  heat — *code by site under* Burn, first degree
  ichthyosiforme congenitum bullous Q80.3
  in diseases classified elsewhere L54
  induratum (nontuberculous) L52
    tuberculous A18.4
  infectiosum B08.3
  intertrigo L30.4
  iris L51.9
  marginatum L53.2
    in (due to) acute rheumatic fever I00
  medicamentosum — *see* Dermatitis, due to, drugs
  migrans A26.0
    chronicum A69.20
    tongue K14.1
  multiforme (major) (minor) L51.9
    bullous, bullosum L51.1
    conjunctiva L51.1
    nonbullous L51.0
    pemphigoides L12.0
    specified NEC L51.8
  napkin L22
  neonatorum P83.88
    toxic P83.1
  nodosum L52
    tuberculous A18.4
  palmar L53.8
  pernio T69.1 ☑
  rash, newborn P83.88
  scarlatiniform (recurrent) (exfoliative) L53.8
  solare L55.0

**Erythema, erythematous** — *continued*
  specified NEC L53.8
  toxic, toxicum NEC L53.0
    newborn P83.1
  tuberculous (primary) A18.4
**Erythematous, erythematosus** — *see* condition
**Erythermalgia** (primary) I73.81
**Erythralgia** I73.81
**Erythrasma** L08.1
**Erythredema** (polyneuropathy) — *see* Poisoning, mercury
**Erythremia** (acute) C94.0- ☑
  chronic D45
  secondary D75.1
**Erythroblastopenia** (*see also* Aplasia, red cell) D60.9
  congenital D61.01
**Erythroblastophthisis** D61.09
**Erythroblastosis** (fetalis) (newborn) P55.9
  due to
    ABO (antibodies) (incompatibility) (isoimmunization) P55.1
    Rh (antibodies) (incompatibility) (isoimmunization) P55.0
**Erythrocyanosis** (crurum) I73.89
**Erythrocythemia** — *see* Erythremia
**Erythrocytosis** (megalosplenic) (secondary) D75.1
  familial D75.0
  oval, hereditary — *see* Elliptocytosis
  secondary D75.1
  stress D75.1
**Erythroderma** (secondary) (*see also* Erythema) L53.9
  bullous ichthyosiform, congenital Q80.3
  desquamativum L21.1
  ichthyosiform, congenital (bullous) Q80.3
  neonatorum P83.88
  psoriaticum L40.8
**Erythrodysesthesia, palmar plantar** (PPE) L27.1
**Erythrogenesis imperfecta** D61.09
**Erythroleukemia** C94.0- ☑
**Erythromelalgia** I73.81
**Erythrophagocytosis** D75.89
**Erythrophobia** F40.298
**Erythroplakia, oral epithelium, and tongue** K13.29
**Erythroplasia** (Queyrat) D07.4
  specified site — *see* Neoplasm, skin, in situ
  unspecified site D07.4
**Escherichia coli** (E. coli), **as cause of disease classified elsewhere** B96.20
  non-O157 Shiga toxin-producing (with known O group) B96.22
  non-Shiga toxin-producing B96.29
  O157 B96.21
  O157 with confirmation of Shiga toxin when H antigen is unknown, or is not H7 B96.21
  O157:H- (nonmotile) with confirmation of Shiga toxin B96.21
  O157:H7 with or without confirmation of Shiga toxin-production B96.21
  Shiga toxin-producing (with unspecified O group) (STEC) B96.23
  specified NEC B96.29
**Esophagismus** K22.4
**Esophagitis** (acute) (alkaline) (chemical) (chronic) (infectional) (necrotic) (peptic) (postoperative) K20.9
  candidal B37.81
  due to gastrointestinal reflux disease K21.0
  eosinophilic K20.0
  reflux K21.0
  specified NEC K20.8
  tuberculous A18.83
  ulcerative K22.10
    with bleeding K22.11
**Esophagocele** K22.5
**Esophagomalacia** K22.8
**Esophagospasm** K22.4
**Esophagostenosis** K22.2
**Esophagostomiasis** B81.8
**Esophagotracheal** — *see* condition
**Esophagus** — *see* condition
**Esophoria** H50.51
  convergence, excess H51.12
  divergence, insufficiency H51.8
**Esotropia** — *see* Strabismus, convergent concomitant
**Espundia** B55.2
**Essential** — *see* condition
**Esthesioneuroblastoma** C30.0
**Esthesioneurocytoma** C30.0

**Esthesioneuroepithelioma** C30.0
**Esthiomene** A55
**Estivo-autumnal malaria** (fever) B50.9
**Estrangement** (marital) Z63.5
  parent-child NEC Z62.890
**Estriasis** — see Myiasis
**Ethanolism** — see Alcoholism
**Etherism** — see Dependence, drug, inhalant
**Ethmoid, ethmoidal** — see condition
**Ethmoiditis** (chronic) (nonpurulent) (purulent) (see also Sinusitis, ethmoidal)
  influenzal — see Influenza, with, respiratory manifestations NEC
  Woakes' J33.1
**Ethylism** — see Alcoholism
**Eulenburg's disease** (congenital paramyotonia) G71.19
**Eumycetoma** B47.0
**Eunuchoidism** E29.1
  hypogonadotropic E23.0
**European blastomycosis** — see Cryptococcosis
**Eustachian** — see condition
**Evaluation** (for) (of)
  development state
    adolescent Z00.3
    period of
      delayed growth in childhood Z00.70
        with abnormal findings Z00.71
      rapid growth in childhood Z00.2
      puberty Z00.3
  growth and developmental state (period of rapid growth) Z00.2
    delayed growth Z00.70
      with abnormal findings Z00.71
  mental health (status) Z00.8
    requested by authority Z04.6
  period of
    delayed growth in childhood Z00.70
      with abnormal findings Z00.71
    rapid growth in childhood Z00.2
  suspected condition — see Observation
**Evans syndrome** D69.41
**Event**
  apparent life threatening in newborn and infant (ALTE) R68.13
  brief resolved unexplained event (BRUE) R68.13
**Eventration** (see also Hernia, ventral)
  colon into chest — see Hernia, diaphragm
  diaphragm (congenital) Q79.1
**Eversion**
  bladder N32.89
  cervix (uteri) N86
    with cervicitis N72
  foot NEC (see also Deformity, valgus, ankle)
    congenital Q66.6
  punctum lacrimale (postinfectional) (senile) H04.52- ☑
  ureter (meatus) N28.89
  urethra (meatus) N36.8
  uterus N81.4
**Evidence**
  cytologic
    of malignancy on anal smear R85.614
    of malignancy on cervical smear R87.614
    of malignancy on vaginal smear R87.624
**Evisceration**
  birth injury P15.8
  traumatic NEC
    eye — see Enucleated eye
**Evulsion** — see Avulsion
**Ewing's sarcoma or tumor** — see Neoplasm, bone, malignant
**Examination** (for) (following) (general) (of) (routine) Z00.00
  with abnormal findings Z00.01
  abuse, physical (alleged), ruled out
    adult Z04.71
    child Z04.72
  adolescent (development state) Z00.3
  alleged rape or sexual assault (victim), ruled out
    adult Z04.41
    child Z04.42
  allergy Z01.82
  annual (adult) (periodic) (physical) Z00.00
    with abnormal findings Z00.01
    gynecological Z01.419
      with abnormal findings Z01.411
  antibody response Z01.84
  blood — see Examination, laboratory
  blood pressure Z01.30

**Examination** — continued
  blood pressure — continued
    with abnormal findings Z01.31
  cancer staging — see Neoplasm, malignant, by site
  cervical Papanicolaou smear Z12.4
    as part of routine gynecological examination Z01.419
      with abnormal findings Z01.411
  child (over 28 days old) Z00.129
    with abnormal findings Z00.121
    under 28 days old — see Newborn, examination
  clinical research control or normal comparison (control) (participant) Z00.6
  contraceptive (drug) maintenance (routine) Z30.8
    device (intrauterine) Z30.431
  dental Z01.20
    with abnormal findings Z01.21
  developmental — see Examination, child
  donor (potential) Z00.5
  ear Z01.10
    with abnormal findings NEC Z01.118
  eye Z01.00
    with abnormal findings Z01.01
  following
    accident NEC Z04.3
      transport Z04.1
      work Z04.2
    assault, alleged, ruled out
      adult Z04.71
      child Z04.72
    motor vehicle accident Z04.1
    treatment (for) Z09
      combined NEC Z09
        fracture Z09
        malignant neoplasm Z08
      malignant neoplasm Z08
      mental disorder Z09
      specified condition NEC Z09
  follow-up (routine) (following) Z09
    chemotherapy NEC Z09
      malignant neoplasm Z08
    fracture Z09
    malignant neoplasm Z08
    postpartum Z39.2
    psychotherapy Z09
    radiotherapy NEC Z09
      malignant neoplasm Z08
    surgery NEC Z09
      malignant neoplasm Z08
  gynecological Z01.419
    with abnormal findings Z01.411
    for contraceptive maintenance Z30.8
  health — see Examination, medical
  hearing Z01.10
    with abnormal findings NEC Z01.118
    following failed hearing screening Z01.110
  immunity status testing Z01.84
  laboratory (as part of a general medical examination) Z00.00
    with abnormal findings Z00.01
    preprocedural Z01.812
  lactating mother Z39.1
  medical (adult) (for) (of) Z00.00
    with abnormal findings Z00.01
    administrative purpose only Z02.9
      specified NEC Z02.89
    admission to
      armed forces Z02.3
      old age home Z02.2
      prison Z02.89
      residential institution Z02.2
      school Z02.0
        following illness or medical treatment Z02.0
      summer camp Z02.89
    adoption Z02.82
    blood alcohol or drug level Z02.83
    camp (summer) Z02.89
    clinical research, normal subject (control) (participant) Z00.6
    control subject in clinical research (normal comparison) (participant) Z00.6
    donor (potential) Z00.5
    driving license Z02.4
    general (adult) Z00.00
      with abnormal findings Z00.01
    immigration Z02.89
    insurance purposes Z02.6
    marriage Z02.89
    medicolegal reasons NEC Z04.8

**Examination** — continued
  medical — continued
    naturalization Z02.89
    participation in sport Z02.5
    paternity testing Z02.81
    population survey Z00.8
    pre-employment Z02.1
    pre-operative — see Examination, pre-procedural
    pre-procedural
      cardiovascular Z01.810
      respiratory Z01.811
      specified NEC Z01.818
    preschool children
      for admission to school Z02.0
    prisoners
      for entrance into prison Z02.89
    recruitment for armed forces Z02.3
    specified NEC Z00.8
    sport competition Z02.5
  medicolegal reason NEC Z04.8
  newborn — see Newborn, examination
  pelvic (annual) (periodic) Z01.419
    with abnormal findings Z01.411
  period of rapid growth in childhood Z00.2
  periodic (adult) (annual) (routine) Z00.00
    with abnormal findings Z00.01
  physical (adult) (see also Examination, medical) Z00.00
    sports Z02.5
  postpartum
    immediately after delivery Z39.0
    routine follow-up Z39.2
  pre-chemotherapy (antineoplastic) Z01.818
  prenatal (normal pregnancy) (see also Pregnancy, normal) Z34.9- ☑
  pre-procedural (pre-operative)
    cardiovascular Z01.810
    laboratory Z01.812
    respiratory Z01.811
    specified NEC Z01.818
  prior to chemotherapy (antineoplastic) Z01.818
  psychiatric NEC Z00.8
    follow-up not needing further care Z09
    requested by authority Z04.6
  radiological (as part of a general medical examination) Z00.00
    with abnormal findings Z00.01
  repeat cervical smear to confirm findings of recent normal smear following initial abnormal smear Z01.42
  skin (hypersensitivity) Z01.82
  special (see also Examination, by type) Z01.89
    specified type NEC Z01.89
  specified type or reason NEC Z04.8
  teeth Z01.20
    with abnormal findings Z01.21
  urine — see Examination, laboratory
  vision Z01.00
    with abnormal findings Z01.01
**Exanthem, exanthema** (see also Rash)
  with enteroviral vesicular stomatitis B08.4
  Boston A88.0
  epidemic with meningitis A88.0 [G02]
  subitum B08.20
    due to human herpesvirus 6 B08.21
    due to human herpesvirus 7 B08.22
  viral, virus B09
    specified type NEC B08.8
**Excess, excessive, excessively**
  alcohol level in blood R78.0
  androgen (ovarian) E28.1
  attrition, tooth, teeth K03.0
  carotene, carotin (dietary) E67.1
  cold, effects of T69.9 ☑
    specified effect NEC T69.8 ☑
  convergence H51.12
  crying
    in child, adolescent, or adult R45.83
    in infant R68.11
  development, breast N62
  divergence H51.8
  drinking (alcohol) NEC (without dependence) F10.10
    habitual (continual) (without remission) F10.20
  eating R63.2
  estrogen E28.0
  fat (see also Obesity)
    in heart — see Degeneration, myocardial
    localized E65
  foreskin N47.8

**Excess, excessive, excessively** — continued
gas R14.0
glucagon E16.3
heat — see Heat
intermaxillary vertical dimension of fully erupted teeth M26.37
interocclusal distance of fully erupted teeth M26.37
kalium E87.5
large
colon K59.39
congenital Q43.8
infant P08.0
organ or site, congenital NEC — see Anomaly, by site
long
organ or site, congenital NEC — see Anomaly, by site
menstruation (with regular cycle) N92.0
with irregular cycle N92.1
napping Z72.821
natrium E87.0
number of teeth K00.1
nutrient (dietary) NEC R63.2
potassium (K) E87.5
salivation K11.7
secretion (see also Hypersecretion)
milk O92.6
sputum R09.3
sweat R61
sexual drive F52.8
short
organ or site, congenital NEC — see Anomaly, by site
umbilical cord in labor or delivery O69.3 ☑
skin L98.7
and subcutaneous tissue L98.7
eyelid (acquired) — see Blepharochalasis
congenital Q10.3
sodium (Na) E87.0
spacing of fully erupted teeth M26.32
sputum R09.3
sweating R61
thirst R63.1
due to deprivation of water T73.1 ☑
tuberosity of jaw M26.07
vitamin
A (dietary) E67.0
administered as drug (prolonged intake) — see Table of Drugs and Chemicals, vitamins, adverse effect
overdose or wrong substance given or taken — see Table of Drugs and Chemicals, vitamins, poisoning
D (dietary) E67.3
administered as drug (prolonged intake) — see Table of Drugs and Chemicals, vitamins, adverse effect
overdose or wrong substance given or taken — see Table of Drugs and Chemicals, vitamins, poisoning
weight
gain R63.5
loss R63.4
**Excitability, abnormal, under minor stress** (personality disorder) F60.3
**Excitation**
anomalous atrioventricular I45.6
psychogenic F30.8
reactive (from emotional stress, psychological trauma) F30.8
**Excitement**
hypomanic F30.8
manic F30.9
mental, reactive (from emotional stress, psychological trauma) F30.8
state, reactive (from emotional stress, psychological trauma) F30.8
**Excoriation** (traumatic) (see also Abrasion)
neurotic L98.1
skin picking disorder F42.4
**Exfoliation**
due to erythematous conditions according to extent of body surface involved L49.0
less than 10 percent of body surface L49.0
10-19 percent of body surface L49.1
20-29 percent of body surface L49.2
30-39 percent of body surface L49.3
40-49 percent of body surface L49.4

**Exfoliation** — continued
due to erythematous conditions according to extent of body surface involved — continued
50-59 percent of body surface L49.5
60-69 percent of body surface L49.6
70-79 percent of body surface L49.7
80-89 percent of body surface L49.8
90-99 percent of body surface L49.9
teeth, due to systemic causes K08.0
**Exfoliative** — see condition
**Exhaustion, exhaustive** (physical NEC) R53.83
battle F43.0
cardiac — see Failure, heart
delirium F43.0
due to
cold T69.8 ☑
excessive exertion T73.3 ☑
exposure T73.2 ☑
neurasthenia F48.8
heart — see Failure, heart
heat (see also Heat, exhaustion) T67.5 ☑
due to
salt depletion T67.4 ☑
water depletion T67.3 ☑
maternal, complicating delivery O75.81
mental F48.8
myocardium, myocardial — see Failure, heart
nervous F48.8
old age R54
psychogenic F48.8
psychosis F43.0
senile R54
vital NEC Z73.0
**Exhibitionism** F65.2
**Exocervicitis** — see Cervicitis
**Exomphalos** Q79.2
meaning hernia — see Hernia, umbilicus
**Exophoria** H50.52
convergence, insufficiency H51.11
divergence, excess H51.8
**Exophthalmos** H05.2- ☑
congenital Q15.8
constant NEC H05.24- ☑
displacement, globe — see Displacement, globe
due to thyrotoxicosis (hyperthyroidism) — see Hyperthyroidism, with, goiter (diffuse)
dysthyroid — see Hyperthyroidism, with, goiter (diffuse)
goiter — see Hyperthyroidism, with, goiter (diffuse)
intermittent NEC H05.25- ☑
malignant — see Hyperthyroidism, with, goiter (diffuse)
orbital
edema — see Edema, orbit
hemorrhage — see Hemorrhage, orbit
pulsating NEC H05.26- ☑
thyrotoxic, thyrotropic — see Hyperthyroidism, with, goiter (diffuse)
**Exostosis** (see also Disorder, bone)
cartilaginous — see Neoplasm, bone, benign
congenital (multiple) Q78.6
external ear canal H61.81- ☑
gonococcal A54.49
jaw (bone) M27.8
multiple, congenital Q78.6
orbit H05.35- ☑
osteocartilaginous — see Neoplasm, bone, benign
syphilitic A52.77
**Exotropia** — see Strabismus, divergent concomitant
**Explanation of**
investigation finding Z71.2
medication Z71.89
**Exposure** (to) (see also Contact, with) T75.89 ☑
acariasis Z20.7
AIDS virus Z20.6
air pollution Z77.110
algae and algae toxins Z77.121
algae bloom Z77.121
anthrax Z20.810
aromatic amines Z77.020
aromatic (hazardous) compounds NEC Z77.028
aromatic dyes NOS Z77.028
arsenic Z77.010
asbestos Z77.090
bacterial disease NEC Z20.818
benzene Z77.021
blue-green algae bloom Z77.121

**Exposure** — continued
body fluids (potentially hazardous) Z77.21
brown tide Z77.121
chemicals (chiefly nonmedicinal) (hazardous) NEC Z77.098
cholera Z20.09
chromium compounds Z77.018
cold, effects of T69.9 ☑
specified effect NEC T69.8 ☑
communicable disease Z20.9
bacterial NEC Z20.818
specified NEC Z20.89
viral NEC Z20.828
cyanobacteria bloom Z77.121
disaster Z65.5
discrimination Z60.5
dyes Z77.098
effects of T73.9 ☑
environmental tobacco smoke (acute) (chronic) Z77.22
Escherichia coli (E. coli) Z20.01
exhaustion due to T73.2 ☑
fiberglass — see Table of Drugs and Chemicals, fiberglass
German measles Z20.4
gonorrhea Z20.2
hazardous metals NEC Z77.018
hazardous substances NEC Z77.29
hazards in the physical environment NEC Z77.128
hazards to health NEC Z77.9
human immunodeficiency virus (HIV) Z20.6
human T-lymphotropic virus type-1 (HTLV-1) Z20.89
implanted
mesh — see Complications, mesh
prosthetic materials NEC — see Complications, prosthetic materials NEC
infestation (parasitic) NEC Z20.7
intestinal infectious disease NEC Z20.09
Escherichia coli (E. coli) Z20.01
lead Z77.011
meningococcus Z20.811
mold (toxic) Z77.120
nickel dust Z77.018
noise Z77.122
occupational
air contaminants NEC Z57.39
dust Z57.2
environmental tobacco smoke Z57.31
extreme temperature Z57.6
noise Z57.0
radiation Z57.1
risk factors Z57.9
specified NEC Z57.8
toxic agents (gases) (liquids) (solids) (vapors) in agriculture Z57.4
toxic agents (gases) (liquids) (solids) (vapors) in industry NEC Z57.5
vibration Z57.7
parasitic disease NEC Z20.7
pediculosis Z20.7
persecution Z60.5
pfiesteria piscicida Z77.121
poliomyelitis Z20.89
pollution
air Z77.110
environmental NEC Z77.118
soil Z77.112
water Z77.111
polycyclic aromatic hydrocarbons Z77.028
prenatal (drugs) (toxic chemicals) — see Newborn, affected by, noxious substances transmitted via placenta or breast milk
rabies Z20.3
radiation, naturally occurring NEC Z77.123
radon Z77.123
red tide (Florida) Z77.121
rubella Z20.4
second hand tobacco smoke (acute) (chronic) Z77.22
in the perinatal period P96.81
sexually-transmitted disease Z20.2
smallpox (laboratory) Z20.89
syphilis Z20.2
terrorism Z65.4
torture Z65.4
tuberculosis Z20.1
uranium Z77.012
varicella Z20.820
venereal disease Z20.2
viral disease NEC Z20.828

☑ **Additional Character Required** — Refer to the Tabular List for Character Selection          ▽ **Subterms under main terms may continue to next column or page**

**Exposure** — *continued*
  war Z65.5
  water pollution Z77.111
**Exsanguination** — *see* Hemorrhage
**Exstrophy**
  abdominal contents Q45.8
  bladder Q64.10
    cloacal Q64.12
    specified type NEC Q64.19
    supravesical fissure Q64.11
**Extensive** — *see* condition
**Extra** (*see also* Accessory)
  marker chromosomes (normal individual) Q92.61
    in abnormal individual Q92.62
  rib Q76.6
    cervical Q76.5
**Extrasystoles** (supraventricular) I49.49
  atrial I49.1
  auricular I49.1
  junctional I49.2
  ventricular I49.3
**Extrauterine gestation or pregnancy** — *see* Pregnancy, by site
**Extravasation**
  blood R58
  chyle into mesentery I89.8
  pelvicalyceal N13.8
  pyelosinus N13.8
  urine (from ureter) R39.0
  vesicant agent
    antineoplastic chemotherapy T80.810 ☑
    other agent NEC T80.818 ☑
**Extremity** — *see* condition, limb
**Extrophy** — *see* Exstrophy
**Extroversion**
  bladder Q64.19
  uterus N81.4
    complicating delivery O71.2
    postpartal (old) N81.4
**Extruded tooth** (teeth) M26.34
**Extrusion**
  breast implant (prosthetic) T85.42 ☑
  eye implant (globe) (ball) T85.328 ☑
  intervertebral disc — *see* Displacement, intervertebral disc
  ocular lens implant (prosthetic) — *see* Complications, intraocular lens
  vitreous — *see* Prolapse, vitreous
**Exudate**
  pleural — *see* Effusion, pleura
  retina H35.89
**Exudative** — *see* condition
**Eye, eyeball, eyelid** — *see* condition
**Eyestrain** — *see* Disturbance, vision, subjective
**Eyeworm disease of Africa** B74.3

# F

**Faber's syndrome** (achlorhydric anemia) D50.9
**Fabry** (-Anderson) **disease** E75.21
**Faciocephalalgia, autonomic** (*see also* Neuropathy, peripheral, autonomic) G90.09
**Factor**(s)
  psychic, associated with diseases classified elsewhere F54
  psychological
    affecting physical conditions F54
    or behavioral
      affecting general medical condition F54
      associated with disorders or diseases classified elsewhere F54
**Fahr disease** (of brain) G23.8
**Fahr Volhard disease** (of kidney) I12.- ☑
**Failure, failed**
  abortion — *see* Abortion, attempted
  aortic (valve) I35.8
    rheumatic I06.8
  attempted abortion — *see* Abortion, attempted
  biventricular I50.82
    due to left heart failure I50.814
  bone marrow — *see* Anemia, aplastic
  cardiac — *see* Failure, heart
  cardiorenal (chronic) (*see also* Failure, renal, and Failure, heart) I50.9
    hypertensive I13.2
  cardiorespiratory (*see also* Failure, heart) R09.2
  cardiovascular (chronic) — *see* Failure, heart

**Failure, failed** — *continued*
  cerebrovascular I67.9
  cervical dilatation in labor O62.0
  circulation, circulatory (peripheral) R57.9
    newborn P29.89
  compensation — *see* Disease, heart
  compliance with medical treatment or regimen — *see* Noncompliance
  congestive — *see* Failure, heart, congestive
  dental implant (endosseous) M27.69
    due to
      failure of dental prosthesis M27.63
      lack of attached gingiva M27.62
      occlusal trauma (poor prosthetic design) M27.62
      parafunctional habits M27.62
      periodontal infection (peri-implantitis) M27.62
      poor oral hygiene M27.62
    osseointegration M27.61
      due to
        complications of systemic disease M27.61
        poor bone quality M27.61
      iatrogenic M27.61
    post-osseointegration
      biological M27.62
      due to complications of systemic disease M27.62
      iatrogenic M27.62
      mechanical M27.63
    pre-integration M27.61
    pre-osseointegration M27.61
    specified NEC M27.69
  descent of head (at term) of pregnancy (mother) O32.4 ☑
  endosseous dental implant — *see* Failure, dental implant
  engagement of head (term of pregnancy) (mother) O32.4 ☑
  erection (penile) (*see also* Dysfunction, sexual, male, erectile) N52.9
    nonorganic F52.21
  examination(s), anxiety concerning Z55.2
  expansion terminal respiratory units (newborn) (primary) P28.0
  forceps NOS (with subsequent cesarean delivery) O66.5
  gain weight (child over 28 days old) R62.51
    adult R62.7
    newborn P92.6
  genital response (male) F52.21
    female F52.22
  heart (acute) (senile) (sudden) I50.9
    with
      acute pulmonary edema — *see* Failure, ventricular, left
      decompensation (*see also* Failure, heart, by type as diastolic or systolic, acute and chronic) I50.9
      dilatation — *see* Disease, heart
      normal ejection fraction — *see* Failure, heart, diastolic
      preserved ejection fraction — *see* Failure, heart, diastolic
      reduced ejection fraction — *see* Failure, heart, systolic
    arteriosclerotic I70.90
    biventricular I50.82
      due to left heart failure I50.814
    combined left-right sided I50.82
      due to left heart failure I50.814
    compensated (*see also* Failure, heart, by type as diastolic or systolic, chronic) I50.9
    complicating
      anesthesia (general) (local) or other sedation in labor and delivery O74.2
      in pregnancy O29.12- ☑
      postpartum, puerperal O89.1
      delivery (cesarean) (instrumental) O75.4
    congestive I50.9
      with rheumatic fever (conditions in I00)
        active I01.8
        inactive or quiescent (with chorea) I09.81
      newborn P29.0
      rheumatic (chronic) (inactive) (with chorea) I09.81
        active or acute I01.8
          with chorea I02.0
    decompensated (*see also* Failure, heart, by type as diastolic or systolic, acute and chronic) I50.9

**Failure, failed** — *continued*
  heart — *continued*
    degenerative — *see* Degeneration, myocardial
    diastolic (congestive) (left ventricular) I50.30
      acute (congestive) I50.31
        and (on) chronic (congestive) I50.33
      chronic (congestive) I50.32
        and (on) acute (congestive) I50.33
      combined with systolic (congestive) I50.40
        acute (congestive) I50.41
          and (on) chronic (congestive) I50.43
        chronic (congestive) I50.42
          and (on) acute (congestive) I50.43
    due to presence of cardiac prosthesis I97.13- ☑
    end stage (*see also* Failure, heart, by type as diastolic or systolic, chronic) I50.84
    following cardiac surgery I97.13- ☑
    high output NOS I50.83
    hypertensive — *see* Hypertension, heart
    left (ventricular) (*see also* Failure, ventricular, left)
      combined diastolic and systolic — *see* Failure, heart, diastolic, combined with systolic
      diastolic — *see* Failure, heart, diastolic
      systolic — *see* Failure, heart, systolic
    low output (syndrome) NOS I50.9
    newborn P29.0
    organic — *see* Disease, heart
    peripartum O90.3
    postprocedural I97.13- ☑
    rheumatic (chronic) (inactive) I09.9
    right (isolated) (ventricular) I50.810
      acute I50.811
        and (on) chronic I50.813
      chronic I50.812
        and acute I50.813
      secondary to left heart failure I50.814
    specified NEC I50.89

> Note: heart failure stages A, B, C, and D are based on the American College of Cardiology and American Heart Association stages of heart failure, which complement and should not be confused with the New York Heart Association Classification of Heart Failure, into Class I, Class II, Class III, and Class IV

    stage A Z91.89
    stage B (*see also* Failure, heart, by type as diastolic or systolic) I50.9
    stage C (*see also* Failure, heart, by type as diastolic or systolic) I50.9
    stage D (*see also* Failure, heart, by type as diastolic or systolic, chronic) I50.84
    systolic (congestive) (left ventricular) I50.20
      acute (congestive) I50.21
        and (on) chronic (congestive) I50.23
      chronic (congestive) I50.22
        and (on) acute (congestive) I50.23
      combined with diastolic (congestive) I50.40
        acute (congestive) I50.41
          and (on) chronic (congestive) I50.43
        chronic (congestive) I50.42
          and (on) acute (congestive) I50.43
    thyrotoxic (*see also* Thyrotoxicosis) E05.90 [I43]
      with
        high output (*see also* Thyrotoxicosis) I50.83
        thyroid storm E05.91 [I43]
          high output (*see also* Thyrotoxicosis) I50.83
    valvular — *see* Endocarditis
  hepatic K72.90
    with coma K72.91
    acute or subacute K72.00
      with coma K72.01
      due to drugs K71.10
        with coma K71.11
    alcoholic (acute) (chronic) (subacute) K70.40
      with coma K70.41
    chronic K72.10
      with coma K72.11
      due to drugs (acute) (subacute) (chronic) K71.10
        with coma K71.11
    due to drugs (acute) (subacute) (chronic) K71.10
      with coma K71.11
    postprocedural K91.82
  hepatorenal K76.7
  induction (of labor) O61.9
    abortion — *see* Abortion, attempted
    by
      oxytocic drugs O61.0

**Failure, failed** — *continued*
  induction — *continued*
    by — *continued*
      prostaglandins O61.0
    instrumental O61.1
    mechanical O61.1
    medical O61.0
    specified NEC O61.8
    surgical O61.1
  intubation during anesthesia T88.4 ☑
    in pregnancy O29.6- ☑
    labor and delivery O74.7
    postpartum, puerperal O89.6
  involution, thymus (gland) E32.0
  kidney (*see also* Disease, kidney, chronic) N19
    acute (*see also* Failure, renal, acute) N17.9
  lactation (complete) O92.3
    partial O92.4
  Leydig's cell, adult E29.1
  liver — *see* Failure, hepatic
  menstruation at puberty N91.0
  mitral I05.8
  myocardial, myocardium (*see also* Failure, heart) I50.9
    chronic (*see also* Failure, heart, congestive) I50.9
    congestive (*see also* Failure, heart, congestive) I50.9
  orgasm (female) (psychogenic) F52.31
    male F52.32
  ovarian (primary) E28.39
    iatrogenic E89.40
      asymptomatic E89.40
      symptomatic E89.41
    postprocedural (postablative) (postirradiation)
      (postsurgical) E89.40
      asymptomatic E89.40
      symptomatic E89.41
  ovulation causing infertility N97.0
  polyglandular, autoimmune E31.0
  prosthetic joint implant — *see* Complications, joint
    prosthesis, mechanical, breakdown, by site
  renal N19
    with
      tubular necrosis (acute) N17.0
    acute N17.9
      with
        cortical necrosis N17.1
        medullary necrosis N17.2
        tubular necrosis N17.0
      specified NEC N17.8
    chronic N18.9
      hypertensive — *see* Hypertension, kidney
    congenital P96.0
    end stage (chronic) N18.6
      due to hypertension I12.0
    following
      abortion — *see* Abortion by type complicated
        by specified condition NEC
      crushing T79.5 ☑
      ectopic or molar pregnancy O08.4
      labor and delivery (acute) O90.4
    hypertensive — *see* Hypertension, kidney
    postprocedural N99.0
  respiration, respiratory J96.90
    with
      hypercapnia J96.92
      hypercarbia J96.02
      hypoxia J96.91
    acute J96.00
      with
        hypercapnia J96.02
        hypercarbia J96.02
        hypoxia J96.01
    acute and (on) chronic J96.20
      with
        hypercapnia J96.22
        hypercarbia J96.22
        hypoxia J96.21
    center G93.89
    chronic J96.10
      with
        hypercapnia J96.12
        hypercarbia J96.12
        hypoxia J96.11
    newborn P28.5
    postprocedural (acute) J95.821
      acute and chronic J95.822
  rotation
    cecum Q43.3
    colon Q43.3

**Failure, failed** — *continued*
  rotation — *continued*
    intestine Q43.3
    kidney Q63.2
  sedation (conscious) (moderate) during procedure
    T88.52 ☑
    history of Z92.83
  segmentation (*see also* Fusion)
    fingers — *see* Syndactylism, complex, fingers
    vertebra Q76.49
      with scoliosis Q76.3
  seminiferous tubule, adult E29.1
  senile (general) R54
  sexual arousal (male) F52.21
    female F52.22
  testicular endocrine function E29.1
  to thrive (child over 28 days old) R62.51
    adult R62.7
    newborn P92.6
  transplant T86.92
    bone T86.831
      marrow T86.02
    cornea T86.841
    heart T86.22
      with lung(s) T86.32
    intestine T86.851
    kidney T86.12
    liver T86.42
    lung(s) T86.811
      with heart T86.32
    pancreas T86.891
    skin (allograft) (autograft) T86.821
    specified organ or tissue NEC T86.891
    stem cell (peripheral blood) (umbilical cord) T86.5
  trial of labor (with subsequent cesarean delivery)
    O66.40
    following previous cesarean delivery O66.41
  tubal ligation N99.89
  urinary — *see* Disease, kidney, chronic
  vacuum extraction NOS (with subsequent cesarean
    delivery) O66.5
  vasectomy N99.89
  ventouse NOS (with subsequent cesarean delivery)
    O66.5
  ventricular (*see also* Failure, heart) I50.9
    left (*see also* Failure, heart, left) I50.1
      with rheumatic fever (conditions in I00)
        active I01.8
          with chorea I02.0
        inactive or quiescent (with chorea) I09.81
        rheumatic (chronic) (inactive) (with chorea)
          I09.81
          active or acute I01.8
            with chorea I02.0
    right — *see* Failure, heart, right
  vital centers, newborn P91.88
**Fainting** (fit) R55
**Fallen arches** — *see* Deformity, limb, flat foot
**Falling, falls** (repeated) R29.6
  any organ or part — *see* Prolapse
**Fallopian**
  insufflation Z31.41
  tube — *see* condition
**Fallot's**
  pentalogy Q21.8
  tetrad or tetralogy Q21.3
  triad or trilogy Q22.3
**False** (*see also* condition)
  croup J38.5
  joint — *see* Nonunion, fracture
  labor (pains) O47.9
    at or after 37 completed weeks of gestation O47.1
    before 37 completed weeks of gestation O47.0- ☑
  passage, urethra (prostatic) N36.5
  pregnancy F45.8
**Family, familial** (*see also* condition)
  disruption Z63.8
    involving divorce or separation Z63.5
  Li-Fraumeni (syndrome) Z15.01
  planning advice Z30.09
  problem Z63.9
    specified NEC Z63.8
  retinoblastoma C69.2- ☑
**Famine** (effects of) T73.0 ☑
  edema — *see* Malnutrition, severe
**Fanconi** (-de Toni)(-Debré) **syndrome** E72.09
  with cystinosis E72.04
**Fanconi's anemia** (congenital pancytopenia) D61.09

**Farber's disease or syndrome** E75.29
**Farcy** A24.0
**Farmer's**
  lung J67.0
  skin L57.8
**Farsightedness** — *see* Hypermetropia
**Fascia** — *see* condition
**Fasciculation** R25.3
**Fasciitis** M72.9
  diffuse (eosinophilic) M35.4
  infective M72.8
    necrotizing M72.6
  necrotizing M72.6
  nodular M72.4
  perirenal (with ureteral obstruction) N13.5
    with infection N13.6
  plantar M72.2
  specified NEC M72.8
  traumatic (old) M72.8
    current — *code by* site under Sprain
**Fascioliasis** B66.3
**Fasciolopsis, fasciolopsiasis** (intestinal) B66.5
**Fascioscapulohumeral myopathy** G71.0
**Fast pulse** R00.0
**Fat**
  embolism — *see* Embolism, fat
  excessive (*see also* Obesity)
    in heart — *see* Degeneration, myocardial
  in stool R19.5
  localized (pad) E65
    heart — *see* Degeneration, myocardial
    knee M79.4
    retropatellar M79.4
  necrosis
    breast N64.1
    mesentery K65.4
    omentum K65.4
  pad E65
    knee M79.4
**Fatigue** R53.83
  auditory deafness — *see* Deafness
  chronic R53.82
  combat F43.0
  general R53.83
    psychogenic F48.8
  heat (transient) T67.6 ☑
  muscle M62.89
  myocardium — *see* Failure, heart
  neoplasm-related R53.0
  nervous, neurosis F48.8
  operational F48.8
  psychogenic (general) F48.8
  senile R54
  voice R49.8
**Fatness** — *see* Obesity
**Fatty** (*see also* condition)
  apron E65
  degeneration — *see* Degeneration, fatty
  heart (enlarged) — *see* Degeneration, myocardial
  liver NEC K76.0
    alcoholic K70.0
    nonalcoholic K76.0
  necrosis — *see* Degeneration, fatty
**Fauces** — *see* condition
**Fauchard's disease** (periodontitis) — *see* Periodontitis
**Faucitis** J02.9
**Favism** (anemia) D55.0
**Favus** — *see* Dermatophytosis
**Fazio-Londe disease or syndrome** G12.1
**Fear complex or reaction** F40.9
**Fear of** — *see* Phobia
**Feared complaint unfounded** Z71.1
**Febris, febrile** (*see also* Fever)
  flava (*see also* Fever, yellow) A95.9
  melitensis A23.0
  pestis — *see* Plague
  recurrens — *see* Fever, relapsing
  rubra A38.9
**Fecal**
  incontinence R15.9
  smearing R15.1
  soiling R15.1
  urgency R15.2
**Fecalith** (impaction) K56.41
  appendix K38.1
  congenital P76.8
**Fede's disease** K14.0

☑ **Additional Character Required** — **Refer to the Tabular List for Character Selection**       ⬙ **Subterms under main terms may continue to next column or page**

**Feeble rapid pulse due to shock following injury**
    T79.4 ☑
**Feeble-minded** F70
**Feeding**
    difficulties R63.3
    problem R63.3
        newborn P92.9
            specified NEC P92.8
        nonorganic (adult) — see Disorder, eating
**Feeling** (of)
    foreign body in throat R09.89
**Feer's disease** — see Poisoning, mercury
**Feet** — see condition
**Feigned illness** Z76.5
**Feil-Klippel syndrome** (brevicollis) Q76.1
**Feinmesser's** (hidrotic) **ectodermal dysplasia** Q82.4
**Felinophobia** F40.218
**Felon** (see also Cellulitis, digit)
    with lymphangitis — see Lymphangitis, acute, digit
**Felty's syndrome** M05.00
    ankle M05.07- ☑
    elbow M05.02- ☑
    foot joint M05.07- ☑
    hand joint M05.04- ☑
    hip M05.05- ☑
    knee M05.06- ☑
    multiple site M05.09
    shoulder M05.01- ☑
    vertebra — see Spondylitis, ankylosing
    wrist M05.03- ☑
**Female genital cutting status** — see Female genital
        mutilation status (FGM)
**Female genital mutilation status** (FGM) N90.810
    specified NEC N90.818
    type I (clitorectomy status) N90.811
    type II (clitorectomy with excision of labia minora sta-
        tus) N90.812
    type III (infibulation status) N90.813
    type IV N90.818
**Femur, femoral** — see condition
**Fenestration, fenestrated** (see also Imperfect, closure)
    aortico-pulmonary Q21.4
    cusps, heart valve NEC Q24.8
        pulmonary Q22.3
    pulmonic cusps Q22.3
**Fernell's disease** (aortic aneurysm) I71.9
**Fertile eunuch syndrome** E23.0
**Fetid**
    breath R19.6
    sweat L75.0
**Fetishism** F65.0
    transvestic F65.1
**Fetus, fetal** (see also condition)
    alcohol syndrome (dysmorphic) Q86.0
    compressus O31.0- ☑
    hydantoin syndrome Q86.1
    lung tissue P28.0
    papyraceous O31.0- ☑
**Fever** (inanition) (of unknown origin) (persistent) (with
        chills) (with rigor) R50.9
    abortus A23.1
    Aden (dengue) A90
    African tick-borne A68.1
    American
        mountain (tick) A93.2
            spotted A77.0
    aphthous B08.8
    arbovirus, arboviral A94
        hemorrhagic A94
        specified NEC A93.8
    Argentinian hemorrhagic A96.0
    Assam B55.0
    Australian Q A78
    Bangkok hemorrhagic A91
    Barmah forest A92.8
    Bartonella A44.0
    bilious, hemoglobinuric B50.8
    blackwater B50.8
    blister B00.1
    Bolivian hemorrhagic A96.1
    Bonvale dam T73.3 ☑
    boutonneuse A77.1
    brain — see Encephalitis
    Brazilian purpuric A48.4
    breakbone A90
    Bullis A77.0
    Bunyamwera A92.8

**Fever** — continued
    Burdwan B55.0
    Bwamba A92.8
    Cameroon — see Malaria
    Canton A75.9
    catarrhal (acute) J00
        chronic J31.0
    cat-scratch A28.1
    Central Asian hemorrhagic A98.0
    cerebral — see Encephalitis
    cerebrospinal meningococcal A39.0
    Chagres B50.9
    Chandipura A92.8
    Changuinola A93.1
    Charcot's (biliary) (hepatic) (intermittent) — see Calcu-
        lus, bile duct
    Chikungunya (viral) (hemorrhagic) A92.0
    Chitral A93.1
    Colombo — see Fever, paratyphoid
    Colorado tick (virus) A93.2
    congestive (remittent) — see Malaria
    Congo virus A98.0
    continued malarial B50.9
    Corsican — see Malaria
    Crimean-Congo hemorrhagic A98.0
    Cyprus — see Brucellosis
    dandy A90
    deer fly — see Tularemia
    dengue (virus) A90
        hemorrhagic A91
        sandfly A93.1
    desert B38.0
    drug induced R50.2
    due to
        conditions classified elsewhere R50.81
        heat T67.0 ☑
    enteric A01.00
    enteroviral exanthematous (Boston exanthem) A88.0
    ephemeral (of unknown origin) R50.9
    epidemic hemorrhagic A98.5
    erysipelatous — see Erysipelas
    estivo-autumnal (malarial) B50.9
    famine A75.0
    five day A79.0
    following delivery O86.4
    Fort Bragg A27.89
    gastroenteric A01.00
    gastromalarial — see Malaria
    Gibraltar — see Brucellosis
    glandular — see Mononucleosis, infectious
    Guama (viral) A92.8
    Haverhill A25.1
    hay (allergic) J30.1
        with asthma (bronchial) J45.909
            with
                exacerbation (acute) J45.901
                status asthmaticus J45.902
            due to
                allergen other than pollen J30.89
                pollen, any plant or tree J30.1
    heat (effects) T67.0 ☑
    hematuric, bilious B50.8
    hemoglobinuric (malarial) (bilious) B50.8
    hemorrhagic (arthropod-borne) NOS A94
        with renal syndrome A98.5
        arenaviral A96.9
            specified NEC A96.8
        Argentinian A96.0
        Bangkok A91
        Bolivian A96.1
        Central Asian A98.0
        Chikungunya A92.0
        Crimean-Congo A98.0
        dengue (virus) A91
        epidemic A98.5
        Junin (virus) A96.0
        Korean A98.5
        Kyasanur forest A98.2
        Machupo (virus) A96.1
        mite-borne A93.8
        mosquito-borne A92.8
        Omsk A98.1
        Philippine A91
        Russian A98.5
        Singapore A91
        Southeast Asia A91
        Thailand A91
        tick-borne NEC A93.8

**Fever** — continued
    hemorrhagic — continued
        viral A99
            specified NEC A98.8
    hepatic — see Cholecystitis
    herpetic — see Herpes
    icterohemorrhagic A27.0
    Indiana A93.8
    infective B99.9
        specified NEC B99.8
    intermittent (bilious) (see also Malaria)
        of unknown origin R50.9
        pernicious B50.9
    iodide R50.2
    Japanese river A75.3
    jungle (see also Malaria)
        yellow A95.0
    Junin (virus) hemorrhagic A96.0
    Katayama B65.2
    kedani A75.3
    Kenya (tick) A77.1
    Kew Garden A79.1
    Korean hemorrhagic A98.5
    Lassa A96.2
    Lone Star A77.0
    Machupo (virus) hemorrhagic A96.1
    malaria, malarial — see Malaria
    Malta A23.9
    Marseilles A77.1
    marsh — see Malaria
    Mayaro (viral) A92.8
    Mediterranean (see also Brucellosis) A23.9
        familial M04.1
        tick A77.1
    meningeal — see Meningitis
    Meuse A79.0
    Mexican A75.2
    mianeh A68.1
    miasmatic — see Malaria
    mosquito-borne (viral) A92.9
        hemorrhagic A92.8
    mountain (see also Brucellosis)
        meaning Rocky Mountain spotted fever A77.0
        tick (American) (Colorado) (viral) A93.2
    Mucambo (viral) A92.8
    mud A27.9
    Neapolitan — see Brucellosis
    neutropenic D70.9
    newborn P81.9
        environmental P81.0
    Nine-Mile A78
    non-exanthematous tick A93.2
    North Asian tick-borne A77.2
    Omsk hemorrhagic A98.1
    O'nyong-nyong (viral) A92.1
    Oropouche (viral) A93.0
    Oroya A44.0
    paludal — see Malaria
    Panama (malarial) B50.9
    Pappataci A93.1
    paratyphoid A01.4
        A A01.1
        B A01.2
        C A01.3
    parrot A70
    periodic (Mediterranean) M04.1
    persistent (of unknown origin) R50.9
    petechial A39.0
    pharyngoconjunctival B30.2
    Philippine hemorrhagic A91
    phlebotomus A93.1
    Piry (virus) A93.8
    Pixuna (viral) A92.8
    Plasmodium ovale B53.0
    polioviral (nonparalytic) A80.4
    Pontiac A48.2
    postimmunization R50.83
    postoperative R50.82
        due to infection T81.4 ☑
    posttransfusion R50.84
    postvaccination R50.83
    presenting with conditions classified elsewhere R50.81
    pretibial A27.89
    puerperal O86.4
    Q A78
    quadrilateral A78
    quartan (malaria) B52.9
    Queensland (coastal) (tick) A77.3

---

**Fever** — *continued*
quintan A79.0
rabbit — *see* Tularemia
rat-bite A25.9
  due to
    Spirillum A25.0
    Streptobacillus moniliformis A25.1
recurrent — *see* Fever, relapsing
relapsing (Borrelia) A68.9
  Carter's (Asiatic) A68.1
  Dutton's (West African) A68.1
  Koch's A68.9
  louse-borne A68.0
  Novy's
    louse-borne A68.0
    tick-borne A68.1
  Obermeyer's (European) A68.0
  tick-borne A68.1
remittent (bilious) (congestive) (gastric) — *see* Malaria
rheumatic (active) (acute) (chronic) (subacute) I00
  with central nervous system involvement I02.9
  active with heart involvement — *see* category
    I01 ☑
  inactive or quiescent with
    cardiac hypertrophy I09.89
    carditis I09.9
    endocarditis I09.1
      aortic (valve) I06.9
        with mitral (valve) disease I08.0
      mitral (valve) I05.9
        with aortic (valve) disease I08.0
      pulmonary (valve) I09.89
      tricuspid (valve) I07.8
    heart disease NEC I09.89
    heart failure (congestive) (conditions in I50.)
      I09.81
    left ventricular failure (conditions in I50.1-I50.4-)
      I09.81
    myocarditis, myocardial degeneration (condi-
      tions in I51.4) I09.0
    pancarditis I09.9
    pericarditis I09.2
Rift Valley (viral) A92.4
Rocky Mountain spotted A77.0
rose J30.1
Ross River B33.1
Russian hemorrhagic A98.5
San Joaquin (Valley) B38.0
sandfly A93.1
Sao Paulo A77.0
scarlet A38.9
seven day (leptospirosis) (autumnal) (Japanese) A27.89
  dengue A90
shin-bone A79.0
Singapore hemorrhagic A91
solar A90
Songo A98.5
sore B00.1
South African tick-bite A68.1
Southeast Asia hemorrhagic A91
spinal — *see* Meningitis
spirillary A25.0
splenic — *see* Anthrax
spotted A77.9
  American A77.0
  Brazilian A77.0
  cerebrospinal meningitis A39.0
  Colombian A77.0
  due to Rickettsia
    australis A77.3
    conorii A77.1
    rickettsii A77.0
    sibirica A77.2
    specified type NEC A77.8
  Ehrlichiosis A77.40
    due to
      E. chafeensis A77.41
        specified organism NEC A77.49
  Rocky Mountain A77.0
steroid R50.2
streptobacillary A25.1
subtertian B50.9
Sumatran mite A75.3
sun A90
swamp A27.9
swine A02.8
sylvatic, yellow A95.0
Tahyna B33.8

**Fever** — *continued*
tertian — *see* Malaria, tertian
Thailand hemorrhagic A91
thermic T67.0 ☑
three-day A93.1
tick
  American mountain A93.2
  Colorado A93.2
  Kemerovo A93.8
  Mediterranean A77.1
  mountain A93.2
  nonexanthematous A93.2
  Quaranfil A93.8
tick-bite NEC A93.8
tick-borne (hemorrhagic) NEC A93.8
trench A79.0
tsutsugamushi A75.3
typhogastric A01.00
typhoid (abortive) (hemorrhagic) (intermittent) (malignant) A01.00
  complicated by
    arthritis A01.04
    heart involvement A01.02
    meningitis A01.01
    osteomyelitis A01.05
    pneumonia A01.03
    specified NEC A01.09
typhomalarial — *see* Malaria
typhus — *see* Typhus (fever)
undulant — *see* Brucellosis
unknown origin R50.9
uveoparotid D86.89
valley B38.0
Venezuelan equine A92.2
vesicular stomatitis A93.8
viral hemorrhagic — *see* Fever, hemorrhagic, by type
  of virus
Volhynian A79.0
Wesselsbron (viral) A92.8
West
  African B50.8
  Nile (viral) A92.30
    with
      complications NEC A92.39
      cranial nerve disorders A92.32
      encephalitis A92.31
      encephalomyelitis A92.31
      neurologic manifestation NEC A92.32
      optic neuritis A92.32
      polyradiculitis A92.32
Whitmore's — *see* Melioidosis
Wolhynian A79.0
worm B83.9
yellow A95.9
  jungle A95.0
  sylvatic A95.0
  urban A95.1
Zika virus A92.5
**Fibrillation**
atrial or auricular (established) I48.91
  chronic I48.2
  paroxysmal I48.0
  permanent I48.2
  persistent I48.1
cardiac I49.8
heart I49.8
muscular M62.89
ventricular I49.01
**Fibrin**
ball or bodies, pleural (sac) J94.1
chamber, anterior (eye) (gelatinous exudate) — *see*
  Iridocyclitis, acute
**Fibrinogenolysis** — *see* Fibrinolysis
**Fibrinogenopenia** D68.8
acquired D65
congenital D68.2
**Fibrinolysis** (hemorrhagic) (acquired) D65
antepartum hemorrhage — *see* Hemorrhage, antepartum, with coagulation defect
following
  abortion — *see* Abortion by type complicated by
    hemorrhage
  ectopic or molar pregnancy O08.1
intrapartum O67.0
newborn, transient P60
postpartum O72.3
**Fibrinopenia** (hereditary) D68.2
acquired D68.4

**Fibrinopurulent** — *see* condition
**Fibrinous** — *see* condition
**Fibroadenoma**
cellular intracanalicular D24- ☑
giant D24- ☑
intracanalicular
  cellular D24- ☑
  giant D24- ☑
  specified site — *see* Neoplasm, benign, by site
  unspecified site D24- ☑
juvenile D24- ☑
pericanalicular
  specified site — *see* Neoplasm, benign, by site
  unspecified site D24- ☑
phyllodes D24- ☑
prostate D29.1
specified site NEC — *see* Neoplasm, benign, by site
unspecified site D24- ☑
**Fibroadenosis, breast** (chronic) (cystic) (diffuse) (periodic) (segmental) N60.2- ☑
**Fibroangioma** (*see also* Neoplasm, benign, by site)
juvenile
  specified site — *see* Neoplasm, benign, by site
  unspecified site D10.6
**Fibrochondrosarcoma** — *see* Neoplasm, cartilage,
  malignant
**Fibrocystic**
disease (*see also* Fibrosis, cystic)
  breast — *see* Mastopathy, cystic
  jaw M27.49
  kidney (congenital) Q61.8
  liver Q44.6
  pancreas E84.9
kidney (congenital) Q61.8
**Fibrodysplasia ossificans progressiva** — *see* Myositis,
  ossificans, progressiva
**Fibroelastosis** (cordis) (endocardial) (endomyocardial)
  I42.4
**Fibroid** (tumor) (*see also* Neoplasm, connective tissue,
  benign)
disease, lung (chronic) — *see* Fibrosis, lung
heart (disease) — *see* Myocarditis
in pregnancy or childbirth O34.1- ☑
  causing obstructed labor O65.5
induration, lung (chronic) — *see* Fibrosis, lung
lung — *see* Fibrosis, lung
pneumonia (chronic) — *see* Fibrosis, lung
uterus (*see also* Leiomyoma, uterus) D25.9
**Fibrolipoma** — *see* Lipoma
**Fibroliposarcoma** — *see* Neoplasm, connective tissue,
  malignant
**Fibroma** (*see also* Neoplasm, connective tissue, benign)
ameloblastic — *see* Cyst, calcifying odontogenic
bone (nonossifying) — *see* Disorder, bone, specified
  type NEC
  ossifying — *see* Neoplasm, bone, benign
cementifying — *see* Neoplasm, bone, benign
chondromyxoid — *see* Neoplasm, bone, benign
desmoplastic — *see* Neoplasm, connective tissue,
  uncertain behavior
durum — *see* Neoplasm, connective tissue, benign
fascial — *see* Neoplasm, connective tissue, benign
invasive — *see* Neoplasm, connective tissue, uncertain
  behavior
molle — *see* Lipoma
myxoid — *see* Neoplasm, connective tissue, benign
nasopharynx, nasopharyngeal (juvenile) D10.6
nonosteogenic (nonossifying) — *see* Dysplasia, fibrous
odontogenic (central) — *see* Cyst, calcifying odontogenic
ossifying — *see* Neoplasm, bone, benign
periosteal — *see* Neoplasm, bone, benign
soft — *see* Lipoma
**Fibromatosis** M72.9
abdominal — *see* Neoplasm, connective tissue, uncertain behavior
aggressive — *see* Neoplasm, connective tissue, uncertain behavior
congenital generalized — *see* Neoplasm, connective
  tissue, uncertain behavior
Dupuytren's M72.0
gingival K06.1
palmar (fascial) M72.0
plantar (fascial) M72.2
pseudosarcomatous (proliferative) (subcutaneous)
  M72.4
retroperitoneal D48.3

**Fibromatosis** — *continued*
  specified NEC M72.8
**Fibromyalgia** M79.7
**Fibromyoma** (*see also* Neoplasm, connective tissue, benign)
  uterus (corpus) (*see also* Leiomyoma, uterus)
    in pregnancy or childbirth — *see* Fibroid, in pregnancy or childbirth
      causing obstructed labor O65.5
**Fibromyositis** M79.7
**Fibromyxolipoma** D17.9
**Fibromyxoma** — *see* Neoplasm, connective tissue, benign
**Fibromyxosarcoma** — *see* Neoplasm, connective tissue, malignant
**Fibro-odontoma, ameloblastic** — *see* Cyst, calcifying odontogenic
**Fibro-osteoma** — *see* Neoplasm, bone, benign
**Fibroplasia, retrolental** H35.17- ☑
**Fibropurulent** — *see* condition
**Fibrosarcoma** (*see also* Neoplasm, connective tissue, malignant)
  ameloblastic C41.1
    upper jaw (bone) C41.0
  congenital — *see* Neoplasm, connective tissue, malignant
  fascial — *see* Neoplasm, connective tissue, malignant
  infantile — *see* Neoplasm, connective tissue, malignant
  odontogenic C41.1
    upper jaw (bone) C41.0
  periosteal — *see* Neoplasm, bone, malignant
**Fibrosclerosis**
  breast N60.3- ☑
  multifocal M35.5
  penis (corpora cavernosa) N48.6
**Fibrosis, fibrotic**
  adrenal (gland) E27.8
  amnion O41.8X- ☑
  anal papillae K62.89
  arteriocapillary — *see* Arteriosclerosis
  bladder N32.89
    interstitial — *see* Cystitis, chronic, interstitial
    localized submucosal — *see* Cystitis, chronic, interstitial
    panmural — *see* Cystitis, chronic, interstitial
  breast — *see* Fibrosclerosis, breast
  capillary (*see also* Arteriosclerosis) I70.90
    lung (chronic) — *see* Fibrosis, lung
  cardiac — *see* Myocarditis
  cervix N88.8
  chorion O41.8X- ☑
  corpus cavernosum (sclerosing) N48.6
  cystic (of pancreas) E84.9
    with
      distal intestinal obstruction syndrome E84.19
      fecal impaction E84.19
      intestinal manifestations NEC E84.19
      pulmonary manifestations E84.0
      specified manifestations NEC E84.8
  due to device, implant or graft (*see also* Complications, by site and type, specified NEC) T85.828 ☑
    arterial graft NEC T82.828 ☑
    breast (implant) T85.828 ☑
    catheter NEC T85.828 ☑
      dialysis (renal) T82.828 ☑
        intraperitoneal T85.828 ☑
      infusion NEC T82.828 ☑
        spinal (epidural) (subdural) T85.820 ☑
      urinary (indwelling) T83.82 ☑
    electronic (electrode) (pulse generator) (stimulator)
      bone T84.82 ☑
      cardiac T82.827 ☑
      nervous system (brain) (peripheral nerve) (spinal) T85.820 ☑
      urinary T83.82 ☑
    fixation, internal (orthopedic) NEC T84.82 ☑
    gastrointestinal (bile duct) (esophagus) T85.828 ☑
    genital NEC T83.82 ☑
    heart NEC T82.827 ☑
    joint prosthesis T84.82 ☑
    ocular (corneal graft) (orbital implant) NEC T85.828 ☑
    orthopedic NEC T84.82 ☑
    specified NEC T85.828 ☑
    urinary NEC T83.82 ☑
    vascular NEC T82.828 ☑

**Fibrosis, fibrotic** — *continued*
  due to device, implant or graft (*see also* Complications, by site and type, specified) — *continued*
    ventricular intracranial shunt T85.820 ☑
  ejaculatory duct N50.89
  endocardium — *see* Endocarditis
  endomyocardial (tropical) I42.3
  epididymis N50.89
  eye muscle — *see* Strabismus, mechanical
  heart — *see* Myocarditis
  hepatic — *see* Fibrosis, liver
  hepatolienal (portal hypertension) K76.6
  hepatosplenic (portal hypertension) K76.6
  infrapatellar fat pad M79.4
  intrascrotal N50.89
  kidney N26.9
  liver K74.0
    with sclerosis K74.2
    alcoholic K70.2
  lung (atrophic) (chronic) (confluent) (massive) (perialveolar) (peribronchial) J84.10
    with
      anthracosilicosis J60
      anthracosis J60
      asbestosis J61
      bagassosis J67.1
      bauxite J63.1
      berylliosis J63.2
      byssinosis J66.0
      calcicosis J62.8
      chalicosis J62.8
      dust reticulation J64
      farmer's lung J67.0
      ganister disease J62.8
      graphite J63.3
      pneumoconiosis NOS J64
      siderosis J63.4
      silicosis J62.8
  capillary J84.10
  congenital P27.8
  diffuse (idiopathic) J84.10
    chemicals, gases, fumes or vapors (inhalation) J68.4
    interstitial J84.10
      acute J84.114
    talc J62.0
  following radiation J70.1
  idiopathic J84.112
  postinflammatory J84.10
  silicotic J62.8
  tuberculous — *see* Tuberculosis, pulmonary
  lymphatic gland I89.8
  median bar — *see* Hyperplasia, prostate
  mediastinum (idiopathic) J98.59
  meninges G96.19
  myocardium, myocardial — *see* Myocarditis
  ovary N83.8
  oviduct N83.8
  pancreas K86.89
  penis NEC N48.6
  pericardium I31.0
  perineum, in pregnancy or childbirth O34.7- ☑
    causing obstructed labor O65.5
  pleura J94.1
  popliteal fat pad M79.4
  prostate (chronic) — *see* Hyperplasia, prostate
  pulmonary (*see also* Fibrosis, lung) J84.10
    congenital P27.8
    idiopathic J84.112
  rectal sphincter K62.89
  retroperitoneal, idiopathic (with ureteral obstruction) N13.5
    with infection N13.6
  sclerosing mesenteric (idiopathic) K65.4
  scrotum N50.89
  seminal vesicle N50.89
  senile R54
  skin L90.5
  spermatic cord N50.89
  spleen D73.89
    in schistosomiasis (bilharziasis) B65.9 [D77]
  subepidermal nodular — *see* Neoplasm, skin, benign
  submucous (oral) (tongue) K13.5
  testis N44.8
    chronic, due to syphilis A52.76
  thymus (gland) E32.8
  tongue, submucous K13.5
  tunica vaginalis N50.89

**Fibrosis, fibrotic** — *continued*
  uterus (non-neoplastic) N85.8
  vagina N89.8
  valve, heart — *see* Endocarditis
  vas deferens N50.89
  vein I87.8
**Fibrositis** (periarticular) M79.7
  nodular, chronic (Jaccoud's) (rheumatoid) — *see* Arthropathy, postrheumatic, chronic
**Fibrothorax** J94.1
**Fibrotic** — *see* Fibrosis
**Fibrous** — *see* condition
**Fibroxanthoma** (*see also* Neoplasm, connective tissue, benign)
  atypical — *see* Neoplasm, connective tissue, uncertain behavior
  malignant — *see* Neoplasm, connective tissue, malignant
**Fibroxanthosarcoma** — *see* Neoplasm, connective tissue, malignant
**Fiedler's**
  disease (icterohemorrhagic leptospirosis) A27.0
  myocarditis (acute) I40.1
**Fifth disease** B08.3
  venereal A55
**Filaria, filarial, filariasis** — *see* Infestation, filarial
**Filatov's disease** — *see* Mononucleosis, infectious
**File-cutter's disease** — *see* Poisoning, lead
**Filling defect**
  biliary tract R93.2
  bladder R93.41
  duodenum R93.3
  gallbladder R93.2
  gastrointestinal tract R93.3
  intestine R93.3
  kidney R93.42- ☑
  stomach R93.3
  ureter R93.41
  urinary organs, specified NEC R93.49
**Fimbrial cyst** Q50.4
**Financial problem affecting care NOS** Z59.9
  bankruptcy Z59.8
  foreclosure on loan Z59.8
**Findings, abnormal, inconclusive, without diagnosis**
  (*see also* Abnormal)
  17-ketosteroids, elevated R82.5
  acetonuria R82.4
  alcohol in blood R78.0
  anisocytosis R71.8
  antenatal screening of mother O28.9
    biochemical O28.1
    chromosomal O28.5
    cytological O28.2
    genetic O28.5
    hematological O28.0
    radiological O28.4
    specified NEC O28.8
    ultrasonic O28.3
  antibody titer, elevated R76.0
  anticardiolipin antibody R76.0
  antiphosphatidylglycerol antibody R76.0
  antiphosphatidylinositol antibody R76.0
  antiphosphatidylserine antibody R76.0
  antiphospholipid antibody R76.0
  bacteriuria R82.71
  bicarbonate E87.8
  bile in urine R82.2
  blood sugar R73.09
    high R73.9
    low (transient) E16.2
  body fluid or substance, specified NEC R88.8
  casts, urine R82.99
  catecholamines R82.5
  cells, urine R82.99
  chloride E87.8
  cholesterol E78.9
    high E78.00
      with high triglycerides E78.2
  chyluria R82.0
  cloudy
    dialysis effluent R88.0
    urine R82.90
  creatinine clearance R94.4
  crystals, urine R82.99
  culture
    blood R78.81
    positive — *see* Positive, culture
  echocardiogram R93.1

**Findings, abnormal, inconclusive, without diagnosis**
— *continued*
- electrolyte level, urinary R82.99
- function study NEC R94.8
  - bladder R94.8
  - endocrine NEC R94.7
    - thyroid R94.6
  - kidney R94.4
  - liver R94.5
  - pancreas R94.8
  - placenta R94.8
  - pulmonary R94.2
  - spleen R94.8
- gallbladder, nonvisualization R93.2
- glucose (tolerance test) (non-fasting) R73.09
- glycosuria R81
- heart
  - shadow R93.1
  - sounds R01.2
- hematinuria R82.3
- hematocrit drop (precipitous) R71.0
- hemoglobinuria R82.3
- human papillomavirus (HPV) DNA test positive
  - cervix
    - high risk R87.810
    - low risk R87.820
  - vagina
    - high risk R87.811
    - low risk R87.821
- in blood (of substance not normally found in blood) R78.9
  - addictive drug NEC R78.4
  - alcohol (excessive level) R78.0
  - cocaine R78.2
  - hallucinogen R78.3
  - heavy metals (abnormal level) R78.79
  - lead R78.71
  - lithium (abnormal level) R78.89
  - opiate drug R78.1
  - psychotropic drug R78.5
  - specified substance NEC R78.89
  - steroid agent R78.6
- indoleacetic acid, elevated R82.5
- ketonuria R82.4
- lactic acid dehydrogenase (LDH) R74.0
- liver function test R79.89
- mammogram NEC R92.8
  - calcification (calculus) R92.1
  - inconclusive result (due to dense breasts) R92.2
  - microcalcification R92.0
- mediastinal shift R93.8
- melanin, urine R82.99
- myoglobinuria R82.1
- neonatal screening P09
- nonvisualization of gallbladder R93.2
- odor of urine NOS R82.90
- Papanicolaou cervix R87.619
  - non-atypical endometrial cells R87.618
- pneumoencephalogram R93.0
- poikilocytosis R71.8
- potassium (deficiency) E87.6
  - excess E87.5
- PPD R76.11
- radiologic (X-ray) R93.8
  - abdomen R93.5
  - biliary tract R93.2
  - breast R92.8
  - gastrointestinal tract R93.3
  - genitourinary organs R93.8
  - head R93.0
  - inconclusive due to excess body fat of patient R93.9
  - intrathoracic organs NEC R93.1
  - placenta R93.8
  - retroperitoneum R93.5
  - skin R93.8
  - skull R93.0
  - subcutaneous tissue R93.8
- red blood cell (count) (morphology) (sickling) (volume) R71.8
- scan NEC R94.8
  - bladder R94.8
  - bone R94.8
  - kidney R94.4
  - liver R93.2
  - lung R94.2
  - pancreas R94.8
  - placental R94.8
  - spleen R94.8
  - thyroid R94.6

**Findings, abnormal, inconclusive, without diagnosis**
— *continued*
- sedimentation rate, elevated R70.0
- SGOT R74.0
- SGPT R74.0
- sodium (deficiency) E87.1
  - excess E87.0
- specified body fluid NEC R88.8
- stress test R94.39
- thyroid (function) (metabolic rate) (scan) (uptake) R94.6
- transaminase (level) R74.0
- triglycerides E78.9
  - high E78.1
    - with high cholesterol E78.2
- tuberculin skin test (without active tuberculosis) R76.11
- urine R82.90
  - acetone R82.4
  - bacteria R82.71
  - bile R82.2
  - casts or cells R82.99
  - chyle R82.0
  - culture positive R82.79
  - glucose R81
  - hemoglobin R82.3
  - ketone R82.4
  - sugar R81
- vanillylmandelic acid (VMA), elevated R82.5
- vectorcardiogram (VCG) R94.39
- ventriculogram R93.0
- white blood cell (count) (differential) (morphology) D72.9
- xerography R92.8

**Finger** — *see* condition
**Fire, Saint Anthony's** — *see* Erysipelas
**Fire-setting**
- pathological (compulsive) F63.1
**Fish hook stomach** K31.89
**Fishmeal-worker's lung** J67.8
**Fissure, fissured**
- anus, anal K60.2
  - acute K60.0
  - chronic K60.1
  - congenital Q43.8
- ear, lobule, congenital Q17.8
- epiglottis (congenital) Q31.8
- larynx J38.7
  - congenital Q31.8
- lip K13.0
  - congenital — *see* Cleft, lip
- nipple N64.0
  - associated with
    - lactation O92.13
    - pregnancy O92.11- ☑
    - puerperium O92.12
- nose Q30.2
- palate (congenital) — *see* Cleft, palate
- skin R23.4
- spine (congenital) (*see also* Spina bifida)
  - with hydrocephalus — *see* Spina bifida, by site, with hydrocephalus
- tongue (acquired) K14.5
  - congenital Q38.3
**Fistula** (cutaneous) L98.8
- abdomen (wall) K63.2
  - bladder N32.2
  - intestine NEC K63.2
  - ureter N28.89
  - uterus N82.5
- abdominorectal K63.2
- abdominosigmoidal K63.2
- abdominothoracic J86.0
- abdominouterine N82.5
  - congenital Q51.7
- abdominovesical N32.2
- accessory sinuses — *see* Sinusitis
- actinomycotic — *see* Actinomycosis
- alveolar antrum — *see* Sinusitis, maxillary
- alveolar process K04.6
- anorectal K60.5
- antrobuccal — *see* Sinusitis, maxillary
- antrum — *see* Sinusitis, maxillary
- anus, anal (recurrent) (infectional) K60.3
  - congenital Q43.6
    - with absence, atresia and stenosis Q42.2
  - tuberculous A18.32
- aorta-duodenal I77.2

**Fistula** — *continued*
- appendix, appendicular K38.3
- arteriovenous (acquired) (nonruptured) I77.0
  - brain I67.1
    - congenital Q28.2
      - ruptured I60.8
    - ruptured I60.8
  - cerebral — *see* Fistula, arteriovenous, brain
  - congenital (peripheral) (*see also* Malformation, arteriovenous)
    - brain Q28.2
      - ruptured I60.8
    - coronary Q24.5
    - pulmonary Q25.72
  - coronary I25.41
    - congenital Q24.5
  - pulmonary I28.0
    - congenital Q25.72
  - surgically created (for dialysis) Z99.2
    - complication — *see* Complication, arteriovenous, fistula, surgically created
  - traumatic — *see* Injury, blood vessel
- artery I77.2
- aural (mastoid) — *see* Mastoiditis, chronic
- auricle (*see also* Disorder, pinna, specified type NEC)
  - congenital Q18.1
- Bartholin's gland N82.8
- bile duct (common) (hepatic) K83.3
  - with calculus, stones — *see* Calculus, bile duct
- biliary (tract) — *see* Fistula, bile duct
- bladder (sphincter) NEC (*see also* Fistula, vesico-) N32.2
  - into seminal vesicle N32.2
- bone (*see also* Disorder, bone, specified type NEC)
  - with osteomyelitis, chronic — *see* Osteomyelitis, chronic, with draining sinus
- brain G93.89
  - arteriovenous (acquired) I67.1
    - congenital Q28.2
- branchial (cleft) Q18.0
- branchiogenous Q18.0
- breast N61.0
  - puerperal, postpartum or gestational, due to mastitis (purulent) — *see* Mastitis, obstetric, purulent
- bronchial J86.0
- bronchocutaneous, bronchomediastinal, bronchopleural, bronchopleuromediastinal (infective) J86.0
  - tuberculous NEC A15.5
- bronchoesophageal J86.0
  - congenital Q39.2
    - with atresia of esophagus Q39.1
- bronchovisceral J86.0
- buccal cavity (infective) K12.2
- cecosigmoidal K63.2
- cecum K63.2
- cerebrospinal (fluid) G96.0
- cervical, lateral Q18.1
- cervicoaural Q18.1
- cervicosigmoidal N82.4
- cervicovesical N82.1
- cervix N82.8
- chest (wall) J86.0
- cholecystenteric — *see* Fistula, gallbladder
- cholecystocolic — *see* Fistula, gallbladder
- cholecystocolonic — *see* Fistula, gallbladder
- cholecystoduodenal — *see* Fistula, gallbladder
- cholecystogastric — *see* Fistula, gallbladder
- cholecystointestinal — *see* Fistula, gallbladder
- choledochoduodenal — *see* Fistula, bile duct
- cholocolic K82.3
- coccyx — *see* Sinus, pilonidal
- colon K63.2
- colostomy K94.09
- common duct — *see* Fistula, bile duct
- congenital, site not listed — *see* Anomaly, by site
- coronary, arteriovenous I25.41
  - congenital Q24.5
- costal region J86.0
- cul-de-sac, Douglas' N82.8
- cystic duct (*see also* Fistula, gallbladder)
  - congenital Q44.5
- dental K04.6
- diaphragm J86.0
- duodenum K31.6
- ear (external) (canal) — *see* Disorder, ear, external, specified type NEC
- enterocolic K63.2
- enterocutaneous K63.2

☑ **Additional Character Required** — Refer to the Tabular List for Character Selection       ▽ Subterms under main terms may continue to next column or page

**Fistula** — *continued*
  enterouterine N82.4
    congenital Q51.7
  enterovaginal N82.4
    congenital Q52.2
    large intestine N82.3
    small intestine N82.2
  enterovesical N32.1
  epididymis N50.89
    tuberculous A18.15
  esophagobronchial J86.0
    congenital Q39.2
      with atresia of esophagus Q39.1
  esophagocutaneous K22.8
  esophagopleural-cutaneous J86.0
  esophagotracheal J86.0
    congenital Q39.2
      with atresia of esophagus Q39.1
  esophagus K22.8
    congenital Q39.2
      with atresia of esophagus Q39.1
  ethmoid — *see* Sinusitis, ethmoidal
  eyeball (cornea) (sclera) — *see* Disorder, globe, hypotony
  eyelid H01.8
  fallopian tube, external N82.5
  fecal K63.2
    congenital Q43.6
  from periapical abscess K04.6
  frontal sinus — *see* Sinusitis, frontal
  gallbladder K82.3
    with calculus, cholelithiasis, stones — *see* Calculus, gallbladder
  gastric K31.6
  gastrocolic K31.6
    congenital Q40.2
    tuberculous A18.32
  gastroenterocolic K31.6
  gastroesophageal K31.6
  gastrojejunal K31.6
  gastrojejunocolic K31.6
  genital tract (female) N82.9
    specified NEC N82.8
    to intestine NEC N82.4
    to skin N82.5
  hepatic artery-portal vein, congenital Q26.6
  hepatopleural J86.0
  hepatopulmonary J86.0
  ileorectal or ileosigmoidal K63.2
  ileovaginal N82.2
  ileovesical N32.1
  ileum K63.2
  in ano K60.3
    tuberculous A18.32
  inner ear (labyrinth) — *see* subcategory H83.1 ☑
  intestine NEC K63.2
  intestinocolonic (abdominal) K63.2
  intestinoureteral N28.89
  intestinouterine N82.4
  intestinovaginal N82.4
    large intestine N82.3
    small intestine N82.2
  intestinovesical N32.1
  ischiorectal (fossa) K61.3
  jejunum K63.2
  joint M25.10
    ankle M25.17- ☑
    elbow M25.12- ☑
    foot joint M25.17- ☑
    hand joint M25.14- ☑
    hip M25.15- ☑
    knee M25.16- ☑
    shoulder M25.11- ☑
    specified joint NEC M25.18
    tuberculous — *see* Tuberculosis, joint
    vertebrae M25.18
    wrist M25.13- ☑
  kidney N28.89
  labium (majus) (minus) N82.8
  labyrinth — *see* subcategory H83.1 ☑
  lacrimal (gland) (sac) H04.61-
  lacrimonasal duct — *see* Fistula, lacrimal
  laryngotracheal, congenital Q34.8
  larynx J38.7
  lip K13.0
    congenital Q38.0
  lumbar, tuberculous A18.01
  lung J86.0

**Fistula** — *continued*
  lymphatic I89.8
  mammary (gland) N61.0
  mastoid (process) (region) — *see* Mastoiditis, chronic
  maxillary J32.0
  medial, face and neck Q18.8
  mediastinal J86.0
  mediastinobronchial J86.0
  mediastinocutaneous J86.0
  middle ear — *see* subcategory H74.8 ☑
  mouth K12.2
  nasal J34.89
    sinus — *see* Sinusitis
  nasopharynx J39.2
  nipple N64.0
  nose J34.89
  oral (cutaneous) K12.2
    maxillary J32.0
    nasal (with cleft palate) — *see* Cleft, palate
  orbit, orbital — *see* Disorder, orbit, specified type NEC
  oroantral J32.0
  oviduct, external N82.5
  palate (hard) M27.8
  pancreatic K86.89
  pancreaticoduodenal K86.89
  parotid (gland) K11.4
    region K12.2
  penis N48.89
  perianal K60.3
  pericardium (pleura) (sac) — *see* Pericarditis
  pericecal K63.2
  perineorectal K60.4
  perineosigmoidal K63.2
  perineum, perineal (with urethral involvement) NEC N36.0
    tuberculous A18.13
    ureter N28.89
  perirectal K60.4
    tuberculous A18.32
  peritoneum K65.9
  pharyngoesophageal J39.2
  pharynx J39.2
    branchial cleft (congenital) Q18.0
  pilonidal (infected) (rectum) — *see* Sinus, pilonidal
  pleura, pleural, pleurocutaneous, pleuroperitoneal J86.0
    tuberculous NEC A15.6
  pleuropericardial I31.8
  portal vein-hepatic artery, congenital Q26.6
  postauricular H70.81- ☑
  postoperative, persistent T81.83 ☑
    specified site — *see* Fistula, by site
  preauricular (congenital) Q18.1
  prostate N42.89
  pulmonary J86.0
    arteriovenous I28.0
      congenital Q25.72
    tuberculous — *see* Tuberculosis, pulmonary
  pulmonoperitoneal J86.0
  rectolabial N82.4
  rectosigmoid (intercommunicating) K63.2
  rectoureteral N28.89
  rectourethral N36.0
    congenital Q64.73
  rectouterine N82.4
    congenital Q51.7
  rectovaginal N82.3
    congenital Q52.2
    tuberculous A18.18
  rectovesical N32.1
    congenital Q64.79
  rectovesicovaginal N82.3
  rectovulval N82.4
    congenital Q52.79
  rectum (to skin) K60.4
    congenital Q43.6
      with absence, atresia and stenosis Q42.0
    tuberculous A18.32
  renal N28.89
  retroauricular — *see* Fistula, postauricular
  salivary duct or gland (any) K11.4
    congenital Q38.4
  scrotum (urinary) N50.89
    tuberculous A18.15
  semicircular canals — *see* subcategory H83.1 ☑
  sigmoid K63.2
    to bladder N32.1
  sinus — *see* Sinusitis

**Fistula** — *continued*
  skin L98.8
    to genital tract (female) N82.5
  splenocolic D73.89
  stercoral K63.2
  stomach K31.6
  sublingual gland K11.4
  submandibular gland K11.4
  submaxillary (gland) K11.4
    region K12.2
  thoracic J86.0
    duct I89.8
  thoracoabdominal J86.0
  thoracogastric J86.0
  thoracointestinal J86.0
  thorax J86.0
  thyroglossal duct Q89.2
  thyroid E07.89
  trachea, congenital (external) (internal) Q32.1
  tracheoesophageal J86.0
    congenital Q39.2
      with atresia of esophagus Q39.1
    following tracheostomy J95.04
  traumatic arteriovenous — *see* Injury, blood vessel, by site
  tuberculous — *code by* site under Tuberculosis
  typhoid A01.09
  umbilicourinary Q64.8
  urachus, congenital Q64.4
  ureter (persistent) N28.89
  ureteroabdominal N28.89
  ureterorectal N28.89
  ureterosigmoido-abdominal N28.89
  ureterovaginal N82.1
  ureterovesical N32.2
  urethra N36.0
    congenital Q64.79
    tuberculous A18.13
  urethroperineal N36.0
  urethroperineovesical N32.2
  urethrorectal N36.0
    congenital Q64.73
  urethroscrotal N50.89
  urethrovaginal N82.1
  urethrovesical N32.2
  urinary (tract) (persistent) (recurrent) N36.0
  uteroabdominal N82.5
    congenital Q51.7
  uteroenteric, uterointestinal N82.4
    congenital Q51.7
  uterorectal N82.4
    congenital Q51.7
  uteroureteric N82.1
  uterourethral Q51.7
  uterovaginal N82.8
  uterovesical N82.1
    congenital Q51.7
  uterus N82.8
  vagina (postpartal) (wall) N82.8
  vaginocutaneous (postpartal) N82.5
  vaginointestinal NEC N82.4
    large intestine N82.3
    small intestine N82.2
  vaginoperineal N82.5
  vasocutaneous, congenital Q55.7
  vesical NEC N32.2
  vesicoabdominal N32.2
  vesicocervicovaginal N82.1
  vesicocolic N32.1
  vesicocutaneous N32.2
  vesicoenteric N32.1
  vesicointestinal N32.1
  vesicometrorectal N82.4
  vesicoperineal N32.2
  vesicorectal N32.1
    congenital Q64.79
  vesicosigmoidal N32.1
  vesicosigmoidovaginal N82.3
  vesicoureteral N32.2
  vesicoureterovaginal N82.1
  vesicourethral N32.2
  vesicourethrorectal N32.1
  vesicouterine N82.1
    congenital Q51.7
  vesicovaginal N82.0
  vulvorectal N82.4
    congenital Q52.79
**Fit** R56.9
  epileptic — *see* Epilepsy

**Fit** — *continued*
fainting R55
hysterical F44.5
newborn P90
**Fitting** (and adjustment) (of)
artificial
arm — *see* Admission, adjustment, artificial, arm
breast Z44.3 ☑
eye Z44.2 ☑
leg — *see* Admission, adjustment, artificial, leg
automatic implantable cardiac defibrillator (with synchronous cardiac pacemaker) Z45.02
brain neuropacemaker Z46.2
implanted Z45.42
cardiac defibrillator — *see* Fitting (and adjustment) (of), automatic implantable cardiac defibrillator
catheter, non-vascular Z46.82
colostomy belt Z46.89
contact lenses Z46.0
CRT-D (resynchronization therapy defibrillator) Z45.02
CRT-P (cardiac resynchronization therapy pacemaker) Z45.018
pulse generator Z45.010
cystostomy device Z46.6
defibrillator, cardiac — *see* Fitting (and adjustment) (of), automatic implantable cardiac defibrillator
dentures Z46.3
device NOS Z46.9
abdominal Z46.89
gastrointestinal NEC Z46.59
implanted NEC Z45.89
nervous system Z46.2
implanted — *see* Admission, adjustment, device, implanted, nervous system
orthodontic Z46.4
orthoptic Z46.0
orthotic Z46.89
prosthetic (external) Z44.9
breast Z44.3 ☑
dental Z46.3
eye Z44.2 ☑
specified NEC Z44.8
specified NEC Z46.89
substitution
auditory Z46.2
implanted — *see* Admission, adjustment, device, implanted, hearing device
nervous system Z46.2
implanted — *see* Admission, adjustment, device, implanted, nervous system
visual Z46.2
implanted Z45.31
urinary Z46.6
gastric lap band Z46.51
gastrointestinal appliance NEC Z46.59
glasses (reading) Z46.0
hearing aid Z46.1
ileostomy device Z46.89
insulin pump Z46.81
intestinal appliance NEC Z46.89
myringotomy device (stent) (tube) Z45.82
neuropacemaker Z46.2
implanted Z45.42
non-vascular catheter Z46.82
orthodontic device Z46.4
orthopedic device (brace) (cast) (corset) (shoes) Z46.89
pacemaker (cardiac) (cardiac resynchronization therapy (CRT-P)) Z45.018
nervous system (brain) (peripheral nerve) (spinal cord) Z46.2
implanted Z45.42
pulse generator Z45.010
portacath (port-a-cath) Z45.2
prosthesis (external) Z44.9
arm — *see* Admission, adjustment, artificial, arm
breast Z44.3 ☑
dental Z46.3
eye Z44.2 ☑
leg — *see* Admission, adjustment, artificial, leg
specified NEC Z44.8
spectacles Z46.0
wheelchair Z46.89
**Fitzhugh-Curtis syndrome**
due to
Chlamydia trachomatis A74.81
Neisseria gonorrhorea (gonococcal peritonitis) A54.85

**Fitz's syndrome** (acute hemorrhagic pancreatitis) (*see also* Pancreatitis, acute) K85.80
**Fixation**
joint — *see* Ankylosis
larynx J38.7
stapes — *see* Ankylosis, ear ossicles
deafness — *see* Deafness, conductive
uterus (acquired) — *see* Malposition, uterus
vocal cord J38.3
**Flabby ridge** K06.8
**Flaccid** (*see also* condition)
palate, congenital Q38.5
**Flail**
chest S22.5 ☑
newborn (birth injury) P13.8
joint (paralytic) M25.20
ankle M25.27- ☑
elbow M25.22- ☑
foot joint M25.27- ☑
hand joint M25.24- ☑
hip M25.25- ☑
knee M25.26- ☑
shoulder M25.21- ☑
specified joint NEC M25.28
wrist M25.23- ☑
**Flajani's disease** — *see* Hyperthyroidism, with, goiter (diffuse)
**Flap, liver** K71.3
**Flashbacks** (residual to hallucinogen use) F16.283
**Flat**
chamber (eye) — *see* Disorder, globe, hypotony, flat anterior chamber
chest, congenital Q67.8
foot (acquired) (fixed type) (painful) (postural) (*see also* Deformity, limb, flat foot)
congenital (rigid) (spastic) (everted) Q66.5- ☑
rachitic sequelae (late effect) E64.3
organ or site, congenital NEC — *see* Anomaly, by site
pelvis M95.5
with disproportion (fetopelvic) O33.0
causing obstructed labor O65.0
congenital Q74.2
**Flatau-Schilder disease** G37.0
**Flatback syndrome** M40.30
lumbar region M40.36
lumbosacral region M40.37
thoracolumbar region M40.35
**Flattening**
head, femur M89.8X5
hip — *see* Coxa, plana
lip (congenital) Q18.8
nose (congenital) Q67.4
acquired M95.0
**Flatulence** R14.3
psychogenic F45.8
**Flatus** R14.3
vaginalis N89.8
**Flax-dresser's disease** J66.1
**Flea bite** — *see* Injury, bite, by site, superficial, insect
**Flecks, glaucomatous** (subcapsular) — *see* Cataract, complicated
**Fleischer** (-Kayser) **ring** (cornea) H18.04- ☑
**Fleshy mole** O02.0
**Flexibilitas cerea** — *see* Catalepsy
**Flexion**
amputation stump (surgical) T87.89
cervix — *see* Malposition, uterus
contracture, joint — *see* Contraction, joint
deformity, joint (*see also* Deformity, limb, flexion) M21.20
hip, congenital Q65.89
uterus (*see also* Malposition, uterus)
lateral — *see* Lateroversion, uterus
**Flexner-Boyd dysentery** A03.2
**Flexner's dysentery** A03.1
**Flexure** — *see* Flexion
**Flint murmur** (aortic insufficiency) I35.1
**Floater, vitreous** — *see* Opacity, vitreous
**Floating**
cartilage (joint) (*see also* Loose, body, joint)
knee — *see* Derangement, knee, loose body
gallbladder, congenital Q44.1
kidney N28.89
congenital Q63.8
spleen D73.89
**Flooding** N92.0
**Floor** — *see* condition

**Floppy**
baby syndrome (nonspecific) P94.2
iris syndrome (intraoperative) (IFIS) H21.81
nonrheumatic mitral valve syndrome I34.1
**Flu** (*see also* Influenza)
avian (*see also* Influenza, due to, identified novel influenza A virus) J09.X2
bird (*see also* Influenza, due to, identified novel influenza A virus) J09.X2
intestinal NEC A08.4
swine (viruses that normally cause infections in pigs) (*see also* Influenza, due to, identified novel influenza A virus) J09.X2
**Fluctuating blood pressure** I99.8
**Fluid**
abdomen R18.8
chest J94.8
heart — *see* Failure, heart, congestive
joint — *see* Effusion, joint
loss (acute) E86.9
lung — *see* Edema, lung
overload E87.70
specified NEC E87.79
peritoneal cavity R18.8
pleural cavity J94.8
retention R60.9
**Flukes NEC** (*see also* Infestation, fluke)
blood NEC — *see* Schistosomiasis
liver B66.3
**Fluor** (vaginalis) N89.8
trichomonal or due to Trichomonas (vaginalis) A59.00
**Fluorosis**
dental K00.3
skeletal M85.10
ankle M85.17- ☑
foot M85.17- ☑
forearm M85.13- ☑
hand M85.14- ☑
lower leg M85.16- ☑
multiple site M85.19
neck M85.18
rib M85.18
shoulder M85.11- ☑
skull M85.18
specified site NEC M85.18
thigh M85.15- ☑
toe M85.17- ☑
upper arm M85.12- ☑
vertebra M85.18
**Flush syndrome** E34.0
**Flushing** R23.2
menopausal N95.1
**Flutter**
atrial or auricular I48.92
atypical I48.4
type I I48.3
type II I48.4
typical I48.3
heart I49.8
atrial or auricular I48.92
atypical I48.4
type I I48.3
type II I48.4
typical I48.3
ventricular I49.02
ventricular I49.02
**FNHTR** (febrile nonhemolytic transfusion reaction) R50.84
**Fochier's abscess** — *code by* site under Abscess
**Focus, Assmann's** — *see* Tuberculosis, pulmonary
**Fogo selvagem** L10.3
**Foix-Alajouanine syndrome** G95.19
**Fold, folds** (anomalous) (*see also* Anomaly, by site)
Descemet's membrane — *see* Change, corneal membrane, Descemet's, fold
epicanthic Q10.3
heart Q24.8
**Folie à deux** F24
**Follicle**
cervix (nabothian) (ruptured) N88.8
graafian, ruptured, with hemorrhage N83.0- ☑
nabothian N88.8
**Follicular** — *see* condition
**Folliculitis** (superficial) L73.9
abscedens et suffodiens L66.3
cyst N83.0- ☑
decalvans L66.2
deep — *see* Furuncle, by site

☑ **Additional Character Required** — **Refer to the Tabular List for Character Selection**      ▽ **Subterms under main terms may continue to next column or page**

**Folliculitis** — *continued*
    gonococcal (acute) (chronic) A54.01
    keloid, keloidalis L73.0
    pustular L01.02
    ulerythematosa reticulata L66.4
**Folliculome lipidique**
    specified site — *see* Neoplasm, benign, by site
    unspecified site
        female D27.9
        male D29.20
**Følling's disease** E70.0
**Follow-up** — *see* Examination, follow-up
**Fong's syndrome** (hereditary osteo-onychodysplasia) Q87.2
**Food**
    allergy L27.2
    asphyxia (from aspiration or inhalation) — *see* Foreign body, by site
    choked on — *see* Foreign body, by site
    deprivation T73.0 ☑
        specified kind of food NEC E63.8
    intoxication — *see* Poisoning, food
    lack of T73.0 ☑
    poisoning — *see* Poisoning, food
    rejection NEC — *see* Disorder, eating
    strangulation or suffocation — *see* Foreign body, by site
    toxemia — *see* Poisoning, food
**Foot** — *see* condition
**Foramen ovale** (nonclosure) (patent) (persistent) Q21.1
**Forbes' glycogen storage disease** E74.03
**Fordyce-Fox disease** L75.2
**Fordyce's disease** (mouth) Q38.6
**Forearm** — *see* condition
**Foreign body**
    with
        laceration — *see* Laceration, by site, with foreign body
        puncture wound — *see* Puncture, by site, with foreign body
    accidentally left following a procedure T81.509 ☑
        aspiration T81.506 ☑
            resulting in
                adhesions T81.516 ☑
                obstruction T81.526 ☑
                perforation T81.536 ☑
                specified complication NEC T81.596 ☑
        cardiac catheterization T81.505 ☑
            resulting in
                acute reaction T81.60 ☑
                    aseptic peritonitis T81.61 ☑
                    specified NEC T81.69 ☑
                adhesions T81.515 ☑
                obstruction T81.525 ☑
                perforation T81.535 ☑
                specified complication NEC T81.595 ☑
        causing
            acute reaction T81.60 ☑
                aseptic peritonitis T81.61 ☑
                specified complication NEC T81.69 ☑
            adhesions T81.519 ☑
            aseptic peritonitis T81.61 ☑
            obstruction T81.529 ☑
            perforation T81.539 ☑
            specified complication NEC T81.599 ☑
        endoscopy T81.504 ☑
            resulting in
                adhesions T81.514 ☑
                obstruction T81.524 ☑
                perforation T81.534 ☑
                specified complication NEC T81.594 ☑
        immunization T81.503 ☑
            resulting in
                adhesions T81.513 ☑
                obstruction T81.523 ☑
                perforation T81.533 ☑
                specified complication NEC T81.593 ☑
        infusion T81.501 ☑
            resulting in
                adhesions T81.511 ☑
                obstruction T81.521 ☑
                perforation T81.531 ☑
                specified complication NEC T81.591 ☑
        injection T81.503 ☑
            resulting in
                adhesions T81.513 ☑

**Foreign body** — *continued*
    accidentally left following a procedure — *continued*
        injection — *continued*
            resulting in — *continued*
                obstruction T81.523 ☑
                perforation T81.533 ☑
                specified complication NEC T81.593 ☑
        kidney dialysis T81.502 ☑
            resulting in
                adhesions T81.512 ☑
                obstruction T81.522 ☑
                perforation T81.532 ☑
                specified complication NEC T81.592 ☑
        packing removal T81.507 ☑
            resulting in
                acute reaction T81.60 ☑
                    aseptic peritonitis T81.61 ☑
                    specified NEC T81.69 ☑
                adhesions T81.517 ☑
                obstruction T81.527 ☑
                perforation T81.537 ☑
                specified complication NEC T81.597 ☑
        puncture T81.506 ☑
            resulting in
                adhesions T81.516 ☑
                obstruction T81.526 ☑
                perforation T81.536 ☑
                specified complication NEC T81.596 ☑
        specified procedure NEC T81.508 ☑
            resulting in
                acute reaction T81.60 ☑
                    aseptic peritonitis T81.61 ☑
                    specified NEC T81.69 ☑
                adhesions T81.518 ☑
                obstruction T81.528 ☑
                perforation T81.538 ☑
                specified complication NEC T81.598 ☑
        surgical operation T81.500 ☑
            resulting in
                acute reaction T81.60 ☑
                    aseptic peritonitis T81.61 ☑
                    specified NEC T81.69 ☑
                adhesions T81.510 ☑
                obstruction T81.520 ☑
                perforation T81.530 ☑
                specified complication NEC T81.590 ☑
        transfusion T81.501 ☑
            resulting in
                adhesions T81.511 ☑
                obstruction T81.521 ☑
                perforation T81.531 ☑
                specified complication NEC T81.591 ☑
    alimentary tract T18.9 ☑
        anus T18.5 ☑
        colon T18.4 ☑
        esophagus — *see* Foreign body, esophagus
        mouth T18.0 ☑
        multiple sites T18.8 ☑
        rectosigmoid (junction) T18.5 ☑
        rectum T18.5 ☑
        small intestine T18.3 ☑
        specified site NEC T18.8 ☑
        stomach T18.2 ☑
    anterior chamber (eye) S05.5- ☑
    auditory canal — *see* Foreign body, entering through orifice, ear
    bronchus T17.508 ☑
        causing
            asphyxiation T17.500 ☑
                food (bone) (seed) T17.520 ☑
                gastric contents (vomitus) T17.510 ☑
                specified type NEC T17.590 ☑
            injury NEC T17.508 ☑
                food (bone) (seed) T17.528 ☑
                gastric contents (vomitus) T17.518 ☑
                specified type NEC T17.598 ☑
    canthus — *see* Foreign body, conjunctival sac
    ciliary body (eye) S05.5- ☑
    conjunctival sac T15.1- ☑
    cornea T15.0- ☑
    entering through orifice
        accessory sinus T17.0 ☑
        alimentary canal T18.9 ☑
            multiple parts T18.8 ☑
            specified part NEC T18.8 ☑

**Foreign body** — *continued*
    entering through orifice — *continued*
        alveolar process T18.0 ☑
        antrum (Highmore's) T17.0 ☑
        anus T18.5 ☑
        appendix T18.4 ☑
        auditory canal — *see* Foreign body, entering through orifice, ear
        auricle — *see* Foreign body, entering through orifice, ear
        bladder T19.1 ☑
        bronchioles — *see* Foreign body, respiratory tract, specified site NEC
        bronchus (main) — *see* Foreign body, bronchus
        buccal cavity T18.0 ☑
        canthus (inner) — *see* Foreign body, conjunctival sac
        cecum T18.4 ☑
        cervix (canal) (uteri) T19.3 ☑
        colon T18.4 ☑
        conjunctival sac — *see* Foreign body, conjunctival sac
        cornea — *see* Foreign body, cornea
        digestive organ or tract NOS T18.9 ☑
            multiple parts T18.8 ☑
            specified part NEC T18.8 ☑
        duodenum T18.3 ☑
        ear (external) T16.- ☑
        esophagus — *see* Foreign body, esophagus
        eye (external) NOS T15.9- ☑
            conjunctival sac — *see* Foreign body, conjunctival sac
            cornea — *see* Foreign body, cornea
            specified part NEC T15.8- ☑
        eyeball (*see also* Foreign body, entering through orifice, eye, specified part NEC)
            with penetrating wound — *see* Puncture, eyeball
        eyelid (*see also* Foreign body, conjunctival sac)
            with
                laceration — *see* Laceration, eyelid, with foreign body
                puncture — *see* Puncture, eyelid, with foreign body
                superficial injury — *see* Foreign body, superficial, eyelid
        gastrointestinal tract T18.9 ☑
            multiple parts T18.8 ☑
            specified part NEC T18.8 ☑
        genitourinary tract T19.9 ☑
            multiple parts T19.8 ☑
            specified part NEC T19.8 ☑
        globe — *see* Foreign body, entering through orifice, eyeball
        gum T18.0 ☑
        Highmore's antrum T17.0 ☑
        hypopharynx — *see* Foreign body, pharynx
        ileum T18.3 ☑
        intestine (small) T18.3 ☑
            large T18.4 ☑
        lacrimal apparatus (punctum) — *see* Foreign body, entering through orifice, eye, specified part NEC
        large intestine T18.4 ☑
        larynx — *see* Foreign body, larynx
        lung — *see* Foreign body, respiratory tract, specified site NEC
        maxillary sinus T17.0 ☑
        mouth T18.0 ☑
        nasal sinus T17.0 ☑
        nasopharynx — *see* Foreign body, pharynx
        nose (passage) T17.1 ☑
        nostril T17.1 ☑
        oral cavity T18.0 ☑
        palate T18.0 ☑
        penis T19.4 ☑
        pharynx — *see* Foreign body, pharynx
        piriform sinus — *see* Foreign body, pharynx
        rectosigmoid (junction) T18.5 ☑
        rectum T18.5 ☑
        respiratory tract — *see* Foreign body, respiratory tract
        sinus (accessory) (frontal) (maxillary) (nasal) T17.0 ☑
            piriform — *see* Foreign body, pharynx
        small intestine T18.3 ☑

**Foreign body** — *continued*
  entering through orifice — *continued*
    stomach T18.2 ☑
    suffocation by — *see* Foreign body, by site
    tear ducts or glands — *see* Foreign body, entering
      through orifice, eye, specified part NEC
    throat — *see* Foreign body, pharynx
    tongue T18.0 ☑
    tonsil, tonsillar (fossa) — *see* Foreign body, pharynx
    trachea — *see* Foreign body, trachea
    ureter T19.8 ☑
    urethra T19.0 ☑
    uterus (any part) T19.3 ☑
    vagina T19.2 ☑
    vulva T19.2 ☑
  esophagus T18.108 ☑
    causing
      injury NEC T18.108 ☑
        food (bone) (seed) T18.128 ☑
        gastric contents (vomitus) T18.118 ☑
        specified type NEC T18.198 ☑
      tracheal compression T18.100 ☑
        food (bone) (seed) T18.120 ☑
        gastric contents (vomitus) T18.110 ☑
        specified type NEC T18.190 ☑
  feeling of, in throat R09.89
  fragment — *see* Retained, foreign body fragments
    (type of)
  genitourinary tract T19.9 ☑
    bladder T19.1 ☑
    multiple parts T19.8 ☑
    penis T19.4 ☑
    specified site NEC T19.8 ☑
    urethra T19.0 ☑
    uterus T19.3 ☑
      IUD Z97.5
    vagina T19.2 ☑
      contraceptive device Z97.5
    vulva T19.2 ☑
  granuloma (old) (soft tissue) (*see also* Granuloma,
    foreign body)
    skin L92.3
  in
    laceration — *see* Laceration, by site, with foreign
      body
    puncture wound — *see* Puncture, by site, with
      foreign body
    soft tissue (residual) M79.5
  inadvertently left in operation wound — *see* Foreign
    body, accidentally left during a procedure
  ingestion, ingested NOS T18.9 ☑
  inhalation or inspiration — *see* Foreign body, by site
  internal organ, not entering through a natural orifice
    — code as specific injury with foreign body
  intraocular S05.5- ☑
    old, retained (nonmagnetic) H44.70- ☑
      anterior chamber H44.71- ☑
      ciliary body H44.72- ☑
      iris H44.72- ☑
      lens H44.73- ☑
      magnetic H44.60- ☑
        anterior chamber H44.61- ☑
        ciliary body H44.62- ☑
        iris H44.62- ☑
        lens H44.63- ☑
        posterior wall H44.64- ☑
        specified site NEC H44.69- ☑
        vitreous body H44.65- ☑
      posterior wall H44.74- ☑
      specified site NEC H44.79- ☑
      vitreous body H44.75- ☑
  iris — *see* Foreign body, intraocular
  lacrimal punctum — *see* Foreign body, entering
    through orifice, eye, specified part NEC
  larynx T17.308 ☑
    causing
      asphyxiation T17.300 ☑
        food (bone) (seed) T17.320 ☑
        gastric contents (vomitus) T17.310 ☑
        specified type NEC T17.390 ☑
      injury NEC T17.308 ☑
        food (bone) (seed) T17.328 ☑
        gastric contents (vomitus) T17.318 ☑
        specified type NEC T17.398 ☑
  lens — *see* Foreign body, intraocular
  ocular muscle S05.4- ☑

**Foreign body** — *continued*
  ocular muscle — *continued*
    old, retained — *see* Foreign body, orbit, old
  old or residual
    soft tissue (residual) M79.5
  operation wound, left accidentally — *see* Foreign
    body, accidentally left during a procedure
  orbit S05.4- ☑
    old, retained H05.5- ☑
  pharynx T17.208 ☑
    causing
      asphyxiation T17.200 ☑
        food (bone) (seed) T17.220 ☑
        gastric contents (vomitus) T17.210 ☑
        specified type NEC T17.290 ☑
      injury NEC T17.208 ☑
        food (bone) (seed) T17.228 ☑
        gastric contents (vomitus) T17.218 ☑
        specified type NEC T17.298 ☑
  respiratory tract T17.908 ☑
    bronchioles — *see* Foreign body, respiratory tract,
      specified site NEC
    bronchus — *see* Foreign body, bronchus
    causing
      asphyxiation T17.900 ☑
        food (bone) (seed) T17.920 ☑
        gastric contents (vomitus) T17.910 ☑
        specified type NEC T17.990 ☑
      injury NEC T17.908 ☑
        food (bone) (seed) T17.928 ☑
        gastric contents (vomitus) T17.918 ☑
        specified type NEC T17.998 ☑
    larynx — *see* Foreign body, larynx
    lung — *see* Foreign body, respiratory tract, speci-
      fied site NEC
    multiple parts — *see* Foreign body, respiratory
      tract, specified site NEC
    nasal sinus T17.0 ☑
    nasopharynx — *see* Foreign body, pharynx
    nose T17.1 ☑
    nostril T17.1 ☑
    pharynx — *see* Foreign body, pharynx
    specified site NEC T17.808 ☑
      causing
        asphyxiation T17.800 ☑
          food (bone) (seed) T17.820 ☑
          gastric contents (vomitus) T17.810 ☑
          specified type NEC T17.890 ☑
        injury NEC T17.808 ☑
          food (bone) (seed) T17.828 ☑
          gastric contents (vomitus) T17.818 ☑
          specified type NEC T17.898 ☑
    throat — *see* Foreign body, pharynx
    trachea — *see* Foreign body, trachea
  retained (old) (nonmagnetic) (in)
    anterior chamber (eye) — *see* Foreign body, intraoc-
      ular, old, retained, anterior chamber
      magnetic — *see* Foreign body, intraocular, old,
        retained, magnetic, anterior chamber
    ciliary body — *see* Foreign body, intraocular, old,
      retained, ciliary body
      magnetic — *see* Foreign body, intraocular, old,
        retained, magnetic, ciliary body
    eyelid H02.819
      left H02.816
        lower H02.815
        upper H02.814
      right H02.813
        lower H02.812
        upper H02.811
    fragments — *see* Retained, foreign body fragments
      (type of)
    globe — *see* Foreign body, intraocular, old, re-
      tained
      magnetic — *see* Foreign body, intraocular, old,
        retained, magnetic
    intraocular — *see* Foreign body, intraocular, old,
      retained
      magnetic — *see* Foreign body, intraocular, old,
        retained, magnetic
    iris — *see* Foreign body, intraocular, old, retained,
      iris
      magnetic — *see* Foreign body, intraocular, old,
        retained, magnetic, iris
    lens — *see* Foreign body, intraocular, old, retained,
      lens

**Foreign body** — *continued*
  retained — *continued*
    lens — *see* Foreign body, intraocular, old, retained,
      lens — *continued*
        magnetic — *see* Foreign body, intraocular, old,
          retained, magnetic, lens
    muscle — *see* Foreign body, retained, soft tissue
    orbit — *see* Foreign body, orbit, old
    posterior wall of globe — *see* Foreign body, intraoc-
      ular, old, retained, posterior wall
      magnetic — *see* Foreign body, intraocular, old,
        retained, magnetic, posterior wall
    retrobulbar — *see* Foreign body, orbit, old,
      retrobulbar
    soft tissue M79.5
    vitreous — *see* Foreign body, intraocular, old, re-
      tained, vitreous body
      magnetic — *see* Foreign body, intraocular, old,
        retained, magnetic, vitreous body
  retina S05.5- ☑
  superficial, without open wound
    abdomen, abdominal (wall) S30.851 ☑
    alveolar process S00.552 ☑
    ankle S90.55- ☑
    antecubital space — *see* Foreign body, superficial,
      forearm
    anus S30.857 ☑
    arm (upper) S40.85- ☑
    auditory canal — *see* Foreign body, superficial, ear
    auricle — *see* Foreign body, superficial, ear
    axilla — *see* Foreign body, superficial, arm
    back, lower S30.850 ☑
    breast S20.15- ☑
    brow S00.85 ☑
    buttock S30.850 ☑
    calf — *see* Foreign body, superficial, leg
    canthus — *see* Foreign body, superficial, eyelid
    cheek S00.85 ☑
      internal S00.552 ☑
    chest wall — *see* Foreign body, superficial, thorax
    chin S00.85 ☑
    clitoris S30.854 ☑
    costal region — *see* Foreign body, superficial,
      thorax
    digit(s)
      foot — *see* Foreign body, superficial, toe
      hand — *see* Foreign body, superficial, finger
    ear S00.45- ☑
    elbow S50.35- ☑
    epididymis S30.853 ☑
    epigastric region S30.851 ☑
    epiglottis S10.15 ☑
    esophagus, cervical S10.15 ☑
    eyebrow — *see* Foreign body, superficial, eyelid
    eyelid S00.25- ☑
    face S00.85 ☑
    finger(s) S60.459 ☑
      index S60.45- ☑
      little S60.45- ☑
      middle S60.45- ☑
      ring S60.45- ☑
    flank S30.851 ☑
    foot (except toe(s) alone) S90.85- ☑
      toe — *see* Foreign body, superficial, toe
    forearm S50.85- ☑
      elbow only — *see* Foreign body, superficial, el-
        bow
    forehead S00.85 ☑
    genital organs, external
      female S30.856 ☑
      male S30.855 ☑
    groin S30.851 ☑
    gum S00.552 ☑
    hand S60.55- ☑
    head S00.95 ☑
      ear — *see* Foreign body, superficial, ear
      eyelid — *see* Foreign body, superficial, eyelid
      lip S00.551 ☑
      nose S00.35 ☑
      oral cavity S00.552 ☑
      scalp S00.05 ☑
      specified site NEC S00.85 ☑
    heel — *see* Foreign body, superficial, foot
    hip S70.25- ☑
    inguinal region S30.851 ☑
    interscapular region S20.459 ☑

☑ **Additional Character Required** — **Refer to the Tabular List for Character Selection**      ▽ **Subterms under main terms may continue to next column or page**

**Foreign body** — *continued*
  superficial, without open wound — *continued*
    jaw S00.85 ☑
    knee S80.25- ☑
    labium (majus) (minus) S30.854 ☑
    larynx S10.15 ☑
    leg (lower) S80.85- ☑
      knee — *see* Foreign body, superficial, knee
      upper — *see* Foreign body, superficial, thigh
    lip S00.551 ☑
    lower back S30.850 ☑
    lumbar region S30.850 ☑
    malar region S00.85 ☑
    mammary — *see* Foreign body, superficial, breast
    mastoid region S00.85 ☑
    mouth S00.552 ☑
    nail
      finger — *see* Foreign body, superficial, finger
      toe — *see* Foreign body, superficial, toe
    nape S10.85 ☑
    nasal S00.35 ☑
    neck S10.95 ☑
      specified site NEC S10.85 ☑
      throat S10.15 ☑
    nose S00.35 ☑
    occipital region S00.05 ☑
    oral cavity S00.552 ☑
    orbital region — *see* Foreign body, superficial, eyelid
    palate S00.552 ☑
    palm — *see* Foreign body, superficial, hand
    parietal region S00.05 ☑
    pelvis S30.850 ☑
    penis S30.852 ☑
    perineum
      female S30.854 ☑
      male S30.850 ☑
    periocular area — *see* Foreign body, superficial, eyelid
    phalanges
      finger — *see* Foreign body, superficial, finger
      toe — *see* Foreign body, superficial, toe
    pharynx S10.15 ☑
    pinna — *see* Foreign body, superficial, ear
    popliteal space — *see* Foreign body, superficial, knee
    prepuce S30.852 ☑
    pubic region S30.850 ☑
    pudendum
      female S30.856 ☑
      male S30.855 ☑
    sacral region S30.850 ☑
    scalp S00.05 ☑
    scapular region — *see* Foreign body, superficial, shoulder
    scrotum S30.853 ☑
    shin — *see* Foreign body, superficial, leg
    shoulder S40.25- ☑
    sternal region S20.359 ☑
    submaxillary region S00.85 ☑
    submental region S00.85 ☑
    subungual
      finger(s) — *see* Foreign body, superficial, finger
      toe(s) — *see* Foreign body, superficial, toe
    supraclavicular fossa S10.85 ☑
    supraorbital S00.85 ☑
    temple S00.85 ☑
    temporal region S00.85 ☑
    testis S30.853 ☑
    thigh S70.35- ☑
    thorax, thoracic (wall) S20.95 ☑
      back S20.45- ☑
      front S20.35- ☑
    throat S10.15 ☑
    thumb S60.35- ☑
    toe(s) (lesser) S90.456 ☑
      great S90.45- ☑
    tongue S00.552 ☑
    trachea S10.15 ☑
    tunica vaginalis S30.853 ☑
    tympanum, tympanic membrane — *see* Foreign body, superficial, ear
    uvula S00.552 ☑
    vagina S30.854 ☑
    vocal cords S10.15 ☑
    vulva S30.854 ☑

**Foreign body** — *continued*
  superficial, without open wound — *continued*
    wrist S60.85- ☑
  swallowed T18.9 ☑
  trachea T17.408 ☑
    causing
      asphyxiation T17.400 ☑
        food (bone) (seed) T17.420 ☑
        gastric contents (vomitus) T17.410 ☑
        specified type NEC T17.490 ☑
      injury NEC T17.408 ☑
        food (bone) (seed) T17.428 ☑
        gastric contents (vomitus) T17.418 ☑
        specified type NEC T17.498 ☑
  type of fragment — *see* Retained, foreign body fragments (type of)
  vitreous (humor) S05.5- ☑
**Forestier's disease** (rhizomelic pseudopolyarthritis) M35.3
  meaning ankylosing hyperostosis — *see* Hyperostosis, ankylosing
**Formation**
  hyalin in cornea — *see* Degeneration, cornea
  sequestrum in bone (due to infection) — *see* Osteomyelitis, chronic
  valve
    colon, congenital Q43.8
    ureter (congenital) Q62.39
**Formication** R20.2
**Fort Bragg fever** A27.89
**Fossa** (*see also* condition)
  pyriform — *see* condition
**Foster-Kennedy syndrome** H47.14- ☑
**Fothergill's**
  disease (trigeminal neuralgia) (*see also* Neuralgia, trigeminal)
  scarlatina anginosa A38.9
**Foul breath** R19.6
**Foundling** Z76.1
**Fournier disease or gangrene** N49.3
  female N76.89
**Fourth**
  cranial nerve — *see* condition
  molar K00.1
**Foville's** (peduncular) **disease or syndrome** G46.3
**Fox** (-Fordyce) disease (apocrine miliaria) L75.2
**Fracture, burst** — *see* Fracture, traumatic, by site
**Fracture, chronic** — *see* Fracture, pathological, by site
**Fracture, insufficiency** — *see* Fracture, pathological, by site
**Fracture, nontraumatic, NEC**
  atypical
    femur M84.750- ☑
      complete
        oblique M84.759 ☑
          left side M84.758 ☑
          right side M84.757 ☑
        transverse M84.756 ☑
          left side M84.755 ☑
          right side M84.754 ☑
      incomplete M84.753 ☑
        left side M84.752 ☑
        right side M84.751 ☑
**Fracture, pathological** (pathologic) (*see also* Fracture, traumatic) M84.40 ☑
  ankle M84.47- ☑
  carpus M84.44- ☑
  clavicle M84.41- ☑
  compression (not due to trauma) (*see also* Collapse, vertebra) M48.50- ☑
  dental implant M27.63
  dental restorative material K08.539
    with loss of material K08.531
    without loss of material K08.530
  due to
    neoplastic disease NEC (*see also* Neoplasm) M84.50 ☑
      ankle M84.57- ☑
      carpus M84.54- ☑
      clavicle M84.51- ☑
      femur M84.55- ☑
      fibula M84.56- ☑
      finger M84.54- ☑
      hip M84.559 ☑
      humerus M84.52- ☑
      ilium M84.550 ☑

**Fracture, pathological** — *continued*
  due to — *continued*
    neoplastic disease (*see also* Neoplasm) — *continued*
      ischium M84.550 ☑
      metacarpus M84.54- ☑
      metatarsus M84.57- ☑
      neck M84.58 ☑
      pelvis M84.550 ☑
      radius M84.53- ☑
      rib M84.58 ☑
      scapula M84.51- ☑
      skull M84.58 ☑
      specified site NEC M84.58 ☑
      tarsus M84.57- ☑
      tibia M84.56- ☑
      toe M84.57- ☑
      ulna M84.53- ☑
      vertebra M84.58 ☑
    osteoporosis M80.00 ☑
      disuse — *see* Osteoporosis, specified type NEC, with pathological fracture
      drug-induced — *see* Osteoporosis, drug-induced, with pathological fracture
      idiopathic — *see* Osteoporosis, specified type NEC, with pathological fracture
      postmenopausal — *see* Osteoporosis, postmenopausal, with pathological fracture
      postoophorectomy — *see* Osteoporosis, postoophorectomy, with pathological fracture
      postsurgical malabsorption — *see* Osteoporosis, specified type NEC, with pathological fracture
      specified cause NEC — *see* Osteoporosis, specified type NEC, with pathological fracture
  specified disease NEC M84.60 ☑
    ankle M84.67- ☑
    carpus M84.64- ☑
    clavicle M84.61- ☑
    femur M84.65- ☑
    fibula M84.66- ☑
    finger M84.64- ☑
    hip M84.65- ☑
    humerus M84.62- ☑
    ilium M84.650 ☑
    ischium M84.650 ☑
    metacarpus M84.64- ☑
    metatarsus M84.67- ☑
    neck M84.68 ☑
    radius M84.63- ☑
    rib M84.68 ☑
    scapula M84.61- ☑
    skull M84.68 ☑
    tarsus M84.67- ☑
    tibia M84.66- ☑
    toe M84.67- ☑
    ulna M84.63- ☑
    vertebra M84.68 ☑
  femur M84.45- ☑
  fibula M84.46- ☑
  finger M84.44- ☑
  hip M84.459 ☑
  humerus M84.42- ☑
  ilium M84.454 ☑
  ischium M84.454 ☑
  joint prosthesis — *see* Complications, joint prosthesis, mechanical, breakdown, by site
    periprosthetic — *see* Fracture, pathological, periprosthetic
  metacarpus M84.44- ☑
  metatarsus M84.47- ☑
  neck M84.48 ☑
  pelvis M84.454 ☑
  periprosthetic M97.9 ☑
    ankle M97.2- ☑
    elbow M97.4- ☑
    finger M97.8 ☑
    hip M97.0- ☑
    knee M97.1- ☑
    other specified joint M97.8 ☑
    shoulder M97.3- ☑
    spinal joint M97.8 ☑
    toe joint M97.8 ☑
    wrist joint M97.8 ☑
  radius M84.43- ☑

**Fracture, pathological** — *continued*
restorative material (dental) K08.539
with loss of material K08.531
without loss of material K08.530
rib M84.48 ☑
scapula M84.41- ☑
skull M84.48 ☑
tarsus M84.47- ☑
tibia M84.46- ☑
toe M84.47- ☑
ulna M84.43- ☑
vertebra M84.48 ☑
**Fracture, traumatic** (abduction) (adduction) (separation)
(*see also* Fracture, pathological) T14.8 ☑
acetabulum S32.40- ☑
column
anterior (displaced) (iliopubic) S32.43- ☑
nondisplaced S32.436
posterior (displaced) (ilioischial) S32.443 ☑
nondisplaced S32.44- ☑
dome (displaced) S32.48- ☑
nondisplaced S32.48 ☑
specified NEC S32.49- ☑
transverse (displaced) S32.45- ☑
with associated posterior wall fracture (displaced) S32.46- ☑
nondisplaced S32.46- ☑
nondisplaced S32.45- ☑
wall
anterior (displaced) S32.41- ☑
nondisplaced S32.41- ☑
medial (displaced) S32.47- ☑
nondisplaced S32.47- ☑
posterior (displaced) S32.42- ☑
with associated transverse fracture (displaced) S32.46- ☑
nondisplaced S32.46- ☑
nondisplaced S32.42- ☑
acromion — *see* Fracture, scapula, acromial process
ankle S82.899 ☑
bimalleolar (displaced) S82.84- ☑
nondisplaced S82.84- ☑
lateral malleolus only (displaced) S82.6- ☑
nondisplaced S82.6- ☑
medial malleolus (displaced) S82.5- ☑
associated with Maisonneuve's fracture — *see* Fracture, Maisonneuve's
nondisplaced S82.5- ☑
talus — *see* Fracture, tarsal, talus
trimalleolar (displaced) S82.85- ☑
nondisplaced S82.85- ☑
arm (upper) (*see also* Fracture, humerus, shaft)
humerus — *see* Fracture, humerus
radius — *see* Fracture, radius
ulna — *see* Fracture, ulna
astragalus — *see* Fracture, tarsal, talus
atlas — *see* Fracture, neck, cervical vertebra, first
axis — *see* Fracture, neck, cervical vertebra, second
back — *see* Fracture, vertebra
Barton's — *see* Barton's fracture
base of skull — *see* Fracture, skull, base
basicervical (basal) (femoral) S72.0 ☑
Bennett's — *see* Bennett's fracture
bimalleolar — *see* Fracture, ankle, bimalleolar
blow-out S02.3- ☑
bone NEC T14.8 ☑
birth injury P13.9
following insertion of orthopedic implant, joint prosthesis or bone plate — *see* Fracture, following insertion of orthopedic implant, joint prosthesis or bone plate
in (due to) neoplastic disease NEC — *see* Fracture, pathological, due to, neoplastic disease
pathological (cause unknown) — *see* Fracture, pathological
breast bone — *see* Fracture, sternum
bucket handle (semilunar cartilage) — *see* Tear, meniscus
burst — *see* Fracture, traumatic, by site
calcaneus — *see* Fracture, tarsal, calcaneus
carpal bone(s) S62.10- ☑
capitate (displaced) S62.13- ☑
nondisplaced S62.13- ☑
cuneiform — *see* Fracture, carpal bone, triquetrum
hamate (body) (displaced) S62.143
hook process (displaced) S62.15- ☑

**Fracture, traumatic** — *continued*
carpal bone(s) — *continued*
hamate — *continued*
hook process — *continued*
nondisplaced S62.15- ☑
nondisplaced S62.14- ☑
larger multangular — *see* Fracture, carpal bones, trapezium
lunate (displaced) S62.12- ☑
nondisplaced S62.12- ☑
navicular S62.00- ☑
distal pole (displaced) S62.01- ☑
nondisplaced S62.01- ☑
middle third (displaced) S62.02- ☑
nondisplaced S62.02- ☑
proximal third (displaced) S62.03- ☑
nondisplaced S62.03- ☑
volar tuberosity — *see* Fracture, carpal bones, navicular, distal pole
os magnum — *see* Fracture, carpal bones, capitate
pisiform (displaced) S62.16- ☑
nondisplaced S62.16- ☑
semilunar — *see* Fracture, carpal bones, lunate
smaller multangular — *see* Fracture, carpal bones, trapezoid
trapezium (displaced) S62.17- ☑
nondisplaced S62.17- ☑
trapezoid (displaced) S62.18- ☑
nondisplaced S62.18- ☑
triquetrum (displaced) S62.11- ☑
nondisplaced S62.11- ☑
unciform — *see* Fracture, carpal bones, hamate
cervical — *see* Fracture, vertebra, cervical
clavicle S42.00- ☑
acromial end (displaced) S42.03- ☑
nondisplaced S42.03- ☑
birth injury P13.4
lateral end — *see* Fracture, clavicle, acromial end
shaft (displaced) S42.02- ☑
nondisplaced S42.02- ☑
sternal end (anterior) (displaced) S42.01- ☑
nondisplaced S42.01- ☑
posterior S42.01- ☑
coccyx S32.2 ☑
collapsed — *see* Collapse, vertebra
collar bone — *see* Fracture, clavicle
Colles' — *see* Colles' fracture
coronoid process — *see* Fracture, ulna, upper end, coronoid process
corpus cavernosum penis S39.840 ☑
costochondral cartilage S23.41 ☑
costochondral, costosternal junction — *see* Fracture, rib
cranium — *see* Fracture, skull
cricoid cartilage S12.8 ☑
cuboid (ankle) — *see* Fracture, tarsal, cuboid
cuneiform
foot — *see* Fracture, tarsal, cuneiform
wrist — *see* Fracture, carpal, triquetrum
delayed union — *see* Delay, union, fracture
dental restorative material K08.539
with loss of material K08.531
without loss of material K08.530
due to
birth injury — *see* Birth, injury, fracture
osteoporosis — *see* Osteoporosis, with fracture
Dupuytren's — *see* Fracture, ankle, lateral malleolus
elbow S42.40- ☑
ethmoid (bone) (sinus) — *see* Fracture, skull, base
face bone S02.92 ☑
fatigue (*see also* Fracture, stress)
vertebra M48.40 ☑
cervical region M48.42 ☑
cervicothoracic region M48.43 ☑
lumbar region M48.46 ☑
lumbosacral region M48.47 ☑
occipito-atlanto-axial region M48.41 ☑
sacrococcygeal region M48.48 ☑
thoracic region M48.44 ☑
thoracolumbar region M48.45 ☑
femur, femoral S72.9- ☑
basicervical (basal) S72.0 ☑
birth injury P13.2
capital epiphyseal S79.01- ☑
condyles, epicondyles — *see* Fracture, femur, lower end

**Fracture, traumatic** — *continued*
femur, femoral — *continued*
distal end — *see* Fracture, femur, lower end
epiphysis
head — *see* Fracture, femur, upper end, epiphysis
lower — *see* Fracture, femur, lower end, epiphysis
upper — *see* Fracture, femur, upper end, epiphysis
following insertion of implant, prosthesis or plate M96.66- ☑
head — *see* Fracture, femur, upper end, head
intertrochanteric — *see* Fracture, femur, trochanteric
intratrochanteric — *see* Fracture, femur, trochanteric
lower end S72.40- ☑
condyle (displaced) S72.41- ☑
lateral (displaced) S72.42- ☑
nondisplaced S72.42- ☑
medial (displaced) S72.43- ☑
nondisplaced S72.43- ☑
nondisplaced S72.41- ☑
epiphysis (displaced) S72.44- ☑
nondisplaced S72.44- ☑
physeal S79.10- ☑
Salter-Harris
Type I S79.11- ☑
Type II S79.12- ☑
Type III S79.13- ☑
Type IV S79.14- ☑
specified NEC S79.19- ☑
specified NEC S72.49- ☑
supracondylar (displaced) S72.45- ☑
with intracondylar extension (displaced) S72.46- ☑
nondisplaced S72.46- ☑
nondisplaced S72.45- ☑
torus S72.47- ☑
neck — *see* Fracture, femur, upper end, neck
pertrochanteric — *see* Fracture, femur, trochanteric
shaft (lower third) (middle third) (upper third) S72.30- ☑
comminuted (displaced) S72.35- ☑
nondisplaced S72.35- ☑
oblique (displaced) S72.33- ☑
nondisplaced S72.33- ☑
segmental (displaced) S72.36- ☑
nondisplaced S72.36- ☑
specified NEC S72.39- ☑
spiral (displaced) S72.34- ☑
nondisplaced S72.34- ☑
transverse (displaced) S72.32- ☑
nondisplaced S72.32- ☑
specified site NEC — *see* subcategory S72.8 ☑
subcapital (displaced) S72.01- ☑
subtrochanteric (region) (section) (displaced) S72.2- ☑
nondisplaced S72.2- ☑
transcervical — *see* Fracture, femur, upper end, neck
transtrochanteric — *see* Fracture, femur, trochanteric
trochanteric S72.10- ☑
apophyseal (displaced) S72.13- ☑
nondisplaced S72.13- ☑
greater trochanter (displaced) S72.11- ☑
nondisplaced S72.11- ☑
intertrochanteric (displaced) S72.14- ☑
nondisplaced S72.14- ☑
lesser trochanter (displaced) S72.12- ☑
nondisplaced S72.12- ☑
upper end S72.00- ☑
apophyseal (displaced) S72.13- ☑
nondisplaced S72.13- ☑
cervicotrochanteric — *see* Fracture, femur, upper end, neck, base
epiphysis (displaced) S72.02- ☑
nondisplaced S72.02- ☑
head S72.05- ☑
articular (displaced) S72.06- ☑
nondisplaced S72.06- ☑
specified NEC S72.09- ☑
intertrochanteric (displaced) S72.14- ☑

☑ **Additional Character Required** — **Refer to the Tabular List for Character Selection**          ▽ Subterms under main terms may continue to next column or page

**Fracture, traumatic** — *continued*
  femur, femoral — *continued*
    upper end — *continued*
      intertrochanteric — *continued*
        nondisplaced S72.14- ☑
      intracapsular S72.01- ☑
      midcervical (displaced) S72.03- ☑
        nondisplaced S72.03- ☑
      neck S72.00- ☑
        base (displaced) S72.04- ☑
          nondisplaced S72.04- ☑
        specified NEC S72.09- ☑
      pertrochanteric — *see* Fracture, femur, upper end, trochanteric
      physeal S79.00- ☑
        Salter-Harris type I S79.01- ☑
        specified NEC S79.09- ☑
      subcapital (displaced) S72.01- ☑
      subtrochanteric (displaced) S72.2- ☑
        nondisplaced S72.2- ☑
      transcervical — *see* Fracture, femur, upper end, midcervical
      trochanteric S72.10- ☑
        greater (displaced) S72.11- ☑
          nondisplaced S72.11- ☑
        lesser (displaced) S72.12- ☑
          nondisplaced S72.12- ☑
  fibula (shaft) (styloid) S82.40- ☑
    comminuted (displaced) S82.45- ☑
      nondisplaced S82.45- ☑
    following insertion of implant, prosthesis or plate M96.67- ☑
    involving ankle or malleolus — *see* Fracture, fibula, lateral malleolus
    lateral malleolus (displaced) S82.6- ☑
      nondisplaced S82.6- ☑
    lower end
      physeal S89.30- ☑
        Salter-Harris
          Type I S89.31- ☑
          Type II S89.32- ☑
        specified NEC S89.39- ☑
      specified NEC S82.83- ☑
      torus S82.82- ☑
    oblique (displaced) S82.43- ☑
      nondisplaced S82.43- ☑
    segmental (displaced) S82.46- ☑
      nondisplaced S82.46- ☑
    specified NEC S82.49- ☑
    spiral (displaced) S82.44- ☑
      nondisplaced S82.44- ☑
    transverse (displaced) S82.42- ☑
      nondisplaced S82.42- ☑
    upper end
      physeal S89.20- ☑
        Salter-Harris
          Type I S89.21- ☑
          Type II S89.22- ☑
        specified NEC S89.29- ☑
      specified NEC S82.83- ☑
      torus S82.81- ☑
  finger (except thumb) S62.60- ☑
    distal phalanx (displaced) S62.63- ☑
      nondisplaced S62.66- ☑
    index S62.60- ☑
      distal phalanx (displaced) S62.63- ☑
        nondisplaced S62.66- ☑
      medial phalanx (displaced) S62.62- ☑
        nondisplaced S62.65- ☑
      proximal phalanx (displaced) S62.61- ☑
        nondisplaced S62.64- ☑
    little S62.60- ☑
      distal phalanx (displaced) S62.63- ☑
        nondisplaced S62.66- ☑
      medial phalanx (displaced) S62.62- ☑
        nondisplaced S62.65- ☑
      proximal phalanx (displaced) S62.61- ☑
        nondisplaced S62.64- ☑
    medial phalanx (displaced) S62.62- ☑
      nondisplaced S62.65- ☑
    middle S62.60- ☑
      distal phalanx (displaced) S62.63- ☑
        nondisplaced S62.66- ☑
      medial phalanx (displaced) S62.62- ☑
        nondisplaced S62.65- ☑
      proximal phalanx (displaced) S62.61- ☑

**Fracture, traumatic** — *continued*
  finger — *continued*
    middle — *continued*
      proximal phalanx — *continued*
        nondisplaced S62.64- ☑
      proximal phalanx (displaced) S62.61- ☑
        nondisplaced S62.64- ☑
    ring S62.60- ☑
      distal phalanx (displaced) S62.63- ☑
        nondisplaced S62.66- ☑
      medial phalanx (displaced) S62.62- ☑
        nondisplaced S62.65- ☑
      proximal phalanx (displaced) S62.61- ☑
        nondisplaced S62.64- ☑
    thumb — *see* Fracture, thumb
  following insertion (intraoperative) (postoperative) of orthopedic implant, joint prosthesis or bone plate M96.69
    femur M96.66- ☑
    fibula M96.67- ☑
    humerus M96.62- ☑
    pelvis M96.65
    radius M96.63- ☑
    specified bone NEC M96.69
    tibia M96.67- ☑
    ulna M96.63- ☑
  foot S92.90- ☑
    astragalus — *see* Fracture, tarsal, talus
    calcaneus — *see* Fracture, tarsal, calcaneus
    cuboid — *see* Fracture, tarsal, cuboid
    cuneiform — *see* Fracture, tarsal, cuneiform
    metatarsal — *see* Fracture, metatarsal
    navicular — *see* Fracture, tarsal, navicular
    sesamoid S92.81- ☑
    specified NEC S92.81- ☑
    talus — *see* Fracture, tarsal, talus
    tarsal — *see* Fracture, tarsal
    toe — *see* Fracture, toe
  forearm S52.9- ☑
    radius — *see* Fracture, radius
    ulna — *see* Fracture, ulna
  fossa (anterior) (middle) (posterior) S02.19 ☑
  frontal (bone) (skull) S02.0 ☑
    sinus S02.19 ☑
  glenoid (cavity) (scapula) — *see* Fracture, scapula, glenoid cavity
  greenstick — *see* Fracture, by site
  hallux — *see* Fracture, toe, great
  hand S62.9- ☑
    carpal — *see* Fracture, carpal bone
    finger (except thumb) — *see* Fracture, finger
    metacarpal — *see* Fracture, metacarpal
    navicular (scaphoid) (hand) — *see* Fracture, carpal bone, navicular
    thumb — *see* Fracture, thumb
  healed or old
    with complications — *code by* Nature of the complication
  heel bone — *see* Fracture, tarsal, calcaneus
  Hill-Sachs S42.29- ☑
  hip — *see* Fracture, femur, neck
  humerus S42.30- ☑
    anatomical neck — *see* Fracture, humerus, upper end
    articular process — *see* Fracture, humerus, lower end
    capitellum — *see* Fracture, humerus, lower end, condyle, lateral
    distal end — *see* Fracture, humerus, lower end
    epiphysis
      lower — *see* Fracture, humerus, lower end, physeal
      upper — *see* Fracture, humerus, upper end, physeal
    external condyle — *see* Fracture, humerus, lower end, condyle, lateral
    following insertion of implant, prosthesis or plate M96.62- ☑
    great tuberosity — *see* Fracture, humerus, upper end, greater tuberosity
    intercondylar — *see* Fracture, humerus, lower end
    internal epicondyle — *see* Fracture, humerus, lower end, epicondyle, medial
    lesser tuberosity — *see* Fracture, humerus, upper end, lesser tuberosity
    lower end S42.40- ☑

**Fracture, traumatic** — *continued*
  humerus — *continued*
    lower end — *continued*
      condyle
        lateral (displaced) S42.45- ☑
          nondisplaced S42.45- ☑
        medial (displaced) S42.46- ☑
          nondisplaced S42.46- ☑
      epicondyle
        lateral (displaced) S42.43- ☑
          nondisplaced S42.43- ☑
        medial (displaced) S42.44- ☑
          incarcerated S42.44- ☑
          nondisplaced S42.44- ☑
      physeal S49.10- ☑
        Salter-Harris
          Type I S49.11- ☑
          Type II S49.12- ☑
          Type III S49.13- ☑
          Type IV S49.14- ☑
        specified NEC S49.19- ☑
      specified NEC (displaced) S42.49- ☑
        nondisplaced S42.49- ☑
      supracondylar (simple) (displaced) S42.41- ☑
        with intercondylar fracture — *see* Fracture, humerus, lower end
        comminuted (displaced) S42.42- ☑
          nondisplaced S42.42- ☑
        nondisplaced S42.41- ☑
      torus S42.48- ☑
      transcondylar (displaced) S42.47- ☑
        nondisplaced S42.47- ☑
    proximal end — *see* Fracture, humerus, upper end
    shaft S42.30- ☑
      comminuted (displaced) S42.35- ☑
        nondisplaced S42.35- ☑
      greenstick S42.31- ☑
      oblique (displaced) S42.33- ☑
        nondisplaced S42.33- ☑
      segmental (displaced) S42.36- ☑
        nondisplaced S42.36- ☑
      specified NEC S42.39- ☑
      spiral (displaced) S42.34- ☑
        nondisplaced S42.34- ☑
      transverse (displaced) S42.32- ☑
        nondisplaced S42.32- ☑
    supracondylar — *see* Fracture, humerus, lower end
    surgical neck — *see* Fracture, humerus, upper end, surgical neck
    trochlea — *see* Fracture, humerus, lower end, condyle, medial
    tuberosity — *see* Fracture, humerus, upper end
    upper end S42.20- ☑
      anatomical neck — *see* Fracture, humerus, upper end, specified NEC
      articular head — *see* Fracture, humerus, upper end, specified NEC
      epiphysis — *see* Fracture, humerus, upper end, physeal
      greater tuberosity (displaced) S42.25- ☑
        nondisplaced S42.25- ☑
      lesser tuberosity (displaced) S42.26- ☑
        nondisplaced S42.26- ☑
      physeal S49.00- ☑
        Salter-Harris
          Type I S49.01- ☑
          Type II S49.02- ☑
          Type III S49.03- ☑
          Type IV S49.04- ☑
        specified NEC S49.09- ☑
      specified NEC (displaced) S42.29- ☑
        nondisplaced S42.29- ☑
      surgical neck (displaced) S42.21- ☑
        four-part S42.24- ☑
        nondisplaced S42.21- ☑
        three-part S42.23- ☑
        two-part (displaced) S42.22- ☑
          nondisplaced S42.22- ☑
      torus S42.27- ☑
      transepiphyseal — *see* Fracture, humerus, upper end, physeal
  hyoid bone S12.8 ☑
  ilium S32.30- ☑
    with disruption of pelvic ring — *see* Disruption, pelvic ring
    avulsion (displaced) S32.31- ☑

**Fracture, traumatic** — *continued*
  ilium — *continued*
    avulsion — *continued*
      nondisplaced S32.31- ☑
    specified NEC S32.39- ☑
  impaction, impacted — *code as* Fracture, by site
  innominate bone — *see* Fracture, ilium
  instep — *see* Fracture, foot
  ischium S32.60- ☑
    with disruption of pelvic ring — *see* Disruption, pelvic ring
    avulsion (displaced) S32.61- ☑
      nondisplaced S32.61- ☑
    specified NEC S32.69- ☑
  jaw (bone) (lower) — *see* Fracture, mandible
    upper — *see* Fracture, maxilla
  joint prosthesis — *see* Complications, joint prosthesis, mechanical, breakdown, by site
    periprosthetic — *see* Fracture, traumatic, periprosthetic
  knee cap — *see* Fracture, patella
  larynx S12.8 ☑
  late effects — *see* Sequelae, fracture
  leg (lower) S82.9- ☑
    ankle — *see* Fracture, ankle
    femur — *see* Fracture, femur
    fibula — *see* Fracture, fibula
    malleolus — *see* Fracture, ankle
    patella — *see* Fracture, patella
    specified site NEC S82.89- ☑
    tibia — *see* Fracture, tibia
  lumbar spine — *see* Fracture, vertebra, lumbar
  lumbosacral spine S32.9 ☑
  Maisonneuve's (displaced) S82.86- ☑
    nondisplaced S82.86- ☑
  malar bone (*see also* Fracture, maxilla) S02.400 ☑
    left side S02.40B ☑
    right side S02.40A ☑
  malleolus — *see* Fracture, ankle
  malunion — *see* Fracture, by site
  mandible (lower jaw (bone)) S02.609 ☑
    alveolus S02.67- ☑
    angle (of jaw) S02.65- ☑
    body, unspecified S02.600 ☑
      left side S02.602 ☑
      right side S02.601 ☑
    condylar process S02.61- ☑
    coronoid process S02.63- ☑
    ramus, unspecified S02.64- ☑
    specified site NEC S02.69 ☑
    subcondylar process S02.62- ☑
    symphysis S02.66 ☑
  manubrium (sterni) S22.21 ☑
    dissociation from sternum S22.23 ☑
  march — *see* Fracture, traumatic, stress, by site
  maxilla, maxillary (bone) (sinus) (superior) (upper jaw) S02.401 ☑
    alveolus S02.42 ☑
    inferior — *see* Fracture, mandible
    LeFort I S02.411 ☑
    LeFort II S02.412 ☑
    LeFort III S02.413 ☑
    left side S02.40D ☑
    right side S02.40C ☑
  metacarpal S62.309 ☑
    base (displaced) S62.319 ☑
      nondisplaced S62.349 ☑
    fifth S62.30- ☑
      base (displaced) S62.31- ☑
        nondisplaced S62.34- ☑
      neck (displaced) S62.33- ☑
        nondisplaced S62.36- ☑
      shaft (displaced) S62.32- ☑
        nondisplaced S62.35- ☑
      specified NEC S62.398 ☑
    first S62.20- ☑
      base NEC (displaced) S62.23- ☑
        nondisplaced S62.23- ☑
      Bennett's — *see* Bennett's fracture
      neck (displaced) S62.25- ☑
        nondisplaced S62.25- ☑
      shaft (displaced) S62.24- ☑
        nondisplaced S62.24- ☑
      specified NEC S62.29- ☑
    fourth S62.30- ☑
      base (displaced) S62.31- ☑

**Fracture, traumatic** — *continued*
  metacarpal — *continued*
    fourth — *continued*
      base — *continued*
        nondisplaced S62.34- ☑
      neck (displaced) S62.33- ☑
        nondisplaced S62.36- ☑
      shaft (displaced) S62.32- ☑
        nondisplaced S62.35- ☑
      specified NEC S62.39- ☑
    neck (displaced) S62.33- ☑
      nondisplaced S62.36- ☑
    Rolando's — *see* Rolando's fracture
    second S62.30- ☑
      base (displaced) S62.31- ☑
        nondisplaced S62.34- ☑
      neck (displaced) S62.33- ☑
        nondisplaced S62.36- ☑
      shaft (displaced) S62.32- ☑
        nondisplaced S62.35- ☑
      specified NEC S62.39- ☑
    shaft (displaced) S62.32- ☑
      nondisplaced S62.35- ☑
    specified NEC S62.399 ☑
    third S62.30- ☑
      base (displaced) S62.31- ☑
        nondisplaced S62.34- ☑
      neck (displaced) S62.33- ☑
        nondisplaced S62.36- ☑
      shaft (displaced) S62.32- ☑
        nondisplaced S62.35- ☑
      specified NEC S62.39- ☑
  metastatic — *see* Fracture, pathological, due to, neoplastic disease (*see also* Neoplasm)
  metatarsal bone S92.30- ☑
    fifth (displaced) S92.35- ☑
      nondisplaced S92.35- ☑
    first (displaced) S92.31- ☑
      nondisplaced S92.31- ☑
    fourth (displaced) S92.34- ☑
      nondisplaced S92.34- ☑
    physeal S99.10- ☑
      Salter-Harris
        Type I S99.11- ☑
        Type II S99.12- ☑
        Type III S99.13- ☑
        Type IV S99.14- ☑
      specified NEC S99.19- ☑
    second (displaced) S92.32- ☑
      nondisplaced S92.32- ☑
    third (displaced) S92.33- ☑
      nondisplaced S92.33- ☑
  Monteggia's — *see* Monteggia's fracture
  multiple
    hand (and wrist) NEC — *see* Fracture, by site
    ribs — *see* Fracture, rib, multiple
  nasal (bone(s)) S02.2 ☑
  navicular (scaphoid) (foot) (*see also* Fracture, tarsal, navicular)
    hand — *see* Fracture, carpal, navicular
  neck S12.9 ☑
    cervical vertebra S12.9 ☑
      fifth (displaced) S12.400 ☑
        nondisplaced S12.401 ☑
        specified type NEC (displaced) S12.490 ☑
          nondisplaced S12.491 ☑
      first (displaced) S12.000 ☑
        burst (stable) S12.01 ☑
          unstable S12.02 ☑
        lateral mass (displaced) S12.040 ☑
          nondisplaced S12.041 ☑
        nondisplaced S12.001 ☑
        posterior arch (displaced) S12.030 ☑
          nondisplaced S12.031 ☑
        specified type NEC (displaced) S12.090 ☑
          nondisplaced S12.091 ☑
      fourth (displaced) S12.300 ☑
        nondisplaced S12.301 ☑
        specified type NEC (displaced) S12.390 ☑
          nondisplaced S12.391 ☑
      second (displaced) S12.100 ☑
        dens (anterior) (displaced) (type II) S12.110 ☑
          nondisplaced S12.112 ☑
          posterior S12.111 ☑

**Fracture, traumatic** — *continued*
  neck — *continued*
    cervical vertebra — *continued*
      second — *continued*
        dens — *continued*
          specified type NEC (displaced) S12.120 ☑
            nondisplaced S12.121 ☑
        nondisplaced S12.101 ☑
        specified type NEC (displaced) S12.190 ☑
          nondisplaced S12.191 ☑
      seventh (displaced) S12.600 ☑
        nondisplaced S12.601 ☑
        specified type NEC (displaced) S12.690 ☑
          nondisplaced S12.691 ☑
      sixth (displaced) S12.500 ☑
        nondisplaced S12.501 ☑
        specified type NEC (displaced) S12.590 ☑
          nondisplaced S12.591 ☑
      third (displaced) S12.200 ☑
        nondisplaced S12.201 ☑
        specified type NEC (displaced) S12.290 ☑
          nondisplaced S12.291 ☑
    hyoid bone S12.8 ☑
    larynx S12.8 ☑
    specified site NEC S12.8 ☑
    thyroid cartilage S12.8 ☑
    trachea S12.8 ☑
  neoplastic NEC — *see* Fracture, pathological, due to, neoplastic disease
  neural arch — *see* Fracture, vertebra
  newborn — *see* Birth, injury, fracture
  nontraumatic — *see* Fracture, pathological
  nonunion — *see* Nonunion, fracture
  nose, nasal (bone) (septum) S02.2 ☑
  occiput — *see* Fracture, skull, base, occiput
  odontoid process — *see* Fracture, neck, cervical vertebra, second
  olecranon (process) (ulna) — *see* Fracture, ulna, upper end, olecranon process
  orbit, orbital (bone) (region) S02.8- ☑
    floor (blow-out) S02.3- ☑
    roof S02.19 ☑
  os
    calcis — *see* Fracture, tarsal, calcaneus
    magnum — *see* Fracture, carpal, capitate
    pubis — *see* Fracture, pubis
  palate S02.8- ☑
  parietal bone (skull) S02.0 ☑
  patella S82.00- ☑
    comminuted (displaced) S82.04- ☑
      nondisplaced S82.04- ☑
    longitudinal (displaced) S82.02- ☑
      nondisplaced S82.02- ☑
    osteochondral (displaced) S82.01- ☑
      nondisplaced S82.01- ☑
    specified NEC S82.09- ☑
    transverse (displaced) S82.03- ☑
      nondisplaced S82.03- ☑
  pedicle (of vertebral arch) — *see* Fracture, vertebra
  pelvis, pelvic (bone) S32.9 ☑
    acetabulum — *see* Fracture, acetabulum
    circle — *see* Disruption, pelvic ring
    following insertion of implant, prosthesis or plate M96.65
    ilium — *see* Fracture, ilium
    ischium — *see* Fracture, ischium
    multiple
      with disruption of pelvic ring (circle) — *see* Disruption, pelvic ring
      without disruption of pelvic ring (circle) S32.82 ☑
    pubis — *see* Fracture, pubis
    sacrum — *see* Fracture, sacrum
    specified site NEC S32.89 ☑
  periprosthetic, around internal prosthetic joint M97.9 ☑
    ankle M97.2- ☑
    elbow M97.4- ☑
    finger M97.8 ☑
    hip M97.0- ☑
    knee M97.1- ☑
    shoulder M97.3- ☑
    specified joint NEC M97.8 ☑
    spine M97.8 ☑
    toe M97.8 ☑

☑ **Additional Character Required** — **Refer to the Tabular List for Character Selection**

▽ **Subterms under main terms may continue to next column or page**

**Fracture, traumatic** — *continued*
 thorax — *continued*
  vertebra — *continued*
   eighth — *continued*
    burst — *continued*
     unstable S22.062 ☑
    specified type NEC S22.068 ☑
    wedge compression S22.060 ☑
   eleventh S22.089 ☑
    burst (stable) S22.081 ☑
     unstable S22.082 ☑
    specified type NEC S22.088 ☑
    wedge compression S22.080 ☑
   fifth S22.059 ☑
    burst (stable) S22.051 ☑
     unstable S22.052 ☑
    specified type NEC S22.058 ☑
    wedge compression S22.050 ☑
   first S22.019 ☑
    burst (stable) S22.011 ☑
     unstable S22.012 ☑
    specified type NEC S22.018 ☑
    wedge compression S22.010 ☑
   fourth S22.049 ☑
    burst (stable) S22.041 ☑
     unstable S22.042 ☑
    specified type NEC S22.048 ☑
    wedge compression S22.040 ☑
   ninth S22.079 ☑
    burst (stable) S22.071 ☑
     unstable S22.072 ☑
    specified type NEC S22.078 ☑
    wedge compression S22.070 ☑
   nondisplaced S22.001 ☑
   second S22.029 ☑
    burst (stable) S22.021 ☑
     unstable S22.022 ☑
    specified type NEC S22.028 ☑
    wedge compression S22.020 ☑
   seventh S22.069 ☑
    burst (stable) S22.061 ☑
     unstable S22.062 ☑
    specified type NEC S22.068 ☑
    wedge compression S22.060 ☑
   sixth S22.059 ☑
    burst (stable) S22.051 ☑
     unstable S22.052 ☑
    specified type NEC S22.058 ☑
    wedge compression S22.050 ☑
   specified type NEC S22.008 ☑
   tenth S22.079 ☑
    burst (stable) S22.071 ☑
     unstable S22.072 ☑
    specified type NEC S22.078 ☑
    wedge compression S22.070 ☑
   third S22.039 ☑
    burst (stable) S22.031 ☑
     unstable S22.032 ☑
    specified type NEC S22.038 ☑
    wedge compression S22.030 ☑
   twelfth S22.089 ☑
    burst (stable) S22.081 ☑
     unstable S22.082 ☑
    specified type NEC S22.088 ☑
    wedge compression S22.080 ☑
   wedge compression S22.000 ☑
 thumb S62.50- ☑
  distal phalanx (displaced) S62.52- ☑
   nondisplaced S62.52- ☑
  proximal phalanx (displaced) S62.51- ☑
   nondisplaced S62.51- ☑
 thyroid cartilage S12.8 ☑
 tibia (shaft) S82.20- ☑
  comminuted (displaced) S82.25- ☑
   nondisplaced S82.25- ☑
  condyles — *see* Fracture, tibia, upper end
  distal end — *see* Fracture, tibia, lower end
  epiphysis
   lower — *see* Fracture, tibia, lower end
   upper — *see* Fracture, tibia, upper end
  following insertion of implant, prosthesis or plate
    M96.67- ☑
  head (involving knee joint) — *see* Fracture, tibia, upper end
  intercondyloid eminence — *see* Fracture, tibia, upper end

**Fracture, traumatic** — *continued*
 tibia — *continued*
  involving ankle or malleolus — *see* Fracture, ankle, medial malleolus
  lower end S82.30- ☑
   physeal S89.10- ☑
    Salter-Harris
     Type I S89.11- ☑
     Type II S89.12- ☑
     Type III S89.13- ☑
     Type IV S89.14- ☑
    specified NEC S89.19- ☑
   pilon (displaced) S82.87- ☑
    nondisplaced S82.87- ☑
   specified NEC S82.39- ☑
   torus S82.31- ☑
  malleolus — *see* Fracture, ankle, medial malleolus
  oblique (displaced) S82.23- ☑
   nondisplaced S82.23- ☑
  pilon — *see* Fracture, tibia, lower end, pilon
  proximal end — *see* Fracture, tibia, upper end
  segmental (displaced) S82.26- ☑
   nondisplaced S82.26- ☑
  specified NEC S82.29- ☑
  spine — *see* Fracture, tibia, upper end, spine
  spiral (displaced) S82.24- ☑
   nondisplaced S82.24- ☑
  transverse (displaced) S82.22- ☑
   nondisplaced S82.22- ☑
  tuberosity — *see* Fracture, tibia, upper end, tuberosity
  upper end S82.10- ☑
   bicondylar (displaced) S82.14- ☑
    nondisplaced S82.14- ☑
   lateral condyle (displaced) S82.12- ☑
    nondisplaced S82.12- ☑
   medial condyle (displaced) S82.13- ☑
    nondisplaced S82.13- ☑
   physeal S89.00- ☑
    Salter-Harris
     Type I S89.01- ☑
     Type II S89.02- ☑
     Type III S89.03- ☑
     Type IV S89.04- ☑
    specified NEC S89.09- ☑
   plateau — *see* Fracture, tibia, upper end, bicondylar
   specified NEC S82.19- ☑
   spine (displaced) S82.11- ☑
    nondisplaced S82.11- ☑
   torus S82.16- ☑
   tuberosity (displaced) S82.15- ☑
    nondisplaced S82.15- ☑
  toe S92.91- ☑
   great (displaced) S92.40- ☑
    distal phalanx (displaced) S92.42- ☑
     nondisplaced S92.42- ☑
    nondisplaced S92.40- ☑
    proximal phalanx (displaced) S92.41- ☑
     nondisplaced S92.41- ☑
    specified NEC S92.49- ☑
   lesser (displaced) S92.50- ☑
    distal phalanx (displaced) S92.53- ☑
     nondisplaced S92.53- ☑
    medial phalanx (displaced) S92.52- ☑
     nondisplaced S92.52- ☑
    nondisplaced S92.50- ☑
    proximal phalanx (displaced) S92.51- ☑
     nondisplaced S92.51- ☑
    specified NEC S92.59- ☑
   physeal
    phalanx S99.20- ☑
     Salter-Harris
      Type I S99.21- ☑
      Type II S99.22- ☑
      Type III S99.23- ☑
      Type IV S99.24- ☑
     specified NEC S99.29- ☑
  tooth (root) S02.5 ☑
  trachea (cartilage) S12.8 ☑
  transverse process — *see* Fracture, vertebra
  trapezium or trapezoid bone — *see* Fracture, carpal
  trimalleolar — *see* Fracture, ankle, trimalleolar
  triquetrum (cuneiform of carpus) — *see* Fracture, carpal, triquetrum
  trochanter — *see* Fracture, femur, trochanteric

**Fracture, traumatic** — *continued*
 tuberosity (external) — *see* Fracture, traumatic, by site
 ulna (shaft) S52.20- ☑
  bent bone S52.28- ☑
  coronoid process — *see* Fracture, ulna, upper end, coronoid process
  distal end — *see* Fracture, ulna, lower end
  following insertion of implant, prosthesis or plate
    M96.63- ☑
  head S52.60- ☑
  lower end S52.60- ☑
   physeal S59.00- ☑
    Salter-Harris
     Type I S59.01- ☑
     Type II S59.02- ☑
     Type III S59.03- ☑
     Type IV S59.04- ☑
    specified NEC S59.09- ☑
   specified NEC S52.69- ☑
   styloid process (displaced) S52.61- ☑
    nondisplaced S52.61- ☑
   torus S52.62- ☑
  proximal end — *see* Fracture, ulna, upper end
  shaft S52.20- ☑
   comminuted (displaced) S52.25- ☑
    nondisplaced S52.25- ☑
   greenstick S52.21- ☑
   Monteggia's — *see* Monteggia's fracture
   oblique (displaced) S52.23- ☑
    nondisplaced S52.23- ☑
   segmental (displaced) S52.26- ☑
    nondisplaced S52.26- ☑
   specified NEC S52.29- ☑
   spiral (displaced) S52.24- ☑
    nondisplaced S52.24- ☑
   transverse (displaced) S52.22- ☑
    nondisplaced S52.22- ☑
  upper end S52.00- ☑
   coronoid process (displaced) S52.04- ☑
    nondisplaced S52.04- ☑
   olecranon process (displaced) S52.02- ☑
    with intraarticular extension S52.03- ☑
    nondisplaced S52.02- ☑
     with intraarticular extension S52.03- ☑
   specified NEC S52.09- ☑
   torus S52.01- ☑
 unciform — *see* Fracture, carpal, hamate
 vault of skull S02.0 ☑
 vertebra, vertebral (arch) (body) (column) (neural arch)
    (pedicle) (spinous process) (transverse process)
  atlas — *see* Fracture, neck, cervical vertebra, first
  axis — *see* Fracture, neck, cervical vertebra, second
  cervical (teardrop) S12.9 ☑
   axis — *see* Fracture, neck, cervical vertebra, second
   first (atlas) — *see* Fracture, neck, cervical vertebra, first
   second (axis) — *see* Fracture, neck, cervical vertebra, second
  chronic M84.48 ☑
  coccyx S32.2 ☑
  dorsal — *see* Fracture, thorax, vertebra
  lumbar S32.009 ☑
   burst (stable) S32.001 ☑
    unstable S32.002 ☑
   fifth S32.059 ☑
    burst (stable) S32.051 ☑
     unstable S32.052 ☑
    specified type NEC S32.058 ☑
    wedge compression S32.050 ☑
   first S32.019 ☑
    burst (stable) S32.011 ☑
     unstable S32.012 ☑
    specified type NEC S32.018 ☑
    wedge compression S32.010 ☑
   fourth S32.049 ☑
    burst (stable) S32.041 ☑
     unstable S32.042 ☑
    specified type NEC S32.048 ☑
    wedge compression S32.040 ☑
   second S32.029 ☑
    burst (stable) S32.021 ☑
     unstable S32.022 ☑
    specified type NEC S32.028 ☑
    wedge compression S32.020 ☑
   specified type NEC S32.008 ☑

☑ **Additional Character Required** — Refer to the Tabular List for Character Selection      ▽ Subterms under main terms may continue to next column or page

**Fracture, traumatic** — *continued*
  vertebra, vertebral — *continued*
    lumbar — *continued*
      third S32.039 ☑
        burst (stable) S32.031 ☑
          unstable S32.032 ☑
        specified type NEC S32.038 ☑
        wedge compression S32.030 ☑
        wedge compression S32.000 ☑
    metastatic — *see* Collapse, vertebra, in, specified disease NEC (*see also* Neoplasm)
    newborn (birth injury) P11.5
    sacrum S32.10 ☑
      specified NEC S32.19 ☑
      Type
        1 S32.14 ☑
        2 S32.15 ☑
        3 S32.16 ☑
        4 S32.17 ☑
      Zone
        I S32.119 ☑
          displaced (minimally) S32.111 ☑
            severely S32.112 ☑
          nondisplaced S32.110 ☑
        II S32.129 ☑
          displaced (minimally) S32.121 ☑
            severely S32.122 ☑
          nondisplaced S32.120 ☑
        III S32.139 ☑
          displaced (minimally) S32.131 ☑
            severely S32.132 ☑
          nondisplaced S32.130 ☑
    thoracic — *see* Fracture, thorax, vertebra
  vertex S02.0 ☑
  vomer (bone) S02.2 ☑
  wrist S62.10- ☑
    carpal — *see* Fracture, carpal bone
    navicular (scaphoid) (hand) — *see* Fracture, carpal, navicular
  xiphisternum, xiphoid (process) S22.24 ☑
  zygoma S02.402 ☑
    left side S02.40F ☑
    right side S02.40E ☑
**Fragile, fragility**
  autosomal site Q95.5
  bone, congenital (with blue sclera) Q78.0
  capillary (hereditary) D69.8
  hair L67.8
  nails L60.3
  non-sex chromosome site Q95.5
  X chromosome Q99.2
**Fragilitas**
  crinium L67.8
  ossium (with blue sclerae) (hereditary) Q78.0
  unguium L60.3
    congenital Q84.6
**Fragments, cataract** (lens), **following cataract surgery** H59.02- ☑
  retained foreign body — *see* Retained, foreign body fragments (type of)
**Frailty** (frail) R54
  mental R41.81
**Frambesia, frambesial** (tropica) (*see also* Yaws)
  initial lesion or ulcer A66.0
  primary A66.0
**Frambeside**
  gummatous A66.4
  of early yaws A66.2
**Frambesioma** A66.1
**Franceschetti-Klein** (-Wildervanck) **disease or syndrome** Q75.4
**Francis' disease** — *see* Tularemia
**Franklin disease** C88.2
**Frank's essential thrombocytopenia** D69.3
**Fraser's syndrome** Q87.0
**Freckle**(s) L81.2
  malignant melanoma in — *see* Melanoma
  melanotic (Hutchinson's) — *see* Melanoma, in situ
  retinal D49.81
**Frederickson's hyperlipoproteinemia, type**
  I and V E78.3
  IIA E78.00
  IIB and III E78.2
  IV E78.1
**Freeman Sheldon syndrome** Q87.0
**Freezing** (*see also* Effect, adverse, cold) T69.9 ☑

**Freiberg's disease** (infraction of metatarsal head or osteochondrosis) — *see* Osteochondrosis, juvenile, metatarsus
**Frei's disease** A55
**Fremitus, friction, cardiac** R01.2
**Frenum, frenulum**
  external os Q51.828
  tongue (shortening) (congenital) Q38.1
**Frequency micturition** (nocturnal) R35.0
  psychogenic F45.8
**Frey's syndrome**
  auriculotemporal G50.8
  hyperhidrosis L74.52
**Friction**
  burn — *see* Burn, by site
  fremitus, cardiac R01.2
  precordial R01.2
  sounds, chest R09.89
**Friderichsen-Waterhouse syndrome or disease** A39.1
**Friedländer's B** (bacillus) **NEC** (*see also* condition) A49.8
**Friedreich's**
  ataxia G11.1
  combined systemic disease G11.1
  facial hemihypertrophy Q67.4
  sclerosis (cerebellum) (spinal cord) G11.1
**Frigidity** F52.22
**Fröhlich's syndrome** E23.6
**Frontal** (*see also* condition)
  lobe syndrome F07.0
**Frostbite** (superficial) T33.90 ☑
  with
    partial thickness skin loss — *see* Frostbite (superficial), by site
    tissue necrosis T34.90 ☑
  abdominal wall T33.3
    with tissue necrosis T34.3 ☑
  ankle T33.81- ☑
    with tissue necrosis T34.81- ☑
  arm T33.4- ☑
    with tissue necrosis T34.4- ☑
    finger(s) — *see* Frostbite, finger
    hand — *see* Frostbite, hand
    wrist — *see* Frostbite, wrist
  ear T33.01- ☑
    with tissue necrosis T34.01- ☑
  face T33.09 ☑
    with tissue necrosis T34.09 ☑
  finger T33.53- ☑
    with tissue necrosis T34.53- ☑
  foot T33.82- ☑
    with tissue necrosis T34.82- ☑
  hand T33.52- ☑
    with tissue necrosis T34.52- ☑
  head T33.09 ☑
    with tissue necrosis T34.09 ☑
    ear — *see* Frostbite, ear
    nose — *see* Frostbite, nose
  hip (and thigh) T33.6- ☑
    with tissue necrosis T34.6- ☑
  knee T33.7- ☑
    with tissue necrosis T34.7- ☑
  leg T33.9- ☑
    with tissue necrosis T34.9- ☑
    ankle — *see* Frostbite, ankle
    foot — *see* Frostbite, foot
    knee — *see* Frostbite, knee
    lower T33.7- ☑
      with tissue necrosis T34.7- ☑
    thigh — *see* Frostbite, hip
    toe — *see* Frostbite, toe
  limb
    lower T33.99 ☑
      with tissue necrosis T34.99 ☑
    upper — *see* Frostbite, arm
  neck T33.1 ☑
    with tissue necrosis T34.1 ☑
  nose T33.02 ☑
    with tissue necrosis T34.02 ☑
  pelvis T33.3 ☑
    with tissue necrosis T34.3 ☑
  specified site NEC T33.99 ☑
    with tissue necrosis T34.99 ☑
  thigh — *see* Frostbite, hip
  thorax T33.2 ☑
    with tissue necrosis T34.2 ☑
  toes T33.83- ☑

**Frostbite** — *continued*
  toes — *continued*
    with tissue necrosis T34.83- ☑
  trunk T33.99 ☑
    with tissue necrosis T34.99 ☑
  wrist T33.51- ☑
    with tissue necrosis T34.51- ☑
**Frotteurism** F65.81
**Frozen** (*see also* Effect, adverse, cold) T69.9 ☑
  pelvis (female) N94.89
    male K66.8
  shoulder — *see* Capsulitis, adhesive
**Fructokinase deficiency** E74.11
**Fructose 1,6 diphosphatase deficiency** E74.19
**Fructosemia** (benign) (essential) E74.12
**Fructosuria** (benign) (essential) E74.11
**Fuchs'**
  black spot (myopic) (*see also* Myopia, degenerative) H44.2- ☑
  dystrophy (corneal endothelium) H18.51
  heterochromic cyclitis — *see* Cyclitis, Fuchs' heterochromic
**Fucosidosis** E77.1
**Fugue** R68.89
  dissociative F44.1
  hysterical (dissociative) F44.1
  postictal in epilepsy — *see* Epilepsy
  reaction to exceptional stress (transient) F43.0
**Fulminant, fulminating** — *see* condition
**Functional** (*see also* condition)
  bleeding (uterus) N93.8
**Functioning, intellectual, borderline** R41.83
**Fundus** — *see* condition
**Fungemia NOS** B49
**Fungus, fungous**
  cerebral G93.89
  disease NOS B49
  infection — *see* Infection, fungus
**Funiculitis** (acute) (chronic) (endemic) N49.1
  gonococcal (acute) (chronic) A54.23
  tuberculous A18.15
**Funnel**
  breast (acquired) M95.4
    congenital Q67.6
    sequelae (late effect) of rickets E64.3
  chest (acquired) M95.4
    congenital Q67.6
    sequelae (late effect) of rickets E64.3
  pelvis (acquired) M95.5
    with disproportion (fetopelvic) O33.3 ☑
      causing obstructed labor O65.3
    congenital Q74.2
**FUO** (fever of unknown origin) R50.9
**Furfur** L21.0
  microsporon B36.0
**Furrier's lung** J67.8
**Furrowed** K14.5
  nail(s) (transverse) L60.4
    congenital Q84.6
  tongue K14.5
    congenital Q38.3
**Furuncle** L02.92
  abdominal wall L02.221
  ankle — *see* Furuncle, lower limb
  antecubital space — *see* Furuncle, upper limb
  anus K61.0
  arm — *see* Furuncle, upper limb
  auditory canal, external — *see* Abscess, ear, external
  auricle (ear) — *see* Abscess, ear, external
  axilla (region) L02.42- ☑
  back (any part) L02.222
  breast N61.1
  buttock L02.32
  cheek (external) L02.02
  chest wall L02.223
  chin L02.02
  corpus cavernosum N48.21
  ear, external — *see* Abscess, ear, external
  external auditory canal — *see* Abscess, ear, external
  eyelid — *see* Abscess, eyelid
  face L02.02
  femoral (region) — *see* Furuncle, lower limb
  finger — *see* Furuncle, hand
  flank L02.221
  foot L02.62- ☑
  forehead L02.02
  gluteal (region) L02.32

**Furuncle** — *continued*
  groin LØ2.224
  hand LØ2.52- ☑
  head LØ2.821
    face LØ2.Ø2
  hip — *see* Furuncle, lower limb
  kidney — *see* Abscess, kidney
  knee — *see* Furuncle, lower limb
  labium (majus) (minus) N76.4
  lacrimal
    gland — *see* Dacryoadenitis
    passages (duct) (sac) — *see* Inflammation, lacrimal,
      passages, acute
  leg (any part) — *see* Furuncle, lower limb
  lower limb LØ2.42- ☑
  malignant A22.Ø
  mouth K12.2
  navel LØ2.226
  neck LØ2.12
  nose J34.Ø
  orbit, orbital — *see* Abscess, orbit
  palmar (space) — *see* Furuncle, hand
  partes posteriores LØ2.32
  pectoral region LØ2.223
  penis N48.21
  perineum LØ2.225
  pinna — *see* Abscess, ear, external
  popliteal — *see* Furuncle, lower limb
  prepatellar — *see* Furuncle, lower limb
  scalp LØ2.821
  seminal vesicle N49.Ø
  shoulder — *see* Furuncle, upper limb
  specified site NEC LØ2.828
  submandibular K12.2
  temple (region) LØ2.Ø2
  thumb — *see* Furuncle, hand
  toe — *see* Furuncle, foot
  trunk LØ2.229
    abdominal wall LØ2.221
    back LØ2.222

**Furuncle** — *continued*
  trunk — *continued*
    chest wall LØ2.223
    groin LØ2.224
    perineum LØ2.225
    umbilicus LØ2.226
  umbilicus LØ2.226
  upper limb LØ2.42- ☑
  vulva N76.4
**Furunculosis** — *see* Furuncle
**Fused** — *see* Fusion, fused
**Fusion, fused** (congenital)
  astragaloscaphoid Q74.2
  atria Q21.1
  auditory canal Q16.1
  auricles, heart Q21.1
  binocular with defective stereopsis H53.32
  bone Q79.8
  cervical spine M43.22
  choanal Q3Ø.Ø
  commissure, mitral valve Q23.2
  cusps, heart valve NEC Q24.8
    mitral Q23.2
    pulmonary Q22.1
    tricuspid Q22.4
  ear ossicles Q16.3
  fingers Q7Ø.Ø ☑
  hymen Q52.3
  joint (acquired) (*see also* Ankylosis)
    congenital Q74.8
  kidneys (incomplete) Q63.1
  labium (majus) (minus) Q52.5
  larynx and trachea Q34.8
  limb, congenital Q74.8
    lower Q74.2
    upper Q74.Ø
  lobes, lung Q33.8
  lumbosacral (acquired) M43.27
    arthrodesis status Z98.1
    congenital Q76.49

**Fusion, fused** — *continued*
  lumbosacral — *continued*
    postprocedural status Z98.1
  nares, nose, nasal, nostril(s) Q3Ø.Ø
  organ or site not listed — *see* Anomaly, by site
  ossicles Q79.9
    auditory Q16.3
  pulmonic cusps Q22.1
  ribs Q76.6
  sacroiliac (joint) (acquired) M43.28
    arthrodesis status Z98.1
    congenital Q74.2
    postprocedural status Z98.1
  spine (acquired) NEC M43.2Ø
    arthrodesis status Z98.1
    cervical region M43.22
    cervicothoracic region M43.23
    congenital Q76.49
    lumbar M43.26
    lumbosacral region M43.27
    occipito-atlanto-axial region M43.21
    postoperative status Z98.1
    sacrococcygeal region M43.28
    thoracic region M43.24
    thoracolumbar region M43.25
  sublingual duct with submaxillary duct at opening in
    mouth Q38.4
  testes Q55.1
  toes Q7Ø.2- ☑
  tooth, teeth KØØ.2
  trachea and esophagus Q39.8
  twins Q89.4
  vagina Q52.4
  ventricles, heart Q21.Ø
  vertebra (arch) — *see* Fusion, spine
  vulva Q52.5
**Fusospirillosis** (mouth) (tongue) (tonsil) A69.1
**Fussy baby** R68.12

☑ **Additional Character Required** — **Refer to the Tabular List for Character Selection**    🔽 **Subterms under main terms may continue to next column or page**

# G

**Gain in weight** (abnormal) (excessive) (*see also* Weight, gain)
**Gaisböck's disease** (polycythemia hypertonica) D75.1
**Gait abnormality** R26.9
  ataxic R26.0
  falling R29.6
  hysterical (ataxic) (staggering) F44.4
  paralytic R26.1
  spastic R26.1
  specified type NEC R26.89
  staggering R26.0
  unsteadiness R26.81
  walking difficulty NEC R26.2
**Galactocele** (breast) N64.89
  puerperal, postpartum O92.79
**Galactokinase deficiency** E74.29
**Galactophoritis** N61.0
  gestational, puerperal, postpartum O91.2- ☑
**Galactorrhea** O92.6
  not associated with childbirth N64.3
**Galactosemia** (classic) (congenital) E74.21
**Galactosuria** E74.29
**Galacturia** R82.0
  schistosomiasis (bilharziasis) B65.0
**GALD** (gestational alloimmune liver disease) P78.84
**Galeazzi's fracture** S52.37- ☑
**Galen's vein** — *see* condition
**Galeophobia** F40.218
**Gall duct** — *see* condition
**Gallbladder** (*see also* condition)
  acute K81.0
**Gallop rhythm** R00.8
**Gallstone** (colic) (cystic duct) (gallbladder) (impacted) (multiple) (*see also* Calculus, gallbladder)
  with
    cholecystitis — *see* Calculus, gallbladder, with cholecystitis
  bile duct (common) (hepatic) — *see* Calculus, bile duct
  causing intestinal obstruction K56.3
  specified NEC K80.80
    with obstruction K80.81
**Gambling** Z72.6
  pathological (compulsive) F63.0
**Gammopathy** (of undetermined significance [MGUS]) D47.2
  associated with lymphoplasmacytic dyscrasia D47.2
  monoclonal D47.2
  polyclonal D89.0
**Gamna's disease** (siderotic splenomegaly) D73.1
**Gamophobia** F40.298
**Gampsodactylia** (congenital) Q66.7
**Gamstorp's disease** (adynamia episodica hereditaria) G72.3
**Gandy-Nanta disease** (siderotic splenomegaly) D73.1
**Gang**
  membership offenses Z72.810
**Gangliocytoma** D36.10
**Ganglioglioma** — *see* Neoplasm, uncertain behavior, by site
**Ganglion** (compound) (diffuse) (joint) (tendon (sheath)) M67.40
  ankle M67.47- ☑
  foot M67.47- ☑
  forearm M67.43- ☑
  hand M67.44- ☑
  lower leg M67.46- ☑
  multiple sites M67.49
  of yaws (early) (late) A66.6
  pelvic region M67.45- ☑
  periosteal — *see* Periostitis
  shoulder region M67.41- ☑
  specified site NEC M67.48
  thigh region M67.45- ☑
  tuberculous A18.09
  upper arm M67.42- ☑
  wrist M67.43- ☑
**Ganglioneuroblastoma** — *see* Neoplasm, nerve, malignant
**Ganglioneuroma** D36.10
  malignant — *see* Neoplasm, nerve, malignant
**Ganglioneuromatosis** D36.10
**Ganglionitis**
  fifth nerve — *see* Neuralgia, trigeminal
  gasserian (postherpetic) (postzoster) B02.21

**Ganglionitis** — *continued*
  geniculate G51.1
    newborn (birth injury) P11.3
    postherpetic, postzoster B02.21
  herpes zoster B02.21
  postherpetic geniculate B02.21
**Gangliosidosis** E75.10
  GM1 E75.19
  GM2 E75.00
    other specified E75.09
    Sandhoff disease E75.01
    Tay-Sachs disease E75.02
  GM3 E75.19
  mucolipidosis IV E75.11
**Gangosa** A66.5
**Gangrene, gangrenous** (connective tissue) (dropsical) (dry) (moist) (skin) (ulcer) (*see also* Necrosis) I96
  with diabetes (mellitus) — *see* Diabetes, gangrene
  abdomen (wall) I96
  alveolar M27.3
  appendix K35.80
    with
      perforation or rupture K35.2
      peritoneal abscess K35.3
      peritonitis NEC K35.3
        generalized (with perforation or rupture) K35.2
        localized (with perforation or rupture) K35.3
  arteriosclerotic (general) (senile) — *see* Arteriosclerosis, extremities, with, gangrene
  auricle I96
  Bacillus welchii A48.0
  bladder (infectious) — *see* Cystitis, specified type NEC
  bowel, cecum, or colon — *see* Gangrene, intestine
  Clostridium perfringens or welchii A48.0
  cornea H18.89- ☑
  corpora cavernosa N48.29
    noninfective N48.89
  cutaneous, spreading I96
  decubital — *see* Ulcer, pressure, by site
  diabetic (any site) — *see* Diabetes, gangrene
  emphysematous — *see* Gangrene, gas
  epidemic — *see* Poisoning, food, noxious, plant
  epididymis (infectional) N45.1
  erysipelas — *see* Erysipelas
  extremity (lower) (upper) I96
  Fournier N49.3
    female N76.89
  fusospirochetal A69.0
  gallbladder — *see* Cholecystitis, acute
  gas (bacillus) A48.0
    following
      abortion — *see* Abortion by type complicated by infection
      ectopic or molar pregnancy O08.0
  glossitis K14.0
  hernia — *see* Hernia, by site, with gangrene
  intestine, intestinal (hemorrhagic) (massive) (*see also* Infarct, intestine) K55.069
    with
      mesenteric embolism (*see also* Infarct, intestine) K55.069
      obstruction — *see* Obstruction, intestine
  laryngitis J04.0
  limb (lower) (upper) I96
  lung J85.0
    spirochetal A69.8
  lymphangitis I89.1
  Meleney's (synergistic) — *see* Ulcer, skin
  mesentery (*see also* Infarct, intestine) K55.069
    with
      embolism (*see also* Infarct, intestine) K55.069
      intestinal obstruction — *see* Obstruction, intestine
  mouth A69.0
  ovary — *see* Oophoritis
  pancreas — *see* Pancreatitis, acute
  penis N48.29
    noninfective N48.89
  perineum I96
  pharynx (*see also* Pharyngitis)
    Vincent's A69.1
  presenile I73.1
  progressive synergistic — *see* Ulcer, skin
  pulmonary J85.0
  pulpal (dental) K04.1
  quinsy J36
  Raynaud's (symmetric gangrene) I73.01

**Gangrene, gangrenous** — *continued*
  retropharyngeal J39.2
  scrotum N49.3
    noninfective N50.89
  senile (atherosclerotic) — *see* Arteriosclerosis, extremities, with, gangrene
  spermatic cord N49.1
    noninfective N50.89
  spine I96
  spirochetal NEC A69.8
  spreading cutaneous I96
  stomatitis A69.0
  symmetrical I73.01
  testis (infectional) N45.2
    noninfective N44.8
  throat (*see also* Pharyngitis)
    diphtheritic A36.0
    Vincent's A69.1
  thyroid (gland) E07.89
  tooth (pulp) K04.1
  tuberculous NEC — *see* Tuberculosis
  tunica vaginalis N49.1
    noninfective N50.89
  umbilicus I96
  uterus — *see* Endometritis
  uvulitis K12.2
  vas deferens N49.1
    noninfective N50.89
  vulva N76.89
**Ganister disease** J62.8
**Ganser's syndrome** (hysterical) F44.89
**Gardner-Diamond syndrome** (autoerythrocyte sensitization) D69.2
**Gargoylism** E76.01
**Garré's disease, osteitis** (sclerosing), osteomyelitis — *see* Osteomyelitis, specified type NEC
**Garrod's pad, knuckle** M72.1
**Gartner's duct**
  cyst Q52.4
  persistent Q50.6
**Gas** R14.3
  asphyxiation, inhalation, poisoning, suffocation NEC — *see* Table of Drugs and Chemicals
  excessive R14.0
  gangrene A48.0
    following
      abortion — *see* Abortion by type complicated by infection
      ectopic or molar pregnancy O08.0
  on stomach R14.0
  pains R14.1
**Gastralgia** (*see also* Pain, abdominal)
**Gastrectasis** K31.0
  psychogenic F45.8
**Gastric** — *see* condition
**Gastrinoma**
  malignant
    pancreas C25.4
    specified site NEC — *see* Neoplasm, malignant, by site
    unspecified site C25.4
  specified site — *see* Neoplasm, uncertain behavior
  unspecified site D37.9
**Gastritis** (simple) K29.70
  with bleeding K29.71
  acute (erosive) K29.00
    with bleeding K29.01
  alcoholic K29.20
    with bleeding K29.21
  allergic K29.60
    with bleeding K29.61
  atrophic (chronic) K29.40
    with bleeding K29.41
  chronic (antral) (fundal) K29.50
    with bleeding K29.51
    atrophic K29.40
      with bleeding K29.41
    superficial K29.30
      with bleeding K29.31
  dietary counseling and surveillance Z71.3
  due to diet deficiency E63.9
  eosinophilic K52.81
  giant hypertrophic K29.60
    with bleeding K29.61
  granulomatous K29.60
    with bleeding K29.61
  hypertrophic (mucosa) K29.60
    with bleeding K29.61

**Gastritis** — *continued*
nervous F54
spastic K29.60
with bleeding K29.61
specified NEC K29.60
with bleeding K29.61
superficial chronic K29.30
with bleeding K29.31
tuberculous A18.83
viral NEC A08.4
**Gastrocarcinoma** — *see* Neoplasm, malignant, stomach
**Gastrocolic** — *see* condition
**Gastrodisciasis, gastrodiscoidiasis** B66.8
**Gastroduodenitis** K29.90
with bleeding K29.91
virus, viral A08.4
specified type NEC A08.39
**Gastrodynia** — *see* Pain, abdominal
**Gastroenteritis** (acute) (chronic) (noninfectious) (*see also* Enteritis) K52.9
allergic K52.29
with
eosinophilic gastritis or gastroenteritis K52.81
food protein-induced enterocolitis syndrome K52.21
food protein-induced enteropathy K52.22
dietetic (*see also* Gastroenteritis, allergic) K52.29
drug-induced K52.1
due to
Cryptosporidium A07.2
drugs K52.1
food poisoning — *see* Intoxication, foodborne
radiation K52.0
eosinophilic K52.81
epidemic (infectious) A09
food hypersensitivity (*see also* Gastroenteritis, allergic) K52.29
infectious — *see* Enteritis, infectious
influenzal — *see* Influenza, with gastroenteritis
noninfectious K52.9
specified NEC K52.89
rotaviral A08.0
Salmonella A02.0
toxic K52.1
viral NEC A08.4
acute infectious A08.39
type Norwalk A08.11
infantile (acute) A08.39
Norwalk agent A08.11
rotaviral A08.0
severe of infants A08.39
specified type NEC A08.39
**Gastroenteropathy** (*see also* Gastroenteritis) K52.9
acute, due to Norovirus A08.11
acute, due to Norwalk agent A08.11
infectious A09
**Gastroenteroptosis** K63.4
**Gastroesophageal laceration- hemorrhage syndrome** K22.6
**Gastrointestinal** — *see* condition
**Gastrojejunal** — *see* condition
**Gastrojejunitis** (*see also* Enteritis) K52.9
**Gastrojejunocolic** — *see* condition
**Gastroliths** K31.89
**Gastromalacia** K31.89
**Gastroparalysis** K31.84
diabetic — *see* Diabetes, gastroparalysis
**Gastroparesis** K31.84
diabetic — *see* Diabetes, by type, with gastroparesis
**Gastropathy** K31.9
congestive portal K31.89
erythematous K29.70
exudative K90.89
portal hypertensive K31.89
**Gastroptosis** K31.89
**Gastrorrhagia** K92.2
psychogenic F45.8
**Gastroschisis** (congenital) Q79.3
**Gastrospasm** (neurogenic) (reflex) K31.89
neurotic F45.8
psychogenic F45.8
**Gastrostaxis** — *see* Gastritis, with bleeding
**Gastrostenosis** K31.89
**Gastrostomy**
attention to Z43.1
status Z93.1
**Gastrosuccorrhea** (continuous) (intermittent) K31.89
neurotic F45.8

**Gastrosuccorrhea** — *continued*
psychogenic F45.8
**Gatophobia** F40.218
**Gaucher's disease or splenomegaly** (adult) (infantile) E75.22
**Gee** (-Herter)(-Thaysen) **disease** (nontropical sprue) K90.0
**Gélineau's syndrome** G47.419
with cataplexy G47.411
**Gemination, tooth, teeth** K00.2
**Gemistocytoma**
specified site — *see* Neoplasm, malignant, by site
unspecified site C71.9
**General, generalized** — *see* condition
**Genetic**
carrier (status)
cystic fibrosis Z14.1
hemophilia A (asymptomatic) Z14.01
symptomatic Z14.02
specified NEC Z14.8
susceptibility to disease NEC Z15.89
malignant neoplasm Z15.09
breast Z15.01
endometrium Z15.04
ovary Z15.02
prostate Z15.03
specified NEC Z15.09
multiple endocrine neoplasia Z15.81
**Genital** — *see* condition
**Genito-anorectal syndrome** A55
**Genitourinary system** — *see* condition
**Genu**
congenital Q74.1
extrorsum (acquired) (*see also* Deformity, varus, knee)
congenital Q74.1
sequelae (late effect) of rickets E64.3
introrsum (acquired) (*see also* Deformity, valgus, knee)
congenital Q74.1
sequelae (late effect) of rickets E64.3
rachitic (old) E64.3
recurvatum (acquired) (*see also* Deformity, limb, specified type NEC, lower leg)
congenital Q68.2
sequelae (late effect) of rickets E64.3
valgum (acquired) (knock-knee) M21.06- ☑
congenital Q74.1
sequelae (late effect) of rickets E64.3
varum (acquired) (bowleg) M21.16- ☑
congenital Q74.1
sequelae (late effect) of rickets E64.3
**Geographic tongue** K14.1
**Geophagia** — *see* Pica
**Geotrichosis** B48.3
stomatitis B48.3
**Gephyrophobia** F40.242
**Gerbode defect** Q21.0
**GERD** (gastroesophageal reflux disease) K21.9
**Gerhardt's**
disease (erythromelalgia) I73.81
syndrome (vocal cord paralysis) J38.00
bilateral J38.02
unilateral J38.01
**German measles** (*see also* Rubella)
exposure to Z20.4
**Germinoblastoma** (diffuse) C85.9- ☑
follicular C82.9- ☑
**Germinoma** — *see* Neoplasm, malignant, by site
**Gerontoxon** — *see* Degeneration, cornea, senile
**Gerstmann's syndrome** R48.8
developmental F81.2
**Gerstmann-Sträussler-Scheinker syndrome** (GSS) A81.82
**Gestation** (period) (*see also* Pregnancy)
ectopic — *see* Pregnancy, by site
multiple O30.9- ☑
greater than quadruplets — *see* Pregnancy, multiple (gestation), specified NEC
specified NEC — *see* Pregnancy, multiple (gestation), specified NEC
**Gestational**
mammary abscess O91.11- ☑
purulent mastitis O91.11- ☑
subareolar abscess O91.11- ☑
**Ghon tubercle, primary infection** A15.7
**Ghost**
teeth K00.4
vessels (cornea) H16.41- ☑
**Ghoul hand** A66.3

**Gianotti-Crosti disease** L44.4
**Giant**
cell
epulis K06.8
peripheral granuloma K06.8
esophagus, congenital Q39.5
kidney, congenital Q63.3
urticaria T78.3 ☑
hereditary D84.1
**Giardiasis** A07.1
**Gibert's disease or pityriasis** L42
**Giddiness** R42
hysterical F44.89
psychogenic F45.8
**Gierke's disease** (glycogenosis I) E74.01
**Gigantism** (cerebral) (hypophyseal) (pituitary) E22.0
constitutional E34.4
**Gilbert's disease or syndrome** E80.4
**Gilchrist's disease** B40.9
**Gilford-Hutchinson disease** E34.8
**Gilles de la Tourette's disease or syndrome** (motor-verbal tic) F95.2
**Gingivitis** K05.10
acute (catarrhal) K05.00
necrotizing A69.1
nonplaque induced K05.01
plaque induced K05.00
chronic (desquamative) (hyperplastic) (simple marginal) (pregnancy associated) (ulcerative) K05.10
nonplaque induced K05.11
plaque induced K05.10
expulsiva — *see* Periodontitis
necrotizing ulcerative (acute) A69.1
pellagrous E52
acute necrotizing A69.1
Vincent's A69.1
**Gingivoglossitis** K14.0
**Gingivopericementitis** — *see* Periodontitis
**Gingivosis** — *see* Gingivitis, chronic
**Gingivostomatitis** K05.10
herpesviral B00.2
necrotizing ulcerative (acute) A69.1
**Gland, glandular** — *see* condition
**Glanders** A24.0
**Glanzmann** (-Naegeli) **disease or thrombasthenia** D69.1
**Glasgow coma scale**
total score
3-8 R40.243 ☑
9-12 R40.242 ☑
13-15 R40.241 ☑
**Glass-blower's disease** (cataract) — *see* Cataract, specified NEC
**Glaucoma** H40.9
with
increased episcleral venous pressure H40.81- ☑
pseudoexfoliation of lens — *see* Glaucoma, open angle, primary, capsular
absolute H44.51- ☑
angle-closure (primary) H40.20- ☑
acute (attack) (crisis) H40.21- ☑
chronic H40.22- ☑
intermittent H40.23- ☑
residual stage H40.24- ☑
borderline H40.00- ☑
capsular (with pseudoexfoliation of lens) — *see* Glaucoma, open angle, primary, capsular
childhood Q15.0
closed angle — *see* Glaucoma, angle-closure
congenital Q15.0
corticosteroid-induced — *see* Glaucoma, secondary, drugs
hypersecretion H40.82- ☑
in (due to)
amyloidosis E85.4 [H42]
aniridia Q13.1 [H42]
concussion of globe — *see* Glaucoma, secondary, trauma
dislocation of lens — *see* Glaucoma, secondary
disorder of lens NEC — *see* Glaucoma, secondary
drugs — *see* Glaucoma, secondary, drugs
endocrine disease NOS E34.9 [H42]
eye
inflammation — *see* Glaucoma, secondary, inflammation
trauma — *see* Glaucoma, secondary, trauma

**Glaucoma** — continued
  in — continued
    hypermature cataract — see Glaucoma, secondary
    iridocyclitis — see Glaucoma, secondary, inflammation
    lens disorder — see Glaucoma, secondary
    Lowe's syndrome E72.03 [H42]
    metabolic disease NOS E88.9 [H42]
    ocular disorders NEC — see Glaucoma, secondary
    onchocerciasis B73.02
    pupillary block — see Glaucoma, secondary
    retinal vein occlusion — see Glaucoma, secondary
    Rieger's anomaly Q13.81 [H42]
    rubeosis of iris — see Glaucoma, secondary
    tumor of globe — see Glaucoma, secondary
  infantile Q15.0
  low tension — see Glaucoma, open angle, primary, low-tension
  malignant H40.83- ☑
  narrow angle — see Glaucoma, angle-closure
  newborn Q15.0
  noncongestive (chronic) — see Glaucoma, open angle
  nonobstructive — see Glaucoma, open angle
  obstructive (see also Glaucoma, angle-closure)
    due to lens changes — see Glaucoma, secondary
  open angle H40.10- ☑
    primary H40.11- ☑
      capsular (with pseudoexfoliation of lens) H40.14- ☑
      low-tension H40.12- ☑
      pigmentary H40.13- ☑
      residual stage H40.15- ☑
  phacolytic — see Glaucoma, secondary
  pigmentary — see Glaucoma, open angle, primary, pigmentary
  postinfectious — see Glaucoma, secondary, inflammation
  secondary (to) H40.5- ☑
    drugs H40.6- ☑
    inflammation H40.4- ☑
    trauma H40.3- ☑
  simple (chronic) H40.11- ☑
  simplex H40.11- ☑
  specified type NEC H40.89
  suspect H40.00- ☑
  syphilitic A52.71
  traumatic (see also Glaucoma, secondary, trauma)
    newborn (birth injury) P15.3
  tuberculous A18.59
**Glaucomatous flecks** (subcapsular) — see Cataract, complicated
**Glazed tongue** K14.4
**Gleet** (gonococcal) A54.01
**Glénard's disease** K63.4
**Glioblastoma** (multiforme)
  with sarcomatous component
    specified site — see Neoplasm, malignant, by site
    unspecified site C71.9
  giant cell
    specified site — see Neoplasm, malignant, by site
    unspecified site C71.9
  specified site — see Neoplasm, malignant, by site
  unspecified site C71.9
**Glioma** (malignant)
  astrocytic
    specified site — see Neoplasm, malignant, by site
    unspecified site C71.9
  mixed
    specified site — see Neoplasm, malignant, by site
    unspecified site C71.9
  nose Q30.8
  specified site NEC — see Neoplasm, malignant, by site
  subependymal D43.2
    specified site — see Neoplasm, uncertain behavior, by site
    unspecified site D43.2
  unspecified site C71.9
**Gliomatosis cerebri** C71.0
**Glioneuroma** — see Neoplasm, uncertain behavior, by site
**Gliosarcoma**
  specified site — see Neoplasm, malignant, by site
  unspecified site C71.9
**Gliosis** (cerebral) G93.89
  spinal G95.89
**Glisson's disease** — see Rickets
**Globinuria** R82.3

**Globus** (hystericus) F45.8
**Glomangioma** D18.00
  intra-abdominal D18.03
  intracranial D18.02
  skin D18.01
  specified site NEC D18.09
**Glomangiomyoma** D18.00
  intra-abdominal D18.03
  intracranial D18.02
  skin D18.01
  specified site NEC D18.09
**Glomangiosarcoma** — see Neoplasm, connective tissue, malignant
**Glomerular**
  disease in syphilis A52.75
  nephritis — see Glomerulonephritis
**Glomerulitis** — see Glomerulonephritis
**Glomerulonephritis** (see also Nephritis) N05.9
  with
    edema — see Nephrosis
    minimal change N05.0
    minor glomerular abnormality N05.0
  acute N00.9
  chronic N03.9
  crescentic (diffuse) NEC (see also N00-N07 with fourth character .7) N05.7
  dense deposit (see also N00-N07 with fourth character .6) N05.6
  diffuse
    crescentic (see also N00-N07 with fourth character .7) N05.7
    endocapillary proliferative (see also N00-N07 with fourth character .4) N05.4
    membranous (see also N00-N07 with fourth character .2) N05.2
    mesangial proliferative (see also N00-N07 with fourth character .3) N05.3
    mesangiocapillary (see also N00-N07 with fourth character .5) N05.5
    sclerosing N18.9
  endocapillary proliferative (diffuse) NEC (see also N00-N07 with fourth character .4) N05.4
  extracapillary NEC (see also N00-N07 with fourth character .7) N05.7
  focal (and segmental) (see also N00-N07 with fourth character .1) N05.1
  hypocomplementemic — see Glomerulonephritis, membranoproliferative
  IgA — see Nephropathy, IgA
  immune complex (circulating) NEC N05.8
  in (due to)
    amyloidosis E85.4 [N08]
    bilharziasis B65.9 [N08]
    cryoglobulinemia D89.1 [N08]
    defibrination syndrome D65 [N08]
    diabetes mellitus — see Diabetes, glomerulosclerosis
    disseminated intravascular coagulation D65 [N08]
    Fabry (-Anderson) disease E75.21 [N08]
    Goodpasture's syndrome M31.0
    hemolytic-uremic syndrome D59.3
    Henoch (-Schönlein) purpura D69.0 [N08]
    lecithin cholesterol acyltransferase deficiency E78.6 [N08]
    microscopic polyangiitis M31.7 [N08]
    multiple myeloma C90.0- ☑ [N08]
    Plasmodium malariae B52.0
    schistosomiasis B65.9 [N08]
    sepsis A41.9 [N08]
      streptococcal A40- ☑ [N08]
    sickle-cell disorders D57.- ☑ [N08]
    strongyloidiasis B78.9 [N08]
    subacute bacterial endocarditis I33.0 [N08]
    syphilis (late) congenital A50.59 [N08]
    systemic lupus erythematosus M32.14
    thrombotic thrombocytopenic purpura M31.1 [N08]
    typhoid fever A01.09
    Waldenström macroglobulinemia C88.0 [N08]
    Wegener's granulomatosis M31.31
  latent or quiescent N03.9
  lobular, lobulonodular — see Glomerulonephritis, membranoproliferative
  membranoproliferative (diffuse)(type 1 or 3) (see also N00-N07 with fourth character .5) N05.5
    dense deposit (type 2) NEC (see also N00-N07 with fourth character .6) N05.6

**Glomerulonephritis** — continued
  membranous (diffuse) NEC (see also N00-N07 with fourth character .2) N05.2
  mesangial
    IgA/IgG — see Nephropathy, IgA
    proliferative (diffuse) NEC (see also N00-N07 with fourth character .3) N05.3
  mesangiocapillary (diffuse) NEC (see also N00-N07 with fourth character .5) N05.5
  necrotic, necrotizing NEC (see also N00- N07 with fourth character .8) N05.8
  nodular — see Glomerulonephritis, membranoproliferative
  poststreptococcal NEC N05.9
    acute N00.9
    chronic N03.9
    rapidly progressive N01.9
  proliferative NEC (see also N00-N07 with fourth character .8) N05.8
    diffuse (lupus) M32.14
  rapidly progressive N01.9
  sclerosing, diffuse N18.9
  specified pathology NEC (see also N00- N07 with fourth character .8) N05.8
  subacute N01.9
**Glomerulopathy** — see Glomerulonephritis
**Glomerulosclerosis** (see also Sclerosis, renal)
  intercapillary (nodular) (with diabetes) — see Diabetes, glomerulosclerosis
  intracapillary — see Diabetes, glomerulosclerosis
**Glossagra** K14.6
**Glossalgia** K14.6
**Glossitis** (chronic superficial) (gangrenous) (Moeller's) K14.0
  areata exfoliativa K14.1
  atrophic K14.4
  benign migratory K14.1
  cortical superficial, sclerotic K14.0
  Hunter's D51.0
  interstitial, sclerous K14.0
  median rhomboid K14.2
  pellagrous E52
  superficial, chronic K14.0
**Glossocele** K14.8
**Glossodynia** K14.6
  exfoliativa K14.4
**Glossoncus** K14.8
**Glossopathy** K14.9
**Glossophytia** K14.3
**Glossoplegia** K14.8
**Glossoptosis** K14.8
**Glossopyrosis** K14.6
**Glossotrichia** K14.3
**Glossy skin** L90.8
**Glottis** — see condition
**Glottitis** (see also Laryngitis) J04.0
**Glucagonoma**
  pancreas
    benign D13.7
    malignant C25.4
    uncertain behavior D37.8
  specified site NEC
    benign — see Neoplasm, benign, by site
    malignant — see Neoplasm, malignant, by site
    uncertain behavior — see Neoplasm, uncertain behavior, by site
  unspecified site
    benign D13.7
    malignant C25.4
    uncertain behavior D37.8
**Glucoglycinuria** E72.51
**Glucose-galactose malabsorption** E74.39
**Glue**
  ear — see Otitis, media, nonsuppurative, chronic, mucoid
  sniffing (airplane) — see Abuse, drug, inhalant
    dependence — see Dependence, drug, inhalant
**Glutaric aciduria** E72.3
**Glutinemia** E72.51
**Glycinuria** (renal) (with ketosis) E72.09
**Glycogen**
  infiltration — see Disease, glycogen storage
  storage disease — see Disease, glycogen storage
**Glycogenosis** (diffuse) (generalized) (see also Disease, glycogen storage)
  cardiac E74.02 [I43]

**Glycogenosis** — *continued*
  diabetic, secondary — *see* Diabetes, glycogenosis, secondary
  pulmonary interstitial J84.842
**Glycopenia** E16.2
**Glycosuria** R81
  renal E74.8
**Gnathostoma spinigerum** (infection) (infestation), **gnathostomiasis** (wandering swelling) B83.1
**Goiter** (plunging) (substernal) E04.9
  with
    hyperthyroidism (recurrent) — *see* Hyperthyroidism, with, goiter
    thyrotoxicosis — *see* Hyperthyroidism, with, goiter
  adenomatous — *see* Goiter, nodular
  cancerous C73
  congenital (nontoxic) E03.0
    diffuse E03.0
    parenchymatous E03.0
    transitory, with normal functioning P72.0
  cystic E04.2
    due to iodine-deficiency E01.1
  due to
    enzyme defect in synthesis of thyroid hormone E07.1
    iodine-deficiency (endemic) E01.2
  dyshormonogenetic (familial) E07.1
  endemic (iodine-deficiency) E01.2
    diffuse E01.0
    multinodular E01.1
  exophthalmic — *see* Hyperthyroidism, with, goiter
  iodine-deficiency (endemic) E01.2
    diffuse E01.0
    multinodular E01.1
    nodular E01.1
  lingual Q89.2
  lymphadenoid E06.3
  malignant C73
  multinodular (cystic) (nontoxic) E04.2
    toxic or with hyperthyroidism E05.20
      with thyroid storm E05.21
  neonatal NEC P72.0
  nodular (nontoxic) (due to) E04.9
    with
      hyperthyroidism E05.20
        with thyroid storm E05.21
      thyrotoxicosis E05.20
        with thyroid storm E05.21
    endemic E01.1
    iodine-deficiency E01.1
    sporadic E04.9
    toxic E05.20
      with thyroid storm E05.21
  nontoxic E04.9
    diffuse (colloid) E04.0
    multinodular E04.2
    simple E04.0
    specified NEC E04.8
    uninodular E04.1
  simple E04.0
  toxic — *see* Hyperthyroidism, with, goiter
  uninodular (nontoxic) E04.1
    toxic or with hyperthyroidism E05.10
      with thyroid storm E05.11
**Goiter-deafness syndrome** E07.1
**Goldberg syndrome** Q89.8
**Goldberg-Maxwell syndrome** E34.51
**Goldblatt's hypertension or kidney** I70.1
**Goldenhar** (-Gorlin) **syndrome** Q87.0
**Goldflam-Erb disease or syndrome** G70.00
  with exacerbation (acute) G70.01
  in crisis G70.01
**Goldscheider's disease** Q81.8
**Goldstein's disease** (familial hemorrhagic telangiectasia) I78.0
**Golfer's elbow** — *see* Epicondylitis, medial
**Gonadoblastoma**
  specified site — *see* Neoplasm, uncertain behavior, by site
  unspecified site
    female D39.10
    male D40.10
**Gonecystitis** — *see* Vesiculitis
**Gongylonemiasis** B83.8
**Goniosynechiae** — *see* Adhesions, iris, goniosynechiae
**Gonococcemia** A54.86
**Gonococcus, gonococcal** (disease) (infection) (*see also* condition) A54.9

**Gonococcus, gonococcal** — *continued*
  anus A54.6
  bursa, bursitis A54.49
  conjunctiva, conjunctivitis (neonatorum) A54.31
  endocardium A54.83
  eye A54.30
    conjunctivitis A54.31
    iridocyclitis A54.32
    keratitis A54.33
    newborn A54.31
    other specified A54.39
  fallopian tubes (acute) (chronic) A54.24
  genitourinary (organ) (system) (tract) (acute)
    lower A54.00
      with abscess (accessory gland) (periurethral) A54.1
    upper (*see also* condition) A54.29
  heart A54.83
  iridocyclitis A54.32
  joint A54.42
  lymphatic (gland) (node) A54.89
  meninges, meningitis A54.81
  musculoskeletal A54.40
    arthritis A54.42
    osteomyelitis A54.43
    other specified A54.49
    spondylopathy A54.41
  pelviperitonitis A54.24
  pelvis (acute) (chronic) A54.24
  pharynx A54.5
  proctitis A54.6
  pyosalpinx (acute) (chronic) A54.24
  rectum A54.6
  skin A54.89
  specified site NEC A54.89
  tendon sheath A54.49
  throat A54.5
  urethra (acute) (chronic) A54.01
    with abscess (accessory gland) (periurethral) A54.1
  vulva (acute) (chronic) A54.02
**Gonocytoma**
  specified site — *see* Neoplasm, uncertain behavior, by site
  unspecified site
    female D39.10
    male D40.10
**Gonorrhea** (acute) (chronic) A54.9
  Bartholin's gland (acute) (chronic) (purulent) A54.02
    with abscess (accessory gland) (periurethral) A54.1
  bladder A54.01
  cervix A54.03
  conjunctiva, conjunctivitis (neonatorum) A54.31
  contact Z20.2
  Cowper's gland (with abscess) A54.1
  exposure to Z20.2
  fallopian tube (acute) (chronic) A54.24
  kidney (acute) (chronic) A54.21
  lower genitourinary tract A54.00
    with abscess (accessory gland) (periurethral) A54.1
  ovary (acute) (chronic) A54.24
  pelvis (acute) (chronic) A54.24
    female pelvic inflammatory disease A54.24
  penis A54.09
  prostate (acute) (chronic) A54.22
  seminal vesicle (acute) (chronic) A54.23
  specified site not listed (*see also* Gonococcus) A54.89
  spermatic cord (acute) (chronic) A54.23
  urethra A54.01
    with abscess (accessory gland) (periurethral) A54.1
  vagina A54.02
  vas deferens (acute) (chronic) A54.23
  vulva A54.02
**Goodall's disease** A08.19
**Goodpasture's syndrome** M31.0
**Gopalan's syndrome** (burning feet) E53.0
**Gorlin-Chaudry-Moss syndrome** Q87.0
**Gottron's papules** L94.4
**Gougerot-Blum syndrome** (pigmented purpuric lichenoid dermatitis) L81.7
**Gougerot-Carteaud disease or syndrome** (confluent reticulate papillomatosis) L83
**Gougerot's syndrome** (trisymptomatic) L81.7
**Gouley's syndrome** (constrictive pericarditis) I31.1
**Goundou** A66.6
**Gout, chronic** (*see also* Gout, gouty) M1A.9 ☑ (*following* M08)
  drug-induced M1A.20 ☑ (*following* M08)
    ankle M1A.27- ☑ (*following* M08)

**Gout, chronic** — *continued*
  drug-induced — *continued*
    elbow M1A.22- ☑ (*following* M08)
    foot joint M1A.27- ☑ (*following* M08)
    hand joint M1A.24- ☑ (*following* M08)
    hip M1A.25- ☑ (*following* M08)
    knee M1A.26- ☑ (*following* M08)
    multiple site M1A.29- ☑ (*following* M08)
    shoulder M1A.21- ☑ (*following* M08)
    vertebrae M1A.28 ☑ (*following* M08)
    wrist M1A.23- ☑ (*following* M08)
  idiopathic M1A.00 ☑ (*following* M08)
    ankle M1A.07- ☑ (*following* M08)
    elbow M1A.02- ☑ (*following* M08)
    foot joint M1A.07- ☑ (*following* M08)
    hand joint M1A.04- ☑ (*following* M08)
    hip M1A.05- ☑ (*following* M08)
    knee M1A.06- ☑ (*following* M08)
    multiple site M1A.09 ☑ (*following* M08)
    shoulder M1A.01- ☑ (*following* M08)
    vertebrae M1A.08 ☑ (*following* M08)
    wrist M1A.03- ☑ (*following* M08)
  in (due to) renal impairment M1A.30 ☑ (*following* M08)
    ankle M1A.37- ☑ (*following* M08)
    elbow M1A.32- ☑ (*following* M08)
    foot joint M1A.37- ☑ (*following* M08)
    hand joint M1A.34- ☑ (*following* M08)
    hip M1A.35- ☑ (*following* M08)
    knee M1A.36- ☑ (*following* M08)
    multiple site M1A.39 ☑ (*following* M08)
    shoulder M1A.31- ☑ (*following* M08)
    vertebrae M1A.38 ☑ (*following* M08)
    wrist M1A.33- ☑ (*following* M08)
  lead-induced M1A.10 ☑ (*following* M08)
    ankle M1A.17- ☑ (*following* M08)
    elbow M1A.12- ☑ (*following* M08)
    foot joint M1A.17- ☑ (*following* M08)
    hand joint M1A.14- ☑ (*following* M08)
    hip M1A.15- ☑ (*following* M08)
    knee M1A.16- ☑ (*following* M08)
    multiple site M1A.19 ☑ (*following* M08)
    shoulder M1A.11- ☑ (*following* M08)
    vertebrae M1A.18 ☑ (*following* M08)
    wrist M1A.13- ☑ (*following* M08)
  primary — *see* Gout, chronic, idiopathic
  saturnine — *see* Gout, chronic, lead-induced
  secondary NEC M1A.40 ☑ (*following* M08)
    ankle M1A.47- ☑ (*following* M08)
    elbow M1A.42- ☑ (*following* M08)
    foot joint M1A.47- ☑ (*following* M08)
    hand joint M1A.44- ☑ (*following* M08)
    hip M1A.45- ☑ (*following* M08)
    knee M1A.46- ☑ (*following* M08)
    multiple site M1A.49 ☑ (*following* M08)
    shoulder M1A.41- ☑ (*following* M08)
    vertebrae M1A.48 ☑ (*following* M08)
    wrist M1A.43- ☑ (*following* M08)
  syphilitic (*see also* subcategory M14.8-) A52.77
  tophi M1A.9 ☑ (*following* M08)
**Gout, gouty** (acute) (attack) (flare) (*see also* Gout, chronic) M10.9
  drug-induced M10.20
    ankle M10.27- ☑
    elbow M10.22- ☑
    foot joint M10.27- ☑
    hand joint M10.24- ☑
    hip M10.25- ☑
    knee M10.26- ☑
    multiple site M10.29
    shoulder M10.21- ☑
    vertebrae M10.28
    wrist M10.23- ☑
  idiopathic M10.00
    ankle M10.07- ☑
    elbow M10.02- ☑
    foot joint M10.07- ☑
    hand joint M10.04- ☑
    hip M10.05- ☑
    knee M10.06- ☑
    multiple site M10.09
    shoulder M10.01- ☑
    vertebrae M10.08
    wrist M10.03- ☑
  in (due to) renal impairment M10.30
    ankle M10.37- ☑

**Gout, gouty** — *continued*
  in renal impairment — *continued*
    elbow M10.32- ☑
    foot joint M10.37- ☑
    hand joint M10.34- ☑
    hip M10.35- ☑
    knee M10.36- ☑
    multiple site M10.39
    shoulder M10.31- ☑
    vertebrae M10.38
    wrist M10.33- ☑
  lead-induced M10.10
    ankle M10.17- ☑
    elbow M10.12- ☑
    foot joint M10.17- ☑
    hand joint M10.14- ☑
    hip M10.15- ☑
    knee M10.16- ☑
    multiple site M10.19
    shoulder M10.11- ☑
    vertebrae M10.18
    wrist M10.13- ☑
  primary — *see* Gout, idiopathic
  saturnine — *see* Gout, lead-induced
  secondary NEC M10.40
    ankle M10.47- ☑
    elbow M10.42- ☑
    foot joint M10.47- ☑
    hand joint M10.44- ☑
    hip M10.45- ☑
    knee M10.46- ☑
    multiple site M10.49
    shoulder M10.41- ☑
    vertebrae M10.48
    wrist M10.43- ☑
  syphilitic (*see also* subcategory M14.8-) A52.77
  tophi — *see* Gout, chronic
**Gower's**
  muscular dystrophy G71.0
  syndrome (vasovagal attack) R55
**Gradenigo's syndrome** — *see* Otitis, media, suppurative, acute
**Graefe's disease** — *see* Strabismus, paralytic, ophthalmoplegia, progressive
**Graft-versus-host disease** D89.813
  acute D89.810
  acute on chronic D89.812
  chronic D89.811
**Grain mite** (itch) B88.0
**Grainhandler's disease or lung** J67.8
**Grand mal** — *see* Epilepsy, generalized, specified NEC
**Grand multipara status only** (not pregnant) Z64.1
  pregnant — *see* Pregnancy, complicated by, grand multiparity
**Granite worker's lung** J62.8
**Granular** (*see also* condition)
  inflammation, pharynx J31.2
  kidney (contracting) — *see* Sclerosis, renal
  liver K74.69
**Granulation tissue** (abnormal) (excessive) L92.9
  postmastoidectomy cavity — *see* Complications, postmastoidectomy, granulation
**Granulocytopenia** (primary) (malignant) — *see* Agranulocytosis
**Granuloma** L92.9
  abdomen K66.8
    from residual foreign body L92.3
    pyogenicum L98.0
  actinic L57.5
  annulare (perforating) L92.0
  apical K04.5
  aural — *see* Otitis, externa, specified NEC
  beryllium (skin) L92.3
  bone
    eosinophilic C96.6
    from residual foreign body — *see* Osteomyelitis, specified type NEC
    lung C96.6
  brain (any site) G06.0
    schistosomiasis B65.9 [G07]
  canaliculus lacrimalis — *see* Granuloma, lacrimal
  candidal (cutaneous) B37.2
  cerebral (any site) G06.0
  coccidioidal (primary) (progressive) B38.7
    lung B38.1
    meninges B38.4
  colon K63.89

**Granuloma** — *continued*
  conjunctiva H11.22- ☑
  dental K04.5
  ear, middle — *see* Cholesteatoma
  eosinophilic C96.6
    bone C96.6
    lung C96.6
    oral mucosa K13.4
    skin L92.2
  eyelid H01.8
  facial (e) L92.2
  foreign body (in soft tissue) NEC M60.20
    ankle M60.27- ☑
    foot M60.27- ☑
    forearm M60.23- ☑
    hand M60.24- ☑
    in operation wound — *see* Foreign body, accidentally left during a procedure
    lower leg M60.26- ☑
    pelvic region M60.25- ☑
    shoulder region M60.21- ☑
    skin L92.3
    specified site NEC M60.28
    subcutaneous tissue L92.3
    thigh M60.25- ☑
    upper arm M60.22- ☑
  gangraenescens M31.2
  genito-inguinale A58
  giant cell (central) (reparative) (jaw) M27.1
    gingiva (peripheral) K06.8
  gland (lymph) I88.8
  hepatic NEC K75.3
    in (due to)
      berylliosis J63.2 [K77]
      sarcoidosis D86.89
  Hodgkin C81.9 ☑
  ileum K63.89
  infectious B99.9
    specified NEC B99.8
  inguinale (Donovan) (venereal) A58
  intestine NEC K63.89
  intracranial (any site) G06.0
  intraspinal (any part) G06.1
  iridocyclitis — *see* Iridocyclitis, chronic
  jaw (bone) (central) M27.1
    reparative giant cell M27.1
  kidney (*see also* Infection, kidney) N15.8
  lacrimal H04.81- ☑
  larynx J38.7
  lethal midline (faciale(e)) M31.2
  liver NEC — *see* Granuloma, hepatic
  lung (infectious) (*see also* Fibrosis, lung)
    coccidioidal B38.1
    eosinophilic C96.6
  Majocchi's B35.8
  malignant (facial(e)) M31.2
  mandible (central) M27.1
  midline (lethal) M31.2
  monilial (cutaneous) B37.2
  nasal sinus — *see* Sinusitis
  operation wound T81.89 ☑
    foreign body — *see* Foreign body, accidentally left during a procedure
    stitch T81.89 ☑
    talc — *see* Foreign body, accidentally left during a procedure
  oral mucosa K13.4
  orbit, orbital H05.11- ☑
  paracoccidioidal B41.8
  penis, venereal A58
  periapical K04.5
  peritoneum K66.8
    due to ova of helminths NOS (*see also* Helminthiasis) B83.9 [K67]
  postmastoidectomy cavity — *see* Complications, postmastoidectomy, recurrent cholesteatoma
  prostate N42.89
  pudendi (ulcerating) A58
  pulp, internal (tooth) K03.3
  pyogenic, pyogenicum (of) (skin) L98.0
    gingiva K06.8
    maxillary alveolar ridge K04.5
    oral mucosa K13.4
  rectum K62.89
  reticulohistiocytic D76.3
  rubrum nasi L74.8
  Schistosoma — *see* Schistosomiasis
  septic (skin) L98.0

**Granuloma** — *continued*
  silica (skin) L92.3
  sinus (accessory) (infective) (nasal) — *see* Sinusitis
  skin L92.9
    from residual foreign body L92.3
    pyogenicum L98.0
  spine
    syphilitic (epidural) A52.19
    tuberculous A18.01
  stitch (postoperative) T81.89 ☑
  suppurative (skin) L98.0
  swimming pool A31.1
  talc (*see also* Granuloma, foreign body)
    in operation wound — *see* Foreign body, accidentally left during a procedure
  telangiectaticum (skin) L98.0
  tracheostomy J95.09
  trichophyticum B35.8
  tropicum A66.4
  umbilical P83.81
  umbilicus P83.81
  urethra N36.8
  uveitis — *see* Iridocyclitis, chronic
  vagina A58
  venereum A58
  vocal cord J38.3
**Granulomatosis** L92.9
  lymphoid C83.8- ☑
  miliary (listerial) A32.89
  necrotizing, respiratory M31.30
  progressive septic D71
  specified NEC L92.8
  Wegener's M31.30
    with renal involvement M31.31
**Granulomatous tissue** (abnormal) (excessive) L92.9
**Granulosis rubra nasi** L74.8
**Graphite fibrosis** (of lung) J63.3
**Graphospasm** F48.8
  organic G25.89
**Grating scapula** M89.8X1
**Gravel** (urinary) — *see* Calculus, urinary
**Graves' disease** — *see* Hyperthyroidism, with, goiter
**Gravis** — *see* condition
**Grawitz tumor** C64.- ☑
**Gray syndrome** (newborn) P93.0
**Grayness, hair** (premature) L67.1
  congenital Q84.2
**Green sickness** D50.8
**Greenfield's disease**
  meaning
    concentric sclerosis (encephalitis periaxialis concentrica) G37.5
    metachromatic leukodystrophy E75.25
**Greenstick fracture** — *code as* Fracture, by site
**Grey syndrome** (newborn) P93.0
**Grief** F43.21
  prolonged F43.29
  reaction (*see also* Disorder, adjustment) F43.20
**Griesinger's disease** B76.9
**Grinder's lung or pneumoconiosis** J62.8
**Grinding, teeth**
  psychogenic F45.8
  sleep related G47.63
**Grip**
  Dabney's B33.0
  devil's B33.0
**Grippe, grippal** (*see also* Influenza)
  Balkan A78
  summer, of Italy A93.1
**Grisel's disease** M43.6
**Groin** — *see* condition
**Grooved tongue** K14.5
**Ground itch** B76.9
**Grover's disease or syndrome** L11.1
**Growing pains, children** R29.898
**Growth** (fungoid) (neoplastic) (new) (*see also* Neoplasm)
  adenoid (vegetative) J35.8
  benign — *see* Neoplasm, benign, by site
  malignant — *see* Neoplasm, malignant, by site
  rapid, childhood Z00.2
  secondary — *see* Neoplasm, secondary, by site
**Gruby's disease** B35.0
**Gubler-Millard paralysis or syndrome** G46.3
**Guerin-Stern syndrome** Q74.3
**Guidance, insufficient anterior** (occlusal) M26.54
**Guillain-Barré disease or syndrome** G61.0
  sequelae G65.0

**Guinea worms** (infection) (infestation) B72
**Guinon's disease** (motor-verbal tic) F95.2
**Gull's disease** E03.4
**Gum** — *see* condition
**Gumboil** K04.7
  with sinus K04.6
**Gumma** (syphilitic) A52.79
  artery A52.09
    cerebral A52.04
  bone A52.77
    of yaws (late) A66.6
  brain A52.19
  cauda equina A52.19
  central nervous system A52.3
  ciliary body A52.71
  congenital A50.59
  eyelid A52.71
  heart A52.06
  intracranial A52.19
  iris A52.71
  kidney A52.75
  larynx A52.73
  leptomeninges A52.19
  liver A52.74
  meninges A52.19
  myocardium A52.06
  nasopharynx A52.73
  neurosyphilitic A52.3
  nose A52.73
  orbit A52.71
  palate (soft) A52.79
  penis A52.76
  pericardium A52.06
  pharynx A52.73
  pituitary A52.79
  scrofulous (tuberculous) A18.4
  skin A52.79
  specified site NEC A52.79
  spinal cord A52.19
  tongue A52.79
  tonsil A52.73
  trachea A52.73
  tuberculous A18.4
  ulcerative due to yaws A66.4
  ureter A52.75
  yaws A66.4
    bone A66.6
**Gunn's syndrome** Q07.8
**Gunshot wound** (*see also* Wound, open)
  fracture — *code as* Fracture, by site
  internal organs — *see* Injury, by site
**Gynandrism** Q56.0
**Gynandroblastoma**
  specified site — *see* Neoplasm, uncertain behavior, by site
  unspecified site
    female D39.10
    male D40.10
**Gynecological examination** (periodic) (routine) Z01.419
  with abnormal findings Z01.411
**Gynecomastia** N62
**Gynephobia** F40.291
**Gyrate scalp** Q82.8

# H

**H** (Hartnup's) **disease** E72.02
**Haas' disease or osteochondrosis** (juvenile) (head of humerus) — *see* Osteochondrosis, juvenile, humerus
**Habit, habituation**
  bad sleep Z72.821
  chorea F95.8
  disturbance, child F98.9
  drug — *see* Dependence, drug
  irregular sleep Z72.821
  laxative F55.2
  spasm — *see* Tic
  tic — *see* Tic
**Haemophilus** (H.) **influenzae, as cause of disease classified elsewhere** B96.3
**Haff disease** — *see* Poisoning, mercury
**Hageman's factor defect, deficiency or disease** D68.2
**Haglund's disease or osteochondrosis** (juvenile) (os tibiale externum) — *see* Osteochondrosis, juvenile, tarsus
**Hailey-Hailey disease** Q82.8

**Hair** (*see also* condition)
  plucking F63.3
    in stereotyped movement disorder F98.4
  tourniquet syndrome (*see also* Constriction, external, by site)
    finger S60.44- ☑
    penis S30.842 ☑
    thumb S60.34- ☑
    toe S90.44- ☑
**Hairball in stomach** T18.2 ☑
**Hair-pulling, pathological** (compulsive) F63.3
**Hairy black tongue** K14.3
**Half vertebra** Q76.49
**Halitosis** R19.6
**Hallerman-Streiff syndrome** Q87.0
**Hallervorden-Spatz disease** G23.0
**Hallopeau's acrodermatitis or disease** L40.2
**Hallucination** R44.3
  auditory R44.0
  gustatory R44.2
  olfactory R44.2
  specified NEC R44.2
  tactile R44.2
  visual R44.1
**Hallucinosis** (chronic) F28
  alcoholic (acute) F10.951
    in
      abuse F10.151
      dependence F10.251
  drug-induced F19.951
    cannabis F12.951
    cocaine F14.951
    hallucinogen F16.151
    in
      abuse F19.151
        cannabis F12.151
        cocaine F14.151
        hallucinogen F16.151
        inhalant F18.151
        opioid F11.151
        sedative, anxiolytic or hypnotic F13.151
        stimulant NEC F15.151
      dependence F19.251
        cannabis F12.251
        cocaine F14.251
        hallucinogen F16.251
        inhalant F18.251
        opioid F11.251
        sedative, anxiolytic or hypnotic F13.251
        stimulant NEC F15.251
    inhalant F18.951
    opioid F11.951
    sedative, anxiolytic or hypnotic F13.951
    stimulant NEC F15.951
  organic F06.0
**Hallux**
  deformity (acquired) NEC M20.5X- ☑
  limitus M20.5X- ☑
  malleus (acquired) NEC M20.3- ☑
  rigidus (acquired) M20.2- ☑
    congenital Q74.2
    sequelae (late effect) of rickets E64.3
  valgus (acquired) M20.1- ☑
    congenital Q66.6
  varus (acquired) M20.3- ☑
    congenital Q66.3
**Halo, visual** H53.19
**Hamartoma, hamartoblastoma** Q85.9
  epithelial (gingival), odontogenic, central or peripheral — *see* Cyst, calcifying odontogenic
**Hamartosis** Q85.9
**Hamman-Rich syndrome** J84.114
**Hammer toe** (acquired) NEC (*see also* Deformity, toe, hammer toe)
  congenital Q66.89
  sequelae (late effect) of rickets E64.3
**Hand** — *see* condition
**Hand-foot syndrome** L27.1
**Handicap, handicapped**
  educational Z55.9
    specified NEC Z55.8
**Hand-Schüller-Christian disease or syndrome** C96.5
**Hanging** (asphyxia) (strangulation) (suffocation) — *see* Asphyxia, traumatic, due to mechanical threat
**Hangnail** (*see also* Cellulitis, digit)
  with lymphangitis — *see* Lymphangitis, acute, digit
**Hangover** (alcohol) F10.129

**Hanhart's syndrome** Q87.0
**Hanot-Chauffard** (-Troisier) **syndrome** E83.19
**Hanot's cirrhosis or disease** K74.3
**Hansen's disease** — *see* Leprosy
**Hantaan virus disease** (Korean hemorrhagic fever) A98.5
**Hantavirus disease** (with renal manifestations) (Dobrava) (Puumala) (Seoul) A98.5
  with pulmonary manifestations (Andes) (Bayou) (Bermejo) (Black Creek Canal) (Choclo) (Juquitiba) (Laguna negra) (Lechiguanas) (New York) (Oran) (Sin nombre) B33.4
**Happy puppet syndrome** Q93.5
**Harada's disease or syndrome** H30.81- ☑
**Hardening**
  artery — *see* Arteriosclerosis
  brain G93.89
**Harelip** (complete) (incomplete) — *see* Cleft, lip
**Harlequin** (newborn) Q80.4
**Harley's disease** D59.6
**Harmful use** (of)
  alcohol F10.10
  anxiolytics — *see* Abuse, drug, sedative
  cannabinoids — *see* Abuse, drug, cannabis
  cocaine — *see* Abuse, drug, cocaine
  drug — *see* Abuse, drug
  hallucinogens — *see* Abuse, drug, hallucinogen
  hypnotics — *see* Abuse, drug, sedative
  opioids — *see* Abuse, drug, opioid
  PCP (phencyclidine) — *see* Abuse, drug, hallucinogen
  sedatives — *see* Abuse, drug, sedative
  stimulants NEC — *see* Abuse, drug, stimulant
**Harris' lines** — *see* Arrest, epiphyseal
**Hartnup's disease** E72.02
**Harvester's lung** J67.0
**Harvesting ovum for in vitro fertilization** Z31.83
**Hashimoto's disease or thyroiditis** E06.3
**Hashitoxicosis** (transient) E06.3
**Hassal-Henle bodies or warts** (cornea) H18.49
**Haut mal** — *see* Epilepsy, generalized, specified NEC
**Haverhill fever** A25.1
**Hay fever** (*see also* Fever, hay) J30.1
**Hayem-Widal syndrome** D59.8
**Haygarth's nodes** M15.8
**Haymaker's lung** J67.0
**Hb** (abnormal)
  Bart's disease D56.0
  disease — *see* Disease, hemoglobin
  trait — *see* Trait
**Head** — *see* condition
**Headache** R51
  allergic NEC G44.89
  associated with sexual activity G44.82
  chronic daily R51
  cluster G44.009
    chronic G44.029
      intractable G44.021
      not intractable G44.029
    episodic G44.019
      intractable G44.011
      not intractable G44.019
    intractable G44.001
    not intractable G44.009
  cough (primary) G44.83
  daily chronic R51
  drug-induced NEC G44.40
    intractable G44.41
    not intractable G44.40
  exertional (primary) G44.84
  histamine G44.009
    intractable G44.001
    not intractable G44.009
  hypnic G44.81
  lumbar puncture G97.1
  medication overuse G44.40
    intractable G44.41
    not intractable G44.40
  menstrual — *see* Migraine, menstrual
  migraine (type) (*see also* Migraine) G43.909
  nasal septum R51
  neuralgiform, short lasting unilateral, with conjunctival injection and tearing (SUNCT) G44.059
    intractable G44.051
    not intractable G44.059
  new daily persistent (NDPH) G44.52
  orgasmic G44.82
  periodic syndromes in adults and children G43.C0 (*following* G43.7)

☑ **Additional Character Required** — Refer to the Tabular List for Character Selection    ▽ **Subterms under main terms may continue to next column or page**

**Headache** — *continued*
  periodic syndromes in adults and children — *continued*
    with refractory migraine G43.C1 (*following* G43.7)
    without refractory migraine G43.C0 (*following* G43.7)
    intractable G43.C1 (*following* G43.7)
    not intractable G43.C0 (*following* G43.7)
  postspinal puncture G97.1
  post-traumatic G44.309
    acute G44.319
      intractable G44.311
      not intractable G44.319
    chronic G44.329
      intractable G44.321
      not intractable G44.329
    intractable G44.301
    not intractable G44.309
  pre-menstrual — *see* Migraine, menstrual
  preorgasmic G44.82
  primary
    cough G44.83
    exertional G44.84
    stabbing G44.85
    thunderclap G44.53
  rebound G44.40
    intractable G44.41
    not intractable G44.40
  short lasting unilateral neuralgiform, with conjunctival injection and tearing (SUNCT) G44.059
    intractable G44.051
    not intractable G44.059
  specified syndrome NEC G44.89
  spinal and epidural anesthesia - induced T88.59 ☑
    in labor and delivery O74.5
    in pregnancy O29.4- ☑
    postpartum, puerperal O89.4
  spinal fluid loss (from puncture) G97.1
  stabbing (primary) G44.85
  tension (-type) G44.209
    chronic G44.229
      intractable G44.221
      not intractable G44.229
    episodic G44.219
      intractable G44.211
      not intractable G44.219
    intractable G44.201
    not intractable G44.209
  thunderclap (primary) G44.53
  vascular NEC G44.1
**Healthy**
  infant
    accompanying sick mother Z76.3
    receiving care Z76.2
  person accompanying sick person Z76.3
**Hearing examination** Z01.10
  with abnormal findings NEC Z01.118
  following failed hearing screening Z01.110
  for hearing conservation and treatment Z01.12
**Heart** — *see* condition
**Heart beat**
  abnormality R00.9
    specified NEC R00.8
  awareness R00.2
  rapid R00.0
  slow R00.1
**Heartburn** R12
  psychogenic F45.8
**Heartland virus disease** A93.8
**Heat** (effects) T67.9 ☑
  apoplexy T67.0 ☑
  burn (*see also* Burn) L55.9
  collapse T67.1 ☑
  cramps T67.2 ☑
  dermatitis or eczema L59.0
  edema T67.7 ☑
  erythema — *code by site under* Burn, first degree
  excessive T67.9 ☑
    specified effect NEC T67.8 ☑
  exhaustion T67.5 ☑
    anhydrotic T67.3 ☑
    due to
      salt (and water) depletion T67.4 ☑
      water depletion T67.3 ☑
        with salt depletion T67.4 ☑
  fatigue (transient) T67.6 ☑
  fever T67.0 ☑
  hyperpyrexia T67.0 ☑

**Heat** — *continued*
  prickly L74.0
  prostration — *see* Heat, exhaustion
  pyrexia T67.0 ☑
  rash L74.0
  specified effect NEC T67.8 ☑
  stroke T67.0 ☑
  sunburn — *see* Sunburn
  syncope T67.1 ☑
**Heavy-for-dates NEC** (infant) (4000g to 4499g) P08.1
  exceptionally (4500g or more) P08.0
**Hebephrenia, hebephrenic** (schizophrenia) F20.1
**Heberden's disease or nodes** (with arthropathy) M15.1
**Hebra's**
  pityriasis L26
  prurigo L28.2
**Heel** — *see* condition
**Heerfordt's disease** D86.89
**Hegglin's anomaly or syndrome** D72.0
**Heilmeyer-Schoner disease** D45
**Heine-Medin disease** A80.9
**Heinz body anemia, congenital** D58.2
**Heliophobia** F40.228
**Heller's disease or syndrome** F84.3
**HELLP syndrome** (hemolysis, elevated liver enzymes and low platelet count) O14.2- ☑
  complicating
    childbirth O14.24
    puerperium O14.25
**Helminthiasis** (*see also* Infestation, helminth)
  Ancylostoma B76.0
  intestinal B82.0
    mixed types (types classifiable to more than one of the titles B65.0-B81.3 and B81.8) B81.4
    specified type NEC B81.8
  mixed types (intestinal) (types classifiable to more than one of the titles B65.0-B81.3 and B81.8) B81.4
  Necator (americanus) B76.1
  specified type NEC B83.8
**Heloma** L84
**Hemangioblastoma** — *see* Neoplasm, connective tissue, uncertain behavior
  malignant — *see* Neoplasm, connective tissue, malignant
**Hemangioendothelioma** (*see also* Neoplasm, uncertain behavior, by site)
  benign D18.00
    intra-abdominal D18.03
    intracranial D18.02
    skin D18.01
    specified site NEC D18.09
  bone (diffuse) — *see* Neoplasm, bone, malignant
  epithelioid (*see also* Neoplasm, uncertain behavior, by site)
    malignant — *see* Neoplasm, malignant, by site
  malignant — *see* Neoplasm, connective tissue, malignant
**Hemangiofibroma** — *see* Neoplasm, benign, by site
**Hemangiolipoma** — *see* Lipoma
**Hemangioma** D18.00
  arteriovenous D18.00
    intra-abdominal D18.03
    intracranial D18.02
    skin D18.01
    specified site NEC D18.09
  capillary D18.00
    intra-abdominal D18.03
    intracranial D18.02
    skin D18.01
    specified site NEC D18.09
  cavernous D18.00
    intra-abdominal D18.03
    intracranial D18.02
    skin D18.01
    specified site NEC D18.09
  epithelioid D18.00
    intra-abdominal D18.03
    intracranial D18.02
    skin D18.01
    specified site NEC D18.09
  histiocytoid D18.00
    intra-abdominal D18.03
    intracranial D18.02
    skin D18.01
    specified site NEC D18.09
  infantile D18.00
    intra-abdominal D18.03

**Hemangioma** — *continued*
  infantile — *continued*
    intracranial D18.02
    skin D18.01
    specified site NEC D18.09
  intra-abdominal D18.03
  intracranial D18.02
  intramuscular D18.00
    intra-abdominal D18.03
    intracranial D18.02
    skin D18.01
    specified site NEC D18.09
  intrathoracic structures D18.09
  juvenile D18.00
  malignant — *see* Neoplasm,connective tissue, malignant
  plexiform D18.00
    intra-abdominal D18.03
    intracranial D18.02
    skin D18.01
    specified site NEC D18.09
  racemose D18.00
    intra-abdominal D18.03
    intracranial D18.02
    skin D18.01
    specified site NEC D18.09
  sclerosing — *see* Neoplasm, skin, benign
  simplex D18.00
    intra-abdominal D18.03
    intracranial D18.02
    skin D18.01
    specified site NEC D18.09
  skin D18.01
  specified site NEC D18.09
  venous D18.00
    intra-abdominal D18.03
    intracranial D18.02
    skin D18.01
    specified site NEC D18.09
  verrucous keratotic D18.00
    intra-abdominal D18.03
    intracranial D18.02
    skin D18.01
    specified site NEC D18.09
**Hemangiomatosis** (systemic) I78.8
  involving single site — *see* Hemangioma
**Hemangiopericytoma** (*see also* Neoplasm, connective tissue, uncertain behavior)
  benign — *see* Neoplasm, connective tissue, benign
  malignant — *see* Neoplasm, connective tissue, malignant
**Hemangiosarcoma** — *see* Neoplasm, connective tissue, malignant
**Hemarthrosis** (nontraumatic) M25.00
  ankle M25.07- ☑
  elbow M25.02- ☑
  foot joint M25.07- ☑
  hand joint M25.04- ☑
  hip M25.05- ☑
  in hemophilic arthropathy — *see* Arthropathy, hemophilic
  knee M25.06- ☑
  shoulder M25.01- ☑
  specified joint NEC M25.08
  traumatic — *see* Sprain, by site
  vertebrae M25.08
  wrist M25.03- ☑
**Hematemesis** K92.0
  with ulcer — *code by site under* Ulcer, with hemorrhage K27.4
  newborn, neonatal P54.0
    due to swallowed maternal blood P78.2
**Hematidrosis** L74.8
**Hematinuria** (*see also* Hemoglobinuria)
  malarial B50.8
**Hematobilia** K83.8
**Hematocele**
  female NEC N94.89
    with ectopic pregnancy O00.90
      with intrauterine pregnancy O00.91
    ovary N83.8
  male N50.1
**Hematochezia** (*see also* Melena) K92.1
**Hematochyluria** (*see also* Infestation, filarial)
  schistosomiasis (bilharziasis) B65.0
**Hematocolpos** (with hematometra or hematosalpinx) N89.7
**Hematocornea** — *see* Pigmentation, cornea, stromal

**Hematogenous** — *see* condition
**Hematoma** (traumatic) (skin surface intact) (*see also*
  Contusion)
  with
    injury of internal organs — *see* Injury, by site
    open wound — *see* Wound, open
  amputation stump (surgical) (late) T87.89
  aorta, dissecting I71.00
    abdominal I71.02
    thoracic I71.01
    thoracoabdominal I71.03
  aortic intramural — *see* Dissection, aorta
  arterial (complicating trauma) — *see* Injury, blood
    vessel, by site
  auricle — *see* Contusion, ear
    nontraumatic — *see* Disorder, pinna, hematoma
  birth injury NEC P15.8
  brain (traumatic)
    with
      cerebral laceration or contusion (diffuse) — *see*
        Injury, intracranial, diffuse
        focal — *see* Injury, intracranial, focal
    cerebellar, traumatic S06.37- ☑
    intracerebral, traumatic — *see* Injury, intracranial,
      intracerebral hemorrhage
    newborn NEC P52.4
      birth injury P10.1
    nontraumatic — *see* Hemorrhage, intracranial
    subarachnoid, arachnoid, traumatic — *see* Injury,
      intracranial, subarachnoid hemorrhage
    subdural, traumatic — *see* Injury, intracranial,
      subdural hemorrhage
  breast (nontraumatic) N64.89
  broad ligament (nontraumatic) N83.7
    traumatic S37.892 ☑
  cerebellar, traumatic S06.37- ☑
  cerebral — *see* Hematoma, brain
  cerebrum S06.36- ☑
    left S06.35- ☑
    right S06.34- ☑
  cesarean delivery wound O90.2
  complicating delivery (perineal) (pelvic) (vagina) (vul-
    va) O71.7
  corpus cavernosum (nontraumatic) N48.89
  epididymis (nontraumatic) N50.1
  epidural (traumatic) — *see* Injury, intracranial, epidural
    hemorrhage
    spinal — *see* Injury, spinal cord, by region
  episiotomy O90.2
  face, birth injury P15.4
  genital organ NEC (nontraumatic)
    female (nonobstetric) N94.89
      traumatic S30.202 ☑
    male N50.1
      traumatic S30.201 ☑
  internal organs — *see* Injury, by site
  intracerebral, traumatic — *see* Injury, intracranial, in-
    tracerebral hemorrhage
  intraoperative — *see* Complications, intraoperative,
    hemorrhage
  labia (nontraumatic) (nonobstetric) N90.89
  liver (subcapsular) (nontraumatic) K76.89
    birth injury P15.0
  mediastinum — *see* Injury, intrathoracic
  mesosalpinx (nontraumatic) N83.7
    traumatic S37.898 ☑
  muscle — code by site under Contusion
  nontraumatic
    muscle M79.81
    soft tissue M79.81
  obstetrical surgical wound O90.2
  orbit, orbital (nontraumatic) (*see also* Hemorrhage,
    orbit)
    traumatic — *see* Contusion, orbit
  pelvis (female) (nontraumatic) (nonobstetric) N94.89
    obstetric O71.7
    traumatic — *see* Injury, by site
  penis (nontraumatic) N48.89
    birth injury P15.5
  perianal (nontraumatic) K64.5
  perineal S30.23 ☑
    complicating delivery O71.7
  perirenal — *see* Injury, kidney
  pinna — *see* Contusion, ear
    nontraumatic — *see* Disorder, pinna, hematoma
  placenta O43.89- ☑

**Hematoma** — *continued*
  postoperative (postprocedural) — *see* Complication,
    postprocedural, hematoma
  retroperitoneal (nontraumatic) K66.1
    traumatic S36.892 ☑
  scrotum, superficial S30.22 ☑
    birth injury P15.5
  seminal vesicle (nontraumatic) N50.1
    traumatic S37.892 ☑
  spermatic cord (traumatic) S37.892 ☑
    nontraumatic N50.1
  spinal (cord) (meninges) (*see also* Injury, spinal cord,
    by region)
    newborn (birth injury) P11.5
  spleen D73.5
    intraoperative — *see* Complications, intraoperative,
      hemorrhage, spleen
    postprocedural (postoperative) — *see* Complica-
      tions, postprocedural, hemorrhage, spleen
  sternocleidomastoid, birth injury P15.2
  sternomastoid, birth injury P15.2
  subarachnoid (traumatic) — *see* Injury, intracranial,
    subarachnoid hemorrhage
    newborn (nontraumatic) P52.5
      due to birth injury P10.3
    nontraumatic — *see* Hemorrhage, intracranial,
      subarachnoid
  subdural (traumatic) — *see* Injury, intracranial, subdu-
    ral hemorrhage
    newborn (localized) P52.8
      birth injury P10.0
    nontraumatic — *see* Hemorrhage, intracranial,
      subdural
  superficial, newborn P54.5
  testis (nontraumatic) N50.1
    birth injury P15.5
  tunica vaginalis (nontraumatic) N50.1
  umbilical cord, complicating delivery O69.5 ☑
  uterine ligament (broad) (nontraumatic) N83.7
    traumatic S37.892 ☑
  vagina (ruptured) (nontraumatic) N89.8
    complicating delivery O71.7
  vas deferens (nontraumatic) N50.1
    traumatic S37.892 ☑
  vitreous — *see* Hemorrhage, vitreous
  vulva (nontraumatic) (nonobstetric) N90.89
    complicating delivery O71.7
    newborn (birth injury) P15.5
**Hematometra** N85.7
  with hematocolpos N89.7
**Hematomyelia** (central) G95.19
  newborn (birth injury) P11.5
  traumatic T14.8 ☑
**Hematomyelitis** G04.90
**Hematoperitoneum** — *see* Hemoperitoneum
**Hematophobia** F40.230
**Hematopneumothorax** (see Hemothorax)
**Hematopoiesis, cyclic** D70.4
**Hematoporphyria** — *see* Porphyria
**Hematorachis, hematorrhachis** G95.19
  newborn (birth injury) P11.5
**Hematosalpinx** N83.6
  with
    hematocolpos N89.7
    hematometra N85.7
      with hematocolpos N89.7
  infectional — *see* Salpingitis
**Hematospermia** R36.1
**Hematothorax** (see Hemothorax)
**Hematuria** R31.9
  benign (familial) (of childhood) (*see also* Hematuria,
    idiopathic)
    essential microscopic R31.1
  due to sulphonamide, sulfonamide — *see* Table of
    Drugs and Chemicals, by drug
  endemic (*see also* Schistosomiasis) B65.0
  gross R31.0
  idiopathic N02.9
    with glomerular lesion
      crescentic (diffuse) glomerulonephritis N02.7
      dense deposit disease N02.6
      endocapillary proliferative glomerulonephritis
        N02.4
      focal and segmental hyalinosis or sclerosis
        N02.1
      membranoproliferative (diffuse) N02.5
      membranous (diffuse) N02.2
      mesangial proliferative (diffuse) N02.3

**Hematuria** — *continued*
  idiopathic — *continued*
    with glomerular lesion — *continued*
      mesangiocapillary (diffuse) N02.5
      minor abnormality N02.0
      proliferative NEC N02.8
      specified pathology NEC N02.8
  intermittent — *see* Hematuria, idiopathic
  malarial B50.8
  microscopic NEC (with symptoms) R31.29
    asymptomatic R31.21
    benign essential R31.1
  paroxysmal (*see also* Hematuria, idiopathic)
    nocturnal D59.5
  persistent — *see* Hematuria, idiopathic
  recurrent — *see* Hematuria, idiopathic
  tropical (*see also* Schistosomiasis) B65.0
  tuberculous A18.13
**Hemeralopia** (day blindness) H53.11
  vitamin A deficiency E50.5
**Hemi-akinesia** R41.4
**Hemianalgesia** R20.0
**Hemianencephaly** Q00.0
**Hemianesthesia** R20.0
**Hemianopia, hemianopsia** (heteronymous) H53.47
  homonymous H53.46- ☑
  syphilitic A52.71
**Hemiathetosis** R25.8
**Hemiatrophy** R68.89
  cerebellar G31.9
  face, facial, progressive (Romberg) G51.8
  tongue K14.8
**Hemiballism** (us) G25.5
**Hemicardia** Q24.8
**Hemicephalus, hemicephaly** Q00.0
**Hemichorea** G25.5
**Hemicolitis, left** — *see* Colitis, left sided
**Hemicrania**
  congenital malformation Q00.0
  continua G44.51
  meaning migraine (*see also* Migraine) G43.909
  paroxysmal G44.039
    chronic G44.049
      intractable G44.041
      not intractable G44.049
    episodic G44.039
      intractable G44.031
      not intractable G44.039
    intractable G44.031
    not intractable G44.039
**Hemidystrophy** — *see* Hemiatrophy
**Hemiectromelia** Q73.8
**Hemihypalgesia** R20.8
**Hemihypesthesia** R20.1
**Hemi-inattention** R41.4
**Hemimelia** Q73.8
  lower limb — *see* Defect, reduction, lower limb, spec-
    ified type NEC
  upper limb — *see* Defect, reduction, upper limb,
    specified type NEC
**Hemiparalysis** — *see* Hemiplegia
**Hemiparesis** — *see* Hemiplegia
**Hemiparesthesia** R20.2
**Hemiparkinsonism** G20
**Hemiplegia** G81.9- ☑
  alternans facialis G83.89
  ascending NEC G81.90
    spinal G95.89
  congenital (cerebral) G80.8
    spastic G80.2
  embolic (current episode) I63.4- ☑
  flaccid G81.0- ☑
  following
    cerebrovascular disease I69.959
      cerebral infarction I69.35- ☑
      intracerebral hemorrhage I69.15- ☑
      nontraumatic intracranial hemorrhage NEC
        I69.25- ☑
      specified disease NEC I69.85- ☑
      stroke NOS I69.35- ☑
      subarachnoid hemorrhage I69.05- ☑
  hysterical F44.4
  newborn NEC P91.88
    birth injury P11.9
  spastic G81.1- ☑
    congenital G80.2
  thrombotic (current episode) I63.3- ☑

**Hemisection, spinal cord** — *see* Injury, spinal cord, by region
**Hemispasm** (facial) R25.2
**Hemisporosis** B48.8
**Hemitremor** R25.1
**Hemivertebra** Q76.49
  failure of segmentation with scoliosis Q76.3
  fusion with scoliosis Q76.3
**Hemochromatosis** E83.119
  with refractory anemia D46.1
  due to repeated red blood cell transfusion E83.111
  hereditary (primary) E83.110
  neonatal P78.84
  primary E83.110
  specified NEC E83.118
**Hemoglobin** (*see also* condition)
  abnormal (disease) — *see* Disease, hemoglobin
  AS genotype D57.3
  Constant Spring D58.2
  E-beta thalassemia D56.5
  fetal, hereditary persistence (HPFH) D56.4
  H Constant Spring D56.0
  low NOS D64.9
  S (Hb S), heterozygous D57.3
**Hemoglobinemia** D59.9
  due to blood transfusion T80.89 ☑
  paroxysmal D59.6
    nocturnal D59.5
**Hemoglobinopathy** (mixed) D58.2
  with thalassemia D56.8
  sickle-cell D57.1
    with thalassemia D57.40
      with crisis (vasoocclusive pain) D57.419
        with
          acute chest syndrome D57.411
          splenic sequestration D57.412
      without crisis D57.40
**Hemoglobinuria** R82.3
  with anemia, hemolytic, acquired (chronic) NEC D59.6
  cold (agglutinin) (paroxysmal) (with Raynaud's syndrome) D59.6
  due to exertion or hemolysis NEC D59.6
  intermittent D59.6
  malarial B50.8
  march D59.6
  nocturnal (paroxysmal) D59.5
  paroxysmal (cold) D59.6
    nocturnal D59.5
**Hemolymphangioma** D18.1
**Hemolysis**
  intravascular
    with
      abortion — *see* Abortion, by type, complicated by, hemorrhage
      ectopic or molar pregnancy O08.1
      hemorrhage
        antepartum — *see* Hemorrhage, antepartum, with coagulation defect
        intrapartum (*see also* Hemorrhage, complicating, delivery) O67.0
      postpartum O72.3
  neonatal (excessive) P58.9
    specified NEC P58.8
**Hemolytic** — *see* condition
**Hemopericardium** I31.2
  following acute myocardial infarction (current complication) I23.0
  newborn P54.8
  traumatic — *see* Injury, heart, with hemopericardium
**Hemoperitoneum** K66.1
  infectional K65.9
  traumatic S36.899 ☑
    with open wound — *see* Wound, open, with penetration into peritoneal cavity
**Hemophilia** (classical) (familial) (hereditary) D66
  A D66
  acquired D68.311
  autoimmune D68.311
  B D67
  C D68.1
  calcipriva (*see also* Defect, coagulation) D68.4
  nonfamilial (*see also* Defect, coagulation) D68.4
  secondary D68.311
  vascular D68.0
**Hemophthalmos** H44.81- ☑
**Hemopneumothorax** (*see also* Hemothorax)
  traumatic S27.2 ☑
**Hemoptysis** R04.2

**Hemoptysis** — *continued*
  newborn P26.9
  tuberculous — *see* Tuberculosis, pulmonary
**Hemorrhage, hemorrhagic** (concealed) R58
  abdomen R58
  accidental antepartum — *see* Hemorrhage, antepartum
  acute idiopathic pulmonary, in infants R04.81
  adenoid J35.8
  adrenal (capsule) (gland) E27.49
    medulla E27.8
    newborn P54.4
  after delivery — *see* Hemorrhage, postpartum
  alveolar
    lung, newborn P26.8
    process K08.89
  alveolus K08.89
  amputation stump (surgical) T87.89
  anemia (chronic) D50.0
    acute D62
  antepartum (with) O46.90
    with coagulation defect O46.00- ☑
      afibrinogenemia O46.01- ☑
      disseminated intravascular coagulation O46.02- ☑
      hypofibrinogenemia O46.01- ☑
      specified defect NEC O46.09- ☑
    before 20 weeks gestation O20.9
      specified type NEC O20.8
      threatened abortion O20.0
    due to
      abruptio placenta (*see also* Abruptio placentae) O45.9-
      leiomyoma, uterus — *see* Hemorrhage, antepartum, specified cause NEC
      placenta previa O44.1- ☑
    specified cause NEC — *see* subcategory O46.8X- ☑
  anus (sphincter) K62.5
  apoplexy (stroke) — *see* Hemorrhage, intracranial, intracerebral
  arachnoid — *see* Hemorrhage, intracranial, subarachnoid
  artery R58
    brain — *see* Hemorrhage, intracranial, intracerebral
  basilar (ganglion) I61.0
  bladder N32.89
  bowel K92.2
    newborn P54.3
  brain (miliary) (nontraumatic) — *see* Hemorrhage, intracranial, intracerebral
    due to
      birth injury P10.1
      syphilis A52.05
    epidural or extradural (traumatic) — *see* Injury, intracranial, epidural hemorrhage
    newborn P52.4
      birth injury P10.1
    subarachnoid — *see* Hemorrhage, intracranial, subarachnoid
    subdural — *see* Hemorrhage, intracranial, subdural
  brainstem (nontraumatic) I61.3
    traumatic S06.38- ☑
  breast N64.59
  bronchial tube — *see* Hemorrhage, lung
  bronchopulmonary — *see* Hemorrhage, lung
  bronchus — *see* Hemorrhage, lung
  bulbar I61.5
  capillary I78.8
    primary D69.8
  cecum K92.2
  cerebellar, cerebellum (nontraumatic) I61.4
    newborn P52.6
    traumatic S06.37- ☑
  cerebral, cerebrum (*see also* Hemorrhage, intracranial, intracerebral)
    lobe I61.1
    newborn (anoxic) P52.4
      birth injury P10.1
  cerebromeningeal I61.8
  cerebrospinal — *see* Hemorrhage, intracranial, intracerebral
  cervix (uteri) (stump) NEC N88.8
  chamber, anterior (eye) — *see* Hyphema
  childbirth — *see* Hemorrhage, complicating, delivery
  choroid H31.30- ☑
    expulsive H31.31- ☑
  ciliary body — *see* Hyphema
  cochlea — *see* subcategory H83.8 ☑

**Hemorrhage, hemorrhagic** — *continued*
  colon K92.2
  complicating
    abortion — *see* Abortion, by type, complicated by, hemorrhage
    delivery O67.9
      associated with coagulation defect (afibrinogenemia) (DIC) (hyperfibrinolysis) O67.0
      specified cause NEC O67.8
    surgical procedure — *see* Hemorrhage, intraoperative
  conjunctiva H11.3- ☑
    newborn P54.8
  cord, newborn (stump) P51.9
  corpus luteum (ruptured) cyst N83.1- ☑
  cortical (brain) I61.1
  cranial — *see* Hemorrhage, intracranial
  cutaneous R23.3
    due to autosensitivity, erythrocyte D69.2
    newborn P54.5
  delayed
    following ectopic or molar pregnancy O08.1
    postpartum O72.2
  diathesis (familial) D69.9
  disease D69.9
    newborn P53
    specified type NEC D69.8
  due to or associated with
    afibrinogenemia or other coagulation defect (conditions in categories D65- D69)
      antepartum — *see* Hemorrhage, antepartum, with coagulation defect
      intrapartum O67.0
  dental implant M27.61
  device, implant or graft (*see also* Complications, by site and type, specified NEC) T85.838 ☑
    arterial graft NEC T82.838 ☑
    breast T85.838 ☑
    catheter NEC T85.838 ☑
      dialysis (renal) T82.838 ☑
        intraperitoneal T85.838 ☑
      infusion NEC T82.838 ☑
        spinal (epidural) (subdural) T85.830 ☑
      urinary (indwelling) T83.83 ☑
    electronic (electrode) (pulse generator) (stimulator)
      bone T84.83 ☑
      cardiac T82.837 ☑
      nervous system (brain) (peripheral nerve) (spinal) T85.830 ☑
      urinary T83.83 ☑
    fixation, internal (orthopedic) NEC T84.83 ☑
    gastrointestinal (bile duct) (esophagus) T85.838 ☑
    genital NEC T83.83 ☑
    heart NEC T82.837 ☑
    joint prosthesis T84.83 ☑
    ocular (corneal graft) (orbital implant) NEC T85.838 ☑
    orthopedic NEC T84.83 ☑
      bone graft T86.838 ☑
    specified NEC T85.838 ☑
    urinary NEC T83.83 ☑
    vascular NEC T82.838 ☑
    ventricular intracranial shunt T85.830 ☑
  duodenum, duodenal K92.2
    ulcer — *see* Ulcer, duodenum, with hemorrhage
  dura mater — *see* Hemorrhage, intracranial, subdural
  endotracheal — *see* Hemorrhage, lung
  epicranial subaponeurotic (massive), birth injury P12.2
  epidural (traumatic) (*see also* Injury, intracranial, epidural hemorrhage)
    nontraumatic I62.1
  esophagus K22.8
    varix I85.01
      secondary I85.11
  excessive, following ectopic gestation (subsequent episode) O08.1
  extradural (traumatic) — *see* Injury, intracranial, epidural hemorrhage
    birth injury P10.8
    newborn (anoxic) (nontraumatic) P52.8
    nontraumatic I62.1
  eye NEC H57.8
    fundus — *see* Hemorrhage, retina
    lid — *see* Disorder, eyelid, specified type NEC
  fallopian tube N83.6

**Hemorrhage, hemorrhagic** — *continued*
  fibrinogenolysis — *see* Fibrinolysis
  fibrinolytic (acquired) — *see* Fibrinolysis
  from
    ear (nontraumatic) — *see* Otorrhagia
    tracheostomy stoma J95.01
  fundus, eye — *see* Hemorrhage, retina
  funis — *see* Hemorrhage, umbilicus, cord
  gastric — *see* Hemorrhage, stomach
  gastroenteric K92.2
    newborn P54.3
  gastrointestinal (tract) K92.2
    newborn P54.3
  genital organ, male N50.1
  genitourinary (tract) NOS R31.9
  gingiva K06.8
  globe (eye) — *see* Hemophthalmos
  graafian follicle cyst (ruptured) N83.0- ☑
  gum K06.8
  heart I51.89
  hypopharyngeal (throat) R04.1
  intermenstrual (regular) N92.3
    irregular N92.1
  internal (organs) NEC R58
    capsule I61.0
    ear — *see* subcategory H83.8 ☑
    newborn P54.8
  intestine K92.2
    newborn P54.3
  intra-abdominal R58
  intra-alveolar (lung), newborn P26.8
  intracerebral (nontraumatic) — *see* Hemorrhage, intracranial, intracerebral
  intracranial (nontraumatic) I62.9
    birth injury P10.9
    epidural, nontraumatic I62.1
    extradural, nontraumatic I62.1
    intracerebral (nontraumatic) (in) I61.9
      brain stem I61.3
      cerebellum I61.4
      hemisphere I61.2
        cortical (superficial) I61.1
        subcortical (deep) I61.0
      intraoperative
        during a nervous system procedure G97.31
        during other procedure G97.32
      intraventricular I61.5
      multiple localized I61.6
      newborn P52.4
        birth injury P10.1
      postprocedural
        following a nervous system procedure G97.51
        following other procedure G97.52
      specified NEC I61.8
      superficial I61.1
      traumatic (diffuse) — *see* Injury, intracranial, diffuse
        focal — *see* Injury, intracranial, focal
    newborn P52.9
      specified NEC P52.8
    subarachnoid (nontraumatic) (from) I60.9
      intracranial (cerebral) artery I60.7
        anterior communicating I60.2
        basilar I60.4
        carotid siphon and bifurcation I60.0- ☑
        communicating I60.7
          anterior I60.2
          posterior I60.3- ☑
        middle cerebral I60.1- ☑
        posterior communicating I60.3- ☑
        specified artery NEC I60.6
        vertebral I60.5- ☑
      newborn P52.5
        birth injury P10.3
      specified NEC I60.8
      traumatic S06.6X- ☑
    subdural (nontraumatic) I62.00
      acute I62.01
      birth injury P10.0
      chronic I62.03
      newborn (anoxic) (hypoxic) P52.8
        birth injury P10.0
      spinal G95.19
      subacute I62.02
      traumatic — *see* Injury, intracranial, subdural hemorrhage

**Hemorrhage, hemorrhagic** — *continued*
  intracranial — *continued*
    traumatic — *see* Injury, intracranial, focal brain injury
  intramedullary NEC G95.19
  intraocular — *see* Hemophthalmos
  intraoperative, intraprocedural — *see* Complication, hemorrhage (hematoma), intraoperative (intraprocedural), by site
  intrapartum — *see* Hemorrhage, complicating, delivery
  intrapelvic
    female N94.89
    male K66.1
  intraperitoneal K66.1
  intrapontine I61.3
  intraprocedural — *see* Complication, hemorrhage (hematoma), intraoperative (intraprocedural), by site
  intrauterine N85.7
    complicating delivery (*see also* Hemorrhage, complicating, delivery) O67.9
    postpartum — *see* Hemorrhage, postpartum
  intraventricular I61.5
    newborn (nontraumatic) (*see also* Newborn, affected by, hemorrhage) P52.3
      due to birth injury P10.2
      grade
        1 P52.0
        2 P52.1
        3 P52.21
        4 P52.22
  intravesical N32.89
  iris (postinfectional) (postinflammatory) (toxic) — *see* Hyphema
  joint (nontraumatic) — *see* Hemarthrosis
  kidney N28.89
  knee (joint) (nontraumatic) — *see* Hemarthrosis, knee
  labyrinth — *see* subcategory H83.8 ☑
  lenticular striate artery I61.0
  ligature, vessel — *see* Hemorrhage, postoperative
  liver K76.89
  lung R04.89
    newborn P26.9
      massive P26.1
      specified NEC P26.8
    tuberculous — *see* Tuberculosis, pulmonary
    massive umbilical, newborn P51.0
  mediastinum — *see* Hemorrhage, lung
  medulla I61.3
  membrane (brain) I60.8
    spinal cord — *see* Hemorrhage, spinal cord
  meninges, meningeal (brain) (middle) I60.8
    spinal cord — *see* Hemorrhage, spinal cord
  mesentery K66.1
  metritis — *see* Endometritis
  mouth K13.79
  mucous membrane NEC R58
    newborn P54.8
  muscle M62.89
  nail (subungual) L60.8
  nasal turbinate R04.0
    newborn P54.8
  navel, newborn P51.9
  newborn P54.9
    specified NEC P54.8
  nipple N64.59
  nose R04.0
    newborn P54.8
  omentum K66.1
  optic nerve (sheath) H47.02- ☑
  orbit, orbital H05.23- ☑
  ovary NEC N83.8
  oviduct N83.6
  pancreas K86.89
  parathyroid (gland) (spontaneous) E21.4
  parturition — *see* Hemorrhage, complicating, delivery
  penis N48.89
  pericardium, pericarditis I31.2
  peritoneum, peritoneal K66.1
  peritonsillar tissue J35.8
    due to infection J36
  petechial R23.3
    due to autosensitivity, erythrocyte D69.2
  pituitary (gland) E23.6
  pleura — *see* Hemorrhage, lung
  polioencephalitis, superior E51.2
  polymyositis — *see* Polymyositis

**Hemorrhage, hemorrhagic** — *continued*
  pons, pontine I61.3
  posterior fossa (nontraumatic) I61.8
    newborn P52.6
  postmenopausal N95.0
  postnasal R04.0
  postoperative — *see* Complications, postprocedural, hemorrhage, by site
  postpartum NEC (following delivery of placenta) O72.1
    delayed or secondary O72.2
      retained placenta O72.0
    third stage O72.0
  pregnancy — *see* Hemorrhage, antepartum
  preretinal — *see* Hemorrhage, retina
  prostate N42.1
  puerperal — *see* Hemorrhage, postpartum
    delayed or secondary O72.2
  pulmonary R04.89
    newborn P26.9
      massive P26.1
      specified NEC P26.8
    tuberculous — *see* Tuberculosis, pulmonary
  purpura (primary) D69.3
  rectum (sphincter) K62.5
    newborn P54.2
  recurring, following initial hemorrhage at time of injury T79.2 ☑
  renal N28.89
  respiratory passage or tract R04.9
    specified NEC R04.89
  retina, retinal (vessels) H35.6- ☑
    diabetic — *see* Diabetes, retinal, hemorrhage
  retroperitoneal R58
  scalp R58
  scrotum N50.1
  secondary (nontraumatic) R58
    following initial hemorrhage at time of injury T79.2 ☑
  seminal vesicle N50.1
  skin R23.3
    newborn P54.5
  slipped umbilical ligature P51.8
  spermatic cord N50.1
  spinal (cord) G95.19
    newborn (birth injury) P11.5
  spleen D73.5
    intraoperative — *see* Complications, intraoperative, hemorrhage, spleen
    postprocedural — *see* Complications, postprocedural, hemorrhage, spleen
  stomach K92.2
    newborn P54.3
    ulcer — *see* Ulcer, stomach, with hemorrhage
  subarachnoid (nontraumatic) — *see* Hemorrhage, intracranial, subarachnoid
  subconjunctival (*see also* Hemorrhage, conjunctiva)
    birth injury P15.3
  subcortical (brain) I61.0
  subcutaneous R23.3
  subdiaphragmatic R58
  subdural (acute) (nontraumatic) — *see* Hemorrhage, intracranial, subdural
  subependymal
    newborn P52.0
      with intraventricular extension P52.1
        and intracerebral extension P52.22
  subgaleal P12.2
  subhyaloid — *see* Hemorrhage, retina
  subperiosteal — *see* Disorder, bone, specified type NEC
  subretinal — *see* Hemorrhage, retina
  subtentorial — *see* Hemorrhage, intracranial, subdural
  subungual L60.8
  suprarenal (capsule) (gland) E27.49
    newborn P54.4
  tentorium (traumatic) NEC — *see* Hemorrhage, brain
    newborn (birth injury) P10.4
  testis N50.1
  third stage (postpartum) O72.0
  thorax — *see* Hemorrhage, lung
  throat R04.1
  thymus (gland) E32.8
  thyroid (cyst) (gland) E07.89
  tongue K14.8
  tonsil J35.8
  trachea — *see* Hemorrhage, lung
  tracheobronchial R04.89
    newborn P26.0

☑ **Additional Character Required** — **Refer to the Tabular List for Character Selection**          ⌐ᴡ Subterms under main terms may continue to next column or page

**Hemorrhage, hemorrhagic** — *continued*
 traumatic — *code to* specific injury
  cerebellar — *see* Hemorrhage, brain
  intracranial — *see* Hemorrhage, brain
  recurring or secondary (following initial hemor-
    rhage at time of injury) T79.2 ☑
 tuberculous NEC (*see also* Tuberculosis, pulmonary)
   A15.0
 tunica vaginalis N50.1
 ulcer — *code by* site under Ulcer, with hemorrhage
   K27.4
 umbilicus, umbilical
  cord
   after birth, newborn P51.9
   complicating delivery O69.5 ☑
  newborn P51.9
   massive P51.0
   slipped ligature P51.8
  stump P51.9
 urethra (idiopathic) N36.8
 uterus, uterine (abnormal) N93.9
  climacteric N92.4
  complicating delivery — *see* Hemorrhage, compli-
    cating, delivery
  dysfunctional or functional N93.8
  intermenstrual (regular) N92.3
   irregular N92.1
  postmenopausal N95.0
  postpartum — *see* Hemorrhage, postpartum
  preclimacteric or premenopausal N92.4
  prepubertal N93.8
  pubertal N92.2
 vagina (abnormal) N93.9
  newborn P54.6
 vas deferens N50.1
 vasa previa O69.4 ☑
 ventricular I61.5
 vesical N32.89
 viscera NEC R58
  newborn P54.8
 vitreous (humor) (intraocular) H43.1- ☑
 vulva N90.89
**Hemorrhoids** (bleeding) (without mention of degree)
   K64.9
 1st degree (grade/stage I) (without prolapse outside
   of anal canal) K64.0
 2nd degree (grade/stage II) (that prolapse with
   straining but retract spontaneously) K64.1
 3rd degree (grade/stage III) (that prolapse with
   straining and require manual replacement back
   inside anal canal) K64.2
 4th degree (grade/stage IV) (with prolapsed tissue that
   cannot be manually replaced) K64.3
 complicating
  pregnancy O22.4 ☑
  puerperium O87.2
 external K64.4
  with
   thrombosis K64.5
 internal (without mention of degree) K64.8
 prolapsed K64.8
 skin tags
  anus K64.4
  residual K64.4
 specified NEC K64.8
 strangulated (*see also* Hemorrhoids, by degree) K64.8
 thrombosed (*see also* Hemorrhoids, by degree) K64.5
 ulcerated (*see also* Hemorrhoids, by degree) K64.8
**Hemosalpinx** N83.6
 with
  hematocolpos N89.7
  hematometra N85.7
   with hematocolpos N89.7
**Hemosiderosis** (dietary) E83.19
 pulmonary, idiopathic E83.1- ☑ [J84.03]
 transfusion T80.89 ☑
**Hemothorax** (bacterial) (nontuberculous) J94.2
 newborn P54.8
 traumatic S27.1 ☑
  with pneumothorax S27.2 ☑
 tuberculous NEC A15.6
**Henoch** (-Schönlein) **disease or syndrome** (purpura)
   D69.0
**Henpue, henpuye** A66.6
**Hepar lobatum** (syphilitic) A52.74
**Hepatalgia** K76.89
**Hepatitis** K75.9
 acute B17.9

**Hepatitis** — *continued*
 acute — *continued*
  with coma K72.01
  with hepatic failure — *see* Failure, hepatic
  alcoholic — *see* Hepatitis, alcoholic
  infectious B17.9
  non-viral K72.0 ☑
  viral B17.9
 alcoholic (acute) (chronic) K70.10
  with ascites K70.11
 amebic — *see* Abscess, liver, amebic
 anicteric, (viral) — *see* Hepatitis, viral
 antigen-associated (HAA) — *see* Hepatitis, B
 Australia-antigen (positive) — *see* Hepatitis, B
 autoimmune K75.4
 B B19.10
  with hepatic coma B19.11
  acute B16.9
   with
    delta-agent (coinfection) (without hepatic
     coma) B16.1
     with hepatic coma B16.0
    hepatic coma (without delta-agent coinfec-
     tion) B16.2
  chronic B18.1
   with delta-agent B18.0
 bacterial NEC K75.89
 C (viral) B19.20
  with hepatic coma B19.21
  acute B17.10
   with hepatic coma B17.11
  chronic B18.2
 catarrhal (acute) B15.9
  with hepatic coma B15.0
 cholangiolitic K75.89
 cholestatic K75.89
 chronic K73.9
  active NEC K73.2
  lobular NEC K73.1
  persistent NEC K73.0
  specified NEC K73.8
 cytomegaloviral B25.1
 due to ethanol (acute) (chronic) — *see* Hepatitis, alcoholic
 epidemic B15.9
  with hepatic coma B15.0
 fulminant NEC (viral) — *see* Hepatitis, viral
 granulomatous NEC K75.3
 herpesviral B00.81
 history of
  B Z86.19
  C Z86.19
 homologous serum — *see* Hepatitis, viral, type B
 in (due to)
  mumps B26.81
  toxoplasmosis (acquired) B58.1
   congenital (active) P37.1 [K77]
 infectious, infective B15.9
  acute (subacute) B17.9
  chronic B18.9
 inoculation — *see* Hepatitis, viral, type B
 interstitial (chronic) K74.69
 lupoid NEC K75.4
 malignant NEC (with hepatic failure) K72.90
  with coma K72.91
 neonatal (idiopathic) (toxic) P59.29
 neonatal giant cell P59.29
 newborn P59.29
 non-viral K72.0 ☑
 postimmunization — *see* Hepatitis, viral, type B
 post-transfusion — *see* Hepatitis, viral, type B
 reactive, nonspecific K75.2
 serum — *see* Hepatitis, viral, type B
 specified type NEC
  with hepatic failure — *see* Failure, hepatic
 syphilitic (late) A52.74
  congenital (early) A50.08 [K77]
   late A50.59 [K77]
  secondary A51.45
 toxic (*see also* Disease, liver, toxic) K71.6
 tuberculous A18.83
 viral, virus B19.9
  with hepatic coma B19.0
  acute B17.9
  chronic B18.9
   specified NEC B18.8
   type
    B B18.1

**Hepatitis** — *continued*
 viral, virus — *continued*
  chronic — *continued*
   type — *continued*
    B — *continued*
     with delta-agent B18.0
    C B18.2
 congenital P35.3
 coxsackie B33.8 [K77]
 cytomegalic inclusion B25.1
 in remission, any type — *code to* Hepatitis, chronic,
   by type
 non-A, non-B B17.8
 specified type NEC (with or without coma) B17.8
 type
  A B15.9
   with hepatic coma B15.0
  B B19.10
   with hepatic coma B19.11
   acute B16.9
    with
     delta-agent (coinfection) (without
      hepatic coma) B16.1
      with hepatic coma B16.0
     hepatic coma (without delta-agent
      coinfection) B16.2
   chronic B18.1
    with delta-agent B18.0
  C B19.20
   with hepatic coma B19.21
   acute B17.10
    with hepatic coma B17.11
   chronic B18.2
  E B17.2
 non-A, non-B B17.8
**Hepatization lung** (acute) — *see* Pneumonia, lobar
**Hepatoblastoma** C22.2
**Hepatocarcinoma** C22.0
**Hepatocholangiocarcinoma** C22.0
**Hepatocholangioma, benign** D13.4
**Hepatocholangitis** K75.89
**Hepatolenticular degeneration** E83.01
**Hepatoma** (malignant) C22.0
 benign D13.4
 embryonal C22.0
**Hepatomegaly** (*see also* Hypertrophy, liver)
 with splenomegaly R16.2
 congenital Q44.7
 in mononucleosis
  gammaherpesviral B27.09
  infectious specified NEC B27.89
**Hepatoptosis** K76.89
**Hepatorenal syndrome following labor and delivery**
   O90.4
**Hepatosis** K76.89
**Hepatosplenomegaly** R16.2
 hyperlipemic (Bürger-Grütz type) E78.3 [K77]
**Hereditary** — *see* condition
**Heredodegeneration, macular** — *see* Dystrophy, retina
**Heredopathia atactica polyneuritiformis** G60.1
**Heredosyphilis** — *see* Syphilis, congenital
**Herlitz' syndrome** Q81.1
**Hermansky-Pudlak syndrome** E70.331
**Hermaphrodite, hermaphroditism** (true) Q56.0
 46,XX with streak gonads Q99.1
 46,XX/46,XY Q99.0
 46,XY with streak gonads Q99.1
 chimera 46,XX/46,XY Q99.0
**Hernia, hernial** (acquired) (recurrent) K46.9
 with
  gangrene — *see* Hernia, by site, with, gangrene
  incarceration — *see* Hernia, by site, with, obstruc-
    tion
  irreducible — *see* Hernia, by site, with, obstruction
  obstruction — *see* Hernia, by site, with, obstruction
  strangulation — *see* Hernia, by site, with, obstruc-
    tion
 abdomen, abdominal K46.9
  with
   gangrene (and obstruction) K46.1
   obstruction K46.0
  femoral — *see* Hernia, femoral
  incisional — *see* Hernia, incisional
  inguinal — *see* Hernia, inguinal
  specified site NEC K45.8
   with
    gangrene (and obstruction) K45.1
    obstruction K45.0

**Hernia, hernial** — *continued*
  abdomen, abdominal — *continued*
    umbilical — *see* Hernia, umbilical
    wall — *see* Hernia, ventral
  appendix — *see* Hernia, abdomen
  bladder (mucosa) (sphincter)
    congenital (female) (male) Q79.51
    female — *see* Cystocele
    male N32.89
  brain, congenital — *see* Encephalocele
  cartilage, vertebra — *see* Displacement, intervertebral disc
  cerebral, congenital (*see also* Encephalocele)
    endaural Q01.8
  ciliary body (traumatic) S05.2- ☑
  colon — *see* Hernia, abdomen
  Cooper's — *see* Hernia, abdomen, specified site NEC
  crural — *see* Hernia, femoral
  diaphragm, diaphragmatic K44.9
    with
      gangrene (and obstruction) K44.1
      obstruction K44.0
    congenital Q79.0
  direct (inguinal) — *see* Hernia, inguinal
  diverticulum, intestine — *see* Hernia, abdomen
  double (inguinal) — *see* Hernia, inguinal, bilateral
  due to adhesions (with obstruction) K56.50
  epigastric (*see also* Hernia, ventral) K43.9
  esophageal hiatus — *see* Hernia, hiatal
  external (inguinal) — *see* Hernia, inguinal
  fallopian tube N83.4- ☑
  fascia M62.89
  femoral K41.90
    with
      gangrene (and obstruction) K41.40
        not specified as recurrent K41.40
        recurrent K41.41
      obstruction K41.30
        not specified as recurrent K41.30
        recurrent K41.31
    bilateral K41.20
      with
        gangrene (and obstruction) K41.10
          not specified as recurrent K41.10
          recurrent K41.11
        obstruction K41.00
          not specified as recurrent K41.00
          recurrent K41.01
      not specified as recurrent K41.20
      recurrent K41.21
    not specified as recurrent K41.90
    recurrent K41.91
    unilateral K41.90
      with
        gangrene (and obstruction) K41.40
          not specified as recurrent K41.40
          recurrent K41.41
        obstruction K41.30
          not specified as recurrent K41.30
          recurrent K41.31
      not specified as recurrent K41.90
      recurrent K41.91
  foramen magnum G93.5
    congenital Q01.8
  funicular (umbilical) (*see also* Hernia, umbilicus)
    spermatic (cord) — *see* Hernia, inguinal
  gastrointestinal tract — *see* Hernia, abdomen
  Hesselbach's — *see* Hernia, femoral, specified site NEC
  hiatal (esophageal) (sliding) K44.9
    with
      gangrene (and obstruction) K44.1
      obstruction K44.0
    congenital Q40.1
  hypogastric — *see* Hernia, ventral
  incarcerated (*see also* Hernia, by site, with obstruction)
    with gangrene — *see* Hernia, by site, with gangrene
  incisional K43.2
    with
      gangrene (and obstruction) K43.1
      obstruction K43.0
  indirect (inguinal) — *see* Hernia, inguinal
  inguinal (direct) (external) (funicular) (indirect) (internal) (oblique) (scrotal) (sliding) K40.90
    with
      gangrene (and obstruction) K40.40
        not specified as recurrent K40.40
        recurrent K40.41

**Hernia, hernial** — *continued*
  inguinal — *continued*
    with — *continued*
      obstruction K40.30
        not specified as recurrent K40.30
        recurrent K40.31
    bilateral K40.20
      with
        gangrene (and obstruction) K40.10
          not specified as recurrent K40.10
          recurrent K40.11
        obstruction K40.00
          not specified as recurrent K40.00
          recurrent K40.01
      not specified as recurrent K40.20
      recurrent K40.21
    not specified as recurrent K40.90
    recurrent K40.91
    unilateral K40.90
      with
        gangrene (and obstruction) K40.40
          not specified as recurrent K40.40
          recurrent K40.41
        obstruction K40.30
          not specified as recurrent K40.30
          recurrent K40.31
      not specified as recurrent K40.90
      recurrent K40.91
  internal (*see also* Hernia, abdomen)
    inguinal — *see* Hernia, inguinal
  interstitial — *see* Hernia, abdomen
  intervertebral cartilage or disc — *see* Displacement, intervertebral disc
  intestine, intestinal — *see* Hernia, by site
  intra-abdominal — *see* Hernia, abdomen
  iris (traumatic) S05.2- ☑
  irreducible (*see also* Hernia, by site, with obstruction)
    with gangrene — *see* Hernia, by site, with gangrene
  ischiatic — *see* Hernia, abdomen, specified site NEC
  ischiorectal — *see* Hernia, abdomen, specified site NEC
  lens (traumatic) S05.2- ☑
  linea (alba) (semilunaris) — *see* Hernia, ventral
  Littre's — *see* Hernia, abdomen
  lumbar — *see* Hernia, abdomen, specified site NEC
  lung (subcutaneous) J98.4
  mediastinum J98.59
  mesenteric (internal) — *see* Hernia, abdomen
  midline — *see* Hernia, ventral
  muscle (sheath) M62.89
  nucleus pulposus — *see* Displacement, intervertebral disc
  oblique (inguinal) — *see* Hernia, inguinal
  obstructive (*see also* Hernia, by site, with obstruction)
    with gangrene — *see* Hernia, by site, with gangrene
  obturator — *see* Hernia, abdomen, specified site NEC
  omental — *see* Hernia, abdomen
  ovary N83.4- ☑
  oviduct N83.4- ☑
  paraesophageal (*see also* Hernia, diaphragm)
    congenital Q40.1
  parastomal K43.5
    with
      gangrene (and obstruction) K43.4
      obstruction K43.3
  paraumbilical — *see* Hernia, umbilicus
  perineal — *see* Hernia, abdomen, specified site NEC
  Petit's — *see* Hernia, abdomen, specified site NEC
  postoperative — *see* Hernia, incisional
  pregnant uterus — *see* Abnormal, uterus in pregnancy or childbirth
  prevesical N32.89
  properitoneal — *see* Hernia, abdomen, specified site NEC
  pudendal — *see* Hernia, abdomen, specified site NEC
  rectovaginal N81.6
  retroperitoneal — *see* Hernia, abdomen, specified site NEC
  Richter's — *see* Hernia, abdomen, with obstruction
  Rieux's, Riex's — *see* Hernia, abdomen, specified site NEC
  sac condition (adhesion) (dropsy) (inflammation) (laceration) (suppuration) — *code by site under* Hernia
  sciatic — *see* Hernia, abdomen, specified site NEC

**Hernia, hernial** — *continued*
  scrotum, scrotal — *see* Hernia, inguinal
  sliding (inguinal) (*see also* Hernia, inguinal)
    hiatus — *see* Hernia, hiatal
  spigelian — *see* Hernia, ventral
  spinal — *see* Spina bifida
  strangulated (*see also* Hernia, by site, with obstruction)
    with gangrene — *see* Hernia, by site, with gangrene
  subxiphoid — *see* Hernia, ventral
  supra-umbilicus — *see* Hernia, ventral
  tendon — *see* Disorder, tendon, specified type NEC
  Treitz's (fossa) — *see* Hernia, abdomen, specified site NEC
  tunica vaginalis Q55.29
  umbilicus, umbilical K42.9
    with
      gangrene (and obstruction) K42.1
      obstruction K42.0
  ureter N28.89
  urethra, congenital Q64.79
  urinary meatus, congenital Q64.79
  uterus N81.4
    pregnant — *see* Abnormal, uterus in pregnancy or childbirth
  vaginal (anterior) (wall) — *see* Cystocele
  Velpeau's — *see* Hernia, femoral
  ventral K43.9
    with
      gangrene (and obstruction) K43.7
      obstruction K43.6
    incisional K43.2
      with
        gangrene (and obstruction) K43.1
        obstruction K43.0
      recurrent — *see* Hernia, incisional
    specified NEC K43.9
      with
        gangrene (and obstruction) K43.7
        obstruction K43.6
  vesical
    congenital (female) (male) Q79.51
    female — *see* Cystocele
    male N32.89
  vitreous (into wound) S05.2- ☑
    into anterior chamber — *see* Prolapse, vitreous
**Herniation** (*see also* Hernia)
  brain (stem) G93.5
  cerebral G93.5
  mediastinum J98.59
  nucleus pulposus — *see* Displacement, intervertebral disc
**Herpangina** B08.5
**Herpes, herpesvirus, herpetic** B00.9
  anogenital A60.9
    perianal skin A60.1
    rectum A60.1
    urogenital tract A60.00
      cervix A60.03
      male genital organ NEC A60.02
      penis A60.01
      specified site NEC A60.09
      vagina A60.04
      vulva A60.04
  blepharitis (zoster) B02.39
    simplex B00.59
  circinatus B35.4
    bullosus L12.0
  conjunctivitis (simplex) B00.53
    zoster B02.31
  cornea B02.33
  encephalitis B00.4
    due to herpesvirus 6 B10.01
    due to herpesvirus 7 B10.09
    specified NEC B10.09
  eye (zoster) B02.30
    simplex B00.50
  eyelid (zoster) B02.39
    simplex B00.59
  facialis B00.1
  febrilis B00.1
  geniculate ganglionitis B02.21
  genital, genitalis A60.00
    female A60.09
    male A60.02
  gestational, gestationis O26.4- ☑
  gingivostomatitis B00.2
  human B00.9

**Herpes, herpesvirus, herpetic** — *continued*
  human — *continued*
    1 — *see* Herpes, simplex
    2 — *see* Herpes, simplex
    3 — *see* Varicella
    4 — *see* Mononucleosis, Epstein-Barr (virus)
    5 — *see* Disease, cytomegalic inclusion (generalized)
    6
      encephalitis B10.01
      specified NEC B10.81
    7
      encephalitis B10.09
      specified NEC B10.82
    8 B10.89
  infection NEC B10.89
    Kaposi's sarcoma associated B10.89
  iridocyclitis (simplex) B00.51
    zoster B02.32
  iris (vesicular erythema multiforme) L51.9
  iritis (simplex) B00.51
  Kaposi's sarcoma associated B10.89
  keratitis (simplex) (dendritic) (disciform) (interstitial) B00.52
    zoster (interstitial) B02.33
  keratoconjunctivitis (simplex) B00.52
    zoster B02.33
  labialis B00.1
  lip B00.1
  meningitis (simplex) B00.3
    zoster B02.1
  ophthalmicus (zoster) NEC B02.30
    simplex B00.50
  penis A60.01
  perianal skin A60.1
  pharyngitis, pharyngotonsillitis B00.2
  rectum A60.1
  scrotum A60.02
  sepsis B00.7
  simplex B00.9
    complicated NEC B00.89
    congenital P35.2
    conjunctivitis B00.53
    external ear B00.1
    eyelid B00.59
    hepatitis B00.81
    keratitis (interstitial) B00.52
    myelitis B00.82
    specified complication NEC B00.89
    visceral B00.89
  stomatitis B00.2
  tonsurans B35.0
  visceral B00.89
  vulva A60.04
  whitlow B00.89
  zoster (*see also* condition) B02.9
    auricularis B02.21
    complicated NEC B02.8
    conjunctivitis B02.31
    disseminated B02.7
    encephalitis B02.0
    eye (lid) B02.39
    geniculate ganglionitis B02.21
    keratitis (interstitial) B02.33
    meningitis B02.1
    myelitis B02.24
    neuritis, neuralgia B02.29
    ophthalmicus NEC B02.30
    oticus B02.21
    polyneuropathy B02.23
    specified complication NEC B02.8
    trigeminal neuralgia B02.22
**Herpesvirus** (human) — *see* Herpes
**Herpetophobia** F40.218
**Herrick's anemia** — *see* Disease, sickle-cell
**Hers' disease** E74.09
**Herter-Gee syndrome** K90.0
**Herxheimer's reaction** R68.89
**Hesitancy**
  of micturition R39.11
  urinary R39.11
**Hesselbach's hernia** — *see* Hernia, femoral, specified site NEC
**Heterochromia** (congenital) Q13.2
  cataract — *see* Cataract, complicated
  cyclitis (Fuchs) — *see* Cyclitis, Fuchs' heterochromic
  hair L67.1
  iritis — *see* Cyclitis, Fuchs' heterochromic

**Heterochromia** — *continued*
  retained metallic foreign body (nonmagnetic) — *see* Foreign body, intraocular, old, retained
    magnetic — *see* Foreign body, intraocular, old, retained, magnetic
  uveitis — *see* Cyclitis, Fuchs' heterochromic
**Heterophoria** — *see* Strabismus, heterophoria
**Heterophyes, heterophyiasis** (small intestine) B66.8
**Heterotopia, heterotopic** (*see also* Malposition, congenital)
  cerebralis Q04.8
**Heterotropia** — *see* Strabismus
**Heubner-Herter disease** K90.0
**Hexadactylism** Q69.9
**HGSIL** (cytology finding) (high grade squamous intraepithelial lesion on cytologic smear) (Pap smear finding)
  anus R85.613
  cervix R87.613
    biopsy (histology) finding — *see* Neoplasia, intraepithelial, cervix, grade II or grade III
  vagina R87.623
    biopsy (histology) finding — *see* Neoplasia, intraepithelial, cervix, grade II or grade III
**Hibernoma** — *see* Lipoma
**Hiccup, hiccough** R06.6
  epidemic B33.0
  psychogenic F45.8
**Hidden penis** (congenital) Q55.64
  acquired N48.83
**Hidradenitis** (axillaris) (suppurative) L73.2
**Hidradenoma** (nodular) (*see also* Neoplasm, skin, benign)
  clear cell — *see* Neoplasm, skin, benign
  papillary — *see* Neoplasm, skin, benign
**Hidrocystoma** — *see* Neoplasm, skin, benign
**High**
  altitude effects T70.20 ☑
    anoxia T70.29 ☑
    on
      ears T70.0 ☑
      sinuses T70.1 ☑
    polycythemia D75.1
  arch
    foot Q66.7
    palate, congenital Q38.5
  arterial tension — *see* Hypertension
  basal metabolic rate R94.8
  blood pressure (*see also* Hypertension)
    borderline R03.0
    reading (incidental) (isolated) (nonspecific), without diagnosis of hypertension R03.0
  cholesterol E78.00
    with high triglycerides E78.2
  diaphragm (congenital) Q79.1
  expressed emotional level within family Z63.8
  head at term O32.4 ☑
  palate, congenital Q38.5
  risk
    infant NEC Z76.2
    sexual behavior (heterosexual) Z72.51
      bisexual Z72.53
      homosexual Z72.52
  scrotal testis, testes
    bilateral Q53.23
    unilateral Q53.13
  temperature (of unknown origin) R50.9
  thoracic rib Q76.6
  triglycerides E78.1
    with high cholesterol E78.2
**Hildenbrand's disease** A75.0
**Hilum** — *see* condition
**Hip** — *see* condition
**Hippel's disease** Q85.8
**Hippophobia** F40.218
**Hippus** H57.09
**Hirschsprung's disease or megacolon** Q43.1
**Hirsutism, hirsuties** L68.0
**Hirudiniasis**
  external B88.3
  internal B83.4
**Hiss-Russell dysentery** A03.1
**Histidinemia, histidinuria** E70.41
**Histiocytoma** (*see also* Neoplasm, skin, benign)
  fibrous (*see also* Neoplasm, skin, benign)
    atypical — *see* Neoplasm, connective tissue, uncertain behavior

**Histiocytoma** — *continued*
  fibrous (*see also* Neoplasm, skin, benign) — *continued*
    malignant — *see* Neoplasm, connective tissue, malignant
**Histiocytosis** D76.3
  acute differentiated progressive C96.0
  Langerhans' cell NEC C96.6
    multifocal X
      multisystemic (disseminated) C96.0
      unisystemic C96.5
    pulmonary, adult (adult PLCH) J84.82
    unifocal (X) C96.6
  lipid, lipoid D76.3
    essential E75.29
  malignant C96.A (*following* C96.6)
  mononuclear phagocytes NEC D76.1
    Langerhans' cells C96.6
  non-Langerhans cell D76.3
  polyostotic sclerosing D76.3
  sinus, with massive lymphadenopathy D76.3
  syndrome NEC D76.3
  X NEC C96.6
    acute (progressive) C96.0
    chronic C96.6
    multifocal C96.5
    multisystemic C96.0
    unifocal C96.6
**Histoplasmosis** B39.9
  with pneumonia NEC B39.2
  African B39.5
  American — *see* Histoplasmosis, capsulati
  capsulati B39.4
    disseminated B39.3
    generalized B39.3
    pulmonary B39.2
      acute B39.0
      chronic B39.1
  Darling's B39.4
  duboisii B39.5
  lung NEC B39.2
**History**
  family (of) (*see also* History, personal (of))
    alcohol abuse Z81.1
    allergy NEC Z84.89
    anemia Z83.2
    arthritis Z82.61
    asthma Z82.5
    blindness Z82.1
    cardiac death (sudden) Z82.41
    carrier of genetic disease Z84.81
    chromosomal anomaly Z82.79
    chronic
      disabling disease NEC Z82.8
      lower respiratory disease Z82.5
    colonic polyps Z83.71
    congenital malformations and deformations Z82.79
      polycystic kidney Z82.71
    consanguinity Z84.3
    deafness Z82.2
    diabetes mellitus Z83.3
    disability NEC Z82.8
    disease or disorder (of)
      allergic NEC Z84.89
      behavioral NEC Z81.8
      blood and blood-forming organs Z83.2
      cardiovascular NEC Z82.49
      chronic disabling NEC Z82.8
      digestive Z83.79
      ear NEC Z83.52
      endocrine NEC Z83.49
      eye NEC Z83.518
        glaucoma Z83.511
      familial hypercholesterolemia Z83.42
      genitourinary NEC Z84.2
      glaucoma Z83.511
      hematological Z83.2
      immune mechanism Z83.2
      infectious NEC Z83.1
      ischemic heart Z82.49
      kidney Z84.1
      mental NEC Z81.8
      metabolic Z83.49
      musculoskeletal NEC Z82.69
      neurological NEC Z82.0
      nutritional Z83.49
      parasitic NEC Z83.1
      psychiatric NEC Z81.8
      respiratory NEC Z83.6

**History** — *continued*
  family (*see also* History, personal) — *continued*
    disease or disorder — *continued*
      skin and subcutaneous tissue NEC Z84.0
        specified NEC Z84.89
      drug abuse NEC Z81.3
      epilepsy Z82.0
      familial hypercholesterolemia Z83.42
      genetic disease carrier Z84.81
      glaucoma Z83.511
      hearing loss Z82.2
      human immunodeficiency virus (HIV) infection Z83.0
      Huntington's chorea Z82.0
      intellectual disability Z81.0
      leukemia Z80.6
      malignant neoplasm (of) NOS Z80.9
        bladder Z80.52
        breast Z80.3
        bronchus Z80.1
        digestive organ Z80.0
        gastrointestinal tract Z80.0
        genital organ Z80.49
          ovary Z80.41
          prostate Z80.42
          specified organ NEC Z80.49
          testis Z80.43
        hematopoietic NEC Z80.7
        intrathoracic organ NEC Z80.2
        kidney Z80.51
        lung Z80.1
        lymphatic NEC Z80.7
        ovary Z80.41
        prostate Z80.42
        respiratory organ NEC Z80.2
        specified site NEC Z80.8
        testis Z80.43
        trachea Z80.1
        urinary organ or tract Z80.59
          bladder Z80.52
          kidney Z80.51
      mental
        disorder NEC Z81.8
      multiple endocrine neoplasia (MEN) syndrome Z83.41
      osteoporosis Z82.62
      polycystic kidney Z82.71
      polyps (colon) Z83.71
      psychiatric disorder Z81.8
      psychoactive substance abuse NEC Z81.3
      respiratory condition NEC Z83.6
        asthma and other lower respiratory conditions Z82.5
      self-harmful behavior Z81.8
      SIDS (sudden infant death syndrome) Z84.82
      skin condition Z84.0
      specified condition NEC Z84.89
      stroke (cerebrovascular) Z82.3
      substance abuse NEC Z81.4
        alcohol Z81.1
        drug NEC Z81.3
        psychoactive NEC Z81.3
        tobacco Z81.2
      sudden
        cardiac death Z82.41
        infant death syndrome (SIDS) Z84.82
      tobacco abuse Z81.2
      violence, violent behavior Z81.8
      visual loss Z82.1
  personal (of) (*see also* History, family (of))
    abuse
      adult Z91.419
        physical and sexual Z91.410
        psychological Z91.411
      childhood Z62.819
        physical Z62.810
        psychological Z62.811
        sexual Z62.810
    alcohol dependence F10.21
    allergy (to) Z88.9
      analgesic agent NEC Z88.6
      anesthetic Z88.4
      antibiotic agent NEC Z88.1
      anti-infective agent NEC Z88.3
      contrast media Z91.041
      drugs, medicaments and biological substances Z88.9
        specified NEC Z88.8
      food Z91.018

**History** — *continued*
  personal (*see also* History, family) — *continued*
    allergy — *continued*
      food — *continued*
        additives Z91.02
        eggs Z91.012
        milk products Z91.011
        peanuts Z91.010
        seafood Z91.013
        specified food NEC Z91.018
      insect Z91.038
        bee Z91.030
      latex Z91.040
      medicinal agents Z88.9
        specified NEC Z88.8
      narcotic agent NEC Z88.5
      nonmedicinal agents Z91.048
      penicillin Z88.0
      serum Z88.7
      specified NEC Z91.09
      sulfonamides Z88.2
      vaccine Z88.7
    anaphylactic shock Z87.892
    anaphylaxis Z87.892
    behavioral disorders Z86.59
    benign carcinoid tumor Z86.012
    benign neoplasm Z86.018
      brain Z86.011
      carcinoid Z86.012
      colonic polyps Z86.010
    brain injury (traumatic) Z87.820
    breast implant removal Z98.86
    calculi, renal Z87.442
    cancer — *see* History, personal (of), malignant neoplasm (of)
    cardiac arrest (death), successfully resuscitated Z86.74
    cerebral infarction without residual deficit Z86.73
    cervical dysplasia Z87.410
    chemotherapy for neoplastic condition Z92.21
    childhood abuse — *see* History, personal (of), abuse
    cleft lip (corrected) Z87.730
    cleft palate (corrected) Z87.730
    collapsed vertebra (healed) Z87.311
      due to osteoporosis Z87.310
    combat and operational stress reaction Z86.51
    congenital malformation (corrected) Z87.798
      circulatory system (corrected) Z87.74
      digestive system (corrected) NEC Z87.738
      ear (corrected) Z87.721
      eye (corrected) Z87.720
      face and neck (corrected) Z87.790
      genitourinary system (corrected) NEC Z87.718
      heart (corrected) Z87.74
      integument (corrected) Z87.76
      limb(s) (corrected) Z87.76
      musculoskeletal system (corrected) Z87.76
      neck (corrected) Z87.790
      nervous system (corrected) NEC Z87.728
      respiratory system (corrected) Z87.75
      sense organs (corrected) NEC Z87.728
      specified NEC Z87.798
    contraception Z92.0
    deployment (military) Z91.82
    diabetic foot ulcer Z86.31
    disease or disorder (of) Z87.898
      anaphylaxis Z87.892
      blood and blood-forming organs Z86.2
      circulatory system Z86.79
        specified condition NEC Z86.79
      connective tissue Z87.39
      digestive system Z87.19
        colonic polyp Z86.010
        peptic ulcer disease Z87.11
        specified condition NEC Z87.19
      ear Z86.69
      endocrine Z86.39
        diabetic foot ulcer Z86.31
        gestational diabetes Z86.32
        specified type NEC Z86.39
      eye Z86.69
      genital (track) system NEC
        female Z87.42
        male Z87.438
      hematological Z86.2
      Hodgkin Z85.71
      immune mechanism Z86.2
      infectious Z86.19

**History** — *continued*
  personal (*see also* History, family) — *continued*
    disease or disorder — *continued*
      infectious — *continued*
        malaria Z86.13
        Methicillin resistant Staphylococcus aureus (MRSA) Z86.14
        poliomyelitis Z86.12
        specified NEC Z86.19
        tuberculosis Z86.11
      mental NEC Z86.59
      metabolic Z86.39
        diabetic foot ulcer Z86.31
        gestational diabetes Z86.32
        specified type NEC Z86.39
      musculoskeletal NEC Z87.39
      nervous system Z86.69
      nutritional Z86.39
      parasitic Z86.19
      respiratory system NEC Z87.09
      sense organs Z86.69
      skin Z87.2
      specified site or type NEC Z87.898
      subcutaneous tissue Z87.2
      trophoblastic Z87.59
      urinary system NEC Z87.448
    drug dependence — *see* Dependence, drug, by type, in remission
    drug therapy
      antineoplastic chemotherapy Z92.21
      estrogen Z92.23
      immunosupression Z92.25
      inhaled steroids Z92.240
      monoclonal drug Z92.22
      specified NEC Z92.29
      steroid Z92.241
      systemic steroids Z92.241
    dysplasia
      cervical (mild) (moderate) Z87.410
        severe (grade III) Z86.001
      prostatic Z87.430
      vaginal (mild) (moderate) Z87.411
        severe (grade III) Z86.008
      vulvar (mild) (moderate) Z87.412
        severe (grade III) Z86.008
    embolism (venous) Z86.718
      pulmonary Z86.711
    encephalitis Z86.61
    estrogen therapy Z92.23
    extracorporeal membrane oxygenation (ECMO) Z92.81
    failed conscious sedation Z92.83
    failed moderate sedation Z92.83
    fall, falling Z91.81
    fracture (healed)
      fatigue Z87.312
      fragility Z87.310
      osteoporosis Z87.310
      pathological NEC Z87.311
      stress Z87.312
      traumatic Z87.81
    gestational diabetes Z86.32
    hepatitis
      B Z86.19
      C Z86.19
    Hodgkin disease Z85.71
    hyperthermia, malignant Z88.4
    hypospadias (corrected) Z87.710
    hysterectomy Z90.710
    immunosupression therapy Z92.25
    in situ neoplasm
      breast Z86.000
      cervix uteri Z86.001
      specified NEC Z86.008
    in utero procedure during pregnancy Z98.870
    in utero procedure while a fetus Z98.871
    infection NEC Z86.19
      central nervous system Z86.61
      Methicillin resistant Staphylococcus aureus (MRSA) Z86.14
      urinary (recurrent) (tract) Z87.440
    injury NEC Z87.828
    irradiation Z92.3
    kidney stones Z87.442
    leukemia Z85.6
    lymphoma (non-Hodgkin) Z85.72
    malignant melanoma (skin) Z85.820
    malignant neoplasm (of) Z85.9
      accessory sinuses Z85.22

☑ **Additional Character Required** — Refer to the Tabular List for Character Selection      ▽ Subterms under main terms may continue to next column or page

**History** — *continued*
  personal (*see also* History, family) — *continued*
    malignant neoplasm — *continued*
      anus NEC Z85.048
        carcinoid Z85.040
      bladder Z85.51
      bone Z85.830
      brain Z85.841
      breast Z85.3
      bronchus NEC Z85.118
        carcinoid Z85.110
      carcinoid — *see* History, personal (of), malignant neoplasm, by site, carcinoid
      cervix Z85.41
      colon NEC Z85.038
        carcinoid Z85.030
      digestive organ Z85.00
        specified NEC Z85.09
      endocrine gland NEC Z85.858
      epididymis Z85.48
      esophagus Z85.01
      eye Z85.840
      gastrointestinal tract — *see* History, malignant neoplasm, digestive organ
      genital organ
        female Z85.40
          specified NEC Z85.44
        male Z85.45
          specified NEC Z85.49
      hematopoietic NEC Z85.79
      intrathoracic organ Z85.20
      kidney NEC Z85.528
        carcinoid Z85.520
      large intestine NEC Z85.038
        carcinoid Z85.030
      larynx Z85.21
      liver Z85.05
      lung NEC Z85.118
        carcinoid Z85.110
      mediastinum Z85.29
      Merkel cell Z85.821
      middle ear Z85.22
      nasal cavities Z85.22
      nervous system NEC Z85.848
      oral cavity Z85.819
        specified site NEC Z85.818
      ovary Z85.43
      pancreas Z85.07
      pelvis Z85.53
      pharynx Z85.819
        specified site NEC Z85.818
      pleura Z85.29
      prostate Z85.46
      rectosigmoid junction NEC Z85.048
        carcinoid Z85.040
      rectum NEC Z85.048
        carcinoid Z85.040
      respiratory organ Z85.20
      sinuses, accessory Z85.22
      skin NEC Z85.828
        melanoma Z85.820
        Merkel cell Z85.821
      small intestine NEC Z85.068
        carcinoid Z85.060
      soft tissue Z85.831
      specified site NEC Z85.89
      stomach NEC Z85.028
        carcinoid Z85.020
      testis Z85.47
      thymus NEC Z85.238
        carcinoid Z85.230
      thyroid Z85.850
      tongue Z85.810
      trachea Z85.12
      urinary organ or tract Z85.50
        specified NEC Z85.59
      uterus Z85.42
  maltreatment Z91.89
  medical treatment NEC Z92.89
  melanoma (malignant) (skin) Z85.820
  meningitis Z86.61
  mental disorder Z86.59
  Merkel cell carcinoma (skin) Z85.821
  Methicillin resistant Staphylococcus aureus (MRSA) Z86.14
  military deployment Z91.82
  military war, peacekeeping and humanitarian deployment (current or past conflict) Z91.82
  myocardial infarction (old) I25.2

**History** — *continued*
  personal (*see also* History, family) — *continued*
    neglect (in)
      adult Z91.412
      childhood Z62.812
    neoplasm
      benign Z86.018
        brain Z86.011
        colon polyp Z86.010
      in situ
        breast Z86.000
        cervix uteri Z86.001
        specified NEC Z86.008
      malignant — *see* History of, malignant neoplasm
      uncertain behavior Z86.03
    nephrotic syndrome Z87.441
    nicotine dependence Z87.891
    noncompliance with medical treatment or regimen — *see* Noncompliance
    nutritional deficiency Z86.39
    obstetric complications Z87.59
      childbirth Z87.59
      pregnancy Z87.59
      pre-term labor Z87.51
      puerperium Z87.59
    osteoporosis fractures Z87.31 ☑
    parasuicide (attempt) Z91.5
    physical trauma NEC Z87.828
      self-harm or suicide attempt Z91.5
    pneumonia (recurrent) Z87.01
    poisoning NEC Z91.89
      self-harm or suicide attempt Z91.5
    poor personal hygiene Z91.89
    preterm labor Z87.51
    procedure during pregnancy Z98.870
    procedure while a fetus Z98.871
    prolonged reversible ischemic neurologic deficit (PRIND) Z86.73
    prostatic dysplasia Z87.430
    psychological
      abuse
        adult Z91.411
        child Z62.811
      trauma, specified NEC Z91.49
    radiation therapy Z92.3
    removal
      implant
        breast Z98.86
    renal calculi Z87.442
    respiratory condition NEC Z87.09
    retained foreign body fully removed Z87.821
    risk factors NEC Z91.89
    self-harm Z91.5
    self-poisoning attempt Z91.5
    sex reassignment Z87.890
    sleep-wake cycle problem Z72.821
    specified NEC Z87.898
    steroid therapy (systemic) Z92.241
      inhaled Z92.240
    stroke without residual deficits Z86.73
    substance abuse NEC F10-F19
    sudden cardiac arrest Z86.74
    sudden cardiac death successfully resuscitated Z86.74
    suicide attempt Z91.5
    surgery NEC Z98.890
      with uterine scar Z98.891
      sex reassignment Z87.890
      transplant — *see* Transplant
    thrombophlebitis Z86.72
    thrombosis (venous) Z86.718
      pulmonary Z86.711
    tobacco dependence Z87.891
    transient ischemic attack (TIA) without residual deficits Z86.73
    trauma (physical) NEC Z87.828
      psychological NEC Z91.49
      self-harm Z91.5
    traumatic brain injury Z87.820
    unhealthy sleep-wake cycle Z72.821
    unintended awareness under general anesthesia Z92.84
    urinary calculi Z87.442
    urinary (recurrent) (tract) infection(s) Z87.440
    uterine scar from previous surgery Z98.891
    vaginal dysplasia Z87.411
    venous thrombosis or embolism Z86.718
      pulmonary Z86.711

**History** — *continued*
  personal (*see also* History, family) — *continued*
    vulvar dysplasia Z87.412
**His-Werner disease** A79.0
**HIV** (*see also* Human, immunodeficiency virus) B20
  laboratory evidence (nonconclusive) R75
  nonconclusive test (in infants) R75
  positive, seropositive Z21
**Hives** (bold) — *see* Urticaria
**Hoarseness** R49.0
**Hobo** Z59.0
**Hodgkin disease** — *see* Lymphoma, Hodgkin
**Hodgson's disease** I71.2
  ruptured I71.1
**Hoffa-Kastert disease** E88.89
**Hoffa's disease** E88.89
**Hoffmann-Bouveret syndrome** I47.9
**Hoffmann's syndrome** E03.9 [G73.7]
**Hole** (round)
  macula H35.34- ☑
  retina (without detachment) — *see* Break, retina, round hole
    with detachment — *see* Detachment, retina, with retinal, break
**Holiday relief care** Z75.5
**Hollenhorst's plaque** — *see* Occlusion, artery, retina
**Hollow foot** (congenital) Q66.7
  acquired — *see* Deformity, limb, foot, specified NEC
**Holoprosencephaly** Q04.2
**Holt-Oram syndrome** Q87.2
**Homelessness** Z59.0
**Homesickness** — *see* Disorder, adjustment
**Homocystinemia, homocystinuria** E72.11
**Homogentisate 1,2-dioxygenase deficiency** E70.29
**Homologous serum hepatitis** (prophylactic) (therapeutic) — *see* Hepatitis, viral, type B
**Honeycomb lung** J98.4
  congenital Q33.0
**Hooded**
  clitoris Q52.6
  penis Q55.69
**Hookworm** (anemia) (disease) (infection) (infestation) B76.9
  specified NEC B76.8
**Hordeolum** (eyelid) (externum) (recurrent) H00.019
  internum H00.029
    left H00.026
      lower H00.025
      upper H00.024
    right H00.023
      lower H00.022
      upper H00.021
  left H00.016
    lower H00.015
    upper H00.014
  right H00.013
    lower H00.012
    upper H00.011
**Horn**
  cutaneous L85.8
  nail L60.2
    congenital Q84.6
**Horner** (-Claude Bernard) **syndrome** G90.2
  traumatic — *see* Injury, nerve, cervical sympathetic
**Horseshoe kidney** (congenital) Q63.1
**Horton's headache or neuralgia** G44.099
  intractable G44.091
  not intractable G44.099
**Hospital hopper syndrome** — *see* Disorder, factitious
**Hospitalism in children** — *see* Disorder, adjustment
**Hostility** R45.5
  towards child Z62.3
**Hot flashes**
  menopausal N95.1
**Hourglass** (contracture) (*see also* Contraction, hourglass)
  stomach K31.89
    congenital Q40.2
    stricture K31.2
**Household, housing circumstance affecting care** Z59.9
  specified NEC Z59.8
**Housemaid's knee** — *see* Bursitis, prepatellar
**Hudson** (-Stähli) **line** (cornea) — *see* Pigmentation, cornea, anterior
**Human**
  bite (open wound) (*see also* Bite)
    intact skin surface — *see* Bite, superficial

**Human** — *continued*
  herpesvirus — *see* Herpes
  immunodeficiency virus (HIV) disease (infection) B20
    asymptomatic status Z21
    contact Z20.6
    counseling Z71.7
    dementia B20 [F02.80]
      with behavioral disturbance B20 [F02.81]
    exposure to Z20.6
    laboratory evidence R75
    type-2 (HIV 2) as cause of disease classified elsewhere B97.35
  papillomavirus (HPV)
    DNA test positive
      high risk
        cervix R87.810
        vagina R87.811
      low risk
        cervix R87.820
        vagina R87.821
    screening for Z11.51
  T-cell lymphotropic virus
    type-1 (HTLV-I) infection B33.3
      as cause of disease classified elsewhere B97.33
      carrier Z22.6
    type-2 (HTLV-II) as cause of disease classified elsewhere B97.34
**Humidifier lung or pneumonitis** J67.7
**Humiliation** (experience) **in childhood** Z62.898
**Humpback** (acquired) — *see* Kyphosis
**Hunchback** (acquired) — *see* Kyphosis
**Hunger** T73.0 ☑
  air, psychogenic F45.8
**Hungry bone syndrome** E83.81
**Hunner's ulcer** — *see* Cystitis, chronic, interstitial
**Hunter's**
  glossitis D51.0
  syndrome E76.1
**Huntington's disease or chorea** G10
  with dementia G10 [F02.80]
    with behavioral disturbance G10 [F02.81]
**Hunt's**
  disease or syndrome (herpetic geniculate ganglionitis) B02.21
    dyssynergia cerebellaris myoclonica G11.1
  neuralgia B02.21
**Hurler** (-Scheie) **disease or syndrome** E76.02
**Hurst's disease** G36.1
**Hurthle cell**
  adenocarcinoma C73
  adenoma D34
  carcinoma C73
  tumor D34
**Hutchinson-Boeck disease or syndrome** — *see* Sarcoidosis
**Hutchinson-Gilford disease or syndrome** E34.8
**Hutchinson's**
  disease, meaning
    angioma serpiginosum L81.7
    pompholyx (cheiropompholyx) L30.1
    prurigo estivalis L56.4
    summer eruption or summer prurigo L56.4
  melanotic freckle — *see* Melanoma, in situ
    malignant melanoma in — *see* Melanoma
  teeth or incisors (congenital syphilis) A50.52
  triad (congenital syphilis) A50.53
**Hyalin plaque, sclera, senile** H15.89
**Hyaline membrane** (disease) (lung) (pulmonary) (newborn) P22.0
**Hyalinosis**
  cutis (et mucosae) E78.89
  focal and segmental (glomerular) (*see also* N00-N07 with fourth character .1) N05.1
**Hyalitis, hyalosis, asteroid** (*see also* Deposit, crystalline)
  syphilitic (late) A52.71
**Hydatid**
  cyst or tumor — *see* Echinococcus
  mole — *see* Hydatidiform mole
  Morgagni
    female Q50.5
    male (epididymal) Q55.4
      testicular Q55.29
**Hydatidiform mole** (benign) (complicating pregnancy) (delivered) (undelivered) O01.9
  classical O01.0
  complete O01.0
  incomplete O01.1
  invasive D39.2

**Hydatidiform mole** — *continued*
  malignant D39.2
  partial O01.1
**Hydatidosis** — *see* Echinococcus
**Hydradenitis** (axillaris) (suppurative) L73.2
**Hydradenoma** — *see* Hidradenoma
**Hydramnios** O40.- ☑
**Hydrancephaly, hydranencephaly** Q04.3
  with spina bifida — *see* Spina bifida, with hydrocephalus
**Hydrargyrism NEC** — *see* Poisoning, mercury
**Hydrarthrosis** (*see also* Effusion, joint)
  gonococcal A54.42
  intermittent M12.40
    ankle M12.47- ☑
    elbow M12.42- ☑
    foot joint M12.47- ☑
    hand joint M12.44- ☑
    hip M12.45- ☑
    knee M12.46- ☑
    multiple site M12.49
    shoulder M12.41- ☑
    specified joint NEC M12.48
    wrist M12.43- ☑
  of yaws (early) (late) (*see also* subcategory M14.8-) A66.6
  syphilitic (late) A52.77
    congenital A50.55 [M12.80]
**Hydremia** D64.89
**Hydrencephalocele** (congenital) — *see* Encephalocele
**Hydrencephalomeningocele** (congenital) — *see* Encephalocele
**Hydroa** R23.8
  aestivale L56.4
  vacciniforme L56.4
**Hydroadenitis** (axillaris) (suppurative) L73.2
**Hydrocalycosis** — *see* Hydronephrosis
**Hydrocele** (spermatic cord) (testis) (tunica vaginalis) N43.3
  canal of Nuck N94.89
  communicating N43.2
    congenital P83.5
  congenital P83.5
  encysted N43.0
  female NEC N94.89
  infected N43.1
  newborn P83.5
  round ligament N94.89
  specified NEC N43.2
  spinalis — *see* Spina bifida
  vulva N90.89
**Hydrocephalus** (acquired) (external) (internal) (malignant) (recurrent) G91.9
  aqueduct Sylvius stricture Q03.0
  causing disproportion O33.6 ☑
    with obstructed labor O66.3
  communicating G91.0
  congenital (external) (internal) Q03.9
    with spina bifida Q05.4
      cervical Q05.0
      dorsal Q05.1
      lumbar Q05.2
      lumbosacral Q05.2
      sacral Q05.3
      thoracic Q05.1
      thoracolumbar Q05.1
    specified NEC Q03.8
  due to toxoplasmosis (congenital) P37.1
  foramen Magendie block (acquired) G91.1
    congenital (*see also* Hydrocephalus, congenital) Q03.1
  in (due to)
    infectious disease NEC B89 [G91.4]
    neoplastic disease NEC (*see also* Neoplasm) G91.4
    parasitic disease B89 [G91.4]
  newborn Q03.9
    with spina bifida — *see* Spina bifida, with hydrocephalus
  noncommunicating G91.1
  normal pressure G91.2
    secondary G91.0
  obstructive G91.1
  otitic G93.2
  post-traumatic NEC G91.3
  secondary G91.4
    post-traumatic G91.3
  specified NEC G91.8
  syphilitic, congenital A50.49

**Hydrocolpos** (congenital) N89.8
**Hydrocystoma** — *see* Neoplasm, skin, benign
**Hydroencephalocele** (congenital) — *see* Encephalocele
**Hydroencephalomeningocele** (congenital) — *see* Encephalocele
**Hydrohematopneumothorax** — *see* Hemothorax
**Hydromeningitis** — *see* Meningitis
**Hydromeningocele** (spinal) (*see also* Spina bifida)
  cranial — *see* Encephalocele
**Hydrometra** N85.8
**Hydrometrocolpos** N89.8
**Hydromicrocephaly** Q02
**Hydromphalos** (since birth) Q45.8
**Hydromyelia** Q06.4
**Hydromyelocele** — *see* Spina bifida
**Hydronephrosis** (atrophic) (early) (functionless) (intermittent) (primary) (secondary) NEC N13.30
  with
    infection N13.6
    obstruction (by) (of)
      renal calculus N13.2
        with infection N13.6
      ureteral NEC N13.1
        with infection N13.6
        calculus N13.2
          with infection N13.6
      ureteropelvic junction (congenital) Q62.11
        acquired N13.0
          with infection N13.6
      ureteral stricture NEC N13.1
        with infection N13.6
  congenital Q62.0
  due to acquired occlusion of ureteropelvic junction N13.0
  specified type NEC N13.39
  tuberculous A18.11
**Hydropericarditis** — *see* Pericarditis
**Hydropericardium** — *see* Pericarditis
**Hydroperitoneum** R18.8
**Hydrophobia** — *see* Rabies
**Hydrophthalmos** Q15.0
**Hydropneumohemothorax** — *see* Hemothorax
**Hydropneumopericarditis** — *see* Pericarditis
**Hydropneumopericardium** — *see* Pericarditis
**Hydropneumothorax** J94.8
  traumatic — *see* Injury, intrathoracic, lung
  tuberculous NEC A15.6
**Hydrops** R60.9
  abdominis R18.8
  articulorum intermittens — *see* Hydrarthrosis, intermittent
  cardiac — *see* Failure, heart, congestive
  causing obstructed labor (mother) O66.3
  endolymphatic H81.0- ☑
  fetal — *see* Pregnancy, complicated by, hydrops, fetalis
  fetalis P83.2
    due to
      ABO isoimmunization P56.0
      alpha thalassemia D56.0
      hemolytic disease P56.90
        specified NEC P56.99
      isoimmunization (ABO) (Rh) P56.0
      other specified nonhemolytic disease NEC P83.2
      Rh incompatibility P56.0
    during pregnancy — *see* Pregnancy, complicated by, hydrops, fetalis
  gallbladder K82.1
  joint — *see* Effusion, joint
  labyrinth H81.0- ☑
  newborn (idiopathic) P83.2
    due to
      ABO isoimmunization P56.0
      alpha thalassemia D56.0
      hemolytic disease P56.90
        specified NEC P56.99
      isoimmunization (ABO) (Rh) P56.0
      Rh incompatibility P56.0
  nutritional — *see* Malnutrition, severe
  pericardium — *see* Pericarditis
  pleura — *see* Hydrothorax
  spermatic cord — *see* Hydrocele
**Hydropyonephrosis** N13.6
**Hydrorachis** Q06.4
**Hydrorrhea** (nasal) J34.89
  pregnancy — *see* Rupture, membranes, premature
**Hydrosadenitis** (axillaris) (suppurative) L73.2
**Hydrosalpinx** (fallopian tube) (follicularis) N70.11

**Hydrothorax** (double) (pleura) J94.8
  chylous (nonfilarial) I89.8
    filarial (*see also* Infestation, filarial) B74.9 [J91.8]
  traumatic — *see* Injury, intrathoracic
  tuberculous NEC (non primary) A15.6
**Hydroureter** (*see also* Hydronephrosis) N13.4
  with infection N13.6
  congenital Q62.39
**Hydroureteronephrosis** — *see* Hydronephrosis
**Hydrourethra** N36.8
**Hydroxykynureninuria** E70.8
**Hydroxylysinemia** E72.3
**Hydroxyprolinemia** E72.59
**Hygiene, sleep**
  abuse Z72.821
  inadequate Z72.821
  poor Z72.821
**Hygroma** (congenital) (cystic) D18.1
  praepatellare, prepatellar — *see* Bursitis, prepatellar
  subdural I62.03
**Hymen** — *see* condition
**Hymenolepis, hymenolepiasis** (diminuta) (infection)
  (infestation) (nana) B71.0
**Hypalgesia** R20.8
**Hyperacidity** (gastric) K31.89
  psychogenic F45.8
**Hyperactive, hyperactivity** F90.9
  basal cell, uterine cervix — *see* Dysplasia, cervix
  bowel sounds R19.12
  cervix epithelial (basal) — *see* Dysplasia, cervix
  child F90.9
    attention deficit — *see* Disorder, attention-deficit
      hyperactivity
  detrusor muscle N32.81
  gastrointestinal K31.89
    psychogenic F45.8
  nasal mucous membrane J34.3
  stomach K31.89
  thyroid (gland) — *see* Hyperthyroidism
**Hyperacusis** H93.23- ☑
**Hyperadrenalism** E27.5
**Hyperadrenocorticism** E24.9
  congenital E25.0
  iatrogenic E24.2
    correct substance properly administered — *see*
      Table of Drugs and Chemicals, by drug, ad-
      verse effect
    overdose or wrong substance given or taken —
      *see* Table of Drugs and Chemicals, by drug,
      poisoning
  not associated with Cushing's syndrome E27.0
  pituitary-dependent E24.0
**Hyperaldosteronism** E26.9
  familial (type I) E26.02
  glucocorticoid-remediable E26.02
  primary (due to (bilateral) adrenal hyperplasia) E26.09
  primary NEC E26.09
  secondary E26.1
  specified NEC E26.89
**Hyperalgesia** R20.8
**Hyperalimentation** R63.2
  carotene, carotin E67.1
  specified NEC E67.8
  vitamin
    A E67.0
    D E67.3
**Hyperaminoaciduria**
  arginine E72.21
  cystine E72.01
  lysine E72.3
  ornithine E72.4
**Hyperammonemia** (congenital) E72.20
**Hyperazotemia** — *see* Uremia
**Hyperbetalipoproteinemia** (familial) E78.00
  with prebetalipoproteinemia E78.2
**Hyperbilirubinemia**
  constitutional E80.6
  familial conjugated E80.6
  neonatal (transient) — *see* Jaundice, newborn
**Hypercalcemia, hypocalciuric, familial** E83.52
**Hypercalciuria, idiopathic** E83.52
**Hypercapnia** R06.89
  newborn P84
**Hypercarotenemia, hypercarotinemia** (dietary) E67.1
**Hypercementosis** K03.4
**Hyperchloremia** E87.8
**Hyperchlorhydria** K31.89

**Hyperchlorhydria** — *continued*
  neurotic F45.8
  psychogenic F45.8
**Hypercholesterinemia** — *see* Hypercholesterolemia
**Hypercholesterolemia** (essential) (primary) (pure)
  E78.00
  with hyperglyceridemia, endogenous E78.2
  dietary counseling and surveillance Z71.3
  familial E78.01
  hereditary E78.01
**Hyperchylia gastrica, psychogenic** F45.8
**Hyperchylomicronemia** (familial) (primary) E78.3
  with hyperbetalipoproteinemia E78.3
**Hypercoagulable** (state) D68.59
  activated protein C resistance D68.51
  antithrombin (III) deficiency D68.59
  factor V Leiden mutation D68.51
  primary NEC D68.59
  protein C deficiency D68.59
  protein S deficiency D68.59
  prothrombin gene mutation D68.52
  secondary D68.69
  specified NEC D68.69
**Hypercoagulation** (state) D68.59
**Hypercorticalism, pituitary-dependent** E24.0
**Hypercorticosolism** — *see* Cushing's, syndrome
**Hypercorticosteronism** E24.2
  correct substance properly administered — *see* Table
    of Drugs and Chemicals, by drug, adverse effect
  overdose or wrong substance given or taken — *see*
    Table of Drugs and Chemicals, by drug, poison-
    ing
**Hypercortisonism** E24.2
  correct substance properly administered — *see* Table
    of Drugs and Chemicals, by drug, adverse effect
  overdose or wrong substance given or taken — *see*
    Table of Drugs and Chemicals, by drug, poison-
    ing
**Hyperekplexia** Q89.8
**Hyperelectrolytemia** E87.8
**Hyperemesis** R11.10
  with nausea R11.2
  gravidarum (mild) O21.0
    with
      carbohydrate depletion O21.1
      dehydration O21.1
      electrolyte imbalance O21.1
      metabolic disturbance O21.1
      severe (with metabolic disturbance) O21.1
  projectile R11.12
  psychogenic F45.8
**Hyperemia** (acute) (passive) R68.89
  anal mucosa K62.89
  bladder N32.89
  cerebral I67.89
  conjunctiva H11.43- ☑
  ear internal, acute — *see* subcategory H83.0 ☑
  enteric K59.8
  eye — *see* Hyperemia, conjunctiva
  eyelid (active) (passive) — *see* Disorder, eyelid, speci-
    fied type NEC
  intestine K59.8
  iris — *see* Disorder, iris, vascular
  kidney N28.89
  labyrinth — *see* subcategory H83.0 ☑
  liver (active) K76.89
  lung (passive) — *see* Edema, lung
  pulmonary (passive) — *see* Edema, lung
  renal N28.89
  retina H35.89
  stomach K31.89
**Hyperesthesia** (body surface) R20.3
  larynx (reflex) J38.7
    hysterical F44.89
  pharynx (reflex) J39.2
    hysterical F44.89
**Hyperestrogenism** (drug-induced) (iatrogenic) E28.0
**Hyperexplexia** Q89.8
**Hyperfibrinolysis** — *see* Fibrinolysis
**Hyperfructosemia** E74.19
**Hyperfunction**
  adrenal cortex, not associated with Cushing's syn-
    drome E27.0
    medulla E27.5
      adrenomedullary E27.5
    virilism E25.9
      congenital E25.0
  ovarian E28.8

**Hyperfunction** — *continued*
  pancreas K86.89
  parathyroid (gland) E21.3
  pituitary (gland) (anterior) E22.9
    specified NEC E22.8
  polyglandular E31.1
  testicular E29.0
**Hypergammaglobulinemia** D89.2
  polyclonal D89.0
  Waldenström D89.0
**Hypergastrinemia** E16.4
**Hyperglobulinemia** R77.1
**Hyperglycemia, hyperglycemic** (transient) R73.9
  coma — *see* Diabetes, by type, with coma
  postpancreatectomy E89.1
**Hyperglyceridemia** (endogenous) (essential) (familial)
  (hereditary) (pure) E78.1
  mixed E78.3
**Hyperglycinemia** (non-ketotic) E72.51
**Hypergonadism**
  ovarian E28.8
  testicular (primary) (infantile) E29.0
**Hyperheparinemia** D68.32
**Hyperhidrosis, hyperidrosis** R61
  focal
    primary L74.519
      axilla L74.510
      face L74.511
      palms L74.512
      soles L74.513
    secondary L74.52
  generalized R61
  localized
    primary L74.519
      axilla L74.510
      face L74.511
      palms L74.512
      soles L74.513
    secondary L74.52
  psychogenic F45.8
  secondary R61
    focal L74.52
**Hyperhistidinemia** E70.41
**Hyperhomocysteinemia** E72.11
**Hyperhydroxyprolinemia** E72.59
**Hyperinsulinism** (functional) E16.1
  with
    coma (hypoglycemic) E15
    encephalopathy E16.1 [G94]
  ectopic E16.1
  therapeutic misadventure (from administration of in-
    sulin) — *see* subcategory T38.3 ☑
**Hyperkalemia** E87.5
**Hyperkeratosis** (*see also* Keratosis) L85.9
  cervix N88.0
  due to yaws (early) (late) (palmar or plantar) A66.3
  follicularis Q82.8
    penetrans (in cutem) L87.0
  palmoplantaris climacterica L85.1
  pinta A67.1
  senile (with pruritus) L57.0
  universalis congenita Q80.8
  vocal cord J38.3
  vulva N90.4
**Hyperkinesia, hyperkinetic** (disease) (reaction) (syn-
    drome) (childhood) (adolescence) (*see also* Disorder,
    attention-deficit hyperactivity)
  heart I51.89
**Hyperleucine-isoleucinemia** E71.19
**Hyperlipemia, hyperlipidemia** E78.5
  combined E78.2
    familial E78.4
  group
    A E78.00
    B E78.1
    C E78.2
    D E78.3
  mixed E78.2
  specified NEC E78.4
**Hyperlipidosis** E75.6
  hereditary NEC E75.5
**Hyperlipoproteinemia** E78.5
  Fredrickson's type
    I E78.3
    IIa E78.00
    IIb E78.2
    III E78.2
    IV E78.1

**Hyperlipoproteinemia** — continued
  Fredrickson's type — continued
    V E78.3
    low-density-lipoprotein-type (LDL) E78.00
    very-low-density-lipoprotein-type (VLDL) E78.1
**Hyperlucent lung, unilateral** J43.0
**Hyperlysinemia** E72.3
**Hypermagnesemia** E83.41
  neonatal P71.8
**Hypermenorrhea** N92.0
**Hypermethioninemia** E72.19
**Hypermetropia** (congenital) H52.0- ☑
**Hypermobility, hypermotility**
  cecum — see Syndrome, irritable bowel
  coccyx — see subcategory M53.2 ☑
  colon — see Syndrome, irritable bowel
    psychogenic F45.8
  ileum K58.9
  intestine (see also Syndrome, irritable bowel) K58.9
    psychogenic F45.8
  meniscus (knee) — see Derangement, knee, meniscus
  scapula — see Instability, joint, shoulder
  stomach K31.89
    psychogenic F45.8
  syndrome M35.7
  urethra N36.41
    with intrinsic sphincter deficiency N36.43
**Hypernasality** R49.21
**Hypernatremia** E87.0
**Hypernephroma** C64.- ☑
**Hyperopia** — see Hypermetropia
**Hyperorexia nervosa** F50.2
**Hyperornithinemia** E72.4
**Hyperosmia** R43.1
**Hyperosmolality** E87.0
**Hyperostosis** (monomelic) (see also Disorder, bone, density and structure, specified NEC)
  ankylosing (spine) M48.10
    cervical region M48.12
    cervicothoracic region M48.13
    lumbar region M48.16
    lumbosacral region M48.17
    multiple sites M48.19
    occipito-atlanto-axial region M48.11
    sacrococcygeal region M48.18
    thoracic region M48.14
    thoracolumbar region M48.15
  cortical (skull) M85.2
    infantile M89.8X- ☑
  frontal, internal of skull M85.2
  interna frontalis M85.2
  skeletal, diffuse idiopathic — see Hyperostosis, ankylosing
  skull M85.2
    congenital Q75.8
  vertebral, ankylosing — see Hyperostosis, ankylosing
**Hyperovarism** E28.8
**Hyperoxaluria** (primary) E72.53
**Hyperparathyroidism** E21.3
  primary E21.0
  secondary (renal) N25.81
    non-renal E21.1
  specified NEC E21.2
  tertiary E21.2
**Hyperpathia** R20.8
**Hyperperistalsis** R19.2
  psychogenic F45.8
**Hyperpermeability, capillary** I78.8
**Hyperphagia** R63.2
**Hyperphenylalaninemia NEC** E70.1
**Hyperphoria** (alternating) H50.53
**Hyperphosphatemia** E83.39
**Hyperpiesis, hyperpiesia** — see Hypertension
**Hyperpigmentation** (see also Pigmentation)
  melanin NEC L81.4
  postinflammatory L81.0
**Hyperpinealism** E34.8
**Hyperpituitarism** E22.9
**Hyperplasia, hyperplastic**
  adenoids J35.2
  adrenal (capsule) (cortex) (gland) E27.8
    with
      sexual precocity (male) E25.9
        congenital E25.0
      virilism, adrenal E25.9
        congenital E25.0
      virilization (female) E25.9

**Hyperplasia, hyperplastic** — continued
  adrenal — continued
    with — continued
      virilization — continued
        congenital E25.0
    congenital E25.0
      salt-losing E25.0
  adrenomedullary E27.5
  angiolymphoid, eosinophilia (ALHE) D18.01
  appendix (lymphoid) K38.0
  artery, fibromuscular I77.3
  bone (see also Hypertrophy, bone)
    marrow D75.89
  breast (see also Hypertrophy, breast)
    ductal (atypical) N60.9- ☑
  C-cell, thyroid E07.0
  cementation (tooth) (teeth) K03.4
  cervical gland R59.0
  cervix (uteri) (basal cell) (endometrium) (polypoid) (see also Dysplasia, cervix)
    congenital Q51.828
  clitoris, congenital Q52.6
  denture K06.2
  endocervicitis N72
  endometrium, endometrial (adenomatous) (benign) (cystic) (glandular) (glandular-cystic) (polypoid) N85.00
    with atypia N85.02
    cervix — see Dysplasia, cervix
    complex (without atypia) N85.01
    simple (without atypia) N85.01
  epithelial L85.9
    focal, oral, including tongue K13.29
    nipple N62
    skin L85.9
    tongue K13.29
    vaginal wall N89.3
  erythroid D75.89
  fibromuscular of artery (carotid) (renal) I77.3
  genital
    female NEC N94.89
    male N50.89
  gingiva K06.1
  glandularis cystica uteri (interstitialis) (see also Hyperplasia, endometrial) N85.00
  gum K06.1
  hymen, congenital Q52.4
  irritative, edentulous (alveolar) K06.2
  jaw M26.09
    alveolar M26.79
    lower M26.03
      alveolar M26.72
    upper M26.01
      alveolar M26.71
  kidney (congenital) Q63.3
  labia N90.69
    epithelial N90.3
  liver (congenital) Q44.7
    nodular, focal K76.89
  lymph gland or node R59.9
  mandible, mandibular M26.03
    alveolar M26.72
    unilateral condylar M27.8
  maxilla, maxillary M26.01
    alveolar M26.71
  myometrium, myometrial N85.2
  neuroendocrine cell, of infancy J84.841
  nose
    lymphoid J34.89
    polypoid J33.9
  oral mucosa (irritative) K13.6
  organ or site, congenital NEC — see Anomaly, by site
  ovary N83.8
  palate, papillary (irritative) K13.6
  pancreatic islet cells E16.9
    alpha E16.8
      with excess
        gastrin E16.4
        glucagon E16.3
    beta E16.1
  parathyroid (gland) E21.0
  pharynx (lymphoid) J39.2
  prostate (adenofibromatous) (nodular) N40.0
    with lower urinary tract symptoms (LUTS) N40.1
    without lower urinary tract symptoms (LUTS) N40.0
  renal artery I77.89
  reticulo-endothelial (cell) D75.89
  salivary gland (any) K11.1

**Hyperplasia, hyperplastic** — continued
  Schimmelbusch's — see Mastopathy, cystic
  suprarenal capsule (gland) E27.8
  thymus (gland) (persistent) E32.0
  thyroid (gland) — see Goiter
  tonsils (faucial) (infective) (lingual) (lymphoid) J35.1
    with adenoids J35.3
  unilateral condylar M27.8
  uterus, uterine N85.2
    endometrium (glandular) (see also Hyperplasia, endometrial) N85.00
  vulva N90.69
    epithelial N90.3
**Hyperpnea** — see Hyperventilation
**Hyperpotassemia** E87.5
**Hyperprebetalipoproteinemia** (familial) E78.1
**Hyperprolactinemia** E22.1
**Hyperprolinemia** (type I) (type II) E72.59
**Hyperproteinemia** E88.09
**Hyperprothrombinemia, causing coagulation factor deficiency** D68.4
**Hyperpyrexia** R50.9
  heat (effects) T67.0 ☑
  malignant, due to anesthetic T88.3 ☑
  rheumatic — see Fever, rheumatic
  unknown origin R50.9
**Hyper-reflexia** R29.2
**Hypersalivation** K11.7
**Hypersecretion**
  ACTH (not associated with Cushing's syndrome) E27.0
    pituitary E24.0
  adrenaline E27.5
  adrenomedullary E27.5
  androgen (testicular) E29.0
    ovarian (drug-induced) (iatrogenic) E28.1
  calcitonin E07.0
  catecholamine E27.5
  corticoadrenal E24.9
  cortisol E24.9
  epinephrine E27.5
  estrogen E28.0
  gastric K31.89
    psychogenic F45.8
  gastrin E16.4
  glucagon E16.3
  hormone(s)
    ACTH (not associated with Cushing's syndrome) E27.0
      pituitary E24.0
    antidiuretic E22.2
    growth E22.0
    intestinal NEC E34.1
    ovarian androgen E28.1
    pituitary E22.9
    testicular E29.0
    thyroid stimulating E05.80
      with thyroid storm E05.81
  insulin — see Hyperinsulinism
  lacrimal glands — see Epiphora
  medulloadrenal E27.5
  milk O92.6
  ovarian androgens E28.1
  salivary gland (any) K11.7
  thyrocalcitonin E07.0
  upper respiratory J39.8
**Hypersegmentation, leukocytic, hereditary** D72.0
**Hypersensitive, hypersensitiveness, hypersensitivity** (see also Allergy)
  carotid sinus G90.01
  colon — see Irritable, colon
  drug T88.7 ☑
  gastrointestinal K52.29
    immediate K52.29
    psychogenic F45.8
  labyrinth — see subcategory H83.2 ☑
  pain R20.8
  pneumonitis — see Pneumonitis, allergic
  reaction T78.40 ☑
    upper respiratory tract NEC J39.3
**Hypersomnia** (organic) G47.10
  due to
    alcohol
      abuse F10.182
      dependence F10.282
      use F10.982
    amphetamines
      abuse F15.182
      dependence F15.282

☑ **Additional Character Required** — Refer to the Tabular List for Character Selection    ▽ Subterms under main terms may continue to next column or page

**Hypersomnia** — *continued*
  due to — *continued*
    amphetamines — *continued*
      use F15.982
    caffeine
      abuse F15.182
      dependence F15.282
      use F15.982
    cocaine
      abuse F14.182
      dependence F14.282
      use F14.982
    drug NEC
      abuse F19.182
      dependence F19.282
      use F19.982
    medical condition G47.14
    mental disorder F51.13
    opioid
      abuse F11.182
      dependence F11.282
      use F11.982
    psychoactive substance NEC
      abuse F19.182
      dependence F19.282
      use F19.982
    sedative, hypnotic, or anxiolytic
      abuse F13.182
      dependence F13.282
      use F13.982
    stimulant NEC
      abuse F15.182
      dependence F15.282
      use F15.982
  idiopathic G47.11
    with long sleep time G47.11
    without long sleep time G47.12
  menstrual related G47.13
  nonorganic origin F51.11
    specified NEC F51.19
  not due to a substance or known physiological condition F51.11
    specified NEC F51.19
  primary F51.11
  recurrent G47.13
  specified NEC G47.19
**Hypersplenia, hypersplenism** D73.1
**Hyperstimulation, ovaries** (associated with induced ovulation) N98.1
**Hypersusceptibility** — *see* Allergy
**Hypertelorism** (ocular) (orbital) Q75.2
**Hypertension, hypertensive** (accelerated) (benign) (essential) (idiopathic) (malignant) (systemic) I10
  with
    heart failure (congestive) I11.0
    heart involvement (conditions in I50.-, I51.4-I51.9 due to hypertension) — *see* Hypertension, heart
    kidney involvement — *see* Hypertension, kidney
  benign, intracranial G93.2
  borderline R03.0
  cardiorenal (disease) I13.10
    with heart failure I13.0
      with stage 1 through stage 4 chronic kidney disease I13.0
      with stage 5 or end stage renal disease I13.2
    without heart failure I13.10
      with stage 1 through stage 4 chronic kidney disease I13.10
      with stage 5 or end stage renal disease I13.11
  cardiovascular
    disease (arteriosclerotic) (sclerotic) — *see* Hypertension, heart
    renal (disease) — *see* Hypertension, cardiorenal
  chronic venous — *see* Hypertension, venous (chronic)
  complicating
    childbirth (labor) O16.4
      pre-existing O10.92
        with
          heart disease O10.12
            with renal disease O10.32
          pre-eclampsia O11.4
          renal disease O10.22
            with heart disease O10.32
          essential O10.02
      secondary O10.42
    pregnancy O16.- ☑
      with edema (*see also* Pre-eclampsia) O14.9- ☑

**Hypertension, hypertensive** — *continued*
  complicating — *continued*
    pregnancy — *continued*
      gestational (pregnancy induced) (without proteinuria) O13.- ☑
        with proteinuria O14.9- ☑
          mild pre-eclampsia O14.0- ☑
          moderate pre-eclampsia O14.0- ☑
          severe pre-eclampsia O14.1- ☑
            with hemolysis, elevated liver enzymes and low platelet count (HELLP) O14.2- ☑
      pre-existing O10.91- ☑
        with
          heart disease O10.11- ☑
            with renal disease O10.31- ☑
          pre-eclampsia — *see* category O11
          renal disease O10.21- ☑
            with heart disease O10.31- ☑
        essential O10.01- ☑
      secondary O10.41- ☑
      transient O13- ☑
    puerperium, pre-existing O16.5
      pre-existing
        with
          heart disease O10.13
            with renal disease O10.33
          pre-eclampsia O11.5
          renal disease O10.23
            with heart disease O10.33
          essential O10.03
      pregnancy-induced O13.9
      secondary O10.43
  crisis I16.9
  due to
    endocrine disorders I15.2
    pheochromocytoma I15.2
    renal disorders NEC I15.1
      arterial I15.0
    renovascular disorders I15.0
    specified disease NEC I15.8
  emergency I16.1
  encephalopathy I67.4
  gestational (without significant proteinuria) (pregnancy-induced) (transient) O13.- ☑
    with significant proteinuria — *see* Pre-eclampsia
  complicating
    delivery O13.4
    puerperium O13.5
  Goldblatt's I70.1
  heart (disease) (conditions in I51.4-I51.9 due to hypertension) I11.9
    with
      heart failure (congestive) I11.0
      kidney disease (chronic) — *see* Hypertension, cardiorenal
  intracranial (benign) G93.2
  kidney I12.9
    with
      heart disease — *see* Hypertension, cardiorenal
      stage 1 through stage 4 chronic kidney disease I12.9
      stage 5 chronic kidney disease (CKD) or end stage renal disease (ESRD) I12.0
  lesser circulation I27.0
  maternal O16- ☑
  newborn P29.2
    pulmonary (persistent) P29.30
  ocular H40.05- ☑
  pancreatic duct — *code to* underlying condition
    with chronic pancreatitis K86.1
  portal (due to chronic liver disease) (idiopathic) K76.6
    gastropathy K31.89
    in (due to) schistosomiasis (bilharziasis) B65.9 [K77]
  postoperative I97.3
  psychogenic F45.8
  pulmonary I27.20
    with
      cor pulmonale (chronic) I27.29
        acute I26.09
      right heart ventricular strain/failure I27.29
        acute I26.09
      right to left shunt related to congenital heart disease I27.83
      unclear multifactorial mechanisms I27.29
    arterial (associated) (drug-induced) (toxin-induced) I27.21
    chronic thromboembolic I27.24

**Hypertension, hypertensive** — *continued*
  pulmonary — *continued*
    due to
      hematologic disorders I27.29
      left heart disease I27.22
      lung diseases and hypoxia I27.23
      metabolic disorders I27.29
      specified systemic disorders I27.29
    group 1 (associated) (drug-induced) (toxin-induced) I27.21
    group 2 I27.22
    group 3 I27.23
    group 4 I27.24
    group 5 I27.29
    of newborn (persistent) P29.30
    primary (idiopathic) I27.0
    secondary
      arterial I27.21
      specified NEC I27.29
  renal — *see* Hypertension, kidney
  renovascular I15.0
  secondary NEC I15.9
    due to
      endocrine disorders I15.2
      pheochromocytoma I15.2
      renal disorders NEC I15.1
        arterial I15.0
      renovascular disorders I15.0
    specified NEC I15.8
  transient, of pregnancy O13- ☑
  urgency I16.0
  venous (chronic)
    due to
      deep vein thrombosis — *see* Syndrome, post-thrombotic
    idiopathic I87.309
      with
        inflammation I87.32- ☑
          with ulcer I87.33- ☑
        specified complication NEC I87.39- ☑
        ulcer I87.31- ☑
          with inflammation I87.33- ☑
      asymptomatic I87.30- ☑
**Hypertensive urgency** — *see* Hypertension
**Hyperthecosis ovary** E28.8
**Hyperthermia** (of unknown origin) (*see also* Hyperpyrexia)
  malignant, due to anesthesia T88.3 ☑
  newborn P81.9
    environmental P81.0
**Hyperthyroid** (recurrent) — *see* Hyperthyroidism
**Hyperthyroidism** (latent) (pre-adult) (recurrent) E05.90
  with
    goiter (diffuse) E05.00
      with thyroid storm E05.01
      nodular (multinodular) E05.20
        with thyroid storm E05.21
        uninodular E05.10
          with thyroid storm E05.11
      storm E05.91
  due to ectopic thyroid tissue E05.30
    with thyroid storm E05.31
  neonatal, transitory P72.1
  specified NEC E05.80
    with thyroid storm E05.81
**Hypertony, hypertonia, hypertonicity**
  bladder N31.8
  congenital P94.1
  stomach K31.89
    psychogenic F45.8
  uterus, uterine (contractions) (complicating delivery) O62.4
**Hypertrichosis** L68.9
  congenital Q84.2
  eyelid H02.869
    left H02.866
      lower H02.865
      upper H02.864
    right H02.863
      lower H02.862
      upper H02.861
  lanuginosa Q84.2
    acquired L68.1
  localized L68.2
  specified NEC L68.8
**Hypertriglyceridemia, essential** E78.1

**Hypertrophy, hypertrophic**
adenofibromatous, prostate — *see* Enlargement, enlarged, prostate
adenoids (infective) J35.2
  with tonsils J35.3
adrenal cortex E27.8
alveolar process or ridge — *see* Anomaly, alveolar
anal papillae K62.89
artery I77.89
  congenital NEC Q27.8
    digestive system Q27.8
    lower limb Q27.8
    specified site NEC Q27.8
    upper limb Q27.8
auricular — *see* Hypertrophy, cardiac
Bartholin's gland N75.8
bile duct (common) (hepatic) K83.8
bladder (sphincter) (trigone) N32.89
bone M89.30
  carpus M89.34- ☑
  clavicle M89.31- ☑
  femur M89.35- ☑
  fibula M89.36- ☑
  finger M89.34- ☑
  humerus M89.32- ☑
  ilium M89.359
  ischium M89.359
  metacarpus M89.34- ☑
  metatarsus M89.37- ☑
  multiple sites M89.39
  neck M89.38
  radius M89.33- ☑
  rib M89.38
  scapula M89.31- ☑
  skull M89.38
  tarsus M89.37- ☑
  tibia M89.36- ☑
  toe M89.37- ☑
  ulna M89.33- ☑
  vertebra M89.38
brain G93.89
breast N62
  cystic — *see* Mastopathy, cystic
  newborn P83.4
  pubertal, massive N62
  puerperal, postpartum — *see* Disorder, breast, specified type NEC
  senile (parenchymatous) N62
cardiac (chronic) (idiopathic) I51.7
  with rheumatic fever (conditions in I00)
    active I01.8
    inactive or quiescent (with chorea) I09.89
  congenital NEC Q24.8
  fatty — *see* Degeneration, myocardial
  hypertensive — *see* Hypertension, heart
  rheumatic (with chorea) I09.89
    active or acute I01.8
      with chorea I02.0
  valve — *see* Endocarditis
cartilage — *see* Disorder, cartilage, specified type NEC
cecum — *see* Megacolon
cervix (uteri) N88.8
  congenital Q51.828
  elongation N88.4
clitoris (cirrhotic) N90.89
  congenital Q52.6
colon (*see also* Megacolon)
  congenital Q43.2
conjunctiva, lymphoid H11.89
corpora cavernosa N48.89
cystic duct K82.8
duodenum K31.89
endometrium (glandular) (*see also* Hyperplasia, endometrial) N85.00
  cervix N88.8
epididymis N50.89
esophageal hiatus (congenital) Q79.1
  with hernia — *see* Hernia, hiatal
eyelid — *see* Disorder, eyelid, specified type NEC
fat pad E65
  knee (infrapatellar) (popliteal) (prepatellar) (retropatellar) M79.4
foot (congenital) Q74.2
frenulum, frenum (tongue) K14.8
  lip K13.0
gallbladder K82.8
gastric mucosa K29.60
  with bleeding K29.61

**Hypertrophy, hypertrophic** — *continued*
gland, glandular R59.9
  generalized R59.1
  localized R59.0
gum (mucous membrane) K06.1
heart (idiopathic) (*see also* Hypertrophy, cardiac)
  valve (*see also* Endocarditis) I38
hemifacial Q67.4
hepatic — *see* Hypertrophy, liver
hiatus (esophageal) Q79.1
hilus gland R59.0
hymen, congenital Q52.4
ileum K63.89
intestine NEC K63.89
jejunum K63.89
kidney (compensatory) N28.81
  congenital Q63.3
labium (majus) (minus) N90.60
ligament — *see* Disorder, ligament
lingual tonsil (infective) J35.1
  with adenoids J35.3
lip K13.0
  congenital Q18.6
liver R16.0
  acute K76.89
  cirrhotic — *see* Cirrhosis, liver
  congenital Q44.7
  fatty — *see* Fatty, liver
lymph, lymphatic gland R59.9
  generalized R59.1
  localized R59.0
  tuberculous — *see* Tuberculosis, lymph gland
mammary gland — *see* Hypertrophy, breast
Meckel's diverticulum (congenital) Q43.0
  malignant — *see* Table of Neoplasms, small intestine, malignant
median bar — *see* Hyperplasia, prostate
meibomian gland — *see* Chalazion
meniscus, knee, congenital Q74.1
metatarsal head — *see* Hypertrophy, bone, metatarsus
metatarsus — *see* Hypertrophy, bone, metatarsus
mucous membrane
  alveolar ridge K06.2
  gum K06.1
  nose (turbinate) J34.3
muscle M62.89
muscular coat, artery I77.89
myocardium (*see also* Hypertrophy, cardiac)
  idiopathic I42.2
myometrium N85.2
nail L60.2
  congenital Q84.5
nasal J34.89
  alae J34.89
  bone J34.89
  cartilage J34.89
  mucous membrane (septum) J34.3
  sinus J34.89
  turbinate J34.3
nasopharynx, lymphoid (infectional) (tissue) (wall) J35.2
nipple N62
organ or site, congenital NEC — *see* Anomaly, by site
ovary N83.8
palate (hard) M27.8
  soft K13.79
pancreas, congenital Q45.3
parathyroid (gland) E21.0
parotid gland K11.1
penis N48.89
pharyngeal tonsil J35.2
pharynx J39.2
  lymphoid (infectional) (tissue) (wall) J35.2
pituitary (anterior) (fossa) (gland) E23.6
prepuce (congenital) N47.8
  female N90.89
prostate — *see* Enlargement, enlarged, prostate
  congenital Q55.4
pseudomuscular G71.0
pylorus (adult) (muscle) (sphincter) K31.1
  congenital or infantile Q40.0
rectal, rectum (sphincter) K62.89
rhinitis (turbinate) J31.0
salivary gland (any) K11.1
  congenital Q38.4
scaphoid (tarsal) — *see* Hypertrophy, bone, tarsus
scar L91.0
scrotum N50.89

**Hypertrophy, hypertrophic** — *continued*
seminal vesicle N50.89
sigmoid — *see* Megacolon
skin L91.9
  specified NEC L91.8
spermatic cord N50.89
spleen — *see* Splenomegaly
spondylitis — *see* Spondylosis
stomach K31.89
sublingual gland K11.1
submandibular gland K11.1
suprarenal cortex (gland) E27.8
synovial NEC M67.20
  acromioclavicular M67.21- ☑
  ankle M67.27- ☑
  elbow M67.22- ☑
  foot M67.27- ☑
  hand M67.24- ☑
  hip M67.25- ☑
  knee M67.26- ☑
  multiple sites M67.29
  specified site NEC M67.28
  wrist M67.23- ☑
tendon — *see* Disorder, tendon, specified type NEC
testis N44.8
  congenital Q55.29
thymic, thymus (gland) (congenital) E32.0
thyroid (gland) — *see* Goiter
toe (congenital) Q74.2
  acquired (*see also* Deformity, toe, specified NEC)
tongue K14.8
  congenital Q38.2
  papillae (foliate) K14.3
tonsils (faucial) (infective) (lingual) (lymphoid) J35.1
  with adenoids J35.3
tunica vaginalis N50.89
ureter N28.89
urethra N36.8
uterus N85.2
  neck (with elongation) N88.4
  puerperal O90.89
uvula K13.79
vagina N89.8
vas deferens N50.89
vein I87.8
ventricle, ventricular (heart) (*see also* Hypertrophy, cardiac)
  congenital Q24.8
  in tetralogy of Fallot Q21.3
verumontanum N36.8
vocal cord J38.3
vulva N90.60
  stasis (nonfilarial) N90.69
**Hypertropia** H50.2- ☑
**Hypertyrosinemia** E70.21
**Hyperuricemia** (asymptomatic) E79.0
**Hypervalinemia** E71.19
**Hyperventilation** (tetany) R06.4
  hysterical F45.8
  psychogenic F45.8
  syndrome F45.8
**Hypervitaminosis** (dietary) NEC E67.8
  A E67.0
    administered as drug (prolonged intake) — *see* Table of Drugs and Chemicals, vitamins, adverse effect
    overdose or wrong substance given or taken — *see* Table of Drugs and Chemicals, vitamins, poisoning
  B6 E67.2
  D E67.3
    administered as drug (prolonged intake) — *see* Table of Drugs and Chemicals, vitamins, adverse effect
    overdose or wrong substance given or taken — *see* Table of Drugs and Chemicals, vitamins, poisoning
  K E67.8
    administered as drug (prolonged intake) — *see* Table of Drugs and Chemicals, vitamins, adverse effect
    overdose or wrong substance given or taken — *see* Table of Drugs and Chemicals, vitamins, poisoning
**Hypervolemia** E87.70
  specified NEC E87.79
**Hypesthesia** R20.1
  cornea — *see* Anesthesia, cornea

☑ **Additional Character Required** — Refer to the Tabular List for Character Selection        ⬇ **Subterms under main terms may continue to next column or page**

**Hyphema** H21.0- ☑
   traumatic S05.1- ☑
**Hypoacidity, gastric** K31.89
   psychogenic F45.8
**Hypoadrenalism, hypoadrenia** E27.40
   primary E27.1
   tuberculous A18.7
**Hypoadrenocorticism** E27.40
   pituitary E23.0
   primary E27.1
**Hypoalbuminemia** E88.09
**Hypoaldosteronism** E27.40
**Hypoalphalipoproteinemia** E78.6
**Hypobarism** T70.29 ☑
**Hypobaropathy** T70.29 ☑
**Hypobetalipoproteinemia** (familial) E78.6
**Hypocalcemia** E83.51
   dietary E58
   neonatal P71.1
      due to cow's milk P71.0
   phosphate-loading (newborn) P71.1
**Hypochloremia** E87.8
**Hypochlorhydria** K31.89
   neurotic F45.8
   psychogenic F45.8
**Hypochondria, hypochondriac, hypochondriasis**
   (reaction) F45.21
   sleep F51.03
**Hypochondrogenesis** Q77.0
**Hypochondroplasia** Q77.4
**Hypochromasia, blood cells** D50.8
**Hypodontia** — *see* Anodontia
**Hypoeosinophilia** D72.89
**Hypoesthesia** R20.1
**Hypofibrinogenemia** D68.8
   acquired D65
   congenital (hereditary) D68.2
**Hypofunction**
   adrenocortical E27.40
      drug-induced E27.3
      postprocedural E89.6
      primary E27.1
   adrenomedullary, postprocedural E89.6
   cerebral R29.818
   corticoadrenal NEC E27.40
   intestinal K59.8
   labyrinth — *see* subcategory H83.2 ☑
   ovary E28.39
   pituitary (gland) (anterior) E23.0
   testicular E29.1
      postprocedural (postsurgical) (postirradiation) (iatrogenic) E89.5
**Hypogalactia** O92.4
**Hypogammaglobulinemia** (*see also* Agammaglobulinemia) D80.1
   hereditary D80.0
   nonfamilial D80.1
   transient, of infancy D80.7
**Hypogenitalism** (congenital) — *see* Hypogonadism
**Hypoglossia** Q38.3
**Hypoglycemia** (spontaneous) E16.2
   coma E15
      diabetic — *see* Diabetes, by type, with hypoglycemia, with coma
   diabetic — *see* Diabetes, hypoglycemia
   dietary counseling and surveillance Z71.3
   drug-induced E16.0
      with coma (nondiabetic) E15
   due to insulin E16.0
      with coma (nondiabetic) E15
      therapeutic misadventure — *see* subcategory T38.3 ☑
   functional, nonhyperinsulinemic E16.1
   iatrogenic E16.0
      with coma (nondiabetic) E15
   in infant of diabetic mother P70.1
      gestational diabetes P70.0
   infantile E16.1
   leucine-induced E71.19
   neonatal (transitory) P70.4
      iatrogenic P70.3
   reactive (not drug-induced) E16.1
   transitory neonatal P70.4
**Hypogonadism**
   female E28.39
   hypogonadotropic E23.0
   male E29.1
   ovarian (primary) E28.39

**Hypogonadism** — *continued*
   pituitary E23.0
   testicular (primary) E29.1
**Hypohidrosis, hypoidrosis** L74.4
**Hypoinsulinemia, postprocedural** E89.1
**Hypokalemia** E87.6
**Hypoleukocytosis** — *see* Agranulocytosis
**Hypolipoproteinemia** (alpha) (beta) E78.6
**Hypomagnesemia** E83.42
   neonatal P71.2
**Hypomania, hypomanic reaction** F30.8
**Hypomenorrhea** — *see* Oligomenorrhea
**Hypometabolism** R63.8
**Hypomotility**
   gastrointestinal (tract) K31.89
      psychogenic F45.8
   intestine K59.8
      psychogenic F45.8
   stomach K31.89
      psychogenic F45.8
**Hyponasality** R49.22
**Hyponatremia** E87.1
**Hypo-osmolality** E87.1
**Hypo-ovarianism, hypo-ovarism** E28.39
**Hypoparathyroidism** E20.9
   familial E20.8
   idiopathic E20.0
   neonatal, transitory P71.4
   postprocedural E89.2
   specified NEC E20.8
**Hypoperfusion** (in)
   newborn P96.89
**Hypopharyngitis** — *see* Laryngopharyngitis
**Hypophoria** H50.53
**Hypophosphatemia, hypophosphatasia** (acquired) (congenital) (renal) E83.39
   familial E83.31
**Hypophyseal, hypophysis** (*see also* condition)
   dwarfism E23.0
   gigantism E22.0
**Hypopiesis** — *see* Hypotension
**Hypopinealism** E34.8
**Hypopituitarism** (juvenile) E23.0
   drug-induced E23.1
   due to
      hypophysectomy E89.3
      radiotherapy E89.3
   iatrogenic NEC E23.1
   postirradiation E89.3
   postpartum O99.285
   postprocedural E89.3
**Hypoplasia, hypoplastic**
   adrenal (gland), congenital Q89.1
   alimentary tract, congenital Q45.8
      upper Q40.8
   anus, anal (canal) Q42.3
      with fistula Q42.2
   aorta, aortic Q25.42
      ascending, in hypoplastic left heart syndrome Q23.4
      valve Q23.1
         in hypoplastic left heart syndrome Q23.4
   areola, congenital Q83.8
   arm (congenital) — *see* Defect, reduction, upper limb
   artery (peripheral) Q27.8
      brain (congenital) Q28.3
      coronary Q24.5
      digestive system Q27.8
      lower limb Q27.8
      pulmonary Q25.79
         functional, unilateral J43.0
      retinal (congenital) Q14.1
      specified site NEC Q27.8
      umbilical Q27.0
      upper limb Q27.8
   auditory canal Q17.8
      causing impairment of hearing Q16.9
   biliary duct or passage Q44.5
   bone NOS Q79.9
      face Q75.8
      marrow D61.9
         megakaryocytic D69.49
      skull — *see* Hypoplasia, skull
   brain Q02
      gyri Q04.3
      part of Q04.3
   breast (areola) N64.82
   bronchus Q32.4

**Hypoplasia, hypoplastic** — *continued*
   cardiac Q24.8
   carpus — *see* Defect, reduction, upper limb, specified type NEC
   cartilage hair Q78.8
   cecum Q42.8
   cementum K00.4
   cephalic Q02
   cerebellum Q04.3
   cervix (uteri), congenital Q51.821
   clavicle (congenital) Q74.0
   coccyx Q76.49
   colon Q42.9
      specified NEC Q42.8
   corpus callosum Q04.0
   cricoid cartilage Q31.2
   digestive organ(s) or tract NEC Q45.8
      upper (congenital) Q40.8
   ear (auricle) (lobe) Q17.2
      middle Q16.4
   enamel of teeth (neonatal) (postnatal) (prenatal) K00.4
   endocrine (gland) NEC Q89.2
   endometrium N85.8
   epididymis (congenital) Q55.4
   epiglottis Q31.2
   erythroid, congenital D61.01
   esophagus (congenital) Q39.8
   eustachian tube Q17.8
   eye Q11.2
   eyelid (congenital) Q10.3
   face Q18.8
      bone(s) Q75.8
   femur (congenital) — *see* Defect, reduction, lower limb, specified type NEC
   fibula (congenital) — *see* Defect, reduction, lower limb, specified type NEC
   finger (congenital) — *see* Defect, reduction, upper limb, specified type NEC
   focal dermal Q82.8
   foot — *see* Defect, reduction, lower limb, specified type NEC
   gallbladder Q44.0
   genitalia, genital organ(s)
      female, congenital Q52.8
         external Q52.79
         internal NEC Q52.8
      in adiposogenital dystrophy E23.6
   glottis Q31.2
   hair Q84.2
   hand (congenital) — *see* Defect, reduction, upper limb, specified type NEC
   heart Q24.8
   humerus (congenital) — *see* Defect, reduction, upper limb, specified type NEC
   intestine (small) Q41.9
      large Q42.9
         specified NEC Q42.8
   jaw M26.09
      alveolar M26.79
      lower M26.04
         alveolar M26.74
      upper M26.02
         alveolar M26.73
   kidney(s) Q60.5
      bilateral Q60.4
      unilateral Q60.3
   labium (majus) (minus), congenital Q52.79
   larynx Q31.2
   left heart syndrome Q23.4
   leg (congenital) — *see* Defect, reduction, lower limb
   limb Q73.8
      lower (congenital) — *see* Defect, reduction, lower limb
      upper (congenital) — *see* Defect, reduction, upper limb
   liver Q44.7
   lung (lobe) (not associated with short gestation) Q33.6
      associated with immaturity, low birth weight, prematurity, or short gestation P28.0
   mammary (areola), congenital Q83.8
   mandible, mandibular M26.04
      alveolar M26.74
      unilateral condylar M27.8
   maxillary M26.02
      alveolar M26.73
   medullary D61.9
   megakaryocytic D69.49

**Hypoplasia, hypoplastic** — *continued*
  metacarpus — *see* Defect, reduction, upper limb, specified type NEC
  metatarsus — *see* Defect, reduction, lower limb, specified type NEC
  muscle Q79.8
  nail(s) Q84.6
  nose, nasal Q30.1
  optic nerve H47.03- ☑
  osseous meatus (ear) Q17.8
  ovary, congenital Q50.39
  pancreas Q45.0
  parathyroid (gland) Q89.2
  parotid gland Q38.4
  patella Q74.1
  pelvis, pelvic girdle Q74.2
  penis (congenital) Q55.62
  peripheral vascular system Q27.8
    digestive system Q27.8
    lower limb Q27.8
    specified site NEC Q27.8
    upper limb Q27.8
  pituitary (gland) (congenital) Q89.2
  pulmonary (not associated with short gestation) Q33.6
    artery, functional J43.0
    associated with short gestation P28.0
  radioulnar — *see* Defect, reduction, upper limb, specified type NEC
  radius — *see* Defect, reduction, upper limb
  rectum Q42.1
    with fistula Q42.0
  respiratory system NEC Q34.8
  rib Q76.6
  right heart syndrome Q22.6
  sacrum Q76.49
  scapula Q74.0
  scrotum Q55.1
  shoulder girdle Q74.0
  skin Q82.8
  skull (bone) Q75.8
    with
      anencephaly Q00.0
      encephalocele — *see* Encephalocele
      hydrocephalus Q03.9
        with spina bifida — *see* Spina bifida, by site, with hydrocephalus
      microcephaly Q02
  spinal (cord) (ventral horn cell) Q06.1
  spine Q76.49
  sternum Q76.7
  tarsus — *see* Defect, reduction, lower limb, specified type NEC
  testis Q55.1
  thymic, with immunodeficiency D82.1
  thymus (gland) Q89.2
    with immunodeficiency D82.1
  thyroid (gland) E03.1
    cartilage Q31.2
  tibiofibular (congenital) — *see* Defect, reduction, lower limb, specified type NEC
  toe — *see* Defect, reduction, lower limb, specified type NEC
  tongue Q38.3
  Turner's K00.4
  ulna (congenital) — *see* Defect, reduction, upper limb
  umbilical artery Q27.0
  unilateral condylar M27.8
  ureter Q62.8
  uterus, congenital Q51.811
  vagina Q52.4
  vascular NEC peripheral Q27.8
    brain Q28.3
    digestive system Q27.8
    lower limb Q27.8
    specified site NEC Q27.8
    upper limb Q27.8
  vein(s) (peripheral) Q27.8
    brain Q28.3
    digestive system Q27.8
    great Q26.8
    lower limb Q27.8
    specified site NEC Q27.8
    upper limb Q27.8
  vena cava (inferior) (superior) Q26.8
  vertebra Q76.49
  vulva, congenital Q52.79
  zonule (ciliary) Q12.8
**Hypopnea, obstructive sleep apnea** G47.33

**Hypopotassemia** E87.6
**Hypoproconvertinemia, congenital** (hereditary) D68.2
**Hypoproteinemia** E77.8
**Hypoprothrombinemia** (congenital) (hereditary) (idiopathic) D68.2
  acquired D68.4
  newborn, transient P61.6
**Hypoptyalism** K11.7
**Hypopyon** (eye) (anterior chamber) — *see* Iridocyclitis, acute, hypopyon
**Hypopyrexia** R68.0
**Hyporeflexia** R29.2
**Hyposecretion**
  ACTH E23.0
  antidiuretic hormone E23.2
  ovary E28.39
  salivary gland (any) K11.7
  vasopressin E23.2
**Hyposegmentation, leukocytic, hereditary** D72.0
**Hyposiderinemia** D50.9
**Hypospadias** Q54.9
  balanic Q54.0
  coronal Q54.0
  glandular Q54.0
  penile Q54.1
  penoscrotal Q54.2
  perineal Q54.3
  specified NEC Q54.8
**Hypospermatogenesis** — *see* Oligospermia
**Hyposplenism** D73.0
**Hypostasis pulmonary, passive** — *see* Edema, lung
**Hypostatic** — *see* condition
**Hyposthenuria** N28.89
**Hypotension** (arterial) (constitutional) I95.9
  chronic I95.89
  drug-induced I95.2
  due to (of) hemodialysis I95.3
  iatrogenic I95.89
  idiopathic (permanent) I95.0
  intracranial, following ventricular shunting (ventriculostomy) G97.2
  intra-dialytic I95.3
  maternal, syndrome (following labor and delivery) O26.5- ☑
  neurogenic, orthostatic G90.3
  orthostatic (chronic) I95.1
    due to drugs I95.2
    neurogenic G90.3
  postoperative I95.81
  postural I95.1
  specified NEC I95.89
**Hypothermia** (accidental) T68 ☑
  due to anesthesia, anesthetic T88.51 ☑
  low environmental temperature T68 ☑
  neonatal P80.9
    environmental (mild) NEC P80.8
    mild P80.8
    severe (chronic) (cold injury syndrome) P80.0
    specified NEC P80.8
  not associated with low environmental temperature R68.0
**Hypothyroidism** (acquired) E03.9
  autoimmune — *see* Thyroiditis, autoimmune
  congenital (without goiter) E03.1
    with goiter (diffuse) E03.0
  due to
    exogenous substance NEC E03.2
    iodine-deficiency, acquired E01.8
      subclinical E02
    irradiation therapy E89.0
    medicament NEC E03.2
    P-aminosalicylic acid (PAS) E03.2
    phenylbutazone E03.2
    resorcinol E03.2
    sulfonamide E03.2
    surgery E89.0
    thiourea group drugs E03.2
  iatrogenic NEC E03.2
  iodine-deficiency (acquired) E01.8
    congenital — *see* Syndrome, iodine- deficiency, congenital
    subclinical E02
  neonatal, transitory P72.2
  postinfectious E03.3
  postirradiation E89.0
  postprocedural E89.0
  postsurgical E89.0
  specified NEC E03.8

**Hypothyroidism** — *continued*
  subclinical, iodine-deficiency related E02
**Hypotonia, hypotonicity, hypotony**
  bladder N31.2
  congenital (benign) P94.2
  eye — *see* Disorder, globe, hypotony
**Hypotrichosis** — *see* Alopecia
**Hypotropia** H50.2- ☑
**Hypoventilation** R06.89
  congenital central alveolar G47.35
  sleep related
    idiopathic nonobstructive alveolar G47.34
    in conditions classified elsewhere G47.36
**Hypovitaminosis** — *see* Deficiency, vitamin
**Hypovolemia** E86.1
  surgical shock T81.19 ☑
  traumatic (shock) T79.4 ☑
**Hypoxemia** R09.02
  newborn P84
  sleep related, in conditions classified elsewhere G47.36
**Hypoxia** (see also Anoxia) R09.02
  cerebral, during a procedure NEC G97.81
    postprocedural NEC G97.82
  intrauterine P84
  myocardial — *see* Insufficiency, coronary
  newborn P84
  sleep-related G47.34
**Hypsarhythmia** — *see* Epilepsy, generalized, specified NEC
**Hysteralgia, pregnant uterus** O26.89- ☑
**Hysteria, hysterical** (conversion) (dissociative state) F44.9
  anxiety F41.8
  convulsions F44.5
  psychosis, acute F44.9
**Hysteroepilepsy** F44.5

# I

**IBDU** (colonic inflammatory bowel dissease unclassified) K52.3
**Ichthyoparasitism due to Vandellia cirrhosa** B88.8
**Ichthyosis** (congenital) Q80.9
  acquired L85.0
  fetalis Q80.4
  hystrix Q80.8
  lamellar Q80.2
  lingual K13.29
  palmaris and plantaris Q82.8
  simplex Q80.0
  vera Q80.8
  vulgaris Q80.0
  X-linked Q80.1
**Ichthyotoxism** — *see* Poisoning, fish
  bacterial — *see* Intoxication, foodborne
**Icteroanemia, hemolytic** (acquired) D59.9
  congenital — *see* Spherocytosis
**Icterus** (see also Jaundice)
  conjunctiva R17
  gravis, newborn P55.0
  hematogenous (acquired) D59.9
  hemolytic (acquired) D59.9
    congenital — *see* Spherocytosis
  hemorrhagic (acute) (leptospiral) (spirochetal) A27.0
    newborn P53
  infectious B15.9
    with hepatic coma B15.0
    leptospiral A27.0
    spirochetal A27.0
  neonatorum — *see* Jaundice, newborn
  newborn P59.9
  spirochetal A27.0
**Ictus solaris, solis** T67.0 ☑
**Id reaction** (due to bacteria) L30.2
**Ideation**
  homicidal R45.850
  suicidal R45.851
**Identity disorder** (child) F64.9
  gender role F64.2
  psychosexual F64.2
**Idioglossia** F80.0
**Idiopathic** — *see* condition
**Idiot, idiocy** (congenital) F73
  amaurotic (Bielschowsky(-Jansky)) (family) (infantile (late)) (juvenile (late)) (Vogt-Spielmeyer) E75.4
  microcephalic Q02
**IgE asthma** J45.909

   ☑ **Additional Character Required** — Refer to the Tabular List for Character Selection    ▽ **Subterms under main terms may continue to next column or page**

**IIAC** (idiopathic infantile arterial calcification) Q28.8
**Ileitis** (chronic) (noninfectious) (see also Enteritis) K52.9
  backwash — see Pancolitis, ulcerative (chronic)
  infectious A09
  regional (ulcerative) — see Enteritis, regional, small intestine
  segmental — see Enteritis, regional
  terminal (ulcerative) — see Enteritis, regional, small intestine
**Ileocolitis** (see also Enteritis) K52.9
  infectious A09
  regional — see Enteritis, regional
  ulcerative K51.0- ☑
**Ileostomy**
  attention to Z43.2
  malfunctioning K94.13
  status Z93.2
    with complication — see Complications, enterostomy
**Ileotyphus** — see Typhoid
**Ileum** — see condition
**Ileus** (bowel) (colon) (inhibitory) (intestine) K56.7
  adynamic K56.0
  due to gallstone (in intestine) K56.3
  duodenal (chronic) K31.5
  gallstone K56.3
  mechanical NEC (see also Obstruction, intestine, specified NEC) K56.699
  meconium P76.0
    in cystic fibrosis E84.11
    meaning meconium plug (without cystic fibrosis) P76.0
  myxedema K59.8
  neurogenic K56.0
    Hirschsprung's disease or megacolon Q43.1
  newborn
    due to meconium P76.0
      in cystic fibrosis E84.11
      meaning meconium plug (without cystic fibrosis) P76.0
    transitory P76.1
  obstructive (see also Obstruction, intestine, specified NEC) K56.699
  paralytic K56.0
  postoperative K91.89
**Iliac** — see condition
**Iliotibial band syndrome** M76.3- ☑
**Illiteracy** Z55.0
**Illness** (see also Disease) R69
  manic-depressive — see Disorder, bipolar
**Imbalance** R26.89
  autonomic G90.8
  constituents of food intake E63.1
  electrolyte E87.8
    with
      abortion — see Abortion by type, complicated by, electrolyte imbalance
      molar pregnancy O08.5
    due to hyperemesis gravidarum O21.1
    following ectopic or molar pregnancy O08.5
    neonatal, transitory NEC P74.4
      potassium P74.3
      sodium P74.2
  endocrine E34.9
  eye muscle NOS H50.9
  hormone E34.9
  hysterical F44.4
  labyrinth — see subcategory H83.2 ☑
  posture R29.3
  protein-energy — see Malnutrition
  sympathetic G90.8
**Imbecile, imbecility** (I.Q. 35-49) F71
**Imbedding, intrauterine device** T83.39 ☑
**Imbibition, cholesterol** (gallbladder) K82.4
**Imbrication, teeth,, fully erupted** M26.30
**Imerslund** (-Gräsbeck) **syndrome** D51.1
**Immature** (see also Immaturity)
  birth (less than 37 completed weeks) — see Preterm, newborn
    extremely (less than 28 completed weeks) — see Immaturity, extreme
  personality F60.89
**Immaturity** (less than 37 completed weeks) (see also Preterm, newborn)
  extreme of newborn (less than 28 completed weeks of gestation) (less than 196 completed days of gestation) (unspecified weeks of gestation) P07.20

**Immaturity** — continued
  extreme of newborn — continued
    gestational age
      less than 23 completed weeks P07.21
      23 completed weeks (23 weeks, 0 days through 23 weeks, 6 days) P07.22
      24 completed weeks (24 weeks, 0 days through 24 weeks, 6 days) P07.23
      25 completed weeks (25 weeks, 0 days through 25 weeks, 6 days) P07.24
      26 completed weeks (26 weeks, 0 days through 26 weeks, 6 days) P07.25
      27 completed weeks (27 weeks, 0 days through 27 weeks, 6 days) P07.26
  fetus or infant light-for-dates — see Light-for-dates
  lung, newborn P28.0
  organ or site NEC — see Hypoplasia
  pulmonary, newborn P28.0
  reaction F60.89
  sexual (female) (male), after puberty E30.0
**Immersion** T75.1 ☑
  foot T69.02- ☑
  hand T69.01- ☑
**Immobile, immobility**
  complete, due to severe physical disability or frailty R53.2
  intestine K59.8
  syndrome (paraplegic) M62.3
**Immune reconstitution** (inflammatory) syndrome [IRIS] D89.3
**Immunization** (see also Vaccination)
  ABO — see Incompatibility, ABO
    in newborn P55.1
  complication — see Complications, vaccination
  encounter for Z23
  not done (not carried out) Z28.9
    because (of)
      acute illness of patient Z28.01
      allergy to vaccine (or component) Z28.04
      caregiver refusal Z28.82
      chronic illness of patient Z28.02
      contraindication NEC Z28.09
      group pressure Z28.1
      guardian refusal Z28.82
      immune compromised state of patient Z28.03
      parent refusal Z28.82
      patient had disease being vaccinated against Z28.81
      patient refusal Z28.21
      patient's belief Z28.1
      religious beliefs of patient Z28.1
      specified reason NEC Z28.89
        of patient Z28.29
      unspecified patient reason Z28.20
  Rh factor
    affecting management of pregnancy NEC O36.09- ☑
    anti-D antibody O36.01- ☑
    from transfusion — see Complication(s), transfusion, incompatibility reaction, Rh (factor)
**Immunocytoma** C83.0- ☑
**Immunodeficiency** D84.9
  with
    adenosine-deaminase deficiency D81.3
    antibody defects D80.9
      specified type NEC D80.8
    hyperimmunoglobulinemia D80.6
    increased immunoglobulin M (IgM) D80.5
    major defect D82.9
      specified type NEC D82.8
    partial albinism D82.8
    short-limbed stature D82.2
    thrombocytopenia and eczema D82.0
  antibody with
    hyperimmunoglobulinemia D80.6
    near-normal immunoglobulins D80.6
  autosomal recessive, Swiss type D80.0
  combined D81.9
    biotin-dependent carboxylase D81.819
      biotinidase D81.810
      holocarboxylase synthetase D81.818
      specified type NEC D81.818
    severe (SCID) D81.9
      with
        low or normal B-cell numbers D81.2
        low T- and B-cell numbers D81.1
        reticular dysgenesis D81.0
    specified type NEC D81.89

**Immunodeficiency** — continued
  common variable D83.9
    with
      abnormalities of B-cell numbers and function D83.0
      autoantibodies to B- or T-cells D83.2
      immunoregulatory T-cell disorders D83.1
      specified type NEC D83.8
  following hereditary defective response to Epstein-Barr virus (EBV) D82.3
  selective, immunoglobulin
    A (IgA) D80.2
    G (IgG) (subclasses) D80.3
    M (IgM) D80.4
  severe combined (SCID) D81.9
  specified type NEC D84.8
  X-linked, with increased IgM D80.5
**Immunotherapy** (encounter for)
  antineoplastic Z51.12
**Impaction, impacted**
  bowel, colon, rectum (see also Impaction, fecal) K56.49
    by gallstone K56.3
  calculus — see Calculus
  cerumen (ear) (external) H61.2- ☑
  cuspid — see Impaction, tooth
  dental (same or adjacent tooth) K01.1
  fecal, feces K56.41
  fracture — see Fracture, by site
  gallbladder — see Calculus, gallbladder
  gallstone(s) — see Calculus, gallbladder
    bile duct (common) (hepatic) — see Calculus, bile duct
    cystic duct — see Calculus, gallbladder
    in intestine, with obstruction (any part) K56.3
  intestine (calculous) NEC (see also Impaction, fecal) K56.49
    gallstone, with ileus K56.3
  intrauterine device (IUD) T83.39 ☑
  molar — see Impaction, tooth
  shoulder, causing obstructed labor O66.0
  tooth, teeth K01.1
  turbinate J34.89
**Impaired, impairment** (function)
  auditory discrimination — see Abnormal, auditory perception
  cognitive, mild, so stated G31.84
  dual sensory Z73.82
  fasting glucose R73.01
  glucose tolerance (oral) R73.02
  hearing — see Deafness
  heart — see Disease, heart
  kidney N28.9
    disorder resulting from N25.9
      specified NEC N25.89
  liver K72.90
    with coma K72.91
  mastication K08.89
  mild cognitive, so stated G31.84
  mobility
    ear ossicles — see Ankylosis, ear ossicles
    requiring care provider Z74.09
  myocardium, myocardial — see Insufficiency, myocardial
  rectal sphincter R19.8
  renal (acute) (chronic) N28.9
    disorder resulting from N25.9
      specified NEC N25.89
  vision NEC H54.7
    both eyes H54.3
**Impediment, speech** R47.9
  psychogenic (childhood) F98.8
  slurring R47.81
  specified NEC R47.89
**Impending**
  coronary syndrome I20.0
  delirium tremens F10.239
  myocardial infarction I20.0
**Imperception auditory** (acquired) (see also Deafness)
  congenital H93.25
**Imperfect**
  aeration, lung (newborn) NEC — see Atelectasis
  closure (congenital)
    alimentary tract NEC Q45.8
      lower Q43.8
      upper Q40.8
    atrioventricular ostium Q21.2
    atrium (secundum) Q21.1
    branchial cleft NOS Q18.2

**Imperfect** — continued
closure — continued
branchial cleft — continued
cyst Q18.0
fistula Q18.0
sinus Q18.0
choroid Q14.3
cricoid cartilage Q31.8
cusps, heart valve NEC Q24.8
pulmonary Q22.3
ductus
arteriosus Q25.0
Botalli Q25.0
ear drum (causing impairment of hearing) Q16.4
esophagus with communication to bronchus or trachea Q39.1
eyelid Q10.3
foramen
botalli Q21.1
ovale Q21.1
genitalia, genital organ(s) or system
female Q52.8
external Q52.79
internal NEC Q52.8
male Q55.8
glottis Q31.8
interatrial ostium or septum Q21.1
interauricular ostium or septum Q21.1
interventricular ostium or septum Q21.0
larynx Q31.8
lip — see Cleft, lip
nasal septum Q30.3
nose Q30.2
omphalomesenteric duct Q43.0
optic nerve entry Q14.2
organ or site not listed — see Anomaly, by site
ostium
interatrial Q21.1
interauricular Q21.1
interventricular Q21.0
palate — see Cleft, palate
preauricular sinus Q18.1
retina Q14.1
roof of orbit Q75.8
sclera Q13.5
septum
aorticopulmonary Q21.4
atrial (secundum) Q21.1
between aorta and pulmonary artery Q21.4
heart Q21.9
interatrial (secundum) Q21.1
interauricular (secundum) Q21.1
interventricular Q21.0
in tetralogy of Fallot Q21.3
nasal Q30.3
ventricular Q21.0
with pulmonary stenosis or atresia, dextraposition of aorta, and hypertrophy of right ventricle Q21.3
in tetralogy of Fallot Q21.3
skull Q75.0
with
anencephaly Q00.0
encephalocele — see Encephalocele
hydrocephalus Q03.9
with spina bifida — see Spina bifida, by site, with hydrocephalus
microcephaly Q02
spine (with meningocele) — see Spina bifida
trachea Q32.1
tympanic membrane (causing impairment of hearing) Q16.4
uterus Q51.818
vitelline duct Q43.0
erection — see Dysfunction, sexual, male, erectile
fusion — see Imperfect, closure
inflation, lung (newborn) — see Atelectasis
posture R29.3
rotation, intestine Q43.3
septum, ventricular Q21.0
**Imperfectly descended testis** — see Cryptorchid
**Imperforate** (congenital) (see also Atresia)
anus Q42.3
with fistula Q42.2
cervix (uteri) Q51.828
esophagus Q39.0
with tracheoesophageal fistula Q39.1
hymen Q52.3

**Imperforate** — continued
jejunum Q41.1
pharynx Q38.8
rectum Q42.1
with fistula Q42.0
urethra Q64.39
vagina Q52.4
**Impervious** (congenital) (see also Atresia)
anus Q42.3
with fistula Q42.2
bile duct Q44.2
esophagus Q39.0
with tracheoesophageal fistula Q39.1
intestine (small) Q41.9
large Q42.9
specified NEC Q42.8
rectum Q42.1
with fistula Q42.0
ureter — see Atresia, ureter
urethra Q64.39
**Impetiginization of dermatoses** L01.1
**Impetigo** (any organism) (any site) (circinate) (contagiosa) (simplex) (vulgaris) L01.00
Bockhart's L01.02
bullous, bullosa L01.03
external ear L01.00 [H62.40]
follicularis L01.02
furfuracea L30.5
herpetiformis L40.1
nonobstetrical L40.1
neonatorum L01.03
nonbullous L01.01
specified type NEC L01.09
ulcerative L01.09
**Impingement** (on teeth)
soft tissue
anterior M26.81
posterior M26.82
**Implant, endometrial** N80.9
**Implantation**
anomalous — see Anomaly, by site
ureter Q62.63
cyst
external area or site (skin) NEC L72.0
iris — see Cyst, iris, implantation
vagina N89.8
vulva N90.7
dermoid (cyst) — see Implantation, cyst
**Impotence** (sexual) N52.9
counseling Z70.1
organic origin (see also Dysfunction, sexual, male, erectile) N52.9
psychogenic F52.21
**Impression, basilar** Q75.8
**Imprisonment, anxiety concerning** Z65.1
**Improper care** (child) (newborn) — see Maltreatment
**Improperly tied umbilical cord** (causing hemorrhage) P51.8
**Impulsiveness** (impulsive) R45.87
**Inability to swallow** — see Aphagia
**Inaccessible, inaccessibility**
health care NEC Z75.3
due to
waiting period Z75.2
for admission to facility elsewhere Z75.1
other helping agencies Z75.4
**Inactive** — see condition
**Inadequate, inadequacy**
aesthetics of dental restoration K08.56
biologic, constitutional, functional, or social F60.7
development
child R62.50
genitalia
after puberty NEC E30.0
congenital
female Q52.8
external Q52.79
internal Q52.8
male Q55.8
lungs Q33.6
associated with short gestation P28.0
organ or site not listed — see Anomaly, by site
diet (causing nutritional deficiency) E63.9
eating habits Z72.4
environment, household Z59.1
family support Z63.8
food (supply) NEC Z59.4
hunger effects T73.0 ☑

**Inadequate, inadequacy** — continued
functional F60.7
household care, due to
family member
handicapped or ill Z74.2
on vacation Z75.5
temporarily away from home Z74.2
technical defects in home Z59.1
temporary absence from home of person rendering care Z74.2
housing (heating) (space) Z59.1
income (financial) Z59.6
intrafamilial communication Z63.8
material resources Z59.9
mental — see Disability, intellectual
parental supervision or control of child Z62.0
personality F60.7
pulmonary
function R06.89
newborn P28.5
ventilation, newborn P28.5
sample of cytologic smear
anus R85.615
cervix R87.615
vagina R87.625
social F60.7
insurance Z59.7
skills NEC Z73.4
supervision of child by parent Z62.0
teaching affecting education Z55.8
welfare support Z59.7
**Inanition** R64
with edema — see Malnutrition, severe
due to
deprivation of food T73.0 ☑
malnutrition — see Malnutrition
fever R50.9
**Inappropriate**
change in quantitative human chorionic gonadotropin (hCG) in early pregnancy O02.81
diet or eating habits Z72.4
level of quantitative human chorionic gonadotropin (hCG) for gestational age in early pregnancy O02.81
secretion
antidiuretic hormone (ADH) (excessive) E22.2
deficiency E23.2
pituitary (posterior) E22.2
**Inattention at or after birth** — see Neglect
**Incarceration, incarcerated**
enterocele K46.0
gangrenous K46.1
epiplocele K46.0
gangrenous K46.1
exomphalos K42.0
gangrenous K42.1
hernia (see also Hernia, by site, with obstruction)
with gangrene — see Hernia, by site, with gangrene
iris, in wound — see Injury, eye, laceration, with prolapse
lens, in wound — see Injury, eye, laceration, with prolapse
omphalocele K42.0
prison, anxiety concerning Z65.1
rupture — see Hernia, by site
sarcoepiplocele K46.0
gangrenous K46.1
sarcoepiplomphalocele K42.0
with gangrene K42.1
uterus N85.8
gravid O34.51- ☑
causing obstructed labor O65.5
**Incised wound**
external — see Laceration
internal organs — see Injury, by site
**Incision, incisional**
hernia K43.2
with
gangrene (and obstruction) K43.1
obstruction K43.0
surgical, complication — see Complications, surgical procedure
traumatic
external — see Laceration
internal organs — see Injury, by site
**Inclusion**
azurophilic leukocytic D72.0

☑ **Additional Character Required** — Refer to the Tabular List for Character Selection          ▽ᵇᵘˡˡ **Subterms under main terms may continue to next column or page**

**Inclusion** — *continued*
  blennorrhea (neonatal) (newborn) P39.1
  gallbladder in liver (congenital) Q44.1
**Incompatibility**
  ABO
    affecting management of pregnancy O36.11- ☑
      anti-A sensitization O36.11- ☑
      anti-B sensitization O36.19- ☑
      specified NEC O36.19- ☑
    infusion or transfusion reaction — *see* Complication(s), transfusion, incompatibility reaction, ABO
    newborn P55.1
  blood (group) (Duffy) (K(ell)) (Kidd) (Lewis) (M) (S) NEC
    affecting management of pregnancy O36.11- ☑
      anti-A sensitization O36.11- ☑
      anti-B sensitization O36.19- ☑
    infusion or transfusion reaction T80.89 ☑
    newborn P55.8
  divorce or estrangement Z63.5
  Rh (blood group) (factor) Z31.82
    affecting management of pregnancy NEC O36.09- ☑
      anti-D antibody O36.01- ☑
    infusion or transfusion reaction — *see* Complication(s), transfusion, incompatibility reaction, Rh (factor)
    newborn P55.0
  rhesus — *see* Incompatibility, Rh
**Incompetency, incompetent, incompetence**
  annular
    aortic (valve) — *see* Insufficiency, aortic
    mitral (valve) I34.0
    pulmonary valve (heart) I37.1
  aortic (valve) — *see* Insufficiency, aortic
  cardiac valve — *see* Endocarditis
  cervix, cervical (os) N88.3
    in pregnancy O34.3- ☑
  chronotropic I45.89
    with
      autonomic dysfunction G90.8
      ischemic heart disease I25.89
      left ventricular dysfunction I51.89
      sinus node dysfunction I49.8
  esophagogastric (junction) (sphincter) K22.0
  mitral (valve) — *see* Insufficiency, mitral
  pelvic fundus N81.89
  pubocervical tissue N81.82
  pulmonary valve (heart) I37.1
    congenital Q22.3
  rectovaginal tissue N81.83
  tricuspid (annular) (valve) — *see* Insufficiency, tricuspid
  valvular — *see* Endocarditis
    congenital Q24.8
  vein, venous (saphenous) (varicose) — *see* Varix, leg
**Incomplete** (*see also* condition)
  bladder, emptying R33.9
  defecation R15.0
  expansion lungs (newborn) NEC — *see* Atelectasis
  rotation, intestine Q43.3
**Inconclusive**
  diagnostic imaging due to excess body fat of patient R93.9
  findings on diagnostic imaging of breast NEC R92.8
  mammogram (due to dense breasts) R92.2
**Incontinence** R32
  anal sphincter R15.9
  coital N39.491
  feces R15.9
    nonorganic origin F98.1
  insensible (urinary) N39.42
  overflow N39.490
  postural (urinary) N39.492
  psychogenic F45.8
  rectal R15.9
  reflex N39.498
  stress (female) (male) N39.3
    and urge N39.46
  urethral sphincter R32
  urge N39.41
    and stress (female) (male) N39.46
  urine (urinary) R32
    continuous N39.45
    due to cognitive impairment, or severe physical disability or immobility R39.81
    functional R39.81
    insensible N39.42
    mixed (stress and urge) N39.46

**Incontinence** — *continued*
  urine — *continued*
    nocturnal N39.44
    nonorganic origin F98.0
    overflow N39.490
    post dribbling N39.43
    postural N39.492
    reflex N39.498
    specified NEC N39.498
    stress (female) (male) N39.3
      and urge N39.46
    total N39.498
    unaware N39.42
    urge N39.41
      and stress (female) (male) N39.46
**Incontinentia pigmenti** Q82.3
**Incoordinate, incoordination**
  esophageal-pharyngeal (newborn) — *see* Dysphagia
  muscular R27.8
  uterus (action) (contractions) (complicating delivery) O62.4
**Increase, increased**
  abnormal, in development R63.8
  androgens (ovarian) E28.1
  anticoagulants (antithrombin) (anti-VIIIa) (anti-IXa) (anti-Xa) (anti-XIa) — *see* Circulating anticoagulants
  cold sense R20.8
  estrogen E28.0
  function
    adrenal
      cortex — *see* Cushing's, syndrome
      medulla E27.5
    pituitary (gland) (anterior) (lobe) E22.9
      posterior E22.2
  heat sense R20.8
  intracranial pressure (benign) G93.2
  permeability, capillaries I78.8
  pressure, intracranial G93.2
  secretion
    gastrin E16.4
    glucagon E16.3
    pancreas, endocrine E16.9
      growth hormone-releasing hormone E16.8
      pancreatic polypeptide E16.8
      somatostatin E16.8
      vasoactive-intestinal polypeptide E16.8
  sphericity, lens Q12.4
  splenic activity D73.1
  venous pressure I87.8
    portal K76.6
**Increta placenta** O43.22- ☑
**Incrustation, cornea, foreign body** (lead)(zinc) — *see* Foreign body, cornea
**Incyclophoria** H50.54
**Incyclotropia** — *see* Cyclotropia
**Indeterminate sex** Q56.4
**India rubber skin** Q82.8
**Indigestion** (acid) (bilious) (functional) K30
  catarrhal K31.89
  due to decomposed food NOS A05.9
  nervous F45.8
  psychogenic F45.8
**Indirect** — *see* condition
**Induratio penis plastica** N48.6
**Induration, indurated**
  brain G93.89
  breast (fibrous) N64.51
    puerperal, postpartum O92.29
  broad ligament N83.8
  chancre
    anus A51.1
    congenital A50.07
    extragenital NEC A51.2
  corpora cavernosa (penis) (plastic) N48.6
  liver (chronic) K76.89
  lung (black) (chronic) (fibroid) (*see also* Fibrosis, lung) J84.10
    essential brown J84.03
  penile (plastic) N48.6
  phlebitic — *see* Phlebitis
  skin R23.4
**Inebriety** (without dependence) — *see* Alcohol, intoxication
**Inefficiency, kidney** N28.9
**Inelasticity, skin** R23.4
**Inequality, leg** (length) (acquired) (*see also* Deformity, limb, unequal length)
  congenital — *see* Defect, reduction, lower limb

**Inequality, leg** — *continued*
  lower leg — *see* Deformity, limb, unequal length
**Inertia**
  bladder (neurogenic) N31.2
  stomach K31.89
    psychogenic F45.8
  uterus, uterine during labor O62.2
    during latent phase of labor O62.0
    primary O62.0
    secondary O62.1
  vesical (neurogenic) N31.2
**Infancy, infantile, infantilism** (*see also* condition)
  celiac K90.0
  genitalia, genitals (after puberty) E30.0
  Herter's (nontropical sprue) K90.0
  intestinal K90.0
  Lorain E23.0
  pancreatic K86.89
  pelvis M95.5
    with disproportion (fetopelvic) O33.1
      causing obstructed labor O65.1
  pituitary E23.0
  renal N25.0
  uterus — *see* Infantile, genitalia
**Infant**(s) (*see also* Infancy)
  excessive crying R68.11
  irritable child R68.12
  lack of care — *see* Neglect
  liveborn (singleton) Z38.2
    born in hospital Z38.00
      by cesarean Z38.01
    born outside hospital Z38.1
    multiple NEC Z38.8
      born in hospital Z38.68
        by cesarean Z38.69
      born outside hospital Z38.7
    quadruplet Z38.8
      born in hospital Z38.63
        by cesarean Z38.64
      born outside hospital Z38.7
    quintuplet Z38.8
      born in hospital Z38.65
        by cesarean Z38.66
      born outside hospital Z38.7
    triplet Z38.8
      born in hospital Z38.61
        by cesarean Z38.62
      born outside hospital Z38.7
    twin Z38.5
      born in hospital Z38.30
        by cesarean Z38.31
      born outside hospital Z38.4
  of diabetic mother (syndrome of) P70.1
    gestational diabetes P70.0
**Infantile** (*see also* condition)
  genitalia, genitals E30.0
  os, uterine E30.0
  penis E30.0
  testis E29.1
  uterus E30.0
**Infantilism** — *see* Infancy
**Infarct, infarction**
  adrenal (capsule) (gland) E27.49
  appendices epiploicae (*see also* Infarct, intestine) K55.069
  bowel (*see also* Infarct, intestine) K55.069
  brain (stem) — *see* Infarct, cerebral
  breast N64.89
  brewer's (kidney) N28.0
  cardiac — *see* Infarct, myocardium
  cerebellar — *see* Infarct, cerebral
  cerebral (*see also* Occlusion, artery cerebral or precerebral, with infarction) I63.9
    aborted I63.9
    cortical I63.9
    due to
      cerebral venous thrombosis, nonpyogenic I63.6
      embolism
        cerebral arteries I63.4- ☑
        precerebral arteries I63.1- ☑
      occlusion NEC
        cerebral arteries I63.5- ☑
        precerebral arteries I63.2- ☑
      stenosis NEC
        cerebral arteries I63.5- ☑
        precerebral arteries I63.2- ☑

Infarct, infarction — continued
- cerebral (see also Occlusion, artery cerebral or precerebral, with infarction) — continued
  - due to — continued
    - thrombosis
      - cerebral artery I63.3- ☑
      - precerebral artery I63.0- ☑
    - intraoperative
      - during cardiac surgery I97.810
      - during other surgery I97.811
    - postprocedural
      - following cardiac surgery I97.820
      - following other surgery I97.821
    - specified NEC I63.8
- colon (acute) (agnogenic) (embolic) (hemorrhagic) (nonocclusive) (nonthrombotic) (occlusive) (segmental) (thrombotic) (with gangrene) (see also Infarct, intestine) K55.049
- coronary artery — see Infarct, myocardium
- embolic — see Embolism
- fallopian tube N83.8
- gallbladder K82.8
- heart — see Infarct, myocardium
- hepatic K76.3
- hypophysis (anterior lobe) E23.6
- impending (myocardium) I20.0
- intestine (acute) (agnogenic) (embolic) (hemorrhagic) (nonocclusive) (nonthrombotic) (occlusive) (thrombotic) (with gangrene) K55.069
  - diffuse K55.062
  - focal K55.061
  - large K55.049
    - diffuse K55.042
    - focal K55.041
  - small K55.029
    - diffuse K55.022
    - focal K55.021
- kidney N28.0
- liver K76.3
- lung (embolic) (thrombotic) — see Embolism, pulmonary
- lymph node I89.8
- mesentery, mesenteric (embolic) (thrombotic) (with gangrene) (see also Infarct, intestine) K55.069
- muscle (ischemic) M62.20
  - ankle M62.27- ☑
  - foot M62.27- ☑
  - forearm M62.23- ☑
  - hand M62.24- ☑
  - lower leg M62.26- ☑
  - pelvic region M62.25- ☑
  - shoulder region M62.21- ☑
  - specified site NEC M62.28
  - thigh M62.25- ☑
  - upper arm M62.22- ☑
- myocardium, myocardial (acute) (with stated duration of 4 weeks or less) I21.9
  - associated with revascularization procedure I21.A9
  - diagnosed on ECG, but presenting no symptoms I25.2
  - due to
    - demand ischemia I21.A1
    - ischemic imbalance I21.A1
  - healed or old I25.2
  - intraoperative (see also Infarct, myocardium, associated with revascularization procedure)
    - during cardiac surgery I97.790
    - during other surgery I97.791
  - non-Q wave I21.4
  - non-ST elevation (NSTEMI) I21.4
    - subsequent I22.2
  - nontransmural I21.4
  - past (diagnosed on ECG or other investigation, but currently presenting no symptoms) I25.2
  - postprocedural (see also Infarct, myocardium, associated with revascularization procedure)
    - following cardiac surgery (see also Infarct, myocardium, type 4 or type 5) I97.190
    - following other surgery I97.191
  - Q wave (see also, Infarct, myocardium, by site) I21.3
  - secondary to
    - demand ischemia I21.A1
    - ischemic imbalance I21.A1
  - ST elevation (STEMI) I21.3
    - anterior (anteroapical) (anterolateral) (anteroseptal) (Q wave) (wall) I21.09
      - subsequent I22.0

Infarct, infarction — continued
- myocardium, myocardial — continued
  - ST elevation — continued
    - inferior (diaphragmatic) (inferolateral) (inferoposterior) (wall) NEC I21.19
      - subsequent I22.1
    - inferoposterior transmural (Q wave) I21.11
    - involving
      - coronary artery of anterior wall NEC I21.09
      - coronary artery of inferior wall NEC I21.19
      - diagonal coronary artery I21.02
      - left anterior descending coronary artery I21.02
      - left circumflex coronary artery I21.21
      - left main coronary artery I21.01
      - oblique marginal coronary artery I21.21
      - right coronary artery I21.11
    - lateral (apical-lateral) (basal-lateral) (high) I21.29
      - subsequent I22.8
    - posterior (posterobasal) (posterolateral) (posteroseptal) (true) I21.29
      - subsequent I22.8
    - septal I21.29
      - subsequent I22.8
    - specified NEC I21.29
      - subsequent I22.8
  - subsequent I22.9
    - anterior (anteroapical) (anterolateral) (anteroseptal) (wall) I22.0
    - diaphragmatic (wall) I22.1
    - inferior (diaphragmatic) (inferolateral) (inferoposterior) (wall) I22.1
    - lateral (apical-lateral) (basal-lateral) (high) I22.8
    - non-ST elevation (NSTEMI) I22.2
    - posterior (posterobasal) (posterolateral) (posteroseptal) (true) I22.8
    - septal I22.8
    - specified NEC I22.8
    - ST elevation I22.9
      - anterior (anteroapical) (anterolateral) (anteroseptal) (wall) I22.0
      - inferior (diaphragmatic) (inferolateral) (inferoposterior) (wall) I22.1
      - specified NEC I22.8
    - subendocardial I22.2
    - transmural I22.9
      - anterior (anteroapical) (anterolateral) (anteroseptal) (wall) I22.0
      - diaphragmatic (wall) I22.1
      - inferior (diaphragmatic) (inferolateral) (inferoposterior) (wall) I22.1
      - lateral (apical-lateral) (basal-lateral) (high) I22.8
      - posterior (posterobasal) (posterolateral) (posteroseptal) (true) I22.8
      - specified NEC I22.8
    - type 1 (see also Infarction, myocardial, subsequent, by site, or by ST elevation or non-ST elevation) I22.9
    - type 2 I21.A1
    - type 3 I21.A9
    - type 4 I21.A9
    - type 5 I21.A9
  - syphilitic A52.06
  - transmural I21.9
    - anterior (anteroapical) (anterolateral) (anteroseptal) (Q wave) (wall) NEC I21.09
    - inferior (diaphragmatic) (inferolateral) (inferoposterior) (Q wave) (wall) NEC I21.19
    - inferoposterior (Q wave) I21.11
    - lateral (apical-lateral) (basal-lateral) (high) NEC I21.29
    - posterior (posterobasal) (posterolateral) (posteroseptal) (true) NEC I21.29
    - septal NEC I21.29
    - specified NEC I21.29
    - type 1 (see also Infarction, myocardial, by site, or by ST elevation or non-ST elevation) I21.9
    - type 2 I21.A1
    - type 3 I21.A9
    - type 4 (a) (b) (c) I21.A9
    - type 5 I21.A9
  - nontransmural I21.4
- omentum (see also Infarct, intestine) K55.069
- ovary N83.8
- pancreas K86.89
- papillary muscle — see Infarct, myocardium

Infarct, infarction — continued
- parathyroid gland E21.4
- pituitary (gland) E23.6
- placenta O43.81- ☑
- prostate N42.89
- pulmonary (artery) (vein) (hemorrhagic) — see Embolism, pulmonary
- renal (embolic) (thrombotic) N28.0
- retina, retinal (artery) — see Occlusion, artery, retina
- spinal (cord) (acute) (embolic) (nonembolic) G95.11
- spleen D73.5
  - embolic or thrombotic I74.8
- subendocardial (acute) (nontransmural) I21.4
- suprarenal (capsule) (gland) E27.49
- testis N50.1
- thrombotic (see also Thrombosis)
  - artery, arterial — see Embolism
- thyroid (gland) E07.89
- ventricle (heart) — see Infarct, myocardium

Infecting — see condition

**Infection, infected, infective** (opportunistic) B99.9
- with
  - drug resistant organism — see Resistance (to), drug (see also specific organism)
  - lymphangitis — see Lymphangitis
  - organ dysfunction (acute) R65.20
    - with septic shock R65.21
- abscess (skin) — code by site under Abscess
- Absidia — see Mucormycosis
- Acanthamoeba — see Acanthamebiasis
- Acanthocheilonema (perstans) (streptocerca) B74.4
- accessory sinus (chronic) — see Sinusitis
- achorion — see Dermatophytosis
- Acremonium falciforme B47.0
- acromioclavicular M00.9
- Actinobacillus (actinomycetem-comitans) A28.8
  - mallei A24.0
  - muris A25.1
- Actinomadura B47.1
- Actinomyces (israelii) (see also Actinomycosis) A42.9
- Actinomycetales — see Actinomycosis
- actinomycotic NOS — see Actinomycosis
- adenoid (and tonsil) J03.90
  - chronic J35.02
- adenovirus NEC
  - as cause of disease classified elsewhere B97.0
  - unspecified nature or site B34.0
- aerogenes capsulatus A48.0
- aertrycke — see Infection, salmonella
- alimentary canal NOS — see Enteritis, infectious
- Allescheria boydii B48.2
- Alternaria B48.8
- alveolus, alveolar (process) K04.7
- Ameba, amebic (histolytica) — see Amebiasis
- amniotic fluid, sac or cavity O41.10- ☑
  - chorioamnionitis O41.12- ☑
  - placentitis O41.14- ☑
- amputation stump (surgical) — see Complication, amputation stump, infection
- Ancylostoma (duodenalis) B76.0
- Anisakiasis, Anisakis larvae B81.0
- anthrax — see Anthrax
- antrum (chronic) — see Sinusitis, maxillary
- anus, anal (papillae) (sphincter) K62.89
- arbovirus (arbor virus) A94
  - specified type NEC A93.8
- artificial insemination N98.0
- Ascaris lumbricoides — see Ascariasis
- Ascomycetes B47.0
- Aspergillus (flavus) (fumigatus) (terreus) — see Aspergillosis
- atypical
  - acid-fast (bacilli) — see Mycobacterium, atypical
  - mycobacteria — see Mycobacterium, atypical
  - virus A81.9
    - specified type NEC A81.89
- auditory meatus (external) — see Otitis, externa, infective
- auricle (ear) — see Otitis, externa, infective
- axillary gland (lymph) L04.2
- Bacillus A49.9
  - abortus A23.1
  - anthracis — see Anthrax
  - Ducrey's (any location) A57
  - Flexner's A03.1
  - Friedländer's NEC A49.8
  - gas (gangrene) A48.0
  - mallei A24.0

**Infection, infected, infective** — *continued*
  Bacillus — *continued*
    melitensis A23.0
    paratyphoid, paratyphosus A01.4
      A A01.1
      B A01.2
      C A01.3
    Shiga (-Kruse) A03.0
    suipestifer — *see* Infection, salmonella
    swimming pool A31.1
    typhosa A01.00
    welchii — *see* Gangrene, gas
  bacterial NOS A49.9
    as cause of disease classified elsewhere B96.89
      Bacteroides fragilis [B. fragilis] B96.6
      Clostridium perfringens [C. perfringens] B96.7
      Enterobacter sakazakii B96.89
      Enterococcus B95.2
      Escherichia coli [E. coli] (*see also* Escherichia coli) B96.20
      Helicobacter pylori [H.pylori] B96.81
      Hemophilus influenzae [H. influenzae] B96.3
      Klebsiella pneumoniae [K. pneumoniae] B96.1
      Mycoplasma pneumoniae [M. pneumoniae] B96.0
      Proteus (mirabilis) (morganii) B96.4
      Pseudomonas (aeruginosa) (mallei) (pseudomallei) B96.5
      Staphylococcus B95.8
        aureus (methicillin susceptible) (MSSA) B95.61
        methicillin resistant (MRSA) B95.62
        specified NEC B95.7
      Streptococcus B95.5
        group A B95.0
        group B B95.1
        pneumoniae B95.3
        specified NEC B95.4
      Vibrio vulnificus B96.82
    specified NEC A48.8
  Bacterium
    paratyphosum A01.4
      A A01.1
      B A01.2
      C A01.3
    typhosum A01.00
  Bacteroides NEC A49.8
    fragilis, as cause of disease classified elsewhere B96.6
  Balantidium coli A07.0
  Bartholin's gland N75.8
  Basidiobolus B46.8
  bile duct (common) (hepatic) — *see* Cholangitis
  bladder — *see* Cystitis
  Blastomyces, blastomycotic (*see also* Blastomycosis)
    brasiliensis — *see* Paracoccidioidomycosis
    dermatitidis — *see* Blastomycosis
    European — *see* Cryptococcosis
    Loboi B48.0
    North American B40.9
    South American — *see* Paracoccidioidomycosis
  bleb, postprocedure — *see* Blebitis
  bone — *see* Osteomyelitis
  Bordetella — *see* Whooping cough
  Borrelia bergdorfi A69.20
  brain (*see also* Encephalitis) G04.90
    membranes — *see* Meningitis
    septic G06.0
      meninges — *see* Meningitis, bacterial
  branchial cyst Q18.0
  breast — *see* Mastitis
  bronchus — *see* Bronchitis
  Brucella A23.9
    abortus A23.1
    canis A23.3
    melitensis A23.0
    mixed A23.8
    specified NEC A23.8
    suis A23.2
  Brugia (malayi) B74.1
    timori B74.2
  bursa — *see* Bursitis, infective
  buttocks (skin) L08.9
  Campylobacter, intestinal A04.5
    as cause of disease classified elsewhere B96.81
  Candida (albicans) (tropicalis) — *see* Candidiasis
  candiru B88.8
  Capillaria (intestinal) B81.1

**Infection, infected, infective** — *continued*
  Capillaria — *continued*
    hepatica B83.8
    philippinensis B81.1
  cartilage — *see* Disorder, cartilage, specified type NEC
  cat liver fluke B66.0
  catheter-related bloodstream (CRBSI) T80.211 ☑
  cellulitis — *code by* site under Cellulitis
  central line-associated T80.219 ☑
    bloodstream (CLABSI) T80.211 ☑
    specified NEC T80.218 ☑
  Cephalosporium falciforme B47.0
  cerebrospinal — *see* Meningitis
  cervical gland (lymph) L04.0
  cervix — *see* Cervicitis
  cesarean delivery wound (puerperal) O86.0
  cestodes — *see* Infestation, cestodes
  chest J22
  Chilomastix (intestinal) A07.8
  Chlamydia, chlamydial A74.9
    anus A56.3
    genitourinary tract A56.2
      lower A56.00
      specified NEC A56.19
    lymphogranuloma A55
    pharynx A56.4
    psittaci A70
    rectum A56.3
    sexually transmitted NEC A56.8
  cholera — *see* Cholera
  Cladosporium
    bantianum (brain abscess) B43.1
    carrionii B43.0
    castellanii B36.1
    trichoides (brain abscess) B43.1
    werneckii B36.1
  Clonorchis (sinensis) (liver) B66.1
  Clostridium NEC
    bifermentans A48.0
    botulinum (food poisoning) A05.1
      infant A48.51
      wound A48.52
    difficile
      as cause of disease classified elsewhere B96.89
      foodborne (disease)
        not specified as recurrent A04.72
        recurrent A04.71
      gas gangrene A48.0
      necrotizing enterocolitis
        not specified as recurrent A04.72
        recurrent A04.71
      sepsis A41.4
    gas-forming NEC A48.0
    histolyticum A48.0
    novyi, causing gas gangrene A48.0
    oedematiens A48.0
    perfringens
      as cause of disease classified elsewhere B96.7
      due to food A05.2
      foodborne (disease) A05.2
      gas gangrene A48.0
      sepsis A41.4
    septicum, causing gas gangrene A48.0
    sordellii, causing gas gangrene A48.0
    welchii
      as cause of disease classified elsewhere B96.7
      foodborne (disease) A05.2
      gas gangrene A48.0
      necrotizing enteritis A05.2
      sepsis A41.4
  Coccidioides (immitis) — *see* Coccidioidomycosis
  colon — *see* Enteritis, infectious
  colostomy K94.02
  common duct — *see* Cholangitis
  congenital P39.9
    Candida (albicans) P37.5
    cytomegalovirus P35.1
    hepatitis, viral P35.3
    herpes simplex P35.2
    infectious or parasitic disease P37.9
      specified NEC P37.8
    listeriosis (disseminated) P37.2
    malaria NEC P37.4
      falciparum P37.3
    Plasmodium falciparum P37.3
    poliomyelitis P35.8
    rubella P35.0
    skin P39.4

**Infection, infected, infective** — *continued*
  congenital — *continued*
    toxoplasmosis (acute) (subacute) (chronic) P37.1
    tuberculosis P37.0
    urinary (tract) P39.3
    vaccinia P35.8
    virus P35.9
      specified type NEC P35.8
  Conidiobolus B46.8
  coronavirus NEC B34.2
    as cause of disease classified elsewhere B97.29
    severe acute respiratory syndrome (SARS associated) B97.21
  corpus luteum — *see* Salpingo-oophoritis
  Corynebacterium diphtheriae — *see* Diphtheria
  cotia virus B08.8
  Coxiella burnetii A78
  coxsackie — *see* Coxsackie
  Cryptococcus neoformans — *see* Cryptococcosis
  Cryptosporidium A07.2
  Cunninghamella — *see* Mucormycosis
  cyst — *see* Cyst
  cystic duct (*see also* Cholecystitis) K81.9
  Cysticercus cellulosae — *see* Cysticercosis
  cytomegalovirus, cytomegaloviral B25.9
    congenital P35.1
    maternal, maternal care for (suspected) damage to fetus O35.3 ☑
    mononucleosis B27.10
      with
        complication NEC B27.19
        meningitis B27.12
        polyneuropathy B27.11
  delta-agent (acute), in hepatitis B carrier B17.0
  dental (pulpal origin) K04.7
  Deuteromycetes B47.0
  Dicrocoelium dendriticum B66.2
  Dipetalonema (perstans) (streptocerca) B74.4
  diphtherial — *see* Diphtheria
  Diphyllobothrium (adult) (latum) (pacificum) B70.0
    larval B70.1
  Diplogonoporus (grandis) B71.8
  Dipylidium caninum B67.4
  Dirofilaria B74.8
  Dracunculus medinensis B72
  Drechslera (hawaiiensis) B43.8
  Ducrey Haemophilus (any location) A57
  due to or resulting from
    artificial insemination N98.0
    central venous catheter T80.219 ☑
      bloodstream T80.211 ☑
      exit or insertion site T80.212 ☑
      localized T80.212 ☑
      port or reservoir T80.212 ☑
      specified NEC T80.218 ☑
      tunnel T80.212 ☑
    device, implant or graft (*see also* Complications, by site and type, infection or inflammation) T85.79 ☑
      arterial graft NEC T82.7 ☑
      breast (implant) T85.79 ☑
      catheter NEC T85.79 ☑
        dialysis (renal) T82.7 ☑
          intraperitoneal T85.71 ☑
        infusion NEC T82.7 ☑
          cranial T85.735 ☑
          intrathecal T85.735 ☑
          spinal (epidural) (subdural) T85.735 ☑
          subarachnoid T85.735 ☑
        urinary T83.518 ☑
          cystostomy T83.510 ☑
          Hopkins T83.518 ☑
          ileostomy T83.518 ☑
          nephrostomy T83.512 ☑
          specified NEC T83.518 ☑
          urethral indwelling T83.511 ☑
          urostomy T83.518 ☑
      electronic (electrode) (pulse generator) (stimulator)
        bone T84.7 ☑
        cardiac T82.7 ☑
        nervous system T85.738 ☑
          brain T85.731 ☑
          cranial nerve T85.732 ☑
          gastric nerve T85.732 ☑
          generator pocket T85.734 ☑
          neurostimulator generator T85.734 ☑

**Infection, infected, infective** — *continued*
  due to or resulting from — *continued*
    device, implant or graft (*see also* Complications, by site and type, infection or inflammation) — *continued*
      electronic — *continued*
        nervous system — *continued*
          peripheral nerve T85.732 ☑
          sacral nerve T85.732 ☑
          spinal cord T85.733 ☑
          vagal nerve T85.732 ☑
          urinary (indwelling) T83.51 ☑
      fixation, internal (orthopedic) NEC — *see* Complication, fixation device, infection
      gastrointestinal (bile duct) (esophagus) T85.79 ☑
        neurostimulator electrode (lead) T85.732 ☑
      genital NEC T83.69 ☑
      heart NEC T82.7 ☑
        valve (prosthesis) T82.6 ☑
          graft T82.7 ☑
      joint prosthesis — *see* Complication, joint prosthesis, infection
      ocular (corneal graft) (orbital implant) NEC T85.79 ☑
      orthopedic NEC T84.7 ☑
      penile (cylinder) (pump) (resevoir) T83.61 ☑
      specified NEC T85.79 ☑
      testicular T83.62 ☑
      urinary NEC T83.598 ☑
        ileal conduit stent T83.593 ☑
        implanted neurostimulation T83.590 ☑
        implanted sphincter T83.591 ☑
        indwelling ureteral stent T83.592 ☑
        nephroureteral stent T83.593 ☑
        specified stent NEC T83.593 ☑
      vascular NEC T82.7 ☑
      ventricular intracranial (communicating) shunt T85.730 ☑
    Hickman catheter T80.219 ☑
      bloodstream T80.211 ☑
      localized T80.212 ☑
      specified NEC T80.218 ☑
    immunization or vaccination T88.0 ☑
    infusion, injection or transfusion NEC T80.29 ☑
    injury NEC — *code by* site under Wound, open
    peripherally inserted central catheter (PICC) T80.219 ☑
      bloodstream T80.211 ☑
      localized T80.212 ☑
      specified NEC T80.218 ☑
    portacath (port-a-cath) T80.219 ☑
      bloodstream T80.211 ☑
      localized T80.212 ☑
      specified NEC T80.218 ☑
    pulmonary artery catheter — *see* Infection, due to or resulting from, central venous catheter
    surgery T81.4 ☑
    Swan Ganz catheter — *see* Infection, due to or resulting from, central venous catheter
    triple lumen catheter T80.219 ☑
      bloodstream T80.211 ☑
      localized T80.212 ☑
      specified NEC T80.218 ☑
    umbilical venous catheter T80.219 ☑
      bloodstream T80.211 ☑
      localized T80.212 ☑
      specified NEC T80.218 ☑
  during labor NEC O75.3
  ear (middle) (*see also* Otitis media)
    external — *see* Otitis, externa, infective
    inner — *see* subcategory H83.0 ☑
  Eberthella typhosa A01.00
  Echinococcus — *see* Echinococcus
  echovirus
    as cause of disease classified elsewhere B97.12
    unspecified nature or site B34.1
  endocardium I33.0
  endocervix — *see* Cervicitis
  Entamoeba — *see* Amebiasis
  enteric — *see* Enteritis, infectious
  Enterobacter sakazakii B96.89
  Enterobius vermicularis B80
  enterostomy K94.12
  enterovirus B34.1
    as cause of disease classified elsewhere B97.10

**Infection, infected, infective** — *continued*
  enterovirus — *continued*
    as cause of disease classified elsewhere — *continued*
      coxsackievirus B97.11
      echovirus B97.12
      specified NEC B97.19
  Entomophthora B46.8
  Epidermophyton — *see* Dermatophytosis
  epididymis — *see* Epididymitis
  episiotomy (puerperal) O86.0
  Erysipelothrix (insidiosa) (rhusiopathiae) — *see* Erysipeloid
  erythema infectiosum B08.3
  Escherichia (E.) coli NEC A49.8
    as cause of disease classified elsewhere (*see also* Escherichia coli) B96.20
    congenital P39.8
      sepsis P36.4
    generalized A41.51
    intestinal — *see* Enteritis, infectious, due to, Escherichia coli
  ethmoidal (chronic) (sinus) — *see* Sinusitis, ethmoidal
  eustachian tube (ear) — *see* Salpingitis, eustachian
  external auditory canal (meatus) NEC — *see* Otitis, externa, infective
  eye (purulent) — *see* Endophthalmitis, purulent
  eyelid — *see* Inflammation, eyelid
  fallopian tube — *see* Salpingo-oophoritis
  Fasciola (gigantica) (hepatica) (indica) B66.3
  Fasciolopsis (buski) B66.5
  filarial — *see* Infestation, filarial
  finger (skin) L08.9
    nail L03.01-
      fungus B35.1
  fish tapeworm B70.0
    larval B70.1
  flagellate, intestinal A07.9
  fluke — *see* Infestation, fluke
  focal
    teeth (pulpal origin) K04.7
    tonsils J35.01
  Fonsecaea (compactum) (pedrosoi) B43.0
  food — *see* Intoxication, foodborne
  foot (skin) L08.9
    dermatophytic fungus B35.3
  Francisella tularensis — *see* Tularemia
  frontal (sinus) (chronic) — *see* Sinusitis, frontal
  fungus NOS B49
    beard B35.0
    dermatophytic — *see* Dermatophytosis
    foot B35.3
    groin B35.6
    hand B35.2
    nail B35.1
    pathogenic to compromised host only B48.8
    perianal (area) B35.6
    scalp B35.0
    skin B36.9
      foot B35.3
      hand B35.2
      toenails B35.1
  Fusarium B48.8
  gallbladder — *see* Cholecystitis
  gas bacillus — *see* Gangrene, gas
  gastrointestinal — *see* Enteritis, infectious
  generalized NEC — *see* Sepsis
  generator pocket, implanted electronic neurostimulator T85.734 ☑
  genital organ or tract
    female — *see* Disease, pelvis, inflammatory
    male N49.9
      multiple sites N49.8
      specified NEC N49.8
  Ghon tubercle, primary A15.7
  Giardia lamblia A07.1
  gingiva (chronic) K05.10
    acute K05.00
      nonplaque induced K05.01
      plaque induced K05.00
    nonplaque induced K05.11
    plaque induced K05.10
  glanders A24.0
  glenosporopsis B48.0
  Gnathostoma (spinigerum) B83.1
  Gongylonema B83.8
  gonococcal — *see* Gonococcus
  gram-negative bacilli NOS A49.9

**Infection, infected, infective** — *continued*
  guinea worm B72
  gum (chronic) K05.10
    acute K05.00
      nonplaque induced K05.01
      plaque induced K05.00
    nonplaque induced K05.11
    plaque induced K05.10
  Haemophilus — *see* Infection, Hemophilus
  heart — *see* Carditis
  Helicobacter pylori A04.8
    as cause of disease classified elsewhere B96.81
  helminths B83.9
    intestinal B82.0
      mixed (types classifiable to more than one of the titles B65.0-B81.3 and B81.8) B81.4
      specified type NEC B81.8
    specified type NEC B83.8
  Hemophilus
    aegyptius, systemic A48.4
    ducrey (any location) A57
    generalized A41.3
    influenzae NEC A49.2
      as cause of disease classified elsewhere B96.3
  herpes (simplex) (*see also* Herpes)
    congenital P35.2
    disseminated B00.7
    zoster B02.9
  herpesvirus, herpesviral — *see* Herpes
  Heterophyes (heterophyes) B66.8
  hip (joint) NEC M00.9
    due to internal joint prosthesis
      left T84.52 ☑
      right T84.51 ☑
    skin NEC L08.9
  Histoplasma — *see* Histoplasmosis
    American B39.4
    capsulatum B39.4
  hookworm B76.9
  human
    papilloma virus A63.0
    T-cell lymphotropic virus type-1 (HTLV-1) B33.3
  hydrocele N43.0
  Hymenolepis B71.0
  hypopharynx — *see* Pharyngitis
  inguinal (lymph) glands L04.1
    due to soft chancre A57
  intervertebral disc, pyogenic M46.30
    cervical region M46.32
    cervicothoracic region M46.33
    lumbar region M46.36
    lumbosacral region M46.37
    multiple sites M46.39
    occipito-atlanto-axial region M46.31
    sacrococcygeal region M46.38
    thoracic region M46.34
    thoracolumbar region M46.35
  intestine, intestinal — *see* Enteritis, infectious
    specified NEC A08.8
  intra-amniotic affecting newborn NEC P39.2
  Isospora belli or hominis A07.3
  Japanese B encephalitis A83.0
  jaw (bone) (lower) (upper) M27.2
  joint NEC M00.9
    due to internal joint prosthesis T84.50 ☑
  kidney (cortex) (hematogenous) N15.9
    with calculus N20.0
      with hydronephrosis N13.6
    following ectopic gestation O08.83
    pelvis and ureter (cystic) N28.85
    puerperal (postpartum) O86.21
    specified NEC N15.8
  Klebsiella (K.) pneumoniae NEC A49.8
    as cause of disease classified elsewhere B96.1
  knee (joint) NEC M00.9
    due to internal joint prosthesis
      left T84.54 ☑
      right T84.53 ☑
    joint M00.9
    skin L08.9
  Koch's — *see* Tuberculosis
  labia (majora) (minora) (acute) — *see* Vulvitis
  lacrimal
    gland — *see* Dacryoadenitis
    passages (duct) (sac) — *see* Inflammation, lacrimal, passages
  lancet fluke B66.2
  larynx NEC J38.7

**Infection, infected, infective** — *continued*
- leg (skin) NOS L08.9
- Legionella pneumophila A48.1
  - nonpneumonic A48.2
- Leishmania (*see also* Leishmaniasis)
  - aethiopica B55.1
  - braziliensis B55.2
  - chagasi B55.0
  - donovani B55.0
  - infantum B55.0
  - major B55.1
  - mexicana B55.1
  - tropica B55.1
- lentivirus, as cause of disease classified elsewhere B97.31
- Leptosphaeria senegalensis B47.0
- Leptospira interrogans A27.9
  - autumnalis A27.89
  - canicola A27.89
  - hebdomadis A27.89
  - icterohaemorrhagiae A27.0
  - pomona A27.89
  - specified type NEC A27.89
- leptospirochetal NEC — *see* Leptospirosis
- Listeria monocytogenes (*see also* Listeriosis)
  - congenital P37.2
- Loa loa B74.3
  - with conjunctival infestation B74.3
  - eyelid B74.3
- Loboa loboi B48.0
- local, skin (staphylococcal) (streptococcal) L08.9
  - abscess — *code by* site under Abscess
  - cellulitis — *code by* site under Cellulitis
  - specified NEC L08.89
  - ulcer — *see* Ulcer, skin
- Loefflerella mallei A24.0
- lung (*see also* Pneumonia) J18.9
  - atypical Mycobacterium A31.0
  - spirochetal A69.8
  - tuberculous — *see* Tuberculosis, pulmonary
  - virus — *see* Pneumonia, viral
- lymph gland (*see also* Lymphadenitis, acute)
  - mesenteric I88.0
- lymphoid tissue, base of tongue or posterior pharynx, NEC (chronic) J35.03
- Madurella (grisea) (mycetomii) B47.0
- major
  - following ectopic or molar pregnancy O08.0
  - puerperal, postpartum, childbirth O85
- Malassezia furfur B36.0
- Malleomyces
  - mallei A24.0
  - pseudomallei (whitmori) — *see* Melioidosis
- mammary gland N61.0
- Mansonella (ozzardi) (perstans) (streptocerca) B74.4
- mastoid — *see* Mastoiditis
- maxilla, maxillary M27.2
  - sinus (chronic) — *see* Sinusitis, maxillary
- mediastinum J98.51
- Medina (worm) B72
- meibomian cyst or gland — *see* Hordeolum
- meninges — *see* Meningitis, bacterial
- meningococcal (*see also* condition) A39.9
  - adrenals A39.1
  - brain A39.81
  - cerebrospinal A39.0
  - conjunctiva A39.89
  - endocardium A39.51
  - heart A39.50
    - endocardium A39.51
    - myocardium A39.52
    - pericardium A39.53
  - joint A39.83
  - meninges A39.0
  - meningococcemia A39.4
    - acute A39.2
    - chronic A39.3
  - myocardium A39.52
  - pericardium A39.53
  - retrobulbar neuritis A39.82
  - specified site NEC A39.89
- mesenteric lymph nodes or glands NEC I88.0
- Metagonimus B66.8
- metatarsophalangeal M00.9
- methicillin
  - resistant Staphylococcus aureus (MRSA) A49.02
  - susceptible Staphylococcus aureus (MSSA) A49.01
- Microsporum, microsporic — *see* Dermatophytosis

**Infection, infected, infective** — *continued*
- mixed flora (bacterial) NEC A49.8
- Monilia — *see* Candidiasis
- Monosporium apiospermum B48.2
- mouth, parasitic B37.0
- Mucor — *see* Mucormycosis
- muscle NEC — *see* Myositis, infective
- mycelium NOS B49
- mycetoma B47.9
  - actinomycotic NEC B47.1
  - mycotic NEC B47.0
- Mycobacterium, mycobacterial — *see* Mycobacterium
- Mycoplasma NEC A49.3
  - pneumoniae, as cause of disease classified elsewhere B96.0
- mycotic NOS B49
  - pathogenic to compromised host only B48.8
  - skin NOS B36.9
- myocardium NEC I40.0
- nail (chronic)
  - with lymphangitis — *see* Lymphangitis, acute, digit
  - finger L03.01- ☑
    - fungus B35.1
    - ingrowing L60.0
  - toe L03.03- ☑
    - fungus B35.1
- nasal sinus (chronic) — *see* Sinusitis
- nasopharynx — *see* Nasopharyngitis
- navel L08.82
- Necator americanus B76.1
- Neisseria — *see* Gonococcus
- Neotestudina rosatii B47.0
- newborn P39.9
  - intra-amniotic NEC P39.2
  - skin P39.4
  - specified type NEC P39.8
- nipple N61.0
  - associated with
    - lactation O91.03
    - pregnancy O91.01- ☑
    - puerperium O91.02
- Nocardia — *see* Nocardiosis
- obstetrical surgical wound (puerperal) O86.0
- Oesophagostomum (apiostomum) B81.8
- Oestrus ovis — *see* Myiasis
- Oidium albicans B37.9
- Onchocerca (volvulus) — *see* Onchocerciasis
- oncovirus, as cause of disease classified elsewhere B97.32
- operation wound T81.4 ☑
- Opisthorchis (felineus) (viverrini) B66.0
- orbit, orbital — *see* Inflammation, orbit
- orthopoxvirus NEC B08.09
- ovary — *see* Salpingo-oophoritis
- Oxyuris vermicularis B80
- pancreas (acute) — *see* Pancreatitis, acute
  - abscess — *see* Pancreatitis, acute
  - specified NEC (*see also* Pancreatitis, acute) K85.80
- papillomavirus, as cause of disease classified elsewhere B97.7
- papovavirus NEC B34.4
- Paracoccidioides brasiliensis — *see* Paracoccidioidomycosis
- Paragonimus (westermani) B66.4
- parainfluenza virus B34.8
- parameningococcus NOS A39.9
- parapoxvirus B08.60
  - specified NEC B08.69
- parasitic B89
- Parastrongylus
  - cantonensis B83.2
  - costaricensis B81.3
  - paratyphoid A01.4
    - Type A A01.1
    - Type B A01.2
    - Type C A01.3
- paraurethral ducts N34.2
- parotid gland — *see* Sialoadenitis
- parvovirus NEC B34.3
  - as cause of disease classified elsewhere B97.6
- Pasteurella NEC A28.9
  - multocida A28.0
  - pestis — *see* Plague
  - pseudotuberculosis A28.2
  - septica (cat bite) (dog bite) A28.0
  - tularensis — *see* Tularemia
- pelvic, female — *see* Disease, pelvis, inflammatory

**Infection, infected, infective** — *continued*
- Penicillium (marneffei) B48.4
- penis (glans) (retention) NEC N48.29
- periapical K04.5
- peridental, periodontal K05.20
  - generalized — *see* Peridontitis, aggressive, generalized
  - localized — *see* Peridontitis, aggressive, localized
- perinatal period P39.9
  - specified type NEC P39.8
- perineal repair (puerperal) O86.0
- periorbital — *see* Inflammation, orbit
- perirectal K62.89
- perirenal — *see* Infection, kidney
- peritoneal — *see* Peritonitis
- periureteral N28.89
- Petriellidium boydii B48.2
- pharynx (*see also* Pharyngitis)
  - coxsackievirus B08.5
  - posterior, lymphoid (chronic) J35.03
- Phialophora
  - gougerotii (subcutaneous abscess or cyst) B43.2
  - jeanselmei (subcutaneous abscess or cyst) B43.2
  - verrucosa (skin) B43.0
- Piedraia hortae B36.3
- pinta A67.9
  - intermediate A67.1
  - late A67.2
  - mixed A67.3
  - primary A67.0
- pinworm B80
- pityrosporum furfur B36.0
- pleuro-pneumonia-like organism (PPLO) NEC A49.3
  - as cause of disease classified elsewhere B96.0
- pneumococcus, pneumococcal NEC A49.1
  - as cause of disease classified elsewhere B95.3
  - generalized (purulent) A40.3
    - with pneumonia J13
- Pneumocystis carinii (pneumonia) B59
- Pneumocystis jiroveci (pneumonia) B59
- port or reservoir T80.212 ☑
- postoperative T81.4 ☑
- postoperative wound T81.4 ☑
- postprocedural T81.4 ☑
- postvaccinal T88.0 ☑
- prepuce NEC N47.7
  - with penile inflammation N47.6
- prion — *see* Disease, prion, central nervous system
- prostate (capsule) — *see* Prostatitis
- Proteus (mirabilis) (morganii) (vulgaris) NEC A49.8
  - as cause of disease classified elsewhere B96.4
- protozoal NEC B64
  - intestinal A07.9
    - specified NEC A07.8
  - specified NEC B60.8
- Pseudoallescheria boydii B48.2
- Pseudomonas NEC A49.8
  - as cause of disease classified elsewhere B96.5
  - mallei A24.0
  - pneumonia J15.1
  - pseudomallei — *see* Melioidosis
- puerperal O86.4
  - genitourinary tract NEC O86.89
  - major or generalized O85
  - minor O86.4
  - specified NEC O86.89
- pulmonary — *see* Infection, lung
- purulent — *see* Abscess
- Pyrenochaeta romeroi B47.0
- Q fever A78
- rectum (sphincter) K62.89
- renal (*see also* Infection, kidney)
  - pelvis and ureter (cystic) N28.85
- reovirus, as cause of disease classified elsewhere B97.5
- respiratory (tract) NEC J98.8
  - acute J22
  - chronic J98.8
  - influenzal (upper) (acute) — *see* Influenza, with, respiratory manifestations NEC
  - lower (acute) J22
    - chronic — *see* Bronchitis, chronic
  - rhinovirus J00
  - syncytial virus, as cause of disease classified elsewhere B97.4
  - upper (acute) NOS J06.9
    - chronic J39.8
    - streptococcal J06.9
    - viral NOS J06.9

---

**Infection, infected, infective** — *continued*
  resulting from
    presence of internal prosthesis, implant, graft —
      *see* Complications, by site and type, infection
  retortamoniasis A07.8
  retroperitoneal NEC K68.9
  retrovirus B33.3
    as cause of disease classified elsewhere B97.30
      human
        immunodeficiency, type 2 (HIV 2) B97.35
        T-cell lymphotropic
          type I (HTLV-I) B97.33
          type II (HTLV-II) B97.34
      lentivirus B97.31
      oncovirus B97.32
      specified NEC B97.39
  Rhinosporidium (seeberi) B48.1
  rhinovirus
    as cause of disease classified elsewhere B97.89
    unspecified nature or site B34.8
  Rhizopus — *see* Mucormycosis
  rickettsial NOS A79.9
  roundworm (large) NEC B82.0
    Ascariasis (*see also* Ascariasis) B77.9
  rubella — *see* Rubella
  Saccharomyces — *see* Candidiasis
  salivary duct or gland (any) — *see* Sialoadenitis
  Salmonella (aertrycke) (arizonae) (callinarum)
    (cholerae-suis) (enteritidis) (suipestifer) (ty-
    phimurium) A02.9
    with
      (gastro)enteritis A02.0
      sepsis A02.1
      specified manifestation NEC A02.8
    due to food (poisoning) A02.9
    hirschfeldii A01.3
    localized A02.20
      arthritis A02.23
      meningitis A02.21
      osteomyelitis A02.24
      pneumonia A02.22
      pyelonephritis A02.25
      specified NEC A02.29
    paratyphi A01.4
      A A01.1
      B A01.2
      C A01.3
    schottmuelleri A01.2
    typhi, typhosa — *see* Typhoid
  Sarcocystis A07.8
  scabies B86
  Schistosoma — *see* Infestation, Schistosoma
  scrotum (acute) NEC N49.2
  seminal vesicle — *see* Vesiculitis
  septic
    localized, skin — *see* Abscess
  sheep liver fluke B66.3
  Shigella A03.9
    boydii A03.2
    dysenteriae A03.0
    flexneri A03.1
    group
      A A03.0
      B A03.1
      C A03.2
      D A03.3
    Schmitz (-Stutzer) A03.0
    schmitzii A03.0
    shigae A03.0
    sonnei A03.3
    specified NEC A03.8
  shoulder (joint) NEC M00.9
    due to internal joint prosthesis T84.59 ☑
    skin NEC L08.9
  sinus (accessory) (chronic) (nasal) (*see also* Sinusitis)
    pilonidal — *see* Sinus, pilonidal
    skin NEC L08.89
  Skene's duct or gland — *see* Urethritis
  skin (local) (staphylococcal) (streptococcal) L08.9
    abscess — *code by* site under Abscess
    cellulitis — *code by* site under Cellulitis
    due to fungus B36.9
      specified type NEC B36.8
    mycotic B36.9
      specified type NEC B36.8
    newborn P39.4
    ulcer — *see* Ulcer, skin
  slow virus A81.9

**Infection, infected, infective** — *continued*
  slow virus — *continued*
    specified NEC A81.89
  Sparganum (mansoni) (proliferum) (baxteri) B70.1
  specific (*see also* Syphilis)
    to perinatal period — *see* Infection, congenital
  specified NEC B99.8
  spermatic cord NEC N49.1
  sphenoidal (sinus) — *see* Sinusitis, sphenoidal
  spinal cord NOS (*see also* Myelitis) G04.91
    abscess G06.1
    meninges — *see* Meningitis
    streptococcal G04.89
  Spirillum A25.0
  spirochetal NOS A69.9
    lung A69.8
    specified NEC A69.8
  Spirometra larvae B70.1
  spleen D73.89
  Sporotrichum, Sporothrix (schenckii) — *see* Sporotri-
    chosis
  staphylococcal, unspecified site
    as cause of disease classified elsewhere B95.8
      aureus (methicillin susceptible) (MSSA) B95.61
        methicillin resistant (MRSA) B95.62
      specified NEC B95.7
    aureus (methicillin susceptible) (MSSA) A49.01
      methicillin resistant (MRSA) A49.02
    food poisoning A05.0
    generalized (purulent) A41.2
    pneumonia — *see* Pneumonia, staphylococcal
  Stellantchasmus falcatus B66.8
  streptobacillus moniliformis A25.1
  streptococcal NEC A49.1
    as cause of disease classified elsewhere B95.5
    B genitourinary complicating
      childbirth O98.82
      pregnancy O98.81- ☑
      puerperium O98.83
    congenital
      sepsis P36.10
        group B P36.0
        specified NEC P36.19
    generalized (purulent) A40.9
  Streptomyces B47.1
  Strongyloides (stercoralis) — *see* Strongyloidiasis
  stump (amputation) (surgical) — *see* Complication,
    amputation stump, infection
  subcutaneous tissue, local L08.9
  suipestifer — *see* Infection, salmonella
  swimming pool bacillus A31.1
  Taenia — *see* Infestation, Taenia
  Taeniarhynchus saginatus B68.1
  tapeworm — *see* Infestation, tapeworm
  tendon (sheath) — *see* Tenosynovitis, infective NEC
  Ternidens diminutus B81.8
  testis — *see* Orchitis
  threadworm B80
  throat — *see* Pharyngitis
  thyroglossal duct K14.8
  toe (skin) L08.9
    cellulitis L03.03- ☑
      fungus B35.1
    nail L03.03- ☑
      fungus B35.1
  tongue NEC K14.0
    parasitic B37.0
  tonsil (and adenoid) (faucial) (lingual) (pharyngeal) —
    *see* Tonsillitis
  tooth, teeth K04.7
    periapical K04.7
    peridental, periodontal K05.20
      generalized — *see* Peridontitis, aggressive,
        generalized
      localized — *see* Peridontitis, aggressive, local-
        ized
    pulp K04.01
      irreversible K04.02
      reversible K04.01
    socket M27.3
  TORCH — *see* Infection, congenital
    without active infection P00.2
  Torula histolytica — *see* Cryptococcosis
  Toxocara (canis) (cati) (felis) B83.0
  Toxoplasma gondii — *see* Toxoplasma
  trachea, chronic J42
  trematode NEC — *see* Infestation, fluke
  trench fever A79.0

**Infection, infected, infective** — *continued*
  Treponema pallidum — *see* Syphilis
  Trichinella (spiralis) B75
  Trichomonas A59.9
    cervix A59.09
    intestine A07.8
    prostate A59.02
    specified site NEC A59.8
    urethra A59.03
    urogenitalis A59.00
    vagina A59.01
    vulva A59.01
  Trichophyton, trichophytic — *see* Dermatophytosis
  Trichosporon (beigelii) cutaneum B36.2
  Trichostrongylus B81.2
  Trichuris (trichiura) B79
  Trombicula (irritans) B88.0
  Trypanosoma
    brucei
      gambiense B56.0
      rhodesiense B56.1
    cruzi — *see* Chagas' disease
  tubal — *see* Salpingo-oophoritis
  tuberculous NEC — *see* Tuberculosis
  tubo-ovarian — *see* Salpingo-oophoritis
  tunica vaginalis N49.1
  tunnel T80.212 ☑
  tympanic membrane NEC — *see* Myringitis
  typhoid (abortive) (ambulant) (bacillus) — *see* Typhoid
  typhus A75.9
    flea-borne A75.2
    mite-borne A75.3
    recrudescent A75.1
    tick-borne A77.9
      African A77.1
      North Asian A77.2
  umbilicus L08.82
  ureter N28.86
  urethra — *see* Urethritis
  urinary (tract) N39.0
    bladder — *see* Cystitis
    complicating
      pregnancy O23.4- ☑
        specified type NEC O23.3- ☑
    kidney — *see* Infection, kidney
    newborn P39.3
    puerperal (postpartum) O86.20
    tuberculous A18.13
    urethra — *see* Urethritis
  uterus, uterine — *see* Endometritis
  vaccination T88.0 ☑
  vaccinia not from vaccination B08.011
  vagina (acute) — *see* Vaginitis
  varicella B01.9
  varicose veins — *see* Varix
  vas deferens NEC N49.1
  vesical — *see* Cystitis
  Vibrio
    cholerae A00.0
      El Tor A00.1
    parahaemolyticus (food poisoning) A05.3
    vulnificus
      as cause of disease classified elsewhere B96.82
      foodborne intoxication A05.5
  Vincent's (gum) (mouth) (tonsil) A69.1
  virus, viral NOS B34.9
    adenovirus
      as cause of disease classified elsewhere B97.0
      unspecified nature or site B34.0
    arbovirus, arbovirus arthropod-borne A94
    as cause of disease classified elsewhere B97.89
      adenovirus B97.0
      coronavirus B97.29
        SARS-associated B97.21
      coxsackievirus B97.11
      echovirus B97.12
      enterovirus B97.10
        coxsackievirus B97.11
        echovirus B97.12
        specified NEC B97.19
      human
        immunodeficiency, type 2 (HIV 2) B97.35
        metapneumovirus B97.81
        T-cell lymphotropic,
          type I (HTLV-I) B97.33
          type II (HTLV-II) B97.34
      papillomavirus B97.7
      parvovirus B97.6

☑ **Additional Character Required** — Refer to the Tabular List for Character Selection    ▽ **Subterms under main terms may continue to next column or page**

**Infection, infected, infective** — *continued*
  virus, viral — *continued*
    as cause of disease classified elsewhere — *continued*
      reovirus B97.5
      respiratory syncytial B97.4
      retrovirus B97.30
        human
          immunodeficiency, type 2 (HIV 2) B97.35
          T-cell lymphotropic,
            type I (HTLV-I) B97.33
            type II (HTLV-II) B97.34
        lentivirus B97.31
        oncovirus B97.32
        specified NEC B97.39
      specified NEC B97.89
    central nervous system A89
      atypical A81.9
        specified NEC A81.89
      enterovirus NEC A88.8
        meningitis A87.0
      slow virus A81.9
        specified NEC A81.89
      specified NEC A88.8
    chest J98.8
    cotia B08.8
    coxsackie (*see also* Infection, coxsackie) B34.1
      as cause of disease classified elsewhere B97.11
    ECHO
      as cause of disease classified elsewhere B97.12
      unspecified nature or site B34.1
    encephalitis, tick-borne A84.9
    enterovirus, as cause of disease classified elsewhere
        B97.10
      coxsackievirus B97.11
      echovirus B97.12
      specified NEC B97.19
    exanthem NOS B09
    human metapneumovirus as cause of disease
        classified elsewhere B97.81
    human papilloma as cause of disease classified
        elsewhere B97.7
    intestine — *see* Enteritis, viral
    respiratory syncytial
      as cause of disease classified elsewhere B97.4
      bronchopneumonia J12.1
      common cold syndrome J00
      nasopharyngitis (acute) J00
    rhinovirus
      as cause of disease classified elsewhere B97.89
      unspecified nature or site B34.8
    slow A81.9
      specified NEC A81.89
    specified type NEC B33.8
      as cause of disease classified elsewhere B97.89
      unspecified nature or site B34.8
    unspecified nature or site B34.9
    West Nile — *see* Virus, West Nile
  vulva (acute) — *see* Vulvitis
  West Nile — *see* Virus, West Nile
  whipworm B79
  worms B83.9
    specified type NEC B83.8
  Wuchereria (bancrofti) B74.0
    malayi B74.1
  yatapoxvirus B08.70
    specified NEC B08.79
  yeast (*see also* Candidiasis) B37.9
  yellow fever — *see* Fever, yellow
  Yersinia
    enterocolitica (intestinal) A04.6
    pestis — *see* Plague
    pseudotuberculosis A28.2
  Zeis' gland — *see* Hordeolum
  Zika virus A92.5
  zoonotic bacterial NOS A28.9
  Zopfia senegalensis B47.0
**Infective, infectious** — *see* condition
**Infertility**
  female N97.9
    age-related N97.8
    associated with
      anovulation N97.0
      cervical (mucus) disease or anomaly N88.3
      congenital anomaly
        cervix N88.3
        fallopian tube N97.1
        uterus N97.2

**Infertility** — *continued*
  female — *continued*
    associated with — *continued*
      congenital anomaly — *continued*
        vagina N97.8
      dysmucorrhea N88.3
      fallopian tube disease or anomaly N97.1
      pituitary-hypothalamic origin E23.0
      specified origin NEC N97.8
      Stein-Leventhal syndrome E28.2
      uterine disease or anomaly N97.2
      vaginal disease or anomaly N97.8
    due to
      cervical anomaly N88.3
      fallopian tube anomaly N97.1
      ovarian failure E28.39
      Stein-Leventhal syndrome E28.2
      uterine anomaly N97.2
      vaginal anomaly N97.8
    nonimplantation N97.2
    origin
      cervical N88.3
      tubal (block) (occlusion) (stenosis) N97.1
      uterine N97.2
      vaginal N97.8
  male N46.9
    azoospermia N46.01
      extratesticular cause N46.029
        drug therapy N46.021
        efferent duct obstruction N46.023
        infection N46.022
        radiation N46.024
        specified cause NEC N46.029
        systemic disease N46.025
    oligospermia N46.11
      extratesticular cause N46.129
        drug therapy N46.121
        efferent duct obstruction N46.123
        infection N46.122
        radiation N46.124
        specified cause NEC N46.129
        systemic disease N46.125
    specified type NEC N46.8
**Infestation** B88.9
  Acanthocheilonema (perstans) (streptocerca) B74.4
  Acariasis B88.0
    demodex folliculorum B88.0
    sarcoptes scabiei B86
    trombiculae B88.0
  Agamofilaria streptocerca B74.4
  Ancylostoma, ankylostoma (braziliense) (caninum)
      (ceylanicum) (duodenale) B76.0
    americanum B76.1
    new world B76.1
  Anisakis larvae, anisakiasis B81.0
  arthropod NEC B88.2
  Ascaris lumbricoides — *see* Ascariasis
  Balantidium coli A07.0
  beef tapeworm B68.1
  Bothriocephalus (latus) B70.0
    larval B70.1
  broad tapeworm B70.0
    larval B70.1
  Brugia (malayi) B74.1
    timori B74.2
  candiru B88.8
  Capillaria
    hepatica B83.8
    philippinensis B81.1
  cat liver fluke B66.0
  cestodes B71.9
    diphyllobothrium — *see* Infestation, diphyllobothrium
    dipylidiasis B71.1
    hymenolepiasis B71.0
    specified type NEC B71.8
  chigger B88.0
  chigo, chigoe B88.1
  Clonorchis (sinensis) (liver) B66.1
  coccidial A07.3
  crab-lice B85.3
  Cysticercus cellulosae — *see* Cysticercosis
  Demodex (folliculorum) B88.0
  Dermanyssus gallinae B88.0
  Dermatobia (hominis) — *see* Myiasis
  Dibothriocephalus (latus) B70.0
    larval B70.1
  Dicrocoelium dendriticum B66.2

**Infestation** — *continued*
  Diphyllobothrium (adult) (latum) (intestinal) (pacificum) B70.0
    larval B70.1
  Diplogonoporus (grandis) B71.8
  Dipylidium caninum B67.4
  Distoma hepaticum B66.3
  dog tapeworm B67.4
  Dracunculus medinensis B72
  dragon worm B72
  dwarf tapeworm B71.0
  Echinococcus — *see* Echinococcus
  Echinostomum ilocanum B66.8
  Entamoeba (histolytica) — *see* Infection, Ameba
  Enterobius vermicularis B80
  eyelid
    in (due to)
      leishmaniasis B55.1
      loiasis B74.3
      onchocerciasis B73.09
      phthiriasis B85.3
    parasitic NOS B89
  eyeworm B74.3
  Fasciola (gigantica) (hepatica) (indica) B66.3
  Fasciolopsis (buski) (intestine) B66.5
  filarial B74.9
    bancroftian B74.0
    conjunctiva B74.9
    due to
      Acanthocheilonema (perstans) (streptocerca)
          B74.4
      Brugia (malayi) B74.1
        timori B74.2
      Dracunculus medinensis B72
      guinea worm B72
      loa loa B74.3
      Mansonella (ozzardi) (perstans) (streptocerca)
          B74.4
      Onchocerca volvulus B73.00
        eye B73.00
        eyelid B73.09
      Wuchereria (bancrofti) B74.0
    Malayan B74.1
    ozzardi B74.4
    specified type NEC B74.8
  fish tapeworm B70.0
    larval B70.1
  fluke B66.9
    blood NOS — *see* Schistosomiasis
    cat liver B66.0
    intestinal B66.5
    lancet B66.2
    liver (sheep) B66.3
      cat B66.0
      Chinese B66.1
      due to clonorchiasis B66.1
      oriental B66.1
    lung (oriental) B66.4
    sheep liver B66.3
    specified type NEC B66.8
  fly larvae — *see* Myiasis
  Gasterophilus (intestinalis) — *see* Myiasis
  Gastrodiscoides hominis B66.8
  Giardia lamblia A07.1
  Gnathostoma (spinigerum) B83.1
  Gongylonema B83.8
  guinea worm B72
  helminth B83.9
    angiostrongyliasis B83.2
      intestinal B81.3
    gnathostomiasis B83.1
    hirudiniasis, internal B83.4
    intestinal B82.0
      angiostrongyliasis B81.3
      anisakiasis B81.0
      ascariasis — *see* Ascariasis
      capillariasis B81.1
      cysticercosis — *see* Cysticercosis
      diphyllobothriasis — *see* Infestation, diphyllobothriasis
      dracunculiasis B72
      echinococcus — *see* Echinococcosis
      enterobiasis B80
      filariasis — *see* Infestation, filarial
      fluke — *see* Infestation, fluke
      hookworm — *see* Infestation, hookworm
      mixed (types classifiable to more than one of
          the titles B65.0-B81.3 and B81.8) B81.4

**Infestation** — *continued*
  helminth — *continued*
    intestinal — *continued*
      onchocerciasis — *see* Onchocerciasis
      schistosomiasis — *see* Infestation, schistosoma
      specified
        cestode NEC — *see* Infestation, cestode
          type NEC B81.8
      strongyloidiasis — *see* Strongyloidiasis
      taenia — *see* Infestation, taenia
      trichinellosis B75
      trichostrongyliasis B81.2
      trichuriasis B79
    specified type NEC B83.8
    syngamiasis B83.3
    visceral larva migrans B83.0
  Heterophyes (heterophyes) B66.8
  hookworm B76.9
    ancylostomiasis B76.0
    necatoriasis B76.1
    specified type NEC B76.8
  Hymenolepis (diminuta) (nana) B71.0
  intestinal NEC B82.9
  leeches (aquatic) (land) — *see* Hirudiniasis
  Leishmania — *see* Leishmaniasis
  lice, louse — *see* Infestation, Pediculus
  Linguatula B88.8
  Liponyssoides sanguineus B88.0
  Loa loa B74.3
    conjunctival B74.3
    eyelid B74.3
  louse — *see* Infestation, Pediculus
  maggots — *see* Myiasis
  Mansonella (ozzardi) (perstans) (streptocerca) B74.4
  Medina (worm) B72
  Metagonimus (yokogawai) B66.8
  microfilaria streptocerca — *see* Onchocerciasis
    eye B73.00
    eyelid B73.09
  mites B88.9
    scabic B86
  Monilia (albicans) — *see* Candidiasis
  mouth B37.0
  Necator americanus B76.1
  nematode NEC (intestinal) B82.0
    Ancylostoma B76.0
    conjunctiva NEC B83.9
    Enterobius vermicularis B80
    Gnathostoma spinigerum B83.1
    physaloptera B80
    specified NEC B81.8
    trichostrongylus B81.2
    trichuris (trichuria) B79
  Oesophagostomum (apiostomum) B81.8
  Oestrus ovis (*see also* Myiasis) B87.9
  Onchocerca (volvulus) — *see* Onchocerciasis
  Opisthorchis (felineus) (viverrini) B66.0
  orbit, parasitic NOS B89
  Oxyuris vermicularis B80
  Paragonimus (westermani) B66.4
  parasite, parasitic B89
    eyelid B89
    intestinal NOS B82.9
    mouth B37.0
    skin B88.9
    tongue B37.0
  Parastrongylus
    cantonensis B83.2
    costaricensis B81.3
  Pediculus B85.2
    body B85.1
    capitis (humanus) (any site) B85.0
    corporis (humanus) (any site) B85.1
    head B85.0
    mixed (classifiable to more than one of the titles
      B85.0 - B85.3) B85.4
    pubis (any site) B85.3
  Pentastoma B88.8
  Phthirus (pubis) (any site) B85.3
    with any infestation classifiable to B85.0 - B85.2
      B85.4
  pinworm B80
  pork tapeworm (adult) B68.0
  protozoal NEC B64
    intestinal A07.9
      specified NEC A07.8
    specified NEC B60.8
  pubic, louse B85.3

**Infestation** — *continued*
  rat tapeworm B71.0
  red bug B88.0
  roundworm (large) NEC B82.0
    Ascariasis (*see also* Ascariasis) B77.9
  sandflea B88.1
  Sarcoptes scabiei B86
  scabies B86
  Schistosoma B65.9
    bovis B65.8
    cercariae B65.3
    haematobium B65.0
    intercalatum B65.8
    japonicum B65.2
    mansoni B65.1
    mattheei B65.8
    mekongi B65.8
    specified type NEC B65.8
    spindale B65.8
  screw worms — *see* Myiasis
  skin NOS B88.9
  Sparganum (mansoni) (proliferum) (baxteri) B70.1
    larval B70.1
  specified type NEC B88.8
  Spirometra larvae B70.1
  Stellantchasmus falcatus B66.8
  Strongyloides stercoralis — *see* Strongyloidiasis
  Taenia B68.9
    diminuta B71.0
    echinococcus — *see* Echinococcus
    mediocanellata B68.1
    nana B71.0
    saginata B68.1
    solium (intestinal form) B68.0
      larval form — *see* Cysticercosis
  Taeniarhynchus saginatus B68.1
  tapeworm B71.9
    beef B68.1
    broad B70.0
      larval B70.1
    dog B67.4
    dwarf B71.0
    fish B70.0
      larval B70.1
    pork B68.0
    rat B71.0
  Ternidens diminutus B81.8
  Tetranychus molestissimus B88.0
  threadworm B80
  tongue B37.0
  Toxocara (canis) (cati) (felis) B83.0
  trematode(s) NEC — *see* Infestation, fluke
  Trichinella (spiralis) B75
  Trichocephalus B79
  Trichomonas — *see* Trichomoniasis
  Trichostrongylus B81.2
  Trichuris (trichiura) B79
  Trombicula (irritans) B88.0
  Tunga penetrans B88.1
  Uncinaria americana B76.1
  Vandellia cirrhosa B88.8
  whipworm B79
  worms B83.9
    intestinal B82.0
  Wuchereria (bancrofti) B74.0
**Infiltrate, infiltration**
  amyloid (generalized) (localized) — *see* Amyloidosis
  calcareous NEC R89.7
    localized — *see* Degeneration, by site
  calcium salt R89.7
  cardiac
    fatty — *see* Degeneration, myocardial
    glycogenic E74.02 [I43]
  corneal — *see* Edema, cornea
  eyelid — *see* Inflammation, eyelid
  glycogen, glycogenic — *see* Disease, glycogen storage
  heart, cardiac
    fatty — *see* Degeneration, myocardial
    glycogenic E74.02 [I43]
  inflammatory in vitreous H43.89
  kidney N28.89
  leukemic — *see* Leukemia
  liver K76.89
    fatty — *see* Fatty, liver NEC
    glycogen (*see also* Disease, glycogen storage)
      E74.03 [K77]
  lung R91.8
    eosinophilic J82

**Infiltrate, infiltration** — *continued*
  lymphatic (*see also* Leukemia, lymphatic) C91.9- ☑
    gland I88.9
  muscle, fatty M62.89
  myocardium, myocardial
    fatty — *see* Degeneration, myocardial
    glycogenic E74.02 [I43]
  on chest x-ray R91.8
  pulmonary R91.8
    with eosinophilia J82
  skin (lymphocytic) L98.6
  thymus (gland) (fatty) E32.8
  urine R39.0
  vesicant agent
    antineoplastic chemotherapy T80.810 ☑
    other agent NEC T80.818 ☑
  vitreous body H43.89
**Infirmity** R68.89
  senile R54
**Inflammation, inflamed, inflammatory** (with exuda-
    tion)
  abducent (nerve) — *see* Strabismus, paralytic, sixth
    nerve
  accessory sinus (chronic) — *see* Sinusitis
  adrenal (gland) E27.8
  alveoli, teeth M27.3
    scorbutic E54
  anal canal, anus K62.89
  antrum (chronic) — *see* Sinusitis, maxillary
  appendix — *see* Appendicitis
  arachnoid — *see* Meningitis
  areola N61.0
    puerperal, postpartum or gestational — *see* Infec-
      tion, nipple
  areolar tissue NOS L08.9
  artery — *see* Arteritis
  auditory meatus (external) — *see* Otitis, externa
  Bartholin's gland N75.8
  bile duct (common) (hepatic) or passage — *see*
    Cholangitis
  bladder — *see* Cystitis
  bone — *see* Osteomyelitis
  brain (*see also* Encephalitis)
    membrane — *see* Meningitis
  breast N61.0
    puerperal, postpartum, gestational — *see* Mastitis,
      obstetric
  broad ligament — *see* Disease, pelvis, inflammatory
  bronchi — *see* Bronchitis
  catarrhal J00
  cecum — *see* Appendicitis
  cerebral (*see also* Encephalitis)
    membrane — *see* Meningitis
  cerebrospinal
    meningococcal A39.0
  cervix (uteri) — *see* Cervicitis
  chest J98.8
  chorioretinal H30.9- ☑
    cyclitis — *see* Cyclitis
    disseminated H30.10- ☑
      generalized H30.13- ☑
      peripheral H30.12- ☑
      posterior pole H30.11- ☑
    epitheliopathy — *see* Epitheliopathy
    focal H30.00- ☑
      juxtapapillary H30.01- ☑
      macular H30.04- ☑
      paramacular — *see* Inflammation, chorioretinal,
        focal, macular
      peripheral H30.03- ☑
      posterior pole H30.02- ☑
    specified type NEC H30.89- ☑
  choroid — *see* Inflammation, chorioretinal
  chronic, postmastoidectomy cavity — *see* Complica-
    tions, postmastoidectomy, inflammation
  colon — *see* Enteritis
  connective tissue (diffuse) NEC — *see* Disorder, soft
    tissue, specified type NEC
  cornea — *see* Keratitis
  corpora cavernosa N48.29
  cranial nerve — *see* Disorder, nerve, cranial
  Douglas' cul-de-sac or pouch (chronic) N73.0
  due to device, implant or graft (*see also* Complications,
    by site and type, infection or inflammation)
    arterial graft T82.7 ☑
    breast (implant) T85.79 ☑
    catheter T85.79 ☑

**Inflammation, inflamed, inflammatory** — *continued*
  due to device, implant or graft (*see also* Complications, by site and type, infection or inflammation) — *continued*
    catheter — *continued*
      dialysis (renal) T82.7 ☑
        intraperitoneal T85.71 ☑
      infusion T82.7 ☑
        cranial T85.735 ☑
        intrathecal T85.735 ☑
        spinal (epidural) (subdural) T85.735 ☑
        subarachnoid T85.735 ☑
      urinary T83.518 ☑
        cystostomy T83.510 ☑
        Hopkins T83.518 ☑
        ileostomy T83.518 ☑
        nephrostomy T83.512 ☑
        specified NEC T83.518 ☑
        urethral indwelling T83.511 ☑
        urostomy T83.518 ☑
    electronic (electrode) (pulse generator) (stimulator)
      bone T84.7 ☑
      cardiac T82.7 ☑
      nervous system T85.738 ☑
        brain T85.731 ☑
        cranial nerve T85.732 ☑
        gastric nerve T85.732 ☑
        neurostimulator generator T85.734 ☑
        peripheral nerve T85.732 ☑
        sacral nerve T85.732 ☑
        spinal cord T85.733 ☑
        vagal nerve T85.732 ☑
      urinary T83.590 ☑
    fixation, internal (orthopedic) NEC — *see* Complication, fixation device, infection
    gastrointestinal (bile duct) (esophagus) T85.79 ☑
      neurostimulator electrode (lead) T85.732 ☑
    genital NEC T83.69 ☑
    heart NEC T82.7 ☑
      valve (prosthesis) T82.6 ☑
        graft T82.7 ☑
    joint prosthesis — *see* Complication, joint prosthesis, infection
    ocular (corneal graft) (orbital implant) NEC T85.79 ☑
    orthopedic NEC T84.7 ☑
    penile (cylinder) (pump) (resevoir) T83.61 ☑
    specified NEC T85.79 ☑
    testicular T83.62 ☑
    urinary NEC T83.598 ☑
      ileal conduit stent T83.593 ☑
      implanted neurostimulation T83.590 ☑
      implanted sphincter T83.591 ☑
      indwelling ureteral stent T83.592 ☑
      nephroureteral stent T83.593 ☑
      specified stent NEC T83.593 ☑
    vascular NEC T82.7 ☑
    ventricular intracranial (communicating) shunt T85.730 ☑
  duodenum K29.80
    with bleeding K29.81
  dura mater — *see* Meningitis
  ear (middle) (*see also* Otitis, media)
    external — *see* Otitis, externa
    inner — *see* subcategory H83.0 ☑
  epididymis — *see* Epididymitis
  esophagus K20.9
  ethmoidal (sinus) (chronic) — *see* Sinusitis, ethmoidal
  eustachian tube (catarrhal) — *see* Salpingitis, eustachian
  eyelid H01.9
    abscess — *see* Abscess, eyelid
    blepharitis — *see* Blepharitis
    chalazion — *see* Chalazion
    dermatosis (noninfectious) — *see* Dermatosis, eyelid
    hordeolum — *see* Hordeolum
    specified NEC H01.8
  fallopian tube — *see* Salpingo-oophoritis
  fascia — *see* Myositis
  follicular, pharynx J31.2
  frontal (sinus) (chronic) — *see* Sinusitis, frontal
  gallbladder — *see* Cholecystitis
  gastric — *see* Gastritis
  gastrointestinal — *see* Enteritis

**Inflammation, inflamed, inflammatory** — *continued*
  genital organ (internal) (diffuse)
    female — *see* Disease, pelvis, inflammatory
    male N49.9
      multiple sites N49.8
      specified NEC N49.8
  gland (lymph) — *see* Lymphadenitis
  glottis — *see* Laryngitis
  granular, pharynx J31.2
  gum K05.10
    nonplaque induced K05.11
    plaque induced K05.10
  heart — *see* Carditis
  hepatic duct — *see* Cholangitis
  ileoanal (internal) pouch K91.850
  ileum (*see also* Enteritis)
    regional or terminal — *see* Enteritis, regional
  intestinal pouch K91.850
  intestine (any part) — *see* Enteritis
  jaw (acute) (bone) (chronic) (lower) (suppurative) (upper) M27.2
  joint NEC — *see* Arthritis
    sacroiliac M46.1
  kidney — *see* Nephritis
  knee (joint) M13.169
    tuberculous A18.02
  labium (majus) (minus) — *see* Vulvitis
  lacrimal
    gland — *see* Dacryoadenitis
    passages (duct) (sac) (*see also* Dacryocystitis)
      canaliculitis — *see* Canaliculitis, lacrimal
  larynx — *see* Laryngitis
  leg NOS L08.9
  lip K13.0
  liver (capsule) (*see also* Hepatitis)
    chronic K73.9
    suppurative K75.0
  lung (acute) (*see also* Pneumonia)
    chronic J98.4
  lymph gland or node — *see* Lymphadenitis
  lymphatic vessel — *see* Lymphangitis
  maxilla, maxillary M27.2
    sinus (chronic) — *see* Sinusitis, maxillary
  membranes of brain or spinal cord — *see* Meningitis
  meninges — *see* Meningitis
  mouth K12.1
  muscle — *see* Myositis
  myocardium — *see* Myocarditis
  nasal sinus (chronic) — *see* Sinusitis
  nasopharynx — *see* Nasopharyngitis
  navel L08.82
  nerve NEC — *see* Neuralgia
  nipple N61.0
    puerperal, postpartum or gestational — *see* Infection, nipple
  nose — *see* Rhinitis
  oculomotor (nerve) — *see* Strabismus, paralytic, third nerve
  optic nerve — *see* Neuritis, optic
  orbit (chronic) H05.10
    acute H05.00
      abscess — *see* Abscess, orbit
      cellulitis — *see* Cellulitis, orbit
      osteomyelitis — *see* Osteomyelitis, orbit
      periostitis — *see* Periostitis, orbital
      tenonitis — *see* Tenonitis, eye
    granuloma — *see* Granuloma, orbit
    myositis — *see* Myositis, orbital
  ovary — *see* Salpingo-oophoritis
  oviduct — *see* Salpingo-oophoritis
  pancreas (acute) — *see* Pancreatitis
  parametrium N73.0
  parotid region L08.9
  pelvis, female — *see* Disease, pelvis, inflammatory
  penis (corpora cavernosa) N48.29
  perianal K62.89
  pericardium — *see* Pericarditis
  perineum (female) (male) L08.9
  perirectal K62.89
  peritoneum — *see* Peritonitis
  periuterine — *see* Disease, pelvis, inflammatory
  perivesical — *see* Cystitis
  petrous bone (acute) (chronic) — *see* Petrositis
  pharynx (acute) — *see* Pharyngitis
  pia mater — *see* Meningitis
  pleura — *see* Pleurisy

**Inflammation, inflamed, inflammatory** — *continued*
  polyp, colon (*see also* Polyp, colon, inflammatory) K51.40
  prostate (*see also* Prostatitis)
    specified type NEC N41.8
  rectosigmoid — *see* Rectosigmoiditis
  rectum (*see also* Proctitis) K62.89
  respiratory, upper (*see also* Infection, respiratory, upper) J06.9
    acute, due to radiation J70.0
    chronic, due to external agent — *see* condition, respiratory, chronic, due to
    due to
      chemicals, gases, fumes or vapors (inhalation) J68.2
      radiation J70.1
  retina — *see* Chorioretinitis
  retrocecal — *see* Appendicitis
  retroperitoneal — *see* Peritonitis
  salivary duct or gland (any) (suppurative) — *see* Sialoadenitis
  scorbutic, alveoli, teeth E54
  scrotum N49.2
  seminal vesicle — *see* Vesiculitis
  sigmoid — *see* Enteritis
  sinus — *see* Sinusitis
  Skene's duct or gland — *see* Urethritis
  skin L08.9
  spermatic cord N49.1
  sphenoidal (sinus) — *see* Sinusitis, sphenoidal
  spinal
    cord — *see* Encephalitis
    membrane — *see* Meningitis
    nerve — *see* Disorder, nerve
  spine — *see* Spondylopathy, inflammatory
  spleen (capsule) D73.89
  stomach — *see* Gastritis
  subcutaneous tissue L08.9
  suprarenal (gland) E27.8
  synovial — *see* Tenosynovitis
  tendon (sheath) NEC — *see* Tenosynovitis
  testis — *see* Orchitis
  throat (acute) — *see* Pharyngitis
  thymus (gland) E32.8
  thyroid (gland) — *see* Thyroiditis
  tongue K14.0
  tonsil — *see* Tonsillitis
  trachea — *see* Tracheitis
  trochlear (nerve) — *see* Strabismus, paralytic, fourth nerve
  tubal — *see* Salpingo-oophoritis
  tuberculous NEC — *see* Tuberculosis
  tubo-ovarian — *see* Salpingo-oophoritis
  tunica vaginalis N49.1
  tympanic membrane — *see* Tympanitis
  umbilicus, umbilical L08.82
  uterine ligament — *see* Disease, pelvis, inflammatory
  uterus (catarrhal) — *see* Endometritis
  uveal tract (anterior) NOS (*see also* Iridocyclitis)
    posterior — *see* Chorioretinitis
  vagina — *see* Vaginitis
  vas deferens N49.1
  vein (*see also* Phlebitis)
    intracranial or intraspinal (septic) G08
    thrombotic I80.9
      leg — *see* Phlebitis, leg
      lower extremity — *see* Phlebitis, leg
  vocal cord J38.3
  vulva — *see* Vulvitis
  Wharton's duct (suppurative) — *see* Sialoadenitis
**Inflation, lung, imperfect** (newborn) — *see* Atelectasis
**Influenza** (bronchial) (epidemic) (respiratory (upper)) (unidentified influenza virus) J11.1
  with
    digestive manifestations J11.2
    encephalopathy J11.81
    enteritis J11.2
    gastroenteritis J11.2
    gastrointestinal manifestations J11.2
    laryngitis J11.1
    myocarditis J11.82
    otitis media J11.83
    pharyngitis J11.1
    pneumonia J11.00
      specified type J11.08
    respiratory manifestations NEC J11.1

**Influenza** — *continued*
 with — *continued*
  specified manifestation NEC J11.89
  A/H5N1 (*see also* Influenza, due to, identified novel
    influenza A virus) J09.X2
  avian (*see also* Influenza, due to, identified novel in-
    fluenza A virus) J09.X2
  bird (*see also* Influenza, due to, identified novel influen-
    za A virus) J09.X2
 due to
  avian (*see also* Influenza, due to, identified novel
    influenza A virus) J09.X2
  identified influenza virus NEC J10.1
   with
    digestive manifestations J10.2
    encephalopathy J10.81
    enteritis J10.2
    gastroenteritis J10.2
    gastrointestinal manifestations J10.2
    laryngitis J10.1
    myocarditis J10.82
    otitis media J10.83
    pharyngitis J10.1
    pneumonia (unspecified type) J10.00
     with same identified influenza virus
      J10.01
     specified type NEC J10.08
    respiratory manifestations NEC J10.1
    specified manifestation NEC J10.89
  identified novel influenza A virus J09.X2
   with
    digestive manifestations J09.X3
    encephalopathy J09.X9
    enteritis J09.X3
    gastroenteritis J09.X3
    gastrointestinal manifestations J09.X3
    laryngitis J09.X2
    myocarditis J09.X9
    otitis media J09.X9
    pharyngitis J09.X2
    pneumonia J09.X1
    respiratory manifestations NEC J09.X2
    specified manifestation NEC J09.X9
    upper respiratory symptoms J09.X2
  novel (2009) H1N1 influenza (*see also* Influenza, due
    to, identified influenza virus NEC) J10.1
  novel influenza A/H1N1 (*see also* Influenza, due to,
    identified influenza virus NEC) J10.1
  of other animal origin, not bird or swine (*see also* In-
    fluenza, due to, identified novel influenza A
    virus) J09.X2
  swine (viruses that normally cause infections in pigs)
    (*see also* Influenza, due to, identified novel in-
    fluenza A virus) J09.X2
**Influenzal** — *see* Influenza
**Influenza-like disease** — *see* Influenza
**Infraction, Freiberg's** (metatarsal head) — *see* Osteochondrosis, juvenile, metatarsus
**Infraeruption of tooth** (teeth) M26.34
**Infusion complication, misadventure, or reaction**
  — *see* Complications, infusion
**Ingestion**
 chemical — *see* Table of Drugs and Chemicals, by
  substance, poisoning
 drug or medicament
  correct substance properly administered — *see*
   Table of Drugs and Chemicals, by drug, adverse effect
  overdose or wrong substance given or taken —
   *see* Table of Drugs and Chemicals, by drug,
   poisoning
 foreign body — *see* Foreign body, alimentary tract
 tularemia A21.3
**Ingrowing**
 hair (beard) L73.1
 nail (finger) (toe) L60.0
**Inguinal** (*see also* condition)
 testicle Q53.9
  bilateral Q53.212
  unilateral Q53.112
**Inhalant-induced**
 anxiety disorder F18.980
 depressive disorder F18.94
 major neurocognitive disorder F18.97
 mild neurocognitive disorder F18.988
 psychotic disorder F18.959
**Inhalation**
 anthrax A22.1

**Inhalation** — *continued*
 flame T27.3
 food or foreign body — *see* Foreign body, by site
 gases, fumes, or vapors NEC T59.9- ☑
  specified agent — *see* Table of Drugs and Chemicals, by substance
 liquid or vomitus — *see* Asphyxia
 meconium (newborn) P24.00
  with
   with respiratory symptoms P24.01
   pneumonia (pneumonitis) P24.01
 mucus — *see* Asphyxia, mucus
 oil or gasoline (causing suffocation) — *see* Foreign
  body, by site
 smoke J70.5
  due to chemicals, gases, fumes and vapors J68.9
 steam — *see* Toxicity, vapors
 stomach contents or secretions — *see* Foreign body,
  by site
  due to anesthesia (general) (local) or other sedation
   T88.59 ☑
   in labor and delivery O74.0
   in pregnancy O29.01- ☑
   postpartum, puerperal O89.01
**Inhibition, orgasm**
 female F52.31
 male F52.32
**Inhibitor, systemic lupus erythematosus** (presence
  of) D68.62
**Iniencephalus, iniencephaly** Q00.2
**Injection, traumatic jet** (air) (industrial) (water) (paint
  or dye) T70.4 ☑
**Injury** (*see also* specified injury type) T14.90 ☑
 abdomen, abdominal S39.91
  blood vessel — *see* Injury, blood vessel, abdomen
  cavity — *see* Injury, intra-abdominal
  contusion S30.1 ☑
  internal — *see* Injury, intra-abdominal
  intra-abdominal organ — *see* Injury, intra-abdominal
  nerve — *see* Injury, nerve, abdomen
  open — *see* Wound, open, abdomen
  specified NEC S39.81 ☑
  superficial — *see* Injury, superficial, abdomen
 Achilles tendon S86.00- ☑
  laceration S86.02- ☑
  specified type NEC S86.09- ☑
  strain S86.01- ☑
 acoustic, resulting in deafness — *see* Injury, nerve,
  acoustic
 adrenal (gland) S37.819 ☑
  contusion S37.812 ☑
  laceration S37.813 ☑
  specified type NEC S37.818 ☑
 alveolar (process) S09.93 ☑
 ankle S99.91- ☑
  contusion — *see* Contusion, ankle
  dislocation — *see* Dislocation, ankle
  fracture — *see* Fracture, ankle
  nerve — *see* Injury, nerve, ankle
  open — *see* Wound, open, ankle
  specified type NEC S99.81- ☑
  sprain — *see* Sprain, ankle
  superficial — *see* Injury, superficial, ankle
 anterior chamber, eye — *see* Injury, eye, specified site
  NEC
 anus — *see* Injury, abdomen
 aorta (thoracic) S25.00 ☑
  abdominal S35.00 ☑
   laceration (minor) (superficial) S35.01 ☑
    major S35.02 ☑
   specified type NEC S35.09 ☑
  laceration (minor) (superficial) S25.01 ☑
   major S25.02 ☑
  specified type NEC S25.09 ☑
 arm (upper) S49.9- ☑
  blood vessel — *see* Injury, blood vessel, arm
  contusion — *see* Contusion, arm, upper
  fracture — *see* Fracture, humerus
  lower — *see* Injury, forearm
  muscle — *see* Injury, muscle, shoulder
  nerve — *see* Injury, nerve, arm
  open — *see* Wound, open, arm
  specified type NEC S49.8- ☑
  superficial — *see* Injury, superficial, arm

**Injury** — *continued*
 artery (complicating trauma) (*see also* Injury, blood
  vessel, by site)
  cerebral or meningeal — *see* Injury, intracranial
 auditory canal (external) (meatus) S09.91 ☑
 auricle, auris, ear S09.91 ☑
 axilla — *see* Injury, shoulder
 back — *see* Injury, back, lower
 bile duct S36.13 ☑
 birth (*see also* Birth, injury) P15.9
 bladder (sphincter) S37.20 ☑
  at delivery O71.5
  contusion S37.22 ☑
  laceration S37.23 ☑
  obstetrical trauma O71.5
  specified type NEC S37.29 ☑
 blast (air) (hydraulic) (immersion) (underwater) NEC
  T14.8 ☑
  acoustic nerve trauma — *see* Injury, nerve, acoustic
  bladder — *see* Injury, bladder
  brain — *see* Concussion
  colon — *see* Injury, intestine, large
  ear (primary) S09.31- ☑
   secondary S09.39- ☑
  generalized T70.8 ☑
  lung — *see* Injury, intrathoracic, lung
  multiple body organs T70.8 ☑
  peritoneum S36.81 ☑
  rectum S36.61 ☑
  retroperitoneum S36.898 ☑
  small intestine S36.419 ☑
   duodenum S36.410 ☑
   specified site NEC S36.418 ☑
  specified
   intra-abdominal organ NEC S36.898 ☑
   pelvic organ NEC S37.899 ☑
 blood vessel NEC T14.8 ☑
  abdomen S35.9 ☑
   aorta — *see* Injury, aorta, abdominal
   celiac artery — *see* Injury, blood vessel, celiac
    artery
   iliac vessel — *see* Injury, blood vessel, iliac
   laceration S35.91 ☑
   mesenteric vessel — *see* Injury, mesenteric
   portal vein — *see* Injury, blood vessel, portal
    vein
   renal vessel — *see* Injury, blood vessel, renal
   specified vessel NEC S35.8X- ☑
   splenic vessel — *see* Injury, blood vessel,
    splenic
   vena cava — *see* Injury, vena cava, inferior
  ankle — *see* Injury, blood vessel, foot
  aorta (abdominal) (thoracic) — *see* Injury, aorta
  arm (upper) NEC S45.90- ☑
   forearm — *see* Injury, blood vessel, forearm
   laceration S45.91- ☑
   specified
    site NEC S45.80- ☑
     laceration S45.81- ☑
     specified type NEC S45.89- ☑
    type NEC S45.99- ☑
   superficial vein S45.30- ☑
    laceration S45.31- ☑
    specified type NEC S45.39- ☑
  axillary
   artery S45.00- ☑
    laceration S45.01- ☑
    specified type NEC S45.09- ☑
   vein S45.20- ☑
    laceration S45.21- ☑
    specified type NEC S45.29- ☑
  azygos vein — *see* Injury, blood vessel, thoracic,
   specified site NEC
  brachial
   artery S45.10- ☑
    laceration S45.11- ☑
    specified type NEC S45.19- ☑
   vein S45.20- ☑
    laceration S45.219 ☑
    specified type NEC S45.29- ☑
  carotid artery (common) (external) (internal, extracranial) S15.00- ☑
   internal, intracranial S06.8- ☑
   laceration (minor) (superficial) S15.01- ☑
    major S15.02- ☑
   specified type NEC S15.09- ☑

**Injury** — *continued*
blood vessel — *continued*
   celiac artery S35.219 ☑
     branch S35.299 ☑
       laceration (minor) (superficial) S35.291 ☑
         major S35.292 ☑
       specified NEC S35.298 ☑
     laceration (minor) (superficial) S35.211 ☑
       major S35.212 ☑
     specified type NEC S35.218 ☑
   cerebral — *see* Injury, intracranial
   deep plantar — *see* Injury, blood vessel, plantar artery
   digital (hand) — *see* Injury, blood vessel, finger
   dorsal
     artery (foot) S95.00- ☑
       laceration S95.01- ☑
       specified type NEC S95.09- ☑
     vein (foot) S95.20- ☑
       laceration S95.21- ☑
       specified type NEC S95.29- ☑
   due to accidental laceration during procedure — *see* Laceration, accidental complicating surgery
   extremity — *see* Injury, blood vessel, limb
   femoral
     artery (common) (superficial) S75.00- ☑
       laceration (minor) (superficial) S75.01- ☑
         major S75.02- ☑
       specified type NEC S75.09- ☑
     vein (hip level) (thigh level) S75.10- ☑
       laceration (minor) (superficial) S75.11- ☑
         major S75.12- ☑
       specified type NEC S75.19- ☑
   finger S65.50- ☑
     index S65.50- ☑
       laceration S65.51- ☑
       specified type NEC S65.59- ☑
     laceration S65.51- ☑
     little S65.50- ☑
       laceration S65.51- ☑
       specified type NEC S65.59- ☑
     middle S65.50- ☑
       laceration S65.51- ☑
       specified type NEC S65.59- ☑
     specified type NEC S65.59- ☑
     thumb — *see* Injury, blood vessel, thumb
   foot S95.90- ☑
     dorsal
       artery — *see* Injury, blood vessel, dorsal, artery
       vein — *see* Injury, blood vessel, dorsal, vein
     laceration S95.91- ☑
     plantar artery — *see* Injury, blood vessel, plantar artery
     specified
       site NEC S95.80- ☑
         laceration S95.81- ☑
         specified type NEC S95.89- ☑
       specified type NEC S95.99- ☑
   forearm S55.90- ☑
     laceration S55.91- ☑
     radial artery — *see* Injury, blood vessel, radial artery
     specified
       site NEC S55.80- ☑
         laceration S55.81- ☑
         specified type NEC S55.89- ☑
       type NEC S55.99- ☑
     ulnar artery — *see* Injury, blood vessel, ulnar artery
     vein S55.20- ☑
       laceration S55.21- ☑
       specified type NEC S55.29- ☑
   gastric
     artery — *see* Injury, mesenteric, artery, branch
     vein — *see* Injury, blood vessel, abdomen
   gastroduodenal artery — *see* Injury, mesenteric, artery, branch
   greater saphenous vein (lower leg level) S85.30- ☑
     hip (and thigh) level S75.20- ☑
       laceration (minor) (superficial) S75.21- ☑
         major S75.22- ☑
       specified type NEC S75.29- ☑
     laceration S85.31- ☑
     specified type NEC S85.39- ☑

**Injury** — *continued*
blood vessel — *continued*
   hand (level) S65.90- ☑
     finger — *see* Injury, blood vessel, finger
     laceration S65.91- ☑
     palmar arch — *see* Injury, blood vessel, palmar arch
     radial artery — *see* Injury, blood vessel, radial artery, hand
     specified
       site NEC S65.80- ☑
         laceration S65.81- ☑
         specified type NEC S65.89- ☑
       type NEC S65.99- ☑
     thumb — *see* Injury, blood vessel, thumb
     ulnar artery — *see* Injury, blood vessel, ulnar artery, hand
   head S09.0 ☑
     intracranial — *see* Injury, intracranial
     multiple S09.0 ☑
   hepatic
     artery — *see* Injury, mesenteric, artery
     vein — *see* Injury, vena cava, inferior
   hip S75.90- ☑
     femoral artery — *see* Injury, blood vessel, femoral, artery
     femoral vein — *see* Injury, blood vessel, femoral, vein
     greater saphenous vein — *see* Injury, blood vessel, greater saphenous, hip level
     laceration S75.91- ☑
     specified
       site NEC S75.80- ☑
         laceration S75.81- ☑
         specified type NEC S75.89- ☑
       type NEC S75.99- ☑
   hypogastric (artery) (vein) — *see* Injury, blood vessel, iliac
   iliac S35.5- ☑
     artery S35.51- ☑
     specified vessel NEC S35.5- ☑
     uterine vessel — *see* Injury, blood vessel, uterine
     vein S35.51- ☑
   innominate — *see* Injury, blood vessel, thoracic, innominate
   intercostal (artery) (vein) — *see* Injury, blood vessel, thoracic, intercostal
   jugular vein (external) S15.20- ☑
     internal S15.30- ☑
       laceration (minor) (superficial) S15.31- ☑
         major S15.32- ☑
       specified type NEC S15.39- ☑
     laceration (minor) (superficial) S15.21- ☑
       major S15.22- ☑
     specified type NEC S15.29- ☑
   leg (level) (lower) S85.90- ☑
     greater saphenous — *see* Injury, blood vessel, greater saphenous
     laceration S85.91- ☑
     lesser saphenous — *see* Injury, blood vessel, lesser saphenous
     peroneal artery — *see* Injury, blood vessel, peroneal artery
     popliteal
       artery — *see* Injury, blood vessel, popliteal, artery
       vein — *see* Injury, blood vessel, popliteal, vein
     specified
       site NEC S85.80- ☑
         laceration S85.81- ☑
         specified type NEC S85.89- ☑
       type NEC S85.99- ☑
     thigh — *see* Injury, blood vessel, hip
     tibial artery — *see* Injury, blood vessel, tibial artery
   lesser saphenous vein (lower leg level) S85.40- ☑
     laceration S85.41- ☑
     specified type NEC S85.49- ☑
   limb
     lower — *see* Injury, blood vessel, leg
     upper — *see* Injury, blood vessel, arm
   lower back — *see* Injury, blood vessel, abdomen
     specified NEC — *see* Injury, blood vessel, abdomen, specified, site NEC

**Injury** — *continued*
blood vessel — *continued*
   mammary (artery) (vein) — *see* Injury, blood vessel, thoracic, specified site NEC
   mesenteric (inferior) (superior)
     artery — *see* Injury, mesenteric, artery
     vein — *see* Injury, blood vessel, mesenteric, vein
   neck S15.9 ☑
     specified site NEC S15.8 ☑
   ovarian (artery) (vein) — *see* subcategory S35.8 ☑
   palmar arch (superficial) S65.20- ☑
     deep S65.30- ☑
       laceration S65.31- ☑
       specified type NEC S65.39- ☑
     laceration S65.21- ☑
     specified type NEC S65.29- ☑
   pelvis — *see* Injury, blood vessel, abdomen
     specified NEC — *see* Injury, blood vessel, abdomen, specified, site NEC
   peroneal artery S85.20- ☑
     laceration S85.21- ☑
     specified type NEC S85.29- ☑
   plantar artery (deep) (foot) S95.10- ☑
     laceration S95.11- ☑
     specified type NEC S95.19- ☑
   popliteal
     artery S85.00- ☑
       laceration S85.01- ☑
       specified type NEC S85.09- ☑
     vein S85.50- ☑
       laceration S85.51- ☑
       specified type NEC S85.59- ☑
   portal vein S35.319 ☑
     laceration S35.311 ☑
     specified type NEC S35.318 ☑
   precerebral — *see* Injury, blood vessel, neck
   pulmonary (artery) (vein) — *see* Injury, blood vessel, thoracic, pulmonary
   radial artery (forearm level) S55.10- ☑
     hand and wrist (level) S65.10- ☑
       laceration S65.11- ☑
       specified type NEC S65.19- ☑
     laceration S55.11- ☑
     specified type NEC S55.19- ☑
   renal
     artery S35.40- ☑
       laceration S35.41- ☑
       specified NEC S35.49- ☑
     vein S35.40- ☑
       laceration S35.41- ☑
       specified NEC S35.49- ☑
   saphenous vein (greater) (lower leg level) — *see* Injury, blood vessel, greater saphenous
     hip and thigh level — *see* Injury, blood vessel, greater saphenous, hip level
     lesser — *see* Injury, blood vessel, lesser saphenous
   shoulder
     specified NEC — *see* Injury, blood vessel, arm, specified site NEC
     superficial vein — *see* Injury, blood vessel, arm, superficial vein
   specified NEC T14.8 ☑
   splenic
     artery — *see* Injury, blood vessel, celiac artery, branch
     vein S35.329 ☑
       laceration S35.321 ☑
       specified NEC S35.328 ☑
   subclavian — *see* Injury, blood vessel, thoracic, innominate
   thigh — *see* Injury, blood vessel, hip
   thoracic S25.90 ☑
     aorta S25.00 ☑
       laceration (minor) (superficial) S25.01 ☑
         major S25.02 ☑
       specified type NEC S25.09 ☑
     azygos vein — *see* Injury, blood vessel, thoracic, specified, site NEC
     innominate
       artery S25.10- ☑
         laceration (minor) (superficial) S25.11- ☑
           major S25.12- ☑
         specified type NEC S25.19- ☑

Index

Injury — Injury

**Injury** — continued
  blood vessel — continued
    thoracic — continued
      innominate — continued
        vein S25.30- ✓
          laceration (minor) (superficial)
            S25.31- ✓
          major S25.32- ✓
          specified type NEC S25.39- ✓
      intercostal S25.50- ✓
        laceration S25.51- ✓
        specified type NEC S25.59- ✓
      laceration S25.91 ✓
      mammary vessel — see Injury, blood vessel,
        thoracic, specified, site NEC
      pulmonary S25.40- ✓
        laceration (minor) (superficial) S25.41- ✓
          major S25.42- ✓
        specified type NEC S25.49- ✓
      specified
        site NEC S25.80- ✓
          laceration S25.81 ✓
          specified type NEC S25.89- ✓
        type NEC S25.99- ✓
      subclavian — see Injury, blood vessel, thoracic,
        innominate
      vena cava (superior) S25.20 ✓
        laceration (minor) (superficial) S25.21- ✓
          major S25.22 ✓
        specified type NEC S25.29 ✓
    thumb S65.40- ✓
      laceration S65.41- ✓
      specified type NEC S65.49- ✓
    tibial artery S85.10- ✓
      anterior S85.13- ✓
        laceration S85.14- ✓
        specified injury NEC S85.15- ✓
      laceration S85.11- ✓
      posterior S85.16- ✓
        laceration S85.17- ✓
        specified injury NEC S85.18- ✓
      specified injury NEC S85.12- ✓
    ulnar artery (forearm level) S55.00- ✓
      hand and wrist (level) S65.00- ✓
        laceration S65.01- ✓
        specified type NEC S65.09- ✓
      laceration S55.01- ✓
      specified type NEC S55.09- ✓
    upper arm (level) — see Injury, blood vessel, arm
    superficial vein — see Injury, blood vessel, arm,
      superficial vein
    uterine S35.5- ✓
      artery S35.53- ✓
      vein S35.53- ✓
    vena cava — see Injury, vena cava
    vertebral artery S15.10- ✓
      laceration (minor) (superficial) S15.11- ✓
        major S15.12- ✓
      specified type NEC S15.19- ✓
    wrist (level) — see Injury, blood vessel, hand
  brachial plexus S14.3 ✓
    newborn P14.3
  brain (traumatic) S06.9- ✓
    diffuse (axonal) S06.2X- ✓
    focal S06.30- ✓
  brainstem S06.38- ✓
  breast NOS S29.9 ✓
  broad ligament — see Injury, pelvic organ, specified
    site NEC
  bronchus, bronchi — see Injury, intrathoracic,
    bronchus
  brow S09.90 ✓
  buttock S39.92 ✓
  canthus, eye S05.90 ✓
  cardiac plexus — see Injury, nerve, thorax, sympathetic
  cauda equina S34.3 ✓
  cavernous sinus — see Injury, intracranial
  cecum — see Injury, colon
  celiac ganglion or plexus — see Injury, nerve, lum-
    bosacral, sympathetic
  cerebellum — see Injury, intracranial
  cerebral — see Injury, intracranial
  cervix (uteri) — see Injury, uterus
  cheek (wall) S09.93 ✓
  chest — see Injury, thorax

**Injury** — continued
  childbirth (newborn) (see also Birth, injury)
    maternal NEC O71.9
  chin S09.93 ✓
  choroid (eye) — see Injury, eye, specified site NEC
  clitoris S39.94 ✓
  coccyx (see also Injury, back, lower)
    complicating delivery O71.6
  colon — see Injury, intestine, large
  common bile duct — see Injury, liver
  conjunctiva (superficial) — see Injury, eye, conjunctiva
  conus medullaris — see Injury, spinal, sacral
  cord
    spermatic (pelvic region) S37.898 ✓
      scrotal region S39.848 ✓
    spinal — see Injury, spinal cord, by region
  cornea — see Injury, eye, specified site NEC
    abrasion — see Injury, eye, cornea, abrasion
  cortex (cerebral) (see also Injury, intracranial)
    visual — see Injury, nerve, optic
  costal region NEC S29.9 ✓
  costochondral NEC S29.9 ✓
  cranial
    cavity — see Injury, intracranial
    nerve — see Injury, nerve, cranial
  crushing — see Crush
  cutaneous sensory nerve
  cystic duct — see Injury, liver
  deep tissue — see Contusion, by site
    meaning pressure ulcer — see Ulcer, pressure, un-
      stageable, by site
  delivery (newborn) P15.9
    maternal NEC O71.9
  Descemet's membrane — see Injury, eyeball, penetrat-
    ing
  diaphragm — see Injury, intrathoracic, diaphragm
  duodenum — see Injury, intestine, small, duodenum
  ear (auricle) (external) (canal) S09.91 ✓
    abrasion — see Abrasion, ear
    bite — see Bite, ear
    blister — see Blister, ear
    bruise — see Contusion, ear
    contusion — see Contusion, ear
    external constriction — see Constriction, external,
      ear
    hematoma — see Hematoma, ear
    inner — see Injury, ear, middle
    laceration — see Laceration, ear
    middle S09.30- ✓
      blast — see Injury, blast, ear
      specified NEC S09.39- ✓
    puncture — see Puncture, ear
    superficial — see Injury, superficial, ear
  eighth cranial nerve (acoustic or auditory) — see Injury,
    nerve, acoustic
  elbow S59.90- ✓
    contusion — see Contusion, elbow
    dislocation — see Dislocation, elbow
    fracture — see Fracture, ulna, upper end
    open — see Wound, open, elbow
    specified NEC S59.80- ✓
    sprain — see Sprain, elbow
    superficial — see Injury, superficial, elbow
  eleventh cranial nerve (accessory) — see Injury, nerve,
    accessory
  epididymis S39.94 ✓
  epigastric region S39.91 ✓
  epiglottis NEC S19.89 ✓
  esophageal plexus — see Injury, nerve, thorax, sympa-
    thetic
  esophagus (thoracic part) (see also Injury, intrathoracic,
    esophagus)
    cervical NEC S19.85 ✓
  eustachian tube S09.30 ✓
  eye S05.9- ✓
    avulsion S05.7- ✓
    ball — see Injury, eyeball
    conjunctiva S05.0- ✓
    cornea
      abrasion S05.0- ✓
    laceration S05.3- ✓
      with prolapse S05.2- ✓
    lacrimal apparatus S05.8X- ✓
    orbit penetration S05.4- ✓
    specified site NEC S05.8X- ✓
  eyeball S05.8X- ✓

**Injury** — continued
  eyeball — continued
    contusion S05.1- ✓
    penetrating S05.6- ✓
      with
        foreign body S05.5- ✓
        prolapse or loss of intraocular tissue
          S05.2- ✓
      without prolapse or loss of intraocular tissue
        S05.3- ✓
    specified type NEC S05.8- ✓
  eyebrow S09.93 ✓
  eyelid S09.93 ✓
    abrasion — see Abrasion, eyelid
    contusion — see Contusion, eyelid
    open — see Wound, open, eyelid
  face S09.93 ✓
  fallopian tube S37.509 ✓
    bilateral S37.502 ✓
      blast injury S37.512 ✓
      contusion S37.522 ✓
      laceration S37.532 ✓
      specified type NEC S37.592 ✓
    blast injury (primary) S37.519 ✓
      bilateral S37.512 ✓
      secondary — see Injury, fallopian tube, speci-
        fied type NEC
      unilateral S37.511 ✓
    contusion S37.529 ✓
      bilateral S37.522 ✓
      unilateral S37.521 ✓
    laceration S37.539 ✓
      bilateral S37.532 ✓
      unilateral S37.531 ✓
    specified type NEC S37.599 ✓
      bilateral S37.592 ✓
      unilateral S37.591 ✓
    unilateral S37.501 ✓
      blast injury S37.511 ✓
      contusion S37.521 ✓
      laceration S37.531 ✓
      specified type NEC S37.591 ✓
  fascia — see Injury, muscle
  fifth cranial nerve (trigeminal) — see Injury, nerve,
    trigeminal
  finger (nail) S69.9- ✓
    blood vessel — see Injury, blood vessel, finger
    contusion — see Contusion, finger
    dislocation — see Dislocation, finger
    fracture — see Fracture, finger
    muscle — see Injury, muscle, finger
    nerve — see Injury, nerve, digital, finger
    open — see Wound, open, finger
    specified NEC S69.8- ✓
    sprain — see Sprain, finger
    superficial — see Injury, superficial, finger
  first cranial nerve (olfactory) — see Injury, nerve, olfac-
    tory
  flank — see Injury, abdomen
  foot S99.92- ✓
    blood vessel — see Injury, blood vessel, foot
    contusion — see Contusion, foot
    dislocation — see Dislocation, foot
    fracture — see Fracture, foot
    muscle — see Injury, muscle, foot
    open — see Wound, open, foot
    specified type NEC S99.82- ✓
    sprain — see Sprain, foot
    superficial — see Injury, superficial, foot
  forceps NOS P15.9
  forearm S59.91- ✓
    blood vessel — see Injury, blood vessel, forearm
    contusion — see Contusion, forearm
    fracture — see Fracture, forearm
    muscle — see Injury, muscle, forearm
    nerve — see Injury, nerve, forearm
    open — see Wound, open, forearm
    specified NEC S59.81- ✓
    superficial — see Injury, superficial, forearm
  forehead S09.90 ✓
  fourth cranial nerve (trochlear) — see Injury, nerve,
    trochlear
  gallbladder S36.129 ✓
    contusion S36.122 ✓
    laceration S36.123 ✓
    specified NEC S36.128 ✓

**Injury** — *continued*
ganglion
  celiac, coeliac — *see* Injury, nerve, lumbosacral, sympathetic
  gasserian — *see* Injury, nerve, trigeminal
  stellate — *see* Injury, nerve, thorax, sympathetic
  thoracic sympathetic — *see* Injury, nerve, thorax, sympathetic
gasserian ganglion — *see* Injury, nerve, trigeminal
gastric artery — *see* Injury, blood vessel, celiac artery, branch
gastroduodenal artery — *see* Injury, blood vessel, celiac artery, branch
gastrointestinal tract — *see* Injury, intra-abdominal
  with open wound into abdominal cavity — *see* Wound, open, with penetration into peritoneal cavity
  colon — *see* Injury, intestine, large
  rectum — *see* Injury, intestine, large, rectum
    with open wound into abdominal cavity S36.61
  small intestine — *see* Injury, intestine, small
  specified site NEC — *see* Injury, intra-abdominal, specified, site NEC
  stomach — *see* Injury, stomach
genital organ(s)
  external S39.94 ☑
    specified NEC S39.848 ☑
  internal S37.90 ☑
    fallopian tube — *see* Injury, fallopian tube
    ovary — *see* Injury, ovary
    prostate — *see* Injury, prostate
    seminal vesicle — *see* Injury, pelvis, organ, specified site NEC
    uterus — *see* Injury, uterus
    vas deferens — *see* Injury, pelvis, organ, specified site NEC
  obstetrical trauma O71.9
gland
  lacrimal laceration — *see* Injury, eye, specified site NEC
  salivary S09.93 ☑
  thyroid NEC S19.84 ☑
globe (eye) S05.90 ☑
  specified NEC S05.8X- ☑
groin — *see* Injury, abdomen
gum S09.90 ☑
hand S69.9- ☑
  blood vessel — *see* Injury, blood vessel, hand
  contusion — *see* Contusion, hand
  fracture — *see* Fracture, hand
  muscle — *see* Injury, muscle, hand
  nerve — *see* Injury, nerve, hand
  open — *see* Wound, open, hand
  specified NEC S69.8- ☑
  sprain — *see* Sprain, hand
  superficial — *see* Injury, superficial, hand
head S09.90 ☑
  with loss of consciousness S06.9- ☑
  specified NEC S09.8 ☑
heart S26.90 ☑
  with hemopericardium S26.00 ☑
    contusion S26.01 ☑
    laceration (mild) S26.020 ☑
      major S26.022 ☑
      moderate S26.021 ☑
    specified type NEC S26.09 ☑
  without hemopericardium S26.10 ☑
    contusion S26.11 ☑
    laceration S26.12 ☑
    specified type NEC S26.19 ☑
  contusion S26.91 ☑
  laceration S26.92 ☑
  specified type NEC S26.99 ☑
heel — *see* Injury, foot
hepatic
  artery — *see* Injury, blood vessel, celiac artery, branch
  duct — *see* Injury, liver
  vein — *see* Injury, vena cava, inferior
hip S79.91- ☑
  blood vessel — *see* Injury, blood vessel, hip
  contusion — *see* Contusion, hip
  dislocation — *see* Dislocation, hip
  fracture — *see* Fracture, femur, neck
  muscle — *see* Injury, muscle, hip

**Injury** — *continued*
hip — *continued*
  nerve — *see* Injury, nerve, hip
  open — *see* Wound, open, hip
  specified NEC S79.81- ☑
  sprain — *see* Sprain, hip
  superficial — *see* Injury, superficial, hip
hymen S39.94 ☑
hypogastric
  blood vessel — *see* Injury, blood vessel, iliac
  plexus — *see* Injury, nerve, lumbosacral, sympathetic
ileum — *see* Injury, intestine, small
iliac region S39.91 ☑
instrumental (during surgery) — *see* Laceration, accidental complicating surgery
  birth injury — *see* Birth, injury
  nonsurgical — *see* Injury, by site
  obstetrical O71.9
    bladder O71.5
    cervix O71.3
    high vaginal O71.4
    perineal NOS O70.9
    urethra O71.5
    uterus O71.5
      with rupture or perforation O71.1
internal T14.8 ☑
  aorta — *see* Injury, aorta
  bladder (sphincter) — *see* Injury, bladder
    with
      ectopic or molar pregnancy O08.6
    following ectopic or molar pregnancy O08.6
    obstetrical trauma O71.5
  bronchus, bronchi — *see* Injury, intrathoracic, bronchus
  cecum — *see* Injury, intestine, large
  cervix (uteri) (*see also* Injury, uterus)
    with ectopic or molar pregnancy O08.6
    following ectopic or molar pregnancy O08.6
    obstetrical trauma O71.3
  chest — *see* Injury, intrathoracic
  gastrointestinal tract — *see* Injury, intra-abdominal
  heart — *see* Injury, heart
  intestine NEC — *see* Injury, intestine
  intrauterine — *see* Injury, uterus
  mesentery — *see* Injury, intra-abdominal, specified, site NEC
  pelvis, pelvic (organ) S37.90 ☑
    following ectopic or molar pregnancy (subsequent episode) O08.6
    obstetrical trauma NEC O71.5
      rupture or perforation O71.1
    specified NEC S39.83 ☑
  rectum — *see* Injury, intestine, large, rectum
  stomach — *see* Injury, stomach
  ureter — *see* Injury, ureter
  urethra (sphincter) following ectopic or molar pregnancy O08.6
  uterus — *see* Injury, uterus
interscapular area — *see* Injury, thorax
intestine
  large S36.509 ☑
    ascending (right) S36.500 ☑
      blast injury (primary) S36.510 ☑
        secondary S36.590 ☑
      contusion S36.520 ☑
      laceration S36.530 ☑
      specified type NEC S36.590 ☑
    blast injury (primary) S36.519 ☑
      ascending (right) S36.510 ☑
      descending (left) S36.512 ☑
      rectum S36.61 ☑
      sigmoid S36.513 ☑
      specified site NEC S36.518 ☑
      transverse S36.511 ☑
    contusion S36.529 ☑
      ascending (right) S36.520 ☑
      descending (left) S36.522 ☑
      rectum S36.62 ☑
      sigmoid S36.523 ☑
      specified site NEC S36.528 ☑
      transverse S36.521 ☑
    descending (left) S36.502 ☑
      blast injury (primary) S36.512 ☑
        secondary S36.592 ☑
      contusion S36.522 ☑
      laceration S36.532 ☑

**Injury** — *continued*
intestine — *continued*
  large — *continued*
    descending — *continued*
      specified type NEC S36.592 ☑
    laceration S36.539 ☑
      ascending (right) S36.530 ☑
      descending (left) S36.532 ☑
      rectum S36.63 ☑
      sigmoid S36.533 ☑
      specified site NEC S36.538 ☑
      transverse S36.531 ☑
    rectum S36.60 ☑
      blast injury (primary) S36.61 ☑
        secondary S36.69 ☑
      contusion S36.62 ☑
      laceration S36.63 ☑
      specified type NEC S36.69 ☑
    sigmoid S36.503 ☑
      blast injury (primary) S36.513 ☑
        secondary S36.593 ☑
      contusion S36.523 ☑
      laceration S36.533 ☑
      specified type NEC S36.593 ☑
    specified
      site NEC S36.508 ☑
        blast injury (primary) S36.518 ☑
          secondary S36.598 ☑
        contusion S36.528 ☑
        laceration S36.538 ☑
        specified type NEC S36.598 ☑
      type NEC S36.599 ☑
        ascending (right) S36.590 ☑
        descending (left) S36.592 ☑
        rectum S36.69 ☑
        sigmoid S36.593 ☑
        specified site NEC S36.598 ☑
        transverse S36.591 ☑
    transverse S36.501 ☑
      blast injury (primary) S36.511 ☑
        secondary S36.591 ☑
      contusion S36.521 ☑
      laceration S36.531 ☑
      specified type NEC S36.591 ☑
  small S36.409 ☑
    blast injury (primary) S36.419 ☑
      duodenum S36.410 ☑
      secondary S36.499 ☑
        duodenum S36.490 ☑
        specified site NEC S36.498 ☑
      specified site NEC S36.418 ☑
    contusion S36.429 ☑
      duodenum S36.420 ☑
      specified site NEC S36.428 ☑
    duodenum S36.400 ☑
      blast injury (primary) S36.410 ☑
        secondary S36.490 ☑
      contusion S36.420 ☑
      laceration S36.430 ☑
      specified NEC S36.490 ☑
    laceration S36.439 ☑
      duodenum S36.430 ☑
      specified site NEC S36.438 ☑
    specified
      site NEC S36.408 ☑
      type NEC S36.499 ☑
        duodenum S36.490 ☑
        specified site NEC S36.498 ☑
intra-abdominal S36.90 ☑
  adrenal gland — *see* Injury, adrenal gland
  bladder — *see* Injury, bladder
  colon — *see* Injury, intestine, large
  contusion S36.92 ☑
  fallopian tube — *see* Injury, fallopian tube
  gallbladder — *see* Injury, gallbladder
  intestine — *see* Injury, intestine
  kidney — *see* Injury, kidney
  laceration S36.93 ☑
  liver — *see* Injury, liver
  ovary — *see* Injury, ovary
  pancreas — *see* Injury, pancreas
  pelvic NOS S37.90 ☑
  peritoneum — *see* Injury, intra-abdominal, specified, site NEC
  prostate — *see* Injury, prostate
  rectum — *see* Injury, intestine, large, rectum

**Injury** — *continued*
  intra-abdominal — *continued*
    retroperitoneum — *see* Injury, intra-abdominal, specified, site NEC
    seminal vesicle — *see* Injury, pelvis, organ, specified site NEC
    small intestine — *see* Injury, intestine, small
    specified
      pelvic S37.90 ☑
        specified
          site NEC S37.899 ☑
            specified type NEC S37.898 ☑
          type NEC S37.99 ☑
      site NEC S36.899 ☑
        contusion S36.892 ☑
        laceration S36.893 ☑
        specified type NEC S36.898 ☑
      type NEC S36.99 ☑
    spleen — *see* Injury, spleen
    stomach — *see* Injury, stomach
    ureter — *see* Injury, ureter
    urethra — *see* Injury, urethra
    uterus — *see* Injury, uterus
    vas deferens — *see* Injury, pelvis, organ, specified site NEC
  intracranial (traumatic) S06.9- ☑
    cerebellar hemorrhage, traumatic — *see* Injury, intracranial, focal
    cerebral edema, traumatic S06.1X- ☑
      diffuse S06.1X- ☑
      focal S06.1X- ☑
    diffuse (axonal) S06.2X- ☑
    epidural hemorrhage (traumatic) S06.4X- ☑
    focal brain injury S06.30- ☑
      contusion — *see* Contusion, cerebral
      laceration — *see* Laceration, cerebral
    intracerebral hemorrhage, traumatic S06.36- ☑
      left side S06.35- ☑
      right side S06.34- ☑
    subarachnoid hemorrhage, traumatic S06.6X- ☑
    subdural hemorrhage, traumatic S06.5X- ☑
  intraocular — *see* Injury, eyeball, penetrating
  intrathoracic S27.9 ☑
    bronchus S27.409 ☑
      bilateral S27.402 ☑
      blast injury (primary) S27.419 ☑
        bilateral S27.412 ☑
        secondary — *see* Injury, intrathoracic, bronchus, specified type NEC
        unilateral S27.411 ☑
      contusion S27.429 ☑
        bilateral S27.422 ☑
        unilateral S27.421 ☑
      laceration S27.439 ☑
        bilateral S27.432 ☑
        unilateral S27.431 ☑
      specified type NEC S27.499 ☑
        bilateral S27.492 ☑
        unilateral S27.491 ☑
      unilateral S27.401 ☑
    diaphragm S27.809 ☑
      contusion S27.802 ☑
      laceration S27.803 ☑
      specified type NEC S27.808 ☑
    esophagus (thoracic) S27.819 ☑
      contusion S27.812 ☑
      laceration S27.813 ☑
      specified type NEC S27.818 ☑
    heart — *see* Injury, heart
    hemopneumothorax S27.2 ☑
    hemothorax S27.1 ☑
    lung S27.309 ☑
      aspiration J69.0
      bilateral S27.302 ☑
      blast injury (primary) S27.319 ☑
        bilateral S27.312 ☑
        secondary — *see* Injury, intrathoracic, lung, specified type NEC
        unilateral S27.311 ☑
      contusion S27.329 ☑
        bilateral S27.322 ☑
        unilateral S27.321 ☑
      laceration S27.339 ☑
        bilateral S27.332 ☑
        unilateral S27.331 ☑
      specified type NEC S27.399 ☑

**Injury** — *continued*
  intrathoracic — *continued*
    lung — *continued*
      specified type — *continued*
        bilateral S27.392 ☑
        unilateral S27.391 ☑
      unilateral S27.301 ☑
    pleura S27.60 ☑
      laceration S27.63 ☑
      specified type NEC S27.69 ☑
    pneumothorax S27.0 ☑
    specified organ NEC S27.899 ☑
      contusion S27.892 ☑
      laceration S27.893 ☑
      specified type NEC S27.898 ☑
    thoracic duct — *see* Injury, intrathoracic, specified organ NEC
    thymus gland — *see* Injury, intrathoracic, specified organ NEC
    trachea, thoracic S27.50 ☑
      blast (primary) S27.51 ☑
      contusion S27.52 ☑
      laceration S27.53 ☑
      specified type NEC S27.59 ☑
  iris — *see* Injury, eye, specified site NEC
    penetrating — *see* Injury, eyeball, penetrating
  jaw S09.93 ☑
  jejunum — *see* Injury, intestine, small
  joint NOS T14.8 ☑
    old or residual — *see* Disorder, joint, specified type NEC
  kidney S37.00- ☑
    acute (nontraumatic) N17.9
    contusion — *see* Contusion, kidney
    laceration — *see* Laceration, kidney
    specified NEC S37.09- ☑
  knee S89.9- ☑
    contusion — *see* Contusion, knee
    dislocation — *see* Dislocation, knee
    meniscus (lateral) (medial) — *see* Sprain, knee, specified site NEC
      old injury or tear — *see* Derangement, knee, meniscus, due to old injury
    open — *see* Wound, open, knee
    specified NEC S89.8- ☑
    sprain — *see* Sprain, knee
    superficial — *see* Injury, superficial, knee
  labium (majus) (minus) S39.94 ☑
  labyrinth, ear S09.30- ☑
  lacrimal apparatus, duct, gland, or sac — *see* Injury, eye, specified site NEC
  larynx NEC S19.81 ☑
  leg (lower) S89.9- ☑
    blood vessel — *see* Injury, blood vessel, leg
    contusion — *see* Contusion, leg
    fracture — *see* Fracture, leg
    muscle — *see* Injury, muscle, leg
    nerve — *see* Injury, nerve, leg
    open — *see* Wound, open, leg
    specified NEC S89.8- ☑
    superficial — *see* Injury, superficial, leg
  lens, eye — *see* Injury, eye, specified site NEC
    penetrating — *see* Injury, eyeball, penetrating
  limb NEC T14.8 ☑
  lip S09.93 ☑
  liver S36.119 ☑
    contusion S36.112 ☑
    laceration S36.113 ☑
      major (stellate) S36.116 ☑
      minor S36.114 ☑
      moderate S36.115 ☑
    specified NEC S36.118 ☑
  lower back S39.92 ☑
    specified NEC S39.82 ☑
  lumbar, lumbosacral (region) S39.92 ☑
    plexus — *see* Injury, lumbosacral plexus
  lumbosacral plexus S34.4 ☑
  lung (*see also* Injury, intrathoracic, lung)
    aspiration J69.0
    transfusion-related (TRALI) J95.84
  lymphatic thoracic duct — *see* Injury, intrathoracic, specified organ NEC
  malar region S09.93 ☑
  mastoid region S09.90 ☑
  maxilla S09.93 ☑

**Injury** — *continued*
  mediastinum — *see* Injury, intrathoracic, specified organ NEC
  membrane, brain — *see* Injury, intracranial
  meningeal artery — *see* Injury, intracranial, subdural hemorrhage
  meninges (cerebral) — *see* Injury, intracranial
  mesenteric
    artery
      branch S35.299 ☑
        laceration (minor) (superficial) S35.291 ☑
          major S35.292 ☑
        specified NEC S35.298 ☑
      inferior S35.239 ☑
        laceration (minor) (superficial) S35.231 ☑
          major S35.232 ☑
        specified NEC S35.238 ☑
      superior S35.229 ☑
        laceration (minor) (superficial) S35.221 ☑
          major S35.222 ☑
        specified NEC S35.228 ☑
    plexus (inferior) (superior) — *see* Injury, nerve, lumbosacral, sympathetic
    vein
      inferior S35.349 ☑
        laceration S35.341 ☑
        specified NEC S35.348 ☑
      superior S35.339 ☑
        laceration S35.331 ☑
        specified NEC S35.338 ☑
  mesentery — *see* Injury, intra-abdominal, specified site NEC
  mesosalpinx — *see* Injury, pelvic organ, specified site NEC
  middle ear S09.30- ☑
  midthoracic region NOS S29.9 ☑
  mouth S09.93 ☑
  multiple NOS T07 ☑
  muscle (and fascia) (and tendon)
    abdomen S39.001 ☑
      laceration S39.021 ☑
      specified type NEC S39.091 ☑
      strain S39.011 ☑
    abductor
      thumb, forearm level — *see* Injury, muscle, thumb, abductor
    adductor
      thigh S76.20- ☑
        laceration S76.22- ☑
        specified type NEC S76.29- ☑
        strain S76.21- ☑
    ankle — *see* Injury, muscle, foot
    anterior muscle group, at leg level (lower) S86.20- ☑
      laceration S86.22- ☑
      specified type NEC S86.29- ☑
      strain S86.21- ☑
    arm (upper) — *see* Injury, muscle, shoulder
    biceps (parts NEC) S46.20- ☑
      laceration S46.22- ☑
      long head S46.10- ☑
        laceration S46.12- ☑
        specified type NEC S46.19- ☑
        strain S46.11- ☑
      specified type NEC S46.29- ☑
      strain S46.21- ☑
    extensor
      finger(s) (other than thumb) — *see* Injury, muscle, finger by site, extensor
      forearm level, specified NEC — *see* Injury, muscle, forearm, extensor
      thumb — *see* Injury, muscle, thumb, extensor
      toe (large) (ankle level) (foot level) — *see* Injury, muscle, toe, extensor
    finger
      extensor (forearm level) S56.40- ☑
        hand level S66.309 ☑
          laceration S66.329 ☑
          specified type NEC S66.399 ☑
          strain S66.319 ☑
        laceration S56.429 ☑
        specified type NEC S56.499 ☑
        strain S56.419 ☑
      flexor (forearm level) S56.10- ☑
        hand level S66.109 ☑
          laceration S66.129 ☑

☑ **Additional Character Required — Refer to the Tabular List for Character Selection**
▽ **Subterms under main terms may continue to next column or page**

**Injury** — *continued*
  muscle — *continued*
    finger — *continued*
      flexor — *continued*
        hand level — *continued*
          specified type NEC S66.199 ☑
          strain S66.119 ☑
        laceration S56.129 ☑
        specified type NEC S56.199 ☑
        strain S56.119 ☑
      index
        extensor (forearm level)
          hand level S66.308 ☑
            laceration S66.32- ☑
            specified type NEC S66.39- ☑
            strain S66.31- ☑
          specified type NEC S56.492- ☑
        flexor (forearm level)
          hand level S66.108 ☑
            laceration S66.12- ☑
            specified type NEC S66.19- ☑
            strain S66.11- ☑
          specified type NEC S56.19- ☑
          strain S56.11- ☑
        intrinsic S66.50- ☑
          laceration S66.52- ☑
          specified type NEC S66.59- ☑
          strain S66.51- ☑
        intrinsic S66.509 ☑
          laceration S66.529 ☑
          specified type NEC S66.599 ☑
          strain S66.519 ☑
      little
        extensor (forearm level)
          hand level S66.30- ☑
            laceration S66.32- ☑
            specified type NEC S66.39- ☑
            strain S66.31- ☑
          laceration S56.42- ☑
          specified type NEC S56.49- ☑
          strain S56.41- ☑
        flexor (forearm level)
          hand level S66.10- ☑
            laceration S66.12- ☑
            specified type NEC S66.19- ☑
            strain S66.11- ☑
          laceration S56.12- ☑
          specified type NEC S56.19- ☑
          strain S56.11- ☑
        intrinsic S66.50- ☑
          laceration S66.52- ☑
          specified type NEC S66.59- ☑
          strain S66.51- ☑
      middle
        extensor (forearm level)
          hand level S66.30- ☑
            laceration S66.32- ☑
            specified type NEC S66.39- ☑
            strain S66.31- ☑
          laceration S56.42- ☑
          specified type NEC S56.49- ☑
          strain S56.41- ☑
        flexor (forearm level)
          hand level S66.10- ☑
            laceration S66.12- ☑
            specified type NEC S66.19- ☑
            strain S66.11- ☑
          laceration S56.12- ☑
          specified type NEC S56.19- ☑
          strain S56.11- ☑
        intrinsic S66.50- ☑
          laceration S66.52- ☑
          specified type NEC S66.59- ☑
          strain S66.51- ☑
      ring
        extensor (forearm level)
          hand level S66.30- ☑
            laceration S66.32- ☑
            specified type NEC S66.39- ☑
            strain S66.31- ☑
          laceration S56.42- ☑
          specified type NEC S56.49- ☑
          strain S56.41- ☑
        flexor (forearm level)
          hand level S66.10- ☑
            laceration S66.12-

---

**Injury** — *continued*
  muscle — *continued*
    finger — *continued*
      ring — *continued*
        flexor — *continued*
          hand level — *continued*
            specified type NEC S66.19- ☑
            strain S66.11- ☑
          laceration S56.12- ☑
          specified type NEC S56.19- ☑
          strain S56.11- ☑
        intrinsic S66.50- ☑
          laceration S66.52- ☑
          specified type NEC S66.59- ☑
          strain S66.51- ☑
    flexor
      finger(s) (other than thumb) — *see* Injury, muscle, finger
      forearm level, specified NEC — *see* Injury, muscle, forearm, flexor
      thumb — *see* Injury, muscle, thumb, flexor
      toe (long) (ankle level) (foot level) — *see* Injury, muscle, toe, flexor
    foot S96.90- ☑
      intrinsic S96.20- ☑
        laceration S96.22- ☑
        specified type NEC S96.29- ☑
        strain S96.21- ☑
      laceration S96.92- ☑
      long extensor, toe — *see* Injury, muscle, toe, extensor
      long flexor, toe — *see* Injury, muscle, toe, flexor
      specified
        site NEC S96.80- ☑
          laceration S96.82- ☑
          specified type NEC S96.89- ☑
          strain S96.81- ☑
        type S96.99- ☑
      strain S96.91- ☑
    forearm (level) S56.90- ☑
      extensor S56.50- ☑
        laceration S56.52- ☑
        specified type NEC S56.59- ☑
        strain S56.51- ☑
      flexor S56.20- ☑
        laceration S56.22- ☑
        specified type NEC S56.29- ☑
        strain S56.21- ☑
      laceration S56.92- ☑
      specified S56.99- ☑
        site NEC S56.80- ☑
          laceration S56.82- ☑
          strain S56.81- ☑
          type NEC S56.89- ☑
      strain S56.91- ☑
    hand (level) S66.90- ☑
      laceration S66.92- ☑
      specified
        site NEC S66.80- ☑
          laceration S66.82- ☑
          specified type NEC S66.89- ☑
          strain S66.81- ☑
          type NEC S66.99- ☑
      strain S66.91- ☑
    head S09.10 ☑
      laceration S09.12 ☑
      specified type NEC S09.19 ☑
      strain S09.11 ☑
    hip NEC S76.00- ☑
      laceration S76.02- ☑
      specified type NEC S76.09- ☑
      strain S76.01- ☑
    intrinsic
      ankle and foot level — *see* Injury, muscle, foot, intrinsic
      finger (other than thumb) — *see* Injury, muscle, finger by site, intrinsic
      foot (level) — *see* Injury, muscle, foot, intrinsic
      thumb — *see* Injury, muscle, thumb, intrinsic
    leg (level) (lower) S86.90- ☑
      Achilles tendon — *see* Injury, Achilles tendon
      anterior muscle group — *see* Injury, muscle, anterior muscle group
      laceration S86.92- ☑
      peroneal muscle group — *see* Injury, muscle, peroneal muscle group

---

**Injury** — *continued*
  muscle — *continued*
    leg — *continued*
      posterior muscle group — *see* Injury, muscle, posterior muscle group, leg level
      specified
        site NEC S86.80- ☑
          laceration S86.82- ☑
          specified type NEC S86.89- ☑
          strain S86.81- ☑
        type NEC S86.99- ☑
      strain S86.91- ☑
    long
      extensor toe, at ankle and foot level — *see* Injury, muscle, toe, extensor
      flexor, toe, at ankle and foot level — *see* Injury, muscle, toe, flexor
      head, biceps — *see* Injury, muscle, biceps, long head
    lower back S39.002 ☑
      laceration S39.022 ☑
      specified type NEC S39.092 ☑
      strain S39.012 ☑
    neck (level) S16.9 ☑
      laceration S16.2 ☑
      specified type NEC S16.8 ☑
      strain S16.1 ☑
    pelvis S39.003 ☑
      laceration S39.023 ☑
      specified type NEC S39.093 ☑
      strain S39.013 ☑
    peroneal muscle group, at leg level (lower) S86.30- ☑
      laceration S86.32- ☑
      specified type NEC S86.39- ☑
      strain S86.31- ☑
    posterior muscle (group)
      leg level (lower) S86.10- ☑
        laceration S86.12- ☑
        specified type NEC S86.19- ☑
        strain S86.11- ☑
      thigh level S76.30- ☑
        laceration S76.32- ☑
        specified type NEC S76.39- ☑
        strain S76.31- ☑
    quadriceps (thigh) S76.10- ☑
      laceration S76.12- ☑
      specified type NEC S76.19- ☑
      strain S76.11- ☑
    shoulder S46.90- ☑
      laceration S46.92- ☑
      rotator cuff — *see* Injury, rotator cuff
      specified site NEC S46.80- ☑
        laceration S46.82- ☑
        specified type NEC S46.89- ☑
        strain S46.81- ☑
      specified type NEC S46.99- ☑
      strain S46.91- ☑
    thigh NEC (level) S76.90- ☑
      adductor — *see* Injury, muscle, adductor, thigh
      laceration S76.92- ☑
      posterior muscle (group) — *see* Injury, muscle, posterior muscle, thigh level
      quadriceps — *see* Injury, muscle, quadriceps
      specified
        site NEC S76.80- ☑
          laceration S76.82- ☑
          specified type NEC S76.89- ☑
          strain S76.81- ☑
        type NEC S76.99- ☑
      strain S76.91- ☑
    thorax (level) S29.009 ☑
      back wall S29.002 ☑
      front wall S29.001 ☑
      laceration S29.029 ☑
        back wall S29.022 ☑
        front wall S29.021 ☑
      specified type NEC S29.099 ☑
        back wall S29.092 ☑
        front wall S29.091 ☑
      strain S29.019 ☑
        back wall S29.012 ☑
        front wall S29.011 ☑
    thumb
      abductor (forearm level) S56.30- ☑
        laceration S56.32- ☑

▽ Subterms under main terms may continue to next column or page     ☑ Additional Character Required — Refer to the Tabular List for Character Selection     195

Index

Injury — Injury

Injury — *continued*
  muscle — *continued*
    thumb — *continued*
      abductor — *continued*
        specified type NEC S56.39- ☑
        strain S56.31- ☑
      extensor (forearm level) S56.30- ☑
        hand level S66.20- ☑
          laceration S66.22- ☑
          specified type NEC S66.29- ☑
          strain S66.21- ☑
        laceration S56.32- ☑
        specified type NEC S56.39- ☑
        strain S56.31- ☑
      flexor (forearm level) S56.00- ☑
        hand level S66.00- ☑
          laceration S66.02- ☑
          specified type NEC S66.09- ☑
          strain S66.01- ☑
        laceration S56.02- ☑
        specified type NEC S56.09- ☑
        strain S56.01- ☑
        wrist level — *see* Injury, muscle, thumb, flexor, hand level
      intrinsic S66.40- ☑
        laceration S66.42- ☑
        specified type NEC S66.49- ☑
        strain S66.41- ☑
    toe (*see also* Injury, muscle, foot)
      extensor, long S96.10- ☑
        laceration S96.12- ☑
        specified type NEC S96.19- ☑
        strain S96.11- ☑
      flexor, long S96.00- ☑
        laceration S96.02- ☑
        specified type NEC S96.09- ☑
        strain S96.01- ☑
    triceps S46.30- ☑
      laceration S46.32- ☑
      specified type NEC S46.39- ☑
      strain S46.31- ☑
    wrist (and hand) level — *see* Injury, muscle, hand
  musculocutaneous nerve — *see* Injury, nerve, musculocutaneous
  myocardium — *see* Injury, heart
  nape — *see* Injury, neck
  nasal (septum) (sinus) S09.92 ☑
  nasopharynx S09.92 ☑
  neck S19.9 ☑
    specified NEC S19.80 ☑
      specified site NEC S19.89 ☑
  nerve NEC T14.8 ☑
    abdomen S34.9 ☑
      peripheral S34.6 ☑
      specified site NEC S34.8 ☑
    abducens S04.4- ☑
      contusion S04.4- ☑
      laceration S04.4- ☑
      specified type NEC S04.4- ☑
    abducent — *see* Injury, nerve, abducens
    accessory S04.7- ☑
      contusion S04.7- ☑
      laceration S04.7- ☑
      specified type NEC S04.7- ☑
    acoustic S04.6- ☑
      contusion S04.6- ☑
      laceration S04.6- ☑
      specified type NEC S04.6- ☑
    ankle S94.9- ☑
      cutaneous sensory S94.3- ☑
      specified site NEC — *see* subcategory S94.8 ☑
    anterior crural, femoral — *see* Injury, nerve, femoral
    arm (upper) S44.9- ☑
      axillary — *see* Injury, nerve, axillary
      cutaneous — *see* Injury, nerve, cutaneous, arm
      median — *see* Injury, nerve, median, upper arm
      musculocutaneous — *see* Injury, nerve, musculocutaneous
      radial — *see* Injury, nerve, radial, upper arm
      specified site NEC — *see* subcategory S44.8 ☑
      ulnar — *see* Injury, nerve, ulnar, arm
    auditory — *see* Injury, nerve, acoustic
    axillary S44.3- ☑
    brachial plexus — *see* Injury, brachial plexus
    cervical sympathetic S14.5 ☑
    cranial S04.9 ☑

Injury — *continued*
  nerve — *continued*
    cranial — *continued*
      contusion S04.9 ☑
      eighth (acoustic or auditory) — *see* Injury, nerve, acoustic
      eleventh (accessory) — *see* Injury, nerve, accessory
      fifth (trigeminal) — *see* Injury, nerve, trigeminal
      first (olfactory) — *see* Injury, nerve, olfactory
      fourth (trochlear) — *see* Injury, nerve, trochlear
      laceration S04.9 ☑
      ninth (glossopharyngeal) — *see* Injury, nerve, glossopharyngeal
      second (optic) — *see* Injury, nerve, optic
      seventh (facial) — *see* Injury, nerve, facial
      sixth (abducent) — *see* Injury, nerve, abducens
      specified
        nerve NEC S04.89- ☑
          contusion S04.89- ☑
          laceration S04.89- ☑
          specified type NEC S04.89- ☑
        type NEC S04.9 ☑
      tenth (pneumogastric or vagus) — *see* Injury, nerve, vagus
      third (oculomotor) — *see* Injury, nerve, oculomotor
      twelfth (hypoglossal) — *see* Injury, nerve, hypoglossal
    cutaneous sensory
      ankle (level) S94.3- ☑
      arm (upper) (level) S44.5- ☑
      foot (level) — *see* Injury, nerve, cutaneous sensory, ankle
      forearm (level) S54.3- ☑
      hip (level) S74.2- ☑
      leg (lower level) S84.2- ☑
      shoulder (level) — *see* Injury, nerve, cutaneous sensory, arm
      thigh (level) — *see* Injury, nerve, cutaneous sensory, hip
    deep peroneal — *see* Injury, nerve, peroneal, foot
    digital
      finger S64.4- ☑
        index S64.49- ☑
        little S64.49- ☑
        middle S64.49- ☑
        ring S64.49- ☑
      thumb S64.3- ☑
      toe — *see* Injury, nerve, ankle, specified site NEC
    eighth cranial (acoustic or auditory) — *see* Injury, nerve, acoustic
    eleventh cranial (accessory) — *see* Injury, nerve, accessory
    facial S04.5- ☑
      contusion S04.5- ☑
      laceration S04.5- ☑
      newborn P11.3
      specified type NEC S04.5- ☑
    femoral (hip level) (thigh level) S74.1- ☑
    fifth cranial (trigeminal) — *see* Injury, nerve, trigeminal
    finger (digital) — *see* Injury, nerve, digital, finger
    first cranial (olfactory) — *see* Injury, nerve, olfactory
    foot S94.9- ☑
      cutaneous sensory S94.3- ☑
      deep peroneal S94.2- ☑
      lateral plantar S94.0- ☑
      medial plantar S94.1- ☑
      specified site NEC — *see* subcategory S94.8 ☑
    forearm (level) S54.9- ☑
      cutaneous sensory — *see* Injury, nerve, cutaneous sensory, forearm
      median — *see* Injury, nerve, median
      radial — *see* Injury, nerve, radial
      specified site NEC — *see* subcategory S54.8 ☑
      ulnar — *see* Injury, nerve, ulnar
    fourth cranial (trochlear) — *see* Injury, nerve, trochlear
    glossopharyngeal S04.89- ☑
      specified type NEC S04.89- ☑
    hand S64.9- ☑
      median — *see* Injury, nerve, median, hand
      radial — *see* Injury, nerve, radial, hand
      specified NEC — *see* subcategory S64.8 ☑

Injury — *continued*
  nerve — *continued*
    hand — *continued*
      ulnar — *see* Injury, nerve, ulnar, hand
    hip (level) S74.9- ☑
      cutaneous sensory — *see* Injury, nerve, cutaneous sensory, hip
      femoral — *see* Injury, nerve, femoral
      sciatic — *see* Injury, nerve, sciatic
      specified site NEC — *see* subcategory S74.8 ☑
    hypoglossal S04.89- ☑
      specified type NEC S04.89- ☑
    lateral plantar S94.0- ☑
    leg (lower) S84.9- ☑
      cutaneous sensory — *see* Injury, nerve, cutaneous sensory, leg
      peroneal — *see* Injury, nerve, peroneal
      specified site NEC — *see* subcategory S84.8 ☑
      tibial — *see* Injury, nerve, tibial
      upper — *see* Injury, nerve, thigh
    lower
      back — *see* Injury, nerve, abdomen, specified site NEC
        peripheral — *see* Injury, nerve, abdomen, peripheral
      limb — *see* Injury, nerve, leg
    lumbar plexus — *see* Injury, nerve, lumbosacral, sympathetic
    lumbar spinal — *see* Injury, nerve, spinal, lumbar
    lumbosacral
      plexus — *see* Injury, nerve, lumbosacral, sympathetic
      sympathetic S34.5 ☑
    medial plantar S94.1- ☑
    median (forearm level) S54.1- ☑
      hand (level) S64.1- ☑
      upper arm (level) S44.1- ☑
      wrist (level) — *see* Injury, nerve, median, hand
    musculocutaneous S44.4- ☑
    musculospiral (upper arm level) — *see* Injury, nerve, radial, upper arm
    neck S14.9 ☑
      peripheral S14.4 ☑
      specified site NEC S14.8 ☑
      sympathetic S14.5 ☑
    ninth cranial (glossopharyngeal) — *see* Injury, nerve, glossopharyngeal
    oculomotor S04.1- ☑
      contusion S04.1- ☑
      laceration S04.1- ☑
      specified type NEC S04.1- ☑
    olfactory S04.81- ☑
      specified type NEC S04.81- ☑
    optic S04.01- ☑
      contusion S04.01- ☑
      laceration S04.01- ☑
      specified type NEC S04.01- ☑
    pelvic girdle — *see* Injury, nerve, hip
    pelvis — *see* Injury, nerve, abdomen, specified site NEC
      peripheral — *see* Injury, nerve, abdomen, peripheral
    peripheral NEC T14.8 ☑
      abdomen — *see* Injury, nerve, abdomen, peripheral
      lower back — *see* Injury, nerve, abdomen, peripheral
      neck — *see* Injury, nerve, neck, peripheral
      pelvis — *see* Injury, nerve, abdomen, peripheral
      specified NEC T14.8 ☑
    peroneal (lower leg level) S84.1- ☑
      foot S94.2- ☑
    plexus
      brachial — *see* Injury, brachial plexus
      celiac, coeliac — *see* Injury, nerve, lumbosacral, sympathetic
      mesenteric, inferior — *see* Injury, nerve, lumbosacral, sympathetic
      sacral — *see* Injury, lumbosacral plexus
      spinal
        brachial — *see* Injury, brachial plexus
        lumbosacral — *see* Injury, lumbosacral plexus
    pneumogastric — *see* Injury, nerve, vagus
    radial (forearm level) S54.2- ☑
      hand (level) S64.2- ☑

☑ Additional Character Required — Refer to the Tabular List for Character Selection    ▽ Subterms under main terms may continue to next column or page

**Injury** — *continued*
  nerve — *continued*
    radial — *continued*
      upper arm (level) S44.2- ☑
      wrist (level) — *see* Injury, nerve, radial, hand
    root — *see* Injury, nerve, spinal, root
    sacral plexus — *see* Injury, lumbosacral plexus
    sacral spinal — *see* Injury, nerve, spinal, sacral
    sciatic (hip level) (thigh level) S74.0- ☑
    second cranial (optic) — *see* Injury, nerve, optic
    seventh cranial (facial) — *see* Injury, nerve, facial
    shoulder — *see* Injury, nerve, arm
    sixth cranial (abducent) — *see* Injury, nerve, abducens
    spinal
      plexus — *see* Injury, nerve, plexus, spinal
      root
        cervical S14.2 ☑
        dorsal S24.2 ☑
        lumbar S34.21 ☑
        sacral S34.22 ☑
        thoracic — *see* Injury, nerve, spinal, root, dorsal
    splanchnic — *see* Injury, nerve, lumbosacral, sympathetic
    sympathetic NEC — *see* Injury, nerve, lumbosacral, sympathetic
      cervical — *see* Injury, nerve, cervical sympathetic
    tenth cranial (pneumogastric or vagus) — *see* Injury, nerve, vagus
    thigh (level) — *see* Injury, nerve, hip
      cutaneous sensory — *see* Injury, nerve, cutaneous sensory, hip
      femoral — *see* Injury, nerve, femoral
      sciatic — *see* Injury, nerve, sciatic
      specified NEC — *see* Injury, nerve, hip
    third cranial (oculomotor) — *see* Injury, nerve, oculomotor
    thorax S24.9 ☑
      peripheral S24.3 ☑
      specified site NEC S24.8 ☑
      sympathetic S24.4 ☑
    thumb, digital — *see* Injury, nerve, digital, thumb
    tibial (lower leg level) (posterior) S84.0- ☑
    toe — *see* Injury, nerve, ankle
    trigeminal S04.3- ☑
      contusion S04.3- ☑
      laceration S04.3- ☑
      specified type NEC S04.3- ☑
    trochlear S04.2- ☑
      contusion S04.2- ☑
      laceration S04.2- ☑
      specified type NEC S04.2- ☑
    twelfth cranial (hypoglossal) — *see* Injury, nerve, hypoglossal
    ulnar (forearm level) S54.0- ☑
      arm (upper) (level) S44.0- ☑
      hand (level) S64.0- ☑
      wrist (level) — *see* Injury, nerve, ulnar, hand
    vagus S04.89- ☑
      specified type NEC S04.89- ☑
    wrist (level) — *see* Injury, nerve, hand
    ninth cranial nerve (glossopharyngeal) — *see* Injury, nerve, glossopharyngeal
  nose (septum) S09.92 ☑
  obstetrical O71.9
    specified NEC O71.89
  occipital (region) (scalp) S09.90 ☑
    lobe — *see* Injury, intracranial
  optic chiasm S04.02 ☑
  optic radiation S04.03- ☑
  optic tract and pathways S04.03- ☑
  orbit, orbital (region) — *see* Injury, eye
    penetrating (with foreign body) — *see* Injury, eye, orbit, penetrating
    specified NEC — *see* Injury, eye, specified site NEC
  ovary, ovarian S37.409 ☑
    bilateral S37.402 ☑
      contusion S37.422 ☑
      laceration S37.432 ☑
      specified type NEC S37.492 ☑
    blood vessel — *see* Injury, blood vessel, ovarian
    contusion S37.429 ☑
      bilateral S37.422 ☑
      unilateral S37.421 ☑

**Injury** — *continued*
  ovary, ovarian — *continued*
    laceration S37.439 ☑
      bilateral S37.432 ☑
      unilateral S37.431 ☑
    specified type NEC S37.499 ☑
      bilateral S37.492 ☑
      unilateral S37.491 ☑
    unilateral S37.401 ☑
      contusion S37.421 ☑
      laceration S37.431 ☑
      specified type NEC S37.491 ☑
  palate (hard) (soft) S09.93 ☑
  pancreas S36.209 ☑
    body S36.201 ☑
      contusion S36.221 ☑
      laceration S36.231 ☑
        major S36.261 ☑
        minor S36.241 ☑
        moderate S36.251 ☑
      specified type NEC S36.291 ☑
    contusion S36.229 ☑
    head S36.200 ☑
      contusion S36.220 ☑
      laceration S36.230 ☑
        major S36.260 ☑
        minor S36.240 ☑
        moderate S36.250 ☑
      specified type NEC S36.290 ☑
    laceration S36.239 ☑
      major S36.269 ☑
      minor S36.249 ☑
      moderate S36.259 ☑
    specified type NEC S36.299 ☑
    tail S36.202 ☑
      contusion S36.222 ☑
      laceration S36.232 ☑
        major S36.262 ☑
        minor S36.242 ☑
        moderate S36.252 ☑
      specified type NEC S36.292 ☑
  parietal (region) (scalp) S09.90 ☑
    lobe — *see* Injury, intracranial
  patellar ligament (tendon) S76.10- ☑
    laceration S76.12- ☑
    specified NEC S76.19- ☑
    strain S76.11- ☑
  pelvis, pelvic (floor) S39.93 ☑
    complicating delivery O70.1
    joint or ligament, complicating delivery O71.6
    organ S37.90 ☑
      with ectopic or molar pregnancy O08.6
      complication of abortion — *see* Abortion
      contusion S37.92 ☑
      following ectopic or molar pregnancy O08.6
      laceration S37.93 ☑
      obstetrical trauma NEC O71.5
      specified
        site NEC S37.899 ☑
          contusion S37.892 ☑
          laceration S37.893 ☑
          specified type NEC S37.898 ☑
        type NEC S37.99 ☑
    specified NEC S39.83 ☑
  penis S39.94 ☑
  perineum S39.94 ☑
  peritoneum S36.81 ☑
    laceration S36.893 ☑
  periurethral tissue — *see* Injury, urethra
    complicating delivery O71.82
  phalanges
    foot — *see* Injury, foot
    hand — *see* Injury, hand
  pharynx NEC S19.85 ☑
  pleura — *see* Injury, intrathoracic, pleura
  plexus
    brachial — *see* Injury, brachial plexus
    cardiac — *see* Injury, nerve, thorax, sympathetic
    celiac, coeliac — *see* Injury, nerve, lumbosacral, sympathetic
    esophageal — *see* Injury, nerve, thorax, sympathetic
    hypogastric — *see* Injury, nerve, lumbosacral, sympathetic
    lumbar, lumbosacral — *see* Injury, lumbosacral plexus

**Injury** — *continued*
  plexus — *continued*
    mesenteric — *see* Injury, nerve, lumbosacral, sympathetic
    pulmonary — *see* Injury, nerve, thorax, sympathetic
  postcardiac surgery (syndrome) I97.0
  prepuce S39.94 ☑
  prostate S37.829 ☑
    contusion S37.822 ☑
    laceration S37.823 ☑
    specified type NEC S37.828 ☑
  pubic region S39.94 ☑
  pudendum S39.94 ☑
  pulmonary plexus — *see* Injury, nerve, thorax, sympathetic
  rectovaginal septum NEC S39.83 ☑
  rectum — *see* Injury, intestine, large, rectum
  retina — *see* Injury, eye, specified site NEC
    penetrating — *see* Injury, eyeball, penetrating
  retroperitoneal — *see* Injury, intra-abdominal, specified site NEC
  rotator cuff (muscle(s)) (tendon(s)) S46.00- ☑
    laceration S46.02- ☑
    specified type NEC S46.09- ☑
    strain S46.01- ☑
  round ligament — *see* Injury, pelvic organ, specified site NEC
  sacral plexus — *see* Injury, lumbosacral plexus
  salivary duct or gland S09.93 ☑
  scalp S09.90 ☑
    newborn (birth injury) P12.9
      due to monitoring (electrode) (sampling incision) P12.4
      specified NEC P12.89
        caput succedaneum P12.81
  scapular region — *see* Injury, shoulder
  sclera — *see* Injury, eye, specified site NEC
    penetrating — *see* Injury, eyeball, penetrating
  scrotum S39.94 ☑
  second cranial nerve (optic) — *see* Injury, nerve, optic
  seminal vesicle — *see* Injury, pelvic organ, specified site NEC
  seventh cranial nerve (facial) — *see* Injury, nerve, facial
  shoulder S49.9- ☑
    blood vessel — *see* Injury, blood vessel, arm
    contusion — *see* Contusion, shoulder
    dislocation — *see* Dislocation, shoulder
    fracture — *see* Fracture, shoulder
    muscle — *see* Injury, muscle, shoulder
    nerve — *see* Injury, nerve, shoulder
    open — *see* Wound, open, shoulder
    specified type NEC S49.8- ☑
    sprain — *see* Sprain, shoulder girdle
    superficial — *see* Injury, superficial, shoulder
  sinus
    cavernous — *see* Injury, intracranial
    nasal S09.92 ☑
  sixth cranial nerve (abducent) — *see* Injury, nerve, abducens
  skeleton, birth injury P13.9
    specified part NEC P13.8
  skin NEC T14.8 ☑
    surface intact — *see* Injury, superficial
  skull NEC S09.90 ☑
  specified NEC T14.8 ☑
  spermatic cord (pelvic region) S37.898 ☑
    scrotal region S39.848 ☑
  spinal (cord)
    cervical (neck) S14.109 ☑
      anterior cord syndrome S14.139 ☑
        C1 level S14.131 ☑
        C2 level S14.132 ☑
        C3 level S14.133 ☑
        C4 level S14.134 ☑
        C5 level S14.135 ☑
        C6 level S14.136 ☑
        C7 level S14.137 ☑
        C8 level S14.138 ☑
      Brown-Séquard syndrome S14.149 ☑
        C1 level S14.141 ☑
        C2 level S14.142 ☑
        C3 level S14.143 ☑
        C4 level S14.144 ☑
        C5 level S14.145 ☑
        C6 level S14.146 ☑

▽ **Subterms under main terms may continue to next column or page**     ☑ **Additional Character Required — Refer to the Tabular List for Character Selection**     **197**

Injury — Injury

☑ **Additional Character Required** — Refer to the Tabular List for Character Selection   ▽ **Subterms under main terms may continue to next column or page**

**Injury** — *continued*
  superficial — *continued*
    face NEC — *see* Injury, superficial, head, specified NEC
    finger(s) S60.949 ☑
      abrasion — *see* Abrasion, finger
      bite — *see* Bite, superficial, finger
      blister — *see* Blister, finger
      contusion — *see* Contusion, finger
      external constriction — *see* Constriction, external, finger
      foreign body — *see* Foreign body, superficial, finger
      index S60.94- ☑
      insect bite — *see* Bite, by site, superficial, insect
      little S60.94- ☑
      middle S60.94- ☑
      ring S60.94- ☑
    flank S30.92 ☑
    foot S90.92- ☑
      abrasion — *see* Abrasion, foot
      bite — *see* Bite, foot
      blister — *see* Blister, foot
      contusion — *see* Contusion, foot
      external constriction — *see* Constriction, external, foot
      foreign body — *see* Foreign body, superficial, foot
    forearm S50.91- ☑
      abrasion — *see* Abrasion, forearm
      bite — *see* Bite, forearm, superficial
      blister — *see* Blister, forearm
      contusion — *see* Contusion, forearm
      elbow only — *see* Injury, superficial, elbow
      external constriction — *see* Constriction, external, forearm
      foreign body — *see* Foreign body, superficial, forearm
    forehead — *see* Injury, superficial, head NEC
    foreign body — *see* Foreign body, superficial
    genital organs, external
      female S30.97 ☑
      male S30.96 ☑
    globe (eye) — *see* Injury, eye, specified site NEC
    groin S30.92 ☑
    gum — *see* Injury, superficial, oral cavity
    hand S60.92- ☑
      abrasion — *see* Abrasion, hand
      bite — *see* Bite, superficial, hand
      contusion — *see* Contusion, hand
      external constriction — *see* Constriction, external, hand
      foreign body — *see* Foreign body, superficial, hand
    head S00.90 ☑
      ear — *see* Injury, superficial, ear
      eyelid — *see* Injury, superficial, eyelid
      nose S00.30 ☑
      oral cavity S00.502 ☑
      scalp S00.00 ☑
      specified site NEC S00.80 ☑
    heel — *see* Injury, superficial, foot
    hip S70.91- ☑
      abrasion — *see* Abrasion, hip
      bite — *see* Bite, superficial, hip
      blister — *see* Blister, hip
      contusion — *see* Contusion, hip
      external constriction — *see* Constriction, external, hip
      foreign body — *see* Foreign body, superficial, hip
    iliac region — *see* Injury, superficial, abdomen
    inguinal region — *see* Injury, superficial, abdomen
    insect bite — *see* Bite, by site, superficial, insect
    interscapular region — *see* Injury, superficial, thorax, back
    jaw — *see* Injury, superficial, head, specified NEC
    knee S80.91- ☑
      abrasion — *see* Abrasion, knee
      bite — *see* Bite, superficial, knee
      blister — *see* Blister, knee
      contusion — *see* Contusion, knee
      external constriction — *see* Constriction, external, knee
      foreign body — *see* Foreign body, superficial, knee

**Injury** — *continued*
  superficial — *continued*
    labium (majus) (minus) S30.95 ☑
    lacrimal (apparatus) (gland) (sac) — *see* Injury, eye, specified site NEC
    larynx — *see* Injury, superficial, throat
    leg (lower) S80.92- ☑
      abrasion — *see* Abrasion, leg
      bite — *see* Bite, superficial, leg
      contusion — *see* Contusion, leg
      external constriction — *see* Constriction, external, leg
      foreign body — *see* Foreign body, superficial, leg
      knee — *see* Injury, superficial, knee
    limb NEC T14.8 ☑
    lip S00.501 ☑
    lower back S30.91 ☑
    lumbar region S30.91 ☑
    malar region — *see* Injury, superficial, head, specified NEC
    mammary — *see* Injury, superficial, breast
    mastoid region — *see* Injury, superficial, head, specified NEC
    mouth — *see* Injury, superficial, oral cavity
    muscle NEC T14.8 ☑
    nail NEC T14.8 ☑
      finger — *see* Injury, superficial, finger
      toe — *see* Injury, superficial, toe
    nasal (septum) — *see* Injury, superficial, nose
    neck S10.90 ☑
      specified site NEC S10.80 ☑
    nose (septum) S00.30 ☑
    occipital region — *see* Injury, superficial, scalp
    oral cavity S00.502 ☑
    orbital region — *see* Injury, superficial, periocular area
    palate — *see* Injury, superficial, oral cavity
    palm — *see* Injury, superficial, hand
    parietal region — *see* Injury, superficial, scalp
    pelvis S30.91 ☑
      girdle — *see* Injury, superficial, hip
    penis S30.93 ☑
    perineum
      female S30.95 ☑
      male S30.91 ☑
    periocular area S00.20- ☑
      abrasion — *see* Abrasion, eyelid
      bite — *see* Bite, superficial, eyelid
      contusion — *see* Contusion, eyelid
      external constriction — *see* Constriction, external, eyelid
      foreign body — *see* Foreign body, superficial, eyelid
    phalanges
      finger — *see* Injury, superficial, finger
      toe — *see* Injury, superficial, toe
    pharynx — *see* Injury, superficial, throat
    pinna — *see* Injury, superficial, ear
    popliteal space — *see* Injury, superficial, knee
    prepuce S30.93 ☑
    pubic region S30.91 ☑
    pudendum
      female S30.97 ☑
      male S30.96 ☑
    sacral region S30.91 ☑
    scalp S00.00 ☑
    scapular region — *see* Injury, superficial, shoulder
    sclera — *see* Injury, eye, specified site NEC
    scrotum S30.94 ☑
    shin — *see* Injury, superficial, leg
    shoulder S40.91- ☑
      abrasion — *see* Abrasion, shoulder
      bite — *see* Bite, superficial, shoulder
      blister — *see* Blister, shoulder
      contusion — *see* Contusion, shoulder
      external constriction — *see* Constriction, external, shoulder
      foreign body — *see* Foreign body, superficial, shoulder
    skin NEC T14.8 ☑
    sternal region — *see* Injury, superficial, thorax, front
    subconjunctival — *see* Injury, eye, specified site NEC
    subcutaneous NEC T14.8 ☑

**Injury** — *continued*
  superficial — *continued*
    submaxillary region — *see* Injury, superficial, head, specified NEC
    submental region — *see* Injury, superficial, head, specified NEC
    subungual
      finger(s) — *see* Injury, superficial, finger
      toe(s) — *see* Injury, superficial, toe
    supraclavicular fossa — *see* Injury, superficial, neck
    supraorbital — *see* Injury, superficial, head, specified NEC
    temple — *see* Injury, superficial, head, specified NEC
    temporal region — *see* Injury, superficial, head, specified NEC
    testis S30.94 ☑
    thigh S70.92- ☑
      abrasion — *see* Abrasion, thigh
      bite — *see* Bite, superficial, thigh
      blister — *see* Blister, thigh
      contusion — *see* Contusion, thigh
      external constriction — *see* Constriction, external, thigh
      foreign body — *see* Foreign body, superficial, thigh
    thorax, thoracic (wall) S20.90 ☑
      abrasion — *see* Abrasion, thorax
      back S20.40- ☑
      bite — *see* Bite, thorax, superficial
      blister — *see* Blister, thorax
      contusion — *see* Contusion, thorax
      external constriction — *see* Constriction, external, thorax
      foreign body — *see* Foreign body, superficial, thorax
      front S20.30- ☑
    throat S10.10 ☑
      abrasion S10.11 ☑
      bite S10.17 ☑
        insect S10.16 ☑
      blister S10.12 ☑
      contusion S10.0 ☑
      external constriction S10.14 ☑
      foreign body S10.15 ☑
    thumb S60.93- ☑
      abrasion — *see* Abrasion, thumb
      bite — *see* Bite, superficial, thumb
      blister — *see* Blister, thumb
      contusion — *see* Contusion, thumb
      external constriction — *see* Constriction, external, thumb
      foreign body — *see* Foreign body, superficial, thumb
      insect bite — *see* Bite, by site, superficial, insect
      specified type NEC S60.39 ☑
    toe(s) S90.93- ☑
      abrasion — *see* Abrasion, toe
      bite — *see* Bite, toe
      blister — *see* Blister, toe
      contusion — *see* Contusion, toe
      external constriction — *see* Constriction, external, toe
      foreign body — *see* Foreign body, superficial, toe
      great S90.93- ☑
    tongue — *see* Injury, superficial, oral cavity
    tooth, teeth — *see* Injury, superficial, oral cavity
    trachea S10.10 ☑
    tunica vaginalis S30.94 ☑
    tympanum, tympanic membrane — *see* Injury, superficial, ear
    uvula — *see* Injury, superficial, oral cavity
    vagina S30.95 ☑
    vocal cords — *see* Injury, superficial, throat
    vulva S30.95 ☑
    wrist S60.91- ☑
  supraclavicular region — *see* Injury, neck
  supraorbital S09.93 ☑
  suprarenal gland (multiple) — *see* Injury, adrenal
  surgical complication (external or internal site) — *see* Laceration, accidental complicating surgery
  temple S09.90 ☑
  temporal region S09.90 ☑
  tendon (*see also* Injury, muscle, by site)
    abdomen — *see* Injury, muscle, abdomen

⏷ Subterms under main terms may continue to next column or page      ☑ Additional Character Required — Refer to the Tabular List for Character Selection      199

Injury — Injury

**Injury** — *continued*
  tendon (*see also* Injury, muscle, by site) — *continued*
    Achilles — *see* Injury, Achilles tendon
    lower back — *see* Injury, muscle, lower back
    pelvic organs — *see* Injury, muscle, pelvis
    tenth cranial nerve (pneumogastric or vagus) — *see* Injury, nerve, vagus
  testis S39.94 ☑
  thigh S79.92- ☑
    blood vessel — *see* Injury, blood vessel, hip
    contusion — *see* Contusion, thigh
    fracture — *see* Fracture, femur
    muscle — *see* Injury, muscle, thigh
    nerve — *see* Injury, nerve, thigh
    open — *see* Wound, open, thigh
    specified NEC S79.82- ☑
    superficial — *see* Injury, superficial, thigh
  third cranial nerve (oculomotor) — *see* Injury, nerve, oculomotor
  thorax, thoracic S29.9 ☑
    blood vessel — *see* Injury, blood vessel, thorax
    cavity — *see* Injury, intrathoracic
    dislocation — *see* Dislocation, thorax
    external (wall) S29.9 ☑
      contusion — *see* Contusion, thorax
      nerve — *see* Injury, nerve, thorax
      open — *see* Wound, open, thorax
      specified NEC S29.8 ☑
      sprain — *see* Sprain, thorax
      superficial — *see* Injury, superficial, thorax
    fracture — *see* Fracture, thorax
    internal — *see* Injury, intrathoracic
    intrathoracic organ — *see* Injury, intrathoracic
    sympathetic ganglion — *see* Injury, nerve, thorax, sympathetic
  throat (*see also* Injury, neck) S19.9 ☑
  thumb S69.9- ☑
    blood vessel — *see* Injury, blood vessel, thumb
    contusion — *see* Contusion, thumb
    dislocation — *see* Dislocation, thumb
    fracture — *see* Fracture, thumb
    muscle — *see* Injury, muscle, thumb
    nerve — *see* Injury, nerve, digital, thumb
    open — *see* Wound, open, thumb
    specified NEC S69.8- ☑
    sprain — *see* Sprain, thumb
    superficial — *see* Injury, superficial, thumb
  thymus (gland) — *see* Injury, intrathoracic, specified organ NEC
  thyroid (gland) NEC S19.84 ☑
  toe S99.92- ☑
    contusion — *see* Contusion, toe
    dislocation — *see* Dislocation, toe
    fracture — *see* Fracture, toe
    muscle — *see* Injury, muscle, toe
    open — *see* Wound, open, toe
    specified type NEC S99.82- ☑
    sprain — *see* Sprain, toe
    superficial — *see* Injury, superficial, toe
  tongue S09.93 ☑
  tonsil S09.93 ☑
  tooth S09.93 ☑
  trachea (cervical) NEC S19.82 ☑
    thoracic — *see* Injury, intrathoracic, trachea, thoracic
  transfusion-related acute lung (TRALI) J95.84
  tunica vaginalis S39.94 ☑
  twelfth cranial nerve (hypoglossal) — *see* Injury, nerve, hypoglossal
  ureter S37.10 ☑
    contusion S37.12 ☑
    laceration S37.13 ☑
    specified type NEC S37.19 ☑
  urethra (sphincter) S37.30 ☑
    at delivery O71.5
    contusion S37.32 ☑
    laceration S37.33 ☑
    specified type NEC S37.39 ☑
  urinary organ S37.90 ☑
    contusion S37.92 ☑
    laceration S37.93 ☑
    specified
      site NEC S37.899 ☑
        contusion S37.892 ☑
        laceration S37.893 ☑

**Injury** — *continued*
  urinary organ — *continued*
    specified — *continued*
      site — *continued*
        specified type NEC S37.898 ☑
      type NEC S37.99 ☑
  uterus, uterine S37.60 ☑
    with ectopic or molar pregnancy O08.6
    blood vessel — *see* Injury, blood vessel, iliac
    contusion S37.62 ☑
    laceration S37.63 ☑
      cervix at delivery O71.3
    rupture associated with obstetrics — *see* Rupture, uterus
    specified type NEC S37.69 ☑
  uvula S09.93 ☑
  vagina S39.93 ☑
    abrasion S30.814 ☑
    bite S31.45 ☑
      insect S30.864 ☑
      superficial NEC S30.874 ☑
    contusion S30.23 ☑
    crush S38.03 ☑
    during delivery — *see* Laceration, vagina, during delivery
    external constriction S30.844 ☑
    insect bite S30.864 ☑
    laceration S31.41 ☑
      with foreign body S31.42 ☑
    open wound S31.40 ☑
    puncture S31.43 ☑
      with foreign body S31.44 ☑
    superficial S30.95 ☑
      foreign body S30.854 ☑
  vas deferens — *see* Injury, pelvic organ, specified site NEC
  vascular NEC T14.8 ☑
  vein — *see* Injury, blood vessel
  vena cava (superior) S25.20 ☑
    inferior S35.10 ☑
      laceration (minor) (superficial) S35.11 ☑
        major S35.12 ☑
      specified type NEC S35.19 ☑
    laceration (minor) (superficial) S25.21 ☑
      major S25.22 ☑
    specified type NEC S25.29 ☑
  vesical (sphincter) — *see* Injury, bladder
  visual cortex S04.04- ☑
  vitreous (humor) S05.90 ☑
    specified NEC S05.8X- ☑
  vocal cord NEC S19.83 ☑
  vulva S39.94 ☑
    abrasion S30.814 ☑
    bite S31.45 ☑
      insect S30.864 ☑
      superficial NEC S30.874 ☑
    contusion S30.23 ☑
    crush S38.03 ☑
    during delivery — *see* Laceration, perineum, female, during delivery
    external constriction S30.844 ☑
    insect bite S30.864 ☑
    laceration S31.41 ☑
      with foreign body S31.42 ☑
    open wound S31.40 ☑
    puncture S31.43 ☑
      with foreign body S31.44 ☑
    superficial S30.95 ☑
      foreign body S30.854 ☑
  whiplash (cervical spine) S13.4 ☑
  wrist S69.9- ☑
    blood vessel — *see* Injury, blood vessel, hand
    contusion — *see* Contusion, wrist
    dislocation — *see* Dislocation, wrist
    fracture — *see* Fracture, wrist
    muscle — *see* Injury, muscle, hand
    nerve — *see* Injury, nerve, hand
    open — *see* Wound, open, wrist
    specified NEC S69.8- ☑
    sprain — *see* Sprain, wrist
    superficial — *see* Injury, superficial, wrist
**Inoculation** (*see also* Vaccination)
  complication or reaction — *see* Complications, vaccination
**Insanity, insane** (*see also* Psychosis)
  adolescent — *see* Schizophrenia

**Insanity, insane** — *continued*
  confusional F28
    acute or subacute F05
  delusional F22
  senile F03 ☑
**Insect**
  bite — *see* Bite, by site, superficial, insect
  venomous, poisoning NEC (by) — *see* Venom, arthropod
**Insensitivity**
  adrenocorticotropin hormone (ACTH) E27.49
  androgen E34.50
    complete E34.51
    partial E34.52
**Insertion**
  cord (umbilical) lateral or velamentous O43.12- ☑
  intrauterine contraceptive device (encounter for) — *see* Intrauterine contraceptive device
**Insolation** (sunstroke) T67.0 ☑
**Insomnia** (organic) G47.00
  without objective findings F51.02
  adjustment F51.02
  adjustment disorder F51.02
  behavioral, of childhood Z73.819
    combined type Z73.812
    limit setting type Z73.811
    sleep-onset association type Z73.810
  childhood Z73.819
  chronic F51.04
    somatized tension F51.04
  conditioned F51.04
  due to
    alcohol
      abuse F10.182
      dependence F10.282
      use F10.982
    amphetamines
      abuse F15.182
      dependence F15.282
      use F15.982
    anxiety disorder F51.05
    caffeine
      abuse F15.182
      dependence F15.282
      use F15.982
    cocaine
      abuse F14.182
      dependence F14.282
      use F14.982
    depression F51.05
    drug NEC
      abuse F19.182
      dependence F19.282
      use F19.982
    medical condition G47.01
    mental disorder NEC F51.05
    opioid
      abuse F11.182
      dependence F11.282
      use F11.982
    psychoactive substance NEC
      abuse F19.182
      dependence F19.182
      use F19.982
    sedative, hypnotic, or anxiolytic
      abuse F13.182
      dependence F13.282
      use F13.982
    stimulant NEC
      abuse F15.182
      dependence F15.282
      use F15.982
  fatal familial (FFI) A81.83
  idiopathic F51.01
  learned F51.3
  nonorganic origin F51.01
  not due to a substance or known physiological condition F51.01
    specified NEC F51.09
  paradoxical F51.03
  primary F51.01
  psychiatric F51.05
  psychophysiologic F51.04
  related to psychopathology F51.05
  short-term F51.02
  specified NEC G47.09
  stress-related F51.02
  transient F51.02

☑ **Additional Character Required** — **Refer to the Tabular List for Character Selection**  ▽ **Subterms under main terms may continue to next column or page**

**Inspiration**
  food or foreign body — *see* Foreign body, by site
  mucus — *see* Asphyxia, mucus
**Inspissated bile syndrome** (newborn) P59.1
**Instability**
  emotional (excessive) F60.3
  joint (post-traumatic) M25.30
    ankle M25.37- ☑
    due to old ligament injury — *see* Disorder, ligament
    elbow M25.32- ☑
    flail — *see* Flail, joint
    foot M25.37- ☑
    hand M25.34- ☑
    hip M25.35- ☑
    knee M25.36- ☑
    lumbosacral — *see* subcategory M53.2 ☑
    prosthesis — *see* Complications, joint prosthesis, mechanical, displacement, by site
    sacroiliac — *see* subcategory M53.2 ☑
    secondary to
      old ligament injury — *see* Disorder, ligament
      removal of joint prosthesis M96.89
    shoulder (region) M25.31- ☑
    spine — *see* subcategory M53.2 ☑
    wrist M25.33- ☑
  knee (chronic) M23.5- ☑
  lumbosacral — *see* subcategory M53.2 ☑
  nervous F48.8
  personality (emotional) F60.3
  spine — *see* Instability, joint, spine
  vasomotor R55
**Institutional syndrome** (childhood) F94.2
**Institutionalization, affecting child** Z62.22
  disinhibited attachment F94.2
**Insufficiency, insufficient**
  accommodation, old age H52.4
  adrenal (gland) E27.40
    primary E27.1
  adrenocortical E27.40
    drug-induced E27.3
    iatrogenic E27.3
    primary E27.1
  anatomic crown height K08.89
  anterior (occlusal) guidance M26.54
  anus K62.89
  aortic (valve) I35.1
    with
      mitral (valve) disease I08.0
        with tricuspid (valve) disease I08.3
      stenosis I35.2
      tricuspid (valve) disease I08.2
        with mitral (valve) disease I08.3
    congenital Q23.1
    rheumatic I06.1
      with
        mitral (valve) disease I08.0
          with tricuspid (valve) disease I08.3
        stenosis I06.2
          with mitral (valve) disease I08.0
            with tricuspid (valve) disease I08.3
        tricuspid (valve) disease I08.2
          with mitral (valve) disease I08.3
    specified cause NEC I35.1
    syphilitic A52.03
  arterial I77.1
    basilar G45.0
    carotid (hemispheric) G45.1
    cerebral I67.81
    coronary (acute or subacute) I24.8
    mesenteric K55.1
    peripheral I73.9
    precerebral (multiple) (bilateral) G45.2
    vertebral G45.0
  arteriovenous I99.8
  biliary K83.8
  cardiac (*see also* Insufficiency, myocardial)
    due to presence of (cardiac) prosthesis I97.11- ☑
    postprocedural I97.11- ☑
  cardiorenal, hypertensive I13.2
  cardiovascular — *see* Disease, cardiovascular
  cerebrovascular (acute) I67.81
    with transient focal neurological signs and symptoms G45.8
  circulatory NEC I99.8
    newborn P29.89
  clinical crown length K08.89
  convergence H51.11

**Insufficiency, insufficient** — *continued*
  coronary (acute or subacute) I24.8
    chronic or with a stated duration of over 4 weeks I25.89
  corticoadrenal E27.40
    primary E27.1
  dietary E63.9
  divergence H51.8
  food T73.0 ☑
  gastroesophageal K22.8
  gonadal
    ovary E28.39
    testis E29.1
  heart (*see also* Insufficiency, myocardial)
    newborn P29.0
    valve — *see* Endocarditis
  hepatic — *see* Failure, hepatic
  idiopathic autonomic G90.09
  interocclusal distance of fully erupted teeth (ridge) M26.36
  kidney N28.9
    acute N28.9
    chronic N18.9
  lacrimal (secretion) H04.12- ☑
    passages — *see* Stenosis, lacrimal
  liver — *see* Failure, hepatic
  lung — *see* Insufficiency, pulmonary
  mental (congenital) — *see* Disability, intellectual
  mesenteric K55.1
  mitral (valve) I34.0
    with
      aortic valve disease I08.0
        with tricuspid (valve) disease I08.3
      obstruction or stenosis I05.2
        with aortic valve disease I08.0
      tricuspid (valve) disease I08.1
        with aortic (valve) disease I08.3
    congenital Q23.3
    rheumatic I05.1
      with
        aortic valve disease I08.0
          with tricuspid (valve) disease I08.3
        obstruction or stenosis I05.2
          with aortic valve disease I08.0
            with tricuspid (valve) disease I08.3
        tricuspid (valve) disease I08.1
          with aortic (valve) disease I08.3
      active or acute I01.1
        with chorea, rheumatic (Sydenham's) I02.0
    specified cause, except rheumatic I34.0
  muscle (*see also* Disease, muscle)
    heart — *see* Insufficiency, myocardial
    ocular NEC H50.9
  myocardial, myocardium (with arteriosclerosis) (*see also* Failure, heart) I50.9
    with
      rheumatic fever (conditions in I00) I09.0
        active, acute or subacute I01.2
          with chorea I02.0
        inactive or quiescent (with chorea) I09.0
    congenital Q24.8
    hypertensive — *see* Hypertension, heart
    newborn P29.0
    rheumatic I09.0
      active, acute, or subacute I01.2
    syphilitic A52.06
  nourishment T73.0 ☑
  pancreatic K86.89
    exocrine K86.81
  parathyroid (gland) E20.9
  peripheral vascular (arterial) I73.9
  pituitary E23.0
  placental (mother) O36.51- ☑
  platelets D69.6
  prenatal care affecting management of pregnancy O09.3- ☑
  progressive pluriglandular E31.0
  pulmonary J98.4
    acute, following surgery (nonthoracic) J95.2
      thoracic J95.1
    chronic, following surgery J95.3
    following
      shock J98.4
      trauma J98.4
    newborn P28.5
    valve I37.1
      with stenosis I37.2
      congenital Q22.2

**Insufficiency, insufficient** — *continued*
  pulmonary — *continued*
    valve — *continued*
      rheumatic I09.89
        with aortic, mitral or tricuspid (valve) disease I08.8
  pyloric K31.89
  renal (acute) N28.9
    chronic N18.9
  respiratory R06.89
    newborn P28.5
  rotation — *see* Malrotation
  sleep syndrome F51.12
  social insurance Z59.7
  suprarenal E27.40
    primary E27.1
  tarso-orbital fascia, congenital Q10.3
  testis E29.1
  thyroid (gland) (acquired) E03.9
    congenital E03.1
  tricuspid (valve) (rheumatic) I07.1
    with
      aortic (valve) disease I08.2
        with mitral (valve) disease I08.3
      mitral (valve) disease I08.1
        with aortic (valve) disease I08.3
      obstruction or stenosis I07.2
        with aortic (valve) disease I08.2
          with mitral (valve) disease I08.3
    congenital Q22.8
    nonrheumatic I36.1
      with stenosis I36.2
  urethral sphincter R32
  valve, valvular (heart) I38
    aortic — *see* Insufficiency, aortic (valve)
    congenital Q24.8
    mitral — *see* Insufficiency, mitral (valve)
    pulmonary — *see* Insufficiency, pulmonary, valve
    tricuspid — *see* Insufficiency, tricuspid (valve)
  vascular I99.8
    intestine K55.9
      acute (*see also* Ischemia, intestine, acute) K55.059
    mesenteric K55.1
    peripheral I73.9
    renal — *see* Hypertension, kidney
  velopharyngeal
    acquired K13.79
    congenital Q38.8
  venous (chronic) (peripheral) I87.2
  ventricular — *see* Insufficiency, myocardial
  welfare support Z59.7
**Insufflation, fallopian** Z31.41
**Insular** — *see* condition
**Insulinoma**
  pancreas
    benign D13.7
    malignant C25.4
    uncertain behavior D37.8
  specified site
    benign — *see* Neoplasm, by site, benign
    malignant — *see* Neoplasm, by site, malignant
    uncertain behavior — *see* Neoplasm, by site, uncertain behavior
  unspecified site
    benign D13.7
    malignant C25.4
    uncertain behavior D37.8
**Insuloma** — *see* Insulinoma
**Interference**
  balancing side M26.56
  non-working side M26.56
**Intermenstrual** — *see* condition
**Intermittent** — *see* condition
**Internal** — *see* condition
**Interrogation**
  cardiac defibrillator (automatic) (implantable) Z45.02
  cardiac pacemaker Z45.018
  cardiac (event) (loop) recorder Z45.09
  infusion pump (implanted) (intrathecal) Z45.1
  neurostimulator Z46.2
**Interruption**
  aortic arch Q25.21
  bundle of His I44.30
  phase-shift, sleep cycle — *see* Disorder, sleep, circadian rhythm
  sleep phase-shift, or 24 hour sleep-wake cycle — *see* Disorder, sleep, circadian rhythm

**Interstitial** — *see* condition
**Intertrigo** L30.4
  labialis K13.0
**Intervertebral disc** — *see* condition
**Intestine, intestinal** — *see* condition
**Intolerance**
  carbohydrate K90.49
  disaccharide, hereditary E73.0
  fat NEC K90.49
    pancreatic K90.3
  food K90.49
    dietary counseling and surveillance Z71.3
  fructose E74.10
    hereditary E74.12
  glucose (-galactose) E74.39
  gluten K90.41
  lactose E73.9
    specified NEC E73.8
  lysine E72.3
  milk NEC K90.49
    lactose E73.9
  protein K90.49
  starch NEC K90.49
  sucrose (-isomaltose) E74.31
**Intoxicated NEC** (without dependence) — *see* Alcohol, intoxication
**Intoxication**
  acid E87.2
  alcoholic (acute) (without dependence) — *see* Alcohol, intoxication
  alimentary canal K52.1
  amphetamine (without dependence) — *see* Abuse, drug, stimulant, with intoxication
    with dependence — *see* Dependence, drug, stimulant, with intoxication
  anxiolytic (acute) (without dependence) — *see* Abuse, drug, sedative, with intoxication
    with dependence — *see* Dependence, drug, sedative, with intoxication
  caffeine F15.929
    with dependence — *see* Dependence, drug, stimulant, with intoxication
  cannabinoids (acute) (without dependence) — *see* Use, cannabis, with intoxication
    with
      abuse — *see* Abuse, drug, cannabis, with intoxication
      dependence — *see* Dependence, drug, cannabis, with intoxication
  chemical — *see* Table of Drugs and Chemicals
    via placenta or breast milk — *see* - Absorption, chemical, through placenta
  cocaine (acute) (without dependence) — *see* Abuse, drug, cocaine, with intoxication
    with dependence — *see* Dependence, drug, cocaine, with intoxication
  drug
    acute (without dependence) — *see* Abuse, drug, by type with intoxication
      with dependence — *see* Dependence, drug, by type with intoxication
    addictive
      via placenta or breast milk — *see* Absorption, drug, addictive, through placenta
    newborn P93.8
      gray baby syndrome P93.0
    overdose or wrong substance given or taken — *see* Table of Drugs and Chemicals, by drug, poisoning
  enteric K52.1
  foodborne A05.9
    bacterial A05.9
    classical (Clostridium botulinum) A05.1
    due to
      Bacillus cereus A05.4
      bacterium A05.9
        specified NEC A05.8
      Clostridium
        botulinum A05.1
        perfringens A05.2
        welchii A05.2
      Salmonella A02.9
        with
          (gastro)enteritis A02.0
          localized infection(s) A02.20
            arthritis A02.23
            meningitis A02.21
            osteomyelitis A02.24

**Intoxication** — *continued*
  foodborne — *continued*
    due to — *continued*
      Salmonella — *continued*
        with — *continued*
          localized infection(s) — *continued*
            pneumonia A02.22
            pyelonephritis A02.25
            specified NEC A02.29
          sepsis A02.1
          specified manifestation NEC A02.8
        Staphylococcus A05.0
        Vibrio
          parahaemolyticus A05.3
          vulnificus A05.5
      enterotoxin, staphylococcal A05.0
      noxious — *see* Poisoning, food, noxious
  gastrointestinal K52.1
  hallucinogenic (without dependence) — *see* Abuse, drug, hallucinogen, with intoxication
    with dependence — *see* Dependence, drug, hallucinogen, with intoxication
  hypnotic (acute) (without dependence) — *see* Abuse, drug, sedative, with intoxication
    with dependence — *see* Dependence, drug, sedative, with intoxication
  inhalant (acute) (without dependence) — *see* Abuse, drug, inhalant, with intoxication
    with dependence — *see* Dependence, drug, inhalant, with intoxication
  meaning
    inebriation — *see* category F10 ☑
    poisoning — *see* Table of Drugs and Chemicals
  methyl alcohol (acute) (without dependence) — *see* Alcohol, intoxication
  opioid (acute) (without dependence) — *see* Abuse, drug, opioid, with intoxication
    with dependence — *see* Dependence, drug, opioid, with intoxication
  pathologic NEC (without dependence) — *see* Alcohol, intoxication
  phencyclidine (without dependence) — *see* Abuse, drug, hallucinogen, with intoxication
    with dependence — *see* Dependence, drug, hallucinogen, with intoxication
  potassium (K) E87.5
  psychoactive substance NEC (without dependence) — *see* Abuse, drug, psychoactive NEC, with intoxication
    with dependence — *see* Dependence, drug, psychoactive NEC, with intoxication
  sedative (acute) (without dependence) — *see* Abuse, drug, sedative, with intoxication
    with dependence — *see* Dependence, drug, sedative, with intoxication
  serum (*see also* Reaction, serum) T80.69 ☑
  uremic — *see* Uremia
  volatile solvents (acute) (without dependence) — *see* Abuse, drug, inhalant, with intoxication
    with dependence — *see* Dependence, drug, inhalant, with intoxication
  water E87.79
**Intraabdominal testis, testes**
  bilateral Q53.211
  unilateral Q53.111
**Intracranial** — *see* condition
**Intrahepatic gallbladder** Q44.1
**Intraligamentous** — *see* condition
**Intrathoracic** (*see also* condition)
  kidney Q63.2
**Intrauterine contraceptive device**
  checking Z30.431
  in situ Z97.5
  insertion Z30.430
    immediately following removal Z30.433
  management Z30.431
  reinsertion Z30.433
  removal Z30.432
  replacement Z30.433
  retention in pregnancy O26.3- ☑
**Intraventricular** — *see* condition
**Intrinsic deformity** — *see* Deformity
**Intubation, difficult or failed** T88.4 ☑
**Intumescence, lens** (eye) (cataract) — *see* Cataract
**Intussusception** (bowel) (colon) (enteric) (ileocecal) (ileocolic) (intestine) ( rectum) K56.1
  appendix K38.8
  congenital Q43.8

**Intussusception** — *continued*
  ureter (with obstruction) N13.5
**Invagination** (bowel, colon, intestine or rectum) K56.1
**Inversion**
  albumin-globulin (A-G) ratio E88.09
  bladder N32.89
  cecum — *see* Intussusception
  cervix N88.8
  chromosome in normal individual Q95.1
  circadian rhythm — *see* Disorder, sleep, circadian rhythm
  nipple N64.59
    congenital Q83.8
    gestational — *see* Retraction, nipple
    puerperal, postpartum — *see* Retraction, nipple
  nyctohemeral rhythm — *see* Disorder, sleep, circadian rhythm
  optic papilla Q14.2
  organ or site, congenital NEC — *see* Anomaly, by site
  sleep rhythm — *see* Disorder, sleep, circadian rhythm
  testis (congenital) Q55.29
  uterus (chronic) (postinfectional) (postpartal, old) N85.5
    postpartum O71.2
  vagina (posthysterectomy) N99.3
  ventricular Q20.5
**Investigation** (*see also* Examination) Z04.9
  clinical research subject (control) (normal comparison) (participant) Z00.6
**Involuntary movement, abnormal** R25.9
**Involution, involutional** (*see also* condition)
  breast, cystic — *see* Dysplasia, mammary, specified type NEC
  depression (single episode) F32.89
    recurrent episode F33.9
  melancholia (single episode) F32.89
    recurrent episode F33.8
  ovary, senile — *see* Atrophy, ovary
  thymus failure E32.8
**I.Q.**
  under 20 F73
  20-34 F72
  35-49 F71
  50-69 F70
**IRDS** (type I) P22.0
  type II P22.1
**Irideremia** Q13.1
**Iridis rubeosis** — *see* Disorder, iris, vascular
**Iridochoroiditis** (panuveitis) — *see* Panuveitis
**Iridocyclitis** H20.9
  acute H20.0- ☑
    hypopyon H20.05- ☑
    primary H20.01- ☑
    recurrent H20.02- ☑
    secondary (noninfectious) H20.04- ☑
      infectious H20.03- ☑
  chronic H20.1- ☑
  due to allergy — *see* Iridocyclitis, acute, secondary
  endogenous — *see* Iridocyclitis, acute, primary
  Fuchs' — *see* Cyclitis, Fuchs' heterochromic
  gonococcal A54.32
  granulomatous — *see* Iridocyclitis, chronic
  herpes, herpetic (simplex) B00.51
    zoster B02.32
  hypopyon — *see* Iridocyclitis, acute, hypopyon
  in (due to)
    ankylosing spondylitis M45.9
    gonococcal infection A54.32
    herpes (simplex) virus B00.51
      zoster B02.32
    infectious disease NOS B99
    parasitic disease NOS B89 [H22]
    sarcoidosis D86.83
    syphilis A51.43
    tuberculosis A18.54
    zoster B02.32
  lens-induced H20.2- ☑
  nongranulomatous — *see* Iridocyclitis, acute
  recurrent — *see* Iridocyclitis, acute, recurrent
  rheumatic — *see* Iridocyclitis, chronic
  subacute — *see* Iridocyclitis, acute
  sympathetic — *see* Uveitis, sympathetic
  syphilitic (secondary) A51.43
  tuberculous (chronic) A18.54
  Vogt-Koyanagi H20.82- ☑
**Iridocyclochoroiditis** (panuveitis) — *see* Panuveitis
**Iridodialysis** H21.53- ☑

☑ **Additional Character Required — Refer to the Tabular List for Character Selection**

🔻 **Subterms under main terms may continue to next column or page**

**Iridodonesis** H21.89
**Iridoplegia** (complete) (partial) (reflex) H57.09
**Iridoschisis** H21.25- ☑
**Iris** (*see also* condition)
  bombé — *see* Membrane, pupillary
**Iritis** (*see also* Iridocyclitis)
  chronic — *see* Iridocyclitis, chronic
  diabetic — *see* E08-E13 with .39
  due to
    herpes simplex B00.51
    leprosy A30.9 [H22]
  gonococcal A54.32
  gouty (*see also* Gout, by type) M10.9 [H22]
  granulomatous — *see* Iridocyclitis, chronic
  lens induced — *see* Iridocyclitis, lens-induced
  papulosa (syphilitic) A52.71
  rheumatic — *see* Iridocyclitis, chronic
  syphilitic (secondary) A51.43
    congenital (early) A50.01
    late A52.71
  tuberculous A18.54
**Iron** — *see* condition
**Iron-miner's lung** J63.4
**Irradiated enamel** (tooth, teeth) K03.89
**Irradiation effects, adverse** T66 ☑
**Irreducible, irreducibility** — *see* condition
**Irregular, irregularity**
  action, heart I49.9
  alveolar process K08.89
  bleeding N92.6
  breathing R06.89
  contour of cornea (acquired) — *see* Deformity, cornea
    congenital Q13.4
  contour, reconstructed breast N65.0
  dentin (in pulp) K04.3
  eye movements H55.89
    nystagmus — *see* Nystagmus
    saccadic H55.81
  labor O62.2
  menstruation (cause unknown) N92.6
  periods N92.6
  prostate N42.9
  pupil — *see* Abnormality, pupillary
  reconstructed breast N65.0
  respiratory R06.89
  septum (nasal) J34.2
  shape, organ or site, congenital NEC — *see* Distortion
  sleep-wake pattern (rhythm) G47.23
**Irritable, irritability** R45.4
  bladder N32.89
  bowel (syndrome) K58.9
    with
      constipation K58.1
      diarrhea K58.0
    mixed K58.2
    psychogenic F45.8
    specified NEC K58.8
  bronchial — *see* Bronchitis
  cerebral, in newborn P91.3
  colon (*see also* Irritable, bowel) K58.9
    with diarrhea K58.0
    psychogenic F45.8
  duodenum K59.8
  heart (psychogenic) F45.8
  hip — *see* Derangement, joint, specified type NEC, hip
  ileum K59.8
  infant R68.12
  jejunum K59.8
  rectum K59.8
  stomach K31.89
    psychogenic F45.8
  sympathetic G90.8
  urethra N36.8
**Irritation**
  anus K62.89
  axillary nerve G54.0
  bladder N32.89
  brachial plexus G54.0
  bronchial — *see* Bronchitis
  cervical plexus G54.2
  cervix — *see* Cervicitis
  choroid, sympathetic — *see* Endophthalmitis
  cranial nerve — *see* Disorder, nerve, cranial
  gastric K31.89
    psychogenic F45.8
  globe, sympathetic — *see* Uveitis, sympathetic
  labyrinth — *see* subcategory H83.2 ☑
  lumbosacral plexus G54.1

**Irritation** — *continued*
  meninges (traumatic) — *see* Injury, intracranial
    nontraumatic — *see* Meningismus
  nerve — *see* Disorder, nerve
  nervous R45.0
  penis N48.89
  perineum NEC L29.3
  peripheral autonomic nervous system G90.8
  peritoneum — *see* Peritonitis
  pharynx J39.2
  plantar nerve — *see* Lesion, nerve, plantar
  spinal (cord) (traumatic) (*see also* Injury, spinal cord, by region)
    nerve G58.9
      root NEC — *see* Radiculopathy
    nontraumatic — *see* Myelopathy
  stomach K31.89
    psychogenic F45.8
  sympathetic nerve NEC G90.8
  ulnar nerve — *see* Lesion, nerve, ulnar
  vagina N89.8
**Ischemia, ischemic** I99.8
  bowel (transient)
    acute (*see also* Ischemia, intestine, acute) K55.059
    chronic K55.1
    due to mesenteric artery insufficiency K55.1
  brain — *see* Ischemia, cerebral
  cardiac (see Disease, heart, ischemic)
  cardiomyopathy I25.5
  cerebral (chronic) (generalized) I67.82
    arteriosclerotic I67.2
    intermittent G45.9
    newborn P91.0
    recurrent focal G45.8
    transient G45.9
  colon chronic (due to mesenteric artery insufficiency) K55.1
  coronary — *see* Disease, heart, ischemic
  demand (coronary) (*see also* Angina) I24.8
    with myocardial infarction I21.A1
    resulting in myocardial infarction I21.A1
  heart (chronic or with a stated duration of over 4 weeks) I25.9
    acute or with a stated duration of 4 weeks or less I24.9
    subacute I24.9
  infarction, muscle — *see* Infarct, muscle
  intestine (large) (small) (transient) K55.9
    acute K55.059
      diffuse K55.052
      focal K55.051
      large K55.039
        diffuse K55.032
        focal K55.031
      small K55.019
        diffuse K55.012
        focal K55.011
    chronic K55.1
    due to mesenteric artery insufficiency K55.1
  kidney N28.0
  mesenteric, acute (*see also* Ischemia, intestine, acute) K55.059
  muscle, traumatic T79.6 ☑
  myocardium, myocardial (chronic or with a stated duration of over 4 weeks) I25.9
    acute, without myocardial infarction I51.3
    silent (asymptomatic) I25.6
    transient of newborn P29.4
  renal N28.0
  retina, retinal — *see* Occlusion, artery, retina
  small bowel
    acute K55.019
      diffuse K55.012
      focal K55.011
    chronic K55.1
    due to mesenteric artery insufficiency K55.1
  spinal cord G95.11
  subendocardial — *see* Insufficiency, coronary
  supply (coronary) (*see also* Angina) I25.9
    due to vasospasm I20.1
**Ischial spine** — *see* condition
**Ischialgia** — *see* Sciatica
**Ischiopagus** Q89.4
**Ischium, ischial** — *see* condition
**Ischuria** R34
**Iselin's disease or osteochondrosis** — *see* Osteochondrosis, juvenile, metatarsus

**Islands of**
  parotid tissue in
    lymph nodes Q38.6
    neck structures Q38.6
  submaxillary glands in
    fascia Q38.6
    lymph nodes Q38.6
    neck muscles Q38.6
**Islet cell tumor, pancreas** D13.7
**Isoimmunization NEC** (*see also* Incompatibility)
  affecting management of pregnancy (ABO) (with hydrops fetalis) O36.11-
    anti-A sensitization O36.11- ☑
    anti-B sensitization O36.19- ☑
    anti-c sensitization O36.09- ☑
    anti-C sensitization O36.09- ☑
    anti-e sensitization O36.09- ☑
    anti-E sensitization O36.09- ☑
    Rh NEC O36.09- ☑
      anti-D antibody O36.01- ☑
    specified NEC O36.19- ☑
  newborn P55.9
    with
      hydrops fetalis P56.0
      kernicterus P57.0
    ABO (blood groups) P55.1
    Rhesus (Rh) factor P55.0
    specified type NEC P55.8
**Isolation, isolated**
  dwelling Z59.8
  family Z63.79
  social Z60.4
**Isoleucinosis** E71.19
**Isomerism atrial appendages** (with asplenia or polysplenia) Q20.6
**Isosporiasis, isosporosis** A07.3
**Isovaleric acidemia** E71.110
**Issue of**
  medical certificate Z02.79
    for disability determination Z02.71
  repeat prescription (appliance) (glasses) (medicinal substance, medicament, medicine) Z76.0
    contraception — *see* Contraception
**Itch, itching** (*see also* Pruritus)
  baker's L23.6
  barber's B35.0
  bricklayer's L24.5
  cheese B88.0
  clam digger's B65.3
  coolie B76.9
  copra B88.0
  dew B76.9
  dhobi B35.6
  filarial — *see* Infestation, filarial
  grain B88.0
  grocer's B88.0
  ground B76.9
  harvest B88.0
  jock B35.6
  Malabar B35.5
    beard B35.0
    foot B35.3
    scalp B35.0
  meaning scabies B86
  Norwegian B86
  perianal L29.0
  poultrymen's B88.0
  sarcoptic B86
  scabies B86
  scrub B88.0
  straw B88.0
  swimmer's B65.3
  water B76.9
  winter L29.8
**Ivemark's syndrome** (asplenia with congenital heart disease) Q89.01
**Ivory bones** Q78.2
**Ixodiasis NEC** B88.8

# J

**Jaccoud's syndrome** — *see* Arthropathy, postrheumatic, chronic
**Jackson's**
  membrane Q43.3
  paralysis or syndrome G83.89
  veil Q43.3
**Jacquet's dermatitis** (diaper dermatitis) L22

**Jadassohn-Pellizari's disease or anetoderma** L90.2
**Jadassohn's**
blue nevus — *see* Nevus
intraepidermal epithelioma — *see* Neoplasm, skin, benign
**Jaffe-Lichtenstein** (-Uehlinger) **syndrome** — *see* Dysplasia, fibrous, bone NEC
**Jakob-Creutzfeldt disease or syndrome** — *see* Creutzfeldt-Jakob disease or syndrome
**Jaksch-Luzet disease** D64.89
**Jamaican**
neuropathy G92
paraplegic tropical ataxic-spastic syndrome G92
**Janet's disease** F48.8
**Janiceps** Q89.4
**Jansky-Bielschowsky amaurotic idiocy** E75.4
**Japanese**
B-type encephalitis A83.0
river fever A75.3
**Jaundice** (yellow) R17
acholuric (familial) (splenomegalic) (*see also* Spherocytosis)
acquired D59.8
breast-milk (inhibitor) P59.3
catarrhal (acute) B15.9
with hepatic coma B15.0
cholestatic (benign) R17
due to or associated with
delayed conjugation P59.8
associated with (due to) preterm delivery P59.0
preterm delivery P59.0
epidemic (catarrhal) B15.9
with hepatic coma B15.0
leptospiral A27.0
spirochetal A27.0
familial nonhemolytic (congenital) (Gilbert) E80.4
Crigler-Najjar E80.5
febrile (acute) B15.9
with hepatic coma B15.0
leptospiral A27.0
spirochetal A27.0
hematogenous D59.9
hemolytic (acquired) D59.9
congenital — *see* Spherocytosis
hemorrhagic (acute) (leptospiral) (spirochetal) A27.0
infectious (acute) (subacute) B15.9
with hepatic coma B15.0
leptospiral A27.0
spirochetal A27.0
leptospiral (hemorrhagic) A27.0
malignant (without coma) K72.90
with coma K72.91
neonatal — *see* Jaundice, newborn
newborn P59.9
due to or associated with
ABO
antibodies P55.1
incompatibility, maternal/fetal P55.1
isoimmunization P55.1
absence or deficiency of enzyme system for bilirubin conjugation (congenital) P59.8
bleeding P58.1
breast milk inhibitors to conjugation P59.3
associated with preterm delivery P59.0
bruising P58.0
Crigler-Najjar syndrome E80.5
delayed conjugation P59.8
associated with preterm delivery P59.0
drugs or toxins
given to newborn P58.42
transmitted from mother P58.41
excessive hemolysis P58.9
due to
bleeding P58.1
bruising P58.0
drugs or toxins
given to newborn P58.42
transmitted from mother P58.41
infection P58.2
polycythemia P58.3
swallowed maternal blood P58.5
specified type NEC P58.8
galactosemia E74.21
Gilbert syndrome E80.4
hemolytic disease P55.9
ABO isoimmunization P55.1
Rh isoimmunization P55.0
specified NEC P55.8

**Jaundice** — *continued*
newborn — *continued*
due to or associated with — *continued*
hepatocellular damage P59.20
specified NEC P59.29
hereditary hemolytic anemia P58.8
hypothyroidism, congenital E03.1
incompatibility, maternal/fetal NOS P55.9
infection P58.2
inspissated bile syndrome P59.1
isoimmunization NOS P55.9
mucoviscidosis E84.9
polycythemia P58.3
preterm delivery P59.0
Rh
antibodies P55.0
incompatibility, maternal/fetal P55.0
isoimmunization P55.0
specified cause NEC P59.8
swallowed maternal blood P58.5
spherocytosis (congenital) D58.0
nonhemolytic congenital familial (Gilbert) E80.4
nuclear, newborn (*see also* Kernicterus of newborn) P57.9
obstructive (*see also* Obstruction, bile duct) K83.1
post-immunization — *see* Hepatitis, viral, type, B
post-transfusion — *see* Hepatitis, viral, type, B
regurgitation (*see also* Obstruction, bile duct) K83.1
serum (homologous) (prophylactic) (therapeutic) — *see* Hepatitis, viral, type, B
spirochetal (hemorrhagic) A27.0
symptomatic R17
newborn P59.9
**Jaw** — *see* condition
**Jaw-winking phenomenon or syndrome** Q07.8
**Jealousy**
alcoholic F10.988
childhood F93.8
sibling F93.8
**Jejunitis** — *see* Enteritis
**Jejunostomy status** Z93.4
**Jejunum, jejunal** — *see* condition
**Jensen's disease** — *see* Inflammation, chorioretinal, focal, juxtapapillary
**Jerks, myoclonic** G25.3
**Jervell-Lange-Nielsen syndrome** I45.81
**Jeune's disease** Q77.2
**Jigger disease** B88.1
**Job's syndrome** (chronic granulomatous disease) D71
**Joint** (*see also* condition)
mice — *see* Loose, body, joint
knee M23.4- ☑
**Jordan's anomaly or syndrome** D72.0
**Joseph-Diamond-Blackfan anemia** (congenital hypoplastic) D61.01
**Jungle yellow fever** A95.0
**Jüngling's disease** — *see* Sarcoidosis
**Juvenile** — *see* condition

# K

**Kahler's disease** C90.0- ☑
**Kakke** E51.11
**Kala-azar** B55.0
**Kallmann's syndrome** E23.0
**Kanner's syndrome** (autism) — *see* Psychosis, childhood
**Kaposi's**
dermatosis (xeroderma pigmentosum) Q82.1
lichen ruber L44.0
acuminatus L44.0
sarcoma
colon C46.4
connective tissue C46.1
gastrointestinal organ C46.4
lung C46.5- ☑
lymph node (multiple) C46.3
palate (hard) (soft) C46.2
rectum C46.4
skin (multiple sites) C46.0
specified site NEC C46.7
stomach C46.4
unspecified site C46.9
varicelliform eruption B00.0
vaccinia T88.1 ☑
**Kartagener's syndrome or triad** (sinusitis, bronchiectasis, situs inversus) Q89.3

**Karyotype**
with abnormality except iso (Xq) Q96.2
45,X Q96.0
46,X
iso (Xq) Q96.1
46,XX Q98.3
with streak gonads Q50.32
hermaphrodite (true) Q99.1
male Q98.3
46,XY
with streak gonads Q56.1
female Q97.3
hermaphrodite (true) Q99.1
47,XXX Q97.0
47,XXY Q98.0
47,XYY Q98.5
**Kaschin-Beck disease** — *see* Disease, Kaschin-Beck
**Katayama's disease or fever** B65.2
**Kawasaki's syndrome** M30.3
**Kayser-Fleischer ring** (cornea) (pseudosclerosis) H18.04- ☑
**Kaznelson's syndrome** (congenital hypoplastic anemia) D61.01
**Kearns-Sayre syndrome** H49.81- ☑
**Kedani fever** A75.3
**Kelis** L91.0
**Kelly** (-Patterson) **syndrome** (sideropenic dysphagia) D50.1
**Keloid, cheloid** L91.0
acne L73.0
Addison's L94.0
cornea — *see* Opacity, cornea
Hawkin's L91.0
scar L91.0
**Keloma** L91.0
**Kenya fever** A77.1
**Keratectasia** (*see also* Ectasia, cornea)
congenital Q13.4
**Keratinization of alveolar ridge mucosa**
excessive K13.23
minimal K13.22
**Keratinized residual ridge mucosa**
excessive K13.23
minimal K13.22
**Keratitis** (nodular) (nonulcerative) (simple) (zonular) H16.9
with ulceration (central) (marginal) (perforated) (ring) — *see* Ulcer, cornea
actinic — *see* Photokeratitis
arborescens (herpes simplex) B00.52
areolar H16.11- ☑
bullosa H16.8
deep H16.309
specified type NEC H16.399
dendritic (a) (herpes simplex) B00.52
disciform (is) (herpes simplex) B00.52
varicella B01.81
filamentary H16.12- ☑
gonococcal (congenital or prenatal) A54.33
herpes, herpetic (simplex) B00.52
zoster B02.33
in (due to)
acanthamebiasis B60.13
adenovirus B30.0
exanthema (*see also* Exanthem) B09
herpes (simplex) virus B00.52
measles B05.81
syphilis A50.31
tuberculosis A18.52
zoster B02.33
interstitial (nonsyphilitic) H16.30- ☑
diffuse H16.32- ☑
herpes, herpetic (simplex) B00.52
zoster B02.33
sclerosing H16.33- ☑
specified type NEC H16.39- ☑
syphilitic (congenital) (late) A50.31
tuberculous A18.52
macular H16.11- ☑
nummular H16.11- ☑
oyster shuckers' H16.8
parenchymatous — *see* Keratitis, interstitial
petrificans H16.8
postmeasles B05.81
punctata
leprosa A30.9 [H16.14-] ☑
syphilitic (profunda) A50.31
punctate H16.14- ☑

**Keratitis** — *continued*
  purulent H16.8
  rosacea L71.8
  sclerosing H16.33- ☑
  specified type NEC H16.8
  stellate H16.11- ☑
  striate H16.11- ☑
  superficial H16.10- ☑
    with conjunctivitis — *see* Keratoconjunctivitis
    due to light — *see* Photokeratitis
  suppurative H16.8
  syphilitic (congenital) (prenatal) A50.31
  trachomatous A71.1
    sequelae B94.0
  tuberculous A18.52
  vesicular H16.8
  xerotic (*see also* Keratomalacia) H16.8
    vitamin A deficiency E50.4
**Keratoacanthoma** L85.8
**Keratocele** — *see* Descemetocele
**Keratoconjunctivitis** H16.20- ☑
  Acanthamoeba B60.13
  adenoviral B30.0
  epidemic B30.0
  exposure H16.21- ☑
  herpes, herpetic (simplex) B00.52
    zoster B02.33
  in exanthema (*see also* Exanthem) B09
  infectious B30.0
  lagophthalmic — *see* Keratoconjunctivitis, specified
    type NEC
  neurotrophic H16.23- ☑
  phlyctenular H16.25- ☑
  postmeasles B05.81
  shipyard B30.0
  sicca (Sjogren's) M35.0- ☑
    not Sjogren's H16.22- ☑
  specified type NEC H16.29- ☑
  tuberculous (phlyctenular) A18.52
  vernal H16.26- ☑
**Keratoconus** H18.60- ☑
  congenital Q13.4
  stable H18.61- ☑
  unstable H18.62- ☑
**Keratocyst** (dental) (odontogenic) — *see* Cyst, calcifying
  odontogenic
**Keratoderma, keratodermia** (congenital) (palmaris et
  plantaris) (symmetrical) Q82.8
  acquired L85.1
    in diseases classified elsewhere L86
  climactericum L85.1
  gonococcal A54.89
  gonorrheal A54.89
  punctata L85.2
  Reiter's — *see* Reiter's disease
**Keratodermatocele** — *see* Descemetocele
**Keratoglobus** H18.79 ☑
  congenital Q15.8
    with glaucoma Q15.0
**Keratohemia** — *see* Pigmentation, cornea, stromal
**Keratoiritis** (*see also* Iridocyclitis)
  syphilitic A50.39
  tuberculous A18.54
**Keratoma** L57.0
  palmaris and plantaris hereditarium Q82.8
  senile L57.0
**Keratomalacia** H18.44- ☑
  vitamin A deficiency E50.4
**Keratomegaly** Q13.4
**Keratomycosis** B49
  nigrans, nigricans (palmaris) B36.1
**Keratopathy** H18.9
  band H18.42- ☑
  bullous (aphakic), following cataract surgery
    H59.01- ☑
  bullous H18.1- ☑
**Keratoscleritis, tuberculous** A18.52
**Keratosis** L57.0
  actinic L57.0
  arsenical L85.8
  congenital, specified NEC Q80.8
  female genital NEC N94.89
  follicularis Q82.8
    acquired L11.0
    congenita Q82.8
    et parafollicularis in cutem penetrans L87.0
    spinulosa (decalvans) Q82.8

**Keratosis** — *continued*
  follicularis — *continued*
    vitamin A deficiency E50.8
  gonococcal A54.89
  male genital (external) N50.89
  nigricans L83
  obturans, external ear (canal) — *see* Cholesteatoma,
    external ear
  palmaris et plantaris (inherited) (symmetrical) Q82.8
    acquired L85.1
  penile N48.89
  pharynx J39.2
  pilaris, acquired L85.8
  punctata (palmaris et plantaris) L85.2
  scrotal N50.89
  seborrheic L82.1
    inflamed L82.0
  senile L57.0
  solar L57.0
  tonsillaris J35.8
  vagina N89.4
  vegetans Q82.8
  vitamin A deficiency E50.8
  vocal cord J38.3
**Kerato-uveitis** — *see* Iridocyclitis
**Kerion** (celsi) B35.0
**Kernicterus of newborn** (not due to isoimmunization)
  P57.9
  due to isoimmunization (conditions in P55.0-P55.9)
    P57.0
  specified type NEC P57.8
**Kerunoparalysis** T75.09 ☑
**Keshan disease** E59
**Ketoacidosis** E87.2
  diabetic — *see* Diabetes, by type, with ketoacidosis
**Ketonuria** R82.4
**Ketosis NEC** E88.89
  diabetic — *see* Diabetes, by type, with with ketoacido-
    sis
**Kew Garden fever** A79.1
**Kidney** — *see* condition
**Kienböck's disease** (*see also* Osteochondrosis, juvenile,
  hand, carpal lunate)
  adult M93.1
**Kimmelstiel** (-Wilson) **disease** — *see* Diabetes, Kimmelstiel (-Wilson) disease
**Kink, kinking**
  artery I77.1
  hair (acquired) L67.8
  ileum or intestine — *see* Obstruction, intestine
  Lane's — *see* Obstruction, intestine
  organ or site, congenital NEC — *see* Anomaly, by site
  ureter (pelvic junction) N13.5
    with
      hydronephrosis N13.1
        with infection N13.6
      pyelonephritis (chronic) N11.1
    congenital Q62.39
  vein(s) I87.8
    caval I87.1
    peripheral I87.1
**Kinnier Wilson's disease** (hepatolenticular degeneration) E83.01
**Kissing spine** M48.20
  cervical region M48.22
  cervicothoracic region M48.23
  lumbar region M48.26
  lumbosacral region M48.27
  occipito-atlanto-axial region M48.21
  thoracic region M48.24
  thoracolumbar region M48.25
**Klatskin's tumor** C22.1
**Klauder's disease** A26.8
**Klebs' disease** (*see also* Glomerulonephritis) N05- ☑
**Klebsiella** (K.) **pneumoniae, as cause of disease**
  **classified elsewhere** B96.1
**Klein** (e)-**Levin syndrome** G47.13
**Kleptomania** F63.2
**Klinefelter's syndrome** Q98.4
  karyotype 47,XXY Q98.0
  male with more than two X chromosomes Q98.1
**Klippel-Feil deficiency, disease, or syndrome** (brevi-
  collis) Q76.1
**Klippel's disease** I67.2
**Klippel-Trenaunay** (-Weber) **syndrome** Q87.2
**Klumpke** (-Déjerine) **palsy, paralysis** (birth) (newborn)
  P14.1
**Knee** — *see* condition

**Knock knee** (acquired) M21.06- ☑
  congenital Q74.1
**Knot**(s)
  intestinal, syndrome (volvulus) K56.2
  surfer S89.8- ☑
  umbilical cord (true) O69.2 ☑
**Knotting** (of)
  hair L67.8
  intestine K56.2
**Knuckle pad** (Garrod's) M72.1
**Koch's**
  infection — *see* Tuberculosis
  relapsing fever A68.9
**Koch-Weeks' conjunctivitis** — *see* Conjunctivitis, acute,
  mucopurulent
**Köebner's syndrome** Q81.8
**Köenig's disease** (osteochondritis dissecans) — *see* Osteochondritis, dissecans
**Köhler-Pellegrini-Steida disease or syndrome** (calcification, knee joint) — *see* Bursitis, tibial collateral
**Köhler's disease**
  patellar — *see* Osteochondrosis, juvenile, patella
  tarsal navicular — *see* Osteochondrosis, juvenile, tarsus
**Koilonychia** L60.3
  congenital Q84.6
**Kojevnikov's, epilepsy** — *see* Kozhevnikof's epilepsy
**Koplik's spots** B05.9
**Kopp's asthma** E32.8
**Korsakoff's** (Wernicke) **disease, psychosis or syn-**
  **drome** (alcoholic) F10.96
  with dependence F10.26
  drug-induced
    due to drug abuse — *see* Abuse, drug, by type,
      with amnestic disorder
    due to drug dependence — *see* Dependence, drug,
      by type, with amnestic disorder
  nonalcoholic F04
**Korsakov's disease, psychosis or syndrome** — *see*
  Korsakoff's disease
**Korsakow's disease, psychosis or syndrome** — *see*
  Korsakoff's disease
**Kostmann's disease or syndrome** (infantile genetic
  agranulocytosis) — *see* Agranulocytosis
**Kozhevnikof's epilepsy** G40.109
  intractable G40.119
    with status epilepticus G40.111
    without status epilepticus G40.119
  not intractable G40.109
    with status epilepticus G40.101
    without status epilepticus G40.109
**Krabbe's**
  disease E75.23
  syndrome, congenital muscle hypoplasia Q79.8
**Kraepelin-Morel disease** — *see* Schizophrenia
**Kraft-Weber-Dimitri disease** Q85.8
**Kraurosis**
  ani K62.89
  penis N48.0
  vagina N89.8
  vulva N90.4
**Kreotoxism** A05.9
**Krukenberg's**
  spindle — *see* Pigmentation, cornea, posterior
  tumor C79.6- ☑
**Kufs' disease** E75.4
**Kugelberg-Welander disease** G12.1
**Kuhnt-Junius degeneration** (*see also* Degeneration,
  macula) H35.32- ☑
**Kümmell's disease or spondylitis** — *see* Spondylopa-
  thy, traumatic
**Kupffer cell sarcoma** C22.3
**Kuru** A81.81
**Kussmaul's**
  disease M30.0
  respiration E87.2
    in diabetic acidosis — *see* Diabetes, by type, with
      ketoacidosis
**Kwashiorkor** E40
  marasmic, marasmus type E42
**Kyasanur Forest disease** A98.2
**Kyphoscoliosis, kyphoscoliotic** (acquired) (*see also*
  Scoliosis) M41.9
  congenital Q67.5
  heart (disease) I27.1
  sequelae of rickets E64.3
  tuberculous A18.01
**Kyphosis, kyphotic** (acquired) M40.209

---

**Kyphosis, kyphotic** — *continued*
cervical region M40.202
cervicothoracic region M40.203
congenital Q76.419
cervical region Q76.412
cervicothoracic region Q76.413
occipito-atlanto-axial region Q76.411
thoracic region Q76.414
thoracolumbar region Q76.415
Morquio-Brailsford type (spinal) (*see also* subcategory M49.8) E76.219
postlaminectomy M96.3
postradiation therapy M96.2
postural (adolescent) M40.00
cervicothoracic region M40.03
thoracic region M40.04
thoracolumbar region M40.05
secondary NEC M40.10
cervical region M40.12
cervicothoracic region M40.13
thoracic region M40.14
thoracolumbar region M40.15
sequelae of rickets E64.3
specified type NEC M40.299
cervical region M40.292
cervicothoracic region M40.293
thoracic region M40.294
thoracolumbar region M40.295
syphilitic, congenital A50.56
thoracic region M40.204
thoracolumbar region M40.205
tuberculous A18.01
**Kyrle disease** L87.0

# L

**Labia, labium** — *see* condition
**Labile**
blood pressure R09.89
vasomotor system I73.9
**Labioglossal paralysis** G12.29
**Labium leporinum** — *see* Cleft, lip
**Labor** — *see* Delivery
**Labored breathing** — *see* Hyperventilation
**Labyrinthitis** (circumscribed) (destructive) (diffuse) (inner ear) (latent) (purulent) (suppurative) (*see also* subcategory) H83.0 ☑
syphilitic A52.79
**Laceration**
with abortion — *see* Abortion, by type, complicated by laceration of pelvic organs
abdomen, abdominal
wall S31.119 ☑
with
foreign body S31.129 ☑
penetration into peritoneal cavity S31.619 ☑
with foreign body S31.629 ☑
epigastric region S31.112 ☑
with
foreign body S31.122 ☑
penetration into peritoneal cavity S31.612 ☑
with foreign body S31.622 ☑
left
lower quadrant S31.114 ☑
with
foreign body S31.124 ☑
penetration into peritoneal cavity S31.614 ☑
with foreign body S31.624 ☑
upper quadrant S31.111 ☑
with
foreign body S31.121 ☑
penetration into peritoneal cavity S31.611 ☑
with foreign body S31.621 ☑
periumbilic region S31.115 ☑
with
foreign body S31.125 ☑
penetration into peritoneal cavity S31.615 ☑
with foreign body S31.625 ☑
right
lower quadrant S31.113 ☑
with
foreign body S31.123 ☑

**Laceration** — *continued*
abdomen, abdominal — *continued*
wall — *continued*
right — *continued*
lower quadrant — *continued*
with — *continued*
penetration into peritoneal cavity S31.613 ☑
with foreign body S31.623 ☑
upper quadrant S31.110 ☑
with
foreign body S31.120 ☑
penetration into peritoneal cavity S31.610 ☑
with foreign body S31.620 ☑
accidental, complicating surgery — *see* Complications, surgical, accidental puncture or laceration
Achilles tendon S86.02- ☑
adrenal gland S37.813 ☑
alveolar (process) — *see* Laceration, oral cavity
ankle S91.01- ☑
with
foreign body S91.02- ☑
antecubital space — *see* Laceration, elbow
anus (sphincter) S31.831 ☑
with
ectopic or molar pregnancy O08.6
foreign body S31.832 ☑
complicating delivery — *see* Delivery, complicated, by, laceration, anus (sphincter)
following ectopic or molar pregnancy O08.6
nontraumatic, nonpuerperal — *see* Fissure, anus
arm (upper) S41.11- ☑
with foreign body S41.12- ☑
lower — *see* Laceration, forearm
auditory canal (external) (meatus) — *see* Laceration, ear
auricle, ear — *see* Laceration, ear
axilla — *see* Laceration, arm
back (*see also* Laceration, thorax, back)
lower S31.010 ☑
with
foreign body S31.020 ☑
with penetration into retroperitoneal space S31.021 ☑
penetration into retroperitoneal space S31.011 ☑
bile duct S36.13 ☑
bladder S37.23 ☑
with ectopic or molar pregnancy O08.6
following ectopic or molar pregnancy O08.6
obstetrical trauma O71.5
blood vessel — *see* Injury, blood vessel
bowel (*see also* Laceration, intestine)
with ectopic or molar pregnancy O08.6
complicating abortion — *see* Abortion, by type, complicated by, specified condition NEC
following ectopic or molar pregnancy O08.6
obstetrical trauma O71.5
brain (any part) (cortex) (diffuse) (membrane) (*see also* Injury, intracranial, diffuse)
during birth P10.8
with hemorrhage P10.1
focal — *see* Injury, intracranial, focal brain injury
brainstem S06.38- ☑
breast S21.01- ☑
with foreign body S21.02- ☑
broad ligament S37.893 ☑
with ectopic or molar pregnancy O08.6
following ectopic or molar pregnancy O08.6
laceration syndrome N83.8
obstetrical trauma O71.6
syndrome (laceration) N83.8
buttock S31.801 ☑
with foreign body S31.802 ☑
left S31.821 ☑
with foreign body S31.822 ☑
right S31.811 ☑
with foreign body S31.812 ☑
calf — *see* Laceration, leg
canaliculus lacrimalis — *see* Laceration, eyelid
canthus, eye — *see* Laceration, eyelid
capsule, joint — *see* Sprain
causing eversion of cervix uteri (old) N86
central (perineal), complicating delivery O70.9
cerebellum, traumatic S06.37- ☑
cerebral S06.33- ☑

**Laceration** — *continued*
cerebral — *continued*
during birth P10.8
with hemorrhage P10.1
left side S06.32- ☑
right side S06.31- ☑
cervix (uteri)
with ectopic or molar pregnancy O08.6
following ectopic or molar pregnancy O08.6
nonpuerperal, nontraumatic N88.1
obstetrical trauma (current) O71.3
old (postpartal) N88.1
traumatic S37.63 ☑
cheek (external) S01.41- ☑
with foreign body S01.42- ☑
internal — *see* Laceration, oral cavity
chest wall — *see* Laceration, thorax
chin — *see* Laceration, head, specified site NEC
chordae tendinae NEC I51.1
concurrent with acute myocardial infarction — *see* Infarct, myocardium
following acute myocardial infarction (current complication) I23.4
clitoris — *see* Laceration, vulva
colon — *see* Laceration, intestine, large, colon
common bile duct S36.13 ☑
cortex (cerebral) — *see* Injury, intracranial, diffuse
costal region — *see* Laceration, thorax
cystic duct S36.13 ☑
diaphragm S27.803 ☑
digit(s)
foot — *see* Laceration, toe
hand — *see* Laceration, finger
duodenum S36.430 ☑
ear (canal) (external) S01.31- ☑
with foreign body S01.32- ☑
drum S09.2- ☑
elbow S51.01- ☑
with
foreign body S51.02- ☑
epididymis — *see* Laceration, testis
epigastric region — *see* Laceration, abdomen, wall, epigastric region
esophagus K22.8
traumatic
cervical S11.21 ☑
with foreign body S11.22 ☑
thoracic S27.813 ☑
eye (ball) S05.3- ☑
with prolapse or loss of intraocular tissue S05.2- ☑
penetrating S05.6- ☑
eyebrow — *see* Laceration, eyelid
eyelid S01.11- ☑
with foreign body S01.12- ☑
face NEC — *see* Laceration, head, specified site NEC
fallopian tube S37.539 ☑
bilateral S37.532 ☑
unilateral S37.531 ☑
finger(s) S61.219 ☑
with
damage to nail S61.319 ☑
with
foreign body S61.329 ☑
foreign body S61.229 ☑
index S61.218 ☑
with
damage to nail S61.318 ☑
with
foreign body S61.328 ☑
foreign body S61.228 ☑
left S61.211 ☑
with
damage to nail S61.311 ☑
with
foreign body S61.321 ☑
foreign body S61.221 ☑
right S61.210 ☑
with
damage to nail S61.310 ☑
with
foreign body S61.320 ☑
foreign body S61.220 ☑
little S61.218 ☑
with
damage to nail S61.318 ☑
with
foreign body S61.328 ☑

**Laceration** — *continued*
  finger(s) — *continued*
    little — *continued*
      with — *continued*
        foreign body S61.228 ☑
      left S61.217 ☑
        with
          damage to nail S61.317 ☑
            with
              foreign body S61.327 ☑
          foreign body S61.227 ☑
      right S61.216 ☑
        with
          damage to nail S61.316 ☑
            with
              foreign body S61.326 ☑
          foreign body S61.226 ☑
    middle S61.218 ☑
      with
        damage to nail S61.318 ☑
          with
            foreign body S61.328 ☑
        foreign body S61.228 ☑
      left S61.213 ☑
        with
          damage to nail S61.313 ☑
            with
              foreign body S61.323 ☑
          foreign body S61.223 ☑
      right S61.212 ☑
        with
          damage to nail S61.312 ☑
            with
              foreign body S61.322 ☑
          foreign body S61.222 ☑
    ring S61.218 ☑
      with
        damage to nail S61.318 ☑
          with
            foreign body S61.328 ☑
        foreign body S61.228 ☑
      left S61.215 ☑
        with
          damage to nail S61.315 ☑
            with
              foreign body S61.325 ☑
          foreign body S61.225 ☑
      right S61.214 ☑
        with
          damage to nail S61.314 ☑
            with
              foreign body S61.324 ☑
          foreign body S61.224 ☑
  flank S31.119 ☑
    with foreign body S31.129 ☑
  foot (except toe(s) alone) S91.319 ☑
    with foreign body S91.329 ☑
    left S91.312 ☑
      with foreign body S91.322 ☑
    right S91.311 ☑
      with foreign body S91.321 ☑
    toe — *see* Laceration, toe
  forearm S51.819 ☑
    with
      foreign body S51.829 ☑
    elbow only — *see* Laceration, elbow
    left S51.812 ☑
      with
        foreign body S51.822 ☑
    right S51.811 ☑
      with
        foreign body S51.821 ☑
  forehead S01.81 ☑
    with foreign body S01.82 ☑
  fourchette O70.0
    with ectopic or molar pregnancy O08.6
    complicating delivery O70.0
    following ectopic or molar pregnancy O08.6
  gallbladder S36.123 ☑
  genital organs, external
    female S31.512 ☑
      with foreign body S31.522 ☑
      vagina — *see* Laceration, vagina
      vulva — *see* Laceration, vulva
    male S31.511 ☑
      with foreign body S31.521 ☑

**Laceration** — *continued*
  genital organs, external — *continued*
    male — *continued*
      penis — *see* Laceration, penis
      scrotum — *see* Laceration, scrotum
      testis — *see* Laceration, testis
  groin — *see* Laceration, abdomen, wall
  gum — *see* Laceration, oral cavity
  hand S61.419 ☑
    with
      foreign body S61.429 ☑
    finger — *see* Laceration, finger
    left S61.412 ☑
      with
        foreign body S61.422 ☑
    right S61.411 ☑
      with
        foreign body S61.421 ☑
    thumb — *see* Laceration, thumb
  head S01.91 ☑
    with foreign body S01.92 ☑
    cheek — *see* Laceration, cheek
    ear — *see* Laceration, ear
    eyelid — *see* Laceration, eyelid
    lip — *see* Laceration, lip
    nose — *see* Laceration, nose
    oral cavity — *see* Laceration, oral cavity
    scalp S01.01 ☑
      with foreign body S01.02 ☑
    specified site NEC S01.81 ☑
      with foreign body S01.82 ☑
    temporomandibular area — *see* Laceration, cheek
  heart — *see* Injury, heart, laceration
  heel — *see* Laceration, foot
  hepatic duct S36.13 ☑
  hip S71.019 ☑
    with foreign body S71.029 ☑
    left S71.012 ☑
      with foreign body S71.022 ☑
    right S71.011 ☑
      with foreign body S71.021 ☑
  hymen — *see* Laceration, vagina
  hypochondrium — *see* Laceration, abdomen, wall
  hypogastric region — *see* Laceration, abdomen, wall
  ileum S36.438 ☑
  inguinal region — *see* Laceration, abdomen, wall
  instep — *see* Laceration, foot
  internal organ — *see* Injury, by site
  interscapular region — *see* Laceration, thorax, back
  intestine
    large
      colon S36.539 ☑
        ascending S36.530 ☑
        descending S36.532 ☑
        sigmoid S36.533 ☑
        specified site NEC S36.538 ☑
      rectum S36.63 ☑
      transverse S36.531 ☑
    small S36.439 ☑
      duodenum S36.430 ☑
      specified site NEC S36.438 ☑
  intra-abdominal organ S36.93 ☑
    intestine — *see* Laceration, intestine
    liver — *see* Laceration, liver
    pancreas — *see* Laceration, pancreas
    peritoneum S36.81 ☑
    specified site NEC S36.893 ☑
    spleen — *see* Laceration, spleen
    stomach — *see* Laceration, stomach
  intracranial NEC (*see also* Injury, intracranial, diffuse)
    birth injury P10.9
  jaw — *see* Laceration, head, specified site NEC
  jejunum S36.438 ☑
  joint capsule — *see* Sprain, by site
  kidney S37.03- ☑
    major (greater than 3 cm) (massive) (stellate) S37.06- ☑
    minor (less than 1 cm) S37.04- ☑
    moderate (1 to 3 cm) S37.05- ☑
      multiple S37.06- ☑
  knee S81.01- ☑
    with foreign body S81.02- ☑
  labium (majus) (minus) — *see* Laceration, vulva
  lacrimal duct — *see* Laceration, eyelid
  large intestine — *see* Laceration, intestine, large
  larynx S11.011 ☑

**Laceration** — *continued*
  larynx — *continued*
    with foreign body S11.012 ☑
  leg (lower) S81.819 ☑
    with foreign body S81.829 ☑
    foot — *see* Laceration, foot
    knee — *see* Laceration, knee
    left S81.812 ☑
      with foreign body S81.822 ☑
    right S81.811 ☑
      with foreign body S81.821 ☑
    upper — *see* Laceration, thigh
  ligament — *see* Sprain
  lip S01.511 ☑
    with foreign body S01.521 ☑
  liver S36.113 ☑
    major (stellate) S36.116 ☑
    minor S36.114 ☑
    moderate S36.115 ☑
  loin — *see* Laceration, abdomen, wall
  lower back — *see* Laceration, back, lower
  lumbar region — *see* Laceration, back, lower
  lung S27.339 ☑
    bilateral S27.332 ☑
    unilateral S27.331 ☑
  malar region — *see* Laceration, head, specified site NEC
  mammary — *see* Laceration, breast
  mastoid region — *see* Laceration, head, specified site NEC
  meninges — *see* Injury, intracranial, diffuse
  meniscus — *see* Tear, meniscus
  mesentery S36.893 ☑
  mesosalpinx S37.893 ☑
  mouth — *see* Laceration, oral cavity
  muscle — *see* Injury, muscle, by site, laceration
  nail
    finger — *see* Laceration, finger, with damage to nail
    toe — *see* Laceration, toe, with damage to nail
  nasal (septum) (sinus) — *see* Laceration, nose
  nasopharynx — *see* Laceration, head, specified site NEC
  neck S11.91 ☑
    with foreign body S11.92 ☑
    involving
      cervical esophagus S11.21 ☑
        with foreign body S11.22 ☑
      larynx — *see* Laceration, larynx
      pharynx — *see* Laceration, pharynx
      thyroid gland — *see* Laceration, thyroid gland
      trachea — *see* Laceration, trachea
    specified site NEC S11.81 ☑
      with foreign body S11.82 ☑
  nerve — *see* Injury, nerve
  nose (septum) (sinus) S01.21 ☑
    with foreign body S01.22 ☑
  ocular NOS S05.3- ☑
    adnexa NOS S01.11- ☑
  oral cavity S01.512 ☑
    with foreign body S01.522 ☑
  orbit (eye) — *see* Wound, open, ocular, orbit
  ovary S37.439 ☑
    bilateral S37.432 ☑
    unilateral S37.431 ☑
  palate — *see* Laceration, oral cavity
  palm — *see* Laceration, hand
  pancreas S36.239 ☑
  pelvic S31.010 ☑
    with
      foreign body S31.020 ☑
        penetration into retroperitoneal cavity S31.021 ☑
      penetration into retroperitoneal cavity S31.011 ☑
    floor (*see also* Laceration, back, lower)
      with ectopic or molar pregnancy O08.6
      complicating delivery O70.1
      following ectopic or molar pregnancy O08.6
      old (postpartal) N81.89
    organ S37.93 ☑
  penis S31.21 ☑
    with foreign body S31.22 ☑
  perineum
    female S31.41 ☑

⏃ Subterms under main terms may continue to next column or page     ☑ Additional Character Required — Refer to the Tabular List for Character Selection     207

Laceration — Laceration

**Laceration** — *continued*
  perineum — *continued*
    female — *continued*
      with
        ectopic or molar pregnancy O08.6
        foreign body S31.42 ☑
      during delivery O70.9
        first degree O70.0
        fourth degree O70.3
        second degree O70.1
        third degree (*see also* Delivery, complicated, by, laceration, perineum, third degree) O70.20
      old (postpartal) N81.89
      postpartal N81.89
      secondary (postpartal) O90.1
    male S31.119 ☑
      with foreign body S31.129 ☑
  periocular area (with or without lacrimal passages) — *see* Laceration, eyelid
  peritoneum S36.893 ☑
  periumbilic region — *see* Laceration, abdomen, wall, periumbilic
  periurethral tissue — *see* Laceration, urethra
  phalanges
    finger — *see* Laceration, finger
    toe — *see* Laceration, toe
  pharynx S11.21 ☑
    with foreign body S11.22 ☑
  pinna — *see* Laceration, ear
  popliteal space — *see* Laceration, knee
  prepuce — *see* Laceration, penis
  prostate S37.823 ☑
  pubic region S31.119 ☑
    with foreign body S31.129 ☑
  pudendum — *see* Laceration, genital organs, external
  rectovaginal septum — *see* Laceration, vagina
  rectum S36.63 ☑
  retroperitoneum S36.893 ☑
  round ligament S37.893 ☑
  sacral region — *see* Laceration, back, lower
  sacroiliac region — *see* Laceration, back, lower
  salivary gland — *see* Laceration, oral cavity
  scalp S01.01 ☑
    with foreign body S01.02 ☑
  scapular region — *see* Laceration, shoulder
  scrotum S31.31 ☑
    with foreign body S31.32 ☑
  seminal vesicle S37.893 ☑
  shin — *see* Laceration, leg
  shoulder S41.019 ☑
    with foreign body S41.029 ☑
    left S41.012 ☑
      with foreign body S41.022 ☑
    right S41.011 ☑
      with foreign body S41.021 ☑
  small intestine — *see* Laceration, intestine, small
  spermatic cord — *see* Laceration, testis
  spinal cord (meninges) (*see also* Injury, spinal cord, by region)
    due to injury at birth P11.5
    newborn (birth injury) P11.5
  spleen S36.039 ☑
    major (massive) (stellate) S36.032 ☑
    moderate S36.031 ☑
    superficial (minor) S36.030 ☑
  sternal region — *see* Laceration, thorax, front
  stomach S36.33 ☑
  submaxillary region — *see* Laceration, head, specified site NEC
  submental region — *see* Laceration, head, specified site NEC
  subungual
    finger(s) — *see* Laceration, finger, with damage to nail
    toe(s) — *see* Laceration, toe, with damage to nail
  suprarenal gland — *see* Laceration, adrenal gland
  temple, temporal region — *see* Laceration, head, specified site NEC
  temporomandibular area — *see* Laceration, cheek
  tendon — *see* Injury, muscle, by site, laceration
    Achilles S86.02- ☑
  tentorium cerebelli — *see* Injury, intracranial, diffuse
  testis S31.31 ☑
    with foreign body S31.32 ☑
  thigh S71.11- ☑
    with foreign body S71.12- ☑

**Laceration** — *continued*
  thorax, thoracic (wall) S21.91 ☑
    with foreign body S21.92 ☑
    back S21.22- ☑
      with penetration into thoracic cavity S21.42- ☑
    front S21.12- ☑
      with penetration into thoracic cavity S21.32- ☑
    back S21.21- ☑
      with
        foreign body S21.22- ☑
          with penetration into thoracic cavity S21.42- ☑
        penetration into thoracic cavity S21.41- ☑
    breast — *see* Laceration, breast
    front S21.11- ☑
      with
        foreign body S21.12- ☑
          with penetration into thoracic cavity S21.32- ☑
        penetration into thoracic cavity S21.31- ☑
  thumb S61.019 ☑
    with
      damage to nail S61.119 ☑
        with
          foreign body S61.129 ☑
      foreign body S61.029 ☑
    left S61.012 ☑
      with
        damage to nail S61.112 ☑
          with
            foreign body S61.122 ☑
        foreign body S61.022 ☑
    right S61.011 ☑
      with
        damage to nail S61.111 ☑
          with
            foreign body S61.121 ☑
        foreign body S61.021 ☑
  thyroid gland S11.11 ☑
    with foreign body S11.12 ☑
  toe(s) S91.119 ☑
    with
      damage to nail S91.219 ☑
        with
          foreign body S91.229 ☑
      foreign body S91.129 ☑
    great S91.113 ☑
      with
        damage to nail S91.213 ☑
          with
            foreign body S91.223 ☑
        foreign body S91.123 ☑
      left S91.112 ☑
        with
          damage to nail S91.212 ☑
            with
              foreign body S91.222 ☑
          foreign body S91.122 ☑
      right S91.111 ☑
        with
          damage to nail S91.211 ☑
            with
              foreign body S91.221 ☑
          foreign body S91.121 ☑
    lesser S91.116 ☑
      with
        damage to nail S91.216 ☑
          with
            foreign body S91.226 ☑
        foreign body S91.126 ☑
      left S91.115 ☑
        with
          damage to nail S91.215 ☑
            with
              foreign body S91.225 ☑
          foreign body S91.125 ☑
      right S91.114 ☑
        with
          damage to nail S91.214 ☑
            with
              foreign body S91.224 ☑
          foreign body S91.124 ☑
  tongue — *see* Laceration, oral cavity
  trachea S11.021 ☑

**Laceration** — *continued*
  trachea — *continued*
    with foreign body S11.022 ☑
  tunica vaginalis — *see* Laceration, testis
  tympanum, tympanic membrane — *see* Laceration, ear, drum
  umbilical region S31.115 ☑
    with foreign body S31.125 ☑
  ureter S37.13 ☑
  urethra S37.33 ☑
    with or following ectopic or molar pregnancy O08.6
    obstetrical trauma O71.5
  urinary organ NEC S37.893 ☑
  uterus S37.63 ☑
    with ectopic or molar pregnancy O08.6
    following ectopic or molar pregnancy O08.6
    nonpuerperal, nontraumatic N85.8
    obstetrical trauma NEC O71.81
    old (postpartal) N85.8
  uvula — *see* Laceration, oral cavity
  vagina S31.41 ☑
    with
      ectopic or molar pregnancy O08.6
      foreign body S31.42 ☑
    during delivery O71.4
      with perineal laceration — *see* Laceration, perineum, female, during delivery
    following ectopic or molar pregnancy O08.6
    nonpuerperal, nontraumatic N89.8
    old (postpartal) N89.8
  vas deferens S37.893 ☑
  vesical — *see* Laceration, bladder
  vocal cords S11.031 ☑
    with foreign body S11.032 ☑
  vulva S31.41 ☑
    with
      ectopic or molar pregnancy O08.6
      foreign body S31.42 ☑
    complicating delivery O70.0
    following ectopic or molar pregnancy O08.6
    nonpuerperal, nontraumatic N90.89
    old (postpartal) N90.89
  wrist S61.519 ☑
    with
      foreign body S61.529 ☑
    left S61.512 ☑
      with
        foreign body S61.522 ☑
    right S61.511 ☑
      with
        foreign body S61.521 ☑

**Lack of**
  achievement in school Z55.3
  adequate
    food Z59.4
    intermaxillary vertical dimension of fully erupted teeth M26.36
    sleep Z72.820
  appetite (see Anorexia) R63.0
  awareness R41.9
  care
    in home Z74.2
    of infant (at or after birth) T76.02 ☑
      confirmed T74.02 ☑
  cognitive functions R41.9
  coordination R27.9
    ataxia R27.0
    specified type NEC R27.8
  development (physiological) R62.50
    failure to thrive (child over 28 days old) R62.51
      adult R62.7
      newborn P92.6
    short stature R62.52
    specified type NEC R62.59
  energy R53.83
  financial resources Z59.6
  food T73.0 ☑
  growth R62.52
  heating Z59.1
  housing (permanent) (temporary) Z59.0
    adequate Z59.1
  learning experiences in childhood Z62.898
  leisure time (affecting life-style) Z73.2
  material resources Z59.9
  memory (*see also* Amnesia)
    mild, following organic brain damage F06.8
  ovulation N97.0
  parental supervision or control of child Z62.0

**Lack of** — *continued*
person able to render necessary care Z74.2
physical exercise Z72.3
play experience in childhood Z62.898
posterior occlusal support Z73.2
relaxation (affecting life-style) Z73.2
sexual
desire F52.0
enjoyment F52.1
shelter Z59.0
sleep (adequate) Z72.820
supervision of child by parent Z62.0
support, posterior occlusal M26.57
water T73.1 ☑
**Lacrimal** — *see* condition
**Lacrimation, abnormal** — *see* Epiphora
**Lacrimonasal duct** — *see* condition
**Lactation, lactating** (breast) (puerperal, postpartum)
associated
cracked nipple O92.13
retracted nipple O92.03
defective O92.4
disorder NEC O92.79
excessive O92.6
failed (complete) O92.3
partial O92.4
mastitis NEC — *see* Mastitis, obstetric
mother (care and/or examination) Z39.1
nonpuerperal N64.3
**Lacticemia, excessive** E87.2
**Lacunar skull** Q75.8
**Laennec's cirrhosis** K70.30
with ascites K70.31
nonalcoholic K74.69
**Lafora's disease** — *see* Epilepsy, generalized, idiopathic
**Lag, lid** (nervous) — *see* Retraction, lid
**Lagophthalmos** (eyelid) (nervous) H02.209
cicatricial H02.219
left H02.216
lower H02.215
upper H02.214
right H02.213
lower H02.212
upper H02.211
keratoconjunctivitis — *see* Keratoconjunctivitis
left H02.206
lower H02.205
upper H02.204
mechanical H02.229
left H02.226
lower H02.225
upper H02.224
right H02.223
lower H02.222
upper H02.221
paralytic H02.239
left H02.236
lower H02.235
upper H02.234
right H02.233
lower H02.232
upper H02.231
right H02.203
lower H02.202
upper H02.201
**Laki-Lorand factor deficiency** — *see* Defect, coagulation, specified type NEC
**Lalling** F80.0
**Lambert-Eaton syndrome** — *see* Syndrome, Lambert-Eaton
**Lambliasis, lambliosis** A07.1
**Landau-Kleffner syndrome** — *see* Epilepsy, specified NEC
**Landouzy-Déjérine dystrophy or facioscapulohumeral atrophy** G71.0
**Landouzy's disease** (icterohemorrhagic leptospirosis) A27.0
**Landry-Guillain-Barré, syndrome or paralysis** G61.0
**Landry's disease or paralysis** G61.0
**Lane's**
band Q43.3
kink — *see* Obstruction, intestine
syndrome K90.2
**Langdon Down syndrome** — *see* Trisomy, 21
**Lapsed immunization schedule status** Z28.3
**Large**
baby (regardless of gestational age) (4000g to 4499g) P08.1

**Large** — *continued*
ear, congenital Q17.1
physiological cup Q14.2
stature R68.89
**Large-for-dates NEC** (infant) (4000g to 4499g) P08.1
affecting management of pregnancy O36.6- ☑
exceptionally (4500g or more) P08.0
**Larsen-Johansson disease orosteochondrosis** — *see* Osteochondrosis, juvenile, patella
**Larsen's syndrome** (flattened facies and multiple congenital dislocations) Q74.8
**Larva migrans**
cutaneous B76.9
Ancylostoma B76.0
visceral B83.0
**Laryngeal** — *see* condition
**Laryngismus** (stridulus) J38.5
congenital P28.89
diphtheritic A36.2
**Laryngitis** (acute) (edematous) (fibrinous) (infective) (infiltrative) (malignant) (membranous) (phlegmonous) (pneumococcal) (pseudomembranous) (septic) (subglottic) (suppurative) (ulcerative) J04.0
with
influenza, flu, or grippe — *see* Influenza, with, laryngitis
tracheitis (acute) — *see* Laryngotracheitis
atrophic J37.0
catarrhal J37.0
chronic J37.0
with tracheitis (chronic) J37.1
diphtheritic A36.2
due to external agent — *see* Inflammation, respiratory, upper, due to
H. influenzae J04.0
Hemophilus influenzae J04.0
hypertrophic J37.0
influenzal — *see* Influenza, with, respiratory manifestations NEC
obstructive J05.0
sicca J37.0
spasmodic J05.0
acute J04.0
streptococcal J04.0
stridulous J05.0
syphilitic (late) A52.73
congenital A50.59 [J99]
early A50.03 [J99]
tuberculous A15.5
Vincent's A69.1
**Laryngocele** (congenital) (ventricular) Q31.3
**Laryngofissure** J38.7
congenital Q31.8
**Laryngomalacia** (congenital) Q31.5
**Laryngopharyngitis** (acute) J06.0
chronic J37.0
due to external agent — *see* Inflammation, respiratory, upper, due to
**Laryngoplegia** J38.00
bilateral J38.02
unilateral J38.01
**Laryngoptosis** J38.7
**Laryngospasm** J38.5
**Laryngostenosis** J38.6
**Laryngotracheitis** (acute) (Infectional) (infective) (viral) J04.2
atrophic J37.1
catarrhal J37.1
chronic J37.1
diphtheritic A36.2
due to external agent — *see* Inflammation, respiratory, upper, due to
Hemophilus influenzae J04.2
hypertrophic J37.1
influenzal — *see* Influenza, with, respiratory manifestations NEC
pachydermic J38.7
sicca J37.1
spasmodic J38.5
acute J05.0
streptococcal J04.2
stridulous J38.5
syphilitic (late) A52.73
congenital A50.59 [J99]
early A50.03 [J99]
tuberculous A15.5
Vincent's A69.1
**Laryngotracheobronchitis** — *see* Bronchitis

**Larynx, laryngeal** — *see* condition
**Lassa fever** A96.2
**Lassitude** — *see* Weakness
**Late**
talker R62.0
walker R62.0
**Late effect**(s) — *see* Sequelae
**Latent** — *see* condition
**Laterocession** — *see* Lateroversion
**Lateroflexion** — *see* Lateroversion
**Lateroversion**
cervix — *see* Lateroversion, uterus
uterus, uterine (cervix) (postinfectional) (postpartal, old) N85.4
congenital Q51.818
in pregnancy or childbirth O34.59- ☑
**Lathyrism** — *see* Poisoning, food, noxious, plant
**Launois' syndrome** (pituitary gigantism) E22.0
**Launois-Bensaude adenolipomatosis** E88.89
**Laurence-Moon** (-Bardet)-**Biedl syndrome** Q87.89
**Lax, laxity** (*see also* Relaxation)
ligament (ous) (*see also* Disorder, ligament)
familial M35.7
knee — *see* Derangement, knee
skin (acquired) L57.4
congenital Q82.8
**Laxative habit** F55.2
**Lazy leukocyte syndrome** D70.8
**Lead miner's lung** J63.6
**Leak, leakage**
air NEC J93.82
postprocedural J95.812
amniotic fluid — *see* Rupture, membranes, premature
blood (microscopic), fetal, into maternal circulation
affecting management of pregnancy — *see* Pregnancy, complicated by
cerebrospinal fluid G96.0
from spinal (lumbar) puncture G97.0
device, implant or graft (*see also* Complications, by site and type, mechanical)
arterial graft NEC — *see* Complication, cardiovascular device, mechanical, vascular
breast (implant) T85.43 ☑
catheter NEC T85.638 ☑
dialysis (renal) T82.43 ☑
intraperitoneal T85.631 ☑
infusion NEC T82.534 ☑
spinal (epidural) (subdural) T85.630 ☑
urinary T83.038 ☑
cystostomy T83.030 ☑
Hopkins T83.038 ☑
ileostomy T83.038 ☑
indwelling T83.031 ☑
nephrostomy T83.032 ☑
specified T83.038 ☑
urostomy T83.038 ☑
gastrointestinal — *see* Complications, prosthetic device, mechanical, gastrointestinal device
genital NEC T83.498 ☑
penile prosthesis (cylinder) (implanted) (pump) (reservoir) T83.490 ☑
testicular prosthesis T83.491 ☑
heart NEC — *see* Complication, cardiovascular device, mechanical
joint prosthesis — *see* Complications, joint prosthesis, mechanical, specified NEC, by site
ocular NEC — *see* Complications, prosthetic device, mechanical, ocular device
orthopedic NEC — *see* Complication, orthopedic, device, mechanical
persistent air J93.82
specified NEC T85.638 ☑
urinary NEC (*see also* Complication, genitourinary, device, urinary, mechanical)
graft T83.23 ☑
vascular NEC — *see* Complication, cardiovascular device, mechanical
ventricular intracranial shunt T85.03 ☑
urine — *see* Incontinence
**Leaky heart** — *see* Endocarditis
**Learning defect** (specific) F81.9
**Leather bottle stomach** C16.9
**Leber's**
congenital amaurosis H35.50
optic atrophy (hereditary) H47.22
**Lederer's anemia** D59.1
**Leeches** (external) — *see* Hirudiniasis

---

▽ Subterms under main terms may continue to next column or page | ☑ Additional Character Required — Refer to the Tabular List for Character Selection | **209**

**Leg** — see condition
**Legg** (-Calvé)-**Perthes disease, syndrome or osteochondrosis** M91.1- ☑
**Legionellosis** A48.1
 nonpneumonic A48.2
**Legionnaires'**
 disease A48.1
  nonpneumonic A48.2
 pneumonia A48.1
**Leigh's disease** G31.82
**Leiner's disease** L21.1
**Leiofibromyoma** — see Leiomyoma
**Leiomyoblastoma** — see Neoplasm, connective tissue,
 benign
**Leiomyofibroma** (see also Neoplasm, connective tissue,
 benign)
 uterus (cervix) (corpus) D25.9
**Leiomyoma** (see also Neoplasm, connective tissue, benign)
 bizarre — see Neoplasm, connective tissue, benign
 cellular — see Neoplasm, connective tissue, benign
 epithelioid — see Neoplasm, connective tissue, benign
 uterus (cervix) (corpus) D25.9
  intramural D25.1
  submucous D25.0
  subserosal D25.2
 vascular — see Neoplasm, connective tissue, benign
**Leiomyoma, leiomyomatosis** (intravascular) — see
 Neoplasm, connective tissue, uncertain behavior
**Leiomyosarcoma** (see also Neoplasm, connective tissue,
 malignant)
 epithelioid — see Neoplasm, connective tissue, malignant
 myxoid — see Neoplasm, connective tissue, malignant
**Leishmaniasis** B55.9
 American (mucocutaneous) B55.2
  cutaneous B55.1
 Asian Desert B55.1
 Brazilian B55.2
 cutaneous (any type) B55.1
 dermal (see also Leishmaniasis, cutaneous)
  post-kala-azar B55.0
 eyelid B55.1
 infantile B55.0
 Mediterranean B55.0
 mucocutaneous (American) (New World) B55.2
 naso-oral B55.2
 nasopharyngeal B55.2
 old world B55.1
 tegumentaria diffusa B55.1
 visceral B55.0
**Leishmanoid, dermal** (see also Leishmaniasis, cutaneous)
 post-kala-azar B55.0
**Lenegre's disease** I44.2
**Lengthening, leg** — see Deformity, limb, unequal length
**Lennert's lymphoma** — see Lymphoma, Lennert's
**Lennox-Gastaut syndrome** G40.812
 intractable G40.814
  with status epilepticus G40.813
  without status epilepticus G40.814
 not intractable G40.812
  with status epilepticus G40.811
  without status epilepticus G40.812
**Lens** — see condition
**Lenticonus** (anterior) (posterior) (congenital) Q12.8
**Lenticular degeneration, progressive** E83.01
**Lentiglobus** (posterior) (congenital) Q12.8
**Lentigo** (congenital) L81.4
 maligna (see also Melanoma, in situ)
  melanoma — see Melanoma
**Lentivirus, as cause of disease classified elsewhere**
 B97.31
**Leontiasis**
 ossium M85.2
 syphilitic (late) A52.78
  congenital A50.59
**Lepothrix** A48.8
**Lepra** — see Leprosy
**Leprechaunism** E34.8
**Leprosy** A30.- ☑
 with muscle disorder A30.9 [M63.80]
  ankle A30.9 [M63.87-] ☑
  foot A30.9 [M63.87-] ☑
  forearm A30.9 [M63.83-] ☑
  hand A30.9 [M63.84-] ☑
  lower leg A30.9 [M63.86-] ☑

**Leprosy** — continued
 with muscle disorder — continued
  multiple sites A30.9 [M63.89]
  pelvic region A30.9 [M63.85-] ☑
  shoulder region A30.9 [M63.81-] ☑
  specified site NEC A30.9 [M63.88]
  thigh A30.9 [M63.85-] ☑
  upper arm A30.9 [M63.82-] ☑
 anesthetic A30.9
 BB A30.3
 BL A30.4
 borderline (infiltrated) (neuritic) A30.3
  lepromatous A30.4
  tuberculoid A30.2
 BT A30.2
 dimorphous (infiltrated) (neuritic) A30.3
 I A30.0
 indeterminate (macular) (neuritic) A30.0
 lepromatous (diffuse) (infiltrated) (macular) (neuritic)
  (nodular) A30.5
 LL A30.5
 macular (early) (neuritic) (simple) A30.9
 maculoanesthetic A30.9
 mixed A30.3
 neural A30.9
 nodular A30.5
 primary neuritic A30.3
 specified type NEC A30.8
 TT A30.1
 tuberculoid (major) (minor) A30.1
**Leptocytosis, hereditary** D56.9
**Leptomeningitis** (chronic) (circumscribed) (hemorrhagic)
 (nonsuppurative) — see Meningitis
**Leptomeningopathy** G96.19
**Leptospiral** — see condition
**Leptospirochetal** — see condition
**Leptospirosis** A27.9
 canicola A27.89
 due to Leptospira interrogans serovar icterohaemorrhagiae A27.0
 icterohemorrhagica A27.0
 pomona A27.89
 Weil's disease A27.0
**Leptus dermatitis** B88.0
**Leriche's syndrome** (aortic bifurcation occlusion) I74.09
**Leri's pleonosteosis** Q78.8
**Leri-Weill syndrome** Q77.8
**Lermoyez' syndrome** — see Vertigo, peripheral NEC
**Lesch-Nyhan syndrome** E79.1
**Leser-Trélat disease** L82.1
 inflamed L82.0
**Lesion**(s) (nontraumatic)
 abducens nerve — see Strabismus, paralytic, sixth
  nerve
 alveolar process K08.9
 angiocentric immunoproliferative D47.Z9 (following
  D47.4)
 anorectal K62.9
 aortic (valve) I35.9
 auditory nerve — see subcategory H93.3 ☑
 basal ganglion G25.9
 bile duct — see Disease, bile duct
 biomechanical M99.9
  specified type NEC M99.89
   abdomen M99.89
   acromioclavicular M99.87
   cervical region M99.81
   cervicothoracic M99.81
   costochondral M99.88
   costovertebral M99.88
   head region M99.80
   hip M99.85
   lower extremity M99.86
   lumbar region M99.83
   lumbosacral M99.83
   occipitocervical M99.80
   pelvic region M99.85
   pubic M99.85
   rib cage M99.88
   sacral region M99.84
   sacrococcygeal M99.84
   sacroiliac M99.84
   specified NEC M99.89
   sternochondral M99.88
   sternoclavicular M99.87
   thoracic region M99.82
   thoracolumbar M99.82
   upper extremity M99.87

**Lesion**(s) — continued
 bladder N32.9
 bone — see Disorder, bone
 brachial plexus G54.0
 brain G93.9
  congenital Q04.9
  vascular I67.9
   degenerative I67.9
   hypertensive I67.4
 buccal cavity K13.79
 calcified — see Calcification
 canthus — see Disorder, eyelid
 carate — see Pinta, lesions
 cardia K31.9
 cardiac (see also Disease, heart) I51.9
  congenital Q24.9
  valvular — see Endocarditis
 cauda equina G83.4
 cecum K63.9
 cerebral — see Lesion, brain
 cerebrovascular I67.9
  degenerative I67.9
  hypertensive I67.4
 cervical (nerve) root NEC G54.2
 chiasmal — see Disorder, optic, chiasm
 chorda tympani G51.8
 coin, lung R91.1
 colon K63.9
 combined periodontic - endodontic K05.5
 congenital — see Anomaly, by site
 conjunctiva H11.9
 conus medullaris — see Injury, conus medullaris
 coronary artery — see Ischemia, heart
 cranial nerve G52.9
  eighth — see Disorder, ear
  eleventh G52.9
  fifth G50.9
  first G52.0
  fourth — see Strabismus, paralytic, fourth nerve
  seventh G51.9
  sixth — see Strabismus, paralytic, sixth nerve
  tenth G52.2
  twelfth G52.3
 cystic — see Cyst
 degenerative — see Degeneration
 duodenum K31.9
 edentulous (alveolar) ridge, associated with trauma,
  due to traumatic occlusion K06.2
 en coup de sabre L94.1
 eyelid — see Disorder, eyelid
 gasserian ganglion G50.8
 gastric K31.9
 gastroduodenal K31.9
 gastrointestinal K63.9
 gingiva, associated with trauma K06.2
 glomerular
  focal and segmental (see also N00-N07 with fourth
   character .1) N05.1
  minimal change (see also N00-N07 with fourth
   character .0) N05.0
 heart (organic) — see Disease, heart
 hyperchromic, due to pinta (carate) A67.1
 hyperkeratotic — see Hyperkeratosis
 hypothalamic E23.7
 ileocecal K63.9
 ileum K63.9
 iliohypogastric nerve G57.8- ☑
 inflammatory — see Inflammation
 intestine K63.9
 intracerebral — see Lesion, brain
 intrachiasmal (optic) — see Disorder, optic, chiasm
 intracranial, space-occupying R90.0
 joint — see Disorder, joint
  sacroiliac (old) M53.3
 keratotic — see Keratosis
 kidney — see Disease, renal
 laryngeal nerve (recurrent) G52.2
 lip K13.0
 liver K76.9
 lumbosacral
  plexus G54.1
  root (nerve) NEC G54.4
 lung (coin) R91.1
 maxillary sinus J32.0
 mitral I05.9
 Morel-Lavallée — see Hematoma, by site
 motor cortex NEC G93.89
 mouth K13.79

☑ **Additional Character Required** — Refer to the Tabular List for Character Selection  ▽ **Subterms under main terms may continue to next column or page**

Lesion(s) — continued
  nerve G58.9
    femoral G57.2- ☑
    median G56.1- ☑
      carpal tunnel syndrome — see Syndrome,
        carpal tunnel
    plantar G57.6- ☑
    popliteal (lateral) G57.3- ☑
      medial G57.4- ☑
    radial G56.3- ☑
    sciatic G57.0- ☑
    spinal — see Injury, nerve, spinal
    ulnar G56.2- ☑
  nervous system, congenital Q07.9
  nonallopathic — see Lesion, biomechanical
  nose (internal) J34.89
  obstructive — see Obstruction
  obturator nerve G57.8- ☑
  oral mucosa K13.70
  organ or site NEC — see Disease, by site
  osteolytic — see Osteolysis
  peptic K27.9
  periodontal, due to traumatic occlusion K05.5
  pharynx J39.2
  pigment, pigmented (skin) L81.9
  pinta — see Pinta, lesions
  polypoid — see Polyp
  prechiasmal (optic) — see Disorder, optic, chiasm
  primary (see also Syphilis, primary) A51.0
    carate A67.0
    pinta A67.0
    yaws A66.0
  pulmonary J98.4
    valve I37.9
  pylorus K31.9
  rectosigmoid K63.9
  retina, retinal H35.9
  sacroiliac (joint) (old) M53.3
  salivary gland K11.9
    benign lymphoepithelial K11.8
  saphenous nerve G57.8- ☑
  sciatic nerve G57.0- ☑
  secondary — see Syphilis, secondary
  shoulder (region) M75.9- ☑
    specified NEC M75.8- ☑
  sigmoid K63.9
  sinus (accessory) (nasal) J34.89
  skin L98.9
    suppurative L08.0
  SLAP S43.43- ☑
  spinal cord G95.9
    congenital Q06.9
  spleen D73.89
  stomach K31.9
  superior glenoid labrum S43.43- ☑
  syphilitic — see Syphilis
  tertiary — see Syphilis, tertiary
  thoracic root (nerve) NEC G54.3
  tonsillar fossa J35.9
  tooth, teeth K08.9
    white spot
      chewing surface K02.51
      pit and fissure surface K02.51
      smooth surface K02.61
  traumatic — see specific type of injury by site
  tricuspid (valve) I07.9
    nonrheumatic I36.9
  trigeminal nerve G50.9
  ulcerated or ulcerative — see Ulcer, skin
  uterus N85.9
  vagus nerve G52.2
  valvular — see Endocarditis
  vascular I99.9
    affecting central nervous system I67.9
    following trauma NEC T14.8 ☑
    umbilical cord, complicating delivery O69.5 ☑
  warty — see Verruca
  white spot (tooth)
    chewing surface K02.51
    pit and fissure surface K02.51
    smooth surface K02.61
Lethargic — see condition
Lethargy R53.83
Letterer-Siwe's disease C96.0
Leukemia, leukemic C95.9- ☑
  acute basophilic C94.8- ☑
  acute bilineal C95.0- ☑

Leukemia, leukemic — continued
  acute erythroid C94.0- ☑
  acute lymphoblastic C91.0- ☑
  acute megakaryoblastic C94.2- ☑
  acute megakaryocytic C94.2- ☑
  acute mixed lineage C95.0- ☑
  acute monoblastic (monoblastic/monocytic) C93.0- ☑
  acute monocytic (monoblastic/monocytic) C93.0- ☑
  acute myeloblastic (minimal differentiation) (with
    maturation) C92.0- ☑
  acute myeloid
    with
      11q23-abnormality C92.6- ☑
      dysplasia of remaining hematopoesis and/or
        myelodysplastic disease in its history
        C92.A- ☑ (following C92.6)
      multilineage dysplasia C92.A- ☑ (following
        C92.6)
      variation of MLL-gene C92.6- ☑
    M6 (a)(b) C94.0- ☑
    M7 C94.2- ☑
  acute myelomonocytic C92.5- ☑
  acute promyelocytic C92.4- ☑
  adult T-cell (HTLV-1-associated) (acute variant)
    (chronic variant) (lymphomatoid variant)
    (smouldering variant) C91.5- ☑
  aggressive NK-cell C94.8- ☑
  AML (1/ETO) (M0) (M1) (M2) (without a FAB classifica-
    tion) C92.0- ☑
  AML M3 C92.4- ☑
  AML M4 (Eo with inv(16) or t(16;16)) C92.5- ☑
  AML M5 C93.0- ☑
  AML M5a C93.0- ☑
  AML M5b C93.0- ☑
  AML Me with t (15;17) and variants C92.4- ☑
  atypical chronic myeloid, BCR/ABL-negative C92.2- ☑
  biphenotypic acute C95.0- ☑
  blast cell C95.0- ☑
  Burkitt-type, mature B-cell C91.A- ☑ (following C91.6)
  chronic lymphocytic, of B-cell type C91.1- ☑
  chronic monocytic C93.1- ☑
  chronic myelogenous (Philadelphia chromosome (Ph1)
    positive) (t(9;22)) (q34;q11) (with crisis of blast
    cells) C92.1- ☑
  chronic myeloid, BCR/ABL-positive C92.1- ☑
    atypical, BCR/ABL-negative C92.2- ☑
  chronic myelomonocytic C93.1- ☑
  chronic neutrophilic D47.1
  CMML (-1) (-2) (with eosinophilia) C93.1- ☑
  granulocytic (see also Category C92) C92.9- ☑
  hairy cell C91.4- ☑
  juvenile myelomonocytic C93.3- ☑
  lymphoid C91.9- ☑
    specified NEC C91.Z- ☑ (following C91.6)
  mast cell C94.3- ☑
  mature B-cell, Burkitt-type C91.A- ☑ (following C91.6)
  monocytic (subacute) C93.9- ☑
    specified NEC C93.Z- ☑ (following C93.3)
  myelogenous (see also Category C92) C92.9- ☑
  myeloid C92.9- ☑
    specified NEC C92.Z- ☑ (following C92.6)
  plasma cell C90.1- ☑
  plasmacytic C90.1- ☑
  prolymphocytic
    of B-cell type C91.3- ☑
    of T-cell type C91.6- ☑
  specified NEC C94.8- ☑
  stem cell, of unclear lineage C95.0- ☑
  subacute lymphocytic C91.9- ☑
  T-cell large granular lymphocytic C91.Z- ☑ (following
    C91.6)
  unspecified cell type C95.9- ☑
    acute C95.0- ☑
    chronic C95.1- ☑
Leukemoid reaction (see also Reaction, leukemoid)
  D72.823
Leukoaraiosis (hypertensive) I67.81
Leukoariosis — see Leukoaraiosis
Leukocoria — see Disorder, globe, degenerated condi-
  tion, leucocoria
Leukocytopenia D72.819
Leukocytosis D72.829
  eosinophilic D72.1
Leukoderma, leukodermia NEC L81.5
  syphilitic A51.39
    late A52.79

Leukodystrophy E75.29
Leukoedema, oral epithelium K13.29
Leukoencephalitis G04.81
  acute (subacute) hemorrhagic G36.1
    postimmunization or postvaccinal G04.02
  postinfectious G04.01
  subacute sclerosing A81.1
  van Bogaert's (sclerosing) A81.1
Leukoencephalopathy (see also Encephalopathy)
  G93.49
  Binswanger's I67.3
  heroin vapor G92
  metachromatic E75.25
  multifocal (progressive) A81.2
  postimmunization and postvaccinal G04.02
  progressive multifocal A81.2
  reversible, posterior G93.6
  van Bogaert's (sclerosing) A81.1
  vascular, progressive I67.3
Leukoerythroblastosis D75.9
Leukokeratosis (see also Leukoplakia)
  mouth K13.21
  nicotina palati K13.24
  oral mucosa K13.21
  tongue K13.21
  vocal cord J38.3
Leukokraurosis vulva (e) N90.4
Leukoma (cornea) (see also Opacity, cornea)
  adherent H17.0- ☑
  interfering with central vision — see Opacity, cornea,
    central
Leukomalacia, cerebral, newborn P91.2
  periventricular P91.2
Leukomelanopathy, hereditary D72.0
Leukonychia (punctata) (striata) L60.8
  congenital Q84.4
Leukopathia unguium L60.8
  congenital Q84.4
Leukopenia D72.819
  basophilic D72.818
  chemotherapy (cancer) induced D70.1
  congenital D70.0
  cyclic D70.0
  drug induced NEC D70.2
    due to cytoreductive cancer chemotherapy D70.1
  eosinophilic D72.818
  familial D70.0
  infantile genetic D70.0
  malignant D70.9
  periodic D70.0
  transitory neonatal P61.5
Leukopenic — see condition
Leukoplakia
  anus K62.89
  bladder (postinfectional) N32.89
  buccal K13.21
  cervix (uteri) N88.0
  esophagus K22.8
  gingiva K13.21
  hairy (oral mucosa) (tongue) K13.3
  kidney (pelvis) N28.89
  larynx J38.7
  lip K13.21
  mouth K13.21
  oral epithelium, including tongue (mucosa) K13.21
  palate K13.21
  pelvis (kidney) N28.89
  penis (infectional) N48.0
  rectum K62.89
  syphilitic (late) A52.79
  tongue K13.21
  ureter (postinfectional) N28.89
  urethra (postinfectional) N36.8
  uterus N85.8
  vagina N89.4
  vocal cord J38.3
  vulva N90.4
Leukorrhea N89.8
  due to Trichomonas (vaginalis) A59.00
  trichomonal A59.00
Leukosarcoma C85.9- ☑
Levocardia (isolated) Q24.1
  with situs inversus Q89.3
Levotransposition Q20.5
Lev's disease or syndrome (acquired complete heart
  block) I44.2
Levulosuria — see Fructosuria
Levurid L30.2

**Lewy body** (ies) (dementia) (disease) G31.83
**Leyden-Moebius dystrophy** G71.0
**Leydig cell**
 carcinoma
  specified site — *see* Neoplasm, malignant, by site
  unspecified site
   female C56.9
   male C62.9- ☑
 tumor
  benign
   specified site — *see* Neoplasm, benign, by site
   unspecified site
    female D27.- ☑
    male D29.2- ☑
  malignant
   specified site — *see* Neoplasm, malignant, by site
   unspecified site
    female C56.- ☑
    male C62.9- ☑
  specified site — *see* Neoplasm, uncertain behavior, by site
  unspecified site
   female D39.1- ☑
   male D40.1- ☑
**Leydig-Sertoli cell tumor**
 specified site — *see* Neoplasm, benign, by site
 unspecified site
  female D27.- ☑
  male D29.2- ☑
**LGSIL** (Low grade squamous intraepithelial lesion on cytologic smear of)
 anus R85.612
 cervix R87.612
 vagina R87.622
**Liar, pathologic** F60.2
**Libido**
 decreased R68.82
**Libman-Sacks disease** M32.11
**Lice** (infestation) B85.2
 body (Pediculus corporis) B85.1
 crab B85.3
 head (Pediculus capitis) B85.0
 mixed (classifiable to more than one of the titles B85.0-B85.3) B85.4
 pubic (Phthirus pubis) B85.3
**Lichen** L28.0
 albus L90.0
  penis N48.0
  vulva N90.4
 amyloidosis E85.4 [L99]
 atrophicus L90.0
  penis N48.0
  vulva N90.4
 congenital Q82.8
 myxedematosus L98.5
 nitidus L44.1
 pilaris Q82.8
  acquired L85.8
 planopilaris L66.1
 planus (chronicus) L43.9
  annularis L43.8
  bullous L43.1
  follicular L66.1
  hypertrophic L43.0
  moniliformis L44.3
  of Wilson L43.9
  specified NEC L43.8
  subacute (active) L43.3
  tropicus L43.3
 ruber
  acuminatus L44.0
  moniliformis L44.3
  planus L43.9
 sclerosus (et atrophicus) L90.0
  penis N48.0
  vulva N90.4
 scrofulosus (primary) (tuberculous) A18.4
 simplex (chronicus) (circumscriptus) L28.0
 striatus L44.2
 urticatus L28.2
**Lichenification** L28.0
**Lichenoides tuberculosis** (primary) A18.4
**Lichtheim's disease or syndrome** — *see* Degeneration, combined
**Lien migrans** D73.89
**Ligament** — *see* condition

**Light**
 for gestational age — *see* Light for dates
 headedness R42
**Light-for-dates** (infant) P05.00
 with weight of
  1000-1249 grams P05.04
  1250-1499 grams P05.05
  1500-1749 grams P05.06
  1750-1999 grams P05.07
  2000-2499 grams P05.08
  2500 grams and over P05.09
  499 grams or less P05.01
  500-749 grams P05.02
  750-999 grams P05.03
 affecting management of pregnancy O36.59- ☑
 and small-for-dates — *see* Small for dates
 specified NEC P05.09
**Lightning** (effects) (stroke) (struck by) T75.00 ☑
 burn — *see* Burn
 foot E53.8
 shock T75.01 ☑
 specified effect NEC T75.09 ☑
**Lightwood-Albright syndrome** N25.89
**Lightwood's disease or syndrome** (renal tubular acidosis) N25.89
**Lignac** (-de Toni) (-Fanconi) (-Debré) **disease or syndrome** E72.09
 with cystinosis E72.04
**Ligneous thyroiditis** E06.5
**Likoff's syndrome** I20.8
**Limb** — *see* condition
**Limbic epilepsy personality syndrome** F07.0
**Limitation, limited**
 activities due to disability Z73.6
 cardiac reserve — *see* Disease, heart
 eye muscle duction, traumatic — *see* Strabismus, mechanical
 mandibular range of motion M26.52
**Lindau** (-von Hippel) **disease** Q85.8
**Line(s)**
 Beau's L60.4
 Harris' — *see* Arrest, epiphyseal
 Hudson's (cornea) — *see* Pigmentation, cornea, anterior
 Stähli's (cornea) — *see* Pigmentation, cornea, anterior
**Linea corneae senilis** — *see* Change, cornea, senile
**Lingua**
 geographica K14.1
 nigra (villosa) K14.3
 plicata K14.5
 tylosis K13.29
**Lingual** — *see* condition
**Linguatulosis** B88.8
**Linitis** (gastric) **plastica** C16.9
**Lip** — *see* condition
**Lipedema** — *see* Edema
**Lipemia** (*see also* Hyperlipidemia)
 retina, retinalis E78.3
**Lipidosis** E75.6
 cerebral (infantile) (juvenile) (late) E75.4
 cerebroretinal E75.4
 cerebroside E75.22
 cholesterol (cerebral) E75.5
 glycolipid E75.21
 hepatosplenomegalic E78.3
 sphingomyelin — *see* Niemann-Pick disease or syndrome
 sulfatide E75.29
**Lipoadenoma** — *see* Neoplasm, benign, by site
**Lipoblastoma** — *see* Lipoma
**Lipoblastomatosis** — *see* Lipoma
**Lipochondrodystrophy** E76.01
**Lipochrome histiocytosis** (familial) D71
**Lipodermatosclerosis** — *see* Varix, leg, with, inflammation
 ulcerated — *see* Varix, leg, with, ulcer, with inflammation by site
**Lipodystrophia progressiva** E88.1
**Lipodystrophy** (progressive) E88.1
 insulin E88.1
 intestinal K90.81
 mesenteric K65.4
**Lipofibroma** — *see* Lipoma
**Lipofuscinosis, neuronal** (with ceroidosis) E75.4
**Lipogranuloma, sclerosing** L92.8
**Lipogranulomatosis** E78.89
**Lipoid** (*see also* condition)

**Lipoid** — *continued*
 histiocytosis D76.3
  essential E75.29
 nephrosis N04.9
 proteinosis of Urbach E78.89
**Lipoidemia** — *see* Hyperlipidemia
**Lipoidosis** — *see* Lipidosis
**Lipoma** D17.9
 fetal D17.9
  fat cell D17.9
 infiltrating D17.9
 intramuscular D17.9
 pleomorphic D17.9
 site classification
  arms (skin) (subcutaneous) D17.2- ☑
  connective tissue D17.30
   intra-abdominal D17.5
   intrathoracic D17.4
   peritoneum D17.79
   retroperitoneum D17.79
   specified site NEC D17.39
   spermatic cord D17.6
  face (skin) (subcutaneous) D17.0
  genitourinary organ NEC D17.72
  head (skin) (subcutaneous) D17.0
  intra-abdominal D17.5
  intrathoracic D17.4
  kidney D17.71
  legs (skin) (subcutaneous) D17.2- ☑
  neck (skin) (subcutaneous) D17.0
  peritoneum D17.79
  retroperitoneum D17.79
  skin D17.30
   specified site NEC D17.39
  specified site NEC D17.79
  spermatic cord D17.6
  subcutaneous D17.30
   specified site NEC D17.39
  trunk (skin) (subcutaneous) D17.1
  unspecified D17.9
 spindle cell D17.9
**Lipomatosis** E88.2
 dolorosa (Dercum) E88.2
 fetal — *see* Lipoma
 Launois-Bensaude E88.89
**Lipomyoma** — *see* Lipoma
**Lipomyxoma** — *see* Lipoma
**Lipomyxosarcoma** — *see* Neoplasm, connective tissue, malignant
**Lipoprotein metabolism disorder** E78.9
**Lipoproteinemia** E78.5
 broad-beta E78.2
 floating-beta E78.2
 hyper-pre-beta E78.1
**Liposarcoma** (*see also* Neoplasm, connective tissue, malignant)
 dedifferentiated — *see* Neoplasm, connective tissue, malignant
 differentiated type — *see* Neoplasm, connective tissue, malignant
 embryonal — *see* Neoplasm, connective tissue, malignant
 mixed type — *see* Neoplasm, connective tissue, malignant
 myxoid — *see* Neoplasm, connective tissue, malignant
 pleomorphic — *see* Neoplasm, connective tissue, malignant
 round cell — *see* Neoplasm, connective tissue, malignant
 well differentiated type — *see* Neoplasm, connective tissue, malignant
**Liposynovitis prepatellaris** E88.89
**Lipping, cervix** N86
**Lipschütz disease or ulcer** N76.6
**Lipuria** R82.0
 schistosomiasis (bilharziasis) B65.0
**Lisping** F80.0
**Lissauer's paralysis** A52.17
**Lissencephalia, lissencephaly** Q04.3
**Listeriosis, listerellosis** A32.9
 congenital (disseminated) P37.2
 cutaneous A32.0
 neonatal, newborn (disseminated) P37.2
 oculoglandular A32.81
 specified NEC A32.89
**Lithemia** E79.0
**Lithiasis** — *see* Calculus
**Lithosis** J62.8

☑ **Additional Character Required — Refer to the Tabular List for Character Selection**

▽ **Subterms under main terms may continue to next column or page**

**Low** — *continued*
   birthweight — *continued*
      extreme — *continued*
         with weight of — *continued*
            750-999 grams P07.03
      for gestational age — *see* Light for dates
   blood pressure (*see also* Hypotension)
      reading (incidental) (isolated) (nonspecific) R03.1
   cardiac reserve — *see* Disease, heart
   function (*see also* Hypofunction)
      kidney N28.9
   hematocrit D64.9
   hemoglobin D64.9
   income Z59.6
   level of literacy Z55.0
   lying
      kidney N28.89
      organ or site, congenital — *see* Malposition, congenital
   output syndrome (cardiac) — *see* Failure, heart
   platelets (blood) — *see* Thrombocytopenia
   reserve, kidney N28.89
   salt syndrome E87.1
   self esteem R45.81
   set ears Q17.4
   vision H54.2X- ☑
      one eye (other eye normal) H54.50
         left (normal vision on right) H54.52A- ☑
            other eye blind — *see* Blindness
         right (normal vision on left) H54.511- ☑
**Low-density-lipoprotein-type** (LDL) **hyperlipoproteinemia** E78.00
**Lowe's syndrome** E72.03
**Lown-Ganong-Levine syndrome** I45.6
**LSD reaction** (acute) (without dependence) F16.90
   with dependence F16.20
**L-shaped kidney** Q63.8
**Ludwig's angina or disease** K12.2
**Lues** (venerea), **luetic** — *see* Syphilis
**Luetscher's syndrome** (dehydration) E86.0
**Lumbago, lumbalgia** M54.5
   with sciatica M54.4- ☑
      due to intervertebral disc disorder M51.17
   due to displacement, intervertebral disc M51.27
      with sciatica M51.17
**Lumbar** — *see* condition
**Lumbarization, vertebra, congenital** Q76.49
**Lumbermen's itch** B88.0
**Lump** (*see also* Mass)
   breast N63.0
      axillary tail
         left N63.32
         right N63.31
      left
         lower inner quadrant N63.24
         lower outer quadrant N63.23
         unspecified quadrant N63.20
         upper inner quadrant N63.22
         upper outer quadrant N63.21
      right
         lower inner quadrant N63.14
         lower outer quadrant N63.13
         unspecified quadrant N63.10
         upper inner quadrant N63.12
         upper outer quadrant N63.11
      subareolar
         left N63.42
         right N63.41
**Lunacy** — *see* Psychosis
**Lung** — *see* condition
**Lupoid** (miliary) **of Boeck** D86.3
**Lupus**
   anticoagulant D68.62
      with
         hemorrhagic disorder D68.312
         hypercoagulable state D68.62
         finding without diagnosis R76.0
   discoid (local) L93.0
   erythematosus (discoid) (local) L93.0
      disseminated — *see* Lupus, erythematosus, systemic
      eyelid H01.129
         left H01.126
            lower H01.125
            upper H01.124
         right H01.123
            lower H01.122
            upper H01.121

**Lupus** — *continued*
   erythematosus — *continued*
      profundus L93.2
      specified NEC L93.2
      subacute cutaneous L93.1
      systemic M32.9
         with organ or system involvement M32.10
            endocarditis M32.11
            lung M32.13
            pericarditis M32.12
            renal (glomerular) M32.14
               tubulo-interstitial M32.15
            specified organ or system NEC M32.19
         drug-induced M32.0
         inhibitor (presence of) D68.62
            with
               hemorrhagic disorder D68.312
               hypercoagulable state D68.62
               finding without diagnosis R76.0
         specified NEC M32.8
      exedens A18.4
      hydralazine M32.0
         correct substance properly administered — *see* Table of Drugs and Chemicals, by drug, adverse effect
         overdose or wrong substance given or taken — *see* Table of Drugs and Chemicals, by drug, poisoning
      nephritis (chronic) M32.14
      nontuberculous, not disseminated L93.0
      panniculitis L93.2
      pernio (Besnier) D86.3
      systemic — *see* Lupus, erythematosus, systemic
      tuberculous A18.4
         eyelid A18.4
      vulgaris A18.4
         eyelid A18.4
**Luteinoma** D27.- ☑
**Lutembacher's disease or syndrome** (atrial septal defect with mitral stenosis) Q21.1
**Luteoma** D27.- ☑
**Lutz** (-Splendore-de Almeida) **disease** — *see* Paracoccidioidomycosis
**Luxation** (*see also* Dislocation)
   eyeball (nontraumatic) — *see* Luxation, globe
      birth injury P15.3
   globe, nontraumatic H44.82- ☑
   lacrimal gland — *see* Dislocation, lacrimal gland
   lens (old) (partial) (spontaneous)
      congenital Q12.1
      syphilitic A50.39
**Lycanthropy** F22
**Lyell's syndrome** L51.2
   due to drug L51.2
      correct substance properly administered — *see* Table of Drugs and Chemicals, by drug, adverse effect
      overdose or wrong substance given or taken — *see* Table of Drugs and Chemicals, by drug, poisoning
**Lyme disease** A69.20
**Lymph**
   gland or node — *see* condition
   scrotum — *see* Infestation, filarial
**Lymphadenitis** I88.9
   with ectopic or molar pregnancy O08.0
   acute L04.9
      axilla L04.2
      face L04.0
      head L04.0
      hip L04.3
      limb
         lower L04.3
         upper L04.2
      neck L04.0
      shoulder L04.2
      specified site NEC L04.8
      trunk L04.1
   anthracosis (occupational) J60
   any site, except mesenteric I88.9
      chronic I88.1
      subacute I88.1
   breast
      gestational — *see* Mastitis, obstetric
      puerperal, postpartum (nonpurulent) O91.22
   chancroidal (congenital) A57
   chronic I88.1
      mesenteric I88.0

**Lymphadenitis** — *continued*
   due to
      Brugia (malayi) B74.1
         timori B74.2
      chlamydial lymphogranuloma A55
      diphtheria (toxin) A36.89
      lymphogranuloma venereum A55
      Wuchereria bancrofti B74.0
   following ectopic or molar pregnancy O08.0
   gonorrheal A54.89
   infective — *see* Lymphadenitis, acute
   mesenteric (acute) (chronic) (nonspecific) (subacute) I88.0
      due to Salmonella typhi A01.09
      tuberculous A18.39
   mycobacterial A31.8
   purulent — *see* Lymphadenitis, acute
   pyogenic — *see* Lymphadenitis, acute
   regional, nonbacterial I88.8
   septic — *see* Lymphadenitis, acute
   subacute, unspecified site I88.1
   suppurative — *see* Lymphadenitis, acute
   syphilitic (early) (secondary) A51.49
      late A52.79
   tuberculous — *see* Tuberculosis, lymph gland
   venereal (chlamydial) A55
**Lymphadenoid goiter** E06.3
**Lymphadenopathy** (generalized) R59.1
   angioimmunoblastic, with dysproteinemia (AILD) C86.5
   due to toxoplasmosis (acquired) B58.89
      congenital (acute) (subacute) (chronic) P37.1
   localized R59.0
   syphilitic (early) (secondary) A51.49
**Lymphadenosis** R59.1
**Lymphangiectasis** I89.0
   conjunctiva H11.89
   postinfectional I89.0
   scrotum I89.0
**Lymphangiectatic elephantiasis, nonfilarial** I89.0
**Lymphangioendothelioma** D18.1
   malignant — *see* Neoplasm, connective tissue, malignant
**Lymphangioleiomyomatosis** J84.81
**Lymphangioma** D18.1
   capillary D18.1
   cavernous D18.1
   cystic D18.1
   malignant — *see* Neoplasm, connective tissue, malignant
**Lymphangiomyoma** D18.1
**Lymphangiomyomatosis** J84.81
**Lymphangiosarcoma** — *see* Neoplasm, connective tissue, malignant
**Lymphangitis** I89.1
   with
      abscess — *code by* site under Abscess
      cellulitis — *code by* site under Cellulitis
      ectopic or molar pregnancy O08.0
   acute L03.91
      abdominal wall L03.321
      ankle — *see* Lymphangitis, acute, lower limb
      arm — *see* Lymphangitis, acute, upper limb
      auricle (ear) — *see* Lymphangitis, acute, ear
      axilla L03.12- ☑
      back (any part) L03.322
      buttock L03.327
      cervical (meaning neck) L03.222
      cheek (external) L03.212
      chest wall L03.323
      digit
         finger — *see* Lymphangitis, acute, finger
         toe — *see* Lymphangitis, acute, toe
      ear (external) H60.1- ☑
      external auditory canal — *see* Lymphangitis, acute, ear
      eyelid — *see* Abscess, eyelid
      face NEC L03.212
      finger (intrathecal) (periosteal) (subcutaneous) (subcuticular) L03.02- ☑
      foot — *see* Lymphangitis, acute, lower limb
      gluteal (region) L03.327
      groin L03.324
      hand — *see* Lymphangitis, acute, upper limb
      head NEC L03.891
         face (any part, except ear, eye and nose) L03.212
      heel — *see* Lymphangitis, acute, lower limb

**Lymphangitis** — *continued*
  acute — *continued*
      hip — *see* Lymphangitis, acute, lower limb
      jaw (region) L03.212
      knee — *see* Lymphangitis, acute, lower limb
      leg — *see* Lymphangitis, acute, lower limb
      lower limb L03.12- ☑
        toe — *see* Lymphangitis, acute, toe
      navel L03.326
      neck (region) L03.222
      orbit, orbital — *see* Cellulitis, orbit
      pectoral (region) L03.323
      perineal, perineum L03.325
      scalp (any part) L03.891
      shoulder — *see* Lymphangitis, acute, upper limb
      specified site NEC L03.898
      thigh — *see* Lymphangitis, acute, lower limb
      thumb (intrathecal) (periosteal) (subcutaneous)
          (subcuticular) — *see* Lymphangitis, acute,
          finger
      toe (intrathecal) (periosteal) (subcutaneous) (sub-
          cuticular) L03.04- ☑
      trunk L03.329
        abdominal wall L03.321
        back (any part) L03.322
        buttock L03.327
        chest wall L03.323
        groin L03.324
        perineal, perineum L03.325
        umbilicus L03.326
      umbilicus L03.326
      upper limb L03.12- ☑
        axilla — *see* Lymphangitis, acute, axilla
        finger — *see* Lymphangitis, acute, finger
        thumb — *see* Lymphangitis, acute, finger
      wrist — *see* Lymphangitis, acute, upper limb
  breast
      gestational — *see* Mastitis, obstetric
  chancroidal A57
  chronic (any site) I89.1
  due to
      Brugia (malayi) B74.1
        timori B74.2
      Wuchereria bancrofti B74.0
  following ectopic or molar pregnancy O08.89
  penis
      acute N48.29
      gonococcal (acute) (chronic) A54.09
  puerperal, postpartum, childbirth O86.89
  strumous, tuberculous A18.2
  subacute (any site) I89.1
  tuberculous — *see* Tuberculosis, lymph gland
**Lymphatic** (vessel) — *see* condition
**Lymphatism** E32.8
**Lymphectasia** I89.0
**Lymphedema** (acquired) (*see also* Elephantiasis)
  congenital Q82.0
  hereditary (chronic) (idiopathic) Q82.0
  postmastectomy I97.2
  praecox I89.0
  secondary I89.0
  surgical NEC I97.89
      postmastectomy (syndrome) I97.2
**Lymphoblastic** — *see* condition
**Lymphoblastoma** (diffuse) — *see* Lymphoma, lym-
      phoblastic (diffuse)
  giant follicular — *see* Lymphoma, lymphoblastic (dif-
      fuse)
  macrofollicular — *see* Lymphoma, lymphoblastic
      (diffuse)
**Lymphocele** I89.8
**Lymphocytic**
  chorioencephalitis (acute) (serous) A87.2
  choriomeningitis (acute) (serous) A87.2
  meningoencephalitis A87.2
**Lymphocytoma, benign cutis** L98.8
**Lymphocytopenia** D72.810
**Lymphocytosis** (symptomatic) D72.820
  infectious (acute) B33.3
**Lymphoepithelioma** — *see* Neoplasm, malignant, by
      site
**Lymphogranuloma** (malignant) (*see also* Lymphoma,
      Hodgkin)
  chlamydial A55
  inguinale A55
  venereum (any site) (chlamydial) (with stricture of
      rectum) A55

**Lymphogranulomatosis** (malignant) (*see also* Lym-
      phoma, Hodgkin)
  benign (Boeck's sarcoid) (Schaumann's) D86.1
**Lymphohistocytosis, hemophagocytic** (familial) D76.1
**Lymphoid** — *see* condition
**Lymphoma** (of) (malignant) C85.90
  adult T-cell (HTLV-1-associated) (acute variant)
      (chronic variant) (lymphomatoid variant)
      (smouldering variant) C91.5-
  anaplastic large cell
      ALK-negative C84.7- ☑
      ALK-positive C84.6- ☑
      CD30-positive C84.6- ☑
      primary cutaneous C86.6
  angioimmunoblastic T-cell C86.5
  BALT C88.4
  B-cell C85.1- ☑
  blastic NK-cell C86.4
  blastic plasmacytoid dendritic cell neoplasm (BPDCN)
      C86.4
  B-precursor C83.5- ☑
  bronchial-associated lymphoid tissue [BALT-lym-
      phoma] C88.4
  Burkitt (atypical) C83.7- ☑
  Burkitt-like C83.7- ☑
  centrocytic C83.1- ☑
  cutaneous follicle center C82.6- ☑
  cutaneous T-cell C84.A- ☑ (*following* C84.7)
  diffuse follicle center C82.5- ☑
  diffuse large cell C83.3- ☑
      anaplastic C83.3- ☑
      B-cell C83.3- ☑
      CD30-positive C83.3- ☑
      centroblastic C83.3- ☑
      immunoblastic C83.3- ☑
      plasmablastic C83.3- ☑
      subtype not specified C83.3- ☑
      T-cell rich C83.3- ☑
  enteropathy-type (associated) (intestinal) T-cell C86.2
  extranodal marginal zone B-cell lymphoma of mucosa-
      associated lymphoid tissue [MALT-lymphoma]
      C88.4
  extranodal NK/T-cell, nasal type C86.0
  follicular C82.9- ☑
      grade
        I C82.0- ☑
        II C82.1- ☑
        III C82.2- ☑
        IIIa C82.3- ☑
        IIIb C82.4- ☑
      specified NEC C82.8- ☑
  hepatosplenic T-cell (alpha-beta) (gamma-delta) C86.1
  histiocytic C85.9- ☑
      true C96.A (*following* C96.6)
  Hodgkin C81.9 ☑
      lymphocyte depleted (classical) C81.3- ☑
      lymphocyte-rich (classical) C81.4- ☑
      mixed cellularity (classical) C81.2- ☑
      nodular
        lymphocyte predominant C81.0- ☑
        sclerosis (classical) C81.1- ☑
      nodular sclerosis (classical) C81.1- ☑
      specified NEC (classical) C81.7- ☑
  intravascular large B-cell C83.8- ☑
  Lennert's C84.4- ☑
  lymphoblastic (diffuse) C83.5- ☑
  lymphoblastic B-cell C83.5- ☑
  lymphoblastic T-cell C83.5- ☑
  lymphoepithelioid C84.4- ☑
  lymphoplasmacytic C83.0- ☑
      with IgM-production C88.0
  MALT C88.4
  mantle cell C83.1- ☑
  mature T-cell NEC C84.4- ☑
  mature T/NK-cell C84.9- ☑
      specified NEC C84.Z- ☑ (*following* C84.7)
  mediastinal (thymic) large B-cell C85.2- ☑
  Mediterranean C88.3
  mucosa-associated lymphoid tissue [MALT-lymphoma]
      C88.4
  NK/T cell C84.9- ☑
  nodal marginal zone C83.0- ☑
  non-follicular (diffuse) C83.9- ☑
      specified NEC C83.8- ☑
  non-Hodgkin (*see also* Lymphoma, by type) C85.9- ☑
      specified NEC C85.8- ☑

**Lymphoma** — *continued*
  non-leukemic variant of B-CLL C83.0- ☑
  peripheral T-cell, not classified C84.4- ☑
  primary cutaneous
      anaplastic large cell C86.6
      CD30-positive large T-cell C86.6
  primary effusion B-cell C83.8- ☑
  SALT C88.4
  skin-associated lymphoid tissue [SALT-lymphoma]
      C88.4
  small cell B-cell C83.0- ☑
  splenic marginal zone C83.0- ☑
  subcutaneous panniculitis-like T-cell C86.3
  T-precursor C83.5- ☑
  true histiocytic C96.A (*following* C96.6)
**Lymphomatosis** — *see* Lymphoma
**Lymphopathia venereum, veneris** A55
**Lymphopenia** D72.810
**Lymphoplasmacytic leukemia** — *see* Leukemia,
      chronic lymphocytic, B-cell type
**Lymphoproliferation, X-linked disease** D82.3
**Lymphoreticulosis, benign** (of inoculation) A28.1
**Lymphorrhea** I89.8
**Lymphosarcoma** (diffuse) (*see also* Lymphoma)
      C85.9- ☑
**Lymphostasis** I89.8
**Lypemania** — *see* Melancholia
**Lysine and hydroxylysine metabolism disorder** E72.3
**Lyssa** — *see* Rabies

# M

**Macacus ear** Q17.3
**Maceration, wet feet, tropical** (syndrome) T69.02- ☑
**MacLeod's syndrome** J43.0
**Macrocephalia, macrocephaly** Q75.3
**Macrocheilia, macrochilia** (congenital) Q18.6
**Macrocolon** (*see also* Megacolon) Q43.1
**Macrocornea** Q15.8
  with glaucoma Q15.0
**Macrocytic** — *see* condition
**Macrocytosis** D75.89
**Macrodactylia, macrodactylism** (fingers) (thumbs)
      Q74.0
  toes Q74.2
**Macrodontia** K00.2
**Macrogenia** M26.05
**Macrogenitosomia** (adrenal) (male) (praecox) E25.9
  congenital E25.0
**Macroglobulinemia** (idiopathic) (primary) C88.0
  monoclonal (essential) D47.2
  Waldenström C88.0
**Macroglossia** (congenital) Q38.2
  acquired K14.8
**Macrognathia, macrognathism** (congenital)
      (mandibular) (maxillary) M26.09
**Macrogyria** Q04.8
**Macrohydrocephalus** — *see* Hydrocephalus
**Macromastia** — *see* Hypertrophy, breast
**Macrophthalmos** Q11.3
  in congenital glaucoma Q15.0
**Macropsia** H53.15
**Macrosigmoid** K59.39
  congenital Q43.2
**Macrospondylitis , acromegalic** E22.0
**Macrostomia** (congenital) Q18.4
**Macrotia** (external ear) (congenital) Q17.1
**Macula**
  cornea, corneal — *see* Opacity, cornea
  degeneration (atrophic) (exudative) (senile) (*see also*
      Degeneration, macula)
      hereditary — *see* Dystrophy, retina
**Maculae ceruleae** B85.1
**Maculopathy, toxic** — *see* Degeneration, macula, toxic
**Madarosis** (eyelid) H02.729
  left H02.726
      lower H02.725
      upper H02.724
  right H02.723
      lower H02.722
      upper H02.721
**Madelung's**
  deformity (radius) Q74.0
  disease
      radial deformity Q74.0
      symmetrical lipomas, neck E88.89
**Madness** — *see* Psychosis

▼ Subterms under main terms may continue to next column or page ☑ Additional Character Required — Refer to the Tabular List for Character Selection

Lymphangitis — Madness

215

**Madura**
  foot B47.9
    actinomycotic B47.1
    mycotic B47.0
**Maduromycosis** B47.0
**Maffucci's syndrome** Q78.4
**Magnesium metabolism disorder** — *see* Disorder, metabolism, magnesium
**Main en griffe** (acquired) (*see also* Deformity, limb, clawhand)
  congenital Q74.0
**Maintenance** (encounter for)
  antineoplastic chemotherapy Z51.11
  antineoplastic radiation therapy Z51.0
  methadone F11.20
**Majocchi's**
  disease L81.7
  granuloma B35.8
**Major** — *see* condition
**Mal de los pintos** — *see* Pinta
**Mal de mer** T75.3 ☑
**Malabar itch** (any site) B35.5
**Malabsorption** K90.9
  calcium K90.89
  carbohydrate K90.49
  disaccharide E73.9
  fat K90.49
  galactose E74.20
  glucose (-galactose) E74.39
  intestinal K90.9
    specified NEC K90.89
  isomaltose E74.31
  lactose E73.9
  methionine E72.19
  monosaccharide E74.39
  postgastrectomy K91.2
  postsurgical K91.2
  protein K90.49
  starch K90.49
  sucrose E74.39
  syndrome K90.9
    postsurgical K91.2
**Malacia, bone** (adult) M83.9
  juvenile — *see* Rickets
**Malacoplakia**
  bladder N32.89
  pelvis (kidney) N28.89
  ureter N28.89
  urethra N36.8
**Malacosteon, juvenile** — *see* Rickets
**Maladaptation** — *see* Maladjustment
**Maladie de Roger** Q21.0
**Maladjustment**
  conjugal Z63.0
    involving divorce or estrangement Z63.5
  educational Z55.4
  family Z63.9
  marital Z63.0
    involving divorce or estrangement Z63.5
  occupational NEC Z56.89
  simple, adult — *see* Disorder, adjustment
  situational — *see* Disorder, adjustment
  social Z60.9
    due to
      acculturation difficulty Z60.3
      discrimination and persecution (perceived) Z60.5
      exclusion and isolation Z60.4
      life-cycle (phase of life) transition Z60.0
      rejection Z60.4
      specified reason NEC Z60.8
**Malaise** R53.81
**Malakoplakia** — *see* Malacoplakia
**Malaria, malarial** (fever) B54
  with
    blackwater fever B50.8
      hemoglobinuric (bilious) B50.8
    hemoglobinuria B50.8
  accidentally induced (therapeutically) — *code by* type under Malaria
  algid B50.9
  cerebral B50.0 [G94]
  clinically diagnosed (without parasitological confirmation) B54
  congenital NEC P37.4
    falciparum P37.3
  congestion, congestive B54
  continued (fever) B50.9

**Malaria, malarial** — *continued*
  estivo-autumnal B50.9
  falciparum B50.9
    with complications NEC B50.8
      cerebral B50.0 [G94]
    severe B50.8
  hemorrhagic B54
  malariae B52.9
    with
      complications NEC B52.8
      glomerular disorder B52.0
  malignant (tertian) — *see* Malaria, falciparum
  mixed infections — *code to* first listed type in B50-B53
  ovale B53.0
  parasitologically confirmed NEC B53.8
  pernicious, acute — *see* Malaria, falciparum
  Plasmodium (P.)
    falciparum NEC — *see* Malaria, falciparum
    malariae NEC B52.9
      with Plasmodium
        falciparum (and or vivax) — *see* Malaria, falciparum
        vivax (*see also* Malaria, vivax)
          and falciparum — *see* Malaria, falciparum
    ovale B53.0
      with Plasmodium malariae (*see also* Malaria, malariae)
        and vivax (*see also* Malaria, vivax)
          and falciparum — *see* Malaria, falciparum
    simian B53.1
      with Plasmodium malariae (*see also* Malaria, malariae)
        and vivax (*see also* Malaria, vivax)
          and falciparum — *see* Malaria, falciparum
    vivax NEC B51.9
      with Plasmodium falciparum — *see* Malaria, falciparum
  quartan — *see* Malaria, malariae
  quotidian — *see* Malaria, falciparum
  recurrent B54
  remittent B54
  specified type NEC (parasitologically confirmed) B53.8
  spleen B54
  subtertian (fever) — *see* Malaria, falciparum
  tertian (benign) (*see also* Malaria, vivax)
    malignant B50.9
  tropical B50.9
  typhoid B54
  vivax B51.9
    with
      complications NEC B51.8
      ruptured spleen B51.0
**Malassez's disease** (cystic) N50.89
**Malassimilation** K90.9
**Maldescent, testis** Q53.9
  bilateral Q53.20
    abdominal Q53.211
    perineal Q53.22
  unilateral Q53.10
    abdominal Q53.111
    perineal Q53.12
**Maldevelopment** (*see also* Anomaly)
  brain Q07.9
  colon Q43.9
  hip Q74.2
    congenital dislocation Q65.2
      bilateral Q65.1
      unilateral Q65.0- ☑
  mastoid process Q75.8
  middle ear Q16.4
    except ossicles Q16.4
    ossicles Q16.3
  ossicles Q16.3
  spine Q76.49
  toe Q74.2
**Male type pelvis** Q74.2
  with disproportion (fetopelvic) O33.3 ☑
    causing obstructed labor O65.3
**Malformation** (congenital) (*see also* Anomaly)
  adrenal gland Q89.1
  affecting multiple systems with skeletal changes NEC Q87.5
  alimentary tract Q45.9
    specified type NEC Q45.8
    upper Q40.9

**Malformation** — *continued*
  alimentary tract — *continued*
    upper — *continued*
      specified type NEC Q40.8
  aorta Q25.40
    absence Q25.41
    aneurysm, congenital Q25.43
    aplasia Q25.41
    atresia Q25.29
      aortic arch Q25.21
    coarctation (preductal) (postductal) Q25.1
    dilatation, congenital Q25.44
    hypoplasia Q25.42
    patent ductus arteriosus Q25.0
    specified type NEC Q25.49
    stenosis Q25.1
      supravalvular Q25.3
  aortic valve Q23.9
    specified NEC Q23.8
  arteriovenous, aneurysmatic (congenital) Q27.30
    brain Q28.2
    cerebral Q28.2
    peripheral Q27.30
      digestive system Q27.33
      lower limb Q27.32
      other specified site Q27.39
      renal vessel Q27.34
      upper limb Q27.31
    precerebral vessels (nonruptured) Q28.0
  auricle
    ear (congenital) Q17.3
      acquired H61.119
        left H61.112
          with right H61.113
        right H61.111
          with left H61.113
  bile duct Q44.5
  bladder Q64.79
    aplasia Q64.5
    diverticulum Q64.6
    exstrophy — *see* Exstrophy, bladder
    neck obstruction Q64.31
  bone Q79.9
    face Q75.9
      specified type NEC Q75.8
    skull Q75.9
      specified type NEC Q75.8
  brain (multiple) Q04.9
    arteriovenous Q28.2
    specified type NEC Q04.8
  branchial cleft Q18.2
  breast Q83.9
    specified type NEC Q83.8
  broad ligament Q50.6
  bronchus Q32.4
  bursa Q79.9
  cardiac
    chambers Q20.9
      specified type NEC Q20.8
    septum Q21.9
      specified type NEC Q21.8
  cerebral Q04.9
    vessels Q28.3
  cervix uteri Q51.9
    specified type NEC Q51.828
  Chiari
    Type I G93.5
    Type II Q07.01
  choroid (congenital) Q14.3
    plexus Q07.8
  circulatory system Q28.9
  cochlea Q16.5
  cornea Q13.4
  coronary vessels Q24.5
  corpus callosum (congenital) Q04.0
  diaphragm Q79.1
  digestive system NEC, specified type NEC Q45.8
  dura Q07.9
    brain Q04.9
    spinal Q06.9
  ear Q17.9
    causing impairment of hearing Q16.9
    external Q17.9
      accessory auricle Q17.0
      causing impairment of hearing Q16.9
        absence of
          auditory canal Q16.1
          auricle Q16.0
      macrotia Q17.1

**Malformation** — *continued*
  ear — *continued*
    external — *continued*
      microtia Q17.2
      misplacement Q17.4
      misshapen NEC Q17.3
      prominence Q17.5
      specified type NEC Q17.8
    inner Q16.5
    middle Q16.4
      absence of eustachian tube Q16.2
      ossicles (fusion) Q16.3
    ossicles Q16.3
    specified type NEC Q17.8
  epididymis Q55.4
  esophagus Q39.9
    specified type NEC Q39.8
  eye Q15.9
    lid Q10.3
    specified NEC Q15.8
  fallopian tube Q50.6
  genital organ — *see* Anomaly, genitalia
  great
    artery Q25.9
      aorta — *see* Malformation, aorta
      pulmonary artery — *see* Malformation, pulmonary, artery
      specified type NEC Q25.8
    vein Q26.9
      anomalous
        portal venous connection Q26.5
        pulmonary venous connection Q26.4
          partial Q26.3
          total Q26.2
      persistent left superior vena cava Q26.1
      portal vein-hepatic artery fistula Q26.6
      specified type NEC Q26.8
      vena cava stenosis, congenital Q26.0
  gum Q38.6
  hair Q84.2
  heart Q24.9
    specified type NEC Q24.8
  integument Q84.9
    specified type NEC Q84.8
  internal ear Q16.5
  intestine Q43.9
    specified type NEC Q43.8
  iris Q13.2
  joint Q74.9
    ankle Q74.2
    lumbosacral Q76.49
    sacroiliac Q74.2
    specified type NEC Q74.8
  kidney Q63.9
    accessory Q63.0
    giant Q63.3
    horseshoe Q63.1
    hydronephrosis Q62.0
    malposition Q63.2
    specified type NEC Q63.8
  lacrimal apparatus Q10.6
  lingual Q38.3
  lip Q38.0
  liver Q44.7
  lung Q33.9
  meninges or membrane (congenital) Q07.9
    cerebral Q04.8
    spinal (cord) Q06.9
  middle ear Q16.4
    ossicles Q16.3
  mitral valve Q23.9
    specified NEC Q23.8
  Mondini's (congenital) (malformation, cochlea) Q16.5
  mouth (congenital) Q38.6
  multiple types NEC Q89.7
  musculoskeletal system Q79.9
  myocardium Q24.8
  nail Q84.6
  nervous system (central) Q07.9
  nose Q30.9
    specified type NEC Q30.8
  optic disc Q14.2
  orbit Q10.7
  ovary Q50.39
  palate Q38.5
  parathyroid gland Q89.2
  pelvic organs or tissues NEC
    in pregnancy or childbirth O34.8- ☑
      causing obstructed labor O65.5

**Malformation** — *continued*
  penis Q55.69
    aplasia Q55.5
    curvature (lateral) Q55.61
    hypoplasia Q55.62
  pericardium Q24.8
  peripheral vascular system Q27.9
    specified type NEC Q27.8
  pharynx Q38.8
  precerebral vessels Q28.1
  prostate Q55.4
  pulmonary
    arteriovenous Q25.72
    artery Q25.9
      atresia Q25.5
      specified type NEC Q25.79
      stenosis Q25.6
    valve Q22.3
  renal artery Q27.2
  respiratory system Q34.9
  retina Q14.1
  scrotum — *see* Malformation, testis and scrotum
  seminal vesicles Q55.4
  sense organs NEC Q07.9
  skin Q82.9
  specified NEC Q89.8
  spinal
    cord Q06.9
    nerve root Q07.8
  spine Q76.49
    kyphosis — *see* Kyphosis, congenital
    lordosis — *see* Lordosis, congenital
  spleen Q89.09
  stomach Q40.3
    specified type NEC Q40.2
  teeth, tooth K00.9
  tendon Q79.9
  testis and scrotum Q55.20
    aplasia Q55.0
    hypoplasia Q55.1
    polyorchism Q55.21
    retractile testis Q55.22
    scrotal transposition Q55.23
    specified NEC Q55.29
  thorax, bony Q76.9
  throat Q38.8
  thyroid gland Q89.2
  tongue (congenital) Q38.3
    hypertrophy Q38.2
    tie Q38.1
  trachea Q32.1
  tricuspid valve Q22.9
    specified type NEC Q22.8
  umbilical cord NEC (complicating delivery) O69.89 ☑
  umbilicus Q89.9
  ureter Q62.8
    agenesis Q62.4
    duplication Q62.5
    malposition — *see* Malposition, congenital, ureter
    obstructive defect — *see* Defect, obstructive, ureter
    vesico-uretero-renal reflux Q62.7
  urethra Q64.79
    aplasia Q64.5
    duplication Q64.74
    posterior valves Q64.2
    prolapse Q64.71
    stricture Q64.32
  urinary system Q64.9
  uterus Q51.9
    specified type NEC Q51.818
  vagina Q52.4
  vas deferens Q55.4
    atresia Q55.3
  vascular system, peripheral Q27.9
  venous — *see* Anomaly, vein(s)
  vulva Q52.70
**Malfunction** (*see also* Dysfunction)
  cardiac electronic device T82.119 ☑
    electrode T82.110 ☑
    pulse generator T82.111 ☑
    specified type NEC T82.118 ☑
  catheter device NEC T85.618 ☑
    cystostomy T83.010 ☑
    dialysis (renal) (vascular) T82.41 ☑
      intraperitoneal T85.611 ☑
    infusion NEC T82.514 ☑
      cranial T85.610 ☑
      epidural T85.610 ☑

**Malfunction** — *continued*
  catheter device — *continued*
    infusion — *continued*
      intrathecal T85.610 ☑
      spinal T85.610 ☑
      subarachnoid T85.610 ☑
      subdural T85.610 ☑
    urinary (*see also* Breakdown, device, catheter) T83.018 ☑
  colostomy K94.03
    valve K94.03
  cystostomy (stoma) N99.512
    catheter T83.010 ☑
  enteric stoma K94.13
  enterostomy K94.13
  esophagostomy K94.33
  gastroenteric K31.89
  gastrostomy K94.23
  ileostomy K94.13
    valve K94.13
  intrathecal infusion pump T85.615 ☑
  jejunostomy K94.13
  nervous system device, implant or graft, specified NEC T85.615 ☑
  pacemaker — *see* Malfunction, cardiac electronic device
  prosthetic device, internal — *see* Complications, prosthetic device, by site, mechanical
  tracheostomy J95.03
  urinary device NEC — *see* Complication, genitourinary, device, urinary, mechanical
  valve
    colostomy K94.03
    heart T82.09 ☑
    ileostomy K94.13
  vascular graft or shunt NEC — *see* Complication, cardiovascular device, mechanical, vascular
  ventricular (communicating shunt) T85.01 ☑
**Malherbe's tumor** — *see* Neoplasm, skin, benign
**Malibu disease** L98.8
**Malignancy** (*see also* Neoplasm, malignant, by site)
  unspecified site (primary) C80.1
**Malignant** — *see* condition
**Malingerer, malingering** Z76.5
**Mallet finger** (acquired) — *see* Deformity, finger, mallet finger
  congenital Q74.0
  sequelae of rickets E64.3
**Malleus** A24.0
**Mallory's bodies** R89.7
**Mallory-Weiss syndrome** K22.6
**Malnutrition** E46
  degree
    first E44.1
      mild (protein) E44.1
      moderate (protein) E44.0
    second E44.0
    severe (protein-energy) E43
      intermediate form E42
        with
          kwashiorkor (and marasmus) E42
          marasmus E41
    third E43
  following gastrointestinal surgery K91.2
  intrauterine
    light-for-dates — *see* Light for dates
    small-for-dates — *see* Small for dates
  lack of care, or neglect (child) (infant) T76.02 ☑
    confirmed T74.02 ☑
  malignant E40
  protein E46
    calorie E46
      mild E44.1
      moderate E44.0
      severe E43
        intermediate form E42
          with
            kwashiorkor (and marasmus) E42
            marasmus E41
    energy E46
      mild E44.1
      moderate E44.0
      severe E43
        intermediate form E42
          with
            kwashiorkor (and marasmus) E42
            marasmus E41
  severe (protein-energy) E43

**Malnutrition** — *continued*
severe — *continued*
  with
    kwashiorkor (and marasmus) E42
    marasmus E41
**Malocclusion** (teeth) M26.4
  Angle's M26.219
    class I M26.211
    class II M26.212
    class III M26.213
  due to
    abnormal swallowing M26.59
    mouth breathing M26.59
    tongue, lip or finger habits M26.59
  temporomandibular (joint) M26.69
**Malposition**
  cervix — *see* Malposition, uterus
  congenital
    adrenal (gland) Q89.1
    alimentary tract Q45.8
      lower Q43.8
      upper Q40.8
    aorta Q25.49
    appendix Q43.8
    arterial trunk Q20.0
    artery (peripheral) Q27.8
      coronary Q24.5
      digestive system Q27.8
      lower limb Q27.8
      pulmonary Q25.79
      specified site NEC Q27.8
      upper limb Q27.8
    auditory canal Q17.8
      causing impairment of hearing Q16.9
    auricle (ear) Q17.4
      causing impairment of hearing Q16.9
      cervical Q18.2
    biliary duct or passage Q44.5
    bladder (mucosa) — *see* Exstrophy, bladder
    brachial plexus Q07.8
    brain tissue Q04.8
    breast Q83.8
    bronchus Q32.4
    cecum Q43.8
    clavicle Q74.0
    colon Q43.8
    digestive organ or tract NEC Q45.8
      lower Q43.8
      upper Q40.8
    ear (auricle) (external) Q17.4
      ossicles Q16.3
    endocrine (gland) NEC Q89.2
    epiglottis Q31.8
    eustachian tube Q17.8
    eye Q15.8
    facial features Q18.8
    fallopian tube Q50.6
    finger(s) Q68.1
      supernumerary Q69.0
    foot Q66.9
    gallbladder Q44.1
    gastrointestinal tract Q45.8
    genitalia, genital organ(s) or tract
      female Q52.8
        external Q52.79
        internal NEC Q52.8
      male Q55.8
    glottis Q31.8
    hand Q68.1
    heart Q24.8
      dextrocardia Q24.0
      with complete transposition of viscera Q89.3
    hepatic duct Q44.5
    hip (joint) Q65.89
    intestine (large) (small) Q43.8
      with anomalous adhesions, fixation or malrotation Q43.3
    joint NEC Q68.8
    kidney Q63.2
    larynx Q31.8
    limb Q68.8
      lower Q68.8
      upper Q68.8
    liver Q44.7
    lung (lobe) Q33.8
    nail(s) Q84.6
    nerve Q07.8
    nervous system NEC Q07.8
    nose, nasal (septum) Q30.8

**Malposition** — *continued*
  congenital — *continued*
    organ or site not listed — *see* Anomaly, by site
    ovary Q50.39
    pancreas Q45.3
    parathyroid (gland) Q89.2
    patella Q74.1
    peripheral vascular system Q27.8
    pituitary (gland) Q89.2
    respiratory organ or system NEC Q34.8
    rib (cage) Q76.6
      supernumerary in cervical region Q76.5
    scapula Q74.0
    shoulder Q74.0
    spinal cord Q06.8
    spleen Q89.09
    sternum NEC Q76.7
    stomach Q40.2
    symphysis pubis Q74.2
    thymus (gland) Q89.2
    thyroid (gland) (tissue) Q89.2
      cartilage Q31.8
    toe(s) Q66.9
      supernumerary Q69.2
    tongue Q38.3
    trachea Q32.1
    ureter Q62.60
      deviation Q62.61
      displacement Q62.62
      ectopia Q62.63
      specified type NEC Q62.69
    uterus Q51.818
    vein(s) (peripheral) Q27.8
      great Q26.8
    vena cava (inferior) (superior) Q26.8
  device, implant or graft (*see also* Complications, by site and type, mechanical) T85.628 ☑
    arterial graft NEC — *see* Complication, cardiovascular device, mechanical, vascular
    breast (implant) T85.42 ☑
    catheter NEC T85.628 ☑
      cystostomy T83.020 ☑
      dialysis (renal) T82.42 ☑
        intraperitoneal T85.621 ☑
      infusion NEC T82.524 ☑
        spinal (epidural) (subdural) T85.620 ☑
      urinary (*see also* Displacement, device, catheter, urinary) T83.028 ☑
    electronic (electrode) (pulse generator) (stimulator)
      bone T84.320 ☑
      cardiac T82.129 ☑
        electrode T82.120 ☑
        pulse generator T82.121 ☑
        specified type NEC T82.128 ☑
      nervous system — *see* Complication, prosthetic device, mechanical, electronic nervous system stimulator
      urinary — *see* Complication, genitourinary, device, urinary, mechanical
    fixation, internal (orthopedic) NEC — *see* Complication, fixation device, mechanical
    gastrointestinal — *see* Complications, prosthetic device, mechanical, gastrointestinal device
    genital NEC T83.428 ☑
      intrauterine contraceptive device (string) T83.32 ☑
      penile prosthesis (cylinder) (implanted) (pump) (reservoir) T83.420 ☑
      testicular prosthesis T83.421 ☑
    heart NEC — *see* Complication, cardiovascular device, mechanical
    joint prosthesis — *see* Complication, joint prosthesis, mechanical
    ocular NEC — *see* Complications, prosthetic device, mechanical, ocular device
    orthopedic NEC — *see* Complication, orthopedic, device, mechanical
    specified NEC T85.628 ☑
    urinary NEC (*see also* Complication, genitourinary, device, urinary, mechanical)
      graft T83.22 ☑
    vascular NEC — *see* Complication, cardiovascular device, mechanical
    ventricular intracranial shunt T85.02 ☑
  fetus — *see* Pregnancy, complicated by (management affected by), presentation, fetal
  gallbladder K82.8

**Malposition** — *continued*
  gastrointestinal tract, congenital Q45.8
  heart, congenital NEC Q24.8
  joint prosthesis — *see* Complications, joint prosthesis, mechanical, displacement, by site
  stomach K31.89
    congenital Q40.2
  tooth, teeth, fully erupted M26.30
  uterus (acute) (acquired) (adherent) (asymptomatic) (postinfectional) (postpartal, old) N85.4
    anteflexion or anteversion N85.4
      congenital Q51.818
    flexion N85.4
      lateral — *see* Lateroversion, uterus
    inversion N85.5
    lateral (flexion) (version) — *see* Lateroversion, uterus
      in pregnancy or childbirth — *see* subcategory O34.5 ☑
    retroflexion or retroversion — *see* Retroversion, uterus
**Malposture** R29.3
**Malrotation**
  cecum Q43.3
  colon Q43.3
  intestine Q43.3
  kidney Q63.2
**Malta fever** — *see* Brucellosis
**Maltreatment**
  adult
    abandonment
      confirmed T74.01 ☑
      suspected T76.01 ☑
    confirmed T74.91 ☑
    history of Z91.419
    neglect
      confirmed T74.01 ☑
      suspected T76.01 ☑
    physical abuse
      confirmed T74.11 ☑
      suspected T76.11 ☑
    psychological abuse
      confirmed T74.31 ☑
      history of Z91.411
      suspected T76.31 ☑
    sexual abuse
      confirmed T74.21 ☑
      suspected T76.21 ☑
    suspected T76.91 ☑
  child
    abandonment
      confirmed of T74.02 ☑
      suspected of T76.02 ☑
    confirmed T74.92 ☑
    history of — *see* History, personal (of), abuse
    neglect
      confirmed T74.02 ☑
      history of — *see* History, personal (of), abuse
      suspected T76.02 ☑
    physical abuse
      confirmed T74.12 ☑
      history of — *see* History, personal (of), abuse
      suspected T76.12 ☑
    psychological abuse
      confirmed T74.32 ☑
      history of — *see* History, personal (of), abuse
      suspected T76.32 ☑
    sexual abuse
      confirmed T74.22 ☑
      history of — *see* History, personal (of), abuse
      suspected T76.22 ☑
    suspected T76.92 ☑
  personal history of Z91.89
**Maltworker's lung** J67.4
**Malunion, fracture** — *see* Fracture, by site
**Mammillitis** N61.0
  puerperal, postpartum O91.02
**Mammitis** — *see* Mastitis
**Mammogram** (examination) Z12.39
  routine Z12.31
**Mammoplasia** N62
**Management** (of)
  bone conduction hearing device (implanted) Z45.320
  cardiac pacemaker NEC Z45.018
  cerebrospinal fluid drainage device Z45.41
  cochlear device (implanted) Z45.321
  contraceptive Z30.9

☑ Additional Character Required — Refer to the Tabular List for Character Selection    ▽ Subterms under main terms may continue to next column or page

**Management** — *continued*
  contraceptive — *continued*
    specified NEC Z30.8
    implanted device Z45.9
      specified NEC Z45.89
  infusion pump Z45.1
  procreative Z31.9
    male factor infertility in female Z31.81
    specified NEC Z31.89
  prosthesis (external) (*see also* Fitting) Z44.9
    implanted Z45.9
      specified NEC Z45.89
  renal dialysis catheter Z49.01
  vascular access device Z45.2
**Mangled** — *see* specified injury by site
**Mania** (monopolar) (*see also* Disorder, mood, manic episode)
  with psychotic symptoms F30.2
  without psychotic symptoms F30.10
    mild F30.11
    moderate F30.12
    severe F30.13
  Bell's F30.8
  chronic (recurrent) F31.89
  hysterical F44.89
  puerperal F30.8
  recurrent F31.89
**Manic depression** F31.9
**Manic-depressive insanity, psychosis, or syndrome** — *see* Disorder, bipolar
**Mannosidosis** E77.1
**Mansonelliasis, mansonellosis** B74.4
**Manson's**
  disease B65.1
  schistosomiasis B65.1
**Manual** — *see* condition
**Maple-bark-stripper's lung** (disease) J67.6
**Maple-syrup-urine disease** E71.0
**Marable's syndrome** (celiac artery compression) I77.4
**Marasmus** E41
  due to malnutrition E41
  intestinal E41
  nutritional E41
  senile R54
  tuberculous NEC — *see* Tuberculosis
**Marble**
  bones Q78.2
  skin R23.8
**Marburg virus disease** A98.3
**March**
  fracture — *see* Fracture, traumatic, stress, by site
  hemoglobinuria D59.6
**Marchesani** (-Weill) **syndrome** Q87.0
**Marchiafava** (-Bignami) **syndrome or disease** G37.1
**Marchiafava-Micheli syndrome** D59.5
**Marcus Gunn's syndrome** Q07.8
**Marfan's syndrome** — *see* Syndrome, Marfan's
**Marie-Bamberger disease** — *see* Osteoarthropathy, hypertrophic, specified NEC
**Marie-Charcot-Tooth neuropathic muscular atrophy** G60.0
**Marie's**
  cerebellar ataxia (late-onset) G11.2
  disease or syndrome (acromegaly) E22.0
**Marie-Strümpell arthritis, disease or spondylitis** — *see* Spondylitis, ankylosing
**Marion's disease** (bladder neck obstruction) N32.0
**Marital conflict** Z63.0
**Mark**
  port wine Q82.5
  raspberry Q82.5
  strawberry Q82.5
  stretch L90.6
  tattoo L81.8
**Marker heterochromatin** — *see* Extra, marker chromosomes
**Maroteaux-Lamy syndrome** (mild) (severe) E76.29
**Marrow** (bone)
  arrest D61.9
  poor function D75.89
**Marseilles fever** A77.1
**Marsh fever** — *see* Malaria
**Marshall's** (hidrotic) **ectodermal dysplasia** Q82.4
**Marsh's disease** (exophthalmic goiter) E05.00
  with storm E05.01
**Masculinization** (female) **with adrenal hyperplasia** E25.9

**Masculinization** (female) **with adrenal hyperplasia** — *continued*
  congenital E25.0
**Masculinovoblastoma** D27.- ☑
**Masochism** (sexual) F65.51
**Mason's lung** J62.8
**Mass**
  abdominal R19.00
    epigastric R19.06
    generalized R19.07
    left lower quadrant R19.04
    left upper quadrant R19.02
    periumbilic R19.05
    right lower quadrant R19.03
    right upper quadrant R19.01
    specified site NEC R19.09
  breast (*see also* Lump, breast) N63.0
  chest R22.2
  cystic — *see* Cyst
  ear H93.8- ☑
  head R22.0
  intra-abdominal (diffuse) (generalized) — *see* Mass, abdominal
  kidney N28.89
  liver R16.0
  localized (skin) R22.9
    chest R22.2
    head R22.0
    limb
      lower R22.4- ☑
      upper R22.3- ☑
    neck R22.1
    trunk R22.2
  lung R91.8
  malignant — *see* Neoplasm, malignant, by site
  neck R22.1
  pelvic (diffuse) (generalized) — *see* Mass, abdominal
  specified organ NEC — *see* Disease, by site
  splenic R16.1
  substernal thyroid — *see* Goiter
  superficial (localized) R22.9
  umbilical (diffuse) (generalized) R19.09
**Massive** — *see* condition
**Mast cell**
  disease, systemic tissue D47.02
  leukemia C94.3- ☑
  neoplasm
    malignant C96.20
      specified type NEC C96.29
    of uncertain behavior NEC D47.09
  sarcoma C96.22
  tumor D47.09
**Mastalgia** N64.4
**Masters-Allen syndrome** N83.8
**Mastitis** (acute) (diffuse) (nonpuerperal) (subacute) N61.0
  with abscess N61.1
  without abscess N61.0
  chronic (cystic) — *see* Mastopathy, cystic
  cystic (Schimmelbusch's type) — *see* Mastopathy, cystic
  fibrocystic — *see* Mastopathy, cystic
  infective N61.0
    newborn P39.0
  interstitial, gestational or puerperal — *see* Mastitis, obstetric
  neonatal (noninfective) P83.4
    infective P39.0
  obstetric (interstitial) (nonpurulent)
    associated with
      lactation O91.23
      pregnancy O91.21- ☑
      puerperium O91.22
    purulent
      associated with
        lactation O91.13
        pregnancy O91.11- ☑
        puerperium O91.12
  periductal — *see* Ectasia, mammary duct
  phlegmonous — *see* Mastopathy, cystic
  plasma cell — *see* Ectasia, mammary duct
**Mastocytoma** (extracutaneous) D47.09
  malignant C96.29
  solitary D47.01
**Mastocytosis** D47.09
  aggressive systemic C96.21
  cutaneous (diffuse) (maculopapular) D47.01
    congenital Q82.8
    of neonatal onset Q82.2

**Mastocytosis** — *continued*
  cutaneous — *continued*
    of newborn onset Q82.2
  indolent systemic D47.02
  isolated bone marrow D47.02
  malignant C96.29
  systemic (indolent) (smoldering)
    with an associated hematological non-mast cell lineage disease (SM-AHNMD) D47.02
**Mastodynia** N64.4
**Mastoid** — *see* condition
**Mastoidalgia** — *see* subcategory H92.0 ☑
**Mastoiditis** (coalescent) (hemorrhagic) (suppurative) H70.9- ☑
  acute, subacute H70.00- ☑
    complicated NEC H70.09- ☑
    subperiosteal H70.01- ☑
  chronic (necrotic) (recurrent) H70.1- ☑
  in (due to)
    infectious disease NEC B99 ☑ [H75.0-] ☑
    parasitic disease NEC B89 [H75.0-] ☑
    tuberculosis A18.03
  petrositis — *see* Petrositis
  postauricular fistula — *see* Fistula, postauricular
  specified NEC H70.89- ☑
  tuberculous A18.03
**Mastopathy, mastopathia** N64.9
  chronica cystica — *see* Mastopathy, cystic
  cystic (chronic) (diffuse) N60.1- ☑
    with epithelial proliferation N60.3- ☑
  diffuse cystic — *see* Mastopathy, cystic
  estrogenic, oestrogenica N64.89
  ovarian origin N64.89
**Mastoplasia, mastoplastia** N62
**Masturbation** (excessive) F98.8
**Maternal care** (for) — *see* Pregnancy (complicated by) (management affected by)
**Matheiu's disease** (leptospiral jaundice) A27.0
**Mauclaire's disease or osteochondrosis** — *see* Osteochondrosis, juvenile, hand, metacarpal
**Maxcy's disease** A75.2
**Maxilla, maxillary** — *see* condition
**May** (-Hegglin) **anomaly or syndrome** D72.0
**McArdle** (-Schmid)(-Pearson) **disease** (glycogen storage) E74.04
**McCune-Albright syndrome** Q78.1
**McQuarrie's syndrome** (idiopathic familial hypoglycemia) E16.2
**Meadow's syndrome** Q86.1
**Measles** (black) (hemorrhagic) (suppressed) B05.9
  with
    complications NEC B05.89
    encephalitis B05.0
    intestinal complications B05.4
    keratitis (keratoconjunctivitis) B05.81
    meningitis B05.1
    otitis media B05.3
    pneumonia B05.2
  French — *see* Rubella
  German — *see* Rubella
  Liberty — *see* Rubella
**Meatitis, urethral** — *see* Urethritis
**Meatus, meatal** — *see* condition
**Meat-wrappers' asthma** J68.9
**Meckel-Gruber syndrome** Q61.9
**Meckel's diverticulitis, diverticulum** (displaced) (hypertrophic) Q43.0
  malignant — *see* Table of Neoplasms, small intestine, malignant
**Meconium**
  ileus, newborn P76.0
    in cystic fibrosis E84.11
    meaning meconium plug (without cystic fibrosis) P76.0
  obstruction, newborn P76.0
    due to fecaliths P76.0
    in mucoviscidosis E84.11
  peritonitis P78.0
  plug syndrome (newborn) NEC P76.0
**Median** (*see also* condition)
  arcuate ligament syndrome I77.4
  bar (prostate) (vesical orifice) — *see* Hyperplasia, prostate
  rhomboid glossitis K14.2
**Mediastinal shift** R93.8
**Mediastinitis** (acute) (chronic) J98.51
  syphilitic A52.73

**Mediastinitis** — *continued*
tuberculous A15.8
**Mediastinopericarditis** (*see also* Pericarditis)
acute I30.9
adhesive I31.0
chronic I31.8
rheumatic I09.2
**Mediastinum, mediastinal** — *see* condition
**Medicine poisoning** — *see* Table of Drugs and Chemicals, by drug, poisoning
**Mediterranean**
fever — *see* Brucellosis
familial M04.1
tick A77.1
kala-azar B55.0
leishmaniasis B55.0
tick fever A77.1
**Medulla** — *see* condition
**Medullary cystic kidney** Q61.5
**Medullated fibers**
optic (nerve) Q14.8
retina Q14.1
**Medulloblastoma**
desmoplastic C71.6
specified site — *see* Neoplasm, malignant, by site
unspecified site C71.6
**Medulloepithelioma** (*see also* Neoplasm, malignant, by site)
teratoid — *see* Neoplasm, malignant, by site
**Medullomyoblastoma**
specified site — *see* Neoplasm, malignant, by site
unspecified site C71.6
**Meekeren-Ehlers-Danlos syndrome** Q79.6
**Megacolon** (acquired) (functional) (not Hirschsprung's disease) (in) K59.39
Chagas' disease B57.32
congenital, congenitum (aganglionic) Q43.1
Hirschsprung's (disease) Q43.1
toxic NEC K59.31
due to Clostridium difficile
not specified as recurrent A04.72
recurrent A04.71
**Megaesophagus** (functional) K22.0
congenital Q39.5
in (due to) Chagas' disease B57.31
**Megalencephaly** Q04.5
**Megalerythema** (epidemic) B08.3
**Megaloappendix** Q43.8
**Megalocephalus, megalocephaly NEC** Q75.3
**Megalocornea** Q15.8
with glaucoma Q15.0
**Megalocytic anemia** D53.1
**Megalodactylia** (fingers) (thumbs) (congenital) Q74.0
toes Q74.2
**Megaloduodenum** Q43.8
**Megaloesophagus** (functional) K22.0
congenital Q39.5
**Megalogastria** (acquired) K31.89
congenital Q40.2
**Megalophthalmos** Q11.3
**Megalopsia** H53.15
**Megalosplenia** — *see* Splenomegaly
**Megaloureter** N28.82
congenital Q62.2
**Megarectum** K62.89
**Megasigmoid** K59.39
congenital Q43.2
**Megaureter** N28.82
congenital Q62.2
**Megavitamin-B6 syndrome** E67.2
**Megrim** — *see* Migraine
**Meibomian**
cyst, infected — *see* Hordeolum
gland — *see* condition
sty, stye — *see* Hordeolum
**Meibomitis** — *see* Hordeolum
**Meige-Milroy disease** (chronic hereditary edema) Q82.0
**Meige's syndrome** Q82.0
**Melalgia, nutritional** E53.8
**Melancholia** F32.9
climacteric (single episode) F32.89
recurrent episode F33.8
hypochondriac F45.29
intermittent (single episode) F32.89
recurrent episode F33.8
involutional (single episode) F32.89
recurrent episode F33.8

**Melancholia** — *continued*
menopausal (single episode) F32.89
recurrent episode F33.8
puerperal F32.89
reactive (emotional stress or trauma) F32.3
recurrent F33.9
senile F03 ☑
stuporous (single episode) F32.89
recurrent episode F33.8
**Melanemia** R79.89
**Melanoameloblastoma** — *see* Neoplasm, bone, benign
**Melanoblastoma** — *see* Melanoma
**Melanocarcinoma** — *see* Melanoma
**Melanocytoma, eyeball** D31.9- ☑
**Melanocytosis, neurocutaneous** Q82.8
**Melanoderma, melanodermia** L81.4
**Melanodontia, infantile** K03.89
**Melanodontoclasia** K03.89
**Melanoepithelioma** — *see* Melanoma
**Melanoma** (malignant) C43.9
acral lentiginous, malignant — *see* Melanoma, skin, by site
amelanotic — *see* Melanoma, skin, by site
balloon cell — *see* Melanoma, skin, by site
benign — *see* Nevus
desmoplastic, malignant — *see* Melanoma, skin, by site
epithelioid cell — *see* Melanoma, skin, by site
with spindle cell, mixed — *see* Melanoma, skin, by site
in
giant pigmented nevus — *see* Melanoma, skin, by site
Hutchinson's melanotic freckle — *see* Melanoma, skin, by site
junctional nevus — *see* Melanoma, skin, by site
precancerous melanosis — *see* Melanoma, skin, by site
in situ D03.9
abdominal wall D03.59
ala nasi D03.39
ankle D03.7- ☑
anus, anal (margin) (skin) D03.51
arm D03.6- ☑
auditory canal D03.2- ☑
auricle (ear) D03.2- ☑
auricular canal (external) D03.2- ☑
axilla, axillary fold D03.59
back D03.59
breast D03.52
brow D03.39
buttock D03.59
canthus (eye) D03.1- ☑
cheek (external) D03.39
chest wall D03.59
chin D03.39
choroid D03.8
conjunctiva D03.8
ear (external) D03.2- ☑
external meatus (ear) D03.2- ☑
eye D03.8
eyebrow D03.39
eyelid (lower) (upper) D03.1- ☑
face D03.30
specified NEC D03.39
female genital organ (external) NEC D03.8
finger D03.6- ☑
flank D03.59
foot D03.7- ☑
forearm D03.6- ☑
forehead D03.39
foreskin D03.8
gluteal region D03.59
groin D03.59
hand D03.6- ☑
heel D03.7- ☑
helix D03.2- ☑
hip D03.7- ☑
interscapular region D03.59
iris D03.8
jaw D03.39
knee D03.7- ☑
labium (majus) (minus) D03.8
lacrimal gland D03.8
leg D03.7- ☑
lip (lower) (upper) D03.0
lower limb NEC D03.7- ☑

**Melanoma** — *continued*
in situ — *continued*
male genital organ (external) NEC D03.8
nail D03.9
finger D03.6- ☑
toe D03.7- ☑
neck D03.4
nose (external) D03.39
orbit D03.8
penis D03.8
perianal skin D03.51
perineum D03.51
pinna D03.2- ☑
popliteal fossa or space D03.7- ☑
prepuce D03.8
pudendum D03.8
retina D03.8
retrobulbar D03.8
scalp D03.4
scrotum D03.8
shoulder D03.6- ☑
specified site NEC D03.8
submammary fold D03.52
temple D03.39
thigh D03.7- ☑
toe D03.7- ☑
trunk NEC D03.59
umbilicus D03.59
upper limb NEC D03.6- ☑
vulva D03.8
juvenile — *see* Nevus
malignant, of soft parts except skin — *see* Neoplasm, connective tissue, malignant
metastatic
breast C79.81
genital organ C79.82
specified site NEC C79.89
neurotropic, malignant — *see* Melanoma, skin, by site
nodular — *see* Melanoma, skin, by site
regressing, malignant — *see* Melanoma, skin, by site
skin C43.9
abdominal wall C43.59
ala nasi C43.31
ankle C43.7- ☑
anus, anal (skin) C43.51
arm C43.6- ☑
auditory canal (external) C43.2- ☑
auricle (ear) C43.2- ☑
auricular canal (external) C43.2- ☑
axilla, axillary fold C43.59
back C43.59
breast (female) (male) C43.52
brow C43.39
buttock C43.59
canthus (eye) C43.1- ☑
cheek (external) C43.39
chest wall C43.59
chin C43.39
ear (external) C43.2- ☑
elbow C43.6- ☑
external meatus (ear) C43.2- ☑
eyebrow C43.39
eyelid (lower) (upper) C43.1- ☑
face C43.30
specified NEC C43.39
female genital organ (external) NEC C51.9
finger C43.6- ☑
flank C43.59
foot C43.7- ☑
forearm C43.6- ☑
forehead C43.39
foreskin C60.0
glabella C43.39
gluteal region C43.59
groin C43.59
hand C43.6- ☑
heel C43.7- ☑
helix C43.2- ☑
hip C43.7- ☑
interscapular region C43.59
jaw (external) C43.39
knee C43.7- ☑
labium C51.9
majus C51.0
minus C51.1
leg C43.7- ☑
lip (lower) (upper) C43.0

☑ **Additional Character Required** — **Refer to the Tabular List for Character Selection**    ▽ **Subterms under main terms may continue to next column or page**

Melanoma — *continued*
  skin — *continued*
    lower limb NEC C43.7- ☑
    male genital organ (external) NEC C63.9
    nail
      finger C43.6- ☑
      toe C43.7- ☑
    nasolabial groove C43.39
    nates C43.59
    neck C43.4
    nose (external) C43.31
    overlapping site C43.8
    palpebra C43.1- ☑
    penis C60.9
    perianal skin C43.51
    perineum C43.51
    pinna C43.2- ☑
    popliteal fossa or space C43.7- ☑
    prepuce C60.0
    pudendum C51.9
    scalp C43.4
    scrotum C63.2
    shoulder C43.6- ☑
    skin NEC C43.9
    submammary fold C43.52
    temple C43.39
    thigh C43.7- ☑
    toe C43.7- ☑
    trunk NEC C43.59
    umbilicus C43.59
    upper limb NEC C43.6- ☑
    vulva C51.9
      overlapping sites C51.8
  spindle cell
    with epithelioid, mixed — *see* Melanoma, skin, by
      site
    type A C69.4- ☑
    type B C69.4- ☑
  superficial spreading — *see* Melanoma, skin, by site
**Melanosarcoma** (*see also* Melanoma)
  epithelioid cell — *see* Melanoma
**Melanosis** L81.4
  addisonian E27.1
    tuberculous A18.7
  adrenal E27.1
  colon K63.89
  conjunctiva — *see* Pigmentation, conjunctiva
    congenital Q13.89
  cornea (presenile) (senile) (*see also* Pigmentation,
    cornea)
    congenital Q13.4
  eye NEC H57.8
    congenital Q15.8
  lenticularis progressiva Q82.1
  liver K76.89
  precancerous (*see also* Melanoma, in situ)
    malignant melanoma in — *see* Melanoma
  Riehl's L81.4
  sclera H15.89
    congenital Q13.89
  suprarenal E27.1
  tar L81.4
  toxic L81.4
**Melanuria** R82.99
**MELAS syndrome** E88.41
**Melasma** L81.1
  adrenal (gland) E27.1
  suprarenal (gland) E27.1
**Melena** K92.1
  with ulcer — *code by* site under Ulcer, with hemor-
    rhage K27.4
  due to swallowed maternal blood P78.2
  newborn, neonatal P54.1
    due to swallowed maternal blood P78.2
**Meleney's**
  gangrene (cutaneous) — *see* Ulcer, skin
  ulcer (chronic undermining) — *see* Ulcer, skin
**Melioidosis** A24.9
  acute A24.1
  chronic A24.2
  fulminating A24.1
  pneumonia A24.1
  pulmonary (chronic) A24.2
    acute A24.1
    subacute A24.2
  sepsis A24.1
  specified NEC A24.3
  subacute A24.2

**Melitensis, febris** A23.0
**Melkersson** (-Rosenthal) **syndrome** G51.2
**Mellitus, diabetes** — *see* Diabetes
**Melorheostosis** (bone) — *see* Disorder, bone, density
  and structure, specified NEC
**Meloschisis** Q18.4
**Melotia** Q17.4
**Membrana**
  capsularis lentis posterior Q13.89
  epipapillaris Q14.2
**Membranacea placenta** O43.19- ☑
**Membranaceous uterus** N85.8
**Membrane**(s), membranous (*see also* condition)
  cyclitic — *see* Membrane, pupillary
  folds, congenital — *see* Web
  Jackson's Q43.3
  over face of newborn P28.9
  premature rupture — *see* Rupture, membranes, pre-
    mature
  pupillary H21.4- ☑
    persistent Q13.89
  retained (with hemorrhage) (complicating delivery)
    O72.2
    without hemorrhage O73.1
  secondary cataract — *see* Cataract, secondary
  unruptured (causing asphyxia) — *see* Asphyxia, new-
    born
  vitreous — *see* Opacity, vitreous, membranes and
    strands
**Membranitis** — *see* Chorioamnionitis
**Memory disturbance, lack or loss** (*see also* Amnesia)
  mild, following organic brain damage F06.8
**Menadione deficiency** E56.1
**Menarche**
  delayed E30.0
  precocious E30.1
**Mendacity, pathologic** F60.2
**Mendelson's syndrome** (due to anesthesia) J95.4
  in labor and delivery O74.0
  in pregnancy O29.01- ☑
  obstetric O74.0
  postpartum, puerperal O89.01
**Ménétrier's disease or syndrome** K29.60
  with bleeding K29.61
**Ménière's disease, syndrome or vertigo** H81.0- ☑
**Meninges, meningeal** — *see* condition
**Meningioma** (*see also* Neoplasm, meninges, benign)
  angioblastic — *see* Neoplasm, meninges, benign
  angiomatous — *see* Neoplasm, meninges, benign
  endotheliomatous — *see* Neoplasm, meninges, benign
  fibroblastic — *see* Neoplasm, meninges, benign
  fibrous — *see* Neoplasm, meninges, benign
  hemangioblastic — *see* Neoplasm, meninges, benign
  hemangiopericytic — *see* Neoplasm, meninges, be-
    nign
  malignant — *see* Neoplasm, meninges, malignant
  meningiothelial — *see* Neoplasm, meninges, benign
  meningotheliomatous — *see* Neoplasm, meninges,
    benign
  mixed — *see* Neoplasm, meninges, benign
  multiple — *see* Neoplasm, meninges, uncertain behav-
    ior
  papillary — *see* Neoplasm, meninges, uncertain behav-
    ior
  psammomatous — *see* Neoplasm, meninges, benign
  syncytial — *see* Neoplasm, meninges, benign
  transitional — *see* Neoplasm, meninges, benign
**Meningiomatosis** (diffuse) — *see* Neoplasm, meninges,
  uncertain behavior
**Meningism** — *see* Meningismus
**Meningismus** (infectional) (pneumococcal) R29.1
  due to serum or vaccine R29.1
  influenzal — *see* Influenza, with, manifestations NEC
**Meningitis** (basal) (basic) (brain) (cerebral) (cervical)
  (congestive) (diffuse) (hemorrhagic) (infantile)
  (membranous) (metastatic) (nonspecific) (pontine)
  (progressive) (simple) (spinal) (subacute) (sympathetic) (toxic) G03.9
  abacterial G03.0
  actinomycotic A42.81
  adenoviral A87.1
  arbovirus A87.8
  aseptic (acute) G03.0
  bacterial G00.9
    Escherichia coli (E. coli) G00.8
    Friedländer (bacillus) G00.8
    gram-negative G00.9

Meningitis — *continued*
  bacterial — *continued*
    H. influenzae G00.0
    Klebsiella G00.8
    pneumococcal G00.1
    specified organism NEC G00.8
    staphylococcal G00.3
    streptococcal (acute) G00.2
  benign recurrent (Mollaret) G03.2
  candidal B37.5
  caseous (tuberculous) A17.0
  cerebrospinal A39.0
  chronic NEC G03.1
  clear cerebrospinal fluid NEC G03.0
  coxsackievirus A87.0
  cryptococcal B45.1
  diplococcal (gram positive) A39.0
  echovirus A87.0
  enteroviral A87.0
  eosinophilic B83.2
  epidemic NEC A39.0
  Escherichia coli (E. coli) G00.8
  fibrinopurulent G00.9
    specified organism NEC G00.8
  Friedländer (bacillus) G00.8
  gonococcal A54.81
  gram-negative cocci G00.9
  gram-positive cocci G00.9
  H. influenzae G00.0
  Haemophilus (influenzae) G00.0
  in (due to)
    adenovirus A87.1
    African trypanosomiasis B56.9 [G02]
    anthrax A22.8
    bacterial disease NEC A48.8 [G01]
    Chagas' disease (chronic) B57.41
    chickenpox B01.0
    coccidioidomycosis B38.4
    Diplococcus pneumoniae G00.1
    enterovirus A87.0
    herpes (simplex) virus B00.3
      zoster B02.1
    infectious mononucleosis B27.92
    leptospirosis A27.81
    Listeria monocytogenes A32.11
    Lyme disease A69.21
    measles B05.1
    mumps (virus) B26.1
    neurosyphilis (late) A52.13
    parasitic disease NEC B89 [G02]
    poliovirus A80.9 [G02]
    preventive immunization, inoculation or vaccina-
      tion G03.8
    rubella B06.02
    Salmonella infection A02.21
    specified cause NEC G03.8
    Streptococcal pneumoniae G00.1
    typhoid fever A01.01
    varicella B01.0
    viral disease NEC A87.8
    whooping cough A37.90
    zoster B02.1
  infectious G00.9
  influenzal (H. influenzae) G00.0
  Klebsiella G00.8
  leptospiral (aseptic) A27.81
  lymphocytic (acute) (benign) (serous) A87.2
  meningococcal A39.0
  Mima polymorpha G00.8
  Mollaret (benign recurrent) G03.2
  monilial B37.5
  mycotic NEC B49 [G02]
  Neisseria A39.0
  nonbacterial G03.0
  nonpyogenic NEC G03.0
  ossificans G96.19
  pneumococcal streptococcus pneumoniae G00.1
  poliovirus A80.9 [G02]
  postmeasles B05.1
  purulent G00.9
    specified organism NEC G00.8
  pyogenic G00.9
    specified organism NEC G00.8
  Salmonella (arizonae) (Cholerae-Suis) (enteritidis) (ty-
    phimurium) A02.21
  septic G00.9
    specified organism NEC G00.8
  serosa circumscripta NEC G03.0
  serous NEC G93.2

⬇ Subterms under main terms may continue to next column or page    ☑ **Additional Character Required — Refer to the Tabular List for Character Selection**    **221**

Melanoma — Meningitis

**Meningitis** — continued
  specified organism NEC G00.8
  sporotrichosis B42.81
  staphylococcal G00.3
  sterile G03.0
  Streptococcal (acute) G00.2
    pneumoniae G00.1
  suppurative G00.9
    specified organism NEC G00.8
  syphilitic (late) (tertiary) A52.13
    acute A51.41
    congenital A50.41
    secondary A51.41
  Torula histolytica (cryptococcal) B45.1
  traumatic (complication of injury) T79.8 ☑
  tuberculous A17.0
  typhoid A01.01
  viral NEC A87.9
  Yersinia pestis A20.3
**Meningocele** (spinal) (see also Spina bifida)
  with hydrocephalus — see Spina bifida, by site, with
    hydrocephalus
  acquired (traumatic) G96.19
  cerebral — see Encephalocele
**Meningocerebritis** — see Meningoencephalitis
**Meningococcemia** A39.4
  acute A39.2
  chronic A39.3
**Meningococcus, meningococcal** (see also condition)
  A39.9
  adrenalitis, hemorrhagic A39.1
  carrier (suspected) of Z22.31
  meningitis (cerebrospinal) A39.0
**Meningoencephalitis** (see also Encephalitis) G04.90
  acute NEC (see also Encephalitis, viral) A86
  bacterial NEC G04.2
  California A83.5
  diphasic A84.1
  eosinophilic B83.2
  epidemic A39.81
  herpesviral, herpetic B00.4
    due to herpesvirus 6 B10.01
    due to herpesvirus 7 B10.09
    specified NEC B10.09
  in (due to)
    blastomycosis NEC B40.81
    diseases classified elsewhere G05.3
    free-living amebae B60.2
    H. influenzae G00.0
    Hemophilus influenzae (H .influenzae) G00.0
    herpes B00.4
      due to herpesvirus 6 B10.01
      due to herpesvirus 7 B10.09
      specified NEC B10.09
    Lyme disease A69.22
    mercury — see subcategory T56.1 ☑
    mumps B26.2
    Naegleria (amebae) (organisms) (fowleri) B60.2
    Parastrongylus cantonensis B83.2
    toxoplasmosis (acquired) B58.2
      congenital P37.1
  infectious (acute) (viral) A86
  influenzal (H. influenzae) G00.0
  Listeria monocytogenes A32.12
  lymphocytic (serous) A87.2
  mumps B26.2
  parasitic NEC B89 [G05.3]
  pneumococcal G04.2
  primary amebic B60.2
  specific (syphilitic) A52.14
  specified organism NEC G04.81
  staphylococcal G04.2
  streptococcal G04.2
  syphilitic A52.14
  toxic NEC G92
    due to mercury — see subcategory T56.1 ☑
  tuberculous A17.82
  virus NEC A86
**Meningoencephalocele** (see also Encephalocele)
  syphilitic A52.19
    congenital A50.49
**Meningoencephalomyelitis** (see also Meningoencephalitis)
  acute NEC (viral) A86
    disseminated G04.00
      postimmunization or postvaccination G04.02
      postinfectious G04.01

**Meningoencephalomyelitis** — continued
  due to
    actinomycosis A42.82
    Torula B45.1
    Toxoplasma or toxoplasmosis (acquired) B58.2
      congenital P37.1
  postimmunization or postvaccination G04.02
**Meningoencephalomyelopathy** G96.9
**Meningoencephalopathy** G96.9
**Meningomyelitis** (see also Meningoencephalitis)
  bacterial NEC G04.2
  blastomycotic NEC B40.81
  cryptococcal B45.1
  in diseases classified elsewhere G05.4
  meningococcal A39.81
  syphilitic A52.14
  tuberculous A17.82
**Meningomyelocele** (see also Spina bifida)
  syphilitic A52.19
**Meningomyeloneuritis** — see Meningoencephalitis
**Meningoradiculitis** — see Meningitis
**Meningovascular** — see condition
**Menkes' disease or syndrome** E83.09
  meaning maple-syrup-urine disease E71.0
**Menometrorrhagia** N92.1
**Menopause, menopausal** (asymptomatic) (state) Z78.0
  arthritis (any site) NEC — see Arthritis, specified form
    NEC
  bleeding N92.4
  depression (single episode) F32.89
    agitated (single episode) F32.2
      recurrent episode F33.9
    psychotic (single episode) F32.89
      recurrent episode F33.9
    recurrent episode F33.8
  melancholia (single episode) F32.89
    recurrent episode F33.8
  paranoid state F22
  premature E28.319
    asymptomatic E28.319
      postirradiation E89.40
      postsurgical E89.40
    symptomatic E28.310
      postirradiation E89.41
      postsurgical E89.41
  psychosis NEC F28
  symptomatic N95.1
  toxic polyarthritis NEC — see Arthritis, specified form
    NEC
**Menorrhagia** (primary) N92.0
  climacteric N92.4
    menopausal N92.4
  menopausal N92.4
  postclimacteric N95.0
  postmenopausal N95.0
  preclimacteric or premenopausal N92.4
  pubertal (menses retained) N92.2
**Menostaxis** N92.0
**Menses, retention** N94.89
**Menstrual** — see Menstruation
**Menstruation**
  absent — see Amenorrhea
  anovulatory N97.0
  cycle, irregular N92.6
  delayed N91.0
  disorder N93.9
    psychogenic F45.8
  during pregnancy O20.8
  excessive (with regular cycle) N92.0
    with irregular cycle N92.1
    at puberty N92.2
  frequent N92.0
  infrequent — see Oligomenorrhea
  irregular N92.6
    specified NEC N92.5
  latent N92.5
  membranous N92.5
  painful (see also Dysmenorrhea) N94.6
    primary N94.4
    psychogenic F45.8
    secondary N94.5
  passage of clots N92.0
  precocious E30.1
  protracted N92.5
  rare — see Oligomenorrhea
  retained N94.89
  retrograde N92.5
  scanty — see Oligomenorrhea

**Menstruation** — continued
  suppression N94.89
  vicarious (nasal) N94.89
**Mental** (see also condition)
  deficiency — see Disability, intellectual
  deterioration — see Psychosis
  disorder — see Disorder, mental
  exhaustion F48.8
  insufficiency (congenital) — see Disability, intellectual
  observation without need for further medical care
    Z03.89
  retardation — see Disability, intellectual
  subnormality — see Disability, intellectuall
  upset — see Disorder, mental
**Meralgia paresthetica** G57.1- ☑
**Mercurial** — see condition
**Mercurialism** — see subcategory T56.1 ☑
**Merkel cell tumor** — see Carcinoma, Merkel cell
**Merocele** — see Hernia, femoral
**Meromelia**
  lower limb — see Defect, reduction, lower limb
    intercalary
      femur — see Defect, reduction, lower limb,
        specified type NEC
        tibiofibular (complete) (incomplete) — see
          Defect, reduction, lower limb
  upper limb — see Defect, reduction, upper limb
    intercalary, humeral, radioulnar — see Agenesis,
      arm, with hand present
**MERRF syndrome** (myoclonic epilepsy associated with
  ragged-red fiber) E88.42
**Merzbacher-Pelizaeus disease** E75.29
**Mesaortitis** — see Aortitis
**Mesarteritis** — see Arteritis
**Mesencephalitis** — see Encephalitis
**Mesenchymoma** (see also Neoplasm, connective tissue,
  uncertain behavior)
  benign — see Neoplasm, connective tissue, benign
  malignant — see Neoplasm, connective tissue, malig-
    nant
**Mesenteritis**
  retractile K65.4
  sclerosing K65.4
**Mesentery, mesenteric** — see condition
**Mesiodens, mesiodentes** K00.1
**Mesio-occlusion** M26.213
**Mesocolon** — see condition
**Mesonephroma** (malignant) — see Neoplasm, malig-
  nant, by site
  benign — see Neoplasm, benign, by site
**Mesophlebitis** — see Phlebitis
**Mesostromal dysgenesis** Q13.89
**Mesothelioma** (malignant) C45.9
  benign
    mesentery D19.1
    mesocolon D19.1
    omentum D19.1
    peritoneum D19.1
    pleura D19.0
    specified site NEC D19.7
    unspecified site D19.9
  biphasic C45.9
    benign
      mesentery D19.1
      mesocolon D19.1
      omentum D19.1
      peritoneum D19.1
      pleura D19.0
      specified site NEC D19.7
      unspecified site D19.9
  cystic D48.4
  epithelioid C45.9
    benign
      mesentery D19.1
      mesocolon D19.1
      omentum D19.1
      peritoneum D19.1
      pleura D19.0
      specified site NEC D19.7
      unspecified site D19.9
  fibrous C45.9
    benign
      mesentery D19.1
      mesocolon D19.1
      omentum D19.1
      peritoneum D19.1
      pleura D19.0
      specified site NEC D19.7

**Mesothelioma** — *continued*
  fibrous — *continued*
    benign — *continued*
      unspecified site D19.9
    site classification
      liver C45.7
      lung C45.7
      mediastinum C45.7
      mesentery C45.1
      mesocolon C45.1
      omentum C45.1
      pericardium C45.2
      peritoneum C45.1
      pleura C45.0
        parietal C45.0
      retroperitoneum C45.7
      specified site NEC C45.7
      unspecified C45.9
**Metabolic syndrome** E88.81
**Metagonimiasis** B66.8
**Metagonimus infestation** (intestine) B66.8
**Metal**
  pigmentation L81.8
  polisher's disease J62.8
**Metamorphopsia** H53.15
**Metaplasia**
  apocrine (breast) — *see* Dysplasia, mammary, specified type NEC
  cervix (squamous) — *see* Dysplasia, cervix
  endometrium (squamous) (uterus) N85.8
  esophagus K22.7- ☑
  kidney (pelvis) (squamous) N28.89
  myelogenous D73.1
  myeloid (agnogenic) (megakaryocytic) D73.1
  spleen D73.1
  squamous cell, bladder N32.89
**Metastasis, metastatic**
  abscess — *see* Abscess
  calcification E83.59
  cancer
    from specified site — *see* Neoplasm, malignant, by site
    to specified site — *see* Neoplasm, secondary, by site
  deposits (in) — *see* Neoplasm, secondary, by site
  disease (*see also* Neoplasm, secondary, by site) C79.9
  spread (to) — *see* Neoplasm, secondary, by site
**Metastrongyliasis** B83.8
**Metatarsalgia** M77.4- ☑
  anterior G57.6- ☑
  Morton's G57.6- ☑
**Metatarsus, metatarsal** (*see also* condition)
  adductus, congenital Q66.22
  valgus (abductus), congenital Q66.6
  varus (congenital) Q66.22
    primus Q66.21
**Methadone use** — *see* Use, opioid
**Methemoglobinemia** D74.9
  acquired (with sulfhemoglobinemia) D74.8
  congenital D74.0
  enzymatic (congenital) D74.0
  Hb M disease D74.0
  hereditary D74.0
  toxic D74.8
**Methemoglobinuria** — *see* Hemoglobinuria
**Methioninemia** E72.19
**Methylmalonic acidemia** E71.120
**Metritis** (catarrhal) (hemorrhagic) (septic) (suppurative) (*see also* Endometritis)
  cervical — *see* Cervicitis
**Metropathia hemorrhagica** N93.8
**Metroperitonitis** — *see* Peritonitis, pelvic, female
**Metrorrhagia** N92.1
  climacteric N92.4
  menopausal N92.4
  postpartum NEC (atonic) (following delivery of placenta) O72.1
    delayed or secondary O72.2
  preclimacteric or premenopausal N92.4
  psychogenic F45.8
**Metrorrhexis** — *see* Rupture, uterus
**Metrosalpingitis** N70.91
**Metrostaxis** N93.8
**Metrovaginitis** — *see* Endometritis
**Meyer-Schwickerath and Weyers syndrome** Q87.0
**Meynert's amentia** (nonalcoholic) F04
  alcoholic F10.96

**Meynert's amentia** — *continued*
  alcoholic — *continued*
    with dependence F10.26
**Mibelli's disease** (porokeratosis) Q82.8
**Mice, joint** — *see* Loose, body, joint
  knee M23.4- ☑
**Micrencephalon, micrencephaly** Q02
**Microalbuminuria** R80.9
**Microaneurysm, retinal** (*see also* Disorder, retina, microaneurysms)
  diabetic — *see* E08-E13 with .31
**Microangiopathy** (peripheral) I73.9
  thrombotic M31.1
**Microcalcifications, breast** R92.0
**Microcephalus, microcephalic, microcephaly** Q02
  due to toxoplasmosis (congenital) P37.1
**Microcheilia** Q18.7
**Microcolon** (congenital) Q43.8
**Microcornea** (congenital) Q13.4
**Microcytic** — *see* condition
**Microdeletions NEC** Q93.88
**Microdontia** K00.2
**Microdrepanocytosis** D57.40
  with crisis (vasoocclusive pain) D57.419
    with
      acute chest syndrome D57.411
      splenic sequestration D57.412
**Microembolism**
  atherothrombotic — *see* Atheroembolism
  retinal — *see* Occlusion, artery, retina
**Microencephalon** Q02
**Microfilaria streptocerca infestation** — *see* Onchocerciasis
**Microgastria** (congenital) Q40.2
**Microgenia** M26.06
**Microgenitalia, congenital**
  female Q52.8
  male Q55.8
**Microglioma** — *see* Lymphoma, non-Hodgkin, specified NEC
**Microglossia** (congenital) Q38.3
**Micrognathia, micrognathism** (congenital) (mandibular) (maxillary) M26.09
**Microgyria** (congenital) Q04.3
**Microinfarct of heart** — *see* Insufficiency, coronary
**Microlentia** (congenital) Q12.8
**Microlithiasis, alveolar, pulmonary** J84.02
**Micromastia** N64.82
**Micromyelia** (congenital) Q06.8
**Micropenis** Q55.62
**Microphakia** (congenital) Q12.8
**Microphthalmos, microphthalmia** (congenital) Q11.2
  due to toxoplasmosis P37.1
**Micropsia** H53.15
**Microscopic polyangiitis** (polyarteritis) M31.7
**Microsporidiosis** B60.8
  intestinal A07.8
**Microsporon furfur infestation** B36.0
**Microsporosis** (*see also* Dermatophytosis)
  nigra B36.1
**Microstomia** (congenital) Q18.5
**Microtia** (congenital) (external ear) Q17.2
**Microtropia** H50.40
**Microvillus inclusion disease** (MVD) (MVID) Q43.8
**Micturition**
  disorder NEC (*see also* Difficulty, micturition) R39.198
    psychogenic F45.8
  frequency R35.0
    psychogenic F45.8
  hesitancy R39.11
  incomplete emptying R39.14
  nocturnal R35.1
  painful R30.9
    dysuria R30.0
    psychogenic F45.8
    tenesmus R30.1
  poor stream R39.12
  position dependent R39.192
  split stream R39.13
  straining R39.16
  urgency R39.15
**Mid plane** — *see* condition
**Middle**
  ear — *see* condition
  lobe (right) syndrome J98.19
**Miescher's elastoma** L87.2
**Mietens' syndrome** Q87.2

**Migraine** (idiopathic) G43.909
  with aura (acute-onset) (prolonged) (typical) (without headache) G43.109
    with refractory migraine G43.119
      with status migrainosus G43.111
      without status migrainosus G43.119
    without mention of refractory migraine G43.109
      with status migrainosus G43.101
      without status migrainosus G43.109
    intractable G43.119
      with status migrainosus G43.111
      without status migrainosus G43.119
    not intractable G43.109
      with status migrainosus G43.101
      without status migrainosus G43.109
    persistent G43.509
      with cerebral infarction G43.609
        with refractory migraine G43.619
          with status migrainosus G43.611
          without status migrainosus G43.619
        without refractory migraine G43.609
          with status migrainosus G43.601
          without status migrainosus G43.609
        intractable G43.619
          with status migrainosus G43.611
          without status migrainosus G43.619
        not intractable G43.609
          with status migrainosus G43.601
          without status migrainosus G43.609
      without cerebral infarction G43.509
        with refractory migraine G43.519
          with status migrainosus G43.511
          without status migrainosus G43.519
        without refractory migraine G43.509
          with status migrainosus G43.501
          without status migrainosus G43.509
        intractable G43.519
          with status migrainosus G43.511
          without status migrainosus G43.519
        not intractable G43.509
          with status migrainosus G43.501
          without status migrainosus G43.509
  with refractory migraine G43.919
    with status migrainosus G43.911
    without status migrainosus G43.919
  without aura G43.009
    with refractory migraine G43.019
      with status migrainosus G43.011
      without status migrainosus G43.019
    without mention of refractory migraine G43.009
      with status migrainosus G43.001
      without status migrainosus G43.009
    chronic G43.709
      with refractory migraine G43.719
        with status migrainosus G43.711
        without status migrainosus G43.719
      without refractory migraine G43.709
        with status migrainosus G43.701
        without status migrainosus G43.709
      intractable
        with status migrainosus G43.711
        without status migrainosus G43.719
      not intractable
        with status migrainosus G43.701
        without status migrainosus G43.709
    intractable
      with status migrainosus G43.011
      without status migrainosus G43.019
    not intractable
      with status migrainosus G43.001
      without status migrainosus G43.009
  without refractory migraine G43.909
    with status migrainosus G43.901
    without status migrainosus G43.919
  abdominal G43.D0 (*following* G43.7)
    with refractory migraine G43.D1 (*following* G43.7)
    without refractory migraine G43.D0 (*following* G43.7)
    intractable G43.D1 (*following* G43.7)
    not intractable G43.D0 (*following* G43.7)
  basilar — *see* Migraine, with aura
  classical — *see* Migraine, with aura
  common — *see* Migraine, without aura
  complicated G43.109
  equivalents — *see* Migraine, with aura
  familiar — *see* Migraine, hemiplegic
  hemiplegic G43.409
    with refractory migraine G43.419
      with status migrainosus G43.411

▼ Subterms under main terms may continue to next column or page    ☑ Additional Character Required — Refer to the Tabular List for Character Selection    **223**

**Mesothelioma — Migraine**

☑ **Additional Character Required** — Refer to the Tabular List for Character Selection      ▽ **Subterms under main terms may continue to next column or page**

**Mononeuropathy** — *continued*
  intercostal G58.0
  lower limb G57.9- ☑
    causalgia — *see* Causalgia, lower limb
    femoral nerve — *see* Lesion, nerve, femoral
    meralgia paresthetica G57.1- ☑
    plantar nerve — *see* Lesion, nerve, plantar
    popliteal nerve — *see* Lesion, nerve, popliteal
    sciatic nerve — *see* Lesion, nerve, sciatic
    specified NEC G57.8- ☑
    tarsal tunnel syndrome — *see* Syndrome, tarsal
      tunnel
  median nerve — *see* Lesion, nerve, median
  multiplex G58.7
  obturator nerve G57.8- ☑
  popliteal nerve — *see* Lesion, nerve, popliteal
  radial nerve — *see* Lesion, nerve, radial
  saphenous nerve G57.8- ☑
  specified NEC G58.8
  tarsal tunnel syndrome — *see* Syndrome, tarsal tunnel
  tuberculous A17.83
  ulnar nerve — *see* Lesion, nerve, ulnar
  upper limb G56.9- ☑
    carpal tunnel syndrome — *see* Syndrome, carpal
      tunnel
    causalgia — *see* Causalgia
    median nerve — *see* Lesion, nerve, median
    radial nerve — *see* Lesion, nerve, radial
    specified site NEC G56.8- ☑
    ulnar nerve — *see* Lesion, nerve, ulnar
**Mononucleosis, infectious** B27.90
  with
    complication NEC B27.99
    meningitis B27.92
    polyneuropathy B27.91
  cytomegaloviral B27.10
    with
      complication NEC B27.19
      meningitis B27.12
      polyneuropathy B27.11
  Epstein-Barr (virus) B27.00
    with
      complication NEC B27.09
      meningitis B27.02
      polyneuropathy B27.01
  gammaherpesviral B27.00
    with
      complication NEC B27.09
      meningitis B27.02
      polyneuropathy B27.01
  specified NEC B27.80
    with
      complication NEC B27.89
      meningitis B27.82
      polyneuropathy B27.81
**Monoplegia** G83.3- ☑
  congenital (cerebral) G80.8
    spastic G80.1
  embolic (current episode) I63.4- ☑
  following
    cerebrovascular disease
      cerebral infarction
        lower limb I69.34- ☑
        upper limb I69.33- ☑
      intracerebral hemorrhage
        lower limb I69.14- ☑
        upper limb I69.13- ☑
      lower limb I69.94- ☑
      nontraumatic intracranial hemorrhage NEC
        lower limb I69.24- ☑
        upper limb I69.23- ☑
      specified disease NEC
        lower limb I69.84- ☑
        upper limb I69.83- ☑
      stroke NOS
        lower limb I69.34- ☑
        upper limb I69.33- ☑
      subarachnoid hemorrhage
        lower limb I69.04- ☑
        upper limb I69.03- ☑
      upper limb I69.93- ☑
  hysterical (transient) F44.4
  lower limb G83.1- ☑
  psychogenic (conversion reaction) F44.4
  thrombotic (current episode) I63.3- ☑
  transient R29.818
  upper limb G83.2- ☑

**Monorchism, monorchidism** Q55.0
**Monosomy** (*see also* Deletion, chromosome) Q93.9
  specified NEC Q93.89
  whole chromosome
    meiotic nondisjunction Q93.0
    mitotic nondisjunction Q93.1
    mosaicism Q93.1
  X Q96.9
**Monster, monstrosity** (single) Q89.7
  acephalic Q00.0
  twin Q89.4
**Monteggia's fracture** (-dislocation) S52.27- ☑
**Mooren's ulcer** (cornea) — *see* Ulcer, cornea, Mooren's
**Moore's syndrome** — *see* Epilepsy, specified NEC
**Mooser-Neill reaction** A75.2
**Mooser's bodies** A75.2
**Morbidity not stated or unknown** R69
**Morbilli** — *see* Measles
**Morbus** (*see also* Disease)
  angelicus, anglorum E55.0
  Beigel B36.2
  caducus — *see* Epilepsy
  celiacus K90.0
  comitialis — *see* Epilepsy
  cordis (*see also* Disease, heart) I51.9
    valvulorum — *see* Endocarditis
  coxae senilis M16.9
    tuberculous A18.02
  hemorrhagicus neonatorum P53
  maculosus neonatorum P54.5
**Morel** (-Stewart)(-Morgagni) **syndrome** M85.2
**Morel-Kraepelin disease** — *see* Schizophrenia
**Morel-Moore syndrome** M85.2
**Morgagni's**
  cyst, organ, hydatid, or appendage
    female Q50.5
    male (epididymal) Q55.4
      testicular Q55.29
  syndrome M85.2
**Morgagni-Stewart-Morel syndrome** M85.2
**Morgagni-Stokes-Adams syndrome** I45.9
**Morgagni-Turner** (-Albright) **syndrome** Q96.9
**Moria** F07.0
**Moron** (I.Q. 50-69) F70
**Morphea** L94.0
**Morphinism** (without remission) F11.20
  with remission F11.21
**Morphinomania** (without remission) F11.20
  with remission F11.21
**Morquio** (-Ullrich)(-Brailsford) **disease or syndrome** —
    *see* Mucopolysaccharidosis
**Mortification** (dry) (moist) — *see* Gangrene
**Morton's metatarsalgia** (neuralgia)(neuroma) (syn-
    drome) G57.6- ☑
**Morvan's disease or syndrome** G60.8
**Mosaicism, mosaic** (autosomal) (chromosomal)
  45,X/46,XX Q96.3
  45,X/other cell lines NEC with abnormal sex chromo-
    some Q96.4
  sex chromosome
    female Q97.8
    lines with various numbers of X chromosomes
      Q97.2
    male Q98.7
  XY Q96.3
**Moschowitz' disease** M31.1
**Mother yaw** A66.0
**Motion sickness** (from travel, any vehicle) (from round-
    abouts or swings) T75.3 ☑
**Mottled, mottling, teeth** (enamel) (endemic) (nonen-
    demic) K00.3
**Mounier-Kuhn syndrome** Q32.4
  with bronchiectasis J47.9
    exacerbation (acute) J47.1
    lower respiratory infection J47.0
  acquired J98.09
    with bronchiectasis J47.9
      with
        exacerbation (acute) J47.1
        lower respiratory infection J47.0
**Mountain**
  sickness T70.29 ☑
    with polycythemia , acquired (acute) D75.1
  tick fever A93.2
**Mouse, joint** — *see* Loose, body, joint
  knee M23.4- ☑
**Mouth** — *see* condition

**Movable**
  coccyx — *see* subcategory M53.2 ☑
  kidney N28.89
    congenital Q63.8
  spleen D73.89
**Movements, dystonic** R25.8
**Moyamoya disease** I67.5
**MRSA** (Methicillin resistant Staphylococcus aureus)
  infection A49.02
    as the cause of diseases classified elsewhere B95.62
  sepsis A41.02
**MSSA** (Methicillin susceptible Staphylococcus aureus)
  infection A49.01
    as the cause of diseases classified elsewhere B95.61
  sepsis A41.01
**Mucha-Habermann disease** L41.0
**Mucinosis** (cutaneous) (focal) (papular) (skin) L98.5
  oral K13.79
**Mucocele**
  appendix K38.8
  buccal cavity K13.79
  gallbladder K82.1
  lacrimal sac, chronic H04.43- ☑
  nasal sinus J34.1
  nose J34.1
  salivary gland (any) K11.6
  sinus (accessory) (nasal) J34.1
  turbinate (bone) (middle) (nasal) J34.1
  uterus N85.8
**Mucolipidosis**
  I E77.1
  II, III E77.0
  IV E75.11
**Mucopolysaccharidosis** E76.3
  beta-gluduronidase deficiency E76.29
  cardiopathy E76.3 [I52]
  Hunter's syndrome E76.1
  Hurler's syndrome E76.01
  Hurler-Scheie syndrome E76.02
  Maroteaux-Lamy syndrome E76.29
  Morquio syndrome E76.219
    A E76.210
    B E76.211
    classic E76.210
  Sanfilippo syndrome E76.22
  Scheie's syndrome E76.03
  specified NEC E76.29
  type
    I
      Hurler's syndrome E76.01
      Hurler-Scheie syndrome E76.02
      Scheie's syndrome E76.03
    II E76.1
    III E76.22
    IV E76.219
    IVA E76.210
    IVB E76.211
    VI E76.29
    VII E76.29
**Mucormycosis** B46.5
  cutaneous B46.3
  disseminated B46.4
  gastrointestinal B46.2
  generalized B46.4
  pulmonary B46.0
  rhinocerebral B46.1
  skin B46.3
  subcutaneous B46.3
**Mucositis** (ulcerative) K12.30
  due to drugs NEC K12.32
  gastrointestinal K92.81
  mouth (oral) (oropharyngeal) K12.30
    due to antineoplastic therapy K12.31
    due to drugs NEC K12.32
    due to radiation K12.33
    specified NEC K12.39
    viral K12.39
  nasal J34.81
  oral cavity — *see* Mucositis, mouth
  oral soft tissues — *see* Mucositis, mouth
  vagina and vulva N76.81
**Mucositis necroticans agranulocytica** — *see* Agranu-
    locytosis
**Mucous** (*see also* condition)
  patches (syphilitic) A51.39
    congenital A50.07
**Mucoviscidosis** E84.9
  with meconium obstruction E84.11

**Mucus**
asphyxia or suffocation — *see* Asphyxia, mucus
in stool R19.5
plug — *see* Asphyxia, mucus
**Muguet** B37.0
**Mulberry molars** (congenital syphilis) A50.52
**Müllerian mixed tumor**
specified site — *see* Neoplasm, malignant, by site
unspecified site C54.9
**Multicystic kidney** (development) Q61.4
**Multiparity** (grand) Z64.1
affecting management of pregnancy, labor and delivery (supervision only) O09.4- ☑
requiring contraceptive management — *see* Contraception
**Multipartita placenta** O43.19- ☑
**Multiple, multiplex** (*see also* condition)
digits (congenital) Q69.9
endocrine neoplasia — *see* Neoplasia, endocrine, multiple (MEN)
personality F44.81
**Mumps** B26.9
arthritis B26.85
complication NEC B26.89
encephalitis B26.2
hepatitis B26.81
meningitis (aseptic) B26.1
meningoencephalitis B26.2
myocarditis B26.82
oophoritis B26.89
orchitis B26.0
pancreatitis B26.3
polyneuropathy B26.84
**Mumu** (*see also* Infestation, filarial) B74.9 [N51]
**Münchhausen's syndrome** — *see* Disorder, factitious
**Münchmeyer's syndrome** — *see* Myositis, ossificans, progressiva
**Mural** — *see* condition
**Murmur** (cardiac) (heart) (organic) R01.1
abdominal R19.15
aortic (valve) — *see* Endocarditis, aortic
benign R01.0
diastolic — *see* Endocarditis
Flint I35.1
functional R01.0
Graham Steell I37.1
innocent R01.0
mitral (valve) — *see* Insufficiency, mitral
nonorganic R01.0
presystolic, mitral — *see* Insufficiency, mitral
pulmonic (valve) I37.8
systolic R01.1
tricuspid (valve) I07.9
valvular — *see* Endocarditis
**Murri's disease** (intermittent hemoglobinuria) D59.6
**Muscle, muscular** (*see also* condition)
carnitine (palmityltransferase) deficiency E71.314
**Musculoneuralgia** — *see* Neuralgia
**Mushrooming hip** — *see* Derangement, joint, specified NEC, hip
**Mushroom-workers'** (pickers') **disease or lung** J67.5
**Mutation**(s)
factor V Leiden D68.51
prothrombin gene D68.52
surfactant, of lung J84.83
**Mutism** (*see also* Aphasia)
deaf (acquired) (congenital) NEC H91.3
elective (adjustment reaction) (childhood) F94.0
hysterical F44.4
selective (childhood) F94.0
**MVD** (microvillus inclusion disease) Q43.8
**MVID** (microvillus inclusion disease) Q43.8
**Myalgia** M79.1
epidemic (cervical) B33.0
traumatic NEC T14.8 ☑
**Myasthenia** G70.9
congenital G70.2
cordis — *see* Failure, heart
developmental G70.2
gravis G70.00
with exacerbation (acute) G70.01
in crisis G70.01
neonatal, transient P94.0
pseudoparalytica G70.00
with exacerbation (acute) G70.01
in crisis G70.01
stomach, psychogenic F45.8

**Myasthenia** — *continued*
syndrome
in
diabetes mellitus — *see* E08-E13 with .44
neoplastic disease (*see also* Neoplasm) D49.9 [G73.3]
pernicious anemia D51.0 [G73.3]
thyrotoxicosis E05.90 [G73.3]
with thyroid storm E05.91 [G73.3]
**Myasthenic** M62.81
**Mycelium infection** B49
**Mycetismus** — *see* Poisoning, food, noxious, mushroom
**Mycetoma** B47.9
actinomycotic B47.1
bone (mycotic) B47.9 [M90.80]
eumycotic B47.0
foot B47.9
actinomycotic B47.1
mycotic B47.0
madurae NEC B47.9
mycotic B47.0
maduromycotic B47.0
mycotic B47.0
nocardial B47.1
**Mycobacteriosis** — *see* Mycobacterium
**Mycobacterium, mycobacterial** (infection) A31.9
anonymous A31.9
atypical A31.9
cutaneous A31.1
pulmonary A31.0
tuberculous — *see* Tuberculosis, pulmonary
specified site NEC A31.8
avium (intracellulare complex) A31.0
balnei A31.1
Battey A31.0
chelonei A31.8
cutaneous A31.1
extrapulmonary systemic A31.8
fortuitum A31.8
intracellulare (Battey bacillus) A31.0
kakaferifu A31.8
kansasii (yellow bacillus) A31.0
kasongo A31.8
leprae (*see also* Leprosy) A30.9
luciflavum A31.1
marinum (M. balnei) A31.1
nonspecific — *see* Mycobacterium, atypical
pulmonary (atypical) A31.0
tuberculous — *see* Tuberculosis, pulmonary
scrofulaceum A31.8
simiae A31.8
systemic, extrapulmonary A31.8
szulgai A31.8
terrae A31.8
triviale A31.8
tuberculosis (human, bovine) — *see* Tuberculosis
ulcerans A31.1
xenopi A31.8
**Mycoplasma** (M.) **pneumoniae, as cause of disease classified elsewhere** B96.0
**Mycosis, mycotic** B49
cutaneous NEC B36.9
ear B36.9
in
aspergillosis B44.89
candidiasis B37.84
moniliasis B37.84
fungoides (extranodal) (solid organ) C84.0- ☑
mouth B37.0
nails B35.1
opportunistic B48.8
skin NEC B36.9
specified NEC B48.8
stomatitis B37.0
vagina, vaginitis (candidal) B37.3
**Mydriasis** (pupil) H57.04
**Myelatelia** Q06.1
**Myelinolysis, pontine, central** G37.2
**Myelitis** (acute) (ascending) (childhood) (chronic) (descending) (diffuse) (disseminated) (idiopathic) (pressure) (progressive) (spinal cord) (subacute) (*see also* Encephalitis) G04.91
herpes simplex B00.82
herpes zoster B02.24
in diseases classified elsewhere G05.4
necrotizing, subacute G37.4
optic neuritis in G36.0
postchickenpox B01.12

**Myelitis** — *continued*
postherpetic B02.24
postimmunization G04.02
postinfectious NEC G04.89
postvaccinal G04.02
specified NEC G04.89
syphilitic (transverse) A52.14
toxic G92
transverse (in demyelinating diseases of central nervous system) G37.3
tuberculous A17.82
varicella B01.12
**Myeloblastic** — *see* condition
**Myeloblastoma**
granular cell (*see also* Neoplasm, connective tissue)
malignant — *see* Neoplasm, connective tissue, malignant
tongue D10.1
**Myelocele** — *see* Spina bifida
**Myelocystocele** — *see* Spina bifida
**Myelocytic** — *see* condition
**Myelodysplasia** D46.9
specified NEC D46.Z (*following* D46.4)
spinal cord (congenital) Q06.1
**Myelodysplastic syndrome** D46.9
with
5q deletion D46.C (*following* D46.2)
isolated del (5q) chromosomal abnormality D46.C (*following* D46.2)
specified NEC D46.Z (*following* D46.4)
**Myeloencephalitis** — *see* Encephalitis
**Myelofibrosis** D75.81
with myeloid metaplasia D47.4
acute C94.4- ☑
idiopathic (chronic) D47.4
primary D47.1
secondary D75.81
in myeloproliferative disease D47.4
**Myelogenous** — *see* condition
**Myeloid** — *see* condition
**Myelokathexis** D70.9
**Myeloleukodystrophy** E75.29
**Myelolipoma** — *see* Lipoma
**Myeloma** (multiple) C90.0- ☑
monostotic C90.3 ☑
plasma cell C90.0- ☑
plasma cell C90.0- ☑
solitary (*see also* Plasmacytoma, solitary) C90.3- ☑
**Myelomalacia** G95.89
**Myelomatosis** C90.0- ☑
**Myelomeningitis** — *see* Meningoencephalitis
**Myelomeningocele** (spinal cord) — *see* Spina bifida
**Myelo-osteo-musculodysplasia hereditaria** Q79.8
**Myelopathic**
anemia D64.89
muscle atrophy — *see* Atrophy, muscle, spinal
pain syndrome G89.0
**Myelopathy** (spinal cord) G95.9
drug-induced G95.89
in (due to)
degeneration or displacement, intervertebral disc NEC — *see* Disorder, disc, with, myelopathy
infection — *see* Encephalitis
intervertebral disc disorder (*see also* Disorder, disc, with, myelopathy)
mercury — *see* subcategory T56.1 ☑
neoplastic disease (*see also* Neoplasm) D49.9 [G99.2]
pernicious anemia D51.0 [G99.2]
spondylosis — *see* Spondylosis, with myelopathy NEC
necrotic (subacute) (vascular) G95.19
radiation-induced G95.89
spondylogenic NEC — *see* Spondylosis, with myelopathy NEC
toxic G95.89
transverse, acute G37.3
vascular G95.19
vitamin B12 E53.8 [G32.0]
**Myelophthisis** D61.82
**Myeloradiculitis** G04.91
**Myeloradiculodysplasia** (spinal) Q06.1
**Myelosarcoma** C92.3- ☑
**Myelosclerosis** D75.89
with myeloid metaplasia D47.4
disseminated, of nervous system G35
megakaryocytic D47.4

**Myelosclerosis** — *continued*
  megakaryocytic — *continued*
    with myeloid metaplasia D47.4
**Myelosis**
  acute C92.0- ☑
  aleukemic C92.9- ☑
  chronic D47.1
  erythremic (acute) C94.0- ☑
  megakaryocytic C94.2- ☑
  nonleukemic D72.828
  subacute C92.9- ☑
**Myiasis** (cavernous) B87.9
  aural B87.4
  creeping B87.0
  cutaneous B87.0
  dermal B87.0
  ear (external) (middle) B87.4
  eye B87.2
  genitourinary B87.81
  intestinal B87.82
  laryngeal B87.3
  nasopharyngeal B87.3
  ocular B87.2
  orbit B87.2
  skin B87.0
  specified site NEC B87.89
  traumatic B87.1
  wound B87.1
**Myoadenoma, prostate** — *see* Hyperplasia, prostate
**Myoblastoma**
  granular cell (*see also* Neoplasm, connective tissue, benign)
    malignant — *see* Neoplasm, connective tissue, malignant
  tongue D10.1
**Myocardial** — *see* condition
**Myocardiopathy** (congestive) (constrictive) (familial) (hypertrophic nonobstructive) (idiopathic) (infiltrative) (obstructive) (primary) (restrictive) (sporadic) (*see also* Cardiomyopathy) I42.9
  alcoholic I42.6
  cobalt-beer I42.6
  glycogen storage E74.02 [I43]
  hypertrophic obstructive I42.1
  in (due to)
    beriberi E51.12
    cardiac glycogenosis E74.02 [I43]
    Friedreich's ataxia G11.1 [I43]
    myotonia atrophica G71.11 [I43]
    progressive muscular dystrophy G71.0 [I43]
  obscure (African) I42.8
  secondary I42.9
  thyrotoxic E05.90 [I43]
    with storm E05.91 [I43]
  toxic NEC I42.7
**Myocarditis** (with arteriosclerosis)(chronic)(fibroid) (interstitial) (old) (progressive) (senile) I51.4
  with
    rheumatic fever (conditions in I00) I09.0
      active — *see* Myocarditis, acute, rheumatic
      inactive or quiescent (with chorea) I09.0
  active I40.9
    rheumatic I01.2
      with chorea (acute) (rheumatic) (Sydenham's) I02.0
  acute or subacute (interstitial) I40.9
    due to
      streptococcus (beta-hemolytic) I01.2
    idiopathic I40.1
    rheumatic I01.2
      with chorea (acute) (rheumatic) (Sydenham's) I02.0
    specified NEC I40.8
  aseptic of newborn B33.22
  bacterial (acute) I40.0
  Coxsackie (virus) B33.22
  diphtheritic A36.81
  eosinophilic I40.1
  epidemic of newborn (Coxsackie) B33.22
  Fiedler's (acute) (isolated) I40.1
  giant cell (acute) (subacute) I40.1
  gonococcal A54.83
  granulomatous (idiopathic) (isolated) (nonspecific) I40.1
  hypertensive — *see* Hypertension, heart
  idiopathic (granulomatous) I40.1
  in (due to)
    diphtheria A36.81

**Myocarditis** — *continued*
  in — *continued*
    epidemic louse-borne typhus A75.0 [I41]
    Lyme disease A69.29
    sarcoidosis D86.85
    scarlet fever A38.1
    toxoplasmosis (acquired) B58.81
    typhoid A01.02
    typhus NEC A75.9 [I41]
  infective I40.0
  influenzal — *see* Influenza, with, myocarditis
  isolated (acute) I40.1
  meningococcal A39.52
  mumps B26.82
  nonrheumatic, active I40.9
  parenchymatous I40.9
  pneumococcal I40.0
  rheumatic (chronic) (inactive) (with chorea) I09.0
    active or acute I01.2
      with chorea (acute) (rheumatic) (Sydenham's) I02.0
  rheumatoid — *see* Rheumatoid, carditis
  septic I40.0
  staphylococcal I40.0
  suppurative I40.0
  syphilitic (chronic) A52.06
  toxic I40.8
    rheumatic — *see* Myocarditis, acute, rheumatic
  tuberculous A18.84
  typhoid A01.02
  valvular — *see* Endocarditis
  virus, viral I40.0
    of newborn (Coxsackie) B33.22
**Myocardium, myocardial** — *see* condition
**Myocardosis** — *see* Cardiomyopathy
**Myoclonus, myoclonic, myoclonia** (familial) (essential) (multifocal) (simplex) G25.3
  drug-induced G25.3
  epilepsy (*see also* Epilepsy, generalized, specified NEC) G40.4- ☑
    familial (progressive) G25.3
  epileptica G40.409
    with status epilepticus G40.401
  facial G51.3
  familial progressive G25.3
  Friedreich's G25.3
  jerks G25.3
  massive G25.3
  palatal G25.3
  pharyngeal G25.3
**Myocytolysis** I51.5
**Myodiastasis** — *see* Diastasis, muscle
**Myoendocarditis** — *see* Endocarditis
**Myoepithelioma** — *see* Neoplasm, benign, by site
**Myofasciitis** (acute) — *see* Myositis
**Myofibroma** (*see also* Neoplasm, connective tissue, benign)
  uterus (cervix) (corpus) — *see* Leiomyoma
**Myofibromatosis** D48.1
  infantile Q89.8
**Myofibrosis** M62.89
  heart — *see* Myocarditis
  scapulohumeral — *see* Lesion, shoulder, specified NEC
**Myofibrositis** M79.7
  scapulohumeral — *see* Lesion, shoulder, specified NEC
**Myoglobulinuria, myoglobinuria** (primary) R82.1
**Myokymia, facial** G51.4
**Myolipoma** — *see* Lipoma
**Myoma** (*see also* Neoplasm, connective tissue, benign)
  malignant — *see* Neoplasm, connective tissue, malignant
  prostate D29.1
  uterus (cervix) (corpus) — *see* Leiomyoma
**Myomalacia** M62.89
**Myometritis** — *see* Endometritis
**Myometrium** — *see* condition
**Myonecrosis, clostridial** A48.0
**Myopathy** G72.9
  acute
    necrotizing G72.81
    quadriplegic G72.81
  alcoholic G72.1
  benign congenital G71.2
  central core G71.2
  centronuclear G71.2
  congenital (benign) G71.2
  critical illness G72.81
  distal G71.0

**Myopathy** — *continued*
  drug-induced G72.0
  endocrine NEC E34.9 [G73.7]
  extraocular muscles H05.82- ☑
  facioscapulohumeral G71.0
  hereditary G71.9
    specified NEC G71.8
  immune NEC G72.49
  in (due to)
    Addison's disease E27.1 [G73.7]
    alcohol G72.1
    amyloidosis E85.0 [G73.7]
    cretinism E00.9 [G73.7]
    Cushing's syndrome E24.9 [G73.7]
    drugs G72.0
    endocrine disease NEC E34.9 [G73.7]
    giant cell arteritis M31.6 [G73.7]
    glycogen storage disease E74.00 [G73.7]
    hyperadrenocorticism E24.9 [G73.7]
    hyperparathyroidism NEC E21.3 [G73.7]
    hypoparathyroidism E20.9 [G73.7]
    hypopituitarism E23.0 [G73.7]
    hypothyroidism E03.9 [G73.7]
    infectious disease NEC B99 ☑ [G73.7]
    lipid storage disease E75.6 [G73.7]
    metabolic disease NEC E88.9 [G73.7]
    myxedema E03.9 [G73.7]
    parasitic disease NEC B89 [G73.7]
    polyarteritis nodosa M30.0 [G73.7]
    rheumatoid arthritis — *see* Rheumatoid, myopathy
    sarcoidosis D86.87
    scleroderma M34.82
    sicca syndrome M35.03
    Sjögren's syndrome M35.03
    systemic lupus erythematosus M32.19
    thyrotoxicosis (hyperthyroidism) E05.90 [G73.7]
      with thyroid storm E05.91 [G73.7]
    toxic agent NEC G72.2
  inflammatory NEC G72.49
  intensive care (ICU) G72.81
  limb-girdle G71.0
  mitochondrial NEC G71.3
  myotubular G71.2
  mytonic, proximal (PROMM) G71.11
  nemaline G71.2
  ocular G71.0
  oculopharyngeal G71.0
  of critical illness G72.81
  primary G71.9
    specified NEC G71.8
  progressive NEC G72.89
  proximal myotonic (PROMM) G71.11
  rod G71.2
  scapulohumeral G71.0
  specified NEC G72.89
  toxic G72.2
**Myopericarditis** (*see also* Pericarditis)
  chronic rheumatic I09.2
**Myopia** (axial) (congenital) H52.1- ☑
  degenerative (malignant) H44.20
    with
      choroidal neovascularization H44.2A- ☑
      foveoschisis H44.2D- ☑
      macular hole H44.2B- ☑
      retinal detachment H44.2C- ☑
      specified maculopathy NEC H44.2E- ☑
    bilateral H44.23
    left eye H44.22
    right eye H44.21
  malignant (*see also* Myopia, degenerative) H44.2- ☑
  pernicious (*see also* Myopia, degenerative) H44.2- ☑
  progressive high (degenerative) (*see also* Myopia, degenerative) H44.2- ☑
**Myosarcoma** — *see* Neoplasm, connective tissue, malignant
**Myosis** (pupil) H57.03
  stromal (endolymphatic) D39.0
**Myositis** M60.9
  clostridial A48.0
  due to posture — *see* Myositis, specified type NEC
  epidemic B33.0
  fibrosa or fibrous (chronic), Volkmann's T79.6 ☑
  foreign body granuloma — *see* Granuloma, foreign body
  in (due to)
    bilharziasis B65.9 [M63.8-] ☑
    cysticercosis B69.81
    leprosy A30.9 [M63.8-] ☑

**Myositis** — *continued*
  in — *continued*
    mycosis B49 [M63.8-] ☑
    sarcoidosis D86.87
    schistosomiasis B65.9 [M63.8-] ☑
    syphilis
      late A52.78
      secondary A51.49
    toxoplasmosis (acquired) B58.82
    trichinellosis B75 [M63.8-] ☑
    tuberculosis A18.09
  inclusion body [IBM] G72.41
  infective M60.009
    arm M60.002
      left M60.001
      right M60.000
    leg M60.005
      left M60.004
      right M60.003
    lower limb M60.005
      ankle M60.07- ☑
      foot M60.07- ☑
      lower leg M60.06- ☑
      thigh M60.05- ☑
      toe M60.07- ☑
    multiple sites M60.09
    specified site NEC M60.08
    upper limb M60.002
      finger M60.04- ☑
      forearm M60.03- ☑
      hand M60.04- ☑
      shoulder region M60.01- ☑
      upper arm M60.02- ☑
  interstitial M60.10
    ankle M60.17- ☑
    foot M60.17- ☑
    forearm M60.13- ☑
    hand M60.14- ☑
    lower leg M60.16- ☑
    multiple sites M60.19
    shoulder region M60.11- ☑
    specified site NEC M60.18
    thigh M60.15- ☑
    upper arm M60.12- ☑
  mycotic B49 [M63.8-] ☑
  orbital, chronic H05.12- ☑
  ossificans or ossifying (circumscripta) (*see also* Ossification, muscle, specified NEC)
    in (due to)
      burns M61.30
        ankle M61.37- ☑
        foot M61.37- ☑
        forearm M61.33- ☑
        hand M61.34- ☑
        lower leg M61.36- ☑
        multiple sites M61.39
        pelvic region M61.35- ☑

**Myositis** — *continued*
  ossificans or ossifying (*see also* Ossification, muscle, specified) — *continued*
    in — *continued*
      burns — *continued*
        shoulder region M61.31- ☑
        specified site NEC M61.38
        thigh M61.35- ☑
        upper arm M61.32- ☑
      quadriplegia or paraplegia M61.20
        ankle M61.27- ☑
        foot M61.27- ☑
        forearm M61.23- ☑
        hand M61.24- ☑
        lower leg M61.26- ☑
        multiple sites M61.29
        pelvic region M61.25- ☑
        shoulder region M61.21- ☑
        specified site NEC M61.28
        thigh M61.25- ☑
        upper arm M61.22- ☑
    progressiva M61.10
      ankle M61.17- ☑
      finger M61.14- ☑
      foot M61.17- ☑
      forearm M61.13- ☑
      hand M61.14- ☑
      lower leg M61.16- ☑
      multiple sites M61.19
      pelvic region M61.15- ☑
      shoulder region M61.11- ☑
      specified site NEC M61.18
      thigh M61.15- ☑
      toe M61.17- ☑
      upper arm M61.12- ☑
    traumatica M61.00
      ankle M61.07- ☑
      foot M61.07- ☑
      forearm M61.03- ☑
      hand M61.04- ☑
      lower leg M61.06- ☑
      multiple sites M61.09
      pelvic region M61.05- ☑
      shoulder region M61.01- ☑
      specified site NEC M61.08
      thigh M61.05- ☑
      upper arm M61.02- ☑
  purulent — *see* Myositis, infective
  specified type NEC M60.80
    ankle M60.87- ☑
    foot M60.87- ☑
    forearm M60.83- ☑
    hand M60.84- ☑
    lower leg M60.86- ☑
    multiple sites M60.89
    pelvic region M60.85- ☑
    shoulder region M60.81- ☑

**Myositis** — *continued*
  specified type — *continued*
    specified site NEC M60.88
    thigh M60.85- ☑
    upper arm M60.82- ☑
  suppurative — *see* Myositis, infective
  traumatic (old) — *see* Myositis, specified type NEC
**Myospasia impulsiva** F95.2
**Myotonia** (acquisita) (intermittens) M62.89
  atrophica G71.11
  chondrodystrophic G71.13
  congenita (acetazolamide responsive) (dominant) (recessive) G71.12
  drug-induced G71.14
  dystrophica G71.11
  fluctuans G71.19
  levior G71.12
  permanens G71.19
  symptomatic G71.19
**Myotonic pupil** — *see* Anomaly, pupil, function, tonic pupil
**Myriapodiasis** B88.2
**Myringitis** H73.2- ☑
  with otitis media — *see* Otitis, media
  acute H73.00- ☑
    bullous H73.01- ☑
    specified NEC H73.09- ☑
  bullous — *see* Myringitis, acute, bullous
  chronic H73.1- ☑
**Mysophobia** F40.228
**Mytilotoxism** — *see* Poisoning, fish
**Myxadenitis labialis** K13.0
**Myxedema** (adult) (idiocy) (infantile) (juvenile) (*see also* Hypothyroidism) E03.9
  circumscribed E05.90
    with storm E05.91
  coma E03.5
  congenital E00.1
  cutis L98.5
  localized (pretibial) E05.90
    with storm E05.91
  papular L98.5
**Myxochondrosarcoma** — *see* Neoplasm, cartilage, malignant
**Myxofibroma** — *see* Neoplasm, connective tissue, benign
  odontogenic — *see* Cyst, calcifying odontogenic
**Myxofibrosarcoma** — *see* Neoplasm, connective tissue, malignant
**Myxolipoma** D17.9
**Myxoliposarcoma** — *see* Neoplasm, connective tissue, malignant
**Myxoma** (*see also* Neoplasm, connective tissue, benign)
  nerve sheath — *see* Neoplasm, nerve, benign
  odontogenic — *see* Cyst, calcifying odontogenic
**Myxosarcoma** — *see* Neoplasm, connective tissue, malignant

☑ **Additional Character Required** — **Refer to the Tabular List for Character Selection**   ▽ **Subterms under main terms may continue to next column or page**

# N

**Naegeli's**
  disease Q82.8
  leukemia, monocytic C93.1- ☑
**Naegleriasis** (with meningoencephalitis) B60.2
**Naffziger's syndrome** G54.0
**Naga sore** — *see* Ulcer, skin
**Nägele's pelvis** M95.5
  with disproportion (fetopelvic) O33.0
    causing obstructed labor O65.0
**Nail** (*see also* condition)
  biting F98.8
  patella syndrome Q87.2
**Nanism, nanosomia** — *see* Dwarfism
**Nanophyetiasis** B66.8
**Nanukayami** A27.89
**Napkin rash** L22
**Narcolepsy** G47.419
  with cataplexy G47.411
  in conditions classified elsewhere G47.429
    with cataplexy G47.421
**Narcosis** R06.89
**Narcotism** — *see* Dependence
**NARP** (Neuropathy, Ataxia and Retinitis pigmentosa)
  syndrome E88.49
**Narrow**
  anterior chamber angle H40.03- ☑
  gingival width (of periodontal soft tissue) K05.5
  pelvis — *see* Contraction, pelvis
**Narrowing** (*see also* Stenosis)
  artery I77.1
    auditory, internal I65.8
    basilar — *see* Occlusion, artery, basilar
    carotid — *see* Occlusion, artery, carotid
    cerebellar — *see* Occlusion, artery, cerebellar
    cerebral — *see* Occlusion artery, cerebral
    choroidal — *see* Occlusion, artery, cerebral, specified NEC
    communicating posterior — *see* Occlusion, artery, cerebral, specified NEC
    coronary (*see also* Disease, heart, ischemic, atherosclerotic)
      congenital Q24.5
        syphilitic A50.54 [I52]
      due to syphilis NEC A52.06
    hypophyseal — *see* Occlusion, artery, cerebral, specified NEC
    pontine — *see* Occlusion, artery, cerebral, specified NEC
    precerebral — *see* Occlusion, artery, precerebral
    vertebral — *see* Occlusion, artery, vertebral
  auditory canal (external) — *see* Stenosis, external ear canal
  eustachian tube — *see* Obstruction, eustachian tube
  eyelid — *see* Disorder, eyelid function
  larynx J38.6
  mesenteric artery (*see also* Ischemia, intestine, acute) K55.059
  palate M26.89
  palpebral fissure — *see* Disorder, eyelid function
  ureter N13.5
    with infection N13.6
  urethra — *see* Stricture, urethra
**Narrowness, abnormal, eyelid** Q10.3
**Nasal** — *see* condition
**Nasolachrymal, nasolacrimal** — *see* condition
**Nasopharyngeal** (*see also* condition)
  pituitary gland Q89.2
  torticollis M43.6
**Nasopharyngitis** (acute) (infective) (streptococcal) (subacute) J00
  chronic (suppurative) (ulcerative) J31.1
**Nasopharynx, nasopharyngeal** — *see* condition
**Natal tooth, teeth** K00.6
**Nausea** (without vomiting) R11.0
  with vomiting R11.2
  gravidarum — *see* Hyperemesis, gravidarum
  marina T75.3 ☑
  navalis T75.3 ☑
**Navel** — *see* condition
**Neapolitan fever** — *see* Brucellosis
**Near drowning** T75.1 ☑
**Nearsightedness** — *see* Myopia
**Near-syncope** R55
**Nebula, cornea** — *see* Opacity, cornea

**Necator americanus infestation** B76.1
**Necatoriasis** B76.1
**Neck** — *see* condition
**Necrobiosis** R68.89
  lipoidica NEC L92.1
    with diabetes — *see* E08-E13 with .620
**Necrolysis, toxic epidermal** L51.2
  due to drug
    correct substance properly administered — *see* Table of Drugs and Chemicals, by drug, adverse effect
    overdose or wrong substance given or taken — *see* Table of Drugs and Chemicals, by drug, poisoning
**Necrophilia** F65.89
**Necrosis, necrotic** (ischemic) (*see also* Gangrene)
  adrenal (capsule) (gland) E27.49
  amputation stump (surgical) (late) T87.50
    arm T87.5- ☑
    leg T87.5- ☑
  antrum J32.0
  aorta (hyaline) (*see also* Aneurysm, aorta)
    cystic medial — *see* Dissection, aorta
  artery I77.5
  bladder (aseptic) (sphincter) N32.89
  bone (*see also* Osteonecrosis) M87.9
    aseptic or avascular — *see* Osteonecrosis
      idiopathic M87.00
    ethmoid J32.2
    jaw M27.2
    tuberculous — *see* Tuberculosis, bone
  brain I67.89
  breast (aseptic) (fat) (segmental) N64.1
  bronchus J98.09
  central nervous system NEC I67.89
  cerebellar I67.89
  cerebral I67.89
  colon (*see also* Infarct, intestine) K55.049
  cornea H18.89- ☑
  cortical (acute) (renal) N17.1
  cystic medial (aorta) — *see* Dissection, aorta
  dental pulp K04.1
  esophagus K22.8
  ethmoid (bone) J32.2
  eyelid — *see* Disorder, eyelid, degenerative
  fat, fatty (generalized) (*see also* Disorder, soft tissue, specified type NEC)
    abdominal wall K65.4
    breast (aseptic) (segmental) N64.1
    localized — *see* Degeneration, by site, fatty
    mesentery K65.4
    omentum K65.4
    pancreas K86.89
    peritoneum K65.4
    skin (subcutaneous), newborn P83.0
    subcutaneous, due to birth injury P15.6
  gallbladder — *see* Cholecystitis, acute
  heart — *see* Infarct, myocardium
  hip, aseptic or avascular — *see* Osteonecrosis, by type, femur
  intestine (acute) (hemorrhagic) (massive) (*see also* Infarct, intestine) K55.069
  jaw M27.2
  kidney (bilateral) N28.0
    acute N17.9
    cortical (acute) (bilateral) N17.1
      with ectopic or molar pregnancy O08.4
    medullary (bilateral) (in acute renal failure) (papillary) N17.2
    papillary (bilateral) (in acute renal failure) N17.2
    tubular N17.0
      with ectopic or molar pregnancy O08.4
      complicating
        abortion — *see* Abortion, by type, complicated by, tubular necrosis
        ectopic or molar pregnancy O08.4
        pregnancy — *see* Pregnancy, complicated by, diseases of, specified type or system NEC
      following ectopic or molar pregnancy O08.4
      traumatic T79.5 ☑
  larynx J38.7
  liver (with hepatic failure) (cell) — *see* Failure, hepatic
    hemorrhagic, central K76.2
  lung J85.0
  lymphatic gland — *see* Lymphadenitis, acute
  mammary gland (fat) (segmental) N64.1
  mastoid (chronic) — *see* Mastoiditis, chronic

**Necrosis, necrotic** — *continued*
  medullary (acute) (renal) N17.2
  mesentery (*see also* Infarct, intestine) K55.069
    fat K65.4
  mitral valve — *see* Insufficiency, mitral
  myocardium, myocardial — *see* Infarct, myocardium
  nose J34.0
  omentum (with mesenteric infarction) (*see also* Infarct, intestine) K55.069
    fat K65.4
  orbit, orbital — *see* Osteomyelitis, orbit
  ossicles, ear — *see* Abnormal, ear ossicles
  ovary N70.92
  pancreas (aseptic) (duct) (fat) K86.89
    acute (infective) — *see* Pancreatitis, acute
    infective — *see* Pancreatitis, acute
  papillary (acute) (renal) N17.2
  perineum N90.89
  peritoneum (with mesenteric infarction) (*see also* Infarct, intestine) K55.069
    fat K65.4
  pharynx J02.9
    in granulocytopenia — *see* Neutropenia
      Vincent's A69.1
  phosphorus — *see* subcategory T54.2 ☑
  pituitary (gland) E23.0
    postpartum O99.285
    Sheehan O99.285
  pressure — *see* Ulcer, pressure, by site
  pulmonary J85.0
  pulp (dental) K04.1
  radiation — *see* Necrosis, by site
  radium — *see* Necrosis, by site
  renal — *see* Necrosis, kidney
  sclera H15.89
  scrotum N50.89
  skin or subcutaneous tissue NEC I96
  spine, spinal (column) (*see also* Osteonecrosis, by type, vertebra)
    cord G95.19
  spleen D73.5
  stomach K31.89
  stomatitis (ulcerative) A69.0
  subcutaneous fat, newborn P83.88
  subendocardial (acute) I21.4
    chronic I25.89
  suprarenal (capsule) (gland) E27.49
  testis N50.89
  thymus (gland) E32.8
  tonsil J35.8
  trachea J39.8
  tuberculous NEC — *see* Tuberculosis
  tubular (acute) (anoxic) (renal) (toxic) N17.0
    postprocedural N99.0
  vagina N89.8
  vertebra (*see also* Osteonecrosis, by type, vertebra)
    tuberculous A18.01
  vulva N90.89
  X-ray — *see* Necrosis, by site
**Necrospermia** — *see* Infertility, male
**Need** (for)
  care provider because (of)
    assistance with personal care Z74.1
    continuous supervision required Z74.3
    impaired mobility Z74.09
    no other household member able to render care Z74.2
    specified reason NEC Z74.8
  immunization — *see* Vaccination
  vaccination — *see* Vaccination
**Neglect**
  adult
    confirmed T74.01 ☑
    history of Z91.412
    suspected T76.01 ☑
  child (childhood)
    confirmed T74.02 ☑
    history of Z62.812
    suspected T76.02 ☑
  emotional, in childhood Z62.898
  hemispatial R41.4
  left-sided R41.4
  sensory R41.4
  visuospatial R41.4
**Neisserian infection NEC** — *see* Gonococcus
**Nelaton's syndrome** G60.8
**Nelson's syndrome** E24.1
**Nematodiasis** (intestinal) B82.0

**Nematodiasis** — *continued*
   Ancylostoma B76.0
**Neonatal** (*see also* Newborn)
   acne L70.4
   bradycardia P29.12
   screening, abnormal findings on P09
   tachycardia P29.11
   tooth, teeth K00.6
**Neonatorum** — *see* condition
**Neoplasia**
   endocrine, multiple (MEN) E31.20
     type I E31.21
     type IIA E31.22
     type IIB E31.23
   intraepithelial (histologically confirmed)
     anal (AIN) (histologically confirmed) K62.82
       grade I K62.82
       grade II K62.82
       severe D01.3
     cervical glandular (histologically confirmed) D06.9
     cervix (uteri) (CIN) (histologically confirmed) N87.9
       glandular D06.9
       grade I N87.0
       grade II N87.1
       grade III (severe dysplasia) (*see also* Carcinoma, cervix uteri, in situ) D06.9
     prostate (histologically confirmed) (PIN) N42.31
       grade I N42.31
       grade II N42.31
       grade III (severe dysplasia) D07.5
     vagina (histologically confirmed) (VAIN) N89.3
       grade I N89.0
       grade II N89.1
       grade III (severe dysplasia) D07.2
     vulva (histologically confirmed) (VIN) N90.3
       grade I N90.0
       grade II N90.1
       grade III (severe dysplasia) D07.1
**Neoplasm, neoplastic** (*see also* Table of Neoplasms)
   lipomatous, benign — *see* Lipoma
   malignant mast cell C96.20
     specified type NEC C96.29
   mast cell, of uncertain behavior NEC D47.09
**Neovascularization**
   ciliary body — *see* Disorder, iris, vascular
   cornea H16.40- ☑
     deep H16.44- ☑
     ghost vessels — *see* Ghost, vessels
     localized H16.43- ☑
     pannus — *see* Pannus
   iris — *see* Disorder, iris, vascular
   retina H35.05- ☑
**Nephralgia** N23
**Nephritis, nephritic** (albuminuric) (azotemic) (congenital) (disseminated) (epithelial) (familial) (focal) (granulomatous) (hemorrhagic) (infantile) (nonsuppurative, excretory) (uremic) N05.9
   with
     dense deposit disease N05.6
     diffuse
       crescentic glomerulonephritis N05.7
       endocapillary proliferative glomerulonephritis N05.4
       membranous glomerulonephritis N05.2
       mesangial proliferative glomerulonephritis N05.3
       mesangiocapillary glomerulonephritis N05.5
     edema — *see* Nephrosis
     focal and segmental glomerular lesions N05.1
     foot process disease N04.9
     glomerular lesion
       diffuse sclerosing N05.8
       hypocomplementemic — *see* Nephritis, membranoproliferative
       IgA — *see* Nephropathy, IgA
       lobular, lobulonodular — *see* Nephritis, membranoproliferative
       nodular — *see* Nephritis, membranoproliferative
     lesion of
       glomerulonephritis, proliferative N05.8
       renal necrosis N05.9
     minor glomerular abnormality N05.0
     specified morphological changes NEC N05.8
   acute N00.9
     with
       dense deposit disease N00.6

**Nephritis, nephritic** — *continued*
   acute — *continued*
     with — *continued*
       diffuse
         crescentic glomerulonephritis N00.7
         endocapillary proliferative glomerulonephritis N00.4
         membranous glomerulonephritis N00.2
         mesangial proliferative glomerulonephritis N00.3
         mesangiocapillary glomerulonephritis N00.5
       focal and segmental glomerular lesions N00.1
       minor glomerular abnormality N00.0
       specified morphological changes NEC N00.8
   amyloid E85.4 [N08]
   antiglomerular basement membrane (anti-GBM) antibody NEC
     in Goodpasture's syndrome M31.0
   antitubular basement membrane (tubulo-interstitial) NEC N12
     toxic — *see* Nephropathy, toxic
   arteriolar — *see* Hypertension, kidney
   arteriosclerotic — *see* Hypertension, kidney
   ascending — *see* Nephritis, tubulo-interstitial
   atrophic N03.9
   Balkan (endemic) N15.0
   calculous, calculus — *see* Calculus, kidney
   cardiac — *see* Hypertension, kidney
   cardiovascular — *see* Hypertension, kidney
   chronic N03.9
     with
       dense deposit disease N03.6
       diffuse
         crescentic glomerulonephritis N03.7
         endocapillary proliferative glomerulonephritis N03.4
         membranous glomerulonephritis N03.2
         mesangial proliferative glomerulonephritis N03.3
         mesangiocapillary glomerulonephritis N03.5
       focal and segmental glomerular lesions N03.1
       minor glomerular abnormality N03.0
       specified morphological changes NEC N03.8
     arteriosclerotic — *see* Hypertension, kidney
   cirrhotic N26.9
   complicating pregnancy O26.83- ☑
   croupous N00.9
   degenerative — *see* Nephrosis
   diffuse sclerosing N05.8
   due to
     diabetes mellitus — *see* E08-E13 with .21
     subacute bacterial endocarditis I33.0
     systemic lupus erythematosus (chronic) M32.14
     typhoid fever A01.09
   gonococcal (acute) (chronic) A54.21
   hypocomplementemic — *see* Nephritis, membranoproliferative
   IgA — *see* Nephropathy, IgA
   infective — *see* Nephritis, tubulo-interstitial
   interstitial — *see* Nephritis, tubulo-interstitial
   lead N14.3
   membranoproliferative (diffuse) (type 1 or 3) (*see also* N00-N07 with fourth character .5) N05.5
     type 2 (*see also* N00-N07 with fourth character .6) N05.6
   minimal change N05.0
   necrotic, necrotizing NEC (*see also* N00-N07 with fourth character .8) N05.8
   nephrotic — *see* Nephrosis
   nodular — *see* Nephritis, membranoproliferative
   polycystic Q61.3
     adult type Q61.2
     autosomal
       dominant Q61.2
       recessive NEC Q61.19
     childhood type NEC Q61.19
     infantile type NEC Q61.19
   poststreptococcal N05.9
     acute N00.9
     chronic N03.9
     rapidly progressive N01.9
   proliferative NEC (*see also* N00-N07 with fourth character .8) N05.8
   purulent — *see* Nephritis, tubulo-interstitial
   rapidly progressive N01.9
     with
       dense deposit disease N01.6

**Nephritis, nephritic** — *continued*
   rapidly progressive — *continued*
     with — *continued*
       diffuse
         crescentic glomerulonephritis N01.7
         endocapillary proliferative glomerulonephritis N01.4
         membranous glomerulonephritis N01.2
         mesangial proliferative glomerulonephritis N01.3
         mesangiocapillary glomerulonephritis N01.5
       focal and segmental glomerular lesions N01.1
       minor glomerular abnormality N01.0
       specified morphological changes NEC N01.8
   salt losing or wasting NEC N28.89
   saturnine N14.3
   sclerosing, diffuse N05.8
   septic — *see* Nephritis, tubulo-interstitial
   specified pathology NEC (*see also* N00-N07 with fourth character .8) N05.8
   subacute N01.9
   suppurative — *see* Nephritis, tubulo-interstitial
   syphilitic (late) A52.75
     congenital A50.59 [N08]
     early (secondary) A51.44
   toxic — *see* Nephropathy, toxic
   tubal, tubular — *see* Nephritis, tubulo-interstitial
   tuberculous A18.11
   tubulo-interstitial (in) N12
     acute (infectious) N10
     chronic (infectious) N11.9
       nonobstructive N11.8
         reflux-associated N11.0
       obstructive N11.1
       specified NEC N11.8
     due to
       brucellosis A23.9 [N16]
       cryoglobulinemia D89.1 [N16]
       glycogen storage disease E74.00 [N16]
       Sjögren's syndrome M35.04
   vascular — *see* Hypertension, kidney
   war N00.9
**Nephroblastoma** (epithelial) (mesenchymal) C64- ☑
**Nephrocalcinosis** E83.59 [N29]
**Nephrocystitis, pustular** — *see* Nephritis, tubulo-interstitial
**Nephrolithiasis** (congenital) (pelvis) (recurrent) (*see also* Calculus, kidney)
**Nephroma** C64- ☑
   mesoblastic D41.0- ☑
**Nephronephritis** — *see* Nephrosis
**Nephronophthisis** Q61.5
**Nephropathia epidemica** A98.5
**Nephropathy** (*see also* Nephritis) N28.9
   with
     edema — *see* Nephrosis
     glomerular lesion — *see* Glomerulonephritis
   amyloid, hereditary E85.0
   analgesic N14.0
     with medullary necrosis, acute N17.2
   Balkan (endemic) N15.0
   chemical — *see* Nephropathy, toxic
   diabetic — *see* E08-E13 with .21
   drug-induced N14.2
     specified NEC N14.1
   focal and segmental hyalinosis or sclerosis N02.1
   heavy metal-induced N14.3
   hereditary NEC N07.9
     with
       dense deposit disease N07.6
       diffuse
         crescentic glomerulonephritis N07.7
         endocapillary proliferative glomerulonephritis N07.4
         membranous glomerulonephritis N07.2
         mesangial proliferative glomerulonephritis N07.3
         mesangiocapillary glomerulonephritis N07.5
       focal and segmental glomerular lesions N07.1
       minor glomerular abnormality N07.0
       specified morphological changes NEC N07.8
   hypercalcemic N25.89
   hypertensive — *see* Hypertension, kidney
   hypokalemic (vacuolar) N25.89
   IgA N02.8
     with glomerular lesion N02.9
       focal and segmental hyalinosis or sclerosis N02.1

**Nephropathy** — *continued*
 IgA — *continued*
  with glomerular lesion — *continued*
   membranoproliferative (diffuse) N02.5
   membranous (diffuse) N02.2
   mesangial proliferative (diffuse) N02.3
   mesangiocapillary (diffuse) N02.5
   proliferative NEC N02.8
   specified pathology NEC N02.8
 lead N14.3
 membranoproliferative (diffuse) N02.5
 membranous (diffuse) N02.2
 mesangial (IgA/IgG) — *see* Nephropathy, IgA
  proliferative (diffuse) N02.3
 mesangiocapillary (diffuse) N02.5
 obstructive N13.8
 phenacetin N17.2
 phosphate-losing N25.0
 potassium depletion N25.89
 pregnancy-related O26.83- ☑
 proliferative NEC (*see also* N00-N07 with fourth character .8) N05.8
 protein-losing N25.89
 saturnine N14.3
 sickle-cell D57.- ☑ [N08]
 toxic NEC N14.4
  due to
   drugs N14.2
    analgesic N14.0
    specified NEC N14.1
   heavy metals N14.3
 vasomotor N17.0
 water-losing N25.89
**Nephroptosis** N28.83
**Nephropyosis** — *see* Abscess, kidney
**Nephrorrhagia** N28.89
**Nephrosclerosis** (arteriolar)(arteriosclerotic) (chronic) (hyaline) (*see also* Hypertension, kidney)
 hyperplastic — *see* Hypertension, kidney
 senile N26.9
**Nephrosis, nephrotic** (Epstein's) (syndrome) (congenital) N04.9
 with
  foot process disease N04.9
  glomerular lesion N04.1
  hypocomplementemic N04.5
 acute N04.9
 anoxic — *see* Nephrosis, tubular
 chemical — *see* Nephrosis, tubular
 cholemic K76.7
 diabetic — *see* E08-E13 with .21
 Finnish type (congenital) Q89.8
 hemoglobin N10
 hemoglobinuric — *see* Nephrosis, tubular
 in
  amyloidosis E85.4 [N08]
  diabetes mellitus — *see* E08-E13 with .21
  epidemic hemorrhagic fever A98.5
  malaria (malariae) B52.0
 ischemic — *see* Nephrosis, tubular
 lipoid N04.9
 lower nephron — *see* Nephrosis, tubular
 malarial (malariae) B52.0
 minimal change N04.0
 myoglobin N10
 necrotizing — *see* Nephrosis, tubular
 osmotic (sucrose) N25.89
 radiation N04.9
 syphilitic (late) A52.75
 toxic — *see* Nephrosis, tubular
 tubular (acute) N17.0
  postprocedural N99.0
  radiation N04.9
**Nephrosonephritis, hemorrhagic** (endemic) A98.5
**Nephrostomy**
 attention to Z43.6
 status Z93.6
**Nerve** (*see also* condition)
 injury — *see* Injury, nerve, by body site
**Nerves** R45.0
**Nervous** (*see also* condition) R45.0
 heart F45.8
 stomach F45.8
 tension R45.0
**Nervousness** R45.0
**Nesidioblastoma**
 pancreas D13.7
 specified site NEC — *see* Neoplasm, benign, by site

**Nesidioblastoma** — *continued*
 unspecified site D13.7
**Nettleship's syndrome** — *see* Urticaria pigmentosa
**Neumann's disease or syndrome** L10.1
**Neuralgia, neuralgic** (acute) M79.2
 accessory (nerve) G52.8
 acoustic (nerve) — *see* subcategory H93.3 ☑
 auditory (nerve) — *see* subcategory H93.3 ☑
 ciliary G44.009
  intractable G44.001
  not intractable G44.009
 cranial
  nerve (*see also* Disorder, nerve, cranial)
   fifth or trigeminal — *see* Neuralgia, trigeminal
  postherpetic, postzoster B02.29
 ear — *see* subcategory H92.0 ☑
 facialis vera G51.1
 Fothergill's — *see* Neuralgia, trigeminal
 glossopharyngeal (nerve) G52.1
 Horton's G44.099
  intractable G44.091
  not intractable G44.099
 Hunt's B02.21
 hypoglossal (nerve) G52.3
 infraorbital — *see* Neuralgia, trigeminal
 malarial — *see* Malaria
 migrainous G44.009
  intractable G44.001
  not intractable G44.009
 Morton's G57.6- ☑
 nerve, cranial — *see* Disorder, nerve, cranial
 nose G52.0
 occipital M54.81
 olfactory G52.0
 penis N48.9
 perineum R10.2
 postherpetic NEC B02.29
  trigeminal B02.22
 pubic region R10.2
 scrotum R10.2
 Sluder's G44.89
 specified nerve NEC G58.8
 spermatic cord R10.2
 sphenopalatine (ganglion) G90.09
 trifacial — *see* Neuralgia, trigeminal
 trigeminal G50.0
  postherpetic, postzoster B02.22
 vagus (nerve) G52.2
 writer's F48.8
  organic G25.89
**Neurapraxia** — *see* Injury, nerve
**Neurasthenia** F48.8
 cardiac F45.8
 gastric F45.8
 heart F45.8
**Neurilemmoma** (*see also* Neoplasm, nerve, benign)
 acoustic (nerve) D33.3
 malignant (*see also* Neoplasm, nerve, malignant)
  acoustic (nerve) C72.4- ☑
**Neurilemmosarcoma** — *see* Neoplasm, nerve, malignant
**Neurinoma** — *see* Neoplasm, nerve, benign
**Neurinomatosis** — *see* Neoplasm, nerve, uncertain behavior
**Neuritis** (rheumatoid) M79.2
 abducens (nerve) — *see* Strabismus, paralytic, sixth nerve
 accessory (nerve) G52.8
 acoustic (nerve) (*see also* subcategory) H93.3 ☑
  in (due to)
   infectious disease NEC B99 ☑ [H94.0-] ☑
   parasitic disease NEC B89 [H94.0-] ☑
  syphilitic A52.15
 alcoholic G62.1
  with psychosis — *see* Psychosis, alcoholic
 amyloid, any site E85.4 [G63]
 auditory (nerve) — *see* subcategory H93.3 ☑
 brachial — *see* Radiculopathy
  due to displacement, intervertebral disc — *see* Disorder, disc, cervical, with neuritis
 cranial nerve
  due to Lyme disease A69.22
  eighth or acoustic or auditory — *see* subcategory H93.3 ☑
  eleventh or accessory G52.8
  fifth or trigeminal G51.0
  first or olfactory G52.0

**Neuritis** — *continued*
 cranial nerve — *continued*
  fourth or trochlear — *see* Strabismus, paralytic, fourth nerve
  second or optic — *see* Neuritis, optic
  seventh or facial G51.8
   newborn (birth injury) P11.3
  sixth or abducent — *see* Strabismus, paralytic, sixth nerve
  tenth or vagus G52.2
  third or oculomotor — *see* Strabismus, paralytic, third nerve
  twelfth or hypoglossal G52.3
 Déjérine-Sottas G60.0
 diabetic (mononeuropathy) — *see* E08-E13 with .41
  polyneuropathy — *see* E08-E13 with .42
 due to
  beriberi E51.11
  displacement, prolapse or rupture, intervertebral disc — *see* Disorder, disc, with, radiculopathy
  herniation, nucleus pulposus M51.9 [G55]
 endemic E51.11
 facial G51.8
  newborn (birth injury) P11.3
 general — *see* Polyneuropathy
 geniculate ganglion G51.1
  due to herpes (zoster) B02.21
 gouty (*see also* Gout, by type) M10.9 [G63]
 hypoglossal (nerve) G52.3
 ilioinguinal (nerve) G57.9- ☑
 infectious (multiple) NEC G61.0
 interstitial hypertrophic progressive G60.0
 lumbar M54.16
 lumbosacral M54.17
 multiple (*see also* Polyneuropathy)
  endemic E51.11
  infective, acute G61.0
 multiplex endemica E51.11
 nerve root — *see* Radiculopathy
 oculomotor (nerve) — *see* Strabismus, paralytic, third nerve
 olfactory nerve G52.0
 optic (nerve) (hereditary) (sympathetic) H46.9
  with demyelination G36.9
  in myelitis G36.0
  nutritional H46.2
  papillitis — *see* Papillitis, optic
  retrobulbar H46.1- ☑
  specified type NEC H46.8
  toxic H46.3
 peripheral (nerve) G62.9
  multiple — *see* Polyneuropathy
  single — *see* Mononeuritis
 pneumogastric (nerve) G52.2
 postherpetic, postzoster B02.29
 progressive hypertrophic interstitial G60.0
 retrobulbar (*see also* Neuritis, optic, retrobulbar)
  in (due to)
   late syphilis A52.15
   meningococcal infection A39.82
  meningococcal A39.82
  syphilitic A52.15
 sciatic (nerve) (*see also* Sciatica)
  due to displacement of intervertebral disc — *see* Disorder, disc, with, radiculopathy
 serum (*see also* Reaction, serum) T80.69 ☑
 shoulder-girdle G54.5
 specified nerve NEC G58.8
 spinal (nerve) root — *see* Radiculopathy
 syphilitic A52.15
 thenar (median) G56.1- ☑
 thoracic M54.14
 toxic NEC G62.2
 trochlear (nerve) — *see* Strabismus, paralytic, fourth nerve
 vagus (nerve) G52.2
**Neuroastrocytoma** — *see* Neoplasm, uncertain behavior, by site
**Neuroavitaminosis** E56.9 [G99.8]
**Neuroblastoma**
 olfactory C30.0
 specified site — *see* Neoplasm, malignant, by site
 unspecified site C74.90
**Neurochorioretinitis** — *see* Chorioretinitis
**Neurocirculatory asthenia** F45.8
**Neurocysticercosis** B69.0
**Neurocytoma** — *see* Neoplasm, benign, by site

**Neurodermatitis** (circumscribed) (circumscripta) (local) L28.0
  atopic L20.81
  diffuse (Brocq) L20.81
  disseminated L20.81
**Neuroencephalomyelopathy, optic** G36.0
**Neuroepithelioma** (see also Neoplasm, malignant, by site)
  olfactory C30.0
**Neurofibroma** (see also Neoplasm, nerve, benign)
  melanotic — see Neoplasm, nerve, benign
  multiple — see Neurofibromatosis
  plexiform — see Neoplasm, nerve, benign
**Neurofibromatosis** (multiple) (nonmalignant) Q85.00
  acoustic Q85.02
  malignant — see Neoplasm, nerve, malignant
  specified NEC Q85.09
  type 1 (von Recklinghausen) Q85.01
  type 2 Q85.02
**Neurofibrosarcoma** — see Neoplasm, nerve, malignant
**Neurogenic** (see also condition)
  bladder (see also Dysfunction, bladder, neuromuscular) N31.9
    cauda equina syndrome G83.4
  bowel NEC K59.2
  heart F45.8
**Neuroglioma** — see Neoplasm, uncertain behavior, by site
**Neurolabyrinthitis** (of Dix and Hallpike) — see Neuronitis, vestibular
**Neurolathyrism** — see Poisoning, food, noxious, plant
**Neuroleprosy** A30.9
**Neuroma** (see also Neoplasm, nerve, benign)
  acoustic (nerve) D33.3
  amputation (stump) (traumatic) (surgical complication) (late) T87.3- ☑
    arm T87.3- ☑
    leg T87.3- ☑
  digital (toe) G57.6- ☑
  interdigital G58.8
    lower limb (toe) G57.8- ☑
    upper limb G56.8- ☑
  intermetatarsal G57.8- ☑
  Morton's G57.6- ☑
  nonneoplastic
    arm G56.9- ☑
    leg G57.9- ☑
    lower extremity G57.9- ☑
    upper extremity G56.9- ☑
  optic (nerve) D33.3
  plantar G57.6- ☑
  plexiform — see Neoplasm, nerve, benign
  surgical (nonneoplastic)
    arm G56.9- ☑
    leg G57.9- ☑
    lower extremity G57.9- ☑
    upper extremity G56.9- ☑
**Neuromyalgia** — see Neuralgia
**Neuromyasthenia** (epidemic) (postinfectious) G93.3
**Neuromyelitis** G36.9
  ascending G61.0
  optica G36.0
**Neuromyopathy** G70.9
  paraneoplastic D49.9 [G13.0]
**Neuromyotonia** (Isaacs) G71.19
**Neuronevus** — see Nevus
**Neuronitis** G58.9
  ascending (acute) G57.2- ☑
  vestibular H81.2- ☑
**Neuroparalytic** — see condition
**Neuropathy, neuropathic** G62.9
  acute motor G62.81
  alcoholic G62.1
    with psychosis — see Psychosis, alcoholic
  arm G56.9- ☑
  autonomic, peripheral — see Neuropathy, peripheral, autonomic
  axillary G56.9- ☑
  bladder N31.9
    atonic (motor) (sensory) N31.2
    autonomous N31.2
    flaccid N31.2
    nonreflex N31.2
    reflex N31.1
    uninhibited N31.0
  brachial plexus G54.0
  cervical plexus G54.2

**Neuropathy, neuropathic** — continued
  chronic
      progressive segmentally demyelinating G62.89
      relapsing demyelinating G62.89
  Déjérine-Sottas G60.0
  diabetic — see E08-E13 with .40
      mononeuropathy — see E08-E13 with .41
      polyneuropathy — see E08-E13 with .42
  entrapment G58.9
      iliohypogastric nerve G57.8- ☑
      ilioinguinal nerve G57.8- ☑
      lateral cutaneous nerve of thigh G57.1- ☑
      median nerve G56.0- ☑
      obturator nerve G57.8- ☑
      peroneal nerve G57.3- ☑
      posterior tibial nerve G57.5- ☑
      saphenous nerve G57.8- ☑
      ulnar nerve G56.2- ☑
  facial nerve G51.9
  hereditary G60.9
      motor and sensory (types I-IV) G60.0
      sensory G60.8
      specified NEC G60.8
  hypertrophic G60.0
      Charcot-Marie-Tooth G60.0
      Déjérine-Sottas G60.0
      interstitial progressive G60.0
      of infancy G60.0
      Refsum G60.1
  idiopathic G60.9
      progressive G60.3
      specified NEC G60.8
  in association with hereditary ataxia G60.2
  intercostal G58.0
  ischemic — see Disorder, nerve
  Jamaica (ginger) G62.2
  leg NEC G57.9- ☑
  lower extremity G57.9- ☑
  lumbar plexus G54.1
  median nerve G56.1- ☑
  motor and sensory (see also Polyneuropathy)
      hereditary (types I-IV) G60.0
  multifocal motor (MMN) G61.82
  multiple (acute) (chronic) — see Polyneuropathy
  optic (nerve) (see also Neuritis, optic)
      ischemic H47.01- ☑
  paraneoplastic (sensorial) (Denny Brown) D49.9 [G13.0]
  peripheral (nerve) (see also Polyneuropathy) G62.9
      autonomic G90.9
          idiopathic G90.09
          in (due to)
              amyloidosis E85.4 [G99.0]
              diabetes mellitus — see E08-E13 with .43
              endocrine disease NEC E34.9 [G99.0]
              gout M10.00 [G99.0]
              hyperthyroidism E05.90 [G99.0]
                  with thyroid storm E05.91 [G99.0]
              metabolic disease NEC E88.9 [G99.0]
      idiopathic G60.9
          progressive G60.3
      in (due to)
          antitetanus serum G62.0
          arsenic G62.2
          drugs NEC G62.0
          lead G62.2
          organophosphate compounds G62.2
          toxic agent NEC G62.2
  plantar nerves G57.6- ☑
  progressive
      hypertrophic interstitial G60.0
      inflammatory G62.81
  radicular NEC — see Radiculopathy
  sacral plexus G54.1
  sciatic G57.0- ☑
  serum G61.1
  toxic NEC G62.2
  trigeminal sensory G50.8
  ulnar nerve G56.2- ☑
  uremic N18.9 [G63]
  vitamin B12 E53.8 [G63]
      with anemia (pernicious) D51.0 [G63]
          due to dietary deficiency D51.3 [G63]
**Neurophthisis** (see also Disorder, nerve)
  peripheral, diabetic — see E08-E13 with .42
**Neuroretinitis** — see Chorioretinitis
**Neuroretinopathy, hereditary optic** H47.22
**Neurosarcoma** — see Neoplasm, nerve, malignant
**Neurosclerosis** — see Disorder, nerve

**Neurosis, neurotic** F48.9
  anankastic F42.8
  anxiety (state) F41.1
      panic type F41.0
  asthenic F48.8
  bladder F45.8
  cardiac (reflex) F45.8
  cardiovascular F45.8
  character F60.9
  colon F45.8
  compensation F68.1 ☑
  compulsive, compulsion F42.8
  conversion F44.9
  craft F48.8
  cutaneous F45.8
  depersonalization F48.1
  depressive (reaction) (type) F34.1
  environmental F48.8
  excoriation L98.1
  fatigue F48.8
  functional — see Disorder, somatoform
  gastric F45.8
  gastrointestinal F45.8
  heart F45.8
  hypochondriacal F45.21
  hysterical F44.9
  incoordination F45.8
      larynx F45.8
      vocal cord F45.8
  intestine F45.8
  larynx (sensory) F45.8
      hysterical F44.4
  mixed NEC F48.8
  musculoskeletal F45.8
  obsessional F42.8
  obsessive-compulsive F42.8
  occupational F48.8
  ocular NEC F45.8
  organ — see Disorder, somatoform
  pharynx F45.8
  phobic F40.9
  posttraumatic (situational) F43.10
      acute F43.11
      chronic F43.12
  psychasthenic (type) F48.8
  railroad F48.8
  rectum F45.8
  respiratory F45.8
  rumination F45.8
  sexual F65.9
  situational F48.8
  social F40.10
      generalized F40.11
  specified type NEC F48.8
  state F48.9
      with depersonalization episode F48.1
  stomach F45.8
  traumatic F43.10
      acute F43.11
      chronic F43.12
  vasomotor F45.8
  visceral F45.8
  war F48.8
**Neurospongioblastosis diffusa** Q85.1
**Neurosyphilis** (arrested) (early) (gumma) (late) (latent) (recurrent) (relapse) A52.3
  with ataxia (cerebellar) (locomotor) (spastic) (spinal) A52.19
  aneurysm (cerebral) A52.05
  arachnoid (adhesive) A52.13
  arteritis (any artery) (cerebral) A52.04
  asymptomatic A52.2
  congenital A50.40
  dura (mater) A52.13
  general paresis A52.17
  hemorrhagic A52.05
  juvenile (asymptomatic) (meningeal) A50.40
  leptomeninges (aseptic) A52.13
  meningeal, meninges (adhesive) A52.13
  meningitis A52.13
  meningovascular (diffuse) A52.13
  optic atrophy A52.15
  parenchymatous (degenerative) A52.19
  paresis, paretic A52.17
      juvenile A50.45
  remission in (sustained) A52.3
  serological (without symptoms) A52.2
  specified nature or site NEC A52.19
  tabes, tabetic (dorsalis) A52.11

**Neurosyphilis** — continued
  tabes, tabetic — continued
    juvenile A50.45
  taboparesis A52.17
    juvenile A50.45
  thrombosis (cerebral) A52.05
  vascular (cerebral) NEC A52.05
**Neurothekeoma** — see Neoplasm, nerve, benign
**Neurotic** — see Neurosis
**Neurotoxemia** — see Toxemia
**Neuroclusion** M26.211
**Neutropenia, neutropenic** (chronic) (genetic) (idiopathic) (immune) (infantile) (malignant) (pernicious) (splenic) D70.9
  congenital (primary) D70.0
  cyclic D70.4
  cytoreductive cancer chemotherapy sequela D70.1
  drug-induced D70.2
    due to cytoreductive cancer chemotherapy D70.1
  due to infection D70.3
  fever D70.9
  neonatal, transitory (isoimmune) (maternal transfer) P61.5
  periodic D70.4
  secondary (cyclic) (periodic) (splenic) D70.4
    drug-induced D70.2
      due to cytoreductive cancer chemotherapy D70.1
  toxic D70.8
**Neutrophilia, hereditary giant** D72.0
**Nevocarcinoma** — see Melanoma
**Nevus** D22.9
  achromic — see Neoplasm, skin, benign
  amelanotic — see Neoplasm, skin, benign
  angiomatous D18.00
    intra-abdominal D18.03
    intracranial D18.02
    skin D18.01
    specified site NEC D18.09
  araneus I78.1
  balloon cell — see Neoplasm, skin, benign
  bathing trunk D48.5
  blue — see Neoplasm, skin, benign
    cellular — see Neoplasm, skin, benign
    giant — see Neoplasm, skin, benign
    Jadassohn's — see Neoplasm, skin, benign
    malignant — see Melanoma
  capillary D18.00
    intra-abdominal D18.03
    intracranial D18.02
    skin D18.01
    specified site NEC D18.09
  cavernous D18.00
    intra-abdominal D18.03
    intracranial D18.02
    skin D18.01
    specified site NEC D18.09
  cellular — see Neoplasm, skin, benign
    blue — see Neoplasm, skin, benign
  choroid D31.3- ☑
  comedonicus Q82.5
  conjunctiva D31.0- ☑
  dermal — see Neoplasm, skin, benign
    with epidermal nevus — see Neoplasm, skin, benign
  dysplastic — see Neoplasm, skin, benign
  eye D31.9- ☑
  flammeus Q82.5
  hemangiomatous D18.00
    intra-abdominal D18.03
    intracranial D18.02
    skin D18.01
    specified site NEC D18.09
  iris D31.4- ☑
  lacrimal gland D31.5- ☑
  lymphatic D18.1
  magnocellular
    specified site — see Neoplasm, benign, by site
    unspecified site D31.40
  malignant — see Melanoma
  meaning hemangioma D18.00
    intra-abdominal D18.03
    intracranial D18.02
    skin D18.01
    specified site NEC D18.09
  mouth (mucosa) D10.30
    specified site NEC D10.39
    white sponge Q38.6

**Nevus** — continued
  multiplex Q85.1
  non-neoplastic I78.1
  oral mucosa D10.30
    specified site NEC D10.39
    white sponge Q38.6
  orbit D31.6- ☑
  pigmented
    giant (see also Neoplasm, skin, uncertain behavior) D48.5
      malignant melanoma in — see Melanoma
  portwine Q82.5
  retina D31.2- ☑
  retrobulbar D31.6- ☑
  sanguineous Q82.5
  senile I78.1
  skin D22.9
    abdominal wall D22.5
    ala nasi D22.39
    ankle D22.7- ☑
    anus, anal D22.5
    arm D22.6- ☑
    auditory canal (external) D22.2- ☑
    auricle (ear) D22.2- ☑
    auricular canal (external) D22.2- ☑
    axilla, axillary fold D22.5
    back D22.5
    breast D22.5
    brow D22.39
    buttock D22.5
    canthus (eye) D22.1- ☑
    cheek (external) D22.39
    chest wall D22.5
    chin D22.39
    ear (external) D22.2- ☑
    external meatus (ear) D22.2- ☑
    eyebrow D22.39
    eyelid (lower) (upper) D22.1- ☑
    face D22.30
      specified NEC D22.39
    female genital organ (external) NEC D28.0
    finger D22.6- ☑
    flank D22.5
    foot D22.7- ☑
    forearm D22.6- ☑
    forehead D22.39
    foreskin D29.0
    genital organ (external) NEC
      female D28.0
      male D29.9
    gluteal region D22.5
    groin D22.5
    hand D22.6- ☑
    heel D22.7- ☑
    helix D22.2- ☑
    hip D22.7- ☑
    interscapular region D22.5
    jaw D22.39
    knee D22.7- ☑
    labium (majus) (minus) D28.0
    leg D22.7- ☑
    lip (lower) (upper) D22.0
    lower limb D22.7- ☑
    male genital organ (external) D29.9
    nail D22.9
      finger D22.6- ☑
      toe D22.7- ☑
    nasolabial groove D22.39
    nates D22.5
    neck D22.4
    nose (external) D22.39
    palpebra D22.1- ☑
    penis D29.0
    perianal skin D22.5
    perineum D22.5
    pinna D22.2- ☑
    popliteal fossa or space D22.7- ☑
    prepuce D29.0
    pudendum D28.0
    scalp D22.4
    scrotum D29.4
    shoulder D22.6- ☑
    submammary fold D22.5
    temple D22.39
    thigh D22.7- ☑
    toe D22.7- ☑
    trunk NEC D22.5

**Nevus** — continued
  skin — continued
    umbilicus D22.5
    upper limb D22.6- ☑
    vulva D28.0
  specified site NEC — see Neoplasm, by site, benign
  spider I78.1
  stellar I78.1
  strawberry Q82.5
  Sutton's benign D22.9
  unius lateris Q82.5
  Unna's Q82.5
  vascular Q82.5
  verrucous Q82.5
**Newborn** (infant) (liveborn) (singleton) Z38.2
  abstinence syndrome P96.1
  acne L70.4
  affected by
    abnormalities of membranes P02.9
      specified NEC P02.8
    abruptio placenta P02.1
    amino-acid metabolic disorder, transitory P74.8
    amniocentesis (while in utero) P00.6
    amnionitis P02.7
    apparent life threatening event (ALTE) R68.13
    bleeding (into)
      cerebral cortex P52.22
      germinal matrix P52.0
      ventricles P52.1
    breech delivery P03.0
    cardiac arrest P29.81
    cardiomyopathy I42.8
      congenital I42.4
    cerebral ischemia P91.0
    Cesarean delivery P03.4
    chemotherapy agents P04.1
    chorioamnionitis P02.7
    cocaine (crack) P04.41
    complications of labor and delivery P03.9
      specified NEC P03.89
    compression of umbilical cord NEC P02.5
    contracted pelvis P03.1
    delivery P03.9
      Cesarean P03.4
      forceps P03.2
      vacuum extractor P03.3
    entanglement (knot) in umbilical cord P02.5
    environmental chemicals P04.6
    fetal (intrauterine)
      growth retardation P05.9
      malnutrition not light or small for gestational age P05.2
    forceps delivery P03.2
    heart rate abnormalities
      bradycardia P29.12
      intrauterine P03.819
        before onset of labor P03.810
        during labor P03.811
      tachycardia P29.11
    hemorrhage (antepartum) P02.1
      cerebellar (nontraumatic) P52.6
      intracerebral (nontraumatic) P52.4
      intracranial (nontraumatic) P52.9
        specified NEC P52.8
      intraventricular (nontraumatic) P52.3
        grade 1 P52.0
        grade 2 P52.1
        grade 3 P52.21
        grade 4 P52.22
      posterior fossa (nontraumatic) P52.6
      subarachnoid (nontraumatic) P52.5
      subependymal P52.0
        with intracerebral extension P52.22
        with intraventricular extension P52.1
          with enlargment of ventricles P52.21
        without intraventricular extension P52.0
    hypoxic ischemic encephalopathy [HIE] P91.60
      mild P91.61
      moderate P91.62
      severe P91.63
    induction of labor P03.89
    intestinal perforation P78.0
    intrauterine (fetal) blood loss P50.9
      due to (from)
        cut end of co-twin cord P50.5
        hemorrhage into
          co-twin P50.3
          maternal circulation P50.4
        placenta P50.2

**Newborn** — *continued*
  affected by — *continued*
    intrauterine blood loss — *continued*
      due to — *continued*
        ruptured cord blood P50.1
        vasa previa P50.0
      specified NEC P50.8
    intrauterine (fetal) hemorrhage P50.9
    intrauterine (in utero) procedure P96.5
    malpresentation (malposition) NEC P03.1
    maternal (complication of) (use of)
      alcohol P04.3
      analgesia (maternal) P04.0
      anesthesia (maternal) P04.0
      blood loss P02.1
      circulatory disease P00.3
      condition P00.9
        specified NEC P00.89
      delivery P03.9
        Cesarean P03.4
        forceps P03.2
        vacuum extractor P03.3
      diabetes mellitus (pre-existing) P70.1
      disorder P00.9
        specified NEC P00.89
      drugs (addictive) (illegal) NEC P04.49
      ectopic pregnancy P01.4
      gestational diabetes P70.0
      hemorrhage P02.1
      hypertensive disorder P00.0
      incompetent cervix P01.0
      infectious disease P00.2
      injury P00.5
      labor and delivery P03.9
      malpresentation before labor P01.7
      maternal death P01.6
      medical procedure P00.7
      medication P04.1
      multiple pregnancy P01.5
      nutritional disorder P00.4
      oligohydramnios P01.2
      parasitic disease P00.2
      periodontal disease P00.81
      placenta previa P02.0
      polyhydramnios P01.3
      precipitate delivery P03.5
      pregnancy P01.9
        specified P01.8
      premature rupture of membranes P01.1
      renal disease P00.1
      respiratory disease P00.3
      surgical procedure P00.6
      urinary tract disease P00.1
      uterine contraction (abnormal) P03.6
    meconium peritonitis P78.0
    medication (legal) (maternal use) (prescribed) P04.1
    membrane abnormalities P02.9
      specified NEC P02.8
    membranitis P02.7
    methamphetamine(s) P04.49
    mixed metabolic and respiratory acidosis P84
    neonatal abstinence syndrome P96.1
    noxious substances transmitted via placenta or breast milk P04.9
      specified NEC P04.8
    nutritional supplements P04.5
    placenta previa P02.0
    placental
      abnormality (functional) (morphological) P02.20
        specified NEC P02.29
      dysfunction P02.29
      infarction P02.29
      insufficiency P02.29
      separation NEC P02.1
      transfusion syndromes P02.3
    placentitis P02.7
    precipitate delivery P03.5
    prolapsed cord P02.4
    respiratory arrest P28.81
    slow intrauterine growth P05.9
    tobacco P04.2
    twin to twin transplacental transfusion P02.3
    umbilical cord (tightly) around neck P02.5
    umbilical cord condition P02.60
      short cord P02.69
      specified NEC P02.69
    uterine contractions (abnormal) P03.6
    vasa previa P02.69

**Newborn** — *continued*
  affected by — *continued*
    vasa previa — *continued*
      from intrauterine blood loss P50.0
  apnea P28.4
    obstructive P28.4
    primary P28.3
    sleep (central) (obstructive) (primary) P28.3
  born in hospital Z38.00
    by cesarean Z38.01
  born outside hospital Z38.1
  breast buds P96.89
  breast engorgement P83.4
  check-up — *see* Newborn, examination
  convulsion P90
  dehydration P74.1
  examination
    8 to 28 days old Z00.111
    under 8 days old Z00.110
  fever P81.9
    environmentally-induced P81.0
  hyperbilirubinemia P59.9
    of prematurity P59.0
  hypernatremia P74.2
  hyponatremia P74.2
  infection P39.9
    candidal P37.5
    specified NEC P39.8
    urinary tract P39.3
  jaundice P59.9
    due to
      breast milk inhibitor P59.3
      hepatocellular damage P59.20
        specified NEC P59.29
      preterm delivery P59.0
    of prematurity P59.0
    specified NEC P59.8
  late metabolic acidosis P74.0
  mastitis P39.0
    infective P39.0
    noninfective P83.4
  multiple born NEC Z38.8
    born in hospital Z38.68
      by cesarean Z38.69
    born outside hospital Z38.7
  omphalitis P38.9
    with mild hemorrhage P38.1
    without hemorrhage P38.9
  post-term P08.21
  prolonged gestation (over 42 completed weeks) P08.22
  quadruplet Z38.8
    born in hospital Z38.63
      by cesarean Z38.64
    born outside hospital Z38.7
  quintuplet Z38.8
    born in hospital Z38.65
      by cesarean Z38.66
    born outside hospital Z38.7
  seizure P90
  sepsis (congenital) P36.9
    due to
      anaerobes NEC P36.5
      Escherichia coli P36.4
      Staphylococcus P36.30
        aureus P36.2
        specified NEC P36.39
      Streptococcus P36.10
        group B P36.0
        specified NEC P36.19
      specified NEC P36.8
  triplet Z38.8
    born in hospital Z38.61
      by cesarean Z38.62
    born outside hospital Z38.7
  twin Z38.5
    born in hospital Z38.30
      by cesarean Z38.31
    born outside hospital Z38.4
  vomiting P92.09
    bilious P92.01
  weight check Z00.111

**Newcastle conjunctivitis or disease** B30.8
**Nezelof's syndrome** (pure alymphocytosis) D81.4
**Niacin** (amide) **deficiency** E52
**Nicolas** (-Durand)-**Favre disease** A55
**Nicotine** — *see* Tobacco
**Nicotinic acid deficiency** E52

**Niemann-Pick disease or syndrome** E75.249
  specified NEC E75.248
  type
    A E75.240
    B E75.241
    C E75.242
    D E75.243
**Night**
  blindness — *see* Blindness, night
  sweats R61
  terrors (child) F51.4
**Nightmares** (REM sleep type) F51.5
**NIHSS** (National Institutes of Health Stroke Scale) **score** R29.7- ☑
**Nipple** — *see* condition
**Nisbet's chancre** A57
**Nishimoto** (-Takeuchi) **disease** I67.5
**Nitritoid crisis or reaction** — *see* Crisis, nitritoid
**Nitrosohemoglobinemia** D74.8
**Njovera** A65
**Nocardiosis, nocardiasis** A43.9
  cutaneous A43.1
  lung A43.0
  pneumonia A43.0
  pulmonary A43.0
  specified site NEC A43.8
**Nocturia** R35.1
  psychogenic F45.8
**Nocturnal** — *see* condition
**Nodal rhythm** I49.8
**Node**(s) (*see also* Nodule)
  Bouchard's (with arthropathy) M15.2
  Haygarth's M15.8
  Heberden's (with arthropathy) M15.1
  larynx J38.7
  lymph — *see* condition
  milker's B08.03
  Osler's I33.0
  Schmorl's — *see* Schmorl's disease
  singer's J38.2
  teacher's J38.2
  tuberculous — *see* Tuberculosis, lymph gland
  vocal cord J38.2
**Nodule**(s), **nodular**
  actinomycotic — *see* Actinomycosis
  breast NEC (*see also* Lump, breast) N63.0
  colloid (cystic), thyroid E04.1
  cutaneous — *see* Swelling, localized
  endometrial (stromal) D26.1
  Haygarth's M15.8
  inflammatory — *see* Inflammation
  juxta-articular
    syphilitic A52.77
    yaws A66.7
  larynx J38.7
  lung, solitary (subsegmental branch of the bronchial tree) R91.1
    multiple R91.8
  milker's B08.03
  prostate N40.2
    with lower urinary tract symptoms (LUTS) N40.3
    without lower urinary tract symtpoms (LUTS) N40.2
  pulmonary, solitary (subsegmental branch of the bronchial tree) R91.1
  retrocardiac R09.89
  rheumatoid M06.30
    ankle M06.37- ☑
    elbow M06.32- ☑
    foot joint M06.37- ☑
    hand joint M06.34- ☑
    hip M06.35- ☑
    knee M06.36- ☑
    multiple site M06.39
    shoulder M06.31- ☑
    vertebra M06.38
    wrist M06.33- ☑
  scrotum (inflammatory) N49.2
  singer's J38.2
  solitary, lung (subsegmental branch of the bronchial tree) R91.1
    multiple R91.8
  subcutaneous — *see* Swelling, localized
  teacher's J38.2
  thyroid (cold) (gland) (nontoxic) E04.1
    with thyrotoxicosis E05.20
      with thyroid storm E05.21
    toxic or with hyperthyroidism E05.20
      with thyroid storm E05.21

**Nodule(s), nodular** — *continued*
  vocal cord J38.2
**Noma** (gangrenous) (hospital) (infective) A69.0
  auricle I96
  mouth A69.0
  pudendi N76.89
  vulvae N76.89
**Nomad, nomadism** Z59.0
**NOMID** (neonatal onset multisystemic inflammatory
    disorder) M04.2
**Nonadherence to medical treatment** Z91.19
**Nonautoimmune hemolytic anemia** D59.4
  drug-induced D59.2
**Nonclosure** (see also Imperfect, closure)
  ductus arteriosus (Botallo's) Q25.0
  foramen
    botalli Q21.1
    ovale Q21.1
**Noncompliance** Z91.19
  with
    dialysis Z91.15
    dietary regimen Z91.11
    medical treatment Z91.19
    medication regimen NEC Z91.14
      underdosing (see also Table of Drugs and
        Chemicals, categories T36-T50, with final
        character 6) Z91.14
        intentional NEC Z91.128
          due to financial hardship of patient
            Z91.120
        unintentional NEC Z91.138
          due to patient's age related debility
            Z91.130
    renal dialysis Z91.15
**Nondescent** (congenital) (see also Malposition, congenital)
  cecum Q43.3
  colon Q43.3
  testicle Q53.9
    bilateral Q53.20
      abdominal Q53.211
      perineal Q53.22
    unilateral Q53.10
      abdominal Q53.111
      perineal Q53.12
**Nondevelopment**
  brain Q02
    part of Q04.3
  heart Q24.8
  organ or site, congenital NEC — see Hypoplasia
**Nonengagement**
  head NEC O32.4 ☑
    in labor, causing obstructed labor O64.8 ☑
**Nonexanthematous tick fever** A93.2
**Nonexpansion, lung** (newborn) P28.0
**Nonfunctioning**
  cystic duct (see also Disease, gallbladder) K82.8
  gallbladder (see also Disease, gallbladder) K82.8
  kidney N28.9
  labyrinth — see subcategory H83.2 ☑
**Non-Hodgkin lymphoma NEC** — see Lymphoma, non-
   Hodgkin
**Nonimplantation, ovum** N97.2
**Noninsufflation, fallopian tube** N97.1
**Non-ketotic hyperglycinemia** E72.51
**Nonne-Milroy syndrome** Q82.0
**Nonovulation** N97.0
**Non-palpable testicle**(s)
  bilateral R39.84
  unilateral R39.83
**Nonpatent fallopian tube** N97.1
**Nonpneumatization, lung NEC** P28.0
**Nonrotation** — see Malrotation
**Nonsecretion, urine** — see Anuria
**Nonunion**
  fracture — see Fracture, by site
  joint, following fusion or arthrodesis M96.0
  organ or site, congenital NEC — see Imperfect, closure
  symphysis pubis, congenital Q74.2
**Nonvisualization, gallbladder** R93.2
**Nonvital, nonvitalized tooth** K04.99
**Non-working side interference** M26.56
**Noonan's syndrome** Q87.1
**Normocytic anemia** (infectional) due to blood loss
   (chronic) D50.0
  acute D62
**Norrie's disease** (congenital) Q15.8

**North American blastomycosis** B40.9
**Norwegian itch** B86
**Nose, nasal** — see condition
**Nosebleed** R04.0
**Nose-picking** F98.8
**Nosomania** F45.21
**Nosophobia** F45.22
**Nostalgia** F43.20
**Notch of iris** Q13.2
**Notching nose, congenital** (tip) Q30.2
**Nothnagel's**
  syndrome — see Strabismus, paralytic, third nerve
  vasomotor acroparesthesia I73.89
**Novy's relapsing fever** A68.9
  louse-borne A68.0
  tick-borne A68.1
**Noxious**
  foodstuffs, poisoning by — see Poisoning, food, nox-
    ious, plant
  substances transmitted through placenta or breast
    milk P04.9
**Nucleus pulposus** — see condition
**Numbness** R20.0
**Nuns' knee** — see Bursitis, prepatellar
**Nursemaid's elbow** S53.03- ☑
**Nutcracker esophagus** K22.4
**Nutmeg liver** K76.1
**Nutrient element deficiency** E61.9
  specified NEC E61.8
**Nutrition deficient or insufficient** (see also Malnutrition) E46
  due to
    insufficient food T73.0 ☑
    lack of
      care (child) T76.02 ☑
        adult T76.01 ☑
      food T73.0 ☑
**Nutritional stunting** E45
**Nyctalopia** (night blindness) — see Blindness, night
**Nycturia** R35.1
  psychogenic F45.8
**Nymphomania** F52.8
**Nystagmus** H55.00
  benign paroxysmal — see Vertigo, benign paroxysmal
  central positional H81.4- ☑
  congenital H55.01
  dissociated H55.04
  latent H55.02
  miners' H55.09
  positional
    benign paroxysmal H81.4- ☑
    central H81.4- ☑
  specified form NEC H55.09
  visual deprivation H55.03

# O

**Obermeyer's relapsing fever** (European) A68.0
**Obesity** E66.9
  with alveolar hypoventilation E66.2
  adrenal E27.8
  complicating
    childbirth O99.214
    pregnancy O99.21- ☑
    puerperium O99.215
  constitutional E66.8
  dietary counseling and surveillance Z71.3
  drug-induced E66.1
  due to
    drug E66.1
    excess calories E66.09
      morbid E66.01
      severe E66.01
  endocrine E66.8
  endogenous E66.8
  exogenous E66.09
  familial E66.8
  glandular E66.8
  hypothyroid — see Hypothyroidism
  hypoventilation syndrome (OHS) E66.2
  morbid E66.01
    with
      alveolar hypoventilation E66.2
      obesity hypoventilation syndrome (OHS) E66.2
    due to excess calories E66.01
  nutritional E66.09
  pituitary E23.6

**Obesity** — *continued*
  severe E66.01
  specified type NEC E66.8
**Oblique** — see condition
**Obliteration**
  appendix (lumen) K38.8
  artery I77.1
  bile duct (noncalculous) K83.1
  common duct (noncalculous) K83.1
  cystic duct — see Obstruction, gallbladder
  disease, arteriolar I77.1
  endometrium N85.8
  eye, anterior chamber — see Disorder, globe, hy-
    potony
  fallopian tube N97.1
  lymphatic vessel I89.0
    due to mastectomy I97.2
  organ or site, congenital NEC — see Atresia, by site
  ureter N13.5
    with infection N13.6
  urethra — see Stricture, urethra
  vein I87.8
  vestibule (oral) K08.89
**Observation** (following) (for) (without need for further
    medical care) Z04.9
  accident NEC Z04.3
    at work Z04.2
    transport Z04.1
  adverse effect of drug Z03.6
  alleged rape or sexual assault (victim), ruled out
    adult Z04.41
    child Z04.42
  criminal assault Z04.8
  development state
    adolescent Z00.3
    period of rapid growth in childhood Z00.2
    puberty Z00.3
  disease, specified NEC Z03.89
  following work accident Z04.2
  growth and development state — see Observation,
    development state
  injuries (accidental) NEC (see also Observation, acci-
    dent)
  newborn (for)
    suspected condition, related to exposure from the
      mother or birth process — see Newborn, af-
      fected by, maternal
      ruled out Z05.9
        cardiac Z05.0
        connective tissue Z05.73
        gastrointestinal Z05.5
        genetic Z05.41
        genitourinary Z05.6
        immunologic Z05.43
        infectious Z05.1
        metabolic Z05.42
        musculoskeletal Z05.72
        neurological Z05.2
        respiratory Z05.3
        skin and subcutaneous tissue Z05.71
        specified condition NEC Z05.8
  postpartum
    immediately after delivery Z39.0
    routine follow-up Z39.2
  pregnancy (normal) (without complication) Z34.9- ☑
    high risk O09.9- ☑
  suicide attempt, alleged NEC Z03.89
    self-poisoning Z03.6
  suspected, ruled out (see also Suspected condition,
    ruled out)
    abuse, physical
      adult Z04.71
      child Z04.72
    accident at work Z04.2
    adult battering victim Z04.71
    child battering victim Z04.72
    condition NEC Z03.89
      newborn (see also Observation, newborn (for),
        suspected condition, ruled out) Z05.9
    drug poisoning or adverse effect Z03.6
    exposure (to)
      anthrax Z03.810
      biological agent NEC Z03.818
    inflicted injury NEC Z04.8
    suicide attempt, alleged Z03.89
      self-poisoning Z03.6
    toxic effects from ingested substance (drug) (poi-
      son) Z03.6

---

**Observation** — continued
　toxic effects from ingested substance (drug) (poison) Z03.6
**Obsession, obsessional state** F42.8
　mixed thoughts and acts F42.2
**Obsessive-compulsive neurosis or reaction** F42.8
**Obstetric embolism, septic** — see Embolism, obstetric, septic
**Obstetrical trauma** (complicating delivery) O71.9
　with or following ectopic or molar pregnancy O08.6
　specified type NEC O71.89
**Obstipation** — see Constipation
**Obstruction, obstructed, obstructive**
　airway J98.8
　　with
　　　allergic alveolitis J67.9
　　　asthma J45.909
　　　　with
　　　　　exacerbation (acute) J45.901
　　　　　status asthmaticus J45.902
　　　bronchiectasis J47.9
　　　　with
　　　　　exacerbation (acute) J47.1
　　　　　lower respiratory infection J47.0
　　　bronchitis (chronic) J44.9
　　　emphysema J43.9
　　chronic J44.9
　　　with
　　　　allergic alveolitis — see Pneumonitis, hypersensitivity
　　　　bronchiectasis J47.9
　　　　　with
　　　　　　exacerbation (acute) J47.1
　　　　　　lower respiratory infection J47.0
　　due to
　　　foreign body — see Foreign body, by site, causing asphyxia
　　　inhalation of fumes or vapors J68.9
　　　laryngospasm J38.5
　ampulla of Vater K83.1
　aortic (heart) (valve) — see Stenosis, aortic
　aortoiliac I74.09
　aqueduct of Sylvius G91.1
　　congenital Q03.0
　　　with spina bifida — see Spina bifida, by site, with hydrocephalus
　Arnold-Chiari — see Arnold-Chiari disease
　artery (see also Atherosclerosis, artery) I70.9 ☑
　　basilar (complete) (partial) — see Occlusion, artery, basilar
　　carotid (complete) (partial) — see Occlusion, artery, carotid
　　cerebellar — see Occlusion, artery, cerebellar
　　cerebral (anterior) (middle) (posterior) — see Occlusion, artery, cerebral
　　precerebral — see Occlusion, artery, precerebral
　　renal N28.0
　　retinal NEC — see Occlusion, artery, retina
　　stent — see Restenosis, stent
　　vertebral (complete) (partial) — see Occlusion, artery, vertebral
　band (intestinal) (see also Obstruction, intestine, specified NEC) K56.699
　bile duct or passage (common) (hepatic) (noncalculous) K83.1
　　with calculus K80.51
　　congenital (causing jaundice) Q44.3
　biliary (duct) (tract) K83.1
　　gallbladder K82.0
　bladder-neck (acquired) N32.0
　　congenital Q64.31
　　due to hyperplasia (hypertrophy) of prostate — see Hyperplasia, prostate
　bowel — see Obstruction, intestine
　bronchus J98.09
　canal, ear — see Stenosis, external ear canal
　cardia K22.2
　caval veins (inferior) (superior) I87.1
　cecum — see Obstruction, intestine
　circulatory I99.8
　colon — see Obstruction, intestine
　common duct (noncalculous) K83.1
　coronary (artery) — see Occlusion, coronary
　cystic duct (see also Obstruction, gallbladder)
　　with calculus K80.21
　device, implant or graft (see also Complications, by site and type, mechanical) T85.698 ☑

**Obstruction, obstructed, obstructive** — continued
　device, implant or graft (see also Complications, by site and type, mechanical) — continued
　　arterial graft NEC — see Complication, cardiovascular device, mechanical, vascular
　　catheter NEC T85.628 ☑
　　　cystostomy T83.090 ☑
　　　dialysis (renal) T82.49 ☑
　　　　intraperitoneal T85.691 ☑
　　　Hopkins T83.098 ☑
　　　ileostomy T83.098 ☑
　　　infusion NEC T82.594 ☑
　　　　spinal (epidural) (subdural) T85.690 ☑
　　　nephrostomy T83.092 ☑
　　　urethral indwelling T83.091 ☑
　　　urinary T83.098 ☑
　　　urostomy T83.098 ☑
　　　due to infection T85.79 ☑
　　gastrointestinal — see Complications, prosthetic device, mechanical, gastrointestinal device
　　genital NEC T83.498 ☑
　　　intrauterine contraceptive device T83.39 ☑
　　　penile prosthesis (cylinder) (implanted) (pump) (resevoir) T83.490 ☑
　　　testicular prosthesis T83.491 ☑
　　heart NEC — see Complication, cardiovascular device, mechanical
　　joint prosthesis — see Complications, joint prosthesis, mechanical, specified NEC, by site
　　orthopedic NEC — see Complication, orthopedic, device, mechanical
　　specified NEC T85.628 ☑
　　urinary NEC (see also Complication, genitourinary, device, urinary, mechanical)
　　　graft T83.29 ☑
　　vascular NEC — see Complication, cardiovascular device, mechanical
　　ventricular intracranial shunt T85.09 ☑
　due to foreign body accidentally left in operative wound T81.529 ☑
　duodenum K31.5
　ejaculatory duct N50.89
　esophagus K22.2
　eustachian tube (complete) (partial) H68.10- ☑
　　cartilagenous (extrinsic) H68.13- ☑
　　　intrinsic H68.12- ☑
　　osseous H68.11- ☑
　fallopian tube (bilateral) N97.1
　fecal K56.41
　　with hernia — see Hernia, by site, with obstruction
　foramen of Monro (congenital) Q03.8
　　with spina bifida — see Spina bifida, by site, with hydrocephalus
　foreign body — see Foreign body
　gallbladder K82.0
　　with calculus, stones K80.21
　　congenital Q44.1
　gastric outlet K31.1
　gastrointestinal — see Obstruction, intestine
　hepatic K76.89
　　duct (noncalculous) K83.1
　ileum — see Obstruction, intestine
　iliofemoral (artery) I74.5
　intestine K56.609
　　with
　　　adhesions (intestinal) (peritoneal) K56.50
　　　　complete K56.52
　　　　incomplete K56.51
　　　　partial K56.51
　　adynamic K56.0
　　by gallstone K56.3
　　complete K56.601
　　congenital (small) Q41.9
　　　large Q42.9
　　　　specified part NEC Q42.8
　　incomplete K56.600
　　neurogenic K56.0
　　　Hirschsprung's disease or megacolon Q43.1
　　newborn P76.9
　　　due to
　　　　fecaliths P76.8
　　　　inspissated milk P76.2
　　　　meconium (plug) P76.0
　　　　　in mucoviscidosis E84.11
　　　　specified NEC P76.8
　　partial K56.600
　　postoperative K91.30

**Obstruction, obstructed, obstructive** — continued
　intestine — continued
　　postoperative — continued
　　　complete K91.32
　　　incomplete K91.31
　　　partial K91.31
　　reflex K56.0
　　specified NEC K56.699
　　　complete K56.691
　　　incomplete K56.690
　　　partial K56.690
　　volvulus K56.2
　intracardiac ball valve prosthesis T82.09 ☑
　jejunum — see Obstruction, intestine
　joint prosthesis — see Complications, joint prosthesis, mechanical, specified NEC, by site
　kidney (calices) N28.89
　labor — see Delivery
　lacrimal (passages) (duct)
　　by
　　　dacryolith — see Dacryolith
　　　stenosis — see Stenosis, lacrimal
　　congenital Q10.5
　　neonatal H04.53- ☑
　lacrimonasal duct — see Obstruction, lacrimal
　lacteal, with steatorrhea K90.2
　laryngitis — see Laryngitis
　larynx NEC J38.6
　　congenital Q31.8
　lung J98.4
　　disease, chronic J44.9
　lymphatic I89.0
　meconium (plug)
　　newborn P76.0
　　　due to fecaliths P76.0
　　　in mucoviscidosis E84.11
　mitral — see Stenosis, mitral
　nasal J34.89
　nasolacrimal duct (see also Obstruction, lacrimal)
　　congenital Q10.5
　nasopharynx J39.2
　nose J34.89
　organ or site, congenital NEC — see Atresia, by site
　pancreatic duct K86.89
　parotid duct or gland K11.8
　pelviureteral junction N13.5
　　with hydronephrosis N13.0
　　congenital Q62.39
　pharynx J39.2
　portal (circulation) (vein) I81
　prostate (see also Hyperplasia, prostate)
　　valve (urinary) N32.0
　pulmonary valve (heart) I37.0
　pyelonephritis (chronic) N11.1
　pylorus
　　adult K31.1
　　congenital or infantile Q40.0
　rectosigmoid — see Obstruction, intestine
　rectum K62.4
　renal N28.89
　　outflow N13.8
　　pelvis, congenital Q62.39
　respiratory J98.8
　　chronic J44.9
　retinal (vessels) H34.9
　salivary duct (any) K11.8
　　with calculus K11.5
　sigmoid — see Obstruction, intestine
　sinus (accessory) (nasal) J34.89
　Stensen's duct K11.8
　stomach NEC K31.89
　　acute K31.0
　　congenital Q40.2
　　due to pylorospasm K31.3
　submandibular duct K11.8
　submaxillary gland K11.8
　　with calculus K11.5
　thoracic duct I89.0
　thrombotic — see Thrombosis
　trachea J39.8
　tracheostomy airway J95.03
　tricuspid (valve) — see Stenosis, tricuspid
　upper respiratory, congenital Q34.8
　ureter (functional) (pelvic junction) NEC N13.5
　　with
　　　hydronephrosis N13.1
　　　　with infection N13.6
　　　pyelonephritis (chronic) N11.1

**Obstruction, obstructed, obstructive** — *continued*
  ureter — *continued*
    congenital Q62.39
    due to calculus — *see* Calculus, ureter
  urethra NEC N36.8
    congenital Q64.39
  urinary (moderate) N13.9
    due to hyperplasia (hypertrophy) of prostate —
      *see* Hyperplasia, prostate
    organ or tract (lower) N13.9
    prostatic valve N32.0
    specified NEC N13.8
  uropathy N13.9
  uterus N85.8
  vagina N89.5
  valvular — *see* Endocarditis
  vein, venous I87.1
    caval (inferior) (superior) I87.1
    thrombotic — *see* Thrombosis
  vena cava (inferior) (superior) I87.1
  vesical NEC N32.0
  vesicourethral orifice N32.0
    congenital Q64.31
  vessel NEC I99.8
    stent — *see* Restenosis, stent
**Obturator** — *see* condition
**Occlusal wear, teeth** K03.0
**Occlusio pupillae** — *see* Membrane, pupillary
**Occlusion, occluded**
  anus K62.4
    congenital Q42.3
      with fistula Q42.2
  aortoiliac (chronic) I74.09
  aqueduct of Sylvius G91.1
    congenital Q03.0
      with spina bifida — *see* Spina bifida, by site,
        with hydrocephalus
  artery (*see also* Atherosclerosis, artery) I70.9 ☑
    auditory, internal I65.8
    basilar I65.1
      with
        infarction I63.22
          due to
            embolism I63.12
            thrombosis I63.02
    brain or cerebral I66.9
      with infarction (due to) I63.5- ☑
        embolism I63.4- ☑
        thrombosis I63.3- ☑
    carotid I65.2- ☑
      with
        infarction I63.23- ☑
          due to
            embolism I63.13- ☑
            thrombosis I63.03- ☑
    cerebellar (anterior inferior) (posterior inferior)
      (superior) I66.3
      with infarction I63.54- ☑
        due to
          embolism I63.44- ☑
          thrombosis I63.34- ☑
    cerebral I66.9
      with infarction I63.50
        due to
          embolism I63.40
            specified NEC I63.49
          thrombosis I63.30
            specified NEC I63.39
      anterior I66.1- ☑
        with infarction I63.52- ☑
          due to
            embolism I63.42- ☑
            thrombosis I63.32- ☑
      middle I66.0- ☑
        with infarction I63.51- ☑
          due to
            embolism I63.41- ☑
            thrombosis I63.31- ☑
      posterior I66.2- ☑
        with infarction I63.53- ☑
          due to
            embolism I63.43- ☑
            thrombosis I63.33- ☑
      specified NEC I66.8
        with infarction I63.59
          due to
            embolism I63.4-

---

**Occlusion, occluded** — *continued*
  artery (*see also* Atherosclerosis, artery) — *contin-*
    *ued*
    cerebral — *continued*
      specified — *continued*
        with infarction — *continued*
          due to — *continued*
            thrombosis I63.3- ☑
    choroidal (anterior) — *see* Occlusion, artery, pre-
      cerebral, specified NEC
    communicating posterior — *see* Occlusion, artery,
      precerebral, specified NEC
    complete
      coronary I25.82
      extremities I70.92
    coronary (acute) (thrombotic) (without myocardial
      infarction) I24.0
      with myocardial infarction — *see* Infarction,
        myocardium
      chronic total I25.82
      complete I25.82
      healed or old I25.2
      total (chronic) I25.82
    hypophyseal — *see* Occlusion, artery, precerebral,
      specified NEC
    iliac I74.5
    lower extremities due to stenosis or stricture I77.1
    mesenteric (embolic) (thrombotic) (*see also* Infarct,
      intestine) K55.069
    perforating — *see* Occlusion, artery, cerebral,
      specified NEC
    peripheral I77.9
      thrombotic or embolic I74.4
    pontine — *see* Occlusion, artery, precerebral,
      specified NEC
    precerebral I65.9
      with infarction I63.20
        due to
          embolism I63.10
            specified NEC I63.19
          thrombosis I63.00
            specified NEC I63.09
        specified NEC I63.29
      basilar — *see* Occlusion, artery, basilar
      carotid — *see* Occlusion, artery, carotid
      puerperal O88.23
      specified NEC I65.8
        with infarction I63.29
          due to
            embolism I63.19
            thrombosis I63.09
      vertebral — *see* Occlusion, artery, vertebral
    renal N28.0
    retinal
      branch H34.23- ☑
      central H34.1- ☑
      partial H34.21- ☑
      transient H34.0- ☑
    spinal — *see* Occlusion, artery, precerebral, verte-
      bral
    total (chronic)
      coronary I25.82
      extremities I70.92
    vertebral I65.0- ☑
      with
        infarction I63.21- ☑
          due to
            embolism I63.11- ☑
            thrombosis I63.01- ☑
  basilar artery — *see* Occlusion, artery, basilar
  bile duct (common) (hepatic) (noncalculous) K83.1
  bowel — *see* Obstruction, intestine
  carotid (artery) (common) (internal) — *see* Occlusion,
    artery, carotid
  centric (of teeth) M26.59
    maximum intercuspation discrepancy M26.55
  cerebellar (artery) — *see* Occlusion, artery, cerebellar
  cerebral (artery) — *see* Occlusion, artery, cerebral
  cerebrovascular (*see also* Occlusion, artery, cerebral)
    with infarction I63.5- ☑
  cervical canal — *see* Stricture, cervix
  cervix (uteri) — *see* Stricture, cervix
  choanal Q30.0
  choroidal (artery) — *see* Occlusion, artery, precerebral,
    specified NEC
  colon — *see* Obstruction, intestine
  communicating posterior artery — *see* Occlusion,
    artery, precerebral, specified NEC

---

**Occlusion, occluded** — *continued*
  coronary (artery) (vein) (thrombotic) (*see also* Infarct,
    myocardium)
    chronic total I25.82
    healed or old I25.2
    not resulting in infarction I24.0
    total (chronic) I25.82
  cystic duct — *see* Obstruction, gallbladder
  embolic — *see* Embolism
  fallopian tube N97.1
    congenital Q50.6
  gallbladder (*see also* Obstruction, gallbladder)
    congenital (causing jaundice) Q44.1
  gingiva, traumatic K06.2
  hymen N89.6
    congenital Q52.3
  hypophyseal (artery) — *see* Occlusion, artery, precere-
    bral, specified NEC
  iliac artery I74.5
  intestine — *see* Obstruction, intestine
  lacrimal passages — *see* Obstruction, lacrimal
  lung J98.4
  lymph or lymphatic channel I89.0
  mammary duct N64.89
  mesenteric artery (embolic) (thrombotic) (*see also* In-
    farct, intestine) K55.069
  nose J34.89
    congenital Q30.0
  organ or site, congenital NEC — *see* Atresia, by site
  oviduct N97.1
    congenital Q50.6
  peripheral arteries
    due to stricture or stenosis I77.1
    upper extremity I74.2
  pontine (artery) — *see* Occlusion, artery, precerebral,
    specified NEC
  posterior lingual, of mandibular teeth M26.29
  precerebral artery — *see* Occlusion, artery, precerebral
  punctum lacrimale — *see* Obstruction, lacrimal
  pupil — *see* Membrane, pupillary
  pylorus, adult (*see also* Stricture, pylorus) K31.1
  renal artery N28.0
  retina, retinal
    artery — *see* Occlusion, artery, retinal
    vein (central) H34.81- ☑
      engorgement H34.82- ☑
      tributary H34.83- ☑
    vessels H34.9
  spinal artery — *see* Occlusion, artery, precerebral,
    vertebral
  teeth (mandibular) (posterior lingual) M26.29
  thoracic duct I89.0
  thrombotic — *see* Thrombosis, artery
  traumatic
    edentulous (alveolar) ridge K06.2
    gingiva K06.2
    periodontal K05.5
  tubal N97.1
  ureter (complete) (partial) N13.5
    congenital Q62.10
  ureteropelvic junction N13.5
    congenital Q62.11
  ureterovesical orifice N13.5
    congenital Q62.12
  urethra — *see* Stricture, urethra
  uterus N85.8
  vagina N89.5
  vascular NEC I99.8
  vein — *see* Thrombosis
    retinal — *see* Occlusion, retinal, vein
  vena cava (inferior) (superior) — *see* Embolism, vena
    cava
  ventricle (brain) NEC G91.1
  vertebral (artery) — *see* Occlusion, artery, vertebral
  vessel (blood) I99.8
  vulva N90.5
**Occult**
  blood in feces (stools) R19.5
**Occupational**
  problems NEC Z56.89
**Ochlophobia** — *see* Agoraphobia
**Ochronosis** (endogenous) E70.29
**Ocular muscle** — *see* condition
**Oculogyric crisis or disturbance** H51.8
  psychogenic F45.8
**Oculomotor syndrome** H51.9
**Oculopathy**
  syphilitic NEC A52.71

---

**Oculopathy** — *continued*
  syphilitic — *continued*
    congenital
      early A50.01
      late A50.30
    early (secondary) A51.43
    late A52.71
**Oddi's sphincter spasm** K83.4
**Odontalgia** K08.89
**Odontoameloblastoma** — *see* Cyst, calcifying odontogenic
**Odontoclasia** K03.89
**Odontodysplasia, regional** K00.4
**Odontogenesis imperfecta** K00.5
**Odontoma** (ameloblastic) (complex) (compound) (fibroameloblastic) — *see* Cyst, calcifying odontogenic
**Odontomyelitis** (closed) (open) K04.01
  irreversible K04.02
  reversible K04.01
**Odontorrhagia** K08.89
**Odontosarcoma, ameloblastic** C41.1
  upper jaw (bone) C41.0
**Oestriasis** — *see* Myiasis
**Oguchi's disease** H53.63
**Ohara's disease** — *see* Tularemia
**OHS** (obesity hypoventilation syndrome) E66.2
**Oidiomycosis** — *see* Candidiasis
**Oidium albicans infection** — *see* Candidiasis
**Old age** (without mention of debility) R54
  dementia F03 ☑
**Old** (previous) **myocardial infarction** I25.2
**Olfactory** — *see* condition
**Oligemia** — *see* Anemia
**Oligoastrocytoma**
  specified site — *see* Neoplasm, malignant, by site
  unspecified site C71.9
**Oligocythemia** D64.9
**Oligodendroblastoma**
  specified site — *see* Neoplasm, malignant
  unspecified site C71.9
**Oligodendroglioma**
  anaplastic type
    specified site — *see* Neoplasm, malignant, by site
    unspecified site C71.9
  specified site — *see* Neoplasm, malignant, by site
  unspecified site C71.9
**Oligodontia** — *see* Anodontia
**Oligoencephalon** Q02
**Oligohidrosis** L74.4
**Oligohydramnios** O41.0- ☑
**Oligohydrosis** L74.4
**Oligomenorrhea** N91.5
  primary N91.3
  secondary N91.4
**Oligophrenia** (*see also* Disability, intellectual)
  phenylpyruvic E70.0
**Oligospermia** N46.11
  due to
    drug therapy N46.121
    efferent duct obstruction N46.123
    infection N46.122
    radiation N46.124
    specified cause NEC N46.129
    systemic disease N46.125
**Oligotrichia** — *see* Alopecia
**Oliguria** R34
  postprocedural N99.0
  with, complicating or following ectopic or molar pregnancy O08.4
**Ollier's disease** Q78.4
**Omenotocele** — *see* Hernia, abdomen, specified site NEC
**Omentitis** — *see* Peritonitis
**Omentum, omental** — *see* condition
**Omphalitis** (congenital) (newborn) P38.9
  with mild hemorrhage P38.1
  without hemorrhage P38.9
  not of newborn L08.82
  tetanus A33
**Omphalocele** Q79.2
**Omphalomesenteric duct, persistent** Q43.0
**Omphalorrhagia, newborn** P51.9
**Omsk hemorrhagic fever** A98.1
**Onanism** (excessive) F98.8
**Onchocerciasis, onchocercosis** B73.1
  with
    eye disease B73.00

**Onchocerciasis, onchocercosis** — *continued*
  with — *continued*
    eye disease — *continued*
      endophthalmitis B73.01
      eyelid B73.09
      glaucoma B73.02
      specified NEC B73.09
    eyelid B73.09
    eye NEC B73.00
**Oncocytoma** — *see* Neoplasm, benign, by site
**Oncovirus, as cause of disease classified elsewhere** B97.32
**Ondine's curse** — *see* Apnea, sleep
**Oneirophrenia** F23
**Onychauxis** L60.2
  congenital Q84.5
**Onychia** (*see also* Cellulitis, digit)
  with lymphangitis — *see* Lymphangitis, acute, digit
  candidal B37.2
  dermatophytic B35.1
**Onychitis** (*see also* Cellulitis, digit)
  with lymphangitis — *see* Lymphangitis, acute, digit
**Onychocryptosis** L60.0
**Onychodystrophy** L60.3
  congenital Q84.6
**Onychogryphosis, onychogryposis** L60.2
**Onycholysis** L60.1
**Onychomadesis** L60.8
**Onychomalacia** L60.3
**Onychomycosis** (finger) (toe) B35.1
**Onycho-osteodysplasia** Q87.2
**Onychophagia** F98.8
**Onychophosis** L60.8
**Onychoptosis** L60.8
**Onychorrhexis** L60.3
  congenital Q84.6
**Onychoschizia** L60.3
**Onyxis** (finger) (toe) L60.0
**Onyxitis** (*see also* Cellulitis, digit)
  with lymphangitis — *see* Lymphangitis, acute, digit
**Oophoritis** (cystic) (infectional) (interstitial) N70.92
  with salpingitis N70.93
  acute N70.02
    with salpingitis N70.03
  chronic N70.12
    with salpingitis N70.13
  complicating abortion — *see* Abortion, by type, complicated by, oophoritis
**Oophorocele** N83.4- ☑
**Opacity, opacities**
  cornea H17.- ☑
    central H17.1- ☑
    congenital Q13.3
    degenerative — *see* Degeneration, cornea
    hereditary — *see* Dystrophy, cornea
    inflammatory — *see* Keratitis
    minor H17.81- ☑
    peripheral H17.82- ☑
    sequelae of trachoma (healed) B94.0
    specified NEC H17.89
  enamel (teeth) (fluoride) (nonfluoride) K00.3
  lens — *see* Cataract
  snowball — *see* Deposit, crystalline
  vitreous (humor) NEC H43.39- ☑
    congenital Q14.0
    membranes and strands H43.31- ☑
**Opalescent dentin** (hereditary) K00.5
**Open, opening**
  abnormal, organ or site, congenital — *see* Imperfect, closure
  angle with
    borderline
      findings
        high risk H40.02- ☑
        low risk H40.01- ☑
      intraocular pressure H40.00- ☑
    cupping of discs H40.01- ☑
    glaucoma (primary) — *see* Glaucoma, open angle
  bite
    anterior M26.220
    posterior M26.221
  false — *see* Imperfect, closure
  margin on tooth restoration K08.51
  restoration margins of tooth K08.51
  wound — *see* Wound, open
**Operational fatigue** F48.8
**Operative** — *see* condition

**Operculitis** — *see* Periodontitis
**Operculum** — *see* Break, retina
**Ophiasis** L63.2
**Ophthalmia** (*see also* Conjunctivitis) H10.9
  actinic rays — *see* Photokeratitis
  allergic (acute) — *see* Conjunctivitis, acute, atopic
  blennorrhagic (gonococcal) (neonatorum) A54.31
  diphtheritic A36.86
  Egyptian A71.1
  electrica — *see* Photokeratitis
  gonococcal (neonatorum) A54.31
  metastatic — *see* Endophthalmitis, purulent
  migraine — *see* Migraine, ophthalmoplegic
  neonatorum, newborn P39.1
    gonococcal A54.31
  nodosa H16.24- ☑
  purulent — *see* Conjunctivitis, acute, mucopurulent
  spring — *see* Conjunctivitis, acute, atopic
  sympathetic — *see* Uveitis, sympathetic
**Ophthalmitis** — *see* Ophthalmia
**Ophthalmocele** (congenital) Q15.8
**Ophthalmoneuromyelitis** G36.0
**Ophthalmoplegia** (*see also* Strabismus, paralytic)
  anterior internuclear — *see* Ophthalmoplegia, internuclear
  ataxia-areflexia G61.0
  diabetic — *see* E08-E13 with .39
  exophthalmic E05.00
    with thyroid storm E05.01
  external H49.88- ☑
    progressive H49.4- ☑
      with pigmentary retinopathy — *see* Kearns-Sayre syndrome
    total H49.3- ☑
  internal (complete) (total) H52.51- ☑
  internuclear H51.2- ☑
  migraine — *see* Migraine, ophthalmoplegic
  Parinaud's H49.88- ☑
  progressive external — *see* Ophthalmoplegia, external, progressive
  supranuclear, progressive G23.1
  total (external) — *see* Ophthalmoplegia, external, total
**Opioid**(s)
  abuse — *see* Abuse, drug, opioids
  dependence — *see* Dependence, drug, opioids
  induced, without use disorder
    anxiety disorder F11.988
    delirium F11.921
    depressive disorder F11.94
    sexual dysfunction F11.981
    sleep disorder F11.982
**Opisthognathism** M26.09
**Opisthorchiasis** (felineus) (viverrini) B66.0
**Opitz' disease** D73.2
**Opiumism** — *see* Dependence, drug, opioid
**Oppenheim's disease** G70.2
**Oppenheim-Urbach disease** (necrobiosis lipoidica diabeticorum) — *see* E08-E13 with .620
**Optic nerve** — *see* condition
**Orbit** — *see* condition
**Orchioblastoma** C62.9- ☑
**Orchitis** (gangrenous) (nonspecific) (septic) (suppurative) N45.2
  blennorrhagic (gonococcal) (acute) (chronic) A54.23
  chlamydial A56.19
  filarial (*see also* Infestation, filarial) B74.9 [N51]
  gonococcal (acute) (chronic) A54.23
  mumps B26.0
  syphilitic A52.76
  tuberculous A18.15
**Orf** (virus disease) B08.02
**Organic** (*see also* condition)
  brain syndrome F09
  heart — *see* Disease, heart
  mental disorder F09
  psychosis F09
**Orgasm**
  anejaculatory N53.13
**Oriental**
  bilharziasis B65.2
  schistosomiasis B65.2
**Orifice** — *see* condition
**Origin of both great vessels from right ventricle** Q20.1
**Ormond's disease** (with ureteral obstruction) N13.5
  with infection N13.6
**Ornithine metabolism disorder** E72.4

☑ **Additional Character Required** — **Refer to the Tabular List for Character Selection**
⌐ **Subterms under main terms may continue to next column or page**

**Ornithinemia** (Type I) (Type II) E72.4
**Ornithosis** A70
**Orotaciduria, oroticaciduria** (congenital) (hereditary) (pyrimidine deficiency) E79.8
   anemia D53.0
**Orthodontics**
   adjustment Z46.4
   fitting Z46.4
**Orthopnea** R06.01
**Orthopoxvirus** B08.09
   specified NEC B08.09
**Os, uterus** — *see* condition
**Osgood-Schlatter disease or osteochondrosis** — *see* Osteochondrosis, juvenile, tibia
**Osler** (-Weber)-**Rendu disease** I78.0
**Osler's nodes** I33.0
**Osmidrosis** L75.0
**Osseous** — *see* condition
**Ossification**
   artery — *see* Arteriosclerosis
   auricle (ear) — *see* Disorder, pinna, specified type NEC
   bronchial J98.09
   cardiac — *see* Degeneration, myocardial
   cartilage (senile) — *see* Disorder, cartilage, specified type NEC
   coronary (artery) — *see* Disease, heart, ischemic, atherosclerotic
   diaphragm J98.6
   ear, middle — *see* Otosclerosis
   falx cerebri G96.19
   fontanel, premature Q75.0
   heart (*see also* Degeneration, myocardial)
      valve — *see* Endocarditis
   larynx J38.7
   ligament — *see* Disorder, tendon, specified type NEC
      posterior longitudinal — *see* Spondylopathy, specified NEC
   meninges (cerebral) (spinal) G96.19
   multiple, eccentric centers — *see* Disorder, bone, development or growth
   muscle (*see also* Calcification, muscle)
      due to burns — *see* Myositis, ossificans, in, burns
      paralytic — *see* Myositis, ossificans, in, quadriplegia
      progressive — *see* Myositis, ossificans, progressiva
      specified NEC M61.50
         ankle M61.57- ☑
         foot M61.57- ☑
         forearm M61.53- ☑
         hand M61.54- ☑
         lower leg M61.56- ☑
         multiple sites M61.59
         pelvic region M61.55- ☑
         shoulder region M61.51- ☑
         specified site NEC M61.58
         thigh M61.55- ☑
         upper arm M61.52- ☑
      traumatic — *see* Myositis, ossificans, traumatica
   myocardium, myocardial — *see* Degeneration, myocardial
   penis N48.89
   periarticular — *see* Disorder, joint, specified type NEC
   pinna — *see* Disorder, pinna, specified type NEC
   rider's bone — *see* Ossification, muscle, specified NEC
   sclera H15.89
   subperiosteal, post-traumatic M89.8X- ☑
   tendon — *see* Disorder, tendon, specified type NEC
   trachea J39.8
   tympanic membrane — *see* Disorder, tympanic membrane, specified NEC
   vitreous (humor) — *see* Deposit, crystalline
**Osteitis** (*see also* Osteomyelitis)
   alveolar M27.3
   condensans M85.30
      ankle M85.37- ☑
      foot M85.37- ☑
      forearm M85.33- ☑
      hand M85.34- ☑
      lower leg M85.36- ☑
      multiple site M85.39
      neck M85.38
      rib M85.38
      shoulder M85.31- ☑
      skull M85.38
      specified site NEC M85.38
      thigh M85.35- ☑
      toe M85.37- ☑
      upper arm M85.32- ☑

**Osteitis** — *continued*
   condensans — *continued*
      vertebra M85.38
   deformans M88.9
      in (due to)
         malignant neoplasm of bone C41.9 [M90.60]
         neoplastic disease (*see also* Neoplasm) D49.9 [M90.60]
            carpus D49.9 [M90.64-] ☑
            clavicle D49.9 [M90.61-] ☑
            femur D49.9 [M90.65-] ☑
            fibula D49.9 [M90.66-] ☑
            finger D49.9 [M90.64-] ☑
            humerus D49.9 [M90.62-] ☑
            ilium D49.9 [M90.65-] ☑
            ischium D49.9 [M90.65-] ☑
            metacarpus D49.9 [M90.64-] ☑
            metatarsus D49.9 [M90.67-] ☑
            multiple sites D49.9 [M90.69]
            neck D49.9 [M90.68]
            radius D49.9 [M90.63-] ☑
            rib D49.9 [M90.68]
            scapula D49.9 [M90.61-] ☑
            skull D49.9 [M90.68]
            tarsus D49.9 [M90.67-] ☑
            tibia D49.9 [M90.66-] ☑
            toe D49.9 [M90.67-] ☑
            ulna D49.9 [M90.63-] ☑
            vertebra D49.9 [M90.68]
      skull M88.0
      specified NEC — *see* Paget's disease, bone, by site
      vertebra M88.1
   due to yaws A66.6
   fibrosa NEC — *see* Cyst, bone, by site
      circumscripta — *see* Dysplasia, fibrous, bone NEC
      cystica (generalisata) E21.0
      disseminata Q78.1
      osteoplastica E21.0
   fragilitans Q78.0
   Garr's (sclerosing) — *see* Osteomyelitis, specified NEC
   jaw (acute) (chronic) (lower) (suppurative) (upper) M27.2
   parathyroid E21.0
   petrous bone (acute) (chronic) — *see* Petrositis
   sclerotic, nonsuppurative — *see* Osteomyelitis, specified type NEC
   tuberculosa A18.09
      cystica D86.89
      multiplex cystoides D86.89
**Osteoarthritis** M19.90
   ankle M19.07- ☑
   elbow M19.02- ☑
   foot joint M19.07- ☑
   generalized M15.9
      erosive M15.4
      primary M15.0
      specified NEC M15.8
   hand joint M19.04- ☑
      first carpometacarpal joint M18.9
   hip M16.1- ☑
      bilateral M16.0
      due to hip dysplasia (unilateral) M16.3- ☑
         bilateral M16.2
   interphalangeal
      distal (Heberden) M15.1
      proximal (Bouchard) M15.2
   knee M17.1- ☑
      bilateral M17.0
   post-traumatic NEC M19.92
      ankle M19.17- ☑
      elbow M19.12- ☑
      foot joint M19.17- ☑
      hand joint M19.14- ☑
         first carpometacarpal joint M18.3- ☑
            bilateral M18.2
      hip M16.5- ☑
         bilateral M16.4
      knee M17.3- ☑
         bilateral M17.2
      shoulder M19.11- ☑
      wrist M19.13- ☑
   primary M19.91
      ankle M19.07- ☑
      elbow M19.02- ☑
      foot joint M19.07- ☑
      hand joint M19.04- ☑

**Osteoarthritis** — *continued*
   primary — *continued*
      hand joint — *continued*
         first carpometacarpal joint M18.1- ☑
            bilateral M18.0
      hip M16.1- ☑
         bilateral M16.0
      knee M17.1- ☑
         bilateral M17.0
      shoulder M19.01- ☑
      spine — *see* Spondylosis
      wrist M19.03- ☑
   secondary M19.93
      ankle M19.27- ☑
      elbow M19.22- ☑
      foot joint M19.27- ☑
      hand joint M19.24- ☑
         first carpometacarpal joint M18.5- ☑
            bilateral M18.4
      hip M16.7
         bilateral M16.6
      knee M17.5
         bilateral M17.4
      multiple M15.3
      shoulder M19.21- ☑
      spine — *see* Spondylosis
      wrist M19.23- ☑
   shoulder M19.01- ☑
   spine — *see* Spondylosis
   wrist M19.03- ☑
**Osteoarthropathy** (hypertrophic) M19.90
   ankle — *see* Osteoarthritis, primary, ankle
   elbow — *see* Osteoarthritis, primary, elbow
   foot joint — *see* Osteoarthritis, primary, foot
   hand joint — *see* Osteoarthritis, primary, hand joint
   knee joint — *see* Osteoarthritis, primary, knee
   multiple site — *see* Osteoarthritis, primary, multiple joint
   pulmonary (*see also* Osteoarthropathy, specified type NEC)
      hypertrophic — *see* Osteoarthropathy, hypertrophic, specified type NEC
   secondary — *see* Osteoarthropathy, specified type NEC
   secondary hypertrophic — *see* Osteoarthropathy, specified type NEC
   shoulder — *see* Osteoarthritis, primary, shoulder
   specified joint NEC — *see* Osteoarthritis, primary, specified joint NEC
   specified type NEC M89.40
      carpus M89.44- ☑
      clavicle M89.41- ☑
      femur M89.45- ☑
      fibula M89.46- ☑
      finger M89.44- ☑
      humerus M89.42- ☑
      ilium M89.459
      ischium M89.459
      metacarpus M89.44- ☑
      metatarsus M89.47- ☑
      multiple sites M89.49
      neck M89.48
      radius M89.43- ☑
      rib M89.48
      scapula M89.41- ☑
      skull M89.48
      tarsus M89.47- ☑
      tibia M89.46- ☑
      toe M89.47- ☑
      ulna M89.43- ☑
      vertebra M89.48
   spine — *see* Spondylosis
   wrist — *see* Osteoarthritis, primary, wrist
**Osteoarthrosis** (degenerative) (hypertrophic) (joint) (*see also* Osteoarthritis)
   deformans alkaptonurica E70.29 [M36.8]
   erosive M15.4
   generalized M15.9
      primary M15.0
   polyarticular M15.9
   spine — *see* Spondylosis
**Osteoblastoma** — *see* Neoplasm, bone, benign
   aggressive — *see* Neoplasm, bone, uncertain behavior
**Osteochondritis** (*see also* Osteochondropathy, by site)
   Brailsford's — *see* Osteochondrosis, juvenile, radius
   dissecans M93.20
      ankle M93.27- ☑

**Osteochondritis** — *continued*
  dissecans — *continued*
    elbow M93.22- ☑
    foot M93.27- ☑
    hand M93.24- ☑
    hip M93.25- ☑
    knee M93.26- ☑
    multiple sites M93.29
    shoulder joint M93.21- ☑
    specified site NEC M93.28
    wrist M93.23- ☑
   juvenile M92.9
    patellar — *see* Osteochondrosis, juvenile, patella
   syphilitic (congenital) (early) A50.02 [M90.80]
    ankle A50.02 [M90.87-] ☑
    elbow A50.02 [M90.82-] ☑
    foot A50.02 [M90.87-] ☑
    forearm A50.02 [M90.83-] ☑
    hand A50.02 [M90.84-] ☑
    hip A50.02 [M90.85-] ☑
    knee A50.02 [M90.86-] ☑
    multiple sites A50.02 [M90.89]
    shoulder joint A50.02 [M90.81-] ☑
    specified site NEC A50.02 [M90.88]
**Osteochondroarthrosis deformans endemica** — *see* Disease, Kaschin-Beck
**Osteochondrodysplasia** Q78.9
  with defects of growth of tubular bones and spine Q77.9
   specified NEC Q77.8
  specified NEC Q78.8
**Osteochondrodystrophy** E78.9
**Osteochondrolysis** — *see* Osteochondritis, dissecans
**Osteochondroma** — *see* Neoplasm, bone, benign
**Osteochondromatosis** D48.0
  syndrome Q78.4
**Osteochondromyxosarcoma** — *see* Neoplasm, bone, malignant
**Osteochondropathy** M93.90
  ankle M93.97- ☑
  elbow M93.92- ☑
  foot M93.97- ☑
  hand M93.94- ☑
  hip M93.95- ☑
  Kienböck's disease of adults M93.1
  knee M93.96- ☑
  multiple joints M93.99
  osteochondritis dissecans — *see* Osteochondritis, dissecans
  osteochondrosis — *see* Osteochondrosis
  shoulder region M93.91- ☑
  slipped upper femoral epiphysis — *see* Slipped, epiphysis, upper femoral
  specified joint NEC M93.98
  specified type NEC M93.80
   ankle M93.87- ☑
   elbow M93.82- ☑
   foot M93.87- ☑
   hand M93.84- ☑
   hip M93.85- ☑
   knee M93.86- ☑
   multiple joints M93.89
   shoulder region M93.81- ☑
   specified joint NEC M93.88
   wrist M93.83- ☑
  syphilitic, congenital
   early A50.02 [M90.80]
   late A50.56 [M90.80]
  wrist M93.93- ☑
**Osteochondrosarcoma** — *see* Neoplasm, bone, malignant
**Osteochondrosis** (*see also* Osteochondropathy, by site)
  acetabulum (juvenile) M91.0
  adult — *see* Osteochondropathy, specified type NEC, by site
  astragalus (juvenile) — *see* Osteochondrosis, juvenile, tarsus
  Blount's — *see* Osteochondrosis, juvenile, tibia
  Buchanan's M91.0
  Burns' — *see* Osteochondrosis, juvenile, ulna
  calcaneus (juvenile) — *see* Osteochondrosis, juvenile, tarsus
  capitular epiphysis (femur) (juvenile) — *see* Legg-Calvé-Perthes disease
  carpal (juvenile) (lunate) (scaphoid) — *see* Osteochondrosis, juvenile, hand, carpal lunate
   adult M93.1

**Osteochondrosis** — *continued*
  coxae juvenilis — *see* Legg-Calvé-Perthes disease
  deformans juvenilis, coxae — *see* Legg-Calvé-Perthes disease
  Diaz's — *see* Osteochondrosis, juvenile, tarsus
  dissecans (knee) (shoulder) — *see* Osteochondritis, dissecans
  femoral capital epiphysis (juvenile) — *see* Legg-Calvé-Perthes disease
  femur (head), juvenile — *see* Legg-Calvé-Perthes disease
  fibula (juvenile) — *see* Osteochondrosis, juvenile, fibula
  foot NEC (juvenile) M92.8
  Freiberg's — *see* Osteochondrosis, juvenile, metatarsus
  Haas' (juvenile) — *see* Osteochondrosis, juvenile, humerus
  Haglund's — *see* Osteochondrosis, juvenile, tarsus
  hip (juvenile) — *see* Legg-Calvé-Perthes disease
  humerus (capitulum) (head) (juvenile) — *see* Osteochondrosis, juvenile, humerus
  ilium, iliac crest (juvenile) M91.0
  ischiopubic synchondrosis M91.0
  Iselin's — *see* Osteochondrosis, juvenile, metatarsus
  juvenile, juvenilis M92.9
   after congenital dislocation of hip reduction — *see* Osteochondrosis, juvenile, hip, specified NEC
   arm — *see* Osteochondrosis, juvenile, upper limb NEC
   capitular epiphysis (femur) — *see* Legg-Calvé-Perthes disease
   clavicle, sternal epiphysis — *see* Osteochondrosis, juvenile, upper limb NEC
   coxae — *see* Legg-Calvé-Perthes disease
   deformans M92.9
   fibula M92.5- ☑
   foot NEC M92.8
   hand M92.20- ☑
    carpal lunate M92.21- ☑
    metacarpal head M92.22- ☑
    specified site NEC M92.29- ☑
   head of femur — *see* Legg-Calvé-Perthes disease
   hip and pelvis M91.9- ☑
    coxa plana — *see* Coxa, plana
    femoral head — *see* Legg-Calvé-Perthes disease
    pelvis M91.0
    pseudocoxalgia — *see* Pseudocoxalgia
    specified NEC M91.8- ☑
   humerus M92.0- ☑
   limb
    lower NEC M92.8
    upper NEC — *see* Osteochondrosis, juvenile, upper limb NEC
   medial cuneiform bone — *see* Osteochondrosis, juvenile, tarsus
   metatarsus M92.7- ☑
   patella M92.4- ☑
   radius M92.1- ☑
   specified site NEC M92.8
   spine M42.00
    cervical region M42.02
    cervicothoracic region M42.03
    lumbar region M42.06
    lumbosacral region M42.07
    multiple sites M42.09
    occipito-atlanto-axial region M42.01
    sacrococcygeal region M42.08
    thoracic region M42.04
    thoracolumbar region M42.05
   tarsus M92.6- ☑
   tibia M92.5- ☑
   ulna M92.1- ☑
   upper limb NEC M92.3- ☑
   vertebra (body) (epiphyseal plates) (Calvé's) (Scheuermann's) — *see* Osteochondrosis, juvenile, spine
  Kienböck's — *see* Osteochondrosis, juvenile, hand, carpal lunate
   adult M93.1
  Köhler's
   patellar — *see* Osteochondrosis, juvenile, patella
   tarsal navicular — *see* Osteochondrosis, juvenile, tarsus
  Legg-Perthes (-Calvé)(-Waldenström) — *see* Legg-Calvé-Perthes disease
  limb
   lower NEC (juvenile) M92.8

**Osteochondrosis** — *continued*
  limb — *continued*
   upper NEC (juvenile) — *see* Osteochondrosis, juvenile, upper limb NEC
  lunate bone (carpal) (juvenile) (*see also* Osteochondrosis, juvenile, hand, carpal lunate)
   adult M93.1
  Mauclaire's — *see* Osteochondrosis, juvenile, hand, metacarpal
  metacarpal (head) (juvenile) — *see* Osteochondrosis, juvenile, hand, metacarpal
  metatarsus (fifth) (head) (juvenile) (second) — *see* Osteochondrosis, juvenile, metatarsus
  navicular (juvenile) — *see* Osteochondrosis, juvenile, tarsus
  os
   calcis (juvenile) — *see* Osteochondrosis, juvenile, tarsus
   tibiale externum (juvenile) — *see* Osteochondrosis, juvenile, tarsus
  Osgood-Schlatter — *see* Osteochondrosis, juvenile, tibia
  Panner's — *see* Osteochondrosis, juvenile, humerus
  patellar center (juvenile) (primary) (secondary) — *see* Osteochondrosis, juvenile, patella
  pelvis (juvenile) M91.0
  Pierson's M91.0
  radius (head) (juvenile) — *see* Osteochondrosis, juvenile, radius
  Scheuermann's — *see* Osteochondrosis, juvenile, spine
  Sever's — *see* Osteochondrosis, juvenile, tarsus
  Sinding-Larsen — *see* Osteochondrosis, juvenile, patella
  spine M42.9
   adult M42.10
    cervical region M42.12
    cervicothoracic region M42.13
    lumbar region M42.16
    lumbosacral region M42.17
    multiple sites M42.19
    occipito-atlanto-axial region M42.11
    sacrococcygeal region M42.18
    thoracic region M42.14
    thoracolumbar region M42.15
   juvenile — *see* Osteochondrosis, juvenile, spine
  symphysis pubis (juvenile) M91.0
  syphilitic (congenital) A50.02
  talus (juvenile) — *see* Osteochondrosis, juvenile, tarsus
  tarsus (navicular) (juvenile) — *see* Osteochondrosis, juvenile, tarsus
  tibia (proximal) (tubercle) (juvenile) — *see* Osteochondrosis, juvenile, tibia
  tuberculous — *see* Tuberculosis, bone
  ulna (lower) (juvenile) — *see* Osteochondrosis, juvenile, ulna
  van Neck's M91.0
  vertebral — *see* Osteochondrosis, spine
**Osteoclastoma** D48.0
  malignant — *see* Neoplasm, bone, malignant
**Osteodynia** — *see* Disorder, bone, specified type NEC
**Osteodystrophy** Q78.9
  azotemic N25.0
  congenital Q78.9
  parathyroid, secondary E21.1
  renal N25.0
**Osteofibroma** — *see* Neoplasm, bone, benign
**Osteofibrosarcoma** — *see* Neoplasm, bone, malignant
**Osteogenesis imperfecta** Q78.0
**Osteogenic** — *see* condition
**Osteolysis** M89.50
  carpus M89.54- ☑
  clavicle M89.51- ☑
  femur M89.55- ☑
  fibula M89.56- ☑
  finger M89.54- ☑
  humerus M89.52- ☑
  ilium M89.559
  ischium M89.559
  joint prosthesis (periprosthetic) — *see* Complications, joint prosthesis, mechanical, periprosthetic, osteolysis, by site
  metacarpus M89.54- ☑
  metatarsus M89.57- ☑
  multiple sites M89.59
  neck M89.58
  periprosthetic — *see* Complications, joint prosthesis, mechanical, periprosthetic, osteolysis, by site

**Osteomyelofibrosis** D47.4
**Osteomyelosclerosis** D75.89
**Osteonecrosis** M87.9
  due to
    drugs — see Osteonecrosis, secondary, due to, drugs
    trauma — see Osteonecrosis, secondary, due to, trauma
  idiopathic aseptic M87.00
    ankle M87.07- ☑
    carpus M87.03- ☑
    clavicle M87.01- ☑
    femur M87.05- ☑
    fibula M87.06- ☑
    finger M87.04- ☑
    humerus M87.02- ☑
    ilium M87.050
    ischium M87.050
    metacarpus M87.04- ☑
    metatarsus M87.07- ☑
    multiple sites M87.09
    neck M87.08
    pelvis M87.050
    radius M87.03- ☑
    rib M87.08
    scapula M87.01- ☑
    skull M87.08
    tarsus M87.07- ☑
    tibia M87.06- ☑
    toe M87.07- ☑
    ulna M87.03- ☑
    vertebra M87.08
  secondary NEC M87.30
    carpus M87.33- ☑
    clavicle M87.31- ☑
    due to
      drugs M87.10
        carpus M87.13- ☑
        clavicle M87.11- ☑
        femur M87.15- ☑
        fibula M87.16- ☑
        finger M87.14- ☑
        humerus M87.12- ☑
        ilium M87.159
        ischium M87.159
        jaw M87.180
        metacarpus M87.14- ☑
        metatarsus M87.17- ☑
        multiple sites M87.19
        neck M87.18
        radius M87.13- ☑
        rib M87.18
        scapula M87.11- ☑
        skull M87.18
        tarsus M87.17- ☑
        tibia M87.16- ☑
        toe M87.17- ☑
        ulna M87.13- ☑
        vertebra M87.18 ☑
      hemoglobinopathy NEC D58.2 [M90.50]
        carpus D58.2 [M90.54-] ☑
        clavicle D58.2 [M90.51-] ☑
        femur D58.2 [M90.55-] ☑
        fibula D58.2 [M90.56-] ☑
        finger D58.2 [M90.54-] ☑
        humerus D58.2 [M90.52-] ☑
        ilium D58.2 [M90.55-] ☑
        ischium D58.2 [M90.55-] ☑
        metacarpus D58.2 [M90.54-] ☑
        metatarsus D58.2 [M90.57-] ☑
        multiple sites D58.2 [M90.58]
        neck D58.2 [M90.58]
        radius D58.2 [M90.53-] ☑
        rib D58.2 [M90.58]
        scapula D58.2 [M90.51-] ☑
        skull D58.2 [M90.58]
        tarsus D58.2 [M90.57-] ☑
        tibia D58.2 [M90.56-] ☑
        toe D58.2 [M90.57-] ☑
        ulna D58.2 [M90.53-] ☑
        vertebra D58.2 [M90.58]
      trauma (previous) M87.20
        carpus M87.23- ☑
        clavicle M87.21- ☑
        femur M87.25- ☑
        fibula M87.26- ☑

**Osteonecrosis** — continued
  secondary — continued
    due to — continued
      trauma — continued
        finger M87.24- ☑
        humerus M87.22- ☑
        ilium M87.25- ☑
        ischium M87.25- ☑
        metacarpus M87.24- ☑
        metatarsus M87.27- ☑
        multiple sites M87.29
        neck M87.28
        radius M87.23- ☑
        rib M87.28
        scapula M87.21- ☑
        skull M87.28
        tarsus M87.27- ☑
        tibia M87.26- ☑
        toe M87.27- ☑
        ulna M87.23- ☑
        vertebra M87.28
    femur M87.35- ☑
    fibula M87.36- ☑
    finger M87.34- ☑
    humerus M87.32- ☑
    ilium M87.350
    in
      caisson disease T70.3 ☑ [M90.50]
        carpus T70.3 ☑ [M90.54-] ☑
        clavicle T70.3 ☑ [M90.51-] ☑
        femur T70.3 ☑ [M90.55-] ☑
        fibula T70.3 ☑ [M90.56-] ☑
        finger T70.3 ☑ [M90.54-] ☑
        humerus T70.3 ☑ [M90.52-] ☑
        ilium T70.3 ☑ [M90.55-] ☑
        ischium T70.3 ☑ [M90.55-] ☑
        metacarpus T70.3 ☑ [M90.54-] ☑
        metatarsus T70.3 ☑ [M90.57-] ☑
        multiple sites T70.3 ☑ [M90.59]
        neck T70.3 ☑ [M90.58]
        radius T70.3 ☑ [M90.53-] ☑
        rib T70.3 ☑ [M90.58]
        scapula T70.3 ☑ [M90.51-] ☑
        skull T70.3 ☑ [M90.58]
        tarsus T70.3 ☑ [M90.57-] ☑
        tibia T70.3 ☑ [M90.56-] ☑
        toe T70.3 ☑ [M90.57-] ☑
        ulna T70.3 ☑ [M90.53-] ☑
        vertebra T70.3 ☑ [M90.58]
    ischium M87.350
    metacarpus M87.34- ☑
    metatarsus M87.37- ☑
    multiple site M87.39
    neck M87.38
    radius M87.33- ☑
    rib M87.38
    scapula M87.319
    skull M87.38
    tarsus M87.379
    tibia M87.366
    toe M87.379
    ulna M87.33- ☑
    vertebra M87.38
  specified type NEC M87.80
    carpus M87.83- ☑
    clavicle M87.81- ☑
    femur M87.85- ☑
    fibula M87.86- ☑
    finger M87.84- ☑
    humerus M87.82- ☑
    ilium M87.85- ☑
    ischium M87.85- ☑
    metacarpus M87.84- ☑
    metatarsus M87.87- ☑
    multiple sites M87.89
    neck M87.88
    radius M87.83- ☑
    rib M87.88
    scapula M87.81- ☑
    skull M87.88
    tarsus M87.87- ☑
    tibia M87.86- ☑
    toe M87.87- ☑
    ulna M87.83- ☑
    vertebra M87.88
**Osteo-onycho-arthro-dysplasia** Q87.2

**Osteo-onychodysplasia, hereditary** Q87.2
**Osteopathia condensans disseminata** Q78.8
**Osteopathy** (see also Osteomyelitis, Osteonecrosis, Osteoporosis)
  after poliomyelitis M89.60
    carpus M89.64- ☑
    clavicle M89.61- ☑
    femur M89.65- ☑
    fibula M89.66- ☑
    finger M89.64- ☑
    humerus M89.62- ☑
    ilium M89.659
    ischium M89.659
    metacarpus M89.64- ☑
    metatarsus M89.67- ☑
    multiple sites M89.69
    neck M89.68
    radius M89.63- ☑
    rib M89.68
    scapula M89.61- ☑
    skull M89.68
    tarsus M89.67- ☑
    tibia M89.66- ☑
    toe M89.67- ☑
    ulna M89.63- ☑
    vertebra M89.68
  in (due to)
    renal osteodystrophy N25.0
    specified diseases classified elsewhere — see subcategory M90.8 ☑
**Osteopenia** M85.8- ☑
  borderline M85.8- ☑
**Osteoperiostitis** — see Osteomyelitis, specified type NEC
**Osteopetrosis** (familial) Q78.2
**Osteophyte** M25.70
  ankle M25.77- ☑
  elbow M25.72- ☑
  foot joint M25.77- ☑
  hand joint M25.74- ☑
  hip M25.75- ☑
  knee M25.76- ☑
  shoulder M25.71- ☑
  spine M25.78
  vertebrae M25.78
  wrist M25.73- ☑
**Osteopoikilosis** Q78.8
**Osteoporosis** (female) (male) M81.0
  with current pathological fracture M80.00 ☑
  age-related M81.0
    with current pathologic fracture M80.00 ☑
      carpus M80.04- ☑
      clavicle M80.01- ☑
      fibula M80.06- ☑
      finger M80.04- ☑
      humerus M80.02- ☑
      ilium M80.05- ☑
      ischium M80.05- ☑
      metacarpus M80.04- ☑
      metatarsus M80.07- ☑
      pelvis M80.05- ☑
      radius M80.03- ☑
      scapula M80.01- ☑
      tarsus M80.07- ☑
      tibia M80.06- ☑
      toe M80.07- ☑
      ulna M80.03- ☑
      vertebra M80.08 ☑
  disuse M81.8
    with current pathological fracture M80.80 ☑
      carpus M80.84- ☑
      clavicle M80.81- ☑
      fibula M80.86- ☑
      finger M80.84- ☑
      humerus M80.82- ☑
      ilium M80.85- ☑
      ischium M80.85- ☑
      metacarpus M80.84- ☑
      metatarsus M80.87- ☑
      pelvis M80.85- ☑
      radius M80.83- ☑
      scapula M80.81- ☑
      tarsus M80.87- ☑
      tibia M80.86- ☑
      toe M80.87- ☑
      ulna M80.83- ☑

**Osteomyelofibrosis — Osteoporosis**    Index

242    ☑ **Additional Character Required** — Refer to the Tabular List for Character Selection      🔻 **Subterms under main terms may continue to next column or page**

**Osteoporosis** — continued
  disuse — continued
    with current pathological fracture — continued
      vertebra M80.88 ☑
  drug-induced — see Osteoporosis, specified type NEC
  idiopathic — see Osteoporosis, specified type NEC
  involutional — see Osteoporosis, age-related
  Lequesne M81.6
  localized M81.6
  postmenopausal M81.0
    with pathological fracture M80.00 ☑
      carpus M80.04- ☑
      clavicle M80.01- ☑
      fibula M80.06- ☑
      finger M80.04- ☑
      humerus M80.02- ☑
      ilium M80.05- ☑
      ischium M80.05- ☑
      metacarpus M80.04- ☑
      metatarsus M80.07- ☑
      pelvis M80.05- ☑
      radius M80.03- ☑
      scapula M80.01- ☑
      tarsus M80.07- ☑
      tibia M80.06- ☑
      toe M80.07- ☑
      ulna M80.03- ☑
      vertebra M80.08 ☑
  postoophorectomy — see Osteoporosis, specified type
    NEC
  postsurgical malabsorption — see Osteoporosis,
    specified type NEC
  post-traumatic — see Osteoporosis, specified type
    NEC
  senile — see Osteoporosis, age-related
  specified type NEC M81.8
    with pathological fracture M80.80 ☑
      carpus M80.84- ☑
      clavicle M80.81- ☑
      fibula M80.86- ☑
      finger M80.84- ☑
      humerus M80.82- ☑
      ilium M80.85- ☑
      ischium M80.85- ☑
      metacarpus M80.84- ☑
      metatarsus M80.87- ☑
      pelvis M80.85- ☑
      radius M80.83- ☑
      scapula M80.81- ☑
      tarsus M80.87- ☑
      tibia M80.86- ☑
      toe M80.87- ☑
      ulna M80.83- ☑
      vertebra M80.88 ☑
**Osteopsathyrosis** (idiopathica) Q78.0
**Osteoradionecrosis, jaw** (acute) (chronic) (lower)
  (suppurative) (upper) M27.2
**Osteosarcoma** (any form) — see Neoplasm, bone, malignant
**Osteosclerosis** Q78.2
  acquired M85.8- ☑
  congenita Q77.4
  fragilitas (generalisata) Q78.2
  myelofibrosis D75.81
**Osteosclerotic anemia** D64.89
**Osteosis**
  cutis L94.2
  renal fibrocystic N25.0
**Österreicher-Turner syndrome** Q87.2
**Ostium**
  atrioventriculare commune Q21.2
  primum (arteriosum) (defect) (persistent) Q21.2
  secundum (arteriosum) (defect) (patent) (persistent)
    Q21.1
**Ostrum-Furst syndrome** Q75.8
**Otalgia** H92.0 ☑
**Otitis** (acute) H66.90
  with effusion (see also Otitis, media, nonsuppurative)
    purulent — see Otitis, media, suppurative
  adhesive — see subcategory H74.1
  chronic (see also Otitis, media, chronic)
    with effusion (see also Otitis, media, nonsuppura-
      tive, chronic)
  externa H60.9-
    abscess — see Abscess, ear, external
    acute (noninfective) H60.50- ☑

**Otitis** — continued
  externa — continued
    acute — continued
      actinic H60.51- ☑
      chemical H60.52- ☑
      contact H60.53- ☑
      eczematoid H60.54- ☑
      infective — see Otitis, externa, infective
      reactive H60.55- ☑
      specified NEC H60.59- ☑
    cellulitis — see Cellulitis, ear
    chronic H60.6- ☑
    diffuse — see Otitis, externa, infective, diffuse
    hemorrhagic — see Otitis, externa, infective,
      hemorrhagic
    in (due to)
      aspergillosis B44.89
      candidiasis B37.84
      erysipelas A46 [H62.40]
      herpes (simplex) virus infection B00.1
        zoster B02.8
      impetigo L01.00 [H62.40]
      infectious disease NEC B99 [H62.4-] ☑
      mycosis NEC B36.9 [H62.40]
      parasitic disease NEC B89 [H62.40]
      viral disease NEC B34.9 [H62.40]
      zoster B02.8
    infective NEC H60.39- ☑
      abscess — see Abscess, ear, external
      cellulitis — see Cellulitis, ear
      diffuse H60.31- ☑
      hemorrhagic H60.32- ☑
      swimmer's ear — see Swimmer's, ear
    malignant H60.2- ☑
    mycotic NEC B36.9 [H62.40]
      in
        aspergillosis B44.89
        candidiasis B37.84
        moniliasis B37.84
    necrotizing — see Otitis, externa, malignant
    Pseudomonas aeruginosa — see Otitis, externa,
      malignant
    reactive — see Otitis, externa, acute, reactive
    specified NEC — see subcategory H60.8 ☑
    tropical NEC B36.9 [H62.40]
      in
        aspergillosis B44.89
        candidiasis B37.84
        moniliasis B37.84
  insidiosa — see Otosclerosis
  interna H83.0 ☑
  media (hemorrhagic) (staphylococcal) (streptococcal)
    H66.9- ☑
    with effusion (nonpurulent) — see Otitis, media,
      nonsuppurative
    acute, subacute H66.90
      allergic — see Otitis, media, nonsuppurative,
        acute, allergic
      exudative — see Otitis, media, suppurative,
        acute
      mucoid — see Otitis, media, nonsuppurative,
        acute
      necrotizing (see also Otitis, media, suppurative,
        acute)
        in
          measles B05.3
          scarlet fever A38.0
      nonsuppurative NEC — see Otitis, media, non-
        suppurative, acute
      purulent — see Otitis, media, suppurative,
        acute
      sanguinous — see Otitis, media, nonsuppura-
        tive, acute
      secretory — see Otitis, media, nonsuppurative,
        acute, serous
      seromucinous — see Otitis, media, nonsuppu-
        rative, acute
      serous — see Otitis, media, nonsuppurative,
        acute, serous
      suppurative — see Otitis, media, suppurative,
        acute
    allergic — see Otitis, media, nonsuppurative
    catarrhal — see Otitis, media, nonsuppurative
    chronic H66.90
      with effusion (nonpurulent) — see Otitis, media,
        nonsuppurative, chronic

**Otitis** — continued
  media — continued
    chronic — continued
      allergic — see Otitis, media, nonsuppurative,
        chronic, allergic
      benign suppurative — see Otitis, media, suppu-
        rative, chronic, tubotympanic
      catarrhal — see Otitis, media, nonsuppurative,
        chronic, serous
      exudative — see Otitis, media, nonsuppurative,
        chronic
      mucinous — see Otitis, media, nonsuppurative,
        chronic, mucoid
      mucoid — see Otitis, media, nonsuppurative,
        chronic, mucoid
      nonsuppurative NEC — see Otitis, media, non-
        suppurative, chronic
      purulent — see Otitis, media, suppurative,
        chronic
      secretory — see Otitis, media, nonsuppurative,
        chronic, mucoid
      seromucinous — see Otitis, media, nonsuppu-
        rative, chronic
      serous — see Otitis, media, nonsuppurative,
        chronic, serous
      suppurative — see Otitis, media, suppurative,
        chronic
      transudative — see Otitis, media, nonsuppura-
        tive, chronic, mucoid
    exudative — see Otitis, media, suppurative
    in (due to) (with)
      influenza — see Influenza, with, otitis media
      measles B05.3
      scarlet fever A38.0
      tuberculosis A18.6
      viral disease NEC B34.- ☑ [H67.-] ☑
    mucoid — see Otitis, media, nonsuppurative
    nonsuppurative H65.9- ☑
      acute or subacute NEC H65.19- ☑
        allergic H65.11- ☑
          recurrent H65.11- ☑
        recurrent H65.19- ☑
        secretory — see Otitis, media, nonsuppura-
          tive, serous
        serous H65.0- ☑
          recurrent H65.0- ☑
      chronic H65.49- ☑
        allergic H65.41- ☑
        mucoid H65.3- ☑
        serous H65.2- ☑
    postmeasles B05.3
    purulent — see Otitis, media, suppurative
    secretory — see Otitis, media, nonsuppurative
    seromucinous — see Otitis, media, nonsuppurative
    serous — see Otitis, media, nonsuppurative
    suppurative H66.4- ☑
      acute H66.00- ☑
        with rupture of ear drum H66.01- ☑
        recurrent H66.00- ☑
          with rupture of ear drum H66.01- ☑
      chronic (see also subcategory) H66.3 ☑
        atticoantral H66.2- ☑
        benign — see Otitis, media, suppurative,
          chronic, tubotympanic
        tubotympanic H66.1- ☑
    transudative — see Otitis, media, nonsuppurative
    tuberculous A18.6
**Otocephaly** Q18.2
**Otolith syndrome** — see subcategory H81.8 ☑
**Otomycosis** (diffuse) NEC B36.9 [H62.40]
  in
    aspergillosis B44.89
    candidiasis B37.84
    moniliasis B37.84
**Otoporosis** — see Otosclerosis
**Otorrhagia** (nontraumatic) H92.2- ☑
  traumatic — code by Type of injury
**Otorrhea** H92.1- ☑
  cerebrospinal G96.0
**Otosclerosis** (general) H80.9- ☑
  cochlear (endosteal) H80.2- ☑
  involving
    otic capsule — see Otosclerosis, cochlear
    oval window
      nonobliterative H80.0- ☑
      obliterative H80.1- ☑
    round window — see Otosclerosis, cochlear

**Otosclerosis** — *continued*
> nonobliterative — *see* Otosclerosis, involving, oval
>> window, nonobliterative
> obliterative — *see* Otosclerosis, involving, oval win-
>> dow, obliterative
> specified NEC H80.8- ☑
**Otospongiosis** — *see* Otosclerosis
**Otto's disease or pelvis** M24.7
**Outcome of delivery** Z37.9
> multiple births Z37.9
>> all liveborn Z37.50
>>> quadruplets Z37.52
>>> quintuplets Z37.53
>>> sextuplets Z37.54
>>> specified number NEC Z37.59
>>> triplets Z37.51
>> all stillborn Z37.7
>> some liveborn Z37.60
>>> quadruplets Z37.62
>>> quintuplets Z37.63
>>> sextuplets Z37.64
>>> specified number NEC Z37.69
>>> triplets Z37.61
> single NEC Z37.9
>> liveborn Z37.0
>> stillborn Z37.1
> twins NEC Z37.9
>> both liveborn Z37.2
>> both stillborn Z37.4
>> one liveborn, one stillborn Z37.3
**Outlet** — *see* condition
**Ovalocytosis** (congenital) (hereditary) — *see* Elliptocyto-
> sis
**Ovarian** — *see* Condition
**Ovariocele** N83.4- ☑
**Ovaritis** (cystic) — *see* Oophoritis
**Ovary, ovarian** (*see also* condition)
> resistant syndrome E28.39
> vein syndrome N13.8
**Overactive** (*see also* Hyperfunction)
> adrenal cortex NEC E27.0
> bladder N32.81
> hypothalamus E23.3
> thyroid — *see* Hyperthyroidism
**Overactivity** R46.3
> child — *see* Disorder, attention-deficit hyperactivity
**Overbite** (deep) (excessive) (horizontal) (vertical) M26.29
**Overbreathing** — *see* Hyperventilation
**Overconscientious personality** F60.5
**Overdevelopment** — *see* Hypertrophy
**Overdistension** — *see* Distension
**Overdose, overdosage** (drug) — *see* Table of Drugs and
> Chemicals, by drug, poisoning
**Overeating** R63.2
> nonorganic origin F50.89
> psychogenic F50.89
**Overexertion** (effects) (exhaustion) T73.3 ☑
**Overexposure** (effects) T73.9 ☑
> exhaustion T73.2 ☑
**Overfeeding** — *see* Overeating
> newborn P92.4
**Overfill, endodontic** M27.52
**Overgrowth, bone** — *see* Hypertrophy, bone
**Overhanging of dental restorative material** (unre-
> pairable) K08.52
**Overheated** (places) (effects) — *see* Heat
**Overjet** (excessive horizontal) M26.23
**Overlaid, overlying** (suffocation) — *see* Asphyxia,
> traumatic, due to mechanical threat
**Overlap, excessive horizontal** (teeth) M26.23
**Overlapping toe** (acquired) (*see also* Deformity, toe,
> specified NEC)
> congenital (fifth toe) Q66.89
**Overload**
> circulatory, due to transfusion (blood) (blood compo-
>> nents) (TACO) E87.71
> fluid E87.70
>> due to transfusion (blood) (blood components)
>>> E87.71
>> specified NEC E87.79
> iron, due to repeated red blood cell transfusions
>> E83.111
> potassium (K) E87.5
> sodium (Na) E87.0
**Overnutrition** — *see* Hyperalimentation
**Overproduction** (*see also* Hypersecretion)
> ACTH E27.0

**Overproduction** — *continued*
> catecholamine E27.5
> growth hormone E22.0
**Overprotection, child by parent** Z62.1
**Overriding**
> aorta Q25.49
> finger (acquired) — *see* Deformity, finger
>> congenital Q68.1
> toe (acquired) (*see also* Deformity, toe, specified NEC)
>> congenital Q66.89
**Overstrained** R53.83
> heart — *see* Hypertrophy, cardiac
**Overuse, muscle NEC** M70.8- ☑
**Overweight** E66.3
**Overworked** R53.83
**Oviduct** — *see* condition
**Ovotestis** Q56.0
**Ovulation** (cycle)
> failure or lack of N97.0
> pain N94.0
**Ovum** — *see* condition
**Owren's disease or syndrome** (parahemophilia) D68.2
**Ox heart** — *see* Hypertrophy, cardiac
**Oxalosis** E72.53
**Oxaluria** E72.53
**Oxycephaly, oxycephalic** Q75.0
> syphilitic, congenital A50.02
**Oxyuriasis** B80
**Oxyuris vermicularis** (infestation) B80
**Ozena** J31.0

# P

**Pachyderma, pachydermia** L85.9
> larynx (verrucosa) J38.7
**Pachydermatocele** (congenital) Q82.8
**Pachydermoperiostosis** (*see also* Osteoarthropathy,
> hypertrophic, specified type NEC)
> clubbed nail M89.40 [L62]
**Pachygyria** Q04.3
**Pachymeningitis** (adhesive) (basal) (brain) (cervical)
> (chronic)(circumscribed) (external) (fibrous) (hem-
> orrhagic) (hypertrophic) (internal) (purulent) (spinal)
> (suppurative) — *see* Meningitis
**Pachyonychia** (congenital) Q84.5
**Pacinian tumor** — *see* Neoplasm, skin, benign
**Pad, knuckle or Garrod's** M72.1
**Paget's disease**
> with infiltrating duct carcinoma — *see* Neoplasm,
>> breast, malignant
> bone M88.9
>> carpus M88.84- ☑
>> clavicle M88.81- ☑
>> femur M88.85- ☑
>> fibula M88.86- ☑
>> finger M88.84- ☑
>> humerus M88.82- ☑
>> ilium M88.85- ☑
>> in neoplastic disease — *see* Osteitis, deformans, in
>>> neoplastic disease
>> ischium M88.85- ☑
>> metacarpus M88.84- ☑
>> metatarsus M88.87- ☑
>> multiple sites M88.89
>> neck M88.88
>> radius M88.83- ☑
>> rib M88.88
>> scapula M88.81- ☑
>> skull M88.0
>> tarsus M88.87- ☑
>> tibia M88.86- ☑
>> toe M88.87- ☑
>> ulna M88.83- ☑
>> vertebra M88.88
> breast (female) C50.01- ☑
>> male C50.02- ☑
> extramammary (*see also* Neoplasm, skin, malignant)
>> anus C21.0
>>> margin C44.590
>>> skin C44.590
> intraductal carcinoma — *see* Neoplasm, breast, malig-
>> nant
> malignant — *see* Neoplasm, skin, malignant
>> breast (female) C50.01- ☑
>>> male C50.02- ☑
>> unspecified site (female) C50.01- ☑
>>> male C50.02- ☑

**Paget's disease** — *continued*
> mammary — *see* Paget's disease, breast
> nipple — *see* Paget's disease, breast
> osteitis deformans — *see* Paget's disease, bone
**Paget-Schroetter syndrome** I82.890
**Pain**(s) (*see also* Painful) R52
> abdominal R10.9
>> colic R10.83
>> generalized R10.84
>>> with acute abdomen R10.0
>> lower R10.30
>>> left quadrant R10.32
>>> pelvic or perineal R10.2
>>> periumbilical R10.33
>>> right quadrant R10.31
>> rebound — *see* Tenderness, abdominal, rebound
>> severe with abdominal rigidity R10.0
>> tenderness — *see* Tenderness, abdominal
>> upper R10.10
>>> epigastric R10.13
>>> left quadrant R10.12
>>> right quadrant R10.11
> acute R52
>> due to trauma G89.11
>> neoplasm related G89.3
>> postprocedural NEC G89.18
>> post-thoracotomy G89.12
>> specified by site — *code to* Pain, by site
> adnexa (uteri) R10.2
> anginoid — *see* Pain, precordial
> anus K62.89
> arm — *see* Pain, limb, upper
> axillary (axilla) M79.62- ☑
> back (postural) M54.9
> bladder R39.89
>> associated with micturition — *see* Micturition,
>>> painful
>> chronic R39.82
> bone — *see* Disorder, bone, specified type NEC
> breast N64.4
> broad ligament R10.2
> cancer associated (acute) (chronic) G89.3
> cecum — *see* Pain, abdominal
> cervicobrachial M53.1
> chest (central) R07.9
>> anterior wall R07.89
>> atypical R07.89
>> ischemic I20.9
>> musculoskeletal R07.89
>> non-cardiac R07.89
>> on breathing R07.1
>> pleurodynia R07.81
>> precordial R07.2
>> wall (anterior) R07.89
> chronic G89.29
>> associated with significant psychosocial dysfunc-
>>> tion G89.4
>> due to trauma G89.21
>> neoplasm related G89.3
>> postoperative NEC G89.28
>> postprocedural NEC G89.28
>> post-thoracotomy G89.22
>> specified NEC G89.29
> coccyx M53.3
> colon — *see* Pain, abdominal
> coronary — *see* Angina
> costochondral R07.1
> diaphragm R07.1
> due to cancer G89.3
> due to device, implant or graft (*see also* Complications,
>> by site and type, specified NEC) T85.848 ☑
>> arterial graft NEC T82.848 ☑
>> breast (implant) T85.848 ☑
>> catheter NEC T85.848 ☑
>>> dialysis (renal) T82.848 ☑
>>>> intraperitoneal T85.848 ☑
>>> infusion NEC T82.848 ☑
>>>> spinal (epidural) (subdural) T85.840 ☑
>>> urinary (indwelling) T83.84 ☑
>> electronic (electrode) (pulse generator) (stimulator)
>>> bone T85.840 ☑
>>> cardiac T82.847 ☑
>>> nervous system (brain) (peripheral nerve)
>>>> (spinal) T85.84 ☑
>>> urinary T83.84 ☑
>> fixation, internal (orthopedic) NEC T84.84 ☑
>> gastrointestinal (bile duct) (esophagus) T85.848 ☑
>> genital NEC T83.84 ☑

☑ **Additional Character Required** — **Refer to the Tabular List for Character Selection**     ▽ **Subterms under main terms may continue to next column or page**

**Pain(s)** — *continued*
  due to device, implant or graft (*see also* Complications,
    by site and type, specified) — *continued*
    heart NEC T82.847 ☑
    infusion NEC T85.848 ☑
    joint prosthesis T84.84 ☑
    ocular (corneal graft) (orbital implant) NEC
      T85.848 ☑
    orthopedic NEC T84.84 ☑
    specified NEC T85.848 ☑
    urinary NEC T83.84 ☑
    vascular NEC T82.848 ☑
    ventricular intracranial shunt T85.840 ☑
  due to malignancy (primary) (secondary) G89.3
  ear — *see* subcategory H92.0 ☑
  epigastric, epigastrium R10.13
  eye — *see* Pain, ocular
  face, facial R51
    atypical G50.1
  female genital organs NEC N94.89
  finger — *see* Pain, limb, upper
  flank — *see* Pain, abdominal
  foot — *see* Pain, limb, lower
  gallbladder K82.9
  gas (intestinal) R14.1
  gastric — *see* Pain, abdominal
  generalized NOS R52
  genital organ
    female N94.89
    male N50.89
  groin — *see* Pain, abdominal, lower
  hand — *see* Pain, limb, upper
  head — *see* Headache
  heart — *see* Pain, precordial
  infra-orbital — *see* Neuralgia, trigeminal
  intercostal R07.82
  intermenstrual N94.0
  jaw R68.84
  joint M25.50
    ankle M25.57- ☑
    elbow M25.52- ☑
    finger M25.54- ☑
    foot M25.57- ☑
    hand M25.54- ☑
    hip M25.55- ☑
    knee M25.56- ☑
    shoulder M25.51- ☑
    toe M25.57- ☑
    wrist M25.53- ☑
  kidney N23
  laryngeal R07.0
  leg — *see* Pain, limb, lower
  limb M79.609
    lower M79.60- ☑
      foot M79.67- ☑
      lower leg M79.66- ☑
      thigh M79.65- ☑
      toe M79.67- ☑
    upper M79.60- ☑
      axilla M79.62- ☑
      finger M79.64- ☑
      forearm M79.63- ☑
      hand M79.64- ☑
      upper arm M79.62- ☑
  loin M54.5
  low back M54.5
  lumbar region M54.5
  mandibular R68.84
  mastoid — *see* subcategory H92.0 ☑
  maxilla R68.84
  menstrual (*see also* Dysmenorrhea) N94.6
  metacarpophalangeal (joint) — *see* Pain, joint, hand
  metatarsophalangeal (joint) — *see* Pain, joint, foot
  mouth K13.79
  muscle — *see* Myalgia
  musculoskeletal (*see also* Pain, by site) M79.1
  myofascial M79.1
  nasal J34.89
  nasopharynx J39.2
  neck NEC M54.2
  nerve NEC — *see* Neuralgia
  neuromuscular — *see* Neuralgia
  nose J34.89
  ocular H57.1- ☑
  ophthalmic — *see* Pain, ocular
  orbital region — *see* Pain, ocular
  ovary N94.89

**Pain(s)** — *continued*
  over heart — *see* Pain, precordial
  ovulation N94.0
  pelvic (female) R10.2
  penis N48.89
  pericardial — *see* Pain, precordial
  perineal, perineum R10.2
  pharynx J39.2
  pleura, pleural, pleuritic R07.81
  postoperative NOS G89.18
  postprocedural NOS G89.18
  post-thoracotomy G89.12
  precordial (region) R07.2
  premenstrual N94.3
  psychogenic (persistent) (any site) F45.41
  radicular (spinal) — *see* Radiculopathy
  rectum K62.89
  respiration R07.1
  retrosternal R07.2
  rheumatoid, muscular — *see* Myalgia
  rib R07.81
  root (spinal) — *see* Radiculopathy
  round ligament (stretch) R10.2
  sacroiliac M53.3
  sciatic — *see* Sciatica
  scrotum N50.82
  seminal vesicle N50.89
  shoulder M25.51- ☑
  spermatic cord N50.89
  spinal root — *see* Radiculopathy
  spine M54.9
    cervical M54.2
    low back M54.5
      with sciatica M54.4- ☑
    thoracic M54.6
  stomach — *see* Pain, abdominal
  substernal R07.2
  temporomandibular (joint) M26.62- ☑
  testis N50.81- ☑
  thoracic spine M54.6
    with radicular and visceral pain M54.14
  throat R07.0
  tibia — *see* Pain, limb, lower
  toe — *see* Pain, limb, lower
  tongue K14.6
  tooth K08.89
  trigeminal — *see* Neuralgia, trigeminal
  tumor associated G89.3
  ureter N23
  urinary (organ) (system) N23
  uterus NEC N94.89
  vagina R10.2
  vertebrogenic (syndrome) M54.89
  vesical R39.89
    associated with micturition — *see* Micturition,
      painful
  vulva R10.2
**Painful** (*see also* Pain)
  coitus
    female N94.10
    male N53.12
    psychogenic F52.6
  ejaculation (semen) N53.12
    psychogenic F52.6
  erection — *see* Priapism
  feet syndrome E53.8
  joint replacement (hip) (knee) T84.84 ☑
  menstruation — *see* Dysmenorrhea
    psychogenic F45.8
  micturition — *see* Micturition, painful
  respiration R07.1
  scar NEC L90.5
  wire sutures T81.89 ☑
**Painter's colic** — *see* subcategory T56.0 ☑
**Palate** — *see* condition
**Palatoplegia** K13.79
**Palatoschisis** — *see* Cleft, palate
**Palilalia** R48.8
**Palliative care** Z51.5
**Pallor** R23.1
  optic disc, temporal — *see* Atrophy, optic
**Palmar** (*see also* condition)
  fascia — *see* condition
**Palpable**
  cecum K63.89
  kidney N28.89
  ovary N83.8
  prostate N42.9

**Palpable** — *continued*
  spleen — *see* Splenomegaly
**Palpitations** (heart) R00.2
  psychogenic F45.8
**Palsy** (*see also* Paralysis) G83.9
  atrophic diffuse (progressive) G12.22
  Bell's (*see also* Palsy, facial)
    newborn P11.3
  brachial plexus NEC G54.0
    newborn (birth injury) P14.3
  brain — *see* Palsy, cerebral
  bulbar (progressive) (chronic) G12.22
    of childhood (Fazio-Londe) G12.1
    pseudo NEC G12.29
    supranuclear (progressive) G23.1
  cerebral (congenital) G80.9
    ataxic G80.4
    athetoid G80.3
    choreathetoid G80.3
    diplegic G80.8
      spastic G80.1
    dyskinetic G80.3
      athetoid G80.3
      choreathetoid G80.3
      distonic G80.3
    dystonic G80.3
    hemiplegic G80.8
      spastic G80.2
    mixed G80.8
    monoplegic G80.8
      spastic G80.1
    paraplegic G80.8
      spastic G80.1
    quadriplegic G80.8
      spastic G80.0
    spastic G80.1
      diplegic G80.1
      hemiplegic G80.2
      monoplegic G80.1
      quadriplegic G80.0
      specified NEC G80.1
      tetrapelgic G80.0
    specified NEC G80.8
    syphilitic A52.12
      congenital A50.49
    tetraplegic G80.8
      spastic G80.0
  cranial nerve (*see also* Disorder, nerve, cranial)
    multiple G52.7
      in
        infectious disease B99 ☑ [G53]
        neoplastic disease (*see also* Neoplasm)
          D49.9 [G53]
        parasitic disease B89 [G53]
        sarcoidosis D86.82
  creeping G12.22
  diver's T70.3 ☑
  Erb's P14.0
  facial G51.0
    newborn (birth injury) P11.3
  glossopharyngeal G52.1
  Klumpke (-Déjérine) P14.1
  lead — *see* subcategory T56.0 ☑
  median nerve (tardy) G56.1- ☑
  nerve G58.9
    specified NEC G58.8
  peroneal nerve (acute) (tardy) G57.3- ☑
  progressive supranuclear G23.1
  pseudobulbar NEC G12.29
  radial nerve (acute) G56.3- ☑
  seventh nerve (*see also* Palsy, facial)
    newborn P11.3
  shaking — *see* Parkinsonism
  spastic (cerebral) (spinal) G80.1
  ulnar nerve (tardy) G56.2- ☑
  wasting G12.29
**Paludism** — *see* Malaria
**Panangiitis** M30.0
**Panaris, panaritium** (*see also* Cellulitis, digit)
  with lymphangitis — *see* Lymphangitis, acute, digit
**Panarteritis nodosa** M30.0
  brain or cerebral I67.7
**Pancake heart** R93.1
  with cor pulmonale (chronic) I27.81
**Pancarditis** (acute) (chronic) I51.89
  rheumatic I09.89
    active or acute I01.8
**Pancoast's syndrome or tumor** C34.1- ☑

**Pancolitis, ulcerative** (chronic) K51.00
  with
    abscess K51.014
    complication K51.019
    fistula K51.013
    obstruction K51.012
    rectal bleeding K51.011
    specified complication NEC K51.018
**Pancreas, pancreatic** — *see* condition
**Pancreatitis** (annular) (apoplectic) (calcareous) (edematous) (hemorrhagic) (malignant) (recurrent) (subacute) (suppurative) K85.90
  with necrosis (uninfected) K85.91
    infected K85.92
  acute (without necrosis or infection) K85.90
    with necrosis (uninfected) K85.91
      infected K85.92
    alcohol induced (without necrosis or infection) K85.20
      with necrosis (uninfected) K85.21
        infected K85.22
    biliary (without necrosis or infection) K85.10
      with necrosis (uninfected) K85.11
        infected K85.12
    drug induced (without necrosis or infection) K85.30
      with necrosis (uninfected) K85.31
        infected K85.32
    gallstone (without necrosis or infection) K85.10
      with necrosis (uninfected) K85.11
        infected K85.12
    idiopathic (without necrosis or infection) K85.00
      with necrosis (uninfected) K85.01
        infected K85.02
    specified NEC (without necrosis or infection) K85.80
      with necrosis (uninfected) K85.81
        infected K85.82
  chronic (infectious) K86.1
    alcohol-induced K86.0
    recurrent K86.1
    relapsing K86.1
  cystic (chronic) K86.1
  cytomegaloviral B25.2
  fibrous (chronic) K86.1
  gallstone (without necrosis or infection) K85.10
    with necrosis (uninfected) K85.11
      infected K85.12
  gangrenous — *see* Pancreatitis, acute
  interstitial (chronic) K86.1
    acute (*see also* Pancreatitis, acute) K85.80
  mumps B26.3
  recurrent (chronic) K86.1
  relapsing, chronic K86.1
  syphilitic A52.74
**Pancreatoblastoma** — *see* Neoplasm, pancreas, malignant
**Pancreolithiasis** K86.89
**Pancytolysis** D75.89
**Pancytopenia** (acquired) D61.818
  with
    malformations D61.09
    myelodysplastic syndrome — *see* Syndrome, myelodysplastic
  antineoplastic chemotherapy induced D61.810
  congenital D61.09
  drug-induced NEC D61.811
**PANDAS** (pediatric autoimmune neuropsychiatric disorders associated with streptococcal infections syndrome) D89.89
**Panencephalitis, subacute, sclerosing** A81.1
**Panhematopenia** D61.9
  congenital D61.09
  constitutional D61.09
  splenic, primary D73.1
**Panhemocytopenia** D61.9
  congenital D61.09
  constitutional D61.09
**Panhypogonadism** E29.1
**Panhypopituitarism** E23.0
  prepubertal E23.0
**Panic** (attack) (state) F41.0
  reaction to exceptional stress (transient) F43.0
**Panmyelopathy, familial, constitutional** D61.09
**Panmyelophthisis** D61.82
  congenital D61.09
**Panmyelosis** (acute) (with myelofibrosis) C94.4- ☑
**Panner's disease** — *see* Osteochondrosis, juvenile, humerus
**Panneuritis endemica** E51.11

**Panniculitis** (nodular) (nonsuppurative) M79.3
  back M54.00
    cervical region M54.02
    cervicothoracic region M54.03
    lumbar region M54.06
    lumbosacral region M54.07
    multiple sites M54.09
    occipito-atlanto-axial region M54.01
    sacrococcygeal region M54.08
    thoracic region M54.04
    thoracolumbar region M54.05
  lupus L93.2
  mesenteric K65.4
  neck M54.02
    cervicothoracic region M54.03
    occipito-atlanto-axial region M54.01
  relapsing M35.6
**Panniculus adiposus** (abdominal) E65
**Pannus** (allergic) (cornea) (degenerativus) (keratic) H16.42- ☑
  abdominal (symptomatic) E65
  trachomatosus, trachomatous (active) A71.1
**Panophthalmitis** H44.01- ☑
**Pansinusitis** (chronic) (hyperplastic) (nonpurulent) (purulent) J32.4
  acute J01.40
    recurrent J01.41
  tuberculous A15.8
**Panuveitis** (sympathetic) H44.11- ☑
**Panvalvular disease** I08.9
  specified NEC I08.8
**PAPA** (pyogenic arthritis, pyoderma gangrenosum, and acne syndrome) M04.8
**Papanicolaou smear, cervix** Z12.4
  as part of routine gynecological examination Z01.419
    with abnormal findings Z01.411
  for suspected neoplasm Z12.4
  nonspecific abnormal finding R87.619
  routine Z01.419
    with abnormal findings Z01.411
**Papilledema** (choked disc) H47.10
  associated with
    decreased ocular pressure H47.12
    increased intracranial pressure H47.11
    retinal disorder H47.13
  Foster-Kennedy syndrome H47.14- ☑
**Papillitis** H46.00
  anus K62.89
  chronic lingual K14.4
  necrotizing, kidney N17.2
  optic H46.0- ☑
  rectum K62.89
  renal, necrotizing N17.2
  tongue K14.0
**Papilloma** (*see also* Neoplasm, benign, by site)
  acuminatum (female) (male) (anogenital) A63.0
  basal cell L82.1
    inflamed L82.0
  benign pinta (primary) A67.0
  bladder (urinary) (transitional cell) D41.4
  choroid plexus (lateral ventricle) (third ventricle) D33.0
    anaplastic C71.5
    fourth ventricle D33.1
    malignant C71.5
  renal pelvis (transitional cell) D41.1- ☑
    benign D30.1- ☑
  Schneiderian
    specified site — *see* Neoplasm, benign, by site
    unspecified site D14.0
  serous surface
    borderline malignancy
      specified site — *see* Neoplasm, uncertain behavior, by site
      unspecified site D39.10
    specified site — *see* Neoplasm, benign, by site
    unspecified site D27.9
  transitional (cell)
    bladder (urinary) D41.4
    inverted type — *see* Neoplasm, uncertain behavior, by site
    renal pelvis D41.1- ☑
    ureter D41.2- ☑
  ureter (transitional cell) D41.2- ☑
    benign D30.2- ☑
  urothelial — *see* Neoplasm, uncertain behavior, by site
  villous — *see* Neoplasm, uncertain behavior, by site

**Papilloma** — *continued*
  villous — *see* Neoplasm, uncertain behavior, by site
    — *continued*
    adenocarcinoma in — *see* Neoplasm, malignant, by site
    in situ — *see* Neoplasm, in situ
  yaws, plantar or palmar A66.1
**Papillomata, multiple, of yaws** A66.1
**Papillomatosis** (*see also* Neoplasm, benign, by site)
  confluent and reticulated L83
  cystic, breast — *see* Mastopathy, cystic
  ductal, breast — *see* Mastopathy, cystic
  intraductal (diffuse) — *see* Neoplasm, benign, by site
  subareolar duct D24- ☑
**Papillomavirus, as cause of disease classified elsewhere** B97.7
**Papillon-Léage and Psaume syndrome** Q87.0
**Papule(s)** R23.8
  carate (primary) A67.0
  fibrous, of nose D22.39
  Gottron's L94.4
  pinta (primary) A67.0
**Papulosis**
  lymphomatoid C86.6
  malignant I77.89
**Papyraceous fetus** O31.0- ☑
**Para-albuminemia** E88.09
**Paracephalus** Q89.7
**Parachute mitral valve** Q23.2
**Paracoccidioidomycosis** B41.9
  disseminated B41.7
  generalized B41.7
  mucocutaneous-lymphangitic B41.8
  pulmonary B41.0
  specified NEC B41.8
  visceral B41.8
**Paradentosis** K05.4
**Paraffinoma** T88.8 ☑
**Paraganglioma** D44.7
  adrenal D35.0- ☑
    malignant C74.1- ☑
  aortic body D44.7
    malignant C75.5
  carotid body D44.6
    malignant C75.4
  chromaffin (*see also* Neoplasm, benign, by site)
    malignant — *see* Neoplasm, malignant, by site
  extra-adrenal D44.7
    malignant C75.5
      specified site — *see* Neoplasm, malignant, by site
      unspecified site C75.5
    specified site — *see* Neoplasm, uncertain behavior, by site
    unspecified site D44.7
  gangliocytic D13.2
    specified site — *see* Neoplasm, benign, by site
    unspecified site D13.2
  glomus jugulare D44.7
    malignant C75.5
  jugular D44.7
  malignant C75.5
    specified site — *see* Neoplasm, malignant, by site
    unspecified site C75.5
  nonchromaffin D44.7
    malignant C75.5
      specified site — *see* Neoplasm, malignant, by site
      unspecified site C75.5
    specified site — *see* Neoplasm, uncertain behavior, by site
    unspecified site D44.7
  parasympathetic D44.7
    specified site — *see* Neoplasm, uncertain behavior, by site
    unspecified site D44.7
  specified site — *see* Neoplasm, uncertain behavior, by site
  sympathetic D44.7
    specified site — *see* Neoplasm, uncertain behavior, by site
    unspecified site D44.7
  unspecified site D44.7
**Parageusia** R43.2
  psychogenic F45.8
**Paragonimiasis** B66.4

**Paragranuloma, Hodgkin** — *see* Lymphoma, Hodgkin, specified NEC
**Parahemophilia** (*see also* Defect, coagulation) D68.2
**Parakeratosis** R23.4
　variegata L41.0
**Paralysis, paralytic** (complete) (incomplete) G83.9
　with
　　syphilis A52.17
　abducens, abducent (nerve) — *see* Strabismus, paralytic, sixth nerve
　abductor, lower extremity G57.9- ☑
　accessory nerve G52.8
　accommodation (*see also* Paresis, of accommodation)
　　hysterical F44.89
　acoustic nerve (except Deafness) H93.3 ☑
　agitans (*see also* Parkinsonism) G20
　　arteriosclerotic G21.4
　alternating (oculomotor) G83.89
　amyotrophic G12.21
　ankle G57.9- ☑
　anus (sphincter) K62.89
　arm — *see* Monoplegia, upper limb
　ascending (spinal), acute G61.0
　association G12.29
　asthenic bulbar G70.00
　　with exacerbation (acute) G70.01
　　in crisis G70.01
　ataxic (hereditary) G11.9
　　general (syphilitic) A52.17
　atrophic G58.9
　　infantile, acute — *see* Poliomyelitis, paralytic
　　progressive G12.22
　　spinal (acute) — *see* Poliomyelitis, paralytic
　axillary G54.0
　Babinski-Nageotte's G83.89
　Bell's G51.0
　　newborn P11.3
　Benedikt's G46.3
　birth injury P14.9
　　spinal cord P11.5
　bladder (neurogenic) (sphincter) N31.2
　bowel, colon or intestine K56.0
　brachial plexus G54.0
　　birth injury P14.3
　　newborn (birth injury) P14.3
　brain G83.9
　　diplegia G83.0
　　triplegia G83.89
　bronchial J98.09
　Brown-Séquard G83.81
　bulbar (chronic) (progressive) G12.22
　　infantile — *see* Poliomyelitis, paralytic
　　poliomyelitic — *see* Poliomyelitis, paralytic
　　pseudo G12.29
　bulbospinal G70.00
　　with exacerbation (acute) G70.01
　　in crisis G70.01
　cardiac (*see also* Failure, heart) I50.9
　cerebrocerebellar, diplegic G80.1
　cervical
　　plexus G54.2
　　sympathetic G90.09
　Cèstan-Chenais G46.3
　Charcot-Marie-Tooth type G60.0
　Clark's G80.9
　colon K56.0
　compressed air T70.3 ☑
　compression
　　arm G56.9- ☑
　　leg G57.9- ☑
　　lower extremity G57.9- ☑
　　upper extremity G56.9- ☑
　congenital (cerebral) — *see* Palsy, cerebral
　conjugate movement (gaze) (of eye) H51.0
　　cortical (nuclear) (supranuclear) H51.0
　cordis — *see* Failure, heart
　cranial or cerebral nerve G52.9
　creeping G12.22
　crossed leg G83.89
　crutch — *see* Injury, brachial plexus
　deglutition R13.0
　　hysterical F44.4
　dementia A52.17
　descending (spinal) NEC G12.29
　diaphragm (flaccid) J98.6
　　due to accidental dissection of phrenic nerve during procedure — *see* Puncture, accidental complicating surgery

**Paralysis, paralytic** — *continued*
　digestive organs NEC K59.8
　diplegic — *see* Diplegia
　divergence (nuclear) H51.8
　diver's T70.3 ☑
　Duchenne's
　　birth injury P14.0
　　due to or associated with
　　　motor neuron disease G12.22
　　　muscular dystrophy G71.0
　due to intracranial or spinal birth injury — *see* Palsy, cerebral
　embolic (current episode) I63.4- ☑
　Erb (-Duchenne) (birth) (newborn) P14.0
　Erb's syphilitic spastic spinal A52.17
　esophagus K22.8
　eye muscle (extrinsic) H49.9
　　intrinsic (*see also* Paresis, of accommodation)
　facial (nerve) G51.0
　　birth injury P11.3
　　congenital P11.3
　　following operation NEC — *see* Puncture, accidental complicating surgery
　　newborn (birth injury) P11.3
　familial (recurrent) (periodic) G72.3
　　spastic G11.4
　fauces J39.2
　finger G56.9- ☑
　gait R26.1
　gastric nerve (nondiabetic) G52.2
　gaze, conjugate H51.0
　general (progressive) (syphilitic) A52.17
　　juvenile A50.45
　glottis J38.00
　　bilateral J38.02
　　unilateral J38.01
　gluteal G54.1
　Gubler (-Millard) G46.3
　hand — *see* Monoplegia, upper limb
　heart — *see* Arrest, cardiac
　hemiplegic — *see* Hemiplegia
　hyperkalemic periodic (familial) G72.3
　hypoglossal (nerve) G52.3
　hypokalemic periodic G72.3
　hysterical F44.4
　ileus K56.0
　infantile (*see also* Poliomyelitis, paralytic) A80.30
　　bulbar — *see* Poliomyelitis, paralytic
　　cerebral — *see* Palsy, cerebral
　　spastic — *see* Palsy, cerebral, spastic
　infective — *see* Poliomyelitis, paralytic
　inferior nuclear G83.9
　internuclear — *see* Ophthalmoplegia, internuclear
　intestine K56.0
　iris H57.09
　　due to diphtheria (toxin) A36.89
　ischemic, Volkmann's (complicating trauma) T79.6 ☑
　Jackson's G83.89
　jake — *see* Poisoning, food, noxious, plant
　Jamaica ginger (jake) G62.2
　juvenile general A50.45
　Klumpke (-Déjérine) (birth) (newborn) P14.1
　labioglossal (laryngeal) (pharyngeal) G12.29
　Landry's G61.0
　laryngeal nerve (recurrent) (superior) (unilateral) J38.00
　　bilateral J38.02
　　unilateral J38.01
　larynx J38.00
　　bilateral J38.02
　　due to diphtheria (toxin) A36.2
　　unilateral J38.01
　lateral G12.23
　lead T56.0 ☑
　left side — *see* Hemiplegia
　leg G83.1- ☑
　　both — *see* Paraplegia
　　crossed G83.89
　　hysterical F44.4
　　psychogenic F44.4
　　transient or transitory R29.818
　　　traumatic NEC — *see* Injury, nerve, leg
　levator palpebrae superioris — *see* Blepharoptosis, paralytic
　limb — *see* Monoplegia
　lip K13.0
　Lissauer's A52.17
　lower limb — *see* Monoplegia, lower limb
　　both — *see* Paraplegia

**Paralysis, paralytic** — *continued*
　lung J98.4
　median nerve G56.1- ☑
　medullary (tegmental) G83.89
　mesencephalic NEC G83.89
　　tegmental G83.89
　middle alternating G83.89
　Millard-Gubler-Foville G46.3
　monoplegic — *see* Monoplegia
　motor G83.9
　muscle, muscular NEC G72.89
　　due to nerve lesion G58.9
　　eye (extrinsic) H49.9
　　　intrinsic — *see* Paresis, of accommodation
　　　oblique — *see* Strabismus, paralytic, fourth nerve
　　iris sphincter H21.9
　　ischemic (Volkmann's) (complicating trauma) T79.6 ☑
　　progressive G12.21
　　pseudohypertrophic G71.0
　musculocutaneous nerve G56.9- ☑
　musculospiral G56.9- ☑
　nerve (*see also* Disorder, nerve)
　　abducent — *see* Strabismus, paralytic, sixth nerve
　　accessory G52.8
　　auditory (except Deafness) H93.3 ☑
　　birth injury P14.9
　　cranial or cerebral G52.9
　　facial G51.0
　　　birth injury P11.3
　　　congenital P11.3
　　　newborn (birth injury) P11.3
　　fourth or trochlear — *see* Strabismus, paralytic, fourth nerve
　　newborn (birth injury) P14.9
　　oculomotor — *see* Strabismus, paralytic, third nerve
　　phrenic (birth injury) P14.2
　　radial G56.3- ☑
　　seventh or facial G51.0
　　　newborn (birth injury) P11.3
　　sixth or abducent — *see* Strabismus, paralytic, sixth nerve
　　syphilitic A52.15
　　third or oculomotor — *see* Strabismus, paralytic, third nerve
　　trigeminal G50.9
　　trochlear — *see* Strabismus, paralytic, fourth nerve
　　ulnar G56.2- ☑
　normokalemic periodic G72.3
　ocular H49.9
　　alternating G83.89
　oculofacial, congenital (Moebius) Q87.0
　oculomotor (external bilateral) (nerve) — *see* Strabismus, paralytic, third nerve
　palate (soft) K13.79
　paratrigeminal G50.9
　periodic (familial) (hyperkalemic) (hypokalemic) (myotonic) (normokalemic) (potassium sensitive) (secondary) G72.3
　peripheral autonomic nervous system — *see* Neuropathy, peripheral, autonomic
　peroneal (nerve) G57.3- ☑
　pharynx J39.2
　phrenic nerve G56.8- ☑
　plantar nerve(s) G57.6- ☑
　pneumogastric nerve G52.2
　poliomyelitis (current) — *see* Poliomyelitis, paralytic
　popliteal nerve G57.3- ☑
　postepileptic transitory G83.84
　progressive (atrophic) (bulbar) (spinal) G12.22
　　general A52.17
　　infantile acute — *see* Poliomyelitis, paralytic
　　supranuclear G23.1
　pseudobulbar G12.29
　pseudohypertrophic (muscle) G71.0
　psychogenic F44.4
　quadriceps G57.9- ☑
　quadriplegic — *see* Tetraplegia
　radial nerve G56.3- ☑
　rectus muscle (eye) H49.9
　recurrent isolated sleep G47.53
　respiratory (muscle) (system) (tract) R06.81
　　center NEC G93.89
　　congenital P28.89
　　newborn P28.89
　right side — *see* Hemiplegia

**Paralysis, paralytic** — *continued*
- saturnine T56.0 ☑
- sciatic nerve G57.0- ☑
- senile G83.9
- shaking — *see* Parkinsonism
- shoulder G56.9- ☑
- sleep, recurrent isolated G47.53
- spastic G83.9
  - cerebral — *see* Palsy, cerebral, spastic
  - congenital (cerebral) — *see* Palsy, cerebral, spastic
  - familial G11.4
  - hereditary G11.4
  - quadriplegic G80.0
  - syphilitic (spinal) A52.17
- sphincter, bladder — *see* Paralysis, bladder
- spinal (cord) G83.9
  - accessory nerve G52.8
  - acute — *see* Poliomyelitis, paralytic
  - ascending acute G61.0
  - atrophic (acute) (*see also* Poliomyelitis, paralytic)
    - spastic, syphilitic A52.17
  - congenital NEC — *see* Palsy, cerebral
  - hereditary G95.89
  - infantile — *see* Poliomyelitis, paralytic
  - progressive G12.21
  - sequelae NEC G83.89
- sternomastoid G52.8
- stomach K31.84
  - diabetic — *see* Diabetes, by type, with gastroparesis
  - nerve G52.2
    - diabetic — *see* Diabetes, by type, with gastroparesis
- stroke — *see* Infarct, brain
- subcapsularis G56.8- ☑
- supranuclear (progressive) G23.1
- sympathetic G90.8
  - cervical G90.09
  - nervous system — *see* Neuropathy, peripheral, autonomic
- syndrome G83.9
  - specified NEC G83.89
- syphilitic spastic spinal (Erb's) A52.17
- thigh G57.9- ☑
- throat J39.2
  - diphtheritic A36.0
  - muscle J39.2
- thrombotic (current episode) I63.3- ☑
- thumb G56.9- ☑
- tick — *see* Toxicity, venom, arthropod, specified NEC
- Todd's (postepileptic transitory paralysis) G83.84
- toe G57.6- ☑
- tongue K14.8
- transient R29.5
  - arm or leg NEC R29.818
  - traumatic NEC — *see* Injury, nerve
- trapezius G52.8
- traumatic, transient NEC — *see* Injury, nerve
- trembling — *see* Parkinsonism
- triceps brachii G56.9- ☑
- trigeminal nerve G50.9
- trochlear (nerve) — *see* Strabismus, paralytic, fourth nerve
- ulnar nerve G56.2- ☑
- upper limb — *see* Monoplegia, upper limb
- uremic N18.9 [G99.8]
- uveoparotitic D86.89
- uvula K13.79
  - postdiphtheritic A36.0
- vagus nerve G52.2
- vasomotor NEC G90.8
- velum palati K13.79
- vesical — *see* Paralysis, bladder
- vestibular nerve (except Vertigo) H93.3 ☑
- vocal cords J38.00
  - bilateral J38.02
  - unilateral J38.01
- Volkmann's (complicating trauma) T79.6- ☑
- wasting G12.29
- Weber's G46.3
- wrist G56.9- ☑

**Paramedial urethrovesical orifice** Q64.79
**Paramenia** N92.6
**Parametritis** (*see also* Disease, pelvis, inflammatory) N73.2
- acute N73.0

**Parametritis** — *continued*
- complicating abortion — *see* Abortion, by type, complicated by, parametritis
**Parametrium, parametric** — *see* condition
**Paramnesia** — *see* Amnesia
**Paramolar** K00.1
**Paramyloidosis** E85.89
**Paramyoclonus multiplex** G25.3
**Paramyotonia** (congenita) G71.19
**Parangi** — *see* Yaws
**Paranoia** (querulans) F22
- senile F03 ☑
**Paranoid**
- dementia (senile) F03 ☑
  - praecox — *see* Schizophrenia
- personality F60.0
- psychosis (climacteric) (involutional) (menopausal) F22
  - psychogenic (acute) F23
  - senile F03 ☑
- reaction (acute) F23
  - chronic F22
- schizophrenia F20.0
- state (climacteric) (involutional) (menopausal) (simple) F22
  - senile F03 ☑
- tendencies F60.0
- traits F60.0
- trends F60.0
- type, psychopathic personality F60.0
**Paraparesis** — *see* Paraplegia
**Paraphasia** R47.02
**Paraphilia** F65.9
**Paraphimosis** (congenital) N47.2
- chancroidal A57
**Paraphrenia, paraphrenic** (late) F22
- schizophrenia F20.0
**Paraplegia** (lower) G82.20
- ataxic — *see* Degeneration, combined, spinal cord
- complete G82.21
- congenital (cerebral) G80.8
  - spastic G80.1
- familial spastic G11.4
- functional (hysterical) F44.4
- hereditary, spastic G11.4
- hysterical F44.4
- incomplete G82.22
- Pott's A18.01
- psychogenic F44.4
- spastic
  - Erb's spinal, syphilitic A52.17
  - hereditary G11.4
  - tropical G04.1
- syphilitic (spastic) A52.17
- tropical spastic G04.1
**Parapoxvirus** B08.60
- specified NEC B08.69
**Paraproteinemia** D89.2
- benign (familial) D89.2
- monoclonal D47.2
- secondary to malignant disease D47.2
**Parapsoriasis** L41.9
- en plaques L41.4
- guttata L41.1
- large plaque L41.4
- retiform, retiformis L41.5
- small plaque L41.3
- specified NEC L41.8
- varioliformis (acuta) L41.0
**Parasitic** (*see also* condition)
- disease NEC B89
- stomatitis B37.0
- sycosis (beard) (scalp) B35.0
- twin Q89.4
**Parasitism** B89
- intestinal B82.9
- skin B88.9
- specified — *see* Infestation
**Parasitophobia** F40.218
**Parasomnia** G47.50
- due to
  - alcohol
    - abuse F10.182
    - dependence F10.282
    - use F10.982
  - amphetamines
    - abuse F15.182
    - dependence F15.282

**Parasomnia** — *continued*
- due to — *continued*
  - amphetamines — *continued*
    - use F15.982
  - caffeine
    - abuse F15.182
    - dependence F15.282
    - use F15.982
  - cocaine
    - abuse F14.182
    - dependence F14.282
    - use F14.982
  - drug NEC
    - abuse F19.182
    - dependence F19.282
    - use F19.982
  - opioid
    - abuse F11.182
    - dependence F11.282
    - use F11.982
  - psychoactive substance NEC
    - abuse F19.182
    - dependence F19.282
    - use F19.982
  - sedative, hypnotic, or anxiolytic
    - abuse F13.182
    - dependence F13.282
    - use F13.982
  - stimulant NEC
    - abuse F15.182
    - dependence F15.282
    - use F15.982
  - in conditions classified elsewhere G47.54
  - nonorganic origin F51.8
  - organic G47.50
  - specified NEC G47.59
**Paraspadias** Q54.9
**Paraspasmus facialis** G51.8
**Parasuicide** (attempt)
- history of (personal) Z91.5
  - in family Z81.8
**Parathyroid gland** — *see* condition
**Parathyroid tetany** E20.9
**Paratrachoma** A74.0
**Paratyphilitis** — *see* Appendicitis
**Paratyphoid** (fever) — *see* Fever, paratyphoid
**Paratyphus** — *see* Fever, paratyphoid
**Paraurethral duct** Q64.79
- nonorganic origin F51.5
**Paraurethritis** (*see also* Urethritis)
- gonococcal (acute) (chronic) (with abscess) A54.1
**Paravaccinia NEC** B08.04
**Paravaginitis** — *see* Vaginitis
**Parencephalitis** (*see also* Encephalitis)
- sequelae G09
**Parent-child conflict** — *see* Conflict, parent-child
- estrangement NEC Z62.890
**Paresis** (*see also* Paralysis)
- accommodation — *see* Paresis, of accommodation
- Bernhardt's G57.1- ☑
- bladder (sphincter) (*see also* Paralysis, bladder)
  - tabetic A52.17
- bowel, colon or intestine K56.0
- extrinsic muscle, eye H49.9
- general (progressive) (syphilitic) A52.17
  - juvenile A50.45
- heart — *see* Failure, heart
- insane (syphilitic) A52.17
- juvenile (general) A50.45
- of accommodation H52.52- ☑
- peripheral progressive (idiopathic) G60.3
- pseudohypertrophic G71.0
- senile G83.9
- syphilitic (general) A52.17
  - congenital A50.45
- vesical NEC N31.2
**Paresthesia** (*see also* Disturbance, sensation, skin) R20.2
- Bernhardt G57.1- ☑
**Paretic** — *see* condition
**Parinaud's**
- conjunctivitis H10.89
- oculoglandular syndrome H10.89
- ophthalmoplegia H49.88- ☑
**Parkinsonism** (idiopathic) (primary) G20
- with neurogenic orthostatic hypotension (symptomatic) G90.3
- arteriosclerotic G21.4
- dementia G31.83 [F02.80]

☑ **Additional Character Required** — Refer to the Tabular List for Character Selection    ▽ **Subterms under main terms may continue to next column or page**

**Parkinsonism** — *continued*
  dementia — *continued*
    with behavioral disturbance G31.83 [F02.81]
  due to
    drugs NEC G21.19
      neuroleptic G21.11
    medication-induced NEC G21.19
  neuroleptic induced G21.11
  postencephalitic G21.3
  secondary G21.9
    due to
      arteriosclerosis G21.4
      drugs NEC G21.19
        neuroleptic G21.11
      encephalitis G21.3
      external agents NEC G21.2
      syphilis A52.19
    specified NEC G21.8
  syphilitic A52.19
  treatment-induced NEC G21.19
  vascular G21.4
**Parkinson's disease, syndrome or tremor** — *see* Parkinsonism
**Parodontitis** — *see* Periodontitis
**Parodontosis** K05.4
**Paronychia** (*see also* Cellulitis, digit)
  with lymphangitis — *see* Lymphangitis, acute, digit
  candidal (chronic) B37.2
  tuberculous (primary) A18.4
**Parorexia** (psychogenic) F50.89
**Parosmia** R43.1
  psychogenic F45.8
**Parotid gland** — *see* condition
**Parotitis, parotiditis** (allergic)(nonspecific toxic) (purulent) (septic) (suppurative) (*see also* Sialoadenitis)
  epidemic — *see* Mumps
  infectious — *see* Mumps
  postoperative K91.89
  surgical K91.89
**Parrot fever** A70
**Parrot's disease** (early congenital syphilitic pseudoparalysis) A50.02
**Parry-Romberg syndrome** G51.8
**Parry's disease or syndrome** E05.00
  with thyroid storm E05.01
**Pars planitis** — *see* Cyclitis
**Parsonage** (-Aldren)-**Turner syndrome** G54.5
**Parson's disease** (exophthalmic goiter) E05.00
  with thyroid storm E05.01
**Particolored infant** Q82.8
**Parturition** — *see* Delivery
**Parulis** K04.7
  with sinus K04.6
**Parvovirus, as cause of disease classified elsewhere** B97.6
**Pasini and Pierini's atrophoderma** L90.3
**Passage**
  false, urethra N36.5
  meconium (newborn) during delivery P03.82
  of sounds or bougies — *see* Attention to, artificial, opening
**Passive** — *see* condition
  smoking Z77.22
**Pasteurella septica** A28.0
**Pasteurellosis** — *see* Infection, Pasteurella
**PAT** (paroxysmal atrial tachycardia) I47.1
**Patau's syndrome** — *see* Trisomy, 13
**Patches**
  mucous (syphilitic) A51.39
    congenital A50.07
  smokers' (mouth) K13.24
**Patellar** — *see* condition
**Patent** (*see also* Imperfect, closure)
  canal of Nuck Q52.4
  cervix N88.3
  ductus arteriosus or Botallo's Q25.0
  foramen
    botalli Q21.1
    ovale Q21.1
  interauricular septum Q21.1
  interventricular septum Q21.0
  omphalomesenteric duct Q43.0
  os (uteri) — *see* Patent, cervix
  ostium secundum Q21.1
  urachus Q64.4
  vitelline duct Q43.0
**Paterson** (-Brown)(-Kelly) **syndrome or web** D50.1

**Pathologic, pathological** (*see also* condition)
  asphyxia R09.01
  fire-setting F63.1
  gambling F63.0
  ovum O02.0
  resorption, tooth K03.3
  stealing F63.2
**Pathology** (of) — *see* Disease
  periradicular, associated with previous endodontic treatment NEC M27.59
**Pattern, sleep-wake, irregular** G47.23
**Patulous** (*see also* Imperfect, closure (congenital))
  alimentary tract Q45.8
    lower Q43.8
    upper Q40.8
  eustachian tube H69.0- ☑
**Pause, sinoatrial** I49.5
**Paxton's disease** B36.2
**Pearl(s)**
  enamel K00.2
  Epstein's K09.8
**Pearl-worker's disease** — *see* Osteomyelitis, specified type NEC
**Pectenosis** K62.4
**Pectoral** — *see* condition
**Pectus**
  carinatum (congenital) Q67.7
    acquired M95.4
    rachitic sequelae (late effect) E64.3
  excavatum (congenital) Q67.6
    acquired M95.4
    rachitic sequelae (late effect) E64.3
  recurvatum (congenital) Q67.6
**Pedatrophia** E41
**Pederosis** F65.4
**Pediculosis** (infestation) B85.2
  capitis (head-louse) (any site) B85.0
  corporis (body-louse) (any site) B85.1
  eyelid B85.0
  mixed (classifiable to more than one of the titles B85.0-B85.3) B85.4
  pubis (pubic louse) (any site) B85.3
  vestimenti B85.1
  vulvae B85.3
**Pediculus** (infestation) — *see* Pediculosis
**Pedophilia** F65.4
**Peg-shaped teeth** K00.2
**Pelade** — *see* Alopecia, areata
**Pelger-Huët anomaly or syndrome** D72.0
**Peliosis** (rheumatica) D69.0
  hepatis K76.4
    with toxic liver disease K71.8
**Pelizaeus-Merzbacher disease** E75.29
**Pellagra** (alcoholic) (with polyneuropathy) E52
**Pellagra-cerebellar-ataxia-renal aminoaciduria syndrome** E72.02
**Pellegrini** (-Stieda) **disease or syndrome** — *see* Bursitis, tibial collateral
**Pellizzi's syndrome** E34.8
**Pel's crisis** A52.11
**Pelvic** (*see also* condition)
  examination (periodic) (routine) Z01.419
    with abnormal findings Z01.411
  kidney, congenital Q63.2
**Pelviolithiasis** — *see* Calculus, kidney
**Pelviperitonitis** (*see also* Peritonitis, pelvic)
  gonococcal A54.24
  puerperal O85
**Pelvis** — *see* condition or type
**Pemphigoid** L12.9
  benign, mucous membrane L12.1
  bullous L12.0
  cicatricial L12.1
  juvenile L12.2
  ocular L12.1
  specified NEC L12.8
**Pemphigus** L10.9
  benign familial (chronic) Q82.8
  Brazilian L10.3
  circinatus L13.0
  conjunctiva L12.1
  drug-induced L10.5
  erythematosus L10.4
  foliaceous L10.2
  gangrenous — *see* Gangrene
  neonatorum L01.03
  ocular L12.1
  paraneoplastic L10.81

**Pemphigus** — *continued*
  specified NEC L10.89
  syphilitic (congenital) A50.06
  vegetans L10.1
  vulgaris L10.0
  wildfire L10.3
**Pendred's syndrome** E07.1
**Pendulous**
  abdomen, in pregnancy — *see* Pregnancy, complicated by, abnormal, pelvic organs or tissues NEC
  breast N64.89
**Penetrating wound** (*see also* Puncture)
  with internal injury — *see* Injury, by site
  eyeball — *see* Puncture, eyeball
  orbit (with or without foreign body) — *see* Puncture, orbit
  uterus by instrument with or following ectopic or molar pregnancy O08.6
**Penicillosis** B48.4
**Penis** — *see* condition
**Penitis** N48.29
**Pentalogy of Fallot** Q21.8
**Pentasomy X syndrome** Q97.1
**Pentosuria** (essential) E74.8
**Percreta placenta** - O43.23 ☑
**Peregrinating patient** — *see* Disorder, factitious
**Perforation, perforated** (nontraumatic) (of)
  accidental during procedure (blood vessel) (nerve) (organ) — *see* Complication, accidental puncture or laceration
  antrum — *see* Sinusitis, maxillary
  appendix K35.2
    with localized peritonitis K35.3
  atrial septum, multiple Q21.1
  attic, ear — *see* Perforation, tympanum, attic
  bile duct (common) (hepatic) K83.2
    cystic K82.2
  bladder (urinary)
    with or following ectopic or molar pregnancy O08.6
    obstetrical trauma O71.5
    traumatic S37.29 ☑
      at delivery O71.5
  bowel K63.1
    with or following ectopic or molar pregnancy O08.6
    newborn P78.0
    obstetrical trauma O71.5
    traumatic — *see* Laceration, intestine
  broad ligament N83.8
    with or following ectopic or molar pregnancy O08.6
    obstetrical trauma O71.6
  by
    device, implant or graft (*see also* Complications, by site and type, mechanical) T85.628 ☑
      arterial graft NEC — *see* Complication, cardiovascular device, mechanical, vascular
      breast (implant) T85.49 ☑
      catheter NEC T85.698 ☑
        cystostomy T83.090 ☑
        dialysis (renal) T82.49 ☑
          intraperitoneal T85.691 ☑
        infusion NEC T82.594 ☑
          spinal (epidural) (subdural) T85.690 ☑
        urinary (*see also* Complications, catheter, urinary T83.098 ☑
      electronic (electrode) (pulse generator) (stimulator)
        bone T84.390 ☑
        cardiac T82.199 ☑
          electrode T82.190 ☑
          pulse generator T82.191 ☑
          specified type NEC T82.198 ☑
        nervous system — *see* Complication, prosthetic device, mechanical, electronic nervous system stimulator
        urinary — *see* Complication, genitourinary, device, urinary, mechanical
      fixation, internal (orthopedic) NEC — *see* Complication, fixation device, mechanical
      gastrointestinal — *see* Complications, prosthetic device, mechanical, gastrointestinal device
      genital NEC T83.498 ☑
        intrauterine contraceptive device T83.39 ☑
        penile prosthesis T83.490 ☑
      heart NEC — *see* Complication, cardiovascular device, mechanical

**Perforation, perforated** — *continued*
  by — *continued*
    device, implant or graft (*see also* Complications, by
      site and type, mechanical) — *continued*
      joint prosthesis — *see* Complications, joint
        prosthesis, mechanical, specified NEC, by
        site
      ocular NEC — *see* Complications, prosthetic
        device, mechanical, ocular device
      orthopedic NEC — *see* Complication, orthope-
        dic, device, mechanical
      specified NEC T85.628 ☑
      urinary NEC (*see also* Complication, genitouri-
        nary, device, urinary, mechanical)
        graft T83.29 ☑
      vascular NEC — *see* Complication, cardiovascu-
        lar device, mechanical
      ventricular intracranial shunt T85.09 ☑
    foreign body left accidentally in operative wound
      T81.539 ☑
    instrument (any) during a procedure, accidental
      — *see* Puncture, accidental complicating
      surgery
  cecum K35.2
    with localized peritonitis K35.3
  cervix (uteri) N88.8
    with or following ectopic or molar pregnancy O08.6
    obstetrical trauma O71.3
  colon K63.1
    newborn P78.0
    obstetrical trauma O71.5
    traumatic — *see* Laceration, intestine, large
  common duct (bile) K83.2
  cornea (due to ulceration) — *see* Ulcer, cornea, perfo-
    rated
  cystic duct K82.2
  diverticulum (intestine) K57.80
    with bleeding K57.81
    large intestine K57.20
      with
        bleeding K57.21
        small intestine K57.40
          with bleeding K57.41
    small intestine K57.00
      with
        bleeding K57.01
        large intestine K57.40
          with bleeding K57.41
  ear drum — *see* Perforation, tympanum
  esophagus K22.3
  ethmoidal sinus — *see* Sinusitis, ethmoidal
  frontal sinus — *see* Sinusitis, frontal
  gallbladder K82.2
  heart valve — *see* Endocarditis
  ileum K63.1
    newborn P78.0
    obstetrical trauma O71.5
    traumatic — *see* Laceration, intestine, small
  instrumental, surgical (accidental) (blood vessel)
    (nerve) (organ) — *see* Puncture, accidental
    complicating surgery
  intestine NEC K63.1
    with ectopic or molar pregnancy O08.6
    newborn P78.0
    obstetrical trauma O71.5
    traumatic — *see* Laceration, intestine
    ulcerative NEC K63.1
      newborn P78.0
  jejunum, jejunal K63.1
    obstetrical trauma O71.5
    traumatic — *see* Laceration, intestine, small
    ulcer — *see* Ulcer, gastrojejunal, with perforation
  joint prosthesis — *see* Complications, joint prosthesis,
    mechanical, specified NEC, by site
  mastoid (antrum) (cell) — *see* Disorder, mastoid,
    specified NEC
  maxillary sinus — *see* Sinusitis, maxillary
  membrana tympani — *see* Perforation, tympanum
  nasal
    septum J34.89
      congenital Q30.3
      syphilitic A52.73
    sinus J34.89
      congenital Q30.8
      due to sinusitis — *see* Sinusitis
  palate (*see also* Cleft, palate) Q35.9
    syphilitic A52.79
  palatine vault (*see also* Cleft, palate, hard) Q35.1

**Perforation, perforated** — *continued*
  palatine vault (*see also* Cleft, palate, hard) — *contin-
    ued*
    syphilitic A52.79
      congenital A50.59
  pars flaccida (ear drum) — *see* Perforation, tympanum,
    attic
  pelvic
    floor S31.030 ☑
      with
        ectopic or molar pregnancy O08.6
        penetration into retroperitoneal space
          S31.031
        retained foreign body S31.040 ☑
          with penetration into retroperitoneal
            space S31.041 ☑
      following ectopic or molar pregnancy O08.6
      obstetrical trauma O70.1
    organ S37.99
      adrenal gland S37.818 ☑
      bladder — *see* Perforation, bladder
      fallopian tube S37.599 ☑
        bilateral S37.592 ☑
        unilateral S37.591 ☑
      kidney S37.09- ☑
      obstetrical trauma O71.5
      ovary S37.499 ☑
        bilateral S37.492 ☑
        unilateral S37.491 ☑
      prostate S37.828 ☑
      specified organ NEC S37.898 ☑
      ureter — *see* Perforation, ureter
      urethra — *see* Perforation, urethra
      uterus — *see* Perforation, uterus
  perineum — *see* Laceration, perineum
  pharynx J39.2
  rectum K63.1
    newborn P78.0
    obstetrical trauma O71.5
    traumatic S36.63 ☑
  root canal space due to endodontic treatment M27.51
  sigmoid K63.1
    newborn P78.0
    obstetrical trauma O71.5
    traumatic S36.533 ☑
  sinus (accessory) (chronic) (nasal) J34.89
  sphenoidal sinus — *see* Sinusitis, sphenoidal
  surgical (accidental) (by instrument) (blood vessel)
    (nerve) (organ) — *see* Puncture, accidental
    complicating surgery
  traumatic
    external — *see* Puncture
    eye — *see* Puncture, eyeball
    internal organ — *see* Injury, by site
  tympanum, tympanic (membrane) (persistent post-
    traumatic) (postinflammatory) H72.9- ☑
    attic H72.1- ☑
      multiple — *see* Perforation, tympanum, multi-
        ple
      total — *see* Perforation, tympanum, total
    central H72.0- ☑
      multiple — *see* Perforation, tympanum, multi-
        ple
      total — *see* Perforation, tympanum, total
    marginal NEC — *see* subcategory H72.2 ☑
    multiple H72.81- ☑
    pars flaccida — *see* Perforation, tympanum, attic
    total H72.82- ☑
    traumatic, current episode S09.2- ☑
  typhoid, gastrointestinal — *see* Typhoid
  ulcer — *see* Ulcer, by site, with perforation
  ureter N28.89
    traumatic S37.19 ☑
  urethra N36.8
    with ectopic or molar pregnancy O08.6
    following ectopic or molar pregnancy O08.6
    obstetrical trauma O71.5
    traumatic S37.39 ☑
      at delivery O71.5
  uterus
    with ectopic or molar pregnancy O08.6
    by intrauterine contraceptive device T83.39 ☑
    following ectopic or molar pregnancy O08.6
    obstetrical trauma O71.1
    traumatic S37.69 ☑
      obstetric O71.1
  uvula K13.79

**Perforation, perforated** — *continued*
  uvula — *continued*
    syphilitic A52.79
  vagina O71.4
    obstetrical trauma O71.4
    other trauma — *see* Puncture, vagina
**Periadenitis mucosa necrotica recurrens** K12.0
**Periappendicitis** (acute) — *see* Appendicitis
**Periarteritis nodosa** (disseminated) (infectious)
  (necrotizing) M30.0
**Periarthritis** (joint) (*see also* Enthesopathy)
  Duplay's M75.0- ☑
  gonococcal A54.42
  humeroscapularis — *see* Capsulitis, adhesive
  scapulohumeral — *see* Capsulitis, adhesive
  shoulder — *see* Capsulitis, adhesive
  wrist M77.2- ☑
**Periarthrosis** (angioneural) — *see* Enthesopathy
**Pericapsulitis, adhesive** (shoulder) — *see* Capsulitis,
  adhesive
**Pericarditis** (with decompensation) (with effusion) I31.9
  with rheumatic fever (conditions in I00)
    active — *see* Pericarditis, rheumatic
    inactive or quiescent I09.2
  acute (hemorrhagic) (nonrheumatic) (Sicca) I30.9
    with chorea (acute) (rheumatic) (Sydenham's) I02.0
    benign I30.8
    nonspecific I30.0
    rheumatic I01.0
      with chorea (acute) (Sydenham's) I02.0
  adhesive or adherent (chronic) (external) (internal)
    I31.0
    acute — *see* Pericarditis, acute
    rheumatic I09.2
  bacterial (acute) (subacute) (with serous or seropuru-
    lent effusion) I30.1
  calcareous I31.1
  cholesterol (chronic) I31.8
    acute I30.9
  chronic (nonrheumatic) I31.9
    rheumatic I09.2
  constrictive (chronic) I31.1
  coxsackie B33.23
  fibrinocaseous (tuberculous) A18.84
  fibrinopurulent I30.1
  fibrinous I30.8
  fibrous I31.0
  gonococcal A54.83
  idiopathic I30.0
  in systemic lupus erythematosus M32.12
  infective I30.1
  meningococcal A39.53
  neoplastic (chronic) I31.8
    acute I30.9
  obliterans, obliterating I31.0
  plastic I31.0
  pneumococcal I30.1
  postinfarction I24.1
  purulent I30.1
  rheumatic (active) (acute) (with effusion) (with pneu-
    monia) I01.0
    with chorea (acute) (rheumatic) (Sydenham's) I02.0
    chronic or inactive (with chorea) I09.2
  rheumatoid — *see* Rheumatoid, carditis
  septic I30.1
  serofibrinous I30.8
  staphylococcal I30.1
  streptococcal I30.1
  suppurative I30.1
  syphilitic A52.06
  tuberculous A18.84
  uremic N18.9 [I32]
  viral I30.1
**Pericardium, pericardial** — *see* condition
**Pericellulitis** — *see* Cellulitis
**Pericementitis** (chronic) (suppurative) (*see also* Periodontitis)
  acute K05.20
    generalized — *see* Peridontitis, aggressive, gener-
      alized
    localized — *see* Peridontitis, aggressive, localized
**Perichondritis**
  auricle — *see* Perichondritis, ear
  bronchus J98.09
  ear (external) H61.00- ☑
    acute H61.01- ☑
    chronic H61.02- ☑
  external auditory canal — *see* Perichondritis, ear

**Perichondritis** — *continued*
  larynx J38.7
    syphilitic A52.73
    typhoid A01.09
  nose J34.89
  pinna — *see* Perichondritis, ear
  trachea J39.8
**Periclasia** K05.4
**Pericoronitis** — *see* Periodontitis
**Pericystitis** N30.90
  with hematuria N30.91
**Peridiverticulitis** (intestine) K57.92
  cecum — *see* Diverticulitis, intestine, large
  colon — *see* Diverticulitis, intestine, large
  duodenum — *see* Diverticulitis, intestine, small
  intestine — *see* Diverticulitis, intestine
  jejunum — *see* Diverticulitis, intestine, small
  rectosigmoid — *see* Diverticulitis, intestine, large
  rectum — *see* Diverticulitis, intestine, large
  sigmoid — *see* Diverticulitis, intestine, large
**Periendocarditis** — *see* Endocarditis
**Periepididymitis** N45.1
**Perifolliculitis** L01.02
  abscedens, caput, scalp L66.3
  capitis, abscedens (et suffodiens) L66.3
  superficial pustular L01.02
**Perihepatitis** K65.8
**Perilabyrinthitis** (acute) — *see* subcategory H83.0 ☑
**Perimeningitis** — *see* Meningitis
**Perimetritis** — *see* Endometritis
**Perimetrosalpingitis** — *see* Salpingo-oophoritis
**Perineocele** N81.81
**Perinephric, perinephritic** — *see* condition
**Perinephritis** (*see also* Infection, kidney)
  purulent — *see* Abscess, kidney
**Perineum, perineal** — *see* condition
**Perineuritis NEC** — *see* Neuralgia
**Periodic** — *see* condition
**Periodontitis** (chronic) (complex) (compound) (local)
    (simplex) K05.30
  acute K05.20
    generalized K05.229
      moderate K05.222
      severe K05.223
      slight K05.221
    localized K05.219
      moderate K05.212
      severe K05.213
      slight K05.211
  apical K04.5
    acute (pulpal origin) K04.4
  generalized K05.329
    moderate K05.322
    severe K05.323
    slight K05.321
  localized K05.319
    moderate K05.312
    severe K05.313
    slight K05.311
**Periodontoclasia** K05.4
**Periodontosis** (juvenile) K05.4
**Periods** (*see also* Menstruation)
  heavy N92.0
  irregular N92.6
  shortened intervals (irregular) N92.1
**Perionychia** (*see also* Cellulitis, digit)
  with lymphangitis — *see* Lymphangitis, acute, digit
**Perioophoritis** — *see* Salpingo-oophoritis
**Periorchitis** N45.2
**Periosteum, periosteal** — *see* condition
**Periostitis** (albuminosa) (circumscribed) (diffuse) (infec-
    tive) (monomelic) (*see also* Osteomyelitis)
  alveolar M27.3
  alveolodental M27.3
  dental M27.3
  gonorrheal A54.43
  jaw (lower) (upper) M27.2
  orbit H05.03- ☑
  syphilitic A52.77
    congenital (early) A50.02 [M90.80]
    secondary A51.46
  tuberculous — *see* Tuberculosis, bone
  yaws (hypertrophic) (early) (late) A66.6 [M90.80]
**Periostosis** (hyperplastic) (*see also* Disorder, bone,
    specified type NEC)
  with osteomyelitis — *see* Osteomyelitis, specified type
    NEC

**Peripartum**
  cardiomyopathy O90.3
**Periphlebitis** — *see* Phlebitis
**Periproctitis** K62.89
**Periprostatitis** — *see* Prostatitis
**Perirectal** — *see* condition
**Perirenal** — *see* condition
**Perisalpingitis** — *see* Salpingo-oophoritis
**Perisplenitis** (infectional) D73.89
**Peristalsis, visible or reversed** R19.2
**Peritendinitis** — *see* Enthesopathy
**Peritoneum, peritoneal** — *see* condition
**Peritonitis** (adhesive) (bacterial) (fibrinous) (hemorrhag-
    ic) (idiopathic) (localized) (perforative) (primary)
    (with adhesions) (with effusion) K65.9
  with or following
    abscess K65.1
    appendicitis K35.3
      with perforation or rupture K35.2
      generalized K35.2
      localized K35.3
    diverticular disease (intestine) K57.80
      with bleeding K57.81
      ectopic or molar pregnancy O08.0
      large intestine K57.20
        with
          bleeding K57.21
          small intestine K57.40
            with bleeding K57.41
      small intestine K57.00
        with
          bleeding K57.01
          large intestine K57.40
            with bleeding K57.41
  acute (generalized) K65.0
  aseptic T81.61 ☑
  bile, biliary K65.3
  chemical T81.61 ☑
  chlamydial A74.81
  chronic proliferative K65.8
  complicating abortion — *see* Abortion, by type, com-
    plicated by, pelvic peritonitis
  congenital P78.1
  diaphragmatic K65.0
  diffuse K65.0
  diphtheritic A36.89
  disseminated K65.0
  due to
    bile K65.3
    foreign
      body or object accidentally left during a proce-
        dure (instrument) (sponge) (swab)
        T81.599 ☑
      substance accidentally left during a procedure
        (chemical) (powder) (talc) T81.61 ☑
    talc T81.61 ☑
    urine K65.8
  eosinophilic K65.8
    acute K65.0
  fibrocaseous (tuberculous) A18.31
  fibropurulent K65.0
  following ectopic or molar pregnancy O08.0
  general (ized) K65.0
  gonococcal A54.85
  meconium (newborn) P78.0
  neonatal P78.1
    meconium P78.0
  pancreatic K65.0
  paroxysmal, familial E85.0
    benign E85.0
  pelvic
    female N73.5
      acute N73.3
      chronic N73.4
        with adhesions N73.6
    male K65.0
  periodic, familial E85.0
  proliferative, chronic K65.8
  puerperal, postpartum, childbirth O85
  purulent K65.0
  septic K65.0
  specified NEC K65.8
  spontaneous bacterial K65.2
  subdiaphragmatic K65.0
  subphrenic K65.0
  suppurative K65.0
  syphilitic A52.74
    congenital (early) A50.08 [K67]

**Peritonitis** — *continued*
  talc T81.61 ☑
  tuberculous A18.31
  urine K65.8
**Peritonsillar** — *see* condition
**Peritonsillitis** J36
**Perityphlitis** K37
**Periureteritis** N28.89
**Periurethral** — *see* condition
**Periurethritis** (gangrenous) — *see* Urethritis
**Periuterine** — *see* condition
**Perivaginitis** — *see* Vaginitis
**Perivasculitis, retinal** H35.06- ☑
**Perivasitis** (chronic) N49.1
**Perivesiculitis** (seminal) — *see* Vesiculitis
**Perlèche NEC** K13.0
  due to
    candidiasis B37.83
    moniliasis B37.83
    riboflavin deficiency E53.0
    vitamin B2 (riboflavin) deficiency E53.0
**Pernicious** — *see* condition
**Pernio, perniosis** T69.1 ☑
**Perpetrator** (of abuse) — *see* Index to External Causes
  of Injury, Perpetrator
**Persecution**
  delusion F22
  social Z60.5
**Perseveration** (tonic) R48.8
**Persistence, persistent** (congenital)
  anal membrane Q42.3
    with fistula Q42.2
  arteria stapedia Q16.3
  atrioventricular canal Q21.2
  branchial cleft NOS Q18.2
    cyst Q18.0
    fistula Q18.0
    sinus Q18.0
  bulbus cordis in left ventricle Q21.8
  canal of Cloquet Q14.0
  capsule (opaque) Q12.8
  cilioretinal artery or vein Q14.8
  cloaca Q43.7
  communication — *see* Fistula, congenital
  convolutions
    aortic arch Q25.46
    fallopian tube Q50.6
    oviduct Q50.6
    uterine tube Q50.6
  double aortic arch Q25.45
  ductus arteriosus (Botalli) Q25.0
  fetal
    circulation P29.38
    form of cervix (uteri) Q51.828
    hemoglobin, hereditary (HPFH) D56.4
  foramen
    Botalli Q21.1
    ovale Q21.1
  Gartner's duct Q52.4
  hemoglobin, fetal (hereditary) (HPFH) D56.4
  hyaloid
    artery (generally incomplete) Q14.0
    system Q14.8
  hymen, in pregnancy or childbirth — *see* Pregnancy,
    complicated by, abnormal, vulva
  lanugo Q84.2
  left
    posterior cardinal vein Q26.8
    root with right arch of aorta Q25.49
    superior vena cava Q26.1
  Meckel's diverticulum Q43.0
    malignant — *see* Table of Neoplasms, small intes-
      tine, malignant
  mucosal disease (middle ear) — *see* Otitis, media,
    suppurative, chronic, tubotympanic
  nail(s), anomalous Q84.6
  omphalomesenteric duct Q43.0
  organ or site not listed — *see* Anomaly, by site
  ostium
    atrioventriculare commune Q21.2
    primum Q21.2
    secundum Q21.1
  ovarian rests in fallopian tube Q50.6
  pancreatic tissue in intestinal tract Q43.8
  primary (deciduous)
    teeth K00.6
  vitreous hyperplasia Q14.0
  pupillary membrane Q13.89

Index

Persistence, persistent — Phlebitis

**Persistence, persistent** — *continued*
  rhesus (Rh) titer — *see* Complication(s), transfusion, incompatibility reaction, Rh (factor)
  right aortic arch Q25.47
  sinus
    urogenitalis
      female Q52.8
      male Q55.8
    venosus with imperfect incorporation in right auricle Q26.8
  thymus (gland) (hyperplasia) E32.0
  thyroglossal duct Q89.2
  thyrolingual duct Q89.2
  truncus arteriosus or communis Q20.0
  tunica vasculosa lentis Q12.2
  umbilical sinus Q64.4
  urachus Q64.4
  vitelline duct Q43.0
**Person** (with)
  admitted for clinical research, as a control subject (normal comparison) (participant) Z00.6
  awaiting admission to adequate facility elsewhere Z75.1
  concern (normal) about sick person in family Z63.6
  consulting on behalf of another Z71.0
  feigning illness Z76.5
  living (in)
    without
      adequate housing (heating) (space) Z59.1
      housing (permanent) (temporary) Z59.0
      person able to render necessary care Z74.2
      shelter Z59.0
    alone Z60.2
    boarding school Z59.3
    residential institution Z59.3
  on waiting list Z75.1
  sick or handicapped in family Z63.6
**Personality** (disorder) F60.9
  accentuation of traits (type A pattern) Z73.1
  affective F34.0
  aggressive F60.3
  amoral F60.2
  anacastic, anankastic F60.5
  antisocial F60.2
  anxious F60.6
  asocial F60.2
  asthenic F60.7
  avoidant F60.6
  borderline F60.3
  change due to organic condition (enduring) F07.0
  compulsive F60.5
  cycloid F34.0
  cyclothymic F34.0
  dependent F60.7
  depressive F34.1
  dissocial F60.2
  dual F44.81
  eccentric F60.89
  emotionally unstable F60.3
  expansive paranoid F60.0
  explosive F60.3
  fanatic F60.0
  haltlose type F60.89
  histrionic F60.4
  hyperthymic F34.0
  hypothymic F34.1
  hysterical F60.4
  immature F60.89
  inadequate F60.7
  labile (emotional) F60.3
  mixed (nonspecific) F60.89
  morally defective F60.2
  multiple F44.81
  narcissistic F60.81
  obsessional F60.5
  obsessive (-compulsive) F60.5
  organic F07.0
  overconscientious F60.5
  paranoid F60.0
  passive (-dependent) F60.7
  passive-aggressive F60.89
  pathologic F60.9
  pattern defect or disturbance F60.9
  pseudopsychopathic (organic) F07.0
  pseudoretarded (organic) F07.0
  psychoinfantile F60.4
  psychoneurotic NEC F60.89
  psychopathic F60.2
  querulant F60.0

**Personality** — *continued*
  sadistic F60.89
  schizoid F60.1
  self-defeating F60.7
  sensitive paranoid F60.0
  sociopathic (amoral) (antisocial) (asocial) (dissocial) F60.2
  specified NEC F60.89
  type A Z73.1
  unstable (emotional) F60.3
**Perthes' disease** — *see* Legg-Calvé-Perthes disease
**Pertussis** (*see also* Whooping cough) A37.90
**Perversion, perverted**
  appetite F50.89
    psychogenic F50.89
  function
    pituitary gland E23.2
      posterior lobe E22.2
  sense of smell and taste R43.8
    psychogenic F45.8
  sexual — *see* Deviation, sexual
**Pervious, congenital** (*see also* Imperfect, closure)
  ductus arteriosus Q25.0
**Pes** (congenital) (*see also* Talipes)
  acquired (*see also* Deformity, limb, foot, specified NEC)
    planus — *see* Deformity, limb, flat foot
  adductus Q66.89
  cavus Q66.7
  deformity NEC, acquired — *see* Deformity, limb, foot, specified NEC
  planus (acquired) (any degree) (*see also* Deformity, limb, flat foot)
    rachitic sequelae (late effect) E64.3
  valgus Q66.6
**Pest, pestis** — *see* Plague
**Petechia, petechiae** R23.3
  newborn P54.5
**Petechial typhus** A75.9
**Peter's anomaly** Q13.4
**Petit mal seizure** — *see* Epilepsy, generalized, specified NEC
**Petit's hernia** — *see* Hernia, abdomen, specified site NEC
**Petrellidosis** B48.2
**Petrositis** H70.20- ☑
  acute H70.21- ☑
  chronic H70.22- ☑
**Peutz-Jeghers disease or syndrome** Q85.8
**Peyronie's disease** N48.6
**PFAPA** (periodic fever, aphthous stomatitis, pharyngitis, and adenopathy syndrome) M04.8
**Pfeiffer's disease** — *see* Mononucleosis, infectious
**Phagedena** (dry) (moist) (sloughing) (*see also* Gangrene)
  geometric L88
  penis N48.29
  tropical — *see* Ulcer, skin
  vulva N76.6
**Phagedenic** — *see* condition
**Phakoma** H35.89
**Phakomatosis** (*see also* specific eponymous syndromes) Q85.9
  Bourneville's Q85.1
  specified NEC Q85.8
**Phantom limb syndrome** (without pain) G54.7
  with pain G54.6
**Pharyngeal pouch syndrome** D82.1
**Pharyngitis** (acute) (catarrhal) (gangrenous) (infective) (malignant) (membranous) (phlegmonous) (pseudomembranous) (simple) (subacute) (suppurative) (ulcerative) (viral) J02.9
  with influenza, flu, or grippe — *see* Influenza, with, pharyngitis
  aphthous B08.5
  atrophic J31.2
  chlamydial A56.4
  chronic (atrophic) (granular) (hypertrophic) J31.2
  coxsackievirus B08.5
  diphtheritic A36.0
  enteroviral vesicular B08.5
  follicular (chronic) J31.2
  fusospirochetal A69.1
  gonococcal A54.5
  granular (chronic) J31.2
  herpesviral B00.2
  hypertrophic J31.2
  infectional, chronic J31.2
  influenzal — *see* Influenza, with, respiratory manifestations NEC

**Pharyngitis** — *continued*
  lymphonodular, acute (enteroviral) B08.8
  pneumococcal J02.8
  purulent J02.9
  putrid J02.9
  septic J02.0
  sicca J31.2
  specified organism NEC J02.8
  staphylococcal J02.8
  streptococcal J02.0
  syphilitic, congenital (early) A50.03
  tuberculous A15.8
  vesicular, enteroviral B08.5
  viral NEC J02.8
**Pharyngoconjunctivitis, viral** B30.2
**Pharyngolaryngitis** (acute) J06.0
  chronic J37.0
**Pharyngoplegia** J39.2
**Pharyngotonsillitis, herpesviral** B00.2
**Pharyngotracheitis, chronic** J42
**Pharynx, pharyngeal** — *see* condition
**Phencyclidine-induced**
  anxiety disorder F16.980
  bipolar and related disorder F16.94
  depressive disorder F16.94
  psychotic disorder F16.959
**Phenomenon**
  Arthus' — *see* Arthus' phenomenon
  jaw-winking Q07.8
  lupus erythematosus (LE) cell M32.9
  Raynaud's (secondary) I73.00
    with gangrene I73.01
  vasomotor R55
  vasospastic I73.9
  vasovagal R55
  Wenckebach's I44.1
**Phenylketonuria** E70.1
  classical E70.0
  maternal E70.1
**Pheochromoblastoma**
  specified site — *see* Neoplasm, malignant, by site
  unspecified site C74.10
**Pheochromocytoma**
  malignant
    specified site — *see* Neoplasm, malignant, by site
    unspecified site C74.10
  specified site — *see* Neoplasm, benign, by site
  unspecified site D35.00
**Pheohyphomycosis** — *see* Chromomycosis
**Pheomycosis** — *see* Chromomycosis
**Phimosis** (congenital) (due to infection) N47.1
  chancroidal A57
**Phlebectasia** (*see also* Varix)
  congenital Q27.4
**Phlebitis** (infective) (pyemic) (septic) (suppurative) I80.9
  antepartum — *see* Thrombophlebitis, antepartum
  blue — *see* Phlebitis, leg, deep
  breast, superficial I80.8
  cavernous (venous) sinus — *see* Phlebitis, intracranial (venous) sinus
  cerebral (venous) sinus — *see* Phlebitis, intracranial (venous) sinus
  chest wall, superficial I80.8
  cranial (venous) sinus — *see* Phlebitis, intracranial (venous) sinus
  deep (vessels) — *see* Phlebitis, leg, deep
  due to implanted device — *see* Complications, by site and type, specified NEC
  during or resulting from a procedure T81.72 ☑
  femoral vein (superficial) I80.1- ☑
  femoropopliteal vein I80.0- ☑
  gestational — *see* Phlebopathy, gestational
  hepatic veins I80.8
  iliofemoral — *see* Phlebitis, femoral vein
  intracranial (venous) sinus (any) G08
    nonpyogenic I67.6
  intraspinal venous sinuses and veins G08
    nonpyogenic G95.19
  lateral (venous) sinus — *see* Phlebitis, intracranial (venous) sinus
  leg I80.3
    antepartum — *see* Thrombophlebitis, antepartum
    deep (vessels) NEC I80.20- ☑
      iliac I80.21- ☑
      popliteal vein I80.22- ☑
      specified vessel NEC I80.29- ☑
      tibial vein I80.23- ☑

**Phlebitis** — *continued*
　leg — *continued*
　　femoral vein (superficial) I80.1- ☑
　　superficial (vessels) I80.0- ☑
　longitudinal sinus — *see* Phlebitis, intracranial (venous) sinus
　lower limb — *see* Phlebitis, leg
　migrans, migrating (superficial) I82.1
　pelvic
　　with ectopic or molar pregnancy O08.0
　　following ectopic or molar pregnancy O08.0
　　puerperal, postpartum O87.1
　popliteal vein — *see* Phlebitis, leg, deep, popliteal
　portal (vein) K75.1
　postoperative T81.72 ☑
　pregnancy — *see* Thrombophlebitis, antepartum
　puerperal, postpartum, childbirth O87.0
　　deep O87.1
　　pelvic O87.1
　　superficial O87.0
　retina — *see* Vasculitis, retina
　saphenous (accessory) (great) (long) (small) — *see* Phlebitis, leg, superficial
　sinus (meninges) — *see* Phlebitis, intracranial (venous) sinus
　specified site NEC I80.8
　syphilitic A52.09
　tibial vein — *see* Phlebitis, leg, deep, tibial
　ulcerative I80.9
　　leg — *see* Phlebitis, leg
　umbilicus I80.8
　uterus (septic) — *see* Endometritis
　varicose (leg) (lower limb) — *see* Varix, leg, with, inflammation
**Phlebofibrosis** I87.8
**Phleboliths** I87.8
**Phlebopathy,**
　gestational O22.9- ☑
　puerperal O87.9
**Phlebosclerosis** I87.8
**Phlebothrombosis** (*see also* Thrombosis)
　antepartum — *see* Thrombophlebitis, antepartum
　pregnancy — *see* Thrombophlebitis, antepartum
　puerperal — *see* Thrombophlebitis, puerperal
**Phlebotomus fever** A93.1
**Phlegmasia**
　alba dolens O87.1
　　nonpuerperal — *see* Phlebitis, femoral vein
　cerulea dolens — *see* Phlebitis, leg, deep
**Phlegmon** — *see* Abscess
**Phlegmonous** — *see* condition
**Phlyctenulosis** (allergic) (keratoconjunctivitis) (nontuberculous) (*see also* Keratoconjunctivitis)
　cornea — *see* Keratoconjunctivitis
　tuberculous A18.52
**Phobia, phobic** F40.9
　animal F40.218
　　spiders F40.210
　examination F40.298
　reaction F40.9
　simple F40.298
　social F40.10
　　generalized F40.11
　specific (isolated) F40.298
　　animal F40.218
　　　spiders F40.210
　　blood F40.230
　　injection F40.231
　　injury F40.233
　　men F40.290
　　natural environment F40.228
　　　thunderstorms F40.220
　　situational F40.248
　　　bridges F40.242
　　　closed in spaces F40.240
　　　flying F40.243
　　　heights F40.241
　　specified focus NEC F40.298
　　transfusion F40.231
　　women F40.291
　specified NEC F40.8
　　medical care NEC F40.232
　state F40.9
**Phocas' disease** — *see* Mastopathy, cystic
**Phocomelia** Q73.1
　lower limb — *see* Agenesis, leg, with foot present
　upper limb — *see* Agenesis, arm, with hand present

**Phoria** H50.50
**Phosphate-losing tubular disorder** N25.0
**Phosphatemia** E83.39
**Phosphaturia** E83.39
**Photodermatitis** (sun) L56.8
　chronic L57.8
　due to drug L56.8
　light other than sun L59.8
**Photokeratitis** H16.13- ☑
**Photophobia** H53.14- ☑
**Photophthalmia** — *see* Photokeratitis
**Photopsia** H53.19
**Photoretinitis** — *see* Retinopathy, solar
**Photosensitivity, photosensitization** (sun) skin L56.8
　light other than sun L59.8
**Phrenitis** — *see* Encephalitis
**Phrynoderma** (vitamin A deficiency) E50.8
**Phthiriasis** (pubis) B85.3
　with any infestation classifiable to B85.0-B85.2 B85.4
**Phthirus infestation** — *see* Phthiriasis
**Phthisis** (*see also* Tuberculosis)
　bulbi (infectional) — *see* Disorder, globe, degenerated condition, atrophy
　eyeball (due to infection) — *see* Disorder, globe, degenerated condition, atrophy
**Phycomycosis** — *see* Zygomycosis
**Physalopteriasis** B81.8
**Physical restraint status** Z78.1
**Phytobezoar** T18.9 ☑
　intestine T18.3 ☑
　stomach T18.2 ☑
**Pian** — *see* Yaws
**Pianoma** A66.1
**Pica** F50.89
　in adults F50.89
　infant or child F98.3
**Picking, nose** F98.8
**Pick-Niemann disease** — *see* Niemann-Pick disease or syndrome
**Pick's**
　cerebral atrophy G31.01 [F02.80]
　　with behavioral disturbance G31.01 [F02.81]
　disease or syndrome (brain) G31.01 [F02.80]
　　with behavioral disturbance G31.01 [F02.81]
　　brain G31.01 [F02.80]
　　　with behavioral disturbance G31.01 [F02.81]
　　pericardium (pericardial pseudocirrhosis of liver) I31.1
　syndrome
　　brain G31.01 [F02.80]
　　　with behavioral disturbance G31.01 [F02.81]
　　of heart (pericardial pseudocirrhosis of liver) I31.1
**Pickwickian syndrome** E66.2
**Piebaldism** E70.39
**Piedra** (beard) (scalp) B36.8
　black B36.3
　white B36.2
**Pierre Robin deformity or syndrome** Q87.0
**Pierson's disease or osteochondrosis** M91.0
**Pig-bel** A05.2
**Pigeon**
　breast or chest (acquired) M95.4
　　congenital Q67.7
　　rachitic sequelae (late effect) E64.3
　breeder's disease or lung J67.2
　fancier's disease or lung J67.2
　toe — *see* Deformity, toe, specified NEC
**Pigmentation** (abnormal) (anomaly) L81.9
　conjunctiva H11.13- ☑
　cornea (anterior) H18.01- ☑
　　posterior H18.05- ☑
　　stromal H18.06- ☑
　diminished melanin formation NEC L81.6
　iron L81.8
　lids, congenital Q82.8
　limbus corneae — *see* Pigmentation, cornea
　metals L81.8
　optic papilla, congenital Q14.2
　retina, congenital (grouped) (nevoid) Q14.1
　scrotum, congenital Q82.8
　tattoo L81.8
**Piles** (*see also* Hemorrhoids) K64.9
**Pili**
　annulati or torti (congenital) Q84.1
　incarnati L73.1
**Pill roller hand** (intrinsic) — *see* Parkinsonism
**Pilomatrixoma** — *see* Neoplasm, skin, benign

**Pilomatrixoma** — *continued*
　malignant — *see* Neoplasm, skin, malignant
**Pilonidal** — *see* condition
**Pimple** R23.8
**PIN** — *see* Neoplasia, intraepithelial, prostate
**Pinched nerve** — *see* Neuropathy, entrapment
**Pindborg tumor** — *see* Cyst, calcifying odontogenic
**Pineal body or gland** — *see* condition
**Pinealoblastoma** C75.3
**Pinealoma** D44.5
　malignant C75.3
**Pineoblastoma** C75.3
**Pineocytoma** D44.5
**Pinguecula** H11.15- ☑
**Pingueculitis** H10.81- ☑
**Pinhole meatus** (*see also* Stricture, urethra) N35.9
**Pink**
　disease — *see* subcategory T56.1 ☑
　eye — *see* Conjunctivitis, acute, mucopurulent
**Pinkus' disease** (lichen nitidus) L44.1
**Pinpoint**
　meatus — *see* Stricture, urethra
　os (uteri) — *see* Stricture, cervix
**Pins and needles** R20.2
**Pinta** A67.9
　cardiovascular lesions A67.2
　chancre (primary) A67.0
　erythematous plaques A67.1
　hyperchromic lesions A67.1
　hyperkeratosis A67.1
　lesions A67.9
　　cardiovascular A67.2
　　hyperchromic A67.1
　　intermediate A67.1
　　late A67.2
　　mixed A67.3
　　primary A67.0
　　skin (achromic) (cicatricial) (dyschromic) A67.2
　　　hyperchromic A67.1
　　　mixed (achromic and hyperchromic) A67.3
　papule (primary) A67.0
　skin lesions (achromic) (cicatricial) (dyschromic) A67.2
　　hyperchromic A67.1
　　mixed (achromic and hyperchromic) A67.3
　vitiligo A67.2
**Pintids** A67.1
**Pinworm** (disease) (infection) (infestation) B80
**Piroplasmosis** B60.0
**Pistol wound** — *see* Gunshot wound
**Pitchers' elbow** — *see* Derangement, joint, specified type NEC, elbow
**Pithecoid pelvis** Q74.2
　with disproportion (fetopelvic) O33.0
　　causing obstructed labor O65.0
**Pithiatism** F48.8
**Pitted** — *see* Pitting
**Pitting** (*see also* Edema) R60.9
　lip R60.0
　nail L60.8
　teeth K00.4
**Pituitary gland** — *see* condition
**Pituitary-snuff-taker's disease** J67.8
**Pityriasis** (capitis) L21.0
　alba L30.5
　circinata (et maculata) L42
　furfuracea L21.0
　Hebra's L26
　lichenoides L41.0
　　chronica L41.1
　　et varioliformis (acuta) L41.0
　maculata (et circinata) L30.5
　nigra B36.1
　pilaris, Hebra's L44.0
　rosea L42
　rotunda L44.8
　rubra (Hebra) pilaris L44.0
　simplex L30.5
　specified type NEC L30.5
　streptogenes L30.5
　versicolor (scrotal) B36.0
**Placenta, placental** — *see* Pregnancy, complicated by (care of) (management affected by), specified condition
**Placentitis** O41.14- ☑
**Plagiocephaly** Q67.3
**Plague** A20.9
　abortive A20.8

☟ **Subterms under main terms may continue to next column or page**　　☑ **Additional Character Required** — **Refer to the Tabular List for Character Selection**　　**253**

Phlebitis — Plague

**Plague** — *continued*
  ambulatory A20.8
  asymptomatic A20.8
  bubonic A20.0
  cellulocutaneous A20.1
  cutaneobubonic A20.1
  lymphatic gland A20.0
  meningitis A20.3
  pharyngeal A20.8
  pneumonic (primary) (secondary) A20.2
  pulmonary, pulmonic A20.2
  septicemic A20.7
  tonsillar A20.8
    septicemic A20.7
**Planning, family**
  contraception Z30.9
  procreation Z31.69
**Plaque(s)**
  artery, arterial — *see* Arteriosclerosis
  calcareous — *see* Calcification
  coronary, lipid rich I25.83
  epicardial I31.8
  erythematous, of pinta A67.1
  Hollenhorst's — *see* Occlusion, artery, retina
  lipid rich, coronary I25.83
  pleural (without asbestos) J92.9
    with asbestos J92.0
  tongue K13.29
**Plasmacytoma** C90.3- ☑
  extramedullary C90.2- ☑
  medullary C90.0- ☑
  solitary C90.3- ☑
**Plasmacytopenia** D72.818
**Plasmacytosis** D72.822
**Plaster ulcer** — *see* Ulcer, pressure, by site
**Plateau iris syndrome** (post-iridectomy) (postprocedural) (without glaucoma) H21.82
  with glaucoma H40.22- ☑
**Platybasia** Q75.8
**Platyonychia** (congenital) Q84.6
  acquired L60.8
**Platypelloid pelvis** M95.5
  with disproportion (fetopelvic) O33.0
    causing obstructed labor O65.0
  congenital Q74.2
**Platyspondylisis** Q76.49
**Plaut** (-Vincent) **disease** (*see also* Vincent's) A69.1
**Plethora** R23.2
  newborn P61.1
**Pleura, pleural** — *see* condition
**Pleuralgia** R07.81
**Pleurisy** (acute) (adhesive) (chronic) (costal) (diaphragmatic) (double) (dry) (fibrinous) (fibrous) (interlobar) (latent) (plastic) (primary) (residual) (sicca) (sterile) (subacute) (unresolved) R09.1
  with
    adherent pleura J86.0
    effusion J90
      chylous, chyliform J94.0
      tuberculous (non primary) A15.6
        primary (progressive) A15.7
    tuberculosis — *see* Pleurisy, tuberculous (non primary)
  encysted — *see* Pleurisy, with effusion
  exudative — *see* Pleurisy, with effusion
  fibrinopurulent, fibropurulent — *see* Pyothorax
  hemorrhagic — *see* Hemothorax
  pneumococcal J90
  purulent — *see* Pyothorax
  septic — *see* Pyothorax
  serofibrinous — *see* Pleurisy, with effusion
  seropurulent — *see* Pyothorax
  serous — *see* Pleurisy, with effusion
  staphylococcal J86.9
  streptococcal J90
  suppurative — *see* Pyothorax
  traumatic (post) (current) — *see* Injury, intrathoracic, pleura
  tuberculous (with effusion) (non primary) A15.6
    primary (progressive) A15.7
**Pleuritis sicca** — *see* Pleurisy
**Pleurobronchopneumonia** — *see* Pneumonia, broncho-
**Pleurodynia** R07.81
  epidemic B33.0
  viral B33.0
**Pleuropericarditis** (*see also* Pericarditis)
  acute I30.9

**Pleuropneumonia** (acute) (bilateral) (double) (septic) (*see also* Pneumonia) J18.8
  chronic — *see* Fibrosis, lung
**Pleuro-pneumonia-like-organism** (PPLO), as cause of disease classified elsewhere B96.0
**Pleurorrhea** — *see* Pleurisy, with effusion
**Plexitis, brachial** G54.0
**Plica**
  polonica B85.0
  syndrome, knee M67.5- ☑
  tonsil J35.8
**Plicated tongue** K14.5
**Plug**
  bronchus NEC J98.09
  meconium (newborn) NEC syndrome P76.0
  mucus — *see* Asphyxia, mucus
**Plumbism** — *see* subcategory T56.0 ☑
**Plummer's disease** E05.20
  with thyroid storm E05.21
**Plummer-Vinson syndrome** D50.1
**Pluricarential syndrome of infancy** E40
**Plus** (and minus) **hand** (intrinsic) — *see* Deformity, limb, specified type NEC, forearm
**Pneumathemia** — *see* Air, embolism
**Pneumatic hammer** (drill) **syndrome** T75.21 ☑
**Pneumatocele** (lung) J98.4
  intracranial G93.89
  tension J44.9
**Pneumatosis**
  cystoides intestinalis K63.89
  intestinalis K63.89
  peritonei K66.8
**Pneumaturia** R39.89
**Pneumoblastoma** — *see* Neoplasm, lung, malignant
**Pneumocephalus** G93.89
**Pneumococcemia** A40.3
**Pneumococcus, pneumococcal** — *see* condition
**Pneumoconiosis** (due to) (inhalation of) J64
  with tuberculosis (any type in A15) J65
  aluminum J63.0
  asbestos J61
  bagasse, bagassosis J67.1
  bauxite J63.1
  beryllium J63.2
  coal miners' (simple) J60
  coalworkers' (simple) J60
  collier's J60
  cotton dust J66.0
  diatomite (diatomaceous earth) J62.8
  dust
    inorganic NEC J63.6
    lime J62.8
    marble J62.8
    organic NEC J66.8
  fumes or vapors (from silo) J68.9
  graphite J63.3
  grinder's J62.8
  kaolin J62.8
  mica J62.8
  millstone maker's J62.8
  mineral fibers NEC J61
  miner's J60
  moldy hay J67.0
  potter's J62.8
  rheumatoid — *see* Rheumatoid, lung
  sandblaster's J62.8
  silica, silicate NEC J62.8
    with carbon J60
  stonemason's J62.8
  talc (dust) J62.0
**Pneumocystis carinii pneumonia** B59
**Pneumocystis jiroveci** (pneumonia) B59
**Pneumocystosis** (with pneumonia) B59
**Pneumohemopericardium** I31.2
**Pneumohemothorax** J94.2
  traumatic S27.2 ☑
**Pneumohydropericardium** — *see* Pericarditis
**Pneumohydrothorax** — *see* Hydrothorax
**Pneumomediastinum** J98.2
  congenital or perinatal P25.2
**Pneumomycosis** B49 [J99]
**Pneumonia** (acute) (double) (migratory) (purulent) (septic) (unresolved) J18.9
  with
    influenza — *see* Influenza, with, pneumonia
    lung abscess J85.1

**Pneumonia** — *continued*
  with — *continued*
    lung abscess — *continued*
      due to specified organism — *see* Pneumonia, in (due to)
  adenoviral J12.0
  adynamic J18.2
  alba A50.04
  allergic (eosinophilic) J82
  alveolar — *see* Pneumonia, lobar
  anaerobes J15.8
  anthrax A22.1
  apex, apical — *see* Pneumonia, lobar
  Ascaris B77.81
  aspiration J69.0
    due to
      aspiration of microorganisms
        bacterial J15.9
        viral J12.9
      food (regurgitated) J69.0
      gastric secretions J69.0
      milk (regurgitated) J69.0
      oils, essences J69.1
      solids, liquids NEC J69.8
      vomitus J69.0
    newborn P24.81
      amniotic fluid (clear) P24.11
      blood P24.21
      food (regurgitated) P24.31
      liquor (amnii) P24.11
      meconium P24.01
      milk P24.31
      mucus P24.11
      specified NEC P24.81
      stomach contents P24.31
    postprocedural J95.4
  atypical NEC J18.9
  bacillus J15.9
    specified NEC J15.8
  bacterial J15.9
    specified NEC J15.8
  Bacteroides (fragilis) (oralis) (melaninogenicus) J15.8
  basal, basic, basilar — *see* Pneumonia, by type
  bronchiolitis obliterans organized (BOOP) J84.89
  broncho-, bronchial (confluent) (croupous) (diffuse) (disseminated) (hemorrhagic) (involving lobes) (lobar) (terminal) J18.0
    allergic (eosinophilic) J82
    aspiration — *see* Pneumonia, aspiration
    bacterial J15.9
      specified NEC J15.8
    chronic — *see* Fibrosis, lung
    diplococcal J13
    Eaton's agent J15.7
    Escherichia coli (E. coli) J15.5
    Friedländer's bacillus J15.0
    Hemophilus influenzae J14
    hypostatic J18.2
    inhalation (*see also* Pneumonia, aspiration)
      due to fumes or vapors (chemical) J68.0
      of oils or essences J69.1
    Klebsiella (pneumoniae) J15.0
    lipid, lipoid J69.1
      endogenous J84.89
    Mycoplasma (pneumoniae) J15.7
    pleuro-pneumonia-like-organisms (PPLO) J15.7
    pneumococcal J13
    Proteus J15.6
    Pseudomonas J15.1
    Serratia marcescens J15.6
    specified organism NEC J16.8
    staphylococcal — *see* Pneumonia, staphylococcal
    streptococcal NEC J15.4
      group B J15.3
      pneumoniae J13
    viral, virus — *see* Pneumonia, viral
  Butyrivibrio (fibrisolvens) J15.8
  Candida B37.1
  caseous — *see* Tuberculosis, pulmonary
  catarrhal — *see* Pneumonia, broncho
  chlamydial J16.0
    congenital P23.1
  cholesterol J84.89
  cirrhotic (chronic) — *see* Fibrosis, lung
  Clostridium (haemolyticum) (novyi) J15.8
  confluent — *see* Pneumonia, broncho
  congenital (infective) P23.9

**Pneumonia** — *continued*
  congenital — *continued*
    due to
      bacterium NEC P23.6
      Chlamydia P23.1
      Escherichia coli P23.4
      Haemophilus influenzae P23.6
      infective organism NEC P23.8
      Klebsiella pneumoniae P23.6
      Mycoplasma P23.6
      Pseudomonas P23.5
      Staphylococcus P23.2
      Streptococcus (except group B) P23.6
        group B P23.3
      viral agent P23.0
    specified NEC P23.8
  croupous — *see* Pneumonia, lobar
  cryptogenic organizing J84.116
  cytomegalic inclusion B25.0
  cytomegaloviral B25.0
  deglutition — *see* Pneumonia, aspiration
  desquamative interstitial J84.117
  diffuse — *see* Pneumonia, broncho
  diplococcal, diplococcus (broncho-) (lobar) J13
  disseminated (focal) — *see* Pneumonia, broncho
  Eaton's agent J15.7
  embolic, embolism — *see* Embolism, pulmonary
  Enterobacter J15.6
  eosinophilic J82
  Escherichia coli (E. coli) J15.5
  Eubacterium J15.8
  fibrinous — *see* Pneumonia, lobar
  fibroid, fibrous (chronic) — *see* Fibrosis, lung
  Friedländer's bacillus J15.0
  Fusobacterium (nucleatum) J15.8
  gangrenous J85.0
  giant cell (measles) B05.2
  gonococcal A54.84
  gram-negative bacteria NEC J15.6
    anaerobic J15.8
  Hemophilus influenzae (broncho) (lobar) J14
  human metapneumovirus J12.3
  hypostatic (broncho) (lobar) J18.2
  in (due to)
    actinomycosis A42.0
    adenovirus J12.0
    anthrax A22.1
    ascariasis B77.81
    aspergillosis B44.9
    Bacillus anthracis A22.1
    Bacterium anitratum J15.6
    candidiasis B37.1
    chickenpox B01.2
    Chlamydia J16.0
      neonatal P23.1
    coccidioidomycosis B38.2
      acute B38.0
      chronic B38.1
    cytomegalovirus disease B25.0
    Diplococcus (pneumoniae) J13
    Eaton's agent J15.7
    Enterobacter J15.6
    Escherichia coli (E. coli) J15.5
    Friedländer's bacillus J15.0
    fumes and vapors (chemical) (inhalation) J68.0
    gonorrhea A54.84
    Hemophilus influenzae (H. influenzae) J14
    Herellea J15.6
    histoplasmosis B39.2
      acute B39.0
      chronic B39.1
    human metapneumovirus J12.3
    Klebsiella (pneumoniae) J15.0
    measles B05.2
    Mycoplasma (pneumoniae) J15.7
    nocardiosis, nocardiasis A43.0
    ornithosis A70
    parainfluenza virus J12.2
    pleuro-pneumonia-like-organism (PPLO) J15.7
    pneumococcus J13
    pneumocystosis (Pneumocystis carinii) (Pneumo-cystis jiroveci) B59
    Proteus J15.6
    Pseudomonas NEC J15.1
      pseudomallei A24.1
    psittacosis A70
    Q fever A78
    respiratory syncytial virus J12.1

**Pneumonia** — *continued*
  in — *continued*
    rheumatic fever I00 [J17]
    rubella B06.81
    Salmonella (infection) A02.22
      typhi A01.03
    schistosomiasis B65.9 [J17]
    Serratia marcescens J15.6
    specified
      bacterium NEC J15.8
      organism NEC J16.8
    spirochetal NEC A69.8
    Staphylococcus J15.20
      aureus (methicillin susceptible) (MSSA) J15.211
        methicillin resistant (MRSA) J15.212
      specified NEC J15.29
    Streptococcus J15.4
      group B J15.3
      pneumoniae J13
      specified NEC J15.4
    toxoplasmosis B58.3
    tularemia A21.2
    typhoid (fever) A01.03
    varicella B01.2
    virus — *see* Pneumonia, viral
    whooping cough A37.91
      due to
        Bordetella parapertussis A37.11
        Bordetella pertussis A37.01
        specified NEC A37.81
    Yersinia pestis A20.2
  inhalation of food or vomit — *see* Pneumonia, aspiration
  interstitial J84.9
    chronic J84.111
    desquamative J84.117
    due to
      collagen vascular disease J84.17
      known underlying cause J84.17
    idiopathic NOS J84.111
    in disease classified elsewhere J84.17
    lymphocytic (due to collagen vascular disease) (in diseases classified elsewhere) J84.17
    lymphoid J84.2
    non-specific J84.89
      due to
        collagen vascular disease J84.17
        known underlying cause J84.17
      idiopathic J84.113
      in diseases classified elsewhere J84.17
    plasma cell B59
    pseudomonas J15.1
    usual J84.112
      due to collagen vascular disease J84.17
      idiopathic J84.112
      in diseases classified elsewhere J84.17
  Klebsiella (pneumoniae) J15.0
  lipid, lipoid (exogenous) J69.1
    endogenous J84.89
  lobar (disseminated) (double) (interstitial) J18.1
    bacterial J15.9
      specified NEC J15.8
    chronic — *see* Fibrosis, lung
    Escherichia coli (E. coli) J15.5
    Friedländer's bacillus J15.0
    Hemophilus influenzae J14
    hypostatic J18.2
    Klebsiella (pneumoniae) J15.0
    pneumococcal J13
    Proteus J15.6
    Pseudomonas J15.1
    specified organism NEC J16.8
    staphylococcal — *see* Pneumonia, staphylococcal
    streptococcal NEC J15.4
    Streptococcus pneumoniae J13
    viral, virus — *see* Pneumonia, viral
  lobular — *see* Pneumonia, broncho
  Löffler's J82
  lymphoid interstitial J84.2
  massive — *see* Pneumonia, lobar
  meconium P24.01
  MRSA (methicillin resistant Staphylococcus aureus) J15.212
  MSSA (methicillin susceptible Staphylococcus aureus) J15.211
  multilobar — *see* Pneumonia, by type
  Mycoplasma (pneumoniae) J15.7
  necrotic J85.0

**Pneumonia** — *continued*
  neonatal P23.9
    aspiration — *see* Aspiration, by substance, with pneumonia
  nitrogen dioxide J68.0
  organizing J84.89
    due to
      collagen vascular disease J84.17
      known underlying cause J84.17
    in diseases classified elsewhere J84.17
  orthostatic J18.2
  parainfluenza virus J12.2
  parenchymatous — *see* Fibrosis, lung
  passive J18.2
  patchy — *see* Pneumonia, broncho
  Peptococcus J15.8
  Peptostreptococcus J15.8
  plasma cell (of infants) B59
  pleurolobar — *see* Pneumonia, lobar
  pleuro-pneumonia-like organism (PPLO) J15.7
  pneumococcal (broncho) (lobar) J13
  Pneumocystis (carinii) (jiroveci) B59
  postinfectional NEC B99 ☑ [J17]
  postmeasles B05.2
  Proteus J15.6
  Pseudomonas J15.1
  psittacosis A70
  radiation J70.0
  respiratory syncytial virus J12.1
  resulting from a procedure J95.89
  rheumatic I00 [J17]
  Salmonella (arizonae) (cholerae-suis) (enteritidis) (ty-phimurium) A02.22
    typhi A01.03
    typhoid fever A01.03
  SARS-associated coronavirus J12.81
  segmented, segmental — *see* Pneumonia, broncho-
  Serratia marcescens J15.6
  specified NEC J18.8
    bacterium NEC J15.8
    organism NEC J16.8
    virus NEC J12.89
  spirochetal NEC A69.8
  staphylococcal (broncho) (lobar) J15.20
    aureus (methicillin susceptible) (MSSA) J15.211
      methicillin resistant (MRSA) J15.212
    specified NEC J15.29
  static, stasis J18.2
  streptococcal NEC (broncho) (lobar) J15.4
    group
      A J15.4
      B J15.3
      specified NEC J15.4
  Streptococcus pneumoniae J13
  syphilitic, congenital (early) A50.04
  traumatic (complication) (early) (secondary) T79.8 ☑
  tuberculous (any) — *see* Tuberculosis, pulmonary
  tularemic A21.2
  varicella B01.2
  Veillonella J15.8
  ventilator associated J95.851
  viral, virus (broncho) (interstitial) (lobar) J12.9
    adenoviral J12.0
    congenital P23.0
    human metapneumovirus J12.3
    parainfluenza J12.2
    respiratory syncytial J12.1
    SARS-associated coronavirus J12.81
    specified NEC J12.89
  white (congenital) A50.04
**Pneumonic** — *see* condition
**Pneumonitis** (acute) (primary) (*see also* Pneumonia)
  air-conditioner J67.7
  allergic (due to) J67.9
    organic dust NEC J67.8
    red cedar dust J67.8
    sequoiosis J67.8
    wood dust J67.8
  aspiration J69.0
    due to
      anesthesia J95.4
        during
          labor and delivery O74.0
          pregnancy O29.01- ☑
          puerperium O89.01
      fumes or gases J68.0
    obstetric O74.0

**Pneumonitis** — continued
   chemical (due to gases, fumes or vapors) (inhalation) J68.0
     due to anesthesia J95.4
   cholesterol J84.89
   chronic — see Fibrosis, lung
   congenital rubella P35.0
   crack (cocaine) J68.0
   due to
     beryllium J68.0
     cadmium J68.0
     crack (cocaine) J68.0
     detergent J69.8
     fluorocarbon-polymer J68.0
     food, vomit (aspiration) J69.0
     fumes or vapors J68.0
     gases, fumes or vapors (inhalation) J68.0
     inhalation
       blood J69.8
       essences J69.1
       food (regurgitated), milk, vomit J69.0
       oils, essences J69.1
       saliva J69.0
       solids, liquids NEC J69.8
     manganese J68.0
     nitrogen dioxide J68.0
     oils, essences J69.1
     solids, liquids NEC J69.8
     toxoplasmosis (acquired) B58.3
       congenital P37.1
     vanadium J68.0
     ventilator J95.851
   eosinophilic J82
   hypersensitivity J67.9
     air conditioner lung J67.7
     bagassosis J67.1
     bird fancier's lung J67.2
     farmer's lung J67.0
     maltworker's lung J67.4
     maple bark-stripper's lung J67.6
     mushroom worker's lung J67.5
     specified organic dust NEC J67.8
     suberosis J67.3
   interstitial (chronic) J84.89
     acute J84.114
     lymphoid J84.2
     non-specific J84.89
       idiopathic J84.113
   lymphoid, interstitial J84.2
   meconium P24.01
   postanesthetic J95.4
     correct substance properly administered — see Table of Drugs and Chemicals, by drug, adverse effect
     in labor and delivery O74.0
     in pregnancy O29.01- ☑
     obstetric O74.0
     overdose or wrong substance given or taken (by accident) — see Table of Drugs and Chemicals, by drug, poisoning
     postpartum, puerperal O89.01
   postoperative J95.4
     obstetric O74.0
   radiation J70.0
   rubella, congenital P35.0
   ventilation (air-conditioning) J67.7
   ventilator associated J95.851
   wood-dust J67.8
**Pneumonoconiosis** — see Pneumoconiosis
**Pneumoparotid** K11.8
**Pneumopathy NEC** J98.4
   alveolar J84.09
   due to organic dust NEC J66.8
   parietoalveolar J84.09
**Pneumopericarditis** (see also Pericarditis)
   acute I30.9
**Pneumopericardium** (see also Pericarditis)
   congenital P25.3
   newborn P25.3
   traumatic (post) — see Injury, heart
**Pneumophagia** (psychogenic) F45.8
**Pneumopleurisy, pneumopleuritis** (see also Pneumonia) J18.8
**Pneumopyopericardium** I30.1
**Pneumopyothorax** — see Pyopneumothorax
   with fistula J86.0
**Pneumorrhagia** (see also Hemorrhage, lung)
   tuberculous — see Tuberculosis, pulmonary

**Pneumothorax NOS** J93.9
   acute J93.83
   chronic J93.81
   congenital P25.1
   perinatal period P25.1
   postprocedural J95.811
   specified NEC J93.83
   spontaneous NOS J93.83
     newborn P25.1
     primary J93.11
     secondary J93.12
     tension J93.0
   tense valvular, infectional J93.0
   tension (spontaneous) J93.0
   traumatic S27.0 ☑
     with hemothorax S27.2 ☑
   tuberculous — see Tuberculosis, pulmonary
**Podagra** (see also Gout) M10.9
**Podencephalus** Q01.9
**Poikilocytosis** R71.8
**Poikiloderma** L81.6
   Civatte's L57.3
   congenital Q82.8
   vasculare atrophicans L94.5
**Poikilodermatomyositis** M33.10
   with
     myopathy M33.12
     respiratory involvement M33.11
     specified organ involvement NEC M33.19
**Pointed ear** (congenital) Q17.3
**Poison ivy, oak, sumac or other plant dermatitis** (allergic) (contact) L23.7
**Poisoning** (acute) (see also Table of Drugs and Chemicals)
   algae and toxins T65.82-
   Bacillus B (aertrycke) (cholerae (suis)) (paratyphosus) (suipestifer) A02.9
     botulinus A05.1
   bacterial toxins A05.9
   berries, noxious — see Poisoning, food, noxious, berries
   botulism A05.1
   ciguatera fish T61.0- ☑
   Clostridium botulinum A05.1
   death-cap (Amanita phalloides) (Amanita verna) — see Poisoning, food, noxious, mushrooms
   drug — see Table of Drugs and Chemicals, by drug, poisoning
   epidemic, fish (noxious) — see Poisoning, seafood
     bacterial A05.9
   fava bean D55.0
   fish (noxious) T61.9- ☑
     bacterial — see Intoxication, foodborne, by agent
     ciguatera fish — see Poisoning, ciguatera fish
     scombroid fish — see Poisoning, scombroid fish
     specified type NEC T61.77- ☑
   food (acute) (diseased) (infected) (noxious) NEC T62.9- ☑
     bacterial — see Intoxication, foodborne, by agent
     due to
       Bacillus (aertrycke) (choleraesuis) (paratyphosus) (suipestifer) A02.9
         botulinus A05.1
       Clostridium (perfringens) (Welchii) A05.2
       salmonella (aertrycke) (callinarum) (choleraesuis) (enteritidis) (paratyphi) (suipestifer) A02.9
         with
           gastroenteritis A02.0
           sepsis A02.1
       staphylococcus A05.0
       Vibrio
         parahaemolyticus A05.3
         vulnificus A05.5
     noxious or naturally toxic T62.9- ☑
       berries — see subcategory T62.1 ☑
       fish — see Poisoning, fish
       mushrooms — see subcategory T62.0X ☑
       plants NEC — see subcategory T62.2X ☑
       seafood — see Poisoning, seafood
       specified NEC — see subcategory T62.8X ☑
   ichthyotoxism — see Poisoning, seafood
   kreotoxism, food A05.9
   latex T65.81- ☑
   lead T56.0- ☑
   mushroom — see Poisoning, food, noxious, mushroom
   mussels (see also Poisoning, shellfish)
     bacterial — see Intoxication, foodborne, by agent

**Poisoning** — continued
   nicotine (tobacco) T65.2- ☑
   noxious foodstuffs — see Poisoning, food, noxious
   plants, noxious — see Poisoning, food, noxious, plants NEC
   ptomaine — see Poisoning, food
   radiation J70.0
   Salmonella (arizonae) (cholerae-suis) (enteritidis) (typhimurium) A02.9
   scombroid fish T61.1-
   seafood (noxious) T61.9- ☑
     bacterial — see Intoxication, foodborne, by agent
     fish — see Poisoning, fish
     shellfish — see Poisoning, shellfish
     specified NEC — see subcategory T61.8X ☑
   shellfish (amnesic) (azaspiracid) (diarrheic) (neurotoxic) (noxious) (paralytic) T61.78-
     bacterial — see Intoxication, foodborne, by agent
     ciguatera mollusk — see Poisoning, ciguatera fish
   specified substance NEC T65.891 ☑
   Staphylococcus, food A05.0
   tobacco (nicotine) T65.2- ☑
   water E87.79
**Poker spine** — see Spondylitis, ankylosing
**Poland syndrome** Q79.8
**Polioencephalitis** (acute) (bulbar) A80.9
   inferior G12.22
   influenzal — see Influenza, with, encephalopathy
   superior hemorrhagic (acute) (Wernicke's) E51.2
   Wernicke's E51.2
**Polioencephalomyelitis** (acute) (anterior) A80.9
   with beriberi E51.2
**Polioencephalopathy, superior hemorrhagic** E51.2
   with
     beriberi E51.11
     pellagra E52
**Poliomeningoencephalitis** — see Meningoencephalitis
**Poliomyelitis** (acute) (anterior) (epidemic) A80.9
   with paralysis (bulbar) — see Poliomyelitis, paralytic
   abortive A80.4
   ascending (progressive) — see Poliomyelitis, paralytic
   bulbar (paralytic) — see Poliomyelitis, paralytic
   congenital P35.8
   nonepidemic A80.9
   nonparalytic A80.4
   paralytic A80.30
     specified NEC A80.39
     vaccine-associated A80.0
     wild virus
       imported A80.1
       indigenous A80.2
   spinal, acute A80.9
**Poliosis** (eyebrow) (eyelashes) L67.1
   circumscripta, acquired L67.1
**Pollakiuria** R35.0
   psychogenic F45.8
**Pollinosis** J30.1
**Pollitzer's disease** L73.2
**Polyadenitis** (see also Lymphadenitis)
   malignant A20.0
**Polyalgia** M79.89
**Polyangiitis** M30.0
   microscopic M31.7
   overlap syndrome M30.8
**Polyarteritis**
   microscopic M31.7
   nodosa M30.0
     with lung involvement M30.1
     juvenile M30.2
     related condition NEC M30.8
**Polyarthralgia** — see Pain, joint
**Polyarthritis, polyarthropathy** (see also Arthritis) M13.0
   due to or associated with other specified conditions — see Arthritis
   epidemic (Australian) (with exanthema) B33.1
   infective — see Arthritis, pyogenic or pyemic
   inflammatory M06.4
   juvenile (chronic) (seronegative) M08.3
   migratory — see Fever, rheumatic
   rheumatic, acute — see Fever, rheumatic
**Polyarthrosis** M15.9
   post-traumatic M15.3
   primary M15.0
   specified NEC M15.8
**Polycarential syndrome of infancy** E40
**Polychondritis** (atrophic) (chronic) (see also Disorder, cartilage, specified type NEC)
   relapsing M94.1

**Polycoria** Q13.2
**Polycystic** (disease)
  degeneration, kidney Q61.3
    autosomal dominant (adult type) Q61.2
    autosomal recessive (infantile type)
      NEC Q61.19
  kidney Q61.3
    autosomal
      dominant Q61.2
      recessive NEC Q61.19
    autosomal dominant (adult type) Q61.2
    autosomal recessive (childhood type) NEC Q61.19
    infantile type NEC Q61.19
  liver Q44.6
  lung J98.4
    congenital Q33.0
  ovary, ovaries E28.2
  spleen Q89.09
**Polycythemia** (secondary) D75.1
  acquired D75.1
  benign (familial) D75.0
  due to
    donor twin P61.1
    erythropoietin D75.1
    fall in plasma volume D75.1
    high altitude D75.1
    maternal-fetal transfusion P61.1
    stress D75.1
  emotional D75.1
  erythropoietin D75.1
  familial (benign) D75.0
  Gaisböck's (hypertonica) D75.1
  high altitude D75.1
  hypertonica D75.1
  hypoxemic D75.1
  neonatorum P61.1
  nephrogenous D75.1
  relative D75.1
  secondary D75.1
  spurious D75.1
  stress D75.1
  vera D45
**Polycytosis cryptogenica** D75.1
**Polydactylism, polydactyly** Q69.9
  toes Q69.2
**Polydipsia** R63.1
**Polydystrophy, pseudo-Hurler** E77.0
**Polyembryoma** — see Neoplasm, malignant, by site
**Polyglandular**
  deficiency E31.0
  dyscrasia E31.9
  dysfunction E31.9
  syndrome E31.8
**Polyhydramnios** O40.- ☑
**Polymastia** Q83.1
**Polymenorrhea** N92.0
**Polymyalgia** M35.3
  arteritica, giant cell M31.5
  rheumatica M35.3
    with giant cell arteritis M31.5
**Polymyositis** (acute) (chronic) (hemorrhagic) M33.20
  with
    myopathy M33.22
    respiratory involvement M33.21
    skin involvement — see Dermatopolymyositis
    specified organ involvement NEC M33.29
  ossificans (generalisata) (progressiva) — see Myositis, ossificans, progressiva
**Polyneuritis, polyneuritic** (see also Polyneuropathy)
  acute (post-)infective G61.0
  alcoholic G62.1
  cranialis G52.7
  demyelinating, chronic inflammatory (CIDP) G61.81
  diabetic — see Diabetes, polyneuropathy
  diphtheritic A36.83
  due to lack of vitamin NEC E56.9 [G63]
  endemic E51.11
  erythredema — see subcategory T56.1 ☑
  febrile, acute G61.0
  hereditary ataxic G60.1
  idiopathic, acute G61.0
  infective (acute) G61.0
  inflammatory, chronic demyelinating (CIDP) G61.81
  nutritional E63.9 [G63]
  postinfective (acute) G61.0
  specified NEC G62.89
**Polyneuropathy** (peripheral) G62.9

**Polyneuropathy** — continued
  alcoholic G62.1
  amyloid (Portuguese) E85.1 [G63]
    transthyretin-related (ATTR) familial E85.1
  arsenical G62.2
  critical illness G62.81
  demyelinating, chronic inflammatory (CIDP) G61.81
  diabetic — see Diabetes, polyneuropathy
  drug-induced G62.0
  hereditary G60.9
    specified NEC G60.8
  idiopathic G60.9
    progressive G60.3
  in (due to)
    alcohol G62.1
      sequelae G65.2
    amyloidosis, familial (Portuguese) E85.1 [G63]
    antitetanus serum G61.1
    arsenic G62.2
      sequelae G65.2
    avitaminosis NEC E56.9 [G63]
    beriberi E51.11
    collagen vascular disease NEC M35.9 [G63]
    deficiency (of)
      B (-complex) vitamins E53.9 [G63]
      vitamin B6 E53.1 [G63]
    diabetes — see Diabetes, polyneuropathy
    diphtheria A36.83
    drug or medicament G62.0
      correct substance properly administered — see Table of Drugs and Chemicals, by drug, adverse effect
      overdose or wrong substance given or taken — see Table of Drugs and Chemicals, by drug, poisoning
    endocrine disease NEC E34.9 [G63]
    herpes zoster B02.23
    hypoglycemia E16.2 [G63]
    infectious
      disease NEC B99 ☑ [G63]
      mononucleosis B27.91
    lack of vitamin NEC E56.9 [G63]
    lead G62.2
      sequelae G65.2
    leprosy A30.9 [G63]
    Lyme disease A69.22
    metabolic disease NEC E88.9 [G63]
    microscopic polyangiitis M31.7 [G63]
    mumps B26.84
    neoplastic disease (see also Neoplasm) D49.9 [G63]
    nutritional deficiency NEC E63.9 [G63]
    organophosphate compounds G62.2
      sequelae G65.2
    parasitic disease NEC B89 [G63]
    pellagra E52 [G63]
    polyarteritis nodosa M30.0
    porphyria E80.20 [G63]
    radiation G62.82
    rheumatoid arthritis — see Rheumatoid, polyneuropathy
    sarcoidosis D86.89
    serum G61.1
    syphilis (late) A52.15
      congenital A50.43
    systemic
      connective tissue disorder M35.9 [G63]
      lupus erythematosus M32.19
    toxic agent NEC G62.2
      sequelae G65.2
  inflammatory G61.9
    chronic demyelinating (CIDP) G61.81
    sequelae G65.1
    specified NEC G61.89
  lead G62.2
    sequelae G65.2
  nutritional NEC E63.9 [G63]
  postherpetic (zoster) B02.23
  progressive G60.3
  radiation-induced G62.82
  sensory (hereditary) (idiopathic) G60.8
  specified NEC G62.89
  syphilitic (late) A52.15
    congenital A50.43
  transthyretin-related (ATTR) familial amyloid E85.1
    triorthocresyl phosphate G62.2
      sequelae G65.2
    tuberculosis A17.89
    uremia N18.9 [G63]

**Polyneuropathy** — continued
  transthyretin-related familial amyloid — continued
    vitamin B12 deficiency E53.8 [G63]
      with anemia (pernicious) D51.0 [G63]
        due to dietary deficiency D51.3 [G63]
    zoster B02.23
**Polyopia** H53.8
**Polyorchism, polyorchidism** Q55.21
**Polyosteoarthritis** (see also Osteoarthritis, generalized) M15.9
  post-traumatic M15.3
  specified NEC M15.8
**Polyostotic fibrous dysplasia** Q78.1
**Polyotia** Q17.0
**Polyp, polypus**
  accessory sinus J33.8
  adenocarcinoma in — see Neoplasm, malignant, by site
  adenocarcinoma in situ in — see Neoplasm, in situ, by site
  adenoid tissue J33.0
  adenomatous (see also Neoplasm, benign, by site)
    adenocarcinoma in — see Neoplasm, malignant, by site
    adenocarcinoma in situ in — see Neoplasm, in situ, by site
    carcinoma in — see Neoplasm, malignant, by site
    carcinoma in situ in — see Neoplasm, in situ, by site
    multiple — see Neoplasm, benign
      adenocarcinoma in — see Neoplasm, malignant, by site
      adenocarcinoma in situ in — see Neoplasm, in situ, by site
  antrum J33.8
  anus, anal (canal) K62.0
  Bartholin's gland N84.3
  bladder D41.4
  carcinoma in — see Neoplasm, malignant, by site
  carcinoma in situ in — see Neoplasm, in situ, by site
  cecum D12.0
  cervix (uteri) N84.1
    in pregnancy or childbirth — see Pregnancy, complicated by, abnormal, cervix
    mucous N84.1
    nonneoplastic N84.1
  choanal J33.0
  cholesterol K82.4
  clitoris N84.3
  colon K63.5
    adenomatous D12.6
    ascending D12.2
    cecum D12.0
    descending D12.4
    inflammatory K51.40
      with
        abscess K51.414
        complication K51.419
          specified NEC K51.418
        fistula K51.413
        intestinal obstruction K51.412
        rectal bleeding K51.411
    sigmoid D12.5
    transverse D12.3
  corpus uteri N84.0
  dental K04.01
    irreversible K04.02
    reversible K04.01
  duodenum K31.7
  ear (middle) H74.4- ☑
  endometrium N84.0
  ethmoidal (sinus) J33.8
  fallopian tube N84.8
  female genital tract N84.9
    specified NEC N84.8
  frontal (sinus) J33.8
  gallbladder K82.4
  gingiva, gum K06.8
  labia, labium (majus) (minus) N84.3
  larynx (mucous) J38.1
    adenomatous D14.1
  malignant — see Neoplasm, malignant, by site
  maxillary (sinus) J33.8
  middle ear — see Polyp, ear (middle)
  myometrium N84.0
  nares
    anterior J33.9
    posterior J33.0

**Polyp, polypus** — continued
nasal (mucous) J33.9
cavity J33.0
septum J33.0
nasopharyngeal J33.0
nose (mucous) J33.9
oviduct N84.8
pharynx J39.2
placenta O90.89
prostate — see Enlargement, enlarged, prostate
pudenda, pudendum N84.3
pulpal (dental) K04.01
irreversible K04.02
reversible K04.01
rectum (nonadenomatous) K62.1
adenomatous — see Polyp, adenomatous
septum (nasal) J33.0
sinus (accessory) (ethmoidal) (frontal) (maxillary) (sphenoidal) J33.8
sphenoidal (sinus) J33.8
stomach K31.7
adenomatous D13.1
tube, fallopian N84.8
turbinate, mucous membrane J33.8
umbilical, newborn P83.6
ureter N28.89
urethra N36.2
uterus (body) (corpus) (mucous) N84.0
cervix N84.1
in pregnancy or childbirth — see Pregnancy, complicated by, tumor, uterus
vagina N84.2
vocal cord (mucous) J38.1
vulva N84.3
**Polyphagia** R63.2
**Polyploidy** Q92.7
**Polypoid** — see condition
**Polyposis** (see also Polyp)
coli (adenomatous) D12.6
adenocarcinoma in C18.9
adenocarcinoma in situ in — see Neoplasm, in situ, by site
carcinoma in C18.9
colon (adenomatous) D12.6
familial D12.6
adenocarcinoma in situ in — see Neoplasm, in situ, by site
intestinal (adenomatous) D12.6
malignant lymphomatous C83.1- ☑
multiple, adenomatous (see also Neoplasm, benign) D36.9
**Polyradiculitis** — see Polyneuropathy
**Polyradiculoneuropathy** (acute) (postinfective) (segmentally demyelinating) G61.0
**Polyserositis**
due to pericarditis I31.1
pericardial I31.1
periodic, familial E85.0
tuberculous A19.9
acute A19.1
chronic A19.8
**Polysplenia syndrome** Q89.09
**Polysyndactyly** (see also Syndactylism, syndactyly) Q70.4
**Polytrichia** L68.3
**Polyunguia** Q84.6
**Polyuria** R35.8
nocturnal R35.1
psychogenic F45.8
**Pompe's disease** (glycogen storage) E74.02
**Pompholyx** L30.1
**Poncet's disease** (tuberculous rheumatism) A18.09
**Pond fracture** — see Fracture, skull
**Ponos** B55.0
**Pons, pontine** — see condition
**Poor**
aesthetic of existing restoration of tooth K08.56
contractions, labor O62.2
gingival margin to tooth restoration K08.51
personal hygiene R46.0
prenatal care, affecting management of pregnancy — see Pregnancy, complicated by, insufficient, prenatal care
sucking reflex (newborn) R29.2
urinary stream R39.12
vision NEC H54.7
**Poradenitis, nostras inguinalis or venerea** A55
**Porencephaly** (congenital) (developmental) (true) Q04.6
acquired G93.0

**Porencephaly** — continued
nondevelopmental G93.0
traumatic (post) F07.89
**Porocephaliasis** B88.8
**Porokeratosis** Q82.8
**Poroma, eccrine** — see Neoplasm, skin, benign
**Porphyria** (South African) E80.20
acquired E80.20
acute intermittent (hepatic) (Swedish) E80.21
cutanea tarda (hereditary) (symptomatic) E80.1
due to drugs E80.20
correct substance properly administered — see Table of Drugs and Chemicals, by drug, adverse effect
overdose or wrong substance given or taken — see Table of Drugs and Chemicals, by drug, poisoning
erythropoietic (congenital) (hereditary) E80.0
hepatocutaneous type E80.1
secondary E80.20
toxic NEC E80.20
variegata E80.20
**Porphyrinuria** — see Porphyria
**Porphyruria** — see Porphyria
**Port wine nevus, mark, or stain** Q82.5
**Portal** — see condition
**Posadas-Wernicke disease** B38.9
**Positive**
culture (nonspecific)
blood R78.81
bronchial washings R84.5
cerebrospinal fluid R83.5
cervix uteri R87.5
nasal secretions R84.5
nipple discharge R89.5
nose R84.5
staphylococcus (Methicillin susceptible) Z22.321
Methicillin resistant Z22.322
peritoneal fluid R85.5
pleural fluid R84.5
prostatic secretions R86.5
saliva R85.5
seminal fluid R86.5
sputum R84.5
synovial fluid R89.5
throat scrapings R84.5
urine R82.79
vagina R87.5
vulva R87.5
wound secretions R89.5
PPD (skin test) R76.11
serology for syphilis A53.0
with signs or symptoms — code as Syphilis, by site and stage
false R76.8
skin test, tuberculin (without active tuberculosis) R76.11
test, human immunodeficiency virus (HIV) R75
VDRL A53.0
with signs or symptoms — code by site and stage under Syphilis A53.9
Wassermann reaction A53.0
**Postcardiotomy syndrome** I97.0
**Postcaval ureter** Q62.62
**Postcholecystectomy syndrome** K91.5
**Postclimacteric bleeding** N95.0
**Postcommissurotomy syndrome** I97.0
**Postconcussional syndrome** F07.81
**Postcontusional syndrome** F07.81
**Postcricoid region** — see condition
**Post-dates** (40-42 weeks) (pregnancy) (mother) O48.0
more than 42 weeks gestation O48.1
**Postencephalitic syndrome** F07.89
**Posterior** — see condition
**Posterolateral sclerosis** (spinal cord) — see Degeneration, combined
**Postexanthematous** — see condition
**Postfebrile** — see condition
**Postgastrectomy dumping syndrome** K91.1
**Posthemiplegic chorea** — see Monoplegia
**Posthemorrhagic anemia** (chronic) D50.0
acute D62
newborn P61.3
**Postherpetic neuralgia** (zoster) B02.29
trigeminal B02.22
**Posthitis** N47.7
**Postimmunization complication or reaction** — see Complications, vaccination

**Postinfectious** — see condition
**Postlaminectomy syndrome NEC** M96.1
**Postleukotomy syndrome** F07.0
**Postmastectomy lymphedema** (syndrome) I97.2
**Postmaturity, postmature** (over 42 weeks)
maternal (over 42 weeks gestation) O48.1
newborn P08.22
**Postmeasles complication NEC** (see also condition) B05.89
**Postmenopausal**
endometrium (atrophic) N95.8
suppurative (see also Endometritis) N71.9
osteoporosis — see Osteoporosis, postmenopausal
**Postnasal drip** R09.82
due to
allergic rhinitis — see Rhinitis, allergic
common cold J00
gastroesophageal reflux — see Reflux, gastroesophageal
nasopharyngitis — see Nasopharyngitis
other known condition — code to condition
sinusitis — see Sinusitis
**Postnatal** — see condition
**Postoperative** (postprocedural) — see Complication, postoperative
pneumothorax, therapeutic Z98.3
state NEC Z98.890
**Postpancreatectomy hyperglycemia** E89.1
**Postpartum** — see Puerperal
**Postphlebitic syndrome** — see Syndrome, postthrombotic
**Postpolio** (myelitic) **syndrome** G14
**Postpoliomyelitic** (see also condition)
osteopathy — see Osteopathy, after poliomyelitis
**Postprocedural** (see also Postoperative)
hypoinsulinemia E89.1
**Postschizophrenic depression** F32.89
**Postsurgery status** (see also Status (post))
pneumothorax, therapeutic Z98.3
**Post-term** (40-42 weeks) (pregnancy) (mother) O48.0
infant P08.21
more than 42 weeks gestation (mother) O48.1
**Post-traumatic brain syndrome, nonpsychotic** F07.81
**Post-typhoid abscess** A01.09
**Postures, hysterical** F44.2
**Postvaccinal reaction or complication** — see Complications, vaccination
**Postvalvulotomy syndrome** I97.0
**Potain's**
disease (pulmonary edema) — see Edema, lung
syndrome (gastrectasis with dyspepsia) K31.0
**Potter's**
asthma J62.8
facies Q60.6
lung J62.8
syndrome (with renal agenesis) Q60.6
**Pott's**
curvature (spinal) A18.01
disease or paraplegia A18.01
spinal curvature A18.01
tumor, puffy — see Osteomyelitis, specified type NEC
**Pouch**
bronchus Q32.4
Douglas' — see condition
esophagus, esophageal, congenital Q39.6
acquired K22.5
gastric K31.4
Hartmann's K82.8
pharynx, pharyngeal (congenital) Q38.7
**Pouchitis** K91.850
**Poultrymen's itch** B88.0
**Poverty NEC** Z59.6
extreme Z59.5
**Poxvirus NEC** B08.8
**Prader-Willi syndrome** Q87.1
**Preauricular appendage or tag** Q17.0
**Prebetalipoproteinemia** (acquired) (essential) (familial) (hereditary) (primary) (secondary) E78.1
with chylomicronemia E78.3
**Precipitate labor or delivery** O62.3
**Preclimacteric bleeding** (menorrhagia) N92.4
**Precocious**
adrenarche E30.1
menarche E30.1
menstruation E30.1
pubarche E30.1
puberty E30.1

☑ Additional Character Required — Refer to the Tabular List for Character Selection    ▽ Subterms under main terms may continue to next column or page

**Precocious** — *continued*
  puberty — *continued*
    central E22.8
    sexual development NEC E30.1
    thelarche E30.8
**Precocity, sexual** (constitutional) (cryptogenic) (female)
  (idiopathic) (male) E30.1
  with adrenal hyperplasia E25.9
    congenital E25.0
**Precordial pain** R07.2
**Predeciduous teeth** K00.2
**Prediabetes, prediabetic** R73.03
  complicating
    pregnancy — *see* Pregnancy, complicated by, diseases of, specified type or system NEC
    puerperium O99.89
**Predislocation status of hip at birth** Q65.6
**Pre-eclampsia** O14.9- ☑
  with pre-existing hypertension — *see* Hypertension, complicating pregnancy, pre-existing, with, pre-eclampsia
  complicating
    childbirth O14.94
    puerperium O14.95
  mild O14.0- ☑
    complicating
      childbirth O14.04
      puerperium O14.05
  moderate O14.0- ☑
    complicating
      childbirth O14.04
      puerperium O14.05
  severe O14.1- ☑
    with hemolysis, elevated liver enzymes and low platelet count (HELLP) O14.2- ☑
      complicating
        childbirth O14.24
        puerperium O14.25
    complicating
      childbirth O14.14
      puerperium O14.15
**Pre-eruptive color change, teeth, tooth** K00.8
**Pre-excitation atrioventricular conduction** I45.6
**Preglaucoma** H40.00- ☑
**Pregnancy** (single) (uterine) (*see also* Delivery and Puerperal)

*Note: The Tabular must be reviewed for assignment of appropriate seventh character for multiple gestation codes in Chapter 15*

*Note: The Tabular must be reviewed for assignment of the appropriate character indicating the trimester of the pregnancy*

  abdominal (ectopic) O00.00
    with intrauterine pregnancy O00.01
    with viable fetus O36.7- ☑
  ampullar O00.10- ☑
    with intrauterine pregnancy O00.11- ☑
  biochemical O02.81
  broad ligament O00.80
    with intrauterine pregnancy O00.81
  cervical O00.8
    with intrauterine pregnancy O00.81
  chemical O02.81
  complicated by (care of) (management affected by)
    abnormal, abnormality
      cervix O34.4- ☑
        causing obstructed labor O65.5
      cord (umbilical) O69.9 ☑
      fetal heart rate or rhythm O36.83- ☑
      findings on antenatal screening of mother O28.9
        biochemical O28.1
        chromosomal O28.5
        cytological O28.2
        genetic O28.5
        hematological O28.0
        radiological O28.4
        specified NEC O28.8
        ultrasonic O28.3
      glucose (tolerance) NEC O99.810
      pelvic organs O34.9- ☑
        specified NEC O34.8- ☑
          causing obstructed labor O65.5
      pelvis (bony) (major) NEC O33.0
      perineum O34.7- ☑

**Pregnancy** — *continued*
  complicated by — *continued*
    abnormal, abnormality — *continued*
      position
        placenta O44.0- ☑
          with hemorrhage O44.1- ☑
        uterus O34.59- ☑
      uterus O34.59- ☑
        causing obstructed labor O65.5
        congenital O34.0- ☑
      vagina O34.6- ☑
        causing obstructed labor O65.5
      vulva O34.7- ☑
        causing obstructed labor O65.5
    abruptio placentae — *see* Abruptio placentae
    abscess or cellulitis
      bladder O23.1- ☑
      breast O91.11- ☑
      genital organ or tract O23.9- ☑
    abuse
      physical O9A.31 ☑ (*following* O99)
      psychological O9A.51 ☑ (*following* O99)
      sexual O9A.41 ☑ (*following* O99)
    adverse effect anesthesia O29.9- ☑
      aspiration pneumonitis O29.01- ☑
      cardiac arrest O29.11- ☑
      cardiac complication NEC O29.19- ☑
      cardiac failure O29.12- ☑
      central nervous system complication NEC O29.29- ☑
      cerebral anoxia O29.21- ☑
      failed or difficult intubation O29.6- ☑
      inhalation of stomach contents or secretions NOS O29.01- ☑
      local, toxic reaction O29.3X ☑
      Mendelson's syndrome O29.01- ☑
      pressure collapse of lung O29.02- ☑
      pulmonary complications NEC O29.09- ☑
      specified NEC O29.8X- ☑
      spinal and epidural type NEC O29.5X ☑
        induced headache O29.4- ☑
    albuminuria (*see also* Proteinuria, gestational) O12.1- ☑
    alcohol use O99.31- ☑
    amnionitis O41.12- ☑
    anaphylactoid syndrome of pregnancy O88.01- ☑
    anemia (conditions in D50-D64) (pre-existing) O99.01- ☑
      complicating the puerperium O99.03
    antepartum hemorrhage O46.9- ☑
      with coagulation defect — *see* Hemorrhage, antepartum, with coagulation defect
      specified NEC O46.8X- ☑
    appendicitis O99.61- ☑
    atrophy (yellow) (acute) liver (subacute) O26.61- ☑
    bariatric surgery status O99.84- ☑
    bicornis or bicornuate uterus O34.0- ☑
    biliary tract problems O26.61- ☑
    breech presentation O32.1 ☑
    cardiovascular diseases (conditions in I00-I09, I20-I52, I70-I99) O99.41- ☑
    cerebrovascular disorders (conditions in I60-I69) O99.41- ☑
    cervical shortening O26.87- ☑
    cervicitis O23.51- ☑
    chloasma (gravidarum) O26.89- ☑
    cholecystitis O99.61- ☑
    cholestasis (intrahepatic) O26.61- ☑
    chorioamnionitis O41.12- ☑
    circulatory system disorder (conditions in I00-I09, I20-I99, O99.41-)
    compound presentation O32.6 ☑
    conjoined twins O30.02- ☑
    connective system disorders (conditions in M00-M99) O99.89
    contracted pelvis (general) O33.1
      inlet O33.2
      outlet O33.3
    convulsions (eclamptic) (uremic) (*see also* Eclampsia) O15.9
    cracked nipple O92.11- ☑
    cystitis O23.1- ☑
    cystocele O34.8- ☑
    death of fetus (near term) O36.4 ☑
      early pregnancy O02.1

**Pregnancy** — *continued*
  complicated by — *continued*
    death of fetus — *continued*
      of one fetus or more in multiple gestation O31.2- ☑
    deciduitis O41.14- ☑
    decreased fetal movement O36.81- ☑
    dental problems O99.61- ☑
    diabetes (mellitus) O24.91- ☑
      gestational (pregnancy induced) — *see* Diabetes, gestational
      pre-existing O24.31- ☑
        specified NEC O24.81- ☑
        type 1 O24.01- ☑
        type 2 O24.11- ☑
    digestive system disorders (conditions in K00-K93) O99.61- ☑
    diseases of — *see* Pregnancy, complicated by, specified body system disease
      biliary tract O26.61- ☑
      blood NEC (conditions in D65-D77) O99.11- ☑
      liver O26.61- ☑
      specified NEC O99.89
    disorders of — *see* Pregnancy, complicated by, specified body system disorder
      amniotic fluid and membranes O41.9- ☑
        specified NEC O41.8X- ☑
      biliary tract O26.61- ☑
      ear and mastoid process (conditions in H60-H95) O99.89
      eye and adnexa (conditions in H00-H59) O99.89
      liver O26.61- ☑
      skin (conditions in L00-L99) O99.71- ☑
      specified NEC O99.89
    displacement, uterus NEC O34.59- ☑
      causing obstructed labor O65.5
    disproportion (due to) O33.9
      fetal (ascites) (hydrops) (meningomyelocele) (sacral teratoma) (tumor) deformities NEC O33.7 ☑
      generally contracted pelvis O33.1
      hydrocephalic fetus O33.6
      inlet contraction of pelvis O33.2
      mixed maternal and fetal origin O33.4 ☑
      specified NEC O33.8
    double uterus O34.0- ☑
      causing obstructed labor O65.5
    drug use (conditions in F11-F19) O99.32- ☑
    eclampsia, eclamptic (coma) (convulsions) (delirium) (nephritis) (uremia) (*see also* Eclampsia) O15.- ☑
    ectopic pregnancy — *see* Pregnancy, ectopic
    edema O12.0- ☑
      with
        gestational hypertension, mild (*see also* Preeclampsia) O14.0- ☑
        proteinuria O12.2- ☑
    effusion, amniotic fluid — *see* Pregnancy, complicated by, premature rupture of membranes
    elderly
      multigravida O09.52- ☑
      primigravida O09.51- ☑
    embolism (*see also* Embolism, obstetric, pregnancy) O88.- ☑
    endocrine diseases NEC O99.28- ☑
    endometritis O86.12
    excessive weight gain O26.0- ☑
    exhaustion O26.81- ☑
      during labor and delivery O75.81
    face presentation O32.3 ☑
    failed induction of labor O61.9
      instrumental O61.1
      mechanical O61.1
      medical O61.0
      specified NEC O61.8
      surgical O61.1
    failed or difficult intubation for anesthesia O29.6- ☑
    false labor (pains) O47.9
      at or after 37 completed weeks of pregnancy O47.1
      before 37 completed weeks of pregnancy O47.0- ☑
    fatigue O26.81- ☑
      during labor and delivery O75.81
    fatty metamorphosis of liver O26.61- ☑
    female genital mutilation O34.8- ☑ [N90.81-] ☑

Index

Pregnancy — Pregnancy

**Pregnancy** — *continued*
  complicated by — *continued*
    placental transfusion syndromes
      fetomaternal O43.01- ☑
      fetus to fetus O43.02- ☑
      maternofetal O43.01- ☑
    placentitis O41.14- ☑
    pneumonia O99.51- ☑
    poisoning (*see also* Table of Drugs and Chemicals) O9A.21 ☑ (*following* O99)
    polyhydramnios O40- ☑
    polymorphic eruption of pregnancy O26.86
    poor obstetric history NEC O09.29- ☑
    postmaturity (post-term) (40 to 42 weeks) O48.0
      more than 42 completed weeks gestation (prolonged) O48.1
    pre-eclampsia O14.9- ☑
      mild O14.0- ☑
      moderate O14.0- ☑
      severe O14.1- ☑
        with hemolysis, elevated liver enzymes and low platelet count (HELLP) O14.2- ☑
    premature labor — *see* Pregnancy, complicated by, preterm labor
    premature rupture of membranes O42.90
      with onset of labor
        after 24 hours O42.10
          at or after 37 weeks gestation, onset of labor more than 24 hours following rupture O42.12
          pre-term (before 37 completed weeks of gestation) O42.11- ☑
        within 24 hours O42.00
          at or after 37 weeks gestation, onset of labor within 24 hours of rupture O42.02
          pre-term (before 37 completed weeks of gestation) O42.01- ☑
      at or after 37 weeks gestation, unspecified as to length of time between rupture and onset of labor O42.92
      full-term, unspecified as to length of time between rupture and onset of labor O42.92
      pre-term (before 37 completed weeks of gestation) O42.91- ☑
    premature separation of placenta (*see also* Abruptio placentae) O45.9- ☑
    presentation, fetal — *see* Delivery, complicated by, malposition
    preterm delivery O60.10 ☑
    preterm labor
      with delivery O60.10 ☑
        preterm O60.10 ☑
        term O60.20 ☑
      without delivery O60.00
        second trimester O60.02
        third trimester O60.03
      second trimester
        with preterm delivery
          second trimester O60.12 ☑
          third trimester O60.13 ☑
        with term delivery O60.22 ☑
        without delivery O60.02
      third trimester
        with term delivery O60.23 ☑
        with third trimester preterm delivery O60.14 ☑
        without delivery O60.03
    previous history of — *see* Pregnancy, supervision of, high-risk
    prolapse, uterus O34.52- ☑
    proteinuria (gestational) (*see also* Proteinuria, gestational) O12.1- ☑
      with edema O12.2- ☑
    pruritic urticarial papules and plaques of pregnancy (PUPPP) O26.86
    pruritus (neurogenic) O26.89- ☑
    psychosis or psychoneurosis (puerperal) F53
    ptyalism O26.89- ☑
    PUPPP (pruritic urticarial papules and plaques of pregnancy) O26.86
    pyelitis O23.0- ☑
    recurrent pregnancy loss O26.2- ☑
    renal disease or failure NEC O26.83- ☑
      with secondary hypertension, pre-existing — *see* Hypertension, complicating, pregnancy, pre-existing, secondary

**Pregnancy** — *continued*
  complicated by — *continued*
    renal disease or failure — *continued*
      hypertensive, pre-existing — *see* Hypertension, complicating, pregnancy, pre-existing, with, renal disease
    respiratory condition (conditions in J00-J99) O99.51- ☑
    retained, retention
      dead ovum O02.0
      intrauterine contraceptive device O26.3- ☑
    retroversion, uterus O34.53- ☑
    Rh immunization, incompatibility or sensitization NEC O36.09- ☑
      anti-D antibody O36.01- ☑
    rupture
      amnion (premature) (*see also* Pregnancy, complicated by, premature rupture of membranes) O42- ☑
      membranes (premature) (*see also* Pregnancy, complicated by, premature rupture of membranes) O42- ☑
      uterus (during labor) O71.1
        before onset of labor O71.0- ☑
    salivation (excessive) O26.89- ☑
    salpingitis O23.52- ☑
    salpingo-oophoritis O23.52- ☑
    sepsis (conditions in A40, A41) O98.81- ☑
    size date discrepancy (uterine) O26.84- ☑
    skin condition (conditions in L00-L99) O99.71- ☑
    smoking (tobacco) O99.33- ☑
    social problem O09.7- ☑
    specified condition NEC O26.89- ☑
    spotting O26.85- ☑
    streptococcus group B (GBS) carrier state O99.820
    subluxation of symphysis (pubis) O26.71- ☑
    syphilis (conditions in A50-A53) O98.11- ☑
    threatened
      abortion O20.0
      labor O47.9
        at or after 37 completed weeks of gestation O47.1
        before 37 completed weeks of gestation O47.0- ☑
    thrombophlebitis (superficial) O22.2- ☑
    thrombosis O22.9- ☑
      cerebral venous O22.5- ☑
      cerebrovenous sinus O22.5- ☑
      deep O22.3- ☑
    tobacco use disorder (smoking) O99.33- ☑
    torsion of uterus O34.59- ☑
    toxemia O14.9- ☑
    transverse lie or presentation O32.2 ☑
    tuberculosis (conditions in A15-A19) O98.01- ☑
    tumor (benign)
      cervix O34.4- ☑
      malignant O9A.11- ☑ (*following* O99)
      uterus O34.1- ☑
    unstable lie O32.0 ☑
    upper respiratory infection O99.51- ☑
    urethritis O23.2- ☑
    uterine size date discrepancy O26.84- ☑
    vaginitis or vulvitis O23.59- ☑
    varicose veins (lower extremities) O22.0- ☑
      genitals O22.1- ☑
      legs O22.0- ☑
      perineal O22.1- ☑
      vaginal or vulval O22.1- ☑
    venereal disease NEC (conditions in A63.8) O98.31- ☑
    venous disorders O22.9- ☑
      specified NEC O22.8X- ☑
    very young mother — *see* Pregnancy, complicated by, young mother
    viral diseases (conditions in A80-B09, B25-B34) O98.51- ☑
    vomiting O21.9
      due to diseases classified elsewhere O21.8
      hyperemesis gravidarum (mild) (*see also* Hyperemesis, gravidarum) O21.0
      late (occurring after 20 weeks of gestation) O21.2
    young mother
      multigravida O09.62- ☑
      primigravida O09.61- ☑
  complicated NOS O26.9- ☑
  concealed O09.3- ☑

**Pregnancy** — *continued*
  continuing following
    elective fetal reduction of one or more fetus O31.3- ☑
    intrauterine death of one or more fetus O31.2- ☑
    spontaneous abortion of one or more fetus O31.1- ☑
  cornual O00.80
    with intrauterine pregnancy O00.81
  ectopic (ruptured) O00.90
    with intrauterine pregnancy O00.91
    abdominal O00.00
      with
        intrauterine pregnancy O00.01
        viable fetus O36.7- ☑
    cervical O00.80
      with intrauterine pregnancy O00.81
    complicated (by) O08.9
      afibrinogenemia O08.1
      cardiac arrest O08.81
      chemical damage of pelvic organ(s) O08.6
      circulatory collapse O08.3
      defibrination syndrome O08.1
      electrolyte imbalance O08.5
      embolism (amniotic fluid) (blood clot) (pulmonary) (septic) O08.2
      endometritis O08.0
      genital tract and pelvic infection O08.0
      hemorrhage (delayed) (excessive) O08.1
      infection
        genital tract or pelvic O08.0
        kidney O08.83
        urinary tract O08.3
      intravascular coagulation O08.1
      laceration of pelvic organ(s) O08.6
      metabolic disorder O08.5
      oliguria O08.4
      oophoritis O08.0
      parametritis O08.0
      pelvic peritonitis O08.0
      perforation of pelvic organ(s) O08.6
      renal failure or shutdown O08.4
      salpingitis or salpingo-oophoritis O08.0
      sepsis O08.82
      shock O08.83
        septic O08.82
      specified condition NEC O08.89
      tubular necrosis (renal) O08.4
      uremia O08.4
      urinary infection O08.83
      venous complication NEC O08.7
        embolism O08.2
    cornual O00.80
      with intrauterine pregnancy O00.81
    intraligamentous O00.80
      with intrauterine pregnancy O00.81
    mural O00.80
      with intrauterine pregnancy O00.81
    ovarian O00.20- ☑
      with intrauterine pregnancy O00.21- ☑
    specified site NEC O00.80
      with intrauterine pregnancy O00.81
    tubal (ruptured) O00.10- ☑
      with intrauterine pregnancy O00.11- ☑
  examination (normal) Z34.9- ☑
    first Z34.0- ☑
    high-risk — *see* Pregnancy, supervision of, high-risk
    specified Z34.8- ☑
  extrauterine — *see* Pregnancy, ectopic
  fallopian O00.10- ☑
    with intrauterine pregnancy O00.11- ☑
  false F45.8
  gestational carrier Z33.3
  hidden O09.3- ☑
  high-risk — *see* Pregnancy, supervision of, high-risk
  incidental finding Z33.1
  interstitial O00.80
    with intrauterine pregnancy O00.81
  intraligamentous O00.80
    with intrauterine pregnancy O00.81
  intramural O00.80
    with intrauterine pregnancy O00.81
  intraperitoneal O00.00
    with intrauterine pregnancy O00.01
  isthmian O00.10- ☑
    with intrauterine pregnancy O00.11- ☑
  mesometric (mural) O00.80

**Prescription of contraceptives** — *continued*
  barrier Z30.018
  diaphragm Z30.018
  emergency (postcoital) Z30.012
  implantable subdermal Z30.017
  injectable Z30.013
  intrauterine contraceptive device Z30.014
  pills Z30.011
  postcoital (emergency) Z30.012
  repeat Z30.40
    barrier Z30.49
    diaphragm Z30.49
    implantable subdermal Z30.46
    injectable Z30.42
    pills Z30.41
    specified type NEC Z30.49
    transdermal patch hormonal Z30.45
    vaginal ring hormonal Z30.44
  specified type NEC Z30.018
    transdermal patch hormonal Z30.016
    vaginal ring hormonal Z30.015
**Presence** (of)
  ankle-joint implant (functional) (prosthesis) Z96.66- ☑
  aortocoronary (bypass) graft Z95.1
  arterial-venous shunt (dialysis) Z99.2
  artificial
    eye (globe) Z97.0
    heart (fully implantable) (mechanical) Z95.812
      valve Z95.2
    larynx Z96.3
    lens (intraocular) Z96.1
    limb (complete) (partial) Z97.1- ☑
      arm Z97.1- ☑
        bilateral Z97.15
      leg Z97.1- ☑
        bilateral Z97.16
  audiological implant (functional) Z96.29
  bladder implant (functional) Z96.0
  bone
    conduction hearing device Z96.29
    implant (functional) NEC Z96.7
    joint (prosthesis) — *see* Presence, joint implant
  cardiac
    defibrillator (functional) (with synchronous cardiac
      pacemaker) Z95.810
    implant or graft Z95.9
      specified type NEC Z95.818
    pacemaker Z95.0
    resynchronization therapy
      defibrillator Z95.810
      pacemaker Z95.0
  cardioverter-defibrillator (ICD) Z95.810
  cerebrospinal fluid drainage device Z98.2
  cochlear implant (functional) Z96.21
  contact lens (es) Z97.3
  coronary artery graft or prosthesis Z95.5
  CRT-D (cardiac resynchronization therapy defibrillator)
    Z95.810
  CRT-P (cardiac resynchronization therapy pacemaker)
    Z95.0
  CSF shunt Z98.2
  dental prosthesis device Z97.2
  dentures Z97.2
  device (external) NEC Z97.8
    cardiac NEC Z95.818
    heart assist Z95.811
    implanted (functional) Z96.9
      specified NEC Z96.89
    prosthetic Z97.8
  ear implant Z96.20
    cochlear implant Z96.21
    myringotomy tube Z96.22
    specified type NEC Z96.29
  elbow-joint implant (functional) (prosthesis)
    Z96.62- ☑
  endocrine implant (functional) NEC Z96.49
  eustachian tube stent or device (functional) Z96.29
  external hearing-aid or device Z97.4
  finger-joint implant (functional) (prosthetic) Z96.69- ☑
  functional implant Z96.9
    specified NEC Z96.89
  graft
    cardiac NEC Z95.818
    vascular NEC Z95.828
  hearing-aid or device (external) Z97.4
    implant (bone) (cochlear) (functional) Z96.21
  heart assist device Z95.811
  heart valve implant (functional) Z95.2

**Presence** — *continued*
  heart valve implant — *continued*
    prosthetic Z95.2
    specified type NEC Z95.4
    xenogenic Z95.3
  hip-joint implant (functional) (prosthesis) Z96.64- ☑
  ICD (cardioverter-defibrillator) Z95.810
  implanted device (artificial) (functional) (prosthetic)
    Z96.9
    automatic cardiac defibrillator (with synchronous
      cardiac pacemaker) Z95.810
    cardiac pacemaker Z95.0
    cochlear Z96.21
    dental Z96.5
    heart Z95.812
    heart valve Z95.2
      prosthetic Z95.2
      specified NEC Z95.4
      xenogenic Z95.3
    insulin pump Z96.41
    intraocular lens Z96.1
    joint Z96.60
      ankle Z96.66- ☑
      elbow Z96.62- ☑
      finger Z96.69- ☑
      hip Z96.64- ☑
      knee Z96.65- ☑
      shoulder Z96.61- ☑
      specified NEC Z96.698
      wrist Z96.63- ☑
    larynx Z96.3
    myringotomy tube Z96.22
    otological Z96.20
      cochlear Z96.21
      eustachian stent Z96.29
      myringotomy Z96.22
      specified NEC Z96.29
      stapes Z96.29
    skin Z96.81
    skull plate Z96.7
    specified NEC Z96.89
    urogenital Z96.0
  insulin pump (functional) Z96.41
  intestinal bypass or anastomosis Z98.0
  intraocular lens (functional) Z96.1
  intrauterine contraceptive device (IUD) Z97.5
  intravascular implant (functional) (prosthetic) NEC
    Z95.9
    coronary artery Z95.5
    defibrillator (with synchronous cardiac pacemaker)
      Z95.810
    peripheral vessel (with angioplasty) Z95.820
  joint implant (prosthetic) (any) Z96.60
    ankle — *see* Presence, ankle joint implant
    elbow — *see* Presence, elbow joint implant
    finger — *see* Presence, finger joint implant
    hip — *see* Presence, hip joint implant
    knee — *see* Presence, knee joint implant
    shoulder — *see* Presence, shoulder joint implant
    specified joint NEC Z96.698
    wrist — *see* Presence, wrist joint implant
  knee-joint implant (functional) (prosthesis) Z96.65- ☑
  laryngeal implant (functional) Z96.3
  mandibular implant (dental) Z96.5
  myringotomy tube(s) Z96.22
  orthopedic-joint implant (prosthetic) (any) — *see*
    Presence, joint implant
  otological implant (functional) Z96.29
  shoulder-joint implant (functional) (prosthesis)
    Z96.61- ☑
  skull-plate implant Z96.7
  spectacles Z97.3
  stapes implant (functional) Z96.29
  systemic lupus erythematosus [SLE] inhibitor D68.62
  tendon implant (functional) (graft) Z96.7
  tooth root(s) implant Z96.5
  ureteral stent Z96.0
  urethral stent Z96.0
  urogenital implant (functional) Z96.0
  vascular implant or device Z95.9
    access port device Z95.828
    specified type NEC Z95.828
  wrist-joint implant (functional) (prosthesis) Z96.63- ☑
**Presenile** (*see also* condition)
  dementia F03 ☑
  premature aging E34.8
**Presentation, fetal** — *see* Delivery, complicated by,
  malposition

**Prespondylolisthesis** (congenital) Q76.2
**Pressure**
  area, skin — *see* Ulcer, pressure, by site
  brachial plexus G54.0
  brain G93.5
    injury at birth NEC P11.1
  cerebral — *see* Pressure, brain
  chest R07.89
  cone, tentorial G93.5
  hyposystolic (*see also* Hypotension)
    incidental reading, without diagnosis of hypoten-
      sion R03.1
  increased
    intracranial (benign) G93.2
      injury at birth P11.0
    intraocular H40.05- ☑
  lumbosacral plexus G54.1
  mediastinum J98.59
  necrosis (chronic) — *see* Ulcer, pressure, by site
  parental, inappropriate (excessive) Z62.6
  sore (chronic) — *see* Ulcer, pressure, by site
  spinal cord G95.20
  ulcer (chronic) — *see* Ulcer, pressure, by site
  venous, increased I87.8
**Pre-syncope** R55
**Preterm**
  delivery (*see also* Pregnancy, complicated by, preterm
    labor) O60.10 ☑
  labor — *see* Pregnancy, complicated by, preterm labor
  newborn (infant) P07.30
    gestational age
      28 completed weeks (28 weeks, 0 days through
        28 weeks, 6 days) P07.31
      29 completed weeks (29 weeks, 0 days through
        29 weeks, 6 days) P07.32
      30 completed weeks (30 weeks, 0 days through
        30 weeks, 6 days) P07.33
      31 completed weeks (31 weeks, 0 days through
        31 weeks, 6 days) P07.34
      32 completed weeks (32 weeks, 0 days through
        32 weeks, 6 days) P07.35
      33 completed weeks (33 weeks, 0 days through
        33 weeks, 6 days) P07.36
      34 completed weeks (34 weeks, 0 days through
        34 weeks, 6 days) P07.37
      35 completed weeks (35 weeks, 0 days through
        35 weeks, 6 days) P07.38
      36 completed weeks (36 weeks, 0 days through
        36 weeks, 6 days) P07.39
**Previa**
  placenta (total) (without hemorrhage) O44.0- ☑
    with hemorrhage O44.1- ☑
    complete O44.0- ☑
      with hemorrhage O44.1- ☑
    low (*see also* Delivery, complicated, by, placenta,
      low) O44.4- ☑
      with hemorrhage O44.5- ☑
    marginal O44.2- ☑
      with hemorrhage O44.3- ☑
    partial O44.2- ☑
      with hemorrhage O44.3- ☑
  vasa O69.4 ☑
**Priapism** N48.30
  due to
    disease classified elsewhere N48.32
    drug N48.33
    specified cause NEC N48.39
    trauma N48.31
**Prickling sensation** (skin) R20.2
**Prickly heat** L74.0
**Primary** — *see* condition
**Primigravida**
  elderly, affecting management of pregnancy, labor
    and delivery (supervision only) — *see* Pregnan-
    cy, complicated by, elderly, primigravida
  older, affecting management of pregnancy, labor and
    delivery (supervision only) — *see* Pregnancy,
    complicated by, elderly, primigravida
  very young, affecting management of pregnancy, labor
    and delivery (supervision only) — *see* Pregnan-
    cy, complicated by, young mother, primigravida
**Primipara**
  elderly, affecting management of pregnancy, labor
    and delivery (supervision only) — *see* Pregnan-
    cy, complicated by, elderly, primigravida

**Primipara** — *continued*
  older, affecting management of pregnancy, labor and delivery (supervision only) — *see* Pregnancy, complicated by, elderly, primigravida
  very young, affecting management of pregnancy, labor and delivery (supervision only) — *see* Pregnancy, complicated by, young mother, primigravida
**Primus varus** (bilateral) Q66.2 ☑
**PRIND** (Prolonged reversible ischemic neurologic deficit) I63.9
**Pringle's disease** (tuberous sclerosis) Q85.1
**Prinzmetal angina** I20.1
**Prizefighter ear** — *see* Cauliflower ear
**Problem** (with) (related to)
  academic Z55.8
  acculturation Z60.3
  adjustment (to)
    change of job Z56.1
    life-cycle transition Z60.0
    pension Z60.0
    retirement Z60.0
  adopted child Z62.821
  alcoholism in family Z63.72
  atypical parenting situation Z62.9
  bankruptcy Z59.8
  behavioral (adult) F69
    drug seeking Z76.5
  birth of sibling affecting child Z62.898
  care (of)
    provider dependency Z74.9
      specified NEC Z74.8
    sick or handicapped person in family or household Z63.6
  child
    abuse (affecting the child) — *see* Maltreatment, child
    custody or support proceedings Z65.3
    in care of non-parental family member Z62.21
    in foster care Z62.21
    in welfare custody Z62.21
    living in orphanage or group home Z62.22
  child-rearing Z62.9
    specified NEC Z62.898
  communication (developmental) F80.9
  conflict or discord (with)
    boss Z56.4
    classmates Z55.4
    counselor Z64.4
    employer Z56.4
    family Z63.9
      specified NEC Z63.8
    probation officer Z64.4
    social worker Z64.4
    teachers Z55.4
    workmates Z56.4
  conviction in legal proceedings Z65.0
    with imprisonment Z65.1
  counselor Z64.4
  creditors Z59.8
  digestive K92.9
  drug addict in family Z63.72
  ear — *see* Disorder, ear
  economic Z59.9
    affecting care Z59.9
    specified NEC Z59.8
  education Z55.9
    specified NEC Z55.8
  employment Z56.9
    change of job Z56.1
    discord Z56.4
    environment Z56.5
    sexual harassment Z56.81
    specified NEC Z56.89
    stressful schedule Z56.3
    stress NEC Z56.6
    threat of job loss Z56.2
    unemployment Z56.0
  enuresis, child F98.0
  eye H57.9
  failed examinations (school) Z55.2
  falling Z91.81
  family (*see also* Disruption, family) Z63.9
    specified NEC Z63.8
  feeding (elderly) (infant) R63.3
    newborn P92.9
      breast P92.5
      overfeeding P92.4
      slow P92.2

**Problem** — *continued*
  feeding — *continued*
    newborn — *continued*
      specified NEC P92.8
      underfeeding P92.3
    nonorganic F50.89
  finance Z59.9
    specified NEC Z59.8
  foreclosure on loan Z59.8
  foster child Z62.822
  frightening experience(s) in childhood Z62.898
  genital NEC
    female N94.9
    male N50.9
  health care Z75.9
    specified NEC Z75.8
  hearing — *see* Deafness
  homelessness Z59.0
  housing Z59.9
    inadequate Z59.1
    isolated Z59.8
    specified NEC Z59.8
  identity (of childhood) F93.8
  illegitimate pregnancy (unwanted) Z64.0
  illiteracy Z55.0
  impaired mobility Z74.09
  imprisonment or incarceration Z65.1
  inadequate teaching affecting education Z55.8
  inappropriate (excessive) parental pressure Z62.6
  influencing health status NEC Z78.9
  in-law Z63.1
  institutionalization, affecting child Z62.22
  intrafamilial communication Z63.8
  jealousy, child F93.8
  landlord Z59.2
  language (developmental) F80.9
  learning (developmental) F81.9
  legal Z65.3
    conviction without imprisonment Z65.0
    imprisonment Z65.1
    release from prison Z65.2
  life-management Z73.9
    specified NEC Z73.89
  life-style Z72.9
    gambling Z72.6
    high-risk sexual behavior (heterosexual) Z72.51
      bisexual Z72.53
      homosexual Z72.52
    inappropriate eating habits Z72.4
    self-damaging behavior NEC Z72.89
    specified NEC Z72.89
    tobacco use Z72.0
  literacy Z55.9
    low level Z55.0
    specified NEC Z55.8
  living alone Z60.2
  lodgers Z59.2
  loss of love relationship in childhood Z62.898
  marital Z63.0
    involving
      divorce Z63.5
      estrangement Z63.5
      gender identity F66
  mastication K08.89
  medical
    care, within family Z63.6
    facilities Z75.9
      specified NEC Z75.8
  mental F48.9
  multiparity K64.1
  negative life events in childhood Z62.9
    altered pattern of family relationships Z62.898
    frightening experience Z62.898
    loss of
      love relationship Z62.898
      self-esteem Z62.898
    physical abuse (alleged) — *see* Maltreatment, child
    removal from home Z62.29
    specified event NEC Z62.898
  neighbor Z59.2
  neurological NEC R29.818
  new step-parent affecting child Z62.898
  none (feared complaint unfounded) Z71.1
  occupational NEC Z56.89
  parent-child — *see* Conflict, parent-child
  personal hygiene Z91.89
  personality F69
  phase-of-life transition, adjustment Z60.0

**Problem** — *continued*
  presence of sick or disabled person in family or household Z63.79
    needing care Z63.6
  primary support group (family) Z63.9
    specified NEC Z63.8
  probation officer Z64.4
  psychiatric F99
  psychosexual (development) F66
  psychosocial Z65.9
    religious or spiritual Z65.8
    specified NEC Z65.8
  relationship Z63.9
    childhood F93.8
  release from prison Z65.2
    religious or spiritual Z65.8
  removal from home affecting child Z62.29
  seeking and accepting known hazardous and harmful
    behavioral or psychological interventions Z65.8
    chemical, nutritional or physical interventions Z65.8
  sexual function (nonorganic) F52.9
  sight H54.7
  sleep disorder, child F51.9
  smell — *see* Disturbance, sensation, smell
  social
    environment Z60.9
      specified NEC Z60.8
    exclusion and rejection Z60.4
    worker Z64.4
  speech R47.9
    developmental F80.9
    specified NEC R47.89
  swallowing — *see* Dysphagia
  taste — *see* Disturbance, sensation, taste
  tic, child F95.0
  underachievement in school Z55.3
  unemployment Z56.0
    threatened Z56.2
  unwanted pregnancy Z64.0
  upbringing Z62.9
    specified NEC Z62.898
  urinary N39.9
  voice production R47.89
  work schedule (stressful) Z56.3
**Procedure** (surgical)
  converted
    arthroscopic to open Z53.33
    laparoscopic to open Z53.31
    specified procedure NEC to open Z53.39
    thoracoscopic to open Z53.32
  for purpose other than remedying health state Z41.9
    specified NEC Z41.8
  not done Z53.9
    because of
      administrative reasons Z53.8
      contraindication Z53.09
        smoking Z53.01
      patient's decision Z53.20
        for reasons of belief or group pressure Z53.1
        left against medical advice (AMA) Z53.21
        specified reason NEC Z53.29
      specified reason NEC Z53.8
**Procidentia** (uteri) N81.3
**Proctalgia** K62.89
  fugax K59.4
  spasmodic K59.4
**Proctitis** K62.89
  amebic (acute) A06.0
  chlamydial A56.3
  gonococcal A54.6
  granulomatous — *see* Enteritis, regional, large intestine
  herpetic A60.1
  radiation K62.7
  tuberculous A18.32
  ulcerative (chronic) K51.20
    with
      complication K51.219
        abscess K51.214
        fistula K51.213
        obstruction K51.212
        rectal bleeding K51.211
        specified NEC K51.218
**Proctocele**
  female (without uterine prolapse) N81.6
    with uterine prolapse N81.2
      complete N81.3
  male K62.3

**Proctocolitis**
food protein-induced K52.82
food-induced eosinophilic K52.82
milk protein-induced K52.82
mucosal — *see* Rectosigmoiditis, ulcerative
**Proctoptosis** K62.3
**Proctorrhagia** K62.5
**Proctosigmoiditis** K63.89
ulcerative (chronic) — *see* Rectosigmoiditis, ulcerative
**Proctospasm** K59.4
psychogenic F45.8
**Profichet's disease** — *see* Disorder, soft tissue, specified type NEC
**Progeria** E34.8
**Prognathism** (mandibular) (maxillary) M26.19
**Progonoma** (melanotic) — *see* Neoplasm, benign, by site
**Progressive** — *see* condition
**Prolactinoma**
specified site — *see* Neoplasm, benign, by site
unspecified site D35.2
**Prolapse, prolapsed**
anus, anal (canal) (sphincter) K62.2
arm or hand O32.2 ☑
causing obstructed labor O64.4 ☑
bladder (mucosa) (sphincter) (acquired)
congenital Q79.4
female — *see* Cystocele
male N32.89
breast implant (prosthetic) T85.49 ☑
cecostomy K94.09
cecum K63.4
cervix, cervical (hypertrophied) N81.2
anterior lip, obstructing labor O65.5
congenital Q51.828
postpartal, old N81.2
stump N81.85
ciliary body (traumatic) — *see* Laceration, eye(ball), with prolapse or loss of interocular tissue
colon (pedunculated) K63.4
colostomy K94.09
disc (intervertebral) — *see* Displacement, intervertebral disc
eye implant (orbital) T85.398 ☑
lens (ocular) — *see* Complications, intraocular lens
fallopian tube N83.4- ☑
gastric (mucosa) K31.89
genital, female N81.9
specified NEC N81.89
globe, nontraumatic — *see* Luxation, globe
ileostomy bud K94.19
intervertebral disc — *see* Displacement, intervertebral disc
intestine (small) K63.4
iris (traumatic) — *see* Laceration, eye(ball), with prolapse or loss of interocular tissue
nontraumatic H21.89
kidney N28.83
congenital Q63.2
laryngeal muscles or ventricle J38.7
liver K76.89
meatus urinarius N36.8
mitral (valve) I34.1
ocular lens implant — *see* Complications, intraocular lens
organ or site, congenital NEC — *see* Malposition, congenital
ovary N83.4- ☑
pelvic floor, female N81.89
perineum, female N81.89
rectum (mucosa) (sphincter) K62.3
due to trichuris trichuria B79
spleen D73.89
stomach K31.89
umbilical cord
complicating delivery O69.0 ☑
urachus, congenital Q64.4
ureter N28.89
with obstruction N13.5
with infection N13.6
ureterovesical orifice N28.89
urethra (acquired) (infected) (mucosa) N36.8
congenital Q64.71
urinary meatus N36.8
congenital Q64.72
uterovaginal N81.4
complete N81.3
incomplete N81.2

**Prolapse, prolapsed** — *continued*
uterus (with prolapse of vagina) N81.4
complete N81.3
congenital Q51.818
first degree N81.2
in pregnancy or childbirth — *see* Pregnancy, complicated by, abnormal, uterus
incomplete N81.2
postpartal (old) N81.4
second degree N81.2
third degree N81.3
uveal (traumatic) — *see* Laceration, eye(ball), with prolapse or loss of interocular tissue
vagina (anterior) (wall) — *see* Cystocele
with prolapse of uterus N81.4
complete N81.3
incomplete N81.2
posterior wall N81.6
posthysterectomy N99.3
vitreous (humor) H43.0- ☑
in wound — *see* Laceration, eye(ball), with prolapse or loss of interocular tissue
womb — *see* Prolapse, uterus
**Prolapsus, female** N81.9
specified NEC N81.89
**Proliferation(s)**
primary cutaneous CD30-positive large T-cell C86.6
prostate, atypical small acinar N42.32
**Proliferative** — *see* condition
**Prolonged, prolongation** (of)
bleeding (time) (idiopathic) R79.1
coagulation (time) R79.1
gestation (over 42 completed weeks)
mother O48.1
newborn P08.22
interval I44.0
labor O63.9
first stage O63.0
second stage O63.1
partial thromboplastin time (PTT) R79.1
pregnancy (more than 42 weeks gestation) O48.1
prothrombin time R79.1
QT interval I45.81
uterine contractions in labor O62.4
**Prominence, prominent**
auricle (congenital) (ear) Q17.5
ischial spine or sacral promontory
with disproportion (fetopelvic) O33.0
causing obstructed labor O65.0
nose (congenital) acquired M95.0
**Promiscuity** — *see* High, risk, sexual behavior
**Pronation**
ankle — *see* Deformity, limb, foot, specified NEC
foot (*see also* Deformity, limb, foot, specified NEC)
congenital Q74.2
**Prophylactic**
administration of
antibiotics, long-term Z79.2
short-term use — *omit code*
drug (*see also* Long-term (current) drug therapy (use of)) Z79.899
medication Z79.899
organ removal (for neoplasia management) Z40.00
breast Z40.01
fallopian tube(s) Z40.03
with ovary(s) Z40.02
ovary(s) Z40.02
specified site NEC Z40.09
surgery Z40.9
for risk factors related to malignant neoplasm — *see* Prophylactic, organ removal
specified NEC Z40.8
vaccination Z23
**Propionic acidemia** E71.121
**Proptosis** (ocular) (*see also* Exophthalmos)
thyroid — *see* Hyperthyroidism, with goiter
**Prosecution, anxiety concerning** Z65.3
**Prosopagnosia** R48.3
**Prostadynia** N42.81
**Prostate, prostatic** — *see* condition
**Prostatism** — *see* Hyperplasia, prostate
**Prostatitis** (congestive) (suppurative) (with cystitis) N41.9
acute N41.0
cavitary N41.8
chronic N41.1
diverticular N41.8
due to Trichomonas (vaginalis) A59.02
fibrous N41.1

**Prostatitis** — *continued*
gonococcal (acute) (chronic) A54.22
granulomatous N41.4
hypertrophic N41.1
subacute N41.1
trichomonal A59.02
tuberculous A18.14
**Prostatocystitis** N41.3
**Prostatorrhea** N42.89
**Prostatosis** N42.82
**Prostration** R53.83
heat (*see also* Heat, exhaustion)
anhydrotic T67.3 ☑
due to
salt (and water) depletion T67.4 ☑
water depletion T67.3 ☑
nervous F48.8
senile R54
**Protanomaly** (anomalous trichromat) H53.54
**Protanopia** (complete) (incomplete) H53.54
**Protection** (against) (from) — *see* Prophylactic
**Protein**
deficiency NEC — *see* Malnutrition
malnutrition — *see* Malnutrition
sickness (*see also* Reaction, serum) T80.69 ☑
**Proteinemia** R77.9
**Proteinosis**
alveolar (pulmonary) J84.01
lipid or lipoid (of Urbach) E78.89
**Proteinuria** R80.9
Bence Jones R80.3
complicating pregnancy — *see* Proteinuria, gestational
gestational
complicating
childbirth O12.14
pregnancy O12.1- ☑
with edema O12.2- ☑
puerperium O12.15
idiopathic R80.0
isolated R80.0
with glomerular lesion N06.9
dense deposit disease N06.6
diffuse
crescentic glomerulonephritis N06.7
endocapillary proliferative glomerulonephritis N06.4
mesangiocapillary glomerulonephritis N06.5
focal and segmental hyalinosis or sclerosis N06.1
membranous (diffuse) N06.2
mesangial proliferative (diffuse) N06.3
minimal change N06.0
specified pathology NEC N06.8
orthostatic R80.2
with glomerular lesion — *see* Proteinuria, isolated, with glomerular lesion
persistent R80.1
with glomerular lesion — *see* Proteinuria, isolated, with glomerular lesion
postural R80.2
with glomerular lesion — *see* Proteinuria, isolated, with glomerular lesion
pre-eclamptic — *see* Pre-eclampsia
puerperal O12.15
specified type NEC R80.8
**Proteolysis, pathologic** D65
**Proteus** (mirabilis) (morganii), **as cause of disease classified elsewhere** B96.4
**Prothrombin gene mutation** D68.52
**Protoporphyria, erythropoietic** E80.0
**Protozoal** (*see also* condition)
disease B64
specified NEC B60.8
**Protrusion, protrusio**
acetabuli M24.7
acetabulum (into pelvis) M24.7
device, implant or graft (*see also* Complications, by site and type, mechanical) T85.698 ☑
arterial graft NEC — *see* Complication, cardiovascular device, mechanical, vascular
breast (implant) T85.49 ☑
catheter NEC T85.698 ☑
cystostomy T83.090 ☑
dialysis (renal) T82.49 ☑
intraperitoneal T85.691 ☑
infusion NEC T82.594 ☑
spinal (epidural) (subdural) T85.690 ☑

**Protrusion, protrusio** — *continued*
  device, implant or graft (*see also* Complications, by site and type, mechanical) — *continued*
    catheter — *continued*
      urinary (*see also* Complications, catheter, urinary) T83.098 ☑
      electronic (electrode) (pulse generator) (stimulator)
        bone T84.390 ☑
        nervous system — *see* Complication, prosthetic device, mechanical, electronic nervous system stimulator
      fixation, internal (orthopedic) NEC — *see* Complication, fixation device, mechanical
      gastrointestinal — *see* Complications, prosthetic device, mechanical, gastrointestinal device
      genital NEC T83.498 ☑
        intrauterine contraceptive device T83.39 ☑
        penile prosthesis (cylinder) (implanted) (pump) (resevoir) T83.490 ☑
        testicular prosthesis T83.491 ☑
      heart NEC — *see* Complication, cardiovascular device, mechanical
      joint prosthesis — *see* Complications, joint prosthesis, mechanical, specified NEC, by site
      ocular NEC — *see* Complications, prosthetic device, mechanical, ocular device
      orthopedic NEC — *see* Complication, orthopedic, device, mechanical
      specified NEC T85.628 ☑
      urinary NEC (*see also* Complication, genitourinary, device, urinary, mechanical)
        graft T83.29 ☑
      vascular NEC — *see* Complication, cardiovascular device, mechanical
      ventricular intracranial shunt T85.09 ☑
  intervertebral disc — *see* Displacement, intervertebral disc
  joint prosthesis — *see* Complications, joint prosthesis, mechanical, specified NEC, by site
  nucleus pulposus — *see* Displacement, intervertebral disc
**Prune belly** (syndrome) Q79.4
**Prurigo** (ferox) (gravis) (Hebrae) (Hebra's) (mitis) (simplex) L28.2
  Besnier's L20.0
  estivalis L56.4
  nodularis L28.1
  psychogenic F45.8
**Pruritus, pruritic** (essential) L29.9
  ani, anus L29.0
    psychogenic F45.8
  anogenital L29.3
    psychogenic F45.8
  due to onchocerca volvulus B73.1
  gravidarum — *see* Pregnancy, complicated by, specified pregnancy-related condition NEC
  hiemalis L29.8
  neurogenic (any site) F45.8
  perianal L29.0
  psychogenic (any site) F45.8
  scroti, scrotum L29.1
    psychogenic F45.8
  senile, senilis L29.8
  specified NEC L29.8
    psychogenic F45.8
  Trichomonas A59.9
  vulva, vulvae L29.2
    psychogenic F45.8
**Pseudarthrosis, pseudoarthrosis** (bone) — *see* Nonunion, fracture
  clavicle, congenital Q74.0
  joint, following fusion or arthrodesis M96.0
**Pseudoaneurysm** — *see* Aneurysm
**Pseudoangina** (pectoris) — *see* Angina
**Pseudoangioma** I81
**Pseudoarteriosus** Q28.8
**Pseudoarthrosis** — *see* Pseudarthrosis
**Pseudobulbar affect** (PBA) F48.2
**Pseudochromhidrosis** L67.8
**Pseudocirrhosis, liver, pericardial** I31.1
**Pseudocowpox** B08.03
**Pseudocoxalgia** M91.3- ☑
**Pseudocroup** J38.5
**Pseudo-Cushing's syndrome, alcohol-induced** E24.4
**Pseudocyesis** F45.8
**Pseudocyst**
  lung J98.4

**Pseudocyst** — *continued*
  pancreas K86.3
  retina — *see* Cyst, retina
**Pseudoelephantiasis neuroarthritica** Q82.0
**Pseudoexfoliation, capsule** (lens) — *see* Cataract, specified NEC
**Pseudofolliculitis barbae** L73.1
**Pseudoglioma** H44.89
**Pseudohemophilia** (Bernuth's) (hereditary) (type B) D68.0
  Type A D69.8
  vascular D69.8
**Pseudohermaphroditism** Q56.3
  adrenal E25.8
  female Q56.2
    with adrenocortical disorder E25.8
    without adrenocortical disorder Q56.2
    adrenal (congenital) E25.0
    unspecified E25.9
  male Q56.1
    with
      5-alpha-reductase deficiency E29.1
      adrenocortical disorder E25.8
      androgen resistance E34.51
      cleft scrotum Q56.1
      feminizing testis E34.51
    without gonadal disorder Q56.1
    adrenal E25.8
    unspecified E25.9
**Pseudo-Hurler's polydystrophy** E77.0
**Pseudohydrocephalus** G93.2
**Pseudohypertrophic muscular dystrophy** (Erb's) G71.0
**Pseudohypertrophy, muscle** G71.0
**Pseudohypoparathyroidism** E20.1
**Pseudoinsomnia** F51.03
**Pseudoleukemia, infantile** D64.89
**Pseudomembranous** — *see* condition
**Pseudomeningocele** (cerebral) (infective) (post-traumatic) G96.19
  postprocedural (spinal) G97.82
**Pseudomenses** (newborn) P54.6
**Pseudomenstruation** (newborn) P54.6
**Pseudomonas**
  aeruginosa, as cause of disease classified elsewhere B96.5
  mallei infection A24.0
    as cause of disease classified elsewhere B96.5
    pseudomallei, as cause of disease classified elsewhere B96.5
**Pseudomyotonia** G71.19
**Pseudomyxoma peritonei** C78.6
**Pseudoneuritis, optic** (nerve) (disc) (papilla), **congenital** Q14.2
**Pseudo-obstruction intestine** (acute) (chronic) (idiopathic) (intermittent secondary) (primary) K59.8
**Pseudopapilledema** H47.33- ☑
  congenital Q14.2
**Pseudoparalysis**
  arm or leg R29.818
  atonic, congenital P94.2
**Pseudopelade** L66.0
**Pseudophakia** Z96.1
**Pseudopolyarthritis, rhizomelic** M35.3
**Pseudopolycythemia** D75.1
**Pseudopseudohypoparathyroidism** E20.1
**Pseudopterygium** H11.81- ☑
**Pseudoptosis** (eyelid) — *see* Blepharochalasis
**Pseudopuberty, precocious**
  female heterosexual E25.8
  male isosexual E25.8
**Pseudorickets** (renal) N25.0
**Pseudorubella** B08.20
**Pseudosclerema, newborn** P83.88
**Pseudosclerosis** (brain)
  Jakob's — *see* Creutzfeldt-Jakob disease or syndrome of Westphal (Strümpell) E83.01
  spastic — *see* Creutzfeldt-Jakob disease or syndrome
**Pseudotetanus** — *see* Convulsions
**Pseudotetany** R29.0
  hysterical F44.5
**Pseudotruncus arteriosus** Q25.49
**Pseudotuberculosis** A28.2
  enterocolitis A04.8
  pasteurella (infection) A28.0
**Pseudotumor**
  cerebri G93.2
  orbital H05.11 ☑

**Pseudoxanthoma elasticum** Q82.8
**Psilosis** (sprue) (tropical) K90.1
  nontropical K90.0
**Psittacosis** A70
**Psoitis** M60.88
**Psoriasis** L40.9
  arthropathic L40.50
    arthritis mutilans L40.52
    distal interphalangeal L40.51
    juvenile L40.54
    other specified L40.59
    spondylitis L40.53
  buccal K13.29
  flexural L40.8
  guttate L40.4
  mouth K13.29
  nummular L40.0
  plaque L40.0
  psychogenic F54
  pustular (generalized) L40.1
    palmaris et plantaris L40.3
  specified NEC L40.8
  vulgaris L40.0
**Psychasthenia** F48.8
**Psychiatric disorder or problem** F99
**Psychogenic** (*see also* condition)
  factors associated with physical conditions F54
**Psychological and behavioral factors affecting medical condition** F59
**Psychoneurosis, psychoneurotic** (*see also* Neurosis)
  anxiety (state) F41.1
  depersonalization F48.1
  hypochondriacal F45.21
  hysteria F44.9
  neurasthenic F48.8
  personality NEC F60.89
**Psychopathy, psychopathic**
  affectionless F94.2
  autistic F84.5
  constitution, post-traumatic F07.81
  personality — *see* Disorder, personality
  sexual — *see* Deviation, sexual
  state F60.2
**Psychosexual identity disorder of childhood** F64.2
**Psychosis, psychotic** F29
  acute (transient) F23
    hysterical F44.9
  affective — *see* Disorder, mood
  alcoholic F10.959
    with
      abuse F10.159
      anxiety disorder F10.980
        with
          abuse F10.180
          dependence F10.280
      delirium tremens F10.231
      delusions F10.950
        with
          abuse F10.150
          dependence F10.250
      dementia F10.97
        with dependence F10.27
      dependence F10.259
      hallucinosis F10.951
        with
          abuse F10.151
          dependence F10.251
      mood disorder F10.94
        with
          abuse F10.14
          dependence F10.24
      paranoia F10.950
        with
          abuse F10.150
          dependence F10.250
      persisting amnesia F10.96
        with dependence F10.26
    amnestic confabulatory F10.96
      with dependence F10.26
    delirium tremens F10.231
    Korsakoff's, Korsakov's, Korsakow's F10.26
    paranoid type F10.950
      with
        abuse F10.150
        dependence F10.250
  anergastic — *see* Psychosis, organic
  arteriosclerotic (simple type) (uncomplicated) F01.50
    with behavioral disturbance F01.51

**Psychosis, psychotic** — *continued*
  childhood F84.0
    atypical F84.8
  climacteric — *see* Psychosis, involutional
  confusional F29
    acute or subacute F05
    reactive F23
  cycloid F23
  depressive — *see* Disorder, depressive
  disintegrative (childhood) F84.3
  drug-induced — *see* F11-F19 with .X59
    paranoid and hallucinatory states — *see* F11-F19
      with .X50 or .X51
  due to or associated with
    addiction, drug — *see* F11-F19 with .X59
    dependence
      alcohol F10.259
      drug — *see* F11-F19 with .X59
    epilepsy F06.8
    Huntington's chorea F06.8
    ischemia, cerebrovascular (generalized) F06.8
    multiple sclerosis F06.8
    physical disease F06.8
    presenile dementia F03 ☑
    senile dementia F03 ☑
    vascular disease (arteriosclerotic) (cerebral) F01.50
      with behavioral disturbance F01.51
  epileptic F06.8
  episode F23
    due to or associated with physical condition F06.8
  exhaustive F43.0
  hallucinatory, chronic F28
  hypomanic F30.8
  hysterical (acute) F44.9
  induced F24
  infantile F84.0
    atypical F84.8
  infective (acute) (subacute) F05
  involutional F28
    depressive — *see* Disorder, depressive
    melancholic — *see* Disorder, depressive
    paranoid (state) F22
  Korsakoff's, Korsakov's, Korsakow's (nonalcoholic) F04
    alcoholic F10.96
      in dependence F10.26
    induced by other psychoactive substance — *see*
      categories F11-F19 with .X5X
  mania, manic (single episode) F30.2
    recurrent type F31.89
  manic-depressive — *see* Disorder, bipolar
  menopausal — *see* Psychosis, involutional
  mixed schizophrenic and affective F25.8
  multi-infarct (cerebrovascular) F01.50
    with behavioral disturbance F01.51
  nonorganic F29
    specified NEC F28
  organic F09
    due to or associated with
      arteriosclerosis (cerebral) — *see* Psychosis, ar-
        teriosclerotic
      cerebrovascular disease, arteriosclerotic — *see*
        Psychosis, arteriosclerotic
      childbirth — *see* Psychosis, puerperal
      Creutzfeldt-Jakob disease or syndrome — *see*
        Creutzfeldt-Jakob disease or syndrome
      dependence, alcohol F10.259
      disease
        alcoholic liver F10.259
        brain, arteriosclerotic — *see* Psychosis, arte-
          riosclerotic
        cerebrovascular F01.50
          with behavioral disturbance F01.51
        Creutzfeldt-Jakob — *see* Creutzfeldt-Jakob
          disease or syndrome
        endocrine or metabolic F06.8
          acute or subacute F05
        liver, alcoholic F10.259
      epilepsy transient (acute) F05
      infection
        brain (intracranial) F06.8
          acute or subacute F05
      intoxication
        alcoholic (acute) F10.259
        drug F11-F19 with .X59
      ischemia, cerebrovascular (generalized) — *see*
        Psychosis, arteriosclerotic
      puerperium — *see* Psychosis, puerperal

**Psychosis, psychotic** — *continued*
  organic — *continued*
    due to or associated with — *continued*
      trauma, brain (birth) (from electric current)
        (surgical) F06.8
        acute or subacute F05
      infective F06.8
        acute or subacute F05
      post-traumatic F06.8
        acute or subacute F05
  paranoiac F22
  paranoid (climacteric) (involutional) (menopausal) F22
    psychogenic (acute) F23
    schizophrenic F20.0
    senile F03 ☑
  postpartum F53
  presbyophrenic (type) F03 ☑
  presenile F03 ☑
  psychogenic (paranoid) F23
    depressive F32.3
  puerperal F53
    specified type — *see* Psychosis, by type
  reactive (brief) (transient) (emotional stress) (psycho-
    logical trauma) F23
    depressive F32.3
      recurrent F33.3
    excitative type F30.8
  schizoaffective F25.9
    depressive type F25.1
    manic type F25.0
  schizophrenia, schizophrenic — *see* Schizophrenia
  schizophrenia-like, in epilepsy F06.2
  schizophreniform F20.81
    affective type F25.9
    brief F23
    confusional type F23
    mixed type F25.0
  senile NEC F03 ☑
    depressed or paranoid type F03 ☑
    simple deterioration F03 ☑
    specified type — *code to* condition
  shared F24
  situational (reactive) F23
  symbiotic (childhood) F84.3
  symptomatic F09
**Psychosomatic** — *see* Disorder, psychosomatic
**Psychosyndrome, organic** F07.9
**Psychotic episode due to or associated with physical condition** F06.8
**Pterygium** (eye) H11.00- ☑
  amyloid H11.01- ☑
  central H11.02- ☑
  colli Q18.3
  double H11.03- ☑
  peripheral
    progressive H11.05- ☑
    stationary H11.04- ☑
  recurrent H11.06- ☑
**Ptilosis** (eyelid) — *see* Madarosis
**Ptomaine** (poisoning) — *see* Poisoning, food
**Ptosis** (*see also* Blepharoptosis)
  adiposa (false) — *see* Blepharoptosis
  breast N64.81
  cecum K63.4
  colon K63.4
  congenital (eyelid) Q10.0
    specified site NEC — *see* Anomaly, by site
  eyelid — *see* Blepharoptosis
    congenital Q10.0
  gastric K31.89
  intestine K63.4
  kidney N28.83
  liver K76.89
  renal N28.83
  splanchnic K63.4
  spleen D73.89
  stomach K31.89
  viscera K63.4
**PTP** D69.51
**Ptyalism** (periodic) K11.7
  hysterical F45.8
  pregnancy — *see* Pregnancy, complicated by, specified
    pregnancy-related condition NEC
  psychogenic F45.8
**Ptyalolithiasis** K11.5
**Pubarche, precocious** E30.1
**Pubertas praecox** E30.1
**Puberty** (development state) Z00.3

**Puberty** — *continued*
  bleeding (excessive) N92.2
  delayed E30.0
  precocious (constitutional) (cryptogenic) (idiopathic)
    E30.1
    central E22.8
    due to
      ovarian hyperfunction E28.1
        estrogen E28.0
      testicular hyperfunction E29.0
  premature E30.1
    due to
      adrenal cortical hyperfunction E25.8
      pineal tumor E34.8
      pituitary (anterior) hyperfunction E22.8
**Puckering, macula** — *see* Degeneration, macula, puckering
**Pudenda, pudendum** — *see* condition
**Puente's disease** (simple glandular cheilitis) K13.0
**Puerperal, puerperium** (complicated by, complications)
  abnormal glucose (tolerance test) O99.815
  abscess
    areola O91.02
      associated with lactation O91.03
    Bartholin's gland O86.19
    breast O91.12
      associated with lactation O91.13
    cervix (uteri) O86.11
    genital organ NEC O86.19
    kidney O86.21
    mammary O91.12
      associated with lactation O91.13
    nipple O91.02
      associated with lactation O91.03
    peritoneum O85
    subareolar O91.12
      associated with lactation O91.13
    urinary tract — *see* Puerperal, infection, urinary
    uterus O86.12
    vagina (wall) O86.13
    vaginorectal O86.13
    vulvovaginal gland O86.13
  adnexitis O86.19
  afibrinogenemia, or other coagulation defect O72.3
  albuminuria (acute) (subacute) — *see* Proteinuria,
    gestational
  alcohol use O99.315
  anemia O90.81
    pre-existing (pre-pregnancy) O99.03
  anesthetic death O89.8
  apoplexy O99.43
  bariatric surgery status O99.845
  blood disorder NEC O99.13
  blood dyscrasia O72.3
  cardiomyopathy O90.3
  cerebrovascular disorder (conditions in I60-I69) O99.43
  cervicitis O86.11
  circulatory system disorder O99.43
  coagulopathy (any) O99.13
    with hemorrhage O72.3
  complications O90.9
    specified NEC O90.89
  convulsions — *see* Eclampsia
  cystitis O86.22
  cystopyelitis O86.29
  delirium NEC F05
  diabetes O24.93
    gestational — *see* Puerperal, gestational diabetes
    pre-existing O24.33
      specified NEC O24.83
      type 1 O24.03
      type 2 O24.13
  digestive system disorder O99.63
  disease O90.9
    breast NEC O92.29
    cerebrovascular (acute) O99.43
    nonobstetric NEC O99.89
    tubo-ovarian O86.19
    Valsuani's O99.03
  disorder O90.9
    biliary tract O26.63
    lactation O92.70
    liver O26.63
    nonobstetric NEC O99.89
  disruption
    cesarean wound O90.0
    episiotomy wound O90.1
    perineal laceration wound O90.1

**Puerperal, puerperium** — *continued*
  drug use O99.325
  eclampsia (with pre-existing hypertension) O15.2
  embolism (pulmonary) (blood clot) — *see* Embolism, obstetric, puerperal
  endocrine, nutritional or metabolic disease NEC O99.285
  endophlebitis — *see* Puerperal, phlebitis
  endotrachelitis O86.11
  failure
    lactation (complete) O92.3
      partial O92.4
    renal, acute O90.4
  fever (of unknown origin) O86.4
    septic O85
  fissure, nipple O92.12
    associated with lactation O92.13
  fistula
    breast (due to mastitis) O91.12
      associated with lactation O91.13
    nipple O91.02
      associated with lactation O91.03
  galactophoritis O91.22
    associated with lactation O91.23
  galactorrhea O92.6
  gastric banding status O99.845
  gastric bypass status O99.845
  gastrointestinal disease NEC O99.63
  gestational
    diabetes O24.439
      diet controlled O24.430
      insulin (and diet) controlled O24.434
      oral drug controlled (antidiabetic) (hypo-glycemic) O24.435
    edema O12.05
      with proteinuria O12.25
    proteinuria O12.15
  gonorrhea O98.23
  hematoma, subdural O99.43
  hemiplegia, cerebral O99.355
    due to cerbrovascular disorder O99.43
  hemorrhage O72.1
    brain O99.43
    bulbar O99.43
    cerebellar O99.43
    cerebral O99.43
    cortical O99.43
    delayed or secondary O72.2
    extradural O99.43
    internal capsule O99.43
    intracranial O99.43
    intrapontine O99.43
    meningeal O99.43
    pontine O99.43
    retained placenta O72.0
    subarachnoid O99.43
    subcortical O99.43
    subdural O99.43
    third stage O72.0
    uterine, delayed O72.2
    ventricular O99.43
  hemorrhoids O87.2
  hepatorenal syndrome O90.4
  hypertension — *see* Hypertension, complicating, puerperium
  hypertrophy, breast O92.29
  induration breast (fibrous) O92.29
  infection O86.4
    cervix O86.11
    generalized O85
    genital tract NEC O86.19
      obstetric surgical wound O86.0
    kidney (bacillus coli) O86.21
    maternal O98.93
      carrier state NEC O99.835
      gonorrhea O98.23
      human immunodeficiency virus (HIV) O98.73
      protozoal O98.63
      sexually transmitted NEC O98.33
      specified NEC O98.83
      streptococcus group B (GBS) carrier state O99.825
      syphilis O98.13
      tuberculosis O98.03
      viral hepatitis O98.43
      viral NEC O98.53
    nipple O91.02
      associated with lactation O91.03
    peritoneum O85

**Puerperal, puerperium** — *continued*
  infection — *continued*
    renal O86.21
    specified NEC O86.89
    urinary (asymptomatic) (tract) NEC O86.20
      bladder O86.22
      kidney O86.21
      specified site NEC O86.29
      urethra O86.22
    vagina O86.13
    vein — *see* Puerperal, phlebitis
  ischemia, cerebral O99.43
  lymphangitis O86.89
    breast O91.22
      associated with lactation O91.23
  malignancy O9A.13 (*following* O99)
  malnutrition O25.3
  mammillitis O91.02
    associated with lactation O91.03
  mammitis O91.22
    associated with lactation O91.23
  mania F30.8
  mastitis O91.22
    associated with lactation O91.23
    purulent O91.12
      associated with lactation O91.13
  melancholia — *see* Disorder, depressive
  mental disorder NEC O99.345
  metroperitonitis O85
  metrorrhagia — *see* Hemorrhage, postpartum
  metrosalpingitis O86.19
  metrovaginitis O86.13
  milk leg O87.1
  monoplegia, cerebral O99.43
  mood disturbance O90.6
  necrosis, liver (acute) (subacute) (conditions in subcat-egory K72.0) O26.63
    with renal failure O90.4
  nervous system disorder O99.355
  obesity (pre-existing prior to pregnancy) O99.215
  obesity surgery status O99.845
  occlusion, precerebral artery O99.43
  paralysis
    bladder (sphincter) O90.89
    cerebral O99.43
  paralytic stroke O99.43
  parametritis O85
  paravaginitis O86.13
  pelviperitonitis O85
  perimetritis O86.12
  perimetrosalpingitis O86.19
  perinephritis O86.21
  periphlebitis — *see* Puerperal phlebitis
  peritoneal infection O85
  peritonitis (pelvic) O85
  perivaginitis O86.13
  phlebitis O87.0
    deep O87.1
    pelvic O87.1
    superficial O87.0
  phlebothrombosis, deep O87.1
  phlegmasia alba dolens O87.1
  placental polyp O90.89
  pneumonia, embolic — *see* Embolism, obstetric, puerperal
  pre-eclampsia — *see* Pre-eclampsia
  psychosis F53
  pyelitis O86.21
  pyelocystitis O86.29
  pyelonephritis O86.21
  pyelonephrosis O86.21
  pyemia O85
  pyocystitis O86.29
  pyohemia O85
  pyometra O86.12
  pyonephritis O86.21
  pyosalpingitis O86.19
  pyrexia (of unknown origin) O86.4
  renal
    disease NEC O90.89
    failure O90.4
  respiratory disease NEC O99.53
  retention
    decidua — *see* Retention, decidua
    placenta O72.0
    secundines — *see* Retention, secundines
  retrated nipple O92.02
  salpingo-ovaritis O86.19

**Puerperal, puerperium** — *continued*
  salpingoperitonitis O85
  secondary perineal tear O90.1
  sepsis (pelvic) O85
  sepsis O85
  septic thrombophlebitis O86.81
  skin disorder NEC O99.73
  specified condition NEC O99.89
  stroke O99.43
  subinvolution (uterus) O90.89
  subluxation of symphysis (pubis) O26.73
  suppuration — *see* Puerperal, abscess
  tetanus A34
  thelitis O91.02
    associated with lactation O91.03
  thrombocytopenia O72.3
  thrombophlebitis (superficial) O87.0
    deep O87.1
    pelvic O87.1
    septic O86.81
  thrombosis (venous) — *see* Thrombosis, puerperal
  thyroiditis O90.5
  toxemia (eclamptic) (pre-eclamptic) (with convulsions) O15.2
  trauma, non-obstetric O9A.23 (*following* O99)
    caused by abuse (physical) (suspected) O9A.33 (*following* O99)
      confirmed O9A.33 (*following* O99)
      psychological (suspected) O9A.53 (*following* O99)
        confirmed O9A.53 (*following* O99)
      sexual (suspected) O9A.43 (*following* O99)
        confirmed O9A.43 (*following* O99)
  uremia (due to renal failure) O90.4
  urethritis O86.22
  vaginitis O86.13
  varicose veins (legs) O87.4
    vulva or perineum O87.8
  venous O87.9
  vulvitis O86.19
  vulvovaginitis O86.13
  white leg O87.1
**Puerperium** — *see* Puerperal
**Pulmolithiasis** J98.4
**Pulmonary** — *see* condition
**Pulpitis** (acute) (anachoretic) (chronic) (hyperplastic) (putrescent) (suppurative) (ulcerative) K04.01
  irreversible K04.02
  reversible K04.01
**Pulpless tooth** K04.99
**Pulse**
  alternating R00.8
  bigeminal R00.8
  fast R00.0
  feeble, rapid due to shock following injury T79.4 ☑
  rapid R00.0
  weak R09.89
**Pulsus alternans or trigeminus** R00.8
**Punch drunk** F07.81
**Punctum lacrimale occlusion** — *see* Obstruction, lacrimal
**Puncture**
  abdomen, abdominal
    wall S31.139 ☑
      with
        foreign body S31.149 ☑
        penetration into peritoneal cavity S31.639 ☑
          with foreign body S31.649 ☑
    epigastric region S31.132 ☑
      with
        foreign body S31.142 ☑
        penetration into peritoneal cavity S31.632 ☑
          with foreign body S31.642 ☑
    left
      lower quadrant S31.134 ☑
        with
          foreign body S31.144 ☑
          penetration into peritoneal cavity S31.634 ☑
            with foreign body S31.644 ☑
      upper quadrant S31.131 ☑
        with
          foreign body S31.141 ☑
          penetration into peritoneal cavity S31.631 ☑
            with foreign body S31.641 ☑

**Puncture** — *continued*
  abdomen, abdominal — *continued*
    wall — *continued*
      periumbilic region S31.135 ☑
        with
          foreign body S31.145 ☑
          penetration into peritoneal cavity
            S31.635 ☑
            with foreign body S31.645 ☑
      right
        lower quadrant S31.133 ☑
          with
            foreign body S31.143 ☑
            penetration into peritoneal cavity
              S31.633 ☑
              with foreign body S31.643 ☑
        upper quadrant S31.130 ☑
          with
            foreign body S31.140 ☑
            penetration into peritoneal cavity
              S31.630 ☑
              with foreign body S31.640 ☑
  accidental, complicating surgery — *see* Complication,
    accidental puncture or laceration
  alveolar (process) — *see* Puncture, oral cavity
  ankle S91.039 ☑
    with
      foreign body S91.049 ☑
    left S91.032 ☑
      with
        foreign body S91.042 ☑
    right S91.031 ☑
      with
        foreign body S91.041 ☑
  anus S31.833 ☑
    with foreign body S31.834 ☑
  arm (upper) S41.139 ☑
    with foreign body S41.149 ☑
    left S41.132 ☑
      with foreign body S41.142 ☑
    lower — *see* Puncture, forearm
    right S41.131 ☑
      with foreign body S41.141 ☑
  auditory canal (external) (meatus) — *see* Puncture,
    ear
  auricle, ear — *see* Puncture, ear
  axilla — *see* Puncture, arm
  back (*see also* Puncture, thorax, back)
    lower S31.030 ☑
      with
        foreign body S31.040 ☑
          with penetration into retroperitoneal
            space S31.041 ☑
        penetration into retroperitoneal space
          S31.031 ☑
  bladder (traumatic) S37.29 ☑
    nontraumatic N32.89
  breast S21.039 ☑
    with foreign body S21.049 ☑
    left S21.032 ☑
      with foreign body S21.042 ☑
    right S21.031 ☑
      with foreign body S21.041 ☑
  buttock S31.803 ☑
    with foreign body S31.804 ☑
    left S31.823 ☑
      with foreign body S31.824 ☑
    right S31.813 ☑
      with foreign body S31.814 ☑
  by
    device, implant or graft — *see* Complications, by
      site and type, mechanical
    foreign body left accidentally in operative wound
      T81.539 ☑
    instrument (any) during a procedure, accidental
      — *see* Puncture, accidental complicating
      surgery
  calf — *see* Puncture, leg
  canaliculus lacrimalis — *see* Puncture, eyelid
  canthus, eye — *see* Puncture, eyelid
  cervical esophagus S11.23 ☑
    with foreign body S11.24 ☑
  cheek (external) S01.439 ☑
    with foreign body S01.449 ☑
    internal — *see* Puncture, oral cavity
    left S01.432 ☑

**Puncture** — *continued*
  cheek — *continued*
    left — *continued*
      with foreign body S01.442 ☑
    right S01.431 ☑
      with foreign body S01.441 ☑
  chest wall — *see* Puncture, thorax
  chin — *see* Puncture, head, specified site NEC
  clitoris — *see* Puncture, vulva
  costal region — *see* Puncture, thorax
  digit(s)
    foot — *see* Puncture, toe
    hand — *see* Puncture, finger
  ear (canal) (external) S01.339 ☑
    with foreign body S01.349 ☑
    drum S09.2- ☑
    left S01.332 ☑
      with foreign body S01.342 ☑
    right S01.331 ☑
      with foreign body S01.341 ☑
  elbow S51.039 ☑
    with
      foreign body S51.049 ☑
    left S51.032 ☑
      with
        foreign body S51.042 ☑
    right S51.031 ☑
      with
        foreign body S51.041 ☑
  epididymis — *see* Puncture, testis
  epigastric region — *see* Puncture, abdomen, wall,
    epigastric
  epiglottis S11.83 ☑
    with foreign body S11.84 ☑
  esophagus
    cervical S11.23 ☑
      with foreign body S11.24 ☑
    thoracic S27.818 ☑
  eyeball S05.6- ☑
    with foreign body S05.5- ☑
  eyebrow — *see* Puncture, eyelid
  eyelid S01.13- ☑
    with foreign body S01.14- ☑
    left S01.132 ☑
      with foreign body S01.142 ☑
    right S01.131 ☑
      with foreign body S01.141 ☑
  face NEC — *see* Puncture, head, specified site NEC
  finger(s) S61.239 ☑
    with
      damage to nail S61.339 ☑
        with
          foreign body S61.349 ☑
      foreign body S61.249 ☑
    index S61.238 ☑
      with
        damage to nail S61.338 ☑
          with
            foreign body S61.348 ☑
        foreign body S61.248 ☑
      left S61.231 ☑
        with
          damage to nail S61.331 ☑
            with
              foreign body S61.341 ☑
          foreign body S61.241 ☑
      right S61.230 ☑
        with
          damage to nail S61.330 ☑
            with
              foreign body S61.340 ☑
          foreign body S61.240 ☑
    little S61.238 ☑
      with
        damage to nail S61.338 ☑
          with
            foreign body S61.348 ☑
        foreign body S61.248 ☑
      left S61.237 ☑
        with
          damage to nail S61.337 ☑
            with
              foreign body S61.347 ☑
          foreign body S61.247 ☑
      right S61.236 ☑

**Puncture** — *continued*
  finger(s) — *continued*
    little — *continued*
      right — *continued*
        with
          damage to nail S61.336 ☑
            with
              foreign body S61.346 ☑
          foreign body S61.246 ☑
    middle S61.238 ☑
      with
        damage to nail S61.338 ☑
          with
            foreign body S61.348 ☑
        foreign body S61.248 ☑
      left S61.233 ☑
        with
          damage to nail S61.333 ☑
            with
              foreign body S61.343 ☑
          foreign body S61.243 ☑
      right S61.232 ☑
        with
          damage to nail S61.332 ☑
            with
              foreign body S61.342 ☑
          foreign body S61.242 ☑
    ring S61.238 ☑
      with
        damage to nail S61.338 ☑
          with
            foreign body S61.348 ☑
        foreign body S61.248 ☑
      left S61.235 ☑
        with
          damage to nail S61.335 ☑
            with
              foreign body S61.345 ☑
          foreign body S61.245 ☑
      right S61.234 ☑
        with
          damage to nail S61.334 ☑
            with
              foreign body S61.344 ☑
          foreign body S61.244 ☑
  flank S31.139 ☑
    with foreign body S31.149 ☑
  foot (except toe(s) alone) S91.339 ☑
    with foreign body S91.349 ☑
    left S91.332 ☑
      with foreign body S91.342 ☑
    right S91.331 ☑
      with foreign body S91.341 ☑
    toe — *see* Puncture, toe
  forearm S51.839 ☑
    with
      foreign body S51.849 ☑
    elbow only — *see* Puncture, elbow
    left S51.832 ☑
      with
        foreign body S51.842 ☑
    right S51.831 ☑
      with
        foreign body S51.841 ☑
  forehead — *see* Puncture, head, specified site NEC
  genital organs, external
    female S31.532 ☑
      with foreign body S31.542 ☑
      vagina — *see* Puncture, vagina
      vulva — *see* Puncture, vulva
    male S31.531 ☑
      with foreign body S31.541 ☑
      penis — *see* Puncture, penis
      scrotum — *see* Puncture, scrotum
      testis — *see* Puncture, testis
  groin — *see* Puncture, abdomen, wall
  gum — *see* Puncture, oral cavity
  hand S61.439 ☑
    with
      foreign body S61.449 ☑
    finger — *see* Puncture, finger
    left S61.432 ☑
      with
        foreign body S61.442 ☑
    right S61.431 ☑

⬛ **Subterms under main terms may continue to next column or page**    ☑ **Additional Character Required — Refer to the Tabular List for Character Selection**    269

Puncture — Puncture

**Puncture** — *continued*

hand — *continued*
  right — *continued*
    with
      foreign body S61.441 ☑
    thumb — *see* Puncture, thumb
head S01.93 ☑
  with foreign body S01.94 ☑
  cheek — *see* Puncture, cheek
  ear — *see* Puncture, ear
  eyelid — *see* Puncture, eyelid
  lip — *see* Puncture, oral cavity
  nose — *see* Puncture, nose
  oral cavity — *see* Puncture, oral cavity
  scalp S01.03 ☑
    with foreign body S01.04 ☑
  specified site NEC S01.83 ☑
    with foreign body S01.84 ☑
  temporomandibular area — *see* Puncture, cheek
heart S26.99 ☑
  with hemopericardium S26.09 ☑
  without hemopericardium S26.19 ☑
heel — *see* Puncture, foot
hip S71.039 ☑
  with foreign body S71.049 ☑
  left S71.032 ☑
    with foreign body S71.042 ☑
  right S71.031 ☑
    with foreign body S71.041 ☑
hymen — *see* Puncture, vagina
hypochondrium — *see* Puncture, abdomen, wall
hypogastric region — *see* Puncture, abdomen, wall
inguinal region — *see* Puncture, abdomen, wall
instep — *see* Puncture, foot
internal organs — *see* Injury, by site
interscapular region — *see* Puncture, thorax, back
intestine
  large
    colon S36.599 ☑
      ascending S36.590 ☑
      descending S36.592 ☑
      sigmoid S36.593 ☑
      specified site NEC S36.598 ☑
      transverse S36.591 ☑
    rectum S36.69 ☑
  small S36.499 ☑
    duodenum S36.490 ☑
    specified site NEC S36.498 ☑
intra-abdominal organ S36.99 ☑
  gallbladder S36.128 ☑
  intestine — *see* Puncture, intestine
  liver S36.118 ☑
  pancreas — *see* Puncture, pancreas
  peritoneum S36.81 ☑
  specified site NEC S36.898 ☑
  spleen S36.09 ☑
  stomach S36.39 ☑
jaw — *see* Puncture, head, specified site NEC
knee S81.039 ☑
  with foreign body S81.049 ☑
  left S81.032 ☑
    with foreign body S81.042 ☑
  right S81.031 ☑
    with foreign body S81.041 ☑
labium (majus) (minus) — *see* Puncture, vulva
lacrimal duct — *see* Puncture, eyelid
larynx S11.013 ☑
  with foreign body S11.014 ☑
leg (lower) S81.839 ☑
  with foreign body S81.849 ☑
  foot — *see* Puncture, foot
  knee — *see* Puncture, knee
  left S81.832 ☑
    with foreign body S81.842 ☑
  right S81.831 ☑
    with foreign body S81.841 ☑
  upper — *see* Puncture, thigh
lip S01.531 ☑
  with foreign body S01.541 ☑
loin — *see* Puncture, abdomen, wall
lower back — *see* Puncture, back, lower
lumbar region — *see* Puncture, back, lower
malar region — *see* Puncture, head, specified site NEC
mammary — *see* Puncture, breast
mastoid region — *see* Puncture, head, specified site NEC

**Puncture** — *continued*

mouth — *see* Puncture, oral cavity
nail
  finger — *see* Puncture, finger, with damage to nail
  toe — *see* Puncture, toe, with damage to nail
nasal (septum) (sinus) — *see* Puncture, nose
nasopharynx — *see* Puncture, head, specified site NEC
neck S11.93 ☑
  with foreign body S11.94 ☑
  involving
    cervical esophagus — *see* Puncture, cervical esophagus
    larynx — *see* Puncture, larynx
    pharynx — *see* Puncture, pharynx
    thyroid gland — *see* Puncture, thyroid gland
    trachea — *see* Puncture, trachea
  specified site NEC S11.83 ☑
    with foreign body S11.84 ☑
nose (septum) (sinus) S01.23 ☑
  with foreign body S01.24 ☑
ocular — *see* Puncture, eyeball
oral cavity S01.532 ☑
  with foreign body S01.542 ☑
orbit S05.4- ☑
palate — *see* Puncture, oral cavity
palm — *see* Puncture, hand
pancreas S36.299 ☑
  body S36.291 ☑
  head S36.290 ☑
  tail S36.292 ☑
pelvis — *see* Puncture, back, lower
penis S31.23 ☑
  with foreign body S31.24 ☑
perineum
  female S31.43 ☑
    with foreign body S31.44 ☑
  male S31.139 ☑
    with foreign body S31.149 ☑
periocular area (with or without lacrimal passages) — *see* Puncture, eyelid
phalanges
  finger — *see* Puncture, finger
  toe — *see* Puncture, toe
pharynx S11.23 ☑
  with foreign body S11.24 ☑
pinna — *see* Puncture, ear
popliteal space — *see* Puncture, knee
prepuce — *see* Puncture, penis
pubic region S31.139 ☑
  with foreign body S31.149 ☑
pudendum — *see* Puncture, genital organs, external
rectovaginal septum — *see* Puncture, vagina
sacral region — *see* Puncture, back, lower
sacroiliac region — *see* Puncture, back, lower
salivary gland — *see* Puncture, oral cavity
scalp S01.03 ☑
  with foreign body S01.04 ☑
scapular region — *see* Puncture, shoulder
scrotum S31.33 ☑
  with foreign body S31.34 ☑
shin — *see* Puncture, leg
shoulder S41.039 ☑
  with foreign body S41.049 ☑
  left S41.032 ☑
    with foreign body S41.042 ☑
  right S41.031 ☑
    with foreign body S41.041 ☑
spermatic cord — *see* Puncture, testis
sternal region — *see* Puncture, thorax, front
submaxillary region — *see* Puncture, head, specified site NEC
submental region — *see* Puncture, head, specified site NEC
subungual
  finger(s) — *see* Puncture, finger, with damage to nail
  toe — *see* Puncture, toe, with damage to nail
supraclavicular fossa — *see* Puncture, neck, specified site NEC
temple, temporal region — *see* Puncture, head, specified site NEC
temporomandibular area — *see* Puncture, cheek
testis S31.33 ☑
  with foreign body S31.34 ☑
thigh S71.139 ☑
  with foreign body S71.149 ☑

**Puncture** — *continued*

thigh — *continued*
  left S71.132 ☑
    with foreign body S71.142 ☑
  right S71.131 ☑
    with foreign body S71.141 ☑
thorax, thoracic (wall) S21.93 ☑
  with foreign body S21.94 ☑
  back S21.23- ☑
    with
      foreign body S21.24- ☑
        with penetration S21.44 ☑
      penetration S21.43 ☑
  breast — *see* Puncture, breast
  front S21.13- ☑
    with
      foreign body S21.14- ☑
        with penetration S21.34 ☑
      penetration S21.33 ☑
throat — *see* Puncture, neck
thumb S61.039 ☑
  with
    damage to nail S61.139 ☑
      with
        foreign body S61.149 ☑
    foreign body S61.049 ☑
  left S61.032 ☑
    with
      damage to nail S61.132 ☑
        with
          foreign body S61.142 ☑
      foreign body S61.042 ☑
  right S61.031 ☑
    with
      damage to nail S61.131 ☑
        with
          foreign body S61.141 ☑
      foreign body S61.041 ☑
thyroid gland S11.13 ☑
  with foreign body S11.14 ☑
toe(s) S91.139 ☑
  with
    damage to nail S91.239 ☑
      with
        foreign body S91.249 ☑
    foreign body S91.149 ☑
  great S91.133 ☑
    with
      damage to nail S91.233 ☑
        with
          foreign body S91.243 ☑
      foreign body S91.143 ☑
    left S91.132 ☑
      with
        damage to nail S91.232 ☑
          with
            foreign body S91.242 ☑
        foreign body S91.142 ☑
    right S91.131 ☑
      with
        damage to nail S91.231 ☑
          with
            foreign body S91.241 ☑
        foreign body S91.141 ☑
  lesser S91.136 ☑
    with
      damage to nail S91.236 ☑
        with
          foreign body S91.246 ☑
      foreign body S91.146 ☑
    left S91.135 ☑
      with
        damage to nail S91.235 ☑
          with
            foreign body S91.245 ☑
        foreign body S91.145 ☑
    right S91.134 ☑
      with
        damage to nail S91.234 ☑
          with
            foreign body S91.244 ☑
        foreign body S91.144 ☑
tongue — *see* Puncture, oral cavity
trachea S11.023 ☑
  with foreign body S11.024 ☑
tunica vaginalis — *see* Puncture, testis

☑ **Additional Character Required — Refer to the Tabular List for Character Selection**     ▽ **Subterms under main terms may continue to next column or page**

**Puncture** — *continued*
    tympanum, tympanic membrane S09.2- ☑
    umbilical region S31.135 ☑
        with foreign body S31.145 ☑
    uvula — *see* Puncture, oral cavity
    vagina S31.43 ☑
        with foreign body S31.44 ☑
    vocal cords S11.033 ☑
        with foreign body S11.034 ☑
    vulva S31.43 ☑
        with foreign body S31.44 ☑
    wrist S61.539 ☑
        with
            foreign body S61.549 ☑
        left S61.532 ☑
            with
                foreign body S61.542 ☑
        right S61.531 ☑
            with
                foreign body S61.541 ☑
**PUO** (pyrexia of unknown origin) R50.9
**Pupillary membrane** (persistent) Q13.89
**Pupillotonia** — *see* Anomaly, pupil, function, tonic pupil
**Purpura** D69.2
    abdominal D69.0
    allergic D69.0
    anaphylactoid D69.0
    annularis telangiectodes L81.7
    arthritic D69.0
    autoerythrocyte sensitization D69.2
    autoimmune D69.0
    bacterial D69.0
    Bateman's (senile) D69.2
    capillary fragility (hereditary) (idiopathic) D69.8
    cryoglobulinemic D89.1
    Devil's pinches D69.2
    fibrinolytic — *see* Fibrinolysis
    fulminans, fulminous D65
    gangrenous D69.0
    hemorrhagic, hemorrhagica D69.3
        not due to thrombocytopenia D69.0
    Henoch (-Schönlein) (allergic) D69.0
    hypergammaglobulinemic (benign) (Waldenström)
        D89.0
    idiopathic (thrombocytopenic) D69.3
        nonthrombocytopenic D69.0
    immune thrombocytopenic D69.3
    infectious D69.0
    malignant D69.0
    neonatorum P54.5
    nervosa D69.0
    newborn P54.5
    nonthrombocytopenic D69.2
        hemorrhagic D69.0
        idiopathic D69.0
    nonthrombopenic D69.2
    peliosis rheumatica D69.0
    posttransfusion (post-transfusion) (from (fresh) whole
        blood or blood products) D69.51
    primary D69.49
    red cell membrane sensitivity D69.2
    rheumatica D69.0
    Schönlein (-Henoch) (allergic) D69.0
    scorbutic E54 [D77]
    senile D69.2
    simplex D69.2
    symptomatica D69.0
    telangiectasia annularis L81.7
    thrombocytopenic D69.49
        congenital D69.42
        hemorrhagic D69.3
        hereditary D69.42
        idiopathic D69.3
        immune D69.3
        neonatal, transitory P61.0
        thrombotic M31.1
    thrombohemolytic — *see* Fibrinolysis
    thrombolytic — *see* Fibrinolysis
    thrombopenic D69.49
    thrombotic, thrombocytopenic M31.1
    toxic D69.0
    vascular D69.0
    visceral symptoms D69.0
**Purpuric spots** R23.3
**Purulent** — *see* condition
**Pus**
    in
        stool R19.5

**Pus** — *continued*
    in — *continued*
        urine N39.0
    tube (rupture) — *see* Salpingo-oophoritis
**Pustular rash** L08.0
**Pustule** (nonmalignant) L08.9
    malignant A22.0
**Pustulosis palmaris et plantaris** L40.3
**Putnam** (-Dana) **disease or syndrome** — *see* Degeneration, combined
**Putrescent pulp** (dental) K04.1
**Pyarthritis, pyarthrosis** — *see* Arthritis, pyogenic or pyemic
    tuberculous — *see* Tuberculosis, joint
**Pyelectasis** — *see* Hydronephrosis
**Pyelitis** (congenital) (uremic) (*see also* Pyelonephritis)
    with
        calculus — *see* category N20 ☑
            with hydronephrosis N13.2
        contracted kidney N11.9
    acute N10
    chronic N11.9
        with calculus — *see* category N20 ☑
            with hydronephrosis N13.2
    cystica N28.84
    puerperal (postpartum) O86.21
    tuberculous A18.11
**Pyelocystitis** — *see* Pyelonephritis
**Pyelonephritis** (*see also* Nephritis, tubulo-interstitial)
    with
        calculus — *see* category N20 ☑
            with hydronephrosis N13.2
        contracted kidney N11.9
    acute N10
    calculous — *see* category N20 ☑
        with hydronephrosis N13.2
    chronic N11.9
        with calculus — *see* category N20 ☑
            with hydronephrosis N13.2
        associated with ureteral obstruction or stricture
            N11.1
        nonobstructive N11.8
            with reflux (vesicoureteral) N11.0
        obstructive N11.1
        specified NEC N11.8
    in (due to)
        brucellosis A23.9 [N16]
        cryoglobulinemia (mixed) D89.1 [N16]
        cystinosis E72.04
        diphtheria A36.84
        glycogen storage disease E74.09 [N16]
        leukemia NEC C95.9- ☑ [N16]
        lymphoma NEC C85.90 [N16]
        multiple myeloma C90.0- ☑ [N16]
        obstruction N11.1
        Salmonella infection A02.25
        sarcoidosis D86.84
        sepsis A41.9 [N16]
        Sjögren's disease M35.04
        toxoplasmosis B58.83
        transplant rejection T86.91 [N16]
        Wilson's disease E83.01 [N16]
    nonobstructive N12
        with reflux (vesicoureteral) N11.0
        chronic N11.8
    syphilitic A52.75
**Pyelonephrosis** (obstructive) N11.1
    chronic N11.9
**Pyelophlebitis** I80.8
**Pyeloureteritis cystica** N28.85
**Pyemia, pyemic** (fever) (infection) (purulent) (*see also*
    Sepsis)
    joint — *see* Arthritis, pyogenic or pyemic
    liver K75.1
    pneumococcal A40.3
    portal K75.1
    postvaccinal T88.0 ☑
    puerperal, postpartum, childbirth O85
    specified organism NEC A41.89
    tuberculous — *see* Tuberculosis, miliary
**Pygopagus** Q89.4
**Pyknoepilepsy** (idiopathic) — *see* Pyknolepsy
**Pyknolepsy** G40.A09 (*following* G40.3)
    intractable G40.A19 (*following* G40.3)
        with status epilepticus G40.A11 (*following* G40.3)
        without status epilepticus G40.A19 (*following*
            G40.3)
    not intractable G40.A09 (*following* G40.3)

**Pyknolepsy** — *continued*
    not intractable — *continued*
        with status epilepticus G40.A01 (*following* G40.3)
        without status epilepticus G40.A09 (*following*
            G40.3)
**Pylephlebitis** K75.1
**Pyle's syndrome** Q78.5
**Pylethrombophlebitis** K75.1
**Pylethrombosis** K75.1
**Pyloritis** K29.90
    with bleeding K29.91
**Pylorospasm** (reflex) **NEC** K31.3
    congenital or infantile Q40.0
    neurotic F45.8
    newborn Q40.0
    psychogenic F45.8
**Pylorus, pyloric** — *see* condition
**Pyoarthrosis** — *see* Arthritis, pyogenic or pyemic
**Pyocele**
    mastoid — *see* Mastoiditis, acute
    sinus (accessory) — *see* Sinusitis
    turbinate (bone) J32.9
    urethra (*see also* Urethritis) N34.0
**Pyocolpos** — *see* Vaginitis
**Pyocystitis** N30.80
    with hematuria N30.81
**Pyoderma, pyodermia** L08.0
    gangrenosum L88
    newborn P39.4
    phagedenic L88
    vegetans L08.81
**Pyodermatitis** L08.0
    vegetans L08.81
**Pyogenic** — *see* condition
**Pyohydronephrosis** N13.6
**Pyometra, pyometrium, pyometritis** — *see* Endometritis
**Pyomyositis** (tropical) — *see* Myositis, infective
**Pyonephritis** N12
**Pyonephrosis** N13.6
    tuberculous A18.11
**Pyo-oophoritis** — *see* Salpingo-oophoritis
**Pyo-ovarium** — *see* Salpingo-oophoritis
**Pyopericarditis, pyopericardium** I30.1
**Pyophlebitis** — *see* Phlebitis
**Pyopneumopericardium** I30.1
**Pyopneumothorax** (infective) J86.9
    with fistula J86.0
    tuberculous NEC A15.6
**Pyosalpinx, pyosalpingitis** (*see also* Salpingo-
    oophoritis)
**Pyothorax** J86.9
    with fistula J86.0
    tuberculous NEC A15.6
**Pyoureter** N28.89
    tuberculous A18.11
**Pyramidopallidonigral syndrome** G20
**Pyrexia** (of unknown origin) R50.9
    atmospheric T67.0 ☑
    during labor NEC O75.2
    heat T67.0 ☑
    newborn P81.9
        environmentally-induced P81.0
    persistent R50.9
    puerperal O86.4
**Pyroglobulinemia NEC** E88.09
**Pyromania** F63.1
**Pyrosis** R12
**Pyuria** (bacterial) N39.0

# Q

**Q fever** A78
    with pneumonia A78
**Quadricuspid aortic valve** Q23.8
**Quadrilateral fever** A78
**Quadriparesis** — *see* Quadriplegia
    meaning muscle weakness M62.81
**Quadriplegia** G82.50
    complete
        C1-C4 level G82.51
        C5-C7 level G82.53
    congenital (cerebral) (spinal) G80.8
        spastic G80.0
    embolic (current episode) I63.4- ☑
    functional R53.2

**Reaction** — *continued*
 nitritoid — *see* Crisis, nitritoid
 nonspecific
  to
   cell mediated immunity measurement of gamma interferon antigen response without active tuberculosis R76.12
   QuantiFERON-TB test (QFT) without active tuberculosis R76.12
   tuberculin test (*see also* Reaction, tuberculin skin test) R76.11
 obsessive-compulsive F42.8
 organic, acute or subacute — *see* Delirium
 paranoid (acute) F23
  chronic F22
  senile F03 ☑
 passive dependency F60.7
 phobic F40.9
 post-traumatic stress, uncomplicated Z73.3
 psychogenic F99
 psychoneurotic (*see also* Neurosis)
  compulsive F42.8
  depersonalization F48.1
  depressive F34.1
  hypochondriacal F45.20
  neurasthenic F48.8
  obsessive F42.8
 psychophysiologic — *see* Disorder, somatoform
 psychosomatic — *see* Disorder, somatoform
 psychotic — *see* Psychosis
 scarlet fever toxin — *see* Complications, vaccination
 schizophrenic F23
  acute (brief) (undifferentiated) F23
  latent F21
  undifferentiated (acute) (brief) F23
 serological for syphilis — *see* Serology for syphilis
 serum T80.69 ☑
  anaphylactic (immediate) (*see also* Shock, anaphylactic) T80.59 ☑
  specified reaction NEC
   due to
    administration of blood and blood products T80.61 ☑
    immunization T80.62 ☑
    serum specified NEC T80.69 ☑
    vaccination T80.62 ☑
 situational — *see* Disorder, adjustment
 somatization — *see* Disorder, somatoform
 spinal puncture G97.1
 stress (severe) F43.9
  acute (agitation) ("daze") (disorientation) (disturbance of consciousness) (flight reaction) (fugue) F43.0
  specified NEC F43.8
 surgical procedure — *see* Complications, surgical procedure
 tetanus antitoxin — *see* Complications, vaccination
 toxic, to local anesthesia T88.59 ☑
  in labor and delivery O74.4
  in pregnancy O29.3X- ☑
  postpartum, puerperal O89.3
 toxin-antitoxin — *see* Complications, vaccination
 transfusion (blood) (bone marrow) (lymphocytes) (allergic) — *see* Complications, transfusion
 tuberculin skin test, abnormal R76.11
 vaccination (any) — *see* Complications, vaccination
 withdrawing, child or adolescent F93.8
**Reactive airway disease** — *see* Asthma
**Reactive depression** — *see* Reaction, depressive
**Rearrangement**
 chromosomal
  balanced (in) Q95.9
   abnormal individual (autosomal) Q95.2
    non-sex (autosomal) chromosomes Q95.2
    sex/non-sex chromosomes Q95.3
   specified NEC Q95.8
**Recalcitrant patient** — *see* Noncompliance
**Recanalization, thrombus** — *see* Thrombosis
**Recession, receding**
 chamber angle (eye) H21.55- ☑
 chin M26.09
 gingival (postinfective) (postoperative)
  generalized K06.020
   minimal K06.021
   moderate K06.022
   severe K06.023
  localized K06.010
   minimal K06.011

**Recession, receding** — *continued*
 gingival — *continued*
  localized — *continued*
   moderate K06.012
   severe K06.013
**Recklinghausen disease** Q85.01
 bones E21.0
**Reclus' disease** (cystic) — *see* Mastopathy, cystic
**Recrudescent typhus** (fever) A75.1
**Recruitment, auditory** H93.21- ☑
**Rectalgia** K62.89
**Rectitis** K62.89
**Rectocele**
 female (without uterine prolapse) N81.6
  with uterine prolapse N81.4
   incomplete N81.2
 in pregnancy — *see* Pregnancy, complicated by, abnormal, pelvic organs or tissues NEC
 male K62.3
**Rectosigmoid junction** — *see* condition
**Rectosigmoiditis** K63.89
 ulcerative (chronic) K51.30
  with
   complication K51.319
    abscess K51.314
    fistula K51.313
    obstruction K51.312
    rectal bleeding K51.311
    specified NEC K51.318
**Rectourethral** — *see* condition
**Rectovaginal** — *see* condition
**Rectovesical** — *see* condition
**Rectum, rectal** — *see* condition
**Recurrent** — *see* condition
 pregnancy loss — *see* Loss (of), pregnancy, recurrent
**Red bugs** B88.0
**Red tide** (*see also* Table of Drugs and Chemicals) T65.82- ☑
**Red-cedar lung or pneumonitis** J67.8
**Reduced**
 mobility Z74.09
 ventilatory or vital capacity R94.2
**Redundant, redundancy**
 anus (congenital) Q43.8
 clitoris N90.89
 colon (congenital) Q43.8
 foreskin (congenital) N47.8
 intestine (congenital) Q43.8
 labia N90.69
 organ or site, congenital NEC — *see* Accessory
 panniculus (abdominal) E65
 prepuce (congenital) N47.8
 pylorus K31.89
 rectum (congenital) Q43.8
 scrotum N50.89
 sigmoid (congenital) Q43.8
 skin L98.7
  and subcutaneous tissue L98.7
  of face L57.4
   eyelids — *see* Blepharochalasis
 stomach K31.89
**Reduplication** — *see* Duplication
**Reflex** R29.2
 hyperactive gag J39.2
 pupillary, abnormal — *see* Anomaly, pupil, function
 vasoconstriction I73.9
 vasovagal R55
**Reflux** K21.9
 acid K21.9
 esophageal K21.9
  with esophagitis K21.0
  newborn P78.83
 gastroesophageal K21.9
  with esophagitis K21.0
 mitral — *see* Insufficiency, mitral
 ureteral — *see* Reflux, vesicoureteral
 vesicoureteral (with scarring) N13.70
  with
   nephropathy N13.729
    with hydroureter N13.739
     bilateral N13.732
     unilateral N13.731
    without hydroureter N13.729
     bilateral N13.722
     unilateral N13.721
   bilateral N13.722
   unilateral N13.721
  pyelonephritis (chronic) N11.0

**Reflux** — *continued*
 vesicoureteral — *continued*
  without nephropathy N13.71
  congenital Q62.7
**Reforming, artificial openings** — *see* Attention to, artificial, opening
**Refractive error** — *see* Disorder, refraction
**Refsum's disease or syndrome** G60.1
**Refusal of**
 food, psychogenic F50.89
 treatment (because of) Z53.20
  left against medical advice (AMA) Z53.21
  patient's decision NEC Z53.29
  reasons of belief or group pressure Z53.1
**Regional** — *see* condition
**Regurgitation** R11.10
 aortic (valve) — *see* Insufficiency, aortic
 food (*see also* Vomiting)
  with reswallowing — *see* Rumination
  newborn P92.1
 gastric contents — *see* Vomiting
 heart — *see* Endocarditis
 mitral (valve) — *see* Insufficiency, mitral
  congenital Q23.3
 myocardial — *see* Endocarditis
 pulmonary (valve) (heart) I37.1
  congenital Q22.2
  syphilitic A52.03
 tricuspid — *see* Insufficiency, tricuspid
 valve, valvular — *see* Endocarditis
  congenital Q24.8
 vesicoureteral — *see* Reflux, vesicoureteral
**Reichmann's disease or syndrome** K31.89
**Reifenstein syndrome** E34.52
**Reinsertion**
 implantable subdermal contraceptive Z30.46
 intrauterine contraceptive device Z30.433
**Reiter's disease, syndrome, or urethritis** M02.30
 ankle M02.37- ☑
 elbow M02.32- ☑
 foot joint M02.37- ☑
 hand joint M02.34- ☑
 hip M02.35- ☑
 knee M02.36- ☑
 multiple site M02.39
 shoulder M02.31- ☑
 vertebra M02.38
 wrist M02.33- ☑
**Rejection**
 food, psychogenic F50.89
 transplant T86.91
  bone T86.830
   marrow T86.01
  cornea T86.840
  heart T86.21
   with lung(s) T86.31
  intestine T86.850
  kidney T86.11
  liver T86.41
  lung(s) T86.810
   with heart T86.31
  organ (immune or nonimmune cause) T86.91
  pancreas T86.890
  skin (allograft) (autograft) T86.820
  specified NEC T86.890
  stem cell (peripheral blood) (umbilical cord) T86.5
**Relapsing fever** A68.9
 Carter's (Asiatic) A68.1
 Dutton's (West African) A68.1
 Koch's A68.9
 louse-borne (epidemic) A68.0
 Novy's (American) A68.1
 Obermeyers's (European) A68.0
 Spirillum A68.9
 tick-borne (endemic) A68.1
**Relationship**
 occlusal
  open anterior M26.220
  open posterior M26.221
**Relaxation**
 anus (sphincter) K62.89
  psychogenic F45.8
 arch (foot) (*see also* Deformity, limb, flat foot)
 back ligaments — *see* Instability, joint, spine
 bladder (sphincter) N31.2
 cardioesophageal K21.9
 cervix — *see* Incompetency, cervix
 diaphragm J98.6

Subterms under main terms may continue to next column or page    ☑ Additional Character Required — Refer to the Tabular List for Character Selection    273

Reaction — Relaxation

**Relaxation** — *continued*
  joint (capsule) (ligament) (paralytic) — *see* Flail, joint
    congenital NEC Q74.8
  lumbosacral (joint) — *see* subcategory M53.2 ☑
  pelvic floor N81.89
  perineum N81.89
  posture R29.3
  rectum (sphincter) K62.89
  sacroiliac (joint) — *see* subcategory M53.2 ☑
  scrotum N50.89
  urethra (sphincter) N36.44
  vesical N31.2
**Release from prison, anxiety concerning** Z65.2
**Remains**
  canal of Cloquet Q14.0
  capsule (opaque) Q14.8
**Remittent fever** (malarial) B54
**Remnant**
  canal of Cloquet Q14.0
  capsule (opaque) Q14.8
  cervix, cervical stump (acquired) (postoperative) N88.8
  cystic duct, postcholecystectomy K91.5
  fingernail L60.8
    congenital Q84.6
  meniscus, knee — *see* Derangement, knee, meniscus,
    specified NEC
  thyroglossal duct Q89.2
  tonsil J35.8
    infected (chronic) J35.01
  urachus Q64.4
**Removal** (from) (of)
  artificial
    arm Z44.00- ☑
      complete Z44.01- ☑
      partial Z44.02- ☑
    eye Z44.2- ☑
    leg Z44.10- ☑
      complete Z44.11- ☑
      partial Z44.12- ☑
  breast implant Z45.81 ☑
  cardiac pulse generator (battery) (end-of-life) Z45.010
  catheter (urinary) (indwelling) Z46.6
    from artificial opening — *see* Attention to, artificial,
      opening
    non-vascular Z46.82
    vascular NEC Z45.2
  device Z46.9
    contraceptive Z30.432
      implantable subdermal Z30.46
    implanted NEC Z45.89
    specified NEC Z46.89
  drains Z48.03
  dressing (nonsurgical) Z48.00
    surgical Z48.01
  external
    fixation device — *code to* fracture with seventh
      character D
    prosthesis, prosthetic device Z44.9
      breast Z44.3- ☑
      specified NEC Z44.8
  home in childhood (to foster home or institution)
    Z62.29
  ileostomy Z43.2
  insulin pump Z46.81
  myringotomy device (stent) (tube) Z45.82
  nervous system device NEC Z46.2
    brain neuropacemaker Z46.2
    visual substitution device Z46.2
      implanted Z45.31
  non-vascular catheter Z46.82
  organ, prophylactic (for neoplasia management) —
    *see* Prophylactic, organ removal
  orthodontic device Z46.4
  staples Z48.02
  stent
    ureteral Z46.6
  suture Z48.02
  urinary device Z46.6
  vascular access device or catheter Z45.2
**Ren**
  arcuatus Q63.1
  mobile, mobilis N28.89
    congenital Q63.8
  unguliformis Q63.1
**Renal** — *see* condition
**Rendu-Osler-Weber disease or syndrome** I78.0
**Reninoma** D41.0- ☑
**Renon-Delille syndrome** E23.3

**Reovirus, as cause of disease classified elsewhere**
    B97.5
**Repeated falls NEC** R29.6
**Replaced chromosome by dicentric ring** Q93.2
**Replacement by artificial or mechanical device or**
    **prosthesis of**
  bladder Z96.0
  blood vessel NEC Z95.828
  bone NEC Z96.7
  cochlea Z96.21
  coronary artery Z95.5
  eustachian tube Z96.29
  eye globe Z97.0
  heart Z95.812
    valve Z95.2
      prosthetic Z95.2
      specified NEC Z95.4
      xenogenic Z95.3
  intestine Z96.89
  joint Z96.60
    hip — *see* Presence, hip joint implant
    knee — *see* Presence, knee joint implant
    specified site NEC Z96.698
  larynx Z96.3
  lens Z96.1
  limb(s) — *see* Presence, artificial, limb
  mandible NEC (for tooth root implant(s)) Z96.5
  organ NEC Z96.89
  peripheral vessel NEC Z95.828
  stapes Z96.29
  teeth Z97.2
  tendon Z96.7
  tissue NEC Z96.89
  tooth root(s) Z96.5
  vessel NEC Z95.828
    coronary (artery) Z95.5
**Request for expert evidence** Z04.8
**Reserve, decreased or low**
  cardiac — *see* Disease, heart
  kidney N28.89
**Residual** (*see also* condition)
  ovary syndrome N99.83
  state, schizophrenic F20.5
  urine R39.198
**Resistance, resistant** (to)
  activated protein C D68.51
  complicating pregnancy O26.89 ☑
  insulin E88.81
  organism(s)
    to
      drug Z16.30
        aminoglycosides Z16.29
        amoxicillin Z16.11
        ampicillin Z16.11
        antibiotic(s) Z16.20
          multiple Z16.24
          specified NEC Z16.29
        antifungal Z16.32
        antimicrobial (single) Z16.30
          multiple Z16.35
          specified NEC Z16.39
        antimycobacterial (single) Z16.341
          multiple Z16.342
        antiparasitic Z16.31
        antiviral Z16.33
        beta lactam antibiotics Z16.10
          specified NEC Z16.19
        cephalosporins Z16.19
        extended beta lactamase (ESBL) Z16.12
        fluoroquinolones Z16.23
        macrolides Z16.29
        methicillin — *see* MRSA
        multiple drugs (MDRO)
          antibiotics Z16.24
          antimicrobial Z16.35
          antimycobacterials Z16.342
        penicillins Z16.11
        quinine (and related compounds) Z16.31
        quinolones Z16.23
        sulfonamides Z16.29
        tetracyclines Z16.29
        tuberculostatics (single) Z16.341
          multiple Z16.342
        vancomycin Z16.21
          related antibiotics Z16.22
  thyroid hormone E07.89
**Resorption**
  dental (roots) K03.3

**Resorption** — *continued*
  dental — *continued*
    alveoli M26.79
  teeth (external) (internal) (pathological) (roots) K03.3
**Respiration**
  Cheyne-Stokes R06.3
  decreased due to shock, following injury T79.4 ☑
  disorder of, psychogenic F45.8
  insufficient, or poor R06.89
    newborn P28.5
  painful R07.1
  sighing, psychogenic F45.8
**Respiratory** (*see also* condition)
  distress syndrome (newborn) (type I) P22.0
    type II P22.1
  syncytial virus, as cause of disease classified elsewhere
    B97.4
**Respite care** Z75.5
**Response** (drug)
  photoallergic L56.1
  phototoxic L56.0
**Restenosis**
  stent
    vascular
      end stent
        adjacent to stent — *see* Arteriosclerosis
        within the stent
          coronary T82.855 ☑
          peripheral T82.856 ☑
      in stent
        coronary vessel T82.855 ☑
        peripheral vessel T82.856 ☑
**Restless legs** (syndrome) G25.81
**Restlessness** R45.1
**Restoration** (of)
  dental
    aesthetically inadequate or displeasing K08.56
    defective K08.50
      specified NEC K08.59
    failure of marginal integrity K08.51
    failure of periodontal anatomical intergrity K08.54
  organ continuity from previous sterilization (tuboplas-
    ty) (vasoplasty) Z31.0
    aftercare Z31.42
  tooth (existing)
    contours biologically incompatible with oral health
      K08.54
    open margins K08.51
    overhanging K08.52
    poor aesthetic K08.56
    poor gingival margins K08.51
  unsatisfactory, of tooth K08.50
    specified NEC K08.59
**Restorative material** (dental)
  allergy to K08.55
  fractured K08.539
    with loss of material K08.531
    without loss of material K08.530
  unrepairable overhanging of K08.52
**Restriction of housing space** Z59.1
**Rests, ovarian, in fallopian tube** Q50.6
**Restzustand** (schizophrenic) F20.5
**Retained** (*see also* Retention)
  cholelithiasis following cholecystectomy K91.86
  foreign body fragments (type of) Z18.9
    acrylics Z18.2
    animal quill(s) or spines Z18.31
    cement Z18.83
    concrete Z18.83
    crystalline Z18.83
    depleted isotope Z18.09
    depleted uranium Z18.01
    diethylhexylphthalates Z18.2
    glass Z18.81
    isocyanate Z18.2
    magnetic metal Z18.11
    metal Z18.10
    nonmagnetic metal Z18.12
    nontherapeutic radioactive Z18.09
    organic NEC Z18.39
    plastic Z18.2
    quill(s) (animal) Z18.31
    radioactive (nontherapeutic) NEC Z18.09
    specified NEC Z18.89
    spine(s) (animal) Z18.31
    stone Z18.83
    tooth (teeth) Z18.32
    wood Z18.33

**Retained** — *continued*
  fragments (type of ) Z18.9
    acrylics Z18.2
    animal quill(s) or spines Z18.31
    cement Z18.83
    concrete Z18.83
    crystalline Z18.83
    depleted isotope Z18.09
    depleted uranium Z18.01
    diethylhexylphthalates Z18.2
    glass Z18.81
    isocyanate Z18.2
    magnetic metal Z18.11
    metal Z18.10
    nonmagnectic metal Z18.12
    nontherapeutic radioactive Z18.09
    organic NEC Z18.39
    plastic Z18.2
    quill(s) (animal) Z18.31
    radioactive (nontherapeutic) NEC Z18.09
    specified NEC Z18.89
    spine(s) (animal) Z18.31
    stone Z18.83
    tooth (teeth) Z18.32
    wood Z18.33
  gallstones, following cholecystectomy K91.86
**Retardation**
  development, developmental, specific — *see* Disorder, developmental
  endochondral bone growth — *see* Disorder, bone, development or growth
  growth R62.50
    due to malnutrition E45
  mental — *see* Disability, intellectual
  motor function, specific F82
  physical (child) R62.52
    due to malnutrition E45
  reading (specific) F81.0
  spelling (specific) (without reading disorder) F81.81
**Retching** — *see* Vomiting
**Retention** (*see also* Retained)
  bladder — *see* Retention, urine
  carbon dioxide E87.2
  cholelithiasis following cholecystectomy K91.86
  cyst — *see* Cyst
  dead
    fetus (at or near term) (mother) O36.4 ☑
      early fetal death O02.1
    ovum O02.0
  decidua (fragments) (following delivery) (with hemorrhage) O72.2
    without hemorrhage O73.1
  deciduous tooth K00.6
  dental root K08.3
  fecal — *see* Constipation
  fetus
    dead O36.4 ☑
      early O02.1
  fluid R60.9
  foreign body (*see also* Foreign body, retained)
    current trauma — *code as* Foreign body, by site or type
  gallstones, following cholecystectomy K91.86
  gastric K31.89
  intrauterine contraceptive device, in pregnancy — *see* Pregnancy, complicated by, retention, intrauterine device
  membranes (complicating delivery) (with hemorrhage) O72.2
    with abortion — *see* Abortion, by type
    without hemorrhage O73.1
  meniscus — *see* Derangement, meniscus
  menses N94.89
  milk (puerperal, postpartum) O92.79
  nitrogen, extrarenal R39.2
  ovary syndrome N99.83
  placenta (total) (with hemorrhage) O72.0
    without hemorrhage O73.0
    portions or fragments (with hemorrhage) O72.2
      without hemorrhage O73.1
  products of conception
    early pregnancy (dead fetus) O02.1
    following
      delivery (with hemorrhage) O72.2
        without hemorrhage O73.1
  secundines (following delivery) (with hemorrhage) O72.0
    without hemorrhage O73.0

**Retention** — *continued*
  secundines — *continued*
    complicating puerperium (delayed hemorrhage) O72.2
    partial O72.2
      without hemorrhage O73.1
  smegma, clitoris N90.89
  urine R33.9
    drug-induced R33.0
    due to hyperplasia (hypertrophy) of prostate — *see* Hyperplasia, prostate
    organic R33.8
      drug-induced R33.0
    psychogenic F45.8
    specified NEC R33.8
  water (in tissues) — *see* Edema
**Reticulation, dust** — *see* Pneumoconiosis
**Reticulocytosis** R70.1
**Reticuloendotheliosis**
  acute infantile C96.0
  leukemic C91.4- ☑
  nonlipid C96.0
**Reticulohistiocytoma** (giant-cell) D76.3
**Reticuloid, actinic** L57.1
**Reticulosis** (skin)
  acute of infancy C96.0
  hemophagocytic, familial D76.1
  histiocytic medullary C96.A (*following* C96.6)
  lipomelanotic I89.8
  malignant (midline) C86.0
  polymorphic C83.8- ☑
  Sézary — *see* Sézary disease
**Retina, retinal** (*see also* condition)
  dark area D49.81
**Retinitis** (*see also* Inflammation, chorioretinal)
  albuminurica N18.9 [H32]
  diabetic — *see* Diabetes, retinitis
  disciformis — *see* Degeneration, macula
  focal — *see* Inflammation, chorioretinal, focal
  gravidarum — *see* Pregnancy, complicated by, specified pregnancy-related condition NEC
  juxtapapillaris — *see* Inflammation, chorioretinal, focal, juxtapapillary
  luetic — *see* Retinitis, syphilitic
  pigmentosa H35.52
  proliferans — *see* Disorder, globe, degenerative, specified type NEC
  proliferating — *see* Disorder, globe, degenerative, specified type NEC
  renal N18.9 [H32]
  syphilitic (early) (secondary) A51.43
    central, recurrent A52.71
    congenital (early) A50.01 [H32]
    late A52.71
  tuberculous A18.53
**Retinoblastoma** C69.2- ☑
  differentiated C69.2- ☑
  undifferentiated C69.2- ☑
**Retinochoroiditis** (*see also* Inflammation, chorioretinal)
  disseminated — *see* Inflammation, chorioretinal, disseminated
    syphilitic A52.71
  focal — *see* Inflammation, chorioretinal
  juxtapapillaris — *see* Inflammation, chorioretinal, focal, juxtapapillary
**Retinopathy** (background) H35.00
  arteriosclerotic I70.8 [H35.0-] ☑
  atherosclerotic I70.8 [H35.0-] ☑
  central serous — *see* Chorioretinopathy, central serous
  Coats H35.02- ☑
  diabetic — *see* Diabetes, retinopathy
  exudative H35.02- ☑
  hypertensive H35.03- ☑
  in (due to)
    diabetes — *see* Diabetes, retinopathy
    sickle-cell disorders D57.- ☑ [H36]
  of prematurity H35.10- ☑
    stage 0 H35.11- ☑
    stage 1 H35.12- ☑
    stage 2 H35.13- ☑
    stage 3 H35.14- ☑
    stage 4 H35.15- ☑
    stage 5 H35.16- ☑
  pigmentary, congenital — *see* Dystrophy, retina
  proliferative NEC H35.2- ☑
    diabetic — *see* Diabetes, retinopathy, proliferative
    sickle-cell D57.- ☑ [H36]

**Retinopathy** — *continued*
  solar H31.02- ☑
**Retinoschisis** H33.10- ☑
  congenital Q14.1
  specified type NEC H33.19- ☑
**Retortamoniasis** A07.8
**Retractile testis** Q55.22
**Retraction**
  cervix — *see* Retroversion, uterus
  drum (membrane) — *see* Disorder, tympanic membrane, specified NEC
  finger — *see* Deformity, finger
  lid H02.539
    left H02.536
      lower H02.535
      upper H02.534
    right H02.533
      lower H02.532
      upper H02.531
  lung J98.4
  mediastinum J98.59
  nipple N64.53
    associated with
      lactation O92.03
      pregnancy O92.01- ☑
      puerperium O92.02
    congenital Q83.8
  palmar fascia M72.0
  pleura — *see* Pleurisy
  ring, uterus (Bandl's) (pathological) O62.4
  sternum (congenital) Q76.7
    acquired M95.4
  uterus — *see* Retroversion, uterus
  valve (heart) — *see* Endocarditis
**Retrobulbar** — *see* condition
**Retrocecal** — *see* condition
**Retrocession** — *see* Retroversion
**Retrodisplacement** — *see* Retroversion
**Retroflection, retroflexion** — *see* Retroversion
**Retrognathia, retrognathism** (mandibular) (maxillary) M26.19
**Retrograde menstruation** N92.5
**Retroperineal** — *see* condition
**Retroperitoneal** — *see* condition
**Retroperitonitis** K68.9
**Retropharyngeal** — *see* condition
**Retroplacental** — *see* condition
**Retroposition** — *see* Retroversion
**Retroprosthetic membrane** T85.398 ☑
**Retrosternal thyroid** (congenital) Q89.2
**Retroversion, retroverted**
  cervix — *see* Retroversion, uterus
  female NEC — *see* Retroversion, uterus
  iris H21.89
  testis (congenital) Q55.29
  uterus (acquired) (acute) (any degree) (asymptomatic) (cervix) (postinfectional) (postpartal, old) N85.4
    congenital Q51.818
    in pregnancy O34.53- ☑
**Retrovirus, as cause of disease classified elsewhere** B97.30
  human
    immunodeficiency, type 2 (HIV 2) B97.35
    T-cell lymphotropic
      type I (HTLV-I) B97.33
      type II (HTLV-II) B97.34
  lentivirus B97.31
  oncovirus B97.32
  specified NEC B97.39
**Retrusion, premaxilla** (developmental) M26.09
**Rett's disease or syndrome** F84.2
**Reverse peristalsis** R19.2
**Reye's syndrome** G93.7
**Rh** (factor)
  hemolytic disease (newborn) P55.0
  incompatibility, immunization or sensitization affecting management of pregnancy NEC O36.09- ☑
    anti-D antibody O36.01- ☑
    newborn P55.0
    transfusion reaction — *see* Complication(s), transfusion, incompatibility reaction, Rh (factor)
  negative mother affecting newborn P55.0
  titer elevated — *see* Complication(s), transfusion, incompatibility reaction, Rh (factor)
  transfusion reaction — *see* Complication(s), transfusion, incompatibility reaction, Rh (factor)

▽ **Subterms under main terms may continue to next column or page**    ☑ **Additional Character Required — Refer to the Tabular List for Character Selection**    **275**

Retained — Rh

**Rhabdomyolysis** (idiopathic) NEC M62.82
  traumatic T79.6 ☑
**Rhabdomyoma** (see also Neoplasm, connective tissue, benign)
  adult — see Neoplasm, connective tissue, benign
  fetal — see Neoplasm, connective tissue, benign
  glycogenic — see Neoplasm, connective tissue, benign
**Rhabdomyosarcoma** (any type) — see Neoplasm, connective tissue, malignant
**Rhabdosarcoma** — see Rhabdomyosarcoma
**Rhesus** (factor) **incompatibility** — see Rh, incompatibility
**Rheumatic** (acute) (subacute) (chronic)
  adherent pericardium I09.2
  coronary arteritis I01.9
  degeneration, myocardium I09.0
  fever (acute) — see Fever, rheumatic
  heart — see Disease, heart, rheumatic
  myocardial degeneration — see Degeneration, myocardium
  myocarditis (chronic) (inactive) (with chorea) I09.0
    with chorea (acute) (rheumatic) (Sydenham's) I02.0
    active or acute I01.2
  pancarditis, acute I01.8
    with chorea (acute) (rheumatic) Sydenham's) I02.0
  pericarditis (active) (acute) (with effusion) (with pneumonia) I01.0
    with chorea (acute) (rheumatic) (Sydenham's) I02.0
    chronic or inactive I09.2
  pneumonia I00 [J17]
  torticollis M43.6
  typhoid fever A01.09
**Rheumatism** (articular) (neuralgic) (nonarticular) M79.0
  gout — see Arthritis, rheumatoid
  intercostal, meaning Tietze's disease M94.0
  palindromic (any site) M12.30
    ankle M12.37- ☑
    elbow M12.32- ☑
    foot joint M12.37- ☑
    hand joint M12.34- ☑
    hip M12.35- ☑
    knee M12.36- ☑
    multiple site M12.39
    shoulder M12.31- ☑
    specified joint NEC M12.38
    vertebrae M12.38
    wrist M12.33- ☑
  sciatic M54.4- ☑
**Rheumatoid** (see also condition)
  arthritis (see also Arthritis, rheumatoid)
    with involvement of organs NEC M05.60
      ankle M05.67- ☑
      elbow M05.62- ☑
      foot joint M05.67- ☑
      hand joint M05.64- ☑
      hip M05.65- ☑
      knee M05.66- ☑
      multiple site M05.69
      shoulder M05.61- ☑
      vertebra — see Spondylitis, ankylosing
      wrist M05.63- ☑
    seronegative — see Arthritis, rheumatoid, seronegative
    seropositive — see Arthritis, rheumatoid, seropositive
  carditis M05.30
    ankle M05.37- ☑
    elbow M05.32- ☑
    foot joint M05.37- ☑
    hand joint M05.34- ☑
    hip M05.35- ☑
    knee M05.36- ☑
    multiple site M05.39
    shoulder M05.31- ☑
    vertebra — see Spondylitis, ankylosing
    wrist M05.33- ☑
  endocarditis — see Rheumatoid, carditis
  lung (disease) M05.10
    ankle M05.17- ☑
    elbow M05.12- ☑
    foot joint M05.17- ☑
    hand joint M05.14- ☑
    hip M05.15- ☑
    knee M05.16- ☑
    multiple site M05.19
    shoulder M05.11- ☑
    vertebra — see Spondylitis, ankylosing

**Rheumatoid** — continued
  lung — continued
    wrist M05.13- ☑
  myocarditis — see Rheumatoid, carditis
  myopathy M05.40
    ankle M05.47- ☑
    elbow M05.42- ☑
    foot joint M05.47- ☑
    hand joint M05.44- ☑
    hip M05.45- ☑
    knee M05.46- ☑
    multiple site M05.49
    shoulder M05.41- ☑
    vertebra — see Spondylitis, ankylosing
    wrist M05.43- ☑
  pericarditis — see Rheumatoid, carditis
  polyarthritis — see Arthritis, rheumatoid
  polyneuropathy M05.50
    ankle M05.57- ☑
    elbow M05.52- ☑
    foot joint M05.57- ☑
    hand joint M05.54- ☑
    hip M05.55- ☑
    knee M05.56- ☑
    multiple site M05.59
    shoulder M05.51- ☑
    vertebra — see Spondylitis, ankylosing
    wrist M05.53- ☑
  vasculitis M05.20
    ankle M05.27- ☑
    elbow M05.22- ☑
    foot joint M05.27- ☑
    hand joint M05.24- ☑
    hip M05.25- ☑
    knee M05.26- ☑
    multiple site M05.29
    shoulder M05.21- ☑
    vertebra — see Spondylitis, ankylosing
    wrist M05.23- ☑
**Rhinitis** (atrophic) (catarrhal) (chronic) (croupous) (fibrinous) (granulomatous) (hyperplastic) (hypertrophic) (membranous) (obstructive) (purulent) (suppurative) (ulcerative) J31.0
  with
    sore throat — see Nasopharyngitis
  acute J00
  allergic J30.9
    with asthma J45.909
      with
        exacerbation (acute) J45.901
        status asthmaticus J45.902
    due to
      food J30.5
      pollen J30.1
    nonseasonal J30.89
    perennial J30.89
    seasonal NEC J30.2
    specified NEC J30.89
  infective J00
  pneumococcal J00
  syphilitic A52.73
    congenital A50.05 [J99]
  tuberculous A15.8
  vasomotor J30.0
**Rhinoantritis** (chronic) — see Sinusitis, maxillary
**Rhinodacryolith** — see Dacryolith
**Rhinolith** (nasal sinus) J34.89
**Rhinomegaly** J34.89
**Rhinopharyngitis** (acute) (subacute) (see also Nasopharyngitis)
  chronic J31.1
  destructive ulcerating A66.5
  mutilans A66.5
**Rhinophyma** L71.1
**Rhinorrhea** J34.89
  cerebrospinal (fluid) G96.0
  paroxysmal — see Rhinitis, allergic
  spasmodic — see Rhinitis, allergic
**Rhinosalpingitis** — see Salpingitis, eustachian
**Rhinoscleroma** A48.8
**Rhinosporidiosis** B48.1
**Rhinovirus infection NEC** B34.8
**Rhizomelic chondrodysplasia punctata** E71.540
**Rhythm**
  atrioventricular nodal I49.8
  disorder I49.9
    coronary sinus I49.8

**Rhythm** — continued
  disorder — continued
    ectopic I49.8
    nodal I49.8
    escape I49.9
    heart, abnormal I49.9
    idioventricular I44.2
    nodal I49.8
    sleep, inversion G47.2- ☑
      nonorganic origin — see Disorder, sleep, circadian rhythm, psychogenic
**Rhytidosis facialis** L98.8
**Rib** (see also condition)
  cervical Q76.5
**Riboflavin deficiency** E53.0
**Rice bodies** (see also Loose, body, joint)
  knee M23.4- ☑
**Richter syndrome** — see Leukemia, chronic lymphocytic, B-cell type
**Richter's hernia** — see Hernia, abdomen, with obstruction
**Ricinism** — see Poisoning, food, noxious, plant
**Rickets** (active) (acute) (adolescent) (chest wall) (congenital) (current) (infantile) (intestinal) E55.0
  adult — see Osteomalacia
  celiac K90.0
  hypophosphatemic with nephrotic-glycosuric dwarfism E72.09
  inactive E64.3
  kidney N25.0
  renal N25.0
  sequelae, any E64.3
  vitamin-D-resistant E83.31 [M90.80]
**Rickettsial disease** A79.9
  specified type NEC A79.89
**Rickettsialpox** (Rickettsia akari) A79.1
**Rickettsiosis** A79.9
  due to
    Ehrlichia sennetsu A79.81
    Rickettsia akari (rickettsialpox) A79.1
  specified type NEC A79.89
  tick-borne A77.9
  vesicular A79.1
**Rider's bone** — see Ossification, muscle, specified NEC
**Ridge, alveolus** (see also condition)
  flabby K06.8
**Ridged ear, congenital** Q17.3
**Riedel's**
  lobe, liver Q44.7
  struma, thyroiditis or disease E06.5
**Rieger's anomaly or syndrome** Q13.81
**Riehl's melanosis** L81.4
**Rietti-Greppi-Micheli anemia** D56.9
**Rieux's hernia** — see Hernia, abdomen, specified site NEC
**Riga** (-Fede) **disease** K14.0
**Riggs' disease** — see Periodontitis
**Right aortic arch** Q25.47
**Right middle lobe syndrome** J98.11
**Rigid, rigidity** (see also condition)
  abdominal R19.30
    with severe abdominal pain R10.0
    epigastric R19.36
    generalized R19.37
    left lower quadrant R19.34
    left upper quadrant R19.32
    periumbilic R19.35
    right lower quadrant R19.33
    right upper quadrant R19.31
  articular, multiple, congenital Q68.8
  cervix (uteri) in pregnancy — see Pregnancy, complicated by, abnormal, cervix
  hymen (acquired) (congenital) N89.6
  nuchal R29.1
  pelvic floor in pregnancy — see Pregnancy, complicated by, abnormal, pelvic organs or tissues NEC
  perineum or vulva in pregnancy — see Pregnancy, complicated by, abnormal, vulva
  spine — see Dorsopathy, specified NEC
  vagina in pregnancy — see Pregnancy, complicated by, abnormal, vagina
**Rigors** R68.89
  with fever R50.9
**Riley-Day syndrome** G90.1
**RIND** (reversible ischemic neurologic deficit) I63.9
**Ring(s)**
  aorta (vascular) Q25.45
  Bandl's O62.4

☑ Additional Character Required — Refer to the Tabular List for Character Selection

▽ Subterms under main terms may continue to next column or page

**Ring(s)** — *continued*
  contraction, complicating delivery O62.4
  esophageal, lower (muscular) K22.2
  Fleischer's (cornea) H18.04- ☑
  hymenal, tight (acquired) (congenital) N89.6
  Kayser-Fleischer (cornea) H18.04- ☑
  retraction, uterus, pathological O62.4
  Schatzki's (esophagus) (lower) K22.2
    congenital Q39.3
  Soemmerring's — *see* Cataract, secondary
  vascular (congenital) Q25.8
    aorta Q25.45
**Ringed hair** (congenital) Q84.1
**Ringworm** B35.9
  beard B35.0
  black dot B35.0
  body B35.4
  Burmese B35.5
  corporeal B35.4
  foot B35.3
  groin B35.6
  hand B35.2
  honeycomb B35.0
  nails B35.1
  perianal (area) B35.6
  scalp B35.0
  specified NEC B35.8
  Tokelau B35.5
**Rise, venous pressure** I87.8
**Rising, PSA following treatment for malignant neoplasm of prostate** R97.21
**Risk**
  for
    dental caries Z91.849
      high Z91.843
      low Z91.841
      moderate Z91.842
  suicidal
    meaning personal history of attempted suicide Z91.5
    meaning suicidal ideation — *see* Ideation, suicidal
**Ritter's disease** L00
**Rivalry, sibling** Z62.891
**Rivalta's disease** A42.2
**River blindness** B73.01
**Robert's pelvis** Q74.2
  with disproportion (fetopelvic) O33.0
    causing obstructed labor O65.0
**Robin** (-Pierre) **syndrome** Q87.0
**Robinow-Silvermann-Smith syndrome** Q87.1
**Robinson's** (hidrotic) **ectodermal dysplasia or syndrome** Q82.4
**Robles' disease** B73.01
**Rocky Mountain** (spotted) **fever** A77.0
**Roetheln** — *see* Rubella
**Roger's disease** Q21.0
**Rokitansky-Aschoff sinuses** (gallbladder) K82.8
**Rolando's fracture** (displaced) S62.22- ☑
  nondisplaced S62.22- ☑
**Romano-Ward** (prolonged QT interval) **syndrome** I45.81
**Romberg's disease or syndrome** G51.8
**Roof, mouth** — *see* condition
**Rosacea** L71.9
  acne L71.9
  keratitis L71.8
  specified NEC L71.8
**Rosary, rachitic** E55.0
**Rose**
  cold J30.1
  fever J30.1
  rash R21
    epidemic B06.9
**Rosenbach's erysipeloid** A26.0
**Rosenthal's disease or syndrome** D68.1
**Roseola** B09
  infantum B08.20
    due to human herpesvirus 6 B08.21
    due to human herpesvirus 7 B08.22
**Ross River disease or fever** B33.1
**Rossbach's disease** K31.89
  psychogenic F45.8
**Rostan's asthma** (cardiac) — *see* Failure, ventricular, left
**Rotation**
  anomalous, incomplete or insufficient, intestine Q43.3
  cecum (congenital) Q43.3
  colon (congenital) Q43.3

**Rotation** — *continued*
  spine, incomplete or insufficient — *see* Dorsopathy, deforming, specified NEC
  tooth, teeth, fully erupted M26.35
  vertebra, incomplete or insufficient — *see* Dorsopathy, deforming, specified NEC
**Rotes Quérol disease or syndrome** — *see* Hyperostosis, ankylosing
**Roth** (-Bernhardt) **disease or syndrome** — *see* Meralgia paraesthetica
**Rothmund** (-Thomson) **syndrome** Q82.8
**Rotor's disease or syndrome** E80.6
**Round**
  back (with wedging of vertebrae) — *see* Kyphosis
    sequelae (late effect) of rickets E64.3
  worms (large) (infestation) NEC B82.0
    Ascariasis (*see also* Ascariasis) B77.9
**Roussy-Lévy syndrome** G60.0
**Rubella** (German measles) B06.9
  complication NEC B06.09
    neurological B06.00
  congenital P35.0
  contact Z20.4
  exposure to Z20.4
  maternal
    care for (suspected) damage to fetus O35.3 ☑
    manifest rubella in infant P35.0
    suspected damage to fetus affecting management of pregnancy O35.3 ☑
  specified complications NEC B06.89
**Rubeola** (meaning measles) — *see* Measles
  meaning rubella — *see* Rubella
**Rubeosis, iris** — *see* Disorder, iris, vascular
**Rubinstein-Taybi syndrome** Q87.2
**Rudimentary** (congenital) (*see also* Agenesis)
  arm — *see* Defect, reduction, upper limb
  bone Q79.9
  cervix uteri Q51.828
  eye Q11.2
  lobule of ear Q17.3
  patella Q74.1
  respiratory organs in thoracopagus Q89.4
  tracheal bronchus Q32.4
  uterus Q51.818
    in male Q56.1
  vagina Q52.0
**Ruled out condition** — *see* Observation, suspected
**Rumination** R11.10
  with nausea R11.2
  disorder of infancy F98.21
  neurotic F42.8
  newborn P92.1
  obsessional F42.8
  psychogenic F42.8
**Runeberg's disease** D51.0
**Runny nose** R09.89
**Rupia** (syphilitic) A51.39
  congenital A50.06
  tertiary A52.79
**Rupture, ruptured**
  abscess (spontaneous) — *code by* site under Abscess
  aneurysm — *see* Aneurysm
  anus (sphincter) — *see* Laceration, anus
  aorta, aortic I71.8
    abdominal I71.3
    arch I71.1
    ascending I71.1
    descending I71.8
      abdominal I71.3
      thoracic I71.1
    syphilitic A52.01
    thoracoabdominal I71.5
    thorax, thoracic I71.1
    transverse I71.1
    traumatic — *see* Injury, aorta, laceration, major
    valve or cusp (*see also* Endocarditis, aortic) I35.8
  appendix (with peritonitis) K35.2
    with localized peritonitis K35.3
  arteriovenous fistula, brain I60.8
  artery I77.2
    brain — *see* Hemorrhage, intracranial, intracerebral
    coronary — *see* Infarct, myocardium
    heart — *see* Infarct, myocardium
    pulmonary I28.8
    traumatic (complication) — *see* Injury, blood vessel
  bile duct (common) (hepatic) K83.2
    cystic K82.2

**Rupture, ruptured** — *continued*
  bladder (sphincter) (nontraumatic) (spontaneous) N32.89
    following ectopic or molar pregnancy O08.6
    obstetrical trauma O71.5
    traumatic S37.29 ☑
  blood vessel (*see also* Hemorrhage)
    brain — *see* Hemorrhage, intracranial, intracerebral
    heart — *see* Infarct, myocardium
    traumatic (complication) — *see* Injury, blood vessel, laceration, major, by site
  bone — *see* Fracture
  bowel (nontraumatic) K63.1
  brain
    aneurysm (congenital) (*see also* Hemorrhage, intracranial, subarachnoid)
      syphilitic A52.05
    hemorrhagic — *see* Hemorrhage, intracranial, intracerebral
  capillaries I78.8
  cardiac (auricle) (ventricle) (wall) I23.3
    with hemopericardium I23.0
    infectional I40.9
    traumatic — *see* Injury, heart
  cartilage (articular) (current) (*see also* Sprain)
    knee S83.3- ☑
    semilunar — *see* Tear, meniscus
  cecum (with peritonitis) K65.0
    with peritoneal abscess K35.3
    traumatic S36.598 ☑
  celiac artery, traumatic — *see* Injury, blood vessel, celiac artery, laceration, major
  cerebral aneurysm (congenital) (*see* Hemorrhage, intracranial, subarachnoid)
  cervix (uteri)
    with ectopic or molar pregnancy O08.6
    following ectopic or molar pregnancy O08.6
    obstetrical trauma O71.3
    traumatic S37.69 ☑
  chordae tendineae NEC I51.1
    concurrent with acute myocardial infarction — *see* Infarct, myocardium
    following acute myocardial infarction (current complication) I23.4
  choroid (direct) (indirect) (traumatic) H31.32- ☑
  circle of Willis I60.6
  colon (nontraumatic) K63.1
    traumatic — *see* Injury, intestine, large
  cornea (traumatic) — *see* Injury, eye, laceration
  coronary (artery) (thrombotic) — *see* Infarct, myocardium
  corpus luteum (infected) (ovary) N83.1- ☑
  cyst — *see* Cyst
  cystic duct K82.2
  Descemet's membrane — *see* Change, corneal membrane, Descemet's, rupture
    traumatic — *see* Injury, eye, laceration
  diaphragm, traumatic — *see* Injury, intrathoracic, diaphragm
  disc — *see* Rupture, intervertebral disc
  diverticulum (intestine) K57.80
    with bleeding K57.81
    bladder N32.3
    large intestine K57.20
      with
        bleeding K57.21
        small intestine K57.40
          with bleeding K57.41
    small intestine K57.00
      with
        bleeding K57.01
        large intestine K57.40
          with bleeding K57.41
  duodenal stump K31.89
  ear drum (nontraumatic) (*see also* Perforation, tympanum)
    traumatic S09.2- ☑
    due to blast injury — *see* Injury, blast, ear
  esophagus K22.3
  eye (without prolapse or loss of intraocular tissue) — *see* Injury, eye, laceration
  fallopian tube NEC (nonobstetric) (nontraumatic) N83.8
    due to pregnancy O00.10- ☑
    with intrauterine pregnancy O00.11- ☑
  fontanel P13.1
  gallbladder K82.2
    traumatic S36.128 ☑

☑ Subterms under main terms may continue to next column or page    ☑ Additional Character Required — Refer to the Tabular List for Character Selection    **277**

Index

Ring(s) — Rupture, ruptured

**Rupture, ruptured** — *continued*
 gastric (*see also* Rupture, stomach)
  vessel K92.2
 globe (eye) (traumatic) — *see* Injury, eye, laceration
 graafian follicle (hematoma) N83.0- ☑
 heart — *see* Rupture, cardiac
 hymen (nontraumatic) (nonintentional) N89.8
 internal organ, traumatic — *see* Injury, by site
 intervertebral disc — *see* Displacement, intervertebral
    disc
  traumatic — *see* Rupture, traumatic, intervertebral
    disc
 intestine NEC (nontraumatic) K63.1
  traumatic — *see* Injury, intestine
 iris (*see also* Abnormality, pupillary)
  traumatic — *see* Injury, eye, laceration
 joint capsule, traumatic — *see* Sprain
 kidney (traumatic) S37.06- ☑
  birth injury P15.8
  nontraumatic N28.89
 lacrimal duct (traumatic) — *see* Injury, eye, specified
    site NEC
 lens (cataract) (traumatic) — *see* Cataract, traumatic
 ligament, traumatic — *see* Rupture, traumatic, liga-
    ment, by site
 liver S36.116 ☑
  birth injury P15.0
 lymphatic vessel I89.8
 marginal sinus (placental) (with hemorrhage) — *see*
    Hemorrhage, antepartum, specified cause NEC
 membrana tympani (nontraumatic) — *see* Perforation,
    tympanum
 membranes (spontaneous)
  artificial
   delayed delivery following O75.5
  delayed delivery following — *see* Pregnancy,
    complicated by, premature rupture of
    membranes
 meningeal artery I60.8
 meniscus (knee) (*see also* Tear, meniscus)
  old — *see* Derangement, meniscus
  site other than knee — *code as* Sprain
 mesenteric artery, traumatic — *see* Injury, mesenteric,
    artery, laceration, major
 mesentery (nontraumatic) K66.8
  traumatic — *see* Injury, intra-abdominal, specified,
    site NEC
 mitral (valve) I34.8
 muscle (traumatic) (*see also* Strain)
  diastasis — *see* Diastasis, muscle
  nontraumatic M62.10
   ankle M62.17- ☑
   foot M62.17- ☑
   forearm M62.13- ☑
   hand M62.14- ☑
   lower leg M62.16- ☑
   pelvic region M62.15- ☑
   shoulder region M62.11- ☑
   specified site NEC M62.18
   thigh M62.15- ☑
   upper arm M62.12- ☑
  traumatic — *see* Strain, by site
 musculotendinous junction NEC, nontraumatic — *see*
    Rupture, tendon, spontaneous
 mycotic aneurysm causing cerebral hemorrhage —
    *see* Hemorrhage, intracranial, subarachnoid
 myocardium, myocardial — *see* Rupture, cardiac
  traumatic — *see* Injury, heart
 nontraumatic, meaning hernia — *see* Hernia
 obstructed — *see* Hernia, by site, obstructed
 operation wound — *see* Disruption, wound, operation
 ovary, ovarian N83.8
  corpus luteum cyst N83.1- ☑
  follicle (graafian) N83.0- ☑
 oviduct (nonobstetric) (nontraumatic) N83.8
  due to pregnancy O00.10- ☑
   with intrauterine pregnancy O00.11- ☑
 pancreas (nontraumatic) K86.89
  traumatic S36.299 ☑
 papillary muscle NEC I51.2
  following acute myocardial infarction (current
    complication) I23.5
 pelvic
  floor, complicating delivery O70.1
  organ NEC, obstetrical trauma O71.5
 perineum (nonobstetric) (nontraumatic) N90.89

**Rupture, ruptured** — *continued*
 perineum — *continued*
  complicating delivery — *see* Delivery, complicated,
    by, laceration, anus (sphincter)
 postoperative wound — *see* Disruption, wound, oper-
    ation
 prostate (traumatic) S37.828 ☑
 pulmonary
  artery I28.8
  valve (heart) I37.8
  vein I28.8
  vessel I28.8
 pus tube — *see* Salpingitis
 pyosalpinx — *see* Salpingitis
 rectum (nontraumatic) K63.1
  traumatic S36.69 ☑
 retina, retinal (traumatic) (without detachment) (*see
    also* Break, retina)
  with detachment — *see* Detachment, retina, with
    retinal, break
 rotator cuff (nontraumatic) M75.10- ☑
  complete M75.12- ☑
  incomplete M75.11- ☑
 sclera — *see* Injury, eye, laceration
 sigmoid (nontraumatic) K63.1
  traumatic S36.593 ☑
 spinal cord (*see also* Injury, spinal cord, by region)
  due to injury at birth P11.5
  newborn (birth injury) P11.5
 spleen (traumatic) S36.09 ☑
  birth injury P15.1
  congenital (birth injury) P15.1
  due to P. vivax malaria B51.0
  nontraumatic D73.5
  spontaneous D73.5
 splenic vein R58
  traumatic — *see* Injury, blood vessel, splenic vein
 stomach (nontraumatic) (spontaneous) K31.89
  traumatic S36.39 ☑
 supraspinatus (complete) (incomplete) (nontraumatic)
    — *see* Tear, rotator cuff
 symphysis pubis
  obstetric O71.6
  traumatic S33.4 ☑
 synovium (cyst) M66.10
  ankle M66.17- ☑
  elbow M66.12- ☑
  finger M66.14- ☑
  foot M66.17- ☑
  forearm M66.13- ☑
  hand M66.14- ☑
  pelvic region M66.15- ☑
  shoulder region M66.11- ☑
  specified site NEC M66.18
  thigh M66.15- ☑
  toe M66.17- ☑
  upper arm M66.12- ☑
  wrist M66.13- ☑
 tendon (traumatic) — *see* Strain
  nontraumatic (spontaneous) M66.9
   ankle M66.87- ☑
   extensor M66.20
    ankle M66.27- ☑
    foot M66.27- ☑
    forearm M66.23- ☑
    hand M66.24- ☑
    lower leg M66.26- ☑
    multiple sites M66.29
    pelvic region M66.25- ☑
    shoulder region M66.21- ☑
    specified site NEC M66.28
    thigh M66.25- ☑
    upper arm M66.22- ☑
   flexor M66.30
    ankle M66.37- ☑
    foot M66.37- ☑
    forearm M66.33- ☑
    hand M66.34- ☑
    lower leg M66.36- ☑
    multiple sites M66.39
    pelvic region M66.35- ☑
    shoulder region M66.31- ☑
    specified site NEC M66.38
    thigh M66.35- ☑
    upper arm M66.32- ☑
   foot M66.87- ☑
   forearm M66.83- ☑

**Rupture, ruptured** — *continued*
 tendon — *see* Strain — *continued*
  nontraumatic — *continued*
   hand M66.84- ☑
   lower leg M66.86- ☑
   multiple sites M66.89
   pelvic region M66.85- ☑
   shoulder region M66.81- ☑
   specified
    site NEC M66.88
    tendon M66.80
   thigh M66.85- ☑
   upper arm M66.82- ☑
 thoracic duct I89.8
 tonsil J35.8
 traumatic
  aorta — *see* Injury, aorta, laceration, major
  diaphragm — *see* Injury, intrathoracic, diaphragm
  external site — *see* Wound, open, by site
  eye — *see* Injury, eye, laceration
  internal organ — *see* Injury, by site
  intervertebral disc
   cervical S13.0 ☑
   lumbar S33.0 ☑
   thoracic S23.0 ☑
  kidney S37.06- ☑
  ligament (*see also* Sprain)
   ankle — *see* Sprain, ankle
   carpus — *see* Rupture, traumatic, ligament,
    wrist
   collateral (hand) — *see* Rupture, traumatic,
    ligament, finger, collateral
   finger (metacarpophalangeal) (interphalangeal)
    S63.40- ☑
    collateral S63.41- ☑
     index S63.41- ☑
     little S63.41- ☑
     middle S63.41- ☑
     ring S63.41- ☑
    index S63.40- ☑
    little S63.40- ☑
    middle S63.40- ☑
    palmar S63.42- ☑
     index S63.42- ☑
     little S63.42- ☑
     middle S63.42- ☑
     ring S63.42- ☑
    ring S63.40- ☑
    specified site NEC S63.499 ☑
     index S63.49- ☑
     little S63.49- ☑
     middle S63.49- ☑
     ring S63.49- ☑
    volar plate S63.43- ☑
     index S63.43- ☑
     little S63.43- ☑
     middle S63.43- ☑
     ring S63.43- ☑
   foot — *see* Sprain, foot
   radial collateral S53.2- ☑
   radiocarpal — *see* Rupture, traumatic, ligament,
    wrist, radiocarpal
   ulnar collateral S53.3- ☑
   ulnocarpal — *see* Rupture, traumatic, ligament,
    wrist, ulnocarpal
   wrist S63.30- ☑
    collateral S63.31- ☑
    radiocarpal S63.32- ☑
    specified site NEC S63.39- ☑
    ulnocarpal (palmar) S63.33- ☑
  liver S36.116 ☑
  membrana tympani — *see* Rupture, ear drum,
    traumatic
  muscle or tendon — *see* Strain
  myocardium — *see* Injury, heart
  pancreas S36.299 ☑
  rectum S36.69 ☑
  sigmoid S36.593 ☑
  spleen S36.09 ☑
  stomach S36.39 ☑
  symphysis pubis S33.4 ☑
  tympanum, tympanic (membrane) — *see* Rupture,
    ear drum, traumatic
  ureter S37.19 ☑
  uterus S37.69 ☑
  vagina — *see* Injury, vagina

**Rupture, ruptured** — continued
  traumatic — continued
    vena cava — see Injury, vena cava, laceration, major
    tricuspid (heart) (valve) I07.8
    tube, tubal (nonobstetric) (nontraumatic) N83.8
      abscess — see Salpingitis
      due to pregnancy O00.10- ☑
        with intrauterine pregnancy O00.11- ☑
    tympanum, tympanic (membrane) (nontraumatic) (see also Perforation, tympanic membrane) H72.9- ☑
      traumatic — see Rupture, ear drum, traumatic
    umbilical cord, complicating delivery O69.89 ☑
    ureter (traumatic) S37.19 ☑
      nontraumatic N28.89
    urethra (nontraumatic) N36.8
      with ectopic or molar pregnancy O08.6
      following ectopic or molar pregnancy O08.6
      obstetrical trauma O71.5
      traumatic S37.39 ☑
    uterosacral ligament (nonobstetric) (nontraumatic) N83.8
    uterus (traumatic) S37.69 ☑
      before labor O71.0- ☑
      during or after labor O71.1
      nonpuerperal, nontraumatic N85.8
      pregnant (during labor) O71.1
        before labor O71.0- ☑
    vagina — see Injury, vagina
    valve, valvular (heart) — see Endocarditis
    varicose vein — see Varix
    varix — see Varix
    vena cava R58
      traumatic — see Injury, vena cava, laceration, major
    vesical (urinary) N32.89
    vessel (blood) R58
      pulmonary I28.8
      traumatic — see Injury, blood vessel
    viscus R19.8
    vulva complicating delivery O70.0
**Russell-Silver syndrome** Q87.1
**Russian spring-summer type encephalitis** A84.0
**Rust's disease** (tuberculous cervical spondylitis) A18.01
**Ruvalcaba-Myhre-Smith syndrome** E71.440
**Rytand-Lipsitch syndrome** I44.2

# S

**Saber, sabre shin or tibia** (syphilitic) A50.56 [M90.8-] ☑
**Sac lacrimal** — see condition
**Saccharomyces infection** B37.9
**Saccharopinuria** E72.3
**Saccular** — see condition
**Sacculation**
  aorta (nonsyphilitic) — see Aneurysm, aorta
  bladder N32.3
  intralaryngeal (congenital) (ventricular) Q31.3
  larynx (congenital) (ventricular) Q31.3
  organ or site, congenital — see Distortion
  pregnant uterus — see Pregnancy, complicated by, abnormal, uterus
  ureter N28.89
  urethra N36.1
  vesical N32.3
**Sachs' amaurotic familial idiocy or disease** E75.02
**Sachs-Tay disease** E75.02
**Sacks-Libman disease** M32.11
**Sacralgia** M53.3
**Sacralization** Q76.49
**Sacrodynia** M53.3
**Sacroiliac joint** — see condition
**Sacroiliitis NEC** M46.1
**Sacrum** — see condition
**Saddle**
  back — see Lordosis
  embolus
    abdominal aorta I74.01
    pulmonary artery I26.92
      with acute cor pulmonale I26.02
  injury — code to condition
  nose M95.0
    due to syphilis A50.57
**Sadism** (sexual) F65.52
**Sadness, postpartal** O90.6
**Sadomasochism** F65.50
**Saemisch's ulcer** (cornea) — see Ulcer, cornea, central

**Sagging**
  skin and subcutaneous tissue (following bariatric surgery weight loss) (following dietary weight loss) L98.7
**Sahib disease** B55.0
**Sailors' skin** L57.8
**Saint**
  Anthony's fire — see Erysipelas
  triad — see Hernia, diaphragm
  Vitus' dance — see Chorea, Sydenham's
**Salaam**
  attack(s) — see Epilepsy, spasms
  tic R25.8
**Salicylism**
  abuse F55.8
  overdose or wrong substance given — see Table of Drugs and Chemicals, by drug, poisoning
**Salivary duct or gland** — see condition
**Salivation, excessive** K11.7
**Salmonella** — see Infection, Salmonella
**Salmonellosis** A02.0
**Salpingitis** (catarrhal) (fallopian tube) (nodular) (pseudofollicular) (purulent) (septic) N70.91
  with oophoritis N70.93
  acute N70.01
    with oophoritis N70.03
  chlamydial A56.11
  chronic N70.11
    with oophoritis N70.13
  complicating abortion — see Abortion, by type, complicated by, salpingitis
  ear — see Salpingitis, eustachian
  eustachian (tube) H68.00- ☑
    acute H68.01- ☑
    chronic H68.02- ☑
  follicularis N70.11
    with oophoritis N70.13
  gonococcal (acute) (chronic) A54.24
  interstitial, chronic N70.11
    with oophoritis N70.13
  isthmica nodosa N70.11
    with oophoritis N70.13
  specific (gonococcal) (acute) (chronic) A54.24
  tuberculous (acute) (chronic) A18.17
  venereal (gonococcal) (acute) (chronic) A54.24
**Salpingocele** N83.4- ☑
**Salpingo-oophoritis** (catarrhal) (purulent) (ruptured) (septic) (suppurative) N70.93
  acute N70.03
    with ectopic or molar pregnancy O08.0
    following ectopic or molar pregnancy O08.0
    gonococcal A54.24
  chronic N70.13
  following ectopic or molar pregnancy O08.0
  gonococcal (acute) (chronic) A54.24
  puerperal O86.19
  specific (gonococcal) (acute) (chronic) A54.24
  subacute N70.03
  tuberculous (acute) (chronic) A18.17
  venereal (gonococcal) (acute) (chronic) A54.24
**Salpingo-ovaritis** — see Salpingo-oophoritis
**Salpingoperitonitis** — see Salpingo-oophoritis
**Salzmann's nodular dystrophy** — see Degeneration, cornea, nodular
**Sampson's cyst or tumor** N80.1
**San Joaquin** (Valley) **fever** B38.0
**Sandblaster's asthma, lung or pneumoconiosis** J62.8
**Sander's disease** (paranoia) F22
**Sandfly fever** A93.1
**Sandhoff's disease** E75.01
**Sanfilippo** (Type B) (Type C) (Type D) **syndrome** E76.22
**Sanger-Brown ataxia** G11.2
**Sao Paulo fever or typhus** A77.0
**Saponification, mesenteric** K65.8
**Sarcocele** (benign)
  syphilitic A52.76
    congenital A50.59
**Sarcocystosis** A07.8
**Sarcoepiplocele** — see Hernia
**Sarcoepiplomphalocele** Q79.2
**Sarcoid** (see also Sarcoidosis)
  arthropathy D86.86
  Boeck's D86.9
  Darier-Roussy D86.3
  iridocyclitis D86.83
  meningitis D86.81
  myocarditis D86.85

**Sarcoid** — continued
  myositis D86.87
  pyelonephritis D86.84
  Spiegler-Fendt L08.89
**Sarcoidosis** D86.9
  with
    cranial nerve palsies D86.82
    hepatic granuloma D86.89
    polyarthritis D86.86
    tubulo-interstitial nephropathy D86.84
  combined sites NEC D86.89
  lung D86.0
    and lymph nodes D86.2
  lymph nodes D86.1
    and lung D86.2
  meninges D86.81
  skin D86.3
  specified type NEC D86.89
**Sarcoma** (of) (see also Neoplasm, connective tissue, malignant)
  alveolar soft part — see Neoplasm, connective tissue, malignant
  ameloblastic C41.1
    upper jaw (bone) C41.0
  botryoid — see Neoplasm, connective tissue, malignant
  botryoides — see Neoplasm, connective tissue, malignant
  cerebellar C71.6
    circumscribed (arachnoidal) C71.6
  circumscribed (arachnoidal) cerebellar C71.6
  clear cell (see also Neoplasm, connective tissue, malignant)
    kidney C64.- ☑
  dendritic cells (accessory cells) C96.4
  embryonal — see Neoplasm, connective tissue, malignant
  endometrial (stromal) C54.1
    isthmus C54.0
  epithelioid (cell) — see Neoplasm, connective tissue, malignant
  Ewing's — see Neoplasm, bone, malignant
  follicular dendritic cell C96.4
  germinoblastic (diffuse) — see Lymphoma, diffuse large cell
    follicular — see Lymphoma, follicular, specified NEC
  giant cell (except of bone) (see also Neoplasm, connective tissue, malignant)
    bone — see Neoplasm, bone, malignant
  glomoid — see Neoplasm, connective tissue, malignant
  granulocytic C92.3- ☑
  hemangioendothelial — see Neoplasm, connective tissue, malignant
  hemorrhagic, multiple — see Sarcoma, Kaposi's
  histiocytic C96.A (following C96.6)
  Hodgkin — see Lymphoma, Hodgkin
  immunoblastic (diffuse) — see Lymphoma, diffuse large cell
  interdigitating dendritic cell C96.4
  Kaposi's
    colon C46.4
    connective tissue C46.1
    gastrointestinal organ C46.4
    lung C46.5- ☑
    lymph node(s) C46.3
    palate (hard) (soft) C46.2
    rectum C46.4
    skin C46.0
    specified site NEC C46.7
    stomach C46.4
    unspecified site C46.9
  Kupffer cell C22.3
  Langerhans cell C96.4
  leptomeningeal — see Neoplasm, meninges, malignant
  liver NEC C22.4
  lymphangioendothelial — see Neoplasm, connective tissue, malignant
  lymphoblastic — see Lymphoma, lymphoblastic (diffuse)
  lymphocytic — see Lymphoma, small cell B-cell
  mast cell C96.22
  melanotic — see Melanoma
  meningeal — see Neoplasm, meninges, malignant
  meningothelial — see Neoplasm, meninges, malignant

**Sarcoma** — *continued*
mesenchymal (*see also* Neoplasm, connective tissue, malignant)
  mixed — *see* Neoplasm, connective tissue, malignant
mesothelial — *see* Mesothelioma
monstrocellular
  specified site — *see* Neoplasm, malignant, by site
  unspecified site C71.9
myeloid C92.3- ☑
neurogenic — *see* Neoplasm, nerve, malignant
odontogenic C41.1
  upper jaw (bone) C41.Ø
osteoblastic — *see* Neoplasm, bone, malignant
osteogenic (*see also* Neoplasm, bone, malignant)
  juxtacortical — *see* Neoplasm, bone, malignant
  periosteal — *see* Neoplasm, bone, malignant
periosteal (*see also* Neoplasm, bone, malignant)
  osteogenic — *see* Neoplasm, bone, malignant
pleomorphic cell — *see* Neoplasm, connective tissue, malignant
reticulum cell (diffuse) — *see* Lymphoma, diffuse large cell
  nodular — *see* Lymphoma, follicular
  pleomorphic cell type — *see* Lymphoma, diffuse large cell
rhabdoid — *see* Neoplasm, malignant, by site
round cell — *see* Neoplasm, connective tissue, malignant
small cell — *see* Neoplasm, connective tissue, malignant
soft tissue — *see* Neoplasm, connective tissue, malignant
spindle cell — *see* Neoplasm, connective tissue, malignant
stromal (endometrial) C54.1
  isthmus C54.Ø
synovial (*see also* Neoplasm, connective tissue, malignant)
  biphasic — *see* Neoplasm, connective tissue, malignant
  epithelioid cell — *see* Neoplasm, connective tissue, malignant
  spindle cell — *see* Neoplasm, connective tissue, malignant
**Sarcomatosis**
meningeal — *see* Neoplasm, meninges, malignant
specified site NEC — *see* Neoplasm, connective tissue, malignant
unspecified site C8Ø.1
**Sarcopenia** (age-related) M62.84
**Sarcosinemia** E72.59
**Sarcosporidiosis** (intestinal) AØ7.8
**Satiety, early** R68.81
**Saturnine** — *see* condition
**Saturnism**
overdose or wrong substance given or taken — *see* Table of Drugs and Chemicals, by drug, poisoning
**Satyriasis** F52.8
**Sauriasis** — *see* Ichthyosis
**SBE** (subacute bacterial endocarditis) I33.Ø
**Scabies** (any site) B86
**Scabs** R23.4
**Scaglietti-Dagnini syndrome** E22.Ø
**Scald** — *see* Burn
**Scalenus anticus** (anterior) **syndrome** G54.Ø
**Scales** R23.4
**Scaling, skin** R23.4
**Scalp** — *see* condition
**Scapegoating affecting child** Z62.3
**Scaphocephaly** Q75.Ø
**Scapulalgia** M89.8X1
**Scapulohumeral myopathy** G71.Ø
**Scar, scarring** (*see also* Cicatrix) L9Ø.5
adherent L9Ø.5
atrophic L9Ø.5
cervix
  in pregnancy or childbirth — *see* Pregnancy, complicated by, abnormal cervix
cheloid L91.Ø
chorioretinal H31.ØØ- ☑
  posterior pole macula H31.Ø1- ☑
  postsurgical H59.81- ☑
  solar retinopathy H31.Ø2- ☑
  specified type NEC H31.Ø9- ☑
choroid — *see* Scar, chorioretinal

**Scar, scarring** — *continued*
conjunctiva H11.24- ☑
cornea H17.9
  xerophthalmic (*see also* Opacity, cornea)
    vitamin A deficiency E5Ø.6
duodenum, obstructive K31.5
hypertrophic L91.Ø
keloid L91.Ø
labia N9Ø.89
lung (base) J98.4
macula — *see* Scar, chorioretinal, posterior pole
muscle M62.89
myocardium, myocardial I25.2
painful L9Ø.5
posterior pole (eye) — *see* Scar, chorioretinal, posterior pole
retina — *see* Scar, chorioretinal
trachea J39.8
transmural uterine, in pregnancy O34.29
uterus N85.8
  in pregnancy O34.29
vagina N89.8
  postoperative N99.2
vulva N9Ø.89
**Scarabiasis** B88.2
**Scarlatina** (anginosa) (maligna) A38.9
myocarditis (acute) A38.1
  old — *see* Myocarditis
otitis media A38.Ø
ulcerosa A38.8
**Scarlet fever** (albuminuria) (angina) A38.9
**Schamberg's disease** (progressive pigmentary dermatosis) L81.7
**Schatzki's ring** (acquired) (esophagus) (lower) K22.2
congenital Q39.3
**Schaufenster krankheit** I2Ø.8
**Schaumann's**
benign lymphogranulomatosis D86.1
disease or syndrome — *see* Sarcoidosis
**Scheie's syndrome** E76.Ø3
**Schenck's disease** B42.1
**Scheuermann's disease or osteochondrosis** — *see* Osteochondrosis, juvenile, spine
**Schilder** (-Flatau) **disease** G37.Ø
**Schilling-type monocytic leukemia** C93.Ø- ☑
**Schimmelbusch's disease, cystic mastitis, or hyperplasia** — *see* Mastopathy, cystic
**Schistosoma infestation** — *see* Infestation, Schistosoma
**Schistosomiasis** B65.9
with muscle disorder B65.9 [M63.8Ø]
  ankle B65.9 [M63.87-] ☑
  foot B65.9 [M63.87-] ☑
  forearm B65.9 [M63.83-] ☑
  hand B65.9 [M63.84-] ☑
  lower leg B65.9 [M63.86-] ☑
  multiple sites B65.9 [M63.89]
  pelvic region B65.9 [M63.85-] ☑
  shoulder region B65.9 [M63.81-] ☑
  specified site NEC B65.9 [M63.88]
  thigh B65.9 [M63.85-] ☑
  upper arm B65.9 [M63.82-] ☑
Asiatic B65.2
bladder B65.Ø
chestermani B65.8
colon B65.1
cutaneous B65.3
due to
  S. haematobium B65.Ø
  S. japonicum B65.2
  S. mansoni B65.1
  S. mattheii B65.8
Eastern B65.2
genitourinary tract B65.Ø
intestinal B65.1
lung NEC B65.9 [J99]
  pneumonia B65.9 [J17]
Manson's (intestinal) B65.1
oriental B65.2
pulmonary NEC B65.9 [J99]
  pneumonia B65.9
Schistosoma
  haematobium B65.Ø
  japonicum B65.2
  mansoni B65.1
specified type NEC B65.8
urinary B65.Ø
vesical B65.Ø
**Schizencephaly** Q04.6

**Schizoaffective psychosis** F25.9
**Schizodontia** KØØ.2
**Schizoid personality** F6Ø.1
**Schizophrenia, schizophrenic** F2Ø.9
acute (brief) (undifferentiated) F23
atypical (form) F2Ø.3
borderline F21
catalepsy F2Ø.2
catatonic (type) (excited) (withdrawn) F2Ø.2
cenesthopathic, cenesthesiopathic F2Ø.89
childhood type F84.5
chronic undifferentiated F2Ø.5
cyclic F25.Ø
disorganized (type) F2Ø.1
flexibilitas cerea F2Ø.2
hebephrenic (type) F2Ø.1
incipient F21
latent F21
negative type F2Ø.5
paranoid (type) F2Ø.Ø
paraphrenic F2Ø.Ø
post-psychotic depression F32.89
prepsychotic F21
prodromal F21
pseudoneurotic F21
pseudopsychopathic F21
reaction F23
residual (state) (type) F2Ø.5
restzustand F2Ø.5
schizoaffective (type) — *see* Psychosis, schizoaffective
simple (type) F2Ø.89
simplex F2Ø.89
specified type NEC F2Ø.89
spectrum and other psychotic disorder F29
  specified NEC F28
stupor F2Ø.2
syndrome of childhood F84.5
undifferentiated (type) F2Ø.3
  chronic F2Ø.5
**Schizothymia** (persistent) F6Ø.1
**Schlatter-Osgood disease or osteochondrosis** — *see* Osteochondrosis, juvenile, tibia
**Schlatter's tibia** — *see* Osteochondrosis, juvenile, tibia
**Schmidt's syndrome** (polyglandular, autoimmune) E31.Ø
**Schmincke's carcinoma or tumor** — *see* Neoplasm, nasopharynx, malignant
**Schmitz** (-Stutzer) **dysentery** AØ3.Ø
**Schmorl's disease or nodes**
lumbar region M51.46
lumbosacral region M51.47
sacrococcygeal region M53.3
thoracic region M51.44
thoracolumbar region M51.45
**Schneiderian**
papilloma — *see* Neoplasm, nasopharynx, benign
  specified site — *see* Neoplasm, benign, by site
  unspecified site D14.Ø
specified site — *see* Neoplasm, malignant, by site
  unspecified site C3Ø.Ø
**Scholte's syndrome** (malignant carcinoid) E34.Ø
**Scholz** (-Bielchowsky-Henneberg) **disease or syndrome** E75.25
**Schönlein** (-Henoch) disease or purpura (primary) (rheumatic) D69.Ø
**Schottmuller's disease** AØ1.4
**Schroeder's syndrome** (endocrine hypertensive) E27.Ø
**Schüller-Christian disease or syndrome** C96.5
**Schultze's type acroparesthesia, simple** I73.89
**Schultz's disease or syndrome** — *see* Agranulocytosis
**Schwalbe-Ziehen-Oppenheim disease** G24.1
**Schwannoma** (*see also* Neoplasm, nerve, benign)
malignant (*see also* Neoplasm, nerve, malignant)
  with rhabdomyoblastic differentiation — *see* Neoplasm, nerve, malignant
melanocytic — *see* Neoplasm, nerve, benign
pigmented — *see* Neoplasm, nerve, benign
**Schwannomatosis** Q85.Ø3
**Schwartz** (-Jampel) **syndrome** G71.13
**Schwartz-Bartter syndrome** E22.2
**Schweniger-Buzzi anetoderma** L9Ø.1
**Sciatic** — *see* condition
**Sciatica** (infective)
with lumbago M54.4- ☑
  due to intervertebral disc disorder — *see* Disorder, disc, with, radiculopathy
  due to displacement of intervertebral disc (with lumbago) — *see* Disorder, disc, with, radiculopathy

☑ **Additional Character Required** — Refer to the Tabular List for Character Selection     ⚑ **Subterms under main terms may continue to next column or page**

**Sciatica** — *continued*
  wallet M54.3- ☑
**Scimitar syndrome** Q26.8
**Sclera** — *see* condition
**Sclerectasia** H15.84- ☑
**Scleredema**
  adultorum — *see* Sclerosis, systemic
  Buschke's — *see* Sclerosis, systemic
  newborn P83.0
**Sclerema** (adiposum) (edematosum) (neonatorum)
  (newborn) P83.0
  adultorum — *see* Sclerosis, systemic
**Scleriasis** — *see* Scleroderma
**Scleritis** H15.00- ☑
  with corneal involvement H15.04- ☑
  anterior H15.01- ☑
  brawny H15.02- ☑
  in (due to) zoster B02.34
  posterior H15.03- ☑
  specified type NEC H15.09- ☑
  syphilitic A52.71
  tuberculous (nodular) A18.51
**Sclerochoroiditis** H31.8
**Scleroconjunctivitis** — *see* Scleritis
**Sclerocystic ovary syndrome** E28.2
**Sclerodactyly, sclerodactylia** L94.3
**Scleroderma, sclerodermia** (acrosclerotic) (diffuse)
  (generalized) (progressive) (pulmonary) (*see also*
  Sclerosis, systemic) M34.9
  circumscribed L94.0
  linear L94.1
  localized L94.0
  newborn P83.88
  systemic M34.9
**Sclerokeratitis** H16.8
  tuberculous A18.52
**Scleroma nasi** A48.8
**Scleromalacia** (perforans) H15.05- ☑
**Scleromyxedema** L98.5
**Sclérose en plaques** G35
**Sclerosis, sclerotic**
  adrenal (gland) E27.8
  Alzheimer's — *see* Disease, Alzheimer's
  amyotrophic (lateral) G12.21
  aorta, aortic I70.0
    valve — *see* Endocarditis, aortic
  artery, arterial, arteriolar, arteriovascular — *see* Arteriosclerosis
  ascending multiple G35
  brain (generalized) (lobular) G37.9
    artery, arterial I67.2
    diffuse G37.0
    disseminated G35
    insular G35
    Krabbe's E75.23
    miliary G35
    multiple G35
    presenile (Alzheimer's) — *see* Disease, Alzheimer's, early onset
    senile (arteriosclerotic) I67.2
    stem, multiple G35
    tuberous Q85.1
  bulbar, multiple G35
  bundle of His I44.39
  cardiac — *see* Disease, heart, ischemic, atherosclerotic
  cardiorenal — *see* Hypertension, cardiorenal
  cardiovascular (*see also* Disease, cardiovascular)
    renal — *see* Hypertension, cardiorenal
  cerebellar — *see* Sclerosis, brain
  cerebral — *see* Sclerosis, brain
  cerebrospinal (disseminated) (multiple) G35
  cerebrovascular I67.2
  choroid — *see* Degeneration, choroid
  combined (spinal cord) (*see also* Degeneration, combined)
    multiple G35
  concentric (Balo) G37.5
  cornea — *see* Opacity, cornea
  coronary (artery) I25.10
    with angina pectoris — *see* Arteriosclerosis, coronary (artery),
  corpus cavernosum
    female N90.89
    male N48.6
  diffuse (brain) (spinal cord) G37.0
  disseminated G35
  dorsal G35

**Sclerosis, sclerotic** — *continued*
  dorsolateral (spinal cord) — *see* Degeneration, combined
  endometrium N85.5
  extrapyramidal G25.9
  eye, nuclear (senile) — *see* Cataract, senile, nuclear
  focal and segmental (glomerular) (*see also* N00-N07 with fourth character .1) N05.1
  Friedreich's (spinal cord) G11.1
  funicular (spermatic cord) N50.89
  general (vascular) — *see* Arteriosclerosis
  gland (lymphatic) I89.8
  hepatic K74.1
    alcoholic K70.2
  hereditary
    cerebellar G11.9
    spinal (Friedreich's ataxia) G11.1
  hippocampal G93.81
  insular G35
  kidney — *see* Sclerosis, renal
  larynx J38.7
  lateral (amyotrophic) (descending) (spinal) G12.21
    primary G12.23
  lens, senile nuclear — *see* Cataract, senile, nuclear
  liver K74.1
    with fibrosis K74.2
      alcoholic K70.2
    alcoholic K70.2
    cardiac K76.1
  lung — *see* Fibrosis, lung
  mastoid — *see* Mastoiditis, chronic
  mesial temporal G93.81
  mitral I05.8
  Mönckeberg's (medial) — *see* Arteriosclerosis, extremities
  multiple (brain stem) (cerebral) (generalized) (spinal cord) G35
  myocardium, myocardial — *see* Disease, heart, ischemic, atherosclerotic
  nuclear (senile), eye — *see* Cataract, senile, nuclear
  ovary N83.8
  pancreas K86.89
  penis N48.6
  peripheral arteries — *see* Arteriosclerosis, extremities
  plaques G35
  pluriglandular E31.8
  polyglandular E31.8
  posterolateral (spinal cord) — *see* Degeneration, combined
  presenile (Alzheimer's) — *see* Disease, Alzheimer's, early onset
  primary, lateral G12.23
  progressive, systemic M34.0
  pulmonary — *see* Fibrosis, lung
    artery I27.0
    valve (heart) — *see* Endocarditis, pulmonary
  renal N26.9
    with
      cystine storage disease E72.09
      hypertensive heart disease (conditions in I11) — *see* Hypertension, cardiorenal
    arteriolar (hyaline) (hyperplastic) — *see* Hypertension, kidney
  retina (senile) (vascular) H35.00
  senile (vascular) — *see* Arteriosclerosis
  spinal (cord) (progressive) G95.89
    ascending G61.0
    combined (*see also* Degeneration, combined)
      multiple G35
      syphilitic A52.11
    disseminated G35
    dorsolateral — *see* Degeneration, combined
    hereditary (Friedreich's) (mixed form) G11.1
    lateral (amyotrophic) G12.23
    multiple G35
    posterior (syphilitic) A52.11
  stomach K31.89
  subendocardial, congenital I42.4
  systemic M34.9
    with
      lung involvement M34.81
      myopathy M34.82
      polyneuropathy M34.83
    drug-induced M34.2
    due to chemicals NEC M34.2
    progressive M34.0
    specified NEC M34.89
  temporal (mesial) G93.81

**Sclerosis, sclerotic** — *continued*
  tricuspid (heart) (valve) I07.8
  tuberous (brain) Q85.1
  tympanic membrane — *see* Disorder, tympanic membrane, specified NEC
  valve, valvular (heart) — *see* Endocarditis
  vascular — *see* Arteriosclerosis
  vein I87.8
**Scoliosis** (acquired) (postural) M41.9
  adolescent (idiopathic) — *see* Scoliosis, idiopathic, adolescent
  congenital Q67.5
    due to bony malformation Q76.3
    failure of segmentation (hemivertebra) Q76.3
    hemivertebra fusion Q76.3
    postural Q67.5
  idiopathic M41.20
    adolescent M41.129
      cervical region M41.122
      cervicothoracic region M41.123
      lumbar region M41.126
      lumbosacral region M41.127
      thoracic region M41.124
      thoracolumbar region M41.125
    cervical region M41.22
    cervicothoracic region M41.23
    infantile M41.00
      cervical region M41.02
      cervicothoracic region M41.03
      lumbar region M41.06
      lumbosacral region M41.07
      sacrococcygeal region M41.08
      thoracic region M41.04
      thoracolumbar region M41.05
    juvenile M41.119
      cervical region M41.112
      cervicothoracic region M41.113
      lumbar region M41.116
      lumbosacral region M41.117
      thoracic region M41.114
      thoracolumbar region M41.115
    lumbar region M41.26
    lumbosacral region M41.27
    thoracic region M41.24
    thoracolumbar region M41.25
  infantile — *see* Scoliosis, idiopathic, infantile
  neuromuscular M41.40
    cervical region M41.42
    cervicothoracic region M41.43
    lumbar region M41.46
    lumbosacral region M41.47
    occipito-atlanto-axial region M41.41
    thoracic region M41.44
    thoracolumbar region M41.45
  paralytic — *see* Scoliosis, neuromuscular
  postradiation therapy M96.5
  rachitic (late effect or sequelae) E64.3 [M49.80]
    cervical region E64.3 [M49.82]
    cervicothoracic region E64.3 [M49.83]
    lumbar region E64.3 [M49.86]
    lumbosacral region E64.3 [M49.87]
    multiple sites E64.3 [M49.89]
    occipito-atlanto-axial region E64.3 [M49.81]
    sacrococcygeal region E64.3 [M49.88]
    thoracic region E64.3 [M49.84]
    thoracolumbar region E64.3 [M49.85]
  sciatic M54.4- ☑
  secondary (to) NEC M41.50
    cerebral palsy, Friedreich's ataxia, poliomyelitis, neuromuscular disorders — *see* Scoliosis, neuromuscular
    cervical region M41.52
    cervicothoracic region M41.53
    lumbar region M41.56
    lumbosacral region M41.57
    thoracic region M41.54
    thoracolumbar region M41.55
  specified form NEC M41.80
    cervical region M41.82
    cervicothoracic region M41.83
    lumbar region M41.86
    lumbosacral region M41.87
    thoracic region M41.84
    thoracolumbar region M41.85
  thoracogenic M41.30
    thoracic region M41.34
    thoracolumbar region M41.35
  tuberculous A18.01

**Scoliotic pelvis**
   with disproportion (fetopelvic) O33.0
      causing obstructed labor O65.0
**Scorbutus, scorbutic** (see also Scurvy)
   anemia D53.2
**Score, NIHSS** (National Institutes of Health Stroke Scale)
   R29.7- ☑
**Scotoma** (arcuate) (Bjerrum) (central) (ring) (see also
   Defect, visual field, localized, scotoma)
   scintillating H53.19
**Scratch** — see Abrasion
**Scratchy throat** R09.89
**Screening** (for) Z13.9
   alcoholism Z13.89
   anemia Z13.0
   anomaly, congenital Z13.89
   antenatal, of mother (see also Encounter, antenatal
      screening) Z36.9
   arterial hypertension Z13.6
   arthropod-borne viral disease NEC Z11.59
   bacteriuria, asymptomatic Z13.89
   behavioral disorder Z13.89
   brain injury, traumatic Z13.850
   bronchitis, chronic Z13.83
   brucellosis Z11.2
   cardiovascular disorder Z13.6
   cataract Z13.5
   chlamydial diseases Z11.8
   cholera Z11.0
   chromosomal abnormalities (nonprocreative) NEC
      Z13.79
   colonoscopy Z12.11
   congenital
      dislocation of hip Z13.89
      eye disorder Z13.5
      malformation or deformation Z13.89
   contamination NEC Z13.88
   cystic fibrosis Z13.228
   dengue fever Z11.59
   dental disorder Z13.84
   depression Z13.89
   developmental handicap Z13.4
      in early childhood Z13.4
      infant Z13.4
   diabetes mellitus Z13.1
   diphtheria Z11.2
   disability, intellectual Z13.4
      infant Z13.4
   disease or disorder Z13.9
      bacterial NEC Z11.2
         intestinal infectious Z11.0
         respiratory tuberculosis Z11.1
      blood or blood-forming organ Z13.0
      cardiovascular Z13.6
      Chagas' Z11.6
      chlamydial Z11.8
      dental Z13.89
      developmental Z13.4
         in child Z13.4
         infant Z13.4
      digestive tract NEC Z13.818
         lower GI Z13.811
         upper GI Z13.810
      ear Z13.5
      endocrine Z13.29
      eye Z13.5
      genitourinary Z13.89
      heart Z13.6
      human immunodeficiency virus (HIV) infection
         Z11.4
      immunity Z13.0
      infection
         intestinal Z11.0
            specified NEC Z11.6
      infectious Z11.9
      mental Z13.89
      metabolic Z13.228
      neurological Z13.89
      nutritional Z13.21
         metabolic Z13.228
            lipoid disorders Z13.220
      protozoal Z11.6
         intestinal Z11.0
      respiratory Z13.83
      rheumatic Z13.828
      rickettsial Z11.8
      sexually-transmitted NEC Z11.3
         human immunodeficiency virus (HIV) Z11.4

**Screening** — continued
   disease or disorder — continued
      sickle-cell (trait) Z13.0
      skin Z13.89
      specified NEC Z13.89
      spirochetal Z11.8
      thyroid Z13.29
      vascular Z13.6
      venereal Z11.3
      viral NEC Z11.59
         human immunodeficiency virus (HIV) Z11.4
         intestinal Z11.0
   elevated titer Z13.89
   emphysema Z13.83
   encephalitis, viral (mosquito- or tick-borne) Z11.59
   exposure to contaminants (toxic) Z13.88
   fever
      dengue Z11.59
      hemorrhagic Z11.59
      yellow Z11.59
   filariasis Z11.6
   galactosemia Z13.228
   gastrointestinal condition Z13.818
   genetic (nonprocreative) - for procreative manage-
      ment — see Testing, genetic, for procreative
      management
      disease carrier status (nonprocreative) Z13.71
      specified NEC (nonprocreative) Z13.79
   genitourinary condition Z13.89
   glaucoma Z13.5
   gonorrhea Z11.3
   gout Z13.89
   helminthiasis (intestinal) Z11.6
   hematopoietic malignancy Z12.89
   hemoglobinopathies NEC Z13.0
   hemorrhagic fever Z11.59
   Hodgkin disease Z12.89
   human immunodeficiency virus (HIV) Z11.4
   human papillomavirus Z11.51
   hypertension Z13.6
   immunity disorders Z13.0
   infection
      mycotic Z11.8
      parasitic Z11.8
   ingestion of radioactive substance Z13.88
   intellectual disability Z13.4
      infant Z13.4
   intestinal
      helminthiasis Z11.6
      infectious disease Z11.0
   leishmaniasis Z11.6
   leprosy Z11.2
   leptospirosis Z11.8
   leukemia Z12.89
   lymphoma Z12.89
   malaria Z11.6
   malnutrition Z13.29
      metabolic Z13.228
      nutritional Z13.21
   measles Z11.59
   mental disorder Z13.89
   metabolic errors, inborn Z13.228
   multiphasic Z13.89
   musculoskeletal disorder Z13.828
      osteoporosis Z13.820
   mycoses Z11.8
   myocardial infarction (acute) Z13.6
   neoplasm (malignant) (of) Z12.9
      bladder Z12.6
      blood Z12.89
      breast Z12.39
         routine mammogram Z12.31
      cervix Z12.4
      colon Z12.11
      genitourinary organs NEC Z12.79
         bladder Z12.6
         cervix Z12.4
         ovary Z12.73
         prostate Z12.5
         testis Z12.71
         vagina Z12.72
      hematopoietic system Z12.89
      intestinal tract Z12.10
         colon Z12.11
         rectum Z12.12
         small intestine Z12.13
      lung Z12.2
      lymph (glands) Z12.89
      nervous system Z12.82

**Screening** — continued
   neoplasm — continued
      oral cavity Z12.81
      prostate Z12.5
      rectum Z12.12
      respiratory organs Z12.2
      skin Z12.83
      small intestine Z12.13
      specified site NEC Z12.89
      stomach Z12.0
   nephropathy Z13.89
   nervous system disorders NEC Z13.858
   neurological condition Z13.89
   osteoporosis Z13.820
   parasitic infestation Z11.9
      specified NEC Z11.8
   phenylketonuria Z13.228
   plague Z11.2
   poisoning (chemical) (heavy metal) Z13.88
   poliomyelitis Z11.59
   postnatal, chromosomal abnormalities Z13.89
   prenatal, of mother (see also Encounter, antenatal
      screening) Z36.9
   protozoal disease Z11.6
      intestinal Z11.0
   pulmonary tuberculosis Z11.1
   radiation exposure Z13.88
   respiratory condition Z13.83
   respiratory tuberculosis Z11.1
   rheumatoid arthritis Z13.828
   rubella Z11.59
   schistosomiasis Z11.6
   sexually-transmitted disease NEC Z11.3
      human immunodeficiency virus (HIV) Z11.4
   sickle-cell disease or trait Z13.0
   skin condition Z13.89
   sleeping sickness Z11.6
   special Z13.9
      specified NEC Z13.89
   syphilis Z11.3
   tetanus Z11.2
   trachoma Z11.8
   traumatic brain injury Z13.850
   trypanosomiasis Z11.6
   tuberculosis, respiratory Z11.1
   venereal disease Z11.3
   viral encephalitis (mosquito- or tick-borne) Z11.59
   whooping cough Z11.2
   worms, intestinal Z11.6
   yaws Z11.8
   yellow fever Z11.59
**Scrofula, scrofulosis** (tuberculosis of cervical lymph
   glands) A18.2
**Scrofulide** (primary) (tuberculous) A18.4
**Scrofuloderma, scrofulodermia** (any site) (primary)
   A18.4
**Scrofulosus lichen** (primary) (tuberculous) A18.4
**Scrofulous** — see condition
**Scrotal tongue** K14.5
**Scrotum** — see condition
**Scurvy, scorbutic** E54
   anemia D53.2
   gum E54
   infantile E54
   rickets E55.0 [M90.80]
**Sealpox** B08.62
**Seasickness** T75.3 ☑
**Seatworm** (infection) (infestation) B80
**Sebaceous** (see also condition)
   cyst — see Cyst, sebaceous
**Seborrhea, seborrheic** L21.9
   capillitii R23.8
   capitis L21.0
   dermatitis L21.9
      infantile L21.1
   eczema L21.9
      infantile L21.1
   sicca L21.0
**Seckel's syndrome** Q87.1
**Seclusion, pupil** — see Membrane, pupillary
**Second hand tobacco smoke exposure** (acute)
   (chronic) Z77.22
   in the perinatal period P96.81
**Secondary**
   dentin (in pulp) K04.3
   neoplasm, secondaries — see Table of Neoplasms,
      secondary

## Secretion
antidiuretic hormone, inappropriate E22.2
catecholamine, by pheochromocytoma E27.5
hormone
    antidiuretic, inappropriate (syndrome) E22.2
    by
        carcinoid tumor E34.0
        pheochromocytoma E27.5
    ectopic NEC E34.2
urinary
    excessive R35.8
    suppression R34

## Section
nerve, traumatic — see Injury, nerve

## Sedative, hypnotic, or anxiolytic-induced
anxiety disorder F13.980
bipolar and related disorder F13.94
delirium F13.921
depressive disorder F13.94
major neurocognitive disorder F13.97
mild neurocognitive disorder F13.988
psychotic disorder F13.959
sexual dysfunction F13.981
sleep disorder F13.982

## Segmentation, incomplete (congenital) (see also Fusion)
bone NEC Q78.8
lumbosacral (joint) (vertebra) Q76.49

## Seitelberger's syndrome (infantile neuraxonal dystrophy) G31.89

## Seizure(s) (see also Convulsions) R56.9
akinetic — see Epilepsy, generalized, specified NEC
atonic — see Epilepsy, generalized, specified NEC
autonomic (hysterical) F44.5
convulsive — see Convulsions
cortical (focal) (motor) — see Epilepsy, localization-related, symptomatic, with simple partial seizures
disorder (see also Epilepsy) G40.909
due to stroke — see Sequelae (of), disease, cerebrovascular, by type, specified NEC
epileptic — see Epilepsy
febrile (simple) R56.00
    with status epilepticus G40.901
    complex (atypical) (complicated) R56.01
        with status epilepticus G40.901
grand mal G40.409
    intractable G40.419
        with status epilepticus G40.411
        without status epilepticus G40.419
    not intractable G40.409
        with status epilepticus G40.401
        without status epilepticus G40.409
heart — see Disease, heart
hysterical F44.5
intractable G40.919
    with status epilepticus G40.911
Jacksonian (focal) (motor type) (sensory type) — see Epilepsy, localization-related, symptomatic, with simple partial seizures
newborn P90
nonspecific epileptic
    atonic — see Epilepsy, generalized, specified NEC
    clonic — see Epilepsy, generalized, specified NEC
    myoclonic — see Epilepsy, generalized, specified NEC
    tonic — see Epilepsy, generalized, specified NEC
    tonic-clonic — see Epilepsy, generalized, specified NEC
partial, developing into secondarily generalized seizures
    complex — see Epilepsy, localization-related, symptomatic, with complex partial seizures
    simple — see Epilepsy, localization-related, symptomatic, with simple partial seizures
petit mal G40.409
    intractable G40.419
        with status epilepticus G40.411
        without status epilepticus G40.419
    not intractable G40.409
        with status epilepticus G40.401
        without status epilepticus G40.409
post traumatic R56.1
recurrent G40.909
specified NEC G40.89
uncinate — see Epilepsy, localization-related, symptomatic, with complex partial seizures

## Selenium deficiency, dietary E59

## Self-damaging behavior (life-style) Z72.89
## Self-harm (attempted)
history (personal) Z91.5
    in family Z81.8
## Self-mutilation (attempted)
history (personal) Z91.5
    in family Z81.8
## Self-poisoning
history (personal) Z91.5
    in family Z81.8
observation following (alleged) attempt Z03.6
## Semicoma R40.1
## Seminal vesiculitis N49.0
## Seminoma C62.9- ☑
specified site — see Neoplasm, malignant, by site
## Senear-Usher disease or syndrome L10.4
## Senectus R54
## Senescence (without mention of psychosis) R54
## Senile, senility (see also condition) R41.81
with
    acute confusional state F05
    mental changes NOS F03 ☑
    psychosis NEC — see Psychosis, senile
asthenia R54
cervix (atrophic) N88.8
debility R54
endometrium (atrophic) N85.8
fallopian tube (atrophic) — see Atrophy, fallopian tube
heart (failure) R54
ovary (atrophic) — see Atrophy, ovary
premature E34.8
vagina, vaginitis (atrophic) N95.2
wart L82.1
## Sensation
burning (skin) R20.8
    tongue K14.6
loss of R20.8
prickling (skin) R20.2
tingling (skin) R20.2
## Sense loss
smell — see Disturbance, sensation, smell
taste — see Disturbance, sensation, taste
touch R20.8
## Sensibility disturbance (cortical) (deep) (vibratory) R20.9
## Sensitive, sensitivity (see also Allergy)
carotid sinus G90.01
child (excessive) F93.8
cold, autoimmune D59.1
dentin K03.89
gluten (non-celiac) K90.41
latex Z91.040
methemoglobin D74.8
tuberculin, without clinical or radiological symptoms R76.11
visual
    glare H53.71
    impaired contrast H53.72
## Sensitiver Beziehungswahn F22
## Sensitization, auto-erythrocytic D69.2
## Separation
anxiety, abnormal (of childhood) F93.0
apophysis, traumatic — code as Fracture, by site
choroid — see Detachment, choroid
epiphysis, epiphyseal
    nontraumatic (see also Osteochondropathy, specified type NEC)
        upper femoral — see Slipped, epiphysis, upper femoral
    traumatic — code as Fracture, by site
fracture — see Fracture
infundibulum cardiac from right ventricle by a partition Q24.3
joint (traumatic) (current) — code by site under Dislocation
pubic bone, obstetrical trauma O71.6
retina, retinal — see Detachment, retina
symphysis pubis, obstetrical trauma O71.6
tracheal ring, incomplete, congenital Q32.1
## Sepsis (generalized) (unspecified organism) A41.9
with
    organ dysfunction (acute) (multiple) R65.20
        with septic shock R65.21
actinomycotic A42.7
adrenal hemorrhage syndrome (meningococcal) A39.1
anaerobic A41.4
Bacillus anthracis A22.7
Brucella (see also Brucellosis) A23.9

## Sepsis — continued
candidal B37.7
cryptogenic A41.9
due to device, implant or graft T85.79 ☑
    arterial graft NEC T82.7 ☑
    breast (implant) T85.79 ☑
    catheter NEC T85.79 ☑
        dialysis (renal) T82.7 ☑
            intraperitoneal T85.71 ☑
        infusion NEC T82.7 ☑
            spinal (cranial) (epidural) (intrathecal) (spinal) (subarachnoid) (subdural) T85.735 ☑
        urethral indwelling T83.511 ☑
        urinary T83.518 ☑
    ectopic or molar pregnancy O08.82
    electronic (electrode) (pulse generator) (stimulator)
        bone T84.7 ☑
        cardiac T82.7 ☑
        nervous system T85.738 ☑
            brain T85.731 ☑
            neurostimulator generator T85.734 ☑
            peripheral nerve T85.732 ☑
            spinal cord T85.733 ☑
        urinary T83.590 ☑
    fixation, internal (orthopedic) — see Complication, fixation device, infection
    gastrointestinal (bile duct) (esophagus) T85.79 ☑
        neurostimulator electrode (lead) T85.732 ☑
    genital T83.69 ☑
    heart NEC T82.7 ☑
        valve (prosthesis) T82.6 ☑
            graft T82.7 ☑
    joint prosthesis — see Complication, joint prosthesis, infection
    ocular (corneal graft) (orbital implant) T85.79 ☑
    orthopedic NEC T84.7 ☑
        fixation device, internal — see Complication, fixation device, infection
    specified NEC T85.79 ☑
    vascular T82.7 ☑
    ventricular intracranial (communicating) shunt T85.730 ☑
during labor O75.3
Enterococcus A41.81
Erysipelothrix (rhusiopathiae) (erysipeloid) A26.7
Escherichia coli (E. coli) A41.5 ☑
extraintestinal yersiniosis A28.2
following
    abortion (subsequent episode) O08.0
        current episode — see Abortion
    ectopic or molar pregnancy O08.82
    immunization T88.0 ☑
    infusion, therapeutic injection or transfusion NEC T80.29 ☑
gangrenous A41.9
gonococcal A54.86
Gram-negative (organism) A41.5 ☑
    anaerobic A41.4
Haemophilus influenzae A41.3
herpesviral B00.7
intra-abdominal K65.1
intraocular — see Endophthalmitis, purulent
Listeria monocytogenes A32.7
localized — code to specific localized infection
    in operation wound T81.4 ☑
    skin — see Abscess
malleus A24.0
melioidosis A24.1
meningeal — see Meningitis
meningococcal A39.4
    acute A39.2
    chronic A39.3
MSSA (Methicillin susceptible Staphylococcus aureus) A41.01
newborn P36.9
    due to
        anaerobes NEC P36.5
        Escherichia coli P36.4
        Staphylococcus P36.30
            aureus P36.2
            specified NEC P36.39
        Streptococcus P36.10
            group B P36.0
            specified NEC P36.19
    specified NEC P36.8
Pasteurella multocida A28.0

▼ Subterms under main terms may continue to next column or page      ☑ Additional Character Required — Refer to the Tabular List for Character Selection      283

Secretion — Sepsis

**Sepsis** — continued
pelvic, puerperal, postpartum, childbirth O85
pneumococcal A40.3
postprocedural T81.4 ☑
puerperal, postpartum, childbirth (pelvic) O85
Salmonella (arizonae) (cholerae-suis) (enteritidis) (ty-phimurium) A02.1
severe R65.20
with septic shock R65.21
Shigella (see also Dysentery, bacillary) A03.9
skin, localized — see Abscess
specified organism NEC A41.89
Staphylococcus, staphylococcal A41.2
aureus (methicillin susceptible) (MSSA) A41.01
methicillin resistant (MRSA) A41.02
coagulase-negative A41.1
specified NEC A41.1
Streptococcus, streptococcal A40.9
agalactiae A40.1
group
A A40.0
B A40.1
D A41.81
neonatal P36.10
group B P36.0
specified NEC P36.19
pneumoniae A40.3
pyogenes A40.0
specified NEC A40.8
tracheostomy stoma J95.02
tularemic A21.7
umbilical, umbilical cord (newborn) — see Sepsis, newborn
Yersinia pestis A20.7
**Septate** — see Septum
**Septic** — see condition
arm — see Cellulitis, upper limb
with lymphangitis — see Lymphangitis, acute, upper limb
embolus — see Embolism
finger — see Cellulitis, digit
with lymphangitis — see Lymphangitis, acute, digit
foot — see Cellulitis, lower limb
with lymphangitis — see Lymphangitis, acute, lower limb
gallbladder (acute) K81.0
hand — see Cellulitis, upper limb
with lymphangitis — see Lymphangitis, acute, upper limb
joint — see Arthritis, pyogenic or pyemic
leg — see Cellulitis, lower limb
with lymphangitis — see Lymphangitis, acute, lower limb
nail (see also Cellulitis, digit)
with lymphangitis — see Lymphangitis, acute, digit
sore (see also Abscess)
throat J02.0
streptococcal J02.0
spleen (acute) D73.89
teeth, tooth (pulpal origin) K04.4
throat — see Pharyngitis
thrombus — see Thrombosis
toe — see Cellulitis, digit
with lymphangitis — see Lymphangitis, acute, digit
tonsils, chronic J35.01
with adenoiditis J35.03
uterus — see Endometritis
**Septicemia** A41.9
meaning sepsis — see Sepsis
**Septum, septate** (congenital) (see also Anomaly, by site)
anal Q42.3
with fistula Q42.2
aqueduct of Sylvius Q03.0
with spina bifida — see Spina bifida, by site, with hydrocephalus
uterus (complete) (partial) Q51.2
vagina Q52.10
in pregnancy — see Pregnancy, complicated by, abnormal vagina
causing obstructed labor O65.5
longitudinal Q52.129
microperforate
left side Q52.124
right side Q52.123
nonobstruction Q52.120

**Septum, septate** — continued
vagina — continued
longitudinal — continued
obstructing Q52.129
left side Q52.122
right side Q52.121
transverse Q52.11
**Sequelae** (of) (see also condition)
abscess, intracranial or intraspinal (conditions in G06) G09
amputation — code to injury with seventh character S
burn and corrosion — code to injury with seventh character S
calcium deficiency E64.8
cerebrovascular disease — see Sequelae, disease, cerebrovascular
childbirth O94
contusion — code to injury with seventh character S
corrosion — see Sequelae, burn and corrosion
crushing injury — code to injury with seventh character S
disease
cerebrovascular I69.90
alteration of sensation I69.998
aphasia I69.920
apraxia I69.990
ataxia I69.993
cognitive deficits I69.91 ☑
disturbance of vision I69.998
dysarthria I69.922
dysphagia I69.991
dysphasia I69.921
facial droop I69.992
facial weakness I69.992
fluency disorder I69.923
hemiplegia I69.95- ☑
hemorrhage
intracerebral — see Sequelae, hemorrhage, intracerebral
intracranial, nontraumatic NEC — see Sequelae, hemorrhage, intracranial, nontraumatic
subarachnoid — see Sequelae, hemorrhage, subarachnoid
language deficit I69.928
monoplegia
lower limb I69.94- ☑
upper limb I69.93- ☑
paralytic syndrome I69.96- ☑
specified effect NEC I69.998
specified type NEC I69.80
alteration of sensation I69.898
aphasia I69.820
apraxia I69.890
ataxia I69.893
cognitive deficits I69.81 ☑
disturbance of vision I69.898
dysarthria I69.822
dysphagia I69.891
dysphasia I69.821
facial droop I69.892
facial weakness I69.892
fluency disorder I69.823
hemiplegia I69.85- ☑
language deficit I69.828
monoplegia
lower limb I69.84- ☑
upper limb I69.83- ☑
paralytic syndrome I69.86- ☑
specified effect NEC I69.898
speech deficit I69.928
speech deficit I69.828
stroke NOS — see Sequelae, stroke NOS
dislocation — code to injury with seventh character S
encephalitis or encephalomyelitis (conditions in G04) G09
in infectious disease NEC B94.8
viral B94.1
external cause — code to injury with seventh character S
foreign body entering natural orifice — code to injury with seventh character S
fracture — code to injury with seventh character S
frostbite — code to injury with seventh character S
Hansen's disease B92
hemorrhage
intracerebral I69.10

**Sequelae** — continued
hemorrhage — continued
intracerebral — continued
alteration of sensation I69.198
aphasia I69.120
apraxia I69.190
ataxia I69.193
cognitive deficits I69.11 ☑
disturbance of vision I69.198
dysarthria I69.122
dysphagia I69.191
dysphasia I69.121
facial droop I69.192
facial weakness I69.192
fluency disorder I69.123
hemiplegia I69.15- ☑
language deficit NEC I69.128
monoplegia
lower limb I69.14- ☑
upper limb I69.13- ☑
paralytic syndrome I69.16- ☑
specified effect NEC I69.198
speech deficit NEC I69.128
intracranial, nontraumatic NEC I69.20
alteration of sensation I69.298
aphasia I69.220
apraxia I69.290
ataxia I69.293
cognitive deficits I69.21 ☑
disturbance of vision I69.298
dysarthria I69.222
dysphagia I69.291
dysphasia I69.221
facial droop I69.292
facial weakness I69.292
fluency disorder I69.223
hemiplegia I69.25- ☑
language deficit NEC I69.228
monoplegia
lower limb I69.24- ☑
upper limb I69.23- ☑
paralytic syndrome I69.26- ☑
specified effect NEC I69.298
speech deficit NEC I69.228
subarachnoid I69.00
alteration of sensation I69.098
aphasia I69.020
apraxia I69.090
ataxia I69.093
cognitive deficits — see subcategory I69.01- ☑
disturbance of vision I69.098
dysarthria I69.022
dysphagia I69.091
dysphasia I69.021
facial droop I69.092
facial weakness I69.092
fluency disorder I69.023
hemiplegia I69.05- ☑
language deficit NEC I69.028
monoplegia
lower limb I69.04- ☑
upper limb I69.03- ☑
paralytic syndrome I69.06- ☑
specified effect NEC I69.098
speech deficit NEC I69.028
hepatitis, viral B94.2
hyperalimentation E68
infarction
cerebral I69.30
alteration of sensation I69.398
aphasia I69.320
apraxia I69.390
ataxia I69.393
cognitive deficits I69.31 ☑
disturbance of vision I69.398
dysarthria I69.322
dysphagia I69.391
dysphasia I69.321
facial droop I69.392
facial weakness I69.392
fluency disorder I69.323
hemiplegia I69.35- ☑
language deficit NEC I69.328
monoplegia
lower limb I69.34- ☑
upper limb I69.33- ☑
paralytic syndrome I69.36- ☑
specified effect NEC I69.398

☑ Additional Character Required — Refer to the Tabular List for Character Selection

▽ Subterms under main terms may continue to next column or page

**Sequelae** — *continued*
  infarction — *continued*
    cerebral — *continued*
      speech deficit NEC I69.328
  infection, pyogenic, intracranial or intraspinal G09
  infectious disease B94.9
    specified NEC B94.8
  injury — *code to* injury with seventh character S
  leprosy B92
  meningitis
    bacterial (conditions in G00) G09
    other or unspecified cause (conditions in G03) G09
  muscle (and tendon) injury — *code to* injury with seventh character S
  myelitis — *see* Sequelae, encephalitis
  niacin deficiency E64.8
  nutritional deficiency E64.9
    specified NEC E64.8
  obstetrical condition O94
  parasitic disease B94.9
  phlebitis or thrombophlebitis of intracranial or intraspinal venous sinuses and veins (conditions in G08) G09
  poisoning — *code to* poisoning with seventh character S
    nonmedicinal substance — *see* Sequelae, toxic effect, nonmedicinal substance
  poliomyelitis (acute) B91
  pregnancy O94
  protein-energy malnutrition E64.0
  puerperium O94
  rickets E64.3
  selenium deficiency E64.8
  sprain and strain — *code to* injury with seventh character S
  stroke NOS I69.30
    alteration in sensation I69.398
    aphasia I69.320
    apraxia I69.390
    ataxia I69.393
    cognitive deficits I69.31 ☑
    disturbance of vision I69.398
    dysarthria I69.322
    dysphagia I69.391
    dysphasia I69.321
    facial droop I69.392
    facial weakness I69.392
    hemiplegia I69.35- ☑
    language deficit NEC I69.328
    monoplegia
      lower limb I69.34- ☑
      upper limb I69.33- ☑
    paralytic syndrome I69.36- ☑
    specified effect NEC I69.398
    speech deficit NEC I69.328
  tendon and muscle injury — *code to* injury with seventh character S
  thiamine deficiency E64.8
  trachoma B94.0
  tuberculosis B90.9
    bones and joints B90.2
    central nervous system B90.0
    genitourinary B90.1
    pulmonary (respiratory) B90.9
    specified organs NEC B90.8
  viral
    encephalitis B94.1
    hepatitis B94.2
  vitamin deficiency NEC E64.8
    A E64.1
    B E64.8
    C E64.2
  wound, open — *code to* injury with seventh character S

**Sequestration** (*see also* Sequestrum)
  disk — *see* Displacement, intervertebral disk
  lung, congenital Q33.2

**Sequestrum**
  bone — *see* Osteomyelitis, chronic
  dental M27.2
  jaw bone M27.2
  orbit — *see* Osteomyelitis, orbit
  sinus (accessory) (nasal) — *see* Sinusitis

**Sequoiosis lung or pneumonitis** J67.8

---

**Serology for syphilis**
  doubtful
    with signs or symptoms — *code by* site and stage under Syphilis
    follow-up of latent syphilis — *see* Syphilis, latent
  negative, with signs or symptoms — *code by* site and stage under Syphilis
  positive A53.0
    with signs or symptoms — *code by* site and stage under Syphilis
  reactivated A53.0

**Seroma** (*see also* Hematoma)
  postprocedural — *see* Complication, postprocedural, seroma
  traumatic, secondary and recurrent T79.2 ☑

**Seropurulent** — *see* condition

**Serositis, multiple** K65.8
  pericardial I31.1
  peritoneal K65.8

**Serous** — *see* condition

**Sertoli cell**
  adenoma
    specified site — *see* Neoplasm, benign, by site
    unspecified site
      female D27.9
      male D29.20
  carcinoma
    specified site — *see* Neoplasm, malignant, by site
    unspecified site (male) C62.9- ☑
      female C56.9
  tumor
    with lipid storage
      specified site — *see* Neoplasm, benign, by site
      unspecified site
        female D27.9
        male D29.20
    specified site — *see* Neoplasm, benign, by site
    unspecified site
      female D27.9
      male D29.20

**Sertoli-Leydig cell tumor** — *see* Neoplasm, benign, by site
  specified site — *see* Neoplasm, benign, by site
  unspecified site
    female D27.9
    male D29.20

**Serum**
  allergy, allergic reaction (*see also* Reaction, serum) T80.69 ☑
    shock (*see also* Shock, anaphylactic) T80.59 ☑
  arthritis (*see also* Reaction, serum) T80.69 ☑
  complication or reaction NEC (*see also* Reaction, serum) T80.69 ☑
  disease NEC (*see also* Reaction, serum) T80.69 ☑
  hepatitis (*see also* Hepatitis, viral, type B)
    carrier (suspected) of B18.1
  intoxication (*see also* Reaction, serum) T80.69 ☑
  neuritis (*see also* Reaction, serum) T80.69 ☑
  neuropathy G61.1
  poisoning NEC (*see also* Reaction, serum) T80.69 ☑
  rash NEC (*see also* Reaction, serum) T80.69 ☑
  reaction NEC (*see also* Reaction, serum) T80.69 ☑
  sickness NEC (*see also* Reaction, serum) T80.69 ☑
  urticaria (*see also* Reaction, serum) T80.69 ☑

**Sesamoiditis** M25.8- ☑

**Severe sepsis** R65.20
  with septic shock R65.21

**Sever's disease or osteochondrosis** — *see* Osteochondrosis, juvenile, tarsus

**Sex**
  chromosome mosaics Q97.8
    lines with various numbers of X chromosomes Q97.2
  education Z70.8
  reassignment surgery status Z87.890

**Sextuplet pregnancy** — *see* Pregnancy, sextuplet

**Sexual**
  function, disorder of (psychogenic) F52.9
  immaturity (female) (male) E30.0
  impotence (psychogenic) organic origin NEC — *see* Dysfunction, sexual, male
  precocity (constitutional) (cryptogenic) (female) (idiopathic) (male) E30.1

**Sexuality, pathologic** — *see* Deviation, sexual

**Sézary disease** C84.1- ☑

**Shadow, lung** R91.8

**Shaking palsy or paralysis** — *see* Parkinsonism

---

**Shallowness, acetabulum** — *see* Derangement, joint, specified type NEC, hip

**Shaver's disease** J63.1

**Sheath** (tendon) — *see* condition

**Sheathing, retinal vessels** H35.01- ☑

**Shedding**
  nail L60.8
  premature, primary (deciduous) teeth K00.6

**Sheehan's disease or syndrome** E23.0

**Shelf, rectal** K62.89

**Shell teeth** K00.5

**Shellshock** (current) F43.0
  lasting state — *see* Disorder, post-traumatic stress

**Shield kidney** Q63.1

**Shift**
  auditory threshold (temporary) H93.24- ☑
  mediastinal R93.8

**Shifting sleep-work schedule** (affecting sleep) G47.26

**Shiga** (-Kruse) **dysentery** A03.0

**Shiga's bacillus** A03.0

**Shigella** (dysentery) — *see* Dysentery, bacillary

**Shigellosis** A03.9
  Group A A03.0
  Group B A03.1
  Group C A03.2
  Group D A03.3

**Shin splints** S86.89- ☑

**Shingles** — *see* Herpes, zoster

**Shipyard disease or eye** B30.0

**Shirodkar suture, in pregnancy** — *see* Pregnancy, complicated by, incompetent cervix

**Shock** R57.9
  with ectopic or molar pregnancy O08.3
  adrenal (cortical) (Addisonian) E27.2
  adverse food reaction (anaphylactic) — *see* Shock, anaphylactic, due to food
  allergic — *see* Shock, anaphylactic
  anaphylactic T78.2 ☑
    chemical — *see* Table of Drugs and Chemicals
    due to drug or medicinal substance
      correct substance properly administered T88.6
      overdose or wrong substance given or taken (by accident) — *see* Table of Drugs and Chemicals, by drug, poisoning
    due to food (nonpoisonous) T78.00 ☑
      additives T78.06 ☑
      dairy products T78.07 ☑
      eggs T78.08 ☑
      fish T78.03 ☑
        shellfish T78.02 ☑
      fruit T78.04 ☑
      milk T78.07 ☑
      nuts T78.05 ☑
        multiple types T78.05 ☑
        peanuts T78.01 ☑
      peanuts T78.01 ☑
      seeds T78.05 ☑
      specified type NEC T78.09 ☑
      vegetable T78.04 ☑
    following sting(s) — *see* Venom
    immunization T80.52 ☑
    serum T80.59 ☑
      blood and blood products T80.51 ☑
      immunization T80.52 ☑
      specified NEC T80.59 ☑
      vaccination T80.52 ☑
  anaphylactoid — *see* Shock, anaphylactic
  anesthetic
    correct substance properly administered T88.2 ☑
    overdose or wrong substance given or taken — *see* Table of Drugs and Chemicals, by drug, poisoning
      specified anesthetic — *see* Table of Drugs and Chemicals, by drug, poisoning
  cardiogenic R57.0
  chemical substance — *see* Table of Drugs and Chemicals
  complicating ectopic or molar pregnancy O08.3
  culture — *see* Disorder, adjustment
  drug
    due to correct substance properly administered T88.6 ☑
    overdose or wrong substance given or taken (by accident) — *see* Table of Drugs and Chemicals, by drug, poisoning
  during or after labor and delivery O75.1

---

**Shock** — continued
- electric T75.4 ☑
  - (taser) T75.4 ☑
- endotoxic R65.21
  - postprocedural (resulting from a procedure, not elsewhere classified) T81.12 ☑
- following
  - ectopic or molar pregnancy O08.3
  - injury (immediate) (delayed) T79.4 ☑
  - labor and delivery O75.1
- food (anaphylactic) — see Shock, anaphylactic, due to food
- from electroshock gun (taser) T75.4 ☑
- gram-negative R65.21
  - postprocedural (resulting from a procedure, not elsewhere classified) T81.12 ☑
- hematologic R57.8
- hemorrhagic R57.8
  - surgery (intraoperative) (postoperative) T81.19 ☑
  - trauma T79.4 ☑
- hypovolemic R57.1
  - surgical T81.19 ☑
  - traumatic T79.4 ☑
- insulin E15
  - therapeutic misadventure — see subcategory T38.3 ☑
- kidney N17.0
  - traumatic (following crushing) T79.5 ☑
- lightning T75.01 ☑
- liver K72.00
- lung J80
- obstetric O75.1
  - with ectopic or molar pregnancy O08.3
  - following ectopic or molar pregnancy O08.3
- pleural (surgical) T81.19 ☑
  - due to trauma T79.4 ☑
- postprocedural (postoperative) T81.10 ☑
  - with ectopic or molar pregnancy O08.3
  - cardiogenic T81.11 ☑
  - endotoxic T81.12 ☑
  - following ectopic or molar pregnancy O08.3
  - gram-negative T81.12 ☑
  - hypovolemic T81.19 ☑
  - septic T81.12 ☑
  - specified type NEC T81.19 ☑
- psychic F43.0
- septic (due to severe sepsis) R65.21
- specified NEC R57.8
- surgical T81.10 ☑
- taser gun (taser) T75.4 ☑
- therapeutic misadventure NEC T81.10 ☑
- thyroxin
  - overdose or wrong substance given or taken — see Table of Drugs and Chemicals, by drug, poisoning
- toxic, syndrome A48.3
- transfusion — see Complications, transfusion
- traumatic (immediate) (delayed) T79.4 ☑

**Shoemaker's chest** M95.4

**Short, shortening, shortness**
- arm (acquired) (see also Deformity, limb, unequal length)
  - congenital Q71.81- ☑
  - forearm — see Deformity, limb, unequal length
- bowel syndrome K91.2
- breath R06.02
- cervical (complicating pregnancy) O26.87- ☑
  - non-gravid uterus N88.3
- common bile duct, congenital Q44.5
- cord (umbilical), complicating delivery O69.3 ☑
- cystic duct, congenital Q44.5
- esophagus (congenital) Q39.8
- femur (acquired) — see Deformity, limb, unequal length, femur
  - congenital — see Defect, reduction, lower limb, longitudinal, femur
- frenum, frenulum, linguae (congenital) Q38.1
- hip (acquired) (see also Deformity, limb, unequal length)
  - congenital Q65.89
- leg (acquired) (see also Deformity, limb, unequal length)
  - congenital Q72.81- ☑
  - lower leg (see also Deformity, limb, unequal length)
- limbed stature, with immunodeficiency D82.2
- lower limb (acquired) (see also Deformity, limb, unequal length)

**Short, shortening, shortness** — continued
- lower limb (see also Deformity, limb, unequal length) — continued
  - congenital Q72.81- ☑
- organ or site, congenital NEC — see Distortion
- palate, congenital Q38.5
- radius (acquired) (see also Deformity, limb, unequal length)
  - congenital — see Defect, reduction, upper limb, longitudinal, radius
- rib syndrome Q77.2
- stature (child) (hereditary) (idiopathic) NEC R62.52
  - constitutional E34.3
  - due to endocrine disorder E34.3
  - Laron-type E34.3
- tendon (see also Contraction, tendon)
  - with contracture of joint — see Contraction, joint
  - Achilles (acquired) M67.0- ☑
    - congenital Q66.89
  - congenital Q79.8
- thigh (acquired) (see also Deformity, limb, unequal length, femur)
  - congenital — see Defect, reduction, lower limb, longitudinal, femur
- tibialis anterior (tendon) — see Contraction, tendon
- umbilical cord
  - complicating delivery O69.3 ☑
- upper limb, congenital — see Defect, reduction, upper limb, specified type NEC
- urethra N36.8
- uvula, congenital Q38.5
- vagina (congenital) Q52.4

**Shortsightedness** — see Myopia

**Shoshin** (acute fulminating beriberi) E51.11

**Shoulder** — see condition

**Shovel-shaped incisors** K00.2

**Shower, thromboembolic** — see Embolism

**Shunt**
- arterial-venous (dialysis) Z99.2
- arteriovenous, pulmonary (acquired) I28.0
  - congenital Q25.72
- cerebral ventricle (communicating) in situ Z98.2
- surgical, prosthetic, with complications — see Complications, cardiovascular, device or implant

**Shutdown, renal** N28.9

**Shy-Drager syndrome** G90.3

**Sialadenitis, sialadenosis** (any gland) (chronic) (periodic) (suppurative) — see Sialoadenitis

**Sialectasia** K11.8

**Sialidosis** E77.1

**Sialitis, silitis** (any gland) (chronic) (suppurative) — see Sialoadenitis

**Sialoadenitis** (any gland) (periodic) (suppurative) K11.20
- acute K11.21
  - recurrent K11.22
- chronic K11.23

**Sialoadenopathy** K11.9

**Sialoangitis** — see Sialoadenitis

**Sialodochitis** (fibrinosa) — see Sialoadenitis

**Sialodocholithiasis** K11.5

**Sialolithiasis** K11.5

**Sialometaplasia, necrotizing** K11.8

**Sialorrhea** (see also Ptyalism)
- periodic — see Sialoadenitis

**Sialosis** K11.7

**Siamese twin** Q89.4

**Sibling rivalry** Z62.891

**Sicard's syndrome** G52.7

**Sicca syndrome** M35.00
- with
  - keratoconjunctivitis M35.01
  - lung involvement M35.02
  - myopathy M35.03
  - renal tubulo-interstitial disorders M35.04
  - specified organ involvement NEC M35.09

**Sick** R69
- or handicapped person in family Z63.79
  - needing care at home Z63.6
- sinus (syndrome) I49.5

**Sick-euthyroid syndrome** E07.81

**Sickle-cell**
- anemia — see Disease, sickle-cell
- trait D57.3

**Sicklemia** (see also Disease, sickle-cell)
- trait D57.3

**Sickness**
- air (travel) T75.3 ☑

**Sickness** — continued
- airplane T75.3 ☑
- alpine T70.20 ☑
- altitude T70.20 ☑
- Andes T70.29 ☑
- aviator's T70.29 ☑
- balloon T70.29 ☑
- car T75.3 ☑
- compressed air T70.3 ☑
- decompression T70.3 ☑
- green D50.8
- milk — see Poisoning, food, noxious
- motion T75.3 ☑
- mountain T70.29 ☑
  - acute D75.1
- protein (see also Reaction, serum) T80.69 ☑
- radiation T66 ☑
- roundabout (motion) T75.3 ☑
- sea T75.3 ☑
- serum NEC (see also Reaction, serum) T80.69 ☑
- sleeping (African) B56.9
  - by Trypanosoma B56.9
    - brucei
      - gambiense B56.0
      - rhodesiense B56.1
    - East African B56.1
    - Gambian B56.0
    - Rhodesian B56.1
    - West African B56.0
- swing (motion) T75.3 ☑
- train (railway) (travel) T75.3 ☑
- travel (any vehicle) T75.3 ☑

**Sideropenia** — see Anemia, iron deficiency

**Siderosilicosis** J62.8

**Siderosis** (lung) J63.4
- eye (globe) — see Disorder, globe, degenerative, siderosis

**Siemens' syndrome** (ectodermal dysplasia) Q82.8

**Sighing** R06.89
- psychogenic F45.8

**Sigmoid** (see also condition)
- flexure — see condition
- kidney Q63.1

**Sigmoiditis** (see also Enteritis) K52.9
- infectious A09
- noninfectious K52.9

**Silfverskiöld's syndrome** Q78.9

**Silicosiderosis** J62.8

**Silicosis, silicotic** (simple) (complicated) J62.8
- with tuberculosis J65

**Silicotuberculosis** J65

**Silo-fillers' disease** J68.8
- bronchitis J68.0
- pneumonitis J68.0
- pulmonary edema J68.1

**Silver's syndrome** Q87.1

**Simian malaria** B53.1

**Simmonds' cachexia or disease** E23.0

**Simons' disease or syndrome** (progressive lipodystrophy) E88.1

**Simple, simplex** — see condition

**Simulation, conscious** (of illness) Z76.5

**Simultanagnosia** (asimultagnosia) R48.3

**Sin Nombre virus disease** (Hantavirus) (cardio)-pulmonary syndrome) B33.4

**Sinding-Larsen disease or osteochondrosis** — see Osteochondrosis, juvenile, patella

**Singapore hemorrhagic fever** A91

**Singer's node or nodule** J38.2

**Single**
- atrium Q21.2
- coronary artery Q24.5
- umbilical artery Q27.0
- ventricle Q20.4

**Singultus** R06.6
- epidemicus B33.0

**Sinus** (see also Fistula)
- abdominal K63.89
- arrest I45.5
- arrhythmia I49.8
- bradycardia R00.1
- branchial cleft (internal) (external) Q18.0
- coccygeal — see Sinus, pilonidal
- dental K04.6
- dermal (congenital) Q06.8
  - with abscess Q06.8
  - coccygeal, pilonidal — see Sinus, coccygeal

☑ **Additional Character Required** — Refer to the Tabular List for Character Selection

▽ **Subterms under main terms may continue to next column or page**

**Sinus** — *continued*
  infected, skin NEC L08.89
  marginal, ruptured or bleeding — *see* Hemorrhage,
    antepartum, specified cause NEC
  medial, face and neck Q18.8
  pause I45.5
  pericranii Q01.9
  pilonidal (infected) (rectum) L05.92
    with abscess L05.02
  preauricular Q18.1
  rectovaginal N82.3
  Rokitansky-Aschoff (gallbladder) K82.8
  sacrococcygeal (dermoid) (infected) — *see* Sinus, pi-
    lonidal
  tachycardia R00.0
    paroxysmal I47.1
  tarsi syndrome M25.57- ☑
  testis N50.89
  tract (postinfective) — *see* Fistula
  urachus Q64.4
**Sinusitis** (accessory) (chronic) (hyperplastic) (nasal)
  (nonpurulent) (purulent) J32.9
  acute J01.90
    ethmoidal J01.20
      recurrent J01.21
    frontal J01.10
      recurrent J01.11
    involving more than one sinus, other than pansi-
      nusitis J01.80
      recurrent J01.81
    maxillary J01.00
      recurrent J01.01
    pansinusitis J01.40
      recurrent J01.41
    recurrent J01.91
    specified NEC J01.80
      recurrent J01.81
    sphenoidal J01.30
      recurrent J01.31
  allergic — *see* Rhinitis, allergic
  due to high altitude T70.1 ☑
  ethmoidal J32.2
    acute J01.20
      recurrent J01.21
  frontal J32.1
    acute J01.10
      recurrent J01.11
  influenzal — *see* Influenza, with, respiratory manifes-
    tations NEC
  involving more than one sinus but not pansinusitis
    J32.8
    acute J01.80
      recurrent J01.81
  maxillary J32.0
    acute J01.00
      recurrent J01.01
  sphenoidal J32.3
    acute J01.30
      recurrent J01.31
  tuberculous, any sinus A15.8
**Sinusitis-bronchiectasis-situs inversus** (syndrome)
  (triad) Q89.3
**Sipple's syndrome** E31.22
**Sirenomelia** (syndrome) Q87.2
**Siriasis** T67.0 ☑
**Sirkari's disease** B55.0
**Siti** A65
**Situation, psychiatric** F99
**Situational**
  disturbance (transient) — *see* Disorder, adjustment
    acute F43.0
  maladjustment — *see* Disorder, adjustment
  reaction — *see* Disorder, adjustment
    acute F43.0
**Situs inversus or transversus** (abdominalis) (thoracic)
  Q89.3
**Sixth disease** B08.20
  due to human herpesvirus 6 B08.21
  due to human herpesvirus 7 B08.22
**Sjögren-Larsson syndrome** Q87.1
**Sjögren's syndrome or disease** — *see* Sicca syndrome
**Skeletal** — *see* condition
**Skene's gland** — *see* condition
**Skenitis** — *see* Urethritis
**Skerljevo** A65
**Skevas-Zerfus disease** — *see* Toxicity, venom, marine
  animal, sea anemone
**Skin** (*see also* condition)

**Skin** — *continued*
  clammy R23.1
  donor — *see* Donor, skin
  hidebound M35.9
**Slate-dressers' or slate-miners' lung** J62.8
**Sleep**
  apnea — *see* Apnea, sleep
  deprivation Z72.820
  disorder or disturbance G47.9
    child F51.9
    nonorganic origin F51.9
    specified NEC G47.8
  disturbance G47.9
    nonorganic origin F51.9
  drunkenness F51.9
  rhythm inversion G47.2- ☑
  terrors F51.4
  walking F51.3
    hysterical F44.89
**Sleep hygiene**
  abuse Z72.821
  inadequate Z72.821
  poor Z72.821
**Sleeping sickness** — *see* Sickness, sleeping
**Sleeplessness** — *see* Insomnia
  menopausal N95.1
**Sleep-wake schedule disorder** G47.20
**Slim disease** (in HIV infection) B20
**Slipped, slipping**
  epiphysis (traumatic) (*see also* Osteochondropathy,
    specified type NEC)
    capital femoral (traumatic)
      acute (on chronic) S79.01- ☑
    current traumatic — *code as* Fracture, by site
    upper femoral (nontraumatic) M93.00- ☑
      acute M93.01- ☑
        on chronic M93.03- ☑
      chronic M93.02- ☑
  intervertebral disc — *see* Displacement, intervertebral
    disc
  ligature, umbilical P51.8
  patella — *see* Disorder, patella, derangement NEC
  rib M89.8X8
  sacroiliac joint — *see* subcategory M53.2 ☑
  tendon — *see* Disorder, tendon
  ulnar nerve, nontraumatic — *see* Lesion, nerve, ulnar
  vertebra NEC — *see* Spondylolisthesis
**Slocumb's syndrome** E27.0
**Sloughing** (multiple) (phagedena) (skin) (*see also* Gangrene)
  abscess — *see* Abscess
  appendix K38.8
  fascia — *see* Disorder, soft tissue, specified type NEC
  scrotum N50.89
  tendon — *see* Disorder, tendon
  transplanted organ — *see* Rejection, transplant
  ulcer — *see* Ulcer, skin
**Slow**
  feeding, newborn P92.2
  flow syndrome, coronary I20.8
  heart (beat) R00.1
**Slowing, urinary stream** R39.198
**Sluder's neuralgia** (syndrome) G44.89
**Slurred, slurring speech** R47.81
**Small** (ness)
  for gestational age — *see* Small for dates
  introitus, vagina N89.6
  kidney (unknown cause) N27.9
    bilateral N27.1
    unilateral N27.0
  ovary (congenital) Q50.39
  pelvis
    with disproportion (fetopelvic) O33.1
      causing obstructed labor O65.1
  uterus N85.8
  white kidney N03.9
**Small-and-light-for-dates** — *see* Small for dates
**Small-for-dates** (infant) P05.10
  with weight of
    499 grams or less P05.11
    500-749 grams P05.12
    750-999 grams P05.13
    1000-1249 grams P05.14
    1250-1499 grams P05.15
    1500-1749 grams P05.16
    1750-1999 grams P05.17
    2000-2499 grams P05.18

**Small-for-dates** — *continued*
  with weight of — *continued*
    2500 grams and over P05.19
    specified NEC P05.19
**Smallpox** B03
**Smearing, fecal** R15.1
**Smith-Lemli-Opitz syndrome** E78.72
**Smith's fracture** S52.54- ☑
**Smoker** — *see* Dependence, drug, nicotine
**Smoker's**
  bronchitis J41.0
  cough J41.0
  palate K13.24
  throat J31.2
  tongue K13.24
**Smoking**
  passive Z77.22
**Smothering spells** R06.81
**Snaggle teeth, tooth** M26.39
**Snapping**
  finger — *see* Trigger finger
  hip — *see* Derangement, joint, specified type NEC, hip
    involving the iliotiblial band M76.3- ☑
  knee — *see* Derangement, knee
    involving the iliotiblial band M76.3- ☑
**Sneddon-Wilkinson disease or syndrome** (sub-corneal
  pustular dermatosis) L13.1
**Sneezing** (intractable) R06.7
**Sniffing**
  cocaine
    abuse — *see* Abuse, drug, cocaine
    dependence — *see* Dependence, drug, cocaine
  gasoline
    abuse — *see* Abuse, drug, inhalant
    dependence — *see* Dependence, drug, inhalant
  glue (airplane)
    abuse — *see* Abuse, drug, inhalant
    drug dependence — *see* Dependence, drug, in-
      halant
**Sniffles**
  newborn P28.89
**Snoring** R06.83
**Snow blindness** — *see* Photokeratitis
**Snuffles** (non-syphilitic) R06.5
  newborn P28.89
  syphilitic (infant) A50.05 [J99]
**Social**
  exclusion Z60.4
    due to discrimination or persecution (perceived)
      Z60.5
  migrant Z59.0
    acculturation difficulty Z60.3
  rejection Z60.4
    due to discrimination or persecution Z60.5
  role conflict NEC Z73.5
  skills inadequacy NEC Z73.4
  transplantation Z60.3
**Sodoku** A25.0
**Soemmerring's ring** — *see* Cataract, secondary
**Soft** (*see also* condition)
  nails L60.3
**Softening**
  bone — *see* Osteomalacia
  brain (necrotic) (progressive) G93.89
    congenital Q04.8
    embolic I63.4- ☑
    hemorrhagic — *see* Hemorrhage, intracranial, in-
      tracerebral
    occlusive I63.5- ☑
    thrombotic I63.3- ☑
  cartilage M94.2- ☑
    patella M22.4- ☑
  cerebellar — *see* Softening, brain
  cerebral — *see* Softening, brain
  cerebrospinal — *see* Softening, brain
  myocardial, heart — *see* Degeneration, myocardial
  spinal cord G95.89
  stomach K31.89
**Soldier's**
  heart F45.8
  patches I31.0
**Solitary**
  cyst, kidney N28.1
  kidney, congenital Q60.0
**Solvent abuse** — *see* Abuse, drug, inhalant
  dependence — *see* Dependence, drug, inhalant

**Somatization reaction, somatic reaction** — *see* Disorder, somatoform
**Somnambulism** F51.3
  hysterical F44.89
**Somnolence** R40.0
  nonorganic origin F51.11
**Sonne dysentery** A03.3
**Soor** B37.0
**Sore**
  bed — *see* Ulcer, pressure, by site
  chiclero B55.1
  Delhi B55.1
  desert — *see* Ulcer, skin
  eye H57.1- ☑
  Lahore B55.1
  mouth K13.79
    canker K12.0
  muscle M79.1
  Naga — *see* Ulcer, skin
  of skin — *see* Ulcer, skin
  oriental B55.1
  pressure — *see* Ulcer, pressure, by site
  skin L98.9
  soft A57
  throat (acute) (*see also* Pharyngitis)
    with influenza, flu, or grippe — *see* Influenza, with, respiratory manifestations NEC
    chronic J31.2
    coxsackie (virus) B08.5
    diphtheritic A36.0
    herpesviral B00.2
    influenzal — *see* Influenza, with, respiratory manifestations NEC
    septic J02.0
    streptococcal (ulcerative) J02.0
    viral NEC J02.8
      coxsackie B08.5
  tropical — *see* Ulcer, skin
  veldt — *see* Ulcer, skin
**Soto's syndrome** (cerebral gigantism) Q87.3
**South African cardiomyopathy syndrome** I42.8
**Southeast Asian hemorrhagic fever** A91
**Spacing**
  abnormal, tooth, teeth, fully erupted M26.30
  excessive, tooth, fully erupted M26.32
**Spade-like hand** (congenital) Q68.1
**Spading nail** L60.8
  congenital Q84.6
**Spanish collar** N47.1
**Sparganosis** B70.1
**Spasm(s), spastic, spasticity** (*see also* condition) R25.2
  accommodation — *see* Spasm, of accommodation
  ampulla of Vater K83.4
  anus, ani (sphincter) (reflex) K59.4
    psychogenic F45.8
  artery I73.9
    cerebral G45.9
  Bell's G51.3
  bladder (sphincter, external or internal) N32.89
    psychogenic F45.8
  bronchus, bronchiole J98.01
  cardia K22.0
  cardiac I20.1
  carpopedal — *see* Tetany
  cerebral (arteries) (vascular) G45.9
  cervix, complicating delivery O62.4
  ciliary body (of accommodation) — *see* Spasm, of accommodation
  colon (*see also* Irritable, bowel) K58.9
    with diarrhea K58.0
    psychogenic F45.8
  common duct K83.8
  compulsive — *see* Tic
  conjugate H51.8
  coronary (artery) I20.1
  diaphragm (reflex) R06.6
    epidemic B33.0
    psychogenic F45.8
  duodenum K59.8
  epidemic diaphragmatic (transient) B33.0
  esophagus (diffuse) K22.4
    psychogenic F45.8
  facial G51.3
  fallopian tube N83.8
  gastrointestinal (tract) K31.89
    psychogenic F45.8
  glottis J38.5
    hysterical F44.4

**Spasm(s), spastic, spasticity** — *continued*
  glottis — *continued*
    psychogenic F45.8
      conversion reaction F44.4
    reflex through recurrent laryngeal nerve J38.5
  habit — *see* Tic
  heart I20.1
  hemifacial (clonic) G51.3
  hourglass — *see* Contraction, hourglass
  hysterical F44.4
  infantile — *see* Epilepsy, spasms
  inferior oblique, eye H51.8
  intestinal (*see also* Syndrome, irritable bowel) K58.9
    psychogenic F45.8
  larynx, laryngeal J38.5
    hysterical F44.4
    psychogenic F45.8
      conversion reaction F44.4
  levator palpebrae superioris — *see* Disorder, eyelid function
  muscle NEC M62.838
    back M62.830
  nerve, trigeminal G51.0
  nervous F45.8
  nodding F98.4
  occupational F48.8
  oculogyric H51.8
    psychogenic F45.8
  of accommodation H52.53- ☑
  ophthalmic artery — *see* Occlusion, artery, retina
  perineal, female N94.89
  peroneo-extensor (*see also* Deformity, limb, flat foot)
  pharynx (reflex) J39.2
    hysterical F45.8
    psychogenic F45.8
  psychogenic F45.8
  pylorus NEC K31.3
    adult hypertrophic K31.89
    congenital or infantile Q40.0
    psychogenic F45.8
  rectum (sphincter) K59.4
    psychogenic F45.8
  retinal (artery) — *see* Occlusion, artery, retina
  sigmoid (*see also* Syndrome, irritable bowel) K58.9
    psychogenic F45.8
  sphincter of Oddi K83.4
  stomach K31.89
    neurotic F45.8
  throat J39.2
    hysterical F45.8
    psychogenic F45.8
  tic F95.9
    chronic F95.1
    transient of childhood F95.0
  tongue K14.8
  torsion (progressive) G24.1
  trigeminal nerve — *see* Neuralgia, trigeminal
  ureter N13.5
  urethra (sphincter) N35.9
  uterus N85.8
    complicating labor O62.4
  vagina N94.2
    psychogenic F52.5
  vascular I73.9
  vasomotor I73.9
  vein NEC I87.8
  viscera — *see* Pain, abdominal
**Spasmodic** — *see* condition
**Spasmophilia** — *see* Tetany
**Spasmus nutans** F98.4
**Spastic, spasticity** (*see also* Spasm)
  child (cerebral) (congenital) (paralysis) G80.1
**Speaker's throat** R49.8
**Specific, specified** — *see* condition
**Speech**
  defect, disorder, disturbance, impediment R47.9
    psychogenic, in childhood and adolescence F98.8
    slurring R47.81
    specified NEC R47.89
**Spencer's disease** A08.19
**Spens' syndrome** (syncope with heart block) I45.9
**Sperm counts** (fertility testing) Z31.41
  postvasectomy Z30.8
    reversal Z31.42
**Spermatic cord** — *see* condition
**Spermatocele** N43.40
  congenital Q55.4
  multiple N43.42

**Spermatocele** — *continued*
  single N43.41
**Spermatocystitis** N49.0
**Spermatocytoma** C62.9- ☑
  specified site — *see* Neoplasm, malignant, by site
**Spermatorrhea** N50.89
**Sphacelus** — *see* Gangrene
**Sphenoidal** — *see* condition
**Sphenoiditis** (chronic) — *see* Sinusitis, sphenoidal
**Sphenopalatine ganglion neuralgia** G90.09
**Sphericity, increased, lens** (congenital) Q12.4
**Spherocytosis** (congenital) (familial) (hereditary) D58.0
  hemoglobin disease D58.0
  sickle-cell (disease) D57.8- ☑
**Spherophakia** Q12.4
**Sphincter** — *see* condition
**Sphincteritis, sphincter of Oddi** — *see* Cholangitis
**Sphingolipidosis** E75.3
  specified NEC E75.29
**Sphingomyelinosis** E75.3
**Spicule tooth** K00.2
**Spider**
  bite — *see* Toxicity, venom, spider
  fingers — *see* Syndrome, Marfan's
  nevus I78.1
  toes — *see* Syndrome, Marfan's
  vascular I78.1
**Spiegler-Fendt**
  benign lymphocytoma L98.8
  sarcoid L08.89
**Spielmeyer-Vogt disease** E75.4
**Spina bifida** (aperta) Q05.9
  with hydrocephalus NEC Q05.4
  cervical Q05.5
    with hydrocephalus Q05.0
  dorsal Q05.6
    with hydrocephalus Q05.1
  lumbar Q05.7
    with hydrocephalus Q05.2
  lumbosacral Q05.7
    with hydrocephalus Q05.2
  occulta Q76.0
  sacral Q05.8
    with hydrocephalus Q05.3
  thoracic Q05.6
    with hydrocephalus Q05.1
  thoracolumbar Q05.6
    with hydrocephalus Q05.1
**Spindle, Krukenberg's** — *see* Pigmentation, cornea, posterior
**Spine, spinal** — *see* condition
**Spiradenoma** (eccrine) — *see* Neoplasm, skin, benign
**Spirillosis** A25.0
**Spirillum**
  minus A25.0
  obermeieri infection A68.0
**Spirochetal** — *see* condition
**Spirochetosis** A69.9
  arthritic, arthritica A69.9
  bronchopulmonary A69.8
  icterohemorrhagic A27.0
  lung A69.8
**Spirometrosis** B70.1
**Spitting blood** — *see* Hemoptysis
**Splanchnoptosis** K63.4
**Spleen, splenic** — *see* condition
**Splenectasis** — *see* Splenomegaly
**Splenitis** (interstitial) (malignant) (nonspecific) D73.89
  malarial (*see also* Malaria) B54 [D77]
  tuberculous A18.85
**Splenocele** D73.89
**Splenomegaly, splenomegalia** (Bengal) (cryptogenic) (idiopathic) (tropical) R16.1
  with hepatomegaly R16.2
  cirrhotic D73.2
  congenital Q89.09
  congestive, chronic D73.2
  Egyptian B65.1
  Gaucher's E75.22
  malarial (*see also* Malaria) B54 [D77]
  neutropenic D73.81
  Niemann-Pick — *see* Niemann-Pick disease or syndrome
  siderotic D73.2
  syphilitic A52.79
    congenital (early) A50.08 [D77]
**Splenopathy** D73.9

**Splenoptosis** D73.89
**Splenosis** D73.89
**Splinter** — *see* Foreign body, superficial, by site
**Split, splitting**
  foot Q72.7- ☑
  hand Q71.6 ☑
  heart sounds R01.2
  lip, congenital — *see* Cleft, lip
  nails L60.3
  urinary stream R39.13
**Spondylarthrosis** — *see* Spondylosis
**Spondylitis** (chronic) (*see also* Spondylopathy, inflammatory)
  ankylopoietica — *see* Spondylitis, ankylosing
  ankylosing (chronic) M45.9
    with lung involvement M45.9 [J99]
    cervical region M45.2
    cervicothoracic region M45.3
    juvenile M08.1
    lumbar region M45.6
    lumbosacral region M45.7
    multiple sites M45.0
    occipito-atlanto-axial region M45.1
    sacrococcygeal region M45.8
    thoracic region M45.4
    thoracolumbar region M45.5
  atrophic (ligamentous) — *see* Spondylitis, ankylosing
  deformans (chronic) — *see* Spondylosis
  gonococcal A54.41
  gouty (*see also* Gout, by type, vertebrae) M10.08
  in (due to)
    brucellosis A23.9 [M49.80]
      cervical region A23.9 [M49.82]
      cervicothoracic region A23.9 [M49.83]
      lumbar region A23.9 [M49.86]
      lumbosacral region A23.9 [M49.87]
      multiple sites A23.9 [M49.89]
      occipito-atlanto-axial region A23.9 [M49.81]
      sacrococcygeal region A23.9 [M49.88]
      thoracic region A23.9 [M49.84]
      thoracolumbar region A23.9 [M49.85]
    enterobacteria (*see also* subcategory M49.8) A04.9
    tuberculosis A18.01
  infectious NEC — *see* Spondylopathy, infective
  juvenile ankylosing (chronic) M08.1
  Kümmell's — *see* Spondylopathy, traumatic
  Marie-Strümpell — *see* Spondylitis, ankylosing
  muscularis — *see* Spondylopathy, specified NEC
  psoriatic L40.53
  rheumatoid — *see* Spondylitis, ankylosing
  rhizomelica — *see* Spondylitis, ankylosing
  sacroiliac NEC M46.1
  senescent, senile — *see* Spondylosis
  traumatic (chronic) or post-traumatic — *see* Spondylopathy, traumatic
  tuberculous A18.01
  typhosa A01.05
**Spondylolisthesis** (acquired) (degenerative) M43.10
  with disproportion (fetopelvic) O33.0
    causing obstructed labor O65.0
  cervical region M43.12
  cervicothoracic region M43.13
  congenital Q76.2
  lumbar region M43.16
  lumbosacral region M43.17
  multiple sites M43.19
  occipito-atlanto-axial region M43.11
  sacrococcygeal region M43.18
  thoracic region M43.14
  thoracolumbar region M43.15
  traumatic (old) M43.10
    acute
      fifth cervical (displaced) S12.430 ☑
        nondisplaced S12.431 ☑
        specified type NEC (displaced) S12.450 ☑
          nondisplaced S12.451 ☑
        type III S12.44 ☑
      fourth cervical (displaced) S12.330 ☑
        nondisplaced S12.331 ☑
        specified type NEC (displaced) S12.350 ☑
          nondisplaced S12.351 ☑
        type III S12.34 ☑
      second cervical (displaced) S12.130 ☑
        nondisplaced S12.131 ☑
        specified type NEC (displaced) S12.150 ☑
          nondisplaced S12.151 ☑
        type III S12.14 ☑

**Spondylolisthesis** — *continued*
  traumatic — *continued*
    acute — *continued*
      seventh cervical (displaced) S12.630 ☑
        nondisplaced S12.631 ☑
        specified type NEC (displaced) S12.650 ☑
          nondisplaced S12.651 ☑
        type III S12.64 ☑
      sixth cervical (displaced) S12.530 ☑
        nondisplaced S12.531 ☑
        specified type NEC (displaced) S12.550 ☑
          nondisplaced S12.551 ☑
        type III S12.54 ☑
      third cervical (displaced) S12.230 ☑
        nondisplaced S12.231 ☑
        specified type NEC (displaced) S12.250 ☑
          nondisplaced S12.251 ☑
        type III S12.24 ☑
**Spondylolysis** (acquired) M43.00
  cervical region M43.02
  cervicothoracic region M43.03
  congenital Q76.2
  lumbar region M43.06
  lumbosacral region M43.07
    with disproportion (fetopelvic) O33.0
      causing obstructed labor O65.8
  multiple sites M43.09
  occipito-atlanto-axial region M43.01
  sacrococcygeal region M43.08
  thoracic region M43.04
  thoracolumbar region M43.05
**Spondylopathy** M48.9
  infective NEC M46.50
    cervical region M46.52
    cervicothoracic region M46.53
    lumbar region M46.56
    lumbosacral region M46.57
    multiple sites M46.59
    occipito-atlanto-axial region M46.51
    sacrococcygeal region M46.58
    thoracic region M46.54
    thoracolumbar region M46.55
  inflammatory M46.90
    cervical region M46.92
    cervicothoracic region M46.93
    lumbar region M46.96
    lumbosacral region M46.97
    multiple sites M46.99
    occipito-atlanto-axial region M46.91
    sacrococcygeal region M46.98
    specified type NEC M46.80
      cervical region M46.82
      cervicothoracic region M46.83
      lumbar region M46.86
      lumbosacral region M46.87
      multiple sites M46.89
      occipito-atlanto-axial region M46.81
      sacrococcygeal region M46.88
      thoracic region M46.84
      thoracolumbar region M46.85
    thoracic region M46.94
    thoracolumbar region M46.95
  neuropathic, in
    syringomyelia and syringobulbia G95.0
    tabes dorsalis A52.11
  specified NEC — *see* subcategory M48.8 ☑
  traumatic M48.30
    cervical region M48.32
    cervicothoracic region M48.33
    lumbar region M48.36
    lumbosacral region M48.37
    occipito-atlanto-axial region M48.31
    sacrococcygeal region M48.38
    thoracic region M48.34
    thoracolumbar region M48.35
**Spondylosis** M47.9
  with
    disproportion (fetopelvic) O33.0
      causing obstructed labor O65.0
    myelopathy NEC M47.10
      cervical region M47.12
      cervicothoracic region M47.13
      lumbar region M47.16
      occipito-atlanto-axial region M47.11
      thoracic region M47.14
      thoracolumbar region M47.15
    radiculopathy M47.20
      cervical region M47.22

**Spondylosis** — *continued*
  with — *continued*
    radiculopathy — *continued*
      cervicothoracic region M47.23
      lumbar region M47.26
      lumbosacral region M47.27
      occipito-atlanto-axial region M47.21
      sacrococcygeal region M47.28
      thoracic region M47.24
      thoracolumbar region M47.25
  without myelopathy or radiculopathy M47.819
    cervical region M47.812
    cervicothoracic region M47.813
    lumbar region M47.816
    lumbosacral region M47.817
    occipito-atlanto-axial region M47.811
    sacrococcygeal region M47.818
    thoracic region M47.814
    thoracolumbar region M47.815
  specified NEC M47.899
    cervical region M47.892
    cervicothoracic region M47.893
    lumbar region M47.896
    lumbosacral region M47.897
    occipito-atlanto-axial region M47.891
    sacrococcygeal region M47.898
    thoracic region M47.894
    thoracolumbar region M47.895
  traumatic — *see* Spondylopathy, traumatic
**Sponge**
  inadvertently left in operation wound — *see* Foreign body, accidentally left during a procedure
  kidney (medullary) Q61.5
**Sponge-diver's disease** — *see* Toxicity, venom, marine animal, sea anemone
**Spongioblastoma** (any type) — *see* Neoplasm, malignant, by site
  specified site — *see* Neoplasm, malignant, by site
  unspecified site C71.9
**Spongioneuroblastoma** — *see* Neoplasm, malignant, by site
**Spontaneous** (*see also* condition)
  fracture (cause unknown) — *see* Fracture, pathological
**Spoon nail** L60.3
  congenital Q84.6
**Sporadic** — *see* condition
**Sporothrix schenckii infection** — *see* Sporotrichosis
**Sporotrichosis** B42.9
  arthritis B42.82
  disseminated B42.7
  generalized B42.7
  lymphocutaneous (fixed) (progressive) B42.1
  pulmonary B42.0
  specified NEC B42.89
**Spots, spotting** (in) (of)
  Bitot's (*see also* Pigmentation, conjunctiva)
    in the young child E50.1
      vitamin A deficiency E50.1
  café, au lait L81.3
  Cayenne pepper I78.1
  cotton wool, retina — *see* Occlusion, artery, retina
  de Morgan's (senile angiomas) I78.1
  Fuchs' black (myopic) (*see also* Myopia, degenerative) H44.2- ☑
  intermenstrual (regular) N92.0
    irregular N92.1
  Koplik's B05.9
  liver L81.4
  pregnancy O26.85- ☑
  purpuric R23.3
  ruby I78.1
**Spotted fever** — *see* Fever, spotted N92.3
**Sprain** (joint) (ligament)
  acromioclavicular joint or ligament S43.5- ☑
  ankle S93.40- ☑
    calcaneofibular ligament S93.41- ☑
    deltoid ligament S93.42- ☑
    internal collateral ligament — *see* Sprain, ankle, specified ligament NEC
    specified ligament NEC S93.49- ☑
    talofibular ligament — *see* Sprain, ankle, specified ligament NEC
    tibiofibular ligament S93.43- ☑
  anterior longitudinal, cervical S13.4 ☑
  atlas, atlanto-axial, atlanto-occipital S13.4 ☑
  breast bone — *see* Sprain, sternum
  calcaneofibular — *see* Sprain, ankle
  carpal — *see* Sprain, wrist

⚐ **Subterms under main terms may continue to next column or page**    ☑ **Additional Character Required — Refer to the Tabular List for Character Selection**    **289**

**Splenoptosis — Sprain**

**Sprain** — *continued*

carpometacarpal — *see* Sprain, hand, specified site NEC

cartilage
 costal S23.41 ☑
 semilunar (knee) — *see* Sprain, knee, specified site NEC
  with current tear — *see* Tear, meniscus
 thyroid region S13.5 ☑
 xiphoid — *see* Sprain, sternum

cervical, cervicodorsal, cervicothoracic S13.4 ☑
chondrosternal S23.421 ☑
coracoclavicular S43.8- ☑
coracohumeral S43.41- ☑
coronary, knee — *see* Sprain, knee, specified site NEC
costal cartilage S23.41 ☑
cricoarytenoid articulation or ligament S13.5 ☑
cricothyroid articulation S13.5 ☑
cruciate, knee — *see* Sprain, knee, cruciate
deltoid, ankle — *see* Sprain, ankle
dorsal (spine) S23.3 ☑

elbow S53.40- ☑
 radial collateral ligament S53.43- ☑
 radiohumeral S53.41- ☑
 rupture
  radial collateral ligament — *see* Rupture, traumatic, ligament, radial collateral
  ulnar collateral ligament — *see* Rupture, traumatic, ligament, ulnar collateral
 specified type NEC S53.49- ☑
 ulnar collateral ligament S53.44- ☑
 ulnohumeral S53.42- ☑

femur, head — *see* Sprain, hip
fibular collateral, knee — *see* Sprain, knee, collateral
fibulocalcaneal — *see* Sprain, ankle

finger(s) S63.61- ☑
 index S63.61- ☑
 interphalangeal (joint) S63.63- ☑
  index S63.63- ☑
  little S63.63- ☑
  middle S63.63- ☑
  ring S63.63- ☑
 little S63.61- ☑
 metacarpophalangeal (joint) S63.65- ☑
 middle S63.61- ☑
 ring S63.61- ☑
 specified site NEC S63.69- ☑
  index S63.69- ☑
  little S63.69- ☑
  middle S63.69- ☑
  ring S63.69- ☑

foot S93.60- ☑
 specified ligament NEC S93.69- ☑
 tarsal ligament S93.61- ☑
 tarsometatarsal ligament S93.62- ☑
 toe — *see* Sprain, toe

hand S63.9- ☑
 finger — *see* Sprain, finger
 specified site NEC — *see* subcategory S63.8 ☑
 thumb — *see* Sprain, thumb

head S03.9 ☑

hip S73.10- ☑
 iliofemoral ligament S73.11- ☑
 ischiocapsular (ligament) S73.12- ☑
 specified NEC S73.19- ☑

iliofemoral — *see* Sprain, hip

innominate
 acetabulum — *see* Sprain, hip
 sacral junction S33.6 ☑

internal
 collateral, ankle — *see* Sprain, ankle
 semilunar cartilage — *see* Sprain, knee, specified site NEC

interphalangeal
 finger — *see* Sprain, finger, interphalangeal (joint)
 toe — *see* Sprain, toe, interphalangeal joint

ischiocapsular — *see* Sprain, hip
ischiofemoral — *see* Sprain, hip
jaw (articular disc) (cartilage) (meniscus) S03.4- ☑
 old M26.69

knee S83.9- ☑
 collateral ligament S83.40- ☑
  lateral (fibular) S83.42- ☑
  medial (tibial) S83.41- ☑
 cruciate ligament S83.50- ☑
  anterior S83.51- ☑

**Sprain** — *continued*

knee — *continued*
 cruciate ligament — *continued*
  posterior S83.52- ☑
 lateral (fibular) collateral ligament S83.42- ☑
 medial (tibial) collateral ligament S83.41- ☑
 patellar ligament S76.11- ☑
 specified site NEC S83.8X- ☑
 superior tibiofibular joint (ligament) S83.6- ☑

lateral collateral, knee — *see* Sprain, knee, collateral
lumbar (spine) S33.5 ☑
lumbosacral S33.9 ☑
mandible (articular disc) S03.4- ☑
 old M26.69
medial collateral, knee — *see* Sprain, knee, collateral

meniscus
 jaw S03.4- ☑
  old M26.69
 knee — *see* Sprain, knee, specified site NEC
  with current tear — *see* Tear, meniscus
   old — *see* Derangement, knee, meniscus, due to old tear
 mandible S03.4- ☑
  old M26.69

metacarpal (distal) (proximal) — *see* Sprain, hand, specified site NEC
metacarpophalangeal — *see* Sprain, finger, metacarpophalangeal (joint)
metatarsophalangeal — *see* Sprain, toe, metatarsophalangeal joint
midcarpal — *see* Sprain, hand, specified site NEC
midtarsal — *see* Sprain, foot, specified site NEC

neck S13.9 ☑
 anterior longitudinal cervical ligament S13.4 ☑
 atlanto-axial joint S13.4 ☑
 atlanto-occipital joint S13.4 ☑
 cervical spine S13.4 ☑
 cricoarytenoid ligament S13.5 ☑
 cricothyroid ligament S13.5 ☑
 specified site NEC S13.8 ☑
 thyroid region (cartilage) S13.5 ☑

nose S03.8 ☑
orbicular, hip — *see* Sprain, hip
patella — *see* Sprain, knee, specified site NEC
patellar ligament S76.11- ☑
pelvis NEC S33.8 ☑

phalanx
 finger — *see* Sprain, finger
 toe — *see* Sprain, toe

pubofemoral — *see* Sprain, hip
radiocarpal — *see* Sprain, wrist
radiohumeral — *see* Sprain, elbow
radius, collateral — *see* Rupture, traumatic, ligament, radial collateral
rib (cage) S23.41 ☑
rotator cuff (capsule) S43.42- ☑

sacroiliac (region)
 chronic or old — *see* subcategory M53.2 ☑
 joint S33.6 ☑

scaphoid (hand) — *see* Sprain, hand, specified site NEC
scapula (r) — *see* Sprain, shoulder girdle, specified site NEC
semilunar cartilage (knee) — *see* Sprain, knee, specified site NEC
 with current tear — *see* Tear, meniscus
  old — *see* Derangement, knee, meniscus, due to old tear

shoulder joint S43.40- ☑
 acromioclavicular joint (ligament) — *see* Sprain, acromioclavicular joint
 blade — *see* Sprain, shoulder, girdle, specified site NEC
 coracoclavicular joint (ligament) — *see* Sprain, coracoclavicular joint
 coracohumeral ligament — *see* Sprain, coracohumeral joint
 girdle S43.9- ☑
  specified site NEC S43.8- ☑
 rotator cuff — *see* Sprain, rotator cuff
 specified site NEC S43.49- ☑
 sternoclavicular joint (ligament) — *see* Sprain, sternoclavicular joint

spine
 cervical S13.4 ☑
 lumbar S33.5 ☑

**Sprain** — *continued*

spine — *continued*
 thoracic S23.3 ☑
sternoclavicular joint S43.6- ☑
sternum S23.429 ☑
 chondrosternal joint S23.421 ☑
 specified site NEC S23.428 ☑
 sternoclavicular (joint) (ligament) S23.420 ☑

symphysis
 jaw S03.4- ☑
  old M26.69
 mandibular S03.4- ☑
  old M26.69

talofibular — *see* Sprain, ankle
tarsal — *see* Sprain, foot, specified site NEC
tarsometatarsal — *see* Sprain, foot, specified site NEC
temporomandibular S03.4- ☑
 old M26.69

thorax S23.9 ☑
 ribs S23.41 ☑
 specified site NEC S23.8 ☑
 spine S23.3 ☑
 sternum — *see* Sprain, sternum

thumb S63.60- ☑
 interphalangeal (joint) S63.62- ☑
 metacarpophalangeal (joint) S63.64- ☑
 specified site NEC S63.68- ☑

thyroid cartilage or region S13.5 ☑
tibia (proximal end) — *see* Sprain, knee, specified site NEC
tibial collateral, knee — *see* Sprain, knee, collateral

tibiofibular
 distal — *see* Sprain, ankle
 superior — *see* Sprain, knee, specified site NEC

toe(s) S93.50- ☑
 great S93.50- ☑
 interphalangeal joint S93.51- ☑
  great S93.51- ☑
  lesser S93.51- ☑
 lesser S93.50- ☑
 metatarsophalangeal joint S93.52- ☑
  great S93.52- ☑
  lesser S93.52- ☑

ulna, collateral — *see* Rupture, traumatic, ligament, ulnar collateral
ulnohumeral — *see* Sprain, elbow

wrist S63.50- ☑
 carpal S63.51- ☑
 radiocarpal S63.52- ☑
 specified site NEC S63.59- ☑

xiphoid cartilage — *see* Sprain, sternum

**Sprengel's deformity** (congenital) Q74.0

**Sprue** (tropical) K90.1
 celiac K90.0
 idiopathic K90.49
 meaning thrush B37.0
 nontropical K90.0

**Spur, bone** (*see also* Enthesopathy)
 calcaneal M77.3-
 iliac crest M76.2-
 nose (septum) J34.89

**Spurway's syndrome** Q78.0

**Sputum**
 abnormal (amount) (color) (odor) (purulent) R09.3
 blood-stained R04.2
 excessive (cause unknown) R09.3

**Squamous** (*see also* condition)
 epithelium in
  cervical canal (congenital) Q51.828
  uterine mucosa (congenital) Q51.818

**Squashed nose** M95.0
 congenital Q67.4

**Squeeze, diver's** T70.3 ☑

**Squint** (*see also* Strabismus)
 accommodative — *see* Strabismus, convergent concomitant

**St. Hubert's disease** A82.9

**Stab** (*see also* Laceration)
 internal organs — *see* Injury, by site

**Stafne's cyst or cavity** M27.0

**Staggering gait** R26.0
 hysterical F44.4

**Staghorn calculus** — *see* Calculus, kidney

**Stähli's line** (cornea) (pigment) — *see* Pigmentation, cornea, anterior

☑ **Additional Character Required** — Refer to the Tabular List for Character Selection  ▼ **Subterms under main terms may continue to next column or page**

**Stain, staining**
  meconium (newborn) P96.83
  port wine Q82.5
  tooth, teeth (hard tissues) (extrinsic) K03.6
    due to
      accretions K03.6
      deposits (betel) (black) (green) (materia alba)
        (orange) (soft) (tobacco) K03.6
      metals (copper) (silver) K03.7
      nicotine K03.6
      pulpal bleeding K03.7
      tobacco K03.6
    intrinsic K00.8
**Stammering** (see also Disorder, fluency) F80.81
**Standstill**
  auricular I45.5
  cardiac — see Arrest, cardiac
  sinoatrial I45.5
  ventricular — see Arrest, cardiac
**Stannosis** J63.5
**Stanton's disease** — see Melioidosis
**Staphylitis** (acute) (catarrhal) (chronic) (gangrenous)
  (membranous) (suppurative) (ulcerative) K12.2
**Staphylococcal scalded skin syndrome** L00
**Staphylococcemia** A41.2
**Staphylococcus, staphylococcal** (see also condition)
  as cause of disease classified elsewhere B95.8
    aureus (methicillin susceptible) (MSSA) B95.61
      methicillin resistant (MRSA) B95.62
    specified NEC, as cause of disease classified elsewhere
      B95.7
**Staphyloma** (sclera)
  cornea H18.72- ☑
  equatorial H15.81- ☑
  localized (anterior) H15.82- ☑
  posticum H15.83- ☑
  ring H15.85- ☑
**Stargardt's disease** — see Dystrophy, retina
**Starvation** (inanition) (due to lack of food) T73.0 ☑
  edema — see Malnutrition, severe
**Stasis**
  bile (noncalculous) K83.1
  bronchus J98.09
    with infection — see Bronchitis
  cardiac — see Failure, heart, congestive
  cecum K59.8
  colon K59.8
  dermatitis I87.2
    with
      varicose ulcer — see Varix, leg, with ulcer, with
        inflammation
      varicose veins — see Varix, leg, with, inflamma-
        tion
    due to postthrombotic syndrome — see Syndrome,
      postthrombotic
  duodenal K31.5
  eczema — see Varix, leg, with, inflammation
  edema — see Hypertension, venous (chronic), idiopath-
    ic
  foot T69.0- ☑
  ileocecal coil K59.8
  ileum K59.8
  intestinal K59.8
  jejunum K59.8
  kidney N19
  liver (cirrhotic) K76.1
  lymphatic I89.8
  pneumonia J18.2
  pulmonary — see Edema, lung
  rectal K59.8
  renal N19
    tubular N17.0
  ulcer — see Varix, leg, with, ulcer
    without varicose veins I87.2
  urine — see Retention, urine
  venous I87.8
**State** (of)
  affective and paranoid, mixed, organic psychotic F06.8
  agitated R45.1
    acute reaction to stress F43.0
  anxiety (neurotic) F41.1
  apprehension F41.1
  burn-out Z73.0
  climacteric, female Z78.0
    symptomatic N95.1
  compulsive F42.8
    mixed with obsessional thoughts F42.2
  confusional (psychogenic) F44.89

**State** — continued
  confusional — continued
    acute (see also Delirium)
      with
        arteriosclerotic dementia F01.50
          with behavioral disturbance F01.51
        senility or dementia F05
      alcoholic F10.231
      epileptic F05
    reactive (from emotional stress, psychological
      trauma) F44.89
    subacute — see Delirium
  convulsive — see Convulsions
  crisis F43.0
  depressive F32.9
    neurotic F34.1
  dissociative F44.9
  emotional shock (stress) R45.7
  hypercoagulation — see Hypercoagulable
  locked-in G83.5
  menopausal Z78.0
    symptomatic N95.1
  neurotic F48.9
    with depersonalization F48.1
  obsessional F42.8
  oneiroid (schizophrenia-like) F23
  organic
    hallucinatory (nonalcoholic) F06.0
    paranoid (-hallucinatory) F06.2
  panic F41.0
  paranoid F22
    climacteric F22
    involutional F22
    menopausal F22
    organic F06.2
    senile F03 ☑
    simple F22
  persistent vegetative R40.3
  phobic F40.9
  postleukotomy F07.0
  pregnant
    gestational carrier Z33.3
    incidental Z33.1
  psychogenic, twilight F44.89
  psychopathic (constitutional) F60.2
  psychotic, organic (see also Psychosis, organic)
    mixed paranoid and affective F06.8
    senile or presenile F03 ☑
    transient NEC F06.8
      with
        depression F06.31
        hallucinations F06.0
  residual schizophrenic F20.5
  restlessness R45.1
  stress (emotional) R45.7
  tension (mental) F48.9
    specified NEC F48.8
  transient organic psychotic NEC F06.8
    depressive type F06.31
    hallucinatory type F06.0
  twilight
    epileptic F05
    psychogenic F44.89
  vegetative, persistent R40.3
  vital exhaustion Z73.0
  withdrawal, — see Withdrawal, state
**Status** (post) (see also Presence (of))
  absence, epileptic — see Epilepsy, by type, with status
    epilepticus
  administration of tPA (rtPA) in a different facility
    within the last 24 hours prior to admission to
    current facility Z92.82
  adrenalectomy (unilateral) (bilateral) E89.6
  anastomosis Z98.0
  anginosus I20.9
  angioplasty (peripheral) Z98.62
    with implant Z95.820
    coronary artery Z98.61
      with implant Z95.5
  aortocoronary bypass Z95.1
  arthrodesis Z98.1
  artificial opening (of) Z93.9
    gastrointestinal tract Z93.4
    specified NEC Z93.8
    urinary tract Z93.6
    vagina Z93.8
  asthmaticus — see Asthma, by type, with status asth-
    maticus

**Status** — continued
  awaiting organ transplant Z76.82
  bariatric surgery Z98.84
  bed confinement Z74.01
  bleb, filtering (vitreous), after glaucoma surgery Z98.83
  breast implant Z98.82
    removal Z98.86
  cataract extraction Z98.4- ☑
  cholecystectomy Z90.49
  clitorectomy N90.811
    with excision of labia minora N90.812
  colectomy (complete) (partial) Z90.49
  colonization — see Carrier (suspected) of
  colostomy Z93.3
  convulsivus idiopathicus — see Epilepsy, by type, with
    status epilepticus
  coronary artery angioplasty — see Status, angioplasty,
    coronary artery
  coronary artery bypass graft Z95.1
  cystectomy (urinary bladder) Z90.6
  cystostomy Z93.50
    appendico-vesicostomy Z93.52
    cutaneous Z93.51
    specified NEC Z93.59
  delinquent immunization Z28.3
  dental Z98.818
    crown Z98.811
    fillings Z98.811
    restoration Z98.811
    sealant Z98.810
    specified NEC Z98.818
  deployment (current) (military) Z56.82
  dialysis (hemodialysis) (peritoneal) Z99.2
  do not resuscitate (DNR) Z66
  donor — see Donor
  embedded fragments — see Retained, foreign body
    fragments (type of)
  embedded splinter — see Retained, foreign body
    fragments (type of)
  enterostomy Z93.4
  epileptic, epilepticus (see also Epilepsy, by type, with
    status epilepticus) G40.901
  estrogen receptor
    negative Z17.1
    positive Z17.0
  female genital cutting — see Female genital mutilation
    status
  female genital mutilation — see Female genital muti-
    lation status
  filtering (vitreous) bleb after glaucoma surgery Z98.83
  gastrectomy (complete) (partial) Z90.3
  gastric banding Z98.84
  gastric bypass for obesity Z98.84
  gastrostomy Z93.1
  human immunodeficiency virus (HIV) infection,
    asymptomatic Z21
  hysterectomy (complete) (total) Z90.710
    partial (with remaining cervial stump) Z90.711
  ileostomy Z93.2
  implant
    breast Z98.82
  infibulation N90.813
  intestinal bypass Z98.0
  jejunostomy Z93.4
  lapsed immunization schedule Z28.3
  laryngectomy Z90.02
  lymphaticus E32.8
  malignancy
    castrate resistant prostate Z19.2
    hormone resistant Z19.2
    hormone sensitive Z19.1
  marmoratus G80.3
  mastectomy (unilateral) (bilateral) Z90.1- ☑
  military deployment status (current) Z56.82
    in theater or in support of military war, peacekeep-
      ing and humanitarian operations Z56.82
  nephrectomy (unilateral) (bilateral) Z90.5
  nephrostomy Z93.6
  obesity surgery Z98.84
  oophorectomy
    bilateral Z90.722
    unilateral Z90.721
  organ replacement
    by artificial or mechanical device or prosthesis of
      artery Z95.828
      bladder Z96.0
      blood vessel Z95.828
      breast Z97.8

☟ **Subterms under main terms may continue to next column or page**     ☑ **Additional Character Required — Refer to the Tabular List for Character Selection**     **291**

Stain, staining — Status

**Status** — continued
  organ replacement — continued
    by artificial or mechanical device or prosthesis of — continued
      eye globe Z97.0
      heart Z95.812
        valve Z95.2
      intestine Z97.8
      joint Z96.60
        hip — see Presence, hip joint implant
        knee — see Presence, knee joint implant
        specified site NEC Z96.698
      kidney Z97.8
      larynx Z96.3
      lens Z96.1
      limbs — see Presence, artificial, limb
      liver Z97.8
      lung Z97.8
      pancreas Z97.8
    by organ transplant (heterologous)(homologous) — see Transplant
  pacemaker
    brain Z96.89
    cardiac Z95.0
    specified NEC Z96.89
  pancreatectomy Z90.410
    complete Z90.410
    partial Z90.411
    total Z90.410
  physical restraint Z78.1
  pneumonectomy (complete) (partial) Z90.2
  pneumothorax, therapeutic Z98.3
  postcommotio cerebri F07.81
  postoperative (postprocedural) NEC Z98.890
    breast implant Z98.82
    dental Z98.818
      crown Z98.811
      fillings Z98.811
      restoration Z98.811
      sealant Z98.810
      specified NEC Z98.818
    pneumothorax, therapeutic Z98.3
    uterine scar Z98.891
  postpartum (routine follow-up) Z39.2
    care immediately after delivery Z39.0
  postsurgical (postprocedural) NEC Z98.890
    pneumothorax, therapeutic Z98.3
  pregnancy, incidental Z33.1
  prosthesis coronary angioplasty Z95.5
  pseudophakia Z96.1
  renal dialysis (hemodialysis) (peritoneal) Z99.2
  retained foreign body — see Retained, foreign body fragments (type of)
  reversed jejunal transposition (for bypass) Z98.0
  salpingo-oophorectomy
    bilateral Z90.722
    unilateral Z90.721
  sex reassignment surgery status Z87.890
  shunt
    arteriovenous (for dialysis) Z99.2
    cerebrospinal fluid Z98.2
    ventricular (communicating) ( for drainage) Z98.2
  splenectomy Z90.81
  thymicolymphaticus E32.8
  thymicus E32.8
  thymolymphaticus E32.8
  thyroidectomy (hypothyroidism) E89.0
  tooth (teeth) extraction (see also Absence, teeth, acquired) K08.409
  tPA (rtPA) administration in a different facility within the last 24 hours prior to admission to current facility Z92.82
  tracheostomy Z93.0
  transplant — see Transplant
    organ removed Z98.85
  tubal ligation Z98.51
  underimmunization Z28.3
  ureterostomy Z93.6
  urethrostomy Z93.6
  vagina, artificial Z93.8
  vasectomy Z98.52
  wheelchair confinement Z99.3
**Stealing**
  child problem F91.8
    in company with others Z72.810
  pathological (compulsive) F63.2
**Steam burn** — see Burn
**Steatocystoma multiplex** L72.2

**Steatohepatitis** (nonalcoholic) (NASH) K75.81
**Steatoma** L72.3
  eyelid (cystic) — see Dermatosis, eyelid
    infected — see Hordeolum
**Steatorrhea** (chronic) K90.9
  with lacteal obstruction K90.2
  idiopathic (adult) (infantile) K90.9
  pancreatic K90.3
  primary K90.0
  tropical K90.1
**Steatosis** E88.89
  heart — see Degeneration, myocardial
  kidney N28.89
  liver NEC K76.0
**Steele-Richardson-Olszewski disease or syndrome** G23.1
**Steinbrocker's syndrome** G90.8
**Steinert's disease** G71.11
**Stein-Leventhal syndrome** E28.2
**Stein's syndrome** E28.2
**STEMI** (see also Infarct, myocardium, ST elevation) I21.3
**Stenocardia** I20.8
**Stenocephaly** Q75.8
**Stenosis, stenotic** (cicatricial) (see also Stricture)
  ampulla of Vater K83.1
  anus, anal (canal) (sphincter) K62.4
    and rectum K62.4
    congenital Q42.3
      with fistula Q42.2
  aorta (ascending) (supraventricular) (congenital) Q25.1
    arteriosclerotic I70.0
    calcified I70.0
    supravalvular Q25.3
  aortic (valve) I35.0
    with insufficiency I35.2
    congenital Q23.0
    rheumatic I06.0
      with
        incompetency, insufficiency or regurgitation I06.2
          with mitral (valve) disease I08.0
            with tricuspid (valve) disease I08.3
          mitral (valve) disease I08.0
            with tricuspid (valve) disease I08.3
          tricuspid (valve) disease I08.2
            with mitral (valve) disease I08.3
    specified cause NEC I35.0
    syphilitic A52.03
  aqueduct of Sylvius (congenital) Q03.0
    with spina bifida — see Spina bifida, by site, with hydrocephalus
    acquired G91.1
  artery NEC (see also Arteriosclerosis) I77.1
    celiac I77.4
    cerebral — see Occlusion, artery, cerebral
    extremities — see Arteriosclerosis, extremities
    precerebral — see Occlusion, artery, precerebral
    pulmonary (congenital) Q25.6
      acquired I28.8
    renal I70.1
    stent
      coronary T82.855 ☑
      peripheral T82.856 ☑
  bile duct (common) (hepatic) K83.1
    congenital Q44.3
  bladder-neck (acquired) N32.0
    congenital Q64.31
  brain G93.89
  bronchus J98.09
    congenital Q32.3
    syphilitic A52.72
  cardia (stomach) K22.2
    congenital Q39.3
  cardiovascular — see Disease, cardiovascular
  caudal M48.08
  cervix, cervical (canal) N88.2
    congenital Q51.828
    in pregnancy or childbirth — see Pregnancy, complicated by, abnormal cervix
  colon (see also Obstruction, intestine)
    congenital Q42.9
      specified NEC Q42.8
  colostomy K94.03
  common (bile) duct K83.1
    congenital Q44.3
  coronary (artery) — see Disease, heart, ischemic, atherosclerotic
  cystic duct — see Obstruction, gallbladder

**Stenosis, stenotic** — continued
  due to presence of device, implant or graft (see also Complications, by site and type, specified NEC) T85.858 ☑
    arterial graft NEC T82.858 ☑
    breast (implant) T85.858 ☑
    catheter T85.858 ☑
      dialysis (renal) T82.858 ☑
        intraperitoneal T85.858 ☑
      infusion NEC T82.858 ☑
        spinal (epidural) (subdural) T85.850 ☑
      urinary (indwelling) T83.85 ☑
    fixation, internal (orthopedic) NEC T84.85 ☑
    gastrointestinal (bile duct) (esophagus) T85.858 ☑
    genital NEC T83.85 ☑
    heart NEC T82.857 ☑
    joint prosthesis T84.85 ☑
    ocular (corneal graft) (orbital implant) NEC T85.858 ☑
    orthopedic NEC T84.85 ☑
    specified NEC T85.858 ☑
    urinary NEC T83.85 ☑
    vascular NEC T82.858 ☑
    ventricular intracranial shunt T85.850 ☑
  duodenum K31.5
    congenital Q41.0
  ejaculatory duct NEC N50.89
    stent
      vascular
        end stent
          adjacent to stent — see Arteriosclerosis
          within the stent
            coronary T82.855 ☑
            peripheral T82.856 ☑
        in stent
          coronary vessel T82.855 ☑
          peripheral vessel T82.856 ☑
  endocervical os — see Stenosis, cervix
  enterostomy K94.13
  esophagus K22.2
    congenital Q39.3
    syphilitic A52.79
      congenital A50.59 [K23]
  eustachian tube — see Obstruction, eustachian tube
  external ear canal (acquired) H61.30- ☑
    congenital Q16.1
    due to
      inflammation H61.32- ☑
      trauma H61.31- ☑
    postprocedural H95.81- ☑
    specified cause NEC H61.39- ☑
  gallbladder — see Obstruction, gallbladder
  glottis J38.6
  heart valve (congenital) Q24.8
    aortic Q23.0
    mitral Q23.2
    pulmonary Q22.1
    tricuspid Q22.4
  hepatic duct K83.1
  hymen N89.6
  hypertrophic subaortic (idiopathic) I42.1
  ileum (see also Obstruction, intestine, specified NEC) K56.699
    congenital Q41.2
  infundibulum cardia Q24.3
  intervertebral foramina (see also Lesion, biomechanical, specified NEC)
    connective tissue M99.79
      abdomen M99.79
      cervical region M99.71
      cervicothoracic M99.71
      head region M99.70
      lumbar region M99.73
      lumbosacral M99.73
      occipitocervical M99.70
      sacral region M99.74
      sacrococcygeal M99.74
      sacroiliac M99.74
      specified NEC M99.79
      thoracic region M99.72
      thoracolumbar M99.72
    disc M99.79
      abdomen M99.79
      cervical region M99.71
      cervicothoracic M99.71
      head region M99.70
      lower extremity M99.76

**Stenosis, stenotic** — *continued*
  intervertebral foramina (*see also* Lesion, biomechanical,
      specified) — *continued*
    disc — *continued*
      lumbar region M99.73
      lumbosacral M99.73
      occipitocervical M99.70
      pelvic M99.75
      rib cage M99.78
      sacral region M99.74
      sacrococcygeal M99.74
      sacroiliac M99.74
      specified NEC M99.79
      thoracic region M99.72
      thoracolumbar M99.72
      upper extremity M99.77
    osseous M99.69
      abdomen M99.69
      cervical region M99.61
      cervicothoracic M99.61
      head region M99.60
      lower extremity M99.66
      lumbar region M99.63
      lumbosacral M99.63
      occipitocervical M99.60
      pelvic M99.65
      rib cage M99.68
      sacral region M99.64
      sacrococcygeal M99.64
      sacroiliac M99.64
      specified NEC M99.69
      thoracic region M99.62
      thoracolumbar M99.62
      upper extremity M99.67
    subluxation — *see* Stenosis, intervertebral foramina, osseous
  intestine (*see also* Obstruction, intestine)
    congenital (small) Q41.9
      large Q42.9
        specified NEC Q42.8
      specified NEC Q41.8
    jejunum (*see also* Obstruction, intestine, specified NEC)
        K56.699
      congenital Q41.1
  lacrimal (passage)
    canaliculi H04.54- ☑
    congenital Q10.5
    duct H04.55- ☑
    punctum H04.56- ☑
    sac H04.57- ☑
  lacrimonasal duct — *see* Stenosis, lacrimal, duct
    congenital Q10.5
  larynx J38.6
    congenital NEC Q31.8
      subglottic Q31.1
    syphilitic A52.73
      congenital A50.59 [J99]
  mitral (chronic) (inactive) (valve) I05.0
    with
      aortic valve disease I08.0
      incompetency, insufficiency or regurgitation
          I05.2
    active or acute I01.1
      with rheumatic or Sydenham's chorea I02.0
    congenital Q23.2
    specified cause, except rheumatic I34.2
    syphilitic A52.03
  myocardium, myocardial (*see also* Degeneration, myocardial)
    hypertrophic subaortic (idiopathic) I42.1
  nares (anterior) (posterior) J34.89
    congenital Q30.0
  nasal duct (*see also* Stenosis, lacrimal, duct)
    congenital Q10.5
  nasolacrimal duct (*see also* Stenosis, lacrimal, duct)
    congenital Q10.5
  neural canal (*see also* Lesion, biomechanical, specified NEC)
    connective tissue M99.49
      abdomen M99.49
      cervical region M99.41
      cervicothoracic M99.41
      head region M99.40
      lower extremity M99.46
      lumbar region M99.43
      lumbosacral M99.43
      occipitocervical M99.40
      pelvic M99.45

**Stenosis, stenotic** — *continued*
  neural canal (*see also* Lesion, biomechanical, specified)
      — *continued*
    connective tissue — *continued*
      rib cage M99.48
      sacral region M99.44
      sacrococcygeal M99.44
      sacroiliac M99.44
      specified NEC M99.49
      thoracic region M99.42
      thoracolumbar M99.42
      upper extremity M99.47
    intervertebral disc M99.59
      abdomen M99.59
      cervical region M99.51
      cervicothoracic M99.51
      head region M99.50
      lower extremity M99.56
      lumbar region M99.53
      lumbosacral M99.53
      occipitocervical M99.50
      pelvic M99.55
      rib cage M99.58
      sacral region M99.54
      sacrococcygeal M99.54
      sacroiliac M99.54
      specified NEC M99.59
      thoracic region M99.52
      thoracolumbar M99.52
      upper extremity M99.57
    osseous M99.39
      abdomen M99.39
      cervical region M99.31
      cervicothoracic M99.31
      head region M99.30
      lower extremity M99.36
      lumbar region M99.33
      lumbosacral M99.33
      occipitocervical M99.30
      pelvic M99.35
      rib cage M99.38
      sacral region M99.34
      sacrococcygeal M99.34
      sacroiliac M99.34
      specified NEC M99.39
      thoracic region M99.32
      thoracolumbar M99.32
      upper extremity M99.37
    subluxation M99.29
      cervical region M99.21
      cervicothoracic M99.21
      head region M99.20
      lower extremity M99.26
      lumbar region M99.23
      lumbosacral M99.23
      occipitocervical M99.20
      pelvic M99.25
      rib cage M99.28
      sacral region M99.24
      sacrococcygeal M99.24
      sacroiliac M99.24
      specified NEC M99.29
      thoracic region M99.22
      thoracolumbar M99.22
      upper extremity M99.27
  organ or site, congenital NEC — *see* Atresia, by site
  papilla of Vater K83.1
  pulmonary (artery) (congenital) Q25.6
    with ventricular septal defect, transposition of
        aorta, and hypertrophy of right ventricle
        Q21.3
    acquired I28.8
    in tetralogy of Fallot Q21.3
    infundibular Q24.3
    subvalvular Q24.3
    supravalvular Q25.6
    valve I37.0
      with insufficiency I37.2
      congenital Q22.1
      rheumatic I09.89
        with aortic, mitral or tricuspid (valve) disease
            I08.8
    vein, acquired I28.8
    vessel NEC I28.8
  pulmonic (congenital) Q22.1
    infundibular Q24.3
    subvalvular Q24.3
  pylorus (hypertrophic) (acquired) K31.1
    adult K31.1

**Stenosis, stenotic** — *continued*
  pylorus — *continued*
    congenital Q40.0
    infantile Q40.0
  rectum (sphincter) — *see* Stricture, rectum
  renal artery I70.1
    congenital Q27.1
  salivary duct (any) K11.8
  sphincter of Oddi K83.1
  spinal M48.00
    cervical region M48.02
    cervicothoracic region M48.03
    lumbar region (NOS) (without neurogenic claudi-
        cation) M48.061
      with neurogenic claudication M48.062
    lumbosacral region M48.07
    occipito-atlanto-axial region M48.01
    sacrococcygeal region M48.08
    thoracic region M48.04
    thoracolumbar region M48.05
  stomach, hourglass K31.2
  subaortic (congenital) Q24.4
    hypertrophic (idiopathic) I42.1
  subglottic J38.6
    congenital Q31.1
    postprocedural J95.5
  trachea J39.8
    congenital Q32.1
    syphilitic A52.73
    tuberculous NEC A15.5
  tracheostomy J95.03
  tricuspid (valve) I07.0
    with
      aortic (valve) disease I08.2
      incompetency, insufficiency or regurgitation
          I07.2
        with aortic (valve) disease I08.2
          with mitral (valve) disease I08.3
      mitral (valve) disease I08.1
        with aortic (valve) disease I08.3
    congenital Q22.4
    nonrheumatic I36.0
      with insufficiency I36.2
  tubal N97.1
  ureter — *see* Atresia, ureter
  ureteropelvic junction, congenital Q62.11
  ureterovesical orifice, congenital Q62.12
  urethra (valve) (*see also* Stricture, urethra)
    congenital Q64.32
  urinary meatus, congenital Q64.33
  vagina N89.5
    congenital Q52.4
    in pregnancy — *see* Pregnancy, complicated by,
        abnormal vagina
      causing obstructed labor O65.5
  valve (cardiac) (heart) (*see also* Endocarditis) I38
    congenital Q24.8
      aortic Q23.0
      mitral Q23.2
      pulmonary Q22.1
      tricuspid Q22.4
  vena cava (inferior) (superior) I87.1
    congenital Q26.0
  vesicourethral orifice Q64.31
  vulva N90.5
**Stent jail** T82.897 ☑
**Stercolith** (impaction) K56.41
  appendix K38.1
**Stercoraceous, stercoral ulcer** K63.3
  anus or rectum K62.6
**Stereotypies NEC** F98.4
**Sterility** — *see* Infertility
**Sterilization** — *see* Encounter (for), sterilization
**Sternalgia** — *see* Angina
**Sternopagus** Q89.4
**Sternum bifidum** Q76.7
**Steroid**
  effects (adverse) (adrenocortical) (iatrogenic)
    cushingoid E24.2
      correct substance properly administered — *see*
          Table of Drugs and Chemicals, by drug,
          adverse effect
      overdose or wrong substance given or taken
          — *see* Table of Drugs and Chemicals, by
          drug, poisoning
    diabetes — *see* subcategory E09 ☑

**Steroid** — *continued*
- effects — *continued*
  - diabetes — *see* subcategory — *continued*
    - correct substance properly administered — *see* Table of Drugs and Chemicals, by drug, adverse effect
    - overdose or wrong substance given or taken — *see* Table of Drugs and Chemicals, by drug, poisoning
  - fever R50.2
  - insufficiency E27.3
    - correct substance properly administered — *see* Table of Drugs and Chemicals, by drug, adverse effect
    - overdose or wrong substance given or taken — *see* Table of Drugs and Chemicals, by drug, poisoning
- responder H40.04- ☑
**Stevens-Johnson disease or syndrome** L51.1
- toxic epidermal necrolysis overlap L51.3
**Stewart-Morel syndrome** M85.2
**Sticker's disease** B08.3
**Sticky eye** — *see* Conjunctivitis, acute, mucopurulent
**Stieda's disease** — *see* Bursitis, tibial collateral
**Stiff neck** — *see* Torticollis
**Stiff-man syndrome** G25.82
**Stiffness, joint NEC** M25.60
- ankle M25.67- ☑
- ankylosis — *see* Ankylosis, joint
- contracture — *see* Contraction, joint
- elbow M25.62- ☑
- foot M25.67- ☑
- hand M25.64- ☑
- hip M25.65- ☑
- knee M25.66- ☑
- shoulder M25.61- ☑
- wrist M25.63- ☑
**Stigmata congenital syphilis** A50.59
**Stillbirth** P95
**Still-Felty syndrome** — *see* Felty's syndrome
**Still's disease or syndrome** (juvenile) M08.20
- adult-onset M06.1
- ankle M08.27- ☑
- elbow M08.22- ☑
- foot joint M08.27- ☑
- hand joint M08.24- ☑
- hip M08.25- ☑
- knee M08.26- ☑
- multiple site M08.29
- shoulder M08.21- ☑
- vertebra M08.28
- wrist M08.23- ☑
**Stimulation, ovary** E28.1
**Sting** (venomous) (with allergic or anaphylactic shock) — *see* Table of Drugs and Chemicals, by animal or substance, poisoning
**Stippled epiphyses** Q78.8
**Stitch**
- abscess T81.4 ☑
- burst (in operation wound) — *see* Disruption, wound, operation
**Stokes' disease** E05.00
- with thyroid storm E05.01
**Stokes-Adams disease or syndrome** I45.9
**Stokvis** (-Talma) **disease** D74.8
**Stoma malfunction**
- colostomy K94.03
- enterostomy K94.13
- gastrostomy K94.23
- ileostomy K94.13
- tracheostomy J95.03
**Stomach** — *see* condition
**Stomatitis** (denture) (ulcerative) K12.1
- angular K13.0
  - due to dietary or vitamin deficiency E53.0
- aphthous K12.0
- bovine B08.61
- candidal B37.0
- catarrhal K12.1
- diphtheritic A36.89
- due to
  - dietary deficiency E53.0
  - thrush B37.0
  - vitamin deficiency
    - B group NEC E53.9
    - B2 (riboflavin) E53.0
- epidemic B08.8

**Stomatitis** — *continued*
- epizootic B08.8
- follicular K12.1
- gangrenous A69.0
- Geotrichum B48.3
- herpesviral, herpetic B00.2
- herpetiformis K12.0
- malignant K12.1
- membranous acute K12.1
- monilial B37.0
- mycotic B37.0
- necrotizing ulcerative A69.0
- parasitic B37.0
- septic K12.1
- spirochetal A69.1
- suppurative (acute) K12.2
- ulceromembranous A69.1
- vesicular K12.1
  - with exanthem (enteroviral) B08.4
  - virus disease A93.8
- Vincent's A69.1
**Stomatocytosis** D58.8
**Stomatomycosis** B37.0
**Stomatorrhagia** K13.79
**Stone(s)** (*see also* Calculus)
- bladder (diverticulum) N21.0
- cystine E72.09
- heart syndrome I50.1
- kidney N20.0
- prostate N42.0
- pulpal (dental) K04.2
- renal N20.0
- salivary gland or duct (any) K11.5
- urethra (impacted) N21.1
- urinary (duct) (impacted) (passage) N20.9
  - bladder (diverticulum) N21.0
  - lower tract N21.9
  - specified NEC N21.8
- xanthine E79.8 [N22]
**Stonecutter's lung** J62.8
**Stonemason's asthma, disease, lung or pneumoconiosis** J62.8
**Stoppage**
- heart — *see* Arrest, cardiac
- urine — *see* Retention, urine
**Storm, thyroid** — *see* Thyrotoxicosis
**Strabismus** (congenital) (nonparalytic) H50.9
- concomitant H50.40
  - convergent — *see* Strabismus, convergent concomitant
  - divergent — *see* Strabismus, divergent concomitant
- convergent concomitant H50.00
  - accommodative component H50.43
  - alternating H50.05
    - with
      - A pattern H50.06
      - specified nonconcomitances NEC H50.08
      - V pattern H50.07
  - monocular H50.01- ☑
    - with
      - A pattern H50.02- ☑
      - specified nonconcomitances NEC H50.04- ☑
      - V pattern H50.03- ☑
    - intermittent H50.31- ☑
      - alternating H50.32
- cyclotropia H50.41 ☑
- divergent concomitant H50.10
  - alternating H50.15
    - with
      - A pattern H50.16
      - specified noncomitances NEC H50.18
      - V pattern H50.17
  - monocular H50.11- ☑
    - with
      - A pattern H50.12- ☑
      - specified noncomitances NEC H50.14- ☑
      - V pattern H50.13- ☑
    - intermittent H50.33 ☑
      - alternating H50.34
- Duane's syndrome H50.81- ☑
- due to adhesions, scars H50.69
- heterophoria H50.50
  - alternating H50.55
  - cyclophoria H50.54
  - esophoria H50.51
  - exophoria H50.52
  - vertical H50.53

**Strabismus** — *continued*
- heterotropia H50.40
  - intermittent H50.30
- hypertropia H50.2- ☑
- hypotropia — *see* Hypertropia
- latent H50.50
- mechanical H50.60
  - Brown's sheath syndrome H50.61- ☑
  - specified type NEC H50.69
- monofixation syndrome H50.42
- paralytic H49.9
  - abducens nerve H49.2- ☑
  - fourth nerve H49.1- ☑
  - Kearns-Sayre syndrome H49.81- ☑
  - ophthalmoplegia (external)
    - progressive H49.4- ☑
      - with pigmentary retinopathy H49.81- ☑
    - total H49.3- ☑
  - sixth nerve H49.2- ☑
  - specified type NEC H49.88- ☑
  - third nerve H49.0- ☑
  - trochlear nerve H49.1- ☑
- specified type NEC H50.89
- vertical H50.2- ☑
**Strain**
- back S39.012 ☑
- cervical S16.1 ☑
- eye NEC — *see* Disturbance, vision, subjective
- heart — *see* Disease, heart
- low back S39.012 ☑
- mental NOS Z73.3
  - work-related Z56.6
- muscle (tendon) — *see* Injury, muscle, by site, strain
- neck S16.1 ☑
- physical NOS Z73.3
  - work-related Z56.6
- postural (*see also* Disorder, soft tissue, due to use)
- psychological NEC Z73.3
- tendon — *see* Injury, muscle, by site, strain
**Straining, on urination** R39.16
**Strand, vitreous** — *see* Opacity, vitreous, membranes and strands
**Strangulation, strangulated** (*see also* Asphyxia, traumatic)
- appendix K38.8
- bladder-neck N32.0
- bowel or colon K56.2
- food or foreign body — *see* Foreign body, by site
- hemorrhoids — *see* Hemorrhoids, with complication
- hernia (*see also* Hernia, by site, with obstruction)
  - with gangrene — *see* Hernia, by site, with gangrene
- intestine (large) (small) K56.2
  - with hernia (*see also* Hernia, by site, with obstruction)
    - with gangrene — *see* Hernia, by site, with gangrene
- mesentery K56.2
- mucus — *see* Asphyxia, mucus
- omentum K56.2
- organ or site, congenital NEC — *see* Atresia, by site
- ovary — *see* Torsion, ovary
- penis N48.89
  - foreign body T19.4 ☑
- rupture — *see* Hernia, by site, with obstruction
- stomach due to hernia (*see also* Hernia, by site, with obstruction)
  - with gangrene — *see* Hernia, by site, with gangrene
- vesicourethral orifice N32.0
**Strangury** R30.0
**Straw itch** B88.0
**Strawberry**
- gallbladder K82.4
- mark Q82.5
- tongue (red) (white) K14.3
**Streak(s)**
- macula, angioid H35.33
- ovarian Q50.32
**Strephosymbolia** F81.0
- secondary to organic lesion R48.8
**Streptobacillary fever** A25.1
**Streptobacillosis** A25.1
**Streptobacillus moniliformis** A25.1
**Streptococcus, streptococcal** (*see also* condition)
- as cause of disease classified elsewhere B95.5

☑ **Additional Character Required** — Refer to the Tabular List for Character Selection ▽ **Subterms under main terms may continue to next column or page**

**Streptococcus, streptococcal** — *continued*
    group
        A, as cause of disease classified elsewhere B95.0
        B, as cause of disease classified elsewhere B95.1
        D, as cause of disease classified elsewhere B95.2
    pneumoniae, as cause of disease classified elsewhere
        B95.3
    specified NEC, as cause of disease classified elsewhere
        B95.4
**Streptomycosis** B47.1
**Streptotrichosis** A48.8
**Stress** F43.9
    family — *see* Disruption, family
    fetal P84
        complicating pregnancy O77.9
            due to drug administration O77.1
    mental NEC Z73.3
        work-related Z56.6
    physical NEC Z73.3
        work-related Z56.6
    polycythemia D75.1
    reaction (*see also* Reaction, stress) F43.9
    work schedule Z56.3
**Stretching, nerve** — *see* Injury, nerve
**Striae albicantes, atrophicae or distensae** (cutis) L90.6
**Stricture** (*see also* Stenosis)
    ampulla of Vater K83.1
    anus (sphincter) K62.4
        congenital Q42.3
            with fistula Q42.2
        infantile Q42.3
            with fistula Q42.2
    aorta (ascending) (congenital) Q25.1
        arteriosclerotic I70.0
        calcified I70.0
        supravalvular, congenital Q25.3
    aortic (valve) — *see* Stenosis, aortic
    aqueduct of Sylvius (congenital) Q03.0
        with spina bifida — *see* Spina bifida, by site, with
            hydrocephalus
        acquired G91.1
    artery I77.1
        basilar — *see* Occlusion, artery, basilar
        carotid — *see* Occlusion, artery, carotid
        celiac I77.4
        congenital (peripheral) Q27.8
            cerebral Q28.3
            coronary Q24.5
            digestive system Q27.8
            lower limb Q27.8
            retinal Q14.1
            specified site NEC Q27.8
            umbilical Q27.0
            upper limb Q27.8
        coronary — *see* Disease, heart, ischemic,
            atherosclerotic
            congenital Q24.5
        precerebral — *see* Occlusion, artery, precerebral
        pulmonary (congenital) Q25.6
            acquired I28.8
        renal I70.1
        vertebral — *see* Occlusion, artery, vertebral
    auditory canal (external) (congenital)
        acquired — *see* Stenosis, external ear canal
    bile duct (common) (hepatic) K83.1
        congenital Q44.3
        postoperative K91.89
    bladder N32.89
        neck N32.0
    bowel — *see* Obstruction, intestine
    brain G93.89
    bronchus J98.09
        congenital Q32.3
        syphilitic A52.72
    cardia (stomach) K22.2
        congenital Q39.3
    cardiac (*see also* Disease, heart)
        orifice (stomach) K22.2
    cecum — *see* Obstruction, intestine
    cervix, cervical (canal) N88.2
        congenital Q51.828
        in pregnancy — *see* Pregnancy, complicated by,
            abnormal cervix
            causing obstructed labor O65.5
    colon (*see also* Obstruction, intestine)
        congenital Q42.9
            specified NEC Q42.8
    colostomy K94.03

**Stricture** — *continued*
    common (bile) duct K83.1
    coronary (artery) — *see* Disease, heart, ischemic,
        atherosclerotic
    cystic duct — *see* Obstruction, gallbladder
    digestive organs NEC, congenital Q45.8
    duodenum K31.5
        congenital Q41.0
    ear canal (external) (congenital) Q16.1
        acquired — *see* Stricture, auditory canal, acquired
    ejaculatory duct N50.89
    enterostomy K94.13
    esophagus K22.2
        congenital Q39.3
        syphilitic A52.79
            congenital A50.59 [K23]
    eustachian tube (*see also* Obstruction, eustachian tube)
        congenital Q17.8
    fallopian tube N97.1
        gonococcal A54.24
        tuberculous A18.17
    gallbladder — *see* Obstruction, gallbladder
    glottis J38.6
    heart (*see also* Disease, heart)
        valve (*see also* Endocarditis) I38
            aortic Q23.0
            mitral Q23.2
            pulmonary Q22.1
            tricuspid Q22.4
    hepatic duct K83.1
    hourglass, of stomach K31.2
    hymen N89.6
    hypopharynx J39.2
    ileum (*see also* Obstruction, intestine, specified NEC)
        K56.699
        congenital Q41.2
    intestine (*see also* Obstruction, intestine)
        congenital (small) Q41.9
            large Q42.9
                specified NEC Q42.8
            specified NEC Q41.8
        ischemic K55.1
    jejunum (*see also* Obstruction, intestine, specified NEC)
        K56.699
        congenital Q41.1
    lacrimal passages (*see also* Stenosis, lacrimal)
        congenital Q10.5
    larynx J38.6
        congenital NEC Q31.8
            subglottic Q31.1
        syphilitic A52.73
            congenital A50.59 [J99]
    meatus
        ear (congenital) Q16.1
            acquired — *see* Stricture, auditory canal, ac-
                quired
        osseous (ear) (congenital) Q16.1
            acquired — *see* Stricture, auditory canal, ac-
                quired
        urinarius (*see also* Stricture, urethra)
            congenital Q64.33
    mitral (valve) — *see* Stenosis, mitral
    myocardium, myocardial I51.5
        hypertrophic subaortic (idiopathic) I42.1
    nares (anterior) (posterior) J34.89
        congenital Q30.0
    nasal duct (*see also* Stenosis, lacrimal, duct)
        congenital Q10.5
    nasolacrimal duct (*see also* Stenosis, lacrimal, duct)
        congenital Q10.5
    nasopharynx J39.2
        syphilitic A52.73
    nose J34.89
        congenital Q30.0
        syphilitic A52.73
            congenital A50.59 [J99]
    nostril (anterior) (posterior) J34.89
        congenital Q30.0
        syphilitic A52.73
            congenital A50.59 [J99]
    organ or site, congenital NEC — *see* Atresia, by site
    os uteri — *see* Stricture, cervix
    osseous meatus (ear) (congenital) Q16.1
        acquired — *see* Stricture, auditory canal, acquired
    oviduct — *see* Stricture, fallopian tube
    pelviureteric junction (congenital) Q62.11
        acquired, with hydronephrosis N13.0
    penis, by foreign body T19.4 ☑
    pharynx J39.2
    prostate N42.89

**Stricture** — *continued*
    pulmonary, pulmonic
        artery (congenital) Q25.6
            acquired I28.8
            noncongenital I28.8
        infundibulum (congenital) Q24.3
        valve I37.0
            congenital Q22.1
        vein, acquired I28.8
        vessel NEC I28.8
    punctum lacrimale (*see also* Stenosis, lacrimal, punc-
        tum)
        congenital Q10.5
    pylorus (hypertrophic) K31.1
        adult K31.1
        congenital Q40.0
        infantile Q40.0
    rectosigmoid (*see also* Obstruction, intestine, specified
        NEC) K56.699
    rectum (sphincter) K62.4
        congenital Q42.1
            with fistula Q42.0
        due to
            chlamydial lymphogranuloma A55
            irradiation K91.89
            lymphogranuloma venereum A55
        gonococcal A54.6
        inflammatory (chlamydial) A55
        syphilitic A52.74
        tuberculous A18.32
    renal artery I70.1
        congenital Q27.1
    salivary duct or gland (any) K11.8
    sigmoid (flexure) — *see* Obstruction, intestine
    spermatic cord N50.89
    stoma (following) (of)
        colostomy K94.03
        enterostomy K94.13
        gastrostomy K94.23
        ileostomy K94.13
        tracheostomy J95.03
    stomach K31.89
        congenital Q40.2
        hourglass K31.2
    subaortic Q24.4
        hypertrophic (acquired) (idiopathic) I42.1
    subglottic J38.6
    syphilitic NEC A52.79
    trachea J39.8
        congenital Q32.1
        syphilitic A52.73
        tuberculous NEC A15.5
    tracheostomy J95.03
    tricuspid (valve) — *see* Stenosis, tricuspid
    tunica vaginalis N50.89
    ureter (postoperative) N13.5
        with
            hydronephrosis N13.1
                with infection N13.6
            pyelonephritis (chronic) N11.1
        congenital — *see* Atresia, ureter
        tuberculous A18.11
    ureteropelvic junction (congenital) Q62.11
        acquired, with hydronephrosis N13.0
    ureterovesical orifice N13.5
        with infection N13.6
    urethra (organic) (spasmodic) N35.9
        associated with schistosomiasis B65.0 [N37]
        congenital Q64.39
            valvular (posterior) Q64.2
        due to
            infection — *see* Stricture, urethra, postinfective
            trauma — *see* Stricture, urethra, post-traumatic
        gonococcal, gonorrheal A54.01
        infective NEC — *see* Stricture, urethra, postinfective
        late effect (sequelae) of injury — *see* Stricture,
            urethra, post-traumatic
        postcatheterization — *see* Stricture, urethra, post-
            procedural
        postinfective NEC
            female N35.12
            male N35.119
                anterior urethra N35.114
                bulbous urethra N35.112
                meatal N35.111
                membranous urethra N35.113
        postobstetric N35.021

**Stricture** — *continued*
 urethra — *continued*
  postoperative — *see* Stricture, urethra, postprocedural
  postprocedural
   female N99.12
   male N99.114
    anterior bulbous urethra N99.113
    bulbous urethra N99.111
    fossa navicularis N99.115
    meatal N99.110
    membranous urethra N99.112
  post-traumatic
   female N35.028
    due to childbirth N35.021
   male N35.014
    anterior urethra N35.013
    bulbous urethra N35.011
    meatal N35.010
    membranous urethra N35.012
  sequela (late effect) of
   childbirth N35.021
   injury — *see* Stricture, urethra, post-traumatic
  specified cause NEC N35.8
  syphilitic A52.76
  traumatic — *see* Stricture, urethra, post-traumatic
  valvular (posterior), congenital Q64.2
 urinary meatus — *see* Stricture, urethra
 uterus, uterine (synechiae) N85.6
  os (external) (internal) — *see* Stricture, cervix
 vagina (outlet) — *see* Stenosis, vagina
 valve (cardiac) (heart) (*see also* Endocarditis)
  congenital
   aortic Q23.0
   mitral Q23.2
   pulmonary Q22.1
   tricuspid Q22.4
 vas deferens N50.89
  congenital Q55.4
 vein I87.1
 vena cava (inferior) (superior) NEC I87.1
  congenital Q26.0
 vesicourethral orifice N32.0
  congenital Q64.31
 vulva (acquired) N90.5
**Stridor** R06.1
 congenital (larynx) P28.89
**Stridulous** — *see* condition
**Stroke** (apoplectic) (brain) (embolic) (ischemic) (paralytic)
  (thrombotic) I63.9
 cryptogenic (*see also* infarction, cerebral) I63.9
 epileptic — *see* Epilepsy
 heat T67.0 ☑
 in evolution I63.9
 intraoperative
  during cardiac surgery I97.810
  during other surgery I97.811
 lightning — *see* Lightning
 meaning
  cerebral hemorrhage — *code to* Hemorrhage, intracranial
  cerebral infarction — *code to* Infarction, cerebral
 postprocedural
  following cardiac surgery I97.820
  following other surgery I97.821
 unspecified (NOS) I63.9
**Stromatosis, endometrial** D39.0
**Strongyloidiasis, strongyloidosis** B78.9
 cutaneous B78.1
 disseminated B78.7
 intestinal B78.0
**Strophulus pruriginosus** L28.2
**Struck by lightning** — *see* Lightning
**Struma** (*see also* Goiter)
 Hashimoto E06.3
 lymphomatosa E06.3
 nodosa (simplex) E04.9
  endemic E01.2
   multinodular E01.1
  multinodular E04.2
   iodine-deficiency related E01.1
  toxic or with hyperthyroidism E05.20
   with thyroid storm E05.21
   multinodular E05.20
    with thyroid storm E05.21
   uninodular E05.10
    with thyroid storm E05.11
  toxicosa E05.20

**Struma** — *continued*
 nodosa — *continued*
  toxicosa — *continued*
   with thyroid storm E05.21
   multinodular E05.20
    with thyroid storm E05.21
   uninodular E05.10
    with thyroid storm E05.11
  uninodular E04.1
 ovarii D27.- ☑
 Riedel's E06.5
**Strumipriva cachexia** E03.4
**Strümpell-Marie spine** — *see* Spondylitis, ankylosing
**Strümpell-Westphal pseudosclerosis** E83.01
**Stuart deficiency disease** (factor X) D68.2
**Stuart-Prower factor deficiency** (factor X) D68.2
**Student's elbow** — *see* Bursitis, elbow, olecranon
**Stump** — *see* Amputation
**Stunting, nutritional** E45
**Stupor** (catatonic) R40.1
 depressive (single episode) F32.89
  recurrent episode F33.8
 dissociative F44.2
 manic F30.2
 manic-depressive F31.89
 psychogenic (anergic) F44.2
 reaction to exceptional stress (transient) F43.0
**Sturge** (-Weber) (-Dimitri) (-Kalischer) **disease or syndrome** Q85.8
**Stuttering** F80.81
 adult onset F98.5
 childhood onset F80.81
 following cerebrovascular disease — *see* Disorder,
  fluency. following cerebrovascular disease
 in conditions classified elsewhere R47.82
**Sty, stye** (external) (internal) (meibomian) (zeisian) —
  *see* Hordeolum
**Subacidity, gastric** K31.89
 psychogenic F45.8
**Subacute** — *see* condition
**Subarachnoid** — *see* condition
**Subcortical** — *see* condition
**Subcostal syndrome, nerve compression** — *see*
  Mononeuropathy, upper limb, specified site NEC
**Subcutaneous, subcuticular** — *see* condition
**Subdural** — *see* condition
**Subendocardium** — *see* condition
**Subependymoma**
 specified site — *see* Neoplasm, uncertain behavior,
  by site
 unspecified site D43.2
**Suberosis** J67.3
**Subglossitis** — *see* Glossitis
**Subhemophilia** D66
**Subinvolution**
 breast (postlactational) (postpuerperal) N64.89
 puerperal O90.89
 uterus (chronic) (nonpuerperal) N85.3
  puerperal O90.89
**Sublingual** — *see* condition
**Sublinguitis** — *see* Sialoadenitis
**Subluxatable hip** Q65.6
**Subluxation** (*see also* Dislocation)
 acromioclavicular S43.11- ☑
 ankle S93.0- ☑
 atlantoaxial, recurrent M43.4
  with myelopathy M43.3
 carpometacarpal (joint) NEC S63.05- ☑
  thumb S63.04- ☑
 complex, vertebral — *see* Complex, subluxation
 congenital (*see also* Malposition, congenital)
  hip — *see* Dislocation, hip, congenital, partial
  joint (excluding hip)
   lower limb Q68.8
   shoulder Q68.8
   upper limb Q68.8
 elbow (traumatic) S53.10- ☑
  anterior S53.11- ☑
  lateral S53.14- ☑
  medial S53.13- ☑
  posterior S53.12- ☑
  specified type NEC S53.19- ☑
 finger S63.20- ☑
  index S63.20- ☑
  interphalangeal S63.22- ☑
   distal S63.24- ☑
    index S63.24- ☑

**Subluxation** — *continued*
 finger — *continued*
  interphalangeal — *continued*
   distal — *continued*
    little S63.24- ☑
    middle S63.24- ☑
    ring S63.24- ☑
   index S63.22- ☑
   little S63.22- ☑
   middle S63.22- ☑
   proximal S63.23- ☑
    index S63.23- ☑
    little S63.23- ☑
    middle S63.23- ☑
    ring S63.23- ☑
   ring S63.22- ☑
  little S63.20- ☑
  metacarpophalangeal S63.21- ☑
   index S63.21- ☑
   little S63.21- ☑
   middle S63.21- ☑
   ring S63.21- ☑
  middle S63.20- ☑
  ring S63.20- ☑
 foot S93.30- ☑
  specified site NEC S93.33- ☑
  tarsal joint S93.31- ☑
  tarsometatarsal joint S93.32- ☑
  toe — *see* Subluxation, toe
 hip S73.00- ☑
  anterior S73.03- ☑
   obturator S73.02- ☑
  central S73.04- ☑
  posterior S73.01- ☑
 interphalangeal (joint)
  finger S63.22- ☑
   distal joint S63.24- ☑
    index S63.24- ☑
    little S63.24- ☑
    middle S63.24- ☑
    ring S63.24- ☑
   index S63.22- ☑
   little S63.22- ☑
   middle S63.22- ☑
   proximal joint S63.23- ☑
    index S63.23- ☑
    little S63.23- ☑
    middle S63.23- ☑
    ring S63.23- ☑
   ring S63.22- ☑
  thumb S63.12- ☑
   distal joint S63.14- ☑
   proximal joint S63.13- ☑
  toe S93.13- ☑
   great S93.13- ☑
   lesser S93.13- ☑
 joint prosthesis — *see* Complications, joint prosthesis,
  mechanical, displacement, by site
 knee S83.10- ☑
  cap — *see* Subluxation, patella
  patella — *see* Subluxation, patella
  proximal tibia
   anteriorly S83.11- ☑
   laterally S83.14- ☑
   medially S83.13- ☑
   posteriorly S83.12- ☑
  specified type NEC S83.19- ☑
 lens — *see* Dislocation, lens, partial
 ligament, traumatic — *see* Sprain, by site
 metacarpal (bone)
  proximal end S63.06- ☑
 metacarpophalangeal (joint)
  finger S63.21- ☑
   index S63.21- ☑
   little S63.21- ☑
   middle S63.21- ☑
   ring S63.21- ☑
  thumb S63.11- ☑
 metatarsophalangeal joint S93.14- ☑
  great toe S93.14- ☑
  lesser toe S93.14- ☑
 midcarpal (joint) S63.03- ☑
 patella S83.00- ☑
  lateral S83.01- ☑
  recurrent (nontraumatic) — *see* Dislocation,
   patella, recurrent, incomplete

☑ **Additional Character Required** — **Refer to the Tabular List for Character Selection**    ▽ **Subterms under main terms may continue to next column or page**

**Subluxation** — *continued*
- patella — *continued*
  - specified type NEC S83.09- ☑
  - pathological — *see* Dislocation, pathological
- radial head S53.00- ☑
  - anterior S53.01- ☑
  - nursemaid's elbow S53.03- ☑
  - posterior S53.02- ☑
  - specified type NEC S53.09- ☑
- radiocarpal (joint) S63.02- ☑
- radioulnar (joint)
  - distal S63.01- ☑
  - proximal — *see* Subluxation, elbow
- shoulder
  - congenital Q68.8
  - girdle S43.30- ☑
    - scapula S43.31- ☑
    - specified site NEC S43.39- ☑
  - traumatic S43.00- ☑
    - anterior S43.01- ☑
    - inferior S43.03- ☑
    - posterior S43.02- ☑
    - specified type NEC S43.08- ☑
- sternoclavicular (joint) S43.20- ☑
  - anterior S43.21- ☑
  - posterior S43.22- ☑
- symphysis (pubis)
- thumb S63.103 ☑
  - interphalangeal joint — *see* Subluxation, interphalangeal (joint), thumb
  - metacarpophalangeal joint — *see* Subluxation, metacarpophalangeal (joint), thumb
- toe(s) S93.10- ☑
  - great S93.10- ☑
    - interphalangeal joint S93.13- ☑
    - metatarsophalangeal joint S93.14- ☑
  - interphalangeal joint S93.13- ☑
  - lesser S93.10- ☑
    - interphalangeal joint S93.13- ☑
    - metatarsophalangeal joint S93.14- ☑
  - metatarsophalangeal joint S93.149 ☑
- ulna
  - distal end S63.07- ☑
  - proximal end — *see* Subluxation, elbow
- ulnohumeral joint — *see* Subluxation, elbow
- vertebral
  - recurrent NEC — *see* subcategory M43.5 ☑
  - traumatic
    - cervical S13.100 ☑
      - atlantoaxial joint S13.120 ☑
      - atlantooccipital joint S13.110 ☑
      - atloidooccipital joint S13.110 ☑
      - joint between
        - C0 and C1 S13.110 ☑
        - C1 and C2 S13.120 ☑
        - C2 and C3 S13.130 ☑
        - C3 and C4 S13.140 ☑
        - C4 and C5 S13.150 ☑
        - C5 and C6 S13.160 ☑
        - C6 and C7 S13.170 ☑
        - C7 and T1 S13.180 ☑
      - occipitoatloid joint S13.110 ☑
    - lumbar S33.100 ☑
      - joint between
        - L1 and L2 S33.110 ☑
        - L2 and L3 S33.120 ☑
        - L3 and L4 S33.130 ☑
        - L4 and L5 S33.140 ☑
    - thoracic S23.100 ☑
      - joint between
        - T1 and T2 S23.110 ☑
        - T2 and T3 S23.120 ☑
        - T3 and T4 S23.122 ☑
        - T4 and T5 S23.130 ☑
        - T5 and T6 S23.132 ☑
        - T6 and T7 S23.140 ☑
        - T7 and T8 S23.142 ☑
        - T8 and T9 S23.150 ☑
        - T9 and T10 S23.152 ☑
        - T10 and T11 S23.160 ☑
        - T11 and T12 S23.162 ☑
        - T12 and L1 S23.170 ☑
- wrist (carpal bone) S63.00- ☑
  - carpometacarpal joint — *see* Subluxation, carpometacarpal (joint)

**Subluxation** — *continued*
- wrist — *continued*
  - distal radioulnar joint — *see* Subluxation, radioulnar (joint), distal
  - metacarpal bone, proximal — *see* Subluxation, metacarpal (bone), proximal end
  - midcarpal — *see* Subluxation, midcarpal (joint)
  - radiocarpal joint — *see* Subluxation, radiocarpal (joint)
  - recurrent — *see* Dislocation, recurrent, wrist
  - specified site NEC S63.09- ☑
  - ulna — *see* Subluxation, ulna, distal end
**Submaxillary** — *see* condition
**Submersion** (fatal) (nonfatal) T75.1 ☑
**Submucous** — *see* condition
**Subnormal, subnormality**
- accommodation (old age) H52.4
- mental — *see* Disability, intellectual
- temperature (accidental) T68 ☑
**Subphrenic** — *see* condition
**Subscapular nerve** — *see* condition
**Subseptus uterus** Q51.2
**Subsiding appendicitis** K36
**Substance** (other psychoactive) **-induced**
- anxiety disorder F19.980
- bipolar and related disorder F19.94
- delirium F19.921
- depressive disorder F19.94
- major neurocognitive disorder F19.97
- mild neurocognitive disorder F19.988
- obsessive-compulsive and related disorder F19.988
- psychotic disorder F19.959
- sexual dysfunction F19.981
- sleep disorder F19.982
**Substernal thyroid** E04.9
- congenital Q89.2
**Substitution disorder** F44.9
**Subtentorial** — *see* condition
**Subthyroidism** (acquired) (*see also* Hypothyroidism)
- congenital E03.1
**Succenturiate placenta** O43.19- ☑
**Sucking thumb, child** (excessive) F98.8
**Sudamen, sudamina** L74.1
**Sudanese kala-azar** B55.0
**Sudden**
- hearing loss — *see* Deafness, sudden
- heart failure — *see* Failure, heart
**Sudeck's atrophy, disease, or syndrome** — *see* Algoneurodystrophy
**Suffocation** — *see* Asphyxia, traumatic
**Sugar**
- blood
  - high (transient) R73.9
  - low (transient) E16.2
- in urine R81
**Suicide, suicidal** (attempted) T14.91 ☑
- by poisoning — *see* Table of Drugs and Chemicals
- history of (personal) Z91.5
  - in family Z81.8
- ideation — *see* Ideation, suicidal
- risk
  - meaning personal history of attempted suicide Z91.5
  - meaning suicidal ideation — *see* Ideation, suicidal
- tendencies
  - meaning personal history of attempted suicide Z91.5
  - meaning suicidal ideation — *see* Ideation, suicidal
- trauma — *see* nature of injury by site
**Suipestifer infection** — *see* Infection, salmonella
**Sulfhemoglobinemia, sulphemoglobinemia** (acquired) (with methemoglobinemia) D74.8
**Sumatran mite fever** A75.3
**Summer** — *see* condition
**Sunburn** L55.9
- due to
  - tanning bed (acute) L56.8
    - chronic L57.8
  - ultraviolet radiation (acute) L56.8
    - chronic L57.8
- first degree L55.0
- second degree L55.1
- third degree L55.2
**SUNCT** (short lasting unilateral neuralgiform headache with conjunctival injection and tearing) G44.059
- intractable G44.051
- not intractable G44.059

**Sundowning** F05
**Sunken acetabulum** — *see* Derangement, joint, specified type NEC, hip
**Sunstroke** T67.0 ☑
**Superfecundation** — *see* Pregnancy, multiple
**Superfetation** — *see* Pregnancy, multiple
**Superinvolution** (uterus) N85.8
**Supernumerary** (congenital)
- aortic cusps Q23.8
- auditory ossicles Q16.3
- bone Q79.8
- breast Q83.1
- carpal bones Q74.0
- cusps, heart valve NEC Q24.8
  - aortic Q23.8
  - mitral Q23.2
  - pulmonary Q22.3
- digit(s) Q69.9
- ear (lobule) Q17.0
- fallopian tube Q50.6
- finger Q69.0
- hymen Q52.4
- kidney Q63.0
- lacrimonasal duct Q10.6
- lobule (ear) Q17.0
- mitral cusps Q23.2
- muscle Q79.8
- nipple(s) Q83.3
- organ or site not listed — *see* Accessory
- ossicles, auditory Q16.3
- ovary Q50.31
- oviduct Q50.6
- pulmonary, pulmonic cusps Q22.3
- rib Q76.6
  - cervical or first (syndrome) Q76.5
- roots (of teeth) K00.2
- spleen Q89.09
- tarsal bones Q74.2
- teeth K00.1
- testis Q55.29
- thumb Q69.1
- toe Q69.2
- uterus Q51.2
- vagina Q52.1 ☑
- vertebra Q76.49
**Supervision** (of)
- contraceptive — *see* Prescription, contraceptives
- dietary (for) Z71.3
  - allergy (food) Z71.3
  - colitis Z71.3
  - diabetes mellitus Z71.3
  - food allergy or intolerance Z71.3
  - gastritis Z71.3
  - hypercholesterolemia Z71.3
  - hypoglycemia Z71.3
  - intolerance (food) Z71.3
  - obesity Z71.3
  - specified NEC Z71.3
- healthy infant or child Z76.2
  - foundling Z76.1
- high-risk pregnancy — *see* Pregnancy, complicated by, high, risk
- lactation Z39.1
- pregnancy — *see* Pregnancy, supervision of
**Supplemental teeth** K00.1
**Suppression**
- binocular vision H53.34
- lactation O92.5
- menstruation N94.89
- ovarian secretion E28.39
- renal N28.9
- urine, urinary secretion R34
**Suppuration, suppurative** (*see also* condition)
- accessory sinus (chronic) — *see* Sinusitis
- adrenal gland
- antrum (chronic) — *see* Sinusitis, maxillary
- bladder — *see* Cystitis
- brain G06.0
  - sequelae G09
- breast N61.1
  - puerperal, postpartum or gestational — *see* Mastitis, obstetric, purulent
- dental periosteum M27.3
- ear (middle) (*see also* Otitis, media)
  - external NEC — *see* Otitis, externa, infective
  - internal — *see* subcategory H83.0 ☑
- ethmoidal (chronic) (sinus) — *see* Sinusitis, ethmoidal
- fallopian tube — *see* Salpingo-oophoritis

**Suppuration, suppurative** — *continued*
  frontal (chronic) (sinus) — *see* Sinusitis, frontal
  gallbladder (acute) K81.0
  gum K05.20
    generalized — *see* Peridontitis, aggressive, generalized
    localized — *see* Peridontitis, aggressive, localized
  intracranial G06.0
  joint — *see* Arthritis, pyogenic or pyemic
  labyrinthine — *see* subcategory H83.0 ☑
  lung — *see* Abscess, lung
  mammary gland N61.1
    puerperal, postpartum O91.12
      associated with lactation O91.13
  maxilla, maxillary M27.2
    sinus (chronic) — *see* Sinusitis, maxillary
  muscle — *see* Myositis, infective
  nasal sinus (chronic) — *see* Sinusitis
  pancreas, acute (*see also* Pancreatitis, acute) K85.80
  parotid gland — *see* Sialoadenitis
  pelvis, pelvic
    female — *see* Disease, pelvis, inflammatory
    male K65.0
  pericranial — *see* Osteomyelitis
  salivary duct or gland (any) — *see* Sialoadenitis
  sinus (accessory) (chronic) (nasal) — *see* Sinusitis
  sphenoidal sinus (chronic) — *see* Sinusitis, sphenoidal
  thymus (gland) E32.1
  thyroid (gland) E06.0
  tonsil — *see* Tonsillitis
  uterus — *see* Endometritis
**Supraeruption of tooth** (teeth) M26.34
**Supraglottitis** J04.30
  with obstruction J04.31
**Suprarenal** (gland) — *see* condition
**Suprascapular nerve** — *see* condition
**Suprasellar** — *see* condition
**Surfer's knots or nodules** S89.8- ☑
**Surgical**
  emphysema T81.82 ☑
  procedures, complication or misadventure — *see* Complications, surgical procedures
  shock T81.10 ☑
**Surveillance** (of) (for) (*see also* Observation)
  alcohol abuse Z71.41
  contraceptive — *see* Prescription, contraceptives
  dietary Z71.3
  drug abuse Z71.51
**Susceptibility to disease, genetic** Z15.89
  malignant neoplasm Z15.09
    breast Z15.01
    endometrium Z15.04
    ovary Z15.02
    prostate Z15.03
    specified NEC Z15.09
  multiple endocrine neoplasia Z15.81
**Suspected condition, ruled out** (*see also* Observation, suspected)
  amniotic cavity and membrane Z03.71
  cervical shortening Z03.75
  fetal anomaly Z03.73
  fetal growth Z03.74
  maternal and fetal conditions NEC Z03.79
  newborn (*see also* Observation, newborn, suspected condition ruled out) Z05.9
  oligohydramnios Z03.71
  placental problem Z03.72
  polyhydramnios Z03.71
**Suspended uterus**
  in pregnancy or childbirth — *see* Pregnancy, complicated by, abnormal uterus
**Sutton's nevus** D22.9
**Suture**
  burst (in operation wound) T81.31 ☑
    external operation wound T81.31 ☑
    internal operation wound T81.32 ☑
  inadvertently left in operation wound — *see* Foreign body, accidentally left during a procedure
  removal Z48.02
**Swab inadvertently left in operation wound** — *see* Foreign body, accidentally left during a procedure
**Swallowed, swallowing**
  difficulty — *see* Dysphagia
  foreign body — *see* Foreign body, alimentary tract
**Swan-neck deformity** (finger) — *see* Deformity, finger, swan-neck
**Swearing, compulsive** F42.8

**Swearing, compulsive** — *continued*
  in Gilles de la Tourette's syndrome F95.2
**Sweat, sweats**
  fetid L75.0
  night R61
**Sweating, excessive** R61
**Sweeley-Klionsky disease** E75.21
**Sweet's disease or dermatosis** L98.2
**Swelling** (of) R60.9
  abdomen, abdominal (not referable to any particular organ) — *see* Mass, abdominal
  ankle — *see* Effusion, joint, ankle
  arm M79.89
    forearm M79.89
  breast (*see also* Lump, breast) N63.0
  Calabar B74.3
  cervical gland R59.0
  chest, localized R22.2
  ear H93.8- ☑
  extremity (lower) (upper) — *see* Disorder, soft tissue, specified type NEC
  finger M79.89
  foot M79.89
  glands R59.9
    generalized R59.1
    localized R59.0
  hand M79.89
  head (localized) R22.0
  inflammatory — *see* Inflammation
  intra-abdominal — *see* Mass, abdominal
  joint — *see* Effusion, joint
  leg M79.89
    lower M79.89
  limb — *see* Disorder, soft tissue, specified type NEC
  localized (skin) R22.9
    chest R22.2
    head R22.0
    limb
      lower — *see* Mass, localized, limb, lower
      upper — *see* Mass, localized, limb, upper
    neck R22.1
    trunk R22.2
  neck (localized) R22.1
  pelvic — *see* Mass, abdominal
  scrotum N50.89
  splenic — *see* Splenomegaly
  testis N50.89
  toe M79.89
  umbilical R19.09
  wandering, due to Gnathostoma (spinigerum) B83.1
  white — *see* Tuberculosis, arthritis
**Swift** (-Feer) **disease**
  overdose or wrong substance given or taken — *see* Table of Drugs and Chemicals, by drug, poisoning
**Swimmer's**
  cramp T75.1 ☑
  ear H60.33- ☑
  itch B65.3
**Swimming in the head** R42
**Swollen** — *see* Swelling
**Swyer syndrome** Q99.1
**Sycosis** L73.8
  barbae (not parasitic) L73.8
  contagiosa (mycotic) B35.0
  lupoides L73.8
  mycotic B35.0
  parasitic B35.0
  vulgaris L73.8
**Sydenham's chorea** — *see* Chorea, Sydenham's
**Sylvatic yellow fever** A95.0
**Sylvest's disease** B33.0
**Symblepharon** H11.23- ☑
  congenital Q10.3
**Symond's syndrome** G93.2
**Sympathetic** — *see* condition
**Sympatheticotonia** G90.8
**Sympathicoblastoma**
  specified site — *see* Neoplasm, malignant, by site
  unspecified site C74.90
**Sympathogonioma** — *see* Sympathicoblastoma
**Symphalangy** (fingers) (toes) Q70.9
**Symptoms NEC** R68.89
  breast NEC N64.59
  cold J00
  development NEC R63.8
  factitious, self-induced — *see* Disorder, factitious

**Symptoms** — *continued*
  genital organs, female R10.2
  involving
    abdomen NEC R19.8
    appearance NEC R46.89
    awareness R41.9
      altered mental status R41.82
      amnesia — *see* Amnesia
      borderline intellectual functioning R41.83
      coma — *see* Coma
      disorientation R41.0
      neurologic neglect syndrome R41.4
      senile cognitive decline R41.81
      specified symptom NEC R41.89
    behavior NEC R46.89
    cardiovascular system NEC R09.89
    chest NEC R09.89
    circulatory system NEC R09.89
    cognitive functions R41.9
      altered mental status R41.82
      amnesia — *see* Amnesia
      borderline intellectual functioning R41.83
      coma — *see* Coma
      disorientation R41.0
      neurologic neglect syndrome R41.4
      senile cognitive decline R41.81
      specified symptom NEC R41.89
    development NEC R62.50
    digestive system NEC R19.8
    emotional state NEC R45.89
      emotional lability R45.86
    food and fluid intake R63.8
    general perceptions and sensations R44.9
      specified NEC R44.8
    musculoskeletal system R29.91
      specified NEC R29.898
    nervous system R29.90
      specified NEC R29.818
    pelvis NEC R19.8
    respiratory system NEC R09.89
    skin and integument R23.9
    urinary system R39.9
  menopausal N95.1
  metabolism NEC R63.8
  neurotic F48.8
  of infancy R68.19
  pelvis NEC, female R10.2
  skin and integument NEC R23.9
  subcutaneous tissue NEC R23.9
  viral cold J00
**Sympus** Q74.2
**Syncephalus** Q89.4
**Synchondrosis**
  abnormal (congenital) Q78.8
  ischiopubic M91.0
**Synchysis** (scintillans) (senile) (vitreous body) H43.89
**Syncope** (near) (pre-) R55
  anginosa I20.8
  bradycardia R00.1
  cardiac R55
  carotid sinus G90.01
  due to spinal (lumbar) puncture G97.1
  heart R55
  heat T67.1 ☑
  laryngeal R05
  psychogenic F48.8
  tussive R05
  vasoconstriction R55
  vasodepressor R55
  vasomotor R55
  vasovagal R55
**Syndactylism, syndactyly** Q70.9
  complex (with synostosis)
    fingers Q70.0- ☑
    toes Q70.2- ☑
  simple (without synostosis)
    fingers Q70.1- ☑
    toes Q70.3- ☑
**Syndrome** (*see also* Disease)
  48,XXXX Q97.1
  49,XXXXX Q97.1
  5q minus NOS D46.C (*following* D46.2)
  abdominal
    acute R10.0
    muscle deficiency Q79.4
  abnormal innervation H02.519
    left H02.516
      lower H02.515

☑ **Additional Character Required** — **Refer to the Tabular List for Character Selection**     ▽ **Subterms under main terms may continue to next column or page**

**Syndrome** — *continued*
  abnormal innervation — *continued*
    left — *continued*
      upper H02.514
    right H02.513
      lower H02.512
      upper H02.511
  abstinence, neonatal P96.1
  acid pulmonary aspiration, obstetric O74.0
  acquired immunodeficiency — *see* Human, immunod-
    eficiency virus (HIV) disease
  acute abdominal R10.0
  acute respiratory distress (adult) (child) J80
    idiopathic J84.114
  Adair-Dighton Q78.0
  Adams-Stokes (-Morgagni) I45.9
  adiposogenital E23.6
  adrenal
    hemorrhage (meningococcal) A39.1
    meningococcic A39.1
  adrenocortical — *see* Cushing's, syndrome
  adrenogenital E25.9
    congenital, associated with enzyme deficiency
      E25.0
  afferent loop NEC K91.89
  Alagille's Q44.7
  alcohol withdrawal (without convulsions) — *see* De-
    pendence, alcohol, with, withdrawal
  Alder's D72.0
  Aldrich (-Wiskott) D82.0
  alien hand R41.4
  Alport Q87.81
  alveolar hypoventilation E66.2
  alveolocapillary block J84.10
  amnesic, amnestic (confabulatory) (due to) — *see*
    Disorder, amnesic
  amyostatic (Wilson's disease) E83.01
  androgen insensitivity E34.50
    complete E34.51
    partial E34.52
  androgen resistance (*see also* Syndrome, androgen
    insensitivity) E34.50
  Angelman Q93.5
  anginal — *see* Angina
  ankyloglossia superior Q38.1
  anterior
    chest wall R07.89
    cord G83.82
    spinal artery G95.19
      compression M47.019
        cervical region M47.012
        cervicothoracic region M47.013
        lumbar region M47.016
        occipito-atlanto-axial region M47.011
        thoracic region M47.014
        thoracolumbar region M47.015
    tibial M76.81- ☑
  antibody deficiency D80.9
    agammaglobulinemic D80.1
      hereditary D80.0
    congenital D80.0
    hypogammaglobulinemic D80.1
      hereditary D80.0
  anticardiolipin (-antibody) D68.61
  antidepressant discontinuation T43.205 ☑
  antiphospholipid (-antibody) D68.61
  aortic
    arch M31.4
    bifurcation I74.09
  aortomesenteric duodenum occlusion K31.5
  apical ballooning (transient left ventricular) I51.81
  arcuate ligament I77.4
  argentaffin, argintaffinoma E34.0
  Arnold-Chiari — *see* Arnold-Chiari disease
  Arrillaga-Ayerza I27.0
  arterial tortuosity Q87.82
  arteriovenous steal T82.898- ☑
  Asherman's N85.6
  aspiration, of newborn — *see* Aspiration, by substance,
    with pneumonia
    meconium P24.01
  ataxia-telangiectasia G11.3
  auriculotemporal G50.8
  autoerythrocyte sensitization (Gardner-Diamond)
    D69.2
  autoimmune lymphoproliferative [ALPS] D89.82
  autoimmune polyglandular E31.0
  autoinflammatory M04.9

**Syndrome** — *continued*
  autoinflammatory — *continued*
    specified type NEC M04.8
  autosomal — *see* Abnormal, autosomes
  Avellis' G46.8
  Ayerza (-Arrillaga) I27.0
  Babinski-Nageotte G83.89
  Bakwin-Krida Q78.5
  bare lymphocyte D81.6
  Barré-Guillain G61.0
  Barré-Liéou M53.0
  Barrett's — *see* Barrett's, esophagus
  Barsony-Polgar K22.4
  Bársony-Teschendorf K22.4
  Barth E78.71
  Bartter's E26.81
  basal cell nevus Q87.89
  Basedow's E05.00
    with thyroid storm E05.01
  basilar artery G45.0
  Batten-Steinert G71.11
  battered
    baby or child — *see* Maltreatment, child, physical
      abuse
    spouse — *see* Maltreatment, adult, physical abuse
  Beals Q87.40
  Beau's I51.5
  Beck's I65.8
  Benedikt's G46.3
  Béquez César (-Steinbrinck-Chédiak-Higashi) E70.330
  Bernhardt-Roth — *see* Meralgia paresthetica
  Bernheim's — *see* Failure, heart, right
  big spleen D73.1
  Bing-Horton's — *see* Horton's headache
  Birt-Hogg-Dube syndrome Q87.89
  Björck (-Thorsen) E34.0
  black
    lung J60
    widow spider bite — *see* Toxicity, venom, spider,
      black widow
  Blackfan-Diamond D61.01
  Blau M04.8
  blind loop K90.2
    congenital Q43.8
    postsurgical K91.2
  blue sclera Q78.0
  blue toe I75.02- ☑
  Boder-Sedgewick G11.3
  Boerhaave's K22.3
  Borjeson Forssman Lehmann Q89.8
  Bouillaud's I01.9
  Bourneville (-Pringle) Q85.1
  Bouveret (-Hoffman) I47.9
  brachial plexus G54.0
  bradycardia-tachycardia I49.5
  brain (nonpsychotic) F09
    with psychosis, psychotic reaction F09
    acute or subacute — *see* Delirium
    congenital — *see* Disability, intellectual
    organic F09
      post-traumatic (nonpsychotic) F07.81
        psychotic F09
      personality change F07.0
    postcontusional F07.81
    post-traumatic, nonpsychotic F07.81
    psycho-organic F09
    psychotic F06.8
  brain stem stroke G46.3
  Brandt's (acrodermatitis enteropathica) E83.2
  broad ligament laceration N83.8
  Brock's J98.11
  bronze baby P83.88
  Brown-Sequard G83.81
  Brugada I49.8
  bubbly lung P27.0
  Buchem's M85.2
  Budd-Chiari I82.0
  bulbar (progressive) G12.22
  Bürger-Grütz E78.3
  Burke's K86.89
  Burnett's (milk-alkali) E83.52
  burning feet E53.9
  Bywaters' T79.5 ☑
  Call-Fleming I67.841
  carbohydrate-deficient glycoprotein (CDGS) E77.8
  carcinogenic thrombophlebitis I82.1
  carcinoid E34.0

**Syndrome** — *continued*
  cardiac asthma I50.1
  cardiacos negros I27.0
  cardiofaciocutaneous Q87.89
  cardiopulmonary-obesity E66.2
  cardiorenal — *see* Hypertension, cardiorenal
  cardiorespiratory distress (idiopathic), newborn P22.0
  cardiovascular renal — *see* Hypertension, cardiorenal
  carotid
    artery (hemispheric) (internal) G45.1
    body G90.01
    sinus G90.01
  carpal tunnel G56.0- ☑
  Cassidy (-Scholte) E34.0
  cat cry Q93.4
  cat eye Q92.8
  cauda equina G83.4
  causalgia — *see* Causalgia
  celiac K90.0
    artery compression I77.4
    axis I77.4
  central pain G89.0
  cerebellar
    hereditary G11.9
    stroke G46.4
  cerebellomedullary malformation — *see* Spina bifida
  cerebral
    artery
      anterior G46.1
      middle G46.0
      posterior G46.2
    gigantism E22.0
  cervical (root) M53.1
    disc — *see* Disorder, disc, cervical, with neuritis
    fusion Q76.1
    posterior, sympathicus M53.0
    rib Q76.5
    sympathetic paralysis G90.2
  cervicobrachial (diffuse) M53.1
  cervicocranial M53.0
  cervicodorsal outlet G54.2
  cervicothoracic outlet G54.0
  Céstan (-Raymond) I65.8
  Charcot's (angina cruris) (intermittent claudication)
    I73.9
  Charcot-Weiss-Baker G90.09
  CHARGE Q89.8
  Chédiak-Higashi (-Steinbrinck) E70.330
  chest wall R07.1
  Chiari's (hepatic vein thrombosis) I82.0
  Chilaiditi's Q43.3
  child maltreatment — *see* Maltreatment, child
  chondrocostal junction M94.0
  chondroectodermal dysplasia Q77.6
  chromosome 4 short arm deletion Q93.3
  chromosome 5 short arm deletion Q93.4
  chronic
    infantile neurological, cutaneous and articular
      (CINCA) M04.2
    pain G89.4
    personality F68.8
  Clarke-Hadfield K86.89
  Clerambault's automatism G93.89
  Clouston's (hidrotic ectodermal dysplasia) Q82.4
  clumsiness, clumsy child F82
  cluster headache G44.009
    intractable G44.001
    not intractable G44.009
  Coffin-Lowry Q89.8
  cold injury (newborn) P80.0
  combined immunity deficiency D81.9
  compartment (deep) (posterior) (traumatic) T79.A0 ☑
    (*following* T79.7)
    abdomen T79.A3 ☑ (*following* T79.7)
    lower extremity (hip, buttock, thigh, leg, foot, toes)
      T79.A2 ☑ (*following* T79.7)
    nontraumatic
      abdomen M79.A3 (*following* M79.7)
      lower extremity (hip, buttock, thigh, leg, foot,
        toes) M79.A2- ☑ (*following* M79.7)
      specified site NEC M79.A9 (*following* M79.7)
      upper extremity (shoulder, arm, forearm, wrist,
        hand, fingers) M79.A1- ☑ (*following*
        M79.7)
    postprocedural — *see* Syndrome, compartment,
      nontraumatic
    specified site NEC T79.A9 ☑ (*following* T79.7)

**Syndrome** — *continued*
  compartment — *continued*
    upper extremity (shoulder, arm, forearm, wrist, hand, fingers) T79.A1 ☑ (*following* T79.7)
  complex regional pain — *see* Syndrome, pain, complex regional
  compression T79.5 ☑
    anterior spinal — *see* Syndrome, anterior, spinal artery, compression
    cauda equina G83.4
    celiac artery I77.4
    vertebral artery M47.029
      cervical region M47.022
      occipito-atlanto-axial region M47.021
  concussion F07.81
  congenital
    affecting multiple systems NEC Q87.89
    central alveolar hypoventilation G47.35
    facial diplegia Q87.0
    muscular hypertrophy-cerebral Q87.89
    oculo-auriculovertebral Q87.0
    oculofacial diplegia (Moebius) Q87.0
    rubella (manifest) P35.0
  congestion-fibrosis (pelvic), female N94.89
  congestive dysmenorrhea N94.6
  connective tissue M35.9
    overlap NEC M35.1
  Conn's E26.01
  conus medullaris G95.81
  cord
    anterior G83.82
    posterior G83.83
  coronary
    acute NEC I24.9
    insufficiency or intermediate I20.0
    slow flow I20.8
  Costen's (complex) M26.69
  costochondral junction M94.0
  costoclavicular G54.0
  costovertebral E22.0
  Cowden Q85.8
  craniovertebral M53.0
  Creutzfeldt-Jakob — *see* Creutzfeldt-Jakob disease or syndrome
  crib death R99
  cricopharyngeal — *see* Dysphagia
  cri-du-chat Q93.4
  croup J05.0
  CRPS I — *see* Syndrome, pain, complex regional I
  crush T79.5 ☑
  cryopyrin-associated perodic M04.2
  cryptophthalmos Q87.0
  cubital tunnel — *see* Lesion, nerve, ulnar
  Curschmann (-Batten) (-Steinert) G71.11
  Cushing's E24.9
    alcohol-induced E24.4
    drug-induced E24.2
    due to
      alcohol
      drugs E24.2
      ectopic ACTH E24.3
      overproduction of pituitary ACTH E24.0
    overdose or wrong substance given or taken — *see* Table of Drugs and Chemicals, by drug, poisoning
    pituitary-dependent E24.0
    specified type NEC E24.8
  cystic duct stump K91.5
  Dana-Putnam D51.0
  Danbolt (-Cross) (acrodermatitis enteropathica) E83.2
  Dandy-Walker Q03.1
    with spina bifida Q07.01
  Danlos' Q79.6
  De Quervain E34.51
  de Toni-Fanconi (-Debré) E72.09
    with cystinosis E72.04
  defibrination (*see also* Fibrinolysis)
    with
      antepartum hemorrhage — *see* Hemorrhage, antepartum, with coagulation defect
      intrapartum hemorrhage — *see* Hemorrhage, complicating, delivery
    newborn P60
    postpartum O72.3
  Degos' I77.89
  Déjérine-Roussy G89.0
  delayed sleep phase G47.21
  demyelinating G37.9

**Syndrome** — *continued*
  dependence — *see* F10-F19 with fourth character .2
  depersonalization (-derealization) F48.1
  di George's D82.1
  diabetes mellitus in newborn infant P70.2
  diabetes mellitus-hypertension-nephrosis — *see* Diabetes, nephrosis
  diabetes-nephrosis — *see* Diabetes, nephrosis
  diabetic amyotrophy — *see* Diabetes, amyotrophy
  dialysis associated steal T82.898- ☑
  Diamond-Blackfan D61.01
  Diamond-Gardner D69.2
  DIC (diffuse or disseminated intravascular coagulopathy) D65
  Dighton's Q78.0
  disequilibrium E87.8
  Döhle body-panmyelopathic D72.0
  dorsolateral medullary G46.4
  double athetosis G80.3
  Down (*see also* Down syndrome) Q90.9
  Dresbach's (elliptocytosis) D58.1
  Dressler's (postmyocardial infarction) I24.1
    postcardiotomy I24.1
  drug withdrawal, infant of dependent mother P96.1
  dry eye H04.12- ☑
  due to abnormality
    chromosomal Q99.9
      sex
        female phenotype Q97.9
        male phenotype Q98.9
        specified NEC Q99.8
  dumping (postgastrectomy) K91.1
    nonsurgical K31.89
  Dupré's (meningism) R29.1
  dysmetabolic X E88.81
  dyspraxia, developmental F82
  Eagle-Barrett Q79.4
  Eaton-Lambert — *see* Syndrome, Lambert-Eaton
  Ebstein's Q22.5
  ectopic ACTH E24.3
  eczema-thrombocytopenia D82.0
  Eddowes' Q78.8
  effort (psychogenic) F45.8
  Ehlers-Danlos Q79.6
  Eisenmenger's I27.83
  Ekman's Q78.8
  electric feet E53.8
  Ellis-van Creveld Q77.6
  empty nest Z60.0
  endocrine-hypertensive E27.0
  entrapment — *see* Neuropathy, entrapment
  eosinophilia-myalgia M35.8
  epileptic (*see also* Epilepsy, by type)
    absence G40.A09 (*following* G40.3)
      intractable G40.A19 (*following* G40.3)
        with status epilepticus G40.A11 (*following* G40.3)
        without status epilepticus G40.A19 (*following* G40.3)
      not intractable G40.A09 (*following* G40.3)
        with status epilepticus G40.A01 (*following* G40.3)
        without status epilepticus G40.A09 (*following* G40.3)
  Erdheim-Chester (ECD) E88.89
  Erdheim's E22.0
  erythrocyte fragmentation D59.4
  Evans D69.41
  exhaustion F48.8
  extrapyramidal G25.9
    specified NEC G25.89
  eye retraction — *see* Strabismus
  eyelid-malar-mandible Q87.0
  Faber's D50.9
  facial pain, paroxysmal G50.0
  Fallot's Q21.3
  familial cold autoinflammatory M04.2
  familial eczema-thrombocytopenia (Wiskott-Aldrich) D82.0
  Fanconi (-de Toni) (-Debré) E72.09
    with cystinosis E72.04
  Fanconi's (anemia) (congenital pancytopenia) D61.09
  fatigue
    chronic R53.82
    psychogenic F48.8
  faulty bowel habit K59.39
  Feil-Klippel (brevicollis) Q76.1
  Felty's — *see* Felty's syndrome

**Syndrome** — *continued*
  fertile eunuch E23.0
  fetal
    alcohol (dysmorphic) Q86.0
    hydantoin Q86.1
  Fiedler's I40.1
  first arch Q87.0
  fish odor E72.8
  Fisher's G61.0
  Fitzhugh-Curtis
    due to
      Chlamydia trachomatis A74.81
      Neisseria gonorrhorea (gonococcal peritonitis) A54.85
  Fitz's (*see also* Pancreatitis, acute) K85.80
  Flajani (-Basedow) E05.00
    with thyroid storm E05.01
  flatback — *see* Flatback syndrome
  floppy
    baby P94.2
    iris (intraoeprative) (IFIS) H21.81
    mitral valve I34.1
  flush E34.0
  Foix-Alajouanine G95.19
  Fong's Q87.2
  food protein-induced enterocolitis K52.21
  foramen magnum G93.5
  Foster-Kennedy H47.14- ☑
  Foville's (peduncular) G46.3
  fragile X Q99.2
  Franceschetti Q75.4
  Frey's
    auriculotemporal G50.8
    hyperhidrosis L74.52
  Friderichsen-Waterhouse A39.1
  Froin's G95.89
  frontal lobe F07.0
  Fukuhara E88.49
  functional
    bowel K59.9
    prepubertal castrate E29.1
  Gaisböck's D75.1
  ganglion (basal ganglia brain) G25.9
    geniculi G51.1
  Gardner-Diamond D69.2
  gastroesophageal
    junction K22.0
    laceration-hemorrhage K22.6
  gastrojejunal loop obstruction K91.89
  Gee-Herter-Heubner K90.0
  Gelineau's G47.419
    with cataplexy G47.411
  genito-anorectal A55
  Gerstmann-Sträussler-Scheinker (GSS) A81.82
  Gianotti-Crosti L44.4
  giant platelet (Bernard-Soulier) D69.1
  Gilles de la Tourette's F95.2
  goiter-deafness E07.1
  Goldberg Q89.8
  Goldberg-Maxwell E34.51
  Good's D83.8
  Gopalan' (burning feet) E53.8
  Gorlin's Q87.89
  Gougerot-Blum L81.7
  Gouley's I31.1
  Gower's R55
  gray or grey (newborn) P93.0
    platelet D69.1
  Gubler-Millard G46.3
  Guillain-Barré (-Strohl) G61.0
  gustatory sweating G50.8
  Hadfield-Clarke K86.89
  hair tourniquet — *see* Constriction, external, by site
  Hamman's J98.19
  hand-foot L27.1
  hand-shoulder G90.8
  hantavirus (cardio)-pulmonary (HPS) (HCPS) B33.4
  happy puppet Q93.5
  Harada's H30.81- ☑
  Hayem-Faber D50.9
  headache NEC G44.89
    complicated NEC G44.59
  Heberden's I20.8
  Hedinger's E34.0
  Hegglin's D72.0
  HELLP (hemolysis, elevated liver enzymes and low platelet count) O14.2- ☑
    complicating
      childbirth O14.24

☑ **Additional Character Required** — **Refer to the Tabular List for Character Selection**     ▽ **Subterms under main terms may continue to next column or page**

**Syndrome** — *continued*
  HELLP — *continued*
    complicating — *continued*
      puerperium O14.25
  hemolytic-uremic D59.3
  hemophagocytic, infection-associated D76.2
  Henoch-Schönlein D69.0
  hepatic flexure K59.8
  hepatopulmonary K76.81
  hepatorenal K76.7
    following delivery O90.4
    postoperative or postprocedural K91.83
    postpartum, puerperal O90.4
  hepatourologic K76.7
  Herter (-Gee) (nontropical sprue) K90.0
  Heubner-Herter K90.0
  Heyd's K76.7
  Hilger's G90.09
  histamine-like (fish poisoning) — *see* Poisoning, fish
  histiocytic D76.3
  histiocytosis NEC D76.3
  HIV infection, acute B20
  Hoffmann-Werdnig G12.0
  Hollander-Simons E88.1
  Hoppe-Goldflam G70.00
    with exacerbation (acute) G70.01
    in crisis G70.01
  Horner's G90.2
  hungry bone E83.81
  hunterian glossitis D51.0
  Hutchinson's triad A50.53
  hyperabduction G54.0
  hyperammonemia-hyperornithinemia-homocitrulline-
    mia E72.4
  hypereosinophilic (idiopathic) D72.1
  hyperimmunoglobulin D M04.1
  hyperimmunoglobulin E (IgE) D82.4
  hyperkalemic E87.5
  hyperkinetic — *see* Hyperkinesia
  hypermobility M35.7
  hypernatremia E87.0
  hyperosmolarity E87.0
  hyperperfusion G97.82
  hypersplenic D73.1
  hypertransfusion, newborn P61.1
  hyperventilation F45.8
  hyperviscosity (of serum)
    polycythemic D75.1
    sclerothymic D58.8
  hypoglycemic (familial) (neonatal) E16.2
  hypokalemic E87.6
  hyponatremic E87.1
  hypopituitarism E23.0
  hypoplastic left-heart Q23.4
  hypopotassemia E87.6
  hyposmolality E87.1
  hypotension, maternal O26.5- ☑
  hypothenar hammer I73.89
  hypoventilation, obesity (OHS) E66.2
  ICF (intravascular coagulation-fibrinolysis) D65
  idiopathic
    cardiorespiratory distress, newborn P22.0
    nephrotic (infantile) N04.9
  iliotibial band M76.3- ☑
  immobility, immobilization (paraplegic) M62.3
  immune reconstitution D89.3
  immune reconstitution inflammatory [IRIS] D89.3
  immunity deficiency, combined D81.9
  immunodeficiency
    acquired — *see* Human, immunodeficiency virus
      (HIV) disease
    combined D81.9
  impending coronary I20.0
  impingement, shoulder M75.4- ☑
  inappropriate secretion of antidiuretic hormone E22.2
  infant
    gestational diabetes P70.0
    of diabetic mother P70.1
  infantilism (pituitary) E23.0
  inferior vena cava I87.1
  inspissated bile (newborn) P59.1
  institutional (childhood) F94.2
  insufficient sleep F51.12
  intermediate coronary (artery) I20.0
  interspinous ligament — *see* Spondylopathy, specified
    NEC
  intestinal
    carcinoid E34.0

**Syndrome** — *continued*
  intestinal — *continued*
    knot K56.2
  intravascular coagulation-fibrinolysis (ICF) D65
  iodine-deficiency, congenital E00.9
    type
      mixed E00.2
      myxedematous E00.1
      neurological E00.0
  IRDS (idiopathic respiratory distress, newborn) P22.0
  irritable
    bowel K58.9
      with
        constipation K58.1
        diarrhea K58.0
      mixed K58.2
      psychogenic F45.8
      specified NEC K58.8
    heart (psychogenic) F45.8
    weakness F48.8
  ischemic
    bowel (transient) K55.9
      chronic K55.1
      due to mesenteric artery insufficiency K55.1
    steal T82.898 ☑
  IVC (intravascular coagulopathy) D65
  Ivemark's Q89.01
  Jaccoud's — *see* Arthropathy, postrheumatic, chronic
  Jackson's G83.89
  Jakob-Creutzfeldt — *see* Creutzfeldt-Jakob disease or
    syndrome
  jaw-winking Q07.8
  Jervell-Lange-Nielsen I45.81
  jet lag G47.25
  Job's D71
  Joseph-Diamond-Blackfan D61.01
  jugular foramen G52.7
  Kabuki Q89.8
  Kanner's (autism) F84.0
  Kartagener's Q89.3
  Kelly's D50.1
  Kimmelstiel-Wilson — *see* Diabetes, specified type,
    with Kimmelstiel-Wilson disease
  Klein (e)-Levine G47.13
  Klippel-Feil (brevicollis) Q76.1
  Köhler-Pellegrini-Steida — *see* Bursitis, tibial collateral
  König's K59.8
  Korsakoff (-Wernicke) (nonalcoholic) F04
    alcoholic F10.26
  Kostmann's D70.0
  Krabbe's congenital muscle hypoplasia Q79.8
  labyrinthine — *see* subcategory H83.2 ☑
  lacunar NEC G46.7
  Lambert-Eaton G70.80
    in
      neoplastic disease G73.1
      specified disease NEC G70.81
  Landau-Kleffner — *see* Epilepsy, specified NEC
  Larsen's Q74.8
  lateral
    cutaneous nerve of thigh G57.1- ☑
    medullary G46.4
  Launois' E22.0
  lazy
    leukocyte D70.8
    posture M62.3
  Lemiere I80.8
  Lennox-Gastaut G40.812
    intractable G40.814
      with status epilepticus G40.813
      without status epilepticus G40.814
    not intractable G40.812
      with status epilepticus G40.811
      without status epilepticus G40.812
  lenticular, progressive E83.01
  Leopold-Levi's E05.90
  Lev's I44.2
  Lichtheim's D51.0
  Li-Fraumeni Z15.01
  Lightwood's N25.89
  Lignac (de Toni) (-Fanconi) (-Debré) E72.09
    with cystinosis E72.04
  Likoff's I20.8
  limbic epilepsy personality F07.0
  liver-kidney K76.7
  lobotomy F07.0
  long arm 18 or 21 deletion Q93.89

**Syndrome** — *continued*
  long QT I45.81
  Louis-Barré G11.3
  low
    atmospheric pressure T70.29 ☑
    back M54.5
    output (cardiac) I50.9
  lower radicular, newborn (birth injury) P14.8
  Luetscher's (dehydration) E86.0
  Lupus anticoagulant D68.62
  Lutembacher's Q21.1
  macrophage activation D76.1
    due to infection D76.2
  magnesium-deficiency R29.0
  Majeed M04.8
  Mal de Debarquement R42
  malabsorption K90.9
    postsurgical K91.2
  malformation, congenital, due to
    alcohol Q86.0
    exogenous cause NEC Q86.8
    hydantoin Q86.1
    warfarin Q86.2
  malignant
    carcinoid E34.0
    neuroleptic G21.0
  Mallory-Weiss K22.6
  mandibulofacial dysostosis Q75.4
  manic-depressive — *see* Disorder, bipolar
  maple-syrup-urine E71.0
  Marable's I77.4
  Marfan's Q87.40
    with
      cardiovascular manifestations Q87.418
        aortic dilation Q87.410
      ocular manifestations Q87.42
      skeletal manifestations Q87.43
  Marie's (acromegaly) E22.0
  mast cell activation — *see* Activation, mast cell
  maternal hypotension — *see* Syndrome, hypotension,
    maternal
  May (-Hegglin) D72.0
  McArdle (-Schmidt) (-Pearson) E74.04
  McQuarrie's E16.2
  meconium plug (newborn) P76.0
  median arcuate ligament I77.4
  Meekeren-Ehlers-Danlos Q79.6
  megavitamin-B6 E67.2
  Meige G24.4
  MELAS E88.41
  Mendelson's O74.0
  MERRF (myoclonic epilepsy associated with ragged-
    red fibers) E88.42
  mesenteric
    artery (superior) K55.1
    vascular insufficiency K55.1
  metabolic E88.81
  metastatic carcinoid E34.0
  micrognathia-glossoptosis Q87.0
  midbrain NEC G93.89
  middle lobe (lung) J98.19
  middle radicular G54.0
  migraine (*see also* Migraine) G43.909
  Mikulicz' K11.8
  milk-alkali E83.52
  Millard-Gubler G46.3
  Miller-Dieker Q93.88
  Miller-Fisher G61.0
  Minkowski-Chauffard D58.0
  Mirizzi's K83.1
  MNGIE (Mitochondrial Neurogastrointestinal En-
    cephalopathy) E88.49
  Möbius, ophthalmoplegic migraine — *see* Migraine,
    ophthalmoplegic
  monofixation H50.42
  Morel-Moore M85.2
  Morel-Morgagni M85.2
  Morgagni (-Morel) (-Stewart) M85.2
  Morgagni-Adams-Stokes I45.9
  Mounier-Kuhn Q32.4
    with bronchiectasis J47.9
      with
        exacerbation (acute) J47.1
        lower respiratory infection J47.0
    acquired J98.09
      with bronchiectasis J47.9
        with
          exacerbation (acute) J47.1
          lower respiratory infection J47.0

**Syndrome** — *continued*
    Muckle-Wells M04.2
    mucocutaneous lymph node (acute febrile) (MCLS)
        M30.3
    multiple endocrine neoplasia (MEN) — *see* Neoplasia,
        endocrine, multiple (MEN)
    multiple operations — *see* Disorder, factitious
    myasthenic G70.9
        in
            diabetes mellitus — *see* Diabetes, amyotrophy
            endocrine disease NEC E34.9 [G73.3]
            neoplastic disease (*see also* Neoplasm)
                D49.9 [G73.3]
            thyrotoxicosis (hyperthyroidism) E05.90 [G73.3]
                with thyroid storm E05.91 [G73.3]
    myelodysplastic D46.9
        with
            5q deletion D46.C (*following* D46.2)
            isolated del (5q) chromosomal abnormality
                D46.C (*following* D46.2)
        lesions, low grade D46.20
        specified NEC D46.Z (*following* D46.4)
    myelopathic pain G89.0
    myeloproliferative (chronic) D47.1
    myofascial pain M79.1
    Naffziger's G54.0
    nail patella Q87.2
    NARP (Neuropathy, Ataxia and Retinitis pigmentosa)
        E88.49
    neonatal abstinence P96.1
    nephritic (*see also* Nephritis)
        with edema — *see* Nephrosis
        acute N00.9
        chronic N03.9
        rapidly progressive N01.9
    nephrotic (congenital) (*see also* Nephrosis) N04.9
        with
            dense deposit disease N04.6
            diffuse
                crescentic glomerulonephritis N04.7
                endocapillary proliferative glomerulonephri-
                    tis N04.4
                membranous glomerulonephritis N04.2
                mesangial proliferative glomerulonephritis
                    N04.3
                mesangiocapillary glomerulonephritis N04.5
            focal and segmental glomerular lesions N04.1
            minor glomerular abnormality N04.0
            specified morphological changes NEC N04.8
        diabetic — *see* Diabetes, nephrosis
    neurologic neglect R41.4
    Nezelof's D81.4
    Nonne-Milroy-Meige Q82.0
    Nothnagel's vasomotor acroparesthesia I73.89
    obesity hypoventilation (OHS) E66.2
    oculomotor H51.9
    ophthalmoplegia-cerebellar ataxia — *see* Strabismus,
        paralytic, third nerve
    oral allergy T78.1 ☑
    oral-facial-digital Q87.0
    organic
        affective F06.30
        amnesic (not alcohol- or drug-induced) F04
        brain F09
        depressive F06.31
        hallucinosis F06.0
        personality F07.0
    Ormond's N13.5
    oro-facial-digital Q87.0
    os trigonum Q68.8
    Osler-Weber-Rendu I78.0
    osteoporosis-osteomalacia M83.8
    Osterreicher-Turner Q87.2
    otolith — *see* subcategory H81.8 ☑
    oto-palatal-digital Q87.0
    outlet (thoracic) G54.0
    ovary
        polycystic E28.2
        resistant E28.39
        sclerocystic E28.2
    Owren's D68.2
    Paget-Schroetter I82.890
    pain (*see also* Pain)
        complex regional I G90.50
            lower limb G90.52- ☑
            specified site NEC G90.59
            upper limb G90.51- ☑
        complex regional II — *see* Causalgia

**Syndrome** — *continued*
    painful
        bruising D69.2
        feet E53.8
        prostate N42.81
    paralysis agitans — *see* Parkinsonism
    paralytic G83.9
        specified NEC G83.89
    Parinaud's H51.0
    parkinsonian — *see* Parkinsonism
    Parkinson's — *see* Parkinsonism
    paroxysmal facial pain G50.0
    Parry's E05.00
        with thyroid storm E05.01
    Parsonage (-Aldren)-Turner G54.5
    patella clunk M25.86- ☑
    Paterson (-Brown) (-Kelly) D50.1
    pectoral girdle I77.89
    pectoralis minor I77.89
    pediatric autoimmune neuropsychiatric disorders as-
        sociated with streptococcal infections (PANDAS)
        D89.89
    Pelger-Huet D72.0
    pellagra-cerebellar ataxia-renal aminoaciduria E72.02
    pellagroid E52
    Pellegrini-Stieda — *see* Bursitis, tibial collateral
    pelvic congestion-fibrosis, female N94.89
    penta X Q97.1
    peptic ulcer — *see* Ulcer, peptic
    perabduction I77.89
    periodic fever M04.1
    periodic fever, aphthous stomatitis, pharyngitis, and
        adenopathy [PFAPA] M04.8
    periodic headache, in adults and children — *see*
        Headache, periodic syndromes in adults and
        children
    periurethral fibrosis N13.5
    phantom limb (without pain) G54.7
        with pain G54.6
    pharyngeal pouch D82.1
    Pick's — *see* Disease, Pick's
    Pickwickian E66.2
    PIE (pulmonary infiltration with eosinophilia) J82
    pigmentary pallidal degeneration (progressive) G23.0
    pineal E34.8
    pituitary E22.0
    placental transfusion — *see* Pregnancy, complicated
        by, placental transfusion syndromes
    plantar fascia M72.2
    plateau iris (post-iridectomy) (postprocedural) H21.82
    Plummer-Vinson D50.1
    pluricarential of infancy E40
    plurideficiency E40
    pluriglandular (compensatory) E31.8
        autoimmune E31.0
    pneumatic hammer T75.21 ☑
    polyangiitis overlap M30.8
    polycarential of infancy E40
    polyglandular E31.8
        autoimmune E31.0
    polysplenia Q89.09
    pontine NEC G93.89
    popliteal
        artery entrapment I77.89
        web Q87.89
    post chemoembolization — *code to* associated condi-
        tions
    postcardiac injury
        postcardiotomy I97.0
        postmyocardial infarction I24.1
    postcardiotomy I97.0
    postcholecystectomy K91.5
    postcommissurotomy I97.0
    postconcussional F07.81
    postcontusional F07.81
    postencephalitic F07.89
    posterior
        cervical sympathetic M53.0
        cord G83.83
        fossa compression G93.5
        reversible encephalopathy (PRES) I67.83
    postgastrectomy (dumping) K91.1
    postgastric surgery K91.1
    postinfarction I24.1
    postlaminectomy NEC M96.1
    postleukotomy F07.0
    postmastectomy lymphedema I97.2
    postmyocardial infarction I24.1

**Syndrome** — *continued*
    postoperative NEC T81.9 ☑
        blind loop K90.2
    postpartum panhypopituitary (Sheehan) E23.0
    postpolio (myelitic) G14
    postthrombotic I87.009
        with
            inflammation I87.02- ☑
                with ulcer I87.03- ☑
            specified complication NEC I87.09- ☑
            ulcer I87.01- ☑
                with inflammation I87.03- ☑
        asymptomatic I87.00- ☑
    postvagotomy K91.1
    postvalvulotomy I97.0
    postviral NEC G93.3
        fatigue G93.3
    Potain's K31.0
    potassium intoxication E87.5
    precerebral artery (multiple) (bilateral) G45.2
    preinfarction I20.0
    preleukemic D46.9
    premature senility E34.8
    premenstrual dysphoric F32.89
    premenstrual tension N94.3
    Prinzmetal-Massumi R07.1
    prune belly Q79.4
    pseudo -Turner's Q87.1
    pseudocarpal tunnel (sublimis) — *see* Syndrome,
        carpal tunnel
    pseudoparalytica G70.00
        with exacerbation (acute) G70.01
        in crisis G70.01
    psycho-organic (nonpsychotic severity) F07.9
        acute or subacute F05
        depressive type F06.31
        hallucinatory type F06.0
        nonpsychotic severity F07.0
        specified NEC F07.89
    pulmonary
        arteriosclerosis I27.0
        dysmaturity (Wilson-Mikity) P27.0
        hypoperfusion (idiopathic) P22.0
        renal (hemorrhagic) (Goodpasture's) M31.0
    pure
        motor lacunar G46.5
        sensory lacunar G46.6
    Putnam-Dana D51.0
    pyogenic arthritis, pyoderma gangrenosum, and acne
        [PAPA] M04.8
    pyramidopallidonigral G20
    pyriformis — *see* Lesion, nerve, sciatic
    QT interval prolongation I45.81
    radicular NEC — *see* Radiculopathy
        upper limbs, newborn (birth injury) P14.3
    rapid time-zone change G47.25
    Rasmussen G04.81
    Raymond (-Céstan) I65.8
    Raynaud's I73.00
        with gangrene I73.01
    RDS (respiratory distress syndrome, newborn) P22.0
    reactive airways dysfunction J68.3
    Refsum's G60.1
    Reifenstein E34.52
    renal glomerulohyalinosis-diabetic — *see* Diabetes,
        nephrosis
    Rendu-Osler-Weber I78.0
    residual ovary N99.83
    resistant ovary E28.39
    respiratory
        distress
            acute J80
                adult J80
                child J80
                idiopathic J84.114
            newborn (idiopathic) (type I) P22.0
                type II P22.1
    restless legs G25.81
    retinoblastoma (familial) C69.2 ☑
    retroperitoneal fibrosis N13.5
    retroviral seroconversion (acute) Z21
    Reye's G93.7
    Richter — *see* Leukemia, chronic lymphocytic, B-cell
        type
    Ridley's I50.1
    right
        heart, hypoplastic Q22.6

☑ **Additional Character Required — Refer to the Tabular List for Character Selection**      ▽ Subterms under main terms may continue to next column or page

**Syndrome** — continued
    right — continued
        ventricular obstruction — see Failure, heart, congestive
    Romano-Ward (prolonged QT interval) I45.81
    rotator cuff, shoulder (see also Tear, rotator cuff) M75.10-
    Rotes Quérol — see Hyperostosis, ankylosing
    Roth — see Meralgia paresthetica
    rubella (congenital) P35.0
    Ruvalcaba-Myhre-Smith E71.440
    Rytand-Lipsitch I44.2
    salt
        depletion E87.1
            due to heat NEC T67.8 ☑
                causing heat exhaustion or prostration T67.4 ☑
        low E87.1
    salt-losing N28.89
    Scaglietti-Dagnini E22.0
    scalenus anticus (anterior) G54.0
    scapulocostal — see Mononeuropathy, upper limb, specified site NEC
    scapuloperoneal G71.0
    schizophrenic, of childhood NEC F84.5
    Schnitzler D47.2
    Scholte's E34.0
    Schroeder's E27.0
    Schüller-Christian C96.5
    Schwachman's — see Syndrome, Shwachman's
    Schwartz (-Jampel) G71.13
    Schwartz-Bartter E22.2
    scimitar Q26.8
    sclerocystic ovary E28.2
    Seitelberger's G31.89
    septicemic adrenal hemorrhage A39.1
    seroconversion, retroviral (acute) Z21
    serous meningitis G93.2
    severe acute respiratory (SARS) J12.81
    shaken infant T74.4 ☑
    shock (traumatic) T79.4 ☑
        kidney N17.0
            following crush injury T79.5 ☑
        toxic A48.3
    shock-lung J80
    Shone's — code to specific anomalies
    short
        bowel K91.2
        rib Q77.2
    shoulder-hand — see Algoneurodystrophy
    Shwachman's D70.4
    sicca — see Sicca syndrome
    sick
        cell E87.1
        sinus I49.5
    sick-euthyroid E07.81
    sideropenic D50.1
    Siemens' ectodermal dysplasia Q82.4
    Silfversköld's Q78.9
    Simons' E88.1
    sinus tarsi M25.57- ☑
    sinusitis-bronchiectasis-situs inversus Q89.3
    Sipple's E31.22
    sirenomelia Q87.2
    Slocumb's E27.0
    slow flow, coronary I20.8
    Sluder's G44.89
    Smith-Magenis Q93.88
    Sneddon-Wilkinson L13.1
    Sotos' Q87.3
    South African cardiomyopathy I42.8
    spasmodic
        upward movement, eyes H51.8
        winking F95.8
    Spen's I45.9
    splenic
        agenesis Q89.01
        flexure K59.8
        neutropenia D73.81
    Spurway's Q78.0
    staphylococcal scalded skin L00
    steal
        arteriovenous T82.898- ☑
        ischemic T82.898- ☑
        subclavian G45.8
    Stein-Leventhal E28.2
    Stein's E28.2
    Stevens-Johnson syndrome L51.1

**Syndrome** — continued
    Stevens-Johnson syndrome — continued
        toxic epidermal necrolysis overlap L51.3
    Stewart-Morel M85.2
    Stickler Q89.8
    stiff baby Q89.8
    stiff man G25.82
    Still-Felty — see Felty's syndrome
    Stokes (-Adams) I45.9
    stone heart I50.1
    straight back, congenital Q76.49
    subclavian steal G45.8
    subcoracoid-pectoralis minor G54.0
    subcostal nerve compression I77.89
    subphrenic interposition Q43.3
    superior
        cerebellar artery I63.8
        mesenteric artery K55.1
        semi-circular canal dehiscence H83.8X- ☑
        vena cava I87.1
    supine hypotensive (maternal) — see Syndrome, hypotension, maternal
    suprarenal cortical E27.0
    supraspinatus (see also Tear, rotator cuff) M75.10- ☑
    Susac G93.49
    swallowed blood P78.2
    sweat retention L74.0
    Swyer Q99.1
    Symond's G93.2
    sympathetic
        cervical paralysis G90.2
        pelvic, female N94.89
    systemic inflammatory response (SIRS), of non-infectious origin (without organ dysfunction) R65.10
        with acute organ dysfunction R65.11
    tachycardia-bradycardia I49.5
    takotsubo I51.81
    TAR (thrombocytopenia with absent radius) Q87.2
    tarsal tunnel G57.5- ☑
    teething K00.7
    tegmental G93.89
    telangiectasic-pigmentation-cataract Q82.8
    temporal pyramidal apex — see Otitis, media, suppurative, acute
    temporomandibular joint-pain-dysfunction M26.62- ☑
    Terry's (see also Myopia, degenerative) H44.2- ☑
    testicular feminization (see also Syndrome, androgen insensitivity) E34.51
    thalamic pain (hyperesthetic) G89.0
    thoracic outlet (compression) G54.0
    Thorson-Björck E34.0
    thrombocytopenia with absent radius (TAR) Q87.2
    thyroid-adrenocortical insufficiency E31.0
    tibial
        anterior M76.81- ☑
        posterior M76.82- ☑
    Tietze's M94.0
    time-zone (rapid) G47.25
    Toni-Fanconi E72.09
        with cystinosis E72.04
    Touraine's Q79.8
    tourniquet — see Constriction, external, by site
    toxic shock A48.3
    transient left ventricular apical ballooning I51.81
    traumatic vasospastic T75.22 ☑
    Treacher Collins Q75.4
    triple X, female Q97.0
    trisomy Q92.9
        13 Q91.7
            meiotic nondisjunction Q91.4
            mitotic nondisjunction Q91.5
            mosaicism Q91.5
            translocation Q91.6
        18 Q91.3
            meiotic nondisjunction Q91.0
            mitotic nondisjunction Q91.1
            mosaicism Q91.1
            translocation Q91.2
        20 (q)(p) Q92.8
        21 Q90.9
            meiotic nondisjunction Q90.0
            mitotic nondisjunction Q90.1
            mosaicism Q90.1
            translocation Q90.2
        22 Q92.8
    tropical wet feet T69.0- ☑
    Trousseau's I82.1

**Syndrome** — continued
    tumor lysis (following antineoplastic chemotherapy) (spontaneous) NEC E88.3
    tumor necrosis factor receptor associated periodic (TRAPS) M04.1
    Twiddler's (due to)
        automatic implantable defibrillator T82.198 ☑
        cardiac pacemaker T82.198 ☑
    Unverricht (-Lundborg) — see Epilepsy, generalized, idiopathic
    upward gaze H51.8
    uremia, chronic (see also Disease, kidney, chronic) N18.9
    urethral N34.3
    urethro-oculo-articular — see Reiter's disease
    urohepatic K76.7
    vago-hypoglossal G52.7
    van Buchem's M85.2
    van der Hoeve's Q78.0
    vascular NEC in cerebrovascular disease G46.8
    vasoconstriction, reversible cerebrovascular I67.841
    vasomotor I73.9
    vasospastic (traumatic) T75.22 ☑
    vasovagal R55
    VATER Q87.2
    velo-cardio-facial Q93.81
    vena cava (inferior) (superior) (obstruction) I87.1
    vertebral
        artery G45.0
            compression — see Syndrome, anterior, spinal artery, compression
        steal G45.0
    vertebro-basilar artery G45.0
    vertebrogenic (pain) M54.89
    vertiginous — see Disorder, vestibular function
    Vinson-Plummer D50.1
    virus B34.9
    visceral larva migrans B83.0
    visual disorientation H53.8
    vitamin B6 deficiency E53.1
    vitreal corneal H59.01- ☑
    vitreous (touch) H59.01- ☑
    Vogt-Koyanagi H20.82- ☑
    Volkmann's T79.6 ☑
    von Schroetter's I82.890
    von Willebrand (-Jürgen) D68.0
    Waldenström-Kjellberg D50.1
    Wallenberg's G46.3
    water retention E87.79
    Waterhouse (-Friderichsen) A39.1
    Weber-Gubler G46.3
    Weber-Leyden G46.3
    Weber's G46.3
    Wegener's M31.30
        with
            kidney involvement M31.31
            lung involvement M31.30
                with kidney involvement M31.31
    Weingarten's (tropical eosinophilia) J82
    Weiss-Baker G90.09
    Werdnig-Hoffman G12.0
    Wermer's E31.21
    Werner's E34.8
    Wernicke-Korsakoff (nonalcoholic) F04
        alcoholic F10.26
    Westphal-Strümpell E83.01
    West's — see Epilepsy, spasms
    wet
        feet (maceration) (tropical) T69.0- ☑
        lung, newborn P22.1
    whiplash S13.4 ☑
    whistling face Q87.0
    Wilkie's K55.1
    Wilkinson-Sneddon L13.1
    Willebrand (-Jürgens) D68.0
    Wilson's (hepatolenticular degeneration) E83.01
    Wiskott-Aldrich D82.0
    withdrawal — see Withdrawal, state
        drug
            infant of dependent mother P96.1
                therapeutic use, newborn P96.2
    Woakes' (ethmoiditis) J33.1
    Wright's (hyperabduction) G54.0
    X I20.9
    XXXX Q97.1
    XXXXX Q97.1
    XXXXY Q98.1
    XXY Q98.0

**Syndrome** — *continued*
   yellow nail L60.5
   Zahorsky's B08.5
   Zellweger syndrome E71.510
   Zellweger-like syndrome E71.541
**Synechia** (anterior) (iris) (posterior) (pupil) (*see also* Adhesions, iris)
   intra-uterine (traumatic) N85.6
**Synesthesia** R20.8
**Syngamiasis, syngamosis** B83.3
**Synodontia** K00.2
**Synorchidism, synorchism** Q55.1
**Synostosis** (congenital) Q78.8
   astragalo-scaphoid Q74.2
   radioulnar Q74.0
**Synovial sarcoma** — *see* Neoplasm, connective tissue, malignant
**Synovioma** (malignant) (*see also* Neoplasm, connective tissue, malignant)
   benign — *see* Neoplasm, connective tissue, benign
**Synoviosarcoma** — *see* Neoplasm, connective tissue, malignant
**Synovitis** (*see also* Tenosynovitis) M65.9
   crepitant
     hand M70.0- ☑
     wrist M70.03- ☑
   gonococcal A54.49
   gouty — *see* Gout
   in (due to)
     crystals M65.8- ☑
     gonorrhea A54.49
     syphilis (late) A52.78
     use, overuse, pressure — *see* Disorder, soft tissue, due to use
   infective NEC — *see* Tenosynovitis, infective NEC
   specified NEC — *see* Tenosynovitis, specified type NEC
   syphilitic A52.78
     congenital (early) A50.02
   toxic — *see* Synovitis, transient
   transient M67.3- ☑
     ankle M67.37- ☑
     elbow M67.32- ☑
     foot joint M67.37- ☑
     hand joint M67.34- ☑
     hip M67.35- ☑
     knee M67.36- ☑
     multiple site M67.39
     pelvic region M67.35- ☑
     shoulder M67.31- ☑
     specified joint NEC M67.38
     wrist M67.33- ☑
   traumatic, current — *see* Sprain
   tuberculous — *see* Tuberculosis, synovitis
   villonodular (pigmented) M12.2- ☑
     ankle M12.27- ☑
     elbow M12.22- ☑
     foot joint M12.27- ☑
     hand joint M12.24- ☑
     hip M12.25- ☑
     knee M12.26- ☑
     multiple site M12.29
     pelvic region M12.25- ☑
     shoulder M12.21- ☑
     specified joint NEC M12.28
     vertebrae M12.28
     wrist M12.23- ☑
**Syphilid** A51.39
   congenital A50.06
   newborn A50.06
   tubercular (late) A52.79
**Syphilis, syphilitic** (acquired) A53.9
   abdomen (late) A52.79
   acoustic nerve A52.15
   adenopathy (secondary) A51.49
   adrenal (gland) (with cortical hypofunction) A52.79
   age under 2 years NOS (*see also* Syphilis, congenital, early)
     acquired A51.9
   alopecia (secondary) A51.32
   anemia (late) A52.79 [D63.8]
   aneurysm (aorta) (ruptured) A52.01
     central nervous system A52.05
     congenital A50.54 [I79.0]
   anus (late) A52.74
     primary A51.1
     secondary A51.39
   aorta (arch) (abdominal) (thoracic) A52.02

**Syphilis, syphilitic** — *continued*
   aorta — *continued*
     aneurysm A52.01
   aortic (insufficiency) (regurgitation) (stenosis) A52.03
     aneurysm A52.01
   arachnoid (adhesive) (cerebral) (spinal) A52.13
   asymptomatic — *see* Syphilis, latent
   ataxia (locomotor) A52.11
   atrophoderma maculatum A51.39
   auricular fibrillation A52.06
   bladder (late) A52.76
   bone A52.77
     secondary A51.46
   brain A52.17
   breast (late) A52.79
   bronchus (late) A52.72
   bubo (primary) A51.0
   bulbar palsy A52.19
   bursa (late) A52.78
   cardiac decompensation A52.06
   cardiovascular A52.00
   central nervous system (late) (recurrent) (relapse) (tertiary) A52.3
     with
       ataxia A52.11
       general paralysis A52.17
         juvenile A50.45
       paresis (general) A52.17
         juvenile A50.45
       tabes (dorsalis) A52.11
         juvenile A50.45
       taboparesis A52.17
         juvenile A50.45
     aneurysm A52.05
     congenital A50.40
     juvenile A50.40
     remission in (sustained) A52.3
     serology doubtful, negative, or positive A52.3
     specified nature or site NEC A52.19
     vascular A52.05
   cerebral A52.17
     meningovascular A52.13
     nerves (multiple palsies) A52.15
     sclerosis A52.17
     thrombosis A52.05
   cerebrospinal (tabetic type) A52.12
   cerebrovascular A52.05
   cervix (late) A52.76
   chancre (multiple) A51.0
     extragenital A51.2
     Rollet's A51.0
   Charcot's joint A52.16
   chorioretinitis A51.43
     congenital A50.01
     late A52.71
     prenatal A50.01
   choroiditis — *see* Syphilitic chorioretinitis
   choroidoretinitis — *see* Syphilitic chorioretinitis
   ciliary body (secondary) A51.43
     late A52.71
   colon (late) A52.74
   combined spinal sclerosis A52.11
   condyloma (latum) A51.31
   congenital A50.9
     with
       paresis (general) A50.45
       tabes (dorsalis) A50.45
       taboparesis A50.45
     early, or less than 2 years after birth NEC A50.2
       with manifestations — *see* Syphilis, congenital, early, symptomatic
       latent (without manifestations) A50.1
         negative spinal fluid test A50.1
         serology positive A50.1
       symptomatic A50.09
         cutaneous A50.06
         mucocutaneous A50.07
         oculopathy A50.01
         osteochondropathy A50.02
         pharyngitis A50.03
         pneumonia A50.04
         rhinitis A50.05
         visceral A50.08
     chorioretinitis, choroiditis A50.01 [H32]
     interstitial keratitis A50.31
     juvenile neurosyphilis A50.45
     late, or 2 years or more after birth NEC A50.7
       chorioretinitis, choroiditis A50.32
       interstitial keratitis A50.31

**Syphilis, syphilitic** — *continued*
   congenital — *continued*
     late, or 2 years or more after birth — *continued*
       juvenile neurosyphilis A50.45
       latent (without manifestations) A50.6
         negative spinal fluid test A50.6
         serology positive A50.6
       symptomatic or with manifestations NEC A50.59
         arthropathy A50.55
         cardiovascular A50.54
         Clutton's joints A50.51
         Hutchinson's teeth A50.52
         Hutchinson's triad A50.53
         osteochondropathy A50.56
         saddle nose A50.57
   conjugal A53.9
     tabes A52.11
   conjunctiva (late) A52.71
   contact Z20.2
   cord bladder A52.19
   cornea, late A52.71
   coronary (artery) (sclerosis) A52.06
   coryza, congenital A50.05
   cranial nerve A52.15
     multiple palsies A52.15
   cutaneous — *see* Syphilis, skin
   dacryocystitis (late) A52.71
   degeneration, spinal cord A52.12
   dementia paralytica A52.17
     juvenilis A50.45
   destruction of bone A52.77
   dilatation, aorta A52.01
   due to blood transfusion A53.9
   dura mater A52.13
   ear A52.79
     inner A52.79
       nerve (eighth) A52.15
       neurorecurrence A52.15
   early A51.9
     cardiovascular A52.00
     central nervous system A52.3
     latent (without manifestations) (less than 2 years after infection) A51.5
       negative spinal fluid test A51.5
       serological relapse after treatment A51.5
       serology positive A51.5
     relapse (treated, untreated) A51.9
     skin A51.39
     symptomatic A51.9
       extragenital chancre A51.2
       primary, except extragenital chancre A51.0
       secondary (*see also* Syphilis, secondary) A51.39
         relapse (treated, untreated) A51.49
     ulcer A51.39
   eighth nerve (neuritis) A52.15
   endemic A65
   endocarditis A52.03
     aortic A52.03
     pulmonary A52.03
   epididymis (late) A52.76
   epiglottis (late) A52.73
   epiphysitis (congenital) (early) A50.02
   episcleritis (late) A52.71
   esophagus A52.79
   eustachian tube A52.73
   exposure to Z20.2
   eye A52.71
   eyelid (late) (with gumma) A52.71
   fallopian tube (late) A52.76
   fracture A52.77
   gallbladder (late) A52.74
   gastric (polyposis) (late) A52.74
   general A53.9
     paralysis A52.17
       juvenile A50.45
   genital (primary) A51.0
   glaucoma A52.71
   gumma NEC A52.79
     cardiovascular system A52.00
     central nervous system A52.3
     congenital A50.59
   heart (block) (decompensation) (disease) (failure) A52.06 [I52]
     valve NEC A52.03
   hemianesthesia A52.19
   hemianopsia A52.71
   hemiparesis A52.17
   hemiplegia A52.17

**Syphiloma** A52.79
  cardiovascular system A52.00
  central nervous system A52.3
  circulatory system A52.00
  congenital A50.59
**Syphilophobia** F45.29
**Syringadenoma** (*see also* Neoplasm, skin, benign)
  papillary — *see* Neoplasm, skin, benign

**Syringobulbia** G95.0
**Syringocystadenoma** — *see* Neoplasm, skin, benign
  papillary — *see* Neoplasm, skin, benign
**Syringoma** (*see also* Neoplasm, skin, benign)
  chondroid — *see* Neoplasm, skin, benign
**Syringomyelia** G95.0
**Syringomyelitis** — *see* Encephalitis
**Syringomyelocele** — *see* Spina bifida

**Syringopontia** G95.0
**System, systemic** (*see also* condition)
  disease, combined — *see* Degeneration, combined
  inflammatory response syndrome (SIRS) of non-infectious origin (without organ dysfunction) R65.10
    with acute organ dysfunction R65.11
  lupus erythematosus M32.9
    inhibitor present D68.62

☑ **Additional Character Required** — **Refer to the Tabular List for Character Selection**     ▽ **Subterms under main terms may continue to next column or page**

# T

**Tabacism, tabacosis, tabagism** (*see also* Poisoning, tobacco)
  meaning dependence (without remission) F17.200
    with
      disorder F17.299
        in remission F17.211
        specified disorder NEC F17.298
        withdrawal F17.203
**Tabardillo** A75.9
  flea-borne A75.2
  louse-borne A75.0
**Tabes, tabetic** A52.10
  with
    central nervous system syphilis A52.10
    Charcot's joint A52.16
    cord bladder A52.19
    crisis, viscera (any) A52.19
    paralysis, general A52.17
    paresis (general) A52.17
    perforating ulcer (foot) A52.19
  arthropathy (Charcot) A52.16
  bladder A52.19
  bone A52.11
  cerebrospinal A52.12
  congenital A50.45
  conjugal A52.10
  dorsalis A52.11
    juvenile A50.49
  juvenile A50.49
  latent A52.19
  mesenterica A18.39
  paralysis, insane, general A52.17
  spasmodic A52.17
  syphilis (cerebrospinal) A52.12
**Taboparalysis** A52.17
**Taboparesis** (remission) A52.17
  juvenile A50.45
**TAC** (trigeminal autonomic cephalgia) **NEC** G44.099
  intractable G44.091
  not intractable G44.099
**Tache noir** S60.22- ☑
**Tachyalimentation** K91.2
**Tachyarrhythmia, tachyrhythmia** — *see* Tachycardia
**Tachycardia** R00.0
  atrial (paroxysmal) I47.1
  auricular I47.1
  AV nodal re-entry (re-entrant) I47.1
  junctional (paroxysmal) I47.1
  newborn P29.11
  nodal (paroxysmal) I47.1
  non-paroxysmal AV nodal I45.89
  paroxysmal (sustained) (nonsustained) I47.9
    with sinus bradycardia I49.5
    atrial (PAT) I47.1
    atrioventricular (AV) (re-entrant) I47.1
      psychogenic F54
    junctional I47.1
      ectopic I47.1
    nodal I47.1
    psychogenic (atrial) (supraventricular) (ventricular) F54
    supraventricular (sustained) I47.1
      psychogenic F54
    ventricular I47.2
      psychogenic F54
  psychogenic F45.8
  sick sinus I49.5
  sinoauricular NOS R00.0
    paroxysmal I47.1
  sinus [sinusal] NOS R00.0
    paroxysmal I47.1
  supraventricular I47.1
  ventricular (paroxysmal) (sustained) I47.2
    psychogenic F54
**Tachygastria** K31.89
**Tachypnea** R06.82
  hysterical F45.8
  newborn (idiopathic) (transitory) P22.1
  psychogenic F45.8
  transitory, of newborn P22.1
**TACO** (transfusion associated circulatory overload) E87.71
**Taenia** (infection) (infestation) B68.9
  diminuta B71.0
  echinococcal infestation B67.90
  mediocanellata B68.1

**Taenia** — *continued*
  nana B71.0
  saginata B68.1
  solium (intestinal form) B68.0
    larval form — *see* Cysticercosis
**Taeniasis** (intestine) — *see* Taenia
**Tag** (hypertrophied skin) (infected) L91.8
  adenoid J35.8
  anus K64.4
  hemorrhoidal K64.4
  hymen N89.8
  perineal N90.89
  preauricular Q17.0
  sentinel K64.4
  skin L91.8
    accessory (congenital) Q82.8
    anus K64.4
    congenital Q82.8
    preauricular Q17.0
  tonsil J35.8
  urethra, urethral N36.8
  vulva N90.89
**Tahyna fever** B33.8
**Takahara's disease** E80.3
**Takayasu's disease or syndrome** M31.4
**Talcosis** (pulmonary) J62.0
**Talipes** (congenital) Q66.89
  acquired, planus — *see* Deformity, limb, flat foot
  asymmetric Q66.89
  calcaneovalgus Q66.4
  calcaneovarus Q66.1
  calcaneus Q66.89
  cavus Q66.7
  equinovalgus Q66.6
  equinovarus Q66.0
  equinus Q66.89
  percavus Q66.7
  planovalgus Q66.6
  planus (acquired) (any degree) (*see also* Deformity, limb, flat foot)
    congenital Q66.5- ☑
    due to rickets (sequelae) E64.3
  valgus Q66.6
  varus Q66.3
**Tall stature, constitutional** E34.4
**Talma's disease** M62.89
**Talon noir** S90.3- ☑
  hand S60.22- ☑
  heel S90.3- ☑
  toe S90.1- ☑
**Tamponade, heart** I31.4
**Tanapox** (virus disease) B08.71
**Tangier disease** E78.6
**Tantrum, child problem** F91.8
**Tapeworm** (infection) (infestation) — *see* Infestation, tapeworm
**Tapia's syndrome** G52.7
**TAR** (thrombocytopenia with absent radius) **syndrome** Q87.2
**Tarral-Besnier disease** L44.0
**Tarsal tunnel syndrome** — *see* Syndrome, tarsal tunnel
**Tarsalgia** — *see* Pain, limb, lower
**Tarsitis** (eyelid) H01.8
  syphilitic A52.71
  tuberculous A18.4
**Tartar** (teeth) (dental calculus) K03.6
**Tattoo** (mark) L81.8
**Tauri's disease** E74.09
**Taurodontism** K00.2
**Taussig-Bing syndrome** Q20.1
**Taybi's syndrome** Q87.2
**Tay-Sachs amaurotic familial idiocy or disease** E75.02
**TBI** (traumatic brain injury) S06.9 ☑
**Teacher's node or nodule** J38.2
**Tear, torn** (traumatic) (*see also* Laceration)
  with abortion — *see* Abortion
  annular fibrosis M51.35
  anus, anal (sphincter) S31.831 ☑
  complicating delivery
    with third degree perineal laceration (*see also* Delivery, complicated, by, laceration, perineum, third degree) O70.20
      with mucosa O70.3
    without third degree perineal laceration O70.4
    nontraumatic (healed) (old) K62.81
  articular cartilage, old — *see* Derangement, joint, articular cartilage, by site

**Tear, torn** — *continued*
  bladder
    with ectopic or molar pregnancy O08.6
    following ectopic or molar pregnancy O08.6
    obstetrical O71.5
    traumatic — *see* Injury, bladder
  bowel
    with ectopic or molar pregnancy O08.6
    following ectopic or molar pregnancy O08.6
    obstetrical trauma O71.5
  broad ligament
    with ectopic or molar pregnancy O08.6
    following ectopic or molar pregnancy O08.6
    obstetrical trauma O71.6
  bucket handle (knee) (meniscus) — *see* Tear, meniscus
  capsule, joint — *see* Sprain
  cartilage (*see also* Sprain)
    articular, old — *see* Derangement, joint, articular cartilage, by site
  cervix
    with ectopic or molar pregnancy O08.6
    following ectopic or molar pregnancy O08.6
    obstetrical trauma (current) O71.3
    old N88.1
    traumatic — *see* Injury, uterus
  dural G97.41
    nontraumatic G96.11
  internal organ — *see* Injury, by site
  knee cartilage
    articular (current) S83.3- ☑
    old — *see* Derangement, knee, meniscus, due to old tear
  ligament — *see* Sprain
  meniscus (knee) (current injury) S83.209 ☑
    bucket-handle S83.20- ☑
    lateral
      bucket-handle S83.25- ☑
      complex S83.27- ☑
      peripheral S83.26- ☑
      specified type NEC S83.28- ☑
    medial
      bucket-handle S83.21- ☑
      complex S83.23- ☑
      peripheral S83.22- ☑
      specified type NEC S83.24- ☑
    old — *see* Derangement, knee, meniscus, due to old tear
    site other than knee — *code as* Sprain
    specified type NEC S83.20- ☑
  muscle — *see* Strain
  pelvic
    floor, complicating delivery O70.1
    organ NEC, obstetrical trauma O71.5
      with ectopic or molar pregnancy O08.6
      following ectopic or molar pregnancy O08.6
  perineal, secondary O90.1
  periurethral tissue, obstetrical trauma O71.82
    with ectopic or molar pregnancy O08.6
    following ectopic or molar pregnancy O08.6
  rectovaginal septum — *see* Laceration, vagina
  retina, retinal (without detachment) (horseshoe) (*see also* Break, retina, horseshoe)
    with detachment — *see* Detachment, retina, with retinal, break
  rotator cuff (nontraumatic) M75.10- ☑
    complete M75.12- ☑
    incomplete M75.11- ☑
    traumatic S46.01- ☑
      capsule S43.42- ☑
  semilunar cartilage, knee — *see* Tear, meniscus
  supraspinatus (complete) (incomplete) (nontraumatic) (*see also* Tear, rotator cuff) M75.10- ☑
  tendon — *see* Strain
  tentorial, at birth P10.4
  umbilical cord
    complicating delivery O69.89 ☑
  urethra
    with ectopic or molar pregnancy O08.6
    following ectopic or molar pregnancy O08.6
    obstetrical trauma O71.5
  uterus — *see* Injury, uterus
  vagina — *see* Laceration, vagina
  vessel, from catheter — *see* Puncture, accidental complicating surgery
  vulva, complicating delivery O70.0
**Tear-stone** — *see* Dacryolith

**Teeth** (*see also* condition)
  grinding
    psychogenic F45.8
    sleep related G47.63
**Teething** (syndrome) K00.7
**Telangiectasia, telangiectasis** (verrucous) I78.1
  ataxic (cerebellar) (Louis-Bar) G11.3
  familial I78.0
  hemorrhagic, hereditary (congenital) (senile) I78.0
  hereditary, hemorrhagic (congenital) (senile) I78.0
  juxtafoveal H35.07- ☑
  macular H35.07- ☑
  macularis eruptiva perstans D47.01
  parafoveal H35.07- ☑
  retinal (idiopathic) (juxtafoveal) (macular) (parafoveal)
    H35.07- ☑
  spider I78.1
**Telephone scatologia** F65.89
**Telescoped bowel or intestine** K56.1
  congenital Q43.8
**Temperature**
  body, high (of unknown origin) R50.9
  cold, trauma from T69.9 ☑
    newborn P80.0
    specified effect NEC T69.8 ☑
**Temple** — *see* condition
**Temporal** — *see* condition
**Temporomandibular joint pain-dysfunction syn-**
    **drome** M26.62- ☑
**Temporosphenoidal** — *see* condition
**Tendency**
  bleeding — *see* Defect, coagulation
  suicide
    meaning personal history of attempted suicide
      Z91.5
    meaning suicidal ideation — *see* Ideation, suicidal
  to fall R29.6
**Tenderness, abdominal** R10.819
  epigastric R10.816
  generalized R10.817
  left lower quadrant R10.814
  left upper quadrant R10.812
  periumbilic R10.815
  rebound R10.829
    epigastric R10.826
    generalized R10.827
    left lower quadrant R10.824
    left upper quadrant R10.822
    periumbilic R10.825
    right lower quadrant R10.823
    right upper quadrant R10.821
  right lower quadrant R10.813
  right upper quadrant R10.811
**Tendinitis, tendonitis** (*see also* Enthesopathy)
  Achilles M76.6- ☑
  adhesive — *see* Tenosynovitis, specified type NEC
    shoulder — *see* Capsulitis, adhesive
  bicipital M75.2- ☑
  calcific M65.2-
    ankle M65.27- ☑
    foot M65.27- ☑
    forearm M65.23- ☑
    hand M65.24- ☑
    lower leg M65.26- ☑
    multiple sites M65.29
    pelvic region M65.25- ☑
    shoulder M75.3- ☑
    specified site NEC M65.28
    thigh M65.25- ☑
    upper arm M65.22- ☑
  due to use, overuse, pressure (*see also* Disorder, soft
    tissue, due to use)
    specified NEC — *see* Disorder, soft tissue, due to
      use, specified NEC
  gluteal M76.0- ☑
  patellar M76.5- ☑
  peroneal M76.7- ☑
  psoas M76.1- ☑
  tibial (posterior) M76.82- ☑
    anterior M76.81- ☑
  trochanteric — *see* Bursitis, hip, trochanteric
**Tendon** — *see* condition
**Tendosynovitis** — *see* Tenosynovitis
**Tenesmus** (rectal) R19.8
  vesical R30.1
**Tennis elbow** — *see* Epicondylitis, lateral

**Tenonitis** (*see also* Tenosynovitis)
  eye (capsule) H05.04- ☑
**Tenontosynovitis** — *see* Tenosynovitis
**Tenontothecitis** — *see* Tenosynovitis
**Tenophyte** — *see* Disorder, synovium, specified type
    NEC
**Tenosynovitis** (*see also* Synovitis) M65.9
  adhesive — *see* Tenosynovitis, specified type NEC
    shoulder — *see* Capsulitis, adhesive
  bicipital (calcifying) — *see* Tendinitis, bicipital
  gonococcal A54.49
  in (due to)
    crystals M65.8- ☑
    gonorrhea A54.49
    syphilis (late) A52.78
    use, overuse, pressure (*see also* Disorder, soft tissue,
      due to use)
      specified NEC — *see* Disorder, soft tissue, due
        to use, specified NEC
  infective NEC M65.1- ☑
    ankle M65.17- ☑
    foot M65.17- ☑
    forearm M65.13- ☑
    hand M65.14- ☑
    lower leg M65.16- ☑
    multiple sites M65.19
    pelvic region M65.15- ☑
    shoulder region M65.11- ☑
    specified site NEC M65.18
    thigh M65.15- ☑
    upper arm M65.12- ☑
  radial styloid M65.4
  shoulder region M65.81- ☑
    adhesive — *see* Capsulitis, adhesive
  specified type NEC M65.88
    ankle M65.87- ☑
    foot M65.87- ☑
    forearm M65.83- ☑
    hand M65.84- ☑
    lower leg M65.86- ☑
    multiple sites M65.89
    pelvic region M65.85- ☑
    shoulder region M65.81- ☑
    specified site NEC M65.88
    thigh M65.85- ☑
    upper arm M65.82- ☑
  tuberculous — *see* Tuberculosis, tenosynovitis
**Tenovaginitis** — *see* Tenosynovitis
**Tension**
  arterial, high (*see also* Hypertension)
    without diagnosis of hypertension R03.0
  headache G44.209
    intractable G44.201
    not intractable G44.209
  nervous R45.0
  pneumothorax J93.0
  premenstrual N94.3
  state (mental) F48.9
**Tentorium** — *see* condition
**Teratencephalus** Q89.8
**Teratism** Q89.7
**Teratoblastoma** (malignant) — *see* Neoplasm, malig-
    nant, by site
**Teratocarcinoma** (*see also* Neoplasm, malignant, by
    site)
  liver C22.7
**Teratoma** (solid) (*see also* Neoplasm, uncertain behavior,
    by site)
  with embryonal carcinoma, mixed — *see* Neoplasm,
    malignant, by site
  with malignant transformation — *see* Neoplasm, ma-
    lignant, by site
  adult (cystic) — *see* Neoplasm, benign, by site
  benign — *see* Neoplasm, benign, by site
  combined with choriocarcinoma — *see* Neoplasm,
    malignant, by site
  cystic (adult) — *see* Neoplasm, benign, by site
  differentiated — *see* Neoplasm, benign, by site
  embryonal (*see also* Neoplasm, malignant, by site)
    liver C22.7
  immature — *see* Neoplasm, malignant, by site
  liver C22.7
    adult, benign, cystic, differentiated type or mature
      D13.4
  malignant (*see also* Neoplasm, malignant, by site)
    anaplastic — *see* Neoplasm, malignant, by site
    intermediate — *see* Neoplasm, malignant, by site

**Teratoma** — *continued*
  malignant (*see also* Neoplasm, malignant, by site) —
    *continued*
    intermediate — *see* Neoplasm, malignant, by site
      — *continued*
      specified site — *see* Neoplasm, malignant, by
        site
      unspecified site C62.90
    undifferentiated — *see* Neoplasm, malignant, by
      site
  mature — *see* Neoplasm, uncertain behavior, by site
    malignant — *see* Neoplasm, by site, malignant, by
      site
  ovary D27.- ☑
    embryonal, immature or malignant C56- ☑
  solid — *see* Neoplasm, uncertain behavior, by site
  testis C62.9- ☑
    adult, benign, cystic, differentiated type or mature
      D29.2- ☑
    scrotal C62.1- ☑
    undescended C62.0- ☑
**Termination**
  anomalous (*see also* Malposition, congenital)
    right pulmonary vein Q26.3
  pregnancy, elective Z33.2
**Ternidens diminutus infestation** B81.8
**Ternidensiasis** B81.8
**Terror(s) night** (child) F51.4
**Terrorism, victim of** Z65.4
**Terry's syndrome** (*see also* Myopia, degenerative)
    H44.2- ☑
**Tertiary** — *see* condition
**Test, tests, testing** (for)
  adequacy (for dialysis)
    hemodialysis Z49.31
    peritoneal Z49.32
  blood pressure Z01.30
    abnormal reading — *see* Blood, pressure
  blood typing Z01.83
    Rh typing Z01.83
  blood-alcohol Z04.8
    positive — *see* Findings, abnormal, in blood
  blood-drug Z04.8
    positive — *see* Findings, abnormal, in blood
  cardiac pulse generator (battery) Z45.010
  fertility Z31.41
  genetic
    disease carrier status for procreative management
      female Z31.430
      male Z31.440
    male partner of patient with recurrent pregnancy
      loss Z31.441
    procreative management NEC
      female Z31.438
      male Z31.448
  hearing Z01.10
    with abnormal findings NEC Z01.118
  HIV (human immunodeficiency virus)
    nonconclusive (in infants) R75
    positive Z21
    seropositive Z21
  immunity status Z01.84
  intelligence NEC Z01.89
  laboratory (as part of a general medical examination)
    Z00.00
    with abnormal finding Z00.01
    for medicolegal reason NEC Z04.8
  male partner of patient with recurrent pregnancy loss
    Z31.441
  Mantoux (for tuberculosis) Z11.1
    abnormal result R76.11
  pregnancy, positive first pregnancy — *see* Pregnancy,
    normal, first
  procreative Z31.49
    fertility Z31.41
  skin, diagnostic
    allergy Z01.82
      special screening examination — *see* Screening,
        by name of disease
    Mantoux Z11.1
    tuberculin Z11.1
    specified NEC Z01.89
    tuberculin Z11.1
      abnormal result R76.11
  vision Z01.00
    with abnormal findings Z01.01
  Wassermann Z11.3
    positive — *see* Serology for syphilis, positive

**Testicle, testicular, testis** (*see also* condition)
  feminization syndrome (*see also* Syndrome, androgen
    insensitivity) E34.51
  migrans Q55.29
**Tetanus, tetanic** (cephalic) (convulsions) A35
  with
    abortion A34
    ectopic or molar pregnancy O08.0
  following ectopic or molar pregnancy O08.0
  inoculation reaction (due to serum) — *see* Complica-
    tions, vaccination
  neonatorum A33
  obstetrical A34
  puerperal, postpartum, childbirth A34
**Tetany** (due to) R29.0
  alkalosis E87.3
  associated with rickets E55.0
  convulsions R29.0
    hysterical F44.5
  functional (hysterical) F44.5
  hyperkinetic R29.0
    hysterical F44.5
  hyperpnea R06.4
    hysterical F44.5
    psychogenic F45.8
  hyperventilation (*see also* Hyperventilation) R06.4
    hysterical F44.5
  neonatal (without calcium or magnesium deficiency)
    P71.3
  parathyroid (gland) E20.9
  parathyroprival E89.2
  post- (para)thyroidectomy E89.2
  postoperative E89.2
  pseudotetany R29.0
  psychogenic (conversion reaction) F44.5
**Tetralogy of Fallot** Q21.3
**Tetraplegia** (chronic) (*see also* Quadriplegia) G82.50
**Thailand hemorrhagic fever** A91
**Thalassanemia** — *see* Thalassemia
**Thalassemia** (anemia) (disease) D56.9
  with other hemoglobinopathy D56.8
  alpha (major) (severe) (triple gene defect) D56.0
    minor D56.3
    silent carrier D56.3
    trait D56.3
  beta (severe) D56.1
    homozygous D56.1
    major D56.1
    minor D56.3
    trait D56.3
  delta-beta (homozygous) D56.2
    minor D56.3
    trait D56.3
  dominant D56.8
  hemoglobin
    C D56.8
    E-beta D56.5
  intermedia D56.1
  major D56.1
  minor D56.3
  mixed D56.8
  sickle-cell — *see* Disease, sickle-cell, thalassemia
  specified type NEC D56.8
  trait D56.3
  variants D56.8
**Thanatophoric dwarfism or short stature** Q77.1
**Thaysen-Gee disease** (nontropical sprue) K90.0
**Thaysen's disease** K90.0
**Thecoma** D27- ☑
  luteinized D27- ☑
  malignant C56- ☑
**Thelarche, premature** E30.8
**Thelaziasis** B83.8
**Thelitis** N61.0
  puerperal, postpartum or gestational — *see* Infection,
    nipple
**Therapeutic** — *see* condition
**Therapy**
  drug, long-term (current) (prophylactic)
    agents affecting estrogen receptors and estrogen
      levels NEC Z79.818
    anastrozole (Arimidex) Z79.811
    antibiotics Z79.2
      short-term use — *omit code*
    anticoagulants Z79.01
    anti-inflammatory Z79.1
    antiplatelet Z79.02
    antithrombotics Z79.02

**Therapy** — *continued*
  drug, long-term — *continued*
    aromatase inhibitors Z79.811
    aspirin Z79.82
    birth control pill or patch Z79.3
    bisphosphonates Z79.83
    contraceptive, oral Z79.3
    drug, specified NEC Z79.899
    estrogen receptor downregulators Z79.818
    Evista Z79.810
    exemestane (Aromasin) Z79.811
    Fareston Z79.810
    fulvestrant (Faslodex) Z79.818
    gonadotropin-releasing hormone (GnRH) agonist
      Z79.818
    goserelin acetate (Zoladex) Z79.818
    hormone replacement Z79.890
    insulin Z79.4
    letrozole (Femara) Z79.811
    leuprolide acetate (leuprorelin) (Lupron) Z79.818
    megestrol acetate (Megace) Z79.818
    methadone
      for pain management Z79.891
      maintenance therapy F11.20
    Nolvadex Z79.810
    opiate analgesic Z79.891
    oral contraceptive Z79.3
    raloxifene (Evista) Z79.810
    selective estrogen receptor modulators (SERMs)
      Z79.810
    short term — *omit code*
    steroids
      inhaled Z79.51
      systemic Z79.52
    tamoxifen (Nolvadex) Z79.810
    toremifene (Fareston) Z79.810
**Thermic** — *see* condition
**Thermography** (abnormal) (*see also* Abnormal, diagnostic imaging) R93.8
  breast R92.8
**Thermoplegia** T67.0 ☑
**Thesaurismosis, glycogen** — *see* Disease, glycogen
  storage
**Thiamin deficiency** E51.9
  specified NEC E51.8
**Thiaminic deficiency with beriberi** E51.11
**Thibierge-Weissenbach syndrome** — *see* Sclerosis,
  systemic
**Thickening**
  bone — *see* Hypertrophy, bone
  breast N64.59
  endometrium R93.8
  epidermal L85.9
    specified NEC L85.8
  hymen N89.6
  larynx J38.7
  nail L60.2
    congenital Q84.5
  periosteal — *see* Hypertrophy, bone
  pleura J92.9
    with asbestos J92.0
  skin R23.4
  subepiglottic J38.7
  tongue K14.8
  valve, heart — *see* Endocarditis
**Thigh** — *see* condition
**Thinning vertebra** — *see* Spondylopathy, specified NEC
**Thirst, excessive** R63.1
  due to deprivation of water T73.1 ☑
**Thomsen disease** G71.12
**Thoracic** (*see also* condition)
  kidney Q63.2
  outlet syndrome G54.0
**Thoracogastroschisis** (congenital) Q79.8
**Thoracopagus** Q89.4
**Thorax** — *see* condition
**Thorn's syndrome** N28.89
**Thorson-Björck syndrome** E34.0
**Threadworm** (infection) (infestation) B80
**Threatened**
  abortion O20.0
    with subsequent abortion O03.9
  job loss, anxiety concerning Z56.2
  labor (without delivery) O47.9
    at or after 37 completed weeks of gestation O47.1
    before 37 completed weeks of gestation O47.0- ☑
  loss of job, anxiety concerning Z56.2
  miscarriage O20.0

**Threatened** — *continued*
  unemployment, anxiety concerning Z56.2
**Three-day fever** A93.1
**Threshers' lung** J67.0
**Thrix annulata** (congenital) Q84.1
**Throat** — *see* condition
**Thrombasthenia** (Glanzmann) (hemorrhagic) (heredi-
  tary) D69.1
**Thromboangiitis** I73.1
  obliterans (general) I73.1
    cerebral I67.89
    vessels
      brain I67.89
      spinal cord I67.89
**Thromboarteritis** — *see* Arteritis
**Thromboasthenia** (Glanzmann) (hemorrhagic) (heredi-
  tary) D69.1
**Thrombocytasthenia** (Glanzmann) D69.1
**Thrombocythemia** (essential) (hemorrhagic) (idiopathic)
  (primary) D47.3
**Thrombocytopathy** (dystrophic) (granulopenic) D69.1
**Thrombocytopenia, thrombocytopenic** D69.6
  with absent radius (TAR) Q87.2
  congenital D69.42
  dilutional D69.59
  due to
    (massive) blood transfusion D69.59
    drugs D69.59
    extracorporeal circulation of blood D69.59
    platelet alloimmunization D69.59
  essential D69.3
  heparin induced (HIT) D75.82
  hereditary D69.42
  idiopathic D69.3
  neonatal, transitory P61.0
    due to
      exchange transfusion P61.0
      idiopathic maternal thrombocytopenia P61.0
      isoimmunization P61.0
  primary NEC D69.49
    idiopathic D69.3
  puerperal, postpartum O72.3
  secondary D69.59
  transient neonatal P61.0
**Thrombocytosis, essential** D47.3
  primary D47.3
**Thromboembolism** — *see* Embolism
**Thrombopathy** (Bernard-Soulier) D69.1
  constitutional D68.0
  Willebrand-Jurgens D68.0
**Thrombopenia** — *see* Thrombocytopenia
**Thrombophilia** D68.59
  primary NEC D68.59
  secondary NEC D68.69
  specified NEC D68.69
**Thrombophlebitis** I80.9
  antepartum O22.2- ☑
    deep O22.3- ☑
    superficial O22.2- ☑
  cavernous (venous) sinus G08
    complicating pregnancy O22.5- ☑
    nonpyogenic I67.6
  cerebral (sinus) (vein) G08
    nonpyogenic I67.6
    sequelae G09
  due to implanted device — *see* Complications, by site
    and type, specified NEC
  during or resulting from a procedure NEC T81.72 ☑
  femoral vein (superficial) I80.1- ☑
  femoropopliteal vein I80.0- ☑
  hepatic (vein) I80.8
  idiopathic, recurrent I82.1
  iliofemoral I80.1- ☑
  intracranial venous sinus (any) G08
    nonpyogenic I67.6
    sequelae G09
  intraspinal venous sinuses and veins G08
    nonpyogenic G95.19
  lateral (venous) sinus G08
    nonpyogenic I67.6
  leg I80.3
    superficial I80.0- ☑
  longitudinal (venous) sinus G08
    nonpyogenic I67.6
  lower extremity I80.299
  migrans, migrating I82.1
  pelvic
    with ectopic or molar pregnancy O08.0

**Thrombophlebitis** — *continued*
- pelvic — *continued*
  - following ectopic or molar pregnancy O08.0
  - puerperal O87.1
- popliteal vein — *see* Phlebitis, leg, deep, popliteal
- portal (vein) K75.1
- postoperative T81.72 ☑
- pregnancy — *see* Thrombophlebitis, antepartum
- puerperal, postpartum, childbirth O87.0
  - deep O87.1
  - pelvic O87.1
  - septic O86.81
  - superficial O87.0
- saphenous (greater) (lesser) I80.0- ☑
- sinus (intracranial) G08
  - nonpyogenic I67.6
- specified site NEC I80.8
- tibial vein I80.23- ☑

**Thrombosis, thrombotic** (bland) (multiple) (progressive) (silent) (vessel) I82.90
- anal K64.5
- antepartum — *see* Thrombophlebitis, antepartum
- aorta, aortic I74.10
  - abdominal I74.09
    - saddle I74.01
  - bifurcation I74.09
  - saddle I74.01
  - specified site NEC I74.19
  - terminal I74.09
  - thoracic I74.11
  - valve — *see* Endocarditis, aortic
- apoplexy I63.3- ☑
- artery, arteries (postinfectional) I74.9
  - auditory, internal — *see* Occlusion, artery, precerebral, specified NEC
  - basilar — *see* Occlusion, artery, basilar
  - carotid (common) (internal) — *see* Occlusion, artery, carotid
  - cerebellar (anterior inferior) (posterior inferior) (superior) — *see* Occlusion, artery, cerebellar
  - cerebral — *see* Occlusion, artery, cerebral
  - choroidal (anterior) — *see* Occlusion, artery, precerebral, specified NEC
  - communicating, posterior — *see* Occlusion, artery, precerebral, specified NEC
  - coronary (*see also* Infarct, myocardium)
    - not resulting in infarction I24.0
  - hepatic I74.8
  - hypophyseal — *see* Occlusion, artery, precerebral, specified NEC
  - iliac I74.5
  - limb I74.4
    - lower I74.3
    - upper I74.2
  - meningeal, anterior or posterior — *see* Occlusion, artery, cerebral, specified NEC
  - mesenteric (with gangrene) (*see also* Infarct, intestine) K55.069
  - ophthalmic — *see* Occlusion, artery, retina
  - pontine — *see* Occlusion, artery, precerebral, specified NEC
  - precerebral — *see* Occlusion, artery, precerebral
  - pulmonary (iatrogenic) — *see* Embolism, pulmonary
  - renal N28.0
  - retinal — *see* Occlusion, artery, retina
  - spinal, anterior or posterior G95.11
  - traumatic NEC T14.8 ☑
  - vertebral — *see* Occlusion, artery, vertebral
- atrium, auricular (*see also* Infarct, myocardium)
  - following acute myocardial infarction (current complication) I23.6
  - not resulting in infarction I51.3
  - old I51.3
- basilar (artery) — *see* Occlusion, artery, basilar
- brain (artery) (stem) (*see also* Occlusion, artery, cerebral)
  - due to syphilis A52.05
  - puerperal O99.43
  - sinus — *see* Thrombosis, intracranial venous sinus
- capillary I78.8
- cardiac (*see also* Infarct, myocardium)
  - not resulting in infarction I51.3
  - old I51.3
  - valve — *see* Endocarditis
- carotid (artery) (common) (internal) — *see* Occlusion, artery, carotid

**Thrombosis, thrombotic** — *continued*
- cavernous (venous) sinus — *see* Thrombosis, intracranial venous sinus
- cerebellar artery (anterior inferior) (posterior inferior) (superior) I66.3
- cerebral (artery) — *see* Occlusion, artery, cerebral
- cerebrovenous sinus (*see also* Thrombosis, intracranial venous sinus)
  - puerperium O87.3
- chronic I82.91
- coronary (artery) (vein) (*see also* Infarct, myocardium)
  - not resulting in infarction I24.0
- corpus cavernosum N48.89
- cortical I66.9
- deep — *see* Embolism, vein, lower extremity
- due to device, implant or graft (*see also* Complications, by site and type, specified NEC) T85.868 ☑
  - arterial graft NEC T82.868 ☑
  - breast (implant) T85.868 ☑
  - catheter NEC T85.868 ☑
    - dialysis (renal) T82.868 ☑
      - intraperitoneal T85.868 ☑
    - infusion NEC T82.868 ☑
      - spinal (epidural) (subdural) T85.860 ☑
    - urinary (indwelling) T83.86 ☑
  - electronic (electrode) (pulse generator) (stimulator)
    - bone T84.86 ☑
    - cardiac T82.867 ☑
    - nervous system (brain) (peripheral nerve) (spinal) T85.860 ☑
    - urinary T83.86 ☑
  - fixation, internal (orthopedic) NEC T84.86 ☑
  - gastrointestinal (bile duct) (esophagus) T85.868 ☑
  - genital NEC T83.86 ☑
  - heart T82.867 ☑
  - joint prosthesis T84.86 ☑
  - ocular (corneal graft) (orbital implant) NEC T85.868 ☑
  - orthopedic NEC T84.86 ☑
  - specified NEC T85.868 ☑
  - urinary NEC T83.86 ☑
  - vascular NEC T82.868 ☑
  - ventricular intracranial shunt T85.860 ☑
- during the puerperium — *see* Thrombosis, puerperal
- endocardial (*see also* Infarct, myocardium)
  - not resulting in infarction I51.3
- eye — *see* Occlusion, retina
- genital organ
  - female NEC N94.89
    - pregnancy — *see* Thrombophlebitis, antepartum
  - male N50.1
- gestational — *see* Phlebopathy, gestational
- heart (chamber) (*see also* Infarct, myocardium)
  - not resulting in infarction I51.3
  - old I51.3
- hepatic (vein) I82.0
  - artery I74.8
- history (of) Z86.718
- intestine (with gangrene) (*see also* Infarct, intestine) K55.069
- intracardiac NEC (apical) (atrial) (auricular) (ventricular) (old) I51.3
- intracranial (arterial) I66.9
  - venous sinus (any) G08
    - nonpyogenic origin I67.6
    - puerperium O87.3
- intramural (*see also* Infarct, myocardium)
  - not resulting in infarction I51.3
  - old I51.3
- intraspinal venous sinuses and veins G08
  - nonpyogenic G95.19
- kidney (artery) N28.0
- lateral (venous) sinus — *see* Thrombosis, intracranial venous sinus
- leg — *see* Thrombosis, vein, lower extremity
  - arterial I74.3
- liver (venous) I82.0
  - artery I74.8
  - portal vein I81
- longitudinal (venous) sinus — *see* Thrombosis, intracranial venous sinus
- lower limb — *see* Thrombosis, vein, lower extremity
- lung (iatrogenic) (postoperative) — *see* Embolism, pulmonary
- meninges (brain) (arterial) I66.8

**Thrombosis, thrombotic** — *continued*
- mesenteric (artery) (with gangrene) (*see also* Infarct, intestine) K55.069
  - vein (inferior) (superior) I81
- mitral I34.8
- mural (*see also* Infarct, myocardium)
  - due to syphilis A52.06
  - not resulting in infarction I51.3
  - old I51.3
- omentum (with gangrene) (*see also* Infarct, intestine) K55.069
- ophthalmic — *see* Occlusion, retina
- pampiniform plexus (male) N50.1
- parietal (*see also* Infarct, myocardium)
  - not resulting in infarction I24.0
- penis, superficial vein N48.81
- perianal venous K64.5
- peripheral arteries I74.4
  - upper I74.2
- personal history (of) Z86.718
- portal I81
  - due to syphilis A52.09
- precerebral artery — *see* Occlusion, artery, precerebral
- puerperal, postpartum O87.0
  - brain (artery) O99.43
    - venous (sinus) O87.3
  - cardiac O99.43
  - cerebral (artery) O99.43
    - venous (sinus) O87.3
  - superficial O87.0
- pulmonary (artery) (iatrogenic) (postoperative) (vein) — *see* Embolism, pulmonary
- renal (artery) N28.0
  - vein I82.3
- resulting from presence of device, implant or graft — *see* Complications, by site and type, specified NEC
- retina, retinal — *see* Occlusion, retina
- scrotum N50.1
- seminal vesicle N50.1
- sigmoid (venous) sinus — *see* Thrombosis, intracranial venous sinus
- sinus, intracranial (any) — *see* Thrombosis, intracranial venous sinus
- specified site NEC I82.890
  - chronic I82.891
- spermatic cord N50.1
- spinal cord (arterial) G95.11
  - due to syphilis A52.09
  - pyogenic origin G06.1
- spleen, splenic D73.5
  - artery I74.8
- testis N50.1
- traumatic NEC T14.8 ☑
- tricuspid I07.8
- tumor — *see* Neoplasm, unspecified behavior, by site
- tunica vaginalis N50.1
- umbilical cord (vessels), complicating delivery O69.5 ☑
- vas deferens N50.1
- vein (acute) I82.90
  - antecubital I82.61- ☑
    - chronic I82.71- ☑
  - axillary I82.A1- ☑ (*following* I82.7)
    - chronic I82.A2- ☑ (*following* I82.7)
  - basilic I82.61- ☑
    - chronic I82.71- ☑
  - brachial I82.62- ☑
    - chronic I82.72- ☑
  - brachiocephalic (innominate) I82.290
    - chronic I82.291
  - cephalic I82.61- ☑
    - chronic I82.71- ☑
  - cerebral, nonpyogenic I67.6
  - chronic I82.91
  - deep (DVT) I82.40- ☑
    - calf I82.4Z- ☑
      - chronic I82.5Z- ☑
    - lower leg I82.4Z- ☑
      - chronic I82.5Z- ☑
    - thigh I82.4Y- ☑
      - chronic I82.5Y- ☑
    - upper leg I82.4Y ☑
      - chronic I82.5Y- ☑
  - femoral I82.41- ☑
    - chronic I82.51- ☑
  - iliac (iliofemoral) I82.42- ☑
    - chronic I82.52- ☑

**Thrombosis, thrombotic** — *continued*
  vein — *continued*
    innominate I82.290
      chronic I82.291
    internal jugular I82.C1- ☑ (*following* I82.7)
      chronic I82.C2- ☑ (*following* I82.7)
    lower extremity
      deep I82.40- ☑
        chronic I82.50- ☑
          specified NEC I82.49- ☑
            chronic NEC I82.59- ☑
      distal
        deep I82.4Z- ☑
      proximal
        deep I82.4Y- ☑
          chronic I82.5Y- ☑
      superficial I82.81- ☑
    perianal K64.5
    popliteal I82.43- ☑
      chronic I82.53- ☑
    radial I82.62- ☑
      chronic I82.72- ☑
    renal I82.3
    saphenous (greater) (lesser) I82.81- ☑
    specified NEC I82.890
      chronic NEC I82.891
    subclavian I82.B1- ☑ (*following* I82.7)
      chronic I82.B2- ☑ (*following* I82.7)
    thoracic NEC I82.290
      chronic I82.291
    tibial I82.44- ☑
      chronic I82.54- ☑
    ulnar I82.62- ☑
      chronic I82.72- ☑
    upper extremity I82.60- ☑
      chronic I82.70- ☑
      deep I82.62- ☑
        chronic I82.72- ☑
      superficial I82.61- ☑
        chronic I82.71- ☑
  vena cava
    inferior I82.220
      chronic I82.221
    superior I82.210
      chronic I82.211
  venous, perianal K64.5
  ventricle (*see also* Infarct, myocardium)
    following acute myocardial infarction (current complication) I23.6
    not resulting in infarction I24.0
    old I51.3
**Thrombus** — *see* Thrombosis
**Thrush** (*see also* Candidiasis)
  newborn P37.5
  oral B37.0
  vaginal B37.3
**Thumb** (*see also* condition)
  sucking (child problem) F98.8
**Thymitis** E32.8
**Thymoma** (benign) D15.0
  malignant C37
**Thymus, thymic** (gland) — *see* condition
**Thyrocele** — *see* Goiter
**Thyroglossal** (*see also* condition)
  cyst Q89.2
  duct, persistent Q89.2
**Thyroid** (gland) (body) (*see also* condition)
  hormone resistance E07.89
  lingual Q89.2
  nodule (cystic) (nontoxic) (single) E04.1
**Thyroiditis** E06.9
  acute (nonsuppurative) (pyogenic) (suppurative) E06.0
  autoimmune E06.3
  chronic (nonspecific) (sclerosing) E06.5
    with thyrotoxicosis, transient E06.2
    fibrous E06.5
    lymphadenoid E06.3
    lymphocytic E06.3
    lymphoid E06.3
  de Quervain's E06.1
  drug-induced E06.4
  fibrous (chronic) E06.5
  giant-cell (follicular) E06.1
  granulomatous (de Quervain) (subacute) E06.1
  Hashimoto's (struma lymphomatosa) E06.3
  iatrogenic E06.4
  ligneous E06.5

**Thyroiditis** — *continued*
  lymphocytic (chronic) E06.3
  lymphoid E06.3
  lymphomatous E06.3
  nonsuppurative E06.1
  postpartum, puerperal O90.5
  pseudotuberculous E06.1
  pyogenic E06.0
  radiation E06.4
  Riedel's E06.5
  subacute (granulomatous) E06.1
  suppurative E06.0
  tuberculous A18.81
  viral E06.1
  woody E06.5
**Thyrolingual duct, persistent** Q89.2
**Thyromegaly** E01.0
**Thyrotoxic**
  crisis — *see* Thyrotoxicosis
  heart disease or failure (*see also* Thyrotoxicosis) E05.90 [I43]
    with thyroid storm E05.91 [I43]
  storm — *see* Thyrotoxicosis
**Thyrotoxicosis** (recurrent) E05.90
  with
    goiter (diffuse) E05.00
      with thyroid storm E05.01
      adenomatous uninodular E05.10
        with thyroid storm E05.11
      multinodular E05.20
        with thyroid storm E05.21
      nodular E05.20
        with thyroid storm E05.21
      uninodular E05.10
        with thyroid storm E05.11
    infiltrative
      dermopathy E05.00
        with thyroid storm E05.01
      ophthalmopathy E05.00
        with thyroid storm E05.01
    single thyroid nodule E05.10
      with thyroid storm E05.11
    thyroid storm E05.91
  due to
    ectopic thyroid nodule or tissue E05.30
      with thyroid storm E05.31
    ingestion of (excessive) thyroid material E05.40
      with thyroid storm E05.41
    overproduction of thyroid-stimulating hormone E05.80
      with thyroid storm E05.81
    specified cause NEC E05.80
      with thyroid storm E05.81
  factitia E05.40
    with thyroid storm E05.41
  heart (*see also* Failure, heart, high-output) E05.90 [I43]
    with thyroid storm (*see also* Failure, heart, high-output) E05.91 [I43]
    failure (*see also* Failure, heart, high-output) E05.90 [I43]
  neonatal (transient) P72.1
  transient with chronic thyroiditis E06.2
**Tibia vara** — *see* Osteochondrosis, juvenile, tibia
**Tic** (disorder) F95.9
  breathing F95.8
  child problem F95.0
  compulsive F95.1
  de la Tourette F95.2
  degenerative (generalized) (localized) G25.69
    facial G25.69
  disorder
    chronic
      motor F95.1
      vocal F95.1
    combined vocal and multiple motor F95.2
    transient F95.0
  douloureux G50.0
    atypical G50.1
    postherpetic, postzoster B02.22
  drug-induced G25.61
  eyelid F95.8
  habit F95.9
    chronic F95.1
    transient of childhood F95.0
  lid, transient of childhood F95.0
  motor-verbal F95.2
  occupational F48.8
  orbicularis F95.8

**Tic** — *continued*
  orbicularis — *continued*
    transient of childhood F95.0
  organic origin G25.69
  postchoreic G25.69
  provisional F95.0
  psychogenic, compulsive F95.1
  salaam R25.8
  spasm (motor or vocal) F95.9
    chronic F95.1
    transient of childhood F95.0
  specified NEC F95.8
**Tick-borne** — *see* condition
**Tietze's disease or syndrome** M94.0
**Tight, tightness**
  anus K62.89
  chest R07.89
  fascia (lata) M62.89
  foreskin (congenital) N47.1
  hymen, hymenal ring N89.6
  introitus (acquired) (congenital) N89.6
  rectal sphincter K62.89
  tendon — *see* Short, tendon
  urethral sphincter N35.9
**Tilting vertebra** — *see* Dorsopathy, deforming, specified NEC
**Timidity, child** F93.8
**Tinea** (intersecta) (tarsi) B35.9
  amiantacea L44.8
  asbestina B35.0
  barbae B35.0
  beard B35.0
  black dot B35.0
  blanca B36.2
  capitis B35.0
  corporis B35.4
  cruris B35.6
  flava B36.0
  foot B35.3
  furfuracea B36.0
  imbricata (Tokelau) B35.5
  kerion B35.0
  manuum B35.2
  microsporic — *see* Dermatophytosis
  nigra B36.1
  nodosa — *see* Piedra
  pedis B35.3
  scalp B35.0
  specified NEC B35.8
  sycosis B35.0
  tonsurans B35.0
  trichophytic — *see* Dermatophytosis
  unguium B35.1
  versicolor B36.0
**Tingling sensation** (skin) R20.2
**Tin-miner's lung** J63.5
**Tinnitus NOS** H93.1- ☑
  audible H93.1- ☑
  aurium H93.1- ☑
  pulsatile H93.A- ☑
  subjective H93.1- ☑
**Tipped tooth** (teeth) M26.33
**Tipping**
  pelvis M95.5
    with disproportion (fetopelvic) O33.0
      causing obstructed labor O65.0
  tooth (teeth), fully erupted M26.33
**Tiredness** R53.83
**Tissue** — *see* condition
**Tobacco** (nicotine)
  abuse — *see* Tobacco, use
  dependence — *see* Dependence, drug, nicotine
  harmful use Z72.0
  heart — *see* Tobacco, toxic effect
  maternal use, affecting newborn P04.2
  toxic effect — *see* Table of Drugs and Chemicals, by substance, poisoning
    chewing tobacco — *see* Table of Drugs and Chemicals, by substance, poisoning
    cigarettes — *see* Table of Drugs and Chemicals, by substance, poisoning
  use Z72.0
    complicating
      childbirth O99.334
      pregnancy O99.33- ☑
      puerperium O99.335
    counseling and surveillance Z71.6
    history Z87.891

**Tobacco** — continued
  withdrawal state (see also Dependence, drug, nicotine)
      F17.203
**Tocopherol deficiency** E56.0
**Todd's**
  cirrhosis K74.3
  paralysis (postepileptic) (transitory) G83.84
**Toe** — see condition
**Toilet, artificial opening** — see Attention to, artificial,
      opening
**Tokelau** (ringworm) B35.5
**Tollwut** — see Rabies
**Tommaselli's disease** R31.9
  correct substance properly administered — see Table
      of Drugs and Chemicals, by drug, adverse effect
  overdose or wrong substance given or taken — see
      Table of Drugs and Chemicals, by drug, poison-
      ing
**Tongue** (see also condition)
  tie Q38.1
**Tonic pupil** — see Anomaly, pupil, function, tonic pupil
**Toni-Fanconi syndrome** (cystinosis) E72.09
  with cystinosis E72.04
**Tonsil** — see condition
**Tonsillitis** (acute) (catarrhal) (croupous) (follicular)
      (gangrenous) (infective) (lacunar) (lingual) (malig-
      nant) (membranous) (parenchymatous) (phleg-
      monous) (pseudomembranous) (purulent) (septic)
      (subacute) (suppurative) (toxic) (ulcerative) (vesicu-
      lar) (viral) J03.90
  chronic J35.01
      with adenoiditis J35.03
  diphtheritic A36.0
  hypertrophic J35.01
      with adenoiditis J35.03
  recurrent J03.91
  specified organism NEC J03.80
      recurrent J03.81
  staphylococcal J03.80
      recurrent J03.81
  streptococcal J03.00
      recurrent J03.01
  tuberculous A15.8
  Vincent's A69.1
**Tooth, teeth** — see condition
**Toothache** K08.89
**Topagnosis** R20.8
**Tophi** — see Gout, chronic
**TORCH infection** — see Infection, congenital
  without active infection P00.2
**Torn** — see Tear
**Tornwaldt's cyst or disease** J39.2
**Torsion**
  accessory tube — see Torsion, fallopian tube
  adnexa (female) — see Torsion, fallopian tube
  aorta, acquired I77.1
  appendix epididymis N44.04
  appendix testis N44.03
  bile duct (common) (hepatic) K83.8
      congenital Q44.5
  bowel, colon or intestine K56.2
  cervix — see Malposition, uterus
  cystic duct K82.8
  dystonia — see Dystonia, torsion
  epididymis (appendix) N44.04
  fallopian tube N83.52- ✔
      with ovary N83.53
  gallbladder K82.8
      congenital Q44.1
  hydatid of Morgagni
      female N83.52- ✔
      male N44.03
  kidney (pedicle) (leading to infarction) N28.0
  Meckel's diverticulum (congenital) Q43.0
      malignant — see Table of Neoplasms, small intes-
          tine, malignant
  mesentery K56.2
  omentum K56.2
  organ or site, congenital NEC — see Anomaly, by site
  ovary (pedicle) N83.51- ✔
      with fallopian tube N83.53
      congenital Q50.2
  oviduct — see Torsion, fallopian tube
  penis (acquired) N48.82
      congenital Q55.63
  spasm — see Dystonia, torsion
  spermatic cord N44.02
      extravaginal N44.01

**Torsion** — continued
  spermatic cord — continued
      intravaginal N44.02
  spleen D73.5
  testis, testicle N44.00
      appendix N44.03
  tibia — see Deformity, limb, specified type NEC, lower
      leg
  uterus — see Malposition, uterus
**Torticollis** (intermittent) (spastic) M43.6
  congenital (sternomastoid) Q68.0
  due to birth injury P15.8
  hysterical F44.4
  ocular R29.891
  psychogenic F45.8
      conversion reaction F44.4
  rheumatic M43.6
  rheumatoid M06.88
  spasmodic G24.3
  traumatic, current S13.4 ✔
**Tortipelvis** G24.1
**Tortuous**
  aortic arch Q25.46
  artery I77.1
  organ or site, congenital NEC — see Distortion
  retinal vessel, congenital Q14.1
  ureter N13.8
  urethra N36.8
  vein — see Varix
**Torture, victim of** Z65.4
**Torula, torular** (histolytica) (infection) — see Cryptococ-
      cosis
**Torulosis** — see Cryptococcosis
**Torus** (mandibularis) (palatinus) M27.0
  fracture — see Fracture, by site, torus
**Touraine's syndrome** Q79.8
**Tourette's syndrome** F95.2
**Tourniquet syndrome** — see Constriction, external, by
      site
**Tower skull** Q75.0
  with exophthalmos Q87.0
**Toxemia** R68.89
  bacterial — see Sepsis
  burn — see Burn
  eclamptic (with pre-existing hypertension) — see
      Eclampsia
  erysipelatous — see Erysipelas
  fatigue R68.89
  food — see Poisoning, food
  gastrointestinal K52.1
  intestinal K52.1
  kidney — see Uremia
  malarial — see Malaria
  myocardial — see Myocarditis, toxic
  of pregnancy — see Pre-eclampsia
  pre-eclamptic — see Pre-eclampsia
  small intestine K52.1
  staphylococcal, due to food A05.0
  stasis R68.89
  uremic — see Uremia
  urinary — see Uremia
**Toxemica cerebropathia psychica** (nonalcoholic) F04
  alcoholic — see Alcohol, amnestic disorder
**Toxic** (poisoning) (see also condition) T65.91 ✔
  effect — see Table of Drugs and Chemicals, by sub-
      stance, poisoning
  shock syndrome A48.3
  thyroid (gland) — see Thyrotoxicosis
**Toxicemia** — see Toxemia
**Toxicity** — see Table of Drugs and Chemicals, by sub-
      stance, poisoning
  fava bean D55.0
  food, noxious — see Poisoning, food
  from drug or nonmedicinal substance — see Table of
      Drugs and Chemicals, by drug
**Toxicosis** (see also Toxemia)
  capillary, hemorrhagic D69.0
**Toxinfection, gastrointestinal** K52.1
**Toxocariasis** B83.0
**Toxoplasma, toxoplasmosis** (acquired) B58.9
  with
      hepatitis B58.1
      meningoencephalitis B58.2
      ocular involvement B58.00
      other organ involvement B58.89
      pneumonia, pneumonitis B58.3
  congenital (acute) (subacute) (chronic) P37.1

**Toxoplasma, toxoplasmosis** — continued
  maternal, manifest toxoplasmosis in infant (acute)
      (subacute) (chronic) P37.1
**tPA** (rtPA) **administation in a different facility within
      the last 24 hours prior to admission to current
      facility** Z92.82
**Trabeculation, bladder** N32.89
**Trachea** — see condition
**Tracheitis** (catarrhal) (infantile) (membranous) (plastic)
      (septal) (suppurative) (viral) J04.10
  with
      bronchitis (15 years of age and above) J40
          acute or subacute — see Bronchitis, acute
          chronic J42
          tuberculous NEC A15.5
          under 15 years of age J20.9
      laryngitis (acute) J04.2
          chronic J37.1
          tuberculous NEC A15.5
  acute J04.10
      with obstruction J04.11
  chronic J42
      with
          bronchitis (chronic) J42
          laryngitis (chronic) J37.1
  diphtheritic (membranous) A36.89
  due to external agent — see Inflammation, respiratory,
      upper, due to
  syphilitic A52.73
  tuberculous A15.5
**Trachelitis** (nonvenereal) — see Cervicitis
**Tracheobronchial** — see condition
**Tracheobronchitis** (15 years of age and above) (see also
      Bronchitis)
  due to
      Bordetella bronchiseptica A37.80
          with pneumonia A37.81
      Francisella tularensis A21.8
**Tracheobronchomegaly** Q32.4
  with bronchiectasis J47.9
      with
          exacerbation (acute) J47.1
          lower respiratory infection J47.0
  acquired J98.09
      with bronchiectasis J47.9
          with
              exacerbation (acute) J47.1
              lower respiratory infection J47.0
**Tracheobronchopneumonitis** — see Pneumonia,
      broncho-
**Tracheocele** (external) (internal) J39.8
  congenital Q32.1
**Tracheomalacia** J39.8
  congenital Q32.0
**Tracheopharyngitis** (acute) J06.9
  chronic J42
  due to external agent — see Inflammation, respiratory,
      upper, due to
**Tracheostenosis** J39.8
**Tracheostomy**
  complication — see Complication, tracheostomy
  status Z93.0
      attention to Z43.0
      malfunctioning J95.03
**Trachoma, trachomatous** A71.9
  active (stage) A71.1
  contraction of conjunctiva A71.1
  dubium A71.0
  healed or sequelae B94.0
  initial (stage) A71.0
  pannus A71.1
  Türck's J37.0
**Traction, vitreomacular** H43.82- ✔
**Train sickness** T75.3 ✔
**Trait**(s)
  Hb-S D57.3
  hemoglobin
      abnormal NEC D58.2
          with thalassemia D56.3
      C — see Disease, hemoglobin C
      S (Hb-S) D57.3
  Lepore D56.3
  personality, accentuated Z73.1
  sickle-cell D57.3
      with elliptocytosis or spherocytosis D57.3
  type A personality Z73.1
**Tramp** Z59.0
**Trance** R41.89

**Trance** — *continued*
  hysterical F44.89
**Transaminasemia** R74.0
**Transection**
  abdomen (partial) S38.3 ☑
  aorta (incomplete) (*see also* Injury, aorta)
    complete — *see* Injury, aorta, laceration, major
  carotid artery (incomplete) (*see also* Injury, blood
    vessel, carotid, laceration)
    complete — *see* Injury, blood vessel, carotid, lacer-
      ation, major
  celiac artery (incomplete) S35.211 ☑
    branch (incomplete) S35.291 ☑
      complete S35.292 ☑
    complete S35.212 ☑
  innominate
    artery (incomplete) (*see also* Injury, blood vessel,
      thoracic, innominate, artery, laceration)
      complete — *see* Injury, blood vessel, thoracic,
        innominate, artery, laceration, major
    vein (incomplete) (*see also* Injury, blood vessel,
      thoracic, innominate, vein, laceration)
      complete — *see* Injury, blood vessel, thoracic,
        innominate, vein, laceration, major
  jugular vein (external) (incomplete) (*see also* Injury,
    blood vessel, jugular vein, laceration)
    complete — *see* Injury, blood vessel, jugular vein,
      laceration, major
    internal (incomplete) (*see also* Injury, blood vessel,
      jugular vein, internal, laceration)
      complete — *see* Injury, blood vessel, jugular
        vein, internal, laceration, major
  mesenteric artery (incomplete) (*see also* Injury,
    mesenteric, artery, laceration)
    complete — *see* Injury, mesenteric artery, lacera-
      tion, major
  pulmonary vessel (incomplete) (*see also* Injury, blood
    vessel, thoracic, pulmonary, laceration)
    complete — *see* Injury, blood vessel, thoracic,
      pulmonary, laceration, major
  subclavian — *see* Transection, innominate
  vena cava (incomplete) (*see also* Injury, vena cava)
    complete — *see* Injury, vena cava, laceration, major
  vertebral artery (incomplete) (*see also* Injury, blood
    vessel, vertebral, laceration)
    complete — *see* Injury, blood vessel, vertebral,
      laceration, major
**Transfusion**
  associated (red blood cell) hemochromatosis E83.111
  blood
    ABO incompatible — *see* Complication(s), transfu-
      sion, incompatibility reaction, ABO
    minor blood group (Duffy) (E) (K(ell)) (Kidd) (Lewis)
      (M) (N) (P) (S) T80.89 ☑
    reaction or complication — *see* Complications,
      transfusion
  fetomaternal (mother) — *see* Pregnancy, complicated
    by, placenta, transfusion syndrome
  maternofetal (mother) — *see* Pregnancy, complicated
    by, placenta, transfusion syndrome
  placental (syndrome) (mother) — *see* Pregnancy,
    complicated by, placenta, transfusion syndrome
  reaction (adverse) — *see* Complications, transfusion
  related acute lung injury (TRALI) J95.84
  twin-to-twin — *see* Pregnancy, complicated by, pla-
    centa, transfusion syndrome, fetus to fetus
**Transient** (meaning homeless) (*see also* condition) Z59.0
**Translocation**
  balanced autosomal Q95.9
    in normal individual Q95.0
  chromosomes NEC Q99.8
    balanced and insertion in normal individual Q95.0
  Down syndrome Q90.2
  trisomy
    13 Q91.6
    18 Q91.2
    21 Q90.2
**Translucency, iris** — *see* Degeneration, iris
**Transmission of chemical substances through the**
  **placenta** — *see* Absorption, chemical, through
  placenta
**Transparency, lung, unilateral** J43.0
**Transplant** (ed) (status) Z94.9
  awaiting organ Z76.82
  bone Z94.6
    marrow Z94.81
  candidate Z76.82

**Transplant** — *continued*
  complication — *see* Complication, transplant
  cornea Z94.7
  heart Z94.1
    and lung(s) Z94.3
    valve Z95.2
      prosthetic Z95.2
      specified NEC Z95.4
      xenogenic Z95.3
  intestine Z94.82
  kidney Z94.0
  liver Z94.4
  lung(s) Z94.2
    and heart Z94.3
  organ (failure) (infection) (rejection) Z94.9
    removal status Z98.85
  pancreas Z94.83
  skin Z94.5
  social Z60.3
  specified organ or tissue NEC Z94.89
  stem cells Z94.84
  tissue Z94.9
**Transplants, ovarian, endometrial** N80.1
**Transposed** — *see* Transposition
**Transposition** (congenital) (*see also* Malposition, congenital)
  abdominal viscera Q89.3
  aorta (dextra) Q20.3
  appendix Q43.8
  colon Q43.8
  corrected Q20.5
  great vessels (complete) (partial) Q20.3
  heart Q24.0
    with complete transposition of viscera Q89.3
  intestine (large) (small) Q43.8
  reversed jejunal (for bypass) (status) Z98.0
  scrotum Q55.23
  stomach Q40.2
    with general transposition of viscera Q89.3
  tooth, teeth, fully erupted M26.30
  vessels, great (complete) (partial) Q20.3
  viscera (abdominal) (thoracic) Q89.3
**Transsexualism** F64.0
**Transverse** (*see also* condition)
  arrest (deep), in labor O64.0 ☑
  lie (mother) O32.2 ☑
    causing obstructed labor O64.8 ☑
**Transvestism, transvestitism** (dual-role) F64.1
  fetishistic F65.1
**Trapped placenta** (with hemorrhage) O72.0
  without hemorrhage O73.0
**TRAPS** (tumor necrosis factor receptor associated periodic
  syndrome) M04.1
**Trauma, traumatism** (*see also* Injury)
  acoustic — *see* subcategory H83.3 ☑
  birth — *see* Birth, injury
  complicating ectopic or molar pregnancy O08.6
  during delivery O71.9
  following ectopic or molar pregnancy O08.6
  obstetric O71.9
    specified NEC O71.89
  occlusal
    primary K08.81
    secondary K08.82
**Traumatic** (*see also* condition)
  brain injury S06.9 ☑
**Treacher Collins syndrome** Q75.4
**Treitz's hernia** — *see* Hernia, abdomen, specified site
  NEC
**Trematode infestation** — *see* Infestation, fluke
**Trematodiasis** — *see* Infestation, fluke
**Trembling paralysis** — *see* Parkinsonism
**Tremor(s)** R25.1
  drug induced G25.1
  essential (benign) G25.0
  familial G25.0
  hereditary G25.0
  hysterical F44.4
  intention G25.2
  medication induced postural G25.1
  mercurial — *see* subcategory T56.1 ☑
  Parkinson's — *see* Parkinsonism
  psychogenic (conversion reaction) F44.4
  senilis R54
  specified type NEC G25.2
**Trench**
  fever A79.0
  foot — *see* Immersion, foot

**Trench** — *continued*
  mouth A69.1
**Treponema pallidum infection** — *see* Syphilis
**Treponematosis**
  due to
    T. pallidum — *see* Syphilis
    T. pertenue — *see* Yaws
**Triad**
  Hutchinson's (congenital syphilis) A50.53
  Kartagener's Q89.3
  Saint's — *see* Hernia, diaphragm
**Trichiasis** (eyelid) H02.059
  with entropion — *see* Entropion
  left H02.056
    lower H02.055
    upper H02.054
  right H02.053
    lower H02.052
    upper H02.051
**Trichinella spiralis** (infection) (infestation) B75
**Trichinellosis, trichiniasis, trichinelliasis, trichinosis**
  B75
  with muscle disorder B75 [M63.80]
    ankle B75 [M63.87-] ☑
    foot B75 [M63.87-] ☑
    forearm B75 [M63.83-] ☑
    hand B75 [M63.84-] ☑
    lower leg B75 [M63.86-] ☑
    multiple sites B75 [M63.89]
    pelvic region B75 [M63.85-] ☑
    shoulder region B75 [M63.81-] ☑
    specified site NEC B75 [M63.88]
    thigh B75 [M63.85-] ☑
    upper arm B75 [M63.82-] ☑
**Trichobezoar** T18.9 ☑
  intestine T18.3 ☑
  stomach T18.2 ☑
**Trichocephaliasis, trichocephalosis** B79
**Trichocephalus infestation** B79
**Trichoclasis** L67.8
**Trichoepithelioma** (*see also* Neoplasm, skin, benign)
  malignant — *see* Neoplasm, skin, malignant
**Trichofolliculoma** — *see* Neoplasm, skin, benign
**Tricholemmoma** — *see* Neoplasm, skin, benign
**Trichomoniasis** A59.9
  bladder A59.03
  cervix A59.09
  intestinal A07.8
  prostate A59.02
  seminal vesicles A59.09
  specified site NEC A59.8
  urethra A59.03
  urogenitalis A59.00
  vagina A59.01
  vulva A59.01
**Trichomycosis**
  axillaris A48.8
  nodosa, nodularis B36.8
**Trichonodosis** L67.8
**Trichophytid, trichophyton infection** — *see* Dermato-
  phytosis
**Trichophytobezoar** T18.9 ☑
  intestine T18.3 ☑
  stomach T18.2 ☑
**Trichophytosis** — *see* Dermatophytosis
**Trichoptilosis** L67.8
**Trichorrhexis** (nodosa) (invaginata) L67.0
**Trichosis axillaris** A48.8
**Trichosporosis nodosa** B36.2
**Trichostasis spinulosa** (congenital) Q84.1
**Trichostrongyliasis, trichostrongylosis** (small intes-
  tine) B81.2
**Trichostrongylus infection** B81.2
**Trichotillomania** F63.3
**Trichromat, trichromatopsia, anomalous** (congenital)
  H53.55
**Trichuriasis** B79
**Trichuris trichiura** (infection) (infestation) (any site) B79
**Tricuspid** (valve) — *see* condition
**Trifid** (*see also* Accessory)
  kidney (pelvis) Q63.8
  tongue Q38.3
**Trigeminal neuralgia** — *see* Neuralgia, trigeminal
**Trigeminy** R00.8
**Trigger finger** (acquired) M65.30
  congenital Q74.0
  index finger M65.32- ☑

▼ **Subterms under main terms may continue to next column or page**      ☑ **Additional Character Required — Refer to the Tabular List for Character Selection**      **313**

Trance — Trigger finger

**Trigger finger** — *continued*
little finger M65.35- ☑
middle finger M65.33- ☑
ring finger M65.34- ☑
thumb M65.31- ☑
**Trigonitis** (bladder) (chronic) (pseudomembranous)
N30.30
with hematuria N30.31
**Trigonocephaly** Q75.0
**Trilocular heart** — *see* Cor triloculare
**Trimethylaminuria** E72.52
**Tripartite placenta** O43.19- ☑
**Triphalangeal thumb** Q74.0
**Triple** (*see also* Accessory)
kidneys Q63.0
uteri Q51.818
X, female Q97.0
**Triplegia** G83.89
congenital G80.8
**Triplet** (newborn) (*see also* Newborn, triplet)
complicating pregnancy — *see* Pregnancy, triplet
**Triplication** — *see* Accessory
**Triploidy** Q92.7
**Trismus** R25.2
neonatorum A33
newborn A33
**Trisomy** (syndrome) Q92.9
13 (partial) Q91.7
meiotic nondisjunction Q91.4
mitotic nondisjunction Q91.5
mosaicism Q91.5
translocation Q91.6
18 (partial) Q91.3
meiotic nondisjunction Q91.0
mitotic nondisjunction Q91.1
mosaicism Q91.1
translocation Q91.2
20 Q92.8
21 (partial) Q90.9
meiotic nondisjunction Q90.0
mitotic nondisjunction Q90.1
mosaicism Q90.1
translocation Q90.2
22 Q92.8
autosomes Q92.9
chromosome specified NEC Q92.8
partial Q92.2
due to unbalanced translocation Q92.5
specified NEC Q92.8
whole (nonsex chromosome)
meiotic nondisjunction Q92.0
mitotic nondisjunction Q92.1
mosaicism Q92.1
due to
dicentrics — *see* Extra, marker chromosomes
extra rings — *see* Extra, marker chromosomes
isochromosomes — *see* Extra, marker chromosomes
specified NEC Q92.8
whole chromosome Q92.9
meiotic nondisjunction Q92.0
mitotic nondisjunction Q92.1
mosaicism Q92.1
partial Q92.9
specified NEC Q92.8
**Tritanomaly, tritanopia** H53.55
**Trombiculosis, trombiculiasis, trombidiosis** B88.0
**Trophedema** (congenital) (hereditary) Q82.0
**Trophoblastic disease** (*see also* Mole, hydatidiform)
O01.9
**Tropholymphedema** Q82.0
**Trophoneurosis NEC** G96.8
disseminated M34.9
**Tropical** — *see* condition
**Trouble** (*see also* Disease)
heart — *see* Disease, heart
kidney — *see* Disease, renal
nervous R45.0
sinus — *see* Sinusitis
**Trousseau's syndrome** (thrombophlebitis migrans) I82.1
**Truancy, childhood**
from school Z72.810
**Truncus**
arteriosus (persistent) Q20.0
communis Q20.0
**Trunk** — *see* condition

**Trypanosomiasis**
African B56.9
by Trypanosoma brucei
gambiense B56.0
rhodesiense B56.1
American — *see* Chagas' disease
Brazilian — *see* Chagas' disease
by Trypanosoma
brucei gambiense B56.0
brucei rhodesiense B56.1
cruzi — *see* Chagas' disease
gambiensis, Gambian B56.0
rhodesiensis, Rhodesian B56.1
South American — *see* Chagas' disease
where
African trypanosomiasis is prevalent B56.9
Chagas' disease is prevalent B57.2
**T-shaped incisors** K00.2
**Tsutsugamushi** (disease) (fever) A75.3
**Tube, tubal, tubular** — *see* condition
**Tubercle** (*see also* Tuberculosis)
brain, solitary A17.81
Darwin's Q17.8
Ghon, primary infection A15.7
**Tuberculid, tuberculide** (indurating, subcutaneous)
(lichenoid) (miliary) (papulonecrotic) (primary) (skin)
A18.4
**Tuberculoma** (*see also* Tuberculosis)
brain A17.81
meninges (cerebral) (spinal) A17.1
spinal cord A17.81
**Tuberculosis, tubercular, tuberculous** (calcification)
(calcified) (caseous) (chromogenic acid-fast bacilli)
(degeneration) (fibrocaseous) (fistula) (interstitial)
(isolated circumscribed lesions) (necrosis)
(parenchymatous) (ulcerative) A15.9
with pneumoconiosis (any condition in J60-J64) J65
abdomen (lymph gland) A18.39
abscess (respiratory) A15.9
bone A18.03
hip A18.02
knee A18.02
sacrum A18.01
specified site NEC A18.03
spinal A18.01
vertebra A18.01
brain A17.81
breast A18.89
Cowper's gland A18.15
dura (mater) (cerebral) (spinal) A17.81
epidural (cerebral) (spinal) A17.81
female pelvis A18.17
frontal sinus A15.8
genital organs NEC A18.10
genitourinary A18.10
gland (lymphatic) — *see* Tuberculosis, lymph gland
hip A18.02
intestine A18.32
ischiorectal A18.32
joint NEC A18.02
hip A18.02
knee A18.02
specified NEC A18.02
vertebral A18.01
kidney A18.11
knee A18.02
latent R76.11
lumbar (spine) A18.01
lung — *see* Tuberculosis, pulmonary
meninges (cerebral) (spinal) A17.0
muscle A18.09
perianal (fistula) A18.32
perinephritic A18.11
perirectal A18.32
rectum A18.32
retropharyngeal A15.8
sacrum A18.01
scrofulous A18.2
scrotum A18.15
skin (primary) A18.4
spinal cord A17.81
spine or vertebra (column) A18.01
subdiaphragmatic A18.31
testis A18.15
urinary A18.13
uterus A18.17
accessory sinus — *see* Tuberculosis, sinus
Addison's disease A18.7

**Tuberculosis, tubercular, tuberculous** — *continued*
adenitis — *see* Tuberculosis, lymph gland
adenoids A15.8
adenopathy — *see* Tuberculosis, lymph gland
adherent pericardium A18.84
adnexa (uteri) A18.17
adrenal (capsule) (gland) A18.7
alimentary canal A18.32
anemia A18.89
ankle (joint) (bone) A18.02
anus A18.32
apex, apical — *see* Tuberculosis, pulmonary
appendicitis, appendix A18.32
arachnoid A17.0
artery, arteritis A18.89
cerebral A18.89
arthritis (chronic) (synovial) A18.02
spine or vertebra (column) A18.01
articular — *see* Tuberculosis, joint
ascites A18.31
asthma — *see* Tuberculosis, pulmonary
axilla, axillary (gland) A18.2
bladder A18.12
bone A18.03
hip A18.02
knee A18.02
limb NEC A18.03
sacrum A18.01
spine or vertebral column A18.01
bowel (miliary) A18.32
brain A17.81
breast A18.89
broad ligament A18.17
bronchi, bronchial, bronchus A15.5
ectasia, ectasis (bronchiectasis) — *see* Tuberculosis, pulmonary
fistula A15.5
primary (progressive) A15.7
gland or node A15.4
primary (progressive) A15.7
lymph gland or node A15.4
primary (progressive) A15.7
bronchiectasis — *see* Tuberculosis, pulmonary
bronchitis A15.5
bronchopleural A15.6
bronchopneumonia, bronchopneumonic — *see* Tuberculosis, pulmonary
bronchorrhagia A15.5
bronchotracheal A15.5
bronze disease A18.7
buccal cavity A18.83
bulbourethral gland A18.15
bursa A18.09
cachexia A15.9
cardiomyopathy A18.84
caries — *see* Tuberculosis, bone
cartilage A18.02
intervertebral A18.01
catarrhal — *see* Tuberculosis, respiratory
cecum A18.32
cellulitis (primary) A18.4
cerebellum A17.81
cerebral, cerebrum A17.81
cerebrospinal A17.81
meninges A17.0
cervical (lymph gland or node) A18.2
cervicitis, cervix (uteri) A18.16
chest — *see* Tuberculosis, respiratory
chorioretinitis A18.53
choroid, choroiditis A18.53
ciliary body A18.54
colitis A18.32
collier's J65
colliquativa (primary) A18.4
colon A18.32
complex, primary A15.7
congenital P37.0
conjunctiva A18.59
connective tissue (systemic) A18.89
contact Z20.1
cornea (ulcer) A18.52
Cowper's gland A18.15
coxae A18.02
coxalgia A18.02
cul-de-sac of Douglas A18.17
curvature, spine A18.01
cutis (colliquativa) (primary) A18.4
cyst, ovary A18.18

☑ **Additional Character Required** — **Refer to the Tabular List for Character Selection**      ᵀᴿᵁᴱ **Subterms under main terms may continue to next column or page**

**Tuberculosis, tubercular, tuberculous** — *continued*

cystitis A18.12
dactylitis A18.03
diarrhea A18.32
diffuse — *see* Tuberculosis, miliary
digestive tract A18.32
disseminated — *see* Tuberculosis, miliary
duodenum A18.32
dura (mater) (cerebral) (spinal) A17.0
   abscess (cerebral) (spinal) A17.81
dysentery A18.32
ear (inner) (middle) A18.6
   bone A18.03
   external (primary) A18.4
   skin (primary) A18.4
elbow A18.02
emphysema — *see* Tuberculosis, pulmonary
empyema A15.6
encephalitis A17.82
endarteritis A18.89
endocarditis A18.84
   aortic A18.84
   mitral A18.84
   pulmonary A18.84
   tricuspid A18.84
endocrine glands NEC A18.82
endometrium A18.17
enteric, enterica, enteritis A18.32
enterocolitis A18.32
epididymis, epididymitis A18.15
epidural abscess (cerebral) (spinal) A17.81
epiglottis A15.5
episcleritis A18.51
erythema (induratum) (nodosum) (primary) A18.4
esophagus A18.83
eustachian tube A18.6
exposure (to) Z20.1
exudative — *see* Tuberculosis, pulmonary
eye A18.50
eyelid (primary) (lupus) A18.4
fallopian tube (acute) (chronic) A18.17
fascia A18.09
fauces A15.8
female pelvic inflammatory disease A18.17
finger A18.03
first infection A15.7
gallbladder A18.83
ganglion A18.09
gastritis A18.83
gastrocolic fistula A18.32
gastroenteritis A18.32
gastrointestinal tract A18.32
general, generalized — *see* Tuberculosis, miliary
genital organs A18.10
genitourinary A18.10
genu A18.02
glandula suprarenalis A18.7
glandular, general A18.2
glottis A15.5
grinder's J65
gum A18.83
hand A18.03
heart A18.84
hematogenous — *see* Tuberculosis, miliary
hemoptysis — *see* Tuberculosis, pulmonary
hemorrhage NEC — *see* Tuberculosis, pulmonary
hemothorax A15.6
hepatitis A18.83
hilar lymph nodes A15.4
   primary (progressive) A15.7
hip (joint) (disease) (bone) A18.02
hydropneumothorax A15.6
hydrothorax A15.6
hypoadrenalism A18.7
hypopharynx A15.8
ileocecal (hyperplastic) A18.32
ileocolitis A18.32
ileum A18.32
iliac spine (superior) A18.03
immunological findings only A15.7
indurativa (primary) A18.4
infantile A15.7
infection A15.9
   without clinical manifestations A15.7
infraclavicular gland A18.2
inguinal gland A18.2
inguinalis A18.2
intestine (any part) A18.32

**Tuberculosis, tubercular, tuberculous** — *continued*

iridocyclitis A18.54
iris, iritis A18.54
ischiorectal A18.32
jaw A18.03
jejunum A18.32
joint A18.02
   vertebral A18.01
keratitis (interstitial) A18.52
keratoconjunctivitis A18.52
kidney A18.11
knee (joint) A18.02
kyphosis, kyphoscoliosis A18.01
laryngitis A15.5
larynx A15.5
latent R76.11
leptomeninges, leptomeningitis (cerebral) (spinal)
   A17.0
lichenoides (primary) A18.4
linguae A18.83
lip A18.83
liver A18.83
lordosis A18.01
lung — *see* Tuberculosis, pulmonary
lupus vulgaris A18.4
lymph gland or node (peripheral) A18.2
   abdomen A18.39
   bronchial A15.4
      primary (progressive) A15.7
   cervical A18.2
   hilar A15.4
      primary (progressive) A15.7
   intrathoracic A15.4
      primary (progressive) A15.7
   mediastinal A15.4
      primary (progressive) A15.7
   mesenteric A18.39
   retroperitoneal A18.39
   tracheobronchial A15.4
      primary (progressive) A15.7
lymphadenitis — *see* Tuberculosis, lymph gland
lymphangitis — *see* Tuberculosis, lymph gland
lymphatic (gland) (vessel) — *see* Tuberculosis, lymph
   gland
mammary gland A18.89
marasmus A15.9
mastoiditis A18.03
mediastinal lymph gland or node A15.4
   primary (progressive) A15.7
mediastinitis A15.8
   primary (progressive) A15.7
mediastinum A15.8
   primary (progressive) A15.7
medulla A17.81
melanosis, Addisonian A18.7
meninges, meningitis (basilar) (cerebral) (cerebrospinal) (spinal) A17.0
meningoencephalitis A17.82
mesentery, mesenteric (gland or node) A18.39
miliary A19.9
   acute A19.2
      multiple sites A19.1
      single specified site A19.0
   chronic A19.8
   specified NEC A19.8
millstone makers' J65
miner's J65
molder's J65
mouth A18.83
multiple A19.9
   acute A19.1
   chronic A19.8
muscle A18.09
myelitis A17.82
myocardium, myocarditis A18.84
nasal (passage) (sinus) A15.8
nasopharynx A15.8
neck gland A18.2
nephritis A18.11
nerve (mononeuropathy) A17.83
nervous system A17.9
nose (septum) A15.8
ocular A18.50
omentum A18.31
oophoritis (acute) (chronic) A18.17
optic (nerve trunk) (papilla) A18.59
orbit A18.59
orchitis A18.15
organ, specified NEC A18.89

**Tuberculosis, tubercular, tuberculous** — *continued*

osseous — *see* Tuberculosis, bone
osteitis — *see* Tuberculosis, bone
osteomyelitis — *see* Tuberculosis, bone
otitis media A18.6
ovary, ovaritis (acute) (chronic) A18.17
oviduct (acute) (chronic) A18.17
pachymeningitis A17.0
palate (soft) A18.83
pancreas A18.83
papulonecrotic (a) (primary) A18.4
parathyroid glands A18.82
paronychia (primary) A18.4
parotid gland or region A18.83
pelvis (bony) A18.03
penis A18.15
peribronchitis A15.5
pericardium, pericarditis A18.84
perichondritis, larynx A15.5
periostitis — *see* Tuberculosis, bone
perirectal fistula A18.32
peritoneum NEC A18.31
peritonitis A18.31
pharynx, pharyngitis A15.8
phlyctenulosis (keratoconjunctivitis) A18.52
phthisis NEC — *see* Tuberculosis, pulmonary
pituitary gland A18.82
pleura, pleural, pleurisy, pleuritis (fibrinous) (obliterative) (purulent) (simple plastic) (with effusion)
   A15.6
   primary (progressive) A15.7
pneumonia, pneumonic — *see* Tuberculosis, pulmonary
pneumothorax (spontaneous) (tense valvular) — *see*
   Tuberculosis, pulmonary
polyneuropathy A17.89
polyserositis A19.9
   acute A19.1
   chronic A19.8
potter's J65
prepuce A18.15
primary (complex) A15.7
proctitis A18.32
prostate, prostatitis A18.14
pulmonalis — *see* Tuberculosis, pulmonary
pulmonary (cavitated) (fibrotic) (infiltrative) (nodular)
   A15.0
   childhood type or first infection A15.7
   primary (complex) A15.7
pyelitis A18.11
pyelonephritis A18.11
pyemia — *see* Tuberculosis, miliary
pyonephrosis A18.11
pyopneumothorax A15.6
pyothorax A15.6
rectum (fistula) (with abscess) A18.32
reinfection stage — *see* Tuberculosis, pulmonary
renal A18.11
renis A18.11
respiratory A15.9
   primary A15.7
   specified site NEC A15.8
retina, retinitis A18.53
retroperitoneal (lymph gland or node) A18.39
rheumatism NEC A18.09
rhinitis A15.8
sacroiliac (joint) A18.01
sacrum A18.01
salivary gland A18.83
salpingitis (acute) (chronic) A18.17
sandblaster's J65
sclera A18.51
scoliosis A18.01
scrofulous A18.2
scrotum A18.15
seminal tract or vesicle A18.15
senile A15.9
septic — *see* Tuberculosis, miliary
shoulder (joint) A18.02
   blade A18.03
sigmoid A18.32
sinus (any nasal) A15.8
   bone A18.03
   epididymis A18.15
skeletal NEC A18.03
skin (any site) (primary) A18.4
small intestine A18.32
soft palate A18.83

**Tuberculosis, tubercular, tuberculous** — *continued*
spermatic cord A18.15
spine, spinal (column) A18.Ø1
   cord A17.81
   medulla A17.81
   membrane A17.Ø
   meninges A17.Ø
spleen, splenitis A18.85
spondylitis A18.Ø1
sternoclavicular joint A18.Ø2
stomach A18.83
stonemason's J65
subcutaneous tissue (cellular) (primary) A18.4
subcutis (primary) A18.4
subdeltoid bursa A18.83
submaxillary (region) A18.83
supraclavicular gland A18.2
suprarenal (capsule) (gland) A18.7
swelling, joint (*see also* category MØ1) (*see also* Tuberculosis, joint) A18.Ø2
symphysis pubis A18.Ø2
synovitis A18.Ø9
   articular A18.Ø2
   spine or vertebra A18.Ø1
systemic — *see* Tuberculosis, miliary
tarsitis A18.4
tendon (sheath) — *see* Tuberculosis, tenosynovitis
tenosynovitis A18.Ø9
   spine or vertebra A18.Ø1
testis A18.15
throat A15.8
thymus gland A18.82
thyroid gland A18.81
tongue A18.83
tonsil, tonsillitis A15.8
trachea, tracheal A15.5
   lymph gland or node A15.4
      primary (progressive) A15.7
tracheobronchial A15.5
   lymph gland or node A15.4
      primary (progressive) A15.7
tubal (acute) (chronic) A18.17
tunica vaginalis A18.15
ulcer (skin) (primary) A18.4
   bowel or intestine A18.32
   specified NEC — *see* Tuberculosis, by site
unspecified site A15.9
ureter A18.11
urethra, urethral (gland) A18.13
urinary organ or tract A18.13
uterus A18.17
uveal tract A18.54
uvula A18.83
vagina A18.18
vas deferens A18.15
verruca, verrucosa (cutis) (primary) A18.4
vertebra (column) A18.Ø1
vesiculitis A18.15
vulva A18.18
wrist (joint) A18.Ø2
**Tuberculum**
Carabelli — *see* Excludes Note at KØØ.2
occlusal — *see* Excludes Note at KØØ.2
paramolare KØØ.2
**Tuberosity, enitre maxillary** M26.Ø7
**Tuberous sclerosis** (brain) Q85.1
**Tubo-ovarian** — *see* condition
**Tuboplasty, after previous sterilization** Z31.Ø
   aftercare Z31.42
**Tubotympanitis, catarrhal** (chronic) — *see* Otitis, media, nonsuppurative, chronic, serous
**Tularemia** A21.9
   with
      conjunctivitis A21.1
      pneumonia A21.2
   abdominal A21.3
   bronchopneumonic A21.2
   conjunctivitis A21.1
   cryptogenic A21.3
   enteric A21.3
   gastrointestinal A21.3
   generalized A21.7
   ingestion A21.3
   intestinal A21.3
   oculoglandular A21.1
   ophthalmic A21.1
   pneumonia (any), pneumonic A21.2
   pulmonary A21.2

**Tularemia** — *continued*
   sepsis A21.7
   specified NEC A21.8
   typhoidal A21.7
   ulceroglandular A21.Ø
**Tularensis conjunctivitis** A21.1
**Tumefaction** (*see also* Swelling)
liver — *see* Hypertrophy, liver
**Tumor** (*see also* Neoplasm, unspecified behavior, by site)
acinar cell — *see* Neoplasm, uncertain behavior, by site
acinic cell — *see* Neoplasm, uncertain behavior, by site
adenocarcinoid — *see* Neoplasm, malignant, by site
adenomatoid (*see also* Neoplasm, benign, by site)
   odontogenic — *see* Cyst, calcifying odontogenic
adnexal (skin) — *see* Neoplasm, skin, benign, by site
adrenal
   cortical (benign) D35.Ø- ☑
      malignant C74.Ø- ☑
   rest — *see* Neoplasm, benign, by site
alpha-cell
   malignant
      pancreas C25.4
      specified site NEC — *see* Neoplasm, malignant, by site
      unspecified site C25.4
   pancreas D13.7
   specified site NEC — *see* Neoplasm, benign, by site
   unspecified site D13.7
aneurysmal — *see* Aneurysm
aortic body D44.7
   malignant C75.5
Askin's — *see* Neoplasm, connective tissue, malignant
basal cell (*see also* Neoplasm, skin, uncertain behavior) D48.5
Bednar — *see* Neoplasm, skin, malignant
benign (unclassified) — *see* Neoplasm, benign, by site
beta-cell
   malignant
      pancreas C25.4
      specified site NEC — *see* Neoplasm, malignant, by site
      unspecified site C25.4
   pancreas D13.7
   specified site NEC — *see* Neoplasm, benign, by site
   unspecified site D13.7
Brenner D27.9
   borderline malignancy D39.1- ☑
   malignant C56- ☑
   proliferating D39.1- ☑
bronchial alveolar, intravascular D38.1
Brooke's — *see* Neoplasm, skin, benign
brown fat — *see* Lipoma
Burkitt — *see* Lymphoma, Burkitt
calcifying epithelial odontogenic — *see* Cyst, calcifying odontogenic
carcinoid
   benign D3A.ØØ (*following* D36)
      appendix D3A.Ø2Ø (*following* D36)
      ascending colon D3A.Ø22 (*following* D36)
      bronchus (lung) D3A.Ø9Ø (*following* D36)
      cecum D3A.Ø21 (*following* D36)
      colon D3A.Ø29 (*following* D36)
      descending colon D3A.Ø24 (*following* D36)
      duodenum D3A.Ø1Ø (*following* D36)
      foregut NOS D3A.Ø94 (*following* D36)
      hindgut NOS D3A.Ø96 (*following* D36)
      ileum D3A.Ø12 (*following* D36)
      jejunum D3A.Ø11 (*following* D36)
      kidney D3A.Ø93 (*following* D36)
      large intestine D3A.Ø29 (*following* D36)
      lung (bronchus) D3A.Ø9Ø (*following* D36)
      midgut NOS D3A.Ø95 (*following* D36)
      rectum D3A.Ø26 (*following* D36)
      sigmoid colon D3A.Ø25 (*following* D36)
      small intestine D3A.Ø19 (*following* D36)
      specified NEC D3A.Ø98 (*following* D36)
      stomach D3A.Ø92 (*following* D36)
      thymus D3A.Ø91 (*following* D36)
      transverse colon D3A.Ø23 (*following* D36)
   malignant C7A.ØØ (*following* C75)
      appendix C7A.Ø2Ø (*following* C75)
      ascending colon C7A.Ø22 (*following* C75)
      bronchus (lung) C7A.Ø9Ø (*following* C75)
      cecum C7A.Ø21 (*following* C75)
      colon C7A.Ø29 (*following* C75)
      descending colon C7A.Ø24 (*following* C75)

**Tumor** — *continued*
   carcinoid — *continued*
      malignant — *continued*
         duodenum C7A.Ø1Ø (*following* C75)
         foregut NOS C7A.Ø94 (*following* C75)
         hindgut NOS C7A.Ø96 (*following* C75)
         ileum C7A.Ø12 (*following* C75)
         jejunum C7A.Ø11 (*following* C75)
         kidney C7A.Ø93 (*following* C75)
         large intestine C7A.Ø29 (*following* C75)
         lung (bronchus) C7A.Ø9Ø (*following* C75)
         midgut NOS C7A.Ø95 (*following* C75)
         rectum C7A.Ø26 (*following* C75)
         sigmoid colon C7A.Ø25 (*following* C75)
         small intestine C7A.Ø19 (*following* C75)
         specified NEC C7A.Ø98 (*following* C75)
         stomach C7A.Ø92 (*following* C75)
         thymus C7A.Ø91 (*following* C75)
         transverse colon C7A.Ø23 (*following* C75)
      mesentery metastasis C7B.Ø4 (*following* C75)
      secondary C7B.ØØ (*following* C75)
         bone C7B.Ø3 (*following* C75)
         distant lymph nodes C7B.Ø1 (*following* C75)
         liver C7B.Ø2 (*following* C75)
         peritoneum C7B.Ø4 (*following* C75)
         specified NEC C7B.Ø9 (*following* C75)
   carotid body D44.6
      malignant C75.4
   cells (*see also* Neoplasm, unspecified behavior, by site)
      benign — *see* Neoplasm, benign, by site
      malignant — *see* Neoplasm, malignant, by site
      uncertain whether benign or malignant — *see* Neoplasm, uncertain behavior, by site
   cervix, in pregnancy or childbirth — *see* Pregnancy, complicated by, tumor, cervix
   chondromatous giant cell — *see* Neoplasm, bone, benign
   chromaffin (*see also* Neoplasm, benign, by site)
      malignant — *see* Neoplasm, malignant, by site
   Cock's peculiar L72.3
   Codman's — *see* Neoplasm, bone, benign
   dentigerous, mixed — *see* Cyst, calcifying odontogenic
   dermoid — *see* Neoplasm, benign, by site
      with malignant transformation C56- ☑
   desmoid (extra-abdominal) (*see also* Neoplasm, connective tissue, uncertain behavior)
      abdominal — *see* Neoplasm, connective tissue, uncertain behavior
   embolus — *see* Neoplasm, secondary, by site
   embryonal (mixed) (*see also* Neoplasm, uncertain behavior, by site)
      liver C22.7
   endodermal sinus
      specified site — *see* Neoplasm, malignant, by site
      unspecified site
         female C56.- ☑
         male C62.9Ø
   epithelial
      benign — *see* Neoplasm, benign, by site
      malignant — *see* Neoplasm, malignant, by site
   Ewing's — *see* Neoplasm, bone, malignant, by site
   fatty — *see* Lipoma
   fibroid — *see* Leiomyoma
   G cell
      malignant
         pancreas C25.4
         specified site NEC — *see* Neoplasm, malignant, by site
         unspecified site C25.4
      specified site — *see* Neoplasm, uncertain behavior, by site
      unspecified site D37.8
   germ cell (*see also* Neoplasm, malignant, by site)
      mixed — *see* Neoplasm, malignant, by site
   ghost cell, odontogenic — *see* Cyst, calcifying odontogenic
   giant cell (*see also* Neoplasm, uncertain behavior, by site)
      bone D48.Ø
         malignant — *see* Neoplasm, bone, malignant
      chondromatous — *see* Neoplasm, bone, benign
      malignant — *see* Neoplasm, malignant, by site
      soft parts — *see* Neoplasm, connective tissue, uncertain behavior
         malignant — *see* Neoplasm, connective tissue, malignant
   glomus D18.ØØ
      intra-abdominal D18.Ø3

**Tumor** — *continued*
  glomus — *continued*
    intracranial D18.02
    jugulare D44.7
      malignant C75.5
    skin D18.01
    specified site NEC D18.09
  gonadal stromal — *see* Neoplasm, uncertain behavior, by site
  granular cell (*see also* Neoplasm, connective tissue, benign)
    malignant — *see* Neoplasm, connective tissue, malignant
  granulosa cell D39.1- ☑
    juvenile D39.1- ☑
    malignant C56- ☑
  granulosa cell-theca cell D39.1- ☑
    malignant C56- ☑
  Grawitz's C64- ☑
  hemorrhoidal — *see* Hemorrhoids
  hilar cell D27- ☑
  hilus cell D27- ☑
  Hurthle cell (benign) D34
    malignant C73
  hydatid — *see* Echinococcus
  hypernephroid (*see also* Neoplasm, uncertain behavior, by site)
  interstitial cell (*see also* Neoplasm, uncertain behavior, by site)
    benign — *see* Neoplasm, benign, by site
    malignant — *see* Neoplasm, malignant, by site
  intravascular bronchial alveolar D38.1
  islet cell — *see* Neoplasm, benign, by site
    malignant — *see* Neoplasm, malignant, by site
      pancreas C25.4
      specified site NEC — *see* Neoplasm, malignant, by site
      unspecified site C25.4
    pancreas D13.7
    specified site NEC — *see* Neoplasm, benign, by site
    unspecified site D13.7
  juxtaglomerular D41.0- ☑
  Klatskin's C22.1
  Krukenberg's C79.6- ☑
  Leydig cell — *see* Neoplasm, uncertain behavior, by site
    benign — *see* Neoplasm, benign, by site
      specified site — *see* Neoplasm, benign, by site
      unspecified site
        female D27.9
        male D29.20
    malignant — *see* Neoplasm, malignant, by site
      specified site — *see* Neoplasm, malignant, by site
      unspecified site
        female C56.9
        male C62.90
    specified site — *see* Neoplasm, uncertain behavior, by site
    unspecified site
      female D39.10
      male D40.10
  lipid cell, ovary D27- ☑
  lipoid cell, ovary D27- ☑
  malignant (*see also* Neoplasm, malignant, by site) C80.1
    fusiform cell (type) C80.1
    giant cell (type) C80.1
    localized, plasma cell — *see* Plasmacytoma, solitary
    mixed NEC C80.1
    small cell (type) C80.1
    spindle cell (type) C80.1
    unclassified C80.1
  mast cell D47.09
  melanotic, neuroectodermal — *see* Neoplasm, benign, by site
  Merkel cell — *see* Carcinoma, Merkel cell
  mesenchymal
    malignant — *see* Neoplasm, connective tissue, malignant
    mixed — *see* Neoplasm, connective tissue, uncertain behavior
  mesodermal, mixed (*see also* Neoplasm, malignant, by site)
    liver C22.4

**Tumor** — *continued*
  mesonephric (*see also* Neoplasm, uncertain behavior, by site)
    malignant — *see* Neoplasm, malignant, by site
  metastatic
    from specified site — *see* Neoplasm, malignant, by site
    of specified site — *see* Neoplasm, malignant, by site
    to specified site — *see* Neoplasm, secondary, by site
  mixed NEC (*see also* Neoplasm, benign, by site)
    malignant — *see* Neoplasm, malignant, by site
  mucinous of low malignant potential
    specified site — *see* Neoplasm, malignant, by site
    unspecified site C56.9
  mucocarcinoid
    specified site — *see* Neoplasm, malignant, by site
    unspecified site C18.1
  mucoepidermoid — *see* Neoplasm, uncertain behavior, by site
  Müllerian, mixed
    specified site — *see* Neoplasm, malignant, by site
    unspecified site C54.9
  myoepithelial — *see* Neoplasm, benign, by site
  neuroectodermal (peripheral) — *see* Neoplasm, malignant, by site
    primitive
      specified site — *see* Neoplasm, malignant, by site
      unspecified site C71.9
  neuroendocrine D3A.8 (*following* D36)
    malignant poorly differentiated C7A.1 (*following* C75)
    secondary NEC C7B.8 (*following* C75)
    specified NEC C7A.8 (*following* C75)
  neurogenic olfactory C30.0
  nonencapsulated sclerosing C73
  odontogenic (adenomatoid) (benign) (calcifying epithelial) (keratocystic) (squamous) — *see* Cyst, calcifying odontogenic
    malignant C41.1
      upper jaw (bone) C41.0
  ovarian stromal D39.1- ☑
  ovary, in pregnancy — *see* Pregnancy, complicated by
  pacinian — *see* Neoplasm, skin, benign
  Pancoast's — *see* Pancoast's syndrome
  papillary (*see also* Papilloma)
    cystic D37.9
    mucinous of low malignant potential C56- ☑
      specified site — *see* Neoplasm, malignant, by site
      unspecified site C56.9
    serous of low malignant potential
      specified site — *see* Neoplasm, malignant, by site
      unspecified site C56.9
  pelvic, in pregnancy or childbirth — *see* Pregnancy, complicated by
  phantom F45.8
  phyllodes D48.6- ☑
    benign D24- ☑
    malignant — *see* Neoplasm, breast, malignant
  Pindborg — *see* Cyst, calcifying odontogenic
  placental site trophoblastic D39.2
  plasma cell (malignant) (localized) — *see* Plasmacytoma, solitary
  polyvesicular vitelline
    specified site — *see* Neoplasm, malignant, by site
    unspecified site
      female C56.9
      male C62.90
  Pott's puffy — *see* Osteomyelitis, specified NEC
  Rathke's pouch D44.3
  retinal anlage — *see* Neoplasm, benign, by site
  salivary gland type, mixed — *see* Neoplasm, salivary gland, benign
    malignant — *see* Neoplasm, salivary gland, malignant
  Sampson's N80.1
  Schmincke's — *see* Neoplasm, nasopharynx, malignant
  sclerosing stromal D27- ☑
  sebaceous — *see* Cyst, sebaceous
  secondary — *see* Neoplasm, secondary, by site
    carcinoid C7B.00 (*following* C75)
      bone C7B.03 (*following* C75)
      distant lymph nodes C7B.01 (*following* C75)

**Tumor** — *continued*
  secondary — *see* Neoplasm, secondary, by site — *continued*
    carcinoid — *continued*
      liver C7B.02 (*following* C75)
      peritoneum C7B.04 (*following* C75)
      specified NEC C7B.09 (*following* C75)
    neuroendocrine NEC C7B.8 (*following* C75)
  serous of low malignant potential
    specified site — *see* Neoplasm, malignant, by site
    unspecified site C56.9
  Sertoli cell — *see* Neoplasm, benign, by site
    with lipid storage
      specified site — *see* Neoplasm, benign, by site
      unspecified site
        female D27.9
        male D29.20
    specified site — *see* Neoplasm, benign, by site
    unspecified site
      female D27.9
      male D29.20
  Sertoli-Leydig cell — *see* Neoplasm, benign, by site
    specified site — *see* Neoplasm, benign, by site
    unspecified site
      female D27.9
      male D29.20
  sex cord (-stromal) — *see* Neoplasm, uncertain behavior, by site
    with annular tubules D39.1- ☑
  skin appendage — *see* Neoplasm, skin, benign
  smooth muscle — *see* Neoplasm, connective tissue, uncertain behavior
  soft tissue
    benign — *see* Neoplasm, connective tissue, benign
    malignant — *see* Neoplasm, connective tissue, malignant
  sternomastoid (congenital) Q68.0
  stromal
    endometrial D39.0
    gastric D48.1
      benign D21.4
      malignant C16.9
      uncertain behavior D48.1
    gastrointestinal C49.A- ☑
      benign D21.4
      esophagus C49.A1
      malignant C49.A0
        colon C49.A4
        duodenum C49.A3
        esophagus C49.A1
        ileum C49.A3
        jejunum C49.A3
        large intestine C49.A4
        Meckel diverticulum C49.A3
        omentum C49.A9
        peritoneum C49.A9
        rectum C49.A5
        small intestine C49.A3
        specified site NEC C49.A9
        stomach C49.A2
      rectum C49.A5
      small intestine C49.A3
      specified site NEC C49.A9
      stomach C49.A2
      uncertain behavior D48.1
    intestine
      benign D21.4
      malignant
        large C49.A4
        small C49.A3
      uncertain behavior D48.1
    ovarian D39.1- ☑
    stomach C49.A2
      benign D21.4
      malignant C49.A2
      uncertain behavior D48.1
  sweat gland (*see also* Neoplasm, skin, uncertain behavior)
    benign — *see* Neoplasm, skin, benign
    malignant — *see* Neoplasm, skin, malignant
  syphilitic, brain A52.17
  testicular D40.10
  testicular stromal D40.1- ☑
  theca cell D27.- ☑
  theca cell-granulosa cell D39.1- ☑
  Triton, malignant — *see* Neoplasm, nerve, malignant
  trophoblastic, placental site D39.2
  turban D23.4

**Tumor** — *continued*
  uterus (body), in pregnancy or childbirth — *see* Pregnancy, complicated by, tumor, uterus
  vagina, in pregnancy or childbirth — *see* Pregnancy, complicated by
  varicose — *see* Varix
  von Recklinghausen's — *see* Neurofibromatosis
  vulva or perineum, in pregnancy or childbirth — *see* Pregnancy, complicated by
    causing obstructed labor O65.5
  Warthin's — *see* Neoplasm, salivary gland, benign
  Wilms' C64- ☑
  yolk sac — *see* Neoplasm, malignant, by site
    specified site — *see* Neoplasm, malignant, by site
    unspecified site
      female C56.9
      male C62.90
**Tumor lysis syndrome** (following antineoplastic chemotherapy) (spontaneous) NEC E88.3
**Tumorlet** — *see* Neoplasm, uncertain behavior, by site
**Tungiasis** B88.1
**Tunica vasculosa lentis** Q12.2
**Turban tumor** D23.4
**Türck's trachoma** J37.0
**Turner-Kieser syndrome** Q87.2
**Turner-like syndrome** Q87.1
**Turner's**
  hypoplasia (tooth) K00.4
  syndrome Q96.9
    specified NEC Q96.8
  tooth K00.4
**Turner-Ullrich syndrome** Q96.9
**Tussis convulsiva** — *see* Whooping cough
**Twiddler's syndrome** (due to)
  automatic implantable defibrillator T82.198
  cardiac pacemaker T82.198 ☑
**Twilight state**
  epileptic F05
  psychogenic F44.89
**Twin** (newborn) (*see also* Newborn, twin)
  conjoined Q89.4
  pregnancy — *see* Pregnancy, twin
**Twinning, teeth** K00.2
**Twist, twisted**
  bowel, colon or intestine K56.2
  hair (congenital) Q84.1
  mesentery K56.2
  omentum K56.2
  organ or site, congenital NEC — *see* Anomaly, by site
  ovarian pedicle — *see* Torsion, ovary
**Twitching** R25.3
**Tylosis** (acquired) L84
  buccalis K13.29
  linguae K13.29
  palmaris et plantaris (congenital) (inherited) Q82.8
    acquired L85.1
**Tympanism** R14.0
**Tympanites** (abdominal) (intestinal) R14.0
**Tympanitis** — *see* Myringitis
**Tympanosclerosis** H74.0 ☑
**Tympanum** — *see* condition
**Tympany**
  abdomen R14.0
  chest R09.89
**Type A behavior pattern** Z73.1
**Typhlitis** — *see* Appendicitis
**Typhoenteritis** — *see* Typhoid
**Typhoid** (abortive) (ambulant) (any site) (clinical) (fever) (hemorrhagic) (infection) (intermittent) (malignant) (rheumatic) (Widal negative) A01.00
  with pneumonia A01.03
  abdominal A01.09
  arthritis A01.04
  carrier (suspected) of Z22.0
  cholecystitis (current) A01.09
  endocarditis A01.02
  heart involvement A01.02
  inoculation reaction — *see* Complications, vaccination
  meningitis A01.01
  mesenteric lymph nodes A01.09
  myocarditis A01.02
  osteomyelitis A01.05
  perichondritis, larynx A01.09
  pneumonia A01.03
  specified NEC A01.09
  spine A01.05
  ulcer (perforating) A01.09

**Typhomalaria** (fever) — *see* Malaria
**Typhomania** A01.00
**Typhoperitonitis** A01.09
**Typhus** (fever) A75.9
  abdominal, abdominalis — *see* Typhoid
  African tick A77.1
  amarillic A95.9
  brain A75.9 [G94]
  cerebral A75.9 [G94]
  classical A75.0
  due to Rickettsia
    prowazekii A75.0
      recrudescent A75.1
    tsutsugamushi A75.3
    typhi A75.2
  endemic (flea-borne) A75.2
  epidemic (louse-borne) A75.0
  exanthematicus SAI A75.0
    brillii SAI A75.1
    mexicanus SAI A75.2
    typhus murinus A75.2
  exanthematic NEC A75.0
  flea-borne A75.2
  India tick A77.1
  Kenya (tick) A77.1
  louse-borne A75.0
  Mexican A75.2
  mite-borne A75.3
  murine A75.2
  North Asian tick-borne A77.2
  petechial A75.9
  Queensland tick A77.3
  rat A75.2
  recrudescent A75.1
  recurrens — *see* Fever, relapsing
  Sao Paulo A77.0
  scrub (China) (India) (Malaysia) (New Guinea) A75.3
  shop (of Malaysia) A75.2
  Siberian tick A77.2
  tick-borne A77.9
  tropical (mite-borne) A75.3
**Tyrosinemia** E70.21
  newborn, transitory P74.5
**Tyrosinosis** E70.21
**Tyrosinuria** E70.29

# U

**Uhl's anomaly or disease** Q24.8
**Ulcer, ulcerated, ulcerating, ulceration, ulcerative**
  alveolar process M27.3
  amebic (intestine) A06.1
    skin A06.7
  anastomotic — *see* Ulcer, gastrojejunal
  anorectal K62.6
  antral — *see* Ulcer, stomach
  anus (sphincter) (solitary) K62.6
  aorta — *see* Aneurysm
  aphthous (oral) (recurrent) K12.0
    genital organ(s)
      female N76.6
      male N50.89
  artery I77.2
  atrophic — *see* Ulcer, skin
    decubitus — *see* Ulcer, pressure, by site
  back L98.429
    with
      bone involvement without evidence of necrosis L98.426
      bone necrosis L98.424
      exposed fat layer L98.422
      muscle involvement without evidence of necrosis L98.425
      muscle necrosis L98.423
      skin breakdown only L98.421
      specified severity NEC L98.428
  Barrett's (esophagus) K22.10
    with bleeding K22.11
  bile duct (common) (hepatic) K83.8
  bladder (solitary) (sphincter) NEC N32.89
    bilharzial B65.9 [N33]
    in schistosomiasis (bilharzial) B65.9 [N33]
    submucosal — *see* Cystitis, interstitial
    tuberculous A18.12
  bleeding K27.4
  bone — *see* Osteomyelitis, specified type NEC
  bowel — *see* Ulcer, intestine
  breast N61.1

**Ulcer, ulcerated, ulcerating, ulceration, ulcerative**
  — *continued*
  bronchus J98.09
  buccal (cavity) (traumatic) K12.1
  Buruli A31.1
  buttock L98.419
    with
      bone involvement without evidence of necrosis L98.416
      bone necrosis L98.414
      exposed fat layer L98.412
      muscle involvement without evidence of necrosis L98.415
      muscle necrosis L98.413
      skin breakdown only L98.411
      specified severity NEC L98.418
  cancerous — *see* Neoplasm, malignant, by site
  cardia K22.10
    with bleeding K22.11
  cardioesophageal (peptic) K22.10
    with bleeding K22.11
  cecum — *see* Ulcer, intestine
  cervix (uteri) (decubitus) (trophic) N86
    with cervicitis N72
  chancroidal A57
  chiclero B55.1
  chronic (cause unknown) — *see* Ulcer, skin
  Cochin-China B55.1
  colon — *see* Ulcer, intestine
  conjunctiva H10.89
  cornea H16.00- ☑
    with hypopyon H16.03- ☑
    central H16.01- ☑
    dendritic (herpes simplex) B00.52
    marginal H16.04- ☑
    Mooren's H16.05- ☑
    mycotic H16.06- ☑
    perforated H16.07- ☑
    ring H16.02- ☑
    tuberculous (phlyctenular) A18.52
  corpus cavernosum (chronic) N48.5
  crural — *see* Ulcer, lower limb
  Curling's — *see* Ulcer, peptic, acute
  Cushing's — *see* Ulcer, peptic, acute
  cystic duct K82.8
  cystitis (interstitial) — *see* Cystitis, interstitial
  decubitus — *see* Ulcer, pressure, by site
  dendritic, cornea (herpes simplex) B00.52
  diabetes, diabetic — *see* Diabetes, ulcer
  Dieulafoy's K25.0
  due to
    infection NEC — *see* Ulcer, skin
    radiation NEC L59.8
    trophic disturbance (any region) — *see* Ulcer, skin
    X-ray L58.1
  duodenum, duodenal (eroded) (peptic) K26.9
    with
      hemorrhage K26.4
        and perforation K26.6
      perforation K26.5
    acute K26.3
      with
        hemorrhage K26.0
          and perforation K26.2
        perforation K26.1
    chronic K26.7
      with
        hemorrhage K26.4
          and perforation K26.6
        perforation K26.5
  dysenteric A09
  elusive — *see* Cystitis, interstitial
  endocarditis (acute) (chronic) (subacute) I28.8
  epiglottis J38.7
  esophagus (peptic) K22.10
    with bleeding K22.11
    due to
      aspirin K22.10
        with bleeding K22.11
      gastrointestinal reflux disease K21.0
      ingestion of chemical or medicament K22.10
        with bleeding K22.11
      fungal K22.10
        with bleeding K22.11
      infective K22.10
        with bleeding K22.11
    varicose — *see* Varix, esophagus
  eyelid (region) H01.8

**Ulcer, ulcerated, ulcerating, ulceration, ulcerative**
— continued
fauces J39.2
Fenwick (-Hunner) (solitary) — see Cystitis, interstitial
fistulous — see Ulcer, skin
foot (indolent) (trophic) — see Ulcer, lower limb
frambesial, initial A66.0
frenum (tongue) K14.0
gallbladder or duct K82.8
gangrenous — see Gangrene
gastric — see Ulcer, stomach
gastrocolic — see Ulcer, gastrojejunal
gastroduodenal — see Ulcer, peptic
gastroesophageal — see Ulcer, stomach
gastrointestinal — see Ulcer, gastrojejunal
gastrojejunal (peptic) K28.9
  with
    hemorrhage K28.4
      and perforation K28.6
      perforation K28.5
  acute K28.3
    with
      hemorrhage K28.0
        and perforation K28.2
        perforation K28.1
  chronic K28.7
    with
      hemorrhage K28.4
        and perforation K28.6
      perforation K28.5
gastrojejunocolic — see Ulcer, gastrojejunal
gingiva K06.8
gingivitis K05.10
  nonplaque induced K05.11
  plaque induced K05.10
glottis J38.7
granuloma of pudenda A58
gum K06.8
gumma, due to yaws A66.4
heel — see Ulcer, lower limb
hemorrhoid (see also Hemorrhoids, by degree) K64.8
Hunner's — see Cystitis, interstitial
hypopharynx J39.2
hypopyon (chronic) (subacute) — see Ulcer, cornea, with hypopyon
hypostaticum — see Ulcer, varicose
ileum — see Ulcer, intestine
intestine, intestinal K63.3
  with perforation K63.1
  amebic A06.1
  duodenal — see Ulcer, duodenum
  granulocytopenic (with hemorrhage) — see Neutropenia
  marginal — see Ulcer, gastrojejunal
  perforating K63.1
    newborn P78.0
  primary, small intestine K63.3
  rectum K62.6
  stercoraceous, stercoral K63.3
  tuberculous A18.32
  typhoid (fever) — see Typhoid
  varicose I86.8
jejunum, jejunal — see Ulcer, gastrojejunal
keratitis — see Ulcer, cornea
knee — see Ulcer, lower limb
labium (majus) (minus) N76.6
laryngitis — see Laryngitis
larynx (aphthous) (contact) J38.7
  diphtheritic A36.2
leg — see Ulcer, lower limb
lip K13.0
Lipschütz's N76.6
lower limb (atrophic) (chronic) (neurogenic) (perforating) (pyogenic) (trophic) (tropical) L97.909
  with
    bone involvement without evidence of necrosis L97.906
    bone necrosis L97.904
    exposed fat layer L97.902
    muscle involvement without evidence of necrosis L97.905
    muscle necrosis L97.903
    skin breakdown only L97.901
    specified severity NEC L97.908
  ankle L97.309
    with
      bone involvement without evidence of necrosis L97.306

**Ulcer, ulcerated, ulcerating, ulceration, ulcerative**
— continued
lower limb — continued
  ankle — continued
    with — continued
      bone necrosis L97.304
      exposed fat layer L97.302
      muscle involvement without evidence of necrosis L97.305
      muscle necrosis L97.303
      skin breakdown only L97.301
      specified severity NEC L97.308
    left L97.329
      with
        bone involvement without evidence of necrosis L97.326
        bone necrosis L97.324
        exposed fat layer L97.322
        muscle involvement without evidence of necrosis L97.325
        muscle necrosis L97.323
        skin breakdown only L97.321
        specified severity NEC L97.328
    right L97.319
      with
        bone involvement without evidence of necrosis L97.316
        bone necrosis L97.314
        exposed fat layer L97.312
        muscle involvement without evidence of necrosis L97.315
        muscle necrosis L97.313
        skin breakdown only L97.311
        specified severity NEC L97.318
  calf L97.209
    with
      bone involvement without evidence of necrosis L97.206
      bone necrosis L97.204
      exposed fat layer L97.202
      muscle involvement without evidence of necrosis L97.205
      muscle necrosis L97.203
      skin breakdown only L97.201
      specified severity NEC L97.208
    left L97.229
      with
        bone involvement without evidence of necrosis L97.226
        bone necrosis L97.224
        exposed fat layer L97.222
        muscle involvement without evidence of necrosis L97.225
        muscle necrosis L97.223
        skin breakdown only L97.221
        specified severity NEC L97.228
    right L97.219
      with
        bone involvement without evidence of necrosis L97.216
        bone necrosis L97.214
        exposed fat layer L97.212
        muscle involvement without evidence of necrosis L97.215
        muscle necrosis L97.213
        skin breakdown only L97.211
        specified severity NEC L97.218
  decubitus — see Ulcer, pressure, by site
  foot specified NEC L97.509
    with
      bone involvement without evidence of necrosis L97.506
      bone necrosis L97.504
      exposed fat layer L97.502
      muscle involvement without evidence of necrosis L97.505
      muscle necrosis L97.503
      skin breakdown only L97.501
      specified severity NEC L97.508
    left L97.529
      with
        bone involvement without evidence of necrosis L97.526
        bone necrosis L97.524
        exposed fat layer L97.522
        muscle involvement without evidence of necrosis L97.525
        muscle necrosis L97.523
        skin breakdown only L97.521

**Ulcer, ulcerated, ulcerating, ulceration, ulcerative**
— continued
lower limb — continued
  foot specified — continued
    left — continued
      with — continued
        specified severity NEC L97.528
    right L97.519
      with
        bone involvement without evidence of necrosis L97.516
        bone necrosis L97.514
        exposed fat layer L97.512
        muscle involvement without evidence of necrosis L97.515
        muscle necrosis L97.513
        skin breakdown only L97.511
        specified severity NEC L97.518
    heel L97.409
      with
        bone involvement without evidence of necrosis L97.406
        bone necrosis L97.404
        exposed fat layer L97.402
        muscle involvement without evidence of necrosis L97.405
        muscle necrosis L97.403
        skin breakdown only L97.401
        specified severity NEC L97.408
      left L97.429
        with
          bone involvement without evidence of necrosis L97.426
          bone necrosis L97.424
          exposed fat layer L97.422
          muscle involvement without evidence of necrosis L97.425
          muscle necrosis L97.423
          skin breakdown only L97.421
          specified severity NEC L97.428
      right L97.419
        with
          bone involvement without evidence of necrosis L97.416
          bone necrosis L97.414
          exposed fat layer L97.412
          muscle involvement without evidence of necrosis L97.415
          muscle necrosis L97.413
          skin breakdown only L97.411
          specified severity NEC L97.418
    left L97.929
      with
        bone involvement without evidence of necrosis L97.926
        bone necrosis L97.924
        exposed fat layer L97.922
        muscle involvement without evidence of necrosis L97.925
        muscle necrosis L97.923
        skin breakdown only L97.921
        specified severity NEC L97.928
  leprous A30.1
  lower leg NOS L97.909
    with
      bone involvement without evidence of necrosis L97.906
      bone necrosis L97.904
      exposed fat layer L97.902
      muscle involvement without evidence of necrosis L97.905
      muscle necrosis L97.903
      skin breakdown only L97.901
      specified severity NEC L97.908
    left L97.929
      with
        bone involvement without evidence of necrosis L97.926
        bone necrosis L97.924
        exposed fat layer L97.922
        muscle involvement without evidence of necrosis L97.925
        muscle necrosis L97.923
        skin breakdown only L97.921
        specified severity NEC L97.928
    right L97.919
      with
        bone involvement without evidence of necrosis L97.916

Index

Ulcer, ulcerated, ulcerating, ulceration, ulcerative — Ulcer, ulcerated, ulcerating, ulceration, ulcerative

lower limb — *continued*
  lower leg — *continued*
    right — *continued*
      with — *continued*
        bone necrosis L97.914
        exposed fat layer L97.912
        muscle involvement without evidence of necrosis L97.915
        muscle necrosis L97.913
        skin breakdown only L97.911
        specified severity NEC L97.918
    specified site NEC L97.809
      with
        bone involvement without evidence of necrosis L97.806
        bone necrosis L97.804
        exposed fat layer L97.802
        muscle involvement without evidence of necrosis L97.805
        muscle necrosis L97.803
        skin breakdown only L97.801
        specified severity NEC L97.808
    left L97.829
      with
        bone involvement without evidence of necrosis L97.826
        bone necrosis L97.824
        exposed fat layer L97.822
        muscle involvement without evidence of necrosis L97.825
        muscle necrosis L97.823
        skin breakdown only L97.821
        specified severity NEC L97.828
    right L97.819
      with
        bone involvement without evidence of necrosis L97.816
        bone necrosis L97.814
        exposed fat layer L97.812
        muscle involvement without evidence of necrosis L97.815
        muscle necrosis L97.813
        skin breakdown only L97.811
        specified severity NEC L97.818
  midfoot L97.409
    with
      bone involvement without evidence of necrosis L97.406
      bone necrosis L97.404
      exposed fat layer L97.402
      muscle involvement without evidence of necrosis L97.405
      muscle necrosis L97.403
      skin breakdown only L97.401
      specified severity NEC L97.408
    left L97.429
      with
        bone involvement without evidence of necrosis L97.426
        bone necrosis L97.424
        exposed fat layer L97.422
        muscle involvement without evidence of necrosis L97.425
        muscle necrosis L97.423
        skin breakdown only L97.421
        specified severity NEC L97.428
    right L97.419
      with
        bone involvement without evidence of necrosis L97.416
        bone necrosis L97.414
        exposed fat layer L97.412
        muscle involvement without evidence of necrosis L97.415
        muscle necrosis L97.413
        skin breakdown only L97.411
        specified severity NEC L97.418
  right L97.919
    with
      bone involvement without evidence of necrosis L97.916
      bone necrosis L97.914
      exposed fat layer L97.912
      muscle involvement without evidence of necrosis L97.915
      muscle necrosis L97.913
      skin breakdown only L97.911

lower limb — *continued*
  right — *continued*
    with — *continued*
      specified severity NEC L97.918
  syphilitic A52.19
  thigh L97.109
    with
      bone involvement without evidence of necrosis L97.106
      bone necrosis L97.104
      exposed fat layer L97.102
      muscle involvement without evidence of necrosis L97.105
      muscle necrosis L97.103
      skin breakdown only L97.101
      specified severity NEC L97.108
    left L97.129
      with
        bone involvement without evidence of necrosis L97.126
        bone necrosis L97.124
        exposed fat layer L97.122
        muscle involvement without evidence of necrosis L97.125
        muscle necrosis L97.123
        skin breakdown only L97.121
        specified severity NEC L97.128
    right L97.119
      with
        bone involvement without evidence of necrosis L97.116
        bone necrosis L97.114
        exposed fat layer L97.112
        muscle involvement without evidence of necrosis L97.115
        muscle necrosis L97.113
        skin breakdown only L97.111
        specified severity NEC L97.118
  toe L97.509
    with
      bone involvement without evidence of necrosis L97.506
      bone necrosis L97.504
      exposed fat layer L97.502
      muscle involvement without evidence of necrosis L97.505
      muscle necrosis L97.503
      skin breakdown only L97.501
      specified severity NEC L97.508
    left L97.529
      with
        bone involvement without evidence of necrosis L97.526
        bone necrosis L97.524
        exposed fat layer L97.522
        muscle involvement without evidence of necrosis L97.525
        muscle necrosis L97.523
        skin breakdown only L97.521
        specified severity NEC L97.528
    right L97.519
      with
        bone involvement without evidence of necrosis L97.516
        bone necrosis L97.514
        exposed fat layer L97.512
        muscle involvement without evidence of necrosis L97.515
        muscle necrosis L97.513
        skin breakdown only L97.511
        specified severity NEC L97.518
  varicose — *see* Varix, leg, with, ulcer
luetic — *see* Ulcer, syphilitic
lung J98.4
  tuberculous — *see* Tuberculosis, pulmonary
malignant — *see* Neoplasm, malignant, by site
marginal NEC — *see* Ulcer, gastrojejunal
meatus (urinarius) N34.2
Meckel's diverticulum Q43.0
  malignant — *see* Table of Neoplasms, small intestine, malignant
Meleney's (chronic undermining) — *see* Ulcer, skin
Mooren's (cornea) — *see* Ulcer, cornea, Mooren's
mycobacterial (skin) A31.1
nasopharynx J39.2
neck, uterus N86

neurogenic NEC — *see* Ulcer, skin
nose, nasal (passage) (infective) (septum) J34.0
  skin — *see* Ulcer, skin
  spirochetal A69.8
  varicose (bleeding) I86.8
oral mucosa (traumatic) K12.1
palate (soft) K12.1
penis (chronic) N48.5
peptic (site unspecified) K27.9
  with
    hemorrhage K27.4
      and perforation K27.6
    perforation K27.5
  acute K27.3
    with
      hemorrhage K27.0
        and perforation K27.2
      perforation K27.1
  chronic K27.7
    with
      hemorrhage K27.4
        and perforation K27.6
      perforation K27.5
  esophagus K22.10
    with bleeding K22.11
  newborn P78.82
perforating K27.5
  skin — *see* Ulcer, skin
peritonsillar J35.8
phagedenic (tropical) — *see* Ulcer, skin
pharynx J39.2
phlebitis — *see* Phlebitis
plaster — *see* Ulcer, pressure, by site
popliteal space — *see* Ulcer, lower limb
postpyloric — *see* Ulcer, duodenum
prepuce N47.7
prepyloric — *see* Ulcer, stomach
pressure (pressure area) L89.9- ☑
  ankle L89.5- ☑
  back L89.1- ☑
  buttock L89.3- ☑
  coccyx L89.15- ☑
  contiguous site of back, buttock, hip L89.4- ☑
  elbow L89.0- ☑
  face L89.81- ☑
  head L89.81- ☑
  heel L89.6- ☑
  hip L89.2- ☑
  sacral region (tailbone) L89.15- ☑
  specified site NEC L89.89- ☑
  stage 1 (healing) (pre-ulcer skin changes limited to persistent focal edema)
    ankle L89.5- ☑
    back L89.1- ☑
    buttock L89.3- ☑
    coccyx L89.15- ☑
    contiguous site of back, buttock, hip L89.4- ☑
    elbow L89.0- ☑
    face L89.81- ☑
    head L89.81- ☑
    heel L89.6- ☑
    hip L89.2- ☑
    sacral region (tailbone) L89.15- ☑
    specified site NEC L89.89- ☑
  stage 2 (healing) (abrasion, blister, partial thickness skin loss involving epidermis and/or dermis)
    ankle L89.5- ☑
    back L89.1- ☑
    buttock L89.3- ☑
    coccyx L89.15- ☑
    contiguous site of back, buttock, hip L89.4- ☑
    elbow L89.0- ☑
    face L89.81- ☑
    head L89.81- ☑
    heel L89.6- ☑
    hip L89.2- ☑
    sacral region (tailbone) L89.15- ☑
    specified site NEC L89.89- ☑
  stage 3 (healing) (full thickness skin loss involving damage or necrosis of subcutaneous tissue)
    ankle L89.5- ☑
    back L89.1- ☑
    buttock L89.3- ☑
    coccyx L89.15- ☑
    contiguous site of back, buttock, hip L89.4- ☑

☑ **Additional Character Required** — Refer to the Tabular List for Character Selection

🔺 Subterms under main terms may continue to next column or page

**Ulcer, ulcerated, ulcerating, ulceration, ulcerative**
— *continued*
pressure — *continued*
stage 3 — *continued*
elbow L89.Ø- ☑
face L89.81- ☑
head L89.81- ☑
heel L89.6- ☑
hip L89.2- ☑
sacral region (tailbone) L89.15- ☑
specified site NEC L89.89- ☑
stage 4 (healing) (necrosis of soft tissues through
to underlying muscle, tendon, or bone)
ankle L89.5- ☑
back L89.1- ☑
buttock L89.3- ☑
coccyx L89.15- ☑
contiguous site of back, buttock, hip L89.4- ☑
elbow L89.Ø- ☑
face L89.81- ☑
head L89.81- ☑
heel L89.6- ☑
hip L89.2- ☑
sacral region (tailbone) L89.15- ☑
specified site NEC L89.89- ☑
unspecified stage
ankle L89.5- ☑
back L89.1- ☑
buttock L89.3- ☑
coccyx L89.15- ☑
contiguous site of back, buttock, hip L89.4- ☑
elbow L89.Ø- ☑
face L89.81- ☑
head L89.81- ☑
heel L89.6- ☑
hip L89.2- ☑
sacral region (tailbone) L89.15- ☑
specified site NEC L89.89- ☑
unstageable
ankle L89.5- ☑
back L89.1- ☑
buttock L89.3- ☑
coccyx L89.15- ☑
contiguous site of back, buttock, hip L89.4- ☑
elbow L89.Ø- ☑
face L89.81- ☑
head L89.81- ☑
heel L89.6- ☑
hip L89.2- ☑
sacral region (tailbone) L89.15- ☑
specified site NEC L89.89- ☑
primary of intestine K63.3
with perforation K63.1
prostate N41.9
pyloric — *see* Ulcer, stomach
rectosigmoid K63.3
with perforation K63.1
rectum (sphincter) (solitary) K62.6
stercoraceous, stercoral K62.6
retina — *see* Inflammation, chorioretinal
rodent (*see also* Neoplasm, skin, malignant)
sclera — *see* Scleritis
scrofulous (tuberculous) A18.2
scrotum N5Ø.89
tuberculous A18.15
varicose I86.1
seminal vesicle N5Ø.89
sigmoid — *see* Ulcer, intestine
skin (atrophic) (chronic) (neurogenic) (non-healing)
(perforating) (pyogenic) (trophic) (tropical)
L98.499
with gangrene — *see* Gangrene
amebic AØ6.7
back — *see* Ulcer, back
buttock — *see* Ulcer, buttock
decubitus — *see* Ulcer, pressure
lower limb — *see* Ulcer, lower limb
mycobacterial A31.1
specified site NEC L98.499
with
bone involvement without evidence of
necrosis L98.496
bone necrosis L98.494
exposed fat layer L98.492
muscle involvement without evidence of
necrosis L98.495
muscle necrosis L98.493

**Ulcer, ulcerated, ulcerating, ulceration, ulcerative**
— *continued*
skin — *continued*
specified site — *continued*
with — *continued*
skin breakdown only L98.491
specified severity NEC L98.498
tuberculous (primary) A18.4
varicose — *see* Ulcer, varicose
sloughing — *see* Ulcer, skin
solitary, anus or rectum (sphincter) K62.6
sore throat JØ2.9
streptococcal JØ2.Ø
spermatic cord N5Ø.89
spine (tuberculous) A18.Ø1
stasis (venous) — *see* Varix, leg, with, ulcer
without varicose veins I87.2
stercoraceous, stercoral K63.3
with perforation K63.1
anus or rectum K62.6
stoma, stomal — *see* Ulcer, gastrojejunal
stomach (eroded) (peptic) (round) K25.9
with
hemorrhage K25.4
and perforation K25.6
perforation K25.5
acute K25.3
with
hemorrhage K25.Ø
and perforation K25.2
perforation K25.1
chronic K25.7
with
hemorrhage K25.4
and perforation K25.6
perforation K25.5
stomal — *see* Ulcer, gastrojejunal
stomatitis K12.1
stress — *see* Ulcer, peptic
strumous (tuberculous) A18.2
submucosal, bladder — *see* Cystitis, interstitial
syphilitic (any site) (early) (secondary) A51.39
late A52.79
perforating A52.79
foot A52.11
testis N5Ø.89
thigh — *see* Ulcer, lower limb
throat J39.2
diphtheritic A36.Ø
toe — *see* Ulcer, lower limb
tongue (traumatic) K14.Ø
tonsil J35.8
diphtheritic A36.Ø
trachea J39.8
trophic — *see* Ulcer, skin
tropical — *see* Ulcer, skin
tuberculous — *see* Tuberculosis, ulcer
tunica vaginalis N5Ø.89
turbinate J34.89
typhoid (perforating) — *see* Typhoid
unspecified site — *see* Ulcer, skin
urethra (meatus) — *see* Urethritis
uterus N85.8
cervix N86
with cervicitis N72
neck N86
with cervicitis N72
vagina N76.5
in Behçet's disease M35.2 [N77.Ø]
pessary N89.8
valve, heart I33.Ø
varicose (lower limb, any part) (*see also* Varix, leg, with,
ulcer)
broad ligament I86.2
esophagus — *see* Varix, esophagus
inflamed or infected — *see* Varix, leg, with ulcer,
with inflammation
nasal septum I86.8
perineum I86.3
scrotum I86.1
specified site NEC I86.8
sublingual I86.Ø
vulva I86.3
vas deferens N5Ø.89
vulva (acute) (infectional) N76.6
in (due to)
Behçet's disease M35.2 [N77.Ø]
herpesviral (herpes simplex) infection A6Ø.Ø4

**Ulcer, ulcerated, ulcerating, ulceration, ulcerative**
— *continued*
vulva — *continued*
in — *continued*
tuberculosis A18.18
vulvobuccal, recurring N76.6
X-ray L58.1
yaws A66.4
**Ulcerosa scarlatina** A38.8
**Ulcus** (*see also* Ulcer)
cutis tuberculosum A18.4
duodeni — *see* Ulcer, duodenum
durum (syphilitic) A51.Ø
extragenital A51.2
gastrojejunale — *see* Ulcer, gastrojejunal
hypostaticum — *see* Ulcer, varicose
molle (cutis) (skin) A57
serpens corneae — *see* Ulcer, cornea, central
ventriculi — *see* Ulcer, stomach
**Ulegyria** QØ4.8
**Ulerythema**
ophryogenes, congenital Q84.2
sycosiforme L73.8
**Ullrich** (-Bonnevie)(-Turner) **syndrome** (*see also* Turner's
syndrome) Q87.1
**Ullrich-Feichtiger syndrome** Q87.Ø
**Ulnar** — *see* condition
**Ulorrhagia, ulorrhea** KØ6.8
**Umbilicus, umbilical** — *see* condition
**Unacceptable**
contours of tooth KØ8.54
morphology of tooth KØ8.54
**Unavailability** (of)
bed at medical facility Z75.1
health service-related agencies Z75.4
medical facilities (at) Z75.3
due to
investigation by social service agency Z75.2
lack of services at home Z75.Ø
remoteness from facility Z75.3
waiting list Z75.1
home Z75.Ø
outpatient clinic Z75.3
schooling Z55.1
social service agencies Z75.4
**Uncinaria americana infestation** B76.1
**Uncinariasis** B76.9
**Uncongenial work** Z56.5
**Unconscious** (ness) — *see* Coma
**Under observation** — *see* Observation
**Underachievement in school** Z55.3
**Underdevelopment** (*see also* Undeveloped)
nose Q3Ø.1
sexual E3Ø.Ø
**Underdosing** (*see also* Table of Drugs and Chemicals,
categories T36-T5Ø, with final character 6) Z91.14
intentional NEC Z91.128
due to financial hardship of patient Z91.12Ø
unintentional NEC Z91.138
due to patient's age related debility Z91.13Ø
**Underfeeding, newborn** P92.3
**Underfill, endodontic** M27.53
**Underimmunization status** Z28.3
**Undernourishment** — *see* Malnutrition
**Undernutrition** — *see* Malnutrition
**Underweight** R63.6
for gestational age — *see* Light for dates
**Underwood's disease** P83.Ø
**Undescended** (*see also* Malposition, congenital)
cecum Q43.3
colon Q43.3
testicle — *see* Cryptorchid
**Undeveloped, undevelopment** (*see also* Hypoplasia)
brain (congenital) QØ2
cerebral (congenital) QØ2
heart Q24.8
lung Q33.6
testis E29.1
uterus E3Ø.Ø
**Undiagnosed** (disease) R69
**Undulant fever** — *see* Brucellosis
**Unemployment, anxiety concerning** Z56.Ø
threatened Z56.2
**Unequal length** (acquired) (limb) (*see also* Deformity,
limb, unequal length)
leg (*see also* Deformity, limb, unequal length)
congenital Q72.9- ☑

**Unextracted dental root** KØ8.3
**Unguis incarnatus** L6Ø.Ø
**Unhappiness** R45.2
**Unicornate uterus** Q51.4
  in pregnancy or childbirth O34.ØØ
**Unilateral** (*see also* condition)
  development, breast N64.89
  organ or site, congenital NEC — *see* Agenesis, by site
**Unilocular heart** Q2Ø.8
**Union, abnormal** (*see also* Fusion)
  larynx and trachea Q34.8
**Universal mesentery** Q43.3
**Unrepairable overhanging of dental restorative materials** KØ8.52
**Unsatisfactory**
  restoration of tooth KØ8.5Ø
    specified NEC KØ8.59
  sample of cytologic smear
    anus R85.615
    cervix R87.615
    vagina R87.625
  surroundings Z59.1
    work Z56.5
**Unsoundness of mind** — *see* Psychosis
**Unstable**
  back NEC — *see* Instability, joint, spine
  hip (congenital) Q65.6
    acquired — *see* Derangement, joint, specified type NEC, hip
  joint — *see* Instability, joint
    secondary to removal of joint prosthesis M96.89
  lie (mother) O32.Ø
  lumbosacral joint (congenital)
    acquired — *see* subcategory M53.2 ☑
  sacroiliac — *see* subcategory M53.2 ☑
  spine NEC — *see* Instability, joint, spine
**Unsteadiness on feet** R26.81
**Untruthfulness, child problem** F91.8
**Unverricht** (-Lundborg) **disease or epilepsy** — *see* Epilepsy, generalized, idiopathic
**Unwanted pregnancy** Z64.Ø
**Upbringing, institutional** Z62.22
  away from parents NEC Z62.29
  in care of non-parental family member Z62.21
  in foster care Z62.21
  in orphanage or group home Z62.22
  in welfare custody Z62.21
**Upper respiratory** — *see* condition
**Upset**
  gastric K3Ø
  gastrointestinal K3Ø
    psychogenic F45.8
  intestinal (large) (small) K59.9
    psychogenic F45.8
  menstruation N93.9
  mental F48.9
  stomach K3Ø
    psychogenic F45.8
**Urachus** (*see also* condition)
  patent or persistent Q64.4
**Urbach-Oppenheim disease** (necrobiosis lipoidica diabeticorum) — *see* EØ8-E13 with .62Ø
**Urbach's lipoid proteinosis** E78.89
**Urbach-Wiethe disease** E78.89
**Urban yellow fever** A95.1
**Urea**
  blood, high — *see* Uremia
  cycle metabolism disorder — *see* Disorder, urea cycle metabolism
**Uremia, uremic** N19
  with
    ectopic or molar pregnancy OØ8.4
    polyneuropathy N18.9 [G63]
  chronic NOS (*see also* Disease, kidney, chronic) N18.9
    due to hypertension — *see* Hypertensive, kidney
  complicating
    ectopic or molar pregnancy OØ8.4
  congenital P96.Ø
  extrarenal R39.2
  following ectopic or molar pregnancy OØ8.4
  newborn P96.Ø
  prerenal R39.2
**Ureter, ureteral** — *see* condition
**Ureteralgia** N23
**Ureterectasis** — *see* Hydroureter
**Ureteritis** N28.89
  cystica N28.86

**Ureteritis** — *continued*
  due to calculus N2Ø.1
    with calculus, kidney N2Ø.2
      with hydronephrosis N13.2
  gonococcal (acute) (chronic) A54.21
  nonspecific N28.89
**Ureterocele** N28.89
  congenital (orthotopic) Q62.31
  ectopic Q62.32
**Ureterolith, ureterolithiasis** — *see* Calculus, ureter
**Ureterostomy**
  attention to Z43.6
  status Z93.6
**Urethra, urethral** — *see* condition
**Urethralgia** R39.89
**Urethritis** (anterior) (posterior) N34.2
  calculous N21.1
  candidal B37.41
  chlamydial A56.Ø1
  diplococcal (gonococcal) A54.Ø1
    with abscess (accessory gland) (periurethral) A54.1
  gonococcal A54.Ø1
    with abscess (accessory gland) (periurethral) A54.1
  nongonococcal N34.1
    Reiter's — *see* Reiter's disease
  nonspecific N34.1
  nonvenereal N34.1
  postmenopausal N34.2
  puerperal O86.22
  Reiter's — *see* Reiter's disease
  specified NEC N34.2
  trichomonal or due to Trichomonas (vaginalis) A59.Ø3
**Urethrocele** N81.Ø
  with
    cystocele — *see* Cystocele
    prolapse of uterus — *see* Prolapse, uterus
**Urethrolithiasis** (with colic or infection) N21.1
**Urethrorectal** — *see* condition
**Urethrorrhagia** N36.8
**Urethrorrhea** R36.9
**Urethrostomy**
  attention to Z43.6
  status Z93.6
**Urethrotrigonitis** — *see* Trigonitis
**Urethrovaginal** — *see* condition
**Urgency**
  fecal R15.2
  hypertensive — *see* Hypertension
  urinary R39.15
**Urhidrosis, uridrosis** L74.8
**Uric acid in blood** (increased) E79.Ø
**Uricacidemia** (asymptomatic) E79.Ø
**Uricemia** (asymptomatic) E79.Ø
**Uricosuria** R82.99
**Urinary** — *see* condition
**Urination**
  frequent R35.Ø
  painful R3Ø.9
**Urine**
  blood in — *see* Hematuria
  discharge, excessive R35.8
  enuresis, nonorganic origin F98.Ø
  extravasation R39.Ø
  frequency R35.Ø
  incontinence R32
    nonorganic origin F98.Ø
  intermittent stream R39.198
  pus in N39.Ø
  retention or stasis R33.9
    organic R33.8
      drug-induced R33.Ø
    psychogenic F45.8
  secretion
    deficient R34
    excessive R35.8
    frequency R35.Ø
  stream
    intermittent R39.198
    slowing R39.198
    splitting R39.13
    weak R39.12
**Urinemia** — *see* Uremia
**Urinoma, urethra** N36.8
**Uroarthritis, infectious** (Reiter's) — *see* Reiter's disease
**Urodialysis** R34
**Urolithiasis** — *see* Calculus, urinary
**Uronephrosis** — *see* Hydronephrosis
**Uropathy** N39.9

**Uropathy** — *continued*
  obstructive N13.9
    specified NEC N13.8
  reflux N13.9
    specified NEC N13.8
  vesicoureteral reflux-associated — *see* Reflux, vesicoureteral
**Urosepsis** — *code to* condition
**Urticaria** L5Ø.9
  with angioneurotic edema T78.3 ☑
    hereditary D84.1
  allergic L5Ø.Ø
  cholinergic L5Ø.5
  chronic L5Ø.8
  cold, familial L5Ø.2
  contact L5Ø.6
  dermatographic L5Ø.3
  due to
    cold or heat L5Ø.2
    drugs L5Ø.Ø
    food L5Ø.Ø
    inhalants L5Ø.Ø
    plants L5Ø.6
    serum (*see also* Reaction, serum) T8Ø.69 ☑
  factitial L5Ø.3
  familial cold MØ4.2
  giant T78.3 ☑
    hereditary D84.1
  gigantea T78.3 ☑
  idiopathic L5Ø.1
  larynx T78.3 ☑
    hereditary D84.1
  neonatorum P83.88
  nonallergic L5Ø.1
  papulosa (Hebra) L28.2
  pigmentosa D47.Ø1
    congenital Q82.2
    of neonatal onset Q82.2
    of newborn onset Q82.2
  recurrent periodic L5Ø.8
  serum (*see also* Reaction, serum) T8Ø.69 ☑
  solar L56.3
  specified type NEC L5Ø.8
  thermal (cold) (heat) L5Ø.2
  vibratory L5Ø.4
  xanthelasmoidea — *see* Urticaria pigmentosa
**Use** (of)
  alcohol Z72.89
    with
      intoxication F1Ø.929
      sleep disorder F1Ø.982
    harmful — *see* Abuse, alcohol
  amphetamines — *see* Use, stimulant NEC
  caffeine — *see* Use, stimulant NEC
  cannabis F12.9Ø
    with
      anxiety disorder F12.98Ø
      intoxication F12.929
        with
          delirium F12.921
          perceptual disturbance F12.922
        uncomplicated F12.92Ø
      other specified disorder F12.988
      psychosis F12.959
        delusions F12.95Ø
        hallucinations F12.951
      unspecified disorder F12.99
  cocaine F14.9Ø
    with
      anxiety disorder F14.98Ø
      intoxication F14.929
        with
          delirium F14.921
          perceptual disturbance F14.922
        uncomplicated F14.92Ø
      other specified disorder F14.988
      psychosis F14.959
        delusions F14.95Ø
        hallucinations F14.951
      sexual dysfunction F14.981
      sleep disorder F14.982
      unspecified disorder F14.99
    harmful — *see* Abuse, drug, cocaine
  drug(s) NEC F19.9Ø
    with sleep disorder F19.982
    harmful — *see* Abuse, drug, by type
  hallucinogen NEC F16.9Ø

☑ **Additional Character Required** — Refer to the Tabular List for Character Selection    Ⓥ **Subterms under main terms may continue to next column or page**

**Use** — *continued*
  hallucinogen — *continued*
    with
      anxiety disorder F16.980
      intoxication F16.929
        with
          delirium F16.921
        uncomplicated F16.920
      mood disorder F16.94
      other specified disorder F16.988
      perception disorder (flashbacks) F16.983
      psychosis F16.959
        delusions F16.950
        hallucinations F16.951
      unspecified disorder F16.99
    harmful — *see* Abuse, drug, hallucinogen NEC
  inhalants F18.90
    with
      anxiety disorder F18.980
      intoxication F18.929
        with delirium F18.921
        uncomplicated F18.920
      mood disorder F18.94
      other specified disorder F18.988
      persisting dementia F18.97
      psychosis F18.959
        delusions F18.950
        hallucinations F18.951
      unspecified disorder F18.99
    harmful — *see* Abuse, drug, inhalant
  methadone — *see* Use, opioid
  nonprescribed drugs F19.90
    harmful — *see* Abuse, non-psychoactive substance
  opioid F11.90
    with
      disorder F11.99
        mood F11.94
        sleep F11.982
        specified type NEC F11.988
      intoxication F11.929
        with
          delirium F11.921
          perceptual disturbance F11.922
        uncomplicated F11.920
      withdrawal F11.93
    harmful — *see* Abuse, drug, opioid
  patent medicines F19.90
    harmful — *see* Abuse, non-psychoactive substance
  psychoactive drug NEC F19.90
    with
      anxiety disorder F19.980
      intoxication F19.929
        with
          delirium F19.921
          perceptual disturbance F19.922
        uncomplicated F19.920
      mood disorder F19.94
      other specified disorder F19.988
      persisting
        amnestic disorder F19.96
        dementia F19.97
      psychosis F19.959
        delusions F19.950
        hallucinations F19.951
      sexual dysfunction F19.981
      sleep disorder F19.982
      unspecified disorder F19.99
      withdrawal F19.939
        with
          delirium F19.931
          perceptual disturbance F19.932
        uncomplicated F19.930
    harmful — *see* Abuse, drug NEC, psychoactive NEC
  sedative, hypnotic, or anxiolytic F13.90
    with
      anxiety disorder F13.980
      intoxication F13.929
        with
          delirium F13.921
        uncomplicated F13.920
      other specified disorder F13.988
      persisting
        amnestic disorder F13.96
        dementia F13.97
      psychosis F13.959
        delusions F13.950
        hallucinations F13.951
      sexual dysfunction F13.981

**Use** — *continued*
  sedative, hypnotic, or anxiolytic — *continued*
    with — *continued*
      sleep disorder F13.982
      unspecified disorder F13.99
    harmful — *see* Abuse, drug, sedative, hypnotic, or anxiolytic
  stimulant NEC F15.90
    with
      anxiety disorder F15.980
      intoxication F15.929
        with
          delirium F15.921
          perceptual disturbance F15.922
        uncomplicated F15.920
      mood disorder F15.94
      other specified disorder F15.988
      psychosis F15.959
        delusions F15.950
        hallucinations F15.951
      sexual dysfunction F15.981
      sleep disorder F15.982
      unspecified disorder F15.99
      withdrawal F15.93
    harmful — *see* Abuse, drug, stimulant NEC
  tobacco Z72.0
    with dependence — *see* Dependence, drug, nicotine
  volatile solvents (*see also* Use, inhalant) F18.90
    harmful — *see* Abuse, drug, inhalant

**Usher-Senear disease or syndrome** L10.4
**Uta** B55.1
**Uteromegaly** N85.2
**Uterovaginal** — *see* condition
**Uterovesical** — *see* condition
**Uveal** — *see* condition
**Uveitis** (anterior) (*see also* Iridocyclitis)
  acute — *see* Iridocyclitis, acute
  chronic — *see* Iridocyclitis, chronic
  due to toxoplasmosis (acquired) B58.09
    congenital P37.1
  granulomatous — *see* Iridocyclitis, chronic
  heterochromic — *see* Cyclitis, Fuchs' heterochromic
  lens-induced — *see* Iridocyclitis, lens-induced
  posterior — *see* Chorioretinitis
  sympathetic H44.13- ☑
  syphilitic (secondary) A51.43
    congenital (early) A50.01
    late A52.71
  tuberculous A18.54
**Uveoencephalitis** — *see* Inflammation, chorioretinal
**Uveokeratitis** — *see* Iridocyclitis
**Uveoparotitis** D86.89
**Uvula** — *see* condition
**Uvulitis** (acute) (catarrhal) (chronic) (membranous) (suppurative) (ulcerative) K12.2

## V

**Vaccination** (prophylactic)
  complication or reaction — *see* Complications, vaccination
  delayed Z28.9
  encounter for Z23
  not done — *see* Immunization, not done, because (of)
**Vaccinia** (generalized) (localized) T88.1 ☑
  without vaccination B08.011
  congenital P35.8
**Vacuum, in sinus** (accessory) (nasal) J34.89
**Vagabond, vagabondage** Z59.0
**Vagabond's disease** B85.1
**Vagina, vaginal** — *see* condition
**Vaginalitis** (tunica) (testis) N49.1
**Vaginismus** (reflex) N94.2
  functional F52.5
  nonorganic F52.5
  psychogenic F52.5
  secondary N94.2
**Vaginitis** (acute) (circumscribed) (diffuse) (emphysematous) (nonvenereal) (ulcerative) N76.0
  with ectopic or molar pregnancy O08.0
  amebic A06.82
  atrophic, postmenopausal N95.2
  bacterial N76.0
  blennorrhagic (gonococcal) A54.02
  candidal B37.3
  chlamydial A56.02

**Vaginitis** — *continued*
  chronic N76.1
  due to Trichomonas (vaginalis) A59.01
  following ectopic or molar pregnancy O08.0
  gonococcal A54.02
    with abscess (accessory gland) (periurethral) A54.1
  granuloma A58
  in (due to)
    candidiasis B37.3
    herpesviral (herpes simplex) infection A60.04
    pinworm infection B80 [N77.1]
  monilial B37.3
  mycotic (candidal) B37.3
  postmenopausal atrophic N95.2
  puerperal (postpartum) O86.13
  senile (atrophic) N95.2
  subacute or chronic N76.1
  syphilitic (early) A51.0
    late A52.76
  trichomonal A59.01
  tuberculous A18.18
**Vaginosis** — *see* Vaginitis
**Vagotonia** G52.2
**Vagrancy** Z59.0
**VAIN** — *see* Neoplasia, intraepithelial, vagina
**Vallecula** — *see* condition
**Valley fever** B38.0
**Valsuani's disease** — *see* Anemia, obstetric
**Valve, valvular** (formation) (*see also* condition)
  cerebral ventricle (communicating) in situ Z98.2
  cervix, internal os Q51.828
  congenital NEC — *see* Atresia, by site
  ureter (pelvic junction) (vesical orifice) Q62.39
  urethra (congenital) (posterior) Q64.2
**Valvulitis** (chronic) — *see* Endocarditis
**Valvulopathy** — *see* Endocarditis
**Van Bogaert's leukoencephalopathy** (sclerosing) (subacute) A81.1
**Van Bogaert-Scherer-Epstein disease or syndrome** E75.5
**Van Buchem's syndrome** M85.2
**Van Creveld-von Gierke disease** E74.01
**Van der Hoeve** (-de Kleyn) **syndrome** Q78.0
**Van der Woude's syndrome** Q38.0
**Van Neck's disease or osteochondrosis** M91.0
**Vanishing lung** J44.9
**Vapor asphyxia or suffocation** T59.9 ☑
  specified agent — *see* Table of Drugs and Chemicals
**Variance, lethal ball, prosthetic heart valve** T82.09 ☑
**Variants, thalassemic** D56.8
**Variations in hair color** L67.1
**Varicella** B01.9
  with
    complications NEC B01.89
    encephalitis B01.11
    encephalomyelitis B01.11
    meningitis B01.0
    myelitis B01.12
    pneumonia B01.2
  congenital P35.8
**Varices** — *see* Varix
**Varicocele** (scrotum) (thrombosed) I86.1
  ovary I86.2
  perineum I86.3
  spermatic cord (ulcerated) I86.1
**Varicose**
  aneurysm (ruptured) I77.0
  dermatitis — *see* Varix, leg, with, inflammation
  eczema — *see* Varix, leg, with, inflammation
  phlebitis — *see* Varix, with, inflammation
  tumor — *see* Varix
  ulcer (lower limb, any part) (*see also* Varix, leg, with, ulcer)
    anus (*see also* Hemorrhoids) K64.8
    esophagus — *see* Varix, esophagus
    inflamed or infected — *see* Varix, leg, with ulcer, with inflammation
    nasal septum I86.8
    perineum I86.3
    scrotum I86.1
    specified site NEC I86.8
  vein — *see* Varix
  vessel — *see* Varix, leg
**Varicosis, varicosities, varicosity** — *see* Varix
**Variola** (major) (minor) B03
**Varioloid** B03
**Varix** (lower limb) (ruptured) I83.90

▼ **Subterms under main terms may continue to next column or page**    ☑ **Additional Character Required — Refer to the Tabular List for Character Selection**     **323**

Use — Varix

**Varix** — *continued*
- with
  - edema I83.899
  - inflammation I83.10
    - with ulcer (venous) I83.209
  - pain I83.819
  - specified complication NEC I83.899
  - stasis dermatitis I83.10
    - with ulcer (venous) I83.209
  - swelling I83.899
  - ulcer I83.009
    - with inflammation I83.209
- aneurysmal I77.0
- asymptomatic I83.9- ☑
- bladder I86.2
- broad ligament I86.2
- complicating
  - childbirth (lower extremity) O87.4
    - anus or rectum O87.2
    - genital (vagina, vulva or perineum) O87.8
  - pregnancy (lower extremity) O22.0- ☑
    - anus or rectum O22.4- ☑
    - genital (vagina, vulva or perineum) O22.1- ☑
  - puerperium (lower extremity) O87.4
    - anus or rectum O87.2
    - genital (vagina, vulva, perineum) O87.8
- congenital (any site) Q27.8
- esophagus (idiopathic) (primary) (ulcerated) I85.00
  - bleeding I85.01
  - congenital Q27.8
  - in (due to)
    - alcoholic liver disease I85.10
      - bleeding I85.11
    - cirrhosis of liver I85.10
      - bleeding I85.11
    - portal hypertension I85.10
      - bleeding I85.11
    - schistosomiasis I85.10
      - bleeding I85.11
    - toxic liver disease I85.10
      - bleeding I85.11
  - secondary I85.10
    - bleeding I85.11
- gastric I86.4
- inflamed or infected I83.10
  - ulcerated I83.209
- labia (majora) I86.3
- leg (asymptomatic) I83.90
  - with
    - edema I83.899
    - inflammation I83.10
      - with ulcer — *see* Varix, leg, with, ulcer, with inflammation by site
    - pain I83.819
    - specified complication NEC I83.899
    - swelling I83.899
    - ulcer I83.009
      - with inflammation I83.209
      - ankle I83.003
        - with inflammation I83.203
      - calf I83.002
        - with inflammation I83.202
      - foot NEC I83.005
        - with inflammation I83.205
      - heel I83.004
        - with inflammation I83.204
      - lower leg NEC I83.008
        - with inflammation I83.208
      - midfoot I83.004
        - with inflammation I83.204
      - thigh I83.001
        - with inflammation I83.201
  - bilateral (asymptomatic) I83.93
    - with
      - edema I83.893
      - pain I83.813
      - specified complication NEC I83.893
      - swelling I83.893
      - ulcer I83.0- ☑
        - with inflammation I83.209
  - left (asymptomatic) I83.92
    - with
      - edema I83.892
      - inflammation I83.12
        - with ulcer — *see* Varix, leg, with, ulcer, with inflammation by site
      - pain I83.812
      - specified complication NEC I83.892

**Varix** — *continued*
- leg — *continued*
  - left — *continued*
    - with — *continued*
      - swelling I83.892
      - ulcer I83.029
        - with inflammation I83.229
        - ankle I83.023
          - with inflammation I83.223
        - calf I83.022
          - with inflammation I83.222
        - foot NEC I83.025
          - with inflammation I83.225
        - heel I83.024
          - with inflammation I83.224
        - lower leg NEC I83.028
          - with inflammation I83.228
        - midfoot I83.024
          - with inflammation I83.224
        - thigh I83.021
          - with inflammation I83.221
  - right (asymptomatic) I83.91
    - with
      - edema I83.891
      - inflammation I83.11
        - with ulcer — *see* Varix, leg, with, ulcer, with inflammation by site
      - pain I83.811
      - specified complication NEC I83.891
      - swelling I83.891
      - ulcer I83.019
        - with inflammation I83.219
        - ankle I83.013
          - with inflammation I83.213
        - calf I83.012
          - with inflammation I83.212
        - foot NEC I83.015
          - with inflammation I83.215
        - heel I83.014
          - with inflammation I83.214
        - lower leg NEC I83.018
          - with inflammation I83.218
        - midfoot I83.014
          - with inflammation I83.214
        - thigh I83.011
          - with inflammation I83.211
- nasal septum I86.8
- orbit I86.8
  - congenital Q27.8
- ovary I86.2
- papillary I78.1
- pelvis I86.2
- perineum I86.3
- pharynx I86.8
- placenta O43.89- ☑
- renal papilla I86.8
- retina H35.09
- scrotum (ulcerated) I86.1
- sigmoid colon I86.8
- specified site NEC I86.8
- spinal (cord) (vessels) I86.8
- spleen, splenic (vein) (with phlebolith) I86.8
- stomach I86.4
- sublingual I86.0
- ulcerated I83.009
  - inflamed or infected I83.209
- uterine ligament I86.2
- vagina I86.8
- vocal cord I86.8
- vulva I86.3

**Vas deferens** — *see* condition
**Vas deferentitis** N49.1
**Vasa previa** O69.4 ☑
- hemorrhage from, affecting newborn P50.0
**Vascular** (*see also* condition)
- loop on optic papilla Q14.2
- spasm I73.9
- spider I78.1
**Vascularization, cornea** — *see* Neovascularization, cornea
**Vasculitis** I77.6
- allergic D69.0
- cryoglobulinemic D89.1
- disseminated I77.6
- hypocomplementemic M31.8
- kidney I77.89
- livedoid L95.0
- nodular L95.8

**Vasculitis** — *continued*
- retina H35.06- ☑
- rheumatic — *see* Fever, rheumatic
- rheumatoid — *see* Rheumatoid, vasculitis
- skin (limited to) L95.9
  - specified NEC L95.8
- systemic M31.8
**Vasculopathy, necrotizing** M31.9
- cardiac allograft T86.290
- specified NEC M31.8
**Vasitis** (nodosa) N49.1
- tuberculous A18.15
**Vasodilation** I73.9
**Vasomotor** — *see* condition
**Vasoplasty, after previous sterilization** Z31.0
- aftercare Z31.42
**Vasospasm** (vasoconstriction) I73.9
- cerebral (cerebrovascular) (artery) I67.848
  - reversible I67.841
- coronary I20.1
- nerve
  - arm — *see* Mononeuropathy, upper limb
  - brachial plexus G54.0
  - cervical plexus G54.2
  - leg — *see* Mononeuropathy, lower limb
- peripheral NOS I73.9
- retina (artery) — *see* Occlusion, artery, retina
**Vasospastic** — *see* condition
**Vasovagal attack** (paroxysmal) R55
- psychogenic F45.8
**VATER syndrome** Q87.2
**Vater's ampulla** — *see* condition
**Vegetation, vegetative**
- adenoid (nasal fossa) J35.8
- endocarditis (acute) (any valve) (subacute) I33.0
- heart (mycotic) (valve) I33.0
**Veil**
- Jackson's Q43.3
**Vein, venous** — *see* condition
**Veldt sore** — *see* Ulcer, skin
**Velpeau's hernia** — *see* Hernia, femoral
**Venereal**
- bubo A55
- disease A64
- granuloma inguinale A58
- lymphogranuloma (Durand-Nicolas-Favre) A55
**Venofibrosis** I87.8
**Venom, venomous** — *see* Table of Drugs and Chemicals, by animal or substance, poisoning
**Venous** — *see* condition
**Ventilator lung, newborn** P27.8
**Ventral** — *see* condition
**Ventricle, ventricular** (*see also* condition)
- escape I49.3
- inversion Q20.5
**Ventriculitis** (cerebral) (*see also* Encephalitis) G04.90
**Ventriculostomy status** Z98.2
**Vernet's syndrome** G52.7
**Verneuil's disease** (syphilitic bursitis) A52.78
**Verruca** (due to HPV) (filiformis) (simplex) (viral) (vulgaris) B07.9
- acuminata A63.0
- necrogenica (primary) (tuberculosa) A18.4
- plana B07.8
- plantaris B07.0
- seborrheica L82.1
  - inflamed L82.0
- senile (seborrheic) L82.1
  - inflamed L82.0
- tuberculosa (primary) A18.4
- venerea A63.0
**Verrucosities** — *see* Verruca
**Verruga peruana, peruviana** A44.1
**Version**
- with extraction
- cervix — *see* Malposition, uterus
- uterus (postinfectional) (postpartal, old) — *see* Malposition, uterus
**Vertebra, vertebral** — *see* condition
**Vertical talus** (congenital) Q66.80
- left foot Q66.82
- right foot Q66.81
**Vertigo** R42
- auditory — *see* Vertigo, aural
- aural H81.31- ☑
- benign paroxysmal (positional) H81.1- ☑
- central (origin) H81.4- ☑

**Vertigo** — *continued*
  cerebral H81.4- ☑
  Dix and Hallpike (epidemic) — *see* Neuronitis,
    vestibular
  due to infrasound T75.23 ☑
  epidemic A88.1
    Dix and Hallpike — *see* Neuronitis, vestibular
    Pedersen's — *see* Neuronitis, vestibular
    vestibular neuronitis — *see* Neuronitis, vestibular
  hysterical F44.89
  infrasound T75.23 ☑
  labyrinthine — *see* subcategory H81.0 ☑
  laryngeal R05
  malignant positional H81.4- ☑
  Ménière's — *see* subcategory H81.0 ☑
  menopausal N95.1
  otogenic — *see* Vertigo, aural
  paroxysmal positional, benign — *see* Vertigo, benign
    paroxysmal
  Pedersen's (epidemic) — *see* Neuronitis, vestibular
  peripheral NEC H81.39- ☑
  positional
    benign paroxysmal — *see* Vertigo, benign parox-
      ysmal
    malignant H81.4- ☑
**Very-low-density-lipoprotein-type** (VLDL) **hyper-**
  **lipoproteinemia** E78.1
**Vesania** — *see* Psychosis
**Vesical** — *see* condition
**Vesicle**
  cutaneous R23.8
  seminal — *see* condition
  skin R23.8
**Vesicocolic** — *see* condition
**Vesicoperineal** — *see* condition
**Vesicorectal** — *see* condition
**Vesicourethrorectal** — *see* condition
**Vesicovaginal** — *see* condition
**Vesicular** — *see* condition
**Vesiculitis** (seminal) N49.0
  amebic A06.82
  gonorrheal (acute) (chronic) A54.23
  trichomonal A59.09
  tuberculous A18.15
**Vestibulitis** (ear) (*see also* subcategory) H83.0 ☑
  nose (external) J34.89
  vulvar N94.810
**Vestibulopathy , acute peripheral** (recurrent) — *see*
  Neuronitis, vestibular
**Vestige, vestigial** (*see also* Persistence)
  branchial Q18.0
  structures in vitreous Q14.0
**Vibration**
  adverse effects T75.20 ☑
    pneumatic hammer syndrome T75.21 ☑
    specified effect NEC T75.29 ☑
    vasospastic syndrome T75.22 ☑
    vertigo from infrasound T75.23 ☑
  exposure (occupational) Z57.7
  vertigo T75.23 ☑
**Vibriosis** A28.9
**Victim** (of)
  crime Z65.4
  disaster Z65.5
  terrorism Z65.4
  torture Z65.4
  war Z65.5
**Vidal's disease** L28.0
**Villaret's syndrome** G52.7
**Villous** — *see* condition
**VIN** — *see* Neoplasia, intraepithelial, vulva
**Vincent's infection** (angina) (gingivitis) A69.1
  stomatitis NEC A69.1
**Vinson-Plummer syndrome** D50.1
**Violence, physical** R45.6
**Viosterol deficiency** — *see* Deficiency, calciferol
**Vipoma** — *see* Neoplasm, malignant, by site
**Viremia** B34.9
**Virilism** (adrenal) E25.9
  congenital E25.0
**Virilization** (female) (suprarenal) E25.9
  congenital E25.0
  isosexual E28.2
**Virulent bubo** A57
**Virus, viral** (*see also* condition)
  as cause of disease classified elsewhere B97.89
  cytomegalovirus B25.9

**Virus, viral** — *continued*
  human immunodeficiency (HIV) — *see* Human, immun-
    odeficiency virus (HIV) disease
  infection — *see* Infection, virus
  specified NEC B34.8
  swine influenza (viruses that normally cause infections
    in pigs) (*see also* Influenza, due to, identified
    novel influenza A virus) J09.X2
  West Nile (fever) A92.30
    with
      complications NEC A92.39
      cranial nerve disorders A92.32
      encephalitis A92.31
      encephalomyelitis A92.31
      neurologic manifestation NEC A92.32
      optic neuritis A92.32
      polyradiculitis A92.32
**Viscera, visceral** — *see* condition
**Visceroptosis** K63.4
**Visible peristalsis** R19.2
**Vision, visual**
  binocular, suppression H53.34
  blurred, blurring H53.8
    hysterical F44.6
  defect, defective NEC H54.7
  disorientation (syndrome) H53.8
  disturbance H53.9
    hysterical F44.6
  double H53.2
  examination Z01.00
    with abnormal findings Z01.01
  field, limitation (defect) — *see* Defect, visual field
  hallucinations R44.1
  halos H53.19
  loss — *see* Loss, vision
    sudden — *see* Disturbance, vision, subjective, loss,
      sudden
  low (both eyes) — *see* Low, vision
  perception, simultaneous without fusion H53.33
**Vitality, lack or want of** R53.83
  newborn P96.89
**Vitamin deficiency** — *see* Deficiency, vitamin
**Vitelline duct, persistent** Q43.0
**Vitiligo** L80
  eyelid H02.739
    left H02.736
      lower H02.735
      upper H02.734
    right H02.733
      lower H02.732
      upper H02.731
  pinta A67.2
  vulva N90.89
**Vitreal corneal syndrome** H59.01- ☑
**Vitreoretinopathy, proliferative** (*see also* Retinopathy,
  proliferative)
  with retinal detachment — *see* Detachment, retina,
    traction
**Vitreous** (*see also* condition)
  touch syndrome — *see* Complication, postprocedural,
    following cataract surgery
**Vocal cord** — *see* condition
**Vogt-Koyanagi syndrome** H20.82- ☑
**Vogt's disease or syndrome** G80.3
**Vogt-Spielmeyer amaurotic idiocy or disease** E75.4
**Voice**
  change R49.9
    specified NEC R49.8
  loss — *see* Aphonia
**Volhynian fever** A79.0
**Volkmann's ischemic contracture or paralysis** (complicating trauma) T79.6 ☑
**Volvulus** (bowel) (colon) (intestine) K56.2
  with perforation K56.2
  congenital Q43.8
  duodenum K31.5
  fallopian tube — *see* Torsion, fallopian tube
  oviduct — *see* Torsion, fallopian tube
  stomach (due to absence of gastrocolic ligament)
    K31.89
**Vomiting** R11.10
  with nausea R11.2
  without nausea R11.11
  asphyxia — *see* Foreign body, by site, causing asphyx-
    ia, gastric contents
  bilious (cause unknown) R11.14
    following gastro-intestinal surgery K91.0
    in newborn P92.01

**Vomiting** — *continued*
  blood — *see* Hematemesis
  causing asphyxia, choking, or suffocation — *see* For-
    eign body, by site
  cyclical G43.A0 (*following* G43.7)
    with refractory migraine G43.A1 (*following* G43.7)
    without refractory migraine G43.A0 (*following*
      G43.7)
    intractable G43.A1 (*following* G43.7)
    not intractable G43.A0 (*following* G43.7)
    psychogenic F50.89
  fecal mater R11.13
  following gastrointestinal surgery K91.0
    psychogenic F50.89
  functional K31.89
  hysterical F50.89
  nervous F50.89
  neurotic F50.89
  newborn NEC P92.09
    bilious P92.01
  periodic R11.10
    psychogenic F50.89
  projectile R11.12
  psychogenic F50.89
  uremic — *see* Uremia
**Vomito negro** — *see* Fever, yellow
**Von Bezold's abscess** — *see* Mastoiditis, acute
**Von Economo-Cruchet disease** A85.8
**Von Eulenburg's disease** G71.19
**Von Gierke's disease** E74.01
**Von Hippel** (-Lindau) **disease or syndrome** Q85.8
**Von Jaksch's anemia or disease** D64.89
**Von Recklinghausen**
  disease (neurofibromatosis) Q85.01
    bones E21.0
**Von Schroetter's syndrome** I82.890
**Von Willebrand** (-Jurgens)(-Minot) **disease or syn-**
  **drome** D68.0
**Von Zumbusch's disease** L40.1
**Voyeurism** F65.3
**Vrolik's disease** Q78.0
**Vulva** — *see* condition
**Vulvismus** N94.2
**Vulvitis** (acute) (allergic) (atrophic) (hypertrophic) (intertriginous) (senile) N76.2
  with ectopic or molar pregnancy O08.0
  adhesive, congenital Q52.79
  blennorrhagic (gonococcal) A54.02
  candidal B37.3
  chlamydial A56.02
  due to Haemophilus ducreyi A57
  following ectopic or molar pregnancy O08.0
  gonococcal A54.02
    with abscess (accessory gland) (periurethral) A54.1
  herpesviral A60.04
  leukoplakic N90.4
  monilial B37.3
  puerperal (postpartum) O86.19
  subacute or chronic N76.3
  syphilitic (early) A51.0
    late A52.76
  trichomonal A59.01
  tuberculous A18.18
**Vulvodynia** N94.819
  specified NEC N94.818
**Vulvorectal** — *see* condition
**Vulvovaginitis** (acute) — *see* Vaginitis

# W

**Waiting list, person on** Z75.1
  for organ transplant Z76.82
  undergoing social agency investigation Z75.2
**Waldenström**
  hypergammaglobulinemia D89.0
  syndrome or macroglobulinemia C88.0
**Waldenström-Kjellberg syndrome** D50.1
**Walking**
  difficulty R26.2
    psychogenic F44.4
  sleep F51.3
    hysterical F44.89
**Wall, abdominal** — *see* condition
**Wallenberg's disease or syndrome** G46.3
**Wallgren's disease** I87.8
**Wandering**
  gallbladder, congenital Q44.1
  in diseases classified elsewhere Z91.83

**Wandering** — *continued*
kidney, congenital Q63.8
organ or site, congenital NEC — *see* Malposition, congenital, by site
pacemaker (heart) I49.8
spleen D73.89
**War neurosis** F48.8
**Wart** (due to HPV) (filiform) (infectious) (viral) B07.9
anogenital region (venereal) A63.0
common B07.8
external genital organs (venereal) A63.0
flat B07.8
Hassal-Henle's (of cornea) H18.49
Peruvian A44.1
plantar B07.0
prosector (tuberculous) A18.4
seborrheic L82.1
inflamed L82.0
senile (seborrheic) L82.1
inflamed L82.0
tuberculous A18.4
venereal A63.0
**Warthin's tumor** — *see* Neoplasm, salivary gland, benign
**Wassilieff's disease** A27.0
**Wasting**
disease R64
due to malnutrition E41
extreme (due to malnutrition) E41
muscle NEC — *see* Atrophy, muscle
**Water**
clefts (senile cataract) — *see* Cataract, senile, incipient
deprivation of T73.1 ☑
intoxication E87.79
itch B76.9
lack of T73.1 ☑
loading E87.70
on
brain — *see* Hydrocephalus
chest J94.8
poisoning E87.79
**Waterbrash** R12
**Waterhouse** (-Friderichsen) **syndrome or disease** (meningococcal) A39.1
**Water-losing nephritis** N25.89
**Watermelon stomach** K31.819
with hemorrhage K31.811
without hemorrhage K31.819
**Watsoniasis** B66.8
**Wax in ear** — *see* Impaction, cerumen
**Weak, weakening, weakness** (generalized) R53.1
arches (acquired) (*see also* Deformity, limb, flat foot)
bladder (sphincter) R32
facial R29.810
following
cerebrovascular disease I69.992
cerebral infarction I69.392
intracerebral hemorrhage I69.192
nontraumatic intracranial hemorrhage NEC I69.292
specified disease NEC I69.892
stroke I69.392
subarachnoid hemorrhage I69.092
foot (double) — *see* Weak, arches
heart, cardiac — *see* Failure, heart
mind F70
muscle M62.81
myocardium — *see* Failure, heart
newborn P96.89
pelvic fundus N81.89
pubocervical tissue N81.82
rectovaginal tissue N81.83
senile R54
urinary stream R39.12
valvular — *see* Endocarditis
**Wear, worn** (with normal or routine use)
articular bearing surface of internal joint prosthesis — *see* Complications, joint prosthesis, mechanical, wear of articular bearing surfaces, by site
device, implant or graft — *see* Complications, by site, mechanical complication
tooth, teeth (approximal) (hard tissues) (interproximal) (occlusal) K03.0
**Weather, weathered**
effects of
cold T69.9 ☑
specified effect NEC T69.8 ☑
hot — *see* Heat
skin L57.8

**Weaver's syndrome** Q87.3
**Web, webbed** (congenital)
duodenal Q43.8
esophagus Q39.4
fingers Q70.1- ☑
larynx (glottic) (subglottic) Q31.0
neck (pterygium colli) Q18.3
Paterson-Kelly D50.1
popliteal syndrome Q87.89
toes Q70.3- ☑
**Weber-Christian disease** M35.6
**Weber-Cockayne syndrome** (epidermolysis bullosa) Q81.8
**Weber-Gubler syndrome** G46.3
**Weber-Leyden syndrome** G46.3
**Weber-Osler syndrome** I78.0
**Weber's paralysis or syndrome** G46.3
**Wedge-shaped or wedging vertebra** — *see* Collapse, vertebra NEC
**Wegener's granulomatosis or syndrome** M31.30
with
kidney involvement M31.31
lung involvement M31.30
with kidney involvement M31.31
**Wegner's disease** A50.02
**Weight**
1000-2499 grams at birth (low) — *see* Low, birth-weight
999 grams or less at birth (extremely low) — *see* Low, birthweight, extreme
and length below 10th percentile for gestational age P05.1- ☑
below but length above 10th percentile for gestational age P05.0- ☑
gain (abnormal) (excessive) R63.5
in pregnancy — *see* Pregnancy, complicated by, excessive weight gain
low — *see* Pregnancy, complicated by, insufficient, weight gain
loss (abnormal) (cause unknown) R63.4
**Weightlessness** (effect of) T75.82 ☑
**Weil** (l)-**Marchesani syndrome** Q87.1
**Weil's disease** A27.0
**Weingarten's syndrome** J82
**Weir Mitchell's disease** I73.81
**Weiss-Baker syndrome** G90.09
**Wells' disease** L98.3
**Wen** — *see* Cyst, sebaceous
**Wenckebach's block or phenomenon** I44.1
**Werdnig-Hoffmann syndrome** (muscular atrophy) G12.0
**Werlhof's disease** D69.3
**Werner's disease or syndrome** E31.21
**Werner-His disease** A79.0
**Werner's disease or syndrome** E34.8
**Wernicke-Korsakoff's syndrome or psychosis** (alcoholic) F10.96
with dependence F10.26
drug-induced
due to drug abuse — *see* Abuse, drug, by type, with amnestic disorder
due to drug dependence — *see* Dependence, drug, by type, with amnestic disorder
nonalcoholic F04
**Wernicke-Posadas disease** B38.9
**Wernicke's**
developmental aphasia F80.2
disease or syndrome E51.2
encephalopathy E51.2
polioencephalitis, superior E51.2
**West African fever** B50.8
**Westphal-Strümpell syndrome** E83.01
**West's syndrome** — *see* Epilepsy, spasms
**Wet**
feet, tropical (maceration) (syndrome) — *see* Immersion, foot
lung (syndrome), newborn P22.1
**Wharton's duct** — *see* condition
**Wheal** — *see* Urticaria
**Wheezing** R06.2
**Whiplash injury** S13.4 ☑
**Whipple's disease** (*see also* subcategory M14.8-) K90.81
**Whipworm** (disease) (infection) (infestation) B79
**Whistling face** Q87.0
**White** (*see also* condition)
kidney, small N03.9
leg, puerperal, postpartum, childbirth O87.1

**White** — *continued*
mouth B37.0
patches of mouth K13.29
spot lesions, teeth
chewing surface K02.51
pit and fissure surface K02.51
smooth surface K02.61
**Whitehead** L70.0
**Whitlow** (*see also* Cellulitis, digit)
with lymphangitis — *see* Lymphangitis, acute, digit
herpesviral B00.89
**Whitmore's disease or fever** — *see* Melioidosis
**Whooping cough** A37.90
with pneumonia A37.91
due to Bordetella
bronchiseptica A37.81
parapertussis A37.11
pertussis A37.01
specified organism NEC A37.81
due to
Bordetella
bronchiseptica A37.80
with pneumonia A37.81
parapertussis A37.10
with pneumonia A37.11
pertussis A37.00
with pneumonia A37.01
specified NEC A37.80
with pneumonia A37.81
**Wichman's asthma** J38.5
**Wide cranial sutures, newborn** P96.3
**Widening aorta** — *see* Ectasia, aorta
with aneurysm — *see* Aneurysm, aorta
**Wilkie's disease or syndrome** K55.1
**Wilkinson-Sneddon disease or syndrome** L13.1
**Willebrand** (-Jürgens) **thrombopathy** D68.0
**Willige-Hunt disease or syndrome** G23.1
**Wilms' tumor** C64- ☑
**Wilson-Mikity syndrome** P27.0
**Wilson's**
disease or syndrome E83.01
hepatolenticular degeneration E83.01
lichen ruber L43.9
**Window** (*see also* Imperfect, closure)
aorticopulmonary Q21.4
**Winter** — *see* condition
**Wiskott-Aldrich syndrome** D82.0
**Withdrawal state** (*see also* Dependence, drug by type, with withdrawal)
alcohol
with perceptual disturbances F10.232
without perceptual disturbances F10.239
caffeine F15.93
cannabis F12.288
newborn
correct therapeutic substance properly administered P96.2
infant of dependent mother P96.1
therapeutic substance, neonatal P96.2
**Witts' anemia** D50.8
**Witzelsucht** F07.0
**Woakes' ethmoiditis or syndrome** J33.1
**Wolff-Hirschorn syndrome** Q93.3
**Wolff-Parkinson-White syndrome** I45.6
**Wolhynian fever** A79.0
**Wolman's disease** E75.5
**Wood lung or pneumonitis** J67.8
**Woolly, wooly hair** (congenital) (nevus) Q84.1
**Woolsorter's disease** A22.1
**Word**
blindness (congenital) (developmental) F81.0
deafness (congenital) (developmental) H93.25
**Worm(s)** (infection) (infestation) (*see also* Infestation, helminth)
guinea B72
in intestine NEC B82.0
**Worm-eaten soles** A66.3
**Worn out** — *see* Exhaustion
cardiac
defibrillator (with synchronous cardiace pacemaker) Z45.02
pacemaker
battery Z45.010
lead Z45.018
device, implant or graft — *see* Complications, by site, mechanical
**Worried well** Z71.1
**Worries** R45.82

☑ **Additional Character Required** — **Refer to the Tabular List for Character Selection**    ⬇ **Subterms under main terms may continue to next column or page**

Index

**Wound check** Z48.0- ☑
    due to injury — *code to* Injury, by site, using appropriate seventh character for subsequent encounter
**Wound, open** T14.8- ☑
    abdomen, abdominal
        wall S31.109 ☑
            with penetration into peritoneal cavity S31.609 ☑
            bite — *see* Bite, abdomen, wall
            epigastric region S31.102 ☑
                with penetration into peritoneal cavity S31.602 ☑
                bite — *see* Bite, abdomen, wall, epigastric region
                laceration — *see* Laceration, abdomen, wall, epigastric region
                puncture — *see* Puncture, abdomen, wall, epigastric region
            laceration — *see* Laceration, abdomen, wall
            left
                lower quadrant S31.104 ☑
                    with penetration into peritoneal cavity S31.604 ☑
                    bite — *see* Bite, abdomen, wall, left, lower quadrant
                    laceration — *see* Laceration, abdomen, wall, left, lower quadrant
                    puncture — *see* Puncture, abdomen, wall, left, lower quadrant
                upper quadrant S31.101 ☑
                    with penetration into peritoneal cavity S31.601 ☑
                    bite — *see* Bite, abdomen, wall, left, upper quadrant
                    laceration — *see* Laceration, abdomen, wall, left, upper quadrant
                    puncture — *see* Puncture, abdomen, wall, left, upper quadrant
            periumbilic region S31.105 ☑
                with penetration into peritoneal cavity S31.605 ☑
                bite — *see* Bite, abdomen, wall, periumbilic region
                laceration — *see* Laceration, abdomen, wall, periumbilic region
                puncture — *see* Puncture, abdomen, wall, periumbilic region
            puncture — *see* Puncture, abdomen, wall
            right
                lower quadrant S31.103 ☑
                    with penetration into peritoneal cavity S31.603 ☑
                    bite — *see* Bite, abdomen, wall, right, lower quadrant
                    laceration — *see* Laceration, abdomen, wall, right, lower quadrant
                    puncture — *see* Puncture, abdomen, wall, right, lower quadrant
                upper quadrant S31.100 ☑
                  with penetration into peritoneal cavity S31.600 ☑
                  bite — *see* Bite, abdomen, wall, right, upper quadrant
                  laceration — *see* Laceration, abdomen, wall, right, upper quadrant
                  puncture — *see* Puncture, abdomen, wall, right, upper quadrant
    alveolar (process) — *see* Wound, open, oral cavity
    ankle S91.00- ☑
        bite — *see* Bite, ankle
        laceration — *see* Laceration, ankle
        puncture — *see* Puncture, ankle
    antecubital space — *see* Wound, open, elbow
    anterior chamber, eye — *see* Wound, open, ocular
    anus S31.839 ☑
        bite S31.835 ☑
        laceration — *see* Laceration, anus
        puncture — *see* Puncture, anus
    arm (upper) S41.10- ☑
        with amputation — *see* Amputation, traumatic, arm
        bite — *see* Bite, arm
        forearm — *see* Wound, open, forearm
        laceration — *see* Laceration, arm
        puncture — *see* Puncture, arm
    auditory canal (external) (meatus) — *see* Wound, open, ear

**Wound, open** — *continued*
    auricle, ear — *see* Wound, open, ear
    axilla — *see* Wound, open, arm
    back (*see also* Wound, open, thorax, back)
        lower S31.000 ☑
            with penetration into retroperitoneal space S31.001 ☑
            bite — *see* Bite, back, lower
            laceration — *see* Laceration, back, lower
            puncture — *see* Puncture, back, lower
    bite — *see* Bite
    blood vessel — *see* Injury, blood vessel
    breast S21.00- ☑
        with amputation — *see* Amputation, traumatic, breast
        bite — *see* Bite, breast
        laceration — *see* Laceration, breast
        puncture — *see* Puncture, breast
    buttock S31.809 ☑
        bite — *see* Bite, buttock
        laceration — *see* Laceration, buttock
        left S31.829 ☑
        puncture — *see* Puncture, buttock
        right S31.819 ☑
    calf — *see* Wound, open, leg
    canaliculus lacrimalis — *see* Wound, open, eyelid
    canthus, eye — *see* Wound, open, eyelid
    cervical esophagus S11.20 ☑
        bite S11.25 ☑
        laceration — *see* Laceration, esophagus, traumatic, cervical
        puncture — *see* Puncture, cervical esophagus
    cheek (external) S01.40- ☑
        bite — *see* Bite, cheek
        internal — *see* Wound, open, oral cavity
        laceration — *see* Laceration, cheek
        puncture — *see* Puncture, cheek
    chest wall — *see* Wound, open, thorax
    chin — *see* Wound, open, head, specified site NEC
    choroid — *see* Wound, open, ocular
    ciliary body (eye) — *see* Wound, open, ocular
    clitoris S31.40 ☑
        with amputation — *see* Amputation, traumatic, clitoris
        bite S31.45 ☑
        laceration — *see* Laceration, vulva
        puncture — *see* Puncture, vulva
    conjunctiva — *see* Wound, open, ocular
    cornea — *see* Wound, open, ocular
    costal region — *see* Wound, open, thorax
    Descemet's membrane — *see* Wound, open, ocular
    digit(s)
        foot — *see* Wound, open, toe
        hand — *see* Wound, open, finger
    ear (canal) (external) S01.30- ☑
        with amputation — *see* Amputation, traumatic, ear
        bite — *see* Bite, ear
        drum S09.2- ☑
        laceration — *see* Laceration, ear
        puncture — *see* Puncture, ear
    elbow S51.00- ☑
        bite — *see* Bite, elbow
        laceration — *see* Laceration, elbow
        puncture — *see* Puncture, elbow
    epididymis — *see* Wound, open, testis
    epigastric region S31.102 ☑
        with penetration into peritoneal cavity S31.602 ☑
        bite — *see* Bite, abdomen, wall, epigastric region
        laceration — *see* Laceration, abdomen, wall, epigastric region
        puncture — *see* Puncture, abdomen, wall, epigastric region
    epiglottis — *see* Wound, open, neck, specified site NEC
    esophagus (thoracic) S27.819 ☑
        cervical — *see* Wound, open, cervical esophagus
        laceration S27.813 ☑
        specified type NEC S27.818 ☑
    eye — *see* Wound, open, ocular
    eyeball — *see* Wound, open, ocular
    eyebrow — *see* Wound, open, eyelid
    eyelid S01.10- ☑
        bite — *see* Bite, eyelid
        laceration — *see* Laceration, eyelid
        puncture — *see* Puncture, eyelid

**Wound, open** — *continued*
    face NEC — *see* Wound, open, head, specified site NEC
    finger(s) S61.209 ☑
        with
            amputation — *see* Amputation, traumatic, finger
            damage to nail S61.309 ☑
        bite — *see* Bite, finger
        index S61.208 ☑
            with
                damage to nail S61.308 ☑
            left S61.201 ☑
                with
                    damage to nail S61.301 ☑
            right S61.200 ☑
                with
                    damage to nail S61.300 ☑
        laceration — *see* Laceration, finger
        little S61.208 ☑
            with
                damage to nail S61.308 ☑
            left S61.207 ☑
                with damage to nail S61.307 ☑
            right S61.206 ☑
                with damage to nail S61.306 ☑
        middle S61.208 ☑
            with
                damage to nail S61.308 ☑
            left S61.203 ☑
                with damage to nail S61.303 ☑
            right S61.202 ☑
                with damage to nail S61.302 ☑
        puncture — *see* Puncture, finger
        ring S61.208 ☑
            with
                damage to nail S61.308 ☑
            left S61.205 ☑
                with damage to nail S61.305 ☑
            right S61.204 ☑
                with damage to nail S61.304 ☑
    flank — *see* Wound, open, abdomen, wall
    foot (except toe(s) alone) S91.30- ☑
        with amputation — *see* Amputation, traumatic, foot
        bite — *see* Bite, foot
        laceration — *see* Laceration, foot
        puncture — *see* Puncture, foot
        toe — *see* Wound, open, toe
    forearm S51.80- ☑
        with
            amputation — *see* Amputation, traumatic, forearm
        bite — *see* Bite, forearm
        elbow only — *see* Wound, open, elbow
        laceration — *see* Laceration, forearm
        puncture — *see* Puncture, forearm
    forehead — *see* Wound, open, head, specified site NEC
    genital organs, external
        with amputation — *see* Amputation, traumatic, genital organs
        bite — *see* Bite, genital organ
        female S31.502 ☑
            vagina S31.40 ☑
            vulva S31.40 ☑
        laceration — *see* Laceration, genital organ
        male S31.501 ☑
            penis S31.20 ☑
            scrotum S31.30 ☑
            testes S31.30 ☑
        puncture — *see* Puncture, genital organ
    globe (eye) — *see* Wound, open, ocular
    groin — *see* Wound, open, abdomen, wall
    gum — *see* Wound, open, oral cavity
    hand S61.40- ☑
        with
            amputation — *see* Amputation, traumatic, hand
        bite — *see* Bite, hand
        finger(s) — *see* Wound, open, finger
        laceration — *see* Laceration, hand
        puncture — *see* Puncture, hand
        thumb — *see* Wound, open, thumb
    head S01.90 ☑
        bite — *see* Bite, head
        cheek — *see* Wound, open, cheek
        ear — *see* Wound, open, ear

Wound, open

ICD-10-CM 2018

**Wound, open** — *continued*
  head — *continued*
    eyelid — *see* Wound, open, eyelid
    laceration — *see* Laceration, head
    lip — *see* Wound, open, lip
    nose S01.20 ☑
    oral cavity — *see* Wound, open, oral cavity
    puncture — *see* Puncture, head
    scalp — *see* Wound, open, scalp
    specified site NEC S01.80 ☑
    temporomandibular area — *see* Wound, open, cheek
  heel — *see* Wound, open, foot
  hip S71.00- ☑
    with amputation — *see* Amputation, traumatic, hip
    bite — *see* Bite, hip
    laceration — *see* Laceration, hip
    puncture — *see* Puncture, hip
  hymen S31.40 ☑
    bite — *see* Bite, vulva
    laceration — *see* Laceration, vagina
    puncture — *see* Puncture, vagina
  hypochondrium S31.109 ☑
    bite — *see* Bite, hypochondrium
    laceration — *see* Laceration, hypochondrium
    puncture — *see* Puncture, hypochondrium
  hypogastric region S31.109 ☑
    bite — *see* Bite, hypogastric region
    laceration — *see* Laceration, hypogastric region
    puncture — *see* Puncture, hypogastric region
  iliac (region) — *see* Wound, open, inguinal region
  inguinal region S31.109 ☑
    bite — *see* Bite, abdomen, wall, lower quadrant
    laceration — *see* Laceration, inguinal region
    puncture — *see* Puncture, inguinal region
  instep — *see* Wound, open, foot
  interscapular region — *see* Wound, open, thorax, back
  intraocular — *see* Wound, open, ocular
  iris — *see* Wound, open, ocular
  jaw — *see* Wound, open, head, specified site NEC
  knee S81.00- ☑
    bite — *see* Bite, knee
    laceration — *see* Laceration, knee
    puncture — *see* Puncture, knee
  labium (majus) (minus) — *see* Wound, open, vulva
  laceration — *see* Laceration, by site
  lacrimal duct — *see* Wound, open, eyelid
  larynx S11.019 ☑
    bite — *see* Bite, larynx
    laceration — *see* Laceration, larynx
    puncture — *see* Puncture, larynx
  left
    lower quadrant S31.104 ☑
      with penetration into peritoneal cavity S31.604 ☑
      bite — *see* Bite, abdomen, wall, left, lower quadrant
      laceration — *see* Laceration, abdomen, wall, left, lower quadrant
      puncture — *see* Puncture, abdomen, wall, left, lower quadrant
    upper quadrant S31.101 ☑
      with penetration into peritoneal cavity S31.601 ☑
      bite — *see* Bite, abdomen, wall, left, upper quadrant
      laceration — *see* Laceration, abdomen, wall, left, upper quadrant
      puncture — *see* Puncture, abdomen, wall, left, upper quadrant
  leg (lower) S81.80- ☑
    with amputation — *see* Amputation, traumatic, leg
    ankle — *see* Wound, open, ankle
    bite — *see* Bite, leg
    foot — *see* Wound, open, foot
    knee — *see* Wound, open, knee
    laceration — *see* Laceration, leg
    puncture — *see* Puncture, leg
    toe — *see* Wound, open, toe
    upper — *see* Wound, open, thigh
  lip S01.501 ☑
    bite — *see* Bite, lip
    laceration — *see* Laceration, lip
    puncture — *see* Puncture, lip

  loin S31.109 ☑
    bite — *see* Bite, abdomen, wall
    laceration — *see* Laceration, loin
    puncture — *see* Puncture, loin
  lower back — *see* Wound, open, back, lower
  lumbar region — *see* Wound, open, back, lower
  malar region — *see* Wound, open, head, specified site NEC
  mammary — *see* Wound, open, breast
  mastoid region — *see* Wound, open, head, specified site NEC
  mouth — *see* Wound, open, oral cavity
  nail
    finger — *see* Wound, open, finger, with damage to nail
    toe — *see* Wound, open, toe, with damage to nail
  nape (neck) — *see* Wound, open, neck
  nasal (septum) (sinus) — *see* Wound, open, nose
  nasopharynx — *see* Wound, open, head, specified site NEC
  neck S11.90 ☑
    bite — *see* Bite, neck
    involving
      cervical esophagus S11.20 ☑
      larynx — *see* Wound, open, larynx
      pharynx S11.20 ☑
      thyroid S11.10 ☑
      trachea (cervical) S11.029 ☑
        bite — *see* Bite, trachea
        laceration S11.021 ☑
          with foreign body S11.022 ☑
        puncture S11.023 ☑
          with foreign body S11.024 ☑
    laceration — *see* Laceration, neck
    puncture — *see* Puncture, neck
    specified site NEC S11.80 ☑
    specified type NEC S11.89 ☑
  nose (septum) (sinus) S01.20 ☑
    with amputation — *see* Amputation, traumatic, nose
    bite — *see* Bite, nose
    laceration — *see* Laceration, nose
    puncture — *see* Puncture, nose
  ocular S05.90 ☑
    avulsion (traumatic enucleation) S05.7- ☑
    eyeball S05.6- ☑
      with foreign body S05.5- ☑
    eyelid — *see* Wound, open, eyelid
    laceration and rupture S05.3- ☑
      with prolapse or loss of intraocular tissue S05.2- ☑
    orbit (penetrating) (with or without foreign body) S05.4- ☑
    periocular area — *see* Wound, open, eyelid
    specified NEC S05.8X- ☑
  oral cavity S01.502 ☑
    bite S01.552 ☑
    laceration — *see* Laceration, oral cavity
    puncture — *see* Puncture, oral cavity
  orbit — *see* Wound, open, ocular, orbit
  palate — *see* Wound, open, oral cavity
  palm — *see* Wound, open, hand
  pelvis, pelvic (*see also* Wound, open, back, lower)
    girdle — *see* Wound, open, hip
  penetrating — *see* Puncture, by site
  penis S31.20 ☑
    with amputation — *see* Amputation, traumatic, penis
    bite S31.25 ☑
    laceration — *see* Laceration, penis
    puncture — *see* Puncture, penis
  perineum
    bite — *see* Bite, perineum
    female S31.502 ☑
    laceration — *see* Laceration, perineum
    male S31.501 ☑
    puncture — *see* Puncture, perineum
  periocular area (with or without lacrimal passages) — *see* Wound, open, eyelid
  periumbilic region S31.105 ☑
    with penetration into peritoneal cavity S31.605 ☑
    bite — *see* Bite, abdomen, wall, periumbilic region
    laceration — *see* Laceration, abdomen, wall, periumbilic region

  periumbilic region — *continued*
    puncture — *see* Puncture, abdomen, wall, periumbilic region
  phalanges
    finger — *see* Wound, open, finger
    toe — *see* Wound, open, toe
  pharynx S11.20 ☑
  pinna — *see* Wound, open, ear
  popliteal space — *see* Wound, open, knee
  prepuce — *see* Wound, open, penis
  pubic region — *see* Wound, open, back, lower
  pudendum — *see* Wound, open, genital organs, external
  puncture wound — *see* Puncture
  rectovaginal septum — *see* Wound, open, vagina
  right
    lower quadrant S31.103 ☑
      with penetration into peritoneal cavity S31.603 ☑
      bite — *see* Bite, abdomen, wall, right, lower quadrant
      laceration — *see* Laceration, abdomen, wall, right, lower quadrant
      puncture — *see* Puncture, abdomen, wall, right, lower quadrant
    upper quadrant S31.100 ☑
      with penetration into peritoneal cavity S31.600 ☑
      bite — *see* Bite, abdomen, wall, right, upper quadrant
      laceration — *see* Laceration, abdomen, wall, right, upper quadrant
      puncture — *see* Puncture, abdomen, wall, right, upper quadrant
  sacral region — *see* Wound, open, back, lower
  sacroiliac region — *see* Wound, open, back, lower
  salivary gland — *see* Wound, open, oral cavity
  scalp S01.00 ☑
    bite S01.05 ☑
    laceration — *see* Laceration, scalp
    puncture — *see* Puncture, scalp
  scalpel, newborn (birth injury) P15.8
  scapular region — *see* Wound, open, shoulder
  sclera — *see* Wound, open, ocular
  scrotum S31.30 ☑
    with amputation — *see* Amputation, traumatic, scrotum
    bite S31.35 ☑
    laceration — *see* Laceration, scrotum
    puncture — *see* Puncture, scrotum
  shin — *see* Wound, open, leg
  shoulder S41.00- ☑
    with amputation — *see* Amputation, traumatic, arm
    bite — *see* Bite, shoulder
    laceration — *see* Laceration, shoulder
    puncture — *see* Puncture, shoulder
  skin NOS T14.8 ☑
  spermatic cord — *see* Wound, open, testis
  sternal region — *see* Wound, open, thorax, front wall
  submaxillary region — *see* Wound, open, head, specified site NEC
  submental region — *see* Wound, open, head, specified site NEC
  subungual
    finger(s) — *see* Wound, open, finger
    toe(s) — *see* Wound, open, toe
  supraclavicular region — *see* Wound, open, neck, specified site NEC
  temple, temporal region — *see* Wound, open, head, specified site NEC
  temporomandibular area — *see* Wound, open, cheek
  testis S31.30 ☑
    with amputation — *see* Amputation, traumatic, testes
    bite S31.35 ☑
    laceration — *see* Laceration, testis
    puncture — *see* Puncture, testis
  thigh S71.10- ☑
    with amputation — *see* Amputation, traumatic, hip
    bite — *see* Bite, thigh
    laceration — *see* Laceration, thigh
    puncture — *see* Puncture, thigh
  thorax, thoracic (wall) S21.90 ☑
    back S21.20- ☑

328    ☑ Additional Character Required — Refer to the Tabular List for Character Selection    ▽ Subterms under main terms may continue to next column or page

**Wound, open** — *continued*
  thorax, thoracic — *continued*
    back — *continued*
      with penetration S21.40 ☑
    bite — *see* Bite, thorax
    breast — *see* Wound, open, breast
    front S21.10- ☑
      with penetration S21.30 ☑
    laceration — *see* Laceration, thorax
    puncture — *see* Puncture, thorax
  throat — *see* Wound, open, neck
  thumb S61.009 ☑
    with
      amputation — *see* Amputation, traumatic, thumb
      damage to nail S61.109 ☑
    bite — *see* Bite, thumb
    laceration — *see* Laceration, thumb
    left S61.002 ☑
      with
        damage to nail S61.102 ☑
    puncture — *see* Puncture, thumb
    right S61.001 ☑
      with
        damage to nail S61.101 ☑
  thyroid (gland) — *see* Wound, open, neck, thyroid
  toe(s) S91.109 ☑
    with
      amputation — *see* Amputation, traumatic, toe
      damage to nail S91.209 ☑
    bite — *see* Bite, toe
    great S91.103 ☑
      with
        damage to nail S91.203 ☑
      left S91.102 ☑
        with
          damage to nail S91.202 ☑
      right S91.101 ☑
        with
          damage to nail S91.201 ☑
    laceration — *see* Laceration, toe
    lesser S91.106 ☑
      with
        damage to nail S91.206 ☑
      left S91.105 ☑
        with
          damage to nail S91.205 ☑
      right S91.104 ☑
        with
          damage to nail S91.204 ☑
    puncture — *see* Puncture, toe
  tongue — *see* Wound, open, oral cavity
  trachea (cervical region) — *see* Wound, open, neck, trachea
  tunica vaginalis — *see* Wound, open, testis
  tympanum, tympanic membrane S09.2- ☑
    laceration — *see* Laceration, ear, drum
    puncture — *see* Puncture, tympanum
  umbilical region — *see* Wound, open, abdomen, wall, periumbilic region
  uvula — *see* Wound, open, oral cavity
  vagina S31.40 ☑
    bite S31.45 ☑
    laceration — *see* Laceration, vagina
    puncture — *see* Puncture, vagina
  vitreous (humor) — *see* Wound, open, ocular
  vocal cord S11.039 ☑
    bite — *see* Bite, vocal cord
    laceration S11.031 ☑
      with foreign body S11.032 ☑
    puncture S11.033 ☑
      with foreign body S11.034 ☑
  vulva S31.40 ☑
    with amputation — *see* Amputation, traumatic, vulva
    bite S31.45 ☑
    laceration — *see* Laceration, vulva
    puncture — *see* Puncture, vulva
  wrist S61.50- ☑
    bite — *see* Bite, wrist
    laceration — *see* Laceration, wrist
    puncture — *see* Puncture, wrist
**Wound, superficial** — *see* Injury (*see also* specified injury type)

**Wright's syndrome** G54.0
**Wrist** — *see* condition
**Wrong drug** (by accident) (given in error) — *see* Table of Drugs and Chemicals, by drug, poisoning
**Wry neck** — *see* Torticollis
**Wuchereria** (bancrofti) **infestation** B74.0
**Wuchereriasis** B74.0
**Wuchernde Struma Langhans** C73

# X

**Xanthelasma** (eyelid) (palpebrarum) H02.60
  left H02.66
    lower H02.65
    upper H02.64
  right H02.63
    lower H02.62
    upper H02.61
**Xanthelasmatosis** (essential) E78.2
**Xanthinuria, hereditary** E79.8
**Xanthoastrocytoma**
  specified site — *see* Neoplasm, malignant, by site
  unspecified site C71.9
**Xanthofibroma** — *see* Neoplasm, connective tissue, benign
**Xanthogranuloma** D76.3
**Xanthoma(s), xanthomatosis** (primary) (familial) (hereditary) E75.5
  with
    hyperlipoproteinemia
      Type I E78.3
      Type III E78.2
      Type IV E78.1
      Type V E78.3
  bone (generalisata) C96.5
  cerebrotendinous E75.5
  cutaneotendinous E75.5
  disseminatum (skin) E78.2
  eruptive E78.2
  hypercholesterinemic E78.00
  hypercholesterolemic E78.00
  hyperlipidemic E78.5
  joint E75.5
  multiple (skin) E78.2
  tendon (sheath) E75.5
  tuberosum E78.2
  tuberous E78.2
  tubo-eruptive E78.2
  verrucous, oral mucosa K13.4
**Xanthosis** R23.8
**Xenophobia** F40.10
**Xeroderma** (*see also* Ichthyosis)
  acquired L85.0
  eyelid H01.149
    left H01.146
      lower H01.145
      upper H01.144
    right H01.143
      lower H01.142
      upper H01.141
  pigmentosum Q82.1
  vitamin A deficiency E50.8
**Xerophthalmia** (vitamin A deficiency) E50.7
  unrelated to vitamin A deficiency — *see* Keratoconjunctivitis
**Xerosis**
  conjunctiva H11.14- ☑
    with Bitot's spots (*see also* Pigmentation, conjunctiva)
      vitamin A deficiency E50.1
    vitamin A deficiency E50.0
  cornea H18.89- ☑
    with ulceration — *see* Ulcer, cornea
      vitamin A deficiency E50.3
    vitamin A deficiency E50.2
  cutis L85.3
  skin L85.3
**Xerostomia** K11.7
**Xiphopagus** Q89.4
**XO syndrome** Q96.9
**X-ray** (of)
  abnormal findings — *see* Abnormal, diagnostic imaging
  breast (mammogram) (routine) Z12.31

**X-ray** — *continued*
  chest
    routine (as part of a general medical examination) Z00.00
      with abnormal findings Z00.01
  routine (as part of a general medical examination) Z00.00
    with abnormal findings Z00.01
**XXXXY syndrome** Q98.1
**XXY syndrome** Q98.0

# Y

**Yaba pox** (virus disease) B08.72
**Yatapoxvirus** B08.70
  specified NEC B08.79
**Yawning** R06.89
  psychogenic F45.8
**Yaws** A66.9
  cutaneous, less than five years after infection A66.2
  bone lesions A66.6
  butter A66.1
  chancre A66.0
  early (cutaneous) (macular) (maculopapular) (micropapular) (papular) A66.2
    frambeside A66.2
    skin lesions NEC A66.2
  eyelid A66.2
  ganglion A66.6
  gangosis, gangosa A66.5
  gumma, gummata A66.4
    bone A66.6
  gummatous
    frambeside A66.4
    osteitis A66.6
    periostitis A66.6
  hydrarthrosis (*see also* subcategory M14.8-) A66.6
  hyperkeratosis (early) (late) A66.3
  initial lesions A66.0
  joint lesions (*see also* subcategory M14.8-) A66.6
  juxta-articular nodules A66.7
  late nodular (ulcerated) A66.4
  latent (without clinical manifestations) (with positive serology) A66.8
  mother A66.0
  mucosal A66.7
  multiple papillomata A66.1
  nodular, late (ulcerated) A66.4
  osteitis A66.6
  papilloma, plantar or palmar A66.1
  periostitis (hypertrophic) A66.6
  specified NEC A66.7
  ulcers A66.4
  wet crab A66.1
**Yeast infection** (*see also* Candidiasis) B37.9
**Yellow**
  atrophy (liver) — *see* Failure, hepatic
  fever — *see* Fever, yellow
  jack — *see* Fever, yellow
  jaundice — *see* Jaundice
  nail syndrome L60.5
**Yersiniosis** (*see also* Infection, Yersinia)
  extraintestinal A28.2
  intestinal A04.6

# Z

**Zahorsky's syndrome** (herpangina) B08.5
**Zellweger's syndrome** Q87.89
**Zenker's diverticulum** (esophagus) K22.5
**Ziehen-Oppenheim disease** G24.1
**Zieve's syndrome** K70.0
**Zika NOS** A92.5
**Zinc**
  deficiency, dietary E60
  metabolism disorder E83.2
**Zollinger-Ellison syndrome** E16.4
**Zona** — *see* Herpes, zoster
**Zoophobia** F40.218
**Zoster** (herpes) — *see* Herpes, zoster
**Zygomycosis** B46.9
  specified NEC B46.8
**Zymotic** — *see* condition

Wound, open — Zymotic

▼ **Subterms under main terms may continue to next column or page**     ☑ **Additional Character Required — Refer to the Tabular List for Character Selection**     **329**

**Note:** The list below gives the code number for neoplasms by anatomical site. For each site there are six possible code numbers according to whether the neoplasm in question is malignant, benign, in situ, of uncertain behavior, or of unspecified nature. The description of the neoplasm will often indicate which of the six columns is appropriate; e.g., malignant melanoma of skin, benign fibroadenoma of breast, carcinoma in situ of cervix uteri. Where such descriptors are not present, the remainder of the Index should be consulted where guidance is given to the appropriate column for each morphological (histological) variety listed; e.g., Mesonephroma – see Neoplasm, malignant; Embryoma (see also Neoplasm, uncertain behavior); Disease, Bowen's – see Neoplasm, skin, in situ. However, the guidance in the Index can be overridden if one of the descriptors mentioned above is present; e.g., malignant adenoma of colon is coded to C18.9 and not to D12.6 as the adjective "malignant" overrides the Index entry "Adenoma (see also Neoplasm, benign, by site)." Codes listed with a dash -, following the code have a required additional character for laterality. The tabular list must be reviewed for the complete code.

| | Malignant Primary | Malignant Secondary | Ca in situ | Benign | Uncertain | Unspecified Behavior |
|---|---|---|---|---|---|---|
| **Neoplasm, neoplastic** | C80.1 | C79.9 | D09.9 | D36.9 | D48.9 | D49.9 |
| abdomen, | | | | | | |
|   abdominal | C76.2 | C79.8-☑ | D09.8 | D36.7 | D48.7 | D49.89 |
|   cavity | C76.2 | C79.8-☑ | D09.8 | D36.7 | D48.7 | D49.89 |
|   organ | C76.2 | C79.8-☑ | D09.8 | D36.7 | D48.7 | D49.89 |
|   viscera | C76.2 | C79.8-☑ | D09.8 | D36.7 | D48.7 | D49.89 |
|   wall — *see also* Neoplasm, abdomen, wall, | | | | | | |
|     skin | C44.509 | C79.2 | D04.5 | D23.5 | D48.5 | D49.2 |
|     connective | | | | | | |
|       tissue | C49.4 | C79.8-☑ | — | D21.4 | D48.1 | D49.2 |
|     skin | C44.509 | — | — | — | — | — |
|       basal cell | | | | | | |
|         carcinoma | C44.519 | — | — | — | — | — |
|       specified type | | | | | | |
|         NEC | C44.599 | — | — | — | — | — |
|       squamous cell | | | | | | |
|         carcinoma | C44.529 | — | — | — | — | — |
| abdominopelvic | C76.8 | C79.8-☑ | — | D36.7 | D48.7 | D49.89 |
| accessory sinus — *see* Neoplasm, sinus | | | | | | |
| acoustic nerve | C72.4-☑ | C79.49 | — | D33.3 | D43.3 | D49.7 |
| adenoid (pharynx) (tissue) | C11.1 | C79.89 | D00.08 | D10.6 | D37.05 | D49.0 |
| adipose tissue — *see also* Neoplasm, connective | | | | | | |
|   tissue | C49.4 | C79.89 | — | D21.9 | D48.1 | D49.2 |
| adnexa (uterine) | C57.4 | C79.89 | D07.39 | D28.7 | D39.8 | D49.59 |
| adrenal | C74.9-☑ | C79.7-☑ | D09.3 | D35.0-☑ | D44.1-☑ | D49.7 |
|   capsule | C74.9-☑ | C79.7-☑ | D09.3 | D35.0-☑ | D44.1-☑ | D49.7 |
|   cortex | C74.0-☑ | C79.7-☑ | D09.3 | D35.0-☑ | D44.1-☑ | D49.7 |
|   gland | C74.9-☑ | C79.7-☑ | D09.3 | D35.0-☑ | D44.1-☑ | D49.7 |
|   medulla | C74.1-☑ | C79.7-☑ | D09.3 | D35.0-☑ | D44.1-☑ | D49.7 |
| ala nasi (external) — *see also* Neoplasm, skin, | | | | | | |
|   nose | C44.301 | C79.2 | D04.39 | D23.39 | D48.5 | D49.2 |
| alimentary canal or tract NEC | C26.9 | C78.80 | D01.9 | D13.9 | D37.9 | D49.0 |
| alveolar | C03.9 | C79.89 | D00.03 | D10.39 | D37.09 | D49.0 |
|   mucosa | C03.9 | C79.89 | D00.03 | D10.39 | D37.09 | D49.0 |
|     lower | C03.1 | C79.89 | D00.03 | D10.39 | D37.09 | D49.0 |
|     upper | C03.0 | C79.89 | D00.03 | D10.39 | D37.09 | D49.0 |
|   ridge or process | C41.1 | C79.51 | — | D16.5 | D48.0 | D49.2 |
|     carcinoma | C03.9 | C79.8-☑ | — | — | — | — |
|       lower | C03.1 | C79.8-☑ | — | — | — | — |
|       upper | C03.0 | C79.8-☑ | — | — | — | — |
|     lower | C41.1 | C79.51 | — | D16.5 | D48.0 | D49.2 |
|       mucosa | C03.9 | C79.89 | D00.03 | D10.39 | D37.09 | D49.0 |
|         lower | C03.1 | C79.89 | D00.03 | D10.39 | D37.09 | D49.0 |
|         upper | C03.0 | C79.89 | D00.03 | D10.39 | D37.09 | D49.0 |
|     upper | C41.0 | C79.51 | — | D16.4 | D48.0 | D49.2 |
|   sulcus | C06.1 | C79.89 | D00.02 | D10.39 | D37.09 | D49.0 |
| alveolus | C03.9 | C79.89 | D00.03 | D10.39 | D37.09 | D49.0 |
|   lower | C03.1 | C79.89 | D00.03 | D10.39 | D37.09 | D49.0 |
|   upper | C03.0 | C79.89 | D00.03 | D10.39 | D37.09 | D49.0 |
| ampulla of Vater | C24.1 | C78.89 | D01.5 | D13.5 | D37.6 | D49.0 |
| ankle NEC | C76.5-☑ | C79.89 | D04.7-☑ | D36.7 | D48.7 | D49.89 |
| anorectum, anorectal (junction) | C21.8 | C78.5 | D01.3 | D12.9 | D37.8 | D49.0 |
| antecubital fossa or space | C76.4-☑ | C79.89 | D04.6-☑ | D36.7 | D48.7 | D49.89 |

| **Neoplasm, neoplastic —** *continued* | Malignant Primary | Malignant Secondary | Ca in situ | Benign | Uncertain | Unspecified Behavior |
|---|---|---|---|---|---|---|
| antrum (Highmore) (maxillary) | C31.0 | C78.39 | D02.3 | D14.0 | D38.5 | D49.1 |
|   pyloric | C16.3 | C78.89 | D00.2 | D13.1 | D37.1 | D49.0 |
|   tympanicum | C30.1 | C78.39 | D02.3 | D14.0 | D38.5 | D49.1 |
| anus, anal | C21.0 | C78.5 | D01.3 | D12.9 | D37.8 | D49.0 |
|   canal | C21.1 | C78.5 | D01.3 | D12.9 | D37.8 | D49.0 |
|   cloacogenic zone | C21.2 | C78.5 | D01.3 | D12.9 | D37.8 | D49.0 |
|   margin — *see also* Neoplasm, anus, | | | | | | |
|     skin | C44.500 | C79.2 | D04.5 | D23.5 | D48.5 | D49.2 |
|   overlapping lesion with rectosigmoid junction or | | | | | | |
|     rectum | C21.8 | — | — | — | — | — |
|   skin | C44.500 | C79.2 | D04.5 | D23.5 | D48.5 | D49.2 |
|     basal cell carcinoma | C44.510 | — | — | — | — | — |
|     specified type NEC | C44.590 | — | — | — | — | — |
|     squamous cell carcinoma | C44.520 | — | — | — | — | — |
|   sphincter | C21.1 | C78.5 | D01.3 | D12.9 | D37.8 | D49.0 |
| aorta (thoracic) | C49.3 | C79.89 | — | D21.3 | D48.1 | D49.2 |
|   abdominal | C49.4 | C79.89 | — | D21.4 | D48.1 | D49.2 |
| aortic body | C75.5 | C79.89 | — | D35.6 | D44.7 | D49.7 |
| aponeurosis | C49.9 | C79.89 | — | D21.9 | D48.1 | D49.2 |
|   palmar | C49.1-☑ | C79.89 | — | D21.1-☑ | D48.1 | D49.2 |
|   plantar | C49.2-☑ | C79.89 | — | D21.2-☑ | D48.1 | D49.2 |
| appendix | C18.1 | C78.5 | D01.0 | D12.1 | D37.3 | D49.0 |
| arachnoid | C70.9 | C79.49 | — | D32.9 | D42.9 | D49.7 |
|   cerebral | C70.0 | C79.32 | — | D32.0 | D42.0 | D49.7 |
|   spinal | C70.1 | C79.49 | — | D32.1 | D42.1 | D49.7 |
| areola | C50.0-☑ | C79.81 | D05-☑ | D24-☑ | D48.6-☑ | D49.3 |
| arm NEC | C76.4-☑ | C79.89 | D04.6-☑ | D36.7 | D48.7 | D49.89 |
| artery — *see* Neoplasm, connective tissue | | | | | | |
| aryepiglottic fold | C13.1 | C79.89 | D00.08 | D10.7 | D37.05 | D49.0 |
|   hypopharyngeal aspect | C13.1 | C79.89 | D00.08 | D10.7 | D37.05 | D49.0 |
|   laryngeal aspect | C32.1 | C78.39 | D02.0 | D14.1 | D38.0 | D49.1 |
|   marginal zone | C13.1 | C79.89 | D00.08 | D10.7 | D37.05 | D49.0 |
| arytenoid (cartilage) | C32.3 | C78.39 | D02.0 | D14.1 | D38.0 | D49.1 |
|   fold — *see* Neoplasm, aryepiglottic | | | | | | |
| associated with transplanted organ | C80.2 | — | — | — | — | — |
| atlas | C41.2 | C79.51 | — | D16.6 | D48.0 | D49.2 |
| atrium, cardiac | C38.0 | C79.89 | — | D15.1 | D48.7 | D49.89 |
| auditory | | | | | | |
|   canal (external) (skin) | C44.20-☑ | C79.2 | D04.2-☑ | D23.2-☑ | D48.5 | D49.2 |
|     internal | C30.1 | C78.39 | D02.3 | D14.0 | D38.5 | D49.1 |
|   nerve | C72.4-☑ | C79.49 | — | D33.3 | D43.3 | D49.7 |
|   tube | C30.1 | C78.39 | D02.3 | D14.0 | D38.5 | D49.1 |
|     opening | C11.2 | C79.89 | D00.08 | D10.6 | D37.05 | D49.0 |
| auricle, ear — *see also* Neoplasm, skin, | | | | | | |
|   ear | C44.20-☑ | C79.2 | D04.2-☑ | D23.2-☑ | D48.5 | D49.2 |
| auricular canal (external) — *see also* Neoplasm, skin, ear | | | | | | |
| | C44.20-☑ | C79.2 | D04.2-☑ | D23.2-☑ | D48.5 | D49.2 |
|   internal | C30.1 | C78.39 | D02.3 | D14.0 | D38.5 | D49.2 |
| autonomic nerve or nervous system NEC (see Neoplasm, nerve, peripheral) | | | | | | |
| axilla, axillary | C76.1 | C79.89 | D09.8 | D36.7 | D48.7 | D49.89 |
|   fold — *see also* Neoplasm, skin, | | | | | | |
|     trunk | C44.509 | C79.2 | D04.5 | D23.5 | D48.5 | D49.2 |
| back NEC | C76.8 | C79.89 | D04.5 | D36.7 | D48.7 | D49.89 |
| Bartholin's gland | C51.0 | C79.82 | D07.1 | D28.0 | D39.8 | D49.59 |
| basal ganglia | C71.0 | C79.31 | — | D33.0 | D43.0 | D49.6 |
| basis pedunculi | C71.7 | C79.31 | — | D33.1 | D43.1 | D49.6 |
| bile or biliary (tract) | C24.9 | C78.89 | D01.5 | D13.5 | D37.6 | D49.0 |
|   canaliculi (biliferi) (intrahepatic) | C22.1 | C78.7 | D01.5 | D13.4 | D37.6 | D49.0 |
|   canals, | | | | | | |
|     interlobular | C22.1 | C78.89 | D01.5 | D13.4 | D37.6 | D49.0 |

**Neoplasm Table** (left margin vertical)

**Neoplasm, bile or biliary — Neoplasm, brain NEC** (left margin vertical)

| | Malignant Primary | Malignant Secondary | Ca in situ | Benign | Uncertain | Unspecified Behavior |
|---|---|---|---|---|---|---|
| Neoplasm, neoplastic — *continued* | | | | | | |
| bile or biliary — *continued* | | | | | | |
| duct or passage (common) (cystic) (extrahepatic) | C24.0 | C78.89 | D01.5 | D13.5 | D37.6 | D49.0 |
| interlobular | C22.1 | C78.89 | D01.5 | D13.4 | D37.6 | D49.0 |
| intrahepatic | C22.1 | C78.7 | D01.5 | D13.4 | D37.6 | D49.0 |
| and extrahepatic | C24.8 | C78.89 | D01.5 | D13.5 | D37.6 | D49.0 |
| bladder (urinary) | C67.9 | C79.11 | D09.0 | D30.3 | D41.4 | D49.4 |
| dome | C67.1 | C79.11 | D09.0 | D30.3 | D41.4 | D49.4 |
| neck | C67.5 | C79.11 | D09.0 | D30.3 | D41.4 | D49.4 |
| orifice | C67.9 | C79.11 | D09.0 | D30.3 | D41.4 | D49.4 |
| ureteric | C67.6 | C79.11 | D09.0 | D30.3 | D41.4 | D49.4 |
| urethral | C67.5 | C79.11 | D09.0 | D30.3 | D41.4 | D49.4 |
| overlapping lesion | C67.8 | — | — | — | — | — |
| sphincter | C67.8 | C79.11 | D09.0 | D30.3 | D41.4 | D49.4 |
| trigone | C67.0 | C79.11 | D09.0 | D30.3 | D41.4 | D49.4 |
| urachus | C67.7 | C79.11 | D09.0 | D30.3 | D41.4 | D49.4 |
| wall | C67.9 | C79.11 | D09.0 | D30.3 | D41.4 | D49.4 |
| anterior | C67.3 | C79.11 | D09.0 | D30.3 | D41.4 | D49.4 |
| lateral | C67.2 | C79.11 | D09.0 | D30.3 | D41.4 | D49.4 |
| posterior | C67.4 | C79.11 | D09.0 | D30.3 | D41.4 | D49.4 |
| blood vessel — *see* Neoplasm, connective tissue | | | | | | |
| bone (periosteum) | C41.9 | C79.51 | — | D16.9 | D48.0 | D49.2 |
| acetabulum | C41.4 | C79.51 | — | D16.8 | D48.0 | D49.2 |
| ankle | C40.3-☑ | C79.51 | — | D16.3-☑ | — | — |
| arm NEC | C40.0-☑ | C79.51 | — | D16.0-☑ | — | — |
| astragalus | C40.3-☑ | C79.51 | — | D16.3-☑ | — | — |
| atlas | C41.2 | C79.51 | — | D16.6 | D48.0 | D49.2 |
| axis | C41.2 | C79.51 | — | D16.6 | D48.0 | D49.2 |
| back NEC | C41.2 | C79.51 | — | D16.6 | D48.0 | D49.2 |
| calcaneus | C40.3-☑ | C79.51 | — | D16.3-☑ | — | — |
| calvarium | C41.0 | C79.51 | — | D16.4 | D48.0 | D49.2 |
| carpus (any) | C40.1-☑ | C79.51 | — | D16.1-☑ | — | — |
| cartilage NEC | C41.9 | C79.51 | — | D16.9 | D48.0 | D49.2 |
| clavicle | C41.3 | C79.51 | — | D16.7 | D48.0 | D49.2 |
| clivus | C41.0 | C79.51 | — | D16.4 | D48.0 | D49.2 |
| coccygeal vertebra | C41.4 | C79.51 | — | D16.8 | D48.0 | D49.2 |
| coccyx | C41.4 | C79.51 | — | D16.8 | D48.0 | D49.2 |
| costal cartilage | C41.3 | C79.51 | — | D16.7 | D48.0 | D49.2 |
| costovertebral joint | C41.3 | C79.51 | — | D16.7 | D48.0 | D49.2 |
| cranial | C41.0 | C79.51 | — | D16.4 | D48.0 | D49.2 |
| cuboid | C40.3-☑ | C79.51 | — | D16.3-☑ | — | — |
| cuneiform | C41.9 | C79.51 | — | D16.9 | D48.0 | D49.2 |
| elbow | C40.0-☑ | C79.51 | — | D16.0-☑ | — | — |
| ethmoid (labyrinth) | C41.0 | C79.51 | — | D16.4 | D48.0 | D49.2 |
| face | C41.0 | C79.51 | — | D16.4 | D48.0 | D49.2 |
| femur (any part) | C40.2-☑ | C79.51 | — | D16.2-☑ | — | — |
| fibula (any part) | C40.2-☑ | C79.51 | — | D16.2-☑ | — | — |
| finger (any) | C40.1-☑ | C79.51 | — | D16.1-☑ | — | — |
| foot | C40.3-☑ | C79.51 | — | D16.3-☑ | — | — |
| forearm | C40.0-☑ | C79.51 | — | D16.0-☑ | — | — |
| frontal | C41.0 | C79.51 | — | D16.4 | D48.0 | D49.2 |
| hand | C40.1-☑ | C79.51 | — | D16.1-☑ | — | — |
| heel | C40.3-☑ | C79.51 | — | D16.3-☑ | — | — |
| hip | C41.4 | C79.51 | — | D16.8 | D48.0 | D49.2 |
| humerus (any part) | C40.0-☑ | C79.51 | — | D16.0-☑ | — | — |
| hyoid | C41.0 | C79.51 | — | D16.4 | D48.0 | D49.2 |
| ilium | C41.4 | C79.51 | — | D16.8 | D48.0 | D49.2 |
| innominate | C41.4 | C79.51 | — | D16.8 | D48.0 | D49.2 |
| intervertebral cartilage or disc | C41.2 | C79.51 | — | D16.6 | D48.0 | D49.2 |
| ischium | C41.4 | C79.51 | — | D16.8 | D48.0 | D49.2 |
| jaw (lower) | C41.1 | C79.51 | — | D16.5 | D48.0 | D49.2 |
| knee | C40.2-☑ | C79.51 | — | D16.2-☑ | — | — |
| leg NEC | C40.2-☑ | C79.51 | — | D16.2-☑ | — | — |
| limb NEC | C40.9-☑ | C79.51 | — | D16.9 | — | — |
| lower (long bones) | C40.2-☑ | C79.51 | — | D16.2-☑ | — | — |
| short bones | C40.3-☑ | C79.51 | — | D16.3-☑ | — | — |
| upper (long bones) | C40.0-☑ | C79.51 | — | D16.0-☑ | — | — |
| short bones | C40.1-☑ | C79.51 | — | D16.1-☑ | — | — |
| malar | C41.0 | C79.51 | — | D16.4 | D48.0 | D49.2 |

| | Malignant Primary | Malignant Secondary | Ca in situ | Benign | Uncertain | Unspecified Behavior |
|---|---|---|---|---|---|---|
| Neoplasm, neoplastic — *continued* | | | | | | |
| bone — *continued* | | | | | | |
| mandible | C41.1 | C79.51 | — | D16.5 | D48.0 | D49.2 |
| marrow NEC (any bone) | C96.9 | C79.52 | — | — | D47.9 | D49.89 |
| mastoid | C41.0 | C79.51 | — | D16.4 | D48.0 | D49.2 |
| maxilla, maxillary (superior) | C41.0 | C79.51 | — | D16.4 | D48.0 | D49.2 |
| inferior | C41.1 | C79.51 | — | D16.5 | D48.0 | D49.2 |
| metacarpus (any) | C40.1-☑ | C79.51 | — | D16.1-☑ | — | — |
| metatarsus (any) | C40.3-☑ | C79.51 | — | D16.3-☑ | — | — |
| navicular | | | | | | |
| ankle | C40.3-☑ | C79.51 | — | — | — | — |
| hand | C40.1-☑ | C79.51 | — | — | — | — |
| nose, nasal | C41.0 | C79.51 | — | D16.4 | D48.0 | D49.2 |
| occipital | C41.0 | C79.51 | — | D16.4 | D48.0 | D49.2 |
| orbit | C41.0 | C79.51 | — | D16.4 | D48.0 | D49.2 |
| overlapping sites | C40.8-☑ | — | — | — | — | — |
| parietal | C41.0 | C79.51 | — | D16.4 | D48.0 | D49.2 |
| patella | C40.2-☑ | C79.51 | — | — | — | — |
| pelvic | C41.4 | C79.51 | — | D16.8 | D48.0 | D49.2 |
| phalanges | | | | | | |
| foot | C40.3-☑ | C79.51 | — | — | — | — |
| hand | C40.1-☑ | C79.51 | — | — | — | — |
| pubic | C41.4 | C79.51 | — | D16.8 | D48.0 | D49.2 |
| radius (any part) | C40.0-☑ | C79.51 | — | D16.0-☑ | — | — |
| rib | C41.3 | C79.51 | — | D16.7 | D48.0 | D49.2 |
| sacral vertebra | C41.4 | C79.51 | — | D16.8 | D48.0 | D49.2 |
| sacrum | C41.4 | C79.51 | — | D16.8 | D48.0 | D49.2 |
| scaphoid | | | | | | |
| of ankle | C40.3-☑ | C79.51 | — | — | — | — |
| of hand | C40.1-☑ | C79.51 | — | — | — | — |
| scapula (any part) | C40.0-☑ | C79.51 | — | D16.0-☑ | — | — |
| sella turcica | C41.0 | C79.51 | — | D16.4 | D48.0 | D49.2 |
| shoulder | C40.0-☑ | C79.51 | — | D16.0-☑ | — | — |
| skull | C41.0 | C79.51 | — | D16.4 | D48.0 | D49.2 |
| sphenoid | C41.0 | C79.51 | — | D16.4 | D48.0 | D49.2 |
| spine, spinal (column) | C41.2 | C79.51 | — | D16.6 | D48.0 | D49.2 |
| coccyx | C41.4 | C79.51 | — | D16.8 | D48.0 | D49.2 |
| sacrum | C41.4 | C79.51 | — | D16.8 | D48.0 | D49.2 |
| sternum | C41.3 | C79.51 | — | D16.7 | D48.0 | D49.2 |
| tarsus (any) | C40.3-☑ | C79.51 | — | — | — | — |
| temporal | C41.0 | C79.51 | — | D16.4 | D48.0 | D49.2 |
| thumb | C40.1-☑ | C79.51 | — | — | — | — |
| tibia (any part) | C40.2-☑ | C79.51 | — | — | — | — |
| toe (any) | C40.3-☑ | C79.51 | — | — | — | — |
| trapezium | C40.1-☑ | C79.51 | — | — | — | — |
| trapezoid | C40.1-☑ | C79.51 | — | — | — | — |
| turbinate | C41.0 | C79.51 | — | D16.4 | D48.0 | D49.2 |
| ulna (any part) | C40.0-☑ | C79.51 | — | D16.0-☑ | — | — |
| unciform | C40.1-☑ | C79.51 | — | — | — | — |
| vertebra (column) | C41.2 | C79.51 | — | D16.6 | D48.0 | D49.2 |
| coccyx | C41.4 | C79.51 | — | D16.8 | D48.0 | D49.2 |
| sacrum | C41.4 | C79.51 | — | D16.8 | D48.0 | D49.2 |
| vomer | C41.0 | C79.51 | — | D16.4 | D48.0 | D49.2 |
| wrist | C40.1-☑ | C79.51 | — | — | — | — |
| xiphoid process | C41.3 | C79.51 | — | D16.7 | D48.0 | D49.2 |
| zygomatic | C41.0 | C79.51 | — | D16.4 | D48.0 | D49.2 |
| book-leaf (mouth) — *ventral surface of tongue and floor of mouth* | C06.89 | C79.89 | D00.00 | D10.39 | D37.09 | D49.0 |
| bowel — *see* Neoplasm, intestine | | | | | | |
| brachial plexus | C47.1-☑ | C79.89 | — | D36.12 | D48.2 | D49.2 |
| brain NEC | C71.9 | C79.31 | — | D33.2 | D43.2 | D49.6 |
| basal ganglia | C71.0 | C79.31 | — | D33.0 | D43.0 | D49.6 |
| cerebellopontine angle | C71.6 | C79.31 | — | D33.1 | D43.1 | D49.6 |
| cerebellum NOS | C71.6 | C79.31 | — | D33.1 | D43.1 | D49.6 |
| cerebrum | C71.0 | C79.31 | — | D33.0 | D43.0 | D49.6 |
| choroid plexus | C71.7 | C79.31 | — | D33.1 | D43.1 | D49.6 |
| corpus callosum | C71.8 | C79.31 | — | D33.2 | D43.2 | D49.6 |
| corpus striatum | C71.0 | C79.31 | — | D33.0 | D43.0 | D49.6 |
| cortex (cerebral) | C71.0 | C79.31 | — | D33.0 | D43.0 | D49.6 |
| frontal lobe | C71.1 | C79.31 | — | D33.0 | D43.0 | D49.6 |
| globus pallidus | C71.0 | C79.31 | — | D33.0 | D43.0 | D49.6 |
| hippocampus | C71.2 | C79.31 | — | D33.0 | D43.0 | D49.6 |
| hypothalamus | C71.0 | C79.31 | — | D33.0 | D43.0 | D49.6 |
| internal capsule | C71.0 | C79.31 | — | D33.0 | D43.0 | D49.6 |

☑ **Additional Character Required — Refer to the Tabular List for Character Selection**  ▽ **Subterms under main terms may continue to next column or page**

**Neoplasm, neoplastic —** *continued*

| | Malignant Primary | Malignant Secondary | Ca in situ | Benign | Uncertain | Unspecified Behavior |
|---|---|---|---|---|---|---|
| brain — *continued* | | | | | | |
| medulla oblongata | C71.7 | C79.31 | — | D33.1 | D43.1 | D49.6 |
| meninges | C70.0 | C79.32 | — | D32.0 | D42.0 | D49.7 |
| midbrain | C71.7 | C79.31 | — | D33.1 | D43.1 | D49.6 |
| occipital lobe | C71.4 | C79.31 | — | D33.0 | D43.0 | D49.6 |
| overlapping lesion | C71.8 | C79.31 | — | — | — | D49.6 |
| parietal lobe | C71.3 | C79.31 | — | D33.0 | D43.0 | D49.6 |
| peduncle | C71.7 | C79.31 | — | D33.1 | D43.1 | D49.6 |
| pons | C71.7 | C79.31 | — | D33.1 | D43.1 | D49.6 |
| stem | C71.7 | C79.31 | — | D33.1 | D43.1 | D49.6 |
| tapetum | C71.8 | C79.31 | — | D33.2 | D43.2 | D49.6 |
| temporal lobe | C71.2 | C79.31 | — | D33.0 | D43.0 | D49.6 |
| thalamus | C71.0 | C79.31 | — | D33.0 | D43.0 | D49.6 |
| uncus | C71.2 | C79.31 | — | D33.0 | D43.0 | D49.6 |
| ventricle (floor) | C71.5 | C79.31 | — | D33.0 | D43.0 | D49.6 |
| fourth | C71.7 | C79.31 | — | D33.1 | D43.1 | D49.6 |
| branchial (cleft) (cyst) (vestiges) | C10.4 | C79.89 | D00.08 | D10.5 | D37.05 | D49.0 |
| breast (connective tissue) (glandular tissue) (soft parts) | C50.9-☑ | C79.81 | D05.-☑ | D24.-☑ | D48.6-☑ | D49.3 |
| areola | C50.0-☑ | C79.81 | D05.-☑ | D24.-☑ | D48.6-☑ | D49.3 |
| axillary tail | C50.6-☑ | C79.81 | D05.-☑ | D24.-☑ | D48.6-☑ | D49.3 |
| central portion | C50.1-☑ | C79.81 | D05.-☑ | D24.-☑ | D48.6-☑ | D49.3 |
| inner | C50.8-☑ | C79.81 | D05.-☑ | D24.-☑ | D48.6-☑ | D49.3 |
| lower | C50.8-☑ | C79.81 | D05.-☑ | D24.-☑ | D48.6-☑ | D49.3 |
| lower-inner quadrant | C50.3-☑ | C79.81 | D05.-☑ | D24.-☑ | D48.6-☑ | D49.3 |
| lower-outer quadrant | C50.5-☑ | C79.81 | D05.-☑ | D24.-☑ | D48.6-☑ | D49.3 |
| mastectomy site (skin) — *see also* Neoplasm, breast, skin | C44.501 | C79.2 | — | — | — | — |
| specified as breast tissue | C50.8-☑ | C79.81 | — | — | — | — |
| midline | C50.8-☑ | C79.81 | D05.-☑ | D24.-☑ | D48.6-☑ | D49.3 |
| nipple | C50.0-☑ | C79.81 | D05.-☑ | D24.-☑ | D48.6-☑ | D49.3 |
| outer | C50.8-☑ | C79.81 | D05.-☑ | D24.-☑ | D48.6-☑ | D49.3 |
| overlapping lesion | C50.8-☑ | — | — | — | — | — |
| skin | C44.501 | C79.2 | D04.5 | D23.5 | D48.5 | D49.2 |
| basal cell carcinoma | C44.511 | — | — | — | — | — |
| specified type NEC | C44.591 | — | — | — | — | — |
| squamous cell carcinoma | C44.521 | — | — | — | — | — |
| tail (axillary) | C50.6-☑ | C79.81 | D05.-☑ | D24.-☑ | D48.6-☑ | D49.3 |
| upper | C50.8-☑ | C79.81 | D05.-☑ | D24.-☑ | D48.6-☑ | D49.3 |
| upper-inner quadrant | C50.2-☑ | C79.81 | D05.-☑ | D24.-☑ | D48.6-☑ | D49.3 |
| upper-outer quadrant | C50.4-☑ | C79.81 | D05.-☑ | D24.-☑ | D48.6-☑ | D49.3 |
| broad ligament | C57.1-☑ | C79.82 | D07.39 | D28.2 | D39.8 | D49.59 |
| bronchiogenic, bronchogenic, (lung) | C34.9-☑ | C78.0-☑ | D02.2-☑ | D14.3-☑ | D38.1 | D49.1 |
| bronchiole | C34.9-☑ | C78.0-☑ | D02.2-☑ | D14.3-☑ | D38.1 | D49.1 |
| bronchus | C34.9-☑ | C78.0-☑ | D02.2-☑ | D14.3-☑ | D38.1 | D49.1 |
| carina | C34.0-☑ | C78.0-☑ | D02.2-☑ | D14.3-☑ | D38.1 | D49.1 |
| lower lobe of lung | C34.3-☑ | C78.0-☑ | D02.2-☑ | D14.3-☑ | D38.1 | D49.1 |
| main | C34.0-☑ | C78.0-☑ | D02.2-☑ | D14.3-☑ | D38.1 | D49.1 |
| middle lobe of lung | C34.2 | C78.0-☑ | D02.21 | D14.31 | D38.1 | D49.1 |
| overlapping lesion | C34.8-☑ | — | — | — | — | — |
| upper lobe of lung | C34.1-☑ | C78.0-☑ | D02.2-☑ | D14.3-☑ | D38.1 | D49.1 |
| brow | C44.309 | C79.2 | D04.39 | D23.39 | D48.5 | D49.2 |
| basal cell carcinoma | C44.319 | — | — | — | — | — |
| specified type NEC | C44.399 | — | — | — | — | — |
| squamous cell carcinoma | C44.329 | — | — | — | — | — |
| buccal (cavity) | C06.9 | C79.89 | D00.00 | D10.39 | D37.09 | D49.0 |
| commissure | C06.0 | C79.89 | D00.02 | D10.39 | D37.09 | D49.0 |
| groove (lower) (upper) | C06.1 | C79.89 | D00.02 | D10.39 | D37.09 | D49.0 |
| mucosa | C06.0 | C79.89 | D00.02 | D10.39 | D37.09 | D49.0 |
| sulcus (lower) (upper) | C06.1 | C79.89 | D00.02 | D10.39 | D37.09 | D49.0 |

**Neoplasm, neoplastic —** *continued*

| | Malignant Primary | Malignant Secondary | Ca in situ | Benign | Uncertain | Unspecified Behavior |
|---|---|---|---|---|---|---|
| bulbourethral gland | C68.0 | C79.19 | D09.19 | D30.4 | D41.3 | D49.59 |
| bursa — *see* Neoplasm, connective tissue | | | | | | |
| buttock NEC | C76.3 | C79.89 | D04.5 | D36.7 | D48.7 | D49.89 |
| calf | C76.5-☑ | C79.89 | D04.7-☑ | D36.7 | D48.7 | D49.89 |
| calvarium | C41.0 | C79.51 | — | D16.4 | D48.0 | D49.2 |
| calyx, renal | C65.-☑ | C79.0-☑ | D09.19 | D30.1-☑ | D41.1-☑ | D49.51-☑ |
| canal | | | | | | |
| anal | C21.1 | C78.5 | D01.3 | D12.9 | D37.8 | D49.0 |
| auditory (external) — *see also* Neoplasm, skin, ear | C44.20-☑ | C79.2 | D04.2-☑ | D23.2-☑ | D48.5 | D49.2 |
| auricular (external) — *see also* Neoplasm, skin, ear | C44.20-☑ | C79.2 | D04.2-☑ | D23.2-☑ | D48.5 | D49.2 |
| canaliculi, biliary (biliferi) (intrahepatic) | C22.1 | C78.7 | D01.5 | D13.4 | D37.6 | D49.0 |
| canthus (eye) (inner) (outer) | C44.10-☑ | C79.2 | D04.1-☑ | D23.1-☑ | D48.5 | D49.2 |
| basal cell carcinoma | C44.11-☑ | — | — | — | — | — |
| specified type NEC | C44.19-☑ | — | — | — | — | — |
| squamous cell carcinoma | C44.12-☑ | — | — | — | — | — |
| capillary — *see* Neoplasm, connective tissue | | | | | | |
| caput coli | C18.0 | C78.5 | D01.0 | D12.0 | D37.4 | D49.0 |
| carcinoid — *see* Tumor, carcinoid | | | | | | |
| cardia (gastric) | C16.0 | C78.89 | D00.2 | D13.1 | D37.1 | D49.0 |
| cardiac orifice (stomach) | C16.0 | C78.89 | D00.2 | D13.1 | D37.1 | D49.0 |
| cardio-esophageal junction | C16.0 | C78.89 | D00.2 | D13.1 | D37.1 | D49.0 |
| cardio-esophagus | C16.0 | C78.89 | D00.2 | D13.1 | D37.1 | D49.0 |
| carina (bronchus) | C34.0-☑ | C78.0-☑ | D02.2-☑ | D14.3-☑ | D38.1 | D49.1 |
| carotid (artery) | C49.0 | C79.89 | — | D21.0 | D48.1 | D49.2 |
| body | C75.4 | C79.89 | — | D35.5 | D44.6 | D49.7 |
| carpus (any bone) | C40.1-☑ | C79.51 | — | D16.1-☑ | — | — |
| cartilage (articular) (joint) NEC — *see also* Neoplasm, bone | C41.9 | C79.51 | — | D16.9 | D48.0 | D49.2 |
| arytenoid | C32.3 | C78.39 | D02.0 | D14.1 | D38.0 | D49.1 |
| auricular | C49.0 | C79.89 | — | D21.0 | D48.1 | D49.2 |
| bronchi | C34.0-☑ | C78.39 | — | D14.3-☑ | D38.1 | D49.1 |
| costal | C41.3 | C79.51 | — | D16.7 | D48.0 | D49.2 |
| cricoid | C32.3 | C78.39 | D02.0 | D14.1 | D38.0 | D49.1 |
| cuneiform | C32.3 | C78.39 | D02.0 | D14.1 | D38.0 | D49.1 |
| ear (external) | C49.0 | C79.89 | — | D21.0 | D48.1 | D49.2 |
| ensiform | C41.3 | C79.51 | — | D16.7 | D48.0 | D49.2 |
| epiglottis | C32.1 | C78.39 | D02.0 | D14.1 | D38.0 | D49.1 |
| anterior surface | C10.1 | C79.89 | D00.08 | D10.5 | D37.05 | D49.0 |
| eyelid | C49.0 | C79.89 | — | D21.0 | D48.1 | D49.2 |
| intervertebral | C41.2 | C79.51 | — | D16.6 | D48.0 | D49.2 |
| larynx, laryngeal | C32.3 | C78.39 | D02.0 | D14.1 | D38.0 | D49.1 |
| nose, nasal | C30.0 | C78.39 | D02.3 | D14.0 | D38.5 | D49.1 |
| pinna | C49.0 | C79.89 | — | D21.0 | D48.1 | D49.2 |
| rib | C41.3 | C79.51 | — | D16.7 | D48.0 | D49.2 |
| semilunar (knee) | C40.2-☑ | C79.51 | — | D16.2-☑ | D48.0 | D49.2 |
| thyroid | C32.3 | C78.39 | D02.0 | D14.1 | D38.0 | D49.1 |
| trachea | C33 | C78.39 | D02.1 | D14.2 | D38.1 | D49.1 |
| cauda equina | C72.1 | C79.49 | — | D33.4 | D43.4 | D49.7 |
| cavity | | | | | | |
| buccal | C06.9 | C79.89 | D00.00 | D10.30 | D37.09 | D49.0 |
| nasal | C30.0 | C78.39 | D02.3 | D14.0 | D38.5 | D49.1 |
| oral | C06.9 | C79.89 | D00.00 | D10.30 | D37.09 | D49.0 |
| peritoneal | C48.2 | C78.6 | — | D20.1 | D48.4 | D49.0 |
| tympanic | C30.1 | C78.39 | D02.3 | D14.0 | D38.5 | D49.1 |
| cecum | C18.0 | C78.5 | D01.0 | D12.0 | D37.4 | D49.0 |
| central nervous system | C72.9 | C79.40 | — | — | — | — |
| cerebellopontine (angle) | C71.6 | C79.31 | — | D33.1 | D43.1 | D49.6 |
| cerebellum, cerebellar | C71.6 | C79.31 | — | D33.1 | D43.1 | D49.6 |
| cerebrum, cerebral (cortex) (hemisphere) (white matter) | C71.0 | C79.31 | — | D33.0 | D43.0 | D49.6 |
| meninges | C70.0 | C79.32 | — | D32.0 | D42.0 | D49.7 |
| peduncle | C71.7 | C79.31 | — | D33.1 | D43.1 | D49.6 |

Neoplasm, cerebrum, cerebral — Neoplasm, connective tissue NEC

**Neoplasm, neoplastic — continued**

| | Malignant Primary | Malignant Secondary | Ca in situ | Benign | Uncertain | Unspecified Behavior |
|---|---|---|---|---|---|---|
| cerebrum, cerebral — continued | | | | | | |
| ventricle | C71.5 | C79.31 | — | D33.0 | D43.0 | D49.6 |
| fourth | C71.7 | C79.31 | — | D33.1 | D43.1 | D49.6 |
| cervical region | C76.0 | C79.89 | D09.8 | D36.7 | D48.7 | D49.89 |
| cervix (cervical) (uteri) (uterus) | C53.9 | C79.82 | D06.9 | D26.0 | D39.0 | D49.59 |
| canal | C53.0 | C79.82 | D06.0 | D26.0 | D39.0 | D49.59 |
| endocervix (canal) (gland) | C53.0 | C79.82 | D06.0 | D26.0 | D39.0 | D49.59 |
| exocervix | C53.1 | C79.82 | D06.1 | D26.0 | D39.0 | D49.59 |
| external os | C53.1 | C79.82 | D06.1 | D26.0 | D39.0 | D49.59 |
| internal os | C53.0 | C79.82 | D06.0 | D26.0 | D39.0 | D49.59 |
| nabothian gland | C53.0 | C79.82 | D06.0 | D26.0 | D39.0 | D49.59 |
| overlapping lesion | C53.8 | — | — | — | — | — |
| squamocolumnar junction | C53.8 | C79.82 | D06.7 | D26.0 | D39.0 | D49.59 |
| stump | C53.8 | C79.82 | D06.7 | D26.0 | D39.0 | D49.59 |
| cheek | C76.0 | C79.89 | D09.8 | D36.7 | D48.7 | D49.89 |
| external | C44.309 | C79.2 | D04.39 | D23.39 | D48.5 | D49.2 |
| basal cell carcinoma | C44.319 | — | — | — | — | — |
| specified type NEC | C44.399 | — | — | — | — | — |
| squamous cell carcinoma | C44.329 | — | — | — | — | — |
| inner aspect | C06.0 | C79.89 | D00.02 | D10.39 | D37.09 | D49.0 |
| internal | C06.0 | C79.89 | D00.02 | D10.39 | D37.09 | D49.0 |
| mucosa | C06.0 | C79.89 | D00.02 | D10.39 | D37.09 | D49.0 |
| chest (wall) NEC | C76.1 | C79.89 | D09.8 | D36.7 | D48.7 | D49.89 |
| chiasma opticum | C72.3-☑ | C79.49 | — | D33.3 | D43.3 | D49.7 |
| chin | C44.309 | C79.2 | D04.39 | D23.39 | D48.5 | D49.2 |
| basal cell carcinoma | C44.319 | — | — | — | — | — |
| specified type NEC | C44.399 | — | — | — | — | — |
| squamous cell carcinoma | C44.329 | — | — | — | — | — |
| choana | C11.3 | C79.89 | D00.08 | D10.6 | D37.05 | D49.0 |
| cholangiole | C22.1 | C78.89 | D01.5 | D13.4 | D37.6 | D49.0 |
| choledochal duct | C24.0 | C78.89 | D01.5 | D13.5 | D37.6 | D49.0 |
| choroid | C69.3-☑ | C79.49 | D09.2-☑ | D31.3-☑ | D48.7 | D49.81 |
| plexus | C71.5 | C79.31 | — | D33.0 | D43.0 | D49.6 |
| ciliary body | C69.4-☑ | C79.49 | D09.2-☑ | D31.4-☑ | D48.7 | D49.89 |
| clavicle | C41.3 | C79.51 | — | D16.7 | D48.0 | D49.2 |
| clitoris | C51.2 | C79.82 | D07.1 | D28.0 | D39.8 | D49.59 |
| clivus | C41.0 | C79.51 | — | D16.4 | D48.0 | D49.2 |
| cloacogenic zone | C21.2 | C78.5 | D01.3 | D12.9 | D37.8 | D49.0 |
| coccygeal | | | | | | |
| body or glomus | C49.5 | C79.89 | — | D21.5 | D48.1 | D49.2 |
| vertebra | C41.4 | C79.51 | — | D16.8 | D48.0 | D49.2 |
| coccyx | C41.4 | C79.51 | — | D16.8 | D48.0 | D49.2 |
| colon — see also Neoplasm, intestine, large | C18.9 | C78.5 | — | — | — | — |
| with rectum | C19 | C78.5 | D01.1 | D12.7 | D37.5 | D49.0 |
| columnella — see also Neoplasm, skin, face | C44.390 | C79.2 | D04.39 | D23.39 | D48.5 | D49.2 |
| column, spinal — see Neoplasm, spine | | | | | | |
| commissure | | | | | | |
| labial, lip | C00.6 | C79.89 | D00.01 | D10.39 | D37.01 | D49.0 |
| laryngeal | C32.0 | C78.39 | D02.0 | D14.1 | D38.0 | D49.1 |
| common (bile) duct | C24.0 | C78.89 | D01.5 | D13.5 | D37.6 | D49.0 |
| concha — see also Neoplasm, skin, | | | | | | |
| ear | C44.20-☑ | C79.2 | D04.2-☑ | D23.2-☑ | D48.5 | D49.2 |
| nose | C30.0 | C78.39 | D02.3 | D14.0 | D38.5 | D49.1 |
| conjunctiva | C69.0-☑ | C79.49 | D09.2-☑ | D31.0-☑ | D48.7 | D49.89 |

**Neoplasm, neoplastic — continued**

| | Malignant Primary | Malignant Secondary | Ca in situ | Benign | Uncertain | Unspecified Behavior |
|---|---|---|---|---|---|---|
| connective tissue NEC | C49.9 | C79.89 | — | D21.9 | D48.1 | D49.2 |

Note: For neoplasms of connective tissue (blood vessel, bursa, fascia, ligament, muscle, peripheral nerves, sympathetic and parasympathetic nerves and ganglia, synovia, tendon, etc.) or of morphological types that indicate connective tissue, code according to the list under "Neoplasm, connective tissue". For sites that do not appear in this list, code to neoplasm of that site; e.g., fibrosarcoma, pancreas (C25.9)

Note: Morphological types that indicate connective tissue appear in their proper place in the alphabetic index with the instruction "see Neoplasm, connective tissue ...."

| | Malignant Primary | Malignant Secondary | Ca in situ | Benign | Uncertain | Unspecified Behavior |
|---|---|---|---|---|---|---|
| abdomen | C49.4 | C79.89 | — | D21.4 | D48.1 | D49.2 |
| abdominal wall | C49.4 | C79.89 | — | D21.4 | D48.1 | D49.2 |
| ankle | C49.2-☑ | C79.89 | — | D21.2-☑ | D48.1 | D49.2 |
| antecubital fossa or space | C49.1-☑ | C79.89 | — | D21.1-☑ | D48.1 | D49.2 |
| arm | C49.1-☑ | C79.89 | — | D21.1-☑ | D48.1 | D49.2 |
| auricle (ear) | C49.0 | C79.89 | — | D21.0 | D48.1 | D49.2 |
| axilla | C49.3 | C79.89 | — | D21.3 | D48.1 | D49.2 |
| back | C49.6 | C79.89 | — | D21.6 | D48.1 | D49.2 |
| breast — see Neoplasm, breast | | | | | | |
| buttock | C49.5 | C79.89 | — | D21.5 | D48.1 | D49.2 |
| calf | C49.2-☑ | C79.89 | — | D21.2-☑ | D48.1 | D49.2 |
| cervical region | C49.0 | C79.89 | — | D21.0 | D48.1 | D49.2 |
| cheek | C49.0 | C79.89 | — | D21.0 | D48.1 | D49.2 |
| chest (wall) | C49.3 | C79.89 | — | D21.3 | D48.1 | D49.2 |
| chin | C49.0 | C79.89 | — | D21.0 | D48.1 | D49.2 |
| diaphragm | C49.3 | C79.89 | — | D21.3 | D48.1 | D49.2 |
| ear (external) | C49.0 | C79.89 | — | D21.0 | D48.1 | D49.2 |
| elbow | C49.1-☑ | C79.89 | — | D21.1-☑ | D48.1 | D49.2 |
| extrarectal | C49.5 | C79.89 | — | D21.5 | D48.1 | D49.2 |
| extremity | C49.9 | C79.89 | — | D21.9 | D48.1 | D49.2 |
| lower | C49.2-☑ | C79.89 | — | D21.2-☑ | D48.1 | D49.2 |
| upper | C49.1-☑ | C79.89 | — | D21.1-☑ | D48.1 | D49.2 |
| eyelid | C49.0 | C79.89 | — | D21.0 | D48.1 | D49.2 |
| face | C49.0 | C79.89 | — | D21.0 | D48.1 | D49.2 |
| finger | C49.1-☑ | C79.89 | — | D21.1-☑ | D48.1 | D49.2 |
| flank | C49.6 | C79.89 | — | D21.6 | D48.1 | D49.2 |
| foot | C49.2-☑ | C79.89 | — | D21.2-☑ | D48.1 | D49.2 |
| forearm | C49.1-☑ | C79.89 | — | D21.1-☑ | D48.1 | D49.2 |
| forehead | C49.0 | C79.89 | — | D21.0 | D48.1 | D49.2 |
| gastric | C49.4 | C79.89 | — | D21.4 | D48.1 | D49.2 |
| gastrointestinal | C49.4 | C79.89 | — | D21.4 | D48.1 | D49.2 |
| gluteal region | C49.5 | C79.89 | — | D21.5 | D48.1 | D49.2 |
| great vessels NEC | C49.3 | C79.89 | — | D21.3 | D48.1 | D49.2 |
| groin | C49.5 | C79.89 | — | D21.5 | D48.1 | D49.2 |
| hand | C49.1-☑ | C79.89 | — | D21.1-☑ | D48.1 | D49.2 |
| head | C49.0 | C79.89 | — | D21.0 | D48.1 | D49.2 |
| heel | C49.2-☑ | C79.89 | — | D21.2-☑ | D48.1 | D49.2 |
| hip | C49.2-☑ | C79.89 | — | D21.2-☑ | D48.1 | D49.2 |
| hypochondrium | C49.4 | C79.89 | — | D21.4 | D48.1 | D49.2 |
| iliopsoas muscle | C49.5 | C79.89 | — | D21.5 | D48.1 | D49.2 |
| infraclavicular region | C49.3 | C79.89 | — | D21.3 | D48.1 | D49.2 |
| inguinal (canal) (region) | C49.5 | C79.89 | — | D21.5 | D48.1 | D49.2 |
| intestinal | C49.4 | C79.89 | — | D21.4 | D48.1 | D49.2 |
| intrathoracic | C49.3 | C79.89 | — | D21.3 | D48.1 | D49.2 |
| ischiorectal fossa | C49.5 | C79.89 | — | D21.5 | D48.1 | D49.2 |
| jaw | C03.9 | C79.89 | D00.03 | D10.39 | D48.1 | D49.0 |
| knee | C49.2-☑ | C79.89 | — | D21.2-☑ | D48.1 | D49.2 |
| leg | C49.2-☑ | C79.89 | — | D21.2-☑ | D48.1 | D49.2 |
| limb NEC | C49.9 | C79.89 | — | D21.9 | D48.1 | D49.2 |
| lower | C49.2-☑ | C79.89 | — | D21.2-☑ | D48.1 | D49.2 |
| upper | C49.1-☑ | C79.89 | — | D21.1-☑ | D48.1 | D49.2 |
| nates | C49.5 | C79.89 | — | D21.5 | D48.1 | D49.2 |
| neck | C49.0 | C79.89 | — | D21.0 | D48.1 | D49.2 |
| orbit | C69.6-☑ | C79.49 | D09.2-☑ | D31.6-☑ | D48.1 | D49.89 |
| overlapping lesion | C49.8 | — | — | — | — | — |
| pararectal | C49.5 | C79.89 | — | D21.5 | D48.1 | D49.2 |
| para-urethral | C49.5 | C79.89 | — | D21.5 | D48.1 | D49.2 |
| paravaginal | C49.5 | C79.89 | — | D21.5 | D48.1 | D49.2 |
| pelvis (floor) | C49.5 | C79.89 | — | D21.5 | D48.1 | D49.2 |
| pelvo-abdominal | C49.8 | C79.89 | — | D21.6 | D48.1 | D49.2 |
| perineum | C49.5 | C79.89 | — | D21.5 | D48.1 | D49.2 |
| perirectal (tissue) | C49.5 | C79.89 | — | D21.5 | D48.1 | D49.2 |

☑ Additional Character Required — Refer to the Tabular List for Character Selection    ▽ Subterms under main terms may continue to next column or page

| Neoplasm, neoplastic — | Malignant Primary | Malignant Secondary | Ca in situ | Benign | Uncertain | Unspecified Behavior |
|---|---|---|---|---|---|---|
| *continued* | | | | | | |
| connective tissue — | | | | | | |
| *continued* | | | | | | |
| periurethral | | | | | | |
| (tissue) | C49.5 | C79.89 | — | D21.5 | D48.1 | D49.2 |
| popliteal fossa or | | | | | | |
| space | C49.2-☑ | C79.89 | — | D21.2-☑ | D48.1 | D49.2 |
| presacral | C49.5 | C79.89 | — | D21.5 | D48.1 | D49.2 |
| psoas muscle | C49.4 | C79.89 | — | D21.4 | D48.1 | D49.2 |
| pterygoid fossa | C49.0 | C79.89 | — | D21.0 | D48.1 | D49.2 |
| rectovaginal septum or | | | | | | |
| wall | C49.5 | C79.89 | — | D21.5 | D48.1 | D49.2 |
| rectovesical | C49.5 | C79.89 | — | D21.5 | D48.1 | D49.2 |
| retroperitoneum | C48.0 | C78.6 | — | D20.0 | D48.3 | D49.0 |
| sacrococcygeal | | | | | | |
| region | C49.5 | C79.89 | — | D21.5 | D48.1 | D49.2 |
| scalp | C49.0 | C79.89 | — | D21.0 | D48.1 | D49.2 |
| scapular region | C49.3 | C79.89 | — | D21.3 | D48.1 | D49.2 |
| shoulder | C49.1-☑ | C79.89 | — | D21.1-☑ | D48.1 | D49.2 |
| skin (dermis) NEC — *see* | | | | | | |
| *also* Neoplasm, skin, | | | | | | |
| by site | C44.90 | C79.2 | D04.9 | D23.9 | D48.5 | D49.2 |
| stomach | C49.4 | C79.89 | — | D21.4 | D48.1 | D49.2 |
| submental | C49.0 | C79.89 | — | D21.0 | D48.1 | D49.2 |
| supraclavicular | | | | | | |
| region | C49.0 | C79.89 | — | D21.0 | D48.1 | D49.2 |
| temple | C49.0 | C79.89 | — | D21.0 | D48.1 | D49.2 |
| temporal region | C49.0 | C79.89 | — | D21.0 | D48.1 | D49.2 |
| thigh | C49.2-☑ | C79.89 | — | D21.2-☑ | D48.1 | D49.2 |
| thoracic (duct) | | | | | | |
| (wall) | C49.3 | C79.89 | — | D21.3 | D48.1 | D49.2 |
| thorax | C49.3 | C79.89 | — | D21.3 | D48.1 | D49.2 |
| thumb | C49.1-☑ | C79.89 | — | D21.1-☑ | D48.1 | D49.2 |
| toe | C49.2-☑ | C79.89 | — | D21.2-☑ | D48.1 | D49.2 |
| trunk | C49.6 | C79.89 | — | D21.6 | D48.1 | D49.2 |
| umbilicus | C49.4 | C79.89 | — | D21.4 | D48.1 | D49.2 |
| vesicorectal | C49.5 | C79.89 | — | D21.5 | D48.1 | D49.2 |
| wrist | C49.1-☑ | C79.89 | — | D21.1-☑ | D48.1 | D49.2 |
| conus medullaris | C72.0 | C79.49 | — | D33.4 | D43.4 | D49.7 |
| cord (true) (vocal) | C32.0 | C78.39 | D02.0 | D14.1 | D38.0 | D49.1 |
| false | C32.1 | C78.39 | D02.0 | D14.1 | D38.0 | D49.1 |
| spermatic | C63.1-☑ | C79.82 | D07.69 | D29.8 | D40.8 | D49.59 |
| spinal (cervical) | | | | | | |
| (lumbar) | | | | | | |
| (thoracic) | C72.0 | C79.49 | — | D33.4 | D43.4 | D49.7 |
| cornea (limbus) | C69.1-☑ | C79.49 | D09.2-☑ | D31.1-☑ | D48.7 | D49.89 |
| corpus | | | | | | |
| albicans | C56.-☑ | C79.6-☑ | D07.39 | D27.-☑ | D39.1-☑ | D49.59 |
| callosum, brain | C71.0 | C79.31 | — | D33.0 | D43.2 | D49.6 |
| cavernosum | C60.2 | C79.82 | D07.4 | D29.0 | D40.8 | D49.59 |
| gastric | C16.2 | C78.89 | D00.2 | D13.1 | D37.1 | D49.0 |
| overlapping sites | C54.8 | — | — | — | — | — |
| penis | C60.2 | C79.82 | D07.4 | D29.0 | D40.8 | D49.59 |
| striatum, | | | | | | |
| cerebrum | C71.0 | C79.31 | — | D33.0 | D43.0 | D49.6 |
| uteri | C54.9 | C79.82 | D07.0 | D26.1 | D39.0 | D49.59 |
| isthmus | C54.0 | C79.82 | D07.0 | D26.1 | D39.0 | D49.59 |
| cortex | | | | | | |
| adrenal | C74.0-☑ | C79.7-☑ | D09.3 | D35.0-☑ | D44.1-☑ | D49.7 |
| cerebral | C71.0 | C79.31 | — | D33.0 | D43.0 | D49.6 |
| costal cartilage | C41.3 | C79.51 | — | D16.7 | D48.0 | D49.2 |
| costovertebral joint | C41.3 | C79.51 | — | D16.7 | D48.0 | D49.2 |
| Cowper's gland | C68.0 | C79.19 | D09.19 | D30.4 | D41.3 | D49.59 |
| cranial (fossa, any) | C71.9 | C79.31 | — | D33.2 | D43.2 | D49.6 |
| meninges | C70.0 | C79.32 | — | D32.0 | D42.0 | D49.7 |
| nerve | C72.50 | C79.49 | — | D33.3 | D43.3 | D49.7 |
| specified NEC | C72.59 | C79.49 | — | D33.3 | D43.3 | D49.7 |
| craniobuccal pouch | C75.2 | C79.89 | D09.3 | D35.2 | D44.3 | D49.7 |
| craniopharyngeal (duct) | | | | | | |
| (pouch) | C75.2 | C79.89 | D09.3 | D35.3 | D44.4 | D49.7 |
| cricoid | C13.0 | C79.89 | D00.08 | D10.7 | D37.05 | D49.0 |
| cartilage | C32.3 | C78.39 | D02.0 | D14.1 | D38.0 | D49.1 |
| cricopharynx | C13.0 | C79.89 | D00.08 | D10.7 | D37.05 | D49.0 |
| crypt of Morgagni | C21.8 | C78.5 | D01.3 | D12.9 | D37.8 | D49.0 |
| crystalline lens | C69.4-☑ | C79.49 | D09.2-☑ | D31.4-☑ | D48.7 | D49.89 |
| cul-de-sac | | | | | | |
| (Douglas') | C48.1 | C78.6 | — | D20.1 | D48.4 | D49.0 |
| cuneiform cartilage | C32.3 | C78.39 | D02.0 | D14.1 | D38.0 | D49.1 |
| cutaneous — *see* | | | | | | |
| Neoplasm, skin | | | | | | |
| cutis — *see* Neoplasm, | | | | | | |
| skin | | | | | | |

| Neoplasm, neoplastic — | Malignant Primary | Malignant Secondary | Ca in situ | Benign | Uncertain | Unspecified Behavior |
|---|---|---|---|---|---|---|
| *continued* | | | | | | |
| cystic (bile) duct | | | | | | |
| (common) | C24.0 | C78.89 | D01.5 | D13.5 | D37.6 | D49.0 |
| dermis — *see* Neoplasm, | | | | | | |
| skin | | | | | | |
| diaphragm | C49.3 | C79.89 | — | D21.3 | D48.1 | D49.2 |
| digestive organs, system, | | | | | | |
| tube, or tract | | | | | | |
| NEC | C26.9 | C78.89 | D01.9 | D13.9 | D37.9 | D49.0 |
| disc, intervertebral | C41.2 | C79.51 | — | D16.6 | D48.0 | D49.2 |
| disease, generalized | C80.0 | — | — | — | — | — |
| disseminated | C80.0 | — | — | — | — | — |
| Douglas' cul-de-sac or | | | | | | |
| pouch | C48.1 | C78.6 | — | D20.1 | D48.4 | D49.0 |
| duodenojejunal | | | | | | |
| junction | C17.8 | C78.4 | D01.49 | D13.39 | D37.2 | D49.0 |
| duodenum | C17.0 | C78.4 | D01.49 | D13.2 | D37.2 | D49.0 |
| dura (cranial) | | | | | | |
| (mater) | C70.9 | C79.49 | — | D32.9 | D42.9 | D49.7 |
| cerebral | C70.0 | C79.32 | — | D32.0 | D42.0 | D49.7 |
| spinal | C70.1 | C79.49 | — | D32.1 | D42.1 | D49.7 |
| ear (external) — *see also* | | | | | | |
| Neoplasm, skin, | | | | | | |
| ear | C44.20-☑ | C79.2 | D04.2-☑ | D23.2-☑ | D48.5 | D49.2 |
| auricle or auris — *see* | | | | | | |
| *also* Neoplasm, skin, | | | | | | |
| ear | C44.20-☑ | C79.2 | D04.2-☑ | D23.2-☑ | D48.5 | D49.2 |
| canal, external — *see* | | | | | | |
| *also* Neoplasm, skin, | | | | | | |
| ear | C44.20-☑ | C79.2 | D04.2-☑ | D23.2-☑ | D48.5 | D49.2 |
| cartilage | C49.0 | C79.89 | — | D21.0 | D48.1 | D49.2 |
| external meatus — *see* | | | | | | |
| *also* Neoplasm, skin, | | | | | | |
| ear | C44.20-☑ | C79.2 | D04.2-☑ | D23.2-☑ | D48.5 | D49.2 |
| inner | C30.1 | C78.39 | D02.3 | D14.0 | D38.5 | D49.1 |
| lobule — *see also* | | | | | | |
| Neoplasm, skin, | | | | | | |
| ear | C44.20-☑ | C79.2 | D04.2-☑ | D23.2-☑ | D48.5 | D49.2 |
| middle | C30.1 | C78.39 | D02.3 | D14.0 | D38.5 | D49.1 |
| overlapping lesion with | | | | | | |
| accessory | | | | | | |
| sinuses | C31.8 | — | — | — | — | — |
| skin | C44.20-☑ | C79.2 | D04.2-☑ | D23.2-☑ | D48.5 | D49.2 |
| basal cell | | | | | | |
| carcinoma | C44.21-☑ | — | — | — | — | — |
| specified type | | | | | | |
| NEC | C44.29-☑ | — | — | — | — | — |
| squamous cell | | | | | | |
| carcinoma | C44.22-☑ | — | — | — | — | — |
| earlobe | C44.20-☑ | C79.2 | D04.2-☑ | D23.2-☑ | D48.5 | D49.2 |
| basal cell | | | | | | |
| carcinoma | C44.21-☑ | — | — | — | — | — |
| specified type NEC | C44.29-☑ | — | — | — | — | — |
| squamous cell | | | | | | |
| carcinoma | C44.22-☑ | — | — | — | — | — |
| ejaculatory duct | C63.7 | C79.82 | D07.69 | D29.8 | D40.8 | D49.59 |
| elbow NEC | C76.4-☑ | C79.89 | D04.6-☑ | D36.7 | D48.7 | D49.89 |
| endocardium | C38.0 | C79.89 | — | D15.1 | D48.7 | D49.89 |
| endocervix (canal) | | | | | | |
| (gland) | C53.0 | C79.82 | D06.0 | D26.0 | D39.0 | D49.59 |
| endocrine gland | | | | | | |
| NEC | C75.9 | C79.89 | D09.3 | D35.9 | D44.9 | D49.7 |
| pluriglandular | C75.8 | C79.89 | D09.3 | D35.7 | D44.9 | D49.7 |
| endometrium (gland) | | | | | | |
| (stroma) | C54.1 | C79.82 | D07.0 | D26.1 | D39.0 | D49.59 |
| ensiform cartilage | C41.3 | C79.51 | — | D16.7 | D48.0 | D49.2 |
| enteric — *see* Neoplasm, | | | | | | |
| intestine | | | | | | |
| ependyma (brain) | C71.5 | C79.31 | — | D33.0 | D43.0 | D49.6 |
| fourth ventricle | C71.7 | C79.31 | — | D33.1 | D43.1 | D49.6 |
| epicardium | C38.0 | C79.89 | — | D15.1 | D48.7 | D49.89 |
| epididymis | C63.0-☑ | C79.82 | D07.69 | D29.3-☑ | D40.8 | D49.59 |
| epidural | C72.9 | C79.49 | — | D33.9 | D43.9 | D49.7 |
| epiglottis | C32.1 | C78.39 | D02.0 | D14.1 | D38.0 | D49.1 |
| anterior aspect or | | | | | | |
| surface | C10.1 | C79.89 | D00.08 | D10.5 | D37.05 | D49.0 |
| cartilage | C32.3 | C78.39 | D02.0 | D14.1 | D38.0 | D49.1 |
| free border | | | | | | |
| (margin) | C10.1 | C79.89 | D00.08 | D10.5 | D37.05 | D49.0 |
| junctional region | C10.8 | C79.89 | D00.08 | D10.5 | D37.05 | D49.0 |
| posterior (laryngeal) | | | | | | |
| surface | C32.1 | C78.39 | D02.0 | D14.1 | D38.0 | D49.1 |

| Neoplasm, neoplastic — *continued* | Malignant Primary | Malignant Secondary | Ca in situ | Benign | Uncertain | Unspecified Behavior |
|---|---|---|---|---|---|---|
| epiglottis — *continued* | | | | | | |
|   suprahyoid | | | | | | |
|     portion | C32.1 | C78.39 | D02.0 | D14.1 | D38.0 | D49.1 |
| esophagogastric | | | | | | |
|   junction | C16.0 | C78.89 | D00.2 | D13.1 | D37.1 | D49.0 |
| esophagus | C15.9 | C78.89 | D00.1 | D13.0 | D37.8 | D49.0 |
|   abdominal | C15.5 | C78.89 | D00.1 | D13.0 | D37.8 | D49.0 |
|   cervical | C15.3 | C78.89 | D00.1 | D13.0 | D37.8 | D49.0 |
|   distal (third) | C15.5 | C78.89 | D00.1 | D13.0 | D37.8 | D49.0 |
|   lower (third) | C15.5 | C78.89 | D00.1 | D13.0 | D37.8 | D49.0 |
|   middle (third) | C15.4 | C78.89 | D00.1 | D13.0 | D37.8 | D49.0 |
|   overlapping lesion | C15.8 | — | — | — | — | — |
|   proximal (third) | C15.3 | C78.89 | D00.1 | D13.0 | D37.8 | D49.0 |
|   thoracic | C15.4 | C78.89 | D00.1 | D13.0 | D37.8 | D49.0 |
|   upper (third) | C15.3 | C78.89 | D00.1 | D13.0 | D37.8 | D49.0 |
| ethmoid (sinus) | C31.1 | C78.39 | D02.3 | D14.0 | D38.5 | D49.1 |
|   bone or labyrinth | C41.0 | C79.51 | — | D16.4 | D48.0 | D49.2 |
| eustachian tube | C30.1 | C78.39 | D02.3 | D14.0 | D38.5 | D49.1 |
| exocervix | C53.1 | C79.82 | D06.1 | D26.0 | D39.0 | D49.59 |
| external | | | | | | |
|   meatus (ear) — *see also* | | | | | | |
|     Neoplasm, skin, | | | | | | |
|     ear | C44.20-☑ | C79.2 | D04.2-☑ | D23.2-☑ | D48.5 | D49.2 |
|   os, cervix uteri | C53.1 | C79.82 | D06.1 | D26.0 | D39.0 | D49.59 |
| extradural | C72.9 | C79.49 | — | D33.9 | D43.9 | D49.7 |
| extrahepatic (bile) | | | | | | |
|   duct | C24.0 | C78.89 | D01.5 | D13.5 | D37.6 | D49.0 |
|   overlapping lesion with | | | | | | |
|     gallbladder | C24.8 | — | — | — | — | — |
| extraocular muscle | C69.6-☑ | C79.49 | D09.2-☑ | D31.6-☑ | D48.7 | D49.89 |
| extrarectal | C76.3 | C79.89 | D09.8 | D36.7 | D48.7 | D49.89 |
| extremity | C76.8 | C79.89 | D04.8 | D36.7 | D48.7 | D49.89 |
|   lower | C76.5-☑ | C79.89 | D04.7-☑ | D36.7 | D48.7 | D49.89 |
|   upper | C76.4-☑ | C79.89 | D04.6-☑ | D36.7 | D48.7 | D49.89 |
| eyeball | C69.9-☑ | C79.49 | D09.2-☑ | D31.9-☑ | D48.7 | D49.89 |
| eyebrow | C44.309 | C79.2 | D04.39 | D23.39 | D48.5 | D49.2 |
|   basal cell | | | | | | |
|     carcinoma | C44.319 | — | — | — | — | — |
|   specified type NEC | C44.399 | — | — | — | — | — |
|   squamous cell | | | | | | |
|     carcinoma | C44.329 | — | — | — | — | — |
| eyelid (lower) (skin) | | | | | | |
|   (upper) | C44.10-☑ | | | | | |
|   basal cell | | | | | | |
|     carcinoma | C44.11-☑ | — | | — | — | — |
|   cartilage | C49.0 | C79.89 | | D21.0 | D48.1 | D49.2 |
|   specified type NEC | C44.19-☑ | | | | | |
|   squamous cell | | | | | | |
|     carcinoma | C44.12-☑ | — | — | — | — | — |
| eye NEC | C69.9-☑ | C79.49 | D09.2-☑ | D31.9-☑ | D48.7 | D49.89 |
|   overlapping sites | C69.8-☑ | — | — | — | — | — |
| face NEC | C76.0 | C79.89 | D04.39 | D36.7 | D48.7 | D49.89 |
| fallopian tube | | | | | | |
|   (accessory) | C57.0-☑ | C79.82 | D07.39 | D28.2 | D39.8 | D49.59 |
| falx (cerebella) | | | | | | |
|   (cerebri) | C70.0 | C79.32 | — | D32.0 | D42.0 | D49.7 |
| fascia — *see also* | | | | | | |
|   Neoplasm, connective | | | | | | |
|   tissue | | | | | | |
|   palmar | C49.1-☑ | C79.89 | — | D21.1-☑ | D48.1 | D49.2 |
|   plantar | C49.2-☑ | C79.89 | — | D21.2-☑ | D48.1 | D49.2 |
| fatty tissue — *see* | | | | | | |
|   Neoplasm, connective | | | | | | |
|   tissue | | | | | | |
| fauces, faucial NEC | C10.9 | C79.89 | D00.08 | D10.5 | D37.05 | D49.0 |
|   pillars | C09.1 | C79.89 | D00.08 | D10.5 | D37.05 | D49.0 |
|   tonsil | C09.9 | C79.89 | D00.08 | D10.5 | D37.05 | D49.0 |
| femur (any part) | C40.2-☑ | — | — | D16.2-☑ | — | — |
| fetal membrane | C58 | C79.82 | D07.0 | D26.7 | D39.2 | D49.59 |
| fibrous tissue — *see* | | | | | | |
|   Neoplasm, connective | | | | | | |
|   tissue | | | | | | |
| fibula (any part) | C40.2-☑ | C79.51 | — | D16.2-☑ | — | — |
| filum terminale | C72.0 | C79.49 | — | D33.4 | D43.4 | D49.7 |
| finger NEC | C76.4-☑ | C79.89 | D04.6-☑ | D36.7 | D48.7 | D49.89 |
| flank NEC | C76.8 | C79.89 | D04.5 | D36.7 | D48.7 | D49.89 |
| follicle, nabothian | C53.0 | C79.82 | D06.0 | D26.0 | D39.0 | D49.59 |
| foot NEC | C76.5-☑ | C79.89 | D04.7-☑ | D36.7 | D48.7 | D49.89 |
| forearm NEC | C76.4-☑ | C79.89 | D04.6-☑ | D36.7 | D48.7 | D49.89 |
| forehead (skin) | C44.309 | C79.2 | D04.39 | D23.39 | D48.5 | D49.2 |

| Neoplasm, neoplastic — *continued* | Malignant Primary | Malignant Secondary | Ca in situ | Benign | Uncertain | Unspecified Behavior |
|---|---|---|---|---|---|---|
| forehead — *continued* | | | | | | |
|   basal cell | | | | | | |
|     carcinoma | C44.319 | — | — | — | — | — |
|   specified type NEC | C44.399 | — | — | — | — | — |
|   squamous cell | | | | | | |
|     carcinoma | C44.329 | — | — | — | — | — |
| foreskin | C60.0 | C79.82 | D07.4 | D29.0 | D40.8 | D49.59 |
| fornix | | | | | | |
|   pharyngeal | C11.3 | C79.89 | D00.08 | D10.6 | D37.05 | D49.0 |
|   vagina | C52 | C79.82 | D07.2 | D28.1 | D39.8 | D49.59 |
| fossa (of) | | | | | | |
|   anterior (cranial) | C71.9 | C79.31 | — | D33.2 | D43.2 | D49.6 |
|   cranial | C71.9 | C79.31 | — | D33.2 | D43.2 | D49.6 |
|   ischiorectal | C76.3 | C79.89 | D09.8 | D36.7 | D48.7 | D49.89 |
|   middle (cranial) | C71.9 | C79.31 | — | D33.2 | D43.2 | D49.6 |
|   piriform | C12 | C79.89 | D00.08 | D10.7 | D37.05 | D49.0 |
|   pituitary | C75.1 | C79.89 | D09.3 | D35.2 | D44.3 | D49.7 |
|   posterior (cranial) | C71.9 | C79.31 | — | D33.2 | D43.2 | D49.6 |
|   pterygoid | C49.0 | C79.89 | — | D21.0 | D48.1 | D49.2 |
|   pyriform | C12 | C79.89 | D00.08 | D10.7 | D37.05 | D49.0 |
|   Rosenmuller | C11.2 | C79.89 | D00.08 | D10.6 | D37.05 | D49.0 |
|   tonsillar | C09.0 | C79.89 | D00.08 | D10.5 | D37.05 | D49.0 |
| fourchette | C51.9 | C79.82 | D07.1 | D28.0 | D39.8 | D49.59 |
| frenulum | | | | | | |
|   labii — *see Neoplasm,* | | | | | | |
|     lip, internal | | | | | | |
|   linguae | C02.2 | C79.89 | D00.07 | D10.1 | D37.02 | D49.0 |
| frontal | | | | | | |
|   bone | C41.0 | C79.51 | — | D16.4 | D48.0 | D49.2 |
|   lobe, brain | C71.1 | C79.31 | — | D33.0 | D43.0 | D49.6 |
|   pole | C71.1 | C79.31 | — | D33.0 | D43.0 | D49.6 |
|   sinus | C31.2 | C78.39 | D02.3 | D14.0 | D38.5 | D49.1 |
| fundus | | | | | | |
|   stomach | C16.1 | C78.89 | D00.2 | D13.1 | D37.1 | D49.0 |
|   uterus | C54.3 | C79.82 | D07.0 | D26.1 | D39.0 | D49.59 |
| gallbladder | C23 | C78.89 | D01.5 | D13.5 | D37.6 | D49.0 |
|   overlapping lesion with | | | | | | |
|     extrahepatic bile | | | | | | |
|     ducts | C24.8 | — | — | — | — | — |
| gall duct | | | | | | |
|   (extrahepatic) | C24.0 | C78.89 | D01.5 | D13.5 | D37.6 | D49.0 |
|   intrahepatic | C22.1 | C78.7 | D01.5 | D13.4 | D37.6 | D49.0 |
| ganglia — *see also* | | | | | | |
|   Neoplasm, nerve, | | | | | | |
|   peripheral | C47.9 | C79.89 | — | D36.10 | D48.2 | D49.2 |
|   basal | C71.0 | C79.31 | — | D33.0 | D43.0 | D49.6 |
|   cranial nerve | C72.50 | C79.49 | — | D33.3 | D43.3 | D49.7 |
| Gartner's duct | C52 | C79.82 | D07.2 | D28.1 | D39.8 | D49.59 |
| gastric — *see Neoplasm,* | | | | | | |
|   stomach | | | | | | |
| gastrocolic | C26.9 | C78.89 | D01.9 | D13.9 | D37.9 | D49.0 |
| gastroesophageal | | | | | | |
|   junction | C16.0 | C78.89 | D00.2 | D13.1 | D37.1 | D49.0 |
| gastrointestinal (tract) | | | | | | |
|   NEC | C26.9 | C78.89 | D01.9 | D13.9 | D37.9 | D49.0 |
| generalized | C80.0 | — | — | — | — | — |
| genital organ or tract | | | | | | |
|   female NEC | C57.9 | C79.82 | D07.30 | D28.9 | D39.9 | D49.59 |
|     overlapping | | | | | | |
|      lesion | C57.8 | — | — | — | — | — |
|     specified site | | | | | | |
|      NEC | C57.7 | C79.82 | D07.39 | D28.7 | D39.8 | D49.59 |
|   male NEC | C63.9 | C79.82 | D07.60 | D29.9 | D40.9 | D49.59 |
|     overlapping | | | | | | |
|      lesion | C63.8 | — | — | — | — | — |
|     specified site | | | | | | |
|      NEC | C63.7 | C79.82 | D07.69 | D29.8 | D40.8 | D49.59 |
| genitourinary tract | | | | | | |
|   female | C57.9 | C79.82 | D07.30 | D28.9 | D39.9 | D49.59 |
|   male | C63.9 | C79.82 | D07.60 | D29.9 | D40.9 | D49.59 |
| gingiva (alveolar) | | | | | | |
|   (marginal) | C03.9 | C79.89 | D00.03 | D10.39 | D37.09 | D49.0 |
|   lower | C03.1 | C79.89 | D00.03 | D10.39 | D37.09 | D49.0 |
|   mandibular | C03.1 | C79.89 | D00.03 | D10.39 | D37.09 | D49.0 |
|   maxillary | C03.0 | C79.89 | D00.03 | D10.39 | D37.09 | D49.0 |
|   upper | C03.0 | C79.89 | D00.03 | D10.39 | D37.09 | D49.0 |
| gland, glandular | | | | | | |
|   (lymphatic) (system) | | | | | | |
|    — *see also Neoplasm,* | | | | | | |
|   lymph gland | | | | | | |
|   endocrine NEC | C75.9 | C79.89 | D09.3 | D35.9 | D44.9 | D49.7 |

| Neoplasm, neoplastic — continued | Malignant Primary | Malignant Secondary | Ca in situ | Benign | Uncertain | Unspecified Behavior |
|---|---|---|---|---|---|---|
| gland, glandular — see also Neoplasm, lymph gland — continued | | | | | | |
| salivary — see Neoplasm, salivary gland | | | | | | |
| glans penis | C60.1 | C79.82 | D07.4 | D29.0 | D40.8 | D49.59 |
| globus pallidus | C71.0 | C79.31 | — | D33.0 | D43.0 | D49.6 |
| glomus | | | | | | |
| coccygeal | C49.5 | C79.89 | — | D21.5 | D48.1 | D49.2 |
| jugularis | C75.5 | C79.89 | — | D35.6 | D44.7 | D49.7 |
| glosso-epiglottic fold(s) | C10.1 | C79.89 | D00.08 | D10.5 | D37.05 | D49.0 |
| glossopalatine fold | C09.1 | C79.89 | D00.08 | D10.5 | D37.05 | D49.0 |
| glossopharyngeal sulcus | C09.0 | C79.89 | D00.08 | D10.5 | D37.05 | D49.0 |
| glottis | C32.0 | C78.39 | D02.0 | D14.1 | D38.0 | D49.1 |
| gluteal region | C76.3 | C79.89 | D04.5 | D36.7 | D48.7 | D49.89 |
| great vessels NEC | C49.3 | C79.89 | — | D21.3 | D48.1 | D49.2 |
| groin NEC | C76.3 | C79.89 | D04.5 | D36.7 | D48.7 | D49.89 |
| gum | C03.9 | C79.89 | D00.03 | D10.39 | D37.09 | D49.0 |
| lower | C03.1 | C79.89 | D00.03 | D10.39 | D37.09 | D49.0 |
| upper | C03.0 | C79.89 | D00.03 | D10.39 | D37.09 | D49.0 |
| hand NEC | C76.4-☑ | C79.89 | D04.6-☑ | D36.7 | D48.7 | D49.89 |
| head NEC | C76.0 | C79.89 | D04.4 | D36.7 | D48.7 | D49.89 |
| heart | C38.0 | C79.89 | — | D15.1 | D48.7 | D49.89 |
| heel NEC | C76.5-☑ | C79.89 | D04.7-☑ | D36.7 | D48.7 | D49.89 |
| helix — see also Neoplasm, skin, ear | C44.20-☑ | C79.2 | D04.2-☑ | D23.2-☑ | D48.5 | D49.2 |
| hematopoietic, hemopoietic tissue NEC | C96.9 | — | — | — | — | — |
| specified NEC | C96.Z | — | — | — | — | — |
| hemisphere, cerebral | C71.0 | C79.31 | — | D33.0 | D43.0 | D49.6 |
| hemorrhoidal zone | C21.1 | C78.5 | D01.3 | D12.9 | D37.8 | D49.0 |
| hepatic — see also Index to disease, by histology | C22.9 | C78.7 | D01.5 | D13.4 | D37.6 | D49.0 |
| duct (bile) | C24.0 | C78.89 | D01.5 | D13.5 | D37.6 | D49.0 |
| flexure (colon) | C18.3 | C78.5 | D01.0 | D12.3 | D37.4 | D49.0 |
| primary | C22.8 | C78.7 | D01.5 | D13.4 | D37.6 | D49.0 |
| hepatobiliary | C24.9 | C78.89 | D01.5 | D13.5 | D37.6 | D49.0 |
| hepatoblastoma | C22.2 | C78.7 | D01.5 | D13.4 | D37.6 | D49.0 |
| hepatoma | C22.0 | C78.7 | D01.5 | D13.4 | D37.6 | D49.0 |
| hilus of lung | C34.0-☑ | C78.0-☑ | D02.2-☑ | D14.3-☑ | D38.1 | D49.1 |
| hippocampus, brain | C71.2 | C79.31 | — | D33.0 | D43.0 | D49.6 |
| hip NEC | C76.5-☑ | C79.89 | D04.7-☑ | D36.7 | D48.7 | D49.89 |
| humerus (any part) | C40.0-☑ | C79.51 | — | D16.0-☑ | — | — |
| hymen | C52 | C79.82 | D07.2 | D28.1 | D39.8 | D49.59 |
| hypopharynx, hypopharyngeal NEC | C13.9 | C79.89 | D00.08 | D10.7 | D37.05 | D49.0 |
| overlapping lesion | C13.8 | — | — | — | — | — |
| postcricoid region | C13.0 | C79.89 | D00.08 | D10.7 | D37.05 | D49.0 |
| posterior wall | C13.2 | C79.89 | D00.08 | D10.7 | D37.05 | D49.0 |
| pyriform fossa (sinus) | C12 | C79.89 | D00.08 | D10.7 | D37.05 | D49.0 |
| hypophysis | C75.1 | C79.89 | D09.3 | D35.2 | D44.3 | D49.7 |
| hypothalamus | C71.0 | C79.31 | — | D33.0 | D43.0 | D49.6 |
| ileocecum, ileocecal (coil) (junction) (valve) | C18.0 | C78.5 | D01.0 | D12.0 | D37.4 | D49.0 |
| ileum | C17.2 | C78.4 | D01.49 | D13.39 | D37.2 | D49.0 |
| ilium | C41.4 | C79.51 | — | D16.8 | D48.0 | D49.2 |
| immunoproliferative NEC | C88.9 | — | — | — | — | — |
| infraclavicular (region) | C76.1 | C79.89 | D04.5 | D36.7 | D48.7 | D49.89 |
| inguinal (region) | C76.3 | C79.89 | D04.5 | D36.7 | D48.7 | D49.89 |
| insula | C71.0 | C79.31 | — | D33.0 | D43.0 | D49.6 |
| insular tissue (pancreas) | C25.4 | C78.89 | D01.7 | D13.7 | D37.8 | D49.0 |
| brain | C71.0 | C79.31 | — | D33.0 | D43.0 | D49.6 |
| interarytenoid fold | C13.1 | C78.39 | D00.08 | D10.7 | D37.05 | D49.0 |
| hypopharyngeal aspect | C13.1 | C79.89 | D00.08 | D10.7 | D37.05 | D49.0 |
| laryngeal aspect | C32.1 | C78.39 | D02.0 | D14.1 | D38.0 | D49.1 |
| marginal zone | C13.1 | C79.89 | D00.08 | D10.7 | D37.05 | D49.0 |
| interdental papillae | C03.9 | C79.89 | D00.03 | D10.39 | D37.09 | D49.0 |

| Neoplasm, neoplastic — continued | Malignant Primary | Malignant Secondary | Ca in situ | Benign | Uncertain | Unspecified Behavior |
|---|---|---|---|---|---|---|
| interdental papillae — continued | | | | | | |
| lower | C03.1 | C79.89 | D00.03 | D10.39 | D37.09 | D49.0 |
| upper | C03.0 | C79.89 | D00.03 | D10.39 | D37.09 | D49.0 |
| internal | | | | | | |
| capsule | C71.0 | C79.31 | — | D33.0 | D43.0 | D49.6 |
| os (cervix) | C53.0 | C79.82 | D06.0 | D26.0 | D39.0 | D49.59 |
| intervertebral cartilage or disc | C41.2 | C79.51 | — | D16.6 | D48.0 | D49.2 |
| intestine, intestinal | C26.0 | C78.80 | D01.40 | D13.9 | D37.8 | D49.0 |
| large | C18.9 | C78.5 | D01.0 | D12.6 | D37.4 | D49.0 |
| appendix | C18.1 | C78.5 | D01.0 | D12.1 | D37.3 | D49.0 |
| caput coli | C18.0 | C78.5 | D01.0 | D12.0 | D37.4 | D49.0 |
| cecum | C18.0 | C78.5 | D01.0 | D12.0 | D37.4 | D49.0 |
| colon | C18.9 | C78.5 | D01.0 | D12.6 | D37.4 | D49.0 |
| and rectum | C19 | C78.5 | D01.1 | D12.7 | D37.5 | D49.0 |
| ascending | C18.2 | C78.5 | D01.0 | D12.2 | D37.4 | D49.0 |
| caput | C18.0 | C78.5 | D01.0 | D12.0 | D37.4 | D49.0 |
| descending | C18.6 | C78.5 | D01.0 | D12.4 | D37.4 | D49.0 |
| distal | C18.6 | C78.5 | D01.0 | D12.4 | D37.4 | D49.0 |
| left | C18.6 | C78.5 | D01.0 | D12.4 | D37.4 | D49.0 |
| overlapping lesion | C18.8 | — | — | — | — | — |
| pelvic | C18.7 | C78.5 | D01.0 | D12.5 | D37.4 | D49.0 |
| right | C18.2 | C78.5 | D01.0 | D12.2 | D37.4 | D49.0 |
| sigmoid (flexure) | C18.7 | C78.5 | D01.0 | D12.5 | D37.4 | D49.0 |
| transverse | C18.4 | C78.5 | D01.0 | D12.3 | D37.4 | D49.0 |
| hepatic flexure | C18.3 | C78.5 | D01.0 | D12.3 | D37.4 | D49.0 |
| ileocecum, ileocecal (coil) (valve) | C18.0 | C78.5 | D01.0 | D12.0 | D37.4 | D49.0 |
| overlapping lesion | C18.8 | — | — | — | — | — |
| sigmoid flexure (lower) (upper) | C18.7 | C78.5 | D01.0 | D12.5 | D37.4 | D49.0 |
| splenic flexure | C18.5 | C78.5 | D01.0 | D12.3 | D37.4 | D49.0 |
| small | C17.9 | C78.4 | D01.40 | D13.30 | D37.2 | D49.0 |
| duodenum | C17.0 | C78.4 | D01.49 | D13.2 | D37.2 | D49.0 |
| ileum | C17.2 | C78.4 | D01.49 | D13.39 | D37.2 | D49.0 |
| jejunum | C17.1 | C78.4 | D01.49 | D13.39 | D37.2 | D49.0 |
| overlapping lesion | C17.8 | — | — | — | — | — |
| tract NEC | C26.0 | C78.89 | D01.40 | D13.9 | D37.8 | D49.0 |
| intra-abdominal | C76.2 | C79.89 | D09.8 | D36.7 | D48.7 | D49.89 |
| intracranial NEC | C71.9 | C79.31 | — | D33.2 | D43.2 | D49.6 |
| intrahepatic (bile) duct | C22.1 | C78.7 | D01.5 | D13.4 | D37.6 | D49.0 |
| intraocular | C69.9-☑ | C79.49 | D09.2-☑ | D31.9-☑ | D48.7 | D49.89 |
| intraorbital | C69.6-☑ | C79.49 | D09.2-☑ | D31.6-☑ | D48.7 | D49.89 |
| intrasellar | C75.1 | C79.89 | D09.3 | D35.2 | D44.3 | D49.7 |
| intrathoracic (cavity) (organs) | C76.1 | C79.89 | D09.8 | D15.9 | D48.7 | D49.89 |
| specified NEC | C76.1 | C79.89 | D09.8 | D15.7 | — | — |
| iris | C69.4-☑ | C79.49 | D09.2-☑ | D31.4-☑ | D48.7 | D49.89 |
| ischiorectal (fossa) | C76.3 | C79.89 | D09.8 | D36.7 | D48.7 | D49.89 |
| ischium | C41.4 | C79.51 | — | D16.8 | D48.0 | D49.2 |
| island of Reil | C71.0 | C79.31 | — | D33.0 | D43.0 | D49.6 |
| islands or islets of Langerhans | C25.4 | C78.89 | D01.7 | D13.7 | D37.8 | D49.0 |
| isthmus uteri | C54.0 | C79.82 | D07.0 | D26.1 | D39.0 | D49.59 |
| jaw | C76.0 | C79.89 | D09.8 | D36.7 | D48.7 | D49.89 |
| bone | C41.1 | C79.51 | — | D16.5 | D48.0 | D49.2 |
| lower | C41.1 | C79.51 | — | D16.5 | — | — |
| upper | C41.0 | C79.51 | — | D16.4 | — | — |
| carcinoma (any type) (lower) (upper) | C76.0 | C79.89 | | — | — | — |
| skin — see also Neoplasm, skin, face | C44.309 | C79.2 | D04.39 | D23.39 | D48.5 | D49.2 |
| soft tissues | C03.9 | C79.89 | D00.03 | D10.39 | D37.09 | D49.0 |
| lower | C03.1 | C79.89 | D00.03 | D10.39 | D37.09 | D49.0 |
| upper | C03.0 | C79.89 | D00.03 | D10.39 | D37.09 | D49.0 |
| jejunum | C17.1 | C78.4 | D01.49 | D13.39 | D37.2 | D49.0 |
| joint NEC — see also Neoplasm, bone | C41.9 | C79.51 | — | D16.9 | D48.0 | D49.2 |
| acromioclavicular | C40.0-☑ | C79.51 | — | D16.0-☑ | — | — |

## Neoplasm, neoplastic — continued (left column)

| | Malignant Primary | Malignant Secondary | Ca in situ | Benign | Uncertain | Unspecified Behavior |
|---|---|---|---|---|---|---|
| joint — see also Neoplasm, bone — continued | | | | | | |
| bursa or synovial membrane — see Neoplasm, connective tissue | | | | | | |
| costovertebral | C41.3 | C79.51 | — | D16.7 | D48.0 | D49.2 |
| sternocostal | C41.3 | C79.51 | — | D16.7 | D48.0 | D49.2 |
| temporomandibular | C41.1 | C79.51 | — | D16.5 | D48.0 | D49.2 |
| junction | | | | | | |
| anorectal | C21.8 | C78.5 | D01.3 | D12.9 | D37.8 | D49.0 |
| cardioesophageal | C16.0 | C78.89 | D00.2 | D13.1 | D37.1 | D49.0 |
| esophagogastric | C16.0 | C78.89 | D00.2 | D13.1 | D37.1 | D49.0 |
| gastroesophageal | C16.0 | C78.89 | D00.2 | D13.1 | D37.1 | D49.0 |
| hard and soft palate | C05.9 | C79.89 | D00.00 | D10.39 | D37.09 | D49.0 |
| ileocecal | C18.0 | C78.5 | D01.0 | D12.0 | D37.4 | D49.0 |
| pelvirectal | C19 | C78.5 | D01.1 | D12.7 | D37.5 | D49.0 |
| pelviureteric | C65.-☑ | C79.0-☑ | D09.19 | D30.1-☑ | D41.1-☑ | D49.59 |
| rectosigmoid | C19 | C78.5 | D01.1 | D12.7 | D37.5 | D49.0 |
| squamocolumnar, of cervix | C53.8 | C79.82 | D06.7 | D26.0 | D39.0 | D49.59 |
| Kaposi's sarcoma — see Kaposi's, sarcoma | | | | | | |
| kidney (parenchymal) | C64.-☑ | C79.0-☑ | D09.19 | D30.0-☑ | D41.0-☑ | D49.51-☑ |
| calyx | C65.-☑ | C79.0-☑ | D09.19 | D30.1-☑ | D41.1-☑ | D49.51-☑ |
| hilus | C65.-☑ | C79.0-☑ | D09.19 | D30.1-☑ | D41.1-☑ | D49.51-☑ |
| pelvis | C65.-☑ | C79.0-☑ | D09.19 | D30.1-☑ | D41.1-☑ | D49.51-☑ |
| knee NEC | C76.5-☑ | C79.89 | D04.7-☑ | D36.7 | D48.7 | D49.89 |
| labia (skin) | C51.9 | C79.82 | D07.1 | D28.0 | D39.8 | D49.59 |
| majora | C51.0 | C79.82 | D07.1 | D28.0 | D39.8 | D49.59 |
| minora | C51.1 | C79.82 | D07.1 | D28.0 | D39.8 | D49.59 |
| labial — see also Neoplasm, lip | C00.9 | C79.89 | D00.01 | D10.0 | D37.01 | D49.0 |
| sulcus (lower) (upper) | C06.1 | C79.89 | D00.02 | D10.39 | D37.09 | D49.0 |
| labium (skin) | C51.9 | C79.82 | D07.1 | D28.0 | D39.8 | D49.59 |
| majus | C51.0 | C79.82 | D07.1 | D28.0 | D39.8 | D49.59 |
| minus | C51.1 | C79.82 | D07.1 | D28.0 | D39.8 | D49.59 |
| lacrimal | | | | | | |
| canaliculi | C69.5-☑ | C79.49 | D09.2-☑ | D31.5-☑ | D48.7 | D49.89 |
| duct (nasal) | C69.5-☑ | C79.49 | D09.2-☑ | D31.5-☑ | D48.7 | D49.89 |
| gland | C69.5-☑ | C79.49 | D09.2-☑ | D31.5-☑ | D48.7 | D49.89 |
| punctum | C69.5-☑ | C79.49 | D09.2-☑ | D31.5-☑ | D48.7 | D49.89 |
| sac | C69.5-☑ | C79.49 | D09.2-☑ | D31.5-☑ | D48.7 | D49.89 |
| Langerhans, islands or islets | C25.4 | C78.89 | D01.7 | D13.7 | D37.8 | D49.0 |
| laryngopharynx | C13.9 | C79.89 | D00.08 | D10.7 | D37.05 | D49.0 |
| larynx, laryngeal NEC | C32.9 | C78.39 | D02.0 | D14.1 | D38.0 | D49.1 |
| aryepiglottic fold | C32.1 | C78.39 | D02.0 | D14.1 | D38.0 | D49.1 |
| cartilage (arytenoid) (cricoid) (cuneiform) (thyroid) | C32.3 | C78.39 | D02.0 | D14.1 | D38.0 | D49.1 |
| commissure (anterior) (posterior) | C32.0 | C78.39 | D02.0 | D14.1 | D38.0 | D49.1 |
| extrinsic NEC | C32.1 | C78.39 | D02.0 | D14.1 | D38.0 | D49.1 |
| meaning hypopharynx | C13.9 | C79.89 | D00.08 | D10.7 | D37.05 | D49.0 |
| interarytenoid fold | C32.1 | C78.39 | D02.0 | D14.1 | D38.0 | D49.1 |
| intrinsic | C32.0 | C78.39 | D02.0 | D14.1 | D38.0 | D49.1 |
| overlapping lesion | C32.8 | — | | | | |
| ventricular band | C32.1 | C78.39 | D02.0 | D14.1 | D38.0 | D49.1 |
| leg NEC | C76.5-☑ | C79.89 | D04.7-☑ | D36.7 | D48.7 | D49.89 |
| lens, crystalline | C69.4-☑ | C79.49 | D09.2-☑ | D31.4-☑ | D48.7 | D49.89 |
| lid (lower) (upper) | C44.10-☑ | C79.2 | D04.1-☑ | D23.1-☑ | D48.5 | D49.2 |
| basal cell carcinoma | C44.11-☑ | — | — | — | — | — |
| specified type NEC | C44.19-☑ | — | — | — | — | — |
| squamous cell carcinoma | C44.12-☑ | — | — | — | — | — |

## Neoplasm, neoplastic — continued (right column)

| | Malignant Primary | Malignant Secondary | Ca in situ | Benign | Uncertain | Unspecified Behavior |
|---|---|---|---|---|---|---|
| ligament — see also Neoplasm, connective tissue | | | | | | |
| broad | C57.1-☑ | C79.82 | D07.39 | D28.2 | D39.8 | D49.59 |
| Mackenrodt's | C57.7 | C79.82 | D07.39 | D28.7 | D39.8 | D49.59 |
| non-uterine — see Neoplasm, connective tissue | | | | | | |
| round | C57.2-☑ | C79.82 | — | D28.2 | D39.8 | D49.59 |
| sacro-uterine | C57.3 | C79.82 | — | D28.2 | D39.8 | D49.59 |
| uterine | C57.3 | C79.82 | — | D28.2 | D39.8 | D49.59 |
| utero-ovarian | C57.7 | C79.82 | D07.39 | D28.2 | D39.8 | D49.59 |
| uterosacral | C57.3 | C79.82 | — | D28.2 | D39.8 | D49.59 |
| limb | C76.8 | C79.89 | D04.8 | D36.7 | D48.7 | D49.89 |
| lower | C76.5-☑ | C79.89 | D04.7-☑ | D36.7 | D48.7 | D49.89 |
| upper | C76.4-☑ | C79.89 | D04.6-☑ | D36.7 | D48.7 | D49.89 |
| limbus of cornea | C69.1-☑ | C79.49 | D09.2-☑ | D31.1-☑ | D48.7 | D49.89 |
| lingual NEC — see also Neoplasm, tongue | C02.9 | C79.89 | D00.07 | D10.1 | D37.02 | D49.0 |
| lingula, lung | C34.1-☑ | C78.0-☑ | D02.2-☑ | D14.3-☑ | D38.1 | D49.1 |
| lip | C00.9 | C79.89 | D00.01 | D10.0 | D37.01 | D49.0 |
| buccal aspect — see Neoplasm, lip, internal | | | | | | |
| commissure | C00.6 | C79.89 | D00.01 | D10.0 | D37.01 | D49.0 |
| external | C00.2 | C79.89 | D00.01 | D10.0 | D37.01 | D49.0 |
| lower | C00.1 | C79.89 | D00.01 | D10.0 | D37.01 | D49.0 |
| upper | C00.0 | C79.89 | D00.01 | D10.0 | D37.01 | D49.0 |
| frenulum — see Neoplasm, lip, internal | | | | | | |
| inner aspect — see Neoplasm, lip, internal | | | | | | |
| internal | C00.5 | C79.89 | D00.01 | D10.0 | D37.01 | D49.0 |
| lower | C00.4 | C79.89 | D00.01 | D10.0 | D37.01 | D49.0 |
| upper | C00.3 | C79.89 | D00.01 | D10.0 | D37.01 | D49.0 |
| lipstick area | C00.2 | C79.89 | D00.01 | D10.0 | D37.01 | D49.0 |
| lower | C00.1 | C79.89 | D00.01 | D10.0 | D37.01 | D49.0 |
| upper | C00.0 | C79.89 | D00.01 | D10.0 | D37.01 | D49.0 |
| lower | C00.1 | C79.89 | D00.01 | D10.0 | D37.01 | D49.0 |
| internal | C00.4 | C79.89 | D00.01 | D10.0 | D37.01 | D49.0 |
| mucosa — see Neoplasm, lip, internal | | | | | | |
| oral aspect — see Neoplasm, lip, internal | | | | | | |
| overlapping lesion | C00.8 | — | — | — | — | — |
| with oral cavity or pharynx | C14.8 | — | — | — | — | — |
| skin (commissure) (lower) (upper) | C44.00 | C79.2 | D04.0 | D23.0 | D48.5 | D49.2 |
| basal cell carcinoma | C44.01 | — | — | — | — | — |
| specified type NEC | C44.09 | — | — | — | — | — |
| squamous cell carcinoma | C44.02 | — | — | — | — | — |
| upper | C00.0 | C79.89 | D00.01 | D10.0 | D37.01 | D49.0 |
| internal | C00.3 | C79.89 | D00.01 | D10.0 | D37.01 | D49.0 |
| vermilion border | C00.2 | C79.89 | D00.01 | D10.0 | D37.01 | D49.0 |
| lower | C00.1 | C79.89 | D00.01 | D10.0 | D37.01 | D49.0 |
| upper | C00.0 | C79.89 | D00.01 | D10.0 | D37.01 | D49.0 |
| lipomatous — see Lipoma, by site | | | | | | |
| liver — see also Index to disease, by histology | C22.9 | C78.7 | D01.5 | D13.4 | D37.6 | D49.0 |
| primary | C22.8 | C78.7 | D01.5 | D13.4 | D37.6 | D49.0 |
| lumbosacral plexus | C47.5 | C79.89 | — | D36.16 | D48.2 | D49.2 |
| lung | C34.9-☑ | C78.0-☑ | D02.2-☑ | D14.3-☑ | D38.1 | D49.1 |
| azygos lobe | C34.1-☑ | C78.0-☑ | D02.2-☑ | D14.3-☑ | D38.1 | D49.1 |
| carina | C34.0-☑ | C78.0-☑ | D02.2-☑ | D14.3-☑ | D38.1 | D49.1 |
| hilus | C34.0-☑ | C78.0-☑ | D02.2-☑ | D14.3-☑ | D38.1 | D49.1 |
| lingula | C34.1-☑ | C78.0-☑ | D02.2-☑ | D14.3-☑ | D38.1 | D49.1 |
| lobe NEC | C34.9-☑ | C78.0-☑ | D02.2-☑ | D14.3-☑ | D38.1 | D49.1 |
| lower lobe | C34.3-☑ | C78.0-☑ | D02.2-☑ | D14.3-☑ | D38.1 | D49.1 |

☑ Additional Character Required — Refer to the Tabular List for Character Selection ▽ Subterms under main terms may continue to next column or page

| Neoplasm, neoplastic — continued | Malignant Primary | Malignant Secondary | Ca in situ | Benign | Uncertain | Unspecified Behavior |
|---|---|---|---|---|---|---|
| lung — continued | | | | | | |
| main bronchus | C34.0-✓ | C78.0-✓ | D02.2-✓ | D14.3-✓ | D38.1 | D49.1 |
| mesothelioma — see Mesothelioma | | | | | | |
| middle lobe | C34.2 | C78.0-✓ | D02.21 | D14.31 | D38.1 | D49.1 |
| overlapping lesion | C34.8-✓ | — | | | | |
| upper lobe | C34.1-✓ | C78.0-✓ | D02.2-✓ | D14.3-✓ | D38.1 | D49.1 |
| lymph, lymphatic channel | | | | | | |
| NEC | C49.9 | C79.89 | — | D21.9 | D48.1 | D49.2 |
| gland (secondary) | — | C77.9 | — | D36.0 | D48.7 | D49.89 |
| abdominal | — | C77.2 | — | D36.0 | D48.7 | D49.89 |
| aortic | — | C77.2 | — | D36.0 | D48.7 | D49.89 |
| arm | — | C77.3 | — | D36.0 | D48.7 | D49.89 |
| auricular (anterior) (posterior) | — | C77.0 | — | D36.0 | D48.7 | D49.89 |
| axilla, axillary | — | C77.3 | — | D36.0 | D48.7 | D49.89 |
| brachial | — | C77.3 | — | D36.0 | D48.7 | D49.89 |
| bronchial | — | C77.1 | — | D36.0 | D48.7 | D49.89 |
| bronchopulmonary | — | C77.1 | — | D36.0 | D48.7 | D49.89 |
| celiac | — | C77.2 | — | D36.0 | D48.7 | D49.89 |
| cervical | — | C77.0 | — | D36.0 | D48.7 | D49.89 |
| cervicofacial | — | C77.0 | — | D36.0 | D48.7 | D49.89 |
| Cloquet | — | C77.4 | — | D36.0 | D48.7 | D49.89 |
| colic | — | C77.2 | — | D36.0 | D48.7 | D49.89 |
| common duct | — | C77.2 | — | D36.0 | D48.7 | D49.89 |
| cubital | — | C77.3 | — | D36.0 | D48.7 | D49.89 |
| diaphragmatic | — | C77.1 | — | D36.0 | D48.7 | D49.89 |
| epigastric, inferior | — | C77.1 | — | D36.0 | D48.7 | D49.89 |
| epitrochlear | — | C77.3 | — | D36.0 | D48.7 | D49.89 |
| esophageal | — | C77.1 | — | D36.0 | D48.7 | D49.89 |
| face | — | C77.0 | — | D36.0 | D48.7 | D49.89 |
| femoral | — | C77.4 | — | D36.0 | D48.7 | D49.89 |
| gastric | — | C77.2 | — | D36.0 | D48.7 | D49.89 |
| groin | — | C77.4 | — | D36.0 | D48.7 | D49.89 |
| head | — | C77.0 | — | D36.0 | D48.7 | D49.89 |
| hepatic | — | C77.2 | — | D36.0 | D48.7 | D49.89 |
| hilar (pulmonary) | — | C77.1 | — | D36.0 | D48.7 | D49.89 |
| splenic | — | C77.2 | — | D36.0 | D48.7 | D49.89 |
| hypogastric | — | C77.5 | — | D36.0 | D48.7 | D49.89 |
| ileocolic | — | C77.2 | — | D36.0 | D48.7 | D49.89 |
| iliac | — | C77.5 | — | D36.0 | D48.7 | D49.89 |
| infraclavicular | — | C77.3 | — | D36.0 | D48.7 | D49.89 |
| inguina, inguinal | — | C77.4 | — | D36.0 | D48.7 | D49.89 |
| innominate | — | C77.1 | — | D36.0 | D48.7 | D49.89 |
| intercostal | — | C77.1 | — | D36.0 | D48.7 | D49.89 |
| intestinal | — | C77.2 | — | D36.0 | D48.7 | D49.89 |
| intrabdominal | — | C77.2 | — | D36.0 | D48.7 | D49.89 |
| intrapelvic | — | C77.5 | — | D36.0 | D48.7 | D49.89 |
| intrathoracic | — | C77.1 | — | D36.0 | D48.7 | D49.89 |
| jugular | — | C77.0 | — | D36.0 | D48.7 | D49.89 |
| leg | — | C77.4 | — | D36.0 | D48.7 | D49.89 |
| limb | | | | | | |
| lower | — | C77.4 | — | D36.0 | D48.7 | D49.89 |
| upper | — | C77.3 | — | D36.0 | D48.7 | D49.89 |
| lower limb | — | C77.4 | — | D36.0 | D48.7 | D49.89 |
| lumbar | — | C77.2 | — | D36.0 | D48.7 | D49.89 |
| mandibular | — | C77.0 | — | D36.0 | D48.7 | D49.89 |
| mediastinal | — | C77.1 | — | D36.0 | D48.7 | D49.89 |
| mesenteric (inferior) (superior) | — | C77.2 | — | D36.0 | D48.7 | D49.89 |
| midcolic | — | C77.2 | — | D36.0 | D48.7 | D49.89 |
| multiple sites in categories C77.0-C77.5 | — | C77.8 | — | D36.0 | D48.7 | D49.89 |
| neck | — | C77.0 | — | D36.0 | D48.7 | D49.89 |
| obturator | — | C77.5 | — | D36.0 | D48.7 | D49.89 |
| occipital | — | C77.0 | — | D36.0 | D48.7 | D49.89 |
| pancreatic | — | C77.2 | — | D36.0 | D48.7 | D49.89 |
| para-aortic | — | C77.2 | — | D36.0 | D48.7 | D49.89 |
| paracervical | — | C77.5 | — | D36.0 | D48.7 | D49.89 |
| parametrial | — | C77.5 | — | D36.0 | D48.7 | D49.89 |
| parasternal | — | C77.1 | — | D36.0 | D48.7 | D49.89 |
| parotid | — | C77.0 | — | D36.0 | D48.7 | D49.89 |
| pectoral | — | C77.3 | — | D36.0 | D48.7 | D49.89 |
| pelvic | — | C77.5 | — | D36.0 | D48.7 | D49.89 |
| peri-aortic | — | C77.2 | — | D36.0 | D48.7 | D49.89 |
| peripancreatic | — | C77.2 | — | D36.0 | D48.7 | D49.89 |
| popliteal | — | C77.4 | — | D36.0 | D48.7 | D49.89 |
| porta hepatis | — | C77.2 | — | D36.0 | D48.7 | D49.89 |

| Neoplasm, neoplastic — continued | Malignant Primary | Malignant Secondary | Ca in situ | Benign | Uncertain | Unspecified Behavior |
|---|---|---|---|---|---|---|
| lymph, lymphatic channel — continued | | | | | | |
| gland — continued | | | | | | |
| portal | — | C77.2 | — | D36.0 | D48.7 | D49.89 |
| preauricular | — | C77.0 | — | D36.0 | D48.7 | D49.89 |
| prelaryngeal | — | C77.0 | — | D36.0 | D48.7 | D49.89 |
| presymphysial | — | C77.5 | — | D36.0 | D48.7 | D49.89 |
| pretracheal | — | C77.0 | — | D36.0 | D48.7 | D49.89 |
| primary (any site) NEC | C96.9 | — | — | — | — | — |
| pulmonary (hiler) | — | C77.1 | — | D36.0 | D48.7 | D49.89 |
| pyloric | — | C77.2 | — | D36.0 | D48.7 | D49.89 |
| retroperitoneal | — | C77.2 | — | D36.0 | D48.7 | D49.89 |
| retropharyngeal | — | C77.0 | — | D36.0 | D48.7 | D49.89 |
| Rosenmuller's | — | C77.4 | — | D36.0 | D48.7 | D49.89 |
| sacral | — | C77.5 | — | D36.0 | D48.7 | D49.89 |
| scalene | — | C77.0 | — | D36.0 | D48.7 | D49.89 |
| site NEC | — | C77.9 | — | D36.0 | D48.7 | D49.89 |
| splenic (hilar) | — | C77.2 | — | D36.0 | D48.7 | D49.89 |
| subclavicular | — | C77.3 | — | D36.0 | D48.7 | D49.89 |
| subinguinal | — | C77.4 | — | D36.0 | D48.7 | D49.89 |
| sublingual | — | C77.0 | — | D36.0 | D48.7 | D49.89 |
| submandibular | — | C77.0 | — | D36.0 | D48.7 | D49.89 |
| submaxillary | — | C77.0 | — | D36.0 | D48.7 | D49.89 |
| submental | — | C77.0 | — | D36.0 | D48.7 | D49.89 |
| subscapular | — | C77.3 | — | D36.0 | D48.7 | D49.89 |
| supraclavicular | — | C77.0 | — | D36.0 | D48.7 | D49.89 |
| thoracic | — | C77.1 | — | D36.0 | D48.7 | D49.89 |
| tibial | — | C77.4 | — | D36.0 | D48.7 | D49.89 |
| tracheal | — | C77.1 | — | D36.0 | D48.7 | D49.89 |
| tracheobronchial | — | C77.1 | — | D36.0 | D48.7 | D49.89 |
| upper limb | — | C77.3 | — | D36.0 | D48.7 | D49.89 |
| Virchow's | — | C77.0 | — | D36.0 | D48.7 | D49.89 |
| node — see also Neoplasm, lymph gland | | | | | | |
| primary NEC | C96.9 | — | — | — | — | — |
| vessel — see also Neoplasm, connective tissue | C49.9 | C79.89 | — | D21.9 | D48.1 | D49.2 |
| Mackenrodt's ligament | C57.7 | C79.82 | D07.39 | D28.7 | D39.8 | D49.59 |
| malar | C41.0 | C79.51 | — | D16.4 | D48.0 | D49.2 |
| region — see Neoplasm, cheek | | | | | | |
| mammary gland — see Neoplasm, breast | | | | | | |
| mandible | C41.1 | C79.51 | — | D16.5 | D48.0 | D49.2 |
| alveolar | | | | | | |
| mucosa (carcinoma) | C03.1 | C79.89 | D00.03 | D10.39 | D37.09 | D49.0 |
| ridge or process | C41.1 | C79.51 | — | D16.5 | D48.0 | D49.2 |
| marrow (bone) NEC | C96.9 | C79.52 | — | — | D47.9 | D49.89 |
| mastectomy site (skin) — see also Neoplasm, breast, skin | C44.501 | C79.2 | — | — | — | — |
| specified as breast tissue | C50.8-✓ | C79.81 | — | — | — | — |
| mastoid (air cells) (antrum) (cavity) | C30.1 | C78.39 | D02.3 | D14.0 | D38.5 | D49.1 |
| bone or process | C41.0 | C79.51 | — | D16.4 | D48.0 | D49.2 |
| maxilla, maxillary (superior) | C41.0 | C79.51 | — | D16.4 | D48.0 | D49.2 |
| alveolar | | | | | | |
| mucosa | C03.0 | C79.89 | D00.03 | D10.39 | D37.09 | D49.0 |
| ridge or process (carcinoma) | C41.0 | C79.51 | — | D16.4 | D48.0 | D49.2 |
| antrum | C31.0 | C78.39 | D02.3 | D14.0 | D38.5 | D49.1 |
| carcinoma | C03.0 | C79.51 | — | — | — | — |
| inferior — see Neoplasm, mandible | | | | | | |
| sinus | C31.0 | C78.39 | D02.3 | D14.0 | D38.5 | D49.1 |
| meatus external (ear) — see also Neoplasm, skin, ear | C44.20-✓ | C79.2 | D04.2-✓ | D23.2-✓ | D48.5 | D49.2 |
| Meckel diverticulum, malignant | C17.3 | C78.4 | D01.49 | D13.39 | D37.2 | D49.0 |
| mediastinum, mediastinal | C38.3 | C78.1 | — | D15.2 | D38.3 | D49.89 |

| | Malignant Primary | Malignant Secondary | Ca in situ | Benign | Uncertain | Unspecified Behavior |
|---|---|---|---|---|---|---|
| **Neoplasm, neoplastic —** | | | | | | |
| *continued* | | | | | | |
| mediastinum, mediastinal | | | | | | |
| *— continued* | | | | | | |
| anterior | C38.1 | C78.1 | — | D15.2 | D38.3 | D49.89 |
| posterior | C38.2 | C78.1 | — | D15.2 | D38.3 | D49.89 |
| medulla | | | | | | |
| adrenal | C74.1-☑ | C79.7-☑ | D09.3 | D35.0-☑ | D44.1-☑ | D49.7 |
| oblongata | C71.7 | C79.31 | | D33.1 | D43.1 | D49.6 |
| meibomian gland | C44.10-☑ | C79.2 | D04.1-☑ | D23.1-☑ | D48.5 | D49.2 |
| basal cell | | | | | | |
| carcinoma | C44.11-☑ | — | — | — | — | — |
| specified type NEC | C44.19-☑ | — | — | — | — | — |
| squamous cell | | | | | | |
| carcinoma | C44.12-☑ | | | | | |
| melanoma — *see* | | | | | | |
| Melanoma | | | | | | |
| meninges | C70.9 | C79.49 | — | D32.9 | D42.9 | D49.7 |
| brain | C70.0 | C79.32 | — | D32.0 | D42.0 | D49.7 |
| cerebral | C70.0 | C79.32 | — | D32.0 | D42.0 | D49.7 |
| crainial | C70.0 | C79.32 | — | D32.0 | D42.0 | D49.7 |
| intracranial | C70.0 | C79.32 | — | D32.0 | D42.0 | D49.7 |
| spinal (cord) | C70.1 | C79.49 | — | D32.1 | D42.1 | D49.7 |
| meniscus, knee joint | | | | | | |
| (lateral) (medial) | C40.2-☑ | C79.51 | | D16.2-☑ | D48.0 | D49.2 |
| Merkel cell — *see* | | | | | | |
| Carcinoma, Merkel | | | | | | |
| cell | | | | | | |
| mesentery, | | | | | | |
| mesenteric | C48.1 | C78.6 | — | D20.1 | D48.4 | D49.0 |
| mesoappendix | C48.1 | C78.6 | — | D20.1 | D48.4 | D49.0 |
| mesocolon | C48.1 | C78.6 | — | D20.1 | D48.4 | D49.0 |
| mesopharynx — *see* | | | | | | |
| Neoplasm, | | | | | | |
| oropharynx | | | | | | |
| mesosalpinx | C57.1-☑ | C79.82 | D07.39 | D28.2 | D39.8 | D49.59 |
| mesothelial tissue — *see* | | | | | | |
| Mesothelioma | | | | | | |
| mesothelioma — *see* | | | | | | |
| Mesothelioma | | | | | | |
| mesovarium | C57.1-☑ | C79.82 | D07.39 | D28.2 | D39.8 | D49.59 |
| metacarpus (any | | | | | | |
| bone) | C40.1-☑ | C79.51 | — | D16.1-☑ | — | — |
| metastatic NEC — *see* | | | | | | |
| *also* Neoplasm, by | | | | | | |
| site, secondary | — | C79.9 | — | — | — | — |
| metatarsus (any | | | | | | |
| bone) | C40.3-☑ | C79.51 | — | D16.3-☑ | — | — |
| midbrain | C71.7 | C79.31 | | D33.1 | D43.1 | D49.6 |
| milk duct — *see* | | | | | | |
| Neoplasm, breast | | | | | | |
| mons | | | | | | |
| pubis | C51.9 | C79.82 | D07.1 | D28.0 | D39.8 | D49.59 |
| veneris | C51.9 | C79.82 | D07.1 | D28.0 | D39.8 | D49.59 |
| motor tract | C72.9 | C79.49 | — | D33.9 | D43.9 | D49.7 |
| brain | C71.9 | C79.31 | — | D33.2 | D43.2 | D49.6 |
| cauda equina | C72.1 | C79.49 | — | D33.4 | D43.4 | D49.7 |
| spinal | C72.0 | C79.49 | — | D33.4 | D43.4 | D49.7 |
| mouth | C06.9 | C79.89 | D00.00 | D10.30 | D37.09 | D49.0 |
| book-leaf | C06.89 | C79.89 | — | — | — | — |
| floor | C04.9 | C79.89 | D00.06 | D10.2 | D37.09 | D49.0 |
| anterior portion | C04.0 | C79.89 | D00.06 | D10.2 | D37.09 | D49.0 |
| lateral portion | C04.1 | C79.89 | D00.06 | D10.2 | D37.09 | D49.0 |
| overlapping | | | | | | |
| lesion | C04.8 | — | — | — | — | — |
| overlapping NEC | C06.80 | — | — | — | — | — |
| roof | C05.9 | C79.89 | D00.00 | D10.39 | D37.09 | D49.0 |
| specified part NEC | C06.89 | C79.89 | D00.00 | D10.39 | D37.09 | D49.0 |
| vestibule | C06.1 | C79.89 | D00.00 | D10.39 | D37.09 | D49.0 |
| mucosa | | | | | | |
| alveolar (ridge or | | | | | | |
| process) | C03.9 | C79.89 | D00.03 | D10.39 | D37.09 | D49.0 |
| lower | C03.1 | C79.89 | D00.03 | D10.39 | D37.09 | D49.0 |
| upper | C03.0 | C79.89 | D00.03 | D10.39 | D37.09 | D49.0 |
| buccal | C06.0 | C79.89 | D00.02 | D10.39 | D37.09 | D49.0 |
| cheek | C06.0 | C79.89 | D00.02 | D10.39 | D37.09 | D49.0 |
| lip — *see* Neoplasm, lip, | | | | | | |
| internal | | | | | | |
| nasal | C30.0 | C78.39 | D02.3 | D14.0 | D38.5 | D49.1 |
| oral | C06.0 | C79.89 | D00.02 | D10.39 | D37.09 | D49.0 |
| Mullerian duct | | | | | | |
| female | C57.7 | C79.82 | D07.39 | D28.7 | D39.8 | D49.59 |
| male | C63.7 | C79.82 | D07.69 | D29.8 | D40.8 | D49.59 |

| | Malignant Primary | Malignant Secondary | Ca in situ | Benign | Uncertain | Unspecified Behavior |
|---|---|---|---|---|---|---|
| **Neoplasm, neoplastic —** | | | | | | |
| *continued* | | | | | | |
| muscle — *see also* | | | | | | |
| Neoplasm, connective | | | | | | |
| tissue | | | | | | |
| extraocular | C69.6-☑ | C79.49 | D09.2-☑ | D31.6-☑ | D48.7 | D49.89 |
| myocardium | C38.0 | C79.89 | — | D15.1 | D48.7 | D49.89 |
| myometrium | C54.2 | C79.82 | D07.0 | D26.1 | D39.0 | D49.59 |
| myopericardium | C38.0 | C79.89 | — | D15.1 | D48.7 | D49.89 |
| nabothian gland | | | | | | |
| (follicle) | C53.0 | C79.82 | D06.0 | D26.0 | D39.0 | D49.59 |
| nail — *see also* Neoplasm, | | | | | | |
| skin, limb | C44.90 | C79.2 | D04.9 | D23.9 | D48.5 | D49.2 |
| finger — *see also* | | | | | | |
| Neoplasm, skin, | | | | | | |
| limb, upper | C44.60-☑ | C79.2 | D04.6-☑ | D23.6-☑ | D48.5 | D49.2 |
| toe — *see also* | | | | | | |
| Neoplasm, skin, | | | | | | |
| limb, lower | C44.70-☑ | C79.2 | D04.7-☑ | D23.7-☑ | D48.5 | D49.2 |
| nares, naris (anterior) | | | | | | |
| (posterior) | C30.0 | C78.39 | D02.3 | D14.0 | D38.5 | D49.1 |
| nasal — *see* Neoplasm, | | | | | | |
| nose | | | | | | |
| nasolabial groove — *see* | | | | | | |
| *also* Neoplasm, skin, | | | | | | |
| face | C44.309 | C79.2 | D04.39 | D23.39 | D48.5 | D49.2 |
| nasolacrimal duct | C69.5-☑ | C79.49 | D09.2-☑ | D31.5-☑ | D48.7 | D49.89 |
| nasopharynx, | | | | | | |
| nasopharyngeal | C11.9 | C79.89 | D00.08 | D10.6 | D37.05 | D49.0 |
| floor | C11.3 | C79.89 | D00.08 | D10.6 | D37.05 | D49.0 |
| overlapping lesion | C11.8 | — | — | — | — | — |
| roof | C11.0 | C79.89 | D00.08 | D10.6 | D37.05 | D49.0 |
| wall | C11.9 | C79.89 | D00.08 | D10.6 | D37.05 | D49.0 |
| anterior | C11.3 | C79.89 | D00.08 | D10.6 | D37.05 | D49.0 |
| lateral | C11.2 | C79.89 | D00.08 | D10.6 | D37.05 | D49.0 |
| posterior | C11.1 | C79.89 | D00.08 | D10.6 | D37.05 | D49.0 |
| superior | C11.0 | C79.89 | D00.08 | D10.6 | D37.05 | D49.0 |
| nates — *see also* | | | | | | |
| Neoplasm, skin, | | | | | | |
| trunk | C44.509 | C79.2 | D04.5 | D23.5 | D48.5 | D49.2 |
| neck NEC | C76.0 | C79.89 | D09.8 | D36.7 | D48.7 | D49.89 |
| skin | C44.40 | — | — | — | — | — |
| basal cell | | | | | | |
| carcinoma | C44.41 | — | — | — | — | — |
| specified type | | | | | | |
| NEC | C44.49 | — | — | — | — | — |
| squamous cell | | | | | | |
| carcinoma | C44.42 | — | — | — | — | — |
| nerve (ganglion) | C47.9 | C79.89 | — | D36.10 | D48.2 | D49.2 |
| abducens | C72.59 | C79.49 | — | D33.3 | D43.3 | D49.7 |
| accessory (spinal) | C72.59 | C79.49 | — | D33.3 | D43.3 | D49.7 |
| acoustic | C72.4-☑ | C79.49 | — | D33.3 | D43.3 | D49.7 |
| auditory | C72.4-☑ | C79.49 | — | D33.3 | | D49.7 |
| autonomic NEC — *see* | | | | | | |
| *also* Neoplasm, | | | | | | |
| nerve, | | | | | | |
| peripheral | C47.9 | C79.89 | — | D36.10 | D48.2 | D49.2 |
| brachial | C47.1-☑ | C79.89 | — | D36.12 | D48.2 | D49.2 |
| cranial | C72.50 | C79.49 | — | D33.3 | D43.3 | D49.7 |
| specified NEC | C72.59 | C79.49 | — | D33.3 | D43.3 | D49.7 |
| facial | C72.59 | C79.49 | — | D33.3 | D43.3 | D49.7 |
| femoral | C47.2-☑ | C79.89 | — | D36.13 | D48.2 | D49.2 |
| ganglion NEC — *see* | | | | | | |
| *also* Neoplasm, | | | | | | |
| nerve, | | | | | | |
| peripheral | C47.9 | C79.89 | — | D36.10 | D48.2 | D49.2 |
| glossopharyngeal | C72.59 | C79.49 | — | D33.3 | D43.3 | D49.7 |
| hypoglossal | C72.59 | C79.49 | — | D33.3 | D43.3 | D49.7 |
| intercostal | C47.3 | C79.89 | — | D36.14 | D48.2 | D49.2 |
| lumbar | C47.6 | C79.89 | — | D36.17 | D48.2 | D49.2 |
| median | C47.1-☑ | C79.89 | — | D36.12 | D48.2 | D49.2 |
| obturator | C47.2-☑ | C79.89 | — | D36.13 | D48.2 | D49.2 |
| oculomotor | C72.59 | C79.49 | — | D33.3 | D43.3 | D49.7 |
| olfactory | C47.2-☑ | C79.49 | — | D33.3 | D43.3 | D49.7 |
| optic | C72.3-☑ | C79.49 | — | D33.3 | D43.3 | D49.7 |
| parasympathetic | | | | | | |
| NEC | C47.9 | C79.89 | — | D36.10 | D48.2 | D49.2 |
| peripheral NEC | C47.9 | C79.89 | — | D36.10 | D48.2 | D49.2 |
| abdomen | C47.4 | C79.89 | — | D36.15 | D48.2 | D49.2 |
| abdominal wall | C47.4 | C79.89 | — | D36.15 | D48.2 | D49.2 |
| ankle | C47.2-☑ | C79.89 | — | D36.13 | D48.2 | D49.2 |
| antecubital fossa or | | | | | | |
| space | C47.1-☑ | C79.89 | — | D36.12 | D48.2 | D49.2 |

    ☑ **Additional Character Required — Refer to the Tabular List for Character Selection**     ▽ Subterms under main terms may continue to next column or page

**Neoplasm, neoplastic — continued**
*nerve — continued*
*peripheral — continued*

| Term | Malignant Primary | Malignant Secondary | Ca in situ | Benign | Uncertain | Unspecified Behavior |
|---|---|---|---|---|---|---|
| arm | C47.1-✓ | C79.89 | — | D36.12 | D48.2 | D49.2 |
| auricle (ear) | C47.0 | C79.89 | — | D36.11 | D48.2 | D49.2 |
| axilla | C47.3 | C79.89 | — | D36.12 | D48.2 | D49.2 |
| back | C47.6 | C79.89 | — | D36.17 | D48.2 | D49.2 |
| buttock | C47.5 | C79.89 | — | D36.16 | D48.2 | D49.2 |
| calf | C47.2-✓ | C79.89 | — | D36.13 | D48.2 | D49.2 |
| cervical region | C47.0 | C79.89 | — | D36.11 | D48.2 | D49.2 |
| cheek | C47.0 | C79.89 | — | D36.11 | D48.2 | D49.2 |
| chest (wall) | C47.3 | C79.89 | — | D36.14 | D48.2 | D49.2 |
| chin | C47.0 | C79.89 | — | D36.11 | D48.2 | D49.2 |
| ear (external) | C47.0 | C79.89 | — | D36.11 | D48.2 | D49.2 |
| elbow | C47.1-✓ | C79.89 | — | D36.12 | D48.2 | D49.2 |
| extrarectal | C47.5 | C79.89 | — | D36.16 | D48.2 | D49.2 |
| extremity | C47.9 | C79.89 | — | D36.10 | D48.2 | D49.2 |
|   lower | C47.2-✓ | C79.89 | — | D36.13 | D48.2 | D49.2 |
|   upper | C47.1-✓ | C79.89 | — | D36.12 | D48.2 | D49.2 |
| eyelid | C47.0 | C79.89 | — | D36.11 | D48.2 | D49.2 |
| face | C47.0 | C79.89 | — | D36.11 | D48.2 | D49.2 |
| finger | C47.1-✓ | C79.89 | — | D36.12 | D48.2 | D49.2 |
| flank | C47.6 | C79.89 | — | D36.17 | D48.2 | D49.2 |
| foot | C47.2-✓ | C79.89 | — | D36.13 | D48.2 | D49.2 |
| forearm | C47.1-✓ | C79.89 | — | D36.12 | D48.2 | D49.2 |
| forehead | C47.0 | C79.89 | — | D36.11 | D48.2 | D49.2 |
| gluteal region | C47.5 | C79.89 | — | D36.16 | D48.2 | D49.2 |
| groin | C47.5 | C79.89 | — | D36.16 | D48.2 | D49.2 |
| hand | C47.1-✓ | C79.89 | — | D36.12 | D48.2 | D49.2 |
| head | C47.0 | C79.89 | — | D36.11 | D48.2 | D49.2 |
| heel | C47.2-✓ | C79.89 | — | D36.13 | D48.2 | D49.2 |
| hip | C47.2-✓ | C79.89 | — | D36.13 | D48.2 | D49.2 |
| infraclavicular region | C47.3 | C79.89 | — | D36.14 | D48.2 | D49.2 |
| inguinal (canal) (region) | C47.5 | C79.89 | — | D36.16 | D48.2 | D49.2 |
| intrathoracic | C47.3 | C79.89 | — | D36.14 | D48.2 | D49.2 |
| ischiorectal fossa | C47.5 | C79.89 | — | D36.16 | D48.2 | D49.2 |
| knee | C47.2-✓ | C79.89 | — | D36.13 | D48.2 | D49.2 |
| leg | C47.2-✓ | C79.89 | — | D36.13 | D48.2 | D49.2 |
| limb NEC | C47.9 | C79.89 | — | D36.10 | D48.2 | D49.2 |
|   lower | C47.2-✓ | C79.89 | — | D36.13 | D48.2 | D49.2 |
|   upper | C47.1-✓ | C79.89 | — | D36.12 | D48.2 | D49.2 |
| nates | C47.5 | C79.89 | — | D36.16 | D48.2 | D49.2 |
| neck | C47.0 | C79.89 | — | D36.11 | D48.2 | D49.2 |
| orbit | C69.6-✓ | C79.49 | — | D31.6-✓ | D48.7 | D49.2 |
| pararectal | C47.5 | C79.89 | — | D36.16 | D48.2 | D49.2 |
| paraurethral | C47.5 | C79.89 | — | D36.16 | D48.2 | D49.2 |
| paravaginal | C47.5 | C79.89 | — | D36.16 | D48.2 | D49.2 |
| pelvis (floor) | C47.5 | C79.89 | — | D36.16 | D48.2 | D49.2 |
| pelvoabdominal | C47.8 | C79.89 | — | D36.17 | D48.2 | D49.2 |
| perineum | C47.5 | C79.89 | — | D36.16 | D48.2 | D49.2 |
| perirectal (tissue) | C47.5 | C79.89 | — | D36.16 | D48.2 | D49.2 |
| periurethral (tissue) | C47.5 | C79.89 | — | D36.16 | D48.2 | D49.2 |
| popliteal fossa or space | C47.2-✓ | C79.89 | — | D36.13 | D48.2 | D49.2 |
| presacral | C47.5 | C79.89 | — | D36.16 | D48.2 | D49.2 |
| pterygoid fossa | C47.0 | C79.89 | — | D36.11 | D48.2 | D49.2 |
| rectovaginal septum or wall | C47.5 | C79.89 | — | D36.16 | D48.2 | D49.2 |
| rectovesical | C47.5 | C79.89 | — | D36.16 | D48.2 | D49.2 |
| sacrococcygeal region | C47.5 | C79.89 | — | D36.16 | D48.2 | D49.2 |
| scalp | C47.0 | C79.89 | — | D36.11 | D48.2 | D49.2 |
| scapular region | C47.3 | C79.89 | — | D36.14 | D48.2 | D49.2 |
| shoulder | C47.1-✓ | C79.89 | — | D36.12 | D48.2 | D49.2 |
| submental | C47.0 | C79.89 | — | D36.11 | D48.2 | D49.2 |
| supraclavicular region | C47.0 | C79.89 | — | D36.11 | D48.2 | D49.2 |
| temple | C47.0 | C79.89 | — | D36.11 | D48.2 | D49.2 |
| temporal region | C47.0 | C79.89 | — | D36.11 | D48.2 | D49.2 |
| thigh | C47.2-✓ | C79.89 | — | D36.13 | D48.2 | D49.2 |
| thoracic (duct) (wall) | C47.3 | C79.89 | — | D36.14 | D48.2 | D49.2 |
| thorax | C47.3 | C79.89 | — | D36.14 | D48.2 | D49.2 |
| thumb | C47.1-✓ | C79.89 | — | D36.12 | D48.2 | D49.2 |
| toe | C47.2-✓ | C79.89 | — | D36.13 | D48.2 | D49.2 |
| trunk | C47.6 | C79.89 | — | D36.17 | D48.2 | D49.2 |

**Neoplasm, neoplastic — continued**
*nerve — continued*
*peripheral — continued*

| Term | Malignant Primary | Malignant Secondary | Ca in situ | Benign | Uncertain | Unspecified Behavior |
|---|---|---|---|---|---|---|
| umbilicus | C47.4 | C79.89 | — | D36.15 | D48.2 | D49.2 |
| vesicorectal | C47.5 | C79.89 | — | D36.16 | D48.2 | D49.2 |
| wrist | C47.1-✓ | C79.89 | — | D36.12 | D48.2 | D49.2 |
| radial | C47.1-✓ | C79.89 | — | D36.12 | D48.2 | D49.2 |
| sacral | C47.5 | C79.89 | — | D36.16 | D48.2 | D49.2 |
| sciatic | C47.2-✓ | C79.89 | — | D36.13 | D48.2 | D49.2 |
| spinal NEC | C47.9 | C79.89 | — | D36.10 | D48.2 | D49.2 |
| accessory | C72.59 | C79.49 | — | D33.3 | D43.3 | D49.7 |
| sympathetic NEC — *see also* Neoplasm, nerve, peripheral | C47.9 | C79.89 | — | D36.10 | D48.2 | D49.2 |
| trigeminal | C72.59 | C79.49 | — | D33.3 | D43.3 | D49.7 |
| trochlear | C72.59 | C79.49 | — | D33.3 | D43.3 | D49.7 |
| ulnar | C47.1-✓ | C79.89 | — | D36.12 | D48.2 | D49.2 |
| vagus | C72.59 | C79.49 | — | D33.3 | D43.3 | D49.7 |
| nervous system (central) | C72.9 | C79.40 | — | D33.9 | D43.9 | D49.7 |
|   autonomic — *see* Neoplasm, nerve, peripheral | | | | | | |
|   parasympathetic — *see* Neoplasm, nerve, peripheral | | | | | | |
|   specified site NEC | — | C79.49 | — | D33.7 | D43.8 | — |
|   sympathetic — *see* Neoplasm, nerve, peripheral | | | | | | |
| nevus — *see* Nevus | | | | | | |
| nipple | C50.0-✓ | C79.81 | D05.-✓ | D24.-✓ | — | — |
| nose, nasal | C76.0 | C79.89 | D09.8 | D36.7 | D48.7 | D49.89 |
|   ala (external) (nasi) — *see also* Neoplasm, nose, skin | C44.301 | C79.2 | D04.39 | D23.39 | D48.5 | D49.2 |
|   bone | C41.0 | C79.51 | — | D16.4 | D48.0 | D49.2 |
|   cartilage | C30.0 | C78.39 | D02.3 | D14.0 | D38.5 | D49.1 |
|   cavity | C30.0 | C78.39 | D02.3 | D14.0 | D38.5 | D49.1 |
|   choana | C11.3 | C79.89 | D00.08 | D10.6 | D37.05 | D49.0 |
|   external (skin) — *see also* Neoplasm, nose, skin | C44.301 | C79.2 | D04.39 | D23.39 | D48.5 | D49.2 |
|   fossa | C30.0 | C78.39 | D02.3 | D14.0 | D38.5 | D49.1 |
|   internal | C30.0 | C78.39 | D02.3 | D14.0 | D38.5 | D49.1 |
|   mucosa | C30.0 | C78.39 | D02.3 | D14.0 | D38.5 | D49.1 |
|   septum | C30.0 | C78.39 | D02.3 | D14.0 | D38.5 | D49.1 |
|     posterior margin | C11.3 | C79.89 | D00.08 | D10.6 | D37.05 | D49.0 |
|   sinus — *see* Neoplasm, sinus | | | | | | |
|   skin | C44.301 | C79.2 | D04.39 | D23.39 | D48.5 | D49.2 |
|     basal cell carcinoma | C44.311 | — | — | — | — | — |
|     specified type NEC | C44.391 | — | — | — | — | — |
|     squamous cell carcinoma | C44.321 | — | — | — | — | — |
|   turbinate (mucosa) | C30.0 | C78.39 | D02.3 | D14.0 | D38.5 | D49.1 |
|     bone | C41.0 | C79.51 | — | D16.4 | D48.0 | D49.2 |
|   vestibule | C30.0 | C78.39 | D02.3 | D14.0 | D38.5 | D49.1 |
| nostril | C30.0 | C78.39 | D02.3 | D14.0 | D38.5 | D49.1 |
| nucleus pulposus | C41.2 | C79.51 | — | D16.6 | D48.0 | D49.2 |
| occipital | | | | | | |
|   bone | C41.0 | C79.51 | — | D16.4 | D48.0 | D49.2 |
|   lobe or pole, brain | C71.4 | C79.31 | — | D33.0 | D43.0 | D49.6 |
| odontogenic — *see* Neoplasm, jaw bone | | | | | | |
| olfactory nerve or bulb | C72.2-✓ | C79.49 | — | D33.3 | D43.3 | D49.7 |
| olive (brain) | C71.7 | C79.31 | — | D33.1 | D43.1 | D49.6 |
| omentum | C48.1 | C78.6 | — | D20.1 | D48.4 | D49.0 |
| operculum (brain) | C71.0 | C79.31 | — | D33.0 | D43.0 | D49.6 |
| optic nerve, chiasm, or tract | C72.3-✓ | C79.49 | — | D33.3 | D43.3 | D49.7 |
| oral (cavity) | C06.9 | C79.89 | D00.00 | D10.30 | D37.09 | D49.0 |
|   ill-defined | C14.8 | C79.89 | D00.00 | D10.30 | D37.09 | D49.0 |
|   mucosa | C06.0 | C79.89 | D00.02 | D10.39 | D37.09 | D49.0 |
| orbit | C69.6-✓ | C79.49 | D09.2-✓ | D31.6-✓ | D48.7 | D49.89 |
|   autonomic nerve | C69.6-✓ | C79.49 | — | D31.6-✓ | D48.7 | D49.2 |
|   bone | C41.0 | C79.51 | — | D16.4 | D48.0 | D49.2 |

| Neoplasm, neoplastic — | Malignant Primary | Malignant Secondary | Ca in situ | Benign | Uncertain | Unspecified Behavior |
|---|---|---|---|---|---|---|
| continued | | | | | | |
| orbit — continued | | | | | | |
| eye | C69.6-☑ | C79.49 | D09.2-☑ | D31.6-☑ | D48.7 | D49.89 |
| peripheral nerves | C69.6-☑ | C79.49 | — | D31.6-☑ | D48.7 | D49.2 |
| soft parts | C69.6-☑ | C79.49 | D09.2-☑ | D31.6-☑ | D48.7 | D49.89 |
| organ of | | | | | | |
| Zuckerkandl | C75.5 | C79.89 | — | D35.6 | D44.7 | D49.7 |
| oropharynx | C10.9 | C79.89 | D00.08 | D10.5 | D37.05 | D49.0 |
| branchial cleft | | | | | | |
| (vestige) | C10.4 | C79.89 | D00.08 | D10.5 | D37.05 | D49.0 |
| junctional region | C10.8 | C79.89 | D00.08 | D10.5 | D37.05 | D49.0 |
| lateral wall | C10.2 | C79.89 | D00.08 | D10.5 | D37.05 | D49.0 |
| overlapping lesion | C10.8 | — | — | — | — | — |
| pillars or fauces | C09.1 | C79.89 | D00.08 | D10.5 | D37.05 | D49.0 |
| posterior wall | C10.3 | C79.89 | D00.08 | D10.5 | D37.05 | D49.0 |
| vallecula | C10.0 | C79.89 | D00.08 | D10.5 | D37.05 | D49.0 |
| os | | | | | | |
| external | C53.1 | C79.82 | D06.1 | D26.0 | D39.0 | D49.59 |
| internal | C53.0 | C79.82 | D06.0 | D26.0 | D39.0 | D49.59 |
| ovary | C56.-☑ | C79.6-☑ | D07.39 | D27.-☑ | D39.1-☑ | D49.59 |
| oviduct | C57.0-☑ | C79.82 | D07.39 | D28.2 | D39.8 | D49.59 |
| palate | C05.9 | C79.89 | D00.00 | D10.39 | D37.09 | D49.0 |
| hard | C05.0 | C79.89 | D00.05 | D10.39 | D37.09 | D49.0 |
| junction of hard and | | | | | | |
| soft palate | C05.9 | C79.89 | D00.00 | D10.39 | D37.09 | D49.0 |
| overlapping | | | | | | |
| lesions | C05.8 | — | — | — | — | — |
| soft | C05.1 | C79.89 | D00.04 | D10.39 | D37.09 | D49.0 |
| nasopharyngeal | | | | | | |
| surface | C11.3 | C79.89 | D00.08 | D10.6 | D37.05 | D49.0 |
| posterior surface | C11.3 | C79.89 | D00.08 | D10.6 | D37.05 | D49.0 |
| superior surface | C11.3 | C79.89 | D00.08 | D10.6 | D37.05 | D49.0 |
| palatoglossal arch | C09.1 | C79.89 | D00.00 | D10.5 | D37.09 | D49.0 |
| palatopharyngeal | | | | | | |
| arch | C09.1 | C79.89 | D00.00 | D10.5 | D37.09 | D49.0 |
| pallium | C71.0 | C79.31 | — | D33.0 | D43.0 | D49.6 |
| palpebra | C44.10-☑ | C79.2 | D04.1-☑ | D23.1-☑ | D48.5 | D49.2 |
| basal cell | | | | | | |
| carcinoma | C44.11-☑ | — | — | — | — | — |
| specified type NEC | C44.19-☑ | — | — | — | — | — |
| squamous cell | | | | | | |
| carcinoma | C44.12-☑ | — | — | — | — | — |
| pancreas | C25.9 | C78.89 | D01.7 | D13.6 | D37.8 | D49.0 |
| body | C25.1 | C78.89 | D01.7 | D13.6 | D37.8 | D49.0 |
| duct (of Santorini) (of | | | | | | |
| Wirsung) | C25.3 | C78.89 | D01.7 | D13.6 | D37.8 | D49.0 |
| ectopic tissue | C25.7 | C78.89 | — | D13.6 | D37.8 | D49.0 |
| head | C25.0 | C78.89 | D01.7 | D13.6 | D37.8 | D49.0 |
| islet cells | C25.4 | C78.89 | D01.7 | D13.7 | D37.8 | D49.0 |
| neck | C25.7 | C78.89 | D01.7 | D13.6 | D37.8 | D49.0 |
| overlapping lesion | C25.8 | — | — | — | — | — |
| tail | C25.2 | C78.89 | D01.7 | D13.6 | D37.8 | D49.0 |
| para-aortic body | C75.5 | C79.89 | — | D35.6 | D44.7 | D49.7 |
| paraganglion NEC | C75.5 | C79.89 | — | D35.6 | D44.7 | D49.7 |
| parametrium | C57.3 | C79.82 | — | D28.2 | D39.8 | D49.59 |
| paranephric | C48.0 | C78.6 | — | D20.0 | D48.3 | D49.0 |
| pararectal | C76.3 | C79.89 | — | D36.7 | D48.7 | D49.89 |
| parasagittal (region) | C76.0 | C79.89 | D09.8 | D36.7 | D48.7 | D49.89 |
| parasellar | C72.9 | C79.49 | — | D33.9 | D43.8 | D49.7 |
| parathyroid (gland) | C75.0 | C79.89 | D09.3 | D35.1 | D44.2 | D49.7 |
| paraurethral | C76.3 | C79.89 | — | D36.7 | D48.7 | D49.89 |
| gland | C68.1 | C79.19 | D09.19 | D30.8 | D41.8 | D49.59 |
| paravaginal | C76.3 | C79.89 | — | D36.7 | D48.7 | D49.89 |
| parenchyma, kidney | C64.-☑ | C79.0-☑ | D09.19 | D30.0-☑ | D41.0-☑ | D49.51-☑ |
| parietal | | | | | | |
| bone | C41.0 | C79.51 | — | D16.4 | D48.0 | D49.2 |
| lobe, brain | C71.3 | C79.31 | — | D33.0 | D43.0 | D49.6 |
| paroophoron | C57.1-☑ | C79.82 | D07.39 | D28.2 | D39.8 | D49.59 |
| parotid (duct) | | | | | | |
| (gland) | C07 | C79.89 | D00.00 | D11.0 | D37.030 | D49.0 |
| parovarium | C57.1-☑ | C79.82 | D07.39 | D28.2 | D39.8 | D49.59 |
| patella | C40.20 | C79.51 | — | | | |
| peduncle, cerebral | C71.7 | C79.31 | — | D33.1 | D43.1 | D49.6 |
| pelvirectal junction | C19 | C78.5 | D01.1 | D12.7 | D37.5 | D49.0 |
| pelvis, pelvic | C76.3 | C79.89 | D09.8 | D36.7 | D48.7 | D49.89 |
| bone | C41.4 | C79.51 | — | D16.8 | D48.0 | D49.2 |
| floor | C76.3 | C79.89 | D09.8 | D36.7 | D48.7 | D49.89 |
| renal | C65.-☑ | C79.0-☑ | D09.19 | D30.1-☑ | D41.1-☑ | D49.51-☑ |
| viscera | C76.3 | C79.89 | D09.8 | D36.7 | D48.7 | D49.89 |
| wall | C76.3 | C79.89 | D09.8 | D36.7 | D48.7 | D49.89 |
| pelvo-abdominal | C76.8 | C79.89 | D09.8 | D36.7 | D48.7 | D49.89 |
| penis | C60.9 | C79.82 | D07.4 | D29.0 | D40.8 | D49.59 |

| Neoplasm, neoplastic — | Malignant Primary | Malignant Secondary | Ca in situ | Benign | Uncertain | Unspecified Behavior |
|---|---|---|---|---|---|---|
| continued | | | | | | |
| penis — continued | | | | | | |
| body | C60.2 | C79.82 | D07.4 | D29.0 | D40.8 | D49.59 |
| corpus | | | | | | |
| (cavernosum) | C60.2 | C79.82 | D07.4 | D29.0 | D40.8 | D49.59 |
| glans | C60.1 | C79.82 | D07.4 | D29.0 | D40.8 | D49.59 |
| overlapping sites | C60.8 | — | — | — | — | — |
| skin NEC | C60.9 | C79.82 | D07.4 | D29.0 | D40.8 | D49.59 |
| periadrenal (tissue) | C48.0 | C78.6 | — | D20.0 | D48.3 | D49.0 |
| perianal (skin) — see also | | | | | | |
| Neoplasm, anus, | | | | | | |
| skin | C44.500 | C79.2 | D04.5 | D23.5 | D48.5 | D49.2 |
| pericardium | C38.0 | C79.89 | — | D15.1 | D48.7 | D49.89 |
| perinephric | C48.0 | C78.6 | — | D20.0 | D48.3 | D49.0 |
| perineum | C76.3 | C79.89 | D09.8 | D36.7 | D48.7 | D49.89 |
| periodontal tissue | | | | | | |
| NEC | C03.9 | C79.89 | D00.03 | D10.39 | D37.09 | D49.0 |
| periosteum — see | | | | | | |
| Neoplasm, bone | | | | | | |
| peripancreatic | C48.0 | C78.6 | — | D20.0 | D48.3 | D49.0 |
| peripheral nerve | | | | | | |
| NEC | C47.9 | C79.89 | — | D36.10 | D48.2 | D49.2 |
| perirectal (tissue) | C76.3 | C79.89 | — | D36.7 | D48.7 | D49.89 |
| perirenal (tissue) | C48.0 | C78.6 | — | D20.0 | D48.3 | D49.0 |
| peritoneum, peritoneal | | | | | | |
| (cavity) | C48.2 | C78.6 | — | D20.1 | D48.4 | D49.0 |
| benign mesothelial | | | | | | |
| tissue — see | | | | | | |
| Mesothelioma, | | | | | | |
| benign | | | | | | |
| overlapping lesion | C48.8 | — | — | — | — | — |
| with digestive | | | | | | |
| organs | C26.9 | — | — | — | — | — |
| parietal | C48.1 | C78.6 | — | D20.1 | D48.4 | D49.0 |
| pelvic | C48.1 | C78.6 | — | D20.1 | D48.4 | D49.0 |
| specified part NEC | C48.1 | C78.6 | — | D20.1 | D48.4 | D49.0 |
| peritonsillar (tissue) | C76.0 | C79.89 | D09.8 | D36.7 | D48.7 | D49.89 |
| periurethral tissue | C76.3 | C79.89 | — | D36.7 | D48.7 | D49.89 |
| phalanges | | | | | | |
| foot | C40.3-☑ | C79.51 | — | D16.3-☑ | — | — |
| hand | C40.1-☑ | C79.51 | — | D16.1-☑ | — | — |
| pharynx, pharyngeal | C14.0 | C79.89 | D00.08 | D10.9 | D37.05 | D49.0 |
| bursa | C11.1 | C79.89 | D00.08 | D10.6 | D37.05 | D49.0 |
| fornix | C11.3 | C79.89 | D00.08 | D10.6 | D37.05 | D49.0 |
| recess | C11.2 | C79.89 | D00.08 | D10.6 | D37.05 | D49.0 |
| region | C14.0 | C79.89 | D00.08 | D10.9 | D37.05 | D49.0 |
| tonsil | C11.1 | C79.89 | D00.08 | D10.6 | D37.05 | D49.0 |
| wall (lateral) | | | | | | |
| (posterior) | C14.0 | C79.89 | D00.08 | D10.9 | D37.05 | D49.0 |
| pia mater | C70.9 | C79.40 | — | D32.9 | D42.9 | D49.7 |
| cerebral | C70.0 | C79.32 | — | D32.0 | D42.0 | D49.7 |
| cranial | C70.0 | C79.32 | — | D32.0 | D42.0 | D49.7 |
| spinal | C70.1 | C79.49 | — | D32.1 | D42.1 | D49.7 |
| pillars of fauces | C09.1 | C79.89 | D00.08 | D10.5 | D37.05 | D49.0 |
| pineal (body) | | | | | | |
| (gland) | C75.3 | C79.89 | D09.3 | D35.4 | D44.5 | D49.7 |
| pinna (ear) NEC — see | | | | | | |
| also Neoplasm, skin, | | | | | | |
| ear | C44.20-☑ | C79.2 | D04.2-☑ | D23.2-☑ | D48.5 | D49.2 |
| piriform fossa or | | | | | | |
| sinus | C12 | C79.89 | D00.08 | D10.7 | D37.05 | D49.0 |
| pituitary (body) (fossa) | | | | | | |
| (gland) (lobe) | C75.1 | C79.89 | D09.3 | D35.2 | D44.3 | D49.7 |
| placenta | C58 | C79.82 | D07.0 | D26.7 | D39.2 | D49.59 |
| pleura, pleural | | | | | | |
| (cavity) | C38.4 | C78.2 | — | D19.0 | D38.2 | D49.1 |
| overlapping lesion with | | | | | | |
| heart or | | | | | | |
| mediastinum | C38.8 | — | — | — | — | — |
| parietal | C38.4 | C78.2 | — | D19.0 | D38.2 | D49.1 |
| visceral | C38.4 | C78.2 | — | D19.0 | D38.2 | D49.1 |
| plexus | | | | | | |
| brachial | C47.1-☑ | C79.89 | — | D36.12 | D48.2 | D49.2 |
| cervical | C47.0 | C79.89 | — | D36.11 | D48.2 | D49.2 |
| choroid | C71.5 | C79.31 | — | D33.0 | D43.0 | D49.6 |
| lumbosacral | C47.5 | C79.89 | — | D36.16 | D48.2 | D49.2 |
| sacral | C47.5 | C79.89 | — | D36.16 | D48.2 | D49.2 |
| pluriendocrine | C75.8 | C79.89 | D09.3 | D35.7 | D44.9 | D49.7 |
| pole | | | | | | |
| frontal | C71.1 | C79.31 | — | D33.0 | D43.0 | D49.6 |
| occipital | C71.4 | C79.31 | — | D33.0 | D43.0 | D49.6 |
| pons (varolii) | C71.7 | C79.31 | — | D33.1 | D43.1 | D49.6 |

## Neoplasm, neoplastic — continued

| | Malignant Primary | Malignant Secondary | Ca in situ | Benign | Uncertain | Unspecified Behavior |
|---|---|---|---|---|---|---|
| popliteal fossa or space | C76.5-✓ | C79.89 | D04.7-✓ | D36.7 | D48.7 | D49.89 |
| postcricoid (region) | C13.0 | C79.89 | D00.08 | D10.7 | D37.05 | D49.0 |
| posterior fossa (cranial) | C71.9 | C79.31 | — | D33.2 | D43.2 | D49.6 |
| postnasal space | C11.9 | C79.89 | D00.08 | D10.6 | D37.05 | D49.0 |
| prepuce | C60.0 | C79.82 | D07.4 | D29.0 | D40.8 | D49.59 |
| prepylorus | C16.4 | C78.89 | D00.2 | D13.1 | D37.1 | D49.0 |
| presacral (region) | C76.3 | C79.89 | — | D36.7 | D48.7 | D49.89 |
| prostate (gland) | C61 | C79.82 | D07.5 | D29.1 | D40.0 | D49.59 |
|   utricle | C68.0 | C79.19 | D09.19 | D30.4 | D41.3 | D49.59 |
| pterygoid fossa | C49.0 | C79.89 | — | D21.0 | D48.1 | D49.2 |
| pubic bone | C41.4 | C79.51 | — | D16.8 | D48.0 | D49.2 |
| pudenda, pudendum (femaie) | C51.9 | C79.82 | D07.1 | D28.0 | D39.8 | D49.59 |
| pulmonary — see also Neoplasm, lung | C34.9-✓ | C78.0-✓ | D02.2-✓ | D14.3-✓ | D38.1 | D49.1 |
| putamen | C71.0 | C79.31 | — | D33.0 | D43.0 | D49.6 |
| pyloric | | | | | | |
|   antrum | C16.3 | C78.89 | D00.2 | D13.1 | D37.1 | D49.0 |
|   canal | C16.4 | C78.89 | D00.2 | D13.1 | D37.1 | D49.0 |
| pylorus | C16.4 | C78.89 | D00.2 | D13.1 | D37.1 | D49.0 |
| pyramid (brain) | C71.7 | C79.31 | — | D33.1 | D43.1 | D49.6 |
| pyriform fossa or sinus | C12 | C79.89 | D00.08 | D10.7 | D37.05 | D49.0 |
| radius (any part) | C40.0-✓ | C79.51 | — | D16.0-✓ | — | — |
| Rathke's pouch | C75.1 | C79.89 | D09.3 | D35.2 | D44.3 | D49.7 |
| rectosigmoid (junction) | C19 | C78.5 | D01.1 | D12.7 | D37.5 | D49.0 |
|   overlapping lesion with anus or rectum | C21.8 | — | — | — | — | — |
| rectouterine pouch | C48.1 | C78.6 | — | D20.1 | D48.4 | D49.0 |
| rectovaginal septum or wall | C76.3 | C79.89 | D09.8 | D36.7 | D48.7 | D49.89 |
| rectovesical septum | C76.3 | C79.89 | D09.8 | D36.7 | D48.7 | D49.89 |
| rectum (ampulla) | C20 | C78.5 | D01.2 | D12.8 | D37.5 | D49.0 |
|   and colon | C19 | C78.5 | D01.1 | D12.7 | D37.5 | D49.0 |
|   overlapping lesion with anus or rectosigmoid junction | C21.8 | — | — | — | — | — |
| renal | C64.-✓ | C79.0-✓ | D09.19 | D30.0-✓ | D41.0-✓ | D49.51-✓ |
|   calyx | C65.-✓ | C79.0-✓ | D09.19 | D30.1-✓ | D41.1-✓ | D49.51-✓ |
|   hilus | C65.-✓ | C79.0-✓ | D09.19 | D30.1-✓ | D41.1-✓ | D49.51-✓ |
|   parenchyma | C64.-✓ | C79.0-✓ | D09.19 | D30.0-✓ | D41.0-✓ | D49.51-✓ |
|   pelvis | C65.-✓ | C79.0-✓ | D09.19 | D30.1-✓ | D41.1-✓ | D49.51-✓ |
| respiratory | | | | | | |
|   organs or system NEC | C39.9 | C78.30 | D02.4 | D14.4 | D38.6 | D49.1 |
|   tract NEC | C39.9 | C78.30 | D02.4 | D14.4 | D38.5 | D49.1 |
|   upper | C39.0 | C78.30 | D02.4 | D14.4 | D38.5 | D49.1 |
| retina | C69.2-✓ | C79.49 | D09.2-✓ | D31.2-✓ | D48.7 | D49.81 |
| retrobulbar | C69.6-✓ | C79.49 | — | D31.6-✓ | D48.7 | D49.89 |
| retrocecal | C48.0 | C78.6 | — | D20.0 | D48.3 | D49.0 |
| retromolar (area) (triangle) (trigone) | C06.2 | C79.89 | D00.00 | D10.39 | D37.09 | D49.0 |
| retro-orbital | C76.0 | C79.89 | D09.8 | D36.7 | D48.7 | D49.89 |
| retroperitoneal (space) (tissue) | C48.0 | C78.6 | — | D20.0 | D48.3 | D49.0 |
| retroperitoneum | C48.0 | C78.6 | — | D20.0 | D48.3 | D49.0 |
| retropharyngeal | C14.0 | C79.89 | D00.08 | D10.9 | D37.05 | D49.0 |
| retrovesical (septum) | C76.3 | C79.89 | D09.8 | D36.7 | D48.7 | D49.89 |
| rhinencephalon | C71.0 | C79.31 | — | D33.0 | D43.0 | D49.6 |
| rib | C41.3 | C79.51 | — | D16.7 | D48.0 | D49.2 |
| Rosenmuller's fossa | C11.2 | C79.89 | D00.08 | D10.6 | D37.05 | D49.0 |
| round ligament | C57.2-✓ | C79.82 | — | D28.2 | D39.8 | D49.59 |
| sacrococcyx, sacrococcygeal | C41.4 | C79.51 | — | D16.8 | D48.0 | D49.2 |
| region | C76.3 | C79.89 | D09.8 | D36.7 | D48.7 | D49.89 |
| sacrouterine ligament | C57.3 | C79.82 | — | D28.2 | D39.8 | D49.59 |
| sacrum, sacral (vertebra) | C41.4 | C79.51 | — | D16.8 | D48.0 | D49.2 |
| salivary gland or duct (major) | C08.9 | C79.89 | D00.00 | D11.9 | D37.039 | D49.0 |
|   minor NEC | C06.9 | C79.89 | D00.00 | D10.39 | D37.04 | D49.0 |
|   overlapping lesion | C08.9 | — | — | — | — | — |
|   parotid | C07 | C79.89 | D00.00 | D11.0 | D37.030 | D49.0 |

## Neoplasm, neoplastic — continued

| | Malignant Primary | Malignant Secondary | Ca in situ | Benign | Uncertain | Unspecified Behavior |
|---|---|---|---|---|---|---|
| salivary gland or duct — continued | | | | | | |
|   pluriglandular | C08.9 | C79.89 | D00.00 | D11.9 | D37.039 | D49.0 |
|   sublingual | C08.1 | C79.89 | D00.00 | D11.7 | D37.031 | D49.0 |
|   submandibular | C08.0 | C79.89 | D00.00 | D11.7 | D37.032 | D49.0 |
|   submaxillary | C08.0 | C79.89 | D00.00 | D11.7 | D37.032 | D49.0 |
| salpinx (uterine) | C57.0-✓ | C79.82 | D07.39 | D28.2 | D39.8 | D49.59 |
| Santorini's duct | C25.3 | C78.89 | D01.7 | D13.6 | D37.8 | D49.0 |
| scalp | C44.40 | C79.2 | D04.4 | D23.4 | D48.5 | D49.2 |
|   basal cell carcinoma | C44.41 | — | — | — | — | — |
|   specified type NEC | C44.49 | — | — | — | — | — |
|   squamous cell carcinoma | C44.42 | — | — | — | — | — |
| scapula (any part) | C40.0-✓ | C79.51 | — | D16.0-✓ | — | — |
| scapular region | C76.1 | C79.89 | D09.8 | D36.7 | D48.7 | D49.89 |
| scar NEC — see also Neoplasm, skin, by site | C44.90 | C79.2 | D04.9 | D23.9 | D48.5 | D49.2 |
| sciatic nerve | C47.2-✓ | C79.89 | — | D36.13 | D48.2 | D49.2 |
| sclera | C69.4-✓ | C79.49 | D09.2-✓ | D31.4-✓ | D48.7 | D49.89 |
| scrotum (skin) | C63.2 | C79.82 | D07.61 | D29.4 | D40.8 | D49.59 |
| sebaceous gland — see Neoplasm, skin | | | | | | |
| sella turcica | C75.1 | C79.89 | D09.3 | D35.2 | D44.3 | D49.7 |
|   bone | C41.0 | C79.51 | — | D16.4 | D48.0 | D49.2 |
| semilunar cartilage (knee) | C40.2-✓ | C79.51 | — | D16.2-✓ | D48.0 | D49.2 |
| seminal vesicle | C63.7 | C79.82 | D07.69 | D29.8 | D40.8 | D49.59 |
| septum | | | | | | |
|   nasal | C30.0 | C78.39 | D02.3 | D14.0 | D38.5 | D49.1 |
|     posterior margin | C11.3 | C79.89 | D00.08 | D10.6 | D37.05 | D49.0 |
|   rectovaginal | C76.3 | C79.89 | D09.8 | D36.7 | D48.7 | D49.89 |
|   rectovesical | C76.3 | C79.89 | D09.8 | D36.7 | D48.7 | D49.89 |
|   urethrovaginal | C57.9 | C79.82 | D07.30 | D28.9 | D39.9 | D49.59 |
|   vesicovaginal | C57.9 | C79.82 | D07.30 | D28.9 | D39.9 | D49.59 |
| shoulder NEC | C76.4-✓ | C79.89 | D04.6-✓ | D36.7 | D48.7 | D49.89 |
| sigmoid flexure (lower) (upper) | C18.7 | C78.5 | D01.0 | D12.5 | D37.4 | D49.0 |
| sinus (accessory) | C31.9 | C78.39 | D02.3 | D14.0 | D38.5 | D49.1 |
|   bone (any) | C41.0 | C79.51 | — | D16.4 | D48.0 | D49.2 |
|   ethmoidal | C31.1 | C78.39 | D02.3 | D14.0 | D38.5 | D49.1 |
|   frontal | C31.2 | C78.39 | D02.3 | D14.0 | D38.5 | D49.1 |
|   maxillary | C31.0 | C78.39 | D02.3 | D14.0 | D38.5 | D49.1 |
|   nasal, paranasal NEC | C31.9 | C78.39 | D02.3 | D14.0 | D38.5 | D49.1 |
|   overlapping lesion | C31.8 | — | — | — | — | — |
|   pyriform | C12 | C79.89 | D00.08 | D10.7 | D37.05 | D49.0 |
|   sphenoid | C31.3 | C78.39 | D02.3 | D14.0 | D38.5 | D49.1 |
| skeleton, skeletal NEC | C41.9 | C79.51 | — | D16.9 | D48.0 | D49.2 |
| Skene's gland | C68.1 | C79.19 | D09.19 | D30.8 | D41.8 | D49.59 |
| skin NOS | C44.90 | C79.2 | D04.9 | D23.9 | D48.5 | D49.2 |
|   abdominal wall | C44.509 | C79.2 | D04.5 | D23.5 | D48.5 | D49.2 |
|     basal cell carcinoma | C44.519 | — | — | — | — | — |
|     specified type NEC | C44.599 | — | — | — | — | — |
|     squamous cell carcinoma | C44.529 | — | — | — | — | — |
|   ala nasi — see also Neoplasm, nose, skin | C44.301 | C79.2 | D04.39 | D23.39 | D48.5 | D49.2 |
|   ankle — see also Neoplasm, skin, limb, lower | C44.70-✓ | C79.2 | D04.7-✓ | D23.7-✓ | D48.5 | D49.2 |
|   antecubital space — see also Neoplasm, skin, limb, upper | C44.60-✓ | C79.2 | D04.6-✓ | D23.6-✓ | D48.5 | D49.2 |
|   anus | C44.500 | C79.2 | D04.5 | D23.5 | D48.5 | D49.2 |
|     basal cell carcinoma | C44.510 | — | — | — | — | — |
|     specified type NEC | C44.590 | — | — | — | — | — |
|     squamous cell carcinoma | C44.520 | — | — | — | — | — |
|   arm — see also Neoplasm, skin, limb, upper | C44.60-✓ | C79.2 | D04.6-✓ | D23.6-✓ | D48.5 | D49.2 |

**Neoplasm, neoplastic — continued**
**skin — continued**

| | Malignant Primary | Malignant Secondary | Ca in situ | Benign | Uncertain | Unspecified Behavior |
|---|---|---|---|---|---|---|
| auditory canal (external) — *see also* Neoplasm, skin, ear | C44.20-☑ | C79.2 | D04.2-☑ | D23.2-☑ | D48.5 | D49.2 |
| auricle (ear) — *see also* Neoplasm, skin, ear | C44.20-☑ | C79.2 | D04.2-☑ | D23.2-☑ | D48.5 | D49.2 |
| auricular canal (external) — *see also* Neoplasm, skin, ear | C44.20-☑ | C79.2 | D04.2-☑ | D23.2-☑ | D48.5 | D49.2 |
| axilla, axillary fold — *see also* Neoplasm, skin, trunk | C44.509 | C79.2 | D04.5 | D23.5 | D48.5 | D49.2 |
| back — *see also* Neoplasm, skin, trunk | C44.509 | C79.2 | D04.5 | D23.5 | D48.5 | D49.2 |
| basal cell carcinoma | C44.91 | — | — | — | — | — |
| breast | C44.501 | C79.2 | D04.5 | D23.5 | D48.5 | D49.2 |
| basal cell carcinoma | C44.511 | — | — | — | — | — |
| specified type NEC | C44.591 | — | — | — | — | — |
| squamous cell carcinoma | C44.521 | — | — | — | — | — |
| brow — *see also* Neoplasm, skin, face | C44.309 | C79.2 | D04.39 | D23.39 | D48.5 | D49.2 |
| buttock — *see also* Neoplasm, skin, trunk | C44.509 | C79.2 | D04.5 | D23.5 | D48.5 | D49.2 |
| calf — *see also* Neoplasm, skin, limb, lower | C44.70-☑ | C79.2 | D04.7-☑ | D23.7-☑ | D48.5 | D49.2 |
| canthus (eye) (inner) (outer) | C44.10-☑ | C79.2 | D04.1-☑ | D23.1-☑ | D48.5 | D49.2 |
| basal cell carcinoma | C44.11-☑ | — | — | — | — | — |
| specified type NEC | C44.19-☑ | — | — | — | — | — |
| squamous cell carcinoma | C44.12-☑ | — | — | — | — | — |
| cervical region — *see also* Neoplasm, skin, neck | C44.40 | C79.2 | D04.4 | D23.4 | D48.5 | D49.2 |
| cheek (external) — *see also* Neoplasm, skin, face | C44.309 | C79.2 | D04.39 | D23.39 | D48.5 | D49.2 |
| chest (wall) — *see also* Neoplasm, skin, trunk | C44.509 | C79.2 | D04.5 | D23.5 | D48.5 | D49.2 |
| chin — *see also* Neoplasm, skin, face | C44.309 | C79.2 | D04.39 | D23.39 | D48.5 | D49.2 |
| clavicular area — *see also* Neoplasm, skin, trunk | C44.509 | C79.2 | D04.5 | D23.5 | D48.5 | D49.2 |
| clitoris | C51.2 | C79.82 | D07.1 | D28.0 | D39.8 | D49.59 |
| columnella — *see also* Neoplasm, skin, face | C44.309 | C79.2 | D04.39 | D23.39 | D48.5 | D49.2 |
| concha — *see also* Neoplasm, skin, ear | C44.20-☑ | C79.2 | D04.2-☑ | D23.2-☑ | D48.5 | D49.2 |
| ear (external) | C44.20-☑ | C79.2 | D04.2-☑ | D23.2-☑ | D48.5 | D49.2 |
| basal cell carcinoma | C44.21-☑ | — | — | — | — | — |
| specified type NEC | C44.29-☑ | — | — | — | — | — |
| squamous cell carcinoma | C44.22-☑ | — | — | — | — | — |
| elbow — *see also* Neoplasm, skin, limb, upper | C44.60-☑ | C79.2 | D04.6-☑ | D23.6-☑ | D48.5 | D49.2 |
| eyebrow — *see also* Neoplasm, skin, face | C44.309 | C79.2 | D04.39 | D23.39 | D48.5 | D49.2 |
| eyelid | C44.10-☑ | C79.2 | D04.1-☑ | D23.1-☑ | D48.5 | D49.2 |

**Neoplasm, neoplastic — continued**
**skin — continued**
**eyelid — continued**

| | Malignant Primary | Malignant Secondary | Ca in situ | Benign | Uncertain | Unspecified Behavior |
|---|---|---|---|---|---|---|
| basal cell carcinoma | C44.11-☑ | — | — | — | — | — |
| specified type NEC | C44.19-☑ | — | — | — | — | — |
| squamous cell carcinoma | C44.12-☑ | — | — | — | — | — |
| face NOS | C44.300 | C79.2 | D04.30 | D23.30 | D48.5 | D49.2 |
| basal cell carcinoma | C44.310 | — | — | — | — | — |
| specified type NEC | C44.390 | — | — | — | — | — |
| squamous cell carcinoma | C44.320 | — | — | — | — | — |
| female genital organs (external) | C51.9 | C79.82 | D07.1 | D28.0 | D39.8 | D49.59 |
| clitoris | C51.2 | C79.82 | D07.1 | D28.0 | D39.8 | D49.59 |
| labium NEC | C51.9 | C79.82 | D07.1 | D28.0 | D39.8 | D49.59 |
| majus | C51.0 | C79.82 | D07.1 | D28.0 | D39.8 | D49.59 |
| minus | C51.1 | C79.82 | D07.1 | D28.0 | D39.8 | D49.59 |
| pudendum | C51.9 | C79.82 | D07.1 | D28.0 | D39.8 | D49.59 |
| vulva | C51.9 | C79.82 | D07.1 | D28.0 | D39.8 | D49.59 |
| finger — *see also* Neoplasm, skin, limb, upper | C44.60-☑ | C79.2 | D04.6-☑ | D23.6-☑ | D48.5 | D49.2 |
| flank — *see also* Neoplasm, skin, trunk | C44.509 | C79.2 | D04.5 | D23.5 | D48.5 | D49.2 |
| foot — *see also* Neoplasm, skin, limb, lower | C44.70-☑ | C79.2 | D04.7-☑ | D23.7-☑ | D48.5 | D49.2 |
| forearm — *see also* Neoplasm, skin, limb, upper | C44.60-☑ | C79.2 | D04.6-☑ | D23.6-☑ | D48.5 | D49.2 |
| forehead — *see also* Neoplasm, skin, face | C44.309 | C79.2 | D04.39 | D23.39 | D48.5 | D49.2 |
| glabella — *see also* Neoplasm, skin, face | C44.309 | C79.2 | D04.39 | D23.39 | D48.5 | D49.2 |
| gluteal region — *see also* Neoplasm, skin, trunk | C44.509 | C79.2 | D04.5 | D23.5 | D48.5 | D49.2 |
| groin — *see also* Neoplasm, skin, trunk | C44.509 | C79.2 | D04.5 | D23.5 | D48.5 | D49.2 |
| hand — *see also* Neoplasm, skin, limb, upper | C44.60-☑ | C79.2 | D04.6-☑ | D23.6-☑ | D48.5 | D49.2 |
| head NEC — *see also* Neoplasm, skin, scalp | C44.40 | C79.2 | D04.4 | D23.4 | D48.5 | D49.2 |
| heel — *see also* Neoplasm, skin, limb, lower | C44.70-☑ | C79.2 | D04.7-☑ | D23.7-☑ | D48.5 | D49.2 |
| helix — *see also* Neoplasm, skin, ear | C44.20-☑ | C79.2 | D04.2-☑ | D23.2-☑ | D48.5 | D49.2 |
| hip — *see also* Neoplasm, skin, limb, lower | C44.70-☑ | C79.2 | D04.7-☑ | D23.7-☑ | D48.5 | D49.2 |
| infraclavicular region — *see also* Neoplasm, skin, trunk | C44.509 | C79.2 | D04.5 | D23.5 | D48.5 | D49.2 |
| inguinal region — *see also* Neoplasm, skin, trunk | C44.509 | C79.2 | D04.5 | D23.5 | D48.5 | D49.2 |
| jaw — *see also* Neoplasm, skin, face | C44.309 | C79.2 | D04.39 | D23.39 | D48.5 | D49.2 |
| Kaposi's sarcoma — *see* Kaposi's, sarcoma, skin | | | | | | |
| knee — *see also* Neoplasm, skin, limb, lower | C44.70-☑ | C79.2 | D04.7-☑ | D23.7-☑ | D48.5 | D49.2 |
| labia | | | | | | |
| majora | C51.0 | C79.82 | D07.1 | D28.0 | D39.8 | D49.59 |
| minora | C51.1 | C79.82 | D07.1 | D28.0 | D39.8 | D49.59 |

☑ **Additional Character Required — Refer to the Tabular List for Character Selection**      🖝 Subterms under main terms may continue to next column or page

| Neoplasm, neoplastic — continued | Malignant Primary | Malignant Secondary | Ca in situ | Benign | Uncertain | Unspecified Behavior |
|---|---|---|---|---|---|---|
| skin — *continued* | | | | | | |
|   leg — *see also* Neoplasm, skin, limb, lower | C44.70-☑ | C79.2 | D04.7-☑ | D23.7-☑ | D48.5 | D49.2 |
|   lid (lower) (upper) | C44.10-☑ | C79.2 | D04.1-☑ | D23.1-☑ | D48.5 | D49.2 |
|     basal cell carcinoma | C44.11-☑ | — | — | — | — | — |
|     specified type NEC | C44.19-☑ | — | — | — | — | — |
|     squamous cell carcinoma | C44.12-☑ | — | — | — | — | — |
|   limb NEC | C44.90 | C79.2 | D04.9 | D23.9 | D48.5 | D49.2 |
|     basal cell carcinoma | C44.91 | — | — | — | — | — |
|     lower | C44.70-☑ | C79.2 | D04.7-☑ | D23.7-☑ | D48.5 | D49.2 |
|       basal cell carcinoma | C44.71-☑ | — | — | — | — | — |
|       specified type NEC | C44.79-☑ | — | — | — | — | — |
|       squamous cell carcinoma | C44.72-☑ | — | — | — | — | — |
|     upper | C44.60-☑ | C79.2 | D04.6-☑ | D23.6-☑ | D48.5 | D49.2 |
|       basal cell carcinoma | C44.61-☑ | — | — | — | — | — |
|       specified type NEC | C44.69-☑ | — | — | — | — | — |
|       squamous cell carcinoma | C44.62-☑ | — | — | — | — | — |
|   lip (lower) (upper) | C44.00 | C79.2 | D04.0 | D23.0 | D48.5 | D49.2 |
|     basal cell carcinoma | C44.01 | — | — | — | — | — |
|     specified type NEC | C44.09 | — | — | — | — | — |
|     squamous cell carcinoma | C44.02 | — | — | — | — | — |
|   male genital organs | C63.9 | C79.82 | D07.60 | D29.9 | D40.8 | D49.59 |
|     penis | C60.9 | C79.82 | D07.4 | D29.0 | D40.8 | D49.59 |
|     prepuce | C60.0 | C79.82 | D07.4 | D29.0 | D40.8 | D49.59 |
|     scrotum | C63.2 | C79.82 | D07.61 | D29.4 | D40.8 | D49.59 |
|   mastectomy site (skin) — *see also* Neoplasm, skin, breast | C44.501 | C79.2 | — | — | — | — |
|     specified as breast tissue | C50.8-☑ | C79.81 | — | — | — | — |
|   meatus, acoustic (external) — *see also* Neoplasm, skin, ear | C44.20-☑ | C79.2 | D04.2-☑ | D23.2-☑ | D48.5 | D49.2 |
|   melanotic — *see* Melanoma | | | | | | |
|   Merkel cell — *see* Carcinoma, Merkel cell | | | | | | |
|   nates — *see also* Neoplasm, skin, trunk | C44.509 | C79.2 | D04.5 | D23.5 | D48.5 | D49.2 |
|   neck | C44.40 | C79.2 | D04.4 | D23.4 | D48.5 | D49.2 |
|     basal cell carcinoma | C44.41 | — | — | — | — | — |
|     specified type NEC | C44.49 | — | — | — | — | — |
|     squamous cell carcinoma | C44.42 | — | — | — | — | — |
|   nevus — *see* Nevus, skin | | | | | | |
|   nose (external) — *see also* Neoplasm, nose, skin | C44.301 | C79.2 | D04.39 | D23.39 | D48.5 | D49.2 |
|   overlapping lesion | C44.80 | — | — | — | — | — |
|     basal cell carcinoma | C44.81 | — | — | — | — | — |
|     specified type NEC | C44.89 | — | — | — | — | — |
|     squamous cell carcinoma | C44.82 | — | — | — | — | — |
|   palm — *see also* Neoplasm, skin, limb, upper | C44.60-☑ | C79.2 | D04.6-☑ | D23.6-☑ | D48.5 | D49.2 |
|   palpebra | C44.10-☑ | C79.2 | D04.1-☑ | D23.1-☑ | D48.5 | D49.2 |
|   palpebra — *continued* | | | | | | |
|     basal cell carcinoma | C44.11-☑ | — | — | — | — | — |
|     specified type NEC | C44.19-☑ | — | — | — | — | — |
|     squamous cell carcinoma | C44.12-☑ | — | — | — | — | — |
|   penis NEC | C60.9 | C79.82 | D07.4 | D29.0 | D40.8 | D49.59 |
|   perianal — *see also* Neoplasm, skin, anus | C44.500 | C79.2 | D04.5 | D23.5 | D48.5 | D49.2 |
|   perineum — *see also* Neoplasm, skin, anus | C44.500 | C79.2 | D04.5 | D23.5 | D48.5 | D49.2 |
|   pinna — *see also* Neoplasm, skin, ear | C44.20-☑ | C79.2 | D04.2-☑ | D23.2-☑ | D48.5 | D49.2 |
|   plantar — *see also* Neoplasm, skin, limb, lower | C44.70-☑ | C79.2 | D04.7-☑ | D23.7-☑ | D48.5 | D49.2 |
|   popliteal fossa or space — *see also* Neoplasm, skin, limb, lower | C44.70-☑ | C79.2 | D04.7-☑ | D23.7-☑ | D48.5 | D49.2 |
|   prepuce | C60.0 | C79.82 | D07.4 | D29.0 | D40.8 | D49.59 |
|   pubes — *see also* Neoplasm, skin, trunk | C44.509 | C79.2 | D04.5 | D23.5 | D48.5 | D49.2 |
|   sacrococcygeal region — *see also* Neoplasm, skin, trunk | C44.509 | C79.2 | D04.5 | D23.5 | D48.5 | D49.2 |
|   scalp | C44.40 | C79.2 | D04.4 | D23.4 | D48.5 | D49.2 |
|     basal cell carcinoma | C44.41 | — | — | — | — | — |
|     specified type NEC | C44.49 | — | — | — | — | — |
|     squamous cell carcinoma | C44.42 | — | — | — | — | — |
|   scapular region — *see also* Neoplasm, skin, trunk | C44.509 | C79.2 | D04.5 | D23.5 | D48.5 | D49.2 |
|   scrotum | C63.2 | C79.82 | D07.61 | D29.4 | D40.8 | D49.59 |
|   shoulder — *see also* Neoplasm, skin, limb, upper | C44.60-☑ | C79.2 | D04.6-☑ | D23.6-☑ | D48.5 | D49.2 |
|   sole (foot) — *see also* Neoplasm, skin, limb, lower | C44.70-☑ | C79.2 | D04.7-☑ | D23.7-☑ | D48.5 | D49.2 |
|   specified sites NEC | C44.80 | C79.2 | D04.8 | D23.9 | D48.5 | D49.2 |
|     basal cell carcinoma | C44.81 | — | — | — | — | — |
|     specified type NEC | C44.89 | — | — | — | — | — |
|     squamous cell carcinoma | C44.82 | — | — | — | — | — |
|   specified type NEC | C44.99 | — | — | — | — | — |
|     squamous cell carcinoma | C44.92 | — | — | — | — | — |
|   submammary fold — *see also* Neoplasm, skin, trunk | C44.509 | C79.2 | D04.5 | D23.5 | D48.5 | D49.2 |
|   supraclavicular region — *see also* Neoplasm, skin, neck | C44.40 | C79.2 | D04.4 | D23.4 | D48.5 | D49.2 |
|   temple — *see also* Neoplasm, skin, face | C44.309 | C79.2 | D04.39 | D23.39 | D48.5 | D49.2 |
|   thigh — *see also* Neoplasm, skin, limb, lower | C44.70-☑ | C79.2 | D04.7-☑ | D23.7-☑ | D48.5 | D49.2 |
|   thoracic wall — *see also* Neoplasm, skin, trunk | C44.509 | C79.2 | D04.5 | D23.5 | D48.5 | D49.2 |
|   thumb — *see also* Neoplasm, skin, limb, upper | C44.60-☑ | C79.2 | D04.6-☑ | D23.6-☑ | D48.5 | D49.2 |
|   toe — *see also* Neoplasm, skin, limb, lower | C44.70-☑ | C79.2 | D04.7-☑ | D23.7-☑ | D48.5 | D49.2 |

| Neoplasm, neoplastic — continued | Malignant Primary | Malignant Secondary | Ca in situ | Benign | Uncertain | Unspecified Behavior |
|---|---|---|---|---|---|---|
| skin — continued | | | | | | |
| tragus — see also Neoplasm, skin, ear | C44.20-☑ | C79.2 | D04.2-☑ | D23.2-☑ | D48.5 | D49.2 |
| trunk | C44.509 | C79.2 | D04.5 | D23.5 | D48.5 | D49.2 |
| basal cell carcinoma | C44.519 | — | — | — | — | — |
| specified type NEC | C44.599 | | | | | |
| squamous cell carcinoma | C44.529 | — | — | — | — | — |
| umbilicus — see also Neoplasm, skin, trunk | C44.509 | C79.2 | D04.5 | D23.5 | D48.5 | D49.2 |
| vulva | C51.9 | C79.82 | D07.1 | D28.0 | D39.8 | D49.59 |
| overlapping lesion | C51.8 | | | | | |
| wrist — see also Neoplasm, skin, limb, upper | C44.60-☑ | C79.2 | D04.6-☑ | D23.6-☑ | D48.5 | D49.2 |
| skull | C41.0 | C79.51 | | D16.4 | D48.0 | D49.2 |
| soft parts or tissues — see Neoplasm, connective tissue | | | | | | |
| specified site NEC | C76.8 | C79.89 | D09.8 | D36.7 | D48.7 | D49.89 |
| spermatic cord | C63.1-☑ | C79.82 | D07.69 | D29.8 | D40.8 | D49.59 |
| sphenoid | C31.3 | C78.39 | D02.3 | D14.0 | D38.5 | D49.1 |
| bone | C41.0 | C79.51 | — | D16.4 | D48.0 | D49.2 |
| sinus | C31.3 | C78.39 | D02.3 | D14.0 | D38.5 | D49.1 |
| sphincter | | | | | | |
| anal | C21.1 | C78.5 | D01.3 | D12.9 | D37.8 | D49.0 |
| of Oddi | C24.0 | C78.89 | D01.5 | D13.5 | D37.6 | D49.0 |
| spine, spinal (column) | C41.2 | C79.51 | — | D16.6 | D48.0 | D49.2 |
| bulb | C71.7 | C79.31 | — | D33.1 | D43.1 | D49.6 |
| coccyx | C41.4 | C79.51 | — | D16.8 | D48.0 | D49.2 |
| cord (cervical) (lumbar) (sacral) | | | | | | |
| (thoracic) | C72.0 | C79.49 | — | D33.4 | D43.4 | D49.7 |
| dura mater | C70.1 | C79.49 | — | D32.1 | D42.1 | D49.7 |
| lumbosacral | C41.2 | C79.51 | — | D16.6 | D48.0 | D49.2 |
| marrow NEC | C96.9 | C79.52 | — | — | D47.9 | D49.89 |
| membrane | C70.1 | C79.49 | — | D32.1 | D42.1 | D49.7 |
| meninges | C70.1 | C79.49 | — | D32.1 | D42.1 | D49.7 |
| nerve (root) | C47.9 | C79.89 | — | D36.10 | D48.2 | D49.2 |
| pia mater | C70.1 | C79.49 | — | D32.1 | D42.1 | D49.7 |
| root | C47.9 | C79.89 | — | D36.10 | D48.2 | D49.2 |
| sacrum | C41.4 | C79.51 | — | D16.8 | D48.0 | D49.2 |
| spleen, splenic NEC | C26.1 | C78.89 | D01.7 | D13.9 | D37.8 | D49.0 |
| flexure (colon) | C18.5 | C78.5 | D01.0 | D12.3 | D37.4 | D49.0 |
| stem, brain | C71.7 | C79.31 | — | D33.1 | D43.1 | D49.6 |
| Stensen's duct | C07 | C79.89 | D00.00 | D11.0 | D37.030 | D49.0 |
| sternum | C41.3 | C79.51 | — | D16.7 | D48.0 | D49.2 |
| stomach | C16.9 | C78.89 | D00.2 | D13.1 | D37.1 | D49.0 |
| antrum (pyloric) | C16.3 | C78.89 | D00.2 | D13.1 | D37.1 | D49.0 |
| body | C16.2 | C78.89 | D00.2 | D13.1 | D37.1 | D49.0 |
| cardia | C16.0 | C78.89 | D00.2 | D13.1 | D37.1 | D49.0 |
| cardiac orifice | C16.0 | C78.89 | D00.2 | D13.1 | D37.1 | D49.0 |
| corpus | C16.2 | C78.89 | D00.2 | D13.1 | D37.1 | D49.0 |
| fundus | C16.1 | C78.89 | D00.2 | D13.1 | D37.1 | D49.0 |
| greater curvature NEC | C16.6 | C78.89 | D00.2 | D13.1 | D37.1 | D49.0 |
| lesser curvature NEC | C16.5 | C78.89 | D00.2 | D13.1 | D37.1 | D49.0 |
| overlapping lesion | C16.8 | — | — | — | — | — |
| prepylorus | C16.4 | C78.89 | D00.2 | D13.1 | D37.1 | D49.0 |
| pylorus | C16.4 | C78.89 | D00.2 | D13.1 | D37.1 | D49.0 |
| wall NEC | C16.9 | C78.89 | D00.2 | D13.1 | D37.1 | D49.0 |
| anterior NEC | C16.8 | C78.89 | D00.2 | D13.1 | D37.1 | D49.0 |
| posterior NEC | C16.8 | C78.89 | D00.2 | D13.1 | D37.1 | D49.0 |
| stroma, endometrial | C54.1 | C79.82 | D07.0 | D26.1 | D39.0 | D49.59 |
| stump, cervical | C53.8 | C79.82 | D06.7 | D26.0 | D39.0 | D49.59 |
| subcutaneous (nodule) (tissue) NEC — see Neoplasm, connective tissue | | | | | | |
| subdural | C70.9 | C79.32 | — | D32.9 | D42.9 | D49.7 |
| subglottis, subglottic | C32.2 | C78.39 | D02.0 | D14.1 | D38.0 | D49.1 |
| sublingual | C04.9 | C79.89 | D00.06 | D10.2 | D37.09 | D49.0 |
| gland or duct | C08.1 | C79.89 | D00.00 | D11.7 | D37.031 | D49.0 |

| Neoplasm, neoplastic — continued | Malignant Primary | Malignant Secondary | Ca in situ | Benign | Uncertain | Unspecified Behavior |
|---|---|---|---|---|---|---|
| submandibular gland | C08.0 | C79.89 | D00.00 | D11.7 | D37.032 | D49.0 |
| submaxillary gland or duct | C08.0 | C79.89 | D00.00 | D11.7 | D37.032 | D49.0 |
| submental | C76.0 | C79.89 | D09.8 | D36.7 | D48.7 | D49.89 |
| subpleural | C34.9-☑ | C78.0-☑ | D02.2-☑ | D14.3-☑ | D38.1 | D49.1 |
| substernal | C38.1 | C78.1 | | D15.2 | D38.3 | D49.89 |
| sudoriferous, sudoriparous gland, site unspecified | C44.90 | C79.2 | D04.9 | D23.9 | D48.5 | D49.2 |
| specified site — see Neoplasm, skin | | | | | | |
| supraclavicular region | C76.0 | C79.89 | D09.8 | D36.7 | D48.7 | D49.89 |
| supraglottis | C32.1 | C78.39 | D02.0 | D14.1 | D38.0 | D49.1 |
| suprarenal | C74.9-☑ | C79.7-☑ | D09.3 | D35.0-☑ | D44.1-☑ | D49.7 |
| capsule | C74.9-☑ | C79.7-☑ | D09.3 | D35.0-☑ | D44.1-☑ | D49.7 |
| cortex | C74.0-☑ | C79.7-☑ | D09.3 | D35.0-☑ | D44.1-☑ | D49.7 |
| gland | C74.9-☑ | C79.7-☑ | D09.3 | D35.0-☑ | D44.1-☑ | D49.7 |
| medulla | C74.1-☑ | C79.7-☑ | D09.3 | D35.0-☑ | D44.1-☑ | D49.7 |
| suprasellar (region) | C71.9 | C79.31 | — | D33.2 | D43.2 | D49.6 |
| supratentorial (brain) NEC | C71.0 | C79.31 | — | D33.0 | D43.0 | D49.6 |
| sweat gland (apocrine) (eccrine), site unspecified | C44.90 | C79.2 | D04.9 | D23.9 | D48.5 | D49.2 |
| specified site — see Neoplasm, skin | | | | | | |
| sympathetic nerve or nervous system NEC | C47.9 | C79.89 | — | D36.10 | D48.2 | D49.2 |
| symphysis pubis | C41.4 | C79.51 | — | D16.8 | D48.0 | D49.2 |
| synovial membrane — see Neoplasm, connective tissue | | | | | | |
| tapetum, brain | C71.8 | C79.31 | — | D33.2 | D43.2 | D49.6 |
| tarsus (any bone) | C40.3-☑ | C79.51 | | D16.3-☑ | — | — |
| temple (skin) — see also Neoplasm, skin, face | C44.309 | C79.2 | D04.39 | D23.39 | D48.5 | D49.2 |
| temporal | | | | | | |
| bone | C41.0 | C79.51 | | D16.4 | D48.0 | D49.2 |
| lobe or pole | C71.2 | C79.31 | — | D33.0 | D43.0 | D49.6 |
| region | C76.0 | C79.89 | D09.8 | D36.7 | D48.7 | D49.89 |
| skin — see also Neoplasm, skin, face | C44.309 | C79.2 | D04.39 | D23.39 | D48.5 | D49.2 |
| tendon (sheath) — see Neoplasm, connective tissue | | | | | | |
| tentorium (cerebelli) | C70.0 | C79.32 | — | D32.0 | D42.0 | D49.7 |
| testis, testes | C62.9-☑ | C79.82 | D07.69 | D29.2-☑ | D40.1-☑ | D49.59 |
| descended | C62.1-☑ | C79.82 | D07.69 | D29.2-☑ | D40.1-☑ | D49.59 |
| ectopic | C62.0-☑ | C79.82 | D07.69 | D29.2-☑ | D40.1-☑ | D49.59 |
| retained | C62.0-☑ | C79.82 | D07.69 | D29.2-☑ | D40.1-☑ | D49.59 |
| scrotal | C62.1-☑ | C79.82 | D07.69 | D29.2-☑ | D40.1-☑ | D49.59 |
| undescended | C62.0-☑ | C79.82 | D07.69 | D29.2-☑ | D40.1-☑ | D49.59 |
| unspecified whether descended or undescended | C62.9-☑ | C79.82 | D07.69 | D29.2-☑ | D40.1-☑ | D49.59 |
| thalamus | C71.0 | C79.31 | — | D33.0 | D43.0 | D49.6 |
| thigh NEC | C76.5-☑ | C79.89 | D04.7-☑ | D36.7 | D48.7 | D49.89 |
| thorax, thoracic (cavity) (organs NEC) | C76.1 | C79.89 | D09.8 | D36.7 | D48.7 | D49.89 |
| duct | C49.3 | C79.89 | — | D21.3 | D48.1 | D49.2 |
| wall NEC | C76.1 | C79.89 | D09.8 | D36.7 | D48.7 | D49.89 |
| throat | C14.0 | C79.89 | D00.08 | D10.9 | D37.05 | D49.0 |
| thumb NEC | C76.4-☑ | C79.89 | D04.6-☑ | D36.7 | D48.7 | D49.89 |
| thymus (gland) | C37 | C79.89 | D09.3 | D15.0 | D38.4 | D49.89 |
| thyroglossal duct | C73 | C79.89 | D09.3 | D34 | D44.0 | D49.7 |
| thyroid (gland) | C73 | C79.89 | D09.3 | D34 | D44.0 | D49.7 |
| cartilage | C32.3 | C78.39 | D02.0 | D14.1 | D38.0 | D49.1 |
| tibia (any part) | C40.2-☑ | C79.51 | — | D16.2-☑ | — | — |
| toe NEC | C76.5-☑ | C79.89 | D04.7-☑ | D36.7 | D48.7 | D49.89 |
| tongue | C02.9 | C79.89 | D00.07 | D10.1 | D37.02 | D49.0 |
| anterior (two-thirds) NEC | C02.3 | C79.89 | D00.07 | D10.1 | D37.02 | D49.0 |
| dorsal surface | C02.0 | C79.89 | D00.07 | D10.1 | D37.02 | D49.0 |
| ventral surface | C02.2 | C79.89 | D00.07 | D10.1 | D37.02 | D49.0 |

☑ Additional Character Required — Refer to the Tabular List for Character Selection ▽ Subterms under main terms may continue to next column or page

| Neoplasm, neoplastic — | Malignant Primary | Malignant Secondary | Ca in situ | Benign | Uncertain | Unspecified Behavior |
|---|---|---|---|---|---|---|
| *continued* | | | | | | |
| tongue — *continued* | | | | | | |
| base (dorsal surface) | C01 | C79.89 | D00.07 | D10.1 | D37.02 | D49.0 |
| border (lateral) | C02.1 | C79.89 | D00.07 | D10.1 | D37.02 | D49.0 |
| dorsal surface NEC | C02.0 | C79.89 | D00.07 | D10.1 | D37.02 | D49.0 |
| fixed part NEC | C01 | C79.89 | D00.07 | D10.1 | D37.02 | D49.0 |
| foreamen cecum | C02.0 | C79.89 | D00.07 | D10.1 | D37.02 | D49.0 |
| frenulum linguae | C02.2 | C79.89 | D00.07 | D10.1 | D37.02 | D49.0 |
| junctional zone | C02.8 | C79.89 | D00.07 | D10.1 | D37.02 | D49.0 |
| margin (lateral) | C02.1 | C79.89 | D00.07 | D10.1 | D37.02 | D49.0 |
| midline NEC | C02.0 | C79.89 | D00.07 | D10.1 | D37.02 | D49.0 |
| mobile part NEC | C02.3 | C79.89 | D00.07 | D10.1 | D37.02 | D49.0 |
| overlapping lesion | C02.8 | — | — | — | — | — |
| posterior (third) | C01 | C79.89 | D00.07 | D10.1 | D37.02 | D49.0 |
| root | C01 | C79.89 | D00.07 | D10.1 | D37.02 | D49.0 |
| surface (dorsal) | C02.0 | C79.89 | D00.07 | D10.1 | D37.02 | D49.0 |
| base | C01 | C79.89 | D00.07 | D10.1 | D37.02 | D49.0 |
| ventral | C02.2 | C79.89 | D00.07 | D10.1 | D37.02 | D49.0 |
| tip | C02.1 | C79.89 | D00.07 | D10.1 | D37.02 | D49.0 |
| tonsil | C02.4 | C79.89 | D00.07 | D10.1 | D37.02 | D49.0 |
| tonsil | C09.9 | C79.89 | D00.08 | D10.4 | D37.05 | D49.0 |
| fauces, faucial | C09.9 | C79.89 | D00.08 | D10.4 | D37.05 | D49.0 |
| lingual | C02.4 | C79.89 | D00.07 | D10.1 | D37.02 | D49.0 |
| overlapping sites | C09.8 | — | — | — | — | — |
| palatine | C09.9 | C79.89 | D00.08 | D10.4 | D37.05 | D49.0 |
| pharyngeal | C11.1 | C79.89 | D00.08 | D10.6 | D37.05 | D49.0 |
| pillar (anterior) (posterior) | C09.1 | C79.89 | D00.08 | D10.5 | D37.05 | D49.0 |
| tonsillar fossa | C09.0 | C79.89 | D00.08 | D10.5 | D37.05 | D49.0 |
| tooth socket NEC | C03.9 | C79.89 | D00.03 | D10.39 | D37.09 | D49.0 |
| trachea (cartilage) (mucosa) | C33 | C78.39 | D02.1 | D14.2 | D38.1 | D49.1 |
| overlapping lesion with bronchus or lung | C34.8-☑ | — | | — | | — |
| tracheobronchial | C34.8-☑ | C78.39 | D02.1 | D14.2 | D38.1 | D49.1 |
| overlapping lesion with lung | C34.8-☑ | — | | — | | — |
| tragus — *see also* Neoplasm, skin, | | | | | | |
| ear | C44.20-☑ | C79.2 | D04.2-☑ | D23.2-☑ | D48.5 | D49.2 |
| trunk NEC | C76.8 | C79.89 | D04.5 | D36.7 | D48.7 | D49.89 |
| tubo-ovarian | C57.8 | C79.82 | D07.39 | D28.7 | D39.8 | D49.59 |
| tunica vaginalis | C63.7 | C79.82 | D07.69 | D29.8 | D40.8 | D49.59 |
| turbinate (bone) | C41.0 | C79.51 | — | D16.4 | D48.0 | D49.2 |
| nasal | C30.0 | C78.39 | D02.3 | D14.0 | D38.5 | D49.1 |
| tympanic cavity | C30.1 | C78.39 | D02.3 | D14.0 | D38.5 | D49.1 |
| ulna (any part) | C40.0-☑ | C79.51 | | D16.0-☑ | | |
| umbilicus, umbilical — *see also* Neoplasm, skin, trunk | C44.509 | C79.2 | D04.5 | D23.5 | D48.5 | D49.2 |
| uncus, brain | C71.2 | C79.31 | — | D33.0 | D43.0 | D49.6 |
| unknown site or unspecified | C80.1 | C79.9 | D09.9 | D36.9 | D48.9 | D49.9 |
| urachus | C67.7 | C79.11 | D09.0 | D30.3 | D41.4 | D49.4 |
| ureter-bladder (junction) | C67.6 | C79.11 | D09.0 | D30.3 | D41.4 | D49.4 |
| ureter, ureteral | C66.-☑ | C79.19 | D09.19 | D30.2-☑ | D41.2-☑ | D49.59 |
| orifice (bladder) | C67.6 | C79.11 | D09.0 | D30.3 | D41.4 | D49.4 |
| urethra, urethral (gland) | C68.0 | C79.19 | D09.19 | D30.4 | D41.3 | D49.59 |
| orifice, internal | C67.5 | C79.11 | D09.0 | D30.3 | D41.4 | D49.4 |
| urethrovaginal (septum) | C57.9 | C79.82 | D07.30 | D28.9 | D39.8 | D49.59 |
| urinary organ or system | C68.9 | C79.10 | D09.10 | D30.9 | D41.9 | D49.59 |
| bladder — *see* Neoplasm, bladder | | | | | | |
| overlapping lesion | C68.8 | — | — | — | — | — |
| specified sites NEC | C68.8 | C79.19 | D09.19 | D30.8 | D41.8 | D49.59 |
| utero-ovarian | C57.8 | C79.82 | D07.39 | D28.7 | D39.8 | D49.59 |
| ligament | C57.1-☑ | C79.82 | D07.39 | D28.2 | D39.8 | D49.59 |
| uterosacral ligament | C57.3 | C79.82 | — | D28.2 | D39.8 | D49.59 |
| uterus, uteri, uterine | C55 | C79.82 | D07.0 | D26.9 | D39.0 | D49.59 |
| adnexa NEC | C57.4 | C79.82 | D07.39 | D28.7 | D39.8 | D49.59 |
| body | C54.9 | C79.82 | D07.0 | D26.1 | D39.0 | D49.59 |
| cervix | C53.9 | C79.82 | D06.9 | D26.0 | D39.0 | D49.59 |
| cornu | C54.9 | C79.82 | D07.0 | D26.1 | D39.0 | D49.59 |
| corpus | C54.9 | C79.82 | D07.0 | D26.1 | D39.0 | D49.59 |
| endocervix (canal) (gland) | C53.0 | C79.82 | D06.0 | D26.0 | D39.0 | D49.59 |

| Neoplasm, neoplastic — | Malignant Primary | Malignant Secondary | Ca in situ | Benign | Uncertain | Unspecified Behavior |
|---|---|---|---|---|---|---|
| *continued* | | | | | | |
| uterus, uteri, uterine — *continued* | | | | | | |
| endometrium | C54.1 | C79.82 | D07.0 | D26.1 | D39.0 | D49.59 |
| exocervix | C53.1 | C79.82 | D06.1 | D26.0 | D39.0 | D49.59 |
| external os | C53.1 | C79.82 | D06.1 | D26.0 | D39.0 | D49.59 |
| fundus | C54.3 | C79.82 | D07.0 | D26.1 | D39.0 | D49.59 |
| internal os | C53.0 | C79.82 | D06.0 | D26.0 | D39.0 | D49.59 |
| isthmus | C54.3 | C79.82 | D07.0 | D26.1 | D39.0 | D49.59 |
| ligament | C57.3 | C79.82 | — | D28.2 | D39.8 | D49.59 |
| broad | C57.1-☑ | C79.82 | D07.39 | D28.2 | D39.8 | D49.59 |
| round | C57.2-☑ | C79.82 | — | D28.2 | D39.8 | D49.59 |
| lower segment | C54.0 | C79.82 | D07.0 | D26.1 | D39.0 | D49.59 |
| myometrium | C54.2 | C79.82 | D07.0 | D26.1 | D39.0 | D49.59 |
| overlapping sites | C54.8 | — | — | — | — | — |
| squamocolumnar junction | C53.8 | C79.82 | D06.7 | D26.0 | D39.0 | D49.59 |
| tube | C57.0-☑ | C79.82 | D07.39 | D28.2 | D39.8 | D49.59 |
| utricle, prostatic | C68.0 | C79.19 | D09.19 | D30.4 | D41.3 | D49.59 |
| uveal tract | C69.4-☑ | C79.49 | D09.2-☑ | D31.4-☑ | D48.7 | D49.89 |
| uvula | C05.2 | C79.89 | D00.04 | D10.39 | D37.09 | D49.0 |
| vagina, vaginal (fornix) (vault) (wall) | C52 | C79.82 | D07.2 | D28.1 | D39.8 | D49.59 |
| vaginovesical | C57.9 | C79.82 | D07.30 | D28.9 | D39.9 | D49.59 |
| septum | C57.9 | C79.82 | D07.30 | D28.9 | D39.9 | D49.59 |
| vallecula (epigiottis) | C10.0 | C79.89 | D00.08 | D10.5 | D37.05 | D49.0 |
| vascular — *see* Neoplasm, connective tissue | | | | | | |
| vas deferens | C63.1-☑ | C79.82 | D07.69 | D29.8 | D40.8 | D49.59 |
| Vater's ampulla | C24.1 | C78.89 | D01.5 | D13.5 | D37.6 | D49.0 |
| vein, venous — *see* Neoplasm, connective tissue | | | | | | |
| vena cava (abdominal) (inferior) | C49.4 | C79.89 | — | D21.4 | D48.1 | D49.2 |
| superior | C49.3 | C79.89 | — | D21.3 | D48.1 | D49.2 |
| ventricle (cerebral) (floor) (lateral) (third) | C71.5 | C79.31 | — | D33.0 | D43.0 | D49.6 |
| cardiac (left) (right) | C38.0 | C79.89 | — | D15.1 | D48.7 | D49.89 |
| fourth | C71.7 | C79.31 | — | D33.1 | D43.1 | D49.6 |
| ventricular band of larynx | C32.1 | C78.39 | D02.0 | D14.1 | D38.0 | D49.1 |
| ventriculus — *see* Neoplasm, stomach | | | | | | |
| vermillion border — *see* Neoplasm, lip | | | | | | |
| vermis, cerebellum | C71.6 | C79.31 | — | D33.1 | D43.1 | D49.6 |
| vertebra (column) | C41.2 | C79.51 | — | D16.6 | D48.0 | D49.2 |
| coccyx | C41.4 | C79.51 | — | D16.8 | D48.0 | D49.2 |
| marrow NEC | C96.9 | C79.52 | — | — | D47.9 | D49.89 |
| sacrum | C41.4 | C79.51 | — | D16.8 | D48.0 | D49.2 |
| vesical — *see* Neoplasm, bladder | | | | | | |
| vesicle, seminal | C63.7 | C79.82 | D07.69 | D29.8 | D40.8 | D49.59 |
| vesicocervical tissue | C57.9 | C79.82 | D07.30 | D28.9 | D39.9 | D49.59 |
| vesicorectal | C76.3 | C79.82 | D09.8 | D36.7 | D48.7 | D49.89 |
| vesicovaginal | C57.9 | C79.82 | D07.30 | D28.9 | D39.9 | D49.59 |
| septum | C57.9 | C79.82 | D07.30 | D28.9 | D39.8 | D49.59 |
| vessel (blood) — *see* Neoplasm, connective tissue | | | | | | |
| vestibular gland, greater | C51.0 | C79.82 | D07.1 | D28.0 | D39.8 | D49.59 |
| vestibule | | | | | | |
| mouth | C06.1 | C79.89 | D00.00 | D10.39 | D37.09 | D49.0 |
| nose | C30.0 | C78.39 | D02.3 | D14.0 | D38.5 | D49.1 |
| Virchow's gland | C77.0 | C77.0 | — | D36.0 | D48.7 | D49.89 |
| viscera NEC | C76.8 | C79.89 | D09.8 | D36.7 | D48.7 | D49.89 |
| vocal cords (true) | C32.0 | C78.39 | D02.0 | D14.1 | D38.0 | D49.1 |
| false | C32.1 | C78.39 | D02.0 | D14.1 | D38.0 | D49.1 |
| vomer | C41.0 | C79.51 | — | D16.4 | D48.0 | D49.2 |
| vulva | C51.9 | C79.82 | D07.1 | D28.0 | D39.8 | D49.59 |
| vulvovaginal gland | C51.0 | C79.82 | D07.1 | D28.0 | D39.8 | D49.59 |
| Waldeyer's ring | C14.2 | C79.89 | D00.08 | D10.9 | D37.05 | D49.0 |
| Wharton's duct | C08.0 | C79.89 | D00.00 | D11.7 | D37.032 | D49.0 |
| white matter (central) (cerebral) | C71.0 | C79.31 | — | D33.0 | D43.0 | D49.6 |
| windpipe | C33 | C78.39 | D02.1 | D14.2 | D38.1 | D49.1 |
| Wirsung's duct | C25.3 | C78.89 | D01.7 | D13.6 | D37.8 | D49.0 |
| wolffian (body) (duct) | | | | | | |
| female | C57.7 | C79.82 | D07.39 | D28.7 | D39.8 | D49.59 |

| | Malignant Primary | Malignant Secondary | Ca in situ | Benign | Uncertain | Unspecified Behavior |
|---|---|---|---|---|---|---|
| **Neoplasm, neoplastic —** *continued* | | | | | | |
| wolffian — *continued* | | | | | | |
|    male | C63.7 | C79.82 | D07.69 | D29.8 | D40.8 | D49.59 |
| womb — *see* Neoplasm, uterus | | | | | | |
| wrist NEC | C76.4-☑ | C79.89 | D04.6-☑ | D36.7 | D48.7 | D49.89 |
| xiphoid process | C41.3 | C79.51 | — | D16.7 | D48.0 | D49.2 |
| Zuckerkandl organ | C75.5 | C79.89 | — | D35.6 | D44.7 | D49.7 |

☑ **Additional Character Required — Refer to the Tabular List for Character Selection**          ▽ Subterms under main terms may continue to next column or page

**Table of Drugs and Chemicals**

| Substance | Poisoning, Accidental (unintentional) | Poisoning, Intentional Self-harm | Poisoning, Assault | Poisoning, Undetermined | Adverse Effect | Underdosing |
|---|---|---|---|---|---|---|
| 14-Hydroxydihydromorphinone | T40.2X1 | T40.2X2 | T40.2X3 | T40.2X4 | T40.2X5 | T40.2X6 |
| 1-Propanol | T51.3X1 | T51.3X2 | T51.3X3 | T51.3X4 | — | — |
| 2,3,7,8-Tetrachlorodibenzo-p-dioxin | T53.7X1 | T53.7X2 | T53.7X3 | T53.7X4 | — | — |
| 2,4,5-T (trichlorophenoxyacetic acid) | T60.1X1 | T60.1X2 | T60.1X3 | T60.1X4 | — | — |
| 2,4,5-Trichlorophenoxyacetic acid | T60.3X1 | T60.3X2 | T60.3X3 | T60.3X4 | — | — |
| 2,4-D (dichlorophenoxyacetic acid) | T60.3X1 | T60.3X2 | T60.3X3 | T60.3X4 | — | — |
| 2,4-Toluene diisocyanate | T65.0X1 | T65.0X2 | T65.0X3 | T65.0X4 | — | — |
| 2-Deoxy-5-fluorouridine | T45.1X1 | T45.1X2 | T45.1X3 | T45.1X4 | T45.1X5 | T45.1X6 |
| 2-Ethoxyethanol | T52.3X1 | T52.3X2 | T52.3X3 | T52.3X4 | — | — |
| 2-Methoxyethanol | T52.3X1 | T52.3X2 | T52.3X3 | T52.3X4 | — | — |
| 2-Propanol | T51.2X1 | T51.2X2 | T51.2X3 | T51.2X4 | — | — |
| 4-Aminobutyric acid | T43.8X1 | T43.8X2 | T43.8X3 | T43.8X4 | T43.8X5 | T43.8X6 |
| 4-Aminophenol derivatives | T39.1X1 | T39.1X2 | T39.1X3 | T39.1X4 | T39.1X5 | T39.1X6 |
| 5-Deoxy-5-fluorouridine | T45.1X1 | T45.1X2 | T45.1X3 | T45.1X4 | T45.1X5 | T45.1X6 |
| 5-Methoxypsoralen (5-MOP) | T50.991 | T50.992 | T50.993 | T50.994 | T50.995 | T50.996 |
| 8-Aminoquinoline drugs | T37.2X1 | T37.2X2 | T37.2X3 | T37.2X4 | T37.2X5 | T37.2X6 |
| 8-Methoxypsoralen (8-MOP) | T50.991 | T50.992 | T50.993 | T50.994 | T50.995 | T50.996 |
| ABOB | T37.5X1 | T37.5X2 | T37.5X3 | T37.5X4 | T37.5X5 | T37.5X6 |
| Abrine | T62.2X1 | T62.2X2 | T62.2X3 | T62.2X4 | — | — |
| Abrus (seed) | T62.2X1 | T62.2X2 | T62.2X3 | T62.2X4 | — | — |
| Absinthe | T51.0X1 | T51.0X2 | T51.0X3 | T51.0X4 | — | — |
|   beverage | T51.0X1 | T51.0X2 | T51.0X3 | T51.0X4 | — | — |
| Acaricide | T60.8X1 | T60.8X2 | T60.8X3 | T60.8X4 | — | — |
| Acebutolol | T44.7X1 | T44.7X2 | T44.7X3 | T44.7X4 | T44.7X5 | T44.7X6 |
| Acecarbromal | T42.6X1 | T42.6X2 | T42.6X3 | T42.6X4 | T42.6X5 | T42.6X6 |
| Aceclidine | T44.1X1 | T44.1X2 | T44.1X3 | T44.1X4 | T44.1X5 | T44.1X6 |
| Acedapsone | T37.0X1 | T37.0X2 | T37.0X3 | T37.0X4 | T37.0X5 | T37.0X6 |
| Acefylline piperazine | T48.6X1 | T48.6X2 | T48.6X3 | T48.6X4 | T48.6X5 | T48.6X6 |
| Acemorphan | T40.2X1 | T40.2X2 | T40.2X3 | T40.2X4 | T40.2X5 | T40.2X6 |
| Acenocoumarin | T45.511 | T45.512 | T45.513 | T45.514 | T45.515 | T45.516 |
| Acenocoumarol | T45.511 | T45.512 | T45.513 | T45.514 | T45.515 | T45.516 |
| Acepifylline | T48.6X1 | T48.6X2 | T48.6X3 | T48.6X4 | T48.6X5 | T48.6X6 |
| Acepromazine | T43.3X1 | T43.3X2 | T43.3X3 | T43.3X4 | T43.3X5 | T43.3X6 |
| Acesulfamethoxypyridazine | T37.0X1 | T37.0X2 | T37.0X3 | T37.0X4 | T37.0X5 | T37.0X6 |
| Acetal | T52.8X1 | T52.8X2 | T52.8X3 | T52.8X4 | — | — |
| Acetaldehyde (vapor) | T52.8X1 | T52.8X2 | T52.8X3 | T52.8X4 | — | — |
|   liquid | T65.891 | T65.892 | T65.893 | T65.894 | — | — |
| Acetaminophen | T39.1X1 | T39.1X2 | T39.1X3 | T39.1X4 | T39.1X5 | T39.1X6 |
| Acetaminosalol | T39.1X1 | T39.1X2 | T39.1X3 | T39.1X4 | T39.1X5 | T39.1X6 |
| Acetanilide | T39.1X1 | T39.1X2 | T39.1X3 | T39.1X4 | T39.1X5 | T39.1X6 |
| Acetarsol | T37.3X1 | T37.3X2 | T37.3X3 | T37.3X4 | T37.3X5 | T37.3X6 |
| Acetazolamide | T50.2X1 | T50.2X2 | T50.2X3 | T50.2X4 | T50.2X5 | T50.2X6 |
| Acetiamine | T45.2X1 | T45.2X2 | T45.2X3 | T45.2X4 | T45.2X5 | T45.2X6 |
| Acetic | | | | | | |
|   acid | T54.2X1 | T54.2X2 | T54.2X3 | T54.2X4 | — | — |
|     with sodium acetate (ointment) | T49.3X1 | T49.3X2 | T49.3X3 | T49.3X4 | T49.3X5 | T49.3X6 |
|     ester (solvent)(vapor) | T52.8X1 | T52.8X2 | T52.8X3 | T52.8X4 | — | — |
|     irrigating solution | T50.3X1 | T50.3X2 | T50.3X3 | T50.3X4 | T50.3X5 | T50.3X6 |
|     medicinal (lotion) | T49.2X1 | T49.2X2 | T49.2X3 | T49.2X4 | T49.2X5 | T49.2X6 |
|   anhydride | T65.891 | T65.892 | T65.893 | T65.894 | — | — |
|   ether (vapor) | T52.8X1 | T52.8X2 | T52.8X3 | T52.8X4 | — | — |
| Acetohexamide | T38.3X1 | T38.3X2 | T38.3X3 | T38.3X4 | T38.3X5 | T38.3X6 |
| Acetohydroxamic acid | T50.991 | T50.992 | T50.993 | T50.994 | T50.995 | T50.996 |
| Acetomenaphthone | T45.7X1 | T45.7X2 | T45.7X3 | T45.7X4 | T45.7X5 | T45.7X6 |
| Acetomorphine | T40.1X1 | T40.1X2 | T40.1X3 | T40.1X4 | — | — |
| Acetone (oils) | T52.4X1 | T52.4X2 | T52.4X3 | T52.4X4 | — | — |
|   chlorinated | T52.4X1 | T52.4X2 | T52.4X3 | T52.4X4 | — | — |
|   vapor | T52.4X1 | T52.4X2 | T52.4X3 | T52.4X4 | — | — |
| Acetonitrile | T52.8X1 | T52.8X2 | T52.8X3 | T52.8X4 | — | — |
| Acetophenazine | T43.3X1 | T43.3X2 | T43.3X3 | T43.3X4 | T43.3X5 | T43.3X6 |
| Acetophenetedin | T39.1X1 | T39.1X2 | T39.1X3 | T39.1X4 | T39.1X5 | T39.1X6 |
| Acetophenone | T52.4X1 | T52.4X2 | T52.4X3 | T52.4X4 | — | — |
| Acetorphine | T40.2X1 | T40.2X2 | T40.2X3 | T40.2X4 | — | — |
| Acetosulfone (sodium) | T37.1X1 | T37.1X2 | T37.1X3 | T37.1X4 | T37.1X5 | T37.1X6 |
| Acetrizoate (sodium) | T50.8X1 | T50.8X2 | T50.8X3 | T50.8X4 | T50.8X5 | T50.8X6 |
| Acetrizoic acid | T50.8X1 | T50.8X2 | T50.8X3 | T50.8X4 | T50.8X5 | T50.8X6 |
| Acetyl | | | | | | |
|   bromide | T53.6X1 | T53.6X2 | T53.6X3 | T53.6X4 | — | — |
|   chloride | T53.6X1 | T53.6X2 | T53.6X3 | T53.6X4 | — | — |
| Acetylcarbromal | T42.6X1 | T42.6X2 | T42.6X3 | T42.6X4 | T42.6X5 | T42.6X6 |
| Acetylcholine | | | | | | |
|   chloride | T44.1X1 | T44.1X2 | T44.1X3 | T44.1X4 | T44.1X5 | T44.1X6 |
|   derivative | T44.1X1 | T44.1X2 | T44.1X3 | T44.1X4 | T44.1X5 | T44.1X6 |
| Acetylcysteine | T48.4X1 | T48.4X2 | T48.4X3 | T48.4X4 | T48.4X5 | T48.4X6 |
| Acetyldigitoxin | T46.0X1 | T46.0X2 | T46.0X3 | T46.0X4 | T46.0X5 | T46.0X6 |
| Acetyldigoxin | T46.0X1 | T46.0X2 | T46.0X3 | T46.0X4 | T46.0X5 | T46.0X6 |

| Substance | Poisoning, Accidental (unintentional) | Poisoning, Intentional Self-harm | Poisoning, Assault | Poisoning, Undetermined | Adverse Effect | Underdosing |
|---|---|---|---|---|---|---|
| Acetyldihydrocodeine | T40.2X1 | T40.2X2 | T40.2X3 | T40.2X4 | — | — |
| Acetyldihydrocodeinone | T40.2X1 | T40.2X2 | T40.2X3 | T40.2X4 | — | — |
| Acetylene (gas) | T59.891 | T59.892 | T59.893 | T59.894 | — | — |
|   dichloride | T53.6X1 | T53.6X2 | T53.6X3 | T53.6X4 | — | — |
|   incomplete combustion of | T58.11 | T58.12 | T58.13 | T58.14 | — | — |
|   industrial | T59.891 | T59.892 | T59.893 | T59.894 | — | — |
|   tetrachloride | T53.6X1 | T53.6X2 | T53.6X3 | T53.6X4 | — | — |
|   vapor | T53.6X1 | T53.6X2 | T53.6X3 | T53.6X4 | — | — |
| Acetylpheneturide | T42.6X1 | T42.6X2 | T42.6X3 | T42.6X4 | T42.6X5 | T42.6X6 |
| Acetylphenylhydrazine | T39.8X1 | T39.8X2 | T39.8X3 | T39.8X4 | T39.8X5 | T39.8X6 |
| Acetylsalicylic acid (salts) | T39.011 | T39.012 | T39.013 | T39.014 | T39.015 | T39.016 |
|   enteric coated | T39.011 | T39.012 | T39.013 | T39.014 | T39.015 | T39.016 |
| Acetylsulfamethoxypyridazine | T37.0X1 | T37.0X2 | T37.0X3 | T37.0X4 | T37.0X5 | T37.0X6 |
| Achromycin | T36.4X1 | T36.4X2 | T36.4X3 | T36.4X4 | T36.4X5 | T36.4X6 |
|   ophthalmic preparation | T49.5X1 | T49.5X2 | T49.5X3 | T49.5X4 | T49.5X5 | T49.5X6 |
|   topical NEC | T49.0X1 | T49.0X2 | T49.0X3 | T49.0X4 | T49.0X5 | T49.0X6 |
| Aciclovir | T37.5X1 | T37.5X2 | T37.5X3 | T37.5X4 | T37.5X5 | T37.5X6 |
| Acidifying agent NEC | T50.901 | T50.902 | T50.903 | T50.904 | T50.905 | T50.906 |
| Acid (corrosive) NEC | T54.2X1 | T54.2X2 | T54.2X3 | T54.2X4 | — | — |
| Acipimox | T46.6X1 | T46.6X2 | T46.6X3 | T46.6X4 | T46.6X5 | T46.6X6 |
| Acitretin | T50.991 | T50.992 | T50.993 | T50.994 | T50.995 | T50.996 |
| Aclarubicin | T45.1X1 | T45.1X2 | T45.1X3 | T45.1X4 | T45.1X5 | T45.1X6 |
| Aclatonium napadisilate | T48.1X1 | T48.1X2 | T48.1X3 | T48.1X4 | T48.1X5 | T48.1X6 |
| Aconite (wild) | T46.991 | T46.992 | T46.993 | T46.994 | T46.995 | T46.996 |
| Aconitine | T46.991 | T46.992 | T46.993 | T46.994 | T46.995 | T46.996 |
| Aconitum ferox | T46.991 | T46.992 | T46.993 | T46.994 | T46.995 | T46.996 |
| Acridine | T65.6X1 | T65.6X2 | T65.6X3 | T65.6X4 | — | — |
|   vapor | T59.891 | T59.892 | T59.893 | T59.894 | — | — |
| Acriflavine | T37.91 | T37.92 | T37.93 | T37.94 | T37.95 | T37.96 |
| Acriflavinium chloride | T49.0X1 | T49.0X2 | T49.0X3 | T49.0X4 | T49.0X5 | T49.0X6 |
| Acrinol | T49.0X1 | T49.0X2 | T49.0X3 | T49.0X4 | T49.0X5 | T49.0X6 |
| Acrisorcin | T49.0X1 | T49.0X2 | T49.0X3 | T49.0X4 | T49.0X5 | T49.0X6 |
| Acrivastine | T45.0X1 | T45.0X2 | T45.0X3 | T45.0X4 | T45.0X5 | T45.0X6 |
| Acrolein (gas) | T59.891 | T59.892 | T59.893 | T59.894 | — | — |
|   liquid | T54.1X1 | T54.1X2 | T54.1X3 | T54.1X4 | — | — |
| Acrylamide | T65.891 | T65.892 | T65.893 | T65.894 | — | — |
| Acrylic resin | T49.3X1 | T49.3X2 | T49.3X3 | T49.3X4 | T49.3X5 | T49.3X6 |
| Acrylonitrile | T65.891 | T65.892 | T65.893 | T65.894 | — | — |
| Actaea spicata | T62.2X1 | T62.2X2 | T62.2X3 | T62.2X4 | — | — |
|   berry | T62.1X1 | T62.1X2 | T62.1X3 | T62.1X4 | — | — |
| Acterol | T37.3X1 | T37.3X2 | T37.3X3 | T37.3X4 | T37.3X5 | T37.3X6 |
| ACTH | T38.811 | T38.812 | T38.813 | T38.814 | T38.815 | T38.816 |
| Actinomycin C | T45.1X1 | T45.1X2 | T45.1X3 | T45.1X4 | T45.1X5 | T45.1X6 |
| Actinomycin D | T45.1X1 | T45.1X2 | T45.1X3 | T45.1X4 | T45.1X5 | T45.1X6 |
| Activated charcoal — see also Charcoal, medicinal | T47.6X1 | T47.6X2 | T47.6X3 | T47.6X4 | T47.6X5 | T47.6X6 |
| Acyclovir | T37.5X1 | T37.5X2 | T37.5X3 | T37.5X4 | T37.5X5 | T37.5X6 |
| Adenine | T45.2X1 | T45.2X2 | T45.2X3 | T45.2X4 | T45.2X5 | T45.2X6 |
|   arabinoside | T37.5X1 | T37.5X2 | T37.5X3 | T37.5X4 | T37.5X5 | T37.5X6 |
| Adenosine (phosphate) | T46.2X1 | T46.2X2 | T46.2X3 | T46.2X4 | T46.2X5 | T46.2X6 |
| ADH | T38.891 | T38.892 | T38.893 | T38.894 | T38.895 | T38.896 |
| Adhesive NEC | T65.891 | T65.892 | T65.893 | T65.894 | — | — |
| Adicillin | T36.0X1 | T36.0X2 | T36.0X3 | T36.0X4 | T36.0X5 | T36.0X6 |
| Adiphenine | T44.3X1 | T44.3X2 | T44.3X3 | T44.3X4 | T44.3X5 | T44.3X6 |
| Adipiodone | T50.8X1 | T50.8X2 | T50.8X3 | T50.8X4 | T50.8X5 | T50.8X6 |
| Adjunct, pharmaceutical | T50.901 | T50.902 | T50.903 | T50.904 | T50.905 | T50.906 |
| Adrenal (extract, cortex or medulla) (glucocorticoids) (hormones) (mineralocorticoids) | T38.0X1 | T38.0X2 | T38.0X3 | T38.0X4 | T38.0X5 | T38.0X6 |
|   ENT agent | T49.6X1 | T49.6X2 | T49.6X3 | T49.6X4 | T49.6X5 | T49.6X6 |
|   ophthalmic preparation | T49.5X1 | T49.5X2 | T49.5X3 | T49.5X4 | T49.5X5 | T49.5X6 |
|   topical NEC | T49.0X1 | T49.0X2 | T49.0X3 | T49.0X4 | T49.0X5 | T49.0X6 |
| Adrenalin — see Adrenaline | | | | | | |
| Adrenaline | T44.5X1 | T44.5X2 | T44.5X3 | T44.5X4 | T44.5X5 | T44.5X6 |
| Adrenergic NEC | T44.901 | T44.902 | T44.903 | T44.904 | T44.905 | T44.906 |
|   blocking agent NEC | T44.8X1 | T44.8X2 | T44.8X3 | T44.8X4 | T44.8X5 | T44.8X6 |
|     beta, heart | T44.7X1 | T44.7X2 | T44.7X3 | T44.7X4 | T44.7X5 | T44.7X6 |
|   specified NEC | T44.991 | T44.992 | T44.993 | T44.994 | T44.995 | T44.996 |
| Adrenochrome | | | | | | |
|   derivative | T46.991 | T46.992 | T46.993 | T46.994 | T46.995 | T46.996 |
|   (mono) semicarbazone | T46.991 | T46.992 | T46.993 | T46.994 | T46.995 | T46.996 |
| Adrenocorticotrophic hormone | T38.811 | T38.812 | T38.813 | T38.814 | T38.815 | T38.816 |
| Adrenocorticotrophin | T38.811 | T38.812 | T38.813 | T38.814 | T38.815 | T38.816 |
| Adriamycin | T45.1X1 | T45.1X2 | T45.1X3 | T45.1X4 | T45.1X5 | T45.1X6 |
| Aerosol spray NEC | T65.91 | T65.92 | T65.93 | T65.94 | — | — |
| Aerosporin | T36.8X1 | T36.8X2 | T36.8X3 | T36.8X4 | T36.8X5 | T36.8X6 |
|   ENT agent | T49.6X1 | T49.6X2 | T49.6X3 | T49.6X4 | T49.6X5 | T49.6X6 |
|   ophthalmic preparation | T49.5X1 | T49.5X2 | T49.5X3 | T49.5X4 | T49.5X5 | T49.5X6 |
|   topical NEC | T49.0X1 | T49.0X2 | T49.0X3 | T49.0X4 | T49.0X5 | T49.0X6 |
| Aethusa cynapium | T62.2X1 | T62.2X2 | T62.2X3 | T62.2X4 | — | — |
| Afghanistan black | T40.7X1 | T40.7X2 | T40.7X3 | T40.7X4 | T40.7X5 | T40.7X6 |

| Substance | Poisoning, Accidental (unintentional) | Poisoning, Intentional Self-harm | Poisoning, Assault | Poisoning, Undetermined | Adverse Effect | Under-dosing |
|---|---|---|---|---|---|---|
| Aflatoxin | T64.01 | T64.02 | T64.03 | T64.04 | | |
| Afloqualone | T42.8X1 | T42.8X2 | T42.8X3 | T42.8X4 | T42.8X5 | T42.8X6 |
| African boxwood | T62.2X1 | T62.2X2 | T62.2X3 | T62.2X4 | | |
| Agar | T47.4X1 | T47.4X2 | T47.4X3 | T47.4X4 | T47.4X5 | T47.4X6 |
| Agonist | | | | | | |
| predominantly | | | | | | |
| alpha-adrenoreceptor | T44.4X1 | T44.4X2 | T44.4X3 | T44.4X4 | T44.4X5 | T44.4X6 |
| beta-adrenoreceptor | T44.5X1 | T44.5X2 | T44.5X3 | T44.5X4 | T44.5X5 | T44.5X6 |
| Agricultural agent NEC | T65.91 | T65.92 | T65.93 | T65.94 | | |
| Agrypnal | T42.3X1 | T42.3X2 | T42.3X3 | T42.3X4 | T42.3X5 | T42.3X6 |
| AHLG | T50.Z11 | T50.Z12 | T50.Z13 | T50.Z14 | T50.Z15 | T50.Z16 |
| Air contaminant(s), source/type NOS | T65.91 | T65.92 | T65.93 | T65.94 | | |
| Ajmaline | T46.2X1 | T46.2X2 | T46.2X3 | T46.2X4 | T46.2X5 | T46.2X6 |
| Akee | T62.1X1 | T62.1X2 | T62.1X3 | T62.1X4 | | |
| Akrinol | T49.0X1 | T49.0X2 | T49.0X3 | T49.0X4 | T49.0X5 | T49.0X6 |
| Akritoin | T37.8X1 | T37.8X2 | T37.8X3 | T37.8X4 | T37.8X5 | T37.8X6 |
| Alacepril | T46.4X1 | T46.4X2 | T46.4X3 | T46.4X4 | T46.4X5 | T46.4X6 |
| Alantolactone | T37.4X1 | T37.4X2 | T37.4X3 | T37.4X4 | T37.4X5 | T37.4X6 |
| Albamycin | T36.8X1 | T36.8X2 | T36.8X3 | T36.8X4 | T36.8X5 | T36.8X6 |
| Albendazole | T37.4X1 | T37.4X2 | T37.4X3 | T37.4X4 | T37.4X5 | T37.4X6 |
| Albumin | | | | | | |
| bovine | T45.8X1 | T45.8X2 | T45.8X3 | T45.8X4 | T45.8X5 | T45.8X6 |
| human serum | T45.8X1 | T45.8X2 | T45.8X3 | T45.8X4 | T45.8X5 | T45.8X6 |
| salt-poor | T45.8X1 | T45.8X2 | T45.8X3 | T45.8X4 | T45.8X5 | T45.8X6 |
| normal human serum | T45.8X1 | T45.8X2 | T45.8X3 | T45.8X4 | T45.8X5 | T45.8X6 |
| Albuterol | T48.6X1 | T48.6X2 | T48.6X3 | T48.6X4 | T48.6X5 | T48.6X6 |
| Albutoin | T42.0X1 | T42.0X2 | T42.0X3 | T42.0X4 | T42.0X5 | T42.0X6 |
| Alclometasone | T49.0X1 | T49.0X2 | T49.0X3 | T49.0X4 | T49.0X5 | T49.0X6 |
| Alcohol | T51.91 | T51.92 | T51.93 | T51.94 | | |
| absolute | T51.0X1 | T51.0X2 | T51.0X3 | T51.0X4 | | |
| beverage | T51.0X1 | T51.0X2 | T51.0X3 | T51.0X4 | | |
| allyl | T51.8X1 | T51.8X2 | T51.8X3 | T51.8X4 | | |
| amyl | T51.3X1 | T51.3X2 | T51.3X3 | T51.3X4 | | |
| antifreeze | T51.1X1 | T51.1X2 | T51.1X3 | T51.1X4 | | |
| beverage | T51.0X1 | T51.0X2 | T51.0X3 | T51.0X4 | | |
| butyl | T51.3X1 | T51.3X2 | T51.3X3 | T51.3X4 | | |
| dehydrated | T51.0X1 | T51.0X2 | T51.0X3 | T51.0X4 | | |
| beverage | T51.0X1 | T51.0X2 | T51.0X3 | T51.0X4 | | |
| denatured | T51.0X1 | T51.0X2 | T51.0X3 | T51.0X4 | | |
| deterrent NEC | T50.6X1 | T50.6X2 | T50.6X3 | T50.6X4 | T50.6X5 | T50.6X6 |
| diagnostic (gastric function) | T50.8X1 | T50.8X2 | T50.8X3 | T50.8X4 | T50.8X5 | T50.8X6 |
| ethyl | T51.0X1 | T51.0X2 | T51.0X3 | T51.0X4 | | |
| beverage | T51.0X1 | T51.0X2 | T51.0X3 | T51.0X4 | | |
| grain | T51.0X1 | T51.0X2 | T51.0X3 | T51.0X4 | | |
| beverage | T51.0X1 | T51.0X2 | T51.0X3 | T51.0X4 | | |
| industrial | T51.0X1 | T51.0X2 | T51.0X3 | T51.0X4 | | |
| isopropyl | T51.2X1 | T51.2X2 | T51.2X3 | T51.2X4 | | |
| methyl | T51.1X1 | T51.1X2 | T51.1X3 | T51.1X4 | | |
| preparation for consumption | T51.0X1 | T51.0X2 | T51.0X3 | T51.0X4 | | |
| propyl | T51.3X1 | T51.3X2 | T51.3X3 | T51.3X4 | | |
| secondary | T51.2X1 | T51.2X2 | T51.2X3 | T51.2X4 | | |
| radiator | T51.1X1 | T51.1X2 | T51.1X3 | T51.1X4 | | |
| rubbing | T51.2X1 | T51.2X2 | T51.2X3 | T51.2X4 | | |
| specified type NEC | T51.8X1 | T51.8X2 | T51.8X3 | T51.8X4 | | |
| surgical | T51.0X1 | T51.0X2 | T51.0X3 | T51.0X4 | | |
| vapor (from any type of Alcohol) | T59.891 | T59.892 | T59.893 | T59.894 | | |
| wood | T51.1X1 | T51.1X2 | T51.1X3 | T51.1X4 | | |
| Alcuronium (chloride) | T48.1X1 | T48.1X2 | T48.1X3 | T48.1X4 | T48.1X5 | T48.1X6 |
| Aldactone | T50.0X1 | T50.0X2 | T50.0X3 | T50.0X4 | T50.0X5 | T50.0X6 |
| Aldesulfone sodium | T37.1X1 | T37.1X2 | T37.1X3 | T37.1X4 | T37.1X5 | T37.1X6 |
| Aldicarb | T60.0X1 | T60.0X2 | T60.0X3 | T60.0X4 | — | — |
| Aldomet | T46.5X1 | T46.5X2 | T46.5X3 | T46.5X4 | T46.5X5 | T46.5X6 |
| Aldosterone | T50.0X1 | T50.0X2 | T50.0X3 | T50.0X4 | T50.0X5 | T50.0X6 |
| Aldrin (dust) | T60.1X1 | T60.1X2 | T60.1X3 | T60.1X4 | — | — |
| Aleve — see Naproxen | | | | | | |
| Alexitol sodium | T47.1X1 | T47.1X2 | T47.1X3 | T47.1X4 | T47.1X5 | T47.1X6 |
| Alfacalcidol | T45.2X1 | T45.2X2 | T45.2X3 | T45.2X4 | T45.2X5 | T45.2X6 |
| Alfadolone | T41.1X1 | T41.1X2 | T41.1X3 | T41.1X4 | T41.1X5 | T41.1X6 |
| Alfaxalone | T41.1X1 | T41.1X2 | T41.1X3 | T41.1X4 | T41.1X5 | T41.1X6 |
| Alfentanil | T40.4X1 | T40.4X2 | T40.4X3 | T40.4X4 | T40.4X5 | T40.4X6 |
| Alfuzosin (hydrochloride) | T44.8X1 | T44.8X2 | T44.8X3 | T44.8X4 | T44.8X5 | T44.8X6 |
| Algae (harmful) (toxin) | T65.821 | T65.822 | T65.823 | T65.824 | — | — |
| Algeldrate | T47.1X1 | T47.1X2 | T47.1X3 | T47.1X4 | T47.1X5 | T47.1X6 |
| Algin | T47.8X1 | T47.8X2 | T47.8X3 | T47.8X4 | T47.8X5 | T47.8X6 |
| Alglucerase | T45.3X1 | T45.3X2 | T45.3X3 | T45.3X4 | T45.3X5 | T45.3X6 |
| Alidase | T45.3X1 | T45.3X2 | T45.3X3 | T45.3X4 | T45.3X5 | T45.3X6 |
| Alimemazine | T43.3X1 | T43.3X2 | T43.3X3 | T43.3X4 | T43.3X5 | T43.3X6 |
| Aliphatic thiocyanates | T65.0X1 | T65.0X2 | T65.0X3 | T65.0X4 | — | — |
| Alizapride | T45.0X1 | T45.0X2 | T45.0X4 | T45.0X5 | T45.0X6 | |

| Substance | Poisoning, Accidental (unintentional) | Poisoning, Intentional Self-harm | Poisoning, Assault | Poisoning, Undetermined | Adverse Effect | Under-dosing |
|---|---|---|---|---|---|---|
| Alkali (caustic) | T54.3X1 | T54.3X2 | T54.3X3 | T54.3X4 | — | — |
| Alkaline antiseptic solution (aromatic) | T49.6X1 | T49.6X2 | T49.6X3 | T49.6X4 | T49.6X5 | T49.6X6 |
| Alkalinizing agents (medicinal) | T50.901 | T50.902 | T50.903 | T50.904 | T50.905 | T50.906 |
| Alkalizing agent NEC | T50.901 | T50.902 | T50.903 | T50.904 | T50.905 | T50.906 |
| Alka-seltzer | T39.011 | T39.012 | T39.013 | T39.014 | T39.015 | T39.016 |
| Alkavervir | T46.5X1 | T46.5X2 | T46.5X3 | T46.5X4 | T46.5X5 | T46.5X6 |
| Alkonium (bromide) | T49.0X1 | T49.0X2 | T49.0X3 | T49.0X4 | T49.0X5 | T49.0X6 |
| Alkylating drug NEC | T45.1X1 | T45.1X2 | T45.1X3 | T45.1X4 | T45.1X5 | T45.1X6 |
| antimyeloproliferative | T45.1X1 | T45.1X2 | T45.1X3 | T45.1X4 | T45.1X5 | T45.1X6 |
| lymphatic | T45.1X1 | T45.1X2 | T45.1X3 | T45.1X4 | T45.1X5 | T45.1X6 |
| Alkylisocyanate | T65.0X1 | T65.0X2 | T65.0X3 | T65.0X4 | | |
| Allantoin | T49.4X1 | T49.4X2 | T49.4X3 | T49.4X4 | T49.4X5 | T49.4X6 |
| Allegron | T43.011 | T43.012 | T43.013 | T43.014 | T43.015 | T43.016 |
| Allethrin | T49.0X1 | T49.0X2 | T49.0X3 | T49.0X4 | T49.0X5 | T49.0X6 |
| Allobarbital | T42.3X1 | T42.3X2 | T42.3X3 | T42.3X4 | T42.3X5 | T42.3X6 |
| Allopurinol | T50.4X1 | T50.4X2 | T50.4X3 | T50.4X4 | T50.4X5 | T50.4X6 |
| Allyl | | | | | | |
| alcohol | T51.8X1 | T51.8X2 | T51.8X3 | T51.8X4 | — | — |
| disulfide | T46.6X1 | T46.6X2 | T46.6X3 | T46.6X4 | T46.6X5 | T46.6X6 |
| Allylestrenol | T38.5X1 | T38.5X2 | T38.5X3 | T38.5X4 | T38.5X5 | T38.5X6 |
| Allylisopropylacetylurea | T42.6X1 | T42.6X2 | T42.6X3 | T42.6X4 | T42.6X5 | T42.6X6 |
| Allylisopropylmalonylurea | T42.3X1 | T42.3X2 | T42.3X3 | T42.3X4 | T42.3X5 | T42.3X6 |
| Allylthiourea | T49.3X1 | T49.3X2 | T49.3X3 | T49.3X4 | T49.3X5 | T49.3X6 |
| Allyltribromide | T42.6X1 | T42.6X2 | T42.6X3 | T42.6X4 | T42.6X5 | T42.6X6 |
| Allypropymal | T42.3X1 | T42.3X2 | T42.3X3 | T42.3X4 | T42.3X5 | T42.3X6 |
| Almagate | T47.1X1 | T47.1X2 | T47.1X3 | T47.1X4 | T47.1X5 | T47.1X6 |
| Almasilate | T47.1X1 | T47.1X2 | T47.1X3 | T47.1X4 | T47.1X5 | T47.1X6 |
| Almitrine | T50.7X1 | T50.7X2 | T50.7X3 | T50.7X4 | T50.7X5 | T50.7X6 |
| Aloes | T47.2X1 | T47.2X2 | T47.2X3 | T47.2X4 | T47.2X5 | T47.2X6 |
| Aloglutamol | T47.1X1 | T47.1X2 | T47.1X3 | T47.1X4 | T47.1X5 | T47.1X6 |
| Aloin | T47.2X1 | T47.2X2 | T47.2X3 | T47.2X4 | T47.2X5 | T47.2X6 |
| Aloxidone | T42.2X1 | T42.2X2 | T42.2X3 | T42.2X4 | T42.2X5 | T42.2X6 |
| Alpha | | | | | | |
| acetyldigoxin | T46.0X1 | T46.0X2 | T46.0X3 | T46.0X4 | T46.0X5 | T46.0X6 |
| adrenergic blocking drug | T44.6X1 | T44.6X2 | T44.6X3 | T44.6X4 | T44.6X5 | T44.6X6 |
| amylase | T45.3X1 | T45.3X2 | T45.3X3 | T45.3X4 | T45.3X5 | T45.3X6 |
| tocoferol (acetate) | T45.2X1 | T45.2X2 | T45.2X3 | T45.2X4 | T45.2X5 | T45.2X6 |
| tocopherol | T45.2X1 | T45.2X2 | T45.2X3 | T45.2X4 | T45.2X5 | T45.2X6 |
| Alphadolone | T41.1X1 | T41.1X2 | T41.1X3 | T41.1X4 | T41.1X5 | T41.1X6 |
| Alphaprodine | T40.4X1 | T40.4X2 | T40.4X3 | T40.4X4 | T40.4X5 | T40.4X6 |
| Alphaxalone | T41.1X1 | T41.1X2 | T41.1X3 | T41.1X4 | T41.1X5 | T41.1X6 |
| Alprazolam | T42.4X1 | T42.4X2 | T42.4X3 | T42.4X4 | T42.4X5 | T42.4X6 |
| Alprenolol | T44.7X1 | T44.7X2 | T44.7X3 | T44.7X4 | T44.7X5 | T44.7X6 |
| Alprostadil | T46.7X1 | T46.7X2 | T46.7X3 | T46.7X4 | T46.7X5 | T46.7X6 |
| Alsactide | T38.811 | T38.812 | T38.813 | T38.814 | T38.815 | T38.816 |
| Alseroxylon | T46.5X1 | T46.5X2 | T46.5X3 | T46.5X4 | T46.5X5 | T46.5X6 |
| Alteplase | T45.611 | T45.612 | T45.613 | T45.614 | T45.615 | T45.616 |
| Altizide | T50.2X1 | T50.2X2 | T50.2X3 | T50.2X4 | T50.2X5 | T50.2X6 |
| Altretamine | T45.1X1 | T45.1X2 | T45.1X3 | T45.1X4 | T45.1X5 | T45.1X6 |
| Alum (medicinal) | T49.4X1 | T49.4X2 | T49.4X3 | T49.4X4 | T49.4X5 | T49.4X6 |
| nonmedicinal (ammonium) (potassium) | T56.891 | T56.892 | T56.893 | T56.894 | — | — |
| Aluminium, aluminum | | | | | | |
| acetate | T49.2X1 | T49.2X2 | T49.2X3 | T49.2X4 | T49.2X5 | T49.2X6 |
| solution | T49.0X1 | T49.0X2 | T49.0X3 | T49.0X4 | T49.0X5 | T49.0X6 |
| aspirin | T39.011 | T39.012 | T39.013 | T39.014 | T39.015 | T39.016 |
| bis (acetylsalicylate) | T39.011 | T39.012 | T39.013 | T39.014 | T39.015 | T39.016 |
| carbonate (gel, basic) | T47.1X1 | T47.1X2 | T47.1X3 | T47.1X4 | T47.1X5 | T47.1X6 |
| chlorhydroxide-complex | T47.1X1 | T47.1X2 | T47.1X3 | T47.1X4 | T47.1X5 | T47.1X6 |
| chloride | T49.2X1 | T49.2X2 | T49.2X3 | T49.2X4 | T49.2X5 | T49.2X6 |
| clofibrate | T46.6X1 | T46.6X2 | T46.6X3 | T46.6X4 | T46.6X5 | T46.6X6 |
| diacetate | T49.2X1 | T49.2X2 | T49.2X3 | T49.2X4 | T49.2X5 | T49.2X6 |
| glycinate | T47.1X1 | T47.1X2 | T47.1X3 | T47.1X4 | T47.1X5 | T47.1X6 |
| hydroxide (gel) | T47.1X1 | T47.1X2 | T47.1X3 | T47.1X4 | T47.1X5 | T47.1X6 |
| hydroxide-magnesium carb. gel | T47.1X1 | T47.1X2 | T47.1X3 | T47.1X4 | T47.1X5 | T47.1X6 |
| magnesium silicate | T47.1X1 | T47.1X2 | T47.1X3 | T47.1X4 | T47.1X5 | T47.1X6 |
| nicotinate | T46.7X1 | T46.7X2 | T46.7X3 | T46.7X4 | T46.7X5 | T46.7X6 |
| ointment (surgical) (topical) | T49.3X1 | T49.3X2 | T49.3X3 | T49.3X4 | T49.3X5 | T49.3X6 |
| phosphate | T47.1X1 | T47.1X2 | T47.1X3 | T47.1X4 | T47.1X5 | T47.1X6 |
| salicylate | T39.091 | T39.092 | T39.093 | T39.094 | T39.095 | T39.096 |
| silicate | T47.1X1 | T47.1X2 | T47.1X3 | T47.1X4 | T47.1X5 | T47.1X6 |
| sodium silicate | T47.1X1 | T47.1X2 | T47.1X3 | T47.1X4 | T47.1X5 | T47.1X6 |
| subacetate | T49.2X1 | T49.2X2 | T49.2X3 | T49.2X4 | T49.2X5 | T49.2X6 |
| sulfate | T49.0X1 | T49.0X2 | T49.0X3 | T49.0X4 | T49.0X5 | T49.0X6 |
| tannate | T47.6X1 | T47.6X2 | T47.6X3 | T47.6X4 | T47.6X5 | T47.6X6 |
| topical NEC | T49.3X1 | T49.3X2 | T49.3X3 | T49.3X4 | T49.3X5 | T49.3X6 |
| Alurate | T42.3X1 | T42.3X2 | T42.3X3 | T42.3X4 | T42.3X5 | T42.3X6 |
| Alverine | T44.3X1 | T44.3X2 | T44.3X3 | T44.3X4 | T44.3X5 | T44.3X6 |
| Alvodine | T40.2X1 | T40.2X2 | T40.2X3 | T40.2X4 | T40.2X5 | T40.2X6 |
| Amanita phalloides | T62.0X1 | T62.0X2 | T62.0X3 | T62.0X4 | — | — |

Additional Character May Be Required — Refer to the Tabular List for Character Selection

▽ Subterms under main terms may continue to next column or page

| Substance | Poisoning, Accidental (unintentional) | Poisoning, Intentional Self-harm | Poisoning, Assault | Poisoning, Undetermined | Adverse Effect | Under-dosing |
|---|---|---|---|---|---|---|
| **Amanitine** | T62.0X1 | T62.0X2 | T62.0X3 | T62.0X4 | — | — |
| **Amantadine** | T42.8X1 | T42.8X2 | T42.8X3 | T42.8X4 | T42.8X5 | T42.8X6 |
| **Ambazone** | T49.6X1 | T49.6X2 | T49.6X3 | T49.6X4 | T49.6X5 | T49.6X6 |
| **Ambenonium** (chloride) | T44.0X1 | T44.0X2 | T44.0X3 | T44.0X4 | T44.0X5 | T44.0X6 |
| **Ambroxol** | T48.4X1 | T48.4X2 | T48.4X3 | T48.4X4 | T48.4X5 | T48.4X6 |
| **Ambuphylline** | T48.6X1 | T48.6X2 | T48.6X3 | T48.6X4 | T48.6X5 | T48.6X6 |
| **Ambutonium bromide** | T44.3X1 | T44.3X2 | T44.3X3 | T44.3X4 | T44.3X5 | T44.3X6 |
| **Amcinonide** | T49.0X1 | T49.0X2 | T49.0X3 | T49.0X4 | T49.0X5 | T49.0X6 |
| **Amdinocilline** | T36.0X1 | T36.0X2 | T36.0X3 | T36.0X4 | T36.0X5 | T36.0X6 |
| **Ametazole** | T50.8X1 | T50.8X2 | T50.8X3 | T50.8X4 | T50.8X5 | T50.8X6 |
| **Amethocaine** | T41.3X1 | T41.3X2 | T41.3X3 | T41.3X4 | T41.3X5 | T41.3X6 |
|   regional | T41.3X1 | T41.3X2 | T41.3X3 | T41.3X4 | T41.3X5 | T41.3X6 |
|   spinal | T41.3X1 | T41.3X2 | T41.3X3 | T41.3X4 | T41.3X5 | T41.3X6 |
| **Amethopterin** | T45.1X1 | T45.1X2 | T45.1X3 | T45.1X4 | T45.1X5 | T45.1X6 |
| **Amezinium metilsulfate** | T44.991 | T44.992 | T44.993 | T44.994 | T44.995 | T44.996 |
| **Amfebutamone** | T43.291 | T43.292 | T43.293 | T43.294 | T43.295 | T43.296 |
| **Amfepramone** | T50.5X1 | T50.5X2 | T50.5X3 | T50.5X4 | T50.5X5 | T50.5X6 |
| **Amfetamine** | T43.621 | T43.622 | T43.623 | T43.624 | T43.625 | T43.626 |
| **Amfetaminil** | T43.621 | T43.622 | T43.623 | T43.624 | T43.625 | T43.626 |
| **Amfomycin** | T36.8X1 | T36.8X2 | T36.8X3 | T36.8X4 | T36.8X5 | T36.8X6 |
| **Amidefrine mesilate** | T48.5X1 | T48.5X2 | T48.5X3 | T48.5X4 | T48.5X5 | T48.5X6 |
| **Amidone** | T40.3X1 | T40.3X2 | T40.3X3 | T40.3X4 | T40.3X5 | T40.3X6 |
| **Amidopyrine** | T39.2X1 | T39.2X2 | T39.2X3 | T39.2X4 | T39.2X5 | T39.2X6 |
| **Amidotrizoate** | T50.8X1 | T50.8X2 | T50.8X3 | T50.8X4 | T50.8X5 | T50.8X6 |
| **Amiflamine** | T43.1X1 | T43.1X2 | T43.1X3 | T43.1X4 | T43.1X5 | T43.1X6 |
| **Amikacin** | T36.5X1 | T36.5X2 | T36.5X3 | T36.5X4 | T36.5X5 | T36.5X6 |
| **Amikhelline** | T46.3X1 | T46.3X2 | T46.3X3 | T46.3X4 | T46.3X5 | T46.3X6 |
| **Amiloride** | T50.2X1 | T50.2X2 | T50.2X3 | T50.2X4 | T50.2X5 | T50.2X6 |
| **Aminacrine** | T49.0X1 | T49.0X2 | T49.0X3 | T49.0X4 | T49.0X5 | T49.0X6 |
| **Amineptine** | T43.011 | T43.012 | T43.013 | T43.014 | T43.015 | T43.016 |
| **Aminitrozole** | T37.3X1 | T37.3X2 | T37.3X3 | T37.3X4 | T37.3X5 | T37.3X6 |
| **Aminoacetic acid** | T50.3X1 | T50.3X2 | T50.3X3 | T50.3X4 | T50.3X5 | T50.3X6 |
|   (derivatives) | | | | | | |
| **Amino acids** | T50.3X1 | T50.3X2 | T50.3X3 | T50.3X4 | T50.3X5 | T50.3X6 |
| **Aminoacridine** | T49.0X1 | T49.0X2 | T49.0X3 | T49.0X4 | T49.0X5 | T49.0X6 |
| **Aminobenzoic acid** (-p) | T49.3X1 | T49.3X2 | T49.3X3 | T49.3X4 | T49.3X5 | T49.3X6 |
| **Aminocaproic acid** | T45.621 | T45.622 | T45.623 | T45.624 | T45.625 | T45.626 |
| **Aminoethylisothiourium** | T45.8X1 | T45.8X2 | T45.8X3 | T45.8X4 | T45.8X5 | T45.8X6 |
| **Aminofenazone** | T39.2X1 | T39.2X2 | T39.2X3 | T39.2X4 | T39.2X5 | T39.2X6 |
| **Aminoglutethimide** | T45.1X1 | T45.1X2 | T45.1X3 | T45.1X4 | T45.1X5 | T45.1X6 |
| **Aminohippuric acid** | T50.8X1 | T50.8X2 | T50.8X3 | T50.8X4 | T50.8X5 | T50.8X6 |
| **Aminomethylbenzoic acid** | T45.691 | T45.692 | T45.693 | T45.694 | T45.695 | T45.696 |
| **Aminometradine** | T50.2X1 | T50.2X2 | T50.2X3 | T50.2X4 | T50.2X5 | T50.2X6 |
| **Aminopentamide** | T44.3X1 | T44.3X2 | T44.3X3 | T44.3X4 | T44.3X5 | T44.3X6 |
| **Aminophenazone** | T39.2X1 | T39.2X2 | T39.2X3 | T39.2X4 | T39.2X5 | T39.2X6 |
| **Aminophenol** | T54.0X1 | T54.0X2 | T54.0X3 | T54.0X4 | — | — |
| **Aminophenylpyridone** | T43.591 | T43.592 | T43.593 | T43.594 | T43.595 | T43.596 |
| **Aminophylline** | T48.6X1 | T48.6X2 | T48.6X3 | T48.6X4 | T48.6X5 | T48.6X6 |
| **Aminopterin sodium** | T45.1X1 | T45.1X2 | T45.1X3 | T45.1X4 | T45.1X5 | T45.1X6 |
| **Aminopyrine** | T39.2X1 | T39.2X2 | T39.2X3 | T39.2X4 | T39.2X5 | T39.2X6 |
| **Aminorex** | T50.5X1 | T50.5X2 | T50.5X3 | T50.5X4 | T50.5X5 | T50.5X6 |
| **Aminosalicylic acid** | T37.1X1 | T37.1X2 | T37.1X3 | T37.1X4 | T37.1X5 | T37.1X6 |
| **Aminosalylum** | T37.1X1 | T37.1X2 | T37.1X3 | T37.1X4 | T37.1X5 | T37.1X6 |
| **Amiodarone** | T46.2X1 | T46.2X2 | T46.2X3 | T46.2X4 | T46.2X5 | T46.2X6 |
| **Amiphenazole** | T50.7X1 | T50.7X2 | T50.7X3 | T50.7X4 | T50.7X5 | T50.7X6 |
| **Amiquinsin** | T46.5X1 | T46.5X2 | T46.5X3 | T46.5X4 | T46.5X5 | T46.5X6 |
| **Amisometradine** | T50.2X1 | T50.2X2 | T50.2X3 | T50.2X4 | T50.2X5 | T50.2X6 |
| **Amisulpride** | T43.591 | T43.592 | T43.593 | T43.594 | T43.595 | T43.596 |
| **Amitriptyline** | T43.011 | T43.012 | T43.013 | T43.014 | T43.015 | T43.016 |
| **Amitriptylinoxide** | T43.011 | T43.012 | T43.013 | T43.014 | T43.015 | T43.016 |
| **Amlexanox** | T48.6X1 | T48.6X2 | T48.6X3 | T48.6X4 | T48.6X5 | T48.6X6 |
| **Ammonia** (fumes) (gas) | T59.891 | T59.892 | T59.893 | T59.894 | — | — |
|   (vapor) | | | | | | |
|   aromatic spirit | T48.991 | T48.992 | T48.993 | T48.994 | T48.995 | T48.996 |
|   liquid (household) | T54.3X1 | T54.3X2 | T54.3X3 | T54.3X4 | — | — |
| **Ammoniated mercury** | T49.0X1 | T49.0X2 | T49.0X3 | T49.0X4 | T49.0X5 | T49.0X6 |
| **Ammonium** | | | | | | |
|   acid tartrate | T49.5X1 | T49.5X2 | T49.5X3 | T49.5X4 | T49.5X5 | T49.5X6 |
|   bromide | T42.6X1 | T42.6X2 | T42.6X3 | T42.6X4 | T42.6X5 | T42.6X6 |
|   carbonate | T54.3X1 | T54.3X2 | T54.3X3 | T54.3X4 | — | — |
|   chloride | T50.991 | T50.992 | T50.993 | T50.994 | T50.995 | T50.996 |
|     expectorant | T48.4X1 | T48.4X2 | T48.4X3 | T48.4X4 | T48.4X5 | T48.4X6 |
|   compounds (household) NEC | T54.3X1 | T54.3X2 | T54.3X3 | T54.3X4 | — | — |
|   fumes (any usage) | T59.891 | T59.892 | T59.893 | T59.894 | — | — |
|   industrial | T54.3X1 | T54.3X2 | T54.3X3 | T54.3X4 | — | — |
|   ichthyosulronate | T49.4X1 | T49.4X2 | T49.4X3 | T49.4X4 | T49.4X5 | T49.4X6 |
|   mandelate | T37.91 | T37.92 | T37.93 | T37.94 | T37.95 | T37.96 |
|   sulfamate | T60.3X1 | T60.3X2 | T60.3X3 | T60.3X4 | — | — |
|   sulfonate resin | T47.8X1 | T47.8X2 | T47.8X3 | T47.8X4 | T47.8X5 | T47.8X6 |
| **Amobarbital** (sodium) | T42.3X1 | T42.3X2 | T42.3X3 | T42.3X4 | T42.3X5 | T42.3X6 |
| **Amodiaquine** | T37.2X1 | T37.2X2 | T37.2X3 | T37.2X4 | T37.2X5 | T37.2X6 |
| **Amopyroquin** (e) | T37.2X1 | T37.2X2 | T37.2X3 | T37.2X4 | T37.2X5 | T37.2X6 |

| Substance | Poisoning, Accidental (unintentional) | Poisoning, Intentional Self-harm | Poisoning, Assault | Poisoning, Undetermined | Adverse Effect | Under-dosing |
|---|---|---|---|---|---|---|
| **Amoxapine** | T43.011 | T43.012 | T43.013 | T43.014 | T43.015 | T43.016 |
| **Amoxicillin** | T36.0X1 | T36.0X2 | T36.0X3 | T36.0X4 | T36.0X5 | T36.0X6 |
| **Amperozide** | T43.591 | T43.592 | T43.593 | T43.595 | T43.595 | T43.596 |
| **Amphenidone** | T43.591 | T43.592 | T43.593 | T43.594 | T43.595 | T43.596 |
| **Amphetamine NEC** | T43.621 | T43.622 | T43.623 | T43.624 | T43.625 | T43.626 |
| **Amphomycin** | T36.8X1 | T36.8X2 | T36.8X3 | T36.8X4 | T36.8X5 | T36.8X6 |
| **Amphotalide** | T37.4X1 | T37.4X2 | T37.4X3 | T37.4X4 | T37.4X5 | T37.4X6 |
| **Amphotericin B** | T36.7X1 | T36.7X2 | T36.7X3 | T36.7X4 | T36.7X5 | T36.7X6 |
|   topical | T49.0X1 | T49.0X2 | T49.0X3 | T49.0X4 | T49.0X5 | T49.0X6 |
| **Ampicillin** | T36.0X1 | T36.0X2 | T36.0X3 | T36.0X4 | T36.0X5 | T36.0X6 |
| **Amprotropine** | T44.3X1 | T44.3X2 | T44.3X3 | T44.3X4 | T44.3X5 | T44.3X6 |
| **Amsacrine** | T45.1X1 | T45.1X2 | T45.1X3 | T45.1X4 | T45.1X5 | T45.1X6 |
| **Amygdaline** | T62.2X1 | T62.2X2 | T62.2X3 | T62.2X4 | — | — |
| **Amyl** | | | | | | |
|   acetate | T52.8X1 | T52.8X2 | T52.8X3 | T52.8X4 | — | — |
|     vapor | T59.891 | T59.892 | T59.893 | T59.894 | — | — |
|   alcohol | T51.3X1 | T51.3X2 | T51.3X3 | T51.3X4 | — | — |
|   chloride | T53.6X1 | T53.6X2 | T53.6X3 | T53.6X4 | — | — |
|   formate | T52.8X1 | T52.8X2 | T52.8X3 | T52.8X4 | — | — |
|   nitrite | T46.3X1 | T46.3X2 | T46.3X3 | T46.3X4 | T46.3X5 | T46.3X6 |
|   propionate | T65.891 | T65.892 | T65.893 | T65.894 | — | — |
| **Amylase** | T47.5X1 | T47.5X2 | T47.5X3 | T47.5X4 | T47.5X5 | T47.5X6 |
| **Amyleine, regional** | T41.3X1 | T41.3X2 | T41.3X3 | T41.3X4 | T41.3X5 | T41.3X6 |
| **Amylene** | | | | | | |
|   dichloride | T53.6X1 | T53.6X2 | T53.6X3 | T53.6X4 | — | — |
|   hydrate | T51.3X1 | T51.3X2 | T51.3X3 | T51.3X4 | — | — |
| **Amylmetacresol** | T49.6X1 | T49.6X2 | T49.6X3 | T49.6X4 | T49.6X5 | T49.6X6 |
| **Amylobarbitone** | T42.3X1 | T42.3X2 | T42.3X3 | T42.3X4 | T42.3X5 | T42.3X6 |
| **Amylocaine, regional** | T41.3X1 | T41.3X2 | T41.3X3 | T41.3X4 | T41.3X5 | T41.3X6 |
|   infiltration (subcutaneous) | T41.3X1 | T41.3X2 | T41.3X3 | T41.3X4 | T41.3X5 | T41.3X6 |
|   nerve block (peripheral) (plexus) | T41.3X1 | T41.3X2 | T41.3X3 | T41.3X4 | T41.3X5 | T41.3X6 |
|   spinal | T41.3X1 | T41.3X2 | T41.3X3 | T41.3X4 | T41.3X5 | T41.3X6 |
|   topical (surface) | T41.3X1 | T41.3X2 | T41.3X3 | T41.3X4 | T41.3X5 | T41.3X6 |
| **Amylopectin** | T47.6X1 | T47.6X2 | T47.6X3 | T47.6X4 | T47.6X5 | T47.6X6 |
| **Amytal** (sodium) | T42.3X1 | T42.3X2 | T42.3X3 | T42.3X4 | T42.3X5 | T42.3X6 |
| **Anabolic steroid** | T38.7X1 | T38.7X2 | T38.7X3 | T38.7X4 | T38.7X5 | T38.7X6 |
| **Analeptic NEC** | T50.7X1 | T50.7X2 | T50.7X3 | T50.7X4 | T50.7X5 | T50.7X6 |
| **Analgesic** | T39.91 | T39.92 | T39.93 | T39.94 | T39.95 | T39.96 |
|   anti-inflammatory NEC | T39.91 | T39.92 | T39.93 | T39.94 | T39.95 | T39.96 |
|     propionic acid derivative | T39.311 | T39.312 | T39.313 | T39.314 | T39.315 | T39.316 |
|   antirheumatic NEC | T39.4X1 | T39.4X2 | T39.4X3 | T39.4X4 | T39.4X5 | T39.4X6 |
|   aromatic NEC | T39.1X1 | T39.1X2 | T39.1X3 | T39.1X4 | T39.1X5 | T39.1X6 |
|   narcotic NEC | T40.601 | T40.602 | T40.603 | T40.604 | T40.605 | T40.606 |
|     combination | T40.601 | T40.602 | T40.603 | T40.604 | T40.605 | T40.606 |
|     obstetric | T40.601 | T40.602 | T40.603 | T40.604 | T40.605 | T40.606 |
|   non-narcotic NEC | T39.91 | T39.92 | T39.93 | T39.94 | T39.95 | T39.96 |
|     combination | T39.91 | T39.92 | T39.93 | T39.94 | T39.95 | T39.96 |
|   pyrazole | T39.2X1 | T39.2X2 | T39.2X3 | T39.2X4 | T39.2X5 | T39.2X6 |
|   specified NEC | T39.8X1 | T39.8X2 | T39.8X3 | T39.8X4 | T39.8X5 | T39.8X6 |
| **Analgin** | T39.2X1 | T39.2X2 | T39.2X3 | T39.2X4 | T39.2X5 | T39.2X6 |
| **Anamirta cocculus** | T62.1X1 | T62.1X2 | T62.1X3 | T62.1X4 | — | — |
| **Ancillin** | T36.0X1 | T36.0X2 | T36.0X3 | T36.0X4 | T36.0X5 | T36.0X6 |
| **Ancrod** | T45.691 | T45.692 | T45.693 | T45.694 | T45.695 | T45.696 |
| **Androgen** | T38.7X1 | T38.7X2 | T38.7X3 | T38.7X4 | T38.7X5 | T38.7X6 |
| **Androgen-estrogen mixture** | T38.7X1 | T38.7X2 | T38.7X3 | T38.7X4 | T38.7X5 | T38.7X6 |
| **Androstalone** | T38.7X1 | T38.7X2 | T38.7X3 | T38.7X4 | T38.7X5 | T38.7X6 |
| **Androstanolone** | T38.7X1 | T38.7X2 | T38.7X3 | T38.7X4 | T38.7X5 | T38.7X6 |
| **Androsterone** | T38.7X1 | T38.7X2 | T38.7X3 | T38.7X4 | T38.7X5 | T38.7X6 |
| **Anemone pulsatilla** | T62.2X1 | T62.2X2 | T62.2X3 | T62.2X4 | — | — |
| **Anesthesia** | | | | | | |
|   caudal | T41.3X1 | T41.3X2 | T41.3X3 | T41.3X4 | T41.3X5 | T41.3X6 |
|   endotracheal | T41.0X1 | T41.0X2 | T41.0X3 | T41.0X4 | T41.0X5 | T41.0X6 |
|   epidural | T41.3X1 | T41.3X2 | T41.3X3 | T41.3X4 | T41.3X5 | T41.3X6 |
|   inhalation | T41.0X1 | T41.0X2 | T41.0X3 | T41.0X4 | T41.0X5 | T41.0X6 |
|   local | T41.3X1 | T41.3X2 | T41.3X3 | T41.3X4 | T41.3X5 | T41.3X6 |
|   mucosal | T41.3X1 | T41.3X2 | T41.3X3 | T41.3X4 | T41.3X5 | T41.3X6 |
|   muscle relaxation | T48.1X1 | T48.1X2 | T48.1X3 | T48.1X4 | T48.1X5 | T48.1X6 |
|   nerve blocking | T41.3X1 | T41.3X2 | T41.3X3 | T41.3X4 | T41.3X5 | T41.3X6 |
|   plexus blocking | T41.3X1 | T41.3X2 | T41.3X3 | T41.3X4 | T41.3X5 | T41.3X6 |
|   potentiated | T41.201 | T41.202 | T41.203 | T41.204 | T41.205 | T41.206 |
|   rectal | T41.201 | T41.202 | T41.203 | T41.204 | T41.205 | T41.206 |
|     general | T41.201 | T41.202 | T41.203 | T41.204 | T41.205 | T41.206 |
|     local | T41.3X1 | T41.3X2 | T41.3X3 | T41.3X4 | T41.3X5 | T41.3X6 |
|   regional | T41.3X1 | T41.3X2 | T41.3X3 | T41.3X4 | T41.3X5 | T41.3X6 |
|   surface | T41.3X1 | T41.3X2 | T41.3X3 | T41.3X4 | T41.3X5 | T41.3X6 |
| **Anesthetic NEC** — see also Anesthesia | T41.41 | T41.42 | T41.43 | T41.44 | T41.45 | T41.46 |
|   with muscle relaxant | T41.201 | T41.202 | T41.203 | T41.204 | T41.205 | T41.206 |
|     general | T41.201 | T41.202 | T41.203 | T41.204 | T41.205 | T41.206 |
|     local | T41.3X1 | T41.3X2 | T41.3X3 | T41.3X4 | T41.3X5 | T41.3X6 |
|   gaseous NEC | T41.0X1 | T41.0X2 | T41.0X3 | T41.0X4 | T41.0X5 | T41.0X6 |

▽ Subterms under main terms may continue to next column or page    Additional Character May Be Required — Refer to the Tabular List for Character Selection    351

Amanitine — Anesthetic NEC

Table of Drugs and Chemicals

| Substance | Poisoning, Accidental (unintentional) | Poisoning, Intentional Self-harm | Poisoning, Assault | Poisoning, Undetermined | Adverse Effect | Under-dosing |
|---|---|---|---|---|---|---|
| **Anesthetic** — *see also* Anesthesia — *continued* | | | | | | |
| general NEC | T41.201 | T41.202 | T41.203 | T41.204 | T41.205 | T41.206 |
| halogenated hydrocarbon derivatives NEC | T41.0X1 | T41.0X2 | T41.0X3 | T41.0X4 | T41.0X5 | T41.0X6 |
| infiltration NEC | T41.3X1 | T41.3X2 | T41.3X3 | T41.3X4 | T41.3X5 | T41.3X6 |
| intravenous NEC | T41.1X1 | T41.1X2 | T41.1X3 | T41.1X4 | T41.1X5 | T41.1X6 |
| local NEC | T41.3X1 | T41.3X2 | T41.3X3 | T41.3X4 | T41.3X5 | T41.3X6 |
| rectal | T41.201 | T41.202 | T41.203 | T41.204 | T41.205 | T41.206 |
| general | T41.201 | T41.202 | T41.203 | T41.204 | T41.205 | T41.206 |
| local | T41.3X1 | T41.3X2 | T41.3X3 | T41.3X4 | T41.3X5 | T41.3X6 |
| regional NEC | T41.3X1 | T41.3X2 | T41.3X3 | T41.3X4 | T41.3X5 | T41.3X6 |
| spinal NEC | T41.3X1 | T41.3X2 | T41.3X3 | T41.3X4 | T41.3X5 | T41.3X6 |
| thiobarbiturate | T41.1X1 | T41.1X2 | T41.1X3 | T41.1X4 | T41.1X5 | T41.1X6 |
| topical | T41.3X1 | T41.3X2 | T41.3X3 | T41.3X4 | T41.3X5 | T41.3X6 |
| **Aneurine** | T45.2X1 | T45.2X2 | T45.2X3 | T45.2X4 | T45.2X5 | T45.2X6 |
| **Angio-Conray** | T50.8X1 | T50.8X2 | T50.8X3 | T50.8X4 | T50.8X5 | T50.8X6 |
| **Angiotensin** | T44.5X1 | T44.5X2 | T44.5X3 | T44.5X4 | T44.5X5 | T44.5X6 |
| **Angiotensinamide** | T44.991 | T44.992 | T44.993 | T44.994 | T44.995 | T44.996 |
| **Anhydrohydroxy-progesterone** | T38.5X1 | T38.5X2 | T38.5X3 | T38.5X4 | T38.5X5 | T38.5X6 |
| **Anhydron** | T50.2X1 | T50.2X2 | T50.2X3 | T50.2X4 | T50.2X5 | T50.2X6 |
| **Anileridine** | T40.4X1 | T40.4X2 | T40.4X3 | T40.4X4 | T40.4X5 | T40.4X6 |
| **Aniline** (dye) (liquid) | T65.3X1 | T65.3X2 | T65.3X3 | T65.3X4 | — | — |
| analgesic | T39.1X1 | T39.1X2 | T39.1X3 | T39.1X4 | T39.1X5 | T39.1X6 |
| derivatives, therapeutic NEC | T39.1X1 | T39.1X2 | T39.1X3 | T39.1X4 | T39.1X5 | T39.1X6 |
| vapor | T65.3X1 | T65.3X2 | T65.3X3 | T65.3X4 | — | — |
| **Aniscoropine** | T44.3X1 | T44.3X2 | T44.3X3 | T44.3X4 | T44.3X5 | T44.3X6 |
| **Anise oil** | T47.5X1 | T47.5X2 | T47.5X3 | T47.5X4 | T47.5X5 | T47.5X6 |
| **Anisidine** | T65.3X1 | T65.3X2 | T65.3X3 | T65.3X4 | — | — |
| **Anisindione** | T45.511 | T45.512 | T45.513 | T45.514 | T45.515 | T45.516 |
| **Anisotropine** methyl-bromide | T44.3X1 | T44.3X2 | T44.3X3 | T44.3X4 | T44.3X5 | T44.3X6 |
| **Anistreplase** | T45.611 | T45.612 | T45.613 | T45.614 | T45.615 | T45.616 |
| **Anorexiant** (central) | T50.5X1 | T50.5X2 | T50.5X3 | T50.5X4 | T50.5X5 | T50.5X6 |
| **Anorexic agents** | T50.5X1 | T50.5X2 | T50.5X3 | T50.5X4 | T50.5X5 | T50.5X6 |
| **Ansamycin** | T36.6X1 | T36.6X2 | T36.6X3 | T36.6X4 | T36.6X5 | T36.6X6 |
| **Ant** (bite) (sting) | T63.421 | T63.422 | T63.423 | T63.424 | — | — |
| **Antabuse** | T50.6X1 | T50.6X2 | T50.6X3 | T50.6X4 | T50.6X5 | T50.6X6 |
| **Antacid NEC** | T47.1X1 | T47.1X2 | T47.1X3 | T47.1X4 | T47.1X5 | T47.1X6 |
| **Antagonist** | | | | | | |
| Aldosterone | T50.0X1 | T50.0X2 | T50.0X3 | T50.0X4 | T50.0X5 | T50.0X6 |
| alpha-adrenoreceptor | T44.6X1 | T44.6X2 | T44.6X3 | T44.6X4 | T44.6X5 | T44.6X6 |
| anticoagulant | T45.7X1 | T45.7X2 | T45.7X3 | T45.7X4 | T45.7X5 | T45.7X6 |
| beta-adrenoreceptor | T44.7X1 | T44.7X2 | T44.7X3 | T44.7X4 | T44.7X5 | T44.7X6 |
| extrapyramidal NEC | T44.3X1 | T44.3X2 | T44.3X3 | T44.3X4 | T44.3X5 | T44.3X6 |
| folic acid | T45.1X1 | T45.1X2 | T45.1X3 | T45.1X4 | T45.1X5 | T45.1X6 |
| H2 receptor | T47.0X1 | T47.0X2 | T47.0X3 | T47.0X4 | T47.0X5 | T47.0X6 |
| heavy metal | T45.8X1 | T45.8X2 | T45.8X3 | T45.8X4 | T45.8X5 | T45.8X6 |
| narcotic analgesic | T50.7X1 | T50.7X2 | T50.7X3 | T50.7X4 | T50.7X5 | T50.7X6 |
| opiate | T50.7X1 | T50.7X2 | T50.7X3 | T50.7X4 | T50.7X5 | T50.7X6 |
| pyrimidine | T45.1X1 | T45.1X2 | T45.1X3 | T45.1X4 | T45.1X5 | T45.1X6 |
| serotonin | T46.5X1 | T46.5X2 | T46.5X3 | T46.5X4 | T46.5X5 | T46.5X6 |
| **Antazolin** (e) | T45.0X1 | T45.0X2 | T45.0X3 | T45.0X4 | T45.0X5 | T45.0X6 |
| **Anterior pituitary hormone NEC** | T38.811 | T38.812 | T38.813 | T38.814 | T38.815 | T38.816 |
| **Anthelmintic NEC** | T37.4X1 | T37.4X2 | T37.4X3 | T37.4X4 | T37.4X5 | T37.4X6 |
| **Anthiolimine** | T37.4X1 | T37.4X2 | T37.4X3 | T37.4X4 | T37.4X5 | T37.4X6 |
| **Anthralin** | T49.4X1 | T49.4X2 | T49.4X3 | T49.4X4 | T49.4X5 | T49.4X6 |
| **Anthramycin** | T45.1X1 | T45.1X2 | T45.1X3 | T45.1X4 | T45.1X5 | T45.1X6 |
| **Antiadrenergic NEC** | T44.8X1 | T44.8X2 | T44.8X3 | T44.8X4 | T44.8X5 | T44.8X6 |
| **Antiallergic NEC** | T45.0X1 | T45.0X2 | T45.0X3 | T45.0X4 | T45.0X5 | T45.0X6 |
| **Antiandrogen NEC** | T38.6X1 | T38.6X2 | T38.6X3 | T38.6X4 | T38.6X5 | T38.6X6 |
| **Anti-anemic** (drug) (preparation) | T45.8X1 | T45.8X2 | T45.8X3 | T45.8X4 | T45.8X5 | T45.8X6 |
| **Antianxiety drug NEC** | T43.501 | T43.502 | T43.503 | T43.504 | T43.505 | T43.506 |
| **Antiaris toxicaria** | T65.891 | T65.892 | T65.893 | T65.894 | — | — |
| **Antiarteriosclerotic drug** | T46.6X1 | T46.6X2 | T46.6X3 | T46.6X4 | T46.6X5 | T46.6X6 |
| **Antiasthmatic drug NEC** | T48.6X1 | T48.6X2 | T48.6X3 | T48.6X4 | T48.6X5 | T48.6X6 |
| **Antibiotic NEC** | T36.91 | T36.92 | T36.93 | T36.94 | T36.95 | T36.96 |
| aminoglycoside | T36.5X1 | T36.5X2 | T36.5X3 | T36.5X4 | T36.5X5 | T36.5X6 |
| anticancer | T45.1X1 | T45.1X2 | T45.1X3 | T45.1X4 | T45.1X5 | T45.1X6 |
| antifungal | T36.7X1 | T36.7X2 | T36.7X3 | T36.7X4 | T36.7X5 | T36.7X6 |
| antimycobacterial | T36.5X1 | T36.5X2 | T36.5X3 | T36.5X4 | T36.5X5 | T36.5X6 |
| antineoplastic | T45.1X1 | T45.1X2 | T45.1X3 | T45.1X4 | T45.1X5 | T45.1X6 |
| b-lactam NEC | T36.1X1 | T36.1X2 | T36.1X3 | T36.1X4 | T36.1X5 | T36.1X6 |
| cephalosporin (group) | T36.1X1 | T36.1X2 | T36.1X3 | T36.1X4 | T36.1X5 | T36.1X6 |
| chloramphenicol (group) | T36.2X1 | T36.2X2 | T36.2X3 | T36.2X4 | T36.2X5 | T36.2X6 |
| ENT | T49.6X1 | T49.6X2 | T49.6X3 | T49.6X4 | T49.6X5 | T49.6X6 |
| eye | T49.5X1 | T49.5X2 | T49.5X3 | T49.5X4 | T49.5X5 | T49.5X6 |
| fungicidal (local) | T49.0X1 | T49.0X2 | T49.0X3 | T49.0X4 | T49.0X5 | T49.0X6 |
| intestinal | T36.8X1 | T36.8X2 | T36.8X3 | T36.8X4 | T36.8X5 | T36.8X6 |
| local | T49.0X1 | T49.0X2 | T49.0X3 | T49.0X4 | T49.0X5 | T49.0X6 |
| **Antibiotic** — *continued* | | | | | | |
| macrolides | T36.3X1 | T36.3X2 | T36.3X3 | T36.3X4 | T36.3X5 | T36.3X6 |
| polypeptide | T36.8X1 | T36.8X2 | T36.8X3 | T36.8X4 | T36.8X5 | T36.8X6 |
| specified NEC | T36.8X1 | T36.8X2 | T36.8X3 | T36.8X4 | T36.8X5 | T36.8X6 |
| tetracycline (group) | T36.4X1 | T36.4X2 | T36.4X3 | T36.4X4 | T36.4X5 | T36.4X6 |
| throat | T49.6X1 | T49.6X2 | T49.6X3 | T49.6X4 | T49.6X5 | T49.6X6 |
| **Anticancer agents NEC** | T45.1X1 | T45.1X2 | T45.1X3 | T45.1X4 | T45.1X5 | T45.1X6 |
| **Anticholesterolemic drug NEC** | T46.6X1 | T46.6X2 | T46.6X3 | T46.6X4 | T46.6X5 | T46.6X6 |
| **Anticholinergic NEC** | T44.3X1 | T44.3X2 | T44.3X3 | T44.3X4 | T44.3X5 | T44.3X6 |
| **Anticholinesterase** | T44.0X1 | T44.0X2 | T44.0X3 | T44.0X4 | T44.0X5 | T44.0X6 |
| organophosphorus | T44.0X1 | T44.0X2 | T44.0X3 | T44.0X4 | T44.0X5 | T44.0X6 |
| insecticide | T60.0X1 | T60.0X2 | T60.0X3 | T60.0X4 | — | — |
| nerve gas | T59.891 | T59.892 | T59.893 | T59.894 | — | — |
| reversible | T44.0X1 | T44.0X2 | T44.0X3 | T44.0X4 | T44.0X5 | T44.0X6 |
| ophthalmological | T49.5X1 | T49.5X2 | T49.5X3 | T49.5X4 | T49.5X5 | T49.5X6 |
| **Anticoagulant NEC** | T45.511 | T45.512 | T45.513 | T45.514 | T45.515 | T45.516 |
| Antagonist | T45.7X1 | T45.7X2 | T45.7X3 | T45.7X4 | T45.7X5 | T45.7X6 |
| **Anti-common-cold drug NEC** | T48.5X1 | T48.5X2 | T48.5X3 | T48.5X4 | T48.5X5 | T48.5X6 |
| **Anticonvulsant** | T42.71 | T42.72 | T42.73 | T42.74 | T42.75 | T42.76 |
| barbiturate | T42.3X1 | T42.3X2 | T42.3X3 | T42.3X4 | T42.3X5 | T42.3X6 |
| combination (with barbiturate) | T42.3X1 | T42.3X2 | T42.3X3 | T42.3X4 | T42.3X5 | T42.3X6 |
| hydantoin | T42.0X1 | T42.0X2 | T42.0X3 | T42.0X4 | T42.0X5 | T42.0X6 |
| hypnotic NEC | T42.6X1 | T42.6X2 | T42.6X3 | T42.6X4 | T42.6X5 | T42.6X6 |
| oxazolidinedione | T42.2X1 | T42.2X2 | T42.2X3 | T42.2X4 | T42.2X5 | T42.2X6 |
| pyrimidinedione | T42.6X1 | T42.6X2 | T42.6X3 | T42.6X4 | T42.6X5 | T42.6X6 |
| specified NEC | T42.6X1 | T42.6X2 | T42.6X3 | T42.6X4 | T42.6X5 | T42.6X6 |
| succinimide | T42.2X1 | T42.2X2 | T42.2X3 | T42.2X4 | T42.2X5 | T42.2X6 |
| **Antidepressant** | T43.201 | T43.202 | T43.203 | T43.204 | T43.205 | T43.206 |
| monoamine oxidase inhibitor | T43.1X1 | T43.1X2 | T43.1X3 | T43.1X4 | T43.1X5 | T43.1X6 |
| selective serotonin norepinephrine reuptake inhibitor | T43.211 | T43.212 | T43.213 | T43.214 | T43.215 | T43.216 |
| selective serotonin reuptake inhibitor | T43.221 | T43.222 | T43.223 | T43.224 | T43.225 | T43.226 |
| specified NEC | T43.291 | T43.292 | T43.293 | T43.294 | T43.295 | T43.296 |
| tetracyclic | T43.021 | T43.022 | T43.023 | T43.024 | T43.025 | T43.026 |
| triazolopyridine | T43.211 | T43.212 | T43.213 | T43.214 | T43.215 | T43.216 |
| tricyclic | T43.011 | T43.012 | T43.013 | T43.014 | T43.015 | T43.016 |
| **Antidiabetic NEC** | T38.3X1 | T38.3X2 | T38.3X3 | T38.3X4 | T38.3X5 | T38.3X6 |
| biguanide | T38.3X1 | T38.3X2 | T38.3X3 | T38.3X4 | T38.3X5 | T38.3X6 |
| and sulfonyl combined | T38.3X1 | T38.3X2 | T38.3X3 | T38.3X4 | T38.3X5 | T38.3X6 |
| combined | T38.3X1 | T38.3X2 | T38.3X3 | T38.3X4 | T38.3X5 | T38.3X6 |
| sulfonylurea | T38.3X1 | T38.3X2 | T38.3X3 | T38.3X4 | T38.3X5 | T38.3X6 |
| **Antidiarrheal drug NEC** | T47.6X1 | T47.6X2 | T47.6X3 | T47.6X4 | T47.6X5 | T47.6X6 |
| absorbent | T47.6X1 | T47.6X2 | T47.6X3 | T47.6X4 | T47.6X5 | T47.6X6 |
| **Anti-D immunoglobulin** (human) | T50.Z11 | T50.Z12 | T50.Z13 | T50.Z14 | T50.Z15 | T50.Z16 |
| **Antidiphtheria serum** | T50.Z11 | T50.Z12 | T50.Z13 | T50.Z14 | T50.Z15 | T50.Z16 |
| **Antidiuretic hormone** | T38.891 | T38.892 | T38.893 | T38.894 | T38.895 | T38.896 |
| **Antidote NEC** | T50.6X1 | T50.6X2 | T50.6X3 | T50.6X4 | T50.6X5 | T50.6X6 |
| heavy metal | T45.8X1 | T45.8X2 | T45.8X3 | T45.8X4 | T45.8X5 | T45.8X6 |
| **Antidysrhythmic NEC** | T46.2X1 | T46.2X2 | T46.2X3 | T46.2X4 | T46.2X5 | T46.2X6 |
| **Antiemetic drug** | T45.0X1 | T45.0X2 | T45.0X3 | T45.0X4 | T45.0X5 | T45.0X6 |
| **Antiepilepsy agent** | T42.71 | T42.72 | T42.73 | T42.74 | T42.75 | T42.76 |
| combination | T42.5X1 | T42.5X2 | T42.5X3 | T42.5X4 | T42.5X5 | T42.5X6 |
| mixed | T42.5X1 | T42.5X2 | T42.5X3 | T42.5X4 | T42.5X5 | T42.5X6 |
| specified, NEC | T42.6X1 | T42.6X2 | T42.6X3 | T42.6X4 | T42.6X5 | T42.6X6 |
| **Antiestrogen NEC** | T38.6X1 | T38.6X2 | T38.6X3 | T38.6X4 | T38.6X5 | T38.6X6 |
| **Antifertility pill** | T38.4X1 | T38.4X2 | T38.4X3 | T38.4X4 | T38.4X5 | T38.4X6 |
| **Antifibrinolytic drug** | T45.621 | T45.622 | T45.623 | T45.624 | T45.625 | T45.626 |
| **Antifilarial drug** | T37.4X1 | T37.4X2 | T37.4X3 | T37.4X4 | T37.4X5 | T37.4X6 |
| **Antiflatulent** | T47.5X1 | T47.5X2 | T47.5X3 | T47.5X4 | T47.5X5 | T47.5X6 |
| **Antifreeze** | T65.91 | T65.92 | T65.93 | T65.94 | — | — |
| alcohol | T51.1X1 | T51.1X2 | T51.1X3 | T51.1X4 | — | — |
| ethylene glycol | T51.8X1 | T51.8X2 | T51.8X3 | T51.8X4 | — | — |
| **Antifungal** | | | | | | |
| antibiotic (systemic) | T36.7X1 | T36.7X2 | T36.7X3 | T36.7X4 | T36.7X5 | T36.7X6 |
| anti-infective NEC | T37.91 | T37.92 | T37.93 | T37.94 | T37.95 | T37.96 |
| disinfectant, local | T49.0X1 | T49.0X2 | T49.0X3 | T49.0X4 | T49.0X5 | T49.0X6 |
| nonmedicinal (spray) | T60.3X1 | T60.3X2 | T60.3X3 | T60.3X4 | — | — |
| topical | T49.0X1 | T49.0X2 | T49.0X3 | T49.0X4 | T49.0X5 | T49.0X6 |
| **Anti-gastric-secretion drug NEC** | T47.1X1 | T47.1X2 | T47.1X3 | T47.1X4 | T47.1X5 | T47.1X6 |
| **Antigonadotrophin NEC** | T38.6X1 | T38.6X2 | T38.6X3 | T38.6X4 | T38.6X5 | T38.6X6 |
| **Antihallucinogen** | T43.501 | T43.502 | T43.503 | T43.504 | T43.505 | T43.506 |
| **Antihelmintics** | T37.4X1 | T37.4X2 | T37.4X3 | T37.4X4 | T37.4X5 | T37.4X6 |
| **Antihemophilic** | | | | | | |
| factor | T45.8X1 | T45.8X2 | T45.8X3 | T45.8X4 | T45.8X5 | T45.8X6 |
| fraction | T45.8X1 | T45.8X2 | T45.8X3 | T45.8X4 | T45.8X5 | T45.8X6 |

Anesthetic NEC — Antihemophilic

**Additional Character May Be Required — Refer to the Tabular List for Character Selection**

▽ **Subterms under main terms may continue to next column or page**

**Table of Drugs and Chemicals**

| Substance | Poisoning, Accidental (unintentional) | Poisoning, Intentional Self-harm | Poisoning, Assault | Poisoning, Undetermined | Adverse Effect | Under-dosing |
|---|---|---|---|---|---|---|
| **Antihemophilic** — *continued* | | | | | | |
| globulin concentrate | T45.7X1 | T45.7X2 | T45.7X3 | T45.7X4 | T45.7X5 | T45.7X6 |
| human plasma | T45.8X1 | T45.8X2 | T45.8X3 | T45.8X4 | T45.8X5 | T45.8X6 |
| plasma, dried | T45.7X1 | T45.7X2 | T45.7X3 | T45.7X4 | T45.7X5 | T45.7X6 |
| **Antihemorrhoidal preparation** | T49.2X1 | T49.2X2 | T49.2X3 | T49.2X4 | T49.2X5 | T49.2X6 |
| **Antiheparin drug** | T45.7X1 | T45.7X2 | T45.7X3 | T45.7X4 | T45.7X5 | T45.7X6 |
| **Antihistamine** | T45.0X1 | T45.0X2 | T45.0X3 | T45.0X4 | T45.0X5 | T45.0X6 |
| **Antihookworm drug** | T37.4X1 | T37.4X2 | T37.4X3 | T37.4X4 | T37.4X5 | T37.4X6 |
| **Anti-human lymphocytic globulin** | T50.Z11 | T50.Z12 | T50.Z13 | T50.Z14 | T50.Z15 | T50.Z16 |
| **Antihyperlipidemic drug** | T46.6X1 | T46.6X2 | T46.6X3 | T46.6X4 | T46.6X5 | T46.6X6 |
| **Antihypertensive drug NEC** | T46.5X1 | T46.5X2 | T46.5X3 | T46.5X4 | T46.5X5 | T46.5X6 |
| **Anti-infective NEC** | T37.91 | T37.92 | T37.93 | T37.94 | T37.95 | T37.96 |
| anthelmintic | T37.4X1 | T37.4X2 | T37.4X3 | T37.4X4 | T37.4X5 | T37.4X6 |
| antibiotics | T36.91 | T36.92 | T36.93 | T36.94 | T36.95 | T36.96 |
| specified NEC | T36.8X1 | T36.8X2 | T36.8X3 | T36.8X4 | T36.8X5 | T36.8X6 |
| antimalarial | T37.2X1 | T37.2X2 | T37.2X3 | T37.2X4 | T37.2X5 | T37.2X6 |
| antimycobacterial NEC | T37.1X1 | T37.1X2 | T37.1X3 | T37.1X4 | T37.1X5 | T37.1X6 |
| antibiotics | T36.5X1 | T36.5X2 | T36.5X3 | T36.5X4 | T36.5X5 | T36.5X6 |
| antiprotozoal NEC | T37.3X1 | T37.3X2 | T37.3X3 | T37.3X4 | T37.3X5 | T37.3X6 |
| blood | T37.2X1 | T37.2X2 | T37.2X3 | T37.2X4 | T37.2X5 | T37.2X6 |
| antiviral | T37.5X1 | T37.5X2 | T37.5X3 | T37.5X4 | T37.5X5 | T37.5X6 |
| arsenical | T37.8X1 | T37.8X2 | T37.8X3 | T37.8X4 | T37.8X5 | T37.8X6 |
| bismuth, local | T49.0X1 | T49.0X2 | T49.0X3 | T49.0X4 | T49.0X5 | T49.0X6 |
| ENT | T49.6X1 | T49.6X2 | T49.6X3 | T49.6X4 | T49.6X5 | T49.6X6 |
| eye NEC | T49.5X1 | T49.5X2 | T49.5X3 | T49.5X4 | T49.5X5 | T49.5X6 |
| heavy metals NEC | T37.8X1 | T37.8X2 | T37.8X3 | T37.8X4 | T37.8X5 | T37.8X6 |
| local NEC | T49.0X1 | T49.0X2 | T49.0X3 | T49.0X4 | T49.0X5 | T49.0X6 |
| specified NEC | T49.0X1 | T49.0X2 | T49.0X3 | T49.0X4 | T49.0X5 | T49.0X6 |
| mixed | T37.91 | T37.92 | T37.93 | T37.94 | T37.95 | T37.96 |
| ophthalmic preparation | T49.5X1 | T49.5X2 | T49.5X3 | T49.5X4 | T49.5X5 | T49.5X6 |
| topical NEC | T49.0X1 | T49.0X2 | T49.0X3 | T49.0X4 | T49.0X5 | T49.0X6 |
| **Anti-inflammatory drug NEC** | T39.391 | T39.392 | T39.393 | T39.394 | T39.395 | T39.396 |
| local | T49.0X1 | T49.0X2 | T49.0X3 | T49.0X4 | T49.0X5 | T49.0X6 |
| nonsteroidal NEC | T39.391 | T39.392 | T39.393 | T39.394 | T39.395 | T39.396 |
| propionic acid derivative | T39.311 | T39.312 | T39.313 | T39.314 | T39.315 | T39.316 |
| specified NEC | T39.391 | T39.392 | T39.393 | T39.394 | T39.395 | T39.396 |
| **Antikaluretic** | T50.3X1 | T50.3X2 | T50.3X3 | T50.3X4 | T50.3X5 | T50.3X6 |
| **Antiknock** (tetraethyl lead) | T56.0X1 | T56.0X2 | T56.0X3 | T56.0X4 | — | — |
| **Antilipemic drug NEC** | T46.6X1 | T46.6X2 | T46.6X3 | T46.6X4 | T46.6X5 | T46.6X6 |
| **Antimalarial** | T37.2X1 | T37.2X2 | T37.2X3 | T37.2X4 | T37.2X5 | T37.2X6 |
| prophylactic NEC | T37.2X1 | T37.2X2 | T37.2X3 | T37.2X4 | T37.2X5 | T37.2X6 |
| pyrimidine derivative | T37.2X1 | T37.2X2 | T37.2X3 | T37.2X4 | T37.2X5 | T37.2X6 |
| **Antimetabolite** | T45.1X1 | T45.1X2 | T45.1X3 | T45.1X4 | T45.1X5 | T45.1X6 |
| **Antimitotic agent** | T45.1X1 | T45.1X2 | T45.1X3 | T45.1X4 | T45.1X5 | T45.1X6 |
| **Antimony** (compounds) (vapor) **NEC** | T56.891 | T56.892 | T56.893 | T56.894 | — | — |
| anti-infectives | T37.8X1 | T37.8X2 | T37.8X3 | T37.8X4 | T37.8X5 | T37.8X6 |
| dimercaptosuccinate | T37.3X1 | T37.3X2 | T37.3X3 | T37.3X4 | T37.3X5 | T37.3X6 |
| hydride | T56.891 | T56.892 | T56.893 | T56.894 | — | — |
| pesticide (vapor) | T60.8X1 | T60.8X2 | T60.8X3 | T60.8X4 | — | — |
| potassium (sodium) tartrate | T37.8X1 | T37.8X2 | T37.8X3 | T37.8X4 | — | T37.8X6 |
| sodium dimercaptosuccinate | T37.3X1 | T37.3X2 | T37.3X3 | T37.3X4 | T37.3X5 | T37.3X6 |
| tartrate | T37.8X1 | T37.8X2 | T37.8X3 | T37.8X4 | T37.8X5 | T37.8X6 |
| **Antimuscarinic NEC** | T44.3X1 | T44.3X2 | T44.3X3 | T44.3X4 | T44.3X5 | T44.3X6 |
| **Antimycobacterial drug NEC** | T37.1X1 | T37.1X2 | T37.1X3 | T37.1X4 | T37.1X5 | T37.1X6 |
| antibiotics | T36.5X1 | T36.5X2 | T36.5X3 | T36.5X4 | T36.5X5 | T36.5X6 |
| combination | T37.1X1 | T37.1X2 | T37.1X3 | T37.1X4 | T37.1X5 | T37.1X6 |
| **Antinausea drug** | T45.0X1 | T45.0X2 | T45.0X3 | T45.0X4 | T45.0X5 | T45.0X6 |
| **Antinematode drug** | T37.4X1 | T37.4X2 | T37.4X3 | T37.4X4 | T37.4X5 | T37.4X6 |
| **Antineoplastic NEC** | T45.1X1 | T45.1X2 | T45.1X3 | T45.1X4 | T45.1X5 | T45.1X6 |
| alkaloidal | T45.1X1 | T45.1X2 | T45.1X3 | T45.1X4 | T45.1X5 | T45.1X6 |
| antibiotics | T45.1X1 | T45.1X2 | T45.1X3 | T45.1X4 | T45.1X5 | T45.1X6 |
| combination | T45.1X1 | T45.1X2 | T45.1X3 | T45.1X4 | T45.1X5 | T45.1X6 |
| estrogen | T38.5X1 | T38.5X2 | T38.5X3 | T38.5X4 | T38.5X5 | T38.5X6 |
| steroid | T38.7X1 | T38.7X2 | T38.7X3 | T38.7X4 | T38.7X5 | T38.7X6 |
| **Antiparasitic drug** (systemic) | T37.91 | T37.92 | T37.93 | T37.94 | T37.95 | T37.96 |
| local | T49.0X1 | T49.0X2 | T49.0X3 | T49.0X4 | T49.0X5 | T49.0X6 |
| specified NEC | T37.8X1 | T37.8X2 | T37.8X3 | T37.8X4 | T37.8X5 | T37.8X6 |
| **Antiparkinsonism drug NEC** | T42.8X1 | T42.8X2 | T42.8X3 | T42.8X4 | T42.8X5 | T42.8X6 |
| **Antiperspirant NEC** | T49.2X1 | T49.2X2 | T49.2X3 | T49.2X4 | T49.2X5 | T49.2X6 |
| **Antiphlogistic NEC** | T39.4X1 | T39.4X2 | T39.4X3 | T39.4X4 | T39.4X5 | T39.4X6 |
| **Antiplatyhelmintic drug** | T37.4X1 | T37.4X2 | T37.4X3 | T37.4X4 | T37.4X5 | T37.4X6 |
| **Antiprotozoal drug NEC** | T37.3X1 | T37.3X2 | T37.3X3 | T37.3X4 | T37.3X5 | T37.3X6 |
| blood | T37.2X1 | T37.2X2 | T37.2X3 | T37.2X4 | T37.2X5 | T37.2X6 |
| local | T49.0X1 | T49.0X2 | T49.0X3 | T49.0X4 | T49.0X5 | T49.0X6 |

| Substance | Poisoning, Accidental (unintentional) | Poisoning, Intentional Self-harm | Poisoning, Assault | Poisoning, Undetermined | Adverse Effect | Under-dosing |
|---|---|---|---|---|---|---|
| **Antipruritic drug NEC** | T49.1X1 | T49.1X2 | T49.1X3 | T49.1X4 | T49.1X5 | T49.1X6 |
| **Antipsychotic drug** | T43.501 | T43.502 | T43.503 | T43.504 | T43.505 | T43.506 |
| specified NEC | T43.591 | T43.592 | T43.593 | T43.594 | T43.595 | T43.596 |
| **Antipyretic** | T39.91 | T39.92 | T39.93 | T39.94 | T39.95 | T39.96 |
| specified NEC | T39.8X1 | T39.8X2 | T39.8X3 | T39.8X4 | T39.8X5 | T39.8X6 |
| **Antipyrine** | T39.2X1 | T39.2X2 | T39.2X3 | T39.2X4 | T39.2X5 | T39.2X6 |
| **Antirabies hyperimmune serum** | T50.Z11 | T50.Z12 | T50.Z13 | T50.Z14 | T50.Z15 | T50.Z16 |
| **Antirheumatic NEC** | T39.4X1 | T39.4X2 | T39.4X3 | T39.4X4 | T39.4X5 | T39.4X6 |
| **Antirigidity drug NEC** | T42.8X1 | T42.8X2 | T42.8X3 | T42.8X4 | T42.8X5 | T42.8X6 |
| **Antischistosomal drug** | T37.4X1 | T37.4X2 | T37.4X3 | T37.4X4 | T37.4X5 | T37.4X6 |
| **Antiscorpion sera** | T50.Z11 | T50.Z12 | T50.Z13 | T50.Z14 | T50.Z15 | T50.Z16 |
| **Antiseborrheics** | T49.4X1 | T49.4X2 | T49.4X3 | T49.4X4 | T49.4X5 | T49.4X6 |
| **Antiseptics** (external) (medicinal) | T49.0X1 | T49.0X2 | T49.0X3 | T49.0X4 | T49.0X5 | T49.0X6 |
| **Antistine** | T45.0X1 | T45.0X2 | T45.0X3 | T45.0X4 | T45.0X5 | T45.0X6 |
| **Antitapeworm drug** | T37.4X1 | T37.4X2 | T37.4X3 | T37.4X4 | T37.4X5 | T37.4X6 |
| **Antitetanus immunoglobulin** | T50.Z11 | T50.Z12 | T50.Z13 | T50.Z14 | T50.Z15 | T50.Z16 |
| **Antithrombotic** | T45.521 | T45.522 | T45.523 | T45.524 | T45.525 | T45.526 |
| **Antithyroid drug NEC** | T38.2X1 | T38.2X2 | T38.2X3 | T38.2X4 | T38.2X5 | T38.2X6 |
| **Antitoxin** | T50.Z11 | T50.Z12 | T50.Z13 | T50.Z14 | T50.Z15 | T50.Z16 |
| diphtheria | T50.Z11 | T50.Z12 | T50.Z13 | T50.Z14 | T50.Z15 | T50.Z16 |
| gas gangrene | T50.Z11 | T50.Z12 | T50.Z13 | T50.Z14 | T50.Z15 | T50.Z16 |
| tetanus | T50.Z11 | T50.Z12 | T50.Z13 | T50.Z14 | T50.Z15 | T50.Z16 |
| **Antitrichomonal drug** | T37.3X1 | T37.3X2 | T37.3X3 | T37.3X4 | T37.3X5 | T37.3X6 |
| **Antituberculars** | T37.1X1 | T37.1X2 | T37.1X3 | T37.1X4 | T37.1X5 | T37.1X6 |
| antibiotics | T36.5X1 | T36.5X2 | T36.5X3 | T36.5X4 | T36.5X5 | T36.5X6 |
| **Antitussive NEC** | T48.3X1 | T48.3X2 | T48.3X3 | T48.3X4 | T48.3X5 | T48.3X6 |
| codeine mixture | T40.2X1 | T40.2X2 | T40.2X3 | T40.2X4 | T40.2X5 | T40.2X6 |
| opiate | T40.2X1 | T40.2X2 | T40.2X3 | T40.2X4 | T40.2X5 | T40.2X6 |
| **Antivaricose drug** | T46.8X1 | T46.8X2 | T46.8X3 | T46.8X4 | T46.8X5 | T46.8X6 |
| **Antivenin, antivenom** (sera) | T50.Z11 | T50.Z12 | T50.Z13 | T50.Z14 | T50.Z15 | T50.Z16 |
| crotaline | T50.Z11 | T50.Z12 | T50.Z13 | T50.Z14 | T50.Z15 | T50.Z16 |
| spider bite | T50.Z11 | T50.Z12 | T50.Z13 | T50.Z14 | T50.Z15 | T50.Z16 |
| **Antivertigo drug** | T45.0X1 | T45.0X2 | T45.0X3 | T45.0X4 | T45.0X5 | T45.0X6 |
| **Antiviral drug NEC** | T37.5X1 | T37.5X2 | T37.5X3 | T37.5X4 | T37.5X5 | T37.5X6 |
| eye | T49.5X1 | T49.5X2 | T49.5X3 | T49.5X4 | T49.5X5 | T49.5X6 |
| **Antiwhipworm drug** | T37.4X1 | T37.4X2 | T37.4X3 | T37.4X4 | T37.4X5 | T37.4X6 |
| **Ant poison** — *see* Insecticide | | | | | | |
| **Antrol** — *see also* by specific chemical substance | T60.91 | T60.92 | T60.93 | T60.94 | — | — |
| fungicide | T60.91 | T60.92 | T60.93 | T60.94 | — | — |
| **ANTU** (alpha naphthylthiourea) | T60.4X1 | T60.4X2 | T60.4X3 | T60.4X4 | — | — |
| **Apalcillin** | T36.0X1 | T36.0X2 | T36.0X3 | T36.0X4 | T36.0X5 | T36.0X6 |
| **APC** | T48.5X1 | T48.5X2 | T48.5X3 | T48.5X4 | T48.5X5 | T48.5X6 |
| **Aplonidine** | T44.4X1 | T44.4X2 | T44.4X3 | T44.4X4 | T44.4X5 | T44.4X6 |
| **Apomorphine** | T47.7X1 | T47.7X2 | T47.7X3 | T47.7X4 | T47.7X5 | T47.7X6 |
| **Appetite depressants, central** | T50.5X1 | T50.5X2 | T50.5X3 | T50.5X4 | T50.5X5 | T50.5X6 |
| **Apraclonidine** (hydrochloride) | T44.4X1 | T44.4X2 | T44.4X3 | T44.4X4 | T44.4X5 | T44.4X6 |
| **Apresoline** | T46.5X1 | T46.5X2 | T46.5X3 | T46.5X4 | T46.5X5 | T46.5X6 |
| **Aprindine** | T46.2X1 | T46.2X2 | T46.2X3 | T46.2X4 | T46.2X5 | T46.2X6 |
| **Aprobarbital** | T42.3X1 | T42.3X2 | T42.3X3 | T42.3X4 | T42.3X5 | T42.3X6 |
| **Apronalide** | T42.6X1 | T42.6X2 | T42.6X3 | T42.6X4 | T42.6X5 | T42.6X6 |
| **Aprotinin** | T45.621 | T45.622 | T45.623 | T45.624 | T45.625 | T45.626 |
| **Aptocaine** | T41.3X1 | T41.3X2 | T41.3X3 | T41.3X4 | T41.3X5 | T41.3X6 |
| **Aqua fortis** | T54.2X1 | T54.2X2 | T54.2X3 | T54.2X4 | — | — |
| **Ara-A** | T37.5X1 | T37.5X2 | T37.5X3 | T37.5X4 | T37.5X5 | T37.5X6 |
| **Ara-C** | T45.1X1 | T45.1X2 | T45.1X3 | T45.1X4 | T45.1X5 | T45.1X6 |
| **Arachis oil** | T49.3X1 | T49.3X2 | T49.3X3 | T49.3X4 | T49.3X5 | T49.3X6 |
| cathartic | T47.4X1 | T47.4X2 | T47.4X3 | T47.4X4 | T47.4X5 | T47.4X6 |
| **Aralen** | T37.2X1 | T37.2X2 | T37.2X3 | T37.2X4 | T37.2X5 | T37.2X6 |
| **Arecoline** | T44.1X1 | T44.1X2 | T44.1X3 | T44.1X4 | T44.1X5 | T44.1X6 |
| **Arginine** | T50.991 | T50.992 | T50.993 | T50.994 | T50.995 | T50.996 |
| glutamate | T50.991 | T50.992 | T50.993 | T50.994 | T50.995 | T50.996 |
| **Argyrol** | T49.0X1 | T49.0X2 | T49.0X3 | T49.0X4 | T49.0X5 | T49.0X6 |
| ENT agent | T49.6X1 | T49.6X2 | T49.6X3 | T49.6X4 | T49.6X5 | T49.6X6 |
| ophthalmic preparation | T49.5X1 | T49.5X2 | T49.5X3 | T49.5X4 | T49.5X5 | T49.5X6 |
| **Aristocort** | T38.0X1 | T38.0X2 | T38.0X3 | T38.0X4 | T38.0X5 | T38.0X6 |
| ENT agent | T49.6X1 | T49.6X2 | T49.6X3 | T49.6X4 | T49.6X5 | T49.6X6 |
| ophthalmic preparation | T49.5X1 | T49.5X2 | T49.5X3 | T49.5X4 | T49.5X5 | T49.5X6 |
| topical NEC | T49.0X1 | T49.0X2 | T49.0X3 | T49.0X4 | T49.0X5 | T49.0X6 |
| **Aromatics, corrosive** | T54.1X1 | T54.1X2 | T54.1X3 | T54.1X4 | — | — |
| disinfectants | T54.1X1 | T54.1X2 | T54.1X3 | T54.1X4 | — | — |
| **Arsenate of lead** | T57.0X1 | T57.0X2 | T57.0X3 | T57.0X4 | — | — |
| herbicide | T57.0X1 | T57.0X2 | T57.0X3 | T57.0X4 | — | — |
| **Arsenic, arsenicals** (compounds) (dust) (vapor) **NEC** | T57.0X1 | T57.0X2 | T57.0X3 | T57.0X4 | — | — |
| anti-infectives | T37.8X1 | T37.8X2 | T37.8X3 | T37.8X4 | T37.8X5 | T37.8X6 |
| pesticide (dust) (fumes) | T57.0X1 | T57.0X2 | T57.0X3 | T57.0X4 | — | — |

Table of Drugs and Chemicals

Arsine — Benzedrex

| Substance | Poisoning, Accidental (unintentional) | Poisoning, Intentional Self-harm | Poisoning, Assault | Poisoning, Undetermined | Adverse Effect | Under-dosing |
|---|---|---|---|---|---|---|
| Arsine (gas) | T57.0X1 | T57.0X2 | T57.0X3 | T57.0X4 | — | — |
| Arsphenamine (silver) | T37.8X1 | T37.8X2 | T37.8X3 | T37.8X4 | T37.8X5 | T37.8X6 |
| Arsthinol | T37.3X1 | T37.3X2 | T37.3X3 | T37.3X4 | T37.3X5 | T37.3X6 |
| Artane | T44.3X1 | T44.3X2 | T44.3X3 | T44.3X4 | T44.3X5 | T44.3X6 |
| Arthropod (venomous) NEC | T63.481 | T63.482 | T63.483 | T63.484 | | |
| Articaine | T41.3X1 | T41.3X2 | T41.3X3 | T41.3X4 | T41.3X5 | T41.3X6 |
| Asbestos | T57.8X1 | T57.8X2 | T57.8X3 | T57.8X4 | | |
| Ascaridole | T37.4X1 | T37.4X2 | T37.4X3 | T37.4X4 | T37.4X5 | T37.4X6 |
| Ascorbic acid | T45.2X1 | T45.2X2 | T45.2X3 | T45.2X4 | T45.2X5 | T45.2X6 |
| Asiaticoside | T49.0X1 | T49.0X2 | T49.0X3 | T49.0X4 | T49.0X5 | T49.0X6 |
| Asparaginase | T45.1X1 | T45.1X2 | T45.1X3 | T45.1X4 | T45.1X5 | T45.1X6 |
| Aspidium (oleoresin) | T37.4X1 | T37.4X2 | T37.4X3 | T37.4X4 | T37.4X5 | T37.4X6 |
| Aspirin (aluminum) (soluble) | T39.011 | T39.012 | T39.013 | T39.014 | T39.015 | T39.016 |
| Aspoxicillin | T36.0X1 | T36.0X2 | T36.0X3 | T36.0X4 | T36.0X5 | T36.0X6 |
| Astemizole | T45.0X1 | T45.0X2 | T45.0X3 | T45.0X4 | T45.0X5 | T45.0X6 |
| Astringent (local) | T49.2X1 | T49.2X2 | T49.2X3 | T49.2X4 | T49.2X5 | T49.2X6 |
| specified NEC | T49.2X1 | T49.2X2 | T49.2X3 | T49.2X4 | T49.2X5 | T49.2X6 |
| Astromicin | T36.5X1 | T36.5X2 | T36.5X3 | T36.5X4 | T36.5X5 | T36.5X6 |
| Ataractic drug NEC | T43.501 | T43.502 | T43.503 | T43.504 | T43.505 | T43.506 |
| Atenolol | T44.7X1 | T44.7X2 | T44.7X3 | T44.7X4 | T44.7X5 | T44.7X6 |
| Atonia drug, intestinal | T47.4X1 | T47.4X2 | T47.4X3 | T47.4X4 | T47.4X5 | T47.4X6 |
| Atophan | T50.4X1 | T50.4X2 | T50.4X3 | T50.4X4 | T50.4X5 | T50.4X6 |
| Atracurium besilate | T48.1X1 | T48.1X2 | T48.1X3 | T48.1X4 | T48.1X5 | T48.1X6 |
| Atropine | T44.3X1 | T44.3X2 | T44.3X3 | T44.3X4 | T44.3X5 | T44.3X6 |
| derivative | T44.3X1 | T44.3X2 | T44.3X3 | T44.3X4 | T44.3X5 | T44.3X6 |
| methonitrate | T44.3X1 | T44.3X2 | T44.3X3 | T44.3X4 | T44.3X5 | T44.3X6 |
| Attapulgite | T47.6X1 | T47.6X2 | T47.6X3 | T47.6X4 | T47.6X5 | T47.6X6 |
| Auramine | T65.891 | T65.892 | T65.893 | T65.894 | — | — |
| dye | T65.6X1 | T65.6X2 | T65.6X3 | T65.6X4 | — | — |
| fungicide | T60.3X1 | T60.3X2 | T60.3X3 | T60.3X4 | — | — |
| Auranofin | T39.4X1 | T39.4X2 | T39.4X3 | T39.4X4 | T39.4X5 | T39.4X6 |
| Aurantiin | T46.991 | T46.992 | T46.993 | T46.994 | T46.995 | T46.996 |
| Aureomycin | T36.4X1 | T36.4X2 | T36.4X3 | T36.4X4 | T36.4X5 | T36.4X6 |
| ophthalmic preparation | T49.5X1 | T49.5X2 | T49.5X3 | T49.5X4 | T49.5X5 | T49.5X6 |
| topical NEC | T49.0X1 | T49.0X2 | T49.0X3 | T49.0X4 | T49.0X5 | T49.0X6 |
| Aurothioglucose | T39.4X1 | T39.4X2 | T39.4X3 | T39.4X4 | T39.4X5 | T39.4X6 |
| Aurothioglycanide | T39.4X1 | T39.4X2 | T39.4X3 | T39.4X4 | T39.4X5 | T39.4X6 |
| Aurothiomalate sodium | T39.4X1 | T39.4X2 | T39.4X3 | T39.4X4 | T39.4X5 | T39.4X6 |
| Aurotioprol | T39.4X1 | T39.4X2 | T39.4X3 | T39.4X4 | T39.4X5 | T39.4X6 |
| Automobile fuel | T52.0X1 | T52.0X2 | T52.0X3 | T52.0X4 | | |
| Autonomic nervous system agent NEC | T44.901 | T44.902 | T44.903 | T44.904 | T44.905 | T44.906 |
| Avlosulfon | T37.1X1 | T37.1X2 | T37.1X3 | T37.1X4 | T37.1X5 | T37.1X6 |
| Avomine | T42.6X1 | T42.6X2 | T42.6X3 | T42.6X4 | T42.6X5 | T42.6X6 |
| Axerophthol | T45.2X1 | T45.2X2 | T45.2X3 | T45.2X4 | T45.2X5 | T45.2X6 |
| Azacitidine | T45.1X1 | T45.1X2 | T45.1X3 | T45.1X4 | T45.1X5 | T45.1X6 |
| Azacyclonol | T43.591 | T43.592 | T43.593 | T43.594 | T43.595 | T43.596 |
| Azadirachta | T60.2X1 | T60.2X2 | T60.2X3 | T60.2X4 | — | — |
| Azanidazole | T37.3X1 | T37.3X2 | T37.3X3 | T37.3X4 | T37.3X5 | T37.3X6 |
| Azapetine | T46.7X1 | T46.7X2 | T46.7X3 | T46.7X4 | T46.7X5 | T46.7X6 |
| Azapropazone | T39.2X1 | T39.2X2 | T39.2X3 | T39.2X4 | T39.2X5 | T39.2X6 |
| Azaribine | T45.1X1 | T45.1X2 | T45.1X3 | T45.1X4 | T45.1X5 | T45.1X6 |
| Azaserine | T45.1X1 | T45.1X2 | T45.1X3 | T45.1X4 | T45.1X5 | T45.1X6 |
| Azatadine | T45.0X1 | T45.0X2 | T45.0X3 | T45.0X4 | T45.0X5 | T45.0X6 |
| Azatepa | T45.1X1 | T45.1X2 | T45.1X3 | T45.1X4 | T45.1X5 | T45.1X6 |
| Azathioprine | T45.1X1 | T45.1X2 | T45.1X3 | T45.1X4 | T45.1X5 | T45.1X6 |
| Azelaic acid | T49.0X1 | T49.0X2 | T49.0X3 | T49.0X4 | T49.0X5 | T49.0X6 |
| Azelastine | T45.0X1 | T45.0X2 | T45.0X3 | T45.0X4 | T45.0X5 | T45.0X6 |
| Azidocillin | T36.0X1 | T36.0X2 | T36.0X3 | T36.0X4 | T36.0X5 | T36.0X6 |
| Azidothymidine | T37.5X1 | T37.5X2 | T37.5X3 | T37.5X4 | T37.5X5 | T37.5X6 |
| Azinphos (ethyl) (methyl) | T60.0X1 | T60.0X2 | T60.0X3 | T60.0X4 | — | — |
| Aziridine (chelating) | T54.1X1 | T54.1X2 | T54.1X3 | T54.1X4 | — | — |
| Azithromycin | T36.3X1 | T36.3X2 | T36.3X3 | T36.3X4 | T36.3X5 | T36.3X6 |
| Azlocillin | T36.0X1 | T36.0X2 | T36.0X3 | T36.0X4 | T36.0X5 | T36.0X6 |
| Azobenzene smoke | T65.3X1 | T65.3X2 | T65.3X3 | T65.3X4 | — | — |
| acaricide | T60.8X1 | T60.8X2 | T60.8X3 | T60.8X4 | — | — |
| Azosulfamide | T37.0X1 | T37.0X2 | T37.0X3 | T37.0X4 | T37.0X5 | T37.0X6 |
| AZT | T37.5X1 | T37.5X2 | T37.5X3 | T37.5X4 | T37.5X5 | T37.5X6 |
| Aztreonam | T36.1X1 | T36.1X2 | T36.1X3 | T36.1X4 | T36.1X5 | T36.1X6 |
| Azulfidine | T37.0X1 | T37.0X2 | T37.0X3 | T37.0X4 | T37.0X5 | T37.0X6 |
| Azuresin | T50.8X1 | T50.8X2 | T50.8X3 | T50.8X4 | T50.8X5 | T50.8X6 |
| b-acetyldigoxin | T46.0X1 | T46.0X2 | T46.0X3 | T46.0X4 | T46.0X5 | T46.0X6 |
| P-Acetamidophenol | T39.1X1 | T39.1X2 | T39.1X3 | T39.1X4 | T39.1X5 | T39.1X6 |
| Bacampicillin | T36.0X1 | T36.0X2 | T36.0X3 | T36.0X4 | T36.0X5 | T36.0X6 |
| Bacillus | | | | | | |
| lactobacillus | T47.8X1 | T47.8X2 | T47.8X3 | T47.8X4 | T47.8X5 | T47.8X6 |
| subtilis | T47.6X1 | T47.6X2 | T47.6X3 | T47.6X4 | T47.6X5 | T47.6X6 |
| Bacimycin | T49.0X1 | T49.0X2 | T49.0X3 | T49.0X4 | T49.0X5 | T49.0X6 |
| ophthalmic preparation | T49.5X1 | T49.5X2 | T49.5X3 | T49.5X4 | T49.5X5 | T49.5X6 |
| Bacitracin zinc | T49.0X1 | T49.0X2 | T49.0X3 | T49.0X4 | T49.0X5 | T49.0X6 |
| with neomycin | T49.0X1 | T49.0X2 | T49.0X3 | T49.0X4 | T49.0X5 | T49.0X6 |
| ENT agent | T49.6X1 | T49.6X2 | T49.6X3 | T49.6X4 | T49.6X5 | T49.6X6 |
| ophthalmic preparation | T49.5X1 | T49.5X2 | T49.5X3 | T49.5X4 | T49.5X5 | T49.5X6 |

| Substance | Poisoning, Accidental (unintentional) | Poisoning, Intentional Self-harm | Poisoning, Assault | Poisoning, Undetermined | Adverse Effect | Under-dosing |
|---|---|---|---|---|---|---|
| Bacitracin zinc — continued | | | | | | |
| topical NEC | T49.0X1 | T49.0X2 | T49.0X3 | T49.0X4 | T49.0X5 | T49.0X6 |
| Baclofen | T42.8X1 | T42.8X2 | T42.8X3 | T42.8X4 | T42.8X5 | T42.8X6 |
| Baking soda | T50.991 | T50.992 | T50.993 | T50.994 | T50.995 | T50.996 |
| BAL | T45.8X1 | T45.8X2 | T45.8X3 | T45.8X4 | T45.8X5 | T45.8X6 |
| Bambuterol | T48.6X1 | T48.6X2 | T48.6X3 | T48.6X4 | T48.6X5 | T48.6X6 |
| Bamethan (sulfate) | T46.7X1 | T46.7X2 | T46.7X3 | T46.7X4 | T46.7X5 | T46.7X6 |
| Bamifylline | T48.6X1 | T48.6X2 | T48.6X3 | T48.6X4 | T48.6X5 | T48.6X6 |
| Bamipine | T45.0X1 | T45.0X2 | T45.0X3 | T45.0X4 | T45.0X5 | T45.0X6 |
| Baneberry — see Actaea spicata | | | | | | |
| Banewort — see Belladonna | | | | | | |
| Barbenyl | T42.3X1 | T42.3X2 | T42.3X3 | T42.3X4 | T42.3X5 | T42.3X6 |
| Barbexaclone | T42.6X1 | T42.6X2 | T42.6X3 | T42.6X4 | T42.6X5 | T42.6X6 |
| Barbital | T42.3X1 | T42.3X2 | T42.3X3 | T42.3X4 | T42.3X5 | T42.3X6 |
| sodium | T42.3X1 | T42.3X2 | T42.3X3 | T42.3X4 | T42.3X5 | T42.3X6 |
| Barbitone | T42.3X1 | T42.3X2 | T42.3X3 | T42.3X4 | T42.3X5 | T42.3X6 |
| Barbiturate NEC | T42.3X1 | T42.3X2 | T42.3X3 | T42.3X4 | T42.3X5 | T42.3X6 |
| with tranquilizer | T42.3X1 | T42.3X2 | T42.3X3 | T42.3X4 | T42.3X5 | T42.3X6 |
| anesthetic (intravenous) | T41.1X1 | T41.1X2 | T41.1X3 | T41.1X4 | T41.1X5 | T41.1X6 |
| Barium (carbonate) (chloride) (sulfate) | T57.8X1 | T57.8X2 | T57.8X3 | T57.8X4 | — | — |
| diagnostic agent | T50.8X1 | T50.8X2 | T50.8X3 | T50.8X4 | T50.8X5 | T50.8X6 |
| pesticide | T60.4X1 | T60.4X2 | T60.4X3 | T60.4X4 | — | — |
| rodenticide | T60.4X1 | T60.4X2 | T60.4X3 | T60.4X4 | — | — |
| sulfate (medicinal) | T50.8X1 | T50.8X2 | T50.8X3 | T50.8X4 | T50.8X5 | T50.8X6 |
| Barrier cream | T49.3X1 | T49.3X2 | T49.3X3 | T49.3X4 | T49.3X5 | T49.3X6 |
| Basic fuchsin | T49.0X1 | T49.0X2 | T49.0X3 | T49.0X4 | T49.0X5 | T49.0X6 |
| Battery acid or fluid | T54.2X1 | T54.2X2 | T54.2X3 | T54.2X4 | | |
| Bay rum | T51.8X1 | T51.8X2 | T51.8X3 | T51.8X4 | | |
| b-benzalbutyramide | T46.6X1 | T46.6X2 | T46.6X3 | T46.6X4 | T46.6X5 | T46.6X6 |
| BCG (vaccine) | T50.A91 | T50.A92 | T50.A93 | T50.A94 | T50.A95 | T50.A96 |
| BCNU | T45.1X1 | T45.1X2 | T45.1X3 | T45.1X4 | T45.1X5 | T45.1X6 |
| Bearsfoot | T62.2X1 | T62.2X2 | T62.2X3 | T62.2X4 | | |
| Beclamide | T42.6X1 | T42.6X2 | T42.6X3 | T42.6X4 | T42.6X5 | T42.6X6 |
| Beclomethasone | T44.5X1 | T44.5X2 | T44.5X3 | T44.5X4 | T44.5X5 | T44.5X6 |
| Bee (sting) (venom) | T63.441 | T63.442 | T63.443 | T63.444 | | |
| Befunolol | T49.5X1 | T49.5X2 | T49.5X3 | T49.5X4 | T49.5X5 | T49.5X6 |
| Bekanamycin | T36.5X1 | T36.5X2 | T36.5X3 | T36.5X4 | T36.5X5 | T36.5X6 |
| Belladonna — see also Nightshade | | | | | | |
| alkaloids | T44.3X1 | T44.3X2 | T44.3X3 | T44.3X4 | T44.3X5 | T44.3X6 |
| extract | T44.3X1 | T44.3X2 | T44.3X3 | T44.3X4 | T44.3X5 | T44.3X6 |
| herb | T44.3X1 | T44.3X2 | T44.3X3 | T44.3X4 | T44.3X5 | T44.3X6 |
| Bemegride | T50.7X1 | T50.7X2 | T50.7X3 | T50.7X4 | T50.7X5 | T50.7X6 |
| Benactyzine | T44.3X1 | T44.3X2 | T44.3X3 | T44.3X4 | T44.3X5 | T44.3X6 |
| Benadryl | T45.0X1 | T45.0X2 | T45.0X3 | T45.0X4 | T45.0X5 | T45.0X6 |
| Benaprizine | T44.3X1 | T44.3X2 | T44.3X3 | T44.3X4 | T44.3X5 | T44.3X6 |
| Benazepril | T46.4X1 | T46.4X2 | T46.4X3 | T46.4X4 | T46.4X5 | T46.4X6 |
| Bencyclane | T46.7X1 | T46.7X2 | T46.7X3 | T46.7X4 | T46.7X5 | T46.7X6 |
| Bendazol | T46.3X1 | T46.3X2 | T46.3X3 | T46.3X4 | T46.3X5 | T46.3X6 |
| Bendrofluazide | T50.2X1 | T50.2X2 | T50.2X3 | T50.2X4 | T50.2X5 | T50.2X6 |
| Bendroflumethiazide | T50.2X1 | T50.2X2 | T50.2X3 | T50.2X4 | T50.2X5 | T50.2X6 |
| Benemid | T50.4X1 | T50.4X2 | T50.4X3 | T50.4X4 | T50.4X5 | T50.4X6 |
| Benethamine penicillin | T36.0X1 | T36.0X2 | T36.0X3 | T36.0X4 | T36.0X5 | T36.0X6 |
| Benexate | T47.1X1 | T47.1X2 | T47.1X3 | T47.1X4 | T47.1X5 | T47.1X6 |
| Benfluorex | T46.6X1 | T46.6X2 | T46.6X3 | T46.6X4 | T46.6X5 | T46.6X6 |
| Benfotiamine | T45.2X1 | T45.2X2 | T45.2X3 | T45.2X4 | T45.2X5 | T45.2X6 |
| Benisone | T49.0X1 | T49.0X2 | T49.0X3 | T49.0X4 | T49.0X5 | T49.0X6 |
| Benomyl | T60.0X1 | T60.0X2 | T60.0X3 | T60.0X4 | | |
| Benoquin | T49.8X1 | T49.8X2 | T49.8X3 | T49.8X4 | T49.8X5 | T49.8X6 |
| Benoxinate | T41.3X1 | T41.3X2 | T41.3X3 | T41.3X4 | T41.3X5 | T41.3X6 |
| Benperidol | T43.4X1 | T43.4X2 | T43.4X3 | T43.4X4 | T43.4X5 | T43.4X6 |
| Benproperine | T48.3X1 | T48.3X2 | T48.3X3 | T48.3X4 | T48.3X5 | T48.3X6 |
| Benserazide | T42.8X1 | T42.8X2 | T42.8X3 | T42.8X4 | T42.8X5 | T42.8X6 |
| Bentazepam | T42.4X1 | T42.4X2 | T42.4X3 | T42.4X4 | T42.4X5 | T42.4X6 |
| Bentiromide | T50.8X1 | T50.8X2 | T50.8X3 | T50.8X4 | T50.8X5 | T50.8X6 |
| Bentonite | T49.3X1 | T49.3X2 | T49.3X3 | T49.3X4 | T49.3X5 | T49.3X6 |
| Benzalbutyramide | T46.6X1 | T46.6X2 | T46.6X3 | T46.6X4 | T46.6X5 | T46.6X6 |
| Benzalkonium (chloride) | T49.0X1 | T49.0X2 | T49.0X3 | T49.0X4 | T49.0X5 | T49.0X6 |
| ophthalmic preparation | T49.5X1 | T49.5X2 | T49.5X3 | T49.5X4 | T49.5X5 | T49.5X6 |
| Benzamidosalicylate (calcium) | T37.1X1 | T37.1X2 | T37.1X3 | T37.1X4 | T37.1X5 | T37.1X6 |
| Benzamine | T41.3X1 | T41.3X2 | T41.3X3 | T41.3X4 | T41.3X5 | T41.3X6 |
| lactate | T49.1X1 | T49.1X2 | T49.1X3 | T49.1X4 | T49.1X5 | T49.1X6 |
| Benzamphetamine | T50.5X1 | T50.5X2 | T50.5X3 | T50.5X4 | T50.5X5 | T50.5X6 |
| Benzapril hydrochloride | T46.5X1 | T46.5X2 | T46.5X3 | T46.5X4 | T46.5X5 | T46.5X6 |
| Benzathine benzylpenicillin | T36.0X1 | T36.0X2 | T36.0X3 | T36.0X4 | T36.0X5 | T36.0X6 |
| Benzathine penicillin | T36.0X1 | T36.0X2 | T36.0X3 | T36.0X4 | T36.0X5 | T36.0X6 |
| Benzatropine | T42.8X1 | T42.8X2 | T42.8X3 | T42.8X4 | T42.8X5 | T42.8X6 |
| Benzbromarone | T50.4X1 | T50.4X2 | T50.4X3 | T50.4X4 | T50.4X5 | T50.4X6 |
| Benzcarbimine | T45.1X1 | T45.1X2 | T45.1X3 | T45.1X4 | T45.1X5 | T45.1X6 |
| Benzedrex | T44.991 | T44.992 | T44.993 | T44.994 | T44.995 | T44.996 |

Additional Character May Be Required — Refer to the Tabular List for Character Selection     ▽ Subterms under main terms may continue to next column or page

| Substance | Poisoning, Accidental (unintentional) | Poisoning, Intentional Self-harm | Poisoning, Assault | Poisoning, Undetermined | Adverse Effect | Underdosing |
|---|---|---|---|---|---|---|
| **Benzedrine** (amphetamine) | T43.621 | T43.622 | T43.623 | T43.624 | T43.625 | T43.626 |
| **Benzenamine** | T65.3X1 | T65.3X2 | T65.3X3 | T65.3X4 | — | — |
| **Benzene** | T52.1X1 | T52.1X2 | T52.1X3 | T52.1X4 | — | — |
| homologues (acetyl) (dimethyl) (methyl) (solvent) | T52.2X1 | T52.2X2 | T52.2X3 | T52.2X4 | — | — |
| **Benzethonium** (chloride) | T49.0X1 | T49.0X2 | T49.0X3 | T49.0X4 | T49.0X5 | T49.0X6 |
| **Benzfetamine** | T50.5X1 | T50.5X2 | T50.5X3 | T50.5X4 | T50.5X5 | T50.5X6 |
| **Benzhexol** | T44.3X1 | T44.3X2 | T44.3X3 | T44.3X4 | T44.3X5 | T44.3X6 |
| **Benzhydramine** (chloride) | T45.0X1 | T45.0X2 | T45.0X3 | T45.0X4 | T45.0X5 | T45.0X6 |
| **Benzidine** | T65.891 | T65.892 | T65.893 | T65.894 | | |
| **Benzilonium bromide** | T44.3X1 | T44.3X2 | T44.3X3 | T44.3X4 | T44.3X5 | T44.3X6 |
| **Benzimidazole** | T60.3X1 | T60.3X2 | T60.3X3 | T60.3X4 | — | — |
| **Benzin** (e) — see Ligroin | | | | | | |
| **Benziodarone** | T46.3X1 | T46.3X2 | T46.3X3 | T46.3X4 | T46.3X5 | T46.3X6 |
| **Benznidazole** | T37.3X1 | T37.3X2 | T37.3X3 | T37.3X4 | T37.3X5 | T37.3X6 |
| **Benzocaine** | T41.3X1 | T41.3X2 | T41.3X3 | T41.3X4 | T41.3X5 | T41.3X6 |
| **Benzodiapin** | T42.4X1 | T42.4X2 | T42.4X3 | T42.4X4 | T42.4X5 | T42.4X6 |
| **Benzodiazepine NEC** | T42.4X1 | T42.4X2 | T42.4X3 | T42.4X4 | T42.4X5 | T42.4X6 |
| **Benzoic acid** | T49.0X1 | T49.0X2 | T49.0X3 | T49.0X4 | T49.0X5 | T49.0X6 |
| with salicylic acid | T49.0X1 | T49.0X2 | T49.0X3 | T49.0X4 | T49.0X5 | T49.0X6 |
| **Benzoin** (tincture) | T48.5X1 | T48.5X2 | T48.5X3 | T48.5X4 | T48.5X5 | T48.5X6 |
| **Benzol** (benzene) | T52.1X1 | T52.1X2 | T52.1X3 | T52.1X4 | — | — |
| vapor | T52.0X1 | T52.0X2 | T52.0X3 | T52.0X4 | — | — |
| **Benzomorphan** | T40.2X1 | T40.2X2 | T40.2X3 | T40.2X4 | T40.2X5 | T40.2X6 |
| **Benzonatate** | T48.3X1 | T48.3X2 | T48.3X3 | T48.3X4 | T48.3X5 | T48.3X6 |
| **Benzophenones** | T49.3X1 | T49.3X2 | T49.3X3 | T49.3X4 | T49.3X5 | T49.3X6 |
| **Benzopyrone** | T46.991 | T46.992 | T46.993 | T46.994 | T46.995 | T46.996 |
| **Benzothiadiazides** | T50.2X1 | T50.2X2 | T50.2X3 | T50.2X4 | T50.2X5 | T50.2X6 |
| **Benzoxonium chloride** | T49.0X1 | T49.0X2 | T49.0X3 | T49.0X4 | T49.0X5 | T49.0X6 |
| **Benzoylpas calcium** | T37.1X1 | T37.1X2 | T37.1X3 | T37.1X4 | T37.1X5 | T37.1X6 |
| **Benzoyl peroxide** | T49.0X1 | T49.0X2 | T49.0X3 | T49.0X4 | T49.0X5 | T49.0X6 |
| **Benzperidin** | T43.591 | T43.592 | T43.593 | T43.594 | T43.595 | T43.596 |
| **Benzperidol** | T43.591 | T43.592 | T43.593 | T43.594 | T43.595 | T43.596 |
| **Benzphetamine** | T50.5X1 | T50.5X2 | T50.5X3 | T50.5X4 | T50.5X5 | T50.5X6 |
| **Benzpyrinium bromide** | T44.1X1 | T44.1X2 | T44.1X3 | T44.1X4 | T44.1X5 | T44.1X6 |
| **Benzquinamide** | T45.0X1 | T45.0X2 | T45.0X3 | T45.0X4 | T45.0X5 | T45.0X6 |
| **Benzthiazide** | T50.2X1 | T50.2X2 | T50.2X3 | T50.2X4 | T50.2X5 | T50.2X6 |
| **Benztropine** | | | | | | |
| anticholinergic | T44.3X1 | T44.3X2 | T44.3X3 | T44.3X4 | T44.3X5 | T44.3X6 |
| antiparkinson | T42.8X1 | T42.8X2 | T42.8X3 | T42.8X4 | T42.8X5 | T42.8X6 |
| **Benzydamine** | T49.0X1 | T49.0X2 | T49.0X3 | T49.0X4 | T49.0X5 | T49.0X6 |
| **Benzyl** | | | | | | |
| acetate | T52.8X1 | T52.8X2 | T52.8X3 | T52.8X4 | — | — |
| alcohol | T49.0X1 | T49.0X2 | T49.0X3 | T49.0X4 | T49.0X5 | T49.0X6 |
| benzoate | T49.0X1 | T49.0X2 | T49.0X3 | T49.0X4 | T49.0X5 | T49.0X6 |
| Benzoic acid | T49.0X1 | T49.0X2 | T49.0X3 | T49.0X4 | T49.0X5 | T49.0X6 |
| morphine | T40.2X1 | T40.2X2 | T40.2X3 | T40.2X4 | | |
| nicotinate | T46.6X1 | T46.6X2 | T46.6X3 | T46.6X4 | T46.6X5 | T46.6X6 |
| penicillin | T36.0X1 | T36.0X2 | T36.0X3 | T36.0X4 | T36.0X5 | T36.0X6 |
| **Benzylhydrochlorthiazide** | T50.2X1 | T50.2X2 | T50.2X3 | T50.2X4 | T50.2X5 | T50.2X6 |
| **Benzylpenicillin** | T36.0X1 | T36.0X2 | T36.0X3 | T36.0X4 | T36.0X5 | T36.0X6 |
| **Benzylthiouracil** | T38.2X1 | T38.2X2 | T38.2X3 | T38.2X4 | T38.2X5 | T38.2X6 |
| **Bephenium hydroxynaphthoate** | T37.4X1 | T37.4X2 | T37.4X3 | T37.4X4 | T37.4X5 | T37.4X6 |
| **Bepridil** | T46.1X1 | T46.1X2 | T46.1X3 | T46.1X4 | T46.1X5 | T46.1X6 |
| **Bergamot oil** | T65.891 | T65.892 | T65.893 | T65.894 | — | — |
| **Bergapten** | T50.991 | T50.992 | T50.993 | T50.994 | T50.995 | T50.996 |
| **Berries, poisonous** | T62.1X1 | T62.1X2 | T62.1X3 | T62.1X4 | — | — |
| **Beryllium** (compounds) | T56.7X1 | T56.7X2 | T56.7X3 | T56.7X4 | — | — |
| **beta adrenergic blocking agent, heart** | T44.7X1 | T44.7X2 | T44.7X3 | T44.7X4 | T44.7X5 | T44.7X6 |
| **Betacarotene** | T45.2X1 | T45.2X2 | T45.2X3 | T45.2X4 | T45.2X5 | T45.2X6 |
| **Beta-Chlor** | T42.6X1 | T42.6X2 | T42.6X3 | T42.6X4 | T42.6X5 | T42.6X6 |
| **Betahistine** | T46.7X1 | T46.7X2 | T46.7X3 | T46.7X4 | T46.7X5 | T46.7X6 |
| **Betaine** | T47.5X1 | T47.5X2 | T47.5X3 | T47.5X4 | T47.5X5 | T47.5X6 |
| **Betamethasone** | T49.0X1 | T49.0X2 | T49.0X3 | T49.0X4 | T49.0X5 | T49.0X6 |
| topical | T49.0X1 | T49.0X2 | T49.0X3 | T49.0X4 | T49.0X5 | T49.0X6 |
| **Betamicin** | T36.8X1 | T36.8X2 | T36.8X3 | T36.8X4 | T36.8X5 | T36.8X6 |
| **Betanidine** | T46.5X1 | T46.5X2 | T46.5X3 | T46.5X4 | T46.5X5 | T46.5X6 |
| **Betaxolol** | T44.7X1 | T44.7X2 | T44.7X3 | T44.7X4 | T44.7X5 | T44.7X6 |
| **Betazole** | T50.8X1 | T50.8X2 | T50.8X3 | T50.8X4 | T50.8X5 | T50.8X6 |
| **Bethanechol** | T44.1X1 | T44.1X2 | T44.1X3 | T44.1X4 | T44.1X5 | T44.1X6 |
| chloride | T44.1X1 | T44.1X2 | T44.1X3 | T44.1X4 | T44.1X5 | T44.1X6 |
| **Bethanidine** | T46.5X1 | T46.5X2 | T46.5X3 | T46.5X4 | T46.5X5 | T46.5X6 |
| **Betoxycaine** | T41.3X1 | T41.3X2 | T41.3X3 | T41.3X4 | T41.3X5 | T41.3X6 |
| **Betula oil** | T49.3X1 | T49.3X2 | T49.3X3 | T49.3X4 | T49.3X5 | T49.3X6 |
| **Bevantolol** | T44.7X1 | T44.7X2 | T44.7X3 | T44.7X4 | T44.7X5 | T44.7X6 |
| **Bevonium metilsulfate** | T44.3X1 | T44.3X2 | T44.3X3 | T44.3X4 | T44.3X5 | T44.3X6 |
| **Bezafibrate** | T46.6X1 | T46.6X2 | T46.6X3 | T46.6X4 | T46.6X5 | T46.6X6 |
| **Bezitramide** | T40.4X1 | T40.4X2 | T40.4X3 | T40.4X4 | T40.4X5 | T40.4X6 |
| **BHA** | T50.991 | T50.992 | T50.993 | T50.994 | T50.995 | T50.996 |
| **Bhang** | T40.7X1 | T40.7X2 | T40.7X3 | T40.7X4 | T40.7X5 | T40.7X6 |
| **BHC** (medicinal) | T49.0X1 | T49.0X2 | T49.0X3 | T49.0X4 | T49.0X5 | T49.0X6 |
| **BHC** — continued | | | | | | |
| nonmedicinal (vapor) | T53.6X1 | T53.6X2 | T53.6X3 | T53.6X4 | — | — |
| **Bialamicol** | T37.3X1 | T37.3X2 | T37.3X3 | T37.3X4 | T37.3X5 | T37.3X6 |
| **Bibenzonium bromide** | T48.3X1 | T48.3X2 | T48.3X3 | T48.3X4 | T48.3X5 | T48.3X6 |
| **Bibrocathol** | T49.5X1 | T49.5X2 | T49.5X3 | T49.5X4 | T49.5X5 | T49.5X6 |
| **Bichloride of mercury** — see Mercury, chloride | | | | | | |
| **Bichromates** (calcium) (potassium)(sodium) (crystals) | T57.8X1 | T57.8X2 | T57.8X3 | T57.8X4 | — | — |
| fumes | T56.2X1 | T56.2X2 | T56.2X3 | T56.2X4 | — | — |
| **Biclotymol** | T49.6X1 | T49.6X2 | T49.6X3 | T49.6X4 | T49.6X5 | T49.6X6 |
| **Bicucculine** | T50.7X1 | T50.7X2 | T50.7X3 | T50.7X4 | T50.7X5 | T50.7X6 |
| **Bifemelane** | T43.291 | T43.292 | T43.293 | T43.294 | T43.295 | T43.296 |
| **Biguanide derivatives, oral** | T38.3X1 | T38.3X2 | T38.3X3 | T38.3X4 | T38.3X5 | T38.3X6 |
| **Bile salts** | T47.5X1 | T47.5X2 | T47.5X3 | T47.5X4 | T47.5X5 | T47.5X6 |
| **Biligrafin** | T50.8X1 | T50.8X2 | T50.8X3 | T50.8X4 | T50.8X5 | T50.8X6 |
| **Bilopaque** | T50.8X1 | T50.8X2 | T50.8X3 | T50.8X4 | T50.8X5 | T50.8X6 |
| **Binifibrate** | T46.6X1 | T46.6X2 | T46.6X3 | T46.6X4 | T46.6X5 | T46.6X6 |
| **Binitrobenzol** | T65.3X1 | T65.3X2 | T65.3X3 | T65.3X4 | | |
| **Bioflavonoid**(s) | T46.991 | T46.992 | T46.993 | T46.994 | T46.995 | T46.996 |
| **Biological substance NEC** | T50.901 | T50.902 | T50.903 | T50.904 | T50.905 | T50.906 |
| **Biotin** | T45.2X1 | T45.2X2 | T45.2X3 | T45.2X4 | T45.2X5 | T45.2X6 |
| **Biperiden** | T44.3X1 | T44.3X2 | T44.3X3 | T44.3X4 | T44.3X5 | T44.3X6 |
| **Bisacodyl** | T47.2X1 | T47.2X2 | T47.2X3 | T47.2X4 | T47.2X5 | T47.2X6 |
| **Bisbentiamine** | T45.2X1 | T45.2X2 | T45.2X3 | T45.2X4 | T45.2X5 | T45.2X6 |
| **Bisbutiamine** | T45.2X1 | T45.2X2 | T45.2X3 | T45.2X4 | T45.2X5 | T45.2X6 |
| **Bisdequalinium** (salts) (diacetate) | T49.6X1 | T49.6X2 | T49.6X3 | T49.6X4 | T49.6X5 | T49.6X6 |
| **Bishydroxycoumarin** | T45.511 | T45.512 | T45.513 | T45.514 | T45.515 | T45.516 |
| **Bismarsen** | T37.8X1 | T37.8X2 | T37.8X3 | T37.8X4 | T37.8X5 | T37.8X6 |
| **Bismuth salts** | T47.6X1 | T47.6X2 | T47.6X3 | T47.6X4 | T47.6X5 | T47.6X6 |
| aluminate | T47.1X1 | T47.1X2 | T47.1X3 | T47.1X4 | T47.1X5 | T47.1X6 |
| anti-infectives | T37.8X1 | T37.8X2 | T37.8X3 | T37.8X4 | T37.8X5 | T37.8X6 |
| formic iodide | T49.0X1 | T49.0X2 | T49.0X3 | T49.0X4 | T49.0X5 | T49.0X6 |
| glycolylarsenate | T49.0X1 | T49.0X2 | T49.0X3 | T49.0X4 | T49.0X5 | T49.0X6 |
| nonmedicinal (compounds) NEC | T65.91 | T65.92 | T65.93 | T65.94 | — | — |
| subcarbonate | T47.6X1 | T47.6X2 | T47.6X3 | T47.6X4 | T47.6X5 | T47.6X6 |
| subsalicylate | T37.8X1 | T37.8X2 | T37.8X3 | T37.8X4 | T37.8X5 | T37.8X6 |
| sulfarsphenamine | T37.8X1 | T37.8X2 | T37.8X3 | T37.8X4 | T37.8X5 | T37.8X6 |
| **Bisoprolol** | T44.7X1 | T44.7X2 | T44.7X3 | T44.7X4 | T44.7X5 | T44.7X6 |
| **Bisoxatin** | T47.2X1 | T47.2X2 | T47.2X3 | T47.2X4 | T47.2X5 | T47.2X6 |
| **Bisulepin** (hydrochloride) | T45.0X1 | T45.0X2 | T45.0X3 | T45.0X4 | T45.0X5 | T45.0X6 |
| **Bithionol** | T37.8X1 | T37.8X2 | T37.8X3 | T37.8X4 | T37.8X5 | T37.8X6 |
| anthelminthic | T37.4X1 | T37.4X2 | T37.4X3 | T37.4X4 | T37.4X5 | T37.4X6 |
| **Bitolterol** | T48.6X1 | T48.6X2 | T48.6X3 | T48.6X4 | T48.6X5 | T48.6X6 |
| **Bitoscanate** | T37.4X1 | T37.4X2 | T37.4X3 | T37.4X4 | T37.4X5 | T37.4X6 |
| **Bitter almond oil** | T62.8X1 | T62.8X2 | T62.8X3 | T62.8X4 | — | — |
| **Bittersweet** | T62.2X1 | T62.2X2 | T62.2X3 | T62.2X4 | — | — |
| **Black** | | | | | | |
| flag | T60.91 | T60.92 | T60.93 | T60.94 | — | — |
| henbane | T62.2X1 | T62.2X2 | T62.2X3 | T62.2X4 | — | — |
| leaf (40) | T60.91 | T60.92 | T60.93 | T60.94 | — | — |
| widow spider (bite) | T63.311 | T63.312 | T63.313 | T63.314 | — | — |
| antivenin | T50.Z11 | T50.Z12 | T50.Z13 | T50.Z14 | T50.Z15 | T50.Z16 |
| **Blast furnace gas** (carbon monoxide from) | T58.8X1 | T58.8X2 | T58.8X3 | T58.8X4 | — | — |
| **Bleach** | T54.91 | T54.92 | T54.93 | T54.94 | — | — |
| **Bleaching agent** (medicinal) | T49.4X1 | T49.4X2 | T49.4X3 | T49.4X4 | T49.4X5 | T49.4X6 |
| **Bleomycin** | T45.1X1 | T45.1X2 | T45.1X3 | T45.1X4 | T45.1X5 | T45.1X6 |
| **Blockain** | T41.3X1 | T41.3X2 | T41.3X3 | T41.3X4 | T41.3X5 | T41.3X6 |
| infiltration (subcutaneous) | T41.3X1 | T41.3X2 | T41.3X3 | T41.3X4 | T41.3X5 | T41.3X6 |
| nerve block (peripheral) (plexus) | T41.3X1 | T41.3X2 | T41.3X3 | T41.3X4 | T41.3X5 | T41.3X6 |
| topical (surface) | T41.3X1 | T41.3X2 | T41.3X3 | T41.3X4 | T41.3X5 | T41.3X6 |
| **Blockers, calcium channel** | T46.1X1 | T46.1X2 | T46.1X3 | T46.1X4 | T46.1X5 | T46.1X6 |
| **Blood** (derivatives) (natural) (plasma) (whole) | T45.8X1 | T45.8X2 | T45.8X3 | T45.8X4 | T45.8X5 | T45.8X6 |
| dried | T45.8X1 | T45.8X2 | T45.8X3 | T45.8X4 | T45.8X5 | T45.8X6 |
| drug affecting NEC | T45.91 | T45.92 | T45.93 | T45.94 | T45.95 | T45.96 |
| expander NEC | T45.8X1 | T45.8X2 | T45.8X3 | T45.8X4 | T45.8X5 | T45.8X6 |
| fraction NEC | T45.8X1 | T45.8X2 | T45.8X3 | T45.8X4 | T45.8X5 | T45.8X6 |
| substitute (macromolecular) | T45.8X1 | T45.8X2 | T45.8X3 | T45.8X4 | T45.8X5 | T45.8X6 |
| **Blue velvet** | T40.2X1 | T40.2X2 | T40.2X3 | T40.2X4 | — | — |
| **Bone meal** | T62.8X1 | T62.8X2 | T62.8X3 | T62.8X4 | — | — |
| **Bonine** | T45.0X1 | T45.0X2 | T45.0X3 | T45.0X4 | T45.0X5 | T45.0X6 |
| **Bopindolol** | T44.7X1 | T44.7X2 | T44.7X3 | T44.7X4 | T44.7X5 | T44.7X6 |
| **Boracic acid** | T49.0X1 | T49.0X2 | T49.0X3 | T49.0X4 | T49.0X5 | T49.0X6 |
| ENT agent | T49.6X1 | T49.6X2 | T49.6X3 | T49.6X4 | T49.6X5 | T49.6X6 |
| ophthalmic preparation | T49.5X1 | T49.5X2 | T49.5X3 | T49.5X4 | T49.5X5 | T49.5X6 |
| **Borane complex** | T57.8X1 | T57.8X2 | T57.8X3 | T57.8X4 | — | — |

Subterms under main terms may continue to next column or page    Additional Character May Be Required — Refer to the Tabular List for Character Selection    355

Benzedrine — Borane complex

| Substance | Poisoning, Accidental (unintentional) | Poisoning, Intentional Self-harm | Poisoning, Assault | Poisoning, Undetermined | Adverse Effect | Under-dosing |
|---|---|---|---|---|---|---|
| **Borate(s)** | T57.8X1 | T57.8X2 | T57.8X3 | T57.8X4 | — | — |
| buffer | T50.991 | T50.992 | T50.993 | T50.994 | T50.995 | T50.996 |
| cleanser | T54.91 | T54.92 | T54.93 | T54.94 | — | — |
| sodium | T57.8X1 | T57.8X2 | T57.8X3 | T57.8X4 | — | — |
| **Borax** (cleanser) | T54.91 | T54.92 | T54.93 | T54.94 | — | — |
| **Bordeaux mixture** | T60.3X1 | T60.3X2 | T60.3X3 | T60.3X4 | — | — |
| **Boric acid** | T49.0X1 | T49.0X2 | T49.0X3 | T49.0X4 | T49.0X5 | T49.0X6 |
| ENT agent | T49.6X1 | T49.6X2 | T49.6X3 | T49.6X4 | T49.6X5 | T49.6X6 |
| ophthalmic preparation | T49.5X1 | T49.5X2 | T49.5X3 | T49.5X4 | T49.5X5 | T49.5X6 |
| **Bornaprine** | T44.3X1 | T44.3X2 | T44.3X3 | T44.3X4 | T44.3X5 | T44.3X6 |
| **Boron** | T57.8X1 | T57.8X2 | T57.8X3 | T57.8X4 | — | — |
| hydride NEC | T57.8X1 | T57.8X2 | T57.8X3 | T57.8X4 | — | — |
| fumes or gas | T57.8X1 | T57.8X2 | T57.8X3 | T57.8X4 | — | — |
| trifluoride | T59.891 | T59.892 | T59.893 | T59.894 | — | — |
| **Botox** | T48.291 | T48.292 | T48.293 | T48.294 | T48.295 | T48.296 |
| **Botulinus anti-toxin** (type A, B) | T50.Z11 | T50.Z12 | T50.Z13 | T50.Z14 | T50.Z15 | T50.Z16 |
| **Brake fluid vapor** | T59.891 | T59.892 | T59.893 | T59.894 | — | — |
| **Brallobarbital** | T42.3X1 | T42.3X2 | T42.3X3 | T42.3X4 | T42.3X5 | T42.3X6 |
| **Bran** (wheat) | T47.4X1 | T47.4X2 | T47.4X3 | T47.4X4 | T47.4X5 | T47.4X6 |
| **Brass** (fumes) | T56.891 | T56.892 | T56.893 | T56.894 | — | — |
| **Brasso** | T52.0X1 | T52.0X2 | T52.0X3 | T52.0X4 | — | — |
| **Bretylium tosilate** | T46.2X1 | T46.2X2 | T46.2X3 | T46.2X4 | T46.2X5 | T46.2X6 |
| **Brevital** (sodium) | T41.1X1 | T41.1X2 | T41.1X3 | T41.1X4 | T41.1X5 | T41.1X6 |
| **Brinase** | T45.3X1 | T45.3X2 | T45.3X3 | T45.3X4 | T45.3X5 | T45.3X6 |
| **British antilewisite** | T45.8X1 | T45.8X2 | T45.8X3 | T45.8X4 | T45.8X5 | T45.8X6 |
| **Brodifacoum** | T60.4X1 | T60.4X2 | T60.4X3 | T60.4X4 | — | — |
| **Bromal** (hydrate) | T42.6X1 | T42.6X2 | T42.6X3 | T42.6X4 | T42.6X5 | T42.6X6 |
| **Bromazepam** | T42.4X1 | T42.4X2 | T42.4X3 | T42.4X4 | T42.4X5 | T42.4X6 |
| **Bromazine** | T45.0X1 | T45.0X2 | T45.0X3 | T45.0X4 | T45.0X5 | T45.0X6 |
| **Brombenzylcyanide** | T59.3X1 | T59.3X2 | T59.3X3 | T59.3X4 | — | — |
| **Bromelains** | T45.3X1 | T45.3X2 | T45.3X3 | T45.3X4 | T45.3X5 | T45.3X6 |
| **Bromethalin** | T60.4X1 | T60.4X2 | T60.4X3 | T60.4X4 | — | — |
| **Bromhexine** | T48.4X1 | T48.4X2 | T48.4X3 | T48.4X4 | T48.4X5 | T48.4X6 |
| **Bromide salts** | T42.6X1 | T42.6X2 | T42.6X3 | T42.6X4 | T42.6X5 | T42.6X6 |
| **Bromindione** | T45.511 | T45.512 | T45.513 | T45.514 | T45.515 | T45.516 |
| **Bromine** | | | | | | |
| compounds (medicinal) | T42.6X1 | T42.6X2 | T42.6X3 | T42.6X4 | T42.6X5 | T42.6X6 |
| sedative | T42.6X1 | T42.6X2 | T42.6X3 | T42.6X4 | T42.6X5 | T42.6X6 |
| vapor | T59.891 | T59.892 | T59.893 | T59.894 | — | — |
| **Bromisoval** | T42.6X1 | T42.6X2 | T42.6X3 | T42.6X4 | T42.6X5 | T42.6X6 |
| **Bromisovalum** | T42.6X1 | T42.6X2 | T42.6X3 | T42.6X4 | T42.6X5 | T42.6X6 |
| **Bromobenzylcyanide** | T59.3X1 | T59.3X2 | T59.3X3 | T59.3X4 | — | — |
| **Bromochlorosalicylani-lide** | T49.0X1 | T49.0X2 | T49.0X3 | T49.0X4 | T49.0X5 | T49.0X6 |
| **Bromocriptine** | T42.8X1 | T42.8X2 | T42.8X3 | T42.8X4 | T42.8X5 | T42.8X6 |
| **Bromodiphenhydramine** | T45.0X1 | T45.0X2 | T45.0X3 | T45.0X4 | T45.0X5 | T45.0X6 |
| **Bromoform** | T42.6X1 | T42.6X2 | T42.6X3 | T42.6X4 | T42.6X5 | T42.6X6 |
| **Bromophenol blue reagent** | T50.991 | T50.992 | T50.993 | T50.994 | T50.995 | T50.996 |
| **Bromopride** | T47.8X1 | T47.8X2 | T47.8X3 | T47.8X4 | T47.8X5 | T47.8X6 |
| **Bromosalicylchloranitide** | T49.0X1 | T49.0X2 | T49.0X3 | T49.0X4 | T49.0X5 | T49.0X6 |
| **Bromosalicylhydroxamic acid** | T37.1X1 | T37.1X2 | T37.1X3 | T37.1X4 | T37.1X5 | T37.1X6 |
| **Bromo-seltzer** | T39.1X1 | T39.1X2 | T39.1X3 | T39.1X4 | T39.1X5 | T39.1X6 |
| **Bromoxynil** | T60.3X1 | T60.3X2 | T60.3X3 | T60.3X4 | — | — |
| **Bromperidol** | T43.4X1 | T43.4X2 | T43.4X3 | T43.4X4 | T43.4X5 | T43.4X6 |
| **Brompheniramine** | T45.0X1 | T45.0X2 | T45.0X3 | T45.0X4 | T45.0X5 | T45.0X6 |
| **Bromsulphthalein** | T50.8X1 | T50.8X2 | T50.8X3 | T50.8X4 | T50.8X5 | T50.8X6 |
| **Bromural** | T42.6X1 | T42.6X2 | T42.6X3 | T42.6X4 | T42.6X5 | T42.6X6 |
| **Bromvaletone** | T42.6X1 | T42.6X2 | T42.6X3 | T42.6X4 | T42.6X5 | T42.6X6 |
| **Bronchodilator NEC** | T48.6X1 | T48.6X2 | T48.6X3 | T48.6X4 | T48.6X5 | T48.6X6 |
| **Brotizolam** | T42.4X1 | T42.4X2 | T42.4X3 | T42.4X4 | T42.4X5 | T42.4X6 |
| **Brovincamine** | T46.7X1 | T46.7X2 | T46.7X3 | T46.7X4 | T46.7X5 | T46.7X6 |
| **Brown recluse spider** (bite) (venom) | T63.331 | T63.332 | T63.333 | T63.334 | — | — |
| **Brown spider** (bite) (venom) | T63.391 | T63.392 | T63.393 | T63.394 | — | — |
| **Broxaterol** | T48.6X1 | T48.6X2 | T48.6X3 | T48.6X4 | T48.6X5 | T48.6X6 |
| **Broxuridine** | T45.1X1 | T45.1X2 | T45.1X3 | T45.1X4 | T45.1X5 | T45.1X6 |
| **Broxyquinoline** | T37.8X1 | T37.8X2 | T37.8X3 | T37.8X4 | T37.8X5 | T37.8X6 |
| **Bruceine** | T48.291 | T48.292 | T48.293 | T48.294 | T48.295 | T48.296 |
| **Brucia** | T62.2X1 | T62.2X2 | T62.2X3 | T62.2X4 | — | — |
| **Brucine** | T65.1X1 | T65.1X2 | T65.1X3 | T65.1X4 | — | — |
| **Brunswick green** — see Copper | | | | | | |
| **Bruten** — see Ibuprofen | | | | | | |
| **Bryonia** | T47.2X1 | T47.2X2 | T47.2X3 | T47.2X4 | T47.2X5 | T47.2X6 |
| **Buclizine** | T45.0X1 | T45.0X2 | T45.0X3 | T45.0X4 | T45.0X5 | T45.0X6 |
| **Buclosamide** | T49.0X1 | T49.0X2 | T49.0X3 | T49.0X4 | T49.0X5 | T49.0X6 |
| **Budesonide** | T44.5X1 | T44.5X2 | T44.5X3 | T44.5X4 | T44.5X5 | T44.5X6 |
| **Budralazine** | T46.5X1 | T46.5X2 | T46.5X3 | T46.5X4 | T46.5X5 | T46.5X6 |
| **Bufferin** | T39.011 | T39.012 | T39.013 | T39.014 | T39.015 | T39.016 |
| **Buflomedil** | T46.7X1 | T46.7X2 | T46.7X3 | T46.7X4 | T46.7X5 | T46.7X6 |
| **Buformin** | T38.3X1 | T38.3X2 | T38.3X3 | T38.3X4 | T38.3X5 | T38.3X6 |
| **Bufotenine** | T40.991 | T40.992 | T40.993 | T40.994 | — | — |
| **Bufrolin** | T48.6X1 | T48.6X2 | T48.6X3 | T48.6X4 | T48.6X5 | T48.6X6 |
| **Bufylline** | T48.6X1 | T48.6X2 | T48.6X3 | T48.6X4 | T48.6X5 | T48.6X6 |
| **Bulk filler** | T50.5X1 | T50.5X2 | T50.5X3 | T50.5X4 | T50.5X5 | T50.5X6 |
| cathartic | T47.4X1 | T47.4X2 | T47.4X3 | T47.4X4 | T47.4X5 | T47.4X6 |
| **Bumetanide** | T50.1X1 | T50.1X2 | T50.1X3 | T50.1X4 | T50.1X5 | T50.1X6 |
| **Bunaftine** | T46.2X1 | T46.2X2 | T46.2X3 | T46.2X4 | T46.2X5 | T46.2X6 |
| **Bunamiodyl** | T50.8X1 | T50.8X2 | T50.8X3 | T50.8X4 | T50.8X5 | T50.8X6 |
| **Bunazosin** | T44.6X1 | T44.6X2 | T44.6X3 | T44.6X4 | T44.6X5 | T44.6X6 |
| **Bunitrolol** | T44.7X1 | T44.7X2 | T44.7X3 | T44.7X4 | T44.7X5 | T44.7X6 |
| **Buphenine** | T46.7X1 | T46.7X2 | T46.7X3 | T46.7X4 | T46.7X5 | T46.7X6 |
| **Bupivacaine** | T41.3X1 | T41.3X2 | T41.3X3 | T41.3X4 | T41.3X5 | T41.3X6 |
| infiltration (subcutaneous) | T41.3X1 | T41.3X2 | T41.3X3 | T41.3X4 | T41.3X5 | T41.3X6 |
| nerve block (peripheral) (plexus) | T41.3X1 | T41.3X2 | T41.3X3 | T41.3X4 | T41.3X5 | T41.3X6 |
| spinal | T41.3X1 | T41.3X2 | T41.3X3 | T41.3X4 | T41.3X5 | T41.3X6 |
| **Bupranolol** | T44.7X1 | T44.7X2 | T44.7X3 | T44.7X4 | T44.7X5 | T44.7X6 |
| **Buprenorphine** | T40.4X1 | T40.4X2 | T40.4X3 | T40.4X4 | T40.4X5 | T40.4X6 |
| **Bupropion** | T43.291 | T43.292 | T43.293 | T43.294 | T43.295 | T43.296 |
| **Burimamide** | T47.1X1 | T47.1X2 | T47.1X3 | T47.1X4 | T47.1X5 | T47.1X6 |
| **Buserelin** | T38.891 | T38.892 | T38.893 | T38.894 | T38.895 | T38.896 |
| **Buspirone** | T43.591 | T43.592 | T43.593 | T43.594 | T43.595 | T43.596 |
| **Busulfan, busulphan** | T45.1X1 | T45.1X2 | T45.1X3 | T45.1X4 | T45.1X5 | T45.1X6 |
| **Butabarbital** (sodium) | T42.3X1 | T42.3X2 | T42.3X3 | T42.3X4 | T42.3X5 | T42.3X6 |
| **Butabarbitone** | T42.3X1 | T42.3X2 | T42.3X3 | T42.3X4 | T42.3X5 | T42.3X6 |
| **Butabarpal** | T42.3X1 | T42.3X2 | T42.3X3 | T42.3X4 | T42.3X5 | T42.3X6 |
| **Butacaine** | T41.3X1 | T41.3X2 | T41.3X3 | T41.3X4 | T41.3X5 | T41.3X6 |
| **Butalamine** | T46.7X1 | T46.7X2 | T46.7X3 | T46.7X4 | T46.7X5 | T46.7X6 |
| **Butalbital** | T42.3X1 | T42.3X2 | T42.3X3 | T42.3X4 | T42.3X5 | T42.3X6 |
| **Butallylonal** | T42.3X1 | T42.3X2 | T42.3X3 | T42.3X4 | T42.3X5 | T42.3X6 |
| **Butamben** | T41.3X1 | T41.3X2 | T41.3X3 | T41.3X4 | T41.3X5 | T41.3X6 |
| **Butamirate** | T48.3X1 | T48.3X2 | T48.3X3 | T48.3X4 | T48.3X5 | T48.3X6 |
| **Butane** (distributed in mobile container) | T59.891 | T59.892 | T59.893 | T59.894 | — | — |
| distributed through pipes | T59.891 | T59.892 | T59.893 | T59.894 | — | — |
| incomplete combustion | T58.11 | T58.12 | T58.13 | T58.14 | — | — |
| **Butanilicaine** | T41.3X1 | T41.3X2 | T41.3X3 | T41.3X4 | T41.3X5 | T41.3X6 |
| **Butanol** | T51.3X1 | T51.3X2 | T51.3X3 | T51.3X4 | — | — |
| **Butanone, 2-butanone** | T52.4X1 | T52.4X2 | T52.4X3 | T52.4X4 | — | — |
| **Butantrone** | T49.4X1 | T49.4X2 | T49.4X3 | T49.4X4 | T49.4X5 | T49.4X6 |
| **Butaperazine** | T43.3X1 | T43.3X2 | T43.3X3 | T43.3X4 | T43.3X5 | T43.3X6 |
| **Butazolidin** | T39.2X1 | T39.2X2 | T39.2X3 | T39.2X4 | T39.2X5 | T39.2X6 |
| **Butetamate** | T48.6X1 | T48.6X2 | T48.6X3 | T48.6X4 | T48.6X5 | T48.6X6 |
| **Butethal** | T42.3X1 | T42.3X2 | T42.3X3 | T42.3X4 | T42.3X5 | T42.3X6 |
| **Butethamate** | T44.3X1 | T44.3X2 | T44.3X3 | T44.3X4 | T44.3X5 | T44.3X6 |
| **Buthalitone** (sodium) | T41.1X1 | T41.1X2 | T41.1X3 | T41.1X4 | T41.1X5 | T41.1X6 |
| **Butisol** (sodium) | T42.3X1 | T42.3X2 | T42.3X3 | T42.3X4 | T42.3X5 | T42.3X6 |
| **Butizide** | T50.2X1 | T50.2X2 | T50.2X3 | T50.2X4 | T50.2X5 | T50.2X6 |
| **Butobarbital** | T42.3X1 | T42.3X2 | T42.3X3 | T42.3X4 | T42.3X5 | T42.3X6 |
| sodium | T42.3X1 | T42.3X2 | T42.3X3 | T42.3X4 | T42.3X5 | T42.3X6 |
| **Butobarbitone** | T42.3X1 | T42.3X2 | T42.3X3 | T42.3X4 | T42.3X5 | T42.3X6 |
| **Butoconazole** (nitrate) | T49.0X1 | T49.0X2 | T49.0X3 | T49.0X4 | T49.0X5 | T49.0X6 |
| **Butorphanol** | T40.4X1 | T40.4X2 | T40.4X3 | T40.4X4 | T40.4X5 | T40.4X6 |
| **Butriptyline** | T43.011 | T43.012 | T43.013 | T43.014 | T43.015 | T43.016 |
| **Butropium bromide** | T44.3X1 | T44.3X2 | T44.3X3 | T44.3X4 | T44.3X5 | T44.3X6 |
| **Buttercups** | T62.2X1 | T62.2X2 | T62.2X3 | T62.2X4 | — | — |
| **Butter of antimony** — see Antimony | | | | | | |
| **Butyl** | | | | | | |
| acetate (secondary) | T52.8X1 | T52.8X2 | T52.8X3 | T52.8X4 | — | — |
| alcohol | T51.3X1 | T51.3X2 | T51.3X3 | T51.3X4 | — | — |
| aminobenzoate | T41.3X1 | T41.3X2 | T41.3X3 | T41.3X4 | T41.3X5 | T41.3X6 |
| butyrate | T52.8X1 | T52.8X2 | T52.8X3 | T52.8X4 | — | — |
| carbinol | T51.3X1 | T51.3X2 | T51.3X3 | T51.3X4 | — | — |
| carbitol | T52.3X1 | T52.3X2 | T52.3X3 | T52.3X4 | — | — |
| cellosolve | T52.3X1 | T52.3X2 | T52.3X3 | T52.3X4 | — | — |
| chloral (hydrate) | T42.6X1 | T42.6X2 | T42.6X3 | T42.6X4 | T42.6X5 | T42.6X6 |
| formate | T52.8X1 | T52.8X2 | T52.8X3 | T52.8X4 | — | — |
| lactate | T52.8X1 | T52.8X2 | T52.8X3 | T52.8X4 | — | — |
| propionate | T52.8X1 | T52.8X2 | T52.8X3 | T52.8X4 | — | — |
| scopolamine bromide | T44.3X1 | T44.3X2 | T44.3X3 | T44.3X4 | T44.3X5 | T44.3X6 |
| thiobarbital sodium | T41.1X1 | T41.1X2 | T41.1X3 | T41.1X4 | T41.1X5 | T41.1X6 |
| **Butylated hydroxyanisole** | T50.991 | T50.992 | T50.993 | T50.994 | T50.995 | T50.996 |
| **Butylchloral hydrate** | T42.6X1 | T42.6X2 | T42.6X3 | T42.6X4 | T42.6X5 | T42.6X6 |
| **Butyltoluene** | T52.2X1 | T52.2X2 | T52.2X3 | T52.2X4 | — | — |
| **Butyn** | T41.3X1 | T41.3X2 | T41.3X3 | T41.3X4 | T41.3X5 | T41.3X6 |
| **Butyrophenone** (-based tranquilizers) | T43.4X1 | T43.4X2 | T43.4X3 | T43.4X4 | T43.4X5 | T43.4X6 |
| **Cabergoline** | T42.8X1 | T42.8X2 | T42.8X3 | T42.8X4 | T42.8X5 | T42.8X6 |
| **Cacodyl, cacodylic acid** | T57.0X1 | T57.0X2 | T57.0X3 | T57.0X4 | — | — |
| **Cactinomycin** | T45.1X1 | T45.1X2 | T45.1X3 | T45.1X4 | T45.1X5 | T45.1X6 |
| **Cade oil** | T49.4X1 | T49.4X2 | T49.4X3 | T49.4X4 | T49.4X5 | T49.4X6 |
| **Cadexomer iodine** | T49.0X1 | T49.0X2 | T49.0X3 | T49.0X4 | T49.0X5 | T49.0X6 |
| **Cadmium** (chloride) (fumes) (oxide) | T56.3X1 | T56.3X2 | T56.3X3 | T56.3X4 | — | — |

| Substance | Poisoning, Accidental (unintentional) | Poisoning, Intentional Self-harm | Poisoning, Assault | Poisoning, Undetermined | Adverse Effect | Under-dosing |
|---|---|---|---|---|---|---|
| **Cadmium** — *continued* | | | | | | |
| sulfide (medicinal) NEC | T49.4X1 | T49.4X2 | T49.4X3 | T49.4X4 | T49.4X5 | T49.4X6 |
| **Cadralazine** | T46.5X1 | T46.5X2 | T46.5X3 | T46.5X4 | T46.5X5 | T46.5X6 |
| **Caffeine** | T43.611 | T43.612 | T43.613 | T43.614 | T43.615 | T43.616 |
| **Calabar bean** | T62.2X1 | T62.2X2 | T62.2X3 | T62.2X4 | — | — |
| **Caladium seguinum** | T62.2X1 | T62.2X2 | T62.2X3 | T62.2X4 | — | — |
| **Calamine** (lotion) | T49.3X1 | T49.3X2 | T49.3X3 | T49.3X4 | T49.3X5 | T49.3X6 |
| **Calcifediol** | T45.2X1 | T45.2X2 | T45.2X3 | T45.2X4 | T45.2X5 | T45.2X6 |
| **Calciferol** | T45.2X1 | T45.2X2 | T45.2X3 | T45.2X4 | T45.2X5 | T45.2X6 |
| **Calcitonin** | T50.991 | T50.992 | T50.993 | T50.994 | T50.995 | T50.996 |
| **Calcitriol** | T45.2X1 | T45.2X2 | T45.2X3 | T45.2X4 | T45.2X5 | T45.2X6 |
| **Calcium** | T50.3X1 | T50.3X2 | T50.3X3 | T50.3X4 | T50.3X5 | T50.3X6 |
| actylsalicylate | T39.011 | T39.012 | T39.013 | T39.014 | T39.015 | T39.016 |
| benzamidosalicylate | T37.1X1 | T37.1X2 | T37.1X3 | T37.1X4 | T37.1X5 | T37.1X6 |
| bromide | T42.6X1 | T42.6X2 | T42.6X3 | T42.6X4 | T42.6X5 | T42.6X6 |
| bromolactobionate | T42.6X1 | T42.6X2 | T42.6X3 | T42.6X4 | T42.6X5 | T42.6X6 |
| carbaspirin | T39.011 | T39.012 | T39.013 | T39.014 | T39.015 | T39.016 |
| carbimide | T50.6X1 | T50.6X2 | T50.6X3 | T50.6X4 | T50.6X5 | T50.6X6 |
| carbonate | T47.1X1 | T47.1X2 | T47.1X3 | T47.1X4 | T47.1X5 | T47.1X6 |
| chloride | T50.992 | T50.992 | T50.993 | T50.994 | T50.995 | T50.996 |
|   anhydrous | T50.991 | T50.992 | T50.993 | T50.994 | T50.995 | T50.996 |
| cyanide | T57.8X1 | T57.8X2 | T57.8X3 | T57.8X4 | — | — |
| dioctyl sulfosuccinate | T47.4X1 | T47.4X2 | T47.4X3 | T47.4X4 | T47.4X5 | T47.4X6 |
| disodium edathamil | T45.8X1 | T45.8X2 | T45.8X3 | T45.8X4 | T45.8X5 | T45.8X6 |
| disodium edetate | T45.8X1 | T45.8X2 | T45.8X3 | T45.8X4 | T45.8X5 | T45.8X6 |
| dobesilate | T46.991 | T46.992 | T46.993 | T46.994 | T46.995 | T46.996 |
| EDTA | T45.8X1 | T45.8X2 | T45.8X3 | T45.8X4 | T45.8X5 | T45.8X6 |
| ferrous citrate | T45.4X1 | T45.4X2 | T45.4X3 | T45.4X4 | T45.4X5 | T45.4X6 |
| folinate | T45.8X1 | T45.8X2 | T45.8X3 | T45.8X4 | T45.8X5 | T45.8X6 |
| glubionate | T50.3X1 | T50.3X2 | T50.3X3 | T50.3X4 | T50.3X5 | T50.3X6 |
| gluconate | T50.3X1 | T50.3X2 | T50.3X3 | T50.3X4 | T50.3X5 | T50.3X6 |
| gluconogalactogluconate | T50.3X1 | T50.3X2 | T50.3X3 | T50.3X4 | T50.3X5 | T50.3X6 |
| hydrate, hydroxide | T54.3X1 | T54.3X2 | T54.3X3 | T54.3X4 | — | — |
| hypochlorite | T54.3X1 | T54.3X2 | T54.3X3 | T54.3X4 | — | — |
| iodide | T48.4X1 | T48.4X2 | T48.4X3 | T48.4X4 | T48.4X5 | T48.4X6 |
| ipodate | T50.8X1 | T50.8X2 | T50.8X3 | T50.8X4 | T50.8X5 | T50.8X6 |
| lactate | T50.3X1 | T50.3X2 | T50.3X3 | T50.3X4 | T50.3X5 | T50.3X6 |
| leucovorin | T45.8X1 | T45.8X2 | T45.8X3 | T45.8X4 | T45.8X5 | T45.8X6 |
| mandelate | T37.91 | T37.92 | T37.93 | T37.94 | T37.95 | T37.96 |
| oxide | T54.3X1 | T54.3X2 | T54.3X3 | T54.3X4 | — | — |
| pantothenate | T45.2X1 | T45.2X2 | T45.2X3 | T45.2X4 | T45.2X5 | T45.2X6 |
| phosphate | T50.3X1 | T50.3X2 | T50.3X3 | T50.3X4 | T50.3X5 | T50.3X6 |
| salicylate | T39.091 | T39.092 | T39.093 | T39.094 | T39.095 | T39.096 |
| salts | T50.3X1 | T50.3X2 | T50.3X3 | T50.3X4 | T50.3X5 | T50.3X6 |
| **Calculus-dissolving drug** | T50.991 | T50.992 | T50.993 | T50.994 | T50.995 | T50.996 |
| **Calomel** | T49.0X1 | T49.0X2 | T49.0X3 | T49.0X4 | T49.0X5 | T49.0X6 |
| **Caloric agent** | T50.3X1 | T50.3X2 | T50.3X3 | T50.3X4 | T50.3X5 | T50.3X6 |
| **Calusterone** | T38.7X1 | T38.7X2 | T38.7X3 | T38.7X4 | T38.7X5 | T38.7X6 |
| **Camazepam** | T42.4X1 | T42.4X2 | T42.4X3 | T42.4X4 | T42.4X5 | T42.4X6 |
| **Camomile** | T49.0X1 | T49.0X2 | T49.0X3 | T49.0X4 | T49.0X5 | T49.0X6 |
| **Camoquin** | T37.2X1 | T37.2X2 | T37.2X3 | T37.2X4 | T37.2X5 | T37.2X6 |
| **Camphor** | | | | | | |
| insecticide | T60.2X1 | T60.2X2 | T60.2X3 | T60.2X4 | — | — |
| medicinal | T49.8X1 | T49.8X2 | T49.8X3 | T49.8X4 | T49.8X5 | T49.8X6 |
| **Camylofin** | T44.3X1 | T44.3X2 | T44.3X3 | T44.3X4 | T44.3X5 | T44.3X6 |
| **Cancer chemotherapy drug regimen** | T45.1X1 | T45.1X2 | T45.1X3 | T45.1X4 | T45.1X5 | T45.1X6 |
| **Candeptin** | T49.0X1 | T49.0X2 | T49.0X3 | T49.0X4 | T49.0X5 | T49.0X6 |
| **Candicidin** | T49.0X1 | T49.0X2 | T49.0X3 | T49.0X4 | T49.0X5 | T49.0X6 |
| **Cannabinol** | T40.7X1 | T40.7X2 | T40.7X3 | T40.7X4 | T40.7X5 | T40.7X6 |
| **Cannabis** (derivatives) | T40.7X1 | T40.7X2 | T40.7X3 | T40.7X4 | T40.7X5 | T40.7X6 |
| **Canned heat** | T51.1X1 | T51.1X2 | T51.1X3 | T51.1X4 | — | — |
| **Canrenoic acid** | T50.0X1 | T50.0X2 | T50.0X3 | T50.0X4 | T50.0X5 | T50.0X6 |
| **Canrenone** | T50.0X1 | T50.0X2 | T50.0X3 | T50.0X4 | T50.0X5 | T50.0X6 |
| **Cantharides, cantharidin, cantharis** | T49.8X1 | T49.8X2 | T49.8X3 | T49.8X4 | T49.8X5 | T49.8X6 |
| **Canthaxanthin** | T50.991 | T50.992 | T50.993 | T50.994 | T50.995 | T50.996 |
| **Capillary-active drug NEC** | T46.901 | T46.902 | T46.903 | T46.904 | T46.905 | T46.906 |
| **Capreomycin** | T36.8X1 | T36.8X2 | T36.8X3 | T36.8X4 | T36.8X5 | T36.8X6 |
| **Capsicum** | T49.4X1 | T49.4X2 | T49.4X3 | T49.4X4 | T49.4X5 | T49.4X6 |
| **Captafol** | T60.3X1 | T60.3X2 | T60.3X3 | T60.3X4 | — | — |
| **Captan** | T60.3X1 | T60.3X2 | T60.3X3 | T60.3X4 | — | — |
| **Captodiame, captodiamine** | T43.591 | T43.592 | T43.593 | T43.594 | T43.595 | T43.596 |
| **Captopril** | T46.4X1 | T46.4X2 | T46.4X3 | T46.4X4 | T46.4X5 | T46.4X6 |
| **Caramiphen** | T44.3X1 | T44.3X2 | T44.3X3 | T44.3X4 | T44.3X5 | T44.3X6 |
| **Carazolol** | T44.7X1 | T44.7X2 | T44.7X3 | T44.7X4 | T44.7X5 | T44.7X6 |
| **Carbachol** | T44.1X1 | T44.1X2 | T44.1X3 | T44.1X4 | T44.1X5 | T44.1X6 |
| **Carbacrylamine** (resin) | T50.3X1 | T50.3X2 | T50.3X3 | T50.3X4 | T50.3X5 | T50.3X6 |
| **Carbamate** (insecticide) | T60.0X1 | T60.0X2 | T60.0X3 | T60.0X4 | — | — |
| **Carbamate** (sedative) | T42.6X1 | T42.6X2 | T42.6X3 | T42.6X4 | T42.6X5 | T42.6X6 |
| herbicide | T60.0X1 | T60.0X2 | T60.0X3 | T60.0X4 | — | — |
| insecticide | T60.0X1 | T60.0X2 | T60.0X3 | T60.0X4 | — | — |
| **Carbamazepine** | T42.1X1 | T42.1X2 | T42.1X3 | T42.1X4 | T42.1X5 | T42.1X6 |

| Substance | Poisoning, Accidental (unintentional) | Poisoning, Intentional Self-harm | Poisoning, Assault | Poisoning, Undetermined | Adverse Effect | Under-dosing |
|---|---|---|---|---|---|---|
| **Carbamide** | T47.3X1 | T47.3X2 | T47.3X3 | T47.3X4 | T47.3X5 | T47.3X6 |
| peroxide | T49.0X1 | T49.0X2 | T49.0X3 | T49.0X4 | T49.0X5 | T49.0X6 |
| topical | T49.8X1 | T49.8X2 | T49.8X3 | T49.8X4 | T49.8X5 | T49.8X6 |
| **Carbamylcholine chloride** | T44.1X1 | T44.1X2 | T44.1X3 | T44.1X4 | T44.1X5 | T44.1X6 |
| **Carbaril** | T60.0X1 | T60.0X2 | T60.0X3 | T60.0X4 | — | — |
| **Carbarsone** | T37.3X1 | T37.3X2 | T37.3X3 | T37.3X4 | T37.3X5 | T37.3X6 |
| **Carbaryl** | T60.0X1 | T60.0X2 | T60.0X3 | T60.0X4 | — | — |
| **Carbaspirin** | T39.011 | T39.012 | T39.013 | T39.014 | T39.015 | T39.016 |
| **Carbazochrome** (salicylate) (sodium sulfonate) | T49.4X1 | T49.4X2 | T49.4X3 | T49.4X4 | T49.4X5 | T49.4X6 |
| **Carbenicillin** | T36.0X1 | T36.0X2 | T36.0X3 | T36.0X4 | T36.0X5 | T36.0X6 |
| **Carbenoxolone** | T47.1X1 | T47.1X2 | T47.1X3 | T47.1X4 | T47.1X5 | T47.1X6 |
| **Carbetapentane** | T48.3X1 | T48.3X2 | T48.3X3 | T48.3X4 | T48.3X5 | T48.3X6 |
| **Carbethyl salicylate** | T39.091 | T39.092 | T39.093 | T39.094 | T39.095 | T39.096 |
| **Carbidopa** (with levodopa) | T42.8X1 | T42.8X2 | T42.8X3 | T42.8X4 | T42.8X5 | T42.8X6 |
| **Carbimazole** | T38.2X1 | T38.2X2 | T38.2X3 | T38.2X4 | T38.2X5 | T38.2X6 |
| **Carbinol** | T51.1X1 | T51.1X2 | T51.1X3 | T51.1X4 | — | — |
| **Carbinoxamine** | T45.0X1 | T45.0X2 | T45.0X3 | T45.0X4 | T45.0X5 | T45.0X6 |
| **Carbiphene** | T39.8X1 | T39.8X2 | T39.8X3 | T39.8X4 | T39.8X5 | T39.8X6 |
| **Carbitol** | T52.3X1 | T52.3X2 | T52.3X3 | T52.3X4 | — | — |
| **Carbocaine** | T41.3X1 | T41.3X2 | T41.3X3 | T41.3X4 | T41.3X5 | T41.3X6 |
| infiltration (subcutaneous) | T41.3X1 | T41.3X2 | T41.3X3 | T41.3X4 | T41.3X5 | T41.3X6 |
| nerve block (peripheral) (plexus) | T41.3X1 | T41.3X2 | T41.3X3 | T41.3X4 | T41.3X5 | T41.3X6 |
| topical (surface) | T41.3X1 | T41.3X2 | T41.3X3 | T41.3X4 | T41.3X5 | T41.3X6 |
| **Carbocisteine** | T48.4X1 | T48.4X2 | T48.4X3 | T48.4X4 | T48.4X5 | T48.4X6 |
| **Carbocromen** | T46.3X1 | T46.3X2 | T46.3X3 | T46.3X4 | T46.3X5 | T46.3X6 |
| **Carbol fuchsin** | T49.0X1 | T49.0X2 | T49.0X3 | T49.0X4 | T49.0X5 | T49.0X6 |
| **Carbolic acid** — *see also* Phenol | T54.0X1 | T54.0X2 | T54.0X3 | T54.0X4 | — | — |
| **Carbolonium** (bromide) | T48.1X1 | T48.1X2 | T48.1X3 | T48.1X4 | T48.1X5 | T48.1X6 |
| **Carbo medicinalis** | T47.6X1 | T47.6X2 | T47.6X3 | T47.6X4 | T47.6X5 | T47.6X6 |
| **Carbomycin** | T36.8X1 | T36.8X2 | T36.8X3 | T36.8X4 | T36.8X5 | T36.8X6 |
| **Carbon** | | | | | | |
| bisulfide (liquid) | T65.4X1 | T65.4X2 | T65.4X3 | T65.4X4 | — | — |
|   vapor | T65.4X1 | T65.4X2 | T65.4X3 | T65.4X4 | — | — |
| dioxide (gas) | T59.7X1 | T59.7X2 | T59.7X3 | T59.7X4 | — | — |
|   medicinal | T41.5X1 | T41.5X2 | T41.5X3 | T41.5X4 | T41.5X5 | T41.5X6 |
|   nonmedicinal | T59.7X1 | T59.7X2 | T59.7X3 | T59.7X4 | — | — |
|   snow | T49.4X1 | T49.4X2 | T49.4X3 | T49.4X4 | T49.4X5 | T49.4X6 |
| disulfide (liquid) | T65.4X1 | T65.4X2 | T65.4X3 | T65.4X4 | — | — |
|   vapor | T65.4X1 | T65.4X2 | T65.4X3 | T65.4X4 | — | — |
| monoxide (from incomplete combustion) | T58.91 | T58.92 | T58.93 | T58.94 | — | — |
|   blast furnace gas | T58.8X1 | T58.8X2 | T58.8X3 | T58.8X4 | — | — |
|   butane (distributed in mobile container) | T58.11 | T58.12 | T58.13 | T58.14 | — | — |
|   distributed through pipes | T58.11 | T58.12 | T58.13 | T58.14 | — | — |
|   charcoal fumes | T58.2X1 | T58.2X2 | T58.2X3 | T58.2X4 | — | — |
|   coal | T58.2X1 | T58.2X2 | T58.2X3 | T58.2X4 | — | — |
|   coke (in domestic stoves, fireplaces) | T58.2X1 | T58.2X2 | T58.2X3 | T58.2X4 | — | — |
|   exhaust gas (motor) not in transit | T58.01 | T58.02 | T58.03 | T58.04 | — | — |
|   combustion engine, any not in watercraft | T58.01 | T58.02 | T58.03 | T58.04 | — | — |
|   farm tractor, not in transit | T58.01 | T58.02 | T58.03 | T58.04 | — | — |
|   gas engine | T58.01 | T58.02 | T58.03 | T58.04 | — | — |
|   motor pump | T58.01 | T58.02 | T58.03 | T58.04 | — | — |
|   motor vehicle, not in transit | T58.01 | T58.02 | T58.03 | T58.04 | — | — |
|   fuel (in domestic use) | T58.2X1 | T58.2X2 | T58.2X3 | T58.2X4 | — | — |
|   gas (piped) | T58.11 | T58.12 | T58.13 | T58.14 | — | — |
|     in mobile container | T58.11 | T58.12 | T58.13 | T58.14 | — | — |
|     piped (natural) | T58.11 | T58.12 | T58.13 | T58.14 | — | — |
|     utility | T58.11 | T58.12 | T58.13 | T58.14 | — | — |
|      in mobile container | T58.11 | T58.12 | T58.13 | T58.14 | — | — |
|   gas (piped) | T58.11 | T58.12 | T58.13 | T58.14 | — | — |
|   illuminating gas | T58.11 | T58.12 | T58.13 | T58.14 | — | — |
|   industrial fuels or gases, any | T58.8X1 | T58.8X2 | T58.8X3 | T58.8X4 | — | — |
|   kerosene (in domestic stoves, fireplaces) | T58.2X1 | T58.2X2 | T58.2X3 | T58.2X4 | — | — |
|   kiln gas or vapor | T58.8X1 | T58.8X2 | T58.8X3 | T58.8X4 | — | — |
|   motor exhaust gas, not in transit | T58.01 | T58.02 | T58.03 | T58.04 | — | — |
|   piped gas (manufactured) (natural) | T58.11 | T58.12 | T58.13 | T58.14 | — | — |
|   producer gas | T58.8X1 | T58.8X2 | T58.8X3 | T58.8X4 | — | — |
|   propane (distributed in mobile container) | T58.11 | T58.12 | T58.13 | T58.14 | — | — |

Table of Drugs and Chemicals

| Substance | Poisoning, Accidental (unintentional) | Poisoning, Intentional Self-harm | Poisoning, Assault | Poisoning, Undetermined | Adverse Effect | Under-dosing |
|---|---|---|---|---|---|---|
| **Carbon** — *continued* | | | | | | |
| monoxide — *continued* | | | | | | |
| propane — *continued* | | | | | | |
| distributed through pipes | T58.11 | T58.12 | T58.13 | T58.14 | — | — |
| solid (in domestic stoves, fireplaces) | T58.2X1 | T58.2X2 | T58.2X3 | T58.2X4 | — | — |
| specified source NEC | T58.8X1 | T58.8X2 | T58.8X3 | T58.8X4 | — | — |
| stove gas | T58.11 | T58.12 | T58.13 | T58.14 | — | — |
| piped | T58.11 | T58.12 | T58.13 | T58.14 | — | — |
| utility gas | T58.11 | T58.12 | T58.13 | T58.14 | — | — |
| piped | T58.11 | T58.12 | T58.13 | T58.14 | — | — |
| water gas | T58.11 | T58.12 | T58.13 | T58.14 | — | — |
| wood (in domestic stoves, fireplaces) | T58.2X1 | T58.2X2 | T58.2X3 | T58.2X4 | — | — |
| tetrachloride (vapor) NEC | T53.0X1 | T53.0X2 | T53.0X3 | T53.0X4 | — | — |
| liquid (cleansing agent) NEC | T53.0X1 | T53.0X2 | T53.0X3 | T53.0X4 | — | — |
| solvent | T53.0X1 | T53.0X2 | T53.0X3 | T53.0X4 | — | — |
| **Carbonic acid gas** | T59.7X1 | T59.7X2 | T59.7X3 | T59.7X4 | — | — |
| anhydrase inhibitor NEC | T50.2X1 | T50.2X2 | T50.2X3 | T50.2X4 | T50.2X5 | T50.2X6 |
| **Carbophenothion** | T60.0X1 | T60.0X2 | T60.0X3 | T60.0X4 | — | — |
| **Carboplatin** | T45.1X1 | T45.1X2 | T45.1X3 | T45.1X4 | T45.1X5 | T45.1X6 |
| **Carboprost** | T48.0X1 | T48.0X2 | T48.0X3 | T48.0X4 | T48.0X5 | T48.0X6 |
| **Carboquone** | T45.1X1 | T45.1X2 | T45.1X3 | T45.1X4 | T45.1X5 | T45.1X6 |
| **Carbowax** | T49.3X1 | T49.3X2 | T49.3X3 | T49.3X4 | T49.3X5 | T49.3X6 |
| **Carboxymethylcellulose** | T47.4X1 | T47.4X2 | T47.4X3 | T47.4X4 | T47.4X5 | T47.4X6 |
| **Carbrital** | T42.3X1 | T42.3X2 | T42.3X3 | T42.3X4 | T42.3X5 | T42.3X6 |
| **Carbromal** | T42.6X1 | T42.6X2 | T42.6X3 | T42.6X4 | T42.6X5 | T42.6X6 |
| **Carbutamide** | T38.3X1 | T38.3X2 | T38.3X3 | T38.3X4 | T38.3X5 | T38.3X6 |
| **Carbuterol** | T48.6X1 | T48.6X2 | T48.6X3 | T48.6X4 | T48.6X5 | T48.6X6 |
| **Cardiac** | | | | | | |
| depressants | T46.2X1 | T46.2X2 | T46.2X3 | T46.2X4 | T46.2X5 | T46.2X6 |
| rhythm regulator | T46.2X1 | T46.2X2 | T46.2X3 | T46.2X4 | T46.2X5 | T46.2X6 |
| specified NEC | T46.2X1 | T46.2X2 | T46.2X3 | T46.2X4 | T46.2X5 | T46.2X6 |
| **Cardiografin** | T50.8X1 | T50.8X2 | T50.8X3 | T50.8X4 | T50.8X5 | T50.8X6 |
| **Cardiogreen** | T50.8X1 | T50.8X2 | T50.8X3 | T50.8X4 | T50.8X5 | T50.8X6 |
| **Cardiotonic** (glycoside) **NEC** | T46.0X1 | T46.0X2 | T46.0X3 | T46.0X4 | T46.0X5 | T46.0X6 |
| **Cardiovascular drug NEC** | T46.901 | T46.902 | T46.903 | T46.904 | T46.905 | T46.906 |
| **Cardrase** | T50.2X1 | T50.2X2 | T50.2X3 | T50.2X4 | T50.2X5 | T50.2X6 |
| **Carfecillin** | T36.0X1 | T36.0X2 | T36.0X3 | T36.0X4 | T36.0X5 | T36.0X6 |
| **Carfenazine** | T43.3X1 | T43.3X2 | T43.3X3 | T43.3X4 | T43.3X5 | T43.3X6 |
| **Carfusin** | T49.0X1 | T49.0X2 | T49.0X3 | T49.0X4 | T49.0X5 | T49.0X6 |
| **Carindacillin** | T36.0X1 | T36.0X2 | T36.0X3 | T36.0X4 | T36.0X5 | T36.0X6 |
| **Carisoprodol** | T42.8X1 | T42.8X2 | T42.8X3 | T42.8X4 | T42.8X5 | T42.8X6 |
| **Carmellose** | T47.4X1 | T47.4X2 | T47.4X3 | T47.4X4 | T47.4X5 | T47.4X6 |
| **Carminative** | T47.5X1 | T47.5X2 | T47.5X3 | T47.5X4 | T47.5X5 | T47.5X6 |
| **Carmofur** | T45.1X1 | T45.1X2 | T45.1X3 | T45.1X4 | T45.1X5 | T45.1X6 |
| **Carmustine** | T45.1X1 | T45.1X2 | T45.1X3 | T45.1X4 | T45.1X5 | T45.1X6 |
| **Carotene** | T45.2X1 | T45.2X2 | T45.2X3 | T45.2X4 | T45.2X5 | T45.2X6 |
| **Carphenazine** | T43.3X1 | T43.3X2 | T43.3X3 | T43.3X4 | T43.3X5 | T43.3X6 |
| **Carpipramine** | T42.4X1 | T42.4X2 | T42.4X3 | T42.4X4 | T42.4X5 | T42.4X6 |
| **Carprofen** | T39.311 | T39.312 | T39.313 | T39.314 | T39.315 | T39.316 |
| **Carpronium chloride** | T44.3X1 | T44.3X2 | T44.3X3 | T44.3X4 | T44.3X5 | T44.3X6 |
| **Carrageenan** | T47.8X1 | T47.8X2 | T47.8X3 | T47.8X4 | T47.8X5 | T47.8X6 |
| **Carteolol** | T44.7X1 | T44.7X2 | T44.7X3 | T44.7X4 | T44.7X5 | T44.7X6 |
| **Carter's Little Pills** | T47.2X1 | T47.2X2 | T47.2X3 | T47.2X4 | T47.2X5 | T47.2X6 |
| **Cascara** (sagrada) | T47.2X1 | T47.2X2 | T47.2X3 | T47.2X4 | T47.2X5 | T47.2X6 |
| **Cassava** | T62.2X1 | T62.2X2 | T62.2X3 | T62.2X4 | — | — |
| **Castellani's paint** | T49.0X1 | T49.0X2 | T49.0X3 | T49.0X4 | T49.0X5 | T49.0X6 |
| **Castor** | | | | | | |
| bean | T62.2X1 | T62.2X2 | T62.2X3 | T62.2X4 | — | — |
| oil | T47.2X1 | T47.2X2 | T47.2X3 | T47.2X4 | T47.2X5 | T47.2X6 |
| **Catalase** | T45.3X1 | T45.3X2 | T45.3X3 | T45.3X4 | T45.3X5 | T45.3X6 |
| **Caterpillar** (sting) | T63.431 | T63.432 | T63.433 | T63.434 | — | — |
| **Catha** (edulis) (tea) | T43.691 | T43.692 | T43.693 | T43.694 | — | — |
| **Cathartic NEC** | T47.4X1 | T47.4X2 | T47.4X3 | T47.4X4 | T47.4X5 | T47.4X6 |
| anthacene derivative | T47.2X1 | T47.2X2 | T47.2X3 | T47.2X4 | T47.2X5 | T47.2X6 |
| bulk | T47.4X1 | T47.4X2 | T47.4X3 | T47.4X4 | T47.4X5 | T47.4X6 |
| contact | T47.2X1 | T47.2X2 | T47.2X3 | T47.2X4 | T47.2X5 | T47.2X6 |
| emollient NEC | T47.4X1 | T47.4X2 | T47.4X3 | T47.4X4 | T47.4X5 | T47.4X6 |
| irritant NEC | T47.2X1 | T47.2X2 | T47.2X3 | T47.2X4 | T47.2X5 | T47.2X6 |
| mucilage | T47.4X1 | T47.4X2 | T47.4X3 | T47.4X4 | T47.4X5 | T47.4X6 |
| saline | T47.3X1 | T47.3X2 | T47.3X3 | T47.3X4 | T47.3X5 | T47.3X6 |
| vegetable | T47.2X1 | T47.2X2 | T47.2X3 | T47.2X4 | T47.2X5 | T47.2X6 |
| **Cathine** | T50.5X1 | T50.5X2 | T50.5X3 | T50.5X4 | T50.5X5 | T50.5X6 |
| **Cathomycin** | T36.8X1 | T36.8X2 | T36.8X3 | T36.8X4 | T36.8X5 | T36.8X6 |
| **Cation exchange resin** | T50.3X1 | T50.3X2 | T50.3X3 | T50.3X4 | T50.3X5 | T50.3X6 |
| **Caustic(s) NEC** | T54.91 | T54.92 | T54.93 | T54.94 | — | — |
| alkali | T54.3X1 | T54.3X2 | T54.3X3 | T54.3X4 | — | — |
| hydroxide | T54.3X1 | T54.3X2 | T54.3X3 | T54.3X4 | — | — |
| potash | T54.3X1 | T54.3X2 | T54.3X3 | T54.3X4 | — | — |
| soda | T54.3X1 | T54.3X2 | T54.3X3 | T54.3X4 | — | — |

| Substance | Poisoning, Accidental (unintentional) | Poisoning, Intentional Self-harm | Poisoning, Assault | Poisoning, Undetermined | Adverse Effect | Under-dosing |
|---|---|---|---|---|---|---|
| **Caustic(s) NEC** — *continued* | | | | | | |
| specified NEC | T54.91 | T54.92 | T54.93 | T54.94 | — | — |
| **Ceepryn** | T49.0X1 | T49.0X2 | T49.0X3 | T49.0X4 | T49.0X5 | T49.0X6 |
| ENT agent | T49.6X1 | T49.6X2 | T49.6X3 | T49.6X4 | T49.6X5 | T49.6X6 |
| lozenges | T49.6X1 | T49.6X2 | T49.6X3 | T49.6X4 | T49.6X5 | T49.6X6 |
| **Cefacetrile** | T36.1X1 | T36.1X2 | T36.1X3 | T36.1X4 | T36.1X5 | T36.1X6 |
| **Cefaclor** | T36.1X1 | T36.1X2 | T36.1X3 | T36.1X4 | T36.1X5 | T36.1X6 |
| **Cefadroxil** | T36.1X1 | T36.1X2 | T36.1X3 | T36.1X4 | T36.1X5 | T36.1X6 |
| **Cefalexin** | T36.1X1 | T36.1X2 | T36.1X3 | T36.1X4 | T36.1X5 | T36.1X6 |
| **Cefaloglycin** | T36.1X1 | T36.1X2 | T36.1X3 | T36.1X4 | T36.1X5 | T36.1X6 |
| **Cefaloridine** | T36.1X1 | T36.1X2 | T36.1X3 | T36.1X4 | T36.1X5 | T36.1X6 |
| **Cefalosporins** | T36.1X1 | T36.1X2 | T36.1X3 | T36.1X4 | T36.1X5 | T36.1X6 |
| **Cefalotin** | T36.1X1 | T36.1X2 | T36.1X3 | T36.1X4 | T36.1X5 | T36.1X6 |
| **Cefamandole** | T36.1X1 | T36.1X2 | T36.1X3 | T36.1X4 | T36.1X5 | T36.1X6 |
| **Cefamycin antibiotic** | T36.1X1 | T36.1X2 | T36.1X3 | T36.1X4 | T36.1X5 | T36.1X6 |
| **Cefapirin** | T36.1X1 | T36.1X2 | T36.1X3 | T36.1X4 | T36.1X5 | T36.1X6 |
| **Cefatrizine** | T36.1X1 | T36.1X2 | T36.1X3 | T36.1X4 | T36.1X5 | T36.1X6 |
| **Cefazedone** | T36.1X1 | T36.1X2 | T36.1X3 | T36.1X4 | T36.1X5 | T36.1X6 |
| **Cefazolin** | T36.1X1 | T36.1X2 | T36.1X3 | T36.1X4 | T36.1X5 | T36.1X6 |
| **Cefbuperazone** | T36.1X1 | T36.1X2 | T36.1X3 | T36.1X4 | T36.1X5 | T36.1X6 |
| **Cefetamet** | T36.1X1 | T36.1X2 | T36.1X3 | T36.1X4 | T36.1X5 | T36.1X6 |
| **Cefixime** | T36.1X1 | T36.1X2 | T36.1X3 | T36.1X4 | T36.1X5 | T36.1X6 |
| **Cefmenoxime** | T36.1X1 | T36.1X2 | T36.1X3 | T36.1X4 | T36.1X5 | T36.1X6 |
| **Cefmetazole** | T36.1X1 | T36.1X2 | T36.1X3 | T36.1X4 | T36.1X5 | T36.1X6 |
| **Cefminox** | T36.1X1 | T36.1X2 | T36.1X3 | T36.1X4 | T36.1X5 | T36.1X6 |
| **Cefonicid** | T36.1X1 | T36.1X2 | T36.1X3 | T36.1X4 | T36.1X5 | T36.1X6 |
| **Cefoperazone** | T36.1X1 | T36.1X2 | T36.1X3 | T36.1X4 | T36.1X5 | T36.1X6 |
| **Ceforanide** | T36.1X1 | T36.1X2 | T36.1X3 | T36.1X4 | T36.1X5 | T36.1X6 |
| **Cefotaxime** | T36.1X1 | T36.1X2 | T36.1X3 | T36.1X4 | T36.1X5 | T36.1X6 |
| **Cefotetan** | T36.1X1 | T36.1X2 | T36.1X3 | T36.1X4 | T36.1X5 | T36.1X6 |
| **Cefotiam** | T36.1X1 | T36.1X2 | T36.1X3 | T36.1X4 | T36.1X5 | T36.1X6 |
| **Cefoxitin** | T36.1X1 | T36.1X2 | T36.1X3 | T36.1X4 | T36.1X5 | T36.1X6 |
| **Cefpimizole** | T36.1X1 | T36.1X2 | T36.1X3 | T36.1X4 | T36.1X5 | T36.1X6 |
| **Cefpiramide** | T36.1X1 | T36.1X2 | T36.1X3 | T36.1X4 | T36.1X5 | T36.1X6 |
| **Cefradine** | T36.1X1 | T36.1X2 | T36.1X3 | T36.1X4 | T36.1X5 | T36.1X6 |
| **Cefroxadine** | T36.1X1 | T36.1X2 | T36.1X3 | T36.1X4 | T36.1X5 | T36.1X6 |
| **Cefsulodin** | T36.1X1 | T36.1X2 | T36.1X3 | T36.1X4 | T36.1X5 | T36.1X6 |
| **Ceftazidime** | T36.1X1 | T36.1X2 | T36.1X3 | T36.1X4 | T36.1X5 | T36.1X6 |
| **Cefteram** | T36.1X1 | T36.1X2 | T36.1X3 | T36.1X4 | T36.1X5 | T36.1X6 |
| **Ceftezole** | T36.1X1 | T36.1X2 | T36.1X3 | T36.1X4 | T36.1X5 | T36.1X6 |
| **Ceftizoxime** | T36.1X1 | T36.1X2 | T36.1X3 | T36.1X4 | T36.1X5 | T36.1X6 |
| **Ceftriaxone** | T36.1X1 | T36.1X2 | T36.1X3 | T36.1X4 | T36.1X5 | T36.1X6 |
| **Cefuroxime** | T36.1X1 | T36.1X2 | T36.1X3 | T36.1X4 | T36.1X5 | T36.1X6 |
| **Cefuzonam** | T36.1X1 | T36.1X2 | T36.1X3 | T36.1X4 | T36.1X5 | T36.1X6 |
| **Celestone** | T38.0X1 | T38.0X2 | T38.0X3 | T38.0X4 | T38.0X5 | T38.0X6 |
| topical | T49.0X1 | T49.0X2 | T49.0X3 | T49.0X4 | T49.0X5 | T49.0X6 |
| **Celiprolol** | T44.7X1 | T44.7X2 | T44.7X3 | T44.7X4 | T44.7X5 | T44.7X6 |
| **Cellosolve** | T52.91 | T52.92 | T52.93 | T52.94 | — | — |
| **Cell stimulants and proliferants** | T49.8X1 | T49.8X2 | T49.8X3 | T49.8X4 | T49.8X5 | T49.8X6 |
| **Cellulose** | | | | | | |
| cathartic | T47.4X1 | T47.4X2 | T47.4X3 | T47.4X4 | T47.4X5 | T47.4X6 |
| hydroxyethyl | T47.4X1 | T47.4X2 | T47.4X3 | T47.4X4 | T47.4X5 | T47.4X6 |
| nitrates (topical) | T49.3X1 | T49.3X2 | T49.3X3 | T49.3X4 | T49.3X5 | T49.3X6 |
| oxidized | T49.4X1 | T49.4X2 | T49.4X3 | T49.4X4 | T49.4X5 | T49.4X6 |
| **Centipede** (bite) | T63.411 | T63.412 | T63.413 | T63.414 | — | — |
| **Central nervous system** | | | | | | |
| depressants | T42.71 | T42.72 | T42.73 | T42.74 | T42.75 | T42.76 |
| anesthetic (general) NEC | T41.201 | T41.202 | T41.203 | T41.204 | T41.205 | T41.206 |
| gases NEC | T41.0X1 | T41.0X2 | T41.0X3 | T41.0X4 | T41.0X5 | T41.0X6 |
| intravenous | T41.1X1 | T41.1X2 | T41.1X3 | T41.1X4 | T41.1X5 | T41.1X6 |
| barbiturates | T42.3X1 | T42.3X2 | T42.3X3 | T42.3X4 | T42.3X5 | T42.3X6 |
| benzodiazepines | T42.4X1 | T42.4X2 | T42.4X3 | T42.4X4 | T42.4X5 | T42.4X6 |
| bromides | T42.6X1 | T42.6X2 | T42.6X3 | T42.6X4 | T42.6X5 | T42.6X6 |
| cannabis sativa | T40.7X1 | T40.7X2 | T40.7X3 | T40.7X4 | T40.7X5 | T40.7X6 |
| chloral hydrate | T42.6X1 | T42.6X2 | T42.6X3 | T42.6X4 | T42.6X5 | T42.6X6 |
| ethanol | T51.0X1 | T51.0X2 | T51.0X3 | T51.0X4 | — | — |
| hallucinogenics | T40.901 | T40.902 | T40.903 | T40.904 | T40.905 | T40.906 |
| hypnotics | T42.71 | T42.72 | T42.73 | T42.74 | T42.75 | T42.76 |
| specified NEC | T42.6X1 | T42.6X2 | T42.6X3 | T42.6X4 | T42.6X5 | T42.6X6 |
| muscle relaxants | T42.8X1 | T42.8X2 | T42.8X3 | T42.8X4 | T42.8X5 | T42.8X6 |
| paraldehyde | T42.6X1 | T42.6X2 | T42.6X3 | T42.6X4 | T42.6X5 | T42.6X6 |
| sedatives | T42.71 | T42.72 | T42.73 | T42.74 | T42.75 | T42.76 |
| sedative-hypnotics | | | | | | |
| mixed NEC | T42.6X1 | T42.6X2 | T42.6X3 | T42.6X4 | T42.6X5 | T42.6X6 |
| specified NEC | T42.6X1 | T42.6X2 | T42.6X3 | T42.6X4 | T42.6X5 | T42.6X6 |
| muscle-tone depressants | T42.8X1 | T42.8X2 | T42.8X3 | T42.8X4 | T42.8X5 | T42.8X6 |
| stimulants | T43.601 | T43.602 | T43.603 | T43.604 | T43.605 | T43.606 |
| amphetamines | T43.621 | T43.622 | T43.623 | T43.624 | T43.625 | T43.626 |
| analeptics | T50.7X1 | T50.7X2 | T50.7X3 | T50.7X4 | T50.7X5 | T50.7X6 |
| antidepressants | T43.201 | T43.202 | T43.203 | T43.204 | T43.205 | T43.206 |
| opiate antagonists | T50.7X1 | T50.7X2 | T50.7X3 | T50.7X4 | T50.7X5 | T50.7X6 |
| specified NEC | T43.691 | T43.692 | T43.693 | T43.694 | T43.695 | T43.696 |

| Substance | Poisoning, Accidental (unintentional) | Poisoning, Intentional Self-harm | Poisoning, Assault | Poisoning, Undetermined | Adverse Effect | Under-dosing |
|---|---|---|---|---|---|---|
| Cephalexin | T36.1X1 | T36.1X2 | T36.1X3 | T36.1X4 | T36.1X5 | T36.1X6 |
| Cephaloglycin | T36.1X1 | T36.1X2 | T36.1X3 | T36.1X4 | T36.1X5 | T36.1X6 |
| Cephaloridine | T36.1X1 | T36.1X2 | T36.1X3 | T36.1X4 | T36.1X5 | T36.1X6 |
| Cephalosporins | T36.1X1 | T36.1X2 | T36.1X3 | T36.1X4 | T36.1X5 | T36.1X6 |
|   N (adicillin) | T36.0X1 | T36.0X2 | T36.0X3 | T36.0X4 | T36.0X5 | T36.0X6 |
| Cephalothin | T36.1X1 | T36.1X2 | T36.1X3 | T36.1X4 | T36.1X5 | T36.1X6 |
| Cephalotin | T36.1X1 | T36.1X2 | T36.1X3 | T36.1X4 | T36.1X5 | T36.1X6 |
| Cephradine | T36.1X1 | T36.1X2 | T36.1X3 | T36.1X4 | T36.1X5 | T36.1X6 |
| Cerbera (odallam) | T62.2X1 | T62.2X2 | T62.2X3 | T62.2X4 | — | — |
| Cerberin | T46.0X1 | T46.0X2 | T46.0X3 | T46.0X4 | T46.0X5 | T46.0X6 |
| Cerebral stimulants | T43.601 | T43.602 | T43.603 | T43.604 | T43.605 | T43.606 |
|   psychotherapeutic | T43.601 | T43.602 | T43.603 | T43.604 | T43.605 | T43.606 |
|   specified NEC | T43.691 | T43.692 | T43.693 | T43.694 | T43.695 | T43.696 |
| Cerium oxalate | T45.0X1 | T45.0X2 | T45.0X3 | T45.0X4 | T45.0X5 | T45.0X6 |
| Cerous oxalate | T45.0X1 | T45.0X2 | T45.0X3 | T45.0X4 | T45.0X5 | T45.0X6 |
| Ceruletide | T50.8X1 | T50.8X2 | T50.8X3 | T50.8X4 | T50.8X5 | T50.8X6 |
| Cetalkonium (chloride) | T49.0X1 | T49.0X2 | T49.0X3 | T49.0X4 | T49.0X5 | T49.0X6 |
| Cethexonium chloride | T49.0X1 | T49.0X2 | T49.0X3 | T49.0X4 | T49.0X5 | T49.0X6 |
| Cetiedil | T46.7X1 | T46.7X2 | T46.7X3 | T46.7X4 | T46.7X5 | T46.7X6 |
| Cetirizine | T45.0X1 | T45.0X2 | T45.0X3 | T45.0X4 | T45.0X5 | T45.0X6 |
| Cetomacrogol | T50.991 | T50.992 | T50.993 | T50.994 | T50.995 | T50.996 |
| Cetotiamine | T45.2X1 | T45.2X2 | T45.2X3 | T45.2X4 | T45.2X5 | T45.2X6 |
| Cetoxime | T45.0X1 | T45.0X2 | T45.0X3 | T45.0X4 | T45.0X5 | T45.0X6 |
| Cetraxate | T47.1X1 | T47.1X2 | T47.1X3 | T47.1X4 | T47.1X5 | T47.1X6 |
| Cetrimide | T49.0X1 | T49.0X2 | T49.0X3 | T49.0X4 | T49.0X5 | T49.0X6 |
| Cetrimonium (bromide) | T49.0X1 | T49.0X2 | T49.0X3 | T49.0X4 | T49.0X5 | T49.0X6 |
| Cetylpyridinium chloride | T49.0X1 | T49.0X2 | T49.0X3 | T49.0X4 | T49.0X5 | T49.0X6 |
|   ENT agent | T49.6X1 | T49.6X2 | T49.6X3 | T49.6X4 | T49.6X5 | T49.6X6 |
|   lozenges | T49.6X1 | T49.6X2 | T49.6X3 | T49.6X4 | T49.6X5 | T49.6X6 |
| Cevadilla — see Sabadilla | | | | | | |
| Cevitamic acid | T45.2X1 | T45.2X2 | T45.2X3 | T45.2X4 | T45.2X5 | T45.2X6 |
| Chalk, precipitated | T47.1X1 | T47.1X2 | T47.1X3 | T47.1X4 | T47.1X5 | T47.1X6 |
| Chamomile | T49.0X1 | T49.0X2 | T49.0X3 | T49.0X4 | T49.0X5 | T49.0X6 |
| Ch'an su | T46.0X1 | T46.0X2 | T46.0X3 | T46.0X4 | T46.0X5 | T46.0X6 |
| Charcoal | T47.6X1 | T47.6X2 | T47.6X3 | T47.6X4 | T47.6X5 | T47.6X6 |
|   activated — see also Charcoal, medicinal | T47.6X1 | T47.6X2 | T47.6X3 | T47.6X4 | T47.6X5 | T47.6X6 |
|   fumes (Carbon monoxide) | T58.2X1 | T58.2X2 | T58.2X3 | T58.2X4 | — | — |
|     industrial | T58.8X1 | T58.8X2 | T58.8X3 | T58.8X4 | — | — |
|   medicinal (activated) | T47.6X1 | T47.6X2 | T47.6X3 | T47.6X4 | T47.6X5 | T47.6X6 |
|     antidiarrheal | T47.6X1 | T47.6X2 | T47.6X3 | T47.6X4 | T47.6X5 | T47.6X6 |
|     poison control | T47.8X1 | T47.8X2 | T47.8X3 | T47.8X4 | T47.8X5 | T47.8X6 |
|     specified use other than for diarrhea | T47.8X1 | T47.8X2 | T47.8X3 | T47.8X4 | T47.8X5 | T47.8X6 |
|   topical | T49.8X1 | T49.8X2 | T49.8X3 | T49.8X4 | T49.8X5 | T49.8X6 |
| Chaulmosulfone | T37.1X1 | T37.1X2 | T37.1X3 | T37.1X4 | T37.1X5 | T37.1X6 |
| Chelating agent NEC | T50.6X1 | T50.6X2 | T50.6X3 | T50.6X4 | T50.6X5 | T50.6X6 |
| Chelidonium majus | T62.2X1 | T62.2X2 | T62.2X3 | T62.2X4 | — | — |
| Chemical substance NEC | T65.91 | T65.92 | T65.93 | T65.94 | — | — |
| Chenodeoxycholic acid | T47.5X1 | T47.5X2 | T47.5X3 | T47.5X4 | T47.5X5 | T47.5X6 |
| Chenodiol | T47.5X1 | T47.5X2 | T47.5X3 | T47.5X4 | T47.5X5 | T47.5X6 |
| Chenopodium | T37.4X1 | T37.4X2 | T37.4X3 | T37.4X4 | T37.4X5 | T37.4X6 |
| Cherry laurel | T62.2X1 | T62.2X2 | T62.2X3 | T62.2X4 | — | — |
| Chinidin (e) | T46.2X1 | T46.2X2 | T46.2X3 | T46.2X4 | T46.2X5 | T46.2X6 |
| Chiniofon | T37.8X1 | T37.8X2 | T37.8X3 | T37.8X4 | T37.8X5 | T37.8X6 |
| Chlophedianol | T48.3X1 | T48.3X2 | T48.3X3 | T48.3X4 | T48.3X5 | T48.3X6 |
| Chloral | T42.6X1 | T42.6X2 | T42.6X3 | T42.6X4 | T42.6X5 | T42.6X6 |
|   derivative | T42.6X1 | T42.6X2 | T42.6X3 | T42.6X4 | T42.6X5 | T42.6X6 |
|   hydrate | T42.6X1 | T42.6X2 | T42.6X3 | T42.6X4 | T42.6X5 | T42.6X6 |
| Chloralamide | T42.6X1 | T42.6X2 | T42.6X3 | T42.6X4 | T42.6X5 | T42.6X6 |
| Chloralodol | T42.6X1 | T42.6X2 | T42.6X3 | T42.6X4 | T42.6X5 | T42.6X6 |
| Chloralose | T60.4X1 | T60.4X2 | T60.4X3 | T60.4X4 | — | — |
| Chlorambucil | T45.1X1 | T45.1X2 | T45.1X3 | T45.1X4 | T45.1X5 | T45.1X6 |
| Chloramine | T57.8X1 | T57.8X2 | T57.8X3 | T57.8X4 | — | — |
|   T | T49.0X1 | T49.0X2 | T49.0X3 | T49.0X4 | T49.0X5 | T49.0X6 |
|   topical | T49.0X1 | T49.0X2 | T49.0X3 | T49.0X4 | T49.0X5 | T49.0X6 |
| Chloramphenicol | T36.2X1 | T36.2X2 | T36.2X3 | T36.2X4 | T36.2X5 | T36.2X6 |
|   ENT agent | T49.6X1 | T49.6X2 | T49.6X3 | T49.6X4 | T49.6X5 | T49.6X6 |
|   ophthalmic preparation | T49.5X1 | T49.5X2 | T49.5X3 | T49.5X4 | T49.5X5 | T49.5X6 |
|   topical NEC | T49.0X1 | T49.0X2 | T49.0X3 | T49.0X4 | T49.0X5 | T49.0X6 |
| Chlorate (potassium) (sodium) NEC | T60.3X1 | T60.3X2 | T60.3X3 | T60.3X4 | — | — |
|   herbicide | T60.3X1 | T60.3X2 | T60.3X3 | T60.3X4 | — | — |
| Chlorazanil | T50.2X1 | T50.2X2 | T50.2X3 | T50.2X4 | T50.2X5 | T50.2X6 |
| Chlorbenzene, chlorbenzol | T53.7X1 | T53.7X2 | T53.7X3 | T53.7X4 | — | — |
| Chlorbenzoxamine | T44.3X1 | T44.3X2 | T44.3X3 | T44.3X4 | T44.3X5 | T44.3X6 |
| Chlorbutol | T42.6X1 | T42.6X2 | T42.6X3 | T42.6X4 | T42.6X5 | T42.6X6 |
| Chlorcyclizine | T45.0X1 | T45.0X2 | T45.0X3 | T45.0X4 | T45.0X5 | T45.0X6 |
| Chlordan (e) (dust) | T60.1X1 | T60.1X2 | T60.1X3 | T60.1X4 | — | — |
| Chlordantoin | T49.0X1 | T49.0X2 | T49.0X3 | T49.0X4 | T49.0X5 | T49.0X6 |
| Chlordiazepoxide | T42.4X1 | T42.4X2 | T42.4X3 | T42.4X4 | T42.4X5 | T42.4X6 |
| Chlordiethyl benzamide | T49.3X1 | T49.3X2 | T49.3X3 | T49.3X4 | T49.3X5 | T49.3X6 |
| Chloresium | T49.8X1 | T49.8X2 | T49.8X3 | T49.8X4 | T49.8X5 | T49.8X6 |
| Chlorethiazol | T42.6X1 | T42.6X2 | T42.6X3 | T42.6X4 | T42.6X5 | T42.6X6 |
| Chlorethyl — see Ethyl chloride | | | | | | |
| Chloretone | T42.6X1 | T42.6X2 | T42.6X3 | T42.6X4 | T42.6X5 | T42.6X6 |
| Chlorex | T53.6X1 | T53.6X2 | T53.6X3 | T53.6X4 | — | — |
|   insecticide | T60.1X1 | T60.1X2 | T60.1X3 | T60.1X4 | — | — |
| Chlorfenvinphos | T60.0X1 | T60.0X2 | T60.0X3 | T60.0X4 | — | — |
| Chlorhexadol | T42.6X1 | T42.6X2 | T42.6X3 | T42.6X4 | T42.6X5 | T42.6X6 |
| Chlorhexamide | T45.1X1 | T45.1X2 | T45.1X3 | T45.1X4 | T45.1X5 | T45.1X6 |
| Chlorhexidine | T49.0X1 | T49.0X2 | T49.0X3 | T49.0X4 | T49.0X5 | T49.0X6 |
| Chlorhydroxyquinolin | T49.0X1 | T49.0X2 | T49.0X3 | T49.0X4 | T49.0X5 | T49.0X6 |
| Chloride of lime (bleach) | T54.3X1 | T54.3X2 | T54.3X3 | T54.3X4 | — | — |
| Chlorimipramine | T43.011 | T43.012 | T43.013 | T43.014 | T43.015 | T43.016 |
| Chlorinated | | | | | | |
|   camphene | T53.6X1 | T53.6X2 | T53.6X3 | T53.6X4 | — | — |
|   diphenyl | T53.7X1 | T53.7X2 | T53.7X3 | T53.7X4 | — | — |
|   hydrocarbons NEC | T53.91 | T53.92 | T53.93 | T53.94 | — | — |
|     solvents | T53.91 | T53.92 | T53.93 | T53.94 | — | — |
|   lime (bleach) | T54.3X1 | T54.3X2 | T54.3X3 | T54.3X4 | — | — |
|     and boric acid solution | T49.0X1 | T49.0X2 | T49.0X3 | T49.0X4 | T49.0X5 | T49.0X6 |
|   naphthalene (insecticide) | T60.1X1 | T60.1X2 | T60.1X3 | T60.1X4 | — | — |
|     industrial (non-pesticide) | T53.7X1 | T53.7X2 | T53.7X3 | T53.7X4 | — | — |
|   pesticide NEC | T60.8X1 | T60.8X2 | T60.8X3 | T60.8X4 | — | — |
|   soda — see also sodium hypochlorite | | | | | | |
|   solution | T49.0X1 | T49.0X2 | T49.0X3 | T49.0X4 | T49.0X5 | T49.0X6 |
| Chlorine (fumes) (gas) | T59.4X1 | T59.4X2 | T59.4X3 | T59.4X4 | — | — |
|   bleach | T54.3X1 | T54.3X2 | T54.3X3 | T54.3X4 | — | — |
|   compound gas NEC | T59.4X1 | T59.4X2 | T59.4X3 | T59.4X4 | — | — |
|   disinfectant | T59.4X1 | T59.4X2 | T59.4X3 | T59.4X4 | — | — |
|   releasing agents NEC | T59.4X1 | T59.4X2 | T59.4X3 | T59.4X4 | — | — |
| Chlorisondamine chloride | T46.991 | T46.992 | T46.993 | T46.994 | T46.995 | T46.996 |
| Chlormadinone | T38.5X1 | T38.5X2 | T38.5X3 | T38.5X4 | T38.5X5 | T38.5X6 |
| Chlormephos | T60.0X1 | T60.0X2 | T60.0X3 | T60.0X4 | — | — |
| Chlormerodrin | T50.2X1 | T50.2X2 | T50.2X3 | T50.2X4 | T50.2X5 | T50.2X6 |
| Chlormethiazole | T42.6X1 | T42.6X2 | T42.6X3 | T42.6X4 | T42.6X5 | T42.6X6 |
| Chlormethine | T45.1X1 | T45.1X2 | T45.1X3 | T45.1X4 | T45.1X5 | T45.1X6 |
| Chlormethylenecycline | T36.4X1 | T36.4X2 | T36.4X3 | T36.4X4 | T36.4X5 | T36.4X6 |
| Chlormezanone | T42.6X1 | T42.6X2 | T42.6X3 | T42.6X4 | T42.6X5 | T42.6X6 |
| Chloroacetic acid | T60.3X1 | T60.3X2 | T60.3X3 | T60.3X4 | — | — |
| Chloroacetone | T59.3X1 | T59.3X2 | T59.3X3 | T59.3X4 | — | — |
| Chloroacetophenone | T59.3X1 | T59.3X2 | T59.3X3 | T59.3X4 | — | — |
| Chloroaniline | T53.7X1 | T53.7X2 | T53.7X3 | T53.7X4 | — | — |
| Chlorobenzene, chlorobenzol | T53.7X1 | T53.7X2 | T53.7X3 | T53.7X4 | — | — |
| Chlorobromomethane (fire extinguisher) | T53.6X1 | T53.6X2 | T53.6X3 | T53.6X4 | — | — |
| Chlorobutanol | T49.0X1 | T49.0X2 | T49.0X3 | T49.0X4 | T49.0X5 | T49.0X6 |
| Chlorocresol | T49.0X1 | T49.0X2 | T49.0X3 | T49.0X4 | T49.0X5 | T49.0X6 |
| Chlorodehydromethyltestosterone | T38.7X1 | T38.7X2 | T38.7X3 | T38.7X4 | T38.7X5 | T38.7X6 |
| Chlorodinitrobenzene | T53.7X1 | T53.7X2 | T53.7X3 | T53.7X4 | — | — |
|   dust or vapor | T53.7X1 | T53.7X2 | T53.7X3 | T53.7X4 | — | — |
| Chlorodiphenyl | T53.7X1 | T53.7X2 | T53.7X3 | T53.7X4 | — | — |
| Chloroethane — see Ethyl chloride | | | | | | |
| Chloroethylene | T53.6X1 | T53.6X2 | T53.6X3 | T53.6X4 | — | — |
| Chlorofluorocarbons | T53.5X1 | T53.5X2 | T53.5X3 | T53.5X4 | — | — |
| Chloroform (fumes) (vapor) | T53.1X1 | T53.1X2 | T53.1X3 | T53.1X4 | — | — |
|   anesthetic | T41.0X1 | T41.0X2 | T41.0X3 | T41.0X4 | T41.0X5 | T41.0X6 |
|   solvent | T53.1X1 | T53.1X2 | T53.1X3 | T53.1X4 | — | — |
|   water, concentrated | T41.0X1 | T41.0X2 | T41.0X3 | T41.0X4 | T41.0X5 | T41.0X6 |
| Chloroguanide | T37.2X1 | T37.2X2 | T37.2X3 | T37.2X4 | T37.2X5 | T37.2X6 |
| Chloromycetin | T36.2X1 | T36.2X2 | T36.2X3 | T36.2X4 | T36.2X5 | T36.2X6 |
|   ENT agent | T49.6X1 | T49.6X2 | T49.6X3 | T49.6X4 | T49.6X5 | T49.6X6 |
|   ophthalmic preparation | T49.5X1 | T49.5X2 | T49.5X3 | T49.5X4 | T49.5X5 | T49.5X6 |
|   otic solution | T49.6X1 | T49.6X2 | T49.6X3 | T49.6X4 | T49.6X5 | T49.6X6 |
|   topical NEC | T49.0X1 | T49.0X2 | T49.0X3 | T49.0X4 | T49.0X5 | T49.0X6 |
| Chloronitrobenzene | T53.7X1 | T53.7X2 | T53.7X3 | T53.7X4 | — | — |
|   dust or vapor | T53.7X1 | T53.7X2 | T53.7X3 | T53.7X4 | — | — |
| Chlorophacinone | T60.4X1 | T60.4X2 | T60.4X3 | T60.4X4 | — | — |
| Chlorophenol | T53.7X1 | T53.7X2 | T53.7X3 | T53.7X4 | — | — |
| Chlorophenothane | T60.1X1 | T60.1X2 | T60.1X3 | T60.1X4 | — | — |
| Chlorophyll | T50.991 | T50.992 | T50.993 | T50.994 | T50.995 | T50.996 |
| Chloropicrin (fumes) | T53.6X1 | T53.6X2 | T53.6X3 | T53.6X4 | — | — |
|   fumigant | T60.8X1 | T60.8X2 | T60.8X3 | T60.8X4 | — | — |
|   fungicide | T60.3X1 | T60.3X2 | T60.3X3 | T60.3X4 | — | — |
|   pesticide | T60.8X1 | T60.8X2 | T60.8X3 | T60.8X4 | — | — |
| Chloroprocaine | T41.3X1 | T41.3X2 | T41.3X3 | T41.3X4 | T41.3X5 | T41.3X6 |
|   infiltration (subcutaneous) | T41.3X1 | T41.3X2 | T41.3X3 | T41.3X4 | T41.3X5 | T41.3X6 |
|   nerve block (peripheral) (plexus) | T41.3X1 | T41.3X2 | T41.3X3 | T41.3X4 | T41.3X5 | T41.3X6 |
|   spinal | T41.3X1 | T41.3X2 | T41.3X3 | T41.3X4 | T41.3X5 | T41.3X6 |
| Chloroptic | T49.5X1 | T49.5X2 | T49.5X3 | T49.5X4 | T49.5X5 | T49.5X6 |
| Chloropurine | T45.1X1 | T45.1X2 | T45.1X3 | T45.1X4 | T45.1X5 | T45.1X6 |

| Substance | Poisoning, Accidental (unintentional) | Poisoning, Intentional Self-harm | Poisoning, Assault | Poisoning, Undetermined | Adverse Effect | Under-dosing |
|---|---|---|---|---|---|---|
| Chloropyramine | T45.0X1 | T45.0X2 | T45.0X3 | T45.0X4 | T45.0X5 | T45.0X6 |
| Chloropyrifos | T60.0X1 | T60.0X2 | T60.0X3 | T60.0X4 | — | — |
| Chloropyrilene | T45.0X1 | T45.0X2 | T45.0X3 | T45.0X4 | T45.0X5 | T45.0X6 |
| Chloroquine | T37.2X1 | T37.2X2 | T37.2X3 | T37.2X4 | T37.2X5 | T37.2X6 |
| Chlorothalonil | T60.3X1 | T60.3X2 | T60.3X3 | T60.3X4 | — | — |
| Chlorothen | T45.0X1 | T45.0X2 | T45.0X3 | T45.0X4 | T45.0X5 | T45.0X6 |
| Chlorothiazide | T50.2X1 | T50.2X2 | T50.2X3 | T50.2X4 | T50.2X5 | T50.2X6 |
| Chlorothymol | T49.4X1 | T49.4X2 | T49.4X3 | T49.4X4 | T49.4X5 | T49.4X6 |
| Chlorotrianisene | T38.5X1 | T38.5X2 | T38.5X3 | T38.5X4 | T38.5X5 | T38.5X6 |
| Chlorovinyldichloroarsine, not in war | T57.0X1 | T57.0X2 | T57.0X3 | T57.0X4 | | |
| Chloroxine | T49.4X1 | T49.4X2 | T49.4X3 | T49.4X4 | T49.4X5 | T49.4X6 |
| Chloroxylenol | T49.0X1 | T49.0X2 | T49.0X3 | T49.0X4 | T49.0X5 | T49.0X6 |
| Chlorphenamine | T45.0X1 | T45.0X2 | T45.0X3 | T45.0X4 | T45.0X5 | T45.0X6 |
| Chlorphenesin | T42.8X1 | T42.8X2 | T42.8X3 | T42.8X4 | T42.8X5 | T42.8X6 |
| topical (antifungal) | T49.0X1 | T49.0X2 | T49.0X3 | T49.0X4 | T49.0X5 | T49.0X6 |
| Chlorpheniramine | T45.0X1 | T45.0X2 | T45.0X3 | T45.0X4 | T45.0X5 | T45.0X6 |
| Chlorphenoxamine | T45.0X1 | T45.0X2 | T45.0X3 | T45.0X4 | T45.0X5 | T45.0X6 |
| Chlorphentermine | T50.5X1 | T50.5X2 | T50.5X3 | T50.5X4 | T50.5X5 | T50.5X6 |
| Chloroprocaine — see Chloroprocaine | | | | | | |
| Chlorproguanil | T37.2X1 | T37.2X2 | T37.2X3 | T37.2X4 | T37.2X5 | T37.2X6 |
| Chlorpromazine | T43.3X1 | T43.3X2 | T43.3X3 | T43.3X4 | T43.3X5 | T43.3X6 |
| Chlorpropamide | T38.3X1 | T38.3X2 | T38.3X3 | T38.3X4 | T38.3X5 | T38.3X6 |
| Chlorprothixene | T43.4X1 | T43.4X2 | T43.4X3 | T43.4X4 | T43.4X5 | T43.4X6 |
| Chlorquinaldol | T49.0X1 | T49.0X2 | T49.0X3 | T49.0X4 | T49.0X5 | T49.0X6 |
| Chlorquinol | T49.0X1 | T49.0X2 | T49.0X3 | T49.0X4 | T49.0X5 | T49.0X6 |
| Chlortalidone | T50.2X1 | T50.2X2 | T50.2X3 | T50.2X4 | T50.2X5 | T50.2X6 |
| Chlortetracycline | T36.4X1 | T36.4X2 | T36.4X3 | T36.4X4 | T36.4X5 | T36.4X6 |
| Chlorthalidone | T50.2X1 | T50.2X2 | T50.2X3 | T50.2X4 | T50.2X5 | T50.2X6 |
| Chlorthion | T60.0X1 | T60.0X2 | T60.0X3 | T60.0X4 | — | — |
| Chlorthiophos | T60.0X1 | T60.0X2 | T60.0X3 | T60.0X4 | — | — |
| Chlortrianisene | T38.5X1 | T38.5X2 | T38.5X3 | T38.5X4 | T38.5X5 | T38.5X6 |
| Chlor-Trimeton | T45.0X1 | T45.0X2 | T45.0X3 | T45.0X4 | T45.0X5 | T45.0X6 |
| Chlorzoxazone | T42.8X1 | T42.8X2 | T42.8X3 | T42.8X4 | T42.8X5 | T42.8X6 |
| Choke damp | T59.7X1 | T59.7X2 | T59.7X3 | T59.7X4 | — | — |
| Cholagogues | T47.5X1 | T47.5X2 | T47.5X3 | T47.5X4 | T47.5X5 | T47.5X6 |
| Cholebrine | T50.8X1 | T50.8X2 | T50.8X3 | T50.8X4 | T50.8X5 | T50.8X6 |
| Cholecalciferol | T45.2X1 | T45.2X2 | T45.2X3 | T45.2X4 | T45.2X5 | T45.2X6 |
| Cholecystokinin | T50.8X1 | T50.8X2 | T50.8X3 | T50.8X4 | T50.8X5 | T50.8X6 |
| Cholera vaccine | T50.A91 | T50.A92 | T50.A93 | T50.A94 | T50.A95 | T50.A96 |
| Choleretic | T47.5X1 | T47.5X2 | T47.5X3 | T47.5X4 | T47.5X5 | T47.5X6 |
| Cholesterol-lowering agents | T46.6X1 | T46.6X2 | T46.6X3 | T46.6X4 | T46.6X5 | T46.6X6 |
| Cholestyramine (resin) | T46.6X1 | T46.6X2 | T46.6X3 | T46.6X4 | T46.6X5 | T46.6X6 |
| Cholic acid | T47.5X1 | T47.5X2 | T47.5X3 | T47.5X4 | T47.5X5 | T47.5X6 |
| Choline | T48.6X1 | T48.6X2 | T48.6X3 | T48.6X4 | T48.6X5 | T48.6X6 |
| chloride | T50.991 | T50.992 | T50.993 | T50.994 | T50.995 | T50.996 |
| dihydrogen citrate | T50.991 | T50.992 | T50.993 | T50.994 | T50.995 | T50.996 |
| salicylate | T39.091 | T39.092 | T39.093 | T39.094 | T39.095 | T39.096 |
| theophyllinate | T48.6X1 | T48.6X2 | T48.6X3 | T48.6X4 | T48.6X5 | T48.6X6 |
| Cholinergic (drug) NEC | T44.1X1 | T44.1X2 | T44.1X3 | T44.1X4 | T44.1X5 | T44.1X6 |
| muscle tone enhancer | T44.1X1 | T44.1X2 | T44.1X3 | T44.1X4 | T44.1X5 | T44.1X6 |
| organophosphorus | T44.0X1 | T44.0X2 | T44.0X3 | T44.0X4 | T44.0X5 | T44.0X6 |
| insecticide | T60.0X1 | T60.0X2 | T60.0X3 | T60.0X4 | — | — |
| nerve gas | T59.891 | T59.892 | T59.893 | T59.894 | — | — |
| trimethyl ammonium propanediol | T44.1X1 | T44.1X2 | T44.1X3 | T44.1X4 | T44.1X5 | T44.1X6 |
| Cholinesterase reactivator | T50.6X1 | T50.6X2 | T50.6X3 | T50.6X4 | T50.6X5 | T50.6X6 |
| Cholografin | T50.8X1 | T50.8X2 | T50.8X3 | T50.8X4 | T50.8X5 | T50.8X6 |
| Chorionic gonadotropin | T38.891 | T38.892 | T38.893 | T38.894 | T38.895 | T38.896 |
| Chromate | T56.2X1 | T56.2X2 | T56.2X3 | T56.2X4 | — | — |
| dust or mist | T56.2X1 | T56.2X2 | T56.2X3 | T56.2X4 | — | — |
| lead — see also lead | T56.0X1 | T56.0X2 | T56.0X3 | T56.0X4 | — | — |
| paint | T56.0X1 | T56.0X2 | T56.0X3 | T56.0X4 | — | — |
| Chromic | | | | | | |
| acid | T56.2X1 | T56.2X2 | T56.2X3 | T56.2X4 | — | — |
| dust or mist | T56.2X1 | T56.2X2 | T56.2X3 | T56.2X4 | — | — |
| phosphate 32P | T45.1X1 | T45.1X2 | T45.1X3 | T45.1X4 | T45.1X5 | T45.1X6 |
| Chromium | T56.2X1 | T56.2X2 | T56.2X3 | T56.2X4 | — | — |
| compounds — see Chromate | | | | | | |
| sesquioxide | T50.8X1 | T50.8X2 | T50.8X3 | T50.8X4 | T50.8X5 | T50.8X6 |
| Chromomycin A3 | T45.1X1 | T45.1X2 | T45.1X3 | T45.1X4 | T45.1X5 | T45.1X6 |
| Chromonar | T46.3X1 | T46.3X2 | T46.3X3 | T46.3X4 | T46.3X5 | T46.3X6 |
| Chromyl chloride | T56.2X1 | T56.2X2 | T56.2X3 | T56.2X4 | — | — |
| Chrysarobin | T49.4X1 | T49.4X2 | T49.4X3 | T49.4X4 | T49.4X5 | T49.4X6 |
| Chrysazin | T47.2X1 | T47.2X2 | T47.2X3 | T47.2X4 | T47.2X5 | T47.2X6 |
| Chymar | T45.3X1 | T45.3X2 | T45.3X3 | T45.3X4 | T45.3X5 | T45.3X6 |
| ophthalmic preparation | T49.5X1 | T49.5X2 | T49.5X3 | T49.5X4 | T49.5X5 | T49.5X6 |
| Chymopapain | T45.3X1 | T45.3X2 | T45.3X3 | T45.3X4 | T45.3X5 | T45.3X6 |
| Chymotrypsin | T45.3X1 | T45.3X2 | T45.3X3 | T45.3X4 | T45.3X5 | T45.3X6 |
| ophthalmic preparation | T49.5X1 | T49.5X2 | T49.5X3 | T49.5X4 | T49.5X5 | T49.5X6 |
| Cianidanol | T50.991 | T50.992 | T50.993 | T50.994 | T50.995 | T50.996 |
| Cianopramine | T43.011 | T43.012 | T43.013 | T43.014 | T43.015 | T43.016 |
| Cibenzoline | T46.2X1 | T46.2X2 | T46.2X3 | T46.2X4 | T46.2X5 | T46.2X6 |
| Ciclacillin | T36.0X1 | T36.0X2 | T36.0X3 | T36.0X4 | T36.0X5 | T36.0X6 |
| Ciclobarbital — see Hexobarbital | | | | | | |
| Ciclonicate | T46.7X1 | T46.7X2 | T46.7X3 | T46.7X4 | T46.7X5 | T46.7X6 |
| Ciclopirox (olamine) | T49.0X1 | T49.0X2 | T49.0X3 | T49.0X4 | T49.0X5 | T49.0X6 |
| Ciclosporin | T45.1X1 | T45.1X2 | T45.1X3 | T45.1X4 | T45.1X5 | T45.1X6 |
| Cicuta maculata or virosa | T62.2X1 | T62.2X2 | T62.2X3 | T62.2X4 | — | — |
| Cicutoxin | T62.2X1 | T62.2X2 | T62.2X3 | T62.2X4 | — | — |
| Cigarette lighter fluid | T52.0X1 | T52.0X2 | T52.0X3 | T52.0X4 | — | — |
| Cigarettes (tobacco) | T65.221 | T65.222 | T65.223 | T65.224 | — | — |
| Ciguatoxin | T61.01 | T61.02 | T61.03 | T61.04 | — | — |
| Cilazapril | T46.4X1 | T46.4X2 | T46.4X3 | T46.4X4 | T46.4X5 | T46.4X6 |
| Cimetidine | T47.0X1 | T47.0X2 | T47.0X3 | T47.0X4 | T47.0X5 | T47.0X6 |
| Cimetropium bromide | T44.3X1 | T44.3X2 | T44.3X3 | T44.3X4 | T44.3X5 | T44.3X6 |
| Cinchocaine | T41.3X1 | T41.3X2 | T41.3X3 | T41.3X4 | T41.3X5 | T41.3X6 |
| topical (surface) | T41.3X1 | T41.3X2 | T41.3X3 | T41.3X4 | T41.3X5 | T41.3X6 |
| Cinchona | T37.2X1 | T37.2X2 | T37.2X3 | T37.2X4 | T37.2X5 | T37.2X6 |
| Cinchonine alkaloids | T37.2X1 | T37.2X2 | T37.2X3 | T37.2X4 | T37.2X5 | T37.2X6 |
| Cinchophen | T50.4X1 | T50.4X2 | T50.4X3 | T50.4X4 | T50.4X5 | T50.4X6 |
| Cinepazide | T46.7X1 | T46.7X2 | T46.7X3 | T46.7X4 | T46.7X5 | T46.7X6 |
| Cinnamedrine | T48.5X1 | T48.5X2 | T48.5X3 | T48.5X4 | T48.5X5 | T48.5X6 |
| Cinnarizine | T45.0X1 | T45.0X2 | T45.0X3 | T45.0X4 | T45.0X5 | T45.0X6 |
| Cinoxacin | T37.8X1 | T37.8X2 | T37.8X3 | T37.8X4 | T37.8X5 | T37.8X6 |
| Ciprofibrate | T46.6X1 | T46.6X2 | T46.6X3 | T46.6X4 | T46.6X5 | T46.6X6 |
| Ciprofloxacin | T36.8X1 | T36.8X2 | T36.8X3 | T36.8X4 | T36.8X5 | T36.8X6 |
| Cisapride | T47.8X1 | T47.8X2 | T47.8X3 | T47.8X4 | T47.8X5 | T47.8X6 |
| Cisplatin | T45.1X1 | T45.1X2 | T45.1X3 | T45.1X4 | T45.1X5 | T45.1X6 |
| Citalopram | T43.221 | T43.222 | T43.223 | T43.224 | T43.225 | T43.226 |
| Citanest | T41.3X1 | T41.3X2 | T41.3X3 | T41.3X4 | T41.3X5 | T41.3X6 |
| infiltration (subcutaneous) | T41.3X1 | T41.3X2 | T41.3X3 | T41.3X4 | T41.3X5 | T41.3X6 |
| nerve block (peripheral) (plexus) | T41.3X1 | T41.3X2 | T41.3X3 | T41.3X4 | T41.3X5 | T41.3X6 |
| Citric acid | T47.5X1 | T47.5X2 | T47.5X3 | T47.5X4 | T47.5X5 | T47.5X6 |
| Citrovorum (factor) | T45.8X1 | T45.8X2 | T45.8X3 | T45.8X4 | T45.8X5 | T45.8X6 |
| Claviceps purpurea | T62.2X1 | T62.2X2 | T62.2X3 | T62.2X4 | — | — |
| Clavulanic acid | T36.1X1 | T36.1X2 | T36.1X3 | T36.1X4 | T36.1X5 | T36.1X6 |
| Cleaner, cleansing agent, type not specified | T65.891 | T65.892 | T65.893 | T65.894 | — | — |
| of paint or varnish | T52.91 | T52.92 | T52.93 | T52.94 | — | — |
| specified type NEC | T65.891 | T65.892 | T65.893 | T65.894 | — | — |
| Clebopride | T47.8X1 | T47.8X2 | T47.8X3 | T47.8X4 | T47.8X5 | T47.8X6 |
| Clefamide | T37.3X1 | T37.3X2 | T37.3X3 | T37.3X4 | T37.3X5 | T37.3X6 |
| Clemastine | T45.0X1 | T45.0X2 | T45.0X3 | T45.0X4 | T45.0X5 | T45.0X6 |
| Clematis vitalba | T62.2X1 | T62.2X2 | T62.2X3 | T62.2X4 | — | — |
| Clemizole | T45.0X1 | T45.0X2 | T45.0X3 | T45.0X4 | T45.0X5 | T45.0X6 |
| penicillin | T36.0X1 | T36.0X2 | T36.0X3 | T36.0X4 | T36.0X5 | T36.0X6 |
| Clenbuterol | T48.6X1 | T48.6X2 | T48.6X3 | T48.6X4 | T48.6X5 | T48.6X6 |
| Clidinium bromide | T44.3X1 | T44.3X2 | T44.3X3 | T44.3X4 | T44.3X5 | T44.3X6 |
| Clindamycin | T36.8X1 | T36.8X2 | T36.8X3 | T36.8X4 | T36.8X5 | T36.8X6 |
| Clinofibrate | T46.6X1 | T46.6X2 | T46.6X3 | T46.6X4 | T46.6X5 | T46.6X6 |
| Clioquinol | T37.8X1 | T37.8X2 | T37.8X3 | T37.8X4 | T37.8X5 | T37.8X6 |
| Cliradon | T40.2X1 | T40.2X2 | T40.2X3 | T40.2X4 | — | — |
| Clobazam | T42.4X1 | T42.4X2 | T42.4X3 | T42.4X4 | T42.4X5 | T42.4X6 |
| Clobenzorex | T50.5X1 | T50.5X2 | T50.5X3 | T50.5X4 | T50.5X5 | T50.5X6 |
| Clobetasol | T49.0X1 | T49.0X2 | T49.0X3 | T49.0X4 | T49.0X5 | T49.0X6 |
| Clobetasone | T49.0X1 | T49.0X2 | T49.0X3 | T49.0X4 | T49.0X5 | T49.0X6 |
| Clobutinol | T48.3X1 | T48.3X2 | T48.3X3 | T48.3X4 | T48.3X5 | T48.3X6 |
| Clocortolone | T38.0X1 | T38.0X2 | T38.0X3 | T38.0X4 | T38.0X5 | T38.0X6 |
| Clodantoin | T49.0X1 | T49.0X2 | T49.0X3 | T49.0X4 | T49.0X5 | T49.0X6 |
| Clodronic acid | T50.991 | T50.992 | T50.993 | T50.994 | T50.995 | T50.996 |
| Clofazimine | T37.1X1 | T37.1X2 | T37.1X3 | T37.1X4 | T37.1X5 | T37.1X6 |
| Clofedanol | T48.3X1 | T48.3X2 | T48.3X3 | T48.3X4 | T48.3X5 | T48.3X6 |
| Clofenamide | T50.2X1 | T50.2X2 | T50.2X3 | T50.2X4 | T50.2X5 | T50.2X6 |
| Clofenotane | T49.0X1 | T49.0X2 | T49.0X3 | T49.0X4 | T49.0X5 | T49.0X6 |
| Clofezone | T39.2X1 | T39.2X2 | T39.2X3 | T39.2X4 | T39.2X5 | T39.2X6 |
| Clofibrate | T46.6X1 | T46.6X2 | T46.6X3 | T46.6X4 | T46.6X5 | T46.6X6 |
| Clofibride | T46.6X1 | T46.6X2 | T46.6X3 | T46.6X4 | T46.6X5 | T46.6X6 |
| Cloforex | T50.5X1 | T50.5X2 | T50.5X3 | T50.5X4 | T50.5X5 | T50.5X6 |
| Clomethiazole | T42.6X1 | T42.6X2 | T42.6X3 | T42.6X4 | T42.6X5 | T42.6X6 |
| Clometocillin | T36.0X1 | T36.0X2 | T36.0X3 | T36.0X4 | T36.0X5 | T36.0X6 |
| Clomifene | T38.5X1 | T38.5X2 | T38.5X3 | T38.5X4 | T38.5X5 | T38.5X6 |
| Clomiphene | T38.5X1 | T38.5X2 | T38.5X3 | T38.5X4 | T38.5X5 | T38.5X6 |
| Clomipramine | T43.011 | T43.012 | T43.013 | T43.014 | T43.015 | T43.016 |
| Clomocycline | T36.4X1 | T36.4X2 | T36.4X3 | T36.4X4 | T36.4X5 | T36.4X6 |
| Clonazepam | T42.4X1 | T42.4X2 | T42.4X3 | T42.4X4 | T42.4X5 | T42.4X6 |
| Clonidine | T46.5X1 | T46.5X2 | T46.5X3 | T46.5X4 | T46.5X5 | T46.5X6 |
| Clonixin | T39.8X1 | T39.8X2 | T39.8X3 | T39.8X4 | T39.8X5 | T39.8X6 |
| Clopamide | T50.2X1 | T50.2X2 | T50.2X3 | T50.2X4 | T50.2X5 | T50.2X6 |
| Clopenthixol | T43.4X1 | T43.4X2 | T43.4X3 | T43.4X4 | T43.4X5 | T43.4X6 |
| Cloperastine | T48.3X1 | T48.3X2 | T48.3X3 | T48.3X4 | T48.3X5 | T48.3X6 |
| Clophedianol | T48.3X1 | T48.3X2 | T48.3X3 | T48.3X4 | T48.3X5 | T48.3X6 |
| Cloponone | T36.2X1 | T36.2X2 | T36.2X3 | T36.2X4 | T36.2X5 | T36.2X6 |

| Substance | Poisoning, Accidental (unintentional) | Poisoning, Intentional Self-harm | Poisoning, Assault | Poisoning, Undetermined | Adverse Effect | Underdosing |
|---|---|---|---|---|---|---|
| **Cloprednol** | T38.0X1 | T38.0X2 | T38.0X3 | T38.0X4 | T38.0X5 | T38.0X6 |
| **Cloral betaine** | T42.6X1 | T42.6X2 | T42.6X3 | T42.6X4 | T42.6X5 | T42.6X6 |
| **Cloramfenicol** | T36.2X1 | T36.2X2 | T36.2X3 | T36.2X4 | T36.2X5 | T36.2X6 |
| **Clorazepate** (dipotassium) | T42.4X1 | T42.4X2 | T42.4X3 | T42.4X4 | T42.4X5 | T42.4X6 |
| **Clorexolone** | T50.2X1 | T50.2X2 | T50.2X3 | T50.2X4 | T50.2X5 | T50.2X6 |
| **Clorfenamine** | T45.0X1 | T45.0X2 | T45.0X3 | T45.0X4 | T45.0X5 | T45.0X6 |
| **Clorgiline** | T43.1X1 | T43.1X2 | T43.1X3 | T43.1X4 | T43.1X5 | T43.1X6 |
| **Clorotepine** | T44.3X1 | T44.3X2 | T44.3X3 | T44.3X4 | T44.3X5 | T44.3X6 |
| **Clorox** (bleach) | T54.91 | T54.92 | T54.93 | T54.94 | — | — |
| **Clorprenaline** | T48.6X1 | T48.6X2 | T48.6X3 | T48.6X4 | T48.6X5 | T48.6X6 |
| **Clortermine** | T50.5X1 | T50.5X2 | T50.5X3 | T50.5X4 | T50.5X5 | T50.5X6 |
| **Clotiapine** | T43.591 | T43.592 | T43.593 | T43.594 | T43.595 | T43.596 |
| **Clotiazepam** | T42.4X1 | T42.4X2 | T42.4X3 | T42.4X4 | T42.4X5 | T42.4X6 |
| **Clotibric acid** | T46.6X1 | T46.6X2 | T46.6X3 | T46.6X4 | T46.6X5 | T46.6X6 |
| **Clotrimazole** | T49.0X1 | T49.0X2 | T49.0X3 | T49.0X4 | T49.0X5 | T49.0X6 |
| **Cloxacillin** | T36.0X1 | T36.0X2 | T36.0X3 | T36.0X4 | T36.0X5 | T36.0X6 |
| **Cloxazolam** | T42.4X1 | T42.4X2 | T42.4X3 | T42.4X4 | T42.4X5 | T42.4X6 |
| **Cloxiquine** | T49.0X1 | T49.0X2 | T49.0X3 | T49.0X4 | T49.0X5 | T49.0X6 |
| **Clozapine** | T42.4X1 | T42.4X2 | T42.4X3 | T42.4X4 | T42.4X5 | T42.4X6 |
| **Coagulant NEC** | T45.7X1 | T45.7X2 | T45.7X3 | T45.7X4 | T45.7X5 | T45.7X6 |
| **Coal** (carbon monoxide from) — *see also* Carbon, monoxide, coal | T58.2X1 | T58.2X2 | T58.2X3 | T58.2X4 | | |
| oil — *see* Kerosene | | | | | | |
| tar | T49.1X1 | T49.1X2 | T49.1X3 | T49.1X4 | T49.1X5 | T49.1X6 |
| fumes | T59.891 | T59.892 | T59.893 | T59.894 | — | — |
| medicinal (ointment) | T49.4X1 | T49.4X2 | T49.4X3 | T49.4X4 | T49.4X5 | T49.4X6 |
| analgesics NEC | T39.2X1 | T39.2X2 | T39.2X3 | T39.2X4 | T39.2X5 | T39.2X6 |
| naphtha (solvent) | T52.0X1 | T52.0X2 | T52.0X3 | T52.0X4 | — | — |
| **Cobalamine** | T45.2X1 | T45.2X2 | T45.2X3 | T45.2X4 | T45.2X5 | T45.2X6 |
| **Cobalt** (nonmedicinal) (fumes) (industrial) | T56.891 | T56.892 | T56.893 | T56.894 | — | — |
| medicinal (trace) (chloride) | T45.8X1 | T45.8X2 | T45.8X3 | T45.8X4 | T45.8X5 | T45.8X6 |
| **Cobra** (venom) | T63.041 | T63.042 | T63.043 | T63.044 | — | — |
| **Coca** (leaf) | T40.5X1 | T40.5X2 | T40.5X3 | T40.5X4 | T40.5X5 | T40.5X6 |
| **Cocaine** | T40.5X1 | T40.5X2 | T40.5X3 | T40.5X4 | T40.5X5 | T40.5X6 |
| topical anesthetic | T41.3X1 | T41.3X2 | T41.3X3 | T41.3X4 | T41.3X5 | T41.3X6 |
| **Cocarboxylase** | T45.3X1 | T45.3X2 | T45.3X3 | T45.3X4 | T45.3X5 | T45.3X6 |
| **Coccidioidin** | T50.8X1 | T50.8X2 | T50.8X3 | T50.8X4 | T50.8X5 | T50.8X6 |
| **Cocculus indicus** | T62.1X1 | T62.1X2 | T62.1X3 | T62.1X4 | — | — |
| **Cochineal** | T65.6X1 | T65.6X2 | T65.6X3 | T65.6X4 | — | — |
| medicinal products | T50.991 | T50.992 | T50.993 | T50.994 | T50.995 | T50.996 |
| **Codeine** | T40.2X1 | T40.2X2 | T40.2X3 | T40.2X4 | T40.2X5 | T40.2X6 |
| **Cod-liver oil** | T45.2X1 | T45.2X2 | T45.2X3 | T45.2X4 | T45.2X5 | T45.2X6 |
| **Coenzyme A** | T50.991 | T50.992 | T50.993 | T50.994 | T50.995 | T50.996 |
| **Coffee** | T62.8X1 | T62.8X2 | T62.8X3 | T62.8X4 | — | — |
| **Cogalactoisomerase** | T50.991 | T50.992 | T50.993 | T50.994 | T50.995 | T50.996 |
| **Cogentin** | T44.3X1 | T44.3X2 | T44.3X3 | T44.3X4 | T44.3X5 | T44.3X6 |
| **Coke fumes or gas** (carbon monoxide) | T58.2X1 | T58.2X2 | T58.2X3 | T58.2X4 | | |
| industrial use | T58.8X1 | T58.8X2 | T58.8X3 | T58.8X4 | — | — |
| **Colace** | T47.4X1 | T47.4X2 | T47.4X3 | T47.4X4 | T47.4X5 | T47.4X6 |
| **Colaspase** | T45.1X1 | T45.1X2 | T45.1X3 | T45.1X4 | T45.1X5 | T45.1X6 |
| **Colchicine** | T50.4X1 | T50.4X2 | T50.4X3 | T50.4X4 | T50.4X5 | T50.4X6 |
| **Colchicum** | T62.2X1 | T62.2X2 | T62.2X3 | T62.2X4 | — | — |
| **Cold cream** | T49.3X1 | T49.3X2 | T49.3X3 | T49.3X4 | T49.3X5 | T49.3X6 |
| **Colecalciferol** | T45.2X1 | T45.2X2 | T45.2X3 | T45.2X4 | T45.2X5 | T45.2X6 |
| **Colestipol** | T46.6X1 | T46.6X2 | T46.6X3 | T46.6X4 | T46.6X5 | T46.6X6 |
| **Colestyramine** | T46.6X1 | T46.6X2 | T46.6X3 | T46.6X4 | T46.6X5 | T46.6X6 |
| **Colimycin** | T36.8X1 | T36.8X2 | T36.8X3 | T36.8X4 | T36.8X5 | T36.8X6 |
| **Colistimethate** | T36.8X1 | T36.8X2 | T36.8X3 | T36.8X4 | T36.8X5 | T36.8X6 |
| **Colistin** | T36.8X1 | T36.8X2 | T36.8X3 | T36.8X4 | T36.8X5 | T36.8X6 |
| sulfate (eye preparation) | T49.5X1 | T49.5X2 | T49.5X3 | T49.5X4 | T49.5X5 | T49.5X6 |
| **Collagen** | T50.991 | T50.992 | T50.993 | T50.994 | T50.995 | T50.996 |
| **Collagenase** | T49.4X1 | T49.4X2 | T49.4X3 | T49.4X4 | T49.4X5 | T49.4X6 |
| **Collodion** | T49.3X1 | T49.3X2 | T49.3X3 | T49.3X4 | T49.3X5 | T49.3X6 |
| **Colocynth** | T47.2X1 | T47.2X2 | T47.2X3 | T47.2X4 | T47.2X5 | T47.2X6 |
| **Colophony adhesive** | T49.3X1 | T49.3X2 | T49.3X3 | T49.3X4 | T49.3X5 | T49.3X6 |
| **Colorant** — *see also* Dye | T50.991 | T50.992 | T50.993 | T50.994 | T50.995 | T50.996 |
| **Coloring matter** — *see* Dye(s) | | | | | | |
| **Combustion gas** (after combustion) — *see* Carbon, monoxide | | | | | | |
| prior to combustion | T59.891 | T59.892 | T59.893 | T59.894 | — | — |
| **Compazine** | T43.3X1 | T43.3X2 | T43.3X3 | T43.3X4 | T43.3X5 | T43.3X6 |
| **Compound** | | | | | | |
| 42 (warfarin) | T60.4X1 | T60.4X2 | T60.4X3 | T60.4X4 | — | — |
| 269 (endrin) | T60.1X1 | T60.1X2 | T60.1X3 | T60.1X4 | — | — |
| 497 (dieldrin) | T60.1X1 | T60.1X2 | T60.1X3 | T60.1X4 | — | — |
| 1080 (sodium fluoroacetate) | T60.4X1 | T60.4X2 | T60.4X3 | T60.4X4 | — | — |
| 3422 (parathion) | T60.0X1 | T60.0X2 | T60.0X3 | T60.0X4 | — | — |
| 3911 (phorate) | T60.0X1 | T60.0X2 | T60.0X3 | T60.0X4 | — | — |
| **Compound** — *continued* | | | | | | |
| 3956 (toxaphene) | T60.1X1 | T60.1X2 | T60.1X3 | T60.1X4 | — | — |
| 4049 (malathion) | T60.0X1 | T60.0X2 | T60.0X3 | T60.0X4 | — | — |
| 4069 (malathion) | T60.0X1 | T60.0X2 | T60.0X3 | T60.0X4 | — | — |
| 4124 (dicapthon) | T60.0X1 | T60.0X2 | T60.0X3 | T60.0X4 | — | — |
| E (cortisone) | T38.0X1 | T38.0X2 | T38.0X3 | T38.0X4 | T38.0X5 | T38.0X6 |
| F (hydrocortisone) | T38.0X1 | T38.0X2 | T38.0X3 | T38.0X4 | T38.0X5 | T38.0X6 |
| **Congener, anabolic** | T38.7X1 | T38.7X2 | T38.7X3 | T38.7X4 | T38.7X5 | T38.7X6 |
| **Congo red** | T50.8X1 | T50.8X2 | T50.8X3 | T50.8X4 | T50.8X5 | T50.8X6 |
| **Coniine, conine** | T62.2X1 | T62.2X2 | T62.2X3 | T62.2X4 | — | — |
| **Conium** (maculatum) | T62.2X1 | T62.2X2 | T62.2X3 | T62.2X4 | — | — |
| **Conjugated estrogenic substances** | T38.5X1 | T38.5X2 | T38.5X3 | T38.5X4 | T38.5X5 | T38.5X6 |
| **Contac** | T48.5X1 | T48.5X2 | T48.5X3 | T48.5X4 | T48.5X5 | T48.5X6 |
| **Contact lens solution** | T49.5X1 | T49.5X2 | T49.5X3 | T49.5X4 | T49.5X5 | T49.5X6 |
| **Contraceptive** (oral) | T38.4X1 | T38.4X2 | T38.4X3 | T38.4X4 | T38.4X5 | T38.4X6 |
| vaginal | T49.8X1 | T49.8X2 | T49.8X3 | T49.8X4 | T49.8X5 | T49.8X6 |
| **Contrast medium, radiography** | T50.8X1 | T50.8X2 | T50.8X3 | T50.8X4 | T50.8X5 | T50.8X6 |
| **Convallaria glycosides** | T46.0X1 | T46.0X2 | T46.0X3 | T46.0X4 | T46.0X5 | T46.0X6 |
| **Convallaria majalis** | T62.2X1 | T62.2X2 | T62.2X3 | T62.2X4 | — | — |
| berry | T62.1X1 | T62.1X2 | T62.1X3 | T62.1X4 | — | — |
| **Copperhead snake** (bite) (venom) | T63.061 | T63.062 | T63.063 | T63.064 | | |
| **Copper** (dust) (fumes) (nonmedicinal) **NEC** | T56.4X1 | T56.4X2 | T56.4X3 | T56.4X4 | | |
| arsenate, arsenite | T57.0X1 | T57.0X2 | T57.0X3 | T57.0X4 | — | — |
| insecticide | T60.2X1 | T60.2X2 | T60.2X3 | T60.2X4 | — | — |
| emetic | T47.7X1 | T47.7X2 | T47.7X3 | T47.7X4 | T47.7X5 | T47.7X6 |
| fungicide | T60.3X1 | T60.3X2 | T60.3X3 | T60.3X4 | — | — |
| gluconate | T49.0X1 | T49.0X2 | T49.0X3 | T49.0X4 | T49.0X5 | T49.0X6 |
| insecticide | T60.2X1 | T60.2X2 | T60.2X3 | T60.2X4 | — | — |
| medicinal (trace) | T45.8X1 | T45.8X2 | T45.8X3 | T45.8X4 | T45.8X5 | T45.8X6 |
| oleate | T49.0X1 | T49.0X2 | T49.0X3 | T49.0X4 | T49.0X5 | T49.0X6 |
| sulfate | T56.4X1 | T56.4X2 | T56.4X3 | T56.4X4 | — | — |
| cupric | T56.4X1 | T56.4X2 | T56.4X3 | T56.4X4 | — | — |
| fungicide | T60.3X1 | T60.3X2 | T60.3X3 | T60.3X4 | — | — |
| medicinal | | | | | | |
| ear | T49.6X1 | T49.6X2 | T49.6X3 | T49.6X4 | T49.6X5 | T49.6X6 |
| emetic | T47.7X1 | T47.7X2 | T47.7X3 | T47.7X4 | T47.7X5 | T47.7X6 |
| eye | T49.5X1 | T49.5X2 | T49.5X3 | T49.5X4 | T49.5X5 | T49.5X6 |
| cuprous | T56.4X1 | T56.4X2 | T56.4X3 | T56.4X4 | — | — |
| fungicide | T60.3X1 | T60.3X2 | T60.3X3 | T60.3X4 | — | — |
| medicinal | | | | | | |
| ear | T49.6X1 | T49.6X2 | T49.6X3 | T49.6X4 | T49.6X5 | T49.6X6 |
| emetic | T47.7X1 | T47.7X2 | T47.7X3 | T47.7X4 | T47.7X5 | T47.7X6 |
| eye | T49.5X1 | T49.5X2 | T49.5X3 | T49.5X4 | T49.5X5 | T49.5X6 |
| **Coral** (sting) | T63.691 | T63.692 | T63.693 | T63.694 | | |
| snake (bite) (venom) | T63.021 | T63.022 | T63.023 | T63.024 | | |
| **Corbadrine** | T49.6X1 | T49.6X2 | T49.6X3 | T49.6X4 | T49.6X5 | T49.6X6 |
| **Cordite** | T65.891 | T65.892 | T65.893 | T65.894 | — | — |
| vapor | T59.891 | T59.892 | T59.893 | T59.894 | | |
| **Cordran** | T49.0X1 | T49.0X2 | T49.0X3 | T49.0X4 | T49.0X5 | T49.0X6 |
| **Corn cures** | T49.4X1 | T49.4X2 | T49.4X3 | T49.4X4 | T49.4X5 | T49.4X6 |
| **Cornhusker's lotion** | T49.3X1 | T49.3X2 | T49.3X3 | T49.3X4 | T49.3X5 | T49.3X6 |
| **Corn starch** | T49.3X1 | T49.3X2 | T49.3X3 | T49.3X4 | T49.3X5 | T49.3X6 |
| **Coronary vasodilator NEC** | T46.3X1 | T46.3X2 | T46.3X3 | T46.3X4 | T46.3X5 | T46.3X6 |
| **Corrosive NEC** | T54.91 | T54.92 | T54.93 | T54.94 | — | — |
| acid NEC | T54.2X1 | T54.2X2 | T54.2X3 | T54.2X4 | — | — |
| aromatics | T54.1X1 | T54.1X2 | T54.1X3 | T54.1X4 | — | — |
| disinfectant | T54.1X1 | T54.1X2 | T54.1X3 | T54.1X4 | — | — |
| fumes NEC | T54.91 | T54.92 | T54.93 | T54.94 | — | — |
| specified NEC | T54.91 | T54.92 | T54.93 | T54.94 | — | — |
| sublimate | T56.1X1 | T56.1X2 | T56.1X3 | T56.1X4 | — | — |
| **Cortate** | T38.0X1 | T38.0X2 | T38.0X3 | T38.0X4 | T38.0X5 | T38.0X6 |
| **Cort-Dome** | T38.0X1 | T38.0X2 | T38.0X3 | T38.0X4 | T38.0X5 | T38.0X6 |
| ENT agent | T49.6X1 | T49.6X2 | T49.6X3 | T49.6X4 | T49.6X5 | T49.6X6 |
| ophthalmic preparation | T49.5X1 | T49.5X2 | T49.5X3 | T49.5X4 | T49.5X5 | T49.5X6 |
| topical NEC | T49.0X1 | T49.0X2 | T49.0X3 | T49.0X4 | T49.0X5 | T49.0X6 |
| **Cortef** | T38.0X1 | T38.0X2 | T38.0X3 | T38.0X4 | T38.0X5 | T38.0X6 |
| ENT agent | T49.6X1 | T49.6X2 | T49.6X3 | T49.6X4 | T49.6X5 | T49.6X6 |
| ophthalmic preparation | T49.5X1 | T49.5X2 | T49.5X3 | T49.5X4 | T49.5X5 | T49.5X6 |
| topical NEC | T49.0X1 | T49.0X2 | T49.0X3 | T49.0X4 | T49.0X5 | T49.0X6 |
| **Corticosteroid** | T38.0X1 | T38.0X2 | T38.0X3 | T38.0X4 | T38.0X5 | T38.0X6 |
| ENT agent | T49.6X1 | T49.6X2 | T49.6X3 | T49.6X4 | T49.6X5 | T49.6X6 |
| mineral | T50.0X1 | T50.0X2 | T50.0X3 | T50.0X4 | T50.0X5 | T50.0X6 |
| ophthalmic | T49.5X1 | T49.5X2 | T49.5X3 | T49.5X4 | T49.5X5 | T49.5X6 |
| topical NEC | T49.0X1 | T49.0X2 | T49.0X3 | T49.0X4 | T49.0X5 | T49.0X6 |
| **Corticotropin** | T38.811 | T38.812 | T38.813 | T38.814 | T38.815 | T38.816 |
| **Cortisol** | T49.0X1 | T49.0X2 | T49.0X3 | T49.0X4 | T49.0X5 | T49.0X6 |
| ENT agent | T49.6X1 | T49.6X2 | T49.6X3 | T49.6X4 | T49.6X5 | T49.6X6 |
| ophthalmic preparation | T49.5X1 | T49.5X2 | T49.5X3 | T49.5X4 | T49.5X5 | T49.5X6 |
| topical NEC | T49.0X1 | T49.0X2 | T49.0X3 | T49.0X4 | T49.0X5 | T49.0X6 |

**Table of Drugs and Chemicals**

| Substance | Poisoning, Accidental (unintentional) | Poisoning, Intentional Self-harm | Poisoning, Assault | Poisoning, Undetermined | Adverse Effect | Under-dosing |
|---|---|---|---|---|---|---|
| **Cortisone** (acetate) | T38.0X1 | T38.0X2 | T38.0X3 | T38.0X4 | T38.0X5 | T38.0X6 |
| ENT agent | T49.6X1 | T49.6X2 | T49.6X3 | T49.6X4 | T49.6X5 | T49.6X6 |
| ophthalmic preparation | T49.5X1 | T49.5X2 | T49.5X3 | T49.5X4 | T49.5X5 | T49.5X6 |
| topical NEC | T49.0X1 | T49.0X2 | T49.0X3 | T49.0X4 | T49.0X5 | T49.0X6 |
| **Cortivazol** | T38.0X1 | T38.0X2 | T38.0X3 | T38.0X4 | T38.0X5 | T38.0X6 |
| **Cortogen** | T38.0X1 | T38.0X2 | T38.0X3 | T38.0X4 | T38.0X5 | T38.0X6 |
| ENT agent | T49.6X1 | T49.6X2 | T49.6X3 | T49.6X4 | T49.6X5 | T49.6X6 |
| ophthalmic preparation | T49.5X1 | T49.5X2 | T49.5X3 | T49.5X4 | T49.5X5 | T49.5X6 |
| **Cortone** | T38.0X1 | T38.0X2 | T38.0X3 | T38.0X4 | T38.0X5 | T38.0X6 |
| ENT agent | T49.6X1 | T49.6X2 | T49.6X3 | T49.6X4 | T49.6X5 | T49.6X6 |
| ophthalmic preparation | T49.5X1 | T49.5X2 | T49.5X3 | T49.5X4 | T49.5X5 | T49.5X6 |
| **Cortril** | T38.0X1 | T38.0X2 | T38.0X3 | T38.0X4 | T38.0X5 | T38.0X6 |
| ENT agent | T49.6X1 | T49.6X2 | T49.6X3 | T49.6X4 | T49.6X5 | T49.6X6 |
| ophthalmic preparation | T49.5X1 | T49.5X2 | T49.5X3 | T49.5X4 | T49.5X5 | T49.5X6 |
| topical NEC | T49.0X1 | T49.0X2 | T49.0X3 | T49.0X4 | T49.0X5 | T49.0X6 |
| **Corynebacterium parvum** | T45.1X1 | T45.1X2 | T45.1X3 | T45.1X4 | T45.1X5 | T45.1X6 |
| **Cosmetic preparation** | T49.8X1 | T49.8X2 | T49.8X3 | T49.8X4 | T49.8X5 | T49.8X6 |
| **Cosmetics** | T49.8X1 | T49.8X2 | T49.8X3 | T49.8X4 | T49.8X5 | T49.8X6 |
| **Cosyntropin** | T38.811 | T38.812 | T38.813 | T38.814 | T38.815 | T38.816 |
| **Cotarnine** | T45.7X1 | T45.7X2 | T45.7X3 | T45.7X4 | T45.7X5 | T45.7X6 |
| **Co-trimoxazole** | T36.8X1 | T36.8X2 | T36.8X3 | T36.8X4 | T36.8X5 | T36.8X6 |
| **Cottonseed oil** | T49.3X1 | T49.3X2 | T49.3X3 | T49.3X4 | T49.3X5 | T49.3X6 |
| **Cough mixture** (syrup) | T48.4X1 | T48.4X2 | T48.4X3 | T48.4X4 | T48.4X5 | T48.4X6 |
| containing opiates | T40.2X1 | T40.2X2 | T40.2X3 | T40.2X4 | T40.2X5 | T40.2X6 |
| expectorants | T48.4X1 | T48.4X2 | T48.4X3 | T48.4X4 | T48.4X5 | T48.4X6 |
| **Coumadin** | T45.511 | T45.512 | T45.513 | T45.514 | T45.515 | T45.516 |
| rodenticide | T60.4X1 | T60.4X2 | T60.4X3 | T60.4X4 | — | — |
| **Coumaphos** | T60.0X1 | T60.0X2 | T60.0X3 | T60.0X4 | — | — |
| **Coumarin** | T45.511 | T45.512 | T45.513 | T45.514 | T45.515 | T45.516 |
| **Coumetarol** | T45.511 | T45.512 | T45.513 | T45.514 | T45.515 | T45.516 |
| **Cowbane** | T62.2X1 | T62.2X2 | T62.2X3 | T62.2X4 | — | — |
| **Cozyme** | T45.2X1 | T45.2X2 | T45.2X3 | T45.2X4 | T45.2X5 | T45.2X6 |
| **Crack** | T40.5X1 | T40.5X2 | T40.5X3 | T40.5X4 | — | — |
| **Crataegus extract** | T46.0X1 | T46.0X2 | T46.0X3 | T46.0X4 | T46.0X5 | T46.0X6 |
| **Creolin** | T54.1X1 | T54.1X2 | T54.1X3 | T54.1X4 | — | — |
| disinfectant | T54.1X1 | T54.1X2 | T54.1X3 | T54.1X4 | — | — |
| **Creosol** (compound) | T49.0X1 | T49.0X2 | T49.0X3 | T49.0X4 | T49.0X5 | T49.0X6 |
| **Creosote** (coal tar) | T49.0X1 | T49.0X2 | T49.0X3 | T49.0X4 | T49.0X5 | T49.0X6 |
| (beechwood) | | | | | | |
| medicinal (expectorant) | T48.4X1 | T48.4X2 | T48.4X3 | T48.4X4 | T48.4X5 | T48.4X6 |
| syrup | T48.4X1 | T48.4X2 | T48.4X3 | T48.4X4 | T48.4X5 | T48.4X6 |
| **Cresol**(s) | T49.0X1 | T49.0X2 | T49.0X3 | T49.0X4 | T49.0X5 | T49.0X6 |
| and soap solution | T49.0X1 | T49.0X2 | T49.0X3 | T49.0X4 | T49.0X5 | T49.0X6 |
| **Cresyl acetate** | T49.0X1 | T49.0X2 | T49.0X3 | T49.0X4 | T49.0X5 | T49.0X6 |
| **Cresylic acid** | T49.0X1 | T49.0X2 | T49.0X3 | T49.0X4 | T49.0X5 | T49.0X6 |
| **Crimidine** | T60.4X1 | T60.4X2 | T60.4X3 | T60.4X4 | — | — |
| **Croconazole** | T37.8X1 | T37.8X2 | T37.8X3 | T37.8X4 | T37.8X5 | T37.8X6 |
| **Cromoglicic acid** | T48.6X1 | T48.6X2 | T48.6X3 | T48.6X4 | T48.6X5 | T48.6X6 |
| **Cromolyn** | T48.6X1 | T48.6X2 | T48.6X3 | T48.6X4 | T48.6X5 | T48.6X6 |
| **Cromonar** | T46.3X1 | T46.3X2 | T46.3X3 | T46.3X4 | T46.3X5 | T46.3X6 |
| **Cropropamide** | T39.8X1 | T39.8X2 | T39.8X3 | T39.8X4 | T39.8X5 | T39.8X6 |
| with crotethamide | T50.7X1 | T50.7X2 | T50.7X3 | T50.7X4 | T50.7X5 | T50.7X6 |
| **Crotamiton** | T49.0X1 | T49.0X2 | T49.0X3 | T49.0X4 | T49.0X5 | T49.0X6 |
| **Crotethamide** | T39.8X1 | T39.8X2 | T39.8X3 | T39.8X4 | T39.8X5 | T39.8X6 |
| with cropropamide | T50.7X1 | T50.7X2 | T50.7X3 | T50.7X4 | T50.7X5 | T50.7X6 |
| **Croton** (oil) | T47.2X1 | T47.2X2 | T47.2X3 | T47.2X4 | T47.2X5 | T47.2X6 |
| chloral | T42.6X1 | T42.6X2 | T42.6X3 | T42.6X4 | T42.6X5 | T42.6X6 |
| **Crude oil** | T52.0X1 | T52.0X2 | T52.0X3 | T52.0X4 | — | — |
| **Cryogenine** | T39.8X1 | T39.8X2 | T39.8X3 | T39.8X4 | T39.8X5 | T39.8X6 |
| **Cryolite** (vapor) | T60.1X1 | T60.1X2 | T60.1X3 | T60.1X4 | — | — |
| insecticide | T60.1X1 | T60.1X2 | T60.1X3 | T60.1X4 | — | — |
| **Cryptenamine** (tannates) | T46.5X1 | T46.5X2 | T46.5X3 | T46.5X4 | T46.5X5 | T46.5X6 |
| **Crystal violet** | T49.0X1 | T49.0X2 | T49.0X3 | T49.0X4 | T49.0X5 | T49.0X6 |
| **Cuckoopint** | T62.2X1 | T62.2X2 | T62.2X3 | T62.2X4 | — | — |
| **Cumetharol** | T45.511 | T45.512 | T45.513 | T45.514 | T45.515 | T45.516 |
| **Cupric** | | | | | | |
| acetate | T60.3X1 | T60.3X2 | T60.3X3 | T60.3X4 | — | — |
| acetoarsenite | T57.0X1 | T57.0X2 | T57.0X3 | T57.0X4 | — | — |
| arsenate | T57.0X1 | T57.0X2 | T57.0X3 | T57.0X4 | — | — |
| gluconate | T49.0X1 | T49.0X2 | T49.0X3 | T49.0X4 | T49.0X5 | T49.0X6 |
| oleate | T49.0X1 | T49.0X2 | T49.0X3 | T49.0X4 | T49.0X5 | T49.0X6 |
| sulfate | T56.4X1 | T56.4X2 | T56.4X3 | T56.4X4 | — | — |
| **Cuprous sulfate** — *see also* | T56.4X1 | T56.4X2 | T56.4X3 | T56.4X4 | — | — |
| Copper sulfate | | | | | | |
| **Curare, curarine** | T48.1X1 | T48.1X2 | T48.1X3 | T48.1X4 | T48.1X5 | T48.1X6 |
| **Cyamemazine** | T43.3X1 | T43.3X2 | T43.3X3 | T43.3X4 | T43.3X5 | T43.3X6 |
| **Cyamopsis tetragonoloba** | T46.6X1 | T46.6X2 | T46.6X3 | T46.6X4 | T46.6X5 | T46.6X6 |
| **Cyanacetyl hydrazide** | T37.1X1 | T37.1X2 | T37.1X3 | T37.1X4 | T37.1X5 | T37.1X6 |
| **Cyanic acid** (gas) | T59.891 | T59.892 | T59.893 | T59.894 | — | — |
| **Cyanide**(s) (compounds) | T65.0X1 | T65.0X2 | T65.0X3 | T65.0X4 | — | — |
| (potassium) (sodium) | | | | | | |
| **NEC** | | | | | | |
| dust or gas (inhalation) NEC | T57.3X1 | T57.3X2 | T57.3X3 | T57.3X4 | — | — |

| Substance | Poisoning, Accidental (unintentional) | Poisoning, Intentional Self-harm | Poisoning, Assault | Poisoning, Undetermined | Adverse Effect | Under-dosing |
|---|---|---|---|---|---|---|
| **Cyanide**(s) (compounds) (potassium) (sodium) **NEC** — *continued* | | | | | | |
| fumigant | T65.0X1 | T65.0X2 | T65.0X3 | T65.0X4 | — | — |
| hydrogen | T57.3X1 | T57.3X2 | T57.3X3 | T57.3X4 | — | — |
| mercuric — *see* Mercury | | | | | | |
| pesticide (dust) (fumes) | T65.0X1 | T65.0X2 | T65.0X3 | T65.0X4 | — | — |
| **Cyanoacrylate adhesive** | T49.3X1 | T49.3X2 | T49.3X3 | T49.3X4 | T49.3X5 | T49.3X6 |
| **Cyanocobalamin** | T45.8X1 | T45.8X2 | T45.8X3 | T45.8X4 | T45.8X5 | T45.8X6 |
| **Cyanogen** (chloride) (gas) **NEC** | T59.891 | T59.892 | T59.893 | T59.894 | — | — |
| **Cyclacillin** | T36.0X1 | T36.0X2 | T36.0X3 | T36.0X4 | T36.0X5 | T36.0X6 |
| **Cyclaine** | T41.3X1 | T41.3X2 | T41.3X3 | T41.3X4 | T41.3X5 | T41.3X6 |
| **Cyclamate** | T50.991 | T50.992 | T50.993 | T50.994 | T50.995 | T50.996 |
| **Cyclamen europaeum** | T62.2X1 | T62.2X2 | T62.2X3 | T62.2X4 | — | — |
| **Cyclandelate** | T46.7X1 | T46.7X2 | T46.7X3 | T46.7X4 | T46.7X5 | T46.7X6 |
| **Cyclazocine** | T50.7X1 | T50.7X2 | T50.7X3 | T50.7X4 | T50.7X5 | T50.7X6 |
| **Cyclizine** | T45.0X1 | T45.0X2 | T45.0X3 | T45.0X4 | T45.0X5 | T45.0X6 |
| **Cyclobarbital** | T42.3X1 | T42.3X2 | T42.3X3 | T42.3X4 | T42.3X5 | T42.3X6 |
| **Cyclobarbitone** | T42.3X1 | T42.3X2 | T42.3X3 | T42.3X4 | T42.3X5 | T42.3X6 |
| **Cyclobenzaprine** | T48.1X1 | T48.1X2 | T48.1X3 | T48.1X4 | T48.1X5 | T48.1X6 |
| **Cyclodrine** | T44.3X1 | T44.3X2 | T44.3X3 | T44.3X4 | T44.3X5 | T44.3X6 |
| **Cycloguanil embonate** | T37.2X1 | T37.2X2 | T37.2X3 | T37.2X4 | T37.2X5 | T37.2X6 |
| **Cyclohexane** | T52.8X1 | T52.8X2 | T52.8X3 | T52.8X4 | — | — |
| **Cyclohexanol** | T51.8X1 | T51.8X2 | T51.8X3 | T51.8X4 | — | — |
| **Cyclohexanone** | T52.4X1 | T52.4X2 | T52.4X3 | T52.4X4 | — | — |
| **Cycloheximide** | T60.3X1 | T60.3X2 | T60.3X3 | T60.3X4 | — | — |
| **Cyclohexyl acetate** | T52.8X1 | T52.8X2 | T52.8X3 | T52.8X4 | — | — |
| **Cycloleucin** | T45.1X1 | T45.1X2 | T45.1X3 | T45.1X4 | T45.1X5 | T45.1X6 |
| **Cyclomethycaine** | T41.3X1 | T41.3X2 | T41.3X3 | T41.3X4 | T41.3X5 | T41.3X6 |
| **Cyclopentamine** | T44.4X1 | T44.4X2 | T44.4X3 | T44.4X4 | T44.4X5 | T44.4X6 |
| **Cyclopenthiazide** | T50.2X1 | T50.2X2 | T50.2X3 | T50.2X4 | T50.2X5 | T50.2X6 |
| **Cyclopentolate** | T44.3X1 | T44.3X2 | T44.3X3 | T44.3X4 | T44.3X5 | T44.3X6 |
| **Cyclophosphamide** | T45.1X1 | T45.1X2 | T45.1X3 | T45.1X4 | T45.1X5 | T45.1X6 |
| **Cycloplegic drug** | T49.5X1 | T49.5X2 | T49.5X3 | T49.5X4 | T49.5X5 | T49.5X6 |
| **Cyclopropane** | T41.291 | T41.292 | T41.293 | T41.294 | T41.295 | T41.296 |
| **Cyclopyrabital** | T39.8X1 | T39.8X2 | T39.8X3 | T39.8X4 | T39.8X5 | T39.8X6 |
| **Cycloserine** | T37.1X1 | T37.1X2 | T37.1X3 | T37.1X4 | T37.1X5 | T37.1X6 |
| **Cyclosporin** | T45.1X1 | T45.1X2 | T45.1X3 | T45.1X4 | T45.1X5 | T45.1X6 |
| **Cyclothiazide** | T50.2X1 | T50.2X2 | T50.2X3 | T50.2X4 | T50.2X5 | T50.2X6 |
| **Cycrimine** | T44.3X1 | T44.3X2 | T44.3X3 | T44.3X4 | T44.3X5 | T44.3X6 |
| **Cyhalothrin** | T60.1X1 | T60.1X2 | T60.1X3 | T60.1X4 | — | — |
| **Cymarin** | T46.0X1 | T46.0X2 | T46.0X3 | T46.0X4 | T46.0X5 | T46.0X6 |
| **Cypermethrin** | T60.1X1 | T60.1X2 | T60.1X3 | T60.1X4 | — | — |
| **Cyphenothrin** | T60.2X1 | T60.2X2 | T60.2X3 | T60.2X4 | — | — |
| **Cyproheptadine** | T45.0X1 | T45.0X2 | T45.0X3 | T45.0X4 | T45.0X5 | T45.0X6 |
| **Cyproterone** | T38.6X1 | T38.6X2 | T38.6X3 | T38.6X4 | T38.6X5 | T38.6X6 |
| **Cysteamine** | T50.6X1 | T50.6X2 | T50.6X3 | T50.6X4 | T50.6X5 | T50.6X6 |
| **Cytarabine** | T45.1X1 | T45.1X2 | T45.1X3 | T45.1X4 | T45.1X5 | T45.1X6 |
| **Cytisus** | | | | | | |
| laburnum | T62.2X1 | T62.2X2 | T62.2X3 | T62.2X4 | — | — |
| scoparius | T62.2X1 | T62.2X2 | T62.2X3 | T62.2X4 | — | — |
| **Cytochrome C** | T47.5X1 | T47.5X2 | T47.5X3 | T47.5X4 | T47.5X5 | T47.5X6 |
| **Cytomel** | T38.1X1 | T38.1X2 | T38.1X3 | T38.1X4 | T38.1X5 | T38.1X6 |
| **Cytosine arabinoside** | T45.1X1 | T45.1X2 | T45.1X3 | T45.1X4 | T45.1X5 | T45.1X6 |
| **Cytoxan** | T45.1X1 | T45.1X2 | T45.1X3 | T45.1X4 | T45.1X5 | T45.1X6 |
| **Cytozyme** | T45.7X1 | T45.7X2 | T45.7X3 | T45.7X4 | T45.7X5 | T45.7X6 |
| **S-Carboxymethylcysteine** | T48.4X1 | T48.4X2 | T48.4X3 | T48.4X4 | T48.4X5 | T48.4X6 |
| **Dacarbazine** | T45.1X1 | T45.1X2 | T45.1X3 | T45.1X4 | T45.1X5 | T45.1X6 |
| **Dactinomycin** | T45.1X1 | T45.1X2 | T45.1X3 | T45.1X4 | T45.1X5 | T45.1X6 |
| **DADPS** | T37.1X1 | T37.1X2 | T37.1X3 | T37.1X4 | T37.1X5 | T37.1X6 |
| **Dakin's solution** | T49.0X1 | T49.0X2 | T49.0X3 | T49.0X4 | T49.0X5 | T49.0X6 |
| **Dalapon** (sodium) | T60.3X1 | T60.3X2 | T60.3X3 | T60.3X4 | — | — |
| **Dalmane** | T42.4X1 | T42.4X2 | T42.4X3 | T42.4X4 | T42.4X5 | T42.4X6 |
| **Danazol** | T38.6X1 | T38.6X2 | T38.6X3 | T38.6X4 | T38.6X5 | T38.6X6 |
| **Danilone** | T45.511 | T45.512 | T45.513 | T45.514 | T45.515 | T45.516 |
| **Danthron** | T47.2X1 | T47.2X2 | T47.2X3 | T47.2X4 | T47.2X5 | T47.2X6 |
| **Dantrolene** | T42.8X1 | T42.8X2 | T42.8X3 | T42.8X4 | T42.8X5 | T42.8X6 |
| **Dantron** | T47.2X1 | T47.2X2 | T47.2X3 | T47.2X4 | T47.2X5 | T47.2X6 |
| **Daphne** (gnidium) (mezereum) | T62.2X1 | T62.2X2 | T62.2X3 | T62.2X4 | — | — |
| berry | T62.1X1 | T62.1X2 | T62.1X3 | T62.1X4 | — | — |
| **Dapsone** | T37.1X1 | T37.1X2 | T37.1X3 | T37.1X4 | T37.1X5 | T37.1X6 |
| **Daraprim** | T37.2X1 | T37.2X2 | T37.2X3 | T37.2X4 | T37.2X5 | T37.2X6 |
| **Darnel** | T62.2X1 | T62.2X2 | T62.2X3 | T62.2X4 | — | — |
| **Darvon** | T39.8X1 | T39.8X2 | T39.8X3 | T39.8X4 | T39.8X5 | T39.8X6 |
| **Daunomycin** | T45.1X1 | T45.1X2 | T45.1X3 | T45.1X4 | T45.1X5 | T45.1X6 |
| **Daunorubicin** | T45.1X1 | T45.1X2 | T45.1X3 | T45.1X4 | T45.1X5 | T45.1X6 |
| **DBI** | T38.3X1 | T38.3X2 | T38.3X3 | T38.3X4 | T38.3X5 | T38.3X6 |
| **D-Con** | T60.91 | T60.92 | T60.93 | T60.94 | — | — |
| insecticide | T60.2X1 | T60.2X2 | T60.2X3 | T60.2X4 | — | — |
| rodenticide | T60.4X1 | T60.4X2 | T60.4X3 | T60.4X4 | — | — |
| **DDAVP** | T38.891 | T38.892 | T38.893 | T38.894 | T38.895 | T38.896 |

| Substance | Poisoning, Accidental (unintentional) | Poisoning, Intentional Self-harm | Poisoning, Assault | Poisoning, Undetermined | Adverse Effect | Under-dosing |
|---|---|---|---|---|---|---|
| **DDE** (bis(chlorophenyl)-dichloroethylene) | T60.2X1 | T60.2X2 | T60.2X3 | T60.2X4 | — | — |
| **DDS** | T37.1X1 | T37.1X2 | T37.1X3 | T37.1X4 | T37.1X5 | T37.1X6 |
| **DDT** (dust) | T60.1X1 | T60.1X2 | T60.1X3 | T60.1X4 | — | — |
| **Deadly nightshade** — see also Belladonna | T62.2X1 | T62.2X2 | T62.2X3 | T62.2X4 | — | — |
| berry | T62.1X1 | T62.1X2 | T62.1X3 | T62.1X4 | — | — |
| **Deamino-D-arginine vasopressin** | T38.891 | T38.892 | T38.893 | T38.894 | T38.895 | T38.896 |
| **Deanol** (aceglumate) | T50.991 | T50.992 | T50.993 | T50.994 | T50.995 | T50.996 |
| **Debrisoquine** | T46.5X1 | T46.5X2 | T46.5X3 | T46.5X4 | T46.5X5 | T46.5X6 |
| **Decaborane** | T57.8X1 | T57.8X2 | T57.8X3 | T57.8X4 | — | — |
| fumes | T59.891 | T59.892 | T59.893 | T59.894 | — | — |
| **Decadron** | T38.0X1 | T38.0X2 | T38.0X3 | T38.0X4 | T38.0X5 | T38.0X6 |
| ENT agent | T49.6X1 | T49.6X2 | T49.6X3 | T49.6X4 | T49.6X5 | T49.6X6 |
| ophthalmic preparation | T49.5X1 | T49.5X2 | T49.5X3 | T49.5X4 | T49.5X5 | T49.5X6 |
| topical NEC | T49.0X1 | T49.0X2 | T49.0X3 | T49.0X4 | T49.0X5 | T49.0X6 |
| **Decahydronaphthalene** | T52.8X1 | T52.8X2 | T52.8X3 | T52.8X4 | — | — |
| **Decalin** | T52.8X1 | T52.8X2 | T52.8X3 | T52.8X4 | — | — |
| **Decamethonium** (bromide) | T48.1X1 | T48.1X2 | T48.1X3 | T48.1X4 | T48.1X5 | T48.1X6 |
| **Decholin** | T47.5X1 | T47.5X2 | T47.5X3 | T47.5X4 | T47.5X5 | T47.5X6 |
| **Declomycin** | T36.4X1 | T36.4X2 | T36.4X3 | T36.4X4 | T36.4X5 | T36.4X6 |
| **Decongestant, nasal** (mucosa) | T48.5X1 | T48.5X2 | T48.5X3 | T48.5X4 | T48.5X5 | T48.5X6 |
| combination | T48.5X1 | T48.5X2 | T48.5X3 | T48.5X4 | T48.5X5 | T48.5X6 |
| **Deet** | T60.8X1 | T60.8X2 | T60.8X3 | T60.8X4 | — | — |
| **Deferoxamine** | T45.8X1 | T45.8X2 | T45.8X3 | T45.8X4 | T45.8X5 | T45.8X6 |
| **Deflazacort** | T38.0X1 | T38.0X2 | T38.0X3 | T38.0X4 | T38.0X5 | T38.0X6 |
| **Deglycyrrhizinized extract of licorice** | T48.4X1 | T48.4X2 | T48.4X3 | T48.4X4 | T48.4X5 | T48.4X6 |
| **Dehydrocholic acid** | T47.5X1 | T47.5X2 | T47.5X3 | T47.5X4 | T47.5X5 | T47.5X6 |
| **Dehydroemetine** | T37.3X1 | T37.3X2 | T37.3X3 | T37.3X4 | T37.3X5 | T37.3X6 |
| **Dekalin** | T52.8X1 | T52.8X2 | T52.8X3 | T52.8X4 | — | — |
| **Delalutin** | T38.5X1 | T38.5X2 | T38.5X3 | T38.5X4 | T38.5X5 | T38.5X6 |
| **Delorazepam** | T42.4X1 | T42.4X2 | T42.4X3 | T42.4X4 | T42.4X5 | T42.4X6 |
| **Delphinium** | T62.2X1 | T62.2X2 | T62.2X3 | T62.2X4 | — | — |
| **Deltamethrin** | T60.1X1 | T60.1X2 | T60.1X3 | T60.1X4 | — | — |
| **Deltasone** | T38.0X1 | T38.0X2 | T38.0X3 | T38.0X4 | T38.0X5 | T38.0X6 |
| **Deltra** | T38.0X1 | T38.0X2 | T38.0X3 | T38.0X4 | T38.0X5 | T38.0X6 |
| **Delvinal** | T42.3X1 | T42.3X2 | T42.3X3 | T42.3X4 | T42.3X5 | T42.3X6 |
| **Demecarium** (bromide) | T49.5X1 | T49.5X2 | T49.5X3 | T49.5X4 | T49.5X5 | T49.5X6 |
| **Demeclocycline** | T36.4X1 | T36.4X2 | T36.4X3 | T36.4X4 | T36.4X5 | T36.4X6 |
| **Demecolcine** | T45.1X1 | T45.1X2 | T45.1X3 | T45.1X4 | T45.1X5 | T45.1X6 |
| **Demegestone** | T38.5X1 | T38.5X2 | T38.5X3 | T38.5X4 | T38.5X5 | T38.5X6 |
| **Demelanizing agents** | T49.8X1 | T49.8X2 | T49.8X3 | T49.8X4 | T49.8X5 | T49.8X6 |
| **Demephion -O and -S** | T60.0X1 | T60.0X2 | T60.0X3 | T60.0X4 | — | — |
| **Demerol** | T40.2X1 | T40.2X2 | T40.2X3 | T40.2X4 | T40.2X5 | T40.2X6 |
| **Demethylchlortetracycline** | T36.4X1 | T36.4X2 | T36.4X3 | T36.4X4 | T36.4X5 | T36.4X6 |
| **Demethyltetracycline** | T36.4X1 | T36.4X2 | T36.4X3 | T36.4X4 | T36.4X5 | T36.4X6 |
| **Demeton -O and -S** | T60.0X1 | T60.0X2 | T60.0X3 | T60.0X4 | — | — |
| **Demulcent** (external) | T49.3X1 | T49.3X2 | T49.3X3 | T49.3X4 | T49.3X5 | T49.3X6 |
| specified NEC | T49.3X1 | T49.3X2 | T49.3X3 | T49.3X4 | T49.3X5 | T49.3X6 |
| **Demulen** | T38.4X1 | T38.4X2 | T38.4X3 | T38.4X4 | T38.4X5 | T38.4X6 |
| **Denatured alcohol** | T51.0X1 | T51.0X2 | T51.0X3 | T51.0X4 | — | — |
| **Dendrid** | T49.5X1 | T49.5X2 | T49.5X3 | T49.5X4 | T49.5X5 | T49.5X6 |
| **Dental drug, topical application NEC** | T49.7X1 | T49.7X2 | T49.7X3 | T49.7X4 | T49.7X5 | T49.7X6 |
| **Dentifrice** | T49.7X1 | T49.7X2 | T49.7X3 | T49.7X4 | T49.7X5 | T49.7X6 |
| **Deodorant spray** (feminine hygiene) | T49.8X1 | T49.8X2 | T49.8X3 | T49.8X4 | T49.8X5 | T49.8X6 |
| **Deoxycortone** | T50.0X1 | T50.0X2 | T50.0X3 | T50.0X4 | T50.0X5 | T50.0X6 |
| **Deoxyribonuclease** (pancreatic) | T45.3X1 | T45.3X2 | T45.3X3 | T45.3X4 | T45.3X5 | T45.3X6 |
| **Depilatory** | T49.4X1 | T49.4X2 | T49.4X3 | T49.4X4 | T49.4X5 | T49.4X6 |
| **Deprenalin** | T42.8X1 | T42.8X2 | T42.8X3 | T42.8X4 | T42.8X5 | T42.8X6 |
| **Deprenyl** | T42.8X1 | T42.8X2 | T42.8X3 | T42.8X4 | T42.8X5 | T42.8X6 |
| **Depressant** | | | | | | |
| appetite (central) | T50.5X1 | T50.5X2 | T50.5X3 | T50.5X4 | T50.5X5 | T50.5X6 |
| cardiac | T46.2X1 | T46.2X2 | T46.2X3 | T46.2X4 | T46.2X5 | T46.2X6 |
| central nervous system (anesthetic) — see also Central nervous system, depressants | T42.71 | T42.72 | T42.73 | T42.74 | T42.75 | T42.76 |
| general anesthetic | T41.201 | T41.202 | T41.203 | T41.204 | T41.205 | T41.206 |
| muscle tone | T42.8X1 | T42.8X2 | T42.8X3 | T42.8X4 | T42.8X5 | T42.8X6 |
| muscle tone, central | T42.8X1 | T42.8X2 | T42.8X3 | T42.8X4 | T42.8X5 | T42.8X6 |
| psychotherapeutic | T43.501 | T43.502 | T43.503 | T43.504 | T43.505 | T43.506 |
| **Depressant, appetite** | T50.5X1 | T50.5X2 | T50.5X3 | T50.5X4 | T50.5X5 | T50.5X6 |
| **Deptropine** | T45.0X1 | T45.0X2 | T45.0X3 | T45.0X4 | T45.0X5 | T45.0X6 |
| **Dequalinium** (chloride) | T49.0X1 | T49.0X2 | T49.0X3 | T49.0X4 | T49.0X5 | T49.0X6 |
| **Derris root** | T60.2X1 | T60.2X2 | T60.2X3 | T60.2X4 | — | — |
| **Deserpidine** | T46.5X1 | T46.5X2 | T46.5X3 | T46.5X4 | T46.5X5 | T46.5X6 |
| **Desferrioxamine** | T45.8X1 | T45.8X2 | T45.8X3 | T45.8X4 | T45.8X5 | T45.8X6 |
| **Desipramine** | T43.011 | T43.012 | T43.013 | T43.014 | T43.015 | T43.016 |
| **Deslanoside** | T46.0X1 | T46.0X2 | T46.0X3 | T46.0X4 | T46.0X5 | T46.0X6 |
| **Desloughing agent** | T49.4X1 | T49.4X2 | T49.4X3 | T49.4X4 | T49.4X5 | T49.4X6 |
| **Desmethylimipramine** | T43.011 | T43.012 | T43.013 | T43.014 | T43.015 | T43.016 |
| **Desmopressin** | T38.891 | T38.892 | T38.893 | T38.894 | T38.895 | T38.896 |
| **Desocodeine** | T40.2X1 | T40.2X2 | T40.2X3 | T40.2X4 | T40.2X5 | T40.2X6 |
| **Desogestrel** | T38.5X1 | T38.5X2 | T38.5X3 | T38.5X4 | T38.5X5 | T38.5X6 |
| **Desomorphine** | T40.2X1 | T40.2X2 | T40.2X3 | T40.2X4 | — | — |
| **Desonide** | T49.0X1 | T49.0X2 | T49.0X3 | T49.0X4 | T49.0X5 | T49.0X6 |
| **Desoximetasone** | T49.0X1 | T49.0X2 | T49.0X3 | T49.0X4 | T49.0X5 | T49.0X6 |
| **Desoxycorticosteroid** | T50.0X1 | T50.0X2 | T50.0X3 | T50.0X4 | T50.0X5 | T50.0X6 |
| **Desoxycortone** | T50.0X1 | T50.0X2 | T50.0X3 | T50.0X4 | T50.0X5 | T50.0X6 |
| **Desoxyephedrine** | T43.621 | T43.622 | T43.623 | T43.624 | T43.625 | T43.626 |
| **Detaxtran** | T46.6X1 | T46.6X2 | T46.6X3 | T46.6X4 | T46.6X5 | T46.6X6 |
| **Detergent** | T49.2X1 | T49.2X2 | T49.2X3 | T49.2X4 | T49.2X5 | T49.2X6 |
| external medication | T49.2X1 | T49.2X2 | T49.2X3 | T49.2X4 | T49.2X5 | T49.2X6 |
| local | T49.2X1 | T49.2X2 | T49.2X3 | T49.2X4 | T49.2X5 | T49.2X6 |
| medicinal | T49.2X1 | T49.2X2 | T49.2X3 | T49.2X4 | T49.2X5 | T49.2X6 |
| nonmedicinal | T55.1X1 | T55.1X2 | T55.1X3 | T55.1X4 | — | — |
| specified NEC | T55.1X1 | T55.1X2 | T55.1X3 | T55.1X4 | — | — |
| **Deterrent, alcohol** | T50.6X1 | T50.6X2 | T50.6X3 | T50.6X4 | T50.6X5 | T50.6X6 |
| **Detoxifying agent** | T50.6X1 | T50.6X2 | T50.6X3 | T50.6X4 | T50.6X5 | T50.6X6 |
| **Detrothyronine** | T38.1X1 | T38.1X2 | T38.1X3 | T38.1X4 | T38.1X5 | T38.1X6 |
| **Dettol** (external medication) | T49.0X1 | T49.0X2 | T49.0X3 | T49.0X4 | T49.0X5 | T49.0X6 |
| **Dexamethasone** | T38.0X1 | T38.0X2 | T38.0X3 | T38.0X4 | T38.0X5 | T38.0X6 |
| ENT agent | T49.6X1 | T49.6X2 | T49.6X3 | T49.6X4 | T49.6X5 | T49.6X6 |
| ophthalmic preparation | T49.5X1 | T49.5X2 | T49.5X3 | T49.5X4 | T49.5X5 | T49.5X6 |
| topical NEC | T49.0X1 | T49.0X2 | T49.0X3 | T49.0X4 | T49.0X5 | T49.0X6 |
| **Dexamfetamine** | T43.621 | T43.622 | T43.623 | T43.624 | T43.625 | T43.626 |
| **Dexamphetamine** | T43.621 | T43.622 | T43.623 | T43.624 | T43.625 | T43.626 |
| **Dexbrompheniramine** | T45.0X1 | T45.0X2 | T45.0X3 | T45.0X4 | T45.0X5 | T45.0X6 |
| **Dexchlorpheniramine** | T45.0X1 | T45.0X2 | T45.0X3 | T45.0X4 | T45.0X5 | T45.0X6 |
| **Dexedrine** | T43.621 | T43.622 | T43.623 | T43.624 | T43.625 | T43.626 |
| **Dexetimide** | T44.3X1 | T44.3X2 | T44.3X3 | T44.3X4 | T44.3X5 | T44.3X6 |
| **Dexfenfluramine** | T50.5X1 | T50.5X2 | T50.5X3 | T50.5X4 | T50.5X5 | T50.5X6 |
| **Dexpanthenol** | T45.2X1 | T45.2X2 | T45.2X3 | T45.2X4 | T45.2X5 | T45.2X6 |
| **Dextran** (40) (70) (150) | T45.8X1 | T45.8X2 | T45.8X3 | T45.8X4 | T45.8X5 | T45.8X6 |
| **Dextriferron** | T45.4X1 | T45.4X2 | T45.4X3 | T45.4X4 | T45.4X5 | T45.4X6 |
| **Dextroamphetamine** | T43.621 | T43.622 | T43.623 | T43.624 | T43.625 | T43.626 |
| **Dextro calcium pantothenate** | T45.2X1 | T45.2X2 | T45.2X3 | T45.2X4 | T45.2X5 | T45.2X6 |
| **Dextromethorphan** | T48.3X1 | T48.3X2 | T48.3X3 | T48.3X4 | T48.3X5 | T48.3X6 |
| **Dextromoramide** | T40.4X1 | T40.4X2 | T40.4X3 | T40.4X4 | — | — |
| topical | T49.8X1 | T49.8X2 | T49.8X3 | T49.8X4 | T49.8X5 | T49.8X6 |
| **Dextro pantothenyl alcohol** | T45.2X1 | T45.2X2 | T45.2X3 | T45.2X4 | T45.2X5 | T45.2X6 |
| **Dextropropoxyphene** | T40.4X1 | T40.4X2 | T40.4X3 | T40.4X4 | T40.4X5 | T40.4X6 |
| **Dextrorphan** | T40.2X1 | T40.2X2 | T40.2X3 | T40.2X4 | T40.2X5 | T40.2X6 |
| **Dextrose** | T50.3X1 | T50.3X2 | T50.3X3 | T50.3X4 | T50.3X5 | T50.3X6 |
| concentrated solution, intravenous | T46.8X1 | T46.8X2 | T46.8X3 | T46.8X4 | T46.8X5 | T46.8X6 |
| **Dextrothyroxin** | T38.1X1 | T38.1X2 | T38.1X3 | T38.1X4 | T38.1X5 | T38.1X6 |
| **Dextrothyroxine sodium** | T38.1X1 | T38.1X2 | T38.1X3 | T38.1X4 | T38.1X5 | T38.1X6 |
| **DFP** | T44.0X1 | T44.0X2 | T44.0X3 | T44.0X4 | T44.0X5 | T44.0X6 |
| **DHE** | T37.3X1 | T37.3X2 | T37.3X3 | T37.3X4 | T37.3X5 | T37.3X6 |
| 45 | T46.5X1 | T46.5X2 | T46.5X3 | T46.5X4 | T46.5X5 | T46.5X6 |
| **Diabinese** | T38.3X1 | T38.3X2 | T38.3X3 | T38.3X4 | T38.3X5 | T38.3X6 |
| **Diacetone alcohol** | T52.4X1 | T52.4X2 | T52.4X3 | T52.4X4 | — | — |
| **Diacetyl monoxime** | T50.991 | T50.992 | T50.993 | T50.994 | — | — |
| **Diacetylmorphine** | T40.1X1 | T40.1X2 | T40.1X3 | T40.1X4 | — | — |
| **Diachylon plaster** | T49.4X1 | T49.4X2 | T49.4X3 | T49.4X4 | T49.4X5 | T49.4X6 |
| **Diaethylstilboestrolum** | T38.5X1 | T38.5X2 | T38.5X3 | T38.5X4 | T38.5X5 | T38.5X6 |
| **Diagnostic agent NEC** | T50.8X1 | T50.8X2 | T50.8X3 | T50.8X4 | T50.8X5 | T50.8X6 |
| **Dial** (soap) | T49.2X1 | T49.2X2 | T49.2X3 | T49.2X4 | T49.2X5 | T49.2X6 |
| sedative | T42.3X1 | T42.3X2 | T42.3X3 | T42.3X4 | T42.3X5 | T42.3X6 |
| **Dialkyl carbonate** | T52.91 | T52.92 | T52.93 | T52.94 | — | — |
| **Diallylbarbituric acid** | T42.3X1 | T42.3X2 | T42.3X3 | T42.3X4 | T42.3X5 | T42.3X6 |
| **Diallymal** | T42.3X1 | T42.3X2 | T42.3X3 | T42.3X4 | T42.3X5 | T42.3X6 |
| **Dialysis solution** (intraperitoneal) | T50.3X1 | T50.3X2 | T50.3X3 | T50.3X4 | T50.3X5 | T50.3X6 |
| **Diaminodiphenylsulfone** | T37.1X1 | T37.1X2 | T37.1X3 | T37.1X4 | T37.1X5 | T37.1X6 |
| **Diamorphine** | T40.1X1 | T40.1X2 | T40.1X3 | T40.1X4 | — | — |
| **Diamox** | T50.2X1 | T50.2X2 | T50.2X3 | T50.2X4 | T50.2X5 | T50.2X6 |
| **Diamthazole** | T49.0X1 | T49.0X2 | T49.0X3 | T49.0X4 | T49.0X5 | T49.0X6 |
| **Dianthone** | T47.2X1 | T47.2X2 | T47.2X3 | T47.2X4 | T47.2X5 | T47.2X6 |
| **Diaphenylsulfone** | T37.0X1 | T37.0X2 | T37.0X3 | T37.0X4 | T37.0X5 | T37.0X6 |
| **Diasone** (sodium) | T37.1X1 | T37.1X2 | T37.1X3 | T37.1X4 | T37.1X5 | T37.1X6 |
| **Diastase** | T47.5X1 | T47.5X2 | T47.5X3 | T47.5X4 | T47.5X5 | T47.5X6 |
| **Diatrizoate** | T50.8X1 | T50.8X2 | T50.8X3 | T50.8X4 | T50.8X5 | T50.8X6 |
| **Diazepam** | T42.4X1 | T42.4X2 | T42.4X3 | T42.4X4 | T42.4X5 | T42.4X6 |
| **Diazinon** | T60.0X1 | T60.0X2 | T60.0X3 | T60.0X4 | — | — |
| **Diazomethane** (gas) | T59.891 | T59.892 | T59.893 | T59.894 | — | — |
| **Diazoxide** | T46.5X1 | T46.5X2 | T46.5X3 | T46.5X4 | T46.5X5 | T46.5X6 |
| **Dibekacin** | T36.5X1 | T36.5X2 | T36.5X3 | T36.5X4 | T36.5X5 | T36.5X6 |

▽ Subterms under main terms may continue to next column or page     Additional Character May Be Required — Refer to the Tabular List for Character Selection     363

DDE — Dibekacin

| Substance | Poisoning, Accidental (unintentional) | Poisoning, Intentional Self-harm | Poisoning, Assault | Poisoning, Undetermined | Adverse Effect | Under-dosing |
|---|---|---|---|---|---|---|
| Dibenamine | T44.6X1 | T44.6X2 | T44.6X3 | T44.6X4 | T44.6X5 | T44.6X6 |
| Dibenzepin | T43.011 | T43.012 | T43.013 | T43.014 | T43.015 | T43.016 |
| Dibenzheptropine | T45.0X1 | T45.0X2 | T45.0X3 | T45.0X4 | T45.0X5 | T45.0X6 |
| Dibenzyline | T44.6X1 | T44.6X2 | T44.6X3 | T44.6X4 | T44.6X5 | T44.6X6 |
| Diborane (gas) | T59.891 | T59.892 | T59.893 | T59.894 | — | — |
| Dibromochloropropane | T60.8X1 | T60.8X2 | T60.8X3 | T60.8X4 | — | — |
| Dibromodulcitol | T45.1X1 | T45.1X2 | T45.1X3 | T45.1X4 | T45.1X5 | T45.1X6 |
| Dibromoethane | T53.6X1 | T53.6X2 | T53.6X3 | T53.6X4 | — | — |
| Dibromomannitol | T45.1X1 | T45.1X2 | T45.1X3 | T45.1X4 | T45.1X5 | T45.1X6 |
| Dibromopropamidine isethionate | T49.0X1 | T49.0X2 | T49.0X3 | T49.0X4 | T49.0X5 | T49.0X6 |
| Dibrompropamidine | T49.0X1 | T49.0X2 | T49.0X3 | T49.0X4 | T49.0X5 | T49.0X6 |
| Dibucaine | T41.3X1 | T41.3X2 | T41.3X3 | T41.3X4 | T41.3X5 | T41.3X6 |
| topical (surface) | T41.3X1 | T41.3X2 | T41.3X3 | T41.3X4 | T41.3X5 | T41.3X6 |
| Dibunate sodium | T48.3X1 | T48.3X2 | T48.3X3 | T48.3X4 | T48.3X5 | T48.3X6 |
| Dibutoline sulfate | T44.3X1 | T44.3X2 | T44.3X3 | T44.3X4 | T44.3X5 | T44.3X6 |
| Dicamba | T60.3X1 | T60.3X2 | T60.3X3 | T60.3X4 | — | — |
| Dicapthon | T60.0X1 | T60.0X2 | T60.0X3 | T60.0X4 | — | — |
| Dichlobenil | T60.3X1 | T60.3X2 | T60.3X3 | T60.3X4 | — | — |
| Dichlone | T60.3X1 | T60.3X2 | T60.3X3 | T60.3X4 | — | — |
| Dichloralphenozone | T42.6X1 | T42.6X2 | T42.6X3 | T42.6X4 | T42.6X5 | T42.6X6 |
| Dichlorbenzidine | T65.3X1 | T65.3X2 | T65.3X3 | T65.3X4 | — | — |
| Dichlorhydrin | T52.8X1 | T52.8X2 | T52.8X3 | T52.8X4 | — | — |
| Dichlorhydroxyquinoline | T37.8X1 | T37.8X2 | T37.8X3 | T37.8X4 | T37.8X5 | T37.8X6 |
| Dichlorobenzene | T53.7X1 | T53.7X2 | T53.7X3 | T53.7X4 | — | — |
| Dichlorobenzyl alcohol | T49.6X1 | T49.6X2 | T49.6X3 | T49.6X4 | T49.6X5 | T49.6X6 |
| Dichlorodifluoromethane | T53.5X1 | T53.5X2 | T53.5X3 | T53.5X4 | — | — |
| Dichloroethane | T52.8X1 | T52.8X2 | T52.8X3 | T52.8X4 | — | — |
| Dichloroethylene | T53.6X1 | T53.6X2 | T53.6X3 | T53.6X4 | — | — |
| Dichloroethyl sulfide, not in war | T59.891 | T59.892 | T59.893 | T59.894 | — | — |
| Dichloroformoxine, not in war | T59.891 | T59.892 | T59.893 | T59.894 | — | — |
| Dichlorohydrin, alpha-dichlorohydrin | T52.8X1 | T52.8X2 | T52.8X3 | T52.8X4 | — | — |
| Dichloromethane (solvent) | T53.4X1 | T53.4X2 | T53.4X3 | T53.4X4 | — | — |
| vapor | T53.4X1 | T53.4X2 | T53.4X3 | T53.4X4 | — | — |
| Dichloronaphthoquinone | T60.3X1 | T60.3X2 | T60.3X3 | T60.3X4 | — | — |
| Dichlorophen | T37.4X1 | T37.4X2 | T37.4X3 | T37.4X4 | T37.4X5 | T37.4X6 |
| Dichloropropene | T60.3X1 | T60.3X2 | T60.3X3 | T60.3X4 | — | — |
| Dichloropropionic acid | T60.3X1 | T60.3X2 | T60.3X3 | T60.3X4 | — | — |
| Dichlorphenamide | T50.2X1 | T50.2X2 | T50.2X3 | T50.2X4 | T50.2X5 | T50.2X6 |
| Dichlorvos | T60.0X1 | T60.0X2 | T60.0X3 | T60.0X4 | — | — |
| Diclofenac | T39.391 | T39.392 | T39.393 | T39.394 | T39.395 | T39.396 |
| Diclofenamide | T50.2X1 | T50.2X2 | T50.2X3 | T50.2X4 | T50.2X5 | T50.2X6 |
| Diclofensine | T43.291 | T43.292 | T43.293 | T43.294 | T43.295 | T43.296 |
| Diclonixine | T39.8X1 | T39.8X2 | T39.8X3 | T39.8X4 | T39.8X5 | T39.8X6 |
| Dicloxacillin | T36.0X1 | T36.0X2 | T36.0X3 | T36.0X4 | T36.0X5 | T36.0X6 |
| Dicophane | T49.0X1 | T49.0X2 | T49.0X3 | T49.0X4 | T49.0X5 | T49.0X6 |
| Dicoumarol, dicoumarin, dicumarol | T45.511 | T45.512 | T45.513 | T45.514 | T45.515 | T45.516 |
| Dicrotophos | T60.0X1 | T60.0X2 | T60.0X3 | T60.0X4 | — | — |
| Dicyanogen (gas) | T65.0X1 | T65.0X2 | T65.0X3 | T65.0X4 | — | — |
| Dicyclomine | T44.3X1 | T44.3X2 | T44.3X3 | T44.3X4 | T44.3X5 | T44.3X6 |
| Dicycloverine | T44.3X1 | T44.3X2 | T44.3X3 | T44.3X4 | T44.3X5 | T44.3X6 |
| Dideoxycytidine | T37.5X1 | T37.5X2 | T37.5X3 | T37.5X4 | T37.5X5 | T37.5X6 |
| Dideoxyinosine | T37.5X1 | T37.5X2 | T37.5X3 | T37.5X4 | T37.5X5 | T37.5X6 |
| Dieldrin (vapor) | T60.1X1 | T60.1X2 | T60.1X3 | T60.1X4 | — | — |
| Diemal | T42.3X1 | T42.3X2 | T42.3X3 | T42.3X4 | T42.3X5 | T42.3X6 |
| Dienestrol | T38.5X1 | T38.5X2 | T38.5X3 | T38.5X4 | T38.5X5 | T38.5X6 |
| Dienoestrol | T38.5X1 | T38.5X2 | T38.5X3 | T38.5X4 | T38.5X5 | T38.5X6 |
| Dietetic drug NEC | T50.901 | T50.902 | T50.903 | T50.904 | T50.905 | T50.906 |
| Diethazine | T42.8X1 | T42.8X2 | T42.8X3 | T42.8X4 | T42.8X5 | T42.8X6 |
| Diethyl | | | | | | |
| barbituric acid | T42.3X1 | T42.3X2 | T42.3X3 | T42.3X4 | T42.3X5 | T42.3X6 |
| carbamazine | T37.4X1 | T37.4X2 | T37.4X3 | T37.4X4 | T37.4X5 | T37.4X6 |
| carbinol | T51.3X1 | T51.3X2 | T51.3X3 | T51.3X4 | — | — |
| carbonate | T52.8X1 | T52.8X2 | T52.8X3 | T52.8X4 | — | — |
| ether (vapor) — see also ether | T41.0X1 | T41.0X2 | T41.0X3 | T41.0X4 | T41.0X5 | T41.0X6 |
| oxide | T52.8X1 | T52.8X2 | T52.8X3 | T52.8X4 | — | — |
| propion | T50.5X1 | T50.5X2 | T50.5X3 | T50.5X4 | T50.5X5 | T50.5X6 |
| stilbestrol | T38.5X1 | T38.5X2 | T38.5X3 | T38.5X4 | T38.5X5 | T38.5X6 |
| toluamide (nonmedicinal) | T60.8X1 | T60.8X2 | T60.8X3 | T60.8X4 | — | — |
| medicinal | T49.3X1 | T49.3X2 | T49.3X3 | T49.3X4 | T49.3X5 | T49.3X6 |
| Diethylcarbamazine | T37.4X1 | T37.4X2 | T37.4X3 | T37.4X4 | T37.4X5 | T37.4X6 |
| Diethylene | | | | | | |
| dioxide | T52.8X1 | T52.8X2 | T52.8X3 | T52.8X4 | — | — |
| glycol (monoacetate) (monobutyl ether) (monoethyl ether) | T52.3X1 | T52.3X2 | T52.3X3 | T52.3X4 | — | — |
| Diethylhexylphthalate | T65.891 | T65.892 | T65.893 | T65.894 | — | — |
| Diethylpropion | T50.5X1 | T50.5X2 | T50.5X3 | T50.5X4 | T50.5X5 | T50.5X6 |
| Diethylstilbestrol | T38.5X1 | T38.5X2 | T38.5X3 | T38.5X4 | T38.5X5 | T38.5X6 |
| Diethylstilboestrol | T38.5X1 | T38.5X2 | T38.5X3 | T38.5X4 | T38.5X5 | T38.5X6 |
| Diethylsulfone-diethylmethane | T42.6X1 | T42.6X2 | T42.6X3 | T42.6X4 | T42.6X5 | T42.6X6 |
| Diethyltoluamide | T49.0X1 | T49.0X2 | T49.0X3 | T49.0X4 | T49.0X5 | T49.0X6 |
| Diethyltryptamine (DET) | T40.991 | T40.992 | T40.993 | T40.994 | — | — |
| Difebarbamate | T42.3X1 | T42.3X2 | T42.3X3 | T42.3X4 | T42.3X5 | T42.3X6 |
| Difencloxacine | T40.2X1 | T40.2X2 | T40.2X3 | T40.2X4 | T40.2X5 | T40.2X6 |
| Difenidol | T45.0X1 | T45.0X2 | T45.0X3 | T45.0X4 | T45.0X5 | T45.0X6 |
| Difenoxin | T47.6X1 | T47.6X2 | T47.6X3 | T47.6X4 | T47.6X5 | T47.6X6 |
| Difetarsone | T37.3X1 | T37.3X2 | T37.3X3 | T37.3X4 | T37.3X5 | T37.3X6 |
| Diffusin | T45.3X1 | T45.3X2 | T45.3X3 | T45.3X4 | T45.3X5 | T45.3X6 |
| Diflorasone | T49.0X1 | T49.0X2 | T49.0X3 | T49.0X4 | T49.0X5 | T49.0X6 |
| Diflos | T44.0X1 | T44.0X2 | T44.0X3 | T44.0X4 | T44.0X5 | T44.0X6 |
| Diflubenzuron | T60.1X1 | T60.1X2 | T60.1X3 | T60.1X4 | — | — |
| Diflucortolone | T49.0X1 | T49.0X2 | T49.0X3 | T49.0X4 | T49.0X5 | T49.0X6 |
| Diflunisal | T39.091 | T39.092 | T39.093 | T39.094 | T39.095 | T39.096 |
| Difluoromethyldopa | T42.8X1 | T42.8X2 | T42.8X3 | T42.8X4 | T42.8X5 | T42.8X6 |
| Difluorophate | T44.0X1 | T44.0X2 | T44.0X3 | T44.0X4 | T44.0X5 | T44.0X6 |
| Digestant NEC | T47.5X1 | T47.5X2 | T47.5X3 | T47.5X4 | T47.5X5 | T47.5X6 |
| Digitalin (e) | T46.0X1 | T46.0X2 | T46.0X3 | T46.0X4 | T46.0X5 | T46.0X6 |
| Digitalis (leaf)(glycoside) | T46.0X1 | T46.0X2 | T46.0X3 | T46.0X4 | T46.0X5 | T46.0X6 |
| lanata | T46.0X1 | T46.0X2 | T46.0X3 | T46.0X4 | T46.0X5 | T46.0X6 |
| purpurea | T46.0X1 | T46.0X2 | T46.0X3 | T46.0X4 | T46.0X5 | T46.0X6 |
| Digitoxin | T46.0X1 | T46.0X2 | T46.0X3 | T46.0X4 | T46.0X5 | T46.0X6 |
| Digitoxose | T46.0X1 | T46.0X2 | T46.0X3 | T46.0X4 | T46.0X5 | T46.0X6 |
| Digoxin | T46.0X1 | T46.0X2 | T46.0X3 | T46.0X4 | T46.0X5 | T46.0X6 |
| Digoxine | T46.0X1 | T46.0X2 | T46.0X3 | T46.0X4 | T46.0X5 | T46.0X6 |
| Dihydralazine | T46.5X1 | T46.5X2 | T46.5X3 | T46.5X4 | T46.5X5 | T46.5X6 |
| Dihydrazine | T46.5X1 | T46.5X2 | T46.5X3 | T46.5X4 | T46.5X5 | T46.5X6 |
| Dihydrocodeine | T40.2X1 | T40.2X2 | T40.2X3 | T40.2X4 | T40.2X5 | T40.2X6 |
| Dihydrocodeinone | T40.2X1 | T40.2X2 | T40.2X3 | T40.2X4 | T40.2X5 | T40.2X6 |
| Dihydroergocornine | T46.7X1 | T46.7X2 | T46.7X3 | T46.7X4 | T46.7X5 | T46.7X6 |
| Dihydroergocristine (mesilate) | T46.7X1 | T46.7X2 | T46.7X3 | T46.7X4 | T46.7X5 | T46.7X6 |
| Dihydroergokryptine | T46.7X1 | T46.7X2 | T46.7X3 | T46.7X4 | T46.7X5 | T46.7X6 |
| Dihydroergotamine | T46.5X1 | T46.5X2 | T46.5X3 | T46.5X4 | T46.5X5 | T46.5X6 |
| Dihydroergotoxine | T46.7X1 | T46.7X2 | T46.7X3 | T46.7X4 | T46.7X5 | T46.7X6 |
| mesilate | T46.7X1 | T46.7X2 | T46.7X3 | T46.7X4 | T46.7X5 | T46.7X6 |
| Dihydrohydroxycodeinone | T40.2X1 | T40.2X2 | T40.2X3 | T40.2X4 | T40.2X5 | T40.2X6 |
| Dihydrohydroxymorphinone | T40.2X1 | T40.2X2 | T40.2X3 | T40.2X4 | T40.2X5 | T40.2X6 |
| Dihydroisocodeine | T40.2X1 | T40.2X2 | T40.2X3 | T40.2X4 | T40.2X5 | T40.2X6 |
| Dihydromorphine | T40.2X1 | T40.2X2 | T40.2X3 | T40.2X4 | — | — |
| Dihydromorphinone | T40.2X1 | T40.2X2 | T40.2X3 | T40.2X4 | T40.2X5 | T40.2X6 |
| Dihydrostreptomycin | T36.5X1 | T36.5X2 | T36.5X3 | T36.5X4 | T36.5X5 | T36.5X6 |
| Dihydrotachysterol | T45.2X1 | T45.2X2 | T45.2X3 | T45.2X4 | T45.2X5 | T45.2X6 |
| Dihydroxyaluminum aminoacetate | T47.1X1 | T47.1X2 | T47.1X3 | T47.1X4 | T47.1X5 | T47.1X6 |
| Dihydroxyaluminum sodium carbonate | T47.1X1 | T47.1X2 | T47.1X3 | T47.1X4 | T47.1X5 | T47.1X6 |
| Dihydroxyanthraquinone | T47.2X1 | T47.2X2 | T47.2X3 | T47.2X4 | T47.2X5 | T47.2X6 |
| Dihydroxycodeinone | T40.2X1 | T40.2X2 | T40.2X3 | T40.2X4 | T40.2X5 | T40.2X6 |
| Dihydroxypropyl theophylline | T50.2X1 | T50.2X2 | T50.2X3 | T50.2X4 | T50.2X5 | T50.2X6 |
| Diiodohydroxyquin | T37.8X1 | T37.8X2 | T37.8X3 | T37.8X4 | T37.8X5 | T37.8X6 |
| topical | T49.0X1 | T49.0X2 | T49.0X3 | T49.0X4 | T49.0X5 | T49.0X6 |
| Diiodohydroxyquinoline | T37.8X1 | T37.8X2 | T37.8X3 | T37.8X4 | T37.8X5 | T37.8X6 |
| Diiodotyrosine | T38.2X1 | T38.2X2 | T38.2X3 | T38.2X4 | T38.2X5 | T38.2X6 |
| Diisopromine | T44.3X1 | T44.3X2 | T44.3X3 | T44.3X4 | T44.3X5 | T44.3X6 |
| Diisopropylamine | T46.3X1 | T46.3X2 | T46.3X3 | T46.3X4 | T46.3X5 | T46.3X6 |
| Diisopropylfluorophosphonate | T44.0X1 | T44.0X2 | T44.0X3 | T44.0X4 | T44.0X5 | T44.0X6 |
| Dilantin | T42.0X1 | T42.0X2 | T42.0X3 | T42.0X4 | T42.0X5 | T42.0X6 |
| Dilaudid | T40.2X1 | T40.2X2 | T40.2X3 | T40.2X4 | T40.2X5 | T40.2X6 |
| Dilazep | T46.3X1 | T46.3X2 | T46.3X3 | T46.3X4 | T46.3X5 | T46.3X6 |
| Dill | T47.5X1 | T47.5X2 | T47.5X3 | T47.5X4 | T47.5X5 | T47.5X6 |
| Diloxanide | T37.3X1 | T37.3X2 | T37.3X3 | T37.3X4 | T37.3X5 | T37.3X6 |
| Diltiazem | T46.1X1 | T46.1X2 | T46.1X3 | T46.1X4 | T46.1X5 | T46.1X6 |
| Dimazole | T49.0X1 | T49.0X2 | T49.0X3 | T49.0X4 | T49.0X5 | T49.0X6 |
| Dimefline | T50.7X1 | T50.7X2 | T50.7X3 | T50.7X4 | T50.7X5 | T50.7X6 |
| Dimefox | T60.0X1 | T60.0X2 | T60.0X3 | T60.0X4 | — | — |
| Dimemorfan | T48.3X1 | T48.3X2 | T48.3X3 | T48.3X4 | T48.3X5 | T48.3X6 |
| Dimenhydrinate | T45.0X1 | T45.0X2 | T45.0X3 | T45.0X4 | T45.0X5 | T45.0X6 |
| Dimercaprol (British anti-lewisite) | T45.8X1 | T45.8X2 | T45.8X3 | T45.8X4 | T45.8X5 | T45.8X6 |
| Dimercaptopropanol | T45.8X1 | T45.8X2 | T45.8X3 | T45.8X4 | T45.8X5 | T45.8X6 |
| Dimestrol | T38.5X1 | T38.5X2 | T38.5X3 | T38.5X4 | T38.5X5 | T38.5X6 |
| Dimetane | T45.0X1 | T45.0X2 | T45.0X3 | T45.0X4 | T45.0X5 | T45.0X6 |
| Dimethicone | T47.1X1 | T47.1X2 | T47.1X3 | T47.1X4 | T47.1X5 | T47.1X6 |
| Dimethindene | T45.0X1 | T45.0X2 | T45.0X3 | T45.0X4 | T45.0X5 | T45.0X6 |
| Dimethisoquin | T49.1X1 | T49.1X2 | T49.1X3 | T49.1X4 | T49.1X5 | T49.1X6 |
| Dimethisterone | T38.5X1 | T38.5X2 | T38.5X3 | T38.5X4 | T38.5X5 | T38.5X6 |
| Dimethoate | T60.0X1 | T60.0X2 | T60.0X3 | T60.0X4 | — | — |
| Dimethocaine | T41.3X1 | T41.3X2 | T41.3X3 | T41.3X4 | T41.3X5 | T41.3X6 |
| Dimethoxanate | T48.3X1 | T48.3X2 | T48.3X3 | T48.3X4 | T48.3X5 | T48.3X6 |

| Substance | Poisoning, Accidental (unintentional) | Poisoning, Intentional Self-harm | Poisoning, Assault | Poisoning, Undetermined | Adverse Effect | Under-dosing |
|---|---|---|---|---|---|---|
| **Dimethyl** | | | | | | |
| arsine, arsinic acid | T57.0X1 | T57.0X2 | T57.0X3 | T57.0X4 | — | — |
| carbinol | T51.2X1 | T51.2X2 | T51.2X3 | T51.2X4 | — | — |
| carbonate | T52.8X1 | T52.8X2 | T52.8X3 | T52.8X4 | — | — |
| diguanide | T38.3X1 | T38.3X2 | T38.3X3 | T38.3X4 | T38.3X5 | T38.3X6 |
| ketone | T52.4X1 | T52.4X2 | T52.4X3 | T52.4X4 | — | — |
| vapor | T52.4X1 | T52.4X2 | T52.4X3 | T52.4X4 | — | — |
| meperidine | T40.2X1 | T40.2X2 | T40.2X3 | T40.2X4 | T40.2X5 | T40.2X6 |
| parathion | T60.0X1 | T60.0X2 | T60.0X3 | T60.0X4 | — | — |
| phthlate | T49.3X1 | T49.3X2 | T49.3X3 | T49.3X4 | T49.3X5 | T49.3X6 |
| polysiloxane | T47.8X1 | T47.8X2 | T47.8X3 | T47.8X4 | T47.8X5 | T47.8X6 |
| sulfate (fumes) | T59.891 | T59.892 | T59.893 | T59.894 | — | — |
| liquid | T65.891 | T65.892 | T65.893 | T65.894 | — | — |
| sulfoxide (nonmedicinal) | T52.8X1 | T52.8X2 | T52.8X3 | T52.8X4 | — | — |
| medicinal | T49.4X1 | T49.4X2 | T49.4X3 | T49.4X4 | T49.4X5 | T49.4X6 |
| tryptamine | T40.991 | T40.992 | T40.993 | T40.994 | — | — |
| tubocurarine | T48.1X1 | T48.1X2 | T48.1X3 | T48.1X4 | T48.1X5 | T48.1X6 |
| **Dimethylamine sulfate** | T49.4X1 | T49.4X2 | T49.4X3 | T49.4X4 | T49.4X5 | T49.4X6 |
| **Dimethylformamide** | T52.8X1 | T52.8X2 | T52.8X3 | T52.8X4 | — | — |
| **Dimethyltubocurarinium chloride** | T48.1X1 | T48.1X2 | T48.1X3 | T48.1X4 | T48.1X5 | T48.1X6 |
| **Dimeticone** | T47.1X1 | T47.1X2 | T47.1X3 | T47.1X4 | T47.1X5 | T47.1X6 |
| **Dimetilan** | T60.0X1 | T60.0X2 | T60.0X3 | T60.0X4 | — | — |
| **Dimetindene** | T45.0X1 | T45.0X2 | T45.0X3 | T45.0X4 | T45.0X5 | T45.0X6 |
| **Dimetotiazine** | T43.3X1 | T43.3X2 | T43.3X3 | T43.3X4 | T43.3X5 | T43.3X6 |
| **Dimorpholamine** | T50.7X1 | T50.7X2 | T50.7X3 | T50.7X4 | T50.7X5 | T50.7X6 |
| **Dimoxyline** | T46.3X1 | T46.3X2 | T46.3X3 | T46.3X4 | T46.3X5 | T46.3X6 |
| **Dinitrobenzene** | T65.3X1 | T65.3X2 | T65.3X3 | T65.3X4 | — | — |
| vapor | T59.891 | T59.892 | T59.893 | T59.894 | — | — |
| **Dinitrobenzol** | T65.3X1 | T65.3X2 | T65.3X3 | T65.3X4 | — | — |
| vapor | T59.891 | T59.892 | T59.893 | T59.894 | — | — |
| **Dinitrobutylphenol** | T65.3X1 | T65.3X2 | T65.3X3 | T65.3X4 | — | — |
| **Dinitro** (-ortho-)cresol (pesticide) (spray) | T65.3X1 | T65.3X2 | T65.3X3 | T65.3X4 | — | — |
| **Dinitrocyclohexylphenol** | T65.3X1 | T65.3X2 | T65.3X3 | T65.3X4 | — | — |
| **Dinitrophenol** | T65.3X1 | T65.3X2 | T65.3X3 | T65.3X4 | — | — |
| **Dinoprost** | T48.0X1 | T48.0X2 | T48.0X3 | T48.0X4 | T48.0X5 | T48.0X6 |
| **Dinoprostone** | T48.0X1 | T48.0X2 | T48.0X3 | T48.0X4 | T48.0X5 | T48.0X6 |
| **Dinoseb** | T60.3X1 | T60.3X2 | T60.3X3 | T60.3X4 | — | — |
| **Dioctyl sulfosuccinate** (calcium) (sodium) | T47.4X1 | T47.4X2 | T47.4X3 | T47.4X4 | T47.4X5 | T47.4X6 |
| **Diodone** | T50.8X1 | T50.8X2 | T50.8X3 | T50.8X4 | T50.8X5 | T50.8X6 |
| **Diodoquin** | T37.8X1 | T37.8X2 | T37.8X3 | T37.8X4 | T37.8X5 | T37.8X6 |
| **Dionin** | T40.2X1 | T40.2X2 | T40.2X3 | T40.2X4 | T40.2X5 | T40.2X6 |
| **Diosmin** | T46.991 | T46.992 | T46.993 | T46.994 | T46.995 | T46.996 |
| **Dioxane** | T52.8X1 | T52.8X2 | T52.8X3 | T52.8X4 | — | — |
| **Dioxathion** | T60.0X1 | T60.0X2 | T60.0X3 | T60.0X4 | — | — |
| **Dioxin** | T53.7X1 | T53.7X2 | T53.7X3 | T53.7X4 | — | — |
| **Dioxopromethazine** | T43.3X1 | T43.3X2 | T43.3X3 | T43.3X4 | T43.3X5 | T43.3X6 |
| **Dioxyline** | T46.3X1 | T46.3X2 | T46.3X3 | T46.3X4 | T46.3X5 | T46.3X6 |
| **Dipentene** | T52.8X1 | T52.8X2 | T52.8X3 | T52.8X4 | — | — |
| **Diperodon** | T41.3X1 | T41.3X2 | T41.3X3 | T41.3X4 | T41.3X5 | T41.3X6 |
| **Diphacinone** | T60.4X1 | T60.4X2 | T60.4X3 | T60.4X4 | — | — |
| **Diphemanil** | T44.3X1 | T44.3X2 | T44.3X3 | T44.3X4 | T44.3X5 | T44.3X6 |
| metilsulfate | T44.3X1 | T44.3X2 | T44.3X3 | T44.3X4 | T44.3X5 | T44.3X6 |
| **Diphenadione** | T45.511 | T45.512 | T45.513 | T45.514 | T45.515 | T45.516 |
| rodenticide | T60.4X1 | T60.4X2 | T60.4X3 | T60.4X4 | — | — |
| **Diphenhydramine** | T45.0X1 | T45.0X2 | T45.0X3 | T45.0X4 | T45.0X5 | T45.0X6 |
| **Diphenidol** | T45.0X1 | T45.0X2 | T45.0X3 | T45.0X4 | T45.0X5 | T45.0X6 |
| **Diphenoxylate** | T47.6X1 | T47.6X2 | T47.6X3 | T47.6X4 | T47.6X5 | T47.6X6 |
| **Diphenylamine** | T65.3X1 | T65.3X2 | T65.3X3 | T65.3X4 | — | — |
| **Diphenylbutazone** | T39.2X1 | T39.2X2 | T39.2X3 | T39.2X4 | T39.2X5 | T39.2X6 |
| **Diphenylchloroarsine, not in war** | T57.0X1 | T57.0X2 | T57.0X3 | T57.0X4 | — | — |
| **Diphenylhydantoin** | T42.0X1 | T42.0X2 | T42.0X3 | T42.0X4 | T42.0X5 | T42.0X6 |
| **Diphenylmethane dye** | T52.1X1 | T52.1X2 | T52.1X3 | T52.1X4 | — | — |
| **Diphenylpyraline** | T45.0X1 | T45.0X2 | T45.0X3 | T45.0X4 | T45.0X5 | T45.0X6 |
| **Diphtheria** | | | | | | |
| antitoxin | T50.Z11 | T50.Z12 | T50.Z13 | T50.Z14 | T50.Z15 | T50.Z16 |
| toxoid | T50.A91 | T50.A92 | T50.A93 | T50.A94 | T50.A95 | T50.A96 |
| with tetanus toxoid | T50.A21 | T50.A22 | T50.A23 | T50.A24 | T50.A25 | T50.A26 |
| with pertussis component | T50.A11 | T50.A12 | T50.A13 | T50.A14 | T50.A15 | T50.A16 |
| vaccine | T50.A91 | T50.A92 | T50.A93 | T50.A94 | T50.A95 | T50.A96 |
| combination | | | | | | |
| without pertussis | T50.A21 | T50.A22 | T50.A23 | T50.A24 | T50.A25 | T50.A26 |
| including pertussis | T50.A11 | T50.A12 | T50.A13 | T50.A14 | T50.A15 | T50.A16 |
| **Diphylline** | T50.2X1 | T50.2X2 | T50.2X3 | T50.2X4 | T50.2X5 | T50.2X6 |
| **Dipipanone** | T40.4X1 | T40.4X2 | T40.4X3 | T40.4X4 | — | — |
| **Dipivefrine** | T49.5X1 | T49.5X2 | T49.5X3 | T49.5X4 | T49.5X5 | T49.5X6 |
| **Diplovax** | T50.B91 | T50.B92 | T50.B93 | T50.B94 | T50.B95 | T50.B96 |
| **Diprophylline** | T50.2X1 | T50.2X2 | T50.2X3 | T50.2X4 | T50.2X5 | T50.2X6 |
| **Dipropyline** | T48.291 | T48.292 | T48.293 | T48.294 | T48.295 | T48.296 |
| **Dipyridamole** | T46.3X1 | T46.3X2 | T46.3X3 | T46.3X4 | T46.3X5 | T46.3X6 |
| **Dipyrone** | T39.2X1 | T39.2X2 | T39.2X3 | T39.2X4 | T39.2X5 | T39.2X6 |
| **Diquat** (dibromide) | T60.3X1 | T60.3X2 | T60.3X3 | T60.3X4 | — | — |
| **Disinfectant** | T65.891 | T65.892 | T65.893 | T65.894 | — | — |
| alkaline | T54.3X1 | T54.3X2 | T54.3X3 | T54.3X4 | — | — |
| aromatic | T54.1X1 | T54.1X2 | T54.1X3 | T54.1X4 | — | — |
| intestinal | T37.8X1 | T37.8X2 | T37.8X3 | T37.8X4 | T37.8X5 | T37.8X6 |
| **Disipal** | T42.8X1 | T42.8X2 | T42.8X3 | T42.8X4 | T42.8X5 | T42.8X6 |
| **Disodium edetate** | T50.6X1 | T50.6X2 | T50.6X3 | T50.6X4 | T50.6X5 | T50.6X6 |
| **Disoprofol** | T41.291 | T41.292 | T41.293 | T41.294 | T41.295 | T41.296 |
| **Disopyramide** | T46.2X1 | T46.2X2 | T46.2X3 | T46.2X4 | T46.2X5 | T46.2X6 |
| **Distigmine** (bromide) | T44.0X1 | T44.0X2 | T44.0X3 | T44.0X4 | T44.0X5 | T44.0X6 |
| **Disulfamide** | T50.2X1 | T50.2X2 | T50.2X3 | T50.2X4 | T50.2X5 | T50.2X6 |
| **Disulfanilamide** | T37.0X1 | T37.0X2 | T37.0X3 | T37.0X4 | T37.0X5 | T37.0X6 |
| **Disulfiram** | T50.6X1 | T50.6X2 | T50.6X3 | T50.6X4 | T50.6X5 | T50.6X6 |
| **Disulfoton** | T60.0X1 | T60.0X2 | T60.0X3 | T60.0X4 | — | — |
| **Dithiazanine iodide** | T37.4X1 | T37.4X2 | T37.4X3 | T37.4X4 | T37.4X5 | T37.4X6 |
| **Dithiocarbamate** | T60.0X1 | T60.0X2 | T60.0X3 | T60.0X4 | — | — |
| **Dithranol** | T49.4X1 | T49.4X2 | T49.4X3 | T49.4X4 | T49.4X5 | T49.4X6 |
| **Diucardin** | T50.2X1 | T50.2X2 | T50.2X3 | T50.2X4 | T50.2X5 | T50.2X6 |
| **Diupres** | T50.2X1 | T50.2X2 | T50.2X3 | T50.2X4 | T50.2X5 | T50.2X6 |
| **Diuretic NEC** | T50.2X1 | T50.2X2 | T50.2X3 | T50.2X4 | T50.2X5 | T50.2X6 |
| benzothiadiazine | T50.2X1 | T50.2X2 | T50.2X3 | T50.2X4 | T50.2X5 | T50.2X6 |
| carbonic acid anhydrase inhibitors | T50.2X1 | T50.2X2 | T50.2X3 | T50.2X4 | T50.2X5 | T50.2X6 |
| furfuryl NEC | T50.2X1 | T50.2X2 | T50.2X3 | T50.2X4 | T50.2X5 | T50.2X6 |
| loop (high-ceiling) | T50.1X1 | T50.1X2 | T50.1X3 | T50.1X4 | T50.1X5 | T50.1X6 |
| mercurial NEC | T50.2X1 | T50.2X2 | T50.2X3 | T50.2X4 | T50.2X5 | T50.2X6 |
| osmotic | T50.2X1 | T50.2X2 | T50.2X3 | T50.2X4 | T50.2X5 | T50.2X6 |
| purine NEC | T50.2X1 | T50.2X2 | T50.2X3 | T50.2X4 | T50.2X5 | T50.2X6 |
| saluretic NEC | T50.2X1 | T50.2X2 | T50.2X3 | T50.2X4 | T50.2X5 | T50.2X6 |
| sulfonamide | T50.2X1 | T50.2X2 | T50.2X3 | T50.2X4 | T50.2X5 | T50.2X6 |
| thiazide NEC | T50.2X1 | T50.2X2 | T50.2X3 | T50.2X4 | T50.2X5 | T50.2X6 |
| xanthine | T50.2X1 | T50.2X2 | T50.2X3 | T50.2X4 | T50.2X5 | T50.2X6 |
| **Diurgin** | T50.2X1 | T50.2X2 | T50.2X3 | T50.2X4 | T50.2X5 | T50.2X6 |
| **Diuril** | T50.2X1 | T50.2X2 | T50.2X3 | T50.2X4 | T50.2X5 | T50.2X6 |
| **Diuron** | T60.3X1 | T60.3X2 | T60.3X3 | T60.3X4 | — | — |
| **Divalproex** | T42.6X1 | T42.6X2 | T42.6X3 | T42.6X4 | T42.6X5 | T42.6X6 |
| **Divinyl ether** | T41.0X1 | T41.0X2 | T41.0X3 | T41.0X4 | T41.0X5 | T41.0X6 |
| **Dixanthogen** | T49.0X1 | T49.0X2 | T49.0X3 | T49.0X4 | T49.0X5 | T49.0X6 |
| **Dixyrazine** | T43.3X1 | T43.3X2 | T43.3X3 | T43.3X4 | T43.3X5 | T43.3X6 |
| **D-lysergic acid diethylamide** | T40.8X1 | T40.8X2 | T40.8X3 | T40.8X4 | — | — |
| **DMCT** | T36.4X1 | T36.4X2 | T36.4X3 | T36.4X4 | T36.4X5 | T36.4X6 |
| **DMSO** — *see* Dimethyl sulfoxide | | | | | | |
| **DNBP** | T60.3X1 | T60.3X2 | T60.3X3 | T60.3X4 | — | — |
| **DNOC** | T65.3X1 | T65.3X2 | T65.3X3 | T65.3X4 | — | — |
| **Dobutamine** | T44.5X1 | T44.5X2 | T44.5X3 | T44.5X4 | T44.5X5 | T44.5X6 |
| **DOCA** | T38.0X1 | T38.0X2 | T38.0X3 | T38.0X4 | T38.0X5 | T38.0X6 |
| **Docusate sodium** | T47.4X1 | T47.4X2 | T47.4X3 | T47.4X4 | T47.4X5 | T47.4X6 |
| **Dodicin** | T49.0X1 | T49.0X2 | T49.0X3 | T49.0X4 | T49.0X5 | T49.0X6 |
| **Dofamium chloride** | T49.0X1 | T49.0X2 | T49.0X3 | T49.0X4 | T49.0X5 | T49.0X6 |
| **Dolophine** | T40.3X1 | T40.3X2 | T40.3X3 | T40.3X4 | T40.3X5 | T40.3X6 |
| **Doloxene** | T39.8X1 | T39.8X2 | T39.8X3 | T39.8X4 | T39.8X5 | T39.8X6 |
| **Domestic gas** (after combustion) — *see* Gas, utility | | | | | | |
| prior to combustion | T59.891 | T59.892 | T59.893 | T59.894 | — | — |
| **Domiodol** | T48.4X1 | T48.4X2 | T48.4X3 | T48.4X4 | T48.4X5 | T48.4X6 |
| **Domiphen** (bromide) | T49.0X1 | T49.0X2 | T49.0X3 | T49.0X4 | T49.0X5 | T49.0X6 |
| **Domperidone** | T45.0X1 | T45.0X2 | T45.0X3 | T45.0X4 | T45.0X5 | T45.0X6 |
| **Dopa** | T42.8X1 | T42.8X2 | T42.8X3 | T42.8X4 | T42.8X5 | T42.8X6 |
| **Dopamine** | T44.991 | T44.992 | T44.993 | T44.994 | T44.995 | T44.996 |
| **Doriden** | T42.6X1 | T42.6X2 | T42.6X3 | T42.6X4 | T42.6X5 | T42.6X6 |
| **Dormiral** | T42.3X1 | T42.3X2 | T42.3X3 | T42.3X4 | T42.3X5 | T42.3X6 |
| **Dormison** | T42.6X1 | T42.6X2 | T42.6X3 | T42.6X4 | T42.6X5 | T42.6X6 |
| **Dornase** | T48.4X1 | T48.4X2 | T48.4X3 | T48.4X4 | T48.4X5 | T48.4X6 |
| **Dorsacaine** | T41.3X1 | T41.3X2 | T41.3X3 | T41.3X4 | T41.3X5 | T41.3X6 |
| **Dosulepin** | T43.011 | T43.012 | T43.013 | T43.014 | T43.015 | T43.016 |
| **Dothiepin** | T43.011 | T43.012 | T43.013 | T43.014 | T43.015 | T43.016 |
| **Doxantrazole** | T48.6X1 | T48.6X2 | T48.6X3 | T48.6X4 | T48.6X5 | T48.6X6 |
| **Doxapram** | T50.7X1 | T50.7X2 | T50.7X3 | T50.7X4 | T50.7X5 | T50.7X6 |
| **Doxazosin** | T44.6X1 | T44.6X2 | T44.6X3 | T44.6X4 | T44.6X5 | T44.6X6 |
| **Doxepin** | T43.011 | T43.012 | T43.013 | T43.014 | T43.015 | T43.016 |
| **Doxifluridine** | T45.1X1 | T45.1X2 | T45.1X3 | T45.1X4 | T45.1X5 | T45.1X6 |
| **Doxorubicin** | T45.1X1 | T45.1X2 | T45.1X3 | T45.1X4 | T45.1X5 | T45.1X6 |
| **Doxycycline** | T36.4X1 | T36.4X2 | T36.4X3 | T36.4X4 | T36.4X5 | T36.4X6 |
| **Doxylamine** | T45.0X1 | T45.0X2 | T45.0X3 | T45.0X4 | T45.0X5 | T45.0X6 |
| **Dramamine** | T45.0X1 | T45.0X2 | T45.0X3 | T45.0X4 | T45.0X5 | T45.0X6 |
| **Drano** (drain cleaner) | T54.3X1 | T54.3X2 | T54.3X3 | T54.3X4 | — | — |
| **Dressing, live pulp** | T49.7X1 | T49.7X2 | T49.7X3 | T49.7X4 | T49.7X5 | T49.7X6 |
| **Drocode** | T40.2X1 | T40.2X2 | T40.2X3 | T40.2X4 | T40.2X5 | T40.2X6 |
| **Dromoran** | T40.2X1 | T40.2X2 | T40.2X3 | T40.2X4 | T40.2X5 | T40.2X6 |
| **Dromostanolone** | T38.7X1 | T38.7X2 | T38.7X3 | T38.7X4 | T38.7X5 | T38.7X6 |

Table of Drugs and Chemicals

Dronabinol — Etambutol

| Substance | Poisoning, Accidental (unintentional) | Poisoning, Intentional Self-harm | Poisoning, Assault | Poisoning, Undetermined | Adverse Effect | Under-dosing |
|---|---|---|---|---|---|---|
| Dronabinol | T40.7X1 | T40.7X2 | T40.7X3 | T40.7X4 | T40.7X5 | T40.7X6 |
| Droperidol | T43.591 | T43.592 | T43.593 | T43.594 | T43.595 | T43.596 |
| Dropropizine | T48.3X1 | T48.3X2 | T48.3X3 | T48.3X4 | T48.3X5 | T48.3X6 |
| Drostanolone | T38.7X1 | T38.7X2 | T38.7X3 | T38.7X4 | T38.7X5 | T38.7X6 |
| Drotaverine | T44.3X1 | T44.3X2 | T44.3X3 | T44.3X4 | T44.3X5 | T44.3X6 |
| Drotrecogin alfa | T45.511 | T45.512 | T45.513 | T45.514 | T45.515 | T45.516 |
| Drug NEC | T50.901 | T50.902 | T50.903 | T50.904 | T50.905 | T50.906 |
| specified NEC | T50.991 | T50.992 | T50.993 | T50.994 | T50.995 | T50.996 |
| DTIC | T45.1X1 | T45.1X2 | T45.1X3 | T45.1X4 | T45.1X5 | T45.1X6 |
| Duboisine | T44.3X1 | T44.3X2 | T44.3X3 | T44.3X4 | T44.3X5 | T44.3X6 |
| Dulcolax | T47.2X1 | T47.2X2 | T47.2X3 | T47.2X4 | T47.2X5 | T47.2X6 |
| Duponol (C) (EP) | T49.2X1 | T49.2X2 | T49.2X3 | T49.2X4 | T49.2X5 | T49.2X6 |
| Durabolin | T38.7X1 | T38.7X2 | T38.7X3 | T38.7X4 | T38.7X5 | T38.7X6 |
| Dyclone | T41.3X1 | T41.3X2 | T41.3X3 | T41.3X4 | T41.3X5 | T41.3X6 |
| Dyclonine | T41.3X1 | T41.3X2 | T41.3X3 | T41.3X4 | T41.3X5 | T41.3X6 |
| Dydrogesterone | T38.5X1 | T38.5X2 | T38.5X3 | T38.5X4 | T38.5X5 | T38.5X6 |
| Dye NEC | T65.6X1 | T65.6X2 | T65.6X3 | T65.6X4 | — | — |
| antiseptic | T49.0X1 | T49.0X2 | T49.0X3 | T49.0X4 | T49.0X5 | T49.0X6 |
| diagnostic agents | T50.8X1 | T50.8X2 | T50.8X3 | T50.8X4 | T50.8X5 | T50.8X6 |
| pharmaceutical NEC | T50.901 | T50.902 | T50.903 | T50.904 | T50.905 | T50.906 |
| Dyflos | T44.0X1 | T44.0X2 | T44.0X3 | T44.0X4 | T44.0X5 | T44.0X6 |
| Dymelor | T38.3X1 | T38.3X2 | T38.3X3 | T38.3X4 | T38.3X5 | T38.3X6 |
| Dynamite | T65.3X1 | T65.3X2 | T65.3X3 | T65.3X4 | — | — |
| fumes | T59.891 | T59.892 | T59.893 | T59.894 | — | — |
| Dyphylline | T44.3X1 | T44.3X2 | T44.3X3 | T44.3X4 | T44.3X5 | T44.3X6 |
| b-eucaine | T49.1X1 | T49.1X2 | T49.1X3 | T49.1X4 | T49.1X5 | T49.1X6 |
| Ear drug NEC | T49.6X1 | T49.6X2 | T49.6X3 | T49.6X4 | T49.6X5 | T49.6X6 |
| Ear preparations | T49.6X1 | T49.6X2 | T49.6X3 | T49.6X4 | T49.6X5 | T49.6X6 |
| Echothiophate, echothiopate, ecothiopate | T49.5X1 | T49.5X2 | T49.5X3 | T49.5X4 | T49.5X5 | T49.5X6 |
| Econazole | T49.0X1 | T49.0X2 | T49.0X3 | T49.0X4 | T49.0X5 | T49.0X6 |
| Ecothiopate iodide | T49.5X1 | T49.5X2 | T49.5X3 | T49.5X4 | T49.5X5 | T49.5X6 |
| Ecstasy | T43.621 | T43.622 | T43.623 | T43.624 | T43.625 | T43.626 |
| Ectylurea | T42.6X1 | T42.6X2 | T42.6X3 | T42.6X4 | T42.6X5 | T42.6X6 |
| Edathamil disodium | T45.8X1 | T45.8X2 | T45.8X3 | T45.8X4 | T45.8X5 | T45.8X6 |
| Edecrin | T50.1X1 | T50.1X2 | T50.1X3 | T50.1X4 | T50.1X5 | T50.1X6 |
| Edetate, disodium (calcium) | T45.8X1 | T45.8X2 | T45.8X3 | T45.8X4 | T45.8X5 | T45.8X6 |
| Edoxudine | T49.5X1 | T49.5X2 | T49.5X3 | T49.5X4 | T49.5X5 | T49.5X6 |
| Edrophonium | T44.0X1 | T44.0X2 | T44.0X3 | T44.0X4 | T44.0X5 | T44.0X6 |
| chloride | T44.0X1 | T44.0X2 | T44.0X3 | T44.0X4 | T44.0X5 | T44.0X6 |
| EDTA | T50.6X1 | T50.6X2 | T50.6X3 | T50.6X4 | T50.6X5 | T50.6X6 |
| Eflornithine | T37.2X1 | T37.2X2 | T37.2X3 | T37.2X4 | T37.2X5 | T37.2X6 |
| Efloxate | T46.3X1 | T46.3X2 | T46.3X3 | T46.3X4 | T46.3X5 | T46.3X6 |
| Elase | T49.8X1 | T49.8X2 | T49.8X3 | T49.8X4 | T49.8X5 | T49.8X6 |
| Elastase | T47.5X1 | T47.5X2 | T47.5X3 | T47.5X4 | T47.5X5 | T47.5X6 |
| Elaterium | T47.2X1 | T47.2X2 | T47.2X3 | T47.2X4 | T47.2X5 | T47.2X6 |
| Elcatonin | T50.991 | T50.992 | T50.993 | T50.994 | T50.995 | T50.996 |
| Elder | T62.2X1 | T62.2X2 | T62.2X3 | T62.2X4 | — | — |
| berry, (unripe) | T62.1X1 | T62.1X2 | T62.1X3 | T62.1X4 | — | — |
| Electrolyte balance drug | T50.3X1 | T50.3X2 | T50.3X3 | T50.3X4 | T50.3X5 | T50.3X6 |
| Electrolytes NEC | T50.3X1 | T50.3X2 | T50.3X3 | T50.3X4 | T50.3X5 | T50.3X6 |
| Electrolytic agent NEC | T50.3X1 | T50.3X2 | T50.3X3 | T50.3X4 | T50.3X5 | T50.3X6 |
| Elemental diet | T50.901 | T50.902 | T50.903 | T50.904 | T50.905 | T50.906 |
| Elliptinium acetate | T45.1X1 | T45.1X2 | T45.1X3 | T45.1X4 | T45.1X5 | T45.1X6 |
| Embramine | T45.0X1 | T45.0X2 | T45.0X3 | T45.0X4 | T45.0X5 | T45.0X6 |
| Emepronium (salts) | T44.3X1 | T44.3X2 | T44.3X3 | T44.3X4 | T44.3X5 | T44.3X6 |
| bromide | T44.3X1 | T44.3X2 | T44.3X3 | T44.3X4 | T44.3X5 | T44.3X6 |
| Emetic NEC | T47.7X1 | T47.7X2 | T47.7X3 | T47.7X4 | T47.7X5 | T47.7X6 |
| Emetine | T37.3X1 | T37.3X2 | T37.3X3 | T37.3X4 | T37.3X5 | T37.3X6 |
| Emollient NEC | T49.3X1 | T49.3X2 | T49.3X3 | T49.3X4 | T49.3X5 | T49.3X6 |
| Emorfazone | T39.8X1 | T39.8X2 | T39.8X3 | T39.8X4 | T39.8X5 | T39.8X6 |
| Emylcamate | T43.591 | T43.592 | T43.593 | T43.594 | T43.595 | T43.596 |
| Enalapril | T46.4X1 | T46.4X2 | T46.4X3 | T46.4X4 | T46.4X5 | T46.4X6 |
| Enalaprilat | T46.4X1 | T46.4X2 | T46.4X3 | T46.4X4 | T46.4X5 | T46.4X6 |
| Encainide | T46.2X1 | T46.2X2 | T46.2X3 | T46.2X4 | T46.2X5 | T46.2X6 |
| Endocaine | T41.3X1 | T41.3X2 | T41.3X3 | T41.3X4 | T41.3X5 | T41.3X6 |
| Endosulfan | T60.2X1 | T60.2X2 | T60.2X3 | T60.2X4 | — | — |
| Endothall | T60.3X1 | T60.3X2 | T60.3X3 | T60.3X4 | — | — |
| Endralazine | T46.5X1 | T46.5X2 | T46.5X3 | T46.5X4 | T46.5X5 | T46.5X6 |
| Endrin | T60.1X1 | T60.1X2 | T60.1X3 | T60.1X4 | — | — |
| Enflurane | T41.0X1 | T41.0X2 | T41.0X3 | T41.0X4 | T41.0X5 | T41.0X6 |
| Enhexymal | T42.3X1 | T42.3X2 | T42.3X3 | T42.3X4 | T42.3X5 | T42.3X6 |
| Enocitabine | T45.1X1 | T45.1X2 | T45.1X3 | T45.1X4 | T45.1X5 | T45.1X6 |
| Enovid | T38.4X1 | T38.4X2 | T38.4X3 | T38.4X4 | T38.4X5 | T38.4X6 |
| Enoxacin | T36.8X1 | T36.8X2 | T36.8X3 | T36.8X4 | T36.8X5 | T36.8X6 |
| Enoxaparin (sodium) | T45.511 | T45.512 | T45.513 | T45.514 | T45.515 | T45.516 |
| Enpiprazole | T43.591 | T43.592 | T43.593 | T43.594 | T43.595 | T43.596 |
| Enprofylline | T48.6X1 | T48.6X2 | T48.6X3 | T48.6X4 | T48.6X5 | T48.6X6 |
| Enprostil | T47.1X1 | T47.1X2 | T47.1X3 | T47.1X4 | T47.1X5 | T47.1X6 |
| Enterogastrone | T38.891 | T38.892 | T38.893 | T38.894 | T38.895 | T38.896 |
| ENT preparations (anti-infectives) | T49.6X1 | T49.6X2 | T49.6X3 | T49.6X4 | T49.6X5 | T49.6X6 |
| Enviomycin | T36.8X1 | T36.8X2 | T36.8X3 | T36.8X4 | T36.8X5 | T36.8X6 |
| Enzodase | T45.3X1 | T45.3X2 | T45.3X3 | T45.3X4 | T45.3X5 | T45.3X6 |
| Enzyme NEC | T45.3X1 | T45.3X2 | T45.3X3 | T45.3X4 | T45.3X5 | T45.3X6 |
| depolymerizing | T49.8X1 | T49.8X2 | T49.8X3 | T49.8X4 | T49.8X5 | T49.8X6 |
| fibrolytic | T45.3X1 | T45.3X2 | T45.3X3 | T45.3X4 | T45.3X5 | T45.3X6 |
| gastric | T47.5X1 | T47.5X2 | T47.5X3 | T47.5X4 | T47.5X5 | T47.5X6 |
| intestinal | T47.5X1 | T47.5X2 | T47.5X3 | T47.5X4 | T47.5X5 | T47.5X6 |
| local action | T49.4X1 | T49.4X2 | T49.4X3 | T49.4X4 | T49.4X5 | T49.4X6 |
| proteolytic | T49.4X1 | T49.4X2 | T49.4X3 | T49.4X4 | T49.4X5 | T49.4X6 |
| thrombolytic | T45.3X1 | T45.3X2 | T45.3X3 | T45.3X4 | T45.3X5 | T45.3X6 |
| EPAB | T41.3X1 | T41.3X2 | T41.3X3 | T41.3X4 | T41.3X5 | T41.3X6 |
| Epanutin | T42.0X1 | T42.0X2 | T42.0X3 | T42.0X4 | T42.0X5 | T42.0X6 |
| Ephedra | T44.991 | T44.992 | T44.993 | T44.994 | T44.995 | T44.996 |
| Ephedrine | T44.991 | T44.992 | T44.993 | T44.994 | T44.995 | T44.996 |
| Epichlorhydrin, epichlorohydrin | T52.8X1 | T52.8X2 | T52.8X3 | T52.8X4 | — | — |
| Epicillin | T36.0X1 | T36.0X2 | T36.0X3 | T36.0X4 | T36.0X5 | T36.0X6 |
| Epiestriol | T38.5X1 | T38.5X2 | T38.5X3 | T38.5X4 | T38.5X5 | T38.5X6 |
| Epilim — see Sodium valproate | | | | | | |
| Epimestrol | T38.5X1 | T38.5X2 | T38.5X3 | T38.5X4 | T38.5X5 | T38.5X6 |
| Epinephrine | T44.5X1 | T44.5X2 | T44.5X3 | T44.5X4 | T44.5X5 | T44.5X6 |
| Epirubicin | T45.1X1 | T45.1X2 | T45.1X3 | T45.1X4 | T45.1X5 | T45.1X6 |
| Epitiostanol | T38.7X1 | T38.7X2 | T38.7X3 | T38.7X4 | T38.7X5 | T38.7X6 |
| Epitizide | T50.2X1 | T50.2X2 | T50.2X3 | T50.2X4 | T50.2X5 | T50.2X6 |
| EPN | T60.0X1 | T60.0X2 | T60.0X3 | T60.0X4 | — | — |
| EPO | T45.8X1 | T45.8X2 | T45.8X3 | T45.8X4 | T45.8X5 | T45.8X6 |
| Epoetin alpha | T45.8X1 | T45.8X2 | T45.8X3 | T45.8X4 | T45.8X5 | T45.8X6 |
| Epomediol | T50.991 | T50.992 | T50.993 | T50.994 | T50.995 | T50.996 |
| Epoprostenol | T45.521 | T45.522 | T45.523 | T45.524 | T45.525 | T45.526 |
| Epoxy resin | T65.891 | T65.892 | T65.893 | T65.894 | — | — |
| Eprazinone | T48.4X1 | T48.4X2 | T48.4X3 | T48.4X4 | T48.4X5 | T48.4X6 |
| Epsilon aminocaproic acid | T45.621 | T45.622 | T45.623 | T45.624 | T45.625 | T45.626 |
| Epsom salt | T47.3X1 | T47.3X2 | T47.3X3 | T47.3X4 | T47.3X5 | T47.3X6 |
| Eptazocine | T40.4X1 | T40.4X2 | T40.4X3 | T40.4X4 | T40.4X5 | T40.4X6 |
| Equanil | T43.591 | T43.592 | T43.593 | T43.594 | T43.595 | T43.596 |
| Equisetum | T62.2X1 | T62.2X2 | T62.2X3 | T62.2X4 | — | — |
| diuretic | T50.2X1 | T50.2X2 | T50.2X3 | T50.2X4 | T50.2X5 | T50.2X6 |
| Ergobasine | T48.0X1 | T48.0X2 | T48.0X3 | T48.0X4 | T48.0X5 | T48.0X6 |
| Ergocalciferol | T45.2X1 | T45.2X2 | T45.2X3 | T45.2X4 | T45.2X5 | T45.2X6 |
| Ergoloid mesylates | T46.7X1 | T46.7X2 | T46.7X3 | T46.7X4 | T46.7X5 | T46.7X6 |
| Ergometrine | T48.0X1 | T48.0X2 | T48.0X3 | T48.0X4 | T48.0X5 | T48.0X6 |
| Ergonovine | T48.0X1 | T48.0X2 | T48.0X3 | T48.0X4 | T48.0X5 | T48.0X6 |
| Ergotamine | T46.5X1 | T46.5X2 | T46.5X3 | T46.5X4 | T46.5X5 | T46.5X6 |
| Ergotocine | T48.0X1 | T48.0X2 | T48.0X3 | T48.0X4 | T48.0X5 | T48.0X6 |
| Ergotrate | T48.0X1 | T48.0X2 | T48.0X3 | T48.0X4 | T48.0X5 | T48.0X6 |
| Ergot NEC | T64.81 | T64.82 | T64.83 | T64.84 | — | — |
| derivative | T48.0X1 | T48.0X2 | T48.0X3 | T48.0X4 | T48.0X5 | T48.0X6 |
| medicinal (alkaloids) | T48.0X1 | T48.0X2 | T48.0X3 | T48.0X4 | T48.0X5 | T48.0X6 |
| prepared | T48.0X1 | T48.0X2 | T48.0X3 | T48.0X4 | T48.0X5 | T48.0X6 |
| Erittrityl tetranitrate | T46.3X1 | T46.3X2 | T46.3X3 | T46.3X4 | T46.3X5 | T46.3X6 |
| Erythrityl tetranitrate | T46.3X1 | T46.3X2 | T46.3X3 | T46.3X4 | T46.3X5 | T46.3X6 |
| Erythrol tetranitrate | T46.3X1 | T46.3X2 | T46.3X3 | T46.3X4 | T46.3X5 | T46.3X6 |
| Erythromycin (salts) | T36.3X1 | T36.3X2 | T36.3X3 | T36.3X4 | T36.3X5 | T36.3X6 |
| ophthalmic preparation | T49.5X1 | T49.5X2 | T49.5X3 | T49.5X4 | T49.5X5 | T49.5X6 |
| topical NEC | T49.0X1 | T49.0X2 | T49.0X3 | T49.0X4 | T49.0X5 | T49.0X6 |
| Erythropoietin | T45.8X1 | T45.8X2 | T45.8X3 | T45.8X4 | T45.8X5 | T45.8X6 |
| human | T45.8X1 | T45.8X2 | T45.8X3 | T45.8X4 | T45.8X5 | T45.8X6 |
| Escin | T46.991 | T46.992 | T46.993 | T46.994 | T46.995 | T46.996 |
| Esculin | T45.2X1 | T45.2X2 | T45.2X3 | T45.2X4 | T45.2X5 | T45.2X6 |
| Esculoside | T45.2X1 | T45.2X2 | T45.2X3 | T45.2X4 | T45.2X5 | T45.2X6 |
| ESDT (ether-soluble tar distillate) | T49.1X1 | T49.1X2 | T49.1X3 | T49.1X4 | T49.1X5 | T49.1X6 |
| Eserine | T49.5X1 | T49.5X2 | T49.5X3 | T49.5X4 | T49.5X5 | T49.5X6 |
| Esflurbiprofen | T39.311 | T39.312 | T39.313 | T39.314 | T39.315 | T39.316 |
| Eskabarb | T42.3X1 | T42.3X2 | T42.3X3 | T42.3X4 | T42.3X5 | T42.3X6 |
| Eskalith | T43.8X1 | T43.8X2 | T43.8X3 | T43.8X4 | T43.8X5 | T43.8X6 |
| Esmolol | T44.7X1 | T44.7X2 | T44.7X3 | T44.7X4 | T44.7X5 | T44.7X6 |
| Estanozolol | T38.7X1 | T38.7X2 | T38.7X3 | T38.7X4 | T38.7X5 | T38.7X6 |
| Estazolam | T42.4X1 | T42.4X2 | T42.4X3 | T42.4X4 | T42.4X5 | T42.4X6 |
| Estradiol | T38.5X1 | T38.5X2 | T38.5X3 | T38.5X4 | T38.5X5 | T38.5X6 |
| with testosterone | T38.7X1 | T38.7X2 | T38.7X3 | T38.7X4 | T38.7X5 | T38.7X6 |
| benzoate | T38.5X1 | T38.5X2 | T38.5X3 | T38.5X4 | T38.5X5 | T38.5X6 |
| Estramustine | T45.1X1 | T45.1X2 | T45.1X3 | T45.1X4 | T45.1X5 | T45.1X6 |
| Estriol | T38.5X1 | T38.5X2 | T38.5X3 | T38.5X4 | T38.5X5 | T38.5X6 |
| Estrogen | T38.5X1 | T38.5X2 | T38.5X3 | T38.5X4 | T38.5X5 | T38.5X6 |
| with progesterone | T38.5X1 | T38.5X2 | T38.5X3 | T38.5X4 | T38.5X5 | T38.5X6 |
| conjugated | T38.5X1 | T38.5X2 | T38.5X3 | T38.5X4 | T38.5X5 | T38.5X6 |
| Estrone | T38.5X1 | T38.5X2 | T38.5X3 | T38.5X4 | T38.5X5 | T38.5X6 |
| Estropipate | T38.5X1 | T38.5X2 | T38.5X3 | T38.5X4 | T38.5X5 | T38.5X6 |
| Etacrynate sodium | T50.1X1 | T50.1X2 | T50.1X3 | T50.1X4 | T50.1X5 | T50.1X6 |
| Etacrynic acid | T50.1X1 | T50.1X2 | T50.1X3 | T50.1X4 | T50.1X5 | T50.1X6 |
| Etafedrine | T48.6X1 | T48.6X2 | T48.6X3 | T48.6X4 | T48.6X5 | T48.6X6 |
| Etafenone | T46.3X1 | T46.3X2 | T46.3X3 | T46.3X4 | T46.3X5 | T46.3X6 |
| Etambutol | T37.1X1 | T37.1X2 | T37.1X3 | T37.1X4 | T37.1X5 | T37.1X6 |

Additional Character May Be Required — Refer to the Tabular List for Character Selection

Subterms under main terms may continue to next column or page

| Substance | Poisoning, Accidental (unintentional) | Poisoning, Intentional Self-harm | Poisoning, Assault | Poisoning, Undetermined | Adverse Effect | Under-dosing |
|---|---|---|---|---|---|---|
| Etamiphyllin | T48.6X1 | T48.6X2 | T48.6X3 | T48.6X4 | T48.6X5 | T48.6X6 |
| Etamivan | T50.7X1 | T50.7X2 | T50.7X3 | T50.7X4 | T50.7X5 | T50.7X6 |
| Etamsylate | T45.7X1 | T45.7X2 | T45.7X3 | T45.7X4 | T45.7X5 | T45.7X6 |
| Etebenecid | T50.4X1 | T50.4X2 | T50.4X3 | T50.4X4 | T50.4X5 | T50.4X6 |
| Ethacridine | T49.0X1 | T49.0X2 | T49.0X3 | T49.0X4 | T49.0X5 | T49.0X6 |
| Ethacrynic acid | T50.1X1 | T50.1X2 | T50.1X3 | T50.1X4 | T50.1X5 | T50.1X6 |
| Ethadione | T42.2X1 | T42.2X2 | T42.2X3 | T42.2X4 | T42.2X5 | T42.2X6 |
| Ethambutol | T37.1X1 | T37.1X2 | T37.1X3 | T37.1X4 | T37.1X5 | T37.1X6 |
| Ethamide | T50.2X1 | T50.2X2 | T50.2X3 | T50.2X4 | T50.2X5 | T50.2X6 |
| Ethamivan | T50.7X1 | T50.7X2 | T50.7X3 | T50.7X4 | T50.7X5 | T50.7X6 |
| Ethamsylate | T45.7X1 | T45.7X2 | T45.7X3 | T45.7X4 | T45.7X5 | T45.7X6 |
| Ethanol | T51.0X1 | T51.0X2 | T51.0X3 | T51.0X4 | — | — |
|   beverage | T51.0X1 | T51.0X2 | T51.0X3 | T51.0X4 | — | — |
| Ethanolamine oleate | T46.8X1 | T46.8X2 | T46.8X3 | T46.8X4 | T46.8X5 | T46.8X6 |
| Ethaverine | T44.3X1 | T44.3X2 | T44.3X3 | T44.3X4 | T44.3X5 | T44.3X6 |
| Ethchlorvynol | T42.6X1 | T42.6X2 | T42.6X3 | T42.6X4 | T42.6X5 | T42.6X6 |
| Ethebenecid | T50.4X1 | T50.4X2 | T50.4X3 | T50.4X4 | T50.4X5 | T50.4X6 |
| Ether (vapor) | T41.0X1 | T41.0X2 | T41.0X3 | T41.0X4 | T41.0X5 | T41.0X6 |
|   anesthetic | T41.0X1 | T41.0X2 | T41.0X3 | T41.0X4 | T41.0X5 | T41.0X6 |
|   divinyl | T41.0X1 | T41.0X2 | T41.0X3 | T41.0X4 | T41.0X5 | T41.0X6 |
|   ethyl (medicinal) | T41.0X1 | T41.0X2 | T41.0X3 | T41.0X4 | T41.0X5 | T41.0X6 |
|     nonmedicinal | T52.8X1 | T52.8X2 | T52.8X3 | T52.8X4 | — | — |
|   petroleum — see Ligroin | | | | | | |
|   solvent | T52.8X1 | T52.8X2 | T52.8X3 | T52.8X4 | — | — |
| Ethiazide | T50.2X1 | T50.2X2 | T50.2X3 | T50.2X4 | T50.2X5 | T50.2X6 |
| Ethidium chloride (vapor) | T59.891 | T59.892 | T59.893 | T59.894 | — | — |
| Ethinamate | T42.6X1 | T42.6X2 | T42.6X3 | T42.6X4 | T42.6X5 | T42.6X6 |
| Ethinylestradiol, ethinyloestradiol | T38.5X1 | T38.5X2 | T38.5X3 | T38.5X4 | T38.5X5 | T38.5X6 |
|   with | | | | | | |
|     levonorgestrel | T38.4X1 | T38.4X2 | T38.4X3 | T38.4X4 | T38.4X5 | T38.4X6 |
|     norethisterone | T38.4X1 | T38.4X2 | T38.4X3 | T38.4X4 | T38.4X5 | T38.4X6 |
| Ethiodized oil (131 I) | T50.8X1 | T50.8X2 | T50.8X3 | T50.8X4 | T50.8X5 | T50.8X6 |
| Ethion | T60.0X1 | T60.0X2 | T60.0X3 | T60.0X4 | — | — |
| Ethionamide | T37.1X1 | T37.1X2 | T37.1X3 | T37.1X4 | T37.1X5 | T37.1X6 |
| Ethioniamide | T37.1X1 | T37.1X2 | T37.1X3 | T37.1X4 | T37.1X5 | T37.1X6 |
| Ethisterone | T38.5X1 | T38.5X2 | T38.5X3 | T38.5X4 | T38.5X5 | T38.5X6 |
| Ethobral | T42.3X1 | T42.3X2 | T42.3X3 | T42.3X4 | T42.3X5 | T42.3X6 |
| Ethocaine (infiltration) (topical) | T41.3X1 | T41.3X2 | T41.3X3 | T41.3X4 | T41.3X5 | T41.3X6 |
|   nerve block (peripheral) (plexus) | T41.3X1 | T41.3X2 | T41.3X3 | T41.3X4 | T41.3X5 | T41.3X6 |
|   spinal | T41.3X1 | T41.3X2 | T41.3X3 | T41.3X4 | T41.3X5 | T41.3X6 |
| Ethoheptazine | T40.4X1 | T40.4X2 | T40.4X3 | T40.4X4 | T40.4X5 | T40.4X6 |
| Ethopropazine | T44.3X1 | T44.3X2 | T44.3X3 | T44.3X4 | T44.3X5 | T44.3X6 |
| Ethosuximide | T42.2X1 | T42.2X2 | T42.2X3 | T42.2X4 | T42.2X5 | T42.2X6 |
| Ethotoin | T42.0X1 | T42.0X2 | T42.0X3 | T42.0X4 | T42.0X5 | T42.0X6 |
| Ethoxazene | T37.91 | T37.92 | T37.93 | T37.94 | T37.95 | T37.96 |
| Ethoxazorutoside | T46.991 | T46.992 | T46.993 | T46.994 | T46.995 | T46.996 |
| Ethoxzolamide | T50.2X1 | T50.2X2 | T50.2X3 | T50.2X4 | T50.2X5 | T50.2X6 |
| Ethyl | | | | | | |
|   acetate | T52.8X1 | T52.8X2 | T52.8X3 | T52.8X4 | — | — |
|   alcohol | T51.0X1 | T51.0X2 | T51.0X3 | T51.0X4 | — | — |
|     beverage | T51.0X1 | T51.0X2 | T51.0X3 | T51.0X4 | — | — |
|   aldehyde (vapor) | T59.891 | T59.892 | T59.893 | T59.894 | — | — |
|     liquid | T52.8X1 | T52.8X2 | T52.8X3 | T52.8X4 | — | — |
|   aminobenzoate | T41.3X1 | T41.3X2 | T41.3X3 | T41.3X4 | T41.3X5 | T41.3X6 |
|   aminophenothiazine | T43.3X1 | T43.3X2 | T43.3X3 | T43.3X4 | T43.3X5 | T43.3X6 |
|   benzoate | T52.8X1 | T52.8X2 | T52.8X3 | T52.8X4 | — | — |
|   biscoumacetate | T45.511 | T45.512 | T45.513 | T45.514 | T45.515 | T45.516 |
|   bromide (anesthetic) | T41.0X1 | T41.0X2 | T41.0X3 | T41.0X4 | T41.0X5 | T41.0X6 |
|   carbamate | T45.1X1 | T45.1X2 | T45.1X3 | T45.1X4 | T45.1X5 | T45.1X6 |
|   carbinol | T51.3X1 | T51.3X2 | T51.3X3 | T51.3X4 | — | — |
|   carbonate | T52.8X1 | T52.8X2 | T52.8X3 | T52.8X4 | — | — |
|   chaulmoograte | T37.1X1 | T37.1X2 | T37.1X3 | T37.1X4 | T37.1X5 | T37.1X6 |
|   chloride (anesthetic) | T41.0X1 | T41.0X2 | T41.0X3 | T41.0X4 | T41.0X5 | T41.0X6 |
|     anesthetic (local) | T41.3X1 | T41.3X2 | T41.3X3 | T41.3X4 | T41.3X5 | T41.3X6 |
|     inhaled | T41.0X1 | T41.0X2 | T41.0X3 | T41.0X4 | T41.0X5 | T41.0X6 |
|     local | T49.4X1 | T49.4X2 | T49.4X3 | T49.4X4 | T49.4X5 | T49.4X6 |
|     solvent | T53.6X1 | T53.6X2 | T53.6X3 | T53.6X4 | — | — |
|   dibunate | T48.3X1 | T48.3X2 | T48.3X3 | T48.3X4 | T48.3X5 | T48.3X6 |
|   dichloroarsine (vapor) | T57.0X1 | T57.0X2 | T57.0X3 | T57.0X4 | — | — |
|   estranol | T38.7X1 | T38.7X2 | T38.7X3 | T38.7X4 | T38.7X5 | T38.7X6 |
|   ether — see also ether | T52.8X1 | T52.8X2 | T52.8X3 | T52.8X4 | — | — |
|   formate NEC (solvent) | T52.0X1 | T52.0X2 | T52.0X3 | T52.0X4 | — | — |
|   fumarate | T49.4X1 | T49.4X2 | T49.4X3 | T49.4X4 | T49.4X5 | T49.4X6 |
|   hydroxyisobutyrate NEC (solvent) | T52.8X1 | T52.8X2 | T52.8X3 | T52.8X4 | — | — |
|   iodoacetate | T59.3X1 | T59.3X2 | T59.3X3 | T59.3X4 | — | — |
|   lactate NEC (solvent) | T52.8X1 | T52.8X2 | T52.8X3 | T52.8X4 | — | — |
|   loflazepate | T42.4X1 | T42.4X2 | T42.4X3 | T42.4X4 | T42.4X5 | T42.4X6 |
|   mercuric chloride | T56.1X1 | T56.1X2 | T56.1X3 | T56.1X4 | — | — |
|   methylcarbinol | T51.8X1 | T51.8X2 | T51.8X3 | T51.8X4 | — | — |
| Ethyl — continued | | | | | | |
|   morphine | T40.2X1 | T40.2X2 | T40.2X3 | T40.2X4 | T40.2X5 | T40.2X6 |
|   noradrenaline | T48.6X1 | T48.6X2 | T48.6X3 | T48.6X4 | T48.6X5 | T48.6X6 |
|   oxybutyrate NEC (solvent) | T52.8X1 | T52.8X2 | T52.8X3 | T52.8X4 | — | — |
| Ethylene (gas) | T59.891 | T59.892 | T59.893 | T59.894 | — | — |
|   anesthetic (general) | T41.0X1 | T41.0X2 | T41.0X3 | T41.0X4 | T41.0X5 | T41.0X6 |
|   chlorohydrin | T52.8X1 | T52.8X2 | T52.8X3 | T52.8X4 | — | — |
|     vapor | T53.6X1 | T53.6X2 | T53.6X3 | T53.6X4 | — | — |
|   dichloride | T52.8X1 | T52.8X2 | T52.8X3 | T52.8X4 | — | — |
|     vapor | T53.6X1 | T53.6X2 | T53.6X3 | T53.6X4 | — | — |
|   dinitrate | T52.3X1 | T52.3X2 | T52.3X3 | T52.3X4 | — | — |
|   glycol(s) | T52.8X1 | T52.8X2 | T52.8X3 | T52.8X4 | — | — |
|     dinitrate | T52.3X1 | T52.3X2 | T52.3X3 | T52.3X4 | — | — |
|     monobutyl ether | T52.3X1 | T52.3X2 | T52.3X3 | T52.3X4 | — | — |
|   imine | T54.1X1 | T54.1X2 | T54.1X3 | T54.1X4 | — | — |
|   oxide (fumigant) | T59.891 | T59.892 | T59.893 | T59.894 | — | — |
|     (nonmedicinal) | | | | | | |
|     medicinal | T49.0X1 | T49.0X2 | T49.0X3 | T49.0X4 | T49.0X5 | T49.0X6 |
| Ethylenediaminetetra-acetic acid | T50.6X1 | T50.6X2 | T50.6X3 | T50.6X4 | T50.6X5 | T50.6X6 |
| Ethylenediamine theophylline | T48.6X1 | T48.6X2 | T48.6X3 | T48.6X4 | T48.6X5 | T48.6X6 |
| Ethylenedinitrilotetra-acetate | T50.6X1 | T50.6X2 | T50.6X3 | T50.6X4 | T50.6X5 | T50.6X6 |
| Ethylestrenol | T38.7X1 | T38.7X2 | T38.7X3 | T38.7X4 | T38.7X5 | T38.7X6 |
| Ethylhydroxycellulose | T47.4X1 | T47.4X2 | T47.4X3 | T47.4X4 | T47.4X5 | T47.4X6 |
| Ethylidene | | | | | | |
|   chloride NEC | T53.6X1 | T53.6X2 | T53.6X3 | T53.6X4 | — | — |
|   diacetate | T60.3X1 | T60.3X2 | T60.3X3 | T60.3X4 | — | — |
|   dicoumarin | T45.511 | T45.512 | T45.513 | T45.514 | T45.515 | T45.516 |
|   dicoumarol | T45.511 | T45.512 | T45.513 | T45.514 | T45.515 | T45.516 |
|   diethyl ether | T52.0X1 | T52.0X2 | T52.0X3 | T52.0X4 | — | — |
| Ethylmorphine | T40.2X1 | T40.2X2 | T40.2X3 | T40.2X4 | T40.2X5 | T40.2X6 |
| Ethylnorepinephrine | T48.6X1 | T48.6X2 | T48.6X3 | T48.6X4 | T48.6X5 | T48.6X6 |
| Ethylparachlorophen-oxyisobutyrate | T46.6X1 | T46.6X2 | T46.6X3 | T46.6X4 | T46.6X5 | T46.6X6 |
| Ethynodiol | T38.4X1 | T38.4X2 | T38.4X3 | T38.4X4 | T38.4X5 | T38.4X6 |
|   with mestranol diacetate | T38.4X1 | T38.4X2 | T38.4X3 | T38.4X4 | T38.4X5 | T38.4X6 |
| Etidocaine | T41.3X1 | T41.3X2 | T41.3X3 | T41.3X4 | T41.3X5 | T41.3X6 |
|   infiltration (subcutaneous) | T41.3X1 | T41.3X2 | T41.3X3 | T41.3X4 | T41.3X5 | T41.3X6 |
|   nerve (peripheral) (plexus) | T41.3X1 | T41.3X2 | T41.3X3 | T41.3X4 | T41.3X5 | T41.3X6 |
| Etidronate | T50.991 | T50.992 | T50.993 | T50.994 | T50.995 | T50.996 |
| Etidronic acid (disodium salt) | T50.991 | T50.992 | T50.993 | T50.994 | T50.995 | T50.996 |
| Etifoxine | T42.6X1 | T42.6X2 | T42.6X3 | T42.6X4 | T42.6X5 | T42.6X6 |
| Etilefrine | T44.4X1 | T44.4X2 | T44.4X3 | T44.4X4 | T44.4X5 | T44.4X6 |
| Etilfen | T42.3X1 | T42.3X2 | T42.3X3 | T42.3X4 | T42.3X5 | T42.3X6 |
| Etinodiol | T38.4X1 | T38.4X2 | T38.4X3 | T38.4X4 | T38.4X5 | T38.4X6 |
| Etiroxate | T46.6X1 | T46.6X2 | T46.6X3 | T46.6X4 | T46.6X5 | T46.6X6 |
| Etizolam | T42.4X1 | T42.4X2 | T42.4X3 | T42.4X4 | T42.4X5 | T42.4X6 |
| Etodolac | T39.391 | T39.392 | T39.393 | T39.394 | T39.395 | T39.396 |
| Etofamide | T37.3X1 | T37.3X2 | T37.3X3 | T37.3X4 | T37.3X5 | T37.3X6 |
| Etofibrate | T46.6X1 | T46.6X2 | T46.6X3 | T46.6X4 | T46.6X5 | T46.6X6 |
| Etofylline | T46.7X1 | T46.7X2 | T46.7X3 | T46.7X4 | T46.7X5 | T46.7X6 |
|   clofibrate | T46.6X1 | T46.6X2 | T46.6X3 | T46.6X4 | T46.6X5 | T46.6X6 |
| Etoglucid | T45.1X1 | T45.1X2 | T45.1X3 | T45.1X4 | T45.1X5 | T45.1X6 |
| Etomidate | T41.1X1 | T41.1X2 | T41.1X3 | T41.1X4 | T41.1X5 | T41.1X6 |
| Etomide | T39.8X1 | T39.8X2 | T39.8X3 | T39.8X4 | T39.8X5 | T39.8X6 |
| Etomidoline | T44.3X1 | T44.3X2 | T44.3X3 | T44.3X4 | T44.3X5 | T44.3X6 |
| Etoposide | T45.1X1 | T45.1X2 | T45.1X3 | T45.1X4 | T45.1X5 | T45.1X6 |
| Etorphine | T40.2X1 | T40.2X2 | T40.2X3 | T40.2X4 | T40.2X5 | T40.2X6 |
| Etoval | T42.3X1 | T42.3X2 | T42.3X3 | T42.3X4 | T42.3X5 | T42.3X6 |
| Etozolin | T50.1X1 | T50.1X2 | T50.1X3 | T50.1X4 | T50.1X5 | T50.1X6 |
| Etretinate | T50.991 | T50.992 | T50.993 | T50.994 | T50.995 | T50.996 |
| Etryptamine | T43.691 | T43.692 | T43.693 | T43.694 | T43.695 | T43.696 |
| Etybenzatropine | T44.3X1 | T44.3X2 | T44.3X3 | T44.3X4 | T44.3X5 | T44.3X6 |
| Etynodiol | T38.4X1 | T38.4X2 | T38.4X3 | T38.4X4 | T38.4X5 | T38.4X6 |
| Eucaine | T41.3X1 | T41.3X2 | T41.3X3 | T41.3X4 | T41.3X5 | T41.3X6 |
| Eucalyptus oil | T49.7X1 | T49.7X2 | T49.7X3 | T49.7X4 | T49.7X5 | T49.7X6 |
| Eucatropine | T49.5X1 | T49.5X2 | T49.5X3 | T49.5X4 | T49.5X5 | T49.5X6 |
| Eucodal | T40.2X1 | T40.2X2 | T40.2X3 | T40.2X4 | T40.2X5 | T40.2X6 |
| Euneryl | T42.3X1 | T42.3X2 | T42.3X3 | T42.3X4 | T42.3X5 | T42.3X6 |
| Euphthalmine | T44.3X1 | T44.3X2 | T44.3X3 | T44.3X4 | T44.3X5 | T44.3X6 |
| Eurax | T49.0X1 | T49.0X2 | T49.0X3 | T49.0X4 | T49.0X5 | T49.0X6 |
| Euresol | T49.4X1 | T49.4X2 | T49.4X3 | T49.4X4 | T49.4X5 | T49.4X6 |
| Euthroid | T38.1X1 | T38.1X2 | T38.1X3 | T38.1X4 | T38.1X5 | T38.1X6 |
| Evans blue | T50.8X1 | T50.8X2 | T50.8X3 | T50.8X4 | T50.8X5 | T50.8X6 |
| Evipal | T42.3X1 | T42.3X2 | T42.3X3 | T42.3X4 | T42.3X5 | T42.3X6 |
|   sodium | T41.1X1 | T41.1X2 | T41.1X3 | T41.1X4 | T41.1X5 | T41.1X6 |
| Evipan | T42.3X1 | T42.3X2 | T42.3X3 | T42.3X4 | T42.3X5 | T42.3X6 |
|   sodium | T41.1X1 | T41.1X2 | T41.1X3 | T41.1X4 | T41.1X5 | T41.1X6 |
| Exalamide | T49.0X1 | T49.0X2 | T49.0X3 | T49.0X4 | T49.0X5 | T49.0X6 |
| Exalgin | T39.1X1 | T39.1X2 | T39.1X3 | T39.1X4 | T39.1X5 | T39.1X6 |
| Excipients, pharmaceutical | T50.901 | T50.902 | T50.903 | T50.904 | T50.905 | T50.906 |

Subterms under main terms may continue to next column or page    Additional Character May Be Required — Refer to the Tabular List for Character Selection    367

Etamiphyllin — Excipients, pharmaceutical

Table of Drugs and Chemicals

Exhaust gas — Fluorinated corticosteroids

| Substance | Poisoning, Accidental (unintentional) | Poisoning, Intentional Self-harm | Poisoning, Assault | Poisoning, Undetermined | Adverse Effect | Under-dosing |
|---|---|---|---|---|---|---|
| Exhaust gas (engine) (motor vehicle) | T58.01 | T58.02 | T58.03 | T58.04 | — | — |
| Ex-Lax (phenolphthalein) | T47.2X1 | T47.2X2 | T47.2X3 | T47.2X4 | T47.2X5 | T47.2X6 |
| Expectorant NEC | T48.4X1 | T48.4X2 | T48.4X3 | T48.4X4 | T48.4X5 | T48.4X6 |
| Extended insulin zinc suspension | T38.3X1 | T38.3X2 | T38.3X3 | T38.3X4 | T38.3X5 | T38.3X6 |
| External medications (skin) (mucous membrane) | T49.91 | T49.92 | T49.93 | T49.94 | T49.95 | T49.96 |
| dental agent | T49.7X1 | T49.7X2 | T49.7X3 | T49.7X4 | T49.7X5 | T49.7X6 |
| ENT agent | T49.6X1 | T49.6X2 | T49.6X3 | T49.6X4 | T49.6X5 | T49.6X6 |
| ophthalmic preparation | T49.5X1 | T49.5X2 | T49.5X3 | T49.5X4 | T49.5X5 | T49.5X6 |
| specified NEC | T49.8X1 | T49.8X2 | T49.8X3 | T49.8X4 | T49.8X5 | T49.8X6 |
| Extrapyramidal antagonist NEC | T44.3X1 | T44.3X2 | T44.3X3 | T44.3X4 | T44.3X5 | T44.3X6 |
| Eye agents (anti-infective) | T49.5X1 | T49.5X2 | T49.5X3 | T49.5X4 | T49.5X5 | T49.5X6 |
| Eye drug NEC | T49.5X1 | T49.5X2 | T49.5X3 | T49.5X4 | T49.5X5 | T49.5X6 |
| FAC (fluorouracil + doxorubicin + cyclophosphamide) | T45.1X1 | T45.1X2 | T45.1X3 | T45.1X4 | T45.1X5 | T45.1X6 |
| Factor | | | | | | |
| I (fibrinogen) | T45.8X1 | T45.8X2 | T45.8X3 | T45.8X4 | T45.8X5 | T45.8X6 |
| III (thromboplastin) | T45.8X1 | T45.8X2 | T45.8X3 | T45.8X4 | T45.8X5 | T45.8X6 |
| VIII (antihemophilic Factor) (concentrate) | T45.8X1 | T45.8X2 | T45.8X3 | T45.8X4 | T45.8X5 | T45.8X6 |
| IX complex | T45.7X1 | T45.7X2 | T45.7X3 | T45.7X4 | T45.7X5 | T45.7X6 |
| human | T45.8X1 | T45.8X2 | T45.8X3 | T45.8X4 | T45.8X5 | T45.8X6 |
| Famotidine | T47.0X1 | T47.0X2 | T47.0X3 | T47.0X4 | T47.0X5 | T47.0X6 |
| Fat suspension, intravenous | T50.991 | T50.992 | T50.993 | T50.994 | T50.995 | T50.996 |
| Fazadinium bromide | T48.1X1 | T48.1X2 | T48.1X3 | T48.1X4 | T48.1X5 | T48.1X6 |
| Febarbamate | T42.3X1 | T42.3X2 | T42.3X3 | T42.3X4 | T42.3X5 | T42.3X6 |
| Fecal softener | T47.4X1 | T47.4X2 | T47.4X3 | T47.4X4 | T47.4X5 | T47.4X6 |
| Fedrilate | T48.3X1 | T48.3X2 | T48.3X3 | T48.3X4 | T48.3X5 | T48.3X6 |
| Felodipine | T46.1X1 | T46.1X2 | T46.1X3 | T46.1X4 | T46.1X5 | T46.1X6 |
| Felypressin | T38.891 | T38.892 | T38.893 | T38.894 | T38.895 | T38.896 |
| Femoxetine | T43.221 | T43.222 | T43.223 | T43.224 | T43.225 | T43.226 |
| Fenalcomine | T46.3X1 | T46.3X2 | T46.3X3 | T46.3X4 | T46.3X5 | T46.3X6 |
| Fenamisal | T37.1X1 | T37.1X2 | T37.1X3 | T37.1X4 | T37.1X5 | T37.1X6 |
| Fenazone | T39.2X1 | T39.2X2 | T39.2X3 | T39.2X4 | T39.2X5 | T39.2X6 |
| Fenbendazole | T37.4X1 | T37.4X2 | T37.4X3 | T37.4X4 | T37.4X5 | T37.4X6 |
| Fenbutrazate | T50.5X1 | T50.5X2 | T50.5X3 | T50.5X4 | T50.5X5 | T50.5X6 |
| Fencamfamine | T43.691 | T43.692 | T43.693 | T43.694 | T43.695 | T43.696 |
| Fendiline | T46.1X1 | T46.1X2 | T46.1X3 | T46.1X4 | T46.1X5 | T46.1X6 |
| Fenetylline | T43.691 | T43.692 | T43.693 | T43.694 | T43.695 | T43.696 |
| Fenflumizole | T39.391 | T39.392 | T39.393 | T39.394 | T39.395 | T39.396 |
| Fenfluramine | T50.5X1 | T50.5X2 | T50.5X3 | T50.5X4 | T50.5X5 | T50.5X6 |
| Fenobarbital | T42.3X1 | T42.3X2 | T42.3X3 | T42.3X4 | T42.3X5 | T42.3X6 |
| Fenofibrate | T46.6X1 | T46.6X2 | T46.6X3 | T46.6X4 | T46.6X5 | T46.6X6 |
| Fenoprofen | T39.311 | T39.312 | T39.313 | T39.314 | T39.315 | T39.316 |
| Fenoterol | T48.6X1 | T48.6X2 | T48.6X3 | T48.6X4 | T48.6X5 | T48.6X6 |
| Fenoverine | T44.3X1 | T44.3X2 | T44.3X3 | T44.3X4 | T44.3X5 | T44.3X6 |
| Fenoxazoline | T48.5X1 | T48.5X2 | T48.5X3 | T48.5X4 | T48.5X5 | T48.5X6 |
| Fenproporex | T50.5X1 | T50.5X2 | T50.5X3 | T50.5X4 | T50.5X5 | T50.5X6 |
| Fenquizone | T50.2X1 | T50.2X2 | T50.2X3 | T50.2X4 | T50.2X5 | T50.2X6 |
| Fentanyl | T40.4X1 | T40.4X2 | T40.4X3 | T40.4X4 | T40.4X5 | T40.4X6 |
| Fentazin | T43.3X1 | T43.3X2 | T43.3X3 | T43.3X4 | T43.3X5 | T43.3X6 |
| Fenthion | T60.0X1 | T60.0X2 | T60.0X3 | T60.0X4 | — | — |
| Fenticlor | T49.0X1 | T49.0X2 | T49.0X3 | T49.0X4 | T49.0X5 | T49.0X6 |
| Fenylbutazone | T39.2X1 | T39.2X2 | T39.2X3 | T39.2X4 | T39.2X5 | T39.2X6 |
| Feprazone | T39.2X1 | T39.2X2 | T39.2X3 | T39.2X4 | T39.2X5 | T39.2X6 |
| Fer de lance (bite) (venom) | T63.061 | T63.062 | T63.063 | T63.064 | — | — |
| Ferric — see also Iron | | | | | | |
| chloride | T45.4X1 | T45.4X2 | T45.4X3 | T45.4X4 | T45.4X5 | T45.4X6 |
| citrate | T45.4X1 | T45.4X2 | T45.4X3 | T45.4X4 | T45.4X5 | T45.4X6 |
| hydroxide | | | | | | |
| colloidal | T45.4X1 | T45.4X2 | T45.4X3 | T45.4X4 | T45.4X5 | T45.4X6 |
| polymaltose | T45.4X1 | T45.4X2 | T45.4X3 | T45.4X4 | T45.4X5 | T45.4X6 |
| pyrophosphate | T45.4X1 | T45.4X2 | T45.4X3 | T45.4X4 | T45.4X5 | T45.4X6 |
| Ferritin | T45.4X1 | T45.4X2 | T45.4X3 | T45.4X4 | T45.4X5 | T45.4X6 |
| Ferrocholinate | T45.4X1 | T45.4X2 | T45.4X3 | T45.4X4 | T45.4X5 | T45.4X6 |
| Ferrodextrane | T45.4X1 | T45.4X2 | T45.4X3 | T45.4X4 | T45.4X5 | T45.4X6 |
| Ferropolimaler | T45.4X1 | T45.4X2 | T45.4X3 | T45.4X4 | T45.4X5 | T45.4X6 |
| Ferrous — see also Iron | | | | | | |
| phosphate | T45.4X1 | T45.4X2 | T45.4X3 | T45.4X4 | T45.4X5 | T45.4X6 |
| salt | T45.4X1 | T45.4X2 | T45.4X3 | T45.4X4 | T45.4X5 | T45.4X6 |
| with folic acid | T45.4X1 | T45.4X2 | T45.4X3 | T45.4X4 | T45.4X5 | T45.4X6 |
| Ferrous fumerate, gluconate, lactate, salt NEC, sulfate (medicinal) | T45.4X1 | T45.4X2 | T45.4X3 | T45.4X4 | T45.4X5 | T45.4X6 |
| Ferrovanadium (fumes) | T59.891 | T59.892 | T59.893 | T59.894 | — | — |
| Ferrum — see Iron | | | | | | |
| Fertilizers NEC | T65.891 | T65.892 | T65.893 | T65.894 | — | — |
| with herbicide mixture | T60.3X1 | T60.3X2 | T60.3X3 | T60.3X4 | — | — |
| Fetoxilate | T47.6X1 | T47.6X2 | T47.6X3 | T47.6X4 | T47.6X5 | T47.6X6 |
| Fiber, dietary | T47.4X1 | T47.4X2 | T47.4X3 | T47.4X4 | T47.4X5 | T47.4X6 |
| Fiberglass | T65.831 | T65.832 | T65.833 | T65.834 | — | — |
| Fibrinogen (human) | T45.8X1 | T45.8X2 | T45.8X3 | T45.8X4 | T45.8X5 | T45.8X6 |
| Fibrinolysin (human) | T45.691 | T45.692 | T45.693 | T45.694 | T45.695 | T45.696 |
| Fibrinolysis | | | | | | |
| affecting drug | T45.601 | T45.602 | T45.603 | T45.604 | T45.605 | T45.606 |
| inhibitor NEC | T45.621 | T45.622 | T45.623 | T45.624 | T45.625 | T45.626 |
| Fibrinolytic drug | T45.611 | T45.612 | T45.613 | T45.614 | T45.615 | T45.616 |
| Filix mas | T37.4X1 | T37.4X2 | T37.4X3 | T37.4X4 | T37.4X5 | T37.4X6 |
| Filtering cream | T49.3X1 | T49.3X2 | T49.3X3 | T49.3X4 | T49.3X5 | T49.3X6 |
| Fiorinal | T39.011 | T39.012 | T39.013 | T39.014 | T39.015 | T39.016 |
| Firedamp | T59.891 | T59.892 | T59.893 | T59.894 | — | — |
| Fish, noxious, nonbacterial | T61.91 | T61.92 | T61.93 | T61.94 | — | — |
| ciguatera | T61.01 | T61.02 | T61.03 | T61.04 | — | — |
| scombroid | T61.11 | T61.12 | T61.13 | T61.14 | — | — |
| shell | T61.781 | T61.782 | T61.783 | T61.784 | — | — |
| specified NEC | T61.771 | T61.772 | T61.773 | T61.774 | — | — |
| Flagyl | T37.3X1 | T37.3X2 | T37.3X3 | T37.3X4 | T37.3X5 | T37.3X6 |
| Flavine adenine dinucleotide | T45.2X1 | T45.2X2 | T45.2X3 | T45.2X4 | T45.2X5 | T45.2X6 |
| Flavodic acid | T46.991 | T46.992 | T46.993 | T46.994 | T46.995 | T46.996 |
| Flavoxate | T44.3X1 | T44.3X2 | T44.3X3 | T44.3X4 | T44.3X5 | T44.3X6 |
| Flaxedil | T48.1X1 | T48.1X2 | T48.1X3 | T48.1X4 | T48.1X5 | T48.1X6 |
| Flaxseed (medicinal) | T49.3X1 | T49.3X2 | T49.3X3 | T49.3X4 | T49.3X5 | T49.3X6 |
| Flecainide | T46.2X1 | T46.2X2 | T46.2X3 | T46.2X4 | T46.2X5 | T46.2X6 |
| Fleroxacin | T36.8X1 | T36.8X2 | T36.8X3 | T36.8X4 | T36.8X5 | T36.8X6 |
| Floctafenine | T39.8X1 | T39.8X2 | T39.8X3 | T39.8X4 | T39.8X5 | T39.8X6 |
| Flomax | T44.6X1 | T44.6X2 | T44.6X3 | T44.6X4 | T44.6X5 | T44.6X6 |
| Flomoxef | T36.1X1 | T36.1X2 | T36.1X3 | T36.1X4 | T36.1X5 | T36.1X6 |
| Flopropione | T44.3X1 | T44.3X2 | T44.3X3 | T44.3X4 | T44.3X5 | T44.3X6 |
| Florantyrone | T47.5X1 | T47.5X2 | T47.5X3 | T47.5X4 | T47.5X5 | T47.5X6 |
| Floraquin | T37.8X1 | T37.8X2 | T37.8X3 | T37.8X4 | T37.8X5 | T37.8X6 |
| Florinef | T38.0X1 | T38.0X2 | T38.0X3 | T38.0X4 | T38.0X5 | T38.0X6 |
| ENT agent | T49.6X1 | T49.6X2 | T49.6X3 | T49.6X4 | T49.6X5 | T49.6X6 |
| ophthalmic preparation | T49.5X1 | T49.5X2 | T49.5X3 | T49.5X4 | T49.5X5 | T49.5X6 |
| topical NEC | T49.0X1 | T49.0X2 | T49.0X3 | T49.0X4 | T49.0X5 | T49.0X6 |
| Flowers of sulfur | T49.4X1 | T49.4X2 | T49.4X3 | T49.4X4 | T49.4X5 | T49.4X6 |
| Floxuridine | T45.1X1 | T45.1X2 | T45.1X3 | T45.1X4 | T45.1X5 | T45.1X6 |
| Fluanisone | T43.4X1 | T43.4X2 | T43.4X3 | T43.4X4 | T43.4X5 | T43.4X6 |
| Flubendazole | T37.4X1 | T37.4X2 | T37.4X3 | T37.4X4 | T37.4X5 | T37.4X6 |
| Fluclorolone acetonide | T49.0X1 | T49.0X2 | T49.0X3 | T49.0X4 | T49.0X5 | T49.0X6 |
| Flucloxacillin | T36.0X1 | T36.0X2 | T36.0X3 | T36.0X4 | T36.0X5 | T36.0X6 |
| Fluconazole | T37.8X1 | T37.8X2 | T37.8X3 | T37.8X4 | T37.8X5 | T37.8X6 |
| Flucytosine | T37.8X1 | T37.8X2 | T37.8X3 | T37.8X4 | T37.8X5 | T37.8X6 |
| Fludeoxyglucose (18F) | T50.8X1 | T50.8X2 | T50.8X3 | T50.8X4 | T50.8X5 | T50.8X6 |
| Fludiazepam | T42.4X1 | T42.4X2 | T42.4X3 | T42.4X4 | T42.4X5 | T42.4X6 |
| Fludrocortisone | T50.0X1 | T50.0X2 | T50.0X3 | T50.0X4 | T50.0X5 | T50.0X6 |
| ENT agent | T49.6X1 | T49.6X2 | T49.6X3 | T49.6X4 | T49.6X5 | T49.6X6 |
| ophthalmic preparation | T49.5X1 | T49.5X2 | T49.5X3 | T49.5X4 | T49.5X5 | T49.5X6 |
| topical NEC | T49.0X1 | T49.0X2 | T49.0X3 | T49.0X4 | T49.0X5 | T49.0X6 |
| Fludroxycortide | T49.0X1 | T49.0X2 | T49.0X3 | T49.0X4 | T49.0X5 | T49.0X6 |
| Flufenamic acid | T39.391 | T39.392 | T39.393 | T39.394 | T39.395 | T39.396 |
| Fluindione | T45.511 | T45.512 | T45.513 | T45.514 | T45.515 | T45.516 |
| Flumequine | T37.8X1 | T37.8X2 | T37.8X3 | T37.8X4 | T37.8X5 | T37.8X6 |
| Flumethasone | T49.0X1 | T49.0X2 | T49.0X3 | T49.0X4 | T49.0X5 | T49.0X6 |
| Flumethiazide | T50.2X1 | T50.2X2 | T50.2X3 | T50.2X4 | T50.2X5 | T50.2X6 |
| Flumidin | T37.5X1 | T37.5X2 | T37.5X3 | T37.5X4 | T37.5X5 | T37.5X6 |
| Flunarizine | T46.7X1 | T46.7X2 | T46.7X3 | T46.7X4 | T46.7X5 | T46.7X6 |
| Flunidazole | T37.8X1 | T37.8X2 | T37.8X3 | T37.8X4 | T37.8X5 | T37.8X6 |
| Flunisolide | T48.6X1 | T48.6X2 | T48.6X3 | T48.6X4 | T48.6X5 | T48.6X6 |
| Flunitrazepam | T42.4X1 | T42.4X2 | T42.4X3 | T42.4X4 | T42.4X5 | T42.4X6 |
| Fluocinolone (acetonide) | T49.0X1 | T49.0X2 | T49.0X3 | T49.0X4 | T49.0X5 | T49.0X6 |
| Fluocinonide | T49.0X1 | T49.0X2 | T49.0X3 | T49.0X4 | T49.0X5 | T49.0X6 |
| Fluocortin (butyl) | T49.0X1 | T49.0X2 | T49.0X3 | T49.0X4 | T49.0X5 | T49.0X6 |
| Fluocortolone | T49.0X1 | T49.0X2 | T49.0X3 | T49.0X4 | T49.0X5 | T49.0X6 |
| Fluohydrocortisone | T38.0X1 | T38.0X2 | T38.0X3 | T38.0X4 | T38.0X5 | T38.0X6 |
| ENT agent | T49.6X1 | T49.6X2 | T49.6X3 | T49.6X4 | T49.6X5 | T49.6X6 |
| ophthalmic preparation | T49.5X1 | T49.5X2 | T49.5X3 | T49.5X4 | T49.5X5 | T49.5X6 |
| topical NEC | T49.0X1 | T49.0X2 | T49.0X3 | T49.0X4 | T49.0X5 | T49.0X6 |
| Fluonid | T49.0X1 | T49.0X2 | T49.0X3 | T49.0X4 | T49.0X5 | T49.0X6 |
| Fluopromazine | T43.3X1 | T43.3X2 | T43.3X3 | T43.3X4 | T43.3X5 | T43.3X6 |
| Fluoracetate | T60.8X1 | T60.8X2 | T60.8X3 | T60.8X4 | — | — |
| Fluorescein | T50.8X1 | T50.8X2 | T50.8X3 | T50.8X4 | T50.8X5 | T50.8X6 |
| Fluorhydrocortisone | T50.0X1 | T50.0X2 | T50.0X3 | T50.0X4 | T50.0X5 | T50.0X6 |
| Fluoride (nonmedicinal) (pesticide) (sodium) NEC | T60.8X1 | T60.8X2 | T60.8X3 | T60.8X4 | — | — |
| hydrogen — see Hydrofluoric acid | | | | | | |
| medicinal NEC | T50.991 | T50.992 | T50.993 | T50.994 | T50.995 | T50.996 |
| dental use | T49.7X1 | T49.7X2 | T49.7X3 | T49.7X4 | T49.7X5 | T49.7X6 |
| not pesticide NEC | T54.91 | T54.92 | T54.93 | T54.94 | — | — |
| stannous | T49.7X1 | T49.7X2 | T49.7X3 | T49.7X4 | T49.7X5 | T49.7X6 |
| Fluorinated corticosteroids | T38.0X1 | T38.0X2 | T38.0X3 | T38.0X4 | T38.0X5 | T38.0X6 |

| Substance | Poisoning, Accidental (unintentional) | Poisoning, Intentional Self-harm | Poisoning, Assault | Poisoning, Undetermined | Adverse Effect | Under-dosing |
|---|---|---|---|---|---|---|
| Fluorine (gas) | T59.5X1 | T59.5X2 | T59.5X3 | T59.5X4 | — | — |
| salt — see Fluoride(s) | | | | | | |
| Fluoristan | T49.7X1 | T49.7X2 | T49.7X3 | T49.7X4 | T49.7X5 | T49.7X6 |
| Fluormetholone | T49.0X1 | T49.0X2 | T49.0X3 | T49.0X4 | T49.0X5 | T49.0X6 |
| Fluoroacetate | T60.8X1 | T60.8X2 | T60.8X3 | T60.8X4 | — | — |
| Fluorocarbon monomer | T53.6X1 | T53.6X2 | T53.6X3 | T53.6X4 | — | — |
| Fluorocytosine | T37.8X1 | T37.8X2 | T37.8X3 | T37.8X4 | T37.8X5 | T37.8X6 |
| Fluorodeoxyuridine | T45.1X1 | T45.1X2 | T45.1X3 | T45.1X4 | T45.1X5 | T45.1X6 |
| Fluorometholone | T49.0X1 | T49.0X2 | T49.0X3 | T49.0X4 | T49.0X5 | T49.0X6 |
| ophthalmic preparation | T49.5X1 | T49.5X2 | T49.5X3 | T49.5X4 | T49.5X5 | T49.5X6 |
| Fluorophosphate insecticide | T60.0X1 | T60.0X2 | T60.0X3 | T60.0X4 | — | — |
| Fluorosol | T46.3X1 | T46.3X2 | T46.3X3 | T46.3X4 | T46.3X5 | T46.3X6 |
| Fluorouracil | T45.1X1 | T45.1X2 | T45.1X3 | T45.1X4 | T45.1X5 | T45.1X6 |
| Fluorphenylalanine | T49.5X1 | T49.5X2 | T49.5X3 | T49.5X4 | T49.5X5 | T49.5X6 |
| Fluothane | T41.0X1 | T41.0X2 | T41.0X3 | T41.0X4 | T41.0X5 | T41.0X6 |
| Fluoxetine | T43.221 | T43.222 | T43.223 | T43.224 | T43.225 | T43.226 |
| Fluoxymesterone | T38.7X1 | T38.7X2 | T38.7X3 | T38.7X4 | T38.7X5 | T38.7X6 |
| Flupenthixol | T43.4X1 | T43.4X2 | T43.4X3 | T43.4X4 | T43.4X5 | T43.4X6 |
| Flupentixol | T43.4X1 | T43.4X2 | T43.4X3 | T43.4X4 | T43.4X5 | T43.4X6 |
| Fluphenazine | T43.3X1 | T43.3X2 | T43.3X3 | T43.3X4 | T43.3X5 | T43.3X6 |
| Fluprednidene | T49.0X1 | T49.0X2 | T49.0X3 | T49.0X4 | T49.0X5 | T49.0X6 |
| Fluprednisolone | T38.0X1 | T38.0X2 | T38.0X3 | T38.0X4 | T38.0X5 | T38.0X6 |
| Fluradoline | T39.8X1 | T39.8X2 | T39.8X3 | T39.8X4 | T39.8X5 | T39.8X6 |
| Flurandrenolide | T49.0X1 | T49.0X2 | T49.0X3 | T49.0X4 | T49.0X5 | T49.0X6 |
| Flurandrenolone | T49.0X1 | T49.0X2 | T49.0X3 | T49.0X4 | T49.0X5 | T49.0X6 |
| Flurazepam | T42.4X1 | T42.4X2 | T42.4X3 | T42.4X4 | T42.4X5 | T42.4X6 |
| Flurbiprofen | T39.311 | T39.312 | T39.313 | T39.314 | T39.315 | T39.316 |
| Flurobate | T49.0X1 | T49.0X2 | T49.0X3 | T49.0X4 | T49.0X5 | T49.0X6 |
| Fluroxene | T41.0X1 | T41.0X2 | T41.0X3 | T41.0X4 | T41.0X5 | T41.0X6 |
| Fluspirilene | T43.591 | T43.592 | T43.593 | T43.594 | T43.595 | T43.596 |
| Flutamide | T38.6X1 | T38.6X2 | T38.6X3 | T38.6X4 | T38.6X5 | T38.6X6 |
| Flutazolam | T38.0X1 | T38.0X2 | T38.0X3 | T38.0X4 | T38.0X5 | T38.0X6 |
| Fluticasone propionate | T38.0X1 | T38.0X2 | T38.0X3 | T38.0X4 | T38.0X5 | T38.0X6 |
| Flutoprazepam | T42.4X1 | T42.4X2 | T42.4X3 | T42.4X4 | T42.4X5 | T42.4X6 |
| Flutropium bromide | T48.6X1 | T48.6X2 | T48.6X3 | T48.6X4 | T48.6X5 | T48.6X6 |
| Fluvoxamine | T43.221 | T43.222 | T43.223 | T43.224 | T43.225 | T43.226 |
| Folacin | T45.8X1 | T45.8X2 | T45.8X3 | T45.8X4 | T45.8X5 | T45.8X6 |
| Folic acid | T45.8X1 | T45.8X2 | T45.8X3 | T45.8X4 | T45.8X5 | T45.8X6 |
| with ferrous salt | T45.2X1 | T45.2X2 | T45.2X3 | T45.2X4 | T45.2X5 | T45.2X6 |
| antagonist | T45.1X1 | T45.1X2 | T45.1X3 | T45.1X4 | T45.1X5 | T45.1X6 |
| Folinic acid | T45.8X1 | T45.8X2 | T45.8X3 | T45.8X4 | T45.8X5 | T45.8X6 |
| Folium stramoniae | T48.6X1 | T48.6X2 | T48.6X3 | T48.6X4 | T48.6X5 | T48.6X6 |
| Follicle-stimulating hormone, human | T38.811 | T38.812 | T38.813 | T38.814 | T38.815 | T38.816 |
| Folpet | T60.3X1 | T60.3X2 | T60.3X3 | T60.3X4 | — | — |
| Fominoben | T48.3X1 | T48.3X2 | T48.3X3 | T48.3X4 | T48.3X5 | T48.3X6 |
| Food, foodstuffs, noxious, nonbacterial, NEC | T62.91 | T62.92 | T62.93 | T62.94 | | |
| berries | T62.1X1 | T62.1X2 | T62.1X3 | T62.1X4 | — | — |
| fish — see also Fish | T61.91 | T61.92 | T61.93 | T61.94 | — | — |
| mushrooms | T62.0X1 | T62.0X2 | T62.0X3 | T62.0X4 | — | — |
| plants | T62.2X1 | T62.2X2 | T62.2X3 | T62.2X4 | — | — |
| seafood | T61.91 | T61.92 | T61.93 | T61.94 | — | — |
| specified NEC | T61.8X1 | T61.8X2 | T61.8X3 | T61.8X4 | — | — |
| seeds | T62.2X1 | T62.2X2 | T62.2X3 | T62.2X4 | — | — |
| shellfish | T61.781 | T61.782 | T61.783 | T61.784 | — | — |
| specified NEC | T62.8X1 | T62.8X2 | T62.8X3 | T62.8X4 | — | — |
| Fool's parsley | T62.2X1 | T62.2X2 | T62.2X3 | T62.2X4 | — | — |
| Formaldehyde (solution), gas or vapor | T59.2X1 | T59.2X2 | T59.2X3 | T59.2X4 | — | — |
| fungicide | T60.3X1 | T60.3X2 | T60.3X3 | T60.3X4 | — | — |
| Formalin | T59.2X1 | T59.2X2 | T59.2X3 | T59.2X4 | — | — |
| fungicide | T60.3X1 | T60.3X2 | T60.3X3 | T60.3X4 | — | — |
| vapor | T59.2X1 | T59.2X2 | T59.2X3 | T59.2X4 | — | — |
| Formic acid | T54.2X1 | T54.2X2 | T54.2X3 | T54.2X4 | — | — |
| vapor | T59.891 | T59.892 | T59.893 | T59.894 | — | — |
| Foscarnet sodium | T37.5X1 | T37.5X2 | T37.5X3 | T37.5X4 | T37.5X5 | T37.5X6 |
| Fosfestrol | T38.5X1 | T38.5X2 | T38.5X3 | T38.5X4 | T38.5X5 | T38.5X6 |
| Fosfomycin | T36.8X1 | T36.8X2 | T36.8X3 | T36.8X4 | T36.8X5 | T36.8X6 |
| Fosfonet sodium | T37.5X1 | T37.5X2 | T37.5X3 | T37.5X4 | T37.5X5 | T37.5X6 |
| Fosinopril | T46.4X1 | T46.4X2 | T46.4X3 | T46.4X4 | T46.4X5 | T46.4X6 |
| sodium | T46.4X1 | T46.4X2 | T46.4X3 | T46.4X4 | T46.4X5 | T46.4X6 |
| Fowler's solution | T57.0X1 | T57.0X2 | T57.0X3 | T57.0X4 | — | — |
| Foxglove | T62.2X1 | T62.2X2 | T62.2X3 | T62.2X4 | — | — |
| Framycetin | T36.5X1 | T36.5X2 | T36.5X3 | T36.5X4 | T36.5X5 | T36.5X6 |
| Frangula | T47.2X1 | T47.2X2 | T47.2X3 | T47.2X4 | T47.2X5 | T47.2X6 |
| extract | T47.2X1 | T47.2X2 | T47.2X3 | T47.2X4 | T47.2X5 | T47.2X6 |
| Frei antigen | T50.8X1 | T50.8X2 | T50.8X3 | T50.8X4 | T50.8X5 | T50.8X6 |
| Freon | T53.5X1 | T53.5X2 | T53.5X3 | T53.5X4 | — | — |
| Fructose | T50.3X1 | T50.3X2 | T50.3X3 | T50.3X4 | T50.3X5 | T50.3X6 |
| Frusemide | T50.1X1 | T50.1X2 | T50.1X3 | T50.1X4 | T50.1X5 | T50.1X6 |
| FSH | T38.811 | T38.812 | T38.813 | T38.814 | T38.815 | T38.816 |

| Substance | Poisoning, Accidental (unintentional) | Poisoning, Intentional Self-harm | Poisoning, Assault | Poisoning, Undetermined | Adverse Effect | Under-dosing |
|---|---|---|---|---|---|---|
| Ftorafur | T45.1X1 | T45.1X2 | T45.1X3 | T45.1X4 | T45.1X5 | T45.1X6 |
| Fuel | | | | | | |
| automobile | T52.0X1 | T52.0X2 | T52.0X3 | T52.0X4 | — | — |
| exhaust gas, not in transit | T58.01 | T58.02 | T58.03 | T58.04 | — | — |
| vapor NEC | T52.0X1 | T52.0X2 | T52.0X3 | T52.0X4 | — | — |
| gas (domestic use) — see also Carbon, monoxide, fuel, utility | T59.891 | T59.892 | T59.893 | T59.894 | — | — |
| utility | T59.891 | T59.892 | T59.893 | T59.894 | — | — |
| incomplete combustion of — see Carbon, monoxide, fuel, utility | | | | | | |
| in mobile container | T59.891 | T59.892 | T59.893 | T59.894 | — | — |
| piped (natural) | T59.891 | T59.892 | T59.893 | T59.894 | — | — |
| industrial, incomplete combustion | T58.8X1 | T58.8X2 | T58.8X3 | T58.8X4 | — | — |
| Fugillin | T36.8X1 | T36.8X2 | T36.8X3 | T36.8X4 | T36.8X5 | T36.8X6 |
| Fulminate of mercury | T56.1X1 | T56.1X2 | T56.1X3 | T56.1X4 | — | — |
| Fulvicin | T36.7X1 | T36.7X2 | T36.7X3 | T36.7X4 | T36.7X5 | T36.7X6 |
| Fumadil | T36.8X1 | T36.8X2 | T36.8X3 | T36.8X4 | T36.8X5 | T36.8X6 |
| Fumagillin | T36.8X1 | T36.8X2 | T36.8X3 | T36.8X4 | T36.8X5 | T36.8X6 |
| Fumaric acid | T49.4X1 | T49.4X2 | T49.4X3 | T49.4X4 | T49.4X5 | T49.4X6 |
| Fumes (from) | T59.91 | T59.92 | T59.93 | T59.94 | — | — |
| carbon monoxide — see Carbon, monoxide | | | | | | |
| charcoal (domestic use) — see Charcoal, fumes | | | | | | |
| chloroform — see Chloroform | | | | | | |
| coke (in domestic stoves, fireplaces) — see Coke fumes | | | | | | |
| corrosive NEC | T54.91 | T54.92 | T54.93 | T54.94 | — | — |
| ether — see ether | | | | | | |
| freons | T53.5X1 | T53.5X2 | T53.5X3 | T53.5X4 | — | — |
| hydrocarbons | T59.891 | T59.892 | T59.893 | T59.894 | — | — |
| petroleum (liquefied) | T59.891 | T59.892 | T59.893 | T59.894 | — | — |
| distributed through pipes (pure or mixed with air) | T59.891 | T59.892 | T59.893 | T59.894 | — | — |
| lead — see lead | | | | | | |
| metal — see Metals, or the specified metal | | | | | | |
| nitrogen dioxide | T59.0X1 | T59.0X2 | T59.0X3 | T59.0X4 | — | — |
| pesticides — see Pesticides | | | | | | |
| petroleum (liquefied) | T59.891 | T59.892 | T59.893 | T59.894 | — | — |
| distributed through pipes (pure or mixed with air) | T59.891 | T59.892 | T59.893 | T59.894 | — | — |
| polyester | T59.891 | T59.892 | T59.893 | T59.894 | — | — |
| specified source NEC — see also substance specified | T59.891 | T59.892 | T59.893 | T59.894 | — | — |
| sulfur dioxide | T59.1X1 | T59.1X2 | T59.1X3 | T59.1X4 | — | — |
| Fumigant NEC | T60.91 | T60.92 | T60.93 | T60.94 | — | — |
| Fungicide NEC (nonmedicinal) | T60.3X1 | T60.3X2 | T60.3X3 | T60.3X4 | — | — |
| Fungi, noxious, used as food | T62.0X1 | T62.0X2 | T62.0X3 | T62.0X4 | — | — |
| Fungizone | T36.7X1 | T36.7X2 | T36.7X3 | T36.7X4 | T36.7X5 | T36.7X6 |
| topical | T49.0X1 | T49.0X2 | T49.0X3 | T49.0X4 | T49.0X5 | T49.0X6 |
| Furacin | T49.0X1 | T49.0X2 | T49.0X3 | T49.0X4 | T49.0X5 | T49.0X6 |
| Furadantin | T37.91 | T37.92 | T37.93 | T37.94 | T37.95 | T37.96 |
| Furazolidone | T37.8X1 | T37.8X2 | T37.8X3 | T37.8X4 | T37.8X5 | T37.8X6 |
| Furazolium chloride | T49.0X1 | T49.0X2 | T49.0X3 | T49.0X4 | T49.0X5 | T49.0X6 |
| Furfural | T52.8X1 | T52.8X2 | T52.8X3 | T52.8X4 | — | — |
| Furfural | T52.8X1 | T52.8X2 | T52.8X3 | T52.8X4 | — | — |
| Furnace (coal burning) (domestic), gas from | T58.2X1 | T58.2X2 | T58.2X3 | T58.2X4 | — | — |
| industrial | T58.8X1 | T58.8X2 | T58.8X3 | T58.8X4 | — | — |
| Furniture polish | T65.891 | T65.892 | T65.893 | T65.894 | — | — |
| Furosemide | T50.1X1 | T50.1X2 | T50.1X3 | T50.1X4 | T50.1X5 | T50.1X6 |
| Furoxone | T37.91 | T37.92 | T37.93 | T37.94 | T37.95 | T37.96 |
| Fursultiamine | T45.2X1 | T45.2X2 | T45.2X3 | T45.2X4 | T45.2X5 | T45.2X6 |
| Fusafungine | T36.8X1 | T36.8X2 | T36.8X3 | T36.8X4 | T36.8X5 | T36.8X6 |
| Fusel oil (any) (amyl) (butyl) (propyl), vapor | T51.3X1 | T51.3X2 | T51.3X3 | T51.3X4 | — | — |
| Fusidate (ethanolamine) (sodium) | T36.8X1 | T36.8X2 | T36.8X3 | T36.8X4 | T36.8X5 | T36.8X6 |
| Fusidic acid | T36.8X1 | T36.8X2 | T36.8X3 | T36.8X4 | T36.8X5 | T36.8X6 |
| Fytic acid, nonasodium | T50.6X1 | T50.6X2 | T50.6X3 | T50.6X4 | T50.6X5 | T50.6X6 |
| b-Galactosidase | T47.5X1 | T47.5X2 | T47.5X3 | T47.5X4 | T47.5X5 | T47.5X6 |
| GABA | T43.8X1 | T43.8X2 | T43.8X3 | T43.8X4 | T43.8X5 | T43.8X6 |
| Gadopentetic acid | T50.8X1 | T50.8X2 | T50.8X3 | T50.8X4 | T50.8X5 | T50.8X6 |
| Galactose | T50.3X1 | T50.3X2 | T50.3X3 | T50.3X4 | T50.3X5 | T50.3X6 |
| Galantamine | T44.0X1 | T44.0X2 | T44.0X3 | T44.0X4 | T44.0X5 | T44.0X6 |

Table of Drugs and Chemicals

| Substance | Poisoning, Accidental (unintentional) | Poisoning, Intentional Self-harm | Poisoning, Assault | Poisoning, Undetermined | Adverse Effect | Under-dosing |
|---|---|---|---|---|---|---|
| **Gallamine** (triethiodide) | T48.1X1 | T48.1X2 | T48.1X3 | T48.1X4 | T48.1X5 | T48.1X6 |
| **Gallium citrate** | T50.991 | T50.992 | T50.993 | T50.994 | T50.995 | T50.996 |
| **Gallopamil** | T46.1X1 | T46.1X2 | T46.1X3 | T46.1X4 | T46.1X5 | T46.1X6 |
| **Gamboge** | T47.2X1 | T47.2X2 | T47.2X3 | T47.2X4 | T47.2X5 | T47.2X6 |
| **Gamimune** | T50.Z11 | T50.Z12 | T50.Z13 | T50.Z14 | T50.Z15 | T50.Z16 |
| **Gamma-aminobutyric acid** | T43.8X1 | T43.8X2 | T43.8X3 | T43.8X4 | T43.8X5 | T43.8X6 |
| **Gamma-benzene hexachloride** (medicinal) | T49.0X1 | T49.0X2 | T49.0X3 | T49.0X4 | T49.0X5 | T49.0X6 |
| nonmedicinal, vapor | T53.6X1 | T53.6X2 | T53.6X3 | T53.6X4 | — | — |
| **Gamma-BHC** (medicinal) — see also Gamma-benzene hexachloride | T49.0X1 | T49.0X2 | T49.0X3 | T49.0X4 | T49.0X5 | T49.0X6 |
| **Gamma globulin** | T50.Z11 | T50.Z12 | T50.Z13 | T50.Z14 | T50.Z15 | T50.Z16 |
| **Gamulin** | T50.Z11 | T50.Z12 | T50.Z13 | T50.Z14 | T50.Z15 | T50.Z16 |
| **Ganciclovir** (sodium) | T37.5X1 | T37.5X2 | T37.5X3 | T37.5X4 | T37.5X5 | T37.5X6 |
| **Ganglionic blocking drug NEC** | T44.2X1 | T44.2X2 | T44.2X3 | T44.2X4 | T44.2X5 | T44.2X6 |
| specified NEC | T44.2X1 | T44.2X2 | T44.2X3 | T44.2X4 | T44.2X5 | T44.2X6 |
| **Ganja** | T40.7X1 | T40.7X2 | T40.7X3 | T40.7X4 | T40.7X5 | T40.7X6 |
| **Garamycin** | T36.5X1 | T36.5X2 | T36.5X3 | T36.5X4 | T36.5X5 | T36.5X6 |
| ophthalmic preparation | T49.5X1 | T49.5X2 | T49.5X3 | T49.5X4 | T49.5X5 | T49.5X6 |
| topical NEC | T49.0X1 | T49.0X2 | T49.0X3 | T49.0X4 | T49.0X5 | T49.0X6 |
| **Gardenal** | T42.3X1 | T42.3X2 | T42.3X3 | T42.3X4 | T42.3X5 | T42.3X6 |
| **Gardepanyl** | T42.3X1 | T42.3X2 | T42.3X3 | T42.3X4 | T42.3X5 | T42.3X6 |
| **Gaseous substance** — see Gas | | | | | | |
| **Gasoline** | T52.0X1 | T52.0X2 | T52.0X3 | T52.0X4 | — | — |
| vapor | T52.0X1 | T52.0X2 | T52.0X3 | T52.0X4 | — | — |
| **Gastric enzymes** | T47.5X1 | T47.5X2 | T47.5X3 | T47.5X4 | T47.5X5 | T47.5X6 |
| **Gastrografin** | T50.8X1 | T50.8X2 | T50.8X3 | T50.8X4 | T50.8X5 | T50.8X6 |
| **Gastrointestinal drug** | T47.91 | T47.92 | T47.93 | T47.94 | T47.95 | T47.96 |
| biological | T47.8X1 | T47.8X2 | T47.8X3 | T47.8X4 | T47.8X5 | T47.8X6 |
| specified NEC | T47.8X1 | T47.8X2 | T47.8X3 | T47.8X4 | T47.8X5 | T47.8X6 |
| **Gas NEC** | T59.91 | T59.92 | T59.93 | T59.94 | — | — |
| acetylene | T59.891 | T59.892 | T59.893 | T59.894 | — | — |
| incomplete combustion of | T58.11 | T58.12 | T58.13 | T58.14 | — | — |
| air contaminants, source or type not specified | T59.91 | T59.92 | T59.93 | T59.94 | — | — |
| anesthetic | T41.0X1 | T41.0X2 | T41.0X3 | T41.0X4 | T41.0X5 | T41.0X6 |
| blast furnace | T58.8X1 | T58.8X2 | T58.8X3 | T58.8X4 | — | — |
| butane — see butane | | | | | | |
| carbon monoxide — see Carbon, monoxide | | | | | | |
| chlorine | T59.4X1 | T59.4X2 | T59.4X3 | T59.4X4 | — | — |
| coal | T58.2X1 | T58.2X2 | T58.2X3 | T58.2X4 | — | — |
| cyanide | T57.3X1 | T57.3X2 | T57.3X3 | T57.3X4 | — | — |
| dicyanogen | T65.0X1 | T65.0X2 | T65.0X3 | T65.0X4 | — | — |
| domestic — see Domestic gas | | | | | | |
| exhaust | T58.01 | T58.02 | T58.03 | T58.04 | — | — |
| from utility (for cooking, heating, or lighting) (after combustion) — see Carbon, monoxide, fuel, utility | | | | | | |
| prior to combustion | T59.891 | T59.892 | T59.893 | T59.894 | — | — |
| from wood- or coal-burning stove or fireplace | T58.2X1 | T58.2X2 | T58.2X3 | T58.2X4 | — | — |
| fuel (domestic use) (after combustion) — see also Carbon, monoxide, fuel | | | | | | |
| industrial use | T58.8X1 | T58.8X2 | T58.8X3 | T58.8X4 | — | — |
| prior to combustion | T59.891 | T59.892 | T59.893 | T59.894 | — | — |
| utility | T59.891 | T59.892 | T59.893 | T59.894 | — | — |
| incomplete combustion of — see Carbon, monoxide, fuel, utility | | | | | | |
| in mobile container | T59.891 | T59.892 | T59.893 | T59.894 | — | — |
| piped (natural) | T59.891 | T59.892 | T59.893 | T59.894 | — | — |
| garage | T58.01 | T58.02 | T58.03 | T58.04 | — | — |
| hydrocarbon NEC | T59.891 | T59.892 | T59.893 | T59.894 | — | — |
| incomplete combustion of — see Carbon, monoxide, fuel, utility | | | | | | |
| liquefied — see butane | | | | | | |
| piped | T59.891 | T59.892 | T59.893 | T59.894 | — | — |
| hydrocyanic acid | T65.0X1 | T65.0X2 | T65.0X3 | T65.0X4 | — | — |
| illuminating (after combustion) | T58.11 | T58.12 | T58.13 | T58.14 | — | — |
| prior to combustion | T59.891 | T59.892 | T59.893 | T59.894 | — | — |
| incomplete combustion, any — see Carbon, monoxide | | | | | | |
| kiln | T58.8X1 | T58.8X2 | T58.8X3 | T58.8X4 | — | — |
| lacrimogenic | T59.3X1 | T59.3X2 | T59.3X3 | T59.3X4 | — | — |

| Substance | Poisoning, Accidental (unintentional) | Poisoning, Intentional Self-harm | Poisoning, Assault | Poisoning, Undetermined | Adverse Effect | Under-dosing |
|---|---|---|---|---|---|---|
| **Gas** — continued | | | | | | |
| liquefied petroleum — see butane | | | | | | |
| marsh | T59.891 | T59.892 | T59.893 | T59.894 | — | — |
| motor exhaust, not in transit | T58.01 | T58.02 | T58.03 | T58.04 | — | — |
| mustard, not in war | T59.891 | T59.892 | T59.893 | T59.894 | — | — |
| natural | T59.891 | T59.892 | T59.893 | T59.894 | — | — |
| nerve, not in war | T59.91 | T59.92 | T59.93 | T59.94 | — | — |
| oil | T52.0X1 | T52.0X2 | T52.0X3 | T52.0X4 | — | — |
| petroleum (liquefied) (distributed in mobile containers) | T59.891 | T59.892 | T59.893 | T59.894 | — | — |
| piped (pure or mixed with air) | T59.891 | T59.892 | T59.893 | T59.894 | — | — |
| piped (manufactured) (natural) NEC | T59.891 | T59.892 | T59.893 | T59.894 | — | — |
| producer | T58.8X1 | T58.8X2 | T58.8X3 | T58.8X4 | — | — |
| propane — see propane | | | | | | |
| refrigerant (chlorofluoro-carbon) | T53.5X1 | T53.5X2 | T53.5X3 | T53.5X4 | — | — |
| not chlorofluoro-carbon | T59.891 | T59.892 | T59.893 | T59.894 | — | — |
| sewer | T59.91 | T59.92 | T59.93 | T59.94 | — | — |
| specified source NEC | T59.91 | T59.92 | T59.93 | T59.94 | — | — |
| stove (after combustion) | T58.11 | T58.12 | T58.13 | T58.14 | — | — |
| prior to combustion | T59.891 | T59.892 | T59.893 | T59.894 | — | — |
| tear | T59.3X1 | T59.3X2 | T59.3X3 | T59.3X4 | — | — |
| therapeutic | T41.5X1 | T41.5X2 | T41.5X3 | T41.5X4 | T41.5X5 | T41.5X6 |
| utility (for cooking, heating, or lighting) (piped) NEC | T59.891 | T59.892 | T59.893 | T59.894 | — | — |
| incomplete combustion of — see Carbon, monoxide, fuel, utilty | | | | | | |
| in mobile container | T59.891 | T59.892 | T59.893 | T59.894 | — | — |
| piped (natural) | T59.891 | T59.892 | T59.893 | T59.894 | — | — |
| water | T58.11 | T58.12 | T58.13 | T58.14 | — | — |
| incomplete combustion of — see Carbon, monoxide, fuel, utility | | | | | | |
| **Gaultheria procumbens** | T62.2X1 | T62.2X2 | T62.2X3 | T62.2X4 | — | — |
| **Gefarnate** | T44.3X1 | T44.3X2 | T44.3X3 | T44.3X4 | T44.3X5 | T44.3X6 |
| **Gelatin** (intravenous) | T45.8X1 | T45.8X2 | T45.8X3 | T45.8X4 | T45.8X5 | T45.8X6 |
| absorbable (sponge) | T45.7X1 | T45.7X2 | T45.7X3 | T45.7X4 | T45.7X5 | T45.7X6 |
| **Gelfilm** | T49.8X1 | T49.8X2 | T49.8X3 | T49.8X4 | T49.8X5 | T49.8X6 |
| **Gelfoam** | T45.7X1 | T45.7X2 | T45.7X3 | T45.7X4 | T45.7X5 | T45.7X6 |
| **Gelsemine** | T50.991 | T50.992 | T50.993 | T50.994 | T50.995 | T50.996 |
| **Gelsemium** (sempervirens) | T62.2X1 | T62.2X2 | T62.2X3 | T62.2X4 | — | — |
| **Gemeprost** | T48.0X1 | T48.0X2 | T48.0X3 | T48.0X4 | T48.0X5 | T48.0X6 |
| **Gemfibrozil** | T46.6X1 | T46.6X2 | T46.6X3 | T46.6X4 | T46.6X5 | T46.6X6 |
| **Gemonil** | T42.3X1 | T42.3X2 | T42.3X3 | T42.3X4 | T42.3X5 | T42.3X6 |
| **Gentamicin** | T36.5X1 | T36.5X2 | T36.5X3 | T36.5X4 | T36.5X5 | T36.5X6 |
| ophthalmic preparation | T49.5X1 | T49.5X2 | T49.5X3 | T49.5X4 | T49.5X5 | T49.5X6 |
| topical NEC | T49.0X1 | T49.0X2 | T49.0X3 | T49.0X4 | T49.0X5 | T49.0X6 |
| **Gentian** | T47.5X1 | T47.5X2 | T47.5X3 | T47.5X4 | T47.5X5 | T47.5X6 |
| violet | T49.0X1 | T49.0X2 | T49.0X3 | T49.0X4 | T49.0X5 | T49.0X6 |
| **Gepefrine** | T44.4X1 | T44.4X2 | T44.4X3 | T44.4X4 | T44.4X5 | T44.4X6 |
| **Gestonorone caproate** | T38.5X1 | T38.5X2 | T38.5X3 | T38.5X4 | T38.5X5 | T38.5X6 |
| **Gexane** | T49.0X1 | T49.0X2 | T49.0X3 | T49.0X4 | T49.0X5 | T49.0X6 |
| **Gila monster** (venom) | T63.111 | T63.112 | T63.113 | T63.114 | — | — |
| **Ginger** | T47.5X1 | T47.5X2 | T47.5X3 | T47.5X4 | T47.5X5 | T47.5X6 |
| Jamaica — see Jamaica, ginger | | | | | | |
| **Gitalin** | T46.0X1 | T46.0X2 | T46.0X3 | T46.0X4 | T46.0X5 | T46.0X6 |
| amorphous | T46.0X1 | T46.0X2 | T46.0X3 | T46.0X4 | T46.0X5 | T46.0X6 |
| **Gitaloxin** | T46.0X1 | T46.0X2 | T46.0X3 | T46.0X4 | T46.0X5 | T46.0X6 |
| **Gitoxin** | T46.0X1 | T46.0X2 | T46.0X3 | T46.0X4 | T46.0X5 | T46.0X6 |
| **Glafenine** | T39.8X1 | T39.8X2 | T39.8X3 | T39.8X4 | T39.8X5 | T39.8X6 |
| **Glandular extract** (medicinal) **NEC** | T50.Z91 | T50.Z92 | T50.Z93 | T50.Z94 | T50.Z95 | T50.Z96 |
| **Glaucarubin** | T37.3X1 | T37.3X2 | T37.3X3 | T37.3X4 | T37.3X5 | T37.3X6 |
| **Glibenclamide** | T38.3X1 | T38.3X2 | T38.3X3 | T38.3X4 | T38.3X5 | T38.3X6 |
| **Glibornuride** | T38.3X1 | T38.3X2 | T38.3X3 | T38.3X4 | T38.3X5 | T38.3X6 |
| **Gliclazide** | T38.3X1 | T38.3X2 | T38.3X3 | T38.3X4 | T38.3X5 | T38.3X6 |
| **Glimidine** | T38.3X1 | T38.3X2 | T38.3X3 | T38.3X4 | T38.3X5 | T38.3X6 |
| **Glipizide** | T38.3X1 | T38.3X2 | T38.3X3 | T38.3X4 | T38.3X5 | T38.3X6 |
| **Gliquidone** | T38.3X1 | T38.3X2 | T38.3X3 | T38.3X4 | T38.3X5 | T38.3X6 |
| **Glisolamide** | T38.3X1 | T38.3X2 | T38.3X3 | T38.3X4 | T38.3X5 | T38.3X6 |
| **Glisoxepide** | T38.3X1 | T38.3X2 | T38.3X3 | T38.3X4 | T38.3X5 | T38.3X6 |
| **Globin zinc insulin** | T38.3X1 | T38.3X2 | T38.3X3 | T38.3X4 | T38.3X5 | T38.3X6 |
| **Globulin** | | | | | | |
| antilymphocytic | T50.Z11 | T50.Z12 | T50.Z13 | T50.Z14 | T50.Z15 | T50.Z16 |
| antirhesus | T50.Z11 | T50.Z12 | T50.Z13 | T50.Z14 | T50.Z15 | T50.Z16 |
| antivenin | T50.Z11 | T50.Z12 | T50.Z13 | T50.Z14 | T50.Z15 | T50.Z16 |
| antiviral | T50.Z11 | T50.Z12 | T50.Z13 | T50.Z14 | T50.Z15 | T50.Z16 |

| Substance | Poisoning, Accidental (unintentional) | Poisoning, Intentional Self-harm | Poisoning, Assault | Poisoning, Undetermined | Adverse Effect | Under-dosing |
|---|---|---|---|---|---|---|
| Glucagon | T38.3X1 | T38.3X2 | T38.3X3 | T38.3X4 | T38.3X5 | T38.3X6 |
| Glucocorticoids | T38.0X1 | T38.0X2 | T38.0X3 | T38.0X4 | T38.0X5 | T38.0X6 |
| Glucocorticosteroid | T38.0X1 | T38.0X2 | T38.0X3 | T38.0X4 | T38.0X5 | T38.0X6 |
| Gluconic acid | T50.991 | T50.992 | T50.993 | T50.994 | T50.995 | T50.996 |
| Glucosamine sulfate | T39.4X1 | T39.4X2 | T39.4X3 | T39.4X4 | T39.4X5 | T39.4X6 |
| Glucose | T50.3X1 | T50.3X2 | T50.3X3 | T50.3X4 | T50.3X5 | T50.3X6 |
|   with sodium chloride | T50.3X1 | T50.3X2 | T50.3X3 | T50.3X4 | T50.3X5 | T50.3X6 |
| Glucosulfone sodium | T37.1X1 | T37.1X2 | T37.1X3 | T37.1X4 | T37.1X5 | T37.1X6 |
| Glucurolactone | T47.8X1 | T47.8X2 | T47.8X3 | T47.8X4 | T47.8X5 | T47.8X6 |
| Glue NEC | T52.8X1 | T52.8X2 | T52.8X3 | T52.8X4 | — | — |
| Glutamic acid | T47.5X1 | T47.5X2 | T47.5X3 | T47.5X4 | T47.5X5 | T47.5X6 |
| Glutaral (medicinal) | T49.0X1 | T49.0X2 | T49.0X3 | T49.0X4 | T49.0X5 | T49.0X6 |
|   nonmedicinal | T65.891 | T65.892 | T65.893 | T65.894 | — | — |
| Glutaraldehyde | T65.891 | T65.892 | T65.893 | T65.894 | — | — |
|   (nonmedicinal) | | | | | | |
|   medicinal | T49.0X1 | T49.0X2 | T49.0X3 | T49.0X4 | T49.0X5 | T49.0X6 |
| Glutathione | T50.6X1 | T50.6X2 | T50.6X3 | T50.6X4 | T50.6X5 | T50.6X6 |
| Glutethimide | T42.6X1 | T42.6X2 | T42.6X3 | T42.6X4 | T42.6X5 | T42.6X6 |
| Glyburide | T38.3X1 | T38.3X2 | T38.3X3 | T38.3X4 | T38.3X5 | T38.3X6 |
| Glycerin | T47.4X1 | T47.4X2 | T47.4X3 | T47.4X4 | T47.4X5 | T47.4X6 |
| Glycerol | T47.4X1 | T47.4X2 | T47.4X3 | T47.4X4 | T47.4X5 | T47.4X6 |
|   borax | T49.6X1 | T49.6X2 | T49.6X3 | T49.6X4 | T49.6X5 | T49.6X6 |
|   intravenous | T50.3X1 | T50.3X2 | T50.3X3 | T50.3X4 | T50.3X5 | T50.3X6 |
|   iodinated | T48.4X1 | T48.4X2 | T48.4X3 | T48.4X4 | T48.4X5 | T48.4X6 |
| Glycerophosphate | T50.991 | T50.992 | T50.993 | T50.994 | T50.995 | T50.996 |
| Glyceryl | | | | | | |
|   gualacolate | T48.4X1 | T48.4X2 | T48.4X3 | T48.4X4 | T48.4X5 | T48.4X6 |
|   nitrate | T46.3X1 | T46.3X2 | T46.3X3 | T46.3X4 | T46.3X5 | T46.3X6 |
|   triacetate (topical) | T49.0X1 | T49.0X2 | T49.0X3 | T49.0X4 | T49.0X5 | T49.0X6 |
|   trinitrate | T46.3X1 | T46.3X2 | T46.3X3 | T46.3X4 | T46.3X5 | T46.3X6 |
| Glycine | T50.3X1 | T50.3X2 | T50.3X3 | T50.3X4 | T50.3X5 | T50.3X6 |
| Glyclopyramide | T38.3X1 | T38.3X2 | T38.3X3 | T38.3X4 | T38.3X5 | T38.3X6 |
| Glycobiarsol | T37.3X1 | T37.3X2 | T37.3X3 | T37.3X4 | T37.3X5 | T37.3X6 |
| Glycols (ether) | T52.3X1 | T52.3X2 | T52.3X3 | T52.3X4 | — | — |
| Glyconiazide | T37.1X1 | T37.1X2 | T37.1X3 | T37.1X4 | T37.1X5 | T37.1X6 |
| Glycopyrrolate | T44.3X1 | T44.3X2 | T44.3X3 | T44.3X4 | T44.3X5 | T44.3X6 |
| Glycopyrronium | T44.3X1 | T44.3X2 | T44.3X3 | T44.3X4 | T44.3X5 | T44.3X6 |
|   bromide | T44.3X1 | T44.3X2 | T44.3X3 | T44.3X4 | T44.3X5 | T44.3X6 |
| Glycoside, cardiac | T46.0X1 | T46.0X2 | T46.0X3 | T46.0X4 | T46.0X5 | T46.0X6 |
|   (stimulant) | | | | | | |
| Glycyclamide | T38.3X1 | T38.3X2 | T38.3X3 | T38.3X4 | T38.3X5 | T38.3X6 |
| Glycyrrhiza extract | T48.4X1 | T48.4X2 | T48.4X3 | T48.4X4 | T48.4X5 | T48.4X6 |
| Glycyrrhizic acid | T48.4X1 | T48.4X2 | T48.4X3 | T48.4X4 | T48.4X5 | T48.4X6 |
| Glycyrrhizinate potassium | T48.4X1 | T48.4X2 | T48.4X3 | T48.4X4 | T48.4X5 | T48.4X6 |
| Glymidine sodium | T38.3X1 | T38.3X2 | T38.3X3 | T38.3X4 | T38.3X5 | T38.3X6 |
| Glyphosate | T60.3X1 | T60.3X2 | T60.3X3 | T60.3X4 | — | — |
| Glyphylline | T48.6X1 | T48.6X2 | T48.6X3 | T48.6X4 | T48.6X5 | T48.6X6 |
| Gold | | | | | | |
|   colloidal (I98Au) | T45.1X1 | T45.1X2 | T45.1X3 | T45.1X4 | T45.1X5 | T45.1X6 |
|   salts | T39.4X1 | T39.4X2 | T39.4X3 | T39.4X4 | T39.4X5 | T39.4X6 |
| Golden sulfide of antimony | T56.891 | T56.892 | T56.893 | T56.894 | — | — |
| Goldylocks | T62.2X1 | T62.2X2 | T62.2X3 | T62.2X4 | — | — |
| Gonadal tissue extract | T38.901 | T38.902 | T38.903 | T38.904 | T38.905 | T38.906 |
|   female | T38.5X1 | T38.5X2 | T38.5X3 | T38.5X4 | T38.5X5 | T38.5X6 |
|   male | T38.7X1 | T38.7X2 | T38.7X3 | T38.7X4 | T38.7X5 | T38.7X6 |
| Gonadorelin | T38.891 | T38.892 | T38.893 | T38.894 | T38.895 | T38.896 |
| Gonadotropin | T38.891 | T38.892 | T38.893 | T38.894 | T38.895 | T38.896 |
|   chorionic | T38.891 | T38.892 | T38.893 | T38.894 | T38.895 | T38.896 |
|   pituitary | T38.811 | T38.812 | T38.813 | T38.814 | T38.815 | T38.816 |
| Goserelin | T45.1X1 | T45.1X2 | T45.1X3 | T45.1X4 | T45.1X5 | T45.1X6 |
| Grain alcohol | T51.0X1 | T51.0X2 | T51.0X3 | T51.0X4 | — | — |
| Gramicidin | T49.0X1 | T49.0X2 | T49.0X3 | T49.0X4 | T49.0X5 | T49.0X6 |
| Granisetron | T45.0X1 | T45.0X2 | T45.0X3 | T45.0X4 | T45.0X5 | T45.0X6 |
| Gratiola officinalis | T62.2X1 | T62.2X2 | T62.2X3 | T62.2X4 | — | — |
| Grease | T65.891 | T65.892 | T65.893 | T65.894 | — | — |
| Green hellebore | T62.2X1 | T62.2X2 | T62.2X3 | T62.2X4 | — | — |
| Green soap | T49.2X1 | T49.2X2 | T49.2X3 | T49.2X4 | T49.2X5 | T49.2X6 |
| Grifulvin | T36.7X1 | T36.7X2 | T36.7X3 | T36.7X4 | T36.7X5 | T36.7X6 |
| Griseofulvin | T36.7X1 | T36.7X2 | T36.7X3 | T36.7X4 | T36.7X5 | T36.7X6 |
| Growth hormone | T38.811 | T38.812 | T38.813 | T38.814 | T38.815 | T38.816 |
| Guaiacol derivatives | T48.4X1 | T48.4X2 | T48.4X3 | T48.4X4 | T48.4X5 | T48.4X6 |
| Guaiac reagent | T50.991 | T50.992 | T50.993 | T50.994 | T50.995 | T50.996 |
| Guaifenesin | T48.4X1 | T48.4X2 | T48.4X3 | T48.4X4 | T48.4X5 | T48.4X6 |
| Guaimesal | T48.4X1 | T48.4X2 | T48.4X3 | T48.4X4 | T48.4X5 | T48.4X6 |
| Guaiphenesin | T48.4X1 | T48.4X2 | T48.4X3 | T48.4X4 | T48.4X5 | T48.4X6 |
| Guamecycline | T36.4X1 | T36.4X2 | T36.4X3 | T36.4X4 | T36.4X5 | T36.4X6 |
| Guanabenz | T46.5X1 | T46.5X2 | T46.5X3 | T46.5X4 | T46.5X5 | T46.5X6 |
| Guanacline | T46.5X1 | T46.5X2 | T46.5X3 | T46.5X4 | T46.5X5 | T46.5X6 |
| Guanadrel | T46.5X1 | T46.5X2 | T46.5X3 | T46.5X4 | T46.5X5 | T46.5X6 |
| Guanatol | T37.2X1 | T37.2X2 | T37.2X3 | T37.2X4 | T37.2X5 | T37.2X6 |
| Guanethidine | T46.5X1 | T46.5X2 | T46.5X3 | T46.5X4 | T46.5X5 | T46.5X6 |
| Guanfacine | T46.5X1 | T46.5X2 | T46.5X3 | T46.5X4 | T46.5X5 | T46.5X6 |
| Guano | T65.891 | T65.892 | T65.893 | T65.894 | — | — |

| Substance | Poisoning, Accidental (unintentional) | Poisoning, Intentional Self-harm | Poisoning, Assault | Poisoning, Undetermined | Adverse Effect | Under-dosing |
|---|---|---|---|---|---|---|
| Guanochlor | T46.5X1 | T46.5X2 | T46.5X3 | T46.5X4 | T46.5X5 | T46.5X6 |
| Guanoclor | T46.5X1 | T46.5X2 | T46.5X3 | T46.5X4 | T46.5X5 | T46.5X6 |
| Guanoctine | T46.5X1 | T46.5X2 | T46.5X3 | T46.5X4 | T46.5X5 | T46.5X6 |
| Guanoxabenz | T46.5X1 | T46.5X2 | T46.5X3 | T46.5X4 | T46.5X5 | T46.5X6 |
| Guanoxan | T46.5X1 | T46.5X2 | T46.5X3 | T46.5X4 | T46.5X5 | T46.5X6 |
| Guar gum (medicinal) | T46.6X1 | T46.6X2 | T46.6X3 | T46.6X4 | T46.6X5 | T46.6X6 |
| Hachimycin | T36.7X1 | T36.7X2 | T36.7X3 | T36.7X4 | T36.7X5 | T36.7X6 |
| Hair | | | | | | |
|   dye | T49.4X1 | T49.4X2 | T49.4X3 | T49.4X4 | T49.4X5 | T49.4X6 |
|   preparation NEC | T49.4X1 | T49.4X2 | T49.4X3 | T49.4X4 | T49.4X5 | T49.4X6 |
| Halazepam | T42.4X1 | T42.4X2 | T42.4X3 | T42.4X4 | T42.4X5 | T42.4X6 |
| Halcinolone | T49.0X1 | T49.0X2 | T49.0X3 | T49.0X4 | T49.0X5 | T49.0X6 |
| Halcinonide | T49.0X1 | T49.0X2 | T49.0X3 | T49.0X4 | T49.0X5 | T49.0X6 |
| Halethazole | T49.0X1 | T49.0X2 | T49.0X3 | T49.0X4 | T49.0X5 | T49.0X6 |
| Hallucinogen NEC | T40.901 | T40.902 | T40.903 | T40.904 | T40.905 | T40.906 |
| Halofantrine | T37.2X1 | T37.2X2 | T37.2X3 | T37.2X4 | T37.2X5 | T37.2X6 |
| Halofenate | T46.6X1 | T46.6X2 | T46.6X3 | T46.6X4 | T46.6X5 | T46.6X6 |
| Halometasone | T49.0X1 | T49.0X2 | T49.0X3 | T49.0X4 | T49.0X5 | T49.0X6 |
| Haloperidol | T43.4X1 | T43.4X2 | T43.4X3 | T43.4X4 | T43.4X5 | T43.4X6 |
| Haloprogin | T49.0X1 | T49.0X2 | T49.0X3 | T49.0X4 | T49.0X5 | T49.0X6 |
| Halotex | T49.0X1 | T49.0X2 | T49.0X3 | T49.0X4 | T49.0X5 | T49.0X6 |
| Halothane | T41.0X1 | T41.0X2 | T41.0X3 | T41.0X4 | T41.0X5 | T41.0X6 |
| Haloxazolam | T42.4X1 | T42.4X2 | T42.4X3 | T42.4X4 | T42.4X5 | T42.4X6 |
| Halquinols | T49.0X1 | T49.0X2 | T49.0X3 | T49.0X4 | T49.0X5 | T49.0X6 |
| Hamamelis | T49.2X1 | T49.2X2 | T49.2X3 | T49.2X4 | T49.2X5 | T49.2X6 |
| Haptendextran | T45.8X1 | T45.8X2 | T45.8X3 | T45.8X4 | T45.8X5 | T45.8X6 |
| Harmonyl | T46.5X1 | T46.5X2 | T46.5X3 | T46.5X4 | T46.5X5 | T46.5X6 |
| Hartmann's solution | T50.3X1 | T50.3X2 | T50.3X3 | T50.3X4 | T50.3X5 | T50.3X6 |
| Hashish | T40.7X1 | T40.7X2 | T40.7X3 | T40.7X4 | T40.7X5 | T40.7X6 |
| Hawaiian Woodrose seeds | T40.991 | T40.992 | T40.993 | T40.994 | — | — |
| HCB | T60.3X1 | T60.3X2 | T60.3X3 | T60.3X4 | — | — |
| HCH | T53.6X1 | T53.6X2 | T53.6X3 | T53.6X4 | — | — |
|   medicinal | T49.0X1 | T49.0X2 | T49.0X3 | T49.0X4 | T49.0X5 | T49.0X6 |
| HCN | T57.3X1 | T57.3X2 | T57.3X3 | T57.3X4 | — | — |
| Headache cures, drugs, powders NEC | T50.901 | T50.902 | T50.903 | T50.904 | T50.905 | T50.906 |
| Heavenly Blue (morning glory) | T40.991 | T40.992 | T40.993 | T40.994 | — | — |
| Heavy metal antidote | T45.8X1 | T45.8X2 | T45.8X3 | T45.8X4 | T45.8X5 | T45.8X6 |
| Hedaquinium | T49.0X1 | T49.0X2 | T49.0X3 | T49.0X4 | T49.0X5 | T49.0X6 |
| Hedge hyssop | T62.2X1 | T62.2X2 | T62.2X3 | T62.2X4 | — | — |
| Heet | T49.8X1 | T49.8X2 | T49.8X3 | T49.8X4 | T49.8X5 | T49.8X6 |
| Helenin | T37.4X1 | T37.4X2 | T37.4X3 | T37.4X4 | T37.4X5 | T37.4X6 |
| Helium (nonmedicinal) NEC | T59.891 | T59.892 | T59.893 | T59.894 | — | — |
|   medicinal | T48.991 | T48.992 | T48.993 | T48.994 | T48.995 | T48.996 |
| Hellebore (black) (green) (white) | T62.2X1 | T62.2X2 | T62.2X3 | T62.2X4 | — | — |
| Hematin | T45.8X1 | T45.8X2 | T45.8X3 | T45.8X4 | T45.8X5 | T45.8X6 |
| Hematinic preparation | T45.8X1 | T45.8X2 | T45.8X3 | T45.8X4 | T45.8X5 | T45.8X6 |
| Hematological agent | T45.91 | T45.92 | T45.93 | T45.94 | T45.95 | T45.96 |
|   specified NEC | T45.8X1 | T45.8X2 | T45.8X3 | T45.8X4 | T45.8X5 | T45.8X6 |
| Hemlock | T62.2X1 | T62.2X2 | T62.2X3 | T62.2X4 | — | — |
| Hemostatic | T45.621 | T45.622 | T45.623 | T45.624 | T45.625 | T45.626 |
|   drug, systemic | T45.621 | T45.622 | T45.623 | T45.624 | T45.625 | T45.626 |
| Hemostyptic | T49.4X1 | T49.4X2 | T49.4X3 | T49.4X4 | T49.4X5 | T49.4X6 |
| Henbane | T62.2X1 | T62.2X2 | T62.2X3 | T62.2X4 | — | — |
| Heparin (sodium) | T45.511 | T45.512 | T45.513 | T45.514 | T45.515 | T45.516 |
|   action reverser | T45.7X1 | T45.7X2 | T45.7X3 | T45.7X4 | T45.7X5 | T45.7X6 |
| Heparin-fraction | T45.511 | T45.512 | T45.513 | T45.514 | T45.515 | T45.516 |
| Heparinoid (systemic) | T45.511 | T45.512 | T45.513 | T45.514 | T45.515 | T45.516 |
| Hepatic secretion stimulant | T47.8X1 | T47.8X2 | T47.8X3 | T47.8X4 | T47.8X5 | T47.8X6 |
| Hepatitis B | | | | | | |
|   immune globulin | T50.Z11 | T50.Z12 | T50.Z13 | T50.Z14 | T50.Z15 | T50.Z16 |
|   vaccine | T50.B91 | T50.B92 | T50.B93 | T50.B94 | T50.B95 | T50.B96 |
| Hepronicate | T46.7X1 | T46.7X2 | T46.7X3 | T46.7X4 | T46.7X5 | T46.7X6 |
| Heptabarb | T42.3X1 | T42.3X2 | T42.3X3 | T42.3X4 | T42.3X5 | T42.3X6 |
| Heptabarbital | T42.3X1 | T42.3X2 | T42.3X3 | T42.3X4 | T42.3X5 | T42.3X6 |
| Heptabarbitone | T42.3X1 | T42.3X2 | T42.3X3 | T42.3X4 | T42.3X5 | T42.3X6 |
| Heptachlor | T60.1X1 | T60.1X2 | T60.1X3 | T60.1X4 | — | — |
| Heptalgin | T40.2X1 | T40.2X2 | T40.2X3 | T40.2X4 | T40.2X5 | T40.2X6 |
| Heptaminol | T46.3X1 | T46.3X2 | T46.3X3 | T46.3X4 | T46.3X5 | T46.3X6 |
| Herbicide NEC | T60.3X1 | T60.3X2 | T60.3X3 | T60.3X4 | — | — |
| Heroin | T40.1X1 | T40.1X2 | T40.1X3 | T40.1X4 | — | — |
| Herplex | T49.5X1 | T49.5X2 | T49.5X3 | T49.5X4 | T49.5X5 | T49.5X6 |
| HES | T45.8X1 | T45.8X2 | T45.8X3 | T45.8X4 | T45.8X5 | T45.8X6 |
| Hesperidin | T46.991 | T46.992 | T46.993 | T46.994 | T46.995 | T46.996 |
| Hetacillin | T36.0X1 | T36.0X2 | T36.0X3 | T36.0X4 | T36.0X5 | T36.0X6 |
| Hetastarch | T45.8X1 | T45.8X2 | T45.8X3 | T45.8X4 | T45.8X5 | T45.8X6 |
| HETP | T60.0X1 | T60.0X2 | T60.0X3 | T60.0X4 | — | — |
| Hexachlorobenzene (vapor) | T60.3X1 | T60.3X2 | T60.3X3 | T60.3X4 | — | — |
| Hexachlorocyclohexane | T53.6X1 | T53.6X2 | T53.6X3 | T53.6X4 | — | — |
| Hexachlorophene | T49.0X1 | T49.0X2 | T49.0X3 | T49.0X4 | T49.0X5 | T49.0X6 |

Table of Drugs and Chemicals

Hexadiline — Hydroxyprogesterone

| Substance | Poisoning, Accidental (unintentional) | Poisoning, Intentional Self-harm | Poisoning, Assault | Poisoning, Undetermined | Adverse Effect | Under-dosing |
|---|---|---|---|---|---|---|
| **Hexadiline** | T46.3X1 | T46.3X2 | T46.3X3 | T46.3X4 | T46.3X5 | T46.3X6 |
| **Hexadimethrine** (bromide) | T45.7X1 | T45.7X2 | T45.7X3 | T45.7X4 | T45.7X5 | T45.7X6 |
| **Hexadylamine** | T46.3X1 | T46.3X2 | T46.3X3 | T46.3X4 | T46.3X5 | T46.3X6 |
| **Hexaethyl tetraphosphate** | T60.0X1 | T60.0X2 | T60.0X3 | T60.0X4 | — | — |
| **Hexafluorenium bromide** | T48.1X1 | T48.1X2 | T48.1X3 | T48.1X4 | T48.1X5 | T48.1X6 |
| **Hexafluronium** (bromide) | T48.1X1 | T48.1X2 | T48.1X3 | T48.1X4 | T48.1X5 | T48.1X6 |
| **Hexa-germ** | T49.2X1 | T49.2X2 | T49.2X3 | T49.2X4 | T49.2X5 | T49.2X6 |
| **Hexahydrobenzol** | T52.8X1 | T52.8X2 | T52.8X3 | T52.8X4 | — | — |
| **Hexahydrocresol**(s) | T51.8X1 | T51.8X2 | T51.8X3 | T51.8X4 | — | — |
|   arsenide | T57.0X1 | T57.0X2 | T57.0X3 | T57.0X4 | — | — |
|   arseniurated | T57.0X1 | T57.0X2 | T57.0X3 | T57.0X4 | — | — |
|   cyanide | T57.3X1 | T57.3X2 | T57.3X3 | T57.3X4 | — | — |
|   gas | T59.891 | T59.892 | T59.893 | T59.894 | — | — |
|   Fluoride (liquid) | T57.8X1 | T57.8X2 | T57.8X3 | T57.8X4 | — | — |
|     vapor | T59.891 | T59.892 | T59.893 | T59.894 | — | — |
|   phophorated | T60.0X1 | T60.0X2 | T60.0X3 | T60.0X4 | — | — |
|   sulfate | T57.8X1 | T57.8X2 | T57.8X3 | T57.8X4 | — | — |
|   sulfide (gas) | T59.6X1 | T59.6X2 | T59.6X3 | T59.6X4 | — | — |
|     arseniurated | T57.0X1 | T57.0X2 | T57.0X3 | T57.0X4 | — | — |
|   sulfurated | T57.8X1 | T57.8X2 | T57.8X3 | T57.8X4 | — | — |
| **Hexahydrophenol** | T51.8X1 | T51.8X2 | T51.8X3 | T51.8X4 | — | — |
| **Hexalen** | T51.8X1 | T51.8X2 | T51.8X3 | T51.8X4 | — | — |
| **Hexamethonium bromide** | T44.2X1 | T44.2X2 | T44.2X3 | T44.2X4 | T44.2X5 | T44.2X6 |
| **Hexamethylene** | T52.8X1 | T52.8X2 | T52.8X3 | T52.8X4 | — | — |
| **Hexamethylmelamine** | T45.1X1 | T45.1X2 | T45.1X3 | T45.1X4 | T45.1X5 | T45.1X6 |
| **Hexamidine** | T49.0X1 | T49.0X2 | T49.0X3 | T49.0X4 | T49.0X5 | T49.0X6 |
| **Hexamine** (mandelate) | T37.8X1 | T37.8X2 | T37.8X3 | T37.8X4 | T37.8X5 | T37.8X6 |
| **Hexanone, 2-hexanone** | T52.4X1 | T52.4X2 | T52.4X3 | T52.4X4 | — | — |
| **Hexanuorenium** | T48.1X1 | T48.1X2 | T48.1X3 | T48.1X4 | T48.1X5 | T48.1X6 |
| **Hexapropymate** | T42.6X1 | T42.6X2 | T42.6X3 | T42.6X4 | T42.6X5 | T42.6X6 |
| **Hexasonium iodide** | T44.3X1 | T44.3X2 | T44.3X3 | T44.3X4 | T44.3X5 | T44.3X6 |
| **Hexcarbacholine bromide** | T48.1X1 | T48.1X2 | T48.1X3 | T48.1X4 | T48.1X5 | T48.1X6 |
| **Hexemal** | T42.3X1 | T42.3X2 | T42.3X3 | T42.3X4 | T42.3X5 | T42.3X6 |
| **Hexestrol** | T38.5X1 | T38.5X2 | T38.5X3 | T38.5X4 | T38.5X5 | T38.5X6 |
| **Hexethal** (sodium) | T42.3X1 | T42.3X2 | T42.3X3 | T42.3X4 | T42.3X5 | T42.3X6 |
| **Hexetidine** | T37.8X1 | T37.8X2 | T37.8X3 | T37.8X4 | T37.8X5 | T37.8X6 |
| **Hexobarbital** | T42.3X1 | T42.3X2 | T42.3X3 | T42.3X4 | T42.3X5 | T42.3X6 |
|   rectal | T41.291 | T41.292 | T41.293 | T41.294 | T41.295 | T41.296 |
|   sodium | T41.1X1 | T41.1X2 | T41.1X3 | T41.1X4 | T41.1X5 | T41.1X6 |
| **Hexobendine** | T46.3X1 | T46.3X2 | T46.3X3 | T46.3X4 | T46.3X5 | T46.3X6 |
| **Hexocyclium** | T44.3X1 | T44.3X2 | T44.3X3 | T44.3X4 | T44.3X5 | T44.3X6 |
|   metilsulfate | T44.3X1 | T44.3X2 | T44.3X3 | T44.3X4 | T44.3X5 | T44.3X6 |
| **Hexoestrol** | T38.5X1 | T38.5X2 | T38.5X3 | T38.5X4 | T38.5X5 | T38.5X6 |
| **Hexone** | T52.4X1 | T52.4X2 | T52.4X3 | T52.4X4 | — | — |
| **Hexoprenaline** | T48.6X1 | T48.6X2 | T48.6X3 | T48.6X4 | T48.6X5 | T48.6X6 |
| **Hexylcaine** | T41.3X1 | T41.3X2 | T41.3X3 | T41.3X4 | T41.3X5 | T41.3X6 |
| **Hexylresorcinol** | T52.2X1 | T52.2X2 | T52.2X3 | T52.2X4 | — | — |
| **HGH** (human growth hormone) | T38.811 | T38.812 | T38.813 | T38.814 | T38.815 | T38.816 |
| **Hinkle's pills** | T47.2X1 | T47.2X2 | T47.2X3 | T47.2X4 | T47.2X5 | T47.2X6 |
| **Histalog** | T50.8X1 | T50.8X2 | T50.8X3 | T50.8X4 | T50.8X5 | T50.8X6 |
| **Histamine** (phosphate) | T50.8X1 | T50.8X2 | T50.8X3 | T50.8X4 | T50.8X5 | T50.8X6 |
| **Histoplasmin** | T50.8X1 | T50.8X2 | T50.8X3 | T50.8X4 | T50.8X5 | T50.8X6 |
| **Holly berries** | T62.2X1 | T62.2X2 | T62.2X3 | T62.2X4 | — | — |
| **Homatropine** | T44.3X1 | T44.3X2 | T44.3X3 | T44.3X4 | T44.3X5 | T44.3X6 |
|   methylbromide | T44.3X1 | T44.3X2 | T44.3X3 | T44.3X4 | T44.3X5 | T44.3X6 |
| **Homochlorcyclizine** | T45.0X1 | T45.0X2 | T45.0X3 | T45.0X4 | T45.0X5 | T45.0X6 |
| **Homosalate** | T49.3X1 | T49.3X2 | T49.3X3 | T49.3X4 | T49.3X5 | T49.3X6 |
| **Homo-tet** | T50.Z11 | T50.Z12 | T50.Z13 | T50.Z14 | T50.Z15 | T50.Z16 |
| **Hormone** | T38.801 | T38.802 | T38.803 | T38.804 | T38.805 | T38.806 |
|   adrenal cortical steroids | T38.0X1 | T38.0X2 | T38.0X3 | T38.0X4 | T38.0X5 | T38.0X6 |
|   androgenic | T38.7X1 | T38.7X2 | T38.7X3 | T38.7X4 | T38.7X5 | T38.7X6 |
|   anterior pituitary NEC | T38.811 | T38.812 | T38.813 | T38.814 | T38.815 | T38.816 |
|   antidiabetic agents | T38.3X1 | T38.3X2 | T38.3X3 | T38.3X4 | T38.3X5 | T38.3X6 |
|   antidiuretic | T38.891 | T38.892 | T38.893 | T38.894 | T38.895 | T38.896 |
|   cancer therapy | T45.1X1 | T45.1X2 | T45.1X3 | T45.1X4 | T45.1X5 | T45.1X6 |
|   follicle stimulating | T38.811 | T38.812 | T38.813 | T38.814 | T38.815 | T38.816 |
|   gonadotropic | T38.891 | T38.892 | T38.893 | T38.894 | T38.895 | T38.896 |
|     pituitary | T38.811 | T38.812 | T38.813 | T38.814 | T38.815 | T38.816 |
|   growth | T38.811 | T38.812 | T38.813 | T38.814 | T38.815 | T38.816 |
|   luteinizing | T38.811 | T38.812 | T38.813 | T38.814 | T38.815 | T38.816 |
|   ovarian | T38.5X1 | T38.5X2 | T38.5X3 | T38.5X4 | T38.5X5 | T38.5X6 |
|   oxytocic | T48.0X1 | T48.0X2 | T48.0X3 | T48.0X4 | T48.0X5 | T48.0X6 |
|   parathyroid (derivatives) | T50.991 | T50.992 | T50.993 | T50.994 | T50.995 | T50.996 |
|   pituitary (posterior) NEC | T38.891 | T38.892 | T38.893 | T38.894 | T38.895 | T38.896 |
|     anterior | T38.811 | T38.812 | T38.813 | T38.814 | T38.815 | T38.816 |
|   specified, NEC | T38.891 | T38.892 | T38.893 | T38.894 | T38.895 | T38.896 |
|   thyroid | T38.1X1 | T38.1X2 | T38.1X3 | T38.1X4 | T38.1X5 | T38.1X6 |
| **Hornet** (sting) | T63.451 | T63.452 | T63.453 | T63.454 | — | — |
| **Horse anti-human lymphocytic serum** | T50.Z11 | T50.Z12 | T50.Z13 | T50.Z14 | T50.Z15 | T50.Z16 |
| **Horticulture agent NEC** | T65.91 | T65.92 | T65.93 | T65.94 | — | — |
|   with pesticide | T60.91 | T60.92 | T60.93 | T60.94 | — | — |

| Substance | Poisoning, Accidental (unintentional) | Poisoning, Intentional Self-harm | Poisoning, Assault | Poisoning, Undetermined | Adverse Effect | Under-dosing |
|---|---|---|---|---|---|---|
| **Human** | | | | | | |
|   albumin | T45.8X1 | T45.8X2 | T45.8X3 | T45.8X4 | T45.8X5 | T45.8X6 |
|   growth hormone (HGH) | T38.811 | T38.812 | T38.813 | T38.814 | T38.815 | T38.816 |
|   immune serum | T50.Z11 | T50.Z12 | T50.Z13 | T50.Z14 | T50.Z15 | T50.Z16 |
| **Hyaluronidase** | T45.3X1 | T45.3X2 | T45.3X3 | T45.3X4 | T45.3X5 | T45.3X6 |
| **Hyazyme** | T45.3X1 | T45.3X2 | T45.3X3 | T45.3X4 | T45.3X5 | T45.3X6 |
| **Hycodan** | T40.2X1 | T40.2X2 | T40.2X3 | T40.2X4 | T40.2X5 | T40.2X6 |
| **Hydantoin derivative NEC** | T42.0X1 | T42.0X2 | T42.0X3 | T42.0X4 | T42.0X5 | T42.0X6 |
| **Hydeltra** | T38.0X1 | T38.0X2 | T38.0X3 | T38.0X4 | T38.0X5 | T38.0X6 |
| **Hydergine** | T44.6X1 | T44.6X2 | T44.6X3 | T44.6X4 | T44.6X5 | T44.6X6 |
| **Hydrabamine penicillin** | T36.0X1 | T36.0X2 | T36.0X3 | T36.0X4 | T36.0X5 | T36.0X6 |
| **Hydralazine** | T46.5X1 | T46.5X2 | T46.5X3 | T46.5X4 | T46.5X5 | T46.5X6 |
| **Hydrargaphen** | T49.0X1 | T49.0X2 | T49.0X3 | T49.0X4 | T49.0X5 | T49.0X6 |
| **Hydrargyri aminochloridum** | T49.0X1 | T49.0X2 | T49.0X3 | T49.0X4 | T49.0X5 | T49.0X6 |
| **Hydrastine** | T48.291 | T48.292 | T48.293 | T48.294 | T48.295 | T48.296 |
| **Hydrazine** | T54.1X1 | T54.1X2 | T54.1X3 | T54.1X4 | — | — |
|   monoamine oxidase inhibitors | T43.1X1 | T43.1X2 | T43.1X3 | T43.1X4 | T43.1X5 | T43.1X6 |
| **Hydrazoic acid, azides** | T54.2X1 | T54.2X2 | T54.2X3 | T54.2X4 | — | — |
| **Hydriodic acid** | T48.4X1 | T48.4X2 | T48.4X3 | T48.4X4 | T48.4X5 | T48.4X6 |
| **Hydrocarbon gas** | T59.891 | T59.892 | T59.893 | T59.894 | — | — |
|   incomplete combustion of — *see* Carbon, monoxide, fuel, utility | | | | | | |
|   liquefied (mobile container) | T59.891 | T59.892 | T59.893 | T59.894 | — | — |
|   piped (natural) | T59.891 | T59.892 | T59.893 | T59.894 | — | — |
| **Hydrochloric acid** (liquid) | T54.2X1 | T54.2X2 | T54.2X3 | T54.2X4 | — | — |
|   medicinal (digestant) | T47.5X1 | T47.5X2 | T47.5X3 | T47.5X4 | T47.5X5 | T47.5X6 |
|   vapor | T59.891 | T59.892 | T59.893 | T59.894 | — | — |
| **Hydrochlorothiazide** | T50.2X1 | T50.2X2 | T50.2X3 | T50.2X4 | T50.2X5 | T50.2X6 |
| **Hydrocodone** | T40.2X1 | T40.2X2 | T40.2X3 | T40.2X4 | T40.2X5 | T40.2X6 |
| **Hydrocortisone** (derivatives) | T38.0X1 | T38.0X2 | T38.0X3 | T38.0X4 | T38.0X5 | T38.0X6 |
|   aceponate | T49.0X1 | T49.0X2 | T49.0X3 | T49.0X4 | T49.0X5 | T49.0X6 |
|   ENT agent | T49.6X1 | T49.6X2 | T49.6X3 | T49.6X4 | T49.6X5 | T49.6X6 |
|   ophthalmic preparation | T49.5X1 | T49.5X2 | T49.5X3 | T49.5X4 | T49.5X5 | T49.5X6 |
|   topical NEC | T49.0X1 | T49.0X2 | T49.0X3 | T49.0X4 | T49.0X5 | T49.0X6 |
| **Hydrocortone** | T38.0X1 | T38.0X2 | T38.0X3 | T38.0X4 | T38.0X5 | T38.0X6 |
|   ENT agent | T49.6X1 | T49.6X2 | T49.6X3 | T49.6X4 | T49.6X5 | T49.6X6 |
|   ophthalmic preparation | T49.5X1 | T49.5X2 | T49.5X3 | T49.5X4 | T49.5X5 | T49.5X6 |
|   topical NEC | T49.0X1 | T49.0X2 | T49.0X3 | T49.0X4 | T49.0X5 | T49.0X6 |
| **Hydrocyanic acid** (liquid) | T57.3X1 | T57.3X2 | T57.3X3 | T57.3X4 | — | — |
|   gas | T65.0X1 | T65.0X2 | T65.0X3 | T65.0X4 | — | — |
| **Hydroflumethiazide** | T50.2X1 | T50.2X2 | T50.2X3 | T50.2X4 | T50.2X5 | T50.2X6 |
| **Hydrofluoric acid** (liquid) | T54.2X1 | T54.2X2 | T54.2X3 | T54.2X4 | — | — |
|   vapor | T59.891 | T59.892 | T59.893 | T59.894 | — | — |
| **Hydrogen** | T59.891 | T59.892 | T59.893 | T59.894 | — | — |
|   arsenide | T57.0X1 | T57.0X2 | T57.0X3 | T57.0X4 | — | — |
|   arseniureted | T57.0X1 | T57.0X2 | T57.0X3 | T57.0X4 | — | — |
|   chloride | T57.8X1 | T57.8X2 | T57.8X3 | T57.8X4 | — | — |
|   cyanide (salts) | T57.3X1 | T57.3X2 | T57.3X3 | T57.3X4 | — | — |
|     gas | T57.3X1 | T57.3X2 | T57.3X3 | T57.3X4 | — | — |
|   Fluoride | T59.5X1 | T59.5X2 | T59.5X3 | T59.5X4 | — | — |
|     vapor | T59.5X1 | T59.5X2 | T59.5X3 | T59.5X4 | — | — |
|   peroxide | T49.0X1 | T49.0X2 | T49.0X3 | T49.0X4 | T49.0X5 | T49.0X6 |
|   phosphureted | T57.1X1 | T57.1X2 | T57.1X3 | T57.1X4 | — | — |
|   sulfide | T59.6X1 | T59.6X2 | T59.6X3 | T59.6X4 | — | — |
|     arseniureted | T57.0X1 | T57.0X2 | T57.0X3 | T57.0X4 | — | — |
|   sulfureted | T59.6X1 | T59.6X2 | T59.6X3 | T59.6X4 | — | — |
| **Hydromethylpyridine** | T46.7X1 | T46.7X2 | T46.7X3 | T46.7X4 | T46.7X5 | T46.7X6 |
| **Hydromorphinol** | T40.2X1 | T40.2X2 | T40.2X3 | T40.2X4 | — | — |
| **Hydromorphinone** | T40.2X1 | T40.2X2 | T40.2X3 | T40.2X4 | T40.2X5 | T40.2X6 |
| **Hydromorphone** | T40.2X1 | T40.2X2 | T40.2X3 | T40.2X4 | T40.2X5 | T40.2X6 |
| **Hydromox** | T50.2X1 | T50.2X2 | T50.2X3 | T50.2X4 | T50.2X5 | T50.2X6 |
| **Hydrophilic lotion** | T49.3X1 | T49.3X2 | T49.3X3 | T49.3X4 | T49.3X5 | T49.3X6 |
| **Hydroquinidine** | T46.2X1 | T46.2X2 | T46.2X3 | T46.2X4 | T46.2X5 | T46.2X6 |
| **Hydroquinone** | T52.2X1 | T52.2X2 | T52.2X3 | T52.2X4 | — | — |
|   vapor | T59.891 | T59.892 | T59.893 | T59.894 | — | — |
| **Hydrosulfuric acid** (gas) | T59.6X1 | T59.6X2 | T59.6X3 | T59.6X4 | — | — |
| **Hydrotalcite** | T47.1X1 | T47.1X2 | T47.1X3 | T47.1X4 | T47.1X5 | T47.1X6 |
| **Hydrous wool fat** | T49.3X1 | T49.3X2 | T49.3X3 | T49.3X4 | T49.3X5 | T49.3X6 |
| **Hydroxide, caustic** | T54.3X1 | T54.3X2 | T54.3X3 | T54.3X4 | — | — |
| **Hydroxocobalamin** | T45.8X1 | T45.8X2 | T45.8X3 | T45.8X4 | T45.8X5 | T45.8X6 |
| **Hydroxyamphetamine** | T49.5X1 | T49.5X2 | T49.5X3 | T49.5X4 | T49.5X5 | T49.5X6 |
| **Hydroxycarbamide** | T45.1X1 | T45.1X2 | T45.1X3 | T45.1X4 | T45.1X5 | T45.1X6 |
| **Hydroxychloroquine** | T37.8X1 | T37.8X2 | T37.8X3 | T37.8X4 | T37.8X5 | T37.8X6 |
| **Hydroxydihydrocodeinone** | T40.2X1 | T40.2X2 | T40.2X3 | T40.2X4 | T40.2X5 | T40.2X6 |
| **Hydroxyestrone** | T38.5X1 | T38.5X2 | T38.5X3 | T38.5X4 | T38.5X5 | T38.5X6 |
| **Hydroxyethyl starch** | T45.8X1 | T45.8X2 | T45.8X3 | T45.8X4 | T45.8X5 | T45.8X6 |
| **Hydroxymethylpentanone** | T52.4X1 | T52.4X2 | T52.4X3 | T52.4X4 | — | — |
| **Hydroxyphenamate** | T43.591 | T43.592 | T43.593 | T43.594 | T43.595 | T43.596 |
| **Hydroxyphenylbutazone** | T39.2X1 | T39.2X2 | T39.2X3 | T39.2X4 | T39.2X5 | T39.2X6 |
| **Hydroxyprogesterone** | T38.5X1 | T38.5X2 | T38.5X3 | T38.5X4 | T38.5X5 | T38.5X6 |

| Substance | Poisoning, Accidental (unintentional) | Poisoning, Intentional Self-harm | Poisoning, Assault | Poisoning, Undetermined | Adverse Effect | Under-dosing |
|---|---|---|---|---|---|---|
| **Hydroxyprogesterone** — *continued* | | | | | | |
| caproate | T38.5X1 | T38.5X2 | T38.5X3 | T38.5X4 | T38.5X5 | T38.5X6 |
| **Hydroxyquinoline** (derivatives) **NEC** | T37.8X1 | T37.8X2 | T37.8X3 | T37.8X4 | T37.8X5 | T37.8X6 |
| **Hydroxystilbamidine** | T37.3X1 | T37.3X2 | T37.3X3 | T37.3X4 | T37.3X5 | T37.3X6 |
| **Hydroxytoluene** (nonmedicinal) | T54.0X1 | T54.0X2 | T54.0X3 | T54.0X4 | — | — |
| medicinal | T49.0X1 | T49.0X2 | T49.0X3 | T49.0X4 | T49.0X5 | T49.0X6 |
| **Hydroxyurea** | T45.1X1 | T45.1X2 | T45.1X3 | T45.1X4 | T45.1X5 | T45.1X6 |
| **Hydroxyzine** | T43.591 | T43.592 | T43.593 | T43.594 | T43.595 | T43.596 |
| **Hyoscine** | T44.3X1 | T44.3X2 | T44.3X3 | T44.3X4 | T44.3X5 | T44.3X6 |
| **Hyoscyamine** | T44.3X1 | T44.3X2 | T44.3X3 | T44.3X4 | T44.3X5 | T44.3X6 |
| **Hyoscyamus** | T44.3X1 | T44.3X2 | T44.3X3 | T44.3X4 | T44.3X5 | T44.3X6 |
| dry extract | T44.3X1 | T44.3X2 | T44.3X3 | T44.3X4 | T44.3X5 | T44.3X6 |
| **Hypaque** | T50.8X1 | T50.8X2 | T50.8X3 | T50.8X4 | T50.8X5 | T50.8X6 |
| **Hypertussis** | T50.Z11 | T50.Z12 | T50.Z13 | T50.Z14 | T50.Z15 | T50.Z16 |
| **Hypnotic** | T42.71 | T42.72 | T42.73 | T42.74 | T42.75 | T42.76 |
| anticonvulsant | T42.71 | T42.72 | T42.73 | T42.74 | T42.75 | T42.76 |
| specified NEC | T42.6X1 | T42.6X2 | T42.6X3 | T42.6X4 | T42.6X5 | T42.6X6 |
| **Hypochlorite** | T49.0X1 | T49.0X2 | T49.0X3 | T49.0X4 | T49.0X5 | T49.0X6 |
| **Hypophysis, posterior** | T38.891 | T38.892 | T38.893 | T38.894 | T38.895 | T38.896 |
| **Hypotensive NEC** | T46.5X1 | T46.5X2 | T46.5X3 | T46.5X4 | T46.5X5 | T46.5X6 |
| **Hypromellose** | T49.5X1 | T49.5X2 | T49.5X3 | T49.5X4 | T49.5X5 | T49.5X6 |
| **Ibacitabine** | T37.5X1 | T37.5X2 | T37.5X3 | T37.5X4 | T37.5X5 | T37.5X6 |
| **Ibopamine** | T44.991 | T44.992 | T44.993 | T44.994 | T44.995 | T44.996 |
| **Ibufenac** | T39.311 | T39.312 | T39.313 | T39.314 | T39.315 | T39.316 |
| **Ibuprofen** | T39.311 | T39.312 | T39.313 | T39.314 | T39.315 | T39.316 |
| **Ibuproxam** | T39.311 | T39.312 | T39.313 | T39.314 | T39.315 | T39.316 |
| **Ibuterol** | T48.6X1 | T48.6X2 | T48.6X3 | T48.6X4 | T48.6X5 | T48.6X6 |
| **Ichthammol** | T49.0X1 | T49.0X2 | T49.0X3 | T49.0X4 | T49.0X5 | T49.0X6 |
| **Ichthyol** | T49.4X1 | T49.4X2 | T49.4X3 | T49.4X4 | T49.4X5 | T49.4X6 |
| **Idarubicin** | T45.1X1 | T45.1X2 | T45.1X3 | T45.1X4 | T45.1X5 | T45.1X6 |
| **Idrocilamide** | T42.8X1 | T42.8X2 | T42.8X3 | T42.8X4 | T42.8X5 | T42.8X6 |
| **Ifenprodil** | T46.7X1 | T46.7X2 | T46.7X3 | T46.7X4 | T46.7X5 | T46.7X6 |
| **Ifosfamide** | T45.1X1 | T45.1X2 | T45.1X3 | T45.1X4 | T45.1X5 | T45.1X6 |
| **Iletin** | T38.3X1 | T38.3X2 | T38.3X3 | T38.3X4 | T38.3X5 | T38.3X6 |
| **Ilex** | T62.2X1 | T62.2X2 | T62.2X3 | T62.2X4 | — | — |
| **Illuminating gas** (after combustion) | T58.11 | T58.12 | T58.13 | T58.14 | — | — |
| prior to combustion | T59.891 | T59.892 | T59.893 | T59.894 | — | — |
| **Ilopan** | T45.2X1 | T45.2X2 | T45.2X3 | T45.2X4 | T45.2X5 | T45.2X6 |
| **Iloprost** | T46.7X1 | T46.7X2 | T46.7X3 | T46.7X4 | T46.7X5 | T46.7X6 |
| **Ilotycin** | T36.3X1 | T36.3X2 | T36.3X3 | T36.3X4 | T36.3X5 | T36.3X6 |
| ophthalmic preparation | T49.5X1 | T49.5X2 | T49.5X3 | T49.5X4 | T49.5X5 | T49.5X6 |
| topical NEC | T49.0X1 | T49.0X2 | T49.0X3 | T49.0X4 | T49.0X5 | T49.0X6 |
| **Imidazole-4-carboxamide** | T45.1X1 | T45.1X2 | T45.1X3 | T45.1X4 | T45.1X5 | T45.1X6 |
| **Iminostilbene** | T42.1X1 | T42.1X2 | T42.1X3 | T42.1X4 | T42.1X5 | T42.1X6 |
| **Imipenem** | T36.0X1 | T36.0X2 | T36.0X3 | T36.0X4 | T36.0X5 | T36.0X6 |
| **Imipramine** | T43.011 | T43.012 | T43.013 | T43.014 | T43.015 | T43.016 |
| **Immu-G** | T50.Z11 | T50.Z12 | T50.Z13 | T50.Z14 | T50.Z15 | T50.Z16 |
| **Immuglobin** | T50.Z11 | T50.Z12 | T50.Z13 | T50.Z14 | T50.Z15 | T50.Z16 |
| **Immune** | | | | | | |
| globulin | T50.Z11 | T50.Z12 | T50.Z13 | T50.Z14 | T50.Z15 | T50.Z16 |
| serum globulin | T50.Z11 | T50.Z12 | T50.Z13 | T50.Z14 | T50.Z15 | T50.Z16 |
| **Immunoglobin human** (intravenous) (normal) | T50.Z11 | T50.Z12 | T50.Z13 | T50.Z14 | T50.Z15 | T50.Z16 |
| unmodified | T50.Z11 | T50.Z12 | T50.Z13 | T50.Z14 | T50.Z15 | T50.Z16 |
| **Immunosuppressive drug** | T45.1X1 | T45.1X2 | T45.1X3 | T45.1X4 | T45.1X5 | T45.1X6 |
| **Immu-tetanus** | T50.Z11 | T50.Z12 | T50.Z13 | T50.Z14 | T50.Z15 | T50.Z16 |
| **Indalpine** | T43.221 | T43.222 | T43.223 | T43.224 | T43.225 | T43.226 |
| **Indanazoline** | T48.5X1 | T48.5X2 | T48.5X3 | T48.5X4 | T48.5X5 | T48.5X6 |
| **Indandione** (derivatives) | T45.511 | T45.512 | T45.513 | T45.514 | T45.515 | T45.516 |
| **Indapamide** | T46.5X1 | T46.5X2 | T46.5X3 | T46.5X4 | T46.5X5 | T46.5X6 |
| **Indendione** (derivatives) | T45.511 | T45.512 | T45.513 | T45.514 | T45.515 | T45.516 |
| **Indenolol** | T44.7X1 | T44.7X2 | T44.7X3 | T44.7X4 | T44.7X5 | T44.7X6 |
| **Inderal** | T44.7X1 | T44.7X2 | T44.7X3 | T44.7X4 | T44.7X5 | T44.7X6 |
| **Indian** | | | | | | |
| hemp | T40.7X1 | T40.7X2 | T40.7X3 | T40.7X4 | T40.7X5 | T40.7X6 |
| tobacco | T62.2X1 | T62.2X2 | T62.2X3 | T62.2X4 | — | — |
| **Indigo carmine** | T50.8X1 | T50.8X2 | T50.8X3 | T50.8X4 | T50.8X5 | T50.8X6 |
| **Indobufen** | T45.521 | T45.522 | T45.523 | T45.524 | T45.525 | T45.526 |
| **Indocin** | T39.2X1 | T39.2X2 | T39.2X3 | T39.2X4 | T39.2X5 | T39.2X6 |
| **Indocyanine green** | T50.8X1 | T50.8X2 | T50.8X3 | T50.8X4 | T50.8X5 | T50.8X6 |
| **Indometacin** | T39.391 | T39.392 | T39.393 | T39.394 | T39.395 | T39.396 |
| **Indomethacin** | T39.391 | T39.392 | T39.393 | T39.394 | T39.395 | T39.396 |
| farnesil | T39.4X1 | T39.4X2 | T39.4X3 | T39.4X4 | T39.4X5 | T39.4X6 |
| **Indoramin** | T44.6X1 | T44.6X2 | T44.6X3 | T44.6X4 | T44.6X5 | T44.6X6 |
| **Industrial** | | | | | | |
| alcohol | T51.0X1 | T51.0X2 | T51.0X3 | T51.0X4 | — | — |
| fumes | T59.891 | T59.892 | T59.893 | T59.894 | — | — |
| solvents (fumes) (vapors) | T52.91 | T52.92 | T52.93 | T52.94 | — | — |
| **Influenza vaccine** | T50.B91 | T50.B92 | T50.B93 | T50.B94 | T50.B95 | T50.B96 |

| Substance | Poisoning, Accidental (unintentional) | Poisoning, Intentional Self-harm | Poisoning, Assault | Poisoning, Undetermined | Adverse Effect | Under-dosing |
|---|---|---|---|---|---|---|
| **Ingested substance NEC** | T65.91 | T65.92 | T65.93 | T65.94 | — | — |
| **INH** | T37.1X1 | T37.1X2 | T37.1X3 | T37.1X4 | T37.1X5 | T37.1X6 |
| **Inhalation, gas** (noxious) — *see* Gas | | | | | | |
| **Inhibitor** | | | | | | |
| angiotensin-converting enzyme | T46.4X1 | T46.4X2 | T46.4X3 | T46.4X4 | T46.4X5 | T46.4X6 |
| carbonic anhydrase | T50.2X1 | T50.2X2 | T50.2X3 | T50.2X4 | T50.2X5 | T50.2X6 |
| fibrinolysis | T45.621 | T45.622 | T45.623 | T45.624 | T45.625 | T45.626 |
| monoamine oxidase NEC | T43.1X1 | T43.1X2 | T43.1X3 | T43.1X4 | T43.1X5 | T43.1X6 |
| hydrazine | T43.1X1 | T43.1X2 | T43.1X3 | T43.1X4 | T43.1X5 | T43.1X6 |
| postsynaptic | T43.8X1 | T43.8X2 | T43.8X3 | T43.8X4 | T43.8X5 | T43.8X6 |
| prothrombin synthesis | T45.511 | T45.512 | T45.513 | T45.514 | T45.515 | T45.516 |
| **Ink** | T65.891 | T65.892 | T65.893 | T65.894 | — | — |
| **Inorganic substance NEC** | T57.91 | T57.92 | T57.93 | T57.94 | — | — |
| **Inosine pranobex** | T37.5X1 | T37.5X2 | T37.5X3 | T37.5X4 | T37.5X5 | T37.5X6 |
| **Inositol** | T50.991 | T50.992 | T50.993 | T50.994 | T50.995 | T50.996 |
| nicotinate | T46.7X1 | T46.7X2 | T46.7X3 | T46.7X4 | T46.7X5 | T46.7X6 |
| **Inproquone** | T45.1X1 | T45.1X2 | T45.1X3 | T45.1X4 | T45.1X5 | T45.1X6 |
| **Insecticide NEC** | T60.91 | T60.92 | T60.93 | T60.94 | — | — |
| carbamate | T60.0X1 | T60.0X2 | T60.0X3 | T60.0X4 | — | — |
| chlorinated | T60.1X1 | T60.1X2 | T60.1X3 | T60.1X4 | — | — |
| mixed | T60.91 | T60.92 | T60.93 | T60.94 | — | — |
| organochlorine | T60.1X1 | T60.1X2 | T60.1X3 | T60.1X4 | — | — |
| organophosphorus | T60.0X1 | T60.0X2 | T60.0X3 | T60.0X4 | — | — |
| **Insect** (sting), venomous | T63.481 | T63.482 | T63.483 | T63.484 | — | — |
| ant | T63.421 | T63.422 | T63.423 | T63.424 | — | — |
| bee | T63.441 | T63.442 | T63.443 | T63.444 | — | — |
| caterpillar | T63.431 | T63.432 | T63.433 | T63.434 | — | — |
| hornet | T63.451 | T63.452 | T63.453 | T63.454 | — | — |
| wasp | T63.461 | T63.462 | T63.463 | T63.464 | — | — |
| **Insular tissue extract** | T38.3X1 | T38.3X2 | T38.3X3 | T38.3X4 | T38.3X5 | T38.3X6 |
| **Insulin** (amorphous) (globin) (isophane) (Lente) (NPH) (Semilente) (Ultralente) | T38.3X1 | T38.3X2 | T38.3X3 | T38.3X4 | T38.3X5 | T38.3X6 |
| defalan | T38.3X1 | T38.3X2 | T38.3X3 | T38.3X4 | T38.3X5 | T38.3X6 |
| human | T38.3X1 | T38.3X2 | T38.3X3 | T38.3X4 | T38.3X5 | T38.3X6 |
| injection, soluble | T38.3X1 | T38.3X2 | T38.3X3 | T38.3X4 | T38.3X5 | T38.3X6 |
| biphasic | T38.3X1 | T38.3X2 | T38.3X3 | T38.3X4 | T38.3X5 | T38.3X6 |
| intermediate acting | T38.3X1 | T38.3X2 | T38.3X3 | T38.3X4 | T38.3X5 | T38.3X6 |
| protamine zinc | T38.3X1 | T38.3X2 | T38.3X3 | T38.3X4 | T38.3X5 | T38.3X6 |
| slow acting | T38.3X1 | T38.3X2 | T38.3X3 | T38.3X4 | T38.3X5 | T38.3X6 |
| zinc | | | | | | |
| protamine injection | T38.3X1 | T38.3X2 | T38.3X3 | T38.3X4 | T38.3X5 | T38.3X6 |
| suspension (amorphous) (crystalline) | T38.3X1 | T38.3X2 | T38.3X3 | T38.3X4 | T38.3X5 | T38.3X6 |
| **Interferon** (alpha) (beta) (gamma) | T37.5X1 | T37.5X2 | T37.5X3 | T37.5X4 | T37.5X5 | T37.5X6 |
| **Intestinal motility control drug** | T47.6X1 | T47.6X2 | T47.6X3 | T47.6X4 | T47.6X5 | T47.6X6 |
| biological | T47.8X1 | T47.8X2 | T47.8X3 | T47.8X4 | T47.8X5 | T47.8X6 |
| **Intranarcon** | T41.1X1 | T41.1X2 | T41.1X3 | T41.1X4 | T41.1X5 | T41.1X6 |
| **Intravenous** | | | | | | |
| amino acids | T50.991 | T50.992 | T50.993 | T50.994 | T50.995 | T50.996 |
| fat suspension | T50.991 | T50.992 | T50.993 | T50.994 | T50.995 | T50.996 |
| **Inulin** | T50.8X1 | T50.8X2 | T50.8X3 | T50.8X4 | T50.8X5 | T50.8X6 |
| **Invert sugar** | T50.3X1 | T50.3X2 | T50.3X3 | T50.3X4 | T50.3X5 | T50.3X6 |
| **Inza** — *see* Naproxen | | | | | | |
| **Iobenzamic acid** | T50.8X1 | T50.8X2 | T50.8X3 | T50.8X4 | T50.8X5 | T50.8X6 |
| **Iocarmic acid** | T50.8X1 | T50.8X2 | T50.8X3 | T50.8X4 | T50.8X5 | T50.8X6 |
| **Iocetamic acid** | T50.8X1 | T50.8X2 | T50.8X3 | T50.8X4 | T50.8X5 | T50.8X6 |
| **Iodamide** | T50.8X1 | T50.8X2 | T50.8X3 | T50.8X4 | T50.8X5 | T50.8X6 |
| **Iodide NEC** — *see also* Iodine | T49.0X1 | T49.0X2 | T49.0X3 | T49.0X4 | T49.0X5 | T49.0X6 |
| mercury (ointment) | T49.0X1 | T49.0X2 | T49.0X3 | T49.0X4 | T49.0X5 | T49.0X6 |
| methylate | T49.0X1 | T49.0X2 | T49.0X3 | T49.0X4 | T49.0X5 | T49.0X6 |
| potassium (expectorant) NEC | T48.4X1 | T48.4X2 | T48.4X3 | T48.4X4 | T48.4X5 | T48.4X6 |
| **Iodinated** | | | | | | |
| contrast medium | T50.8X1 | T50.8X2 | T50.8X3 | T50.8X4 | T50.8X5 | T50.8X6 |
| glycerol | T48.4X1 | T48.4X2 | T48.4X3 | T48.4X4 | T48.4X5 | T48.4X6 |
| human serum albumin (131I) | T50.8X1 | T50.8X2 | T50.8X3 | T50.8X4 | T50.8X5 | T50.8X6 |
| **Iodine** (antiseptic, external) (tincture) **NEC** | T49.0X1 | T49.0X2 | T49.0X3 | T49.0X4 | T49.0X5 | T49.0X6 |
| 125 — *see also* Radiation sickness, and Exposure to radioactivce isotopes | T50.8X1 | T50.8X2 | T50.8X3 | T50.8X4 | T50.8X5 | T50.8X6 |
| therapeutic | T50.991 | T50.992 | T50.993 | T50.994 | T50.995 | T50.996 |
| 131 — *see also* Radiation sickness, and Exposure to radioactivce isotopes | T50.8X1 | T50.8X2 | T50.8X3 | T50.8X4 | T50.8X5 | T50.8X6 |
| therapeutic | T38.2X1 | T38.2X2 | T38.2X3 | T38.2X4 | T38.2X5 | T38.2X6 |
| diagnostic | T50.8X1 | T50.8X2 | T50.8X3 | T50.8X4 | T50.8X5 | T50.8X6 |

▽ Subterms under main terms may continue to next column or page          Additional Character May Be Required — Refer to the Tabular List for Character Selection          373

Hydroxyprogesterone — Iodine

Table of Drugs and Chemicals

| Substance | Poisoning, Accidental (unintentional) | Poisoning, Intentional Self-harm | Poisoning, Assault | Poisoning, Undetermined | Adverse Effect | Under-dosing |
|---|---|---|---|---|---|---|
| **Iodine** (antiseptic, external) (tincture) **NEC** — *continued* | | | | | | |
| for thyroid conditions (antithyroid) | T38.2X1 | T38.2X2 | T38.2X3 | T38.2X4 | T38.2X5 | T38.2X6 |
| solution | T49.0X1 | T49.0X2 | T49.0X3 | T49.0X4 | T49.0X5 | T49.0X6 |
| vapor | T59.891 | T59.892 | T59.893 | T59.894 | — | — |
| **Iodipamide** | T50.8X1 | T50.8X2 | T50.8X3 | T50.8X4 | T50.8X5 | T50.8X6 |
| **Iodized** (poppy seed) oil | T50.8X1 | T50.8X2 | T50.8X3 | T50.8X4 | T50.8X5 | T50.8X6 |
| **Iodobismitol** | T37.8X1 | T37.8X2 | T37.8X3 | T37.8X4 | T37.8X5 | T37.8X6 |
| **Iodochlorhydroxyquin** | T37.8X1 | T37.8X2 | T37.8X3 | T37.8X4 | T37.8X5 | T37.8X6 |
| topical | T49.0X1 | T49.0X2 | T49.0X3 | T49.0X4 | T49.0X5 | T49.0X6 |
| **Iodochlorhydroxyquinoline** | T37.8X1 | T37.8X2 | T37.8X3 | T37.8X4 | T37.8X5 | T37.8X6 |
| **Iodocholesterol** (131I) | T50.8X1 | T50.8X2 | T50.8X3 | T50.8X4 | T50.8X5 | T50.8X6 |
| **Iodoform** | T49.0X1 | T49.0X2 | T49.0X3 | T49.0X4 | T49.0X5 | T49.0X6 |
| **Iodohippuric acid** | T50.8X1 | T50.8X2 | T50.8X3 | T50.8X4 | T50.8X5 | T50.8X6 |
| **Iodopanoic acid** | T50.8X1 | T50.8X2 | T50.8X3 | T50.8X4 | T50.8X5 | T50.8X6 |
| **Iodophthalein** (sodium) | T50.8X1 | T50.8X2 | T50.8X3 | T50.8X4 | T50.8X5 | T50.8X6 |
| **Iodopyracet** | T50.8X1 | T50.8X2 | T50.8X3 | T50.8X4 | T50.8X5 | T50.8X6 |
| **Iodoquinol** | T37.8X1 | T37.8X2 | T37.8X3 | T37.8X4 | T37.8X5 | T37.8X6 |
| **Iodoxamic acid** | T50.8X1 | T50.8X2 | T50.8X3 | T50.8X4 | T50.8X5 | T50.8X6 |
| **Iofendylate** | T50.8X1 | T50.8X2 | T50.8X3 | T50.8X4 | T50.8X5 | T50.8X6 |
| **Ioglycamic acid** | T50.8X1 | T50.8X2 | T50.8X3 | T50.8X4 | T50.8X5 | T50.8X6 |
| **Iohexol** | T50.8X1 | T50.8X2 | T50.8X3 | T50.8X4 | T50.8X5 | T50.8X6 |
| **Ion exchange resin** | | | | | | |
| anion | T47.8X1 | T47.8X2 | T47.8X3 | T47.8X4 | T47.8X5 | T47.8X6 |
| cation | T50.3X1 | T50.3X2 | T50.3X3 | T50.3X4 | T50.3X5 | T50.3X6 |
| cholestyramine | T46.6X1 | T46.6X2 | T46.6X3 | T46.6X4 | T46.6X5 | T46.6X6 |
| intestinal | T47.8X1 | T47.8X2 | T47.8X3 | T47.8X4 | T47.8X5 | T47.8X6 |
| **Iopamidol** | T50.8X1 | T50.8X2 | T50.8X3 | T50.8X4 | T50.8X5 | T50.8X6 |
| **Iopanoic acid** | T50.8X1 | T50.8X2 | T50.8X3 | T50.8X4 | T50.8X5 | T50.8X6 |
| **Iophenoic acid** | T50.8X1 | T50.8X2 | T50.8X3 | T50.8X4 | T50.8X5 | T50.8X6 |
| **Iopodate, sodium** | T50.8X1 | T50.8X2 | T50.8X3 | T50.8X4 | T50.8X5 | T50.8X6 |
| **Iopodic acid** | T50.8X1 | T50.8X2 | T50.8X3 | T50.8X4 | T50.8X5 | T50.8X6 |
| **Iopromide** | T50.8X1 | T50.8X2 | T50.8X3 | T50.8X4 | T50.8X5 | T50.8X6 |
| **Iopydol** | T50.8X1 | T50.8X2 | T50.8X3 | T50.8X4 | T50.8X5 | T50.8X6 |
| **Iotalamic acid** | T50.8X1 | T50.8X2 | T50.8X3 | T50.8X4 | T50.8X5 | T50.8X6 |
| **Iothalamate** | T50.8X1 | T50.8X2 | T50.8X3 | T50.8X4 | T50.8X5 | T50.8X6 |
| **Iothiouracil** | T38.2X1 | T38.2X2 | T38.2X3 | T38.2X4 | T38.2X5 | T38.2X6 |
| **Iotrol** | T50.8X1 | T50.8X2 | T50.8X3 | T50.8X4 | T50.8X5 | T50.8X6 |
| **Iotrolan** | T50.8X1 | T50.8X2 | T50.8X3 | T50.8X4 | T50.8X5 | T50.8X6 |
| **Iotroxate** | T50.8X1 | T50.8X2 | T50.8X3 | T50.8X4 | T50.8X5 | T50.8X6 |
| **Iotroxic acid** | T50.8X1 | T50.8X2 | T50.8X3 | T50.8X4 | T50.8X5 | T50.8X6 |
| **Ioversol** | T50.8X1 | T50.8X2 | T50.8X3 | T50.8X4 | T50.8X5 | T50.8X6 |
| **Ioxaglate** | T50.8X1 | T50.8X2 | T50.8X3 | T50.8X4 | T50.8X5 | T50.8X6 |
| **Ioxaglic acid** | T50.8X1 | T50.8X2 | T50.8X3 | T50.8X4 | T50.8X5 | T50.8X6 |
| **Ioxitalamic acid** | T50.8X1 | T50.8X2 | T50.8X3 | T50.8X4 | T50.8X5 | T50.8X6 |
| **Ipecac** | T47.7X1 | T47.7X2 | T47.7X3 | T47.7X4 | T47.7X5 | T47.7X6 |
| **Ipecacuanha** | T48.4X1 | T48.4X2 | T48.4X3 | T48.4X4 | T48.4X5 | T48.4X6 |
| **Ipodate, calcium** | T50.8X1 | T50.8X2 | T50.8X3 | T50.8X4 | T50.8X5 | T50.8X6 |
| **Ipral** | T42.3X1 | T42.3X2 | T42.3X3 | T42.3X4 | T42.3X5 | T42.3X6 |
| **Ipratropium** (bromide) | T48.6X1 | T48.6X2 | T48.6X3 | T48.6X4 | T48.6X5 | T48.6X6 |
| **Ipriflavone** | T46.3X1 | T46.3X2 | T46.3X3 | T46.3X4 | T46.3X5 | T46.3X6 |
| **Iprindole** | T43.011 | T43.012 | T43.013 | T43.014 | T43.015 | T43.016 |
| **Iproclozide** | T43.1X1 | T43.1X2 | T43.1X3 | T43.1X4 | T43.1X5 | T43.1X6 |
| **Iprofenin** | T50.8X1 | T50.8X2 | T50.8X3 | T50.8X4 | T50.8X5 | T50.8X6 |
| **Iproheptine** | T49.2X1 | T49.2X2 | T49.2X3 | T49.2X4 | T49.2X5 | T49.2X6 |
| **Iproniazid** | T43.1X1 | T43.1X2 | T43.1X3 | T43.1X4 | T43.1X5 | T43.1X6 |
| **Iproplatin** | T45.1X1 | T45.1X2 | T45.1X3 | T45.1X4 | T45.1X5 | T45.1X6 |
| **Iproveratril** | T46.1X1 | T46.1X2 | T46.1X3 | T46.1X4 | T46.1X5 | T46.1X6 |
| **Iron** (compounds) (medicinal) **NEC** | T45.4X1 | T45.4X2 | T45.4X3 | T45.4X4 | T45.4X5 | T45.4X6 |
| ammonium | T45.4X1 | T45.4X2 | T45.4X3 | T45.4X4 | T45.4X5 | T45.4X6 |
| dextran injection | T45.4X1 | T45.4X2 | T45.4X3 | T45.4X4 | T45.4X5 | T45.4X6 |
| nonmedicinal | T56.891 | T56.892 | T56.893 | T56.894 | — | — |
| salts | T45.4X1 | T45.4X2 | T45.4X3 | T45.4X4 | T45.4X5 | T45.4X6 |
| sorbitex | T45.4X1 | T45.4X2 | T45.4X3 | T45.4X4 | T45.4X5 | T45.4X6 |
| sorbitol citric acid complex | T45.4X1 | T45.4X2 | T45.4X3 | T45.4X4 | T45.4X5 | T45.4X6 |
| **Irrigating fluid** (vaginal) | T49.8X1 | T49.8X2 | T49.8X3 | T49.8X4 | T49.8X5 | T49.8X6 |
| eye | T49.5X1 | T49.5X2 | T49.5X3 | T49.5X4 | T49.5X5 | T49.5X6 |
| **Isepamicin** | T36.5X1 | T36.5X2 | T36.5X3 | T36.5X4 | T36.5X5 | T36.5X6 |
| **Isoaminile** (citrate) | T48.3X1 | T48.3X2 | T48.3X3 | T48.3X4 | T48.3X5 | T48.3X6 |
| **Isoamyl nitrite** | T46.3X1 | T46.3X2 | T46.3X3 | T46.3X4 | T46.3X5 | T46.3X6 |
| **Isobenzan** | T60.1X1 | T60.1X2 | T60.1X3 | T60.1X4 | — | — |
| **Isobutyl acetate** | T52.8X1 | T52.8X2 | T52.8X3 | T52.8X4 | — | — |
| **Isocarboxazid** | T43.1X1 | T43.1X2 | T43.1X3 | T43.1X4 | T43.1X5 | T43.1X6 |
| **Isoconazole** | T49.0X1 | T49.0X2 | T49.0X3 | T49.0X4 | T49.0X5 | T49.0X6 |
| **Isocyanate** | T65.0X1 | T65.0X2 | T65.0X3 | T65.0X4 | — | — |
| **Isoephedrine** | T44.991 | T44.992 | T44.993 | T44.994 | T44.995 | T44.996 |
| **Isoetarine** | T48.6X1 | T48.6X2 | T48.6X3 | T48.6X4 | T48.6X5 | T48.6X6 |
| **Isoethadione** | T42.2X1 | T42.2X2 | T42.2X3 | T42.2X4 | T42.2X5 | T42.2X6 |
| **Isoetharine** | T44.5X1 | T44.5X2 | T44.5X3 | T44.5X4 | T44.5X5 | T44.5X6 |
| **Isoflurane** | T41.0X1 | T41.0X2 | T41.0X3 | T41.0X4 | T41.0X5 | T41.0X6 |
| **Isoflurophate** | T44.0X1 | T44.0X2 | T44.0X3 | T44.0X4 | T44.0X5 | T44.0X6 |
| **Isomaltose, ferric complex** | T45.4X1 | T45.4X2 | T45.4X3 | T45.4X4 | T45.4X5 | T45.4X6 |
| **Isometheptene** | T44.3X1 | T44.3X2 | T44.3X3 | T44.3X4 | T44.3X5 | T44.3X6 |
| **Isoniazid** | T37.1X1 | T37.1X2 | T37.1X3 | T37.1X4 | T37.1X5 | T37.1X6 |
| with rifampicin | T36.6X1 | T36.6X2 | T36.6X3 | T36.6X4 | T36.6X5 | T36.6X6 |
| thioacetazone | T37.1X1 | T37.1X2 | T37.1X3 | T37.1X4 | T37.1X5 | T37.1X6 |
| **Isonicotinic acid hydrazide** | T37.1X1 | T37.1X2 | T37.1X3 | T37.1X4 | T37.1X5 | T37.1X6 |
| **Isonipecaine** | T40.4X1 | T40.4X2 | T40.4X3 | T40.4X4 | T40.4X5 | T40.4X6 |
| **Isopentaquine** | T37.2X1 | T37.2X2 | T37.2X3 | T37.2X4 | T37.2X5 | T37.2X6 |
| **Isophane insulin** | T38.3X1 | T38.3X2 | T38.3X3 | T38.3X4 | T38.3X5 | T38.3X6 |
| **Isophorone** | T65.891 | T65.892 | T65.893 | T65.894 | — | — |
| **Isophosphamide** | T45.1X1 | T45.1X2 | T45.1X3 | T45.1X4 | T45.1X5 | T45.1X6 |
| **Isopregnenone** | T38.5X1 | T38.5X2 | T38.5X3 | T38.5X4 | T38.5X5 | T38.5X6 |
| **Isoprenaline** | T48.6X1 | T48.6X2 | T48.6X3 | T48.6X4 | T48.6X5 | T48.6X6 |
| **Isopromethazine** | T43.3X1 | T43.3X2 | T43.3X3 | T43.3X4 | T43.3X5 | T43.3X6 |
| **Isopropamide** | T44.3X1 | T44.3X2 | T44.3X3 | T44.3X4 | T44.3X5 | T44.3X6 |
| iodide | T44.3X1 | T44.3X2 | T44.3X3 | T44.3X4 | T44.3X5 | T44.3X6 |
| **Isopropanol** | T51.2X1 | T51.2X2 | T51.2X3 | T51.2X4 | — | — |
| **Isopropyl** | | | | | | |
| acetate | T52.8X1 | T52.8X2 | T52.8X3 | T52.8X4 | — | — |
| alcohol | T51.2X1 | T51.2X2 | T51.2X3 | T51.2X4 | — | — |
| medicinal | T49.4X1 | T49.4X2 | T49.4X3 | T49.4X4 | T49.4X5 | T49.4X6 |
| ether | T52.8X1 | T52.8X2 | T52.8X3 | T52.8X4 | — | — |
| **Isopropylaminophenazone** | T39.2X1 | T39.2X2 | T39.2X3 | T39.2X4 | T39.2X5 | T39.2X6 |
| **Isoproterenol** | T48.6X1 | T48.6X2 | T48.6X3 | T48.6X4 | T48.6X5 | T48.6X6 |
| **Isosorbide dinitrate** | T46.3X1 | T46.3X2 | T46.3X3 | T46.3X4 | T46.3X5 | T46.3X6 |
| **Isothipendyl** | T45.0X1 | T45.0X2 | T45.0X3 | T45.0X4 | T45.0X5 | T45.0X6 |
| **Isotretinoin** | T50.991 | T50.992 | T50.993 | T50.994 | T50.995 | T50.996 |
| **Isoxazolyl penicillin** | T36.0X1 | T36.0X2 | T36.0X3 | T36.0X4 | T36.0X5 | T36.0X6 |
| **Isoxicam** | T39.391 | T39.392 | T39.393 | T39.394 | T39.395 | T39.396 |
| **Isoxsuprine** | T46.7X1 | T46.7X2 | T46.7X3 | T46.7X4 | T46.7X5 | T46.7X6 |
| **Ispagula** | T47.4X1 | T47.4X2 | T47.4X3 | T47.4X4 | T47.4X5 | T47.4X6 |
| husk | T47.4X1 | T47.4X2 | T47.4X3 | T47.4X4 | T47.4X5 | T47.4X6 |
| **Isradipine** | T46.1X1 | T46.1X2 | T46.1X3 | T46.1X4 | T46.1X5 | T46.1X6 |
| **I-thyroxine sodium** | T38.1X1 | T38.1X2 | T38.1X3 | T38.1X4 | T38.1X5 | T38.1X6 |
| **Itraconazole** | T37.8X1 | T37.8X2 | T37.8X3 | T37.8X4 | T37.8X5 | T37.8X6 |
| **Itramin tosilate** | T46.3X1 | T46.3X2 | T46.3X3 | T46.3X4 | T46.3X5 | T46.3X6 |
| **Ivermectin** | T37.4X1 | T37.4X2 | T37.4X3 | T37.4X4 | T37.4X5 | T37.4X6 |
| **Izoniazid** | T37.1X1 | T37.1X2 | T37.1X3 | T37.1X4 | T37.1X5 | T37.1X6 |
| with thioacetazone | T37.1X1 | T37.1X2 | T37.1X3 | T37.1X4 | T37.1X5 | T37.1X6 |
| **Jalap** | T47.2X1 | T47.2X2 | T47.2X3 | T47.2X4 | T47.2X5 | T47.2X6 |
| **Jamaica** | | | | | | |
| dogwood (bark) | T39.8X1 | T39.8X2 | T39.8X3 | T39.8X4 | T39.8X5 | T39.8X6 |
| ginger | T65.891 | T65.892 | T65.893 | T65.894 | — | — |
| root | T62.2X1 | T62.2X2 | T62.2X3 | T62.2X4 | — | — |
| **Jatropha** | T62.2X1 | T62.2X2 | T62.2X3 | T62.2X4 | — | — |
| curcas | T62.2X1 | T62.2X2 | T62.2X3 | T62.2X4 | — | — |
| **Jectofer** | T45.4X1 | T45.4X2 | T45.4X3 | T45.4X4 | T45.4X5 | T45.4X6 |
| **Jellyfish** (sting) | T63.621 | T63.622 | T63.623 | T63.624 | — | — |
| **Jequirity** (bean) | T62.2X1 | T62.2X2 | T62.2X3 | T62.2X4 | — | — |
| **Jimson weed** (stramonium) | T62.2X1 | T62.2X2 | T62.2X3 | T62.2X4 | — | — |
| seeds | T62.2X1 | T62.2X2 | T62.2X3 | T62.2X4 | — | — |
| **Josamycin** | T36.3X1 | T36.3X2 | T36.3X3 | T36.3X4 | T36.3X5 | T36.3X6 |
| **Juniper tar** | T49.1X1 | T49.1X2 | T49.1X3 | T49.1X4 | T49.1X5 | T49.1X6 |
| **Kallidinogenase** | T46.7X1 | T46.7X2 | T46.7X3 | T46.7X4 | T46.7X5 | T46.7X6 |
| **Kallikrein** | T46.7X1 | T46.7X2 | T46.7X3 | T46.7X4 | T46.7X5 | T46.7X6 |
| **Kanamycin** | T36.5X1 | T36.5X2 | T36.5X3 | T36.5X4 | T36.5X5 | T36.5X6 |
| **Kantrex** | T36.5X1 | T36.5X2 | T36.5X3 | T36.5X4 | T36.5X5 | T36.5X6 |
| **Kaolin** | T47.6X1 | T47.6X2 | T47.6X3 | T47.6X4 | T47.6X5 | T47.6X6 |
| light | T47.6X1 | T47.6X2 | T47.6X3 | T47.6X4 | T47.6X5 | T47.6X6 |
| **Karaya** (gum) | T47.4X1 | T47.4X2 | T47.4X3 | T47.4X4 | T47.4X5 | T47.4X6 |
| **Kebuzone** | T39.2X1 | T39.2X2 | T39.2X3 | T39.2X4 | T39.2X5 | T39.2X6 |
| **Kelevan** | T60.1X1 | T60.1X2 | T60.1X3 | T60.1X4 | — | — |
| **Kemithal** | T41.1X1 | T41.1X2 | T41.1X3 | T41.1X4 | T41.1X5 | T41.1X6 |
| **Kenacort** | T38.0X1 | T38.0X2 | T38.0X3 | T38.0X4 | T38.0X5 | T38.0X6 |
| **Keratolytic drug NEC** | T49.4X1 | T49.4X2 | T49.4X3 | T49.4X4 | T49.4X5 | T49.4X6 |
| anthracene | T49.4X1 | T49.4X2 | T49.4X3 | T49.4X4 | T49.4X5 | T49.4X6 |
| **Keratoplastic NEC** | T49.4X1 | T49.4X2 | T49.4X3 | T49.4X4 | T49.4X5 | T49.4X6 |
| **Kerosene, kerosine** (fuel) (solvent) **NEC** | T52.0X1 | T52.0X2 | T52.0X3 | T52.0X4 | — | — |
| insecticide | T52.0X1 | T52.0X2 | T52.0X3 | T52.0X4 | — | — |
| vapor | T52.0X1 | T52.0X2 | T52.0X3 | T52.0X4 | — | — |
| **Ketamine** | T41.291 | T41.292 | T41.293 | T41.294 | T41.295 | T41.296 |
| **Ketazolam** | T42.4X1 | T42.4X2 | T42.4X3 | T42.4X4 | T42.4X5 | T42.4X6 |
| **Ketazon** | T39.2X1 | T39.2X2 | T39.2X3 | T39.2X4 | T39.2X5 | T39.2X6 |
| **Ketobemidone** | T40.4X1 | T40.4X2 | T40.4X3 | T40.4X4 | — | — |
| **Ketoconazole** | T49.0X1 | T49.0X2 | T49.0X3 | T49.0X4 | T49.0X5 | T49.0X6 |
| **Ketols** | T52.4X1 | T52.4X2 | T52.4X3 | T52.4X4 | — | — |
| **Ketone oils** | T52.4X1 | T52.4X2 | T52.4X3 | T52.4X4 | — | — |
| **Ketoprofen** | T39.311 | T39.312 | T39.313 | T39.314 | T39.315 | T39.316 |
| **Ketorolac** | T39.8X1 | T39.8X2 | T39.8X3 | T39.8X4 | T39.8X5 | T39.8X6 |
| **Ketotifen** | T45.0X1 | T45.0X2 | T45.0X3 | T45.0X4 | T45.0X5 | T45.0X6 |
| **Khat** | T43.691 | T43.692 | T43.693 | T43.694 | — | — |

Iodine — Khat

| Substance | Poisoning, Accidental (unintentional) | Poisoning, Intentional Self-harm | Poisoning, Assault | Poisoning, Undetermined | Adverse Effect | Under-dosing |
|---|---|---|---|---|---|---|
| **Khellin** | T46.3X1 | T46.3X2 | T46.3X3 | T46.3X4 | T46.3X5 | T46.3X6 |
| **Khelloside** | T46.3X1 | T46.3X2 | T46.3X3 | T46.3X4 | T46.3X5 | T46.3X6 |
| **Kiln gas or vapor** (carbon monoxide) | T58.8X1 | T58.8X2 | T58.8X3 | T58.8X4 | — | — |
| **Kitasamycin** | T36.3X1 | T36.3X2 | T36.3X3 | T36.3X4 | T36.3X5 | T36.3X6 |
| **Konsyl** | T47.4X1 | T47.4X2 | T47.4X3 | T47.4X4 | T47.4X5 | T47.4X6 |
| **Kosam seed** | T62.2X1 | T62.2X2 | T62.2X3 | T62.2X4 | — | — |
| **Krait** (venom) | T63.091 | T63.092 | T63.093 | T63.094 | — | — |
| **Kwell** (insecticide) | T60.1X1 | T60.1X2 | T60.1X3 | T60.1X4 | — | — |
|   anti-infective (topical) | T49.0X1 | T49.0X2 | T49.0X3 | T49.0X4 | T49.0X5 | T49.0X6 |
| **Labetalol** | T44.8X1 | T44.8X2 | T44.8X3 | T44.8X4 | T44.8X5 | T44.8X6 |
| **Laburnum** (seeds) | T62.2X1 | T62.2X2 | T62.2X3 | T62.2X4 | — | — |
|   leaves | T62.2X1 | T62.2X2 | T62.2X3 | T62.2X4 | — | — |
| **Lachesine** | T49.5X1 | T49.5X2 | T49.5X3 | T49.5X4 | T49.5X5 | T49.5X6 |
| **Lacidipine** | T46.5X1 | T46.5X2 | T46.5X3 | T46.5X4 | T46.5X5 | T46.5X6 |
| **Lacquer** | T65.6X1 | T65.6X2 | T65.6X3 | T65.6X4 | — | — |
| **Lacrimogenic gas** | T59.3X1 | T59.3X2 | T59.3X3 | T59.3X4 | — | — |
| **Lactated potassic saline** | T50.3X1 | T50.3X2 | T50.3X3 | T50.3X4 | T50.3X5 | T50.3X6 |
| **Lactic acid** | T49.8X1 | T49.8X2 | T49.8X3 | T49.8X4 | T49.8X5 | T49.8X6 |
| **Lactobacillus** | | | | | | |
|   acidophilus | T47.6X1 | T47.6X2 | T47.6X3 | T47.6X4 | T47.6X5 | T47.6X6 |
|     compound | T47.6X1 | T47.6X2 | T47.6X3 | T47.6X4 | T47.6X5 | T47.6X6 |
|   bifidus, lyophilized | T47.6X1 | T47.6X2 | T47.6X3 | T47.6X4 | T47.6X5 | T47.6X6 |
|   bulgaricus | T47.6X1 | T47.6X2 | T47.6X3 | T47.6X4 | T47.6X5 | T47.6X6 |
|   sporogenes | T47.6X1 | T47.6X2 | T47.6X3 | T47.6X4 | T47.6X5 | T47.6X6 |
| **Lactoflavin** | T45.2X1 | T45.2X2 | T45.2X3 | T45.2X4 | T45.2X5 | T45.2X6 |
| **Lactose** (as excipient) | T50.901 | T50.902 | T50.903 | T50.904 | T50.905 | T50.906 |
| **Lactuca** (virosa) (extract) | T42.6X1 | T42.6X2 | T42.6X3 | T42.6X4 | T42.6X5 | T42.6X6 |
| **Lactucarium** | T42.6X1 | T42.6X2 | T42.6X3 | T42.6X4 | T42.6X5 | T42.6X6 |
| **Lactulose** | T47.3X1 | T47.3X2 | T47.3X3 | T47.3X4 | T47.3X5 | T47.3X6 |
| **Laevo** — *see* Levo- | | | | | | |
| **Lanatosides** | T46.0X1 | T46.0X2 | T46.0X3 | T46.0X4 | T46.0X5 | T46.0X6 |
| **Lanolin** | T49.3X1 | T49.3X2 | T49.3X3 | T49.3X4 | T49.3X5 | T49.3X6 |
| **Largactil** | T43.3X1 | T43.3X2 | T43.3X3 | T43.3X4 | T43.3X5 | T43.3X6 |
| **Larkspur** | T62.2X1 | T62.2X2 | T62.2X3 | T62.2X4 | — | — |
| **Laroxyl** | T43.011 | T43.012 | T43.013 | T43.014 | T43.015 | T43.016 |
| **Lasix** | T50.1X1 | T50.1X2 | T50.1X3 | T50.1X4 | T50.1X5 | T50.1X6 |
| **Lassar's paste** | T49.4X1 | T49.4X2 | T49.4X3 | T49.4X4 | T49.4X5 | T49.4X6 |
| **Latamoxef** | T36.1X1 | T36.1X2 | T36.1X3 | T36.1X4 | T36.1X5 | T36.1X6 |
| **Latex** | T65.811 | T65.812 | T65.813 | T65.814 | — | — |
| **Lathyrus** (seed) | T62.2X1 | T62.2X2 | T62.2X3 | T62.2X4 | — | — |
| **Laudanum** | T40.0X1 | T40.0X2 | T40.0X3 | T40.0X4 | T40.0X5 | T40.0X6 |
| **Laudexium** | T48.1X1 | T48.1X2 | T48.1X3 | T48.1X4 | T48.1X5 | T48.1X6 |
| **Laughing gas** | T41.0X1 | T41.0X2 | T41.0X3 | T41.0X4 | T41.0X5 | T41.0X6 |
| **Laurel, black or cherry** | T62.2X1 | T62.2X2 | T62.2X3 | T62.2X4 | — | — |
| **Laurolinium** | T49.0X1 | T49.0X2 | T49.0X3 | T49.0X4 | T49.0X5 | T49.0X6 |
| **Lauryl sulfoacetate** | T49.2X1 | T49.2X2 | T49.2X3 | T49.2X4 | T49.2X5 | T49.2X6 |
| **Laxative NEC** | T47.4X1 | T47.4X2 | T47.4X3 | T47.4X4 | T47.4X5 | T47.4X6 |
|   osmotic | T47.3X1 | T47.3X2 | T47.3X3 | T47.3X4 | T47.3X5 | T47.3X6 |
|   saline | T47.3X1 | T47.3X2 | T47.3X3 | T47.3X4 | T47.3X5 | T47.3X6 |
|   stimulant | T47.2X1 | T47.2X2 | T47.2X3 | T47.2X4 | T47.2X5 | T47.2X6 |
| **L-dopa** | T42.8X1 | T42.8X2 | T42.8X3 | T42.8X4 | T42.8X5 | T42.8X6 |
| **Lead** (dust) (fumes) (vapor) | T56.0X1 | T56.0X2 | T56.0X3 | T56.0X4 | — | — |
|   **NEC** | | | | | | |
|   acetate | T49.2X1 | T49.2X2 | T49.2X3 | T49.2X4 | T49.2X5 | T49.2X6 |
|   alkyl (fuel additive) | T56.0X1 | T56.0X2 | T56.0X3 | T56.0X4 | — | — |
|   anti-infectives | T37.8X1 | T37.8X2 | T37.8X3 | T37.8X4 | T37.8X5 | T37.8X6 |
|   antiknock compound (tetraethyl) | T56.0X1 | T56.0X2 | T56.0X3 | T56.0X4 | — | — |
|   arsenate, arsenite (dust)(herbicide) (insecticide) (vapor) | T57.0X1 | T57.0X2 | T57.0X3 | T57.0X4 | — | — |
|   carbonate | T56.0X1 | T56.0X2 | T56.0X3 | T56.0X4 | — | — |
|     paint | T56.0X1 | T56.0X2 | T56.0X3 | T56.0X4 | — | — |
|   chromate | T56.0X1 | T56.0X2 | T56.0X3 | T56.0X4 | — | — |
|     paint | T56.0X1 | T56.0X2 | T56.0X3 | T56.0X4 | — | — |
|   dioxide | T56.0X1 | T56.0X2 | T56.0X3 | T56.0X4 | — | — |
|   inorganic | T56.0X1 | T56.0X2 | T56.0X3 | T56.0X4 | — | — |
|   iodide | T56.0X1 | T56.0X2 | T56.0X3 | T56.0X4 | — | — |
|     pigment (paint) | T56.0X1 | T56.0X2 | T56.0X3 | T56.0X4 | — | — |
|   monoxide (dust) | T56.0X1 | T56.0X2 | T56.0X3 | T56.0X4 | — | — |
|     paint | T56.0X1 | T56.0X2 | T56.0X3 | T56.0X4 | — | — |
|   organic | T56.0X1 | T56.0X2 | T56.0X3 | T56.0X4 | — | — |
|   oxide | T56.0X1 | T56.0X2 | T56.0X3 | T56.0X4 | — | — |
|     paint | T56.0X1 | T56.0X2 | T56.0X3 | T56.0X4 | — | — |
|   paint | T56.0X1 | T56.0X2 | T56.0X3 | T56.0X4 | — | — |
|   salts | T56.0X1 | T56.0X2 | T56.0X3 | T56.0X4 | — | — |
|   specified compound NEC | T56.0X1 | T56.0X2 | T56.0X3 | T56.0X4 | — | — |
|   tetra-ethyl | T56.0X1 | T56.0X2 | T56.0X3 | T56.0X4 | — | — |
| **Lebanese red** | T40.7X1 | T40.7X2 | T40.7X3 | T40.7X4 | T40.7X5 | T40.7X6 |
| **Lefetamine** | T39.8X1 | T39.8X2 | T39.8X3 | T39.8X4 | T39.8X5 | T39.8X6 |
| **Lenperone** | T43.4X1 | T43.4X2 | T43.4X3 | T43.4X4 | T43.4X5 | T43.4X6 |
| **Lente lietin** (insulin) | T38.3X1 | T38.3X2 | T38.3X3 | T38.3X4 | T38.3X5 | T38.3X6 |

| Substance | Poisoning, Accidental (unintentional) | Poisoning, Intentional Self-harm | Poisoning, Assault | Poisoning, Undetermined | Adverse Effect | Under-dosing |
|---|---|---|---|---|---|---|
| **Leptazol** | T50.7X1 | T50.7X2 | T50.7X3 | T50.7X4 | T50.7X5 | T50.7X6 |
| **Leptophos** | T60.0X1 | T60.0X2 | T60.0X3 | T60.0X4 | — | — |
| **Leritine** | T40.2X1 | T40.2X2 | T40.2X3 | T40.2X4 | T40.2X5 | T40.2X6 |
| **Letosteine** | T48.4X1 | T48.4X2 | T48.4X3 | T48.4X4 | T48.4X5 | T48.4X6 |
| **Letter** | T38.1X1 | T38.1X2 | T38.1X3 | T38.1X4 | T38.1X5 | T38.1X6 |
| **Lettuce opium** | T42.6X1 | T42.6X2 | T42.6X3 | T42.6X4 | T42.6X5 | T42.6X6 |
| **Leucinocaine** | T41.3X1 | T41.3X2 | T41.3X3 | T41.3X4 | T41.3X5 | T41.3X6 |
| **Leucocianidol** | T46.991 | T46.992 | T46.993 | T46.994 | T46.995 | T46.996 |
| **Leucovorin** (factor) | T45.8X1 | T45.8X2 | T45.8X3 | T45.8X4 | T45.8X5 | T45.8X6 |
| **Leukeran** | T45.1X1 | T45.1X2 | T45.1X3 | T45.1X4 | T45.1X5 | T45.1X6 |
| **Leuprolide** | T38.891 | T38.892 | T38.893 | T38.894 | T38.895 | T38.896 |
| **Levalbuterol** | T48.6X1 | T48.6X2 | T48.6X3 | T48.6X4 | T48.6X5 | T48.6X6 |
| **Levallorphan** | T50.7X1 | T50.7X2 | T50.7X3 | T50.7X4 | T50.7X5 | T50.7X6 |
| **Levamisole** | T37.4X1 | T37.4X2 | T37.4X3 | T37.4X4 | T37.4X5 | T37.4X6 |
| **Levanil** | T42.6X1 | T42.6X2 | T42.6X3 | T42.6X4 | T42.6X5 | T42.6X6 |
| **Levarterenol** | T44.4X1 | T44.4X2 | T44.4X3 | T44.4X4 | T44.4X5 | T44.4X6 |
| **Levdropropizine** | T48.3X1 | T48.3X2 | T48.3X3 | T48.3X4 | T48.3X5 | T48.3X6 |
| **Levobunolol** | T49.5X1 | T49.5X2 | T49.5X3 | T49.5X4 | T49.5X5 | T49.5X6 |
| **Levocabastine** (hydrochloride) | T45.0X1 | T45.0X2 | T45.0X3 | T45.0X4 | T45.0X5 | T45.0X6 |
| **Levocarnitine** | T50.991 | T50.992 | T50.993 | T50.994 | T50.995 | T50.996 |
| **Levodopa** | T42.8X1 | T42.8X2 | T42.8X3 | T42.8X4 | T42.8X5 | T42.8X6 |
|   with carbidopa | T42.8X1 | T42.8X2 | T42.8X3 | T42.8X4 | T42.8X5 | T42.8X6 |
| **Levo-dromoran** | T40.2X1 | T40.2X2 | T40.2X3 | T40.2X4 | T40.2X5 | T40.2X6 |
| **Levoglutamide** | T50.991 | T50.992 | T50.993 | T50.994 | T50.995 | T50.996 |
| **Levoid** | T38.1X1 | T38.1X2 | T38.1X3 | T38.1X4 | T38.1X5 | T38.1X6 |
| **Levo-isomethadone** | T40.3X1 | T40.3X2 | T40.3X3 | T40.3X4 | T40.3X5 | T40.3X6 |
| **Levomepromazine** | T43.3X1 | T43.3X2 | T43.3X3 | T43.3X4 | T43.3X5 | T43.3X6 |
| **Levonordefrin** | T49.6X1 | T49.6X2 | T49.6X3 | T49.6X4 | T49.6X5 | T49.6X6 |
| **Levonorgestrel** | T38.4X1 | T38.4X2 | T38.4X3 | T38.4X4 | T38.4X5 | T38.4X6 |
|   with ethinylestradiol | T38.5X1 | T38.5X2 | T38.5X3 | T38.5X4 | T38.5X5 | T38.5X6 |
| **Levopromazine** | T43.3X1 | T43.3X2 | T43.3X3 | T43.3X4 | T43.3X5 | T43.3X6 |
| **Levoprome** | T42.6X1 | T42.6X2 | T42.6X3 | T42.6X4 | T42.6X5 | T42.6X6 |
| **Levopropoxyphene** | T40.4X1 | T40.4X2 | T40.4X3 | T40.4X4 | T40.4X5 | T40.4X6 |
| **Levopropylhexedrine** | T50.5X1 | T50.5X2 | T50.5X3 | T50.5X4 | T50.5X5 | T50.5X6 |
| **Levopropylhexedrine** | T48.6X1 | T48.6X2 | T48.6X3 | T48.6X4 | T48.6X5 | T48.6X6 |
| **Levorphanol** | T40.4X1 | T40.4X2 | T40.4X3 | T40.4X4 | T40.4X5 | T40.4X6 |
| **Levothyroxine** | T38.1X1 | T38.1X2 | T38.1X3 | T38.1X4 | T38.1X5 | T38.1X6 |
|   sodium | T38.1X1 | T38.1X2 | T38.1X3 | T38.1X4 | T38.1X5 | T38.1X6 |
| **Levsin** | T44.3X1 | T44.3X2 | T44.3X3 | T44.3X4 | T44.3X5 | T44.3X6 |
| **Levulose** | T50.3X1 | T50.3X2 | T50.3X3 | T50.3X4 | T50.3X5 | T50.3X6 |
| **Lewisite** (gas), not in war | T57.0X1 | T57.0X2 | T57.0X3 | T57.0X4 | — | — |
| **Librium** | T42.4X1 | T42.4X2 | T42.4X3 | T42.4X4 | T42.4X5 | T42.4X6 |
| **Lidex** | T49.0X1 | T49.0X2 | T49.0X3 | T49.0X4 | T49.0X5 | T49.0X6 |
| **Lidocaine** | T41.3X1 | T41.3X2 | T41.3X3 | T41.3X4 | T41.3X5 | T41.3X6 |
|   regional | T41.3X1 | T41.3X2 | T41.3X3 | T41.3X4 | T41.3X5 | T41.3X6 |
|   spinal | T41.3X1 | T41.3X2 | T41.3X3 | T41.3X4 | T41.3X5 | T41.3X6 |
| **Lidofenin** | T50.8X1 | T50.8X2 | T50.8X3 | T50.8X4 | T50.8X5 | T50.8X6 |
| **Lidoflazine** | T46.1X1 | T46.1X2 | T46.1X3 | T46.1X4 | T46.1X5 | T46.1X6 |
| **Lighter fluid** | T52.0X1 | T52.0X2 | T52.0X3 | T52.0X4 | — | — |
| **Lignin hemicellulose** | T47.6X1 | T47.6X2 | T47.6X3 | T47.6X4 | T47.6X5 | T47.6X6 |
| **Lignocaine** | T41.3X1 | T41.3X2 | T41.3X3 | T41.3X4 | T41.3X5 | T41.3X6 |
|   regional | T41.3X1 | T41.3X2 | T41.3X3 | T41.3X4 | T41.3X5 | T41.3X6 |
|   spinal | T41.3X1 | T41.3X2 | T41.3X3 | T41.3X4 | T41.3X5 | T41.3X6 |
| **Ligroin** (e) (solvent) | T52.0X1 | T52.0X2 | T52.0X3 | T52.0X4 | — | — |
|   vapor | T59.891 | T59.892 | T59.893 | T59.894 | — | — |
| **Ligustrum vulgare** | T62.2X1 | T62.2X2 | T62.2X3 | T62.2X4 | — | — |
| **Lily of the valley** | T62.2X1 | T62.2X2 | T62.2X3 | T62.2X4 | — | — |
| **Lime** (chloride) | T54.3X1 | T54.3X2 | T54.3X3 | T54.3X4 | — | — |
| **Limonene** | T52.8X1 | T52.8X2 | T52.8X3 | T52.8X4 | — | — |
| **Lincomycin** | T36.8X1 | T36.8X2 | T36.8X3 | T36.8X4 | T36.8X5 | T36.8X6 |
| **Lindane** (insecticide) (nonmedicinal) (vapor) | T53.6X1 | T53.6X2 | T53.6X3 | T53.6X4 | — | — |
|   medicinal | T49.0X1 | T49.0X2 | T49.0X3 | T49.0X4 | T49.0X5 | T49.0X6 |
| **Liniments NEC** | T49.91 | T49.92 | T49.93 | T49.94 | T49.95 | T49.96 |
| **Linoleic acid** | T46.6X1 | T46.6X2 | T46.6X3 | T46.6X4 | T46.6X5 | T46.6X6 |
| **Linolenic acid** | T46.6X1 | T46.6X2 | T46.6X3 | T46.6X4 | T46.6X5 | T46.6X6 |
| **Linseed** | T47.4X1 | T47.4X2 | T47.4X3 | T47.4X4 | T47.4X5 | T47.4X6 |
| **Liothyronine** | T38.1X1 | T38.1X2 | T38.1X3 | T38.1X4 | T38.1X5 | T38.1X6 |
| **Liotrix** | T38.1X1 | T38.1X2 | T38.1X3 | T38.1X4 | T38.1X5 | T38.1X6 |
| **Lipancreatin** | T47.5X1 | T47.5X2 | T47.5X3 | T47.5X4 | T47.5X5 | T47.5X6 |
| **Lipo-alprostadil** | T46.7X1 | T46.7X2 | T46.7X3 | T46.7X4 | T46.7X5 | T46.7X6 |
| **Lipo-Lutin** | T38.5X1 | T38.5X2 | T38.5X3 | T38.5X4 | T38.5X5 | T38.5X6 |
| **Lipotropic drug NEC** | T50.901 | T50.902 | T50.903 | T50.904 | T50.905 | T50.906 |
| **Liquefied petroleum gases** | T59.891 | T59.892 | T59.893 | T59.894 | — | — |
|   piped (pure or mixed with air) | T59.891 | T59.892 | T59.893 | T59.894 | — | — |
| **Liquid** | | | | | | |
|   paraffin | T47.4X1 | T47.4X2 | T47.4X3 | T47.4X4 | T47.4X5 | T47.4X6 |
|   petrolatum | T47.4X1 | T47.4X2 | T47.4X3 | T47.4X4 | T47.4X5 | T47.4X6 |
|     topical | T49.3X1 | T49.3X2 | T49.3X3 | T49.3X4 | T49.3X5 | T49.3X6 |
|   specified NEC | T65.891 | T65.892 | T65.893 | T65.894 | — | — |
|   substance | T65.91 | T65.92 | T65.93 | T65.94 | — | — |

▽ Subterms under main terms may continue to next column or page     Additional Character May Be Required — Refer to the Tabular List for Character Selection     **375**

**Khellin — Liquid**

| Substance | Poisoning, Accidental (unintentional) | Poisoning, Intentional Self-harm | Poisoning, Assault | Poisoning, Undetermined | Adverse Effect | Under-dosing |
|---|---|---|---|---|---|---|
| Liquor creosolis compositus | T65.891 | T65.892 | T65.893 | T65.894 | — | — |
| Liquorice | T48.4X1 | T48.4X2 | T48.4X3 | T48.4X4 | T48.4X5 | T48.4X6 |
| extract | T47.8X1 | T47.8X2 | T47.8X3 | T47.8X4 | T47.8X5 | T47.8X6 |
| Lisinopril | T46.4X1 | T46.4X2 | T46.4X3 | T46.4X4 | T46.4X5 | T46.4X6 |
| Lisuride | T42.8X1 | T42.8X2 | T42.8X3 | T42.8X4 | T42.8X5 | T42.8X6 |
| Lithane | T43.8X1 | T43.8X2 | T43.8X3 | T43.8X4 | T43.8X5 | T43.8X6 |
| Lithium | T56.891 | T56.892 | T56.893 | T56.894 | — | — |
| gluconate | T43.591 | T43.592 | T43.593 | T43.594 | T43.595 | T43.596 |
| salts (carbonate) | T43.591 | T43.592 | T43.593 | T43.594 | T43.595 | T43.596 |
| Lithonate | T43.8X1 | T43.8X2 | T43.8X3 | T43.8X4 | T43.8X5 | T43.8X6 |
| Liver | | | | | | |
| extract | T45.8X1 | T45.8X2 | T45.8X3 | T45.8X4 | T45.8X5 | T45.8X6 |
| for parenteral use | T45.8X1 | T45.8X2 | T45.8X3 | T45.8X4 | T45.8X5 | T45.8X6 |
| fraction 1 | T45.8X1 | T45.8X2 | T45.8X3 | T45.8X4 | T45.8X5 | T45.8X6 |
| hydrolysate | T45.8X1 | T45.8X2 | T45.8X3 | T45.8X4 | T45.8X5 | T45.8X6 |
| Lizard (bite) (venom) | T63.121 | T63.122 | T63.123 | T63.124 | — | — |
| LMD | T45.8X1 | T45.8X2 | T45.8X3 | T45.8X4 | T45.8X5 | T45.8X6 |
| Lobelia | T62.2X1 | T62.2X2 | T62.2X3 | T62.2X4 | — | — |
| Lobeline | T50.7X1 | T50.7X2 | T50.7X3 | T50.7X4 | T50.7X5 | T50.7X6 |
| Local action drug NEC | T49.8X1 | T49.8X2 | T49.8X3 | T49.8X4 | T49.8X5 | T49.8X6 |
| Locorten | T49.0X1 | T49.0X2 | T49.0X3 | T49.0X4 | T49.0X5 | T49.0X6 |
| Lofepramine | T43.011 | T43.012 | T43.013 | T43.014 | T43.015 | T43.016 |
| Lolium temulentum | T62.2X1 | T62.2X2 | T62.2X3 | T62.2X4 | — | — |
| Lomotil | T47.6X1 | T47.6X2 | T47.6X3 | T47.6X4 | T47.6X5 | T47.6X6 |
| Lomustine | T45.1X1 | T45.1X2 | T45.1X3 | T45.1X4 | T45.1X5 | T45.1X6 |
| Lonidamine | T45.1X1 | T45.1X2 | T45.1X3 | T45.1X4 | T45.1X5 | T45.1X6 |
| Loperamide | T47.6X1 | T47.6X2 | T47.6X3 | T47.6X4 | T47.6X5 | T47.6X6 |
| Loprazolam | T42.4X1 | T42.4X2 | T42.4X3 | T42.4X4 | T42.4X5 | T42.4X6 |
| Lorajmine | T46.2X1 | T46.2X2 | T46.2X3 | T46.2X4 | T46.2X5 | T46.2X6 |
| Loratidine | T45.0X1 | T45.0X2 | T45.0X3 | T45.0X4 | T45.0X5 | T45.0X6 |
| Lorazepam | T42.4X1 | T42.4X2 | T42.4X3 | T42.4X4 | T42.4X5 | T42.4X6 |
| Lorcainide | T46.2X1 | T46.2X2 | T46.2X3 | T46.2X4 | T46.2X5 | T46.2X6 |
| Lormetazepam | T42.4X1 | T42.4X2 | T42.4X3 | T42.4X4 | T42.4X5 | T42.4X6 |
| Lotions NEC | T49.91 | T49.92 | T49.93 | T49.94 | T49.95 | T49.96 |
| Lotusate | T42.3X1 | T42.3X2 | T42.3X3 | T42.3X4 | T42.3X5 | T42.3X6 |
| Lovastatin | T46.6X1 | T46.6X2 | T46.6X3 | T46.6X4 | T46.6X5 | T46.6X6 |
| Lowila | T49.2X1 | T49.2X2 | T49.2X3 | T49.2X4 | T49.2X5 | T49.2X6 |
| Loxapine | T43.591 | T43.592 | T43.593 | T43.594 | T43.595 | T43.596 |
| Lozenges (throat) | T49.6X1 | T49.6X2 | T49.6X3 | T49.6X4 | T49.6X5 | T49.6X6 |
| LSD | T40.8X1 | T40.8X2 | T40.8X3 | T40.8X4 | — | — |
| L-Tryptophan — see amino acid | | | | | | |
| Lubricant, eye | T49.5X1 | T49.5X2 | T49.5X3 | T49.5X4 | T49.5X5 | T49.5X6 |
| Lubricating oil NEC | T52.0X1 | T52.0X2 | T52.0X3 | T52.0X4 | — | — |
| Lucanthone | T37.4X1 | T37.4X2 | T37.4X3 | T37.4X4 | T37.4X5 | T37.4X6 |
| Luminal | T42.3X1 | T42.3X2 | T42.3X3 | T42.3X4 | T42.3X5 | T42.3X6 |
| Lung irritant (gas) NEC | T59.91 | T59.92 | T59.93 | T59.94 | — | — |
| Luteinizing hormone | T38.811 | T38.812 | T38.813 | T38.814 | T38.815 | T38.816 |
| Lutocylol | T38.5X1 | T38.5X2 | T38.5X3 | T38.5X4 | T38.5X5 | T38.5X6 |
| Lutromone | T38.5X1 | T38.5X2 | T38.5X3 | T38.5X4 | T38.5X5 | T38.5X6 |
| Lututrin | T48.291 | T48.292 | T48.293 | T48.294 | T48.295 | T48.296 |
| Lye (concentrated) | T54.3X1 | T54.3X2 | T54.3X3 | T54.3X4 | — | — |
| Lygranum (skin test) | T50.8X1 | T50.8X2 | T50.8X3 | T50.8X4 | T50.8X5 | T50.8X6 |
| Lymecycline | T36.4X1 | T36.4X2 | T36.4X3 | T36.4X4 | T36.4X5 | T36.4X6 |
| Lymphogranuloma venereum antigen | T50.8X1 | T50.8X2 | T50.8X3 | T50.8X4 | T50.8X5 | T50.8X6 |
| Lynestrenol | T38.4X1 | T38.4X2 | T38.4X3 | T38.4X4 | T38.4X5 | T38.4X6 |
| Lyovac Sodium Edecrin | T50.1X1 | T50.1X2 | T50.1X3 | T50.1X4 | T50.1X5 | T50.1X6 |
| Lypressin | T38.891 | T38.892 | T38.893 | T38.894 | T38.895 | T38.896 |
| Lysergic acid diethylamide | T40.8X1 | T40.8X2 | T40.8X3 | T40.8X4 | — | — |
| Lysergide | T40.8X1 | T40.8X2 | T40.8X3 | T40.8X4 | — | — |
| Lysine vasopressin | T38.891 | T38.892 | T38.893 | T38.894 | T38.895 | T38.896 |
| Lysol | T54.1X1 | T54.1X2 | T54.1X3 | T54.1X4 | — | — |
| Lysozyme | T49.0X1 | T49.0X2 | T49.0X3 | T49.0X4 | T49.0X5 | T49.0X6 |
| Lytta (vitatta) | T49.8X1 | T49.8X2 | T49.8X3 | T49.8X4 | T49.8X5 | T49.8X6 |
| Mace | T59.3X1 | T59.3X2 | T59.3X3 | T59.3X4 | — | — |
| Macrogol | T50.991 | T50.992 | T50.993 | T50.994 | T50.995 | T50.996 |
| Macrolide | | | | | | |
| anabolic drug | T38.7X1 | T38.7X2 | T38.7X3 | T38.7X4 | T38.7X5 | T38.7X6 |
| antibiotic | T36.3X1 | T36.3X2 | T36.3X3 | T36.3X4 | T36.3X5 | T36.3X6 |
| Mafenide | T49.0X1 | T49.0X2 | T49.0X3 | T49.0X4 | T49.0X5 | T49.0X6 |
| Magaldrate | T47.1X1 | T47.1X2 | T47.1X3 | T47.1X4 | T47.1X5 | T47.1X6 |
| Magic mushroom | T40.991 | T40.992 | T40.993 | T40.994 | — | — |
| Magnamycin | T36.8X1 | T36.8X2 | T36.8X3 | T36.8X4 | T36.8X5 | T36.8X6 |
| Magnesia magma | T47.1X1 | T47.1X2 | T47.1X3 | T47.1X4 | T47.1X5 | T47.1X6 |
| Magnesium NEC | T56.891 | T56.892 | T56.893 | T56.894 | — | — |
| carbonate | T47.1X1 | T47.1X2 | T47.1X3 | T47.1X4 | T47.1X5 | T47.1X6 |
| citrate | T47.4X1 | T47.4X2 | T47.4X3 | T47.4X4 | T47.4X5 | T47.4X6 |
| hydroxide | T47.1X1 | T47.1X2 | T47.1X3 | T47.1X4 | T47.1X5 | T47.1X6 |
| oxide | T47.1X1 | T47.1X2 | T47.1X3 | T47.1X4 | T47.1X5 | T47.1X6 |
| peroxide | T49.0X1 | T49.0X2 | T49.0X3 | T49.0X4 | T49.0X5 | T49.0X6 |
| salicylate | T39.091 | T39.092 | T39.093 | T39.094 | T39.095 | T39.096 |
| silicofluoride | T50.3X1 | T50.3X2 | T50.3X4 | T50.3X4 | T50.3X5 | T50.3X6 |

| Substance | Poisoning, Accidental (unintentional) | Poisoning, Intentional Self-harm | Poisoning, Assault | Poisoning, Undetermined | Adverse Effect | Under-dosing |
|---|---|---|---|---|---|---|
| Magnesium — continued | | | | | | |
| sulfate | T47.4X1 | T47.4X2 | T47.4X3 | T47.4X4 | T47.4X5 | T47.4X6 |
| thiosulfate | T45.0X1 | T45.0X2 | T45.0X3 | T45.0X4 | T45.0X5 | T45.0X6 |
| trisilicate | T47.1X1 | T47.1X2 | T47.1X3 | T47.1X4 | T47.1X5 | T47.1X6 |
| Malathion (medicinal) | T49.0X1 | T49.0X2 | T49.0X3 | T49.0X4 | T49.0X5 | T49.0X6 |
| insecticide | T60.0X1 | T60.0X2 | T60.0X3 | T60.0X4 | — | — |
| Male fern extract | T37.4X1 | T37.4X2 | T37.4X3 | T37.4X4 | T37.4X5 | T37.4X6 |
| M-AMSA | T45.1X1 | T45.1X2 | T45.1X3 | T45.1X4 | T45.1X5 | T45.1X6 |
| Mandelic acid | T37.8X1 | T37.8X2 | T37.8X3 | T37.8X4 | T37.8X5 | T37.8X6 |
| Manganese (dioxide) (salts) | T57.2X1 | T57.2X2 | T57.2X3 | T57.2X4 | — | — |
| medicinal | T50.991 | T50.992 | T50.993 | T50.994 | T50.995 | T50.996 |
| Mannitol | T47.3X1 | T47.3X2 | T47.3X3 | T47.3X4 | T47.3X5 | T47.3X6 |
| hexanitrate | T46.3X1 | T46.3X2 | T46.3X3 | T46.3X4 | T46.3X5 | T46.3X6 |
| Mannomustine | T45.1X1 | T45.1X2 | T45.1X3 | T45.1X4 | T45.1X5 | T45.1X6 |
| MAO inhibitors | T43.1X1 | T43.1X2 | T43.1X3 | T43.1X4 | T43.1X5 | T43.1X6 |
| Mapharsen | T37.8X1 | T37.8X2 | T37.8X3 | T37.8X4 | T37.8X5 | T37.8X6 |
| Maphenide | T49.0X1 | T49.0X2 | T49.0X3 | T49.0X4 | T49.0X5 | T49.0X6 |
| Maprotiline | T43.021 | T43.022 | T43.023 | T43.024 | T43.025 | T43.026 |
| Marcaine | T41.3X1 | T41.3X2 | T41.3X3 | T41.3X4 | T41.3X5 | T41.3X6 |
| infiltration (subcutaneous) | T41.3X1 | T41.3X2 | T41.3X3 | T41.3X4 | T41.3X5 | T41.3X6 |
| nerve block (peripheral) (plexus) | T41.3X1 | T41.3X2 | T41.3X3 | T41.3X4 | T41.3X5 | T41.3X6 |
| Marezine | T45.0X1 | T45.0X2 | T45.0X3 | T45.0X4 | T45.0X5 | T45.0X6 |
| Marihuana | T40.7X1 | T40.7X2 | T40.7X3 | T40.7X4 | T40.7X5 | T40.7X6 |
| Marijuana | T40.7X1 | T40.7X2 | T40.7X3 | T40.7X4 | T40.7X5 | T40.7X6 |
| Marine (sting) | T63.691 | T63.692 | T63.693 | T63.694 | — | — |
| animals (sting) | T63.691 | T63.692 | T63.693 | T63.694 | — | — |
| plants (sting) | T63.711 | T63.712 | T63.713 | T63.714 | — | — |
| Marplan | T43.1X1 | T43.1X2 | T43.1X3 | T43.1X4 | T43.1X5 | T43.1X6 |
| Marsh gas | T59.891 | T59.892 | T59.893 | T59.894 | — | — |
| Marsilid | T43.1X1 | T43.1X2 | T43.1X3 | T43.1X4 | T43.1X5 | T43.1X6 |
| Matulane | T45.1X1 | T45.1X2 | T45.1X3 | T45.1X4 | T45.1X5 | T45.1X6 |
| Mazindol | T50.5X1 | T50.5X2 | T50.5X3 | T50.5X4 | T50.5X5 | T50.5X6 |
| MCPA | T60.3X1 | T60.3X2 | T60.3X3 | T60.3X4 | — | — |
| MDMA | T43.621 | T43.622 | T43.623 | T43.624 | T43.625 | T43.626 |
| Meadow saffron | T62.2X1 | T62.2X2 | T62.2X3 | T62.2X4 | — | — |
| Measles virus vaccine (attenuated) | T50.B91 | T50.B92 | T50.B93 | T50.B94 | T50.B95 | T50.B96 |
| Meat, noxious | T62.8X1 | T62.8X2 | T62.8X3 | T62.8X4 | — | — |
| Meballymal | T42.3X1 | T42.3X2 | T42.3X3 | T42.3X4 | T42.3X5 | T42.3X6 |
| Mebanazine | T43.1X1 | T43.1X2 | T43.1X3 | T43.1X4 | T43.1X5 | T43.1X6 |
| Mebaral | T42.3X1 | T42.3X2 | T42.3X3 | T42.3X4 | T42.3X5 | T42.3X6 |
| Mebendazole | T37.4X1 | T37.4X2 | T37.4X3 | T37.4X4 | T37.4X5 | T37.4X6 |
| Mebeverine | T44.3X1 | T44.3X2 | T44.3X3 | T44.3X4 | T44.3X5 | T44.3X6 |
| Mebhydrolin | T45.0X1 | T45.0X2 | T45.0X3 | T45.0X4 | T45.0X5 | T45.0X6 |
| Mebumal | T42.3X1 | T42.3X2 | T42.3X3 | T42.3X4 | T42.3X5 | T42.3X6 |
| Mebutamate | T43.591 | T43.592 | T43.593 | T43.594 | T43.595 | T43.596 |
| Mecamylamine | T44.2X1 | T44.2X2 | T44.2X3 | T44.2X4 | T44.2X5 | T44.2X6 |
| Mechlorethamine | T45.1X1 | T45.1X2 | T45.1X3 | T45.1X4 | T45.1X5 | T45.1X6 |
| Mecillinam | T36.0X1 | T36.0X2 | T36.0X3 | T36.0X4 | T36.0X5 | T36.0X6 |
| Meclizine (hydrochloride) | T45.0X1 | T45.0X2 | T45.0X3 | T45.0X4 | T45.0X5 | T45.0X6 |
| Meclocycline | T36.4X1 | T36.4X2 | T36.4X3 | T36.4X4 | T36.4X5 | T36.4X6 |
| Meclofenamate | T39.391 | T39.392 | T39.393 | T39.394 | T39.395 | T39.396 |
| Meclofenamic acid | T39.391 | T39.392 | T39.393 | T39.394 | T39.395 | T39.396 |
| Meclofenoxate | T43.691 | T43.692 | T43.693 | T43.694 | T43.695 | T43.696 |
| Meclozine | T45.0X1 | T45.0X2 | T45.0X3 | T45.0X4 | T45.0X5 | T45.0X6 |
| Mecobalamin | T45.8X1 | T45.8X2 | T45.8X3 | T45.8X4 | T45.8X5 | T45.8X6 |
| Mecoprop | T60.3X1 | T60.3X2 | T60.3X3 | T60.3X4 | — | — |
| Mecrilate | T49.3X1 | T49.3X2 | T49.3X3 | T49.3X4 | T49.3X5 | T49.3X6 |
| Mecysteine | T48.4X1 | T48.4X2 | T48.4X3 | T48.4X4 | T48.4X5 | T48.4X6 |
| Medazepam | T42.4X1 | T42.4X2 | T42.4X3 | T42.4X4 | T42.4X5 | T42.4X6 |
| Medicament NEC | T50.901 | T50.902 | T50.903 | T50.904 | T50.905 | T50.906 |
| Medinal | T42.3X1 | T42.3X2 | T42.3X3 | T42.3X4 | T42.3X5 | T42.3X6 |
| Medomin | T42.3X1 | T42.3X2 | T42.3X3 | T42.3X4 | T42.3X5 | T42.3X6 |
| Medrogestone | T38.5X1 | T38.5X2 | T38.5X3 | T38.5X4 | T38.5X5 | T38.5X6 |
| Medroxalol | T44.8X1 | T44.8X2 | T44.8X3 | T44.8X4 | T44.8X5 | T44.8X6 |
| Medroxyprogesterone acetate (depot) | T38.5X1 | T38.5X2 | T38.5X3 | T38.5X4 | T38.5X5 | T38.5X6 |
| Medrysone | T49.0X1 | T49.0X2 | T49.0X3 | T49.0X4 | T49.0X5 | T49.0X6 |
| Mefenamic acid | T39.391 | T39.392 | T39.393 | T39.394 | T39.395 | T39.396 |
| Mefenorex | T50.5X1 | T50.5X2 | T50.5X3 | T50.5X4 | T50.5X5 | T50.5X6 |
| Mefloquine | T37.2X1 | T37.2X2 | T37.2X3 | T37.2X4 | T37.2X5 | T37.2X6 |
| Mefruside | T50.2X1 | T50.2X2 | T50.2X3 | T50.2X4 | T50.2X5 | T50.2X6 |
| Megahallucinogen | T40.901 | T40.902 | T40.903 | T40.904 | T40.905 | T40.906 |
| Megestrol | T38.5X1 | T38.5X2 | T38.5X3 | T38.5X4 | T38.5X5 | T38.5X6 |
| Meglumine | | | | | | |
| antimoniate | T37.8X1 | T37.8X2 | T37.8X3 | T37.8X4 | T37.8X5 | T37.8X6 |
| diatrizoate | T50.8X1 | T50.8X2 | T50.8X3 | T50.8X4 | T50.8X5 | T50.8X6 |
| iodipamide | T50.8X1 | T50.8X2 | T50.8X3 | T50.8X4 | T50.8X5 | T50.8X6 |
| iotroxate | T50.8X1 | T50.8X2 | T50.8X3 | T50.8X4 | T50.8X5 | T50.8X6 |
| MEK (methyl ethyl ketone) | T52.4X1 | T52.4X2 | T52.4X3 | T52.4X4 | — | — |
| Meladinin | T49.3X1 | T49.3X2 | T49.3X3 | T49.3X4 | T49.3X5 | T49.3X6 |
| Meladrazine | T44.3X1 | T44.3X2 | T44.3X3 | T44.3X4 | T44.3X5 | T44.3X6 |

Additional Character May Be Required — Refer to the Tabular List for Character Selection     ▽ Subterms under main terms may continue to next column or page

| Substance | Poisoning, Accidental (unintentional) | Poisoning, Intentional Self-harm | Poisoning, Assault | Poisoning, Undetermined | Adverse Effect | Under-dosing |
|---|---|---|---|---|---|---|
| Melaleuca alternifolia oil | T49.0X1 | T49.0X2 | T49.0X3 | T49.0X4 | T49.0X5 | T49.0X6 |
| Melanizing agents | T49.3X1 | T49.3X2 | T49.3X3 | T49.3X4 | T49.3X5 | T49.3X6 |
| Melanocyte-stimulating hormone | T38.891 | T38.892 | T38.893 | T38.894 | T38.895 | T38.896 |
| Melarsonyl potassium | T37.3X1 | T37.3X2 | T37.3X3 | T37.3X4 | T37.3X5 | T37.3X6 |
| Melarsoprol | T37.3X1 | T37.3X2 | T37.3X3 | T37.3X4 | T37.3X5 | T37.3X6 |
| Melia azedarach | T62.2X1 | T62.2X2 | T62.2X3 | T62.2X4 | — | — |
| Melitracen | T43.011 | T43.012 | T43.013 | T43.014 | T43.015 | T43.016 |
| Mellaril | T43.3X1 | T43.3X2 | T43.3X3 | T43.3X4 | T43.3X5 | T43.3X6 |
| Meloxine | T49.3X1 | T49.3X2 | T49.3X3 | T49.3X4 | T49.3X5 | T49.3X6 |
| Melperone | T43.4X1 | T43.4X2 | T43.4X3 | T43.4X4 | T43.4X5 | T43.4X6 |
| Melphalan | T45.1X1 | T45.1X2 | T45.1X3 | T45.1X4 | T45.1X5 | T45.1X6 |
| Memantine | T43.8X1 | T43.8X2 | T43.8X3 | T43.8X4 | T43.8X5 | T43.8X6 |
| Menadiol | T45.7X1 | T45.7X2 | T45.7X3 | T45.7X4 | T45.7X5 | T45.7X6 |
|   sodium sulfate | T45.7X1 | T45.7X2 | T45.7X3 | T45.7X4 | T45.7X5 | T45.7X6 |
| Menadione | T45.7X1 | T45.7X2 | T45.7X3 | T45.7X4 | T45.7X5 | T45.7X6 |
|   sodium bisulfite | T45.7X1 | T45.7X2 | T45.7X3 | T45.7X4 | T45.7X5 | T45.7X6 |
| Menaphthone | T45.7X1 | T45.7X2 | T45.7X3 | T45.7X4 | T45.7X5 | T45.7X6 |
| Menaquinone | T45.7X1 | T45.7X2 | T45.7X3 | T45.7X4 | T45.7X5 | T45.7X6 |
| Menatetrenone | T45.7X1 | T45.7X2 | T45.7X3 | T45.7X4 | T45.7X5 | T45.7X6 |
| Meningococcal vaccine | T50.A91 | T50.A92 | T50.A93 | T50.A94 | T50.A95 | T50.A96 |
| Menningovax (-AC) (-C) | T50.A91 | T50.A92 | T50.A93 | T50.A94 | T50.A95 | T50.A96 |
| Menotropins | T38.811 | T38.812 | T38.813 | T38.814 | T38.815 | T38.816 |
| Menthol | T48.5X1 | T48.5X2 | T48.5X3 | T48.5X4 | T48.5X5 | T48.5X6 |
| Mepacrine | T37.2X1 | T37.2X2 | T37.2X3 | T37.2X4 | T37.2X5 | T37.2X6 |
| Meparfynol | T42.6X1 | T42.6X2 | T42.6X3 | T42.6X4 | T42.6X5 | T42.6X6 |
| Mepartricin | T36.7X1 | T36.7X2 | T36.7X3 | T36.7X4 | T36.7X5 | T36.7X6 |
| Mepazine | T43.3X1 | T43.3X2 | T43.3X3 | T43.3X4 | T43.3X5 | T43.3X6 |
| Mepenzolate | T44.3X1 | T44.3X2 | T44.3X3 | T44.3X4 | T44.3X5 | T44.3X6 |
|   bromide | T44.3X1 | T44.3X2 | T44.3X3 | T44.3X4 | T44.3X5 | T44.3X6 |
| Meperidine | T40.4X1 | T40.4X2 | T40.4X3 | T40.4X4 | T40.4X5 | T40.4X6 |
| Mephebarbital | T42.3X1 | T42.3X2 | T42.3X3 | T42.3X4 | T42.3X5 | T42.3X6 |
| Mephenamin (e) | T42.8X1 | T42.8X2 | T42.8X3 | T42.8X4 | T42.8X5 | T42.8X6 |
| Mephenesin | T42.8X1 | T42.8X2 | T42.8X3 | T42.8X4 | T42.8X5 | T42.8X6 |
| Mephenhydramine | T45.0X1 | T45.0X2 | T45.0X3 | T45.0X4 | T45.0X5 | T45.0X6 |
| Mephenoxalone | T42.8X1 | T42.8X2 | T42.8X3 | T42.8X4 | T42.8X5 | T42.8X6 |
| Mephentermine | T44.991 | T44.992 | T44.993 | T44.994 | T44.995 | T44.996 |
| Mephenytoin | T42.0X1 | T42.0X2 | T42.0X3 | T42.0X4 | T42.0X5 | T42.0X6 |
|   with phenobarbital | T42.3X1 | T42.3X2 | T42.3X3 | T42.3X4 | T42.3X5 | T42.3X6 |
| Mephobarbital | T42.3X1 | T42.3X2 | T42.3X3 | T42.3X4 | T42.3X5 | T42.3X6 |
| Mephosfolan | T60.0X1 | T60.0X2 | T60.0X3 | T60.0X4 | — | — |
| Mepindolol | T44.7X1 | T44.7X2 | T44.7X3 | T44.7X4 | T44.7X5 | T44.7X6 |
| Mepiperphenidol | T44.3X1 | T44.3X2 | T44.3X3 | T44.3X4 | T44.3X5 | T44.3X6 |
| Mepitiostane | T38.7X1 | T38.7X2 | T38.7X3 | T38.7X4 | T38.7X5 | T38.7X6 |
| Mepivacaine | T41.3X1 | T41.3X2 | T41.3X3 | T41.3X4 | T41.3X5 | T41.3X6 |
|   epidural | T41.3X1 | T41.3X2 | T41.3X3 | T41.3X4 | T41.3X5 | T41.3X6 |
| Meprednisone | T38.0X1 | T38.0X2 | T38.0X3 | T38.0X4 | T38.0X5 | T38.0X6 |
| Meprobam | T43.591 | T43.592 | T43.593 | T43.594 | T43.595 | T43.596 |
| Meprobamate | T43.591 | T43.592 | T43.593 | T43.594 | T43.595 | T43.596 |
| Meproscillarin | T46.0X1 | T46.0X2 | T46.0X3 | T46.0X4 | T46.0X5 | T46.0X6 |
| Meprylcaine | T41.3X1 | T41.3X2 | T41.3X3 | T41.3X4 | T41.3X5 | T41.3X6 |
| Meptazinol | T39.8X1 | T39.8X2 | T39.8X3 | T39.8X4 | T39.8X5 | T39.8X6 |
| Mepyramine | T45.0X1 | T45.0X2 | T45.0X3 | T45.0X4 | T45.0X5 | T45.0X6 |
| Mequitazine | T43.3X1 | T43.3X2 | T43.3X3 | T43.3X4 | T43.3X5 | T43.3X6 |
| Meralluride | T50.2X1 | T50.2X2 | T50.2X3 | T50.2X4 | T50.2X5 | T50.2X6 |
| Merbaphen | T50.2X1 | T50.2X2 | T50.2X3 | T50.2X4 | T50.2X5 | T50.2X6 |
| Merbromin | T49.0X1 | T49.0X2 | T49.0X3 | T49.0X4 | T49.0X5 | T49.0X6 |
| Mercaptobenzothiazole salts | T49.0X1 | T49.0X2 | T49.0X3 | T49.0X4 | T49.0X5 | T49.0X6 |
| Mercaptomerin | T50.2X1 | T50.2X2 | T50.2X3 | T50.2X4 | T50.2X5 | T50.2X6 |
| Mercaptopurine | T45.1X1 | T45.1X2 | T45.1X3 | T45.1X4 | T45.1X5 | T45.1X6 |
| Mercumatilin | T50.2X1 | T50.2X2 | T50.2X3 | T50.2X4 | T50.2X5 | T50.2X6 |
| Mercuramide | T50.2X1 | T50.2X2 | T50.2X3 | T50.2X4 | T50.2X5 | T50.2X6 |
| Mercurochrome | T49.0X1 | T49.0X2 | T49.0X3 | T49.0X4 | T49.0X5 | T49.0X6 |
| Mercurophylline | T50.2X1 | T50.2X2 | T50.2X3 | T50.2X4 | T50.2X5 | T50.2X6 |
| Mercury, mercurial, mercuric, mercurous (compounds) (cyanide) (fumes) (nonmedicinal) (vapor) NEC | T56.1X1 | T56.1X2 | T56.1X3 | T56.1X4 | — | — |
|   ammoniated | T49.0X1 | T49.0X2 | T49.0X3 | T49.0X4 | T49.0X5 | T49.0X6 |
|   anti-infective | | | | | | |
|     local | T49.0X1 | T49.0X2 | T49.0X3 | T49.0X4 | T49.0X5 | T49.0X6 |
|     systemic | T37.8X1 | T37.8X2 | T37.8X3 | T37.8X4 | T37.8X5 | T37.8X6 |
|     topical | T49.0X1 | T49.0X2 | T49.0X3 | T49.0X4 | T49.0X5 | T49.0X6 |
|   chloride (ammoniated) | T49.0X1 | T49.0X2 | T49.0X3 | T49.0X4 | T49.0X5 | T49.0X6 |
|     fungicide | T56.1X1 | T56.1X2 | T56.1X3 | T56.1X4 | — | — |
|   diuretic NEC | T50.2X1 | T50.2X2 | T50.2X3 | T50.2X4 | T50.2X5 | T50.2X6 |
|   fungicide | T56.1X1 | T56.1X2 | T56.1X3 | T56.1X4 | — | — |
|   organic (fungicide) | T56.1X1 | T56.1X2 | T56.1X3 | T56.1X4 | — | — |
|   oxide, yellow | T49.0X1 | T49.0X2 | T49.0X3 | T49.0X4 | T49.0X5 | T49.0X6 |
| Mersalyl | T50.2X1 | T50.2X2 | T50.2X3 | T50.2X4 | T50.2X5 | T50.2X6 |
| Merthiolate | T49.0X1 | T49.0X2 | T49.0X3 | T49.0X4 | T49.0X5 | T49.0X6 |

| Substance | Poisoning, Accidental (unintentional) | Poisoning, Intentional Self-harm | Poisoning, Assault | Poisoning, Undetermined | Adverse Effect | Under-dosing |
|---|---|---|---|---|---|---|
| Merthiolate — continued | | | | | | |
|   ophthalmic preparation | T49.5X1 | T49.5X2 | T49.5X3 | T49.5X4 | T49.5X5 | T49.5X6 |
| Meruvax | T50.B91 | T50.B92 | T50.B93 | T50.B94 | T50.B95 | T50.B96 |
| Mesalazine | T47.8X1 | T47.8X2 | T47.8X3 | T47.8X4 | T47.8X5 | T47.8X6 |
| Mescal buttons | T40.991 | T40.992 | T40.993 | T40.994 | — | — |
| Mescaline | T40.991 | T40.992 | T40.993 | T40.994 | — | — |
| Mesna | T48.4X1 | T48.4X2 | T48.4X3 | T48.4X4 | T48.4X5 | T48.4X6 |
| Mesoglycan | T46.6X1 | T46.6X2 | T46.6X3 | T46.6X4 | T46.6X5 | T46.6X6 |
| Mesoridazine | T43.3X1 | T43.3X2 | T43.3X3 | T43.3X4 | T43.3X5 | T43.3X6 |
| Mestanolone | T38.7X1 | T38.7X2 | T38.7X3 | T38.7X4 | T38.7X5 | T38.7X6 |
| Mesterolone | T38.7X1 | T38.7X2 | T38.7X3 | T38.7X4 | T38.7X5 | T38.7X6 |
| Mestranol | T38.5X1 | T38.5X2 | T38.5X3 | T38.5X4 | T38.5X5 | T38.5X6 |
| Mesulergine | T42.8X1 | T42.8X2 | T42.8X3 | T42.8X4 | T42.8X5 | T42.8X6 |
| Mesulfen | T49.0X1 | T49.0X2 | T49.0X3 | T49.0X4 | T49.0X5 | T49.0X6 |
| Mesuximide | T42.2X1 | T42.2X2 | T42.2X3 | T42.2X4 | T42.2X5 | T42.2X6 |
| Metabutethamine | T41.3X1 | T41.3X2 | T41.3X3 | T41.3X4 | T41.3X5 | T41.3X6 |
| Metactesylacetate | T49.0X1 | T49.0X2 | T49.0X3 | T49.0X4 | T49.0X5 | T49.0X6 |
| Metacycline | T36.4X1 | T36.4X2 | T36.4X3 | T36.4X4 | T36.4X5 | T36.4X6 |
| Metaldehyde (snail killer) NEC | T60.8X1 | T60.8X2 | T60.8X3 | T60.8X4 | — | — |
| Metals (heavy) (nonmedicinal) | T56.91 | T56.92 | T56.93 | T56.94 | — | — |
|   dust, fumes, or vapor NEC | T56.91 | T56.92 | T56.93 | T56.94 | — | — |
|   light NEC | T56.91 | T56.92 | T56.93 | T56.94 | — | — |
|     dust, fumes, or vapor NEC | T56.91 | T56.92 | T56.93 | T56.94 | — | — |
|   specified NEC | T56.891 | T56.892 | T56.893 | T56.894 | — | — |
|   thallium | T56.811 | T56.812 | T56.813 | T56.814 | — | — |
| Metamfetamine | T43.621 | T43.622 | T43.623 | T43.624 | T43.625 | T43.626 |
| Metamizole sodium | T39.2X1 | T39.2X2 | T39.2X3 | T39.2X4 | T39.2X5 | T39.2X6 |
| Metampicillin | T36.0X1 | T36.0X2 | T36.0X3 | T36.0X4 | T36.0X5 | T36.0X6 |
| Metamucil | T47.4X1 | T47.4X2 | T47.4X3 | T47.4X4 | T47.4X5 | T47.4X6 |
| Metandienone | T38.7X1 | T38.7X2 | T38.7X3 | T38.7X4 | T38.7X5 | T38.7X6 |
| Metandrostenolone | T38.7X1 | T38.7X2 | T38.7X3 | T38.7X4 | T38.7X5 | T38.7X6 |
| Metaphen | T49.0X1 | T49.0X2 | T49.0X3 | T49.0X4 | T49.0X5 | T49.0X6 |
| Metaphos | T60.0X1 | T60.0X2 | T60.0X3 | T60.0X4 | — | — |
| Metapramine | T43.011 | T43.012 | T43.013 | T43.014 | T43.015 | T43.016 |
| Metaproterenol | T48.291 | T48.292 | T48.293 | T48.294 | T48.295 | T48.296 |
| Metaraminol | T44.4X1 | T44.4X2 | T44.4X3 | T44.4X4 | T44.4X5 | T44.4X6 |
| Metaxalone | T42.8X1 | T42.8X2 | T42.8X3 | T42.8X4 | T42.8X5 | T42.8X6 |
| Metenolone | T38.7X1 | T38.7X2 | T38.7X3 | T38.7X4 | T38.7X5 | T38.7X6 |
| Metergoline | T42.8X1 | T42.8X2 | T42.8X3 | T42.8X4 | T42.8X5 | T42.8X6 |
| Metescufylline | T46.991 | T46.992 | T46.993 | T46.994 | T46.995 | T46.996 |
| Metetoin | T42.0X1 | T42.0X2 | T42.0X3 | T42.0X4 | T42.0X5 | T42.0X6 |
| Metformin | T38.3X1 | T38.3X2 | T38.3X3 | T38.3X4 | T38.3X5 | T38.3X6 |
| Methacholine | T44.1X1 | T44.1X2 | T44.1X3 | T44.1X4 | T44.1X5 | T44.1X6 |
| Methacycline | T36.4X1 | T36.4X2 | T36.4X3 | T36.4X4 | T36.4X5 | T36.4X6 |
| Methadone | T40.3X1 | T40.3X2 | T40.3X3 | T40.3X4 | T40.3X5 | T40.3X6 |
| Methallenestril | T38.5X1 | T38.5X2 | T38.5X3 | T38.5X4 | T38.5X5 | T38.5X6 |
| Methallenoestril | T38.5X1 | T38.5X2 | T38.5X3 | T38.5X4 | T38.5X5 | T38.5X6 |
| Methamphetamine | T43.621 | T43.622 | T43.623 | T43.624 | T43.625 | T43.626 |
| Methampyrone | T39.2X1 | T39.2X2 | T39.2X3 | T39.2X4 | T39.2X5 | T39.2X6 |
| Methandienone | T38.7X1 | T38.7X2 | T38.7X3 | T38.7X4 | T38.7X5 | T38.7X6 |
| Methandriol | T38.7X1 | T38.7X2 | T38.7X3 | T38.7X4 | T38.7X5 | T38.7X6 |
| Methandrostenolone | T38.7X1 | T38.7X2 | T38.7X3 | T38.7X4 | T38.7X5 | T38.7X6 |
| Methane | T59.891 | T59.892 | T59.893 | T59.894 | — | — |
| Methanethiol | T59.891 | T59.892 | T59.893 | T59.894 | — | — |
| Methaniazide | T37.1X1 | T37.1X2 | T37.1X3 | T37.1X4 | T37.1X5 | T37.1X6 |
| Methanol (vapor) | T51.1X1 | T51.1X2 | T51.1X3 | T51.1X4 | — | — |
| Methantheline | T44.3X1 | T44.3X2 | T44.3X3 | T44.3X4 | T44.3X5 | T44.3X6 |
| Methanthelinium bromide | T44.3X1 | T44.3X2 | T44.3X3 | T44.3X4 | T44.3X5 | T44.3X6 |
| Methaphenilene | T45.0X1 | T45.0X2 | T45.0X3 | T45.0X4 | T45.0X5 | T45.0X6 |
| Methapyrilene | T45.0X1 | T45.0X2 | T45.0X3 | T45.0X4 | T45.0X5 | T45.0X6 |
| Methaqualone (compound) | T42.6X1 | T42.6X2 | T42.6X3 | T42.6X4 | T42.6X5 | T42.6X6 |
| Metharbital | T42.3X1 | T42.3X2 | T42.3X3 | T42.3X4 | T42.3X5 | T42.3X6 |
| Methazolamide | T50.2X1 | T50.2X2 | T50.2X3 | T50.2X4 | T50.2X5 | T50.2X6 |
| Methdilazine | T43.3X1 | T43.3X2 | T43.3X3 | T43.3X4 | T43.3X5 | T43.3X6 |
| Methedrine | T43.621 | T43.622 | T43.623 | T43.624 | T43.625 | T43.626 |
| Methenamine (mandelate) | T37.8X1 | T37.8X2 | T37.8X3 | T37.8X4 | T37.8X5 | T37.8X6 |
| Methenolone | T38.7X1 | T38.7X2 | T38.7X3 | T38.7X4 | T38.7X5 | T38.7X6 |
| Methergine | T48.0X1 | T48.0X2 | T48.0X3 | T48.0X4 | T48.0X5 | T48.0X6 |
| Methetoin | T42.0X1 | T42.0X2 | T42.0X3 | T42.0X4 | T42.0X5 | T42.0X6 |
| Methiacil | T38.2X1 | T38.2X2 | T38.2X3 | T38.2X4 | T38.2X5 | T38.2X6 |
| Methicillin | T36.0X1 | T36.0X2 | T36.0X3 | T36.0X4 | T36.0X5 | T36.0X6 |
| Methimazole | T38.2X1 | T38.2X2 | T38.2X3 | T38.2X4 | T38.2X5 | T38.2X6 |
| Methiodal sodium | T50.8X1 | T50.8X2 | T50.8X3 | T50.8X4 | T50.8X5 | T50.8X6 |
| Methionine | T50.991 | T50.992 | T50.993 | T50.994 | T50.995 | T50.996 |
| Methisazone | T37.5X1 | T37.5X2 | T37.5X3 | T37.5X4 | T37.5X5 | T37.5X6 |
| Methisoprinol | T37.5X1 | T37.5X2 | T37.5X3 | T37.5X4 | T37.5X5 | T37.5X6 |
| Methitural | T42.3X1 | T42.3X2 | T42.3X3 | T42.3X4 | T42.3X5 | T42.3X6 |
| Methixene | T44.3X1 | T44.3X2 | T44.3X3 | T44.3X4 | T44.3X5 | T44.3X6 |
| Methobarbital, methobarbitone | T42.3X1 | T42.3X2 | T42.3X3 | T42.3X4 | T42.3X5 | T42.3X6 |
| Methocarbamol | T42.8X1 | T42.8X2 | T42.8X3 | T42.8X4 | T42.8X5 | T42.8X6 |

| Substance | Poisoning, Accidental (unintentional) | Poisoning, Intentional Self-harm | Poisoning, Assault | Poisoning, Undetermined | Adverse Effect | Under-dosing |
|---|---|---|---|---|---|---|
| **Methocarbamol** — *continued* | | | | | | |
| skeletal muscle relaxant | T48.1X1 | T48.1X2 | T48.1X3 | T48.1X4 | T48.1X5 | T48.1X6 |
| **Methohexital** | T41.1X1 | T41.1X2 | T41.1X3 | T41.1X4 | T41.1X5 | T41.1X6 |
| **Methohexitone** | T41.1X1 | T41.1X2 | T41.1X3 | T41.1X4 | T41.1X5 | T41.1X6 |
| **Methoin** | T42.0X1 | T42.0X2 | T42.0X3 | T42.0X4 | T42.0X5 | T42.0X6 |
| **Methopholine** | T39.8X1 | T39.8X2 | T39.8X3 | T39.8X4 | T39.8X5 | T39.8X6 |
| **Methopromazine** | T43.3X1 | T43.3X2 | T43.3X3 | T43.3X4 | T43.3X5 | T43.3X6 |
| **Methorate** | T48.3X1 | T48.3X2 | T48.3X3 | T48.3X4 | T48.3X5 | T48.3X6 |
| **Methoserpidine** | T46.5X1 | T46.5X2 | T46.5X3 | T46.5X4 | T46.5X5 | T46.5X6 |
| **Methotrexate** | T45.1X1 | T45.1X2 | T45.1X3 | T45.1X4 | T45.1X5 | T45.1X6 |
| **Methotrimeprazine** | T43.3X1 | T43.3X2 | T43.3X3 | T43.3X4 | T43.3X5 | T43.3X6 |
| **Methoxa-Dome** | T49.3X1 | T49.3X2 | T49.3X3 | T49.3X4 | T49.3X5 | T49.3X6 |
| **Methoxamine** | T44.4X1 | T44.4X2 | T44.4X3 | T44.4X4 | T44.4X5 | T44.4X6 |
| **Methoxsalen** | T50.991 | T50.992 | T50.993 | T50.994 | T50.995 | T50.996 |
| **Methoxyaniline** | T65.3X1 | T65.3X2 | T65.3X3 | T65.3X4 | — | — |
| **Methoxybenzyl penicillin** | T36.0X1 | T36.0X2 | T36.0X3 | T36.0X4 | T36.0X5 | T36.0X6 |
| **Methoxychlor** | T53.7X1 | T53.7X2 | T53.7X3 | T53.7X4 | — | — |
| **Methoxy-DDT** | T53.7X1 | T53.7X2 | T53.7X3 | T53.7X4 | — | — |
| **Methoxyflurane** | T41.0X1 | T41.0X2 | T41.0X3 | T41.0X4 | T41.0X5 | T41.0X6 |
| **Methoxyphenamine** | T48.6X1 | T48.6X2 | T48.6X3 | T48.6X4 | T48.6X5 | T48.6X6 |
| **Methoxypromazine** | T43.3X1 | T43.3X2 | T43.3X3 | T43.3X4 | T43.3X5 | T43.3X6 |
| **Methscopolamine bromide** | T44.3X1 | T44.3X2 | T44.3X3 | T44.3X4 | T44.3X5 | T44.3X6 |
| **Methsuximide** | T42.2X1 | T42.2X2 | T42.2X3 | T42.2X4 | T42.2X5 | T42.2X6 |
| **Methyclothiazide** | T50.2X1 | T50.2X2 | T50.2X3 | T50.2X4 | T50.2X5 | T50.2X6 |
| **Methyl** | | | | | | |
| acetate | T52.4X1 | T52.4X2 | T52.4X3 | T52.4X4 | — | — |
| acetone | T52.4X1 | T52.4X2 | T52.4X3 | T52.4X4 | — | — |
| acrylate | T65.891 | T65.892 | T65.893 | T65.894 | — | — |
| alcohol | T51.1X1 | T51.1X2 | T51.1X3 | T51.1X4 | — | — |
| aminophenol | T65.3X1 | T65.3X2 | T65.3X3 | T65.3X4 | — | — |
| amphetamine | T43.621 | T43.622 | T43.623 | T43.624 | T43.625 | T43.626 |
| androstanolone | T38.7X1 | T38.7X2 | T38.7X3 | T38.7X4 | T38.7X5 | T38.7X6 |
| atropine | T44.3X1 | T44.3X2 | T44.3X3 | T44.3X4 | T44.3X5 | T44.3X6 |
| benzene | T52.2X1 | T52.2X2 | T52.2X3 | T52.2X4 | — | — |
| benzoate | T52.8X1 | T52.8X2 | T52.8X3 | T52.8X4 | — | — |
| benzol | T52.2X1 | T52.2X2 | T52.2X3 | T52.2X4 | — | — |
| bromide (gas) | T59.891 | T59.892 | T59.893 | T59.894 | — | — |
| fumigant | T60.8X1 | T60.8X2 | T60.8X3 | T60.8X4 | — | — |
| butanol | T51.3X1 | T51.3X2 | T51.3X3 | T51.3X4 | — | — |
| carbinol | T51.1X1 | T51.1X2 | T51.1X3 | T51.1X4 | — | — |
| carbonate | T52.8X1 | T52.8X2 | T52.8X3 | T52.8X4 | — | — |
| CCNU | T45.1X1 | T45.1X2 | T45.1X3 | T45.1X4 | T45.1X5 | T45.1X6 |
| cellosolve | T52.91 | T52.92 | T52.93 | T52.94 | — | — |
| cellulose | T47.4X1 | T47.4X2 | T47.4X3 | T47.4X4 | T47.4X5 | T47.4X6 |
| chloride (gas) | T59.891 | T59.892 | T59.893 | T59.894 | — | — |
| chloroformate | T59.3X1 | T59.3X2 | T59.3X3 | T59.3X4 | — | — |
| cyclohexane | T52.8X1 | T52.8X2 | T52.8X3 | T52.8X4 | — | — |
| cyclohexanol | T51.8X1 | T51.8X2 | T51.8X3 | T51.8X4 | — | — |
| cyclohexanone | T52.8X1 | T52.8X2 | T52.8X3 | T52.8X4 | — | — |
| cyclohexyl acetate | T52.8X1 | T52.8X2 | T52.8X3 | T52.8X4 | — | — |
| demeton | T60.0X1 | T60.0X2 | T60.0X3 | T60.0X4 | — | — |
| dihydromorphinone | T40.2X1 | T40.2X2 | T40.2X3 | T40.2X4 | T40.2X5 | T40.2X6 |
| ergometrine | T48.0X1 | T48.0X2 | T48.0X3 | T48.0X4 | T48.0X5 | T48.0X6 |
| ergonovine | T48.0X1 | T48.0X2 | T48.0X3 | T48.0X4 | T48.0X5 | T48.0X6 |
| ethyl ketone | T52.4X1 | T52.4X2 | T52.4X3 | T52.4X4 | — | — |
| glucamine antimonate | T37.8X1 | T37.8X2 | T37.8X3 | T37.8X4 | T37.8X5 | T37.8X6 |
| hydrazine | T65.891 | T65.892 | T65.893 | T65.894 | — | — |
| iodide | T65.891 | T65.892 | T65.893 | T65.894 | — | — |
| isobutyl ketone | T52.4X1 | T52.4X2 | T52.4X3 | T52.4X4 | — | — |
| isothiocyanate | T60.3X1 | T60.3X2 | T60.3X3 | T60.3X4 | — | — |
| mercaptan | T59.891 | T59.892 | T59.893 | T59.894 | — | — |
| morphine NEC | T40.2X1 | T40.2X2 | T40.2X3 | T40.2X4 | T40.2X5 | T40.2X6 |
| nicotinate | T49.4X1 | T49.4X2 | T49.4X3 | T49.4X4 | T49.4X5 | T49.4X6 |
| paraben | T49.0X1 | T49.0X2 | T49.0X3 | T49.0X4 | T49.0X5 | T49.0X6 |
| parafynol | T42.6X1 | T42.6X2 | T42.6X3 | T42.6X4 | T42.6X5 | T42.6X6 |
| parathion | T60.0X1 | T60.0X2 | T60.0X3 | T60.0X4 | — | — |
| peridol | T43.4X1 | T43.4X2 | T43.4X3 | T43.4X4 | T43.4X5 | T43.4X6 |
| phenidate | T43.631 | T43.632 | T43.633 | T43.634 | T43.635 | T43.636 |
| prednisolone | T38.0X1 | T38.0X2 | T38.0X3 | T38.0X4 | T38.0X5 | T38.0X6 |
| ENT agent | T49.6X1 | T49.6X2 | T49.6X3 | T49.6X4 | T49.6X5 | T49.6X6 |
| ophthalmic preparation | T49.5X1 | T49.5X2 | T49.5X3 | T49.5X4 | T49.5X5 | T49.5X6 |
| topical NEC | T49.0X1 | T49.0X2 | T49.0X3 | T49.0X4 | T49.0X5 | T49.0X6 |
| propylcarbinol | T51.3X1 | T51.3X2 | T51.3X3 | T51.3X4 | — | — |
| rosaniline NEC | T49.0X1 | T49.0X2 | T49.0X3 | T49.0X4 | T49.0X5 | T49.0X6 |
| salicylate | T49.2X1 | T49.2X2 | T49.2X3 | T49.2X4 | T49.2X5 | T49.2X6 |
| sulfate (fumes) | T59.891 | T59.892 | T59.893 | T59.894 | — | — |
| liquid | T52.8X1 | T52.8X2 | T52.8X3 | T52.8X4 | — | — |
| sulfonal | T42.6X1 | T42.6X2 | T42.6X3 | T42.6X4 | T42.6X5 | T42.6X6 |
| testosterone | T38.7X1 | T38.7X2 | T38.7X3 | T38.7X4 | T38.7X5 | T38.7X6 |
| thiouracil | T38.2X1 | T38.2X2 | T38.2X3 | T38.2X4 | T38.2X5 | T38.2X6 |
| **Methylamphetamine** | T43.621 | T43.622 | T43.623 | T43.624 | T43.625 | T43.626 |
| **Methylated spirit** | T51.1X1 | T51.1X2 | T51.1X3 | T51.1X4 | — | — |
| **Methylatropine nitrate** | T44.3X1 | T44.3X2 | T44.3X3 | T44.3X4 | T44.3X5 | T44.3X6 |

| Substance | Poisoning, Accidental (unintentional) | Poisoning, Intentional Self-harm | Poisoning, Assault | Poisoning, Undetermined | Adverse Effect | Under-dosing |
|---|---|---|---|---|---|---|
| **Methylbenactyzium bromide** | T44.3X1 | T44.3X2 | T44.3X3 | T44.3X4 | T44.3X5 | T44.3X6 |
| **Methylbenzethonium chloride** | T49.0X1 | T49.0X2 | T49.0X3 | T49.0X4 | T49.0X5 | T49.0X6 |
| **Methylcellulose** | T47.4X1 | T47.4X2 | T47.4X3 | T47.4X4 | T47.4X5 | T47.4X6 |
| laxative | T47.4X1 | T47.4X2 | T47.4X3 | T47.4X4 | T47.4X5 | T47.4X6 |
| **Methylchlorophenoxyacetic acid** | T60.3X1 | T60.3X2 | T60.3X3 | T60.3X4 | — | — |
| **Methyldopa** | T46.5X1 | T46.5X2 | T46.5X3 | T46.5X4 | T46.5X5 | T46.5X6 |
| **Methyldopate** | T46.5X1 | T46.5X2 | T46.5X3 | T46.5X4 | T46.5X5 | T46.5X6 |
| **Methylene** | | | | | | |
| blue | T50.6X1 | T50.6X2 | T50.6X3 | T50.6X4 | T50.6X5 | T50.6X6 |
| chloride or dichloride (solvent) NEC | T53.4X1 | T53.4X2 | T53.4X3 | T53.4X4 | — | — |
| **Methylenedioxyamphetamine** | T43.621 | T43.622 | T43.623 | T43.624 | T43.625 | T43.626 |
| **Methylenedioxymethamphetamine** | T43.621 | T43.622 | T43.623 | T43.624 | T43.625 | T43.626 |
| **Methylergometrine** | T48.0X1 | T48.0X2 | T48.0X3 | T48.0X4 | T48.0X5 | T48.0X6 |
| **Methylergonovine** | T48.0X1 | T48.0X2 | T48.0X3 | T48.0X4 | T48.0X5 | T48.0X6 |
| **Methylestrenolone** | T38.5X1 | T38.5X2 | T38.5X3 | T38.5X4 | T38.5X5 | T38.5X6 |
| **Methylethyl cellulose** | T50.991 | T50.992 | T50.993 | T50.994 | T50.995 | T50.996 |
| **Methylhexabital** | T42.3X1 | T42.3X2 | T42.3X3 | T42.3X4 | T42.3X5 | T42.3X6 |
| **Methylmorphine** | T40.2X1 | T40.2X2 | T40.2X3 | T40.2X4 | T40.2X5 | T40.2X6 |
| **Methylparaben** (ophthalmic) | T49.5X1 | T49.5X2 | T49.5X3 | T49.5X4 | T49.5X5 | T49.5X6 |
| **Methylparafynol** | T42.6X1 | T42.6X2 | T42.6X3 | T42.6X4 | T42.6X5 | T42.6X6 |
| **Methylpentynol, methylpenthynol** | T42.6X1 | T42.6X2 | T42.6X3 | T42.6X4 | T42.6X5 | T42.6X6 |
| **Methylphenidate** | T43.631 | T43.632 | T43.633 | T43.634 | T43.635 | T43.636 |
| **Methylphenobarbital** | T42.3X1 | T42.3X2 | T42.3X3 | T42.3X4 | T42.3X5 | T42.3X6 |
| **Methylpolysiloxane** | T47.1X1 | T47.1X2 | T47.1X3 | T47.1X4 | T47.1X5 | T47.1X6 |
| **Methylprednisolone** — *see* Methyl, prednisolone | | | | | | |
| **Methylrosaniline** | T49.0X1 | T49.0X2 | T49.0X3 | T49.0X4 | T49.0X5 | T49.0X6 |
| **Methylrosanilinium chloride** | T49.0X1 | T49.0X2 | T49.0X3 | T49.0X4 | T49.0X5 | T49.0X6 |
| **Methyltestosterone** | T38.7X1 | T38.7X2 | T38.7X3 | T38.7X4 | T38.7X5 | T38.7X6 |
| **Methylthionine chloride** | T50.6X1 | T50.6X2 | T50.6X3 | T50.6X4 | T50.6X5 | T50.6X6 |
| **Methylthioninium chloride** | T50.6X1 | T50.6X2 | T50.6X3 | T50.6X4 | T50.6X5 | T50.6X6 |
| **Methylthiouracil** | T38.2X1 | T38.2X2 | T38.2X3 | T38.2X4 | T38.2X5 | T38.2X6 |
| **Methyprylon** | T42.6X1 | T42.6X2 | T42.6X3 | T42.6X4 | T42.6X5 | T42.6X6 |
| **Methysergide** | T46.5X1 | T46.5X2 | T46.5X3 | T46.5X4 | T46.5X5 | T46.5X6 |
| **Metiamide** | T47.1X1 | T47.1X2 | T47.1X3 | T47.1X4 | T47.1X5 | T47.1X6 |
| **Meticillin** | T36.0X1 | T36.0X2 | T36.0X3 | T36.0X4 | T36.0X5 | T36.0X6 |
| **Meticrane** | T50.2X1 | T50.2X2 | T50.2X3 | T50.2X4 | T50.2X5 | T50.2X6 |
| **Metildigoxin** | T46.0X1 | T46.0X2 | T46.0X3 | T46.0X4 | T46.0X5 | T46.0X6 |
| **Metipranolol** | T49.5X1 | T49.5X2 | T49.5X3 | T49.5X4 | T49.5X5 | T49.5X6 |
| **Metirosine** | T46.5X1 | T46.5X2 | T46.5X3 | T46.5X4 | T46.5X5 | T46.5X6 |
| **Metisazone** | T37.5X1 | T37.5X2 | T37.5X3 | T37.5X4 | T37.5X5 | T37.5X6 |
| **Metixene** | T44.3X1 | T44.3X2 | T44.3X3 | T44.3X4 | T44.3X5 | T44.3X6 |
| **Metizoline** | T48.5X1 | T48.5X2 | T48.5X3 | T48.5X4 | T48.5X5 | T48.5X6 |
| **Metoclopramide** | T45.0X1 | T45.0X2 | T45.0X3 | T45.0X4 | T45.0X5 | T45.0X6 |
| **Metofenazate** | T43.3X1 | T43.3X2 | T43.3X3 | T43.3X4 | T43.3X5 | T43.3X6 |
| **Metofoline** | T39.8X1 | T39.8X2 | T39.8X3 | T39.8X4 | T39.8X5 | T39.8X6 |
| **Metolazone** | T50.2X1 | T50.2X2 | T50.2X3 | T50.2X4 | T50.2X5 | T50.2X6 |
| **Metopon** | T40.2X1 | T40.2X2 | T40.2X3 | T40.2X4 | T40.2X5 | T40.2X6 |
| **Metoprine** | T45.1X1 | T45.1X2 | T45.1X3 | T45.1X4 | T45.1X5 | T45.1X6 |
| **Metoprolol** | T44.7X1 | T44.7X2 | T44.7X3 | T44.7X4 | T44.7X5 | T44.7X6 |
| **Metrifonate** | T60.0X1 | T60.0X2 | T60.0X3 | T60.0X4 | — | — |
| **Metrizamide** | T50.8X1 | T50.8X2 | T50.8X3 | T50.8X4 | T50.8X5 | T50.8X6 |
| **Metrizoic acid** | T50.8X1 | T50.8X2 | T50.8X3 | T50.8X4 | T50.8X5 | T50.8X6 |
| **Metronidazole** | T37.8X1 | T37.8X2 | T37.8X3 | T37.8X4 | T37.8X5 | T37.8X6 |
| **Metycaine** | T41.3X1 | T41.3X2 | T41.3X3 | T41.3X4 | T41.3X5 | T41.3X6 |
| infiltration (subcutaneous) | T41.3X1 | T41.3X2 | T41.3X3 | T41.3X4 | T41.3X5 | T41.3X6 |
| nerve block (peripheral) (plexus) | T41.3X1 | T41.3X2 | T41.3X3 | T41.3X4 | T41.3X5 | T41.3X6 |
| topical (surface) | T41.3X1 | T41.3X2 | T41.3X3 | T41.3X4 | T41.3X5 | T41.3X6 |
| **Metyrapone** | T50.8X1 | T50.8X2 | T50.8X3 | T50.8X4 | T50.8X5 | T50.8X6 |
| **Mevinphos** | T60.0X1 | T60.0X2 | T60.0X3 | T60.0X4 | — | — |
| **Mexazolam** | T42.4X1 | T42.4X2 | T42.4X3 | T42.4X4 | T42.4X5 | T42.4X6 |
| **Mexenone** | T49.3X1 | T49.3X2 | T49.3X3 | T49.3X4 | T49.3X5 | T49.3X6 |
| **Mexiletine** | T46.2X1 | T46.2X2 | T46.2X3 | T46.2X4 | T46.2X5 | T46.2X6 |
| **Mezereon** | T62.2X1 | T62.2X2 | T62.2X3 | T62.2X4 | — | — |
| berries | T62.1X1 | T62.1X2 | T62.1X3 | T62.1X4 | — | — |
| **Mezlocillin** | T36.0X1 | T36.0X2 | T36.0X3 | T36.0X4 | T36.0X5 | T36.0X6 |
| **Mianserin** | T43.021 | T43.022 | T43.023 | T43.024 | T43.025 | T43.026 |
| **Micatin** | T49.0X1 | T49.0X2 | T49.0X3 | T49.0X4 | T49.0X5 | T49.0X6 |
| **Miconazole** | T49.0X1 | T49.0X2 | T49.0X3 | T49.0X4 | T49.0X5 | T49.0X6 |
| **Micronomicin** | T36.5X1 | T36.5X2 | T36.5X3 | T36.5X4 | T36.5X5 | T36.5X6 |
| **Midazolam** | T42.4X1 | T42.4X2 | T42.4X3 | T42.4X4 | T42.4X5 | T42.4X6 |
| **Midecamycin** | T36.3X1 | T36.3X2 | T36.3X3 | T36.3X4 | T36.3X5 | T36.3X6 |
| **Mifepristone** | T38.6X1 | T38.6X2 | T38.6X3 | T38.6X4 | T38.6X5 | T38.6X6 |
| **Milk of magnesia** | T47.1X1 | T47.1X2 | T47.1X3 | T47.1X4 | T47.1X5 | T47.1X6 |

| Substance | Poisoning, Accidental (unintentional) | Poisoning, Intentional Self-harm | Poisoning, Assault | Poisoning, Undetermined | Adverse Effect | Under-dosing |
|---|---|---|---|---|---|---|
| Millipede (tropical) | T63.411 | T63.412 | T63.413 | T63.414 | — | — |
| (venomous) | | | | | | |
| Miltown | T43.591 | T43.592 | T43.593 | T43.594 | T43.595 | T43.596 |
| Milverine | T44.3X1 | T44.3X2 | T44.3X3 | T44.3X4 | T44.3X5 | T44.3X6 |
| Minaprine | T43.291 | T43.292 | T43.293 | T43.294 | T43.295 | T43.296 |
| Minaxolone | T41.291 | T41.292 | T41.293 | T41.294 | T41.295 | T41.296 |
| Mineral | | | | | | |
| acids | T54.2X1 | T54.2X2 | T54.2X3 | T54.2X4 | | |
| oil (laxative)(medicinal) | T47.4X1 | T47.4X2 | T47.4X3 | T47.4X4 | T47.4X5 | T47.4X6 |
| emulsion | T47.2X1 | T47.2X2 | T47.2X3 | T47.2X4 | T47.2X5 | T47.2X6 |
| nonmedicinal | T52.0X1 | T52.0X2 | T52.0X3 | T52.0X4 | — | — |
| topical | T49.3X1 | T49.3X2 | T49.3X3 | T49.3X4 | T49.3X5 | T49.3X6 |
| salt NEC | T50.3X1 | T50.3X2 | T50.3X3 | T50.3X4 | T50.3X5 | T50.3X6 |
| spirits | T52.0X1 | T52.0X2 | T52.0X3 | T52.0X4 | — | — |
| Mineralocorticosteroid | T50.0X1 | T50.0X2 | T50.0X3 | T50.0X4 | T50.0X5 | T50.0X6 |
| Minocycline | T36.4X1 | T36.4X2 | T36.4X3 | T36.4X4 | T36.4X5 | T36.4X6 |
| Minoxidil | T46.7X1 | T46.7X2 | T46.7X3 | T46.7X4 | T46.7X5 | T46.7X6 |
| Miokamycin | T36.3X1 | T36.3X2 | T36.3X3 | T36.3X4 | T36.3X5 | T36.3X6 |
| Miotic drug | T49.5X1 | T49.5X2 | T49.5X3 | T49.5X4 | T49.5X5 | T49.5X6 |
| Mipafox | T60.0X1 | T60.0X2 | T60.0X3 | T60.0X4 | — | — |
| Mirex | T60.1X1 | T60.1X2 | T60.1X3 | T60.1X4 | — | — |
| Mirtazapine | T43.021 | T43.022 | T43.023 | T43.024 | T43.025 | T43.026 |
| Misonidazole | T37.3X1 | T37.3X2 | T37.3X3 | T37.3X4 | T37.3X5 | T37.3X6 |
| Misoprostol | T47.1X1 | T47.1X2 | T47.1X3 | T47.1X4 | T47.1X5 | T47.1X6 |
| Mithramycin | T45.1X1 | T45.1X2 | T45.1X3 | T45.1X4 | T45.1X5 | T45.1X6 |
| Mitobronitol | T45.1X1 | T45.1X2 | T45.1X3 | T45.1X4 | T45.1X5 | T45.1X6 |
| Mitoguazone | T45.1X1 | T45.1X2 | T45.1X3 | T45.1X4 | T45.1X5 | T45.1X6 |
| Mitolactol | T45.1X1 | T45.1X2 | T45.1X3 | T45.1X4 | T45.1X5 | T45.1X6 |
| Mitomycin | T45.1X1 | T45.1X2 | T45.1X3 | T45.1X4 | T45.1X5 | T45.1X6 |
| Mitopodozide | T45.1X1 | T45.1X2 | T45.1X3 | T45.1X4 | T45.1X5 | T45.1X6 |
| Mitotane | T45.1X1 | T45.1X2 | T45.1X3 | T45.1X4 | T45.1X5 | T45.1X6 |
| Mitoxantrone | T45.1X1 | T45.1X2 | T45.1X3 | T45.1X4 | T45.1X5 | T45.1X6 |
| Mivacurium chloride | T48.1X1 | T48.1X2 | T48.1X3 | T48.1X4 | T48.1X5 | T48.1X6 |
| Miyari bacteria | T47.6X1 | T47.6X2 | T47.6X3 | T47.6X4 | T47.6X5 | T47.6X6 |
| Moclobemide | T43.1X1 | T43.1X2 | T43.1X3 | T43.1X4 | T43.1X5 | T43.1X6 |
| Moderil | T46.5X1 | T46.5X2 | T46.5X3 | T46.5X4 | T46.5X5 | T46.5X6 |
| Mofebutazone | T39.2X1 | T39.2X2 | T39.2X3 | T39.2X4 | T39.2X5 | T39.2X6 |
| Mogadon — see Nitrazepam | | | | | | |
| Molindone | T43.591 | T43.592 | T43.593 | T43.594 | T43.595 | T43.596 |
| Molsidomine | T46.3X1 | T46.3X2 | T46.3X3 | T46.3X4 | T46.3X5 | T46.3X6 |
| Mometasone | T49.0X1 | T49.0X2 | T49.0X3 | T49.0X4 | T49.0X5 | T49.0X6 |
| Monistat | T49.0X1 | T49.0X2 | T49.0X3 | T49.0X4 | T49.0X5 | T49.0X6 |
| Monkshood | T62.2X1 | T62.2X2 | T62.2X3 | T62.2X4 | — | — |
| Monoamine oxidase inhibitor NEC | T43.1X1 | T43.1X2 | T43.1X3 | T43.1X4 | T43.1X5 | T43.1X6 |
| hydrazine | T43.1X1 | T43.1X2 | T43.1X3 | T43.1X4 | T43.1X5 | T43.1X6 |
| Monobenzone | T49.4X1 | T49.4X2 | T49.4X3 | T49.4X4 | T49.4X5 | T49.4X6 |
| Monochloroacetic acid | T60.3X1 | T60.3X2 | T60.3X3 | T60.3X4 | — | — |
| Monochlorobenzene | T53.7X1 | T53.7X2 | T53.7X3 | T53.7X4 | — | — |
| Monoethanolamine | T46.8X1 | T46.8X2 | T46.8X3 | T46.8X4 | T46.8X5 | T46.8X6 |
| oleate | T46.8X1 | T46.8X2 | T46.8X3 | T46.8X4 | T46.8X5 | T46.8X6 |
| Monooctanoin | T50.991 | T50.992 | T50.993 | T50.994 | T50.995 | T50.996 |
| Monophenylbutazone | T39.2X1 | T39.2X2 | T39.2X3 | T39.2X4 | T39.2X5 | T39.2X6 |
| Monosodium glutamate | T65.891 | T65.892 | T65.893 | T65.894 | — | — |
| Monosulfiram | T49.0X1 | T49.0X2 | T49.0X3 | T49.0X4 | T49.0X5 | T49.0X6 |
| Monoxide, carbon — see Carbon, monoxide | | | | | | |
| Monoxidine hydrochloride | T46.1X1 | T46.1X2 | T46.1X3 | T46.1X4 | T46.1X5 | T46.1X6 |
| Monuron | T60.3X1 | T60.3X2 | T60.3X3 | T60.3X4 | — | — |
| Moperone | T43.4X1 | T43.4X2 | T43.4X3 | T43.4X4 | T43.4X5 | T43.4X6 |
| Mopidamol | T45.1X1 | T45.1X2 | T45.1X3 | T45.1X4 | T45.1X5 | T45.1X6 |
| MOPP (mechloreth-amine + vincristine + prednisone + procarba-zine) | T45.1X1 | T45.1X2 | T45.1X3 | T45.1X4 | T45.1X5 | T45.1X6 |
| Morfin | T40.2X1 | T40.2X2 | T40.2X3 | T40.2X4 | T40.2X5 | T40.2X6 |
| Morinamide | T37.1X1 | T37.1X2 | T37.1X3 | T37.1X4 | T37.1X5 | T37.1X6 |
| Morning glory seeds | T40.991 | T40.992 | T40.993 | T40.994 | — | — |
| Moroxydine | T37.5X1 | T37.5X2 | T37.5X3 | T37.5X4 | T37.5X5 | T37.5X6 |
| Morphazinamide | T37.1X1 | T37.1X2 | T37.1X3 | T37.1X4 | T37.1X5 | T37.1X6 |
| Morphine | T40.2X1 | T40.2X2 | T40.2X3 | T40.2X4 | T40.2X5 | T40.2X6 |
| antagonist | T50.7X1 | T50.7X2 | T50.7X3 | T50.7X4 | T50.7X5 | T50.7X6 |
| Morpholinylethylmorphine | T40.2X1 | T40.2X2 | T40.2X3 | T40.2X4 | | |
| Morsuximide | T42.2X1 | T42.2X2 | T42.2X3 | T42.2X4 | T42.2X5 | T42.2X6 |
| Mosapramine | T43.591 | T43.592 | T43.593 | T43.594 | T43.595 | T43.596 |
| Moth balls — see also Pesticides | T60.2X1 | T60.2X2 | T60.2X3 | T60.2X4 | — | — |
| naphthalene | T60.2X1 | T60.2X2 | T60.2X3 | T60.2X4 | — | — |
| paradichlorobenzene | T60.1X1 | T60.1X2 | T60.1X3 | T60.1X4 | — | — |
| Motor exhaust gas | T58.01 | T58.02 | T58.03 | T58.04 | — | — |
| Mouthwash (antiseptic) (zinc chloride) | T49.6X1 | T49.6X2 | T49.6X3 | T49.6X4 | T49.6X5 | T49.6X6 |
| Moxastine | T45.0X1 | T45.0X2 | T45.0X3 | T45.0X4 | T45.0X5 | T45.0X6 |
| Moxaverine | T44.3X1 | T44.3X2 | T44.3X3 | T44.3X4 | T44.3X5 | T44.3X6 |
| Moxisylyte | T46.7X1 | T46.7X2 | T46.7X3 | T46.7X4 | T46.7X5 | T46.7X6 |
| Mucilage, plant | T47.4X1 | T47.4X2 | T47.4X3 | T47.4X4 | T47.4X5 | T47.4X6 |
| Mucolytic drug | T48.4X1 | T48.4X2 | T48.4X3 | T48.4X4 | T48.4X5 | T48.4X6 |
| Mucomyst | T48.4X1 | T48.4X2 | T48.4X3 | T48.4X4 | T48.4X5 | T48.4X6 |
| Mucous membrane agents | T49.91 | T49.92 | T49.93 | T49.94 | T49.95 | T49.96 |
| (external) | | | | | | |
| specified NEC | T49.8X1 | T49.8X2 | T49.8X3 | T49.8X4 | T49.8X5 | T49.8X6 |
| Mumps | | | | | | |
| immune globulin (human) | T50.Z11 | T50.Z12 | T50.Z13 | T50.Z14 | T50.Z15 | T50.Z16 |
| skin test antigen | T50.8X1 | T50.8X2 | T50.8X3 | T50.8X4 | T50.8X5 | T50.8X6 |
| vaccine | T50.B91 | T50.B92 | T50.B93 | T50.B94 | T50.B95 | T50.B96 |
| Mumpsvax | T50.B91 | T50.B92 | T50.B93 | T50.B94 | T50.B95 | T50.B96 |
| Mupirocin | T49.0X1 | T49.0X2 | T49.0X3 | T49.0X4 | T49.0X5 | T49.0X6 |
| Muriatic acid — see Hydrochloric acid | | | | | | |
| Muromonab-CD3 | T45.1X1 | T45.1X2 | T45.1X3 | T45.1X4 | T45.1X5 | T45.1X6 |
| Muscle-action drug NEC | T48.201 | T48.202 | T48.203 | T48.204 | T48.205 | T48.206 |
| Muscle affecting agents NEC | T48.201 | T48.202 | T48.203 | T48.204 | T48.205 | T48.206 |
| oxytocic | T48.0X1 | T48.0X2 | T48.0X3 | T48.0X4 | T48.0X5 | T48.0X6 |
| relaxants | T48.201 | T48.202 | T48.203 | T48.204 | T48.205 | T48.206 |
| central nervous system | T42.8X1 | T42.8X2 | T42.8X3 | T42.8X4 | T42.8X5 | T42.8X6 |
| skeletal | T48.1X1 | T48.1X2 | T48.1X3 | T48.1X4 | T48.1X5 | T48.1X6 |
| smooth | T44.3X1 | T44.3X2 | T44.3X3 | T44.3X4 | T44.3X5 | T44.3X6 |
| Muscle relaxant — see Relaxant, muscle | | | | | | |
| Muscle-tone depressant, central NEC | T42.8X1 | T42.8X2 | T42.8X3 | T42.8X4 | T42.8X5 | T42.8X6 |
| specified NEC | T42.8X1 | T42.8X2 | T42.8X3 | T42.8X4 | T42.8X5 | T42.8X6 |
| Mushroom, noxious | T62.0X1 | T62.0X2 | T62.0X3 | T62.0X4 | — | — |
| Mussel, noxious | T61.781 | T61.782 | T61.783 | T61.784 | — | — |
| Mustard (emetic) | T47.7X1 | T47.7X2 | T47.7X3 | T47.7X4 | T47.7X5 | T47.7X6 |
| black | T47.7X1 | T47.7X2 | T47.7X3 | T47.7X4 | T47.7X5 | T47.7X6 |
| gas, not in war | T59.91 | T59.92 | T59.93 | T59.94 | — | — |
| nitrogen | T45.1X1 | T45.1X2 | T45.1X3 | T45.1X4 | T45.1X5 | T45.1X6 |
| Mustine | T45.1X1 | T45.1X2 | T45.1X3 | T45.1X4 | T45.1X5 | T45.1X6 |
| Mycifradin | T36.5X1 | T36.5X2 | T36.5X3 | T36.5X4 | T36.5X5 | T36.5X6 |
| topical | T49.0X1 | T49.0X2 | T49.0X3 | T49.0X4 | T49.0X5 | T49.0X6 |
| Mycitracin | T36.8X1 | T36.8X2 | T36.8X3 | T36.8X4 | T36.8X5 | T36.8X6 |
| ophthalmic preparation | T49.5X1 | T49.5X2 | T49.5X3 | T49.5X4 | T49.5X5 | T49.5X6 |
| Mycostatin | T36.7X1 | T36.7X2 | T36.7X3 | T36.7X4 | T36.7X5 | T36.7X6 |
| topical | T49.0X1 | T49.0X2 | T49.0X3 | T49.0X4 | T49.0X5 | T49.0X6 |
| Mycotoxins | T64.81 | T64.82 | T64.83 | T64.84 | — | — |
| aflatoxin | T64.01 | T64.02 | T64.03 | T64.04 | — | — |
| specified NEC | T64.81 | T64.82 | T64.83 | T64.84 | — | — |
| Mydriacyl | T44.3X1 | T44.3X2 | T44.3X3 | T44.3X4 | T44.3X5 | T44.3X6 |
| Mydriatic drug | T49.5X1 | T49.5X2 | T49.5X3 | T49.5X4 | T49.5X5 | T49.5X6 |
| Myelobromal | T45.1X1 | T45.1X2 | T45.1X3 | T45.1X4 | T45.1X5 | T45.1X6 |
| Myleran | T45.1X1 | T45.1X2 | T45.1X3 | T45.1X4 | T45.1X5 | T45.1X6 |
| Myochrysin (e) | T39.2X1 | T39.2X2 | T39.2X3 | T39.2X4 | T39.2X5 | T39.2X6 |
| Myoneural blocking agents | T48.1X1 | T48.1X2 | T48.1X3 | T48.1X4 | T48.1X5 | T48.1X6 |
| Myralact | T49.0X1 | T49.0X2 | T49.0X3 | T49.0X4 | T49.0X5 | T49.0X6 |
| Myristica fragrans | T62.2X1 | T62.2X2 | T62.2X3 | T62.2X4 | — | — |
| Myristicin | T65.891 | T65.892 | T65.893 | T65.894 | — | — |
| Mysoline | T42.3X1 | T42.3X2 | T42.3X3 | T42.3X4 | T42.3X5 | T42.3X6 |
| Nabilone | T40.7X1 | T40.7X2 | T40.7X3 | T40.7X4 | T40.7X5 | T40.7X6 |
| Nabumetone | T39.391 | T39.392 | T39.393 | T39.394 | T39.395 | T39.396 |
| Nadolol | T44.7X1 | T44.7X2 | T44.7X3 | T44.7X4 | T44.7X5 | T44.7X6 |
| Nafcillin | T36.0X1 | T36.0X2 | T36.0X3 | T36.0X4 | T36.0X5 | T36.0X6 |
| Nafoxidine | T38.6X1 | T38.6X2 | T38.6X3 | T38.6X4 | T38.6X5 | T38.6X6 |
| Naftazone | T46.991 | T46.992 | T46.993 | T46.994 | T46.995 | T46.996 |
| Naftidrofuryl (oxalate) | T46.7X1 | T46.7X2 | T46.7X3 | T46.7X4 | T46.7X5 | T46.7X6 |
| Naftifine | T49.0X1 | T49.0X2 | T49.0X3 | T49.0X4 | T49.0X5 | T49.0X6 |
| Nail polish remover | T52.91 | T52.92 | T52.93 | T52.94 | | |
| Nalbuphine | T40.4X1 | T40.4X2 | T40.4X3 | T40.4X4 | T40.4X5 | T40.4X6 |
| Naled | T60.0X1 | T60.0X2 | T60.0X3 | T60.0X4 | — | — |
| Nalidixic acid | T37.8X1 | T37.8X2 | T37.8X3 | T37.8X4 | T37.8X5 | T37.8X6 |
| Nalorphine | T50.7X1 | T50.7X2 | T50.7X3 | T50.7X4 | T50.7X5 | T50.7X6 |
| Naloxone | T50.7X1 | T50.7X2 | T50.7X3 | T50.7X4 | T50.7X5 | T50.7X6 |
| Naltrexone | T50.7X1 | T50.7X2 | T50.7X3 | T50.7X4 | T50.7X5 | T50.7X6 |
| Namenda | T43.8X1 | T43.8X2 | T43.8X3 | T43.8X4 | T43.8X5 | T43.8X6 |
| Nandrolone | T38.7X1 | T38.7X2 | T38.7X3 | T38.7X4 | T38.7X5 | T38.7X6 |
| Naphazoline | T48.5X1 | T48.5X2 | T48.5X3 | T48.5X4 | T48.5X5 | T48.5X6 |
| Naphtha (painters') (petroleum) | T52.0X1 | T52.0X2 | T52.0X3 | T52.0X4 | — | — |
| solvent | T52.0X1 | T52.0X2 | T52.0X3 | T52.0X4 | — | — |
| vapor | T52.0X1 | T52.0X2 | T52.0X3 | T52.0X4 | — | — |
| Naphthalene (non-chlorinated) | T60.2X1 | T60.2X2 | T60.2X3 | T60.2X4 | — | — |
| chlorinated | T60.1X1 | T60.1X2 | T60.1X3 | T60.1X4 | — | — |
| vapor | T60.1X1 | T60.1X2 | T60.1X3 | T60.1X4 | — | — |

| Substance | Poisoning, Accidental (unintentional) | Poisoning, Intentional Self-harm | Poisoning, Assault | Poisoning, Undetermined | Adverse Effect | Under-dosing |
|---|---|---|---|---|---|---|
| **Naphthalene** — *continued* | | | | | | |
| insecticide or moth | T60.2X1 | T60.2X2 | T60.2X3 | T60.2X4 | — | — |
| repellent | | | | | | |
| chlorinated | T60.1X1 | T60.1X2 | T60.1X3 | T60.1X4 | — | — |
| vapor | T60.2X1 | T60.2X2 | T60.2X3 | T60.2X4 | — | — |
| chlorinated | T60.1X1 | T60.1X2 | T60.1X3 | T60.1X4 | — | — |
| **Naphthol** | T65.891 | T65.892 | T65.893 | T65.894 | — | — |
| **Naphthylamine** | T65.891 | T65.892 | T65.893 | T65.894 | — | — |
| **Naphthylthiourea** (ANTU) | T60.4X1 | T60.4X2 | T60.4X3 | T60.4X4 | — | — |
| **Naprosyn** — *see* Naproxen | | | | | | |
| **Naproxen** | T39.311 | T39.312 | T39.313 | T39.314 | T39.315 | T39.316 |
| **Narcotic** (drug) | T40.601 | T40.602 | T40.603 | T40.604 | T40.605 | T40.606 |
| analgesic NEC | T40.601 | T40.602 | T40.603 | T40.604 | T40.605 | T40.606 |
| antagonist | T50.7X1 | T50.7X2 | T50.7X3 | T50.7X4 | T50.7X5 | T50.7X6 |
| specified NEC | T40.691 | T40.692 | T40.693 | T40.694 | T40.695 | T40.696 |
| synthetic | T40.4X1 | T40.4X2 | T40.4X3 | T40.4X4 | T40.4X5 | T40.4X6 |
| **Narcotine** | T48.3X1 | T48.3X2 | T48.3X3 | T48.3X4 | T48.3X5 | T48.3X6 |
| **Nardil** | T43.1X1 | T43.1X2 | T43.1X3 | T43.1X4 | T43.1X5 | T43.1X6 |
| **Nasal drug NEC** | T49.6X1 | T49.6X2 | T49.6X3 | T49.6X4 | T49.6X5 | T49.6X6 |
| **Natamycin** | T49.0X1 | T49.0X2 | T49.0X3 | T49.0X4 | T49.0X5 | T49.0X6 |
| **Natrium cyanide** — *see* Cyanide(s) | | | | | | |
| **Natural** | | | | | | |
| blood (product) | T45.8X1 | T45.8X2 | T45.8X3 | T45.8X4 | T45.8X5 | T45.8X6 |
| gas (piped) | T59.891 | T59.892 | T59.893 | T59.894 | — | — |
| incomplete combustion | T58.11 | T58.12 | T58.13 | T58.14 | — | — |
| **Nealbarbital** | T42.3X1 | T42.3X2 | T42.3X3 | T42.3X4 | T42.3X5 | T42.3X6 |
| **Nectadon** | T48.3X1 | T48.3X2 | T48.3X3 | T48.3X4 | T48.3X5 | T48.3X6 |
| **Nedocromil** | T48.6X1 | T48.6X2 | T48.6X3 | T48.6X4 | T48.6X5 | T48.6X6 |
| **Nefopam** | T39.8X1 | T39.8X2 | T39.8X3 | T39.8X4 | T39.8X5 | T39.8X6 |
| **Nematocyst** (sting) | T63.691 | T63.692 | T63.693 | T63.694 | — | — |
| **Nembutal** | T42.3X1 | T42.3X2 | T42.3X3 | T42.3X4 | T42.3X5 | T42.3X6 |
| **Nemonapride** | T43.591 | T43.592 | T43.593 | T43.594 | T43.595 | T43.596 |
| **Neoarsphenamine** | T37.8X1 | T37.8X2 | T37.8X3 | T37.8X4 | T37.8X5 | T37.8X6 |
| **Neocinchophen** | T50.4X1 | T50.4X2 | T50.4X3 | T50.4X4 | T50.4X5 | T50.4X6 |
| **Neomycin** (derivatives) | T36.5X1 | T36.5X2 | T36.5X3 | T36.5X4 | T36.5X5 | T36.5X6 |
| with | | | | | | |
| bacitracin | T49.0X1 | T49.0X2 | T49.0X3 | T49.0X4 | T49.0X5 | T49.0X6 |
| neostigmine | T44.0X1 | T44.0X2 | T44.0X3 | T44.0X4 | T44.0X5 | T44.0X6 |
| ENT agent | T49.6X1 | T49.6X2 | T49.6X3 | T49.6X4 | T49.6X5 | T49.6X6 |
| ophthalmic preparation | T49.5X1 | T49.5X2 | T49.5X3 | T49.5X4 | T49.5X5 | T49.5X6 |
| topical NEC | T49.0X1 | T49.0X2 | T49.0X3 | T49.0X4 | T49.0X5 | T49.0X6 |
| **Neonal** | T42.3X1 | T42.3X2 | T42.3X3 | T42.3X4 | T42.3X5 | T42.3X6 |
| **Neoprontosil** | T37.0X1 | T37.0X2 | T37.0X3 | T37.0X4 | T37.0X5 | T37.0X6 |
| **Neosalvarsan** | T37.8X1 | T37.8X2 | T37.8X3 | T37.8X4 | T37.8X5 | T37.8X6 |
| **Neosilversalvarsan** | T37.8X1 | T37.8X2 | T37.8X3 | T37.8X4 | T37.8X5 | T37.8X6 |
| **Neosporin** | T36.8X1 | T36.8X2 | T36.8X3 | T36.8X4 | T36.8X5 | T36.8X6 |
| ENT agent | T49.6X1 | T49.6X2 | T49.6X3 | T49.6X4 | T49.6X5 | T49.6X6 |
| opthalmic preparation | T49.5X1 | T49.5X2 | T49.5X3 | T49.5X4 | T49.5X5 | T49.5X6 |
| topical NEC | T49.0X1 | T49.0X2 | T49.0X3 | T49.0X4 | T49.0X5 | T49.0X6 |
| **Neostigmine bromide** | T44.0X1 | T44.0X2 | T44.0X3 | T44.0X4 | T44.0X5 | T44.0X6 |
| **Neraval** | T42.3X1 | T42.3X2 | T42.3X3 | T42.3X4 | T42.3X5 | T42.3X6 |
| **Neravan** | T42.3X1 | T42.3X2 | T42.3X3 | T42.3X4 | T42.3X5 | T42.3X6 |
| **Nerium oleander** | T62.2X1 | T62.2X2 | T62.2X3 | T62.2X4 | — | — |
| **Nerve gas, not in war** | T59.91 | T59.92 | T59.93 | T59.94 | — | — |
| **Nesacaine** | T41.3X1 | T41.3X2 | T41.3X3 | T41.3X4 | T41.3X5 | T41.3X6 |
| infiltration (subcutaneous) | T41.3X1 | T41.3X2 | T41.3X3 | T41.3X4 | T41.3X5 | T41.3X6 |
| nerve block (peripheral) (plexus) | T41.3X1 | T41.3X2 | T41.3X3 | T41.3X4 | T41.3X5 | T41.3X6 |
| **Netilmicin** | T36.5X1 | T36.5X2 | T36.5X3 | T36.5X4 | T36.5X5 | T36.5X6 |
| **Neurobarb** | T42.3X1 | T42.3X2 | T42.3X3 | T42.3X4 | T42.3X5 | T42.3X6 |
| **Neuroleptic drug NEC** | T43.501 | T43.502 | T43.503 | T43.504 | T43.505 | T43.506 |
| **Neuromuscular blocking drug** | T48.1X1 | T48.1X2 | T48.1X3 | T48.1X4 | T48.1X5 | T48.1X6 |
| **Neutral insulin injection** | T38.3X1 | T38.3X2 | T38.3X3 | T38.3X4 | T38.3X5 | T38.3X6 |
| **Neutral spirits** | T51.0X1 | T51.0X2 | T51.0X3 | T51.0X4 | — | — |
| beverage | T51.0X1 | T51.0X2 | T51.0X3 | T51.0X4 | — | — |
| **Niacin** | T46.7X1 | T46.7X2 | T46.7X3 | T46.7X4 | T46.7X5 | T46.7X6 |
| **Niacinamide** | T45.2X1 | T45.2X2 | T45.2X3 | T45.2X4 | T45.2X5 | T45.2X6 |
| **Nialamide** | T43.1X1 | T43.1X2 | T43.1X3 | T43.1X4 | T43.1X5 | T43.1X6 |
| **Niaprazine** | T42.6X1 | T42.6X2 | T42.6X3 | T42.6X4 | T42.6X5 | T42.6X6 |
| **Nicametate** | T46.7X1 | T46.7X2 | T46.7X3 | T46.7X4 | T46.7X5 | T46.7X6 |
| **Nicardipine** | T46.1X1 | T46.1X2 | T46.1X3 | T46.1X4 | T46.1X5 | T46.1X6 |
| **Nicergoline** | T46.7X1 | T46.7X2 | T46.7X3 | T46.7X4 | T46.7X5 | T46.7X6 |
| **Nickel** (carbonyl) (tetra-carbonyl) (fumes) (vapor) | T56.891 | T56.892 | T56.893 | T56.894 | — | — |
| **Nickelocene** | T56.891 | T56.892 | T56.893 | T56.894 | — | — |
| **Niclosamide** | T37.4X1 | T37.4X2 | T37.4X3 | T37.4X4 | T37.4X5 | T37.4X6 |
| **Nicofuranose** | T46.7X1 | T46.7X2 | T46.7X3 | T46.7X4 | T46.7X5 | T46.7X6 |
| **Nicomorphine** | T40.2X1 | T40.2X2 | T40.2X3 | T40.2X4 | — | — |
| **Nicorandil** | T46.3X1 | T46.3X2 | T46.3X3 | T46.3X4 | T46.3X5 | T46.3X6 |
| **Nicotiana** (plant) | T62.2X1 | T62.2X2 | T62.2X3 | T62.2X4 | — | — |
| **Nicotinamide** | T45.2X1 | T45.2X2 | T45.2X3 | T45.2X4 | T45.2X5 | T45.2X6 |

| Substance | Poisoning, Accidental (unintentional) | Poisoning, Intentional Self-harm | Poisoning, Assault | Poisoning, Undetermined | Adverse Effect | Under-dosing |
|---|---|---|---|---|---|---|
| **Nicotine** (insecticide) (spray) (sulfate) NEC | T60.2X1 | T60.2X2 | T60.2X3 | T60.2X4 | — | — |
| from tobacco | T65.291 | T65.292 | T65.293 | T65.294 | — | — |
| cigarettes | T65.221 | T65.222 | T65.223 | T65.224 | — | — |
| not insecticide | T65.291 | T65.292 | T65.293 | T65.294 | — | — |
| **Nicotinic acid** | T46.7X1 | T46.7X2 | T46.7X3 | T46.7X4 | T46.7X5 | T46.7X6 |
| **Nicotinyl alcohol** | T46.7X1 | T46.7X2 | T46.7X3 | T46.7X4 | T46.7X5 | T46.7X6 |
| **Nicoumalone** | T45.511 | T45.512 | T45.513 | T45.514 | T45.515 | T45.516 |
| **Nifedipine** | T46.1X1 | T46.1X2 | T46.1X3 | T46.1X4 | T46.1X5 | T46.1X6 |
| **Nifenazone** | T39.2X1 | T39.2X2 | T39.2X3 | T39.2X4 | T39.2X5 | T39.2X6 |
| **Nifuraldezone** | T37.91 | T37.92 | T37.93 | T37.94 | T37.95 | T37.96 |
| **Nifuratel** | T37.8X1 | T37.8X2 | T37.8X3 | T37.8X4 | T37.8X5 | T37.8X6 |
| **Nifurtimox** | T37.3X1 | T37.3X2 | T37.3X3 | T37.3X4 | T37.3X5 | T37.3X6 |
| **Nifurtoinol** | T37.8X1 | T37.8X2 | T37.8X3 | T37.8X4 | T37.8X5 | T37.8X6 |
| **Nightshade, deadly** (solanum) — *see also* Belladonna | T62.2X1 | T62.2X2 | T62.2X3 | T62.2X4 | — | — |
| berry | T62.1X1 | T62.1X2 | T62.1X3 | T62.1X4 | — | — |
| **Nikethamide** | T50.7X1 | T50.7X2 | T50.7X3 | T50.7X4 | T50.7X5 | T50.7X6 |
| **Nilstat** | T36.7X1 | T36.7X2 | T36.7X3 | T36.7X4 | T36.7X5 | T36.7X6 |
| topical | T49.0X1 | T49.0X2 | T49.0X3 | T49.0X4 | T49.0X5 | T49.0X6 |
| **Nilutamide** | T38.6X1 | T38.6X2 | T38.6X3 | T38.6X4 | T38.6X5 | T38.6X6 |
| **Nimesulide** | T39.391 | T39.392 | T39.393 | T39.394 | T39.395 | T39.396 |
| **Nimetazepam** | T42.4X1 | T42.4X2 | T42.4X3 | T42.4X4 | T42.4X5 | T42.4X6 |
| **Nimodipine** | T46.1X1 | T46.1X2 | T46.1X3 | T46.1X4 | T46.1X5 | T46.1X6 |
| **Nimorazole** | T37.3X1 | T37.3X2 | T37.3X3 | T37.3X4 | T37.3X5 | T37.3X6 |
| **Nimustine** | T45.1X1 | T45.1X2 | T45.1X3 | T45.1X4 | T45.1X5 | T45.1X6 |
| **Niridazole** | T37.4X1 | T37.4X2 | T37.4X3 | T37.4X4 | T37.4X5 | T37.4X6 |
| **Nisentil** | T40.2X1 | T40.2X2 | T40.2X3 | T40.2X4 | T40.2X5 | T40.2X6 |
| **Nisoldipine** | T46.1X1 | T46.1X2 | T46.1X3 | T46.1X4 | T46.1X5 | T46.1X6 |
| **Nitramine** | T65.3X1 | T65.3X2 | T65.3X3 | T65.3X4 | — | — |
| **Nitrate, organic** | T46.3X1 | T46.3X2 | T46.3X3 | T46.3X4 | T46.3X5 | T46.3X6 |
| **Nitrazepam** | T42.4X1 | T42.4X2 | T42.4X3 | T42.4X4 | T42.4X5 | T42.4X6 |
| **Nitrefazole** | T50.6X1 | T50.6X2 | T50.6X3 | T50.6X4 | T50.6X5 | T50.6X6 |
| **Nitrendipine** | T46.1X1 | T46.1X2 | T46.1X3 | T46.1X4 | T46.1X5 | T46.1X6 |
| **Nitric** | | | | | | |
| acid (liquid) | T54.2X1 | T54.2X2 | T54.2X3 | T54.2X4 | — | — |
| vapor | T59.891 | T59.892 | T59.893 | T59.894 | — | — |
| oxide (gas) | T59.0X1 | T59.0X2 | T59.0X3 | T59.0X4 | — | — |
| **Nitrimidazine** | T37.3X1 | T37.3X2 | T37.3X3 | T37.3X4 | T37.3X5 | T37.3X6 |
| **Nitrite, amyl** (medicinal) | T46.3X1 | T46.3X2 | T46.3X3 | T46.3X4 | T46.3X5 | T46.3X6 |
| (vapor) | | | | | | |
| **Nitroaniline** | T65.3X1 | T65.3X2 | T65.3X3 | T65.3X4 | — | — |
| vapor | T59.891 | T59.892 | T59.893 | T59.894 | — | — |
| **Nitrobenzene, nitrobenzol** | T65.3X1 | T65.3X2 | T65.3X3 | T65.3X4 | — | — |
| vapor | T65.3X1 | T65.3X2 | T65.3X3 | T65.3X4 | — | — |
| **Nitrocellulose** | T65.891 | T65.892 | T65.893 | T65.894 | — | — |
| lacquer | T65.891 | T65.892 | T65.893 | T65.894 | — | — |
| **Nitrodiphenyl** | T65.3X1 | T65.3X2 | T65.3X3 | T65.3X4 | — | — |
| **Nitrofural** | T49.0X1 | T49.0X2 | T49.0X3 | T49.0X4 | T49.0X5 | T49.0X6 |
| **Nitrofurantoin** | T37.8X1 | T37.8X2 | T37.8X3 | T37.8X4 | T37.8X5 | T37.8X6 |
| **Nitrofurazone** | T49.0X1 | T49.0X2 | T49.0X3 | T49.0X4 | T49.0X5 | T49.0X6 |
| **Nitrogen** | T59.0X1 | T59.0X2 | T59.0X3 | T59.0X4 | — | — |
| mustard | T45.1X1 | T45.1X2 | T45.1X3 | T45.1X4 | T45.1X5 | T45.1X6 |
| **Nitroglycerin, nitroglycerol** (medicinal) | T46.3X1 | T46.3X2 | T46.3X3 | T46.3X4 | T46.3X5 | T46.3X6 |
| nonmedicinal | T65.5X1 | T65.5X2 | T65.5X3 | T65.5X4 | — | — |
| fumes | T65.5X1 | T65.5X2 | T65.5X3 | T65.5X4 | — | — |
| **Nitroglycol** | T52.3X1 | T52.3X2 | T52.3X3 | T52.3X4 | — | — |
| **Nitrohydrochloric acid** | T54.2X1 | T54.2X2 | T54.2X3 | T54.2X4 | — | — |
| **Nitromersol** | T49.0X1 | T49.0X2 | T49.0X3 | T49.0X4 | T49.0X5 | T49.0X6 |
| **Nitronaphthalene** | T65.891 | T65.892 | T65.893 | T65.894 | — | — |
| **Nitrophenol** | T54.0X1 | T54.0X2 | T54.0X3 | T54.0X4 | — | — |
| **Nitropropane** | T52.8X1 | T52.8X2 | T52.8X3 | T52.8X4 | — | — |
| **Nitroprusside** | T46.5X1 | T46.5X2 | T46.5X3 | T46.5X4 | T46.5X5 | T46.5X6 |
| **Nitrosodimethylamine** | T65.3X1 | T65.3X2 | T65.3X3 | T65.3X4 | — | — |
| **Nitrothiazol** | T37.4X1 | T37.4X2 | T37.4X3 | T37.4X4 | T37.4X5 | T37.4X6 |
| **Nitrotoluene, nitrotoluol** | T65.3X1 | T65.3X2 | T65.3X3 | T65.3X4 | — | — |
| vapor | T65.3X1 | T65.3X2 | T65.3X3 | T65.3X4 | — | — |
| **Nitrous** | | | | | | |
| acid (liquid) | T54.2X1 | T54.2X2 | T54.2X3 | T54.2X4 | — | — |
| fumes | T59.891 | T59.892 | T59.893 | T59.894 | — | — |
| ether spirit | T46.3X1 | T46.3X2 | T46.3X3 | T46.3X4 | T46.3X5 | T46.3X6 |
| oxide | T41.0X1 | T41.0X2 | T41.0X3 | T41.0X4 | T41.0X5 | T41.0X6 |
| **Nitroxoline** | T37.8X1 | T37.8X2 | T37.8X3 | T37.8X4 | T37.8X5 | T37.8X6 |
| **Nitrozone** | T49.0X1 | T49.0X2 | T49.0X3 | T49.0X4 | T49.0X5 | T49.0X6 |
| **Nizatidine** | T47.0X1 | T47.0X2 | T47.0X3 | T47.0X4 | T47.0X5 | T47.0X6 |
| **Nizofenone** | T43.8X1 | T43.8X2 | T43.8X3 | T43.8X4 | T43.8X5 | T43.8X6 |
| **Noctec** | T42.6X1 | T42.6X2 | T42.6X3 | T42.6X4 | T42.6X5 | T42.6X6 |
| **Noludar** | T42.6X1 | T42.6X2 | T42.6X3 | T42.6X4 | T42.6X5 | T42.6X6 |
| **Nomegestrol** | T38.5X1 | T38.5X2 | T38.5X3 | T38.5X4 | T38.5X5 | T38.5X6 |
| **Nomifensine** | T43.291 | T43.292 | T43.293 | T43.294 | T43.295 | T43.296 |
| **Nonoxinol** | T49.8X1 | T49.8X2 | T49.8X3 | T49.8X4 | T49.8X5 | T49.8X6 |

**Additional Character May Be Required — Refer to the Tabular List for Character Selection**  ▽ **Subterms under main terms may continue to next column or page**

| Substance | Poisoning, Accidental (unintentional) | Poisoning, Intentional Self-harm | Poisoning, Assault | Poisoning, Undetermined | Adverse Effect | Under-dosing |
|---|---|---|---|---|---|---|
| Nonylphenoxy | T49.8X1 | T49.8X2 | T49.8X3 | T49.8X4 | T49.8X5 | T49.8X6 |
| (polyethoxyethanol) | | | | | | |
| Noptil | T42.3X1 | T42.3X2 | T42.3X3 | T42.3X4 | T42.3X5 | T42.3X6 |
| Noradrenaline | T44.4X1 | T44.4X2 | T44.4X3 | T44.4X4 | T44.4X5 | T44.4X6 |
| Noramidopyrine | T39.2X1 | T39.2X2 | T39.2X3 | T39.2X4 | T39.2X5 | T39.2X6 |
| methanesulfonate sodium | T39.2X1 | T39.2X2 | T39.2X3 | T39.2X4 | T39.2X5 | T39.2X6 |
| Norbormide | T60.4X1 | T60.4X2 | T60.4X3 | T60.4X4 | — | — |
| Nordazepam | T42.4X1 | T42.4X2 | T42.4X3 | T42.4X4 | T42.4X5 | T42.4X6 |
| Norepinephrine | T44.4X1 | T44.4X2 | T44.4X3 | T44.4X4 | T44.4X5 | T44.4X6 |
| Norethandrolone | T38.7X1 | T38.7X2 | T38.7X3 | T38.7X4 | T38.7X5 | T38.7X6 |
| Norethindrone | T38.4X1 | T38.4X2 | T38.4X3 | T38.4X4 | T38.4X5 | T38.4X6 |
| Norethisterone (acetate) | T38.4X1 | T38.4X2 | T38.4X3 | T38.4X4 | T38.4X5 | T38.4X6 |
| (enantate) | | | | | | |
| with ethinylestradiol | T38.5X1 | T38.5X2 | T38.5X3 | T38.5X4 | T38.5X5 | T38.5X6 |
| Noretynodrel | T38.5X1 | T38.5X2 | T38.5X3 | T38.5X4 | T38.5X5 | T38.5X6 |
| Norfenefrine | T44.4X1 | T44.4X2 | T44.4X3 | T44.4X4 | T44.4X5 | T44.4X6 |
| Norfloxacin | T36.8X1 | T36.8X2 | T36.8X3 | T36.8X4 | T36.8X5 | T36.8X6 |
| Norgestrel | T38.4X1 | T38.4X2 | T38.4X3 | T38.4X4 | T38.4X5 | T38.4X6 |
| Norgestrienone | T38.4X1 | T38.4X2 | T38.4X3 | T38.4X4 | T38.4X5 | T38.4X6 |
| Norlestrin | T38.4X1 | T38.4X2 | T38.4X3 | T38.4X4 | T38.4X5 | T38.4X6 |
| Norlutin | T38.4X1 | T38.4X2 | T38.4X3 | T38.4X4 | T38.4X5 | T38.4X6 |
| Normal serum albumin (human), | T45.8X1 | T45.8X2 | T45.8X3 | T45.8X4 | T45.8X5 | T45.8X6 |
| salt-poor | | | | | | |
| Normethandrone | T38.5X1 | T38.5X2 | T38.5X3 | T38.5X4 | T38.5X5 | T38.5X6 |
| Normison — see Benzodiazepines | | | | | | |
| Normorphine | T40.2X1 | T40.2X2 | T40.2X3 | T40.2X4 | — | — |
| Norpseudoephedrine | T50.5X1 | T50.5X2 | T50.5X3 | T50.5X4 | T50.5X5 | T50.5X6 |
| Nortestosterone | T38.7X1 | T38.7X2 | T38.7X3 | T38.7X4 | T38.7X5 | T38.7X6 |
| (furanpropionate) | | | | | | |
| Nortriptyline | T43.011 | T43.012 | T43.013 | T43.014 | T43.015 | T43.016 |
| Noscapine | T48.3X1 | T48.3X2 | T48.3X3 | T48.3X4 | T48.3X5 | T48.3X6 |
| Nose preparations | T49.6X1 | T49.6X2 | T49.6X3 | T49.6X4 | T49.6X5 | T49.6X6 |
| Novobiocin | T36.5X1 | T36.5X2 | T36.5X3 | T36.5X4 | T36.5X5 | T36.5X6 |
| Novocain (infiltration) | T41.3X1 | T41.3X2 | T41.3X3 | T41.3X4 | T41.3X5 | T41.3X6 |
| (topical) | | | | | | |
| nerve block (peripheral) (plexus) | T41.3X1 | T41.3X2 | T41.3X3 | T41.3X4 | T41.3X5 | T41.3X6 |
| spinal | T41.3X1 | T41.3X2 | T41.3X3 | T41.3X4 | T41.3X5 | T41.3X6 |
| Noxious foodstuff | T62.91 | T62.92 | T62.93 | T62.94 | — | — |
| specified NEC | T62.8X1 | T62.8X2 | T62.8X3 | T62.8X4 | — | — |
| Noxiptiline | T43.011 | T43.012 | T43.013 | T43.014 | T43.015 | T43.016 |
| Noxytiolin | T49.0X1 | T49.0X2 | T49.0X3 | T49.0X4 | T49.0X5 | T49.0X6 |
| NPH Iletin (insulin) | T38.3X1 | T38.3X2 | T38.3X3 | T38.3X4 | T38.3X5 | T38.3X6 |
| Numorphan | T40.2X1 | T40.2X2 | T40.2X3 | T40.2X4 | T40.2X5 | T40.2X6 |
| Nunol | T42.3X1 | T42.3X2 | T42.3X3 | T42.3X4 | T42.3X5 | T42.3X6 |
| Nupercaine (spinal anesthetic) | T41.3X1 | T41.3X2 | T41.3X3 | T41.3X4 | T41.3X5 | T41.3X6 |
| topical (surface) | T41.3X1 | T41.3X2 | T41.3X3 | T41.3X4 | T41.3X5 | T41.3X6 |
| Nutmeg oil (liniment) | T49.3X1 | T49.3X2 | T49.3X3 | T49.3X4 | T49.3X5 | T49.3X6 |
| Nutritional supplement | T50.901 | T50.902 | T50.903 | T50.904 | T50.905 | T50.906 |
| Nux vomica | T65.1X1 | T65.1X2 | T65.1X3 | T65.1X4 | — | — |
| Nydrazid | T37.1X1 | T37.1X2 | T37.1X3 | T37.1X4 | T37.1X5 | T37.1X6 |
| Nylidrin | T46.7X1 | T46.7X2 | T46.7X3 | T46.7X4 | T46.7X5 | T46.7X6 |
| Nystatin | T36.7X1 | T36.7X2 | T36.7X3 | T36.7X4 | T36.7X5 | T36.7X6 |
| topical | T49.0X1 | T49.0X2 | T49.0X3 | T49.0X4 | T49.0X5 | T49.0X6 |
| Nytol | T45.0X1 | T45.0X2 | T45.0X3 | T45.0X4 | T45.0X5 | T45.0X6 |
| Obidoxime chloride | T50.6X1 | T50.6X2 | T50.6X3 | T50.6X4 | T50.6X5 | T50.6X6 |
| Octafonium (chloride) | T49.3X1 | T49.3X2 | T49.3X3 | T49.3X4 | T49.3X5 | T49.3X6 |
| Octamethyl pyrophosphoramide | T60.0X1 | T60.0X2 | T60.0X3 | T60.0X4 | — | — |
| Octanoin | T50.991 | T50.992 | T50.993 | T50.994 | T50.995 | T50.996 |
| Octatropine methylbromide | T44.3X1 | T44.3X2 | T44.3X3 | T44.3X4 | T44.3X5 | T44.3X6 |
| Octotiamine | T45.2X1 | T45.2X2 | T45.2X3 | T45.2X4 | T45.2X5 | T45.2X6 |
| Octoxinol (9) | T49.8X1 | T49.8X2 | T49.8X3 | T49.8X4 | T49.8X5 | T49.8X6 |
| Octreotide | T38.991 | T38.992 | T38.993 | T38.994 | T38.995 | T38.996 |
| Octyl nitrite | T46.3X1 | T46.3X2 | T46.3X3 | T46.3X4 | T46.3X5 | T46.3X6 |
| Oestradiol | T38.5X1 | T38.5X2 | T38.5X3 | T38.5X4 | T38.5X5 | T38.5X6 |
| Oestriol | T38.5X1 | T38.5X2 | T38.5X3 | T38.5X4 | T38.5X5 | T38.5X6 |
| Oestrogen | T38.5X1 | T38.5X2 | T38.5X3 | T38.5X4 | T38.5X5 | T38.5X6 |
| Oestrone | T38.5X1 | T38.5X2 | T38.5X3 | T38.5X4 | T38.5X5 | T38.5X6 |
| Ofloxacin | T36.8X1 | T36.8X2 | T36.8X3 | T36.8X4 | T36.8X5 | T36.8X6 |
| Oil (of) | T65.891 | T65.892 | T65.893 | T65.894 | — | — |
| bitter almond | T62.8X1 | T62.8X2 | T62.8X3 | T62.8X4 | — | — |
| cloves | T49.7X1 | T49.7X2 | T49.7X3 | T49.7X4 | T49.7X5 | T49.7X6 |
| colors | T65.6X1 | T65.6X2 | T65.6X3 | T65.6X4 | — | — |
| fumes | T59.891 | T59.892 | T59.893 | T59.894 | — | — |
| lubricating | T52.0X1 | T52.0X2 | T52.0X3 | T52.0X4 | — | — |
| Niobe | T52.8X1 | T52.8X2 | T52.8X3 | T52.8X4 | — | — |
| vitriol (liquid) | T54.2X1 | T54.2X2 | T54.2X3 | T54.2X4 | — | — |
| fumes | T54.2X1 | T54.2X2 | T54.2X3 | T54.2X4 | — | — |
| wintergreen (bitter) NEC | T49.3X1 | T49.3X2 | T49.3X3 | T49.3X4 | T49.3X5 | T49.3X6 |
| Oily preparation (for skin) | T49.3X1 | T49.3X2 | T49.3X3 | T49.3X4 | T49.3X5 | T49.3X6 |
| Ointment NEC | T49.3X1 | T49.3X2 | T49.3X3 | T49.3X4 | T49.3X5 | T49.3X6 |
| Olanzapine | T43.591 | T43.592 | T43.593 | T43.594 | T43.595 | T43.596 |
| Oleander | T62.2X1 | T62.2X2 | T62.2X3 | T62.2X4 | — | — |
| Oleandomycin | T36.3X1 | T36.3X2 | T36.3X3 | T36.3X4 | T36.3X5 | T36.3X6 |
| Oleandrin | T46.0X1 | T46.0X2 | T46.0X3 | T46.0X4 | T46.0X5 | T46.0X6 |
| Oleic acid | T46.6X1 | T46.6X2 | T46.6X3 | T46.6X4 | T46.6X5 | T46.6X6 |
| Oleovitamin A | T45.2X1 | T45.2X2 | T45.2X3 | T45.2X4 | T45.2X5 | T45.2X6 |
| Oleum ricini | T47.2X1 | T47.2X2 | T47.2X3 | T47.2X4 | T47.2X5 | T47.2X6 |
| Olive oil (medicinal) NEC | T47.4X1 | T47.4X2 | T47.4X3 | T47.4X4 | T47.4X5 | T47.4X6 |
| Olivomycin | T45.1X1 | T45.1X2 | T45.1X3 | T45.1X4 | T45.1X5 | T45.1X6 |
| Olsalazine | T47.8X1 | T47.8X2 | T47.8X3 | T47.8X4 | T47.8X5 | T47.8X6 |
| Omeprazole | T47.1X1 | T47.1X2 | T47.1X3 | T47.1X4 | T47.1X5 | T47.1X6 |
| OMPA | T60.0X1 | T60.0X2 | T60.0X3 | T60.0X4 | — | — |
| Oncovin | T45.1X1 | T45.1X2 | T45.1X3 | T45.1X4 | T45.1X5 | T45.1X6 |
| Ondansetron | T45.0X1 | T45.0X2 | T45.0X3 | T45.0X4 | T45.0X5 | T45.0X6 |
| Ophthaine | T41.3X1 | T41.3X2 | T41.3X3 | T41.3X4 | T41.3X5 | T41.3X6 |
| Ophthetic | T41.3X1 | T41.3X2 | T41.3X3 | T41.3X4 | T41.3X5 | T41.3X6 |
| Opiate NEC | T40.601 | T40.602 | T40.603 | T40.604 | T40.605 | T40.606 |
| antagonists | T50.7X1 | T50.7X2 | T50.7X3 | T50.7X4 | T50.7X5 | T50.7X6 |
| Opioid NEC | T40.2X1 | T40.2X2 | T40.2X3 | T40.2X4 | T40.2X5 | T40.2X6 |
| Opipramol | T43.011 | T43.012 | T43.013 | T43.014 | T43.015 | T43.016 |
| Opium alkaloids (total) | T40.0X1 | T40.0X2 | T40.0X3 | T40.0X4 | T40.0X5 | T40.0X6 |
| standardized powdered | T40.0X1 | T40.0X2 | T40.0X3 | T40.0X4 | T40.0X5 | T40.0X6 |
| tincture (camphorated) | T40.0X1 | T40.0X2 | T40.0X3 | T40.0X4 | T40.0X5 | T40.0X6 |
| Oracon | T38.4X1 | T38.4X2 | T38.4X3 | T38.4X4 | T38.4X5 | T38.4X6 |
| Oragrafin | T50.8X1 | T50.8X2 | T50.8X3 | T50.8X4 | T50.8X5 | T50.8X6 |
| Oral contraceptives | T38.4X1 | T38.4X2 | T38.4X3 | T38.4X4 | T38.4X5 | T38.4X6 |
| Oral rehydration salts | T50.3X1 | T50.3X2 | T50.3X3 | T50.3X4 | T50.3X5 | T50.3X6 |
| Orazamide | T50.991 | T50.992 | T50.993 | T50.994 | T50.995 | T50.996 |
| Orciprenaline | T48.291 | T48.292 | T48.293 | T48.294 | T48.295 | T48.296 |
| Organidin | T48.4X1 | T48.4X2 | T48.4X3 | T48.4X4 | T48.4X5 | T48.4X6 |
| Organonitrate NEC | T46.3X1 | T46.3X2 | T46.3X3 | T46.3X4 | T46.3X5 | T46.3X6 |
| Organophosphates | T60.0X1 | T60.0X2 | T60.0X3 | T60.0X4 | — | — |
| Orimune | T50.B91 | T50.B92 | T50.B93 | T50.B94 | T50.B95 | T50.B96 |
| Orinase | T38.3X1 | T38.3X2 | T38.3X3 | T38.3X4 | T38.3X5 | T38.3X6 |
| Ormeloxifene | T38.6X1 | T38.6X2 | T38.6X3 | T38.6X4 | T38.6X5 | T38.6X6 |
| Ornidazole | T37.3X1 | T37.3X2 | T37.3X3 | T37.3X4 | T37.3X5 | T37.3X6 |
| Ornithine aspartate | T50.991 | T50.992 | T50.993 | T50.994 | T50.995 | T50.996 |
| Ornoprostil | T47.1X1 | T47.1X2 | T47.1X3 | T47.1X4 | T47.1X5 | T47.1X6 |
| Orphenadrine (hydrochloride) | T42.8X1 | T42.8X2 | T42.8X3 | T42.8X4 | T42.8X5 | T42.8X6 |
| Ortal (sodium) | T42.3X1 | T42.3X2 | T42.3X3 | T42.3X4 | T42.3X5 | T42.3X6 |
| Orthoboric acid | T49.0X1 | T49.0X2 | T49.0X3 | T49.0X4 | T49.0X5 | T49.0X6 |
| ENT agent | T49.6X1 | T49.6X2 | T49.6X3 | T49.6X4 | T49.6X5 | T49.6X6 |
| ophthalmic preparation | T49.5X1 | T49.5X2 | T49.5X3 | T49.5X4 | T49.5X5 | T49.5X6 |
| Orthocaine | T41.3X1 | T41.3X2 | T41.3X3 | T41.3X4 | T41.3X5 | T41.3X6 |
| Orthodichlorobenzene | T53.7X1 | T53.7X2 | T53.7X3 | T53.7X4 | — | — |
| Ortho-Novum | T38.4X1 | T38.4X2 | T38.4X3 | T38.4X4 | T38.4X5 | T38.4X6 |
| Orthotolidine (reagent) | T54.2X1 | T54.2X2 | T54.2X3 | T54.2X4 | — | — |
| Osmic acid (liquid) | T54.2X1 | T54.2X2 | T54.2X3 | T54.2X4 | — | — |
| fumes | T54.2X1 | T54.2X2 | T54.2X3 | T54.2X4 | — | — |
| Osmotic diuretics | T50.2X1 | T50.2X2 | T50.2X3 | T50.2X4 | T50.2X5 | T50.2X6 |
| Otilonium bromide | T44.3X1 | T44.3X2 | T44.3X3 | T44.3X4 | T44.3X5 | T44.3X6 |
| Otorhinolaryngological drug NEC | T49.6X1 | T49.6X2 | T49.6X3 | T49.6X4 | T49.6X5 | T49.6X6 |
| Ouabain (e) | T46.0X1 | T46.0X2 | T46.0X3 | T46.0X4 | T46.0X5 | T46.0X6 |
| Ovarian hormone | T38.5X1 | T38.5X2 | T38.5X3 | T38.5X4 | T38.5X5 | T38.5X6 |
| stimulant | T38.5X1 | T38.5X2 | T38.5X3 | T38.5X4 | T38.5X5 | T38.5X6 |
| Ovral | T38.4X1 | T38.4X2 | T38.4X3 | T38.4X4 | T38.4X5 | T38.4X6 |
| Ovulen | T38.4X1 | T38.4X2 | T38.4X3 | T38.4X4 | T38.4X5 | T38.4X6 |
| Oxacillin | T36.0X1 | T36.0X2 | T36.0X3 | T36.0X4 | T36.0X5 | T36.0X6 |
| Oxalic acid | T54.2X1 | T54.2X2 | T54.2X3 | T54.2X4 | — | — |
| ammonium salt | T50.991 | T50.992 | T50.993 | T50.994 | T50.995 | T50.996 |
| Oxamniquine | T37.4X1 | T37.4X2 | T37.4X3 | T37.4X4 | T37.4X5 | T37.4X6 |
| Oxanamide | T43.591 | T43.592 | T43.593 | T43.594 | T43.595 | T43.596 |
| Oxandrolone | T38.7X1 | T38.7X2 | T38.7X3 | T38.7X4 | T38.7X5 | T38.7X6 |
| Oxantel | T37.4X1 | T37.4X2 | T37.4X3 | T37.4X4 | T37.4X5 | T37.4X6 |
| Oxapium iodide | T44.3X1 | T44.3X2 | T44.3X3 | T44.3X4 | T44.3X5 | T44.3X6 |
| Oxaprotiline | T43.021 | T43.022 | T43.023 | T43.024 | T43.025 | T43.026 |
| Oxaprozin | T39.311 | T39.312 | T39.313 | T39.314 | T39.315 | T39.316 |
| Oxatomide | T45.0X1 | T45.0X2 | T45.0X3 | T45.0X4 | T45.0X5 | T45.0X6 |
| Oxazepam | T42.4X1 | T42.4X2 | T42.4X3 | T42.4X4 | T42.4X5 | T42.4X6 |
| Oxazimedrine | T50.5X1 | T50.5X2 | T50.5X3 | T50.5X4 | T50.5X5 | T50.5X6 |
| Oxazolam | T42.4X1 | T42.4X2 | T42.4X3 | T42.4X4 | T42.4X5 | T42.4X6 |
| Oxazolidine derivatives | T42.2X1 | T42.2X2 | T42.2X3 | T42.2X4 | T42.2X5 | T42.2X6 |
| Oxazolidinedione (derivative) | T42.2X1 | T42.2X2 | T42.2X3 | T42.2X4 | T42.2X5 | T42.2X6 |
| Ox bile extract | T47.5X1 | T47.5X2 | T47.5X3 | T47.5X4 | T47.5X5 | T47.5X6 |
| Oxcarbazepine | T42.1X1 | T42.1X2 | T42.1X3 | T42.1X4 | T42.1X5 | T42.1X6 |
| Oxedrine | T44.4X1 | T44.4X2 | T44.4X3 | T44.4X4 | T44.4X5 | T44.4X6 |
| Oxeladin (citrate) | T48.3X1 | T48.3X2 | T48.3X3 | T48.3X4 | T48.3X5 | T48.3X6 |

Subterms under main terms may continue to next column or page    Additional Character May Be Required — Refer to the Tabular List for Character Selection    381

Nonylphenoxy — Oxeladin

**Table of Drugs and Chemicals**

**Oxendolone — Pentaquine**

| Substance | Poisoning, Accidental (unintentional) | Poisoning, Intentional Self-harm | Poisoning, Assault | Poisoning, Undetermined | Adverse Effect | Under-dosing |
|---|---|---|---|---|---|---|
| Oxendolone | T38.5X1 | T38.5X2 | T38.5X3 | T38.5X4 | T38.5X5 | T38.5X6 |
| Oxetacaine | T41.3X1 | T41.3X2 | T41.3X3 | T41.3X4 | T41.3X5 | T41.3X6 |
| Oxethazine | T41.3X1 | T41.3X2 | T41.3X3 | T41.3X4 | T41.3X5 | T41.3X6 |
| Oxetorone | T39.8X1 | T39.8X2 | T39.8X3 | T39.8X4 | T39.8X5 | T39.8X6 |
| Oxiconazole | T49.0X1 | T49.0X2 | T49.0X3 | T49.0X4 | T49.0X5 | T49.0X6 |
| Oxidizing agent NEC | T54.91 | T54.92 | T54.93 | T54.94 | — | — |
| Oxipurinol | T50.4X1 | T50.4X2 | T50.4X3 | T50.4X4 | T50.4X5 | T50.4X6 |
| Oxitriptan | T43.291 | T43.292 | T43.293 | T43.294 | T43.295 | T43.296 |
| Oxitropium bromide | T48.6X1 | T48.6X2 | T48.6X3 | T48.6X4 | T48.6X5 | T48.6X6 |
| Oxodipine | T46.1X1 | T46.1X2 | T46.1X3 | T46.1X4 | T46.1X5 | T46.1X6 |
| Oxolamine | T48.3X1 | T48.3X2 | T48.3X3 | T48.3X4 | T48.3X5 | T48.3X6 |
| Oxolinic acid | T37.8X1 | T37.8X2 | T37.8X3 | T37.8X4 | T37.8X5 | T37.8X6 |
| Oxomemazine | T43.3X1 | T43.3X2 | T43.3X3 | T43.3X4 | T43.3X5 | T43.3X6 |
| Oxophenarsine | T37.3X1 | T37.3X2 | T37.3X3 | T37.3X4 | T37.3X5 | T37.3X6 |
| Oxprenolol | T44.7X1 | T44.7X2 | T44.7X3 | T44.7X4 | T44.7X5 | T44.7X6 |
| Oxsoralen | T49.3X1 | T49.3X2 | T49.3X3 | T49.3X4 | T49.3X5 | T49.3X6 |
| Oxtriphylline | T48.6X1 | T48.6X2 | T48.6X3 | T48.6X4 | T48.6X5 | T48.6X6 |
| Oxybate sodium | T41.291 | T41.292 | T41.293 | T41.294 | T41.295 | T41.296 |
| Oxybuprocaine | T41.3X1 | T41.3X2 | T41.3X3 | T41.3X4 | T41.3X5 | T41.3X6 |
| Oxybutynin | T44.3X1 | T44.3X2 | T44.3X3 | T44.3X4 | T44.3X5 | T44.3X6 |
| Oxychlorosene | T49.0X1 | T49.0X2 | T49.0X3 | T49.0X4 | T49.0X5 | T49.0X6 |
| Oxycodone | T40.2X1 | T40.2X2 | T40.2X3 | T40.2X4 | T40.2X5 | T40.2X6 |
| Oxyfedrine | T46.3X1 | T46.3X2 | T46.3X3 | T46.3X4 | T46.3X5 | T46.3X6 |
| Oxygen | T41.5X1 | T41.5X2 | T41.5X3 | T41.5X4 | T41.5X5 | T41.5X6 |
| Oxylone | T49.0X1 | T49.0X2 | T49.0X3 | T49.0X4 | T49.0X5 | T49.0X6 |
|   ophthalmic preparation | T49.5X1 | T49.5X2 | T49.5X3 | T49.5X4 | T49.5X5 | T49.5X6 |
| Oxymesterone | T38.7X1 | T38.7X2 | T38.7X3 | T38.7X4 | T38.7X5 | T38.7X6 |
| Oxymetazoline | T48.5X1 | T48.5X2 | T48.5X3 | T48.5X4 | T48.5X5 | T48.5X6 |
| Oxymetholone | T38.7X1 | T38.7X2 | T38.7X3 | T38.7X4 | T38.7X5 | T38.7X6 |
| Oxymorphone | T40.2X1 | T40.2X2 | T40.2X3 | T40.2X4 | T40.2X5 | T40.2X6 |
| Oxypertine | T43.591 | T43.592 | T43.593 | T43.594 | T43.595 | T43.596 |
| Oxyphenbutazone | T39.2X1 | T39.2X2 | T39.2X3 | T39.2X4 | T39.2X5 | T39.2X6 |
| Oxyphencyclimine | T44.3X1 | T44.3X2 | T44.3X3 | T44.3X4 | T44.3X5 | T44.3X6 |
| Oxyphenisatine | T47.2X1 | T47.2X2 | T47.2X3 | T47.2X4 | T47.2X5 | T47.2X6 |
| Oxyphenonium bromide | T44.3X1 | T44.3X2 | T44.3X3 | T44.3X4 | T44.3X5 | T44.3X6 |
| Oxypolygelatin | T45.8X1 | T45.8X2 | T45.8X3 | T45.8X4 | T45.8X5 | T45.8X6 |
| Oxyquinoline (derivatives) | T37.8X1 | T37.8X2 | T37.8X3 | T37.8X4 | T37.8X5 | T37.8X6 |
| Oxytetracycline | T36.4X1 | T36.4X2 | T36.4X3 | T36.4X4 | T36.4X5 | T36.4X6 |
| Oxytocic drug NEC | T48.0X1 | T48.0X2 | T48.0X3 | T48.0X4 | T48.0X5 | T48.0X6 |
| Oxytocin (synthetic) | T48.0X1 | T48.0X2 | T48.0X3 | T48.0X4 | T48.0X5 | T48.0X6 |
| Ozone | T59.891 | T59.892 | T59.893 | T59.894 | — | — |
| PABA | T49.3X1 | T49.3X2 | T49.3X3 | T49.3X4 | T49.3X5 | T49.3X6 |
| Packed red cells | T45.8X1 | T45.8X2 | T45.8X3 | T45.8X4 | T45.8X5 | T45.8X6 |
| Padimate | T49.3X1 | T49.3X2 | T49.3X3 | T49.3X4 | T49.3X5 | T49.3X6 |
| Paint NEC | T65.6X1 | T65.6X2 | T65.6X3 | T65.6X4 | — | — |
|   cleaner | T52.91 | T52.92 | T52.93 | T52.94 | — | — |
|   fumes NEC | T59.891 | T59.892 | T59.893 | T59.894 | — | — |
|   lead (fumes) | T56.0X1 | T56.0X2 | T56.0X3 | T56.0X4 | — | — |
|   solvent NEC | T52.8X1 | T52.8X2 | T52.8X3 | T52.8X4 | — | — |
|   stripper | T52.8X1 | T52.8X2 | T52.8X3 | T52.8X4 | — | — |
| Palfium | T40.2X1 | T40.2X2 | T40.2X3 | T40.2X4 | — | — |
| Palm kernel oil | T50.991 | T50.992 | T50.993 | T50.994 | T50.995 | T50.996 |
| Paludrine | T37.2X1 | T37.2X2 | T37.2X3 | T37.2X4 | T37.2X5 | T37.2X6 |
| PAM (pralidoxime) | T50.6X1 | T50.6X2 | T50.6X3 | T50.6X4 | T50.6X5 | T50.6X6 |
| Pamaquine (naphthoute) | T37.2X1 | T37.2X2 | T37.2X3 | T37.2X4 | T37.2X5 | T37.2X6 |
| Panadol | T39.1X1 | T39.1X2 | T39.1X3 | T39.1X4 | T39.1X5 | T39.1X6 |
| Pancreatic | | | | | | |
|   digestive secretion stimulant | T47.8X1 | T47.8X2 | T47.8X3 | T47.8X4 | T47.8X5 | T47.8X6 |
|   dornase | T45.3X1 | T45.3X2 | T45.3X3 | T45.3X4 | T45.3X5 | T45.3X6 |
| Pancreatin | T47.5X1 | T47.5X2 | T47.5X3 | T47.5X4 | T47.5X5 | T47.5X6 |
| Pancrelipase | T47.5X1 | T47.5X2 | T47.5X3 | T47.5X4 | T47.5X5 | T47.5X6 |
| Pancuronium (bromide) | T48.1X1 | T48.1X2 | T48.1X3 | T48.1X4 | T48.1X5 | T48.1X6 |
| Pangamic acid | T45.2X1 | T45.2X2 | T45.2X3 | T45.2X4 | T45.2X5 | T45.2X6 |
| Panthenol | T45.2X1 | T45.2X2 | T45.2X3 | T45.2X4 | T45.2X5 | T45.2X6 |
|   topical | T49.8X1 | T49.8X2 | T49.8X3 | T49.8X4 | T49.8X5 | T49.8X6 |
| Pantopon | T40.0X1 | T40.0X2 | T40.0X3 | T40.0X4 | T40.0X5 | T40.0X6 |
| Pantothenic acid | T45.2X1 | T45.2X2 | T45.2X3 | T45.2X4 | T45.2X5 | T45.2X6 |
| Panwarfin | T45.511 | T45.512 | T45.513 | T45.514 | T45.515 | T45.516 |
| Papain | T47.5X1 | T47.5X2 | T47.5X3 | T47.5X4 | T47.5X5 | T47.5X6 |
|   digestant | T47.5X1 | T47.5X2 | T47.5X3 | T47.5X4 | T47.5X5 | T47.5X6 |
| Papaveretum | T40.0X1 | T40.0X2 | T40.0X3 | T40.0X4 | T40.0X5 | T40.0X6 |
| Papaverine | T44.3X1 | T44.3X2 | T44.3X3 | T44.3X4 | T44.3X5 | T44.3X6 |
| Para-acetamidophenol | T39.1X1 | T39.1X2 | T39.1X3 | T39.1X4 | T39.1X5 | T39.1X6 |
| Para-aminobenzoic acid | T49.3X1 | T49.3X2 | T49.3X3 | T49.3X4 | T49.3X5 | T49.3X6 |
| Para-aminophenol derivatives | T39.1X1 | T39.1X2 | T39.1X3 | T39.1X4 | T39.1X5 | T39.1X6 |
| Para-aminosalicylic acid | T37.1X1 | T37.1X2 | T37.1X3 | T37.1X4 | T37.1X5 | T37.1X6 |
| Paracetaldehyde | T42.6X1 | T42.6X2 | T42.6X3 | T42.6X4 | T42.6X5 | T42.6X6 |
| Paracetamol | T39.1X1 | T39.1X2 | T39.1X3 | T39.1X4 | T39.1X5 | T39.1X6 |
| Parachlorophenol (camphorated) | T49.0X1 | T49.0X2 | T49.0X3 | T49.0X4 | T49.0X5 | T49.0X6 |
| Paracodin | T40.2X1 | T40.2X2 | T40.2X3 | T40.2X4 | T40.2X5 | T40.2X6 |
| Paradione | T42.2X1 | T42.2X2 | T42.2X3 | T42.2X4 | T42.2X5 | T42.2X6 |
| Paraffin(s) (wax) | T52.0X1 | T52.0X2 | T52.0X3 | T52.0X4 | — | — |
|   liquid (medicinal) | T47.4X1 | T47.4X2 | T47.4X3 | T47.4X4 | T47.4X5 | T47.4X6 |
|   nonmedicinal | T52.0X1 | T52.0X2 | T52.0X3 | T52.0X4 | — | — |
| Paraformaldehyde | T60.3X1 | T60.3X2 | T60.3X3 | T60.3X4 | — | — |
| Paraldehyde | T42.6X1 | T42.6X2 | T42.6X3 | T42.6X4 | T42.6X5 | T42.6X6 |
| Paramethadione | T42.2X1 | T42.2X2 | T42.2X3 | T42.2X4 | T42.2X5 | T42.2X6 |
| Paramethasone | T38.0X1 | T38.0X2 | T38.0X3 | T38.0X4 | T38.0X5 | T38.0X6 |
|   acetate | T49.0X1 | T49.0X2 | T49.0X3 | T49.0X4 | T49.0X5 | T49.0X6 |
| Paraoxon | T60.0X1 | T60.0X2 | T60.0X3 | T60.0X4 | — | — |
| Paraquat | T60.3X1 | T60.3X2 | T60.3X3 | T60.3X4 | — | — |
| Parasympatholytic NEC | T44.3X1 | T44.3X2 | T44.3X3 | T44.3X4 | T44.3X5 | T44.3X6 |
| Parasympathomimetic drug NEC | T44.1X1 | T44.1X2 | T44.1X3 | T44.1X4 | T44.1X5 | T44.1X6 |
| Parathion | T60.0X1 | T60.0X2 | T60.0X3 | T60.0X4 | — | — |
| Parathormone | T50.991 | T50.992 | T50.993 | T50.994 | T50.995 | T50.996 |
| Parathyroid extract | T50.991 | T50.992 | T50.993 | T50.994 | T50.995 | T50.996 |
| Paratyphoid vaccine | T50.A91 | T50.A92 | T50.A93 | T50.A94 | T50.A95 | T50.A96 |
| Paredrine | T44.4X1 | T44.4X2 | T44.4X3 | T44.4X4 | T44.4X5 | T44.4X6 |
| Paregoric | T40.0X1 | T40.0X2 | T40.0X3 | T40.0X4 | T40.0X5 | T40.0X6 |
| Pargyline | T46.5X1 | T46.5X2 | T46.5X3 | T46.5X4 | T46.5X5 | T46.5X6 |
| Paris green | T57.0X1 | T57.0X2 | T57.0X3 | T57.0X4 | — | — |
|   insecticide | T57.0X1 | T57.0X2 | T57.0X3 | T57.0X4 | — | — |
| Parnate | T43.1X1 | T43.1X2 | T43.1X3 | T43.1X4 | T43.1X5 | T43.1X6 |
| Paromomycin | T36.5X1 | T36.5X2 | T36.5X3 | T36.5X4 | T36.5X5 | T36.5X6 |
| Paroxypropione | T45.1X1 | T45.1X2 | T45.1X3 | T45.1X4 | T45.1X5 | T45.1X6 |
| Parzone | T40.2X1 | T40.2X2 | T40.2X3 | T40.2X4 | T40.2X5 | T40.2X6 |
| PAS | T37.1X1 | T37.1X2 | T37.1X3 | T37.1X4 | T37.1X5 | T37.1X6 |
| Pasiniazid | T37.1X1 | T37.1X2 | T37.1X3 | T37.1X4 | T37.1X5 | T37.1X6 |
| PBB (polybrominated biphenyls) | T65.891 | T65.892 | T65.893 | T65.894 | — | — |
| PCB | T65.891 | T65.892 | T65.893 | T65.894 | — | — |
| PCP | | | | | | |
|   meaning pentachlorophenol | | | | | | |
|     fungicide | T60.3X1 | T60.3X2 | T60.3X3 | T60.3X4 | — | — |
|     herbicide | T60.3X1 | T60.3X2 | T60.3X3 | T60.3X4 | — | — |
|     insecticide | T60.1X1 | T60.1X2 | T60.1X3 | T60.1X4 | — | — |
|   meaning phencyclidine | T40.991 | T40.992 | T40.993 | T40.994 | — | — |
| Peach kernel oil (emulsion) | T47.4X1 | T47.4X2 | T47.4X3 | T47.4X4 | T47.4X5 | T47.4X6 |
| Peanut oil (emulsion) NEC | T47.4X1 | T47.4X2 | T47.4X3 | T47.4X4 | T47.4X5 | T47.4X6 |
|   topical | T49.3X1 | T49.3X2 | T49.3X3 | T49.3X4 | T49.3X5 | T49.3X6 |
| Pearly Gates (morning glory seeds) | T40.991 | T40.992 | T40.993 | T40.994 | — | — |
| Pecazine | T43.3X1 | T43.3X2 | T43.3X3 | T43.3X4 | T43.3X5 | T43.3X6 |
| Pectin | T47.6X1 | T47.6X2 | T47.6X3 | T47.6X4 | T47.6X5 | T47.6X6 |
| Pefloxacin | T37.8X1 | T37.8X2 | T37.8X3 | T37.8X4 | T37.8X5 | T37.8X6 |
| Pegademase, bovine | T50.Z91 | T50.Z92 | T50.Z93 | T50.Z94 | T50.Z95 | T50.Z96 |
| Pelletierine tannate | T37.4X1 | T37.4X2 | T37.4X3 | T37.4X4 | T37.4X5 | T37.4X6 |
| Pemirolast (potassium) | T48.6X1 | T48.6X2 | T48.6X3 | T48.6X4 | T48.6X5 | T48.6X6 |
| Pemoline | T50.7X1 | T50.7X2 | T50.7X3 | T50.7X4 | T50.7X5 | T50.7X6 |
| Pempidine | T44.2X1 | T44.2X2 | T44.2X3 | T44.2X4 | T44.2X5 | T44.2X6 |
| Penamecillin | T36.0X1 | T36.0X2 | T36.0X3 | T36.0X4 | T36.0X5 | T36.0X6 |
| Penbutolol | T44.7X1 | T44.7X2 | T44.7X3 | T44.7X4 | T44.7X5 | T44.7X6 |
| Penethamate | T36.0X1 | T36.0X2 | T36.0X3 | T36.0X4 | T36.0X5 | T36.0X6 |
| Penfluridol | T43.591 | T43.592 | T43.593 | T43.594 | T43.595 | T43.596 |
| Penflutizide | T50.2X1 | T50.2X2 | T50.2X3 | T50.2X4 | T50.2X5 | T50.2X6 |
| Pengitoxin | T46.0X1 | T46.0X2 | T46.0X3 | T46.0X4 | T46.0X5 | T46.0X6 |
| Penicillamine | T50.6X1 | T50.6X2 | T50.6X3 | T50.6X4 | T50.6X5 | T50.6X6 |
| Penicillin (any) | T36.0X1 | T36.0X2 | T36.0X3 | T36.0X4 | T36.0X5 | T36.0X6 |
| Penicillinase | T45.3X1 | T45.3X2 | T45.3X3 | T45.3X4 | T45.3X5 | T45.3X6 |
| Penicilloyl polylysine | T50.8X1 | T50.8X2 | T50.8X3 | T50.8X4 | T50.8X5 | T50.8X6 |
| Penimepicycline | T36.4X1 | T36.4X2 | T36.4X3 | T36.4X4 | T36.4X5 | T36.4X6 |
| Pentachloroethane | T53.6X1 | T53.6X2 | T53.6X3 | T53.6X4 | — | — |
| Pentachloronaphthalene | T53.7X1 | T53.7X2 | T53.7X3 | T53.7X4 | — | — |
| Pentachlorophenol (pesticide) | T60.1X1 | T60.1X2 | T60.1X3 | T60.1X4 | — | — |
|   fungicide | T60.3X1 | T60.3X2 | T60.3X3 | T60.3X4 | — | — |
|   herbicide | T60.3X1 | T60.3X2 | T60.3X3 | T60.3X4 | — | — |
|   insecticide | T60.1X1 | T60.1X2 | T60.1X3 | T60.1X4 | — | — |
| Pentaerythritol | T46.3X1 | T46.3X2 | T46.3X3 | T46.3X4 | T46.3X5 | T46.3X6 |
|   chloral | T42.6X1 | T42.6X2 | T42.6X3 | T42.6X4 | T42.6X5 | T42.6X6 |
|   tetranitrate NEC | T46.3X1 | T46.3X2 | T46.3X3 | T46.3X4 | T46.3X5 | T46.3X6 |
| Pentaerythrityl tetranitrate | T46.3X1 | T46.3X2 | T46.3X3 | T46.3X4 | T46.3X5 | T46.3X6 |
| Pentagastrin | T50.8X1 | T50.8X2 | T50.8X3 | T50.8X4 | T50.8X5 | T50.8X6 |
| Pentalin | T53.6X1 | T53.6X2 | T53.6X3 | T53.6X4 | — | — |
| Pentamethonium bromide | T44.2X1 | T44.2X2 | T44.2X3 | T44.2X4 | T44.2X5 | T44.2X6 |
| Pentamidine | T37.3X1 | T37.3X2 | T37.3X3 | T37.3X4 | T37.3X5 | T37.3X6 |
| Pentanol | T51.3X1 | T51.3X2 | T51.3X3 | T51.3X4 | — | — |
| Pentapyrrolinium (bitartrate) | T44.2X1 | T44.2X2 | T44.2X3 | T44.2X4 | T44.2X5 | T44.2X6 |
| Pentaquine | T37.2X1 | T37.2X2 | T37.2X3 | T37.2X4 | T37.2X5 | T37.2X6 |

Additional Character May Be Required — Refer to the Tabular List for Character Selection    ▽ Subterms under main terms may continue to next column or page

**Table of Drugs and Chemicals**

| Substance | Poisoning, Accidental (unintentional) | Poisoning, Intentional Self-harm | Poisoning, Assault | Poisoning, Undetermined | Adverse Effect | Under-dosing |
|---|---|---|---|---|---|---|
| Pentazocine | T40.4X1 | T40.4X2 | T40.4X3 | T40.4X4 | T40.4X5 | T40.4X6 |
| Pentetrazole | T50.7X1 | T50.7X2 | T50.7X3 | T50.7X4 | T50.7X5 | T50.7X6 |
| Penthienate bromide | T44.3X1 | T44.3X2 | T44.3X3 | T44.3X4 | T44.3X5 | T44.3X6 |
| Pentifylline | T46.7X1 | T46.7X2 | T46.7X3 | T46.7X4 | T46.7X5 | T46.7X6 |
| Pentobarbital | T42.3X1 | T42.3X2 | T42.3X3 | T42.3X4 | T42.3X5 | T42.3X6 |
|   sodium | T42.3X1 | T42.3X2 | T42.3X3 | T42.3X4 | T42.3X5 | T42.3X6 |
| Pentobarbitone | T42.3X1 | T42.3X2 | T42.3X3 | T42.3X4 | T42.3X5 | T42.3X6 |
| Pentolonium tartrate | T44.2X1 | T44.2X2 | T44.2X3 | T44.2X4 | T44.2X5 | T44.2X6 |
| Pentosan polysulfate (sodium) | T39.8X1 | T39.8X2 | T39.8X3 | T39.8X4 | T39.8X5 | T39.8X6 |
| Pentostatin | T45.1X1 | T45.1X2 | T45.1X3 | T45.1X4 | T45.1X5 | T45.1X6 |
| Pentothal | T41.1X1 | T41.1X2 | T41.1X3 | T41.1X4 | T41.1X5 | T41.1X6 |
| Pentoxifylline | T46.7X1 | T46.7X2 | T46.7X3 | T46.7X4 | T46.7X5 | T46.7X6 |
| Pentoxyverine | T48.3X1 | T48.3X2 | T48.3X3 | T48.3X4 | T48.3X5 | T48.3X6 |
| Pentrinat | T46.3X1 | T46.3X2 | T46.3X3 | T46.3X4 | T46.3X5 | T46.3X6 |
| Pentylenetetrazole | T50.7X1 | T50.7X2 | T50.7X3 | T50.7X4 | T50.7X5 | T50.7X6 |
| Pentylsalicylamide | T37.1X1 | T37.1X2 | T37.1X3 | T37.1X4 | T37.1X5 | T37.1X6 |
| Pentymal | T42.3X1 | T42.3X2 | T42.3X3 | T42.3X4 | T42.3X5 | T42.3X6 |
| Peplomycin | T45.1X1 | T45.1X2 | T45.1X3 | T45.1X4 | T45.1X5 | T45.1X6 |
| Peppermint (oil) | T47.5X1 | T47.5X2 | T47.5X3 | T47.5X4 | T47.5X5 | T47.5X6 |
| Pepsin | T47.5X1 | T47.5X2 | T47.5X3 | T47.5X4 | T47.5X5 | T47.5X6 |
|   digestant | T47.5X1 | T47.5X2 | T47.5X3 | T47.5X4 | T47.5X5 | T47.5X6 |
| Pepstatin | T47.1X1 | T47.1X2 | T47.1X3 | T47.1X4 | T47.1X5 | T47.1X6 |
| Peptavlon | T50.8X1 | T50.8X2 | T50.8X3 | T50.8X4 | T50.8X5 | T50.8X6 |
| Perazine | T43.3X1 | T43.3X2 | T43.3X3 | T43.3X4 | T43.3X5 | T43.3X6 |
| Percaine (spinal) | T41.3X1 | T41.3X2 | T41.3X3 | T41.3X4 | T41.3X5 | T41.3X6 |
|   topical (surface) | T41.3X1 | T41.3X2 | T41.3X3 | T41.3X4 | T41.3X5 | T41.3X6 |
| Perchloroethylene | T53.5X1 | T53.5X2 | T53.5X3 | T53.5X4 | — | — |
|   medicinal | T37.4X1 | T37.4X2 | T37.4X3 | T37.4X4 | T37.4X5 | T37.4X6 |
|   vapor | T53.3X1 | T53.3X2 | T53.3X3 | T53.3X4 | — | — |
| Percodan | T40.2X1 | T40.2X2 | T40.2X3 | T40.2X4 | T40.2X5 | T40.2X6 |
| Percogesic — see also acetaminophen | T45.0X1 | T45.0X2 | T45.0X3 | T45.0X4 | T45.0X5 | T45.0X6 |
| Percorten | T38.0X1 | T38.0X2 | T38.0X3 | T38.0X4 | T38.0X5 | T38.0X6 |
| Pergolide | T42.8X1 | T42.8X2 | T42.8X3 | T42.8X4 | T42.8X5 | T42.8X6 |
| Pergonal | T38.811 | T38.812 | T38.813 | T38.814 | T38.815 | T38.816 |
| Perhexilene | T46.3X1 | T46.3X2 | T46.3X3 | T46.3X4 | T46.3X5 | T46.3X6 |
| Perhexiline (maleate) | T46.3X1 | T46.3X2 | T46.3X3 | T46.3X4 | T46.3X5 | T46.3X6 |
| Periactin | T45.0X1 | T45.0X2 | T45.0X3 | T45.0X4 | T45.0X5 | T45.0X6 |
| Periciazine | T43.3X1 | T43.3X2 | T43.3X3 | T43.3X4 | T43.3X5 | T43.3X6 |
| Periclor | T42.6X1 | T42.6X2 | T42.6X3 | T42.6X4 | T42.6X5 | T42.6X6 |
| Perindopril | T46.4X1 | T46.4X2 | T46.4X3 | T46.4X4 | T46.4X5 | T46.4X6 |
| Perisoxal | T39.8X1 | T39.8X2 | T39.8X3 | T39.8X4 | T39.8X5 | T39.8X6 |
| Peritoneal dialysis solution | T50.3X1 | T50.3X2 | T50.3X3 | T50.3X4 | T50.3X5 | T50.3X6 |
| Peritrate | T46.3X1 | T46.3X2 | T46.3X3 | T46.3X4 | T46.3X5 | T46.3X6 |
| Perlapine | T42.4X1 | T42.4X2 | T42.4X3 | T42.4X4 | T42.4X5 | T42.4X6 |
| Permanganate | T65.891 | T65.892 | T65.893 | T65.894 | — | — |
| Permethrin | T60.1X1 | T60.1X2 | T60.1X3 | T60.1X4 | — | — |
| Pernocton | T42.3X1 | T42.3X2 | T42.3X3 | T42.3X4 | T42.3X5 | T42.3X6 |
| Pernoston | T42.3X1 | T42.3X2 | T42.3X3 | T42.3X4 | T42.3X5 | T42.3X6 |
| Peronine | T40.2X1 | T40.2X2 | T40.2X3 | T40.2X4 | — | — |
| Perphenazine | T43.3X1 | T43.3X2 | T43.3X3 | T43.3X4 | T43.3X5 | T43.3X6 |
| Pertofrane | T43.011 | T43.012 | T43.013 | T43.014 | T43.015 | T43.016 |
| Pertussis | | | | | | |
|   immune serum (human) | T50.Z11 | T50.Z12 | T50.Z13 | T50.Z14 | T50.Z15 | T50.Z16 |
|   vaccine (with diphtheria toxoid) (with tetanus toxoid) | T50.A11 | T50.A12 | T50.A13 | T50.A14 | T50.A15 | T50.A16 |
| Peruvian balsam | T49.0X1 | T49.0X2 | T49.0X3 | T49.0X4 | T49.0X5 | T49.0X6 |
| Peruvoside | T46.0X1 | T46.0X2 | T46.0X3 | T46.0X4 | T46.0X5 | T46.0X6 |
| Pesticide (dust) (fumes) (vapor) | T60.91 | T60.92 | T60.93 | T60.94 | — | — |
|   NEC | | | | | | |
|   arsenic | T57.0X1 | T57.0X2 | T57.0X3 | T57.0X4 | — | — |
|   chlorinated | T60.1X1 | T60.1X2 | T60.1X3 | T60.1X4 | — | — |
|   cyanide | T65.0X1 | T65.0X2 | T65.0X3 | T65.0X4 | — | — |
|   kerosene | T52.0X1 | T52.0X2 | T52.0X3 | T52.0X4 | — | — |
|   mixture (of compounds) | T60.91 | T60.92 | T60.93 | T60.94 | — | — |
|   naphthalene | T60.2X1 | T60.2X2 | T60.2X3 | T60.2X4 | — | — |
|   organochlorine (compounds) | T60.1X1 | T60.1X2 | T60.1X3 | T60.1X4 | — | — |
|   petroleum (distillate) (products) NEC | T60.8X1 | T60.8X2 | T60.8X3 | T60.8X4 | — | — |
|   specified ingredient NEC | T60.8X1 | T60.8X2 | T60.8X3 | T60.8X4 | — | — |
|   strychnine | T65.1X1 | T65.1X2 | T65.1X3 | T65.1X4 | — | — |
|   thallium | T60.4X1 | T60.4X2 | T60.4X3 | T60.4X4 | — | — |
| Pethidine | T40.4X1 | T40.4X2 | T40.4X3 | T40.4X4 | T40.4X5 | T40.4X6 |
| Petrichloral | T42.6X1 | T42.6X2 | T42.6X3 | T42.6X4 | T42.6X5 | T42.6X6 |
| Petrol | T52.0X1 | T52.0X2 | T52.0X3 | T52.0X4 | — | — |
|   vapor | T52.0X1 | T52.0X2 | T52.0X3 | T52.0X4 | — | — |
| Petrolatum | T49.3X1 | T49.3X2 | T49.3X3 | T49.3X4 | T49.3X5 | T49.3X6 |
|   hydrophilic | T49.3X1 | T49.3X2 | T49.3X3 | T49.3X4 | T49.3X5 | T49.3X6 |
|   liquid | T47.4X1 | T47.4X2 | T47.4X3 | T47.4X4 | T47.4X5 | T47.4X6 |
|     topical | T49.3X1 | T49.3X2 | T49.3X3 | T49.3X4 | T49.3X5 | T49.3X6 |
|   nonmedicinal | T52.0X1 | T52.0X2 | T52.0X3 | T52.0X4 | — | — |
| Petrolatum — continued | | | | | | |
|   red veterinary | T49.3X1 | T49.3X2 | T49.3X3 | T49.3X4 | T49.3X5 | T49.3X6 |
|   white | T49.3X1 | T49.3X2 | T49.3X3 | T49.3X4 | T49.3X5 | T49.3X6 |
| Petroleum (products) NEC | T52.0X1 | T52.0X2 | T52.0X3 | T52.0X4 | — | — |
|   benzine(s) — see Ligroin | | | | | | |
|   ether — see Ligroin | | | | | | |
|   jelly — see Petrolatum | | | | | | |
|   naphtha — see Ligroin | | | | | | |
|   pesticide | T60.8X1 | T60.8X2 | T60.8X3 | T60.8X4 | — | — |
|   solids | T52.0X1 | T52.0X2 | T52.0X3 | T52.0X4 | — | — |
|   solvents | T52.0X1 | T52.0X2 | T52.0X3 | T52.0X4 | — | — |
|   vapor | T52.0X1 | T52.0X2 | T52.0X3 | T52.0X4 | — | — |
| Peyote | T40.991 | T40.992 | T40.993 | T40.994 | — | — |
| Phanodorm, phanodorn | T42.3X1 | T42.3X2 | T42.3X3 | T42.3X4 | T42.3X5 | T42.3X6 |
| Phanquinone | T37.3X1 | T37.3X2 | T37.3X3 | T37.3X4 | T37.3X5 | T37.3X6 |
| Phanquone | T37.3X1 | T37.3X2 | T37.3X3 | T37.3X4 | T37.3X5 | T37.3X6 |
| Pharmaceutical | | | | | | |
|   adjunct NEC | T50.901 | T50.902 | T50.903 | T50.904 | T50.905 | T50.906 |
|   excipient NEC | T50.901 | T50.902 | T50.903 | T50.904 | T50.905 | T50.906 |
|   sweetener | T50.901 | T50.902 | T50.903 | T50.904 | T50.905 | T50.906 |
|   viscous agent | T50.901 | T50.902 | T50.903 | T50.904 | T50.905 | T50.906 |
| Phemitone | T42.3X1 | T42.3X2 | T42.3X3 | T42.3X4 | T42.3X5 | T42.3X6 |
| Phenacaine | T41.3X1 | T41.3X2 | T41.3X3 | T41.3X4 | T41.3X5 | T41.3X6 |
| Phenacemide | T42.6X1 | T42.6X2 | T42.6X3 | T42.6X4 | T42.6X5 | T42.6X6 |
| Phenacetin | T39.1X1 | T39.1X2 | T39.1X3 | T39.1X4 | T39.1X5 | T39.1X6 |
| Phenadoxone | T40.2X1 | T40.2X2 | T40.2X3 | T40.2X4 | — | — |
| Phenaglycodol | T43.591 | T43.592 | T43.593 | T43.594 | T43.595 | T43.596 |
| Phenantoin | T42.0X1 | T42.0X2 | T42.0X3 | T42.0X4 | T42.0X5 | T42.0X6 |
| Phenaphthazine reagent | T50.991 | T50.992 | T50.993 | T50.994 | T50.995 | T50.996 |
| Phenazocine | T40.4X1 | T40.4X2 | T40.4X3 | T40.4X4 | T40.4X5 | T40.4X6 |
| Phenazone | T39.2X1 | T39.2X2 | T39.2X3 | T39.2X4 | T39.2X5 | T39.2X6 |
| Phenazopyridine | T39.8X1 | T39.8X2 | T39.8X3 | T39.8X4 | T39.8X5 | T39.8X6 |
| Phenbenicillin | T36.0X1 | T36.0X2 | T36.0X3 | T36.0X4 | T36.0X5 | T36.0X6 |
| Phenbutrazate | T50.5X1 | T50.5X2 | T50.5X3 | T50.5X4 | T50.5X5 | T50.5X6 |
| Phencyclidine | T40.991 | T40.992 | T40.993 | T40.994 | T40.995 | T40.996 |
| Phendimetrazine | T50.5X1 | T50.5X2 | T50.5X3 | T50.5X4 | T50.5X5 | T50.5X6 |
| Phenelzine | T43.1X1 | T43.1X2 | T43.1X3 | T43.1X4 | T43.1X5 | T43.1X6 |
| Phenemal | T42.3X1 | T42.3X2 | T42.3X3 | T42.3X4 | T42.3X5 | T42.3X6 |
| Phenergan | T42.6X1 | T42.6X2 | T42.6X3 | T42.6X4 | T42.6X5 | T42.6X6 |
| Pheneticillin | T36.0X1 | T36.0X2 | T36.0X3 | T36.0X4 | T36.0X5 | T36.0X6 |
| Pheneturide | T42.6X1 | T42.6X2 | T42.6X3 | T42.6X4 | T42.6X5 | T42.6X6 |
| Phenformin | T38.3X1 | T38.3X2 | T38.3X3 | T38.3X4 | T38.3X5 | T38.3X6 |
| Phenglutarimide | T44.3X1 | T44.3X2 | T44.3X3 | T44.3X4 | T44.3X5 | T44.3X6 |
| Phenicarbazide | T39.8X1 | T39.8X2 | T39.8X3 | T39.8X4 | T39.8X5 | T39.8X6 |
| Phenindamine | T45.0X1 | T45.0X2 | T45.0X3 | T45.0X4 | T45.0X5 | T45.0X6 |
| Phenindione | T45.511 | T45.512 | T45.513 | T45.514 | T45.515 | T45.516 |
| Pheniprazine | T43.1X1 | T43.1X2 | T43.1X3 | T43.1X4 | T43.1X5 | T43.1X6 |
| Pheniramine | T45.0X1 | T45.0X2 | T45.0X3 | T45.0X4 | T45.0X5 | T45.0X6 |
| Phenisatin | T47.2X1 | T47.2X2 | T47.2X3 | T47.2X4 | T47.2X5 | T47.2X6 |
| Phenmetrazine | T50.5X1 | T50.5X2 | T50.5X3 | T50.5X4 | T50.5X5 | T50.5X6 |
| Phenobal | T42.3X1 | T42.3X2 | T42.3X3 | T42.3X4 | T42.3X5 | T42.3X6 |
| Phenobarbital | | | | | | |
|   with | | | | | | |
|     mephenytoin | T42.3X1 | T42.3X2 | T42.3X3 | T42.3X4 | T42.3X5 | T42.3X6 |
|     phenytoin | T42.3X1 | T42.3X2 | T42.3X3 | T42.3X4 | T42.3X5 | T42.3X6 |
|   sodium | T42.3X1 | T42.3X2 | T42.3X3 | T42.3X4 | T42.3X5 | T42.3X6 |
| Phenobarbitone | T42.3X1 | T42.3X2 | T42.3X3 | T42.3X4 | T42.3X5 | T42.3X6 |
| Phenobutiodil | T50.8X1 | T50.8X2 | T50.8X3 | T50.8X4 | T50.8X5 | T50.8X6 |
| Phenoctide | T49.0X1 | T49.0X2 | T49.0X3 | T49.0X4 | T49.0X5 | T49.0X6 |
| Phenol | T49.0X1 | T49.0X2 | T49.0X3 | T49.0X4 | T49.0X5 | T49.0X6 |
|   disinfectant | T54.0X1 | T54.0X2 | T54.0X3 | T54.0X4 | — | — |
|   in oil injection | T46.8X1 | T46.8X2 | T46.8X3 | T46.8X4 | T46.8X5 | T46.8X6 |
|   medicinal | T49.1X1 | T49.1X2 | T49.1X3 | T49.1X4 | T49.1X5 | T49.1X6 |
|   nonmedicinal NEC | T54.0X1 | T54.0X2 | T54.0X3 | T54.0X4 | — | — |
|   pesticide | T60.8X1 | T60.8X2 | T60.8X3 | T60.8X4 | — | — |
|   red | T50.8X1 | T50.8X2 | T50.8X3 | T50.8X4 | T50.8X5 | T50.8X6 |
| Phenolic preparation | T49.1X1 | T49.1X2 | T49.1X3 | T49.1X4 | T49.1X5 | T49.1X6 |
| Phenolphthalein | T47.2X1 | T47.2X2 | T47.2X3 | T47.2X4 | T47.2X5 | T47.2X6 |
| Phenolsulfonphthalein | T50.8X1 | T50.8X2 | T50.8X3 | T50.8X4 | T50.8X5 | T50.8X6 |
| Phenomorphan | T40.2X1 | T40.2X2 | T40.2X3 | T40.2X4 | — | — |
| Phenonyl | T42.3X1 | T42.3X2 | T42.3X3 | T42.3X4 | T42.3X5 | T42.3X6 |
| Phenoperidine | T40.4X1 | T40.4X2 | T40.4X3 | T40.4X4 | — | — |
| Phenopyrazone | T46.991 | T46.992 | T46.993 | T46.994 | T46.995 | T46.996 |
| Phenoquin | T50.4X1 | T50.4X2 | T50.4X3 | T50.4X4 | T50.4X5 | T50.4X6 |
| Phenothiazine (psychotropic) | T43.3X1 | T43.3X2 | T43.3X3 | T43.3X4 | T43.3X5 | T43.3X6 |
|   NEC | | | | | | |
|   insecticide | T60.2X1 | T60.2X2 | T60.2X3 | T60.2X4 | — | — |
| Phenothrin | T49.0X1 | T49.0X2 | T49.0X3 | T49.0X4 | T49.0X5 | T49.0X6 |
| Phenoxybenzamine | T46.7X1 | T46.7X2 | T46.7X3 | T46.7X4 | T46.7X5 | T46.7X6 |
| Phenoxyethanol | T49.0X1 | T49.0X2 | T49.0X3 | T49.0X4 | T49.0X5 | T49.0X6 |
| Phenoxymethyl penicillin | T36.0X1 | T36.0X2 | T36.0X3 | T36.0X4 | T36.0X5 | T36.0X6 |
| Phenprobamate | T42.8X1 | T42.8X2 | T42.8X3 | T42.8X4 | T42.8X5 | T42.8X6 |
| Phenprocoumon | T45.511 | T45.512 | T45.513 | T45.514 | T45.515 | T45.516 |

| Substance | Poisoning, Accidental (unintentional) | Poisoning, Intentional Self-harm | Poisoning, Assault | Poisoning, Undetermined | Adverse Effect | Under-dosing |
|---|---|---|---|---|---|---|
| Phensuximide | T42.2X1 | T42.2X2 | T42.2X3 | T42.2X4 | T42.2X5 | T42.2X6 |
| Phentermine | T50.5X1 | T50.5X2 | T50.5X3 | T50.5X4 | T50.5X5 | T50.5X6 |
| Phenthicillin | T36.0X1 | T36.0X2 | T36.0X3 | T36.0X4 | T36.0X5 | T36.0X6 |
| Phentolamine | T46.7X1 | T46.7X2 | T46.7X3 | T46.7X4 | T46.7X5 | T46.7X6 |
| Phenyl | | | | | | |
|   butazone | T39.2X1 | T39.2X2 | T39.2X3 | T39.2X4 | T39.2X5 | T39.2X6 |
|   enediamine | T65.3X1 | T65.3X2 | T65.3X3 | T65.3X4 | — | — |
|   hydrazine | T65.3X1 | T65.3X2 | T65.3X3 | T65.3X4 | — | — |
|     antineoplastic | T45.1X1 | T45.1X2 | T45.1X3 | T45.1X4 | T45.1X5 | T45.1X6 |
|   mercuric compounds — see Mercury | | | | | | |
|   salicylate | T49.3X1 | T49.3X2 | T49.3X3 | T49.3X4 | T49.3X5 | T49.3X6 |
| Phenylalanine mustard | T45.1X1 | T45.1X2 | T45.1X3 | T45.1X4 | T45.1X5 | T45.1X6 |
| Phenylbutazone | T39.2X1 | T39.2X2 | T39.2X3 | T39.2X4 | T39.2X5 | T39.2X6 |
| Phenylenediamine | T65.3X1 | T65.3X2 | T65.3X3 | T65.3X4 | — | — |
| Phenylephrine | T44.4X1 | T44.4X2 | T44.4X3 | T44.4X4 | T44.4X5 | T44.4X6 |
| Phenylethylbiguanide | T38.3X1 | T38.3X2 | T38.3X3 | T38.3X4 | T38.3X5 | T38.3X6 |
| Phenylmercuric | | | | | | |
|   acetate | T49.0X1 | T49.0X2 | T49.0X3 | T49.0X4 | T49.0X5 | T49.0X6 |
|   borate | T49.0X1 | T49.0X2 | T49.0X3 | T49.0X4 | T49.0X5 | T49.0X6 |
|   nitrate | T49.0X1 | T49.0X2 | T49.0X3 | T49.0X4 | T49.0X5 | T49.0X6 |
| Phenylmethylbarbitone | T42.3X1 | T42.3X2 | T42.3X3 | T42.3X4 | T42.3X5 | T42.3X6 |
| Phenylpropanol | T47.5X1 | T47.5X2 | T47.5X3 | T47.5X4 | T47.5X5 | T47.5X6 |
| Phenylpropanolamine | T44.991 | T44.992 | T44.993 | T44.994 | T44.995 | T44.996 |
| Phenylsulfthion | T60.0X1 | T60.0X2 | T60.0X3 | T60.0X4 | — | — |
| Phenyltoloxamine | T45.0X1 | T45.0X2 | T45.0X3 | T45.0X4 | T45.0X5 | T45.0X6 |
| Phenyramidol, phenyramidon | T39.8X1 | T39.8X2 | T39.8X3 | T39.8X4 | T39.8X5 | T39.8X6 |
| Phenytoin | T42.0X1 | T42.0X2 | T42.0X3 | T42.0X4 | T42.0X5 | T42.0X6 |
|   with Phenobarbital | T42.3X1 | T42.3X2 | T42.3X3 | T42.3X4 | T42.3X5 | T42.3X6 |
| pHisoHex | T49.2X1 | T49.2X2 | T49.2X3 | T49.2X4 | T49.2X5 | T49.2X6 |
| Pholcodine | T48.3X1 | T48.3X2 | T48.3X3 | T48.3X4 | T48.3X5 | T48.3X6 |
| Pholedrine | T46.991 | T46.992 | T46.993 | T46.994 | T46.995 | T46.996 |
| Phorate | T60.0X1 | T60.0X2 | T60.0X3 | T60.0X4 | — | — |
| Phosdrin | T60.0X1 | T60.0X2 | T60.0X3 | T60.0X4 | — | — |
| Phosfolan | T60.0X1 | T60.0X2 | T60.0X3 | T60.0X4 | — | — |
| Phosgene (gas) | T59.891 | T59.892 | T59.893 | T59.894 | — | — |
| Phosphamidon | T60.0X1 | T60.0X2 | T60.0X3 | T60.0X4 | — | — |
| Phosphate | T65.891 | T65.892 | T65.893 | T65.894 | — | — |
|   laxative | T47.4X1 | T47.4X2 | T47.4X3 | T47.4X4 | T47.4X5 | T47.4X6 |
|   organic | T60.0X1 | T60.0X2 | T60.0X3 | T60.0X4 | — | — |
|   solvent | T52.91 | T52.92 | T52.93 | T52.94 | — | — |
|   tricresyl | T65.891 | T65.892 | T65.893 | T65.894 | — | — |
| Phosphine | T57.1X1 | T57.1X2 | T57.1X3 | T57.1X4 | — | — |
|   fumigant | T57.1X1 | T57.1X2 | T57.1X3 | T57.1X4 | — | — |
| Phospholine | T49.5X1 | T49.5X2 | T49.5X3 | T49.5X4 | T49.5X5 | T49.5X6 |
| Phosphoric acid | T54.2X1 | T54.2X2 | T54.2X3 | T54.2X4 | — | — |
| Phosphorus (compound) NEC | T57.1X1 | T57.1X2 | T57.1X3 | T57.1X4 | — | — |
|   pesticide | T60.0X1 | T60.0X2 | T60.0X3 | T60.0X4 | — | — |
| Phthalates | T65.891 | T65.892 | T65.893 | T65.894 | — | — |
| Phthalic anhydride | T65.891 | T65.892 | T65.893 | T65.894 | — | — |
| Phthalimidoglutarimide | T42.6X1 | T42.6X2 | T42.6X3 | T42.6X4 | T42.6X5 | T42.6X6 |
| Phthalylsulfathiazole | T37.0X1 | T37.0X2 | T37.0X3 | T37.0X4 | T37.0X5 | T37.0X6 |
| Phylloquinone | T45.7X1 | T45.7X2 | T45.7X3 | T45.7X4 | T45.7X5 | T45.7X6 |
| Physeptone | T40.3X1 | T40.3X2 | T40.3X3 | T40.3X4 | T40.3X5 | T40.3X6 |
| Physostigma venenosum | T62.2X1 | T62.2X2 | T62.2X3 | T62.2X4 | — | — |
| Physostigmine | T49.5X1 | T49.5X2 | T49.5X3 | T49.5X4 | T49.5X5 | T49.5X6 |
| Phytolacca decandra | T62.2X1 | T62.2X2 | T62.2X3 | T62.2X4 | — | — |
|   berries | T62.1X1 | T62.1X2 | T62.1X3 | T62.1X4 | — | — |
| Phytomenadione | T45.7X1 | T45.7X2 | T45.7X3 | T45.7X4 | T45.7X5 | T45.7X6 |
| Phytonadione | T45.7X1 | T45.7X2 | T45.7X3 | T45.7X4 | T45.7X5 | T45.7X6 |
| Picoperine | T48.3X1 | T48.3X2 | T48.3X3 | T48.3X4 | T48.3X5 | T48.3X6 |
| Picosulfate (sodium) | T47.2X1 | T47.2X2 | T47.2X3 | T47.2X4 | T47.2X5 | T47.2X6 |
| Picric (acid) | T54.2X1 | T54.2X2 | T54.2X3 | T54.2X4 | — | — |
| Picrotoxin | T50.7X1 | T50.7X2 | T50.7X3 | T50.7X4 | T50.7X5 | T50.7X6 |
| Piketoprofen | T49.0X1 | T49.0X2 | T49.0X3 | T49.0X4 | T49.0X5 | T49.0X6 |
| Pilocarpine | T44.1X1 | T44.1X2 | T44.1X3 | T44.1X4 | T44.1X5 | T44.1X6 |
| Pilocarpus (jaborandi) | T44.1X1 | T44.1X2 | T44.1X3 | T44.1X4 | T44.1X5 | T44.1X6 |
|   extract | | | | | | |
| Pilsicainide (hydrochloride) | T46.2X1 | T46.2X2 | T46.2X3 | T46.2X4 | T46.2X5 | T46.2X6 |
| Pimaricin | T36.7X1 | T36.7X2 | T36.7X3 | T36.7X4 | T36.7X5 | T36.7X6 |
| Pimeclone | T50.7X1 | T50.7X2 | T50.7X3 | T50.7X4 | T50.7X5 | T50.7X6 |
| Pimelic ketone | T52.8X1 | T52.8X2 | T52.8X3 | T52.8X4 | — | — |
| Pimethixene | T45.0X1 | T45.0X2 | T45.0X3 | T45.0X4 | T45.0X5 | T45.0X6 |
| Piminodine | T40.2X1 | T40.2X2 | T40.2X3 | T40.2X4 | T40.2X5 | T40.2X6 |
| Pimozide | T43.591 | T43.592 | T43.593 | T43.594 | T43.595 | T43.596 |
| Pinacidil | T46.5X1 | T46.5X2 | T46.5X3 | T46.5X4 | T46.5X5 | T46.5X6 |
| Pinaverium bromide | T44.3X1 | T44.3X2 | T44.3X3 | T44.3X4 | T44.3X5 | T44.3X6 |
| Pinazepam | T42.4X1 | T42.4X2 | T42.4X3 | T42.4X4 | T42.4X5 | T42.4X6 |
| Pindolol | T44.7X1 | T44.7X2 | T44.7X3 | T44.7X4 | T44.7X5 | T44.7X6 |
| Pindone | T60.4X1 | T60.4X2 | T60.4X3 | T60.4X4 | — | — |
| Pine oil (disinfectant) | T65.891 | T65.892 | T65.893 | T65.894 | — | — |
| Pinkroot | T37.4X1 | T37.4X2 | T37.4X3 | T37.4X4 | T37.4X5 | T37.4X6 |
| Pipadone | T40.2X1 | T40.2X2 | T40.2X3 | T40.2X4 | — | — |
| Pipamazine | T45.0X1 | T45.0X2 | T45.0X3 | T45.0X4 | T45.0X5 | T45.0X6 |
| Pipamperone | T43.4X1 | T43.4X2 | T43.4X3 | T43.4X4 | T43.4X5 | T43.4X6 |
| Pipazetate | T48.3X1 | T48.3X2 | T48.3X3 | T48.3X4 | T48.3X5 | T48.3X6 |
| Pipemidic acid | T37.8X1 | T37.8X2 | T37.8X3 | T37.8X4 | T37.8X5 | T37.8X6 |
| Pipenzolate bromide | T44.3X1 | T44.3X2 | T44.3X3 | T44.3X4 | T44.3X5 | T44.3X6 |
| Piperacetazine | T43.3X1 | T43.3X2 | T43.3X3 | T43.3X4 | T43.3X5 | T43.3X6 |
| Piperacillin | T36.0X1 | T36.0X2 | T36.0X3 | T36.0X4 | T36.0X5 | T36.0X6 |
| Piperazine | T37.4X1 | T37.4X2 | T37.4X3 | T37.4X4 | T37.4X5 | T37.4X6 |
|   estrone sulfate | T38.5X1 | T38.5X2 | T38.5X3 | T38.5X4 | T38.5X5 | T38.5X6 |
| Piper cubeba | T62.2X1 | T62.2X2 | T62.2X3 | T62.2X4 | — | — |
| Piperidione | T48.3X1 | T48.3X2 | T48.3X3 | T48.3X4 | T48.3X5 | T48.3X6 |
| Piperidolate | T44.3X1 | T44.3X2 | T44.3X3 | T44.3X4 | T44.3X5 | T44.3X6 |
| Piperocaine | T41.3X1 | T41.3X2 | T41.3X3 | T41.3X4 | T41.3X5 | T41.3X6 |
|   infiltration (subcutaneous) | T41.3X1 | T41.3X2 | T41.3X3 | T41.3X4 | T41.3X5 | T41.3X6 |
|   nerve block (peripheral) (plexus) | T41.3X1 | T41.3X2 | T41.3X3 | T41.3X4 | T41.3X5 | T41.3X6 |
|   topical (surface) | T41.3X1 | T41.3X2 | T41.3X3 | T41.3X4 | T41.3X5 | T41.3X6 |
| Piperonyl butoxide | T60.8X1 | T60.8X2 | T60.8X3 | T60.8X4 | — | — |
| Pipethanate | T44.3X1 | T44.3X2 | T44.3X3 | T44.3X4 | T44.3X5 | T44.3X6 |
| Pipobroman | T45.1X1 | T45.1X2 | T45.1X3 | T45.1X4 | T45.1X5 | T45.1X6 |
| Pipotiazine | T43.3X1 | T43.3X2 | T43.3X3 | T43.3X4 | T43.3X5 | T43.3X6 |
| Pipoxizine | T45.0X1 | T45.0X2 | T45.0X3 | T45.0X4 | T45.0X5 | T45.0X6 |
| Pipradrol | T43.691 | T43.692 | T43.693 | T43.694 | T43.695 | T43.696 |
| Piprinhydrinate | T45.0X1 | T45.0X2 | T45.0X3 | T45.0X4 | T45.0X5 | T45.0X6 |
| Pirarubicin | T45.1X1 | T45.1X2 | T45.1X3 | T45.1X4 | T45.1X5 | T45.1X6 |
| Pirazinamide | T37.1X1 | T37.1X2 | T37.1X3 | T37.1X4 | T37.1X5 | T37.1X6 |
| Pirbuterol | T48.6X1 | T48.6X2 | T48.6X3 | T48.6X4 | T48.6X5 | T48.6X6 |
| Pirenzepine | T47.1X1 | T47.1X2 | T47.1X3 | T47.1X4 | T47.1X5 | T47.1X6 |
| Piretanide | T50.1X1 | T50.1X2 | T50.1X3 | T50.1X4 | T50.1X5 | T50.1X6 |
| Piribedil | T42.8X1 | T42.8X2 | T42.8X3 | T42.8X4 | T42.8X5 | T42.8X6 |
| Piridoxilate | T46.3X1 | T46.3X2 | T46.3X3 | T46.3X4 | T46.3X5 | T46.3X6 |
| Piritramide | T40.4X1 | T40.4X2 | T40.4X3 | T40.4X4 | — | — |
| Piromidic acid | T37.8X1 | T37.8X2 | T37.8X3 | T37.8X4 | T37.8X5 | T37.8X6 |
| Piroxicam | T39.391 | T39.392 | T39.393 | T39.394 | T39.395 | T39.396 |
|   beta-cyclodextrin complex | T39.8X1 | T39.8X2 | T39.8X3 | T39.8X4 | T39.8X5 | T39.8X6 |
| Pirozadil | T46.6X1 | T46.6X2 | T46.6X3 | T46.6X4 | T46.6X5 | T46.6X6 |
| Piscidia (bark) (erythrina) | T39.8X1 | T39.8X2 | T39.8X3 | T39.8X4 | T39.8X5 | T39.8X6 |
| Pitch | T65.891 | T65.892 | T65.893 | T65.894 | — | — |
| Pitkin's solution | T41.3X1 | T41.3X2 | T41.3X3 | T41.3X4 | T41.3X5 | T41.3X6 |
| Pitocin | T48.0X1 | T48.0X2 | T48.0X3 | T48.0X4 | T48.0X5 | T48.0X6 |
| Pitressin (tannate) | T38.891 | T38.892 | T38.893 | T38.894 | T38.895 | T38.896 |
| Pituitary extracts (posterior) | T38.891 | T38.892 | T38.893 | T38.894 | T38.895 | T38.896 |
|   anterior | T38.811 | T38.812 | T38.813 | T38.814 | T38.815 | T38.816 |
| Pituitrin | T38.891 | T38.892 | T38.893 | T38.894 | T38.895 | T38.896 |
| Pivampicillin | T36.0X1 | T36.0X2 | T36.0X3 | T36.0X4 | T36.0X5 | T36.0X6 |
| Pivmecillinam | T36.0X1 | T36.0X2 | T36.0X3 | T36.0X4 | T36.0X5 | T36.0X6 |
| Placental hormone | T38.891 | T38.892 | T38.893 | T38.894 | T38.895 | T38.896 |
| Placidyl | T42.6X1 | T42.6X2 | T42.6X3 | T42.6X4 | T42.6X5 | T42.6X6 |
| Plague vaccine | T50.A91 | T50.A92 | T50.A93 | T50.A94 | T50.A95 | T50.A96 |
| Plant | | | | | | |
|   food or fertilizer NEC | T65.891 | T65.892 | T65.893 | T65.894 | — | — |
|     containing herbicide | T60.3X1 | T60.3X2 | T60.3X3 | T60.3X4 | — | — |
|   noxious, used as food | T62.2X1 | T62.2X2 | T62.2X3 | T62.2X4 | — | — |
|     berries | T62.1X1 | T62.1X2 | T62.1X3 | T62.1X4 | — | — |
|     seeds | T62.2X1 | T62.2X2 | T62.2X3 | T62.2X4 | — | — |
|     specified type NEC | T62.2X1 | T62.2X2 | T62.2X3 | T62.2X4 | — | — |
| Plasma | T45.8X1 | T45.8X2 | T45.8X3 | T45.8X4 | T45.8X5 | T45.8X6 |
|   expander NEC | T45.8X1 | T45.8X2 | T45.8X3 | T45.8X4 | T45.8X5 | T45.8X6 |
|   protein fraction (human) | T45.8X1 | T45.8X2 | T45.8X3 | T45.8X4 | T45.8X5 | T45.8X6 |
| Plasmanate | T45.8X1 | T45.8X2 | T45.8X3 | T45.8X4 | T45.8X5 | T45.8X6 |
| Plasminogen (tissue) activator | T45.611 | T45.612 | T45.613 | T45.614 | T45.615 | T45.616 |
| Plaster dressing | T49.3X1 | T49.3X2 | T49.3X3 | T49.3X4 | T49.3X5 | T49.3X6 |
| Plastic dressing | T49.3X1 | T49.3X2 | T49.3X3 | T49.3X4 | T49.3X5 | T49.3X6 |
| Plegicil | T43.3X1 | T43.3X2 | T43.3X3 | T43.3X4 | T43.3X5 | T43.3X6 |
| Plicamycin | T45.1X1 | T45.1X2 | T45.1X3 | T45.1X4 | T45.1X5 | T45.1X6 |
| Podophyllotoxin | T49.8X1 | T49.8X2 | T49.8X3 | T49.8X4 | T49.8X5 | T49.8X6 |
| Podophyllum (resin) | T49.4X1 | T49.4X2 | T49.4X3 | T49.4X4 | T49.4X5 | T49.4X6 |
| Poisonous berries | T62.1X1 | T62.1X2 | T62.1X3 | T62.1X4 | — | — |
| Poison NEC | T65.91 | T65.92 | T65.93 | T65.94 | — | — |
| Pokeweed (any part) | T62.2X1 | T62.2X2 | T62.2X3 | T62.2X4 | — | — |
| Poldine metilsulfate | T44.3X1 | T44.3X2 | T44.3X3 | T44.3X4 | T44.3X5 | T44.3X6 |
| Polidexide (sulfate) | T46.6X1 | T46.6X2 | T46.6X3 | T46.6X4 | T46.6X5 | T46.6X6 |
| Polidocanol | T46.8X1 | T46.8X2 | T46.8X3 | T46.8X4 | T46.8X5 | T46.8X6 |
| Poliomyelitis vaccine | T50.B91 | T50.B92 | T50.B93 | T50.B94 | T50.B95 | T50.B96 |
| Polish (car) (floor) (furniture) (metal) (porcelain) (silver) | T65.891 | T65.892 | T65.893 | T65.894 | — | — |
|   abrasive | T65.891 | T65.892 | T65.893 | T65.894 | — | — |
|   porcelain | T65.891 | T65.892 | T65.893 | T65.894 | — | — |
| Poloxalkol | T47.4X1 | T47.4X2 | T47.4X3 | T47.4X4 | T47.4X5 | T47.4X6 |
| Poloxamer | T47.4X1 | T47.4X2 | T47.4X3 | T47.4X4 | T47.4X5 | T47.4X6 |

| Substance | Poisoning, Accidental (unintentional) | Poisoning, Intentional Self-harm | Poisoning, Assault | Poisoning, Undetermined | Adverse Effect | Under-dosing |
|---|---|---|---|---|---|---|
| Polyaminostyrene resins | T50.3X1 | T50.3X2 | T50.3X3 | T50.3X4 | T50.3X5 | T50.3X6 |
| Polycarbophil | T47.4X1 | T47.4X2 | T47.4X3 | T47.4X4 | T47.4X5 | T47.4X6 |
| Polychlorinated biphenyl | T65.891 | T65.892 | T65.893 | T65.894 | — | — |
| Polycycline | T36.4X1 | T36.4X2 | T36.4X3 | T36.4X4 | T36.4X5 | T36.4X6 |
| Polyester fumes | T59.891 | T59.892 | T59.893 | T59.894 | — | — |
| Polyester resin hardener | T52.91 | T52.92 | T52.93 | T52.94 | — | — |
|   fumes | T59.891 | T59.892 | T59.893 | T59.894 | — | — |
| Polyestradiol phosphate | T38.5X1 | T38.5X2 | T38.5X3 | T38.5X4 | T38.5X5 | T38.5X6 |
| Polyethanolamine alkyl sulfate | T49.2X1 | T49.2X2 | T49.2X3 | T49.2X4 | T49.2X5 | T49.2X6 |
| Polyethylene adhesive | T49.3X1 | T49.3X2 | T49.3X3 | T49.3X4 | T49.3X5 | T49.3X6 |
| Polyferose | T45.4X1 | T45.4X2 | T45.4X3 | T45.4X4 | T45.4X5 | T45.4X6 |
| Polygeline | T45.8X1 | T45.8X2 | T45.8X3 | T45.8X4 | T45.8X5 | T45.8X6 |
| Polymyxin | T36.8X1 | T36.8X2 | T36.8X3 | T36.8X4 | T36.8X5 | T36.8X6 |
|   B | T36.8X1 | T36.8X2 | T36.8X3 | T36.8X4 | T36.8X5 | T36.8X6 |
|     ENT agent | T49.6X1 | T49.6X2 | T49.6X3 | T49.6X4 | T49.6X5 | T49.6X6 |
|     ophthalmic preparation | T49.5X1 | T49.5X2 | T49.5X3 | T49.5X4 | T49.5X5 | T49.5X6 |
|     topical NEC | T49.0X1 | T49.0X2 | T49.0X3 | T49.0X4 | T49.0X6 | T49.0X6 |
|   E sulfate (eye preparation) | T49.5X1 | T49.5X2 | T49.5X3 | T49.5X4 | T49.5X5 | T49.5X6 |
| Polynoxylin | T49.0X1 | T49.0X2 | T49.0X3 | T49.0X4 | T49.0X5 | T49.0X6 |
| Polyoestradiol phosphate | T38.5X1 | T38.5X2 | T38.5X3 | T38.5X4 | T38.5X5 | T38.5X6 |
| Polyoxymethyleneurea | T49.0X1 | T49.0X2 | T49.0X3 | T49.0X4 | T49.0X5 | T49.0X6 |
| Polysilane | T47.8X1 | T47.8X2 | T47.8X3 | T47.8X4 | T47.8X5 | T47.8X6 |
| Polytetrafluoroethylene (inhaled) | T59.891 | T59.892 | T59.893 | T59.894 | — | — |
| Polythiazide | T50.2X1 | T50.2X2 | T50.2X3 | T50.2X4 | T50.2X5 | T50.2X6 |
| Polyvidone | T45.8X1 | T45.8X2 | T45.8X3 | T45.8X4 | T45.8X5 | T45.8X6 |
| Polyvinylpyrrolidone | T45.8X1 | T45.8X2 | T45.8X3 | T45.8X4 | T45.8X5 | T45.8X6 |
| Pontocaine (hydrochloride) (infiltration) (topical) | T41.3X1 | T41.3X2 | T41.3X3 | T41.3X4 | T41.3X5 | T41.3X6 |
|   nerve block (peripheral) (plexus) | T41.3X1 | T41.3X2 | T41.3X3 | T41.3X4 | T41.3X5 | T41.3X6 |
|   spinal | T41.3X1 | T41.3X2 | T41.3X3 | T41.3X4 | T41.3X5 | T41.3X6 |
| Porfiromycin | T45.1X1 | T45.1X2 | T45.1X3 | T45.1X4 | T45.1X5 | T45.1X6 |
| Posterior pituitary hormone NEC | T38.891 | T38.892 | T38.893 | T38.894 | T38.895 | T38.896 |
| Pot | T40.7X1 | T40.7X2 | T40.7X3 | T40.7X4 | T40.7X5 | T40.7X6 |
| Potash (caustic) | T54.3X1 | T54.3X2 | T54.3X3 | T54.3X4 | — | — |
| Potassic saline injection (lactated) | T50.3X1 | T50.3X2 | T50.3X3 | T50.3X4 | T50.3X5 | T50.3X6 |
| Potassium-removing resin | T50.3X1 | T50.3X2 | T50.3X3 | T50.3X4 | T50.3X5 | T50.3X6 |
| Potassium-retaining drug | T50.3X1 | T50.3X2 | T50.3X3 | T50.3X4 | T50.3X5 | T50.3X6 |
| Potassium (salts) NEC | T50.3X1 | T50.3X2 | T50.3X3 | T50.3X4 | T50.3X5 | T50.3X6 |
|   aminobenzoate | T45.8X1 | T45.8X2 | T45.8X3 | T45.8X4 | T45.8X5 | T45.8X6 |
|   aminosalicylate | T37.1X1 | T37.1X2 | T37.1X3 | T37.1X4 | T37.1X5 | T37.1X6 |
|   antimony ' tartrate' | T37.8X1 | T37.8X2 | T37.8X3 | T37.8X4 | T37.8X5 | T37.8X6 |
|   arsenite (solution) | T57.0X1 | T57.0X2 | T57.0X3 | T57.0X4 | — | — |
|   bichromate | T56.2X1 | T56.2X2 | T56.2X3 | T56.2X4 | — | — |
|   bisulfate | T47.3X1 | T47.3X2 | T47.3X3 | T47.3X4 | T47.3X5 | T47.3X6 |
|   bromide | T42.6X1 | T42.6X2 | T42.6X3 | T42.6X4 | T42.6X5 | T42.6X6 |
|   canrenoate | T50.0X1 | T50.0X2 | T50.0X3 | T50.0X4 | T50.0X5 | T50.0X6 |
|   carbonate | T54.3X1 | T54.3X2 | T54.3X3 | T54.3X4 | — | — |
|   chlorate NEC | T65.891 | T65.892 | T65.893 | T65.894 | — | — |
|   chloride | T50.3X1 | T50.3X2 | T50.3X3 | T50.3X4 | T50.3X5 | T50.3X6 |
|   citrate | T50.991 | T50.992 | T50.993 | T50.994 | T50.995 | T50.996 |
|   cyanide | T65.0X1 | T65.0X2 | T65.0X3 | T65.0X4 | — | — |
|   ferric hexacyanoferrate (medicinal) | T50.6X1 | T50.6X2 | T50.6X3 | T50.6X4 | T50.6X5 | T50.6X6 |
|     nonmedicinal | T65.891 | T65.892 | T65.893 | T65.894 | — | — |
|   Fluoride | T57.8X1 | T57.8X2 | T57.8X3 | T57.8X4 | — | — |
|   glucaldrate | T47.1X1 | T47.1X2 | T47.1X3 | T47.1X4 | T47.1X5 | T47.1X6 |
|   hydroxide | T54.3X1 | T54.3X2 | T54.3X3 | T54.3X4 | — | — |
|   iodate | T49.0X1 | T49.0X2 | T49.0X3 | T49.0X4 | T49.0X5 | T49.0X6 |
|   iodide | T48.4X1 | T48.4X2 | T48.4X3 | T48.4X4 | T48.4X5 | T48.4X6 |
|   nitrate | T57.8X1 | T57.8X2 | T57.8X3 | T57.8X4 | — | — |
|   oxalate | T65.891 | T65.892 | T65.893 | T65.894 | — | — |
|   perchlorate (nonmedicinal) NEC | T65.891 | T65.892 | T65.893 | T65.894 | — | — |
|     antithyroid | T38.2X1 | T38.2X2 | T38.2X3 | T38.2X4 | T38.2X5 | T38.2X6 |
|     medicinal | T38.2X1 | T38.2X2 | T38.2X3 | T38.2X4 | T38.2X5 | T38.2X6 |
|   Permanganate (nonmedicinal) | T65.891 | T65.892 | T65.893 | T65.894 | — | — |
|     medicinal | T49.0X1 | T49.0X2 | T49.0X3 | T49.0X4 | T49.0X5 | T49.0X6 |
|   sulfate | T47.2X1 | T47.2X2 | T47.2X3 | T47.2X4 | T47.2X5 | T47.2X6 |
| Povidone | T45.8X1 | T45.8X2 | T45.8X3 | T45.8X4 | T45.8X5 | T45.8X6 |
|   iodine | T49.0X1 | T49.0X2 | T49.0X3 | T49.0X4 | T49.0X5 | T49.0X6 |
| Practolol | T44.7X1 | T44.7X2 | T44.7X3 | T44.7X4 | T44.7X5 | T44.7X6 |
| Prajmalium bitartrate | T46.2X1 | T46.2X2 | T46.2X3 | T46.2X4 | T46.2X5 | T46.2X6 |
| Pralidoxime (iodide) | T50.6X1 | T50.6X2 | T50.6X3 | T50.6X4 | T50.6X5 | T50.6X6 |
|   chloride | T50.6X1 | T50.6X2 | T50.6X3 | T50.6X4 | T50.6X5 | T50.6X6 |
| Pramiverine | T44.3X1 | T44.3X2 | T44.3X3 | T44.3X4 | T44.3X5 | T44.3X6 |
| Pramocaine | T49.1X1 | T49.1X2 | T49.1X3 | T49.1X4 | T49.1X5 | T49.1X6 |
| Pramoxine | T49.1X1 | T49.1X2 | T49.1X3 | T49.1X4 | T49.1X5 | T49.1X6 |

| Substance | Poisoning, Accidental (unintentional) | Poisoning, Intentional Self-harm | Poisoning, Assault | Poisoning, Undetermined | Adverse Effect | Under-dosing |
|---|---|---|---|---|---|---|
| Prasterone | T38.7X1 | T38.7X2 | T38.7X3 | T38.7X4 | T38.7X5 | T38.7X6 |
| Pravastatin | T46.6X1 | T46.6X2 | T46.6X3 | T46.6X4 | T46.6X5 | T46.6X6 |
| Prazepam | T42.4X1 | T42.4X2 | T42.4X3 | T42.4X4 | T42.4X5 | T42.4X6 |
| Praziquantel | T37.4X1 | T37.4X2 | T37.4X3 | T37.4X4 | T37.4X5 | T37.4X6 |
| Prazitone | T43.291 | T43.292 | T43.293 | T43.294 | T43.295 | T43.296 |
| Prazosin | T44.6X1 | T44.6X2 | T44.6X3 | T44.6X4 | T44.6X5 | T44.6X6 |
| Prednicarbate | T49.0X1 | T49.0X2 | T49.0X3 | T49.0X4 | T49.0X5 | T49.0X6 |
| Prednimustine | T45.1X1 | T45.1X2 | T45.1X3 | T45.1X4 | T45.1X5 | T45.1X6 |
| Prednisolone | T38.0X1 | T38.0X2 | T38.0X3 | T38.0X4 | T38.0X5 | T38.0X6 |
|   ENT agent | T49.6X1 | T49.6X2 | T49.6X3 | T49.6X4 | T49.6X5 | T49.6X6 |
|   ophthalmic preparation | T49.5X1 | T49.5X2 | T49.5X3 | T49.5X4 | T49.5X5 | T49.5X6 |
|   steaglate | T49.0X1 | T49.0X2 | T49.0X3 | T49.0X4 | T49.0X5 | T49.0X6 |
|   topical NEC | T49.0X1 | T49.0X2 | T49.0X3 | T49.0X4 | T49.0X5 | T49.0X6 |
| Prednisone | T38.0X1 | T38.0X2 | T38.0X3 | T38.0X4 | T38.0X5 | T38.0X6 |
| Prednylidene | T38.0X1 | T38.0X2 | T38.0X3 | T38.0X4 | T38.0X5 | T38.0X6 |
| Pregnandiol | T38.5X1 | T38.5X2 | T38.5X3 | T38.5X4 | T38.5X5 | T38.5X6 |
| Pregneninolone | T38.5X1 | T38.5X2 | T38.5X3 | T38.5X4 | T38.5X5 | T38.5X6 |
| Preludin | T43.691 | T43.692 | T43.693 | T43.694 | T43.695 | T43.696 |
| Premarin | T38.5X1 | T38.5X2 | T38.5X3 | T38.5X4 | T38.5X5 | T38.5X6 |
| Premedication anesthetic | T41.201 | T41.202 | T41.203 | T41.204 | T41.205 | T41.206 |
| Prenalterol | T44.5X1 | T44.5X2 | T44.5X3 | T44.5X4 | T44.5X5 | T44.5X6 |
| Prenoxdiazine | T48.3X1 | T48.3X2 | T48.3X3 | T48.3X4 | T48.3X5 | T48.3X6 |
| Prenylamine | T46.3X1 | T46.3X2 | T46.3X3 | T46.3X4 | T46.3X5 | T46.3X6 |
| Preparation H | T49.8X1 | T49.8X2 | T49.8X3 | T49.8X4 | T49.8X5 | T49.8X6 |
| Preparation, local | T49.4X1 | T49.4X2 | T49.4X3 | T49.4X4 | T49.4X5 | T49.4X6 |
| Preservative (nonmedicinal) | T65.891 | T65.892 | T65.893 | T65.894 | — | — |
|   medicinal | T50.901 | T50.902 | T50.903 | T50.904 | T50.905 | T50.906 |
|   wood | T60.91 | T60.92 | T60.93 | T60.94 | — | — |
| Prethcamide | T50.7X1 | T50.7X2 | T50.7X3 | T50.7X4 | T50.7X5 | T50.7X6 |
| Pride of China | T62.2X1 | T62.2X2 | T62.2X3 | T62.2X4 | — | — |
| Pridinol | T44.3X1 | T44.3X2 | T44.3X3 | T44.3X4 | T44.3X5 | T44.3X6 |
| Prifinium bromide | T44.3X1 | T44.3X2 | T44.3X3 | T44.3X4 | T44.3X5 | T44.3X6 |
| Prilocaine | T41.3X1 | T41.3X2 | T41.3X3 | T41.3X4 | T41.3X5 | T41.3X6 |
|   infiltration (subcutaneous) | T41.3X1 | T41.3X2 | T41.3X3 | T41.3X4 | T41.3X5 | T41.3X6 |
|   nerve block (peripheral) (plexus) | T41.3X1 | T41.3X2 | T41.3X3 | T41.3X4 | T41.3X5 | T41.3X6 |
|   regional | T41.3X1 | T41.3X2 | T41.3X3 | T41.3X4 | T41.3X5 | T41.3X6 |
| Primaquine | T37.2X1 | T37.2X2 | T37.2X3 | T37.2X4 | T37.2X5 | T37.2X6 |
| Primidone | T42.6X1 | T42.6X2 | T42.6X3 | T42.6X4 | T42.6X5 | T42.6X6 |
| Primula (veris) | T62.2X1 | T62.2X2 | T62.2X3 | T62.2X4 | — | — |
| Prinadol | T40.2X1 | T40.2X2 | T40.2X3 | T40.2X4 | T40.2X5 | T40.2X6 |
| Priscol, Priscoline | T44.6X1 | T44.6X2 | T44.6X3 | T44.6X4 | T44.6X5 | T44.6X6 |
| Pristinamycin | T36.3X1 | T36.3X2 | T36.3X3 | T36.3X4 | T36.3X5 | T36.3X6 |
| Privet | T62.2X1 | T62.2X2 | T62.2X3 | T62.2X4 | — | — |
|   berries | T62.1X1 | T62.1X2 | T62.1X3 | T62.1X4 | — | — |
| Privine | T44.4X1 | T44.4X2 | T44.4X3 | T44.4X4 | T44.4X5 | T44.4X6 |
| Pro-Banthine | T44.3X1 | T44.3X2 | T44.3X3 | T44.3X4 | T44.3X5 | T44.3X6 |
| Probarbital | T42.3X1 | T42.3X2 | T42.3X3 | T42.3X4 | T42.3X5 | T42.3X6 |
| Probenecid | T50.4X1 | T50.4X2 | T50.4X3 | T50.4X4 | T50.4X5 | T50.4X6 |
| Probucol | T46.6X1 | T46.6X2 | T46.6X3 | T46.6X4 | T46.6X5 | T46.6X6 |
| Procainamide | T46.2X1 | T46.2X2 | T46.2X3 | T46.2X4 | T46.2X5 | T46.2X6 |
| Procaine | T41.3X1 | T41.3X2 | T41.3X3 | T41.3X4 | T41.3X5 | T41.3X6 |
|   benzylpenicillin | T36.0X1 | T36.0X2 | T36.0X3 | T36.0X4 | T36.0X5 | T36.0X6 |
|   nerve block (periphreal) (plexus) | T41.3X1 | T41.3X2 | T41.3X3 | T41.3X4 | T41.3X5 | T41.3X6 |
|   penicillin G | T36.0X1 | T36.0X2 | T36.0X3 | T36.0X4 | T36.0X5 | T36.0X6 |
|   regional | T41.3X1 | T41.3X2 | T41.3X3 | T41.3X4 | T41.3X5 | T41.3X6 |
|   spinal | T41.3X1 | T41.3X2 | T41.3X3 | T41.3X4 | T41.3X5 | T41.3X6 |
| Procalmidol | T43.591 | T43.592 | T43.593 | T43.594 | T43.595 | T43.596 |
| Procarbazine | T45.1X1 | T45.1X2 | T45.1X3 | T45.1X4 | T45.1X5 | T45.1X6 |
| Procaterol | T44.5X1 | T44.5X2 | T44.5X3 | T44.5X4 | T44.5X5 | T44.5X6 |
| Prochlorperazine | T43.3X1 | T43.3X2 | T43.3X3 | T43.3X4 | T43.3X5 | T43.3X6 |
| Procyclidine | T44.3X1 | T44.3X2 | T44.3X3 | T44.3X4 | T44.3X5 | T44.3X6 |
| Producer gas | T58.8X1 | T58.8X2 | T58.8X3 | T58.8X4 | — | — |
| Profadol | T40.4X1 | T40.4X2 | T40.4X3 | T40.4X4 | T40.4X5 | T40.4X6 |
| Profenamine | T44.3X1 | T44.3X2 | T44.3X3 | T44.3X4 | T44.3X5 | T44.3X6 |
| Profenil | T44.3X1 | T44.3X2 | T44.3X3 | T44.3X4 | T44.3X5 | T44.3X6 |
| Proflavine | T49.0X1 | T49.0X2 | T49.0X3 | T49.0X4 | T49.0X5 | T49.0X6 |
| Progabide | T42.6X1 | T42.6X2 | T42.6X3 | T42.6X4 | T42.6X5 | T42.6X6 |
| Progesterone | T38.5X1 | T38.5X2 | T38.5X3 | T38.5X4 | T38.5X5 | T38.5X6 |
| Progestin | T38.5X1 | T38.5X2 | T38.5X3 | T38.5X4 | T38.5X5 | T38.5X6 |
|   oral contraceptive | T38.4X1 | T38.4X2 | T38.4X3 | T38.4X4 | T38.4X5 | T38.4X6 |
| Progestogen NEC | T38.5X1 | T38.5X2 | T38.5X3 | T38.5X4 | T38.5X5 | T38.5X6 |
| Progestone | T38.5X1 | T38.5X2 | T38.5X3 | T38.5X4 | T38.5X5 | T38.5X6 |
| Proglumide | T47.1X1 | T47.1X2 | T47.1X3 | T47.1X4 | T47.1X5 | T47.1X6 |
| Proguanil | T37.2X1 | T37.2X2 | T37.2X3 | T37.2X4 | T37.2X5 | T37.2X6 |
| Prolactin | T38.811 | T38.812 | T38.813 | T38.814 | T38.815 | T38.816 |
| Prolintane | T43.691 | T43.692 | T43.693 | T43.694 | T43.695 | T43.696 |
| Proloid | T38.1X1 | T38.1X2 | T38.1X3 | T38.1X4 | T38.1X5 | T38.1X6 |
| Proluton | T38.5X1 | T38.5X2 | T38.5X3 | T38.5X4 | T38.5X5 | T38.5X6 |
| Promacetin | T37.1X1 | T37.1X2 | T37.1X3 | T37.1X4 | T37.1X5 | T37.1X6 |
| Promazine | T43.3X1 | T43.3X2 | T43.3X3 | T43.3X4 | T43.3X5 | T43.3X6 |
| Promedol | T40.2X1 | T40.2X2 | T40.2X3 | T40.2X4 | — | — |

| Substance | Poisoning, Accidental (unintentional) | Poisoning, Intentional Self-harm | Poisoning, Assault | Poisoning, Undetermined | Adverse Effect | Under-dosing |
|---|---|---|---|---|---|---|
| Promegestone | T38.5X1 | T38.5X2 | T38.5X3 | T38.5X4 | T38.5X5 | T38.5X6 |
| Promethazine (teoclate) | T43.3X1 | T43.3X2 | T43.3X3 | T43.3X4 | T43.3X5 | T43.3X6 |
| Promin | T37.1X1 | T37.1X2 | T37.1X3 | T37.1X4 | T37.1X5 | T37.1X6 |
| Pronase | T45.3X1 | T45.3X2 | T45.3X3 | T45.3X4 | T45.3X5 | T45.3X6 |
| Pronestyl (hydrochloride) | T46.2X1 | T46.2X2 | T46.2X3 | T46.2X4 | T46.2X5 | T46.2X6 |
| Pronetalol | T44.7X1 | T44.7X2 | T44.7X3 | T44.7X4 | T44.7X5 | T44.7X6 |
| Prontosil | T37.0X1 | T37.0X2 | T37.0X3 | T37.0X4 | T37.0X5 | T37.0X6 |
| Propachlor | T60.3X1 | T60.3X2 | T60.3X3 | T60.3X4 | — | — |
| Propafenone | T46.2X1 | T46.2X2 | T46.2X3 | T46.2X4 | T46.2X5 | T46.2X6 |
| Propallylonal | T42.3X1 | T42.3X2 | T42.3X3 | T42.3X4 | T42.3X5 | T42.3X6 |
| Propamidine | T49.0X1 | T49.0X2 | T49.0X3 | T49.0X4 | T49.0X5 | T49.0X6 |
| Propane (distributed in mobile container) | T59.891 | T59.892 | T59.893 | T59.894 | | |
|   distributed through pipes | T59.891 | T59.892 | T59.893 | T59.894 | — | — |
|   incomplete combustion | T58.11 | T58.12 | T58.13 | T58.14 | — | — |
| Propanidid | T41.291 | T41.292 | T41.293 | T41.294 | T41.295 | T41.296 |
| Propanil | T60.3X1 | T60.3X2 | T60.3X3 | T60.3X4 | — | — |
| Propantheline | T44.3X1 | T44.3X2 | T44.3X3 | T44.3X4 | T44.3X5 | T44.3X6 |
|   bromide | T44.3X1 | T44.3X2 | T44.3X3 | T44.3X4 | T44.3X5 | T44.3X6 |
| Proparacaine | T41.3X1 | T41.3X2 | T41.3X3 | T41.3X4 | T41.3X5 | T41.3X6 |
| Propatylnitrate | T46.3X1 | T46.3X2 | T46.3X3 | T46.3X4 | T46.3X5 | T46.3X6 |
| Propicillin | T36.0X1 | T36.0X2 | T36.0X3 | T36.0X4 | T36.0X5 | T36.0X6 |
| Propiolactone | T49.0X1 | T49.0X2 | T49.0X3 | T49.0X4 | T49.0X5 | T49.0X6 |
| Propiomazine | T45.0X1 | T45.0X2 | T45.0X3 | T45.0X4 | T45.0X5 | T45.0X6 |
| Propionaldehyde (medicinal) | T42.6X1 | T42.6X2 | T42.6X3 | T42.6X4 | T42.6X5 | T42.6X6 |
| Propionate (calcium) (sodium) | T49.0X1 | T49.0X2 | T49.0X3 | T49.0X4 | T49.0X5 | T49.0X6 |
| Propion gel | T49.0X1 | T49.0X2 | T49.0X3 | T49.0X4 | T49.0X5 | T49.0X6 |
| Propitocaine | T41.3X1 | T41.3X2 | T41.3X3 | T41.3X4 | T41.3X5 | T41.3X6 |
|   infiltration (subcutaneous) | T41.3X1 | T41.3X2 | T41.3X3 | T41.3X4 | T41.3X5 | T41.3X6 |
|   nerve block (peripheral) (plexus) | T41.3X1 | T41.3X2 | T41.3X3 | T41.3X4 | T41.3X5 | T41.3X6 |
| Propofol | T41.291 | T41.292 | T41.293 | T41.294 | T41.295 | T41.296 |
| Propoxur | T60.0X1 | T60.0X2 | T60.0X3 | T60.0X4 | — | — |
| Propoxycaine | T41.3X1 | T41.3X2 | T41.3X3 | T41.3X4 | T41.3X5 | T41.3X6 |
|   infiltration (subcutaneous) | T41.3X1 | T41.3X2 | T41.3X3 | T41.3X4 | T41.3X5 | T41.3X6 |
|   nerve block (peripheral) (plexus) | T41.3X1 | T41.3X2 | T41.3X3 | T41.3X4 | T41.3X5 | T41.3X6 |
|   topical (surface) | T41.3X1 | T41.3X2 | T41.3X3 | T41.3X4 | T41.3X5 | T41.3X6 |
| Propoxyphene | T40.4X1 | T40.4X2 | T40.4X3 | T40.4X4 | T40.4X5 | T40.4X6 |
| Propranolol | T44.7X1 | T44.7X2 | T44.7X3 | T44.7X4 | T44.7X5 | T44.7X6 |
| Propyl | | | | | | |
|   alcohol | T51.3X1 | T51.3X2 | T51.3X3 | T51.3X4 | — | — |
|   carbinol | T51.3X1 | T51.3X2 | T51.3X3 | T51.3X4 | — | — |
|   hexadrine | T44.4X1 | T44.4X2 | T44.4X3 | T44.4X4 | T44.4X5 | T44.4X6 |
|   iodone | T50.8X1 | T50.8X2 | T50.8X3 | T50.8X4 | T50.8X5 | T50.8X6 |
|   thiouracil | T38.2X1 | T38.2X2 | T38.2X3 | T38.2X4 | T38.2X5 | T38.2X6 |
| Propylaminophenothiazine | T43.3X1 | T43.3X2 | T43.3X3 | T43.3X4 | T43.3X5 | T43.3X6 |
| Propylene | T59.891 | T59.892 | T59.893 | T59.894 | — | — |
| Propylhexedrine | T48.5X1 | T48.5X2 | T48.5X3 | T48.5X4 | T48.5X5 | T48.5X6 |
| Propyliodone | T50.8X1 | T50.8X2 | T50.8X3 | T50.8X4 | T50.8X5 | T50.8X6 |
| Propylparaben (ophthalmic) | T49.5X1 | T49.5X2 | T49.5X3 | T49.5X4 | T49.5X5 | T49.5X6 |
| Propylthiouracil | T38.2X1 | T38.2X2 | T38.2X3 | T38.2X4 | T38.2X5 | T38.2X6 |
| Propyphenazone | T39.2X1 | T39.2X2 | T39.2X3 | T39.2X4 | T39.2X5 | T39.2X6 |
| Proquazone | T39.391 | T39.392 | T39.393 | T39.394 | T39.395 | T39.396 |
| Proscillaridin | T46.0X1 | T46.0X2 | T46.0X3 | T46.0X4 | T46.0X5 | T46.0X6 |
| Prostacyclin | T45.521 | T45.522 | T45.523 | T45.524 | T45.525 | T45.526 |
| Prostaglandin (I2) | T45.521 | T45.522 | T45.523 | T45.524 | T45.525 | T45.526 |
|   E1 | T46.7X1 | T46.7X2 | T46.7X3 | T46.7X4 | T46.7X5 | T46.7X6 |
|   E2 | T48.0X1 | T48.0X2 | T48.0X3 | T48.0X4 | T48.0X5 | T48.0X6 |
|   F2 alpha | T48.0X1 | T48.0X2 | T48.0X3 | T48.0X4 | T48.0X5 | T48.0X6 |
| Prostigmin | T44.0X1 | T44.0X2 | T44.0X3 | T44.0X4 | T44.0X5 | T44.0X6 |
| Prosultiamine | T45.2X1 | T45.2X2 | T45.2X3 | T45.2X4 | T45.2X5 | T45.2X6 |
| Protamine sulfate | T45.7X1 | T45.7X2 | T45.7X3 | T45.7X4 | T45.7X5 | T45.7X6 |
|   zinc insulin | T38.3X1 | T38.3X2 | T38.3X3 | T38.3X4 | T38.3X5 | T38.3X6 |
| Protease | T47.5X1 | T47.5X2 | T47.5X3 | T47.5X4 | T47.5X5 | T47.5X6 |
| Protectant, skin NEC | T49.3X1 | T49.3X2 | T49.3X3 | T49.3X4 | T49.3X5 | T49.3X6 |
| Protein hydrolysate | T50.991 | T50.992 | T50.993 | T50.994 | T50.995 | T50.996 |
| Prothiaden — see Dothiepin hydrochloride | | | | | | |
| Prothionamide | T37.1X1 | T37.1X2 | T37.1X3 | T37.1X4 | T37.1X5 | T37.1X6 |
| Prothipendyl | T43.591 | T43.592 | T43.593 | T43.594 | T43.595 | T43.596 |
| Prothoate | T60.0X1 | T60.0X2 | T60.0X3 | T60.0X4 | — | — |
| Prothrombin | | | | | | |
|   activator | T45.7X1 | T45.7X2 | T45.7X3 | T45.7X4 | T45.7X5 | T45.7X6 |
|   synthesis inhibitor | T45.511 | T45.512 | T45.513 | T45.514 | T45.515 | T45.516 |
| Protionamide | T37.1X1 | T37.1X2 | T37.1X3 | T37.1X4 | T37.1X5 | T37.1X6 |
| Protirelin | T38.891 | T38.892 | T38.893 | T38.894 | T38.895 | T38.896 |
| Protokylol | T48.6X1 | T48.6X2 | T48.6X3 | T48.6X4 | T48.6X5 | T48.6X6 |
| Protopam | T50.6X1 | T50.6X2 | T50.6X3 | T50.6X4 | T50.6X5 | T50.6X6 |
| Protoveratrine(s) (A) (B) | T46.5X1 | T46.5X2 | T46.5X3 | T46.5X4 | T46.5X5 | T46.5X6 |
| Protriptyline | T43.011 | T43.012 | T43.013 | T43.014 | T43.015 | T43.016 |
| Provera | T38.5X1 | T38.5X2 | T38.5X3 | T38.5X4 | T38.5X5 | T38.5X6 |
| Provitamin A | T45.2X1 | T45.2X2 | T45.2X3 | T45.2X4 | T45.2X5 | T45.2X6 |
| Proxibarbal | T42.3X1 | T42.3X2 | T42.3X3 | T42.3X4 | T42.3X5 | T42.3X6 |
| Proxymetacaine | T41.3X1 | T41.3X2 | T41.3X3 | T41.3X4 | T41.3X5 | T41.3X6 |
| Proxyphylline | T48.6X1 | T48.6X2 | T48.6X3 | T48.6X4 | T48.6X5 | T48.6X6 |
| Prozac — see Fluoxetine hydrochloride | | | | | | |
| Prunus | | | | | | |
|   laurocerasus | T62.2X1 | T62.2X2 | T62.2X3 | T62.2X4 | — | — |
|   virginiana | T62.2X1 | T62.2X2 | T62.2X3 | T62.2X4 | — | — |
| Prussian blue | | | | | | |
|   commercial | T65.891 | T65.892 | T65.893 | T65.894 | — | — |
|   therapeutic | T50.6X1 | T50.6X2 | T50.6X3 | T50.6X4 | T50.6X5 | T50.6X6 |
| Prussic acid | T65.0X1 | T65.0X2 | T65.0X3 | T65.0X4 | — | — |
|   vapor | T57.3X1 | T57.3X2 | T57.3X3 | T57.3X4 | — | — |
| Pseudoephedrine | T44.991 | T44.992 | T44.993 | T44.994 | T44.995 | T44.996 |
| Psilocin | T40.991 | T40.992 | T40.993 | T40.994 | — | — |
| Psilocybin | T40.991 | T40.992 | T40.993 | T40.994 | — | — |
| Psilocybine | T40.991 | T40.992 | T40.993 | T40.994 | — | — |
| Psoralene (nonmedicinal) | T65.891 | T65.892 | T65.893 | T65.894 | — | — |
| Psoralens (medicinal) | T50.991 | T50.992 | T50.993 | T50.994 | T50.995 | T50.996 |
| PSP (phenolsulfonphthalein) | T50.8X1 | T50.8X2 | T50.8X3 | T50.8X4 | T50.8X5 | T50.8X6 |
| Psychodysleptic drug NEC | T40.901 | T40.902 | T40.903 | T40.904 | T40.905 | T40.906 |
| Psychostimulant | T43.601 | T43.602 | T43.603 | T43.604 | T43.605 | T43.606 |
|   amphetamine | T43.621 | T43.622 | T43.623 | T43.624 | T43.625 | T43.626 |
|   caffeine | T43.611 | T43.612 | T43.613 | T43.614 | T43.615 | T43.616 |
|   methylphenidate | T43.631 | T43.632 | T43.633 | T43.634 | T43.635 | T43.636 |
|   specified NEC | T43.691 | T43.692 | T43.693 | T43.694 | T43.695 | T43.696 |
| Psychotherapeutic drug NEC | T43.91 | T43.92 | T43.93 | T43.94 | T43.95 | T43.96 |
|   antidepressants — see also Antidepressant | T43.201 | T43.202 | T43.203 | T43.204 | T43.205 | T43.206 |
|   specified NEC | T43.8X1 | T43.8X2 | T43.8X3 | T43.8X4 | T43.8X5 | T43.8X6 |
|   tranquilizers NEC | T43.501 | T43.502 | T43.503 | T43.504 | T43.505 | T43.506 |
| Psychotomimetic agents | T40.901 | T40.902 | T40.903 | T40.904 | T40.905 | T40.906 |
| Psychotropic drug NEC | T43.91 | T43.92 | T43.93 | T43.94 | T43.95 | T43.96 |
|   specified NEC | T43.8X1 | T43.8X2 | T43.8X3 | T43.8X4 | T43.8X5 | T43.8X6 |
| Psyllium hydrophilic mucilloid | T47.4X1 | T47.4X2 | T47.4X3 | T47.4X4 | T47.4X5 | T47.4X6 |
| Pteroylglutamic acid | T45.8X1 | T45.8X2 | T45.8X3 | T45.8X4 | T45.8X5 | T45.8X6 |
| Pteroyltriglutamate | T45.1X1 | T45.1X2 | T45.1X3 | T45.1X4 | T45.1X5 | T45.1X6 |
| PTFE — see Polytetrafluoroethylene | | | | | | |
| Pulp | | | | | | |
|   devitalizing paste | T49.7X1 | T49.7X2 | T49.7X3 | T49.7X4 | T49.7X5 | T49.7X6 |
|   dressing | T49.7X1 | T49.7X2 | T49.7X3 | T49.7X4 | T49.7X5 | T49.7X6 |
| Pulsatilla | T62.2X1 | T62.2X2 | T62.2X3 | T62.2X4 | — | — |
| Pumpkin seed extract | T37.4X1 | T37.4X2 | T37.4X3 | T37.4X4 | — | T37.4X6 |
| Purex (bleach) | T54.91 | T54.92 | T54.93 | T54.94 | — | — |
| Purgative NEC — see also Cathartic | T47.4X1 | T47.4X2 | T47.4X3 | T47.4X4 | T47.4X5 | T47.4X6 |
| Purine analogue (antineoplastic) | T45.1X1 | T45.1X2 | T45.1X3 | T45.1X4 | T45.1X5 | T45.1X6 |
| Purine diuretics | T50.2X1 | T50.2X2 | T50.2X3 | T50.2X4 | T50.2X5 | T50.2X6 |
| Purinethol | T45.1X1 | T45.1X2 | T45.1X3 | T45.1X4 | T45.1X5 | T45.1X6 |
| PVP | T45.8X1 | T45.8X2 | T45.8X3 | T45.8X4 | T45.8X5 | T45.8X6 |
| Pyrabital | T39.8X1 | T39.8X2 | T39.8X3 | T39.8X4 | T39.8X5 | T39.8X6 |
| Pyramidon | T39.2X1 | T39.2X2 | T39.2X3 | T39.2X4 | T39.2X5 | T39.2X6 |
| Pyrantel | T37.4X1 | T37.4X2 | T37.4X3 | T37.4X4 | T37.4X5 | T37.4X6 |
| Pyrathiazine | T45.0X1 | T45.0X2 | T45.0X3 | T45.0X4 | T45.0X5 | T45.0X6 |
| Pyrazinamide | T37.1X1 | T37.1X2 | T37.1X3 | T37.1X4 | T37.1X5 | T37.1X6 |
| Pyrazinoic acid (amide) | T37.1X1 | T37.1X2 | T37.1X3 | T37.1X4 | T37.1X5 | T37.1X6 |
| Pyrazole (derivatives) | T39.2X1 | T39.2X2 | T39.2X3 | T39.2X4 | T39.2X5 | T39.2X6 |
| Pyrazolone analgesic NEC | T39.2X1 | T39.2X2 | T39.2X3 | T39.2X4 | T39.2X5 | T39.2X6 |
| Pyrethrin, pyrethrum (nonmedicinal) | T60.2X1 | T60.2X2 | T60.2X3 | T60.2X4 | — | — |
| Pyrethrum extract | T49.0X1 | T49.0X2 | T49.0X3 | T49.0X4 | T49.0X5 | T49.0X6 |
| Pyribenzamine | T45.0X1 | T45.0X2 | T45.0X3 | T45.0X4 | T45.0X5 | T45.0X6 |
| Pyridine | T52.8X1 | T52.8X2 | T52.8X3 | T52.8X4 | — | — |
|   aldoxime methiodide | T50.6X1 | T50.6X2 | T50.6X3 | T50.6X4 | T50.6X5 | T50.6X6 |
|   aldoxime methyl chloride | T50.6X1 | T50.6X2 | T50.6X3 | T50.6X4 | T50.6X5 | T50.6X6 |
|   vapor | T59.891 | T59.892 | T59.893 | T59.894 | — | — |
| Pyridium | T39.8X1 | T39.8X2 | T39.8X3 | T39.8X4 | T39.8X5 | T39.8X6 |
| Pyridostigmine bromide | T44.0X1 | T44.0X2 | T44.0X3 | T44.0X4 | T44.0X5 | T44.0X6 |
| Pyridoxal phosphate | T45.2X1 | T45.2X2 | T45.2X3 | T45.2X4 | T45.2X5 | T45.2X6 |
| Pyridoxine | T45.2X1 | T45.2X2 | T45.2X3 | T45.2X4 | T45.2X5 | T45.2X6 |
| Pyrilamine | T45.0X1 | T45.0X2 | T45.0X3 | T45.0X4 | T45.0X5 | T45.0X6 |
| Pyrimethamine | T37.2X1 | T37.2X2 | T37.2X3 | T37.2X4 | T37.2X5 | T37.2X6 |
|   with sulfadoxine | T37.2X1 | T37.2X2 | T37.2X3 | T37.2X4 | T37.2X5 | T37.2X6 |
| Pyrimidine antagonist | T45.1X1 | T45.1X2 | T45.1X3 | T45.1X4 | T45.1X5 | T45.1X6 |
| Pyriminil | T60.4X1 | T60.4X2 | T60.4X3 | T60.4X4 | — | — |
| Pyrithione zinc | T49.4X1 | T49.4X2 | T49.4X3 | T49.4X4 | T49.4X5 | T49.4X6 |
| Pyrithyldione | T42.6X1 | T42.6X2 | T42.6X3 | T42.6X4 | T42.6X5 | T42.6X6 |

| Substance | Poisoning, Accidental (unintentional) | Poisoning, Intentional Self-harm | Poisoning, Assault | Poisoning, Undetermined | Adverse Effect | Under-dosing |
|---|---|---|---|---|---|---|
| Pyrogallic acid | T49.0X1 | T49.0X2 | T49.0X3 | T49.0X4 | T49.0X5 | T49.0X6 |
| Pyrogallol | T49.0X1 | T49.0X2 | T49.0X3 | T49.0X4 | T49.0X5 | T49.0X6 |
| Pyroxylin | T49.3X1 | T49.3X2 | T49.3X3 | T49.3X4 | T49.3X5 | T49.3X6 |
| Pyrrobutamine | T45.0X1 | T45.0X2 | T45.0X3 | T45.0X4 | T45.0X5 | T45.0X6 |
| Pyrrolizidine alkaloids | T62.8X1 | T62.8X2 | T62.8X3 | T62.8X4 | — | — |
| Pyrvinium chloride | T37.4X1 | T37.4X2 | T37.4X3 | T37.4X4 | T37.4X5 | T37.4X6 |
| PZI | T38.3X1 | T38.3X2 | T38.3X3 | T38.3X4 | T38.3X5 | T38.3X6 |
| Quaalude | T42.6X1 | T42.6X2 | T42.6X3 | T42.6X4 | T42.6X5 | T42.6X6 |
| Quaternary ammonium | | | | | | |
|   anti-infective | T49.0X1 | T49.0X2 | T49.0X3 | T49.0X4 | T49.0X5 | T49.0X6 |
|   ganglion blocking | T44.2X1 | T44.2X2 | T44.2X3 | T44.2X4 | T44.2X5 | T44.2X6 |
|   parasympatholytic | T44.3X1 | T44.3X2 | T44.3X3 | T44.3X4 | T44.3X5 | T44.3X6 |
| Quazepam | T42.4X1 | T42.4X2 | T42.4X3 | T42.4X4 | T42.4X5 | T42.4X6 |
| Quicklime | T54.3X1 | T54.3X2 | T54.3X3 | T54.3X4 | — | — |
| Quillaja extract | T48.4X1 | T48.4X2 | T48.4X3 | T48.4X4 | T48.4X5 | T48.4X6 |
| Quinacrine | T37.2X1 | T37.2X2 | T37.2X3 | T37.2X4 | T37.2X5 | T37.2X6 |
| Quinaglute | T46.2X1 | T46.2X2 | T46.2X3 | T46.2X4 | T46.2X5 | T46.2X6 |
| Quinalbarbital | T42.3X1 | T42.3X2 | T42.3X3 | T42.3X4 | T42.3X5 | T42.3X6 |
| Quinalbarbitone sodium | T42.3X1 | T42.3X2 | T42.3X3 | T42.3X4 | T42.3X5 | T42.3X6 |
| Quinalphos | T60.0X1 | T60.0X2 | T60.0X3 | T60.0X4 | — | — |
| Quinapril | T46.4X1 | T46.4X2 | T46.4X3 | T46.4X4 | T46.4X5 | T46.4X6 |
| Quinestradiol | T38.5X1 | T38.5X2 | T38.5X3 | T38.5X4 | T38.5X5 | T38.5X6 |
| Quinestradol | T38.5X1 | T38.5X2 | T38.5X3 | T38.5X4 | T38.5X5 | T38.5X6 |
| Quinestrol | T38.5X1 | T38.5X2 | T38.5X3 | T38.5X4 | T38.5X5 | T38.5X6 |
| Quinethazone | T50.2X1 | T50.2X2 | T50.2X3 | T50.2X4 | T50.2X5 | T50.2X6 |
| Quingestanol | T38.4X1 | T38.4X2 | T38.4X3 | T38.4X4 | T38.4X5 | T38.4X6 |
| Quinidine | T46.2X1 | T46.2X2 | T46.2X3 | T46.2X4 | T46.2X5 | T46.2X6 |
| Quinine | T37.2X1 | T37.2X2 | T37.2X3 | T37.2X4 | T37.2X5 | T37.2X6 |
| Quiniobine | T37.8X1 | T37.8X2 | T37.8X3 | T37.8X4 | T37.8X5 | T37.8X6 |
| Quinisocaine | T49.1X1 | T49.1X2 | T49.1X3 | T49.1X4 | T49.1X5 | T49.1X6 |
| Quinocide | T37.2X1 | T37.2X2 | T37.2X3 | T37.2X4 | T37.2X5 | T37.2X6 |
| Quinoline (derivatives) NEC | T37.8X1 | T37.8X2 | T37.8X3 | T37.8X4 | T37.8X5 | T37.8X6 |
| Quinupramine | T43.011 | T43.012 | T43.013 | T43.014 | T43.015 | T43.016 |
| Quotane | T41.3X1 | T41.3X2 | T41.3X3 | T41.3X4 | T41.3X5 | T41.3X6 |
| Rabies | | | | | | |
|   immune globulin (human) | T50.Z11 | T50.Z12 | T50.Z13 | T50.Z14 | T50.Z15 | T50.Z16 |
|   vaccine | T50.B91 | T50.B92 | T50.B93 | T50.B94 | T50.B95 | T50.B96 |
| Racemoramide | T40.2X1 | T40.2X2 | T40.2X3 | T40.2X4 | — | — |
| Racemorphan | T40.2X1 | T40.2X2 | T40.2X3 | T40.2X4 | T40.2X5 | T40.2X6 |
| Racepinefrin | T44.5X1 | T44.5X2 | T44.5X3 | T44.5X4 | T44.5X5 | T44.5X6 |
| Raclopride | T43.591 | T43.592 | T43.593 | T43.594 | T43.595 | T43.596 |
| Radiator alcohol | T51.1X1 | T51.1X2 | T51.1X3 | T51.1X4 | | |
| Radioactive drug NEC | T50.8X1 | T50.8X2 | T50.8X3 | T50.8X4 | T50.8X5 | T50.8X6 |
| Radio-opaque (drugs) (materials) | T50.8X1 | T50.8X2 | T50.8X3 | T50.8X4 | T50.8X5 | T50.8X6 |
| Ramifenazone | T39.2X1 | T39.2X2 | T39.2X3 | T39.2X4 | T39.2X5 | T39.2X6 |
| Ramipril | T46.4X1 | T46.4X2 | T46.4X3 | T46.4X4 | T46.4X5 | T46.4X6 |
| Ranitidine | T47.0X1 | T47.0X2 | T47.0X3 | T47.0X4 | T47.0X5 | T47.0X6 |
| Ranunculus | T62.2X1 | T62.2X2 | T62.2X3 | T62.2X4 | — | — |
| Rat poison NEC | T60.4X1 | T60.4X2 | T60.4X3 | T60.4X4 | — | — |
| Rattlesnake (venom) | T63.011 | T63.012 | T63.013 | T63.014 | — | — |
| Raubasine | T46.7X1 | T46.7X2 | T46.7X3 | T46.7X4 | T46.7X5 | T46.7X6 |
| Raudixin | T46.5X1 | T46.5X2 | T46.5X3 | T46.5X4 | T46.5X5 | T46.5X6 |
| Rautensin | T46.5X1 | T46.5X2 | T46.5X3 | T46.5X4 | T46.5X5 | T46.5X6 |
| Rautina | T46.5X1 | T46.5X2 | T46.5X3 | T46.5X4 | T46.5X5 | T46.5X6 |
| Rautotal | T46.5X1 | T46.5X2 | T46.5X3 | T46.5X4 | T46.5X5 | T46.5X6 |
| Rauwiloid | T46.5X1 | T46.5X2 | T46.5X3 | T46.5X4 | T46.5X5 | T46.5X6 |
| Rauwoldin | T46.5X1 | T46.5X2 | T46.5X3 | T46.5X4 | T46.5X5 | T46.5X6 |
| Rauwolfia (alkaloids) | T46.5X1 | T46.5X2 | T46.5X3 | T46.5X4 | T46.5X5 | T46.5X6 |
| Razoxane | T45.1X1 | T45.1X2 | T45.1X3 | T45.1X4 | T45.1X5 | T45.1X6 |
| Realgar | T57.0X1 | T57.0X2 | T57.0X3 | T57.0X4 | — | — |
| Recombinant (R) — see specific protein | | | | | | |
| Red blood cells, packed | T45.8X1 | T45.8X2 | T45.8X3 | T45.8X4 | T45.8X5 | T45.8X6 |
| Red squill (scilliroside) | T60.4X1 | T60.4X2 | T60.4X3 | T60.4X4 | — | — |
| Reducing agent, industrial NEC | T65.891 | T65.892 | T65.893 | T65.894 | — | — |
| Refrigerant gas (chlorofluorocarbon) | T53.5X1 | T53.5X2 | T53.5X3 | T53.5X4 | | |
|   not chlorofluorocarbon | T59.891 | T59.892 | T59.893 | T59.894 | — | — |
| Regroton | T50.2X1 | T50.2X2 | T50.2X3 | T50.2X4 | T50.2X5 | T50.2X6 |
| Rehydration salts (oral) | T50.3X1 | T50.3X2 | T50.3X3 | T50.3X4 | T50.3X5 | T50.3X6 |
| Rela | T42.8X1 | T42.8X2 | T42.8X3 | T42.8X4 | T42.8X5 | T42.8X6 |
| Relaxant, muscle | | | | | | |
|   anesthetic | T48.1X1 | T48.1X2 | T48.1X3 | T48.1X4 | T48.1X5 | T48.1X6 |
|   central nervous system | T42.8X1 | T42.8X2 | T42.8X3 | T42.8X4 | T42.8X5 | T42.8X6 |
|   skeletal NEC | T48.1X1 | T48.1X2 | T48.1X3 | T48.1X4 | T48.1X5 | T48.1X6 |
|   smooth NEC | T44.3X1 | T44.3X2 | T44.3X3 | T44.3X4 | T44.3X5 | T44.3X6 |
| Remoxipride | T43.591 | T43.592 | T43.593 | T43.594 | T43.595 | T43.596 |
| Renese | T50.2X1 | T50.2X2 | T50.2X3 | T50.2X4 | T50.2X5 | T50.2X6 |
| Renografin | T50.8X1 | T50.8X2 | T50.8X3 | T50.8X4 | T50.8X5 | T50.8X6 |
| Replacement solution | T50.3X1 | T50.3X2 | T50.3X3 | T50.3X4 | T50.3X5 | T50.3X6 |
| Reproterol | T48.6X1 | T48.6X2 | T48.6X3 | T48.6X4 | T48.6X5 | T48.6X6 |

| Substance | Poisoning, Accidental (unintentional) | Poisoning, Intentional Self-harm | Poisoning, Assault | Poisoning, Undetermined | Adverse Effect | Under-dosing |
|---|---|---|---|---|---|---|
| Rescinnamine | T46.5X1 | T46.5X2 | T46.5X3 | T46.5X4 | T46.5X5 | T46.5X6 |
| Reserpin (e) | T46.5X1 | T46.5X2 | T46.5X3 | T46.5X4 | T46.5X5 | T46.5X6 |
| Resorcin, resorcinol (nonmedicinal) | T65.891 | T65.892 | T65.893 | T65.894 | — | — |
|   medicinal | T49.4X1 | T49.4X2 | T49.4X3 | T49.4X4 | T49.4X5 | T49.4X6 |
| Respaire | T48.4X1 | T48.4X2 | T48.4X3 | T48.4X4 | T48.4X5 | T48.4X6 |
| Respiratory drug NEC | T48.901 | T48.902 | T48.903 | T48.904 | T48.905 | T48.906 |
|   antiasthmatic NEC | T48.6X1 | T48.6X2 | T48.6X3 | T48.6X4 | T48.6X5 | T48.6X6 |
|   anti-common-cold NEC | T48.5X1 | T48.5X2 | T48.5X3 | T48.5X4 | T48.5X5 | T48.5X6 |
|   expectorant NEC | T48.4X1 | T48.4X2 | T48.4X3 | T48.4X4 | T48.4X5 | T48.4X6 |
|   stimulant | T48.901 | T48.902 | T48.903 | T48.904 | T48.905 | T48.906 |
| Retinoic acid | T49.0X1 | T49.0X2 | T49.0X3 | T49.0X4 | T49.0X5 | T49.0X6 |
| Retinol | T45.2X1 | T45.2X2 | T45.2X3 | T45.2X4 | T45.2X5 | T45.2X6 |
| Rh (D) immune globulin (human) | T50.Z11 | T50.Z12 | T50.Z13 | T50.Z14 | T50.Z15 | T50.Z16 |
| Rhodine | T39.011 | T39.012 | T39.013 | T39.014 | T39.015 | T39.016 |
| RhoGAM | T50.Z11 | T50.Z12 | T50.Z13 | T50.Z14 | T50.Z15 | T50.Z16 |
| Rhubarb | | | | | | |
|   dry extract | T47.2X1 | T47.2X2 | T47.2X3 | T47.2X4 | T47.2X5 | T47.2X6 |
|   tincture, compound | T47.2X1 | T47.2X2 | T47.2X3 | T47.2X4 | T47.2X5 | T47.2X6 |
| Ribavirin | T37.5X1 | T37.5X2 | T37.5X3 | T37.5X4 | T37.5X5 | T37.5X6 |
| Riboflavin | T45.2X1 | T45.2X2 | T45.2X3 | T45.2X4 | T45.2X5 | T45.2X6 |
| Ribostamycin | T36.5X1 | T36.5X2 | T36.5X3 | T36.5X4 | T36.5X5 | T36.5X6 |
| Ricin | T62.2X1 | T62.2X2 | T62.2X3 | T62.2X4 | | |
| Ricinus communis | T62.2X1 | T62.2X2 | T62.2X3 | T62.2X4 | — | — |
| Rickettsial vaccine NEC | T50.A91 | T50.A92 | T50.A93 | T50.A94 | T50.A95 | T50.A96 |
| Rifabutin | T36.6X1 | T36.6X2 | T36.6X3 | T36.6X4 | T36.6X5 | T36.6X6 |
| Rifamide | T36.6X1 | T36.6X2 | T36.6X3 | T36.6X4 | T36.6X5 | T36.6X6 |
| Rifampicin | T36.6X1 | T36.6X2 | T36.6X3 | T36.6X4 | T36.6X5 | T36.6X6 |
|   with isoniazid | T37.1X1 | T37.1X2 | T37.1X3 | T37.1X4 | T37.1X5 | T37.1X6 |
| Rifampin | T36.6X1 | T36.6X2 | T36.6X3 | T36.6X4 | T36.6X5 | T36.6X6 |
| Rifamycin | T36.6X1 | T36.6X2 | T36.6X3 | T36.6X4 | T36.6X5 | T36.6X6 |
| Rifaximin | T36.6X1 | T36.6X2 | T36.6X3 | T36.6X4 | T36.6X5 | T36.6X6 |
| Rimantadine | T37.5X1 | T37.5X2 | T37.5X3 | T37.5X4 | T37.5X5 | T37.5X6 |
| Rimazolium metilsulfate | T39.8X1 | T39.8X2 | T39.8X3 | T39.8X4 | T39.8X5 | T39.8X6 |
| Rimifon | T37.1X1 | T37.1X2 | T37.1X3 | T37.1X4 | T37.1X5 | T37.1X6 |
| Rimiterol | T48.6X1 | T48.6X2 | T48.6X3 | T48.6X4 | T48.6X5 | T48.6X6 |
| Ringer (lactate) solution | T50.3X1 | T50.3X2 | T50.3X3 | T50.3X4 | T50.3X5 | T50.3X6 |
| Ristocetin | T36.8X1 | T36.8X2 | T36.8X3 | T36.8X4 | T36.8X5 | T36.8X6 |
| Ritalin | T43.631 | T43.632 | T43.633 | T43.634 | T43.635 | T43.636 |
| Ritodrine | T44.5X1 | T44.5X2 | T44.5X3 | T44.5X4 | T44.5X5 | T44.5X6 |
| Roach killer — see Insecticide | | | | | | |
| Rociverine | T44.3X1 | T44.3X2 | T44.3X3 | T44.3X4 | T44.3X5 | T44.3X6 |
| Rocky Mountain spotted fever vaccine | T50.A91 | T50.A92 | T50.A93 | T50.A94 | T50.A95 | T50.A96 |
| Rodenticide NEC | T60.4X1 | T60.4X2 | T60.4X3 | T60.4X4 | — | — |
| Rohypnol | T42.4X1 | T42.4X2 | T42.4X3 | T42.4X4 | T42.4X5 | T42.4X6 |
| Rokitamycin | T36.3X1 | T36.3X2 | T36.3X3 | T36.3X4 | T36.3X5 | T36.3X6 |
| Rolaids | T47.1X1 | T47.1X2 | T47.1X3 | T47.1X4 | T47.1X5 | T47.1X6 |
| Rolitetracycline | T36.4X1 | T36.4X2 | T36.4X3 | T36.4X4 | T36.4X5 | T36.4X6 |
| Romilar | T48.3X1 | T48.3X2 | T48.3X3 | T48.3X4 | T48.3X5 | T48.3X6 |
| Ronifibrate | T46.6X1 | T46.6X2 | T46.6X3 | T46.6X4 | T46.6X5 | T46.6X6 |
| Rosaprostol | T47.1X1 | T47.1X2 | T47.1X3 | T47.1X4 | T47.1X5 | T47.1X6 |
| Rose bengal sodium (131I) | T50.8X1 | T50.8X2 | T50.8X3 | T50.8X4 | T50.8X5 | T50.8X6 |
| Rose water ointment | T49.3X1 | T49.3X2 | T49.3X3 | T49.3X4 | T49.3X5 | T49.3X6 |
| Rosoxacin | T37.8X1 | T37.8X2 | T37.8X3 | T37.8X4 | T37.8X5 | T37.8X6 |
| Rotenone | T60.2X1 | T60.2X2 | T60.2X3 | T60.2X4 | — | — |
| Rotoxamine | T45.0X1 | T45.0X2 | T45.0X3 | T45.0X4 | T45.0X5 | T45.0X6 |
| Rough-on-rats | T60.4X1 | T60.4X2 | T60.4X3 | T60.4X4 | — | — |
| Roxatidine | T47.0X1 | T47.0X2 | T47.0X3 | T47.0X4 | T47.0X5 | T47.0X6 |
| Roxithromycin | T36.3X1 | T36.3X2 | T36.3X3 | T36.3X4 | T36.3X5 | T36.3X6 |
| Rt-PA | T45.611 | T45.612 | T45.613 | T45.614 | T45.615 | T45.616 |
| Rubbing alcohol | T51.2X1 | T51.2X2 | T51.2X3 | T51.2X4 | | |
| Rubefacient | T49.4X1 | T49.4X2 | T49.4X3 | T49.4X4 | T49.4X5 | T49.4X6 |
| Rubella vaccine | T50.B91 | T50.B92 | T50.B93 | T50.B94 | T50.B95 | T50.B96 |
| Rubeola vaccine | T50.B91 | T50.B92 | T50.B93 | T50.B94 | T50.B95 | T50.B96 |
| Rubidium chloride Rb82 | T50.8X1 | T50.8X2 | T50.8X3 | T50.8X4 | T50.8X5 | T50.8X6 |
| Rubidomycin | T45.1X1 | T45.1X2 | T45.1X3 | T45.1X4 | T45.1X5 | T45.1X6 |
| Rue | T62.2X1 | T62.2X2 | T62.2X3 | T62.2X4 | — | — |
| Rufocromomycin | T45.1X1 | T45.1X2 | T45.1X3 | T45.1X4 | T45.1X5 | T45.1X6 |
| Russel's viper venin | T45.7X1 | T45.7X2 | T45.7X3 | T45.7X4 | T45.7X5 | T45.7X6 |
| Ruta (graveolens) | T62.2X1 | T62.2X2 | T62.2X3 | T62.2X4 | — | — |
| Rutinum | T46.991 | T46.992 | T46.993 | T46.994 | T46.995 | T46.996 |
| Rutoside | T46.991 | T46.992 | T46.993 | T46.994 | T46.995 | T46.996 |
| b-sitosterol(s) | T46.6X1 | T46.6X2 | T46.6X3 | T46.6X4 | T46.6X5 | T46.6X6 |
| Sabadilla (plant) | T62.2X1 | T62.2X2 | T62.2X3 | T62.2X4 | — | — |
|   pesticide | T60.2X1 | T60.2X2 | T60.2X3 | T60.2X4 | — | — |
| Saccharated iron oxide | T45.8X1 | T45.8X2 | T45.8X3 | T45.8X4 | T45.8X5 | T45.8X6 |
| Saccharin | T50.901 | T50.902 | T50.903 | T50.904 | T50.905 | T50.906 |
| Saccharomyces boulardii | T47.6X1 | T47.6X2 | T47.6X3 | T47.6X4 | T47.6X5 | T47.6X6 |
| Safflower oil | T46.6X1 | T46.6X2 | T46.6X3 | T46.6X4 | T46.6X5 | T46.6X6 |
| Safrazine | T43.1X1 | T43.1X2 | T43.1X3 | T43.1X4 | T43.1X5 | T43.1X6 |
| Salazosulfapyridine | T37.0X1 | T37.0X2 | T37.0X3 | T37.0X4 | T37.0X5 | T37.0X6 |

▽ Subterms under main terms may continue to next column or page    Additional Character May Be Required — Refer to the Tabular List for Character Selection    387

Pyrogallic acid — Salazosulfapyridine

| Substance | Poisoning, Accidental (unintentional) | Poisoning, Intentional Self-harm | Poisoning, Assault | Poisoning, Undetermined | Adverse Effect | Under-dosing |
|---|---|---|---|---|---|---|
| **Salbutamol** | T48.6X1 | T48.6X2 | T48.6X3 | T48.6X4 | T48.6X5 | T48.6X6 |
| **Salicylamide** | T39.091 | T39.092 | T39.093 | T39.094 | T39.095 | T39.096 |
| **Salicylate NEC** | T39.091 | T39.092 | T39.093 | T39.094 | T39.095 | T39.096 |
| methyl | T49.3X1 | T49.3X2 | T49.3X3 | T49.3X4 | T49.3X5 | T49.3X6 |
| theobromine calcium | T50.2X1 | T50.2X2 | T50.2X3 | T50.2X4 | T50.2X5 | T50.2X6 |
| **Salicylazosulfapyridine** | T37.0X1 | T37.0X2 | T37.0X3 | T37.0X4 | T37.0X5 | T37.0X6 |
| **Salicylhydroxamic acid** | T49.0X1 | T49.0X2 | T49.0X3 | T49.0X4 | T49.0X5 | T49.0X6 |
| **Salicylic acid** | T49.4X1 | T49.4X2 | T49.4X3 | T49.4X4 | T49.4X5 | T49.4X6 |
| with benzoic acid | T49.4X1 | T49.4X2 | T49.4X3 | T49.4X4 | T49.4X5 | T49.4X6 |
| congeners | T39.091 | T39.092 | T39.093 | T39.094 | T39.095 | T39.096 |
| derivative | T39.091 | T39.092 | T39.093 | T39.094 | T39.095 | T39.096 |
| salts | T39.091 | T39.092 | T39.093 | T39.094 | T39.095 | T39.096 |
| **Salinazid** | T37.1X1 | T37.1X2 | T37.1X3 | T37.1X4 | T37.1X5 | T37.1X6 |
| **Salmeterol** | T48.6X1 | T48.6X2 | T48.6X3 | T48.6X4 | T48.6X5 | T48.6X6 |
| **Salol** | T49.3X1 | T49.3X2 | T49.3X3 | T49.3X4 | T49.3X5 | T49.3X6 |
| **Salsalate** | T39.091 | T39.092 | T39.093 | T39.094 | T39.095 | T39.096 |
| **Salt-replacing drug** | T50.901 | T50.902 | T50.903 | T50.904 | T50.905 | T50.906 |
| **Salt-retaining mineralocorticoid** | T50.0X1 | T50.0X2 | T50.0X3 | T50.0X4 | T50.0X5 | T50.0X6 |
| **Salt substitute** | T50.901 | T50.902 | T50.903 | T50.904 | T50.905 | T50.906 |
| **Saluretic NEC** | T50.2X1 | T50.2X2 | T50.2X3 | T50.2X4 | T50.2X5 | T50.2X6 |
| **Saluron** | T50.2X1 | T50.2X2 | T50.2X3 | T50.2X4 | T50.2X5 | T50.2X6 |
| **Salvarsan 606** (neosilver) (silver) | T37.8X1 | T37.8X2 | T37.8X3 | T37.8X4 | T37.8X5 | T37.8X6 |
| **Sambucus canadensis** | T62.2X1 | T62.2X2 | T62.2X3 | T62.2X4 | — | — |
| berry | T62.1X1 | T62.1X2 | T62.1X3 | T62.1X4 | — | — |
| **Sandril** | T46.5X1 | T46.5X2 | T46.5X3 | T46.5X4 | T46.5X5 | T46.5X6 |
| **Sanguinaria canadensis** | T62.2X1 | T62.2X2 | T62.2X3 | T62.2X4 | — | — |
| **Saniflush** (cleaner) | T54.2X1 | T54.2X2 | T54.2X3 | T54.2X4 | — | — |
| **Santonin** | T37.4X1 | T37.4X2 | T37.4X3 | T37.4X4 | T37.4X5 | T37.4X6 |
| **Santyl** | T49.8X1 | T49.8X2 | T49.8X3 | T49.8X4 | T49.8X5 | T49.8X6 |
| **Saralasin** | T46.5X1 | T46.5X2 | T46.5X3 | T46.5X4 | T46.5X5 | T46.5X6 |
| **Sarcolysin** | T45.1X1 | T45.1X2 | T45.1X3 | T45.1X4 | T45.1X5 | T45.1X6 |
| **Sarkomycin** | T45.1X1 | T45.1X2 | T45.1X3 | T45.1X4 | T45.1X5 | T45.1X6 |
| **Saroten** | T43.011 | T43.012 | T43.013 | T43.014 | T43.015 | T43.016 |
| **Saturnine** — see Lead | | | | | | |
| **Savin** (oil) | T49.4X1 | T49.4X2 | T49.4X3 | T49.4X4 | T49.4X5 | T49.4X6 |
| **Scammony** | T47.2X1 | T47.2X2 | T47.2X3 | T47.2X4 | T47.2X5 | T47.2X6 |
| **Scarlet red** | T49.8X1 | T49.8X2 | T49.8X3 | T49.8X4 | T49.8X5 | T49.8X6 |
| **Scheele's green** | T57.0X1 | T57.0X2 | T57.0X3 | T57.0X4 | — | — |
| insecticide | T57.0X1 | T57.0X2 | T57.0X3 | T57.0X4 | — | — |
| **Schizontozide** (blood) (tissue) | T37.2X1 | T37.2X2 | T37.2X3 | T37.2X4 | T37.2X5 | T37.2X6 |
| **Schradan** | T60.0X1 | T60.0X2 | T60.0X3 | T60.0X4 | — | — |
| **Schweinfurth green** | T57.0X1 | T57.0X2 | T57.0X3 | T57.0X4 | — | — |
| insecticide | T57.0X1 | T57.0X2 | T57.0X3 | T57.0X4 | — | — |
| **Scilla, rat poison** | T60.4X1 | T60.4X2 | T60.4X3 | T60.4X4 | — | — |
| **Scillaren** | T60.4X1 | T60.4X2 | T60.4X3 | T60.4X4 | — | — |
| **Sclerosing agent** | T46.8X1 | T46.8X2 | T46.8X3 | T46.8X4 | T46.8X5 | T46.8X6 |
| **Scombrotoxin** | T61.11 | T61.12 | T61.13 | T61.14 | | |
| **Scopolamine** | T44.3X1 | T44.3X2 | T44.3X3 | T44.3X4 | T44.3X5 | T44.3X6 |
| **Scopolia extract** | T44.3X1 | T44.3X2 | T44.3X3 | T44.3X4 | T44.3X5 | T44.3X6 |
| **Scouring powder** | T65.891 | T65.892 | T65.893 | T65.894 | — | — |
| **Sea** | | | | | | |
| anemone (sting) | T63.631 | T63.632 | T63.633 | T63.634 | | |
| cucumber (sting) | T63.691 | T63.692 | T63.693 | T63.694 | | |
| snake (bite) (venom) | T63.091 | T63.092 | T63.093 | T63.094 | — | — |
| urchin spine (puncture) | T63.691 | T63.692 | T63.693 | T63.694 | — | — |
| **Seafood** | T61.91 | T61.92 | T61.93 | T61.94 | — | — |
| specified NEC | T61.8X1 | T61.8X2 | T61.8X3 | T61.8X4 | — | — |
| **Secbutabarbital** | T42.3X1 | T42.3X2 | T42.3X3 | T42.3X4 | T42.3X5 | T42.3X6 |
| **Secbutabarbitone** | T42.3X1 | T42.3X2 | T42.3X3 | T42.3X4 | T42.3X5 | T42.3X6 |
| **Secnidazole** | T37.3X1 | T37.3X2 | T37.3X3 | T37.3X4 | T37.3X5 | T37.3X6 |
| **Secobarbital** | T42.3X1 | T42.3X2 | T42.3X3 | T42.3X4 | T42.3X5 | T42.3X6 |
| **Seconal** | T42.3X1 | T42.3X2 | T42.3X3 | T42.3X4 | T42.3X5 | T42.3X6 |
| **Secretin** | T50.8X1 | T50.8X2 | T50.8X3 | T50.8X4 | T50.8X5 | T50.8X6 |
| **Sedative NEC** | T42.71 | T42.72 | T42.73 | T42.74 | T42.75 | T42.76 |
| mixed NEC | T42.6X1 | T42.6X2 | T42.6X3 | T42.6X4 | T42.6X5 | T42.6X6 |
| **Sedormid** | T42.6X1 | T42.6X2 | T42.6X3 | T42.6X4 | T42.6X5 | T42.6X6 |
| **Seed disinfectant or dressing** | T60.8X1 | T60.8X2 | T60.8X3 | T60.8X4 | — | — |
| **Seeds** (poisonous) | T62.2X1 | T62.2X2 | T62.2X3 | T62.2X4 | — | — |
| **Selegiline** | T42.8X1 | T42.8X2 | T42.8X3 | T42.8X4 | T42.8X5 | T42.8X6 |
| **Selenium NEC** | T56.891 | T56.892 | T56.893 | T56.894 | — | — |
| disulfide or sulfide | T49.4X1 | T49.4X2 | T49.4X3 | T49.4X4 | T49.4X5 | T49.4X6 |
| fumes | T59.891 | T59.892 | T59.893 | T59.894 | — | — |
| sulfide | T49.4X1 | T49.4X2 | T49.4X3 | T49.4X4 | T49.4X5 | T49.4X6 |
| **Selenomethionine** (75Se) | T50.8X1 | T50.8X2 | T50.8X3 | T50.8X4 | T50.8X5 | T50.8X6 |
| **Selsun** | T49.4X1 | T49.4X2 | T49.4X3 | T49.4X4 | T49.4X5 | T49.4X6 |
| **Semustine** | T45.1X1 | T45.1X2 | T45.1X3 | T45.1X4 | T45.1X5 | T45.1X6 |
| **Senega syrup** | T48.4X1 | T48.4X2 | T48.4X3 | T48.4X4 | T48.4X5 | T48.4X6 |
| **Senna** | T47.2X1 | T47.2X2 | T47.2X3 | T47.2X4 | T47.2X5 | T47.2X6 |
| **Sennoside A+B** | T47.2X1 | T47.2X2 | T47.2X3 | T47.2X4 | T47.2X5 | T47.2X6 |

| Substance | Poisoning, Accidental (unintentional) | Poisoning, Intentional Self-harm | Poisoning, Assault | Poisoning, Undetermined | Adverse Effect | Under-dosing |
|---|---|---|---|---|---|---|
| **Septisol** | T49.2X1 | T49.2X2 | T49.2X3 | T49.2X4 | T49.2X5 | T49.2X6 |
| **Seractide** | T38.811 | T38.812 | T38.813 | T38.814 | T38.815 | T38.816 |
| **Serax** | T42.4X1 | T42.4X2 | T42.4X3 | T42.4X4 | T42.4X5 | T42.4X6 |
| **Serenesil** | T42.6X1 | T42.6X2 | T42.6X3 | T42.6X4 | T42.6X5 | T42.6X6 |
| **Serenium** (hydrochloride) | T37.91 | T37.92 | T37.93 | T37.94 | T37.95 | T37.96 |
| **Serepax** — see Oxazepam | | | | | | |
| **Sermorelin** | T38.891 | T38.892 | T38.893 | T38.894 | T38.895 | T38.896 |
| **Sernyl** | T41.1X1 | T41.1X2 | T41.1X3 | T41.1X4 | T41.1X5 | T41.1X6 |
| **Serotonin** | T50.991 | T50.992 | T50.993 | T50.994 | T50.995 | T50.996 |
| **Serpasil** | T46.5X1 | T46.5X2 | T46.5X3 | T46.5X4 | T46.5X5 | T46.5X6 |
| **Serrapeptase** | T45.3X1 | T45.3X2 | T45.3X3 | T45.3X4 | T45.3X5 | T45.3X6 |
| **Serum** | | | | | | |
| antibotulinus | T50.Z11 | T50.Z12 | T50.Z13 | T50.Z14 | T50.Z15 | T50.Z16 |
| anticytotoxic | T50.Z11 | T50.Z12 | T50.Z13 | T50.Z14 | T50.Z15 | T50.Z16 |
| antidiphtheria | T50.Z11 | T50.Z12 | T50.Z13 | T50.Z14 | T50.Z15 | T50.Z16 |
| antimeningococcus | T50.Z11 | T50.Z12 | T50.Z13 | T50.Z14 | T50.Z15 | T50.Z16 |
| anti-Rh | T50.Z11 | T50.Z12 | T50.Z13 | T50.Z14 | T50.Z15 | T50.Z16 |
| anti-snake-bite | T50.Z11 | T50.Z12 | T50.Z13 | T50.Z14 | T50.Z15 | T50.Z16 |
| antitetanic | T50.Z11 | T50.Z12 | T50.Z13 | T50.Z14 | T50.Z15 | T50.Z16 |
| antitoxic | T50.Z11 | T50.Z12 | T50.Z13 | T50.Z14 | T50.Z15 | T50.Z16 |
| complement (inhibitor) | T45.8X1 | T45.8X2 | T45.8X3 | T45.8X4 | T45.8X5 | T45.8X6 |
| convalescent | T50.Z11 | T50.Z12 | T50.Z13 | T50.Z14 | T50.Z15 | T50.Z16 |
| hemolytic complement | T45.8X1 | T45.8X2 | T45.8X3 | T45.8X4 | T45.8X5 | T45.8X6 |
| immune (human) | T50.Z11 | T50.Z12 | T50.Z13 | T50.Z14 | T50.Z15 | T50.Z16 |
| protective NEC | T50.Z11 | T50.Z12 | T50.Z13 | T50.Z14 | T50.Z15 | T50.Z16 |
| **Setastine** | T45.0X1 | T45.0X2 | T45.0X3 | T45.0X4 | T45.0X5 | T45.0X6 |
| **Setoperone** | T43.591 | T43.592 | T43.593 | T43.594 | T43.595 | T43.596 |
| **Sewer gas** | T59.91 | T59.92 | T59.93 | T59.94 | | |
| **Shampoo** | T55.0X1 | T55.0X2 | T55.0X3 | T55.0X4 | | |
| **Shellfish, noxious, nonbacterial** | T61.781 | T61.782 | T61.783 | T61.784 | | |
| **Sildenafil** | T46.7X1 | T46.7X2 | T46.7X3 | T46.7X4 | T46.7X5 | T46.7X6 |
| **Silibinin** | T50.991 | T50.992 | T50.993 | T50.994 | T50.995 | T50.996 |
| **Silicone NEC** | T65.891 | T65.892 | T65.893 | T65.894 | — | — |
| medicinal | T49.3X1 | T49.3X2 | T49.3X3 | T49.3X4 | T49.3X5 | T49.3X6 |
| **Silvadene** | T49.0X1 | T49.0X2 | T49.0X3 | T49.0X4 | T49.0X5 | T49.0X6 |
| **Silver** | T49.0X1 | T49.0X2 | T49.0X3 | T49.0X4 | T49.0X5 | T49.0X6 |
| anti-infectives | T49.0X1 | T49.0X2 | T49.0X3 | T49.0X4 | T49.0X5 | T49.0X6 |
| arsphenamine | T37.8X1 | T37.8X2 | T37.8X3 | T37.8X4 | T37.8X5 | T37.8X6 |
| colloidal | T49.0X1 | T49.0X2 | T49.0X3 | T49.0X4 | T49.0X5 | T49.0X6 |
| nitrate | T49.0X1 | T49.0X2 | T49.0X3 | T49.0X4 | T49.0X5 | T49.0X6 |
| ophthalmic preparation | T49.5X1 | T49.5X2 | T49.5X3 | T49.5X4 | T49.5X5 | T49.5X6 |
| toughened (keratolytic) | T49.4X1 | T49.4X2 | T49.4X3 | T49.4X4 | T49.4X5 | T49.4X6 |
| nonmedicinal (dust) | T56.891 | T56.892 | T56.893 | T56.894 | — | — |
| protein | T49.5X1 | T49.5X2 | T49.5X3 | T49.5X4 | T49.5X5 | T49.5X6 |
| salvarsan | T37.8X1 | T37.8X2 | T37.8X3 | T37.8X4 | T37.8X5 | T37.8X6 |
| sulfadiazine | T49.4X1 | T49.4X2 | T49.4X3 | T49.4X4 | T49.4X5 | T49.4X6 |
| **Silymarin** | T50.991 | T50.992 | T50.993 | T50.994 | T50.995 | T50.996 |
| **Simaldrate** | T47.1X1 | T47.1X2 | T47.1X3 | T47.1X4 | T47.1X5 | T47.1X6 |
| **Simazine** | T60.3X1 | T60.3X2 | T60.3X3 | T60.3X4 | — | — |
| **Simethicone** | T47.1X1 | T47.1X2 | T47.1X3 | T47.1X4 | T47.1X5 | T47.1X6 |
| **Simfibrate** | T46.6X1 | T46.6X2 | T46.6X3 | T46.6X4 | T46.6X5 | T46.6X6 |
| **Simvastatin** | T46.6X1 | T46.6X2 | T46.6X3 | T46.6X4 | T46.6X5 | T46.6X6 |
| **Sincalide** | T50.8X1 | T50.8X2 | T50.8X3 | T50.8X4 | T50.8X5 | T50.8X6 |
| **Sinequan** | T43.011 | T43.012 | T43.013 | T43.014 | T43.015 | T43.016 |
| **Singoserp** | T46.5X1 | T46.5X2 | T46.5X3 | T46.5X4 | T46.5X5 | T46.5X6 |
| **Sintrom** | T45.511 | T45.512 | T45.513 | T45.514 | T45.515 | T45.516 |
| **Sisomicin** | T36.5X1 | T36.5X2 | T36.5X3 | T36.5X4 | T36.5X5 | T36.5X6 |
| **Sitosterols** | T46.6X1 | T46.6X2 | T46.6X3 | T46.6X4 | T46.6X5 | T46.6X6 |
| **Skeletal muscle relaxants** | T48.1X1 | T48.1X2 | T48.1X3 | T48.1X4 | T48.1X5 | T48.1X6 |
| **Skin** | | | | | | |
| agents (external) | T49.91 | T49.92 | T49.93 | T49.94 | T49.95 | T49.96 |
| specified NEC | T49.8X1 | T49.8X2 | T49.8X3 | T49.8X4 | T49.8X5 | T49.8X6 |
| test antigen | T50.8X1 | T50.8X2 | T50.8X3 | T50.8X4 | T50.8X5 | T50.8X6 |
| **Sleep-eze** | T45.0X1 | T45.0X2 | T45.0X3 | T45.0X4 | T45.0X5 | T45.0X6 |
| **Sleeping draught, pill** | T42.71 | T42.72 | T42.73 | T42.74 | T42.75 | T42.76 |
| **Smallpox vaccine** | T50.B11 | T50.B12 | T50.B13 | T50.B14 | T50.B15 | T50.B16 |
| **Smelter fumes NEC** | T56.91 | T56.92 | T56.93 | T56.94 | — | — |
| **Smog** | T59.1X1 | T59.1X2 | T59.1X3 | T59.1X4 | — | — |
| **Smoke NEC** | T59.811 | T59.812 | T59.813 | T59.814 | — | — |
| **Smooth muscle relaxant** | T44.3X1 | T44.3X2 | T44.3X3 | T44.3X4 | T44.3X5 | T44.3X6 |
| **Snail killer NEC** | T60.8X1 | T60.8X2 | T60.8X3 | T60.8X4 | — | — |
| **Snake venom or bite** | T63.001 | T63.002 | T63.003 | T63.004 | — | — |
| hemocoagulase | T45.7X1 | T45.7X2 | T45.7X3 | T45.7X4 | T45.7X5 | T45.7X6 |
| **Snuff** | T65.211 | T65.212 | T65.213 | T65.214 | — | — |
| **Soap** (powder) (product) | T55.0X1 | T55.0X2 | T55.0X3 | T55.0X4 | — | — |
| enema | T47.4X1 | T47.4X2 | T47.4X3 | T47.4X4 | T47.4X5 | T47.4X6 |
| medicinal, soft | T49.2X1 | T49.2X2 | T49.2X3 | T49.2X4 | T49.2X5 | T49.2X6 |
| superfatted | T49.2X1 | T49.2X2 | T49.2X3 | T49.2X4 | T49.2X5 | T49.2X6 |
| **Sobrerol** | T48.4X1 | T48.4X2 | T48.4X3 | T48.4X4 | T48.4X5 | T48.4X6 |
| **Soda** (caustic) | T54.3X1 | T54.3X2 | T54.3X3 | T54.3X4 | | |
| bicarb | T47.1X1 | T47.1X2 | T47.1X3 | T47.1X4 | T47.1X5 | T47.1X6 |

Additional Character May Be Required — Refer to the Tabular List for Character Selection      ▽ Subterms under main terms may continue to next column or page

| Substance | Poisoning, Accidental (unintentional) | Poisoning, Intentional Self-harm | Poisoning, Assault | Poisoning, Undetermined | Adverse Effect | Under-dosing |
|---|---|---|---|---|---|---|
| **Soda** — *continued* | | | | | | |
| chlorinated — *see* Sodium, hypochlorite | | | | | | |
| **Sodium** | | | | | | |
| acetosulfone | T37.1X1 | T37.1X2 | T37.1X3 | T37.1X4 | T37.1X5 | T37.1X6 |
| acetrizoate | T50.8X1 | T50.8X2 | T50.8X3 | T50.8X4 | T50.8X5 | T50.8X6 |
| acid phosphate | T50.3X1 | T50.3X2 | T50.3X3 | T50.3X4 | T50.3X5 | T50.3X6 |
| alginate | T47.8X1 | T47.8X2 | T47.8X3 | T47.8X4 | T47.8X5 | T47.8X6 |
| amidotrizoate | T50.8X1 | T50.8X2 | T50.8X3 | T50.8X4 | T50.8X5 | T50.8X6 |
| aminopterin | T45.1X1 | T45.1X2 | T45.1X3 | T45.1X4 | T45.1X5 | T45.1X6 |
| amylosulfate | T47.8X1 | T47.8X2 | T47.8X3 | T47.8X4 | T47.8X5 | T47.8X6 |
| amytal | T42.3X1 | T42.3X2 | T42.3X3 | T42.3X4 | T42.3X5 | T42.3X6 |
| antimony gluconate | T37.3X1 | T37.3X2 | T37.3X3 | T37.3X4 | T37.3X5 | T37.3X6 |
| arsenate | T57.0X1 | T57.0X2 | T57.0X3 | T57.0X4 | — | — |
| aurothiomalate | T39.4X1 | T39.4X2 | T39.4X3 | T39.4X4 | T39.4X5 | T39.4X6 |
| aurothiosulfate | T39.4X1 | T39.4X2 | T39.4X3 | T39.4X4 | T39.4X5 | T39.4X6 |
| barbiturate | T42.3X1 | T42.3X2 | T42.3X3 | T42.3X4 | T42.3X5 | T42.3X6 |
| basic phosphate | T47.4X1 | T47.4X2 | T47.4X3 | T47.4X4 | T47.4X5 | T47.4X6 |
| bicarbonate | T47.1X1 | T47.1X2 | T47.1X3 | T47.1X4 | T47.1X5 | T47.1X6 |
| bichromate | T57.8X1 | T57.8X2 | T57.8X3 | T57.8X4 | — | — |
| biphosphate | T50.3X1 | T50.3X2 | T50.3X3 | T50.3X4 | T50.3X5 | T50.3X6 |
| bisulfate | T65.891 | T65.892 | T65.893 | T65.894 | — | — |
| borate | | | | | | |
| cleanser | T57.8X1 | T57.8X2 | T57.8X3 | T57.8X4 | — | — |
| eye | T49.5X1 | T49.5X2 | T49.5X3 | T49.5X4 | T49.5X5 | T49.5X6 |
| therapeutic | T49.8X1 | T49.8X2 | T49.8X3 | T49.8X4 | T49.8X5 | T49.8X6 |
| bromide | T42.6X1 | T42.6X2 | T42.6X3 | T42.6X4 | T42.6X5 | T42.6X6 |
| cacodylate (nonmedicinal) NEC | T50.8X1 | T50.8X2 | T50.8X3 | T50.8X4 | T50.8X5 | T50.8X6 |
| anti-infective | T37.8X1 | T37.8X2 | T37.8X3 | T37.8X4 | T37.8X5 | T37.8X6 |
| herbicide | T60.3X1 | T60.3X2 | T60.3X3 | T60.3X4 | — | — |
| calcium edetate | T45.8X1 | T45.8X2 | T45.8X3 | T45.8X4 | T45.8X5 | T45.8X6 |
| carbonate NEC | T54.3X1 | T54.3X2 | T54.3X3 | T54.3X4 | — | — |
| chlorate NEC | T65.891 | T65.892 | T65.893 | T65.894 | — | — |
| herbicide | T54.91 | T54.92 | T54.93 | T54.94 | — | — |
| chloride | T50.3X1 | T50.3X2 | T50.3X3 | T50.3X4 | T50.3X5 | T50.3X6 |
| with glucose | T50.3X1 | T50.3X2 | T50.3X3 | T50.3X4 | T50.3X5 | T50.3X6 |
| chromate | T65.891 | T65.892 | T65.893 | T65.894 | — | — |
| citrate | T50.991 | T50.992 | T50.993 | T50.994 | T50.995 | T50.996 |
| cromoglicate | T48.6X1 | T48.6X2 | T48.6X3 | T48.6X4 | T48.6X5 | T48.6X6 |
| cyanide | T65.0X1 | T65.0X2 | T65.0X3 | T65.0X4 | — | — |
| cyclamate | T50.3X1 | T50.3X2 | T50.3X3 | T50.3X4 | T50.3X5 | T50.3X6 |
| dehydrocholate | T45.8X1 | T45.8X2 | T45.8X3 | T45.8X4 | T45.8X5 | T45.8X6 |
| diatrizoate | T50.8X1 | T50.8X2 | T50.8X3 | T50.8X4 | T50.8X5 | T50.8X6 |
| dibunate | T48.4X1 | T48.4X2 | T48.4X3 | T48.4X4 | T48.4X5 | T48.4X6 |
| dioctyl sulfosuccinate | T47.4X1 | T47.4X2 | T47.4X3 | T47.4X4 | T47.4X5 | T47.4X6 |
| dipantoyl ferrate | T45.8X1 | T45.8X2 | T45.8X3 | T45.8X4 | T45.8X5 | T45.8X6 |
| edetate | T45.8X1 | T45.8X2 | T45.8X3 | T45.8X4 | T45.8X5 | T45.8X6 |
| ethacrynate | T50.1X1 | T50.1X2 | T50.1X3 | T50.1X4 | T50.1X5 | T50.1X6 |
| feredetate | T45.8X1 | T45.8X2 | T45.8X3 | T45.8X4 | T45.8X5 | T45.8X6 |
| Fluoride — *see* Fluoride | | | | | | |
| fluoroacetate (dust) (pesticide) | T60.4X1 | T60.4X2 | T60.4X3 | T60.4X4 | — | — |
| free salt | T50.3X1 | T50.3X2 | T50.3X3 | T50.3X4 | T50.3X5 | T50.3X6 |
| fusidate | T36.8X1 | T36.8X2 | T36.8X3 | T36.8X4 | T36.8X5 | T36.8X6 |
| glucaldrate | T47.1X1 | T47.1X2 | T47.1X3 | T47.1X4 | T47.1X5 | T47.1X6 |
| glucosulfone | T37.1X1 | T37.1X2 | T37.1X3 | T37.1X4 | T37.1X5 | T37.1X6 |
| glutamate | T45.8X1 | T45.8X2 | T45.8X3 | T45.8X4 | T45.8X5 | T45.8X6 |
| hydrogen carbonate | T50.3X1 | T50.3X2 | T50.3X3 | T50.3X4 | T50.3X5 | T50.3X6 |
| hydroxide | T54.3X1 | T54.3X2 | T54.3X3 | T54.3X4 | — | — |
| hypochlorite (bleach) NEC | T54.3X1 | T54.3X2 | T54.3X3 | T54.3X4 | — | — |
| disinfectant | T54.3X1 | T54.3X2 | T54.3X3 | T54.3X4 | — | — |
| medicinal (anti-infective) (external) | T49.0X1 | T49.0X2 | T49.0X3 | T49.0X4 | T49.0X5 | T49.0X6 |
| vapor | T54.3X1 | T54.3X2 | T54.3X3 | T54.3X4 | — | — |
| hyposulfite | T49.0X1 | T49.0X2 | T49.0X3 | T49.0X4 | T49.0X5 | T49.0X6 |
| indigotin disulfonate | T50.8X1 | T50.8X2 | T50.8X3 | T50.8X4 | T50.8X5 | T50.8X6 |
| iodide | T50.991 | T50.992 | T50.993 | T50.994 | T50.995 | T50.996 |
| I-131 | T50.8X1 | T50.8X2 | T50.8X3 | T50.8X4 | T50.8X5 | T50.8X6 |
| therapeutic | T38.2X1 | T38.2X2 | T38.2X3 | T38.2X4 | T38.2X5 | T38.2X6 |
| iodohippurate (131I) | T50.8X1 | T50.8X2 | T50.8X3 | T50.8X4 | T50.8X5 | T50.8X6 |
| iopodate | T50.8X1 | T50.8X2 | T50.8X3 | T50.8X4 | T50.8X5 | T50.8X6 |
| iothalamate | T50.8X1 | T50.8X2 | T50.8X3 | T50.8X4 | T50.8X5 | T50.8X6 |
| iron edetate | T45.4X1 | T45.4X2 | T45.4X3 | T45.4X4 | T45.4X5 | T45.4X6 |
| lactate (compound solution) | T45.8X1 | T45.8X2 | T45.8X3 | T45.8X4 | T45.8X5 | T45.8X6 |
| lauryl (sulfate) | T49.2X1 | T49.2X2 | T49.2X3 | T49.2X4 | T49.2X5 | T49.2X6 |
| L-triiodothyronine | T38.1X1 | T38.1X2 | T38.1X3 | T38.1X4 | T38.1X5 | T38.1X6 |
| magnesium citrate | T50.991 | T50.992 | T50.993 | T50.994 | T50.995 | T50.996 |
| mersalate | T50.2X1 | T50.2X2 | T50.2X3 | T50.2X4 | T50.2X5 | T50.2X6 |
| metasilicate | T65.891 | T65.892 | T65.893 | T65.894 | — | — |
| metrizoate | T50.8X1 | T50.8X2 | T50.8X3 | T50.8X4 | T50.8X5 | T50.8X6 |
| **Sodium** — *continued* | | | | | | |
| monofluoroacetate (pesticide) | T60.1X1 | T60.1X2 | T60.1X3 | T60.1X4 | | |
| morrhuate | T46.8X1 | T46.8X2 | T46.8X3 | T46.8X4 | T46.8X5 | T46.8X6 |
| nafcillin | T36.0X1 | T36.0X2 | T36.0X3 | T36.0X4 | T36.0X5 | T36.0X6 |
| nitrate (oxidizing agent) | T65.891 | T65.892 | T65.893 | T65.894 | — | — |
| nitrite | T50.6X1 | T50.6X2 | T50.6X3 | T50.6X4 | T50.6X5 | T50.6X6 |
| nitroferricyanide | T46.5X1 | T46.5X2 | T46.5X3 | T46.5X4 | T46.5X5 | T46.5X6 |
| nitroprusside | T46.5X1 | T46.5X2 | T46.5X3 | T46.5X4 | T46.5X5 | T46.5X6 |
| oxalate | T65.891 | T65.892 | T65.893 | T65.894 | — | — |
| oxide/peroxide | T65.891 | T65.892 | T65.893 | T65.894 | — | — |
| oxybate | T41.291 | T41.292 | T41.293 | T41.294 | T41.295 | T41.296 |
| para-aminohippurate | T50.8X1 | T50.8X2 | T50.8X3 | T50.8X4 | T50.8X5 | T50.8X6 |
| perborate (nonmedicinal) NEC | T65.891 | T65.892 | T65.893 | T65.894 | — | — |
| medicinal | T49.0X1 | T49.0X2 | T49.0X3 | T49.0X4 | T49.0X5 | T49.0X6 |
| soap | T55.0X1 | T55.0X2 | T55.0X3 | T55.0X4 | — | — |
| percarbonate — *see* Sodium, perborate | | | | | | |
| pertechnetate Tc99m | T50.8X1 | T50.8X2 | T50.8X3 | T50.8X4 | T50.8X5 | T50.8X6 |
| phosphate | | | | | | |
| cellulose | T45.8X1 | T45.8X2 | T45.8X3 | T45.8X4 | T45.8X5 | T45.8X6 |
| dibasic | T47.2X1 | T47.2X2 | T47.2X3 | T47.2X4 | T47.2X5 | T47.2X6 |
| monobasic | T47.2X1 | T47.2X2 | T47.2X3 | T47.2X4 | T47.2X5 | T47.2X6 |
| phytate | T50.6X1 | T50.6X2 | T50.6X3 | T50.6X4 | T50.6X5 | T50.6X6 |
| picosulfate | T47.2X1 | T47.2X2 | T47.2X3 | T47.2X4 | T47.2X5 | T47.2X6 |
| polyhydroxyaluminium monocarbonate | T47.1X1 | T47.1X2 | T47.1X3 | T47.1X4 | T47.1X5 | T47.1X6 |
| polystyrene sulfonate | T50.3X1 | T50.3X2 | T50.3X3 | T50.3X4 | T50.3X5 | T50.3X6 |
| propionate | T49.0X1 | T49.0X2 | T49.0X3 | T49.0X4 | T49.0X5 | T49.0X6 |
| propyl hydroxybenzoate | T50.991 | T50.992 | T50.993 | T50.994 | T50.995 | T50.996 |
| psylliate | T46.8X1 | T46.8X2 | T46.8X3 | T46.8X4 | T46.8X5 | T46.8X6 |
| removing resins | T50.3X1 | T50.3X2 | T50.3X3 | T50.3X4 | T50.3X5 | T50.3X6 |
| salicylate | T39.091 | T39.092 | T39.093 | T39.094 | T39.095 | T39.096 |
| salt NEC | T50.3X1 | T50.3X2 | T50.3X3 | T50.3X4 | T50.3X5 | T50.3X6 |
| selenate | T60.2X1 | T60.2X2 | T60.2X3 | T60.2X4 | — | — |
| stibogluconate | T37.3X1 | T37.3X2 | T37.3X3 | T37.3X4 | T37.3X5 | T37.3X6 |
| sulfate | T47.4X1 | T47.4X2 | T47.4X3 | T47.4X4 | T47.4X5 | T47.4X6 |
| sulfoxone | T37.1X1 | T37.1X2 | T37.1X3 | T37.1X4 | T37.1X5 | T37.1X6 |
| tetradecyl sulfate | T46.8X1 | T46.8X2 | T46.8X3 | T46.8X4 | T46.8X5 | T46.8X6 |
| thiopental | T41.1X1 | T41.1X2 | T41.1X3 | T41.1X4 | T41.1X5 | T41.1X6 |
| thiosalicylate | T39.091 | T39.092 | T39.093 | T39.094 | T39.095 | T39.096 |
| thiosulfate | T50.6X1 | T50.6X2 | T50.6X3 | T50.6X4 | T50.6X5 | T50.6X6 |
| tolbutamide | T38.3X1 | T38.3X2 | T38.3X3 | T38.3X4 | T38.3X5 | T38.3X6 |
| (L)-triiodothyronine | T38.1X1 | T38.1X2 | T38.1X3 | T38.1X4 | T38.1X5 | T38.1X6 |
| tyropanoate | T50.8X1 | T50.8X2 | T50.8X3 | T50.8X4 | T50.8X5 | T50.8X6 |
| valproate | T42.6X1 | T42.6X2 | T42.6X3 | T42.6X4 | T42.6X5 | T42.6X6 |
| versenate | T50.6X1 | T50.6X2 | T50.6X3 | T50.6X4 | T50.6X5 | T50.6X6 |
| **Sodium-free salt** | T50.901 | T50.902 | T50.903 | T50.904 | T50.905 | T50.906 |
| **Sodium-removing resin** | T50.3X1 | T50.3X2 | T50.3X3 | T50.3X4 | T50.3X5 | T50.3X6 |
| **Soft soap** | T55.0X1 | T55.0X2 | T55.0X3 | T55.0X4 | — | — |
| **Solanine** | T62.2X1 | T62.2X2 | T62.2X3 | T62.2X4 | — | — |
| berries | T62.1X1 | T62.1X2 | T62.1X3 | T62.1X4 | — | — |
| **Solanum dulcamara** | T62.2X1 | T62.2X2 | T62.2X3 | T62.2X4 | — | — |
| berries | T62.1X1 | T62.1X2 | T62.1X3 | T62.1X4 | — | — |
| **Solapsone** | T37.1X1 | T37.1X2 | T37.1X3 | T37.1X4 | T37.1X5 | T37.1X6 |
| **Solar lotion** | T49.3X1 | T49.3X2 | T49.3X3 | T49.3X4 | T49.3X5 | T49.3X6 |
| **Solasulfone** | T37.1X1 | T37.1X2 | T37.1X3 | T37.1X4 | T37.1X5 | T37.1X6 |
| **Soldering fluid** | T65.891 | T65.892 | T65.893 | T65.894 | — | — |
| **Solid substance** | T65.91 | T65.92 | T65.93 | T65.94 | — | — |
| specified NEC | T65.891 | T65.892 | T65.893 | T65.894 | — | — |
| **Solvent, industrial NEC** | T52.91 | T52.92 | T52.93 | T52.94 | — | — |
| naphtha | T52.0X1 | T52.0X2 | T52.0X3 | T52.0X4 | — | — |
| petroleum | T52.0X1 | T52.0X2 | T52.0X3 | T52.0X4 | — | — |
| specified NEC | T52.8X1 | T52.8X2 | T52.8X3 | T52.8X4 | — | — |
| **Soma** | T42.8X1 | T42.8X2 | T42.8X3 | T42.8X4 | T42.8X5 | T42.8X6 |
| **Somatorelin** | T38.891 | T38.892 | T38.893 | T38.894 | T38.895 | T38.896 |
| **Somatostatin** | T38.991 | T38.992 | T38.993 | T38.994 | T38.995 | T38.996 |
| **Somatotropin** | T38.811 | T38.812 | T38.813 | T38.814 | T38.815 | T38.816 |
| **Somatrem** | T38.811 | T38.812 | T38.813 | T38.814 | T38.815 | T38.816 |
| **Somatropin** | T38.811 | T38.812 | T38.813 | T38.814 | T38.815 | T38.816 |
| **Sominex** | T45.0X1 | T45.0X2 | T45.0X3 | T45.0X4 | T45.0X5 | T45.0X6 |
| **Somnos** | T42.6X1 | T42.6X2 | T42.6X3 | T42.6X4 | T42.6X5 | T42.6X6 |
| **Somonal** | T42.3X1 | T42.3X2 | T42.3X3 | T42.3X4 | T42.3X5 | T42.3X6 |
| **Soneryl** | T42.3X1 | T42.3X2 | T42.3X3 | T42.3X4 | T42.3X5 | T42.3X6 |
| **Soothing syrup** | T50.901 | T50.902 | T50.903 | T50.904 | T50.905 | T50.906 |
| **Sopor** | T42.6X1 | T42.6X2 | T42.6X3 | T42.6X4 | T42.6X5 | T42.6X6 |
| **Soporific** | T42.71 | T42.72 | T42.73 | T42.74 | T42.75 | T42.76 |
| **Soporific drug** | T42.71 | T42.72 | T42.73 | T42.74 | T42.75 | T42.76 |
| specified type NEC | T42.6X1 | T42.6X2 | T42.6X3 | T42.6X4 | T42.6X5 | T42.6X6 |
| **Sorbide nitrate** | T46.3X1 | T46.3X2 | T46.3X3 | T46.3X4 | T46.3X5 | T46.3X6 |
| **Sorbitol** | T47.4X1 | T47.4X2 | T47.4X3 | T47.4X4 | T47.4X5 | T47.4X6 |
| **Sotalol** | T44.7X1 | T44.7X2 | T44.7X3 | T44.7X4 | T44.7X5 | T44.7X6 |

Table of Drugs and Chemicals

Sotradecol — Sulfanilylguanidine

| Substance | Poisoning, Accidental (unintentional) | Poisoning, Intentional Self-harm | Poisoning, Assault | Poisoning, Undetermined | Adverse Effect | Under-dosing |
|---|---|---|---|---|---|---|
| Sotradecol | T46.8X1 | T46.8X2 | T46.8X3 | T46.8X4 | T46.8X5 | T46.8X6 |
| Soysterol | T46.6X1 | T46.6X2 | T46.6X3 | T46.6X4 | T46.6X5 | T46.6X6 |
| Spacoline | T44.3X1 | T44.3X2 | T44.3X3 | T44.3X4 | T44.3X5 | T44.3X6 |
| Spanish fly | T49.8X1 | T49.8X2 | T49.8X3 | T49.8X4 | T49.8X5 | T49.8X6 |
| Sparine | T43.3X1 | T43.3X2 | T43.3X3 | T43.3X4 | T43.3X5 | T43.3X6 |
| Sparteine | T48.0X1 | T48.0X2 | T48.0X3 | T48.0X4 | T48.0X5 | T48.0X6 |
| Spasmolytic | | | | | | |
|   anticholinergics | T44.3X1 | T44.3X2 | T44.3X3 | T44.3X4 | T44.3X5 | T44.3X6 |
|   autonomic | T44.3X1 | T44.3X2 | T44.3X3 | T44.3X4 | T44.3X5 | T44.3X6 |
|   bronchial NEC | T48.6X1 | T48.6X2 | T48.6X3 | T48.6X4 | T48.6X5 | T48.6X6 |
|   quaternary ammonium | T44.3X1 | T44.3X2 | T44.3X3 | T44.3X4 | T44.3X5 | T44.3X6 |
|   skeletal muscle NEC | T48.1X1 | T48.1X2 | T48.1X3 | T48.1X4 | T48.1X5 | T48.1X6 |
| Spectinomycin | T36.5X1 | T36.5X2 | T36.5X3 | T36.5X4 | T36.5X5 | T36.5X6 |
| Speed | T43.621 | T43.622 | T43.623 | T43.624 | T43.625 | T43.626 |
| Spermicide | T49.8X1 | T49.8X2 | T49.8X3 | T49.8X4 | T49.8X5 | T49.8X6 |
| Spider (bite) (venom) | T63.391 | T63.392 | T63.393 | T63.394 | — | — |
|   antivenin | T50.Z11 | T50.Z12 | T50.Z13 | T50.Z14 | T50.Z15 | T50.Z16 |
| Spigelia (root) | T37.4X1 | T37.4X2 | T37.4X3 | T37.4X4 | T37.4X5 | T37.4X6 |
| Spindle inactivator | T50.4X1 | T50.4X2 | T50.4X3 | T50.4X4 | T50.4X5 | T50.4X6 |
| Spiperone | T43.4X1 | T43.4X2 | T43.4X3 | T43.4X4 | T43.4X5 | T43.4X6 |
| Spiramycin | T36.3X1 | T36.3X2 | T36.3X3 | T36.3X4 | T36.3X5 | T36.3X6 |
| Spirapril | T46.4X1 | T46.4X2 | T46.4X3 | T46.4X4 | T46.4X5 | T46.4X6 |
| Spirilene | T43.591 | T43.592 | T43.593 | T43.594 | T43.595 | T43.596 |
| Spirit(s) (neutral) NEC | T51.0X1 | T51.0X2 | T51.0X3 | T51.0X4 | — | — |
|   beverage | T51.0X1 | T51.0X2 | T51.0X3 | T51.0X4 | — | — |
|   industrial | T51.0X1 | T51.0X2 | T51.0X3 | T51.0X4 | — | — |
|   mineral | T52.0X1 | T52.0X2 | T52.0X3 | T52.0X4 | — | — |
|   of salt — see Hydrochloric acid | | | | | | |
|   surgical | T51.0X1 | T51.0X2 | T51.0X3 | T51.0X4 | — | — |
| Spironolactone | T50.0X1 | T50.0X2 | T50.0X3 | T50.0X4 | T50.0X5 | T50.0X6 |
| Spiroperidol | T43.4X1 | T43.4X2 | T43.4X3 | T43.4X4 | T43.4X5 | T43.4X6 |
| Sponge, absorbable | T45.7X1 | T45.7X2 | T45.7X3 | T45.7X4 | T45.7X5 | T45.7X6 |
|   (gelatin) | | | | | | |
| Sporostacin | T49.0X1 | T49.0X2 | T49.0X3 | T49.0X4 | T49.0X5 | T49.0X6 |
| Spray (aerosol) | T65.91 | T65.92 | T65.93 | T65.94 | — | — |
|   cosmetic | T65.891 | T65.892 | T65.893 | T65.894 | — | — |
|   medicinal NEC | T50.901 | T50.902 | T50.903 | T50.904 | T50.905 | T50.906 |
|   pesticides — see Pesticides | | | | | | |
|   specified content — see specific | | | | | | |
|     substance | | | | | | |
| Spurge flax | T62.2X1 | T62.2X2 | T62.2X3 | T62.2X4 | — | — |
| Spurges | T62.2X1 | T62.2X2 | T62.2X3 | T62.2X4 | — | — |
| Sputum viscosity-lowering | T48.4X1 | T48.4X2 | T48.4X3 | T48.4X4 | T48.4X5 | T48.4X6 |
|   drug | | | | | | |
| Squill | T46.0X1 | T46.0X2 | T46.0X3 | T46.0X4 | T46.0X5 | T46.0X6 |
|   rat poison | T60.4X1 | T60.4X2 | T60.4X3 | T60.4X4 | — | — |
| Squirting cucumber | T47.2X1 | T47.2X2 | T47.2X3 | T47.2X4 | T47.2X5 | T47.2X6 |
|   (cathartic) | | | | | | |
| Stains | T65.6X1 | T65.6X2 | T65.6X3 | T65.6X4 | — | — |
| Stannous fluoride | T49.7X1 | T49.7X2 | T49.7X3 | T49.7X4 | T49.7X5 | T49.7X6 |
| Stanolone | T38.7X1 | T38.7X2 | T38.7X3 | T38.7X4 | T38.7X5 | T38.7X6 |
| Stanozolol | T38.7X1 | T38.7X2 | T38.7X3 | T38.7X4 | T38.7X5 | T38.7X6 |
| Staphisagria or stavesacre | T49.0X1 | T49.0X2 | T49.0X3 | T49.0X4 | T49.0X5 | T49.0X6 |
|   (pediculicide) | | | | | | |
| Starch | T50.901 | T50.902 | T50.903 | T50.904 | T50.905 | T50.906 |
| Stelazine | T43.3X1 | T43.3X2 | T43.3X3 | T43.3X4 | T43.3X5 | T43.3X6 |
| Stemetil | T43.3X1 | T43.3X2 | T43.3X3 | T43.3X4 | T43.3X5 | T43.3X6 |
| Stepronin | T48.4X1 | T48.4X2 | T48.4X3 | T48.4X4 | T48.4X5 | T48.4X6 |
| Sterculia | T47.4X1 | T47.4X2 | T47.4X3 | T47.4X4 | T47.4X5 | T47.4X6 |
| Sternutator gas | T59.891 | T59.892 | T59.893 | T59.894 | — | — |
| Steroid | T38.0X1 | T38.0X2 | T38.0X3 | T38.0X4 | T38.0X5 | T38.0X6 |
|   anabolic | T38.7X1 | T38.7X2 | T38.7X3 | T38.7X4 | T38.7X5 | T38.7X6 |
|   androgenic | T38.7X1 | T38.7X2 | T38.7X3 | T38.7X4 | T38.7X5 | T38.7X6 |
|   antineoplastic, hormone | T38.7X1 | T38.7X2 | T38.7X3 | T38.7X4 | T38.7X5 | T38.7X6 |
|   estrogen | T38.5X1 | T38.5X2 | T38.5X3 | T38.5X4 | T38.5X5 | T38.5X6 |
|   ENT agent | T49.6X1 | T49.6X2 | T49.6X3 | T49.6X4 | T49.6X5 | T49.6X6 |
|   ophthalmic preparation | T49.5X1 | T49.5X2 | T49.5X3 | T49.5X4 | T49.5X5 | T49.5X6 |
|   topical NEC | T49.0X1 | T49.0X2 | T49.0X3 | T49.0X4 | T49.0X5 | T49.0X6 |
| Stibine | T56.891 | T56.892 | T56.893 | T56.894 | — | — |
| Stibogluconate | T37.3X1 | T37.3X2 | T37.3X3 | T37.3X4 | T37.3X5 | T37.3X6 |
| Stibophen | T37.4X1 | T37.4X2 | T37.4X3 | T37.4X4 | T37.4X5 | T37.4X6 |
| Stilbamidine (isetionate) | T37.3X1 | T37.3X2 | T37.3X3 | T37.3X4 | T37.3X5 | T37.3X6 |
| Stilbestrol | T38.5X1 | T38.5X2 | T38.5X3 | T38.5X4 | T38.5X5 | T38.5X6 |
| Stilboestrol | T38.5X1 | T38.5X2 | T38.5X3 | T38.5X4 | T38.5X5 | T38.5X6 |
| Stimulant | | | | | | |
|   central nervous system — see | T43.601 | T43.602 | T43.603 | T43.604 | T43.605 | T43.606 |
|     also Psychostimulant | | | | | | |
|   analeptics | T50.7X1 | T50.7X2 | T50.7X3 | T50.7X4 | T50.7X5 | T50.7X6 |
|   opiate antagonist | T50.7X1 | T50.7X2 | T50.7X3 | T50.7X4 | T50.7X5 | T50.7X6 |
|   psychotherapeutic NEC — see | T43.601 | T43.602 | T43.603 | T43.604 | T43.605 | T43.606 |
|     also Psychotherapeutic | | | | | | |
|     drug | | | | | | |
|   specified NEC | T43.691 | T43.692 | T43.693 | T43.694 | T43.695 | T43.696 |

| Substance | Poisoning, Accidental (unintentional) | Poisoning, Intentional Self-harm | Poisoning, Assault | Poisoning, Undetermined | Adverse Effect | Under-dosing |
|---|---|---|---|---|---|---|
| Stimulant — continued | | | | | | |
|   respiratory | T48.901 | T48.902 | T48.903 | T48.904 | T48.905 | T48.906 |
| Stone-dissolving drug | T50.901 | T50.902 | T50.903 | T50.904 | T50.905 | T50.906 |
| Storage battery (cells) (acid) | T54.2X1 | T54.2X2 | T54.2X3 | T54.2X4 | — | — |
| Stovaine | T41.3X1 | T41.3X2 | T41.3X3 | T41.3X4 | T41.3X5 | T41.3X6 |
|   infiltration (subcutaneous) | T41.3X1 | T41.3X2 | T41.3X3 | T41.3X4 | T41.3X5 | T41.3X6 |
|   nerve block (peripheral) | T41.3X1 | T41.3X2 | T41.3X3 | T41.3X4 | T41.3X5 | T41.3X6 |
|     (plexus) | | | | | | |
|   spinal | T41.3X1 | T41.3X2 | T41.3X3 | T41.3X4 | T41.3X5 | T41.3X6 |
|   topical (surface) | T41.3X1 | T41.3X2 | T41.3X3 | T41.3X4 | T41.3X5 | T41.3X6 |
| Stovarsal | T37.8X1 | T37.8X2 | T37.8X3 | T37.8X4 | T37.8X5 | T37.8X6 |
| Stove gas — see Gas, stove | | | | | | |
| Stoxil | T49.5X1 | T49.5X2 | T49.5X3 | T49.5X4 | T49.5X5 | T49.5X6 |
| Stramonium | T48.6X1 | T48.6X2 | T48.6X3 | T48.6X4 | T48.6X5 | T48.6X6 |
|   natural state | T62.2X1 | T62.2X2 | T62.2X3 | T62.2X4 | — | — |
| Streptodornase | T45.3X1 | T45.3X2 | T45.3X3 | T45.3X4 | T45.3X5 | T45.3X6 |
| Streptoduocin | T36.5X1 | T36.5X2 | T36.5X3 | T36.5X4 | T36.5X5 | T36.5X6 |
| Streptokinase | T45.611 | T45.612 | T45.613 | T45.614 | T45.615 | T45.616 |
| Streptomycin (derivative) | T36.5X1 | T36.5X2 | T36.5X3 | T36.5X4 | T36.5X5 | T36.5X6 |
| Streptonivicin | T36.5X1 | T36.5X2 | T36.5X3 | T36.5X4 | T36.5X5 | T36.5X6 |
| Streptovarycin | T36.5X1 | T36.5X2 | T36.5X3 | T36.5X4 | T36.5X5 | T36.5X6 |
| Streptozocin | T45.1X1 | T45.1X2 | T45.1X3 | T45.1X4 | T45.1X5 | T45.1X6 |
| Streptozotocin | T45.1X1 | T45.1X2 | T45.1X3 | T45.1X4 | T45.1X5 | T45.1X6 |
| Stripper (paint) (solvent) | T52.8X1 | T52.8X2 | T52.8X3 | T52.8X4 | — | — |
| Strobane | T60.1X1 | T60.1X2 | T60.1X3 | T60.1X4 | — | — |
| Strofantina | T46.0X1 | T46.0X2 | T46.0X3 | T46.0X4 | T46.0X5 | T46.0X6 |
| Strophanthin (g) (k) | T46.0X1 | T46.0X2 | T46.0X3 | T46.0X4 | T46.0X5 | T46.0X6 |
| Strophanthus | T46.0X1 | T46.0X2 | T46.0X3 | T46.0X4 | T46.0X5 | T46.0X6 |
| Strophantin | T46.0X1 | T46.0X2 | T46.0X3 | T46.0X4 | T46.0X5 | T46.0X6 |
| Strophantin-g | T46.0X1 | T46.0X2 | T46.0X3 | T46.0X4 | T46.0X5 | T46.0X6 |
| Strychnine (nonmedicinal) | T65.1X1 | T65.1X2 | T65.1X3 | T65.1X4 | — | — |
|   (pesticide) (salts) | | | | | | |
|   medicinal | T48.291 | T48.292 | T48.293 | T48.294 | T48.295 | T48.296 |
| Strychnos (ignatii) — see | | | | | | |
|   Strychnine | | | | | | |
| Styramate | T42.8X1 | T42.8X2 | T42.8X3 | T42.8X4 | T42.8X5 | T42.8X6 |
| Styrene | T65.891 | T65.892 | T65.893 | T65.894 | — | — |
| Succinimide, antiepileptic or | T42.2X1 | T42.2X2 | T42.2X3 | T42.2X4 | T42.2X5 | T42.2X6 |
|   anticonvulsant | | | | | | |
|   mercuric — see Mercury | | | | | | |
| Succinylcholine | T48.1X1 | T48.1X2 | T48.1X3 | T48.1X4 | T48.1X5 | T48.1X6 |
| Succinylsulfathiazole | T37.0X1 | T37.0X2 | T37.0X3 | T37.0X4 | T37.0X5 | T37.0X6 |
| Sucralfate | T47.1X1 | T47.1X2 | T47.1X3 | T47.1X4 | T47.1X5 | T47.1X6 |
| Sucrose | T50.3X1 | T50.3X2 | T50.3X3 | T50.3X4 | T50.3X5 | T50.3X6 |
| Sufentanil | T40.4X1 | T40.4X2 | T40.4X3 | T40.4X4 | T40.4X5 | T40.4X6 |
| Sulbactam | T36.0X1 | T36.0X2 | T36.0X3 | T36.0X4 | T36.0X5 | T36.0X6 |
| Sulbenicillin | T36.0X1 | T36.0X2 | T36.0X3 | T36.0X4 | T36.0X5 | T36.0X6 |
| Sulbentine | T49.0X1 | T49.0X2 | T49.0X3 | T49.0X4 | T49.0X5 | T49.0X6 |
| Sulfacetamide | T49.0X1 | T49.0X2 | T49.0X3 | T49.0X4 | T49.0X5 | T49.0X6 |
|   ophthalmic preparation | T49.5X1 | T49.5X2 | T49.5X3 | T49.5X4 | T49.5X5 | T49.5X6 |
| Sulfachlorpyridazine | T37.0X1 | T37.0X2 | T37.0X3 | T37.0X4 | T37.0X5 | T37.0X6 |
| Sulfacitine | T37.0X1 | T37.0X2 | T37.0X3 | T37.0X4 | T37.0X5 | T37.0X6 |
| Sulfadiasulfone sodium | T37.0X1 | T37.0X2 | T37.0X3 | T37.0X4 | T37.0X5 | T37.0X6 |
| Sulfadiazine | T37.0X1 | T37.0X2 | T37.0X3 | T37.0X4 | T37.0X5 | T37.0X6 |
|   silver (topical) | T49.0X1 | T49.0X2 | T49.0X3 | T49.0X4 | T49.0X5 | T49.0X6 |
| Sulfadimethoxine | T37.0X1 | T37.0X2 | T37.0X3 | T37.0X4 | T37.0X5 | T37.0X6 |
| Sulfadimidine | T37.0X1 | T37.0X2 | T37.0X3 | T37.0X4 | T37.0X5 | T37.0X6 |
| Sulfadoxine | T37.0X1 | T37.0X2 | T37.0X3 | T37.0X4 | T37.0X5 | T37.0X6 |
|   with pyrimethamine | T37.2X1 | T37.2X2 | T37.2X3 | T37.2X4 | T37.2X5 | T37.2X6 |
| Sulfaethidole | T37.0X1 | T37.0X2 | T37.0X3 | T37.0X4 | T37.0X5 | T37.0X6 |
| Sulfafurazole | T37.0X1 | T37.0X2 | T37.0X3 | T37.0X4 | T37.0X5 | T37.0X6 |
| Sulfaguanidine | T37.0X1 | T37.0X2 | T37.0X3 | T37.0X4 | T37.0X5 | T37.0X6 |
| Sulfalene | T37.0X1 | T37.0X2 | T37.0X3 | T37.0X4 | T37.0X5 | T37.0X6 |
| Sulfaloxate | T37.0X1 | T37.0X2 | T37.0X3 | T37.0X4 | T37.0X5 | T37.0X6 |
| Sulfaloxic acid | T37.0X1 | T37.0X2 | T37.0X3 | T37.0X4 | T37.0X5 | T37.0X6 |
| Sulfamazone | T39.2X1 | T39.2X2 | T39.2X3 | T39.2X4 | T39.2X5 | T39.2X6 |
| Sulfamerazine | T37.0X1 | T37.0X2 | T37.0X3 | T37.0X4 | T37.0X5 | T37.0X6 |
| Sulfameter | T37.0X1 | T37.0X2 | T37.0X3 | T37.0X4 | T37.0X5 | T37.0X6 |
| Sulfamethazine | T37.0X1 | T37.0X2 | T37.0X3 | T37.0X4 | T37.0X5 | T37.0X6 |
| Sulfamethizole | T37.0X1 | T37.0X2 | T37.0X3 | T37.0X4 | T37.0X5 | T37.0X6 |
| Sulfamethoxazole | T37.0X1 | T37.0X2 | T37.0X3 | T37.0X4 | T37.0X5 | T37.0X6 |
|   with trimethoprim | T36.8X1 | T36.8X2 | T36.8X3 | T36.8X4 | T36.8X5 | T36.8X6 |
| Sulfamethoxydiazine | T37.0X1 | T37.0X2 | T37.0X3 | T37.0X4 | T37.0X5 | T37.0X6 |
| Sulfamethoxypyridazine | T37.0X1 | T37.0X2 | T37.0X3 | T37.0X4 | T37.0X5 | T37.0X6 |
| Sulfamethylthiazole | T37.0X1 | T37.0X2 | T37.0X3 | T37.0X4 | T37.0X5 | T37.0X6 |
| Sulfametoxydiazine | T37.0X1 | T37.0X2 | T37.0X3 | T37.0X4 | T37.0X5 | T37.0X6 |
| Sulfamidopyrine | T39.2X1 | T39.2X2 | T39.2X3 | T39.2X4 | T39.2X5 | T39.2X6 |
| Sulfamonomethoxine | T37.0X1 | T37.0X2 | T37.0X3 | T37.0X4 | T37.0X5 | T37.0X6 |
| Sulfamoxole | T37.0X1 | T37.0X2 | T37.0X3 | T37.0X4 | T37.0X5 | T37.0X6 |
| Sulfamylon | T49.0X1 | T49.0X2 | T49.0X3 | T49.0X4 | T49.0X5 | T49.0X6 |
| Sulfan blue (diagnostic dye) | T50.8X1 | T50.8X2 | T50.8X3 | T50.8X4 | T50.8X5 | T50.8X6 |
| Sulfanilamide | T37.0X1 | T37.0X2 | T37.0X3 | T37.0X4 | T37.0X5 | T37.0X6 |
| Sulfanilylguanidine | T37.0X1 | T37.0X2 | T37.0X3 | T37.0X4 | T37.0X5 | T37.0X6 |

**Additional Character May Be Required — Refer to the Tabular List for Character Selection** ▽ Subterms under main terms may continue to next column or page

| Substance | Poisoning, Accidental (unintentional) | Poisoning, Intentional Self-harm | Poisoning, Assault | Poisoning, Undetermined | Adverse Effect | Under-dosing |
|---|---|---|---|---|---|---|
| Sulfaperin | T37.0X1 | T37.0X2 | T37.0X3 | T37.0X4 | T37.0X5 | T37.0X6 |
| Sulfaphenazole | T37.0X1 | T37.0X2 | T37.0X3 | T37.0X4 | T37.0X5 | T37.0X6 |
| Sulfaphenylthiazole | T37.0X1 | T37.0X2 | T37.0X3 | T37.0X4 | T37.0X5 | T37.0X6 |
| Sulfaproxyline | T37.0X1 | T37.0X2 | T37.0X3 | T37.0X4 | T37.0X5 | T37.0X6 |
| Sulfapyridine | T37.0X1 | T37.0X2 | T37.0X3 | T37.0X4 | T37.0X5 | T37.0X6 |
| Sulfapyrimidine | T37.0X1 | T37.0X2 | T37.0X3 | T37.0X4 | T37.0X5 | T37.0X6 |
| Sulfarsphenamine | T37.8X1 | T37.8X2 | T37.8X3 | T37.8X4 | T37.8X5 | T37.8X6 |
| Sulfasalazine | T37.0X1 | T37.0X2 | T37.0X3 | T37.0X4 | T37.0X5 | T37.0X6 |
| Sulfasuxidine | T37.0X1 | T37.0X2 | T37.0X3 | T37.0X4 | T37.0X5 | T37.0X6 |
| Sulfasymazine | T37.0X1 | T37.0X2 | T37.0X3 | T37.0X4 | T37.0X5 | T37.0X6 |
| Sulfated amylopectin | T47.8X1 | T47.8X2 | T47.8X3 | T47.8X4 | T47.8X5 | T47.8X6 |
| Sulfathiazole | T37.0X1 | T37.0X2 | T37.0X3 | T37.0X4 | T37.0X5 | T37.0X6 |
| Sulfatostearate | T49.2X1 | T49.2X2 | T49.2X3 | T49.2X4 | T49.2X5 | T49.2X6 |
| Sulfinpyrazone | T50.4X1 | T50.4X2 | T50.4X3 | T50.4X4 | T50.4X5 | T50.4X6 |
| Sulfiram | T49.0X1 | T49.0X2 | T49.0X3 | T49.0X4 | T49.0X5 | T49.0X6 |
| Sulfisomidine | T37.0X1 | T37.0X2 | T37.0X3 | T37.0X4 | T37.0X5 | T37.0X6 |
| Sulfisoxazole | T37.0X1 | T37.0X2 | T37.0X3 | T37.0X4 | T37.0X5 | T37.0X6 |
|   ophthalmic preparation | T49.5X1 | T49.5X2 | T49.5X3 | T49.5X4 | T49.5X5 | T49.5X6 |
| Sulfobromophthalein (sodium) | T50.8X1 | T50.8X2 | T50.8X3 | T50.8X4 | T50.8X5 | T50.8X6 |
| Sulfobromphthalein | T50.8X1 | T50.8X2 | T50.8X3 | T50.8X4 | T50.8X5 | T50.8X6 |
| Sulfogaiacol | T48.4X1 | T48.4X2 | T48.4X3 | T48.4X4 | T48.4X5 | T48.4X6 |
| Sulfomyxin | T36.8X1 | T36.8X2 | T36.8X3 | T36.8X4 | T36.8X5 | T36.8X6 |
| Sulfonal | T42.6X1 | T42.6X2 | T42.6X3 | T42.6X4 | T42.6X5 | T42.6X6 |
| Sulfonamide NEC | T37.0X1 | T37.0X2 | T37.0X3 | T37.0X4 | T37.0X5 | T37.0X6 |
|   eye | T49.5X1 | T49.5X2 | T49.5X3 | T49.5X4 | T49.5X5 | T49.5X6 |
| Sulfonazide | T37.1X1 | T37.1X2 | T37.1X3 | T37.1X4 | T37.1X5 | T37.1X6 |
| Sulfones | T37.1X1 | T37.1X2 | T37.1X3 | T37.1X4 | T37.1X5 | T37.1X6 |
| Sulfonethylmethane | T42.6X1 | T42.6X2 | T42.6X3 | T42.6X4 | T42.6X5 | T42.6X6 |
| Sulfonmethane | T42.6X1 | T42.6X2 | T42.6X3 | T42.6X4 | T42.6X5 | T42.6X6 |
| Sulfonphthal, sulfonphthol | T50.8X1 | T50.8X2 | T50.8X3 | T50.8X4 | T50.8X5 | T50.8X6 |
| Sulfonylurea derivatives, oral | T38.3X1 | T38.3X2 | T38.3X3 | T38.3X4 | T38.3X5 | T38.3X6 |
| Sulforidazine | T43.3X1 | T43.3X2 | T43.3X3 | T43.3X4 | T43.3X5 | T43.3X6 |
| Sulfoxone | T37.1X1 | T37.1X2 | T37.1X3 | T37.1X4 | T37.1X5 | T37.1X6 |
| Sulfuric acid | T54.2X1 | T54.2X2 | T54.2X3 | T54.2X4 | — | — |
| Sulfur, sulfurated, sulfuric, sulfurous, sulfuryl (compounds NEC) (medicinal) | T49.4X1 | T49.4X2 | T49.4X3 | T49.4X4 | T49.4X5 | T49.4X6 |
|   acid | T54.2X1 | T54.2X2 | T54.2X3 | T54.2X4 | — | — |
|   dioxide (gas) | T59.1X1 | T59.1X2 | T59.1X3 | T59.1X4 | — | — |
|   ether — see Ether(s) | | | | | | |
|   hydrogen | T59.6X1 | T59.6X2 | T59.6X3 | T59.6X4 | — | — |
|   medicinal (keratolytic) (ointment) NEC | T49.4X1 | T49.4X2 | T49.4X3 | T49.4X4 | T49.4X5 | T49.4X6 |
|   ointment | T49.0X1 | T49.0X2 | T49.0X3 | T49.0X4 | T49.0X5 | T49.0X6 |
|   pesticide (vapor) | T60.91 | T60.92 | T60.93 | T60.94 | — | — |
|   vapor NEC | T59.891 | T59.892 | T59.893 | T59.894 | — | — |
| Sulglicotide | T47.1X1 | T47.1X2 | T47.1X3 | T47.1X4 | T47.1X5 | T47.1X6 |
| Sulindac | T39.391 | T39.392 | T39.393 | T39.394 | T39.395 | T39.396 |
| Sulisatin | T47.2X1 | T47.2X2 | T47.2X3 | T47.2X4 | T47.2X5 | T47.2X6 |
| Sulisobenzone | T49.3X1 | T49.3X2 | T49.3X3 | T49.3X4 | T49.3X5 | T49.3X6 |
| Sulkowitch's reagent | T50.8X1 | T50.8X2 | T50.8X3 | T50.8X4 | T50.8X5 | T50.8X6 |
| Sulmetozine | T44.3X1 | T44.3X2 | T44.3X3 | T44.3X4 | T44.3X5 | T44.3X6 |
| Suloctidil | T46.7X1 | T46.7X2 | T46.7X3 | T46.7X4 | T46.7X5 | T46.7X6 |
| Sulph- — see also Sulf- | | | | | | |
| Sulphadiazine | T37.0X1 | T37.0X2 | T37.0X3 | T37.0X4 | T37.0X5 | T37.0X6 |
| Sulphadimethoxine | T37.0X1 | T37.0X2 | T37.0X3 | T37.0X4 | T37.0X5 | T37.0X6 |
| Sulphadimidine | T37.0X1 | T37.0X2 | T37.0X3 | T37.0X4 | T37.0X5 | T37.0X6 |
| Sulphadione | T37.1X1 | T37.1X2 | T37.1X3 | T37.1X4 | T37.1X5 | T37.1X6 |
| Sulphafurazole | T37.0X1 | T37.0X2 | T37.0X3 | T37.0X4 | T37.0X5 | T37.0X6 |
| Sulphamethizole | T37.0X1 | T37.0X2 | T37.0X3 | T37.0X4 | T37.0X5 | T37.0X6 |
| Sulphamethoxazole | T37.0X1 | T37.0X2 | T37.0X3 | T37.0X4 | T37.0X5 | T37.0X6 |
| Sulphan blue | T50.8X1 | T50.8X2 | T50.8X3 | T50.8X4 | T50.8X5 | T50.8X6 |
| Sulphaphenazole | T37.0X1 | T37.0X2 | T37.0X3 | T37.0X4 | T37.0X5 | T37.0X6 |
| Sulphapyridine | T37.0X1 | T37.0X2 | T37.0X3 | T37.0X4 | T37.0X5 | T37.0X6 |
| Sulphasalazine | T37.0X1 | T37.0X2 | T37.0X3 | T37.0X4 | T37.0X5 | T37.0X6 |
| Sulphinpyrazone | T50.4X1 | T50.4X2 | T50.4X3 | T50.4X4 | T50.4X5 | T50.4X6 |
| Sulpiride | T43.591 | T43.592 | T43.593 | T43.594 | T43.595 | T43.596 |
| Sulprostone | T48.0X1 | T48.0X2 | T48.0X3 | T48.0X4 | T48.0X5 | T48.0X6 |
| Sulpyrine | T39.2X1 | T39.2X2 | T39.2X3 | T39.2X4 | T39.2X5 | T39.2X6 |
| Sultamicillin | T36.0X1 | T36.0X2 | T36.0X3 | T36.0X4 | T36.0X5 | T36.0X6 |
| Sulthiame | T42.6X1 | T42.6X2 | T42.6X3 | T42.6X4 | T42.6X5 | T42.6X6 |
| Sultiame | T42.6X1 | T42.6X2 | T42.6X3 | T42.6X4 | T42.6X5 | T42.6X6 |
| Sultopride | T43.591 | T43.592 | T43.593 | T43.594 | T43.595 | T43.596 |
| Sumatriptan | T39.8X1 | T39.8X2 | T39.8X3 | T39.8X4 | T39.8X5 | T39.8X6 |
| Sunflower seed oil | T46.6X1 | T46.6X2 | T46.6X3 | T46.6X4 | T46.6X5 | T46.6X6 |
| Superinone | T48.4X1 | T48.4X2 | T48.4X3 | T48.4X4 | T48.4X5 | T48.4X6 |
| Suprofen | T39.311 | T39.312 | T39.313 | T39.314 | T39.315 | T39.316 |
| Suramin (sodium) | T37.4X1 | T37.4X2 | T37.4X3 | T37.4X4 | T37.4X5 | T37.4X6 |
| Surfacaine | T41.3X1 | T41.3X2 | T41.3X3 | T41.3X4 | T41.3X5 | T41.3X6 |
| Surital | T41.1X1 | T41.1X2 | T41.1X3 | T41.1X4 | T41.1X5 | T41.1X6 |

| Substance | Poisoning, Accidental (unintentional) | Poisoning, Intentional Self-harm | Poisoning, Assault | Poisoning, Undetermined | Adverse Effect | Under-dosing |
|---|---|---|---|---|---|---|
| Sutilains | T45.3X1 | T45.3X2 | T45.3X3 | T45.3X4 | T45.3X5 | T45.3X6 |
| Suxamethonium (chloride) | T48.1X1 | T48.1X2 | T48.1X3 | T48.1X4 | T48.1X5 | T48.1X6 |
| Suxethonium (chloride) | T48.1X1 | T48.1X2 | T48.1X3 | T48.1X4 | T48.1X5 | T48.1X6 |
| Suxibuzone | T39.2X1 | T39.2X2 | T39.2X3 | T39.2X4 | T39.2X5 | T39.2X6 |
| Sweetener | T50.901 | T50.902 | T50.903 | T50.904 | T50.905 | T50.906 |
| Sweet niter spirit | T46.3X1 | T46.3X2 | T46.3X3 | T46.3X4 | T46.3X5 | T46.3X6 |
| Sweet oil (birch) | T49.3X1 | T49.3X2 | T49.3X3 | T49.3X4 | T49.3X5 | T49.3X6 |
| Sym-dichloroethyl ether | T53.6X1 | T53.6X2 | T53.6X3 | T53.6X4 | — | — |
| Sympatholytic NEC | T44.8X1 | T44.8X2 | T44.8X3 | T44.8X4 | T44.8X5 | T44.8X6 |
|   haloalkylamine | T44.8X1 | T44.8X2 | T44.8X3 | T44.8X4 | T44.8X5 | T44.8X6 |
| Sympathomimetic NEC | T44.901 | T44.902 | T44.903 | T44.904 | T44.905 | T44.906 |
|   anti-common-cold | T48.5X1 | T48.5X2 | T48.5X3 | T48.5X4 | T48.5X5 | T48.5X6 |
|   bronchodilator | T48.6X1 | T48.6X2 | T48.6X3 | T48.6X4 | T48.6X5 | T48.6X6 |
|   specified NEC | T44.991 | T44.992 | T44.993 | T44.994 | T44.995 | T44.996 |
| Synagis | T50.B91 | T50.B92 | T50.B93 | T50.B94 | T50.B95 | T50.B96 |
| Synalar | T49.0X1 | T49.0X2 | T49.0X3 | T49.0X4 | T49.0X5 | T49.0X6 |
| Synthroid | T38.1X1 | T38.1X2 | T38.1X3 | T38.1X4 | T38.1X5 | T38.1X6 |
| Syntocinon | T48.0X1 | T48.0X2 | T48.0X3 | T48.0X4 | T48.0X5 | T48.0X6 |
| Syrosingopine | T46.5X1 | T46.5X2 | T46.5X3 | T46.5X4 | T46.5X5 | T46.5X6 |
| Systemic drug | T45.91 | T45.92 | T45.93 | T45.94 | T45.95 | T45.96 |
|   specified NEC | T45.8X1 | T45.8X2 | T45.8X3 | T45.8X4 | T45.8X5 | T45.8X6 |
| Tablets — see also specified substance | T50.901 | T50.902 | T50.903 | T50.904 | T50.905 | T50.906 |
| Tace | T38.5X1 | T38.5X2 | T38.5X3 | T38.5X4 | T38.5X5 | T38.5X6 |
| Tacrine | T44.0X1 | T44.0X2 | T44.0X3 | T44.0X4 | T44.0X5 | T44.0X6 |
| Tadalafil | T46.7X1 | T46.7X2 | T46.7X3 | T46.7X4 | T46.7X5 | T46.7X6 |
| Talampicillin | T36.0X1 | T36.0X2 | T36.0X3 | T36.0X4 | T36.0X5 | T36.0X6 |
| Talbutal | T42.3X1 | T42.3X2 | T42.3X3 | T42.3X4 | T42.3X5 | T42.3X6 |
| Talc powder | T49.3X1 | T49.3X2 | T49.3X3 | T49.3X4 | T49.3X5 | T49.3X6 |
| Talcum | T49.3X1 | T49.3X2 | T49.3X3 | T49.3X4 | T49.3X5 | T49.3X6 |
| Taleranol | T38.6X1 | T38.6X2 | T38.6X3 | T38.6X4 | T38.6X5 | T38.6X6 |
| Tamoxifen | T38.6X1 | T38.6X2 | T38.6X3 | T38.6X4 | T38.6X5 | T38.6X6 |
| Tamsulosin | T44.6X1 | T44.6X2 | T44.6X3 | T44.6X4 | T44.6X5 | T44.6X6 |
| Tandearil, tanderil | T39.2X1 | T39.2X2 | T39.2X3 | T39.2X4 | T39.2X5 | T39.2X6 |
| Tannic acid | T49.2X1 | T49.2X2 | T49.2X3 | T49.2X4 | T49.2X5 | T49.2X6 |
|   medicinal (astringent) | T49.2X1 | T49.2X2 | T49.2X3 | T49.2X4 | T49.2X5 | T49.2X6 |
| Tannin — see Tannic acid | | | | | | |
| Tansy | T62.2X1 | T62.2X2 | T62.2X3 | T62.2X4 | — | — |
| TAO | T36.3X1 | T36.3X2 | T36.3X3 | T36.3X4 | T36.3X5 | T36.3X6 |
| Tapazole | T38.2X1 | T38.2X2 | T38.2X3 | T38.2X4 | T38.2X5 | T38.2X6 |
| Taractan | T43.591 | T43.592 | T43.593 | T43.594 | T43.595 | T43.596 |
| Tarantula (venomous) | T63.321 | T63.322 | T63.323 | T63.324 | — | — |
| Tartar emetic | T37.8X1 | T37.8X2 | T37.8X3 | T37.8X4 | T37.8X5 | T37.8X6 |
| Tartaric acid | T65.891 | T65.892 | T65.893 | T65.894 | — | — |
| Tartrated antimony (anti-infective) | T37.8X1 | T37.8X2 | T37.8X3 | T37.8X4 | T37.8X5 | T37.8X6 |
| Tartrate, laxative | T47.4X1 | T47.4X2 | T47.4X3 | T47.4X4 | T47.4X5 | T47.4X6 |
| Tar NEC | T52.0X1 | T52.0X2 | T52.0X3 | T52.0X4 | — | — |
|   camphor | T60.1X1 | T60.1X2 | T60.1X3 | T60.1X4 | — | — |
|   distillate | T49.1X1 | T49.1X2 | T49.1X3 | T49.1X4 | T49.1X5 | T49.1X6 |
|   fumes | T59.891 | T59.892 | T59.893 | T59.894 | — | — |
|   medicinal | T49.1X1 | T49.1X2 | T49.1X3 | T49.1X4 | T49.1X5 | T49.1X6 |
|   ointment | T49.1X1 | T49.1X2 | T49.1X3 | T49.1X4 | T49.1X5 | T49.1X6 |
| Tauromustine | T45.1X1 | T45.1X2 | T45.1X3 | T45.1X4 | T45.1X5 | T45.1X6 |
| TCA — see Trichloroacetic acid | | | | | | |
| TCDD | T53.7X1 | T53.7X2 | T53.7X3 | T53.7X4 | — | — |
| TDI (vapor) | T65.0X1 | T65.0X2 | T65.0X3 | T65.0X4 | — | — |
| Tear | | | | | | |
|   gas | T59.3X1 | T59.3X2 | T59.3X3 | T59.3X4 | — | — |
|   solution | T49.5X1 | T49.5X2 | T49.5X3 | T49.5X4 | T49.5X5 | T49.5X6 |
| Teclothiazide | T50.2X1 | T50.2X2 | T50.2X3 | T50.2X4 | T50.2X5 | T50.2X6 |
| Teclozan | T37.3X1 | T37.3X2 | T37.3X3 | T37.3X4 | T37.3X5 | T37.3X6 |
| Tegafur | T45.1X1 | T45.1X2 | T45.1X3 | T45.1X4 | T45.1X5 | T45.1X6 |
| Tegretol | T42.1X1 | T42.1X2 | T42.1X3 | T42.1X4 | T42.1X5 | T42.1X6 |
| Teicoplanin | T36.8X1 | T36.8X2 | T36.8X3 | T36.8X4 | T36.8X5 | T36.8X6 |
| Telepaque | T50.8X1 | T50.8X2 | T50.8X3 | T50.8X4 | T50.8X5 | T50.8X6 |
| Tellurium | T56.891 | T56.892 | T56.893 | T56.894 | — | — |
|   fumes | T56.891 | T56.892 | T56.893 | T56.894 | — | — |
| TEM | T45.1X1 | T45.1X2 | T45.1X3 | T45.1X4 | T45.1X5 | T45.1X6 |
| Temazepam | T42.4X1 | T42.4X2 | T42.4X3 | T42.4X4 | T42.4X5 | T42.4X6 |
| Temocillin | T36.0X1 | T36.0X2 | T36.0X3 | T36.0X4 | T36.0X5 | T36.0X6 |
| Tenamfetamine | T43.621 | T43.622 | T43.623 | T43.624 | T43.625 | T43.626 |
| Teniposide | T45.1X1 | T45.1X2 | T45.1X3 | T45.1X4 | T45.1X5 | T45.1X6 |
| Tenitramine | T46.3X1 | T46.3X2 | T46.3X3 | T46.3X4 | T46.3X5 | T46.3X6 |
| Tenoglicin | T48.4X1 | T48.4X2 | T48.4X3 | T48.4X4 | T48.4X5 | T48.4X6 |
| Tenonitrozole | T37.3X1 | T37.3X2 | T37.3X3 | T37.3X4 | T37.3X5 | T37.3X6 |
| Tenoxicam | T39.391 | T39.392 | T39.393 | T39.394 | T39.395 | T39.396 |
| TEPA | T45.1X1 | T45.1X2 | T45.1X3 | T45.1X4 | T45.1X5 | T45.1X6 |
| TEPP | T60.0X1 | T60.0X2 | T60.0X3 | T60.0X4 | — | — |
| Teprotide | T46.5X1 | T46.5X2 | T46.5X3 | T46.5X4 | T46.5X5 | T46.5X6 |
| Terazosin | T44.6X1 | T44.6X2 | T44.6X3 | T44.6X4 | T44.6X5 | T44.6X6 |
| Terbufos | T60.0X1 | T60.0X2 | T60.0X3 | T60.0X4 | — | — |
| Terbutaline | T48.6X1 | T48.6X2 | T48.6X3 | T48.6X4 | T48.6X5 | T48.6X6 |

▽ Subterms under main terms may continue to next column or page    Additional Character May Be Required — Refer to the Tabular List for Character Selection    391

Sulfaperin — Terbutaline

| Substance | Poisoning, Accidental (unintentional) | Poisoning, Intentional Self-harm | Poisoning, Assault | Poisoning, Undetermined | Adverse Effect | Under-dosing |
|---|---|---|---|---|---|---|
| Terconazole | T49.0X1 | T49.0X2 | T49.0X3 | T49.0X4 | T49.0X5 | T49.0X6 |
| Terfenadine | T45.0X1 | T45.0X2 | T45.0X3 | T45.0X4 | T45.0X5 | T45.0X6 |
| Teriparatide (acetate) | T50.991 | T50.992 | T50.993 | T50.994 | T50.995 | T50.996 |
| Terizidone | T37.1X1 | T37.1X2 | T37.1X3 | T37.1X4 | T37.1X5 | T37.1X6 |
| Terlipressin | T38.891 | T38.892 | T38.893 | T38.894 | T38.895 | T38.896 |
| Terodiline | T46.3X1 | T46.3X2 | T46.3X3 | T46.3X4 | T46.3X5 | T46.3X6 |
| Teroxalene | T37.4X1 | T37.4X2 | T37.4X3 | T37.4X4 | T37.4X5 | T37.4X6 |
| Terpin (cis) hydrate | T48.4X1 | T48.4X2 | T48.4X3 | T48.4X4 | T48.4X5 | T48.4X6 |
| Terramycin | T36.4X1 | T36.4X2 | T36.4X3 | T36.4X4 | T36.4X5 | T36.4X6 |
| Tertatolol | T44.7X1 | T44.7X2 | T44.7X3 | T44.7X4 | T44.7X5 | T44.7X6 |
| Tessalon | T48.3X1 | T48.3X2 | T48.3X3 | T48.3X4 | T48.3X5 | T48.3X6 |
| Testolactone | T38.7X1 | T38.7X2 | T38.7X3 | T38.7X4 | T38.7X5 | T38.7X6 |
| Testosterone | T38.7X1 | T38.7X2 | T38.7X3 | T38.7X4 | T38.7X5 | T38.7X6 |
| Tetanus toxoid or vaccine | T50.A91 | T50.A92 | T50.A93 | T50.A94 | T50.A95 | T50.A96 |
| antitoxin | T50.Z11 | T50.Z12 | T50.Z13 | T50.Z14 | T50.Z15 | T50.Z16 |
| immune globulin (human) | T50.Z11 | T50.Z12 | T50.Z13 | T50.Z14 | T50.Z15 | T50.Z16 |
| toxoid | T50.A91 | T50.A92 | T50.A93 | T50.A94 | T50.A95 | T50.A96 |
| with diphtheria toxoid | T50.A21 | T50.A22 | T50.A23 | T50.A24 | T50.A25 | T50.A26 |
| with pertussis | T50.A11 | T50.A12 | T50.A13 | T50.A14 | T50.A15 | T50.A16 |
| Tetrabenazine | T43.591 | T43.592 | T43.593 | T43.594 | T43.595 | T43.596 |
| Tetracaine | T41.3X1 | T41.3X2 | T41.3X3 | T41.3X4 | T41.3X5 | T41.3X6 |
| nerve block (peripheral) (plexus) | T41.3X1 | T41.3X2 | T41.3X3 | T41.3X4 | T41.3X5 | T41.3X6 |
| regional | T41.3X1 | T41.3X2 | T41.3X3 | T41.3X4 | T41.3X5 | T41.3X6 |
| spinal | T41.3X1 | T41.3X2 | T41.3X3 | T41.3X4 | T41.3X5 | T41.3X6 |
| Tetrachlorethylene — see Tetrachloroethylene | | | | | | |
| Tetrachlormethiazide | T50.2X1 | T50.2X2 | T50.2X3 | T50.2X4 | T50.2X5 | T50.2X6 |
| Tetrachloroethane | T53.6X1 | T53.6X2 | T53.6X3 | T53.6X4 | — | — |
| vapor | T53.6X1 | T53.6X2 | T53.6X3 | T53.6X4 | — | — |
| paint or varnish | T53.6X1 | T53.6X2 | T53.6X3 | T53.6X4 | — | — |
| Tetrachloroethylene (liquid) | T53.3X1 | T53.3X2 | T53.3X3 | T53.3X4 | — | — |
| medicinal | T37.4X1 | T37.4X2 | T37.4X3 | T37.4X4 | T37.4X5 | T37.4X6 |
| vapor | T53.3X1 | T53.3X2 | T53.3X3 | T53.3X4 | — | — |
| Tetrachloromethane — see Carbon tetrachloride | | | | | | |
| Tetracosactide | T38.811 | T38.812 | T38.813 | T38.814 | T38.815 | T38.816 |
| Tetracosactrin | T38.811 | T38.812 | T38.813 | T38.814 | T38.815 | T38.816 |
| Tetracycline | T36.4X1 | T36.4X2 | T36.4X3 | T36.4X4 | T36.4X5 | T36.4X6 |
| ophthalmic preparation | T49.5X1 | T49.5X2 | T49.5X3 | T49.5X4 | T49.5X5 | T49.5X6 |
| topical NEC | T49.0X1 | T49.0X2 | T49.0X3 | T49.0X4 | T49.0X5 | T49.0X6 |
| Tetradifon | T60.8X1 | T60.8X2 | T60.8X3 | T60.8X4 | — | — |
| Tetradotoxin | T61.771 | T61.772 | T61.773 | T61.774 | — | — |
| Tetraethyl | | | | | | |
| lead | T56.0X1 | T56.0X2 | T56.0X3 | T56.0X4 | — | — |
| pyrophosphate | T60.0X1 | T60.0X2 | T60.0X3 | T60.0X4 | — | — |
| Tetraethylammonium chloride | T44.2X1 | T44.2X2 | T44.2X3 | T44.2X4 | T44.2X5 | T44.2X6 |
| Tetraethylthiuram disulfide | T50.6X1 | T50.6X2 | T50.6X3 | T50.6X4 | T50.6X5 | T50.6X6 |
| Tetrahydroaminoacridine | T44.0X1 | T44.0X2 | T44.0X3 | T44.0X4 | T44.0X5 | T44.0X6 |
| Tetrahydrocannabinol | T40.7X1 | T40.7X2 | T40.7X3 | T40.7X4 | T40.7X5 | T40.7X6 |
| Tetrahydrofuran | T52.8X1 | T52.8X2 | T52.8X3 | T52.8X4 | — | — |
| Tetrahydronaphthalene | T52.8X1 | T52.8X2 | T52.8X3 | T52.8X4 | — | — |
| Tetrahydrozoline | T49.5X1 | T49.5X2 | T49.5X3 | T49.5X4 | T49.5X5 | T49.5X6 |
| Tetralin | T52.8X1 | T52.8X2 | T52.8X3 | T52.8X4 | — | — |
| Tetramethrin | T60.2X1 | T60.2X2 | T60.2X3 | T60.2X4 | — | — |
| Tetramethylthiuram (disulfide) NEC | T60.3X1 | T60.3X2 | T60.3X3 | T60.3X4 | — | — |
| medicinal | T49.0X1 | T49.0X2 | T49.0X3 | T49.0X4 | T49.0X5 | T49.0X6 |
| Tetramisole | T37.4X1 | T37.4X2 | T37.4X3 | T37.4X4 | T37.4X5 | T37.4X6 |
| Tetranicotinoyl fructose | T46.7X1 | T46.7X2 | T46.7X3 | T46.7X4 | T46.7X5 | T46.7X6 |
| Tetrazepam | T42.4X1 | T42.4X2 | T42.4X3 | T42.4X4 | T42.4X5 | T42.4X6 |
| Tetronal | T42.6X1 | T42.6X2 | T42.6X3 | T42.6X4 | T42.6X5 | T42.6X6 |
| Tetryl | T65.3X1 | T65.3X2 | T65.3X3 | T65.3X4 | — | — |
| Tetrylammonium chloride | T44.2X1 | T44.2X2 | T44.2X3 | T44.2X4 | T44.2X5 | T44.2X6 |
| Tetryzoline | T49.5X1 | T49.5X2 | T49.5X3 | T49.5X4 | T49.5X5 | T49.5X6 |
| Thalidomide | T45.1X1 | T45.1X2 | T45.1X3 | T45.1X4 | T45.1X5 | T45.1X6 |
| Thallium (compounds) (dust) NEC | T56.811 | T56.812 | T56.813 | T56.814 | — | — |
| pesticide | T60.4X1 | T60.4X2 | T60.4X3 | T60.4X4 | — | — |
| THC | T40.7X1 | T40.7X2 | T40.7X3 | T40.7X4 | T40.7X5 | T40.7X6 |
| Thebacon | T48.3X1 | T48.3X2 | T48.3X3 | T48.3X4 | T48.3X5 | T48.3X6 |
| Thebaine | T40.2X1 | T40.2X2 | T40.2X3 | T40.2X4 | T40.2X5 | T40.2X6 |
| Thenoic acid | T49.6X1 | T49.6X2 | T49.6X3 | T49.6X4 | T49.6X5 | T49.6X6 |
| Thenyldiamine | T45.0X1 | T45.0X2 | T45.0X3 | T45.0X4 | T45.0X5 | T45.0X6 |
| Theobromine (calcium salicylate) | T48.6X1 | T48.6X2 | T48.6X3 | T48.6X4 | T48.6X5 | T48.6X6 |
| sodium salicylate | T48.6X1 | T48.6X2 | T48.6X3 | T48.6X4 | T48.6X5 | T48.6X6 |
| Theophyllamine | T48.6X1 | T48.6X2 | T48.6X3 | T48.6X4 | T48.6X5 | T48.6X6 |
| Theophylline | T48.6X1 | T48.6X2 | T48.6X3 | T48.6X4 | T48.6X5 | T48.6X6 |
| aminobenzoic acid | T48.6X1 | T48.6X2 | T48.6X3 | T48.6X4 | T48.6X5 | T48.6X6 |

| Substance | Poisoning, Accidental (unintentional) | Poisoning, Intentional Self-harm | Poisoning, Assault | Poisoning, Undetermined | Adverse Effect | Under-dosing |
|---|---|---|---|---|---|---|
| Theophylline — continued | | | | | | |
| ethylenediamine | T48.6X1 | T48.6X2 | T48.6X3 | T48.6X4 | T48.6X5 | T48.6X6 |
| piperazine p-amino-benzoate | T48.6X1 | T48.6X2 | T48.6X3 | T48.6X4 | T48.6X5 | T48.6X6 |
| Thiabendazole | T37.4X1 | T37.4X2 | T37.4X3 | T37.4X4 | T37.4X5 | T37.4X6 |
| Thialbarbital | T41.1X1 | T41.1X2 | T41.1X3 | T41.1X4 | T41.1X5 | T41.1X6 |
| Thiamazole | T38.2X1 | T38.2X2 | T38.2X3 | T38.2X4 | T38.2X5 | T38.2X6 |
| Thiambutosine | T37.1X1 | T37.1X2 | T37.1X3 | T37.1X4 | T37.1X5 | T37.1X6 |
| Thiamine | T45.2X1 | T45.2X2 | T45.2X3 | T45.2X4 | T45.2X5 | T45.2X6 |
| Thiamphenicol | T36.2X1 | T36.2X2 | T36.2X3 | T36.2X4 | T36.2X5 | T36.2X6 |
| Thiamylal | T41.1X1 | T41.1X2 | T41.1X3 | T41.1X4 | T41.1X5 | T41.1X6 |
| sodium | T41.1X1 | T41.1X2 | T41.1X3 | T41.1X4 | T41.1X5 | T41.1X6 |
| Thiazesim | T43.291 | T43.292 | T43.293 | T43.294 | T43.295 | T43.296 |
| Thiazides (diuretics) | T50.2X1 | T50.2X2 | T50.2X3 | T50.2X4 | T50.2X5 | T50.2X6 |
| Thiazinamium metilsulfate | T43.3X1 | T43.3X2 | T43.3X3 | T43.3X4 | T43.3X5 | T43.3X6 |
| Thiethylperazine | T43.3X1 | T43.3X2 | T43.3X3 | T43.3X4 | T43.3X5 | T43.3X6 |
| Thimerosal | T49.0X1 | T49.0X2 | T49.0X3 | T49.0X4 | T49.0X5 | T49.0X6 |
| ophthalmic preparation | T49.5X1 | T49.5X2 | T49.5X3 | T49.5X4 | T49.5X5 | T49.5X6 |
| Thioacetazone | T37.1X1 | T37.1X2 | T37.1X3 | T37.1X4 | T37.1X5 | T37.1X6 |
| with isoniazid | T37.1X1 | T37.1X2 | T37.1X3 | T37.1X4 | T37.1X5 | T37.1X6 |
| Thiobarbital sodium | T41.1X1 | T41.1X2 | T41.1X3 | T41.1X4 | T41.1X5 | T41.1X6 |
| Thiobarbiturate anesthetic | T41.1X1 | T41.1X2 | T41.1X3 | T41.1X4 | T41.1X5 | T41.1X6 |
| Thiobismol | T37.8X1 | T37.8X2 | T37.8X3 | T37.8X4 | T37.8X5 | T37.8X6 |
| Thiobutabarbital sodium | T41.1X1 | T41.1X2 | T41.1X3 | T41.1X4 | T41.1X5 | T41.1X6 |
| Thiocarbamate (insecticide) | T60.0X1 | T60.0X2 | T60.0X3 | T60.0X4 | — | — |
| Thiocarbamide | T38.2X1 | T38.2X2 | T38.2X3 | T38.2X4 | T38.2X5 | T38.2X6 |
| Thiocarbarsone | T37.8X1 | T37.8X2 | T37.8X3 | T37.8X4 | T37.8X5 | T37.8X6 |
| Thiocarlide | T37.1X1 | T37.1X2 | T37.1X3 | T37.1X4 | T37.1X5 | T37.1X6 |
| Thioctamide | T50.991 | T50.992 | T50.993 | T50.994 | T50.995 | T50.996 |
| Thioctic acid | T50.991 | T50.992 | T50.993 | T50.994 | T50.995 | T50.996 |
| Thiofos | T60.0X1 | T60.0X2 | T60.0X3 | T60.0X4 | — | — |
| Thioglycolate | T49.4X1 | T49.4X2 | T49.4X3 | T49.4X4 | T49.4X5 | T49.4X6 |
| Thioglycolic acid | T65.891 | T65.892 | T65.893 | T65.894 | — | — |
| Thioguanine | T45.1X1 | T45.1X2 | T45.1X3 | T45.1X4 | T45.1X5 | T45.1X6 |
| Thiomercaptomerin | T50.2X1 | T50.2X2 | T50.2X3 | T50.2X4 | T50.2X5 | T50.2X6 |
| Thiomerin | T50.2X1 | T50.2X2 | T50.2X3 | T50.2X4 | T50.2X5 | T50.2X6 |
| Thiomersal | T49.0X1 | T49.0X2 | T49.0X3 | T49.0X4 | T49.0X5 | T49.0X6 |
| Thionazin | T60.0X1 | T60.0X2 | T60.0X3 | T60.0X4 | — | — |
| Thiopental (sodium) | T41.1X1 | T41.1X2 | T41.1X3 | T41.1X4 | T41.1X5 | T41.1X6 |
| Thiopentone (sodium) | T41.1X1 | T41.1X2 | T41.1X3 | T41.1X4 | T41.1X5 | T41.1X6 |
| Thiopropazate | T43.3X1 | T43.3X2 | T43.3X3 | T43.3X4 | T43.3X5 | T43.3X6 |
| Thioproperazine | T43.3X1 | T43.3X2 | T43.3X3 | T43.3X4 | T43.3X5 | T43.3X6 |
| Thioridazine | T43.3X1 | T43.3X2 | T43.3X3 | T43.3X4 | T43.3X5 | T43.3X6 |
| Thiosinamine | T49.3X1 | T49.3X2 | T49.3X3 | T49.3X4 | T49.3X5 | T49.3X6 |
| Thiotepa | T45.1X1 | T45.1X2 | T45.1X3 | T45.1X4 | T45.1X5 | T45.1X6 |
| Thiothixene | T43.4X1 | T43.4X2 | T43.4X3 | T43.4X4 | T43.4X5 | T43.4X6 |
| Thiouracil (benzyl) (methyl) (propyl) | T38.2X1 | T38.2X2 | T38.2X3 | T38.2X4 | T38.2X5 | T38.2X6 |
| Thiourea | T38.2X1 | T38.2X2 | T38.2X3 | T38.2X4 | T38.2X5 | T38.2X6 |
| Thiphenamil | T44.3X1 | T44.3X2 | T44.3X3 | T44.3X4 | T44.3X5 | T44.3X6 |
| Thiram | T60.3X1 | T60.3X2 | T60.3X3 | T60.3X4 | — | — |
| medicinal | T49.2X1 | T49.2X2 | T49.2X3 | T49.2X4 | T49.2X5 | T49.2X6 |
| Thonzylamine (systemic) | T45.0X1 | T45.0X2 | T45.0X3 | T45.0X4 | T45.0X5 | T45.0X6 |
| mucosal decongestant | T48.5X1 | T48.5X2 | T48.5X3 | T48.5X4 | T48.5X5 | T48.5X6 |
| Thorazine | T43.3X1 | T43.3X2 | T43.3X3 | T43.3X4 | T43.3X5 | T43.3X6 |
| Thorium dioxide suspension | T50.8X1 | T50.8X2 | T50.8X3 | T50.8X4 | T50.8X5 | T50.8X6 |
| Thornapple | T62.2X1 | T62.2X2 | T62.2X3 | T62.2X4 | — | — |
| Throat drug NEC | T49.6X1 | T49.6X2 | T49.6X3 | T49.6X4 | T49.6X5 | T49.6X6 |
| Thrombin | T45.7X1 | T45.7X2 | T45.7X3 | T45.7X4 | T45.7X5 | T45.7X6 |
| Thrombolysin | T45.611 | T45.612 | T45.613 | T45.614 | T45.615 | T45.616 |
| Thromboplastin | T45.7X1 | T45.7X2 | T45.7X3 | T45.7X4 | T45.7X5 | T45.7X6 |
| Thurfyl nicotinate | T46.7X1 | T46.7X2 | T46.7X3 | T46.7X4 | T46.7X5 | T46.7X6 |
| Thymol | T49.0X1 | T49.0X2 | T49.0X3 | T49.0X4 | T49.0X5 | T49.0X6 |
| Thymopentin | T37.5X1 | T37.5X2 | T37.5X3 | T37.5X4 | T37.5X5 | T37.5X6 |
| Thymoxamine | T46.7X1 | T46.7X2 | T46.7X3 | T46.7X4 | T46.7X5 | T46.7X6 |
| Thymus extract | T38.891 | T38.892 | T38.893 | T38.894 | T38.895 | T38.896 |
| Thyreotrophic hormone | T38.811 | T38.812 | T38.813 | T38.814 | T38.815 | T38.816 |
| Thyroglobulin | T38.1X1 | T38.1X2 | T38.1X3 | T38.1X4 | T38.1X5 | T38.1X6 |
| Thyroid (hormone) | T38.1X1 | T38.1X2 | T38.1X3 | T38.1X4 | T38.1X5 | T38.1X6 |
| Thyrolar | T38.1X1 | T38.1X2 | T38.1X3 | T38.1X4 | T38.1X5 | T38.1X6 |
| Thyrotrophin | T38.811 | T38.812 | T38.813 | T38.814 | T38.815 | T38.816 |
| Thyrotropic hormone | T38.811 | T38.812 | T38.813 | T38.814 | T38.815 | T38.816 |
| Thyroxine | T38.1X1 | T38.1X2 | T38.1X3 | T38.1X4 | T38.1X5 | T38.1X6 |
| Tiabendazole | T37.4X1 | T37.4X2 | T37.4X3 | T37.4X4 | T37.4X5 | T37.4X6 |
| Tiamizide | T50.2X1 | T50.2X2 | T50.2X3 | T50.2X4 | T50.2X5 | T50.2X6 |
| Tianeptine | T43.291 | T43.292 | T43.293 | T43.294 | T43.295 | T43.296 |
| Tiapamil | T46.1X1 | T46.1X2 | T46.1X3 | T46.1X4 | T46.1X5 | T46.1X6 |
| Tiapride | T43.591 | T43.592 | T43.593 | T43.594 | T43.595 | T43.596 |
| Tiaprofenic acid | T39.311 | T39.312 | T39.313 | T39.314 | T39.315 | T39.316 |
| Tiaramide | T39.8X1 | T39.8X2 | T39.8X3 | T39.8X4 | T39.8X5 | T39.8X6 |
| Ticarcillin | T36.0X1 | T36.0X2 | T36.0X3 | T36.0X4 | T36.0X5 | T36.0X6 |
| Ticlatone | T49.0X1 | T49.0X2 | T49.0X3 | T49.0X4 | T49.0X5 | T49.0X6 |

Additional Character May Be Required — Refer to the Tabular List for Character Selection

⏷ Subterms under main terms may continue to next column or page

| Substance | Poisoning, Accidental (unintentional) | Poisoning, Intentional Self-harm | Poisoning, Assault | Poisoning, Undetermined | Adverse Effect | Under-dosing |
|---|---|---|---|---|---|---|
| Ticlopidine | T45.521 | T45.522 | T45.523 | T45.524 | T45.525 | T45.526 |
| Ticrynafen | T50.1X1 | T50.1X2 | T50.1X3 | T50.1X4 | T50.1X5 | T50.1X6 |
| Tidiacic | T50.991 | T50.992 | T50.993 | T50.994 | T50.995 | T50.996 |
| Tiemonium | T44.3X1 | T44.3X2 | T44.3X3 | T44.3X4 | T44.3X5 | T44.3X6 |
| iodide | T44.3X1 | T44.3X2 | T44.3X3 | T44.3X4 | T44.3X5 | T44.3X6 |
| Tienilic acid | T50.1X1 | T50.1X2 | T50.1X3 | T50.1X4 | T50.1X5 | T50.1X6 |
| Tifenamil | T44.3X1 | T44.3X2 | T44.3X3 | T44.3X4 | T44.3X5 | T44.3X6 |
| Tigan | T45.0X1 | T45.0X2 | T45.0X3 | T45.0X4 | T45.0X5 | T45.0X6 |
| Tigloidine | T44.3X1 | T44.3X2 | T44.3X3 | T44.3X4 | T44.3X5 | T44.3X6 |
| Tilactase | T47.5X1 | T47.5X2 | T47.5X3 | T47.5X4 | T47.5X5 | T47.5X6 |
| Tiletamine | T41.291 | T41.292 | T41.293 | T41.294 | T41.295 | T41.296 |
| Tilidine | T40.4X1 | T40.4X2 | T40.4X3 | T40.4X4 | — | — |
| Timepidium bromide | T44.3X1 | T44.3X2 | T44.3X3 | T44.3X4 | T44.3X5 | T44.3X6 |
| Timiperone | T43.4X1 | T43.4X2 | T43.4X3 | T43.4X4 | T43.4X5 | T43.4X6 |
| Timolol | T44.7X1 | T44.7X2 | T44.7X3 | T44.7X4 | T44.7X5 | T44.7X6 |
| Tincture, iodine — see Iodine | | | | | | |
| Tindal | T43.3X1 | T43.3X2 | T43.3X3 | T43.3X4 | T43.3X5 | T43.3X6 |
| Tinidazole | T37.3X1 | T37.3X2 | T37.3X3 | T37.3X4 | T37.3X5 | T37.3X6 |
| Tinoridine | T39.8X1 | T39.8X2 | T39.8X3 | T39.8X4 | T39.8X5 | T39.8X6 |
| Tin (chloride) (dust) (oxide) NEC | T56.6X1 | T56.6X2 | T56.6X3 | T56.6X4 | — | — |
| anti-infectives | T37.8X1 | T37.8X2 | T37.8X3 | T37.8X4 | T37.8X5 | T37.8X6 |
| Tiocarlide | T37.1X1 | T37.1X2 | T37.1X3 | T37.1X4 | T37.1X5 | T37.1X6 |
| Tioclomarol | T45.511 | T45.512 | T45.513 | T45.514 | T45.515 | T45.516 |
| Tioconazole | T49.0X1 | T49.0X2 | T49.0X3 | T49.0X4 | T49.0X5 | T49.0X6 |
| Tioguanine | T45.1X1 | T45.1X2 | T45.1X3 | T45.1X4 | T45.1X5 | T45.1X6 |
| Tiopronin | T50.991 | T50.992 | T50.993 | T50.994 | T50.995 | T50.996 |
| Tiotixene | T43.4X1 | T43.4X2 | T43.4X3 | T43.4X4 | T43.4X5 | T43.4X6 |
| Tioxolone | T49.4X1 | T49.4X2 | T49.4X3 | T49.4X4 | T49.4X5 | T49.4X6 |
| Tipepidine | T48.3X1 | T48.3X2 | T48.3X3 | T48.3X4 | T48.3X5 | T48.3X6 |
| Tiquizium bromide | T44.3X1 | T44.3X2 | T44.3X3 | T44.3X4 | T44.3X5 | T44.3X6 |
| Tiratricol | T38.1X1 | T38.1X2 | T38.1X3 | T38.1X4 | T38.1X5 | T38.1X6 |
| Tisopurine | T50.4X1 | T50.4X2 | T50.4X3 | T50.4X4 | T50.4X5 | T50.4X6 |
| Titanium (compounds) (vapor) | T56.891 | T56.892 | T56.893 | T56.894 | — | — |
| dioxide | T49.3X1 | T49.3X2 | T49.3X3 | T49.3X4 | T49.3X5 | T49.3X6 |
| ointment | T49.3X1 | T49.3X2 | T49.3X3 | T49.3X4 | T49.3X5 | T49.3X6 |
| oxide | T49.3X1 | T49.3X2 | T49.3X3 | T49.3X4 | T49.3X5 | T49.3X6 |
| tetrachloride | T56.891 | T56.892 | T56.893 | T56.894 | — | — |
| Titanocene | T56.891 | T56.892 | T56.893 | T56.894 | — | — |
| Titroid | T38.1X1 | T38.1X2 | T38.1X3 | T38.1X4 | T38.1X5 | T38.1X6 |
| Tizanidine | T42.8X1 | T42.8X2 | T42.8X3 | T42.8X4 | T42.8X5 | T42.8X6 |
| TMTD | T60.3X1 | T60.3X2 | T60.3X3 | T60.3X4 | — | — |
| TNT (fumes) | T65.3X1 | T65.3X2 | T65.3X3 | T65.3X4 | — | — |
| Toadstool | T62.0X1 | T62.0X2 | T62.0X3 | T62.0X4 | — | — |
| Tobacco NEC | T65.291 | T65.292 | T65.293 | T65.294 | — | — |
| cigarettes | T65.221 | T65.222 | T65.223 | T65.224 | — | — |
| Indian | T62.2X1 | T62.2X2 | T62.2X3 | T62.2X4 | — | — |
| smoke, second-hand | T65.221 | T65.222 | T65.223 | T65.224 | — | — |
| Tobramycin | T36.5X1 | T36.5X2 | T36.5X3 | T36.5X4 | T36.5X5 | T36.5X6 |
| Tocainide | T46.2X1 | T46.2X2 | T46.2X3 | T46.2X4 | T46.2X5 | T46.2X6 |
| Tocoferol | T45.2X1 | T45.2X2 | T45.2X3 | T45.2X4 | T45.2X5 | T45.2X6 |
| Tocopherol | T45.2X1 | T45.2X2 | T45.2X3 | T45.2X4 | T45.2X5 | T45.2X6 |
| acetate | T45.2X1 | T45.2X2 | T45.2X3 | T45.2X4 | T45.2X5 | T45.2X6 |
| Tocosamine | T48.0X1 | T48.0X2 | T48.0X3 | T48.0X4 | T48.0X5 | T48.0X6 |
| Todralazine | T46.5X1 | T46.5X2 | T46.5X3 | T46.5X4 | T46.5X5 | T46.5X6 |
| Tofisopam | T42.4X1 | T42.4X2 | T42.4X3 | T42.4X4 | T42.4X5 | T42.4X6 |
| Tofranil | T43.011 | T43.012 | T43.013 | T43.014 | T43.015 | T43.016 |
| Toilet deodorizer | T65.891 | T65.892 | T65.893 | T65.894 | — | — |
| Tolamolol | T44.7X1 | T44.7X2 | T44.7X3 | T44.7X4 | T44.7X5 | T44.7X6 |
| Tolazamide | T38.3X1 | T38.3X2 | T38.3X3 | T38.3X4 | T38.3X5 | T38.3X6 |
| Tolazoline | T46.7X1 | T46.7X2 | T46.7X3 | T46.7X4 | T46.7X5 | T46.7X6 |
| Tolbutamide (sodium) | T38.3X1 | T38.3X2 | T38.3X3 | T38.3X4 | T38.3X5 | T38.3X6 |
| Tolciclate | T49.0X1 | T49.0X2 | T49.0X3 | T49.0X4 | T49.0X5 | T49.0X6 |
| Tolmetin | T39.391 | T39.392 | T39.393 | T39.394 | T39.395 | T39.396 |
| Tolnaftate | T49.0X1 | T49.0X2 | T49.0X3 | T49.0X4 | T49.0X5 | T49.0X6 |
| Tolonidine | T46.5X1 | T46.5X2 | T46.5X3 | T46.5X4 | T46.5X5 | T46.5X6 |
| Toloxatone | T42.6X1 | T42.6X2 | T42.6X3 | T42.6X4 | T42.6X5 | T42.6X6 |
| Tolperisone | T44.3X1 | T44.3X2 | T44.3X3 | T44.3X4 | T44.3X5 | T44.3X6 |
| Tolserol | T42.8X1 | T42.8X2 | T42.8X3 | T42.8X4 | T42.8X5 | T42.8X6 |
| Toluene (liquid) | T52.2X1 | T52.2X2 | T52.2X3 | T52.2X4 | — | — |
| diisocyanate | T65.0X1 | T65.0X2 | T65.0X3 | T65.0X4 | — | — |
| Toluidine | T65.891 | T65.892 | T65.893 | T65.894 | — | — |
| vapor | T59.891 | T59.892 | T59.893 | T59.894 | — | — |
| Toluol (liquid) | T52.2X1 | T52.2X2 | T52.2X3 | T52.2X4 | — | — |
| vapor | T52.2X1 | T52.2X2 | T52.2X3 | T52.2X4 | — | — |
| Toluylenediamine | T65.3X1 | T65.3X2 | T65.3X3 | T65.3X4 | — | — |
| Tolylene-2,4-diisocyanate | T65.0X1 | T65.0X2 | T65.0X3 | T65.0X4 | — | — |
| Tonic NEC | T50.901 | T50.902 | T50.903 | T50.904 | T50.905 | T50.906 |
| Topical action drug NEC | T49.91 | T49.92 | T49.93 | T49.94 | T49.95 | T49.96 |
| ear, nose or throat | T49.6X1 | T49.6X2 | T49.6X3 | T49.6X4 | T49.6X5 | T49.6X6 |
| eye | T49.5X1 | T49.5X2 | T49.5X3 | T49.5X4 | T49.5X5 | T49.5X6 |
| skin | T49.91 | T49.92 | T49.93 | T49.94 | T49.95 | T49.96 |

| Substance | Poisoning, Accidental (unintentional) | Poisoning, Intentional Self-harm | Poisoning, Assault | Poisoning, Undetermined | Adverse Effect | Under-dosing |
|---|---|---|---|---|---|---|
| Topical action drug — *continued* | | | | | | |
| specified NEC | T49.8X1 | T49.8X2 | T49.8X3 | T49.8X4 | T49.8X5 | T49.8X6 |
| Toquizine | T44.3X1 | T44.3X2 | T44.3X3 | T44.3X4 | T44.3X5 | T44.3X6 |
| Toremifene | T38.6X1 | T38.6X2 | T38.6X3 | T38.6X4 | T38.6X5 | T38.6X6 |
| Tosylchloramide sodium | T49.8X1 | T49.8X2 | T49.8X3 | T49.8X4 | T49.8X5 | T49.8X6 |
| Toxaphene (dust) (spray) | T60.1X1 | T60.1X2 | T60.1X3 | T60.1X4 | — | — |
| Toxin, diphtheria (Schick Test) | T50.8X1 | T50.8X2 | T50.8X3 | T50.8X4 | T50.8X5 | T50.8X6 |
| Toxoid | | | | | | |
| combined | T50.A21 | T50.A22 | T50.A23 | T50.A24 | T50.A25 | T50.A26 |
| diphtheria | T50.A91 | T50.A92 | T50.A93 | T50.A94 | T50.A95 | T50.A96 |
| tetanus | T50.A91 | T50.A92 | T50.A93 | T50.A94 | T50.A95 | T50.A96 |
| Trace element NEC | T45.8X1 | T45.8X2 | T45.8X3 | T45.8X4 | T45.8X5 | T45.8X6 |
| Tractor fuel NEC | T52.0X1 | T52.0X2 | T52.0X3 | T52.0X4 | — | — |
| Tragacanth | T50.991 | T50.992 | T50.993 | T50.994 | T50.995 | T50.996 |
| Tramadol | T40.4X1 | T40.4X2 | T40.4X3 | T40.4X4 | T40.4X5 | T40.4X6 |
| Tramazoline | T48.5X1 | T48.5X2 | T48.5X3 | T48.5X4 | T48.5X5 | T48.5X6 |
| Tranexamic acid | T45.621 | T45.622 | T45.623 | T45.624 | T45.625 | T45.626 |
| Tranilast | T45.0X1 | T45.0X2 | T45.0X3 | T45.0X4 | T45.0X5 | T45.0X6 |
| Tranquilizer NEC | T43.501 | T43.502 | T43.503 | T43.504 | T43.505 | T43.506 |
| with hypnotic or sedative | T42.6X1 | T42.6X2 | T42.6X3 | T42.6X4 | T42.6X5 | T42.6X6 |
| benzodiazepine NEC | T42.4X1 | T42.4X2 | T42.4X3 | T42.4X4 | T42.4X5 | T42.4X6 |
| butyrophenone NEC | T43.4X1 | T43.4X2 | T43.4X3 | T43.4X4 | T43.4X5 | T43.4X6 |
| carbamate | T43.591 | T43.592 | T43.593 | T43.594 | T43.595 | T43.596 |
| dimethylamine | T43.3X1 | T43.3X2 | T43.3X3 | T43.3X4 | T43.3X5 | T43.3X6 |
| ethylamine | T43.3X1 | T43.3X2 | T43.3X3 | T43.3X4 | T43.3X5 | T43.3X6 |
| hydroxyzine | T43.591 | T43.592 | T43.593 | T43.594 | T43.595 | T43.596 |
| major NEC | T43.501 | T43.502 | T43.503 | T43.504 | T43.505 | T43.506 |
| penothiazine NEC | T43.3X1 | T43.3X2 | T43.3X3 | T43.3X4 | T43.3X5 | T43.3X6 |
| phenothiazine-based | T43.3X1 | T43.3X2 | T43.3X3 | T43.3X4 | T43.3X5 | T43.3X6 |
| piperazine NEC | T43.3X1 | T43.3X2 | T43.3X3 | T43.3X4 | T43.3X5 | T43.3X6 |
| piperidine | T43.3X1 | T43.3X2 | T43.3X3 | T43.3X4 | T43.3X5 | T43.3X6 |
| propylamine | T43.3X1 | T43.3X2 | T43.3X3 | T43.3X4 | T43.3X5 | T43.3X6 |
| specified NEC | T43.591 | T43.592 | T43.593 | T43.594 | T43.595 | T43.596 |
| thioxanthene NEC | T43.591 | T43.592 | T43.593 | T43.594 | T43.595 | T43.596 |
| Tranxene | T42.4X1 | T42.4X2 | T42.4X3 | T42.4X4 | T42.4X5 | T42.4X6 |
| Tranylcypromine | T43.1X1 | T43.1X2 | T43.1X3 | T43.1X4 | T43.1X5 | T43.1X6 |
| Trapidil | T46.3X1 | T46.3X2 | T46.3X3 | T46.3X4 | T46.3X5 | T46.3X6 |
| Trasentine | T44.3X1 | T44.3X2 | T44.3X3 | T44.3X4 | T44.3X5 | T44.3X6 |
| Travert | T50.3X1 | T50.3X2 | T50.3X3 | T50.3X4 | T50.3X5 | T50.3X6 |
| Trazodone | T43.211 | T43.212 | T43.213 | T43.214 | T43.215 | T43.216 |
| Trecator | T37.1X1 | T37.1X2 | T37.1X3 | T37.1X4 | T37.1X5 | T37.1X6 |
| Treosulfan | T45.1X1 | T45.1X2 | T45.1X3 | T45.1X4 | T45.1X5 | T45.1X6 |
| Tretamine | T45.1X1 | T45.1X2 | T45.1X3 | T45.1X4 | T45.1X5 | T45.1X6 |
| Tretinoin | T49.0X1 | T49.0X2 | T49.0X3 | T49.0X4 | T49.0X5 | T49.0X6 |
| Tretoquinol | T48.6X1 | T48.6X2 | T48.6X3 | T48.6X4 | T48.6X5 | T48.6X6 |
| Triacetin | T49.0X1 | T49.0X2 | T49.0X3 | T49.0X4 | T49.0X5 | T49.0X6 |
| Triacetoxyanthracene | T49.4X1 | T49.4X2 | T49.4X3 | T49.4X4 | T49.4X5 | T49.4X6 |
| Triacetyloleandomycin | T36.3X1 | T36.3X2 | T36.3X3 | T36.3X4 | T36.3X5 | T36.3X6 |
| Triamcinolone | T38.0X1 | T38.0X2 | T38.0X3 | T38.0X4 | T38.0X5 | T38.0X6 |
| ENT agent | T49.6X1 | T49.6X2 | T49.6X3 | T49.6X4 | T49.6X5 | T49.6X6 |
| hexacetonide | T49.0X1 | T49.0X2 | T49.0X3 | T49.0X4 | T49.0X5 | T49.0X6 |
| ophthalmic preparation | T49.5X1 | T49.5X2 | T49.5X3 | T49.5X4 | T49.5X5 | T49.5X6 |
| topical NEC | T49.0X1 | T49.0X2 | T49.0X3 | T49.0X4 | T49.0X5 | T49.0X6 |
| Triampyzine | T44.3X1 | T44.3X2 | T44.3X3 | T44.3X4 | T44.3X5 | T44.3X6 |
| Triamterene | T50.2X1 | T50.2X2 | T50.2X3 | T50.2X4 | T50.2X5 | T50.2X6 |
| Triazine (herbicide) | T60.3X1 | T60.3X2 | T60.3X3 | T60.3X4 | — | — |
| Triaziquone | T45.1X1 | T45.1X2 | T45.1X3 | T45.1X4 | T45.1X5 | T45.1X6 |
| Triazolam | T42.4X1 | T42.4X2 | T42.4X3 | T42.4X4 | T42.4X5 | T42.4X6 |
| Triazole (herbicide) | T60.3X1 | T60.3X2 | T60.3X3 | T60.3X4 | — | — |
| Tribenoside | T46.991 | T46.992 | T46.993 | T46.994 | T46.995 | T46.996 |
| Tribromacetaldehyde | T42.6X1 | T42.6X2 | T42.6X3 | T42.6X4 | T42.6X5 | T42.6X6 |
| Tribromoethanol, rectal | T41.291 | T41.292 | T41.293 | T41.294 | T41.295 | T41.296 |
| Tribromomethane | T42.6X1 | T42.6X2 | T42.6X3 | T42.6X4 | T42.6X5 | T42.6X6 |
| Trichlorethane | T53.2X1 | T53.2X2 | T53.2X3 | T53.2X4 | — | — |
| Trichlorethylene | T53.2X1 | T53.2X2 | T53.2X3 | T53.2X4 | — | — |
| Trichlorfon | T60.0X1 | T60.0X2 | T60.0X3 | T60.0X4 | — | — |
| Trichlormethiazide | T50.2X1 | T50.2X2 | T50.2X3 | T50.2X4 | T50.2X5 | T50.2X6 |
| Trichlormethine | T45.1X1 | T45.1X2 | T45.1X3 | T45.1X4 | T45.1X5 | T45.1X6 |
| Trichloroacetic acid, Trichloracetic acid | T54.2X1 | T54.2X2 | T54.2X3 | T54.2X4 | — | — |
| medicinal | T49.4X1 | T49.4X2 | T49.4X3 | T49.4X4 | T49.4X5 | T49.4X6 |
| Trichloroethane | T53.2X1 | T53.2X2 | T53.2X3 | T53.2X4 | — | — |
| Trichloroethanol | T42.6X1 | T42.6X2 | T42.6X3 | T42.6X4 | T42.6X5 | T42.6X6 |
| Trichloroethylene (liquid) (vapor) | T53.2X1 | T53.2X2 | T53.2X3 | T53.2X4 | — | — |
| anesthetic (gas) | T41.0X1 | T41.0X2 | T41.0X3 | T41.0X4 | T41.0X5 | T41.0X6 |
| vapor NEC | T53.2X1 | T53.2X2 | T53.2X3 | T53.2X4 | — | — |
| Trichloroethyl phosphate | T42.6X1 | T42.6X2 | T42.6X3 | T42.6X4 | T42.6X5 | T42.6X6 |
| Trichlorofluoromethane NEC | T53.5X1 | T53.5X2 | T53.5X3 | T53.5X4 | — | — |
| Trichloronate | T60.0X1 | T60.0X2 | T60.0X3 | T60.0X4 | — | — |
| Trichloropropane | T53.6X1 | T53.6X2 | T53.6X3 | T53.6X4 | — | — |

| Substance | Poisoning, Accidental (unintentional) | Poisoning, Intentional Self-harm | Poisoning, Assault | Poisoning, Undetermined | Adverse Effect | Under-dosing |
|---|---|---|---|---|---|---|
| Trichlorotriethylamine | T45.1X1 | T45.1X2 | T45.1X3 | T45.1X4 | T45.1X5 | T45.1X6 |
| Trichomonacides NEC | T37.3X1 | T37.3X2 | T37.3X3 | T37.3X4 | T37.3X5 | T37.3X6 |
| Trichomycin | T36.7X1 | T36.7X2 | T36.7X3 | T36.7X4 | T36.7X5 | T36.7X6 |
| Triclobisonium chloride | T49.0X1 | T49.0X2 | T49.0X3 | T49.0X4 | T49.0X5 | T49.0X6 |
| Triclocarban | T49.0X1 | T49.0X2 | T49.0X3 | T49.0X4 | T49.0X5 | T49.0X6 |
| Triclofos | T42.6X1 | T42.6X2 | T42.6X3 | T42.6X4 | T42.6X5 | T42.6X6 |
| Triclosan | T49.0X1 | T49.0X2 | T49.0X3 | T49.0X4 | T49.0X5 | T49.0X6 |
| Tricresyl phosphate | T65.891 | T65.892 | T65.893 | T65.894 | — | — |
|   solvent | T52.91 | T52.92 | T52.93 | T52.94 | | |
| Tricyclamol chloride | T44.3X1 | T44.3X2 | T44.3X3 | T44.3X4 | T44.3X5 | T44.3X6 |
| Tridesilon | T49.0X1 | T49.0X2 | T49.0X3 | T49.0X4 | T49.0X5 | T49.0X6 |
| Tridihexethyl iodide | T44.3X1 | T44.3X2 | T44.3X3 | T44.3X4 | T44.3X5 | T44.3X6 |
| Tridione | T42.2X1 | T42.2X2 | T42.2X3 | T42.2X4 | T42.2X5 | T42.2X6 |
| Trientine | T45.8X1 | T45.8X2 | T45.8X3 | T45.8X4 | T45.8X5 | T45.8X6 |
| Triethanolamine NEC | T54.3X1 | T54.3X2 | T54.3X3 | T54.3X4 | — | — |
|   detergent | T54.3X1 | T54.3X2 | T54.3X3 | T54.3X4 | | |
|   trinitrate (biphosphate) | T46.3X1 | T46.3X2 | T46.3X3 | T46.3X4 | T46.3X5 | T46.3X6 |
| Triethanomelamine | T45.1X1 | T45.1X2 | T45.1X3 | T45.1X4 | T45.1X5 | T45.1X6 |
| Triethylenemelamine | T45.1X1 | T45.1X2 | T45.1X3 | T45.1X4 | T45.1X5 | T45.1X6 |
| Triethylenephosphoramide | T45.1X1 | T45.1X2 | T45.1X3 | T45.1X4 | T45.1X5 | T45.1X6 |
| Triethylenethiophosphoramide | T45.1X1 | T45.1X2 | T45.1X3 | T45.1X4 | T45.1X5 | T45.1X6 |
| Trifluoperazine | T43.3X1 | T43.3X2 | T43.3X3 | T43.3X4 | T43.3X5 | T43.3X6 |
| Trifluoroethyl vinyl ether | T41.0X1 | T41.0X2 | T41.0X3 | T41.0X4 | T41.0X5 | T41.0X6 |
| Trifluperidol | T43.4X1 | T43.4X2 | T43.4X3 | T43.4X4 | T43.4X5 | T43.4X6 |
| Triflupromazine | T43.3X1 | T43.3X2 | T43.3X3 | T43.3X4 | T43.3X5 | T43.3X6 |
| Trifluridine | T37.5X1 | T37.5X2 | T37.5X3 | T37.5X4 | T37.5X5 | T37.5X6 |
| Triflusal | T45.521 | T45.522 | T45.523 | T45.524 | T45.525 | T45.526 |
| Trihexyphenidyl | T44.3X1 | T44.3X2 | T44.3X3 | T44.3X4 | T44.3X5 | T44.3X6 |
| Triiodothyronine | T38.1X1 | T38.1X2 | T38.1X3 | T38.1X4 | T38.1X5 | T38.1X6 |
| Trilene | T41.0X1 | T41.0X2 | T41.0X3 | T41.0X4 | T41.0X5 | T41.0X6 |
| Trilostane | T38.991 | T38.992 | T38.993 | T38.994 | T38.995 | T38.996 |
| Trimebutine | T44.3X1 | T44.3X2 | T44.3X3 | T44.3X4 | T44.3X5 | T44.3X6 |
| Trimecaine | T41.3X1 | T41.3X2 | T41.3X3 | T41.3X4 | T41.3X5 | T41.3X6 |
| Trimeprazine (tartrate) | T44.3X1 | T44.3X2 | T44.3X3 | T44.3X4 | T44.3X5 | T44.3X6 |
| Trimetaphan camsilate | T44.2X1 | T44.2X2 | T44.2X3 | T44.2X4 | T44.2X5 | T44.2X6 |
| Trimetazidine | T46.7X1 | T46.7X2 | T46.7X3 | T46.7X4 | T46.7X5 | T46.7X6 |
| Trimethadione | T42.2X1 | T42.2X2 | T42.2X3 | T42.2X4 | T42.2X5 | T42.2X6 |
| Trimethaphan | T44.2X1 | T44.2X2 | T44.2X3 | T44.2X4 | T44.2X5 | T44.2X6 |
| Trimethidinium | T44.2X1 | T44.2X2 | T44.2X3 | T44.2X4 | T44.2X5 | T44.2X6 |
| Trimethobenzamide | T45.0X1 | T45.0X2 | T45.0X3 | T45.0X4 | T45.0X5 | T45.0X6 |
| Trimethoprim | T37.8X1 | T37.8X2 | T37.8X3 | T37.8X4 | T37.8X5 | T37.8X6 |
|   with sulfamethoxazole | T36.8X1 | T36.8X2 | T36.8X3 | T36.8X4 | T36.8X5 | T36.8X6 |
| Trimethylcarbinol | T51.3X1 | T51.3X2 | T51.3X3 | T51.3X4 | | |
| Trimethylpsoralen | T49.3X1 | T49.3X2 | T49.3X3 | T49.3X4 | T49.3X5 | T49.3X6 |
| Trimeton | T45.0X1 | T45.0X2 | T45.0X3 | T45.0X4 | T45.0X5 | T45.0X6 |
| Trimetrexate | T45.1X1 | T45.1X2 | T45.1X3 | T45.1X4 | T45.1X5 | T45.1X6 |
| Trimipramine | T43.011 | T43.012 | T43.013 | T43.014 | T43.015 | T43.016 |
| Trimustine | T45.1X1 | T45.1X2 | T45.1X3 | T45.1X4 | T45.1X5 | T45.1X6 |
| Trinitrine | T46.3X1 | T46.3X2 | T46.3X3 | T46.3X4 | T46.3X5 | T46.3X6 |
| Trinitrobenzol | T65.3X1 | T65.3X2 | T65.3X3 | T65.3X4 | — | — |
| Trinitrophenol | T65.3X1 | T65.3X2 | T65.3X3 | T65.3X4 | — | — |
| Trinitrotoluene (fumes) | T65.3X1 | T65.3X2 | T65.3X3 | T65.3X4 | — | — |
| Trional | T42.6X1 | T42.6X2 | T42.6X3 | T42.6X4 | T42.6X5 | T42.6X6 |
| Triorthocresyl phosphate | T65.891 | T65.892 | T65.893 | T65.894 | — | — |
| Trioxide of arsenic | T57.0X1 | T57.0X2 | T57.0X3 | T57.0X4 | — | — |
| Trioxysalen | T49.4X1 | T49.4X2 | T49.4X3 | T49.4X4 | T49.4X5 | T49.4X6 |
| Tripamide | T50.2X1 | T50.2X2 | T50.2X3 | T50.2X4 | T50.2X5 | T50.2X6 |
| Triparanol | T46.6X1 | T46.6X2 | T46.6X3 | T46.6X4 | T46.6X5 | T46.6X6 |
| Tripelennamine | T45.0X1 | T45.0X2 | T45.0X3 | T45.0X4 | T45.0X5 | T45.0X6 |
| Triperiden | T44.3X1 | T44.3X2 | T44.3X3 | T44.3X4 | T44.3X5 | T44.3X6 |
| Triperidol | T43.4X1 | T43.4X2 | T43.4X3 | T43.4X4 | T43.4X5 | T43.4X6 |
| Triphenylphosphate | T65.891 | T65.892 | T65.893 | T65.894 | — | — |
| Triple | | | | | | |
|   bromides | T42.6X1 | T42.6X2 | T42.6X3 | T42.6X4 | T42.6X5 | T42.6X6 |
|   carbonate | T47.1X1 | T47.1X2 | T47.1X3 | T47.1X4 | T47.1X5 | T47.1X6 |
|   vaccine | | | | | | |
|     DPT | T50.A11 | T50.A12 | T50.A13 | T50.A14 | T50.A15 | T50.A16 |
|     including pertussis | T50.A11 | T50.A12 | T50.A13 | T50.A14 | T50.A15 | T50.A16 |
|     MMR | T50.B91 | T50.B92 | T50.B93 | T50.B94 | T50.B95 | T50.B96 |
| Triprolidine | T45.0X1 | T45.0X2 | T45.0X3 | T45.0X4 | T45.0X5 | T45.0X6 |
| Trisodium hydrogen edetate | T50.6X1 | T50.6X2 | T50.6X3 | T50.6X4 | T50.6X5 | T50.6X6 |
| Trisoralen | T49.3X1 | T49.3X2 | T49.3X3 | T49.3X4 | T49.3X5 | T49.3X6 |
| Trisulfapyrimidines | T37.0X1 | T37.0X2 | T37.0X3 | T37.0X4 | T37.0X5 | T37.0X6 |
| Trithiozine | T44.3X1 | T44.3X2 | T44.3X3 | T44.3X4 | T44.3X5 | T44.3X6 |
| Tritiozine | T44.3X1 | T44.3X2 | T44.3X3 | T44.3X4 | T44.3X5 | T44.3X6 |
| Tritoqualine | T45.0X1 | T45.0X2 | T45.0X3 | T45.0X4 | T45.0X5 | T45.0X6 |
| Trofosfamide | T45.1X1 | T45.1X2 | T45.1X3 | T45.1X4 | T45.1X5 | T45.1X6 |
| Troleandomycin | T36.3X1 | T36.3X2 | T36.3X3 | T36.3X4 | T36.3X5 | T36.3X6 |
| Trolnitrate (phosphate) | T46.3X1 | T46.3X2 | T46.3X3 | T46.3X4 | T46.3X5 | T46.3X6 |
| Tromantadine | T37.5X1 | T37.5X2 | T37.5X3 | T37.5X4 | T37.5X5 | T37.5X6 |
| Trometamol | T50.2X1 | T50.2X2 | T50.2X3 | T50.2X4 | T50.2X5 | T50.2X6 |
| Tromethamine | T50.2X1 | T50.2X2 | T50.2X3 | T50.2X4 | T50.2X5 | T50.2X6 |

| Substance | Poisoning, Accidental (unintentional) | Poisoning, Intentional Self-harm | Poisoning, Assault | Poisoning, Undetermined | Adverse Effect | Under-dosing |
|---|---|---|---|---|---|---|
| Tronothane | T41.3X1 | T41.3X2 | T41.3X3 | T41.3X4 | T41.3X5 | T41.3X6 |
| Tropacine | T44.3X1 | T44.3X2 | T44.3X3 | T44.3X4 | T44.3X5 | T44.3X6 |
| Tropatepine | T44.3X1 | T44.3X2 | T44.3X3 | T44.3X4 | T44.3X5 | T44.3X6 |
| Tropicamide | T44.3X1 | T44.3X2 | T44.3X3 | T44.3X4 | T44.3X5 | T44.3X6 |
| Trospium chloride | T44.3X1 | T44.3X2 | T44.3X3 | T44.3X4 | T44.3X5 | T44.3X6 |
| Troxerutin | T46.991 | T46.992 | T46.993 | T46.994 | T46.995 | T46.996 |
| Troxidone | T42.2X1 | T42.2X2 | T42.2X3 | T42.2X4 | T42.2X5 | T42.2X6 |
| Tryparsamide | T37.3X1 | T37.3X2 | T37.3X3 | T37.3X4 | T37.3X5 | T37.3X6 |
| Trypsin | T45.3X1 | T45.3X2 | T45.3X3 | T45.3X4 | T45.3X5 | T45.3X6 |
| Tryptizol | T43.011 | T43.012 | T43.013 | T43.014 | T43.015 | T43.016 |
| TSH | T38.811 | T38.812 | T38.813 | T38.814 | T38.815 | T38.816 |
| Tuaminoheptane | T48.5X1 | T48.5X2 | T48.5X3 | T48.5X4 | T48.5X5 | T48.5X6 |
| Tuberculin, purified protein derivative (PPD) | T50.8X1 | T50.8X2 | T50.8X3 | T50.8X4 | T50.8X5 | T50.8X6 |
| Tubocurare | T48.1X1 | T48.1X2 | T48.1X3 | T48.1X4 | T48.1X5 | T48.1X6 |
| Tubocurarine (chloride) | T48.1X1 | T48.1X2 | T48.1X3 | T48.1X4 | T48.1X5 | T48.1X6 |
| Tulobuterol | T48.6X1 | T48.6X2 | T48.6X3 | T48.6X4 | T48.6X5 | T48.6X6 |
| Turpentine (spirits of) | T52.8X1 | T52.8X2 | T52.8X3 | T52.8X4 | — | — |
|   vapor | T52.8X1 | T52.8X2 | T52.8X3 | T52.8X4 | — | — |
| Tybamate | T43.591 | T43.592 | T43.593 | T43.594 | T43.595 | T43.596 |
| Tyloxapol | T48.4X1 | T48.4X2 | T48.4X3 | T48.4X4 | T48.4X5 | T48.4X6 |
| Tymazoline | T48.5X1 | T48.5X2 | T48.5X3 | T48.5X4 | T48.5X5 | T48.5X6 |
| Typhoid-paratyphoid vaccine | T50.A91 | T50.A92 | T50.A93 | T50.A94 | T50.A95 | T50.A96 |
| Typhus vaccine | T50.A91 | T50.A92 | T50.A93 | T50.A94 | T50.A95 | T50.A96 |
| Tyropanoate | T50.8X1 | T50.8X2 | T50.8X3 | T50.8X4 | T50.8X5 | T50.8X6 |
| Tyrothricin | T49.6X1 | T49.6X2 | T49.6X3 | T49.6X4 | T49.6X5 | T49.6X6 |
|   ENT agent | T49.6X1 | T49.6X2 | T49.6X3 | T49.6X4 | T49.6X5 | T49.6X6 |
|   ophthalmic preparation | T49.5X1 | T49.5X2 | T49.5X3 | T49.5X4 | T49.5X5 | T49.5X6 |
| Ufenamate | T39.391 | T39.392 | T39.393 | T39.394 | T39.395 | T39.396 |
| Ultraviolet light protectant | T49.3X1 | T49.3X2 | T49.3X3 | T49.3X4 | T49.3X5 | T49.3X6 |
| Undecenoic acid | T49.0X1 | T49.0X2 | T49.0X3 | T49.0X4 | T49.0X5 | T49.0X6 |
| Undecoylium | T49.0X1 | T49.0X2 | T49.0X3 | T49.0X4 | T49.0X5 | T49.0X6 |
| Undecylenic acid (derivatives) | T49.0X1 | T49.0X2 | T49.0X3 | T49.0X4 | T49.0X5 | T49.0X6 |
| Unna's boot | T49.3X1 | T49.3X2 | T49.3X3 | T49.3X4 | T49.3X5 | T49.3X6 |
| Unsaturated fatty acid | T46.6X1 | T46.6X2 | T46.6X3 | T46.6X4 | T46.6X5 | T46.6X6 |
| Uracil mustard | T45.1X1 | T45.1X2 | T45.1X3 | T45.1X4 | T45.1X5 | T45.1X6 |
| Uramustine | T45.1X1 | T45.1X2 | T45.1X3 | T45.1X4 | T45.1X5 | T45.1X6 |
| Urapidil | T46.5X1 | T46.5X2 | T46.5X3 | T46.5X4 | T46.5X5 | T46.5X6 |
| Urari | T48.1X1 | T48.1X2 | T48.1X3 | T48.1X4 | T48.1X5 | T48.1X6 |
| Urate oxidase | T50.4X1 | T50.4X2 | T50.4X3 | T50.4X4 | T50.4X5 | T50.4X6 |
| Urea | T47.3X1 | T47.3X2 | T47.3X3 | T47.3X4 | T47.3X5 | T47.3X6 |
|   peroxide | T49.0X1 | T49.0X2 | T49.0X3 | T49.0X4 | T49.0X5 | T49.0X6 |
|   stibamine | T37.4X1 | T37.4X2 | T37.4X3 | T37.4X4 | T37.4X5 | T37.4X6 |
|   topical | T49.8X1 | T49.8X2 | T49.8X3 | T49.8X4 | T49.8X5 | T49.8X6 |
| Urethane | T45.1X1 | T45.1X2 | T45.1X3 | T45.1X4 | T45.1X5 | T45.1X6 |
| Urginea (maritima) (scilla) — see Squill | | | | | | |
| Uric acid metabolism drug NEC | T50.4X1 | T50.4X2 | T50.4X3 | T50.4X4 | T50.4X5 | T50.4X6 |
| Uricosuric agent | T50.4X1 | T50.4X2 | T50.4X3 | T50.4X4 | T50.4X5 | T50.4X6 |
| Urinary anti-infective | T37.8X1 | T37.8X2 | T37.8X3 | T37.8X4 | T37.8X5 | T37.8X6 |
| Urofollitropin | T38.811 | T38.812 | T38.813 | T38.814 | T38.815 | T38.816 |
| Urokinase | T45.611 | T45.612 | T45.613 | T45.614 | T45.615 | T45.616 |
| Urokon | T50.8X1 | T50.8X2 | T50.8X3 | T50.8X4 | T50.8X5 | T50.8X6 |
| Ursodeoxycholic acid | T50.991 | T50.992 | T50.993 | T50.994 | T50.995 | T50.996 |
| Ursodiol | T50.991 | T50.992 | T50.993 | T50.994 | T50.995 | T50.996 |
| Urtica | T62.2X1 | T62.2X2 | T62.2X3 | T62.2X4 | — | — |
| Utility gas — see Gas, utility | | | | | | |
| Vaccine NEC | T50.Z91 | T50.Z92 | T50.Z93 | T50.Z94 | T50.Z95 | T50.Z96 |
|   antineoplastic | T50.Z91 | T50.Z92 | T50.Z93 | T50.Z94 | T50.Z95 | T50.Z96 |
|   bacterial NEC | T50.A91 | T50.A92 | T50.A93 | T50.A94 | T50.A95 | T50.A96 |
|     with | | | | | | |
|       other bacterial component | T50.A21 | T50.A22 | T50.A23 | T50.A24 | T50.A25 | T50.A26 |
|       pertussis component | T50.A11 | T50.A12 | T50.A13 | T50.A14 | T50.A15 | T50.A16 |
|       viral-rickettsial component | T50.A21 | T50.A22 | T50.A23 | T50.A24 | T50.A25 | T50.A26 |
|     mixed NEC | T50.A21 | T50.A22 | T50.A23 | T50.A24 | T50.A25 | T50.A26 |
|   BCG | T50.A91 | T50.A92 | T50.A93 | T50.A94 | T50.A95 | T50.A96 |
|   cholera | T50.A91 | T50.A92 | T50.A93 | T50.A94 | T50.A95 | T50.A96 |
|   diphtheria | T50.A91 | T50.A92 | T50.A93 | T50.A94 | T50.A95 | T50.A96 |
|     with tetanus | T50.A21 | T50.A22 | T50.A23 | T50.A24 | T50.A25 | T50.A26 |
|       and pertussis | T50.A11 | T50.A12 | T50.A13 | T50.A14 | T50.A15 | T50.A16 |
|   influenza | T50.B91 | T50.B92 | T50.B93 | T50.B94 | T50.B95 | T50.B96 |
|   measles | T50.B91 | T50.B92 | T50.B93 | T50.B94 | T50.B95 | T50.B96 |
|     with mumps and rubella | T50.B91 | T50.B92 | T50.B93 | T50.B94 | T50.B95 | T50.B96 |
|   meningococcal | T50.A91 | T50.A92 | T50.A93 | T50.A94 | T50.A95 | T50.A96 |
|   mumps | T50.B91 | T50.B92 | T50.B93 | T50.B94 | T50.B95 | T50.B96 |
|   paratyphoid | T50.A91 | T50.A92 | T50.A93 | T50.A94 | T50.A95 | T50.A96 |
|   pertussis | T50.A11 | T50.A12 | T50.A13 | T50.A14 | T50.A15 | T50.A16 |
|     with diphtheria | T50.A11 | T50.A12 | T50.A13 | T50.A14 | T50.A15 | T50.A16 |

**Additional Character May Be Required — Refer to the Tabular List for Character Selection**

▽ Subterms under main terms may continue to next column or page

| Substance | Poisoning, Accidental (unintentional) | Poisoning, Intentional Self-harm | Poisoning, Assault | Poisoning, Undetermined | Adverse Effect | Under-dosing |
|---|---|---|---|---|---|---|
| Vaccine — continued | | | | | | |
| pertussis — continued | | | | | | |
| with diphtheria — continued | | | | | | |
| and tetanus | T50.A11 | T50.A12 | T50.A13 | T50.A14 | T50.A15 | T50.A16 |
| with other component | T50.A11 | T50.A12 | T50.A13 | T50.A14 | T50.A15 | T50.A16 |
| plague | T50.A91 | T50.A92 | T50.A93 | T50.A94 | T50.A95 | T50.A96 |
| poliomyelitis | T50.B91 | T50.B92 | T50.B93 | T50.B94 | T50.B95 | T50.B96 |
| poliovirus | T50.B91 | T50.B92 | T50.B93 | T50.B94 | T50.B95 | T50.B96 |
| rabies | T50.B91 | T50.B92 | T50.B93 | T50.B94 | T50.B95 | T50.B96 |
| respiratory syncytial virus | T50.B91 | T50.B92 | T50.B93 | T50.B94 | T50.B95 | T50.B96 |
| rickettsial NEC | T50.A91 | T50.A92 | T50.A93 | T50.A94 | T50.A95 | T50.A96 |
| with | | | | | | |
| bacterial component | T50.A21 | T50.A22 | T50.A23 | T50.A24 | T50.A25 | T50.A26 |
| Rocky Mountain spotted | T50.A91 | T50.A92 | T50.A93 | T50.A94 | T50.A95 | T50.A96 |
| fever | | | | | | |
| rubella | T50.B91 | T50.B92 | T50.B93 | T50.B94 | T50.B95 | T50.B96 |
| sabin oral | T50.B91 | T50.B92 | T50.B93 | T50.B94 | T50.B95 | T50.B96 |
| smallpox | T50.B11 | T50.B12 | T50.B13 | T50.B14 | T50.B15 | T50.B16 |
| TAB | T50.A91 | T50.A92 | T50.A93 | T50.A94 | T50.A95 | T50.A96 |
| tetanus | T50.A91 | T50.A92 | T50.A93 | T50.A94 | T50.A95 | T50.A96 |
| typhoid | T50.A91 | T50.A92 | T50.A93 | T50.A94 | T50.A95 | T50.A96 |
| typhus | T50.A91 | T50.A92 | T50.A93 | T50.A94 | T50.A95 | T50.A96 |
| viral NEC | T50.B91 | T50.B92 | T50.B93 | T50.B94 | T50.B95 | T50.B96 |
| yellow fever | T50.B91 | T50.B92 | T50.B93 | T50.B94 | T50.B95 | T50.B96 |
| Vaccinia immune globulin | T50.Z11 | T50.Z12 | T50.Z13 | T50.Z14 | T50.Z15 | T50.Z16 |
| Vaginal contraceptives | T49.8X1 | T49.8X2 | T49.8X3 | T49.8X4 | T49.8X5 | T49.8X6 |
| Valerian | | | | | | |
| root | T42.6X1 | T42.6X2 | T42.6X3 | T42.6X4 | T42.6X5 | T42.6X6 |
| tincture | T42.6X1 | T42.6X2 | T42.6X3 | T42.6X4 | T42.6X5 | T42.6X6 |
| Valethamate bromide | T44.3X1 | T44.3X2 | T44.3X3 | T44.3X4 | T44.3X5 | T44.3X6 |
| Valisone | T49.0X1 | T49.0X2 | T49.0X3 | T49.0X4 | T49.0X5 | T49.0X6 |
| Valium | T42.4X1 | T42.4X2 | T42.4X3 | T42.4X4 | T42.4X5 | T42.4X6 |
| Valmid | T42.6X1 | T42.6X2 | T42.6X3 | T42.6X4 | T42.6X5 | T42.6X6 |
| Valnoctamide | T42.6X1 | T42.6X2 | T42.6X3 | T42.6X4 | T42.6X5 | T42.6X6 |
| Valproate (sodium) | T42.6X1 | T42.6X2 | T42.6X3 | T42.6X4 | T42.6X5 | T42.6X6 |
| Valproic acid | T42.6X1 | T42.6X2 | T42.6X3 | T42.6X4 | T42.6X5 | T42.6X6 |
| Valpromide | T42.6X1 | T42.6X2 | T42.6X3 | T42.6X4 | T42.6X5 | T42.6X6 |
| Vanadium | T56.891 | T56.892 | T56.893 | T56.894 | — | — |
| Vancomycin | T36.8X1 | T36.8X2 | T36.8X3 | T36.8X4 | T36.8X5 | T36.8X6 |
| Vapor — see also Gas | T59.91 | T59.92 | T59.93 | T59.94 | — | — |
| kiln (carbon monoxide) | T58.8X1 | T58.8X2 | T58.8X3 | T58.8X4 | — | — |
| lead — see lead | | | | | | |
| specified source NEC | T59.891 | T59.892 | T59.893 | T59.894 | — | — |
| Vardenafil | T46.7X1 | T46.7X2 | T46.7X3 | T46.7X4 | T46.7X5 | T46.7X6 |
| Varicose reduction drug | T46.8X1 | T46.8X2 | T46.8X3 | T46.8X4 | T46.8X5 | T46.8X6 |
| Varnish | T65.4X1 | T65.4X2 | T65.4X3 | T65.4X4 | — | — |
| cleaner | T52.91 | T52.92 | T52.93 | T52.94 | — | — |
| Vaseline | T49.3X1 | T49.3X2 | T49.3X3 | T49.3X4 | T49.3X5 | T49.3X6 |
| Vasodilan | T46.7X1 | T46.7X2 | T46.7X3 | T46.7X4 | T46.7X5 | T46.7X6 |
| Vasodilator | | | | | | |
| coronary NEC | T46.3X1 | T46.3X2 | T46.3X3 | T46.3X4 | T46.3X5 | T46.3X6 |
| peripheral NEC | T46.7X1 | T46.7X2 | T46.7X3 | T46.7X4 | T46.7X5 | T46.7X6 |
| Vasopressin | T38.891 | T38.892 | T38.893 | T38.894 | T38.895 | T38.896 |
| Vasopressor drugs | T38.891 | T38.892 | T38.893 | T38.894 | T38.895 | T38.896 |
| Vecuronium bromide | T48.1X1 | T48.1X2 | T48.1X3 | T48.1X4 | T48.1X5 | T48.1X6 |
| Vegetable extract, astringent | T49.2X1 | T49.2X2 | T49.2X3 | T49.2X4 | T49.2X5 | T49.2X6 |
| Venlafaxine | T43.211 | T43.212 | T43.213 | T43.214 | T43.215 | T43.216 |
| Venom, venomous (bite) (sting) | T63.91 | T63.92 | T63.93 | T63.94 | — | — |
| amphibian NEC | T63.831 | T63.832 | T63.833 | T63.834 | — | — |
| animal NEC | T63.891 | T63.892 | T63.893 | T63.894 | — | — |
| ant | T63.421 | T63.422 | T63.423 | T63.424 | — | — |
| arthropod NEC | T63.481 | T63.482 | T63.483 | T63.484 | — | — |
| bee | T63.441 | T63.442 | T63.443 | T63.444 | — | — |
| centipede | T63.411 | T63.412 | T63.413 | T63.414 | — | — |
| fish | T63.591 | T63.592 | T63.593 | T63.594 | — | — |
| frog | T63.811 | T63.812 | T63.813 | T63.814 | — | — |
| hornet | T63.451 | T63.452 | T63.453 | T63.454 | — | — |
| insect NEC | T63.481 | T63.482 | T63.483 | T63.484 | — | — |
| lizard | T63.121 | T63.122 | T63.123 | T63.124 | — | — |
| marine | | | | | | |
| animals | T63.691 | T63.692 | T63.693 | T63.694 | — | — |
| bluebottle | T63.611 | T63.612 | T63.613 | T63.614 | — | — |
| jellyfish NEC | T63.621 | T63.622 | T63.623 | T63.624 | — | — |
| Portugese Man-o-war | T63.611 | T63.612 | T63.613 | T63.614 | — | — |
| sea anemone | T63.631 | T63.632 | T63.633 | T63.634 | — | — |
| specified NEC | T63.691 | T63.692 | T63.693 | T63.694 | — | — |
| fish | T63.591 | T63.592 | T63.593 | T63.594 | — | — |
| plants | T63.711 | T63.712 | T63.713 | T63.714 | — | — |
| sting ray | T63.511 | T63.512 | T63.513 | T63.514 | — | — |
| millipede (tropical) | T63.411 | T63.412 | T63.413 | T63.414 | — | — |
| plant NEC | T63.791 | T63.792 | T63.793 | T63.794 | — | — |

| Substance | Poisoning, Accidental (unintentional) | Poisoning, Intentional Self-harm | Poisoning, Assault | Poisoning, Undetermined | Adverse Effect | Under-dosing |
|---|---|---|---|---|---|---|
| Venom, venomous — continued | | | | | | |
| plant — continued | | | | | | |
| marine | T63.711 | T63.712 | T63.713 | T63.714 | — | — |
| reptile | T63.191 | T63.192 | T63.193 | T63.194 | — | — |
| gila monster | T63.111 | T63.112 | T63.113 | T63.114 | — | — |
| lizard NEC | T63.121 | T63.122 | T63.123 | T63.124 | — | — |
| scorpion | T63.2X1 | T63.2X2 | T63.2X3 | T63.2X4 | — | — |
| snake | T63.001 | T63.002 | T63.003 | T63.004 | — | — |
| African NEC | T63.081 | T63.082 | T63.083 | T63.084 | — | — |
| American (North) (South) NEC | T63.061 | T63.062 | T63.063 | T63.064 | — | — |
| Asian | T63.081 | T63.082 | T63.083 | T63.084 | — | — |
| Australian | T63.071 | T63.072 | T63.073 | T63.074 | — | — |
| cobra | T63.041 | T63.042 | T63.043 | T63.044 | — | — |
| coral snake | T63.021 | T63.022 | T63.023 | T63.024 | — | — |
| rattlesnake | T63.011 | T63.012 | T63.013 | T63.014 | — | — |
| specified NEC | T63.091 | T63.092 | T63.093 | T63.094 | — | — |
| taipan | T63.031 | T63.032 | T63.033 | T63.034 | — | — |
| specified NEC | T63.891 | T63.892 | T63.893 | T63.894 | — | — |
| spider | T63.301 | T63.302 | T63.303 | T63.304 | — | — |
| black widow | T63.311 | T63.312 | T63.313 | T63.314 | — | — |
| brown recluse | T63.331 | T63.332 | T63.333 | T63.334 | — | — |
| specified NEC | T63.391 | T63.392 | T63.393 | T63.394 | — | — |
| tarantula | T63.321 | T63.322 | T63.323 | T63.324 | — | — |
| sting ray | T63.511 | T63.512 | T63.513 | T63.514 | — | — |
| toad | T63.821 | T63.822 | T63.823 | T63.824 | — | — |
| wasp | T63.461 | T63.462 | T63.463 | T63.464 | — | — |
| Venous sclerosing drug NEC | T46.8X1 | T46.8X2 | T46.8X3 | T46.8X4 | T46.8X5 | T46.8X6 |
| Ventolin — see Albuterol | | | | | | |
| Veramon | T42.3X1 | T42.3X2 | T42.3X3 | T42.3X4 | T42.3X5 | T42.3X6 |
| Verapamil | T46.1X1 | T46.1X2 | T46.1X3 | T46.1X4 | T46.1X5 | T46.1X6 |
| Veratrine | T46.5X1 | T46.5X2 | T46.5X3 | T46.5X4 | T46.5X5 | T46.5X6 |
| Veratrum | | | | | | |
| album | T62.2X1 | T62.2X2 | T62.2X3 | T62.2X4 | — | — |
| alkaloids | T46.5X1 | T46.5X2 | T46.5X3 | T46.5X4 | T46.5X5 | T46.5X6 |
| viride | T62.2X1 | T62.2X2 | T62.2X3 | T62.2X4 | — | — |
| Verdigris | T60.3X1 | T60.3X2 | T60.3X3 | T60.3X4 | — | — |
| Veronal | T42.3X1 | T42.3X2 | T42.3X3 | T42.3X4 | T42.3X5 | T42.3X6 |
| Veroxil | T37.4X1 | T37.4X2 | T37.4X3 | T37.4X4 | T37.4X5 | T37.4X6 |
| Versenate | T50.6X1 | T50.6X2 | T50.6X3 | T50.6X4 | T50.6X5 | T50.6X6 |
| Versidyne | T39.8X1 | T39.8X2 | T39.8X3 | T39.8X4 | T39.8X5 | T39.8X6 |
| Vetrabutine | T48.0X1 | T48.0X2 | T48.0X3 | T48.0X4 | T48.0X5 | T48.0X6 |
| Vidarabine | T37.5X1 | T37.5X2 | T37.5X3 | T37.5X4 | T37.5X5 | T37.5X6 |
| Vienna | | | | | | |
| green | T57.0X1 | T57.0X2 | T57.0X3 | T57.0X4 | — | — |
| insecticide | T60.2X1 | T60.2X2 | T60.2X3 | T60.2X4 | — | — |
| red | T57.0X1 | T57.0X2 | T57.0X3 | T57.0X4 | — | — |
| pharmaceutical dye | T50.991 | T50.992 | T50.993 | T50.994 | T50.995 | T50.996 |
| Vigabatrin | T42.6X1 | T42.6X2 | T42.6X3 | T42.6X4 | T42.6X5 | T42.6X6 |
| Viloxazine | T43.291 | T43.292 | T43.293 | T43.294 | T43.295 | T43.296 |
| Viminol | T39.8X1 | T39.8X2 | T39.8X3 | T39.8X4 | T39.8X5 | T39.8X6 |
| Vinbarbital, vinbarbitone | T42.3X1 | T42.3X2 | T42.3X3 | T42.3X4 | T42.3X5 | T42.3X6 |
| Vinblastine | T45.1X1 | T45.1X2 | T45.1X3 | T45.1X4 | T45.1X5 | T45.1X6 |
| Vinburnine | T46.7X1 | T46.7X2 | T46.7X3 | T46.7X4 | T46.7X5 | T46.7X6 |
| Vincamine | T45.1X1 | T45.1X2 | T45.1X3 | T45.1X4 | T45.1X5 | T45.1X6 |
| Vincristine | T45.1X1 | T45.1X2 | T45.1X3 | T45.1X4 | T45.1X5 | T45.1X6 |
| Vindesine | T45.1X1 | T45.1X2 | T45.1X3 | T45.1X4 | T45.1X5 | T45.1X6 |
| Vinesthene, vinethene | T41.0X1 | T41.0X2 | T41.0X3 | T41.0X4 | T41.0X5 | T41.0X6 |
| Vinorelbine tartrate | T45.1X1 | T45.1X2 | T45.1X3 | T45.1X4 | T45.1X5 | T45.1X6 |
| Vinpocetine | T46.7X1 | T46.7X2 | T46.7X3 | T46.7X4 | T46.7X5 | T46.7X6 |
| Vinyl | | | | | | |
| acetate | T65.891 | T65.892 | T65.893 | T65.894 | — | — |
| bital | T42.3X1 | T42.3X2 | T42.3X3 | T42.3X4 | T42.3X5 | T42.3X6 |
| bromide | T65.891 | T65.892 | T65.893 | T65.894 | — | — |
| chloride | T59.891 | T59.892 | T59.893 | T59.894 | — | — |
| ether | T41.0X1 | T41.0X2 | T41.0X3 | T41.0X4 | T41.0X5 | T41.0X6 |
| Vinylbital | T42.3X1 | T42.3X2 | T42.3X3 | T42.3X4 | T42.3X5 | T42.3X6 |
| Vinylidene chloride | T65.891 | T65.892 | T65.893 | T65.894 | — | — |
| Vioform | T37.8X1 | T37.8X2 | T37.8X3 | T37.8X4 | T37.8X5 | T37.8X6 |
| topical | T49.0X1 | T49.0X2 | T49.0X3 | T49.0X4 | T49.0X5 | T49.0X6 |
| Viomycin | T36.8X1 | T36.8X2 | T36.8X3 | T36.8X4 | T36.8X5 | T36.8X6 |
| Viosterol | T45.2X1 | T45.2X2 | T45.2X3 | T45.2X4 | T45.2X5 | T45.2X6 |
| Viper (venom) | T63.091 | T63.092 | T63.093 | T63.094 | | |
| Viprynium | T37.4X1 | T37.4X2 | T37.4X3 | T37.4X4 | T37.4X5 | T37.4X6 |
| Viquidil | T46.7X1 | T46.7X2 | T46.7X3 | T46.7X4 | T46.7X5 | T46.7X6 |
| Viral vaccine NEC | T50.B91 | T50.B92 | T50.B93 | T50.B94 | T50.B95 | T50.B96 |
| Virginiamycin | T36.8X1 | T36.8X2 | T36.8X3 | T36.8X4 | T36.8X5 | T36.8X6 |
| Virugon | T37.5X1 | T37.5X2 | T37.5X3 | T37.5X4 | T37.5X5 | T37.5X6 |
| Viscous agent | T50.901 | T50.902 | T50.903 | T50.904 | T50.905 | T50.906 |
| Visine | T49.5X1 | T49.5X2 | T49.5X3 | T49.5X4 | T49.5X5 | T49.5X6 |
| Visnadine | T46.3X1 | T46.3X2 | T46.3X3 | T46.3X4 | T46.3X5 | T46.3X6 |
| **Vitamin NEC** | T45.2X1 | T45.2X2 | T45.2X3 | T45.2X4 | T45.2X5 | T45.2X6 |

| Substance | Poisoning, Accidental (unintentional) | Poisoning, Intentional Self-harm | Poisoning, Assault | Poisoning, Undetermined | Adverse Effect | Underdosing |
|---|---|---|---|---|---|---|
| **Vitamin** — *continued* | | | | | | |
| A | T45.2X1 | T45.2X2 | T45.2X3 | T45.2X4 | T45.2X5 | T45.2X6 |
| B1 | T45.2X1 | T45.2X2 | T45.2X3 | T45.2X4 | T45.2X5 | T45.2X6 |
| B2 | T45.2X1 | T45.2X2 | T45.2X3 | T45.2X4 | T45.2X5 | T45.2X6 |
| B6 | T45.2X1 | T45.2X2 | T45.2X3 | T45.2X4 | T45.2X5 | T45.2X6 |
| B12 | T45.2X1 | T45.2X2 | T45.2X3 | T45.2X4 | T45.2X5 | T45.2X6 |
| B15 | T45.2X1 | T45.2X2 | T45.2X3 | T45.2X4 | T45.2X5 | T45.2X6 |
| B NEC | T45.2X1 | T45.2X2 | T45.2X3 | T45.2X4 | T45.2X5 | T45.2X6 |
| nicotinic acid | T46.7X1 | T46.7X2 | T46.7X3 | T46.7X4 | T46.7X5 | T46.7X6 |
| C | T45.2X1 | T45.2X2 | T45.2X3 | T45.2X4 | T45.2X5 | T45.2X6 |
| D | T45.2X1 | T45.2X2 | T45.2X3 | T45.2X4 | T45.2X5 | T45.2X6 |
| D2 | T45.2X1 | T45.2X2 | T45.2X3 | T45.2X4 | T45.2X5 | T45.2X6 |
| D3 | T45.2X1 | T45.2X2 | T45.2X3 | T45.2X4 | T45.2X5 | T45.2X6 |
| E | T45.2X1 | T45.2X2 | T45.2X3 | T45.2X4 | T45.2X5 | T45.2X6 |
| E acetate | T45.2X1 | T45.2X2 | T45.2X3 | T45.2X4 | T45.2X5 | T45.2X6 |
| hematopoietic | T45.8X1 | T45.8X2 | T45.8X3 | T45.8X4 | T45.8X5 | T45.8X6 |
| K1 | T45.7X1 | T45.7X2 | T45.7X3 | T45.7X4 | T45.7X5 | T45.7X6 |
| K2 | T45.7X1 | T45.7X2 | T45.7X3 | T45.7X4 | T45.7X5 | T45.7X6 |
| K NEC | T45.7X1 | T45.7X2 | T45.7X3 | T45.7X4 | T45.7X5 | T45.7X6 |
| PP | T45.2X1 | T45.2X2 | T45.2X3 | T45.2X4 | T45.2X5 | T45.2X6 |
| ulceroprotectant | T47.1X1 | T47.1X2 | T47.1X3 | T47.1X4 | T47.1X5 | T47.1X6 |
| **Vleminckx's solution** | T49.4X1 | T49.4X2 | T49.4X3 | T49.4X4 | T49.4X5 | T49.4X6 |
| **Voltaren** — *see* Diclofenac | | | | | | |
| sodium | | | | | | |
| **Warfarin** | T45.511 | T45.512 | T45.513 | T45.514 | T45.515 | T45.516 |
| rodenticide | T45.511 | T45.512 | T45.513 | T45.514 | T45.515 | T45.516 |
| sodium | T45.511 | T45.512 | T45.513 | T45.514 | T45.515 | T45.516 |
| **Wasp** (sting) | T63.461 | T63.462 | T63.463 | T63.464 | — | — |
| **Water** | | | | | | |
| balance drug | T50.3X1 | T50.3X2 | T50.3X3 | T50.3X4 | T50.3X5 | T50.3X6 |
| distilled | T50.3X1 | T50.3X2 | T50.3X3 | T50.3X4 | T50.3X5 | T50.3X6 |
| gas — *see* Gas, water | | | | | | |
| incomplete combustion of — | | | | | | |
| *see* Carbon, monoxide, | | | | | | |
| fuel, utility | | | | | | |
| hemlock | T62.2X1 | T62.2X2 | T62.2X3 | T62.2X4 | — | — |
| moccasin (venom) | T63.061 | T63.062 | T63.063 | T63.064 | — | — |
| purified | T50.3X1 | T50.3X2 | T50.3X3 | T50.3X4 | T50.3X5 | T50.3X6 |
| **Wax** (paraffin) (petroleum) | T52.0X1 | T52.0X2 | T52.0X3 | T52.0X4 | — | — |
| automobile | T65.891 | T65.892 | T65.893 | T65.894 | — | — |
| floor | T52.0X1 | T52.0X2 | T52.0X3 | T52.0X4 | — | — |
| **Weed killers NEC** | T60.3X1 | T60.3X2 | T60.3X3 | T60.3X4 | — | — |
| **Welldorm** | T42.6X1 | T42.6X2 | T42.6X3 | T42.6X4 | T42.6X5 | T42.6X6 |
| **White** | | | | | | |
| arsenic | T57.0X1 | T57.0X2 | T57.0X3 | T57.0X4 | — | — |
| hellebore | T62.2X1 | T62.2X2 | T62.2X3 | T62.2X4 | — | — |
| lotion (keratolytic) | T49.4X1 | T49.4X2 | T49.4X3 | T49.4X4 | T49.4X5 | T49.4X6 |
| spirit | T52.0X1 | T52.0X2 | T52.0X3 | T52.0X4 | — | — |
| **Whitewash** | T65.891 | T65.892 | T65.893 | T65.894 | — | — |
| **Whole blood** (human) | T45.8X1 | T45.8X2 | T45.8X3 | T45.8X4 | T45.8X5 | T45.8X6 |
| **Wild** | | | | | | |
| black cherry | T62.2X1 | T62.2X2 | T62.2X3 | T62.2X4 | — | — |
| poisonous plants NEC | T62.2X1 | T62.2X2 | T62.2X3 | T62.2X4 | — | — |
| **Window cleaning fluid** | T65.891 | T65.892 | T65.893 | T65.894 | — | — |
| **Wintergreen** (oil) | T49.3X1 | T49.3X2 | T49.3X3 | T49.3X4 | T49.3X5 | T49.3X6 |
| **Wisterine** | T62.2X1 | T62.2X2 | T62.2X3 | T62.2X4 | — | — |
| **Witch hazel** | T49.2X1 | T49.2X2 | T49.2X3 | T49.2X4 | T49.2X5 | T49.2X6 |
| **Wood alcohol or spirit** | T51.1X1 | T51.1X2 | T51.1X3 | T51.1X4 | — | — |
| **Wool fat** (hydrous) | T49.3X1 | T49.3X2 | T49.3X3 | T49.3X4 | T49.3X5 | T49.3X6 |
| **Woorali** | T48.1X1 | T48.1X2 | T48.1X3 | T48.1X4 | T48.1X5 | T48.1X6 |
| **Wormseed, American** | T37.4X1 | T37.4X2 | T37.4X3 | T37.4X4 | T37.4X5 | T37.4X6 |
| **Xamoterol** | T44.5X1 | T44.5X2 | T44.5X3 | T44.5X4 | T44.5X5 | T44.5X6 |
| **Xanthine diuretics** | T50.2X1 | T50.2X2 | T50.2X3 | T50.2X4 | T50.2X5 | T50.2X6 |
| **Xanthinol nicotinate** | T46.7X1 | T46.7X2 | T46.7X3 | T46.7X4 | T46.7X5 | T46.7X6 |
| **Xanthotoxin** | T49.3X1 | T49.3X2 | T49.3X3 | T49.3X4 | T49.3X5 | T49.3X6 |
| **Xantinol nicotinate** | T46.7X1 | T46.7X2 | T46.7X3 | T46.7X4 | T46.7X5 | T46.7X6 |
| **Xantocillin** | T36.0X1 | T36.0X2 | T36.0X3 | T36.0X4 | T36.0X5 | T36.0X6 |
| **Xenon** (127Xe) (133Xe) | T50.8X1 | T50.8X2 | T50.8X3 | T50.8X4 | T50.8X5 | T50.8X6 |
| **Xenysalate** | T49.4X1 | T49.4X2 | T49.4X3 | T49.4X4 | T49.4X5 | T49.4X6 |
| **Xibornol** | T37.8X1 | T37.8X2 | T37.8X3 | T37.8X4 | T37.8X5 | T37.8X6 |
| **Xigris** | T45.511 | T45.512 | T45.513 | T45.514 | T45.515 | T45.516 |
| **Xipamide** | T50.2X1 | T50.2X2 | T50.2X3 | T50.2X4 | T50.2X5 | T50.2X6 |
| **Xylene** (vapor) | T52.2X1 | T52.2X2 | T52.2X3 | T52.2X4 | — | — |
| **Xylocaine** (infiltration) (topical) | T41.3X1 | T41.3X2 | T41.3X3 | T41.3X4 | T41.3X5 | T41.3X6 |
| nerve block (peripheral) (plexus) | T41.3X1 | T41.3X2 | T41.3X3 | T41.3X4 | T41.3X5 | T41.3X6 |
| spinal | T41.3X1 | T41.3X2 | T41.3X3 | T41.3X4 | T41.3X5 | T41.3X6 |
| **Xylol** (vapor) | T52.2X1 | T52.2X2 | T52.2X3 | T52.2X4 | — | — |
| **Xylometazoline** | T48.5X1 | T48.5X2 | T48.5X3 | T48.5X4 | T48.5X5 | T48.5X6 |
| **Yeast** | T45.2X1 | T45.2X2 | T45.2X3 | T45.2X4 | T45.2X5 | T45.2X6 |
| dried | T45.2X1 | T45.2X2 | T45.2X3 | T45.2X4 | T45.2X5 | T45.2X6 |

| Substance | Poisoning, Accidental (unintentional) | Poisoning, Intentional Self-harm | Poisoning, Assault | Poisoning, Undetermined | Adverse Effect | Underdosing |
|---|---|---|---|---|---|---|
| **Yellow** | | | | | | |
| fever vaccine | T50.B91 | T50.B92 | T50.B93 | T50.B94 | T50.B95 | T50.B96 |
| jasmine | T62.2X1 | T62.2X2 | T62.2X3 | T62.2X4 | | |
| phenolphthalein | T47.2X1 | T47.2X2 | T47.2X3 | T47.2X4 | T47.2X5 | T47.2X6 |
| **Yew** | T62.2X1 | T62.2X2 | T62.2X3 | T62.2X4 | | |
| **Yohimbic acid** | T40.991 | T40.992 | T40.993 | T40.994 | T40.995 | T40.996 |
| **Zactane** | T39.8X1 | T39.8X2 | T39.8X3 | T39.8X4 | T39.8X5 | T39.8X6 |
| **Zalcitabine** | T37.5X1 | T37.5X2 | T37.5X3 | T37.5X4 | T37.5X5 | T37.5X6 |
| **Zaroxolyn** | T50.2X1 | T50.2X2 | T50.2X3 | T50.2X4 | T50.2X5 | T50.2X6 |
| **Zephiran** (topical) | T49.0X1 | T49.0X2 | T49.0X3 | T49.0X4 | T49.0X5 | T49.0X6 |
| ophthalmic preparation | T49.5X1 | T49.5X2 | T49.5X3 | T49.5X4 | T49.5X5 | T49.5X6 |
| **Zeranol** | T38.7X1 | T38.7X2 | T38.7X3 | T38.7X4 | T38.7X5 | T38.7X6 |
| **Zerone** | T51.1X1 | T51.1X2 | T51.1X3 | T51.1X4 | — | — |
| **Zidovudine** | T37.5X1 | T37.5X2 | T37.5X3 | T37.5X4 | T37.5X5 | T37.5X6 |
| **Zimeldine** | T43.221 | T43.222 | T43.223 | T43.224 | T43.225 | T43.226 |
| **Zinc** (compounds) (fumes) (vapor) | T56.5X1 | T56.5X2 | T56.5X3 | T56.5X4 | — | — |
| **NEC** | | | | | | |
| anti-infectives | T49.0X1 | T49.0X2 | T49.0X3 | T49.0X4 | T49.0X5 | T49.0X6 |
| antivaricose | T46.8X1 | T46.8X2 | T46.8X3 | T46.8X4 | T46.8X5 | T46.8X6 |
| bacitracin | T49.0X1 | T49.0X2 | T49.0X3 | T49.0X4 | T49.0X5 | T49.0X6 |
| chloride (mouthwash) | T49.6X1 | T49.6X2 | T49.6X3 | T49.6X4 | T49.6X5 | T49.6X6 |
| chromate | T56.5X1 | T56.5X2 | T56.5X3 | T56.5X4 | — | — |
| gelatin | T49.3X1 | T49.3X2 | T49.3X3 | T49.3X4 | T49.3X5 | T49.3X6 |
| oxide | T49.3X1 | T49.3X2 | T49.3X3 | T49.3X4 | T49.3X5 | T49.3X6 |
| plaster | T49.3X1 | T49.3X2 | T49.3X3 | T49.3X4 | T49.3X5 | T49.3X6 |
| peroxide | T49.0X1 | T49.0X2 | T49.0X3 | T49.0X4 | T49.0X5 | T49.0X6 |
| pesticides | T56.5X1 | T56.5X2 | T56.5X3 | T56.5X4 | — | — |
| phosphide | T60.4X1 | T60.4X2 | T60.4X3 | T60.4X4 | — | — |
| pyrithionate | T49.4X1 | T49.4X2 | T49.4X3 | T49.4X4 | T49.4X5 | T49.4X6 |
| stearate | T49.3X1 | T49.3X2 | T49.3X3 | T49.3X4 | T49.3X5 | T49.3X6 |
| sulfate | T49.5X1 | T49.5X2 | T49.5X3 | T49.5X4 | T49.5X5 | T49.5X6 |
| ENT agent | T49.6X1 | T49.6X2 | T49.6X3 | T49.6X4 | T49.6X5 | T49.6X6 |
| ophthalmic solution | T49.5X1 | T49.5X2 | T49.5X3 | T49.5X4 | T49.5X5 | T49.5X6 |
| topical NEC | T49.0X1 | T49.0X2 | T49.0X3 | T49.0X4 | T49.0X5 | T49.0X6 |
| undecylenate | T49.0X1 | T49.0X2 | T49.0X3 | T49.0X4 | T49.0X5 | T49.0X6 |
| **Zineb** | T60.0X1 | T60.0X2 | T60.0X3 | T60.0X4 | — | — |
| **Zinostatin** | T45.1X1 | T45.1X2 | T45.1X3 | T45.1X4 | T45.1X5 | T45.1X6 |
| **Zipeprol** | T48.3X1 | T48.3X2 | T48.3X3 | T48.3X4 | T48.3X5 | T48.3X6 |
| **Zofenopril** | T46.4X1 | T46.4X2 | T46.4X3 | T46.4X4 | T46.4X5 | T46.4X6 |
| **Zolpidem** | T42.6X1 | T42.6X2 | T42.6X3 | T42.6X4 | T42.6X5 | T42.6X6 |
| **Zomepirac** | T39.391 | T39.392 | T39.393 | T39.394 | T39.395 | T39.396 |
| **Zopiclone** | T42.6X1 | T42.6X2 | T42.6X3 | T42.6X4 | T42.6X5 | T42.6X6 |
| **Zorubicin** | T45.1X1 | T45.1X2 | T45.1X3 | T45.1X4 | T45.1X5 | T45.1X6 |
| **Zotepine** | T43.591 | T43.592 | T43.593 | T43.594 | | T43.596 |
| **Zovant** | T45.511 | T45.512 | T45.513 | T45.514 | T45.515 | T45.516 |
| **Zoxazolamine** | T42.8X1 | T42.8X2 | T42.8X3 | T42.8X4 | T42.8X5 | T42.8X6 |
| **Zuclopenthixol** | T43.4X1 | T43.4X2 | T43.4X3 | T43.4X4 | T43.4X5 | T43.4X6 |
| **Zygadenus** (venenosus) | T62.2X1 | T62.2X2 | T62.2X3 | T62.2X4 | — | — |
| **Zyprexa** | T43.591 | T43.592 | T43.593 | T43.594 | T43.595 | T43.596 |

Additional Character May Be Required — Refer to the Tabular List for Character Selection ▽ Subterms under main terms may continue to next column or page

# A

**Abandonment** (causing exposure to weather conditions) (with intent to injure or kill) NEC X58 ☑
**Abuse** (adult) (child) (mental) (physical) (sexual) X58 ☑
**Accident** (to) X58 ☑
 aircraft (in transit) (powered) (*see also* Accident, transport, aircraft)
  due to, caused by cataclysm — *see* Forces of nature, by type
 animal-drawn vehicle — *see* Accident, transport, animal-drawn vehicle occupant
 animal-rider — *see* Accident, transport, animal-rider
 automobile — *see* Accident, transport, car occupant
 bare foot water skier V94.4 ☑
 boat, boating (*see also* Accident, watercraft)
  striking swimmer
   powered V94.11 ☑
   unpowered V94.12 ☑
 bus — *see* Accident, transport, bus occupant
 cable car, not on rails V98.0 ☑
  on rails — *see* Accident, transport, streetcar occupant
 car — *see* Accident, transport, car occupant
 caused by, due to
  animal NEC W64 ☑
  chain hoist W24.0 ☑
  cold (excessive) — *see* Exposure, cold
  corrosive liquid, substance — *see* Table of Drugs and Chemicals
  cutting or piercing instrument — *see* Contact, with, by type of instrument
  drive belt W24.0 ☑
  electric
   current — *see* Exposure, electric current
   motor (*see also* Contact, with, by type of machine) W31.3 ☑
   current (of) W86.8 ☑
  environmental factor NEC X58 ☑
  explosive material — *see* Explosion
  fire, flames — *see* Exposure, fire
  firearm missile — *see* Discharge, firearm by type
  heat (excessive) — *see* Heat
  hot — *see* Contact, with, hot
  ignition — *see* Ignition
  lifting device W24.0 ☑
  lightning — *see* subcategory T75.0 ☑
   causing fire — *see* Exposure, fire
  machine, machinery — *see* Contact, with, by type of machine
  natural factor NEC X58 ☑
  pulley (block) W24.0 ☑
  radiation — *see* Radiation
  steam X13.1 ☑
   inhalation X13.0 ☑
   pipe X16 ☑
  thunderbolt — *see* subcategory T75.0 ☑
   causing fire — *see* Exposure, fire
  transmission device W24.1 ☑
 coach — *see* Accident, transport, bus occupant
 coal car — *see* Accident, transport, industrial vehicle occupant
 diving (*see also* Fall, into, water)
  with
   drowning or submersion — *see* Drowning
 forklift — *see* Accident, transport, industrial vehicle occupant
 heavy transport vehicle NOS — *see* Accident, transport, truck occupant
 ice yacht V98.2 ☑
 in
  medical, surgical procedure
   as, or due to misadventure — *see* Misadventure
   causing an abnormal reaction or later complication without mention of misadventure (*see also* Complication of or following, by type of procedure) Y84.9
 land yacht V98.1 ☑
 late effect of — *see* W00-X58 with 7th character S
 logging car — *see* Accident, transport, industrial vehicle occupant
 machine, machinery (*see also* Contact, with, by type of machine)
  on board watercraft V93.69 ☑
   explosion — *see* Explosion, in, watercraft

**Accident** — *continued*
 machine, machinery (*see also* Contact, with, by type of machine) — *continued*
  on board watercraft — *continued*
   fire — *see* Burn, on board watercraft
   powered craft V93.63 ☑
    ferry boat V93.61 ☑
    fishing boat V93.62 ☑
    jetskis V93.63 ☑
    liner V93.61 ☑
    merchant ship V93.60 ☑
    passenger ship V93.61 ☑
    sailboat V93.64 ☑
 mine tram — *see* Accident, transport, industrial vehicle occupant
 mobility scooter (motorized) — *see* Accident, transport, pedestrian, conveyance, specified type NEC
 motor scooter — *see* Accident, transport, motorcyclist
 motor vehicle NOS (traffic) (*see also* Accident, transport) V89.2 ☑
  nontraffic V89.0 ☑
  three-wheeled NOS — *see* Accident, transport, three-wheeled motor vehicle occupant
 motorcycle NOS — *see* Accident, transport, motorcyclist
 nonmotor vehicle NOS (nontraffic) (*see also* Accident, transport) V89.1 ☑
  traffic NOS V89.3 ☑
 nontraffic (victim's mode of transport NOS) V88.9 ☑
  collision (between) V88.7 ☑
   bus and truck V88.5 ☑
   car and:
    bus V88.3 ☑
    pickup V88.2 ☑
    three-wheeled motor vehicle V88.0 ☑
    train V88.6 ☑
    truck V88.4 ☑
    two-wheeled motor vehicle V88.0 ☑
    van V88.2 ☑
   specified vehicle NEC and:
    three-wheeled motor vehicle V88.1 ☑
    two-wheeled motor vehicle V88.1 ☑
  known mode of transport — *see* Accident, transport, by type of vehicle
  noncollision V88.8 ☑
 on board watercraft V93.89 ☑
  powered craft V93.83 ☑
   ferry boat V93.81 ☑
   fishing boat V93.82 ☑
   jetskis V93.83 ☑
   liner V93.81 ☑
   merchant ship V93.80 ☑
   passenger ship V93.81 ☑
  unpowered craft V93.88 ☑
   canoe V93.85 ☑
   inflatable V93.86 ☑
    in tow
     recreational V94.31 ☑
     specified NEC V94.32 ☑
   kayak V93.85 ☑
   sailboat V93.84 ☑
   surf-board V93.88 ☑
   water skis V93.87 ☑
   windsurfer V93.88 ☑
 parachutist V97.29 ☑
  entangled in object V97.21 ☑
  injured on landing V97.22 ☑
 pedal cycle — *see* Accident, transport, pedal cyclist
 pedestrian (on foot)
  with
   another pedestrian W51 ☑
    with fall W03 ☑
     due to ice or snow W00.0 ☑
    on pedestrian conveyance NEC V00.09 ☑
   roller skater (in-line) V00.01 ☑
   skate boarder V00.02 ☑
   transport vehicle — *see* Accident, transport
  on pedestrian conveyance — *see* Accident, transport, pedestrian, conveyance
 pick-up truck or van — *see* Accident, transport, pickup truck occupant
 quarry truck — *see* Accident, transport, industrial vehicle occupant
 railway vehicle (any) (in motion) — *see* Accident, transport, railway vehicle occupant
  due to cataclysm — *see* Forces of nature, by type

**Accident** — *continued*
 scooter (non-motorized) — *see* Accident, transport, pedestrian, conveyance, scooter
 sequelae of — *see* categories W00-X58 with 7th character S
 skateboard — *see* Accident, transport, pedestrian, conveyance, skateboard
 ski(ing) — *see* Accident, transport, pedestrian, conveyance
  lift V98.3 ☑
 specified cause NEC X58 ☑
 streetcar — *see* Accident, transport, streetcar occupant
 traffic (victim's mode of transport NOS) V87.9 ☑
  collision (between) V87.7 ☑
   bus and truck V87.5 ☑
   car and:
    bus V87.3 ☑
    pickup V87.2 ☑
    three-wheeled motor vehicle V87.0 ☑
    train V87.6 ☑
    truck V87.4 ☑
    two-wheeled motor vehicle V87.0 ☑
    van V87.2 ☑
   specified vehicle NEC and:
    three-wheeled motor vehicle V87.1 ☑
    two-wheeled motor vehicle V87.1 ☑
  known mode of transport — *see* Accident, transport, by type of vehicle
  noncollision V87.8 ☑
 transport (involving injury to) V99 ☑
  18 wheeler — *see* Accident, transport, truck occupant
  agricultural vehicle occupant (nontraffic) V84.9 ☑
   driver V84.5 ☑
   hanger-on V84.7 ☑
   passenger V84.6 ☑
   traffic V84.3 ☑
    driver V84.0 ☑
    hanger-on V84.2 ☑
    passenger V84.1 ☑
   while boarding or alighting V84.4 ☑
  aircraft NEC V97.89 ☑
   military NEC V97.818 ☑
    with civlian aircraft V97.810 ☑
    civilian injured by V97.811 ☑
   occupant injured (in)
    nonpowered craft accident V96.9 ☑
     balloon V96.00 ☑
      collision V96.03 ☑
      crash V96.01 ☑
      explosion V96.05 ☑
      fire V96.04 ☑
      forced landing V96.02 ☑
      specified type NEC V96.09 ☑
     glider V96.20 ☑
      collision V96.23 ☑
      crash V96.21 ☑
      explosion V96.25 ☑
      fire V96.24 ☑
      forced landing V96.22 ☑
      specified type NEC V96.29 ☑
     hang glider V96.10 ☑
      collision V96.13 ☑
      crash V96.11 ☑
      explosion V96.15 ☑
      fire V96.14 ☑
      forced landing V96.12 ☑
      specified type NEC V96.19 ☑
     specified craft NEC V96.8 ☑
    powered craft accident V95.9 ☑
     fixed wing NEC
      commercial V95.30 ☑
       collision V95.33 ☑
       crash V95.31 ☑
       explosion V95.35 ☑
       fire V95.34 ☑
       forced landing V95.32 ☑
       specified type NEC V95.39 ☑
      private V95.20 ☑
       collision V95.23 ☑
       crash V95.21 ☑
       explosion V95.25 ☑
       fire V95.24 ☑
       forced landing V95.22 ☑
       specified type NEC V95.29 ☑
     glider V95.10 ☑

**Accident** — *continued*
  transport — *continued*
    aircraft — *continued*
      occupant injured — *continued*
        powered craft accident — *continued*
          glider — *continued*
            collision V95.13 ☑
            crash V95.11 ☑
            explosion V95.15 ☑
            fire V95.14 ☑
            forced landing V95.12 ☑
            specified type NEC V95.19 ☑
          helicopter V95.00 ☑
            collision V95.03 ☑
            crash V95.01 ☑
            explosion V95.05 ☑
            fire V95.04 ☑
            forced landing V95.02 ☑
            specified type NEC V95.09 ☑
          spacecraft V95.40 ☑
            collision V95.43 ☑
            crash V95.41 ☑
            explosion V95.45 ☑
            fire V95.44 ☑
            forced landing V95.42 ☑
            specified type NEC V95.49 ☑
          specified craft NEC V95.8 ☑
          ultralight V95.10 ☑
            collision V95.13 ☑
            crash V95.11 ☑
            explosion V95.15 ☑
            fire V95.14 ☑
            forced landing V95.12 ☑
            specified type NEC V95.19 ☑
        specified accident NEC V97.0 ☑
        while boarding or alighting V97.1 ☑
      person (injured by)
        falling from, in or on aircraft V97.0 ☑
        machinery on aircraft V97.89 ☑
        on ground with aircraft involvement
          V97.39 ☑
        rotating propeller V97.32 ☑
        struck by object falling from aircraft
          V97.31 ☑
        sucked into aircraft jet V97.33 ☑
        while boarding or alighting aircraft V97.1 ☑
      airport (battery-powered) passenger vehicle —
        *see* Accident, transport, industrial vehicle
        occupant
      all-terrain vehicle occupant (nontraffic) V86.95 ☑
        driver V86.55 ☑
        dune buggy — *see* Accident, transport, dune
          buggy occupant
        hanger-on V86.75 ☑
        passenger V86.65 ☑
        snowmobile — *see* Accident, transport, snow-
          mobile occupant
        specified type NEC V86.99 ☑
        traffic V86.35 ☑
          driver V86.05 ☑
          hanger-on V86.25 ☑
          passenger V86.15 ☑
        while boarding or alighting V86.45 ☑
      ambulance occupant (traffic) V86.31 ☑
        driver V86.01 ☑
        hanger-on V86.21 ☑
        nontraffic V86.91 ☑
          driver V86.51 ☑
          hanger-on V86.71 ☑
          passenger V86.61 ☑
        passenger V86.11 ☑
        while boarding or alighting V86.41 ☑
      animal-drawn vehicle occupant (in) V80.929 ☑
        collision (with)
          animal V80.12 ☑
            being ridden V80.711 ☑
          animal-drawn vehicle V80.721 ☑
          bus V80.42 ☑
          car V80.42 ☑
          fixed or stationary object V80.82 ☑
          military vehicle V80.920 ☑
          nonmotor vehicle V80.791 ☑
          pedal cycle V80.22 ☑
          pedestrian V80.12 ☑
          pickup V80.42 ☑
          railway train or vehicle V80.62 ☑

**Accident** — *continued*
  transport — *continued*
    animal-drawn vehicle occupant — *continued*
      collision — *continued*
        specified motor vehicle NEC V80.52 ☑
        streetcar V80.731 ☑
        truck V80.42 ☑
        two- or three-wheeled motor vehicle
          V80.32 ☑
        van V80.42 ☑
      noncollision V80.02 ☑
      specified circumstance NEC V80.928 ☑
    animal-rider V80.919 ☑
      collision (with)
        animal V80.11 ☑
          being ridden V80.710 ☑
        animal-drawn vehicle V80.720 ☑
        bus V80.41 ☑
        car V80.41 ☑
        fixed or stationary object V80.81 ☑
        military vehicle V80.910 ☑
        nonmotor vehicle V80.790 ☑
        pedal cycle V80.21 ☑
        pedestrian V80.11 ☑
        pickup V80.41 ☑
        railway train or vehicle V80.61 ☑
        specified motor vehicle NEC V80.51 ☑
        streetcar V80.730 ☑
        truck V80.41 ☑
        two- or three-wheeled motor vehicle
          V80.31 ☑
        van V80.41 ☑
      noncollision V80.018 ☑
        specified as horse rider V80.010 ☑
      specified circumstance NEC V80.918 ☑
    armored car — *see* Accident, transport, truck occu-
      pant
    battery-powered truck (baggage) (mail) — *see*
      Accident, transport, industrial vehicle occu-
      pant
    bus occupant V79.9 ☑
      collision (with)
        animal (traffic) V70.9 ☑
          being ridden (traffic) V76.9 ☑
            nontraffic V76.3 ☑
            while boarding or alighting V76.4 ☑
          nontraffic V70.3 ☑
          while boarding or alighting V70.4 ☑
        animal-drawn vehicle (traffic) V76.9 ☑
          nontraffic V76.3 ☑
          while boarding or alighting V76.4 ☑
        bus (traffic) V74.9 ☑
          nontraffic V74.3 ☑
          while boarding or alighting V74.4 ☑
        car (traffic) V73.9 ☑
          nontraffic V73.3 ☑
          while boarding or alighting V73.4 ☑
        motor vehicle NOS (traffic) V79.60 ☑
          nontraffic V79.20 ☑
          specified type NEC (traffic) V79.69 ☑
            nontraffic V79.29 ☑
        pedal cycle (traffic) V71.9 ☑
          nontraffic V71.3 ☑
          while boarding or alighting V71.4 ☑
        pickup truck (traffic) V73.9 ☑
          nontraffic V73.3 ☑
          while boarding or alighting V73.4 ☑
        railway vehicle (traffic) V75.9 ☑
          nontraffic V75.3 ☑
          while boarding or alighting V75.4 ☑
        specified vehicle NEC (traffic) V76.9 ☑
          nontraffic V76.3 ☑
          while boarding or alighting V76.4 ☑
        stationary object (traffic) V77.9 ☑
          nontraffic V77.3 ☑
          while boarding or alighting V77.4 ☑
        streetcar (traffic) V76.9 ☑
          nontraffic V76.3 ☑
          while boarding or alighting V76.4 ☑
        three wheeled motor vehicle (traffic)
          V72.9 ☑
          nontraffic V72.3 ☑
          while boarding or alighting V72.4 ☑
        truck (traffic) V74.9 ☑
          nontraffic V74.3 ☑
          while boarding or alighting V74.4 ☑

**Accident** — *continued*
  transport — *continued*
    bus occupant — *continued*
      collision — *continued*
        two wheeled motor vehicle (traffic) V72.9 ☑
          nontraffic V72.3 ☑
          while boarding or alighting V72.4 ☑
        van (traffic) V73.9 ☑
          nontraffic V73.3 ☑
          while boarding or alighting V73.4 ☑
      driver
        collision (with)
          animal (traffic) V70.5 ☑
            being ridden (traffic) V76.5 ☑
              nontraffic V76.0 ☑
            nontraffic V70.0 ☑
          animal-drawn vehicle (traffic) V76.5 ☑
            nontraffic V76.0 ☑
          bus (traffic) V74.5 ☑
            nontraffic V74.0 ☑
          car (traffic) V73.5 ☑
            nontraffic V73.0 ☑
          motor vehicle NOS (traffic) V79.40 ☑
            nontraffic V79.00 ☑
            specified type NEC (traffic) V79.49 ☑
              nontraffic V79.09 ☑
          pedal cycle (traffic) V71.5 ☑
            nontraffic V71.0 ☑
          pickup truck (traffic) V73.5 ☑
            nontraffic V73.0 ☑
          railway vehicle (traffic) V75.5 ☑
            nontraffic V75.0 ☑
          specified vehicle NEC (traffic) V76.5 ☑
            nontraffic V76.0 ☑
          stationary object (traffic) V77.5 ☑
            nontraffic V77.0 ☑
          streetcar (traffic) V76.5 ☑
            nontraffic V76.0 ☑
          three wheeled motor vehicle (traffic)
            V72.5 ☑
            nontraffic V72.0 ☑
          truck (traffic) V74.5 ☑
            nontraffic V74.0 ☑
          two wheeled motor vehicle (traffic)
            V72.5 ☑
            nontraffic V72.0 ☑
          van (traffic) V73.5 ☑
            nontraffic V73.0 ☑
        noncollision accident (traffic) V78.5 ☑
          nontraffic V78.0 ☑
      hanger-on
        collision (with)
          animal (traffic) V70.7 ☑
            being ridden (traffic) V76.7 ☑
              nontraffic V76.2 ☑
            nontraffic V70.2 ☑
          animal-drawn vehicle (traffic) V76.7 ☑
            nontraffic V76.2 ☑
          bus (traffic) V74.7 ☑
            nontraffic V74.2 ☑
          car (traffic) V73.7 ☑
            nontraffic V73.2 ☑
          pedal cycle (traffic) V71.7 ☑
            nontraffic V71.2 ☑
          pickup truck (traffic) V73.7 ☑
            nontraffic V73.2 ☑
          railway vehicle (traffic) V75.7 ☑
            nontraffic V75.2 ☑
          specified vehicle NEC (traffic) V76.7 ☑
            nontraffic V76.2 ☑
          stationary object (traffic) V77.7 ☑
            nontraffic V77.2 ☑
          streetcar (traffic) V76.7 ☑
            nontraffic V76.2 ☑
          three wheeled motor vehicle (traffic)
            V72.7 ☑
            nontraffic V72.2 ☑
          truck (traffic) V74.7 ☑
            nontraffic V74.2 ☑
          two wheeled motor vehicle (traffic)
            V72.7 ☑
            nontraffic V72.2 ☑
          van (traffic) V73.7 ☑
            nontraffic V73.2 ☑
        noncollision accident (traffic) V78.7 ☑
          nontraffic V78.2 ☑

☑ **Additional Character Required** — **Refer to the Tabular List for Character Selection** ▽ **Subterms under main terms may continue to next column or page**

**Accident** — *continued*
  transport — *continued*
    bus occupant — *continued*
      noncollision accident (traffic) V78.9 ☑
        nontraffic V78.3 ☑
        while boarding or alighting V78.4 ☑
      nontraffic V79.3 ☑
      passenger
        collision (with)
          animal (traffic) V70.6 ☑
            being ridden (traffic) V76.6 ☑
              nontraffic V76.1 ☑
            nontraffic V70.1 ☑
          animal-drawn vehicle (traffic) V76.6 ☑
            nontraffic V76.1 ☑
          bus (traffic) V74.6 ☑
            nontraffic V74.1 ☑
          car (traffic) V73.6 ☑
            nontraffic V73.1 ☑
          motor vehicle NOS (traffic) V79.50 ☑
            nontraffic V79.10 ☑
            specified type NEC (traffic) V79.59 ☑
              nontraffic V79.19 ☑
          pedal cycle (traffic) V71.6 ☑
            nontraffic V71.1 ☑
          pickup truck (traffic) V73.6 ☑
            nontraffic V73.1 ☑
          railway vehicle (traffic) V75.6 ☑
            nontraffic V75.1 ☑
          specified vehicle NEC (traffic) V76.6 ☑
            nontraffic V76.1 ☑
          stationary object (traffic) V77.6 ☑
            nontraffic V77.1 ☑
          streetcar (traffic) V76.6 ☑
            nontraffic V76.1 ☑
          three wheeled motor vehicle (traffic)
            V72.6 ☑
            nontraffic V72.1 ☑
          truck (traffic) V74.6 ☑
            nontraffic V74.1 ☑
          two wheeled motor vehicle (traffic)
            V72.6 ☑
            nontraffic V72.1 ☑
          van (traffic) V73.6 ☑
            nontraffic V73.1 ☑
        noncollision accident (traffic) V78.6 ☑
          nontraffic V78.1 ☑
      specified type NEC V79.88 ☑
      military vehicle V79.81 ☑
    cable car, not on rails V98.0 ☑
      on rails — *see* Accident, transport, streetcar
        occupant
    car occupant V49.9 ☑
      ambulance occupant — *see* Accident, transport,
        ambulance occupant
      collision (with)
        animal (traffic) V40.9 ☑
          being ridden (traffic) V46.9 ☑
            nontraffic V46.3 ☑
            while boarding or alighting V46.4 ☑
          nontraffic V40.3 ☑
          while boarding or alighting V40.4 ☑
        animal-drawn vehicle (traffic) V46.9 ☑
          nontraffic V46.3 ☑
          while boarding or alighting V46.4 ☑
        bus (traffic) V44.9 ☑
          nontraffic V44.3 ☑
          while boarding or alighting V44.4 ☑
        car (traffic) V43.92 ☑
          nontraffic V43.32 ☑
          while boarding or alighting V43.42 ☑
        motor vehicle NOS (traffic) V49.60 ☑
          nontraffic V49.20 ☑
          specified type NEC (traffic) V49.69 ☑
            nontraffic V49.29 ☑
        pedal cycle (traffic) V41.9 ☑
          nontraffic V41.3 ☑
          while boarding or alighting V41.4 ☑
        pickup truck (traffic) V43.93 ☑
          nontraffic V43.33 ☑
          while boarding or alighting V43.43 ☑
        railway vehicle (traffic) V45.9 ☑
          nontraffic V45.3 ☑
          while boarding or alighting V45.4 ☑
        specified vehicle NEC (traffic) V46.9 ☑
          nontraffic V46.3 ☑

**Accident** — *continued*
  transport — *continued*
    car occupant — *continued*
      collision — *continued*
        specified vehicle — *continued*
          while boarding or alighting V46.4 ☑
        sport utility vehicle (traffic) V43.91 ☑
          nontraffic V43.31 ☑
          while boarding or alighting V43.41 ☑
        stationary object (traffic) V47.9 ☑
          nontraffic V47.3 ☑
          while boarding or alighting V47.4 ☑
        streetcar (traffic) V46.9 ☑
          nontraffic V46.3 ☑
          while boarding or alighting V46.4 ☑
        three wheeled motor vehicle (traffic)
          V42.9 ☑
          nontraffic V42.3 ☑
          while boarding or alighting V42.4 ☑
        truck (traffic) V44.9 ☑
          nontraffic V44.3 ☑
          while boarding or alighting V44.4 ☑
        two wheeled motor vehicle (traffic) V42.9 ☑
          nontraffic V42.3 ☑
          while boarding or alighting V42.4 ☑
        van (traffic) V43.94 ☑
          nontraffic V43.34 ☑
          while boarding or alighting V43.44 ☑
      driver
        collision (with)
          animal (traffic) V40.5 ☑
            being ridden (traffic) V46.5 ☑
              nontraffic V46.0 ☑
            nontraffic V40.0 ☑
          animal-drawn vehicle (traffic) V46.5 ☑
            nontraffic V46.0 ☑
          bus (traffic) V44.5 ☑
            nontraffic V44.0 ☑
          car (traffic) V43.52 ☑
            nontraffic V43.02 ☑
          motor vehicle NOS (traffic) V49.40 ☑
            nontraffic V49.00 ☑
            specified type NEC (traffic) V49.49 ☑
              nontraffic V49.09 ☑
          pedal cycle (traffic) V41.5 ☑
            nontraffic V41.0 ☑
          pickup truck (traffic) V43.53 ☑
            nontraffic V43.03 ☑
          railway vehicle (traffic) V45.5 ☑
            nontraffic V45.0 ☑
          specified vehicle NEC (traffic) V46.5 ☑
            nontraffic V46.0 ☑
          sport utility vehicle (traffic) V43.51 ☑
            nontraffic V43.01 ☑
          stationary object (traffic) V47.5 ☑
            nontraffic V47.0 ☑
          streetcar (traffic) V46.5 ☑
            nontraffic V46.0 ☑
          three wheeled motor vehicle (traffic)
            V42.5 ☑
            nontraffic V42.0 ☑
          truck (traffic) V44.5 ☑
            nontraffic V44.0 ☑
          two wheeled motor vehicle (traffic)
            V42.5 ☑
            nontraffic V42.0 ☑
          van (traffic) V43.54 ☑
            nontraffic V43.04 ☑
        noncollision accident (traffic) V48.5 ☑
          nontraffic V48.0 ☑
      hanger-on
        collision (with)
          animal (traffic) V40.7 ☑
            being ridden (traffic) V46.7 ☑
              nontraffic V46.2 ☑
            nontraffic V40.2 ☑
          animal-drawn vehicle (traffic) V46.7 ☑
            nontraffic V46.2 ☑
          bus (traffic) V44.7 ☑
            nontraffic V44.2 ☑
          car (traffic) V43.72 ☑
            nontraffic V43.22 ☑
          pedal cycle (traffic) V41.7 ☑
            nontraffic V41.2 ☑
          pickup truck (traffic) V43.73 ☑
            nontraffic V43.23 ☑

**Accident** — *continued*
  transport — *continued*
    car occupant — *continued*
      hanger-on — *continued*
        collision — *continued*
          railway vehicle (traffic) V45.7 ☑
            nontraffic V45.2 ☑
          specified vehicle NEC (traffic) V46.7 ☑
            nontraffic V46.2 ☑
          sport utility vehicle (traffic) V43.71 ☑
            nontraffic V43.21 ☑
          stationary object (traffic) V47.7 ☑
            nontraffic V47.2 ☑
          streetcar (traffic) V46.7 ☑
            nontraffic V46.2 ☑
          three wheeled motor vehicle (traffic)
            V42.7 ☑
            nontraffic V42.2 ☑
          truck (traffic) V44.7 ☑
            nontraffic V44.2 ☑
          two wheeled motor vehicle (traffic)
            V42.7 ☑
            nontraffic V42.2 ☑
          van (traffic) V43.74 ☑
            nontraffic V43.24 ☑
        noncollision accident (traffic) V48.7 ☑
          nontraffic V48.2 ☑
      noncollision accident (traffic) V48.9 ☑
        nontraffic V48.3 ☑
        while boarding or alighting V48.4 ☑
      nontraffic V49.3 ☑
      passenger
        collision (with)
          animal (traffic) V40.6 ☑
            being ridden (traffic) V46.6 ☑
              nontraffic V46.1 ☑
            nontraffic V40.1 ☑
          animal-drawn vehicle (traffic) V46.6 ☑
            nontraffic V46.1 ☑
          bus (traffic) V44.6 ☑
            nontraffic V44.1 ☑
          car (traffic) V43.62 ☑
            nontraffic V43.12 ☑
          motor vehicle NOS (traffic) V49.50 ☑
            nontraffic V49.10 ☑
            specified type NEC (traffic) V49.59 ☑
              nontraffic V49.19 ☑
          pedal cycle (traffic) V41.6 ☑
            nontraffic V41.1 ☑
          pickup truck (traffic) V43.63 ☑
            nontraffic V43.13 ☑
          railway vehicle (traffic) V45.6 ☑
            nontraffic V45.1 ☑
          specified vehicle NEC (traffic) V46.6 ☑
            nontraffic V46.1 ☑
          sport utility vehicle (traffic) V43.61 ☑
            nontraffic V43.11 ☑
          stationary object (traffic) V47.6 ☑
            nontraffic V47.1 ☑
          streetcar (traffic) V46.6 ☑
            nontraffic V46.1 ☑
          three wheeled motor vehicle (traffic)
            V42.6 ☑
            nontraffic V42.1 ☑
          truck (traffic) V44.6 ☑
            nontraffic V44.1 ☑
          two wheeled motor vehicle (traffic)
            V42.6 ☑
            nontraffic V42.1 ☑
          van (traffic) V43.64 ☑
            nontraffic V43.14 ☑
        noncollision accident (traffic) V48.6 ☑
          nontraffic V48.1 ☑
      specified type NEC V49.88 ☑
      military vehicle V49.81 ☑
    coal car — *see* Accident, transport, industrial vehicle occupant
    construction vehicle occupant (nontraffic) V85.9 ☑
      driver V85.5 ☑
      hanger-on V85.7 ☑
      passenger V85.6 ☑
      traffic V85.3 ☑
        driver V85.0 ☑
        hanger-on V85.2 ☑
        passenger V85.1 ☑
      while boarding or alighting V85.4 ☑

**Accident** — *continued*
    transport — *continued*
        dirt bike rider (nontraffic) V86.96 ☑
            driver V86.56 ☑
            hanger-on V86.76 ☑
            passenger V86.66 ☑
            traffic V86.36 ☑
                driver V86.06 ☑
                hanger-on V86.26 ☑
                passenger V86.16 ☑
            while boarding or alighting V86.46 ☑
        due to cataclysm — *see* Forces of nature, by type
        dune buggy occupant (nontraffic) V86.93 ☑
            driver V86.53 ☑
            hanger-on V86.73 ☑
            passenger V86.63 ☑
            traffic V86.33 ☑
                driver V86.03 ☑
                hanger-on V86.23 ☑
                passenger V86.13 ☑
            while boarding or alighting V86.43 ☑
        forklift — *see* Accident, transport, industrial vehicle occupant
        go cart — *see* Accident, transport, all-terrain vehicle occupant
        golf cart — *see* Accident, transport, all-terrain vehicle occupant
        heavy transport vehicle occupant — *see* Accident, transport, truck occupant
        ice yacht V98.2 ☑
        industrial vehicle occupant (nontraffic) V83.9 ☑
            driver V83.5 ☑
            hanger-on V83.7 ☑
            passenger V83.6 ☑
            traffic V83.3 ☑
                driver V83.0 ☑
                hanger-on V83.2 ☑
                passenger V83.1 ☑
            while boarding or alighting V83.4 ☑
        interurban electric car — *see* Accident, transport, streetcar
        land yacht V98.1 ☑
        logging car — *see* Accident, transport, industrial vehicle occupant
        military vehicle occupant (traffic) V86.34 ☑
            driver V86.04 ☑
            hanger-on V86.24 ☑
            nontraffic V86.94 ☑
                driver V86.54 ☑
                hanger-on V86.74 ☑
                passenger V86.64 ☑
            passenger V86.14 ☑
            while boarding or alighting V86.44 ☑
        mine tram — *see* Accident, transport, industrial vehicle occupant
        motor vehicle NEC occupant (traffic) V89.2 ☑
        motorcoach — *see* Accident, transport, bus occupant
        motor/cross bike rider (*see also* Accident, transport, dirt bike rider) V86.96 ☑
        motorcyclist V29.9 ☑
            collision (with)
                animal (traffic) V20.9 ☑
                    being ridden (traffic) V26.9 ☑
                        nontraffic V26.2 ☑
                            while boarding or alighting V26.3 ☑
                    nontraffic V20.2 ☑
                    while boarding or alighting V20.3 ☑
                animal-drawn vehicle (traffic) V26.9 ☑
                    nontraffic V26.2 ☑
                    while boarding or alighting V26.3 ☑
                bus (traffic) V24.9 ☑
                    nontraffic V24.2 ☑
                    while boarding or alighting V24.3 ☑
                car (traffic) V23.9 ☑
                    nontraffic V23.2 ☑
                    while boarding or alighting V23.3 ☑
                motor vehicle NOS (traffic) V29.60 ☑
                    nontraffic V29.20 ☑
                    specified type NEC (traffic) V29.69 ☑
                        nontraffic V29.29 ☑
                pedal cycle (traffic) V21.9 ☑
                    nontraffic V21.2 ☑
                    while boarding or alighting V21.3 ☑
                pickup truck (traffic) V23.9 ☑
                    nontraffic V23.2 ☑

**Accident** — *continued*
    transport — *continued*
        motorcyclist — *continued*
            collision — *continued*
                pickup truck — *continued*
                    while boarding or alighting V23.3 ☑
                railway vehicle (traffic) V25.9 ☑
                    nontraffic V25.2 ☑
                    while boarding or alighting V25.3 ☑
                specified vehicle NEC (traffic) V26.9 ☑
                    nontraffic V26.2 ☑
                    while boarding or alighting V26.3 ☑
                stationary object (traffic) V27.9 ☑
                    nontraffic V27.2 ☑
                    while boarding or alighting V27.3 ☑
                streetcar (traffic) V26.9 ☑
                    nontraffic V26.2 ☑
                    while boarding or alighting V26.3 ☑
                three wheeled motor vehicle (traffic) V22.9 ☑
                    nontraffic V22.2 ☑
                    while boarding or alighting V22.3 ☑
                truck (traffic) V24.9 ☑
                    nontraffic V24.2 ☑
                    while boarding or alighting V24.3 ☑
                two wheeled motor vehicle (traffic) V22.9 ☑
                    nontraffic V22.2 ☑
                    while boarding or alighting V22.3 ☑
                van (traffic) V23.9 ☑
                    nontraffic V23.2 ☑
                    while boarding or alighting V23.3 ☑
            driver
                collision (with)
                    animal (traffic) V20.4 ☑
                        being ridden (traffic) V26.4 ☑
                            nontraffic V26.0 ☑
                        nontraffic V20.0 ☑
                    animal-drawn vehicle (traffic) V26.4 ☑
                        nontraffic V26.0 ☑
                    bus (traffic) V24.4 ☑
                        nontraffic V24.0 ☑
                    car (traffic) V23.4 ☑
                        nontraffic V23.0 ☑
                    motor vehicle NOS (traffic) V29.40 ☑
                        nontraffic V29.00 ☑
                        specified type NEC (traffic) V29.49 ☑
                            nontraffic V29.09 ☑
                    pedal cycle (traffic) V21.4 ☑
                        nontraffic V21.0 ☑
                    pickup truck (traffic) V23.4 ☑
                        nontraffic V23.0 ☑
                    railway vehicle (traffic) V25.4 ☑
                        nontraffic V25.0 ☑
                    specified vehicle NEC (traffic) V26.4 ☑
                        nontraffic V26.0 ☑
                    stationary object (traffic) V27.4 ☑
                        nontraffic V27.0 ☑
                    streetcar (traffic) V26.4 ☑
                        nontraffic V26.0 ☑
                    three wheeled motor vehicle (traffic) V22.4 ☑
                        nontraffic V22.0 ☑
                    truck (traffic) V24.4 ☑
                        nontraffic V24.0 ☑
                    two wheeled motor vehicle (traffic) V22.4 ☑
                        nontraffic V22.0 ☑
                    van (traffic) V23.4 ☑
                        nontraffic V23.0 ☑
                    noncollision accident (traffic) V28.4 ☑
                        nontraffic V28.0 ☑
                noncollision accident (traffic) V28.9 ☑
                    nontraffic V28.2 ☑
                    while boarding or alighting V28.3 ☑
            nontraffic V29.3 ☑
            passenger
                collision (with)
                    animal (traffic) V20.5 ☑
                        being ridden (traffic) V26.5 ☑
                            nontraffic V26.1 ☑
                        nontraffic V20.1 ☑
                    animal-drawn vehicle (traffic) V26.5 ☑
                        nontraffic V26.1 ☑
                    bus (traffic) V24.5 ☑
                        nontraffic V24.1 ☑
                    car (traffic) V23.5 ☑

**Accident** — *continued*
    transport — *continued*
        motorcyclist — *continued*
            passenger — *continued*
                collision — *continued*
                    car — *continued*
                        nontraffic V23.1 ☑
                    motor vehicle NOS (traffic) V29.50 ☑
                        nontraffic V29.10 ☑
                        specified type NEC (traffic) V29.59 ☑
                            nontraffic V29.19 ☑
                    pedal cycle (traffic) V21.5 ☑
                        nontraffic V21.1 ☑
                    pickup truck (traffic) V23.5 ☑
                        nontraffic V23.1 ☑
                    railway vehicle (traffic) V25.5 ☑
                        nontraffic V25.1 ☑
                    specified vehicle NEC (traffic) V26.5 ☑
                        nontraffic V26.1 ☑
                    stationary object (traffic) V27.5 ☑
                        nontraffic V27.1 ☑
                    streetcar (traffic) V26.5 ☑
                        nontraffic V26.1 ☑
                    three wheeled motor vehicle (traffic) V22.5 ☑
                        nontraffic V22.1 ☑
                    truck (traffic) V24.5 ☑
                        nontraffic V24.1 ☑
                    two wheeled motor vehicle (traffic) V22.5 ☑
                        nontraffic V22.1 ☑
                    van (traffic) V23.5 ☑
                        nontraffic V23.1 ☑
                noncollision accident (traffic) V28.5 ☑
                    nontraffic V28.1 ☑
            specified type NEC V29.88 ☑
            military vehicle V29.81 ☑
        occupant (of)
            aircraft (powered) V95.9 ☑
                fixed wing
                    commercial — *see* Accident, transport, aircraft, occupant, powered, fixed wing, commercial
                    private — *see* Accident, transport, aircraft, occupant, powered, fixed wing, private
                nonpowered V96.9 ☑
                specified NEC V95.8 ☑
            airport battery-powered vehicle — *see* Accident, transport, industrial vehicle occupant
            all-terrain vehicle (ATV) — *see* Accident, transport, all-terrain vehicle occupant
            animal-drawn vehicle — *see* Accident, transport, animal-drawn vehicle occupant
            automobile — *see* Accident, transport, car occupant
            balloon V96.00 ☑
            battery-powered vehicle — *see* Accident, transport, industrial vehicle occupant
            bicycle — *see* Accident, transport, pedal cyclist
                motorized — *see* Accident, transport, motorcycle rider
            boat NEC — *see* Accident, watercraft
            bulldozer — *see* Accident, transport, construction vehicle occupant
            bus — *see* Accident, transport, bus occupant
            cable car (on rails) (*see also* Accident, transport, streetcar occupant)
                not on rails V98.0 ☑
            car (*see also* Accident, transport, car occupant)
                cable (on rails) (*see also* Accident, transport, streetcar occupant)
                    not on rails V98.0 ☑
            coach — *see* Accident, transport, bus occupant
            coal-car — *see* Accident, transport, industrial vehicle occupant
            digger — *see* Accident, transport, construction vehicle occupant
            dump truck — *see* Accident, transport, construction vehicle occupant
            earth-leveler — *see* Accident, transport, construction vehicle occupant
            farm machinery (self-propelled) — *see* Accident, transport, agricultural vehicle occupant

**Accident** — *continued*
  transport — *continued*
    occupant — *continued*
      forklift — *see* Accident, transport, industrial vehicle occupant
      glider (unpowered) V96.20 ☑
        hang V96.10 ☑
        powered (microlight) (ultralight) — *see* Accident, transport, aircraft, occupant, powered, glider
      glider (unpowered) NEC V96.20 ☑
      hang-glider V96.10 ☑
      harvester — *see* Accident, transport, agricultural vehicle occupant
      heavy (transport) vehicle — *see* Accident, transport, truck occupant
      helicopter — *see* Accident, transport, aircraft, occupant, helicopter
      ice-yacht V98.2 ☑
      kite (carrying person) V96.8 ☑
      land-yacht V98.1 ☑
      logging car — *see* Accident, transport, industrial vehicle occupant
      mechanical shovel — *see* Accident, transport, construction vehicle occupant
      microlight — *see* Accident, transport, aircraft, occupant, powered, glider
      minibus — *see* Accident, transport, pickup truck occupant
      minivan — *see* Accident, transport, pickup truck occupant
      moped — *see* Accident, transport, motorcycle
      motor scooter — *see* Accident, transport, motorcycle
      motorcycle (with sidecar) — *see* Accident, transport, motorcycle
      off-road motor-vehicle (*see also* Accident, transport, all-terrain vehicle occupant) V86.99 ☑
      pedal cycle (*see also* Accident, transport, pedal cyclist)
      pick-up (truck) — *see* Accident, transport, pickup truck occupant
      railway (train) (vehicle) (subterranean) (elevated) — *see* Accident, transport, railway vehicle occupant
      rickshaw — *see* Accident, transport, pedal cycle
        motorized — *see* Accident, transport, three-wheeled motor vehicle
        pedal driven — *see* Accident, transport, pedal cyclist
      road-roller — *see* Accident, transport, construction vehicle occupant
      ship NOS V94.9 ☑
      ski-lift (chair) (gondola) V98.3 ☑
      snowmobile — *see* Accident, transport, snowmobile occupant
      spacecraft, spaceship — *see* Accident, transport, aircraft, occupant, spacecraft
      sport utility vehicle — *see* Accident, transport, pickup truck occupant
      streetcar (interurban) (operating on public street or highway) — *see* Accident, transport, streetcar occupant
      SUV — *see* Accident, transport, pickup truck occupant
      téléférique V98.0 ☑
      three-wheeled vehicle (motorized) (*see also* Accident, transport, three-wheeled motor vehicle occupant)
        nonmotorized — *see* Accident, transport, pedal cycle
      tractor (farm) (and trailer) — *see* Accident, transport, agricultural vehicle occupant
      train — *see* Accident, transport, railway vehicle occupant
      tram — *see* Accident, transport, streetcar occupant
        in mine or quarry — *see* Accident, transport, industrial vehicle occupant
      tricycle — *see* Accident, transport, pedal cycle
        motorized — *see* Accident, transport, three-wheeled motor vehicle
      trolley — *see* Accident, transport, streetcar occupant
        in mine or quarry — *see* Accident, transport, industrial vehicle occupant

**Accident** — *continued*
  transport — *continued*
    occupant — *continued*
      tub, in mine or quarry — *see* Accident, transport, industrial vehicle occupant
      ultralight — *see* Accident, transport, aircraft, occupant, powered, glider
      van — *see* Accident, transport, van occupant
      vehicle NEC V89.9 ☑
        heavy transport — *see* Accident, transport, truck occupant
        motor (traffic) NEC V89.2 ☑
        nontraffic NEC V89.0 ☑
      watercraft NOS V94.9 ☑
        causing drowning — *see* Drowning, resulting from accident to boat
      off-road motor-vehicle (*see also* Accident, transport, all-terrain vehicle occupant) V86.99 ☑
    parachutist V97.29 ☑
      after accident to aircraft — *see* Accident, transport, aircraft
      entangled in object V97.21 ☑
      injured on landing V97.22 ☑
    pedal cyclist V19.9 ☑
      collision (with)
        animal (traffic) V10.9 ☑
          being ridden (traffic) V16.9 ☑
            nontraffic V16.2 ☑
            while boarding or alighting V16.3 ☑
          nontraffic V10.2 ☑
          while boarding or alighting V10.3 ☑
        animal-drawn vehicle (traffic) V16.9 ☑
          nontraffic V16.2 ☑
          while boarding or alighting V16.3 ☑
        bus (traffic) V14.9 ☑
          nontraffic V14.2 ☑
          while boarding or alighting V14.3 ☑
        car (traffic) V13.9 ☑
          nontraffic V13.2 ☑
          while boarding or alighting V13.3 ☑
        motor vehicle NOS (traffic) V19.60 ☑
          nontraffic V19.20 ☑
          specified type NEC (traffic) V19.69 ☑
            nontraffic V19.29 ☑
        pedal cycle (traffic) V11.9 ☑
          nontraffic V11.2 ☑
          while boarding or alighting V11.3 ☑
        pickup truck (traffic) V13.9 ☑
          nontraffic V13.2 ☑
          while boarding or alighting V13.3 ☑
        railway vehicle (traffic) V15.9 ☑
          nontraffic V15.2 ☑
          while boarding or alighting V15.3 ☑
        specified vehicle NEC (traffic) V16.9 ☑
          nontraffic V16.2 ☑
          while boarding or alighting V16.3 ☑
        stationary object (traffic) V17.9 ☑
          nontraffic V17.2 ☑
          while boarding or alighting V17.3 ☑
        streetcar (traffic) V16.9 ☑
          nontraffic V16.2 ☑
          while boarding or alighting V16.3 ☑
        three wheeled motor vehicle (traffic) V12.9 ☑
          nontraffic V12.2 ☑
          while boarding or alighting V12.3 ☑
        truck (traffic) V14.9 ☑
          nontraffic V14.2 ☑
          while boarding or alighting V14.3 ☑
        two wheeled motor vehicle (traffic) V12.9 ☑
          nontraffic V12.2 ☑
          while boarding or alighting V12.3 ☑
        van (traffic) V13.9 ☑
          nontraffic V13.2 ☑
          while boarding or alighting V13.3 ☑
      driver
        collision (with)
          animal (traffic) V10.4 ☑
            being ridden (traffic) V16.4 ☑
              nontraffic V16.0 ☑
            nontraffic V10.0 ☑
          animal-drawn vehicle (traffic) V16.4 ☑
            nontraffic V16.0 ☑
          bus (traffic) V14.4 ☑
            nontraffic V14.0 ☑
          car (traffic) V13.4 ☑

**Accident** — *continued*
  transport — *continued*
    pedal cyclist — *continued*
      driver — *continued*
        collision — *continued*
          car — *continued*
            nontraffic V13.0 ☑
          motor vehicle NOS (traffic) V19.40 ☑
            nontraffic V19.00 ☑
            specified type NEC (traffic) V19.49 ☑
              nontraffic V19.09 ☑
          pedal cycle (traffic) V11.4 ☑
            nontraffic V11.0 ☑
          pickup truck (traffic) V13.4 ☑
            nontraffic V13.0 ☑
          railway vehicle (traffic) V15.4 ☑
            nontraffic V15.0 ☑
          specified vehicle NEC (traffic) V16.4 ☑
            nontraffic V16.0 ☑
          stationary object (traffic) V17.4 ☑
            nontraffic V17.0 ☑
          streetcar (traffic) V16.4 ☑
            nontraffic V16.0 ☑
          three wheeled motor vehicle (traffic) V12.4 ☑
            nontraffic V12.0 ☑
          truck (traffic) V14.4 ☑
            nontraffic V14.0 ☑
          two wheeled motor vehicle (traffic) V12.4 ☑
            nontraffic V12.0 ☑
          van (traffic) V13.4 ☑
            nontraffic V13.0 ☑
        noncollision accident (traffic) V18.4 ☑
          nontraffic V18.0 ☑
      noncollision accident (traffic) V18.9 ☑
        nontraffic V18.2 ☑
        while boarding or alighting V18.3 ☑
      nontraffic V19.3 ☑
      passenger
        collision (with)
          animal (traffic) V10.5 ☑
            being ridden (traffic) V16.5 ☑
              nontraffic V16.1 ☑
            nontraffic V10.1 ☑
          animal-drawn vehicle (traffic) V16.5 ☑
            nontraffic V16.1 ☑
          bus (traffic) V14.5 ☑
            nontraffic V14.1 ☑
          car (traffic) V13.5 ☑
            nontraffic V13.1 ☑
          motor vehicle NOS (traffic) V19.50 ☑
            nontraffic V19.10 ☑
            specified type NEC (traffic) V19.59 ☑
              nontraffic V19.19 ☑
          pedal cycle (traffic) V11.5 ☑
            nontraffic V11.1 ☑
          pickup truck (traffic) V13.5 ☑
            nontraffic V13.1 ☑
          railway vehicle (traffic) V15.5 ☑
            nontraffic V15.1 ☑
          specified vehicle NEC (traffic) V16.5 ☑
            nontraffic V16.1 ☑
          stationary object (traffic) V17.5 ☑
            nontraffic V17.1 ☑
          streetcar (traffic) V16.5 ☑
            nontraffic V16.1 ☑
          three wheeled motor vehicle (traffic) V12.5 ☑
            nontraffic V12.1 ☑
          truck (traffic) V14.5 ☑
            nontraffic V14.1 ☑
          two wheeled motor vehicle (traffic) V12.5 ☑
            nontraffic V12.1 ☑
          van (traffic) V13.5 ☑
            nontraffic V13.1 ☑
        noncollision accident (traffic) V18.5 ☑
          nontraffic V18.1 ☑
      specified type NEC V19.88 ☑
        military vehicle V19.81 ☑
    pedestrian
      conveyance (occupant) V09.9 ☑
        babystroller V00.828 ☑
        collision (with) V09.9 ☑

**Accident** — *continued*
  transport — *continued*
    pedestrian — *continued*
      conveyance — *continued*
        babystroller — *continued*
          collision — *continued*
            animal being ridden or animal drawn vehicle V06.99 ☑
              nontraffic V06.09 ☑
              traffic V06.19 ☑
            bus or heavy transport V04.99 ☑
              nontraffic V04.09 ☑
              traffic V04.19 ☑
            car V03.99 ☑
              nontraffic V03.09 ☑
              traffic V03.19 ☑
            pedal cycle V01.99 ☑
              nontraffic V01.09 ☑
              traffic V01.19 ☑
            pick-up truck or van V03.99 ☑
              nontraffic V03.09 ☑
              traffic V03.19 ☑
            railway (train) (vehicle) V05.99 ☑
              nontraffic V05.09 ☑
              traffic V05.19 ☑
            stationary object V00.822 ☑
            streetcar V06.99 ☑
              nontraffic V06.09 ☑
              traffic V06.19 ☑
            two- or three-wheeled motor vehicle V02.99 ☑
              nontraffic V02.09 ☑
              traffic V02.19 ☑
            vehicle V09.9 ☑
              animal-drawn V06.99 ☑
                nontraffic V06.09 ☑
                traffic V06.19 ☑
              motor
                nontraffic V09.00 ☑
                traffic V09.20 ☑
           fall V00.821 ☑
          nontraffic V09.1 ☑
            involving motor vehicle NEC V09.00 ☑
          traffic V09.3 ☑
            involving motor vehicle NEC V09.20 ☑
         flat-bottomed NEC V00.388 ☑
          collision (with) V09.9 ☑
            animal being ridden or animal drawn vehicle V06.99 ☑
              nontraffic V06.09 ☑
              traffic V06.19 ☑
            bus or heavy transport V04.99 ☑
              nontraffic V04.09 ☑
              traffic V04.19 ☑
            car V03.99 ☑
              nontraffic V03.09 ☑
              traffic V03.19 ☑
            pedal cycle V01.99 ☑
              nontraffic V01.09 ☑
              traffic V01.19 ☑
            pick-up truck or van V03.99 ☑
              nontraffic V03.09 ☑
              traffic V03.19 ☑
            railway (train) (vehicle) V05.99 ☑
              nontraffic V05.09 ☑
              traffic V05.19 ☑
            stationary object V00.382 ☑
            streetcar V06.99 ☑
              nontraffic V06.09 ☑
              traffic V06.19 ☑
            two- or three-wheeled motor vehicle V02.99 ☑
              nontraffic V02.09 ☑
              traffic V02.19 ☑
            vehicle V09.9 ☑
              animal-drawn V06.99 ☑
                nontraffic V06.09 ☑
                traffic V06.19 ☑
              motor
                nontraffic V09.00 ☑
                traffic V09.20 ☑
           fall V00.381 ☑
          nontraffic V09.1 ☑

---

**Accident** — *continued*
  transport — *continued*
    pedestrian — *continued*
      conveyance — *continued*
        flat-bottomed — *continued*
          nontraffic — *continued*
            involving motor vehicle NEC V09.00 ☑
          snow
            board — *see* Accident, transport, pedestrian, conveyance, snow board
            ski — *see* Accident, transport, pedestrian, conveyance, skis (snow)
          traffic V09.3 ☑
            involving motor vehicle NEC V09.20 ☑
        gliding type NEC V00.288 ☑
          collision (with) V09.9 ☑
            animal being ridden or animal drawn vehicle V06.99 ☑
              nontraffic V06.09 ☑
              traffic V06.19 ☑
            bus or heavy transport V04.99 ☑
              nontraffic V04.09 ☑
              traffic V04.19 ☑
            car V03.99 ☑
              nontraffic V03.09 ☑
              traffic V03.19 ☑
            pedal cycle V01.99 ☑
              nontraffic V01.09 ☑
              traffic V01.19 ☑
            pick-up truck or van V03.99 ☑
              nontraffic V03.09 ☑
              traffic V03.19 ☑
            railway (train) (vehicle) V05.99 ☑
              nontraffic V05.09 ☑
              traffic V05.19 ☑
            stationary object V00.282 ☑
            streetcar V06.99 ☑
              nontraffic V06.09 ☑
              traffic V02.19 ☑
            two- or three-wheeled motor vehicle V02.99 ☑
              nontraffic V02.09 ☑
              traffic V02.19 ☑
            vehicle V09.9 ☑
              animal-drawn V06.99 ☑
                nontraffic V06.09 ☑
                traffic V06.19 ☑
              motor
                nontraffic V09.00 ☑
                traffic V09.20 ☑
         fall V00.281 ☑
        heelies — *see* Accident, transport, pedestrian, conveyance, heelies
        ice skate — *see* Accident, transport, pedestrian, conveyance, ice skate
        nontraffic V09.1 ☑
          involving motor vehicle NEC V09.00 ☑
        sled — *see* Accident, transport, pedestrian, conveyance, sled
        traffic V09.3 ☑
          involving motor vehicle NEC V09.20 ☑
        wheelies — *see* Accident, transport, pedestrian, conveyance, heelies
      heelies V00.158 ☑
        colliding with stationary object V00.152 ☑
        fall V00.151 ☑
      ice skates V00.218 ☑
        collision (with) V09.9 ☑
          animal being ridden or animal drawn vehicle V06.99 ☑
            nontraffic V06.09 ☑
            traffic V06.19 ☑
          bus or heavy transport V04.99 ☑
            nontraffic V04.09 ☑
            traffic V04.19 ☑
          car V03.99 ☑
            nontraffic V03.09 ☑
            traffic V03.19 ☑

---

**Accident** — *continued*
  transport — *continued*
    pedestrian — *continued*
      conveyance — *continued*
        ice skates — *continued*
          collision — *continued*
            pedal cycle V01.99 ☑
              nontraffic V01.09 ☑
              traffic V01.19 ☑
            pick-up truck or van V03.99 ☑
              nontraffic V03.09 ☑
              traffic V03.19 ☑
            railway (train) (vehicle) V05.99 ☑
              nontraffic V05.09 ☑
              traffic V05.19 ☑
            stationary object V00.212 ☑
            streetcar V06.99 ☑
              nontraffic V06.09 ☑
              traffic V06.19 ☑
            two- or three-wheeled motor vehicle V02.99 ☑
              nontraffic V02.09 ☑
              traffic V02.19 ☑
            vehicle V09.9 ☑
              animal-drawn V06.99 ☑
                nontraffic V06.09 ☑
                traffic V06.19 ☑
              motor
                nontraffic V09.00 ☑
                traffic V09.20 ☑
           fall V00.211 ☑
          nontraffic V09.1 ☑
            involving motor vehicle NEC V09.00 ☑
          traffic V09.3 ☑
            involving motor vehicle NEC V09.20 ☑
        motorized mobility scooter V00.838 ☑
          collision with stationary object V00.832 ☑
          fall from V00.831 ☑
        nontraffic V09.1 ☑
          involving motor vehicle V09.00 ☑
            military V09.01 ☑
            specified type NEC V09.09 ☑
        roller skates (non in-line) V00.128 ☑
          collision (with) V09.9 ☑
            animal being ridden or animal drawn vehicle V06.91 ☑
              nontraffic V06.01 ☑
              traffic V06.11 ☑
            bus or heavy transport V04.91 ☑
              nontraffic V04.01 ☑
              traffic V04.11 ☑
            car V03.91 ☑
              nontraffic V03.01 ☑
              traffic V03.11 ☑
            pedal cycle V01.91 ☑
              nontraffic V01.01 ☑
              traffic V01.11 ☑
            pick-up truck or van V03.91 ☑
              nontraffic V03.01 ☑
              traffic V03.11 ☑
            railway (train) (vehicle) V05.91 ☑
              nontraffic V05.01 ☑
              traffic V05.11 ☑
            stationary object V00.122 ☑
            streetcar V06.91 ☑
              nontraffic V06.01 ☑
              traffic V06.11 ☑
            two- or three-wheeled motor vehicle V02.91 ☑
              nontraffic V02.01 ☑
              traffic V02.11 ☑
            vehicle V09.9 ☑
              animal-drawn V06.91 ☑
                nontraffic V06.01 ☑
                traffic V06.11 ☑
              motor
                nontraffic V09.00 ☑
                traffic V09.20 ☑
           fall V00.121 ☑
          in-line V00.118 ☑

☑ Additional Character Required — Refer to the Tabular List for Character Selection    ▽ Subterms under main terms may continue to next column or page

Accident — *continued*
  transport — *continued*
    pedestrian — *continued*
      conveyance — *continued*
        roller skates — *continued*
          in-line — *continued*
            collision — *see also* Accident, transport, pedestrian, conveyance occupant, roller skates, collision
              with stationary object V00.112 ☑
            fall V00.111 ☑
            nontraffic V09.1 ☑
              involving motor vehicle NEC V09.00 ☑
            traffic V09.3 ☑
              involving motor vehicle NEC V09.20 ☑
        rolling shoes V00.158 ☑
          colliding with stationary object V00.152 ☑
          fall V00.151 ☑
        rolling type NEC V00.188 ☑
          collision (with) V09.9 ☑
            animal being ridden or animal drawn vehicle V06.99 ☑
              nontraffic V06.09 ☑
              traffic V06.19 ☑
            bus or heavy transport V04.99 ☑
              nontraffic V04.09 ☑
              traffic V04.19 ☑
            car V03.99 ☑
              nontraffic V03.09 ☑
              traffic V03.19 ☑
            pedal cycle V01.99 ☑
              nontraffic V01.09 ☑
              traffic V01.19 ☑
            pick-up truck or van V03.99 ☑
              nontraffic V03.09 ☑
              traffic V03.19 ☑
            railway (train) (vehicle) V05.99 ☑
              nontraffic V05.09 ☑
              traffic V05.19 ☑
            stationary object V00.182 ☑
            streetcar V06.99 ☑
              nontraffic V06.09 ☑
              traffic V06.19 ☑
            two- or three-wheeled motor vehicle V02.99 ☑
              nontraffic V02.09 ☑
              traffic V02.19 ☑
            vehicle V09.9 ☑
              animal-drawn V06.99 ☑
                nontraffic V06.09 ☑
                traffic V06.19 ☑
              motor
                nontraffic V09.00 ☑
                traffic V09.20 ☑
          fall V00.181 ☑
        in-line roller skate — *see* Accident, transport, pedestrian, conveyance, roller skate, in-line
          nontraffic V09.1 ☑
            involving motor vehicle NEC V09.00 ☑
        roller skate — *see* Accident, transport, pedestrian, conveyance, roller skate
        scooter (non-motorized) — *see* Accident, transport, pedestrian, conveyance, scooter
        skateboard — *see* Accident, transport, pedestrian, conveyance, skateboard
          traffic V09.3 ☑
            involving motor vehicle NEC V09.20 ☑
        scooter (non-motorized) V00.148 ☑
          collision (with) V09.9 ☑
            animal being ridden or animal drawn vehicle V06.99 ☑
              nontraffic V06.09 ☑
              traffic V06.19 ☑
            bus or heavy transport V04.99 ☑
              nontraffic V04.09 ☑
              traffic V04.19 ☑

Accident — *continued*
  transport — *continued*
    pedestrian — *continued*
      conveyance — *continued*
        scooter — *continued*
          collision — *continued*
            car V03.99 ☑
              nontraffic V03.09 ☑
              traffic V03.19 ☑
            pedal cycle V01.99 ☑
              nontraffic V01.09 ☑
              traffic V01.19 ☑
            pick-up truck or van V03.99 ☑
              nontraffic V03.09 ☑
              traffic V03.19 ☑
            railway (train) (vehicle) V05.99 ☑
              nontraffic V05.09 ☑
              traffic V05.19 ☑
            stationary object V00.142 ☑
            streetcar V06.99 ☑
              nontraffic V06.09 ☑
              traffic V06.19 ☑
            two- or three-wheeled motor vehicle V02.99 ☑
              nontraffic V02.09 ☑
              traffic V02.19 ☑
            vehicle V09.9 ☑
              animal-drawn V06.99 ☑
                nontraffic V06.09 ☑
                traffic V06.19 ☑
              motor
                nontraffic V09.00 ☑
                traffic V09.20 ☑
          fall V00.141 ☑
          nontraffic V09.1 ☑
            involving motor vehicle NEC V09.00 ☑
          traffic V09.3 ☑
            involving motor vehicle NEC V09.20 ☑
        skate board V00.138 ☑
          collision (with) V09.9 ☑
            animal being ridden or animal drawn vehicle V06.92 ☑
              nontraffic V06.02 ☑
              traffic V06.12 ☑
            bus or heavy transport V04.92 ☑
              nontraffic V04.02 ☑
              traffic V04.12 ☑
            car V03.92 ☑
              nontraffic V03.02 ☑
              traffic V03.12 ☑
            pedal cycle V01.92 ☑
              nontraffic V01.02 ☑
              traffic V01.12 ☑
            pick-up truck or van V03.92 ☑
              nontraffic V03.02 ☑
              traffic V03.12 ☑
            railway (train) (vehicle) V05.92 ☑
              nontraffic V05.02 ☑
              traffic V05.12 ☑
            stationary object V00.132 ☑
            streetcar V06.92 ☑
              nontraffic V06.02 ☑
              traffic V06.12 ☑
            two- or three-wheeled motor vehicle V02.92 ☑
              nontraffic V02.02 ☑
              traffic V02.12 ☑
            vehicle V09.9 ☑
              animal-drawn V06.92 ☑
                nontraffic V06.02 ☑
                traffic V06.12 ☑
              motor
                nontraffic V09.00 ☑
                traffic V09.20 ☑
          fall V00.131 ☑
          nontraffic V09.1 ☑
            involving motor vehicle NEC V09.00 ☑
          traffic V09.3 ☑
            involving motor vehicle NEC V09.20 ☑
        skis (snow) V00.328 ☑
          collision (with) V09.9 ☑

Accident — *continued*
  transport — *continued*
    pedestrian — *continued*
      conveyance — *continued*
        skis — *continued*
          collision — *continued*
            animal being ridden or animal drawn vehicle V06.99 ☑
              nontraffic V06.09 ☑
              traffic V06.19 ☑
            bus or heavy transport V04.99 ☑
              nontraffic V04.09 ☑
              traffic V04.19 ☑
            car V03.99 ☑
              nontraffic V03.09 ☑
              traffic V03.19 ☑
            pedal cycle V01.99 ☑
              nontraffic V01.09 ☑
              traffic V01.19 ☑
            pick-up truck or van V03.99 ☑
              nontraffic V03.09 ☑
              traffic V03.19 ☑
            railway (train) (vehicle) V05.99 ☑
              nontraffic V05.09 ☑
              traffic V05.19 ☑
            stationary object V00.322 ☑
            streetcar V06.99 ☑
              nontraffic V06.09 ☑
              traffic V06.19 ☑
            two- or three-wheeled motor vehicle V02.99 ☑
              nontraffic V02.09 ☑
              traffic V02.19 ☑
            vehicle V09.9 ☑
              animal-drawn V06.99 ☑
                nontraffic V06.09 ☑
                traffic V06.19 ☑
              motor
                nontraffic V09.00 ☑
                traffic V09.20 ☑
          fall V00.321 ☑
          nontraffic V09.1 ☑
            involving motor vehicle NEC V09.00 ☑
          traffic V09.3 ☑
            involving motor vehicle NEC V09.20 ☑
        sled V00.228 ☑
          collision (with) V09.9 ☑
            animal being ridden or animal drawn vehicle V06.99 ☑
              nontraffic V06.09 ☑
              traffic V06.19 ☑
            bus or heavy transport V04.99 ☑
              nontraffic V04.09 ☑
              traffic V04.19 ☑
            car V03.99 ☑
              nontraffic V03.09 ☑
              traffic V03.19 ☑
            pedal cycle V01.99 ☑
              nontraffic V01.09 ☑
              traffic V01.19 ☑
            pick-up truck or van V03.99 ☑
              nontraffic V03.09 ☑
              traffic V03.19 ☑
            railway (train) (vehicle) V05.99 ☑
              nontraffic V05.09 ☑
              traffic V05.19 ☑
            stationary object V00.222 ☑
            streetcar V06.99 ☑
              nontraffic V06.09 ☑
              traffic V06.19 ☑
            two- or three-wheeled motor vehicle V02.99 ☑
              nontraffic V02.09 ☑
              traffic V02.19 ☑
            vehicle V09.9 ☑
              animal-drawn V06.99 ☑
                nontraffic V06.09 ☑
                traffic V06.19 ☑
              motor
                nontraffic V09.00 ☑
                traffic V09.20 ☑
          fall V00.221 ☑
          nontraffic V09.1 ☑

**Accident** — *continued*
  transport — *continued*
    pedestrian — *continued*
      conveyance — *continued*
        sled — *continued*
          nontraffic — *continued*
            involving motor vehicle NEC
              V09.00 ☑
          traffic V09.3 ☑
            involving motor vehicle NEC
              V09.20 ☑
        snow board V00.318 ☑
          collision (with) V09.9 ☑
            animal being ridden or animal drawn
              vehicle V06.99 ☑
              nontraffic V06.09 ☑
              traffic V06.19 ☑
            bus or heavy transport V04.99 ☑
              nontraffic V04.09 ☑
              traffic V04.19 ☑
            car V03.99 ☑
              nontraffic V03.09 ☑
              traffic V03.19 ☑
            pedal cycle V01.99 ☑
              nontraffic V01.09 ☑
              traffic V01.19 ☑
            pick-up truck or van V03.99 ☑
              nontraffic V03.09 ☑
              traffic V03.19 ☑
            railway (train) (vehicle) V05.99 ☑
              nontraffic V05.09 ☑
              traffic V05.19 ☑
            stationary object V00.312 ☑
            streetcar V06.99 ☑
              nontraffic V06.09 ☑
              traffic V06.19 ☑
            two- or three-wheeled motor vehicle
              V02.99 ☑
              nontraffic V02.09 ☑
              traffic V02.19 ☑
            vehicle V09.9 ☑
              animal-drawn V06.99 ☑
                nontraffic V06.09 ☑
                traffic V06.19 ☑
              motor
                nontraffic V09.00 ☑
                traffic V09.20 ☑
           fall V00.311 ☑
          nontraffic V09.1 ☑
            involving motor vehicle NEC
              V09.00 ☑
          traffic V09.3 ☑
            involving motor vehicle NEC
              V09.20 ☑
        specified type NEC V00.898 ☑
          collision (with) V09.9 ☑
            animal being ridden or animal drawn
              vehicle V06.99 ☑
              nontraffic V06.09 ☑
              traffic V06.19 ☑
            bus or heavy transport V04.99 ☑
              nontraffic V04.09 ☑
              traffic V04.19 ☑
            car V03.99 ☑
              nontraffic V03.09 ☑
              traffic V03.19 ☑
            pedal cycle V01.99 ☑
              nontraffic V01.09 ☑
              traffic V01.19 ☑
            pick-up truck or van V03.99 ☑
              nontraffic V03.09 ☑
              traffic V03.19 ☑
            railway (train) (vehicle) V05.99 ☑
              nontraffic V05.09 ☑
              traffic V05.19 ☑
            stationary object V00.892 ☑
            streetcar V06.99 ☑
              nontraffic V06.09 ☑
              traffic V06.19 ☑
            two- or three-wheeled motor vehicle
              V02.99 ☑
              nontraffic V02.09 ☑
              traffic V02.19 ☑
            vehicle V09.9 ☑
              animal-drawn V06.99 ☑
                nontraffic V06.09 ☑

---

**Accident** — *continued*
  transport — *continued*
    pedestrian — *continued*
      conveyance — *continued*
        specified type — *continued*
          collision — *continued*
            vehicle — *continued*
              animal-drawn — *continued*
                traffic V06.19 ☑
              motor
                nontraffic V09.00 ☑
                traffic V09.20 ☑
           fall V00.891 ☑
          nontraffic V09.1 ☑
            involving motor vehicle NEC
              V09.00 ☑
          traffic V09.3 ☑
            involving motor vehicle NEC
              V09.20 ☑
        traffic V09.3 ☑
          involving motor vehicle V09.20 ☑
            military V09.21 ☑
            specified type NEC V09.29 ☑
        wheelchair (powered) V00.818 ☑
          collision (with) V09.9 ☑
            animal being ridden or animal drawn
              vehicle V06.99 ☑
              nontraffic V06.09 ☑
              traffic V06.19 ☑
            bus or heavy transport V04.99 ☑
              nontraffic V04.09 ☑
              traffic V04.19 ☑
            car V03.99 ☑
              nontraffic V03.09 ☑
              traffic V03.19 ☑
            pedal cycle V01.99 ☑
              nontraffic V01.09 ☑
              traffic V01.19 ☑
            pick-up truck or van V03.99 ☑
              nontraffic V03.09 ☑
              traffic V03.19 ☑
            railway (train) (vehicle) V05.99 ☑
              nontraffic V05.09 ☑
              traffic V05.19 ☑
            stationary object V00.812 ☑
            streetcar V06.99 ☑
              nontraffic V06.09 ☑
              traffic V06.19 ☑
            two- or three-wheeled motor vehicle
              V02.99 ☑
              nontraffic V02.09 ☑
              traffic V02.19 ☑
            vehicle V09.9 ☑
              animal-drawn V06.99 ☑
                nontraffic V06.09 ☑
                traffic V06.19 ☑
              motor
                nontraffic V09.00 ☑
                traffic V09.20 ☑
           fall V00.811 ☑
          nontraffic V09.1 ☑
            involving motor vehicle NEC
              V09.00 ☑
          traffic V09.3 ☑
            involving motor vehicle NEC
              V09.20 ☑
        wheeled shoe V00.158 ☑
          colliding with stationary object
            V00.152 ☑
          fall V00.151 ☑
      on foot (*see also* Accident, pedestrian)
        collision (with)
          animal being ridden or animal drawn
            vehicle V06.90 ☑
            nontraffic V06.00 ☑
            traffic V06.10 ☑
          bus or heavy transport V04.90 ☑
            nontraffic V04.00 ☑
            traffic V04.10 ☑
          car V03.90 ☑
            nontraffic V03.00 ☑
            traffic V03.10 ☑
          pedal cycle V01.90 ☑
            nontraffic V01.00 ☑
            traffic V01.10 ☑
          pick-up truck or van V03.90 ☑

---

**Accident** — *continued*
  transport — *continued*
    pedestrian — *continued*
      on foot (*see also* Accident, pedestrian) — con-
        tinued
        collision — *continued*
          pick-up truck or van — *continued*
            nontraffic V03.00 ☑
            traffic V03.10 ☑
          railway (train) (vehicle) V05.90 ☑
            nontraffic V05.00 ☑
            traffic V05.10 ☑
          streetcar V06.90 ☑
            nontraffic V06.00 ☑
            traffic V06.10 ☑
          two- or three-wheeled motor vehicle
            V02.90 ☑
            nontraffic V02.00 ☑
            traffic V02.10 ☑
          vehicle V09.9 ☑
            animal-drawn V06.90 ☑
              nontraffic V06.00 ☑
              traffic V06.10 ☑
            motor
        nontraffic V09.1 ☑
          involving motor vehicle V09.00 ☑
            military V09.01 ☑
            specified type NEC V09.09 ☑
        traffic V09.3 ☑
          involving motor vehicle V09.20 ☑
            military V09.21 ☑
            specified type NEC V09.29 ☑
    person NEC (unknown way or transportation)
      V99 ☑
    collision (between)
      bus (with)
        heavy transport vehicle (traffic) V87.5 ☑
          nontraffic V88.5 ☑
      car (with)
        bus (traffic) V87.3 ☑
          nontraffic V88.3 ☑
        heavy transport vehicle (traffic) V87.4 ☑
          nontraffic V88.4 ☑
        nontraffic V88.5 ☑
        pick-up truck or van (traffic) V87.2 ☑
          nontraffic V88.2 ☑
        train or railway vehicle (traffic) V87.6 ☑
          nontraffic V88.6 ☑
        two- or three-wheeled motor vehicle
          (traffic) V87.0 ☑
          nontraffic V88.0 ☑
      motor vehicle (traffic) NEC V87.7 ☑
        nontraffic V88.7 ☑
      two- or three-wheeled vehicle (with) (traffic)
        motor vehicle NEC V87.1 ☑
          nontraffic V88.1 ☑
      nonmotor vehicle (collision) (noncollision)
        (traffic) V87.9 ☑
        nontraffic V88.9 ☑
    pickup truck occupant V59.9 ☑
      collision (with)
        animal (traffic) V50.9 ☑
          being ridden (traffic) V56.9 ☑
            nontraffic V56.3 ☑
            while boarding or alighting V56.4 ☑
          nontraffic V50.3 ☑
          while boarding or alighting V50.4 ☑
        animal-drawn vehicle (traffic) V56.9 ☑
          nontraffic V56.3 ☑
          while boarding or alighting V56.4 ☑
        bus (traffic) V54.9 ☑
          nontraffic V54.3 ☑
          while boarding or alighting V54.4 ☑
        car (traffic) V53.9 ☑
          nontraffic V53.3 ☑
          while boarding or alighting V53.4 ☑
        motor vehicle NOS (traffic) V59.60 ☑
          nontraffic V59.20 ☑
          specified type NEC (traffic) V59.69 ☑
           nontraffic V59.29 ☑
        pedal cycle (traffic) V51.9 ☑
          nontraffic V51.3 ☑
          while boarding or alighting V51.4 ☑
        pickup truck (traffic) V53.9 ☑
          nontraffic V53.3 ☑
          while boarding or alighting V53.4 ☑

☑ **Additional Character Required — Refer to the Tabular List for Character Selection**      ▽ **Subterms under main terms may continue to next column or page**

**Accident** — *continued*
  transport — *continued*
    pickup truck occupant — *continued*
      collision — *continued*
        railway vehicle (traffic) V55.9 ☑
          nontraffic V55.3 ☑
          while boarding or alighting V55.4 ☑
        specified vehicle NEC (traffic) V56.9 ☑
          nontraffic V56.3 ☑
          while boarding or alighting V56.4 ☑
        stationary object (traffic) V57.9 ☑
          nontraffic V57.3 ☑
          while boarding or alighting V57.4 ☑
        streetcar (traffic) V56.9 ☑
          nontraffic V56.3 ☑
          while boarding or alighting V56.4 ☑
        three wheeled motor vehicle (traffic) V52.9 ☑
          nontraffic V52.3 ☑
          while boarding or alighting V52.4 ☑
        truck (traffic) V54.9 ☑
          nontraffic V54.3 ☑
          while boarding or alighting V54.4 ☑
        two wheeled motor vehicle (traffic) V52.9 ☑
          nontraffic V52.3 ☑
          while boarding or alighting V52.4 ☑
        van (traffic) V53.9 ☑
          nontraffic V53.3 ☑
          while boarding or alighting V53.4 ☑
      driver
        collision (with)
          animal (traffic) V50.5 ☑
            being ridden (traffic) V56.5 ☑
              nontraffic V56.0 ☑
            nontraffic V50.0 ☑
          animal-drawn vehicle (traffic) V56.5 ☑
            nontraffic V56.0 ☑
          bus (traffic) V54.5 ☑
            nontraffic V54.0 ☑
          car (traffic) V53.5 ☑
            nontraffic V53.0 ☑
          motor vehicle NOS (traffic) V59.40 ☑
            nontraffic V59.00 ☑
            specified type NEC (traffic) V59.49 ☑
              nontraffic V59.09 ☑
          pedal cycle (traffic) V51.5 ☑
            nontraffic V51.0 ☑
          pickup truck (traffic) V53.5 ☑
            nontraffic V53.0 ☑
          railway vehicle (traffic) V55.5 ☑
            nontraffic V55.0 ☑
          specified vehicle NEC (traffic) V56.5 ☑
            nontraffic V56.0 ☑
          stationary object (traffic) V57.5 ☑
            nontraffic V57.0 ☑
          streetcar (traffic) V56.5 ☑
            nontraffic V56.0 ☑
          three wheeled motor vehicle (traffic) V52.5 ☑
            nontraffic V52.0 ☑
          truck (traffic) V54.5 ☑
            nontraffic V54.0 ☑
          two wheeled motor vehicle (traffic) V52.5 ☑
            nontraffic V52.0 ☑
          van (traffic) V53.5 ☑
            nontraffic V53.0 ☑
        noncollision accident (traffic) V58.5 ☑
          nontraffic V58.0 ☑
      hanger-on
        collision (with)
          animal (traffic) V50.7 ☑
            being ridden (traffic) V56.7 ☑
              nontraffic V56.2 ☑
            nontraffic V50.2 ☑
          animal-drawn vehicle (traffic) V56.7 ☑
            nontraffic V56.2 ☑
          bus (traffic) V54.7 ☑
            nontraffic V54.2 ☑
          car (traffic) V53.7 ☑
            nontraffic V53.2 ☑
          pedal cycle (traffic) V51.7 ☑
            nontraffic V51.2 ☑
          pickup truck (traffic) V53.7 ☑
            nontraffic V53.2 ☑
          railway vehicle (traffic) V55.7 ☑

---

**Accident** — *continued*
  transport — *continued*
    pickup truck occupant — *continued*
      hanger-on — *continued*
        collision — *continued*
          railway vehicle — *continued*
            nontraffic V55.2 ☑
          specified vehicle NEC (traffic) V56.7 ☑
            nontraffic V56.2 ☑
          stationary object (traffic) V57.7 ☑
            nontraffic V57.2 ☑
          streetcar (traffic) V56.7 ☑
            nontraffic V56.2 ☑
          three wheeled motor vehicle (traffic) V52.7 ☑
            nontraffic V52.2 ☑
          truck (traffic) V54.7 ☑
            nontraffic V54.2 ☑
          two wheeled motor vehicle (traffic) V52.7 ☑
            nontraffic V52.2 ☑
          van (traffic) V53.7 ☑
            nontraffic V53.2 ☑
        noncollision accident (traffic) V58.7 ☑
          nontraffic V58.2 ☑
      noncollision accident (traffic) V58.9 ☑
        nontraffic V58.3 ☑
        while boarding or alighting V58.4 ☑
      nontraffic V59.3 ☑
      passenger
        collision (with)
          animal (traffic) V50.6 ☑
            being ridden (traffic) V56.6 ☑
              nontraffic V56.1 ☑
            nontraffic V50.1 ☑
          animal-drawn vehicle (traffic) V56.6 ☑
            nontraffic V56.1 ☑
          bus (traffic) V54.6 ☑
            nontraffic V54.1 ☑
          car (traffic) V53.6 ☑
            nontraffic V53.1 ☑
          motor vehicle NOS (traffic) V59.50 ☑
            nontraffic V59.10 ☑
            specified type NEC (traffic) V59.59 ☑
              nontraffic V59.19 ☑
          pedal cycle (traffic) V51.6 ☑
            nontraffic V51.1 ☑
          pickup truck (traffic) V53.6 ☑
            nontraffic V53.1 ☑
          railway vehicle (traffic) V55.6 ☑
            nontraffic V55.1 ☑
          specified vehicle NEC (traffic) V56.6 ☑
            nontraffic V56.1 ☑
          stationary object (traffic) V57.6 ☑
            nontraffic V57.1 ☑
          streetcar (traffic) V56.6 ☑
            nontraffic V56.1 ☑
          three wheeled motor vehicle (traffic) V52.6 ☑
            nontraffic V52.1 ☑
          truck (traffic) V54.6 ☑
            nontraffic V54.1 ☑
          two wheeled motor vehicle (traffic) V52.6 ☑
            nontraffic V52.1 ☑
          van (traffic) V53.6 ☑
            nontraffic V53.1 ☑
        noncollision accident (traffic) V58.6 ☑
          nontraffic V58.1 ☑
      specified type NEC V59.88 ☑
      military vehicle V59.81 ☑
    quarry truck — *see* Accident, transport, industrial vehicle occupant
    race car — *see* Accident, transport, motor vehicle NEC occupant
    railway vehicle occupant V81.9 ☑
      collision (with) V81.3 ☑
        motor vehicle (non-military) (traffic) V81.1 ☑
          military V81.83 ☑
          nontraffic V81.0 ☑
        rolling stock V81.2 ☑
        specified object NEC V81.3 ☑
      during derailment V81.7 ☑

---

**Accident** — *continued*
  transport — *continued*
    railway vehicle occupant — *continued*
      during derailment — *continued*
        with antecedent collision — *see* Accident, transport, railway vehicle occupant, collision
      explosion V81.81 ☑
      fall (in railway vehicle) V81.5 ☑
        during derailment V81.7 ☑
          with antecedent collision — *see* Accident, transport, railway vehicle occupant, collision
        from railway vehicle V81.6 ☑
          during derailment V81.7 ☑
            with antecedent collision — *see* Accident, transport, railway vehicle occupant, collision
        while boarding or alighting V81.4 ☑
      fire V81.81 ☑
      object falling onto train V81.82 ☑
      specified type NEC V81.89 ☑
      while boarding or alighting V81.4 ☑
    ski lift V98.3 ☑
    snowmobile occupant (nontraffic) V86.92 ☑
      driver V86.52 ☑
      hanger-on V86.72 ☑
      passenger V86.62 ☑
      traffic V86.32 ☑
        driver V86.02 ☑
        hanger-on V86.22 ☑
        passenger V86.12 ☑
      while boarding or alighting V86.42 ☑
    specified NEC V98.8 ☑
    sport utility vehicle occupant (*see also* Accident, transport, pickup truck occupant)
    streetcar occupant V82.9 ☑
      collision (with) V82.3 ☑
        motor vehicle (traffic) V82.1 ☑
          nontraffic V82.0 ☑
        rolling stock V82.2 ☑
      during derailment V82.7 ☑
        with antecedent collision — *see* Accident, transport, streetcar occupant, collision
      fall (in streetcar) V82.5 ☑
        during derailment V82.7 ☑
          with antecedent collision — *see* Accident, transport, streetcar occupant, collision
        from streetcar V82.6 ☑
          during derailment V82.7 ☑
            with antecedent collision — *see* Accident, transport, streetcar occupant, collision
        while boarding or alighting V82.4 ☑
      while boarding or alighting V82.4 ☑
      specified type NEC V82.8 ☑
      while boarding or alighting V82.4 ☑
    three-wheeled motor vehicle occupant V39.9 ☑
      collision (with)
        animal (traffic) V30.9 ☑
          being ridden (traffic) V36.9 ☑
            nontraffic V36.3 ☑
            while boarding or alighting V36.4 ☑
          nontraffic V30.3 ☑
            while boarding or alighting V30.4 ☑
        animal-drawn vehicle (traffic) V36.9 ☑
          nontraffic V36.3 ☑
          while boarding or alighting V36.4 ☑
        bus (traffic) V34.9 ☑
          nontraffic V34.3 ☑
          while boarding or alighting V34.4 ☑
        car (traffic) V33.9 ☑
          nontraffic V33.3 ☑
          while boarding or alighting V33.4 ☑
        motor vehicle NOS (traffic) V39.60 ☑
          nontraffic V39.20 ☑
          specified type NEC (traffic) V39.69 ☑
            nontraffic V39.29 ☑
        pedal cycle (traffic) V31.9 ☑
          nontraffic V31.3 ☑
          while boarding or alighting V31.4 ☑
        pickup truck (traffic) V33.9 ☑
          nontraffic V33.3 ☑
          while boarding or alighting V33.4 ☑
        railway vehicle (traffic) V35.9 ☑

**Accident** — continued
  transport — continued
    three-wheeled motor vehicle occupant — continued
      collision — continued
        railway vehicle — continued
          nontraffic V35.3 ☑
          while boarding or alighting V35.4 ☑
        specified vehicle NEC (traffic) V36.9 ☑
          nontraffic V36.3 ☑
          while boarding or alighting V36.4 ☑
        stationary object (traffic) V37.9 ☑
          nontraffic V37.3 ☑
          while boarding or alighting V37.4 ☑
        streetcar (traffic) V36.9 ☑
          nontraffic V36.3 ☑
          while boarding or alighting V36.4 ☑
        three wheeled motor vehicle (traffic) V32.9 ☑
          nontraffic V32.3 ☑
          while boarding or alighting V32.4 ☑
         truck (traffic) V34.9 ☑
          nontraffic V34.3 ☑
          while boarding or alighting V34.4 ☑
        two wheeled motor vehicle (traffic) V32.9 ☑
          nontraffic V32.3 ☑
          while boarding or alighting V32.4 ☑
        van (traffic) V33.9 ☑
          nontraffic V33.3 ☑
          while boarding or alighting V33.4 ☑
      driver
        collision (with)
          animal (traffic) V30.5 ☑
            being ridden (traffic) V36.5 ☑
              nontraffic V36.0 ☑
            nontraffic V30.0 ☑
          animal-drawn vehicle (traffic) V36.5 ☑
            nontraffic V36.0 ☑
          bus (traffic) V34.5 ☑
            nontraffic V34.0 ☑
          car (traffic) V33.5 ☑
            nontraffic V33.0 ☑
          motor vehicle NOS (traffic) V39.40 ☑
            nontraffic V39.00 ☑
            specified type NEC (traffic) V39.49 ☑
              nontraffic V39.09 ☑
          pedal cycle (traffic) V31.5 ☑
            nontraffic V31.0 ☑
          pickup truck (traffic) V33.5 ☑
            nontraffic V33.0 ☑
          railway vehicle (traffic) V35.5 ☑
            nontraffic V35.0 ☑
          specified vehicle NEC (traffic) V36.5 ☑
            nontraffic V36.0 ☑
          stationary object (traffic) V37.5 ☑
            nontraffic V37.0 ☑
          streetcar (traffic) V36.5 ☑
            nontraffic V36.0 ☑
          three wheeled motor vehicle (traffic) V32.5 ☑
            nontraffic V32.0 ☑
          truck (traffic) V34.5 ☑
            nontraffic V34.0 ☑
          two wheeled motor vehicle (traffic) V32.5 ☑
            nontraffic V32.0 ☑
          van (traffic) V33.5 ☑
            nontraffic V33.0 ☑
        noncollision accident (traffic) V38.5 ☑
          nontraffic V38.0 ☑
      hanger-on
        collision (with)
          animal (traffic) V30.7 ☑
            being ridden (traffic) V36.7 ☑
              nontraffic V36.2 ☑
            nontraffic V30.2 ☑
          animal-drawn vehicle (traffic) V36.7 ☑
            nontraffic V36.2 ☑
          bus (traffic) V34.7 ☑
            nontraffic V34.2 ☑
          car (traffic) V33.7 ☑
            nontraffic V33.2 ☑
          pedal cycle (traffic) V31.7 ☑
            nontraffic V31.2 ☑
          pickup truck (traffic) V33.7 ☑
            nontraffic V33.2 ☑

**Accident** — continued
  transport — continued
    three-wheeled motor vehicle occupant — continued
      hanger-on — continued
        collision — continued
          railway vehicle (traffic) V35.7 ☑
            nontraffic V35.2 ☑
          specified vehicle NEC (traffic) V36.7 ☑
            nontraffic V36.2 ☑
          stationary object (traffic) V37.7 ☑
            nontraffic V37.2 ☑
          streetcar (traffic) V36.7 ☑
            nontraffic V36.2 ☑
          three wheeled motor vehicle (traffic) V32.7 ☑
            nontraffic V32.2 ☑
          truck (traffic) V34.7 ☑
            nontraffic V34.2 ☑
          two wheeled motor vehicle (traffic) V32.7 ☑
            nontraffic V32.2 ☑
          van (traffic) V33.7 ☑
            nontraffic V33.2 ☑
        noncollision accident (traffic) V38.7 ☑
          nontraffic V38.2 ☑
      noncollision accident (traffic) V38.9 ☑
        nontraffic V38.3 ☑
        while boarding or alighting V38.4 ☑
      nontraffic V39.3 ☑
      passenger
        collision (with)
          animal (traffic) V30.6 ☑
            being ridden (traffic) V36.6 ☑
              nontraffic V36.1 ☑
            nontraffic V30.1 ☑
          animal-drawn vehicle (traffic) V36.6 ☑
            nontraffic V36.1 ☑
          bus (traffic) V34.6 ☑
            nontraffic V34.1 ☑
          car (traffic) V33.6 ☑
            nontraffic V33.1 ☑
          motor vehicle NOS (traffic) V39.50 ☑
            nontraffic V39.10 ☑
            specified type NEC (traffic) V39.59 ☑
              nontraffic V39.19 ☑
          pedal cycle (traffic) V31.6 ☑
            nontraffic V31.1 ☑
          pickup truck (traffic) V33.6 ☑
            nontraffic V33.1 ☑
          railway vehicle (traffic) V35.6 ☑
            nontraffic V35.1 ☑
          specified vehicle NEC (traffic) V36.6 ☑
            nontraffic V36.1 ☑
          stationary object (traffic) V37.6 ☑
            nontraffic V37.1 ☑
          streetcar (traffic) V36.6 ☑
            nontraffic V36.1 ☑
          three wheeled motor vehicle (traffic) V32.6 ☑
            nontraffic V32.1 ☑
          truck (traffic) V34.6 ☑
            nontraffic V34.1 ☑
          two wheeled motor vehicle (traffic) V32.6 ☑
            nontraffic V32.1 ☑
          van (traffic) V33.6 ☑
            nontraffic V33.1 ☑
        noncollision accident (traffic) V38.6 ☑
          nontraffic V38.1 ☑
      specified type NEC V39.89 ☑
        military vehicle V39.81 ☑
      tractor (farm) (and trailer) — see Accident, transport, agricultural vehicle occupant
      tram — see Accident, transport, streetcar
        in mine or quarry — see Accident, transport, industrial vehicle occupant
      trolley — see Accident, transport, streetcar
        in mine or quarry — see Accident, transport, industrial vehicle occupant
    truck (heavy) occupant V69.9 ☑
      collision (with)
        animal (traffic) V60.9 ☑
          being ridden (traffic) V66.9 ☑
            nontraffic V66.3 ☑
            while boarding or alighting V66.4 ☑

**Accident** — continued
  transport — continued
    truck occupant — continued
      collision — continued
        animal — continued
          nontraffic V60.3 ☑
          while boarding or alighting V60.4 ☑
        animal-drawn vehicle (traffic) V66.9 ☑
          nontraffic V66.3 ☑
          while boarding or alighting V66.4 ☑
        bus (traffic) V64.9 ☑
          nontraffic V64.3 ☑
          while boarding or alighting V64.4 ☑
        car (traffic) V63.9 ☑
          nontraffic V63.3 ☑
          while boarding or alighting V63.4 ☑
        motor vehicle NOS (traffic) V69.60 ☑
          nontraffic V69.20 ☑
          specified type NEC (traffic) V69.69 ☑
            nontraffic V69.29 ☑
        pedal cycle (traffic) V61.9 ☑
          nontraffic V61.3 ☑
          while boarding or alighting V61.4 ☑
        pickup truck (traffic) V63.9 ☑
          nontraffic V63.3 ☑
          while boarding or alighting V63.4 ☑
        railway vehicle (traffic) V65.9 ☑
          nontraffic V65.3 ☑
          while boarding or alighting V65.4 ☑
        specified vehicle NEC (traffic) V66.9 ☑
          nontraffic V66.3 ☑
          while boarding or alighting V66.4 ☑
        stationary object (traffic) V67.9 ☑
          nontraffic V67.3 ☑
          while boarding or alighting V67.4 ☑
        streetcar (traffic) V66.9 ☑
          nontraffic V66.3 ☑
          while boarding or alighting V66.4 ☑
        three wheeled motor vehicle (traffic) V62.9 ☑
          nontraffic V62.3 ☑
          while boarding or alighting V62.4 ☑
        truck (traffic) V64.9 ☑
          nontraffic V64.3 ☑
          while boarding or alighting V64.4 ☑
        two wheeled motor vehicle (traffic) V62.9 ☑
          nontraffic V62.3 ☑
          while boarding or alighting V62.4 ☑
        van (traffic) V63.9 ☑
          nontraffic V63.3 ☑
          while boarding or alighting V63.4 ☑
    driver
      collision (with)
        animal (traffic) V60.5 ☑
          being ridden (traffic) V66.5 ☑
            nontraffic V66.0 ☑
          nontraffic V60.0 ☑
        animal-drawn vehicle (traffic) V66.5 ☑
          nontraffic V66.0 ☑
        bus (traffic) V64.5 ☑
          nontraffic V64.0 ☑
        car (traffic) V63.5 ☑
          nontraffic V63.0 ☑
        motor vehicle NOS (traffic) V69.40 ☑
          nontraffic V69.00 ☑
          specified type NEC (traffic) V69.49 ☑
            nontraffic V69.09 ☑
        pedal cycle (traffic) V61.5 ☑
          nontraffic V61.0 ☑
        pickup truck (traffic) V63.5 ☑
          nontraffic V63.0 ☑
        railway vehicle (traffic) V65.5 ☑
          nontraffic V65.0 ☑
        specified vehicle NEC (traffic) V66.5 ☑
          nontraffic V66.0 ☑
        stationary object (traffic) V67.5 ☑
          nontraffic V67.0 ☑
        streetcar (traffic) V66.5 ☑
          nontraffic V66.0 ☑
        three wheeled motor vehicle (traffic) V62.5 ☑
          nontraffic V62.0 ☑
        truck (traffic) V64.5 ☑
          nontraffic V64.0 ☑
        two wheeled motor vehicle (traffic) V62.5 ☑

☑ **Additional Character Required** — Refer to the Tabular List for Character Selection      ▽ **Subterms under main terms may continue to next column or page**

**Accident** — *continued*
  transport — *continued*
    truck occupant — *continued*
      driver — *continued*
        collision — *continued*
          two wheeled motor vehicle — *continued*
            nontraffic V62.0 ☑
          van (traffic) V63.5 ☑
            nontraffic V63.0 ☑
        noncollision accident (traffic) V68.5 ☑
          nontraffic V68.0 ☑
      dump — *see* Accident, transport, construction vehicle occupant
      hanger-on
        collision (with)
          animal (traffic) V60.7 ☑
            being ridden (traffic) V66.7 ☑
              nontraffic V66.2 ☑
            nontraffic V60.2 ☑
          animal-drawn vehicle (traffic) V66.7 ☑
            nontraffic V66.2 ☑
          bus (traffic) V64.7 ☑
            nontraffic V64.2 ☑
          car (traffic) V63.7 ☑
            nontraffic V63.2 ☑
          pedal cycle (traffic) V61.7 ☑
            nontraffic V61.2 ☑
          pickup truck (traffic) V63.7 ☑
            nontraffic V63.2 ☑
          railway vehicle (traffic) V65.7 ☑
            nontraffic V65.2 ☑
          specified vehicle NEC (traffic) V66.7 ☑
            nontraffic V66.2 ☑
          stationary object (traffic) V67.7 ☑
            nontraffic V67.2 ☑
          streetcar (traffic) V66.7 ☑
            nontraffic V66.2 ☑
          three wheeled motor vehicle (traffic) V62.7 ☑
            nontraffic V62.2 ☑
          truck (traffic) V64.7 ☑
            nontraffic V64.2 ☑
          two wheeled motor vehicle (traffic) V62.7 ☑
            nontraffic V62.2 ☑
          van (traffic) V63.7 ☑
            nontraffic V63.2 ☑
        noncollision accident (traffic) V68.7 ☑
          nontraffic V68.2 ☑
      noncollision accident (traffic) V68.9 ☑
        nontraffic V68.3 ☑
        while boarding or alighting V68.4 ☑
      nontraffic V69.3 ☑
      passenger
        collision (with)
          animal (traffic) V60.6 ☑
            being ridden (traffic) V66.6 ☑
              nontraffic V66.1- ☑
            nontraffic V60.1 ☑
          animal-drawn vehicle (traffic) V66.6 ☑
            nontraffic V66.1 ☑
          bus (traffic) V64.6 ☑
            nontraffic V64.1 ☑
          car (traffic) V63.6 ☑
            nontraffic V63.1 ☑
          motor vehicle NOS (traffic) V69.50 ☑
            nontraffic V69.10 ☑
            specified type NEC (traffic) V69.59 ☑
              nontraffic V69.19 ☑
          pedal cycle (traffic) V61.6 ☑
            nontraffic V61.1 ☑
          pickup truck (traffic) V63.6 ☑
            nontraffic V63.1 ☑
          railway vehicle (traffic) V65.6 ☑
            nontraffic V65.1 ☑
          specified vehicle NEC (traffic) V66.6 ☑
            nontraffic V66.1 ☑
          stationary object (traffic) V67.6 ☑
            nontraffic V67.1 ☑
          streetcar (traffic) V66.6 ☑
            nontraffic V66.1 ☑
          three wheeled motor vehicle (traffic) V62.6 ☑
            nontraffic V62.1 ☑
          truck (traffic) V64.6 ☑

**Accident** — *continued*
  transport — *continued*
    truck occupant — *continued*
      passenger — *continued*
        collision — *continued*
          truck — *continued*
            nontraffic V64.1 ☑
          two wheeled motor vehicle (traffic) V62.6 ☑
            nontraffic V62.1 ☑
          van (traffic) V63.6 ☑
            nontraffic V63.1 ☑
        noncollision accident (traffic) V68.6 ☑
          nontraffic V68.1 ☑
      pickup — *see* Accident, transport, pickup truck occupant
      specified type NEC V69.88 ☑
        military vehicle V69.81 ☑
    van occupant V59.9 ☑
      collision (with)
        animal (traffic) V50.9 ☑
          being ridden (traffic) V56.9 ☑
            nontraffic V56.3 ☑
            while boarding or alighting V56.4 ☑
          nontraffic V50.3 ☑
          while boarding or alighting V50.4 ☑
        animal-drawn vehicle (traffic) V56.9 ☑
          nontraffic V56.3 ☑
          while boarding or alighting V56.4 ☑
        bus (traffic) V54.9 ☑
          nontraffic V54.3 ☑
          while boarding or alighting V54.4 ☑
        car (traffic) V53.9 ☑
          nontraffic V53.3 ☑
          while boarding or alighting V53.4 ☑
        motor vehicle NOS (traffic) V59.60 ☑
          nontraffic V59.20 ☑
          specified type NEC (traffic) V59.69 ☑
            nontraffic V59.29 ☑
        pedal cycle (traffic) V51.9 ☑
          nontraffic V51.3 ☑
          while boarding or alighting V51.4 ☑
        pickup truck (traffic) V53.9 ☑
          nontraffic V53.3 ☑
          while boarding or alighting V53.4 ☑
        railway vehicle (traffic) V55.9 ☑
          nontraffic V55.3 ☑
          while boarding or alighting V55.4 ☑
        specified vehicle NEC (traffic) V56.9 ☑
          nontraffic V56.3 ☑
          while boarding or alighting V56.4 ☑
        stationary object (traffic) V57.9 ☑
          nontraffic V57.3 ☑
          while boarding or alighting V57.4 ☑
        streetcar (traffic) V56.9 ☑
          nontraffic V56.3 ☑
          while boarding or alighting V56.4 ☑
        three wheeled motor vehicle (traffic) V52.9 ☑
          nontraffic V52.3 ☑
          while boarding or alighting V52.4 ☑
        truck (traffic) V54.9 ☑
          nontraffic V54.3 ☑
          while boarding or alighting V54.4 ☑
        two wheeled motor vehicle (traffic) V52.9 ☑
          nontraffic V52.3 ☑
          while boarding or alighting V52.4 ☑
        van (traffic) V53.9 ☑
          nontraffic V53.3 ☑
          while boarding or alighting V53.4 ☑
      driver
        collision (with)
          animal (traffic) V50.5 ☑
           being ridden (traffic) V56.5 ☑
            nontraffic V56.0 ☑
           nontraffic V50.0 ☑
          animal-drawn vehicle (traffic) V56.5 ☑
           nontraffic V56.0 ☑
          bus (traffic) V54.5 ☑
           nontraffic V54.0 ☑
          car (traffic) V53.5 ☑
           nontraffic V53.0 ☑
          motor vehicle NOS (traffic) V59.40 ☑
           nontraffic V59.00 ☑
           specified type NEC (traffic) V59.49 ☑
            nontraffic V59.09 ☑

**Accident** — *continued*
  transport — *continued*
    van occupant — *continued*
      driver — *continued*
        collision — *continued*
          pedal cycle (traffic) V51.5 ☑
           nontraffic V51.0 ☑
          pickup truck (traffic) V53.5 ☑
           nontraffic V53.0 ☑
          railway vehicle (traffic) V55.5 ☑
           nontraffic V55.0 ☑
          specified vehicle NEC (traffic) V56.5 ☑
           nontraffic V56.0 ☑
          stationary object (traffic) V57.5 ☑
           nontraffic V57.0 ☑
          streetcar (traffic) V56.5 ☑
           nontraffic V56.0 ☑
          three wheeled motor vehicle (traffic) V52.5 ☑
           nontraffic V52.0 ☑
          truck (traffic) V54.5 ☑
           nontraffic V54.0 ☑
          two wheeled motor vehicle (traffic) V52.5 ☑
           nontraffic V52.0 ☑
          van (traffic) V53.5 ☑
           nontraffic V53.0 ☑
        noncollision accident (traffic) V58.5 ☑
          nontraffic V58.0 ☑
      hanger-on
        collision (with)
          animal (traffic) V50.7 ☑
           being ridden (traffic) V56.7 ☑
            nontraffic V56.2 ☑
           nontraffic V50.2 ☑
          animal-drawn vehicle (traffic) V56.7 ☑
           nontraffic V56.2 ☑
          bus (traffic) V54.7 ☑
           nontraffic V54.2 ☑
          car (traffic) V53.7 ☑
           nontraffic V53.2 ☑
          pedal cycle (traffic) V51.7 ☑
           nontraffic V51.2 ☑
          pickup truck (traffic) V53.7 ☑
           nontraffic V53.2 ☑
          railway vehicle (traffic) V55.7 ☑
           nontraffic V55.2 ☑
          specified vehicle NEC (traffic) V56.7 ☑
           nontraffic V56.2 ☑
          stationary object (traffic) V57.7 ☑
           nontraffic V57.2 ☑
          streetcar (traffic) V56.7 ☑
           nontraffic V56.2 ☑
          three wheeled motor vehicle (traffic) V52.7 ☑
           nontraffic V52.2 ☑
          truck (traffic) V54.7 ☑
           nontraffic V54.2 ☑
          two wheeled motor vehicle (traffic) V52.7 ☑
           nontraffic V52.2 ☑
          van (traffic) V53.7 ☑
           nontraffic V53.2 ☑
        noncollision accident (traffic) V58.7 ☑
          nontraffic V58.2 ☑
      noncollision accident (traffic) V58.9 ☑
        nontraffic V58.3 ☑
        while boarding or alighting V58.4 ☑
      nontraffic V59.3 ☑
      passenger
        collision (with)
          animal (traffic) V50.6 ☑
           being ridden (traffic) V56.6 ☑
            nontraffic V56.1 ☑
           nontraffic V50.1 ☑
          animal-drawn vehicle (traffic) V56.6 ☑
           nontraffic V56.1 ☑
          bus (traffic) V54.6 ☑
           nontraffic V54.1 ☑
          car (traffic) V53.6 ☑
           nontraffic V53.1 ☑
          motor vehicle NOS (traffic) V59.50 ☑
           nontraffic V59.10 ☑
           specified type NEC (traffic) V59.59 ☑
            nontraffic V59.19 ☑
          pedal cycle (traffic) V51.6 ☑

▽ **Subterms under main terms may continue to next column or page**     ☑ **Additional Character Required — Refer to the Tabular List for Character Selection**     **407**

Accident — Accident

**Accident** — *continued*
  transport — *continued*
    van occupant — *continued*
      passenger — *continued*
        collision — *continued*
          pedal cycle — *continued*
            nontraffic V51.1 ☑
          pickup truck (traffic) V53.6 ☑
            nontraffic V53.1 ☑
          railway vehicle (traffic) V55.6 ☑
            nontraffic V55.1 ☑
          specified vehicle NEC (traffic) V56.6 ☑
            nontraffic V56.1 ☑
          stationary object (traffic) V57.6 ☑
            nontraffic V57.1 ☑
          streetcar (traffic) V56.6 ☑
            nontraffic V56.1 ☑
          three wheeled motor vehicle (traffic)
            V52.6 ☑
            nontraffic V52.1 ☑
          truck (traffic) V54.6 ☑
            nontraffic V54.1 ☑
          two wheeled motor vehicle (traffic)
            V52.6 ☑
            nontraffic V52.1 ☑
          van (traffic) V53.6 ☑
            nontraffic V53.1 ☑
        noncollision accident (traffic) V58.6 ☑
          nontraffic V58.1 ☑
      specified type NEC V59.88 ☑
      military vehicle V59.81 ☑
    watercraft occupant — *see* Accident, watercraft
  vehicle NEC V89.9 ☑
    animal-drawn NEC — *see* Accident, transport, ani-
      mal-drawn vehicle occupant
    special
      agricultural — *see* Accident, transport, agricul-
        tural vehicle occupant
      construction — *see* Accident, transport, con-
        struction vehicle occupant
      industrial — *see* Accident, transport, industrial
        vehicle occupant
      three-wheeled NEC (motorized) — *see* Accident,
        transport, three-wheeled motor vehicle oc-
        cupant
  watercraft V94.9 ☑
    causing
      drowning — *see* Drowning, due to, accident
        to, watercraft
      injury NEC V91.89 ☑
        crushed between craft and object V91.19 ☑
          powered craft V91.13 ☑
            ferry boat V91.11 ☑
            fishing boat V91.12 ☑
            jetskis V91.13 ☑
            liner V91.11 ☑
            merchant ship V91.10 ☑
            passenger ship V91.11 ☑
          unpowered craft V91.18 ☑
            canoe V91.15 ☑
            inflatable V91.16 ☑
            kayak V91.15 ☑
            sailboat V91.14 ☑
            surf-board V91.18 ☑
            windsurfer V91.18 ☑
        fall on board V91.29 ☑
          powered craft V91.23 ☑
            ferry boat V91.21 ☑
            fishing boat V91.22 ☑
            jetskis V91.23 ☑
            liner V91.21 ☑
            merchant ship V91.20 ☑
            passenger ship V91.21 ☑
          unpowered craft
            canoe V91.25 ☑
            inflatable V91.26 ☑
            kayak V91.25 ☑
            sailboat V91.24 ☑
        fire on board causing burn V91.09 ☑
          powered craft V91.03 ☑
            ferry boat V91.01 ☑
            fishing boat V91.02 ☑
            jetskis V91.03 ☑
            liner V91.01 ☑
            merchant ship V91.00 ☑
            passenger ship V91.01 ☑

**Accident** — *continued*
  watercraft — *continued*
    causing — *continued*
      injury — *continued*
        fire on board causing burn — *continued*
          unpowered craft V91.08 ☑
            canoe V91.05 ☑
            inflatable V91.06 ☑
            kayak V91.05 ☑
            sailboat V91.04 ☑
            surf-board V91.08 ☑
            water skis V91.07 ☑
            windsurfer V91.08 ☑
        hit by falling object V91.39 ☑
          powered craft V91.33 ☑
            ferry boat V91.31 ☑
            fishing boat V91.32 ☑
            jetskis V91.33 ☑
            liner V91.31 ☑
            merchant ship V91.30 ☑
            passenger ship V91.31 ☑
          unpowered craft V91.38 ☑
            canoe V91.35 ☑
            inflatable V91.36 ☑
            kayak V91.35 ☑
            sailboat V91.34 ☑
            surf-board V91.38 ☑
            water skis V91.37 ☑
            windsurfer V91.38 ☑
        specified type NEC V91.89 ☑
          powered craft V91.83 ☑
            ferry boat V91.81 ☑
            fishing boat V91.82 ☑
            jetskis V91.83 ☑
            liner V91.81 ☑
            merchant ship V91.80 ☑
            passenger ship V91.81 ☑
          unpowered craft V91.88 ☑
            canoe V91.85 ☑
            inflatable V91.86 ☑
            kayak V91.85 ☑
            sailboat V91.84 ☑
            surf-board V91.88 ☑
            water skis V91.87 ☑
            windsurfer V91.88 ☑
    due to, caused by cataclysm — *see* Forces of na-
      ture, by type
    military NEC V94.818 ☑
      with civilian watercraft V94.810 ☑
        civilian in water injured by V94.811 ☑
    nonpowered, struck by
      nonpowered vessel V94.22 ☑
      powered vessel V94.21 ☑
    specified type NEC V94.89 ☑
    striking swimmer
      powered V94.11 ☑
      unpowered V94.12 ☑

**Acid throwing** (assault) Y08.89 ☑
**Activity** (involving) (of victim at time of event) Y93.9
  aerobic and step exercise (class) Y93.A3 (*following*
    Y93.7)
  alpine skiing Y93.23
  animal care NEC Y93.K9 (*following* Y93.7)
  arts and handcrafts NEC Y93.D9 (*following* Y93.7)
  athletics played as a team or group NEC Y93.69
  athletics played individually NEC Y93.59
  athletics NEC Y93.79
  baking Y93.G3 (*following* Y93.7)
  ballet Y93.41
  barbells Y93.B3 (*following* Y93.7)
  BASE (Building, Antenna, Span, Earth) jumping Y93.33
  baseball Y93.64
  basketball Y93.67
  bathing (personal) Y93.E1 (*following* Y93.7)
  beach volleyball Y93.68
  bike riding Y93.55
  blackout game Y93.85
  boogie boarding Y93.18
  bowling Y93.54
  boxing Y93.71
  brass instrument playing Y93.J4 (*following* Y93.7)
  building construction Y93.H3 (*following* Y93.7)
  bungee jumping Y93.34
  calisthenics Y93.A2 (*following* Y93.7)
  canoeing (in calm and turbulent water) Y93.16
  capture the flag Y93.6A
  cardiorespiratory exercise NEC Y93.A9 (*following* Y93.7)

**Activity** — *continued*
  caregiving (providing) NEC Y93.F9 (*following* Y93.7)
    bathing Y93.F1 (*following* Y93.7)
    lifting Y93.F2 (*following* Y93.7)
  cellular
    communication device Y93.C2 (*following* Y93.7)
    telephone Y93.C2 (*following* Y93.7)
  challenge course Y93.A5 (*following* Y93.7)
  cheerleading Y93.45
  choking game Y93.85
  circuit training Y93.A4 (*following* Y93.7)
  cleaning
    floor Y93.E5 (*following* Y93.7)
  climbing NEC Y93.39
    mountain Y93.31
    rock Y93.31
    wall Y93.31
  clothing care and maintenance NEC Y93.E9 (*following*
    Y93.7)
  combatives Y93.75
  computer
    keyboarding Y93.C1 (*following* Y93.7)
    technology NEC Y93.C9 (*following* Y93.7)
  confidence course Y93.A5 (*following* Y93.7)
  construction (building) Y93.H3 (*following* Y93.7)
  cooking and baking Y93.G3 (*following* Y93.7)
  cool down exercises Y93.A2 (*following* Y93.7)
  cricket Y93.69
  crocheting Y93.D1 (*following* Y93.7)
  cross country skiing Y93.24
  dancing (all types) Y93.41
  digging
    dirt Y93.H1 (*following* Y93.7)
  dirt digging Y93.H1 (*following* Y93.7)
  dishwashing Y93.G1 (*following* Y93.7)
  diving (platform) (springboard) Y93.12
    underwater Y93.15
  dodge ball Y93.6A
  downhill skiing Y93.23
  drum playing Y93.J2 (*following* Y93.7)
  dumbbells Y93.B3 (*following* Y93.7)
  electronic
    devices NEC Y93.C9 (*following* Y93.7)
      hand held interactive Y93.C2 (*following* Y93.7)
    game playing (using) (with)
      interactive device Y93.C2 (*following* Y93.7)
      keyboard or other stationary device Y93.C1
        (*following* Y93.7)
  elliptical machine Y93.A1 (*following* Y93.7)
  exercise(s)
    machines ((primarily) for)
      cardiorespiratory conditioning Y93.A1 (*follow-
        ing* Y93.7)
      muscle strengthening Y93.B1 (*following* Y93.7)
    muscle strengthening (non-machine) NEC Y93.B9
      (*following* Y93.7)
  external motion NEC Y93.I9 (*following* Y93.7)
    rollercoaster Y93.I1 (*following* Y93.7)
  fainting game Y93.85
  field hockey Y93.65
  figure skating (pairs) (singles) Y93.21
  flag football Y93.62
  floor mopping and cleaning Y93.E5 (*following* Y93.7)
  food preparation and clean up Y93.G1 (*following* Y93.7)
  football (American) NOS Y93.61
    flag Y93.62
    tackle Y93.61
    touch Y93.62
  four square Y93.6A
  free weights Y93.B3 (*following* Y93.7)
  frisbee (ultimate) Y93.74
  furniture
    building Y93.D3 (*following* Y93.7)
    finishing Y93.D3 (*following* Y93.7)
    repair Y93.D3 (*following* Y93.7)
  game playing (electronic)
    using interactive device Y93.C2 (*following* Y93.7)
    using keyboard or other stationary device Y93.C1
      (*following* Y93.7)
  gardening Y93.H2 (*following* Y93.7)
  golf Y93.53
  grass drills Y93.A6 (*following* Y93.7)
  grilling and smoking food Y93.G2 (*following* Y93.7)
  grooming and shearing an animal Y93.K3 (*following*
    Y93.7)
  guerilla drills Y93.A6 (*following* Y93.7)
  gymnastics (rhythmic) Y93.43
  hand held interactive electronic device Y93.C2 (*follow-
    ing* Y93.7)

**Activity** — *continued*
handball Y93.73
handcrafts NEC Y93.D9 (*following* Y93.7)
hang gliding Y93.35
hiking (on level or elevated terrain) Y93.Ø1
hockey (ice) Y93.22
　field Y93.65
horseback riding Y93.52
household (interior) maintenance NEC Y93.E9 (*follow-ing* Y93.7)
ice NEC Y93.29
　dancing Y93.21
　hockey Y93.22
　skating Y93.21
inline roller skating Y93.51
ironing Y93.E4 (*following* Y93.7)
judo Y93.75
jumping jacks Y93.A2 (*following* Y93.7)
jumping rope Y93.56
jumping (off) NEC Y93.39
　BASE (Building, Antenna, Span, Earth) Y93.33
　bungee Y93.34
　jacks Y93.A2 (*following* Y93.7)
　rope Y93.56
karate Y93.75
kayaking (in calm and turbulent water) Y93.16
keyboarding (computer) Y93.C1 (*following* Y93.7)
kickball Y93.6A
knitting Y93.D1 (*following* Y93.7)
lacrosse Y93.65
land maintenance NEC Y93.H9 (*following* Y93.7)
landscaping Y93.H2 (*following* Y93.7)
laundry Y93.E2 (*following* Y93.7)
machines (exercise)
　primarily for cardiorespiratory conditioning Y93.A1 (*following* Y93.7)
　primarily for muscle strengthening Y93.B1 (*follow-ing* Y93.7)
maintenance
　exterior building NEC Y93.H9 (*following* Y93.7)
　household (interior) NEC Y93.E9 (*following* Y93.7)
　land Y93.H9 (*following* Y93.7)
　property Y93.H9 (*following* Y93.7)
marching (on level or elevated terrain) Y93.Ø1
martial arts Y93.75
microwave oven Y93.G3 (*following* Y93.7)
milking an animal Y93.K2 (*following* Y93.7)
mopping (floor) Y93.E5 (*following* Y93.7)
mountain climbing Y93.31
muscle strengthening
　exercises (non-machine) NEC Y93.B9 (*following* Y93.7)
　machines Y93.B1 (*following* Y93.7)
musical keyboard (electronic) playing Y93.J1 (*following* Y93.7)
nordic skiing Y93.24
obstacle course Y93.A5 (*following* Y93.7)
oven (microwave) Y93.G3 (*following* Y93.7)
packing up and unpacking in moving to a new resi-dence Y93.E6 (*following* Y93.7)
parasailing Y93.19
pass out game Y93.85
percussion instrument playing NEC Y93.J2 (*following* Y93.7)
personal
　bathing and showering Y93.E1 (*following* Y93.7)
　hygiene NEC Y93.E8 (*following* Y93.7)
　showering Y93.E1 (*following* Y93.7)
physical games generally associated with school re-cess, summer camp and children Y93.6A
physical training NEC Y93.A9 (*following* Y93.7)
piano playing Y93.J1 (*following* Y93.7)
pilates Y93.B4 (*following* Y93.7)
platform diving Y93.12
playing musical instrument
　brass instrument Y93.J4 (*following* Y93.7)
　drum Y93.J2 (*following* Y93.7)
　musical keyboard (electronic) Y93.J1 (*following* Y93.7)
　percussion instrument NEC Y93.J2 (*following* Y93.7)
　piano Y93.J1 (*following* Y93.7)
　string instrument Y93.J3 (*following* Y93.7)
　winds instrument Y93.J4 (*following* Y93.7)
property maintenance
　exterior NEC Y93.H9 (*following* Y93.7)
　interior NEC Y93.E9 (*following* Y93.7)
pruning (garden and lawn) Y93.H2 (*following* Y93.7)
pull-ups Y93.B2 (*following* Y93.7)
push-ups Y93.B2 (*following* Y93.7)

**Activity** — *continued*
racquetball Y93.73
rafting (in calm and turbulent water) Y93.16
raking (leaves) Y93.H1 (*following* Y93.7)
rappelling Y93.32
refereeing a sports activity Y93.81
residential relocation Y93.E6 (*following* Y93.7)
rhythmic gymnastics Y93.43
rhythmic movement NEC Y93.49
riding
　horseback Y93.52
　rollercoaster Y93.I1 (*following* Y93.7)
rock climbing Y93.31
roller skating (inline) Y93.51
rollercoaster riding Y93.I1 (*following* Y93.7)
rough housing and horseplay Y93.83
rowing (in calm and turbulent water) Y93.16
rugby Y93.63
running Y93.Ø2
SCUBA diving Y93.15
sewing Y93.D2 (*following* Y93.7)
shoveling Y93.H1 (*following* Y93.7)
　dirt Y93.H1 (*following* Y93.7)
　snow Y93.H1 (*following* Y93.7)
showering (personal) Y93.E1 (*following* Y93.7)
sit-ups Y93.B2 (*following* Y93.7)
skateboarding Y93.51
skating (ice) Y93.21
　roller Y93.51
skiing (alpine) (downhill) Y93.23
　cross country Y93.24
　nordic Y93.24
　water Y93.17
sledding (snow) Y93.23
sleeping (sleep) Y93.84
smoking and grilling food Y93.G2 (*following* Y93.7)
snorkeling Y93.15
snow NEC Y93.29
　boarding Y93.23
　shoveling Y93.H1 (*following* Y93.7)
　sledding Y93.23
　tubing Y93.23
soccer Y93.66
softball Y93.64
specified NEC Y93.89
spectator at an event Y93.82
sports NEC Y93.79
　sports played as a team or group NEC Y93.69
　sports played individually NEC Y93.59
springboard diving Y93.12
squash Y93.73
stationary bike Y93.A1 (*following* Y93.7)
step (stepping) exercise (class) Y93.A3 (*following* Y93.7)
stepper machine Y93.A1 (*following* Y93.7)
stove Y93.G3 (*following* Y93.7)
string instrument playing Y93.J3 (*following* Y93.7)
surfing Y93.18
　wind Y93.18
swimming Y93.11
tackle football Y93.61
tap dancing Y93.41
tennis Y93.73
tobogganing Y93.23
touch football Y93.62
track and field events (non-running) Y93.57
　running Y93.Ø2
trampoline Y93.44
treadmill Y93.A1 (*following* Y93.7)
trimming shrubs Y93.H2 (*following* Y93.7)
tubing (in calm and turbulent water) Y93.16
　snow Y93.23
ultimate frisbee Y93.74
underwater diving Y93.15
unpacking in moving to a new residence Y93.E6 (*fol-lowing* Y93.7)
use of stove, oven and microwave oven Y93.G3 (*follow-ing* Y93.7)
vacuuming Y93.E3 (*following* Y93.7)
volleyball (beach) (court) Y93.68
wake boarding Y93.17
walking (on level or elevated terrain) Y93.Ø1
　an animal Y93.K1 (*following* Y93.7)
walking an animal Y93.K1 (*following* Y93.7)
wall climbing Y93.31
warm up and cool down exercises Y93.A2 (*following* Y93.7)
water NEC Y93.19
　aerobics Y93.14
　craft NEC Y93.19

**Activity** — *continued*
water — *continued*
　exercise Y93.14
　polo Y93.13
　skiing Y93.17
　sliding Y93.18
　survival training and testing Y93.19
weeding (garden and lawn) Y93.H2 (*following* Y93.7)
wind instrument playing Y93.J4 (*following* Y93.7)
windsurfing Y93.18
wrestling Y93.72
yoga Y93.42
**Adverse effect of drugs** — *see* Table of Drugs and Chemicals
**Aerosinusitis** — *see* Air, pressure
**After-effect, late** — *see* Sequelae
**Air**
　blast in war operations — *see* War operations, air blast
　pressure
　　change, rapid
　　　during
　　　　ascent W94.29 ☑
　　　　　while (in) (surfacing from)
　　　　　　aircraft W94.23 ☑
　　　　　　deep water diving W94.21 ☑
　　　　　　underground W94.22 ☑
　　　　descent W94.39 ☑
　　　　　in
　　　　　　aircraft W94.31 ☑
　　　　　　water W94.32 ☑
　　high, prolonged W94.Ø ☑
　　low, prolonged W94.12 ☑
　　　due to residence or long visit at high altitude W94.11 ☑
**Alpine sickness** W94.11 ☑
**Altitude sickness** W94.11 ☑
**Anaphylactic shock, anaphylaxis** — *see* Table of Drugs and Chemicals
**Andes disease** W94.11 ☑
**Arachnidism, arachnoidism** X58 ☑
**Arson** (with intent to injure or kill) X97 ☑
**Asphyxia, asphyxiation**
　by
　　food (bone) (seed) — *see* categories T17 and T18 ☑
　　gas (*see also* Table of Drugs and Chemicals)
　　　legal
　　　　execution — *see* Legal, intervention, gas
　　　　intervention — *see* Legal, intervention, gas
　from
　　fire (*see also* Exposure, fire)
　　　in war operations — *see* War operations, fire
　　ignition — *see* Ignition
　　vomitus T17.81 ☑
　in war operations — *see* War operations, restriction of airway
**Aspiration**
　food (any type) (into respiratory tract) (with asphyxia, obstruction respiratory tract, suffocation) — *see* categories T17 and T18 ☑
　foreign body — *see* Foreign body, aspiration
　vomitus (with asphyxia, obstruction respiratory tract, suffocation) T17.81 ☑
**Assassination** (attempt) — *see* Assault
**Assault** (homicidal) (by) (in) YØ9
　arson X97 ☑
　bite (of human being) YØ4.1 ☑
　bodily force YØ4.8 ☑
　　bite YØ4.1 ☑
　　bumping into YØ4.2 ☑
　　sexual — *see* subcategories T74.Ø, T76.Ø ☑
　　unarmed fight YØ4.Ø ☑
　bomb X96.9 ☑
　　antipersonnel X96.Ø ☑
　　fertilizer X96.3 ☑
　　gasoline X96.1 ☑
　　letter X96.2 ☑
　　petrol X96.1 ☑
　　pipe X96.3 ☑
　　specified NEC X96.8 ☑
　brawl (hand) (fists) (foot) (unarmed) YØ4.Ø ☑
　burning, burns (by fire) NEC X97 ☑
　　acid YØ8.89 ☑
　　caustic, corrosive substance YØ8.89 ☑
　　chemical from swallowing caustic, corrosive sub-stance — *see* Table of Drugs and Chemicals

**Assault** — *continued*
  burning, burns — *continued*
    cigarette(s) X97 ☑
    hot object X98.9 ☑
      fluid NEC X98.2 ☑
      household appliance X98.3 ☑
      specified NEC X98.8 ☑
      steam X98.0 ☑
      tap water X98.1 ☑
      vapors X98.0 ☑
    scalding — *see* Assault, burning
    steam X98.0 ☑
    vitriol Y08.89 ☑
  caustic, corrosive substance (gas) Y08.89 ☑
  crashing of
    aircraft Y08.81 ☑
    motor vehicle Y03.8 ☑
      pushed in front of Y02.0 ☑
      run over Y03.0 ☑
      specified NEC Y03.8 ☑
  cutting or piercing instrument X99.9 ☑
    dagger X99.2 ☑
    glass X99.0 ☑
    knife X99.1 ☑
    specified NEC X99.8 ☑
    sword X99.2 ☑
  dagger X99.2 ☑
  drowning (in) X92.9 ☑
    bathtub X92.0 ☑
    natural water X92.3 ☑
    specified NEC X92.8 ☑
    swimming pool X92.1 ☑
      following fall X92.2 ☑
  dynamite X96.8 ☑
  explosive(s) (material) X96.9 ☑
  fight (hand) (fists) (foot) (unarmed) Y04.0 ☑
    with weapon — *see* Assault, by type of weapon
  fire X97 ☑
  firearm X95.9 ☑
    airgun X95.01 ☑
    handgun X93 ☑
    hunting rifle X94.1 ☑
    larger X94.9 ☑
      specified NEC X94.8 ☑
    machine gun X94.2 ☑
    shotgun X94.0 ☑
    specified NEC X95.8 ☑
  from high place Y01 ☑
  gunshot (wound) NEC — *see* Assault, firearm, by type
  incendiary device X97 ☑
  injury Y09 ☑
    to child due to criminal abortion attempt NEC Y08.89 ☑
  knife X99.1 ☑
  late effect of — *see* categories X92-Y08 with 7th character S
  placing before moving object NEC Y02.8 ☑
    motor vehicle Y02.0 ☑
  poisoning — *see* categories T36-T65 with 7th character S
  puncture, any part of body — *see* Assault, cutting or piercing instrument
  pushing
    before moving object NEC Y02.8 ☑
      motor vehicle Y02.0 ☑
      subway train Y02.1 ☑
      train Y02.1 ☑
    from high place Y01 ☑
  rape T74.2- ☑
  scalding — *see* Assault, burning
  sequelae of — *see* categories X92-Y08 with 7th character S
  sexual (by bodily force) T74.2- ☑
  shooting — *see* Assault, firearm
  specified means NEC Y08.89 ☑
  stab, any part of body — *see* Assault, cutting or piercing instrument
  steam X98.0 ☑
  striking against
    other person Y04.2 ☑
    sports equipment Y08.09 ☑
      baseball bat Y08.02 ☑
      hockey stick Y08.01 ☑
  struck by
    sports equipment Y08.09 ☑
      baseball bat Y08.02 ☑

**Assault** — *continued*
  struck by — *continued*
    sports equipment — *continued*
      hockey stick Y08.01 ☑
  submersion — *see* Assault, drowning
  violence Y09 ☑
  weapon Y09 ☑
    blunt Y00 ☑
    cutting or piercing — *see* Assault, cutting or piercing instrument
    firearm — *see* Assault, firearm
  wound Y09 ☑
    cutting — *see* Assault, cutting or piercing instrument
    gunshot — *see* Assault, firearm
    knife X99.1 ☑
    piercing — *see* Assault, cutting or piercing instrument
    puncture — *see* Assault, cutting or piercing instrument
    stab — *see* Assault, cutting or piercing instrument
**Attack by mammals NEC** W55.89 ☑
**Avalanche** — *see* Landslide
**Aviator's disease** — *see* Air, pressure

# B

**Barotitis, barodontalgia, barosinusitis, barotrauma** (otitic) (sinus) — *see* Air, pressure
**Battered** (baby) (child) (person) (syndrome) X58 ☑
**Bayonet wound** W26.1 ☑
  in
    legal intervention — *see* Legal, intervention, sharp object, bayonet
    war operations — *see* War operations, combat
  stated as undetermined whether accidental or intentional Y28.8 ☑
  suicide (attempt) X78.2 ☑
**Bean in nose** — *see* categories T17 and T18 ☑
**Bed set on fire NEC** — *see* Exposure, fire, uncontrolled, building, bed
**Beheading** (by guillotine)
  homicide X99.9 ☑
  legal execution — *see* Legal, intervention
**Bending, injury in** (prolonged) (static) X50.1 ☑
**Bends** — *see* Air, pressure, change
**Bite, bitten by**
  alligator W58.01 ☑
  arthropod (nonvenomous) NEC W57 ☑
  bull W55.21 ☑
  cat W55.01 ☑
  cow W55.21 ☑
  crocodile W58.11 ☑
  dog W54.0 ☑
  goat W55.31 ☑
  hoof stock NEC W55.31 ☑
  horse W55.11 ☑
  human being (accidentally) W50.3 ☑
    with intent to injure or kill Y04.1 ☑
    as, or caused by, a crowd or human stampede (with fall) W52 ☑
    assault Y04.1 ☑
    homicide (attempt) Y04.1 ☑
    in
      fight Y04.1 ☑
  insect (nonvenomous) W57 ☑
  lizard (nonvenomous) W59.01 ☑
  mammal NEC W55.81 ☑
    marine W56.31 ☑
  marine animal (nonvenomous) W56.81 ☑
  millipede W57 ☑
  moray eel W56.51 ☑
  mouse W53.01 ☑
  person(s) (accidentally) W50.3 ☑
    with intent to injure or kill Y04.1 ☑
    as, or caused by, a crowd or human stampede (with fall) W52 ☑
    assault Y04.1 ☑
    homicide (attempt) Y04.1 ☑
    in
      fight Y04.1 ☑
  pig W55.41 ☑
  raccoon W55.51 ☑
  rat W53.11 ☑
  reptile W59.81 ☑
    lizard W59.01 ☑

**Bite, bitten by** — *continued*
  reptile — *continued*
    snake W59.11 ☑
    turtle W59.21 ☑
      terrestrial W59.81 ☑
  rodent W53.81 ☑
    mouse W53.01 ☑
    rat W53.11 ☑
    specified NEC W53.81 ☑
    squirrel W53.21 ☑
  shark W56.41 ☑
  sheep W55.31 ☑
  snake (nonvenomous) W59.11 ☑
  spider (nonvenomous) W57 ☑
  squirrel W53.21 ☑
**Blast** (air) in war operations — *see* War operations, blast
**Blizzard** X37.2 ☑
**Blood alcohol level** Y90.9
  less than 20mg/100ml Y90.0
  20-39mg/100ml Y90.1
  40-59mg/100ml Y90.2
  60-79mg/100ml Y90.3
  80-99mg/100ml Y90.4
  100-119mg/100ml Y90.5
  120-199mg/100ml Y90.6
  200-239mg/100ml Y90.7
  presence in blood, level not specified Y90.9
**Blow** X58 ☑
  by law-enforcing agent, police (on duty) — *see* Legal, intervention, manhandling
  blunt object — *see* Legal, intervention, blunt object
**Blowing up** — *see* Explosion
**Brawl** (hand) (fists) (foot) Y04.0 ☑
**Breakage** (accidental) (part of)
  ladder (causing fall) W11 ☑
  scaffolding (causing fall) W12 ☑
**Broken**
  glass, contact with — *see* Contact, with, glass
  power line (causing electric shock) W85 ☑
**Bumping against, into** (accidentally)
  object NEC W22.8 ☑
    with fall — *see* Fall, due to, bumping against, object
    caused by crowd or human stampede (with fall) W52 ☑
    sports equipment W21.9 ☑
  person(s) W51 ☑
    with fall W03 ☑
      due to ice or snow W00.0 ☑
    assault Y04.2 ☑
    caused by, a crowd or human stampede (with fall) W52 ☑
    homicide (attempt) Y04.2 ☑
  sports equipment W21.9 ☑
**Burn, burned, burning** (accidental) (by) (from) (on)
  acid NEC — *see* Table of Drugs and Chemicals
  bed linen — *see* Exposure, fire, uncontrolled, in building, bed
  blowtorch X08.8 ☑
    with ignition of clothing NEC X06.2 ☑
      nightwear X05 ☑
  bonfire, campfire (controlled) (*see also* Exposure, fire, controlled, not in building)
    uncontrolled — *see* Exposure, fire, uncontrolled, not in building
  candle X08.8 ☑
    with ignition of clothing NEC X06.2 ☑
      nightwear X05 ☑
  caustic liquid, substance (external) (internal) NEC — *see* Table of Drugs and Chemicals
  chemical (external) (internal) (*see also* Table of Drugs and Chemicals)
    in war operations — *see* War operations. fire
  cigar(s) or cigarette(s) X08.8 ☑
    with ignition of clothing NEC X06.2 ☑
      nightwear X05 ☑
  clothes, clothing NEC (from controlled fire) X06.2 ☑
    with conflagration — *see* Exposure, fire, uncontrolled, building
    not in building or structure — *see* Exposure, fire, uncontrolled, not in building
  cooker (hot) X15.8 ☑
    stated as undetermined whether accidental or intentional Y27.3 ☑
    suicide (attempt) X77.3 ☑
  electric blanket X16 ☑

**Burn, burned, burning** — *continued*
  engine (hot) X17 ☑
  fire, flames — *see* Exposure, fire
  flare, Very pistol — *see* Discharge, firearm NEC
  heat
    from appliance (electrical) (household) X15.8 ☑
      cooker X15.8 ☑
      hotplate X15.2 ☑
      kettle X15.8 ☑
      light bulb X15.8 ☑
      saucepan X15.3 ☑
      skillet X15.3 ☑
      stated as undetermined whether accidental or intentional Y27.3 ☑
      stove X15.0 ☑
      suicide (attempt) X77.3 ☑
      toaster X15.1 ☑
    in local application or packing during medical or surgical procedure Y63.5
  heating
    appliance, radiator or pipe X16 ☑
  homicide (attempt) — *see* Assault, burning
  hot
    air X14.1 ☑
    cooker X15.8 ☑
    drink X10.0 ☑
    engine X17 ☑
    fat X10.2 ☑
    fluid NEC X12 ☑
    food X10.1 ☑
    gases X14.1 ☑
    heating appliance X16 ☑
    household appliance NEC X15.8 ☑
    kettle X15.8 ☑
    liquid NEC X12 ☑
    machinery X17 ☑
    metal (molten) (liquid) NEC X18 ☑
    object (not producing fire or flames) NEC X19 ☑
    oil (cooking) X10.2 ☑
    pipe(s) X16 ☑
    radiator X16 ☑
    saucepan (glass) (metal) X15.3 ☑
    stove (kitchen) X15.0 ☑
    substance NEC X19 ☑
      caustic or corrosive NEC — *see* Table of Drugs and Chemicals
    toaster X15.1 ☑
    tool X17 ☑
    vapor X13.1 ☑
    water (tap) — *see* Contact, with, hot, tap water
  hotplate X15.2 ☑
    suicide (attempt) X77.3 ☑
  ignition — *see* Ignition
  in war operations — *see* War operations, fire
  inflicted by other person X97 ☑
    by hot objects, hot vapor, and steam — *see* Assault, burning, hot object
  internal, from swallowed caustic, corrosive liquid, substance — *see* Table of Drugs and Chemicals
  iron (hot) X15.8 ☑
    stated as undetermined whether accidental or intentional Y27.3 ☑
    suicide (attempt) X77.3 ☑
  kettle (hot) X15.8 ☑
    stated as undetermined whether accidental or intentional Y27.3 ☑
    suicide (attempt) X77.3 ☑
  lamp (flame) X08.8 ☑
    with ignition of clothing NEC X06.2 ☑
      nightwear X05 ☑
  lighter (cigar) (cigarette) X08.8 ☑
    with ignition of clothing NEC X06.2 ☑
      nightwear X05 ☑
  lightning — *see* subcategory T75.0 ☑
    causing fire — *see* Exposure, fire
  liquid (boiling) (hot) NEC X12 ☑
    stated as undetermined whether accidental or intentional Y27.2 ☑
    suicide (attempt) X77.2 ☑
  local application of externally applied substance in medical or surgical care Y63.5
  machinery (hot) X17 ☑
  matches X08.8 ☑
    with ignition of clothing NEC X06.2 ☑
      nightwear X05 ☑

**Burn, burned, burning** — *continued*
  mattress — *see* Exposure, fire, uncontrolled, building, bed
  medicament, externally applied Y63.5
  metal (hot) (liquid) (molten) NEC X18 ☑
  nightwear (nightclothes, nightdress, gown, pajamas, robe) X05 ☑
  object (hot) NEC X19 ☑
  on board watercraft
    due to
      accident to watercraft V91.09 ☑
        powered craft V91.03 ☑
          ferry boat V91.01 ☑
          fishing boat V91.02 ☑
          jetskis V91.03 ☑
          liner V91.01 ☑
          merchant ship V91.00 ☑
          passenger ship V91.01 ☑
        unpowered craft V91.08 ☑
          canoe V91.05 ☑
          inflatable V91.06 ☑
          kayak V91.05 ☑
          sailboat V91.04 ☑
          surf-board V91.08 ☑
          water skis V91.07 ☑
          windsurfer V91.08 ☑
      fire on board V93.09 ☑
        ferry boat V93.01 ☑
        fishing boat V93.02 ☑
        jetskis V93.03 ☑
        liner V93.01 ☑
        merchant ship V93.00 ☑
        passenger ship V93.01 ☑
        powered craft NEC V93.03 ☑
        sailboat V93.04 ☑
      specified heat source NEC on board V93.19 ☑
        ferry boat V93.11 ☑
        fishing boat V93.12 ☑
        jetskis V93.13 ☑
        liner V93.11 ☑
        merchant ship V93.10 ☑
        passenger ship V93.11 ☑
        powered craft NEC V93.13 ☑
        sailboat V93.14 ☑
  pipe (hot) X16 ☑
    smoking X08.8 ☑
      with ignition of clothing NEC X06.2 ☑
        nightwear X05 ☑
  powder — *see* Powder burn
  radiator (hot) X16 ☑
  saucepan (hot) (glass) (metal) X15.3 ☑
    stated as undetermined whether accidental or intentional Y27.3 ☑
    suicide (attempt) X77.3 ☑
  self-inflicted X76 ☑
    stated as undetermined whether accidental or intentional Y26 ☑
  stated as undetermined whether accidental or intentional Y27.0 ☑
  steam X13.1 ☑
    pipe X16 ☑
      stated as undetermined whether accidental or intentional Y27.8 ☑
    stated as undetermined whether accidental or intentional Y27.0 ☑
    suicide (attempt) X77.0 ☑
  stove (hot) (kitchen) X15.0 ☑
    stated as undetermined whether accidental or intentional Y27.3 ☑
    suicide (attempt) X77.3 ☑
  substance (hot) NEC X19 ☑
    boiling X12 ☑
      stated as undetermined whether accidental or intentional Y27.2 ☑
      suicide (attempt) X77.2 ☑
    molten (metal) X18 ☑
  suicide (attempt) NEC X76 ☑
    hot
      household appliance X77.3 ☑
      object X77.9 ☑
  therapeutic misadventure
    heat in local application or packing during medical or surgical procedure Y63.5
    overdose of radiation Y63.2
  toaster (hot) X15.1 ☑

**Burn, burned, burning** — *continued*
  toaster — *continued*
    stated as undetermined whether accidental or intentional Y27.3 ☑
    suicide (attempt) X77.3 ☑
  tool (hot) X17 ☑
  torch, welding X08.8 ☑
    with ignition of clothing NEC X06.2 ☑
      nightwear X05 ☑
  trash fire (controlled) — *see* Exposure, fire, controlled, not in building
    uncontrolled — *see* Exposure, fire, uncontrolled, not in building
  vapor (hot) X13.1 ☑
    stated as undetermined whether accidental or intentional Y27.0 ☑
    suicide (attempt) X77.0 ☑
  Very pistol — *see* Discharge, firearm NEC
**Butted by animal** W55.82 ☑
  bull W55.22 ☑
  cow W55.22 ☑
  goat W55.32 ☑
  horse W55.12 ☑
  pig W55.42 ☑
  sheep W55.32 ☑

# C

**Caisson disease** — *see* Air, pressure, change
**Campfire** (exposure to) (controlled) (*see also* Exposure, fire, controlled, not in building)
  uncontrolled — *see* Exposure, fire, uncontrolled, not in building
**Capital punishment** (any means) — *see* Legal, intervention
**Car sickness** T75.3 ☑
**Casualty** (not due to war) NEC X58 ☑
  war — *see* War operations
**Cat**
  bite W55.01 ☑
  scratch W55.03 ☑
**Cataclysm, cataclysmic** (any injury) NEC — *see* Forces of nature
**Catching fire** — *see* Exposure, fire
**Caught**
  between
    folding object W23.0 ☑
    objects (moving) (stationary and moving) W23.0 ☑
      and machinery — *see* Contact, with, by type of machine
      stationary W23.1 ☑
    sliding door and door frame W23.0 ☑
  by, in
    machinery (moving parts of) — *see* Contact, with, by type of machine
    washing-machine wringer W23.0 ☑
  under packing crate (due to losing grip) W23.1 ☑
**Cave-in caused by cataclysmic earth surface movement or eruption** — *see* Landslide
**Change**(s) in air pressure — *see* Air, pressure, change
**Choked, choking** (on) (any object except food or vomitus)
  food (bone) (seed) — *see* categories T17 and T18 ☑
  vomitus T17.81- ☑
**Civil insurrection** — *see* War operations
**Cloudburst** (any injury) X37.8 ☑
**Cold, exposure to** (accidental) (excessive) (extreme) (natural) (place) NEC — *see* Exposure, cold
**Collapse**
  building W20.1 ☑
    burning (uncontrolled fire) X00.2 ☑
  dam or man-made structure (causing earth movement) X36.0 ☑
  machinery — *see* Contact, with, by type of machine
  structure W20.1 ☑
    burning (uncontrolled fire) X00.2 ☑
**Collision** (accidental) NEC (*see also* Accident, transport) V89.9 ☑
  pedestrian W51 ☑
    with fall W03 ☑
      due to ice or snow W00.0 ☑
        involving pedestrian conveyance — *see* Accident, transport, pedestrian, conveyance
    and
      crowd or human stampede (with fall) W52 ☑
      object W22.8 ☑

**Collision** — *continued*
  pedestrian — *continued*
    and — *continued*
      object — *continued*
        with fall — *see* Fall, due to, bumping against, object
  person(s) — *see* Collision, pedestrian
  transport vehicle NEC V89.9 ☑
    and
      avalanche, fallen or not moving — *see* Accident, transport
        falling or moving — *see* Landslide
      landslide, fallen or not moving — *see* Accident, transport
        falling or moving — *see* Landslide
      due to cataclysm — *see* Forces of nature, by type
      intentional, purposeful suicide (attempt) — *see* Suicide, collision
**Combustion, spontaneous** — *see* Ignition
**Complication** (delayed) **of or following** (medical or surgical procedure) Y84.9
  with misadventure — *see* Misadventure
  amputation of limb(s) Y83.5
  anastomosis (arteriovenous) (blood vessel) (gastrojejunal) (tendon) (natural or artificial material) Y83.2
  aspiration (of fluid) Y84.4
    tissue Y84.8
  biopsy Y84.8
  blood
    sampling Y84.7
    transfusion
      procedure Y84.8
  bypass Y83.2
  catheterization (urinary) Y84.6
    cardiac Y84.0
  colostomy Y83.3
  cystostomy Y83.3
  dialysis (kidney) Y84.1
  drug — *see* Table of Drugs and Chemicals
  due to misadventure — *see* Misadventure
  duodenostomy Y83.3
  electroshock therapy Y84.3
  external stoma, creation of Y83.3
  formation of external stoma Y83.3
  gastrostomy Y83.3
  graft Y83.2
  hypothermia (medically-induced) Y84.8
  implant, implantation (of)
    artificial
      internal device (cardiac pacemaker) (electrodes in brain) (heart valve prosthesis) (orthopedic) Y83.1
      material or tissue (for anastomosis or bypass) Y83.2
        with creation of external stoma Y83.3
      natural tissues (for anastomosis or bypass) Y83.2
        with creation of external stoma Y83.3
  infusion
    procedure Y84.8
  injection — *see* Table of Drugs and Chemicals
    procedure Y84.8
  insertion of gastric or duodenal sound Y84.5
  insulin-shock therapy Y84.3
  paracentesis (abdominal) (thoracic) (aspirative) Y84.4
  procedures other than surgical operation — *see* Complication of or following, by type of procedure
  radiological procedure or therapy Y84.2
  removal of organ (partial) (total) NEC Y83.6
  sampling
    blood Y84.7
    fluid NEC Y84.4
    tissue Y84.8
  shock therapy Y84.3
  surgical operation NEC (*see also* Complication of or following, by type of operation) Y83.9
    reconstructive NEC Y83.4
      with
        anastomosis, bypass or graft Y83.2
        formation of external stoma Y83.3
    specified NEC Y83.8
  transfusion (*see also* Table of Drugs and Chemicals)
    procedure Y84.8
  transplant, transplantation (heart) (kidney) (liver) (whole organ, any) Y83.0
    partial organ Y83.4
  ureterostomy Y83.3

**Complication** (delayed) **of or following** — *continued*
  vaccination (*see also* Table of Drugs and Chemicals)
    procedure Y84.8
**Compression**
  divers' squeeze — *see* Air, pressure, change
  trachea by
    food (lodged in esophagus) — *see* categories T17 and T18 ☑
    vomitus (lodged in esophagus) T17.81- ☑
**Conflagration** — *see* Exposure, fire, uncontrolled
**Constriction** (external)
  hair W49.01 ☑
  jewelry W49.04 ☑
  ring W49.04 ☑
  rubber band W49.03 ☑
  specified item NEC W49.09 ☑
  string W49.02 ☑
  thread W49.02 ☑
**Contact** (accidental)
  with
    abrasive wheel (metalworking) W31.1 ☑
    alligator W58.09 ☑
      bite W58.01 ☑
      crushing W58.03 ☑
      strike W58.02 ☑
    amphibian W62.9 ☑
      frog W62.0 ☑
      toad W62.1 ☑
    animal (nonvenomous) NEC W64 ☑
      marine W56.89 ☑
        bite W56.81 ☑
        dolphin — *see* Contact, with, dolphin
        fish NEC — *see* Contact, with, fish
        mammal — *see* Contact, with, mammal, marine
        orca — *see* Contact, with, orca
        sea lion — *see* Contact, with, sea lion
        shark — *see* Contact, with, shark
        strike W56.82 ☑
    animate mechanical force NEC W64 ☑
    arrow W21.89 ☑
      not thrown, projected or falling W45.8 ☑
    arthropods (nonvenomous) W57 ☑
    axe W27.0 ☑
    band-saw (industrial) W31.2 ☑
    bayonet — *see* Bayonet wound
    bee(s) X58 ☑
    bench-saw (industrial) W31.2 ☑
    bird W61.99 ☑
      bite W61.91 ☑
      chicken — *see* Contact, with, chicken
      duck — *see* Contact, with, duck
      goose — *see* Contact, with, goose
      macaw — *see* Contact, with, macaw
      parrot — *see* Contact, with, parrot
      psittacine — *see* Contact, with, psittacine
      strike W61.92 ☑
      turkey — *see* Contact, with, turkey
    blender W29.0 ☑
    boiling water X12 ☑
      stated as undetermined whether accidental or intentional Y27.2 ☑
      suicide (attempt) X77.2 ☑
    bore, earth-drilling or mining (land) (seabed) W31.0 ☑
    buffalo — *see* Contact, with, hoof stock NEC
    bull W55.29 ☑
      bite W55.21 ☑
      gored W55.22 ☑
      strike W55.22 ☑
    bumper cars W31.81 ☑
    camel — *see* Contact, with, hoof stock NEC
    can
      lid W26.8 ☑
      opener W27.4 ☑
        powered W29.0 ☑
    cat W55.09 ☑
      bite W55.01 ☑
      scratch W55.03 ☑
    caterpillar (venomous) X58 ☑
    centipede (venomous) X58 ☑
    chain
      hoist W24.0 ☑
        agricultural operations W30.89 ☑
      saw W29.3 ☑

**Contact** — *continued*
  with — *continued*
    chicken W61.39 ☑
      peck W61.33 ☑
      strike W61.32 ☑
    chisel W27.0 ☑
    circular saw W31.2 ☑
    cobra X58 ☑
    combine (harvester) W30.0 ☑
    conveyer belt W24.1 ☑
    cooker (hot) X15.8 ☑
      stated as undetermined whether accidental or intentional Y27.3 ☑
      suicide (attempt) X77.3 ☑
    coral X58 ☑
    cotton gin W31.82 ☑
    cow W55.29 ☑
      bite W55.21 ☑
      strike W55.22 ☑
    crane W24.0 ☑
      agricultural operations W30.89 ☑
    crocodile W58.19 ☑
      bite W58.11 ☑
      crushing W58.13 ☑
      strike W58.12 ☑
    dagger W26.1 ☑
      stated as undetermined whether accidental or intentional Y28.2 ☑
      suicide (attempt) X78.2 ☑
    dairy equipment W31.82 ☑
    dart W21.89 ☑
      not thrown, projected or falling W45.8 ☑
    deer — *see* Contact, with, hoof stock NEC
    derrick W24.0 ☑
      agricultural operations W30.89 ☑
        hay W30.2 ☑
    dog W54.8 ☑
      bite W54.0 ☑
      strike W54.1 ☑
    dolphin W56.09 ☑
      bite W56.01 ☑
      strike W56.02 ☑
    donkey — *see* Contact, with, hoof stock NEC
    drill (powered) W29.8 ☑
      earth (land) (seabed) W31.0 ☑
      nonpowered W27.8 ☑
    drive belt W24.0 ☑
      agricultural operations W30.89 ☑
    dry ice — *see* Exposure, cold, man-made
    dryer (clothes) (powered) (spin) W29.2 ☑
    duck W61.69 ☑
      bite W61.61 ☑
      strike W61.62 ☑
    earth (-)
      drilling machine (industrial) W31.0 ☑
      scraping machine in stationary use W31.83 ☑
    edge of stiff paper W26.2 ☑
    electric
      beater W29.0 ☑
      blanket X16 ☑
      fan W29.2 ☑
        commercial W31.82 ☑
      knife W29.1 ☑
      mixer W29.0 ☑
    elevator (building) W24.0 ☑
      agricultural operations W30.89 ☑
        grain W30.3 ☑
    engine(s), hot NEC X17 ☑
    excavating machine W31.0 ☑
    farm machine W30.9 ☑
    feces — *see* Contact, with, by type of animal
    fer de lance X58 ☑
    fish W56.59 ☑
      bite W56.51 ☑
      shark — *see* Contact, with, shark
      strike W56.52 ☑
    flying horses W31.81 ☑
    forging (metalworking) machine W31.1 ☑
    fork W27.4 ☑
    forklift (truck) W24.0 ☑
      agricultural operations W30.89 ☑
    frog W62.0 ☑
    garden
      cultivator (powered) W29.3 ☑
        riding W30.89 ☑
      fork W27.1 ☑

**Contact** — *continued*
 with — *continued*
  gas turbine W31.3 ☑
  Gila monster X58 ☑
  giraffe — *see* Contact, with, hoof stock NEC
  glass (sharp) (broken) W25 ☑
   with subsequent fall W18.02 ☑
   assault X99.0 ☑
   due to fall — *see* Fall, by type
   stated as undetermined whether accidental or
     intentional Y28.0 ☑
   suicide (attempt) X78.0 ☑
  goat W55.39 ☑
   bite W55.31 ☑
   strike W55.32 ☑
  goose W61.59 ☑
   bite W61.51 ☑
   strike W61.52 ☑
  hand
   saw W27.0 ☑
   tool (not powered) NEC W27.8 ☑
    powered W29.8 ☑
  harvester W30.0 ☑
  hay-derrick W30.2 ☑
  heating
   appliance (hot) X16 ☑
   pad (electric) X16 ☑
  heat NEC X19 ☑
   from appliance (electrical) (household) — *see*
     Contact, with, hot, household appliance
     heating appliance X16 ☑
  hedge-trimmer (powered) W29.3 ☑
  hoe W27.1 ☑
  hoist (chain) (shaft) NEC W24.0 ☑
   agricultural W30.89 ☑
  hoof stock NEC W55.39 ☑
   bite W55.31 ☑
   strike W55.32 ☑
  hornet(s) X58 ☑
  horse W55.19 ☑
   bite W55.11 ☑
   strike W55.12 ☑
  hot
   air X14.1 ☑
    inhalation X14.0 ☑
   cooker X15.8 ☑
   drinks X10.0 ☑
   engine X17 ☑
   fats X10.2 ☑
   fluids NEC X12 ☑
    assault X98.2 ☑
    suicide (attempt) X77.2 ☑
    undetermined whether accidental or inten-
      tional Y27.2 ☑
   food X10.1 ☑
   gases X14.1 ☑
    inhalation X14.0 ☑
   heating appliance X16 ☑
   household appliance X15.8 ☑
    assault X98.3 ☑
    cooker X15.8 ☑
    hotplate X15.2 ☑
    kettle X15.8 ☑
    light bulb X15.8 ☑
    object NEC X19 ☑
     assault X98.8 ☑
     stated as undetermined whether acciden-
       tal or intentional Y27.9 ☑
     suicide (attempt) X77.8 ☑
    saucepan X15.3 ☑
    skillet X15.3 ☑
    stated as undetermined whether accidental
      or intentional Y27.3 ☑
    stove X15.0 ☑
    suicide (attempt) X77.3 ☑
    toaster X15.1 ☑
   kettle X15.8 ☑
   light bulb X15.8 ☑
   liquid NEC (*see also* Burn) X12 ☑
    drinks X10.0 ☑
    stated as undetermined whether accidental
      or intentional Y27.2 ☑
    suicide (attempt) X77.2 ☑
    tap water X11.8 ☑
     stated as undetermined whether acciden-
       tal or intentional Y27.1 ☑

**Contact** — *continued*
 with — *continued*
  hot — *continued*
   liquid (*see also* Burn) — *continued*
    tap water — *continued*
     suicide (attempt) X77.1 ☑
   machinery X17 ☑
   metal (molten) (liquid) NEC X18 ☑
   object (not producing fire or flames) NEC X19 ☑
   oil (cooking) X10.2 ☑
   pipe X16 ☑
   plate X15.2 ☑
   radiator X16 ☑
   saucepan (glass) (metal) X15.3 ☑
   skillet X15.3 ☑
   stove (kitchen) X15.0 ☑
   substance NEC X19 ☑
   tap-water X11.8 ☑
    assault X98.1 ☑
    heated on stove X12 ☑
     stated as undetermined whether acciden-
       tal or intentional Y27.2 ☑
     suicide (attempt) X77.2 ☑
    in bathtub X11.0 ☑
    running X11.1 ☑
    stated as undetermined whether accidental
      or intentional Y27.1 ☑
    suicide (attempt) X77.1 ☑
   toaster X15.1 ☑
   tool X17 ☑
   vapors X13.1 ☑
    inhalation X13.0 ☑
   water (tap) X11.8 ☑
    boiling X12 ☑
     stated as undetermined whether acciden-
       tal or intentional Y27.2 ☑
     suicide (attempt) X77.2 ☑
    heated on stove X12 ☑
     stated as undetermined whether acciden-
       tal or intentional Y27.2 ☑
     suicide (attempt) X77.2 ☑
    in bathtub X11.0 ☑
    running X11.1 ☑
    stated as undetermined whether accidental
      or intentional Y27.1 ☑
    suicide (attempt) X77.1 ☑
  hotplate X15.2 ☑
  ice-pick W27.4 ☑
  insect (nonvenomous) NEC W57 ☑
  kettle (hot) X15.8 ☑
  knife W26.0 ☑
   assault X99.1 ☑
   electric W29.1 ☑
   stated as undetermined whether accidental or
     intentional Y28.1 ☑
   suicide (attempt) X78.1 ☑
  lathe (metalworking) W31.1 ☑
   turnings W45.8 ☑
   woodworking W31.2 ☑
  lawnmower (powered) (ridden) W28 ☑
   causing electrocution W86.8 ☑
    suicide (attempt) X83.1 ☑
   unpowered W27.1 ☑
  lift, lifting (devices) W24.0 ☑
   agricultural operations W30.89 ☑
   shaft W24.0 ☑
  liquefied gas — *see* Exposure, cold, man-made
  liquid air, hydrogen, nitrogen — *see* Exposure, cold,
    man-made
  lizard (nonvenomous) W59.09 ☑
   bite W59.01 ☑
   strike W59.02 ☑
  llama — *see* Contact, with, hoof stock NEC
  macaw W61.19 ☑
   bite W61.11 ☑
   strike W61.12 ☑
  machine, machinery W31.9 ☑
   abrasive wheel W31.1 ☑
   agricultural including animal-powered
     W30.9 ☑
    combine harvester W30.0 ☑
    grain storage elevator W30.3 ☑
    hay derrick W30.2 ☑
    power take-off device W30.1 ☑
    reaper W30.0 ☑
    specified NEC W30.89 ☑

**Contact** — *continued*
 with — *continued*
  machine, machinery — *continued*
   agricultural including animal-powered — *con-
     tinued*
    thresher W30.0 ☑
    transport vehicle, stationary W30.81 ☑
   band saw W31.2 ☑
   bench saw W31.2 ☑
   circular saw W31.2 ☑
   commercial NEC W31.82 ☑
   drilling, metal (industrial) W31.1 ☑
   earth-drilling W31.0 ☑
   earthmoving or scraping W31.89 ☑
   excavating W31.89 ☑
   forging machine W31.1 ☑
   gas turbine W31.3 ☑
   hot X17 ☑
   internal combustion engine W31.3 ☑
   land drill W31.0 ☑
   lathe W31.1 ☑
   lifting (devices) W24.0 ☑
   metal drill W31.1 ☑
   metalworking (industrial) W31.1 ☑
   milling, metal W31.1 ☑
   mining W31.0 ☑
   molding W31.2 ☑
   overhead plane W31.2 ☑
   power press, metal W31.1 ☑
   prime mover W31.3 ☑
   printing W31.89 ☑
   radial saw W31.2 ☑
   recreational W31.81 ☑
   roller-coaster W31.81 ☑
   rolling mill, metal W31.1 ☑
   sander W31.2 ☑
   seabed drill W31.0 ☑
   shaft
    hoist W31.0 ☑
    lift W31.0 ☑
   specified NEC W31.89 ☑
   spinning W31.89 ☑
   steam engine W31.3 ☑
   transmission W24.1 ☑
   undercutter W31.0 ☑
   water driven turbine W31.3 ☑
   weaving W31.89 ☑
   woodworking or forming (industrial) W31.2 ☑
  mammal (feces) (urine) W55.89 ☑
   bull — *see* Contact, with, bull
   cat — *see* Contact, with, cat
   cow — *see* Contact, with, cow
   goat — *see* Contact, with, goat
   hoof stock — *see* Contact, with, hoof stock
   horse — *see* Contact, with, horse
   marine W56.39 ☑
    dolphin — *see* Contact, with, dolphin
    orca — *see* Contact, with, orca
    sea lion — *see* Contact, with, sea lion
    specified NEC W56.39 ☑
     bite W56.31 ☑
     strike W56.32 ☑
   pig — *see* Contact, with, pig
   raccoon — *see* Contact, with, raccoon
   rodent — *see* Contact, with, rodent
   sheep — *see* Contact, with, sheep
   specified NEC W55.89 ☑
    bite W55.81 ☑
    strike W55.82 ☑
  marine
   animal W56.89 ☑
    bite W56.81 ☑
    dolphin — *see* Contact, with, dolphin
    fish NEC — *see* Contact, with, fish
    mammal — *see* Contact, with, mammal,
      marine
    orca — *see* Contact, with, orca
    sea lion — *see* Contact, with, sea lion
    shark — *see* Contact, with, shark
    strike W56.82 ☑
  meat
   grinder (domestic) W29.0 ☑
    industrial W31.82 ☑
    nonpowered W27.4 ☑
   slicer (domestic) W29.0 ☑
    industrial W31.82 ☑

**Contact** — *continued*
 with — *continued*
  merry go round W31.81 ☑
  metal, hot (liquid) (molten) NEC X18 ☑
  millipede W57 ☑
  nail W45.0 ☑
   gun W29.4 ☑
  needle (sewing) W27.3 ☑
   hypodermic W46.0 ☑
    contaminated W46.1 ☑
  object (blunt) NEC
   hot NEC X19 ☑
   legal intervention — *see* Legal, intervention, blunt object
   sharp NEC W45.8 ☑
    inflicted by other person NEC W45.8 ☑
     stated as
      intentional homicide (attempt) — *see* Assault, cutting or piercing instrument
     legal intervention — *see* Legal, intervention, sharp object
     self-inflicted X78.9 ☑
  orca W56.29 ☑
   bite W56.21 ☑
   strike W56.22 ☑
  overhead plane W31.2 ☑
  paper (as sharp object) W26.2 ☑
  paper-cutter W27.5 ☑
  parrot W61.09 ☑
   bite W61.01 ☑
   strike W61.02 ☑
  pig W55.49 ☑
   bite W55.41 ☑
   strike W55.42 ☑
  pipe, hot X16 ☑
  pitchfork W27.1 ☑
  plane (metal) (wood) W27.0 ☑
   overhead W31.2 ☑
  plant thorns, spines, sharp leaves or other mechanisms W60 ☑
  powered
   garden cultivator W29.3 ☑
   household appliance, implement, or machine W29.8 ☑
   saw (industrial) W31.2 ☑
    hand W29.8 ☑
  printing machine W31.89 ☑
  psittacine bird W61.29 ☑
   bite W61.21 ☑
   macaw — *see* Contact, with, macaw
   parrot — *see* Contact, with, parrot
   strike W61.22 ☑
  pulley (block) (transmission) W24.0 ☑
   agricultural operations W30.89 ☑
  raccoon W55.59 ☑
   bite W55.51 ☑
   strike W55.52 ☑
  radial-saw (industrial) W31.2 ☑
  radiator (hot) X16 ☑
  rake W27.1 ☑
  rattlesnake X58 ☑
  reaper W30.0 ☑
  reptile W59.89 ☑
   lizard — *see* Contact, with, lizard
   snake — *see* Contact, with, snake
   specified NEC W59.89 ☑
    bite W59.81 ☑
    crushing W59.83 ☑
    strike W59.82 ☑
   turtle — *see* Contact, with, turtle
  rivet gun (powered) W29.4 ☑
  road scraper — *see* Accident, transport, construction vehicle
  rodent (feces) (urine) W53.89 ☑
   bite W53.81 ☑
   mouse W53.09 ☑
    bite W53.01 ☑
   rat W53.19 ☑
    bite W53.11 ☑
   specified NEC W53.89 ☑
    bite W53.81 ☑
   squirrel W53.29 ☑
    bite W53.21 ☑
  roller coaster W31.81 ☑
  rope NEC W24.0 ☑

**Contact** — *continued*
 with — *continued*
  rope — *continued*
   agricultural operations W30.89 ☑
  saliva — *see* Contact, with, by type of animal
  sander W29.8 ☑
   industrial W31.2 ☑
  saucepan (hot) (glass) (metal) X15.3 ☑
  saw W27.0 ☑
   band (industrial) W31.2 ☑
   bench (industrial) W31.2 ☑
   chain W29.3 ☑
   hand W27.0 ☑
  sawing machine, metal W31.1 ☑
  scissors W27.2 ☑
  scorpion X58 ☑
  screwdriver W27.0 ☑
   powered W29.8 ☑
  sea
   anemone, cucumber or urchin (spine) X58 ☑
   lion W56.19 ☑
    bite W56.11 ☑
    strike W56.12 ☑
  serpent — *see* Contact, with, snake, by type
  sewing-machine (electric) (powered) W29.2 ☑
   not powered W27.8 ☑
  shaft (hoist) (lift) (transmission) NEC W24.0 ☑
   agricultural W30.89 ☑
  shark W56.49 ☑
   bite W56.41 ☑
   strike W56.42 ☑
  sharp object(s) W26.9 ☑
   specified NEC W26.8 ☑
  shears (hand) W27.2 ☑
   powered (industrial) W31.1 ☑
    domestic W29.2 ☑
  sheep W55.39 ☑
   bite W55.31 ☑
   strike W55.32 ☑
  shovel W27.8 ☑
   steam — *see* Accident, transport, construction vehicle
  snake (nonvenomous) W59.19 ☑
   bite W59.11 ☑
   crushing W59.13 ☑
   strike W59.12 ☑
  spade W27.1 ☑
  spider (venomous) X58 ☑
  spin-drier W29.2 ☑
  spinning machine W31.89 ☑
  splinter W45.8 ☑
  sports equipment W21.9 ☑
  staple gun (powered) W29.8 ☑
  steam X13.1 ☑
   engine W31.3 ☑
   inhalation X13.0 ☑
   pipe X16 ☑
   shovel W31.89 ☑
  stove (hot) (kitchen) X15.0 ☑
  substance, hot NEC X19 ☑
   molten (metal) X18 ☑
  sword W26.1 ☑
   assault X99.2 ☑
   stated as undetermined whether accidental or intentional Y28.2 ☑
   suicide (attempt) X78.2 ☑
  tarantula X58 ☑
  thresher W30.0 ☑
  tin can lid W26.8 ☑
  toad W62.1 ☑
  toaster (hot) X15.1 ☑
  tool W27.8 ☑
   hand (not powered) W27.8 ☑
    auger W27.0 ☑
    axe W27.0 ☑
    can opener W27.4 ☑
    chisel W27.0 ☑
    fork W27.4 ☑
    garden W27.1 ☑
    handsaw W27.0 ☑
    hoe W27.1 ☑
    ice-pick W27.4 ☑
    kitchen utensil W27.4 ☑
    manual
     lawn mower W27.1 ☑
     sewing machine W27.8 ☑

**Contact** — *continued*
 with — *continued*
  tool — *continued*
   hand — *continued*
    meat grinder W27.4 ☑
    needle (sewing) W27.3 ☑
     hypodermic W46.0 ☑
      contaminated W46.1 ☑
    paper cutter W27.5 ☑
    pitchfork W27.1 ☑
    rake W27.1 ☑
    scissors W27.2 ☑
    screwdriver W27.0 ☑
    specified NEC W27.8 ☑
    workbench W27.0 ☑
   hot X17 ☑
   powered W29.8 ☑
    blender W29.0 ☑
     commercial W31.82 ☑
    can opener W29.0 ☑
     commercial W31.82 ☑
    chainsaw W29.3 ☑
    clothes dryer W29.2 ☑
     commercial W31.82 ☑
    dishwasher W29.2 ☑
     commercial W31.82 ☑
    edger W29.3 ☑
    electric fan W29.2 ☑
     commercial W31.82 ☑
    electric knife W29.1 ☑
    food processor W29.0 ☑
     commercial W31.82 ☑
    garbage disposal W29.0 ☑
     commercial W31.82 ☑
    garden tool W29.3 ☑
    hedge trimmer W29.3 ☑
    ice maker W29.0 ☑
     commercial W31.82 ☑
    kitchen appliance W29.0 ☑
     commercial W31.82 ☑
    lawn mower W28 ☑
    meat grinder W29.0 ☑
     commercial W31.82 ☑
    mixer W29.0 ☑
     commercial W31.82 ☑
    rototiller W29.3 ☑
    sewing machine W29.2 ☑
     commercial W31.82 ☑
    washing machine W29.2 ☑
     commercial W31.82 ☑
  transmission device (belt, cable, chain, gear, pinion, shaft) W24.1 ☑
   agricultural operations W30.89 ☑
  turbine (gas) (water-driven) W31.3 ☑
  turkey W61.49 ☑
   peck W61.43 ☑
   strike W61.42 ☑
  turtle (nonvenomous) W59.29 ☑
   bite W59.21 ☑
   strike W59.22 ☑
   terrestrial W59.89 ☑
    bite W59.81 ☑
    crushing W59.83 ☑
    strike W59.82 ☑
  under-cutter W31.0 ☑
  urine — *see* Contact, with, by type of animal
  vehicle
   agricultural use (transport) — *see* Accident, transport, agricultural vehicle
    not on public highway W30.81 ☑
   industrial use (transport) — *see* Accident, transport, industrial vehicle
    not on public highway W31.83 ☑
   off-road use (transport) — *see* Accident, transport, all-terrain or off-road vehicle
    not on public highway W31.83 ☑
   special construction use (transport) — *see* Accident, transport, construction vehicle
    not on public highway W31.83 ☑
  venomous
   animal X58 ☑
   arthropods X58 ☑
   lizard X58 ☑
   marine animal NEC X58 ☑
   marine plant NEC X58 ☑
   millipedes (tropical) X58 ☑

**Contact** — *continued*
  with — *continued*
    venomous — *continued*
      plant(s) X58 ☑
      snake X58 ☑
      spider X58 ☑
      viper X58 ☑
      washing-machine (powered) W29.2 ☑
      wasp X58 ☑
      weaving-machine W31.89 ☑
      winch W24.0 ☑
        agricultural operations W30.89 ☑
      wire NEC W24.0 ☑
        agricultural operations W30.89 ☑
      wood slivers W45.8 ☑
      yellow jacket X58 ☑
      zebra — *see* Contact, with, hoof stock NEC
    pressure X50.9 ☑
    stress X50.9 ☑
**Coup de soleil** X32 ☑
**Crash**
  aircraft (in transit) (powered) V95.9 ☑
    balloon V96.01 ☑
    fixed wing NEC (private) V95.21 ☑
      commercial V95.31 ☑
    glider V96.21 ☑
      hang V96.11 ☑
      powered V95.11 ☑
    helicopter V95.01 ☑
    in war operations — *see* War operations, destruction of aircraft
    microlight V95.11 ☑
    nonpowered V96.9 ☑
      specified NEC V96.8 ☑
    powered NEC V95.8 ☑
    stated as
      homicide (attempt) Y08.81 ☑
      suicide (attempt) X83.0 ☑
    ultralight V95.11 ☑
    spacecraft V95.41 ☑
    transport vehicle NEC (*see also* Accident, transport) V89.9 ☑
      homicide (attempt) Y03.8 ☑
      motor NEC (traffic) V89.2 ☑
        homicide (attempt) Y03.8 ☑
      suicide (attempt) — *see* Suicide, collision
**Cruelty** (mental) (physical) (sexual) X58 ☑
**Crushed** (accidentally) X58 ☑
  between objects (moving) (stationary and moving) W23.0 ☑
    stationary W23.1 ☑
  by
    alligator W58.03 ☑
    avalanche NEC — *see* Landslide
    cave-in W20.0 ☑
      caused by cataclysmic earth surface movement — *see* Landslide
    crocodile W58.13 ☑
    crowd or human stampede W52 ☑
    falling
      aircraft V97.39 ☑
        in war operations — *see* War operations, destruction of aircraft
      earth, material W20.0 ☑
        caused by cataclysmic earth surface movement — *see* Landslide
      object NEC W20.8 ☑
    landslide NEC — *see* Landslide
    lizard (nonvenomous) W59.09 ☑
    machinery — *see* Contact, with, by type of machine
    reptile NEC W59.89 ☑
    snake (nonvenomous) W59.13 ☑
  in
    machinery — *see* Contact, with, by type of machine
**Cut, cutting** (any part of body) (accidental) (*see also* Contact, with, by object or machine)
  during medical or surgical treatment as misadventure — *see* Index to Diseases and Injuries, Complications
  homicide (attempt) — *see* Assault, cutting or piercing instrument
  inflicted by other person — *see* Assault, cutting or piercing instrument
  legal
    execution — *see* Legal, intervention

**Cut, cutting** — *continued*
  legal — *continued*
    intervention — *see* Legal, intervention, sharp object
  machine NEC (*see also* Contact, with, by type of machine) W31.9 ☑
  self-inflicted — *see* Suicide, cutting or piercing instrument
  suicide (attempt) — *see* Suicide, cutting or piercing instrument
**Cyclone** (any injury) X37.1 ☑

# D

**Decapitation** (accidental circumstances) NEC X58 ☑
  homicide X99.9 ☑
  legal execution — *see* Legal, intervention
**Dehydration from lack of water** X58 ☑
**Deprivation** X58 ☑
**Derailment** (accidental)
  railway (rolling stock) (train) (vehicle) (without antecedent collision) V81.7 ☑
    with antecedent collision — *see* Accident, transport, railway vehicle occupant
  streetcar (without antecedent collision) V82.7 ☑
    with antecedent collision — *see* Accident, transport, streetcar occupant
**Descent**
  parachute (voluntary) (without accident to aircraft) V97.29 ☑
    due to accident to aircraft — *see* Accident, transport, aircraft
**Desertion** X58 ☑
**Destitution** X58 ☑
**Disability, late effect or sequela of injury** — *see* Sequelae
**Discharge** (accidental)
  airgun W34.010 ☑
    assault X95.01 ☑
    homicide (attempt) X95.01 ☑
    stated as undetermined whether accidental or intentional Y24.0 ☑
    suicide (attempt) X74.01 ☑
  BB gun — *see* Discharge, airgun
  firearm (accidental) W34.00 ☑
    assault X95.9 ☑
    handgun (pistol) (revolver) W32.0 ☑
      assault X93
      homicide (attempt) X93
      legal intervention — *see* Legal, intervention, firearm, handgun
      stated as undetermined whether accidental or intentional Y22 ☑
      suicide (attempt) X72 ☑
    homicide (attempt) X95.9 ☑
    hunting rifle W33.02 ☑
      assault X94.1 ☑
      homicide (attempt) X94.1 ☑
      legal intervention
        injuring
          bystander Y35.032 ☑
          law enforcement personnel Y35.031 ☑
          suspect Y35.033 ☑
      stated as undetermined whether accidental or intentional Y23.1 ☑
      suicide (attempt) X73.1 ☑
    larger W33.00 ☑
      assault X94.9 ☑
      homicide (attempt) X94.9 ☑
      hunting rifle — *see* Discharge, firearm, hunting rifle
      legal intervention — *see* Legal, intervention, firearm by type of firearm
      machine gun — *see* Discharge, firearm, machine gun
      shotgun — *see* Discharge, firearm, shotgun
      specified NEC W33.09 ☑
        assault X94.8 ☑
        homicide (attempt) X94.8 ☑
        legal intervention
          injuring
            bystander Y35.092 ☑
            law enforcement personnel Y35.091 ☑
            suspect Y35.093 ☑

**Discharge** — *continued*
  firearm — *continued*
    larger — *continued*
      specified — *continued*
        stated as undetermined whether accidental or intentional Y23.8 ☑
        suicide (attempt) X73.8 ☑
      stated as undetermined whether accidental or intentional Y23.9 ☑
      suicide (attempt) X73.9 ☑
    legal intervention
      injuring
        bystander Y35.002 ☑
        law enforcement personnel Y35.001 ☑
        suspect Y35.03 ☑
      using rubber bullet
        injuring
          bystander Y35.042 ☑
          law enforcement personnel Y35.041 ☑
          suspect Y35.043 ☑
    machine gun W33.03 ☑
      assault X94.2 ☑
      homicide (attempt) X94.2 ☑
      legal intervention — *see* Legal, intervention, firearm, machine gun
      stated as undetermined whether accidental or intentional Y23.3 ☑
      suicide (attempt) X73.2 ☑
    pellet gun — *see* Discharge, airgun
    shotgun W33.01 ☑
      assault X94.0 ☑
      homicide (attempt) X94.0 ☑
      legal intervention — *see* Legal, intervention, firearm, specified NEC
      stated as undetermined whether accidental or intentional Y23.0 ☑
      suicide (attempt) X73.0 ☑
    specified NEC W34.09 ☑
      assault X95.8 ☑
      homicide (attempt) X95.8 ☑
      legal intervention — *see* Legal, intervention, firearm, specified NEC
      stated as undetermined whether accidental or intentional Y24.8 ☑
      suicide (attempt) X74.8 ☑
    stated as undetermined whether accidental or intentional Y24.9 ☑
    suicide (attempt) X74.9 ☑
    Very pistol W34.09 ☑
      assault X95.8 ☑
      homicide (attempt) X95.8 ☑
      stated as undetermined whether accidental or intentional Y24.8 ☑
      suicide (attempt) X74.8 ☑
  firework(s) W39 ☑
    stated as undetermined whether accidental or intentional Y25 ☑
  gas-operated gun NEC W34.018 ☑
    airgun — *see* Discharge, airgun
    assault X95.09 ☑
    homicide (attempt) X95.09 ☑
    paintball gun — *see* Discharge, paintball gun
    stated as undetermined whether accidental or intentional Y24.8 ☑
    suicide (attempt) X74.09 ☑
  gun NEC (*see also* Discharge, firearm NEC)
    air — *see* Discharge, airgun
    BB — *see* Discharge, airgun
    for single hand use — *see* Discharge, firearm, handgun
    hand — *see* Discharge, firearm, handgun
    machine — *see* Discharge, firearm, machine gun
    other specified — *see* Discharge, firearm NEC
    paintball — *see* Discharge, paintball gun
    pellet — *see* Discharge, airgun
  handgun — *see* Discharge, firearm, handgun
  machine gun — *see* Discharge, firearm, machine gun
  paintball gun W34.011 ☑
    assault X95.02 ☑
    homicide (attempt) X95.02 ☑
    stated as undetermined whether accidental or intentional Y24.8 ☑
    suicide (attempt) X74.02 ☑
  pistol — *see* Discharge, firearm, handgun
    flare — *see* Discharge, firearm, Very pistol
    pellet — *see* Discharge, airgun

---

**Discharge** — *continued*
   pistol — *see* Discharge, firearm, handgun — *continued*
      Very — *see* Discharge, firearm, Very pistol
   revolver — *see* Discharge, firearm, handgun
   rifle (hunting) — *see* Discharge, firearm, hunting rifle
   shotgun — *see* Discharge, firearm, shotgun
   spring-operated gun NEC W34.018 ☑
      assault X95.09 ☑
      homicide (attempt) X95.09 ☑
      stated as undetermined whether accidental or intentional Y24.8 ☑
      suicide (attempt) X74.09 ☑
**Disease**
   Andes W94.11 ☑
   aviator's — *see* Air, pressure
   range W94.11 ☑
**Diver's disease, palsy, paralysis, squeeze** — *see* Air, pressure
**Diving** (into water) — *see* Accident, diving
**Dog bite** W54.0 ☑
**Dragged by transport vehicle NEC** (*see also* Accident, transport) V09.9 ☑
**Drinking poison** (accidental) — *see* Table of Drugs and Chemicals
**Dropped** (accidentally) **while being carried or supported by other person** W04 ☑
**Drowning** (accidental) W74 ☑
   assault X92.9 ☑
   due to
      accident (to)
         machinery — *see* Contact, with, by type of machine
         watercraft V90.89 ☑
            burning V90.29 ☑
               powered V90.23 ☑
                  fishing boat V90.22 ☑
                  jetskis V90.23 ☑
                  merchant ship V90.20 ☑
                  passenger ship V90.21 ☑
               unpowered V90.28 ☑
                  canoe V90.25 ☑
                  inflatable V90.26 ☑
                  kayak V90.25 ☑
                  sailboat V90.24 ☑
                  water skis V90.27 ☑
            crushed V90.39 ☑
               powered V90.33 ☑
                  fishing boat V90.32 ☑
                  jetskis V90.33 ☑
                  merchant ship V90.30 ☑
                  passenger ship V90.31 ☑
               unpowered V90.38 ☑
                  canoe V90.35 ☑
                  inflatable V90.36 ☑
                  kayak V90.35 ☑
                  sailboat V90.34 ☑
                  water skis V90.37 ☑
            overturning V90.09 ☑
               powered V90.03 ☑
                  fishing boat V90.02 ☑
                  jetskis V90.03 ☑
                  merchant ship V90.00 ☑
                  passenger ship V90.01 ☑
               unpowered V90.08 ☑
                  canoe V90.05 ☑
                  inflatable V90.06 ☑
                  kayak V90.05 ☑
                  sailboat V90.04 ☑
            sinking V90.19 ☑
               powered V90.13 ☑
                  fishing boat V90.12 ☑
                  jetskis V90.13 ☑
                  merchant ship V90.10 ☑
                  passenger ship V90.11 ☑
               unpowered V90.18 ☑
                  canoe V90.15 ☑
                  inflatable V90.16 ☑
                  kayak V90.15 ☑
                  sailboat V90.14 ☑
            specified type NEC V90.89 ☑
               powered V90.83 ☑
                  fishing boat V90.82 ☑
                  jetskis V90.83 ☑
                  merchant ship V90.80 ☑
                  passenger ship V90.81 ☑

**Drowning** — *continued*
   due to — *continued*
      accident — *continued*
         watercraft — *continued*
            specified type — *continued*
               unpowered V90.88 ☑
                  canoe V90.85 ☑
                  inflatable V90.86 ☑
                  kayak V90.85 ☑
                  sailboat V90.84 ☑
                  water skis V90.87 ☑
      avalanche — *see* Landslide
      cataclysmic
         earth surface movement NEC — *see* Forces of nature, earth movement
         storm — *see* Forces of nature, cataclysmic storm
      cloudburst X37.8 ☑
      cyclone X37.1 ☑
      fall overboard (from) V92.09 ☑
         powered craft V92.03 ☑
            ferry boat V92.01 ☑
            fishing boat V92.02 ☑
            jetskis V92.03 ☑
            liner V92.01 ☑
            merchant ship V92.00 ☑
            passenger ship V92.01 ☑
         resulting from
            accident to watercraft — *see* Drowning, due to, accident to, watercraft
            being washed overboard (from) V92.29 ☑
               powered craft V92.23 ☑
                  ferry boat V92.21 ☑
                  fishing boat V92.22 ☑
                  jetskis V92.23 ☑
                  liner V92.21 ☑
                  merchant ship V92.20 ☑
                  passenger ship V92.21 ☑
               unpowered craft V92.28 ☑
                  canoe V92.25 ☑
                  inflatable V92.26 ☑
                  kayak V92.25 ☑
                  sailboat V92.24 ☑
                  surf-board V92.28 ☑
                  water skis V92.27 ☑
                  windsurfer V92.28 ☑
            motion of watercraft V92.19 ☑
               powered craft V92.13 ☑
                  ferry boat V92.11 ☑
                  fishing boat V92.12 ☑
                  jetskis V92.13 ☑
                  liner V92.11 ☑
                  merchant ship V92.10 ☑
                  passenger ship V92.11 ☑
               unpowered craft
                  canoe V92.15 ☑
                  inflatable V92.16 ☑
                  kayak V92.15 ☑
                  sailboat V92.14 ☑
         unpowered craft V92.08 ☑
            canoe V92.05 ☑
            inflatable V92.06 ☑
            kayak V92.05 ☑
            sailboat V92.04 ☑
            surf-board V92.08 ☑
            water skis V92.07 ☑
            windsurfer V92.08 ☑
      hurricane X37.0 ☑
      jumping into water from watercraft (involved in accident) (*see also* Drowning, due to, accident to, watercraft)
         without accident to or on watercraft W16.711 ☑
      tidal wave NEC — *see* Forces of nature, tidal wave
      torrential rain X37.8 ☑
   following
      fall
         into
            bathtub W16.211 ☑
            bucket W16.221 ☑
            fountain — *see* Drowning, following, fall, into, water, specified NEC
            quarry — *see* Drowning, following, fall, into, water, specified NEC
            reservoir — *see* Drowning, following, fall, into, water, specified NEC

**Drowning** — *continued*
   following — *continued*
      fall — *continued*
         into — *continued*
            swimming-pool W16.011 ☑
               stated as undetermined whether accidental or intentional Y21.3 ☑
               striking
                  bottom W16.021 ☑
                  wall W16.031 ☑
               suicide (attempt) X71.2 ☑
            water NOS W16.41 ☑
               natural (lake) (open sea) (river) (stream) (pond) W16.111 ☑
                  striking
                     bottom W16.121 ☑
                     side W16.131 ☑
               specified NEC W16.311 ☑
                  striking
                     bottom W16.321 ☑
                     wall W16.331 ☑
      overboard NEC — *see* Drowning, due to, fall overboard
   jump or dive
      from boat W16.711 ☑
         striking bottom W16.721 ☑
      into
         fountain — *see* Drowning, following, jump or dive, into, water, specified NEC
         quarry — *see* Drowning, following, jump or dive, into, water, specified NEC
         reservoir — *see* Drowning, following, jump or dive, into, water, specified NEC
         swimming-pool W16.511 ☑
            striking
               bottom W16.521 ☑
               wall W16.531 ☑
            suicide (attempt) X71.2 ☑
         water NOS W16.91 ☑
            natural (lake) (open sea) (river) (stream) (pond) W16.611 ☑
            specified NEC W16.811 ☑
               bottom W16.821 ☑
               striking
                  bottom W16.821 ☑
                  wall W16.831 ☑
            striking
               bottom W16.821 ☑
               wall W16.831 ☑
            striking bottom W16.621 ☑
   homicide (attempt) X92.9 ☑
   in
      bathtub (accidental) W65 ☑
         assault X92.0 ☑
         following fall W16.211 ☑
            stated as undetermined whether accidental or intentional Y21.1 ☑
         stated as undetermined whether accidental or intentional Y21.0 ☑
         suicide (attempt) X71.0 ☑
      lake — *see* Drowning, in, natural water
      natural water (lake) (open sea) (river) (stream) (pond) W69 ☑
         assault X92.3 ☑
         following
            dive or jump W16.611 ☑
               striking bottom W16.621 ☑
            fall W16.111 ☑
               striking
                  bottom W16.121 ☑
                  side W16.131 ☑
         stated as undetermined whether accidental or intentional Y21.4 ☑
         suicide (attempt) X71.3 ☑
      quarry — *see* Drowning, in, specified place NEC
      quenching tank — *see* Drowning, in, specified place NEC
      reservoir — *see* Drowning, in, specified place NEC
      river — *see* Drowning, in, natural water
      sea — *see* Drowning, in, natural water
      specified place NEC W73 ☑
         assault X92.8 ☑
         following
            dive or jump W16.811 ☑
               striking
                  bottom W16.821 ☑
                  wall W16.831 ☑

**Drowning** — continued
- in — continued
  - specified place — continued
    - following — continued
      - fall W16.311 ☑
        - striking
          - bottom W16.321 ☑
          - wall W16.331 ☑
      - stated as undetermined whether accidental or intentional Y21.8 ☑
      - suicide (attempt) X71.8 ☑
  - stream — see Drowning, in, natural water
  - swimming-pool W67 ☑
    - assault X92.1 ☑
      - following fall X92.2 ☑
    - following
      - dive or jump W16.511 ☑
        - striking
          - bottom W16.521 ☑
          - wall W16.531 ☑
      - fall W16.011 ☑
        - striking
          - bottom W16.021 ☑
          - wall W16.031 ☑
    - stated as undetermined whether accidental or intentional Y21.2 ☑
      - following fall Y21.3 ☑
    - suicide (attempt) X71.1 ☑
      - following fall X71.2 ☑
  - war operations — see War operations, restriction of airway
- resulting from accident to watercraft — see Drowning, due to, accident, watercraft
- self-inflicted X71.9 ☑
- stated as undetermined whether accidental or intentional Y21.9 ☑
- suicide (attempt) X71.9 ☑

# E

**Earth falling** (on) W20.0 ☑
- caused by cataclysmic earth surface movement or eruption — see Landslide

**Earth** (surface) **movement NEC** — see Forces of nature, earth movement

**Earthquake** (any injury) X34 ☑

**Effect**(s) (adverse) **of**
- air pressure (any) — see Air, pressure
- cold, excessive (exposure to) — see Exposure, cold
- heat (excessive) — see Heat
- hot place (weather) — see Heat
- insolation X30 ☑
- late — see Sequelae
- motion — see Motion
- nuclear explosion or weapon in war operations — see War operations, nuclear weapon
- radiation — see Radiation
- travel — see Travel

**Electric shock** (accidental) (by) (in) — see Exposure, electric current

**Electrocution** (accidental) — see Exposure, electric current

**Endotracheal tube wrongly placed during anesthetic procedure**

**Entanglement**
- in
  - bed linen, causing suffocation T71 ☑
  - wheel of pedal cycle V19.88 ☑

**Entry of foreign body or material** — see Foreign body

**Environmental pollution related condition** — see
- category Z57 ☑

**Execution, legal** (any method) — see Legal, intervention

**Exhaustion**
- cold — see Exposure, cold
- due to excessive exertion (see also Overexertion) X50.9 ☑
- heat — see Heat

**Explosion** (accidental) (of) (with secondary fire) W40.9 ☑
- acetylene W40.1 ☑
- aerosol can W36.1 ☑
- air tank (compressed) (in machinery) W36.2 ☑
- aircraft (in transit) (powered) NEC V95.9 ☑
  - balloon V96.05 ☑
  - fixed wing NEC (private) V95.25 ☑
    - commercial V95.35 ☑
  - glider V96.25 ☑

**Explosion** — continued
- aircraft — continued
  - glider — continued
    - hang V96.15 ☑
    - powered V95.15 ☑
  - helicopter V95.05 ☑
  - in war operations — see War operations, destruction of aircraft
  - microlight V95.15 ☑
  - nonpowered V96.9 ☑
    - specified NEC V96.8 ☑
  - powered NEC V95.8 ☑
  - stated as
    - homicide (attempt) Y03.8 ☑
    - suicide (attempt) X83.0 ☑
  - ultralight V95.15 ☑
- anesthetic gas in operating room W40.1 ☑
- antipersonnel bomb W40.8 ☑
  - assault X96.0 ☑
  - homicide (attempt) X96.0 ☑
  - suicide (attempt) X75 ☑
- assault X96.9 ☑
- bicycle tire W37.0 ☑
- blasting (cap) (materials) W40.0 ☑
- boiler (machinery), not on transport vehicle W35 ☑
  - on watercraft — see Explosion, in, watercraft
- butane W40.1 ☑
- caused by other person X96.9 ☑
- coal gas W40.1 ☑
- detonator W40.0 ☑
- dump (munitions) W40.8 ☑
- dynamite W40.0 ☑
  - in
    - assault X96.8 ☑
    - homicide (attempt) X96.8 ☑
    - legal intervention
      - injuring
        - bystander Y35.112 ☑
        - law enforcement personnel Y35.111 ☑
        - suspect Y35.113 ☑
    - suicide (attempt) X75 ☑
- explosive (material) W40.9 ☑
  - gas W40.1 ☑
  - in blasting operation W40.0 ☑
  - specified NEC W40.8 ☑
    - in
      - assault X96.8 ☑
      - homicide (attempt) X96.8 ☑
      - legal intervention
        - injuring
          - bystander Y35.192 ☑
          - law enforcement personnel Y35.191 ☑
          - suspect Y35.193 ☑
      - suicide (attempt) X75 ☑
- factory (munitions) W40.8 ☑
- fertilizer bomb W40.8 ☑
  - assault X96.3 ☑
  - homicide (attempt) X96.3 ☑
  - suicide (attempt) X75 ☑
- firearm (parts) NEC W34.19 ☑
  - airgun W34.110 ☑
  - BB gun W34.110 ☑
  - gas, air or spring-operated gun NEC W34.118 ☑
  - hangun W32.1 ☑
  - hunting rifle W33.12 ☑
  - larger firearm W33.10 ☑
    - specified NEC W33.19 ☑
  - machine gun W33.13 ☑
  - paintball gun W34.111 ☑
  - pellet gun W34.110 ☑
  - shotgun W33.11 ☑
  - Very pistol [flare] W34.19 ☑
- fire-damp W40.1 ☑
- fireworks W39 ☑
- gas (coal) (explosive) W40.1 ☑
  - cylinder W36.9 ☑
    - aerosol can W36.1 ☑
    - air tank W36.2 ☑
    - pressurized W36.3 ☑
    - specified NEC W36.8 ☑
- gasoline (fumes) (tank) not in moving motor vehicle W40.1 ☑
  - bomb W40.8 ☑
    - assault X96.1 ☑
    - homicide (attempt) X96.1 ☑

**Explosion** — continued
- gasoline not in moving motor vehicle — continued
  - bomb — continued
    - suicide (attempt) X75 ☑
  - in motor vehicle — see Accident, transport, by type of vehicle
- grain store W40.8 ☑
- grenade W40.8 ☑
  - in
    - assault X96.8 ☑
    - homicide (attempt) X96.8 ☑
    - legal intervention
      - injuring
        - bystander Y35.192 ☑
        - law enforcement personnel Y35.191 ☑
        - suspect Y35.193 ☑
    - suicide (attempt) X75 ☑
- handgun (parts) — see Explosion, firearm, hangun (parts)
- homicide (attempt) X96.9 ☑
  - antipersonnel bomb — see Explosion, antipersonnel bomb
  - fertilizer bomb — see Explosion, fertilizer bomb
  - gasoline bomb — see Explosion, gasoline bomb
  - letter bomb — see Explosion, letter bomb
  - pipe bomb — see Explosion, pipe bomb
  - specified NEC X96.8 ☑
- hose, pressurized W37.8 ☑
- hot water heater, tank (in machinery) W35 ☑
  - on watercraft — see Explosion, in, watercraft
- in, on
  - dump W40.8 ☑
  - factory W40.8 ☑
  - mine (of explosive gases) NEC W40.1 ☑
  - watercraft V93.59 ☑
    - powered craft V93.53 ☑
      - ferry boat V93.51 ☑
      - fishing boat V93.52 ☑
      - jetskis V93.53 ☑
      - liner V93.51 ☑
      - merchant ship V93.50 ☑
      - passenger ship V93.51 ☑
      - sailboat V93.54 ☑
- letter bomb W40.8 ☑
  - assault X96.2 ☑
  - homicide (attempt) X96.2 ☑
  - suicide (attempt) X75 ☑
- machinery (see also Contact, with, by type of machine)
  - on board watercraft — see Explosion, in, watercraft
  - pressure vessel — see Explosion, by type of vessel
- methane W40.1 ☑
- mine W40.1 ☑
- missile NEC W40.8 ☑
- mortar bomb W40.8 ☑
  - in
    - assault X96.8 ☑
    - homicide (attempt) X96.8 ☑
    - legal intervention
      - injuring
        - bystander Y35.192 ☑
        - law enforcement personnel Y35.191 ☑
        - suspect Y35.193 ☑
    - suicide (attempt) X75 ☑
- munitions (dump) (factory) W40.8 ☑
- pipe, pressurized W37.8 ☑
  - bomb W40.8 ☑
    - assault X96.4 ☑
    - homicide (attempt) X96.4 ☑
    - suicide (attempt) X75 ☑
- pressure, pressurized
  - cooker W38 ☑
  - gas tank (in machinery) W36.3 ☑
  - hose W37.8 ☑
  - pipe W37.8 ☑
  - specified device NEC W38 ☑
  - tire W37.8 ☑
    - bicycle W37.0 ☑
  - vessel (in machinery) W38 ☑
- propane W40.1 ☑
- self-inflicted X75 ☑
- shell (artillery) NEC W40.8 ☑
  - during war operations — see War operations, explosion

**Explosion** — *continued*
　shell — *continued*
　　in
　　　legal intervention
　　　　injuring
　　　　　bystander Y35.122 ☑
　　　　　law enforcement personnel Y35.121 ☑
　　　　　suspect Y35.123 ☑
　　　war — *see* War operations, explosion
　spacecraft V95.45 ☑
　stated as undetermined whether accidental or intentional Y25 ☑
　steam or water lines (in machinery) W37.8 ☑
　stove W40.9 ☑
　suicide (attempt) X75 ☑
　tire, pressurized W37.8 ☑
　　bicycle W37.0 ☑
　undetermined whether accidental or intentional Y25 ☑
　vehicle tire NEC W37.8 ☑
　　bicycle W37.0 ☑
　war operations — *see* War operations, explosion
**Exposure** (to) X58 ☑
　air pressure change — *see* Air, pressure
　cold (accidental) (excessive) (extreme) (natural) (place) X31 ☑
　　assault Y08.89 ☑
　　due to
　　　man-made conditions W93.8 ☑
　　　　dry ice (contact) W93.01 ☑
　　　　　inhalation W93.02 ☑
　　　　liquid air (contact) (hydrogen) (nitrogen) W93.11 ☑
　　　　　inhalation W93.12 ☑
　　　　refrigeration unit (deep freeze) W93.2 ☑
　　　　suicide (attempt) X83.2 ☑
　　　weather (conditions) X31 ☑
　　homicide (attempt) Y08.89 ☑
　　self-inflicted X83.2 ☑
　due to abandonment or neglect X58 ☑
　electric current W86.8 ☑
　　appliance (faulty) W86.8 ☑
　　　domestic W86.0 ☑
　　caused by other person Y08.89 ☑
　　conductor (faulty) W86.1 ☑
　　control apparatus (faulty) W86.1 ☑
　　electric power generating plant, distribution station W86.1 ☑
　　electroshock gun — *see* Exposure, electric current, taser
　　high-voltage cable W85 ☑
　　homicide (attempt) Y08.89 ☑
　　legal execution — *see* Legal, intervention, specified means NEC
　　lightning — *see* subcategory T75.0 ☑
　　live rail W86.8 ☑
　　misadventure in medical or surgical procedure in electroshock therapy Y63.4
　　motor (electric) (faulty) W86.8 ☑
　　　domestic W86.0 ☑
　　self-inflicted X83.1 ☑
　　specified NEC W86.8 ☑
　　　domestic W86.0 ☑
　　stun gun — *see* Exposure, electric current, taser
　　suicide (attempt) X83.1 ☑
　　taser W86.8 ☑
　　　assault Y08.89 ☑
　　　legal intervention — *see* category Y35 ☑
　　　self-harm (intentional) X83.8 ☑
　　　undetermined intent Y33 ☑
　　third rail W86.8 ☑
　　transformer (faulty) W86.1 ☑
　　transmission lines W85 ☑
　environmental tobacco smoke X58 ☑
　excessive
　　cold — *see* Exposure, cold
　　heat (natural) NEC X30 ☑
　　　man-made W92 ☑
　factor(s) NOS X58 ☑
　　environmental NEC X58 ☑
　　　man-made NEC W99 ☑
　　　natural NEC — *see* Forces of nature
　　specified NEC X58 ☑
　fire, flames (accidental) X08.8 ☑
　　assault X97 ☑

　fire, flames — *continued*
　　campfire — *see* Exposure, fire, controlled, not in building
　　controlled (in)
　　　with ignition (of) clothing (*see also* Ignition, clothes) X06.2 ☑
　　　　nightwear X05 ☑
　　　bonfire — *see* Exposure, fire, controlled, not in building
　　　brazier (in building or structure) (*see also* Exposure, fire, controlled, building)
　　　　not in building or structure — *see* Exposure, fire, controlled, not in building
　　　building or structure X02.0 ☑
　　　　with
　　　　　fall from building X02.3 ☑
　　　　　from building X02.5 ☑
　　　　　injury due to building collapse X02.2 ☑
　　　　　smoke inhalation X02.1 ☑
　　　　　hit by object from building X02.4 ☑
　　　　　specified mode of injury NEC X02.8 ☑
　　　fireplace, furnace or stove — *see* Exposure, fire, controlled, building
　　　not in building or structure X03.0 ☑
　　　　with
　　　　　fall X03.3 ☑
　　　　　smoke inhalation X03.1 ☑
　　　　　hit by object X03.4 ☑
　　　　　specified mode of injury NEC X03.8 ☑
　　　trash — *see* Exposure, fire, controlled, not in building
　　fireplace — *see* Exposure, fire, controlled, building
　　fittings or furniture (in building or structure) (uncontrolled) — *see* Exposure, fire, uncontrolled, building
　　forest (uncontrolled) — *see* Exposure, fire, uncontrolled, not in building
　　grass (uncontrolled) — *see* Exposure, fire, uncontrolled, not in building
　　hay (uncontrolled) — *see* Exposure, fire, uncontrolled, not in building
　　homicide (attempt) X97 ☑
　　ignition of highly flammable material X04 ☑
　　in, of, on, starting in
　　　machinery — *see* Contact, with, by type of machine
　　　motor vehicle (in motion) (*see also* Accident, transport, occupant by type of vehicle) V87.8 ☑
　　　　with collision — *see* Collision
　　　railway rolling stock, train, vehicle V81.81 ☑
　　　　with collision — *see* Accident, transport, railway vehicle occupant
　　　street car (in motion) V82.8 ☑
　　　　with collision — *see* Accident, transport, streetcar occupant
　　　transport vehicle NEC (*see also* Accident, transport)
　　　　with collision — *see* Collision
　　　war operations (*see also* War operations, fire)
　　　　from nuclear explosion — *see* War operations, nuclear weapons
　　　watercraft (in transit) (not in transit) V91.09 ☑
　　　　localized — *see* Burn, on board watercraft, due to, fire on board
　　　　powered craft V91.03 ☑
　　　　　ferry boat V91.01 ☑
　　　　　fishing boat V91.02 ☑
　　　　　jet skis V91.03 ☑
　　　　　liner V91.01 ☑
　　　　　merchant ship V91.00 ☑
　　　　　passenger ship V91.01 ☑
　　　　unpowered craft V91.08 ☑
　　　　　canoe V91.05 ☑
　　　　　inflatable V91.06 ☑
　　　　　kayak V91.05 ☑
　　　　　sailboat V91.04 ☑
　　　　　surf-board V91.08 ☑
　　　　　waterskis V91.07 ☑
　　　　　windsurfer V91.08 ☑
　　lumber (uncontrolled) — *see* Exposure, fire, uncontrolled, not in building
　　mine (uncontrolled) — *see* Exposure, fire, uncontrolled, not in building
　　prairie (uncontrolled) — *see* Exposure, fire, uncontrolled, not in building

　fire, flames — *continued*
　　resulting from
　　　explosion — *see* Explosion
　　　lightning X08.8 ☑
　　self-inflicted X76 ☑
　　specified NEC X08.8 ☑
　　started by other person X97 ☑
　　stated as undetermined whether accidental or intentional Y26 ☑
　　stove — *see* Exposure, fire, controlled, building
　　suicide (attempt) X76 ☑
　　tunnel (uncontrolled) — *see* Exposure, fire, uncontrolled, not in building
　　uncontrolled
　　　in building or structure X00.0 ☑
　　　　with
　　　　　fall from building X00.3 ☑
　　　　　injury due to building collapse X00.2 ☑
　　　　　jump from building X00.5 ☑
　　　　　smoke inhalation X00.1 ☑
　　　　bed X08.00 ☑
　　　　　due to
　　　　　　cigarette X08.01 ☑
　　　　　　specified material NEC X08.09 ☑
　　　　furniture NEC X08.20 ☑
　　　　　due to
　　　　　　cigarette X08.21 ☑
　　　　　　specified material NEC X08.29 ☑
　　　　hit by object from building X00.4 ☑
　　　　sofa X08.10 ☑
　　　　　due to
　　　　　　cigarette X08.11 ☑
　　　　　　specified material NEC X08.19 ☑
　　　　specified mode of injury NEC X00.8 ☑
　　　not in building or structure (any) X01.0 ☑
　　　　with
　　　　　fall X01.3 ☑
　　　　　smoke inhalation X01.1 ☑
　　　　　hit by object X01.4 ☑
　　　　　specified mode of injury NEC X01.8 ☑
　　　undetermined whether accidental or intentional Y26 ☑
　forces of nature NEC — *see* Forces of nature
　G-forces (abnormal) W49.9 ☑
　gravitational forces (abnormal) W49.9 ☑
　heat (natural) NEC — *see* Heat
　high-pressure jet (hydraulic) (pneumatic) W49.9 ☑
　hydraulic jet W49.9 ☑
　inanimate mechanical force W49.9 ☑
　jet, high-pressure (hydraulic) (pneumatic) W49.9 ☑
　lightning — *see* subcategory T75.0 ☑
　　causing fire — *see* Exposure, fire
　mechanical forces NEC W49.9 ☑
　　animate NEC W64
　　inanimate NEC W49.9 ☑
　noise W42.9 ☑
　　supersonic W42.0 ☑
　noxious substance — *see* Table of Drugs and Chemicals
　pneumatic jet W49.9 ☑
　prolonged in deep-freeze unit or refrigerator W93.2 ☑
　radiation — *see* Radiation
　smoke (*see also* Exposure, fire)
　　tobacco, second hand Z77.22
　specified factors NEC X58 ☑
　sunlight X32 ☑
　　man-made (sun lamp) W89.8 ☑
　　　tanning bed W89.1 ☑
　supersonic waves W42.0 ☑
　transmission line(s), electric W85 ☑
　vibration W49.9 ☑
　waves
　　infrasound W49.9 ☑
　　sound W42.9 ☑
　　supersonic W42.0 ☑
　weather NEC — *see* Forces of nature
**External cause status** Y99.9
　child assisting in compensated work for family Y99.8
　civilian activity done for financial or other compensation Y99.0
　civilian activity done for income or pay Y99.0
　family member assisting in compensated work for other family member Y99.8
　hobby not done for income Y99.8
　leisure activity Y99.8

**External cause status** — *continued*
military activity Y99.1
off-duty activity of military personnel Y99.8
recreation or sport not for income or while a student Y99.8
specified NEC Y99.8
student activity Y99.8
volunteer activity Y99.2

# F

**Factors, supplemental**
alcohol
blood level
less than 20mg/100ml Y90.0
20-39mg/100ml Y90.1
40-59mg/100ml Y90.2
60-79mg/100ml Y90.3
80-99mg/100ml Y90.4
100-119mg/100ml Y90.5
120-199mg/100ml Y90.6
200-239mg/100ml Y90.7
240mg/100ml or more Y90.8
presence in blood, level not specified Y90.9
presence in blood, but level not specified Y90.9
environmental-pollution-related condition- see Z57
nosocomial condition Y95
work-related condition Y99.0
**Failure**
in suture or ligature during surgical procedure Y65.2
mechanical, of instrument or apparatus (any) (during any medical or surgical procedure) Y65.8
sterile precautions (during medical and surgical care) — *see* Misadventure, failure, sterile precautions, by type of procedure
to
introduce tube or instrument Y65.4
endotracheal tube during anesthesia Y65.3
make curve (transport vehicle) NEC — *see* Accident, transport
remove tube or instrument Y65.4
**Fall, falling** (accidental) W19 ☑
building W20.1 ☑
burning (uncontrolled fire) X00.3 ☑
down
embankment W17.81 ☑
escalator W10.0 ☑
hill W17.81 ☑
ladder W11 ☑
ramp W10.2 ☑
stairs, steps W10.9 ☑
due to
bumping against
object W18.00 ☑
sharp glass W18.02 ☑
specified NEC W18.09 ☑
sports equipment W18.01 ☑
person W03 ☑
due to ice or snow W00.0 ☑
on pedestrian conveyance — *see* Accident, transport, pedestrian, conveyance
collision with another person W03 ☑
due to ice or snow W00.0 ☑
involving pedestrian conveyance — *see* Accident, transport, pedestrian, conveyance
grocery cart tipping over W17.82 ☑
ice or snow W00.9 ☑
from one level to another W00.2 ☑
on stairs or steps W00.1 ☑
involving pedestrian conveyance — *see* Accident, transport, pedestrian, conveyance
on same level W00.0 ☑
slipping (on moving sidewalk) W01.0 ☑
with subsequent striking against object W01.10 ☑
furniture W01.190 ☑
sharp object W01.119 ☑
glass W01.110 ☑
power tool or machine W01.111 ☑
specified NEC W01.118 ☑
specified NEC W01.198 ☑
striking against
object W18.00 ☑
sharp glass W18.02 ☑
specified NEC W18.09 ☑
sports equipment W18.01 ☑
person W03 ☑

**Fall, falling** — *continued*
due to — *continued*
striking against — *continued*
person — *continued*
due to ice or snow W00.0 ☑
on pedestrian conveyance — *see* Accident, transport, pedestrian, conveyance
earth (with asphyxia or suffocation (by pressure)) — *see* Earth, falling
from, off, out of
aircraft NEC (with accident to aircraft NEC) V97.0 ☑
while boarding or alighting V97.1 ☑
balcony W13.0 ☑
bed W06 ☑
boat, ship, watercraft NEC (with drowning or submersion) — *see* Drowning, due to, fall overboard
with hitting bottom or object V94.0 ☑
bridge W13.1 ☑
building W13.9 ☑
burning (uncontrolled fire) X00.3 ☑
cavity W17.2 ☑
chair W07 ☑
cherry picker W17.89 ☑
cliff W15 ☑
dock W17.4 ☑
embankment W17.81 ☑
escalator W10.0 ☑
flagpole W13.8 ☑
furniture NEC W08 ☑
grocery cart W17.82 ☑
haystack W17.89 ☑
high place NEC W17.89 ☑
stated as undetermined whether accidental or intentional Y30 ☑
hole W17.2 ☑
incline W10.2 ☑
ladder W11 ☑
lifting device W17.89 ☑
machine, machinery (*see also* Contact, with, by type of machine)
not in operation W17.89 ☑
manhole W17.1 ☑
mobile elevated work platform [MEWP] W17.89 ☑
motorized mobility scooter W05.2 ☑
one level to another NEC W17.89 ☑
intentional, purposeful, suicide (attempt) X80 ☑
stated as undetermined whether accidental or intentional Y30 ☑
pit W17.2 ☑
playground equipment W09.8 ☑
jungle gym W09.2 ☑
slide W09.0 ☑
swing W09.1 ☑
quarry W17.89 ☑
railing W13.9 ☑
ramp W10.2 ☑
roof W13.2 ☑
scaffolding W12 ☑
scooter (nonmotorized) W05.1 ☑
motorized mobility W05.2 ☑
sky lift W17.89 ☑
stairs, steps W10.9 ☑
curb W10.1 ☑
due to ice or snow W00.1 ☑
escalator W10.0 ☑
incline W10.2 ☑
ramp W10.2 ☑
sidewalk curb W10.1 ☑
specified NEC W10.8 ☑
stepladder W11 ☑
storm drain W17.1 ☑
streetcar NEC V82.6 ☑
with antecedent collision — *see* Accident, transport, streetcar occupant
while boarding or alighting V82.4 ☑
structure NEC W13.8 ☑
burning (uncontrolled fire) X00.3 ☑
table W08 ☑
toilet W18.11 ☑
with subsequent striking against object W18.12 ☑
train NEC V81.6 ☑
during derailment (without antecedent collision) V81.7 ☑

**Fall, falling** — *continued*
from, off, out of — *continued*
train — *continued*
during derailment — *continued*
with antecedent collision — *see* Accident, transport, railway vehicle occupant
while boarding or alighting V81.4 ☑
transport vehicle after collision — *see* Accident, transport, by type of vehicle, collision
tree W14 ☑
vehicle (in motion) NEC (*see also* Accident, transport) V89.9 ☑
motor NEC (*see also* Accident, transport, occupant, by type of vehicle) V87.8 ☑
stationary W17.89 ☑
while boarding or alighting — *see* Accident, transport, by type of vehicle, while boarding or alighting
viaduct W13.8 ☑
wall W13.8 ☑
watercraft (*see also* Drowning, due to, fall overboard)
with hitting bottom or object V94.0 ☑
well W17.0 ☑
wheelchair, non-moving W05.0 ☑
powered — *see* Accident, transport, pedestrian, conveyance occupant, specified type NEC
window W13.4 ☑
in, on
aircraft NEC V97.0 ☑
with accident to aircraft V97.0 ☑
while boarding or alighting V97.1 ☑
bathtub (empty) W18.2 ☑
filled W16.212 ☑
causing drowning W16.211 ☑
escalator W10.0 ☑
incline W10.2 ☑
ladder W11 ☑
machine, machinery — *see* Contact, with, by type of machine
object, edged, pointed or sharp (with cut) — *see* Fall, by type
playground equipment W09.8 ☑
jungle gym W09.2 ☑
slide W09.0 ☑
swing W09.1 ☑
ramp W10.2 ☑
scaffolding W12 ☑
shower W18.2 ☑
causing drowning W16.211 ☑
staircase, stairs, steps W10.9 ☑
curb W10.1 ☑
due to ice or snow W00.1 ☑
escalator W10.0 ☑
incline W10.2 ☑
specified NEC W10.8 ☑
streetcar (without antecedent collision) V82.5 ☑
with antecedent collision — *see* Accident, transport, streetcar occupant
while boarding or alighting V82.4 ☑
train (without antecedent collision) V81.5 ☑
with antecedent collision — *see* Accident, transport, railway vehicle occupant
during derailment (without antecedent collision) V81.7 ☑
with antecedent collision — *see* Accident, transport, railway vehicle occupant
while boarding or alighting V81.4 ☑
transport vehicle after collision — *see* Accident, transport, by type of vehicle, collision
watercraft V93.39 ☑
due to
accident to craft V91.29 ☑
powered craft V91.23 ☑
ferry boat V91.21 ☑
fishing boat V91.22 ☑
jetskis V91.23 ☑
liner V91.21 ☑
merchant ship V91.20 ☑
passenger ship V91.21 ☑
unpowered craft
canoe V91.25 ☑
inflatable V91.26 ☑
kayak V91.25 ☑
sailboat V91.24 ☑
powered craft V93.33 ☑

**Fall, falling** — *continued*
  in, on — *continued*
    watercraft — *continued*
      powered craft — *continued*
        ferry boat V93.31 ☑
        fishing boat V93.32 ☑
        jetskis V93.33 ☑
        liner V93.31 ☑
        merchant ship V93.30 ☑
        passenger ship V93.31 ☑
      unpowered craft V93.38 ☑
        canoe V93.35 ☑
        inflatable V93.36 ☑
        kayak V93.35 ☑
        sailboat V93.34 ☑
        surf-board V93.38 ☑
        windsurfer V93.38 ☑
  into
    cavity W17.2 ☑
    dock W17.4 ☑
    fire — *see* Exposure, fire, by type
    haystack W17.89 ☑
    hole W17.2 ☑
    lake — *see* Fall, into, water
    manhole W17.1 ☑
    moving part of machinery — *see* Contact, with, by
      type of machine
    ocean — *see* Fall, into, water
    opening in surface NEC W17.89 ☑
    pit W17.2 ☑
    pond — *see* Fall, into, water
    quarry W17.89 ☑
    river — *see* Fall, into, water
    shaft W17.89 ☑
    storm drain W17.1 ☑
    stream — *see* Fall, into, water
    swimming pool (*see also* Fall, into, water, in,
      swimming pool)
      empty W17.3 ☑
    tank W17.89 ☑
    water W16.42 ☑
      causing drowning W16.41 ☑
      from watercraft — *see* Drowning, due to, fall
        overboard
      hitting diving board W21.4 ☑
      in
        bathtub W16.212 ☑
          causing drowning W16.211 ☑
        bucket W16.222 ☑
          causing drowning W16.221 ☑
        natural body of water W16.112 ☑
          causing drowning W16.111 ☑
          striking
            bottom W16.122 ☑
              causing drowning W16.121 ☑
            side W16.132 ☑
              causing drowning W16.131 ☑
        specified water NEC W16.312 ☑
          causing drowning W16.311 ☑
          striking
            bottom W16.322 ☑
              causing drowning W16.321 ☑
            wall W16.332 ☑
              causing drowning W16.331 ☑
        swimming pool W16.012 ☑
          causing drowning W16.011 ☑
          striking
            bottom W16.022 ☑
              causing drowning W16.031 ☑
            wall W16.032 ☑
              causing drowning W16.021 ☑
        utility bucket W16.222 ☑
          causing drowning W16.221 ☑
    well W17.0 ☑
  involving
    bed W06 ☑
    chair W07 ☑
    furniture NEC W08 ☑
    glass — *see* Fall, by type
    playground equipment W09.8 ☑
      jungle gym W09.2 ☑
      slide W09.0 ☑
      swing W09.1 ☑
    roller blades — *see* Accident, transport, pedestrian,
      conveyance

**Fall, falling** — *continued*
  involving — *continued*
    skateboard(s) — *see* Accident, transport, pedestri-
      an, conveyance
    skates (ice) (in line) (roller) — *see* Accident, trans-
      port, pedestrian, conveyance
    skis — *see* Accident, transport, pedestrian, con-
      veyance
    table W08 ☑
    wheelchair, non-moving W05.0 ☑
      powered — *see* Accident, transport, pedestrian,
        conveyance, specified type NEC
  object — *see* Struck by, object, falling
  off
    toilet W18.11 ☑
      with subsequent striking against object
        W18.12 ☑
  on same level W18.30 ☑
    due to
      specified NEC W18.39 ☑
      stepping on an object W18.31 ☑
  out of
    bed W06 ☑
    building NEC W13.8 ☑
    chair W07 ☑
    furniture NEC W08 ☑
    wheelchair, non-moving W05.0 ☑
      powered — *see* Accident, transport, pedestrian,
        conveyance, specified type NEC
    window W13.4 ☑
  over
    animal W01.0 ☑
    cliff W15 ☑
    embankment W17.81 ☑
    small object W01.0 ☑
  rock W20.8 ☑
  same level W18.30 ☑
    from
      being crushed, pushed, or stepped on by a
        crowd or human stampede W52 ☑
      collision, pushing, shoving, by or with other
        person W03 ☑
      slipping, stumbling, tripping W01.0 ☑
    involving ice or snow W00.0 ☑
      involving skates (ice) (roller), skateboard, skis
        — *see* Accident, transport, pedestrian,
        conveyance
  snowslide (avalanche) — *see* Landslide
  stone W20.8 ☑
  structure W20.1 ☑
    burning (uncontrolled fire) X00.3 ☑
  through
    bridge W13.1 ☑
    floor W13.3 ☑
    roof W13.2 ☑
    wall W13.8 ☑
    window W13.4 ☑
  timber W20.8 ☑
  tree (caused by lightning) W20.8 ☑
  while being carried or supported by other person(s)
    W04 ☑
**Fallen on by**
  animal (not being ridden) NEC W55.89 ☑
**Felo-de-se** — *see* Suicide
**Fight** (hand) (fists) (foot) — *see* Assault, fight
**Fire** (accidental) — *see* Exposure, fire
**Firearm discharge** — *see* Discharge, firearm
**Fireball effects from nuclear explosion in war oper-**
  **ations** — *see* War operations, nuclear weapons
**Fireworks** (explosion) W39 ☑
**Flash burns from explosion** — *see* Explosion
**Flood** (any injury) (caused by) X38 ☑
  collapse of man-made structure causing earth move-
    ment X36.0 ☑
  tidal wave — *see* Forces of nature, tidal wave
**Food** (any type) **in**
  air passages (with asphyxia, obstruction, or suffoca-
    tion) — *see* categories T17 and T18 ☑
  alimentary tract causing asphyxia (due to compression
    of trachea) — *see* categories T17 and T18 ☑
**Forces of nature** X39.8 ☑
  avalanche X36.1 ☑
    causing transport accident — *see* Accident, trans-
      port, by type of vehicle
  blizzard X37.2 ☑
  cataclysmic storm X37.9 ☑

**Forces of nature** — *continued*
  cataclysmic storm — *continued*
    with flood X38 ☑
    blizzard X37.2 ☑
    cloudburst X37.8 ☑
    cyclone X37.1 ☑
    dust storm X37.3 ☑
    hurricane X37.0 ☑
    specified storm NEC X37.8 ☑
    storm surge X37.0 ☑
    tornado X37.1 ☑
    twister X37.1 ☑
    typhoon X37.0 ☑
  cloudburst X37.8 ☑
  cold (natural) X31 ☑
  cyclone X37.1 ☑
  dam collapse causing earth movement X36.0 ☑
  dust storm X37.3 ☑
  earth movement X36.1 ☑
    caused by dam or structure collapse X36.0 ☑
    earthquake X34 ☑
  earthquake X34 ☑
  flood (caused by) X38 ☑
    dam collapse X36.0 ☑
    tidal wave — *see* Forces of nature, tidal wave
  heat (natural) X30 ☑
  hurricane X37.0 ☑
  landslide X36.1 ☑
    causing transport accident — *see* Accident, trans-
      port, by type of vehicle
  lightning — *see* subcategory T75.0 ☑
    causing fire — *see* Exposure, fire
  mudslide X36.1 ☑
    causing transport accident — *see* Accident, trans-
      port, by type of vehicle
  radiation (natural) X39.08 ☑
    radon X39.01 ☑
  radon X39.01 ☑
  specified force NEC X39.8 ☑
  storm surge X37.0 ☑
  structure collapse causing earth movement X36.0 ☑
  sunlight X32 ☑
  tidal wave X37.41 ☑
    due to
      earthquake X37.41 ☑
      landslide X37.43 ☑
      storm X37.42 ☑
      volcanic eruption X37.41 ☑
  tornado X37.1 ☑
  tsunami X37.41 ☑
  twister X37.1 ☑
  typhoon X37.0 ☑
  volcanic eruption X35 ☑
**Foreign body**
  aspiration — *see* Index to Diseases and Injuries, For-
    eign body, respiratory tract
  embedded in skin W45 ☑
  entering through skin W45.8 ☑
    can lid W26.8 ☑
    nail W45.0 ☑
    paper W26.2 ☑
    specified NEC W45.8 ☑
    splinter W45.8 ☑
**Forest fire** (exposure to) — *see* Exposure, fire, uncontrolled, not in building
**Found injured** X58 ☑
  from exposure (to) — *see* Exposure
  on
    highway, road(way), street V89.9 ☑
    railway right of way V81.9 ☑
**Fracture** (circumstances unknown or unspecified) X58 ☑
  due to specified cause NEC X58 ☑
**Freezing** — *see* Exposure, cold
**Frostbite** X31 ☑
  due to man-made conditions — *see* Exposure, cold,
    man-made
**Frozen** — *see* Exposure, cold

# G

**Gored by bull** W55.22 ☑
**Gunshot wound** W34.00 ☑

# H

**Hailstones, injured by** X39.8 ☑

**Hanged herself or himself** — see Hanging, self-inflicted
**Hanging** (accidental) (see also category) T71 ☑
  legal execution — see Legal, intervention, specified
      means NEC
**Heat** (effects of) (excessive) X30 ☑
  due to
    man-made conditions W92 ☑
      on board watercraft V93.29 ☑
        fishing boat V93.22 ☑
        merchant ship V93.20 ☑
        passenger ship V93.21 ☑
        sailboat V93.24 ☑
        specified powered craft NEC V93.23 ☑
    weather (conditions) X30 ☑
  from
    electric heating apparatus causing burning X16 ☑
    nuclear explosion in war operations — see War
      operations, nuclear weapons
  inappropriate in local application or packing in medical
    or surgical procedure Y63.5
**Hemorrhage**
  delayed following medical or surgical treatment
    without mention of misadventure — see Index
      to Diseases and Injuries, Complication(s)
  during medical or surgical treatment as misadventure
    — see Index to Diseases and Injuries, Complica-
    tion(s)
**High**
  altitude (effects) — see Air, pressure, low
  level of radioactivity, effects — see Radiation
  pressure (effects) — see Air, pressure, high
  temperature, effects — see Heat
**Hit, hitting** (accidental) by — see Struck by
**Hitting against** — see Striking against
**Homicide** (attempt) (justifiable) — see Assault
**Hot**
  place, effects (see also Heat)
  weather, effects X30 ☑
**House fire** (uncontrolled) — see Exposure, fire, uncon-
  trolled, building
**Humidity, causing problem** X39.8 ☑
**Hunger** X58 ☑
**Hurricane** (any injury) X37.0 ☑
**Hypobarism, hypobaropathy** — see Air, pressure, low

**I**

**Ictus**
  caloris (see also Heat)
  solaris X30 ☑
**Ignition** (accidental) (see also Exposure, fire) X08.8 ☑
  anesthetic gas in operating room W40.1 ☑
  apparel X06.2 ☑
    from highly flammable material X04 ☑
    nightwear X05 ☑
  bed linen (sheets) (spreads) (pillows) (mattress) — see
    Exposure, fire, uncontrolled, building, bed
  benzine X04 ☑
  clothes, clothing NEC (from controlled fire) X06.2 ☑
    from
      highly flammable material X04 ☑
  ether X04 ☑
    in operating room W40.1 ☑
  explosive material — see Explosion
  gasoline X04 ☑
  jewelry (plastic) (any) X06.0 ☑
  kerosene X04 ☑
  material
    explosive — see Explosion
    highly flammable with secondary explosion X04 ☑
  nightwear X05 ☑
  paraffin X04 ☑
  petrol X04 ☑
**Immersion** (accidental) (see also Drowning)
  hand or foot due to cold (excessive) X31 ☑
**Implantation of quills of porcupine** W55.89 ☑
**Inanition** (from) (hunger) X58 ☑
  thirst X58 ☑
**Inappropriate operation performed**
  correct operation on wrong side or body part (wrong
    side) (wrong site) Y65.53
  operation intended for another patient done on wrong
    patient Y65.52
  wrong operation performed on correct patient Y65.51
**Inattention after, at birth** (homicidal intent) (infantici-
  dal intent) X58 ☑

**Incident, adverse**
  device
    anesthesiology Y70.8
      accessory Y70.2
      diagnostic Y70.0
      miscellaneous Y70.8
      monitoring Y70.0
      prosthetic Y70.2
      rehabilitative Y70.1
      surgical Y70.3
      therapeutic Y70.1
    cardiovascular Y71.8
      accessory Y71.2
      diagnostic Y71.0
      miscellaneous Y71.8
      monitoring Y71.0
      prosthetic Y71.2
      rehabilitative Y71.1
      surgical Y71.3
      therapeutic Y71.1
    gastroenterology Y73.8
      accessory Y73.2
      diagnostic Y73.0
      miscellaneous Y73.8
      monitoring Y73.0
      prosthetic Y73.2
      rehabilitative Y73.1
      surgical Y73.3
      therapeutic Y73.1
    general
      hospital Y74.8
        accessory Y74.2
        diagnostic Y74.0
        miscellaneous Y74.8
        monitoring Y74.0
        prosthetic Y74.2
        rehabilitative Y74.1
        surgical Y74.3
        therapeutic Y74.1
      surgical Y81.8
        accessory Y81.2
        diagnostic Y81.0
        miscellaneous Y81.8
        monitoring Y81.0
        prosthetic Y81.2
        rehabilitative Y81.1
        surgical Y81.3
        therapeutic Y81.1
    gynecological Y76.8
      accessory Y76.2
      diagnostic Y76.0
      miscellaneous Y76.8
      monitoring Y76.0
      prosthetic Y76.2
      rehabilitative Y76.1
      surgical Y76.3
      therapeutic Y76.1
    medical Y82.9
      specified type NEC Y82.8
    neurological Y75.8
      accessory Y75.2
      diagnostic Y75.0
      miscellaneous Y75.8
      monitoring Y75.0
      prosthetic Y75.2
      rehabilitative Y75.1
      surgical Y75.3
      therapeutic Y75.1
    obstetrical Y76.8
      accessory Y76.2
      diagnostic Y76.0
      miscellaneous Y76.8
      monitoring Y76.0
      prosthetic Y76.2
      rehabilitative Y76.1
      surgical Y76.3
      therapeutic Y76.1
    ophthalmic Y77.8
      accessory Y77.2
      diagnostic Y77.0
      miscellaneous Y77.8
      monitoring Y77.0
      prosthetic Y77.2
      rehabilitative Y77.1
      surgical Y77.3
      therapeutic Y77.1
    orthopedic Y79.8
      accessory Y79.2
      diagnostic Y79.0

**Incident, adverse** — continued
  device — continued
    orthopedic — continued
      miscellaneous Y79.8
      monitoring Y79.0
      prosthetic Y79.2
      rehabilitative Y79.1
      surgical Y79.3
      therapeutic Y79.1
    otorhinolaryngological Y72.8
      accessory Y72.2
      diagnostic Y72.0
      miscellaneous Y72.8
      monitoring Y72.0
      prosthetic Y72.2
      rehabilitative Y72.1
      surgical Y72.3
      therapeutic Y72.1
    personal use Y74.8
      accessory Y74.2
      diagnostic Y74.0
      miscellaneous Y74.8
      monitoring Y74.0
      prosthetic Y74.2
      rehabilitative Y74.1
      surgical Y74.3
      therapeutic Y74.1
    physical medicine Y80.8
      accessory Y80.2
      diagnostic Y80.0
      miscellaneous Y80.8
      monitoring Y80.0
      prosthetic Y80.2
      rehabilitative Y80.1
      surgical Y80.3
      therapeutic Y80.1
    plastic surgical Y81.8
      accessory Y81.2
      diagnostic Y81.0
      miscellaneous Y81.8
      monitoring Y81.0
      prosthetic Y81.2
      rehabilitative Y81.1
      surgical Y81.3
      therapeutic Y81.1
    radiological Y78.8
      accessory Y78.2
      diagnostic Y78.0
      miscellaneous Y78.8
      monitoring Y78.0
      prosthetic Y78.2
      rehabilitative Y78.1
      surgical Y78.3
      therapeutic Y78.1
    urology Y73.8
      accessory Y73.2
      diagnostic Y73.0
      miscellaneous Y73.8
      monitoring Y73.0
      prosthetic Y73.2
      rehabilitative Y73.1
      surgical Y73.3
      therapeutic Y73.1
**Incineration** (accidental) — see Exposure, fire
**Infanticide** — see Assault
**Infrasound waves** (causing injury) W49.9 ☑
**Ingestion**
  foreign body (causing injury) (with obstruction) — see
    Foreign body, alimentary canal
  poisonous
    plant(s) X58 ☑
    substance NEC — see Table of Drugs and Chemicals
**Inhalation**
  excessively cold substance, man-made — see Expo-
    sure, cold, man-made
  food (any type) (into respiratory tract) (with asphyxia,
    obstruction respiratory tract, suffocation) — see
    categories T17 and T18
  foreign body — see Foreign body, aspiration
  gastric contents (with asphyxia, obstruction respiratory
    passage, suffocation) T17.81- ☑
  hot air or gases X14.0 ☑
  liquid air, hydrogen, nitrogen W93.12 ☑
    suicide (attempt) X83.2 ☑
  steam X13.0 ☑
    assault X98.0 ☑
    stated as undetermined whether accidental or in-
      tentional Y27.0 ☑

**Inhalation** — *continued*
  steam — *continued*
    suicide (attempt) X77.0 ☑
  toxic gas — *see* Table of Drugs and Chemicals
  vomitus (with asphyxia, obstruction respiratory passage, suffocation) T17.81-
**Injury, injured** (accidental(ly)) NOS X58 ☑
  by, caused by, from
    assault — *see* Assault
    law-enforcing agent, police, in course of legal intervention — *see* Legal intervention
    suicide (attempt) X83.8 ☑
  due to, in
    civil insurrection — *see* War operations
    fight (*see also* Assault, fight) Y04.0 ☑
    war operations — *see* War operations
  homicide (*see also* Assault) Y09
  inflicted (by)
    in course of arrest (attempted), suppression of disturbance, maintenance of order, by law-enforcing agents — *see* Legal intervention
    other person
      stated as
        accidental X58 ☑
        intentional, homicide (attempt) — *see* Assault
        undetermined whether accidental or intentional Y33 ☑
  purposely (inflicted) by other person(s) — *see* Assault
  self-inflicted X83.8 ☑
    stated as accidental X58 ☑
  specified cause NEC X58 ☑
  undetermined whether accidental or intentional Y33 ☑
**Insolation, effects** X30 ☑
**Insufficient nourishment** X58 ☑
**Interruption of respiration** (by)
  food (lodged in esophagus) — *see* categories T17 and T18 ☑
  vomitus (lodged in esophagus) T17.81- ☑
**Intervention, legal** — *see* Legal intervention
**Intoxication**
  drug — *see* Table of Drugs and Chemicals
  poison — *see* Table of Drugs and Chemicals

## J

**Jammed** (accidentally)
  between objects (moving) (stationary and moving) W23.0 ☑
  stationary W23.1 ☑
**Jumped, jumping**
  before moving object NEC X81.8 ☑
    motor vehicle X81.0 ☑
    subway train X81.1 ☑
    train X81.1 ☑
    undetermined whether accidental or intentional Y31 ☑
  from
    boat (into water) voluntarily, without accident (to or on boat) W16.712 ☑
      with
        accident to or on boat — *see* Accident, watercraft
        drowning or submersion W16.711 ☑
          suicide (attempt) X71.3 ☑
        striking bottom W16.722 ☑
          causing drowning W16.721 ☑
    building (*see also* Jumped, from, high place) W13.9 ☑
      burning (uncontrolled fire) X00.5 ☑
    high place NEC W17.89 ☑
      suicide (attempt) X80 ☑
      undetermined whether accidental or intentional Y30 ☑
    structure (*see also* Jumped, from, high place) W13.9 ☑
      burning (uncontrolled fire) X00.5 ☑
  into water W16.92 ☑
    causing drowning W16.91 ☑
    from, off watercraft — *see* Jumped, from, boat
    in
      natural body W16.612 ☑
        causing drowning W16.611 ☑
        striking bottom W16.622 ☑
          causing drowning W16.621 ☑

**Jumped, jumping** — *continued*
  into water — *continued*
    in — *continued*
      specified place NEC W16.812 ☑
        causing drowning W16.811 ☑
        striking
          bottom W16.822 ☑
            causing drowning W16.821 ☑
          wall W16.832 ☑
            causing drowning W16.831 ☑
      swimming pool W16.512 ☑
        causing drowning W16.511 ☑
        striking
          bottom W16.522 ☑
            causing drowning W16.521 ☑
          wall W16.532 ☑
            causing drowning W16.531 ☑
    suicide (attempt) X71.3 ☑

## K

**Kicked by**
  animal NEC W55.82 ☑
  person(s) (accidentally) W50.1 ☑
    with intent to injure or kill Y04.0 ☑
    as, or caused by, a crowd or human stampede (with fall) W52 ☑
    assault Y04.0 ☑
    homicide (attempt) Y04.0 ☑
    in
      fight Y04.0 ☑
      legal intervention
        injuring
          bystander Y35.812 ☑
          law enforcement personnel Y35.811 ☑
          suspect Y35.813 ☑
**Kicking**
  against
    object W22.8 ☑
      sports equipment W21.9 ☑
      stationary W22.09 ☑
        sports equipment W21.89 ☑
    person — *see* Striking against, person
    sports equipment W21.9 ☑
  carpet stretcher with knee X50.3 ☑
**Killed, killing** (accidentally) NOS (*see also* Injury) X58 ☑
  in
    action — *see* War operations
    brawl, fight (hand) (fists) (foot) Y04.0 ☑
      by weapon (*see also* Assault)
        cutting, piercing — *see* Assault, cutting or piercing instrument
        firearm — *see* Discharge, firearm, by type, homicide
  self
    stated as
      accident NOS X58 ☑
      suicide — *see* Suicide
      undetermined whether accidental or intentional Y33 ☑
**Kneeling** (prolonged (static)) X50.1 ☑
**Knocked down** (accidentally) (by) NOS X58 ☑
  animal (not being ridden) NEC (*see also* Struck by, by type of animal)
  crowd or human stampede W52 ☑
  person W51 ☑
    in brawl, fight Y04.0 ☑
  transport vehicle NEC (*see also* Accident, transport) V09.9 ☑

## L

**Laceration NEC** — *see* Injury
**Lack of**
  care (helpless person) (infant) (newborn) X58 ☑
  food except as result of abandonment or neglect X58 ☑
    due to abandonment or neglect X58 ☑
  water except as result of transport accident X58 ☑
    due to transport accident — *see* Accident, transport, by type
    helpless person, infant, newborn X58 ☑
**Landslide** (falling on transport vehicle) X36.1 ☑
  caused by collapse of man-made structure X36.0 ☑
**Late effect** — *see* Sequelae

**Legal**
  execution (any method) — *see* Legal, intervention
  intervention (by)
    baton — *see* Legal, intervention, blunt object, baton
    bayonet — *see* Legal, intervention, sharp object, bayonet
    blow — *see* Legal, intervention, manhandling
    blunt object
      baton
        injuring
          bystander Y35.312 ☑
          law enforcement personnel Y35.311 ☑
          suspect Y35.313 ☑
        injuring
          bystander Y35.302 ☑
          law enforcement personnel Y35.301 ☑
          suspect Y35.303 ☑
      specified NEC
        injuring
          bystander Y35.392 ☑
          law enforcement personnel Y35.391 ☑
          suspect Y35.393 ☑
      stave
        injuring
          bystander Y35.392 ☑
          law enforcement personnel Y35.391 ☑
          suspect Y35.393 ☑
    bomb — *see* Legal, intervention, explosive
    cutting or piercing instrument — *see* Legal, intervention, sharp object
    dynamite — *see* Legal, intervention, explosive, dynamite
    explosive(s)
      dynamite
        injuring
          bystander Y35.112 ☑
          law enforcement personnel Y35.111 ☑
          suspect Y35.113 ☑
      grenade
        injuring
          bystander Y35.192 ☑
          law enforcement personnel Y35.191 ☑
          suspect Y35.193 ☑
      injuring
        bystander Y35.102 ☑
        law enforcement personnel Y35.101 ☑
        suspect Y35.103 ☑
      mortar bomb
        injuring
          bystander Y35.192 ☑
          law enforcement personnel Y35.191 ☑
          suspect Y35.193 ☑
      shell
        injuring
          bystander Y35.122 ☑
          law enforcement personnel Y35.121 ☑
          suspect Y35.123 ☑
      specified NEC
        injuring
          bystander Y35.192 ☑
          law enforcement personnel Y35.191 ☑
          suspect Y35.193 ☑
    firearm(s) (discharge)
      handgun
        injuring
          bystander Y35.022 ☑
          law enforcement personnel Y35.021 ☑
          suspect Y35.023 ☑
      injuring
        bystander Y35.002 ☑
        law enforcement personnel Y35.001 ☑
        suspect Y35.003 ☑
      machine gun
        injuring
          bystander Y35.012 ☑
          law enforcement personnel Y35.011 ☑
          suspect Y35.013 ☑
      rifle pellet
        injuring
          bystander Y35.032 ☑
          law enforcement personnel Y35.031 ☑
          suspect Y35.033 ☑
      rubber bullet
        injuring
          bystander Y35.042 ☑
          law enforcement personnel Y35.041 ☑

**Legal** — *continued*
  intervention — *continued*
    firearm(s) — *continued*
      rubber bullet — *continued*
        injuring — *continued*
          suspect Y35.043 ☑
      shotgun — *see* Legal, intervention, firearm, specified NEC
      specified NEC
        injuring
          bystander Y35.092 ☑
          law enforcement personnel Y35.091 ☑
          suspect Y35.093 ☑
    gas (asphyxiation) (poisoning)
      injuring
        bystander Y35.202 ☑
        law enforcement personnel Y35.201 ☑
        suspect Y35.203 ☑
      specified NEC
        injuring
          bystander Y35.292 ☑
          law enforcement personnel Y35.291 ☑
          suspect Y35.293 ☑
      tear gas
        injuring
          bystander Y35.212 ☑
          law enforcement personnel Y35.211 ☑
          suspect Y35.213 ☑
    grenade — *see* Legal, intervention, explosive, grenade
    injuring
      bystander Y35.92 ☑
      law enforcement personnel Y35.91 ☑
      suspect Y35.93 ☑
    late effect (of) — *see* with 7th character S Y35
    manhandling
      injuring
        bystander Y35.812 ☑
        law enforcement personnel Y35.811 ☑
        suspect Y35.813 ☑
    sequelae (of) — *see* with 7th character S Y35
    sharp objects
      bayonet
        injuring
          bystander Y35.412 ☑
          law enforcement personnel Y35.411 ☑
          suspect Y35.413 ☑
      injuring
        bystander Y35.402 ☑
        law enforcement personnel Y35.401 ☑
        suspect Y35.403 ☑
      specified NEC
        injuring
          bystander Y35.492 ☑
          law enforcement personnel Y35.491 ☑
          suspect Y35.493 ☑
    specified means NEC
      injuring
        bystander Y35.892 ☑
        law enforcement personnel Y35.891 ☑
        suspect Y35.893 ☑
    stabbing — *see* Legal, intervention, sharp object
    stave — *see* Legal, intervention, blunt object, stave
    tear gas — *see* Legal, intervention, gas, tear gas
    truncheon — *see* Legal, intervention, blunt object, stave

**Lifting** — *see also* Overexertion
  heavy objects X50.0 ☑
  weights X50.0 ☑
**Lightning** (shock) (stroke) (struck by) — *see* subcategory T75.0 ☑
  causing fire — *see* Exposure, fire
**Loss of control** (transport vehicle) NEC — *see* Accident, transport
**Lost at sea NOS** — *see* Drowning, due to, fall overboard
**Low**
  pressure (effects) — *see* Air, pressure, low
  temperature (effects) — *see* Exposure, cold
**Lying before train, vehicle or other moving object** X81.8 ☑
  subway train X81.1 ☑
  train X81.1 ☑
  undetermined whether accidental or intentional Y31 ☑
**Lynching** — *see* Assault

# M

**Malfunction** (mechanism or component) (of)
  firearm W34.10 ☑
    airgun W34.110 ☑
    BB gun W34.110 ☑
    gas, air or spring-operated gun NEC W34.118 ☑
    handgun W32.1 ☑
    hunting rifle W33.12 ☑
    larger firearm W33.10 ☑
      specified NEC W33.19 ☑
    machine gun W33.13 ☑
    paintball gun W34.111 ☑
    pellet gun W34.110 ☑
    shotgun W33.11 ☑
    specified NEC W34.19 ☑
    Very pistol [flare] W34.19 ☑
  handgun — *see* Malfunction, firearm, handgun
**Maltreatment** — *see* Perpetrator
**Mangled** (accidentally) NOS X58 ☑
**Manhandling** (in brawl, fight) Y04.0 ☑
  legal intervention — *see* Legal, intervention, manhandling
**Manslaughter** (nonaccidental) — *see* Assault
**Mauled by animal NEC** W55.89 ☑
**Medical procedure, complication of** (delayed or as an abnormal reaction without mention of misadventure) — *see* Complication of or following, by specified type of procedure
  due to or as a result of misadventure — *see* Misadventure
**Melting** (due to fire) (*see also* Exposure, fire)
  apparel NEC X06.3 ☑
  clothes, clothing NEC X06.3 ☑
    nightwear X05 ☑
  fittings or furniture (burning building) (uncontrolled fire) X00.8 ☑
  nightwear X05 ☑
  plastic jewelry X06.1 ☑
**Mental cruelty** X58 ☑
**Military operations** (injuries to military and civilians occuring during peacetime on military property and during routine military exercises and operations) (by) (from) (involving) Y37.90- ☑
  air blast Y37.20- ☑
  aircraft
    destruction — *see* Military operations, destruction of aircraft
    airway restriction — *see* Military operations, restriction of airways
    asphyxiation — *see* Military operations, restriction of airways
  biological weapons Y37.6X- ☑
  blast Y37.20- ☑
  blast fragments Y37.20- ☑
  blast wave Y37.20- ☑
  blast wind Y37.20- ☑
  bomb Y37.20- ☑
    dirty Y37.50- ☑
    gasoline Y37.31- ☑
    incendiary Y37.31- ☑
    petrol Y37.31- ☑
  bullet Y37.43- ☑
    incendiary Y37.32- ☑
    rubber Y37.41- ☑
  chemical weapons Y37.7X- ☑
  combat
    hand to hand (unarmed) combat Y37.44- ☑
    using blunt or piercing object Y37.45- ☑
  conflagration — *see* Military operations, fire
  conventional warfare NEC Y37.49- ☑
  depth-charge Y37.01- ☑
  destruction of aircraft Y37.10- ☑
    due to
      air to air missile Y37.11- ☑
      collision with other aircraft Y37.12- ☑
      detonation (accidental) of onboard munitions and explosives Y37.14- ☑
      enemy fire or explosives Y37.11- ☑
      explosive placed on aircraft Y37.11- ☑
      onboard fire Y37.13- ☑
      rocket propelled grenade [RPG] Y37.11- ☑
      small arms fire Y37.11- ☑
      surface to air missile Y37.11- ☑
    specified NEC Y37.19- ☑

**Military operations** — *continued*
  detonation (accidental) of
    onboard marine weapons Y37.05- ☑
    own munitions or munitions launch device Y37.24- ☑
  dirty bomb Y37.50- ☑
  explosion (of) Y37.20- ☑
    aerial bomb Y37.21- ☑
    bomb NOS (*see also* Military operations, bomb(s)) Y37.20- ☑
    fragments Y37.20- ☑
    grenade Y37.29- ☑
    guided missile Y37.22- ☑
    improvised explosive device [IED] (person-borne) (roadside) (vehicle-borne) Y37.23- ☑
    land mine Y37.29- ☑
    marine mine (at sea) (in harbor) Y37.02- ☑
    marine weapon Y37.00- ☑
      specified NEC Y37.09- ☑
    own munitions or munitions launch device (accidental) Y37.24- ☑
    sea-based artillery shell Y37.03- ☑
    specified NEC Y37.29- ☑
    torpedo Y37.04- ☑
  fire Y37.30- ☑
    specified NEC Y37.39- ☑
  firearms
    discharge Y37.43- ☑
    pellets Y37.42- ☑
  flamethrower Y37.33- ☑
  fragments (from) (of)
    improvised explosive device [IED] (person-borne) (roadside) (vehicle-borne) Y37.26- ☑
    munitions Y37.25- ☑
    specified NEC Y37.29- ☑
    weapons Y37.27- ☑
  friendly fire Y37.92- ☑
  hand to hand (unarmed) combat Y37.44- ☑
  hot substances — *see* Military operations, fire
  incendiary bullet Y37.32- ☑
  nuclear weapon (effects of) Y37.50- ☑
    acute radiation exposure Y37.54- ☑
    blast pressure Y37.51- ☑
    direct blast Y37.51- ☑
    direct heat Y37.53- ☑
    fallout exposure Y37.54- ☑
    fireball Y37.53- ☑
    indirect blast (struck or crushed by blast debris) (being thrown by blast) Y37.52- ☑
    ionizing radiation (immediate exposure) Y37.54- ☑
    nuclear radiation Y37.54- ☑
    radiation
      ionizing (immediate exposure) Y37.54- ☑
      nuclear Y37.54- ☑
      thermal Y37.53- ☑
    secondary effects Y37.54- ☑
    specified NEC Y37.59- ☑
    thermal radiation Y37.53- ☑
  restriction of air (airway)
    intentional Y37.46- ☑
    unintentional Y37.47- ☑
  rubber bullets Y37.41- ☑
  shrapnel NOS Y37.29- ☑
  suffocation — *see* Military operations, restriction of airways
  unconventional warfare NEC Y37.7X- ☑
  underwater blast NOS Y37.00- ☑
  warfare
    conventional NEC Y37.49- ☑
    unconventional NEC Y37.7X- ☑
  weapon of mass destruction [WMD] Y37.91- ☑
  weapons
    biological weapons Y37.6X- ☑
    chemical Y37.7X- ☑
    nuclear (effects of ) Y37.50- ☑
      acute radiation exposure Y37.54- ☑
      blast pressure Y37.51- ☑
      direct blast Y37.51- ☑
      direct heat Y37.53- ☑
      fallout exposure Y37.54- ☑
      fireball Y37.53- ☑
      radiation
        ionizing (immediate exposure) Y37.54- ☑
        nuclear Y37.54- ☑
        thermal Y37.53- ☑
      secondary effects Y37.54- ☑

**Military operations** — *continued*
  weapons — *continued*
    nuclear — *continued*
      specified NEC Y37.59- ☑
    of mass destruction [WMD] Y37.91- ☑
**Misadventure(s) to patient(s) during surgical or medical care** Y69
  contaminated medical or biological substance (blood, drug, fluid) Y64.9
    administered (by) NEC Y64.9
      immunization Y64.1
      infusion Y64.0
      injection Y64.1
      specified means NEC Y64.8
      transfusion Y64.0
      vaccination Y64.1
  excessive amount of blood or other fluid during transfusion or infusion Y63.0
  failure
    in dosage Y63.9
      electroshock therapy Y63.4
      inappropriate temperature (too hot or too cold) in local application and packing Y63.5
      infusion
        excessive amount of fluid Y63.0
        incorrect dilution of fluid Y63.1
      insulin-shock therapy Y63.4
      nonadministration of necessary drug or biological substance Y63.6
      overdose — *see* Table of Drugs and Chemicals
        radiation, in therapy Y63.2
      radiation
        overdose Y63.2
      specified procedure NEC Y63.8
      transfusion
        excessive amount of blood Y63.0
    mechanical, of instrument or apparatus (any) (during any procedure) Y65.8
    sterile precautions (during procedure) Y62.9
      aspiration of fluid or tissue (by puncture or catheterization, except heart) Y62.6
      biopsy (except needle aspiration) Y62.8
        needle (aspirating) Y62.6
      blood sampling Y62.6
      catheterization Y62.6
        heart Y62.5
      dialysis (kidney) Y62.2
      endoscopic examination Y62.4
      enema Y62.8
      immunization Y62.3
      infusion Y62.1
      injection Y62.3
      needle biopsy Y62.6
      paracentesis (abdominal) (thoracic) Y62.6
      perfusion Y62.2
      puncture (lumbar) Y62.6
      removal of catheter or packing Y62.8
      specified procedure NEC Y62.8
      surgical operation Y62.0
      transfusion Y62.1
      vaccination Y62.3
    suture or ligature during surgical procedure Y65.2
    to introduce or to remove tube or instrument — *see* Failure, to
  hemorrhage — *see* Index to Diseases and Injuries, Complication(s)
  inadvertent exposure of patient to radiation Y63.3
  inappropriate
    operation performed — *see* Inappropriate operation performed
    temperature (too hot or too cold) in local application or packing Y63.5
  infusion (*see also* Misadventure, by type, infusion) Y69
    excessive amount of fluid Y63.0
    incorrect dilution of fluid Y63.1
    wrong fluid Y65.1
  mismatched blood in transfusion Y65.0
  nonadministration of necessary drug or biological substance Y63.6
  overdose — *see* Table of Drugs and Chemicals
    radiation (in therapy) Y63.2
  perforation — *see* Index to Diseases and Injuries, Complication(s)
  performance of inappropriate operation — *see* Inappropriate operation performed
  puncture — *see* Index to Diseases and Injuries, Complication(s)
  specified type NEC Y65.8

**Misadventure(s) to patient(s) during surgical or medical care** — *continued*
  specified type — *continued*
    failure
      suture or ligature during surgical operation Y65.2
      to introduce or to remove tube or instrument — *see* Failure, to
    infusion of wrong fluid Y65.1
    performance of inappropriate operation — *see* Inappropriate operation performed
    transfusion of mismatched blood Y65.0
    wrong
      fluid in infusion Y65.1
      placement of endotracheal tube during anesthetic procedure Y65.3
    transfusion — *see* Misadventure, by type, transfusion
      excessive amount of blood Y63.0
      mismatched blood Y65.0
    wrong
      drug given in error — *see* Table of Drugs and Chemicals
      fluid in infusion Y65.1
      placement of endotracheal tube during anesthetic procedure Y65.3
**Mismatched blood in transfusion** Y65.0
**Motion sickness** T75.3 ☑
**Mountain sickness** W94.11 ☑
**Mudslide** (of cataclysmic nature) — *see* Landslide
**Murder** (attempt) — *see* Assault

# N

**Nail**
  contact with W45.0 ☑
    gun W29.4 ☑
  embedded in skin W45.0 ☑
**Neglect** (criminal) (homicidal intent) X58 ☑
**Noise** (causing injury) (pollution) W42.9 ☑
  supersonic W42.0 ☑
**Nonadministration** (of)
  drug or biological substance (necessary) Y63.6
  surgical and medical care Y66
**Nosocomial condition** Y95

# O

**Object**
  falling
    from, in, on, hitting
      machinery — *see* Contact, with, by type of machine
  set in motion by
    accidental explosion or rupture of pressure vessel W38 ☑
    firearm — *see* Discharge, firearm, by type
    machine(ry) — *see* Contact, with, by type of machine
**Overdose** (drug) — *see* Table of Drugs and Chemicals
  radiation Y63.2
**Overexertion** X50.9 ☑
  from
    prolonged static or awkward postures X50.1 ☑
    repetitive movements X50.3 ☑
    specified strenuous movements or postures NEC X50.9 ☑
    strenuous movement or load X50.0 ☑
**Overexposure** (accidental) (to)
  cold (*see also* Exposure, cold) X31 ☑
    due to man-made conditions — *see* Exposure, cold, man-made
  heat (*see also* Heat) X30 ☑
  radiation — *see* Radiation
  radioactivity W88.0 ☑
  sun (sunburn) X32 ☑
  weather NEC — *see* Forces of nature
  wind NEC — *see* Forces of nature
**Overheated** — *see* Heat
**Overturning** (accidental)
  machinery — *see* Contact, with, by type of machine
  transport vehicle NEC (*see also* Accident, transport) V89.9 ☑
  watercraft (causing drowning, submersion) (*see also* Drowning, due to, accident to, watercraft, overturning)
    causing injury except drowning or submersion — *see* Accident, watercraft, causing, injury NEC

# P

**Parachute descent** (voluntary) (without accident to aircraft) V97.29 ☑
  due to accident to aircraft — *see* Accident, transport, aircraft
**Pecked by bird** W61.99 ☑
**Perforation during medical or surgical treatment as misadventure** — *see* Index to Diseases and Injuries, Complication(s)
**Perpetrator, perpetration, of assault, maltreatment and neglect** (by) Y07.9
  boyfriend Y07.03
  brother Y07.410
    stepbrother Y07.435
  coach Y07.53
  cousin
    female Y07.491
    male Y07.490
  daycare provider Y07.519
    at-home
      adult care Y07.512
      childcare Y07.510
    care center
      adult care Y07.513
      childcare Y07.511
  family member NEC Y07.499
  father Y07.11
    adoptive Y07.13
    foster Y07.420
    stepfather Y07.430
  foster father Y07.420
  foster mother Y07.421
  girl friend Y07.04
  healthcare provider Y07.529
    mental health Y07.521
    specified NEC Y07.528
  husband Y07.01
  instructor Y07.53
  mother Y07.12
    adoptive Y07.14
    foster Y07.421
    stepmother Y07.433
  nonfamily member Y07.50
    specified NEC Y07.59
  nurse Y07.528
  occupational therapist Y07.528
  partner of parent
    female Y07.434
    male Y07.432
  physical therapist Y07.528
  sister Y07.411
  speech therapist Y07.528
  stepbrother Y07.435
  stepfather Y07.430
  stepmother Y07.433
  stepsister Y07.436
  teacher Y07.53
  wife Y07.02
**Piercing** — *see* Contact, with, by type of object or machine
**Pinched**
  between objects (moving) (stationary and moving) W23.0 ☑
  stationary W23.1 ☑
**Pinned under machine**(ry) — *see* Contact, with, by type of machine
**Place of occurrence** Y92.9
  abandoned house Y92.89
  airplane Y92.813
  airport Y92.520
  ambulatory health services establishment NEC Y92.538
  ambulatory surgery center Y92.530
  amusement park Y92.831
  apartment (co-op) — *see* Place of occurrence, residence, apartment
  assembly hall Y92.29
  bank Y92.510
  barn Y92.71
  baseball field Y92.320
  basketball court Y92.310
  beach Y92.832
  boarding house — *see* Place of occurrence, residence, boarding house
  boat Y92.814
  bowling alley Y92.39
  bridge Y92.89

424
☑ **Additional Character Required** — Refer to the Tabular List for Character Selection
▽ Subterms under main terms may continue to next column or page

**Place of occurrence** — *continued*
- building under construction Y92.61
- bus Y92.811
  - station Y92.521
- cafe Y92.511
- campsite Y92.833
- campus — *see* Place of occurrence, school
- canal Y92.89
- car Y92.810
- casino Y92.59
- children's home — *see* Place of occurrence, residence, institutional, orphanage
- church Y92.22
- cinema Y92.26
- clubhouse Y92.29
- coal pit Y92.64
- college (community) Y92.214
- condominium — *see* Place of occurrence, residence, apartment
- construction area — *see* Place of occurrence, industrial and construction area
- convalescent home — *see* Place of occurrence, residence, institutional, nursing home
- court-house Y92.240
- cricket ground Y92.328
- cultural building Y92.258
  - art gallery Y92.250
  - museum Y92.251
  - music hall Y92.252
  - opera house Y92.253
  - specified NEC Y92.258
  - theater Y92.254
- dancehall Y92.252
- day nursery Y92.210
- dentist office Y92.531
- derelict house Y92.89
- desert Y92.820
- dockyard Y92.62
- dock NOS Y92.89
- doctor's office Y92.531
- dormitory — *see* Place of occurrence, residence, institutional, school dormitory
- dry dock Y92.62
- factory (building) (premises) Y92.63
- farm (land under cultivation) (outbuildings) Y92.79
  - barn Y92.71
  - chicken coop Y92.72
  - field Y92.73
  - hen house Y92.72
  - house — *see* Place of occurrence, residence, house
  - orchard Y92.74
  - specified NEC Y92.79
- football field Y92.321
- forest Y92.821
- freeway Y92.411
- gallery Y92.250
- garage (commercial) Y92.59
  - boarding house Y92.044
  - military base Y92.135
  - mobile home Y92.025
  - nursing home Y92.124
  - orphanage Y92.114
  - private house Y92.015
  - reform school Y92.155
- gas station Y92.524
- gasworks Y92.69
- golf course Y92.39
- gravel pit Y92.64
- grocery Y92.512
- gymnasium Y92.39
- handball court Y92.318
- harbor Y92.89
- harness racing course Y92.39
- healthcare provider office Y92.531
- highway (interstate) Y92.411
- hill Y92.828
- hockey rink Y92.330
- home — *see* Place of occurrence, residence
- hospice — *see* Place of occurrence, residence, institutional, nursing home
- hospital Y92.239
  - cafeteria Y92.233
  - corridor Y92.232
  - operating room Y92.234
  - patient
    - bathroom Y92.231
    - room Y92.230
  - specified NEC Y92.238

- hotel Y92.59
- house (*see also* Place of occurrence, residence)
  - abandoned Y92.89
  - under construction Y92.61
- industrial and construction area (yard) Y92.69
  - building under construction Y92.61
  - dock Y92.62
  - dry dock Y92.62
  - factory Y92.63
  - gasworks Y92.69
  - mine Y92.64
  - oil rig Y92.65
  - pit Y92.64
  - power station Y92.69
  - shipyard Y92.62
  - specified NEC Y92.69
  - tunnel under construction Y92.69
  - workshop Y92.69
- kindergarten Y92.211
- lacrosse field Y92.328
- lake Y92.828
- library Y92.241
- mall Y92.59
- market Y92.512
- marsh Y92.828
- military
  - base — *see* Place of occurrence, residence, institutional, military base
  - training ground Y92.84
- mine Y92.64
- mosque Y92.22
- motel Y92.59
- motorway (interstate) Y92.411
- mountain Y92.828
- movie-house Y92.26
- museum Y92.251
- music-hall Y92.252
- not applicable Y92.9
- nuclear power station Y92.69
- nursing home — *see* Place of occurrence, residence, institutional, nursing home
- office building Y92.59
- offshore installation Y92.65
- oil rig Y92.65
- old people's home — *see* Place of occurrence, residence, institutional, specified NEC
- opera-house Y92.253
- orphanage — *see* Place of occurrence, residence, institutional, orphanage
- outpatient surgery center Y92.530
- park (public) Y92.830
  - amusement Y92.831
- parking garage Y92.89
  - lot Y92.481
- pavement Y92.480
- physician office Y92.531
- polo field Y92.328
- pond Y92.828
- post office Y92.242
- power station Y92.69
- prairie Y92.828
- prison — *see* Place of occurrence, residence, institutional, prison
- public
  - administration building Y92.248
    - city hall Y92.243
    - courthouse Y92.240
    - library Y92.241
    - post office Y92.242
    - specified NEC Y92.248
  - building NEC Y92.29
  - hall Y92.29
  - place NOS Y92.89
- race course Y92.39
- radio station Y92.59
- railway line (bridge) Y92.85
- ranch (outbuildings) — *see* Place of occurrence, farm
- recreation area Y92.838
  - amusement park Y92.831
  - beach Y92.832
  - campsite Y92.833
  - park (public) Y92.830
  - seashore Y92.832
  - specified NEC Y92.838
- reform school — *see* Place of occurrence, residence, institutional, reform school
- religious institution Y92.22

**Place of occurrence** — *continued*
- residence (non-institutional) (private) Y92.009
  - apartment Y92.039
    - bathroom Y92.031
    - bedroom Y92.032
    - kitchen Y92.030
    - specified NEC Y92.038
  - bathroom Y92.002
  - bedroom Y92.003
  - boarding house Y92.049
    - bathroom Y92.041
    - bedroom Y92.042
    - driveway Y92.043
    - garage Y92.044
    - garden Y92.046
    - kitchen Y92.040
    - specified NEC Y92.048
    - swimming pool Y92.045
    - yard Y92.046
  - dining room Y92.001
  - garden Y92.007
  - home Y92.009
  - house, single family Y92.019
    - bathroom Y92.012
    - bedroom Y92.013
    - dining room Y92.011
    - driveway Y92.014
    - garage Y92.015
    - garden Y92.017
    - kitchen Y92.010
    - specified NEC Y92.018
    - swimming pool Y92.016
    - yard Y92.017
  - institutional Y92.10
    - children's home — *see* Place of occurrence, residence, institutional, orphanage
    - hospice — *see* Place of occurrence, residence, institutional, nursing home
    - military base Y92.139
      - barracks Y92.133
      - garage Y92.135
      - garden Y92.137
      - kitchen Y92.130
      - mess hall Y92.131
      - specified NEC Y92.138
      - swimming pool Y92.136
      - yard Y92.137
    - nursing home Y92.129
      - bathroom Y92.121
      - bedroom Y92.122
      - driveway Y92.123
      - garage Y92.124
      - garden Y92.126
      - kitchen Y92.120
      - specified NEC Y92.128
      - swimming pool Y92.125
      - yard Y92.126
    - orphanage Y92.119
      - bathroom Y92.111
      - bedroom Y92.112
      - driveway Y92.113
      - garage Y92.114
      - garden Y92.116
      - kitchen Y92.110
      - specified NEC Y92.118
      - swimming pool Y92.115
      - yard Y92.116
    - prison Y92.149
      - bathroom Y92.142
      - cell Y92.143
      - courtyard Y92.147
      - dining room Y92.141
      - kitchen Y92.140
      - specified NEC Y92.148
      - swimming pool Y92.146
    - reform school Y92.159
      - bathroom Y92.152
      - bedroom Y92.153
      - dining room Y92.151
      - driveway Y92.154
      - garage Y92.155
      - garden Y92.157
      - kitchen Y92.150
      - specified NEC Y92.158
      - swimming pool Y92.156
      - yard Y92.157
    - school dormitory Y92.169
      - bathroom Y92.162
      - bedroom Y92.163

**Place of occurrence** — *continued*
  residence — *continued*
    institutional — *continued*
      school dormitory — *continued*
        dining room Y92.161
        kitchen Y92.160
        specified NEC Y92.168
      specified NEC Y92.199
        bathroom Y92.192
        bedroom Y92.193
        dining room Y92.191
        driveway Y92.194
        garage Y92.195
        garden Y92.197
        kitchen Y92.190
        specified NEC Y92.198
        swimming pool Y92.196
        yard Y92.197
    kitchen Y92.000
    mobile home Y92.029
      bathroom Y92.022
      bedroom Y92.023
      dining room Y92.021
      driveway Y92.024
      garage Y92.025
      garden Y92.027
      kitchen Y92.020
      specified NEC Y92.028
      swimming pool Y92.026
      yard Y92.027
    specified place in residence NEC Y92.008
    specified residence type NEC Y92.099
      bathroom Y92.091
      bedroom Y92.092
      driveway Y92.093
      garage Y92.094
      garden Y92.096
      kitchen Y92.090
      specified NEC Y92.098
      swimming pool Y92.095
      yard Y92.096
  restaurant Y92.511
  riding school Y92.39
  river Y92.828
  road Y92.488
  rodeo ring Y92.39
  rugby field Y92.328
  same day surgery center Y92.530
  sand pit Y92.64
  school (private) (public) (state) Y92.219
    college Y92.214
    daycare center Y92.210
    elementary school Y92.211
    high school Y92.213
    kindergarten Y92.211
    middle school Y92.212
    specified NEC Y92.218
    trace school Y92.215
    university Y92.214
    vocational school Y92.215
  sea (shore) Y92.832
  senior citizen center Y92.29
  service area
    airport Y92.520
    bus station Y92.521
    gas station Y92.524
    highway rest stop Y92.523
    railway station Y92.522
  shipyard Y92.62
  shop (commercial) Y92.513
  sidewalk Y92.480
  silo Y92.79
  skating rink (roller) Y92.331
    ice Y92.330
  slaughter house Y92.86
  soccer field Y92.322
  specified place NEC Y92.89
  sports area Y92.39
    athletic
      court Y92.318
        basketball Y92.310
        specified NEC Y92.318
        squash Y92.311
        tennis Y92.312
      field Y92.328
        baseball Y92.320
        cricket ground Y92.328
        football Y92.321
        hockey Y92.328

**Place of occurrence** — *continued*
  sports area — *continued*
    athletic — *continued*
      field — *continued*
        soccer Y92.322
        specified NEC Y92.328
    golf course Y92.39
    gymnasium Y92.39
    riding school Y92.39
    skating rink (roller) Y92.331
      ice Y92.330
    stadium Y92.39
    swimming pool Y92.34
  squash court Y92.311
  stadium Y92.39
  steeplechasing course Y92.39
  store Y92.512
  stream Y92.828
  street and highway Y92.410
    bike path Y92.482
    freeway Y92.411
    highway ramp Y92.415
    interstate highway Y92.411
    local residential or business street Y92.414
    motorway Y92.411
    parking lot Y92.481
    parkway Y92.412
    sidewalk Y92.480
    specified NEC Y92.488
    state road Y92.413
  subway car Y92.816
  supermarket Y92.512
  swamp Y92.828
  swimming pool (public) Y92.34
    private (at) Y92.095
      boarding house Y92.045
      military base Y92.136
      mobile home Y92.026
      nursing home Y92.125
      orphanage Y92.115
      prison Y92.146
      reform school Y92.156
      single family residence Y92.016
  synagogue Y92.22
  television station Y92.59
  tennis court Y92.312
  theater Y92.254
  trade area Y92.59
    bank Y92.510
    cafe Y92.511
    casino Y92.59
    garage Y92.59
    hotel Y92.59
    market Y92.512
    office building Y92.59
    radio station Y92.59
    restaurant Y92.511
    shop Y92.513
    shopping mall Y92.59
    store Y92.512
    supermarket Y92.512
    television station Y92.59
    warehouse Y92.59
  trailer park, residential — *see* Place of occurrence, residence, mobile home
  trailer site NOS Y92.89
  train Y92.815
    station Y92.522
  truck Y92.812
  tunnel under construction Y92.69
  university Y92.214
  urgent (health) care center Y92.532
  vehicle (transport) Y92.818
    airplane Y92.813
    boat Y92.814
    bus Y92.811
    car Y92.810
    specified NEC Y92.818
    subway car Y92.816
    train Y92.815
    truck Y92.812
  warehouse Y92.59
  water reservoir Y92.89
  wilderness area Y92.828
    desert Y92.820
    forest Y92.821
    marsh Y92.828
    mountain Y92.828
    prairie Y92.828

**Place of occurrence** — *continued*
  wilderness area — *continued*
    specified NEC Y92.828
    swamp Y92.828
  workshop Y92.69
  yard, private Y92.096
    boarding house Y92.046
    mobile home Y92.027
    single family house Y92.017
  youth center Y92.29
  zoo (zoological garden) Y92.834
**Plumbism** — *see* Table of Drugs and Chemicals, lead
**Poisoning** (accidental) (by) (*see also* Table of Drugs and Chemicals)
  by plant, thorns, spines, sharp leaves or other mechanisms NEC X58 ☑
  carbon monoxide
    generated by
      motor vehicle — *see* Accident, transport
      watercraft (in transit) (not in transit) V93.89 ☑
        ferry boat V93.81 ☑
        fishing boat V93.82 ☑
        jet skis V93.83 ☑
        liner V93.81 ☑
        merchant ship V93.80 ☑
        passenger ship V93.81 ☑
        powered craft NEC V93.83 ☑
  caused by injection of poisons into skin by plant thorns, spines, sharp leaves X58 ☑
    marine or sea plants (venomous) X58 ☑
  execution — *see* Legal, intervention, gas
    intervention
      by gas — *see* Legal, intervention, gas
      other specified means — *see* Legal, intervention, specified means NEC
  exhaust gas
    generated by
      motor vehicle — *see* Accident, transport
      watercraft (in transit) (not in transit) V93.89 ☑
        ferry boat V93.81 ☑
        fishing boat V93.82 ☑
        jet skis V93.83 ☑
        liner V93.81 ☑
        merchant ship V93.80 ☑
        passenger ship V93.81 ☑
        powered craft NEC V93.83 ☑
  fumes or smoke due to
    explosion (*see also* Explosion) W40.9 ☑
    fire — *see* Exposure, fire
    ignition — *see* Ignition
  gas
    in legal intervention — *see* Legal, intervention, gas
    legal execution — *see* Legal, intervention, gas
  in war operations — *see* War operations
  legal
**Powder burn** (by) (from)
  airgun W34.110 ☑
  BB gun W34.110 ☑
  firearm NEC W34.19 ☑
  gas, air or spring-operated gun NEC W34.118 ☑
  handgun W32.1 ☑
  hunting rifle W33.12 ☑
  larger firearm W33.10 ☑
    specified NEC W33.19 ☑
  machine gun W33.13 ☑
  paintball gun W34.111 ☑
  pellet gun W34.110 ☑
  shotgun W33.11 ☑
  Very pistol [flare] W34.19 ☑
**Premature cessation** (of) **surgical and medical care** Y66
**Privation** (food) (water) X58 ☑
**Procedure** (operation)
  correct, on wrong side or body part (wrong side) (wrong site) Y65.53
  intended for another patient done on wrong patient Y65.52
  performed on patient not scheduled for surgery Y65.52
  performed on wrong patient Y65.52
  wrong, performed on correct patient Y65.51
**Prolonged**
  sitting in transport vehicle — *see* Travel, by type of vehicle
  stay in
    high altitude as cause of anoxia, barodontalgia, barotitis or hypoxia W94.11 ☑
    weightless environment X52 ☑

☑ **Additional Character Required** — Refer to the Tabular List for Character Selection      ▽ **Subterms under main terms may continue to next column or page**

**Pulling, excessive** (see also Overexertion) X50.9- ☑
**Puncture, puncturing** (see also Contact, with, by type of object or machine)
  by
    plant thorns, spines, sharp leaves or other mechanisms NEC W60 ☑
  during medical or surgical treatment as misadventure — see Index to Diseases and Injuries, Complication(s)
**Pushed, pushing** (accidental) (injury in)
  by other person(s) (accidental) W51 ☑
    with fall W03 ☑
      due to ice or snow W00.0 ☑
    as, or caused by, a crowd or human stampede (with fall) W52 ☑
    before moving object NEC Y02.8 ☑
      motor vehicle Y02.0 ☑
      subway train Y02.1 ☑
      train Y02.1 ☑
    from
      high place NEC
        in accidental circumstances W17.89 ☑
        stated as
          intentional, homicide (attempt) Y01
          undetermined whether accidental or intentional Y30
      transport vehicle NEC (see also Accident, transport) V89.9 ☑
        stated as
          intentional, homicide (attempt) Y08.89 ☑
  overexertion X50.9 ☑

# R

**Radiation** (exposure to)
  arc lamps W89.0 ☑
  atomic power plant (malfunction) NEC W88.1 ☑
  complication of or abnormal reaction to medical radiotherapy Y84.2
  electromagnetic, ionizing W88.0 ☑
  gamma rays W88.1 ☑
  in
    war operations (from or following nuclear explosion) — see War operations
  inadvertent exposure of patient (receiving test or therapy) Y63.3
  infrared (heaters and lamps) W90.1 ☑
    excessive heat from W92 ☑
  ionized, ionizing (particles, artificially accelerated) W88.0 ☑
    radioisotopes W88.1 ☑
    specified NEC W88.8 ☑
    x-rays W88.0 ☑
  isotopes, radioactive — see Radiation, radioactive isotopes
  laser(s) W90.2 ☑
    in war operations — see War operations
    misadventure in medical care Y63.2
  light sources (man-made visible and ultraviolet) W89.9 ☑
    natural X32 ☑
    specified NEC W89.8 ☑
    tanning bed W89.1 ☑
    welding light W89.0 ☑
  man-made visible light W89.9 ☑
    specified NEC W89.8 ☑
    tanning bed W89.1 ☑
    welding light W89.0 ☑
  microwave W90.8 ☑
  misadventure in medical or surgical procedure Y63.2
  natural NEC X39.08 ☑
    radon X39.01 ☑
  overdose (in medical or surgical procedure) Y63.2
  radar W90.0 ☑
  radioactive isotopes (any) W88.1 ☑
    atomic power plant malfunction W88.1 ☑
    misadventure in medical or surgical treatment Y63.2
  radiofrequency W90.0 ☑
  radium NEC W88.1 ☑
  sun X32 ☑
  ultraviolet (light) (man-made) W89.9 ☑
    natural X32 ☑
    specified NEC W89.8 ☑
    tanning bed W89.1 ☑
    welding light W89.0 ☑

**Radiation** — continued
  welding arc, torch, or light W89.0 ☑
    excessive heat from W92 ☑
  x-rays (hard) (soft) W88.0 ☑
**Range disease** W94.11 ☑
**Rape** (attempted) T74.2- ☑
**Rat bite** W53.11 ☑
**Reaching** (prolonged) (static) X50.1 ☑
**Reaction, abnormal to medical procedure** (see also Complication of or following, by type of procedure) Y84.9
  with misadventure — see Misadventure
  biologicals — see Table of Drugs and Chemicals
  drugs — see Table of Drugs and Chemicals
  vaccine — see Table of Drugs and Chemicals
**Recoil**
  airgun W34.110 ☑
  BB gun W34.110 ☑
  firearm NEC W34.19 ☑
  gas, air or spring-operated gun NEC W34.118 ☑
  handgun W32.1 ☑
  hunting rifle W33.12 ☑
  larger firearm W33.10 ☑
    specified NEC W33.19 ☑
  machine gun W33.13 ☑
  paintball gun W34.111 ☑
  pellet W34.110 ☑
  shotgun W33.11 ☑
  Very pistol [flare] W34.19 ☑
**Reduction in**
  atmospheric pressure — see Air, pressure, change
**Rock falling on or hitting** (accidentally) (person) W20.8 ☑
  in cave-in W20.0 ☑
**Run over** (accidentally) (by)
  animal (not being ridden) NEC W55.89 ☑
  machinery — see Contact, with, by specified type of machine
  transport vehicle NEC (see also Accident, transport) V09.9 ☑
    intentional homicide (attempt) Y03.0 ☑
    motor NEC V09.20 ☑
      intentional homicide (attempt) Y03.0 ☑
**Running**
  before moving object X81.8 ☑
    motor vehicle X81.0 ☑
**Running off, away**
  animal (being ridden) (see also Accident, transport) V80.918 ☑
    not being ridden W55.89 ☑
  animal-drawn vehicle NEC (see also Accident, transport) V80.928 ☑
  highway, road(way), street
    transport vehicle NEC (see also Accident, transport) V89.9 ☑
**Rupture pressurized devices** — see Explosion, by type of device

# S

**Saturnism** — see Table of Drugs and Chemicals, lead
**Scald, scalding** (accidental) (by) (from) (in) X19 ☑
  air (hot) X14.1 ☑
  gases (hot) X14.1 ☑
  homicide (attempt) — see Assault, burning, hot object
  inflicted by other person
    stated as intentional, homicide (attempt) — see Assault, burning, hot object
  liquid (boiling) (hot) NEC X12 ☑
    stated as undetermined whether accidental or intentional Y27.2 ☑
    suicide (attempt) X77.2 ☑
  local application of externally applied substance in medical or surgical care Y63.5
  metal (molten) (liquid) (hot) NEC X18 ☑
  self-inflicted X77.9 ☑
  stated as undetermined whether accidental or intentional Y27.8 ☑
  steam X13.1 ☑
    assault X98.0 ☑
    stated as undetermined whether accidental or intentional Y27.0 ☑
    suicide (attempt) X77.0 ☑
  suicide (attempt) X77.9 ☑
  vapor (hot) X13.1 ☑
    assault X98.0 ☑

**Scald, scalding** — continued
  vapor — continued
    stated as undetermined whether accidental or intentional Y27.0 ☑
    suicide (attempt) X77.0 ☑
**Scratched by**
  cat W55.03 ☑
  person(s) (accidentally) W50.4 ☑
    with intent to injure or kill Y04.0 ☑
    as, or caused by, a crowd or human stampede (with fall) W52 ☑
    assault Y04.0 ☑
    homicide (attempt) Y04.0 ☑
    in
      fight Y04.0 ☑
      legal intervention
        injuring
          bystander Y35.892 ☑
          law enforcement personnel Y35.891 ☑
          suspect Y35.893 ☑
**Seasickness** T75.3
**Self-harm NEC** (see also External cause by type, undetermined whether accidental or intentional)
  intentional — see Suicide
  poisoning NEC — see Table of Drugs and Chemicals, poisoning, accidental
**Self-inflicted** (injury) **NEC** (see also External cause by type, undetermined whether accidental or intentional)
  intentional — see Suicide
  poisoning NEC — see Table of Drugs and Chemicals, poisoning, accidental
**Sequelae** (of)
  accident NEC — see W00-X58 with 7th character S
  assault (homicidal) (any means) — see X92-Y08 with 7th character S
  homicide, attempt (any means) — see X92-Y08 with 7th character S
  injury undetermined whether accidentally or purposely inflicted — see Y21-Y33 with 7th character S
  intentional self-harm (classifiable to X71-X83) — see X71-X83 with 7th character S
  legal intervention — see with 7th character S Y35 ☑
  motor vehicle accident — see V00-V99 with 7th character S
  suicide, attempt (any means) — see X71-X83 with 7th character S
  transport accident — see V00-V99 with 7th character S
  war operations — see War operations
**Shock**
  electric — see Exposure, electric current
  from electric appliance (any) (faulty) W86.8 ☑
    domestic W86.0 ☑
    suicide (attempt) X83.1 ☑
**Shooting, shot** (accidental(ly)) (see also Discharge, firearm, by type)
  herself or himself — see Discharge, firearm by type, self-inflicted
  homicide (attempt) — see Discharge, firearm by type, homicide
  in war operations — see War operations
  inflicted by other person — see Discharge, firearm by type, homicide
    accidental — see Discharge, firearm, by type of firearm
  legal
    execution — see Legal, intervention, firearm
    intervention — see Legal, intervention, firearm
  self-inflicted — see Discharge, firearm by type, suicide
    accidental — see Discharge, firearm, by type of firearm
  suicide (attempt) — see Discharge, firearm by type, suicide
**Shoving** (accidentally) **by other person** — see Pushed, by other person
**Sickness**
  alpine W94.11 ☑
  motion — see Motion
  mountain W94.11 ☑
**Sinking** (accidental)
  watercraft (causing drowning, submersion) (see also Drowning, due to, accident to, watercraft, sinking)
    causing injury except drowning or submersion — see Accident, watercraft, causing, injury NEC
**Siriasis** X32 ☑

---

**Sitting** (prolonged) (static) X50.1 ☑
**Slashed wrists** — *see* Cut, self-inflicted
**Slipping** (accidental) (on same level) (with fall) W01.0 ☑
  without fall W18.40 ☑
    due to
      specified NEC W18.49 ☑
      stepping from one level to another W18.43 ☑
      stepping into hole or opening W18.42 ☑
      stepping on object W18.41 ☑
  on
    ice W00.0 ☑
      with skates — *see* Accident, transport, pedestri-
        an, conveyance
    mud W01.0 ☑
    oil W01.0 ☑
    snow W00.0 ☑
      with skis — *see* Accident, transport, pedestrian,
        conveyance
    surface (slippery) (wet) NEC W01.0 ☑
**Sliver, wood, contact with** W45.8 ☑
**Smoldering** (due to fire) — *see* Exposure, fire
**Sodomy** (attempted) **by force** T74.2 ☑
**Sound waves** (causing injury) W42.9 ☑
  supersonic W42.0 ☑
**Splinter, contact with** W45.8 ☑
**Stab, stabbing** — *see* Cut
**Standing** (prolonged) (static) X50.1 ☑
**Starvation** X58 ☑
**Status of external cause** Y99.9
  child assisting in compensated work for family Y99.8
  civilian activity done for financial or other compensa-
    tion Y99.0
  civilian activity done for income or pay Y99.0
  family member assisting in compensated work for
    other family member Y99.8
  hobby not done for income Y99.8
  leisure activity Y99.8
  military activity Y99.1
  off-duty activity of military personnel Y99.8
  recreation or sport not for income or while a student
    Y99.8
  specified NEC Y99.8
  student activity Y99.8
  volunteer activity Y99.2
**Stepped on**
  by
    animal (not being ridden) NEC W55.89 ☑
    crowd or human stampede W52 ☑
    person W50.0 ☑
**Stepping on**
  object W22.8 ☑
    with fall W18.31 ☑
    sports equipment W21.9 ☑
    stationary W22.09 ☑
      sports equipment W21.89 ☑
  person W51 ☑
    by crowd or human stampede W52 ☑
  sports equipment W21.9 ☑
**Sting**
  arthropod, nonvenomous W57 ☑
  insect, nonvenomous W57 ☑
**Storm** (cataclysmic) — *see* Forces of nature, cataclysmic
    storm
**Straining, excessive** (*see also* Overexertion) X50.9 ☑
**Strangling** — *see* Strangulation
**Strangulation** (accidental) T71 ☑
**Strenuous movements** (*see also* Overexertion) X50.9 ☑
**Striking against**
  airbag (automobile) W22.10 ☑
    driver side W22.11 ☑
    front passenger side W22.12 ☑
    specified NEC W22.19 ☑
  bottom when
    diving or jumping into water (in) W16.822 ☑
      causing drowning W16.821 ☑
      from boat W16.722 ☑
        causing drowning W16.721 ☑
      natural body W16.622 ☑
        causing drowning W16.821 ☑
      swimming pool W16.522 ☑
        causing drowning W16.521 ☑
    falling into water (in) W16.322 ☑
      causing drowning W16.321 ☑
      fountain — *see* Striking against, bottom when,
        falling into water, specified NEC
      natural body W16.122 ☑

**Striking against** — *continued*
  bottom when — *continued*
    falling into water — *continued*
      natural body — *continued*
        causing drowning W16.121 ☑
      reservoir — *see* Striking against, bottom when,
        falling into water, specified NEC
      specified NEC W16.322 ☑
        causing drowning W16.321 ☑
      swimming pool W16.022 ☑
        causing drowning W16.021 ☑
  diving board (swimming-pool) W21.4 ☑
  object W22.8 ☑
    with
      drowning or submersion — *see* Drowning
      fall — *see* Fall, due to, bumping against, object
      caused by crowd or human stampede (with fall)
        W52 ☑
    furniture W22.03 ☑
    lamppost W22.02 ☑
    sports equipment W21.9 ☑
    stationary W22.09 ☑
      sports equipment W21.89 ☑
    wall W22.01 ☑
  person(s) W51 ☑
    with fall W03 ☑
      due to ice or snow W00.0 ☑
    as, or caused by, a crowd or human stampede (with
      fall) W52 ☑
    assault Y04.2 ☑
    homicide (attempt) Y04.2 ☑
  sports equipment W21.9 ☑
  wall (when) W22.01 ☑
    diving or jumping into water (in) W16.832 ☑
      causing drowning W16.831 ☑
      swimming pool W16.532 ☑
        causing drowning W16.531 ☑
    falling into water (in) W16.332 ☑
      causing drowning W16.331 ☑
      fountain — *see* Striking against, wall when,
        falling into water, specified NEC
      natural body W16.132 ☑
        causing drowning W16.131 ☑
      reservoir — *see* Striking against, wall when,
        falling into water, specified NEC
      specified NEC W16.332 ☑
        causing drowning W16.331 ☑
      swimming pool W16.032 ☑
        causing drowning W16.031 ☑
    swimming pool (when) W22.042 ☑
      causing drowning W22.041 ☑
      diving or jumping into water W16.532 ☑
        causing drowning W16.531 ☑
      falling into water W16.032 ☑
        causing drowning W16.031 ☑
**Struck** (accidentally) **by**
  airbag (automobile) W22.10 ☑
    driver side W22.11 ☑
    front passenger side W22.12 ☑
    specified NEC W22.19 ☑
  alligator W58.02 ☑
  animal (not being ridden) NEC W55.89 ☑
  avalanche — *see* Landslide
  ball (hit) (thrown) W21.00 ☑
    assault Y08.09 ☑
    baseball W21.03 ☑
    basketball W21.05 ☑
    football W21.01 ☑
    golf ball W21.04 ☑
    soccer W21.02 ☑
    softball W21.07 ☑
    specified NEC W21.09 ☑
    volleyball W21.06 ☑
  bat or racquet
    baseball bat W21.11 ☑
      assault Y08.02 ☑
    golf club W21.13 ☑
      assault Y08.09 ☑
    specified NEC W21.19 ☑
      assault Y08.09 ☑
    tennis racquet W21.12 ☑
      assault Y08.09 ☑
  bullet (*see also* Discharge, firearm by type)
    in war operations — *see* War operations
  crocodile W58.12 ☑
  dog W54.1 ☑

**Struck** (accidentally) **by** — *continued*
  flare, Very pistol — *see* Discharge, firearm NEC
  hailstones X39.8 ☑
  hockey (ice)
    field
      puck W21.221 ☑
      stick W21.211 ☑
    puck W21.220 ☑
    stick W21.210 ☑
    assault Y08.01 ☑
  landslide — *see* Landslide
  law-enforcement agent (on duty) — *see* Legal, inter-
    vention, manhandling
    with blunt object — *see* Legal, intervention, blunt
      object
  lightning T75.0 ☑
    causing fire — *see* Exposure, fire
  machine — *see* Contact, with, by type of machine
  mammal NEC W55.89 ☑
    marine W56.32 ☑
  marine animal W56.82 ☑
  missile
    firearm — *see* Discharge, firearm by type
    in war operations — *see* War operations, missile
  object W22.8 ☑
    blunt W22.8 ☑
      assault Y00 ☑
      suicide (attempt) X79 ☑
      undetermined whether accidental or intention-
        al Y29 ☑
    falling W20.8 ☑
      from, in, on
        building W20.1 ☑
          burning (uncontrolled fire) X00.4 ☑
        cataclysmic
          earth surface movement NEC — *see*
            Landslide
          storm — *see* Forces of nature, cata-
            clysmic storm
        cave-in W20.0 ☑
        earthquake X34 ☑
        machine (in operation) — *see* Contact, with,
          by type of machine
        structure W20.1 ☑
          burning X00.4 ☑
        transport vehicle (in motion) — *see* Acci-
          dent, transport, by type of vehicle
        watercraft V93.49 ☑
          due to
            accident to craft V91.39 ☑
              powered craft V91.33 ☑
                ferry boat V91.31 ☑
                fishing boat V91.32 ☑
                jetskis V91.33 ☑
                liner V91.31 ☑
                merchant ship V91.30 ☑
                passenger ship V91.31 ☑
              unpowered craft V91.38 ☑
                canoe V91.35 ☑
                inflatable V91.36 ☑
                kayak V91.35 ☑
                sailboat V91.34 ☑
                surf-board V91.38 ☑
                windsurfer V91.38 ☑
            powered craft V93.43 ☑
              ferry boat V93.41 ☑
              fishing boat V93.42 ☑
              jetskis V93.43 ☑
              liner V93.41 ☑
              merchant ship V93.40 ☑
              passenger ship V93.41 ☑
            unpowered craft V93.48 ☑
              sailboat V93.44 ☑
              surf-board V93.48 ☑
              windsurfer V93.48 ☑
    moving NEC W20.8 ☑
    projected W20.8 ☑
      assault Y00 ☑
      in sports W21.9 ☑
        assault Y08.09 ☑
        ball W21.00 ☑
          baseball W21.03 ☑
          basketball W21.05 ☑
          football W21.01 ☑
          golf ball W21.04 ☑
          soccer W21.02 ☑

**Struck** (accidentally) **by** — *continued*
  object — *continued*
    projected — *continued*
      in sports — *continued*
        ball — *continued*
          softball W21.07 ☑
          specified NEC W21.09 ☑
          volleyball W21.06 ☑
        bat or racquet
          baseball bat W21.11 ☑
            assault Y08.02 ☑
          golf club W21.13 ☑
            assault Y08.09 ☑
          specified NEC W21.19 ☑
            assault Y08.09 ☑
          tennis racquet W21.12 ☑
            assault Y08.09 ☑
        hockey (ice)
          field
            puck W21.221 ☑
            stick W21.211 ☑
          puck W21.220 ☑
          stick W21.210 ☑
            assault Y08.01 ☑
        specified NEC W21.89 ☑
    set in motion by explosion — *see* Explosion
    thrown W20.8 ☑
      assault Y00 ☑
      in sports W21.9 ☑
        assault Y08.09 ☑
        ball W21.00 ☑
          baseball W21.03 ☑
          basketball W21.05 ☑
          football W21.01 ☑
          golf ball W21.04 ☑
          soccer W21.02 ☑
          soft ball W21.07 ☑
          specified NEC W21.09 ☑
          volleyball W21.06 ☑
        bat or racquet
          baseball bat W21.11 ☑
            assault Y08.02 ☑
          golf club W21.13 ☑
            assault Y08.09 ☑
          specified NEC W21.19 ☑
            assault Y08.09 ☑
          tennis racquet W21.12 ☑
            assault Y08.09 ☑
        hockey (ice)
          field
            puck W21.221 ☑
            stick W21.211 ☑
          puck W21.220 ☑
          stick W21.210 ☑
            assault Y08.01 ☑
        specified NEC W21.89 ☑
  other person(s) W50.0 ☑
    with
      blunt object W22.8 ☑
      intentional, homicide (attempt) Y00 ☑
      sports equipment W21.9 ☑
      undetermined whether accidental or intentional Y29 ☑
    fall W03 ☑
      due to ice or snow W00.0 ☑
    as, or caused by, a crowd or human stampede (with fall) W52 ☑
    assault Y04.2 ☑
    homicide (attempt) Y04.2 ☑
    in legal intervention
      injuring
        bystander Y35.812 ☑
        law enforcement personnel Y35.811 ☑
        suspect Y35.813 ☑
    sports equipment W21.9 ☑
  police (on duty) — *see* Legal, intervention, manhandling
    with blunt object — *see* Legal, intervention, blunt object
  sports equipment W21.9 ☑
    assault Y08.09 ☑
    ball W21.00 ☑
      baseball W21.03 ☑
      basketball W21.05 ☑
      football W21.01 ☑
      golf ball W21.04 ☑

**Struck** (accidentally) **by** — *continued*
  sports equipment — *continued*
    ball — *continued*
      soccer W21.02 ☑
      soft ball W21.07 ☑
      specified NEC W21.09 ☑
      volleyball W21.06 ☑
    bat or racquet
      baseball bat W21.11 ☑
        assault Y08.02 ☑
      golf club W21.13 ☑
        assault Y08.09 ☑
      specified NEC W21.19 ☑
      tennis racquet W21.12 ☑
        assault Y08.09 ☑
    cleats (shoe) W21.31 ☑
    foot wear NEC W21.39 ☑
    football helmet W21.81 ☑
    hockey (ice)
      field
        puck W21.221 ☑
        stick W21.211 ☑
      puck W21.220 ☑
      stick W21.210 ☑
        assault Y08.01 ☑
    skate blades W21.32 ☑
    specified NEC W21.89 ☑
      assault Y08.09 ☑
  thunderbolt — *see* subcategory T75.0 ☑
  causing fire — *see* Exposure, fire
  transport vehicle NEC (*see also* Accident, transport) V09.9 ☑
    intentional, homicide (attempt) Y03.0 ☑
    motor NEC (*see also* Accident, transport) V09.20 ☑
      homicide Y03.0 ☑
  vehicle (transport) NEC — *see* Accident, transport, by type of vehicle
  stationary (falling from jack, hydraulic lift, ramp) W20.8 ☑

**Stumbling**
  without fall W18.40 ☑
    due to
      specified NEC W18.49 ☑
      stepping from one level to another W18.43 ☑
      stepping into hole or opening W18.42 ☑
      stepping on object W18.41 ☑
    over
      animal NEC W01.0 ☑
      with fall W18.09 ☑
    carpet, rug or (small) object W22.8 ☑
      with fall W18.09 ☑
    person W51 ☑
      with fall W03 ☑
        due to ice or snow W00.0 ☑
**Submersion** (accidental) — *see* Drowning
**Suffocation** (accidental) (by external means) (by pressure) (mechanical) (*see also* category) T71 ☑
  due to, by
    avalanche — *see* Landslide
    explosion — *see* Explosion
    fire — *see* Exposure, fire
    food, any type (aspiration) (ingestion) (inhalation) — *see* categories T17 and T18 ☑
    ignition — *see* Ignition
    landslide — *see* Landslide
    machine(ry) — *see* Contact, with, by type of machine
    vomitus (aspiration) (inhalation) T17.81- ☑
  in
    burning building X00.8 ☑
**Suicide, suicidal** (attempted) (by) X83.8 ☑
  blunt object X79 ☑
  burning, burns X76 ☑
    hot object X77.9 ☑
      fluid NEC X77.2 ☑
      household appliance X77.3 ☑
      specified NEC X77.8 ☑
      steam X77.0 ☑
      tap water X77.1 ☑
      vapors X77.0 ☑
  caustic substance — *see* Table of Drugs and Chemicals
  cold, extreme X83.2 ☑
  collision of motor vehicle with
    motor vehicle X82.0 ☑
    specified NEC X82.8 ☑
    train X82.1 ☑

**Suicide, suicidal** — *continued*
  collision of motor vehicle with — *continued*
    tree X82.2 ☑
  crashing of aircraft X83.0 ☑
  cut (any part of body) X78.9 ☑
  cutting or piercing instrument X78.9 ☑
    dagger X78.2 ☑
    glass X78.0 ☑
    knife X78.1 ☑
    specified NEC X78.8 ☑
    sword X78.2 ☑
  drowning (in) X71.9 ☑
    bathtub X71.0 ☑
    natural water X71.3 ☑
    specified NEC X71.8 ☑
    swimming pool X71.1 ☑
      following fall X71.2 ☑
  electrocution X83.1 ☑
  explosive(s) (material) X75 ☑
  fire, flames X76 ☑
  firearm X74.9 ☑
    airgun X74.01 ☑
    handgun X72 ☑
    hunting rifle X73.1 ☑
    larger X73.9 ☑
      specified NEC X73.8 ☑
    machine gun X73.2 ☑
    shotgun X73.0 ☑
    specified NEC X74.8 ☑
  hanging X83.8 ☑
  hot object — *see* Suicide, burning, hot object
  jumping
    before moving object X81.8 ☑
      motor vehicle X81.0 ☑
      subway train X81.1 ☑
      train X81.1 ☑
    from high place X80 ☑
  late effect of attempt — *see* X71-X83 with 7th character S
  lying before moving object, train, vehicle X81.8 ☑
  poisoning — *see* Table of Drugs and Chemicals
  puncture (any part of body) — *see* Suicide, cutting or piercing instrument
  scald — *see* Suicide, burning, hot object
  sequelae of attempt — *see* X71-X83 with 7th character S
  sharp object (any) — *see* Suicide, cutting or piercing instrument
  shooting — *see* Suicide, firearm
  specified means NEC X83.8 ☑
  stab (any part of body) — *see* Suicide, cutting or piercing instrument
  steam, hot vapors X77.0 ☑
  strangulation X83.8 ☑
  submersion — *see* Suicide, drowning
  suffocation X83.8 ☑
  wound NEC X83.8 ☑
**Sunstroke** X32 ☑
**Supersonic waves** (causing injury) W42.0 ☑
**Surgical procedure, complication of** (delayed or as an abnormal reaction without mention of misadventure) (*see also* Complication of or following, by type of procedure)
  due to or as a result of misadventure — *see* Misadventure
**Swallowed, swallowing**
  foreign body — *see* Foreign body, alimentary canal
  poison — *see* Table of Drugs and Chemicals
  substance
    caustic or corrosive — *see* Table of Drugs and Chemicals
    poisonous — *see* Table of Drugs and Chemicals

# T

**Tackle in sport** W03 ☑
**Terrorism** (involving) Y38.80 ☑
  biological weapons Y38.6X- ☑
  chemical weapons Y38.7X- ☑
  conflagration Y38.3X- ☑
  drowning and submersion Y38.89- ☑
  explosion Y38.2X- ☑
    destruction of aircraft Y38.1X- ☑
    marine weapons Y38.0X- ☑
  fire Y38.3X- ☑
  firearms Y38.4X- ☑

**Terrorism** — *continued*
  hot substances Y38.3X- ☑
  lasers Y38.89- ☑
  nuclear weapons Y38.5X- ☑
  piercing or stabbing instruments Y38.89- ☑
  secondary effects Y38.9X- ☑
  specified method NEC Y38.89- ☑
  suicide bomber Y38.81- ☑
**Thirst** X58 ☑
**Threat to breathing**
  aspiration — *see* Aspiration
  due to cave-in, falling earth or substance NEC T71 ☑
**Thrown** (accidentally)
  against part (any) of or object in transport vehicle (in motion) NEC (*see also* Accident, transport)
  from
    high place, homicide (attempt) Y01 ☑
    machinery — *see* Contact, with, by type of machine
    transport vehicle NEC (*see also* Accident, transport) V89.9 ☑
  off — *see* Thrown, from
**Thunderbolt** — *see* subcategory T75.0 ☑
  causing fire — *see* Exposure, fire
**Tidal wave** (any injury) **NEC** — *see* Forces of nature, tidal wave
**Took**
  overdose (drug) — *see* Table of Drugs and Chemicals
  poison — *see* Table of Drugs and Chemicals
**Tornado** (any injury) X37.1 ☑
**Torrential rain** (any injury) X37.8 ☑
**Torture** X58 ☑
**Trampled by animal NEC** W55.89 ☑
**Trapped** (accidentally)
  between objects (moving) (stationary and moving) — *see* Caught
  by part (any) of
    motorcycle V29.88 ☑
    pedal cycle V19.88 ☑
    transport vehicle NEC (*see also* Accident, transport) V89.9 ☑
**Travel** (effects) (sickness) T75.3 ☑
**Tree falling on or hitting** (accidentally) (person) W20.8 ☑
**Tripping**
  without fall W18.40 ☑
    due to
      specified NEC W18.49 ☑
      stepping from one level to another W18.43 ☑
      stepping into hole or opening W18.42 ☑
      stepping on object W18.41 ☑
    over
      animal W01.0 ☑
        with fall W01.0 ☑
      carpet, rug or (small) object W22.8 ☑
        with fall W18.09 ☑
      person W51 ☑
        with fall W03 ☑
          due to ice or snow W00.0 ☑
**Twisted by person**(s) (accidentally) W50.2 ☑
  with intent to injure or kill Y04.0 ☑
  as, or caused by, a crowd or human stampede (with fall) W52 ☑
  assault Y04.0 ☑
  homicide (attempt) Y04.0 ☑
  in
    fight Y04.0 ☑
    legal intervention — *see* Legal, intervention, manhandling
**Twisting** (prolonged) (static) X50.1- ☑

# U

**Underdosing of necessary drugs, medicaments or biological substances** Y63.6
**Undetermined intent** (contact) (exposure)
  automobile collision Y32 ☑
  blunt object Y29 ☑
  drowning (submersion) (in) Y21.9 ☑
    bathtub Y21.0 ☑
      after fall Y21.1 ☑
    natural water (lake) (ocean) (pond) (river) (stream) Y21.4 ☑
    specified place NEC Y21.8 ☑
    swimming pool Y21.2 ☑
      after fall Y21.3 ☑
  explosive material Y25 ☑

**Undetermined intent** — *continued*
  fall, jump or push from high place Y30 ☑
  falling, lying or running before moving object Y31 ☑
  fire Y26 ☑
  firearm discharge Y24.9 ☑
    airgun (BB) (pellet) Y24.0 ☑
    handgun (pistol) (revolver) Y22 ☑
    hunting rifle Y23.1 ☑
    larger Y23.9 ☑
      hunting rifle Y23.1 ☑
      machine gun Y23.3 ☑
      military Y23.2 ☑
      shotgun Y23.0 ☑
      specified type NEC Y23.8 ☑
    machine gun Y23.3 ☑
    military Y23.2 ☑
    shotgun Y23.0 ☑
    specified type NEC Y24.8 ☑
    Very pistol Y24.8 ☑
  hot object Y27.9 ☑
    fluid NEC Y27.2 ☑
    household appliance Y27.3 ☑
    specified object NEC Y27.8 ☑
    steam Y27.0 ☑
    tap water Y27.1 ☑
    vapor Y27.0 ☑
  jump, fall or push from high place Y30 ☑
  lying, falling or running before moving object Y31 ☑
  motor vehicle crash Y32 ☑
  push, fall or jump from high place Y30 ☑
  running, falling or lying before moving object Y31 ☑
  sharp object Y28.9 ☑
    dagger Y28.2 ☑
    glass Y28.0 ☑
    knife Y28.1 ☑
    specified object NEC Y28.8 ☑
    sword Y28.2 ☑
  smoke Y26 ☑
  specified event NEC Y33 ☑
**Use of hand as hammer** X50.3 ☑

# V

**Vibration** (causing injury) W49.9 ☑
**Victim** (of)
  avalanche — *see* Landslide
  earth movements NEC — *see* Forces of nature, earth movement
  earthquake X34 ☑
  flood — *see* Flood
  landslide — *see* Landslide
  lightning — *see* subcategory T75.0 ☑
    causing fire — *see* Exposure, fire
  storm (cataclysmic) NEC — *see* Forces of nature, cataclysmic storm
  volcanic eruption X35 ☑
**Volcanic eruption** (any injury) X35 ☑
**Vomitus, gastric contents in air passages** (with asphyxia, obstruction or suffocation) T17.81- ☑

# W

**Walked into stationary object** (any) W22.09 ☑
  furniture W22.03 ☑
  lamppost W22.02 ☑
  wall W22.01 ☑
**War operations** (injuries to military personnel and civilians during war, civil insurrection and peacekeeping missions) (by) (from) (involving) Y36.90 ☑
  after cessation of hostilities Y36.89- ☑
    explosion (of)
      bomb placed during war operations Y36.82- ☑
      mine placed during war operations Y36.81- ☑
      specified NEC Y36.88- ☑
  air blast Y36.20- ☑
  aircraft
    destruction — *see* War operations, destruction of aircraft
    airway restriction — *see* War operations, restriction of airways
  asphyxiation — *see* War operations, restriction of airways
  biological weapons Y36.6X- ☑
  blast Y36.20- ☑
  blast fragments Y36.20- ☑
  blast wave Y36.20- ☑

**War operations** — *continued*
  blast wind Y36.20- ☑
  bomb Y36.20- ☑
    dirty Y36.50- ☑
    gasoline Y36.31- ☑
    incendiary Y36.31- ☑
    petrol Y36.31- ☑
  bullet Y36.43- ☑
    incendiary Y36.32- ☑
    rubber Y36.41- ☑
  chemical weapons Y36.7X- ☑
  combat
    hand to hand (unarmed) combat Y36.44- ☑
    using blunt or piercing object Y36.45- ☑
  conflagration — *see* War operations, fire
  conventional warfare NEC Y36.49- ☑
  depth-charge Y36.01- ☑
  destruction of aircraft Y36.10- ☑
    due to
      air to air missile Y36.11- ☑
      collision with other aircraft Y36.12- ☑
      detonation (accidental) of onboard munitions and explosives Y36.14- ☑
      enemy fire or explosives Y36.11- ☑
      explosive placed on aircraft Y36.11- ☑
      onboard fire Y36.13- ☑
      rocket propelled grenade [RPG] Y36.11- ☑
      small arms fire Y36.11- ☑
      surface to air missile Y36.11- ☑
    specified NEC Y36.19- ☑
  detonation (accidental) of
    onboard marine weapons Y36.05- ☑
    own munitions or munitions launch device Y36.24- ☑
  dirty bomb Y36.50- ☑
  explosion (of) Y36.20- ☑
    aerial bomb Y36.21- ☑
    after cessation of hostilities
      bomb placed during war operations Y36.82- ☑
      mine placed during war operations Y36.81- ☑
    bomb NOS (*see also* War operations, bomb(s)) Y36.20- ☑
    fragments Y36.20- ☑
    grenade Y36.29- ☑
    guided missile Y36.22- ☑
    improvised explosive device [IED] (person-borne) (roadside) (vehicle-borne) Y36.23- ☑
    land mine Y36.29- ☑
    marine mine (at sea) (in harbor) Y36.02- ☑
    marine weapon Y36.00- ☑
      specified NEC Y36.09- ☑
    own munitions or munitions launch device (accidental) Y36.24- ☑
    sea-based artillery shell Y36.03- ☑
    specified NEC Y36.29- ☑
    torpedo Y36.04- ☑
  fire Y36.30- ☑
    specified NEC Y36.39- ☑
  firearms
    discharge Y36.43- ☑
    pellets Y36.42- ☑
  flamethrower Y36.33- ☑
  fragments (from) (of)
    improvised explosive device [IED] (person-borne) (roadside) (vehicle-borne) Y36.26- ☑
    munitions Y36.25- ☑
    specified NEC Y36.29- ☑
    weapons Y36.27- ☑
  friendly fire Y36.92 ☑
  hand to hand (unarmed) combat Y36.44- ☑
  hot substances — *see* War operations, fire
  incendiary bullet Y36.32- ☑
  nuclear weapon (effects of) Y36.50- ☑
    acute radiation exposure Y36.54- ☑
    blast pressure Y36.51- ☑
    direct blast Y36.51- ☑
    direct heat Y36.53- ☑
    fallout exposure Y36.54- ☑
    fireball Y36.53- ☑
    indirect blast (struck or crushed by blast debris) (being thrown by blast) Y36.52- ☑
    ionizing radiation (immediate exposure) Y36.54- ☑
    nuclear radiation Y36.54- ☑
    radiation
      ionizing (immediate exposure) Y36.54- ☑
      nuclear Y36.54- ☑

☑ **Additional Character Required** — **Refer to the Tabular List for Character Selection**
▽ **Subterms under main terms may continue to next column or page**

**War operations** — *continued*
  nuclear weapon — *continued*
    radiation — *continued*
      thermal Y36.53- ☑
      secondary effects Y36.54- ☑
      specified NEC Y36.59- ☑
      thermal radiation Y36.53- ☑
    restriction of air (airway)
      intentional Y36.46- ☑
      unintentional Y36.47- ☑
    rubber bullets Y36.41- ☑
    shrapnel NOS Y36.29- ☑
    suffocation — *see* War operations, restriction of airways
    unconventional warfare NEC Y36.7X- ☑
    underwater blast NOS Y36.00- ☑
    warfare
      conventional NEC Y36.49- ☑
      unconventional NEC Y36.7X- ☑

**War operations** — *continued*
  weapon of mass destruction [WMD] Y36.91 ☑
  weapons
    biological weapons Y36.6X- ☑
    chemical Y36.7X- ☑
    nuclear (effects of) Y36.50- ☑
      acute radiation exposure Y36.54- ☑
      blast pressure Y36.51- ☑
      direct blast Y36.51- ☑
      direct heat Y36.53- ☑
      fallout exposure Y36.54- ☑
      fireball Y36.53- ☑
      radiation
        ionizing (immediate exposure) Y36.54- ☑
        nuclear Y36.54- ☑
        thermal Y36.53- ☑
      secondary effects Y36.54- ☑
      specified NEC Y36.59- ☑
  of mass destruction [WMD] Y36.91 ☑

**Washed**
  away by flood — *see* Flood
  off road by storm (transport vehicle) — *see* Forces of nature, cataclysmic storm
**Weather exposure NEC** — *see* Forces of nature
**Weightlessness** (causing injury) (effects of) (in spacecraft, real or simulated) X52 ☑
**Work related condition** Y99.0
**Wound** (accidental) NEC (*see also* Injury) X58 ☑
  battle (*see also* War operations) Y36.90 ☑
  gunshot — *see* Discharge, firearm by type
**Wreck transport vehicle NEC** (*see also* Accident, transport) V89.9 ☑
**Wrong**
  device implanted into correct surgical site Y65.51
  fluid in infusion Y65.1
  patient, procedure performed on Y65.52
  procedure (operation) on correct patient Y65.51

# ICD-10-CM Tabular List of Diseases and Injuries

## Chapter 1. Certain Infectious and Parasitic Diseases (AØØ–B99)

### Chapter Specific Guidelines with Coding Examples

The chapter specific guidelines from the ICD-10-CM Official Guidelines for Coding and Reporting have been provided below. Along with these guidelines are coding examples, contained in the shaded boxes, that have been developed to help illustrate the coding and/or sequencing guidance found in these guidelines.

#### a. Human immunodeficiency virus (HIV) infections

##### 1) Code only confirmed cases

Code only confirmed cases of HIV infection/illness. This is an exception to the hospital inpatient guideline Section II, H.

In this context, "confirmation" does not require documentation of positive serology or culture for HIV; the provider's diagnostic statement that the patient is HIV positive, or has an HIV-related illness is sufficient.

> Patient admitted with anemia with possible HIV infection
>
> **D64.9**     **Anemia, unspecified**
>
> *Explanation:* Only the anemia is coded in this scenario because it has not been confirmed that an HIV infection is present. This is an exception to the guideline Section II, H for hospital inpatient coding.

##### 2) Selection and sequencing of HIV codes

###### (a) Patient admitted for HIV-related condition

If a patient is admitted for an HIV-related condition, the principal diagnosis should be B2Ø, Human immunodeficiency virus [HIV] disease followed by additional diagnosis codes for all reported HIV-related conditions.

> HIV with PCP
>
> **B2Ø**     **Human immunodeficiency virus [HIV] disease**
>
> **B59**     **Pneumocystosis**
>
> *Explanation:* Pneumonia due to *Pneumocystis carinii* is an HIV related condition, so the HIV diagnosis code is reported first, followed by the code for the pneumonia.

###### (b) Patient with HIV disease admitted for unrelated condition

If a patient with HIV disease is admitted for an unrelated condition (such as a traumatic injury), the code for the unrelated condition (e.g., the nature of injury code) should be the principal diagnosis. Other diagnoses would be B2Ø followed by additional diagnosis codes for all reported HIV-related conditions.

> Unstable angina, native coronary artery atherosclerosis, HIV
>
> **I25.11Ø**     **Atherosclerotic heart disease of native coronary artery with unstable angina pectoris**
>
> **B2Ø**     **Human immunodeficiency virus [HIV] disease**
>
> *Explanation:* The arteriosclerotic coronary artery disease and the unstable angina are not related to HIV, so those conditions are reported first using a combination code, and HIV is reported secondarily.

###### (c) Whether the patient is newly diagnosed

Whether the patient is newly diagnosed or has had previous admissions/encounters for HIV conditions is irrelevant to the sequencing decision.

> Newly diagnosed multiple cutaneous Kaposi's sarcoma lesions in previously diagnosed HIV disease
>
> **B2Ø**     **Human immunodeficiency virus [HIV] disease**
>
> **C46.Ø**     **Kaposi's sarcoma of skin**
>
> *Explanation:* Even though the HIV was diagnosed on a previous encounter, it is still sequenced first when coded with an HIV related condition. Kaposi's sarcoma is an HIV-related condition.

###### (d) Asymptomatic human immunodeficiency virus

Z21, Asymptomatic human immunodeficiency virus [HIV] infection status, is to be applied when the patient without any documentation of symptoms is listed as being "HIV positive," "known HIV," "HIV test positive," or similar terminology. Do not use this code if the term "AIDS" is used or if the patient is treated for any HIV-related illness or is described as having any condition(s) resulting from his/her HIV positive status; use B20 in these cases.

> Patient admitted with acute appendicitis. Status positive HIV test on Atripla, with no prior symptoms
>
> **K35.8Ø**     **Unspecified acute appendicitis**
>
> **Z21**     **Asymptomatic human immunodeficiency virus [HIV] infection status**
>
> *Explanation:* Code Z21 is sequenced second since documentation indicates that the patient has had a positive HIV test but has been asymptomatic. Being on medication for HIV is not an indication that code B20 is used instead of Z21. Unless there has been documentation that the patient has had current or prior symptoms or HIV-related complications, code B20 is not used. The appendicitis is not an AIDS-related complication and is sequenced first.

###### (e) Patients with inconclusive HIV serology

Patients with inconclusive HIV serology, but no definitive diagnosis or manifestations of the illness, may be assigned code R75, Inconclusive laboratory evidence of human immunodeficiency virus [HIV].

###### (f) Previously diagnosed HIV-related illness

Patients with any known prior diagnosis of an HIV-related illness should be coded to B2Ø. Once a patient has developed an HIV-related illness, the patient should always be assigned code B2Ø on every subsequent admission/encounter. Patients previously diagnosed with any HIV illness (B2Ø) should never be assigned to R75 or Z21, Asymptomatic human immunodeficiency virus [HIV] infection status.

###### (g) HIV infection in pregnancy, childbirth and the puerperium

During pregnancy, childbirth or the puerperium, a patient admitted (or presenting for a health care encounter) because of an HIV-related illness should receive a principal diagnosis code of O98.7-, Human immunodeficiency [HIV] disease complicating pregnancy, childbirth and the puerperium, followed by B2Ø and the code(s) for the HIV-related illness(es). Codes from Chapter 15 always take sequencing priority.

Patients with asymptomatic HIV infection status admitted (or presenting for a health care encounter) during pregnancy, childbirth, or the puerperium should receive codes of O98.7- and Z21.

###### (h) Encounters for testing for HIV

If a patient is being seen to determine his/her HIV status, use code Z11.4, Encounter for screening for human immunodeficiency virus [HIV]. Use additional codes for any associated high risk behavior.

If a patient with signs or symptoms is being seen for HIV testing, code the signs and symptoms. An additional counseling code Z71.7, Human immunodeficiency virus [HIV] counseling, may be used if counseling is provided during the encounter for the test.

When a patient returns to be informed of his/her HIV test results and the test result is negative, use code Z71.7, Human immunodeficiency virus [HIV] counseling.

If the results are positive, see previous guidelines and assign codes as appropriate.

#### b. Infectious agents as the cause of diseases classified to other chapters

Certain infections are classified in chapters other than Chapter 1 and no organism is identified as part of the infection code. In these instances, it is necessary to use an additional code from Chapter 1 to identify the organism. A code from category B95, Streptococcus, Staphylococcus, and Enterococcus as the cause of diseases classified to other chapters, B96, Other bacterial agents as the cause of diseases classified to other chapters, or B97, Viral agents as the cause of diseases classified to other chapters, is to be used as an additional code to identify the organism. An instructional note will be found at the infection code advising that an additional organism code is required.

*E. coli* UTI

| N39.Ø | Urinary tract infection, site not specified |
|---|---|
| B96.2Ø | Unspecified Escherichia coli [E.coli] as the cause of diseases classified elsewhere |

*Explanation:* An instructional note under the code for the urinary tract infection indicates to code also the specific organism.

#### c. Infections resistant to antibiotics

Many bacterial infections are resistant to current antibiotics. It is necessary to identify all infections documented as antibiotic resistant. Assign a code from category Z16, Resistance to antimicrobial drugs, following the infection code only if the infection code does not identify drug resistance.

#### d. Sepsis, severe sepsis, and septic shock

##### 1) Coding of Sepsis and Severe Sepsis

###### (a) Sepsis

For a diagnosis of sepsis, assign the appropriate code for the underlying systemic infection. If the type of infection or causal organism is not further specified, assign code A41.9, Sepsis, unspecified organism.

A code from subcategory R65.2, Severe sepsis, should not be assigned unless severe sepsis or an associated acute organ dysfunction is documented.

Gram-negative sepsis

| A41.5Ø | Gram-negative sepsis, unspecified |
|---|---|

Staphylococcal sepsis

| A41.2 | Sepsis due to unspecified staphylococcus |
|---|---|

*Explanation:* In both examples above the organism causing the sepsis is identified, therefore A41.9 Sepsis, unspecified organism, would not be appropriate as this code would not capture the highest degree of specificity found in the documentation. Do not use an additional code for severe sepsis unless an acute organ dysfunction was also documented as "associated with" or "due to" the sepsis or the sepsis was documented as "severe."

###### (i) Negative or inconclusive blood cultures and sepsis

Negative or inconclusive blood cultures do not preclude a diagnosis of sepsis in patients with clinical evidence of the condition; however, the provider should be queried.

###### (ii) Urosepsis

The term urosepsis is a nonspecific term. It is not to be considered synonymous with sepsis. It has no default code in the Alphabetic Index. Should a provider use this term, he/she must be queried for clarification.

###### (iii) Sepsis with organ dysfunction

If a patient has sepsis and associated acute organ dysfunction or multiple organ dysfunction (MOD), follow the instructions for coding severe sepsis.

###### (iv) Acute organ dysfunction that is not clearly associated with the sepsis

If a patient has sepsis and an acute organ dysfunction, but the medical record documentation indicates that the acute organ dysfunction is related to a medical condition other than the sepsis, do not assign a code from subcategory R65.2, Severe sepsis. An acute organ dysfunction must be associated with the sepsis in order to assign the severe sepsis code. If the documentation is not clear as to whether an acute organ dysfunction is related to the sepsis or another medical condition, query the provider.

Sepsis and acute respiratory failure due to COPD exacerbation

| A41.9 | Sepsis, unspecified organism |
|---|---|
| J44.1 | Chronic obstructive pulmonary disease with (acute) exacerbation |
| J96.ØØ | Acute respiratory failure, unspecified whether with hypoxia or hypercapnia |

*Explanation:* Although acute organ dysfunction is present in the form of acute respiratory failure, severe sepsis (R65.2) is not coded in this example, as the acute respiratory failure is attributed to the COPD exacerbation rather than the sepsis. Sequencing of these codes would be determined by the circumstances of the admission.

###### (b) Severe sepsis

The coding of severe sepsis requires a minimum of 2 codes: first a code for the underlying systemic infection, followed by a code from subcategory R65.2, Severe sepsis. If the causal organism is not documented, assign code A41.9, Sepsis, unspecified organism, for the infection. Additional code(s) for the associated acute organ dysfunction are also required.

Due to the complex nature of severe sepsis, some cases may require querying the provider prior to assignment of the codes.

##### 2) Septic shock

###### (a) Septic shock generally refers to circulatory failure associated with severe sepsis, and therefore, it represents a type of acute organ dysfunction.

For cases of septic shock, the code for the systemic infection should be sequenced first, followed by code R65.21, Severe sepsis with septic shock or code T81.12, Postprocedural septic shock. Any additional codes for the other acute organ dysfunctions should also be assigned. As noted in the sequencing instructions in the Tabular List, the code for septic shock cannot be assigned as a principal diagnosis.

Sepsis with septic shock

| A41.9 | Sepsis, unspecified organism |
|---|---|
| R65.21 | Severe sepsis with septic shock |

*Explanation:* Documentation of septic shock automatically implies severe sepsis as it is a form of acute organ dysfunction. Septic shock is not coded as the principal diagnosis; it is always preceded by the code for the systemic infection.

##### 3) Sequencing of severe sepsis

If severe sepsis is present on admission, and meets the definition of principal diagnosis, the underlying systemic infection should be assigned as principal diagnosis followed by the appropriate code from subcategory R65.2 as required by the sequencing rules in the Tabular List. A code from subcategory R65.2 can never be assigned as a principal diagnosis.

When severe sepsis develops during an encounter (it was not present on admission), the underlying systemic infection and the appropriate code from subcategory R65.2 should be assigned as secondary diagnoses.

Severe sepsis may be present on admission, but the diagnosis may not be confirmed until sometime after admission. If the documentation is not clear whether severe sepsis was present on admission, the provider should be queried.

##### 4) Sepsis and severe sepsis with a localized infection

If the reason for admission is both sepsis or severe sepsis and a localized infection, such as pneumonia or cellulitis, a code(s) for the underlying systemic infection should be assigned first and the code for the localized infection should be assigned as a secondary diagnosis. If the patient has severe sepsis, a code from subcategory R65.2 should also be assigned as a secondary diagnosis. If the patient is admitted with a localized infection, such as pneumonia, and sepsis/severe sepsis doesn't develop until after admission, the localized infection should be assigned first, followed by the appropriate sepsis/severe sepsis codes.

Patient presents with acute renal failure due to severe sepsis from *Pseudomonas pneumonia*

| A41.9 | Sepsis, unspecified organism |
|---|---|
| J15.1 | Pneumonia due to Pseudomonas |
| R65.2Ø | Severe sepsis without septic shock |
| N17.9 | Acute kidney failure, unspecified |

*Explanation:* If all conditions are present on admission, the systemic infection (sepsis) is sequenced first followed by the codes for the localized infection (pneumonia), severe sepsis and any organ dysfunction. If only the pneumonia was present on admission with the sepsis and resulting renal failure developing later in the admission, then the pneumonia would be sequenced first.

##### 5) Sepsis due to a postprocedural infection

###### (a) Documentation of causal relationship

As with all postprocedural complications, code assignment is based on the provider's documentation of the relationship between the infection and the procedure.

###### (b) Sepsis due to a postprocedural infection

For such cases, the postprocedural infection code, such as T80.2, Infections following infusion, transfusion, and therapeutic injection, T81.4, Infection following a procedure, T88.Ø, Infection following immunization, or O86.Ø, Infection of obstetric surgical wound, should be coded first, followed by the code for the specific infection. If the patient has severe sepsis, the appropriate code from subcategory R65.2 should also be assigned with the additional code(s) for any acute organ dysfunction.

#### (c) Postprocedural infection and postprocedural septic shock

In cases where a postprocedural infection has occurred and has resulted in severe sepsis the code for the precipitating complication such as code T81.4, Infection following a procedure, or O86.0, Infection of obstetrical surgical wound should be coded first followed by code R65.20, Severe sepsis without septic shock. A code for the systemic infection should also be assigned.

If a postprocedural infection has resulted in postprocedural septic shock, the code for the precipitating complication such as code T81.4, Infection following a procedure, or O86.0, Infection of obstetrical surgical wound should be coded first followed by code T81.12-, Postprocedural septic shock. A code for the systemic infection should also be assigned.

#### 6) Sepsis and severe sepsis associated with a noninfectious process (condition)

In some cases a noninfectious process (condition), such as trauma, may lead to an infection which can result in sepsis or severe sepsis. If sepsis or severe sepsis is documented as associated with a noninfectious condition, such as a burn or serious injury, and this condition meets the definition for principal diagnosis, the code for the noninfectious condition should be sequenced first, followed by the code for the resulting infection. If severe sepsis is present, a code from subcategory R65.2 should also be assigned with any associated organ dysfunction(s) codes. It is not necessary to assign a code from subcategory R65.1, Systemic inflammatory response syndrome (SIRS) of non-infectious origin, for these cases.

If the infection meets the definition of principal diagnosis, it should be sequenced before the non-infectious condition. When both the associated non-infectious condition and the infection meet the definition of principal diagnosis, either may be assigned as principal diagnosis.

Only one code from category R65, Symptoms and signs specifically associated with systemic inflammation and infection, should be assigned. Therefore, when a non-infectious condition leads to an infection resulting in severe sepsis, assign the appropriate code from subcategory R65.2, Severe sepsis. Do not additionally assign a code from subcategory R65.1, Systemic inflammatory response syndrome (SIRS) of non-infectious origin.

*See Section I.C.18. SIRS due to non-infectious process*

---

Patient admitted with multiple third-degree burns of right upper arm develops severe MSSA sepsis with septic shock, three days into admission

**T22.391A**   **Burn of third degree of multiple sites of right shoulder and upper arm limb, except wrist and hand, initial encounter**

**A41.01**   **Sepsis due to Methicillin susceptible Staphylococcus aureus**

**R65.21**   **Severe sepsis with septic shock**

*Explanation:* Severe sepsis is coded rather than SIRS from R65 because it is documented as a severe systemic infectious response with septic shock to a noninfectious condition. The code for the systemic infection is not used as the principal diagnosis because it was not present on admission. The patient was admitted for the burn injury.

---

#### 7) Sepsis and septic shock complicating abortion, pregnancy, childbirth, and the puerperium

*See Section I.C.15. Sepsis and septic shock complicating abortion, pregnancy, childbirth and the puerperium*

#### 8) Newborn sepsis

*See Section I.C.16. f. Bacterial sepsis of Newborn*

### e. Methicillin resistant *Staphylococcus aureus* (MRSA) conditions

#### 1) Selection and sequencing of MRSA codes

##### (a) Combination codes for MRSA infection

When a patient is diagnosed with an infection that is due to methicillin resistant *Staphylococcus aureus* (MRSA), and that infection has a combination code that includes the causal organism (e.g., sepsis, pneumonia) assign the appropriate combination code for the condition (e.g., code A41.02, Sepsis due to Methicillin resistant Staphylococcus aureus or code J15.212, Pneumonia due to Methicillin resistant Staphylococcus aureus). Do not assign code B95.62, Methicillin resistant Staphylococcus aureus infection as the cause of diseases classified elsewhere, as an additional code, because the

combination code includes the type of infection and the MRSA organism. Do not assign a code from subcategory Z16.11, Resistance to penicillins, as an additional diagnosis.

*See Section C.1. for instructions on coding and sequencing of sepsis and severe sepsis.*

##### (b) Other codes for MRSA infection

When there is documentation of a current infection (e.g., wound infection, stitch abscess, urinary tract infection) due to MRSA, and that infection does not have a combination code that includes the causal organism, assign the appropriate code to identify the condition along with code B95.62, Methicillin resistant Staphylococcus aureus infection as the cause of diseases classified elsewhere for the MRSA infection. Do not assign a code from subcategory Z16.11, Resistance to penicillins.

##### (c) Methicillin susceptible Staphylococcus aureus (MSSA) and MRSA colonization

The condition or state of being colonized or carrying MSSA or MRSA is called colonization or carriage, while an individual person is described as being colonized or being a carrier. Colonization means that MSSA or MSRA is present on or in the body without necessarily causing illness. A positive MRSA colonization test might be documented by the provider as "MRSA screen positive" or "MRSA nasal swab positive".

Assign code Z22.322, Carrier or suspected carrier of Methicillin resistant Staphylococcus aureus, for patients documented as having MRSA colonization. Assign code Z22.321, Carrier or suspected carrier of Methicillin susceptible Staphylococcus aureus, for patient documented as having MSSA colonization. Colonization is not necessarily indicative of a disease process or as the cause of a specific condition the patient may have unless documented as such by the provider.

##### (d) MRSA colonization and infection

If a patient is documented as having both MRSA colonization and infection during a hospital admission, code Z22.322, Carrier or suspected carrier of Methicillin resistant Staphylococcus aureus, and a code for the MRSA infection may both be assigned.

### f. Zika virus infections

#### 1) Code only confirmed cases

Code only a confirmed diagnosis of Zika virus (A92.5, Zika virus disease) as documented by the provider. This is an exception to the hospital inpatient guideline Section II, H.

In this context, "confirmation" does not require documentation of the type of test performed; the physician's diagnostic statement that the condition is confirmed is sufficient. This code should be assigned regardless of the stated mode of transmission.

If the provider documents "suspected", "possible" or "probable" Zika, do not assign code A92.5. Assign a code(s) explaining the reason for encounter (such as fever, rash, or joint pain) or Z20.828, Contact with and (suspected) exposure to other viral communicable diseases.

---

A 45-year-old female recently returned from a Caribbean vacation complaining of fever, headache, joint and muscle aches and is admitted for suspected influenza. Infectious Disease consult diagnoses Zika virus. Patient discharged with Zika virus disease and instructions for hydration, rest, acetaminophen, and follow-up with Infectious Disease.

**A92.5**   **Zika virus disease**

*Explanation:* Although only a confirmed diagnosis should be coded, when a provider documents a diagnosis of Zika virus, code A92.5 Zika virus disease, is reported whether or not there is any indication of the type of tests performed. If the patient is pregnant, code first a code from category O98.5- Other viral diseases complicating pregnancy, childbirth and the puerperium, followed by code (A92.5) for the confirmed Zika virus. See also guideline 1.C.15.a.1.

---

# Chapter 1. Certain Infectious and Parasitic Diseases (A00-B99)

**INCLUDES** diseases generally recognized as communicable or transmissible

Use additional code to identify resistance to antimicrobial drugs (Z16.-)

**EXCLUDES 1** certain localized infections—see body system-related chapters

**EXCLUDES 2** carrier or suspected carrier of infectious disease (Z22.-)

infectious and parasitic diseases complicating pregnancy, childbirth and the puerperium (O98.-)

infectious and parasitic diseases specific to the perinatal period (P35-P39)

influenza and other acute respiratory infections (J00-J22)

This chapter contains the following blocks:

A00-A09    Intestinal infectious diseases
A15-A19    Tuberculosis
A20-A28    Certain zoonotic bacterial diseases
A30-A49    Other bacterial diseases
A50-A64    Infections with a predominantly sexual mode of transmission
A65-A69    Other spirochetal diseases
A70-A74    Other diseases caused by chlamydiae
A75-A79    Rickettsioses
A80-A89    Viral infections of the central nervous system
A90-A99    Arthropod-borne viral fevers and viral hemorrhagic fevers
B00-B09    Viral infections characterized by skin and mucous membrane lesions
B10    Other human herpesviruses
B15-B19    Viral hepatitis
B20    Human immunodeficiency virus [HIV] disease
B25-B34    Other viral diseases
B35-B49    Mycoses
B50-B64    Protozoal diseases
B65-B83    Helminthiases
B85-B89    Pediculosis, acariasis and other infestations
B90-B94    Sequelae of infectious and parasitic diseases
B95-B97    Bacterial and viral infectious agents
B99    Other infectious diseases

## Intestinal Infectious Diseases (A00-A09)

### ✓4th A00   Cholera

**CC Excl: For CC codes in category A00:** PDX collection 2

**A00.0   Cholera due to Vibrio cholerae 01, biovar cholerae**   `CC`
Classical cholera

**A00.1   Cholera due to Vibrio cholerae 01, biovar eltor**   `CC`
Cholera eltor

**A00.9   Cholera, unspecified**   `CC`

### ✓4th A01   Typhoid and paratyphoid fevers

**DEF:** Typhoid fever: An acute generalized illness caused by *Salmonella typhi*; clinical features are fever, headache, abdominal pain, cough, toxemia, leukopenia, abnormal pulse, rose spots on the skin, bacteremia, hyperplasia of intestinal lymph nodes, mesenteric lymphadenopathy, and Peyer's patches in the intestines.

**DEF:** Paratyphoid fever: A prolonged febrile illness, caused by *Salmonella* serotypes other than *S. typhi*, especially *S. enterica* serotypes paratyphi A, B, and C.

**CC Excl: For CC codes in category A01:** PDX collection 3

**✓5th A01.0   Typhoid fever**
Infection due to Salmonella typhi

    **A01.00   Typhoid fever, unspecified**   `CC`
    **A01.01   Typhoid meningitis**   `CC`
    **A01.02   Typhoid fever with heart involvement**   `CC`
      Typhoid endocarditis    Typhoid myocarditis
    **A01.03   Typhoid pneumonia**   `CC` `HCC`
    **A01.04   Typhoid arthritis**   `CC` `HCC`
    **A01.05   Typhoid osteomyelitis**   `CC` `HCC`
    **A01.09   Typhoid fever with other complications**   `CC`

**A01.1   Paratyphoid fever A**   `CC`
**A01.2   Paratyphoid fever B**   `CC`
**A01.3   Paratyphoid fever C**   `CC`
**A01.4   Paratyphoid fever, unspecified**   `CC`
    Infection due to Salmonella paratyphi NOS

### ✓4th A02   Other salmonella infections

**INCLUDES** infection or foodborne intoxication due to any Salmonella species other than S. typhi and S. paratyphi

**A02.0   Salmonella enteritis**   `CC`
Salmonellosis
**CC Excl:** PDX collection 4

**A02.1   Salmonella sepsis**   `HIV` `MCC` `HCC`
**CC Excl:** PDX collection 5

### ✓5th A02.2   Localized salmonella infections

    **A02.20   Localized salmonella infection, unspecified**   `HIV`
    **A02.21   Salmonella meningitis**   `HIV` `MCC`
      **CC Excl:** PDX collection 6
    **A02.22   Salmonella pneumonia**   `HIV` `MCC` `HCC`
      **CC Excl:** PDX collection 7
    **A02.23   Salmonella arthritis**   `HIV` `CC` `HCC`
      **CC Excl:** PDX collection 8
    **A02.24   Salmonella osteomyelitis**   `HIV` `CC` `HCC`
      **CC Excl:** PDX collection 9
    **A02.25   Salmonella pyelonephritis**   `HIV` `CC`
      Salmonella tubulo-interstitial nephropathy
      **CC Excl:** PDX collection 10
    **A02.29   Salmonella with other localized infection**   `HIV` `CC`
      **CC Excl:** PDX collection 10

**A02.8   Other specified salmonella infections**   `HIV` `CC`
    **CC Excl:** PDX collection 11

**A02.9   Salmonella infection, unspecified**   `HIV` `CC`
    **CC Excl:** PDX collection 12

### ✓4th A03   Shigellosis

**DEF:** Infection caused by the genus *Shigella*, of the family *Enterobacteriaceae*; known to cause an acute dysenteric infection of the bowel with fever, drowsiness, anorexia, nausea, vomiting, bloody diarrhea, abdominal cramps, and distention.

**A03.0   Shigellosis due to Shigella dysenteriae**   `CC`
    Group A shigellosis [Shiga-Kruse dysentery]
    **CC Excl:** PDX collection 13

**A03.1   Shigellosis due to Shigella flexneri**
    Group B shigellosis

**A03.2   Shigellosis due to Shigella boydii**
    Group C shigellosis

**A03.3   Shigellosis due to Shigella sonnei**
    Group D shigellosis

**A03.8   Other shigellosis**

**A03.9   Shigellosis, unspecified**
    Bacillary dysentery NOS

### ✓4th A04   Other bacterial intestinal infections

**EXCLUDES 1** bacterial foodborne intoxications, NEC (A05.-)
tuberculous enteritis (A18.32)

**CC Excl: For CC codes in category A04, unless otherwise noted:**
**For codes A04.0-A04.4:** PDX collection 14
**For codes A04.5-A04.8:** PDX collection 15

**A04.0   Enteropathogenic Escherichia coli infection**   `CC`
**A04.1   Enterotoxigenic Escherichia coli infection**   `CC`
**A04.2   Enteroinvasive Escherichia coli infection**   `CC`
**A04.3   Enterohemorrhagic Escherichia coli infection**   `CC`
    **DEF:** *E. coli* infection penetrating the intestinal mucosa, producing microscopic ulceration and bleeding.
**A04.4   Other intestinal Escherichia coli infections**   `CC`
    Escherichia coli enteritis NOS
**A04.5   Campylobacter enteritis**   `CC`
**A04.6   Enteritis due to Yersinia enterocolitica**   `CC`
    **EXCLUDES 1** extraintestinal yersiniosis (A28.2)

**✓5th A04.7   Enterocolitis due to Clostridium difficile**
    Foodborne intoxication by Clostridium difficile
    Pseudomembranous colitis

 •     **A04.71   Enterocolitis due to Clostridium difficile, recurrent**   `CC`

 •     **A04.72   Enterocolitis due to Clostridium difficile, not specified as recurrent**   `CC`

**A04.8   Other specified bacterial intestinal infections**   `CC`
**A04.9   Bacterial intestinal infection, unspecified**   `CC`
    Bacterial enteritis NOS
    **CC Excl:** PDX collection 16

### ✓4th A05   Other bacterial foodborne intoxications, not elsewhere classified

**EXCLUDES 1** Clostridium difficile foodborne intoxication and infection ►(A04.7-)◄
Escherichia coli infection (A04.0-A04.4)
listeriosis (A32.-)
salmonella foodborne intoxication and infection (A02.-)
toxic effect of noxious foodstuffs (T61-T62)

**A05.0   Foodborne staphylococcal intoxication**   `CC`
    **CC Excl:** PDX collection 17

N Newborn: 0   P Pediatric: 0-17   M Maternity: 12-55   A Adult: 15-124   MCC Major CC Condition   PDxMCC PDx acts as own MCC   CC CC Condition   PDxCC PDx acts as own CC

**436**                                          ICD-10-CM 2018

**A05.1**　**Botulism food poisoning**　`CC`
　　Botulism NOS
　　Classical foodborne intoxication due to Clostridium botulinum
　　*EXCLUDES 1*　infant botulism (A48.51)
　　　　　　wound botulism (A48.52)
　　**CC Excl:** PDX collection 18

**A05.2**　**Foodborne Clostridium perfringens [Clostridium welchii] intoxication**　`CC`
　　Enteritis necroticans
　　Pig-bel
　　**CC Excl:** PDX collection 19

**A05.3**　**Foodborne Vibrio parahaemolyticus intoxication**　`CC`
　　**CC Excl:** PDX collection 17

**A05.4**　**Foodborne Bacillus cereus intoxication**　`CC`
　　**CC Excl:** PDX collection 17

**A05.5**　**Foodborne Vibrio vulnificus intoxication**　`CC`
　　**CC Excl:** PDX collection 17

**A05.8**　**Other specified bacterial foodborne intoxications**　`CC`
　　**CC Excl:** PDX collection 17

**A05.9**　**Bacterial foodborne intoxication, unspecified**

**✓4ᵗʰ A06**　**Amebiasis**
　　`INCLUDES`　infection due to Entamoeba histolytica
　　*EXCLUDES 1*　other protozoal intestinal diseases (A07.-)
　　*EXCLUDES 2*　acanthamebiasis (B60.1-)
　　　　　　Naegleriasis (B60.2)

**A06.0**　**Acute amebic dysentery**　`CC`
　　Acute amebiasis
　　Intestinal amebiasis NOS
　　**CC Excl:** PDX collection 20

**A06.1**　**Chronic intestinal amebiasis**　`CC`
　　**CC Excl:** PDX collection 20

**A06.2**　**Amebic nondysenteric colitis**　`CC`
　　**CC Excl:** PDX collection 21

**A06.3**　**Ameboma of intestine**　`CC`
　　Ameboma NOS
　　**CC Excl:** PDX collection 22

**A06.4**　**Amebic liver abscess**　`MCC`
　　Hepatic amebiasis
　　**CC Excl:** PDX collection 23

**A06.5**　**Amebic lung abscess**　`MCC` `HCC`
　　Amebic abscess of lung (and liver)
　　**CC Excl:** PDX collection 24

**A06.6**　**Amebic brain abscess**　`MCC`
　　Amebic abscess of brain (and liver) (and lung)
　　**CC Excl:** PDX collection 25

**A06.7**　**Cutaneous amebiasis**

**✓5ᵗʰ A06.8**　**Amebic infection of other sites**

　　**CC Excl: For CC codes in subcategory A06.8:**
　　**PDX collection 22**

　　**A06.81**　**Amebic cystitis**　`CC`

　　**A06.82**　**Other amebic genitourinary infections**　`CC`
　　　　Amebic balanitis
　　　　Amebic vesiculitis
　　　　Amebic vulvovaginitis

　　**A06.89**　**Other amebic infections**　`CC`
　　　　Amebic appendicitis
　　　　Amebic splenic abscess

**A06.9**　**Amebiasis, unspecified**

**✓4ᵗʰ A07**　**Other protozoal intestinal diseases**

　　**CC Excl: For CC codes in category A07, unless otherwise noted:**
　　**PDX collection 26**

**A07.0**　**Balantidiasis**
　　Balantidial dysentery

**A07.1**　**Giardiasis [lambliasis]**　`CC`

**A07.2**　**Cryptosporidiosis**　`CC` `HCC`

**A07.3**　**Isosporiasis**　`HIV` `CC`
　　Infection due to Isospora belli and Isospora hominis
　　Intestinal coccidiosis
　　Isosporosis

**A07.4**　**Cyclosporiasis**　`CC`
　　**CC Excl:** PDX collection 27

**A07.8**　**Other specified protozoal intestinal diseases**　`CC`
　　Intestinal microsporidiosis　Sarcocystosis
　　Intestinal trichomoniasis　Sarcosporidiosis

**A07.9**　**Protozoal intestinal disease, unspecified**　`CC`
　　Flagellate diarrhea　　Protozoal diarrhea
　　Protozoal colitis　　Protozoal dysentery

**✓4ᵗʰ A08**　**Viral and other specified intestinal infections**
　　*EXCLUDES 1*　influenza with involvement of gastrointestinal tract (J09.X3, J10.2, J11.2)

　　**CC Excl: For CC codes in category A08:** PDX collection 28

**A08.0**　**Rotaviral enteritis**　`CC`

**✓5ᵗʰ A08.1**　**Acute gastroenteropathy due to Norwalk agent and other small round viruses**

　　**A08.11**　**Acute gastroenteropathy due to Norwalk agent**　`CC`
　　　　Acute gastroenteropathy due to Norovirus
　　　　Acute gastroenteropathy due to Norwalk-like agent

　　**A08.19**　**Acute gastroenteropathy due to other small round viruses**　`CC`
　　　　Acute gastroenteropathy due to small round virus [SRV] NOS

**A08.2**　**Adenoviral enteritis**　`CC`

**✓5ᵗʰ A08.3**　**Other viral enteritis**

　　**A08.31**　**Calicivirus enteritis**　`CC`

　　**A08.32**　**Astrovirus enteritis**　`CC`

　　**A08.39**　**Other viral enteritis**　`CC`
　　　　Coxsackie virus enteritis
　　　　Echovirus enteritis
　　　　Enterovirus enteritis NEC
　　　　Torovirus enteritis

**A08.4**　**Viral intestinal infection, unspecified**
　　Viral enteritis NOS　　Viral gastroenteropathy NOS
　　Viral gastroenteritis NOS
　　**AHA:** 2016, 3Q, 12

**A08.8**　**Other specified intestinal infections**

**A09**　**Infectious gastroenteritis and colitis, unspecified**　`CC`
　　Infectious colitis NOS
　　Infectious enteritis NOS
　　Infectious gastroenteritis NOS
　　*EXCLUDES 1*　colitis NOS (K52.9)
　　　　　diarrhea NOS (R19.7)
　　　　　enteritis NOS (K52.9)
　　　　　gastroenteritis NOS (K52.9)
　　　　　noninfective gastroenteritis and colitis, unspecified (K52.9)
　　**DEF:** Colitis: An inflammation of mucous membranes of the colon.
　　**DEF:** Enteritis: An inflammation of mucous membranes of the small intestine.
　　**DEF:** Gastroenteritis: An inflammation of mucous membranes of stomach and intestines.
　　**CC Excl:** PDX collection 17

### Tuberculosis (A15-A19)

　　`INCLUDES`　infections due to Mycobacterium tuberculosis and Mycobacterium bovis
　　*EXCLUDES 1*　congenital tuberculosis (P37.0)
　　　　nonspecific reaction to test for tuberculosis without active tuberculosis (R76.1-)
　　　　pneumoconiosis associated with tuberculosis, any type in A15 (J65)
　　　　positive PPD (R76.11)
　　　　positive tuberculin skin test without active tuberculosis (R76.11)
　　　　sequelae of tuberculosis (B90.-)
　　　　silicotuberculosis (J65)

**✓4ᵗʰ A15**　**Respiratory tuberculosis**

**A15.0**　**Tuberculosis of lung**　`HIV` `CC`
　　Tuberculous bronchiectasis
　　Tuberculous fibrosis of lung
　　Tuberculous pneumonia
　　Tuberculous pneumothorax
　　**CC Excl:** PDX collection 29

**A15.4**　**Tuberculosis of intrathoracic lymph nodes**　`HIV` `CC`
　　Tuberculosis of hilar lymph nodes
　　Tuberculosis of mediastinal lymph nodes
　　Tuberculosis of tracheobronchial lymph nodes
　　*EXCLUDES 1*　tuberculosis specified as primary (A15.7)
　　**CC Excl:** PDX collection 29

✔Additional Character Req　✔7ᵗʰ Placeholder Alert　Unacceptable PDx　Manifestation　`H1`-`H14` HAC　`HCC` CMS-HCC Condition　*EXCLUDES 1* Not Coded Here　*EXCLUDES 2* Not Included Here

ICD-10-CM 2018　　　　437

**Tuberculosis of Lung**

Granulomas from Mycobacterium tuberculosis

**A15.5 Tuberculosis of larynx, trachea and bronchus** `HIV` `CC`
　　Tuberculosis of bronchus
　　Tuberculosis of glottis
　　Tuberculosis of larynx
　　Tuberculosis of trachea
　　**CC Excl:** PDX collection 29

**A15.6 Tuberculous pleurisy** `HIV` `CC`
　　Tuberculosis of pleura Tuberculous empyema
　　*EXCLUDES 1* 　primary respiratory tuberculosis (A15.7)
　　**CC Excl:** PDX collection 29

**A15.7 Primary respiratory tuberculosis** `HIV` `CC`
　　**CC Excl:** PDX collection 30

**A15.8 Other respiratory tuberculosis** `HIV` `CC`
　　Mediastinal tuberculosis
　　Nasopharyngeal tuberculosis
　　Tuberculosis of nose
　　Tuberculosis of sinus [any nasal]
　　**CC Excl:** PDX collection 31

**A15.9 Respiratory tuberculosis unspecified** `HIV` `CC`
　　**CC Excl:** PDX collection 31

**✓4ᵗʰ A17 Tuberculosis of nervous system**

　**A17.0 Tuberculous meningitis** `HIV` `MCC`
　　　Tuberculosis of meninges (cerebral)(spinal)
　　　Tuberculous leptomeningitis
　　　*EXCLUDES 1* 　tuberculous meningoencephalitis (A17.82)
　　　**CC Excl:** PDX collection 32

　**A17.1 Meningeal tuberculoma** `HIV` `MCC`
　　　Tuberculoma of meninges (cerebral) (spinal)
　　　*EXCLUDES 2* 　tuberculoma of brain and spinal cord (A17.81)
　　　**CC Excl:** PDX collection 32

　**✓5ᵗʰ A17.8 Other tuberculosis of nervous system**

　　　**A17.81 Tuberculoma of brain and spinal cord** `HIV` `MCC`
　　　　　Tuberculous abscess of brain and spinal cord
　　　　　**CC Excl:** PDX collection 33

　　　**A17.82 Tuberculous meningoencephalitis** `HIV` `MCC`
　　　　　Tuberculous myelitis
　　　　　**CC Excl:** PDX collection 33

　　　**A17.83 Tuberculous neuritis** `HIV` `MCC`
　　　　　Tuberculous mononeuropathy
　　　　　**CC Excl:** No Excl

　　　**A17.89 Other tuberculosis of nervous system** `HIV` `MCC`
　　　　　Tuberculous polyneuropathy
　　　　　**CC Excl:** PDX collection 34

　**A17.9 Tuberculosis of nervous system, unspecified** `HIV` `CC`
　　　**CC Excl:** PDX collection 35

**✓4ᵗʰ A18 Tuberculosis of other organs**

　**✓5ᵗʰ A18.0 Tuberculosis of bones and joints**

　　　**A18.01 Tuberculosis of spine** `HIV` `CC`
　　　　　Pott's disease or curvature of spine
　　　　　Tuberculous arthritis
　　　　　Tuberculous osteomyelitis of spine
　　　　　Tuberculous spondylitis
　　　　　**CC Excl:** PDX collection 36

　　　**A18.02 Tuberculous arthritis of other joints** `HIV` `CC`
　　　　　Tuberculosis of hip (joint)
　　　　　Tuberculosis of knee (joint)
　　　　　**CC Excl:** PDX collection 37

　　　**A18.03 Tuberculosis of other bones** `HIV` `CC`
　　　　　Tuberculous mastoiditis
　　　　　Tuberculous osteomyelitis
　　　　　**CC Excl:** PDX collection 38

　　　**A18.09 Other musculoskeletal tuberculosis** `HIV` `CC`
　　　　　Tuberculous myositis
　　　　　Tuberculous synovitis
　　　　　Tuberculous tenosynovitis
　　　　　**CC Excl:** PDX collection 39

　**✓5ᵗʰ A18.1 Tuberculosis of genitourinary system**

　　　**A18.10 Tuberculosis of genitourinary system, unspecified** `HIV` `CC`
　　　　　**CC Excl:** PDX collection 40

　　　**A18.11 Tuberculosis of kidney and ureter** `HIV` `CC`
　　　　　**CC Excl:** PDX collection 41

　　　**A18.12 Tuberculosis of bladder** `HIV` `CC`
　　　　　**CC Excl:** PDX collection 41

　　　**A18.13 Tuberculosis of other urinary organs** `HIV` `CC`
　　　　　Tuberculous urethritis
　　　　　**CC Excl:** PDX collection 41

　　　**A18.14 Tuberculosis of prostate** `HIV` `CC` `A` ♂
　　　　　**CC Excl:** PDX collection 42

　　　**A18.15 Tuberculosis of other male genital organs** `HIV` `CC` ♂
　　　　　**CC Excl:** PDX collection 42

　　　**A18.16 Tuberculosis of cervix** `HIV` `CC` ♀
　　　　　**CC Excl:** PDX collection 43

　　　**A18.17 Tuberculous female pelvic inflammatory disease** `HIV` `CC` ♀
　　　　　Tuberculous endometritis
　　　　　Tuberculous oophoritis and salpingitis
　　　　　**CC Excl:** PDX collection 43

　　　**A18.18 Tuberculosis of other female genital organs** `HIV` `CC` ♀
　　　　　Tuberculous ulceration of vulva
　　　　　**CC Excl:** PDX collection 43

　**A18.2 Tuberculous peripheral lymphadenopathy** `HIV` `CC`
　　　Tuberculous adenitis
　　　*EXCLUDES 2* 　tuberculosis of bronchial and mediastinal lymph nodes (A15.4)
　　　　　tuberculosis of mesenteric and retroperitoneal lymph nodes (A18.39)
　　　　　tuberculous tracheobronchial adenopathy (A15.4)
　　　**CC Excl:** PDX collection 44

　**✓5ᵗʰ A18.3 Tuberculosis of intestines, peritoneum and mesenteric glands**

　　　**CC Excl: For CC/MCC codes in subcategory A18.3, unless otherwise noted:** PDX collection 45

　　　**A18.31 Tuberculous peritonitis** `HIV` `MCC`
　　　　　Tuberculous ascites
　　　　　**DEF:** Tuberculous inflammation of the membrane lining the abdomen.

　　　**A18.32 Tuberculous enteritis** `HIV` `CC`
　　　　　Tuberculosis of anus and rectum
　　　　　Tuberculosis of intestine (large) (small)

　　　**A18.39 Retroperitoneal tuberculosis** `HIV` `CC`
　　　　　Tuberculosis of mesenteric glands
　　　　　Tuberculosis of retroperitoneal (lymph glands)

　**A18.4 Tuberculosis of skin and subcutaneous tissue** `HIV` `CC`
　　　Erythema induratum, tuberculous
　　　Lupus excedens
　　　Lupus vulgaris NOS
　　　Lupus vulgaris of eyelid
　　　Scrofuloderma
　　　Tuberculosis of external ear
　　　*EXCLUDES 2* 　lupus erythematosus (L93.-)
　　　　　lupus NOS (M32.9)
　　　　　systemic (M32.-)
　　　**CC Excl:** PDX collection 30

　**✓5ᵗʰ A18.5 Tuberculosis of eye**
　　　*EXCLUDES 2* 　lupus vulgaris of eyelid (A18.4)

　　　**CC Excl: For CC codes in subcategory A18.5, unless otherwise noted:** PDX collection 46

　　　**A18.50 Tuberculosis of eye, unspecified** `HIV` `CC`
　　　**A18.51 Tuberculous episcleritis** `HIV` `CC`
　　　**A18.52 Tuberculous keratitis** `HIV` `CC`
　　　　　Tuberculous interstitial keratitis
　　　　　Tuberculous keratoconjunctivitis (interstitial) (phlyctenular)

　　　**A18.53 Tuberculous chorioretinitis** `HIV` `CC`
　　　**A18.54 Tuberculous iridocyclitis** `HIV` `CC`

`N` Newborn: 0　`P` Pediatric: 0-17　`M` Maternity: 12-55　`A` Adult: 15-124　`MCC` Major CC Condition　`PDxMCC` PDx acts as own MCC　`CC` CC Condition　`PDxCC` PDx acts as own CC

**438**　　　　ICD-10-CM 2018

      **A18.59**  **Other tuberculosis of eye**   `HIV` `CC`
          Tuberculous conjunctivitis

**A18.6**  **Tuberculosis of (inner) (middle) ear**   `HIV` `CC`
    Tuberculous otitis media
    *EXCLUDES 2*  tuberculosis of external ear (A18.4)
                tuberculous mastoiditis (A18.03)
    **CC Excl:** PDX collection 47

**A18.7**  **Tuberculosis of adrenal glands**   `HIV` `CC`
    Tuberculous Addison's disease
    **CC Excl:** PDX collection 48

✓5ᵗʰ **A18.8**  **Tuberculosis of other specified organs**

      **A18.81**  **Tuberculosis of thyroid gland**   `HIV` `CC`
          **CC Excl:** PDX collection 49

      **A18.82**  **Tuberculosis of other endocrine glands**   `HIV` `CC`
          Tuberculosis of pituitary gland
          Tuberculosis of thymus gland
          **CC Excl:** PDX collection 35

      **A18.83**  **Tuberculosis of digestive tract organs, not elsewhere classified**   `HIV` `CC`
          *EXCLUDES 1*  tuberculosis of intestine (A18.32)
          **CC Excl:** PDX collection 45

      **A18.84**  **Tuberculosis of heart**   `HIV` `CC`
          Tuberculous cardiomyopathy
          Tuberculous endocarditis
          Tuberculous myocarditis
          Tuberculous pericarditis
          **CC Excl:** PDX collection 35

      **A18.85**  **Tuberculosis of spleen**   `HIV` `CC`
          **CC Excl:** PDX collection 50

      **A18.89**  **Tuberculosis of other sites**   `HIV` `CC`
          Tuberculosis of muscle
          Tuberculous cerebral arteritis
          **CC Excl:** PDX collection 35

✓4ᵗʰ **A19**  **Miliary tuberculosis**
    INCLUDES  disseminated tuberculosis
              generalized tuberculosis
              tuberculous polyserositis

    **CC Excl: For MCC codes in category A19:** PDX collection 51

**A19.0**  **Acute miliary tuberculosis of a single specified site**   `HIV` `MCC`

**A19.1**  **Acute miliary tuberculosis of multiple sites**   `HIV` `MCC`

**A19.2**  **Acute miliary tuberculosis, unspecified**   `HIV` `MCC`

**A19.8**  **Other miliary tuberculosis**   `HIV` `MCC`

**A19.9**  **Miliary tuberculosis, unspecified**   `HIV` `MCC`

## Certain zoonotic bacterial diseases (A20-A28)

✓4ᵗʰ **A20**  **Plague**
    INCLUDES  infection due to Yersinia pestis

**A20.0**  **Bubonic plague**   `MCC`
    **CC Excl:** PDX collection 52

**A20.1**  **Cellulocutaneous plague**   `MCC`
    **CC Excl:** PDX collection 52

**A20.2**  **Pneumonic plague**   `MCC` `HCC`
    **CC Excl:** PDX collection 53

**A20.3**  **Plague meningitis**   `MCC`
    **CC Excl:** PDX collection 54

**A20.7**  **Septicemic plague**   `MCC` `HCC`
    **CC Excl:** PDX collection 55

**A20.8**  **Other forms of plague**   `MCC`
    Abortive plague
    Asymptomatic plague
    Pestis minor
    **CC Excl:** PDX collection 54

**A20.9**  **Plague, unspecified**   `MCC`
    **CC Excl:** PDX collection 56

✓4ᵗʰ **A21**  **Tularemia**
    INCLUDES  deer-fly fever
              infection due to Francisella tularensis
              rabbit fever
    **DEF:** A febrile disease transmitted to humans by the bites of deer flies, fleas, and ticks; by inhaling aerosolized *F. tularensis*; or by ingesting contaminated food or water. Patients quickly develop fever, chills, weakness, headache, backache, and malaise.

**A21.0**  **Ulceroglandular tularemia**   `CC`
    **CC Excl:** PDX collection 57

**A21.1**  **Oculoglandular tularemia**   `CC`
    Ophthalmic tularemia
    **CC Excl:** PDX collection 58

**A21.2**  **Pulmonary tularemia**   `CC` `HCC`
    **CC Excl:** PDX collection 59

**A21.3**  **Gastrointestinal tularemia**   `CC`
    Abdominal tularemia
    **CC Excl:** PDX collection 60

**A21.7**  **Generalized tularemia**   `CC`
    **CC Excl:** PDX collection 61

**A21.8**  **Other forms of tularemia**   `CC`
    **CC Excl:** PDX collection 61

**A21.9**  **Tulamirea, unspecified**   `CC`
    **CC Excl:** PDX collection 61

✓4ᵗʰ **A22**  **Anthrax**
    INCLUDES  infection due to Bacillus anthracis

**A22.0**  **Cutaneous anthrax**   `CC`
    Malignant carbuncle
    Malignant pustule
    **CC Excl:** PDX collection 62

**A22.1**  **Pulmonary anthrax**   `MCC` `HCC`
    Inhalation anthrax
    Ragpicker's disease
    Woolsorter's disease
    **CC Excl:** PDX collection 63

**A22.2**  **Gastrointestinal anthrax**   `CC`
    **CC Excl:** PDX collection 64

**A22.7**  **Anthrax sepsis**   `PDxMCC` `MCC` `HCC`
    **CC Excl:** PDX collection 5

**A22.8**  **Other forms of anthrax**   `CC`
    Anthrax meningitis
    **CC Excl:** PDX collection 65

**A22.9**  **Anthrax, unspecified**   `CC`
    **CC Excl:** PDX collection 66

✓4ᵗʰ **A23**  **Brucellosis**
    INCLUDES  Malta fever
              Mediterranean fever
              undulant fever

**A23.0**  **Brucellosis due to Brucella melitensis**

**A23.1**  **Brucellosis due to Brucella abortus**

**A23.2**  **Brucellosis due to Brucella suis**

**A23.3**  **Brucellosis due to Brucella canis**

**A23.8**  **Other brucellosis**   `CC`
    **CC Excl:** PDX collection 67

**A23.9**  **Brucellosis, unspecified**   `CC`
    **CC Excl:** PDX collection 67

✓4ᵗʰ **A24**  **Glanders and melioidosis**

    **CC Excl: For CC codes in category A24, unless otherwise noted:** PDX collection 69

**A24.0**  **Glanders**   `CC`
    Infection due to Pseudomonas mallei
    Malleus
    **CC Excl:** PDX collection 68

**A24.1**  **Acute and fulminating melioidosis**   `CC`
    Melioidosis pneumonia
    Melioidosis sepsis

**A24.2**  **Subacute and chronic melioidosis**   `CC`

**A24.3**  **Other melioidosis**   `CC`

**A24.9**  **Melioidosis, unspecified**   `CC`
    Infection due to Pseudomonas pseudomallei NOS
    Whitmore's disease

✓4ᵗʰ **A25**  **Rat-bite fevers**

    **CC Excl: For CC codes in category A25, unless otherwise noted:** PDX collection 70

**A25.0**  **Spirillosis**   `CC`
    Sodoku

**A25.1**  **Streptobacillosis**   `CC`
    Epidemic arthritic erythema     Streptobacillary rat-bite fever
    Haverhill fever

**A25.9**  **Rat-bite fever, unspecified**   `CC`

✓4ᵗʰ **A26**  **Erysipeloid**

**A26.0**  **Cutaneous erysipeloid**
    Erythema migrans

**A26.7**  **Erysipelothrix sepsis**   `PDxMCC` `MCC` `HCC`
    **CC Excl:** PDX collection 71

**A26.8**  **Other forms of erysipeloid**

**A26.9**  **Erysipeloid, unspecified**

---

✓ Additional Character Req   ✓×7ᵗʰ Placeholder Alert   Unacceptable PDx   Manifestation   `H1`-`H14` HAC   `HCC` CMS-HCC Condition   *EXCLUDES 1* Not Coded Here   *EXCLUDES 2* Not Included Here

ICD-10-CM 2018         **439**

A18.59–A26.9

Chapter 1. Certain Infectious and Parasitic Diseases

A27–A37.81

## ✓4ᵗʰ A27 Leptospirosis

**CC Excl:** For CC codes in category A27, unless otherwise noted:
PDX collection 72

**A27.0 Leptospirosis icterohemorrhagica** `CC`
Leptospiral or spirochetal jaundice (hemorrhagic)
Weil's disease

✓5ᵗʰ **A27.8 Other forms of leptospirosis**
**A27.81 Aseptic meningitis in leptospirosis** `MCC`
**CC Excl:** PDX collection 73

**A27.89 Other forms of leptospirosis** `CC`

**A27.9 Leptospirosis, unspecified** `CC`

## ✓4ᵗʰ A28 Other zoonotic bacterial diseases, not elsewhere classified

**CC Excl:** For CC codes in category A28, unless otherwise noted:
PDX collection 74

**A28.0 Pasteurellosis** `CC`

**A28.1 Cat-scratch disease** `CC`
Cat-scratch fever
**CC Excl:** PDX collection 75

**A28.2 Extraintestinal yersiniosis** `CC`
*EXCLUDES 1* enteritis due to Yersinia enterocolitica (A04.6)
plague (A20.-)

**A28.8 Other specified zoonotic bacterial diseases, not elsewhere classified** `CC`

**A28.9 Zoonotic bacterial disease, unspecified** `CC`

### Other bacterial diseases (A30-A49)
**AHA:** 2016, 3Q, 8-14

## ✓4ᵗʰ A30 Leprosy [Hansen's disease]
*INCLUDES* infection due to Mycobacterium leprae
*EXCLUDES 1* sequelae of leprosy (B92)

**A30.0 Indeterminate leprosy** `CC`
I leprosy
**CC Excl:** PDX collection 76

**A30.1 Tuberculoid leprosy** `CC`
TT leprosy
**CC Excl:** PDX collection 77

**A30.2 Borderline tuberculoid leprosy** `CC`
BT leprosy
**CC Excl:** PDX collection 78

**A30.3 Borderline leprosy** `CC`
BB leprosy
**CC Excl:** PDX collection 78

**A30.4 Borderline lepromatous leprosy** `CC`
BL leprosy
**CC Excl:** PDX collection 78

**A30.5 Lepromatous leprosy** `CC`
LL leprosy
**CC Excl:** PDX collection 79

**A30.8 Other forms of leprosy** `CC`
**CC Excl:** PDX collection 80

**A30.9 Leprosy, unspecified** `CC`
**CC Excl:** PDX collection 81

## ✓4ᵗʰ A31 Infection due to other mycobacteria
*EXCLUDES 2* leprosy (A30.-)
tuberculosis (A15-A19)

**CC Excl:** For CC codes in category A31, unless otherwise noted:
PDX collection 83

**A31.0 Pulmonary mycobacterial infection** `CC` `HCC`
Infection due to Mycobacterium avium
Infection due to Mycobacterium intracellulare [Battey bacillus]
Infection due to Mycobacterium kansasii
**CC Excl:** PDX collection 82

**A31.1 Cutaneous mycobacterial infection** `CC`
Buruli ulcer
Infection due to Mycobacterium marinum
Infection due to Mycobacterium ulcerans

**A31.2 Disseminated mycobacterium avium-intracellulare complex (DMAC)** `HIV` `CC` `HCC`
MAC sepsis

**A31.8 Other mycobacterial infections** `HIV` `CC`

**A31.9 Mycobacterial infection, unspecified** `HIV` `CC`
Atypical mycobacterial infection NOS
Mycobacteriosis NOS

## ✓4ᵗʰ A32 Listeriosis
*INCLUDES* listerial foodborne infection
*EXCLUDES 1* neonatal (disseminated) listeriosis (P37.2)

**CC Excl:** For CC codes in category A32, unless otherwise noted:
PDX collection 74

**A32.0 Cutaneous listeriosis** `CC`

✓5ᵗʰ **A32.1 Listerial meningitis and meningoencephalitis**
**A32.11 Listerial meningitis** `CC`
**A32.12 Listerial meningoencephalitis** `CC`

**A32.7 Listerial sepsis** `PDxMCC` `MCC` `HCC`
**CC Excl:** PDX collection 71

✓5ᵗʰ **A32.8 Other forms of listeriosis**
**A32.81 Oculoglandular listeriosis** `CC`
**A32.82 Listerial endocarditis** `CC`
**A32.89 Other forms of listeriosis** `CC`
Listerial cerebral arteritis

**A32.9 Listeriosis, unspecified** `CC`

## A33 Tetanus neonatorum `MCC` `N`
**CC Excl:** PDX collection 84

## A34 Obstetrical tetanus `CC` `M` `♀`
**CC Excl:** PDX collection 85

## A35 Other tetanus `MCC`
Tetanus NOS
*EXCLUDES 1* obstetrical tetanus (A34)
tetanus neonatorum (A33)
**CC Excl:** PDX collection 86

## ✓4ᵗʰ A36 Diphtheria

**CC Excl:** For CC codes in category A36, unless otherwise noted:
PDX collection 87

**A36.0 Pharyngeal diphtheria** `CC`
Diphtheritic membranous angina
Tonsillar diphtheria

**A36.1 Nasopharyngeal diphtheria** `CC`

**A36.2 Laryngeal diphtheria** `CC`
Diphtheritic laryngotracheitis

**A36.3 Cutaneous diphtheria** `CC`
*EXCLUDES 2* erythrasma (L08.1)

✓5ᵗʰ **A36.8 Other diphtheria**
**A36.81 Diphtheritic cardiomyopathy** `CC` `HCC`
Diphtheritic myocarditis
**CC Excl:** PDX collection 88

**A36.82 Diphtheritic radiculomyelitis** `CC`
**A36.83 Diphtheritic polyneuritis** `CC`
**A36.84 Diphtheritic tubulo-interstitial nephropathy** `CC`
**A36.85 Diphtheritic cystitis** `CC`
**A36.86 Diphtheritic conjunctivitis** `CC`
**A36.89 Other diphtheritic complications** `CC`
Diphtheritic peritonitis

**A36.9 Diphtheria, unspecified** `CC`

## ✓4ᵗʰ A37 Whooping cough

**CC Excl:** For CC codes in category A37, unless otherwise noted:
PDX collection 89
For MCC codes in category A37, unless otherwise noted:
PDX collection 90

✓5ᵗʰ **A37.0 Whooping cough due to Bordetella pertussis**
**A37.00 Whooping cough due to Bordetella pertussis without pneumonia** `CC`
**A37.01 Whooping cough due to Bordetella pertussis with pneumonia** `PDxMCC` `MCC`

✓5ᵗʰ **A37.1 Whooping cough due to Bordetella parapertussis**
**A37.10 Whooping cough due to Bordetella parapertussis without pneumonia** `CC`
**A37.11 Whooping cough due to Bordetella parapertussis with pneumonia** `PDxMCC` `MCC`

✓5ᵗʰ **A37.8 Whooping cough due to other Bordetella species**
**A37.80 Whooping cough due to other Bordetella species without pneumonia** `CC`
**A37.81 Whooping cough due to other Bordetella species with pneumonia** `PDxMCC` `MCC`

`N` Newborn: 0   `P` Pediatric: 0-17   `M` Maternity: 12-55   `A` Adult: 15-124   `MCC` Major CC Condition   `PDxMCC` PDx acts as own MCC   `CC` CC Condition   `PDxCC` PDx acts as own CC

440

ICD-10-CM 2018

✓5ᵗʰ **A37.9 Whooping cough, unspecified species**

     **A37.90 Whooping cough, unspecified species** without `CC` pneumonia

     **A37.91 Whooping cough, unspecified species** `PDxMCC` `MCC` with pneumonia

✓4ᵗʰ **A38 Scarlet fever**

     `INCLUDES` scarlatina

     `EXCLUDES 2` streptococcal sore throat (J02.0)

     **CC Excl: For CC codes in category A38:** PDX collection 91

     **A38.0 Scarlet fever with** otitis media `CC`

     **A38.1 Scarlet fever with** myocarditis `CC`

     **A38.8 Scarlet fever with** other complications `CC`

     **A38.9 Scarlet fever,** uncomplicated `CC`
         Scarlet fever, NOS

✓4ᵗʰ **A39 Meningococcal infection**

     **A39.0 Meningococcal** meningitis `MCC`
         **CC Excl:** PDX collection 92

     **A39.1 Waterhouse-Friderichsen syndrome** `MCC` `HCC`
         Meningococcal hemorrhagic adrenalitis
         Meningococcic adrenal syndrome
         **CC Excl:** PDX collection 93

     **A39.2 Acute meningococcemia** `MCC` `HCC`
         **CC Excl:** PDX collection 94

     **A39.3 Chronic meningococcemia** `MCC` `HCC`
         **CC Excl:** PDX collection 94

     **A39.4 Meningococcemia,** unspecified `MCC` `HCC`
         **CC Excl:** PDX collection 94

✓5ᵗʰ **A39.5 Meningococcal** heart disease

     **A39.50 Meningococcal carditis,** unspecified `MCC`
         **CC Excl:** PDX collection 95

     **A39.51 Meningococcal** endocarditis `MCC`
         **CC Excl:** PDX collection 96

     **A39.52 Meningococcal** myocarditis `MCC`
         **CC Excl:** PDX collection 97

     **A39.53 Meningococcal** pericarditis `MCC`
         **CC Excl:** PDX collection 98

✓5ᵗʰ **A39.8 Other meningococcal infections**

     **A39.81 Meningococcal** encephalitis `MCC`
         **CC Excl:** PDX collection 99

     **A39.82 Meningococcal retrobulbar neuritis** `CC`
         **CC Excl:** PDX collection 100

     **A39.83 Meningococcal** arthritis `CC` `HCC`
         **CC Excl:** PDX collection 101

     **A39.84 Postmeningococcal** arthritis `CC` `HCC`
         **CC Excl:** PDX collection 101

     **A39.89 Other meningococcal infections** `CC`
         Meningococcal conjunctivitis
         **CC Excl:** PDX collection 102

     **A39.9 Meningococcal infection,** unspecified `CC`
         Meningococcal disease NOS
         **CC Excl:** PDX collection 102

✓4ᵗʰ **A40 Streptococcal sepsis**

     Code first: postprocedural streptococcal sepsis (T81.4-)
         streptococcal sepsis during labor (O75.3)
         streptococcal sepsis following abortion or ectopic or molar
           pregnancy (O03-O07, O08.0)
         streptococcal sepsis following immunization (T88.0)
         streptococcal sepsis following infusion, transfusion or
           therapeutic injection (T80.2-)

     `EXCLUDES 1` neonatal (P36.0-P36.1)
         puerperal sepsis (O85)
         sepsis due to Streptococcus, group D (A41.81)

     **AHA:** 2016, 1Q, 32

     **CC Excl: For MCC codes in category A40:** PDX collection 71

     **A40.0 Sepsis due to streptococcus,** group A `MCC` `HCC`

     **A40.1 Sepsis due to streptococcus,** group B `MCC` `HCC`

     **A40.3 Sepsis due to Streptococcus** pneumoniae `MCC` `HCC`
         Pneumococcal sepsis
         **CC Excl:** No Excl

     **A40.8 Other** streptococcal sepsis `MCC` `HCC`

     **A40.9 Streptococcal sepsis,** unspecified `HIV` `MCC` `HCC`

✓4ᵗʰ **A41 Other sepsis**

     Code first: postprocedural sepsis (T81.4-)sepsis during labor (O75.3)
         sepsis following abortion, ectopic or molar pregnancy
           (O03-O07, O08.0)
         sepsis following immunization (T88.0)
         sepsis following infusion, transfusion or therapeutic injection
           (T80.2-)

     `EXCLUDES 1` bacteremia NOS (R78.81)
         neonatal (P36.-)
         puerperal sepsis (O85)
         streptococcal sepsis (A40.-)

     `EXCLUDES 2` sepsis (due to) (in) actinomycotic (A42.7)
         sepsis (due to) (in) anthrax (A22.7)
         sepsis (due to) (in) candidal (B37.7)
         sepsis (due to) (in) Erysipelothrix (A26.7)
         sepsis (due to) (in) extraintestinal yersiniosis (A28.2)
         sepsis (due to) (in) gonococcal (A54.86)
         sepsis (due to) (in) herpesviral (B00.7)
         sepsis (due to) (in) listerial (A32.7)
         sepsis (due to) (in) melioidosis (A24.1)
         sepsis (due to) (in) meningococcal (A39.2-A39.4)
         sepsis (due to) (in) plague (A20.7)
         sepsis (due to) (in) tularemia (A21.7)
         toxic shock syndrome (A48.3)

     **AHA:** 2016, 1Q, 32; 2014, 2Q, 13

     **CC Excl: For MCC codes in category A41:** PDX collection 71

✓5ᵗʰ **A41.0 Sepsis due to** Staphylococcus aureus

     **A41.01 Sepsis due to** Methicillin susceptible `HIV` `MCC` `HCC`
         **Staphylococcus aureus**
         MSSA sepsis
         Staphylococcus aureus sepsis NOS

     **A41.02 Sepsis due to** Methicillin resistant `HIV` `MCC` `HCC`
         **Staphylococcus aureus**

     **A41.1 Sepsis due to** other specified **staphylococcus** `HIV` `MCC` `HCC`
         Coagulase negative staphylococcus sepsis

     **A41.2 Sepsis due to** unspecified **staphylococcus** `HIV` `MCC` `HCC`

     **A41.3 Sepsis due to** Hemophilus influenzae `HIV` `MCC` `HCC`

     **A41.4 Sepsis due to** anaerobes `HIV` `MCC` `HCC`
         `EXCLUDES 1` gas gangrene (A48.0)

✓5ᵗʰ **A41.5 Sepsis due to other** Gram-negative organisms

     **A41.50 Gram-negative sepsis,** unspecified `HIV` `MCC` `HCC`
         Gram-negative sepsis NOS

     **A41.51 Sepsis due to** Escherichia coli [E. coli] `HIV` `MCC` `HCC`

     **A41.52 Sepsis due to** Pseudomonas `HIV` `MCC` `HCC`
         Pseudomonas aeroginosa

     **A41.53 Sepsis due to** Serratia `HIV` `MCC` `HCC`

     **A41.59 Other** Gram-negative sepsis `HIV` `MCC` `HCC`

✓5ᵗʰ **A41.8 Other** specified sepsis

     **A41.81 Sepsis due to** Enterococcus `HIV` `MCC` `HCC`

     **A41.89 Other** specified sepsis `HIV` `MCC` `HCC`
         **AHA:** 2017, 1Q, 51; 2016, 3Q, 8-14

     **A41.9 Sepsis,** unspecified organism `HIV` `MCC` `HCC`
         Septicemia NOS

✓4ᵗʰ **A42 Actinomycosis**

     `EXCLUDES 1` actinomycetoma (B47.1)

     **A42.0 Pulmonary actinomycosis** `HIV` `CC` `HCC`
         **CC Excl:** PDX collection 103

     **A42.1 Abdominal actinomycosis** `HIV` `CC`
         **CC Excl:** PDX collection 104

     **A42.2 Cervicofacial actinomycosis** `HIV` `CC`
         **CC Excl:** PDX collection 105

     **A42.7 Actinomycotic** sepsis `HIV` `MCC` `HCC`
         **CC Excl:** PDX collection 71

✓5ᵗʰ **A42.8 Other forms of actinomycosis**

     **CC Excl: For CC codes in subcategory A42.8:** PDX
     collection 106

     **A42.81 Actinomycotic** meningitis `HIV` `CC`

     **A42.82 Actinomycotic** encephalitis `HIV` `CC`

     **A42.89 Other forms of actinomycosis** `HIV` `CC`

     **A42.9 Actinomycosis,** unspecified `HIV` `CC`
         **CC Excl:** PDX collection 106

---

☑ Additional Character Req   ✓7ᵗʰ Placeholder Alert   Unacceptable PDx   Manifestation   `H1`-`H14` HAC   `HCC` CMS-HCC Condition   *EXCLUDES 1* Not Coded Here   *EXCLUDES 2* Not Included Here

ICD-10-CM 2018      **441**

**Chapter 1. Certain Infectious and Parasitic Diseases**

## ✓4ᵗʰ A43 Nocardiosis

**A43.0 Pulmonary nocardiosis**    `HIV` `CC` `HCC`
CC Excl: PDX collection 103

**A43.1 Cutaneous nocardiosis**    `HIV` `CC`
CC Excl: PDX collection 107

**A43.8 Other forms of nocardiosis**    `HIV` `CC`
CC Excl: PDX collection 106

**A43.9 Nocardiosis, unspecified**    `HIV` `CC`
CC Excl: PDX collection 106

## ✓4ᵗʰ A44 Bartonellosis

CC Excl: For CC codes in category A44: PDX collection 108

**A44.0 Systemic bartonellosis**    `CC`
Oroya fever

**A44.1 Cutaneous and mucocutaneous bartonellosis**    `CC`
Verruga peruana

**A44.8 Other forms of bartonellosis**    `CC`

**A44.9 Bartonellosis, unspecified**    `CC`

## A46 Erysipelas

*EXCLUDES 1*   *postpartum or puerperal erysipelas (O86.89)*
**DEF:** A skin infection affecting the upper dermis and superficial dermal lymphatics; lesion edges are well demarcated with distinct raised borders; it is often caused by group A *Streptococci*.

## ✓4ᵗʰ A48 Other bacterial diseases, not elsewhere classified

*EXCLUDES 1*   *actinomycetoma (B47.1)*

**A48.0 Gas gangrene**    `MCC` `HCC`
Clostridial cellulitis
Clostridial myonecrosis
CC Excl: PDX collection 109

**A48.1 Legionnaires' disease**    `HIV` `MCC` `HCC`
**DEF:** Severe and often fatal infection by *Legionella pneumophila*; symptoms include high fever, gastrointestinal pain, headache, myalgia, dry cough, and pneumonia; usually transmitted through airborne water droplets via air conditioning systems or hot tubs.
CC Excl: PDX collection 110

**A48.2 Nonpneumonic Legionnaires' disease [Pontiac fever]**

**A48.3 Toxic shock syndrome**    `MCC` `HCC`
Use additional code to identify the organism (B95, B96)
*EXCLUDES 1*   *endotoxic shock NOS (R57.8)*
     *sepsis NOS (A41.9)*
CC Excl: PDX collection 111

**A48.4 Brazilian purpuric fever**
Systemic Hemophilus aegyptius infection

**✓5ᵗʰ A48.5 Other specified botulism**
Non-foodborne intoxication due to toxins of Clostridium botulinum [C. botulinum]
*EXCLUDES 1*   *food poisoning due to toxins of Clostridium botulinum (A05.1)*

CC Excl: For CC codes in subcategory A48.5: PDX collection 18

**A48.51 Infant botulism**    `CC` `P`

**A48.52 Wound botulism**    `CC`
Non-foodborne botulism NOS
Use additional code for associated wound

**A48.8 Other specified bacterial diseases**

## ✓4ᵗʰ A49 Bacterial infection of unspecified site

*EXCLUDES 1*   *bacterial agents as the cause of diseases classified elsewhere (B95-B96)*
     *chlamydial infection NOS (A74.9)*
     *meningococcal infection NOS (A39.9)*
     *rickettsial infection NOS (A79.9)*
     *spirochetal infection NOS (A69.9)*

**✓5ᵗʰ A49.0 Staphylococcal infection, unspecified site**

**A49.01 Methicillin susceptible Staphylococcus aureus infection, unspecified site**
Methicillin susceptible Staphylococcus aureus (MSSA) infection
Staphylococcus aureus infection NOS

**A49.02 Methicillin resistant Staphylococcus aureus infection, unspecified site**
Methicillin resistant Staphylococcus aureus (MRSA) infection

**A49.1 Streptococcal infection, unspecified site**

**A49.2 Hemophilus influenzae infection, unspecified site**

**A49.3 Mycoplasma infection, unspecified site**

**A49.8 Other bacterial infections of unspecified site**

**A49.9 Bacterial infection, unspecified**
*EXCLUDES 1*   *bacteremia NOS (R78.81)*

## Infections with a predominantly sexual mode of transmission (A50-A64)

*EXCLUDES 1*   *human immunodeficiency virus [HIV] disease (B20)*
     *nonspecific and nongonococcal urethritis (N34.1)*
     *Reiter's disease (M02.3-)*

## ✓4ᵗʰ A50 Congenital syphilis

**✓5ᵗʰ A50.0 Early congenital syphilis, symptomatic**
Any congenital syphilitic condition specified as early or manifest less than two years after birth.

CC Excl: For CC codes in subcategory A50.0: PDX collection 112

**A50.01 Early congenital syphilitic oculopathy**    `CC`

**A50.02 Early congenital syphilitic osteochondropathy**    `CC`

**A50.03 Early congenital syphilitic pharyngitis**    `CC`
Early congenital syphilitic laryngitis

**A50.04 Early congenital syphilitic pneumonia**    `CC`

**A50.05 Early congenital syphilitic rhinitis**    `CC`

**A50.06 Early cutaneous congenital syphilis**    `CC`

**A50.07 Early mucocutaneous congenital syphilis**    `CC`

**A50.08 Early visceral congenital syphilis**    `CC`

**A50.09 Other early congenital syphilis, symptomatic**    `CC`

**A50.1 Early congenital syphilis, latent**
Congenital syphilis without clinical manifestations, with positive serological reaction and negative spinal fluid test, less than two years after birth.

**A50.2 Early congenital syphilis, unspecified**    `CC`
Congenital syphilis NOS less than two years after birth.
CC Excl: PDX collection 113

**✓5ᵗʰ A50.3 Late congenital syphilitic oculopathy**
*EXCLUDES 1*   *Hutchinson's triad (A50.53)*

CC Excl: For CC/MCC codes in subcategory A50.3, unless otherwise noted: PDX collection 112

**A50.30 Late congenital syphilitic oculopathy, unspecified**    `CC`

**A50.31 Late congenital syphilitic interstitial keratitis**    `CC`

**A50.32 Late congenital syphilitic chorioretinitis**    `CC`

**A50.39 Other late congenital syphilitic oculopathy**    `CC`

**✓5ᵗʰ A50.4 Late congenital neurosyphilis [juvenile neurosyphilis]**
Use additional code to identify any associated mental disorder
*EXCLUDES 1*   *Hutchinson's triad (A50.53)*

**A50.40 Late congenital neurosyphilis, unspecified**    `CC`
Juvenile neurosyphilis NOS
CC Excl: PDX collection 114

**A50.41 Late congenital syphilitic meningitis**    `MCC`
CC Excl: PDX collection 115

**A50.42 Late congenital syphilitic encephalitis**    `MCC`
CC Excl: PDX collection 114

**A50.43 Late congenital syphilitic polyneuropathy**    `CC`
CC Excl: PDX collection 114

**A50.44 Late congenital syphilitic optic nerve atrophy**    `CC`
CC Excl: PDX collection 112

**A50.45 Juvenile general paresis**    `CC`
Dementia paralytica juvenilis
Juvenile tabetoparetic neurosyphilis
CC Excl: PDX collection 114

**A50.49 Other late congenital neurosyphilis**    `CC`
Juvenile tabes dorsalis
CC Excl: PDX collection 114

**✓5ᵗʰ A50.5 Other late congenital syphilis, symptomatic**
Any congenital syphilitic condition specified as late or manifest two years or more after birth.

CC Excl: For CC codes in subcategory A50.5: PDX collection 112

**A50.51 Clutton's joints**    `CC`

**A50.52 Hutchinson's teeth**    `CC`

**A50.53 Hutchinson's triad**    `CC`

**A50.54 Late congenital cardiovascular syphilis**    `CC`

**A50.55 Late congenital syphilitic arthropathy**    `CC` `HCC`

**A50.56 Late congenital syphilitic osteochondropathy**    `CC`

`N` Newborn: 0   `P` Pediatric: 0-17   `M` Maternity: 12-55   `A` Adult: 15-124   `MCC` Major CC Condition   `PDxMCC` PDx acts as own MCC   `CC` CC Condition   `PDxCC` PDx acts as own CC

442      ICD-10-CM 2018

**A50.57**   **Syphilitic saddle nose**   `CC`

**A50.59**   **Other late congenital syphilis, symptomatic**   `CC`

**A50.6**   **Late congenital syphilis, latent**
Congenital syphilis without clinical manifestations, with positive serological reaction and negative spinal fluid test, two years or more after birth.

**A50.7**   **Late congenital syphilis, unspecified**
Congenital syphilis NOS two years or more after birth.

**A50.9**   **Congenital syphilis, unspecified**

✓4ᵗʰ **A51**   **Early syphilis**

**A51.0**   **Primary genital syphilis**
Syphilitic chancre NOS

**A51.1**   **Primary anal syphilis**

**A51.2**   **Primary syphilis of other sites**

✓5ᵗʰ **A51.3**   **Secondary syphilis of skin and mucous membranes**
**DEF:** Transitory or chronic cutaneous eruptions that present within two to 10 weeks following initial syphilis infection that may include nontender lymphadenopathy along with alopecia and condylomata lata.

  **A51.31**   **Condyloma latum**   `CC`
    CC Excl: PDX collection 112

  **A51.32**   **Syphilitic alopecia**   `CC`
    CC Excl: PDX collection 116

  **A51.39**   **Other secondary syphilis of skin**   `CC`
    Syphilitic leukoderma
    Syphilitic mucous patch
    *EXCLUDES 1*   late syphilitic leukoderma (A52.79)
    CC Excl: PDX collection 112

✓5ᵗʰ **A51.4**   **Other secondary syphilis**

  **A51.41**   **Secondary syphilitic meningitis**   `MCC`
    CC Excl: PDX collection 117

  **A51.42**   **Secondary syphilitic female pelvic disease**   `CC`♀
    CC Excl: PDX collection 113

  **A51.43**   **Secondary syphilitic oculopathy**   `CC`
    Secondary syphilitic chorioretinitis
    Secondary syphilitic iridocyclitis, iritis
    Secondary syphilitic uveitis
    CC Excl: PDX collection 112

  **A51.44**   **Secondary syphilitic nephritis**   `CC`
    CC Excl: PDX collection 113

  **A51.45**   **Secondary syphilitic hepatitis**   `CC`
    CC Excl: PDX collection 118

  **A51.46**   **Secondary syphilitic osteopathy**   `CC`
    CC Excl: PDX collection 119

  **A51.49**   **Other secondary syphilitic conditions**   `CC`
    Secondary syphilitic lymphadenopathy
    Secondary syphilitic myositis
    CC Excl: No Excl

**A51.5**   **Early syphilis, latent**
Syphilis (acquired) without clinical manifestations, with positive serological reaction and negative spinal fluid test, less than two years after infection.

**A51.9**   **Early syphilis, unspecified**

✓4ᵗʰ **A52**   **Late syphilis**

✓5ᵗʰ **A52.0**   **Cardiovascular and cerebrovascular syphilis**

  CC Excl: For CC codes in subcategory A52.0:
  PDX collection 114

  **A52.00**   **Cardiovascular syphilis, unspecified**   `CC`

  **A52.01**   **Syphilitic aneurysm of aorta**   `CC`

  **A52.02**   **Syphilitic aortitis**   `CC`

  **A52.03**   **Syphilitic endocarditis**   `CC`
    Syphilitic aortic valve incompetence or stenosis
    Syphilitic mitral valve stenosis
    Syphilitic pulmonary valve regurgitation

  **A52.04**   **Syphilitic cerebral arteritis**   `CC`

  **A52.05**   **Other cerebrovascular syphilis**   `CC`
    Syphilitic cerebral aneurysm (ruptured) (non-ruptured)
    Syphilitic cerebral thrombosis

  **A52.06**   **Other syphilitic heart involvement**   `CC`
    Syphilitic coronary artery disease
    Syphilitic myocarditis
    Syphilitic pericarditis

  **A52.09**   **Other cardiovascular syphilis**   `CC`

✓5ᵗʰ **A52.1**   **Symptomatic neurosyphilis**

  CC Excl: For CC/MCC codes in subcategory A52.1, unless otherwise noted: PDX collection 114

  **A52.10**   **Symptomatic neurosyphilis, unspecified**   `CC`

  **A52.11**   **Tabes dorsalis**   `CC`
    Locomotor ataxia (progressive)
    Tabetic neurosyphilis

  **A52.12**   **Other cerebrospinal syphilis**   `CC`

  **A52.13**   **Late syphilitic meningitis**   `MCC`
    CC Excl: PDX collection 115

  **A52.14**   **Late syphilitic encephalitis**   `MCC`

  **A52.15**   **Late syphilitic neuropathy**   `CC`
    Late syphilitic acoustic neuritis
    Late syphilitic optic (nerve) atrophy
    Late syphilitic polyneuropathy
    Late syphilitic retrobulbar neuritis

  **A52.16**   **Charcôt's arthropathy (tabetic)**   `CC`

  **A52.17**   **General paresis**   `CC`
    Dementia paralytica

  **A52.19**   **Other symptomatic neurosyphilis**   `CC`
    Syphilitic parkinsonism

**A52.2**   **Asymptomatic neurosyphilis**   `CC`
  CC Excl: PDX collection 114

**A52.3**   **Neurosyphilis, unspecified**   `CC`
  Gumma (syphilitic)
  Syphilis (late)
  Syphiloma
  CC Excl: PDX collection 114

✓5ᵗʰ **A52.7**   **Other symptomatic late syphilis**

  CC Excl: For CC codes in subcategory A52.7, unless otherwise noted: PDX collection 116

  **A52.71**   **Late syphilitic oculopathy**   `CC`
    Late syphilitic chorioretinitis
    Late syphilitic episcleritis
    CC Excl: PDX collection 120

  **A52.72**   **Syphilis of lung and bronchus**   `CC`

  **A52.73**   **Symptomatic late syphilis of other respiratory organs**   `CC`

  **A52.74**   **Syphilis of liver and other viscera**   `CC`
    Late syphilitic peritonitis

  **A52.75**   **Syphilis of kidney and ureter**   `CC`
    Syphilitic glomerular disease

  **A52.76**   **Other genitourinary symptomatic late syphilis**   `CC`
    Late syphilitic female pelvic inflammatory disease

  **A52.77**   **Syphilis of bone and joint**   `CC`

  **A52.78**   **Syphilis of other musculoskeletal tissue**   `CC`
    Late syphilitic bursitis
    Syphilis [stage unspecified] of bursa
    Syphilis [stage unspecified] of muscle
    Syphilis [stage unspecified] of synovium
    Syphilis [stage unspecified] of tendon

  **A52.79**   **Other symptomatic late syphilis**   `CC`
    Late syphilitic leukoderma
    Syphilis of adrenal gland
    Syphilis of pituitary gland
    Syphilis of thyroid gland
    Syphilitic splenomegaly
    *EXCLUDES 1*   syphilitic leukoderma (secondary) (A51.39)

**A52.8**   **Late syphilis, latent**
Syphilis (acquired) without clinical manifestations, with positive serological reaction and negative spinal fluid test, two years or more after infection

**A52.9**   **Late syphilis, unspecified**

✓4ᵗʰ **A53**   **Other and unspecified syphilis**

**A53.0**   **Latent syphilis, unspecified as early or late**
Latent syphilis NOS    Positive serological reaction for syphilis

**A53.9**   **Syphilis, unspecified**
Infection due to Treponema pallidum NOS
Syphilis (acquired) NOS
*EXCLUDES 1*   syphilis NOS under two years of age (A50.2)

✓Additional Character Req   ✓x7ᵗʰ Placeholder Alert   Unacceptable PDx   Manifestation   `H1`-`H14` HAC   `HCC` CMS-HCC Condition   *EXCLUDES 1* Not Coded Here   *EXCLUDES 2* Not Included Here

ICD-10-CM 2018       443

✓4th **A54 Gonococcal infection**

✓5th **A54.0 Gonococcal infection of lower genitourinary tract without periurethral or accessory gland abscess**

**EXCLUDES 1**    *gonococcal infection with genitourinary gland abscess (A54.1)*
         *gonococcal infection with periurethral abscess (A54.1)*

**CC Excl: For CC codes in subcategory A54.0:**
PDX collection 121

  **A54.00 Gonococcal infection of lower genitourinary tract, unspecified**    CC

  **A54.01 Gonococcal cystitis and urethritis, unspecified**    CC

  **A54.02 Gonococcal vulvovaginitis, unspecified**    CC ♀

  **A54.03 Gonococcal cervicitis, unspecified**    CC ♀

  **A54.09 Other gonococcal infection of lower genitourinary tract**    CC

**A54.1 Gonococcal infection of lower genitourinary tract with periurethral and accessory gland abscess**    CC
Gonococcal Bartholin's gland abscess
**CC Excl:** PDX collection 121

✓5th **A54.2 Gonococcal pelviperitonitis and other gonococcal genitourinary infection**

**CC Excl: For CC codes in subcategory A54.2:**
PDX collection 121

  **A54.21 Gonococcal infection of kidney and ureter**    CC

  **A54.22 Gonococcal prostatitis**    CC ♂

  **A54.23 Gonococcal infection of other male genital organs**    CC ♂
Gonococcal epididymitis     Gonococcal orchitis

  **A54.24 Gonococcal female pelvic inflammatory disease**    CC ♀
Gonococcal pelviperitonitis
**EXCLUDES 1** *gonococcal peritonitis (A54.85)*

  **A54.29 Other gonococcal genitourinary infections**    CC

✓5th **A54.3 Gonococcal infection of eye**

**CC Excl: For CC codes in subcategory A54.3:**
PDX collection 116

  **A54.30 Gonococcal infection of eye, unspecified**    CC

  **A54.31 Gonococcal conjunctivitis**    CC
Ophthalmia neonatorum due to gonococcus

  **A54.32 Gonococcal iridocyclitis**    CC

  **A54.33 Gonococcal keratitis**    CC

  **A54.39 Other gonococcal eye infection**    CC
Gonococcal endophthalmia

✓5th **A54.4 Gonococcal infection of musculoskeletal system**

**CC Excl: For CC codes in subcategory A54.4:**
PDX collection 122

  **A54.40 Gonococcal infection of musculoskeletal system, unspecified**    CC HCC

  **A54.41 Gonococcal spondylopathy**    CC HCC

  **A54.42 Gonococcal arthritis**    CC HCC
**EXCLUDES 2** *gonococcal infection of spine (A54.41)*

  **A54.43 Gonococcal osteomyelitis**    CC HCC
**EXCLUDES 2** *gonococcal infection of spine (A54.41)*

  **A54.49 Gonococcal infection of other musculoskeletal tissue**    CC HCC
Gonococcal bursitis
Gonococcal myositis
Gonococcal synovitis
Gonococcal tenosynovitis

**A54.5 Gonococcal pharyngitis**

**A54.6 Gonococcal infection of anus and rectum**

✓5th **A54.8 Other gonococcal infections**

  **A54.81 Gonococcal meningitis**    MCC
**CC Excl:** PDX collection 117

  **A54.82 Gonococcal brain abscess**    CC
**CC Excl:** PDX collection 123

  **A54.83 Gonococcal heart infection**    CC
Gonococcal endocarditis
Gonococcal myocarditis
Gonococcal pericarditis
**CC Excl:** PDX collection 124

  **A54.84 Gonococcal pneumonia**    CC HCC
**CC Excl:** PDX collection 123

  **A54.85 Gonococcal peritonitis**    CC HCC
**EXCLUDES 1** *gonococcal pelviperitonitis (A54.24)*
**CC Excl:** PDX collection 125

  **A54.86 Gonococcal sepsis**    PDxMCC MCC HCC
**CC Excl:** PDX collection 71

  **A54.89 Other gonococcal infections**    CC
Gonococcal keratoderma
Gonococcal lymphadenitis
**CC Excl:** PDX collection 123

**A54.9 Gonococcal infection, unspecified**    CC
**CC Excl:** PDX collection 123

**A55 Chlamydial lymphogranuloma (venereum)**
Climatic or tropical bubo
Durand-Nicolas-Favre disease
Esthiomene
Lymphogranuloma inguinale

✓4th **A56 Other sexually transmitted chlamydial diseases**
**INCLUDES** sexually transmitted diseases due to Chlamydia trachomatis
**EXCLUDES 1** *neonatal chlamydial conjunctivitis (P39.1)*
         *neonatal chlamydial pneumonia (P23.1)*
**EXCLUDES 2** *chlamydial lymphogranuloma (A55)*
         *conditions classified to A74-*

✓5th **A56.0 Chlamydial infection of lower genitourinary tract**

  **A56.00 Chlamydial infection of lower genitourinary tract, unspecified**

  **A56.01 Chlamydial cystitis and urethritis**

  **A56.02 Chlamydial vulvovaginitis**    ♀

  **A56.09 Other chlamydial infection of lower genitourinary tract**
Chlamydial cervicitis

✓5th **A56.1 Chlamydial infection of pelviperitoneum and other genitourinary organs**

  **A56.11 Chlamydial female pelvic inflammatory disease**    ♀

  **A56.19 Other chlamydial genitourinary infection**
Chlamydial epididymitis
Chlamydial orchitis

**A56.2 Chlamydial infection of genitourinary tract, unspecified**

**A56.3 Chlamydial infection of anus and rectum**

**A56.4 Chlamydial infection of pharynx**

**A56.8 Sexually transmitted chlamydial infection of other sites**

**A57 Chancroid**
Ulcus molle

**A58 Granuloma inguinale**
Donovanosis

✓4th **A59 Trichomoniasis**
**EXCLUDES 2** *intestinal trichomoniasis (A07.8)*

✓5th **A59.0 Urogenital trichomoniasis**

  **A59.00 Urogenital trichomoniasis, unspecified**
Fluor (vaginalis) due to Trichomonas
Leukorrhea (vaginalis) due to Trichomonas

  **A59.01 Trichomonal vulvovaginitis**    ♀

  **A59.02 Trichomonal prostatitis**    ♂

  **A59.03 Trichomonal cystitis and urethritis**

  **A59.09 Other urogenital trichomoniasis**
Trichomonas cervicitis

**A59.8 Trichomoniasis of other sites**

**A59.9 Trichomoniasis, unspecified**

✓4th **A60 Anogenital herpesviral [herpes simplex] infections**

✓5th **A60.0 Herpesviral infection of genitalia and urogenital tract**

  **A60.00 Herpesviral infection of urogenital system, unspecified**    HIV

  **A60.01 Herpesviral infection of penis**    HIV ♂

  **A60.02 Herpesviral infection of other male genital organs**    ♂

  **A60.03 Herpesviral cervicitis**    ♀

  **A60.04 Herpesviral vulvovaginitis**    HIV ♀
Herpesviral [herpes simplex] ulceration
Herpesviral [herpes simplex] vaginitis
Herpesviral [herpes simplex] vulvitis

  **A60.09 Herpesviral infection of other urogenital tract**    HIV

**A60.1 Herpesviral infection of perianal skin and rectum**    HIV

**A60.9 Anogenital herpesviral infection, unspecified**    HIV

N Newborn: 0   P Pediatric: 0-17   M Maternity: 12-55   A Adult: 15-124   MCC Major CC Condition   PDxMCC PDx acts as own MCC   CC CC Condition   PDxCC PDx acts as own CC

444                                           ICD-10-CM 2018

✓4ᵗʰ **A63**   **Other predominantly sexually transmitted diseases, not elsewhere classified**

> *EXCLUDES 2*   molluscum contagiosum (B08.1)
>               papilloma of cervix (D26.0)

**A63.0**   **Anogenital (venereal) warts**
     Anogenital warts due to (human) papillomavirus [HPV]
     Condyloma acuminatum

**A63.8**   **Other specified predominantly sexually transmitted diseases**

**A64**   **Unspecified sexually transmitted disease**

### Other spirochetal diseases (A65-A69)

> *EXCLUDES 2*   leptospirosis (A27.-)
>               syphilis (A50-A53)

**A65**   **Nonvenereal syphilis**
     Bejel
     Endemic syphilis
     Njovera

✓4ᵗʰ **A66**   **Yaws**

> *INCLUDES*   bouba
>             frambesia (tropica)
>             pian

**A66.0**   **Initial lesions of yaws**
     Chancre of yaws
     Frambesia, initial or primary
     Initial frambesial ulcer
     Mother yaw

**A66.1**   **Multiple papillomata and wet crab yaws**
     Frambesioma
     Pianoma
     Plantar or palmar papilloma of yaws

**A66.2**   **Other early skin lesions of yaws**
     Cutaneous yaws, less than five years after infection
     Early yaws (cutaneous) (macular) (maculopapular)
         (micropapular) (papular)
     Frambeside of early yaws

**A66.3**   **Hyperkeratosis of yaws**
     Ghoul hand
     Hyperkeratosis, palmar or plantar (early) (late) due to yaws
     Worm-eaten soles

**A66.4**   **Gummata and ulcers of yaws**
     Gummatous frambeside
     Nodular late yaws (ulcerated)

**A66.5**   **Gangosa**
     Rhinopharyngitis mutilans

**A66.6**   **Bone and joint lesions of yaws**   `HCC`
     Yaws ganglion
     Yaws goundou
     Yaws gumma, bone
     Yaws gummatous osteitis or periostitis
     Yaws hydrarthrosis
     Yaws osteitis
     Yaws periostitis (hypertrophic)

**A66.7**   **Other manifestations of yaws**
     Juxta-articular nodules of yaws
     Mucosal yaws

**A66.8**   **Latent yaws**
     Yaws without clinical manifestations, with positive serology

**A66.9**   **Yaws, unspecified**

✓4ᵗʰ **A67**   **Pinta [carate]**

**A67.0**   **Primary lesions of pinta**
     Chancre (primary) of pinta
     Papule (primary) of pinta

**A67.1**   **Intermediate lesions of pinta**
     Erythematous plaques of pinta
     Hyperchromic lesions of pinta
     Hyperkeratosis of pinta
     Pintids

**A67.2**   **Late lesions of pinta**
     Achromic skin lesions of pinta
     Cicatricial skin lesions of pinta
     Dyschromic skin lesions of pinta

**A67.3**   **Mixed lesions of pinta**
     Achromic with hyperchromic skin lesions of pinta [carate]

**A67.9**   **Pinta, unspecified**

✓4ᵗʰ **A68**   **Relapsing fevers**

> *INCLUDES*   recurrent fever
> *EXCLUDES 2*   Lyme disease (A69.2-)

> **CC Excl: For CC codes in category A68:** PDX collection 108

**A68.0**   **Louse-borne relapsing fever**   `CC`
     Relapsing fever due to Borrelia recurrentis

**A68.1**   **Tick-borne relapsing fever**   `CC`
     Relapsing fever due to any Borrelia species other than Borrelia recurrentis

**A68.9**   **Relapsing fever, unspecified**   `CC`

✓4ᵗʰ **A69**   **Other spirochetal infections**

**A69.0**   **Necrotizing ulcerative stomatitis**
     Cancrum oris            Noma
     Fusospirochetal gangrene    Stomatitis gangrenosa

**A69.1**   **Other Vincent's infections**   `CC`
     Fusospirochetal pharyngitis
     Necrotizing ulcerative (acute) gingivitis
     Necrotizing ulcerative (acute) gingivostomatitis
     Spirochetal stomatitis
     Trench mouth
     Vincent's angina
     Vincent's gingivitis
     **CC Excl:** PDX collection 126

✓5ᵗʰ **A69.2**   **Lyme disease**
     Erythema chronicum migrans due to Borrelia burgdorferi
     **DEF:** A recurrent multisystem disorder through tick bites; begins with lesions of erythema chronicum migrans; followed by arthritis of the large joints, myalgia, malaise, and neurological and cardiac manifestations.

> **CC Excl: For CC codes in subcategory A69.2:** PDX collection 108

**A69.20**   **Lyme disease, unspecified**   `CC`

**A69.21**   **Meningitis due to Lyme disease**   `CC`

**A69.22**   **Other neurologic disorders in Lyme disease**   `CC`
     Cranial neuritis
     Meningoencephalitis
     Polyneuropathy

**A69.23**   **Arthritis due to Lyme disease**   `CC` `HCC`

**A69.29**   **Other conditions associated with Lyme disease**   `CC`
     Myopericarditis due to Lyme disease
     **AHA:** 2016, 3Q, 12

**A69.8**   **Other specified spirochetal infections**

**A69.9**   **Spirochetal infection, unspecified**

### Other diseases caused by chlamydiae (A70-A74)

> *EXCLUDES 1*   sexually transmitted chlamydial diseases (A55-A56)

**A70**   **Chlamydia psittaci infections**   `CC`
     Ornithosis
     Parrot fever
     Psittacosis
     **CC Excl:** PDX collection 127

✓4ᵗʰ **A71**   **Trachoma**

> *EXCLUDES 1*   sequelae of trachoma (B94.0)

**A71.0**   **Initial stage of trachoma**
     Trachoma dubium

**A71.1**   **Active stage of trachoma**
     Granular conjunctivitis (trachomatous)
     Trachomatous follicular conjunctivitis
     Trachomatous pannus

**A71.9**   **Trachoma, unspecified**

✓4ᵗʰ **A74**   **Other diseases caused by chlamydiae**

> *EXCLUDES 1*   neonatal chlamydial conjunctivitis (P39.1)
>               neonatal chlamydial pneumonia (P23.1)
>               Reiter's disease (M02.3-)
>               sexually transmitted chlamydial diseases (A55-A56)
> *EXCLUDES 2*   chlamydial pneumonia (J16.0)

**A74.0**   **Chlamydial conjunctivitis**
     Paratrachoma

✓5ᵗʰ **A74.8**   **Other chlamydial diseases**

**A74.81**   **Chlamydial peritonitis**

**A74.89**   **Other chlamydial diseases**

**A74.9**   **Chlamydial infection, unspecified**
     Chlamydiosis NOS

☑ Additional Character Req   ✓x7ᵗʰ Placeholder Alert   Unacceptable PDx   Manifestation   **H1**-**H14** HAC   `HCC` CMS-HCC Condition   *EXCLUDES 1* Not Coded Here   *EXCLUDES 2* Not Included Here

ICD-10-CM 2018                                         **445**

**Chapter 1. Certain Infectious and Parasitic Diseases**

**A75–A83.9**

## Rickettsioses (A75-A79)

**✓4ᵗʰ A75 Typhus fever**

> EXCLUDES 1   rickettsiosis due to Ehrlichia sennetsu (A79.81)

> **CC Excl:** For CC codes in category A75, unless otherwise noted: PDX collection 108

**A75.0 Epidemic louse-borne typhus fever due to Rickettsia prowazekii**   CC
Classical typhus (fever)
Epidemic (louse-borne) typhus

**A75.1 Recrudescent typhus [Brill's disease]**   CC
Brill-Zinsser disease

**A75.2 Typhus fever due to Rickettsia typhi**   CC
Murine (flea-borne) typhus

**A75.3 Typhus fever due to Rickettsia tsutsugamushi**   CC
Scrub (mite-borne) typhus
Tsutsugamushi fever

**A75.9 Typhus fever, unspecified**   CC
Typhus (fever) NOS
**CC Excl:** PDX collection 128

**✓4ᵗʰ A77 Spotted fever [tick-borne rickettsioses]**

> **CC Excl:** For CC codes in category A77: PDX collection 108

**A77.0 Spotted fever due to Rickettsia rickettsii**   CC
Rocky Mountain spotted fever
Sao Paulo fever

**A77.1 Spotted fever due to Rickettsia conorii**   CC
African tick typhus
Boutonneuse fever
India tick typhus
Kenya tick typhus
Marseilles fever
Mediterranean tick fever

**A77.2 Spotted fever due to Rickettsia siberica**   CC
North Asian tick fever
Siberian tick typhus

**A77.3 Spotted fever due to Rickettsia australis**   CC
Queensland tick typhus

**✓5ᵗʰ A77.4 Ehrlichiosis**
> EXCLUDES 1   Rickettsiosis due to Ehrlichia sennetsu (A79.81)

   **A77.40 Ehrlichiosis, unspecified**   CC

   **A77.41 Ehrlichiosis chaffeensis [E. chaffeensis]**   CC

   **A77.49 Other ehrlichiosis**   CC

**A77.8 Other spotted fevers**   CC

**A77.9 Spotted fever, unspecified**   CC
Tick-borne typhus NOS

**A78 Q fever**   CC
Infection due to Coxiella burnetii
Nine Mile fever
Quadrilateral fever
**CC Excl:** PDX collection 108

**✓4ᵗʰ A79 Other rickettsioses**

> **CC Excl:** For CC codes in category A79, unless otherwise noted: PDX collection 129

**A79.0 Trench fever**   CC
Quintan fever
Wolhynian fever
**CC Excl:** PDX collection 108

**A79.1 Rickettsialpox due to Rickettsia akari**   CC
Kew Garden fever
Vesicular rickettsiosis

**✓5ᵗʰ A79.8 Other specified rickettsioses**

   **A79.81 Rickettsiosis due to Ehrlichia sennetsu**   CC

   **A79.89 Other specified rickettsioses**   CC

**A79.9 Rickettsiosis, unspecified**   CC
Rickettsial infection NOS

## Viral and prion infections of the central nervous system (A80-A89)

> EXCLUDES 1   postpolio syndrome (G14)
> sequelae of poliomyelitis (B91)
> sequelae of viral encephalitis (B94.1)

**✓4ᵗʰ A80 Acute poliomyelitis**

> **CC Excl:** For MCC codes in category A80: PDX collection 130

**A80.0 Acute paralytic poliomyelitis, vaccine-associated**   MCC

**A80.1 Acute paralytic poliomyelitis, wild virus, imported**   MCC

**A80.2 Acute paralytic poliomyelitis, wild virus, indigenous**   MCC

**✓5ᵗʰ A80.3 Acute paralytic poliomyelitis, other and unspecified**

   **A80.30 Acute paralytic poliomyelitis, unspecified**   MCC

   **A80.39 Other acute paralytic poliomyelitis**   MCC

**A80.4 Acute nonparalytic poliomyelitis**

**A80.9 Acute poliomyelitis, unspecified**

**✓4ᵗʰ A81 Atypical virus infections of central nervous system**
> INCLUDES   diseases of the central nervous system caused by prions
> Use additional code to identify:
> dementia with behavioral disturbance (F02.81)
> dementia without behavioral disturbance (F02.80)

**✓5ᵗʰ A81.0 Creutzfeldt-Jakob disease**

> **CC Excl:** For codes in subcategory A81.0: PDX collection 131

   **A81.00 Creutzfeldt-Jakob disease, unspecified**   CC
Jakob-Creutzfeldt disease, unspecified

   **A81.01 Variant Creutzfeldt-Jakob disease**   CC
vCJD

   **A81.09 Other Creutzfeldt-Jakob disease**   CC
CJD
Familial Creutzfeldt-Jakob disease
Iatrogenic Creutzfeldt-Jakob disease
Sporadic Creutzfeldt-Jakob disease
Subacute spongiform encephalopathy (with dementia)

**A81.1 Subacute sclerosing panencephalitis**   CC
Dawson's inclusion body encephalitis
Van Bogaert's sclerosing leukoencephalopathy
**CC Excl:** PDX collection 132

**A81.2 Progressive multifocal leukoencephalopathy**   HIV CC
Multifocal leukoencephalopathy NOS
**CC Excl:** PDX collection 133

**✓5ᵗʰ A81.8 Other atypical virus infections of central nervous system**

   **A81.81 Kuru**   CC
**CC Excl:** PDX collection 134

   **A81.82 Gerstmann-Sträussler-Scheinker syndrome**   HIV CC
GSS syndrome
**CC Excl:** PDX collection 135

   **A81.83 Fatal familial insomnia**   HIV CC
FFI
**CC Excl:** PDX collection 135

   **A81.89 Other atypical virus infections of central nervous system**   HIV CC
**CC Excl:** PDX collection 135

**A81.9 Atypical virus infection of central nervous system, unspecified**   HIV CC
Prion diseases of the central nervous system NOS
**CC Excl:** PDX collection 134

**✓4ᵗʰ A82 Rabies**

> **CC Excl:** For CC codes in category A82: PDX collection 136

**A82.0 Sylvatic rabies**   CC

**A82.1 Urban rabies**   CC

**A82.9 Rabies, unspecified**   CC

**✓4ᵗʰ A83 Mosquito-borne viral encephalitis**
> INCLUDES   mosquito-borne viral meningoencephalitis
> EXCLUDES 2   Venezuelan equine encephalitis (A92.2)
> West Nile fever (A92.3-)
> West Nile virus (A92.3-)

> **CC Excl:** For MCC codes in category A83: PDX collection 137

**A83.0 Japanese encephalitis**   MCC

**A83.1 Western equine encephalitis**   MCC

**A83.2 Eastern equine encephalitis**   MCC

**A83.3 St Louis encephalitis**   MCC

**A83.4 Australian encephalitis**   MCC
Kunjin virus disease

**A83.5 California encephalitis**   MCC
California meningoencephalitis
La Crosse encephalitis

**A83.6 Rocio virus disease**   MCC

**A83.8 Other mosquito-borne viral encephalitis**   MCC

**A83.9 Mosquito-borne viral encephalitis, unspecified**   MCC

N Newborn: 0   P Pediatric: 0-17   M Maternity: 12-55   A Adult: 15-124   MCC Major CC Condition   PDxMCC PDx acts as own MCC   CC CC Condition   PDxCC PDx acts as own CC

446      ICD-10-CM 2018

✓4ᵗʰ **A84　Tick-borne viral encephalitis**
　　INCLUDES　tick-borne viral meningoencephalitis

　　CC Excl: For MCC codes in category A84: PDX collection 137

　　**A84.0　Far Eastern tick-borne encephalitis [Russian** 　MCC
　　　　　　**spring-summer encephalitis]**
　　**A84.1　Central European tick-borne encephalitis** 　MCC
　　**A84.8　Other tick-borne viral encephalitis** 　MCC
　　　　　　Louping ill
　　　　　　Powassan virus disease
　　**A84.9　Tick-borne viral encephalitis, unspecified** 　MCC

✓4ᵗʰ **A85　Other viral encephalitis, not elsewhere classified**
　　INCLUDES　specified viral encephalomyelitis NEC
　　　　　　　specified viral meningoencephalitis NEC
　　EXCLUDES 1　benign myalgic encephalomyelitis (G93.3)
　　　　　　　encephalitis due to cytomegalovirus (B25.8)
　　　　　　　encephalitis due to herpesvirus NEC (B10.0-)
　　　　　　　encephalitis due to herpesvirus [herpes simplex] (B00.4)
　　　　　　　encephalitis due to measles virus (B05.0)
　　　　　　　encephalitis due to mumps virus (B26.2)
　　　　　　　encephalitis due to poliomyelitis virus (A80.-)
　　　　　　　encephalitis due to zoster (B02.0)
　　　　　　　lymphocytic choriomeningitis (A87.2)

　　CC Excl: For CC codes in category A85, unless otherwise noted:
　　PDX collection 138

　　**A85.0　Enteroviral encephalitis** 　HIV CC
　　　　　　Enteroviral encephalomyelitis
　　**A85.1　Adenoviral encephalitis** 　HIV CC
　　　　　　Adenoviral meningoencephalitis
　　**A85.2　Arthropod-borne viral encephalitis, unspecified** 　MCC
　　　　　　EXCLUDES 1　West nile virus with encephalitis (A92.31)
　　　　　　CC Excl: PDX collection 137
　　**A85.8　Other specified viral encephalitis** 　HIV CC
　　　　　　Encephalitis lethargica
　　　　　　Von Economo-Cruchet disease

**A86　Unspecified viral encephalitis** 　HIV CC
　　Viral encephalomyelitis NOS
　　Viral meningoencephalitis NOS
　　CC Excl: PDX collection 139

✓4ᵗʰ **A87　Viral meningitis**
　　EXCLUDES 1　meningitis due to herpesvirus [herpes simplex] (B00.3)
　　　　　　　meningitis due to measles virus (B05.1)
　　　　　　　meningitis due to mumps virus (B26.1)
　　　　　　　meningitis due to poliomyelitis virus (A80.-)
　　　　　　　meningitis due to zoster (B02.1)

　　CC Excl: For CC codes in category A87, unless otherwise noted:
　　PDX collection 140

　　**A87.0　Enteroviral meningitis** 　CC
　　　　　　Coxsackievirus meningitis
　　　　　　Echovirus meningitis
　　**A87.1　Adenoviral meningitis** 　CC
　　**A87.2　Lymphocytic choriomeningitis** 　CC
　　　　　　Lymphocytic meningoencephalitis
　　　　　　CC Excl: PDX collection 141
　　**A87.8　Other viral meningitis** 　CC
　　**A87.9　Viral meningitis, unspecified** 　CC

✓4ᵗʰ **A88　Other viral infections of central nervous system, not elsewhere classified**
　　EXCLUDES 1　viral encephalitis NOS (A86)
　　　　　　　viral meningitis NOS (A87.9)
　　**A88.0　Enteroviral exanthematous fever [Boston exanthem]** 　CC
　　　　　　CC Excl: PDX collection 137
　　**A88.1　Epidemic vertigo**
　　**A88.8　Other specified viral infections of central nervous** 　HIV CC
　　　　　　**system**
　　　　　　CC Excl: PDX collection 138

**A89　Unspecified viral infection of central nervous system** 　HIV CC
　　CC Excl: PDX collection 139

### Arthropod-borne viral fevers and viral hemorrhagic fevers (A90-A99)

**A90　Dengue fever [classical dengue]** 　CC
　　EXCLUDES 1　dengue hemorrhagic fever (A91)
　　AHA: 2016, 3Q, 13
　　CC Excl: PDX collection 142

**A91　Dengue hemorrhagic fever** 　CC
　　CC Excl: PDX collection 143

✓4ᵗʰ **A92　Other mosquito-borne viral fevers**
　　EXCLUDES 1　Ross River disease (B33.1)
　　**A92.0　Chikungunya virus disease** 　CC
　　　　　　Chikungunya (hemorrhagic) fever
　　　　　　CC Excl: PDX collection 143
　　**A92.1　O'nyong-nyong fever** 　CC
　　　　　　CC Excl: PDX collection 144
　　**A92.2　Venezuelan equine fever** 　CC
　　　　　　Venezuelan equine encephalitis
　　　　　　Venezuelan equine encephalomyelitis virus disease
　　　　　　CC Excl: PDX collection 144
✓5ᵗʰ **A92.3　West Nile virus infection**
　　　　　　West Nile fever
　　　　　　AHA: 2016, 3Q, 12

　　　　　　CC Excl: For MCC codes in subcategory A92.3:
　　　　　　PDX collection 145

　　　　**A92.30　West Nile virus infection, unspecified** 　MCC
　　　　　　　West Nile fever NOS
　　　　　　　West Nile fever without complications
　　　　　　　West Nile virus NOS
　　　　**A92.31　West Nile virus infection with encephalitis** 　MCC
　　　　　　　West Nile encephalitis
　　　　　　　West Nile encephalomyelitis
　　　　**A92.32　West Nile virus infection with other neurologic** 　MCC
　　　　　　　**manifestation**
　　　　　　　Use additional code to specify the neurologic
　　　　　　　manifestation
　　　　**A92.39　West Nile virus infection with other** 　MCC
　　　　　　　**complications**
　　　　　　　Use additional code to specify the other conditions
　　**A92.4　Rift Valley fever** 　CC
　　　　　　CC Excl: PDX collection 144
　　**A92.5　Zika virus disease** 　CC
　　　　　　Zika virus fever
　　　　　　Zika virus infection
　　　　　　Zika NOS
　　　　　　CC Excl: PDX collection 144
　　**A92.8　Other specified mosquito-borne viral fevers** 　CC
　　　　　　CC Excl: PDX collection 144
　　**A92.9　Mosquito-borne viral fever, unspecified** 　CC
　　　　　　CC Excl: PDX collection 143

✓4ᵗʰ **A93　Other arthropod-borne viral fevers, not elsewhere classified**

　　CC Excl: For CC codes in category A93, unless otherwise noted:
　　PDX collection 143

　　**A93.0　Oropouche virus disease** 　CC
　　　　　　Oropouche fever
　　　　　　CC Excl: PDX collection 144
　　**A93.1　Sandfly fever** 　CC
　　　　　　Pappataci fever
　　　　　　Phlebotomus fever
　　**A93.2　Colorado tick fever** 　CC
　　**A93.8　Other specified arthropod-borne viral fevers** 　CC
　　　　　　Piry virus disease
　　　　　　Vesicular stomatitis virus disease [Indiana fever]

**A94　Unspecified arthropod-borne viral fever** 　CC
　　Arboviral fever NOS
　　Arbovirus infection NOS
　　CC Excl: PDX collection 143

✓4ᵗʰ **A95　Yellow fever**

　　CC Excl: For CC codes in category A95: PDX collection 146

　　**A95.0　Sylvatic yellow fever** 　CC
　　　　　　Jungle yellow fever
　　**A95.1　Urban yellow fever** 　CC
　　**A95.9　Yellow fever, unspecified** 　CC

✓4ᵗʰ **A96　Arenaviral hemorrhagic feverr**

　　CC Excl: For CC codes in category A96: PDX collection 147

　　**A96.0　Junin hemorrhagic fever** 　CC
　　　　　　Argentinian hemorrhagic fever
　　**A96.1　Machupo hemorrhagic fever** 　CC
　　　　　　Bolivian hemorrhagic fever
　　**A96.2　Lassa fever**
　　**A96.8　Other arenaviral hemorrhagic fevers** 　CC
　　**A96.9　Arenaviral hemorrhagic fever, unspecified** 　CC

**Chapter 1. Certain Infectious and Parasitic Diseases**

**A84–A96.9**

**Chapter 1. Certain Infectious and Parasitic Diseases**

✓4th **A98 Other viral hemorrhagic fevers, not elsewhere classified**
- **EXCLUDES 1**   chikungunya hemorrhagic fever (A92.0)
      dengue hemorrhagic fever (A91)

**CC Excl: For CC codes in category A98, unless otherwise noted:** PDX collection 143

**A98.0 Crimean-Congo hemorrhagic fever** `CC`
    Central Asian hemorrhagic fever

**A98.1 Omsk hemorrhagic fever** `CC`

**A98.2 Kyasanur Forest disease** `CC`

**A98.3 Marburg virus disease**

**A98.4 Ebola virus disease**

**A98.5 Hemorrhagic fever with renal syndrome** `CC`
    Epidemic hemorrhagic fever
    Korean hemorrhagic fever
    Russian hemorrhagic fever
    Hantaan virus disease
    Hantavirus disease with renal manifestations
    Nephropathia epidemica
    Songo fever
    **EXCLUDES 1**   hantavirus (cardio)-pulmonary syndrome (B33.4)
    **CC Excl:** PDX collection 148

**A98.8 Other specified viral hemorrhagic fevers** `CC`

**A99 Unspecified viral hemorrhagic fever** `CC`
    **CC Excl:** PDX collection 143

## Viral infections characterized by skin and mucous membrane lesions (B00-B09)

✓4th **B00 Herpesviral [herpes simplex] infections**
- **EXCLUDES 1**   congenital herpesviral infections (P35.2)
- **EXCLUDES 2**   anogenital herpesviral infection (A60.-)
      gammaherpesviral mononucleosis (B27.0-)
      herpangina (B08.5)

**B00.0 Eczema herpeticum** `HIV`
    Kaposi's varicelliform eruption

**B00.1 Herpesviral vesicular dermatitis** `HIV`
    Herpes simplex facialis
    Herpes simplex labialis
    Herpes simplex otitis externa
    Vesicular dermatitis of ear
    Vesicular dermatitis of lip

**B00.2 Herpesviral gingivostomatitis and pharyngotonsillitis** `HIV` `CC`
    Herpesviral pharyngitis
    **CC Excl:** PDX collection 149

**B00.3 Herpesviral meningitis** `HIV` `MCC`
    **CC Excl:** PDX collection 150

**B00.4 Herpesviral encephalitis** `HIV` `MCC`
    Herpesviral meningoencephalitis
    Simian B disease
    **EXCLUDES 1**   herpesviral encephalitis due to herpesvirus 6 and 7 (B10.01, B10.09)
       non-simplex herpesviral encephalitis (B10.0-)
    **CC Excl:** PDX collection 151

✓5th **B00.5 Herpesviral ocular disease**

**CC Excl: For CC codes in subcategory B00.5:** PDX collection 152

**B00.50 Herpesviral ocular disease, unspecified** `HIV` `CC`

**B00.51 Herpesviral iridocyclitis** `HIV` `CC`
    Herpesviral iritis
    Herpesviral uveitis, anterior

**B00.52 Herpesviral keratitis** `HIV` `CC`
    Herpesviral keratoconjunctivitis

**B00.53 Herpesviral conjunctivitis** `HIV` `CC`

**B00.59 Other herpesviral disease of eye** `HIV` `CC`
    Herpesviral dermatitis of eyelid

**B00.7 Disseminated herpesviral disease** `HIV` `MCC` `HCC`
    Herpesviral sepsis
    **CC Excl:** PDX collection 153

✓5th **B00.8 Other forms of herpesviral infections**

**B00.81 Herpesviral hepatitis** `HIV` `CC`
    **CC Excl:** PDX collection 154

**B00.82 Herpes simplex myelitis** `MCC` `HCC`
    **CC Excl:** PDX collection 155

**B00.89 Other herpesviral infection** `HIV` `CC`
    Herpesviral whitlow
    **CC Excl:** PDX collection 156

**B00.9 Herpesviral infection, unspecified** `HIV`
    Herpes simplex infection NOS

✓4th **B01 Varicella [chickenpox]**

**B01.0 Varicella meningitis** `CC`
    **CC Excl:** PDX collection 157

✓5th **B01.1 Varicella encephalitis, myelitis and encephalomyelitis**
    Postchickenpox encephalitis, myelitis and encephalomyelitis

**B01.11 Varicella encephalitis and encephalomyelitis** `MCC`
    Postchickenpox encephalitis and encephalomyelitis
    **CC Excl:** PDX collection 158

**B01.12 Varicella myelitis** `MCC` `HCC`
    Postchickenpox myelitis
    **CC Excl:** PDX collection 159

**B01.2 Varicella pneumonia** `MCC`
    **CC Excl:** PDX collection 160

✓5th **B01.8 Varicella with other complications**

**B01.81 Varicella keratitis** `CC`
    **CC Excl:** PDX collection 157

**B01.89 Other varicella complications** `CC`
    **CC Excl:** PDX collection 157

**B01.9 Varicella without complication** `CC`
    Varicella NOS
    **CC Excl:** PDX collection 157

✓4th **B02 Zoster [herpes zoster]**
- **INCLUDES**   shingles
      zona

**B02.0 Zoster encephalitis** `HIV` `CC`
    Zoster meningoencephalitis
    **CC Excl:** PDX collection 161

**B02.1 Zoster meningitis** `HIV` `MCC`
    **CC Excl:** PDX collection 162

✓5th **B02.2 Zoster with other nervous system involvement**

**CC Excl: For CC codes in subcategory B02.2, unless otherwise noted:** PDX collection 161

**B02.21 Postherpetic geniculate ganglionitis** `HIV` `CC`

**B02.22 Postherpetic trigeminal neuralgia** `HIV` `CC`

**B02.23 Postherpetic polyneuropathy** `HIV` `CC`

**B02.24 Postherpetic myelitis** `MCC` `HCC`
    Herpes zoster myelitis
    **CC Excl:** PDX collection 163

**B02.29 Other postherpetic nervous system involvement** `HIV` `CC`
    Postherpetic radiculopathy

✓5th **B02.3 Zoster ocular disease**

**CC Excl: For CC codes in subcategory B02.3:** PDX collection 164

**B02.30 Zoster ocular disease, unspecified** `HIV` `CC`

**B02.31 Zoster conjunctivitis** `HIV` `CC`

**B02.32 Zoster iridocyclitis** `HIV` `CC`

**B02.33 Zoster keratitis** `HIV` `CC`
    Herpes zoster keratoconjunctivitis

**B02.34 Zoster scleritis** `HIV` `CC`

**B02.39 Other herpes zoster eye disease** `HIV` `CC`
    Zoster blepharitis

**B02.7 Disseminated zoster** `HIV` `CC`
    **CC Excl:** PDX collection 165

**B02.8 Zoster with other complications** `HIV` `CC`
    Herpes zoster otitis externa
    **CC Excl:** PDX collection 165

**B02.9 Zoster without complications** `HIV`
    Zoster NOS

**B03 Smallpox** `CC`
    **NOTE**   In 1980 the 33rd World Health Assembly declared that smallpox had been eradicated.
       The classification is maintained for surveillance purposes.
    **CC Excl:** PDX collection 166

**B04 Monkeypox** `CC`
    **CC Excl:** PDX collection 167

✓4th **B05 Measles**
- **INCLUDES**   morbilli
- **EXCLUDES 1**   subacute sclerosing panencephalitis (A81.1)

**B05.0 Measles complicated by encephalitis** `MCC`
    Postmeasles encephalitis
    **CC Excl:** PDX collection 168

**B05.1 Measles complicated by meningitis** `CC`
    Postmeasles meningitis
    **CC Excl:** PDX collection 169

N Newborn: 0   P Pediatric: 0-17   M Maternity: 12-55   A Adult: 15-124   MCC Major CC Condition   PDxMCC PDx acts as own MCC   CC CC Condition   PDxCC PDx acts as own CC

448              ICD-10-CM 2018

**B05.2 Measles complicated by pneumonia**    `MCC`
Postmeasles pneumonia
**CC Excl:** PDX collection 170

**B05.3 Measles complicated by otitis media**
Postmeasles otitis media

**B05.4 Measles with intestinal complications**    `CC`
**CC Excl:** PDX collection 169

✓5ᵗʰ **B05.8 Measles with other complications**

     **B05.81 Measles keratitis and keratoconjunctivitis**    `CC`
       **CC Excl:** PDX collection 171

     **B05.89 Other measles complications**    `CC`
       **CC Excl:** PDX collection 169

**B05.9 Measles without complication**
Measles NOS

✓4ᵗʰ **B06 Rubella [German measles]**
     `EXCLUDES 1`   congenital rubella (P35.0)

✓5ᵗʰ **B06.0 Rubella with neurological complications**

     **CC Excl: For CC/MCC codes in subcategory B06.0:**
     PDX collection 172

     **B06.00 Rubella with neurological complication,**    `CC`
       **unspecified**

     **B06.01 Rubella encephalitis**    `MCC`
       Rubella meningoencephalitis

     **B06.02 Rubella meningitis**    `CC`

     **B06.09 Other neurological complications of rubella**    `CC`

✓5ᵗʰ **B06.8 Rubella with other complications**

     **B06.81 Rubella pneumonia**    `CC`
       **CC Excl:** PDX collection 172

     **B06.82 Rubella arthritis**    `CC` `HCC`
       **CC Excl:** PDX collection 173

     **B06.89 Other rubella complications**    `CC`
       **CC Excl:** PDX collection 172

**B06.9 Rubella without complication**
Rubella NOS

✓4ᵗʰ **B07 Viral warts**
     `INCLUDES`   verruca simplex
             verruca vulgaris
             viral warts due to human papillomavirus
     `EXCLUDES 2`   anogenital (venereal) warts (A63.0)
             papilloma of bladder (D41.4)
             papilloma of cervix (D26.0)
             papilloma larynx (D14.1)

**B07.0 Plantar wart**
Verruca plantaris

**B07.8 Other viral warts**
Common wart
Flat wart
Verruca plana

**B07.9 Viral wart, unspecified**

✓4ᵗʰ **B08 Other viral infections characterized by skin and mucous membrane lesions, not elsewhere classified**
     `EXCLUDES 1`   vesicular stomatitis virus disease (A93.8)

✓5ᵗʰ **B08.0 Other orthopoxvirus infections**
     `EXCLUDES 2`   monkeypox (B04)

     ✓6ᵗʰ **B08.01 Cowpox and vaccinia not from vaccine**

       **B08.010 Cowpox**
         **DEF:** A disease contracted by milking infected cows; vesicles usually appear on the fingers, hands and adjacent areas and usually disappear without scarring; other symptoms: local edema, lymphangitis, and regional lymphadenitis with or without fever.

       **B08.011 Vaccinia not from vaccine**
         `EXCLUDES 1`   vaccinia (from vaccination) (generalized) (T88.1)

     **B08.02 Orf virus disease**
       Contagious pustular dermatitis
       Ecthyma contagiosum

     **B08.03 Pseudocowpox [milker's node]**

     **B08.04 Paravaccinia, unspecified**

     **B08.09 Other orthopoxvirus infections**
       Orthopoxvirus infection NOS

**B08.1 Molluscum contagiosum**
     **DEF:** Benign poxvirus infection causing small bumps on the skin or conjunctiva; transmitted by close contact.

**B08.2 Exanthema subitum [sixth disease]**
Roseola infantum

     **B08.20 Exanthema subitum [sixth disease], unspecified**    `P`
       Roseola infantum, unspecified

     **B08.21 Exanthema subitum [sixth disease] due to human**    `P`
       **herpesvirus 6**
       Roseola infantum due to human herpesvirus 6

     **B08.22 Exanthema subitum [sixth disease] due to human**    `P`
       **herpesvirus 7**
       Roseola infantum due to human herpesvirus 7

**B08.3 Erythema infectiosum [fifth disease]**    `CC`
**CC Excl:** PDX collection 174

**B08.4 Enteroviral vesicular stomatitis with exanthem**
Hand, foot and mouth disease

**B08.5 Enteroviral vesicular pharyngitis**
Herpangina
**DEF:** Acute infectious Coxsackie virus infection causing throat lesions, fever, and vomiting; generally affects children in summer.

✓5ᵗʰ **B08.6 Parapoxvirus infections**

     **B08.60 Parapoxvirus infection, unspecified**

     **B08.61 Bovine stomatitis**

     **B08.62 Sealpox**

     **B08.69 Other parapoxvirus infections**

✓5ᵗʰ **B08.7 Yatapoxvirus infections**

     **B08.70 Yatapoxvirus infection, unspecified**

     **B08.71 Tanapox virus disease**    `CC`
       **CC Excl:** PDX collection 167

     **B08.72 Yaba pox virus disease**
       Yaba monkey tumor disease

     **B08.79 Other yatapoxvirus infections**

**B08.8 Other specified viral infections characterized by skin and mucous membrane lesions**
Enteroviral lymphonodular pharyngitis
Foot-and-mouth disease
Poxvirus NEC

**B09 Unspecified viral infection characterized by skin and mucous membrane lesions**
Viral enanthema NOS
Viral exanthema NOS

### Other human herpesviruses (B10)

✓4ᵗʰ **B10 Other human herpesviruses**
     `EXCLUDES 2`   cytomegalovirus (B25.9)
             Epstein-Barr virus (B27.0-)
             herpes NOS (B00.9)
             herpes simplex (B00.-)
             herpes zoster (B02.-)
             human herpesvirus NOS (B00.-)
             human herpesvirus 1 and 2 (B00.-)
             human herpesvirus 3 (B01.-, B02.-)
             human herpesvirus 4 (B27.0-)
             human herpesvirus 5 (B25.-)
             varicella (B01.-)
             zoster (B02.-)

✓5ᵗʰ **B10.0 Other human herpesvirus encephalitis**
     `EXCLUDES 2`   herpes encephalitis NOS (B00.4)
             herpes simplex encephalitis (B00.4)
             human herpesvirus encephalitis (B00.4)
             simian B herpes virus encephalitis (B00.4)

     **B10.01 Human herpesvirus 6 encephalitis**    `HIV` `MCC`
       **CC Excl:** PDX collection 151

     **B10.09 Other human herpesvirus encephalitis**    `HIV` `MCC`
       Human herpesvirus 7 encephalitis
       **CC Excl:** PDX collection 151

✓5ᵗʰ **B10.8 Other human herpesvirus infection**

     **B10.81 Human herpesvirus 6 infection**

     **B10.82 Human herpesvirus 7 infection**

     **B10.89 Other human herpesvirus infection**
       Human herpesvirus 8 infection
       Kaposi's sarcoma-associated herpesvirus infection

**Chapter 1. Certain Infectious and Parasitic Diseases**

B15–B27.09

## Viral hepatitis (B15-B19)

**EXCLUDES 1**   *sequelae of viral hepatitis (B94.2)*
**EXCLUDES 2**   *cytomegaloviral hepatitis (B25.1)*
     *herpesviral [herpes simplex] hepatitis (B00.81)*

**DEF:** Hepatitis A: HAV infection is self-limiting with flulike symptoms; transmission, fecal-oral.
**DEF:** Hepatitis B: HBV infection can be chronic and systemic; transmission, bodily fluids.
**DEF:** Hepatitis C: HCV infection can be chronic and systemic; transmission, blood transfusion and unidentified agents.
**DEF:** Hepatitis D (delta): HDV occurs only in the presence of hepatitis B virus; transmission, contaminated blood in contact with mucous membranes.
**DEF:** Hepatitis E: HEV is epidemic form; transmission, fecal-oral, most often from contaminated water.

✓4th **B15**   **Acute hepatitis A**

     **B15.0**   **Hepatitis A** with hepatic coma    `MCC`
         **CC Excl:** PDX collection 175

     **B15.9**   **Hepatitis A** without hepatic coma    `CC`
         Hepatitis A (acute)(viral) NOS
         **CC Excl:** PDX collection 175

✓4th **B16**   **Acute hepatitis B**
     AHA: 2016, 3Q, 13

     **CC Excl: For CC/MCC codes in category B16:** PDX collection 175

     **B16.0**   **Acute hepatitis B** with delta-agent with hepatic coma    `MCC`

     **B16.1**   **Acute hepatitis B** with delta-agent without hepatic coma    `CC`

     **B16.2**   **Acute hepatitis B** without delta-agent with hepatic coma    `MCC`

     **B16.9**   **Acute hepatitis B** without delta-agent and without hepatic coma    `CC`
         Hepatitis B (acute) (viral) NOS

✓4th **B17**   **Other acute viral hepatitis**

     **CC Excl: For CC/MCC codes in category B17:** PDX collection 175

     **B17.0**   **Acute delta-(super) infection of hepatitis B carrier**    `CC`

 ✓5th **B17.1**   **Acute hepatitis C**

         **B17.10**   **Acute hepatitis C** without hepatic coma    `CC`
                 Acute hepatitis C NOS

         **B17.11**   **Acute hepatitis C** with hepatic coma    `MCC`

     **B17.2**   **Acute hepatitis E**    `CC`

     **B17.8**   **Other specified acute viral hepatitis**    `CC`
         Hepatitis non-A non-B (acute) (viral) NEC

     **B17.9**   **Acute viral hepatitis, unspecified**    `CC`
         Acute hepatitis NOS
         Acute infectious hepatitis NOSb

✓4th **B18**   **Chronic viral hepatitis**
     **INCLUDES**   carrier of viral hepatitis
     AHA: 2017, 1Q, 41

     **CC Excl: For CC codes in category B18:** PDX collection 175

     **B18.0**   **Chronic viral hepatitis B** with delta-agent    `CC` `HCC`

     **B18.1**   **Chronic viral hepatitis B** without delta-agent    `CC` `HCC`
         Carrier of viral hepatitis B
         Chronic (viral) hepatitis B

     **B18.2**   **Chronic viral hepatitis C**    `HCC`
         Carrier of viral hepatitis C

     **B18.8**   **Other chronic viral hepatitis**    `CC` `HCC`
         Carrier of other viral hepatitis

     **B18.9**   **Chronic viral hepatitis, unspecified**    `CC` `HCC`
         Carrier of unspecified viral hepatitis

✓4th **B19**   **Unspecified viral hepatitis**

     **CC Excl: For CC/MCC codes in category B19:** PDX collection 175

     **B19.0**   **Unspecified viral hepatitis** with hepatic coma    `MCC`

 ✓5th **B19.1**   **Unspecified viral hepatitis B**

         **B19.10**   **Unspecified viral hepatitis B** without hepatic coma    `CC`
                 Unspecified viral hepatitis B NOS

         **B19.11**   **Unspecified viral hepatitis B** with hepatic coma    `MCC`

 ✓5th **B19.2**   **Unspecified viral hepatitis C**

         **B19.20**   **Unspecified viral hepatitis C** without hepatic coma
                 Viral hepatitis C NOS

         **B19.21**   **Unspecified viral hepatitis C** with hepatic coma    `MCC`

     **B19.9**   **Unspecified viral hepatitis** without hepatic coma    `CC`
         Viral hepatitis NOS

## Human immunodeficiency virus [HIV] disease (B20)

**B20**   **Human immunodeficiency virus [HIV] disease**    `MCC` `HCC`
     **INCLUDES**   acquired immune deficiency syndrome [AIDS]
               AIDS-related complex [ARC]
               HIV infection, symptomatic
     Code first human immunodeficiency virus [HIV] disease complicating pregnancy, childbirth and the puerperium, if applicable (O98.7-)
     Use additional code(s) to identify all manifestations of HIV infection
     **EXCLUDES 1**   *asymptomatic human immunodeficiency virus [HIV] infection status (Z21)*
               *exposure to HIV virus (Z20.6)*
               *inconclusive serologic evidence of HIV (R75)*
     **CC Excl:** PDX collection 176

## Other viral diseases (B25-B34)

✓4th **B25**   **Cytomegaloviral disease**
     **EXCLUDES 1**   *congenital cytomegalovirus infection (P35.1)*
               *cytomegaloviral mononucleosis (B27.1-)*

     **B25.0**   **Cytomegaloviral pneumonitis**    `PDxMCC` `MCC` `HCC`
         **CC Excl:** PDX collection 110

     **B25.1**   **Cytomegaloviral hepatitis**    `PDxCC` `CC` `HCC`
         **CC Excl:** No Excl

     **B25.2**   **Cytomegaloviral pancreatitis**    `PDxMCC` `MCC` `HCC`
         **CC Excl:** PDX collection 177

     **B25.8**   **Other cytomegaloviral diseases**    `HIV` `CC` `HCC`
         Cytomegaloviral encephalitis
         **CC Excl:** PDX collection 178

     **B25.9**   **Cytomegaloviral disease, unspecified**    `HIV` `CC` `HCC`
         **CC Excl:** PDX collection 178

✓4th **B26**   **Mumps**
     **INCLUDES**   epidemic parotitis
               infectious parotitis

     **B26.0**   **Mumps orchitis**    `CC` ♂
         **CC Excl:** PDX collection 179

     **B26.1**   **Mumps meningitis**    `MCC`
         **CC Excl:** PDX collection 180

     **B26.2**   **Mumps encephalitis**    `MCC`
         **CC Excl:** PDX collection 181

     **B26.3**   **Mumps pancreatitis**    `CC`
         **CC Excl:** PDX collection 182

 ✓5th **B26.8**   **Mumps with other complications**

         **B26.81**   **Mumps hepatitis**    `CC`
                 **CC Excl:** PDX collection 183

         **B26.82**   **Mumps myocarditis**    `CC`
                 **CC Excl:** PDX collection 184

         **B26.83**   **Mumps nephritis**    `CC`
                 **CC Excl:** PDX collection 184

         **B26.84**   **Mumps polyneuropathy**    `CC`
                 **CC Excl:** PDX collection 185

         **B26.85**   **Mumps arthritis**    `CC` `HCC`
                 **CC Excl:** PDX collection 184

         **B26.89**   **Other mumps complications**    `CC`
                 **CC Excl:** PDX collection 184

     **B26.9**   **Mumps without complication**
         Mumps NOS
         Mumps parotitis NOS

✓4th **B27**   **Infectious mononucleosis**
     **INCLUDES**   glandular fever
               monocytic angina
               Pfeiffer's disease

 ✓5th **B27.0**   **Gammaherpesviral mononucleosis**
         Mononucleosis due to Epstein-Barr virus

         **B27.00**   **Gammaherpesviral mononucleosis** without complication

         **B27.01**   **Gammaherpesviral mononucleosis** with polyneuropathy

         **B27.02**   **Gammaherpesviral mononucleosis** with meningitis

         **B27.09**   **Gammaherpesviral mononucleosis** with other complications
                 Hepatomegaly in gammaherpesviral mononucleosis

N Newborn: 0    P Pediatric: 0-17    M Maternity: 12-55    A Adult: 15-124    `MCC` Major CC Condition    `PDxMCC` PDx acts as own MCC    `CC` CC Condition    `PDxCC` PDx acts as own CC

450      ICD-10-CM 2018

✓5ᵗʰ **B27.1** **Cytomegaloviral** mononucleosis

  **B27.10** **Cytomegaloviral mononucleosis** without complications

  **B27.11** **Cytomegaloviral mononucleosis** with polyneuropathy

  **B27.12** **Cytomegaloviral mononucleosis** with meningitis

  **B27.19** **Cytomegaloviral mononucleosis** with other complication
      Hepatomegaly in cytomegaloviral mononucleosis

✓5ᵗʰ **B27.8** **Other** infectious mononucleosis

  **B27.80** **Other infectious mononucleosis** without complication

  **B27.81** **Other infectious mononucleosis** with polyneuropathy

  **B27.82** **Other infectious mononucleosis** with meningitis

  **B27.89** **Other infectious mononucleosis** with other complication
      Hepatomegaly in other infectious mononucleosis

✓5ᵗʰ **B27.9** **Infectious mononucleosis,** unspecified

  **B27.90** **Infectious mononucleosis, unspecified** without complication

  **B27.91** **Infectious mononucleosis, unspecified** with polyneuropathy

  **B27.92** **Infectious mononucleosis, unspecified** with meningitis

  **B27.99** **Infectious mononucleosis, unspecified** with other complication
      Hepatomegaly in unspecified infectious mononucleosis

✓4ᵗʰ **B30** **Viral conjunctivitis**

  **EXCLUDES 1** *herpesviral [herpes simplex] ocular disease (B00.5)*
      *ocular zoster (B02.3)*

  **B30.0** **Keratoconjunctivitis** due to **adenovirus**
    Epidemic keratoconjunctivitis
    Shipyard eye

  **B30.1** **Conjunctivitis** due to **adenovirus**
    Acute adenoviral follicular conjunctivitis
    Swimming-pool conjunctivitis

  **B30.2** **Viral pharyngoconjunctivitis**

  **B30.3** **Acute epidemic hemorrhagic conjunctivitis (enteroviral)**
    Conjunctivitis due to coxsackievirus 24
    Conjunctivitis due to enterovirus 70
    Hemorrhagic conjunctivitis (acute)(epidemic)

  **B30.8** **Other viral conjunctivitis**
    Newcastle conjunctivitis

  **B30.9** **Viral conjunctivitis,** unspecified

✓4ᵗʰ **B33** **Other viral diseases,** not elsewhere classified

  **B33.0** **Epidemic myalgia**
    Bornholm disease

  **B33.1** **Ross River disease**    **CC**
    Epidemic polyarthritis and exanthema
    Ross River fever
    **CC Excl:** PDX collection 144

### Viral Conjunctivitis

Normal conjunctiva

Inflamed conjunctiva

✓5ᵗʰ **B33.2** **Viral carditis**
    Coxsackie (virus) carditis

  **B33.20** **Viral carditis,** unspecified    **CC**
    **CC Excl:** PDX collection 186

  **B33.21** **Viral endocarditis**    **CC**
    **CC Excl:** PDX collection 187

  **B33.22** **Viral myocarditis**    **CC**
    **CC Excl:** PDX collection 186

  **B33.23** **Viral pericarditis**    **CC**
    **CC Excl:** PDX collection 188

  **B33.24** **Viral cardiomyopathy**    **HCC**

  **B33.3** **Retrovirus infections,** not elsewhere classified
    Retrovirus infection NOS

  **B33.4** **Hantavirus (cardio)-pulmonary syndrome [HPS] [HCPS]**    **CC**
    Hantavirus disease with pulmonary manifestations
    Sin nombre virus disease
    Use additional code to identify any associated acute kidney failure (N17.9)
    **EXCLUDES 1** *hantavirus disease with renal manifestations (A98.5)*
      *hemorrhagic fever with renal manifestations (A98.5)*
    **CC Excl:** PDX collection 189

  **B33.8** **Other specified viral diseases**
    **EXCLUDES 1** *anogenital human papillomavirus infection (A63.0)*
      *viral warts due to human papillomavirus infection (B07)*

✓4ᵗʰ **B34** **Viral infection of unspecified site**

  **EXCLUDES 1** *anogenital human papillomavirus infection (A63.0)*
    *cytomegaloviral disease NOS (B25.9)*
    *herpesvirus [herpes simplex] infection NOS (B00.9)*
    *retrovirus infection NOS (B33.3)*
    *viral agents as the cause of diseases classified elsewhere (B97.-)*
    *viral warts due to human papillomavirus infection (B07)*

  **B34.0** **Adenovirus** infection, unspecified

  **B34.1** **Enterovirus** infection, unspecified
    Coxsackievirus infection NOS
    Echovirus infection NOS

  **B34.2** **Coronavirus** infection, unspecified
    **EXCLUDES 1** *pneumonia due to SARS-associated coronavirus (J12.81)*

  **B34.3** **Parvovirus** infection, unspecified    **CC**
    **CC Excl:** PDX collection 174

  **B34.4** **Papovavirus** infection, unspecified

  **B34.8** **Other viral infections of unspecified site**

  **B34.9** **Viral infection,** unspecified
    Viremia NOS
    **AHA:** 2016, 3Q, 10

### Mycoses (B35-B49)

**EXCLUDES 2** *hypersensitivity pneumonitis due to organic dust (J67.-)*
  *mycosis fungoides (C84.0-)*

✓4ᵗʰ **B35** **Dermatophytosis**

  **INCLUDES** favus
    infections due to species of Epidermophyton, Micro-sporum and Trichophyton
    tinea, any type except those in B36-
  **DEF:** Contagious superficial fungal infection of the skin that invades and grows in dead keratin.

  **B35.0** **Tinea barbae and tinea capitis**
    Beard ringworm
    Kerion
    Scalp ringworm
    Sycosis, mycotic

  **B35.1** **Tinea unguium**
    Dermatophytic onychia
    Dermatophytosis of nail
    Onychomycosis
    Ringworm of nails

  **B35.2** **Tinea manuum**
    Dermatophytosis of hand
    Hand ringworm

  **B35.3** **Tinea pedis**
    Athlete's foot
    Dermatophytosis of foot
    Foot ringworm

  **B35.4** **Tinea corporis**
    Ringworm of the body

  **B35.5** **Tinea imbricata**
    Tokelau

✓ Additional Character Req    ✓x7ᵗʰ Placeholder Alert    Unacceptable PDx    Manifestation    **H1**-**H4** HAC    **HCC** CMS-HCC Condition    *EXCLUDES 1* Not Coded Here    *EXCLUDES 2* Not Included Here

ICD-10-CM 2018      **451**

B27.1–B35.5

**B35.6** **Tinea** cruris
Dhobi itch
Groin ringworm
Jock itch

**B35.8** **Other** dermatophytoses
Disseminated dermatophytosis
Granulomatous dermatophytosis

**B35.9** **Dermatophytosis,** unspecified
Ringworm NOS

✓4ᵗʰ **B36** **Other superficial mycoses**

**B36.0** **Pityriasis versicolor**
Tinea flava
Tinea versicolor

**B36.1** **Tinea nigra**
Keratomycosis nigricans palmaris
Microsporosis nigra
Pityriasis nigra

**B36.2** **White piedra**
Tinea blanca

**B36.3** **Black piedra**

**B36.8** **Other specified superficial mycoses**

**B36.9** **Superficial mycosis, unspecified**

✓4ᵗʰ **B37** **Candidiasis**
INCLUDES  candidosis
moniliasis
EXCLUDES 1  neonatal candidiasis (P37.5)

**B37.0** **Candidal** stomatitis          HIV CC
Oral thrush
**CC Excl:** PDX collection 190

**B37.1** **Pulmonary candidiasis**          HIV MCC HCC
Candidal bronchitis
Candidal pneumonia
**CC Excl:** PDX collection 190

**B37.2** **Candidiasis of** skin and nail          HIV
Candidal onychia
Candidal paronychia
EXCLUDES 2  diaper dermatitis (L22)

**B37.3** **Candidiasis of** vulva and vagina          ♀
Candidal vulvovaginitis
Monilial vulvovaginitis
Vaginal thrush

✓5ᵗʰ **B37.4** **Candidiasis of** other urogenital sites

**B37.41** **Candidal** cystitis and urethritis          CC H6
**CC Excl:** PDX collection 191

**B37.42** **Candidal** balanitis          ♂

**B37.49** **Other** urogenital candidiasis          CC H6
Candidal pyelonephritis
**CC Excl:** PDX collection 191

**B37.5** **Candidal** meningitis          HIV MCC
**CC Excl:** PDX collection 192

**B37.6** **Candidal** endocarditis          HIV MCC
**CC Excl:** PDX collection 190

**B37.7** **Candidal** sepsis          PDxMCC MCC HCC
Disseminated candidiasis
Systemic candidiasis
**AHA:** 2014, 4Q, 46
**CC Excl:** PDX collection 193

✓5ᵗʰ **B37.8** **Candidiasis of** other sites

**CC Excl: For CC codes in subcategory B37.8, unless otherwise noted:** PDX collection 190

**B37.81** **Candidal** esophagitis          HIV CC HCC

**B37.82** **Candidal** enteritis          HIV CC
Candidal proctitis

**B37.83** **Candidal** cheilitis          HIV CC

**B37.84** **Candidal** otitis externa          HIV CC

**B37.89** **Other** sites of candidiasis          HIV CC
Candidal osteomyelitis
**CC Excl:** PDX collection 194

**B37.9** **Candidiasis,** unspecified          HIV
Thrush NOS

✓4ᵗʰ **B38** **Coccidioidomycosis**

**B38.0** **Acute pulmonary coccidioidomycosis**          HIV CC HCC
**CC Excl:** PDX collection 195

**B38.1** **Chronic pulmonary coccidioidomycosis**          HIV CC HCC
**CC Excl:** PDX collection 196

**B38.2** **Pulmonary coccidioidomycosis,** unspecified          HIV CC HCC
**CC Excl:** PDX collection 196

**B38.3** **Cutaneous coccidioidomycosis**          HIV CC
**CC Excl:** PDX collection 197

**B38.4** **Coccidioidomycosis** meningitis          HIV MCC
**DEF:** *Coccidioides immitis* infection of the lining of the brain and/or spinal cord.
**CC Excl:** PDX collection 198

**B38.7** **Disseminated coccidioidomycosis**          HIV CC
Generalized coccidioidomycosis
**CC Excl:** PDX collection 199

✓5ᵗʰ **B38.8** **Other forms of coccidioidomycosis**

**B38.81** **Prostatic coccidioidomycosis**          HIV CC ♂
**CC Excl:** PDX collection 197

**B38.89** **Other forms of coccidioidomycosis**          HIV CC
**CC Excl:** PDX collection 199

**B38.9** **Coccidioidomycosis,** unspecified          HIV CC
**CC Excl:** PDX collection 199

✓4ᵗʰ **B39** **Histoplasmosis**
Code first associated AIDS (B20)
Use additional code for any associated manifestations, such as:
endocarditis (I39)
meningitis (G02)
pericarditis (I32)
retinitits (H32)
**DEF:** Type of lung infection caused by breathing in fungal spores often found in the droppings of bats and birds or soil contaminated by their droppings.

**CC Excl: For MCC codes in category B39, unless otherwise noted:** PDX collection 200

**B39.0** **Acute pulmonary histoplasmosis capsulati**          HIV MCC HCC

**B39.1** **Chronic pulmonary histoplasmosis capsulati**          HIV MCC HCC

**B39.2** **Pulmonary histoplasmosis capsulati,** unspecified          HIV MCC HCC

**B39.3** **Disseminated histoplasmosis capsulati**          HIV CC
Generalized histoplasmosis capsulati
**CC Excl:** PDX collection 201

**B39.4** **Histoplasmosis** capsulati, unspecified          HIV
American histoplasmosis

**B39.5** **Histoplasmosis** duboisii          HIV
African histoplasmosis

**B39.9** **Histoplasmosis,** unspecified          HIV

✓4ᵗʰ **B40** **Blastomycosis**
EXCLUDES 1  Brazilian blastomycosis (B41.-)
keloidal blastomycosis (B48.0)

**CC Excl: For CC codes in category B40:** PDX collection 202

**B40.0** **Acute pulmonary blastomycosis**          CC HCC

**B40.1** **Chronic pulmonary blastomycosis**          CC HCC

**B40.2** **Pulmonary blastomycosis,** unspecified          CC HCC

**B40.3** **Cutaneous blastomycosis**          CC

**Histoplasmosis**

Histoplasma capsulatum spores

Spores

**B40.7** **Disseminated blastomycosis** `CC`
Generalized blastomycosis

✓5th **B40.8** **Other forms of blastomycosis**

**B40.81** **Blastomycotic meningoencephalitis** `CC`
Meningomyelitis due to blastomycosis

**B40.89** **Other forms of blastomycosis** `CC`

**B40.9** **Blastomycosis, unspecified** `CC`

✓4th **B41** **Paracoccidioidomycosis**
INCLUDES Brazilian blastomycosis
Lutz' disease

CC Excl: For CC codes in category B41: PDX collection 203

**B41.0** **Pulmonary paracoccidioidomycosis** `CC` `HCC`

**B41.7** **Disseminated paracoccidioidomycosis** `CC`
Generalized paracoccidioidomycosis

**B41.8** **Other forms of paracoccidioidomycosis** `CC`

**B41.9** **Paracoccidioidomycosis, unspecified** `CC`

✓4th **B42** **Sporotrichosis**

**B42.0** **Pulmonary sporotrichosis**

**B42.1** **Lymphocutaneous sporotrichosis**

**B42.7** **Disseminated sporotrichosis**
Generalized sporotrichosis

✓5th **B42.8** **Other forms of sporotrichosis**

**B42.81** **Cerebral sporotrichosis**
Meningitis due to sporotrichosis

**B42.82** **Sporotrichosis arthritis** `HCC`

**B42.89** **Other forms of sporotrichosis**

**B42.9** **Sporotrichosis, unspecified**

✓4th **B43** **Chromomycosis and pheomycotic abscess**

**B43.0** **Cutaneous chromomycosis**
Dermatitis verrucosa

**B43.1** **Pheomycotic brain abscess**
Cerebral chromomycosis

**B43.2** **Subcutaneous pheomycotic abscess and cyst**

**B43.8** **Other forms of chromomycosis**

**B43.9** **Chromomycosis, unspecified**

✓4th **B44** **Aspergillosis**
INCLUDES aspergilloma

CC Excl: For CC codes in category B44, unless otherwise noted:
PDX collection 204

**B44.0** **Invasive pulmonary aspergillosis** `PDxMCC` `MCC` `HCC`
CC Excl: PDX collection 110

**B44.1** **Other pulmonary aspergillosis** `CC` `HCC`

**B44.2** **Tonsillar aspergillosis** `CC` `HCC`

**B44.7** **Disseminated aspergillosis** `CC` `HCC`
Generalized aspergillosis

✓5th **B44.8** **Other forms of aspergillosis**

**B44.81** **Allergic bronchopulmonary aspergillosis** `CC` `HCC`
CC Excl: PDX collection 205

**B44.89** **Other forms of aspergillosis** `CC` `HCC`

**B44.9** **Aspergillosis, unspecified** `CC` `HCC`

✓4th **B45** **Cryptococcosis**

CC Excl: For CC codes in category B45, unless otherwise noted:
PDX collection 206

**B45.0** **Pulmonary cryptococcosis** `HIV` `CC` `HCC`

**B45.1** **Cerebral cryptococcosis** `PDxMCC` `MCC` `HCC`
Cryptococcal meningitis
Cryptococcosis meningocerebralis
CC Excl: PDX collection 207

**B45.2** **Cutaneous cryptococcosis** `HIV` `CC` `HCC`

**B45.3** **Osseous cryptococcosis** `HIV` `CC` `HCC`

**B45.7** **Disseminated cryptococcosis** `HIV` `CC` `HCC`
Generalized cryptococcosis

**B45.8** **Other forms of cryptococcosis** `HIV` `CC` `HCC`

**B45.9** **Cryptococcosis, unspecified** `HIV` `CC` `HCC`

✓4th **B46** **Zygomycosis**

CC Excl: For MCC codes in category B46: PDX collection 208

**B46.0** **Pulmonary mucormycosis** `MCC` `HCC`

**B46.1** **Rhinocerebral mucormycosis** `MCC` `HCC`

**B46.2** **Gastrointestinal mucormycosis** `MCC` `HCC`

**B46.3** **Cutaneous mucormycosis** `MCC` `HCC`
Subcutaneous mucormycosis

**B46.4** **Disseminated mucormycosis** `MCC` `HCC`
Generalized mucormycosis

**B46.5** **Mucormycosis, unspecified** `MCC` `HCC`

**B46.8** **Other zygomycoses** `MCC` `HCC`
Entomophthoromycosis

**B46.9** **Zygomycosis, unspecified** `MCC` `HCC`
Phycomycosis NOS

✓4th **B47** **Mycetoma**

**B47.0** **Eumycetoma** `CC`
Madura foot, mycotic
Maduromycosis
CC Excl: PDX collection 209

**B47.1** **Actinomycetoma** `HIV` `CC`
CC Excl: PDX collection 106

**B47.9** **Mycetoma, unspecified** `HIV` `CC`
Madura foot NOS
CC Excl: PDX collection 210

✓4th **B48** **Other mycoses, not elsewhere classified**

**B48.0** **Lobomycosis**
Keloidal blastomycosis
Lobo's disease

**B48.1** **Rhinosporidiosis**

**B48.2** **Allescheriasis** `CC`
Infection due to Pseudallescheria boydii
EXCLUDES 1 eumycetoma (B47.0)
CC Excl: PDX collection 211

**B48.3** **Geotrichosis** `CC`
Geotrichum stomatitis
CC Excl: PDX collection 212

**B48.4** **Penicillosis** `CC` `HCC`
CC Excl: PDX collection 204

**B48.8** **Other specified mycoses** `HIV` `CC` `HCC`
Adiaspiromycosis
Infection of tissue and organs by Alternaria
Infection of tissue and organs by Drechslera
Infection of tissue and organs by Fusarium
Infection of tissue and organs by saprophytic fungi NEC
AHA: 2014, 4Q, 46; 2014, 2Q, 13
CC Excl: PDX collection 213

**B49** **Unspecified mycosis** `CC`
Fungemia NOS
CC Excl: PDX collection 212

## Protozoal diseases (B50-B64)

EXCLUDES 1 amebiasis (A06.-)
other protozoal intestinal diseases (A07.-)

✓4th **B50** **Plasmodium falciparum malaria**
INCLUDES mixed infections of Plasmodium falciparum with any other
Plasmodium species

CC Excl: For CC/MCC codes in category B50: PDX collection 214

**B50.0** **Plasmodium falciparum malaria with cerebral complications** `CC`
Cerebral malaria NOS

**B50.8** **Other severe and complicated Plasmodium falciparum malaria** `CC`
Severe or complicated Plasmodium falciparum malaria NOS

**B50.9** **Plasmodium falciparum malaria, unspecified** `MCC`

✓4th **B51** **Plasmodium vivax malaria**
INCLUDES mixed infections of Plasmodium vivax with other
Plasmodium species, except Plasmodium falciparum
EXCLUDES 1 plasmodium vivax with Plasmodium falciparum (B50.-)

CC Excl: For CC codes in category B51, unless otherwise noted:
PDX collection 214

**B51.0** **Plasmodium vivax malaria with rupture of spleen** `CC`

**B51.8** **Plasmodium vivax malaria with other complications** `CC`

**B51.9** **Plasmodium vivax malaria without complication** `CC`
Plasmodium vivax malaria NOS
CC Excl: PDX collection 215

✓4ᵗʰ **B52** **Plasmodium** malariae **malaria**

INCLUDES   mixed infections of Plasmodium malariae with other Plasmodium species, except Plasmodium falciparum and Plasmodium vivax

EXCLUDES 1   *Plasmodium falciparum (B50.-)*
*Plasmodium vivax (B51.-)*

CC Excl: For CC codes in category B52, unless otherwise noted: PDX collection 214

**B52.0** **Plasmodium malariae malaria with** nephropathy   PDxCC CC
CC Excl: PDX collection 216

**B52.8** **Plasmodium malariae malaria with** other complications   CC

**B52.9** **Plasmodium malariae malaria** without complication   CC
Plasmodium malariae malaria NOS

✓4ᵗʰ **B53** Other **specified malaria**

CC Excl: For CC codes in subcategory B53: PDX collection 214

**B53.0** Plasmodium ovale **malaria**   CC
EXCLUDES 1   *Plasmodium ovale with Plasmodium falciparum (B50.-)*
*Plasmodium ovale with Plasmodium malariae (B52.-)*
*Plasmodium ovale with Plasmodium vivax (B51.-)*

**B53.1** **Malaria due to** simian plasmodia   CC
EXCLUDES 1   *Malaria due to simian plasmodia with Plasmodium falciparum (B50.-)*
*Malaria due to simian plasmodia with Plasmodium malariae (B52.-)*
*Malaria due to simian plasmodia with Plasmodium ovale (B53.0)*
*Malaria due to simian plasmodia with Plasmodium vivax (B51.-)*

**B53.8** Other **malaria, not elsewhere classified**   CC

**B54** Unspecified **malaria**   CC
CC Excl: PDX collection 217

✓4ᵗʰ **B55** **Leishmaniasis**

CC Excl: For CC codes in category B55: PDX collection 218

**B55.0** Visceral **leishmaniasis**
Kala-azar
Post-kala-azar dermal leishmaniasis

**B55.1** Cutaneous **leishmaniasis**   CC

**B55.2** Mucocutaneous **leishmaniasis**   CC

**B55.9** **Leishmaniasis,** unspecified   CC

✓4ᵗʰ **B56** African **trypanosomiasis**

CC Excl: For CC codes in category B56: PDX collection 218

**B56.0** Gambiense **trypanosomiasis**   CC
Infection due to Trypanosoma brucei gambiense
West African sleeping sickness

**B56.1** Rhodesiense **trypanosomiasis**   CC
East African sleeping sickness
Infection due to Trypanosoma brucei rhodesiense

**B56.9** African **trypanosomiasis,** unspecified   CC
Sleeping sickness NOS

✓4ᵗʰ **B57** **Chagas' disease**
INCLUDES   American trypanosomiasis
infection due to Trypanosoma cruzi

CC Excl: For CC codes in category B57, unless otherwise noted: PDX collection 218

**B57.0** Acute **Chagas' disease with heart involvement**   CC
Acute Chagas' disease with myocarditis
CC Excl: PDX collection 219

**B57.1** Acute **Chagas' disease** without heart **involvement**   CC
Acute Chagas' disease NOS

**B57.2** **Chagas' disease** (chronic) **with heart involvement**   CC
American trypanosomiasis NOS
Chagas' disease (chronic) NOS
Chagas' disease (chronic) with myocarditis
Trypanosomiasis NOS
CC Excl: PDX collection 219

✓5ᵗʰ **B57.3** **Chagas' disease** (chronic) **with** digestive system **involvement**

**B57.30** **Chagas' disease with digestive system involvement,** unspecified   CC

**B57.31** Megaesophagus **in Chagas' disease**   CC

**B57.32** Megacolon **in Chagas' disease**   CC

**B57.39** Other **digestive system involvement in Chagas' disease**   CC

✓5ᵗʰ **B57.4** **Chagas' disease** (chronic) **with** nervous system **involvement**

**B57.40** **Chagas' disease with nervous system involvement,** unspecified   CC

**B57.41** Meningitis **in Chagas' disease**   CC

**B57.42** Meningoencephalitis **in Chagas' disease**   CC

**B57.49** Other **nervous system involvement in Chagas' disease**   CC

**B57.5** **Chagas' disease** (chronic) **with other organ involvement**   CC

✓4ᵗʰ **B58** **Toxoplasmosis**
INCLUDES   infection due to Toxoplasma gondii
EXCLUDES 1   *congenital toxoplasmosis (P37.1)*

✓5ᵗʰ **B58.0** **Toxoplasma** oculopathy

**B58.00** **Toxoplasma oculopathy,** unspecified   HIV CC
CC Excl: PDX collection 220

**B58.01** **Toxoplasma** chorioretinitis   HIV CC
CC Excl: PDX collection 221

**B58.09** Other **toxoplasma oculopathy**   HIV CC
Toxoplasma uveitis
CC Excl: PDX collection 222

**B58.1** **Toxoplasma** hepatitis   HIV CC
CC Excl: PDX collection 223

**B58.2** **Toxoplasma** meningoencephalitis   HIV MCC HCC
CC Excl: PDX collection 224

**B58.3** Pulmonary **toxoplasmosis**   HIV MCC HCC
CC Excl: PDX collection 225

✓5ᵗʰ **B58.8** **Toxoplasmosis with** other organ involvement

CC Excl: For CC codes in subcategory B58.8, unless otherwise noted: PDX collection 220

**B58.81** **Toxoplasma** myocarditis   HIV MCC
CC Excl: PDX collection 226

**B58.82** **Toxoplasma** myositis   HIV CC

**B58.83** **Toxoplasma** tubulo-interstitial nephropathy   HIV CC
Toxoplasma pyelonephritis

**B58.89** **Toxoplasmosis with** other **organ involvement**   HIV CC

**B58.9** **Toxoplasmosis,** unspecified   HIV CC
CC Excl: PDX collection 227

**B59** **Pneumocystosis**   HIV MCC HCC
Pneumonia due to Pneumocystis carinii
Pneumonia due to Pneumocystis jiroveci
CC Excl: PDX collection 228

✓4ᵗʰ **B60** **Other protozoal diseases, not elsewhere classified**
EXCLUDES 1   *cryptosporidiosis (A07.2)*
*intestinal microsporidiosis (A07.8)*
*isosporiasis (A07.3)*

**B60.0** **Babesiosis**   CC
Piroplasmosis
CC Excl: PDX collection 218

✓5ᵗʰ **B60.1** **Acanthamebiasis**

**B60.10** **Acanthamebiasis,** unspecified   CC
CC Excl: PDX collection 229

**B60.11** Meningoencephalitis **due to Acanthamoeba (culbertsoni)**

**B60.12** Conjunctivitis **due to Acanthamoeba**

**B60.13** Keratoconjunctivitis **due to Acanthamoeba**

**B60.19** Other **acanthamebic disease**   CC
CC Excl: PDX collection 229

**B60.2** **Naegleriasis**   CC
Primary amebic meningoencephalitis
CC Excl: PDX collection 229

**B60.8** **Other specified protozoal diseases**   HIV
Microsporidiosis

**B64** **Unspecified protozoal disease**

## Helminthiases (B65-B83)

✓4ᵗʰ **B65** **Schistosomiasis [bilharziasis]**
INCLUDES   snail fever

CC Excl: For CC codes in category B65: PDX collection 230

**B65.0** **Schistosomiasis due to** Schistosoma haematobium **[urinary schistosomiasis]**   CC

**B65.1** **Schistosomiasis due to** Schistosoma mansoni **[intestinal schistosomiasis]**   CC

**B65.2** **Schistosomiasis due to** Schistosoma japonicum   CC
Asiatic schistosomiasis

N Newborn: 0   P Pediatric: 0-17   M Maternity: 12-55   A Adult: 15-124   MCC Major CC Condition   PDxMCC PDx acts as own MCC   CC CC Condition   PDxCC PDx acts as own CC

454      ICD-10-CM 2018

**B65.3 Cercarial dermatitis** `CC`
Swimmer's itch

**B65.8 Other schistosomiasis** `CC`
Infection due to Schistosoma intercalatum
Infection due to Schistosoma mattheei
Infection due to Schistosoma mekongi

**B65.9 Schistosomiasis, unspecified** `CC`

✓4th **B66 Other fluke infections**

**CC Excl: For CC codes in category B66:** PDX collection 231

**B66.0 Opisthorchiasis** `CC`
Infection due to cat liver fluke
Infection due to Opisthorchis (felineus)(viverrini)

**B66.1 Clonorchiasis** `CC`
Chinese liver fluke disease
Infection due to Clonorchis sinensis
Oriental liver fluke disease

**B66.2 Dicroceliasis** `CC`
Infection due to Dicrocoelium dendriticum
Lancet fluke infection

**B66.3 Fascioliasis** `CC`
Infection due to Fasciola gigantica
Infection due to Fasciola hepatica
Infection due to Fasciola indica
Sheep liver fluke disease

**B66.4 Paragonimiasis** `CC` `HCC`
Infection due to Paragonimus species
Lung fluke disease
Pulmonary distomiasis

**B66.5 Fasciolopsiasis** `CC`
Infection due to Fasciolopsis buski
Intestinal distomiasis

**B66.8 Other specified fluke infections** `CC`
Echinostomiasis    Nanophyetiasis
Heterophyiasis    Watsoniasis
Metagonimiasis

**B66.9 Fluke infection, unspecified**

✓4th **B67 Echinococcosis**
`INCLUDES` hydatidosis

**B67.0 Echinococcus granulosus infection of liver** `CC`
**CC Excl:** PDX collection 232

**B67.1 Echinococcus granulosus infection of lung** `CC` `HCC`
**CC Excl:** PDX collection 233

**B67.2 Echinococcus granulosus infection of bone** `CC`
**CC Excl:** PDX collection 234

✓5th **B67.3 Echinococcus granulosus infection, other and multiple sites**

**B67.31 Echinococcus granulosus infection, thyroid gland** `CC`
**CC Excl:** PDX collection 235

**B67.32 Echinococcus granulosus infection, multiple sites** `CC`
**CC Excl:** PDX collection 234

**B67.39 Echinococcus granulosus infection, other sites** `CC`
**CC Excl:** PDX collection 234

**B67.4 Echinococcus granulosus infection, unspecified** `CC`
Dog tapeworm (infection)
**CC Excl:** PDX collection 236

**B67.5 Echinococcus multilocularis infection of liver** `CC`
**CC Excl:** PDX collection 237

✓5th **B67.6 Echinococcus multilocularis infection, other and multiple sites**

**B67.61 Echinococcus multilocularis infection, multiple sites** `CC`
**CC Excl:** PDX collection 238

**B67.69 Echinococcus multilocularis infection, other sites** `CC`
**CC Excl:** PDX collection 238

**B67.7 Echinococcus multilocularis infection, unspecified** `CC`
**CC Excl:** PDX collection 239

**B67.8 Echinococcosis, unspecified, of liver** `CC`
**CC Excl:** PDX collection 240

✓5th **B67.9 Echinococcosis, other and unspecified**

**B67.90 Echinococcosis, unspecified** `CC`
Echinococcosis NOS
**CC Excl:** PDX collection 240

**B67.99 Other echinococcosis** `CC`
**CC Excl:** PDX collection 240

✓4th **B68 Taeniasis**
`EXCLUDES 1` cysticercosis (B69.-)

**B68.0 Taenia solium taeniasis** `CC`
Pork tapeworm (infection)
**CC Excl:** PDX collection 241

**B68.1 Taenia saginata taeniasis** `CC`
Beef tapeworm (infection)
Infection due to adult tapeworm Taenia saginata
**CC Excl:** PDX collection 242

**B68.9 Taeniasis, unspecified** `CC`
**CC Excl:** PDX collection 242

✓4th **B69 Cysticercosis**
`INCLUDES` cysticerciasis infection due to larval form of Taenia solium

**CC Excl: For CC codes in category B69:** PDX collection 242

**B69.0 Cysticercosis of central nervous system** `CC`

**B69.1 Cysticercosis of eye** `CC`

✓5th **B69.8 Cysticercosis of other sites**

**B69.81 Myositis in cysticercosis** `CC`

**B69.89 Cysticercosis of other sites** `CC`

**B69.9 Cysticercosis, unspecified** `CC`

✓4th **B70 Diphyllobothriasis and sparganosis**

**CC Excl: For CC codes in category B70:** PDX collection 242

**B70.0 Diphyllobothriasis** `CC`
Diphyllobothrium (adult) (latum) (pacificum) infection
Fish tapeworm (infection)
`EXCLUDES 2` larval diphyllobothriasis (B70.1)

**B70.1 Sparganosis** `CC`
Infection due to Sparganum (mansoni) (proliferum)
Infection due to Spirometra larva
Larval diphyllobothriasis
Spirometrosis

✓4th **B71 Other cestode infections**

**CC Excl: For CC codes in category B71:** PDX collection 242

**B71.0 Hymenolepiasis** `CC`
Dwarf tapeworm infection
Rat tapeworm (infection)

**B71.1 Dipylidiasis** `CC`

**B71.8 Other specified cestode infections** `CC`
Coenurosis

**B71.9 Cestode infection, unspecified**
Tapeworm (infection) NOS

**B72 Dracunculiasis** `CC`
`INCLUDES` guinea worm infection
infection due to Dracunculus medinensis
**CC Excl:** PDX collection 243

✓4th **B73 Onchocerciasis**
`INCLUDES` onchocerca volvulus infection
onchocercosis
river blindness

**CC Excl: For CC codes in category B73:** PDX collection 243

✓5th **B73.0 Onchocerciasis with eye disease**

**B73.00 Onchocerciasis with eye involvement, unspecified** `CC`

**B73.01 Onchocerciasis with endophthalmitis** `CC`

**B73.02 Onchocerciasis with glaucoma** `CC`

**B73.09 Onchocerciasis with other eye involvement** `CC`
Infestation of eyelid due to onchocerciasis

**B73.1 Onchocerciasis without eye disease** `CC`

✓4th **B74 Filariasis**
`EXCLUDES 2` onchocerciasis (B73)
tropical (pulmonary) eosinophilia NOS (J82)

**CC Excl: For CC codes in category B74:** PDX collection 243

**B74.0 Filariasis due to Wuchereria bancrofti** `CC`
Bancroftian elephantiasis
Bancroftian filariasis

**B74.1 Filariasis due to Brugia malayi** `CC`

**B74.2 Filariasis due to Brugia timori** `CC`

**B74.3 Loiasis**
Calabar swelling
Eyeworm disease of Africa
Loa loa infection

**B74.4 Mansonelliasis** `CC`
Infection due to Mansonella ozzardi
Infection due to Mansonella perstans
Infection due to Mansonella streptocerca

**B74.8 Other filariases** `CC`
Dirofilariasis

**B74.9 Filariasis, unspecified** `CC`

**B75 Trichinellosis** `CC`
`INCLUDES` infection due to Trichinella species
trichiniasis
**CC Excl:** PDX collection 244

`✓4th` **B76 Hookworm diseases**
`INCLUDES` uncinariasis

> **CC Excl: For CC codes in category B76:** PDX collection 245

**B76.0 Ancylostomiasis** `CC`
Infection due to Ancylostoma species

**B76.1 Necatoriasis** `CC`
Infection due to Necator americanus

**B76.8 Other hookworm diseases** `CC`

**B76.9 Hookworm disease, unspecified** `CC`
Cutaneous larva migrans NOS

`✓4th` **B77 Ascariasis**
`INCLUDES` ascaridiasis
roundworm infection

> **CC Excl: For CC codes in category B77, unless otherwise noted:** PDX collection 246

**B77.0 Ascariasis with intestinal complications** `CC`

`✓5th` **B77.8 Ascariasis with other complications**

     **B77.81 Ascariasis pneumonia** `PDxMCC` `MCC`
        **CC Excl:** PDX collection 247

     **B77.89 Ascariasis with other complications** `CC`

**B77.9 Ascariasis, unspecified** `CC`

`✓4th` **B78 Strongyloidiasis**
`EXCLUDES 1` *trichostrongyliasis (B81.2)*

> **CC Excl: For CC codes in category B78:** PDX collection 246

**B78.0 Intestinal strongyloidiasis** `HIV` `CC`
**B78.1 Cutaneous strongyloidiasis**
**B78.7 Disseminated strongyloidiasis** `HIV` `CC`
**B78.9 Strongyloidiasis, unspecified** `HIV` `CC`

**B79 Trichuriasis** `CC`
`INCLUDES` trichocephaliasis
whipworm (disease)(infection)
**CC Excl:** PDX collection 246

**B80 Enterobiasis** `CC`
`INCLUDES` oxyuriasis
pinworm infection
threadworm infection
**CC Excl:** PDX collection 246

`✓4th` **B81 Other intestinal helminthiases, not elsewhere classified**
`EXCLUDES 1` ▶*angiostrongyliasis due to:*
*angiostrongylus cantonensis (B83.2)*
*parastrongylus cantonensis (B83.2)* ◄

**B81.0 Anisakiasis** `CC`
Infection due to Anisakis larva
**CC Excl:** PDX collection 246

**B81.1 Intestinal capillariasis** `CC`
Capillariasis NOS
Infection due to Capillaria philippinensis
`EXCLUDES 2` *hepatic capillariasis (B83.8)*
**CC Excl:** PDX collection 246

**B81.2 Trichostrongyliasis** `CC`
**CC Excl:** PDX collection 246

**B81.3 Intestinal angiostrongyliasis** `CC`
▶Angiostrongyliasis due to:
angiostrongylus costaricensis
parastrongylus costaricensis◄
**CC Excl:** PDX collection 248

**B81.4 Mixed intestinal helminthiases** `CC`
Infection due to intestinal helminths classified to more than one of the categories B65.0-B81.3 and B81.8
Mixed helminthiasis NOS
**CC Excl:** PDX collection 248

**B81.8 Other specified intestinal helminthiases** `CC`
Infection due to Oesophagostomum species [esophagostomiasis]
Infection due to Ternidens diminutus [ternidensiasis]
**CC Excl:** PDX collection 248

`✓4th` **B82 Unspecified intestinal parasitism**

**B82.0 Intestinal helminthiasis, unspecified** `CC`
**CC Excl:** PDX collection 248

**B82.9 Intestinal parasitism, unspecified**

`✓4th` **B83 Other helminthiases**
`EXCLUDES 1` *capillariasis NOS (B81.1)*
`EXCLUDES 2` *intestinal capillariasis (B81.1)*

**B83.0 Visceral larva migrans**
Toxocariasis

**B83.1 Gnathostomiasis**
Wandering swelling

**B83.2 Angiostrongyliasis due to Parastrongylus cantonensis**
Eosinophilic meningoencephalitis due to Parastrongylus cantonensis
`EXCLUDES 2` *intestinal angiostrongyliasis (B81.3)*

**B83.3 Syngamiasis**
Syngamosis

**B83.4 Internal hirudiniasis**
`EXCLUDES 2` *external hirudiniasis (B88.3)*

**B83.8 Other specified helminthiases**
Acanthocephaliasis     Metastrongyliasis
Gongylonemiasis     Thelaziasis
Hepatic capillariasis

**B83.9 Helminthiasis, unspecified**
Worms NOS
`EXCLUDES 1` *intestinal helminthiasis NOS (B82.0)*

### Pediculosis, acariasis and other infestations (B85-B89)

`✓4th` **B85 Pediculosis and phthiriasis**

**B85.0 Pediculosis due to Pediculus humanus capitis**
Head-louse infestation

**B85.1 Pediculosis due to Pediculus humanus corporis**
Body-louse infestation

**B85.2 Pediculosis, unspecified**

**B85.3 Phthiriasis**
Infestation by crab-louse
Infestation by Phthirus pubis

**B85.4 Mixed pediculosis and phthiriasis**
Infestation classifiable to more than one of the categories B85.0-B85.3

**B86 Scabies**
Sarcoptic itch

`✓4th` **B87 Myiasis**
`INCLUDES` infestation by larva of flies

**B87.0 Cutaneous myiasis**
Creeping myiasis

**B87.1 Wound myiasis**
Traumatic myiasis

**B87.2 Ocular myiasis**

**B87.3 Nasopharyngeal myiasis**
Laryngeal myiasis

**B87.4 Aural myiasis**

`✓5th` **B87.8 Myiasis of other sites**

     **B87.81 Genitourinary myiasis**

     **B87.82 Intestinal myiasis**

     **B87.89 Myiasis of other sites**

**B87.9 Myiasis, unspecified**

`✓4th` **B88 Other infestations**

**B88.0 Other acariasis**
Acarine dermatitis
Dermatitis due to Demodex species
Dermatitis due to Dermanyssus gallinae
Dermatitis due to Liponyssoides sanguineus
Trombiculosis
`EXCLUDES 2` *scabies (B86)*

**B88.1 Tungiasis [sandflea infestation]**

**B88.2 Other arthropod infestations**
Scarabiasis

`N` Newborn: 0   `P` Pediatric: 0-17   `M` Maternity: 12-55   `A` Adult: 15-124   `MCC` Major CC Condition   `PDxMCC` PDx acts as own MCC   `CC` CC Condition   `PDxCC` PDx acts as own CC

456

ICD-10-CM 2018

B74.4–B88.2

**B88.3  External hirudiniasis**
Leech infestation NOS
*EXCLUDES 2* internal hirudiniasis (B83.4)

**B88.8  Other specified infestations**
Ichthyoparasitism due to Vandellia cirrhosa
Linguatulosis
Porocephaliasis

**B88.9  Infestation, unspecified**
Infestation (skin) NOS        Skin parasites NOS
Infestation by mites NOS

**B89  Unspecified parasitic disease**

### Sequelae of infectious and parasitic diseases (B90-B94)

**NOTE**  Categories B90-B94 are to be used to indicate conditions in categories A00-B89 as the cause of sequelae, which are themselves classified elsewhere. The "sequelae" include conditions specified as such; they also include residuals of diseases classifiable to the above categories if there is evidence that the disease itself is no longer present. Codes from these categories are not to be used for chronic infections. Code chronic current infections to active infectious disease as appropriate.

Code first condition resulting from (sequela) the infectious or parasitic disease

**B90  Sequelae of tuberculosis**
**B90.0  Sequelae of central nervous system tuberculosis**
**B90.1  Sequelae of genitourinary tuberculosis**
**B90.2  Sequelae of tuberculosis of bones and joints**
**B90.8  Sequelae of tuberculosis of other organs**
*EXCLUDES 2* sequelae of respiratory tuberculosis (B90.9)
**B90.9  Sequelae of respiratory and unspecified tuberculosis**
Sequelae of tuberculosis NOS

**B91  Sequelae of poliomyelitis**
*EXCLUDES 1* postpolio syndrome (G14)

**B92  Sequelae of leprosy**

**B94  Sequelae of other and unspecified infectious and parasitic diseases**
**B94.0  Sequelae of trachoma**
**B94.1  Sequelae of viral encephalitis**
**B94.2  Sequelae of viral hepatitis**
**B94.8  Sequelae of other specified infectious and parasitic diseases**
**B94.9  Sequelae of unspecified infectious and parasitic disease**

### Bacterial and viral infectious agents (B95-B97)

**NOTE**  These categories are provided for use as supplementary or additional codes to identify the infectious agent(s) in diseases classified elsewhere.

**B95  Streptococcus, Staphylococcus, and Enterococcus as the cause of diseases classified elsewhere**
**B95.0  Streptococcus, group A, as the cause of diseases classified elsewhere**
**B95.1  Streptococcus, group B, as the cause of diseases classified elsewhere**
**B95.2  Enterococcus as the cause of diseases classified elsewhere**
**B95.3  Streptococcus pneumoniae as the cause of diseases classified elsewhere**
**B95.4  Other streptococcus as the cause of diseases classified elsewhere**
**B95.5  Unspecified streptococcus as the cause of diseases classified elsewhere**
**B95.6  Staphylococcus aureus as the cause of diseases classified elsewhere**
**B95.61  Methicillin susceptible Staphylococcus aureus infection as the cause of diseases classified elsewhere**
Methicillin susceptible Staphylococcus aureus (MSSA) infection as the cause of diseases classified elsewhere
Staphylococcus aureus infection NOS as the cause of diseases classified elsewhere
**B95.62  Methicillin resistant Staphylococcus aureus infection as the cause of diseases classified elsewhere**
Methicillin resistant Staphylococcus aureus (MRSA) infection as the cause of diseases classified elsewhere
**AHA:** 2016, 1Q, 12

**B95.7  Other staphylococcus as the cause of diseases classified elsewhere**
**B95.8  Unspecified staphylococcus as the cause of diseases classified elsewhere**

**B96  Other bacterial agents as the cause of diseases classified elsewhere**
**B96.0  Mycoplasma pneumoniae [M. pneumoniae] as the cause of diseases classified elsewhere**
Pleuro-pneumonia-like-organism [PPLO]
**B96.1  Klebsiella pneumoniae [K. pneumoniae] as the cause of diseases classified elsewhere**
**B96.2  Escherichia coli [E. coli] as the cause of diseases classified elsewhere**
**B96.20  Unspecified Escherichia coli [E. coli] as the cause of diseases classified elsewhere**
Escherichia coli [E. coli] NOS
**B96.21  Shiga toxin-producing Escherichia coli [E. coli] (STEC) O157 as the cause of diseases classified elsewhere**
E. coli O157:H- (nonmotile) with confirmation of Shiga toxin
E. coli O157 with confirmation of Shiga toxin when H antigen is unknown, or is not H7
O157:H7 Escherichia coli [E.coli] with or without confirmation of Shiga toxin-production
Shiga toxin-producing Escherichia coli [E.coli] O157:H7 with or without confirmation of Shiga toxin-production
STEC O157:H7 with or without confirmation of Shiga toxin-production
**B96.22  Other specified Shiga toxin-producing Escherichia coli [E. coli] (STEC) as the cause of diseases classified elsewhere**
Non-O157 Shiga toxin-producing Escherichia coli [E.coli]
Non-O157 Shiga toxin-producing Escherichia coli [E.coli] with known O group
**B96.23  Unspecified Shiga toxin-producing Escherichia coli [E. coli] (STEC) as the cause of diseases classified elsewhere**
Shiga toxin-producing Escherichia coli [E. coli] with unspecified O group
STEC NOS
**B96.29  Other Escherichia coli [E. coli] as the cause of diseases classified elsewhere**
Non-Shiga toxin-producing E. coli
**B96.3  Hemophilus influenzae [H. influenzae] as the cause of diseases classified elsewhere**
**B96.4  Proteus (mirabilis) (morganii) as the cause of diseases classified elsewhere**
**B96.5  Pseudomonas (aeruginosa) (mallei) (pseudomallei) as the cause of diseases classified elsewhere**
**AHA:** 2015, 1Q, 18
**B96.6  Bacteroides fragilis [B. fragilis] as the cause of diseases classified elsewhere**
**B96.7  Clostridium perfringens [C. perfringens] as the cause of diseases classified elsewhere**
**B96.8  Other specified bacterial agents as the cause of diseases classified elsewhere**
**B96.81  Helicobacter pylori [H. pylori] as the cause of diseases classified elsewhere**
**B96.82  Vibrio vulnificus as the cause of diseases classified elsewhere**
**B96.89  Other specified bacterial agents as the cause of diseases classified elsewhere**

**B97  Viral agents as the cause of diseases classified elsewhere**
**AHA:** 2016, 3Q, 8-10, 14
**B97.0  Adenovirus as the cause of diseases classified elsewhere**
**B97.1  Enterovirus as the cause of diseases classified elsewhere**
**B97.10  Unspecified enterovirus as the cause of diseases classified elsewhere**
**B97.11  Coxsackievirus as the cause of diseases classified elsewhere**
**B97.12  Echovirus as the cause of diseases classified elsewhere**
**B97.19  Other enterovirus as the cause of diseases classified elsewhere**

---

✔Additional Character Req    ✔x7ᵗʰ Placeholder Alert    Unacceptable PDx    Manifestation    **H1 - H14** HAC    **HCC** CMS-HCC Condition    *EXCLUDES 1* Not Coded Here    *EXCLUDES 2* Not Included Here

**Chapter 1. Certain Infectious and Parasitic Diseases**

✓5ᵗʰ **B97.2 Coronavirus as the cause of diseases classified elsewhere**

     **B97.21 SARS-associated coronavirus as the cause of diseases classified elsewhere**    CC

         *EXCLUDES 1*   pneumonia due to SARS-associated coronavirus (J12.81)

         **CC Excl:** PDX collection 249

     **B97.29 Other coronavirus as the cause of diseases classified elsewhere**

✓5ᵗʰ **B97.3 Retrovirus as the cause of diseases classified elsewhere**

         *EXCLUDES 1*   human immunodeficiency virus [HIV] disease (B20)

     **B97.30 Unspecified retrovirus as the cause of diseases classified elsewhere**

     **B97.31 Lentivirus as the cause of diseases classified elsewhere**

     **B97.32 Oncovirus as the cause of diseases classified elsewhere**

     **B97.33 Human T-cell lymphotrophic virus, type I [HTLV-I] as the cause of diseases classified elsewhere**    CC

         **CC Excl:** PDX collection 250

     **B97.34 Human T-cell lymphotrophic virus, type II [HTLV-II] as the cause of diseases classified elsewhere**    CC

         **CC Excl:** PDX collection 251

     **B97.35 Human immunodeficiency virus, type 2 [HIV 2] as the cause of diseases classified elsewhere**    CC HCC

         **CC Excl:** PDX collection 252

     **B97.39 Other retrovirus as the cause of diseases classified elsewhere**

**B97.4 Respiratory syncytial virus as the cause of diseases classified elsewhere**

**B97.5 Reovirus as the cause of diseases classified elsewhere**

**B97.6 Parvovirus as the cause of diseases classified elsewhere**

**B97.7 Papillomavirus as the cause of diseases classified elsewhere**

✓5ᵗʰ **B97.8 Other viral agents as the cause of diseases classified elsewhere**

     **B97.81 Human metapneumovirus as the cause of diseases classified elsewhere**

     **B97.89 Other viral agents as the cause of diseases classified elsewhere**

### Other infectious diseases (B99)

✓4ᵗʰ **B99 Other and unspecified infectious diseases**

     **B99.8 Other infectious disease**    HIV

     **B99.9 Unspecified infectious disease**

N Newborn: 0    P Pediatric: 0-17    M Maternity: 12-55    A Adult: 15-124    MCC Major CC Condition    PDx MCC PDx acts as own MCC    CC CC Condition    PDx CC PDx acts as own CC

**458**            ICD-10-CM 2018

# Chapter 2. Neoplasms (C00–D49)

## Chapter Specific Guidelines with Coding Examples

The chapter specific guidelines from the ICD-10-CM Official Guidelines for Coding and Reporting have been provided below. Along with these guidelines are coding examples, contained in the shaded boxes, that have been developed to help illustrate the coding and/or sequencing guidance found in these guidelines.

### General guidelines

Chapter 2 of the ICD-10-CM contains the codes for most benign and all malignant neoplasms. Certain benign neoplasms, such as prostatic adenomas, may be found in the specific body system chapters. To properly code a neoplasm it is necessary to determine from the record if the neoplasm is benign, in-situ, malignant, or of uncertain histologic behavior. If malignant, any secondary (metastatic) sites should also be determined.

Primary malignant neoplasms overlapping site boundaries

> A primary malignant neoplasm that overlaps two or more contiguous (next to each other) sites should be classified to the subcategory/code .8 ('overlapping lesion'), unless the combination is specifically indexed elsewhere. For multiple neoplasms of the same site that are not contiguous such as tumors in different quadrants of the same breast, codes for each site should be assigned.

> A 73-year-old white female with a large rapidly growing malignant tumor in the left breast extending from the upper outer quadrant into the axillary tail
>
> **C50.812**     **Malignant neoplasm of overlapping sites of left female breast**
>
> *Explanation*: Because this is a single large tumor that overlaps two contiguous sites, a single code for overlapping sites is assigned.

> A 52-year old white female with two distinct lesions of the right breast, one (0.5 cm) in the upper outer quadrant and a second (1.5 cm) in the lower outer quadrant; path report indicates both lesions are malignant
>
> **C50.411**     **Malignant neoplasm of upper-outer quadrant of right female breast**
>
> **C50.511**     **Malignant neoplasm of lower-outer quadrant of right female breast**
>
> *Explanation*: This patient has two distinct malignant lesions of right breast in adjacent quadrants. Because the lesions are not contiguous, two codes are reported.

Malignant neoplasm of ectopic tissue

> Malignant neoplasms of ectopic tissue are to be coded to the site of origin mentioned, e.g., ectopic pancreatic malignant neoplasms involving the stomach are coded to pancreas, unspecified (C25.9).

The neoplasm table in the Alphabetic Index should be referenced first. However, if the histological term is documented, that term should be referenced first, rather than going immediately to the Neoplasm Table, in order to determine which column in the Neoplasm Table is appropriate. For example, if the documentation indicates "adenoma," refer to the term in the Alphabetic Index to review the entries under this term and the instructional note to "see also neoplasm, by site, benign." The table provides the proper code based on the type of neoplasm and the site. It is important to select the proper column in the table that corresponds to the type of neoplasm. The Tabular List should then be referenced to verify that the correct code has been selected from the table and that a more specific site code does not exist.

*See Section I.C.21. Factors influencing health status and contact with health services, Status, for information regarding Z15.0, codes for genetic susceptibility to cancer.*

### a. Treatment directed at the malignancy

> If the treatment is directed at the malignancy, designate the malignancy as the principal diagnosis.

> The only exception to this guideline is if a patient admission/encounter is solely for the administration of chemotherapy, immunotherapy or radiation therapy, assign the appropriate Z51.-- code as the first-listed or principal diagnosis, and the diagnosis or problem for which the service is being performed as a secondary diagnosis.

### b. Treatment of secondary site

> When a patient is admitted because of a primary neoplasm with metastasis and treatment is directed toward the secondary site only, the secondary neoplasm is designated as the principal diagnosis even though the primary malignancy is still present.

> Patient with primary prostate cancer with metastasis to lungs admitted for wedge resection of mass in right lung
>
> **C78.01**     **Secondary malignant neoplasm of right lung**
>
> **C61**       **Malignant neoplasm of prostate**
>
> *Explanation*: Since the admission is for treatment of the lung metastasis, the secondary lung metastasis is sequenced before the primary prostate cancer.

### c. Coding and sequencing of complications

Coding and sequencing of complications associated with the malignancies or with the therapy thereof are subject to the following guidelines:

#### 1) Anemia associated with malignancy

> When admission/encounter is for management of an anemia associated with the malignancy, and the treatment is only for anemia, the appropriate code for the malignancy is sequenced as the principal or first-listed diagnosis followed by the appropriate code for the anemia (such as code D63.0, Anemia in neoplastic disease).

> Patient is admitted for treatment of anemia in advanced colon cancer
>
> **C18.9**     **Malignant neoplasm of colon, unspecified**
>
> **D63.0**     **Anemia in neoplastic disease**
>
> *Explanation*: Even though the admission was solely to treat the anemia, this guideline indicates that the code for the malignancy is sequenced first.

#### 2) Anemia associated with chemotherapy, immunotherapy and radiation therapy

> When the admission/encounter is for management of an anemia associated with an adverse effect of the administration of chemotherapy or immunotherapy and the only treatment is for the anemia, the anemia code is sequenced first followed by the appropriate codes for the neoplasm and the adverse effect (T45.1X5, Adverse effect of antineoplastic and immunosuppressive drugs).

> A 56-year-old Hispanic male with grade II follicular lymphoma involving multiple lymph node sites referred for blood transfusion to treat anemia due to chemotherapy
>
> **D64.81**     **Anemia due to antineoplastic chemotherapy**
>
> **C82.18**     **Follicular lymphoma grade II, lymph nodes of multiple sites**
>
> **T45.1X5A**   **Adverse effect of antineoplastic and immunosuppressive drugs, initial encounter**
>
> *Explanation*: The code for the anemia is sequenced first followed by the code for the malignant neoplasm and lastly the code for the adverse effect.

> When the admission/encounter is for management of an anemia associated with an adverse effect of radiotherapy, the anemia code should be sequenced first, followed by the appropriate neoplasm code and code Y84.2, Radiological procedure and radiotherapy as the cause of abnormal reaction of the patient, or of later complication, without mention of misadventure at the time of the procedure.

**Chapter 2. Neoplasms**

A 55-year-old male with a large malignant rectal tumor has been receiving external radiation therapy to shrink the tumor prior to planned surgery. He is admitted today for a blood transfusion to treat anemia related to radiation therapy.

| | |
|---|---|
| **D64.89** | **Other specified anemias** |
| **C20** | **Malignant neoplasm of rectum** |
| **Y84.2** | **Radiological procedure and radiotherapy as the cause of abnormal reaction of the patient, or of later complication, without mention of misadventure at the time of the procedure** |

*Explanation*: The code for the anemia is sequenced first, followed by the code for the malignancy, and lastly the code for the abnormal reaction due to radiotherapy.

**3) Management of dehydration due to the malignancy**

When the admission/encounter is for management of dehydration due to the malignancy and only the dehydration is being treated (intravenous rehydration), the dehydration is sequenced first, followed by the code(s) for the malignancy.

**4) Treatment of a complication resulting from a surgical procedure**

When the admission/encounter is for treatment of a complication resulting from a surgical procedure, designate the complication as the principal or first-listed diagnosis if treatment is directed at resolving the complication.

**d. Primary malignancy previously excised**

When a primary malignancy has been previously excised or eradicated from its site and there is no further treatment directed to that site and there is no evidence of any existing primary malignancy, a code from category Z85, Personal history of malignant neoplasm, should be used to indicate the former site of the malignancy. Any mention of extension, invasion, or metastasis to another site is coded as a secondary malignant neoplasm to that site. The secondary site may be the principal or first-listed with the Z85 code used as a secondary code.

History of breast cancer, left radical mastectomy 18 months ago with no current treatment; bronchoscopy with lung biopsy shows metastatic disease in the right lung

| | |
|---|---|
| **C78.01** | **Secondary malignant neoplasm of right lung** |
| **Z85.3** | **Personal history of malignant neoplasm of breast** |

*Explanation*: The patient has undergone a diagnostic procedure that revealed metastatic breast cancer in the right lung. The code for the secondary (metastatic) site is sequenced first followed by a personal history code to identify the former site of the primary malignancy.

**e. Admissions/encounters involving chemotherapy, immunotherapy and radiation therapy**

**1) Episode of care involves surgical removal of neoplasm**

When an episode of care involves the surgical removal of a neoplasm, primary or secondary site, followed by adjunct chemotherapy or radiation treatment during the same episode of care, the code for the neoplasm should be assigned as principal or first-listed diagnosis.

**2) Patient admission/encounter solely for administration of chemotherapy, immunotherapy and radiation therapy**

If a patient admission/encounter is solely for the administration of chemotherapy, immunotherapy or radiation therapy assign code Z51.0, Encounter for antineoplastic radiation therapy, or Z51.11, Encounter for antineoplastic chemotherapy, or Z51.12, Encounter for antineoplastic immunotherapy as the first-listed or principal diagnosis. If a patient receives more than one of these therapies during the same admission more than one of these codes may be assigned, in any sequence.

The malignancy for which the therapy is being administered should be assigned as a secondary diagnosis.

Patient is admitted for second round of rituximab and fludarabine for his chronic B cell lymphocytic leukemia

| | |
|---|---|
| **Z51.11** | **Encounter for antineoplastic chemotherapy** |
| **Z51.12** | **Encounter for antineoplastic immunotherapy** |
| **C91.10** | **Chronic lymphocytic leukemia of B-cell type not having achieved remission** |

*Explanation*: Rituximab is an antineoplastic immunotherapy while fludarabine is an antineoplastic chemotherapy. The two treatments are often used together. The admission was solely for the purpose of administering this treatment and either can be sequenced first, before the neoplastic condition.

**3) Patient admitted for radiation therapy, chemotherapy or immunotherapy and develops complications**

When a patient is admitted for the purpose of radiotherapy, immunotherapy or chemotherapy and develops complications such as uncontrolled nausea and vomiting or dehydration, the principal or first-listed diagnosis is Z51.0, Encounter for antineoplastic radiation therapy, or Z51.11, Encounter for antineoplastic chemotherapy, or Z51.12, Encounter for antineoplastic immunotherapy followed by any codes for the complications.

**f. Admission/encounter to determine extent of malignancy**

When the reason for admission/encounter is to determine the extent of the malignancy, or for a procedure such as paracentesis or thoracentesis, the primary malignancy or appropriate metastatic site is designated as the principal or first-listed diagnosis, even though chemotherapy or radiotherapy is administered.

Patient with left lung cancer with malignant pleural effusion admitted for paracentesis and initiation/administration of chemotherapy

| | |
|---|---|
| **C34.92** | **Malignant neoplasm of unspecified part of left bronchus or lung** |
| **J91.0** | **Malignant pleural effusion** |
| **Z51.11** | **Encounter for antineoplastic chemotherapy** |

*Explanation*: The lung cancer is sequenced before the chemotherapy in this instance because the paracentesis for the malignant effusion is also being performed. An instructional note under the malignant effusion instructs that the lung cancer be sequenced first.

**g. Symptoms, signs, and abnormal findings listed in Chapter 18 associated with neoplasms**

Symptoms, signs, and ill-defined conditions listed in Chapter 18 characteristic of, or associated with, an existing primary or secondary site malignancy cannot be used to replace the malignancy as principal or first-listed diagnosis, regardless of the number of admissions or encounters for treatment and care of the neoplasm.

*See Section I.C.21. Factors influencing health status and contact with health services, Encounter for prophylactic organ removal.*

**h. Admission/encounter for pain control/management**

*See Section I.C.6. for information on coding admission/encounter for pain control/management.*

**i. Malignancy in two or more noncontiguous sites**

A patient may have more than one malignant tumor in the same organ. These tumors may represent different primaries or metastatic disease, depending on the site. Should the documentation be unclear, the provider should be queried as to the status of each tumor so that the correct codes can be assigned.

**j. Disseminated malignant neoplasm, unspecified**

Code C80.0, Disseminated malignant neoplasm, unspecified, is for use only in those cases where the patient has advanced metastatic disease and no known primary or secondary sites are specified. It should not be used in place of assigning codes for the primary site and all known secondary sites.

Patient who has had no medical care for many years is seen today and diagnosed with carcinomatosis

| | |
|---|---|
| **C80.0** | **Disseminated malignant neoplasm, unspecified** |

*Explanation*: Carcinomatosis NOS is an "includes" note under this code. Should seldom be used but is available for use in cases such as this.

### k. Malignant neoplasm without specification of site

Code C80.1, Malignant (primary) neoplasm, unspecified, equates to Cancer, unspecified. This code should only be used when no determination can be made as to the primary site of a malignancy. This code should rarely be used in the inpatient setting.

> Evaluation of painful hip leads to diagnosis of a metastatic bone lesion from an unknown primary neoplasm source
>
> **C79.51**     **Secondary malignant neoplasm of bone**
>
> **C80.1**     **Malignant (primary) neoplasm, unspecified**
>
> *Explanation*: If only the secondary site is known, use code C80.1 for the unknown primary site.

### l. Sequencing of neoplasm codes

#### 1) Encounter for treatment of primary malignancy

If the reason for the encounter is for treatment of a primary malignancy, assign the malignancy as the principal/first-listed diagnosis. The primary site is to be sequenced first, followed by any metastatic sites.

#### 2) Encounter for treatment of secondary malignancy

When an encounter is for a primary malignancy with metastasis and treatment is directed toward the metastatic (secondary) site(s) only, the metastatic site(s) is designated as the principal/first-listed diagnosis. The primary malignancy is coded as an additional code.

> Patient has primary colon cancer with metastasis to rib and is evaluated for possible excision of portion of rib bone
>
> **C79.51**     **Secondary malignant neoplasm of bone**
>
> **C18.9**     **Malignant neoplasm of colon, unspecified**
>
> *Explanation*: The treatment for this encounter is focused on the metastasis to the rib bone rather than the primary colon cancer, thus indicating that the bone metastasis is sequenced as the first-listed code.

#### 3) Malignant neoplasm in a pregnant patient

When a pregnant woman has a malignant neoplasm, a code from subcategory O9A.1-, Malignant neoplasm complicating pregnancy, childbirth, and the puerperium, should be sequenced first, followed by the appropriate code from Chapter 2 to indicate the type of neoplasm.

> A 30-year-old pregnant female in second trimester evaluated for thyroid malignancy
>
> **O9A.112**     **Malignant neoplasm complicating pregnancy, second trimester**
>
> **C73**     **Malignant neoplasm of thyroid gland**
>
> *Explanation*: Codes from chapter 15 describing complications of pregnancy are sequenced as first-listed codes, further specified by codes from other chapters such as neoplastic, unless the pregnancy is documented as incidental to the condition. See also guideline 1.C.15.a.1.

#### 4) Encounter for complication associated with a neoplasm

When an encounter is for management of a complication associated with a neoplasm, such as dehydration, and the treatment is only for the complication, the complication is coded first, followed by the appropriate code(s) for the neoplasm.

The exception to this guideline is anemia. When the admission/encounter is for management of an anemia associated with the malignancy, and the treatment is only for anemia, the appropriate code for the malignancy is sequenced as the principal or first-listed diagnosis followed by code D63.0, Anemia in neoplastic disease.

> Patient with pancreatic cancer is seen for initiation of TPN for cancer-related moderate protein-calorie malnutrition
>
> **E44.0**     **Moderate protein-calorie malnutrition**
>
> **C25.9**     **Malignant neoplasm of pancreas, unspecified**
>
> *Explanation*: The encounter is to initiate treatment for malnutrition, a common complication of many types of neoplasms, and is sequenced first.

#### 5) Complication from surgical procedure for treatment of a neoplasm

When an encounter is for treatment of a complication resulting from a surgical procedure performed for the treatment of the neoplasm, designate the complication as the principal/first-listed diagnosis. See guideline regarding the coding of a current malignancy versus personal history to determine if the code for the neoplasm should also be assigned.

#### 6) Pathologic fracture due to a neoplasm

When an encounter is for a pathological fracture due to a neoplasm, and the focus of treatment is the fracture, a code from subcategory M84.5, Pathological fracture in neoplastic disease, should be sequenced first, followed by the code for the neoplasm.

If the focus of treatment is the neoplasm with an associated pathological fracture, the neoplasm code should be sequenced first, followed by a code from M84.5 for the pathological fracture.

### m. Current malignancy versus personal history of malignancy

When a primary malignancy has been excised but further treatment, such as an additional surgery for the malignancy, radiation therapy or chemotherapy is directed to that site, the primary malignancy code should be used until treatment is completed.

When a primary malignancy has been previously excised or eradicated from its site, there is no further treatment (of the malignancy) directed to that site, and there is no evidence of any existing primary malignancy, a code from category Z85, Personal history of malignant neoplasm, should be used to indicate the former site of the malignancy.

*See Section I.C.21. Factors influencing health status and contact with health services, History (of)*

> Female patient with ongoing chemotherapy after right mastectomy for breast cancer
>
> **C50.911**     **Malignant neoplasm of unspecified site of right female breast**
>
> **Z90.11**     **Acquired absence of right breast and nipple**
>
> *Explanation*: Even though the breast has been removed, the breast cancer is still being treated with chemotherapy and therefore is still coded as a current condition rather than personal history.

### n. Leukemia, multiple myeloma, and malignant plasma cell neoplasms in remission versus personal history

The categories for leukemia, and category C90, Multiple myeloma and malignant plasma cell neoplasms, have codes indicating whether or not the leukemia has achieved remission. There are also codes Z85.6, Personal history of leukemia, and Z85.79, Personal history of other malignant neoplasms of lymphoid, hematopoietic and related tissues. If the documentation is unclear as to whether the leukemia has achieved remission, the provider should be queried.

*See Section I.C.21. Factors influencing health status and contact with health services, History (of)*

### o. Aftercare following surgery for neoplasm

*See Section I.C.21. Factors influencing health status and contact with health services, Aftercare*

### p. Follow-up care for completed treatment of a malignancy

*See Section I.C.21. Factors influencing health status and contact with health services, Follow-up*

### q. Prophylactic organ removal for prevention of malignancy

*See Section I.C. 21, Factors influencing health status and contact with health services, Prophylactic organ removal*

### r. Malignant neoplasm associated with transplanted organ

A malignant neoplasm of a transplanted organ should be coded as a transplant complication. Assign first the appropriate code from category T86.-, Complications of transplanted organs and tissue, followed by code C80.2, Malignant neoplasm associated with transplanted organ. Use an additional code for the specific malignancy.

# Chapter 2. Neoplasms (C00-D49)

**NOTE**

**Functional activity**

All neoplasms are classified in this chapter, whether they are functionally active or not. An additional code from Chapter 4 may be used, to identify functional activity associated with any neoplasm.

**Morphology [Histology]**

Chapter 2 classifies neoplasms primarily by site (topography), with broad groupings for behavior, malignant, in situ, benign, etc. The Table of Neoplasms should be used to identify the correct topography code. In a few cases, such as for malignant melanoma and certain neuroendocrine tumors, the morphology (histologic type) is included in the category and codes.

**Primary malignant neoplasms overlapping site boundaries**

A primary malignant neoplasm that overlaps two or more contiguous (next to each other) sites should be classified to the subcategory/code 8 ("overlapping lesion"), unless the combination is specifically indexed elsewhere. For multiple neoplasms of the same site that are not contiguous, such as tumors in different quadrants of the same breast, codes for each site should be assigned.

**Malignant neoplasm of ectopic tissue**

Malignant neoplasms of ectopic tissue are to be coded to the site mentioned, e.g., ectopic pancreatic malignant neoplasms are coded to pancreas, unspecified (C25.9).

**AHA:** 2017, 1Q, 4, 5-6, 8

This chapter contains the following blocks:

| | |
|---|---|
| C00-C14 | Malignant neoplasms of lip, oral cavity and pharynx |
| C15-C26 | Malignant neoplasms of digestive organs |
| C30-C39 | Malignant neoplasms of respiratory and intrathoracic organs |
| C40-C41 | Malignant neoplasms of bone and articular cartilage |
| C43-C44 | Melanoma and other malignant neoplasms of skin |
| C45-C49 | Malignant neoplasms of mesothelial and soft tissue |
| C50 | Malignant neoplasms of breast |
| C51-C58 | Malignant neoplasms of female genital organs |
| C60-C63 | Malignant neoplasms of male genital organs |
| C64-C68 | Malignant neoplasms of urinary tract |
| C69-C72 | Malignant neoplasms of eye, brain and other parts of central nervous system |
| C73-C75 | Malignant neoplasms of thyroid and other endocrine glands |
| C7A | Malignant neuroendocrine tumors |
| C7B | Secondary neuroendocrine tumors |
| C76-C80 | Malignant neoplasms of ill-defined, other secondary and unspecified sites |
| C81-C96 | Malignant neoplasms of lymphoid, hematopoietic and related tissue |
| D00-D09 | In situ neoplasms |
| D10-D36 | Benign neoplasms, except benign neuroendocrine tumors |
| D3A | Benign neuroendocrine tumors |
| D37-D48 | Neoplasms of uncertain behavior, polycythemia vera and myelodysplastic syndromes |
| D49 | Neoplasms of unspecified behavior |

## MALIGNANT NEOPLASMS (C00-C96)

Malignant neoplasms, stated or presumed to be primary (of specified sites), and certain specified histologies, except neuroendocrine, and of lymphoid, hematopoietic and related tissue (C00-C75)

## Malignant neoplasms of lip, oral cavity and pharynx (C00-C14)

**☑4th C00 Malignant neoplasm of lip**

Use additional code to identify:
  alcohol abuse and dependence (F10.-)
  history of tobacco dependence (Z87.891)
  tobacco dependence (F17.-)
  tobacco use (Z72.0)

**EXCLUDES 1** *malignant melanoma of lip (C43.0)*
*Merkel cell carcinoma of lip (C4A.0)*
*other and unspecified malignant neoplasm of skin of lip (C44.0-)*

**C00.0 Malignant neoplasm of external upper lip**
  Malignant neoplasm of lipstick area of upper lip
  Malignant neoplasm of upper lip NOS
  Malignant neoplasm of vermilion border of upper lip

**C00.1 Malignant neoplasm of external lower lip**
  Malignant neoplasm of lower lip NOS
  Malignant neoplasm of lipstick area of lower lip
  Malignant neoplasm of vermilion border of lower lip

**C00.2 Malignant neoplasm of external lip, unspecified**
  Malignant neoplasm of vermilion border of lip NOS

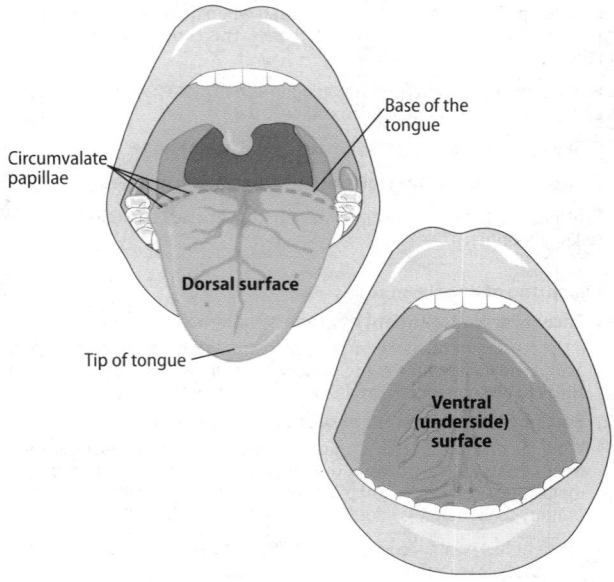

**Malignant Neoplasm of Tongue**

Base of the tongue · Circumvalate papillae · Dorsal surface · Tip of tongue · Ventral (underside) surface

**C00.3 Malignant neoplasm of upper lip, inner aspect**
  Malignant neoplasm of buccal aspect of upper lip
  Malignant neoplasm of frenulum of upper lip
  Malignant neoplasm of mucosa of upper lip
  Malignant neoplasm of oral aspect of upper lip

**C00.4 Malignant neoplasm of lower lip, inner aspect**
  Malignant neoplasm of buccal aspect of lower lip
  Malignant neoplasm of frenulum of lower lip
  Malignant neoplasm of mucosa of lower lip
  Malignant neoplasm of oral aspect of lower lip

**C00.5 Malignant neoplasm of lip, unspecified, inner aspect**
  Malignant neoplasm of buccal aspect of lip, unspecified
  Malignant neoplasm of frenulum of lip, unspecified
  Malignant neoplasm of mucosa of lip, unspecified
  Malignant neoplasm of oral aspect of lip, unspecified

**C00.6 Malignant neoplasm of commissure of lip, unspecified**

**C00.8 Malignant neoplasm of overlapping sites of lip**

**C00.9 Malignant neoplasm of lip, unspecified**

**C01 Malignant neoplasm of base of tongue**    HCC
  Malignant neoplasm of dorsal surface of base of tongue
  Malignant neoplasm of fixed part of tongue NOS
  Malignant neoplasm of posterior third of tongue
  Use additional code to identify:
    alcohol abuse and dependence (F10.-)
    history of tobacco dependence (Z87.891)
    tobacco dependence (F17.-)
    tobacco use (Z72.0)

**☑4th C02 Malignant neoplasm of other and unspecified parts of tongue**
  Use additional code to identify:
    alcohol abuse and dependence (F10.-)
    history of tobacco dependence (Z87.891)
    tobacco dependence (F17.-)
    tobacco use (Z72.0)

**C02.0 Malignant neoplasm of dorsal surface of tongue**    HCC
  Malignant neoplasm of anterior two-thirds of tongue, dorsal surface
  **EXCLUDES 2** *malignant neoplasm of dorsal surface of base of tongue (C01)*

**C02.1 Malignant neoplasm of border of tongue**    HCC
  Malignant neoplasm of tip of tongue

**C02.2 Malignant neoplasm of ventral surface of tongue**    HCC
  Malignant neoplasm of anterior two-thirds of tongue, ventral surface
  Malignant neoplasm of frenulum linguae

**C02.3 Malignant neoplasm of anterior two-thirds of tongue, part unspecified**    HCC
  Malignant neoplasm of middle third of tongue NOS
  Malignant neoplasm of mobile part of tongue NOS

**C02.4 Malignant neoplasm of lingual tonsil**    HCC
  **EXCLUDES 2** *malignant neoplasm of tonsil NOS (C09.9)*

N Newborn: 0   P Pediatric: 0-17   M Maternity: 12-55   A Adult: 15-124   MCC Major CC Condition   PDx MCC PDx acts as own MCC   CC CC Condition   PDx CC PDx acts as own CC

462             ICD-10-CM 2018

**C02.8**    **Malignant neoplasm of overlapping sites of tongue**   HCC
     Malignant neoplasm of two or more contiguous sites of tongue

**C02.9**    **Malignant neoplasm of tongue, unspecified**   HCC

✓4ᵗʰ **C03**    **Malignant neoplasm of gum**
     INCLUDES    malignant neoplasm of alveolar (ridge) mucosa
           malignant neoplasm of gingiva
     Use additional code to identify:
       alcohol abuse and dependence (F10.-)
       history of tobacco dependence (Z87.891)
       tobacco dependence (F17.-)
       tobacco use (Z72.0)
     EXCLUDES 2   malignant odontogenic neoplasms (C41.0-C41.1)

**C03.0**    **Malignant neoplasm of upper gum**   HCC
**C03.1**    **Malignant neoplasm of lower gum**   HCC
**C03.9**    **Malignant neoplasm of gum, unspecified**   HCC

✓4ᵗʰ **C04**    **Malignant neoplasm of floor of mouth**
     Use additional code to identify:
       alcohol abuse and dependence (F10.-)
       history of tobacco dependence (Z87.891)
       tobacco dependence (F17.-)
       tobacco use (Z72.0)

**C04.0**    **Malignant neoplasm of anterior floor of mouth**   HCC
     Malignant neoplasm of anterior to the premolar-canine junction

**C04.1**    **Malignant neoplasm of lateral floor of mouth**   HCC
**C04.8**    **Malignant neoplasm of overlapping sites of floor of mouth**   HCC
**C04.9**    **Malignant neoplasm of floor of mouth, unspecified**   HCC

✓4ᵗʰ **C05**    **Malignant neoplasm of palate**
     Use additional code to identify:
       alcohol abuse and dependence (F10.-)
       history of tobacco dependence (Z87.891)tobacco dependence (F17.-)
       tobacco use (Z72.0)
     EXCLUDES 1   Kaposi's sarcoma of palate (C46.2)

**C05.0**    **Malignant neoplasm of hard palate**   HCC
**C05.1**    **Malignant neoplasm of soft palate**   HCC
     EXCLUDES 2   malignant neoplasm of nasopharyngeal surface of soft palate (C11.3)

**C05.2**    **Malignant neoplasm of uvula**   HCC
**C05.8**    **Malignant neoplasm of overlapping sites of palate**   HCC
**C05.9**    **Malignant neoplasm of palate, unspecified**   HCC
     Malignant neoplasm of roof of mouth

✓4ᵗʰ **C06**    **Malignant neoplasm of other and unspecified parts of mouth**
     Use additional code to identify:
       alcohol abuse and dependence (F10.-)
       history of tobacco dependence (Z87.891)
       tobacco dependence (F17.-)
       tobacco use (Z72.0)

**C06.0**    **Malignant neoplasm of cheek mucosa**   HCC
     Malignant neoplasm of buccal mucosa NOS
     Malignant neoplasm of internal cheek

**C06.1**    **Malignant neoplasm of vestibule of mouth**   HCC
     Malignant neoplasm of buccal sulcus (upper) (lower)
     Malignant neoplasm of labial sulcus (upper) (lower)

**C06.2**    **Malignant neoplasm of retromolar area**   HCC

✓5ᵗʰ **C06.8**    **Malignant neoplasm of overlapping sites of other and unspecified parts of mouth**

     **C06.80**    **Malignant neoplasm of overlapping sites of unspecified parts of mouth**   HCC

     **C06.89**    **Malignant neoplasm of overlapping sites of other parts of mouth**   HCC
       "book leaf" neoplasm [ventral surface of tongue and floor of mouth]

**C06.9**    **Malignant neoplasm of mouth, unspecified**   HCC
     Malignant neoplasm of minor salivary gland, unspecified site
     Malignant neoplasm of oral cavity NOS

**C07**    **Malignant neoplasm of parotid gland**   HCC
     Use additional code to identify:
       alcohol abuse and dependence (F10.-)
       exposure to environmental tobacco smoke (Z77.22)
       exposure to tobacco smoke in the perinatal period (P96.81)
       history of tobacco dependence (Z87.891)
       occupational exposure to environmental tobacco smoke (Z57.31)
       tobacco dependence (F17.-)
       tobacco use (Z72.0)

✓4ᵗʰ **C08**    **Malignant neoplasm of other and unspecified major salivary glands**
     INCLUDES    malignant neoplasm of salivary ducts
     Use additional code to identify:
       alcohol abuse and dependence (F10.-)
       exposure to environmental tobacco smoke (Z77.22)
       exposure to tobacco smoke in the perinatal period (P96.81)
       history of tobacco dependence (Z87.891)
       occupational exposure to environmental tobacco smoke (Z57.31)
       tobacco dependence (F17.-)
       tobacco use (Z72.0)
     EXCLUDES 1   malignant neoplasms of specified minor salivary glands which are classified according to their anatomical location
     EXCLUDES 2   malignant neoplasms of minor salivary glands NOS (C06.9)
           malignant neoplasm of parotid gland (C07)

**C08.0**    **Malignant neoplasm of submandibular gland**   HCC
     Malignant neoplasm of submaxillary gland

**C08.1**    **Malignant neoplasm of sublingual gland**   HCC

**C08.9**    **Malignant neoplasm of major salivary gland, unspecified** HCC
     Malignant neoplasm of salivary gland (major) NOS

✓4ᵗʰ **C09**    **Malignant neoplasm of tonsil**
     Use additional code to identify:
       alcohol abuse and dependence (F10.-)
       exposure to environmental tobacco smoke (Z77.22)
       exposure to tobacco smoke in the perinatal period (P96.81)
       history of tobacco dependence (Z87.891)
       occupational exposure to environmental tobacco smoke (Z57.31)
       tobacco dependence (F17.-)
       tobacco use (Z72.0)
     EXCLUDES 2   malignant neoplasm of lingual tonsil (C02.4)
           malignant neoplasm of pharyngeal tonsil (C11.1)

**C09.0**    **Malignant neoplasm of tonsillar fossa**   HCC
**C09.1**    **Malignant neoplasm of tonsillar pillar (anterior) (posterior)**   HCC
**C09.8**    **Malignant neoplasm of overlapping sites of tonsil**   HCC
**C09.9**    **Malignant neoplasm of tonsil, unspecified**   HCC
     Malignant neoplasm of tonsil NOS
     Malignant neoplasm of faucial tonsils
     Malignant neoplasm of palatine tonsils

✓4ᵗʰ **C10**    **Malignant neoplasm of oropharynx**
     Use additional code to identify:
       alcohol abuse and dependence (F10.-)
       exposure to environmental tobacco smoke (Z77.22)
       exposure to tobacco smoke in the perinatal period (P96.81)
       history of tobacco dependence (Z87.891)
       occupational exposure to environmental tobacco smoke (Z57.31)
       tobacco dependence (F17.-)
       tobacco use (Z72.0)
     EXCLUDES 2   malignant neoplasm of tonsil (C09.-)

**C10.0**    **Malignant neoplasm of vallecula**   HCC
**C10.1**    **Malignant neoplasm of anterior surface of epiglottis**   HCC
     Malignant neoplasm of epiglottis, free border [margin]
     Malignant neoplasm of glossoepiglottic fold(s)
     EXCLUDES 2   malignant neoplasm of epiglottis (suprahyoid portion) NOS (C32.1)

**C10.2**    **Malignant neoplasm of lateral wall of oropharynx**   HCC
**C10.3**    **Malignant neoplasm of posterior wall of oropharynx**   HCC
**C10.4**    **Malignant neoplasm of branchial cleft**   HCC
     Malignant neoplasm of branchial cyst [site of neoplasm]

**C10.8**    **Malignant neoplasm of overlapping sites of oropharynx**   HCC
     Malignant neoplasm of junctional region of oropharynx

**C10.9**    **Malignant neoplasm of oropharynx, unspecified**   HCC

✓4ᵗʰ **C11**    **Malignant neoplasm of nasopharynx**
     Use additional code to identify:
       exposure to environmental tobacco smoke (Z77.22)
       exposure to tobacco smoke in the perinatal period (P96.81)
       history of tobacco dependence (Z87.891)
       occupational exposure to environmental tobacco smoke (Z57.31)
       tobacco dependence (F17.-)
       tobacco use (Z72.0)

**C11.0**    **Malignant neoplasm of superior wall of nasopharynx**   HCC
     Malignant neoplasm of roof of nasopharynx

**C11.1**    **Malignant neoplasm of posterior wall of nasopharynx**   HCC
     Malignant neoplasm of adenoid
     Malignant neoplasm of pharyngeal tonsil

**C11.2**    **Malignant neoplasm of lateral wall of nasopharynx**   HCC
     Malignant neoplasm of fossa of Rosenmüller
     Malignant neoplasm of opening of auditory tube
     Malignant neoplasm of pharyngeal recess

✓ Additional Character Req   ✓x7ᵗʰ Placeholder Alert   Unacceptable PDx   Manifestation   H1-H14 HAC   HCC CMS-HCC Condition   EXCLUDES 1 Not Coded Here   EXCLUDES 2 Not Included Here

ICD-10-CM 2018                                             463

**Chapter 2. Neoplasms**

**C11.3** **Malignant neoplasm of anterior wall of nasopharynx** `HCC`
Malignant neoplasm of floor of nasopharynx
Malignant neoplasm of nasopharyngeal (anterior) (posterior) surface of soft palate
Malignant neoplasm of posterior margin of nasal choana
Malignant neoplasm of posterior margin of nasal septum

**C11.8** **Malignant neoplasm of overlapping sites of nasopharynx** `HCC`

**C11.9** **Malignant neoplasm of nasopharynx, unspecified** `HCC`
Malignant neoplasm of nasopharyngeal wall NOS

**C12** **Malignant neoplasm of pyriform sinus** `HCC`
Malignant neoplasm of pyriform fossa
Use additional code to identify:
exposure to environmental tobacco smoke (Z77.22)
exposure to tobacco smoke in the perinatal period (P96.81)
history of tobacco dependence (Z87.891)
occupational exposure to environmental tobacco smoke (Z57.31)
tobacco dependence (F17.-)
tobacco use (Z72.0)

✓4ᵗʰ **C13** **Malignant neoplasm of hypopharynx**
Use additional code to identify:
exposure to environmental tobacco smoke (Z77.22)
exposure to tobacco smoke in the perinatal period (P96.81)
history of tobacco dependence (Z87.891)
occupational exposure to environmental tobacco smoke (Z57.31)
tobacco dependence (F17.-)
tobacco use (Z72.0)
*EXCLUDES 2*   *malignant neoplasm of pyriform sinus (C12)*

**C13.0** **Malignant neoplasm of postcricoid region** `HCC`

**C13.1** **Malignant neoplasm of aryepiglottic fold, hypopharyngeal aspect** `HCC`
Malignant neoplasm of aryepiglottic fold, marginal zone
Malignant neoplasm of aryepiglottic fold NOS
Malignant neoplasm of interarytenoid fold, marginal zone
Malignant neoplasm of interarytenoid fold NOS
*EXCLUDES 2*   *malignant neoplasm of aryepiglottic fold or interarytenoid fold, laryngeal aspect (C32.1)*

**C13.2** **Malignant neoplasm of posterior wall of hypopharynx** `HCC`

**C13.8** **Malignant neoplasm of overlapping sites of hypopharynx** `HCC`

**C13.9** **Malignant neoplasm of hypopharynx, unspecified** `HCC`
Malignant neoplasm of hypopharyngeal wall NOS

✓4ᵗʰ **C14** **Malignant neoplasm of other and ill-defined sites in the lip, oral cavity and pharynx**
Use additional code to identify:
alcohol abuse and dependence (F10.-)
exposure to environmental tobacco smoke (Z77.22)
exposure to tobacco smoke in the perinatal period (P96.81)
history of tobacco dependence (Z87.891)
occupational exposure to environmental tobacco smoke (Z57.31)
tobacco dependence (F17.-)
tobacco use (Z72.0)
*EXCLUDES 1*   *malignant neoplasm of oral cavity NOS (C06.9)*

**C14.0** **Malignant neoplasm of pharynx, unspecified** `HCC`

**C14.2** **Malignant neoplasm of Waldeyer's ring** `HCC`

**C14.8** **Malignant neoplasm of overlapping sites of lip, oral cavity and pharynx** `HCC`
Primary malignant neoplasm of two or more contiguous sites of lip, oral cavity and pharynx
*EXCLUDES 1*   *"book leaf" neoplasm [ventral surface of tongue and floor of mouth] (C06.89)*

## Malignant neoplasms of digestive organs (C15-C26)

*EXCLUDES 1*   *Kaposi's sarcoma of gastrointestinal sites (C46.4)*
*EXCLUDES 2*   *gastrointestinal stromal tumors (C49.A-)*

✓4ᵗʰ **C15** **Malignant neoplasm of esophagus**
Use additional code to identify:
alcohol abuse and dependence (F10.-)

**CC Excl: For CC codes in category C15:** PDX collection 253

**C15.3** **Malignant neoplasm of upper third of esophagus** `CC` `HCC`

**C15.4** **Malignant neoplasm of middle third of esophagus** `CC` `HCC`

**C15.5** **Malignant neoplasm of lower third of esophagus** `CC` `HCC`
*EXCLUDES 1*   *malignant neoplasm of cardio-esophageal junction (C16.0)*

**C15.8** **Malignant neoplasm of overlapping sites of esophagus** `CC` `HCC`

**C15.9** **Malignant neoplasm of esophagus, unspecified** `CC` `HCC`

✓4ᵗʰ **C16** **Malignant neoplasm of stomach**
Use additional code to identify:
alcohol abuse and dependence (F10.-)
*EXCLUDES 2*   *malignant carcinoid tumor of the stomach (C7A.092)*

**CC Excl: For CC codes in category C16:** PDX collection 254

**C16.0** **Malignant neoplasm of cardia** `CC` `HCC`
Malignant neoplasm of cardiac orifice
Malignant neoplasm of cardio-esophageal junction
Malignant neoplasm of esophagus and stomach
Malignant neoplasm of gastro-esophageal junction

**C16.1** **Malignant neoplasm of fundus of stomach** `CC` `HCC`

**C16.2** **Malignant neoplasm of body of stomach** `CC` `HCC`

**C16.3** **Malignant neoplasm of pyloric antrum** `CC` `HCC`
Malignant neoplasm of gastric antrum

**C16.4** **Malignant neoplasm of pylorus** `CC` `HCC`
Malignant neoplasm of prepylorus
Malignant neoplasm of pyloric canal

**C16.5** **Malignant neoplasm of lesser curvature of stomach, unspecified** `CC` `HCC`
Malignant neoplasm of lesser curvature of stomach, not classifiable to C16.1-C16.4

**C16.6** **Malignant neoplasm of greater curvature of stomach, unspecified** `CC` `HCC`
Malignant neoplasm of greater curvature of stomach, not classifiable to C16.0-C16.4

**C16.8** **Malignant neoplasm of overlapping sites of stomach** `CC` `HCC`

**C16.9** **Malignant neoplasm of stomach, unspecified** `CC` `HCC`
Gastric cancer NOS

✓4ᵗʰ **C17** **Malignant neoplasm of small intestine**
*EXCLUDES 1*   *malignant carcinoid tumors of the small intestine (C7A.01)*
**AHA:** 2016, 1Q, 19

**C17.0** **Malignant neoplasm of duodenum** `CC` `HCC`
**CC Excl:** PDX collection 255

**C17.1** **Malignant neoplasm of jejunum** `CC` `HCC`
**CC Excl:** PDX collection 256

**C17.2** **Malignant neoplasm of ileum** `CC` `HCC`
*EXCLUDES 1*   *malignant neoplasm of ileocecal valve (C18.0)*
**CC Excl:** PDX collection 257

**C17.3** **Meckel's diverticulum, malignant** `CC` `HCC`
*EXCLUDES 1*   *Meckel's diverticulum, congenital (Q43.0)*
**CC Excl:** PDX collection 258

**C17.8** **Malignant neoplasm of overlapping sites of small intestine** `CC` `HCC`
**CC Excl:** PDX collection 259

**C17.9** **Malignant neoplasm of small intestine, unspecified** `CC` `HCC`
**CC Excl:** PDX collection 259

✓4ᵗʰ **C18** **Malignant neoplasm of colon**
*EXCLUDES 1*   *malignant carcinoid tumors of the colon (C7A.02-)*

**C18.0** **Malignant neoplasm of cecum** `CC` `HCC`
Malignant neoplasm of ileocecal valve
**CC Excl:** PDX collection 260

**C18.1** **Malignant neoplasm of appendix** `CC` `HCC`
**CC Excl:** PDX collection 261

**C18.2** **Malignant neoplasm of ascending colon** `CC` `HCC`
**CC Excl:** PDX collection 262

**C18.3** **Malignant neoplasm of hepatic flexure** `CC` `HCC`
**CC Excl:** PDX collection 263

**C18.4** **Malignant neoplasm of transverse colon** `CC` `HCC`
**CC Excl:** PDX collection 264

**C18.5** **Malignant neoplasm of splenic flexure** `CC` `HCC`
**CC Excl:** PDX collection 265

**C18.6** **Malignant neoplasm of descending colon** `CC` `HCC`
**CC Excl:** PDX collection 266

**C18.7** **Malignant neoplasm of sigmoid colon** `CC` `HCC`
Malignant neoplasm of sigmoid (flexure)
*EXCLUDES 1*   *malignant neoplasm of rectosigmoid junction (C19)*
**CC Excl:** PDX collection 267

**C18.8** **Malignant neoplasm of overlapping sites of colon** `CC` `HCC`
**CC Excl:** PDX collection 268

**C18.9** **Malignant neoplasm of colon, unspecified** `CC` `HCC`
Malignant neoplasm of large intestine NOS
**CC Excl:** PDX collection 268

**C19** **Malignant neoplasm of rectosigmoid junction** `CC` `HCC`
Malignant neoplasm of colon with rectum
Malignant neoplasm of rectosigmoid (colon)
*EXCLUDES 1*   *malignant carcinoid tumors of the colon (C7A.02-)*
**CC Excl:** PDX collection 269

---

N Newborn: 0    P Pediatric: 0-17    M Maternity: 12-55    A Adult: 15-124    **MCC** Major CC Condition    **PDx•MCC** PDx acts as own MCC    **CC** CC Condition    **PDx•CC** PDx acts as own CC

**Colon**

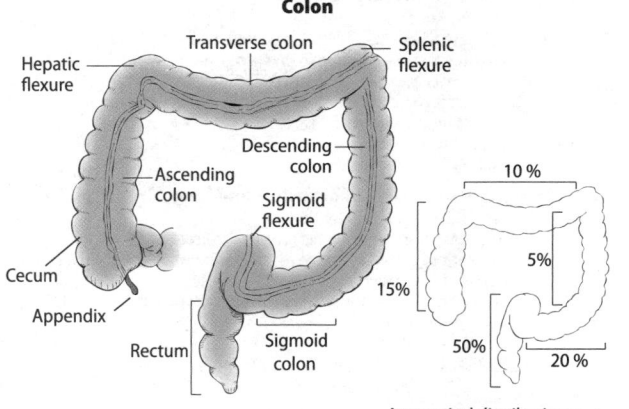

Anatomical distribution
of large bowel cancers

**C20 Malignant neoplasm of rectum** `CC` `HCC`
Malignant neoplasm of rectal ampulla
> **EXCLUDES 1**   malignant carcinoid tumor of the rectum (C7A.026)
> **CC Excl:** PDX collection 270

**✓4ᵗʰ C21 Malignant neoplasm of anus and anal canal**
> **EXCLUDES 2**   malignant carcinoid tumors of the colon (C7A.02-)
> malignant melanoma of anal margin (C43.51)
> malignant melanoma of anal skin (C43.51)
> malignant melanoma of perianal skin (C43.51)
> other and unspecified malignant neoplasm of anal margin
>   (C44.500, C44.510, C44.520, C44.590)
> other and unspecified malignant neoplasm of anal skin
>   (C44.500, C44.510, C44.520, C44.590)
> other and unspecified malignant neoplasm of perianal skin
>   (C44.500, C44.510, C44.520, C44.590)

   **C21.0 Malignant neoplasm of anus, unspecified** `CC` `HCC`
      **CC Excl:** PDX collection 271

   **C21.1 Malignant neoplasm of anal canal** `CC` `HCC`
      Malignant neoplasm of anal sphincter
      **CC Excl:** PDX collection 271

   **C21.2 Malignant neoplasm of cloacogenic zone** `CC` `HCC`
      **CC Excl:** PDX collection 272

   **C21.8 Malignant neoplasm of overlapping sites of rectum, anus and anal canal** `CC` `HCC`
      Malignant neoplasm of anorectal junction
      Malignant neoplasm of anorectum
      Primary malignant neoplasm of two or more contiguous sites of
        rectum, anus and anal canal
      **CC Excl:** PDX collection 272

**✓4ᵗʰ C22 Malignant neoplasm of liver and intrahepatic bile ducts**
> Use additional code to identify:
>   alcohol abuse and dependence (F10.-)
>   hepatitis B (B16.-, B18.0-B18.1)
>   hepatitis C (B17.1-, B18.2)
> **EXCLUDES 1**   malignant neoplasm of biliary tract NOS (C24.9)
> secondary malignant neoplasm of liver and intrahepatic bile
>   duct (C78.7)

   **CC Excl: For CC codes in category C22:** PDX collection 273

   **C22.0 Liver cell carcinoma** `CC` `HCC`
      Hepatocellular carcinoma
      Hepatoma
      **AHA:** 2016, 1Q, 18

   **C22.1 Intrahepatic bile duct carcinoma** `CC` `HCC`
      Cholangiocarcinoma
      > **EXCLUDES 1**   malignant neoplasm of hepatic duct (C24.0)

   **C22.2 Hepatoblastoma** `CC` `HCC`

   **C22.3 Angiosarcoma of liver** `CC` `HCC`
      Kupffer cell sarcoma

   **C22.4 Other sarcomas of liver** `CC` `HCC`

   **C22.7 Other specified carcinomas of liver** `CC` `HCC`

   **C22.8 Malignant neoplasm of liver, primary, unspecified as to type** `CC` `HCC`

   **C22.9 Malignant neoplasm of liver, not specified as primary or secondary** `CC` `HCC`

**C23 Malignant neoplasm of gallbladder** `CC` `HCC`
     **CC Excl:** PDX collection 274

**✓4ᵗʰ C24 Malignant neoplasm of other and unspecified parts of biliary tract**
> **EXCLUDES 1**   malignant neoplasm of intrahepatic bile duct (C22.1)

   **C24.0 Malignant neoplasm of extrahepatic bile duct** `CC` `HCC`
      Malignant neoplasm of biliary duct or passage NOS
      Malignant neoplasm of common bile duct
      Malignant neoplasm of cystic duct
      Malignant neoplasm of hepatic duct
      **CC Excl:** PDX collection 275

   **C24.1 Malignant neoplasm of ampulla of Vater** `CC` `HCC`
      **DEF:** Malignant neoplasm in the area of dilation at the juncture of
      the common bile and pancreatic ducts near the opening into the
      lumen of the duodenum.
      **CC Excl:** PDX collection 276

   **C24.8 Malignant neoplasm of overlapping sites of biliary tract** `CC` `HCC`
      Malignant neoplasm involving both intrahepatic and
        extrahepatic bile ducts
      Primary malignant neoplasm of two or more contiguous sites of
        biliary tract
      **CC Excl:** PDX collection 277

   **C24.9 Malignant neoplasm of biliary tract, unspecified** `CC` `HCC`
      **CC Excl:** PDX collection 277

**✓4ᵗʰ C25 Malignant neoplasm of pancreas**
> Code also exocrine pancreatic insufficiency (K86.81)
> Use additional code to identify:
>   alcohol abuse and dependence (F10.-)

   **CC Excl: For CC codes in category C25:** PDX collection 278

   **C25.0 Malignant neoplasm of head of pancreas** `CC` `HCC`

   **C25.1 Malignant neoplasm of body of pancreas** `CC` `HCC`

   **C25.2 Malignant neoplasm of tail of pancreas** `CC` `HCC`

   **C25.3 Malignant neoplasm of pancreatic duct** `CC` `HCC`

   **C25.4 Malignant neoplasm of endocrine pancreas** `CC` `HCC`
      Malignant neoplasm of islets of Langerhans
      Use additional code to identify any functional activity

   **C25.7 Malignant neoplasm of other parts of pancreas** `CC` `HCC`
      Malignant neoplasm of neck of pancreas

   **C25.8 Malignant neoplasm of overlapping sites of pancreas** `CC` `HCC`

   **C25.9 Malignant neoplasm of pancreas, unspecified** `CC` `HCC`

**✓4ᵗʰ C26 Malignant neoplasm of other and ill-defined digestive organs**
> **EXCLUDES 1**   malignant neoplasm of peritoneum and
>   retroperitoneum (C48.-)

   **C26.0 Malignant neoplasm of intestinal tract, part unspecified** `HCC`
      Malignant neoplasm of intestine NOS

   **C26.1 Malignant neoplasm of spleen** `HCC`
      > **EXCLUDES 1**   Hodgkin lymphoma (C81.-)
>   non-Hodgkin lymphoma (C82-C85)

   **C26.9 Malignant neoplasm of ill-defined sites within the digestive system** `HCC`
      Malignant neoplasm of alimentary canal or tract NOS
      Malignant neoplasm of gastrointestinal tract NOS
      > **EXCLUDES 1**   malignant neoplasm of abdominal NOS (C76.2)
>   malignant neoplasm of intra-abdominal NOS (C76.2)

**Pancreas**

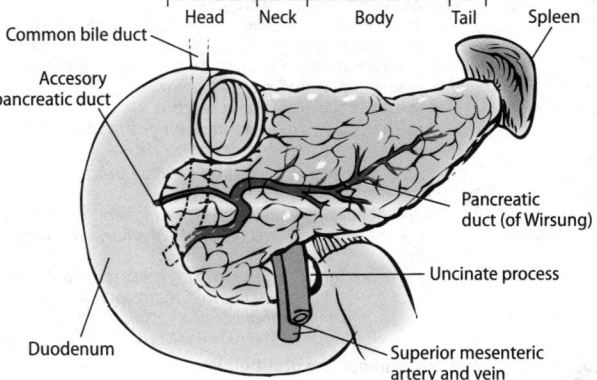

**Chapter 2. Neoplasms**

**C30–C37**

## Malignant neoplasms of respiratory and intrathoracic organs (C30-C39)

> **INCLUDES**    malignant neoplasm of middle ear
> **EXCLUDES 1**    *mesothelioma (C45.-)*

### ✓4th C30   Malignant neoplasm of nasal cavity and middle ear

**C30.0**   **Malignant neoplasm of nasal cavity**    HCC
Malignant neoplasm of cartilage of nose
Malignant neoplasm of nasal concha
Malignant neoplasm of internal nose
Malignant neoplasm of septum of nose
Malignant neoplasm of vestibule of nose
> **EXCLUDES 1**   *malignant melanoma of skin of nose (C43.31)*
> *malignant neoplasm of nasal bone (C41.0)*
> *malignant neoplasm of nose NOS (C76.0)*
> *malignant neoplasm of olfactory bulb (C72.2-)*
> *malignant neoplasm of posterior margin of nasal septum and choana (C11.3)*
> *malignant neoplasm of turbinates (C41.0)*
> *other and unspecified malignant neoplasm of skin of nose (C44.301, C44.311, C44.321, C44.391)*

**C30.1**   **Malignant neoplasm of middle ear**    HCC
Malignant neoplasm of antrum tympanicum
Malignant neoplasm of auditory tube
Malignant neoplasm of eustachian tube
Malignant neoplasm of inner ear
Malignant neoplasm of mastoid air cells
Malignant neoplasm of tympanic cavity
> **EXCLUDES 1**   *malignant melanoma of skin of (external) ear (C43.2-)*
> *malignant neoplasm of auricular canal (external) (C43.2-,C44.2-)*
> *malignant neoplasm of bone of ear (meatus) (C41.0)*
> *malignant neoplasm of cartilage of ear (C49.0)*
> *other and unspecified malignant neoplasm of skin of (external) ear (C44.2-)*

### ✓4th C31   Malignant neoplasm of accessory sinuses

**C31.0**   **Malignant neoplasm of maxillary sinus**    HCC
Malignant neoplasm of antrum (Highmore) (maxillary)

**C31.1**   **Malignant neoplasm of ethmoidal sinus**    HCC

**C31.2**   **Malignant neoplasm of frontal sinus**    HCC

**C31.3**   **Malignant neoplasm of sphenoid sinus**    HCC

**C31.8**   **Malignant neoplasm of overlapping sites of accessory sinuses**    HCC

**C31.9**   **Malignant neoplasm of accessory sinus, unspecified**    HCC

### ✓4th C32   Malignant neoplasm of larynx

Use additional code to identify:
alcohol abuse and dependence (F10.-)
exposure to environmental tobacco smoke (Z77.22)
exposure to tobacco smoke in the perinatal period (P96.81)
history of tobacco dependence (Z87.891)
occupational exposure to environmental tobacco smoke (Z57.31)
tobacco dependence (F17.-)
tobacco use (Z72.0)

**C32.0**   **Malignant neoplasm of glottis**    HCC
Malignant neoplasm of intrinsic larynx
Malignant neoplasm of laryngeal commissure (anterior)(posterior)
Malignant neoplasm of vocal cord (true) NOS

**C32.1**   **Malignant neoplasm of supraglottis**    HCC
Malignant neoplasm of aryepiglottic fold or interarytenoid fold, laryngeal aspect
Malignant neoplasm of epiglottis (suprahyoid portion) NOS
Malignant neoplasm of extrinsic larynx
Malignant neoplasm of false vocal cord
Malignant neoplasm of posterior (laryngeal) surface of epiglottis
Malignant neoplasm of ventricular bands
> **EXCLUDES 2**   *malignant neoplasm of anterior surface of epiglottis (C10.1)*
> *malignant neoplasm of aryepiglottic fold or interarytenoid fold, hypopharyngeal aspect (C13.1)*
> *malignant neoplasm of aryepiglottic fold or interarytenoid fold, marginal zone (C13.1)*
> *malignant neoplasm of aryepiglottic fold or interarytenoid fold NOS (C13.1)*

**C32.2**   **Malignant neoplasm of subglottis**    HCC

**C32.3**   **Malignant neoplasm of laryngeal cartilage**    HCC

**C32.8**   **Malignant neoplasm of overlapping sites of larynx**    HCC

**C32.9**   **Malignant neoplasm of larynx, unspecified**    HCC

### C33   Malignant neoplasm of trachea    CC   HCC

Use additional code to identify:
exposure to environmental tobacco smoke (Z77.22)
exposure to tobacco smoke in the perinatal period (P96.81)
history of tobacco dependence (Z87.891)
occupational exposure to environmental tobacco smoke (Z57.31)
tobacco dependence (F17.-)
tobacco use (Z72.0)
**CC Excl:** PDX collection 279

### ✓4th C34   Malignant neoplasm of bronchus and lung

Use additional code to identify:
exposure to environmental tobacco smoke (Z77.22)
exposure to tobacco smoke in the perinatal period (P96.81)
history of tobacco dependence (Z87.891)
occupational exposure to environmental tobacco smoke (Z57.31)
tobacco dependence (F17.-)
tobacco use (Z72.0)
> **EXCLUDES 1**   *Kaposi's sarcoma of lung (C46.5-)*
> *malignant carcinoid tumor of the bronchus and lung (C7A.090)*

**✓5th C34.0**   **Malignant neoplasm of main bronchus**
Malignant neoplasm of carina
Malignant neoplasm of hilus (of lung)

> **CC Excl: For CC codes in subcategory C34.0:**
> PDX collection 280

**C34.00**   **Malignant neoplasm of unspecified main bronchus**    CC   HCC

**C34.01**   **Malignant neoplasm of right main bronchus**    CC   HCC

**C34.02**   **Malignant neoplasm of left main bronchus**    CC   HCC

**✓5th C34.1**   **Malignant neoplasm of upper lobe, bronchus or lung**

> **CC Excl: For CC codes in subcategory C34.1:**
> PDX collection 281

**C34.10**   **Malignant neoplasm of upper lobe, unspecified bronchus or lung**    CC   HCC

**C34.11**   **Malignant neoplasm of upper lobe, right bronchus or lung**    CC   HCC

**C34.12**   **Malignant neoplasm of upper lobe, left bronchus or lung**    CC   HCC

**C34.2**   **Malignant neoplasm of middle lobe, bronchus or lung**    CC   HCC
**CC Excl:** PDX collection 282

**✓5th C34.3**   **Malignant neoplasm of lower lobe, bronchus or lung**

> **CC Excl: For CC codes in subcategory C34.3:**
> PDX collection 283

**C34.30**   **Malignant neoplasm of lower lobe, unspecified bronchus or lung**    CC   HCC

**C34.31**   **Malignant neoplasm of lower lobe, right bronchus or lung**    CC   HCC

**C34.32**   **Malignant neoplasm of lower lobe, left bronchus or lung**    CC   HCC

**✓5th C34.8**   **Malignant neoplasm of overlapping sites of bronchus and lung**

> **CC Excl: For CC codes in subcategory C34.8:**
> PDX collection 284

**C34.80**   **Malignant neoplasm of overlapping sites of unspecified bronchus and lung**    CC   HCC

**C34.81**   **Malignant neoplasm of overlapping sites of right bronchus and lung**    CC   HCC

**C34.82**   **Malignant neoplasm of overlapping sites of left bronchus and lung**    CC   HCC

**✓5th C34.9**   **Malignant neoplasm of unspecified part of bronchus or lung**

> **CC Excl: For CC codes in subcategory C34.9:**
> PDX collection 284

**C34.90**   **Malignant neoplasm of unspecified part of unspecified bronchus or lung**    CC   HCC
Lung cancer NOS

**C34.91**   **Malignant neoplasm of unspecified part of right bronchus or lung**    CC   HCC

**C34.92**   **Malignant neoplasm of unspecified part of left bronchus or lung**    CC   HCC

### C37   Malignant neoplasm of thymus    CC   HCC
> **EXCLUDES 1**   *malignant carcinoid tumor of the thymus (C7A.091)*
> **CC Excl:** PDX collection 285

---

Ⓝ Newborn: 0    Ⓟ Pediatric: 0-17    Ⓜ Maternity: 12-55    Ⓐ Adult: 15-124    MCC Major CC Condition    PDx MCC PDx acts as own MCC    CC CC Condition    PDx CC PDx acts as own CC

466
ICD-10-CM 2018

✅4ᵗʰ **C38** **Malignant neoplasm of heart, mediastinum and pleura**
     *EXCLUDES 1*   mesothelioma (C45.-)

     **CC Excl: For CC codes in category C38, unless otherwise noted:**
     PDX collection 287

     **C38.0**   **Malignant neoplasm of heart**    `CC` `HCC`
         Malignant neoplasm of pericardium
         *EXCLUDES 1*   malignant neoplasm of great vessels (C49.3)
         CC Excl: PDX collection 286

     **C38.1**   **Malignant neoplasm of anterior mediastinum**   `CC` `HCC`

     **C38.2**   **Malignant neoplasm of posterior mediastinum**   `CC` `HCC`

     **C38.3**   **Malignant neoplasm of mediastinum, part unspecified**   `CC` `HCC`

     **C38.4**   **Malignant neoplasm of pleura**   `CC` `HCC`

     **C38.8**   **Malignant neoplasm of overlapping sites of heart, mediastinum and pleura**   `CC` `HCC`

✅4ᵗʰ **C39** **Malignant neoplasm of other and ill-defined sites in the respiratory system and intrathoracic organs**
     Use additional code to identify:
       exposure to environmental tobacco smoke (Z77.22)
       exposure to tobacco smoke in the perinatal period (P96.81)
       history of tobacco dependence (Z87.891)
       occupational exposure to environmental tobacco smoke (Z57.31)
       tobacco dependence (F17.-)
       tobacco use (Z72.0)
     *EXCLUDES 1*   intrathoracic malignant neoplasm NOS (C76.1)
              thoracic malignant neoplasm NOS (C76.1)

     **C39.0**   **Malignant neoplasm of upper respiratory tract, part unspecified**   `HCC`

     **C39.9**   **Malignant neoplasm of lower respiratory tract, part unspecified**   `HCC`
         Malignant neoplasm of respiratory tract NOS

---

## Malignant neoplasms of bone and articular cartilage (C40-C41)

     *INCLUDES*   malignant neoplasm of cartilage (articular) (joint)
             malignant neoplasm of periosteum
     *EXCLUDES 1*   malignant neoplasm of bone marrow NOS (C96.9)
              malignant neoplasm of synovia (C49.-)

✅4ᵗʰ **C40** **Malignant neoplasm of bone and articular cartilage of limbs**
     Use additional code to identify major osseous defect, if applicable
     (M89.7-)

✅5ᵗʰ   **C40.0**   **Malignant neoplasm of scapula and long bones of upper limb**

     **CC Excl: For CC codes in subcategory C40.0:**
     PDX collection 289

     **C40.00**   **Malignant neoplasm of scapula and long bones of unspecified upper limb**   `CC` `HCC`

     **C40.01**   **Malignant neoplasm of scapula and long bones of right upper limb**   `CC` `HCC`

     **C40.02**   **Malignant neoplasm of scapula and long bones of left upper limb**   `CC` `HCC`

✅5ᵗʰ   **C40.1**   **Malignant neoplasm of short bones of upper limb**

     **CC Excl: For CC codes in subcategory C40.1:**
     PDX collection 290

     **C40.10**   **Malignant neoplasm of short bones of unspecified upper limb**   `CC` `HCC`

     **C40.11**   **Malignant neoplasm of short bones of right upper limb**   `CC` `HCC`

     **C40.12**   **Malignant neoplasm of short bones of left upper limb**   `CC` `HCC`

✅5ᵗʰ   **C40.2**   **Malignant neoplasm of long bones of lower limb**

     **CC Excl: For CC codes in subcategory C40.2:**
     PDX collection 291

     **C40.20**   **Malignant neoplasm of long bones of unspecified lower limb**   `CC` `HCC`

     **C40.21**   **Malignant neoplasm of long bones of right lower limb**   `CC` `HCC`

     **C40.22**   **Malignant neoplasm of long bones of left lower limb**   `CC` `HCC`

✅5ᵗʰ   **C40.3**   **Malignant neoplasm of short bones of lower limb**

     **CC Excl: For CC codes in subcategory C40.3:**
     PDX collection 292

     **C40.30**   **Malignant neoplasm of short bones of unspecified lower limb**   `CC` `HCC`

     **C40.31**   **Malignant neoplasm of short bones of right lower limb**   `CC` `HCC`

---

     **C40.32**   **Malignant neoplasm of short bones of left lower limb**

✅5ᵗʰ   **C40.8**   **Malignant neoplasm of overlapping sites of bone and articular cartilage of limb**

     **CC Excl: For CC codes in subcategory C40.8:**
     PDX collection 293

     **C40.80**   **Malignant neoplasm of overlapping sites of bone and articular cartilage of unspecified limb**   `CC` `HCC`

     **C40.81**   **Malignant neoplasm of overlapping sites of bone and articular cartilage of right limb**   `CC` `HCC`

     **C40.82**   **Malignant neoplasm of overlapping sites of bone and articular cartilage of left limb**   `CC` `HCC`

✅5ᵗʰ   **C40.9**   **Malignant neoplasm of unspecified bones and articular cartilage of limb**

     **CC Excl: For CC codes in subcategory C40.9:**
     PDX collection 293

     **C40.90**   **Malignant neoplasm of unspecified bones and articular cartilage of unspecified limb**   `CC` `HCC`

     **C40.91**   **Malignant neoplasm of unspecified bones and articular cartilage of right limb**   `CC` `HCC`

     **C40.92**   **Malignant neoplasm of unspecified bones and articular cartilage of left limb**   `CC` `HCC`

✅4ᵗʰ **C41** **Malignant neoplasm of bone and articular cartilage of other and unspecified sites**
     *EXCLUDES 1*   malignant neoplasm of bones of limbs (C40.-)
              malignant neoplasm of cartilage of ear (C49.0)
              malignant neoplasm of cartilage of eyelid (C49.0)
              malignant neoplasm of cartilage of larynx (C32.3)
              malignant neoplasm of cartilage of limbs (C40.-)
              malignant neoplasm of cartilage of nose (C30.0)

     **C41.0**   **Malignant neoplasm of bones of skull and face**   `CC` `HCC`
         Malignant neoplasm of maxilla (superior)
         Malignant neoplasm of orbital bone
         *EXCLUDES 2*   carcinoma, any type except intraosseous or
                  odontogenic of:
                    maxillary sinus (C31.0)
                    upper jaw (C03.0)
                  malignant neoplasm of jaw bone (lower) (C41.1)
         CC Excl: PDX collection 294

     **C41.1**   **Malignant neoplasm of mandible**   `CC` `HCC`
         Malignant neoplasm of inferior maxilla
         Malignant neoplasm of lower jaw bone
         *EXCLUDES 2*   carcinoma, any type except intraosseous or
                  odontogenic of:
                    jaw NOS (C03.9)
                    lower (C03.1)
                  malignant neoplasm of upper jaw bone (C41.0)
         CC Excl: PDX collection 295

     **C41.2**   **Malignant neoplasm of vertebral column**   `CC` `HCC`
         *EXCLUDES 1*   malignant neoplasm of sacrum and coccyx (C41.4)
         CC Excl: PDX collection 296

     **C41.3**   **Malignant neoplasm of ribs, sternum and clavicle**   `CC` `HCC`
         CC Excl: PDX collection 297

     **C41.4**   **Malignant neoplasm of pelvic bones, sacrum and coccyx**   `CC` `HCC`
         CC Excl: PDX collection 298

     **C41.9**   **Malignant neoplasm of bone and articular cartilage, unspecified**   `CC` `HCC`
         CC Excl: PDX collection 293

---

## Melanoma and other malignant neoplasms of skin (C43-C44)

✅4ᵗʰ **C43** **Malignant melanoma of skin**
     *EXCLUDES 1*   melanoma in situ (D03.-)
     *EXCLUDES 2*   malignant melanoma of skin of genital organs (C51-C52, C60.-,
              C63.-)
              Merkel cell carcinoma (C4A.-)
              sites other than skin—code to malignant neoplasm of the site

     **C43.0**   **Malignant melanoma of lip**   `HCC`
         *EXCLUDES 1*   malignant neoplasm of vermilion border of lip (C00.0-
                  C00.2)

✅5ᵗʰ   **C43.1**   **Malignant melanoma of eyelid, including canthus**

     **C43.10**   **Malignant melanoma of unspecified eyelid, including canthus**   `HCC`

     **C43.11**   **Malignant melanoma of right eyelid, including canthus**   `HCC`

     **C43.12**   **Malignant melanoma of left eyelid, including canthus**   `HCC`

---

✅Additional Character Req   ✅x 7ᵗʰ Placeholder Alert   Unacceptable PDx   Manifestation   `H1`-`H14` HAC   `HCC` CMS-HCC Condition   *EXCLUDES 1* Not Coded Here   *EXCLUDES 2* Not Included Here

ICD-10-CM 2018                **467**

**Chapter 2. Neoplasms**

✓5ᵗʰ **C43.2 Malignant melanoma of ear and external auricular canal**

     **C43.20 Malignant melanoma of unspecified ear and external auricular canal** `HCC`

     **C43.21 Malignant melanoma of right ear and external auricular canal** `HCC`

     **C43.22 Malignant melanoma of left ear and external auricular canal** `HCC`

✓5ᵗʰ **C43.3 Malignant melanoma of other and unspecified parts of face**

     **C43.30 Malignant melanoma of unspecified part of face** `HCC`

     **C43.31 Malignant melanoma of nose** `HCC`

     **C43.39 Malignant melanoma of other parts of face** `HCC`

   **C43.4 Malignant melanoma of scalp and neck** `HCC`

✓5ᵗʰ **C43.5 Malignant melanoma of trunk**

     **EXCLUDES 2**   *malignant neoplasm of anus NOS (C21.0)*
                *malignant neoplasm of scrotum (C63.2)*

     **C43.51 Malignant melanoma of anal skin** `HCC`
          Malignant melanoma of anal margin
          Malignant melanoma of perianal skin

     **C43.52 Malignant melanoma of skin of breast** `HCC`

     **C43.59 Malignant melanoma of other part of trunk** `HCC`

✓5ᵗʰ **C43.6 Malignant melanoma of upper limb, including shoulder**

     **C43.60 Malignant melanoma of unspecified upper limb, including shoulder** `HCC`

     **C43.61 Malignant melanoma of right upper limb, including shoulder** `HCC`

     **C43.62 Malignant melanoma of left upper limb, including shoulder** `HCC`

✓5ᵗʰ **C43.7 Malignant melanoma of lower limb, including hip**

     **C43.70 Malignant melanoma of unspecified lower limb, including hip** `HCC`

     **C43.71 Malignant melanoma of right lower limb, including hip** `HCC`

     **C43.72 Malignant melanoma of left lower limb, including hip** `HCC`

   **C43.8 Malignant melanoma of overlapping sites of skin** `HCC`

   **C43.9 Malignant melanoma of skin, unspecified** `HCC`
      Malignant melanoma of unspecified site of skin
      Melanoma (malignant) NOS

✓4ᵗʰ **C4A Merkel cell carcinoma**

    **DEF:** Malignant cutaneous cancer predominantly found in elderly patients with sun exposure that usually presents as a flesh-colored or bluish-red lump typically seen on the neck, head and face.

   **C4A.0 Merkel cell carcinoma of lip** `HCC`

     **EXCLUDES 1**   *malignant neoplasm of vermilion border of lip (C00.0-C00.2)*

✓5ᵗʰ **C4A.1 Merkel cell carcinoma of eyelid, including canthus**

     **C4A.10 Merkel cell carcinoma of unspecified eyelid, including canthus** `HCC`

     **C4A.11 Merkel cell carcinoma of right eyelid, including canthus** `HCC`

     **C4A.12 Merkel cell carcinoma of left eyelid, including canthus** `HCC`

✓5ᵗʰ **C4A.2 Merkel cell carcinoma of ear and external auricular canal**

     **C4A.20 Merkel cell carcinoma of unspecified ear and external auricular canal** `HCC`

     **C4A.21 Merkel cell carcinoma of right ear and external auricular canal** `HCC`

     **C4A.22 Merkel cell carcinoma of left ear and external auricular canal** `HCC`

✓5ᵗʰ **C4A.3 Merkel cell carcinoma of other and unspecified parts of face**

     **C4A.30 Merkel cell carcinoma of unspecified part of face** `HCC`

     **C4A.31 Merkel cell carcinoma of nose** `HCC`

     **C4A.39 Merkel cell carcinoma of other parts of face** `HCC`

   **C4A.4 Merkel cell carcinoma of scalp and neck** `HCC`

✓5ᵗʰ **C4A.5 Merkel cell carcinoma of trunk**

     **EXCLUDES 2**   *malignant neoplasm of anus NOS (C21.0)*
                *malignant neoplasm of scrotum (C63.2)*

     **C4A.51 Merkel cell carcinoma of anal skin** `HCC`
          Merkel cell carcinoma of anal margin
          Merkel cell carcinoma of perianal skin

     **C4A.52 Merkel cell carcinoma of skin of breast** `HCC`

     **C4A.59 Merkel cell carcinoma of other part of trunk** `HCC`

✓5ᵗʰ **C4A.6 Merkel cell carcinoma of upper limb, including shoulder**

     **C4A.60 Merkel cell carcinoma of unspecified upper limb, including shoulder** `HCC`

     **C4A.61 Merkel cell carcinoma of right upper limb, including shoulder** `HCC`

     **C4A.62 Merkel cell carcinoma of left upper limb, including shoulder** `HCC`

✓5ᵗʰ **C4A.7 Merkel cell carcinoma of lower limb, including hip**

     **C4A.70 Merkel cell carcinoma of unspecified lower limb, including hip** `HCC`

     **C4A.71 Merkel cell carcinoma of right lower limb, including hip** `HCC`

     **C4A.72 Merkel cell carcinoma of left lower limb, including hip** `HCC`

   **C4A.8 Merkel cell carcinoma of overlapping sites** `HCC`

   **C4A.9 Merkel cell carcinoma, unspecified** `HCC`
      Merkel cell carcinoma of unspecified site
      Merkel cell carcinoma (NOS)

✓4ᵗʰ **C44 Other and unspecified malignant neoplasm of skin**

    **INCLUDES**   malignant neoplasm of sebaceous glands
              malignant neoplasm of sweat glands

    **EXCLUDES 1**   *Kaposi's sarcoma of skin (C46.0)*
             *malignant melanoma of skin (C43.-)*
             *malignant neoplasm of skin of genital organs (C51-C52, C60-, C63.2)*
             *Merkel cell carcinoma (C4A.-)*

    **DEF:** Basal cell carcinoma: An abnormal growth of skin cells that arises from the deepest layer of the epidermis and may present as an open sore, red patches, pink growth, or scar. One of the most common forms of skin cancer, typically caused by sun exposure.

    **DEF:** Squamous cell carcinoma: An uncontrolled growth of abnormal skin cells that arises from the skin's outer layers (epidermis) and may present as an open sore; firm, red nodule; elevated growth with a central depression; or flat sore with a scaly crust.

✓5ᵗʰ **C44.0 Other and unspecified malignant neoplasm of skin of lip**

     **EXCLUDES 1**   *malignant neoplasm of lip (C00.-)*

     **C44.00 Unspecified malignant neoplasm of skin of lip**

     **C44.01 Basal cell carcinoma of skin of lip**

     **C44.02 Squamous cell carcinoma of skin of lip**

     **C44.09 Other specified malignant neoplasm of skin of lip**

✓5ᵗʰ **C44.1 Other and unspecified malignant neoplasm of skin of eyelid, including canthus**

     **EXCLUDES 1**   *connective tissue of eyelid (C49.0)*

   ✓6ᵗʰ **C44.10 Unspecified malignant neoplasm of skin of eyelid, including canthus**

     **C44.101 Unspecified malignant neoplasm of skin of unspecified eyelid, including canthus**

     **C44.102 Unspecified malignant neoplasm of skin of right eyelid, including canthus**

     **C44.109 Unspecified malignant neoplasm of skin of left eyelid, including canthus**

   ✓6ᵗʰ **C44.11 Basal cell carcinoma of skin of eyelid, including canthus**

     **C44.111 Basal cell carcinoma of skin of unspecified eyelid, including canthus**

     **C44.112 Basal cell carcinoma of skin of right eyelid, including canthus**

     **C44.119 Basal cell carcinoma of skin of left eyelid, including canthus**

   ✓6ᵗʰ **C44.12 Squamous cell carcinoma of skin of eyelid, including canthus**

     **C44.121 Squamous cell carcinoma of skin of unspecified eyelid, including canthus**

     **C44.122 Squamous cell carcinoma of skin of right eyelid, including canthus**

     **C44.129 Squamous cell carcinoma of skin of left eyelid, including canthus**

   ✓6ᵗʰ **C44.19 Other specified malignant neoplasm of skin of eyelid, including canthus**

     **C44.191 Other specified malignant neoplasm of skin of unspecified eyelid, including canthus**

     **C44.192 Other specified malignant neoplasm of skin of right eyelid, including canthus**

     **C44.199 Other specified malignant neoplasm of skin of left eyelid, including canthus**

N Newborn: 0   P Pediatric: 0-17   M Maternity: 12-55   A Adult: 15-124   **MCC** Major CC Condition   **PDxMCC** PDx acts as own MCC   **CC** CC Condition   **PDxCC** PDx acts as own CC

468                                               ICD-10-CM 2018

✔5ᵗʰ **C44.2** **Other and unspecified malignant neoplasm of** skin of ear and external auricular canal
  *EXCLUDES 1* *connective tissue of ear (C49.0)*

  ✔6ᵗʰ **C44.20** **Unspecified malignant neoplasm of skin of ear and external auricular canal**
  **C44.201** **Unspecified malignant neoplasm of skin of** unspecified **ear and external auricular canal**
  **C44.202** **Unspecified malignant neoplasm of skin of** right **ear and external auricular canal**
  **C44.209** **Unspecified malignant neoplasm of skin of** left **ear and external auricular canal**

  ✔6ᵗʰ **C44.21** Basal cell carcinoma **of skin of ear and external auricular canal**
  **C44.211** **Basal cell carcinoma of skin of** unspecified **ear and external auricular canal**
  **C44.212** **Basal cell carcinoma of skin of** right **ear and external auricular canal**
  **C44.219** **Basal cell carcinoma of skin of** left **ear and external auricular canal**

  ✔6ᵗʰ **C44.22** Squamous cell carcinoma **of skin of ear and external auricular canal**
  **C44.221** **Squamous cell carcinoma of skin of** unspecified **ear and external auricular canal**
  **C44.222** **Squamous cell carcinoma of skin of** right **ear and external auricular canal**
  **C44.229** **Squamous cell carcinoma of skin of** left **ear and external auricular canal**

  ✔6ᵗʰ **C44.29** Other **specified malignant neoplasm of skin of ear and external auricular canal**
  **C44.291** **Other specified malignant neoplasm of skin of** unspecified **ear and external auricular canal**
  **C44.292** **Other specified malignant neoplasm of skin of** right **ear and external auricular canal**
  **C44.299** **Other specified malignant neoplasm of skin of** left **ear and external auricular canal**

✔5ᵗʰ **C44.3** **Other and unspecified malignant neoplasm of skin of** other and unspecified parts of face

  ✔6ᵗʰ **C44.30** Unspecified **malignant neoplasm of skin of other and unspecified parts of face**
  **C44.300** **Unspecified malignant neoplasm of skin of** unspecified **part of face**
  **C44.301** **Unspecified malignant neoplasm of skin of** nose
  **C44.309** **Unspecified malignant neoplasm of skin of** other **parts of face**

  ✔6ᵗʰ **C44.31** Basal cell carcinoma **of skin of other and unspecified parts of face**
  **C44.310** **Basal cell carcinoma of skin of** unspecified **parts of face**
  **C44.311** **Basal cell carcinoma of skin of** nose
  **C44.319** **Basal cell carcinoma of skin of** other **parts of face**

  ✔6ᵗʰ **C44.32** Squamous cell carcinoma **of skin of other and unspecified parts of face**
  **C44.320** **Squamous cell carcinoma of skin of** unspecified **parts of face**
  **C44.321** **Squamous cell carcinoma of skin of** nose
  **C44.329** **Squamous cell carcinoma of skin of** other **parts of face**

  ✔6ᵗʰ **C44.39** Other **specified malignant neoplasm of skin of other and unspecified parts of face**
  **C44.390** **Other specified malignant neoplasm of skin of** unspecified **parts of face**
  **C44.391** **Other specified malignant neoplasm of skin of** nose
  **C44.399** **Other specified malignant neoplasm of skin of** other **parts of face**

✔5ᵗʰ **C44.4** **Other and unspecified malignant neoplasm of skin of** scalp and neck

  **C44.40** Unspecified **malignant neoplasm of skin of scalp and neck**
  **C44.41** Basal cell carcinoma **of skin of scalp and neck**
  **C44.42** Squamous cell carcinoma **of skin of scalp and neck**

**C44.49** **Other specified malignant neoplasm of skin of scalp and neck**

✔5ᵗʰ **C44.5** **Other and unspecified malignant neoplasm of** skin of trunk
  *EXCLUDES 1* *anus NOS (C21.0)*
  *scrotum (C63.2)*

  ✔6ᵗʰ **C44.50** Unspecified **malignant neoplasm of skin of trunk**
  **C44.500** **Unspecified malignant neoplasm of** anal skin
  Unspecified malignant neoplasm of anal margin
  Unspecified malignant neoplasm of perianal skin
  **C44.501** **Unspecified malignant neoplasm of** skin of breast
  **C44.509** **Unspecified malignant neoplasm of skin of** other **part of trunk**

  ✔6ᵗʰ **C44.51** Basal cell carcinoma **of skin of trunk**
  **C44.510** **Basal cell carcinoma of** anal skin
  Basal cell carcinoma of anal margin
  Basal cell carcinoma of perianal skin
  **C44.511** **Basal cell carcinoma of** skin of breast
  **C44.519** **Basal cell carcinoma of skin of** other **part of trunk**

  ✔6ᵗʰ **C44.52** Squamous cell carcinoma **of skin of trunk**
  **C44.520** **Squamous cell carcinoma of** anal skin
  Squamous cell carcinoma of anal margin
  Squamous cell carcinoma of perianal skin
  **C44.521** **Squamous cell carcinoma of** skin of breast
  **C44.529** **Squamous cell carcinoma of skin of** other **part of trunk**

  ✔6ᵗʰ **C44.59** Other **specified malignant neoplasm of skin of trunk**
  **C44.590** **Other specified malignant neoplasm of** anal skin
  Other specified malignant neoplasm of anal margin
  Other specified malignant neoplasm of perianal skin
  **C44.591** **Other specified malignant neoplasm of** skin of breast
  **C44.599** **Other specified malignant neoplasm of skin of** other **part of trunk**

✔5ᵗʰ **C44.6** **Other and unspecified malignant neoplasm of skin of** upper limb, including shoulder

  ✔6ᵗʰ **C44.60** Unspecified **malignant neoplasm of skin of upper limb, including shoulder**
  **C44.601** **Unspecified malignant neoplasm of skin of** unspecified **upper limb, including shoulder**
  **C44.602** **Unspecified malignant neoplasm of skin of** right **upper limb, including shoulder**
  **C44.609** **Unspecified malignant neoplasm of skin of** left **upper limb, including shoulder**

  ✔6ᵗʰ **C44.61** Basal cell carcinoma **of skin of upper limb, including shoulder**
  **C44.611** **Basal cell carcinoma of skin of** unspecified **upper limb, including shoulder**
  **C44.612** **Basal cell carcinoma of skin of** right **upper limb, including shoulder**
  **C44.619** **Basal cell carcinoma of skin of** left **upper limb, including shoulder**

  ✔6ᵗʰ **C44.62** Squamous cell carcinoma **of skin of upper limb, including shoulder**
  **C44.621** **Squamous cell carcinoma of skin of** unspecified **upper limb, including shoulder**
  **C44.622** **Squamous cell carcinoma of skin of** right **upper limb, including shoulder**
  **C44.629** **Squamous cell carcinoma of skin of** left **upper limb, including shoulder**

  ✔6ᵗʰ **C44.69** Other **specified malignant neoplasm of skin of upper limb, including shoulder**
  **C44.691** **Other specified malignant neoplasm of skin of** unspecified **upper limb, including shoulder**
  **C44.692** **Other specified malignant neoplasm of skin of** right **upper limb, including shoulder**
  **C44.699** **Other specified malignant neoplasm of skin of** left **upper limb, including shoulder**

**Chapter 2. Neoplasms**

✓5ᵗʰ **C44.7** **Other and unspecified malignant neoplasm of skin of lower limb, including hip**

  ✓6ᵗʰ **C44.70** **Unspecified malignant neoplasm of skin of lower limb, including hip**

    **C44.701** **Unspecified malignant neoplasm of skin of unspecified lower limb, including hip**

    **C44.702** **Unspecified malignant neoplasm of skin of right lower limb, including hip**

    **C44.709** **Unspecified malignant neoplasm of skin of left lower limb, including hip**

  ✓6ᵗʰ **C44.71** **Basal cell carcinoma of skin of lower limb, including hip**

    **C44.711** **Basal cell carcinoma of skin of unspecified lower limb, including hip**

    **C44.712** **Basal cell carcinoma of skin of right lower limb, including hip**

    **C44.719** **Basal cell carcinoma of skin of left lower limb, including hip**

  ✓6ᵗʰ **C44.72** **Squamous cell carcinoma of skin of lower limb, including hip**

    **C44.721** **Squamous cell carcinoma of skin of unspecified lower limb, including hip**

    **C44.722** **Squamous cell carcinoma of skin of right lower limb, including hip**

    **C44.729** **Squamous cell carcinoma of skin of left lower limb, including hip**

  ✓6ᵗʰ **C44.79** **Other specified malignant neoplasm of skin of lower limb, including hip**

    **C44.791** **Other specified malignant neoplasm of skin of unspecified lower limb, including hip**

    **C44.792** **Other specified malignant neoplasm of skin of right lower limb, including hip**

    **C44.799** **Other specified malignant neoplasm of skin of left lower limb, including hip**

✓5ᵗʰ **C44.8** **Other and unspecified malignant neoplasm of overlapping sites of skin**

  **C44.80** **Unspecified malignant neoplasm of overlapping sites of skin**

  **C44.81** **Basal cell carcinoma of overlapping sites of skin**

  **C44.82** **Squamous cell carcinoma of overlapping sites of skin**

  **C44.89** **Other specified malignant neoplasm of overlapping sites of skin**

✓5ᵗʰ **C44.9** **Other and unspecified malignant neoplasm of skin, unspecified**

  **C44.90** **Unspecified malignant neoplasm of skin, unspecified**

    Malignant neoplasm of unspecified site of skin

  **C44.91** **Basal cell carcinoma of skin, unspecified**

  **C44.92** **Squamous cell carcinoma of skin, unspecified**

  **C44.99** **Other specified malignant neoplasm of skin, unspecified**

## Malignant neoplasms of mesothelial and soft tissue (C45-C49)

✓4ᵗʰ **C45** **Mesothelioma**

  **DEF:** Rare type of cancer that forms in the thin layer of protective tissue that covers the majority of internal organs (mesothelium).

  **C45.0** **Mesothelioma of pleura**    CC HCC

    *EXCLUDES 1*   *other malignant neoplasm of pleura (C38.4)*

    **AHA:** 2017, 2Q, 11

    **CC Excl:** PDX collection 288

  **C45.1** **Mesothelioma of peritoneum**    CC HCC

    Mesothelioma of cul-de-sac

    Mesothelioma of mesentery

    Mesothelioma of mesocolon

    Mesothelioma of omentum

    Mesothelioma of peritoneum (parietal) (pelvic)

    *EXCLUDES 1*   *other malignant neoplasm of soft tissue of peritoneum (C48.-)*

    **CC Excl:** PDX collection 299

  **C45.2** **Mesothelioma of pericardium**    CC HCC

    *EXCLUDES 1*   *other malignant neoplasm of pericardium (C38.0)*

    **CC Excl:** PDX collection 286

  **C45.7** **Mesothelioma of other sites**    HCC

  **C45.9** **Mesothelioma, unspecified**    HCC

✓4ᵗʰ **C46** **Kaposi's sarcoma**

  Code first any human immunodeficiency virus [HIV] disease (B20)

  **DEF:** Malignant neoplasm that causes patches of abnormal tissue to grow under the skin, in the lining of the mouth, nose, and throat, in lymph nodes, or in other visceral organs. Kaposi's sarcoma is caused by human herpesvirus8 (HHV8).

  **C46.0** **Kaposi's sarcoma of skin**    HIV CC HCC

    **CC Excl:** PDX collection 300

  **C46.1** **Kaposi's sarcoma of soft tissue**    HIV CC HCC

    Kaposi's sarcoma of blood vessel

    Kaposi's sarcoma of connective tissue

    Kaposi's sarcoma of fascia

    Kaposi's sarcoma of ligament

    Kaposi's sarcoma of lymphatic(s) NEC

    Kaposi's sarcoma of muscle

    *EXCLUDES 2*   *Kaposi's sarcoma of lymph glands and nodes (C46.3)*

    **CC Excl:** PDX collection 301

  **C46.2** **Kaposi's sarcoma of palate**    HIV CC HCC

    **CC Excl:** PDX collection 302

  **C46.3** **Kaposi's sarcoma of lymph nodes**    HIV CC HCC

    **CC Excl:** PDX collection 303

  **C46.4** **Kaposi's sarcoma of gastrointestinal sites**    HIV CC HCC

    **CC Excl:** PDX collection 304

✓5ᵗʰ **C46.5** **Kaposi's sarcoma of lung**

    **CC Excl: For CC codes in subcategory C46.5:** PDX collection 284

  **C46.50** **Kaposi's sarcoma of unspecified lung**    HIV CC HCC

  **C46.51** **Kaposi's sarcoma of right lung**    HIV CC HCC

  **C46.52** **Kaposi's sarcoma of left lung**    HIV CC HCC

  **C46.7** **Kaposi's sarcoma of other sites**    HIV CC HCC

    **CC Excl:** PDX collection 305

  **C46.9** **Kaposi's sarcoma, unspecified**    HIV CC HCC

    Kaposi's sarcoma of unspecified site

    **CC Excl:** PDX collection 306

✓4ᵗʰ **C47** **Malignant neoplasm of peripheral nerves and autonomic nervous system**

  *INCLUDES*   malignant neoplasm of sympathetic and parasympathetic nerves and ganglia

  *EXCLUDES 1*   *Kaposi's sarcoma of soft tissue (C46.1)*

  **CC Excl: For CC codes in category C47:** PDX collection 307

  **C47.0** **Malignant neoplasm of peripheral nerves of head, face and neck**    CC HCC

    *EXCLUDES 1*   *malignant neoplasm of peripheral nerves of orbit (C69.6-)*

✓5ᵗʰ **C47.1** **Malignant neoplasm of peripheral nerves of upper limb, including shoulder**

  **C47.10** **Malignant neoplasm of peripheral nerves of unspecified upper limb, including shoulder**    CC HCC

  **C47.11** **Malignant neoplasm of peripheral nerves of right upper limb, including shoulder**    CC HCC

  **C47.12** **Malignant neoplasm of peripheral nerves of left upper limb, including shoulder**    CC HCC

✓5ᵗʰ **C47.2** **Malignant neoplasm of peripheral nerves of lower limb, including hip**

  **C47.20** **Malignant neoplasm of peripheral nerves of unspecified lower limb, including hip**    CC HCC

  **C47.21** **Malignant neoplasm of peripheral nerves of right lower limb, including hip**    CC HCC

  **C47.22** **Malignant neoplasm of peripheral nerves of left lower limb, including hip**    CC HCC

  **C47.3** **Malignant neoplasm of peripheral nerves of thorax**    CC HCC

  **C47.4** **Malignant neoplasm of peripheral nerves of abdomen**    CC HCC

  **C47.5** **Malignant neoplasm of peripheral nerves of pelvis**    CC HCC

  **C47.6** **Malignant neoplasm of peripheral nerves of trunk, unspecified**    CC HCC

    Malignant neoplasm of peripheral nerves of unspecified part of trunk

  **C47.8** **Malignant neoplasm of overlapping sites of peripheral nerves and autonomic nervous system**    CC HCC

  **C47.9** **Malignant neoplasm of peripheral nerves and nervous autonomic system, unspecified**    CC HCC

    Malignant neoplasm of unspecified site of peripheral nerves and autonomic nervous system

N Newborn: 0    P Pediatric: 0-17    M Maternity: 12-55    A Adult: 15-124    MCC Major CC Condition    PDx MCC PDx acts as own MCC    CC CC Condition    PDx CC PDx acts as own CC

470                          ICD-10-CM 2018

**✓4th C48** **Malignant neoplasm of** retroperitoneum and peritoneum
  EXCLUDES 1 *Kaposi's sarcoma of connective tissue (C46.1)*
       *mesothelioma (C45.-)*

  **CC Excl: For CC codes in category C48, unless otherwise noted:**
  PDX collection 299

  **C48.0** **Malignant neoplasm of** retroperitoneum   CC HCC
        **CC Excl:** PDX collection 308
  **C48.1** **Malignant neoplasm of** specified parts of peritoneum   CC HCC
        Malignant neoplasm of cul-de-sac
        Malignant neoplasm of mesentery
        Malignant neoplasm of mesocolon
        Malignant neoplasm of omentum
        Malignant neoplasm of parietal peritoneum
        Malignant neoplasm of pelvic peritoneum
  **C48.2** **Malignant neoplasm of** peritoneum, unspecified   CC HCC
  **C48.8** **Malignant neoplasm of** overlapping sites of   CC HCC
        retroperitoneum and peritoneum

**✓4th C49** **Malignant neoplasm of** other connective and soft tissue
  INCLUDES   malignant neoplasm of blood vessel
        malignant neoplasm of bursa
        malignant neoplasm of cartilage
        malignant neoplasm of fascia
        malignant neoplasm of fat
        malignant neoplasm of ligament, except uterine
        malignant neoplasm of lymphatic vessel
        malignant neoplasm of muscle
        malignant neoplasm of synovia
        malignant neoplasm of tendon (sheath)
  EXCLUDES 1 *malignant neoplasm of cartilage (of):*
       *articular (C40-C41)    larynx (C32.3)    nose (C30.0)*
       *malignant neoplasm of connective tissue of breast (C50.-)*
  EXCLUDES 2 *Kaposi's sarcoma of soft tissue (C46.1)*
       *malignant neoplasm of heart (C38.0)*
       *malignant neoplasm of peripheral nerves and autonomic*
         *nervous system (C47.-)*
       *malignant neoplasm of peritoneum (C48.2)*
       *malignant neoplasm of retroperitoneum (C48.0)*
       *malignant neoplasm of uterine ligament (C57.3)*
       *mesothelioma (C45.-)*

  **CC Excl: For CC codes in category C49, unless otherwise noted:**
  PDX collection 307

  **C49.0** **Malignant neoplasm of** connective and soft tissue   CC HCC
        of head, face and neck
        Malignant neoplasm of connective tissue of ear
        Malignant neoplasm of connective tissue of eyelid
        EXCLUDES 1   *connective tissue of orbit (C69.6-)*
  **✓5th C49.1** **Malignant neoplasm of** connective and soft tissue of upper
        limb, including shoulder
    **C49.10** **Malignant neoplasm of** connective and soft   CC HCC
          tissue of unspecified upper limb, including
          shoulder
    **C49.11** **Malignant neoplasm of** connective and soft   CC HCC
          tissue of right upper limb, including shoulder
    **C49.12** **Malignant neoplasm of** connective and soft   CC HCC
          tissue of left upper limb, including shoulder
  **✓5th C49.2** **Malignant neoplasm of** connective and soft tissue of lower
        limb, including hip
    **C49.20** **Malignant neoplasm of** connective and soft   CC HCC
          tissue of unspecified lower limb, including hip
    **C49.21** **Malignant neoplasm of** connective and soft   CC HCC
          tissue of right lower limb, including hip
    **C49.22** **Malignant neoplasm of** connective and soft   CC HCC
          tissue of left lower limb, including hip
  **C49.3** **Malignant neoplasm of** connective and soft tissue of   CC HCC
        thorax
        Malignant neoplasm of axilla
        Malignant neoplasm of diaphragm
        Malignant neoplasm of great vessels
        EXCLUDES 1   *malignant neoplasm of breast (C50.-)*
           *malignant neoplasm of heart (C38.0)*
           *malignant neoplasm of mediastinum (C38.1-C38.3)*
           *malignant neoplasm of thymus (C37)*
        **AHA:** 2015, 3Q, 19
  **C49.4** **Malignant neoplasm of** connective and soft tissue of   CC HCC
        abdomen
        Malignant neoplasm of abdominal wall
        Malignant neoplasm of hypochondrium

  **C49.5** **Malignant neoplasm of** connective and soft tissue of   CC HCC
        pelvis
        Malignant neoplasm of buttock
        Malignant neoplasm of groin
        Malignant neoplasm of perineum
  **C49.6** **Malignant neoplasm of** connective and soft tissue of   CC HCC
        trunk, unspecified
        Malignant neoplasm of back NOS
  **C49.8** **Malignant neoplasm of** overlapping sites of   CC HCC
        connective and soft tissue
        Primary malignant neoplasm of two or more contiguous sites of
        connective and soft tissue
  **C49.9** **Malignant neoplasm of** connective and soft tissue,   CC HCC
        unspecified
  **✓5th C49.A** **Gastrointestinal stromal tumor**
    **C49.A0** **Gastrointestinal stromal tumor,**   CC HCC
          **unspecified site**
    **C49.A1** **Gastrointestinal stromal tumor of**   CC HCC
          **esophagus**
    **C49.A2** **Gastrointestinal stromal tumor of** stomach   CC HCC
          **CC Excl:** PDX collection 511
    **C49.A3** **Gastrointestinal stromal tumor of** small   CC HCC
          **intestine**
    **C49.A4** **Gastrointestinal stromal tumor of** large   CC HCC
          **intestine**
    **C49.A5** **Gastrointestinal stromal tumor of** rectum   CC HCC
    **C49.A9** **Gastrointestinal stromal tumor of** other sites   CC HCC

### Malignant neoplasms of breast (C50)

**✓4th C50** **Malignant neoplasm of** breast
  INCLUDES   connective tissue of breast
        Paget's disease of breast
        Paget's disease of nipple
  Use additional code to identify estrogen receptor status (Z17.0, Z17.1)
  EXCLUDES 1 *skin of breast (C44.501, C44.511, C44.521, C44.591)*

  **✓5th C50.0** **Malignant neoplasm of** nipple and areola
    **✓6th C50.01** **Malignant neoplasm of** nipple and areola, female
        **C50.011** **Malignant neoplasm of** nipple and   HCC ♀
              areola, right female breast
        **C50.012** **Malignant neoplasm of** nipple and   HCC ♀
              areola, left female breast
        **C50.019** **Malignant neoplasm of** nipple and   HCC ♀
              areola, unspecified female breast
    **✓6th C50.02** **Malignant neoplasm of** nipple and areola, male
        **C50.021** **Malignant neoplasm of** nipple and   HCC ♂
              areola, right male breast
        **C50.022** **Malignant neoplasm of** nipple and   HCC ♂
              areola, left male breast
        **C50.029** **Malignant neoplasm of** nipple and   HCC ♂
              areola, unspecified male breast
  **✓5th C50.1** **Malignant neoplasm of** central portion of breast
    **✓6th C50.11** **Malignant neoplasm of** central portion of breast,
          female
        **C50.111** **Malignant neoplasm of** central   HCC ♀
              portion of right female breast
        **C50.112** **Malignant neoplasm of** central   HCC ♀
              portion of left female breast
        **C50.119** **Malignant neoplasm of** central   HCC ♀
              portion of unspecified female breast
    **✓6th C50.12** **Malignant neoplasm of** central portion of breast,
          male
        **C50.121** **Malignant neoplasm of** central   HCC ♂
              portion of right male breast
        **C50.122** **Malignant neoplasm of** central   HCC ♂
              portion of left male breast
        **C50.129** **Malignant neoplasm of** central   HCC ♂
              portion of unspecified male breast
  **✓5th C50.2** **Malignant neoplasm of** upper-inner quadrant of breast
    **✓6th C50.21** **Malignant neoplasm of** upper-inner quadrant of
          breast, female
        **C50.211** **Malignant neoplasm of** upper-inner   HCC ♀
              quadrant of right female breast
        **C50.212** **Malignant neoplasm of** upper-inner   HCC ♀
              quadrant of left female breast
        **C50.219** **Malignant neoplasm of** upper-inner   HCC ♀
              quadrant of unspecified female breast

**Female Breast**

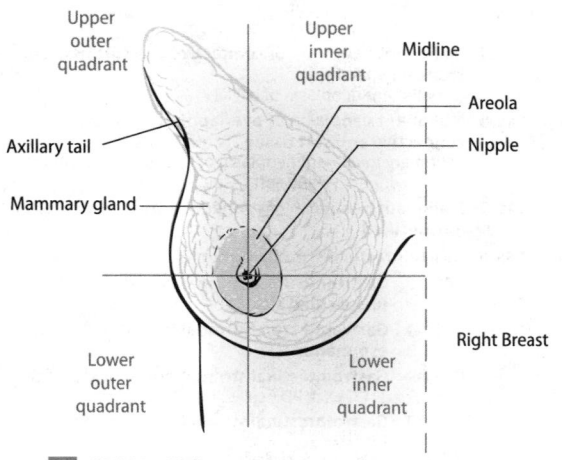

Upper outer quadrant
Upper inner quadrant
Midline
Areola
Nipple
Axillary tail
Mammary gland
Lower outer quadrant
Lower inner quadrant
Right Breast

✓6ᵗʰ **C50.22**   **Malignant neoplasm of upper-inner quadrant of breast,** male
   **C50.221**   Malignant neoplasm of upper-inner ᴴᶜᶜ♂ quadrant of right male breast
   **C50.222**   Malignant neoplasm of upper-inner ᴴᶜᶜ♂ quadrant of left male breast
   **C50.229**   Malignant neoplasm of upper-inner ᴴᶜᶜ♂ quadrant of unspecified male breast

✓5ᵗʰ **C50.3**   **Malignant neoplasm of** lower-inner quadrant **of breast**
   ✓6ᵗʰ **C50.31**   **Malignant neoplasm of lower-inner quadrant of breast,** female
     **C50.311**   Malignant neoplasm of lower-inner ᴴᶜᶜ♀ quadrant of right female breast
     **C50.312**   Malignant neoplasm of lower-inner ᴴᶜᶜ♀ quadrant of left female breast
     **C50.319**   Malignant neoplasm of lower-inner ᴴᶜᶜ♀ quadrant of unspecified female breast
   ✓6ᵗʰ **C50.32**   **Malignant neoplasm of lower-inner quadrant of breast,** male
     **C50.321**   Malignant neoplasm of lower-inner ᴴᶜᶜ♂ quadrant of right male breast
     **C50.322**   Malignant neoplasm of lower-inner ᴴᶜᶜ♂ quadrant of left male breast
     **C50.329**   Malignant neoplasm of lower-inner ᴴᶜᶜ♂ quadrant of unspecified male breast

✓5ᵗʰ **C50.4**   **Malignant neoplasm of** upper-outer quadrant **of breast**
   ✓6ᵗʰ **C50.41**   **Malignant neoplasm of upper-outer quadrant of breast,** female
     **C50.411**   Malignant neoplasm of upper-outer ᴴᶜᶜ♀ quadrant of right female breast
     **C50.412**   Malignant neoplasm of upper-outer ᴴᶜᶜ♀ quadrant of left female breast
     **C50.419**   Malignant neoplasm of upper-outer ᴴᶜᶜ♀ quadrant of unspecified female breast
   ✓6ᵗʰ **C50.42**   **Malignant neoplasm of upper-outer quadrant of breast,** male
     **C50.421**   Malignant neoplasm of upper-outer ᴴᶜᶜ♂ quadrant of right male breast
     **C50.422**   Malignant neoplasm of upper-outer ᴴᶜᶜ♂ quadrant of left male breast
     **C50.429**   Malignant neoplasm of upper-outer ᴴᶜᶜ♂ quadrant of unspecified male breast

✓5ᵗʰ **C50.5**   **Malignant neoplasm of** lower-outer quadrant **of breast**
   ✓6ᵗʰ **C50.51**   **Malignant neoplasm of lower-outer quadrant of breast,** female
     **C50.511**   Malignant neoplasm of lower-outer ᴴᶜᶜ♀ quadrant of right female breast
     **C50.512**   Malignant neoplasm of lower-outer ᴴᶜᶜ♀ quadrant of left female breast
     **C50.519**   Malignant neoplasm of lower-outer ᴴᶜᶜ♀ quadrant of unspecified female breast
   ✓6ᵗʰ **C50.52**   **Malignant neoplasm of lower-outer quadrant of breast,** male
     **C50.521**   Malignant neoplasm of lower-outer ᴴᶜᶜ♂ quadrant of right male breast

     **C50.522**   Malignant neoplasm of lower-outer ᴴᶜᶜ♂ quadrant of left male breast
     **C50.529**   Malignant neoplasm of lower-outer ᴴᶜᶜ♂ quadrant of unspecified male breast

✓5ᵗʰ **C50.6**   **Malignant neoplasm of** axillary tail **of breast**
   ✓6ᵗʰ **C50.61**   **Malignant neoplasm of axillary tail of breast,** female
     **C50.611**   Malignant neoplasm of axillary tail ᴴᶜᶜ♀ of right female breast
     **C50.612**   Malignant neoplasm of axillary tail ᴴᶜᶜ♀ of left female breast
     **C50.619**   Malignant neoplasm of axillary tail ᴴᶜᶜ♀ of unspecified female breast
   ✓6ᵗʰ **C50.62**   **Malignant neoplasm of axillary tail of breast,** male
     **C50.621**   Malignant neoplasm of axillary tail ᴴᶜᶜ♂ of right male breast
     **C50.622**   Malignant neoplasm of axillary tail ᴴᶜᶜ♂ of left male breast
     **C50.629**   Malignant neoplasm of axillary tail ᴴᶜᶜ♂ of unspecified male breast

✓5ᵗʰ **C50.8**   **Malignant neoplasm of** overlapping sites **of breast**
   ✓6ᵗʰ **C50.81**   **Malignant neoplasm of overlapping sites of breast,** female
     **C50.811**   Malignant neoplasm of overlapping ᴴᶜᶜ♀ sites of right female breast
     **C50.812**   Malignant neoplasm of overlapping ᴴᶜᶜ♀ sites of left female breast
     **C50.819**   Malignant neoplasm of overlapping ᴴᶜᶜ♀ sites of unspecified female breast
   ✓6ᵗʰ **C50.82**   **Malignant neoplasm of overlapping sites of breast,** male
     **C50.821**   Malignant neoplasm of overlapping ᴴᶜᶜ♂ sites of right male breast
     **C50.822**   Malignant neoplasm of overlapping ᴴᶜᶜ♂ sites of left male breast
     **C50.829**   Malignant neoplasm of overlapping ᴴᶜᶜ♂ sites of unspecified male breast

✓5ᵗʰ **C50.9**   **Malignant neoplasm of breast of** unspecified site
   ✓6ᵗʰ **C50.91**   **Malignant neoplasm of breast of unspecified site,** female
     **C50.911**   Malignant neoplasm of unspecified ᴴᶜᶜ♀ site of right female breast
     **C50.912**   Malignant neoplasm of unspecified ᴴᶜᶜ♀ site of left female breast
     **C50.919**   Malignant neoplasm of unspecified ᴴᶜᶜ♀ site of unspecified female breast
   ✓6ᵗʰ **C50.92**   **Malignant neoplasm of breast of unspecified site,** male
     **C50.921**   Malignant neoplasm of unspecified ᴴᶜᶜ♂ site of right male breast
     **C50.922**   Malignant neoplasm of unspecified ᴴᶜᶜ♂ site of left male breast
     **C50.929**   Malignant neoplasm of unspecified ᴴᶜᶜ♂ site of unspecified male breast

## Malignant neoplasms of female genital organs (C51-C58)

**INCLUDES**   malignant neoplasm of skin of female genital organs

✓4ᵗʰ **C51**   **Malignant neoplasm of** vulva
   **EXCLUDES 1**   carcinoma in situ of vulva (D07.1)
   **C51.0**   **Malignant neoplasm of** labium majus    ᴴᶜᶜ♀
     Malignant neoplasm of Bartholin's [greater vestibular] gland
   **C51.1**   **Malignant neoplasm of** labium minus    ᴴᶜᶜ♀
   **C51.2**   **Malignant neoplasm of** clitoris    ᴴᶜᶜ♀
   **C51.8**   **Malignant neoplasm of** overlapping sites **of vulva**    ᴴᶜᶜ♀
   **C51.9**   **Malignant neoplasm of vulva,** unspecified    ᴴᶜᶜ♀
     Malignant neoplasm of external female genitalia NOS
     Malignant neoplasm of pudendum

**C52**   **Malignant neoplasm of** vagina    ᴴᶜᶜ♀
   **EXCLUDES 1**   carcinoma in situ of vagina (D07.2)

✓4ᵗʰ **C53**   **Malignant neoplasm of** cervix uteri
   **EXCLUDES 1**   carcinoma in situ of cervix uteri (D06.-)
   **C53.0**   **Malignant neoplasm of** endocervix    ᴴᶜᶜ♀
   **C53.1**   **Malignant neoplasm of** exocervix    ᴴᶜᶜ♀
   **C53.8**   **Malignant neoplasm of** overlapping sites **of cervix uteri**    ᴴᶜᶜ♀
   **C53.9**   **Malignant neoplasm of cervix uteri,** unspecified    ᴴᶜᶜ♀

Ⓝ Newborn: 0   Ⓟ Pediatric: 0-17   Ⓜ Maternity: 12-55   Ⓐ Adult: 15-124   **MCC** Major CC Condition   **PDx MCC** PDx acts as own MCC   **CC** CC Condition   **PDx CC** PDx acts as own CC

**472**          ICD-10-CM 2018

**✓4ᵗʰ C54**   **Malignant neoplasm of corpus uteri**

     **C54.0**   **Malignant neoplasm of isthmus uteri**   HCC ♀
         Malignant neoplasm of lower uterine segment

     **C54.1**   **Malignant neoplasm of endometrium**   HCC ♀

     **C54.2**   **Malignant neoplasm of myometrium**   HCC ♀

     **C54.3**   **Malignant neoplasm of fundus uteri**   HCC ♀

     **C54.8**   **Malignant neoplasm of overlapping sites of corpus uteri**   HCC ♀

     **C54.9**   **Malignant neoplasm of corpus uteri, unspecified**   HCC ♀

**C55**   **Malignant neoplasm of uterus, part unspecified**   HCC ♀

**✓4ᵗʰ C56**   **Malignant neoplasm of ovary**
     Use additional code to identify any functional activity

     **CC Excl: For CC codes in category C56:** PDX collection 309

     **C56.1**   **Malignant neoplasm of right ovary**   CC HCC ♀

     **C56.2**   **Malignant neoplasm of left ovary**   CC HCC ♀

     **C56.9**   **Malignant neoplasm of unspecified ovary**   CC HCC ♀

**✓4ᵗʰ C57**   **Malignant neoplasm of other and unspecified female genital organs**

     **✓5ᵗʰ C57.0**   **Malignant neoplasm of fallopian tube**
         Malignant neoplasm of oviduct
         Malignant neoplasm of uterine tube

         **C57.00**   **Malignant neoplasm of unspecified fallopian tube**   HCC ♀

         **C57.01**   **Malignant neoplasm of right fallopian tube**   HCC ♀

         **C57.02**   **Malignant neoplasm of left fallopian tube**   HCC ♀

     **✓5ᵗʰ C57.1**   **Malignant neoplasm of broad ligament**

         **C57.10**   **Malignant neoplasm of unspecified broad ligament**   HCC ♀

         **C57.11**   **Malignant neoplasm of right broad ligament**   HCC ♀

         **C57.12**   **Malignant neoplasm of left broad ligament**   HCC ♀

     **✓5ᵗʰ C57.2**   **Malignant neoplasm of round ligament**

         **C57.20**   **Malignant neoplasm of unspecified round ligament**   HCC ♀

         **C57.21**   **Malignant neoplasm of right round ligament**   HCC ♀

         **C57.22**   **Malignant neoplasm of left round ligament**   HCC ♀

     **C57.3**   **Malignant neoplasm of parametrium**   HCC ♀
         Malignant neoplasm of uterine ligament NOS

     **C57.4**   **Malignant neoplasm of uterine adnexa, unspecified**   HCC ♀

     **C57.7**   **Malignant neoplasm of other specified female genital organs**   HCC ♀
         Malignant neoplasm of wolffian body or duct

     **C57.8**   **Malignant neoplasm of overlapping sites of female genital organs**   HCC ♀
         Primary malignant neoplasm of two or more contiguous sites of the female genital organs whose point of origin cannot be determined
         Primary tubo-ovarian malignant neoplasm whose point of origin cannot be determined
         Primary utero-ovarian malignant neoplasm whose point of origin cannot be determined

     **C57.9**   **Malignant neoplasm of female genital organ, unspecified**   HCC ♀
         Malignant neoplasm of female genitourinary tract NOS

**C58**   **Malignant neoplasm of placenta**   HCC M ♀
     **INCLUDES**   choriocarcinoma NOS
                chorionepithelioma NOS
     **EXCLUDES 1**   *chorioadenoma (destruens) (D39.2)*
                *hydatidiform mole NOS (O01.9)*
                *invasive hydatidiform mole (D39.2)*
                *male choriocarcinoma NOS (C62.9-)*
                *malignant hydatidiform mole (D39.2)*

### Malignant neoplasms of male genital organs (C60-C63)
     **INCLUDES**   malignant neoplasm of skin of male genital organs

**✓4ᵗʰ C60**   **Malignant neoplasm of penis**

     **C60.0**   **Malignant neoplasm of prepuce**   HCC ♂
         Malignant neoplasm of foreskin

     **C60.1**   **Malignant neoplasm of glans penis**   HCC ♂

     **C60.2**   **Malignant neoplasm of body of penis**   HCC ♂
         Malignant neoplasm of corpus cavernosum

     **C60.8**   **Malignant neoplasm of overlapping sites of penis**   HCC ♂

     **C60.9**   **Malignant neoplasm of penis, unspecified**   HCC ♂
         Malignant neoplasm of skin of penis NOS

**C61**   **Malignant neoplasm of prostate**   HCC ♂
     Use additional code to identify:
         hormone sensitivity status (Z19.1-Z19.2)
         rising PSA following treatment for malignant neoplasm of prostate (R97.21)
     **EXCLUDES 1**   *malignant neoplasm of seminal vesicle (C63.7)*
     **AHA:** 2017, 1Q, 17

**✓4ᵗʰ C62**   **Malignant neoplasm of testis**
     Use additional code to identify any functional activity

     **✓5ᵗʰ C62.0**   **Malignant neoplasm of undescended testis**
         Malignant neoplasm of ectopic testis
         Malignant neoplasm of retained testis

         **C62.00**   **Malignant neoplasm of unspecified undescended testis**   HCC ♂

         **C62.01**   **Malignant neoplasm of undescended right testis**   HCC ♂

         **C62.02**   **Malignant neoplasm of undescended left testis**   HCC ♂

     **✓5ᵗʰ C62.1**   **Malignant neoplasm of descended testis**
         Malignant neoplasm of scrotal testis

         **C62.10**   **Malignant neoplasm of unspecified descended testis**   HCC ♂

         **C62.11**   **Malignant neoplasm of descended right testis**   HCC ♂

         **C62.12**   **Malignant neoplasm of descended left testis**   HCC ♂

     **✓5ᵗʰ C62.9**   **Malignant neoplasm of testis, unspecified whether descended or undescended**

         **C62.90**   **Malignant neoplasm of unspecified testis, unspecified whether descended or undescended**   HCC ♂
                Malignant neoplasm of testis NOS

         **C62.91**   **Malignant neoplasm of right testis, unspecified whether descended or undescended**   HCC ♂

         **C62.92**   **Malignant neoplasm of left testis, unspecified whether descended or undescended**   HCC ♂

**✓4ᵗʰ C63**   **Malignant neoplasm of other and unspecified male genital organs**

     **✓5ᵗʰ C63.0**   **Malignant neoplasm of epididymis**

         **C63.00**   **Malignant neoplasm of unspecified epididymis**   HCC ♂

         **C63.01**   **Malignant neoplasm of right epididymis**   HCC ♂

         **C63.02**   **Malignant neoplasm of left epididymis**   HCC ♂

     **✓5ᵗʰ C63.1**   **Malignant neoplasm of spermatic cord**

         **C63.10**   **Malignant neoplasm of unspecified spermatic cord**   HCC ♂

         **C63.11**   **Malignant neoplasm of right spermatic cord**   HCC ♂

         **C63.12**   **Malignant neoplasm of left spermatic cord**   HCC ♂

     **C63.2**   **Malignant neoplasm of scrotum**   HCC ♂
         Malignant neoplasm of skin of scrotum

     **C63.7**   **Malignant neoplasm of other specified male genital organs**   HCC ♂
         Malignant neoplasm of seminal vesicle
         Malignant neoplasm of tunica vaginalis

     **C63.8**   **Malignant neoplasm of overlapping sites of male genital organs**   HCC ♂
         Primary malignant neoplasm of two or more contiguous sites of male genital organs whose point of origin cannot be determined

     **C63.9**   **Malignant neoplasm of male genital organ, unspecified**   HCC ♂
         Malignant neoplasm of male genitourinary tract NOS

### Malignant neoplasms of urinary tract (C64-C68)

**✓4ᵗʰ C64**   **Malignant neoplasm of kidney, except renal pelvis**
     **EXCLUDES 1**   *malignant carcinoid tumor of the kidney (C7A.093)*
                *malignant neoplasm of renal calyces (C65.-)*
                *malignant neoplasm of renal pelvis (C65.-)*

     **CC Excl: For CC codes in category C64:** PDX collection 310

     **C64.1**   **Malignant neoplasm of right kidney, except renal pelvis**   HCC CC

     **C64.2**   **Malignant neoplasm of left kidney, except renal pelvis**   HCC CC

     **C64.9**   **Malignant neoplasm of unspecified kidney, except renal pelvis**   HCC CC

✓ Additional Character Req   ✓x7ᵗʰ Placeholder Alert   Unacceptable PDx   Manifestation   H1-H14 HAC   HCC CMS-HCC Condition   EXCLUDES 1 Not Coded Here   EXCLUDES 2 Not Included Here

ICD-10-CM 2018          **473**

C54–C64.9

**Chapter 2. Neoplasms**

**C65–C71.9**

✓4ᵗʰ **C65 Malignant neoplasm of renal pelvis**
      INCLUDES   malignant neoplasm of pelviureteric junction
                  malignant neoplasm of renal calyces

      CC Excl: For CC codes in category C65: PDX collection 310

      **C65.1 Malignant neoplasm of right renal pelvis** CC HCC
      **C65.2 Malignant neoplasm of left renal pelvis** CC HCC
      **C65.9 Malignant neoplasm of unspecified renal pelvis** CC HCC

✓4ᵗʰ **C66 Malignant neoplasm of ureter**
      EXCLUDES 1   malignant neoplasm of ureteric orifice of bladder (C67.6)

      CC Excl: For CC codes in category C66: PDX collection 311

      **C66.1 Malignant neoplasm of right ureter** CC HCC
      **C66.2 Malignant neoplasm of left ureter** CC HCC
      **C66.9 Malignant neoplasm of unspecified ureter** CC HCC

✓4ᵗʰ **C67 Malignant neoplasm of bladder**
      **C67.0 Malignant neoplasm of trigone of bladder** HCC
      **C67.1 Malignant neoplasm of dome of bladder** HCC
      **C67.2 Malignant neoplasm of lateral wall of bladder** HCC
      **C67.3 Malignant neoplasm of anterior wall of bladder** HCC
      **C67.4 Malignant neoplasm of posterior wall of bladder** HCC
      **C67.5 Malignant neoplasm of bladder neck** HCC
           Malignant neoplasm of internal urethral orifice
      **C67.6 Malignant neoplasm of ureteric orifice** HCC
      **C67.7 Malignant neoplasm of urachus** HCC
      **C67.8 Malignant neoplasm of overlapping sites of bladder** HCC
      **C67.9 Malignant neoplasm of bladder, unspecified** HCC
           **AHA:** 2016, 1Q, 19

✓4ᵗʰ **C68 Malignant neoplasm of other and unspecified urinary organs**
      EXCLUDES 1   malignant neoplasm of female genitourinary tract NOS (C57.9)
                  malignant neoplasm of male genitourinary tract NOS (C63.9)

      **C68.0 Malignant neoplasm of urethra** CC HCC
           EXCLUDES 1   malignant neoplasm of urethral orifice of bladder
                       (C67.5)
           CC Excl: PDX collection 312
      **C68.1 Malignant neoplasm of paraurethral glands** CC HCC
           CC Excl: PDX collection 312
      **C68.8 Malignant neoplasm of overlapping sites of urinary organs** CC HCC
           Primary malignant neoplasm of two or more contiguous sites of
             urinary organs whose point of origin cannot be determined
           CC Excl: PDX collection 313
      **C68.9 Malignant neoplasm of urinary organ, unspecified** CC HCC
           Malignant neoplasm of urinary system NOS
           CC Excl: PDX collection 313

### Malignant neoplasms of eye, brain and other parts of central nervous system (C69-C72)

✓4ᵗʰ **C69 Malignant neoplasm of eye and adnexa**
      EXCLUDES 1   malignant neoplasm of connective tissue of eyelid (C49.0)
                  malignant neoplasm of eyelid (skin) (C43.1-, C44.1-)
                  malignant neoplasm of optic nerve (C72.3-)

 ✓5ᵗʰ **C69.0 Malignant neoplasm of conjunctiva**
           **C69.00 Malignant neoplasm of unspecified conjunctiva** HCC
           **C69.01 Malignant neoplasm of right conjunctiva** HCC
           **C69.02 Malignant neoplasm of left conjunctiva** HCC
 ✓5ᵗʰ **C69.1 Malignant neoplasm of cornea**
           **C69.10 Malignant neoplasm of unspecified cornea** HCC
           **C69.11 Malignant neoplasm of right cornea** HCC
           **C69.12 Malignant neoplasm of left cornea** HCC
 ✓5ᵗʰ **C69.2 Malignant neoplasm of retina**
           EXCLUDES 1   dark area on retina (D49.81)
                     neoplasm of unspecified behavior of retina and
                         choroid (D49.81)
                     retinal freckle (D49.81)
           **C69.20 Malignant neoplasm of unspecified retina** HCC
           **C69.21 Malignant neoplasm of right retina** HCC
           **C69.22 Malignant neoplasm of left retina** HCC
 ✓5ᵗʰ **C69.3 Malignant neoplasm of choroid**
           **C69.30 Malignant neoplasm of unspecified choroid** HCC
           **C69.31 Malignant neoplasm of right choroid** HCC
           **C69.32 Malignant neoplasm of left choroid** HCC

✓5ᵗʰ **C69.4 Malignant neoplasm of ciliary body**
      **C69.40 Malignant neoplasm of unspecified ciliary body** HCC
      **C69.41 Malignant neoplasm of right ciliary body** HCC
      **C69.42 Malignant neoplasm of left ciliary body** HCC

✓5ᵗʰ **C69.5 Malignant neoplasm of lacrimal gland and duct**
      Malignant neoplasm of lacrimal sac
      Malignant neoplasm of nasolacrimal duct
      **C69.50 Malignant neoplasm of unspecified lacrimal gland and duct** HCC
      **C69.51 Malignant neoplasm of right lacrimal gland and duct** HCC
      **C69.52 Malignant neoplasm of left lacrimal gland and duct** HCC

✓5ᵗʰ **C69.6 Malignant neoplasm of orbit**
      Malignant neoplasm of connective tissue of orbit
      Malignant neoplasm of extraocular muscle
      Malignant neoplasm of peripheral nerves of orbit
      Malignant neoplasm of retrobulbar tissue
      Malignant neoplasm of retro-ocular tissue
      EXCLUDES 1   malignant neoplasm of orbital bone (C41.0)
      **C69.60 Malignant neoplasm of unspecified orbit** HCC
      **C69.61 Malignant neoplasm of right orbit** HCC
      **C69.62 Malignant neoplasm of left orbit** HCC

✓5ᵗʰ **C69.8 Malignant neoplasm of overlapping sites of eye and adnexa**
      **C69.80 Malignant neoplasm of overlapping sites of unspecified eye and adnexa** HCC
      **C69.81 Malignant neoplasm of overlapping sites of right eye and adnexa** HCC
      **C69.82 Malignant neoplasm of overlapping sites of left eye and adnexa** HCC

✓5ᵗʰ **C69.9 Malignant neoplasm of unspecified site of eye**
      Malignant neoplasm of eyeball
      **C69.90 Malignant neoplasm of unspecified site of unspecified eye** HCC
      **C69.91 Malignant neoplasm of unspecified site of right eye** HCC
      **C69.92 Malignant neoplasm of unspecified site of left eye** HCC

✓4ᵗʰ **C70 Malignant neoplasm of meninges**
      **C70.0 Malignant neoplasm of cerebral meninges** CC HCC
           CC Excl: PDX collection 314
      **C70.1 Malignant neoplasm of spinal meninges** CC HCC
           CC Excl: PDX collection 315
      **C70.9 Malignant neoplasm of meninges, unspecified** CC HCC
           CC Excl: PDX collection 314

✓4ᵗʰ **C71 Malignant neoplasm of brain**
      EXCLUDES 1   malignant neoplasm of cranial nerves (C72.2-C72.5)
                  retrobulbar malignant neoplasm (C69.6-)

      CC Excl: For CC codes in category C71: PDX collection 316

      **C71.0 Malignant neoplasm of cerebrum, except lobes and ventricles** CC HCC
           Malignant neoplasm of supratentorial NOS
      **C71.1 Malignant neoplasm of frontal lobe** CC HCC
      **C71.2 Malignant neoplasm of temporal lobe** CC HCC
      **C71.3 Malignant neoplasm of parietal lobe** CC HCC
      **C71.4 Malignant neoplasm of occipital lobe** CC HCC
      **C71.5 Malignant neoplasm of cerebral ventricle** CC HCC
           EXCLUDES 1   malignant neoplasm of fourth cerebral ventricle
                       (C71.7)
      **C71.6 Malignant neoplasm of cerebellum** CC HCC
      **C71.7 Malignant neoplasm of brain stem** CC HCC
           Malignant neoplasm of fourth cerebral ventricle
           Infratentorial malignant neoplasm NOS
      **C71.8 Malignant neoplasm of overlapping sites of brain** CC HCC
      **C71.9 Malignant neoplasm of brain, unspecified** CC HCC
           **AHA:** 2014, 3Q, 3

N Newborn: 0   P Pediatric: 0-17   M Maternity: 12-55   A Adult: 15-124   MCC Major CC Condition   PDxMCC PDx acts as own MCC   CC CC Condition   PDxCC PDx acts as own CC

**474**                                                                           ICD-10-CM 2018

**Lobes of the Brain**

Frontal lobe
Parietal lobe
Occipital lobe
Temporal lobe
Brain stem
Cerebellum

✓4ᵗʰ **C72** **Malignant neoplasm of** spinal cord, cranial nerves and other parts of central nervous system

> EXCLUDES 1   *malignant neoplasm of meninges (C70.-)*
> *malignant neoplasm of peripheral nerves and autonomic nervous system (C47.-)*

**CC Excl: For CC codes in category C72, unless otherwise noted:** PDX collection 318

**C72.0** **Malignant neoplasm of** spinal cord   CC HCC
    CC Excl: PDX collection 317

**C72.1** **Malignant neoplasm of** cauda equina   CC HCC
    CC Excl: PDX collection 317

✓5ᵗʰ **C72.2** **Malignant neoplasm of** olfactory nerve
    Malignant neoplasm of olfactory bulb

    **C72.20** **Malignant neoplasm of** unspecified olfactory nerve   CC HCC

    **C72.21** **Malignant neoplasm of** right olfactory nerve   CC HCC

    **C72.22** **Malignant neoplasm of** left olfactory nerve   CC HCC

✓5ᵗʰ **C72.3** **Malignant neoplasm of** optic nerve

    **C72.30** **Malignant neoplasm of** unspecified optic nerve   CC HCC

    **C72.31** **Malignant neoplasm of** right optic nerve   CC HCC

    **C72.32** **Malignant neoplasm of** left optic nerve   CC HCC

✓5ᵗʰ **C72.4** **Malignant neoplasm of** acoustic nerve

    **C72.40** **Malignant neoplasm of** unspecified acoustic nerve   CC HCC

    **C72.41** **Malignant neoplasm of** right acoustic nerve   CC HCC

    **C72.42** **Malignant neoplasm of** left acoustic nerve   CC HCC

✓5ᵗʰ **C72.5** **Malignant neoplasm of** other and unspecified cranial nerves

    **C72.50** **Malignant neoplasm of** unspecified cranial nerve   CC HCC
       Malignant neoplasm of cranial nerve NOS

    **C72.59** **Malignant neoplasm of** other cranial nerves   CC HCC

**C72.9** **Malignant neoplasm of** central nervous system, unspecified   CC HCC
    Malignant neoplasm of unspecified site of central nervous system
    Malignant neoplasm of nervous system NOS
    **CC Excl:** PDX collection 319

### Malignant neoplasms of thyroid and other endocrine glands (C73-C75)

**C73** **Malignant neoplasm of** thyroid gland   HCC
    Use additional code to identify any functional activity

✓4ᵗʰ **C74** **Malignant neoplasm of** adrenal gland

**CC Excl: For CC codes in category C74:** PDX collection 320

✓5ᵗʰ **C74.0** **Malignant neoplasm of** cortex of adrenal gland

    **C74.00** **Malignant neoplasm of** cortex of unspecified adrenal gland   CC HCC

    **C74.01** **Malignant neoplasm of** cortex of right adrenal gland   CC HCC

    **C74.02** **Malignant neoplasm of** cortex of left adrenal gland   CC HCC

✓5ᵗʰ **C74.1** **Malignant neoplasm of** medulla of adrenal gland

    **C74.10** **Malignant neoplasm of** medulla of unspecified adrenal gland   CC HCC

    **C74.11** **Malignant neoplasm of** medulla of right adrenal gland   CC HCC

    **C74.12** **Malignant neoplasm of** medulla of left adrenal gland   CC HCC

✓5ᵗʰ **C74.9** **Malignant neoplasm of** unspecified part of adrenal gland

    **C74.90** **Malignant neoplasm of** unspecified part of unspecified adrenal gland   CC HCC

    **C74.91** **Malignant neoplasm of** unspecified part of right adrenal gland   CC HCC

    **C74.92** **Malignant neoplasm of** unspecified part of left adrenal gland   CC HCC

✓4ᵗʰ **C75** **Malignant neoplasm of** other endocrine glands and related structures

> EXCLUDES 1   *malignant carcinoid tumors (C7A.0-)*
> *malignant neoplasm of adrenal gland (C74.-)*
> *malignant neoplasm of endocrine pancreas (C25.4)*
> *malignant neoplasm of islets of Langerhans (C25.4)*
> *malignant neoplasm of ovary (C56.-)*
> *malignant neoplasm of testis (C62.-)*
> *malignant neoplasm of thymus (C37)*
> *malignant neoplasm of thyroid gland (C73)*
> *malignant neuroendocrine tumors (C7A.-)*

**C75.0** **Malignant neoplasm of** parathyroid gland   CC HCC
    **CC Excl:** PDX collection 321

**C75.1** **Malignant neoplasm of** pituitary gland   CC HCC
    **CC Excl:** PDX collection 322

**C75.2** **Malignant neoplasm of** craniopharyngeal duct   CC HCC
    **CC Excl:** PDX collection 322

**C75.3** **Malignant neoplasm of** pineal gland   CC HCC
    **CC Excl:** PDX collection 323

**C75.4** **Malignant neoplasm of** carotid body   CC HCC
    **CC Excl:** PDX collection 324

**C75.5** **Malignant neoplasm of** aortic body and other paraganglia   CC HCC
    **CC Excl:** PDX collection 325

**C75.8** **Malignant neoplasm with** pluriglandular involvement, unspecified   CC HCC
    **CC Excl:** PDX collection 326

**C75.9** **Malignant neoplasm of** endocrine gland, unspecified   CC HCC
    **CC Excl:** PDX collection 326

### Malignant neuroendocrine tumors (C7A)

✓4ᵗʰ **C7A** **Malignant** neuroendocrine tumors
    Code also any associated multiple endocrine neoplasia [MEN] syndromes (E31.2-)
    Use additional code to identify any associated endocrine syndrome, such as:
       carcinoid syndrome (E34.0)

> EXCLUDES 2   *malignant pancreatic islet cell tumors (C25.4)*
> *Merkel cell carcinoma (C4A.-)*

✓5ᵗʰ **C7A.0** **Malignant** carcinoid tumors

    **C7A.00** **Malignant carcinoid tumor of** unspecified site   CC HCC
       **CC Excl:** PDX collection 346

    ✓6ᵗʰ **C7A.01** **Malignant carcinoid tumors of the** small intestine

       **C7A.010** **Malignant carcinoid tumor of the** duodenum   CC HCC
         **CC Excl:** PDX collection 347

       **C7A.011** **Malignant carcinoid tumor of the** jejunum   CC HCC
         **CC Excl:** PDX collection 348

       **C7A.012** **Malignant carcinoid tumor of the** ileum   CC HCC
         **CC Excl:** PDX collection 349

       **C7A.019** **Malignant carcinoid tumor of the** small intestine, unspecified portion   CC HCC
         **CC Excl:** PDX collection 350

    ✓6ᵗʰ **C7A.02** **Malignant carcinoid tumors of the** appendix, large intestine, and rectum

       **C7A.020** **Malignant carcinoid tumor of the** appendix   CC HCC
         **CC Excl:** PDX collection 351

       **C7A.021** **Malignant carcinoid tumor of the** cecum   CC HCC
         **CC Excl:** PDX collection 352

**C7A.Ø22** **Malignant carcinoid tumor of the ascending colon** `CC` `HCC`
    **CC Excl:** PDX collection 353

**C7A.Ø23** **Malignant carcinoid tumor of the transverse colon** `CC` `HCC`
    **CC Excl:** PDX collection 354

**C7A.Ø24** **Malignant carcinoid tumor of the descending colon** `CC` `HCC`
    **CC Excl:** PDX collection 355

**C7A.Ø25** **Malignant carcinoid tumor of the sigmoid colon** `CC` `HCC`
    **CC Excl:** PDX collection 356

**C7A.Ø26** **Malignant carcinoid tumor of the rectum** `CC` `HCC`
    **CC Excl:** PDX collection 357

**C7A.Ø29** **Malignant carcinoid tumor of the large, intestine, unspecified portion** `CC` `HCC`
    Malignant carcinoid tumor of the colon NOS
    **CC Excl:** PDX collection 358

✓6ᵗʰ **C7A.Ø9** **Malignant carcinoid tumors of** other sites

**C7A.Ø9Ø** **Malignant carcinoid tumor of the bronchus and lung** `CC` `HCC`
    **CC Excl:** PDX collection 359

**C7A.Ø91** **Malignant carcinoid tumor of the thymus** `CC` `HCC`
    **CC Excl:** PDX collection 360

**C7A.Ø92** **Malignant carcinoid tumor of the stomach** `CC` `HCC`
    **CC Excl:** PDX collection 361

**C7A.Ø93** **Malignant carcinoid tumor of the kidney** `CC` `HCC`
    **CC Excl:** PDX collection 362

**C7A.Ø94** **Malignant carcinoid tumor of the foregut, unspecified** `CC` `HCC`
    **CC Excl:** PDX collection 361

**C7A.Ø95** **Malignant carcinoid tumor of the midgut, unspecified** `CC` `HCC`
    **CC Excl:** PDX collection 361

**C7A.Ø96** **Malignant carcinoid tumor of the hindgut, unspecified** `CC` `HCC`
    **CC Excl:** PDX collection 361

**C7A.Ø98** **Malignant carcinoid tumors of other sites** `CC` `HCC`
    **CC Excl:** PDX collection 346

**C7A.1** **Malignant** poorly differentiated **neuroendocrine tumors** `CC` `HCC`
    High grade neuroendocrine carcinoma, any site
    Malignant poorly differentiated neuroendocrine tumor NOS
    Malignant poorly differentiated neuroendocrine carcinoma, any site
    **CC Excl:** PDX collection 346

**C7A.8** **Other** malignant neuroendocrine tumors `CC` `HCC`
    **CC Excl:** PDX collection 346

### Secondary neuroendocrine tumors (C7B)

✓4ᵗʰ **C7B** **Secondary** neuroendocrine tumors
Use additional code to identify any functional activity

✓5ᵗʰ **C7B.Ø** **Secondary** carcinoid tumors

**C7B.ØØ** **Secondary carcinoid tumors, unspecified** site `HCC`

**C7B.Ø1** **Secondary carcinoid tumors of distant lymph nodes** `CC` `HCC`
    **CC Excl:** PDX collection 363

**C7B.Ø2** **Secondary carcinoid tumors of liver** `CC` `HCC`
    **CC Excl:** PDX collection 364

**C7B.Ø3** **Secondary carcinoid tumors of bone** `CC` `HCC`
    **CC Excl:** PDX collection 365

**C7B.Ø4** **Secondary carcinoid tumors of peritoneum** `CC` `HCC`
    Mesentery metastasis of carcinoid tumor
    **CC Excl:** CPDX collection 366

**C7B.Ø9** **Secondary carcinoid tumors of** other sites `CC` `HCC`
    **CC Excl:** PDX collection 367

**C7B.1** **Secondary** Merkel cell carcinoma `HCC`
    Merkel cell carcinoma nodal presentation
    Merkel cell carcinoma visceral metastatic presentation

**C7B.8** **Other** secondary neuroendocrine tumors `CC` `HCC`
    **CC Excl:** PDX collection 367

### Malignant neoplasms of ill-defined, other secondary and unspecified sites (C76-C8Ø)

✓4ᵗʰ **C76** **Malignant neoplasm of** other and ill-defined sites
    **EXCLUDES 1**   *malignant neoplasm of female genitourinary tract NOS (C57.9)*
        *malignant neoplasm of male genitourinary tract NOS (C63.9)*
        *malignant neoplasm of lymphoid, hematopoietic and related tissue (C81-C96)*
        *malignant neoplasm of skin (C44.-)*
        *malignant neoplasm of unspecified site NOS (C80.1)*

**C76.Ø** **Malignant neoplasm of** head, face and neck `HCC`
    Malignant neoplasm of cheek NOS
    Malignant neoplasm of nose NOS

**C76.1** **Malignant neoplasm of** thorax `HCC`
    Intrathoracic malignant neoplasm NOS
    Malignant neoplasm of axilla NOS
    Thoracic malignant neoplasm NOS

**C76.2** **Malignant neoplasm of** abdomen `HCC`

**C76.3** **Malignant neoplasm of** pelvis `HCC`
    Malignant neoplasm of groin NOS
    Malignant neoplasm of sites overlapping systems within the pelvis
    Rectovaginal (septum) malignant neoplasm
    Rectovesical (septum) malignant neoplasm

✓5ᵗʰ **C76.4** **Malignant neoplasm of** upper limb

**C76.4Ø** **Malignant neoplasm of** unspecified **upper limb** `HCC`

**C76.41** **Malignant neoplasm of** right **upper limb** `HCC`

**C76.42** **Malignant neoplasm of** left **upper limb** `HCC`

✓5ᵗʰ **C76.5** **Malignant neoplasm of** lower limb

**C76.5Ø** **Malignant neoplasm of** unspecified **lower limb** `HCC`

**C76.51** **Malignant neoplasm of** right **lower limb** `HCC`

**C76.52** **Malignant neoplasm of** left **lower limb** `HCC`

**C76.8** **Malignant neoplasm of** other specified ill-defined sites
    Malignant neoplasm of overlapping ill-defined sites

✓4ᵗʰ **C77** **Secondary and unspecified** malignant neoplasm of lymph nodes
    **EXCLUDES 1**   *malignant neoplasm of lymph nodes, specified as primary (C81-C86, C88, C96.-)*
        *mesentery metastasis of carcinoid tumor (C7B.Ø4)*
        *secondary carcinoid tumors of distant lymph nodes (C7B.Ø1)*

**CC Excl: For CC codes in category C77:** PDX collection 3Ø3

**C77.Ø** **Secondary and unspecified malignant neoplasm of** head, face and neck `CC` `HCC`
    Secondary and unspecified malignant neoplasm of supraclavicular lymph nodes

**C77.1** **Secondary and unspecified malignant neoplasm of** intrathoracic **lymph nodes** `CC` `HCC`

**C77.2** **Secondary and unspecified malignant neoplasm of** intra-abdominal **lymph nodes** `CC` `HCC`

**C77.3** **Secondary and unspecified malignant neoplasm of** axilla and upper limb **lymph nodes** `CC` `HCC`
    Secondary and unspecified malignant neoplasm of pectoral lymph nodes

**C77.4** **Secondary and unspecified malignant neoplasm of** inguinal and lower limb **lymph nodes** `CC` `HCC`

**C77.5** **Secondary and unspecified malignant neoplasm of** intrapelvic **lymph nodes** `CC` `HCC`

**C77.8** **Secondary and unspecified malignant neoplasm of** lymph nodes of multiple regions `CC` `HCC`

**C77.9** **Secondary and unspecified malignant neoplasm of** lymph node, unspecified `CC` `HCC`

✓4ᵗʰ **C78** **Secondary** malignant neoplasm of respiratory and digestive organs
    **EXCLUDES 1**   *secondary carcinoid tumors of liver (C7B.Ø2)*
        *secondary carcinoid tumors of peritoneum (C7B.Ø4)*
    **EXCLUDES 2**   *lymph node metastases (C77.Ø)*

✓5ᵗʰ **C78.Ø** **Secondary malignant neoplasm of** lung

**C78.ØØ** **Secondary malignant neoplasm of** unspecified **lung** `CC` `HCC`
    **CC Excl:** PDX collection 327

**C78.Ø1** **Secondary malignant neoplasm of** right **lung** `CC` `HCC`
    **CC Excl:** PDX collection 327

**C78.Ø2** **Secondary malignant neoplasm of** left **lung** `CC` `HCC`
    **CC Excl:** PDX collection 327

**C78.1** **Secondary malignant neoplasm of** mediastinum `CC` `HCC`
    **CC Excl:** PDX collection 328

**C78.2** **Secondary malignant neoplasm of** pleura `CC` `HCC`
    **CC Excl:** PDX collection 329

N Newborn: 0   P Pediatric: 0-17   M Maternity: 12-55   A Adult: 15-124   MCC Major CC Condition   PDxMCC PDx acts as own MCC   CC CC Condition   PDxCC PDx acts as own CC

476      ICD-10-CM 2018

✓5ᵗʰ **C78.3** **Secondary malignant neoplasm of** other and unspecified respiratory organs

    **C78.30** **Secondary malignant neoplasm of** unspecified **respiratory organ** `CC` `HCC`
        CC Excl: PDX collection 330

    **C78.39** **Secondary malignant neoplasm of** other respiratory organs `CC` `HCC`
        CC Excl: PDX collection 330

**C78.4** **Secondary malignant neoplasm of** small intestine `CC` `HCC`
    CC Excl: PDX collection 331

**C78.5** **Secondary malignant neoplasm of** large intestine and `CC` `HCC` rectum
    CC Excl: PDX collection 332

**C78.6** **Secondary malignant neoplasm of** retroperitoneum `CC` `HCC` and peritoneum
    **AHA:** 2017, 2Q, 12
    CC Excl: PDX collection 333

**C78.7** **Secondary malignant neoplasm of** liver and `CC` `HCC` intrahepatic bile duct
    CC Excl: PDX collection 334

✓5ᵗʰ **C78.8** **Secondary malignant neoplasm of** other and unspecified digestive organs

    **C78.80** **Secondary malignant neoplasm of** digestive unspecified **organ** `CC` `HCC`
        CC Excl: PDX collection 335

    **C78.89** **Secondary malignant neoplasm of** other digestive organs `CC` `HCC`
        Code also exocrine pancreatic insufficiency (K86.81)
        CC Excl: PDX collection 335

✓4ᵗʰ **C79** **Secondary malignant neoplasm of** other and unspecified sites
    *EXCLUDES 1*   secondary carcinoid tumors (C7B.-)
               secondary neuroendocrine tumors (C7B.-)
    *EXCLUDES 2*   ~~lymph node metastases (C77.0)~~

✓5ᵗʰ **C79.0** **Secondary malignant neoplasm of** kidney and renal pelvis

    **CC Excl: For CC codes in subcategory C79.0:** PDX collection 336

    **C79.00** **Secondary malignant neoplasm of** unspecified **kidney and renal pelvis** `CC` `HCC`

    **C79.01** **Secondary malignant neoplasm of** right **kidney and renal pelvis** `CC` `HCC`

    **C79.02** **Secondary malignant neoplasm of** left **kidney and renal pelvis** `CC` `HCC`

✓5ᵗʰ **C79.1** **Secondary malignant neoplasm of** bladder and other and unspecified urinary organs

    **CC Excl: For CC codes in subcategory C79.1:** PDX collection 336

    **C79.10** **Secondary malignant neoplasm of** unspecified **urinary organs** `CC` `HCC`

    **C79.11** **Secondary malignant neoplasm of** bladder `CC` `HCC`
        *EXCLUDES 2* ▶lymph node metastases (C77.0)◀

    **C79.19** **Secondary malignant neoplasm of** other urinary organs `CC` `HCC`

**C79.2** **Secondary malignant neoplasm of** skin `CC` `HCC`
    *EXCLUDES 1*   secondary Merkel cell carcinoma (C7B.1)
    CC Excl: PDX collection 337

✓5ᵗʰ **C79.3** **Secondary malignant neoplasm of** brain and cerebral meninges

    **C79.31** **Secondary malignant neoplasm of** brain `CC` `HCC`
        CC Excl: PDX collection 338

    **C79.32** **Secondary malignant neoplasm of** cerebral meninges `CC` `HCC`
        CC Excl: PDX collection 339

✓5ᵗʰ **C79.4** **Secondary malignant neoplasm of** other and unspecified parts of nervous system

    **C79.40** **Secondary malignant neoplasm of** unspecified **part of nervous system** `CC` `HCC`
        CC Excl: PDX collection 339

    **C79.49** **Secondary malignant neoplasm of** other parts of nervous system `CC` `HCC`
        CC Excl: PDX collection 339

✓5ᵗʰ **C79.5** **Secondary malignant neoplasm of** bone and bone marrow
    *EXCLUDES 1*   secondary carcinoid tumors of bone (C7B.03)

    **C79.51** **Secondary malignant neoplasm of** bone `CC` `HCC`
        CC Excl: PDX collection 340

    **C79.52** **Secondary malignant neoplasm of** bone marrow `CC` `HCC`
        CC Excl: PDX collection 340

---

✓5ᵗʰ **C79.6** **Secondary malignant neoplasm of** ovary

    **CC Excl: For CC codes in subcategory C79.6:** PDX collection 341

    **C79.60** **Secondary malignant neoplasm of** unspecified **ovary** `CC` `HCC` ♀

    **C79.61** **Secondary malignant neoplasm of** right **ovary** `CC` `HCC` ♀

    **C79.62** **Secondary malignant neoplasm of** left **ovary** `CC` `HCC` ♀

✓5ᵗʰ **C79.7** **Secondary malignant neoplasm of** adrenal gland

    **CC Excl: For CC codes in subcategory C79.7:** PDX collection 342

    **C79.70** **Secondary malignant neoplasm of** unspecified **adrenal gland** `CC` `HCC`

    **C79.71** **Secondary malignant neoplasm of** right **adrenal gland** `CC` `HCC`

    **C79.72** **Secondary malignant neoplasm of** left **adrenal gland** `CC` `HCC`

✓5ᵗʰ **C79.8** **Secondary malignant neoplasm of** other specified sites

    **C79.81** **Secondary malignant neoplasm of** breast `CC` `HCC`
        CC Excl: PDX collection 343

    **C79.82** **Secondary malignant neoplasm of** genital organs `CC` `HCC`
        CC Excl: PDX collection 344

    **C79.89** **Secondary malignant neoplasm of** other specified sites `CC` `HCC`
        **AHA:** 2017, 2Q, 11
        CC Excl: PDX collection 345

**C79.9** **Secondary malignant neoplasm of** unspecified site `CC` `HCC`
    Metastatic cancer NOS
    Metastatic disease NOS
    *EXCLUDES 1*   carcinomatosis NOS (C80.0)
               generalized cancer NOS (C80.0)
               malignant (primary) neoplasm of unspecified site (C80.1)
    CC Excl: PDX collection 345

✓4ᵗʰ **C80** **Malignant neoplasm** without specification of site
    *EXCLUDES 1*   malignant carcinoid tumor of unspecified site (C7A.00)
               malignant neoplasm of specified multiple sites—code to each site

**C80.0** **Disseminated malignant neoplasm, unspecified** `CC` `HCC`
    Carcinomatosis NOS
    Generalized cancer, unspecified site (primary) (secondary)
    Generalized malignancy, unspecified site (primary) (secondary)
    CC Excl: PDX collection 345

**C80.1** **Malignant** (primary) **neoplasm, unspecified** `HCC`
    Cancer NOS
    Cancer unspecified site (primary)
    Carcinoma unspecified site (primary)
    Malignancy unspecified site (primary)
    *EXCLUDES 1*   secondary malignant neoplasm of unspecified site (C79.9)

**C80.2** **Malignant neoplasm associated with transplanted organ** `CC` `HCC`
    Code first complication of transplanted organ (T86.-)
    Use additional code to identify the specific malignancy
    CC Excl: PDX collection 345

## Malignant neoplasms of lymphoid, hematopoietic and related tissue (C81-C96)

    *EXCLUDES 2*   Kaposi's sarcoma of lymph nodes (C46.3)
               secondary and unspecified neoplasm of lymph nodes (C77.-)
               secondary neoplasm of bone marrow (C79.52)
               secondary neoplasm of spleen (C78.89)

✓4ᵗʰ **C81** **Hodgkin lymphoma**
    *EXCLUDES 1*   personal history of Hodgkin lymphoma (Z85.71)

✓5ᵗʰ **C81.0** **Nodular lymphocyte predominant Hodgkin lymphoma**

    **C81.00** **Nodular lymphocyte predominant Hodgkin lymphoma, unspecified site** `CC` `HCC`
        CC Excl: PDX collection 368

    **C81.01** **Nodular lymphocyte predominant Hodgkin lymphoma, lymph nodes of** head, face, and neck `CC` `HCC`
        CC Excl: PDX collection 369

    **C81.02** **Nodular lymphocyte predominant Hodgkin lymphoma, intrathoracic lymph nodes** `CC` `HCC`
        CC Excl: PDX collection 370

---

✓ Additional Character Req   ✓x7ᵗʰ Placeholder Alert   Unacceptable PDx   Manifestation   `H1`-`H14` HAC   `HCC` CMS-HCC Condition   *EXCLUDES 1* Not Coded Here   *EXCLUDES 2* Not Included Here

ICD-10-CM 2018                                                  **477**

C78.3–C81.02

**C81.03** Nodular lymphocyte predominant Hodgkin lymphoma, intra-abdominal lymph nodes `CC` `HCC`
CC Excl: PDX collection 371

**C81.04** Nodular lymphocyte predominant Hodgkin lymphoma, lymph nodes of axilla and upper limb `CC` `HCC`
CC Excl: PDX collection 372

**C81.05** Nodular lymphocyte predominant Hodgkin lymphoma, lymph nodes of inguinal region and lower limb `CC` `HCC`
CC Excl: PDX collection 373

**C81.06** Nodular lymphocyte predominant Hodgkin lymphoma, intrapelvic lymph nodes `CC` `HCC`
CC Excl: PDX collection 374

**C81.07** Nodular lymphocyte predominant Hodgkin lymphoma, spleen `CC` `HCC`
CC Excl: PDX collection 375

**C81.08** Nodular lymphocyte predominant Hodgkin lymphoma, lymph nodes of multiple sites `CC` `HCC`
CC Excl: PDX collection 368

**C81.09** Nodular lymphocyte predominant Hodgkin lymphoma, extranodal and solid organ sites `CC` `HCC`
CC Excl: PDX collection 368

✓5ᵗʰ **C81.1 Nodular sclerosis Hodgkin lymphoma**
Nodular sclerosis classical Hodgkin lymphoma

**C81.10** Nodular sclerosis Hodgkin lymphoma, unspecified site `CC` `HCC`
CC Excl: PDX collection 376

**C81.11** Nodular sclerosis Hodgkin lymphoma, lymph nodes of head, face, and neck `CC` `HCC`
CC Excl: PDX collection 377

**C81.12** Nodular sclerosis Hodgkin lymphoma, intrathoracic lymph nodes `CC` `HCC`
CC Excl: PDX collection 378

**C81.13** Nodular sclerosis Hodgkin lymphoma, intra-abdominal lymph nodes `CC` `HCC`
CC Excl: PDX collection 379

**C81.14** Nodular sclerosis Hodgkin lymphoma, lymph nodes of axilla and upper limb `CC` `HCC`
CC Excl: PDX collection 380

**C81.15** Nodular sclerosis Hodgkin lymphoma, lymph nodes of inguinal region and lower limb `CC` `HCC`
CC Excl: PDX collection 381

**C81.16** Nodular sclerosis Hodgkin lymphoma, intrapelvic lymph nodes `CC` `HCC`
CC Excl: PDX collection 382

**C81.17** Nodular sclerosis Hodgkin lymphoma, spleen `CC` `HCC`
CC Excl: PDX collection 383

**C81.18** Nodular sclerosis Hodgkin lymphoma, lymph nodes of multiple sites `CC` `HCC`
CC Excl: PDX collection 376

**C81.19** Nodular sclerosis Hodgkin lymphoma, extranodal and solid organ sites `CC` `HCC`
CC Excl: PDX collection 376

✓5ᵗʰ **C81.2 Mixed cellularity Hodgkin lymphoma**
Mixed cellularity classical Hodgkin lymphoma

**C81.20** Mixed cellularity Hodgkin lymphoma, unspecified site `CC` `HCC`
CC Excl: PDX collection 384

**C81.21** Mixed cellularity Hodgkin lymphoma, lymph nodes of head, face, and neck `CC` `HCC`
CC Excl: PDX collection 385

**C81.22** Mixed cellularity Hodgkin lymphoma, intrathoracic lymph nodes `CC` `HCC`
CC Excl: PDX collection 386

**C81.23** Mixed cellularity Hodgkin lymphoma, intra-abdominal lymph nodes `CC` `HCC`
CC Excl: PDX collection 387

**C81.24** Mixed cellularity Hodgkin lymphoma, lymph nodes of axilla and upper limb `CC` `HCC`
CC Excl: PDX collection 388

**C81.25** Mixed cellularity Hodgkin lymphoma, lymph nodes of inguinal region and lower limb `CC` `HCC`
CC Excl: PDX collection 389

**C81.26** Mixed cellularity Hodgkin lymphoma, intrapelvic lymph nodes `CC` `HCC`
CC Excl: CPDX collection 390

**C81.27** Mixed cellularity Hodgkin lymphoma, spleen `CC` `HCC`
CC Excl: PDX collection 391

**C81.28** Mixed cellularity Hodgkin lymphoma, lymph nodes of multiple sites `CC` `HCC`
CC Excl: PDX collection 384

**C81.29** Mixed cellularity Hodgkin lymphoma, extranodal and solid organ sites `CC` `HCC`
CC Excl: PDX collection 384

✓5ᵗʰ **C81.3 Lymphocyte depleted Hodgkin lymphoma**
Lymphocyte depleted classical Hodgkin lymphoma

**C81.30** Lymphocyte depleted Hodgkin lymphoma, unspecified site `CC` `HCC`
CC Excl: PDX collection 392

**C81.31** Lymphocyte depleted Hodgkin lymphoma, lymph nodes of head, face, and neck `CC` `HCC`
CC Excl: PDX collection 393

**C81.32** Lymphocyte depleted Hodgkin lymphoma, intrathoracic lymph nodes `CC` `HCC`
CC Excl: PDX collection 394

**C81.33** Lymphocyte depleted Hodgkin lymphoma, intra-abdominal lymph nodes `CC` `HCC`
CC Excl: PDX collection 395

**C81.34** Lymphocyte depleted Hodgkin lymphoma, lymph nodes of axilla and upper limb `CC` `HCC`
CC Excl: PDX collection 396

**C81.35** Lymphocyte depleted Hodgkin lymphoma, lymph nodes of inguinal region and lower limb `CC` `HCC`
CC Excl: PDX collection 397

**C81.36** Lymphocyte depleted Hodgkin lymphoma, intrapelvic lymph nodes `CC` `HCC`
CC Excl: PDX collection 398

**C81.37** Lymphocyte depleted Hodgkin lymphoma, spleen `CC` `HCC`
CC Excl: PDX collection 399

**C81.38** Lymphocyte depleted Hodgkin lymphoma, lymph nodes of multiple sites `CC` `HCC`
CC Excl: PDX collection 400

**C81.39** Lymphocyte depleted Hodgkin lymphoma, extranodal and solid organ sites `CC` `HCC`
CC Excl: PDX collection 392

✓5ᵗʰ **C81.4 Lymphocyte-rich Hodgkin lymphoma**
Lymphocyte-rich classical Hodgkin lymphoma
**EXCLUDES 1**    nodular lymphocyte predominant Hodgkin lymphoma (C81.0-)

**C81.40** Lymphocyte-rich Hodgkin lymphoma, unspecified site `CC` `HCC`
CC Excl: PDX collection 368

**C81.41** Lymphocyte-rich Hodgkin lymphoma, lymph nodes of head, face, and neck `CC` `HCC`
CC Excl: PDX collection 369

**C81.42** Lymphocyte-rich Hodgkin lymphoma, intrathoracic lymph nodes `CC` `HCC`
CC Excl: PDX collection 370

**C81.43** Lymphocyte-rich Hodgkin lymphoma, intra-abdominal lymph nodes `CC` `HCC`
CC Excl: PDX collection 371

**C81.44** Lymphocyte-rich Hodgkin lymphoma, lymph nodes of axilla and upper limb `CC` `HCC`
CC Excl: PDX collection 372

**C81.45** Lymphocyte-rich Hodgkin lymphoma, lymph nodes of inguinal region and lower limb `CC` `HCC`
CC Excl: PDX collection 373

**C81.46** Lymphocyte-rich Hodgkin lymphoma, intrapelvic lymph nodes `CC` `HCC`
CC Excl: PDX collection 374

**C81.47** Lymphocyte-rich Hodgkin lymphoma, spleen `CC` `HCC`
CC Excl: CPDX collection 375

**C81.48** Lymphocyte-rich Hodgkin lymphoma, lymph nodes of multiple sites `CC` `HCC`
CC Excl: PDX collection 368

**C81.49** Lymphocyte-rich Hodgkin lymphoma, extranodal and solid organ sites `CC` `HCC`
CC Excl: PDX collection 368

✓5ᵗʰ **C81.7 Other Hodgkin lymphoma**
Classical Hodgkin lymphoma NOS
Other classical Hodgkin lymphoma

**C81.70** Other Hodgkin lymphoma, unspecified site `CC` `HCC`
CC Excl: PDX collection 401

**C81.71** Other Hodgkin lymphoma, lymph nodes of head, face, and neck `CC` `HCC`
CC Excl: PDX collection 402

**C81.72** Other Hodgkin lymphoma, intrathoracic lymph nodes `CC` `HCC`
CC Excl: PDX collection 403

Ⓝ Newborn: 0   Ⓟ Pediatric: 0-17   Ⓜ Maternity: 12-55   Ⓐ Adult: 15-124   `MCC` Major CC Condition   `PDxMCC` PDx acts as own MCC   `CC` CC Condition   `PDxCC` PDx acts as own CC

478      ICD-10-CM 2018

C81.73  **Other Hodgkin lymphoma, intra-abdominal** `CC` `HCC`
**lymph nodes**
**CC Excl:** PDX collection 404

C81.74  **Other Hodgkin lymphoma, lymph nodes of** `CC` `HCC`
**axilla and upper limb**
**CC Excl:** PDX collection 405

C81.75  **Other Hodgkin lymphoma, lymph** `CC` `HCC`
**nodes of inguinal region and lower limb**
**CC Excl:** PDX collection 406

C81.76  **Other Hodgkin lymphoma, intrapelvic** `CC` `HCC`
**lymph nodes**
**CC Excl:** PDX collection 407

C81.77  **Other Hodgkin lymphoma, spleen** `CC` `HCC`
**CC Excl:** PDX collection 408

C81.78  **Other Hodgkin lymphoma, lymph** `CC` `HCC`
**nodes of multiple sites**
**CC Excl:** PDX collection 401

C81.79  **Other Hodgkin lymphoma, extranodal** `CC` `HCC`
**and solid organ sites**
**CC Excl:** PDX collection 401

✓5ᵗʰ  **C81.9  Hodgkin lymphoma, unspecified**

C81.90  **Hodgkin lymphoma, unspecified, unspecified** `CC` `HCC`
**site**
**CC Excl:** PDX collection 409

C81.91  **Hodgkin lymphoma, unspecified, lymph** `CC` `HCC`
**nodes of head, face, and neck**
**CC Excl:** PDX collection 410

C81.92  **Hodgkin lymphoma, unspecified,** `CC` `HCC`
**intrathoracic lymph nodes**
**CC Excl:** PDX collection 411

C81.93  **Hodgkin lymphoma, unspecified,** `CC` `HCC`
**intra-abdominal lymph nodes**
**CC Excl:** PDX collection 412

C81.94  **Hodgkin lymphoma, unspecified, lymph** `CC` `HCC`
**nodes of axilla and upper limb**
**CC Excl:** PDX collection 413

C81.95  **Hodgkin lymphoma, unspecified, lymph** `CC` `HCC`
**nodes of inguinal region and lower limb**
**CC Excl:** PDX collection 414

C81.96  **Hodgkin lymphoma, unspecified, intrapelvic** `CC` `HCC`
**lymph nodes**
**CC Excl:** PDX collection 415

C81.97  **Hodgkin lymphoma, unspecified, spleen** `CC` `HCC`
**CC Excl:** PDX collection 416

C81.98  **Hodgkin lymphoma, unspecified, lymph** `CC` `HCC`
**nodes of multiple sites**
**CC Excl:** SPDX collection 409

C81.99  **Hodgkin lymphoma, unspecified, extranodal** `CC` `HCC`
**and solid organ sites**
**CC Excl:** No Excl

✓4ᵗʰ  **C82  Follicular lymphoma**
`INCLUDES`  follicular lymphoma with or without diffuse areas
`EXCLUDES 1`  mature T/NK-cell lymphomas (C84.-)
personal history of non-Hodgkin lymphoma (Z85.72)

✓5ᵗʰ  **C82.0  Follicular lymphoma grade I**

C82.00  **Follicular lymphoma grade I, unspecified site** `CC` `HCC`
**CC Excl:** PDX collection 417

C82.01  **Follicular lymphoma grade I, lymph nodes of** `CC` `HCC`
**head, face, and neck**
**CC Excl:** PDX collection 418

C82.02  **Follicular lymphoma grade I, intrathoracic** `CC` `HCC`
**lymph nodes**
**CC Excl:** PDX collection 419

C82.03  **Follicular lymphoma grade I,** `CC` `HCC`
**intra-abdominal lymph nodes**
**CC Excl:** PDX collection 420

C82.04  **Follicular lymphoma grade I, lymph nodes of** `CC` `HCC`
**axilla and upper limb**
**CC Excl:** PDX collection 421

C82.05  **Follicular lymphoma grade I, lymph nodes of** `CC` `HCC`
**inguinal region and lower limb**
**CC Excl:** PDX collection 422

C82.06  **Follicular lymphoma grade I, intrapelvic** `CC` `HCC`
**lymph nodes**
**CC Excl:** PDX collection 423

C82.07  **Follicular lymphoma grade I, spleen** `CC` `HCC`
**CC Excl:** PDX collection 424

C82.08  **Follicular lymphoma grade I, lymph nodes of** `CC` `HCC`
**multiple sites**
**CC Excl:** PDX collection 425

C82.09  **Follicular lymphoma grade I, extranodal and** `CC` `HCC`
**solid organ sites**
**CC Excl:** PDX collection 417

✓5ᵗʰ  **C82.1  Follicular lymphoma grade II**

C82.10  **Follicular lymphoma grade II, unspecified site** `CC` `HCC`
**CC Excl:** PDX collection 417

C82.11  **Follicular lymphoma grade II, lymph nodes** `CC` `HCC`
**of head, face, and neck**
**CC Excl:** PDX collection 418

C82.12  **Follicular lymphoma grade II, intrathoracic** `CC` `HCC`
**lymph nodes**
**CC Excl:** PDX collection 419

C82.13  **Follicular lymphoma grade II,** `CC` `HCC`
**intra-abdominal lymph nodes**
**CC Excl:** PDX collection 420

C82.14  **Follicular lymphoma grade II, lymph nodes** `CC` `HCC`
**of axilla and upper limb**
**CC Excl:** PDX collection 421

C82.15  **Follicular lymphoma grade II, lymph nodes** `CC` `HCC`
**of inguinal region and lower limb**
**CC Excl:** PDX collection 422

C82.16  **Follicular lymphoma grade II, intrapelvic** `CC` `HCC`
**lymph nodes**
**CC Excl:** PDX collection 423

C82.17  **Follicular lymphoma grade II, spleen** `CC` `HCC`
**CC Excl:** PDX collection 424

C82.18  **Follicular lymphoma grade II, lymph nodes** `CC` `HCC`
**of multiple sites**
**CC Excl:** PDX collection 425

C82.19  **Follicular lymphoma grade II, extranodal** `CC` `HCC`
**and solid organ sites**
**CC Excl:** PDX collection 417

✓5ᵗʰ  **C82.2  Follicular lymphoma grade III, unspecified**

C82.20  **Follicular lymphoma grade III, unspecified,** `CC` `HCC`
**unspecified site**
**CC Excl:** PDX collection 417

C82.21  **Follicular lymphoma grade III, unspecified,** `CC` `HCC`
**lymph nodes of head, face, and neck**
**CC Excl:** PDX collection 418

C82.22  **Follicular lymphoma grade III, unspecified,** `CC` `HCC`
**intrathoracic lymph nodes**
**CC Excl:** PDX collection 419

C82.23  **Follicular lymphoma grade III, unspecified,** `CC` `HCC`
**intra-abdominal lymph nodes**
**CC Excl:** PDX collection 420

C82.24  **Follicular lymphoma grade III, unspecified,** `CC` `HCC`
**lymph nodes of axilla and upper limb**
**CC Excl:** PDX collection 421

C82.25  **Follicular lymphoma grade III, unspecified,** `CC` `HCC`
**lymph nodes of inguinal region and lower limb**
**CC Excl:** PDX collection 422

C82.26  **Follicular lymphoma grade III, unspecified,** `CC` `HCC`
**intrapelvic lymph nodes**
**CC Excl:** PDX collection 423

C82.27  **Follicular lymphoma grade III, unspecified,** `CC` `HCC`
**spleen**
**CC Excl:** PDX collection 424

C82.28  **Follicular lymphoma grade III, unspecified,** `CC` `HCC`
**lymph nodes of multiple sites**
**CC Excl:** PDX collection 425

C82.29  **Follicular lymphoma grade III, unspecified,** `CC` `HCC`
**extranodal and solid organ sites**
**CC Excl:** PDX collection 417

✓5ᵗʰ  **C82.3  Follicular lymphoma grade IIIa**

C82.30  **Follicular lymphoma grade IIIa, unspecified** `CC` `HCC`
**sitespleen**
**CC Excl:** PDX collection 417

C82.31  **Follicular lymphoma grade IIIa, lymph nodes** `CC` `HCC`
**of head, face, and neck**
**CC Excl:** PDX collection 418

C82.32  **Follicular lymphoma grade IIIa, intrathoracic** `CC` `HCC`
**lymph nodes**
**CC Excl:** PDX collection 419

C82.33  **Follicular lymphoma grade IIIa,** `CC` `HCC`
**intra-abdominal lymph nodes**
**CC Excl:** PDX collection 420

C82.34  **Follicular lymphoma grade IIIa, lymph nodes** `CC` `HCC`
**of axilla and upper limb**
**CC Excl:** PDX collection 421

✓Additional Character Req  `✓x7ᵗʰ` Placeholder Alert  Unacceptable PDx  Manifestation  `H1`-`H14` HAC  `HCC` CMS-HCC Condition  `EXCLUDES 1` Not Coded Here  `EXCLUDES 2` Not Included Here

ICD-10-CM 2018  **479**

**Chapter 2. Neoplasms**

**C82.35–C82.98**

**C82.35** Follicular lymphoma grade IIIa, lymph nodes `CC` `HCC`
of inguinal region and lower limb
**CC Excl:** PDX collection 422

**C82.36** Follicular lymphoma grade IIIa, intrapelvic `CC` `HCC`
lymph nodes
**CC Excl:** PDX collection 423

**C82.37** Follicular lymphoma grade IIIa, spleen `CC` `HCC`
**CC Excl:** PDX collection 424

**C82.38** Follicular lymphoma grade IIIa, lymph nodes `CC` `HCC`
of multiple sites
**CC Excl:** PDX collection 425

**C82.39** Follicular lymphoma grade IIIa, extranodal `CC` `HCC`
and solid organ sites
**CC Excl:** PDX collection 417

✓5ᵗʰ **C82.4** Follicular lymphoma grade IIIb

**C82.40** Follicular lymphoma grade IIIb, `CC` `HCC`
unspecified site
**CC Excl:** PDX collection 417

**C82.41** Follicular lymphoma grade IIIb, lymph nodes `CC` `HCC`
of head, face, and neck
**CC Excl:** PDX collection 418

**C82.42** Follicular lymphoma grade IIIb, intrathoracic `CC` `HCC`
lymph nodes
**CC Excl:** PDX collection 419

**C82.43** Follicular lymphoma grade IIIb, `CC` `HCC`
intra-abdominal lymph nodes
**CC Excl:** PDX collection 420

**C82.44** Follicular lymphoma grade IIIb, lymph nodes `CC` `HCC`
of axilla and upper limb
**CC Excl:** PDX collection 421

**C82.45** Follicular lymphoma grade IIIb, lymph `CC` `HCC`
nodes of inguinal region and lower limb
**CC Excl:** PDX collection 422

**C82.46** Follicular lymphoma grade IIIb, intrapelvic `CC` `HCC`
lymph nodes
**CC Excl:** PDX collection 423

**C82.47** Follicular lymphoma grade IIIb, spleen `CC` `HCC`
**CC Excl:** PDX collection 424

**C82.48** Follicular lymphoma grade IIIb, lymph nodes `CC` `HCC`
of multiple sites
**CC Excl:** PDX collection 425

**C82.49** Follicular lymphoma grade IIIb, extranodal `CC` `HCC`
and solid organ sites
**CC Excl:** PDX collection 417

✓5ᵗʰ **C82.5** Diffuse follicle center lymphoma

**C82.50** Diffuse follicle center lymphoma, `HIV` `CC` `HCC`
unspecified site
**CC Excl:** PDX collection 426

**C82.51** Diffuse follicle center lymphoma, lymph `HIV` `CC` `HCC`
nodes of head, face, and neck
**CC Excl:** PDX collection 427

**C82.52** Diffuse follicle center lymphoma, `HIV` `CC` `HCC`
intrathoracic lymph nodes
**CC Excl:** PDX collection 428

**C82.53** Diffuse follicle center lymphoma, intra- `HIV` `CC` `HCC`
abdominal lymph nodes
**CC Excl:** PDX collection 429

**C82.54** Diffuse follicle center lymphoma, lymph `HIV` `CC` `HCC`
nodes of axilla and upper limb
**CC Excl:** PDX collection 430

**C82.55** Diffuse follicle center lymphoma, lymph `HIV` `CC` `HCC`
nodes of inguinal region and lower limb
**CC Excl:** PDX collection 431

**C82.56** Diffuse follicle center lymphoma, `HIV` `CC` `HCC`
intrapelvic lymph nodes
**CC Excl:** PDX collection 432

**C82.57** Diffuse follicle center lymphoma, spleen `HIV` `CC` `HCC`
**CC Excl:** PDX collection 433

**C82.58** Diffuse follicle center lymphoma, lymph `HIV` `CC` `HCC`
nodes of multiple sites
**CC Excl:** PDX collection 434

**C82.59** Diffuse follicle center lymphoma, `HIV` `CC` `HCC`
extranodal and solid organ sites
**CC Excl:** PDX collection 426

✓5ᵗʰ **C82.6** Cutaneous follicle center lymphoma

**C82.60** Cutaneous follicle center lymphoma, `CC` `HCC`
unspecified site
**CC Excl:** PDX collection 417

**C82.61** Cutaneous follicle center lymphoma, lymph `CC` `HCC`
nodes of head, face, and neck
**CC Excl:** PDX collection 418

**C82.62** Cutaneous follicle center lymphoma, `CC` `HCC`
intrathoracic lymph nodes
**CC Excl:** PDX collection 419

**C82.63** Cutaneous follicle center lymphoma, `CC` `HCC`
intra-abdominal lymph nodes
**CC Excl:** PDX collection 420

**C82.64** Cutaneous follicle center lymphoma, lymph `CC` `HCC`
nodes of axilla and upper limb
**CC Excl:** PDX collection 421

**C82.65** Cutaneous follicle center lymphoma, lymph `CC` `HCC`
nodes of inguinal region and lower limb
**CC Excl:** PDX collection 422

**C82.66** Cutaneous follicle center lymphoma, `CC` `HCC`
intrapelvic lymph nodes
**CC Excl:** PDX collection 423

**C82.67** Cutaneous follicle center lymphoma, spleen `CC` `HCC`
**CC Excl:** PDX collection 424

**C82.68** Cutaneous follicle center lymphoma, lymph `CC` `HCC`
nodes of multiple sites
**CC Excl:** PDX collection 425

**C82.69** Cutaneous follicle center lymphoma, `CC` `HCC`
extranodal and solid organ sites
**CC Excl:** PDX collection 417

✓5ᵗʰ **C82.8** Other types of follicular lymphoma

**C82.80** Other types of follicular lymphoma, `CC` `HCC`
unspecified site
**CC Excl:** PDX collection 417

**C82.81** Other types of follicular lymphoma, lymph `CC` `HCC`
nodes of head, face, and neck
**CC Excl:** PDX collection 418

**C82.82** Other types of follicular lymphoma, `CC` `HCC`
intrathoracic lymph nodes
**CC Excl:** PDX collection 419

**C82.83** Other types of follicular lymphoma, `CC` `HCC`
intra-abdominal lymph nodes
**CC Excl:** PDX collection 420

**C82.84** Other types of follicular lymphoma, lymph `CC` `HCC`
nodes of axilla and upper limb
**CC Excl:** PDX collection 421

**C82.85** Other types of follicular lymphoma, lymph `CC` `HCC`
nodes of inguinal region and lower limb
**CC Excl:** PDX collection 422

**C82.86** Other types of follicular lymphoma, `CC` `HCC`
intrapelvic lymph nodes
**CC Excl:** PDX collection 423

**C82.87** Other types of follicular lymphoma, spleen `CC` `HCC`
**CC Excl:** PDX collection 424

**C82.88** Other types of follicular lymphoma, lymph `CC` `HCC`
nodes of multiple sites
**CC Excl:** PDX collection 425

**C82.89** Other types of follicular lymphoma, `CC` `HCC`
extranodal and solid organ sites
**CC Excl:** PDX collection 417

✓5ᵗʰ **C82.9** Follicular lymphoma, unspecified

**C82.90** Follicular lymphoma, unspecified, `CC` `HCC`
unspecified site
**CC Excl:** PDX collection 417

**C82.91** Follicular lymphoma, unspecified, lymph `CC` `HCC`
nodes of head, face, and neck
**CC Excl:** PDX collection 418

**C82.92** Follicular lymphoma, unspecified, `CC` `HCC`
intrathoracic lymph nodes
**CC Excl:** PDX collection 419

**C82.93** Follicular lymphoma, unspecified, intra- `CC` `HCC`
abdominal lymph nodes
**CC Excl:** PDX collection 420

**C82.94** Follicular lymphoma, unspecified, lymph `CC` `HCC`
nodes of axilla and upper limb
**CC Excl:** PDX collection 421

**C82.95** Follicular lymphoma, unspecified, lymph `CC` `HCC`
nodes of inguinal region and lower limb
**CC Excl:** PDX collection 422

**C82.96** Follicular lymphoma, unspecified, `CC` `HCC`
intrapelvic lymph nodes
**CC Excl:** PDX collection 423

**C82.97** Follicular lymphoma, unspecified, spleen `CC` `HCC`
**CC Excl:** PDX collection 424

**C82.98** Follicular lymphoma, unspecified, lymph `CC` `HCC`
nodes of multiple sites
**CC Excl:** PDX collection 425

---

`N` Newborn: 0    `P` Pediatric: 0-17    `M` Maternity: 12-55    `A` Adult: 15-124    `MCC` Major CC Condition    `PDxMCC` PDx acts as own MCC    `CC` CC Condition    `PDxCC` PDx acts as own CC

**C82.99**    **Follicular lymphoma, unspecified,**    `CC` `HCC`
**extranodal and solid organ sites**
     CC Excl: PDX collection 417

**C83**   **Non-follicular lymphoma**
     *EXCLUDES 1*    *personal history of non-Hodgkin lymphoma (Z85.72)*

   **C83.0**   **Small cell B-cell lymphoma**
       Lymphoplasmacytic lymphoma
       Nodal marginal zone lymphoma
       Non-leukemic variant of B-CLL
       Splenic marginal zone lymphoma
       *EXCLUDES 1*   *chronic lymphocytic leukemia (C91.1)*
               *mature T/NK-cell lymphomas (C84.-)*
               *Waldenström macroglobulinemia (C88.0)*

     **C83.00**   **Small cell B-cell lymphoma, unspecified**   `HIV` `CC` `HCC`
**site**
        CC Excl: PDX collection 435

     **C83.01**   **Small cell B-cell lymphoma, lymph nodes**   `HIV` `CC` `HCC`
**of head, face, and neck**
        CC Excl: PDX collection 436

     **C83.02**   **Small cell B-cell lymphoma, intrathoracic**   `HIV` `CC` `HCC`
**lymph nodes**
        CC Excl: PDX collection 437

     **C83.03**   **Small cell B-cell lymphoma, intra-**   `HIV` `CC` `HCC`
**abdominal lymph nodes**
        CC Excl: PDX collection 438

     **C83.04**   **Small cell B-cell lymphoma, lymph nodes**   `HIV` `CC` `HCC`
**of axilla and upper limb**
        CC Excl: PDX collection 439

     **C83.05**   **Small cell B-cell lymphoma, lymph nodes**   `HIV` `CC` `HCC`
**of inguinal region and lower limb**
        CC Excl: CPDX collection 440

     **C83.06**   **Small cell B-cell lymphoma, intrapelvic**   `HIV` `CC` `HCC`
**lymph nodes**
        CC Excl: PDX collection 441

     **C83.07**   **Small cell B-cell lymphoma, spleen**   `HIV` `CC` `HCC`
        CC Excl: PDX collection 442

     **C83.08**   **Small cell B-cell lymphoma, lymph nodes**   `HIV` `CC` `HCC`
**of multiple sites**
        CC Excl: PDX collection 435

     **C83.09**   **Small cell B-cell lymphoma, extranodal**   `HIV` `CC` `HCC`
**and solid organ sites**
        CC Excl: PDX collection 435

   **C83.1**   **Mantle cell lymphoma**
       Centrocytic lymphoma
       Malignant lymphomatous polyposis
       **DEF:** Rare form of B-cell non-Hodgkin lymphoma named for the
       location of tumor cell production, the mantle zone of the lymph
       nodes.

     **C83.10**   **Mantle cell lymphoma, unspecified site**   `HIV` `CC` `HCC`
        CC Excl: PDX collection 426

     **C83.11**   **Mantle cell lymphoma, lymph nodes of**   `HIV` `CC` `HCC`
**head, face, and neck**
        CC Excl: PDX collection 427

     **C83.12**   **Mantle cell lymphoma, intrathoracic**   `HIV` `CC` `HCC`
**lymph nodes**
        CC Excl: PDX collection 428

     **C83.13**   **Mantle cell lymphoma, intra-abdominal**   `HIV` `CC` `HCC`
**lymph nodes**
        CC Excl: PDX collection 429

     **C83.14**   **Mantle cell lymphoma, lymph nodes of**   `HIV` `CC` `HCC`
**axilla and upper limb**
        CC Excl: PDX collection 430

     **C83.15**   **Mantle cell lymphoma, lymph nodes of**   `HIV` `CC` `HCC`
**inguinal region and lower limb**
        CC Excl: PDX collection 431

     **C83.16**   **Mantle cell lymphoma, intrapelvic lymph**   `HIV` `CC` `HCC`
**nodes**
        CC Excl: PDX collection 432

     **C83.17**   **Mantle cell lymphoma, spleen**   `HIV` `CC` `HCC`
        CC Excl: PDX collection 433

     **C83.18**   **Mantle cell lymphoma, lymph nodes of**   `HIV` `CC` `HCC`
**multiple sites**
        CC Excl: PDX collection 434

     **C83.19**   **Mantle cell lymphoma, extranodal and**   `HIV` `CC` `HCC`
**solid organ sites**
        CC Excl: PDX collection 426

   **C83.3**   **Diffuse large B-cell lymphoma**
       Anaplastic diffuse large B-cell lymphoma
       CD30-positive diffuse large B-cell lymphoma
       Centroblastic diffuse large B-cell lymphoma
       Diffuse large B-cell lymphoma, subtype not specified
       Immunoblastic diffuse large B-cell lymphoma
       Plasmablastic diffuse large B-cell lymphoma
       T-cell rich diffuse large B-cell lymphoma
       *EXCLUDES 1*   *mature T/NK-cell lymphomas (C84.-)*
               *mediastinal (thymic) large B-cell lymphoma (C85.2-)*

     **C83.30**   **Diffuse large B-cell lymphoma,**   `HIV` `CC` `HCC`
**unspecified site**
        CC Excl: PDX collection 443

     **C83.31**   **Diffuse large B-cell lymphoma, lymph**   `HIV` `CC` `HCC`
**nodes of head, face, and neck**
        CC Excl: PDX collection 444

     **C83.32**   **Diffuse large B-cell lymphoma,**   `HIV` `CC` `HCC`
**intrathoracic lymph nodes**
        CC Excl: PDX collection 445

     **C83.33**   **Diffuse large B-cell lymphoma, intra-**   `HIV` `CC` `HCC`
**abdominal lymph nodes**
        CC Excl: PDX collection 446

     **C83.34**   **Diffuse large B-cell lymphoma, lymph**   `HIV` `CC` `HCC`
**nodes of axilla and upper limb**
        CC Excl: PDX collection 447

     **C83.35**   **Diffuse large B-cell lymphoma, lymph**   `HIV` `CC` `HCC`
**nodes of inguinal region and lower limb**
        CC Excl: PDX collection 448

     **C83.36**   **Diffuse large B-cell lymphoma,**   `HIV` `CC` `HCC`
**intrapelvic lymph nodes**
        CC Excl: PDX collection 449

     **C83.37**   **Diffuse large B-cell lymphoma, spleen**   `HIV` `CC` `HCC`
        CC Excl: PDX collection 450

     **C83.38**   **Diffuse large B-cell lymphoma, lymph**   `HIV` `CC` `HCC`
**nodes of multiple sites**
        CC Excl: PDX collection 443

     **C83.39**   **Diffuse large B-cell lymphoma, extranodal**   `HIV` `CC` `HCC`
**and solid organ sites**
        CC Excl: PDX collection 443

   **C83.5**   **Lymphoblastic (diffuse) lymphoma**
       B-precursor lymphoma
       Lymphoblastic B-cell lymphoma
       Lymphoblastic lymphoma NOS
       Lymphoblastic T-cell lymphoma
       T-precursor lymphoma

     **C83.50**   **Lymphoblastic (diffuse) lymphoma,**   `CC` `HCC`
**unspecified site**
        CC Excl: PDX collection 451

     **C83.51**   **Lymphoblastic (diffuse) lymphoma, lymph**   `CC` `HCC`
**nodes of head, face, and neck**
        CC Excl: PDX collection 452

     **C83.52**   **Lymphoblastic (diffuse) lymphoma,**   `CC` `HCC`
**intrathoracic lymph nodes**
        CC Excl: PDX collection 453

     **C83.53**   **Lymphoblastic (diffuse) lymphoma,**   `CC` `HCC`
**intra-abdominal lymph nodes**
        CC Excl: PDX collection 454

     **C83.54**   **Lymphoblastic (diffuse) lymphoma, lymph**   `CC` `HCC`
**nodes of axilla and upper limb**
        CC Excl: PDX collection 455

     **C83.55**   **Lymphoblastic (diffuse) lymphoma, lymph**   `CC` `HCC`
**nodes of inguinal region and lower limb**
        CC Excl: PDX collection 456

     **C83.56**   **Lymphoblastic (diffuse) lymphoma,**   `CC` `HCC`
**intrapelvic lymph nodes**
        CC Excl: PDX collection 457

     **C83.57**   **Lymphoblastic (diffuse) lymphoma, spleen**   `CC` `HCC`
        CC Excl: PDX collection 458

     **C83.58**   **Lymphoblastic (diffuse) lymphoma, lymph**   `CC` `HCC`
**nodes of multiple sites**
        CC Excl: PDX collection 451

     **C83.59**   **Lymphoblastic (diffuse) lymphoma,**   `CC` `HCC`
**extranodal and solid organ sites**
        CC Excl: PDX collection 451

✓ Additional Character Req    ✓×7th Placeholder Alert    Unacceptable PDx    Manifestation    `H1`-`H14` HAC    `HCC` CMS-HCC Condition    *EXCLUDES 1* Not Coded Here    *EXCLUDES 2* Not Included Here

ICD-10-CM 2018                                               **481**

✓5th **C83.7　Burkitt lymphoma**
Atypical Burkitt lymphoma
Burkitt-like lymphoma
*EXCLUDES 1*　mature B-cell leukemia Burkitt type (C91.A-)
**DEF:** Malignancy of the lymphatic system, most often seen as a large bone-deteriorating lesion within the jaw or as an abdominal mass. It is a form of non-Hodgkin's lymphoma and is recognized as the fastest growing human tumor.

**C83.70　Burkitt lymphoma, unspecified site**　HIV CC HCC
CC Excl: PDX collection 459

**C83.71　Burkitt lymphoma, lymph nodes of head, face, and neck**　HIV CC HCC
CC Excl: PDX collection 460

**C83.72　Burkitt lymphoma, intrathoracic lymph nodes**　HIV CC HCC
CC Excl: PDX collection 461

**C83.73　Burkitt lymphoma, intra-abdominal lymph nodes**　HIV CC HCC
CC Excl: PDX collection 462

**C83.74　Burkitt lymphoma, lymph nodes of axilla and upper limb**　HIV CC HCC
CC Excl: PDX collection 463

**C83.75　Burkitt lymphoma, lymph nodes of inguinal region and lower limb**　HIV CC HCC
CC Excl: PDX collection 464

**C83.76　Burkitt lymphoma, intrapelvic lymph nodes**　HIV CC HCC
CC Excl: PDX collection 465

**C83.77　Burkitt lymphoma, spleen**　HIV CC HCC
CC Excl: PDX collection 466

**C83.78　Burkitt lymphoma, lymph nodes of multiple sites**　HIV CC HCC
CC Excl: PDX collection 459

**C83.79　Burkitt lymphoma, extranodal and solid organ sites**　HIV CC HCC
CC Excl: PDX collection 459

✓5th **C83.8　Other non-follicular lymphoma**
Intravascular large B-cell lymphoma
Lymphoid granulomatosis
Primary effusion B-cell lymphoma
*EXCLUDES 1*　mediastinal (thymic) large B-cell lymphoma (C85.2-)
　　　　　　T-cell rich B-cell lymphoma (C83.3-)

**C83.80　Other non-follicular lymphoma, unspecified site**　HIV CC HCC
CC Excl: PDX collection 435

**C83.81　Other non-follicular lymphoma, lymph nodes of head, face, and neck**　HIV CC HCC
CC Excl: PDX collection 436

**C83.82　Other non-follicular lymphoma, intrathoracic lymph nodes**　HIV CC HCC
CC Excl: PDX collection 437

**C83.83　Other non-follicular lymphoma, intra-abdominal lymph nodes**　HIV CC HCC
CC Excl: PDX collection 438

**C83.84　Other non-follicular lymphoma, lymph nodes of axilla and upper limb**　HIV CC HCC
CC Excl: PDX collection 439

**C83.85　Other non-follicular lymphoma, lymph nodes of inguinal region and lower limb**　HIV CC HCC
CC Excl: PDX collection 440

**C83.86　Other non-follicular lymphoma, intrapelvic lymph nodes**　HIV CC HCC
CC Excl: PDX collection 441

**C83.87　Other non-follicular lymphoma, spleen**　HIV CC HCC
CC Excl: PDX collection 442

**C83.88　Other non-follicular lymphoma, lymph nodes of multiple sites**　HIV CC HCC
CC Excl: PDX collection 435

**C83.89　Other non-follicular lymphoma, extranodal and solid organ sites**　HIV CC HCC
CC Excl: SPDX collection 435

✓5th **C83.9　Non-follicular (diffuse) lymphoma, unspecified**

**C83.90　Non-follicular (diffuse) lymphoma, unspecified, unspecified site**　HIV CC HCC
CC Excl: PDX collection 435

**C83.91　Non-follicular (diffuse) lymphoma, unspecified, lymph nodes of head, face, and neck**　HIV CC HCC
CC Excl: PDX collection 436

**C83.92　Non-follicular (diffuse) lymphoma, unspecified, intrathoracic lymph nodes**　HIV CC HCC
CC Excl: PDX collection 437

**C83.93　Non-follicular (diffuse) lymphoma, unspecified, intra-abdominal lymph nodes**　HIV CC HCC
CC Excl: PDX collection 438

**C83.94　Non-follicular (diffuse) lymphoma, unspecified, lymph nodes of axilla and upper limb**　HIV CC HCC
CC Excl: PDX collection 439

**C83.95　Non-follicular (diffuse) lymphoma, unspecified, lymph nodes of inguinal region and lower limb**　HIV CC HCC
CC Excl: PDX collection 440

**C83.96　Non-follicular (diffuse) lymphoma, unspecified, intrapelvic lymph nodes**　HIV CC HCC
CC Excl: PDX collection 441

**C83.97　Non-follicular (diffuse) lymphoma, unspecified, spleen**　HIV CC HCC
CC Excl: PDX collection 442

**C83.98　Non-follicular (diffuse) lymphoma, unspecified, lymph nodes of multiple sites**　HIV CC HCC
CC Excl: PDX collection 435

**C83.99　Non-follicular (diffuse) lymphoma, unspecified, extranodal and solid organ sites**　HIV CC HCC
CC Excl: PDX collection 435

✓4th **C84　Mature T/NK-cell lymphomas**
*EXCLUDES 1*　personal history of non-Hodgkin lymphoma (Z85.72)

✓5th **C84.0　Mycosis fungoides**
*EXCLUDES 1*　peripheral T-cell lymphoma, not classified (C84.4-)
**DEF:** Most common form of cutaneous T-cell lymphoma, also known as Alibert-Bazin syndrome. A type of non-Hodgkin lymphoma in which white blood cells become cancerous and affect the skin and sometimes internal organs.

**C84.00　Mycosis fungoides, unspecified site**　CC HCC
CC Excl: PDX collection 467

**C84.01　Mycosis fungoides, lymph nodes of head, face, and neck**　CC HCC
CC Excl: PDX collection 468

**C84.02　Mycosis fungoides, intrathoracic lymph nodes**　CC HCC
CC Excl: PDX collection 469

**C84.03　Mycosis fungoides, intra-abdominal lymph nodes**　CC HCC
CC Excl: PDX collection 470

**C84.04　Mycosis fungoides, lymph nodes of axilla and upper limb**　CC HCC
CC Excl: PDX collection 471

**C84.05　Mycosis fungoides, lymph nodes of inguinal region and lower limb**　CC HCC
CC Excl: PDX collection 472

**C84.06　Mycosis fungoides, intrapelvic lymph nodes**　CC HCC
CC Excl: PDX collection 473

**C84.07　Mycosis fungoides, spleen**　CC HCC
CC Excl: PDX collection 474

**C84.08　Mycosis fungoides, lymph nodes of multiple sites**　CC HCC
CC Excl: PDX collection 475

**C84.09　Mycosis fungoides, extranodal and solid organ sites**　CC HCC
CC Excl: PDX collection 467

✓5th **C84.1　Sézary disease**

**C84.10　Sézary disease, unspecified site**　CC HCC
CC Excl: PDX collection 476

**C84.11　Sézary disease, lymph nodes of head, face, and neck**　CC HCC
CC Excl: PDX collection 477

**C84.12　Sézary disease, intrathoracic lymph nodes**　CC HCC
CC Excl: PDX collection 478

**C84.13　Sézary disease, intra-abdominal lymph nodes**　CC HCC
CC Excl: PDX collection 479

**C84.14　Sézary disease, lymph nodes of axilla and upper limb**　CC HCC
CC Excl: PDX collection 480

**C84.15　Sézary disease, lymph nodes of inguinal region and lower limb**　CC HCC
CC Excl: PDX collection 481

**C84.16　Sézary disease, intrapelvic lymph nodes**　CC HCC
CC Excl: PDX collection 482

**C84.17　Sézary disease, spleen**　CC HCC
CC Excl: PDX collection 483

**C84.18　Sézary disease, lymph nodes of multiple sites**　CC HCC
CC Excl: PDX collection 484

**C84.19**    **Sézary disease,** extranodal and solid organ sites   `CC` `HCC`
     **CC Excl:** PDX collection 476

✓5th   **C84.4**   **Peripheral T-cell lymphoma, not classified**
     Lennert's lymphoma
     Lymphoepithelioid lymphoma
     Mature T-cell lymphoma, not elsewhere classified

     **C84.40**   **Peripheral T-cell lymphoma, not**   `HIV` `CC` `HCC`
         **classified,** unspecified site
         **CC Excl:** PDX collection 426

     **C84.41**   **Peripheral T-cell lymphoma, not**   `HIV` `CC` `HCC`
         **classified, lymph nodes of** head, face, and neck
         **CC Excl:** PDX collection 427

     **C84.42**   **Peripheral T-cell lymphoma, not**   `HIV` `CC` `HCC`
         **classified,** intrathoracic **lymph nodes**
         **CC Excl:** PDX collection 428

     **C84.43**   **Peripheral T-cell lymphoma, not**   `HIV` `CC` `HCC`
         **classified,** intra-abdominal **lymph nodes**
         **CC Excl:** PDX collection 429

     **C84.44**   **Peripheral T-cell lymphoma, not**   `HIV` `CC` `HCC`
         **classified, lymph nodes of** axilla and upper limb
         **CC Excl:** PDX collection 430

     **C84.45**   **Peripheral T-cell lymphoma, not**   `HIV` `CC` `HCC`
         **classified, lymph nodes of** inguinal region
         and lower limb
         **CC Excl:** PDX collection 431

     **C84.46**   **Peripheral T-cell lymphoma, not**   `HIV` `CC` `HCC`
         **classified,** intrapelvic **lymph nodes**
         **CC Excl:** PDX collection 432

     **C84.47**   **Peripheral T-cell lymphoma, not**   `HIV` `CC` `HCC`
         **classified,** spleen
         **CC Excl:** PDX collection 433

     **C84.48**   **Peripheral T-cell lymphoma, not**   `HIV` `CC` `HCC`
         **classified, lymph nodes of** multiple sites
         **CC Excl:** PDX collection 434

     **C84.49**   **Peripheral T-cell lymphoma, not**   `HIV` `CC` `HCC`
         **classified,** extranodal and solid organ sites
         **CC Excl:** PDX collection 426

✓5th   **C84.6**   **Anaplastic large cell lymphoma,** ALK-positive
     Anaplastic large cell lymphoma, CD30-positive

     **C84.60**   **Anaplastic large cell lymphoma,**   `HIV` `CC` `HCC`
         **ALK-positive,** unspecified site
         **CC Excl:** PDX collection 426

     **C84.61**   **Anaplastic large cell lymphoma,**   `HIV` `CC` `HCC`
         **ALK-positive, lymph nodes of** head, face, and neck
         **CC Excl:** PDX collection 427

     **C84.62**   **Anaplastic large cell lymphoma,**   `HIV` `CC` `HCC`
         **ALK-positive,** intrathoracic **lymph nodes**
         **CC Excl:** PDX collection 428

     **C84.63**   **Anaplastic large cell lymphoma,**   `HIV` `CC` `HCC`
         **ALK-positive,** intra-abdominal **lymph nodes**
         **CC Excl:** PDX collection 429

     **C84.64**   **Anaplastic large cell lymphoma,**   `HIV` `CC` `HCC`
         **ALK-positive, lymph nodes of** axilla and
         upper limb
         **CC Excl:** PDX collection 430

     **C84.65**   **Anaplastic large cell lymphoma,**   `HIV` `CC` `HCC`
         **ALK-positive, lymph nodes of** inguinal region
         and lower limb
         **CC Excl:** PDX collection 431

     **C84.66**   **Anaplastic large cell lymphoma,**   `HIV` `CC` `HCC`
         **ALK-positive,** intrapelvic **lymph nodes**
         **CC Excl:** PDX collection 432

     **C84.67**   **Anaplastic large cell lymphoma,**   `HIV` `CC` `HCC`
         **ALK-positive,** spleen
         **CC Excl:** PDX collection 433

     **C84.68**   **Anaplastic large cell lymphoma,**   `HIV` `CC` `HCC`
         **ALK-positive, lymph nodes of** multiple sites
         **CC Excl:** PDX collection 434

     **C84.69**   **Anaplastic large cell lymphoma,**   `HIV` `CC` `HCC`
         **ALK-positive,** extranodal and solid organ sites
         **CC Excl:** PDX collection 426

✓5th   **C84.7**   **Anaplastic large cell lymphoma,** ALK-negative
     *EXCLUDES 1*   *primary cutaneous CD30-positive T-cell proliferations (C86.6-)*

     **C84.70**   **Anaplastic large cell lymphoma,**   `HIV` `CC` `HCC`
         **ALK-negative,** unspecified site
         **CC Excl:** PDX collection 426

     **C84.71**   **Anaplastic large cell lymphoma,**   `HIV` `CC` `HCC`
         **ALK-negative, lymph nodes of** head,
         face, and neck
         **CC Excl:** PDX collection 427

**C84.72**   **Anaplastic large cell lymphoma,**   `HIV` `CC` `HCC`
     **ALK-negative, intrathoracic lymph nodes**
     **CC Excl:** PDX collection 428

**C84.73**   **Anaplastic large cell lymphoma,**   `HIV` `CC` `HCC`
     **ALK-negative, intra-abdominal lymph nodes**
     **CC Excl:** PDX collection 429

**C84.74**   **Anaplastic large cell lymphoma,**   `HIV` `CC` `HCC`
     **ALK-negative, lymph nodes of** axilla
     and upper limb
     **CC Excl:** PDX collection 430

**C84.75**   **Anaplastic large cell lymphoma,**   `HIV` `CC` `HCC`
     **ALK-negative, lymph nodes of** inguinal
     region and lower limb
     **CC Excl:** PDX collection 431

**C84.76**   **Anaplastic large cell lymphoma,**   `HIV` `CC` `HCC`
     **ALK-negative, intrapelvic lymph nodes**
     **CC Excl:** PDX collection 432

**C84.77**   **Anaplastic large cell lymphoma,**   `HIV` `CC` `HCC`
     **ALK-negative, spleen**
     **CC Excl:** PDX collection 433

**C84.78**   **Anaplastic large cell lymphoma,**   `HIV` `CC` `HCC`
     **ALK-negative, lymph nodes of** multiple sites
     **CC Excl:** PDX collection 434

**C84.79**   **Anaplastic large cell lymphoma,**   `HIV` `CC` `HCC`
     **ALK-negative,** extranodal and solid organ sites
     **CC Excl:** PDX collection 426

✓5th   **C84.A**   **Cutaneous T-cell lymphoma, unspecified**

     **C84.A0**   **Cutaneous T-cell lymphoma, unspecified,**   `HIV` `CC` `HCC`
         unspecified site
         **CC Excl:** PDX collection 426

     **C84.A1**   **Cutaneous T-cell lymphoma, unspecified**   `HIV` `CC` `HCC`
         **lymph nodes of** head, face, and neck
         **CC Excl:** PDX collection 427

     **C84.A2**   **Cutaneous T-cell lymphoma, unspecified,**   `HIV` `CC` `HCC`
         intrathoracic **lymph nodes**
         **CC Excl:** PDX collection 428

     **C84.A3**   **Cutaneous T-cell lymphoma, unspecified,**   `HIV` `CC` `HCC`
         intra-abdominal **lymph nodes**
         **CC Excl:** PDX collection 429

     **C84.A4**   **Cutaneous T-cell lymphoma, unspecified,**   `HIV` `CC` `HCC`
         **lymph nodes of** axilla and upper limb
         **CC Excl:** PDX collection 430

     **C84.A5**   **Cutaneous T-cell lymphoma, unspecified,**   `HIV` `CC` `HCC`
         **lymph nodes of** inguinal region and lower limb
         **CC Excl:** PDX collection 431

     **C84.A6**   **Cutaneous T-cell lymphoma, unspecified,**   `HIV` `CC` `HCC`
         intrapelvic **lymph nodes**
         **CC Excl:** PDX collection 432

     **C84.A7**   **Cutaneous T-cell lymphoma, unspecified,**   `HIV` `CC` `HCC`
         spleen
         **CC Excl:** PDX collection 433

     **C84.A8**   **Cutaneous T-cell lymphoma, unspecified,**   `HIV` `CC` `HCC`
         **lymph nodes of** multiple sites
         **CC Excl:** PDX collection 434

     **C84.A9**   **Cutaneous T-cell lymphoma, unspecified,**   `HIV` `CC` `HCC`
         extranodal and solid organ sites
         **CC Excl:** PDX collection 426

✓5th   **C84.Z**   **Other mature T/NK-cell lymphomas**
     `NOTE`   If T-cell lineage or involvement is mentioned in conjunction with a specific lymphoma, code to the more specific description.
     *EXCLUDES 1*   *angioimmunoblastic T-cell lymphoma (C86.5)*
         *blastic NK-cell lymphoma (C86.4)*
         *enteropathy-type T-cell lymphoma (C86.2)*
         *extranodal NK-cell lymphoma, nasal type (C86.0)*
         *hepatosplenic T-cell lymphoma (C86.1)*
         *primary cutaneous CD30-positive T-cell proliferations (C86.6)*
         *subcutaneous panniculitis-like T-cell lymphoma (C86.3)*
         *T-cell leukemia (C91.1-)*

     **C84.Z0**   **Other mature T/NK-cell lymphomas,**   `HIV` `CC` `HCC`
         unspecified site
         **CC Excl:** PDX collection 426

     **C84.Z1**   **Other mature T/NK-cell lymphomas,**   `HIV` `CC` `HCC`
         **lymph nodes of** head, face, and neck
         **CC Excl:** PDX collection 427

     **C84.Z2**   **Other mature T/NK-cell lymphomas,**   `HIV` `CC` `HCC`
         intrathoracic **lymph nodes**
         **CC Excl:** PDX collection 428

☑ Additional Character Req    ✓x7th Placeholder Alert    Unacceptable PDx    Manifestation    `H1`-`H14` HAC    `HCC` CMS-HCC Condition    *EXCLUDES 1* Not Coded Here    *EXCLUDES 2* Not Included Here

**ICD-10-CM 2018**      **483**

**Chapter 2. Neoplasms**

**C84.Z3** **Other mature T/NK-cell lymphomas, intra-** `HIV` `CC` `HCC`
**abdominal lymph nodes**
    CC Excl: PDX collection 429

**C84.Z4** **Other mature T/NK-cell lymphomas,** `HIV` `CC` `HCC`
**lymph nodes of axilla and upper limb**
    CC Excl: PDX collection 430

**C84.Z5** **Other mature T/NK-cell lymphomas,** `HIV` `CC` `HCC`
**lymph nodes of inguinal region and lower limb**
    CC Excl: PDX collection 431

**C84.Z6** **Other mature T/NK-cell lymphomas,** `HIV` `CC` `HCC`
**intrapelvic lymph nodes**
    CC Excl: PDX collection 432

**C84.Z7** **Other mature T/NK-cell lymphomas,** `HIV` `CC` `HCC`
**spleen**
    CC Excl: PDX collection 433

**C84.Z8** **Other mature T/NK-cell lymphomas,** `HIV` `CC` `HCC`
**lymph ndoes of multiple sites**
    CC Excl: PDX collection 434

**C84.Z9** **Other mature T/NK-cell lymphomas,** `HIV` `CC` `HCC`
**extranodal and solid organ sites**
    CC Excl: PDX collection 426

✓5th **C84.9** **Mature T/NK-cell lymphomas, unspecified**
NK/T cell lymphoma NOS
> **EXCLUDES 1**   mature T-cell lymphoma, not elsewhere classified
> (C84.4-)

**C84.90** **Mature T/NK-cell lymphomas, unspecified,** `HIV` `CC` `HCC`
**unspecified site**
    CC Excl: PDX collection 426

**C84.91** **Mature T/NK-cell lymphomas,** `HIV` `CC` `HCC`
**unspecified, lymph nodes of head, face, and neck**
    CC Excl: PDX collection 427

**C84.92** **Mature T/NK-cell lymphomas, unspecified,** `HIV` `CC` `HCC`
**intrathoracic lymph nodes**
    CC Excl: PDX collection 428

**C84.93** **Mature T/NK-cell lymphomas, unspecified,** `HIV` `CC` `HCC`
**intra-abdominal lymph nodes**
    CC Excl: PDX collection 429

**C84.94** **Mature T/NK-cell lymphomas,** `HIV` `CC` `HCC`
**unspecified, lymph nodes of axilla and upper limb**
    CC Excl: PDX collection 430

**C84.95** **Mature T/NK-cell lymphomas,** `HIV` `CC` `HCC`
**unspecified, lymph nodes of inguinal**
**region and lower limb**
    CC Excl: PDX collection 431

**C84.96** **Mature T/NK-cell lymphomas, unspecified,** `HIV` `CC` `HCC`
**intrapelvic lymph nodes**
    CC Excl: PDX collection 432

**C84.97** **Mature T/NK-cell lymphomas,** `HIV` `CC` `HCC`
**unspecified, spleen**
    CC Excl: PDX collection 433

**C84.98** **Mature T/NK-cell lymphomas,** `HIV` `CC` `HCC`
**unspecified, lymph nodes of multiple sites**
    CC Excl: PDX collection 434

**C84.99** **Mature T/NK-cell lymphomas, unspecified,** `HIV` `CC` `HCC`
**extranodal and solid organ sites**
    CC Excl: PDX collection 426

✓4th **C85** **Other specified and unspecified types of non-Hodgkin**
**lymphoma**
> **EXCLUDES 1**   other specified types of T/NK-cell lymphoma (C86.-)
> personal history of non-Hodgkin lymphoma (Z85.72)

✓5th **C85.1** **Unspecified B-cell lymphoma**
> **NOTE**   If B-cell lineage or involvement is mentioned in
> conjunction with a specific lymphoma, code to the
> more specific description.

**C85.10** **Unspecified B-cell lymphoma,** `HIV` `CC` `HCC`
**unspecified site**
    CC Excl: PDX collection 426

**C85.11** **Unspecified B-cell lymphoma, lymph** `HIV` `CC` `HCC`
**nodes of head, face, and neck**
    CC Excl: PDX collection 427

**C85.12** **Unspecified B-cell lymphoma,** `HIV` `CC` `HCC`
**intrathoracic lymph nodes**
    CC Excl: PDX collection 428

**C85.13** **Unspecified B-cell lymphoma,** `HIV` `CC` `HCC`
**intra-abdominal lymph nodes**
    CC Excl: PDX collection 429

**C85.14** **Unspecified B-cell lymphoma, lymph** `HIV` `CC` `HCC`
**nodes of axilla and upper limb**
    CC Excl: PDX collection 430

**C85.15** **Unspecified B-cell lymphoma, lymph** `HIV` `CC` `HCC`
**nodes of inguinal region and lower limb**
    CC Excl: PDX collection 431

**C85.16** **Unspecified B-cell lymphoma, intrapelvic** `HIV` `CC` `HCC`
**lymph nodes**
    CC Excl: PDX collection 432

**C85.17** **Unspecified B-cell lymphoma, spleen** `HIV` `CC` `HCC`
    CC Excl: PDX collection 433

**C85.18** **Unspecified B-cell lymphoma, lymph** `HIV` `CC` `HCC`
**nodes of multiple sites**
    CC Excl: PDX collection 434

**C85.19** **Unspecified B-cell lymphoma, extranodal** `HIV` `CC` `HCC`
**and solid organ sites**
    CC Excl: PDX collection 426

✓5th **C85.2** **Mediastinal (thymic) large B-cell lymphoma**

**C85.20** **Mediastinal (thymic) large B-cell** `HIV` `CC` `HCC`
**lymphoma, unspecified site**
    CC Excl: PDX collection 426

**C85.21** **Mediastinal (thymic) large B-cell** `HIV` `CC` `HCC`
**lymphoma, lymph nodes of head, face, and neck**
    CC Excl: PDX collection 427

**C85.22** **Mediastinal (thymic) large B-cell** `HIV` `CC` `HCC`
**lymphoma, intrathoracic lymph nodes**
    CC Excl: PDX collection 428

**C85.23** **Mediastinal (thymic) large B-cell** `HIV` `CC` `HCC`
**lymphoma, intra-abdominal lymph nodes**
    CC Excl: PDX collection 429

**C85.24** **Mediastinal (thymic) large B-cell** `HIV` `CC` `HCC`
**lymphoma, lymph nodes of axilla and upper limb**
    CC Excl: PDX collection 430

**C85.25** **Mediastinal (thymic) large B-cell** `HIV` `CC` `HCC`
**lymphoma, lymph nodes of inguinal**
**region and lower limb**
    CC Excl: PDX collection 431

**C85.26** **Mediastinal (thymic) large B-cell** `HIV` `CC` `HCC`
**lymphoma, intrapelvic lymph nodes**
    CC Excl: PDX collection 432

**C85.27** **Mediastinal (thymic) large B-cell** `HIV` `CC` `HCC`
**lymphoma, spleen**
    CC Excl: PDX collection 433

**C85.28** **Mediastinal (thymic) large B-cell** `HIV` `CC` `HCC`
**lymphoma, lymph nodes of multiple sites**
    CC Excl: PDX collection 434

**C85.29** **Mediastinal (thymic) large B-cell** `HIV` `CC` `HCC`
**lymphoma, extranodal and solid organ sites**
    CC Excl: PDX collection 426

✓5th **C85.8** **Other specified types of non-Hodgkin lymphoma**

**C85.80** **Other specified types of non-Hodgkin** `HIV` `CC` `HCC`
**lymphoma, unspecified site**
    CC Excl: PDX collection 426

**C85.81** **Other specified types of non-Hodgkin** `HIV` `CC` `HCC`
**lymphoma, lymph nodes of head, face, and neck**
    CC Excl: PDX collection 427

**C85.82** **Other specified types of non-Hodgkin** `HIV` `CC` `HCC`
**lymphoma, intrathoracic lymph nodes**
    CC Excl: PDX collection 428

**C85.83** **Other specified types of non-Hodgkin** `HIV` `CC` `HCC`
**lymphoma, intra-abdominal lymph nodes**
    CC Excl: PDX collection 429

**C85.84** **Other specified types of non-Hodgkin** `HIV` `CC` `HCC`
**lymphoma, lymph nodes of axilla and upper limb**
    CC Excl: PDX collection 430

**C85.85** **Other specified types of non-Hodgkin** `HIV` `CC` `HCC`
**lymphoma, lymph nodes of inguinal region**
**and lower limb**
    CC Excl: PDX collection 431

**C85.86** **Other specified types of non-Hodgkin** `HIV` `CC` `HCC`
**lymphoma, intrapelvic lymph nodes**
    CC Excl: PDX collection 432

**C85.87** **Other specified types of non-Hodgkin** `HIV` `CC` `HCC`
**lymphoma, spleen**
    CC Excl: PDX collection 433

**C85.88** **Other specified types of non-Hodgkin** `HIV` `CC` `HCC`
**lymphoma, lymph nodes of multiple sites**
    CC Excl: PDX collection 434

**C85.89** **Other specified types of non-Hodgkin** `HIV` `CC` `HCC`
**lymphoma, extranodal and solid organ sites**
    CC Excl: PDX collection 426

N Newborn: 0   P Pediatric: 0-17   M Maternity: 12-55   A Adult: 15-124   `MCC` Major CC Condition   `PDxMCC` PDx acts as own MCC   `CC` CC Condition   `PDxCC` PDx acts as own CC

**484**                                            ICD-10-CM 2018

☑5ᵗʰ **C85.9 Non-Hodgkin lymphoma, unspecified**
Lymphoma NOS
Malignant lymphoma NOS
Non-Hodgkin lymphoma NOS

**C85.90 Non-Hodgkin lymphoma, unspecified, unspecified site** `HIV` `CC` `HCC`
CC Excl: PDX collection 426

**C85.91 Non-Hodgkin lymphoma, unspecified, lymph nodes of head, face, and neck** `HIV` `CC` `HCC`
CC Excl: PDX collection 427

**C85.92 Non-Hodgkin lymphoma, unspecified, intrathoracic lymph nodes** `HIV` `CC` `HCC`
CC Excl: PDX collection 428

**C85.93 Non-Hodgkin lymphoma, unspecified, intra-abdominal lymph nodes** `HIV` `CC` `HCC`
CC Excl: PDX collection 429

**C85.94 Non-Hodgkin lymphoma, unspecified, lymph nodes of axilla and upper limb** `HIV` `CC` `HCC`
CC Excl: PDX collection 430

**C85.95 Non-Hodgkin lymphoma, unspecified, lymph nodes of inguinal region and lower limb** `HIV` `CC` `HCC`
CC Excl: PDX collection 431

**C85.96 Non-Hodgkin lymphoma, unspecified, intrapelvic lymph nodes** `HIV` `CC` `HCC`
CC Excl: PDX collection 432

**C85.97 Non-Hodgkin lymphoma, unspecified, spleen** `HIV` `CC` `HCC`
CC Excl: PDX collection 433

**C85.98 Non-Hodgkin lymphoma, unspecified, lymph nodes of multiple sites** `HIV` `CC` `HCC`
CC Excl: PDX collection 434

**C85.99 Non-Hodgkin lymphoma, unspecified, extranodal and solid organ sites** `HIV` `CC` `HCC`
CC Excl: PDX collection 426

☑4ᵗʰ **C86 Other specified types of T/NK-cell lymphoma**
*EXCLUDES 1*   anaplastic large cell lymphoma, ALK negative (C84.7-)
anaplastic large cell lymphoma, ALK positive (C84.6-)
mature T/NK-cell lymphomas (C84.-)
other specified types of non-Hodgkin lymphoma (C85.8-)

**C86.0 Extranodal NK/T-cell lymphoma, nasal type** `HIV` `CC` `HCC`
CC Excl: PDX collection 427

**C86.1 Hepatosplenic T-cell lymphoma** `HIV` `CC` `HCC`
Alpha-beta and gamma delta types
CC Excl: PDX collection 433

**C86.2 Enteropathy-type (intestinal) T-cell lymphoma** `HIV` `CC` `HCC`
Enteropathy associated T-cell lymphoma
CC Excl: PDX collection 429

**C86.3 Subcutaneous panniculitis-like T-cell lymphoma** `HIV` `CC` `HCC`
CC Excl: PDX collection 429

**C86.4 Blastic NK-cell lymphoma** `HIV` `CC` `HCC`
▶Blastic plasmacytoid dendritic cell neoplasm (BPDCN)◀
CC Excl: PDX collection 426

**C86.5 Angioimmunoblastic T-cell lymphoma** `HIV` `CC` `HCC`
Angioimmunoblastic lymphadenopathy with dysproteinemia [AILD]
CC Excl: PDX collection 435

**C86.6 Primary cutaneous CD30-positive T-cell proliferations** `HIV` `CC` `HCC`
Lymphomatoid papulosis
Primary cutaneous anaplastic large cell lymphoma
Primary cutaneous CD30-positive large T-cell lymphoma
CC Excl: PDX collection 435

☑4ᵗʰ **C88 Malignant immunoproliferative diseases and certain other B-cell lymphomas**
*EXCLUDES 1*   B-cell lymphoma, unspecified (C85.1-)
personal history of other malignant neoplasms of lymphoid, hematopoietic and related tissues (Z85.79)

**C88.0 Waldenström macroglobulinemia** `HCC`
Lymphoplasmacytic lymphoma with IgM-production
Macroglobulinemia (idiopathic) (primary)
*EXCLUDES 1*   small cell B-cell lymphoma (C83.0)

**C88.2 Heavy chain disease** `CC` `HCC`
Franklin disease
Gamma heavy chain disease
Mu heavy chain disease
CC Excl: PDX collection 485

**C88.3 Immunoproliferative small intestinal disease** `CC` `HCC`
Alpha heavy chain disease
Mediterranean lymphoma
CC Excl: PDX collection 485

**C88.4 Extranodal marginal zone B-cell lymphoma of mucosa-associated lymphoid tissue [MALT-lymphoma]** `HIV` `CC` `HCC`
Lymphoma of skin-associated lymphoid tissue [SALT-lymphoma]
Lymphoma of bronchial-associated lymphoid tissue [BALT-lymphoma]
*EXCLUDES 1*   high malignant (diffuse large B-cell) lymphoma (C83.3-)
CC Excl: PDX collection 426

**C88.8 Other malignant immunoproliferative diseases** `CC` `HCC`
CC Excl: PDX collection 486

**C88.9 Malignant immunoproliferative disease, unspecified** `CC` `HCC`
Immunoproliferative disease NOS
CC Excl: PDX collection 485

☑4ᵗʰ **C90 Multiple myeloma and malignant plasma cell neoplasms**
*EXCLUDES 1*   personal history of other malignant neoplasms of lymphoid, hematopoietic and related tissues (Z85.79)

> **CC Excl: For CC codes in category C90:** PDX collection 485

☑5ᵗʰ **C90.0 Multiple myeloma**
Kahler's disease
Medullary plasmacytoma
Myelomatosis
Plasma cell myeloma
*EXCLUDES 1*   solitary myeloma (C90.3-)
solitary plasmacytoma (C90.3-)

**C90.00 Multiple myeloma not having achieved remission** `CC` `HCC`
Multiple myeloma with failed remission
Multiple myeloma NOS

**C90.01 Multiple myeloma in remission** `CC` `HCC`
**C90.02 Multiple myeloma in relapse** `CC` `HCC`

☑5ᵗʰ **C90.1 Plasma cell leukemia**
Plasmacytic leukemia

**C90.10 Plasma cell leukemia not having achieved remission** `CC` `HCC`
Plasma cell leukemia with failed remission
Plasma cell leukemia NOS

**C90.11 Plasma cell leukemia in remission** `CC` `HCC`
**C90.12 Plasma cell leukemia in relapse** `CC` `HCC`

☑5ᵗʰ **C90.2 Extramedullary plasmacytoma**

**C90.20 Extramedullary plasmacytoma not having achieved remission** `CC` `HCC`
Extramedullary plasmacytoma with failed remission
Extramedullary plasmacytoma NOS

**C90.21 Extramedullary plasmacytoma in remission** `CC` `HCC`
**C90.22 Extramedullary plasmacytoma in relapse** `CC` `HCC`

☑5ᵗʰ **C90.3 Solitary plasmacytoma**
Localized malignant plasma cell tumor NOS
Plasmacytoma NOS
Solitary myeloma

**C90.30 Solitary plasmacytoma not having achieved remission** `CC` `HCC`
Solitary plasmacytoma with failed remission
Solitary plasmacytoma NOS

**C90.31 Solitary plasmacytoma in remission** `CC` `HCC`
**C90.32 Solitary plasmacytoma in relapse** `CC` `HCC`

☑4ᵗʰ **C91 Lymphoid leukemia**
*EXCLUDES 1*   personal history of leukemia (Z85.6)

> **CC Excl: For CC codes in category C91, unless otherwise noted:** PDX collection 485

☑5ᵗʰ **C91.0 Acute lymphoblastic leukemia [ALL]**
**NOTE**   Code C91.0 should only be used for T-cell and B-cell precursor leukemia

**C91.00 Acute lymphoblastic leukemia not having achieved remission** `CC` `HCC`
Acute lymphoblastic leukemia with failed remission
Acute lymphoblastic leukemia NOS

**C91.01 Acute lymphoblastic leukemia, in remission** `CC` `HCC`
**C91.02 Acute lymphoblastic leukemia, in relapse** `CC` `HCC`

---

☑ Additional Character Req   ☑x7ᵗʰ Placeholder Alert   Unacceptable PDx   Manifestation   `H1`-`H14` HAC   `HCC` CMS-HCC Condition   *EXCLUDES 1* Not Coded Here   *EXCLUDES 2* Not Included Here

ICD-10-CM 2018        485

C85.9–C91.02

✓5ᵗʰ **C91.1** Chronic lymphocytic **leukemia of** B-cell type
Lymphoplasmacytic leukemia
Richter syndrome
**EXCLUDES 1** *lymphoplasmacytic lymphoma (C83.0-)*

    **C91.10** **Chronic lymphocytic leukemia of B-cell type** CC HCC
**not having achieved remission**
Chronic lymphocytic leukemia of B-cell type with
failed remission
Chronic lymphocytic leukemia of B-cell type NOS

    **C91.11** **Chronic lymphocytic leukemia of B-cell type** CC HCC
**in remission**

    **C91.12** **Chronic lymphocytic leukemia of B-cell type** CC HCC
**in relapse**

✓5ᵗʰ **C91.3** Prolymphocytic **leukemia of** B-cell type

    **C91.30** **Prolymphocytic leukemia of B-cell type not** CC HCC
**having achieved remission**
Prolymphocytic leukemia of B-cell type with failed
remission
Prolymphocytic leukemia of B-cell type NOS

    **C91.31** **Prolymphocytic leukemia of B-cell type, in** CC HCC
**remission**

    **C91.32** **Prolymphocytic leukemia of B-cell type, in** CC HCC
**relapse**

✓5ᵗʰ **C91.4** Hairy cell **leukemia**
Leukemic reticuloendotheliosis

**CC Excl: For CC codes in subcategory C91.4:**
PDX collection 487

    **C91.40** **Hairy cell leukemia not having achieved** CC HCC
**remission**
Hairy cell leukemia with failed remission
Hairy cell leukemia NOS

    **C91.41** **Hairy cell leukemia, in remission** CC HCC

    **C91.42** **Hairy cell leukemia, in relapse** CC HCC

✓5ᵗʰ **C91.5** Adult T-cell **lymphoma/leukemia (HTLV-1-associated)**
Acute variant of adult T-cell lymphoma/leukemia (HTLV-1-
associated)
Chronic variant of adult T-cell lymphoma/leukemia (HTLV-1-
associated)
Lymphomatoid variant of adult T-cell lymphoma/leukemia
(HTLV-1-associated)
Smouldering variant of adult T-cell lymphoma/leukemia (HTLV-
1-associated)

    **C91.50** **Adult T-cell lymphoma/leukemia (HTLV-1-** CC HCC A
**associated) not having achieved remission**
Adult T-cell lymphoma/leukemia (HTLV-1-associated)
with failed remission
Adult T-cell lymphoma/leukemia (HTLV-1-associated)
NOS

    **C91.51** **Adult T-cell lymphoma/leukemia** CC HCC A
**(HTLV-1-associated), in remission**

    **C91.52** **Adult T-cell lymphoma/leukemia** CC HCC A
**(HTLV-1-associated), in relapse**

✓5ᵗʰ **C91.6** Prolymphocytic **leukemia of** T-cell type

    **C91.60** **Prolymphocytic leukemia of T-cell type not** CC HCC
**having achieved remission**
Prolymphocytic leukemia of T-cell type with failed
remission
Prolymphocytic leukemia of T-cell type NOS

    **C91.61** **Prolymphocytic leukemia of T-cell type, in** CC HCC
**remission**

    **C91.62** **Prolymphocytic leukemia of T-cell type, in** CC HCC
**relapse**

✓5ᵗʰ **C91.A** Mature B-cell **leukemia** Burkitt-type
**EXCLUDES 1** *Burkitt lymphoma (C83.7-)*

    **C91.A0** **Mature B-cell leukemia Burkitt-type not** CC HCC
**having achieved remission**
Mature B-cell leukemia Burkitt-type with failed
remission
Mature B-cell leukemia Burkitt-type NOS

    **C91.A1** **Mature B-cell leukemia Burkitt-type, in** CC HCC
**remission**

    **C91.A2** **Mature B-cell leukemia Burkitt-type,** CC HCC
**in relapse**

✓5ᵗʰ **C91.Z** Other **lymphoid leukemia**
T-cell large granular lymphocytic leukemia (associated with
rheumatoid arthritis)

    **C91.Z0** **Other lymphoid leukemia not having** CC HCC
**achieved remission**
Other lymphoid leukemia with failed remission
Other lymphoid leukemia NOS

    **C91.Z1** **Other lymphoid leukemia, in remission** CC HCC

    **C91.Z2** **Other lymphoid leukemia, in relapse** CC HCC

✓5ᵗʰ **C91.9** Lymphoid leukemia, **unspecified**

    **C91.90** **Lymphoid leukemia, unspecified not having** CC HCC
**achieved remission**
Lymphoid leukemia with failed remission
Lymphoid leukemia NOS

    **C91.91** **Lymphoid leukemia, unspecified,** CC HCC
**in remission**

    **C91.92** **Lymphoid leukemia, unspecified, in relapse** CC HCC

✓4ᵗʰ **C92** **Myeloid leukemia**
**INCLUDES** granulocytic leukemia
myelogenous leukemia
**EXCLUDES 1** *personal history of leukemia (Z85.6)*

**CC Excl: For CC codes in category C92:** PDX collection 485

✓5ᵗʰ **C92.0** Acute myeloblastic **leukemia**
Acute myeloblastic leukemia, minimal differentiation
Acute myeloblastic leukemia (with maturation)
Acute myeloblastic leukemia 1/ETO
Acute myeloblastic leukemia M0
Acute myeloblastic leukemia M1
Acute myeloblastic leukemia M2
Acute myeloblastic leukemia with t(8;21)
Acute myeloblastic leukemia (without a FAB classification) NOS
Refractory anemia with excess blasts in transformation [RAEB T]
**EXCLUDES 1** *acute exacerbation of chronic myeloid leukemia*
*(C92.10)*
*refractory anemia with excess of blasts not in*
*transformation (D46.2-)*

    **C92.00** **Acute myeloblastic leukemia, not having** CC HCC
**achieved remission**
Acute myeloblastic leukemia with failed remission
Acute myeloblastic leukemia NOS

    **C92.01** **Acute myeloblastic leukemia, in remission** CC HCC

    **C92.02** **Acute myeloblastic leukemia, in relapse** CC HCC

✓5ᵗʰ **C92.1** Chronic **myeloid leukemia,** BCR/ABL-positive
Chronic myelogenous leukemia, Philadelphia chromosome
(Ph1) positive
Chronic myelogenous leukemia, t(9;22) (q34;q11)
Chronic myelogenous leukemia with crisis of blast cells
**EXCLUDES 1** *atypical chronic myeloid leukemia BCR/ABL-negative*
*(C92.2-)*
*chronic myelomonocytic leukemia (C93.1-)*
*chronic myeloproliferative disease (D47.1)*

    **C92.10** **Chronic myeloid leukemia, BCR/ABL-positive,** CC HCC
**not having achieved remission**
Chronic myeloid leukemia, BCR/ABL-positive with
failed remission
Chronic myeloid leukemia, BCR/ABL-positive NOS

    **C92.11** **Chronic myeloid leukemia, BCR/ABL-positive,** CC HCC
**in remission**

    **C92.12** **Chronic myeloid leukemia, BCR/ABL-positive,** CC HCC
**in relapse**

✓5ᵗʰ **C92.2** Atypical chronic **myeloid leukemia,** BCR/ABL-negative

    **C92.20** **Atypical chronic myeloid leukemia,** CC HCC
**BCR/ABL-negative, not having achieved remission**
Atypical chronic myeloid leukemia, BCR/ABL-
negative with failed remission
Atypical chronic myeloid leukemia, BCR/ABL-
negative NOS

    **C92.21** **Atypical chronic myeloid leukemia,** CC HCC
**BCR/ABL-negative, in remission**

    **C92.22** **Atypical chronic myeloid leukemia,** CC HCC
**BCR/ABL-negative, in relapse**

✓5ᵗʰ **C92.3** Myeloid **sarcoma**
A malignant tumor of immature myeloid cells
Chloroma
Granulocytic sarcoma

    **C92.30** **Myeloid sarcoma, not having achieved** CC HCC
**remission**
Myeloid sarcoma with failed remission
Myeloid sarcoma NOS

N Newborn: 0   P Pediatric: 0-17   M Maternity: 12-55   A Adult: 15-124   MCC Major CC Condition   PDxMCC PDx acts as own MCC   CC CC Condition   PDxCC PDx acts as own CC

486                                                 ICD-10-CM 2018

**C92.31**    Myeloid sarcoma, in remission    `CC` `HCC`

**C92.32**    Myeloid sarcoma, in relapse    `CC` `HCC`

√5th **C92.4**   Acute promyelocytic leukemia
AML M3
AML Me with t(15;17) and variants

**C92.40**    Acute promyelocytic leukemia, not having achieved remission    `CC` `HCC`
Acute promyelocytic leukemia with failed remission
Acute promyelocytic leukemia NOS

**C92.41**    Acute promyelocytic leukemia, in remission    `CC` `HCC`

**C92.42**    Acute promyelocytic leukemia, in relapse    `CC` `HCC`

√5th **C92.5**   Acute myelomonocytic leukemia
AML M4
AML M4 Eo with inv(16) or t(16;16)

**C92.50**    Acute myelomonocytic leukemia, not having achieved remission    `CC` `HCC`
Acute myelomonocytic leukemia with failed remission
Acute myelomonocytic leukemia NOS

**C92.51**    Acute myelomonocytic leukemia, in remission    `CC` `HCC`

**C92.52**    Acute myelomonocytic leukemia, in relapse    `CC` `HCC`

√5th **C92.6**   Acute myeloid leukemia with 11q23-abnormality
Acute myeloid leukemia with variation of MLL-gene

**C92.60**    Acute myeloid leukemia with 11q23-abnormality not having achieved remission    `CC` `HCC`
Acute myeloid leukemia with 11q23-abnormality with failed remission
Acute myeloid leukemia with 11q23-abnormality NOS

**C92.61**    Acute myeloid leukemia with 11q23-abnormality in remission    `CC` `HCC`

**C92.62**    Acute myeloid leukemia with 11q23-abnormality in relapse    `CC` `HCC`

√5th **C92.A**   Acute myeloid leukemia with multilineage dysplasia
Acute myeloid leukemia with dysplasia of remaining hematopoesis and/or myelodysplastic disease in its history

**C92.A0**    Acute myeloid leukemia with multilineage dysplasia, not having achieved remission    `CC` `HCC`
Acute myeloid leukemia with multilineage dysplasia with failed remission
Acute myeloid leukemia with multilineage dysplasia NOS

**C92.A1**    Acute myeloid leukemia with multilineage dysplasia, in remission    `CC` `HCC`

**C92.A2**    Acute myeloid leukemia with multilineage dysplasia, in relapse    `CC` `HCC`

√5th **C92.Z**   Other myeloid leukemia

**C92.Z0**    Other myeloid leukemia not having achieved remission    `CC` `HCC`
Myeloid leukemia NEC with failed remission
Myeloid leukemia NEC

**C92.Z1**    Other myeloid leukemia, in remission    `CC` `HCC`

**C92.Z2**    Other myeloid leukemia, in relapse    `CC` `HCC`

√5th **C92.9**   Myeloid leukemia, unspecified

**C92.90**    Myeloid leukemia, unspecified, not having achieved remission    `CC` `HCC`
Myeloid leukemia, unspecified with failed remission
Myeloid leukemia, unspecified NOS

**C92.91**    Myeloid leukemia, unspecified in remission    `CC` `HCC`

**C92.92**    Myeloid leukemia, unspecified in relapse    `CC` `HCC`

√4th **C93**   Monocytic leukemia
`INCLUDES`   monocytoid leukemia
`EXCLUDES 1`   personal history of leukemia (Z85.6))

CC Excl: For CC codes in category C93: PDX collection 485

√5th **C93.0**   Acute monoblastic/monocytic leukemia
AML M5      AML M5b
AML M5a

**C93.00**    Acute monoblastic/monocytic leukemia, not having achieved remission    `CC` `HCC`
Acute monoblastic/monocytic leukemia with failed remission
Acute monoblastic/monocytic leukemia NOS

**C93.01**    Acute monoblastic/monocytic leukemia, in remission    `CC` `HCC`

**C93.02**    Acute monoblastic/monocytic leukemia, in relapse    `CC` `HCC`

√5th **C93.1**   Chronic myelomonocytic leukemia
Chronic monocytic leukemia
CMML-1
CMML-2
CMML with eosinophilia

**C93.10**    Chronic myelomonocytic leukemia not having achieved remission    `CC` `HCC`
Chronic myelomonocytic leukemia with failed remission
Chronic myelomonocytic leukemia NOS

**C93.11**    Chronic myelomonocytic leukemia, in remission    `CC` `HCC`

**C93.12**    Chronic myelomonocytic leukemia, in relapse    `CC` `HCC`

√5th **C93.3**   Juvenile myelomonocytic leukemia

**C93.30**    Juvenile myelomonocytic leukemia, not having achieved remission    `CC` `HCC` `P`
Juvenile myelomonocytic leukemia with failed remission
Juvenile myelomonocytic leukemia NOS

**C93.31**    Juvenile myelomonocytic leukemia, in remission    `CC` `HCC` `P`

**C93.32**    Juvenile myelomonocytic leukemia, in relapse    `CC` `HCC` `P`

√5th **C93.Z**   Other monocytic leukemia

**C93.Z0**    Other monocytic leukemia, not having achieved remission    `CC` `HCC`
Other monocytic leukemia NOS

**C93.Z1**    Other monocytic leukemia, in remission    `CC` `HCC`

**C93.Z2**    Other monocytic leukemia, in relapse    `CC` `HCC`

√5th **C93.9**   Monocytic leukemia, unspecified

**C93.90**    Monocytic leukemia, unspecified, not having achieved remission    `CC` `HCC`
Monocytic leukemia, unspecified with failed remission
Monocytic leukemia, unspecified NOS

**C93.91**    Monocytic leukemia, unspecified in remission    `CC` `HCC`

**C93.92**    Monocytic leukemia, unspecified in relapse    `CC` `HCC`

√4th **C94**   Other leukemias of specified cell type
`EXCLUDES 1`   leukemic reticuloendotheliosis (C91.4-)
      myelodysplastic syndromes (D46.-)
      personal history of leukemia (Z85.6)
      plasma cell leukemia (C90.1-)

CC Excl: For CC codes in category C94, unless otherwise noted:
PDX collection 485

√5th **C94.0**   Acute erythroid leukemia
Acute myeloid leukemia M6(a)(b)
Erythroleukemia
**DEF:** Erythroleukemia: A malignant blood dyscrasia (a myeloproliferative disorder).

**C94.00**    Acute erythroid leukemia, not having achieved remission    `CC` `HCC`
Acute erythroid leukemia with failed remission
Acute erythroid leukemia NOS

**C94.01**    Acute erythroid leukemia, in remission    `CC` `HCC`

**C94.02**    Acute erythroid leukemia, in relapse    `CC` `HCC`

√5th **C94.2**   Acute megakaryoblastic leukemia
Acute myeloid leukemia M7
Acute megakaryocytic leukemia

**C94.20**    Acute megakaryoblastic leukemia not having achieved remission    `CC` `HCC`
Acute megakaryoblastic leukemia with failed remission
Acute megakaryoblastic leukemia NOS

**C94.21**    Acute megakaryoblastic leukemia, in remission    `CC` `HCC`

**C94.22**    Acute megakaryoblastic leukemia, in relapse    `CC` `HCC`

√5th **C94.3**   Mast cell leukemia

**C94.30**    Mast cell leukemia not having achieved remission    `CC` `HCC`
Mast cell leukemia with failed remission
Mast cell leukemia NOS

**C94.31**    Mast cell leukemia, in remission    `CC` `HCC`

**C94.32**    Mast cell leukemia, in relapse    `CC` `HCC`

☑ Additional Character Req   √7th Placeholder Alert   Unacceptable PDx   Manifestation   H1-H14 HAC   HCC CMS-HCC Condition   EXCLUDES 1 Not Coded Here   EXCLUDES 2 Not Included Here

ICD-10-CM 2018         487

**Chapter 2. Neoplasms**

**C94.4–D00.07**

✓5ᵗʰ **C94.4** **Acute panmyelosis with myelofibrosis**
Acute myelofibrosis
EXCLUDES 1    myelofibrosis NOS (D75.81)
         secondary myelofibrosis NOS (D75.81)

     **C94.40** **Acute panmyelosis with myelofibrosis not having achieved remission**   CC HCC
         Acute myelofibrosis NOS
         Acute panmyelosis with myelofibrosis with failed remission
         Acute panmyelosis NOS
         **CC Excl:** PDX collection 488

     **C94.41** **Acute panmyelosis with myelofibrosis, in remission**   CC HCC
         **CC Excl:** PDX collection 488

     **C94.42** **Acute panmyelosis with myelofibrosis, in relapse**   CC HCC
         **CC Excl:** PDX collection 488

  **C94.6** **Myelodysplastic disease, not classified**   CC HCC
     Myeloproliferative disease, not classified
     **CC Excl:** PDX collection 488

✓5ᵗʰ **C94.8** **Other specified leukemias**
Aggressive NK-cell leukemia
Acute basophilic leukemia

     **C94.80** **Other specified leukemias not having achieved remission**   CC HCC
         Other specified leukemia with failed remission
         Other specified leukemias NOS

     **C94.81** **Other specified leukemias, in remission**   CC HCC

     **C94.82** **Other specified leukemias, in relapse**   CC HCC

✓4ᵗʰ **C95** **Leukemia of unspecified cell type**
EXCLUDES 1   personal history of leukemia (Z85.6)

**CC Excl: For CC codes in category C95:** PDX collection 485

✓5ᵗʰ **C95.0** **Acute leukemia of unspecified cell type**
Acute bilineal leukemia
Acute mixed lineage leukemia
Biphenotypic acute leukemia
Stem cell leukemia of unclear lineage
EXCLUDES 1   acute exacerbation of unspecified chronic leukemia (C95.10)

     **C95.00** **Acute leukemia of unspecified cell type not having achieved remission**   CC HCC
         Acute leukemia of unspecified cell type with failed remission
         Acute leukemia NOS

     **C95.01** **Acute leukemia of unspecified cell type, in remission**   CC HCC

     **C95.02** **Acute leukemia of unspecified cell type, in relapse**   CC HCC

✓5ᵗʰ **C95.1** **Chronic leukemia of unspecified cell type**

     **C95.10** **Chronic leukemia of unspecified cell type not having achieved remission**   CC HCC
         Chronic leukemia of unspecified cell type with failed remission
         Chronic leukemia NOS

     **C95.11** **Chronic leukemia of unspecified cell type, in remission**   CC HCC

     **C95.12** **Chronic leukemia of unspecified cell type, in relapse**   CC HCC

✓5ᵗʰ **C95.9** **Leukemia, unspecified**

     **C95.90** **Leukemia, unspecified not having achieved remission**   CC HCC
         Leukemia, unspecified with failed remission
         Leukemia NOS

     **C95.91** **Leukemia, unspecified, in remission**   CC HCC

     **C95.92** **Leukemia, unspecified, in relapse**   CC HCC

✓4ᵗʰ **C96** **Other and unspecified malignant neoplasms of lymphoid, hematopoietic and related tissue**
EXCLUDES 1   personal history of other malignant neoplasms of lymphoid, hematopoietic and related tissues (Z85.79)

  **C96.0** **Multifocal and multisystemic (disseminated) Langerhans-cell histiocytosis**   CC HCC
     Histiocytosis X, multisystemic
     Letterer-Siwe disease
     EXCLUDES 1   adult pulmonary Langerhans cell histiocytosis (J84.82)
          multifocal and unisystemic Langerhans-cell histiocytosis (C96.5)
          unifocal Langerhans-cell histiocytosis (C96.6)
     **CC Excl:** PDX collection 489

▲ ✓5ᵗʰ **C96.2** **Malignant mast cell neoplasm**
~~Aggressive systemic mastocytosis~~
~~Mast cell sarcoma~~
EXCLUDES 1   indolent mastocytosis ▶(D47.02)◄
         mast cell leukemia (C94.30)
         mastocytosis (congenital) (cutaneous) (Q82.2)

**CC Excl: For codes in subcategory C96.2:** PDX collection 490

●      **C96.20** **Malignant mast cell neoplasm, unspecified**   CC
●      **C96.21** **Aggressive systemic mastocytosis**   CC
●      **C96.22** **Mast cell sarcoma**   CC
●      **C96.29** **Other malignant mast cell neoplasm**   CC

  **C96.4** **Sarcoma of dendritic cells (accessory cells)**   CC HCC
     Follicular dendritic cell sarcoma
     Interdigitating dendritic cell sarcoma
     Langerhans cell sarcoma
     **CC Excl:** PDX collection 491

  **C96.5** **Multifocal and unisystemic Langerhans-cell histiocytosis**   CC HCC
     Hand-Schüller-Christian disease
     Histiocytosis X, multifocal
     EXCLUDES 1   multifocal and multisystemic (disseminated) Langerhans-cell histiocytosis (C96.0)
          unifocal Langerhans-cell histiocytosis (C96.6)
     **CC Excl:** PDX collection 492

  **C96.6** **Unifocal Langerhans-cell histiocytosis**   CC HCC
     Eosinophilic granuloma
     Histiocytosis X, unifocal
     Histiocytosis X NOS
     Langerhans-cell histiocytosis NOS
     EXCLUDES 1   multifocal and multisysemic (disseminated) Langerhans-cell histiocytosis (C96.0)
          multifocal and unisystemic Langerhans-cell histiocytosis (C96.5)
     **CC Excl:** PDX collection 492

  **C96.A** **Histiocytic sarcoma**   CC HCC
     Malignant histiocytosis
     **CC Excl:** PDX collection 493

  **C96.Z** **Other specified malignant neoplasms of lymphoid, hematopoietic and related tissue**   CC HCC
     **CC Excl:** PDX collection 491

  **C96.9** **Malignant neoplasm of lymphoid, hematopoietic and related tissue, unspecified**   CC HCC
     **CC Excl:** PDX collection 491

### In situ neoplasms (D00-D09)

INCLUDES   Bowen's disease
         erythroplasia
         grade III intraepithelial neoplasia
         Queyrat's erythroplasia

✓4ᵗʰ **D00** **Carcinoma in situ of oral cavity, esophagus and stomach**
EXCLUDES 1   melanoma in situ (D03.-)

✓5ᵗʰ **D00.0** **Carcinoma in situ of lip, oral cavity and pharynx**
     Use additional code to identify:
     exposure to environmental tobacco smoke (Z77.22)
     exposure to tobacco smoke in the perinatal period (P96.81)
     history of tobacco dependence (Z87.891)
     occupational exposure to environmental tobacco smoke (Z57.31)
     tobacco dependence (F17.-)
     tobacco use (Z72.0)
     EXCLUDES 1   carcinoma in situ of aryepiglottic fold or interarytenoid fold, laryngeal aspect (D02.0)
          carcinoma in situ of epiglottis NOS (D02.0)
          carcinoma in situ of epiglottis suprahyoid portion (D02.0)
          carcinoma in situ of skin of lip (D03.0, D04.0)

     **D00.00** **Carcinoma in situ of oral cavity, unspecified site**

     **D00.01** **Carcinoma in situ of labial mucosa and vermilion border**

     **D00.02** **Carcinoma in situ of buccal mucosa**

     **D00.03** **Carcinoma in situ of gingiva and edentulous alveolar ridge**

     **D00.04** **Carcinoma in situ of soft palate**

     **D00.05** **Carcinoma in situ of hard palate**

     **D00.06** **Carcinoma in situ of floor of mouth**

     **D00.07** **Carcinoma in situ of tongue**

N Newborn: 0   P Pediatric: 0-17   M Maternity: 12-55   A Adult: 15-124   MCC Major CC Condition   PDx MCC PDx acts as own MCC   CC CC Condition   PDx CC PDx acts as own CC

488          ICD-10-CM 2018

**D00.08**   **Carcinoma in situ of** pharynx
Carcinoma in situ of aryepiglottic fold NOS
Carcinoma in situ of hypopharyngeal aspect of
aryepiglottic fold
Carcinoma in situ of marginal zone of aryepiglottic
fold

**D00.1**   **Carcinoma in situ of** esophagus

**D00.2**   **Carcinoma in situ of** stomach

✓4ᵗʰ **D01**   **Carcinoma in situ of** other and unspecified digestive organs
     *EXCLUDES 1*   *melanoma in situ (D03.-)*

   **D01.0**   **Carcinoma in situ of** colon
      *EXCLUDES 1*   *carcinoma in situ of rectosigmoid junction (D01.1)*

   **D01.1**   **Carcinoma in situ of** rectosigmoid junction

   **D01.2**   **Carcinoma in situ of** rectum

   **D01.3**   **Carcinoma in situ of** anus and anal canal
     Anal intraepithelial neoplasia III [AIN III]
     Severe dysplasia of anus
      *EXCLUDES 1*   *anal intraepithelial neoplasia I and II [AIN I and AIN II]*
           *(K62.82)*
           *carcinoma in situ of anal margin (D04.5)*
           *carcinoma in situ of anal skin (D04.5)*
           *carcinoma in situ of perianal skin (D04.5)*

   ✓5ᵗʰ **D01.4**   **Carcinoma in situ of other and unspecified parts of** intestine
      *EXCLUDES 1*   *carcinoma in situ of ampulla of Vater (D01.5)*

     **D01.40**   **Carcinoma in situ of** unspecified **part of intestine**

     **D01.49**   **Carcinoma in situ of** other **parts of intestine**

   **D01.5**   **Carcinoma in situ of** liver, gallbladder and bile ducts
     Carcinoma in situ of ampulla of Vater

   **D01.7**   **Carcinoma in situ of** other **specified digestive organs**
     Carcinoma in situ of pancreas

   **D01.9**   **Carcinoma in situ of digestive organ,** unspecified

✓4ᵗʰ **D02**   **Carcinoma in situ of** middle ear and respiratory system
     Use additional code to identify:
     exposure to environmental tobacco smoke (Z77.22)
     exposure to tobacco smoke in the perinatal period (P96.81)
     history of tobacco dependence (Z87.891)
     occupational exposure to environmental tobacco smoke (Z57.31)
     tobacco dependence (F17.-)
     tobacco use (Z72.0)
     *EXCLUDES 1*   *melanoma in situ (D03.-)*

   **D02.0**   **Carcinoma in situ of** larynx
     Carcinoma in situ of aryepiglottic fold or interarytenoid fold,
     laryngeal aspect
     Carcinoma in situ of epiglottis (suprahyoid portion)
      *EXCLUDES 1*   *carcinoma in situ of aryepiglottic fold or interarytenoid*
           *fold NOS (D00.08)*
           *carcinoma in situ of hypopharyngeal aspect (D00.08)*
           *carcinoma in situ of marginal zone (D00.08)*

   **D02.1**   **Carcinoma in situ of** trachea

   ✓5ᵗʰ **D02.2**   **Carcinoma in situ of** bronchus and lung

     **D02.20**   **Carcinoma in situ of** unspecified **bronchus and lung**

     **D02.21**   **Carcinoma in situ of** right **bronchus and lung**

     **D02.22**   **Carcinoma in situ of** left **bronchus and lung**

   **D02.3**   **Carcinoma in situ of** other **parts of respiratory system**
     Carcinoma in situ of accessory sinuses
     Carcinoma in situ of middle ear
     Carcinoma in situ of nasal cavities
      *EXCLUDES 1*   *carcinoma in situ of ear (external) (skin) (D04.2-)*
           *carcinoma in situ of nose NOS (D09.8)*
           *carcinoma in situ of skin of nose (D04.3)*

   **D02.4**   **Carcinoma in situ of respiratory system,** unspecified

✓4ᵗʰ **D03**   Melanoma **in situ**

   **D03.0**   **Melanoma in situ of** lip        `HCC`

   ✓5ᵗʰ **D03.1**   **Melanoma in situ of** eyelid, including canthus

     **D03.10**   **Melanoma in situ of** unspecified **eyelid,**    `HCC`
           **including canthus**

     **D03.11**   **Melanoma in situ of** right **eyelid, including**    `HCC`
           **canthus**

     **D03.12**   **Melanoma in situ of** left **eyelid, including**    `HCC`
           **canthus**

   ✓5ᵗʰ **D03.2**   **Melanoma in situ of** ear and external auricular canal

     **D03.20**   **Melanoma in situ of** unspecified **ear and**    `HCC`
           **external auricular canal**

     **D03.21**   **Melanoma in situ of** right **ear and external**    `HCC`
           **auricular canal**

**D03.22**   **Melanoma in situ of** left **ear and external**    `HCC`
      **auricular canal**

   ✓5ᵗʰ **D03.3**   **Melanoma in situ of** other and unspecified parts of face

     **D03.30**   **Melanoma in situ of** unspecified **part of face**   `HCC`

     **D03.39**   **Melanoma in situ of** other **parts of face**   `HCC`

   **D03.4**   **Melanoma in situ of** scalp and neck     `HCC`

   ✓5ᵗʰ **D03.5**   **Melanoma in situ of** trunk

     **D03.51**   **Melanoma in situ of** anal skin     `HCC`
           Melanoma in situ of anal margin
           Melanoma in situ of perianal skin

     **D03.52**   **Melanoma in situ of** breast (skin) (soft tissue)   `HCC`

     **D03.59**   **Melanoma in situ of** other part of trunk   `HCC`

   ✓5ᵗʰ **D03.6**   **Melanoma in situ of** upper limb, including shoulder

     **D03.60**   **Melanoma in situ of** unspecified **upper limb,**   `HCC`
           **including shoulder**

     **D03.61**   **Melanoma in situ of** right **upper limb, including**   `HCC`
           **shoulder**

     **D03.62**   **Melanoma in situ of** left **upper limb, including**   `HCC`
           **shoulder**

   ✓5ᵗʰ **D03.7**   **Melanoma in situ of** lower limb, including hip

     **D03.70**   **Melanoma in situ of** unspecified **lower limb,**   `HCC`
           **including hip**

     **D03.71**   **Melanoma in situ of** right **lower limb,**   `HCC`
           **including hip**

     **D03.72**   **Melanoma in situ of** left **lower limb,**   `HCC`
           **including hip**

   **D03.8**   **Melanoma in situ of** other sites     `HCC`
     Melanoma in situ of scrotum
      *EXCLUDES 1*   *carcinoma in situ of scrotum (D07.61)*

   **D03.9**   **Melanoma in situ,** unspecified     `HCC`

✓4ᵗʰ **D04**   **Carcinoma in situ of** skin
     *EXCLUDES 1*   *erythroplasia of Queyrat (penis) NOS (D07.4)*
           *melanoma in situ (D03.-)*

   **D04.0**   **Carcinoma in situ of skin of** lip
      *EXCLUDES 1*   *carcinoma in situ of vermilion border of lip (D00.01)*

   ✓5ᵗʰ **D04.1**   **Carcinoma in situ of skin of** eyelid, including canthus

     **D04.10**   **Carcinoma in situ of skin of** unspecified **eyelid,**
           **including canthus**

     **D04.11**   **Carcinoma in situ of skin of** right **eyelid, including**
           **canthus**

     **D04.12**   **Carcinoma in situ of skin of** left **eyelid, including**
           **canthus**

   ✓5ᵗʰ **D04.2**   **Carcinoma in situ of skin of** ear and external auricular canal

     **D04.20**   **Carcinoma in situ of skin of** unspecified **ear and**
           **external auricular canal**

     **D04.21**   **Carcinoma in situ of skin of** right **ear and external**
           **auricular canal**

     **D04.22**   **Carcinoma in situ of skin of** left **ear and external**
           **auricular canal**

   ✓5ᵗʰ **D04.3**   **Carcinoma in situ of skin of** other and unspecified parts of
     face

     **D04.30**   **Carcinoma in situ of skin of** unspecified **part of face**

     **D04.39**   **Carcinoma in situ of skin of** other **parts of face**

   **D04.4**   **Carcinoma in situ of skin of** scalp and neck

   **D04.5**   **Carcinoma in situ of skin of** trunk
     Carcinoma in situ of anal margin
     Carcinoma in situ of anal skin
     Carcinoma in situ of perianal skin
     Carcinoma in situ of skin of breast
      *EXCLUDES 1*   *carcinoma in situ of anus NOS (D01.3)*
           *carcinoma in situ of scrotum (D07.61)*
           *carcinoma in situ of skin of genital organs (D07.-)*

   ✓5ᵗʰ **D04.6**   **Carcinoma in situ of skin of** upper limb, including shoulder

     **D04.60**   **Carcinoma in situ of skin of** unspecified **upper limb,**
           **including shoulder**

     **D04.61**   **Carcinoma in situ of skin of** right **upper limb,**
           **including shoulder**

     **D04.62**   **Carcinoma in situ of skin of** left **upper limb, including**
           **shoulder**

   ✓5ᵗʰ **D04.7**   **Carcinoma in situ of skin of** lower limb, including hip

     **D04.70**   **Carcinoma in situ of skin of** unspecified **lower limb,**
           **including hip**

     **D04.71**   **Carcinoma in situ of skin of** right **lower limb,**
           **including hip**

---

☑ Additional Character Req    ✓x7ᵗʰ Placeholder Alert    Unacceptable PDx    Manifestation    H1-H14 HAC    HCC CMS-HCC Condition    *EXCLUDES 1* Not Coded Here    *EXCLUDES 2* Not Included Here

ICD-10-CM 2018                                    **489**

      **D04.72** Carcinoma in situ of skin of left lower limb, including hip

**D04.8** Carcinoma in situ of skin of other sites

**D04.9** Carcinoma in situ of skin, unspecified

✓4ᵗʰ **D05 Carcinoma in situ of breast**
> EXCLUDES 1    carcinoma in situ of skin of breast (D04.5)
> melanoma in situ of breast (skin) (D03.5)
> Paget's disease of breast or nipple (C50.-)

✓5ᵗʰ **D05.0 Lobular carcinoma in situ of breast**

    **D05.00** Lobular carcinoma in situ of unspecified breast

    **D05.01** Lobular carcinoma in situ of right breast

    **D05.02** Lobular carcinoma in situ of left breast

✓5ᵗʰ **D05.1 Intraductal carcinoma in situ of breast**

    **D05.10** Intraductal carcinoma in situ of unspecified breast

    **D05.11** Intraductal carcinoma in situ of right breast

    **D05.12** Intraductal carcinoma in situ of left breast

✓5ᵗʰ **D05.8 Other specified type of carcinoma in situ of breast**

    **D05.80** Other specified type of carcinoma in situ of unspecified breast

    **D05.81** Other specified type of carcinoma in situ of right breast

    **D05.82** Other specified type of carcinoma in situ of left breast

✓5ᵗʰ **D05.9 Unspecified type of carcinoma in situ of breast**

    **D05.90** Unspecified type of carcinoma in situ of unspecified breast

    **D05.91** Unspecified type of carcinoma in situ of right breast

    **D05.92** Unspecified type of carcinoma in situ of left breast

✓4ᵗʰ **D06 Carcinoma in situ of cervix uteri**
> INCLUDES    cervical adenocarcinoma in situ
> cervical intraepithelial glandular neoplasia
> cervical intraepithelial neoplasia III [CIN III]
> severe dysplasia of cervix uteri

> EXCLUDES 1    cervical intraepithelial neoplasia II [CIN II] (N87.1)
> cytologic evidence of malignancy of cervix without histologic confirmation (R87.614)
> high grade squamous intraepithelial lesion (HGSIL) of cervix (R87.613)
> melanoma in situ of cervix (D03.5)
> moderate cervical dysplasia (N87.1)

    **D06.0** Carcinoma in situ of endocervix     ♀

    **D06.1** Carcinoma in situ of exocervix     ♀

    **D06.7** Carcinoma in situ of other parts of cervix     ♀

    **D06.9** Carcinoma in situ of cervix, unspecified     ♀

✓4ᵗʰ **D07 Carcinoma in situ of other and unspecified genital organs**
> EXCLUDES 1    melanoma in situ of trunk (D03.5)

    **D07.0** Carcinoma in situ of endometrium     ♀

    **D07.1** Carcinoma in situ of vulva     ♀
       Severe dysplasia of vulva
       Vulvar intraepithelial neoplasia III [VIN III]
> EXCLUDES 1    moderate dysplasia of vulva (N90.1)
> vulvar intraepithelial neoplasia II [VIN II] (N90.1)

    **D07.2** Carcinoma in situ of vagina     ♀
       Severe dysplasia of vagina
       Vaginal intraepithelial neoplasia III [VAIN III ]
> EXCLUDES 1    moderate dysplasia of vagina (N89.1)
> vaginal intraepithelial neoplasia II [VIN II] (N89.1)

✓5ᵗʰ **D07.3 Carcinoma in situ of other and unspecified female genital organs**

    **D07.30** Carcinoma in situ of unspecified female genital organs     ♀

    **D07.39** Carcinoma in situ of other female genital organs     ♀

    **D07.4** Carcinoma in situ of penis     ♂
       Erythroplasia of Queyrat NOS

    **D07.5** Carcinoma in situ of prostate     ♂
       Prostatic intraepithelial neoplasia III (PIN III)
       Severe dysplasia of prostate
> EXCLUDES 1    dysplasia (mild) (moderate) of prostate (N42.3-)
> prostatic intraepithelial neoplasia II [PIN II] (N42.3-)

✓5ᵗʰ **D07.6 Carcinoma in situ of other and unspecified male genital organs**

    **D07.60** Carcinoma in situ of unspecified male genital organs     ♂

    **D07.61** Carcinoma in situ of scrotum     ♂

    **D07.69** Carcinoma in situ of other male genital organs     ♂

✓4ᵗʰ **D09 Carcinoma in situ of other and unspecified sites**
> EXCLUDES 1    melanoma in situ (D03.-)

    **D09.0** Carcinoma in situ of bladder

✓5ᵗʰ **D09.1 Carcinoma in situ of other and unspecified urinary organs**

    **D09.10** Carcinoma in situ of unspecified urinary organ

    **D09.19** Carcinoma in situ of other urinary organs

✓5ᵗʰ **D09.2 Carcinoma in situ of eye**
> EXCLUDES 1    carcinoma in situ of skin of eyelid (D04.1-)

    **D09.20** Carcinoma in situ of unspecified eye

    **D09.21** Carcinoma in situ of right eye

    **D09.22** Carcinoma in situ of left eye

    **D09.3** Carcinoma in situ of thyroid and other endocrine glands
> EXCLUDES 1    carcinoma in situ of endocrine pancreas (D01.7)
> carcinoma in situ of ovary (D07.39)
> carcinoma in situ of testis (D07.69)

    **D09.8** Carcinoma in situ of other specified sites

    **D09.9** Carcinoma in situ, unspecified

## Benign neoplasms, except benign neuroendocrine tumors (D10-D36)

✓4ᵗʰ **D10 Benign neoplasm of mouth and pharynx**

    **D10.0** Benign neoplasm of lip
       Benign neoplasm of lip (frenulum) (inner aspect) (mucosa) (vermilion border)
> EXCLUDES 1    benign neoplasm of skin of lip (D22.0, D23.0)

    **D10.1** Benign neoplasm of tongue
       Benign neoplasm of lingual tonsil

    **D10.2** Benign neoplasm of floor of mouth

✓5ᵗʰ **D10.3 Benign neoplasm of other and unspecified parts of mouth**

    **D10.30** Benign neoplasm of unspecified part of mouth

    **D10.39** Benign neoplasm of other parts of mouth
       Benign neoplasm of minor salivary gland NOS
> EXCLUDES 1    benign odontogenic neoplasms (D16.4-D16.5)
> benign neoplasm of mucosa of lip (D10.0)
> benign neoplasm of nasopharyngeal surface of soft palate (D10.6)

    **D10.4** Benign neoplasm of tonsil
       Benign neoplasm of tonsil (faucial) (palatine)
> EXCLUDES 1    benign neoplasm of lingual tonsil (D10.1)
> benign neoplasm of pharyngeal tonsil (D10.6)
> benign neoplasm of tonsillar fossa (D10.5)
> benign neoplasm of tonsillar pillars (D10.5)

    **D10.5** Benign neoplasm of other parts of oropharynx
       Benign neoplasm of epiglottis, anterior aspect
       Benign neoplasm of tonsillar fossa
       Benign neoplasm of tonsillar pillars
       Benign neoplasm of vallecula
> EXCLUDES 1    benign neoplasm of epiglottis NOS (D14.1)
> benign neoplasm of epiglottis, suprahyoid portion (D14.1)

    **D10.6** Benign neoplasm of nasopharynx
       Benign neoplasm of pharyngeal tonsil
       Benign neoplasm of posterior margin of septum and choanae

    **D10.7** Benign neoplasm of hypopharynx

    **D10.9** Benign neoplasm of pharynx, unspecified

✓4ᵗʰ **D11 Benign neoplasm of major salivary glands**
> EXCLUDES 1    benign neoplasms of specified minor salivary glands which are classified according to their anatomical location
> benign neoplasms of minor salivary glands NOS (D10.39)

    **D11.0** Benign neoplasm of parotid gland

    **D11.7** Benign neoplasm of other major salivary glands
       Benign neoplasm of sublingual salivary gland
       Benign neoplasm of submandibular salivary gland

    **D11.9** Benign neoplasm of major salivary gland, unspecified

✓4ᵗʰ **D12 Benign neoplasm of colon, rectum, anus and anal canal**
> EXCLUDES 1    benign carcinoid tumors of the large intestine, and rectum (D3A.02-)

    **AHA:** 2017, 1Q, 15; 2015, 2Q, 14

    **D12.0** Benign neoplasm of cecum
       Benign neoplasm of ileocecal valve

    **D12.1** Benign neoplasm of appendix
> EXCLUDES 1    benign carcinoid tumor of the appendix (D3A.020)

    **D12.2** Benign neoplasm of ascending colon

N Newborn: 0   P Pediatric: 0-17   M Maternity: 12-55   A Adult: 15-124   MCC Major CC Condition   PDxMCC PDx acts as own MCC   CC CC Condition   PDxCC PDx acts as own CC

490

ICD-10-CM 2018

**D12.3**   **Benign neoplasm of** transverse colon
     Benign neoplasm of hepatic flexure
     Benign neoplasm of splenic flexure
     AHA: 2017, 1Q, 16

**D12.4**   **Benign neoplasm of** descending colon

**D12.5**   **Benign neoplasm of** sigmoid colon

**D12.6**   **Benign neoplasm of colon,** unspecified
     Adenomatosis of colon
     Benign neoplasm of large intestine NOS
     Polyposis (hereditary) of colon
     *EXCLUDES 1*   *inflammatory polyp of colon (K51.4-)*
                *polyp of colon NOS (K63.5)*

**D12.7**   **Benign neoplasm of** rectosigmoid junction

**D12.8**   **Benign neoplasm of** rectum
     *EXCLUDES 1*   *benign carcinoid tumor of the rectum (D3A.Ø26)*

**D12.9**   **Benign neoplasm of** anus and anal canal
     Benign neoplasm of anus NOS
     *EXCLUDES 1*   *benign neoplasm of anal margin (D22.5, D23.5)*
                *benign neoplasm of anal skin (D22.5, D23.5)*
                *benign neoplasm of perianal skin (D22.5, D23.5)*

✓4ᵗʰ **D13**   **Benign neoplasm of** other and ill-defined parts of digestive system
     *EXCLUDES 1*   *benign stromal tumors of digestive system (D21.4)*

**D13.Ø**   **Benign neoplasm of** esophagus

**D13.1**   **Benign neoplasm of** stomach
     *EXCLUDES 1*   *benign carcinoid tumor of the stomach (D3A.Ø92)*

**D13.2**   **Benign neoplasm of** duodenum
     *EXCLUDES 1*   *benign carcinoid tumor of the duodenum (D3A.Ø10)*

✓5ᵗʰ **D13.3**   **Benign neoplasm of other and unspecified parts of** small intestine
     *EXCLUDES 1*   *benign carcinoid tumors of the small intestine (D3A.Ø1)*
                *benign neoplasm of ileocecal valve (D12.0)*

     **D13.3Ø**   **Benign neoplasm of** unspecified part **of small intestine**

     **D13.39**   **Benign neoplasm of** other parts **of small intestine**

**D13.4**   **Benign neoplasm of** liver
     Benign neoplasm of intrahepatic bile ducts

**D13.5**   **Benign neoplasm of** extrahepatic bile ducts

**D13.6**   **Benign neoplasm of** pancreas
     *EXCLUDES 1*   *benign neoplasm of endocrine pancreas (D13.7)*

**D13.7**   **Benign neoplasm of** endocrine pancreas
     Islet cell tumor
     Benign neoplasm of islets of Langerhans
     Use additional code to identify any functional activity

**D13.9**   **Benign neoplasm of** ill-defined sites **within the digestive system**
     Benign neoplasm of digestive system NOS
     Benign neoplasm of intestine NOS
     Benign neoplasm of spleen

✓4ᵗʰ **D14**   **Benign neoplasm of** middle ear and respiratory system

**D14.Ø**   **Benign neoplasm of** middle ear, nasal cavity and accessory sinuses
     Benign neoplasm of cartilage of nose
     *EXCLUDES 1*   *benign neoplasm of auricular canal (external) (D22.2-, D23.2-)*
                *benign neoplasm of bone of ear (D16.4)*
                *benign neoplasm of bone of nose (D16.4)*
                *benign neoplasm of cartilage of ear (D21.Ø)*
                *benign neoplasm of ear (external)(skin) (D22.2-, D23.2-)*
                *benign neoplasm of nose NOS (D36.7)*
                *benign neoplasm of skin of nose (D22.39, D23.39)*
                *benign neoplasm of olfactory bulb (D33.3)*
                *benign neoplasm of posterior margin of septum and choanae (D10.6)*
                *polyp of accessory sinus (J33.8)*
                *polyp of ear (middle) (H74.4)*
                *polyp of nasal (cavity) (J33.-)*

**D14.1**   **Benign neoplasm of** larynx
     Adenomatous polyp of larynx
     Benign neoplasm of epiglottis (suprahyoid portion)
     *EXCLUDES 1*   *benign neoplasm of epiglottis, anterior aspect (D10.5)*
                *polyp (nonadenomatous) of vocal cord or larynx (J38.1)*

**D14.2**   **Benign neoplasm of** trachea

✓5ᵗʰ **D14.3**   **Benign neoplasm of** bronchus and lung
     *EXCLUDES 1*   *benign carcinoid tumor of the bronchus and lung (D3A.Ø90)*

     **D14.3Ø**   **Benign neoplasm of** unspecified **bronchus and lung**

     **D14.31**   **Benign neoplasm of** right **bronchus and lung**

     **D14.32**   **Benign neoplasm of** left **bronchus and lung**

**D14.4**   **Benign neoplasm of respiratory system,** unspecified

✓4ᵗʰ **D15**   **Benign neoplasm of** other and unspecified intrathoracic organs
     *EXCLUDES 1*   *benign neoplasm of mesothelial tissue (D19.-)*

**D15.Ø**   **Benign neoplasm of** thymus
     *EXCLUDES 1*   *benign carcinoid tumor of the thymus (D3A.Ø91)*

**D15.1**   **Benign neoplasm of** heart
     *EXCLUDES 1*   *benign neoplasm of great vessels (D21.3)*

**D15.2**   **Benign neoplasm of** mediastinum

**D15.7**   **Benign neoplasm of** other specified **intrathoracic organs**

**D15.9**   **Benign neoplasm of intrathoracic organ,** unspecified

✓4ᵗʰ **D16**   **Benign neoplasm of** bone and articular cartilage
     *EXCLUDES 1*   *benign neoplasm of connective tissue of ear (D21.Ø)*
                *benign neoplasm of connective tissue of eyelid (D21.Ø)*
                *benign neoplasm of connective tissue of larynx (D14.1)*
                *benign neoplasm of connective tissue of nose (D14.Ø)*
                *benign neoplasm of synovia (D21.-)*

✓5ᵗʰ **D16.Ø**   **Benign neoplasm of** scapula and long bones of upper limb

     **D16.ØØ**   **Benign neoplasm of scapula and long bones of** unspecified **upper limb**

     **D16.Ø1**   **Benign neoplasm of scapula and long bones of** right **upper limb**

     **D16.Ø2**   **Benign neoplasm of scapula and long bones of** left **upper limb**

✓5ᵗʰ **D16.1**   **Benign neoplasm of** short bones of upper limb

     **D16.1Ø**   **Benign neoplasm of short bones of** unspecified **upper limb**

     **D16.11**   **Benign neoplasm of short bones of** right **upper limb**

     **D16.12**   **Benign neoplasm of short bones of** left **upper limb**

✓5ᵗʰ **D16.2**   **Benign neoplasm of** long bones of lower limb

     **D16.2Ø**   **Benign neoplasm of long bones of** unspecified **lower limb**

     **D16.21**   **Benign neoplasm of long bones of** right **lower limb**

     **D16.22**   **Benign neoplasm of long bones of** left **lower limb**

✓5ᵗʰ **D16.3**   **Benign neoplasm of** short bones of lower limb

     **D16.3Ø**   **Benign neoplasm of short bones of** unspecified **lower limb**

     **D16.31**   **Benign neoplasm of short bones of** right **lower limb**

     **D16.32**   **Benign neoplasm of short bones of** left **lower limb**

**D16.4**   **Benign neoplasm of bones of** skull and face
     Benign neoplasm of maxilla (superior)
     Benign neoplasm of orbital bone
     Keratocyst of maxilla
     Keratocystic odontogenic tumor of maxilla
     *EXCLUDES 2*   *benign neoplasm of lower jaw bone (D16.5)*

**D16.5**   **Benign neoplasm of** lower jaw bone
     Keratocyst of mandible
     Keratocystic odontogenic tumor of mandible

**D16.6**   **Benign neoplasm of** vertebral column
     *EXCLUDES 1*   *benign neoplasm of sacrum and coccyx (D16.8)*

**D16.7**   **Benign neoplasm of** ribs, sternum and clavicle

**D16.8**   **Benign neoplasm of** pelvic bones, sacrum and coccyx

**D16.9**   **Benign neoplasm of bone and articular cartilage,** unspecified

✓4ᵗʰ **D17**   **Benign** lipomatous **neoplasm**

**D17.Ø**   **Benign lipomatous neoplasm of** skin and subcutaneous tissue of head, face and neck

**D17.1**   **Benign lipomatous neoplasm of** skin and subcutaneous tissue of trunk

✓5ᵗʰ **D17.2**   **Benign lipomatous neoplasm of** skin and subcutaneous tissue of limb

     **D17.2Ø**   **Benign lipomatous neoplasm of skin and subcutaneous tissue of** unspecified **limb**

     **D17.21**   **Benign lipomatous neoplasm of skin and subcutaneous tissue of** right arm

     **D17.22**   **Benign lipomatous neoplasm of skin and subcutaneous tissue of** left arm

     **D17.23**   **Benign lipomatous neoplasm of skin and subcutaneous tissue of** right leg

✓ Additional Character Req   ✓x7ᵗʰ Placeholder Alert   Unacceptable PDx   Manifestation   H1-H14 HAC   HCC CMS-HCC Condition   *EXCLUDES 1* Not Coded Here   *EXCLUDES 2* Not Included Here

ICD-10-CM 2018                                                **491**

D17.24    **Benign lipomatous neoplasm of skin and subcutaneous tissue of** left leg

✓5th **D17.3**    **Benign lipomatous neoplasm of** skin and subcutaneous tissue of other and unspecified sites

     D17.30    **Benign lipomatous neoplasm of skin and subcutaneous tissue of** unspecified sites

     D17.39    **Benign lipomatous neoplasm of skin and subcutaneous tissue of** other sites

**D17.4**    **Benign lipomatous neoplasm of** intrathoracic organs

**D17.5**    **Benign lipomatous neoplasm of** intra-abdominal organs

     EXCLUDES 1    *benign lipomatous neoplasm of peritoneum and retroperitoneum (D17.79)*

**D17.6**    **Benign lipomatous neoplasm of** spermatic cord    ♂

✓5th **D17.7**    **Benign lipomatous neoplasm of** other sites

     D17.71    **Benign lipomatous neoplasm of** kidney

     D17.72    **Benign lipomatous neoplasm of** other genitourinary organ

     D17.79    **Benign lipomatous neoplasm of** other sites
       Benign lipomatous neoplasm of peritoneum
       Benign lipomatous neoplasm of retroperitoneum

**D17.9**    **Benign lipomatous neoplasm, unspecified**
     Lipoma NOS

✓4th **D18**    **Hemangioma and lymphangioma, any site**
     EXCLUDES 1    *benign neoplasm of glomus jugulare (D35.6)*
       *blue or pigmented nevus (D22.-)*
       *nevus NOS (D22.-)*
       *vascular nevus (Q82.5)*

✓5th **D18.0**    **Hemangioma**
     Angioma NOS
     Cavernous nevus
     **DEF:** A common benign tumor usually occurring in infancy; composed of newly formed blood vessels due to malformation of angioblastic tissue.

     D18.00    **Hemangioma** unspecified site

     D18.01    **Hemangioma of** skin and subcutaneous tissue

     D18.02    **Hemangioma of** intracranial structures    HCC

     D18.03    **Hemangioma of** intra-abdominal structures

     D18.09    **Hemangioma of** other sites

**D18.1**    **Lymphangioma, any site**

✓4th **D19**    **Benign neoplasm of** mesothelial tissue

**D19.0**    **Benign neoplasm of mesothelial tissue of** pleura

**D19.1**    **Benign neoplasm of mesothelial tissue of** peritoneum

**D19.7**    **Benign neoplasm of mesothelial tissue of** other sites

**D19.9**    **Benign neoplasm of mesothelial tissue,** unspecified
     Benign mesothelioma NOS

✓4th **D20**    **Benign neoplasm of soft tissue of** retroperitoneum and peritoneum
     EXCLUDES 1    *benign lipomatous neoplasm of peritoneum and retroperitoneum (D17.79)*
       *benign neoplasm of mesothelial tissue (D19.-)*

**D20.0**    **Benign neoplasm of soft tissue of** retroperitoneum

**D20.1**    **Benign neoplasm of soft tissue of** peritoneum

✓4th **D21**    **Other benign neoplasms of** connective and other soft tissue
     INCLUDES    benign neoplasm of blood vessel
       benign neoplasm of bursa
       benign neoplasm of cartilage
       benign neoplasm of fascia
       benign neoplasm of fat
       benign neoplasm of ligament, except uterine
       benign neoplasm of lymphatic channel
       benign neoplasm of muscle
       benign neoplasm of synovia
       benign neoplasm of tendon (sheath)
       benign stromal tumors

     EXCLUDES 1    *benign neoplasm of articular cartilage (D16.-)*
       *benign neoplasm of cartilage of larynx (D14.1)*
       *benign neoplasm of cartilage of nose (D14.0)*
       *benign neoplasm of connective tissue of breast (D24.-)*
       *benign neoplasm of peripheral nerves and autonomic nervous system (D36.1-)*
       *benign neoplasm of peritoneum (D20.1)*
       *benign neoplasm of retroperitoneum (D20.0)*
       *benign neoplasm of uterine ligament, any (D28.2)*
       *benign neoplasm of vascular tissue (D18.-)*
       *hemangioma (D18.0-)*
       *lipomatous neoplasm (D17.-)*
       *lymphangioma (D18.1)*
       *uterine leiomyoma (D25.-)*

**D21.0**    **Benign neoplasm of connective and other soft tissue of** head, face and neck
     Benign neoplasm of connective tissue of ear
     Benign neoplasm of connective tissue of eyelid
     EXCLUDES 1    *benign neoplasm of connective tissue of orbit (D31.6-)*

✓5th **D21.1**    **Benign neoplasm of connective and other soft tissue of** upper limb, including shoulder

     D21.10    **Benign neoplasm of connective and other soft tissue of** unspecified upper limb, including shoulder

     D21.11    **Benign neoplasm of connective and other soft tissue of** right upper limb, including shoulder

     D21.12    **Benign neoplasm of connective and other soft tissue of** left upper limb, including shoulder

✓5th **D21.2**    **Benign neoplasm of connective and other soft tissue of** lower limb, including hip

     D21.20    **Benign neoplasm of connective and other soft tissue of** unspecified lower limb, including hip

     D21.21    **Benign neoplasm of connective and other soft tissue of** right lower limb, including hip

     D21.22    **Benign neoplasm of connective and other soft tissue of** left lower limb, including hip

**D21.3**    **Benign neoplasm of connective and other soft tissue of** thorax
     Benign neoplasm of axilla
     Benign neoplasm of diaphragm
     Benign neoplasm of great vessels
     EXCLUDES 1    *benign neoplasm of heart (D15.1)*
       *benign neoplasm of mediastinum (D15.2)*
       *benign neoplasm of thymus (D15.0)*

**D21.4**    **Benign neoplasm of connective and other soft tissue of** abdomen
     Benign stromal tumors of abdomen

**D21.5**    **Benign neoplasm of connective and other soft tissue of** pelvis
     EXCLUDES 1    *benign neoplasm of any uterine ligament (D28.2)*
       *uterine leiomyoma (D25.-)*

**D21.6**    **Benign neoplasm of connective and other soft tissue of** trunk, unspecified
     Benign neoplasm of back NOS

**D21.9**    **Benign neoplasm of connective and other soft tissue,** unspecified

✓4th **D22**    **Melanocytic nevi**
     INCLUDES    atypical nevus
       blue hairy pigmented nevus
       nevus NOS

**D22.0**    **Melanocytic nevi of** lip

✓5th **D22.1**    **Melanocytic nevi of** eyelid, including canthus

     D22.10    **Melanocytic nevi of** unspecified eyelid, including canthus

     D22.11    **Melanocytic nevi of** right eyelid, including canthus

     D22.12    **Melanocytic nevi of** left eyelid, including canthus

N Newborn: 0    P Pediatric: 0-17    M Maternity: 12-55    A Adult: 15-124    MCC Major CC Condition    PDxMCC PDx acts as own MCC    CC CC Condition    PDxCC PDx acts as own CC

**492**      ICD-10-CM 2018

D17.24–D22.12

✓5th **D22.2 Melanocytic nevi of** ear and external auricular canal

    **D22.20 Melanocytic nevi of** unspecified **ear and external auricular canal**

    **D22.21 Melanocytic nevi of** right **ear and external auricular canal**

    **D22.22 Melanocytic nevi of** left **ear and external auricular canal**

✓5th **D22.3 Melanocytic nevi of** other and unspecified parts of face

    **D22.30 Melanocytic nevi of** unspecified **part of face**

    **D22.39 Melanocytic nevi of** other **parts of face**

**D22.4 Melanocytic nevi of** scalp and neck

**D22.5 Melanocytic nevi of** trunk
Melanocytic nevi of anal margin
Melanocytic nevi of anal skin
Melanocytic nevi of perianal skin
Melanocytic nevi of skin of breast

✓5th **D22.6 Melanocytic nevi of** upper limb, including shoulder

    **D22.60 Melanocytic nevi of** unspecified **upper limb, including shoulder**

    **D22.61 Melanocytic nevi of** right **upper limb, including shoulder**

    **D22.62 Melanocytic nevi of** left **upper limb, including shoulder**

✓5th **D22.7 Melanocytic nevi of** lower limb, including hip

    **D22.70 Melanocytic nevi of** unspecified **lower limb, including hip**

    **D22.71 Melanocytic nevi of** right **lower limb, including hip**

    **D22.72 Melanocytic nevi of** left **lower limb, including hip**

**D22.9 Melanocytic nevi, unspecified**

✓4th **D23 Other benign neoplasms of** skin

  INCLUDES  benign neoplasm of hair follicles
benign neoplasm of sebaceous glands
benign neoplasm of sweat glands

  EXCLUDES 1  benign lipomatous neoplasms of skin (D17.0-D17.3)
melanocytic nevi (D22.-)

**D23.0 Other benign neoplasm of skin of** lip

    EXCLUDES 1  benign neoplasm of vermilion border of lip (D10.0)

✓5th **D23.1 Other benign neoplasm of skin of** eyelid, including canthus

    **D23.10 Other benign neoplasm of skin of** unspecified **eyelid, including canthus**

    **D23.11 Other benign neoplasm of skin of** right **eyelid, including canthus**

    **D23.12 Other benign neoplasm of skin of** left **eyelid, including canthus**

✓5th **D23.2 Other benign neoplasm of skin of** ear and external auricular canal

    **D23.20 Other benign neoplasm of skin of** unspecified **ear and external auricular canal**

    **D23.21 Other benign neoplasm of skin of** right **ear and external auricular canal**

    **D23.22 Other benign neoplasm of skin of** left **ear and external auricular canal**

✓5th **D23.3 Other benign neoplasm of skin of** other and unspecified parts of face

    **D23.30 Other benign neoplasm of skin of** unspecified **part of face**

    **D23.39 Other benign neoplasm of skin of** other **parts of face**

**D23.4 Other benign neoplasm of skin of** scalp and neck

**D23.5 Other benign neoplasm of skin of** trunk
Other benign neoplasm of anal margin
Other benign neoplasm of anal skin
Other benign neoplasm of perianal skin
Other benign neoplasm of skin of breast

    EXCLUDES 1  benign neoplasm of anus NOS (D12.9)

✓5th **D23.6 Other benign neoplasm of skin of** upper limb, including shoulder

    **D23.60 Other benign neoplasm of skin of** unspecified **upper limb, including shoulder**

    **D23.61 Other benign neoplasm of skin of** right **upper limb, including shoulder**

    **D23.62 Other benign neoplasm of skin of** left **upper limb, including shoulder**

✓5th **D23.7 Other benign neoplasm of skin of** lower limb, including hip

    **D23.70 Other benign neoplasm of skin of** unspecified **lower limb, including hip**

    **D23.71 Other benign neoplasm of skin of** right **lower limb, including hip**

    **D23.72 Other benign neoplasm of skin of** left **lower limb, including hip**

**D23.9 Other benign neoplasm of skin, unspecified**

✓4th **D24 Benign neoplasm of** breast

  INCLUDES  benign neoplasm of connective tissue of breast
benign neoplasm of soft parts of breast
fibroadenoma of breast

  EXCLUDES 2  adenofibrosis of breast (N60.2)
benign cyst of breast (N60.-)
benign mammary dysplasia (N60.-)
benign neoplasm of skin of breast (D22.5, D23.5)
fibrocystic disease of breast (N60.-)

**D24.1 Benign neoplasm of** right **breast**

**D24.2 Benign neoplasm of** left **breast**

**D24.9 Benign neoplasm of** unspecified **breast**

✓4th **D25 Leiomyoma of uterus**

  INCLUDES  uterine fibroid
uterine fibromyoma
uterine myoma

**D25.0 Submucous leiomyoma of uterus** ♀

**D25.1 Intramural leiomyoma of uterus** ♀
Interstitial leiomyoma of uterus

**D25.2 Subserosal leiomyoma of uterus** ♀
Subperitoneal leiomyoma of uterus

**D25.9 Leiomyoma of uterus, unspecified** ♀

✓4th **D26 Other benign neoplasms of uterus**

**D26.0 Other benign neoplasm of cervix uteri** ♀

**D26.1 Other benign neoplasm of corpus uteri** ♀

**D26.7 Other benign neoplasm of other parts of uterus** ♀

**D26.9 Other benign neoplasm of uterus, unspecified** ♀

✓4th **D27 Benign neoplasm of ovary**

Use additional code to identify any functional activity

  EXCLUDES 2  corpus albicans cyst (N83.2-)
corpus luteum cyst (N83.1-)
endometrial cyst (N80.1)
follicular (atretic) cyst (N83.0-)
graafian follicle cyst (N83.0-)
ovarian cyst NEC (N83.2-)
ovarian retention cyst (N83.2-)

**D27.0 Benign neoplasm of right ovary** ♀

**D27.1 Benign neoplasm of left ovary** ♀

**D27.9 Benign neoplasm of unspecified ovary** ♀

**Uterine Leiomyomas (Fibroids)**

| Cornual | Pedunculated |
| Uterine cavity | Intramural |
| Subserosal | Submucosal |
| | Cervical |

✓ Additional Character Req    ✓x7th Placeholder Alert    Unacceptable PDx    Manifestation    H1-H14 HAC    HCC CMS-HCC Condition    EXCLUDES 1 Not Coded Here    EXCLUDES 2 Not Included Here

ICD-10-CM 2018         493

D22.2–D27.9

**Chapter 2. Neoplasms**

☑4ᵗʰ **D28 Benign neoplasm of other and unspecified female genital organs**

INCLUDES   adenomatous polyp
benign neoplasm of skin of female genital organs
benign teratoma

EXCLUDES 1   *epoophoron cyst (Q50.5)*
*fimbrial cyst (Q50.4)*
*Gartner's duct cyst (Q52.4)*
*parovarian cyst (Q50.5)*

D28.0 **Benign neoplasm of vulva**   ♀

D28.1 **Benign neoplasm of vagina**   ♀

D28.2 **Benign neoplasm of uterine tubes and ligaments**   ♀
Benign neoplasm of fallopian tube
Benign neoplasm of uterine ligament (broad) (round)

D28.7 **Benign neoplasm of other specified female genital organs**   ♀

D28.9 **Benign neoplasm of female genital organ, unspecified**   ♀

☑4ᵗʰ **D29 Benign neoplasm of male genital organs**

INCLUDES   benign neoplasm of skin of male genital organs

D29.0 **Benign neoplasm of penis**   ♂

D29.1 **Benign neoplasm of prostate**   ♂
EXCLUDES 1   *enlarged prostate (N40.-)*

☑5ᵗʰ D29.2 **Benign neoplasm of testis**
Use additional code to identify any functional activity

D29.20 **Benign neoplasm of unspecified testis**   ♂

D29.21 **Benign neoplasm of right testis**   ♂

D29.22 **Benign neoplasm of left testis**   ♂

☑5ᵗʰ D29.3 **Benign neoplasm of epididymis**

D29.30 **Benign neoplasm of unspecified epididymis**   ♂

D29.31 **Benign neoplasm of right epididymis**   ♂

D29.32 **Benign neoplasm of left epididymis**   ♂

D29.4 **Benign neoplasm of scrotum**   ♂
Benign neoplasm of skin of scrotum

D29.8 **Benign neoplasm of other specified male genital organs**   ♂
Benign neoplasm of seminal vesicle
Benign neoplasm of spermatic cord
Benign neoplasm of tunica vaginalis

D29.9 **Benign neoplasm of male genital organ, unspecified**   ♂

☑4ᵗʰ **D30 Benign neoplasm of urinary organs**

☑5ᵗʰ D30.0 **Benign neoplasm of kidney**
EXCLUDES 1   *benign carcinoid tumor of the kidney (D3A.093)*
*benign neoplasm of renal calyces (D30.1-)*
*benign neoplasm of renal pelvis (D30.1-)*

D30.00 **Benign neoplasm of unspecified kidney**

D30.01 **Benign neoplasm of right kidney**

D30.02 **Benign neoplasm of left kidney**

☑5ᵗʰ D30.1 **Benign neoplasm of renal pelvis**

D30.10 **Benign neoplasm of unspecified renal pelvis**

D30.11 **Benign neoplasm of right renal pelvis**

D30.12 **Benign neoplasm of left renal pelvis**

☑5ᵗʰ D30.2 **Benign neoplasm of ureter**
EXCLUDES 1   *benign neoplasm of ureteric orifice of bladder (D30.3)*

D30.20 **Benign neoplasm of unspecified ureter**

D30.21 **Benign neoplasm of right ureter**

D30.22 **Benign neoplasm of left ureter**

D30.3 **Benign neoplasm of bladder**
Benign neoplasm of ureteric orifice of bladder
Benign neoplasm of urethral orifice of bladder

D30.4 **Benign neoplasm of urethra**
EXCLUDES 1   *benign neoplasm of urethral orifice of bladder (D30.3)*

D30.8 **Benign neoplasm of other specified urinary organs**
Benign neoplasm of paraurethral glands

D30.9 **Benign neoplasm of urinary organ, unspecified**
Benign neoplasm of urinary system NOS

☑4ᵗʰ **D31 Benign neoplasm of eye and adnexa**
EXCLUDES 1   *benign neoplasm of connective tissue of eyelid (D21.0)*
*benign neoplasm of optic nerve (D33.3)*
*benign neoplasm of skin of eyelid (D22.1-, D23.1-)*

☑5ᵗʰ D31.0 **Benign neoplasm of conjunctiva**

D31.00 **Benign neoplasm of unspecified conjunctiva**

D31.01 **Benign neoplasm of right conjunctiva**

D31.02 **Benign neoplasm of left conjunctiva**

☑5ᵗʰ D31.1 **Benign neoplasm of cornea**

D31.10 **Benign neoplasm of unspecified cornea**

D31.11 **Benign neoplasm of right cornea**

D31.12 **Benign neoplasm of left cornea**

☑5ᵗʰ D31.2 **Benign neoplasm of retina**
EXCLUDES 1   *dark area on retina (D49.81)*
*hemangioma of retina (D49.81)*
*neoplasm of unspecified behavior of retina and choroid (D49.81)*
*retinal freckle (D49.81)*

D31.20 **Benign neoplasm of unspecified retina**

D31.21 **Benign neoplasm of right retina**

D31.22 **Benign neoplasm of left retina**

☑5ᵗʰ D31.3 **Benign neoplasm of choroid**

D31.30 **Benign neoplasm of unspecified choroid**

D31.31 **Benign neoplasm of right choroid**

D31.32 **Benign neoplasm of left choroid**

☑5ᵗʰ D31.4 **Benign neoplasm of ciliary body**

D31.40 **Benign neoplasm of unspecified ciliary body**

D31.41 **Benign neoplasm of right ciliary body**

D31.42 **Benign neoplasm of left ciliary body**

☑5ᵗʰ D31.5 **Benign neoplasm of lacrimal gland and duct**
Benign neoplasm of lacrimal sac
Benign neoplasm of nasolacrimal duct

D31.50 **Benign neoplasm of unspecified lacrimal gland and duct**

D31.51 **Benign neoplasm of right lacrimal gland and duct**

D31.52 **Benign neoplasm of left lacrimal gland and duct**

☑5ᵗʰ D31.6 **Benign neoplasm of unspecified site of orbit**
Benign neoplasm of connective tissue of orbit
Benign neoplasm of extraocular muscle
Benign neoplasm of peripheral nerves of orbit
Benign neoplasm of retrobulbar tissue
Benign neoplasm of retro-ocular tissue
EXCLUDES 1   *benign neoplasm of orbital bone (D16.4)*

D31.60 **Benign neoplasm of unspecified site of unspecified orbit**

D31.61 **Benign neoplasm of unspecified site of right orbit**

D31.62 **Benign neoplasm of unspecified site of left orbit**

☑5ᵗʰ D31.9 **Benign neoplasm of unspecified part of eye**
Benign neoplasm of eyeball

D31.90 **Benign neoplasm of unspecified part of unspecified eye**

D31.91 **Benign neoplasm of unspecified part of right eye**

D31.92 **Benign neoplasm of unspecified part of left eye**

☑4ᵗʰ **D32 Benign neoplasm of meninges**

D32.0 **Benign neoplasm of cerebral meninges**   HCC

D32.1 **Benign neoplasm of spinal meninges**   HCC

D32.9 **Benign neoplasm of meninges, unspecified**   HCC
Meningioma NOS

☑4ᵗʰ **D33 Benign neoplasm of brain and other parts of central nervous system**
EXCLUDES 1   *angioma (D18.0-)*
*benign neoplasm of meninges (D32.-)*
*benign neoplasm of peripheral nerves and autonomic nervous system (D36.1-)*
*hemangioma (D18.0-)*
*neurofibromatosis (Q85.0-)*
*retro-ocular benign neoplasm (D31.6-)*

D33.0 **Benign neoplasm of brain, supratentorial**   HCC
Benign neoplasm of cerebral ventricle
Benign neoplasm of cerebrum
Benign neoplasm of frontal lobe
Benign neoplasm of occipital lobe
Benign neoplasm of parietal lobe
Benign neoplasm of temporal lobe
EXCLUDES 1   *benign neoplasm of fourth ventricle (D33.1)*

D33.1 **Benign neoplasm of brain, infratentorial**   HCC
Benign neoplasm of brain stem
Benign neoplasm of cerebellum
Benign neoplasm of fourth ventricle

D33.2 **Benign neoplasm of brain, unspecified**   HCC

D33.3 **Benign neoplasm of cranial nerves**   HCC
Benign neoplasm of olfactory bulb

D33.4 **Benign neoplasm of spinal cord**   HCC

N Newborn: 0   P Pediatric: 0-17   M Maternity: 12-55   A Adult: 15-124   MCC Major CC Condition   PDx MCC PDx acts as own MCC   CC CC Condition   PDx CC PDx acts as own CC

494

ICD-10-CM 2018

D33.7   **Benign neoplasm of** other specified parts of central nervous system   `HCC`

D33.9   **Benign neoplasm of central nervous system,** unspecified `HCC`
    Benign neoplasm of nervous system (central) NOS

**D34   Benign neoplasm of** thyroid gland
    Use additional code to identify any functional activity

`✓4ᵗʰ` **D35   Benign neoplasm of** other and unspecified endocrine glands
    Use additional code to identify any functional activity
    `EXCLUDES 1`   *benign neoplasm of endocrine pancreas (D13.7)*
           *benign neoplasm of ovary (D27.-)*
           *benign neoplasm of testis (D29.2-)*
           *benign neoplasm of thymus (D15.0)*

   `✓5ᵗʰ` **D35.0   Benign neoplasm of** adrenal gland
      **D35.00   Benign neoplasm of** unspecified **adrenal gland**
      **D35.01   Benign neoplasm of** right **adrenal gland**
      **D35.02   Benign neoplasm of** left **adrenal gland**

   **D35.1   Benign neoplasm of parathyroid gland**

   **D35.2   Benign neoplasm of** pituitary gland   `HCC`
      AHA: 2014, 3Q, 22

   **D35.3   Benign neoplasm of** craniopharyngeal duct   `HCC`

   **D35.4   Benign neoplasm of** pineal gland   `HCC`

   **D35.5   Benign neoplasm of carotid body**

   **D35.6   Benign neoplasm of aortic body and other paraganglia**
      Benign tumor of glomus jugulare

   **D35.7   Benign neoplasm of** other **specified endocrine glands**

   **D35.9   Benign neoplasm of endocrine gland,** unspecified
      Benign neoplasm of unspecified endocrine gland

`✓4ᵗʰ` **D36   Benign neoplasm of** other and unspecified sites

   **D36.0   Benign neoplasm of lymph nodes**
      `EXCLUDES 1`   *lymphangioma (D18.1)*

   `✓5ᵗʰ` **D36.1   Benign neoplasm of** peripheral nerves and autonomic nervous system
      `EXCLUDES 1`   *benign neoplasm of peripheral nerves of orbit (D31.6-)*
             *neurofibromatosis (Q85.0-)*

      **D36.10   Benign neoplasm of peripheral nerves and autonomic nervous system,** unspecified

      **D36.11   Benign neoplasm of peripheral nerves and autonomic nervous system of** face, head, and neck

      **D36.12   Benign neoplasm of peripheral nerves and autonomic nervous system,** upper limb, including shoulder

      **D36.13   Benign neoplasm of peripheral nerves and autonomic nervous system of** lower limb, including hip

      **D36.14   Benign neoplasm of peripheral nerves and autonomic nervous system of** thorax

      **D36.15   Benign neoplasm of peripheral nerves and autonomic nervous system of** abdomen

      **D36.16   Benign neoplasm of peripheral nerves and autonomic nervous system of** pelvis

      **D36.17   Benign neoplasm of peripheral nerves and autonomic nervous system of** trunk, unspecified

   **D36.7   Benign neoplasm of** other **specified sites**
      Benign neoplasm of nose NOS

   **D36.9   Benign neoplasm,** unspecified site

### Benign neuroendocrine tumors (D3A)

`✓4ᵗʰ` **D3A   Benign neuroendocrine tumors**
    Code also any associated multiple endocrine neoplasia [MEN] syndromes (E31.2-)
    Use additional code to identify any associated endocrine syndrome, such as:
      carcinoid syndrome (E34.0)
    `EXCLUDES 2`   *benign pancreatic islet cell tumors (D13.7)*

   `✓5ᵗʰ` **D3A.0   Benign** carcinoid tumors
      **D3A.00   Benign carcinoid tumor of** unspecified site
         Carcinoid tumor NOS

     `✓6ᵗʰ` **D3A.01   Benign carcinoid tumors of the** small intestine
        **D3A.010   Benign carcinoid tumor of the** duodenum
        **D3A.011   Benign carcinoid tumor of the** jejunum
        **D3A.012   Benign carcinoid tumor of the** ileum
        **D3A.019   Benign carcinoid tumor of the small intestine,** unspecified portion

     `✓6ᵗʰ` **D3A.02   Benign carcinoid tumors of the** appendix, large intestine, and rectum
        **D3A.020   Benign carcinoid tumor of the** appendix
        **D3A.021   Benign carcinoid tumor of the** cecum
        **D3A.022   Benign carcinoid tumor of the** ascending colon
        **D3A.023   Benign carcinoid tumor of the** transverse colon
        **D3A.024   Benign carcinoid tumor of the** descending colon
        **D3A.025   Benign carcinoid tumor of the** sigmoid colon
        **D3A.026   Benign carcinoid tumor of the** rectum
        **D3A.029   Benign carcinoid tumor of the** large intestine, unspecified portion
          Benign carcinoid tumor of the colon NOS

     `✓6ᵗʰ` **D3A.09   Benign carcinoid tumors of** other **sites**
        **D3A.090   Benign carcinoid tumor of the** bronchus and lung
        **D3A.091   Benign carcinoid tumor of the** thymus
        **D3A.092   Benign carcinoid tumor of the** stomach
        **D3A.093   Benign carcinoid tumor of the** kidney
        **D3A.094   Benign carcinoid tumor of the** foregut, unspecified
        **D3A.095   Benign carcinoid tumor of the** midgut, unspecified
        **D3A.096   Benign carcinoid tumor of the** hindgut, unspecified
        **D3A.098   Benign carcinoid tumors of** other sites

   **D3A.8   Other benign neuroendocrine tumors**
      Neuroendocrine tumor NOS

### Neoplasms of uncertain behavior, polycythemia vera and myelodysplastic syndromes (D37-D48)

   `NOTE`   Categories D37-D44, and D48 classify by site neoplasms of uncertain behavior, i.e., histologic confirmation whether the neoplasm is malignant or benign cannot be made.
   `EXCLUDES 1`   *neoplasms of unspecified behavior (D49.-)*

`✓4ᵗʰ` **D37   Neoplasm of uncertain behavior of** oral cavity and digestive organs
    `EXCLUDES 1`   *stromal tumors of uncertain behavior of digestive system (D48.1)*

   `✓5ᵗʰ` **D37.0   Neoplasm of uncertain behavior of** lip, oral cavity and pharynx
      `EXCLUDES 1`   *neoplasm of uncertain behavior of aryepiglottic fold or interarytenoid fold, laryngeal aspect (D38.0)*
             *neoplasm of uncertain behavior of epiglottis NOS (D38.0)*
             *neoplasm of uncertain behavior of skin of lip (D48.5)*
             *neoplasm of uncertain behavior of suprahyoid portion of epiglottis (D38.0)*

      **D37.01   Neoplasm of uncertain behavior of** lip
         Neoplasm of uncertain behavior of vermilion border of lip

      **D37.02   Neoplasm of uncertain behavior of** tongue

     `✓6ᵗʰ` **D37.03   Neoplasm of uncertain behavior of the** major salivary glands
        **D37.030   Neoplasm of uncertain behavior of the** parotid **salivary glands**
        **D37.031   Neoplasm of uncertain behavior of the** sublingual **salivary glands**
        **D37.032   Neoplasm of uncertain behavior of the** submandibular **salivary glands**
        **D37.039   Neoplasm of uncertain behavior of the** major salivary glands, unspecified

      **D37.04   Neoplasm of uncertain behavior of the** minor salivary glands
         Neoplasm of uncertain behavior of submucosal salivary glands of lip
         Neoplasm of uncertain behavior of submucosal salivary glands of cheek
         Neoplasm of uncertain behavior of submucosal salivary glands of hard palate
         Neoplasm of uncertain behavior of submucosal salivary glands of soft palate

Chapter 2. Neoplasms

D37.05–D43.9

     **D37.05** **Neoplasm of uncertain behavior of** pharynx
         Neoplasm of uncertain behavior of aryepiglottic fold of pharynx NOS
         Neoplasm of uncertain behavior of hypopharyngeal aspect of aryepiglottic fold of pharynx
         Neoplasm of uncertain behavior of marginal zone of aryepiglottic fold of pharynx

     **D37.09** **Neoplasm of uncertain behavior of** other **specified sites of the oral cavity**

**D37.1** **Neoplasm of uncertain behavior of** stomach

**D37.2** **Neoplasm of uncertain behavior of** small intestine

**D37.3** **Neoplasm of uncertain behavior of** appendix

**D37.4** **Neoplasm of uncertain behavior of** colon

**D37.5** **Neoplasm of uncertain behavior of** rectum
     Neoplasm of uncertain behavior of rectosigmoid junction

**D37.6** **Neoplasm of uncertain behavior of** liver, gallbladder and bile ducts
     Neoplasm of uncertain behavior of ampulla of Vater

**D37.8** **Neoplasm of uncertain behavior of** other **specified digestive organs**
     Neoplasm of uncertain behavior of anal canal
     Neoplasm of uncertain behavior of anal sphincter
     Neoplasm of uncertain behavior of anus NOS
     Neoplasm of uncertain behavior of esophagus
     Neoplasm of uncertain behavior of intestine NOS
     Neoplasm of uncertain behavior of pancreas
     **EXCLUDES 1**   *neoplasm of uncertain behavior of anal margin (D48.5)*
           *neoplasm of uncertain behavior of anal skin (D48.5)*
           *neoplasm of uncertain behavior of perianal skin (D48.5)*

**D37.9** **Neoplasm of uncertain behavior of** digestive organ, unspecified

✓4ᵗʰ **D38** **Neoplasm of uncertain behavior of** middle ear and respiratory and intrathoracic organs
     **EXCLUDES 1**   *neoplasm of uncertain behavior of heart (D48.7)*

**D38.0** **Neoplasm of uncertain behavior of** larynx
     Neoplasm of uncertain behavior of aryepiglottic fold or interarytenoid fold, laryngeal aspect
     Neoplasm of uncertain behavior of epiglottis (suprahyoid portion)
     **EXCLUDES 1**   *neoplasm of uncertain behavior of aryepiglottic fold or interarytenoid fold NOS (D37.05)*
           *neoplasm of uncertain behavior of hypopharyngeal aspect of aryepiglottic fold (D37.05)*
           *neoplasm of uncertain behavior of marginal zone of aryepiglottic fold (D37.05)*

**D38.1** **Neoplasm of uncertain behavior of** trachea, bronchus and lung

**D38.2** **Neoplasm of uncertain behavior of** pleura

**D38.3** **Neoplasm of uncertain behavior of** mediastinum

**D38.4** **Neoplasm of uncertain behavior of** thymus

**D38.5** **Neoplasm of uncertain behavior of** other respiratory organs
     Neoplasm of uncertain behavior of accessory sinuses
     Neoplasm of uncertain behavior of cartilage of nose
     Neoplasm of uncertain behavior of middle ear
     Neoplasm of uncertain behavior of nasal cavities
     **EXCLUDES 1**   *neoplasm of uncertain behavior of ear (external) (skin) (D48.5)*
           *neoplasm of uncertain behavior of nose NOS (D48.7)*
           *neoplasm of uncertain behavior of skin of nose (D48.5)*

**D38.6** **Neoplasm of uncertain behavior of** respiratory organ, unspecified

✓4ᵗʰ **D39** **Neoplasm of uncertain behavior of** female genital organs

**D39.0** **Neoplasm of uncertain behavior of** uterus      ♀

✓5ᵗʰ **D39.1** **Neoplasm of uncertain behavior of** ovary
     Use additional code to identify any functional activity

     **D39.10** **Neoplasm of uncertain behavior of** unspecified ovary      ♀

     **D39.11** **Neoplasm of uncertain behavior of** right ovary      ♀

     **D39.12** **Neoplasm of uncertain behavior of** left ovary      ♀

**D39.2** **Neoplasm of uncertain behavior of** placenta      M ♀
     Chorioadenoma destruens
     Invasive hydatidiform mole
     Malignant hydatidiform mole
     **EXCLUDES 1**   *hydatidiform mole NOS (O01.9)*

**D39.8** **Neoplasm of uncertain behavior of** other specified female genital organs      ♀
     Neoplasm of uncertain behavior of skin of female genital organs

**D39.9** **Neoplasm of uncertain behavior of** female genital organ, unspecified      ♀

✓4ᵗʰ **D40** **Neoplasm of uncertain behavior of** male genital organs

**D40.0** **Neoplasm of uncertain behavior of** prostate      ♂

✓5ᵗʰ **D40.1** **Neoplasm of uncertain behavior of** testis

     **D40.10** **Neoplasm of uncertain behavior of** unspecified testis      ♂

     **D40.11** **Neoplasm of uncertain behavior of** right testis      ♂

     **D40.12** **Neoplasm of uncertain behavior of** left testis      ♂

**D40.8** **Neoplasm of uncertain behavior of** other specified male genital organs      ♂
     Neoplasm of uncertain behavior of skin of male genital organs

**D40.9** **Neoplasm of uncertain behavior of** male genital organ, unspecified      ♂

✓4ᵗʰ **D41** **Neoplasm of uncertain behavior of** urinary organs

✓5ᵗʰ **D41.0** **Neoplasm of uncertain behavior of** kidney
     **EXCLUDES 1**   *neoplasm of uncertain behavior of renal pelvis (D41.1-)*

     **D41.00** **Neoplasm of uncertain behavior of** unspecified kidney

     **D41.01** **Neoplasm of uncertain behavior of** right kidney

     **D41.02** **Neoplasm of uncertain behavior of** left kidney

✓5ᵗʰ **D41.1** **Neoplasm of uncertain behavior of** renal pelvis

     **D41.10** **Neoplasm of uncertain behavior of** unspecified renal pelvis

     **D41.11** **Neoplasm of uncertain behavior of** right renal pelvis

     **D41.12** **Neoplasm of uncertain behavior of** left renal pelvis

✓5ᵗʰ **D41.2** **Neoplasm of uncertain behavior of** ureter

     **D41.20** **Neoplasm of uncertain behavior of** unspecified ureter

     **D41.21** **Neoplasm of uncertain behavior of** right ureter

     **D41.22** **Neoplasm of uncertain behavior of** left ureter

**D41.3** **Neoplasm of uncertain behavior of** urethra

**D41.4** **Neoplasm of uncertain behavior of** bladder

**D41.8** **Neoplasm of uncertain behavior of** other specified urinary organs

**D41.9** **Neoplasm of uncertain behavior of** unspecified urinary organ

✓4ᵗʰ **D42** **Neoplasm of uncertain behavior of** meninges

**D42.0** **Neoplasm of uncertain behavior of** cerebral meninges      HCC

**D42.1** **Neoplasm of uncertain behavior of** spinal meninges      HCC

**D42.9** **Neoplasm of uncertain behavior of** meninges, unspecified      HCC

✓4ᵗʰ **D43** **Neoplasm of uncertain behavior of** brain and central nervous system
     **EXCLUDES 1**   *neoplasm of uncertain behavior of peripheral nerves and autonomic nervous system (D48.2)*

**D43.0** **Neoplasm of uncertain behavior of** brain, supratentorial      HCC
     Neoplasm of uncertain behavior of cerebral ventricle
     Neoplasm of uncertain behavior of cerebrum
     Neoplasm of uncertain behavior of frontal lobe
     Neoplasm of uncertain behavior of occipital lobe
     Neoplasm of uncertain behavior of parietal lobe
     Neoplasm of uncertain behavior of temporal lobe
     **EXCLUDES 1**   *neoplasm of uncertain behavior of fourth ventricle (D43.1)*

**D43.1** **Neoplasm of uncertain behavior of** brain, infratentorial      HCC
     Neoplasm of uncertain behavior of brain stem
     Neoplasm of uncertain behavior of cerebellum
     Neoplasm of uncertain behavior of fourth ventricle

**D43.2** **Neoplasm of uncertain behavior of** brain, unspecified      HCC

**D43.3** **Neoplasm of uncertain behavior of** cranial nerves      HCC

**D43.4** **Neoplasm of uncertain behavior of** spinal cord      HCC

**D43.8** **Neoplasm of uncertain behavior of** other specified parts of central nervous system      HCC

**D43.9** **Neoplasm of uncertain behavior of** central nervous system, unspecified      HCC
     Neoplasm of uncertain behavior of nervous system (central) NOS

**N** Newborn: 0   **P** Pediatric: 0-17   **M** Maternity: 12-55   **A** Adult: 15-124   **MCC** Major CC Condition   **PDxMCC** PDx acts as own MCC   **CC** CC Condition   **PDxCC** PDx acts as own CC

**496**            ICD-10-CM 2018

☑4ᵗʰ **D44  Neoplasm of uncertain behavior of** endocrine glands
- EXCLUDES 1   *multiple endocrine adenomatosis (E31.2-)*
  *multiple endocrine neoplasia (E31.2-)*
  *neoplasm of uncertain behavior of endocrine pancreas (D37.8)*
  *neoplasm of uncertain behavior of ovary (D39.1-)*
  *neoplasm of uncertain behavior of testis (D40.1-)*
  *neoplasm of uncertain behavior of thymus (D38.4)*

**D44.0  Neoplasm of uncertain behavior of** thyroid gland

☑5ᵗʰ **D44.1  Neoplasm of uncertain behavior of** adrenal gland
- Use additional code to identify any functional activity

**D44.10  Neoplasm of uncertain behavior of** unspecified adrenal gland

**D44.11  Neoplasm of uncertain behavior of** right adrenal gland

**D44.12  Neoplasm of uncertain behavior of** left adrenal gland

**D44.2  Neoplasm of uncertain behavior of** parathyroid gland

**D44.3  Neoplasm of uncertain behavior of** pituitary gland   HCC
- Use additional code to identify any functional activity

**D44.4  Neoplasm of uncertain behavior of** craniopharyngeal duct   HCC

**D44.5  Neoplasm of uncertain behavior of** pineal gland   HCC

**D44.6  Neoplasm of uncertain behavior of** carotid body   HCC

**D44.7  Neoplasm of uncertain behavior of** aortic body and other paraganglia   HCC

**D44.9  Neoplasm of uncertain behavior of** unspecified endocrine gland

**D45  Polycythemia vera**   HCC
- EXCLUDES 1   *familial polycythemia (D75.0)*
  *secondary polycythemia (D75.1)*
- **DEF:** Abnormal proliferation of all bone marrow elements, increased red cell mass, and total blood volume; unknown etiology, frequently associated with splenomegaly, leukocytosis, and thrombocythemia.

☑4ᵗʰ **D46  Myelodysplastic syndromes**
- Use additional code for adverse effect, if applicable, to identify drug (T36-T50 with fifth or sixth character 5)
- EXCLUDES 2   *drug-induced aplastic anemia (D61.1)*

**D46.0  Refractory anemia without ring sideroblasts, so stated**   HCC
- Refractory anemia without sideroblasts, without excess of blasts

**D46.1  Refractory anemia with ring sideroblasts**   HCC
- RARS

☑5ᵗʰ **D46.2  Refractory anemia with excess of blasts [RAEB]**

**D46.20  Refractory anemia with excess of blasts, unspecified**   HCC
- RAEB NOS

**D46.21  Refractory anemia with excess of blasts 1**   HCC
- RAEB 1

**D46.22  Refractory anemia with excess of blasts 2**   CC HCC
- RAEB 2
- CC Excl: PDX collection 488

**D46.A  Refractory** cytopenia with multilineage dysplasia   HCC

**D46.B  Refractory** cytopenia with multilineage dysplasia and ring sideroblasts   HCC
- RCMD RS

**D46.C  Myelodysplastic syndrome** with isolated del(5q) chromosomal abnormality   CC HCC
- Myelodysplastic syndrome with 5q deletion
- 5q minus syndrome NOS
- CC Excl: PDX collection 488

**D46.4  Refractory anemia, unspecified**   HCC

**D46.Z  Other myelodysplastic syndromes**   HCC
- EXCLUDES 1   *chronic myelomonocytic leukemia (C93.1-)*

**D46.9  Myelodysplastic syndrome, unspecified**   HCC
- Myelodysplasia NOS

☑4ᵗʰ **D47  Other neoplasms of uncertain behavior of** lymphoid, hematopoietic and related tissue

CC Excl: For CC codes in category D47, unless otherwise noted: PDX collection 488

▲ ☑5ᵗʰ **D47.0  Mast cell neoplasms of uncertain behavior**
- ~~Indolent systemic mastocytosis~~
- ~~Mast cell tumor NOS~~
- ~~Mastocytoma NOS~~
- EXCLUDES 1   ►*congenital cutaneous mastocytosis (Q82.2-)*
  *histiocytic neoplasms of uncertain behavior (D47.Z9)*
  *malignant mast cell neoplasm (C96.2-)*◄
  ~~*mastocytosis (congenital) (cutaneous) (Q82.2)*~~

CC Excl: For codes in subcategory D47.0: PDX collection 494

**D47.01  Cutaneous mastocytosis**   CC
- Diffuse cutaneous mastocytosis
- Maculopapular cutaneous mastocytosis
- Solitary mastocytoma
- Telangiectasia macularis eruptiva perstans
- Urticaria pigmentosa
- EXCLUDES 1   *congenital (diffuse) (maculopapular) cutaneous mastocytosis (Q82.2)*
  *congenital urticaria pigmentosa (Q82.2)*
  *extracutaneous mastocytoma (D47.09)*

**D47.02  Systemic mastocytosis**   CC
- Indolent systemic mastocytosis
- Isolated bone marrow mastocytosis
- Smoldering systemic mastocytosis
- Systemic mastocytosis, with an associated hematological non-mast cell lineage disease (SM-AHNMD)
- Code also, if applicable, any associated hematological non-mast cell lineage disease, such as:
  - acute myeloid leukemia (C92.6-, C92.A-)
  - chronic myelomonocytic leukemia (C93.1-)
  - essential thrombocytosis (D47.3)
  - hypereosinophilic syndrome (D72.1)
  - myelodysplastic syndrome (D46.9)
  - myeloproliferative syndrome (D47.1)
  - non-Hodgkin lymphoma (C82-C85)
  - plasma cell myeloma (C90.0-)
  - polycythemia vera (D45)
- EXCLUDES 1   *aggressive systemic mastocytosis (C96.21)*
  *mast cell leukemia (C94.3-)*

**D47.09  Other mast cell neoplasms of uncertain behavior**   CC
- Extracutaneous mastocytoma
- Mast cell tumor NOS
- Mastocytoma NOS
- Mastocytosis NOS

**D47.1  Chronic myeloproliferative disease**   CC HCC
- Chronic neutrophilic leukemia
- Myeloproliferative disease, unspecified
- EXCLUDES 1   *atypical chronic myeloid leukemia BCR/ABL-negative (C92.2-)*
  *chronic myeloid leukemia BCR/ABL-positive (C92.1-)*
  *myelofibrosis NOS (D75.81)*
  *myelophthisic anemia (D61.82)*
  *myelophthisis (D61.82)*
  *secondary myelofibrosis NOS (D75.81)*

**D47.2  Monoclonal gammopathy**
- Monoclonal gammopathy of undetermined significance [MGUS]

**D47.3  Essential (hemorrhagic) thrombocythemia**   HCC
- Essential thrombocytosis
- Idiopathic hemorrhagic thrombocythemia

**D47.4  Osteomyelofibrosis**   HCC
- Chronic idiopathic myelofibrosis
- Myelofibrosis (idiopathic) (with myeloid metaplasia)
- Myelosclerosis (megakaryocytic) with myeloid metaplasia
- Secondary myelofibrosis in myeloproliferative disease
- EXCLUDES 1   *acute myelofibrosis (C94.4-)*

☑5ᵗʰ **D47.Z  Other specified neoplasms of uncertain behavior of** lymphoid, hematopoietic and related tissue

**D47.Z1  Post-transplant lymphoproliferative disorder (PTLD)**   CC HCC
- Code first complications of transplanted organs and tissue (T86.-)
- **DEF:** Excessive proliferation of B-cell lymphocytes following Epstein-Barr virus infection in organ transplant patients; may progress to non-Hodgkin lymphoma.
- CC Excl: PDX collection 495

---

☑ Additional Character Req   ✓ₓ7ᵗʰ Placeholder Alert   Unacceptable PDx   Manifestation   H1 - H14 HAC   HCC CMS-HCC Condition   EXCLUDES 1 Not Coded Here   EXCLUDES 2 Not Included Here

**D47.Z2 Castleman disease**   CC HCC
Code also if applicable human herpesvirus 8 infection (B10.89)
*EXCLUDES 2*   *Kaposi's sarcoma (C46-)*

**D47.Z9 Other specified neoplasms of uncertain behavior of lymphoid, hematopoietic and related tissue**   CC HCC
Histiocytic tumors of uncertain behavior

**D47.9 Neoplasm of uncertain behavior of lymphoid, hematopoietic and related tissue, unspecified**   CC HCC
Lymphoproliferative disease NOS

**✓4ᵗʰ D48 Neoplasm of uncertain behavior of other and unspecified sites**
*EXCLUDES 1*   *neurofibromatosis (nonmalignant) (Q85.0-)*

**D48.0 Neoplasm of uncertain behavior of bone and articular cartilage**
*EXCLUDES 1*   *neoplasm of uncertain behavior of cartilage of ear (D48.1)*
*neoplasm of uncertain behavior of cartilage of larynx (D38.0)*
*neoplasm of uncertain behavior of cartilage of nose (D38.5)*
*neoplasm of uncertain behavior of connective tissue of eyelid (D48.1)*
*neoplasm of uncertain behavior of synovia (D48.1)*

**D48.1 Neoplasm of uncertain behavior of connective and other soft tissue**
Neoplasm of uncertain behavior of connective tissue of ear
Neoplasm of uncertain behavior of connective tissue of eyelid
Stromal tumors of uncertain behavior of digestive system
*EXCLUDES 1*   *neoplasm of uncertain behavior of articular cartilage (D48.0)*
*neoplasm of uncertain behavior of cartilage of larynx (D38.0)*
*neoplasm of uncertain behavior of cartilage of nose (D38.5)*
*neoplasm of uncertain behavior of connective tissue of breast (D48.6-)*

**D48.2 Neoplasm of uncertain behavior of peripheral nerves and autonomic nervous system**
*EXCLUDES 1*   *neoplasm of uncertain behavior of peripheral nerves of orbit (D48.7)*

**D48.3 Neoplasm of uncertain behavior of retroperitoneum**

**D48.4 Neoplasm of uncertain behavior of peritoneum**

**D48.5 Neoplasm of uncertain behavior of skin**
Neoplasm of uncertain behavior of anal margin
Neoplasm of uncertain behavior of anal skin
Neoplasm of uncertain behavior of perianal skin
Neoplasm of uncertain behavior of skin of breast
*EXCLUDES 1*   *neoplasm of uncertain behavior of anus NOS (D37.8)*
*neoplasm of uncertain behavior of skin of genital organs (D39.8, D40.8)*
*neoplasm of uncertain behavior of vermilion border of lip (D37.0)*

**✓5ᵗʰ D48.6 Neoplasm of uncertain behavior of breast**
Neoplasm of uncertain behavior of connective tissue of breast
Cystosarcoma phyllodes
*EXCLUDES 1*   *neoplasm of uncertain behavior of skin of breast (D48.5)*

**D48.60 Neoplasm of uncertain behavior of unspecified breast**

**D48.61 Neoplasm of uncertain behavior of right breast**

**D48.62 Neoplasm of uncertain behavior of left breast**

**D48.7 Neoplasm of uncertain behavior of other specified sites**
Neoplasm of uncertain behavior of eye
Neoplasm of uncertain behavior of heart
Neoplasm of uncertain behavior of peripheral nerves of orbit
*EXCLUDES 1*   *neoplasm of uncertain behavior of connective tissue (D48.1)*
*neoplasm of uncertain behavior of skin of eyelid (D48.5)*

**D48.9 Neoplasm of uncertain behavior, unspecified**

## Neoplasms of unspecified behavior (D49)

**✓4ᵗʰ D49 Neoplasms of unspecified behavior**
*NOTE*   Category D49 classifies by site neoplasms of unspecified morphology and behavior. The term "mass", unless otherwise stated, is not to be regarded as a neoplastic growth.
*INCLUDES*   "growth" NOS
neoplasm NOS
new growth NOS
tumor NOS
*EXCLUDES 1*   *neoplasms of uncertain behavior (D37-D44, D48)*

**D49.0 Neoplasm of unspecified behavior of digestive system**
*EXCLUDES 1*   *neoplasm of unspecified behavior of margin of anus (D49.2)*
*neoplasm of unspecified behavior of perianal skin (D49.2)*
*neoplasm of unspecified behavior of skin of anus (D49.2)*

**D49.1 Neoplasm of unspecified behavior of respiratory system**

**D49.2 Neoplasm of unspecified behavior of bone, soft tissue, and skin**
*EXCLUDES 1*   *neoplasm of unspecified behavior of anal canal (D49.0)*
*neoplasm of unspecified behavior of anus NOS (D49.0)*
*neoplasm of unspecified behavior of bone marrow (D49.89)*
*neoplasm of unspecified behavior of cartilage of larynx (D49.1)*
*neoplasm of unspecified behavior of cartilage of nose (D49.1)*
*neoplasm of unspecified behavior of connective tissue of breast (D49.3)*
*neoplasm of unspecified behavior of skin of genital organs (D49.59)*
*neoplasm of unspecified behavior of vermilion border of lip (D49.0)*

**D49.3 Neoplasm of unspecified behavior of breast**
*EXCLUDES 1*   *neoplasm of unspecified behavior of skin of breast (D49.2)*

**D49.4 Neoplasm of unspecified behavior of bladder**

**✓5ᵗʰ D49.5 Neoplasm of unspecified behavior of other genitourinary organs**

**✓6ᵗʰ D49.51 Neoplasm of unspecified behavior of kidney**

**D49.511 Neoplasm of unspecified behavior of right kidney**

**D49.512 Neoplasm of unspecified behavior of left kidney**

**D49.519 Neoplasm of unspecified behavior of unspecified kidney**

**D49.59 Neoplasm of unspecified behavior of other genitourinary organ**

**D49.6 Neoplasm of unspecified behavior of brain**   HCC
*EXCLUDES 1*   *neoplasm of unspecified behavior of cerebral meninges (D49.7)*
*neoplasm of unspecified behavior of cranial nerves (D49.7)*

**D49.7 Neoplasm of unspecified behavior of endocrine glands and other parts of nervous system**
*EXCLUDES 1*   *neoplasm of unspecified behavior of peripheral, sympathetic, and parasympathetic nerves and ganglia (D49.2)*

**✓5ᵗʰ D49.8 Neoplasm of unspecified behavior of other specified sites**
*EXCLUDES 1*   *neoplasm of unspecified behavior of eyelid (skin) (D49.2)*
*neoplasm of unspecified behavior of eyelid cartilage (D49.2)*
*neoplasm of unspecified behavior of great vessels (D49.2)*
*neoplasm of unspecified behavior of optic nerve (D49.7)*

**D49.81 Neoplasm of unspecified behavior of retina and choroid**
Dark area on retina
Retinal freckle

**D49.89 Neoplasm of unspecified behavior of other specified sites**

**D49.9 Neoplasm of unspecified behavior of unspecified site**

N Newborn: 0   P Pediatric: 0-17   M Maternity: 12-55   A Adult: 15-124   MCC Major CC Condition   PDxMCC PDx acts as own MCC   CC CC Condition   PDxCC PDx acts as own CC

**498**

ICD-10-CM 2018

# Chapter 3. Diseases of the Blood and Blood-forming Organs and Certain Disorders Involving the Immune Mechanism (D5Ø–D89)

**Chapter Specific Coding Guidelines and Examples**
Reserved for future guideline expansion

# Chapter 3. Diseases of the Blood and Blood-forming Organs and Certain Disorders Involving the Immune Mechanism (D50-D89)

**EXCLUDES 2**   *autoimmune disease (systemic) NOS (M35.9)*
*certain conditions originating in the perinatal period (P00-P96)*
*complications of pregnancy, childbirth and the puerperium (O00-O9A)*
*congenital malformations, deformations and chromosomal abnormalities (Q00-Q99)*
*endocrine, nutritional and metabolic diseases (E00-E88)*
*human immunodeficiency virus [HIV] disease (B20)*
*injury, poisoning and certain other consequences of external causes (S00-T88)*
*neoplasms (C00-D49)*
*symptoms, signs and abnormal clinical and laboratory findings, not elsewhere classified (R00-R94)*

This chapter contains the following blocks:

| | |
|---|---|
| D50-D53 | Nutritional anemias |
| D55-D59 | Hemolytic anemias |
| D60-D64 | Aplastic and other anemias and other bone marrow failure syndromes |
| D65-D69 | Coagulation defects, purpura and other hemorrhagic conditions |
| D70-D77 | Other disorders of blood and blood-forming organs |
| D78 | Intraoperative and postprocedural complications of the spleen |
| D80-D89 | Certain disorders involving the immune mechanism |

## Nutritional anemias (D50-D53)

### ✓4th D50 Iron deficiency anemia
**INCLUDES**   asiderotic anemia
hypochromic anemia

**D50.0 Iron deficiency anemia secondary to blood loss (chronic)**
Posthemorrhagic anemia (chronic)
**EXCLUDES 1**   *acute posthemorrhagic anemia (D62)*
*congenital anemia from fetal blood loss (P61.3)*

**D50.1 Sideropenic dysphagia**
Kelly-Paterson syndrome    Plummer-Vinson syndrome

**D50.8 Other iron deficiency anemias**
Iron deficiency anemia due to inadequate dietary iron intake

**D50.9 Iron deficiency anemia, unspecified**

### ✓4th D51 Vitamin B12 deficiency anemia
**EXCLUDES 1**   *vitamin B12 deficiency (E53.8)*

**D51.0 Vitamin B12 deficiency anemia due to intrinsic factor deficiency**
Addison anemia    Pernicious (congenital) anemia
Biermer anemia    Congenital intrinsic factor deficiency
**DEF:** Chronic progressive anemia due to vitamin B12 malabsorption; caused by lack of secretion of intrinsic factor, which is produced by the gastric mucosa of the stomach.

**D51.1 Vitamin B12 deficiency anemia due to selective vitamin B12 malabsorption with proteinuria**
Imerslund (Gräsbeck) syndrome
Megaloblastic hereditary anemia

**D51.2 Transcobalamin II deficiency**

**D51.3 Other dietary vitamin B12 deficiency anemia**
Vegan anemia

**D51.8 Other vitamin B12 deficiency anemias**

**D51.9 Vitamin B12 deficiency anemia, unspecified**

### ✓4th D52 Folate deficiency anemia
**EXCLUDES 1**   *folate deficiency without anemia (E53.8)*

**D52.0 Dietary folate deficiency anemia**
Nutritional megaloblastic anemia
**DEF:** The result of a poor diet with inadequate intake of folate, which is needed to produce healthy red blood cells.

**D52.1 Drug-induced folate deficiency anemia**
Use additional code for adverse effect, if applicable, to identify drug (T36-T50 with fifth or sixth character 5)

**D52.8 Other folate deficiency anemias**

**D52.9 Folate deficiency anemia, unspecified**
Folic acid deficiency anemia NOS

### ✓4th D53 Other nutritional anemias
**INCLUDES**   megaloblastic anemia unresponsive to vitamin B12 or folate therapy

**D53.0 Protein deficiency anemia**
Amino-acid deficiency anemia
Orotaciduric anemia
**EXCLUDES 1**   *Lesch-Nyhan syndrome (E79.1)*

**D53.1 Other megaloblastic anemias, not elsewhere classified**
Megaloblastic anemia NOS
**EXCLUDES 1**   *Di Guglielmo's disease (C94.0)*

**D53.2 Scorbutic anemia**
**EXCLUDES 1**   *scurvy (E54)*

**D53.8 Other specified nutritional anemias**
Anemia associated with deficiency of copper
Anemia associated with deficiency of molybdenum
Anemia associated with deficiency of zinc
**EXCLUDES 1**   *nutritional deficiencies without anemia, such as:*
*copper deficiency NOS (E61.0)*
*molybdenum deficiency NOS (E61.5)*
*zinc deficiency NOS (E60)*

**D53.9 Nutritional anemia, unspecified**
Simple chronic anemia
**EXCLUDES 1**   *anemia NOS (D64.9)*

## Hemolytic anemias (D55-D59)

### ✓4th D55 Anemia due to enzyme disorders
**EXCLUDES 1**   *drug-induced enzyme deficiency anemia (D59.2)*

**D55.0 Anemia due to glucose-6-phosphate dehydrogenase [G6PD] deficiency**   HCC
Favism
G6PD deficiency anemia

**D55.1 Anemia due to other disorders of glutathione metabolism**   HCC
Anemia (due to) enzyme deficiencies, except G6PD, related to the hexose monophosphate [HMP] shunt pathway
Anemia (due to) hemolytic nonspherocytic (hereditary), type I

**D55.2 Anemia due to disorders of glycolytic enzymes**   HCC
Hemolytic nonspherocytic (hereditary) anemia, type II
Hexokinase deficiency anemia
Pyruvate kinase [PK] deficiency anemia
Triose-phosphate isomerase deficiency anemia
**EXCLUDES 1**   *disorders of glycolysis not associated with anemia (E74.8)*

**D55.3 Anemia due to disorders of nucleotide metabolism**   HCC

**D55.8 Other anemias due to enzyme disorders**   HCC

**D55.9 Anemia due to enzyme disorder, unspecified**   HCC

### ✓4th D56 Thalassemia
**EXCLUDES 1**   *sickle-cell thalassemia (D57.4-)*

**D56.0 Alpha thalassemia**   HCC
Alpha thalassemia major
Hemoglobin H Constant Spring
Hemoglobin H disease
Hydrops fetalis due to alpha thalassemia
Severe alpha thalassemia
Triple gene defect alpha thalassemia
Use additional code, if applicable, for hydrops fetalis due to alpha thalassemia (P56.99)
**EXCLUDES 1**   *alpha thalassemia trait or minor (D56.3)*
*asymptomatic alpha thalassemia (D56.3)*
*hydrops fetalis due to isoimmunization (P56.0)*
*hydrops fetalis not due to immune hemolysis (P83.2)*
**DEF:** HBA1 and HBA2 genetic variant of chromosome 16 prevalent among those of African and Southeast Asian descent; associated with a wide spectrum of anemic presentation; includes hemoglobin H disease subtypes.

**Thalassemia**

Misshapen RBC

Misshapen RBC

Healthy RBC

N Newborn: 0   P Pediatric: 0-17   M Maternity: 12-55   A Adult: 15-124   MCC Major CC Condition   PDx MCC PDx acts as own MCC   CC CC Condition   PDx CC PDx acts as own CC

500      ICD-10-CM 2018

**D56.1**   Beta thalassemia   `HCC`
Beta thalassemia major    Severe beta thalassemia
Cooley's anemia    Thalassemia intermedia
Homozygous beta thalassemia    Thalassemia major
   `EXCLUDES 1`   *beta thalassemia minor (D56.3)*
*beta thalassemia trait (D56.3)*
*delta-beta thalassemia (D56.2)*
*hemoglobin E-beta thalassemia (D56.5)*
*sickle-cell beta thalassemia (D57.4-)*

**D56.2**   Delta-beta thalassemia   `HCC`
Homozygous delta-beta thalassemia
   `EXCLUDES 1`   *delta-beta thalassemia minor (D56.3)*
*delta-beta thalassemia trait (D56.3)*

**D56.3**   Thalassemia minor
Alpha thalassemia minor
Alpha thalassemia silent carrier
Alpha thalassemia trait
Beta thalassemia minor
Beta thalassemia trait
Delta-beta thalassemia minor
Delta-beta thalassemia trait
Thalassemia trait NOS
   `EXCLUDES 1`   *alpha thalassemia (D56.Ø)*
*beta thalassemia (D56.1)*
*delta-beta thalassemia (D56.2)*
*hemoglobin E-beta thalassemia (D56.5)*
*sickle-cell trait (D57.3)*
   **DEF:** Solitary abnormal gene that identifies a carrier of the disease, yet with an absence of symptoms or a clinically mild anemic presentation.

**D56.4**   Hereditary persistence of fetal hemoglobin [HPFH]   `HCC`

**D56.5**   Hemoglobin E-beta thalassemia   `HCC`
   `EXCLUDES 1`   *beta thalassemia (D56.1)*
*beta thalassemia minor (D56.3)*
*beta thalassemia trait (D56.3)*
*delta-beta thalassemia (D56.2)*
*delta-beta thalassemia trait (D56.3)*
*hemoglobin E disease (D58.2)*
*other hemoglobinopathies (D58.2)*
*sickle-cell beta thalassemia (D57.4-)*

**D56.8**   Other thalassemias   `HCC`
Dominant thalassemia
Hemoglobin C thalassemia
Mixed thalassemia
Thalassemia with other hemoglobinopathy
   `EXCLUDES 1`   *hemoglobin C disease (D58.2)*
*hemoglobin E disease (D58.2)*
*other hemoglobinopathies (D58.2)*
*sickle-cell anemia (D57.-)*
*sickle-cell thalassemia (D57.4)*

**D56.9**   Thalassemia, unspecified
Mediterranean anemia (with other hemoglobinopathy)

✓4th **D57**   **Sickle-cell disorders**
Use additional code for any associated fever (R50.81)
   `EXCLUDES 1`   *other hemoglobinopathies (D58.-)*

   **CC Excl: For MCC codes in category D57:** PDX collection 496

✓5th **D57.Ø**   Hb-SS disease with crisis
Sickle-cell disease NOS with crisis
Hb-SS disease with vasoocclusive pain
   **D57.ØØ**   Hb-SS disease with crisis, unspecified   `MCC` `HCC`
   **D57.Ø1**   Hb-SS disease with acute chest syndrome   `MCC` `HCC`
   **D57.Ø2**   Hb-SS disease with splenic sequestration   `MCC` `HCC`

### Sickle cell

Sickle cells

Normal RBCs

**D57.1**   Sickle-cell disease without crisis   `HCC`
Hb-SS disease without crisis
Sickle-cell anemia NOS
Sickle-cell disease NOS
Sickle-cell disorder NOS

✓5th **D57.2**   Sickle-cell/Hb-C disease
Hb-SC disease
Hb-S/Hb-C disease
   **D57.2Ø**   Sickle-cell/Hb-C disease without crisis   `HCC`
   ✓6th **D57.21**   Sickle-cell/Hb-C disease with crisis
     **D57.211**   Sickle-cell/Hb-C disease with acute chest syndrome   `PDx CC` `MCC` `HCC`
     **D57.212**   Sickle-cell/Hb-C disease with splenic sequestration   `MCC` `HCC`
     **D57.219**   Sickle-cell/Hb-C disease with crisis, unspecified   `MCC` `HCC`
Sickle-cell/Hb-C disease with crisis NOS

**D57.3**   Sickle-cell trait   `HCC`
Hb-S trait
Heterozygous hemoglobin S
   **DEF:** Heterozygous genetic makeup characterized by one gene for normal hemoglobin and one for sickle-cell hemoglobin; clinical disease rarely present.

✓5th **D57.4**   Sickle-cell thalassemia
Sickle-cell beta thalassemia
Thalassemia Hb-S disease
   **D57.4Ø**   Sickle-cell thalassemia without crisis   `HCC`
Microdrepanocytosis
Sickle-cell thalassemia NOS
   ✓6th **D57.41**   Sickle-cell thalassemia with crisis
Sickle-cell thalassemia with vasoocclusive pain
     **D57.411**   Sickle-cell thalassemia with acute chest syndrome   `PDx CC` `MCC` `HCC`
     **D57.412**   Sickle-cell thalassemia with splenic sequestration   `MCC` `HCC`
     **D57.419**   Sickle-cell thalassemia with crisis, unspecified   `MCC` `HCC`
Sickle-cell thalassemia with crisis NOS

✓5th **D57.8**   Other sickle-cell disorders
Hb-SD disease
Hb-SE disease
   **D57.8Ø**   Other sickle-cell disorders without crisis   `HCC`
   ✓6th **D57.81**   Other sickle-cell disorders with crisis
     **D57.811**   Other sickle-cell disorders with acute chest syndrome   `MCC` `HCC`
     **D57.812**   Other sickle-cell disorders with splenic sequestration   `MCC` `HCC`
     **D57.819**   Other sickle-cell disorders with crisis, unspecified   `MCC` `HCC`
Other sickle-cell disorders with crisis NOS

✓4th **D58**   **Other hereditary hemolytic anemias**
   `EXCLUDES 1`   *hemolytic anemia of the newborn (P55.-)*

**D58.Ø**   Hereditary spherocytosis   `HCC`
Acholuric (familial) jaundice
Congenital (spherocytic) hemolytic icterus
Minkowski-Chauffard syndrome

**D58.1**   Hereditary elliptocytosis   `HCC`
Elliptocytosis (congenital)
Ovalocytosis (congenital) (hereditary)

**D58.2**   Other hemoglobinopathies   `HCC`
Abnormal hemoglobin NOS
Congenital Heinz body anemia
Hb-C disease
Hb-D disease
Hb-E disease
Hemoglobinopathy NOS
Unstable hemoglobin hemolytic disease
   `EXCLUDES 1`   *familial polycythemia (D75.Ø)*
*Hb-M disease (D74.Ø)*
*hemoglobin E-beta thalassemia (D56.5)*
*hereditary persistence of fetal hemoglobin [HPFH] (D56.4)*
*high-altitude polycythemia (D75.1)*
*methemoglobinemia (D74.-)*
*other hemoglobinopathies with thalassemia (D56.8)*

**D58.8**   Other specified hereditary hemolytic anemias   `CC` `HCC`
Stomatocytosis
   **CC Excl:** PDX collection 497

**D58.9**   Hereditary hemolytic anemia, unspecified   `CC` `HCC`
   **CC Excl:** PDX collection 497

✓ Additional Character Req   ✓x7th Placeholder Alert   Unacceptable PDx   Manifestation   `H1`-`H14` HAC   `HCC` CMS-HCC Condition   `EXCLUDES 1` Not Coded Here   `EXCLUDES 2` Not Included Here

**Chapter 3. Diseases of the Blood and Blood-forming Organs**

**D59–D63.1**

### ☑4ᵗʰ D59 Acquired hemolytic anemia

**DEF:** Non-hereditary anemia characterized by premature destruction of red blood cells; caused by infectious organisms, poisons, and physical agents.

> **CC Excl:** For CC/MCC codes in category D59, unless otherwise noted: PDX collection 496

**D59.0 Drug-induced autoimmune hemolytic anemia** CC HCC
Use additional code for adverse effect, if applicable, to identify drug (T36-T50 with fifth or sixth character 5)

**D59.1 Other autoimmune hemolytic anemias** CC HCC
Autoimmune hemolytic disease (cold type) (warm type)
Chronic cold hemagglutinin disease
Cold agglutinin disease
Cold agglutinin hemoglobinuria
Cold type (secondary) (symptomatic) hemolytic anemia
Warm type (secondary) (symptomatic) hemolytic anemia
> *EXCLUDES 1*   *Evans syndrome (D69.41)*
>       *hemolytic disease of newborn (P55.-)*
>       *paroxysmal cold hemoglobinuria (D59.6)*

**D59.2 Drug-induced nonautoimmune hemolytic anemia** CC HCC
Drug-induced enzyme deficiency anemia
Use additional code for adverse effect, if applicable, to identify drug (T36-T50 with fifth or sixth character 5)

**D59.3 Hemolytic-uremic syndrome** MCC HCC
Use additional code to identify associated:
E. coli infection (B96.2-)
Pneumococcal pneumonia (J13)
Shigella dysenteriae (A03.9)

**D59.4 Other nonautoimmune hemolytic anemias** CC HCC
Mechanical hemolytic anemia
Microangiopathic hemolytic anemia
Toxic hemolytic anemia

**D59.5 Paroxysmal nocturnal hemoglobinuria [Marchiafava-Micheli]** HCC
> *EXCLUDES 1*   *hemoglobinuria NOS (R82.3)*

**D59.6 Hemoglobinuria due to hemolysis from other external causes** HCC
Hemoglobinuria from exertion
March hemoglobinuria
Paroxysmal cold hemoglobinuria
Use additional code (Chapter 20) to identify external cause
> *EXCLUDES 1*   *hemoglobinuria NOS (R82.3)*

**D59.8 Other acquired hemolytic anemias** HCC

**D59.9 Acquired hemolytic anemia, unspecified** CC HCC
Idiopathic hemolytic anemia, chronic

## Aplastic and other anemias and other bone marrow failure syndromes (D60-D64)

### ☑4ᵗʰ D60 Acquired pure red cell aplasia [erythroblastopenia]
> **INCLUDES**   red cell aplasia (acquired) (adult) (with thymoma)
> *EXCLUDES 1*   *congenital red cell aplasia (D61.01)*

> **CC Excl:** For MCC codes in category D60: PDX collection 496

**D60.0 Chronic acquired pure red cell aplasia** MCC HCC

**D60.1 Transient acquired pure red cell aplasia** MCC HCC

**D60.8 Other acquired pure red cell aplasias** MCC HCC

**D60.9 Acquired pure red cell aplasia, unspecified** MCC HCC

### ☑4ᵗʰ D61 Other aplastic anemias and other bone marrow failure syndromes
> *EXCLUDES 1*   *neutropenia (D70.-)*
> **AHA:** 2014, 4Q, 22

### ☑5ᵗʰ D61.0 Constitutional aplastic anemia

**D61.01 Constitutional (pure) red blood cell aplasia** CC HCC
Blackfan-Diamond syndrome
Congenital (pure) red cell aplasia
Familial hypoplastic anemia
Primary (pure) red cell aplasia
Red cell (pure) aplasia of infants
> *EXCLUDES 1*   *acquired red cell aplasia (D60.9)*
> **CC Excl:** PDX collection 498

**D61.09 Other constitutional aplastic anemia** CC HCC
Fanconi's anemia
Pancytopenia with malformations
> **CC Excl:** PDX collection 499

**D61.1 Drug-induced aplastic anemia** MCC HCC
Use additional code for adverse effect, if applicable, to identify drug (T36-T50 with fifth or sixth character 5)
> **CC Excl:** PDX collection 496

**D61.2 Aplastic anemia due to other external agents** MCC HCC
Code first, if applicable, toxic effects of substances chiefly nonmedicinal as to source (T51-T65)
> **CC Excl:** PDX collection 496

**D61.3 Idiopathic aplastic anemia** MCC HCC

### ☑5ᵗʰ D61.8 Other specified aplastic anemias and other bone marrow failure syndromes

> **CC Excl:** For CC/MCC codes in subcategory D61.8: PDX collection 500

### ☑6ᵗʰ D61.81 Pancytopenia
> *EXCLUDES 1*   *pancytopenia (due to) (with) aplastic anemia (D61.9)*
>       *pancytopenia (due to) (with) bone marrow infiltration (D61.82)*
>       *pancytopenia (due to) (with) congenital (pure) red cell aplasia (D61.01)*
>       *pancytopenia (due to) (with) hairy cell leukemia (C91.4-)*
>       *pancytopenia (due to) (with) human immunodeficiency virus disease (B20)*
>       *pancytopenia (due to) (with) leukoerythroblastic anemia (D61.82)*
>       *pancytopenia (due to) (with) myeloproliferative disease (D47.1)*
> *EXCLUDES 2*   *pancytopenia (due to) (with) myelodysplastic syndromes (D46.-)*
> **DEF:** Occurs when a person has a shortage of all three blood cells: white, red, and platelets.

**D61.810 Antineoplastic chemotherapy induced pancytopenia** MCC HCC
> *EXCLUDES 2*   *aplastic anemia due to antineoplastic chemotherapy (D61.1)*

**D61.811 Other drug-induced pancytopenia** MCC HCC
> *EXCLUDES 2*   *aplastic anemia due to drugs (D61.1)*

**D61.818 Other pancytopenia** CC HCC

**D61.82 Myelophthisis** CC HCC
Leukoerythroblastic anemia
Myelophthisic anemia
Panmyelophthisis
Code also the underlying disorder, such as:
malignant neoplasm of breast (C50.-)
tuberculosis (A15.-)
> *EXCLUDES 1*   *idiopathic myelofibrosis (D47.1)*
>       *myelofibrosis NOS (D75.81)*
>       *myelofibrosis with myeloid metaplasia (D47.4)*
>       *primary myelofibrosis (D47.1)*
>       *secondary myelofibrosis (D75.81)*

**D61.89 Other specified aplastic anemias and other bone marrow failure syndromes** MCC HCC
> **CC Excl:** PDX collection 496

**D61.9 Aplastic anemia, unspecified** CC HCC
Hypoplastic anemia NOS
Medullary hypoplasia
> **CC Excl:** PDX collection 496

### D62 Acute posthemorrhagic anemia     CC
> *EXCLUDES 1*   *anemia due to chronic blood loss (D50.0)*
>       *blood loss anemia NOS (D50.0)*
>       *congenital anemia from fetal blood loss (P61.3)*
> **CC Excl:** PDX collection 501

### ☑4ᵗʰ D63 Anemia in chronic diseases classified elsewhere

**D63.0 Anemia in neoplastic disease**
Code first neoplasm (C00-D49)
> *EXCLUDES 1*   ~~*anemia due to antineoplastic chemotherapy (D64.81)*~~
>       *aplastic anemia due to antineoplastic chemotherapy (D61.1)*
> *EXCLUDES 2*   ▶*anemia due to antineoplastic chemotherapy (D64.81)*◀

**D63.1 Anemia in chronic kidney disease**
Erythropoietin resistant anemia (EPO resistant anemia)
Code first underlying chronic kidney disease (CKD) (N18.-)

N Newborn: 0   P Pediatric: 0-17   M Maternity: 12-55   A Adult: 15-124   **MCC** Major CC Condition   **PDx MCC** PDx acts as own MCC   **CC** CC Condition   **PDx CC** PDx acts as own CC

502        ICD-10-CM 2018

**D63.8 Anemia in other chronic diseases classified elsewhere**
Code first underlying disease, such as:
diphyllobothriasis (B70.0)
hookworm disease (B76.0-B76.9)
hypothyroidism (E00.0-E03.9)
malaria (B50.0-B54)
symptomatic late syphilis (A52.79)
tuberculosis (A18.89)

✓4th **D64 Other anemias**
*EXCLUDES 1*   refractory anemia (D46.-)
refractory anemia with excess blasts in transformation [RAEB T] (C92.0-)

**D64.0 Hereditary sideroblastic anemia**    HCC
Sex-linked hypochromic sideroblastic anemia

*D64.1 Secondary sideroblastic anemia due to disease*    HCC
Code first underlying disease

**D64.2 Secondary sideroblastic anemia due to drugs and toxins**   HCC
Code first poisoning due to drug or toxin, if applicable (T36-T65 with fifth or sixth character 1-4 or 6)
Use additional code for adverse effect, if applicable, to identify drug (T36-T50 with fifth or sixth character 5)

**D64.3 Other sideroblastic anemias**    HCC
Sideroblastic anemia NOS
Pyridoxine-responsive sideroblastic anemia NEC

**D64.4 Congenital dyserythropoietic anemia**
Dyshematopoietic anemia (congenital)
*EXCLUDES 1*   Blackfan-Diamond syndrome (D61.01)
Di Guglielmo's disease (C94.0)

✓5th **D64.8 Other specified anemias**
**D64.81 Anemia due to antineoplastic chemotherapy**
Antineoplastic chemotherapy induced anemia
*EXCLUDES 1*   aplastic anemia due to antineoplastic chemotherapy (D61.1)
*EXCLUDES 2*   anemia in neoplastic disease (D63.0)
**AHA:** 2014, 4Q, 22
**DEF:** Reversible adverse effect of chemotherapy, causing inhibition of bone marrow production; decrease in red blood cell production prevents adequate oxygenation of the tissues and organs causing fatigue, SOB, and exacerbation of other medical conditions.

**D64.89 Other specified anemias**
Infantile pseudoleukemia

**D64.9 Anemia, unspecified**
**AHA:** 2017, 1Q, 7

## Coagulation defects, purpura and other hemorrhagic conditions (D65-D69)

**D65 Disseminated intravascular coagulation [defibrination syndrome]**    MCC HCC
Afibrinogenemia, acquired
Consumption coagulopathy
Diffuse or disseminated intravascular coagulation [DIC]
Fibrinolytic hemorrhage, acquired
Fibrinolytic purpura
Purpura fulminans
*EXCLUDES 1*   disseminated intravascular coagulation (complicating):
abortion or ectopic or molar pregnancy (O00-O07, O08.1)
in newborn (P60)
pregnancy, childbirth and the puerperium (O45.0, O46.0, O67.0, O72.3)
**CC Excl:** PDX collection 502

**D66 Hereditary factor VIII deficiency**    MCC HCC
Classical hemophilia
Deficiency factor VIII (with functional defect)
Hemophilia A
Hemophilia NOS
*EXCLUDES 1*   factor VIII deficiency with vascular defect (D68.0)
**DEF:** Hereditary, sex-linked lack of antihemophilic globulin (AHG) (factor VIII); causes abnormal coagulation characterized by increased bleeding, large bruises of skin, bleeding in mouth, nose, gastrointestinal tract; hemorrhages into joints, resulting in swelling and impaired function.
**CC Excl:** PDX collection 502

**Coagulation**

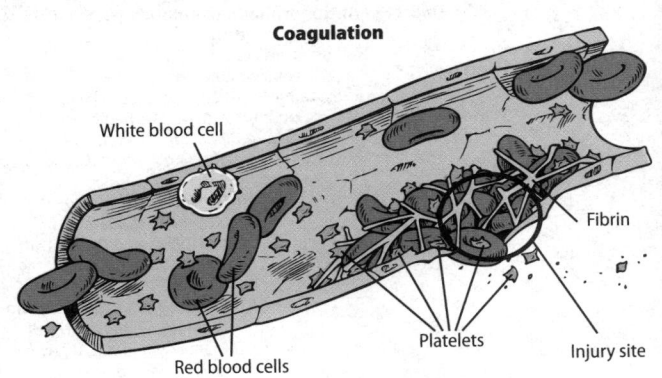

White blood cell
Fibrin
Platelets
Injury site
Red blood cells

**D67 Hereditary factor IX deficiency**    MCC HCC
Christmas disease
Factor IX deficiency (with functional defect)
Hemophilia B
Plasma thromboplastin component [PTC] deficiency
**CC Excl:** PDX collection 502

✓4th **D68 Other coagulation defects**
*EXCLUDES 1*   abnormal coagulation profile (R79.1)
coagulation defects complicating abortion or ectopic or molar pregnancy (O00-O07, O08.1)
coagulation defects complicating pregnancy, childbirth and the puerperium (O45.0, O46.0, O67.0, O72.3)
**AHA:** 2016, 1Q, 14

**CC Excl: For CC codes in category D68, unless otherwise noted:**
PDX collection 502

**D68.0 Von Willebrand's disease**    CC HCC
Angiohemophilia
Factor VIII deficiency with vascular defect
Vascular hemophilia
*EXCLUDES 1*   capillary fragility (hereditary) (D69.8)
factor VIII deficiency NOS (D66)
factor VIII deficiency with functional defect (D66)
**DEF:** Abnormal blood coagulation caused by deficient blood factor VII; congenital; symptoms include excess or prolonged bleeding.

**D68.1 Hereditary factor XI deficiency**    CC HCC
Hemophilia C
Plasma thromboplastin antecedent [PTA] deficiency
Rosenthal's disease

**D68.2 Hereditary deficiency of other clotting factors**    CC HCC
AC globulin deficiency
Congenital afibrinogenemia
Deficiency of factor I [fibrinogen]
Deficiency of factor II [prothrombin]
Deficiency of factor V [labile]
Deficiency of factor VII [stable]
Deficiency of factor X [Stuart-Prower]
Deficiency of factor XII [Hageman]
Deficiency of factor XIII [fibrin stabilizing]
Dysfibrinogenemia (congenital)
Hypoproconvertinemia
Owren's disease
Proaccelerin deficiency

✓5th **D68.3 Hemorrhagic disorder due to circulating anticoagulants**
✓6th **D68.31 Hemorrhagic disorder due to intrinsic circulating anticoagulants, antibodies, or inhibitors**
**D68.311 Acquired hemophilia**    CC HCC
Autoimmune hemophilia
Autoimmune inhibitors to clotting factors
Secondary hemophilia
**CC Excl:** PDX collection 503

**D68.312** **Antiphospholipid antibody with** CC HCC
**hemorrhagic disorder**
Lupus anticoagulant (LAC) with
hemorrhagic disorder
Systemic lupus erythematosus [SLE]
inhibitor with hemorrhagic disorder
EXCLUDES 1   *antiphospholipid antibody,*
*finding without diagnosis*
*(R76.0)*
*antiphospholipid antibody syn-*
*drome (D68.61)*
*antiphospholipid antibody with*
*hypercoagulable state*
*(D68.61)*
*lupus anticoagulant (LAC) finding*
*without diagnosis (R76.0)*
*lupus anticoagulant (LAC) with*
*hypercoagulable state*
*(D68.62)*
*systemic lupus erythematosus*
*[SLE] inhibitor finding with-*
*out diagnosis (R76.0)*
*systemic lupus erythematosus*
*[SLE] inhibitor with hyperco-*
*agulable state (D68.62)*
**CC Excl:** PDX collection 504

**D68.318** **Other hemorrhagic disorder due to** CC HCC
**intrinsic circulating anticoagulants,**
**antibodies, or inhibitors**
Antithromboplastinemia
Antithromboplastinogenemia
Hemorrhagic disorder due to intrinsic
increase in antithrombin
Hemorrhagic disorder due to intrinsic
increase in anti-VIIIa
Hemorrhagic disorder due to intrinsic
increase in anti-IXa
Hemorrhagic disorder due to intrinsic
increase in anti-XIa
**CC Excl:** PDX collection 503

**D68.32** **Hemorrhagic disorder due to extrinsic** CC HCC
**circulating anticoagulants**
Drug-induced hemorrhagic disorder
Hemorrhagic disorder due to increase in anti-IIa
Hemorrhagic disorder due to increase in anti-Xa
Hyperheparinemia
Use additional code for adverse effect, if applicable, to
identify drug (T45.515, T45.525)
**AHA:** 2016, 1Q, 14-15

**D68.4** **Acquired coagulation factor deficiency** CC HCC
Deficiency of coagulation factor due to liver disease
Deficiency of coagulation factor due to vitamin K deficiency
EXCLUDES 1   *vitamin K deficiency of newborn (P53)*

✓5ᵗʰ **D68.5** **Primary thrombophilia**
Primary hypercoagulable states
EXCLUDES 1   *antiphospholipid syndrome (D68.61)*
*lupus anticoagulant (D68.62)*
*secondary activated protein C resistance (D68.69)*
*secondary antiphospholipid antibody syndrome*
*(D68.69)*
*secondary lupus anticoagulant with hypercoagulable*
*state (D68.69)*
*secondary systemic lupus erythematosus [SLE]*
*inhibitor with hypercoagulable state (D68.69)*
*systemic lupus erythematosus [SLE] inhibitor finding*
*without diagnosis (R76.0)*
*systemic lupus erythematosus [SLE] inhibitor with*
*hemorrhagic disorder (D68.312)*
*thrombotic thrombocytopenic purpura (M31.1)*

**CC Excl: For CC codes in subcategory D68.5:**
PDX collection 505

**D68.51** **Activated protein C resistance** CC HCC
Factor V Leiden mutation

**D68.52** **Prothrombin gene mutation** CC HCC

**D68.59** **Other primary thrombophilia** CC HCC
Antithrombin III deficiency
Hypercoagulable state NOS
Primary hypercoagulable state NEC
Primary thrombophilia NEC
Protein C deficiency
Protein S deficiency
Thrombophilia NOS

✓5ᵗʰ **D68.6** **Other thrombophilia**
Other hypercoagulable states
EXCLUDES 1   *diffuse or disseminated intravascular coagulation*
*[DIC] (D65)*
*heparin induced thrombocytopenia (HIT) (D75.82)*
*hyperhomocysteinemia (E72.11)*

**CC Excl: For CC codes in subcategory D68.6:**
PDX collection 505

**D68.61** **Antiphospholipid syndrome** CC HCC
Anticardiolipin syndrome
Antiphospholipid antibody syndrome
EXCLUDES 1   *antiphospholipid antibody, finding without*
*diagnosis (R76.0)*
*antiphospholipid antibody with hemorrhagic*
*disorder (D68.312)*
*lupus anticoagulant syndrome (D68.62)*

**D68.62** **Lupus anticoagulant syndrome** CC HCC
Lupus anticoagulant
Presence of systemic lupus erythematosus [SLE]
inhibitor
EXCLUDES 1   *anticardiolipin syndrome (D68.61)*
*antiphospholipid syndrome (D68.61)*
*lupus anticoagulant (LAC) finding without*
*diagnosis (R76.0)*
*lupus anticoagulant (LAC) with hemorrhagic*
*disorder (D68.312)*

**D68.69** **Other thrombophilia** CC HCC
Hypercoagulable states NEC
Secondary hypercoagulable state NOS

**D68.8** **Other specified coagulation defects** CC HCC
EXCLUDES 1   *hemorrhagic disease of newborn (P53)*

**D68.9** **Coagulation defect, unspecified** CC HCC

✓4ᵗʰ **D69** **Purpura and other hemorrhagic conditions**
EXCLUDES 1   *benign hypergammaglobulinemic purpura (D89.0)*
*cryoglobulinemic purpura (D89.1)*
*essential (hemorrhagic) thrombocythemia (D47.3)*
*hemorrhagic thrombocythemia (D47.3)*
*purpura fulminans (D65)*
*thrombotic thrombocytopenic purpura (M31.1)*
*Waldenström hypergammaglobulinemic purpura (D89.0)*

**CC Excl: For CC codes in category D69:** PDX collection 502

**D69.0** **Allergic purpura** CC HCC
Allergic vasculitis
Nonthrombocytopenic hemorrhagic purpura
Nonthrombocytopenic idiopathic purpura
Purpura anaphylactoid
Purpura Henoch(-Schönlein)
Purpura rheumatica
Vascular purpura
EXCLUDES 1   *thrombocytopenic hemorrhagic purpura (D69.3)*
**DEF:** Any hemorrhagic condition, thrombocytic or
nonthrombocytopenic in origin, caused by a presumed allergic
reaction.

**D69.1** **Qualitative platelet defects** HCC
Bernard-Soulier [giant platelet] syndrome
Glanzmann's disease
Grey platelet syndrome
Thromboasthenia (hemorrhagic) (hereditary)
Thrombocytopathy
EXCLUDES 1   *von Willebrand's disease (D68.0)*

**D69.2** **Other nonthrombocytopenic purpura** HCC
Purpura NOS
Purpura simplex
Senile purpura

**D69.3** **Immune thrombocytopenic purpura** CC HCC
Hemorrhagic (thrombocytopenic) purpura
Idiopathic thrombocytopenic purpura
Tidal platelet dysgenesis
**DEF:** Tidal platelet dysgenesis: Platelet counts fluctuate from
normal to very low within periods of 20 to 40 days and may
involve autoimmune platelet destruction.

✓5ᵗʰ **D69.4** **Other primary thrombocytopenia**
EXCLUDES 1   *transient neonatal thrombocytopenia (P61.0)*
*Wiskott-Aldrich syndrome (D82.0)*

**D69.41** **Evans syndrome** CC HCC

N Newborn: 0   P Pediatric: 0-17   M Maternity: 12-55   A Adult: 15-124   MCC Major CC Condition   PDxMCC PDx acts as own MCC   CC CC Condition   PDxCC PDx acts as own CC

504      ICD-10-CM 2018

**D69.42 Congenital and hereditary thrombocytopenia purpura** `CC` `HCC`
Congenital thrombocytopenia
Hereditary thrombocytopenia
Code first congenital or hereditary disorder, such as:
thrombocytopenia with absent radius (TAR syndrome) (Q87.2)

**D69.49 Other primary thrombocytopenia** `HCC`
Megakaryocytic hypoplasia
Primary thrombocytopenia NOS

✓5th **D69.5 Secondary thrombocytopenia**
*EXCLUDES 1*   *heparin induced thrombocytopenia (HIT) (D75.82)*
*transient thrombocytopenia of newborn (P61.0)*

**D69.51 Posttransfusion purpura**
Posttransfusion purpura from whole blood (fresh) or blood products
PTP

**D69.59 Other secondary thrombocytopenia**
AHA: 2014, 4Q, 22

**D69.6 Thrombocytopenia, unspecified** `HCC`
**D69.8 Other specified hemorrhagic conditions** `HCC`
Capillary fragility (hereditary)
Vascular pseudohemophilia

**D69.9 Hemorrhagic condition, unspecified** `HCC`

## Other disorders of blood and blood-forming organs (D70-D77)

✓4th **D70 Neutropenia**
`INCLUDES`   agranulocytosis
decreased absolute neurophile count (ANC)
Use additional code for any associated:
fever (R50.81)
mucositis (J34.81, K12.3-, K92.81, N76.81)
*EXCLUDES 1*   *neutropenic splenomegaly (D73.81)*
*transient neonatal neutropenia (P61.5)*

**D70.0 Congenital agranulocytosis** `HCC`
Congenital neutropenia
Infantile genetic agranulocytosis
Kostmann's disease

**D70.1 Agranulocytosis secondary to cancer chemotherapy** `HCC`
Code also underlying neoplasm
Use additional code for adverse effect, if applicable, to identify drug (T45.1X5)
AHA: 2014, 4Q, 22

**D70.2 Other drug-induced agranulocytosis** `HCC`
Use additional code for adverse effect, if applicable, to identify drug (T36-T50 with fifth or sixth character 5)

**D70.3 Neutropenia due to infection** `HCC`
**D70.4 Cyclic neutropenia** `HCC`
Cyclic hematopoiesis
Periodic neutropenia

**D70.8 Other neutropenia** `HCC`
**D70.9 Neutropenia, unspecified** `HCC`

**D71 Functional disorders of polymorphonuclear neutrophils** `HCC`
Cell membrane receptor complex [CR3] defect
Chronic (childhood) granulomatous disease
Congenital dysphagocytosis
Progressive septic granulomatosis

✓4th **D72 Other disorders of white blood cells**
*EXCLUDES 1*   *basophilia (D72.824)*
*immunity disorders (D80-D89)*
*neutropenia (D70)*
*preleukemia (syndrome) (D46.9)*

**D72.0 Genetic anomalies of leukocytes** `HCC`
Alder (granulation) (granulocyte) anomaly
Alder syndrome
Hereditary leukocytic hypersegmentation
Hereditary leukocytic hyposegmentation
Hereditary leukomelanopathy
May-Hegglin (granulation) (granulocyte) anomaly
May-Hegglin syndrome
Pelger-Huët (granulation) (granulocyte) anomaly
Pelger-Huët syndrome
*EXCLUDES 1*   *Chédiak (-Steinbrinck)-Higashi syndrome (E70.330)*

**D72.1 Eosinophilia**
Allergic eosinophilia
Hereditary eosinophilia
*EXCLUDES 1*   *Löffler's syndrome (J82)*
*pulmonary eosinophilia (J82)*

✓5th **D72.8 Other specified disorders of white blood cells**
*EXCLUDES 1*   *leukemia (C91-C95)*

✓6th **D72.81 Decreased white blood cell count**
*EXCLUDES 1*   *neutropenia (D70.-)*

**D72.810 Lymphocytopenia**
Decreased lymphocytes

**D72.818 Other decreased white blood cell count**
Basophilic leukopenia
Eosinophilic leukopenia
Monocytopenia
Other decreased leukocytes
Plasmacytopenia

**D72.819 Decreased white blood cell count, unspecified**
Decreased leukocytes, unspecified
Leukocytopenia, unspecified
Leukopenia
*EXCLUDES 1*   *malignant leukopenia (D70.9)*

✓6th **D72.82 Elevated white blood cell count**
*EXCLUDES 1*   *eosinophilia (D72.1)*

**D72.820 Lymphocytosis (symptomatic)**
Elevated lymphocytes

**D72.821 Monocytosis (symptomatic)**
*EXCLUDES 1*   *infectious mononucleosis (B27.-)*

**D72.822 Plasmacytosis**

**D72.823 Leukemoid reaction**
Basophilic leukemoid reaction
Leukemoid reaction NOS
Lymphocytic leukemoid reaction
Monocytic leukemoid reaction
Myelocytic leukemoid reaction
Neutrophilic leukemoid reaction

**D72.824 Basophilia**

**D72.825 Bandemia**
Bandemia without diagnosis of specific infection
*EXCLUDES 1*   *confirmed infection—code to infection*
*leukemia (C91.-, C92.-, C93.-, C94.-, C95.-)*
**DEF:** Increase in early neutrophil cells, called band cells; may indicate infection.

**D72.828 Other elevated white blood cell count**

**D72.829 Elevated white blood cell count, unspecified**
Elevated leukocytes, unspecified
Leukocytosis, unspecified

**D72.89 Other specified disorders of white blood cells**
Abnormality of white blood cells NEC

**D72.9 Disorder of white blood cells, unspecified**
Abnormal leukocyte differential NOS

✓4th **D73 Diseases of spleen**
**D73.0 Hyposplenism**
Atrophy of spleen
*EXCLUDES 1*   *asplenia (congenital) (Q89.01)*
*postsurgical absence of spleen (Z90.81)*

**D73.1 Hypersplenism**
*EXCLUDES 1*   *neutropenic splenomegaly (D73.81)*
*primary splenic neutropenia (D73.81)*
*splenitis, splenomegaly in late syphilis (A52.79)*
*splenitis, splenomegaly in tuberculosis (A18.85)*
*splenomegaly NOS (R16.1)*
*splenomegaly congenital (Q89.0)*

**D73.2 Chronic congestive splenomegaly**
**D73.3 Abscess of spleen**
**D73.4 Cyst of spleen**
**D73.5 Infarction of spleen**
Splenic rupture, nontraumatic
Torsion of spleen
*EXCLUDES 1*   *rupture of spleen due to Plasmodium vivax malaria (B51.0)*
*traumatic rupture of spleen (S36.03-)*

✓5th **D73.8 Other diseases of spleen**
**D73.81 Neutropenic splenomegaly**
Werner-Schultz disease

**D73.89 Other diseases of spleen**
Fibrosis of spleen NOS
Perisplenitis
Splenitis NOS

☑ Additional Character Req   ✓x7th Placeholder Alert   Unacceptable PDx   Manifestation   `H1` - `H14` HAC   `HCC` CMS-HCC Condition   *EXCLUDES 1* Not Coded Here   *EXCLUDES 2* Not Included Here

ICD-10-CM 2018      505

Chapter 3. Diseases of the Blood and Blood-forming Organs

D69.42–D73.89

**D73.9    Disease of spleen, unspecified**

✓4th **D74    Methemoglobinemia**

> **CC Excl: For CC codes in category D74:** PDX collection 506

> **D74.0    Congenital methemoglobinemia**    CC
> Congenital NADH-methemoglobin reductase deficiency
> Hemoglobin-M [Hb-M] disease
> Methemoglobinemia, hereditary

> **D74.8    Other methemoglobinemias**    CC
> Acquired methemoglobinemia (with sulfhemoglobinemia)
> Toxic methemoglobinemia

> **D74.9    Methemoglobinemia, unspecified**    CC

✓4th **D75    Other and unspecified diseases of blood and blood-forming organs**

> EXCLUDES2    acute lymphadenitis (L04.-)
> chronic lymphadenitis (I88.1)
> enlarged lymph nodes (R59.-)
> hypergammaglobulinemia NOS (D89.2)
> lymphadenitis NOS (I88.9)
> mesenteric lymphadenitis (acute) (chronic) (I88.0)

> **D75.0    Familial erythrocytosis**
> Benign polycythemia
> Familial polycythemia
> EXCLUDES1    hereditary ovalocytosis (D58.1)

> **D75.1    Secondary polycythemia**
> Acquired polycythemia
> Emotional polycythemia
> Erythrocytosis NOS
> Hypoxemic polycythemia
> Nephrogenous polycythemia
> Polycythemia due to erythropoietin
> Polycythemia due to fall in plasma volume
> Polycythemia due to high altitude
> Polycythemia due to stress
> Polycythemia NOS
> Relative polycythemia
> EXCLUDES1    polycythemia neonatorum (P61.1)
> polycythemia vera (D45)
> **DEF:** Elevated number of red blood cells in circulating blood as a result of reduced oxygen supply to the tissues.

✓5th **D75.8    Other specified diseases of blood and blood-forming organs**

> **D75.81    Myelofibrosis**    CC HCC
> Myelofibrosis NOS
> Secondary myelofibrosis NOS
> Code first the underlying disorder, such as:
> malignant neoplasm of breast (C50.-)
> Use additional code, if applicable, for associated therapy-related myelodysplastic syndrome (D46.-)
> Use additional code for adverse effect, if applicable, to identify drug (T45.1X5)
> EXCLUDES1    acute myelofibrosis (C94.4-)
> idiopathic myelofibrosis (D47.1)
> leukoerythroblastic anemia (D61.82)
> myelofibrosis with myeloid metaplasia (D47.4)
> myelophthisic anemia (D61.82)
> myelophthisis (D61.82)
> primary myelofibrosis (D47.1)
> **CC Excl:** PDX collection 488

> **D75.82    Heparin induced thrombocytopenia (HIT)**    HCC
> **DEF:** Immune-mediated reaction to heparin therapy causing an abrupt fall in platelet count and serious complications such as pulmonary embolism, stroke, AMI, or DVT.

> **D75.89    Other specified diseases of blood and blood-forming organs**

> **D75.9    Disease of blood and blood-forming organs, unspecified**

✓4th **D76    Other specified diseases with participation of lymphoreticular and reticulohistiocytic tissue**

> EXCLUDES1    (Abt-) Letterer-Siwe disease (C96.0)
> eosinophilic granuloma (C96.6)
> Hand-Schüller-Christian disease (C96.5)
> histiocytic medullary reticulosis (C96.9)
> histiocytic sarcoma (C96.A)
> histiocytosis X, multifocal (C96.5)
> histiocytosis X, unifocal (C96.6)
> Langerhans-cell histiocytosis, multifocal (C96.5)
> Langerhans-cell histiocytosis NOS (C96.6)
> Langerhans-cell histiocytosis, unifocal (C96.6)
> leukemic reticuloendotheliosis (C91.4-)
> lipomelanotic reticulosis (I89.8)
> malignant histiocytosis (C96.A)
> malignant reticulosis (C86.0)
> nonlipid reticuloendotheliosis (C96.0)

> **CC Excl: For CC codes in category D76, unless otherwise noted:** PDX collection 507

> **D76.1    Hemophagocytic lymphohistiocytosis**    CC HCC
> Familial hemophagocytic reticulosis
> Histiocytoses of mononuclear phagocytes

> **D76.2    Hemophagocytic syndrome, infection-associated**    CC HCC
> Use additional code to identify infectious agent or disease

> **D76.3    Other histiocytosis syndromes**    CC HCC
> Reticulohistiocytoma (giant-cell)
> Sinus histiocytosis with massive lymphadenopathy
> Xanthogranuloma

**D77    Other disorders of blood and blood-forming organs in diseases classified elsewhere**

> Code first underlying disease, such as:
> amyloidosis (E85.-)
> congenital early syphilis (A50.0)
> echinococcosis (B67.0-B67.9)
> malaria (B50.0-B54)
> schistosomiasis [bilharziasis] (B65.0-B65.9)
> vitamin C deficiency (E54)
> EXCLUDES1    rupture of spleen due to Plasmodium vivax malaria (B51.0)
> splenitis, splenomegaly in late syphilis (A52.79)
> splenitis, splenomegaly in tuberculosis (A18.85)

## Intraoperative and postprocedural complications of the spleen (D78)

✓4th **D78    Intraoperative and postprocedural complications of the spleen**

> **CC Excl: For CC codes in category D78, unless otherwise noted:** PDX collection 508

✓5th **D78.0    Intraoperative hemorrhage and hematoma of the spleen complicating a procedure**

> EXCLUDES1    intraoperative hemorrhage and hematoma of the spleen due to accidental puncture or laceration during a procedure (D78.1-)

> **D78.01    Intraoperative hemorrhage and hematoma of the spleen complicating a procedure on the spleen**    CC

> **D78.02    Intraoperative hemorrhage and hematoma of the spleen complicating other procedure**    CC

✓5th **D78.1    Accidental puncture and laceration of the spleen during a procedure**

> **D78.11    Accidental puncture and laceration of the spleen during a procedure on the spleen**    CC
> **CC Excl:** PDX collection 509

> **D78.12    Accidental puncture and laceration of the spleen during other procedure**    CC
> **CC Excl:** PDX collection 509

✓5th **D78.2    Postprocedural hemorrhage of the spleen following a procedure**

> **D78.21    Postprocedural hemorrhage of the spleen following a procedure on the spleen**    CC

> **D78.22    Postprocedural hemorrhage of the spleen following other procedure**    CC

✓5th **D78.3    Postprocedural hematoma and seroma of the spleen following a procedure**

> **D78.31    Postprocedural hematoma of the spleen following a procedure on the spleen**    CC

> **D78.32    Postprocedural hematoma of the spleen following other procedure**    CC

> **D78.33    Postprocedural seroma of the spleen following a procedure on the spleen**    CC

**D78.34**   **Postprocedural seroma of the spleen following**   `CC`
other procedure

✓5ᵗʰ **D78.8**   Other **intraoperative and postprocedural complications of the spleen**
Use additional code, if applicable, to further specify disorder

**D78.81**   **Other intraoperative complications**   `CC`
**of the spleen**
**CC Excl:** PDX collection 510

**D78.89**   **Other postprocedural complications**   `CC`
**of the spleen**
**CC Excl:** PDX collection 510

## Certain disorders involving the immune mechanism (D80-D89)

`INCLUDES`   defects in the complement system
immunodeficiency disorders, except human immunodeficiency virus [HIV] disease
sarcoidosis

`EXCLUDES 1`   autoimmune disease (systemic) NOS (M35.9)
functional disorders of polymorphonuclear neutrophils (D71)
human immunodeficiency virus [HIV] disease (B20)

✓4ᵗʰ **D80**   **Immunodeficiency with predominantly antibody defects**

**CC Excl: For CC codes in category D80, unless otherwise noted:**
PDX collection 511

**D80.0**   **Hereditary hypogammaglobulinemia**   `CC` `HCC`
Autosomal recessive agammaglobulinemia (Swiss type)
X-linked agammaglobulinemia [Bruton] (with growth hormone deficiency)

**D80.1**   **Nonfamilial hypogammaglobulinemia**   `CC` `HCC`
Agammaglobulinemia with immunoglobulin-bearing B-lymphocytes
Common variable agammaglobulinemia [CVAgamma]
Hypogammaglobulinemia NOS
**CC Excl:** PDX collection 512

**D80.2**   **Selective deficiency of immunoglobulin A [IgA]**   `CC` `HCC`
**CC Excl:** PDX collection 512

**D80.3**   **Selective deficiency of immunoglobulin G [IgG]**   `CC` `HCC`
**subclasses**

**D80.4**   **Selective deficiency of immunoglobulin M [IgM]**   `CC` `HCC`

**D80.5**   **Immunodeficiency with increased immunoglobulin M**   `CC` `HCC`
**[IgM]**

**D80.6**   **Antibody deficiency with near-normal**   `CC` `HCC`
**immunoglobulins or with hyperimmunoglobulinemia**

**D80.7**   **Transient hypogammaglobulinemia of infancy**   `CC` `HCC`

**D80.8**   **Other immunodeficiencies with predominantly**   `CC` `HCC`
**antibody defects**
Kappa light chain deficiency

**D80.9**   **Immunodeficiency with predominantly antibody**   `CC` `HCC`
**defects, unspecified**

✓4ᵗʰ **D81**   **Combined immunodeficiencies**
`EXCLUDES 1`   autosomal recessive agammaglobulinemia (Swiss type) (D80.0)

**CC Excl: For CC codes in category D81, unless otherwise noted:**
PDX collection 511

**D81.0**   **Severe combined immunodeficiency [SCID] with**   `CC` `HCC`
**reticular dysgenesis**

**D81.1**   **Severe combined immunodeficiency [SCID] with low**   `CC` `HCC`
**T- and B-cell numbers**

**D81.2**   **Severe combined immunodeficiency [SCID] with low**   `CC` `HCC`
**or normal B-cell numbers**

**D81.3**   **Adenosine deaminase [ADA] deficiency**   `CC` `HCC`
**CC Excl:** PDX collection 513

**D81.4**   **Nezelof's syndrome**   `CC` `HCC`

**D81.5**   **Purine nucleoside phosphorylase [PNP] deficiency**   `CC` `HCC`
**CC Excl:** PDX collection 513

**D81.6**   **Major histocompatibility complex class I deficiency**   `CC` `HCC`
Bare lymphocyte syndrome

**D81.7**   **Major histocompatibility complex class II deficiency**   `CC` `HCC`

✓5ᵗʰ **D81.8**   **Other combined immunodeficiencies**

✓6ᵗʰ **D81.81**   **Biotin-dependent carboxylase deficiency**
Multiple carboxylase deficiency
`EXCLUDES 1`   biotin-dependent carboxylase deficiency due to dietary deficiency of biotin (E53.8)

**D81.810**   **Biotinidase deficiency**

**D81.818**   **Other biotin-dependent carboxylase deficiency**
Holocarboxylase synthetase deficiency
Other multiple carboxylase deficiency

**D81.819**   **Biotin-dependent carboxylase deficiency, unspecified**
Multiple carboxylase deficiency, unspecified

**D81.89**   **Other combined immunodeficiencies**   `CC` `HCC`

**D81.9**   **Combined immunodeficiency, unspecified**   `CC` `HCC`
Severe combined immunodeficiency disorder [SCID] NOS

✓4ᵗʰ **D82**   **Immunodeficiency associated with other major defects**
`EXCLUDES 1`   ataxia telangiectasia [Louis-Bar] (G11.3)

**D82.0**   **Wiskott-Aldrich syndrome**   `CC` `HCC`
Immunodeficiency with thrombocytopenia and eczema
**CC Excl:** PDX collection 511

**D82.1**   **Di George's syndrome**   `CC` `HCC`
Pharyngeal pouch syndrome
Thymic alymphoplasia
Thymic aplasia or hypoplasia with immunodeficiency
**CC Excl:** PDX collection 511

**D82.2**   **Immunodeficiency with short-limbed stature**   `HCC`

**D82.3**   **Immunodeficiency following hereditary defective**   `HCC`
**response to Epstein-Barr virus**
X-linked lymphoproliferative disease

**D82.4**   **Hyperimmunoglobulin E [IgE] syndrome**   `HCC`

**D82.8**   **Immunodeficiency associated with other specified**   `HCC`
**major defects**

**D82.9**   **Immunodeficiency associated with major defect,**   `HCC`
**unspecified**

✓4ᵗʰ **D83**   **Common variable immunodeficiency**

**CC Excl: For CC codes in category D83:** PDX collection 511

**D83.0**   **Common variable immunodeficiency with**   `CC` `HCC`
**predominant abnormalities of B-cell numbers and function**

**D83.1**   **Common variable immunodeficiency with**   `CC` `HCC`
**predominant immunoregulatory T-cell disorders**

**D83.2**   **Common variable immunodeficiency with**   `CC` `HCC`
**autoantibodies to B- or T-cells**

**D83.8**   **Other common variable immunodeficiencies**   `CC` `HCC`

**D83.9**   **Common variable immunodeficiency, unspecified**   `CC` `HCC`

✓4ᵗʰ **D84**   **Other immunodeficiencies**

**D84.0**   **Lymphocyte function antigen-1 [LFA-1] defect**   `HCC`

**D84.1**   **Defects in the complement system**   `HCC`
C1 esterase inhibitor [C1-INH] deficiency

**D84.8**   **Other specified immunodeficiencies**   `CC` `HCC`
**CC Excl:** PDX collection 511

**D84.9**   **Immunodeficiency, unspecified**   `CC` `HCC`
**CC Excl:** PDX collection 511

✓4ᵗʰ **D86**   **Sarcoidosis**

**D86.0**   **Sarcoidosis of lung**   `HCC`

**D86.1**   **Sarcoidosis of lymph nodes**

**D86.2**   **Sarcoidosis of lung with sarcoidosis of lymph nodes**   `HCC`

**D86.3**   **Sarcoidosis of skin**

✓5ᵗʰ **D86.8**   **Sarcoidosis of other sites**

**D86.81**   **Sarcoid meningitis**

**D86.82**   **Multiple cranial nerve palsies in sarcoidosis**   `HCC`

**D86.83**   **Sarcoid iridocyclitis**

**D86.84**   **Sarcoid pyelonephritis**
Tubulo-interstitial nephropathy in sarcoidosis

**D86.85**   **Sarcoid myocarditis**

**D86.86**   **Sarcoid arthropathy**
Polyarthritis in sarcoidosis

**D86.87**   **Sarcoid myositis**

**D86.89**   **Sarcoidosis of other sites**
Hepatic granuloma
Uveoparotid fever [Heerfordt]

**D86.9**   **Sarcoidosis, unspecified**

✓4ᵗʰ **D89**   **Other disorders involving the immune mechanism, not elsewhere classified**
`EXCLUDES 1`   hyperglobulinemia NOS (R77.1)
monoclonal gammopathy (of undetermined significance) (D47.2)
`EXCLUDES 2`   transplant failure and rejection (T86.-)

**D89.0**   **Polyclonal hypergammaglobulinemia**
Benign hypergammaglobulinemic purpura
Polyclonal gammopathy NOS

---

✓ Additional Character Req   ✓x7ᵗʰ Placeholder Alert   Unacceptable PDx   Manifestation   `H1`-`H14` HAC   `HCC` CMS-HCC Condition   `EXCLUDES 1` Not Coded Here   `EXCLUDES 2` Not Included Here

ICD-10-CM 2018          **507**

**Chapter 3. Diseases of the Blood and Blood-forming Organs**

**D89.1** **Cryoglobulinemia**    HCC
     Cryoglobulinemic purpura
     Cryoglobulinemic vasculitis
     Essential cryoglobulinemia
     Idiopathic cryoglobulinemia
     Mixed cryoglobulinemia
     Primary cryoglobulinemia
     Secondary cryoglobulinemia

**D89.2** **Hypergammaglobulinemia, unspecified**

**D89.3** **Immune reconstitution syndrome**    HCC
     Immune reconstitution inflammatory syndrome [IRIS]
     Use additional code for adverse effect, if applicable, to identify drug (T36-T50 with fifth or sixth character 5)

**✓5th** **D89.4** **Mast cell activation syndrome and related disorders**
     **EXCLUDES 1**    *aggressive systemic mastocytosis ▶(C96.21)◀*
         *▶congenital cutaneous mastocytosis◀ (Q82.2)*
         *▶(non-congenital) cutaneous mastocytosis (D47.01)*
         *(indolent) systemic mastocytosis (D47.02)*
         *malignant mast cell neoplasm (C96.2-)◀*
         *malignant mastocytoma ▶(C96.29)◀*
         *mast cell leukemia (C94.3-)*
         *▶mast cell sarcoma (C96.22)*
         *mastocytoma NOS (D47.09)*
         *other mast cell neoplasms of uncertain behavior (D47.09)◀*
         *systemic mastocytosis associated with a clonal hematologic non-mast cell lineage disease (SM-AHNMD)▶(D47.02)◀*

**D89.40** **Mast cell activation, unspecified**    HCC
     Mast cell activation disorder, unspecified
     Mast cell activation syndrome, NOS

**D89.41** **Monoclonal mast cell activation syndrome**    HCC

**D89.42** **Idiopathic mast cell activation syndrome**    HCC

**D89.43** **Secondary mast cell activation**    HCC
     Secondary mast cell activation syndrome
     Code also underlying etiology, if known

**D89.49** **Other mast cell activation disorder**    HCC
     Other mast cell activation syndrome

**✓5th** **D89.8** **Other specified disorders involving the immune mechanism, not elsewhere classified**

**✓6th** **D89.81** **Graft-versus-host disease**
     Code first underlying cause, such as:
         complications of transplanted organs and tissue (T86.-)
         complications of blood transfusion (T80.89)
     Use additional code to identify associated manifestations, such as:
         desquamative dermatitis (L30.8)
         diarrhea (R19.7)
         elevated bilirubin (R17)
         hair loss (L65.9)

     **CC Excl: For CC codes in subcategory D89.81:**
     PDX collection 514

**D89.810** **Acute graft-versus-host disease**    CC HCC

**D89.811** **Chronic graft-versus-host disease**    CC HCC

**D89.812** **Acute on chronic graft-versus-host disease**    CC HCC

**D89.813** **Graft-versus-host disease, unspecified**    CC HCC

**D89.82** **Autoimmune lymphoproliferative syndrome [ALPS]**    HCC
     **DEF:** Rare genetic alteration of the Fas protein; impairs normal cellular apoptosis (normal cell death), causing abnormal accumulation of lymphocytes in the lymph glands, liver, and spleen; symptoms include neutropenia, anemia, and thrombocytopenia.

**D89.89** **Other specified disorders involving the immune mechanism, not elsewhere classified**    HCC
     **EXCLUDES 1**    *human immunodeficiency virus disease (B20)*

**D89.9** **Disorder involving the immune mechanism, unspecified**    HCC
     Immune disease NOS
     **AHA:** 2015, 3Q, 22

**N** Newborn: 0    **P** Pediatric: 0-17    **M** Maternity: 12-55    **A** Adult: 15-124    **MCC** Major CC Condition    **PDxMCC** PDx acts as own MCC    **CC** CC Condition    **PDxCC** PDx acts as own CC

**508**

**ICD-10-CM 2018**

# Chapter 4. Endocrine, Nutritional and Metabolic Diseases (E00–E89)

## Chapter Specific Guidelines with Coding Examples

The chapter specific guidelines from the ICD-10-CM Official Guidelines for Coding and Reporting have been provided below. Along with these guidelines are coding examples, contained in the shaded boxes, that have been developed to help illustrate the coding and/or sequencing guidance found in these guidelines.

### a. Diabetes mellitus

The diabetes mellitus codes are combination codes that include the type of diabetes mellitus, the body system affected, and the complications affecting that body system. As many codes within a particular category as are necessary to describe all of the complications of the disease may be used. They should be sequenced based on the reason for a particular encounter. Assign as many codes from categories E08–E13 as needed to identify all of the associated conditions that the patient has.

---

Patient is seen for poorly controlled diabetes, type 2, with diabetic polyneuropathy and diabetic retinopathy with macular edema

**E11.65**    **Type 2 diabetes mellitus with hyperglycemia**

**E11.311**    **Type 2 diabetes mellitus with unspecified diabetic retinopathy with macular edema**

**E11.42**    **Type 2 diabetes mellitus with diabetic polyneuropathy**

*Explanation*: Use as many codes to describe the diabetic complications as needed. Many are combination codes that describe more than one condition. Code first the reason for the encounter. "Poorly controlled" is described as "with hyperglycemia." Diabetes documented as "uncontrolled" is not assumed to be hyperglycemic but can be classified to either hyperglycemia or hypoglycemia. If documentation is not clear, the provider must be queried so that the appropriate code can be reported.

---

### 1) Type of diabetes

The age of a patient is not the sole determining factor, though most type 1 diabetics develop the condition before reaching puberty. For this reason type 1 diabetes mellitus is also referred to as juvenile diabetes.

---

A 45-year-old patient is diagnosed with type 1 diabetes

**E10.9**    **Type 1 diabetes mellitus without complications**

*Explanation*: Although most type 1 diabetics are diagnosed in childhood or adolescence, it can also begin in adults.

---

### 2) Type of diabetes mellitus not documented

If the type of diabetes mellitus is not documented in the medical record the default is E11.-, Type 2 diabetes mellitus.

---

H & P lists diabetes and hypertension on patient problem list

**E11.9**    **Type 2 diabetes mellitus without complications**

**I10**    **Essential (primary) hypertension**

*Explanation*: Since the type of diabetes was not documented and no complications were noted, the default code is E11.9.

---

### 3) Diabetes mellitus and the use of insulin and oral hypoglycemics

If the documentation in a medical record does not indicate the type of diabetes but does indicate that the patient uses insulin, code E11, Type 2 diabetes mellitus, should be assigned. Code Z79.4, Long-term (current) use of insulin, or Z79.84, Long term (current) use of oral hypoglycemic drugs, should also be assigned to indicate that the patient uses insulin or hypoglycemic drugs. Code Z79.4 should not be assigned if insulin is given temporarily to bring a type 2 patient's blood sugar under control during an encounter.

---

The H & P lists chronic diabetes and the use of daily metformin and nightly insulin.

**E11.9**    **Type 2 diabetes mellitus without complications**

**Z79.4**    **Long term (current) use of insulin**

**Z79.84**    **Long term (current) use of oral hypoglycemic drugs**

*Explanation*: Do not assume that a patient on insulin must have type 1 diabetes. The default for diabetes without further specification defaults to type 2. Patients with DM 2 often are prescribed both insulin and an oral hypoglycemic agent. Report both codes for the long-term use of the drugs.

---

### 4) Diabetes mellitus in pregnancy and gestational diabetes

*See Section I.C.15. Diabetes mellitus in pregnancy.*

*See Section I.C.15. Gestational (pregnancy induced) diabetes*

### 5) Complications due to insulin pump malfunction

#### (a) Underdose of insulin due to insulin pump failure

An underdose of insulin due to an insulin pump failure should be assigned to a code from subcategory T85.6, Mechanical complication of other specified internal and external prosthetic devices, implants and grafts, that specifies the type of pump malfunction, as the principal or first-listed code, followed by code T38.3X6-, Underdosing of insulin and oral hypoglycemic [antidiabetic] drugs. Additional codes for the type of diabetes mellitus and any associated complications due to the underdosing should also be assigned.

---

A 24-year-old type 1 diabetic male treated in ED for hyperglycemia; insulin pump found to be malfunctioning and underdosing

**T85.614A**    **Breakdown (mechanical) of insulin pump, initial encounter**

**T38.3X6A**    **Underdosing of insulin and oral hypoglycemic [antidiabetic] drugs, initial encounter**

**E10.65**    **Type 1 diabetes mellitus with hyperglycemia**

*Explanation*: The complication code for the mechanical breakdown of the pump is sequenced first, followed by the underdosing code and type of diabetes with complication. Code all other diabetic complication codes necessary to describe the patient's condition.

---

#### (b) Overdose of insulin due to insulin pump failure

The principal or first-listed code for an encounter due to an insulin pump malfunction resulting in an overdose of insulin, should also be T85.6-, Mechanical complication of other specified internal and external prosthetic devices, implants and grafts, followed by code T38.3X1-, Poisoning by insulin and oral hypoglycemic [antidiabetic] drugs, accidental (unintentional).

---

A 24-year-old type 1 diabetic male found down with diabetic coma, brought into ED and treated for hypoglycemia; insulin pump found to be malfunctioning and overdosing

**T85.614A**    **Breakdown (mechanical) of insulin pump, initial encounter**

**T38.3X1A**    **Poisoning by insulin and oral hypoglycemic [antidiabetic] drugs, accidental (unintentional), initial encounter**

**E10.641**    **Type 1 diabetes mellitus with hypoglycemia with coma**

*Explanation*: The complication code for the mechanical breakdown of the pump is sequenced first, followed by the poisoning code and type of diabetes with complication. All the characters in the combination code must be used to form a valid code and to fully describe the type of diabetes, the hypoglycemia, and the coma.

---

### 6) Secondary diabetes mellitus

Codes under categories E08, Diabetes mellitus due to underlying condition, E09, Drug or chemical induced diabetes mellitus, and E13, Other specified diabetes mellitus, identify complications/manifestations associated with secondary diabetes mellitus. Secondary diabetes is always caused by another condition or event (e.g., cystic fibrosis, malignant neoplasm of pancreas, pancreatectomy, adverse effect of drug, or poisoning).

#### (a) Secondary diabetes mellitus and the use of insulin or hypoglycemic drugs

For patients who routinely use insulin or hypoglycemic drugs, code Z79.4, Long-term (current) use of insulin, or Z79.84, Long term (current) use of oral hypoglycemic drugs should also be assigned. Code Z79.4 should not be assigned if insulin is given temporarily to bring a patient's blood sugar under control during an encounter.

Type 2 diabetic with no complications, normally only on oral metformin, is given insulin for three days to maintain glucose control while in the hospital recovering from surgery

**E11.9**      **Type 2 diabetes mellitus without complications**

**Z79.84**      **Long term (current) use of oral hypoglycemic drugs**

*Explanation*: Although the patient was given insulin for a short time during his hospital stay, the intent was only to maintain the patient's glucose levels while off his regular oral hypoglycemic medication, not for long term use. No code is needed for long term use of insulin, but a Z code for long term use of an oral hypoglycemic should be added to identify the chronic use of this drug.

---

Type 2 diabetic with diabetic polyneuropathy on insulin

**E11.42**      **Type 2 diabetes mellitus with diabetic polyneuropathy**

**Z79.4**      **Long term (current) use of insulin**

*Explanation*: Add the Z code for the long term use of insulin because the insulin is taken chronically.

**(b) Assigning and sequencing secondary diabetes codes and its causes**

The sequencing of the secondary diabetes codes in relationship to codes for the cause of the diabetes is based on the Tabular List instructions for categories E08, E09 and E13.

**(i) Secondary diabetes mellitus due to pancreatectomy**

For postpancreatectomy diabetes mellitus (lack of insulin due to the surgical removal of all or part of the pancreas), assign code E89.1, Postprocedural hypoinsulinemia. Assign a code from category E13 and a code from subcategory Z90.41-, Acquired absence of pancreas, as additional codes.

---

Patient with newly diagnosed diabetes after surgical removal of part of pancreas is discharged with referral for consult to initiate insulin.

**E89.1**      **Postprocedural hypoinsulinemia**

**E13.9**      **Other specified diabetes mellitus without complications**

**Z90.411**      **Acquired partial absence of pancreas**

*Explanation*: Sequence the postprocedural complication of the hypoinsulinemia due to the partial removal of the pancreas as the first-listed code, followed by the other specified diabetes (NEC) with or without complications and the partial or total acquired absence of the pancreas. Code Z79.4 Long term (current) use of insulin, is not added because the insulin has not yet been started.

**(ii) Secondary diabetes due to drugs**

Secondary diabetes may be caused by an adverse effect of correctly administered medications, poisoning or sequela of poisoning.

*See section I.C.19.e for coding of adverse effects and poisoning, and section I.C.20 for external cause code reporting.*

---

Initial encounter for corticosteroid-induced diabetes mellitus

**E09.9**      **Drug or chemical induced diabetes mellitus without complications**

**T38.0X5A**      **Adverse effect of glucocorticoids and synthetic analogues, initial encounter**

*Explanation*: If the diabetes is caused by an adverse effect of a drug, the diabetic condition is coded first. If it occurs from a poisoning or overdose, the poisoning code causing the diabetes is sequenced first.

# Chapter 4. Endocrine, Nutritional and Metabolic Diseases (E00-E89)

**NOTE** All neoplasms, whether functionally active or not, are classified in Chapter 2. Appropriate codes in this chapter (i.e. E05.8, E07.0, E16-E31, E34-) may be used as additional codes to indicate either functional activity by neoplasms and ectopic endocrine tissue or hyperfunction and hypofunction of endocrine glands associated with neoplasms and other conditions classified elsewhere.

**EXCLUDES 1** *transitory endocrine and metabolic disorders specific to newborn (P70-P74)*

This chapter contains the following blocks:

| | |
|---|---|
| E00-E07 | Disorders of thyroid gland |
| E08-E13 | Diabetes mellitus |
| E15-E16 | Other disorders of glucose regulation and pancreatic internal secretion |
| E20-E35 | Disorders of other endocrine glands |
| E36 | Intraoperative complications of endocrine system |
| E40-E46 | Malnutrition |
| E50-E64 | Other nutritional deficiencies |
| E65-E68 | Overweight, obesity and other hyperalimentation |
| E70-E88 | Metabolic disorders |
| E89 | Postprocedural endocrine and metabolic complications and disorders, not elsewhere classified |

## Disorders of thyroid gland (E00-E07)

### ✓4ᵗʰ E00 Congenital iodine-deficiency syndrome

Use additional code (F70-F79) to identify associated intellectual disabilities

**EXCLUDES 1** *subclinical iodine-deficiency hypothyroidism (E02)*

**E00.0 Congenital iodine-deficiency syndrome, neurological type**
Endemic cretinism, neurological type

**E00.1 Congenital iodine-deficiency syndrome, myxedematous type**
Endemic hypothyroid cretinism
Endemic cretinism, myxedematous type

**E00.2 Congenital iodine-deficiency syndrome, mixed type**
Endemic cretinism, mixed type

**E00.9 Congenital iodine-deficiency syndrome, unspecified**
Congenital iodine-deficiency hypothyroidism NOS
Endemic cretinism NOS

### ✓4ᵗʰ E01 Iodine-deficiency related thyroid disorders and allied conditions

**EXCLUDES 1** *congenital iodine-deficiency syndrome (E00.-)*
*subclinical iodine-deficiency hypothyroidism (E02)*

**E01.0 Iodine-deficiency related diffuse (endemic) goiter**

**E01.1 Iodine-deficiency related multinodular (endemic) goiter**
Iodine-deficiency related nodular goiter

**E01.2 Iodine-deficiency related (endemic) goiter, unspecified**
Endemic goiter NOS

**E01.8 Other iodine-deficiency related thyroid disorders and allied conditions**
Acquired iodine-deficiency hypothyroidism NOS

### E02 Subclinical iodine-deficiency hypothyroidism

### ✓4ᵗʰ E03 Other hypothyroidism

**EXCLUDES 1** *iodine-deficiency related hypothyroidism (E00-E02)*
*postprocedural hypothyroidism (E89.0)*

**E03.0 Congenital hypothyroidism with diffuse goiter**
Congenital parenchymatous goiter (nontoxic)
Congenital goiter (nontoxic) NOS
**EXCLUDES 1** *transitory congenital goiter with normal function (P72.0)*

**E03.1 Congenital hypothyroidism without goiter**
Aplasia of thyroid (with myxedema)
Congenital atrophy of thyroid
Congenital hypothyroidism NOS

**E03.2 Hypothyroidism due to medicaments and other exogenous substances**
Code first poisoning due to drug or toxin, if applicable (T36-T65 with fifth or sixth character 1-4 or 6)
Use additional code for adverse effect, if applicable, to identify drug (T36-T50 with fifth or sixth character 5)

**E03.3 Postinfectious hypothyroidism**

**E03.4 Atrophy of thyroid (acquired)**
**EXCLUDES 1** *congenital atrophy of thyroid (E03.1)*

**E03.5 Myxedema coma**    **MCC** **HCC**
CC Excl: PDX collection 515

**E03.8 Other specified hypothyroidism**

**E03.9 Hypothyroidism, unspecified**
Myxedema NOS

### ✓4ᵗʰ E04 Other nontoxic goiter

**EXCLUDES 1** *congenital goiter (NOS) (diffuse) (parenchymatous) (E03.0)*
*iodine-deficiency related goiter (E00-E02)*

**E04.0 Nontoxic diffuse goiter**
Diffuse (colloid) nontoxic goiter
Simple nontoxic goiter

**E04.1 Nontoxic single thyroid nodule**
Colloid nodule (cystic) (thyroid)    Thyroid (cystic) nodule NOS
Nontoxic uninodular goiter
**DEF:** Enlarged thyroid, commonly due to decreased thyroid production, with single nodule; no clinical hypothyroidism.

**E04.2 Nontoxic multinodular goiter**
Cystic goiter NOS
Multinodular (cystic) goiter NOS
**DEF:** Enlarged thyroid, commonly due to decreased thyroid production with multiple nodules; no clinical hypothyroidism.

**E04.8 Other specified nontoxic goiter**

**E04.9 Nontoxic goiter, unspecified**
Goiter NOS
Nodular goiter (nontoxic) NOS

### ✓4ᵗʰ E05 Thyrotoxicosis [hyperthyroidism]

**EXCLUDES 1** *chronic thyroiditis with transient thyrotoxicosis (E06.2)*
*neonatal thyrotoxicosis (P72.1)*

**CC Excl: For MCC codes in category E05:** PDX collection 516

**✓5ᵗʰ E05.0 Thyrotoxicosis with diffuse goiter**
Exophthalmic or toxic goiter NOS
Graves' disease
Toxic diffuse goiter
**DEF:** Diffuse thyroid enlargement accompanied by hyperthyroidism, bulging eyes, and dermopathy.

**E05.00 Thyrotoxicosis with diffuse goiter without thyrotoxic crisis or storm**

**E05.01 Thyrotoxicosis with diffuse goiter with thyrotoxic crisis or storm**    **MCC**

**✓5ᵗʰ E05.1 Thyrotoxicosis with toxic single thyroid nodule**
Thyrotoxicosis with toxic uninodular goiter
**DEF:** Symptomatic hyperthyroidism with a single nodule on the enlarged thyroid gland. Abrupt onset of symptoms include extreme nervousness, insomnia, weight loss, tremors, and psychosis or coma.

**E05.10 Thyrotoxicosis with toxic single thyroid nodule without thyrotoxic crisis or storm**

**E05.11 Thyrotoxicosis with toxic single thyroid nodule with thyrotoxic crisis or storm**    **MCC**

**✓5ᵗʰ E05.2 Thyrotoxicosis with toxic multinodular goiter**
Toxic nodular goiter NOS

**E05.20 Thyrotoxicosis with toxic multinodular goiter without thyrotoxic crisis or storm**

**E05.21 Thyrotoxicosis with toxic multinodular goiter with thyrotoxic crisis or storm**    **MCC**

**✓5ᵗʰ E05.3 Thyrotoxicosis from ectopic thyroid tissue**

**E05.30 Thyrotoxicosis from ectopic thyroid tissue without thyrotoxic crisis or storm**

**E05.31 Thyrotoxicosis from ectopic thyroid tissue with thyrotoxic crisis or storm**    **MCC**

**Goiter**

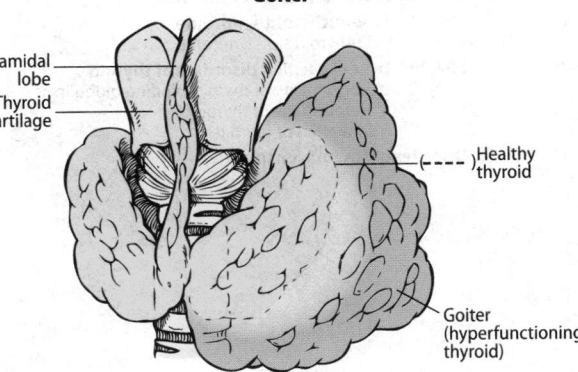

Pyramidal lobe
Thyroid cartilage
Healthy thyroid
Goiter (hyperfunctioning thyroid)

---

☑ Additional Character Req   ✓x7ᵗʰ Placeholder Alert   Unacceptable PDx   Manifestation   **H1** **H14** HAC   **HCC** CMS-HCC Condition   **EXCLUDES 1** Not Coded Here   **EXCLUDES 2** Not Included Here

ICD-10-CM 2018      **511**

**Chapter 4. Endocrine, Nutritional and Metabolic Diseases**

✓5ᵗʰ **E05.4** **Thyrotoxicosis factitia**

**E05.40** **Thyrotoxicosis factitia** without thyrotoxic crisis or storm

**E05.41** **Thyrotoxicosis factitia** with thyrotoxic crisis or storm　MCC

✓5ᵗʰ **E05.8** **Other thyrotoxicosis**
Overproduction of thyroid-stimulating hormone

**E05.80** **Other thyrotoxicosis** without thyrotoxic crisis or storm

**E05.81** **Other thyrotoxicosis** with thyrotoxic crisis or storm　MCC

✓5ᵗʰ **E05.9** **Thyrotoxicosis,** unspecified
Hyperthyroidism NOS

**E05.90** **Thyrotoxicosis, unspecified** without thyrotoxic crisis or storm

**E05.91** **Thyrotoxicosis, unspecified** with thyrotoxic crisis or storm　MCC

✓4ᵗʰ **E06** **Thyroiditis**
EXCLUDES 1　postpartum thyroiditis (O90.5)

**E06.0** **Acute thyroiditis**　CC
Abscess of thyroid
Pyogenic thyroiditis
Suppurative thyroiditis
Use additional code (B95-B97) to identify infectious agent
**CC Excl:** PDX collection 517

**E06.1** **Subacute thyroiditis**
de Quervain thyroiditis
Giant-cell thyroiditis
Granulomatous thyroiditis
Nonsuppurative thyroiditis
Viral thyroiditis
EXCLUDES 1　autoimmune thyroiditis (E06.3)

**E06.2** **Chronic thyroiditis** with transient thyrotoxicosis
EXCLUDES 1　autoimmune thyroiditis (E06.3)

**E06.3** **Autoimmune thyroiditis**
Hashimoto's thyroiditis
Hashitoxicosis (transient)
Lymphadenoid goiter
Lymphocytic thyroiditis
Struma lymphomatosa

**E06.4** **Drug-induced thyroiditis**
Use additional code for adverse effect, if applicable, to identify drug (T36-T50 with fifth or sixth character 5)

**E06.5** **Other chronic thyroiditis**
Chronic fibrous thyroiditis
Chronic thyroiditis NOS
Ligneous thyroiditis
Riedel thyroiditis

**E06.9** **Thyroiditis,** unspecified

✓4ᵗʰ **E07** **Other disorders of thyroid**

**E07.0** **Hypersecretion of calcitonin**
C-cell hyperplasia of thyroid
Hypersecretion of thyrocalcitonin

**E07.1** **Dyshormogenetic goiter**
Familial dyshormogenetic goiter
Pendred's syndrome
EXCLUDES 1　transitory congenital goiter with normal function (P72.0)

✓5ᵗʰ **E07.8** **Other specified disorders of thyroid**

**E07.81** **Sick-euthyroid syndrome**
Euthyroid sick-syndrome

**E07.89** **Other specified disorders of thyroid**
Abnormality of thyroid-binding globulin
Hemorrhage of thyroid
Infarction of thyroid

**E07.9** **Disorder of thyroid, unspecified**

## Diabetes mellitus (E08-E13)
**AHA:** 2017, 1Q, 42; 2016, 2Q, 36; 2016, 1Q, 11-13

✓4ᵗʰ **E08** **Diabetes mellitus** due to underlying condition
Code first the underlying condition, such as:
congenital rubella (P35.0)
cushing's syndrome (E24.-)
cystic fibrosis (E84.-)
malignant neoplasm (C00-C96)
malnutrition (E40-E46)
pancreatitis and other diseases of the pancreas (K85.-, K86.-)
Use additional code to identify control using:
insulin (Z79.4)
oral antidiabetic drugs (Z79.84)
oral hypoglycemic drugs (Z79.84)
EXCLUDES 1　drug or chemical induced diabetes mellitus (E09.-)
gestational diabetes (O24.4-)
neonatal diabetes mellitus (P70.2)
postpancreatectomy diabetes mellitus (E13.-)
postprocedural diabetes mellitus (E13.-)
secondary diabetes mellitus NEC (E13.-)
type 1 diabetes mellitus (E10.-)\
type 2 diabetes mellitus (E11.-)
**AHA:** 2013, 4Q, 114; 2013, 3Q, 20

**CC Excl: For MCC codes in category E08, unless otherwise noted:** PDX collection 518

✓5ᵗʰ **E08.0** **Diabetes mellitus due to underlying condition with hyperosmolarity**

**E08.00** *Diabetes mellitus due to underlying condition with hyperosmolarity without nonketotic hyperglycemic-hyperosmolar coma (NKHHC)*　MCC H9 HCC

**E08.01** *Diabetes mellitus due to underlying condition with hyperosmolarity with coma*　MCC H9 HCC

✓5ᵗʰ **E08.1** **Diabetes mellitus due to underlying condition with ketoacidosis**

**E08.10** *Diabetes mellitus due to underlying condition with ketoacidosis without coma*　MCC H9 HCC

**E08.11** *Diabetes mellitus due to underlying condition with ketoacidosis with coma*　MCC HCC

✓5ᵗʰ **E08.2** **Diabetes mellitus due to underlying condition with kidney complications**

**E08.21** *Diabetes mellitus due to underlying condition with diabetic nephropathy*　HCC
Diabetes mellitus due to underlying condition with intercapillary glomerulosclerosis
Diabetes mellitus due to underlying condition with intracapillary glomerulonephrosis
Diabetes mellitus due to underlying condition with Kimmelstiel-Wilson disease

**E08.22** *Diabetes mellitus due to underlying condition with diabetic chronic kidney disease*　HCC
Use additional code to identify stage of chronic kidney disease (N18.1-N18.6)

**E08.29** *Diabetes mellitus due to underlying condition with other diabetic kidney complication*　HCC
Renal tubular degeneration in diabetes mellitus due to underlying condition

✓5ᵗʰ **E08.3** **Diabetes mellitus due to underlying condition with ophthalmic complications**

One of the following 7th characters is to be assigned to codes in subcategories E08.32, E08.33, E08.34, E08.35, and E08.37 to designate laterality of the disease:
1　right eye
2　left eye
3　bilateral
9　unspecified eye

✓6ᵗʰ **E08.31** **Diabetes mellitus due to underlying condition with unspecified diabetic retinopathy**

**E08.311** *Diabetes mellitus due to underlying condition with unspecified diabetic retinopathy with macular edema*　HCC

**E08.319** *Diabetes mellitus due to underlying condition with unspecified diabetic retinopathy without macular edema*　HCC

N Newborn: 0　P Pediatric: 0-17　M Maternity: 12-55　A Adult: 15-124　MCC Major CC Condition　PDxMCC PDx acts as own MCC　CC CC Condition　PDxCC PDx acts as own CC

512　　ICD-10-CM 2018

√6ᵗʰ **E08.32** **Diabetes mellitus due to underlying condition with mild nonproliferative diabetic retinopathy**
Diabetes mellitus due to underlying condition with nonproliferative diabetic retinopathy NOS

√7ᵗʰ *E08.321*   *Diabetes mellitus due to underlying condition with mild nonproliferative diabetic retinopathy with macular edema*   HCC

√7ᵗʰ *E08.329*   *Diabetes mellitus due to underlying condition with mild nonproliferative diabetic retinopathy without macular edema*   HCC

√6ᵗʰ **E08.33** **Diabetes mellitus due to underlying condition with moderate nonproliferative diabetic retinopathy**

√7ᵗʰ *E08.331*   *Diabetes mellitus due to underlying condition with moderate nonproliferative diabetic retinopathy with macular edema*   HCC

√7ᵗʰ *E08.339*   *Diabetes mellitus due to underlying condition with moderate nonproliferative diabetic retinopathy without macular edema*   HCC

√6ᵗʰ **E08.34** **Diabetes mellitus due to underlying condition with severe nonproliferative diabetic retinopathy**

√7ᵗʰ *E08.341*   *Diabetes mellitus due to underlying condition with severe nonproliferative diabetic retinopathy with macular edema*   HCC

√7ᵗʰ *E08.349*   *Diabetes mellitus due to underlying condition with severe nonproliferative diabetic retinopathy without macular edema*   HCC

√6ᵗʰ **E08.35** **Diabetes mellitus due to underlying condition with proliferative diabetic retinopathy**

√7ᵗʰ *E08.351*   *Diabetes mellitus due to underlying condition with proliferative diabetic retinopathy with macular edema*   HCC

√7ᵗʰ *E08.352*   *Diabetes mellitus due to underlying condition with proliferative diabetic retinopathy with traction retinal detachment involving the macula*   HCC

√7ᵗʰ *E08.353*   *Diabetes mellitus due to underlying condition with proliferative diabetic retinopathy with traction retinal detachment not involving the macula*   HCC

√7ᵗʰ *E08.354*   *Diabetes mellitus due to underlying condition with proliferative diabetic retinopathy with combined traction retinal detachment and rhegmatogenous retinal detachment*   HCC

√7ᵗʰ *E08.355*   *Diabetes mellitus due to underlying condition with stable proliferative diabetic retinopathy*   HCC

√7ᵗʰ *E08.359*   *Diabetes mellitus due to underlying condition with proliferative diabetic retinopathy without macular edema*   HCC

*E08.36*   *Diabetes mellitus due to underlying condition with diabetic cataract*   HCC
AHA: 2016, 4Q, 142

√x7ᵗʰ *E08.37*   *Diabetes mellitus due to underlying condition with diabetic macular edema, resolved following treatment*   HCC

*E08.39*   *Diabetes mellitus due to underlying condition with other diabetic ophthalmic complication*   HCC
Use additional code to identify manifestation, such as: diabetic glaucoma (H40-H42)

√5ᵗʰ **E08.4** **Diabetes mellitus due to underlying condition with neurological complications**

*E08.40*   *Diabetes mellitus due to underlying condition with diabetic neuropathy, unspecified*   HCC

*E08.41*   *Diabetes mellitus due to underlying condition with diabetic mononeuropathy*   HCC

*E08.42*   *Diabetes mellitus due to underlying condition with diabetic polyneuropathy*   HCC
Diabetes mellitus due to underlying condition with diabetic neuralgia

*E08.43*   *Diabetes mellitus due to underlying condition with diabetic autonomic (poly)neuropathy*   HCC
Diabetes mellitus due to underlying condition with diabetic gastroparesis
AHA: 2013, 4Q, 114

*E08.44*   *Diabetes mellitus due to underlying condition with diabetic amyotrophy*   HCC

*E08.49*   *Diabetes mellitus due to underlying condition with other diabetic neurological complication*   HCC

√5ᵗʰ **E08.5** **Diabetes mellitus due to underlying condition with circulatory complications**

*E08.51*   *Diabetes mellitus due to underlying condition with diabetic peripheral angiopathy without gangrene*   HCC

*E08.52*   *Diabetes mellitus due to underlying condition with diabetic peripheral angiopathy with gangrene*   PDxCC CC HCC
Diabetes mellitus due to underlying condition with diabetic gangrene
**CC Excl:** PDX collection 519

*E08.59*   *Diabetes mellitus due to underlying condition with other circulatory complications*   HCC

√5ᵗʰ **E08.6** **Diabetes mellitus due to underlying condition with other specified complications**

√6ᵗʰ **E08.61** **Diabetes mellitus due to underlying condition with diabetic arthropathy**

*E08.610*   *Diabetes mellitus due to underlying condition with diabetic neuropathic arthropathy*   HCC
Diabetes mellitus due to underlying condition with Charcôt's joints

*E08.618*   *Diabetes mellitus due to underlying condition with other diabetic arthropathy*   HCC

√6ᵗʰ **E08.62** **Diabetes mellitus due to underlying condition with skin complications**

*E08.620*   *Diabetes mellitus due to underlying condition with diabetic dermatitis*   HCC
Diabetes mellitus due to underlying condition with diabetic necrobiosis lipoidica

*E08.621*   *Diabetes mellitus due to underlying condition with foot ulcer*   HCC
Use additional code to identify site of ulcer (L97.4-, L97.5-)

*E08.622*   *Diabetes mellitus due to underlying condition with other skin ulcer*   HCC
Use additional code to identify site of ulcer (L97.1-L97.9, L98.41-L98.49)

*E08.628*   *Diabetes mellitus due to underlying condition with other skin complications*   HCC

√6ᵗʰ **E08.63** **Diabetes mellitus due to underlying condition with oral complications**

*E08.630*   *Diabetes mellitus due to underlying condition with periodontal disease*   HCC

*E08.638*   *Diabetes mellitus due to underlying condition with other oral complications*   HCC

√6ᵗʰ **E08.64** **Diabetes mellitus due to underlying condition with hypoglycemia**

*E08.641*   *Diabetes mellitus due to underlying condition with hypoglycemia with coma*   MCC HCC

*E08.649*   *Diabetes mellitus due to underlying condition with hypoglycemia without coma*   HCC
AHA: 2016, 3Q, 42; 2015, 3Q, 21

*E08.65*   *Diabetes mellitus due to underlying condition with hyperglycemia*   HCC

*E08.69*   *Diabetes mellitus due to underlying condition with other specified complication*   HCC
Use additional code to identify complication
AHA: 2016, 4Q, 141; 2016, 1Q, 13

*E08.8*   *Diabetes mellitus due to underlying condition with unspecified complications*   HCC

*E08.9*   *Diabetes mellitus due to underlying condition without complications*   HCC

✓ Additional Character Req    √x7ᵗʰ Placeholder Alert    Unacceptable PDx    Manifestation    H1 - H14 HAC    HCC CMS-HCC Condition    *EXCLUDES 1* Not Coded Here    *EXCLUDES 2* Not Included Here

ICD-10-CM 2018      513

✓4ᵗʰ **E09**   **Drug or chemical induced diabetes mellitus**

Code first poisoning due to drug or toxin, if applicable (T36-T65 with fifth or sixth character 1-4 or 6)

Use additional code for adverse effect, if applicable, to identify drug (T36-T50 with fifth or sixth character 5)

Use additional code to identify control using:
insulin (Z79.4)
oral antidiabetic drugs (Z79.84)
oral hypoglycemic drugs (Z79.84)

**EXCLUDES 1**   diabetes mellitus due to underlying condition (E08.-)
gestational diabetes (O24.4-)
neonatal diabetes mellitus (P70.2)
postpancreatectomy diabetes mellitus (E13.-)
postprocedural diabetes mellitus (E13.-)
secondary diabetes mellitus NEC (E13.-)
type 1 diabetes mellitus (E10.-)
type 2 diabetes mellitus (E11.-)

**AHA:** 2016, 1Q, 11-13; 2013, 4Q, 114; 2013, 3Q, 20

**CC Excl: For MCC codes in category E09, unless otherwise noted:** PDX collection 518

✓5ᵗʰ **E09.0**   **Drug or chemical induced diabetes mellitus with hyperosmolarity**

    **E09.00**   **Drug or chemical induced diabetes mellitus with hyperosmolarity** without nonketotic hyperglycemic-hyperosmolar coma **(NKHHC)**    MCC H9 HCC

    **E09.01**   **Drug or chemical induced diabetes mellitus with hyperosmolarity** with coma    MCC H9 HCC

✓5ᵗʰ **E09.1**   **Drug or chemical induced diabetes mellitus with ketoacidosis**

    **E09.10**   **Drug or chemical induced diabetes mellitus with ketoacidosis** without coma    MCC H9 HCC

    **E09.11**   **Drug or chemical induced diabetes mellitus with ketoacidosis** with coma    MCC HCC

✓5ᵗʰ **E09.2**   **Drug or chemical induced diabetes mellitus with kidney complications**

    **E09.21**   **Drug or chemical induced diabetes mellitus with diabetic nephropathy**    HCC
Drug or chemical induced diabetes mellitus with intercapillary glomerulosclerosis
Drug or chemical induced diabetes mellitus with intracapillary glomerulonephrosis
Drug or chemical induced diabetes mellitus with Kimmelstiel-Wilson disease

    **E09.22**   **Drug or chemical induced diabetes mellitus with diabetic chronic kidney disease**    HCC
Use additional code to identify stage of chronic kidney disease (N18.1-N18.6)

    **E09.29**   **Drug or chemical induced diabetes mellitus with other diabetic kidney complication**    HCC
Drug or chemical induced diabetes mellitus with renal tubular degeneration

✓5ᵗʰ **E09.3**   **Drug or chemical induced diabetes mellitus with ophthalmic complications**

One of the following 7th characters is to be assigned to codes in subcategories E09.32, E09.33, E09.34, E09.35, and E09.37 to designate laterality of the disease:
1    right eye
2    left eye
3    bilateral
9    unspecified eye

✓6ᵗʰ **E09.31**   **Drug or chemical induced diabetes mellitus with unspecified diabetic retinopathy**

    **E09.311**   **Drug or chemical induced diabetes mellitus with unspecified diabetic retinopathy** with macular edema    HCC

    **E09.319**   **Drug or chemical induced diabetes mellitus with unspecified diabetic retinopathy** without macular edema    HCC

✓6ᵗʰ **E09.32**   **Drug or chemical induced diabetes mellitus with mild nonproliferative diabetic retinopathy**
Drug or chemical induced diabetes mellitus with nonproliferative diabetic retinopathy NOS

    ✓7ᵗʰ **E09.321**   **Drug or chemical induced diabetes mellitus with mild nonproliferative diabetic retinopathy** with macular edema    HCC

    ✓7ᵗʰ **E09.329**   **Drug or chemical induced diabetes mellitus with mild nonproliferative diabetic retinopathy** without macular edema    HCC

✓6ᵗʰ **E09.33**   **Drug or chemical induced diabetes mellitus with moderate nonproliferative diabetic retinopathy**

    ✓7ᵗʰ **E09.331**   **Drug or chemical induced diabetes mellitus with moderate nonproliferative diabetic retinopathy** with macular edema    HCC

    ✓7ᵗʰ **E09.339**   **Drug or chemical induced diabetes mellitus with moderate nonproliferative diabetic retinopathy** without macular edema    HCC

✓6ᵗʰ **E09.34**   **Drug or chemical induced diabetes mellitus with severe nonproliferative diabetic retinopathy**

    ✓7ᵗʰ **E09.341**   **Drug or chemical induced diabetes mellitus with severe nonproliferative diabetic retinopathy** with macular edema    HCC

    ✓7ᵗʰ **E09.349**   **Drug or chemical induced diabetes mellitus with severe nonproliferative diabetic retinopathy** without macular edema    HCC

✓6ᵗʰ **E09.35**   **Drug or chemical induced diabetes mellitus with proliferative diabetic retinopathy**

    ✓7ᵗʰ **E09.351**   **Drug or chemical induced diabetes mellitus with proliferative diabetic retinopathy** with macular edema    HCC

    ✓7ᵗʰ **E09.352**   **Drug or chemical induced diabetes mellitus with proliferative diabetic retinopathy** with traction retinal detachment involving the macula    HCC

    ✓7ᵗʰ **E09.353**   **Drug or chemical induced diabetes mellitus with proliferative diabetic retinopathy** with traction retinal detachment not involving the macula    HCC

    ✓7ᵗʰ **E09.354**   **Drug or chemical induced diabetes mellitus with proliferative diabetic retinopathy** with combined traction retinal detachment and rhegmatogenous retinal detachment    HCC

    ✓7ᵗʰ **E09.355**   **Drug or chemical induced diabetes mellitus with stable proliferative diabetic retinopathy**    HCC

    ✓7ᵗʰ **E09.359**   **Drug or chemical induced diabetes mellitus with proliferative diabetic retinopathy** without macular edema    HCC

    **E09.36**   **Drug or chemical induced diabetes mellitus with diabetic cataract**    HCC
**AHA:** 2016, 4Q, 142

✓x7ᵗʰ **E09.37**   **Drug or chemical induced diabetes mellitus with diabetic macular edema, resolved following treatment**    HCC

    **E09.39**   **Drug or chemical induced diabetes mellitus with other diabetic ophthalmic complication**    HCC
Use additional code to identify manifestation, such as: diabetic glaucoma (H40-H42)

✓5ᵗʰ **E09.4**   **Drug or chemical induced diabetes mellitus with neurological complications**

    **E09.40**   **Drug or chemical induced diabetes mellitus with neurological complications with diabetic neuropathy, unspecified**    HCC

    **E09.41**   **Drug or chemical induced diabetes mellitus with neurological complications with diabetic mononeuropathy**    HCC

    **E09.42**   **Drug or chemical induced diabetes mellitus with neurological complications with diabetic polyneuropathy**    HCC
Drug or chemical induced diabetes mellitus with diabetic neuralgia

    **E09.43**   **Drug or chemical induced diabetes mellitus with neurological complications with diabetic autonomic (poly)neuropathy**    HCC
Drug or chemical induced diabetes mellitus with diabetic gastroparesis
**AHA:** 2013, 4Q, 114

    **E09.44**   **Drug or chemical induced diabetes mellitus with neurological complications with diabetic amyotrophy**    HCC

    **E09.49**   **Drug or chemical induced diabetes mellitus with neurological complications with other diabetic neurological complication**    HCC

✓5th **E09.5  Drug or chemical induced diabetes mellitus with circulatory complications**

   **E09.51  Drug or chemical induced diabetes mellitus with diabetic peripheral angiopathy without gangrene** HCC

   **E09.52  Drug or chemical induced diabetes mellitus with diabetic peripheral angiopathy with gangrene** PDxCC CC HCC
      Drug or chemical induced diabetes mellitus with diabetic gangrene
      **CC Excl:** PDX collection 519

   **E09.59  Drug or chemical induced diabetes mellitus with other circulatory complications** HCC

✓5th **E09.6  Drug or chemical induced diabetes mellitus with other specified complications**

   ✓6th **E09.61  Drug or chemical induced diabetes mellitus with diabetic arthropathy**

      **E09.610  Drug or chemical induced diabetes mellitus with diabetic neuropathic arthropathy** HCC
         Drug or chemical induced diabetes mellitus with Charcôt's joints

      **E09.618  Drug or chemical induced diabetes mellitus with other diabetic arthropathy** HCC

   ✓6th **E09.62  Drug or chemical induced diabetes mellitus with skin complications**

      **E09.620  Drug or chemical induced diabetes mellitus with diabetic dermatitis** HCC
         Drug or chemical induced diabetes mellitus with diabetic necrobiosis lipoidica

      **E09.621  Drug or chemical induced diabetes mellitus with foot ulcer** HCC
         Use additional code to identify site of ulcer (L97.4-, L97.5-)

      **E09.622  Drug or chemical induced diabetes mellitus with other skin ulcer** HCC
         Use additional code to identify site of ulcer (L97.1-L97.9, L98.41-L98.49)

      **E09.628  Drug or chemical induced diabetes mellitus with other skin complications** HCC

   ✓6th **E09.63  Drug or chemical induced diabetes mellitus with oral complications**

      **E09.630  Drug or chemical induced diabetes mellitus with periodontal disease** HCC

      **E09.638  Drug or chemical induced diabetes mellitus with other oral complications** HCC

   ✓6th **E09.64  Drug or chemical induced diabetes mellitus with hypoglycemia**

      **E09.641  Drug or chemical induced diabetes mellitus with hypoglycemia with coma** MCC HCC

      **E09.649  Drug or chemical induced diabetes mellitus with hypoglycemia without coma** HCC
         **AHA:** 2016, 3Q, 42; 2015, 3Q, 21

   **E09.65  Drug or chemical induced diabetes mellitus with hyperglycemia** HCC

   **E09.69  Drug or chemical induced diabetes mellitus with other specified complication** HCC
      Use additional code to identify complication
      **AHA:** 2016, 4Q, 141; 2016, 1Q, 13

**E09.8  Drug or chemical induced diabetes mellitus with unspecified complications** HCC

**E09.9  Drug or chemical induced diabetes mellitus without complications** HCC

---

✓4th **E10  Type 1 diabetes mellitus**
   [INCLUDES]  brittle diabetes (mellitus)
      diabetes (mellitus) due to autoimmune process
      diabetes (mellitus) due to immune mediated pancreatic islet beta-cell destruction
      idiopathic diabetes (mellitus)
      juvenile onset diabetes (mellitus)
      ketosis-prone diabetes (mellitus)
   *EXCLUDES 1*  *diabetes mellitus due to underlying condition (E08.-)*
      *drug or chemical induced diabetes mellitus (E09.-)*
      *gestational diabetes (O24.4-)*
      *hyperglycemia NOS (R73.9)*
      *neonatal diabetes mellitus (P70.2)*
      *postpancreatectomy diabetes mellitus (E13.-)*
      *postprocedural diabetes mellitus (E13.-)*
      *secondary diabetes mellitus NEC (E13.-)*
      *type 2 diabetes mellitus (E11.-)*
   **AHA:** 2016, 1Q, 11-13; 2013, 4Q, 114; 2013, 3Q, 20

   **CC Excl: For MCC codes in category E10, unless otherwise noted:** PDX collection 520

   ✓5th **E10.1  Type 1 diabetes mellitus with ketoacidosis**
      **AHA:** 2013, 3Q, 20

      **E10.10  Type 1 diabetes mellitus with ketoacidosis without coma** MCC H9 HCC

      **E10.11  Type 1 diabetes mellitus with ketoacidosis with coma** MCC HCC

   ✓5th **E10.2  Type 1 diabetes mellitus with kidney complications**

      **E10.21  Type 1 diabetes mellitus with diabetic nephropathy** HCC
         Type 1 diabetes mellitus with intercapillary glomerulosclerosis
         Type 1 diabetes mellitus with intracapillary glomerulonephrosis
         Type 1 diabetes mellitus with Kimmelstiel-Wilson disease

      **E10.22  Type 1 diabetes mellitus with diabetic chronic kidney disease** HCC
         Use additional code to identify stage of chronic kidney disease (N18.1-N18.6)

      **E10.29  Type 1 diabetes mellitus with other diabetic kidney complication** HCC
         Type 1 diabetes mellitus with renal tubular degeneration
         **AHA:** 2016, 1Q, 13

   ✓5th **E10.3  Type 1 diabetes mellitus with ophthalmic complications**

      One of the following 7th characters is to be assigned to codes in subcategories E10.32, E10.33, E10.34, E10.35, and E10.37 to designate laterality of the disease:
      1    right eye
      2    left eye
      3    bilateral
      9    unspecified eye

      ✓6th **E10.31  Type 1 diabetes mellitus with unspecified diabetic retinopathy**

         **E10.311  Type 1 diabetes mellitus with unspecified diabetic retinopathy with macular edema** HCC

         **E10.319  Type 1 diabetes mellitus with unspecified diabetic retinopathy without macular edema** HCC

      ✓6th **E10.32  Type 1 diabetes mellitus with mild nonproliferative diabetic retinopathy**
         Type 1 diabetes mellitus with nonproliferative diabetic retinopathy NOS

         ✓7th **E10.321  Type 1 diabetes mellitus with mild nonproliferative diabetic retinopathy with macular edema** HCC

         ✓7th **E10.329  Type 1 diabetes mellitus with mild nonproliferative diabetic retinopathy without macular edema** HCC

      ✓6th **E10.33  Type 1 diabetes mellitus with moderate nonproliferative diabetic retinopathy**

         ✓7th **E10.331  Type 1 diabetes mellitus with moderate nonproliferative diabetic retinopathy with macular edema** HCC

         ✓7th **E10.339  Type 1 diabetes mellitus with moderate nonproliferative diabetic retinopathy without macular edema** HCC

---

**E10.34**   Type 1 diabetes mellitus with severe nonproliferative diabetic retinopathy

> **E10.341**   Type 1 diabetes mellitus with severe nonproliferative diabetic retinopathy with macular edema   HCC
>
> **E10.349**   Type 1 diabetes mellitus with severe nonproliferative diabetic retinopathy without macular edema   HCC

**E10.35**   Type 1 diabetes mellitus with proliferative diabetic retinopathy

> **E10.351**   Type 1 diabetes mellitus with proliferative diabetic retinopathy with macular edema   HCC
>
> **E10.352**   Type 1 diabetes mellitus with proliferative diabetic retinopathy with traction retinal detachment involving the macula   HCC
>
> **E10.353**   Type 1 diabetes mellitus with proliferative diabetic retinopathy with traction retinal detachment not involving the macula   HCC
>
> **E10.354**   Type 1 diabetes mellitus with proliferative diabetic retinopathy with combined traction retinal detachment and rhegmatogenous retinal detachment   HCC
>
> **E10.355**   Type 1 diabetes mellitus with stable proliferative diabetic retinopathy   HCC
>
> **E10.359**   Type 1 diabetes mellitus with proliferative diabetic retinopathy without macular edema   HCC

**E10.36**   Type 1 diabetes mellitus with diabetic cataract   HCC
> AHA: 2016, 4Q, 142

**E10.37**   Type 1 diabetes mellitus with diabetic macular edema, resolved following treatment   HCC

**E10.39**   Type 1 diabetes mellitus with other diabetic ophthalmic complication   HCC
> Use additional code to identify manifestation, such as:
> diabetic glaucoma (H40-H42)

**E10.4**   Type 1 diabetes mellitus with neurological complications

> **E10.40**   Type 1 diabetes mellitus with diabetic neuropathy, unspecified   HCC
>
> **E10.41**   Type 1 diabetes mellitus with diabetic mononeuropathy   HCC
>
> **E10.42**   Type 1 diabetes mellitus with diabetic polyneuropathy   HCC
> > Type 1 diabetes mellitus with diabetic neuralgia
>
> **E10.43**   Type 1 diabetes mellitus with diabetic autonomic (poly)neuropathy   HCC
> > Type 1 diabetes mellitus with diabetic gastroparesis
> > AHA: 2013, 4Q, 114
>
> **E10.44**   Type 1 diabetes mellitus with diabetic amyotrophy   HCC
>
> **E10.49**   Type 1 diabetes mellitus with other diabetic neurological complication   HCC

**E10.5**   Type 1 diabetes mellitus with circulatory complications

> **E10.51**   Type 1 diabetes mellitus with diabetic peripheral angiopathy without gangrene   HCC
>
> **E10.52**   Type 1 diabetes mellitus with diabetic peripheral angiopathy with gangrene   PDxCC CC HCC
> > Type 1 diabetes mellitus with diabetic gangrene
> > CC Excl: PDX collection 519
>
> **E10.59**   Type 1 diabetes mellitus with other circulatory complications   HCC

**E10.6**   Type 1 diabetes mellitus with other specified complications

> **E10.61**   Type 1 diabetes mellitus with diabetic arthropathy
>
> > **E10.610**   Type 1 diabetes mellitus with diabetic neuropathic arthropathy   HCC
> > > Type 1 diabetes mellitus with Charcôt's joints
> >
> > **E10.618**   Type 1 diabetes mellitus with other diabetic arthropathy   HCC
>
> **E10.62**   Type 1 diabetes mellitus with skin complications
>
> > **E10.620**   Type 1 diabetes mellitus with diabetic dermatitis   HCC
> > > Type 1 diabetes mellitus with diabetic necrobiosis lipoidica

> **E10.621**   Type 1 diabetes mellitus with foot ulcer   HCC
> > Use additional code to identify site of ulcer (L97.4-, L97.5-)
>
> **E10.622**   Type 1 diabetes mellitus with other skin ulcer   HCC
> > Use additional code to identify site of ulcer (L97.1-L97.9, L98.41-L98.49)
>
> **E10.628**   Type 1 diabetes mellitus with other skin complications   HCC

**E10.63**   Type 1 diabetes mellitus with oral complications

> **E10.630**   Type 1 diabetes mellitus with periodontal disease   HCC
>
> **E10.638**   Type 1 diabetes mellitus with other oral complications   HCC

**E10.64**   Type 1 diabetes mellitus with hypoglycemia

> **E10.641**   Type 1 diabetes mellitus with hypoglycemia with coma   MCC HCC
>
> **E10.649**   Type 1 diabetes mellitus with hypoglycemia without coma   HCC
> > AHA: 2016, 3Q, 42; 2016, 1Q, 13; 2015, 3Q, 21

**E10.65**   Type 1 diabetes mellitus with hyperglycemia   HCC
> AHA: 2013, 3Q, 20

**E10.69**   Type 1 diabetes mellitus with other specified complication   HCC
> Use additional code to identify complication
> AHA: 2016, 4Q, 141; 2016, 1Q, 13

**E10.8**   Type 1 diabetes mellitus with unspecified complications   HCC

**E10.9**   Type 1 diabetes mellitus without complications   HCC

## E11   Type 2 diabetes mellitus

> **INCLUDES**   diabetes (mellitus) due to insulin secretory defect
> diabetes NOS
> insulin resistant diabetes (mellitus)
>
> Use additional code to identify control using:
> insulin (Z79.4)
> oral antidiabetic drugs (Z79.84)
> oral hypoglycemic drugs (Z79.84)
>
> **EXCLUDES 1**   diabetes mellitus due to underlying condition (E08.-)
> drug or chemical induced diabetes mellitus (E09.-)
> gestational diabetes (O24.4-)
> neonatal diabetes mellitus (P70.2)
> postpancreatectomy diabetes mellitus (E13.-)
> postprocedural diabetes mellitus (E13.-)
> secondary diabetes mellitus NEC (E13.-)
> type 1 diabetes mellitus (E10.-)
>
> AHA: 2016, 2Q, 10; 2016, 1Q, 11-13; 2013, 4Q, 114; 2013, 3Q, 20; 2013, 1Q, 26

> **CC Excl: For MCC codes in category E11, unless otherwise noted:** PDX collection 518

**E11.0**   Type 2 diabetes mellitus with hyperosmolarity

> **E11.00**   Type 2 diabetes mellitus with hyperosmolarity without nonketotic hyperglycemic-hyperosmolar coma (NKHHC)   MCC H9 HCC
>
> **E11.01**   Type 2 diabetes mellitus with hyperosmolarity with coma   MCC H9 HCC

**E11.1**   Type 2 diabetes mellitus with ketoacidosis

> **E11.10**   Type 2 diabetes mellitus with ketoacidosis without coma   MCC
>
> **E11.11**   Type 2 diabetes mellitus with ketoacidosis with coma   MCC

**E11.2**   Type 2 diabetes mellitus with kidney complications

> **E11.21**   Type 2 diabetes mellitus with diabetic nephropathy   HCC
> > Type 2 diabetes mellitus with intercapillary glomerulosclerosis
> > Type 2 diabetes mellitus with intracapillary glomerulonephrosis
> > Type 2 diabetes mellitus with Kimmelstiel-Wilson disease
>
> **E11.22**   Type 2 diabetes mellitus with diabetic chronic kidney disease   HCC
> > Use additional code to identify stage of chronic kidney disease (N18.1-N18.6)
> > AHA: 2016, 1Q, 12
>
> **E11.29**   Type 2 diabetes mellitus with other diabetic kidney complication   HCC
> > Type 2 diabetes mellitus with renal tubular degeneration

N Newborn: 0   P Pediatric: 0-17   M Maternity: 12-55   A Adult: 15-124   MCC Major CC Condition   PDxMCC PDx acts as own MCC   CC CC Condition   PDxCC PDx acts as own CC

516     ICD-10-CM 2018

✓5ᵗʰ **E11.3**   **Type 2 diabetes mellitus with ophthalmic complications**

One of the following 7th characters is to be assigned to codes in subcategories E11.32, E11.33, E11.34, E11.35, and E11.37 to designate laterality of the disease:
1   right eye
2   left eye
3   bilateral
9   unspecified eye

✓6ᵗʰ **E11.31**   **Type 2 diabetes mellitus with unspecified diabetic retinopathy**

     **E11.311**   **Type 2 diabetes mellitus with unspecified diabetic retinopathy with macular edema**   HCC

     **E11.319**   **Type 2 diabetes mellitus with unspecified diabetic retinopathy without macular edema**   HCC

✓6ᵗʰ **E11.32**   **Type 2 diabetes mellitus with mild nonproliferative diabetic retinopathy**
Type 2 diabetes mellitus with nonproliferative diabetic retinopathy NOS

     ✓7ᵗʰ **E11.321**   **Type 2 diabetes mellitus with mild nonproliferative diabetic retinopathy with macular edema**   HCC

     ✓7ᵗʰ **E11.329**   **Type 2 diabetes mellitus with mild nonproliferative diabetic retinopathy without macular edema**   HCC

✓6ᵗʰ **E11.33**   **Type 2 diabetes mellitus with moderate nonproliferative diabetic retinopathy**

     ✓7ᵗʰ **E11.331**   **Type 2 diabetes mellitus with moderate nonproliferative diabetic retinopathy with macular edema**   HCC

     ✓7ᵗʰ **E11.339**   **Type 2 diabetes mellitus with moderate nonproliferative diabetic retinopathy without macular edema**   HCC

✓6ᵗʰ **E11.34**   **Type 2 diabetes mellitus with severe nonproliferative diabetic retinopathy**

     ✓7ᵗʰ **E11.341**   **Type 2 diabetes mellitus with severe nonproliferative diabetic retinopathy with macular edema**   HCC

     ✓7ᵗʰ **E11.349**   **Type 2 diabetes mellitus with severe nonproliferative diabetic retinopathy without macular edema**   HCC

✓6ᵗʰ **E11.35**   **Type 2 diabetes mellitus with proliferative diabetic retinopathy**

     ✓7ᵗʰ **E11.351**   **Type 2 diabetes mellitus with proliferative diabetic retinopathy with macular edema**   HCC

     ✓7ᵗʰ **E11.352**   **Type 2 diabetes mellitus with proliferative diabetic retinopathy with traction retinal detachment involving the macula**   HCC

     ✓7ᵗʰ **E11.353**   **Type 2 diabetes mellitus with proliferative diabetic retinopathy with traction retinal detachment not involving the macula**   HCC

     ✓7ᵗʰ **E11.354**   **Type 2 diabetes mellitus with proliferative diabetic retinopathy with combined traction retinal detachment and rhegmatogenous retinal detachment**   HCC

     ✓7ᵗʰ **E11.355**   **Type 2 diabetes mellitus with stable proliferative diabetic retinopathy**   HCC

     ✓7ᵗʰ **E11.359**   **Type 2 diabetes mellitus with proliferative diabetic retinopathy without macular edema**   HCC

     **E11.36**   **Type 2 diabetes mellitus with diabetic cataract**   HCC
     **AHA:** 2016, 4Q, 142

     ✓x7ᵗʰ **E11.37**   **Type 2 diabetes mellitus with diabetic macular edema, resolved following treatment**   HCC

     **E11.39**   **Type 2 diabetes mellitus with other diabetic ophthalmic complication**   HCC
Use additional code to identify manifestation, such as: diabetic glaucoma (H40-H42)

✓5ᵗʰ **E11.4**   **Type 2 diabetes mellitus with neurological complications**

     **E11.40**   **Type 2 diabetes mellitus with diabetic neuropathy, unspecified**   HCC
     **AHA:** 2013, 4Q, 129

     **E11.41**   **Type 2 diabetes mellitus with diabetic mononeuropathy**   HCC

     **E11.42**   **Type 2 diabetes mellitus with diabetic polyneuropathy**   HCC
Type 2 diabetes mellitus with diabetic neuralgia
     **AHA:** 2016, 1Q, 12

     **E11.43**   **Type 2 diabetes mellitus with diabetic autonomic (poly)neuropathy**   HCC
Type 2 diabetes mellitus with diabetic gastroparesis
     **AHA:** 2013, 4Q, 114

     **E11.44**   **Type 2 diabetes mellitus with diabetic amyotrophy**   HCC

     **E11.49**   **Type 2 diabetes mellitus with other diabetic neurological complication**   HCC

✓5ᵗʰ **E11.5**   **Type 2 diabetes mellitus with circulatory complications**

     **E11.51**   **Type 2 diabetes mellitus with diabetic peripheral angiopathy without gangrene**   HCC

     **E11.52**   **Type 2 diabetes mellitus with diabetic peripheral angiopathy with gangrene**   PDxCC CC HCC
Type 2 diabetes mellitus with diabetic gangrene
     **CC Excl:** PDX collection 519

     **E11.59**   **Type 2 diabetes mellitus with other circulatory complications**   HCC

✓5ᵗʰ **E11.6**   **Type 2 diabetes mellitus with other specified complications**

     ✓6ᵗʰ **E11.61**   **Type 2 diabetes mellitus with diabetic arthropathy**

         **E11.610**   **Type 2 diabetes mellitus with diabetic neuropathic arthropathy**   HCC
Type 2 diabetes mellitus with Charcôt's joints

         **E11.618**   **Type 2 diabetes mellitus with other diabetic arthropathy**   HCC

     ✓6ᵗʰ **E11.62**   **Type 2 diabetes mellitus with skin complications**

         **E11.620**   **Type 2 diabetes mellitus with diabetic dermatitis**   HCC
Type 2 diabetes mellitus with diabetic necrobiosis lipoidica

         **E11.621**   **Type 2 diabetes mellitus with foot ulcer**   HCC
Use additional code to identify site of ulcer (L97.4-, L97.5-)
         **AHA:** 2016, 1Q, 12

         **E11.622**   **Type 2 diabetes mellitus with other skin ulcer**   HCC
Use additional code to identify site of ulcer (L97.1-L97.9, L98.41-L98.49)

         **E11.628**   **Type 2 diabetes mellitus with other skin complications**   HCC

     ✓6ᵗʰ **E11.63**   **Type 2 diabetes mellitus with oral complications**

         **E11.630**   **Type 2 diabetes mellitus with periodontal disease**   HCC

         **E11.638**   **Type 2 diabetes mellitus with other oral complications**   HCC

     ✓6ᵗʰ **E11.64**   **Type 2 diabetes mellitus with hypoglycemia**

         **E11.641**   **Type 2 diabetes mellitus with hypoglycemia with coma**   MCC HCC

         **E11.649**   **Type 2 diabetes mellitus with hypoglycemia without coma**   HCC
         **AHA:** 2016, 3Q, 42; 2015, 3Q, 21

     **E11.65**   **Type 2 diabetes mellitus with hyperglycemia**   HCC
     **AHA:** 2013, 3Q, 20

     **E11.69**   **Type 2 diabetes mellitus with other specified complication**   HCC
Use additional code to identify complication
     **AHA:** 2016, 4Q, 141; 2016, 1Q, 13

**E11.8**   **Type 2 diabetes mellitus with unspecified complications**   HCC

⁴ **E11.9**   **Type 2 diabetes mellitus without complications**   HCC

---

⁴   Questionable admission when used as PDx.

✓ Additional Character Req    ✓x7ᵗʰ Placeholder Alert    Unacceptable PDx    Manifestation    H1-H14 HAC    HCC CMS-HCC Condition    EXCLUDES 1 Not Coded Here    EXCLUDES 2 Not Included Here

**✓4ᵗʰ E13 Other specified diabetes mellitus**

INCLUDES   diabetes mellitus due to genetic defects of beta-cell function
diabetes mellitus due to genetic defects in insulin action
postpancreatectomy diabetes mellitus
postprocedural diabetes mellitus
secondary diabetes mellitus NEC

Use additional code to identify control using:
insulin (Z79.4)
oral antidiabetic drugs (Z79.84)
oral hypoglycemic drugs (Z79.84)

EXCLUDES 1   *diabetes (mellitus) due to autoimmune process (E10.-)*
*diabetes (mellitus) due to immune mediated pancreatic islet*
  *beta-cell destruction (E10.-)*
*diabetes mellitus due to underlying condition (E08.-)*
*drug or chemical induced diabetes mellitus (E09.-)*
*gestational diabetes (O24.4-)*
*neonatal diabetes mellitus (P70.2)*
*type 1 diabetes mellitus (E10.-)*
~~*type 2 diabetes mellitus (E11.-)*~~

AHA: 2016, 1Q, 11-13; 2013, 4Q, 114; 2013, 3Q, 20

CC Excl: For MCC codes in category E13, unless otherwise noted: PDX collection 518

**✓5ᵗʰ E13.0 Other specified diabetes mellitus with** hyperosmolarity

    **E13.00 Other specified diabetes mellitus with**   MCC   H9   HCC
        **hyperosmolarity** without nonketotic
        hyperglycemic-hyperosmolar coma (NKHHC)
        EXCLUDES 2 ▶*type 2 diabetes mellitus (E11.-)*◀

    **E13.01 Other specified diabetes mellitus with**   MCC   H9   HCC
        **hyperosmolarity** with coma

**✓5ᵗʰ E13.1 Other specified diabetes mellitus with** ketoacidosis
    AHA: 2016, 2Q, 10; 2013, 1Q, 26

    **E13.10 Other specified diabetes mellitus with**   MCC   H9   HCC
        **ketoacidosis** without coma

    **E13.11 Other specified diabetes mellitus with**   MCC   HCC
        **ketoacidosis** with coma

**✓5ᵗʰ E13.2 Other specified diabetes mellitus with** kidney complications

    **E13.21 Other specified diabetes mellitus with diabetic**   HCC
        **nephropathy**
        Other specified diabetes mellitus with intercapillary
          glomerulosclerosis
        Other specified diabetes mellitus with intracapillary
          glomerulonephrosis
        Other specified diabetes mellitus with Kimmelstiel-
          Wilson disease

    **E13.22 Other specified diabetes mellitus with diabetic**   HCC
        **chronic kidney disease**
        Use additional code to identify stage of chronic kidney
          disease (N18.1-N18.6)

    **E13.29 Other specified diabetes mellitus with other**   HCC
        **diabetic kidney complication**
        Other specified diabetes mellitus with renal tubular
          degeneration

**✓5ᵗʰ E13.3 Other specified diabetes mellitus with** ophthalmic complications

    One of the following 7th characters is to be assigned to codes
    in subcategories E13.32, E13.33, E13.34, E13.35, and E13.37 to
    designate laterality of the disease:
    1    right eye
    2    left eye
    3    bilateral
    9    unspecified eye

  **✓6ᵗʰ E13.31 Other specified diabetes mellitus with** unspecified diabetic retinopathy

      **E13.311 Other specified diabetes mellitus with** HCC
          **unspecified diabetic retinopathy** with
          **macular edema**

      **E13.319 Other specified diabetes mellitus with** HCC
          **unspecified diabetic retinopathy**
          **without macular edema**

  **✓6ᵗʰ E13.32 Other specified diabetes mellitus with** mild nonproliferative **diabetic** retinopathy
      Other specified diabetes mellitus with nonproliferative
        diabetic retinopathy NOS

      **✓7ᵗʰ E13.321 Other specified diabetes mellitus with** HCC
          **mild nonproliferative diabetic**
          **retinopathy** with macular edema

      **✓7ᵗʰ E13.329 Other specified diabetes mellitus with** HCC
          **mild nonproliferative diabetic**
          **retinopathy** without macular edema

  **✓6ᵗʰ E13.33 Other specified diabetes mellitus with** moderate nonproliferative **diabetic** retinopathy

      **✓7ᵗʰ E13.331 Other specified diabetes mellitus with** HCC
          **moderate nonproliferative diabetic**
          **retinopathy** with macular edema

      **✓7ᵗʰ E13.339 Other specified diabetes mellitus with** HCC
          **moderate nonproliferative diabetic**
          **retinopathy** without macular edema

  **✓6ᵗʰ E13.34 Other specified diabetes mellitus with** severe nonproliferative **diabetic** retinopathy

      **✓7ᵗʰ E13.341 Other specified diabetes mellitus with** HCC
          **severe nonproliferative diabetic**
          **retinopathy** with macular edema

      **✓7ᵗʰ E13.349 Other specified diabetes mellitus with** HCC
          **severe nonproliferative diabetic**
          **retinopathy** without macular edema

  **✓6ᵗʰ E13.35 Other specified diabetes mellitus with** proliferative **diabetic** retinopathy

      **✓7ᵗʰ E13.351 Other specified diabetes mellitus with** HCC
          **proliferative diabetic retinopathy** with
          **macular edema**

      **✓7ᵗʰ E13.352 Other specified diabetes mellitus with** HCC
          **proliferative diabetic retinopathy** with
          **traction retinal detachment involving the**
          **macula**

      **✓7ᵗʰ E13.353 Other specified diabetes mellitus with** HCC
          **proliferative diabetic retinopathy** with
          **traction retinal detachment not involving**
          **the macula**

      **✓7ᵗʰ E13.354 Other specified diabetes mellitus with** HCC
          **proliferative diabetic retinopathy** with
          **combined traction retinal detachment and**
          **rhegmatogenous retinal detachment**

      **✓7ᵗʰ E13.355 Other specified diabetes mellitus with** HCC
          **stable proliferative diabetic retinopathy**

      **✓7ᵗʰ E13.359 Other specified diabetes mellitus with** HCC
          **proliferative diabetic retinopathy** without
          **macular edema**

    **E13.36 Other specified diabetes mellitus with** diabetic   HCC
        **cataract**
        AHA: 2016, 4Q, 142

  **✓x7ᵗʰ E13.37 Other specified diabetes mellitus with** diabetic   HCC
        **macular edema, resolved following treatment**

    **E13.39 Other specified diabetes mellitus with** other   HCC
        **diabetic ophthalmic complication**
        Use additional code to identify manifestation, such as:
          diabetic glaucoma (H40-H42)

**✓5ᵗʰ E13.4 Other specified diabetes mellitus with** neurological complications

    **E13.40 Other specified diabetes mellitus with diabetic**   HCC
        **neuropathy, unspecified**

    **E13.41 Other specified diabetes mellitus with diabetic**   HCC
        **mononeuropathy**

    **E13.42 Other specified diabetes mellitus with diabetic**   HCC
        **polyneuropathy**
        Other specified diabetes mellitus with diabetic
          neuralgia

    **E13.43 Other specified diabetes mellitus with diabetic**   HCC
        **autonomic (poly)neuropathy**
        Other specified diabetes mellitus with diabetic
          gastroparesis
        AHA: 2013, 4Q, 114

    **E13.44 Other specified diabetes mellitus with diabetic**   HCC
        **amyotrophy**

    **E13.49 Other specified diabetes mellitus with** other   HCC
        **diabetic neurological complication**

**✓5ᵗʰ E13.5 Other specified diabetes mellitus with** circulatory complications

    **E13.51 Other specified diabetes mellitus with diabetic**   HCC
        **peripheral angiopathy without gangrene**

    **E13.52 Other specified diabetes mellitus with**   PDxCC   CC   HCC
        **diabetic peripheral angiopathy with gangrene**
        Other specified diabetes mellitus with diabetic
          gangrene
        CC Excl: PDX collection 519

    **E13.59 Other specified diabetes mellitus with** other   HCC
        **circulatory complications**

Ⓝ Newborn: 0    Ⓟ Pediatric: 0-17    Ⓜ Maternity: 12-55    Ⓐ Adult: 15-124    MCC Major CC Condition    PDxMCC PDx acts as own MCC    CC CC Condition    PDxCC PDx acts as own CC

518                                                        ICD-10-CM 2018

✓5ᵗʰ **E13.6** **Other specified diabetes mellitus with** other specified complications

✓6ᵗʰ **E13.61** **Other specified diabetes mellitus with** skin complications
- **E13.610** **Other specified diabetes mellitus with** HCC diabetic **neuropathic** arthropathy
  Other specified diabetes mellitus with Charcôt's joints
- **E13.618** **Other specified diabetes mellitus with** HCC other **diabetic arthropathy**

✓6ᵗʰ **E13.62** **Other specified diabetes mellitus with** skin complications
- **E13.620** **Other specified diabetes mellitus with** HCC diabetic **dermatitis**
  Other specified diabetes mellitus with diabetic necrobiosis lipoidica
- **E13.621** **Other specified diabetes mellitus with** HCC foot ulcer
  Use additional code to identify site of ulcer (L97.4-, L97.5-)
- **E13.622** **Other specified diabetes mellitus with** HCC other skin ulcer
  Use additional code to identify site of ulcer (L97.1-L97.9, L98.41-L98.49)
- **E13.628** **Other specified diabetes mellitus with** HCC other **skin complications**

✓6ᵗʰ **E13.63** **Other specified diabetes mellitus with** oral complications
- **E13.630** **Other specified diabetes mellitus with** HCC periodontal **disease**
- **E13.638** **Other specified diabetes mellitus with** HCC other oral complications

✓6ᵗʰ **E13.64** **Other specified diabetes mellitus with** hypoglycemia
- **E13.641** **Other specified diabetes mellitus** MCC HCC with hypoglycemia with coma
- **E13.649** **Other specified diabetes mellitus with** HCC hypoglycemia without coma
  **AHA:** 2016, 3Q, 42; 2015, 3Q, 21

- **E13.65** **Other specified diabetes mellitus with** HCC hyperglycemia

- **E13.69** **Other specified diabetes mellitus with** other HCC specified complication
  Use additional code to identify complication
  **AHA:** 2016, 4Q, 141; 2016, 1Q, 13

**E13.8** **Other specified diabetes mellitus with** unspecified HCC complications

4 **E13.9** **Other specified diabetes mellitus** without complications HCC

## Other disorders of glucose regulation and pancreatic internal secretion (E15-E16)

**E15** **Nondiabetic hypoglycemic coma**    CC H9 HCC
INCLUDES   drug-induced insulin coma in nondiabetic
hyperinsulinism with hypoglycemic coma
hypoglycemic coma NOS
**CC Excl:** PDX collection 520

✓4ᵗʰ **E16** **Other disorders of pancreatic internal secretion**

**E16.0** **Drug-induced hypoglycemia without coma**
Use additional code for adverse effect, if applicable, to identify drug (T36-T50 with fifth or sixth character 5)
EXCLUDES 1   diabetes with hypoglycemia without coma ▶(E09.649)◀

**E16.1** **Other hypoglycemia**
Functional hyperinsulinism
Functional nonhyperinsulinemic hypoglycemia
Hyperinsulinism NOS
Hyperplasia of pancreatic islet beta cells NOS
EXCLUDES 1   diabetes with hypoglycemia (E08.649, E10.649, E11.649, E13.649)
hypoglycemia in infant of diabetic mother (P70.1)
neonatal hypoglycemia (P70.4)

**E16.2** **Hypoglycemia, unspecified**
EXCLUDES 1   diabetes with hypoglycemia (E08.649, E10.649, E11.649, E13.649)
**AHA:** 2016, 3Q, 42

**E16.3** **Increased secretion of glucagon**
Hyperplasia of pancreatic endocrine cells with glucagon excess

**E16.4** **Increased secretion of gastrin**
Hypergastrinemia
Hyperplasia of pancreatic endocrine cells with gastrin excess
Zollinger-Ellison syndrome

**E16.8** **Other specified disorders of pancreatic internal secretion**
Increased secretion from endocrine pancreas of growth hormone-releasing hormone
Increased secretion from endocrine pancreas of pancreatic polypeptide
Increased secretion from endocrine pancreas of somatostatin
Increased secretion from endocrine pancreas of vasoactive-intestinal polypeptide

**E16.9** **Disorder of pancreatic internal secretion, unspecified**
Islet-cell hyperplasia NOS
Pancreatic endocrine cell hyperplasia NOS

## Disorders of other endocrine glands (E20-E35)

EXCLUDES 1   galactorrhea (N64.3)
gynecomastia (N62)

✓4ᵗʰ **E20** **Hypoparathyroidism**
EXCLUDES 1   Di George's syndrome (D82.1)
postprocedural hypoparathyroidism (E89.2)
tetany NOS (R29.0)
transitory neonatal hypoparathyroidism (P71.4)

**E20.0** **Idiopathic hypoparathyroidism**   HCC
**DEF:** Abnormally low secretion of parathyroid hormones, with unknown cause, which causes decreased calcium and increased phosphorus in the blood, resulting in muscle cramps, tetany, tingling, or burning in lips, fingers, and toes, and cataracts.

**E20.1** **Pseudohypoparathyroidism**

**E20.8** **Other hypoparathyroidism**   HCC

**E20.9** **Hypoparathyroidism, unspecified**   HCC
Parathyroid tetany

✓4ᵗʰ **E21** **Hyperparathyroidism and other disorders of parathyroid gland**
EXCLUDES 1   adult osteomalacia (M83.-)
ectopic hyperparathyroidism (E34.2)
familial hypocalciuric hypercalcemia (E83.52)
hungry bone syndrome (E83.81)
infantile and juvenile osteomalacia (E55.0)

**E21.0** **Primary hyperparathyroidism**   HCC
Hyperplasia of parathyroid
Osteitis fibrosa cystica generalisata [von Recklinghausen's disease of bone]
**DEF:** Parathyroid dysfunction commonly caused by hyperplasia of two or more glands; characteristic hypercalcemia and increased parathyroid hormone levels.

**E21.1** **Secondary hyperparathyroidism, not elsewhere classified** HCC
EXCLUDES 1   secondary hyperparathyroidism of renal origin (N25.81)

**E21.2** **Other hyperparathyroidism**   HCC
Tertiary hyperparathyroidism
EXCLUDES 1   familial hypocalciuric hypercalcemia (E83.52)

**E21.3** **Hyperparathyroidism, unspecified**   HCC

**E21.4** **Other specified disorders of parathyroid gland**   HCC

**E21.5** **Disorder of parathyroid gland, unspecified**   HCC

✓4ᵗʰ **E22** **Hyperfunction of pituitary gland**
EXCLUDES 1   Cushing's syndrome (E24.-)
Nelson's syndrome (E24.1)
overproduction of ACTH not associated with Cushing's disease (E27.0)
overproduction of pituitary ACTH (E24.0)
overproduction of thyroid-stimulating hormone (E05.8-)

**CC Excl: For CC codes in category E22, unless otherwise noted:**
PDX collection 521

**E22.0** **Acromegaly and pituitary gigantism**   HCC
Overproduction of growth hormone
EXCLUDES 1   constitutional gigantism (E34.4)
constitutional tall stature (E34.4)
increased secretion from endocrine pancreas of growth hormone-releasing hormone (E16.8)

**E22.1** **Hyperprolactinemia**   CC HCC
Use additional code for adverse effect, if applicable, to identify drug (T36-T50 with fifth or sixth character 5)

**E22.2** **Syndrome of inappropriate secretion of antidiuretic** CC HCC **hormone**
**CC Excl:** PDX collection 522

---

4   Questionable admission when used as PDx.

*Chapter 4. Endocrine, Nutritional and Metabolic Diseases*

**E22.8**   **Other hyperfunction of pituitary gland**    `CC` `HCC`
Central precocious puberty

**E22.9**   **Hyperfunction of pituitary gland, unspecified**    `CC` `HCC`

✓4ᵗʰ **E23**   **Hypofunction and other disorders of the pituitary gland**
> **INCLUDES**   the listed conditions whether the disorder is in the pituitary or the hypothalamus
> **EXCLUDES 1**   *postprocedural hypopituitarism (E89.3)*

**E23.0**   **Hypopituitarism**    `CC` `HCC`
Fertile eunuch syndrome
Hypogonadotropic hypogonadism
Idiopathic growth hormone deficiency
Isolated deficiency of gonadotropin
Isolated deficiency of growth hormone
Isolated deficiency of pituitary hormone
Kallmann's syndrome
Lorain-Levi short stature
Necrosis of pituitary gland (postpartum)
Panhypopituitarism
Pituitary cachexia
Pituitary insufficiency NOS
Pituitary short stature
Sheehan's syndrome
Simmonds' disease
**CC Excl:** PDX collection 523

**E23.1**   **Drug-induced hypopituitarism**    `HCC`
Use additional code for adverse effect, if applicable, to identify drug (T36-T50 with fifth or sixth character 5)

**E23.2**   **Diabetes insipidus**    `CC` `HCC`
> **EXCLUDES 1**   *nephrogenic diabetes insipidus (N25.1)*
**CC Excl:** PDX collection 524

**E23.3**   **Hypothalamic dysfunction, not elsewhere classified**    `HCC`
> **EXCLUDES 1**   *Prader-Willi syndrome (Q87.1)*
> *Russell-Silver syndrome (Q87.1)*

**E23.6**   **Other disorders of pituitary gland**    `HCC`
Abscess of pituitary
Adiposogenital dystrophy

**E23.7**   **Disorder of pituitary gland, unspecified**    `HCC`

✓4ᵗʰ **E24**   **Cushing's syndrome**
> **EXCLUDES 1**   *congenital adrenal hyperplasia (E25.0)*

**CC Excl: For CC codes in category E24:** PDX collection 525

**E24.0**   **Pituitary-dependent Cushing's disease**    `CC` `HCC`
Overproduction of pituitary ACTH
Pituitary-dependent hypercorticalism

**E24.1**   **Nelson's syndrome**    `HCC`

**E24.2**   **Drug-induced Cushing's syndrome**    `CC` `HCC`
Use additional code for adverse effect, if applicable, to identify drug (T36-T50 with fifth or sixth character 5)

**E24.3**   **Ectopic ACTH syndrome**    `CC` `HCC`

**E24.4**   **Alcohol-induced pseudo-Cushing's syndrome**    `CC` `HCC`

**E24.8**   **Other Cushing's syndrome**    `CC` `HCC`

**E24.9**   **Cushing's syndrome, unspecified**    `CC` `HCC`

✓4ᵗʰ **E25**   **Adrenogenital disorders**
> **INCLUDES**   adrenogenital syndromes, virilizing or feminizing, whether acquired or due to adrenal hyperplasia consequent on inborn enzyme defects in hormone synthesis
> female adrenal pseudohermaphroditism
> female heterosexual precocious pseudopuberty
> male isosexual precocious pseudopuberty
> male macrogenitosomia praecox
> male sexual precocity with adrenal hyperplasia
> male virilization (female)
> **EXCLUDES 1**   *indeterminate sex and pseudohermaphroditism (Q56)*
> *chromosomal abnormalities (Q90-Q99)*

**E25.0**   **Congenital adrenogenital disorders associated with enzyme deficiency**    `HCC`
Congenital adrenal hyperplasia
21-Hydroxylase deficiency
Salt-losing congenital adrenal hyperplasia

**E25.8**   **Other adrenogenital disorders**    `HCC`
Idiopathic adrenogenital disorder
Use additional code for adverse effect, if applicable, to identify drug (T36-T50 with fifth or sixth character 5)

**E25.9**   **Adrenogenital disorder, unspecified**    `HCC`
Adrenogenital syndrome NOS

✓4ᵗʰ **E26**   **Hyperaldosteronism**

✓5ᵗʰ **E26.0**   **Primary hyperaldosteronism**

**E26.01**   **Conn's syndrome**    `HCC`
Code also adrenal adenoma (D35.0-)

**E26.02**   **Glucocorticoid-remediable aldosteronism**    `HCC`
Familial aldosteronism type I
**DEF:** Rare autosomal dominant familial form of primary aldosteronism in which the secretion of aldosterone is under the influence of adrenocorticotrophic hormone (ACTH) rather than the renin-angiotensin mechanism; moderate hypersecretion of aldosterone and suppressed plasma renin activity that are rapidly reversed by administration of glucosteroids; symptoms include hypertension and mild hypokalemia.

**E26.09**   **Other primary hyperaldosteronism**    `HCC`
Primary aldosteronism due to adrenal hyperplasia (bilateral)

**E26.1**   **Secondary hyperaldosteronism**    `HCC`

✓5ᵗʰ **E26.8**   **Other hyperaldosteronism**

**E26.81**   **Bartter's syndrome**    `HCC`

**E26.89**   **Other hyperaldosteronism**    `HCC`

**E26.9**   **Hyperaldosteronism, unspecified**    `HCC`
Aldosteronism NOS
Hyperaldosteronism NOS

✓4ᵗʰ **E27**   **Other disorders of adrenal gland**

**CC Excl: For CC codes in category E27:** PDX collection 526

**E27.0**   **Other adrenocortical overactivity**    `CC` `HCC`
Overproduction of ACTH, not associated with Cushing's disease
Premature adrenarche
> **EXCLUDES 1**   *Cushing's syndrome (E24.-)*

**E27.1**   **Primary adrenocortical insufficiency**    `CC` `HCC`
Addison's disease
Autoimmune adrenalitis
> **EXCLUDES 1**   *Addison only phenotype adrenoleukodystrophy (E71.528)*
> *amyloidosis (E85.-)*
> *tuberculous Addison's disease (A18.7)*
> *Waterhouse-Friderichsen syndrome (A39.1)*

**E27.2**   **Addisonian crisis**    `CC` `HCC`
Adrenal crisis
Adrenocortical crisis

**E27.3**   **Drug-induced adrenocortical insufficiency**    `CC` `HCC`
Use additional code for adverse effect, if applicable, to identify drug (T36-T50 with fifth or sixth character 5)

✓5ᵗʰ **E27.4**   **Other and unspecified adrenocortical insufficiency**
> **EXCLUDES 1**   *adrenoleukodystrophy [Addison-Schilder] (E71.528)*
> *Waterhouse-Friderichsen syndrome (A39.1)*

**E27.40**   **Unspecified adrenocortical insufficiency**    `CC` `HCC`
Adrenocortical insufficiency NOS
Hypoaldosteronism

**E27.49**   **Other adrenocortical insufficiency**    `CC` `HCC`
Adrenal hemorrhage
Adrenal infarction

**E27.5**   **Adrenomedullary hyperfunction**    `CC` `HCC`
Adrenomedullary hyperplasia
Catecholamine hypersecretion

**E27.8**   **Other specified disorders of adrenal gland**    `HCC`
Abnormality of cortisol-binding globulin

**E27.9**   **Disorder of adrenal gland, unspecified**    `HCC`

✓4ᵗʰ **E28**   **Ovarian dysfunction**
> **EXCLUDES 1**   *isolated gonadotropin deficiency (E23.0)*
> *postprocedural ovarian failure (E89.4-)*

**E28.0**   **Estrogen excess**    ♀
Use additional code for adverse effect, if applicable, to identify drug (T36-T50 with fifth or sixth character 5)

**E28.1**   **Androgen excess**    ♀
Hypersecretion of ovarian androgens
Use additional code for adverse effect, if applicable, to identify drug (T36-T50 with fifth or sixth character 5)

**E28.2**   **Polycystic ovarian syndrome**    ♀
Sclerocystic ovary syndrome
Stein-Leventhal syndrome

---

`N` Newborn: 0   `P` Pediatric: 0-17   `M` Maternity: 12-55   `A` Adult: 15-124   `MCC` Major CC Condition   `PDxMCC` PDx acts as own MCC   `CC` CC Condition   `PDxCC` PDx acts as own CC

**520**

ICD-10-CM 2018

☑5ᵗʰ **E28.3 Primary ovarian failure**
> *EXCLUDES 1*   *pure gonadal dysgenesis (Q99.1)*
> *Turner's syndrome (Q96.-)*

  ☑6ᵗʰ **E28.31 Premature menopause**

    **E28.310 Symptomatic premature menopause** Ⓐ ♀
      Symptoms such as flushing, sleeplessness, headache, lack of concentration, associated with premature menopause

    **E28.319 Asymptomatic premature menopause** Ⓐ ♀
      Premature menopause NOS

  **E28.39 Other primary ovarian failure**   ♀
    Decreased estrogen
    Resistant ovary syndrome

**E28.8 Other ovarian dysfunction**   ♀
  Ovarian hyperfunction NOS
> *EXCLUDES 1*   *postprocedural ovarian failure (E89.4-)*

**E28.9 Ovarian dysfunction, unspecified**   ♀

☑4ᵗʰ **E29 Testicular dysfunction**
> *EXCLUDES 1*   *androgen insensitivity syndrome (E34.5-)*
> *azoospermia or oligospermia NOS (N46.0-N46.1)*
> *isolated gonadotropin deficiency (E23.0)*
> *Klinefelter's syndrome (Q98.0-Q98.1, Q98.4)*

**E29.0 Testicular hyperfunction**   ♂
  Hypersecretion of testicular hormones

**E29.1 Testicular hypofunction**   ♂
  Defective biosynthesis of testicular androgen NOS
  5-delta-Reductase deficiency (with male pseudohermaphroditism)
  Testicular hypogonadism NOS
  Use additional code for adverse effect, if applicable, to identify drug (T36-T50 with fifth or sixth character 5)
> *EXCLUDES 1*   *postprocedural testicular hypofunction (E89.5)*

**E29.8 Other testicular dysfunction**   ♂

**E29.9 Testicular dysfunction, unspecified**   ♂

☑4ᵗʰ **E30 Disorders of puberty, not elsewhere classified**

**E30.0 Delayed puberty**
  Constitutional delay of puberty
  Delayed sexual development

**E30.1 Precocious puberty**   Ⓟ
  Precocious menstruation
> *EXCLUDES 1*   *Albright (-McCune) (-Sternberg) syndrome (Q78.1)*
> *central precocious puberty (E22.8)*
> *congenital adrenal hyperplasia (E25.0)*
> *female heterosexual precocious pseudopuberty (E25.-)*
> *male isosexual precocious pseudopuberty (E25.-)*

**E30.8 Other disorders of puberty**   Ⓟ
  Premature thelarche

**E30.9 Disorder of puberty, unspecified**

☑4ᵗʰ **E31 Polyglandular dysfunction**
> *EXCLUDES 1*   *ataxia telangiectasia [Louis-Bar] (G11.3)*
> *dystrophia myotonica [Steinert] (G71.11)*
> *pseudohypoparathyroidism (E20.1)*

**E31.0 Autoimmune polyglandular failure**   HCC
  Schmidt's syndrome

**E31.1 Polyglandular hyperfunction**   HCC
> *EXCLUDES 1*   *multiple endocrine adenomatosis (E31.2-)*
> *multiple endocrine neoplasia (E31.2-)*

☑5ᵗʰ **E31.2 Multiple endocrine neoplasia [MEN] syndromes**
  Multiple endocrine adenomatosis
  Code also any associated malignancies and other conditions associated with the syndromes

  **E31.20 Multiple endocrine neoplasia [MEN] syndrome, unspecified**   HCC
    Multiple endocrine adenomatosis NOS
    Multiple endocrine neoplasia [MEN] syndrome NOS

  **E31.21 Multiple endocrine neoplasia [MEN] type I**   HCC
    Wermer's syndrome

  **E31.22 Multiple endocrine neoplasia [MEN] type IIA**   HCC
    Sipple's syndrome

  **E31.23 Multiple endocrine neoplasia [MEN] type IIB**   HCC

**E31.8 Other polyglandular dysfunction**   HCC

**E31.9 Polyglandular dysfunction, unspecified**   HCC

---

☑4ᵗʰ **E32 Diseases of thymus**
> *EXCLUDES 1*   *aplasia or hypoplasia of thymus with immunodeficiency (D82.1)*
> *myasthenia gravis (G70.0)*

**E32.0 Persistent hyperplasia of thymus**   HCC
  Hypertrophy of thymus

**E32.1 Abscess of thymus**   CC HCC
  **CC Excl:** PDX collection 527

**E32.8 Other diseases of thymus**   HCC
> *EXCLUDES 1*   *aplasia or hypoplasia with immunodeficiency (D82.1)*
> *thymoma (D15.0)*

**E32.9 Disease of thymus, unspecified**   HCC

☑4ᵗʰ **E34 Other endocrine disorders**
> *EXCLUDES 1*   *pseudohypoparathyroidism (E20.1)*

**E34.0 Carcinoid syndrome**   CC HCC
> *NOTE*   May be used as an additional code to identify functional activity associated with a carcinoid tumor.
  **CC Excl:** PDX collection 528

**E34.1 Other hypersecretion of intestinal hormones**

**E34.2 Ectopic hormone secretion, not elsewhere classified**
> *EXCLUDES 1*   *ectopic ACTH syndrome (E24.3)*

**E34.3 Short stature due to endocrine disorder**
  Constitutional short stature
  Laron-type short stature
> *EXCLUDES 1*   *achondroplastic short stature (Q77.4)*
> *hypochondroplastic short stature (Q77.4)*
> *nutritional short stature (E45)*
> *pituitary short stature (E23.0)*
> *progeria (E34.8)*
> *renal short stature (N25.0)*
> *Russell-Silver syndrome (Q87.1)*
> *short-limbed stature with immunodeficiency (D82.2)*
> *short stature in specific dysmorphic syndromes— code to syndrome—see Alphabetical Index*
> *short stature NOS (R62.52)*

**E34.4 Constitutional tall stature**   HCC
  Constitutional gigantism

☑5ᵗʰ **E34.5 Androgen insensitivity syndrome**

  **E34.50 Androgen insensitivity syndrome, unspecified**
    Androgen insensitivity NOS

  **E34.51 Complete androgen insensitivity syndrome**
    Complete androgen insensitivity
    de Quervain syndrome
    Goldberg-Maxwell syndrome

  **E34.52 Partial androgen insensitivity syndrome**
    Partial androgen insensitivity
    Reifenstein syndrome

**E34.8 Other specified endocrine disorders**
  Pineal gland dysfunction      Progeria
> *EXCLUDES 2*   *pseudohypoparathyroidism (E20.1)*

**E34.9 Endocrine disorder, unspecified**
  Endocrine disturbance NOS
  Hormone disturbance NOS

*E35* *Disorders of endocrine glands in diseases classified elsewhere*
  Code first underlying disease, such as:
    late congenital syphilis of thymus gland [Dubois disease] (A50.5)
  Use additional code, if applicable, to identify:
    sequelae of tuberculosis of other organs (B90.8)
> *EXCLUDES 1*   *Echinococcus granulosus infection of thyroid gland (B67.3)*
> *meningococcal hemorrhagic adrenalitis (A39.1)*
> *syphilis of endocrine gland (A52.79)*
> *tuberculosis of adrenal gland, except calcification (A18.7)*
> *tuberculosis of endocrine gland NEC (A18.82)*
> *tuberculosis of thyroid gland (A18.81)*
> *Waterhouse-Friderichsen syndrome (A39.1)*

## Intraoperative Complications of Endocrine System (E36)

☑4ᵗʰ **E36 Intraoperative complications of endocrine system**
> *EXCLUDES 2*   *postprocedural endocrine and metabolic complications and disorders, not elsewhere classified (E89.-)*

☑5ᵗʰ **E36.0 Intraoperative hemorrhage and hematoma of an endocrine system organ or structure complicating a procedure**
> *EXCLUDES 1*   *intraoperative hemorrhage and hematoma of an endocrine system organ or structure due to accidental puncture or laceration during a procedure (E36.1-)*

  **E36.01 Intraoperative hemorrhage and hematoma of an endocrine system organ or structure complicating an endocrine system procedure**   CC
    **CC Excl:** PDX collection 529

---

☑ Additional Character Req   ☑✔7ᵗʰ Placeholder Alert   Unacceptable PDx   Manifestation   H1-H14 HAC   HCC CMS-HCC Condition   *EXCLUDES 1* Not Coded Here   *EXCLUDES 2* Not Included Here

**Chapter 4. Endocrine, Nutritional and Metabolic Diseases**

**E36.02   Intraoperative hemorrhage and hematoma of an endocrine system organ or structure complicating** other procedure    `CC`
     CC Excl: PDX collection 529

✓5ᵗʰ **E36.1   Accidental puncture and laceration of an endocrine system organ or structure during a procedure**

     **E36.11   Accidental puncture and laceration of an endocrine system organ or structure during an endocrine system procedure**    `CC`
       CC Excl: PDX collection 509

     **E36.12   Accidental puncture and laceration of an endocrine system organ or structure during other procedure**    `CC`
       CC Excl: PDX collection 509

**E36.8   Other intraoperative complications of endocrine system**
     Use additional code, if applicable, to further specify disorder

## Malnutrition (E40-E46)

EXCLUDES 1   *intestinal malabsorption (K90.-)*
           *sequelae of protein-calorie malnutrition (E64.0)*
EXCLUDES 2   *nutritional anemias (D50-D53)*
           *starvation (T73.0)*

**E40   Kwashiorkor**    `MCC` `HCC`
     Severe malnutrition with nutritional edema with dyspigmentation of skin and hair
     EXCLUDES 1   *marasmic kwashiorkor (E42)*
     CC Excl: PDX collection 530

**E41   Nutritional marasmus**    `MCC` `HCC`
     Severe malnutrition with marasmus
     EXCLUDES 1   *marasmic kwashiorkor (E42)*
     DEF: Protein-calorie malabsorption or malnutrition in children; characterized by tissue wasting, dehydration, and subcutaneous fat depletion; may occur with infectious disease; also called infantile atrophy.
     CC Excl: PDX collection 530

**E42   Marasmic kwashiorkor**    `MCC` `HCC`
     Intermediate form severe protein-calorie malnutrition
     Severe protein-calorie malnutrition with signs of both kwashiorkor and marasmus
     CC Excl: PDX collection 530

**E43   Unspecified severe protein-calorie malnutrition**    `MCC` `HCC`
     Starvation edema
     CC Excl: PDX collection 530

✓4ᵗʰ **E44   Protein-calorie malnutrition of moderate and mild degree**
     **E44.0   Moderate protein-calorie malnutrition**    `CC` `HCC`
       CC Excl: PDX collection 530

     **E44.1   Mild protein-calorie malnutrition**    `CC` `HCC`
       CC Excl: PDX collection 530

**E45   Retarded development following protein-calorie malnutrition**    `CC` `HCC`
     Nutritional short stature
     Nutritional stunting
     Physical retardation due to malnutrition
     CC Excl: PDX collection 530

**E46   Unspecified protein-calorie malnutrition**    `CC` `HCC`
     Malnutrition NOS
     Protein-calorie imbalance NOS
     EXCLUDES 1   *nutritional deficiency NOS (E63.9)*
     CC Excl: PDX collection 530

## Other nutritional deficiencies (E50-E64)

EXCLUDES 2   *nutritional anemias (D50-D53)*

✓4ᵗʰ **E50   Vitamin A deficiency**
     EXCLUDES 1   *sequelae of vitamin A deficiency (E64.1)*

     **E50.0   Vitamin A deficiency with conjunctival xerosis**

     **E50.1   Vitamin A deficiency with Bitot's spot and conjunctival xerosis**
       Bitot's spot in the young child
       DEF: Vitamin A deficiency with conjunctival dryness, superficial spots of keratinized epithelium.

     **E50.2   Vitamin A deficiency with corneal xerosis**

     **E50.3   Vitamin A deficiency with corneal ulceration and xerosis**

     **E50.4   Vitamin A deficiency with keratomalacia**
       DEF: Vitamin A deficiency creating corneal dryness; progresses to corneal insensitivity, softness, and necrosis; usually bilateral.

     **E50.5   Vitamin A deficiency with night blindness**

     **E50.6   Vitamin A deficiency with xerophthalmic scars of cornea**

     **E50.7   Other ocular manifestations of vitamin A deficiency**
       Xerophthalmia NOS

     **E50.8   Other manifestations of vitamin A deficiency**
       Follicular keratosis
       Xeroderma

     **E50.9   Vitamin A deficiency, unspecified**
       Hypovitaminosis A NOS

✓4ᵗʰ **E51   Thiamine deficiency**
     EXCLUDES 1   *sequelae of thiamine deficiency (E64.8)*

     **CC Excl: For CC codes in category E51: PDX collection 531**

✓5ᵗʰ   **E51.1   Beriberi**
     **E51.11   Dry beriberi**    `CC`
       Beriberi NOS
       Beriberi with polyneuropathy

     **E51.12   Wet beriberi**    `CC`
       Beriberi with cardiovascular manifestations
       Cardiovascular beriberi
       Shoshin disease

     **E51.2   Wernicke's encephalopathy**    `CC`

     **E51.8   Other manifestations of thiamine deficiency**    `CC`

     **E51.9   Thiamine deficiency, unspecified**    `CC`

**E52   Niacin deficiency [pellagra]**
     Niacin (-tryptophan) deficiency
     Nicotinamide deficiency
     Pellagra (alcoholic)
     EXCLUDES 1   *sequelae of niacin deficiency (E64.8)*

✓4ᵗʰ **E53   Deficiency of other B group vitamins**
     EXCLUDES 1   *sequelae of vitamin B deficiency (E64.8)*

     **E53.0   Riboflavin deficiency**    `CC`
       Ariboflavinosis
       Vitamin B2 deficiency
       CC Excl: PDX collection 531

     **E53.1   Pyridoxine deficiency**
       Vitamin B6 deficiency
       EXCLUDES 1   *pyridoxine-responsive sideroblastic anemia (D64.3)*

     **E53.8   Deficiency of other specified B group vitamins**
       Biotin deficiency
       Cyanocobalamin deficiency
       Folate deficiency
       Folic acid deficiency
       Pantothenic acid deficiency
       Vitamin B12 deficiency
       EXCLUDES 1   *folate deficiency anemia (D52.-)*
            *vitamin B12 deficiency anemia (D51.-)*

     **E53.9   Vitamin B deficiency, unspecified**

**E54   Ascorbic acid deficiency**
     Deficiency of vitamin C
     Scurvy
     EXCLUDES 1   *scorbutic anemia (D53.2)*
            *sequelae of vitamin C deficiency (E64.2)*
     DEF: Vitamin C deficiency causing swollen gums, myalgia, weight loss, and weakness.

✓4ᵗʰ **E55   Vitamin D deficiency**
     EXCLUDES 1   *adult osteomalacia (M83.-)*
            *osteoporosis (M80.-)*
            *sequelae of rickets (E64.3)*

     **E55.0   Rickets, active**    `CC`
       Infantile osteomalacia
       Juvenile osteomalacia
       EXCLUDES 1   *celiac rickets (K90.0)*
            *Crohn's rickets (K50.-)*
            *hereditary vitamin D-dependent rickets (E83.32)*
            *inactive rickets (E64.3)*
            *renal rickets (N25.0)*
            *sequelae of rickets (E64.3)*
            *vitamin D-resistant rickets (E83.31)*
       CC Excl: PDX collection 532

     **E55.9   Vitamin D deficiency, unspecified**
       Avitaminosis D

✓4ᵗʰ **E56   Other vitamin deficiencies**
     EXCLUDES 1   *sequelae of other vitamin deficiencies (E64.8)*

     **E56.0   Deficiency of vitamin E**

     **E56.1   Deficiency of vitamin K**
       EXCLUDES 1   *deficiency of coagulation factor due to vitamin K deficiency (D68.4)*
            *vitamin K deficiency of newborn (P53)*

     **E56.8   Deficiency of other vitamins**

     **E56.9   Vitamin deficiency, unspecified**

🅝 Newborn: 0   🅟 Pediatric: 0-17   🅜 Maternity: 12-55   🅐 Adult: 15-124   `MCC` Major CC Condition   `PDxMCC` PDx acts as own MCC   `CC` CC Condition   `PDxCC` PDx acts as own CC

522             ICD-10-CM 2018

**E58   Dietary calcium deficiency**
> *EXCLUDES 1*   *disorders of calcium metabolism (E83.5-)*
> *sequelae of calcium deficiency (E64.8)*

**E59   Dietary selenium deficiency**
Keshan disease
> *EXCLUDES 1*   *sequelae of selenium deficiency (E64.8)*

**E60   Dietary zinc deficiency**

✓4th **E61   Deficiency of other nutrient elements**
> Use additional code for adverse effect, if applicable, to identify drug (T36-T50 with fifth or sixth character 5)
> *EXCLUDES 1*   *disorders of mineral metabolism (E83.-)*
> *iodine deficiency related thyroid disorders (E00-E02)*
> *sequelae of malnutrition and other nutritional deficiencies (E64.-)*

**E61.0   Copper deficiency**
**E61.1   Iron deficiency**
> *EXCLUDES 1*   *iron deficiency anemia (D50.-)*

**E61.2   Magnesium deficiency**
**E61.3   Manganese deficiency**
**E61.4   Chromium deficiency**
**E61.5   Molybdenum deficiency**
**E61.6   Vanadium deficiency**
**E61.7   Deficiency of multiple nutrient elements**
**E61.8   Deficiency of other specified nutrient elements**
**E61.9   Deficiency of nutrient element, unspecified**

✓4th **E63   Other nutritional deficiencies**
> *EXCLUDES 1*   *dehydration (E86.0)*
> *failure to thrive, adult (R62.7)*
> *failure to thrive, child (R62.51)*
> *feeding problems in newborn (P92.-)*
> *sequelae of malnutrition and other nutritional deficiencies (E64.-)*

**E63.0   Essential fatty acid [EFA] deficiency**
**E63.1   Imbalance of constituents of food intake**
**E63.8   Other specified nutritional deficiencies**
**E63.9   Nutritional deficiency, unspecified**

✓4th **E64   Sequelae of malnutrition and other nutritional deficiencies**
> **NOTE**   This category is to be used to indicate conditions in categories E43, E44, E46, E50-E63 as the cause of sequelae, which are themselves classified elsewhere. The 'sequelae' include conditions specified as such; they also include the late effects of diseases classifiable to the above categories if the disease itself is no longer present
>
> Code first condition resulting from (sequela) of malnutrition and other nutritional deficiencies

**E64.0   Sequelae of protein-calorie malnutrition**   CC HCC
> *EXCLUDES 2*   *retarded development following protein-calorie malnutrition (E45)*
> **CC Excl:** PDX collection 530

**E64.1   Sequelae of vitamin A deficiency**
**E64.2   Sequelae of vitamin C deficiency**
**E64.3   Sequelae of rickets**
**E64.8   Sequelae of other nutritional deficiencies**
**E64.9   Sequelae of unspecified nutritional deficiency**

## Overweight, obesity and other hyperalimentation (E65-E68)

**E65   Localized adiposity**
Fat pad

✓4th **E66   Overweight and obesity**
> Code first obesity complicating pregnancy, childbirth and the puerperium, if applicable (O99.21-)
> Use additional code to identify body mass index (BMI), if known (Z68.-)
> *EXCLUDES 1*   *adiposogenital dystrophy (E23.6)*
> *lipomatosis NOS (E88.2)*
> *lipomatosis dolorosa [Dercum] (E88.2)*
> *Prader-Willi syndrome (Q87.1)*

✓5th **E66.0   Obesity due to excess calories**
> **E66.01   Morbid (severe) obesity due to excess calories**   H11 HCC
> > *EXCLUDES 1*   *morbid (severe) obesity with alveolar hypoventilation (E66.2)*
>
> 4 **E66.09   Other obesity due to excess calories**

4 **E66.1   Drug-induced obesity**
> Use additional code for adverse effect, if applicable, to identify drug (T36-T50 with fifth or sixth character 5)

**E66.2   Morbid (severe) obesity with alveolar hypoventilation**   CC HCC
Obesity hypoventilation syndrome (OHS)
Pickwickian syndrome
**CC Excl:** PDX collection 533

**E66.3   Overweight**
4 **E66.8   Other obesity**
4 **E66.9   Obesity, unspecified**
Obesity NOS

✓4th **E67   Other hyperalimentation**
> *EXCLUDES 1*   *hyperalimentation NOS (R63.2)*
> *sequelae of hyperalimentation (E68)*

**E67.0   Hypervitaminosis A**
**E67.1   Hypercarotinemia**
**E67.2   Megavitamin-B6 syndrome**
**E67.3   Hypervitaminosis D**
**E67.8   Other specified hyperalimentation**

**E68   Sequelae of hyperalimentation**
> Code first condition resulting from (sequela) of hyperalimentation

## Metabolic disorders (E70-E88)

> *EXCLUDES 1*   *androgen insensitivity syndrome (E34.5-)*
> *congenital adrenal hyperplasia (E25.0)*
> *Ehlers-Danlos syndrome (Q79.6)*
> *hemolytic anemias attributable to enzyme disorders (D55.-)*
> *Marfan's syndrome (Q87.4)*
> *5-alpha-reductase deficiency (E29.1)*

✓4th **E70   Disorders of aromatic amino-acid metabolism**

> **CC Excl: For CC codes in category E70:** PDX collection 534

**E70.0   Classical phenylketonuria**   CC HCC
**E70.1   Other hyperphenylalaninemias**   CC HCC

✓5th **E70.2   Disorders of tyrosine metabolism**
> *EXCLUDES 1*   *transitory tyrosinemia of newborn (P74.5)*
>
> **E70.20   Disorder of tyrosine metabolism, unspecified**   CC HCC
> **E70.21   Tyrosinemia**   CC HCC
> Hypertyrosinemia
> **E70.29   Other disorders of tyrosine metabolism**   CC HCC
> Alkaptonuria
> Ochronosis

✓5th **E70.3   Albinism**
> **E70.30   Albinism, unspecified**   CC HCC
> ✓6th **E70.31   Ocular albinism**
> > **E70.310   X-linked ocular albinism**   CC HCC
> > **E70.311   Autosomal recessive ocular albinism**   CC HCC
> > **E70.318   Other ocular albinism**   CC HCC
> > **E70.319   Ocular albinism, unspecified**
>
> ✓6th **E70.32   Oculocutaneous albinism**
> > *EXCLUDES 1*   *Chediak-Higashi syndrome (E70.330)*
> > *Hermansky-Pudlak syndrome (E70.331)*
> >
> > **E70.320   Tyrosinase negative oculocutaneous albinism**   CC HCC
> > Albinism I
> > Oculocutaneous albinism ty-neg
> > **E70.321   Tyrosinase positive oculocutaneous albinism**   CC HCC
> > Albinism II
> > Oculocutaneous albinism ty-pos
> > **E70.328   Other oculocutaneous albinism**   CC HCC
> > Cross syndrome
> > **E70.329   Oculocutaneous albinism, unspecified**   CC HCC
>
> ✓6th **E70.33   Albinism with hematologic abnormality**
> > **E70.330   Chediak-Higashi syndrome**   CC HCC
> > **E70.331   Hermansky-Pudlak syndrome**   CC HCC
> > **E70.338   Other albinism with hematologic abnormality**   CC HCC
> > **E70.339   Albinism with hematologic abnormality, unspecified**   CC HCC
>
> **E70.39   Other specified albinism**   CC HCC
> Piebaldism

---

4   Questionable admission when used as PDx.

✓ Additional Character Req   √x7th Placeholder Alert   Unacceptable PDx   Manifestation   H1 - H14 HAC   HCC CMS-HCC Condition   *EXCLUDES 1* Not Coded Here   *EXCLUDES 2* Not Included Here

ICD-10-CM 2018   **523**

√5ᵗʰ **E70.4** **Disorders of** histidine **metabolism**

    **E70.40** **Disorders of histidine metabolism,** `CC` `HCC`
        **unspecified**

    **E70.41** **Histidinemia** `CC` `HCC`

    **E70.49** **Other disorders of histidine metabolism** `CC` `HCC`

**E70.5** **Disorders of** tryptophan **metabolism** `CC` `HCC`

**E70.8** **Other disorders of aromatic amino-acid metabolism** `CC` `HCC`

**E70.9** **Disorder of aromatic amino-acid metabolism,** `CC` `HCC`
  **unspecified**

√4ᵗʰ **E71** **Disorders of branched-chain amino-acid metabolism and fatty-acid metabolism**

  **E71.0** **Maple-syrup-urine disease** `CC` `HCC`
    CC Excl: PDX collection 534

√5ᵗʰ **E71.1** **Other disorders of** branched-chain amino-acid **metabolism**

> CC Excl: For CC codes in subcategory E71.1: PDX collection 534

  √6ᵗʰ **E71.11** **Branched-chain** organic acidurias

    **E71.110** **Isovaleric acidemia** `CC` `HCC`

    **E71.111** **3-methylglutaconic aciduria** `CC` `HCC`

    **E71.118** **Other branched-chain organic** `CC` `HCC`
          **acidurias**

  √6ᵗʰ **E71.12** **Disorders of propionate metabolism**

    **E71.120** **Methylmalonic acidemia** `CC` `HCC`

    **E71.121** **Propionic acidemia** `CC` `HCC`

    **E71.128** **Other disorders of propionate** `CC` `HCC`
          **metabolism**

  **E71.19** **Other disorders of branched-chain** `CC` `HCC`
    **amino-acid metabolism**
      Hyperleucine-isoleucinemia
      Hypervalinemia

**E71.2** **Disorder of branched-chain amino-acid metabolism,** `CC` `HCC`
  **unspecified**
    CC Excl: PDX collection 534

√5ᵗʰ **E71.3** **Disorders of fatty-acid metabolism**

> EXCLUDES 1   peroxisomal disorders (E71.5)
>        Refsum's disease (G60.1)
>        Schilder's disease (G37.0)
> EXCLUDES 2   carnitine deficiency due to inborn error of metabolism
>        (E71.42)

> CC Excl: For CC codes in subcategory E71.3, unless otherwise noted: PDX collection 535

  **E71.30** **Disorder of fatty-acid metabolism, unspecified**

  √6ᵗʰ **E71.31** **Disorders of fatty-acid** oxidation

    **E71.310** **Long chain/very long chain acyl** `CC` `HCC`
          **CoA dehydrogenase deficiency**
           LCAD
           VLCAD

    **E71.311** **Medium chain acyl CoA** `CC` `HCC`
          **dehydrogenase deficiency**
           MCAD

    **E71.312** **Short chain acyl CoA** `CC` `HCC`
          **dehydrogenase deficiency**
           SCAD

    **E71.313** **Glutaric aciduria type II** `CC` `HCC`
          Glutaric aciduria type II A
          Glutaric aciduria type II B
          Glutaric aciduria type II C
          EXCLUDES 1   glutaric aciduria (type 1) NOS
               (E72.3)

    **E71.314** **Muscle carnitine** `CC` `HCC`
          **palmitoyltransferase deficiency**

    **E71.318** **Other disorders of fatty-acid** `CC` `HCC`
          **oxidation**

  **E71.32** **Disorders of ketone metabolism** `CC` `HCC`

  **E71.39** **Other disorders of fatty-acid metabolism** `CC` `HCC`
    CC Excl: PDX collection 492

√5ᵗʰ **E71.4** **Disorders of** carnitine **metabolism**

> EXCLUDES 1   muscle carnitine palmitoyltransferase deficiency
>        (E71.314)

  **E71.40** **Disorder of carnitine metabolism,** unspecified `HCC`

  **E71.41** **Primary carnitine deficiency** `HCC`

  **E71.42** **Carnitine deficiency due to** inborn errors of `HCC`
    **metabolism**
      Code also associated inborn error or metabolism

  **E71.43** **Iatrogenic carnitine deficiency** `HCC`
      Carnitine deficiency due to hemodialysis
      Carnitine deficiency due to Valproic acid therapy

  √6ᵗʰ **E71.44** **Other secondary carnitine deficiency**

    **E71.440** **Ruvalcaba-Myhre-Smith syndrome** `HCC`

    **E71.448** **Other secondary carnitine deficiency** `HCC`

√5ᵗʰ **E71.5** **Peroxisomal disorders**

> EXCLUDES 1   Schilder's disease (G37.0)

> CC Excl: For CC codes in subcategory E71.5: PDX collection 536

  **E71.50** **Peroxisomal disorder, unspecified** `CC` `HCC`

  √6ᵗʰ **E71.51** **Disorders of peroxisome** biogenesis
      Group 1 peroxisomal disorders
      EXCLUDES 1   Refsum's disease (G60.1)

    **E71.510** **Zellweger syndrome** `CC` `HCC`

    **E71.511** **Neonatal adrenoleukodystrophy** `CC` `HCC`
          EXCLUDES 1   X-linked adrenoleukodystrophy
               (E71.52-)

    **E71.518** **Other disorders of peroxisome** `CC` `HCC`
          **biogenesis**

  √6ᵗʰ **E71.52** **X-linked adrenoleukodystrophy**

    **E71.520** **Childhood cerebral X-linked** `CC` `HCC`
          **adrenoleukodystrophy**

    **E71.521** **Adolescent X-linked** `CC` `HCC`
          **adrenoleukodystrophy**

    **E71.522** **Adrenomyeloneuropathy** `CC` `HCC`

    **E71.528** **Other X-linked** `CC` `HCC`
          **adrenoleukodystrophy**
           Addison only phenotype
             adrenoleukodystrophy
           Addison-Schilder adrenoleukodystrophy

    **E71.529** **X-linked adrenoleukodystrophy,** `CC` `HCC`
          **unspecified type**

  **E71.53** **Other group 2 peroxisomal disorders** `CC` `HCC`

  √6ᵗʰ **E71.54** **Other peroxisomal disorders**

    **E71.540** **Rhizomelic chondrodysplasia** `CC` `HCC`
          **punctata**
          EXCLUDES 1   chondrodysplasia punctata NOS
               (Q77.3)

    **E71.541** **Zellweger-like syndrome** `CC` `HCC`

    **E71.542** **Other group 3 peroxisomal** `CC` `HCC`
          **disorders**

    **E71.548** **Other peroxisomal disorders** `CC` `HCC`

√4ᵗʰ **E72** **Other disorders of amino-acid metabolism**

> EXCLUDES 1   disorders of:
>        aromatic amino-acid metabolism (E70.-)
>        branched-chain amino-acid metabolism (E71.0-E71.2)
>        fatty-acid metabolism (E71.3)
>        purine and pyrimidine metabolism (E79.-)
>      gout ( M1A.-, M10.-)

> CC Excl: For CC codes in category E72, unless otherwise noted: PDX collection 534

√5ᵗʰ **E72.0** **Disorders of amino-acid** transport

> EXCLUDES 1   disorders of tryptophan metabolism (E70.5)

  **E72.00** **Disorders of amino-acid transport,** `CC` `HCC`
    **unspecified**

  **E72.01** **Cystinuria** `CC` `HCC`

  **E72.02** **Hartnup's disease** `CC` `HCC`

  **E72.03** **Lowe's syndrome** `CC` `HCC`
      Use additional code for associated glaucoma (H42)
    CC Excl: No Excl

  **E72.04** **Cystinosis** `CC` `HCC`
      Fanconi (-de Toni) (-Debré) syndrome with cystinosis
    EXCLUDES 1   Fanconi (-de Toni) (-Debré) syndrome
            without cystinosis (E72.09)

  **E72.09** **Other disorders of amino-acid transport** `CC` `HCC`
      Fanconi (-de Toni) (-Debré) syndrome, unspecified

Ⓝ Newborn: 0   Ⓟ Pediatric: 0-17   Ⓜ Maternity: 12-55   Ⓐ Adult: 15-124   `MCC` Major CC Condition   `PDxMCC` PDx acts as own MCC   `CC` CC Condition   `PDxCC` PDx acts as own CC

**524**

ICD-10-CM 2018

✓5th **E72.1** **Disorders of sulfur-bearing amino-acid metabolism**
     *EXCLUDES 1*   cystinosis (E72.04)
                cystinuria (E72.01)
                transcobalamin II deficiency (D51.2)

     **E72.10**   **Disorders of sulfur-bearing amino-acid metabolism, unspecified**   CC HCC

     **E72.11**   **Homocystinuria**   CC HCC
                Cystathionine synthase deficiency

     **E72.12**   **Methylenetetrahydrofolate reductase deficiency**   CC HCC

     **E72.19**   **Other disorders of sulfur-bearing amino-acid metabolism**   CC HCC
                Cystathioninuria
                Methioninemia
                Sulfite oxidase deficiency

✓5th **E72.2** **Disorders of urea cycle metabolism**
     *EXCLUDES 1*   disorders of ornithine metabolism (E72.4)

     **E72.20**   **Disorder of urea cycle metabolism, unspecified**   CC HCC
                Hyperammonemia
                *EXCLUDES 1*   hyperammonemia- hyperornithinemia-homocitrullinemia syndrome (E72.4)
                            transient hyperammonemia of newborn (P74.6)

     **E72.21**   **Argininemia**   CC HCC

     **E72.22**   **Arginosuccinic aciduria**   CC HCC

     **E72.23**   **Citrullinemia**   CC HCC

     **E72.29**   **Other disorders of urea cycle metabolism**   CC HCC

**E72.3** **Disorders of lysine and hydroxylysine metabolism**   CC HCC
     Glutaric aciduria NOS
     Glutaric aciduria (type I)
     Hydroxylysinemia
     Hyperlysinemia
     *EXCLUDES 1*   glutaric aciduria type II (E71.313)
                Refsum's disease (G60.1)
                Zellweger syndrome (E71.510)

**E72.4** **Disorders of ornithine metabolism**   CC HCC
     Hyperammonemia-hyperornithinemia-homocitrullinemia syndrome
     Ornithinemia (types I, II)
     Ornithine transcarbamylase deficiency
     *EXCLUDES 1*   hereditary choroidal dystrophy (H31.2-)

✓5th **E72.5** **Disorders of glycine metabolism**
     **E72.50**   **Disorder of glycine metabolism, unspecified**   CC HCC
     **E72.51**   **Non-ketotic hyperglycinemia**   CC HCC
     **E72.52**   **Trimethylaminuria**   CC HCC
     **E72.53**   **Hyperoxaluria**   CC HCC
                Oxalosis
                Oxaluria
     **E72.59**   **Other disorders of glycine metabolism**   CC HCC
                D-glycericacidemia
                Hyperhydroxyprolinemia
                Hyperprolinemia (types I, II)
                Sarcosinemia

**E72.8** **Other specified disorders of amino-acid metabolism**   CC HCC
     Disorders of beta-amino-acid metabolism
     Disorders of gamma-glutamyl cycle

**E72.9** **Disorder of amino-acid metabolism, unspecified**   CC HCC

✓4th **E73** **Lactose intolerance**
     **E73.0**   **Congenital lactase deficiency**
     **E73.1**   **Secondary lactase deficiency**
     **E73.8**   **Other lactose intolerance**
     **E73.9**   **Lactose intolerance, unspecified**

✓4th **E74** **Other disorders of carbohydrate metabolism**
     *EXCLUDES 1*   diabetes mellitus (E08-E13)
                hypoglycemia NOS (E16.2)
                increased secretion of glucagon (E16.3)
                mucopolysaccharidosis (E76.0-E76.3)

     **CC Excl:** For CC codes in category E74: PDX collection 534

✓5th **E74.0** **Glycogen storage disease**
     **E74.00**   **Glycogen storage disease, unspecified**   CC HCC
     **E74.01**   **von Gierke disease**   CC HCC
                Type I glycogen storage disease
     **E74.02**   **Pompe disease**   CC HCC
                Cardiac glycogenosis
                Type II glycogen storage disease
     **E74.03**   **Cori disease**   CC HCC
                Forbes disease
                Type III glycogen storage disease
     **E74.04**   **McArdle disease**   CC HCC
                Type V glycogen storage disease
     **E74.09**   **Other glycogen storage disease**   CC HCC
                Andersen disease
                Hers disease
                Tauri disease
                Glycogen storage disease, types 0, IV, VI-XI
                Liver phosphorylase deficiency
                Muscle phosphofructokinase deficiency

✓5th **E74.1** **Disorders of fructose metabolism**
     *EXCLUDES 1*   muscle phosphofructokinase deficiency (E74.09)
     **E74.10**   **Disorder of fructose metabolism, unspecified**
     **E74.11**   **Essential fructosuria**
                Fructokinase deficiency
     **E74.12**   **Hereditary fructose intolerance**
                Fructosemia
     **E74.19**   **Other disorders of fructose metabolism**
                Fructose-1, 6-diphosphatase deficiency

✓5th **E74.2** **Disorders of galactose metabolism**
     **E74.20**   **Disorders of galactose metabolism, unspecified**   CC HCC
     **E74.21**   **Galactosemia**   CC HCC
                **DEF:** Any of three genetic disorders due to defective galactose metabolism; symptoms include failure to thrive in infancy, jaundice, liver and spleen damage, cataracts, and mental retardation.
     **E74.29**   **Other disorders of galactose metabolism**   CC HCC
                Galactokinase deficiency

✓5th **E74.3** **Other disorders of intestinal carbohydrate absorption**
     *EXCLUDES 2*   lactose intolerance (E73.-)
     **E74.31**   **Sucrase-isomaltase deficiency**
     **E74.39**   **Other disorders of intestinal carbohydrate absorption**
                Disorder of intestinal carbohydrate absorption NOS
                Glucose-galactose malabsorption
                Sucrase deficiency

**E74.4** **Disorders of pyruvate metabolism and gluconeogenesis**   CC HCC
     Deficiency of phosphoenolpyruvate carboxykinase
     Deficiency of pyruvate carboxylase
     Deficiency of pyruvate dehydrogenase
     *EXCLUDES 1*   disorders of pyruvate metabolism and gluconeogenesis with anemia (D55.-)
                          Leigh's syndrome (G31.82)

**E74.8** **Other specified disorders of carbohydrate metabolism**   CC HCC
     Essential pentosuria
     Renal glycosuria

**E74.9** **Disorder of carbohydrate metabolism, unspecified**   HCC

✓ Additional Character Req    ✓x7th Placeholder Alert    Unacceptable PDx    Manifestation    H1-H14 HAC    HCC CMS-HCC Condition    *EXCLUDES 1* Not Coded Here    *EXCLUDES 2* Not Included Here

ICD-10-CM 2018            **525**

**Chapter 4. Endocrine, Nutritional and Metabolic Diseases**

**E75–E78.1**

### Tay-Sachs Disease

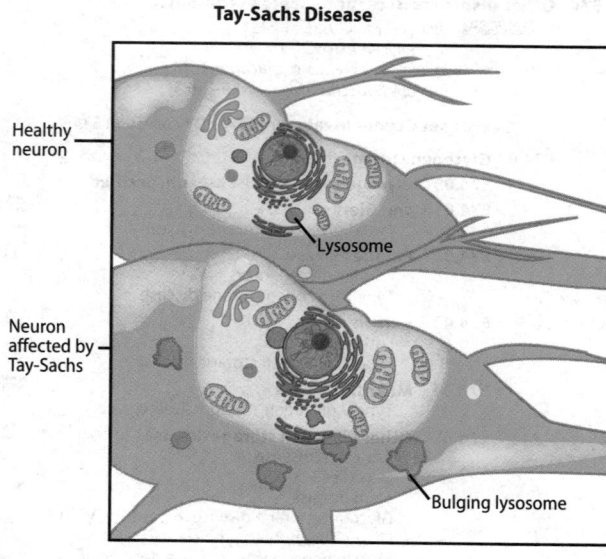

Healthy neuron

Lysosome

Neuron affected by Tay-Sachs

Bulging lysosome

✓4ᵗʰ **E75**   **Disorders of sphingolipid metabolism and other lipid storage disorders**

*EXCLUDES 1*   mucolipidosis, types I-III (E77.0-E77.1)
Refsum's disease (G60.1)

✓5ᵗʰ   **E75.0**   **GM2 gangliosidosis**

**CC Excl: For CC codes in subcategory E75.0:**
PDX collection 537

   **E75.00**   **GM2 gangliosidosis, unspecified**    `CC`

   **E75.01**   **Sandhoff disease**    `CC`

   **E75.02**   **Tay-Sachs disease**    `CC`
       **DEF:** Genetic mutation of the HEXA gene that inhibits the breakdown of a toxic substance called ganglioside. The accumulation of ganglioside results in destruction of the neurons in the brain and spinal cord.

   **E75.09**   **Other GM2 gangliosidosis**    `CC`
       Adult GM2 gangliosidosis
       Juvenile GM2 gangliosidosis

✓5ᵗʰ   **E75.1**   **Other and unspecified gangliosidosis**

**CC Excl: For CC codes in subcategory E75.1:**
PDX collection 537

   **E75.10**   **Unspecified gangliosidosis**    `CC`
       Gangliosidosis NOS

   **E75.11**   **Mucolipidosis IV**    `CC`

   **E75.19**   **Other gangliosidosis**    `CC`
       GM1 gangliosidosis
       GM3 gangliosidosis

✓5ᵗʰ   **E75.2**   **Other sphingolipidosis**

*EXCLUDES 1*   adrenoleukodystrophy [Addison-Schilder] (E71.528)

**CC Excl: For CC codes in subcategory E75.2:**
PDX collection 538

   **E75.21**   **Fabry (-Anderson) disease**    `HCC`

   **E75.22**   **Gaucher disease**    `HCC`

   **E75.23**   **Krabbe disease**    `CC`

✓6ᵗʰ   **E75.24**   **Niemann-Pick disease**

     **E75.240**   **Niemann-Pick disease** type A    `HCC`

     **E75.241**   **Niemann-Pick disease** type B    `HCC`

     **E75.242**   **Niemann-Pick disease** type C    `HCC`

     **E75.243**   **Niemann-Pick disease** type D    `HCC`

     **E75.248**   **Other Niemann-Pick disease**    `HCC`

     **E75.249**   **Niemann-Pick disease, unspecified**    `HCC`

   **E75.25**   **Metachromatic leukodystrophy**    `CC`

   **E75.29**   **Other sphingolipidosis**    `CC`
       Farber's syndrome
       Sulfatase deficiency
       Sulfatide lipidosis

   **E75.3**   **Sphingolipidosis, unspecified**    `HCC`

   **E75.4**   **Neuronal ceroid lipofuscinosis**    `CC`
       Batten disease
       Bielschowsky-Jansky disease
       Kufs disease
       Spielmeyer-Vogt disease
       **CC Excl:** PDX collection 537

   **E75.5**   **Other lipid storage disorders**
       Cerebrotendinous cholesterosis [van Bogaert-Scherer-Epstein]
       Wolman's disease

   **E75.6**   **Lipid storage disorder, unspecified**

✓4ᵗʰ **E76**   **Disorders of glycosaminoglycan metabolism**

**CC Excl: For CC codes in category E76:** PDX collection 539

✓5ᵗʰ   **E76.0**   **Mucopolysaccharidosis, type I**

     **E76.01**   **Hurler's syndrome**    `CC` `HCC`

     **E76.02**   **Hurler-Scheie syndrome**    `CC` `HCC`

     **E76.03**   **Scheie's syndrome**    `CC` `HCC`

   **E76.1**   **Mucopolysaccharidosis, type II**    `CC` `HCC`
       Hunter's syndrome

✓5ᵗʰ   **E76.2**   **Other mucopolysaccharidoses**

✓6ᵗʰ    **E76.21**   **Morquio mucopolysaccharidoses**

       **E76.210**   **Morquio A mucopolysaccharidoses**    `CC` `HCC`
          Classic Morquio syndrome
          Morquio syndrome A
          Mucopolysaccharidosis, type IVA

       **E76.211**   **Morquio B mucopolysaccharidoses**    `CC` `HCC`
          Morquio-like mucopolysaccharidoses
          Morquio-like syndrome
          Morquio syndrome B
          Mucopolysaccharidosis, type IVB

       **E76.219**   **Morquio mucopolysaccharidoses, unspecified**    `CC` `HCC`
          Morquio syndrome
          Mucopolysaccharidosis, type IV

     **E76.22**   **Sanfilippo mucopolysaccharidoses**    `CC` `HCC`
       Mucopolysaccharidosis, type III (A) (B) (C) (D)
       Sanfilippo A syndrome
       Sanfilippo B syndrome
       Sanfilippo C syndrome
       Sanfilippo D syndrome

     **E76.29**   **Other mucopolysaccharidoses**    `CC` `HCC`
       beta-Glucuronidase deficiency
       Maroteaux-Lamy (mild) (severe) syndrome
       Mucopolysaccharidosis, types VI, VII

   **E76.3**   **Mucopolysaccharidosis, unspecified**    `CC` `HCC`

   **E76.8**   **Other disorders of glucosaminoglycan metabolism**    `CC` `HCC`

   **E76.9**   **Glucosaminoglycan metabolism disorder, unspecified**    `CC` `HCC`

✓4ᵗʰ **E77**   **Disorders of glycoprotein metabolism**

   **E77.0**   **Defects in post-translational modification of lysosomal enzymes**    `HCC`
       Mucolipidosis II [I-cell disease]
       Mucolipidosis III [pseudo-Hurler polydystrophy]

   **E77.1**   **Defects in glycoprotein degradation**    `HCC`
       Aspartylglucosaminuria
       Fucosidosis
       Mannosidosis
       Sialidosis [mucolipidosis I]

   **E77.8**   **Other disorders of glycoprotein metabolism**    `HCC`

   **E77.9**   **Disorder of glycoprotein metabolism, unspecified**    `HCC`

✓4ᵗʰ **E78**   **Disorders of lipoprotein metabolism and other lipidemias**

*EXCLUDES 1*   sphingolipidosis (E75.0-E75.3)

✓5ᵗʰ   **E78.0**   **Pure hypercholesterolemia**

     **E78.00**   **Pure hypercholesterolemia, unspecified**
       Fredrickson's hyperlipoproteinemia, type IIa
       Hyperbetalipoproteinemia
       Low-density-lipoprotein-type [LDL] hyperlipoproteinemia
       ▶(Pure) hypercholesterolemia NOS◀

     **E78.01**   **Familial hypercholesterolemia**

   **E78.1**   **Pure hyperglyceridemia**
       Elevated fasting triglycerides
       Endogenous hyperglyceridemia
       Fredrickson's hyperlipoproteinemia, type IV
       Hyperlipidemia, group B
       Hyperprebetalipoproteinemia
       Very-low-density-lipoprotein-type [VLDL] hyperlipoproteinemia

N Newborn: 0   P Pediatric: 0-17   M Maternity: 12-55   A Adult: 15-124   MCC Major CC Condition   PDxMCC PDx acts as own MCC   CC CC Condition   PDxCC PDx acts as own CC

**526**

ICD-10-CM 2018

E78.2 **Mixed hyperlipidemia**
Broad- or floating-betalipoproteinemia
Combined hyperlipidemia NOS
Elevated cholesterol with elevated triglycerides NEC
Fredrickson's hyperlipoproteinemia, type IIb or III
Hyperbetalipoproteinemia with prebetalipoproteinemia
Hypercholesteremia with endogenous hyperglyceridemia
Hyperlipidemia, group C
Tubo-eruptive xanthoma
Xanthoma tuberosum

> EXCLUDES 1    cerebrotendinous cholesterosis [van Bogaert-Scherer-Epstein] (E75.5)
> familial combined hyperlipidemia (E78.4)

E78.3 **Hyperchylomicronemia**
Chylomicron retention disease
Fredrickson's hyperlipoproteinemia, type I or V
Hyperlipidemia, group D
Mixed hyperglyceridemia

E78.4 **Other hyperlipidemia**
Familial combined hyperlipidemia

E78.5 **Hyperlipidemia, unspecified**

E78.6 **Lipoprotein deficiency**
Abetalipoproteinemia
Depressed HDL cholesterol
High-density lipoprotein deficiency
Hypoalphalipoproteinemia
Hypobetalipoproteinemia (familial)
Lecithin cholesterol acyltransferase deficiency
Tangier disease

√5th E78.7 **Disorders of bile acid and cholesterol metabolism**
> EXCLUDES 1    Niemann-Pick disease type C (E75.242)

E78.70 **Disorder of bile acid and cholesterol metabolism, unspecified**

E78.71 **Barth syndrome**                              CC
**CC Excl:** PDX collection 540

E78.72 **Smith-Lemli-Opitz syndrome**                  CC
**CC Excl:** PDX collection 540

E78.79 **Other disorders of bile acid and cholesterol metabolism**

√5th E78.8 **Other disorders of lipoprotein metabolism**

E78.81 **Lipoid dermatoarthritis**

E78.89 **Other lipoprotein metabolism disorders**

E78.9 **Disorder of lipoprotein metabolism, unspecified**

√4th E79 **Disorders of purine and pyrimidine metabolism**
> EXCLUDES 1    Ataxia-telangiectasia (Q87.1)
> Bloom's syndrome (Q82.8)
> Cockayne's syndrome (Q87.1)
> calculus of kidney (N20.0)
> combined immunodeficiency disorders (D81.-)
> Fanconi's anemia (D61.09)
> gout ( M1A.-, M10.-)
> orotaciduric anemia (D53.0)
> progeria (E34.8)
> Werner's syndrome (E34.8)
> xeroderma pigmentosum (Q82.1)

**CC Excl: For CC codes in category E79:** PDX collection 513

E79.0 **Hyperuricemia without signs of inflammatory arthritis and tophaceous disease**
Asymptomatic hyperuricemia

E79.1 **Lesch-Nyhan syndrome**                         CC HCC
HGPRT deficiency

E79.2 **Myoadenylate deaminase deficiency**            CC HCC

E79.8 **Other disorders of purine and pyrimidine metabolism**  CC HCC
Hereditary xanthinuria

E79.9 **Disorder of purine and pyrimidine metabolism, unspecified**  CC HCC

√4th E80 **Disorders of porphyrin and bilirubin metabolism**
INCLUDES    defects of catalase and peroxidase

**CC Excl: For CC codes in category E80, unless otherwise noted:** PDX collection 513

E80.0 **Hereditary erythropoietic porphyria**          CC HCC
Congenital erythropoietic porphyria
Erythropoietic protoporphyria

E80.1 **Porphyria cutanea tarda**                      CC HCC

√5th E80.2 **Other and unspecified porphyria**

E80.20 **Unspecified porphyria**                       CC HCC
Porphyria NOS

E80.21 **Acute intermittent (hepatic) porphyria**      CC HCC

E80.29 **Other porphyria**                             CC HCC
Hereditary coproporphyria

E80.3 **Defects of catalase and peroxidase**           CC HCC
Acatalasia [Takahara]
**CC Excl:** PDX collection 492

E80.4 **Gilbert syndrome**

E80.5 **Crigler-Najjar syndrome**

E80.6 **Other disorders of bilirubin metabolism**
Dubin-Johnson syndrome
Rotor's syndrome

E80.7 **Disorder of bilirubin metabolism, unspecified**

√4th E83 **Disorders of mineral metabolism**
> EXCLUDES 1    dietary mineral deficiency (E58-E61)
> parathyroid disorders (E20-E21)
> vitamin D deficiency (E55.-)

√5th E83.0 **Disorders of copper metabolism**

E83.00 **Disorder of copper metabolism, unspecified**

E83.01 **Wilson's disease**
Code also associated Kayser Fleischer ring (H18.04-)

E83.09 **Other disorders of copper metabolism**
Menkes' (kinky hair) (steely hair) disease

√5th E83.1 **Disorders of iron metabolism**
> EXCLUDES 1    iron deficiency anemia (D50.-)
> sideroblastic anemia (D64.0-D64.3)

E83.10 **Disorder of iron metabolism, unspecified**

√6th E83.11 **Hemochromatosis**
> EXCLUDES 1    ▶GALD (P78.84)
> gestational alloimmune liver disease (P78.84)
> neonatal hemochromatosis (P78.84)◄

E83.110 **Hereditary hemochromatosis**                 HCC
Bronzed diabetes
Pigmentary cirrhosis (of liver)
Primary (hereditary) hemochromatosis

E83.111 **Hemochromatosis due to repeated red blood cell transfusions**
Iron overload due to repeated red blood cell transfusions
Transfusion (red blood cell) associated hemochromatosis

E83.118 **Other hemochromatosis**

E83.119 **Hemochromatosis, unspecified**

E83.19 **Other disorders of iron metabolism**
Use additional code, if applicable, for idiopathic pulmonary hemosiderosis (J84.03)

E83.2 **Disorders of zinc metabolism**
Acrodermatitis enteropathica

√5th E83.3 **Disorders of phosphorus metabolism and phosphatases**
> EXCLUDES 1    adult osteomalacia (M83.-)
> osteoporosis (M80.-)

E83.30 **Disorder of phosphorus metabolism, unspecified**

E83.31 **Familial hypophosphatemia**
Vitamin D-resistant osteomalacia
Vitamin D-resistant rickets
> EXCLUDES 1    vitamin D-deficiency rickets (E55.0)

E83.32 **Hereditary vitamin D-dependent rickets (type 1) (type 2)**
25-hydroxyvitamin D 1-alpha-hydroxylase deficiency
Pseudovitamin D deficiency
Vitamin D receptor defect

E83.39 **Other disorders of phosphorus metabolism**
Acid phosphatase deficiency
Hypophosphatasia

√5th E83.4 **Disorders of magnesium metabolism**

E83.40 **Disorders of magnesium metabolism, unspecified**

E83.41 **Hypermagnesemia**

E83.42 **Hypomagnesemia**

E83.49 **Other disorders of magnesium metabolism**

√5th E83.5 **Disorders of calcium metabolism**
> EXCLUDES 1    chondrocalcinosis (M11.1-M11.2)
> hungry bone syndrome (E83.81)
> hyperparathyroidism (E21.0-E21.3)

E83.50 **Unspecified disorder of calcium metabolism**

**Chapter 4. Endocrine, Nutritional and Metabolic Diseases**

E83.51–E88.2

E83.51 **Hypocalcemia**

E83.52 **Hypercalcemia**
Familial hypocalciuric hypercalcemia

E83.59 **Other disorders of calcium metabolism**
Idiopathic hypercalciuria

✓5th E83.8 **Other disorders of mineral metabolism**

E83.81 **Hungry bone syndrome**

E83.89 **Other disorders of mineral metabolism**

E83.9 **Disorder of mineral metabolism, unspecified**

✓4th E84 **Cystic fibrosis**
INCLUDES mucoviscidosis
Code also exocrine pancreatic insufficiency (K86.81)

CC Excl: For CC/MCC codes in category E84: PDX collection 541

E84.0 **Cystic fibrosis with pulmonary manifestations** MCC HCC
Use additional code to identify any infectious organism present, such as:
Pseudomonas (B96.5)

✓5th E84.1 **Cystic fibrosis with intestinal manifestations**

E84.11 **Meconium ileus in cystic fibrosis** MCC HCC N
EXCLUDES 1 meconium ileus not due to cystic fibrosis (P76.0)

E84.19 **Cystic fibrosis with other intestinal manifestations** CC HCC
Distal intestinal obstruction syndrome

E84.8 **Cystic fibrosis with other manifestations** CC HCC

E84.9 **Cystic fibrosis, unspecified** CC HCC

✓4th E85 **Amyloidosis**
EXCLUDES 1 Alzheimer's disease (G30.0-)
EXCLUDES 2 ▶Alzheimer's disease (G30.0-)◀
**DEF:** Conditions of diverse etiologies characterized by the accumulation of insoluble fibrillar proteins (amyloid) in various organs and tissues of the body, compromising vital functions.

CC Excl: For CC codes in category E85: PDX collection 542

E85.0 **Non-neuropathic heredofamilial amyloidosis** CC HCC
Hereditary amyloid nephropathy
▶Code also associated disorders, such as:
autoinflammatory syndromes (M04.-)◀
EXCLUDES 2 ▶transthyretin-related (ATTR) familial amyloid cardiomyopathy (E85.4)◀

E85.1 **Neuropathic heredofamilial amyloidosis** CC HCC
Amyloid polyneuropathy (Portuguese)
▶Transthyretin-related (ATTR) familial amyloid polyneuropathy◀
AHA: 2012, 4Q, 99

E85.2 **Heredofamilial amyloidosis, unspecified** CC HCC

E85.3 **Secondary systemic amyloidosis** CC HCC
Hemodialysis-associated amyloidosis

E85.4 **Organ-limited amyloidosis** CC HCC
Localized amyloidosis
▶Transthyretin-related (ATTR) familial amyloid cardiomyopathy◀

✓5th E85.8 **Other amyloidosis**

- E85.81 **Light chain (AL) amyloidosis** CC

- E85.82 **Wild-type transthyretin-related (ATTR) amyloidosis** CC
Senile systemic amyloidosis (SSA)

- E85.89 **Other amyloidosis** CC

E85.9 **Amyloidosis, unspecified** CC HCC

✓4th E86 **Volume depletion**
Use additional code(s) for any associated disorders of electrolyte and acid-base balance (E87.-)
EXCLUDES 1 dehydration of newborn (P74.1)
hypovolemic shock NOS (R57.1)
postprocedural hypovolemic shock (T81.19)
traumatic hypovolemic shock (T79.4)

E86.0 **Dehydration**
AHA: 2014, 1Q, 7

E86.1 **Hypovolemia**
Depletion of volume of plasma

E86.9 **Volume depletion, unspecified**
**DEF:** Depletion of total body water (dehydration) and/or contraction of total intravascular plasma (hypovolemia).

✓4th E87 **Other disorders of fluid, electrolyte and acid-base balance**
EXCLUDES 1 diabetes insipidus (E23.2)
electrolyte imbalance associated with hyperemesis gravidarum (O21.1)
electrolyte imbalance following ectopic or molar pregnancy (O08.5)
familial periodic paralysis (G72.3)

CC Excl: For CC codes in category E87: PDX collection 543

E87.0 **Hyperosmolality and hypernatremia** CC
Sodium [Na] excess
Sodium [Na] overload
AHA: 2014, 1Q, 7

E87.1 **Hypo-osmolality and hyponatremia** CC
Sodium [Na] deficiency
EXCLUDES 1 syndrome of inappropriate secretion of antidiuretic hormone (E22.2)
AHA: 2014, 1Q, 7

E87.2 **Acidosis** CC
Acidosis NOS
Lactic acidosis
Metabolic acidosis
Respiratory acidosis
EXCLUDES 1 diabetic acidosis see categories E08-E10, E13 with ketoacidosis

E87.3 **Alkalosis** CC
Alkalosis NOS
Metabolic alkalosis
Respiratory alkalosis

E87.4 **Mixed disorder of acid-base balance** CC

E87.5 **Hyperkalemia**
Potassium [K] excess
Potassium [K] overload

E87.6 **Hypokalemia**
Potassium [K] deficiency

✓5th E87.7 **Fluid overload**
EXCLUDES 1 edema NOS (R60.9)
fluid retention (R60.9)

E87.70 **Fluid overload, unspecified**

E87.71 **Transfusion associated circulatory overload**
Fluid overload due to transfusion (blood) (blood components)
TACO

E87.79 **Other fluid overload**

E87.8 **Other disorders of electrolyte and fluid balance, not elsewhere classified**
Electrolyte imbalance NOS
Hyperchloremia
Hypochloremia

✓4th E88 **Other and unspecified metabolic disorders**
Use additional codes for associated conditions
EXCLUDES 1 histiocytosis X (chronic) (C96.6)

✓5th E88.0 **Disorders of plasma-protein metabolism, not elsewhere classified**
EXCLUDES 1 disorder of lipoprotein metabolism (E78.-)
monoclonal gammopathy (of undetermined significance) (D47.2)
polyclonal hypergammaglobulinemia (D89.0)
Waldenström's macroglobulinemia (C88.0)

E88.01 **Alpha-1-antitrypsin deficiency** HCC
AAT deficiency

E88.09 **Other disorders of plasma-protein metabolism, not elsewhere classified**
Bisalbuminemia

E88.1 **Lipodystrophy, not elsewhere classified**
Lipodystrophy NOS
EXCLUDES 1 Whipple's disease (K90.81)

E88.2 **Lipomatosis, not elsewhere classified**
Lipomatosis NOS
Lipomatosis (Check) dolorosa [Dercum]

N Newborn: 0   P Pediatric: 0-17   M Maternity: 12-55   A Adult: 15-124   MCC Major CC Condition   PDxMCC PDx acts as own MCC   CC CC Condition   PDxCC PDx acts as own CC

528         ICD-10-CM 2018

**E88.3  Tumor lysis syndrome**          `MCC`
Tumor lysis syndrome (spontaneous)
Tumor lysis syndrome following antineoplastic drug
chemotherapy
Use additional code for adverse effect, if applicable, to identify
drug (T45.1X5)
**DEF:** A potentially fatal metabolic complication of tumor necrosis
caused by either spontaneous or treatment-related accumulation
of byproducts from dying cancer cells; symptoms include
hyperkalemia, hyperphosphatemia, hypocalcemia, hyperuricemia,
and hyperuricosuria.
**CC Excl:** PDX collection 544

✓5ᵗʰ **E88.4  Mitochondrial metabolism disorders**
    *EXCLUDES 1*    *disorders of pyruvate metabolism (E74.4)*
        *Kearns-Sayre syndrome (H49.81)*
        *Leber's disease (H47.22)*
        *Leigh's encephalopathy (G31.82)*
        *Mitochondrial myopathy, NEC (G71.3)*
        *Reye's syndrome (G93.7)*

> **CC Excl: For CC codes in subcategory E88.4:**
> PDX collection 545

    **E88.40  Mitochondrial metabolism disorder,**          `CC` `HCC`
          **unspecified**

    **E88.41  MELAS syndrome**          `CC` `HCC`
          Mitochondrial myopathy, encephalopathy, lactic
          acidosis and stroke-like episodes

    **E88.42  MERRF syndrome**          `CC` `HCC`
          Myoclonic epilepsy associated with ragged-red fibers
          Code also progressive myoclonic epilepsy (G40.3-)

    **E88.49  Other mitochondrial metabolism disorders**          `CC` `HCC`

✓5ᵗʰ **E88.8  Other specified metabolic disorders**
    **E88.81  Metabolic syndrome**
          Dysmetabolic syndrome X
          Use additional codes for associated manifestations,
             such as:
             obesity (E66.-)

    **E88.89  Other specified metabolic disorders**          `HCC`
          Launois-Bensaude adenolipomatosis
          *EXCLUDES 1*  *adult pulmonary Langerhans cell*
                  *histiocytosis (J84.82)*

**E88.9  Metabolic disorder, unspecified**

## Postprocedural endocrine and metabolic complications and disorders, not elsewhere classified (E89)

✓4ᵗʰ **E89  Postprocedural endocrine and metabolic complications and
disorders, not elsewhere classified**
    *EXCLUDES 2*  *intraoperative complications of endocrine system organ or*
            *structure (E36.0-, E36.1-, E36.8)*

**E89.0  Postprocedural hypothyroidism**
Postirradiation hypothyroidism
Postsurgical hypothyroidism

**E89.1  Postprocedural hypoinsulinemia**          `CC`
Postpancreatectomy hyperglycemia
Postsurgical hypoinsulinemia
Use additional code, if applicable, to identify:
    acquired absence of pancreas (Z90.41-)
    diabetes mellitus (postpancreatectomy) (postprocedural)
        (E13.-)
    insulin use (Z79.4)
    *EXCLUDES 1*  *transient postprocedural hyperglycemia (R73.9)*
             *transient postprocedural hypoglycemia (E16.2)*
**CC Excl:** PDX collection 520

**E89.2  Postprocedural hypoparathyroidism**          `HCC`
Parathyroprival tetany

**E89.3  Postprocedural hypopituitarism**          `HCC`
Postirradiation hypopituitarism

✓5ᵗʰ **E89.4  Postprocedural ovarian failure**
    **E89.40  Asymptomatic postprocedural ovarian failure**          ♀
          Postprocedural ovarian failure NOS

    **E89.41  Symptomatic postprocedural ovarian failure**          ♀
          Symptoms such as flushing, sleeplessness, headache,
          lack of concentration, associated with
          postprocedural menopause

**E89.5  Postprocedural testicular hypofunction**          ♂

**E89.6  Postprocedural adrenocortical (-medullary)**          `CC` `HCC`
**hypofunction**
**CC Excl:** PDX collection 526

✓5ᵗʰ **E89.8  Other postprocedural endocrine and metabolic complications
and disorders**

> **CC Excl: For CC codes in subcategory E89.8, unless
> otherwise noted:** PDX collection 546

✓6ᵗʰ **E89.81  Postprocedural hemorrhage of an endocrine system
organ or structure following a procedure**
    **E89.810  Postprocedural hemorrhage of an**          `CC`
          **endocrine system organ or structure**
          **following an endocrine system procedure**

    **E89.811  Postprocedural hemorrhage of an**          `CC`
          **endocrine system organ or structure**
          **following other procedure**

✓6ᵗʰ **E89.82  Postprocedural hematoma and seroma of an
endocrine system organ or structure**
    **E89.820  Postprocedural hematoma of an**          `CC`
          **endocrine system organ or structure**
          **following an endocrine system procedure**

    **E89.821  Postprocedural hematoma of an**          `CC`
          **endocrine system organ or structure**
          **following other procedure**

    **E89.822  Postprocedural seroma of an**          `CC`
          **endocrine system organ or structure**
          **following an endocrine system procedure**

    **E89.823  Postprocedural seroma of an**          `CC`
          **endocrine system organ or structure**
          **following other procedure**

**E89.89  Other postprocedural endocrine and metabolic**          `CC`
**complications and disorders**
Use additional code, if applicable, to further specify
disorder

---

# Chapter 5. Mental, Behavioral and Neurodevelopmental Disorders (FØ1–F99)

## Chapter Specific Guidelines with Coding Examples

The chapter specific guidelines from the ICD-10-CM Official Guidelines for Coding and Reporting have been provided below. Along with these guidelines are coding examples, contained in the shaded boxes, that have been developed to help illustrate the coding and/or sequencing guidance found in these guidelines.

### a. Pain disorders related to psychological factors

Assign code F45.41, for pain that is exclusively related to psychological disorders. As indicated by the Excludes 1 note under category G89, a code from category G89 should not be assigned with code F45.41.

> Perceived abdominal pain determined to be persistent somatoform pain disorder
>
> **F45.41      Pain disorder exclusively related to psychological factors**
>
> *Explanation*: This pain was diagnosed as being exclusively psychological; therefore, no code from category G89 is added.

Code F45.42, Pain disorders with related psychological factors, should be used with a code from category G89, Pain, not elsewhere classified, if there is documentation of a psychological component for a patient with acute or chronic pain.
*See Section I.C.6. Pain*

### b. Mental and behavioral disorders due to psychoactive substance use

#### 1) In remission

Selection of codes for "in remission" for categories F10-F19, Mental and behavioral disorders due to psychoactive substance use (categories F10-F19 with -.21) requires the provider's clinical judgment. The appropriate codes for "in remission" are assigned only on the basis of provider documentation (as defined in the Official Guidelines for Coding and Reporting).

> Medical history: Opioid dependence in remission
>
> **F11.21      Opioid dependence, in remission**
>
> *Explanation*: The "in remission" codes are assigned when the provider documents the remission.

#### 2) Psychoactive substance use, abuse and dependence

When the provider documentation refers to use, abuse and dependence of the same substance (e.g. alcohol, opioid, cannabis, etc.), only one code should be assigned to identify the pattern of use based on the following hierarchy:

- If both use and abuse are documented, assign only the code for abuse
- If both abuse and dependence are documented, assign only the code for dependence
- If use, abuse and dependence are all documented, assign only the code for dependence
- If both use and dependence are documented, assign only the code for dependence.

> History and physical notes cannabis dependence; progress note says cannabis abuse
>
> **F12.2Ø      Cannabis dependence, uncomplicated**
>
> *Explanation*: In the hierarchy, the dependence code is used if both abuse and dependence are documented.

> Discharge summary says cocaine abuse; progress notes list cocaine use
>
> **F14.1Ø      Cocaine abuse, uncomplicated**
>
> *Explanation*: In the hierarchy, the abuse code is used if both abuse and use are documented.

#### 3) Psychoactive substance use

As with all other diagnoses, the codes for psychoactive substance use (F1Ø.9-, F11.9-, F12.9-, F13.9-, F14.9-, F15.9-, F16.9-) should only be assigned based on provider documentation and when they meet the definition of a reportable diagnosis (see Section III, Reporting Additional Diagnoses). The codes are to be used only when the psychoactive substance use is associated with a mental or behavioral disorder, and such a relationship is documented by the provider.

> ED reports that a 27-year-old female tripped and broke her right ankle. Her friends reported that they were drinking and dancing at a nightclub.
>
> **S82.891A      Other fracture of right lower leg, initial encounter for closed fracture**
>
> **WØ1.ØXXA      Fall on same level from slipping, tripping and stumbling, without subsequent striking against object, initial encounter**
>
> **Y92.252      Music hall as the place of occurrence of the external cause**
>
> **Y93.41      Activity, dancing**
>
> *Explanation*: Note that no code was added for alcohol use or abuse. Unless it is specifically associated with a diagnosis by provider documentation and meets the definition of a reportable diagnosis, it is not assigned. However, if the documentation from the provider stated: "The patient tripped, fell and fractured her right ankle while dancing due to her elevated blood alcohol, consistent with her ongoing alcohol abuse," the following code would be added:
>
> **F1Ø.1Ø      Alcohol abuse, uncomplicated**

**Chapter 5. Mental, Behavioral and Neurodevelopmental Disorders (F01-F99)**

INCLUDES   disorders of psychological development
EXCLUDES 2   symptoms, signs and abnormal clinical laboratory findings, not elsewhere classified (R00-R99)

This chapter contains the following blocks:

F01-F09   Mental disorders due to known physiological conditions
F10-F19   Mental and behavioral disorders due to psychoactive substance use
F20-F29   Schizophrenia, schizotypal, delusional, and other non-mood psychotic disorders
F30-F39   Mood [affective] disorders
F40-F48   Anxiety, dissociative, stress-related, somatoform and other nonpsychotic mental disorders
F50-F59   Behavioral syndromes associated with physiological disturbances and physical factors
F60-F69   Disorders of adult personality and behavior
F70-F79   Intellectual disabilities
F80-F89   Pervasive and specific developmental disorders
F90-F98   Behavioral and emotional disorders with onset usually occurring in childhood and adolescence
F99   Unspecified mental disorder

## Mental disorders due to known physiological conditions (F01-F09)

NOTE   This block comprises a range of mental disorders grouped together on the basis of their having in common a demonstrable etiology in cerebral disease, brain injury, or other insult leading to cerebral dysfunction. The dysfunction may be primary, as in diseases, injuries, and insults that affect the brain directly and selectively; or secondary, as in systemic diseases and disorders that attack the brain only as one of the multiple organs or systems of the body that are involved.

### ✓4th F01   Vascular dementia

Vascular dementia as a result of infarction of the brain due to vascular disease, including hypertensive cerebrovascular disease.
INCLUDES   arteriosclerotic dementia
Code first the underlying physiological condition or sequelae of cerebrovascular disease.

#### ✓5th F01.5   Vascular dementia

F01.50   **Vascular dementia** without behavioral disturbance    A
    Major neurocognitive disorder without behavioral disturbance

F01.51   **Vascular dementia** with behavioral disturbance    CC A
    Major neurocognitive disorder due to vascular disease, with behavioral disturbance
    Major neurocognitive disorder with aggressive behavior
    Major neurocognitive disorder with combative behavior
    Major neurocognitive disorder with violent behavior
    Vascular dementia with aggressive behavior
    Vascular dementia with combative behavior
    Vascular dementia with violent behavior
    Use additional code, if applicable, to identify wandering in vascular dementia (Z91.83)
    **CC Excl:** PDX collection 547

### ✓4th F02   Dementia in other diseases classified elsewhere

INCLUDES   major neurocognitive disorder in other diseases classified elsewhere

Code first the underlying physiological condition, such as:
    Alzheimer's (G30.-)
    cerebral lipidosis (E75.4)
    Creutzfeldt-Jakob disease (A81.0-)
    dementia with Lewy bodies (G31.83)
    dementia with Parkinsonism (G31.83)
    epilepsy and recurrent seizures (G40.-)
    frontotemporal dementia (G31.09)
    hepatolenticular degeneration (E83.0)
    human immunodeficiency virus [HIV] disease (B20)
    Huntington's disease (G10)
    hypercalcemia (E83.52)
    hypothyroidism, acquired (E00-E03.-)
    intoxications (T36-T65)
    Jakob-Creutzfeldt disease (A81.0-)
    multiple sclerosis (G35)
    neurosyphilis (A52.17)
    niacin deficiency [pellagra] (E52)
    Parkinson's disease (G20)
    Pick's disease (G31.01)
    polyarteritis nodosa (M30.0)
    prion disease (A81.9)
    systemic lupus erythematosus (M32.-)
    traumatic brain injury (S06.-)
    trypanosomiasis (B56.-, B57.-)
    vitamin B deficiency (E53.8)
EXCLUDES 2   dementia in alcohol and psychoactive substance disorders (F10-F19, with .17, .27, .97)
    vascular dementia (F01.5-)

#### ✓5th F02.8   Dementia in other diseases classified elsewhere
    **AHA:** 2017, 2Q, 7; 2016, 4Q, 141; 2016, 2Q, 6

F02.80   *Dementia in other diseases classified elsewhere without behavioral disturbance*
    Dementia in other diseases classified elsewhere NOS
    Major neurocognitive disorder in other diseases classified elsewhere

F02.81   *Dementia in other diseases classified elsewhere with behavioral disturbance*    CC
    Dementia in other diseases classified elsewhere with aggressive behavior
    Dementia in other diseases classified elsewhere with combative behavior
    Dementia in other diseases classified elsewhere with violent behavior
    Major neurocognitive disorder in other diseases classified elsewhere with aggressive behavior
    Major neurocognitive disorder in other diseases classified elsewhere with combative behavior
    Major neurocognitive disorder in other diseases classified elsewhere with violent behavior
    Use additional code, if applicable, to identify wandering in dementia in conditions classified elsewhere (Z91.83)
    **CC Excl:** PDX collection 548

### ✓4th F03   Unspecified dementia

Presenile dementia NOS     Senile dementia NOS
Presenile psychosis NOS     Senile dementia depressed
Primary degenerative dementia NOS     or paranoid type
Senile dementia NOS     Senile psychosis NOS

EXCLUDES 1   senility NOS (R41.81)
EXCLUDES 2   mild memory disturbance due to known physiological condition (F06.8)
    senile dementia with delirium or acute confusional state (F05)

#### ✓5th F03.9   Unspecified dementia

F03.90   **Unspecified dementia** without behavioral disturbance    HIV A
    Dementia NOS
    **AHA:** 2012, 4Q, 92

F03.91   **Unspecified dementia** with behavioral disturbance    CC A
    Unspecified dementia with aggressive behavior
    Unspecified dementia with combative behavior
    Unspecified dementia with violent behavior
    Use additional code, if applicable, to identify wandering in unspecified dementia (Z91.83)
    **CC Excl:** PDX collection 548

N Newborn: 0    P Pediatric: 0-17    M Maternity: 12-55    A Adult: 15-124    MCC Major CC Condition    PDx MCC PDx acts as own MCC    CC CC Condition    PDx CC PDx acts as own CC

532                   ICD-10-CM 2018

**F04**    **Amnestic disorder due to known physiological condition**
Korsakov's psychosis or syndrome, nonalcoholic
Code first the underlying physiological condition

> *EXCLUDES 1*    amnesia NOS (R41.3)
> anterograde amnesia (R41.1)
> dissociative amnesia (F44.0)
> retrograde amnesia (R41.2)

> *EXCLUDES 2*    alcohol-induced or unspecified Korsakov's syndrome (F10.26, F10.96)
> Korsakov's syndrome induced by other psychoactive substances (F13.26, F13.96, F19.16, F19.26, F19.96)

**F05**    **Delirium due to known physiological condition**    `CC`
Acute or subacute brain syndrome
Acute or subacute confusional state (nonalcoholic)
Acute or subacute infective psychosis
Acute or subacute organic reaction
Acute or subacute psycho-organic syndrome
Delirium of mixed etiology
Delirium superimposed on dementia
Sundowning
Code first the underlying physiological condition

> *EXCLUDES 1*    delirium NOS (R41.0)
> *EXCLUDES 2*    delirium tremens alcohol-induced or unspecified (F10.231, F10.921)

**CC Excl:** PDX collection 549

✓4ᵗʰ **F06**    **Other mental disorders due to known physiological condition**

> `INCLUDES`    mental disorders due to endocrine disorder
> mental disorders due to exogenous hormone
> mental disorders due to exogenous toxic substance
> mental disorders due to primary cerebral disease
> mental disorders due to somatic illness
> mental disorders due to systemic disease affecting the brain

Code first the underlying physiological condition

> *EXCLUDES 1*    unspecified dementia (F03)
> *EXCLUDES 2*    delirium due to known physiological condition (F05)
> dementia as classified in F01-F02
> other mental disorders associated with alcohol and other psychoactive substances (F10-F19)

**F06.0**    **Psychotic disorder with hallucinations due to known**    `CC`
**physiological condition**
Organic hallucinatory state (nonalcoholic)

> *EXCLUDES 2*    hallucinations and perceptual disturbance induced by alcohol and other psychoactive substances (F10-F19 with .151, .251, .951)
> schizophrenia (F20.-)

**CC Excl:** PDX collection 550

**F06.1**    **Catatonic disorder due to known physiological condition**
Catatonia associated with another mental disorder
Catatonia NOS

> *EXCLUDES 1*    catatonic stupor (R40.1)
> stupor NOS (R40.1)

> *EXCLUDES 2*    catatonic schizophrenia (F20.2)
> dissociative stupor (F44.2)

**F06.2**    **Psychotic disorder with delusions due to known**    `CC`
**physiological condition**
Paranoid and paranoid-hallucinatory organic states
Schizophrenia-like psychosis in epilepsy

> *EXCLUDES 2*    alcohol and drug-induced psychotic disorder (F10-F19 with .150, .250, .950)
> brief psychotic disorder (F23)
> delusional disorder (F22)
> schizophrenia (F20.-)

**CC Excl:** PDX collection 550

✓5ᵗʰ **F06.3**    **Mood disorder due to known physiological condition**

> *EXCLUDES 2*    mood disorders due to alcohol and other psychoactive substances (F10-F19 with .14, .24, .94)
> mood disorders, not due to known physiological condition or unspecified (F30-F39)

**F06.30**    **Mood disorder due to known physiological condition, unspecified**

**F06.31**    **Mood disorder due to known physiological condition with depressive features**
▶Depressive disorder due to known physiological condition, with depressive features◀

**F06.32**    **Mood disorder due to known physiological condition with major depressive-like episode**
▶Depressive disorder due to known physiological condition, with major depressive–like episode◀

**F06.33**    **Mood disorder due to known physiological condition with manic features**
▶Bipolar and related disorder due to a known physiological condition, with manic features
Bipolar and related disorder due to known physiological condition, with manic- or hypomanic-like episodes◀

**F06.34**    **Mood disorder due to known physiological condition with mixed features**
▶Bipolar and related disorder due to known physiological condition, with mixed features
Depressive disorder due to known physiological condition, with mixed features◀

**F06.4**    **Anxiety disorder due to known physiological condition**

> *EXCLUDES 2*    anxiety disorders due to alcohol and other psychoactive substances (F10-F19 with .180, .280, .980)
> anxiety disorders, not due to known physiological condition or unspecified (F40.-, F41.-)

**F06.8**    **Other specified mental disorders due to known**    `HIV`
**physiological condition**
Epileptic psychosis NOS
▶Obsessive-compulsive and related disorder due to a known physiological condition◀
Organic dissociative disorder
Organic emotionally labile [asthenic] disorder

✓4ᵗʰ **F07**    **Personality and behavioral disorders due to known physiological condition**
Code first the underlying physiological condition

**F07.0**    **Personality change due to known physiological condition**
Frontal lobe syndrome
Limbic epilepsy personality syndrome
Lobotomy syndrome
Organic personality disorder
Organic pseudopsychopathic personality
Organic pseudoretarded personality
Postleucotomy syndrome
Code first underlying physiological condition

> *EXCLUDES 1*    mild cognitive impairment (G31.84)
> postconcussional syndrome (F07.81)
> postencephalitic syndrome (F07.89)
> signs and symptoms involving emotional state (R45.-)

> *EXCLUDES 2*    specific personality disorder (F60.-)

✓5ᵗʰ **F07.8**    **Other personality and behavioral disorders due to known physiological condition**

**F07.81**    **Postconcussional syndrome**
Postcontusional syndrome (encephalopathy)
Post-traumatic brain syndrome, nonpsychotic
Use additional code to identify associated post-traumatic headache, if applicable (G44.3-)

> *EXCLUDES 1*    current concussion (brain) (S06.0-)
> postencephalitic syndrome (F07.89)

**F07.89**    **Other personality and behavioral disorders due to known physiological condition**
Postencephalitic syndrome
Right hemispheric organic affective disorder

**F07.9**    **Unspecified personality and behavioral disorder due to**    `HIV`
**known physiological condition**
Organic psychosyndrome

**F09**    **Unspecified mental disorder due to known physiological**    `HIV`
**condition**
Mental disorder NOS due to known physiological condition
Organic brain syndrome NOS
Organic mental disorder NOS
Organic psychosis NOS
Symptomatic psychosis NOS
Code first the underlying physiological condition

> *EXCLUDES 1*    psychosis NOS (F29)

✓ Additional Character Req    ✓7ᵗʰ Placeholder Alert    Unacceptable PDx    Manifestation    `H1`-`H14` HAC    `HCC` CMS-HCC Condition    *EXCLUDES 1* Not Coded Here    *EXCLUDES 2* Not Included Here

ICD-10-CM 2018    **533**

**Chapter 5. Mental, Behavioral and Neurodevelopmental Disorders**

## Mental and behavioral disorders due to psychoactive substance use (F10-F19)

**AHA:** 2017, 2Q, 27

✓4th **F10 Alcohol related disorders**
Use additional code for blood alcohol level, if applicable (Y90.-)

> **CC Excl:** For CC codes in category F10: PDX collection 550

✓5th **F10.1 Alcohol abuse**
> *EXCLUDES 1*   alcohol dependence (F10.2-)
> alcohol use, unspecified (F10.9-)

**AHA:** 2015, 2Q, 15

**F10.10   Alcohol abuse, uncomplicated**
Alcohol use disorder, mild

**F10.11   Alcohol abuse, in remission**
Alcohol use disorder, mild, in early remission
Alcohol use disorder, mild, in sustained remission

✓6th **F10.12   Alcohol abuse with intoxication**
**F10.120   Alcohol abuse with intoxication, uncomplicated**   `HCC`
**F10.121   Alcohol abuse with intoxication delirium**   `CC` `HCC`
**F10.129   Alcohol abuse with intoxication, unspecified**   `HCC`

**F10.14   Alcohol abuse with alcohol-induced mood disorder**   `CC` `HCC`
Alcohol use disorder, mild, with alcohol-induced bipolar or related disorder
Alcohol use disorder, mild, with alcohol-induced depressive disorder

✓6th **F10.15   Alcohol abuse with alcohol-induced psychotic disorder**
**F10.150   Alcohol abuse with alcohol-induced psychotic disorder with delusions**   `HCC`
**F10.151   Alcohol abuse with alcohol-induced psychotic disorder with hallucinations**   `CC` `HCC`
> **DEF:** Psychosis lasting less than six months with slight or no clouding of consciousness in which auditory hallucinations predominate.

**F10.159   Alcohol abuse with alcohol-induced psychotic disorder, unspecified**   `CC` `HCC`

✓6th **F10.18   Alcohol abuse with other alcohol-induced disorders**
**F10.180   Alcohol abuse with alcohol-induced anxiety disorder**   `CC` `HCC`
**F10.181   Alcohol abuse with alcohol-induced sexual dysfunction**   `CC` `HCC`
**F10.182   Alcohol abuse with alcohol-induced sleep disorder**   `CC` `HCC`
**F10.188   Alcohol abuse with other alcohol-induced disorder**   `CC` `HCC`

**F10.19   Alcohol abuse with unspecified alcohol-induced disorder**   `CC` `HCC`

✓5th **F10.2 Alcohol dependence**
> *EXCLUDES 1*   alcohol abuse (F10.1-)
> alcohol use, unspecified (F10.9-)
> *EXCLUDES 2*   toxic effect of alcohol (T51.0-)

**F10.20   Alcohol dependence, uncomplicated**   `HCC`
Alcohol use disorder, moderate
Alcohol use disorder, severe

**F10.21   Alcohol dependence, in remission**   `HCC`
▶Alcohol use disorder, moderate, in early remission
Alcohol use disorder, moderate, in sustained remission
Alcohol use disorder, severe, in early remission
Alcohol use disorder, severe, in sustained remission◀

✓6th **F10.22   Alcohol dependence with intoxication**
Acute drunkenness (in alcoholism)
> *EXCLUDES 2*   alcohol dependence with withdrawal (F10.23-)

**F10.220   Alcohol dependence with intoxication, uncomplicated**   `HCC`
**F10.221   Alcohol dependence with intoxication delirium**   `CC` `HCC`
**F10.229   Alcohol dependence with intoxication, unspecified**   `HCC`

✓6th **F10.23   Alcohol dependence with withdrawal**
> *EXCLUDES 2*   alcohol dependence with intoxication (F10.22-)

**AHA:** 2015, 2Q, 15

**F10.230   Alcohol dependence with withdrawal, uncomplicated**   `CC` `HCC`
**F10.231   Alcohol dependence with withdrawal delirium**   `CC` `HCC`
**F10.232   Alcohol dependence with withdrawal with perceptual disturbance**   `CC` `HCC`
**F10.239   Alcohol dependence with withdrawal, unspecified**   `CC` `HCC`

**F10.24   Alcohol dependence with alcohol-induced mood disorder**   `CC` `HCC`
Alcohol use disorder, moderate, with alcohol-induced bipolar or related disorder
Alcohol use disorder, moderate, with alcohol-induced depressive disorder
Alcohol use disorder, severe, with alcohol-induced bipolar or related disorder
Alcohol use disorder, severe, with alcohol-induced depressive disorder

✓6th **F10.25   Alcohol dependence with alcohol-induced psychotic disorder**
**F10.250   Alcohol dependence with alcohol-induced psychotic disorder with delusions**   `HCC`
**F10.251   Alcohol dependence with alcohol-induced psychotic disorder with hallucinations**   `CC` `HCC`
**F10.259   Alcohol dependence with alcohol-induced psychotic disorder, unspecified**   `CC` `HCC`

**F10.26   Alcohol dependence with alcohol-induced persisting amnestic disorder**   `HCC`
Alcohol use disorder, moderate, with alcohol-induced major neurocognitive disorder, amnestic-confabulatory type
Alcohol use disorder, severe, with alcohol-induced major neurocognitive disorder, amnestic-confabulatory type
> **DEF:** Prominent and lasting reduced memory span, disordered time appreciation and confabulation, occurs in alcoholics as sequel to acute alcoholic psychosis.

**F10.27   Alcohol dependence with alcohol-induced persisting dementia**   `CC` `HCC`
Alcohol use disorder, moderate, with alcohol-induced major neurocognitive disorder, nonamnestic-confabulatory type
Alcohol use disorder, severe, with alcohol-induced major neurocognitive disorder, nonamnestic-confabulatory type

✓6th **F10.28   Alcohol dependence with other alcohol-induced disorders**
**F10.280   Alcohol dependence with alcohol-induced anxiety disorder**   `CC` `HCC`
**F10.281   Alcohol dependence with alcohol-induced sexual dysfunction**   `CC` `HCC`
**F10.282   Alcohol dependence with alcohol-induced sleep disorder**   `HCC`
**F10.288   Alcohol dependence with other alcohol-induced disorder**   `CC` `HCC`
Alcohol use disorder, moderate, with alcohol-induced mild neurocognitive disorder
Alcohol use disorder, severe, with alcohol-induced mild neurocognitive disorder

**F10.29   Alcohol dependence with unspecified alcohol-induced disorder**   `CC` `HCC`

✓5th **F10.9 Alcohol use, unspecified**
> *EXCLUDES 1*   alcohol abuse (F10.1-)
> alcohol dependence (F10.2-)

✓6th **F10.92   Alcohol use, unspecified with intoxication**
**F10.920   Alcohol use, unspecified with intoxication, uncomplicated**   `HCC`
**F10.921   Alcohol use, unspecified with intoxication delirium**   `CC` `HCC`
**F10.929   Alcohol use, unspecified with intoxication, unspecified**   `HCC`

---

N Newborn: 0    P Pediatric: 0-17    M Maternity: 12-55    A Adult: 15-124    `MCC` Major CC Condition    `PDxMCC` PDx acts as own MCC    `CC` CC Condition    `PDxCC` PDx acts as own CC

**F10.94** **Alcohol use, unspecified with alcohol-induced** mood disorder          `CC` `HCC`
    Alcohol induced bipolar or related disorder, without use disorder
    Alcohol induced depressive disorder, without use disorder

✓6ᵗʰ **F10.95** **Alcohol use, unspecified with alcohol-induced psychotic disorder**
    **F10.950** **Alcohol use, unspecified with alcohol-induced psychotic disorder with** delusions          `HCC`
    **F10.951** **Alcohol use, unspecified with alcohol-induced psychotic disorder with** hallucinations          `CC` `HCC`
    **F10.959** **Alcohol use, unspecified with alcohol-induced psychotic disorder, unspecified**          `CC` `HCC`
        Alcohol-induced psychotic disorder without use disorder

**F10.96** **Alcohol use, unspecified with alcohol-induced persisting amnestic disorder**          `HCC`
    Alcohol-induced major neurocognitive disorder, amnestic-confabulatory type, without use disorder

**F10.97** **Alcohol use, unspecified with alcohol-induced persisting dementia**          `HCC`
    Alcohol-induced major neurocognitive disorder, nonamnestic-confabulatory type, without use disorder

✓6ᵗʰ **F10.98** **Alcohol use, unspecified with other alcohol-induced disorders**
    **F10.980** **Alcohol use, unspecified with alcohol-induced** anxiety disorder          `CC` `HCC`
        Alcohol induced anxiety disorder, without use disorder
    **F10.981** **Alcohol use, unspecified with alcohol-induced** sexual dysfunction          `CC` `HCC`
        Alcohol induced sexual dysfunction, without use disorder
    **F10.982** **Alcohol use, unspecified with alcohol-induced** sleep disorder          `HCC`
        Alcohol induced sleep disorder, without use disorder
    **F10.988** **Alcohol use, unspecified with other alcohol-induced disorder**          `CC` `HCC`
        Alcohol induced mild neurocognitive disorder, without use disorder

**F10.99** **Alcohol use, unspecified with** unspecified **alcohol-induced disorder**          `CC` `HCC`

✓4ᵗʰ **F11** **Opioid related disorders**

> **CC Excl: For CC codes in category F11, unless otherwise noted:** PDX collection 550

✓5ᵗʰ **F11.1** **Opioid** abuse
    *EXCLUDES 1*    opioid dependence (F11.2-)
                 opioid use, unspecified (F11.9-)

    **F11.10** **Opioid abuse,** uncomplicated
        Opioid use disorder, mild

●     **F11.11** **Opioid abuse,** in remission
        Opioid use disorder, mild, in early remission
        Opioid use disorder, mild, in sustained remission

✓6ᵗʰ **F11.12** **Opioid abuse with** intoxication
    **F11.120** **Opioid abuse with intoxication, uncomplicated**          `HCC`
    **F11.121** **Opioid abuse with intoxication delirium**          `CC` `HCC`
    **F11.122** **Opioid abuse with intoxication with perceptual disturbance**          `HCC`
    **F11.129** **Opioid abuse with intoxication, unspecified**          `HCC`

**F11.14** **Opioid abuse with opioid-induced** mood disorder          `HCC`
    Opioid use disorder, mild, with opioid-induced depressive disorder

✓6ᵗʰ **F11.15** **Opioid abuse with opioid-induced** psychotic disorder
    **F11.150** **Opioid abuse with opioid-induced psychotic disorder with** delusions          `CC` `HCC`
    **F11.151** **Opioid abuse with opioid-induced psychotic disorder with** hallucinations          `CC` `HCC`

**F11.159** **Opioid abuse with opioid-induced psychotic disorder,** unspecified          `HCC`

✓6ᵗʰ **F11.18** **Opioid abuse with** other **opioid-induced disorder**
    **F11.181** **Opioid abuse with opioid-induced sexual dysfunction**          `HCC`
    **F11.182** **Opioid abuse with opioid-induced sleep disorder**          `HCC`
    **F11.188** **Opioid abuse with** other **opioid-induced disorder**          `HCC`

**F11.19** **Opioid abuse with** unspecified **opioid-induced disorder**          `HCC`

✓5ᵗʰ **F11.2** **Opioid** dependence
    *EXCLUDES 1*    opioid abuse (F11.1-)
                 opioid use, unspecified (F11.9-)
    *EXCLUDES 2*    opioid poisoning (T40.0-T40.2-)

    **F11.20** **Opioid dependence,** uncomplicated          `CC` `HCC`
        Opioid use disorder, moderate
        Opioid use disorder, severe
        **CC Excl:** No excl

    **F11.21** **Opioid dependence, in remission**          `HCC`
        ▶Opioid use disorder, moderate, in early remission
        Opioid use disorder, moderate, in sustained remission
        Opioid use disorder, severe, in early remission
        Opioid use disorder, severe, in sustained remission◀

✓6ᵗʰ **F11.22** **Opioid dependence with** intoxication
    *EXCLUDES 1*    opioid dependence with withdrawal (F11.23)
    **F11.220** **Opioid dependence with intoxication, uncomplicated**          `HCC`
    **F11.221** **Opioid dependence with intoxication** delirium          `CC` `HCC`
    **F11.222** **Opioid dependence with intoxication with** perceptual disturbance          `CC` `HCC`
        **CC Excl:** No excl
    **F11.229** **Opioid dependence with intoxication, unspecified**          `HCC`

**F11.23** **Opioid dependence with** withdrawal          `CC` `HCC`
    *EXCLUDES 1*    opioid dependence with intoxication (F11.22-)

**F11.24** **Opioid dependence with opioid-induced** mood disorder          `HCC`
    Opioid use disorder, moderate, with opioid induced depressive disorder

✓6ᵗʰ **F11.25** **Opioid dependence with opioid-induced psychotic disorder**
    **F11.250** **Opioid dependence with opioid-induced psychotic disorder with** delusions          `CC` `HCC`
    **F11.251** **Opioid dependence with opioid-induced psychotic disorder with** hallucinations          `CC` `HCC`
    **F11.259** **Opioid dependence with opioid-induced psychotic disorder,** unspecified          `CC` `HCC`
        **CC Excl:** No excl

✓6ᵗʰ **F11.28** **Opioid dependence with** other **opioid-induced disorder**
    **F11.281** **Opioid dependence with opioid-induced** sexual dysfunction          `CC` `HCC`
        **CC Excl:** No excl
    **F11.282** **Opioid dependence with opioid-induced** sleep disorder          `CC` `HCC`
        **CC Excl:** No excl
    **F11.288** **Opioid dependence with** other **opioid-induced disorder**          `CC` `HCC`
        **CC Excl:** No excl

**F11.29** **Opioid dependence with** unspecified **opioid-induced disorder**          `HCC`

✓5ᵗʰ **F11.9** **Opioid use,** unspecified
    *EXCLUDES 1*    opioid abuse (F11.1-)
                 opioid dependence (F11.2-)

    **F11.90** **Opioid use, unspecified,** uncomplicated

✓6ᵗʰ **F11.92** **Opioid use, unspecified with** intoxication
    *EXCLUDES 1*    opioid use, unspecified with withdrawal (F11.93)
    **F11.920** **Opioid use, unspecified with intoxication,** uncomplicated          `HCC`
    **F11.921** **Opioid use, unspecified with intoxication** delirium          `CC` `HCC`
        Opioid-induced delirium

*Chapter 5. Mental, Behavioral and Neurodevelopmental Disorders*

*F10.94–F11.921*

---

✓ Additional Character Req    ✓x7ᵗʰ Placeholder Alert    Unacceptable PDx    Manifestation    **H1**-**H14** HAC    `HCC` CMS-HCC Condition    *EXCLUDES 1* Not Coded Here    *EXCLUDES 2* Not Included Here

**Chapter 5. Mental, Behavioral and Neurodevelopmental Disorders**

**F11.922    Opioid use, unspecified with** `HCC`
     **intoxication with** perceptual disturbance

**F11.929    Opioid use, unspecified with** `HCC`
     **intoxication,** unspecified

**F11.93    Opioid use, unspecified with** withdrawal   `CC` `HCC`
     **EXCLUDES 1**   opioid use, unspecified with intoxication (F11.92-)

**F11.94    Opioid use, unspecified with opioid-induced** `HCC`
     **mood disorder**
     Opioid induced depressive disorder, without use disorder

✓6ᵗʰ **F11.95    Opioid use, unspecified with opioid-induced**
     **psychotic disorder**

     **F11.950    Opioid use, unspecified with** `CC` `HCC`
         **opioid-induced psychotic disorder**
         **with** delusions

     **F11.951    Opioid use, unspecified with** `CC` `HCC`
         **opioid-induced psychotic disorder**
         **with** hallucinations

     **F11.959    Opioid use, unspecified with** `HCC`
         **opioid-induced psychotic disorder,**
         **unspecified**

✓6ᵗʰ **F11.98    Opioid use, unspecified with** other **specified opioid-induced disorder**

     **F11.981    Opioid use, unspecified with opioid-** `HCC`
         **induced** sexual dysfunction
         Opioid induced sexual dysfunction, without use disorder

     **F11.982    Opioid use, unspecified with opioid-** `HCC`
         **induced** sleep disorder
         Opioid induced sleep disorder, without use disorder

     **F11.988    Opioid use, unspecified with** other `HCC`
         **opioid-induced disorder**
         Opioid induced anxiety disorder, without use disorder

**F11.99    Opioid use, unspecified with** unspecified `HCC`
     **opioid-induced disorder**

✓4ᵗʰ **F12   Cannabis related disorders**
     **INCLUDES**   marijuana

> **CC Excl: For CC codes in category F12:** PDX collection 550

✓5ᵗʰ **F12.1    Cannabis** abuse
     **EXCLUDES 1**   cannabis dependence (F12.2-)
               cannabis use, unspecified (F12.9-)

     **F12.10    Cannabis abuse,** uncomplicated
         Cannabis use disorder, mild

     **F12.11    Cannabis abuse,** in remission
         Cannabis use disorder, mild, in early remission
         Cannabis use disorder, mild, in sustained remission

✓6ᵗʰ **F12.12    Cannabis abuse with** intoxication

     **F12.120    Cannabis abuse with intoxication,** `HCC`
         **uncomplicated**

     **F12.121    Cannabis abuse with intoxication** `CC` `HCC`
         **delirium**

     **F12.122    Cannabis abuse with intoxication** `HCC`
         **with** perceptual disturbance

     **F12.129    Cannabis abuse with intoxication,** `HCC`
         **unspecified**

✓6ᵗʰ **F12.15    Cannabis abuse with** psychotic disorder

     **F12.150    Cannabis abuse with psychotic** `CC` `HCC`
         **disorder with** delusions

     **F12.151    Cannabis abuse with psychotic** `CC` `HCC`
         **disorder with** hallucinations

     **F12.159    Cannabis abuse with psychotic** `HCC`
         **disorder,** unspecified

✓6ᵗʰ **F12.18    Cannabis abuse with** other **cannabis-induced disorder**

     **F12.180    Cannabis abuse with cannabis-** `HCC`
         **induced** anxiety disorder

     **F12.188    Cannabis abuse with** other **cannabis-** `HCC`
         **induced disorder**
         Cannabis use disorder, mild, with cannabis-induced sleep disorder

     **F12.19    Cannabis abuse with** unspecified **cannabis-** `HCC`
     **induced disorder**

✓5ᵗʰ **F12.2    Cannabis** dependence
     **EXCLUDES 1**   cannabis abuse (F12.1-)
               cannabis use, unspecified (F12.9-)
     **EXCLUDES 2**   cannabis poisoning (T40.7-)

     **F12.20    Cannabis dependence,** uncomplicated   `HCC`
         Cannabis use disorder, moderate
         Cannabis use disorder, severe

     **F12.21    Cannabis dependence,** in remission   `HCC`
         ▶Cannabis use disorder, moderate, in early remission
         Cannabis use disorder, moderate, in sustained remission
         Cannabis use disorder, severe, in early remission
         Cannabis use disorder, severe, in sustained remission◀

✓6ᵗʰ **F12.22    Cannabis dependence with** intoxication

     **F12.220    Cannabis dependence with** `HCC`
         **intoxication, uncomplicated**

     **F12.221    Cannabis dependence with** `CC` `HCC`
         **intoxication** delirium

     **F12.222    Cannabis dependence with** `HCC`
         **intoxication with** perceptual disturbance

     **F12.229    Cannabis dependence with** `HCC`
         **intoxication,** unspecified

✓6ᵗʰ **F12.25    Cannabis dependence with** psychotic disorder

     **F12.250    Cannabis dependence with** `CC` `HCC`
         **psychotic disorder with** delusions

     **F12.251    Cannabis dependence with** `CC` `HCC`
         **psychotic disorder with** hallucinations

     **F12.259    Cannabis dependence with psychotic** `HCC`
         **disorder,** unspecified

✓6ᵗʰ **F12.28    Cannabis dependence with** other **cannabis-induced disorder**

     **F12.280    Cannabis dependence with cannabis-** `HCC`
         **induced** anxiety disorder

     **F12.288    Cannabis dependence with** other `HCC`
         **cannabis-induced disorder**
         Cannabis use disorder, moderate, with cannabis-induced sleep disorder
         Cannabis use disorder, severe, with cannabis-induced sleep disorder
         Cannabis withdrawal

     **F12.29    Cannabis dependence with** unspecified `HCC`
     **cannabis-induced disorder**

✓5ᵗʰ **F12.9    Cannabis use,** unspecified
     **EXCLUDES 1**   cannabis abuse (F12.1-)
               cannabis dependence (F12.2-)

     **F12.90    Cannabis use, unspecified,** uncomplicated

✓6ᵗʰ **F12.92    Cannabis use, unspecified with** intoxication

     **F12.920    Cannabis use, unspecified with** `HCC`
         **intoxication,** uncomplicated

     **F12.921    Cannabis use, unspecified with** `CC` `HCC`
         **intoxication** delirium

     **F12.922    Cannabis use, unspecified with** `HCC`
         **intoxication with** perceptual disturbance

     **F12.929    Cannabis use, unspecified with** `HCC`
         **intoxication,** unspecified

✓6ᵗʰ **F12.95    Cannabis use, unspecified with** psychotic disorder

     **F12.950    Cannabis use, unspecified with** `CC` `HCC`
         **psychotic disorder with** delusions

     **F12.951    Cannabis use, unspecified with** `CC` `HCC`
         **psychotic disorder with** hallucinations

     **F12.959    Cannabis use, unspecified with** `HCC`
         **psychotic disorder,** unspecified
         Cannabis induced psychotic disorder, without use disorder

✓6ᵗʰ **F12.98    Cannabis use, unspecified with** other **cannabis-induced disorder**

     **F12.980    Cannabis use, unspecified with** `HCC`
         anxiety disorder
         Cannabis induced anxiety disorder, without use disorder

     **F12.988    Cannabis use, unspecified with** other `HCC`
         **cannabis-induced disorder**
         Cannabis induced sleep disorder, without use disorder

     **F12.99    Cannabis use, unspecified with** unspecified `HCC`
     **cannabis-induced disorder**

Ⓝ Newborn: 0    Ⓟ Pediatric: 0-17    Ⓜ Maternity: 12-55    Ⓐ Adult: 15-124    `MCC` Major CC Condition    `PDxMCC` PDx acts as own MCC    `CC` CC Condition    `PDxCC` PDx acts as own CC

**536**      ICD-10-CM 2018

☑4ᵗʰ **F13**   **Sedative, hypnotic, or anxiolytic** related disorders

> **CC Excl: For CC codes in category F13, unless otherwise noted:**
> PDX collection 550

☑5ᵗʰ   **F13.1**   **Sedative, hypnotic or anxiolytic-related** abuse
> *EXCLUDES 1*   sedative, hypnotic or anxiolytic-related dependence
> (F13.2-)
> sedative, hypnotic, or anxiolytic use, unspecified
> (F13.9-)

     **F13.10**   **Sedative, hypnotic or anxiolytic abuse, uncomplicated**
         Sedative, hypnotic, or anxiolytic use disorder, mild

     **F13.11**   **Sedative, hypnotic or anxiolytic abuse, in remission**
         Sedative, hypnotic or anxiolytic use disorder, mild, in early remission
         Sedative, hypnotic or anxiolytic use disorder, mild, in sustained remission

☑6ᵗʰ   **F13.12**   **Sedative, hypnotic or anxiolytic abuse with intoxication**
     **F13.120**   **Sedative, hypnotic or anxiolytic abuse** HCC **with intoxication, uncomplicated**
     **F13.121**   **Sedative, hypnotic or anxiolytic** CC HCC **abuse with intoxication delirium**
     **F13.129**   **Sedative, hypnotic or anxiolytic abuse** HCC **with intoxication, unspecified**

     **F13.14**   **Sedative, hypnotic or anxiolytic abuse with** HCC **sedative, hypnotic or anxiolytic-induced mood disorder**
     ▸Sedative, hypnotic, or anxiolytic use disorder, mild, with sedative, hypnotic, or anxiolytic-induced bipolar or related disorder
         Sedative, hypnotic, or anxiolytic use disorder, mild, with sedative, hypnotic, or anxiolytic-induced depressive disorder◂

☑6ᵗʰ   **F13.15**   **Sedative, hypnotic or anxiolytic abuse with sedative, hypnotic or anxiolytic-induced psychotic disorder**
     **F13.150**   **Sedative, hypnotic or anxiolytic** CC HCC **abuse with sedative, hypnotic or anxiolytic-induced psychotic disorder with delusions**
     **F13.151**   **Sedative, hypnotic or anxiolytic** CC HCC **abuse with sedative, hypnotic or anxiolytic-induced psychotic disorder with hallucinations**
     **F13.159**   **Sedative, hypnotic or anxiolytic abuse** HCC **with sedative, hypnotic or anxiolytic-induced psychotic disorder, unspecified**

☑6ᵗʰ   **F13.18**   **Sedative, hypnotic or anxiolytic abuse with other sedative, hypnotic or anxiolytic-induced disorders**
     **F13.180**   **Sedative, hypnotic or anxiolytic** HCC **abuse with sedative, hypnotic or anxiolytic-induced anxiety disorder**
     **F13.181**   **Sedative, hypnotic or anxiolytic** HCC **abuse with sedative, hypnotic or anxiolytic-induced sexual dysfunction**
     **F13.182**   **Sedative, hypnotic or anxiolytic** HCC **abuse with sedative, hypnotic or anxiolytic-induced sleep disorder**
     **F13.188**   **Sedative, hypnotic or anxiolytic** HCC **abuse with other sedative, hypnotic or anxiolytic-induced disorder**

     **F13.19**   **Sedative, hypnotic or anxiolytic abuse with** HCC **unspecified sedative, hypnotic or anxiolytic-induced disorder**

☑5ᵗʰ   **F13.2**   **Sedative, hypnotic or anxiolytic-related** dependence
> *EXCLUDES 1*   sedative, hypnotic or anxiolytic-related abuse (F13.1-)
> sedative, hypnotic, or anxiolytic use, unspecified
> (F13.9-)
> *EXCLUDES 2*   sedative, hypnotic, or anxiolytic poisoning (T42.-)

     **F13.20**   **Sedative, hypnotic or anxiolytic dependence,** CC HCC **uncomplicated**
         **CC Excl: No excl**

     **F13.21**   **Sedative, hypnotic or anxiolytic dependence, in** HCC **remission**
     ▸Sedative, hypnotic or anxiolytic use disorder, moderate, in early remission
         Sedative, hypnotic or anxiolytic use disorder, moderate, in sustained remission
         Sedative, hypnotic or anxiolytic use disorder, severe, in early remission
         Sedative, hypnotic or anxiolytic use disorder, severe, in sustained remission◂

☑6ᵗʰ   **F13.22**   **Sedative, hypnotic or anxiolytic dependence with intoxication**
> *EXCLUDES 1*   sedative, hypnotic or anxiolytic dependence
> with withdrawal (F13.23-)

     **F13.220**   **Sedative, hypnotic or anxiolytic dependence with intoxication, uncomplicated**
     **F13.221**   **Sedative, hypnotic or anxiolytic** CC HCC **dependence with intoxication delirium**
     **F13.229**   **Sedative, hypnotic or anxiolytic** HCC **dependence with intoxication, unspecified**

☑6ᵗʰ   **F13.23**   **Sedative, hypnotic or anxiolytic dependence with withdrawal**
     Sedative, hypnotic, or anxiolytic use disorder, moderate
     Sedative, hypnotic, or anxiolytic use disorder, severe
> *EXCLUDES 1*   sedative, hypnotic or anxiolytic dependence
> with intoxication (F13.22-)

     **F13.230**   **Sedative, hypnotic or anxiolytic** CC HCC **dependence with withdrawal, uncomplicated**
     **F13.231**   **Sedative, hypnotic or anxiolytic** CC HCC **dependence with withdrawal delirium**
     **F13.232**   **Sedative, hypnotic or anxiolytic** CC HCC **dependence with withdrawal with perceptual disturbance**
         Sedative, hypnotic, or anxiolytic withdrawal with perceptual disturbances
     **F13.239**   **Sedative, hypnotic or anxiolytic** CC HCC **dependence with withdrawal, unspecified**
         Sedative, hypnotic, or anxiolytic withdrawal without perceptual disturbances

     **F13.24**   **Sedative, hypnotic or anxiolytic dependence** HCC **with sedative, hypnotic or anxiolytic-induced mood disorder**
     ▸Sedative, hypnotic, or anxiolytic use disorder, moderate, with sedative, hypnotic, or anxiolytic-induced bipolar or related disorder
         Sedative, hypnotic, or anxiolytic use disorder, moderate, with sedative, hypnotic, or anxiolytic-induced depressive disorder◂
         Sedative, hypnotic, or anxiolytic use disorder, severe, with sedative, hypnotic, or anxiolytic-induced bipolar or related disorder
     ▸Sedative, hypnotic, or anxiolytic use disorder, severe, with sedative, hypnotic, or anxiolytic-induced depressive disorder◂

☑6ᵗʰ   **F13.25**   **Sedative, hypnotic or anxiolytic dependence with sedative, hypnotic or anxiolytic-induced psychotic disorder**
     **F13.250**   **Sedative, hypnotic or anxiolytic** CC HCC **dependence with sedative, hypnotic or anxiolytic-induced psychotic disorder with delusions**
     **F13.251**   **Sedative, hypnotic or anxiolytic** CC HCC **dependence with sedative, hypnotic or anxiolytic-induced psychotic disorder with hallucinations**
     **F13.259**   **Sedative, hypnotic or anxiolytic** CC HCC **dependence with sedative, hypnotic or anxiolytic-induced psychotic disorder, unspecified**
         **CC Excl: No Excl**

     **F13.26**   **Sedative, hypnotic or anxiolytic dependence** CC HCC **with sedative, hypnotic or anxiolytic-induced persisting amnestic disorder**
         **CC Excl: No Excl**

☑ Additional Character Req   ☑x7ᵗʰ Placeholder Alert   Unacceptable PDx   Manifestation   H1-H14 HAC   HCC CMS-HCC Condition   *EXCLUDES 1* Not Coded Here   *EXCLUDES 2* Not Included Here

**ICD-10-CM 2018**      **537**

**Chapter 5. Mental, Behavioral and Neurodevelopmental Disorders**

**F13.27**   **Sedative, hypnotic or anxiolytic dependence** `CC` `HCC` **with sedative, hypnotic or anxiolytic-induced persisting dementia**
▶Sedative, hypnotic, or anxiolytic use disorder, moderate, with sedative, hypnotic, or anxiolytic-induced major neurocognitive disorder◀
Sedative, hypnotic, or anxiolytic use disorder, severe, with sedative, hypnotic, or anxiolytic-induced major neurocognitive disorder

✓6th **F13.28**   **Sedative, hypnotic or anxiolytic dependence with other sedative, hypnotic or anxiolytic-induced disorders**

     **F13.280**   **Sedative, hypnotic or anxiolytic** `CC` `HCC` **dependence with sedative, hypnotic or anxiolytic-induced anxiety disorder**
        **CC Excl:** No Excl

     **F13.281**   **Sedative, hypnotic or anxiolytic** `CC` `HCC` **dependence with sedative, hypnotic or anxiolytic-induced sexual dysfunction**
        **CC Excl:** No Excl

     **F13.282**   **Sedative, hypnotic or anxiolytic** `CC` `HCC` **dependence with sedative, hypnotic or anxiolytic-induced sleep disorder**
        **CC Excl:** No Excl

     **F13.288**   **Sedative, hypnotic or anxiolytic** `CC` `HCC` **dependence with other sedative, hypnotic or anxiolytic-induced disorder**
▶Sedative, hypnotic, or anxiolytic use disorder, moderate, with sedative, hypnotic, or anxiolytic-induced mild neurocognitive disorder
Sedative, hypnotic, or anxiolytic use disorder, severe, with sedative, hypnotic, or anxiolytic-induced mild neurocognitive disorder◀
        **CC Excl:** No Excl

**F13.29**   **Sedative, hypnotic or anxiolytic dependence** `HCC` **with unspecified sedative, hypnotic or anxiolytic-induced disorder**

✓5th **F13.9**   **Sedative, hypnotic or anxiolytic-related use, unspecified**
     **EXCLUDES 1**   *sedative, hypnotic or anxiolytic-related abuse (F13.1-)*
          *sedative, hypnotic or anxiolytic-related dependence (F13.2-)*

     **F13.90**   **Sedative, hypnotic, or anxiolytic use, unspecified, uncomplicated**

✓6th **F13.92**   **Sedative, hypnotic or anxiolytic use, unspecified with intoxication**
     **EXCLUDES 1**   *sedative, hypnotic or anxiolytic use, unspecified with withdrawal (F13.93-)*

     **F13.920**   **Sedative, hypnotic or anxiolytic use,** `HCC` **unspecified with intoxication, uncomplicated**

     **F13.921**   **Sedative, hypnotic or anxiolytic** `CC` `HCC` **use, unspecified with intoxication delirium**
Sedative, hypnotic, or anxiolytic-induced delirium

     **F13.929**   **Sedative, hypnotic or anxiolytic use,** `HCC` **unspecified with intoxication, unspecified**

✓6th **F13.93**   **Sedative, hypnotic or anxiolytic use, unspecified with withdrawal**
     **EXCLUDES 1**   *sedative, hypnotic or anxiolytic use, unspecified with intoxication (F13.92-)*

     **F13.930**   **Sedative, hypnotic or anxiolytic** `CC` `HCC` **use, unspecified with withdrawal, uncomplicated**

     **F13.931**   **Sedative, hypnotic or anxiolytic** `CC` `HCC` **use, unspecified with withdrawal delirium**

     **F13.932**   **Sedative, hypnotic or anxiolytic** `CC` `HCC` **use, unspecified with withdrawal with perceptual disturbances**

     **F13.939**   **Sedative, hypnotic or anxiolytic** `CC` `HCC` **use, unspecified with withdrawal, unspecified**

**F13.94**   **Sedative, hypnotic or anxiolytic use,** `HCC` **unspecified with sedative, hypnotic or anxiolytic-induced mood disorder**
Sedative, hypnotic, or anxiolytic-induced bipolar or related disorder, without use disorder
Sedative, hypnotic, or anxiolytic-induced depressive disorder, without use disorder

✓6th **F13.95**   **Sedative, hypnotic or anxiolytic use, unspecified with sedative, hypnotic or anxiolytic-induced psychotic disorder**

     **F13.950**   **Sedative, hypnotic or anxiolytic** `CC` `HCC` **use, unspecified with sedative, hypnotic or anxiolytic-induced psychotic disorder with delusions**

     **F13.951**   **Sedative, hypnotic or anxiolytic** `CC` `HCC` **use, unspecified with sedative, hypnotic or anxiolytic-induced psychotic disorder with hallucinations**

     **F13.959**   **Sedative, hypnotic or anxiolytic use,** `HCC` **unspecified with sedative, hypnotic or anxiolytic-induced psychotic disorder, unspecified**
▶Sedative, hypnotic, or anxiolytic-induced psychotic disorder, without use disorder◀

**F13.96**   **Sedative, hypnotic or anxiolytic use, unspecified** `HCC` **with sedative, hypnotic or anxiolytic-induced persisting amnestic disorder**

**F13.97**   **Sedative, hypnotic or anxiolytic use,** `CC` `HCC` **unspecified with sedative, hypnotic or anxiolytic-induced persisting dementia**
▶Sedative, hypnotic, or anxiolytic-induced major neurocognitive disorder, without use disorder◀

✓6th **F13.98**   **Sedative, hypnotic or anxiolytic use, unspecified with other sedative, hypnotic or anxiolytic-induced disorders**

     **F13.980**   **Sedative, hypnotic or anxiolytic use,** `HCC` **unspecified with sedative, hypnotic or anxiolytic-induced anxiety disorder**
▶Sedative, hypnotic, or anxiolytic-induced anxiety disorder, without use disorder◀

     **F13.981**   **Sedative, hypnotic or anxiolytic use,** `HCC` **unspecified with sedative, hypnotic or anxiolytic-induced sexual dysfunction**
▶Sedative, hypnotic, or anxiolytic-induced sexual dysfunction disorder, without use disorder◀

     **F13.982**   **Sedative, hypnotic or anxiolytic use,** `HCC` **unspecified with sedative, hypnotic or anxiolytic-induced sleep disorder**
▶Sedative, hypnotic, or anxiolytic-induced sleep disorder, without use disorder◀

     **F13.988**   **Sedative, hypnotic or anxiolytic use,** `HCC` **unspecified with other sedative, hypnotic or anxiolytic-induced disorder**
▶Sedative, hypnotic, or anxiolytic-induced mild neurocognitive disorder◀

**F13.99**   **Sedative, hypnotic or anxiolytic use, unspecified** `HCC` **with unspecified sedative, hypnotic or anxiolytic-induced disorder**

✓4th **F14**   **Cocaine related disorders**
     **EXCLUDES 2**   *other stimulant-related disorders (F15.-)*

     **CC Excl: For CC codes in category F14, unless otherwise noted:** PDX collection 550

✓5th **F14.1**   **Cocaine abuse**
     **EXCLUDES 1**   *cocaine dependence (F14.2-)*
          *cocaine use, unspecified (F14.9-)*

     **F14.10**   **Cocaine abuse, uncomplicated**
Cocaine use disorder, mild

●      **F14.11**   **Cocaine abuse, in remission**
Cocaine use disorder, mild, in early remission
Cocaine use disorder, mild, in sustained remission

✓6th **F14.12**   **Cocaine abuse with intoxication**

     **F14.120**   **Cocaine abuse with intoxication, uncomplicated**

     **F14.121**   **Cocaine abuse with intoxication** `CC` `HCC` **with delirium**

     **F14.122**   **Cocaine abuse with intoxication** `HCC` **with perceptual disturbance**

`N` Newborn: 0   `P` Pediatric: 0-17   `M` Maternity: 12-55   `A` Adult: 15-124   `MCC` Major CC Condition   `PDxMCC` PDx acts as own MCC   `CC` CC Condition   `PDxCC` PDx acts as own CC

538      ICD-10-CM 2018

**F14.129**  **Cocaine abuse with intoxication, unspecified** `HCC`

**F14.14**  **Cocaine abuse with cocaine-induced mood disorder** `HCC`
> Cocaine use disorder, mild, with cocaine-induced bipolar or related disorder
> Cocaine use disorder, mild, with cocaine-induced depressive disorder

√6ᵗʰ **F14.15**  **Cocaine abuse with cocaine-induced psychotic disorder**

**F14.150**  **Cocaine abuse with cocaine-induced psychotic disorder with delusions** `CC` `HCC`

**F14.151**  **Cocaine abuse with cocaine-induced psychotic disorder with hallucinations** `CC` `HCC`

**F14.159**  **Cocaine abuse with cocaine-induced psychotic disorder, unspecified** `HCC`

√6ᵗʰ **F14.18**  **Cocaine abuse with other cocaine-induced disorder**

**F14.180**  **Cocaine abuse with cocaine-induced anxiety disorder** `HCC`

**F14.181**  **Cocaine abuse with cocaine-induced sexual dysfunction** `HCC`

**F14.182**  **Cocaine abuse with cocaine-induced sleep disorder** `HCC`

**F14.188**  **Cocaine abuse with other cocaine-induced disorder** `HCC`
> Cocaine use disorder, mild, with cocaine-induced obsessive compulsive or related disorder

**F14.19**  **Cocaine abuse with unspecified cocaine-induced disorder** `HCC`

√5ᵗʰ **F14.2**  **Cocaine dependence**
> *EXCLUDES 1*   cocaine abuse (F14.1-)
> cocaine use, unspecified (F14.9-)
> *EXCLUDES 2*   cocaine poisoning (T40.5-)

**F14.20**  **Cocaine dependence, uncomplicated** `CC` `HCC`
> Cocaine use disorder, moderate
> Cocaine use disorder, severe
> **CC Excl:** No Excl

**F14.21**  **Cocaine dependence, in remission** `HCC`
> ▶Cocaine use disorder, moderate, in early remission
> Cocaine use disorder, moderate, in sustained remission
> Cocaine use disorder, severe, in early remission
> Cocaine use disorder, severe, in sustained remission◀

√6ᵗʰ **F14.22**  **Cocaine dependence with intoxication**
> *EXCLUDES 1*   cocaine dependence with withdrawal (F14.23)

**F14.220**  **Cocaine dependence with intoxication, uncomplicated** `HCC`

**F14.221**  **Cocaine dependence with intoxication delirium** `CC` `HCC`

**F14.222**  **Cocaine dependence with intoxication with perceptual disturbance** `CC` `HCC`
> **CC Excl:** No Excl

**F14.229**  **Cocaine dependence with intoxication, unspecified** `CC` `HCC`
> **CC Excl:** No Excl

**F14.23**  **Cocaine dependence with withdrawal** `CC` `HCC`
> *EXCLUDES 1*   cocaine dependence with intoxication (F14.22-)

**F14.24**  **Cocaine dependence with cocaine-induced mood disorder** `HCC`
> Cocaine use disorder, moderate, with cocaine-induced bipolar or related disorder
> Cocaine use disorder, moderate, with cocaine-induced depressive disorder
> Cocaine use disorder, severe, with cocaine-induced bipolar or related disorder
> Cocaine use disorder, severe, with cocaine-induced depressive disorder

√6ᵗʰ **F14.25**  **Cocaine dependence with cocaine-induced psychotic disorder**

**F14.250**  **Cocaine dependence with cocaine-induced psychotic disorder with delusions** `CC` `HCC`

**F14.251**  **Cocaine dependence with cocaine-induced psychotic disorder with hallucinations** `CC` `HCC`

**F14.259**  **Cocaine dependence with cocaine-induced psychotic disorder, unspecified** `CC` `HCC`
> **CC Excl:** No Excl

√6ᵗʰ **F14.28**  **Cocaine dependence with other cocaine-induced disorder**

**F14.280**  **Cocaine dependence with cocaine-induced anxiety disorder** `CC` `HCC`
> **CC Excl:** No Excl

**F14.281**  **Cocaine dependence with cocaine-induced sexual dysfunction** `CC` `HCC`
> **CC Excl:** No Excl

**F14.282**  **Cocaine dependence with cocaine-induced sleep disorder** `CC` `HCC`
> **CC Excl:** No Excl

**F14.288**  **Cocaine dependence with other cocaine-induced disorder** `CC` `HCC`
> Cocaine use disorder, moderate, with cocaine-induced obsessive compulsive or related disorder
> Cocaine use disorder, severe, with cocaine-induced obsessive compulsive or related disorder
> **CC Excl:** No Excl

**F14.29**  **Cocaine dependence with unspecified cocaine-induced disorder** `HCC`

√5ᵗʰ **F14.9**  **Cocaine use, unspecified**
> *EXCLUDES 1*   cocaine abuse (F14.1-)
> cocaine dependence (F14.2-)

**F14.90**  **Cocaine use, unspecified, uncomplicated**

√6ᵗʰ **F14.92**  **Cocaine use, unspecified with intoxication**

**F14.920**  **Cocaine use, unspecified with intoxication, uncomplicated** `HCC`

**F14.921**  **Cocaine use, unspecified with intoxication delirium** `CC` `HCC`

**F14.922**  **Cocaine use, unspecified with intoxication with perceptual disturbance** `HCC`

**F14.929**  **Cocaine use, unspecified with intoxication, unspecified** `HCC`

**F14.94**  **Cocaine use, unspecified with cocaine-induced mood disorder** `HCC`
> Cocaine induced bipolar or related disorder, without use disorder
> Cocaine induced depressive disorder, without use disorder

√6ᵗʰ **F14.95**  **Cocaine use, unspecified with cocaine-induced psychotic disorder**

**F14.950**  **Cocaine use, unspecified with cocaine-induced psychotic disorder with delusions** `CC` `HCC`

**F14.951**  **Cocaine use, unspecified with cocaine-induced psychotic disorder with hallucinations** `CC` `HCC`

**F14.959**  **Cocaine use, unspecified with cocaine-induced psychotic disorder, unspecified** `HCC`
> Cocaine induced psychotic disorder, without use disorder

√6ᵗʰ **F14.98**  **Cocaine use, unspecified with other specified cocaine-induced disorder**

**F14.980**  **Cocaine use, unspecified with cocaine-induced anxiety disorder** `HCC`
> Cocaine induced anxiety disorder, without use disorder

**F14.981**  **Cocaine use, unspecified with cocaine-induced sexual dysfunction** `HCC`
> Cocaine induced sexual dysfunction, without use disorder

**F14.982**  **Cocaine use, unspecified with cocaine-induced sleep disorder** `HCC`
> Cocaine induced sleep disorder, without use disorder

**F14.988**  **Cocaine use, unspecified with other cocaine-induced disorder** `HCC`
> Cocaine induced obsessive compulsive or related disorder

**F14.99**  **Cocaine use, unspecified with unspecified cocaine-induced disorder** `HCC`

☑ Additional Character Req  √x7ᵗʰ Placeholder Alert  Unacceptable PDx  Manifestation  **H1**-**H14** HAC  `HCC` CMS-HCC Condition  *EXCLUDES 1* Not Coded Here  *EXCLUDES 2* Not Included Here

ICD-10-CM 2018  **539**

✓4ᵗʰ **F15** **Other stimulant related disorders**
> INCLUDES   amphetamine-related disorders
> caffeine
> EXCLUDES 2   *cocaine-related disorders (F14.-)*

> **CC Excl: For CC codes in category F15, unless otherwise noted:**
> PDX collection 550

✓5ᵗʰ **F15.1** **Other stimulant abuse**
> EXCLUDES 1   *other stimulant dependence (F15.2-)*
> *other stimulant use, unspecified (F15.9-)*

    **F15.10** **Other stimulant abuse, uncomplicated**
> Amphetamine type substance use disorder, mild
> Other or unspecified stimulant use disorder, mild

    **F15.11** **Other stimulant abuse, in remission**
> Amphetamine type substance use disorder, mild, in early remission
> Amphetamine type substance use disorder, mild, in sustained remission
> Other or unspecified stimulant use disorder, mild, in early remission
> Other or unspecified stimulant use disorder, mild, in sustained remission

✓6ᵗʰ   **F15.12** **Other stimulant abuse with intoxication**
        **F15.120** **Other stimulant abuse with**   HCC
             **intoxication, uncomplicated**
        **F15.121** **Other stimulant abuse with**   CC HCC
             **intoxication delirium**
        **F15.122** **Other stimulant abuse with**   HCC
             **intoxication with perceptual disturbance**
> Amphetamine or other stimulant use disorder, mild, with amphetamine or other stimulant intoxication, with perceptual disturbances

        **F15.129** **Other stimulant abuse with**   HCC
             **intoxication, unspecified**
> Amphetamine or other stimulant use disorder, mild, with amphetamine or other stimulant intoxication, without perceptual disturbances

    **F15.14** **Other stimulant abuse with stimulant-induced**   HCC
    **mood disorder**
> Amphetamine or other stimulant use disorder, mild, with amphetamine or other stimulant induced bipolar or related disorder
> Amphetamine or other stimulant use disorder, mild, with amphetamine or other stimulant induced depressive disorder

✓6ᵗʰ   **F15.15** **Other stimulant abuse with stimulant-induced psychotic disorder**
        **F15.150** **Other stimulant abuse with**   CC HCC
             **stimulant-induced psychotic disorder with delusions**
        **F15.151** **Other stimulant abuse with**   CC HCC
             **stimulant-induced psychotic disorder with hallucinations**
        **F15.159** **Other stimulant abuse with**   HCC
             **stimulant-induced psychotic disorder, unspecified**

✓6ᵗʰ   **F15.18** **Other stimulant abuse with other stimulant-induced disorder**
        **F15.180** **Other stimulant abuse with**   HCC
             **stimulant-induced anxiety disorder**
        **F15.181** **Other stimulant abuse with**   HCC
             **stimulant-induced sexual dysfunction**
        **F15.182** **Other stimulant abuse with**   HCC
             **stimulant-induced sleep disorder**
        **F15.188** **Other stimulant abuse with other**   HCC
             **stimulant-induced disorder**
> Amphetamine or other stimulant use disorder, mild, with amphetamine or other stimulant induced obsessive-compulsive or related disorder

    **F15.19** **Other stimulant abuse with unspecified**   HCC
    **stimulant-induced disorder**

✓5ᵗʰ **F15.2** **Other stimulant dependence**
> EXCLUDES 1   *other stimulant abuse (F15.1-)*
> *other stimulant use, unspecified (F15.9-)*

    **F15.20** **Other stimulant dependence, uncomplicated**   CC HCC
> Amphetamine type substance use disorder, moderate
> Amphetamine type substance use disorder, severe
> Other or unspecified stimulant use disorder, moderate
> Other or unspecified stimulant use disorder, severe
> **CC Excl: No Excl**

    **F15.21** **Other stimulant dependence, in remission**   HCC
> ▶Amphetamine type substance use disorder, moderate, in early remission
> Amphetamine type substance use disorder, moderate, in sustained remission
> Amphetamine type substance use disorder, severe, in early remission
> Amphetamine type substance use disorder, severe, in sustained remission
> Other or unspecified stimulant use disorder, moderate, in early remission
> Other or unspecified stimulant use disorder, moderate, in sustained remission
> Other or unspecified stimulant use disorder, severe, in early remission
> Other or unspecified stimulant use disorder, severe, in sustained remission◀

✓6ᵗʰ   **F15.22** **Other stimulant dependence with intoxication**
> EXCLUDES 1   *other stimulant dependence with withdrawal (F15.23)*

        **F15.220** **Other stimulant dependence with**   HCC
             **intoxication, uncomplicated**
        **F15.221** **Other stimulant dependence with**   CC HCC
             **intoxication delirium**
        **F15.222** **Other stimulant dependence with**   CC HCC
             **intoxication with perceptual disturbance**
> Amphetamine or other stimulant use disorder, moderate, with amphetamine or other stimulant intoxication, with perceptual disturbances
> Amphetamine or other stimulant use disorder, severe, with amphetamine or other stimulant intoxication, with perceptual disturbances
> **CC Excl: No Excl**

        **F15.229** **Other stimulant dependence with**   HCC
             **intoxication, unspecified**
> Amphetamine or other stimulant use disorder, moderate, with amphetamine or other stimulant intoxication, without perceptual disturbances
> Amphetamine or other stimulant use disorder, severe, with amphetamine or other stimulant intoxication, without perceptual disturbances

    **F15.23** **Other stimulant dependence with**   CC HCC
    **withdrawal**
> Amphetamine or other stimulant withdrawal
> EXCLUDES 1   *other stimulant dependence with intoxication (F15.22-)*

    **F15.24** **Other stimulant dependence with stimulant-**   HCC
    **induced mood disorder**
> Amphetamine or other stimulant use disorder, moderate, with amphetamine or other stimulant-induced bipolar or related disorder
> Amphetamine or other stimulant use disorder, moderate, with amphetamine or other stimulant induced depressive disorder
> Amphetamine or other stimulant use disorder, severe, with amphetamine or other stimulant-induced bipolar or related disorder
> Amphetamine or other stimulant use disorder, severe, with amphetamine or other stimulant-induced depressive disorder

✓6ᵗʰ   **F15.25** **Other stimulant dependence with stimulant-induced psychotic disorder**
        **F15.250** **Other stimulant dependence with**   CC HCC
             **stimulant-induced psychotic disorder with delusions**
        **F15.251** **Other stimulant dependence with**   CC HCC
             **stimulant-induced psychotic disorder with hallucinations**

N Newborn: 0   P Pediatric: 0-17   M Maternity: 12-55   A Adult: 15-124   MCC Major CC Condition   PDxMCC PDx acts as own MCC   CC CC Condition   PDxCC PDx acts as own CC

**540**                                                    ICD-10-CM 2018

**F15.259**  **Other stimulant dependence with** `CC` `HCC`
    **stimulant-induced psychotic disorder,**
    **unspecified**
    CC Excl: No Excl

✓6ᵗʰ **F15.28**  **Other stimulant dependence with** other stimulant-
    induced disorder

    **F15.280**  **Other stimulant dependence with** `CC` `HCC`
       **stimulant-induced** anxiety disorder
       CC Excl: No Excl

    **F15.281**  **Other stimulant dependence with** `CC` `HCC`
       **stimulant-induced** sexual dysfunction
       CC Excl: No Excl

    **F15.282**  **Other stimulant dependence with** `CC` `HCC`
       **stimulant-induced** sleep disorder
       CC Excl: No Excl

    **F15.288**  **Other stimulant dependence with** `CC` `HCC`
       **other stimulant-induced disorder**
       ▶Amphetamine or other stimulant use
        disorder, moderate, with
        amphetamine or other stimulant
        induced obsessive compulsive or
        related disorder
       Amphetamine or other stimulant use
        disorder, severe, with amphetamine or
        other stimulant induced obsessive
        compulsive or related disorder◀
       CC Excl: No Excl

  **F15.29**  **Other stimulant dependence with** unspecified `HCC`
    stimulant-induced disorder

✓5ᵗʰ **F15.9**  **Other stimulant use, unspecified**
    *EXCLUDES 1*   *other stimulant abuse (F15.1-)*
          *other stimulant dependence (F15.2-)*

  **F15.90**  **Other stimulant use, unspecified, uncomplicated**

✓6ᵗʰ **F15.92**  **Other stimulant use, unspecified** with intoxication
    *EXCLUDES 1*   *other stimulant use, unspecified with*
          *withdrawal (F15.93)*

    **F15.920**  **Other stimulant use, unspecified with** `HCC`
       **intoxication, uncomplicated**

    **F15.921**  **Other stimulant use, unspecified** `CC` `HCC`
       **with intoxication** delirium
       Amphetamine or other stimulant-induced
        delirium

    **F15.922**  **Other stimulant use, unspecified with** `HCC`
       **intoxication with** perceptual disturbance

    **F15.929**  **Other stimulant use, unspecified with** `HCC`
       **intoxication, unspecified**
       Caffeine intoxication

  **F15.93**  **Other stimulant use, unspecified with** `CC` `HCC`
    **withdrawal**
    Caffeine withdrawal
    *EXCLUDES 1*   *other stimulant use, unspecified with*
          *intoxication (F15.92-)*

  **F15.94**  **Other stimulant use, unspecified with** `HCC`
    **stimulant-induced** mood disorder
    Amphetamine or other stimulant-induced bipolar or
     related disorder, without use disorder
    Amphetamine or other stimulant-induced depressive
     disorder, without use disorder

✓6ᵗʰ **F15.95**  **Other stimulant use, unspecified with stimulant-**
    **induced** psychotic disorder

    **F15.950**  **Other stimulant use, unspecified** `CC` `HCC`
       **with stimulant-induced psychotic**
       **disorder with** delusions

    **F15.951**  **Other stimulant use, unspecified** `CC` `HCC`
       **with stimulant-induced psychotic**
       **disorder with** hallucinations

    **F15.959**  **Other stimulant use, unspecified with** `HCC`
       **stimulant-induced psychotic disorder,**
       **unspecified**
       ▶Amphetamine or other stimulant-induced
        psychotic disorder, without use
        disorder◀

✓6ᵗʰ **F15.98**  **Other stimulant use, unspecified with** other
    stimulant-induced disorder

    **F15.980**  **Other stimulant use, unspecified** `HCC`
       **with stimulant-induced** anxiety disorder
       Amphetamine or other stimulant-induced
        anxiety disorder, without use disorder
       Caffeine induced anxiety disorder, without
        use disorder

    **F15.981**  **Other stimulant use, unspecified** `HCC`
       **with stimulant-induced** sexual
       **dysfunction**
       Amphetamine or other stimulant-induced
        sexual dysfunction, without use
        disorder

    **F15.982**  **Other stimulant use, unspecified** `HCC`
       **with stimulant-induced** sleep disorder
       Amphetamine or other stimulant-induced
        sleep disorder, without use disorder
       Caffeine induced sleep disorder, without
        use disorder

    **F15.988**  **Other stimulant use, unspecified with** `HCC`
       **other stimulant-induced disorder**
       Amphetamine or other stimulant-induced
        obsessive compulsive or related
        disorder, without use disorder

  **F15.99**  **Other stimulant use, unspecified with** `HCC`
    **unspecified stimulant-induced disorder**

✓4ᵗʰ **F16**  **Hallucinogen related disorders**
    *INCLUDES*   ecstasy
          PCP
          phencyclidine

    **CC Excl: For CC codes in category F16, unless otherwise noted:**
    PDX collection 550

✓5ᵗʰ **F16.1**  **Hallucinogen abuse**
    *EXCLUDES 1*   *hallucinogen dependence (F16.2-)*
          *hallucinogen use, unspecified (F16.9-)*

  **F16.10**  **Hallucinogen abuse, uncomplicated**
    Other hallucinogen use disorder, mild
    Phencyclidine use disorder, mild

  **F16.11**  **Hallucinogen abuse, in remission**
    Other hallucinogen use disorder, mild, in early
     remission
    Other hallucinogen use disorder, mild, in sustained
     remission
    Phencyclidine use disorder, mild, in early remission
    Phencyclidine use disorder, mild, in sustained
     remission

✓6ᵗʰ **F16.12**  **Hallucinogen abuse with** intoxication

    **F16.120**  **Hallucinogen abuse with intoxication,** `HCC`
       **uncomplicated**

    **F16.121**  **Hallucinogen abuse with** `CC` `HCC`
       **intoxication with** delirium

    **F16.122**  **Hallucinogen abuse with intoxication** `HCC`
       **with** perceptual disturbance

    **F16.129**  **Hallucinogen abuse with intoxication,** `HCC`
       **unspecified**

  **F16.14**  **Hallucinogen abuse with hallucinogen-induced** `HCC`
    **mood disorder**
    Other hallucinogen use disorder, mild, with other
     hallucinogen induced bipolar or related disorder
    Other hallucinogen use disorder, mild, with other
     hallucinogen induced depressive disorder
    Phencyclidine use disorder, mild, with phencyclidine
     induced bipolar or related disorder
    Phencyclidine use disorder, mild, with phencyclidine
     induced depressive disorder

✓6ᵗʰ **F16.15**  **Hallucinogen abuse with hallucinogen-induced**
    **psychotic disorder**

    **F16.150**  **Hallucinogen abuse with** `CC` `HCC`
       **hallucinogen-induced psychotic**
       **disorder with** delusions

    **F16.151**  **Hallucinogen abuse with** `CC` `HCC`
       **hallucinogen-induced psychotic**
       **disorder with** hallucinations

    **F16.159**  **Hallucinogen abuse with** `HCC`
       **hallucinogen-induced psychotic**
       **disorder, unspecified**

✓6ᵗʰ **F16.18**  **Hallucinogen abuse with** other hallucinogen-
    induced disorder

    **F16.180**  **Hallucinogen abuse with** `HCC`
       **hallucinogen-induced** anxiety disorder

    **F16.183**  **Hallucinogen abuse with** `HCC`
       **hallucinogen-induced** persisting
       **perception disorder (flashbacks)**

    **F16.188**  **Hallucinogen abuse with** other `HCC`
       **hallucinogen-induced disorder**

  **F16.19**  **Hallucinogen abuse with** unspecified `HCC`
    **hallucinogen-induced disorder**

✓5ᵗʰ **F16.2 Hallucinogen** dependence
> EXCLUDES 1 *hallucinogen abuse (F16.1-)*
> *hallucinoge n use, unspecified (F16.9-)*

**F16.20 Hallucinogen dependence, uncomplicated** CC HCC
Other hallucinogen use disorder, moderate
Other hallucinogen use disorder, severe
Phencyclidine use disorder, moderate
Phencyclidine use disorder, severe
**CC Excl:** No Excl

**F16.21 Hallucinogen dependence, in remission** HCC
▶Other hallucinogen use disorder, moderate, in early remission
Other hallucinogen use disorder, moderate, in sustained remission
Other hallucinogen use disorder, severe, in early remission
Other hallucinogen use disorder, severe, in sustained remission
Phencyclidine use disorder, moderate, in early remission
Phencyclidine use disorder, moderate, in sustained remission
Phencyclidine use disorder, severe, in early remission
Phencyclidine use disorder, severe, in sustained remission◀

✓6ᵗʰ **F16.22 Hallucinogen dependence with intoxication**

**F16.220 Hallucinogen dependence with intoxication, uncomplicated** HCC

**F16.221 Hallucinogen dependence with intoxication with delirium** CC HCC

**F16.229 Hallucinogen dependence with intoxication, unspecified** HCC

**F16.24 Hallucinogen dependence with hallucinogen-induced mood disorder** HCC
Other hallucinogen use disorder, moderate, with other hallucinogen induced bipolar or related disorder
Other hallucinogen use disorder, moderate, with other hallucinogen induced depressive disorder
Other hallucinogen use disorder, severe, with other hallucinogen-induced bipolar or related disorder
Other hallucinogen use disorder, severe, with other hallucinogen-induced depressive disorder
Phencyclidine use disorder, moderate, with phencyclidine induced bipolar or related disorder
Phencyclidine use disorder, moderate, with phencyclidine induced depressive disorder
Phencyclidine use disorder, severe, with phencyclidine induced bipolar or related disorder
Phencyclidine use disorder, severe, with phencyclidine-induced depressive disorder

✓6ᵗʰ **F16.25 Hallucinogen dependence with hallucinogen-induced psychotic disorder**

**F16.250 Hallucinogen dependence with hallucinogen-induced psychotic disorder with delusions** CC HCC

**F16.251 Hallucinogen dependence with hallucinogen-induced psychotic disorder with hallucinations** CC HCC

**F16.259 Hallucinogen dependence with hallucinogen-induced psychotic disorder, unspecified** CC HCC
**CC Excl:** No Excl

✓6ᵗʰ **F16.28 Hallucinogen dependence with other hallucinogen-induced disorder**

**F16.280 Hallucinogen dependence with hallucinogen-induced anxiety disorder** CC HCC
**CC Excl:** No Excl

**F16.283 Hallucinogen dependence with hallucinogen persisting perception disorder (flashbacks)** CC HCC
**CC Excl:** No Excl

**F16.288 Hallucinogen dependence with other hallucinogen-induced disorder** CC HCC
**CC Excl:** No Excl

**F16.29 Hallucinogen dependence with unspecified hallucinogen-induced disorder** HCC

✓5ᵗʰ **F16.9 Hallucinogen use, unspecified**
> EXCLUDES 1 *hallucinogen abuse (F16.1-)*
> *hallucinogen dependence (F16.2-)*

**F16.90 Hallucinogen use, unspecified, uncomplicated**

✓6ᵗʰ **F16.92 Hallucinogen use, unspecified with intoxication**

**F16.920 Hallucinogen use, unspecified with intoxication, uncomplicated** HCC

**F16.921 Hallucinogen use, unspecified with intoxication with delirium** CC HCC
Other hallucinogen intoxication delirium

**F16.929 Hallucinogen use, unspecified with intoxication, unspecified** HCC

**F16.94 Hallucinogen use, unspecified with hallucinogen-induced mood disorder** HCC
Other hallucinogen induced bipolar or related disorder, without use disorder
Other hallucinogen induced depressive disorder, without use disorder
Phencyclidine induced bipolar or related disorder, without use disorder
Phencyclidine induced depressive disorder, without use disorder

✓6ᵗʰ **F16.95 Hallucinogen use, unspecified with hallucinogen-induced psychotic disorder**

**F16.950 Hallucinogen use, unspecified with hallucinogen-induced psychotic disorder with delusions** CC HCC

**F16.951 Hallucinogen use, unspecified with hallucinogen-induced psychotic disorder with hallucinations** CC HCC

**F16.959 Hallucinogen use, unspecified with hallucinogen-induced psychotic disorder, unspecified** HCC
Other hallucinogen induced psychotic disorder, without use disorder
Phencyclidine induced psychotic disorder, without use disorder

✓6ᵗʰ **F16.98 Hallucinogen use, unspecified with other specified hallucinogen-induced disorder**

**F16.980 Hallucinogen use, unspecified with hallucinogen-induced anxiety disorder** HCC
Other hallucinogen-induced anxiety disorder, without use disorder
Phencyclidine induced anxiety disorder, without use disorder

**F16.983 Hallucinogen use, unspecified with hallucinogen persisting perception disorder (flashbacks)** HCC

**F16.988 Hallucinogen use, unspecified with other hallucinogen-induced disorder** HCC

**F16.99 Hallucinogen use, unspecified with unspecified hallucinogen-induced disorder** HCC

✓4ᵗʰ **F17 Nicotine dependence**
> EXCLUDES 1 *history of tobacco dependence (Z87.891)*
> *tobacco use NOS (Z72.0)*
> EXCLUDES 2 *tobacco use (smoking) during pregnancy, childbirth and the puerperium (O99.33-)*
> *toxic effect of nicotine (T65.2-)*
> **AHA:** 2013, 4Q, 108-109

**CC Excl: For CC codes in category F17:** PDX collection 550

✓5ᵗʰ **F17.2 Nicotine dependence**

✓6ᵗʰ **F17.20 Nicotine dependence, unspecified**

**F17.200 Nicotine dependence, unspecified, uncomplicated**
Tobacco use disorder, mild
Tobacco use disorder, moderate
Tobacco use disorder, severe
**AHA:** 2016, 1Q, 36

**F17.201 Nicotine dependence, unspecified, in remission**
▶Tobacco use disorder, mild, in early remission
Tobacco use disorder, mild, in sustained remission
Tobacco use disorder, moderate, in early remission
Tobacco use disorder, moderate, in sustained remission
Tobacco use disorder, severe, in early remission
Tobacco use disorder, severe, in sustained remission◀

**F17.203 Nicotine dependence unspecified, withdrawal** CC
Tobacco withdrawal

N Newborn: 0  P Pediatric: 0-17  M Maternity: 12-55  A Adult: 15-124  MCC Major CC Condition  PDxMCC PDx acts as own MCC  CC CC Condition  PDxCC PDx acts as own CC

542  ICD-10-CM 2018

**F17.208**   **Nicotine dependence, unspecified, with other nicotine-induced disorders**

**F17.209**   **Nicotine dependence, unspecified, with unspecified nicotine-induced disorders**

√6ᵗʰ   **F17.21**   **Nicotine dependence, cigarettes**

**F17.210**   **Nicotine dependence, cigarettes, uncomplicated**
     **AHA:** 2017, 2Q, 28-29

**F17.211**   **Nicotine dependence, cigarettes, in remission**
     ▶Tobacco use disorder, cigarettes, mild, in early remission
     Tobacco use disorder, cigarettes, mild, in sustained remission
     Tobacco use disorder, cigarettes, moderate, in early remission
     Tobacco use disorder, cigarettes, moderate, in sustained remission
     Tobacco use disorder, cigarettes, severe, in early remission
     Tobacco use disorder, cigarettes, severe, in sustained remission◀

**F17.213**   **Nicotine dependence, cigarettes, with withdrawal**   CC

**F17.218**   **Nicotine dependence, cigarettes, with other nicotine-induced disorders**

**F17.219**   **Nicotine dependence, cigarettes, with unspecified nicotine-induced disorders**

√6ᵗʰ   **F17.22**   **Nicotine dependence, chewing tobacco**

**F17.220**   **Nicotine dependence, chewing tobacco, uncomplicated**

**F17.221**   **Nicotine dependence, chewing tobacco, in remission**
     ▶Tobacco use disorder, chewing tobacco, mild, in early remission
     Tobacco use disorder, chewing tobacco, mild, in sustained remission
     Tobacco use disorder, chewing tobacco, moderate, in early remission
     Tobacco use disorder, chewing tobacco, moderate, in sustained remission
     Tobacco use disorder, chewing tobacco, severe, in early remission
     Tobacco use disorder, chewing tobacco, severe, in sustained remission◀

**F17.223**   **Nicotine dependence, chewing tobacco, with withdrawal**   CC

**F17.228**   **Nicotine dependence, chewing tobacco, with other nicotine-induced disorders**

**F17.229**   **Nicotine dependence, chewing tobacco, with unspecified nicotine-induced disorders**

√6ᵗʰ   **F17.29**   **Nicotine dependence, other tobacco product**

**F17.290**   **Nicotine dependence, other tobacco product, uncomplicated**
     **AHA:** 2017, 2Q, 28-29

**F17.291**   **Nicotine dependence, other tobacco product, in remission**
     ▶Tobacco use disorder, other tobacco product, mild, in early remission
     Tobacco use disorder, other tobacco product, mild, in sustained remission
     Tobacco use disorder, other tobacco product, moderate, in early remission
     Tobacco use disorder, other tobacco product, moderate, in sustained remission
     Tobacco use disorder, other tobacco product, severe, in early remission
     Tobacco use disorder, other tobacco product, severe, in sustained remission◀

**F17.293**   **Nicotine dependence, other tobacco product, with withdrawal**   CC

**F17.298**   **Nicotine dependence, other tobacco product, with other nicotine-induced disorders**

**F17.299**   **Nicotine dependence, other tobacco product, with unspecified nicotine-induced disorders**

√4ᵗʰ   **F18**   **Inhalant related disorders**
     INCLUDES   volatile solvents

     **CC Excl: For CC codes in category F18, unless otherwise noted:** PDX collection 550

√5ᵗʰ   **F18.1**   **Inhalant abuse**
     EXCLUDES 1   inhalant dependence (F18.2-)
           inhalant use, unspecified (F18.9-)

**F18.10**   **Inhalant abuse, uncomplicated**
     Inhalant use disorder, mild

●   **F18.11**   **Inhalant abuse, in remission**
     Inhalant use disorder, mild, in early remission
     Inhalant use disorder, mild, in sustained remission

√6ᵗʰ   **F18.12**   **Inhalant abuse with intoxication**

**F18.120**   **Inhalant abuse with intoxication, uncomplicated**   HCC

**F18.121**   **Inhalant abuse with intoxication delirium**   CC HCC

**F18.129**   **Inhalant abuse with intoxication, unspecified**   HCC

**F18.14**   **Inhalant abuse with inhalant-induced mood disorder**   HCC
     Inhalant use disorder, mild, with inhalant induced depressive disorder

√6ᵗʰ   **F18.15**   **Inhalant abuse with inhalant-induced psychotic disorder**

**F18.150**   **Inhalant abuse with inhalant-induced psychotic disorder with delusions**   CC HCC

**F18.151**   **Inhalant abuse with inhalant-induced psychotic disorder with hallucinations**   CC HCC

**F18.159**   **Inhalant abuse with inhalant-induced psychotic disorder, unspecified**   HCC

**F18.17**   **Inhalant abuse with inhalant-induced dementia**   CC HCC
     Inhalant use disorder, mild, with inhalant induced major neurocognitive disorder

√6ᵗʰ   **F18.18**   **Inhalant abuse with other inhalant-induced disorders**

**F18.180**   **Inhalant abuse with inhalant-induced anxiety disorder**   HCC

**F18.188**   **Inhalant abuse with other inhalant-induced disorder**   HCC
     Inhalant use disorder, mild, with inhalant induced mild neurocognitive disorder

**F18.19**   **Inhalant abuse with unspecified inhalant-induced disorder**   HCC

√5ᵗʰ   **F18.2**   **Inhalant dependence**
     EXCLUDES 1   inhalant abuse (F18.1-)
           inhalant use, unspecified (F18.9-)

**F18.20**   **Inhalant dependence, uncomplicated**   CC HCC
     Inhalant use disorder, moderate
     Inhalant use disorder, severe
     **CC Excl:** No Excl

**F18.21**   **Inhalant dependence, in remission**   HCC
     ▶Inhalant use disorder, moderate, in early remission
     Inhalant use disorder, moderate, in sustained remission
     Inhalant use disorder, severe, in early remission
     Inhalant use disorder, severe, in sustained remission◀

√6ᵗʰ   **F18.22**   **Inhalant dependence with intoxication**

**F18.220**   **Inhalant dependence with intoxication, uncomplicated**   HCC

**F18.221**   **Inhalant dependence with intoxication delirium**   CC HCC

**F18.229**   **Inhalant dependence with intoxication, unspecified**   HCC

**F18.24**   **Inhalant dependence with inhalant-induced mood disorder**   HCC
     Inhalant use disorder, moderate, with inhalant induced depressive disorder
     Inhalant use disorder, severe, with inhalant induced depressive disorder

√6ᵗʰ   **F18.25**   **Inhalant dependence with inhalant-induced psychotic disorder**

**F18.250**   **Inhalant dependence with inhalant-induced psychotic disorder with delusions**   CC HCC

✓ Additional Character Req   √x7ᵗʰ Placeholder Alert   Unacceptable PDx   Manifestation   H1 - H14 HAC   HCC CMS-HCC Condition   EXCLUDES 1 Not Coded Here   EXCLUDES 2 Not Included Here

ICD-10-CM 2018      543

**Chapter 5. Mental, Behavioral and Neurodevelopmental Disorders**

**F18.251**   **Inhalant dependence with** `CC` `HCC`
     **inhalant-induced psychotic disorder
with hallucinations**

**F18.259**   **Inhalant dependence with** `CC` `HCC`
     **inhalant-induced psychotic disorder,
unspecified**
     **CC Excl:** No Excl

**F18.27**   **Inhalant dependence with inhalant-induced** `CC` `HCC`
   **dementia**
     Inhalant use disorder, moderate, with inhalant
      induced major neurocognitive disorder
     Inhalant use disorder, severe, with inhalant induced
      major neurocognitive disorder

✓6th **F18.28**   **Inhalant dependence with other inhalant-induced
disorders**

**F18.280**   **Inhalant dependence with** `CC` `HCC`
     **inhalant-induced anxiety disorder**
     **CC Excl:** No Excl

**F18.288**   **Inhalant dependence with other** `CC` `HCC`
     **inhalant-induced disorder**
     Inhalant use disorder, moderate, with
      inhalant-induced mild neurocognitive
      disorder
     Inhalant use disorder, severe, with
      inhalant-induced mild neurocognitive
      disorder
     **CC Excl:** No Excl

**F18.29**   **Inhalant dependence with unspecified** `HCC`
   **inhalant-induced disorder**

✓5th **F18.9**   **Inhalant use, unspecified**
     `EXCLUDES 1`   inhalant abuse (F18.1-)
              inhalant dependence (F18.2-)

**F18.90**   **Inhalant use, unspecified, uncomplicated**

✓6th **F18.92**   **Inhalant use, unspecified with intoxication**

**F18.920**   **Inhalant use, unspecified with** `HCC`
     **intoxication, uncomplicated**

**F18.921**   **Inhalant use, unspecified with** `CC` `HCC`
     **intoxication with delirium**

**F18.929**   **Inhalant use, unspecified with** `HCC`
     **intoxication, unspecified**

**F18.94**   **Inhalant use, unspecified with inhalant-induced** `HCC`
   **mood disorder**
     Inhalant induced depressive disorder

✓6th **F18.95**   **Inhalant use, unspecified with inhalant-induced
psychotic disorder**

**F18.950**   **Inhalant use, unspecified with** `CC` `HCC`
     **inhalant-induced psychotic disorder
with delusions**

**F18.951**   **Inhalant use, unspecified with** `CC` `HCC`
     **inhalant-induced psychotic disorder
with hallucinations**

**F18.959**   **Inhalant use, unspecified with** `HCC`
     **inhalant-induced psychotic disorder,
unspecified**

**F18.97**   **Inhalant use, unspecified with inhalant-** `CC` `HCC`
   **induced persisting dementia**
     Inhalant-induced major neurocognitive disorder

✓6th **F18.98**   **Inhalant use, unspecified with other inhalant-
induced disorders**

**F18.980**   **Inhalant use, unspecified with** `HCC`
     **inhalant-induced anxiety disorder**

**F18.988**   **Inhalant use, unspecified with other** `HCC`
     **inhalant-induced disorder**
     Inhalant-induced mild neurocognitive
      disorder

**F18.99**   **Inhalant use, unspecified with unspecified** `HCC`
   **inhalant-induced disorder**

✓4th **F19**   **Other psychoactive substance related disorders**
     `INCLUDES`   polysubstance drug use (indiscriminate drug use)

     **CC Excl: For CC codes in category F19, unless otherwise noted:**
     PDX collection 550

✓5th **F19.1**   **Other psychoactive substance abuse**
     `EXCLUDES 1`   other psychoactive substance dependence (F19.2-)
              other psychoactive substance use, unspecified (F19.9-)

**F19.10**   **Other psychoactive substance abuse, uncomplicated**
     Other (or unknown) substance use disorder, mild

● **F19.11**   **Other psychoactive substance abuse, in remission**
     Other (or unknown) substance use disorder, mild, in
      early remission
     Other (or unknown) substance use disorder, mild, in
      sustained remission

✓6th **F19.12**   **Other psychoactive substance abuse with
intoxication**

**F19.120**   **Other psychoactive substance abuse with
intoxication, uncomplicated**

**F19.121**   **Other psychoactive substance** `CC` `HCC`
     **abuse with intoxication delirium**

**F19.122**   **Other psychoactive substance abuse** `HCC`
     **with intoxication with perceptual
disturbances**

**F19.129**   **Other psychoactive substance abuse** `HCC`
     **with intoxication, unspecified**

**F19.14**   **Other psychoactive substance abuse with** `HCC`
   **psychoactive substance-induced mood disorder**
     Other (or unknown) substance use disorder, mild, with
      other (or unknown) substance-induced bipolar or
      related disorder
     Other (or unknown) substance use disorder, mild, with
      other (or unknown) substance-induced
      depressive disorder

✓6th **F19.15**   **Other psychoactive substance abuse with
psychoactive substance-induced psychotic disorder**

**F19.150**   **Other psychoactive substance** `CC` `HCC`
     **abuse with psychoactive substance-
induced psychotic disorder with delusions**

**F19.151**   **Other psychoactive substance** `CC` `HCC`
     **abuse with psychoactive substance-
induced psychotic disorder with
hallucinations**

**F19.159**   **Other psychoactive substance abuse** `HCC`
     **with psychoactive substance-induced
psychotic disorder, unspecified**

**F19.16**   **Other psychoactive substance abuse with** `HCC`
   **psychoactive substance-induced
persisting amnestic disorder**

**F19.17**   **Other psychoactive substance abuse with** `CC` `HCC`
   **psychoactive substance-induced persisting
dementia**
     Other (or unknown) substance use disorder, mild, with
      other (or unknown) substance-induced major
      neurocognitive disorder

✓6th **F19.18**   **Other psychoactive substance abuse with other
psychoactive substance-induced disorders**

**F19.180**   **Other psychoactive substance abuse** `HCC`
     **with psychoactive substance-induced
anxiety disorder**

**F19.181**   **Other psychoactive substance abuse** `HCC`
     **with psychoactive substance-induced
sexual dysfunction**

**F19.182**   **Other psychoactive substance abuse** `HCC`
     **with psychoactive substance-induced
sleep disorder**

**F19.188**   **Other psychoactive substance abuse** `HCC`
     **with other psychoactive substance-
induced disorder**
     Other (or unknown) substance use
      disorder, mild, with other (or
      unknown) substance induced mild
      neurocognitive disorder
     Other (or unknown) substance use
      disorder, mild, with other (or
      unknown) substance induced
      obsessive-compulsive or related
      disorder

**F19.19**   **Other psychoactive substance abuse with** `HCC`
   **unspecified psychoactive substance-induced
disorder**

✓5th **F19.2**   **Other psychoactive substance dependence**
     `EXCLUDES 1`   other psychoactive substance abuse (F19.1-)
              other psychoactive substance use, unspecified (F19.9-)

**F19.20**   **Other psychoactive substance dependence,** `CC` `HCC`
   **uncomplicated**
     Other (or unknown) substance use disorder, moderate
     Other (or unknown) substance use disorder, severe
     **CC Excl:** No Excl

`N` Newborn: 0    `P` Pediatric: 0-17    `M` Maternity: 12-55    `A` Adult: 15-124    `MCC` Major CC Condition    `PDxMCC` PDx acts as own MCC    `CC` CC Condition    `PDxCC` PDx acts as own CC

**544**      ICD-10-CM 2018

F18.251–F19.20

**F19.21**   **Other psychoactive substance dependence, in** HCC **remission**
> ▶Other (or unknown) substance use disorder, moderate, in early remission
> Other (or unknown) substance use disorder, moderate, in sustained remission
> Other (or unknown) substance use disorder, severe, in early remission
> Other (or unknown) substance use, severe, in sustained remission◀

✓6ᵗʰ **F19.22**   **Other psychoactive substance dependence with intoxication**
> *EXCLUDES 1*   other psychoactive substance dependence with withdrawal (F19.23-)

    **F19.220**   **Other psychoactive substance dependence with intoxication, uncomplicated** HCC

    **F19.221**   **Other psychoactive substance** CC HCC **dependence with intoxication delirium**

    **F19.222**   **Other psychoactive substance** CC HCC **dependence with intoxication with perceptual disturbance**
> CC Excl: No Excl

    **F19.229**   **Other psychoactive substance** HCC **dependence with intoxication, unspecified**

✓6ᵗʰ **F19.23**   **Other psychoactive substance dependence with withdrawal**
> *EXCLUDES 1*   other psychoactive substance dependence with intoxication (F19.22-)

    **F19.230**   **Other psychoactive substance** CC HCC **dependence with withdrawal, uncomplicated**

    **F19.231**   **Other psychoactive substance** CC HCC **dependence with withdrawal delirium**

    **F19.232**   **Other psychoactive substance** CC HCC **dependence with withdrawal with perceptual disturbance**

    **F19.239**   **Other psychoactive substance** CC HCC **dependence with withdrawal, unspecified**

**F19.24**   **Other psychoactive substance dependence** HCC **with psychoactive substance-induced mood disorder**
> Other (or unknown) substance use disorder, moderate, with other (or unknown) substance induced bipolar or related disorder
> Other (or unknown) substance use disorder, moderate, with other (or unknown) substance induced depressive disorder
> Other (or unknown) substance use disorder, severe, with other (or unknown) substance induced bipolar or related disorder
> Other (or unknown) substance use disorder, severe, with other (or unknown) substance induced depressive disorder

✓6ᵗʰ **F19.25**   **Other psychoactive substance dependence with psychoactive substance-induced psychotic disorder**

    **F19.250**   **Other psychoactive substance** CC HCC **dependence with psychoactive substance-induced psychotic disorder with delusions**

    **F19.251**   **Other psychoactive substance** CC HCC **dependence with psychoactive substance-induced psychotic disorder with hallucinations**

    **F19.259**   **Other psychoactive substance** CC HCC **dependence with psychoactive substance-induced psychotic disorder, unspecified**
> CC Excl: No Excl

**F19.26**   **Other psychoactive substance dependence** CC HCC **with psychoactive substance-induced persisting amnestic disorder**
> CC Excl: No Excl

**F19.27**   **Other psychoactive substance dependence** CC HCC **with psychoactive substance-induced persisting dementia**
> Other (or unknown) substance use disorder, moderate, with other (or unknown) substance induced major neurocognitive disorder
> Other (or unknown) substance use disorder, severe, with other (or unknown) substance induced major neurocognitive disorder

✓6ᵗʰ **F19.28**   **Other psychoactive substance dependence with other psychoactive substance-induced disorders**

    **F19.280**   **Other psychoactive substance** CC HCC **dependence with psychoactive substance-induced anxiety disorder**
> CC Excl: No Excl

    **F19.281**   **Other psychoactive substance** CC HCC **dependence with psychoactive substance-induced sexual dysfunction**
> CC Excl: No Excl

    **F19.282**   **Other psychoactive substance** CC HCC **dependence with psychoactive substance-induced sleep disorder**
> CC Excl: No Excl

    **F19.288**   **Other psychoactive substance** CC HCC **dependence with other psychoactive substance-induced disorder**
> Other (or unknown) substance use disorder, moderate, with other (or unknown) substance induced mild neurocognitive disorder
> Other (or unknown) substance use disorder, severe, with other (or unknown) substance induced mild neurocognitive disorder
> Other (or unknown) substance use disorder, moderate, with other (or unknown) substance induced obsessive compulsive or related disorder
> Other (or unknown) substance use disorder, severe, with other (or unknown) substance induced obsessive-compulsive or related disorder
> CC Excl: No Excl

**F19.29**   **Other psychoactive substance dependence** HCC **with unspecified psychoactive substance-induced disorder**

✓5ᵗʰ **F19.9**   **Other psychoactive substance use, unspecified**
> *EXCLUDES 1*   other psychoactive substance abuse (F19.1-)
>     other psychoactive substance dependence (F19.2-)

**F19.90**   **Other psychoactive substance use, unspecified, uncomplicated**

✓6ᵗʰ **F19.92**   **Other psychoactive substance use, unspecified with intoxication**
> *EXCLUDES 1*   other psychoactive substance use, unspecified with withdrawal (F19.93)

    **F19.920**   **Other psychoactive substance use,** HCC **unspecified with intoxication, uncomplicated**

    **F19.921**   **Other psychoactive substance use,** CC HCC **unspecified with intoxication with delirium**
> Other (or unknown) substance-induced delirium

    **F19.922**   **Other psychoactive substance use,** HCC **unspecified with intoxication with perceptual disturbance**

    **F19.929**   **Other psychoactive substance use,** HCC **unspecified with intoxication, unspecified**

✓6ᵗʰ **F19.93**   **Other psychoactive substance use, unspecified with withdrawal**
> *EXCLUDES 1*   other psychoactive substance use, unspecified with intoxication (F19.92-)

    **F19.930**   **Other psychoactive substance use,** CC HCC **unspecified with withdrawal, uncomplicated**

    **F19.931**   **Other psychoactive substance use,** CC HCC **unspecified with withdrawal delirium**

    **F19.932**   **Other psychoactive substance use,** CC HCC **unspecified with withdrawal with perceptual disturbance**

    **F19.939**   **Other psychoactive substance use,** CC HCC **unspecified with withdrawal, unspecified**

**F19.94**   **Other psychoactive substance use, unspecified** HCC **with psychoactive substance-induced mood disorder**
> Other (or unknown) substance-induced bipolar or related disorder, without use disorder
> Other (or unknown) substance-induced depressive disorder, without use disorder

☑ Additional Character Req    ✓ₓ7ᵗʰ Placeholder Alert    Unacceptable PDx    Manifestation    H1-H14 HAC    HCC CMS-HCC Condition    *EXCLUDES 1* Not Coded Here    *EXCLUDES 2* Not Included Here

ICD-10-CM 2018        545

**✓6ᵗʰ F19.95 Other psychoactive substance use, unspecified with psychoactive substance-induced psychotic disorder**

**F19.950 Other psychoactive substance use,** CC HCC **unspecified with psychoactive substance-induced psychotic disorder with delusions**

**F19.951 Other psychoactive substance use,** CC HCC **unspecified with psychoactive substance-induced psychotic disorder with hallucinations**

**F19.959 Other psychoactive substance use,** HCC **unspecified with psychoactive substance-induced psychotic disorder, unspecified**
     Other or unknown substance-induced psychotic disorder, without use disorder

**F19.96 Other psychoactive substance use, unspecified** HCC **with psychoactive substance-induced persisting amnestic disorder**

**F19.97 Other psychoactive substance use,** CC HCC **unspecified with psychoactive substance-induced persisting dementia**
     Other (or unknown) substance-induced major neurocognitive disorder, without use disorder

**✓6ᵗʰ F19.98 Other psychoactive substance use, unspecified with other psychoactive substance-induced disorders**

**F19.980 Other psychoactive substance use,** HCC **unspecified with psychoactive substance-induced anxiety disorder**
     Other (or unknown) substance-induced anxiety disorder, without use disorder

**F19.981 Other psychoactive substance use,** HCC **unspecified with psychoactive substance-induced sexual dysfunction**
     Other (or unknown) substance-induced sexual dysfunction, without use disorder

**F19.982 Other psychoactive substance use,** HCC **unspecified with psychoactive substance-induced sleep disorder**
     Other (or unknown) substance-induced sleep disorder, without use disorder

**F19.988 Other psychoactive substance use,** HCC **unspecified with other psychoactive substance-induced disorder**
     Other (or unknown) substance-induced mild neurocognitive disorder, without use disorder
     Other (or unknown) substance-induced obsessive-compulsive or related disorder, without use disorder

**F19.99 Other psychoactive substance use, unspecified** HCC **with unspecified psychoactive substance-induced disorder**

### Schizophrenia, schizotypal, delusional, and other non-mood psychotic disorders (F20-F29)

**✓4ᵗʰ F20 Schizophrenia**
     *EXCLUDES 1*   brief psychotic disorder (F23)
         cyclic schizophrenia (F25.0)
         mood [affective] disorders with psychotic symptoms (F30.2, F31.2, F31.5, F31.64, F32.3, F33.3)
         schizoaffective disorder (F25.-)
         schizophrenic reaction NOS (F23)
     *EXCLUDES 2*   schizophrenic reaction in:
         alcoholism (F10.15-, F10.25-, F10.95-)
         brain disease (F06.2)
         epilepsy (F06.2)
         psychoactive drug use (F11-F19 with .15..25, .95)
         schizotypal disorder (F21)
     **DEF:** Group of disorders with disturbances in thought (delusions, hallucinations), mood (blunted, flattened, inappropriate affect), sense of self; also bizarre, purposeless behavior, repetitive activity, or inactivity.

     **CC Excl: For CC codes in category F20:** PDX collection 551

**F20.0 Paranoid schizophrenia** CC HCC
     Paraphrenic schizophrenia
     *EXCLUDES 1*   involutional paranoid state (F22)
         paranoia (F22)
     **DEF:** Preoccupied with delusional suspicions and auditory hallucinations related to single theme; usually hostile, grandiose, threatening, persecutory, occasionally hypochondriacal.

**F20.1 Disorganized schizophrenia** CC HCC
     Hebephrenic schizophrenia
     Hebephrenia

**F20.2 Catatonic schizophrenia** CC HCC
     Schizophrenic catalepsy
     Schizophrenic catatonia
     Schizophrenic flexibilitas cerea
     *EXCLUDES 1*   catatonic stupor (R40.1)
     **DEF:** Extreme changes in motor activity; one extreme is decreased response or reaction to the environment and the other is spontaneous activity.

**F20.3 Undifferentiated schizophrenia** HCC
     Atypical schizophrenia
     *EXCLUDES 1*   acute schizophrenia-like psychotic disorder (F23)
     *EXCLUDES 2*   post-schizophrenic depression (F32.89)

**F20.5 Residual schizophrenia** CC HCC
     Restzustand (schizophrenic)
     Schizophrenic residual state

**✓5ᵗʰ F20.8 Other schizophrenia**

**F20.81 Schizophreniform disorder** CC HCC
     Schizophreniform psychosis NOS

**F20.89 Other schizophrenia** CC HCC
     Cenesthopathic schizophrenia
     Simple schizophrenia

**F20.9 Schizophrenia, unspecified** HCC

**F21 Schizotypal disorder**
     Borderline schizophrenia
     Latent schizophrenia
     Latent schizophrenic reaction
     Prepsychotic schizophrenia
     Prodromal schizophrenia
     Pseudoneurotic schizophrenia
     Pseudopsychopathic schizophrenia
     Schizotypal personality disorder
     *EXCLUDES 2*   Asperger's syndrome (F84.5)
         schizoid personality disorder (F60.1)

**F22 Delusional disorders** HCC
     Delusional dysmorphophobia
     Involutional paranoid state
     Paranoia
     Paranoia querulans
     Paranoid psychosis
     Paranoid state
     Paraphrenia (late)
     Sensitiver Beziehungswahn
     *EXCLUDES 1*   mood [affective] disorders with psychotic symptoms (F30.2, F31.2, F31.5, F31.64, F32.3, F33.3)
         paranoid schizophrenia (F20.0)
     *EXCLUDES 2*   paranoid personality disorder (F60.0)
         paranoid psychosis, psychogenic (F23)
         paranoid reaction (F23)

**F23 Brief psychotic disorder** CC
     Paranoid reaction
     Psychogenic paranoid psychosis
     *EXCLUDES 2*   mood [affective] disorders with psychotic symptoms (F30.2, F31.2, F31.5, F31.64, F32.3, F33.3)
     **CC Excl: No Excl**

**F24 Shared psychotic disorder** HCC
     Folie à deux
     Induced paranoid disorder
     Induced psychotic disorder

**✓4ᵗʰ F25 Schizoaffective disorders**
     *EXCLUDES 1*   mood [affective] disorders with psychotic symptoms (F30.2, F31.2, F31.5, F31.64, F32.3, F33.3)
         schizophrenia (F20.-)

**F25.0 Schizoaffective disorder, bipolar type** HCC
     Cyclic schizophrenia
     Schizoaffective disorder, manic type
     Schizoaffective disorder, mixed type
     Schizoaffective psychosis, bipolar type
     ~~Schizophreniform psychosis, manic type~~

**F25.1 Schizoaffective disorder, depressive type** HCC
     Schizoaffective psychosis, depressive type
     ~~Schizophreniform psychosis, depressive type~~

**F25.8 Other schizoaffective disorders** HCC

**F25.9 Schizoaffective disorder, unspecified** HCC
     Schizoaffective psychosis NOS

---

N Newborn: 0   P Pediatric: 0-17   M Maternity: 12-55   A Adult: 15-124   **MCC** Major CC Condition   **PDx MCC** PDx acts as own MCC   **CC** CC Condition   **PDx CC** PDx acts as own CC

546      ICD-10-CM 2018

**F28** **Other psychotic disorder not due to a substance or known** `HIV`
**physiological condition**
Chronic hallucinatory psychosis
▶Other specified schizophrenia spectrum and other psychotic disorder◀

**F29** **Unspecified psychosis not due to a substance or known** `HIV`
**physiological condition**
Chronic hallucinatory psychosis
▶Unspecified schizophrenia spectrum and other psychotic disorder◀
`EXCLUDES 1` *mental disorder NOS (F99)*
*unspecified mental disorder due to known physiological*
*condition (F09)*

## Mood [affective] disorders (F30-F39)

`✓4ᵗʰ` **F30** **Manic episode**
`INCLUDES` bipolar disorder, single manic episode
mixed affective episode
`EXCLUDES 1` *bipolar disorder (F31.-)*
*major depressive disorder, recurrent (F33.-)*
*major depressive disorder, single episode (F32.-)*

**CC Excl: For CC codes in category F30, unless otherwise noted:**
PDX collection 551

`✓5ᵗʰ` **F30.1** **Manic episode without psychotic symptoms**
**F30.10** **Manic episode without psychotic symptoms,** `CC` `HCC`
**unspecified**
**F30.11** **Manic episode without psychotic symptoms,** `CC` `HCC`
**mild**
**F30.12** **Manic episode without psychotic symptoms,** `CC` `HCC`
**moderate**
**F30.13** **Manic episode, severe, without psychotic** `CC` `HCC`
**symptoms**
**CC Excl:** PDX collection 552

**F30.2** **Manic episode, severe with psychotic symptoms** `CC` `HCC`
Manic stupor
Mania with mood-congruent psychotic symptoms
Mania with mood-incongruent psychotic symptoms

**F30.3** **Manic episode in partial remission** `HCC`

**F30.4** **Manic episode in full remission** `HCC`

**F30.8** **Other manic episodes** `HCC`
Hypomania

**F30.9** **Manic episode, unspecified** `CC` `HCC`
Mania NOS

`✓4ᵗʰ` **F31** **Bipolar disorder**
`INCLUDES` ▶bipolar I disorder
bipolar type I disorder◀
manic-depressive illness
manic-depressive psychosis
manic-depressive reaction
`EXCLUDES 1` *bipolar disorder, single manic episode (F30.-)*
*major depressive disorder, single episode (F32.-)*
*major depressive disorder, recurrent (F33.-)*
`EXCLUDES 2` *cyclothymia (F34.0)*

**CC Excl: For CC codes in category F31, unless otherwise noted:**
PDX collection 551

**F31.0** **Bipolar disorder, current episode hypomanic** `CC` `HCC`

`✓5ᵗʰ` **F31.1** **Bipolar disorder, current episode manic without psychotic**
**features**
• **F31.10** **Bipolar disorder, current episode manic** `CC` `HCC`
**without psychotic features, unspecified**
**F31.11** **Bipolar disorder, current episode manic** `CC` `HCC`
**without psychotic features, mild**
**F31.12** **Bipolar disorder, current episode manic** `CC` `HCC`
**without psychotic features, moderate**
**F31.13** **Bipolar disorder, current episode manic** `CC` `HCC`
**without psychotic features, severe**
**CC Excl:** PDX collection 553

**F31.2** **Bipolar disorder, current episode manic severe with** `CC` `HCC`
**psychotic features**
Bipolar disorder, current episode manic with mood-congruent
psychotic symptoms
Bipolar disorder, current episode manic with mood-incongruent
psychotic symptoms
▶Bipolar I disorder, current or most recent episode manic with
psychotic features◀

`✓5ᵗʰ` **F31.3** **Bipolar disorder, current episode depressed, mild or**
**moderate severity**
**F31.30** **Bipolar disorder, current episode depressed,** `CC` `HCC`
**mild or moderate severity, unspecified**

**F31.31** **Bipolar disorder, current episode depressed,** `CC` `HCC`
**mild**
**F31.32** **Bipolar disorder, current episode depressed,** `CC` `HCC`
**moderate**

**F31.4** **Bipolar disorder, current episode depressed, severe,** `CC` `HCC`
**without psychotic features**
**CC Excl:** PDX collection 554

**F31.5** **Bipolar disorder, current episode depressed, severe,** `CC` `HCC`
**with psychotic features**
Bipolar disorder, current episode depressed with mood-
incongruent psychotic symptoms
Bipolar disorder, current episode depressed with mood-
congruent psychotic symptoms
▶Bipolar I disorder, current or most recent episode depressed, with
psychotic features◀

`✓5ᵗʰ` **F31.6** **Bipolar disorder, current episode mixed**
**F31.60** **Bipolar disorder, current episode mixed,** `CC` `HCC`
**unspecified**
**F31.61** **Bipolar disorder, current episode mixed,** `CC` `HCC`
**mild**
**F31.62** **Bipolar disorder, current episode mixed,** `CC` `HCC`
**moderate**
**F31.63** **Bipolar disorder, current episode mixed,** `CC` `HCC`
**severe, without psychotic features**
**CC Excl:** PDX collection 554
**F31.64** **Bipolar disorder, current episode mixed,** `CC` `HCC`
**severe, with psychotic features**
Bipolar disorder, current episode mixed with mood-
congruent psychotic symptoms
Bipolar disorder, current episode mixed with mood-
incongruent psychotic symptoms

`✓5ᵗʰ` **F31.7** **Bipolar disorder, currently in remission**
**F31.70** **Bipolar disorder, currently in remission, most** `HCC`
**recent episode unspecified**
**F31.71** **Bipolar disorder, in partial remission, most** `HCC`
**recent episode hypomanic**
**F31.72** **Bipolar disorder, in full remission, most** `HCC`
**recent episode hypomanic**
**F31.73** **Bipolar disorder, in partial remission, most** `HCC`
**recent episode manic**
**F31.74** **Bipolar disorder, in full remission, most** `HCC`
**recent episode manic**
**F31.75** **Bipolar disorder, in partial remission, most** `HCC`
**recent episode depressed**
**F31.76** **Bipolar disorder, in full remission, most** `HCC`
**recent episode depressed**
**F31.77** **Bipolar disorder, in partial remission, most** `HCC`
**recent episode mixed**
**F31.78** **Bipolar disorder, in full remission, most** `HCC`
**recent episode mixed**

`✓5ᵗʰ` **F31.8** **Other bipolar disorders**
**F31.81** **Bipolar II disorder** `CC` `HCC`
▶Bipolar disorder, type 2◀
**F31.89** **Other bipolar disorder** `CC` `HCC`
Recurrent manic episodes NOS

**F31.9** **Bipolar disorder, unspecified** `HCC`
▶Manic depression◀

`✓4ᵗʰ` **F32** **Major depressive disorder, single episode**
`INCLUDES` single episode of agitated depression
single episode of depressive reaction
single episode of major depression
single episode of psychogenic depression
single episode of reactive depression
single episode of vital depression
`EXCLUDES 1` *bipolar disorder (F31.-)*
*manic episode (F30.-)*
*recurrent depressive disorder (F33.-)*
`EXCLUDES 2` *adjustment disorder (F43.2)*
**DEF:** Mood disorder that produces depression; may exhibit as sadness, low
self-esteem, or guilt feelings; other manifestations may be withdrawal
from friends and family and interrupted sleep.

**CC Excl: For CC codes in category F32:** PDX collection 555

**F32.0** **Major depressive disorder, single episode, mild** `CC` `HCC`
**F32.1** **Major depressive disorder, single episode, moderate** `CC` `HCC`
**F32.2** **Major depressive disorder, single episode, severe** `CC` `HCC`
**without psychotic features**

**Chapter 5. Mental, Behavioral and Neurodevelopmental Disorders**

**F32.3   Major depressive disorder, single episode, severe with psychotic features**   CC HCC
Single episode of major depression with mood-congruent psychotic symptoms
Single episode of major depression with mood-incongruent psychotic symptoms
Single episode of major depression with psychotic symptoms
Single episode of psychogenic depressive psychosis
Single episode of psychotic depression
Single episode of reactive depressive psychosis

**F32.4   Major depressive disorder, single episode, in partial remission**   HCC

**F32.5   Major depressive disorder, single episode, in full remission**   HCC

✓5ᵗʰ **F32.8   Other depressive episodes**

     **F32.81   Premenstrual dysphoric disorder**   ♀
        *EXCLUDES 1*   premenstrual tension syndrome (N94.3)

     **F32.89   Other specified depressive episodes**
        Atypical depression
        Post-schizophrenic depression
        Single episode of 'masked' depression NOS

**F32.9   Major depressive disorder, single episode, unspecified**
Depression NOS
Depressive disorder NOS
Major depression NOS
**AHA:** 2013, 4Q, 107

✓4ᵗʰ **F33   Major depressive disorder, recurrent**
   *INCLUDES*   recurrent episodes of depressive reaction
          recurrent episodes of endogenous depression
          recurrent episodes of major depression
          recurrent episodes of psychogenic depression
          recurrent episodes of reactive depression
          recurrent episodes of seasonal depressive disorder
          recurrent episodes of vital depression
   *EXCLUDES 1*   bipolar disorder (F31.-)
           manic episode (F30.-)

   **CC Excl: For CC codes in category F33, unless otherwise noted:** PDX collection 555

**F33.0   Major depressive disorder, recurrent, mild**   CC HCC

**F33.1   Major depressive disorder, recurrent, moderate**   CC HCC

**F33.2   Major depressive disorder, recurrent, severe without psychotic features**   CC HCC

**F33.3   Major depressive disorder, recurrent, severe with psychotic symptoms**   CC HCC
Endogenous depression with psychotic symptoms
▶Major depressive disorder, recurrent, with psychotic features◀
Recurrent severe episodes of major depression with mood-congruent psychotic symptoms
Recurrent severe episodes of major depression with mood-incongruent psychotic symptoms
Recurrent severe episodes of major depression with psychotic symptoms
Recurrent severe episodes of psychogenic depressive psychosis
Recurrent severe episodes of psychotic depression
Recurrent severe episodes of reactive depression psychosis
**CC Excl:** PDX collection 551

✓5ᵗʰ **F33.4   Major depressive disorder, recurrent, in remission**

     **F33.40   Major depressive disorder, recurrent, in remission, unspecified**   CC HCC

     **F33.41   Major depressive disorder, recurrent, in partial remission**   HCC

     **F33.42   Major depressive disorder, recurrent, in full remission**   HCC

**F33.8   Other recurrent depressive disorders**   HCC
Recurrent brief depressive episodes
**CC Excl:** PDX collection 551

**F33.9   Major depressive disorder, recurrent, unspecified**   CC HCC
Monopolar depression NOS

✓4ᵗʰ **F34   Persistent mood [affective] disorders**

**F34.0   Cyclothymic disorder**
Affective personality disorder
Cycloid personality
Cyclothymia
Cyclothymic personality

**F34.1   Dysthymic disorder**
Depressive neurosis
Depressive personality disorder
Dysthymia
Neurotic depression
Persistent anxiety depression
Persistent depressive disorder
   *EXCLUDES 2*   anxiety depression (mild or not persistent) (F41.8)
**DEF:** Depression without psychosis; less severe but persistent depression; is considered a mild to moderate chronic form of depression.

✓5ᵗʰ **F34.8   Other persistent mood [affective] disorders**

     **F34.81   Disruptive mood dysregulation disorder**   CC HCC
          **CC Excl:** PDX collection 551

     **F34.89   Other specified persistent mood disorders**   CC HCC
          **CC Excl:** PDX collection 551

**F34.9   Persistent mood [affective] disorder, unspecified**   CC HCC
**CC Excl:** PDX collection 551

**F39   Unspecified mood [affective] disorder**   HCC
Affective psychosis NOS

## Anxiety, dissociative, stress-related, somatoform and other nonpsychotic mental disorders (F40-F48)

✓4ᵗʰ **F40   Phobic anxiety disorders**

✓5ᵗʰ **F40.0   Agoraphobia**
**DEF:** Profound anxiety or fear of leaving familiar settings like home, or being in unfamiliar locations or with strangers or crowds; may or may not be preceded by recurrent panic attacks.

     **F40.00   Agoraphobia, unspecified**

     **F40.01   Agoraphobia with panic disorder**
        Panic disorder with agoraphobia
        *EXCLUDES 1*   panic disorder without agoraphobia (F41.0)

     **F40.02   Agoraphobia without panic disorder**

✓5ᵗʰ **F40.1   Social phobias**
Anthropophobia
▶Social anxiety disorder◀
Social anxiety disorder of childhood
Social neurosis

     **F40.10   Social phobia, unspecified**

     **F40.11   Social phobia, generalized**

✓5ᵗʰ **F40.2   Specific (isolated) phobias**
   *EXCLUDES 2*   dysmorphophobia (nondelusional) (F45.22)
           nosophobia (F45.22)

  ✓6ᵗʰ **F40.21   Animal type phobia**
       **F40.210   Arachnophobia**
           Fear of spiders
       **F40.218   Other animal type phobia**

  ✓6ᵗʰ **F40.22   Natural environment type phobia**
       **F40.220   Fear of thunderstorms**
       **F40.228   Other natural environment type phobia**

  ✓6ᵗʰ **F40.23   Blood, injection, injury type phobia**
       **F40.230   Fear of blood**
       **F40.231   Fear of injections and transfusions**
       **F40.232   Fear of other medical care**
       **F40.233   Fear of injury**

  ✓6ᵗʰ **F40.24   Situational type phobia**
       **F40.240   Claustrophobia**
       **F40.241   Acrophobia**
       **F40.242   Fear of bridges**
       **F40.243   Fear of flying**
       **F40.248   Other situational type phobia**

  ✓6ᵗʰ **F40.29   Other specified phobia**
       **F40.290   Androphobia**
           Fear of men
       **F40.291   Gynephobia**
           Fear of women
       **F40.298   Other specified phobia**

**F40.8   Other phobic anxiety disorders**
Phobic anxiety disorder of childhood

**F40.9   Phobic anxiety disorder, unspecified**
Phobia NOS
Phobic state NOS

N Newborn: 0   P Pediatric: 0-17   M Maternity: 12-55   A Adult: 15-124   MCC Major CC Condition   PDxMCC PDx acts as own MCC   CC CC Condition   PDxCC PDx acts as own CC

548          ICD-10-CM 2018

## ☑4ᵗʰ F41 Other anxiety disorders

EXCLUDES 2    anxiety in:
      acute stress reaction (F43.Ø)
      transient adjustment reaction (F43.2)
      neurasthenia (F48.8)
      psychophysiologic disorders (F45.-)
      separation anxiety (F93.Ø)

▲    **F41.Ø**   Panic disorder [episodic paroxysmal anxiety]
       Panic attack
       Panic state
       EXCLUDES 1   panic disorder with agoraphobia (F40.Ø1)
       **DEF:** Neurotic disorder characterized by recurrent panic or anxiety, apprehension, fear, or terror; symptoms include shortness of breath, palpitations, dizziness, shakiness; fear of dying may persist.

**F41.1**   Generalized anxiety disorder
       Anxiety neurosis
       Anxiety reaction
       Anxiety state
       Overanxious disorder
       EXCLUDES 2   neurasthenia (F48.8)

**F41.3**   Other mixed anxiety disorders

**F41.8**   Other specified anxiety disorders
       Anxiety depression (mild or not persistent)
       Anxiety hysteria
       Mixed anxiety and depressive disorder

**F41.9**   Anxiety disorder, unspecified
       Anxiety NOS

## ☑4ᵗʰ F42 Obsessive-compulsive disorder

EXCLUDES 2   obsessive-compulsive personality (disorder) (F60.5)
      obsessive-compulsive symptoms occurring in depression (F32-F33)
      obsessive-compulsive symptoms occurring in schizophrenia (F20.-)

**F42.2**   Mixed obsessional thoughts and acts

**F42.3**   Hoarding disorder

**F42.4**   Excoriation (skin-picking) disorder
       EXCLUDES 1   factitial dermatitis (L98.1)
           other specified behavioral and emotional disorders with onset usually occurring in early childhood and adolescence (F98.8)

**F42.8**   Other obsessive-compulsive disorder
       Anancastic neurosis
       Obsessive-compulsive neurosis

**F42.9**   Obsessive-compulsive disorder, unspecified

## ☑4ᵗʰ F43 Reaction to severe stress, and adjustment disorders

**F43.Ø**   Acute stress reaction
       Acute crisis reaction
       Acute reaction to stress
       Combat and operational stress reaction
       Combat fatigue
       Crisis state
       Psychic shock

☑5ᵗʰ **F43.1**   Post-traumatic stress disorder (PTSD)
       Traumatic neurosis
       **DEF:** Preoccupation with traumatic events beyond normal experience; i.e., rape, personal assault, etc.; also recurring flashbacks of trauma; symptoms include difficulty remembering, sleeping, or concentrating, and guilt feelings for surviving.

     **F43.10**   Post-traumatic stress disorder, unspecified

     **F43.11**   Post-traumatic stress disorder, acute

     **F43.12**   Post-traumatic stress disorder, chronic

☑5ᵗʰ **F43.2**   Adjustment disorders
       Culture shock
       Grief reaction
       Hospitalism in children
       EXCLUDES 2   separation anxiety disorder of childhood (F93.Ø)

     **F43.20**   Adjustment disorder, unspecified

     **F43.21**   Adjustment disorder with depressed mood
           **AHA:** 2014, 1Q, 25

     **F43.22**   Adjustment disorder with anxiety

     **F43.23**   Adjustment disorder with mixed anxiety and depressed mood

     **F43.24**   Adjustment disorder with disturbance of conduct

     **F43.25**   Adjustment disorder with mixed disturbance of emotions and conduct

     **F43.29**   Adjustment disorder with other symptoms

**F43.8**   Other reactions to severe stress
       Other specified trauma and stressor-related disorder

**F43.9**   Reaction to severe stress, unspecified
       Trauma and stressor-related disorder, NOS

## ☑4ᵗʰ F44 Dissociative and conversion disorders

INCLUDES    conversion hysteria
      conversion reaction
      hysteria
      hysterical psychosis
EXCLUDES 2   malingering [conscious simulation] (Z76.5)

**F44.Ø**   Dissociative amnesia
       EXCLUDES 1   amnesia NOS (R41.3)
           anterograde amnesia (R41.1)
           dissociative amnesia with dissociative fugue (F44.1)
           retrograde amnesia (R41.2)
       EXCLUDES 2   alcohol-or other psychoactive substance-induced amnestic disorder (F1Ø, F13, F19 with .26, .96)
           amnestic disorder due to known physiological condition (FØ4)
           postictal amnesia in epilepsy (G4Ø.-)

**F44.1**   Dissociative fugue
       Dissociative amnesia with dissociative fugue
       EXCLUDES 2   postictal fugue in epilepsy (G4Ø.-)
       **DEF:** Dissociative hysteria; identified by loss of memory, flight from familiar surroundings to a completely separate environment, episodes may last hours or days; conscious activity is not associated with perception of surroundings and there is no later memory of episode.

**F44.2**   Dissociative stupor
       EXCLUDES 1   catatonic stupor (R4Ø.1)
           stupor NOS (R4Ø.1)
       EXCLUDES 2   catatonic disorder due to known physiological condition (FØ6.1)
           depressive stupor (F32, F33)
           manic stupor (F3Ø, F31)

**F44.4**   Conversion disorder with motor symptom or deficit
       ▶Conversion disorder with abnormal movement
       Conversion disorder with speech symptoms
       Conversion disorder with swallowing symptoms
       Conversion disorder with weakness/paralysis◀
       Dissociative motor disorders
       Psychogenic aphonia
       Psychogenic dysphonia

**F44.5**   Conversion disorder with seizures or convulsions
       ▶Conversion disorder with attacks or seizures◀
       Dissociative convulsions

**F44.6**   Conversion disorder with sensory symptom or deficit
       ▶Conversion disorder with anesthesia or sensory loss
       Conversion disorder with special sensory symptoms◀
       Dissociative anesthesia and sensory loss
       Psychogenic deafness

**F44.7**   Conversion disorder with mixed symptom presentation

☑5ᵗʰ **F44.8**   Other dissociative and conversion disorders

     **F44.81**   Dissociative identity disorder
           Multiple personality disorder

     **F44.89**   Other dissociative and conversion disorders
           Ganser's syndrome
           Psychogenic confusion
           Psychogenic twilight state
           Trance and possession disorders

**F44.9**   Dissociative and conversion disorder, unspecified
       Dissociative disorder NOS

## ☑4ᵗʰ F45 Somatoform disorders

EXCLUDES 2   dissociative and conversion disorders (F44.-)
      factitious disorders (F68.1-)
      hair-plucking (F63.3)
      lalling (F8Ø.Ø)
      lisping (F8Ø.Ø)
      malingering [conscious simulation] (Z76.5)
      nail-biting (F98.8)
      psychological or behavioral factors associated with disorders or diseases classified elsewhere (F54)
      sexual dysfunction, not due to a substance or known physiological condition (F52.-)
      thumb-sucking (F98.8)
      tic disorders (in childhood and adolescence) (F95.-)
      Tourette's syndrome (F95.2)
      trichotillomania (F63.3)

**F45.Ø**   Somatization disorder
       Briquet's disorder
       Multiple psychosomatic disorder

**F45.1 Undifferentiated somatoform disorder**
Somatic symptom disorder
Undifferentiated psychosomatic disorder

✓5th **F45.2 Hypochondriacal disorders**
EXCLUDES 2 *delusional dysmorphophobia (F22)*
*fixed delusions about bodily functions or shape (F22)*

**F45.20 Hypochondriacal disorder, unspecified**

**F45.21 Hypochondriasis**
Hypochondriacal neurosis
Illness anxiety disorder

**F45.22 Body dysmorphic disorder**
Dysmorphophobia (nondelusional)
Nosophobia

**F45.29 Other hypochondriacal disorders**

✓5th **F45.4 Pain disorders related to psychological factors**
EXCLUDES 1 *pain NOS (R52)*

**F45.41 Pain disorder exclusively related to psychological factors**
Somatoform pain disorder (persistent)

**F45.42 Pain disorder with related psychological factors**
Code also associated acute or chronic pain (G89.-)

**F45.8 Other somatoform disorders**
Psychogenic dysmenorrhea
Psychogenic dysphagia, including "globus hystericus"
Psychogenic pruritus
Psychogenic torticollis
Somatoform autonomic dysfunction
Teeth grinding
EXCLUDES 1 *sleep related teeth grinding (G47.63)*

**F45.9 Somatoform disorder, unspecified**
Psychosomatic disorder NOS

✓4th **F48 Other nonpsychotic mental disorders**

**F48.1 Depersonalization-derealization syndrome**

**F48.2 Pseudobulbar affect**
Involuntary emotional expression disorder
Code first underlying cause, if known, such as:
amyotrophic lateral sclerosis (G12.21)
multiple sclerosis (G35)
sequelae of cerebrovascular disease (I69.-)
sequelae of traumatic intracranial injury (S06.-)

**F48.8 Other specified nonpsychotic mental disorders**
Dhat syndrome
Neurasthenia
Occupational neurosis, including writer's cramp
Psychasthenia
Psychasthenic neurosis
Psychogenic syncope

**F48.9 Nonpsychotic mental disorder, unspecified**
Neurosis NOS

## Behavioral syndromes associated with physiological disturbances and physical factors (F50-F59)

✓4th **F50 Eating disorders**
EXCLUDES 1 *anorexia NOS (R63.0)*
*feeding difficulties (R63.3)*
▶*feeding problems of newborn (P92.-)*◀
*polyphagia (R63.2)*
EXCLUDES 2 *feeding disorder in infancy or childhood (F98.2-)*

**CC Excl: For CC codes in category F50, unless otherwise noted:**
PDX collection 556

✓5th **F50.0 Anorexia nervosa**
EXCLUDES 1 *loss of appetite (R63.0)*
*psychogenic loss of appetite (F50.89)*

**F50.00 Anorexia nervosa, unspecified** CC

**F50.01 Anorexia nervosa, restricting type** CC

**F50.02 Anorexia nervosa, binge eating/purging type** CC
EXCLUDES 1 *bulimia nervosa (F50.2)*

**F50.2 Bulimia nervosa** CC
Bulimia NOS
Hyperorexia nervosa
EXCLUDES 1 *anorexia nervosa, binge eating/purging type (F50.02)*
**CC Excl: PDX collection 557**

✓5th **F50.8 Other eating disorders**
EXCLUDES 2 *pica of infancy and childhood (F98.3)*

**F50.81 Binge eating disorder**

**F50.82 Avoidant/restrictive food intake disorder**

**F50.89 Other specified eating disorder**
Pica in adults
Psychogenic loss of appetite

**F50.9 Eating disorder, unspecified**
Atypical anorexia nervosa
Atypical bulimia nervosa
▶Feeding or eating disorder, unspecified
Other specified feeding disorder ◀

✓4th **F51 Sleep disorders not due to a substance or known physiological condition**
EXCLUDES 2 *organic sleep disorders (G47.-)*

✓5th **F51.0 Insomnia not due to a substance or known physiological condition**
EXCLUDES 2 *alcohol related insomnia (F10.182, F10.282, F10.982)*
*drug-related insomnia (F11.182, F11.282, F11.982, F13.182, F13.282, F13.982, F14.182, F14.282, F14.982, F15.182, F15.282, F15.982, F19.182, F19.282, F19.982)*
*insomnia NOS (G47.0-)*
*insomnia due to known physiological condition (G47.0-)*
*organic insomnia (G47.0-)*
*sleep deprivation (Z72.820)*

**F51.01 Primary insomnia**
Idiopathic insomnia

**F51.02 Adjustment insomnia**

**F51.03 Paradoxical insomnia**

**F51.04 Psychophysiologic insomnia**

**F51.05 Insomnia due to other mental disorder**
Code also associated mental disorder

**F51.09 Other insomnia not due to a substance or known physiological condition**

✓5th **F51.1 Hypersomnia not due to a substance or known physiological condition**
EXCLUDES 2 *alcohol related hypersomnia (F10.182, F10.282, F10.982)*
*drug-related hypersomnia (F11.182, F11.282, F11.982, F13.182, F13.282, F13.982, F14.182, F14.282, F14.982, F15.182, F15.282, F15.982, F19.182, F19.282, F19.982)*
*hypersomnia NOS (G47.10)*
*hypersomnia due to known physiological condition (G47.10)*
*idiopathic hypersomnia (G47.11, G47.12)*
*narcolepsy (G47.4-)*

**F51.11 Primary hypersomnia**

**F51.12 Insufficient sleep syndrome**
EXCLUDES 1 *sleep deprivation (Z72.820)*

**F51.13 Hypersomnia due to other mental disorder**
Code also associated mental disorder

**F51.19 Other hypersomnia not due to a substance or known physiological condition**

**F51.3 Sleepwalking [somnambulism]**
▶Non–rapid eye movement sleep arousal disorders, sleepwalking type◀

**F51.4 Sleep terrors [night terrors]**
▶Non–rapid eye movement sleep arousal disorders, sleep terror type◀

**F51.5 Nightmare disorder**
Dream anxiety disorder

**F51.8 Other sleep disorders not due to a substance or known physiological condition**

**F51.9 Sleep disorder not due to a substance or known physiological condition, unspecified**
Emotional sleep disorder NOS

✓4th **F52 Sexual dysfunction not due to a substance or known physiological condition**
EXCLUDES 2 *Dhat syndrome (F48.8)*

**F52.0 Hypoactive sexual desire disorder**
Lack or loss of sexual desire
▶Male hypoactive sexual desire disorder◀
Sexual anhedonia
EXCLUDES 1 *decreased libido (R68.82)*

**F52.1 Sexual aversion disorder**
Sexual aversion and lack of sexual enjoyment

✓5th **F52.2 Sexual arousal disorders**
Failure of genital response

**F52.21**    Male **erectile disorder**        ♂
- ►Erectile disorder◄
- Psychogenic impotence
  - *EXCLUDES 1*   *impotence of organic origin (N52.-)*
  - *impotence NOS (N52.-)*

**F52.22**    Female **sexual arousal disorder**       ♀
- ►Female sexual interest/arousal disorder◄

✓5th   **F52.3**   **Orgasmic disorder**
- Inhibited orgasm
- Psychogenic anorgasmy

**F52.31**    Female **orgasmic disorder**       ♀

**F52.32**    Male **orgasmic disorder**       ♂
- Delayed ejaculation

**F52.4**   **Premature ejaculation**       ♂

**F52.5**   **Vaginismus not due to a substance or known**       ♀
**physiological condition**
- Psychogenic vaginismus
  - *EXCLUDES 2*   *vaginismus (due to a known physiological condition) (N94.2)*
- **DEF:** Psychogenic response resulting in painful contractions of vaginal canal muscles; can be severe enough to prevent sexual intercourse.

**F52.6**   **Dyspareunia not due to a substance or known physiological condition**
- Genito-pelvic pain penetration disorderPsychogenic dyspareunia
  - *EXCLUDES 2*   *dyspareunia (due to a known physiological condition) (N94.1-)*

**F52.8**   **Other sexual dysfunction not due to a substance or known physiological condition**
- Excessive sexual drive
- Nymphomania
- Satyriasis

**F52.9**   **Unspecified sexual dysfunction not due to a substance or known physiological condition**
- Sexual dysfunction NOS

**F53**   **Puerperal psychosis**       M ♀
- Postpartum depression
  - *EXCLUDES 1*   *mood disorders with psychotic features (F30.2, F31.2, F31.5, F31.64, F32.3, F33.3)*
  - *postpartum dysphoria (O90.6)*
  - *psychosis in schizophrenia, schizotypal, delusional, and other psychotic disorders (F20-F29)*

**F54**   *Psychological and behavioral factors associated with disorders or diseases classified elsewhere*
- Psychological factors affecting physical conditions
- Code first the associated physical disorder, such as:
  - asthma (J45.-)
  - dermatitis (L23-L25)
  - gastric ulcer (K25.-)
  - mucous colitis (K58.-)
  - ulcerative colitis (K51.-)
  - urticaria (L50.-)
  - *EXCLUDES 2*   *tension-type headache (G44.2)*

✓4th   **F55**   **Abuse of non-psychoactive substances**
- *EXCLUDES 2*   *abuse of psychoactive substances (F10-F19)*

**F55.0**   **Abuse of** antacids

**F55.1**   **Abuse of** herbal or folk remedies

**F55.2**   **Abuse of** laxatives

**F55.3**   **Abuse of** steroids or hormones

**F55.4**   **Abuse of** vitamins

**F55.8**   **Abuse of** other non-psychoactive substances

**F59**   **Unspecified behavioral syndromes associated with physiological disturbances and physical factors**
- Psychogenic physiological dysfunction NOS

## Disorders of adult personality and behavior (F60-F69)

✓4th   **F60**   **Specific personality disorders**

**F60.0**   **Paranoid personality disorder**
- Expansive paranoid personality (disorder)
- Fanatic personality (disorder)
- Paranoid personality (disorder)
- Querulant personality (disorder)
- Sensitive paranoid personality (disorder)
  - *EXCLUDES 2*   *paranoia (F22)*
  - *paranoia querulans (F22)*
  - *paranoid psychosis (F22)*
  - *paranoid schizophrenia (F20.0)*
  - *paranoid state (F22)*

**F60.1**   **Schizoid personality disorder**
- *EXCLUDES 2*   *Asperger's syndrome (F84.5)*
- *delusional disorder (F22)*
- *schizoid disorder of childhood (F84.5)*
- *schizophrenia (F20.-)*
- *schizotypal disorder (F21)*

**F60.2**   **Antisocial personality disorder**
- Amoral personality (disorder)
- Asocial personality (disorder)
- Dissocial personality disorder
- Psychopathic personality (disorder)
- Sociopathic personality (disorder)
  - *EXCLUDES 1*   *conduct disorders (F91.-)*
  - *EXCLUDES 2*   *borderline personality disorder (F60.3)*

**F60.3**   **Borderline personality disorder**
- Aggressive personality (disorder)
- Emotionally unstable personality disorder
- Explosive personality (disorder)
  - *EXCLUDES 2*   *antisocial personality disorder (F60.2)*

**F60.4**   **Histrionic personality disorder**
- Hysterical personality (disorder)
- Psychoinfantile personality (disorder)

**F60.5**   **Obsessive-compulsive personality disorder**
- Anankastic personality (disorder)
- Compulsive personality (disorder)
- Obsessional personality (disorder)
  - *EXCLUDES 2*   *obsessive-compulsive disorder (F42-)*

**F60.6**   **Avoidant personality disorder**
- Anxious personality disorder

**F60.7**   **Dependent personality disorder**
- Asthenic personality (disorder)
- Inadequate personality (disorder)
- Passive personality (disorder)

✓5th   **F60.8**   **Other specific personality disorders**

**F60.81**   **Narcissistic personality disorder**

**F60.89**   **Other specific personality disorders**
- Eccentric personality disorder
- "Haltlose" type personality disorder
- Immature personality disorder
- Passive-aggressive personality disorder
- Psychoneurotic personality disorder
- Self-defeating personality disorder

**F60.9**   **Personality disorder, unspecified**
- Character disorder NOS
- Character neurosis NOS
- Pathological personality NOS

✓4th   **F63**   **Impulse disorders**
- *EXCLUDES 2*   *habitual excessive use of alcohol or psychoactive substances (F10-F19)*
- *impulse disorders involving sexual behavior (F65.-)*

**F63.0**   **Pathological gambling**
- Compulsive gambling
- ►Gambling disorder◄
  - *EXCLUDES 1*   *gambling and betting NOS (Z72.6)*
  - *EXCLUDES 2*   *excessive gambling by manic patients (F30, F31)*
  - *gambling in antisocial personality disorder (F60.2)*

**F63.1**   **Pyromania**
- Pathological fire-setting
  - *EXCLUDES 2*   *fire-setting (by) (in):*
    - *adult with antisocial personality disorder (F60.2)*
    - *alcohol or psychoactive substance intoxication (F10-F19)*
    - *conduct disorders (F91.-)*
    - *mental disorders due to known physiological condition (F01-F09)*
    - *schizophrenia (F20.-)*

---

✓ Additional Character Req    ✓x7th Placeholder Alert    Unacceptable PDx    Manifestation    H1-H14 HAC    HCC CMS-HCC Condition    *EXCLUDES 1* Not Coded Here    *EXCLUDES 2* Not Included Here

**F63.2   Kleptomania**
Pathological stealing
> *EXCLUDES 1*   shoplifting as the reason for observation for suspected mental disorder (Z03.8)
> *EXCLUDES 2*   depressive disorder with stealing (F31-F33)
> stealing due to underlying mental condition—code to mental condition
> stealing in mental disorders due to known physiological condition (F01-F09)

**F63.3   Trichotillomania**
Hair plucking
> *EXCLUDES 2*   other stereotyped movement disorder (F98.4)

√5th **F63.8   Other impulse disorders**
    **F63.81   Intermittent explosive disorder**
    **F63.89   Other impulse disorders**

**F63.9   Impulse disorder, unspecified**
Impulse control disorder NOS

√4th **F64   Gender identity disorders**
    **F64.0   Transsexualism**
       Gender identity disorder in adolescence and adulthood
       Gender dysphoria in adolescents and adults

    **F64.1   Dual role transvestism**
       Use additional code to identify sex reassignment status (Z87.890)
> *EXCLUDES 1*   gender identity disorder in childhood (F64.2)
> *EXCLUDES 2*   fetishistic transvestism (F65.1)

    **F64.2   Gender identity disorder of childhood**   P
       Gender dysphoria in children
> *EXCLUDES 1*   gender identity disorder in adolescence and adulthood (F64.0)
> *EXCLUDES 2*   sexual maturation disorder (F66)

    **F64.8   Other gender identity disorders**
       ►Other specified gender dysphoria◄

    **F64.9   Gender identity disorder, unspecified**
       ►Gender dysphoria, unspecified◄
       Gender-role disorder NOS

√4th **F65   Paraphilias**
    **F65.0   Fetishism**
       ►Fetishistic disorder◄

    **F65.1   Transvestic fetishism**
       Fetishistic transvestism
       ►Transvestic disorder◄

    **F65.2   Exhibitionism**
       ►Exhibitionistic disorder◄

    **F65.3   Voyeurism**
       ►Voyeuristic disorder◄

    **F65.4   Pedophilia**
       ►Pedophilic disorder◄

√5th **F65.5   Sadomasochism**
    **F65.50   Sadomasochism, unspecified**
    **F65.51   Sexual masochism**
       ►Sexual masochism disorder◄
    **F65.52   Sexual sadism**
       ►Sexual sadism disorder◄

√5th **F65.8   Other paraphilias**
    **F65.81   Frotteurism**
       ►Frotteuristic disorder◄
    **F65.89   Other paraphilias**
       Necrophilia
       ►Other specified paraphilic disorder◄

    **F65.9   Paraphilia, unspecified**
       ►Paraphilic disorder, unspecified◄
       Sexual deviation NOS

**F66   Other sexual disorders**
Sexual maturation disorder
Sexual relationship disorder

√4th **F68   Other disorders of adult personality and behavior**
√5th **F68.1   Factitious disorder**
       Compensation neurosis
       Elaboration of physical symptoms for psychological reasons
       Hospital hopper syndrome
       Münchhausen's syndrome
       Peregrinating patient
> *EXCLUDES 2*   factitial dermatitis (L98.1)
> person feigning illness (with obvious motivation) (Z76.5)

**F68.10   Factitious disorder, unspecified**   CC
       **CC Excl:** PDX collection 551

**F68.11   Factitious disorder with predominantly psychological signs and symptoms**

**F68.12   Factitious disorder with predominantly physical signs and symptoms**   CC
       **CC Excl:** PDX collection 551

**F68.13   Factitious disorder with combined psychological and physical signs and symptoms**

**F68.8   Other specified disorders of adult personality and behavior**

**F69   Unspecified disorder of adult personality and behavior**   A

### Intellectual Disabilities (F70-F79)

Code first any associated physical or developmental disorders
> *EXCLUDES 1*   borderline intellectual functioning, IQ above 70 to 84 (R41.83)

**F70   Mild intellectual disabilities**
IQ level 50-55 to approximately 70
Mild mental subnormality

**F71   Moderate intellectual disabilities**
IQ level 35-40 to 50-55
Moderate mental subnormality

**F72   Severe intellectual disabilities**   CC
IQ 20-25 to 35-40
Severe mental subnormality
**CC Excl:** PDX collection 558

**F73   Profound intellectual disabilities**   CC
IQ level below 20-25
Profound mental subnormality
**CC Excl:** PDX collection 558

**F78   Other intellectual disabilities**

**F79   Unspecified intellectual disabilities**
Mental deficiency NOS
Mental subnormality NOS

### Pervasive and specific developmental disorders (F80-F89)

√4th **F80   Specific developmental disorders of speech and language**
    **F80.0   Phonological disorder**
       Dyslalia
       Functional speech articulation disorder
       Lalling
       Lisping
       Phonological developmental disorder
       Speech articulation developmental disorder
       Speech-sound disorder
> *EXCLUDES 1*   speech articulation impairment due to aphasia NOS (R47.01)
> speech articulation impairment due to apraxia (R48.2)
> *EXCLUDES 2*   speech articulation impairment due to hearing loss (F80.4)
> speech articulation impairment due to intellectual disabilities (F70-F79)
> speech articulation impairment with expressive language developmental disorder (F80.1)
> speech articulation impairment with mixed receptive expressive language developmental disorder (F80.2)

    **F80.1   Expressive language disorder**
       Developmental dysphasia or aphasia, expressive type
> *EXCLUDES 1*   dysphasia and aphasia NOS (R47.-)
> mixed receptive-expressive language disorder (F80.2)
> *EXCLUDES 2*   acquired aphasia with epilepsy [Landau-Kleffner] (G40.80-)
> intellectual disabilities (F70-F79)
> pervasive developmental disorders (F84.-)
> selective mutism (F94.0)

    **F80.2   Mixed receptive-expressive language disorder**
       Developmental dysphasia or aphasia, receptive type
       Developmental Wernicke's aphasia
> *EXCLUDES 1*   central auditory processing disorder (H93.25)
> dysphasia or aphasia NOS (R47.-)
> expressive language disorder (F80.1)
> expressive type dysphasia or aphasia (F80.1)
> word deafness (H93.25)
> *EXCLUDES 2*   acquired aphasia with epilepsy [Landau-Kleffner] (G40.80-)
> intellectual disabilities (F70-F79)
> pervasive developmental disorders (F84.-)
> selective mutism (F94.0)

N Newborn: 0    P Pediatric: 0-17    M Maternity: 12-55    A Adult: 15-124    MCC Major CC Condition    PDx MCC PDx acts as own MCC    CC CC Condition    PDx CC PDx acts as own CC

552                                         ICD-10-CM 2018

**F80.4**   **Speech and language development delay** due to hearing loss
Code also type of hearing loss (H90.-, H91.-)

✓5ᵗʰ **F80.8**   **Other developmental disorders of speech and language**
AHA: 2017, 1Q, 27

     **F80.81**   **Childhood onset fluency disorder**
Cluttering NOS
Stuttering NOS
**EXCLUDES 1**   *adult onset fluency disorder (F98.5)*
*fluency disorder in conditions classified elsewhere (R47.82)*
*fluency disorder (stuttering) following cerebrovascular disease (I69. with final characters-23)*

     **F80.82**   **Social pragmatic communication disorder**
**EXCLUDES 1**   *Asperger's syndrome (F84.5)*
*autistic disorder (F84.0)*

     **F80.89**   **Other developmental disorders of speech and language**

**F80.9**   **Developmental disorder of speech and language,** unspecified
Communication disorder NOS
Language disorder NOS

✓4ᵗʰ **F81**   **Specific developmental disorders of scholastic skills**

**F81.0**   **Specific reading disorder**
"Backward reading"
Developmental dyslexia
▶Specific learning disorder, with impairment in reading◀
Specific reading retardation
**EXCLUDES 1**   *alexia NOS (R48.0)*
*dyslexia NOS (R48.0)*
**DEF:** Serious impairment of reading skills unexplained in relation to general intelligence and teaching processes.

**F81.2**   **Mathematics disorder**
Developmental acalculia
Developmental arithmetical disorder
Developmental Gerstmann's syndrome
▶Specific learning disorder, with impairment in mathmatics◀
**EXCLUDES 1**   *acalculia NOS (R48.8)*
**EXCLUDES 2**   *arithmetical difficulties associated with a reading disorder (F81.0)*
*arithmetical difficulties associated with a spelling disorder (F81.81)*
*arithmetical difficulties due to inadequate teaching (Z55.8)*

✓5ᵗʰ **F81.8**   **Other developmental disorders of scholastic skills**

     **F81.81**   **Disorder of written expression**
▶Specific learning disorder, with impairment in written expression◀
Specific spelling disorder

     **F81.89**   **Other developmental disorders of scholastic skills**

**F81.9**   **Developmental disorder of scholastic skills, unspecified**
Knowledge acquisition disability NOS
Learning disability NOS
Learning disorder NOS

**F82**   **Specific developmental disorder of motor function**
Clumsy child syndrome
Developmental coordination disorder
Developmental dyspraxia
**EXCLUDES 1**   *abnormalities of gait and mobility (R26.-)*
*lack of coordination (R27.-)*
**EXCLUDES 2**   *lack of coordination secondary to intellectual disabilities (F70-F79)*

✓4ᵗʰ **F84**   **Pervasive developmental disorders**
Use additional code to identify any associated medical condition and intellectual disabilities

**CC Excl: For CC codes in category F84, unless otherwise noted:**
PDX collection 551

**F84.0**   **Autistic disorder**   `CC`
Autism spectrum disorder
Infantile autism
Infantile psychosis
Kanner's syndrome
**EXCLUDES 1**   *Asperger's syndrome (F84.5)*
AHA: 2017, 1Q, 27

**F84.2**   **Rett's syndrome**   `CC`
**EXCLUDES 1**   *Asperger's syndrome (F84.5)*
*Autistic disorder (F84.0)*
*Other childhood disintegrative disorder (F84.3)*
**CC Excl:** PDX collection 537

**F84.3**   **Other childhood disintegrative disorder**   `CC` `P`
Dementia infantilis
Disintegrative psychosis
Heller's syndrome
Symbiotic psychosis
Use additional code to identify any associated neurological condition
**EXCLUDES 1**   *Asperger's syndrome (F84.5)*
*Autistic disorder (F84.0)*
*Rett's syndrome (F84.2)*

**F84.5**   **Asperger's syndrome**   `CC`
Asperger's disorder
Autistic psychopathy
Schizoid disorder of childhood

**F84.8**   **Other pervasive developmental disorders**   `CC`
Overactive disorder associated with intellectual disabilities and stereotyped movements

**F84.9**   **Pervasive developmental disorder, unspecified**   `CC`
Atypical autism

**F88**   **Other disorders of psychological development**
Developmental agnosia
Global development delay
Other specified neurodevelopmental disorder

**F89**   **Unspecified disorder of psychological development**
Developmental disorder NOS
Neurodevelopmental disorder NOS

## Behavioral and emotional disorders with onset usually occurring in childhood and adolescence (F90-F98)

**NOTE**   Codes within categories F90-F98 may be used regardless of the age of a patient. These disorders generally have onset within the childhood or adolescent years, but may continue throughout life or not be diagnosed until adulthood

✓4ᵗʰ **F90**   **Attention-deficit hyperactivity disorders**
**INCLUDES**   attention deficit disorder with hyperactivity
attention deficit syndrome with hyperactivity
**EXCLUDES 2**   *anxiety disorders (F40.-, F41.-)*
*mood [affective] disorders (F30-F39)*
*pervasive developmental disorders (F84.-)*
*schizophrenia (F20.-)*

**F90.0**   **Attention-deficit hyperactivity disorder, predominantly inattentive type**
▶Attention-deficit/hyperactivity disorder, predominantly inattentive presentation◀

**F90.1**   **Attention-deficit hyperactivity disorder, predominantly hyperactive type**
▶Attention-deficit/hyperactivity disorder, predominantly hyperactive impulsive presentation◀

**F90.2**   **Attention-deficit hyperactivity disorder, combined type**
▶Attention-deficit/hyperactivity disorder, combined presentation◀

**F90.8**   **Attention-deficit hyperactivity disorder, other type**

**F90.9**   **Attention-deficit hyperactivity disorder, unspecified type**
Attention-deficit hyperactivity disorder of childhood or adolescence NOS
Attention-deficit hyperactivity disorder NOS

✓4ᵗʰ **F91**   **Conduct disorders**
**EXCLUDES 1**   *antisocial behavior (Z72.81-)*
*antisocial personality disorder (F60.2)*
**EXCLUDES 2**   *conduct problems associated with attention-deficit hyperactivity disorder (F90.-)*
*mood [affective] disorders (F30-F39)*
*pervasive developmental disorders (F84.-)*
*schizophrenia (F20.-)*

**F91.0**   **Conduct disorder confined to family context**

**F91.1**   **Conduct disorder, childhood-onset type**
Unsocialized conduct disorder
Conduct disorder, solitary aggressive type
Unsocialized aggressive disorder

**F91.2**   **Conduct disorder, adolescent-onset type**
Socialized conduct disorder
Conduct disorder, group type

**F91.3**   **Oppositional defiant disorder**

**F91.8**   **Other conduct disorders**
Other specified conduct disorder
Other specified disruptive disorder

✓ Additional Character Req   ✓x7ᵗʰ Placeholder Alert   Unacceptable PDx   Manifestation   **H1**-**H14** HAC   **HCC** CMS-HCC Condition   **EXCLUDES 1** Not Coded Here   **EXCLUDES 2** Not Included Here

ICD-10-CM 2018      **553**

**F91.9   Conduct disorder,** unspecified
     Behavioral disorder NOS
     Conduct disorder NOS
     Disruptive behavior disorder NOS
     Disruptive disorder NOS

✓4ᵗʰ **F93   Emotional disorders with onset specific to childhood**

**F93.0   Separation anxiety disorder of childhood**
     *EXCLUDES 2*   *mood [affective] disorders (F30-F39)*
                *nonpsychotic mental disorders (F40-F48)*
                *phobic anxiety disorder of childhood (F40.8)*
                *social phobia (F40.1)*

**F93.8   Other childhood emotional disorders**
     Identity disorder
     *EXCLUDES 2*   *gender identity disorder of childhood (F64.2)*

**F93.9   Childhood emotional disorder, unspecified**

✓4ᵗʰ **F94   Disorders of social functioning with onset specific to childhood and adolescence**

**F94.0   Selective mutism**
     Elective mutism
     *EXCLUDES 2*   *pervasive developmental disorders (F84.-)*
                *schizophrenia (F20.-)*
                *specific developmental disorders of speech and language (F80.-)*
                *transient mutism as part of separation anxiety in young children (F93.0)*

**F94.1   Reactive attachment disorder of childhood**
     Use additional code to identify any associated failure to thrive or growth retardation
     *EXCLUDES 1*   *disinhibited attachment disorder of childhood (F94.1)*
                *normal variation in pattern of selective attachment*
     *EXCLUDES 2*   *Asperger's syndrome (F84.5)*
                *maltreatment syndromes (T74.-)*
                *sexual or physical abuse in childhood, resulting in psychosocial problems (Z62.81-)*

**F94.2   Disinhibited attachment disorder of childhood**
     Affectionless psychopathy
     Institutional syndrome
     *EXCLUDES 1*   *reactive attachment disorder of childhood (F94.1)*
     *EXCLUDES 2*   *Asperger's syndrome (F84.5)*
                *attention-deficit hyperactivity disorders (F90.-)*
                *hospitalism in children (F43.2-)*

**F94.8   Other childhood disorders of social functioning**

**F94.9   Childhood disorder of social functioning, unspecified**

✓4ᵗʰ **F95   Tic disorder**

**F95.0   Transient tic disorder**
     Provisional tic disorder

**F95.1   Chronic motor or vocal tic disorder**

**F95.2   Tourette's disorder**
     Combined vocal and multiple motor tic disorder [de la Tourette]
     Tourette's syndrome

**F95.8   Other tic disorders**

**F95.9   Tic disorder, unspecified**
     Tic NOS

✓4ᵗʰ **F98   Other behavioral and emotional disorders with onset usually occurring in childhood and adolescence**
     *EXCLUDES 2*   *breath-holding spells (R06.89)*
                *gender identity disorder of childhood (F64.2)*
                *Kleine-Levin syndrome (G47.13)*
                *obsessive-compulsive disorder (F42-)*
                *sleep disorders not due to a substance or known physiological condition (F51.-)*

**F98.0   Enuresis not due to a substance or known physiological condition**
     Enuresis (primary) (secondary) of nonorganic origin
     Functional enuresis
     Psychogenic enuresis
     Urinary incontinence of nonorganic origin
     *EXCLUDES 1*   *enuresis NOS (R32)*

**F98.1   Encopresis not due to a substance or known physiological condition**
     Functional encopresis
     Incontinence of feces of nonorganic origin
     Psychogenic encopresis
     Use additional code to identify the cause of any coexisting constipation
     *EXCLUDES 1*   *encopresis NOS (R15.-)*

✓5ᵗʰ **F98.2   Other feeding disorders of infancy and childhood**
     *EXCLUDES 1*   *feeding difficulties (R63.3)*
     *EXCLUDES 2*   *anorexia nervosa and other eating disorders (F50.-)*
                *feeding problems of newborn (P92.-)*
                *pica of infancy or childhood (F98.3)*

**F98.21   Rumination disorder of infancy**

**F98.29   Other feeding disorders of infancy and early childhood**

**F98.3   Pica of infancy and childhood**

**F98.4   Stereotyped movement disorders**
     Stereotype/habit disorder
     *EXCLUDES 1*   *abnormal involuntary movements (R25.-)*
     *EXCLUDES 2*   *compulsions in obsessive-compulsive disorder (F42-)*
                *hair plucking (F63.3)*
                *movement disorders of organic origin (G20-G25)*
                *nail-biting (F98.8)*
                *nose-picking (F98.8)*
                *stereotypies that are part of a broader psychiatric condition (F01-F95)*
                *thumb-sucking (F98.8)*
                *tic disorders (F95.-)*
                *trichotillomania (F63.3)*

**F98.5   Adult onset fluency disorder**
     *EXCLUDES 1*   *childhood onset fluency disorder (F80.81)*
                *dysphasia (R47.02)*
                *fluency disorder in conditions classified elsewhere (R47.82)*
                *fluency disorder (stuttering) following cerebrovascular disease (I69. with final characters -23)*
                *tic disorders (F95.-)*

**F98.8   Other specified behavioral and emotional disorders with onset usually occurring in childhood and adolescence**
     Excessive masturbation
     Nail-biting
     Nose-picking
     Thumb-sucking

**F98.9   Unspecified behavioral and emotional disorders with onset usually occurring in childhood and adolescence**

### Unspecified mental disorder (F99)

**F99   Mental disorder, not otherwise specified**
     Mental illness NOS
     *EXCLUDES 1*   *unspecified mental disorder due to known physiological condition (F09)*

N Newborn: 0   P Pediatric: 0-17   M Maternity: 12-55   A Adult: 15-124   MCC Major CC Condition   PDxMCC PDx acts as own MCC   CC CC Condition   PDxCC PDx acts as own CC

554      ICD-10-CM 2018

# Chapter 6. Diseases of the Nervous System (G00-G99)

## Chapter Specific Guidelines with Coding Examples

The chapter specific guidelines from the ICD-10-CM Official Guidelines for Coding and Reporting have been provided below. Along with these guidelines are coding examples, contained in the shaded boxes, that have been developed to help illustrate the coding and/or sequencing guidance found in these guidelines.

### a. Dominant/nondominant side

Codes from category G81, Hemiplegia and hemiparesis, and subcategories G83.1, Monoplegia of lower limb, G83.2, Monoplegia of upper limb, and G83.3, Monoplegia, unspecified, identify whether the dominant or nondominant side is affected. Should the affected side be documented, but not specified as dominant or nondominant, and the classification system does not indicate a default, code selection is as follows:

- For ambidextrous patients, the default should be dominant.
- If the left side is affected, the default is non-dominant.
- If the right side is affected, the default is dominant.

> Hemiplegia affecting left side of ambidextrous patient
>
> **G81.92**      **Hemiplegia, unspecified affecting left dominant side**
>
> *Explanation*: Documentation states that the left side is affected and dominant is used for ambidextrous persons.

> Right spastic hemiplegia, unknown whether patient is right- or left-handed
>
> **G81.11**      **Spastic hemiplegia affecting right dominant side**
>
> *Explanation*: Since it is unknown whether the patient is right- or left-handed, if the right side is affected, the default is dominant.

### b. Pain—Category G89

#### 1) General coding information

Codes in category G89, Pain, not elsewhere classified, may be used in conjunction with codes from other categories and chapters to provide more detail about acute or chronic pain and neoplasm-related pain, unless otherwise indicated below.

If the pain is not specified as acute or chronic, post-thoracotomy, postprocedural, or neoplasm-related, do not assign codes from category G89.

A code from category G89 should not be assigned if the underlying (definitive) diagnosis is known, unless the reason for the encounter is pain control/ management and not management of the underlying condition.

When an admission or encounter is for a procedure aimed at treating the underlying condition (e.g., spinal fusion, kyphoplasty), a code for the underlying condition (e.g., vertebral fracture, spinal stenosis) should be assigned as the principal diagnosis. No code from category G89 should be assigned.

> Elderly patient with back pain is admitted for kyphoplasty for age-related osteopathic compression fracture at vertebra T3
>
> **M80.08XA**      **Age-related osteoporosis with current pathological fracture, vertebra(e), initial encounter for fracture**
>
> *Explanation*: No code is assigned for the pain as it is inherent in the underlying condition being treated.

#### (a) Category G89 codes as principal or first-listed diagnosis

Category G89 codes are acceptable as principal diagnosis or the first-listed code:

- When pain control or pain management is the reason for the admission/encounter (e.g., a patient with displaced intervertebral disc, nerve impingement and severe back pain presents for injection of steroid into the spinal canal). The underlying cause of the pain should be reported as an additional diagnosis, if known.

- When a patient is admitted for the insertion of a neurostimulator for pain control, assign the appropriate pain code as the principal or first-listed diagnosis. When an admission or encounter is for a procedure aimed at treating the underlying condition and a neurostimulator is inserted for pain control during the same admission/encounter, a code for the underlying condition should be assigned as the principal diagnosis and the appropriate pain code should be assigned as a secondary diagnosis.

> Patient with chronic pain from lumbar spondylosis with radiculopathy not relieved by surgery is admitted for insertion of neurostimulator.
>
> **G89.29**      **Other chronic pain**
>
> **M47.26**      **Other spondylosis with radiculopathy, lumbar region**
>
> *Explanation*: Since the patient is admitted specifically for a neurostimulator implantation for pain management and not to treat the underlying spondylosis, the chronic pain code is sequenced first, followed by the underlying condition. Neither code M54.16 nor M54.5 is necessary because M47.26 describes the radiculopathy and the site.

#### (b) Use of category G89 codes in conjunction with site specific pain codes

#### (i) Assigning category G89 and site-specific pain codes

Codes from category G89 may be used in conjunction with codes that identify the site of pain (including codes from chapter 18) if the category G89 code provides additional information. For example, if the code describes the site of the pain, but does not fully describe whether the pain is acute or chronic, then both codes should be assigned.

> During hospital stay, patient is seen by orthopaedics to evaluate chronic left shoulder pain.
>
> **M25.512**      **Pain in left shoulder**
>
> **G89.29**      **Other chronic pain**
>
> *Explanation*: No underlying condition has been determined yet so the pain would be the reason for the visit. The M25 pain code in this instance does not fully describe the condition as it does not represent that the pain is chronic. The G89 chronic pain code is assigned to provide specificity.

#### (ii) Sequencing of category G89 codes with site-specific pain codes

The sequencing of category G89 codes with site-specific pain codes (including chapter 18 codes), is dependent on the circumstances of the encounter/admission as follows:

- If the encounter is for pain control or pain management, assign the code from category G89 followed by the code identifying the specific site of pain (e.g., encounter for pain management for acute neck pain from trauma is assigned code G89.11, Acute pain due to trauma, followed by code M54.2, Cervicalgia, to identify the site of pain).

> Management of acute, traumatic right knee pain
>
> **G89.11**      **Acute pain due to trauma**
>
> **M25.561**      **Pain in right knee**
>
> *Explanation*: The reason for the encounter is to manage or control the pain, not to treat or evaluate an underlying condition. The G89 pain code is assigned as the principal diagnosis but in this instance does not fully describe the condition as it does not include the site and laterality. The M25 pain code is added to provide this information.

- If the encounter is for any other reason except pain control or pain management, and a related definitive diagnosis has not been established (confirmed) by the provider, assign the code for the specific site of pain first, followed by the appropriate code from category G89.

Tests are performed to investigate the source of the patient's chronic epigastric abdominal pain

**R10.13      Epigastric pain**

**G89.29      Other chronic pain**

*Explanation*: In this instance the patient's epigastric pain is not being treated; rather the source of the pain is being investigated. A code from chapter 18 for epigastric pain is sequenced before the additional specificity of the G89 code for the chronic pain.

**2)  Pain due to devices, implants and grafts**

*See Section I.C.19. Pain due to medical devices*

**3)  Postoperative Pain**

The provider's documentation should be used to guide the coding of postoperative pain, as well as *Section III. Reporting Additional Diagnoses* and *Section IV. Diagnostic Coding and Reporting in the Outpatient Setting.*

The default for post-thoracotomy and other postoperative pain not specified as acute or chronic is the code for the acute form.

Routine or expected postoperative pain immediately after surgery should not be coded.

Pain pump dose is increased for the patient's unexpected, extreme pain post-thoracotomy

**G89.12      Acute post-thoracotomy pain**

*Explanation*: When acute or chronic is not documented, default to acute. The use of "unexpected, extreme" and the increase of medication dosage indicate that the pain was more than routine or expected.

**(a)  Postoperative pain not associated with specific postoperative complication**

Postoperative pain not associated with a specific postoperative complication is assigned to the appropriate postoperative pain code in category G89.

**(b)  Postoperative pain associated with specific postoperative complication**

Postoperative pain associated with a specific postoperative complication (such as painful wire sutures) is assigned to the appropriate code(s) found in Chapter 19, Injury, poisoning, and certain other consequences of external causes. If appropriate, use additional code(s) from category G89 to identify acute or chronic pain (G89.18 or G89.28).

**4)  Chronic pain**

Chronic pain is classified to subcategory G89.2. There is no time frame defining when pain becomes chronic pain. The provider's documentation should be used to guide use of these codes.

**5)  Neoplasm related pain**

Code G89.3 is assigned to pain documented as being related, associated or due to cancer, primary or secondary malignancy, or tumor. This code is assigned regardless of whether the pain is acute or chronic.

This code may be assigned as the principal or first-listed code when the stated reason for the admission/encounter is documented as pain control/pain management. The underlying neoplasm should be reported as an additional diagnosis.

Pain medication adjustment for chronic pain from bone metastasis

**G89.3       Neoplasm related pain (acute)(chronic)**

**C79.51      Secondary malignant neoplasm of bone**

*Explanation*: Since the encounter was for pain medication management, the pain, rather than the neoplasm, was the reason for the encounter and is sequenced first. This "neoplasm-related pain" code includes both acute and chronic pain.

When the reason for the admission/encounter is management of the neoplasm and the pain associated with the neoplasm is also documented, code G89.3 may be assigned as an additional diagnosis. It is not necessary to assign an additional code for the site of the pain.

*See Section I.C.2 for instructions on the sequencing of neoplasms for all other stated reasons for the admission/encounter (except for pain control/pain management).*

Patient with lung cancer presents with acute hip pain and is evaluated and found to have iliac bone metastasis

**C79.51      Secondary malignant neoplasm of bone**

**C34.90      Malignant neoplasm of unspecified part of unspecified bronchus or lung**

**G89.3       Neoplasm related pain (acute)(chronic)**

*Explanation*: The reason for the encounter was the evaluation and diagnosis of the bone metastasis, whose code would be assigned as first-listed, followed by codes for the primary neoplasm and the pain due to the iliac bone metastasis.

**6)  Chronic pain syndrome**

Central pain syndrome (G89.0) and chronic pain syndrome (G89.4) are different than the term "chronic pain," and therefore codes should only be used when the provider has specifically documented this condition.

*See Section I.C.5. Pain disorders related to psychological factors*

# Chapter 6. Diseases of the Nervous System (G00-G99)

> **EXCLUDES 2**   *certain conditions originating in the perinatal period (P04-P96)*
> *certain infectious and parasitic diseases (A00-B99)*
> *complications of pregnancy, childbirth and the puerperium (O00-O9A)*
> *congenital malformations, deformations, and chromosomal abnormalities (Q00-Q99)*
> *endocrine, nutritional and metabolic diseases (E00-E88)*
> *injury, poisoning and certain other consequences of external causes (S00-T88)*
> *neoplasms (C00-D49)*
> *symptoms, signs and abnormal clinical and laboratory findings, not elsewhere classified (R00-R94)*

This chapter contains the following blocks:

| | |
|---|---|
| G00-G09 | Inflammatory diseases of the central nervous system |
| G10-G14 | Systemic atrophies primarily affecting the central nervous system |
| G20-G26 | Extrapyramidal and movement disorders |
| G30-G32 | Other degenerative diseases of the nervous system |
| G35-G37 | Demyelinating diseases of the central nervous system |
| G40-G47 | Episodic and paroxysmal disorders |
| G50-G59 | Nerve, nerve root and plexus disorders |
| G60-G65 | Polyneuropathies and other disorders of the peripheral nervous system |
| G70-G73 | Diseases of myoneural junction and muscle |
| G80-G83 | Cerebral palsy and other paralytic syndromes |
| G89-G99 | Other disorders of the nervous system |

## Inflammatory diseases of the central nervous system (G00-G09)

### ✓4ᵗʰ G00   Bacterial **meningitis, not elsewhere classified**

> **INCLUDES**   bacterial arachnoiditis
> bacterial leptomeningitis
> bacterial meningitis
> bacterial pachymeningitis
>
> **EXCLUDES 1** ▶*bacterial meningoencephalitis* ◀ *(G04.2)*
> ▶*bacterial meningomyelitis* ◀ *(G04.2)*

> **CC Excl: For MCC codes in category G00:** PDX collection 207

**G00.0   Hemophilus meningitis**   `MCC`
Meningitis due to Hemophilus influenzae

**G00.1   Pneumococcal meningitis**   `MCC`
Meningtitis due to Streptococcal pneumoniae

**G00.2   Streptococcal meningitis**   `MCC`
Use additional code to further identify organism (B95.0-B95.5)

**G00.3   Staphylococcal meningitis**   `MCC`
Use additional code to further identify organism (B95.61-B95.8)

**G00.8   Other bacterial meningitis**   `MCC`
Meningitis due to Escherichia coli
Meningitis due to Friedländer's bacillus
Meningitis due to Klebsiella
Use additional code to further identify organism (B96.-)

**G00.9   Bacterial meningitis, unspecified**   `MCC`
Meningitis due to gram-negative bacteria, unspecified
Purulent meningitis NOS
Pyogenic meningitis NOS
Suppurative meningitis NOS

### G01   *Meningitis in bacterial diseases classified elsewhere*   `MCC`

> Code first underlying disease
>
> **EXCLUDES 1**   *meningitis (in):*
> *gonococcal (A54.81)*
> *leptospirosis (A27.81)*
> *listeriosis (A32.11)*
> *Lyme disease (A69.21)*
> *meningococcal (A39.0)*
> *neurosyphilis (A52.13)*
> *tuberculosis (A17.0)*
> *meningoencephalitis and meningomyelitis in bacterial diseases classified elsewhere (G05)*

> **CC Excl:** PDX collection 207

### G02   *Meningitis in other infectious and parasitic diseases classified elsewhere*   `MCC`

> Code first underlying disease, such as:
> African trypanosomiasis (B56.-)
> poliovirus infection (A80.-)
>
> **EXCLUDES 1**   *candidal meningitis (B37.5)*
> *coccidioidomycosis meningitis (B38.4)*
> *cryptococcal meningitis (B45.1)*
> *herpesviral [herpes simplex] meningitis (B00.3)*
> *infectious mononucleosis complicated by meningitis (B27.- with fourth character 2)*
> *measles complicated by meningitis (B05.1)*
> *meningoencephalitis and meningomyelitis in other infectious and parasitic diseases classified elsewhere (G05)*
> *mumps meningitis (B26.1)*
> *rubella meningitis (B06.02)*
> *varicella [chickenpox] meningitis (B01.0)*
> *zoster meningitis (B02.1)*

> **CC Excl:** PDX collection 559

### ✓4ᵗʰ G03   **Meningitis due to** other and unspecified causes

> **INCLUDES**   arachnoiditis NOS
> leptomeningitis NOS
> meningitis NOS
> pachymeningitis NOS
>
> **EXCLUDES 1**   *meningoencephalitis (G04.-)*
> *meningomyelitis (G04.-)*

> **CC Excl: For CC/MCC codes in category G03, unless otherwise noted:** PDX collection 207

**G03.0   Nonpyogenic meningitis**   `MCC`
Aseptic meningitis
Nonbacterial meningitis

**G03.1   Chronic meningitis**   `CC`

**G03.2   Benign recurrent meningitis [Mollaret]**   `CC`
**CC Excl:** PDX collection 140

**G03.8   Meningitis due to other specified causes**   `MCC`

**G03.9   Meningitis, unspecified**   `MCC`
Arachnoiditis (spinal) NOS

### ✓4ᵗʰ G04   **Encephalitis, myelitis and encephalomyelitis**

> **INCLUDES**   acute ascending myelitis
> meningoencephalitis
> meningomyelitis
>
> **EXCLUDES 1**   *encephalopathy NOS (G93.40)*
>
> **EXCLUDES 2**   *acute transverse myelitis (G37.3-)*
> *alcoholic encephalopathy (G31.2)*
> *benign myalgic encephalomyelitis (G93.3)*
> *multiple sclerosis (G35)*
> *subacute necrotizing myelitis (G37.4)*
> *toxic encephalitis (G92)*
> *toxic encephalopathy (G92)*

#### ✓5ᵗʰ G04.0   **Acute disseminated encephalitis and encephalomyelitis (ADEM)**

> **EXCLUDES 1**   *acute necrotizing hemorrhagic encephalopathy (G04.3-)*
> *other noninfectious acute disseminated encephalomyelitis (noninfectious ADEM) (G04.81)*

**G04.00   Acute disseminated encephalitis and encephalomyelitis, unspecified**   `MCC`
**CC Excl:** PDX collection 560

**G04.01   Postinfectious acute disseminated encephalitis and encephalomyelitis (postinfectious ADEM)**   `MCC`
> **EXCLUDES 1**   *post chickenpox encephalitis (B01.1)*
> *post measles encephalitis (B05.0)*
> *post measles myelitis (B05.1)*
**CC Excl:** PDX collection 560

**G04.02   Postimmunization acute disseminated encephalitis, myelitis and encephalomyelitis**   `MCC`
Encephalitis, postimmunization
Encephalomyelitis, postimmunization
Use additional code to identify the vaccine (T50.A-, T50.B-, T50Z-)
**CC Excl:** No Excl

**G04.1   Tropical spastic paraplegia**   `CC` `HCC`
**CC Excl:** PDX collection 561

**G04.2   Bacterial meningoencephalitis and meningomyelitis, not elsewhere classified**   `MCC`
**CC Excl:** PDX collection 207

---

✓ Additional Character Req   ✓x7ᵗʰ Placeholder Alert   Unacceptable PDx   **Manifestation**   `H1`–`H14` HAC   `HCC` CMS-HCC Condition   *EXCLUDES 1* Not Coded Here   *EXCLUDES 2* Not Included Here

✓5ᵗʰ **G04.3 Acute necrotizing hemorrhagic encephalopathy**
> EXCLUDES 1   *acute disseminated encephalitis and encephalomyelitis (G04.0-)*

    **G04.30 Acute necrotizing hemorrhagic encephalopathy, unspecified**    MCC
>     **CC Excl:** No Excl

    **G04.31 Postinfectious acute necrotizing hemorrhagic encephalopathy**    MCC
>     **CC Excl:** PDX collection 560

    **G04.32 Postimmunization acute necrotizing hemorrhagic encephalopathy**    MCC
>     Use additional code to identify the vaccine (T50.A-, T50.B-, T50Z-)
>     **CC Excl:** No Excl

    **G04.39 Other acute necrotizing hemorrhagic encephalopathy**    MCC
>     Code also underlying etiology, if applicable
>     **CC Excl:** No Excl

✓5ᵗʰ **G04.8 Other encephalitis, myelitis and encephalomyelitis**
> Code also any associated seizure (G40.-, R56.9)

    **G04.81 Other encephalitis and encephalomyelitis**    HIV MCC
>     Noninfectious acute disseminated encephalomyelitis (noninfectious ADEM)
>     **CC Excl:** PDX collection 560

    **G04.89 Other myelitis**    HIV MCC HCC
>     **CC Excl:** PDX collection 560

✓5ᵗʰ **G04.9 Encephalitis, myelitis and encephalomyelitis, unspecified**

    **G04.90 Encephalitis and encephalomyelitis, unspecified**    HIV MCC
>     Ventriculitis (cerebral) NOS
>     **CC Excl:** PDX collection 562

    **G04.91 Myelitis, unspecified**    HIV MCC HCC
>     **CC Excl:** PDX collection 562

✓4ᵗʰ **G05 Encephalitis, myelitis and encephalomyelitis in diseases classified elsewhere**
> Code first underlying disease, such as:
>     human immunodeficiency virus [HIV] disease (B20)
>     poliovirus (A80.-)
>     suppurative otitis media (H66.01-H66.4)
>     trichinellosis (B75)
> EXCLUDES 1   *adenoviral encephalitis, myelitis and encephalomyelitis (A85.1)*
>     *congenital toxoplasmosis encephalitis, myelitis and encephalomyelitis (P37.1)*
>     *cytomegaloviral encephalitis, myelitis and encephalomyelitis (B25.8)*
>     *encephalitis, myelitis and encephalomyelitis (in) measles (B05.0)*
>     *encephalitis, myelitis and encephalomyelitis (in) systemic lupus erythematosus (M32.19)*
>     *enteroviral encephalitis, myelitis and encephalomyelitis (A85.0)*
>     *eosinophilic meningoencephalitis (B83.2)*
>     *herpesviral [herpes simplex] encephalitis, myelitis and encephalomyelitis (B00.4)*
>     *listerial encephalitis, myelitis and encephalomyelitis (A32.12)*
>     *meningococcal encephalitis, myelitis and encephalomyelitis (A39.81)*
>     *mumps encephalitis, myelitis and encephalomyelitis (B26.2)*
>     *postchickenpox encephalitis, myelitis and encephalomyelitis (B01.1-)*
>     *rubella encephalitis, myelitis and encephalomyelitis (B06.01)*
>     *toxoplasmosis encephalitis, myelitis and encephalomyelitis (B58.2)*
>     *zoster encephalitis, myelitis and encephalomyelitis (B02.0)*

    **G05.3 *Encephalitis and encephalomyelitis in diseases classified elsewhere***    MCC
>     Meningoencephalitis in diseases classified elsewhere
>     **CC Excl:** PDX collection 560

    **G05.4 *Myelitis in diseases classified elsewhere***    MCC HCC
>     Meningomyelitis in diseases classified elsewhere
>     **CC Excl:** PDX collection 560

✓4ᵗʰ **G06 Intracranial and intraspinal abscess and granuloma**
> Use additional code (B95-B97) to identify infectious agent

    **G06.0 Intracranial abscess and granuloma**    MCC
>     Brain [any part] abscess (embolic)
>     Cerebellar abscess (embolic)
>     Cerebral abscess (embolic)
>     Intracranial epidural abscess or granuloma
>     Intracranial extradural abscess or granuloma
>     Intracranial subdural abscess or granuloma
>     Otogenic abscess (embolic)
> EXCLUDES 1   *tuberculous intracranial abscess and granuloma (A17.81)*
>     **CC Excl:** PDX collection 563

    **G06.1 Intraspinal abscess and granuloma**    MCC
>     Abscess (embolic) of spinal cord [any part]
>     Intraspinal epidural abscess or granuloma
>     Intraspinal extradural abscess or granuloma
>     Intraspinal subdural abscess or granuloma
> EXCLUDES 1   *tuberculous intraspinal abscess and granuloma (A17.81)*
>     **CC Excl:** PDX collection 564

    **G06.2 Extradural and subdural abscess, unspecified**    MCC
>     **CC Excl:** PDX collection 565

**G07 *Intracranial and intraspinal abscess and granuloma in diseases classified elsewhere***    MCC
> Code first underlying disease, such as:
>     schistosomiasis granuloma of brain (B65.-)
> EXCLUDES 1   *abscess of brain:*
>     *amebic (A06.6)*
>     *chromomycotic (B43.1)*
>     *gonococcal (A54.82)*
>     *tuberculous (A17.81)*
>     *tuberculoma of meninges (A17.1)*
> **CC Excl:** PDX collection 565

**G08 Intracranial and intraspinal phlebitis and thrombophlebitis**    MCC
> Septic embolism of intracranial or intraspinal venous sinuses and veins
> Septic endophlebitis of intracranial or intraspinal venous sinuses and veins
> Septic phlebitis of intracranial or intraspinal venous sinuses and veins
> Septic thrombophlebitis of intracranial or intraspinal venous sinuses and veins
> Septic thrombosis of intracranial or intraspinal venous sinuses and veins
> EXCLUDES 1   *intracranial phlebitis and thrombophlebitis complicating:*
>     *abortion, ectopic or molar pregnancy (O00-O07, O08.7)*
>     *pregnancy, childbirth and the puerperium (O22.5, O87.3)*
>     *nonpyogenic intracranial phlebitis and thrombophlebitis (I67.6)*
> EXCLUDES 2   *intracranial phlebitis and thrombophlebitis complicating*
>     *nonpyogenic intraspinal phlebitis and thrombophlebitis (G95.1)*
> **DEF:** Inflammation and formation of blood clot in a vein within the brain or spine, or their linings.
> **CC Excl:** PDX collection 565

**G09 Sequelae of inflammatory diseases of central nervous system**
> NOTE   Category G09 is to be used to indicate conditions whose primary classification is to G00-G08 as the cause of sequelae, themselves classifiable elsewhere. The "sequelae" include conditions specified as residuals.
> Code first condition resulting from (sequela) of inflammatory diseases of central nervous system

## Systemic atrophies primarily affecting the central nervous system (G10-G14)

**G10 Huntington's disease**    CC HCC
> Huntington's chorea
> Huntington's dementia
> ▶Code also dementia in other diseases classified elsewhere without behavioral disturbance (F02.80)◀
> **DEF:** Genetic disease caused by degeneration of nerve cells in the brain, characterized by chronic progressive mental deterioration; dementia and death within 15 to 20 years of onset.
> **CC Excl:** PDX collection 566

✓4ᵗʰ **G11 Hereditary ataxia**
> EXCLUDES 2   *cerebral palsy (G80.-)*
>     *hereditary and idiopathic neuropathy (G60.-)*
>     *metabolic disorders (E70-E88)*
>
> **CC Excl: For CC codes in category G11, unless otherwise noted:** PDX collection 567

    **G11.0 Congenital nonprogressive ataxia**    CC HCC

N Newborn: 0   P Pediatric: 0-17   M Maternity: 12-55   A Adult: 15-124   MCC Major CC Condition   PDxMCC PDx acts as own MCC   CC CC Condition   PDxCC PDx acts as own CC

558      ICD-10-CM 2018

**G11.1** **Early-onset cerebellar ataxia** `CC` `HCC`
Early-onset cerebellar ataxia with essential tremor
Early-onset cerebellar ataxia with myoclonus [Hunt's ataxia]
Early-onset cerebellar ataxia with retained tendon reflexes
Friedreich's ataxia (autosomal recessive)
X-linked recessive spinocerebellar ataxia

**G11.2** **Late-onset cerebellar ataxia** `CC` `HCC` `A`

**G11.3** **Cerebellar ataxia with defective DNA repair** `CC` `HCC`
Ataxia telangiectasia [Louis-Bar]
*EXCLUDES 2*   *Cockayne's syndrome (Q87.1)*
*other disorders of purine and pyrimidine metabolism (E79.-)*
*xeroderma pigmentosum (Q82.1)*

**G11.4** **Hereditary spastic paraplegia** `CC` `HCC`
**CC Excl:** PDX collection 568

**G11.8** **Other hereditary ataxias** `CC` `HCC`

**G11.9** **Hereditary ataxia, unspecified** `CC` `HCC`
Hereditary cerebellar ataxia NOS
Hereditary cerebellar degeneration
Hereditary cerebellar disease
Hereditary cerebellar syndrome
**CC Excl:** PDX collection 569

✓4ᵗʰ **G12** **Spinal muscular atrophy and related syndromes**

> **CC Excl: For CC codes in category G12:** PDX collection 570

**G12.0** **Infantile spinal muscular atrophy, type I [Werdnig-Hoffman]** `CC` `HCC`

**G12.1** **Other inherited spinal muscular atrophy** `CC` `HCC`
Adult form spinal muscular atrophy
Childhood form, type II spinal muscular atrophy
Distal spinal muscular atrophy
Juvenile form, type III spinal muscular atrophy [Kugelberg-Welander]
Progressive bulbar palsy of childhood [Fazio-Londe]
Scapuloperoneal form spinal muscular atrophy

✓5ᵗʰ **G12.2** **Motor neuron disease**

**G12.20** **Motor neuron disease, unspecified** `CC` `HCC`

**G12.21** **Amyotrophic lateral sclerosis** `CC` `HCC` `A`
~~Progressive spinal muscle atrophy~~

**G12.22** **Progressive bulbar palsy** `CC` `HCC`

● **G12.23** **Primary lateral sclerosis** `CC`

● **G12.24** **Familial motor neuron disease** `CC`

● **G12.25** **Progressive spinal muscle atrophy** `CC`

**G12.29** **Other motor neuron disease** `CC` `HCC`
~~Familial motor neuron disease~~
~~Primary lateral sclerosis~~

**G12.8** **Other spinal muscular atrophies and related syndromes** `CC` `HCC`

**G12.9** **Spinal muscular atrophy, unspecified** `CC` `HCC`

✓4ᵗʰ **G13** **Systemic atrophies primarily affecting central nervous system in diseases classified elsewhere**

*G13.0* *Paraneoplastic neuromyopathy and neuropathy* `HCC`
Carcinomatous neuromyopathy
Sensorial paraneoplastic neuropathy [Denny Brown]
Code first underlying neoplasm (C00-D49)

*G13.1* *Other systemic atrophy primarily affecting central nervous system in neoplastic disease* `HCC`
Paraneoplastic limbic encephalopathy
Code first underlying neoplasm (C00-D49)

*G13.2* *Systemic atrophy primarily affecting the central nervous system in myxedema*
Code first underlying disease, such as:
hypothyroidism (E03.-)
myxedematous congenital iodine deficiency (E00.1)

*G13.8* *Systemic atrophy primarily affecting central nervous system in other diseases classified elsewhere*
Code first underlying disease

**G14** **Postpolio syndrome**
*INCLUDES*   postpolio myelitic syndrome
*EXCLUDES 1*   *sequelae of poliomyelitis (B91)*

## Extrapyramidal and movement disorders (G20-G26)

**G20** **Parkinson's disease** `HCC`
Hemiparkinsonism
Idiopathic Parkinsonism or Parkinson's disease
Paralysis agitans
Parkinsonism or Parkinson's disease NOS
Primary Parkinsonism or Parkinson's disease
*EXCLUDES 1*   *dementia with Parkinsonism (G31.83)*
**AHA:** 2017, 2Q, 7; 2016, 2Q, 6

✓4ᵗʰ **G21** **Secondary parkinsonism**
*EXCLUDES 1*   *dementia with Parkinsonism (G31.83)*
*Huntington's disease (G10)*
*Shy-Drager syndrome (G90.3)*
*syphilitic Parkinsonism (A52.19)*

> **CC Excl: For CC codes in category G21, unless otherwise noted:**
> PDX collection 572

**G21.0** **Malignant neuroleptic syndrome** `MCC`
Use additional code for adverse effect, if applicable, to identify drug (T43.3X5, T43.4X5, T43.505, T43.595)
*EXCLUDES 1*   *neuroleptic induced parkinsonism (G21.11)*
**CC Excl:** PDX collection 571

✓5ᵗʰ **G21.1** **Other drug-induced secondary parkinsonism**

**G21.11** **Neuroleptic induced parkinsonism** `CC` `HCC`
Use additional code for adverse effect, if applicable, to identify drug (T43.3X5, T43.4X5, T43.505, T43.595)
*EXCLUDES 1*   *malignant neuroleptic syndrome (G21.0)*

**G21.19** **Other drug induced secondary parkinsonism** `CC` `HCC`
▶Other medication-induced parkinsonism◀
Use additional code for adverse effect, if applicable, to identify drug (T36-T50 with fifth or sixth character 5)

**G21.2** **Secondary parkinsonism due to other external agents** `CC` `HCC`
Code first (T51-T65) to identify external agent

**G21.3** **Postencephalitic parkinsonism** `CC` `HCC`

**G21.4** **Vascular parkinsonism** `HCC`

**G21.8** **Other secondary parkinsonism** `CC` `HCC`

**G21.9** **Secondary parkinsonism, unspecified** `CC` `HCC`

✓4ᵗʰ **G23** **Other degenerative diseases of basal ganglia**
*EXCLUDES 2*   *multi-system degeneration of the autonomic nervous system (G90.3)*

> **CC Excl: For CC codes in category G23:** PDX collection 573

**G23.0** **Hallervorden-Spatz disease** `CC` `HCC`
Pigmentary pallidal degeneration

**G23.1** **Progressive supranuclear ophthalmoplegia [Steele-Richardson-Olszewski]** `CC` `HCC`
Progressive supranuclear palsy

**G23.2** **Striatonigral degeneration** `CC` `HCC`

**G23.8** **Other specified degenerative diseases of basal ganglia** `CC` `HCC`
Calcification of basal ganglia

**G23.9** **Degenerative disease of basal ganglia, unspecified** `CC` `HCC`

✓4ᵗʰ **G24** **Dystonia**
*INCLUDES*   dyskinesia
*EXCLUDES 2*   *athetoid cerebral palsy (G80.3)*

> **CC Excl: For CC codes in category G24:** PDX collection 574

✓5ᵗʰ **G24.0** **Drug induced dystonia**
Use additional code for adverse effect, if applicable, to identify drug (T36-T50 with fifth or sixth character 5)

**G24.01** **Drug induced subacute dyskinesia**
Drug induced blepharospasm
Drug induced orofacial dyskinesia
Neuroleptic induced tardive dyskinesia
Tardive dyskinesia

**G24.02** **Drug induced acute dystonia** `CC`
Acute dystonic reaction to drugs
Neuroleptic induced acute dystonia

**G24.09** **Other drug induced dystonia** `CC`

**G24.1** **Genetic torsion dystonia**
Dystonia deformans progressiva
Dystonia musculorum deformans
Familial torsion dystonia
Idiopathic familial dystonia
Idiopathic (torsion) dystonia NOS
(Schwalbe-) Ziehen-Oppenheim disease

✓Additional Character Req   ✓x7ᵗʰ Placeholder Alert   Unacceptable PDx   Manifestation   `H1`-`H14` HAC   `HCC` CMS-HCC Condition   *EXCLUDES 1* Not Coded Here   *EXCLUDES 2* Not Included Here

ICD-10-CM 2018     **559**

**Chapter 6. Diseases of the Nervous System**

**G24.2  Idiopathic nonfamilial dystonia**  `CC`

**G24.3  Spasmodic torticollis**
> EXCLUDES 1  congenital torticollis (Q68.0)
> hysterical torticollis (F44.4)
> ocular torticollis (R29.891)
> psychogenic torticollis (F45.8)
> torticollis NOS (M43.6)
> traumatic recurrent torticollis (S13.4)

**G24.4  Idiopathic orofacial dystonia**
Orofacial dyskinesia
> EXCLUDES 1  drug induced orofacial dyskinesia (G24.01)

**G24.5  Blepharospasm**
> EXCLUDES 1  drug induced blepharospasm (G24.01)

**G24.8  Other dystonia**  `CC`
Acquired torsion dystonia NOS

**G24.9  Dystonia, unspecified**
Dyskinesia NOS

✓4th **G25  Other extrapyramidal and movement disorders**
> EXCLUDES 2  sleep related movement disorders (G47.6-)

**G25.0  Essential tremor**
Familial tremor
> EXCLUDES 1  tremor NOS (R25.1)

**G25.1  Drug-induced tremor**
> Use additional code for adverse effect, if applicable, to identify drug (T36-T50 with fifth or sixth character 5)

**G25.2  Other specified forms of tremor**
Intention tremor

**G25.3  Myoclonus**
Drug-induced myoclonus
Palatal myoclonus
> Use additional code for adverse effect, if applicable, to identify drug (T36-T50 with fifth or sixth character 5)
> EXCLUDES 1  facial myokymia (G51.4)
> myoclonic epilepsy (G40.-)

**G25.4  Drug-induced chorea**
> Use additional code for adverse effect, if applicable, to identify drug (T36-T50 with fifth or sixth character 5)

**G25.5  Other chorea**
Chorea NOS
> EXCLUDES 1  chorea NOS with heart involvement (I02.0)
> Huntington's chorea (G10)
> rheumatic chorea (I02.-)
> Sydenham's chorea (I02.-)

✓5th **G25.6  Drug induced tics and other tics of organic origin**
**G25.61  Drug induced tics**
> Use additional code for adverse effect, if applicable, to identify drug (T36-T50 with fifth or sixth character 5)

**G25.69  Other tics of organic origin**
> EXCLUDES 1  habit spasm (F95.9)
> tic NOS (F95.9)
> Tourette's syndrome (F95.2)

✓5th **G25.7  Other and unspecified drug induced movement disorders**
> Use additional code for adverse effect, if applicable, to identify drug (T36-T50 with fifth or sixth character 5)

**G25.70  Drug induced movement disorder, unspecified**

**G25.71  Drug induced akathisia**
Drug induced acathisia
Neuroleptic induced acute akathisia
▶Tardive akathisia◀

**G25.79  Other drug induced movement disorders**

✓5th **G25.8  Other specified extrapyramidal and movement disorders**
**G25.81  Restless legs syndrome**
> DEF: Neurological disorder of unknown etiology creating an irresistible urge to move the legs, which may temporarily relieve the symptoms; is accompanied by motor restlessness and sensations of pain, burning, prickling, or tingling.

**G25.82  Stiff-man syndrome**  `CC`
> CC Excl: PDX collection 575

**G25.83  Benign shuddering attacks**

**G25.89  Other specified extrapyramidal and movement disorders**

**G25.9  Extrapyramidal and movement disorder, unspecified**  `CC`
> CC Excl: PDX collection 575

*G26  Extrapyramidal and movement disorders in diseases classified elsewhere*
> Code first underlying disease

## Other degenerative diseases of the nervous system (G30-G32)

✓4th **G30  Alzheimer's disease**
> INCLUDES  Alzheimer's dementia senile and presenile forms
> Use additional code to identify:
> delirium, if applicable (F05)
> dementia with behavioral disturbance (F02.81)
> dementia without behavioral disturbance (F02.80)
> EXCLUDES 1  senile degeneration of brain NEC (G31.1)
> senile dementia NOS (F03)
> senility NOS (R41.81)
> AHA: 2017, 1Q, 43

**G30.0  Alzheimer's disease with early onset**

**G30.1  Alzheimer's disease with late onset**  `A`

**G30.8  Other Alzheimer's disease**

**G30.9  Alzheimer's disease, unspecified**
> AHA: 2016, 2Q, 6; 2012, 4Q, 95

✓4th **G31  Other degenerative diseases of nervous system, not elsewhere classified**
> Use additional code to identify:
> dementia with behavioral disturbance (F02.81)
> dementia without behavioral disturbance (F02.80)
> EXCLUDES 2  Reye's syndrome (G93.7)

✓5th **G31.0  Frontotemporal dementia**
**G31.01  Pick's disease**
Primary progressive aphasia
Progressive isolated aphasia
> DEF: A progressive frontotemporal dementia with asymmetrical atrophy of the frontal and temporal regions of the cerebral cortex, abnormal rounded brain cells called Pick cells with the presence of abnormal staining of protein (called tau); symptoms include prominent apathy, behavioral changes such as disinhibition and restlessness, echolalia, impairment of language, memory, and intellect, increased carelessness, poor personal hygiene, and decreased attention span.

**G31.09  Other frontotemporal dementia**
Frontal dementia

**G31.1  Senile degeneration of brain, not elsewhere classified**
> EXCLUDES 1  Alzheimer's disease (G30.-)
> senility NOS (R41.81)

**G31.2  Degeneration of nervous system due to alcohol**
Alcoholic cerebellar ataxia
Alcoholic cerebellar degeneration
Alcoholic cerebral degeneration
Alcoholic encephalopathy
Dysfunction of the autonomic nervous system due to alcohol
> Code also associated alcoholism (F10.-)

✓5th **G31.8  Other specified degenerative diseases of nervous system**

> CC Excl: For CC codes in subcategory G31.8:
> PDX collection 537

**G31.81  Alpers disease**  `CC`
Grey-matter degeneration

**G31.82  Leigh's disease**  `CC`
Subacute necrotizing encephalopathy

**G31.83  Dementia with Lewy bodies**
Dementia with Parkinsonism
Lewy body disease
Lewy body dementia
> AHA: 2017, 2Q, 7; 2016, 4Q, 141
> DEF: A cerebral dementia with neurophysiologic changes, increased hippocampal volume, hypoperfusion in the occipital lobes, beta amyloid deposits with neurofibrillary tangles, and atrophy of cortex and brainstem. Hallmark neuropsychological characteristics include fluctuating cognition with pronounced variation in attention and alertness; recurrent hallucinations; and Parkinsonism.

N Newborn: 0   P Pediatric: 0-17   M Maternity: 12-55   A Adult: 15-124   MCC Major CC Condition   PDxMCC PDx acts as own MCC   CC CC Condition   PDxCC PDx acts as own CC

560                                                                                                    ICD-10-CM 2018

G31.84 **Mild cognitive impairment, so stated**
▶Mild neurocognitive disorder◀
> *EXCLUDES 1*   age related cognitive decline (R41.81)
> altered mental status (R41.82)
> cerebral degeneration (G31.9)
> change in mental status (R41.82)
> cognitive deficits following (sequelae of)
>      cerebral hemorrhage or infarction
>      (I69.01-, I69.11-, I69.21-, I69.31-, I69.81-,
>      I69.91-)
> cognitive impairment due to intracranial or
>      head injury (S06.-)
> dementia (F01.-, F02.-, F03)
> mild memory disturbance (F06.8)
> neurologic neglect syndrome (R41.4)
> personality change, nonpsychotic (F68.8)

G31.85 **Corticobasal degeneration**

G31.89 **Other specified degenerative diseases of nervous system**

G31.9 **Degenerative disease of nervous system, unspecified**

✓4ᵗʰ **G32 Other degenerative disorders of nervous system in diseases classified elsewhere**

     *G32.0*   *Subacute combined degeneration of spinal cord in* `CC` `HCC`
         *diseases classified elsewhere*
         Dana-Putnam syndrome
         Sclerosis of spinal cord (combined) (dorsolateral) (posterolateral)
         Code first underlying disease, such as:
             anemia (D51.9)
             dietary (D51.3)
             pernicious (D51.0)
             vitamin B12 deficiency (E53.8)
> *EXCLUDES 1*   syphilitic combined degeneration of spinal cord
>      (A52.11)

         **CC Excl:** PDX collection 576

✓5ᵗʰ   **G32.8 Other specified degenerative disorders of nervous system in diseases classified elsewhere**
         Code first underlying disease, such as:
             amyloidosis cerebral degeneration (E85.-)
             cerebral degeneration (due to) hypothyroidism (E00.0-E03.9)
             cerebral degeneration (due to) neoplasm (C00-D49)
             cerebral degeneration (due to) vitamin B deficiency, except
                 thiamine (E52-E53.-)
> *EXCLUDES 1*   superior hemorrhagic polioencephalitis [Wernicke's
>      encephalopathy] (E51.2)

     *G32.81*   *Cerebellar ataxia in diseases classified* `CC` `HCC`
         *elsewhere*
         Code first underlying disease, such as:
             celiac disease (with gluten ataxia) (K90.0)
             cerebellar ataxia (in) neoplastic disease (para-
                 neoplastic cerebellar degeneration) (C00-D49)
             non-celiac gluten ataxia (M35.9)
> *EXCLUDES 1*   systemic atrophy primarily affecting the
>      central nervous system in alcoholic
>      cerebellar ataxia (G31.2)
> systemic atrophy primarily affecting the
>      central nervous system in myxedema
>      (G13.2)

         **CC Excl:** PDX collection 567

     *G32.89*   *Other specified degenerative disorders of nervous*
         *system in diseases classified elsewhere*
         Degenerative encephalopathy in diseases classified
         elsewhere

## Demyelinating diseases of the central nervous system (G35-G37)

**G35 Multiple sclerosis** `HCC`
     Disseminated multiple sclerosis
     Generalized multiple sclerosis
     Multiple sclerosis NOS
     Multiple sclerosis of brain stem
     Multiple sclerosis of cord

✓4ᵗʰ **G36 Other acute disseminated demyelination**
> *EXCLUDES 1*   postinfectious encephalitis and encephalomyelitis NOS
>      (G04.01)

     **CC Excl: For CC codes in category G36, unless otherwise noted:**
     PDX collection 578

     G36.0 **Neuromyelitis optica [Devic]** `CC` `HCC`
         Demyelination in optic neuritis
> *EXCLUDES 1*   optic neuritis NOS (H46)

         **CC Excl:** PDX collection 577

G36.1 **Acute and subacute hemorrhagic leukoencephalitis** `CC` `HCC`
     **[Hurst]**

G36.8 **Other specified acute disseminated demyelination** `CC` `HCC`

G36.9 **Acute disseminated demyelination, unspecified** `HIV` `CC` `HCC`

✓4ᵗʰ **G37 Other demyelinating diseases of central nervous system**

     G37.0 **Diffuse sclerosis of central nervous system** `CC` `HCC`
         Periaxial encephalitis
         Schilder's disease
> *EXCLUDES 1*   X linked adrenoleukodystrophy (E71.52-)

         **CC Excl:** PDX collection 579

     G37.1 **Central demyelination of corpus callosum** `CC` `HCC`
         **CC Excl:** PDX collection 578

     G37.2 **Central pontine myelinolysis** `CC` `HCC`
         **CC Excl:** PDX collection 578

     G37.3 **Acute transverse myelitis in demyelinating disease of** `CC` `HCC`
         **central nervous system**
         Acute transverse myelitis NOS
         Acute transverse myelopathy
> *EXCLUDES 1*   multiple sclerosis (G35)
> neuromyelitis optica [Devic] (G36.0)

         **CC Excl:** PDX collection 580

     G37.4 **Subacute necrotizing myelitis of central nervous** `HIV` `MCC` `HCC`
         **system**
         **CC Excl:** PDX collection 562

     G37.5 **Concentric sclerosis [Balo] of central nervous system** `CC` `HCC`
         **CC Excl:** PDX collection 579

     G37.8 **Other specified demyelinating diseases of central** `CC` `HCC`
         **nervous system**
         **CC Excl:** PDX collection 578

     G37.9 **Demyelinating disease of central nervous system,** `HIV` `CC` `HCC`
         **unspecified**
         **CC Excl:** PDX collection 578

## Episodic and paroxysmal disorders (G40-G47)

✓4ᵗʰ **G40 Epilepsy and recurrent seizures**
     **NOTE**   The following terms are to be considered equivalent to
         intractable: pharmacoresistant (pharmacologically resistant),
         treatment resistant, refractory (medically) and poorly
         controlled
> *EXCLUDES 1*   conversion disorder with seizures (F44.5)
> convulsions NOS (R56.9)
> post traumatic seizures (R56.1)
> seizure (convulsive) NOS (R56.9)
> seizure of newborn (P90)

> *EXCLUDES 2*   hippocampal sclerosis (G93.81)
> mesial temporal sclerosis (G93.81)
> temporal sclerosis (G93.81)
> Todd's paralysis (G83.84)

✓5ᵗʰ   **G40.0 Localization-related (focal) (partial) idiopathic epilepsy and epileptic syndromes with seizures of localized onset**
         Benign childhood epilepsy with centrotemporal EEG spikes
         Childhood epilepsy with occipital EEG paroxysms
> *EXCLUDES 1*   adult onset localization-related epilepsy
>      (G40.1-, G40.2-)

     ✓6ᵗʰ   **G40.00 Localization-related (focal) (partial) idiopathic epilepsy and epileptic syndromes with seizures of localized onset, not intractable**
         Localization-related (focal) (partial) idiopathic epilepsy
         and epileptic syndromes with seizures of
         localized onset without intractability

         **CC Excl: For CC codes in subcategory G40.00, unless otherwise noted:** PDX collection 581

         G40.001 **Localization-related (focal)** `CC` `HCC`
             **(partial) idiopathic epilepsy and**
             **epileptic syndromes with seizures of**
             **localized onset, not intractable,**
             **with status epilepticus**

         G40.009 **Localization-related (focal)** `CC` `HCC`
             **(partial) idiopathic epilepsy and**
             **epileptic syndromes with seizures of**
             **localized onset, not intractable,**
             **without status epilepticus**
             Localization-related (focal) (partial)
             idiopathic epilepsy and epileptic
             syndromes with seizures of localized
             onset NOS

**Chapter 6. Diseases of the Nervous System**

**G40.01–G40.B11**

✓6th **G40.01** **Localization-related (focal) (partial) idiopathic epilepsy and epileptic syndromes with seizures of localized onset, intractable**

> **CC Excl: For CC codes in subcategory G40.01:**
> PDX collection 582

     **G40.011** **Localization-related (focal)** `CC` `HCC`
> **(partial) idiopathic epilepsy and epileptic syndromes with seizures of localized onset, intractable, with status epilepticus**

     **G40.019** **Localization-related (focal)** `CC` `HCC`
> **(partial) idiopathic epilepsy and epileptic syndromes with seizures of localized onset, intractable, without status epilepticus**

✓5th **G40.1** **Localization-related (focal) (partial) symptomatic epilepsy and epileptic syndromes with simple partial seizures**
Attacks without alteration of consciousness
Epilepsia partialis continua [Kozhevnikof]
Simple partial seizures developing into secondarily generalized seizures

✓6th **G40.10** **Localization-related (focal) (partial) symptomatic epilepsy and epileptic syndromes with simple partial seizures, not intractable**
Localization-related (focal) (partial) symptomatic epilepsy and epileptic syndromes with simple partial seizures without intractability

> **CC Excl: For CC codes in subcategory G40.10:**
> PDX collection 581

     **G40.101** **Localization-related (focal)** `CC` `HCC`
> **(partial) symptomatic epilepsy and epileptic syndromes with simple partial seizures, not intractable, with status epilepticus**

     **G40.109** **Localization-related (focal)** `CC` `HCC`
> **(partial) symptomatic epilepsy and epileptic syndromes with simple partial seizures, not intractable, without status epilepticus**
> Localization-related (focal) (partial) symptomatic epilepsy and epileptic syndromes with simple partial seizures NOS

✓6th **G40.11** **Localization-related (focal) (partial) symptomatic epilepsy and epileptic syndromes with simple partial seizures, intractable**

> **CC Excl: For CC codes in subcategory G40.11:**
> PDX collection 582

     **G40.111** **Localization-related (focal)** `CC` `HCC`
> **(partial) symptomatic epilepsy and epileptic syndromes with simple partial seizures, intractable, with status epilepticus**

     **G40.119** **Localization-related (focal)** `CC` `HCC`
> **(partial) symptomatic epilepsy and epileptic syndromes with simple partial seizures, intractable, without status epilepticus**

✓5th **G40.2** **Localization-related (focal) (partial) symptomatic epilepsy and epileptic syndromes with complex partial seizures**
Attacks with alteration of consciousness, often with automatisms
Complex partial seizures developing into secondarily generalized seizures

✓6th **G40.20** **Localization-related (focal) (partial) symptomatic epilepsy and epileptic syndromes with complex partial seizures, not intractable**
Localization-related (focal) (partial) symptomatic epilepsy and epileptic syndromes with complex partial seizures without intractability

> **CC Excl: For CC codes in subcategory G40.20:**
> PDX collection 581

     **G40.201** **Localization-related (focal)** `CC` `HCC`
> **(partial) symptomatic epilepsy and epileptic syndromes with complex partial seizures, not intractable, with status epilepticus**

     **G40.209** **Localization-related (focal)** `CC` `HCC`
> **(partial) symptomatic epilepsy and epileptic syndromes with complex partial seizures, not intractable, without status epilepticus**
> Localization-related (focal) (partial) symptomatic epilepsy and epileptic syndromes with complex partial seizures NOS

✓6th **G40.21** **Localization-related (focal) (partial) symptomatic epilepsy and epileptic syndromes with complex partial seizures, intractable**

> **CC Excl: For CC codes in subcategory G40.21:**
> PDX collection 582

     **G40.211** **Localization-related (focal)** `CC` `HCC`
> **(partial) symptomatic epilepsy and epileptic syndromes with complex partial seizures, intractable, with status epilepticus**

     **G40.219** **Localization-related (focal)** `CC` `HCC`
> **(partial) symptomatic epilepsy and epileptic syndromes with complex partial seizures, intractable, without status epilepticus**

✓5th **G40.3** **Generalized idiopathic epilepsy and epileptic syndromes**
Code also MERRF syndrome, if applicable (E88.42)

> **CC Excl: For MCC codes in subcategory G40.3:**
> PDX collection 583

✓6th **G40.30** **Generalized idiopathic epilepsy and epileptic syndromes, not intractable**
Generalized idiopathic epilepsy and epileptic syndromes without intractability

     **G40.301** **Generalized idiopathic epilepsy** `MCC` `HCC`
> **and epileptic syndromes, not intractable, with status epilepticus**

     **G40.309** **Generalized idiopathic epilepsy and** `HCC`
> **epileptic syndromes, not intractable, without status epilepticus**
> Generalized idiopathic epilepsy and epileptic syndromes NOS

✓6th **G40.31** **Generalized idiopathic epilepsy and epileptic syndromes, intractable**

     **G40.311** **Generalized idiopathic epilepsy** `MCC` `HCC`
> **and epileptic syndromes, intractable, with status epilepticus**

     **G40.319** **Generalized idiopathic epilepsy** `MCC` `HCC`
> **and epileptic syndromes, intractable, without status epilepticus**

✓5th **G40.A** **Absence epileptic syndrome**
Childhood absence epilepsy [pyknolepsy]
Juvenile absence epilepsy
Absence epileptic syndrome, NOS

> **CC Excl: For CC codes in subcategory G40.A:**
> PDX collection 582

✓6th **G40.A0** **Absence epileptic syndrome, not intractable**

     **G40.A01** **Absence epileptic syndrome, not** `HCC`
> **intractable, with status epilepticus**

     **G40.A09** **Absence epileptic syndrome, not** `HCC`
> **intractable, without status epilepticus**

✓6th **G40.A1** **Absence epileptic syndrome, intractable**

     **G40.A11** **Absence epileptic syndrome,** `CC` `HCC`
> **intractable, with status epilepticus**

     **G40.A19** **Absence epileptic syndrome,** `CC` `HCC`
> **intractable, without status epilepticus**

✓5th **G40.B** **Juvenile myoclonic epilepsy [impulsive petit mal]**

> **CC Excl: For CC codes in subcategory G40.B:**
> PDX collection 582

✓6th **G40.B0** **Juvenile myoclonic epilepsy, not intractable**

     **G40.B01** **Juvenile myoclonic epilepsy, not** `CC` `HCC`
> **intractable, with status epilepticus**

     **G40.B09** **Juvenile myoclonic epilepsy, not** `CC` `HCC`
> **intractable, without status epilepticus**

✓6th **G40.B1** **Juvenile myoclonic epilepsy, intractable**

     **G40.B11** **Juvenile myoclonic epilepsy,** `CC` `HCC`
> **intractable, with status epilepticus**

N Newborn: 0    P Pediatric: 0-17    M Maternity: 12-55    A Adult: 15-124    `MCC` Major CC Condition    `PDxMCC` PDx acts as own MCC    `CC` CC Condition    `PDxCC` PDx acts as own CC

**562**          ICD-10-CM 2018

    **G40.B19**  **Juvenile myoclonic epilepsy,** CC HCC
            **intractable, without status epilepticus**

✓5th **G40.4**  **Other generalized epilepsy and epileptic syndromes**
       Epilepsy with grand mal seizures on awakening
       Epilepsy with myoclonic absences
       Epilepsy with myoclonic-astatic seizures
       Grand mal seizure NOS
       Nonspecific atonic epileptic seizures
       Nonspecific clonic epileptic seizures
       Nonspecific myoclonic epileptic seizures
       Nonspecific tonic epileptic seizures
       Nonspecific tonic-clonic epileptic seizures
       Symptomatic early myoclonic encephalopathy

   ✓6th **G40.40**  **Other generalized epilepsy and epileptic syndromes, not intractable**
        Other generalized epilepsy and epileptic syndromes without intractability
        Other generalized epilepsy and epileptic syndromes NOS

       **G40.401**  **Other generalized epilepsy and** HCC
             **epileptic syndromes, not intractable, with status epilepticus**

       **G40.409**  **Other generalized epilepsy and** HCC
             **epileptic syndromes, not intractable, without status epilepticus**

   ✓6th **G40.41**  **Other generalized epilepsy and epileptic syndromes, intractable**

       **CC Excl: For CC codes in subcategory G40.41:** PDX collection 582

       **G40.411**  **Other generalized epilepsy and** CC HCC
             **epileptic syndromes, intractable, with status epilepticus**

       **G40.419**  **Other generalized epilepsy and** CC HCC
             **epileptic syndromes, intractable, without status epilepticus**

✓5th **G40.5**  **Epileptic seizures related to external causes**
       Epileptic seizures related to alcohol
       Epileptic seizures related to drugs
       Epileptic seizures related to hormonal changes
       Epileptic seizures related to sleep deprivation
       Epileptic seizures related to stress
       Use additional code for adverse effect, if applicable, to identify drug (T36-T50 with fifth or sixth character 5)
       Code also, if applicable, associated epilepsy and recurrent seizures (G40.-)

       **CC Excl: For CC codes in subcategory G40.5:** PDX collection 582

   ✓6th **G40.50**  **Epileptic seizures related to external causes, not intractable**

       **G40.501**  **Epileptic seizures related to** CC HCC
             **external causes, not intractable, with status epilepticus**

       **G40.509**  **Epileptic seizures related to** CC HCC
             **external causes, not intractable, without status epilepticus**
            Epileptic seizures related to external causes, NOS

✓5th **G40.8**  **Other epilepsy and recurrent seizures**
       Epilepsies and epileptic syndromes undetermined as to whether they are focal or generalized
       Landau-Kleffner syndrome

       **CC Excl: For CC codes in subcategory G40.8, unless otherwise noted:** PDX collection 582

   ✓6th **G40.80**  **Other epilepsy**
       **G40.801**  **Other epilepsy, not intractable,** CC HCC
             **with status epilepticus**
             Other epilepsy without intractability with status epilepticus

       **G40.802**  **Other epilepsy, not intractable,** CC HCC
             **without status epilepticus**
             Other epilepsy without intractability without status epilepticus

       **G40.803**  **Other epilepsy, intractable,** CC HCC
             **with status epilepticus**

       **G40.804**  **Other epilepsy, intractable,** CC HCC
             **without status epilepticus**

   ✓6th **G40.81**  **Lennox-Gastaut syndrome**
       **G40.811**  **Lennox-Gastaut syndrome, not** CC HCC
             **intractable, with status epilepticus**

       **G40.812**  **Lennox-Gastaut syndrome, not** CC HCC
             **intractable, without status epilepticus**

       **G40.813**  **Lennox-Gastaut syndrome,** CC HCC
             **intractable, with status epilepticus**

       **G40.814**  **Lennox-Gastaut syndrome,** CC HCC
             **intractable, without status epilepticus**

   ✓6th **G40.82**  **Epileptic spasms**
       Infantile spasms
       Salaam attacks
       West's syndrome

       **G40.821**  **Epileptic spasms, not intractable,** CC HCC
             **with status epilepticus**
             **CC Excl:** PDX collection 581

       **G40.822**  **Epileptic spasms, not intractable,** CC HCC
             **without status epilepticus**
             **CC Excl:** PDX collection 581

       **G40.823**  **Epileptic spasms, intractable,** CC HCC
             **with status epilepticus**

       **G40.824**  **Epileptic spasms, intractable,** CC HCC
             **without status epilepticus**

    **G40.89**  **Other seizures** CC HCC
        *EXCLUDES 1*  *post traumatic seizures (R56.1)*
             *recurrent seizures NOS (G40.909)*
             *seizure NOS (R56.9)*

✓5th **G40.9**  **Epilepsy, unspecified**
   ✓6th **G40.90**  **Epilepsy, unspecified, not intractable**
       Epilepsy, unspecified, without intractability

       **G40.901**  **Epilepsy, unspecified, not intractable,** HCC
             **with status epilepticus**

       **G40.909**  **Epilepsy, unspecified, not intractable,** HCC
             **without status epilepticus**
             Epilepsy NOS
             Epileptic convulsions NOS
             Epileptic fits NOS
             Epileptic seizures NOS
             Recurrent seizures NOS
             Seizure disorder NOS

   ✓6th **G40.91**  **Epilepsy, unspecified, intractable**
       Intractable seizure disorder NOS

       **G40.911**  **Epilepsy, unspecified, intractable,** CC HCC
             **with status epilepticus**
             **CC Excl:** PDX collection 582

       **G40.919**  **Epilepsy, unspecified, intractable,** CC HCC
             **without status epilepticus**
             **CC Excl:** PDX collection 582

✓4th **G43**  **Migraine**
    **NOTE**  The following terms are to be considered equivalent to intractable: pharmacoresistant (pharmacologically resistant), treatment resistant, refractory (medically) and poorly controlled
    Use additional code for adverse effect, if applicable, to identify drug (T36-T50 with fifth or sixth character 5)
    *EXCLUDES 1*  *headache NOS (R51)*
           *lower half migraine (G44.00)*
    *EXCLUDES 2*  *headache syndromes (G44.-)*

✓5th **G43.0**  **Migraine without aura**
       Common migraine
       *EXCLUDES 1*  *chronic migraine without aura (G43.7-)*

   ✓6th **G43.00**  **Migraine without aura, not intractable**
       Migraine without aura without mention of refractory migraine

       **G43.001**  **Migraine without aura, not intractable, with status migrainosus**

       **G43.009**  **Migraine without aura, not intractable, without status migrainosus**
             Migraine without aura NOS

   ✓6th **G43.01**  **Migraine without aura, intractable**
       Migraine without aura with refractory migraine

       **G43.011**  **Migraine without aura, intractable, with status migrainosus**

       **G43.019**  **Migraine without aura, intractable, without status migrainosus**

√5th **G43.1** **Migraine with aura**
Basilar migraine
Classical migraine
Migraine equivalents
Migraine preceded or accompanied by transient focal
neurological phenomena
Migraine triggered seizures
Migraine with acute-onset aura
Migraine with aura without headache (migraine equivalents)
Migraine with prolonged aura
Migraine with typical aura
Retinal migraine
Code also any associated seizure (G40.-, R56.9)
EXCLUDES 1     persistent migraine aura (G43.5-, G43.6-)

√6th **G43.10** **Migraine with aura, not intractable**
Migraine with aura without mention of refractory
migraine

**G43.101** **Migraine with aura, not intractable, with
status migrainosus**

**G43.109** **Migraine with aura, not intractable,
without status migrainosus**
Migraine with aura NOS

√6th **G43.11** **Migraine with aura, intractable**
Migraine with aura with refractory migraine

**G43.111** **Migraine with aura, intractable, with
status migrainosus**

**G43.119** **Migraine with aura, intractable, without
status migrainosus**

√5th **G43.4** **Hemiplegic migraine**
Familial migraine
Sporadic migraine

√6th **G43.40** **Hemiplegic migraine, not intractable**
Hemiplegic migraine without refractory migraine

**G43.401** **Hemiplegic migraine, not intractable, with
status migrainosus**

**G43.409** **Hemiplegic migraine, not intractable,
without status migrainosus**
Hemiplegic migraine NOS

√6th **G43.41** **Hemiplegic migraine, intractable**
Hemiplegic migraine with refractory migraine

**G43.411** **Hemiplegic migraine, intractable, with
status migrainosus**

**G43.419** **Hemiplegic migraine, intractable, without
status migrainosus**

√5th **G43.5** **Persistent migraine aura without cerebral infarction**

√6th **G43.50** **Persistent migraine aura without cerebral infarction,
not intractable**
Persistent migraine aura without cerebral infarction,
without refractory migraine

**G43.501** **Persistent migraine aura without cerebral
infarction, not intractable, with status
migrainosus**

**G43.509** **Persistent migraine aura without cerebral
infarction, not intractable, without status
migrainosus**
Persistent migraine aura NOS

√6th **G43.51** **Persistent migraine aura without cerebral infarction,
intractable**
Persistent migraine aura without cerebral infarction,
with refractory migraine

**G43.511** **Persistent migraine aura without cerebral
infarction, intractable, with status
migrainosus**

**G43.519** **Persistent migraine aura without cerebral
infarction, intractable, without status
migrainosus**

√5th **G43.6** **Persistent migraine aura with cerebral infarction**
Code also the type of cerebral infarction (I63.-)

**CC Excl: For CC codes in subcategory G43.6, unless
otherwise noted:** PDX collection 584

√6th **G43.60** **Persistent migraine aura with cerebral infarction,
not intractable**
Persistent migraine aura with cerebral infarction,
without refractory migraine

**G43.601** **Persistent migraine aura with cerebral** CC
**infarction, not intractable, with status
migrainosus**

**G43.609** **Persistent migraine aura with cerebral** CC
**infarction, not intractable, without status
migrainosus**
**CC Excl:** PDX collection 585

√6th **G43.61** **Persistent migraine aura with cerebral infarction,
intractable**
Persistent migraine aura with cerebral infarction, with
refractory migraine

**G43.611** **Persistent migraine aura with cerebral** CC
**infarction, intractable, with status
migrainosus**

**G43.619** **Persistent migraine aura with cerebral** CC
**infarction, intractable, without status
migrainosus**

√5th **G43.7** **Chronic migraine without aura**
Transformed migraine
EXCLUDES 1     migraine without aura (G43.0-)

√6th **G43.70** **Chronic migraine without aura, not intractable**
Chronic migraine without aura, without refractory
migraine

**G43.701** **Chronic migraine without aura, not
intractable, with status migrainosus**

**G43.709** **Chronic migraine without aura, not
intractable, without status migrainosus**
Chronic migraine without aura NOS

√6th **G43.71** **Chronic migraine without aura, intractable**
Chronic migraine without aura, with refractory
migraine

**G43.711** **Chronic migraine without aura,
intractable, with status migrainosus**

**G43.719** **Chronic migraine without aura,
intractable, without status migrainosus**

√5th **G43.A** **Cyclical vomiting**

**G43.A0** **Cyclical vomiting, not intractable**
Cyclical vomiting, without refractory migraine

**G43.A1** **Cyclical vomiting, intractable**
Cyclical vomiting, with refractory migraine

√5th **G43.B** **Ophthalmoplegic migraine**

**G43.B0** **Ophthalmoplegic migraine, not intractable**
Ophthalmoplegic migraine, without refractory
migraine

**G43.B1** **Ophthalmoplegic migraine, intractable**
Ophthalmoplegic migraine, with refractory migraine

√5th **G43.C** **Periodic headache syndromes in child or adult**

**G43.C0** **Periodic headache syndromes in child or adult, not
intractable**
Periodic headache syndromes in child or adult,
without refractory migraine

**G43.C1** **Periodic headache syndromes in child or adult,
intractable**
Periodic headache syndromes in child or adult, with
refractory migraine

√5th **G43.D** **Abdominal migraine**

**G43.D0** **Abdominal migraine, not intractable**
Abdominal migraine, without refractory migraine

**G43.D1** **Abdominal migraine, intractable**
Abdominal migraine, with refractory migraine

√5th **G43.8** **Other migraine**

√6th **G43.80** **Other migraine, not intractable**
Other migraine, without refractory migraine

**G43.801** **Other migraine, not intractable, with
status migrainosus**

**G43.809** **Other migraine, not intractable, without
status migrainosus**

√6th **G43.81** **Other migraine, intractable**
Other migraine, with refractory migraine

**G43.811** **Other migraine, intractable, with status
migrainosus**

**G43.819** **Other migraine, intractable, without
status migrainosus**

N Newborn: 0   P Pediatric: 0-17   M Maternity: 12-55   A Adult: 15-124   MCC Major CC Condition   PDxMCC PDx acts as own MCC   CC CC Condition   PDxCC PDx acts as own CC

564                                                                                                                                                          ICD-10-CM 2018

✓6ᵗʰ **G43.82** **Menstrual migraine, not intractable**
Menstrual headache, not intractable
Menstrual migraine, without refractory migraine
Menstrually related migraine, not intractable
Pre-menstrual headache, not intractable
Pre-menstrual migraine, not intractable
Pure menstrual migraine, not intractable
Code also associated premenstrual tension syndrome (N94.3)

**G43.821** **Menstrual migraine, not intractable,** ♀
**with status migrainosus**

**G43.829** **Menstrual migraine, not intractable,** ♀
**without status migrainosus**
Menstrual migraine NOS

✓6ᵗʰ **G43.83** **Menstrual migraine, intractable**
Menstrual headache, intractable
Menstrual migraine, with refractory migraine
Menstrually related migraine, intractable
Pre-menstrual headache, intractable
Pre-menstrual migraine, intractable
Pure menstrual migraine, intractable
Code also associated premenstrual tension syndrome (N94.3)

**G43.831** **Menstrual migraine, intractable, with** ♀
**status migrainosus**

**G43.839** **Menstrual migraine, intractable,** ♀
**without status migrainosus**

✓5ᵗʰ **G43.9** **Migraine,** unspecified

✓6ᵗʰ **G43.90** **Migraine, unspecified, not intractable**
Migraine, unspecified, without refractory migraine

**G43.901** **Migraine, unspecified, not intractable,**
**with status migrainosus**
Status migrainosus NOS

**G43.909** **Migraine, unspecified, not intractable,**
**without status migrainosus**
Migraine NOS

✓6ᵗʰ **G43.91** **Migraine, unspecified, intractable**
Migraine, unspecified, with refractory migraine

**G43.911** **Migraine, unspecified, intractable, with**
**status migrainosus**

**G43.919** **Migraine, unspecified, intractable,**
**without status migrainosus**

✓4ᵗʰ **G44** **Other headache syndromes**
EXCLUDES 1    headache NOS (R51)
EXCLUDES 2    atypical facial pain (G50.1)
headache due to lumbar puncture (G97.1)
migraines (G43.-)
trigeminal neuralgia (G50.0)

✓5ᵗʰ **G44.0** **Cluster headaches and other trigeminal autonomic**
**cephalgias (TAC)**

✓6ᵗʰ **G44.00** **Cluster headache syndrome,** unspecified
Ciliary neuralgia                 Lower half migraine
Cluster headache NOS      Migrainous neuralgia
Histamine cephalgia

**G44.001** **Cluster headache syndrome, unspecified,**
**intractable**

**G44.009** **Cluster headache syndrome, unspecified,**
**not intractable**
Cluster headache syndrome NOS

✓6ᵗʰ **G44.01** **Episodic cluster headache**

**G44.011** **Episodic cluster headache, intractable**

**G44.019** **Episodic cluster headache,** not intractable
Episodic cluster headache NOS

✓6ᵗʰ **G44.02** **Chronic cluster headache**

**G44.021** **Chronic cluster headache, intractable**

**G44.029** **Chronic cluster headache,** not intractable
Chronic cluster headache NOS

✓6ᵗʰ **G44.03** **Episodic paroxysmal hemicrania**
Paroxysmal hemicrania NOS

**G44.031** **Episodic paroxysmal hemicrania,**
**intractable**

**G44.039** **Episodic paroxysmal hemicrania,** not
**intractable**
Episodic paroxysmal hemicrania NOS

✓6ᵗʰ **G44.04** **Chronic paroxysmal hemicrania**

**G44.041** **Chronic paroxysmal hemicrania,**
**intractable**

**G44.049** **Chronic paroxysmal hemicrania,** not
**intractable**
Chronic paroxysmal hemicrania NOS

✓6ᵗʰ **G44.05** **Short lasting unilateral neuralgiform headache with**
**conjunctival injection and tearing (SUNCT)**

**G44.051** **Short lasting unilateral neuralgiform**
**headache with conjunctival injection and**
**tearing (SUNCT), intractable**

**G44.059** **Short lasting unilateral neuralgiform**
**headache with conjunctival injection and**
**tearing (SUNCT), not intractable**
Short lasting unilateral neuralgiform
headache with conjunctival injection
and tearing (SUNCT) NOS

✓6ᵗʰ **G44.09** **Other** trigeminal autonomic cephalgias (TAC)

**G44.091** **Other trigeminal autonomic cephalgias**
**(TAC), intractable**

**G44.099** **Other trigeminal autonomic cephalgias**
**syndrome (TAC), not intractable**

**G44.1** **Vascular** headache, not elsewhere classified
EXCLUDES 2    cluster headache (G44.0)
complicated headache syndromes (G44.5-)
drug-induced headache (G44.4-)
migraine (G43.-)
other specified headache syndromes (G44.8-)
post-traumatic headache (G44.3-)
tension-type headache (G44.2-)

✓5ᵗʰ **G44.2** **Tension-type headache**

✓6ᵗʰ **G44.20** **Tension-type headache,** unspecified

**G44.201** **Tension-type headache, unspecified,**
**intractable**

**G44.209** **Tension-type headache, unspecified, not**
**intractable**
Tension headache NOS

✓6ᵗʰ **G44.21** **Episodic tension-type headache**

**G44.211** **Episodic tension-type headache,**
**intractable**

**G44.219** **Episodic tension-type headache,** not
**intractable**
Episodic tension-type headache NOS

✓6ᵗʰ **G44.22** **Chronic tension-type headache**

**G44.221** **Chronic tension-type headache,**
**intractable**

**G44.229** **Chronic tension-type headache,** not
**intractable**
Chronic tension-type headache NOS

✓5ᵗʰ **G44.3** **Post-traumatic** headache

✓6ᵗʰ **G44.30** **Post-traumatic headache,** unspecified

**G44.301** **Post-traumatic headache, unspecified,**
**intractable**

**G44.309** **Post-traumatic headache, unspecified,** not
**intractable**
Post-traumatic headache NOS

✓6ᵗʰ **G44.31** **Acute post-traumatic headache**

**G44.311** **Acute post-traumatic headache,**
**intractable**

**G44.319** **Acute post-traumatic headache,** not
**intractable**
Acute post-traumatic headache NOS

✓6ᵗʰ **G44.32** **Chronic post-traumatic headache**

**G44.321** **Chronic post-traumatic headache,**
**intractable**

**G44.329** **Chronic post-traumatic headache,** not
**intractable**
Chronic post-traumatic headache NOS

✓5ᵗʰ **G44.4** **Drug-induced** headache, not elsewhere classified
Medication overuse headache
Use additional code for adverse effect, if applicable, to identify
drug (T36-T50 with fifth or sixth character 5)

**G44.40** **Drug-induced headache, not elsewhere classified,**
**not intractable**

**G44.41** **Drug-induced headache, not elsewhere classified,**
**intractable**

✓5ᵗʰ **G44.5** **Complicated headache syndromes**

**G44.51** **Hemicrania continua**

**G44.52** **New daily persistent headache (NDPH)**

**G44.53** **Primary thunderclap** headache

---

✓ Additional Character Req    ✓x7ᵗʰ Placeholder Alert   Unacceptable PDx    Manifestation    H1 - H14 HAC   HCC CMS-HCC Condition    EXCLUDES 1 Not Coded Here    EXCLUDES 2 Not Included Here

**Chapter 6. Diseases of the Nervous System**

**G44.59**   Other complicated **headache** syndrome

☑5ᵗʰ **G44.8**   Other specified **headache** syndromes

    **G44.81**   Hypnic **headache**

    **G44.82**   **Headache** associated with **sexual activity**
        Orgasmic headache
        Preorgasmic headache

    **G44.83**   Primary **cough headache**

    **G44.84**   Primary **exertional headache**

    **G44.85**   Primary **stabbing headache**

    **G44.89**   Other **headache** syndrome

☑4ᵗʰ **G45**   **Transient cerebral ischemic attacks and related syndromes**

    *EXCLUDES 1*   neonatal cerebral ischemia (P91.0)
              transient retinal artery occlusion (H34.0-)

> **CC Excl: For CC codes in category G45, unless otherwise noted:**
> PDX collection 586

    **G45.0**   Vertebro-basilar artery syndrome     `CC`

    **G45.1**   Carotid artery syndrome (hemispheric)   `CC`

    **G45.2**   Multiple and bilateral precerebral artery syndromes   `CC`

    **G45.3**   Amaurosis fugax     `CC`
        **CC Excl:** PDX collection 587

    **G45.4**   Transient global amnesia
        *EXCLUDES 1*   amnesia NOS (R41.3)

    **G45.8**   Other transient cerebral ischemic attacks and related syndromes   `CC`

    **G45.9**   Transient cerebral ischemic attack, unspecified   `CC`
        Spasm of cerebral artery
        TIA
        Transient cerebral ischemia NOS

☑4ᵗʰ **G46**   **Vascular syndromes of brain in cerebrovascular diseases**
    Code first underlying cerebrovascular disease (I60-I69)

> **CC Excl: For CC codes in category G46:** PDX collection 586

    **G46.0**   Middle **cerebral artery syndrome**   `CC`

    **G46.1**   Anterior **cerebral artery syndrome**   `CC`

    **G46.2**   Posterior **cerebral artery syndrome**   `CC`

    **G46.3**   Brain stem stroke **syndrome**
        Benedikt syndrome     Millard-Gubler syndrome
        Claude syndrome       Wallenberg syndrome
        Foville syndrome       Weber syndrome

    **G46.4**   Cerebellar stroke **syndrome**

    **G46.5**   Pure motor lacunar **syndrome**

    **G46.6**   Pure sensory lacunar **syndrome**

    **G46.7**   Other lacunar **syndromes**

    **G46.8**   Other **vascular syndromes of brain in cerebrovascular diseases**

☑4ᵗʰ **G47**   **Sleep disorders**
    *EXCLUDES 2*   nightmares (F51.5)
              nonorganic sleep disorders (F51.-)
              sleep terrors (F51.4)
              sleepwalking (F51.3)

☑5ᵗʰ **G47.0**   Insomnia
    *EXCLUDES 2*   alcohol related insomnia (F10.182, F10.282, F10.982)
              drug-related insomnia (F11.182, F11.282, F11.982,
                  F13.182, F13.282, F13.982, F14.182,
                  F14.282,F14.982, F15.182, F15.282, F15.982,
                  F19.182, F19.282, F19.982)
              idiopathic insomnia (F51.01)
              insomnia due to a mental disorder (F51.05)
              insomnia not due to a substance or known
                  physiological condition (F51.0-)
              nonorganic insomnia (F51.0-)
              primary insomnia (F51.01)
              sleep apnea (G47.3-)

    **G47.00**   Insomnia, unspecified
        Insomnia NOS

    **G47.01**   Insomnia due to medical condition
        Code also associated medical condition

    **G47.09**   Other insomnia

☑5ᵗʰ **G47.1**   Hypersomnia
    *EXCLUDES 2*   alcohol-related hypersomnia (F10.182, F10.282,
                  F10.982)
              drug-related hypersomnia (F11.182, F11.282, F11.982,
                  F13.182, F13.282, F13.982, F14.182,F14.282,
                  F14.982, F15.182, F15.282, F15.982, F19.182,
                  F19.282, F19.982)
              hypersomnia due to a mental disorder (F51.13)
              hypersomnia not due to a substance or known
                  physiological condition (F51.1-)
              primary hypersomnia (F51.11)
              sleep apnea (G47.3-)

    **G47.10**   Hypersomnia, unspecified
        Hypersomnia NOS

    **G47.11**   Idiopathic **hypersomnia** with long sleep time
        Idiopathic hypersomnia NOS

    **G47.12**   Idiopathic **hypersomnia** without long sleep time

    **G47.13**   Recurrent **hypersomnia**
        Kleine-Levin syndrome
        Menstrual related hypersomnia

    **G47.14**   Hypersomnia due to medical condition
        Code also associated medical condition

    **G47.19**   Other **hypersomnia**

☑5ᵗʰ **G47.2**   Circadian rhythm sleep disorders
    Disorders of the sleep wake schedule
    Inversion of nyctohemeral rhythm
    Inversion of sleep rhythm

    **G47.20**   Circadian rhythm sleep disorder, unspecified type
        Sleep wake schedule disorder NOS

    **G47.21**   Circadian rhythm sleep disorder, delayed sleep phase type
        Delayed sleep phase syndrome

    **G47.22**   Circadian rhythm sleep disorder, advanced sleep phase type

    **G47.23**   Circadian rhythm sleep disorder, irregular sleep wake type
        Irregular sleep-wake pattern

    **G47.24**   Circadian rhythm sleep disorder, free running type
        ► Circadian rhythm sleep disorder, non-24-hour
           sleep-wake type ◄

    **G47.25**   Circadian rhythm sleep disorder, jet lag type

    **G47.26**   Circadian rhythm sleep disorder, shift work type

    **G47.27**   *Circadian rhythm sleep disorder in conditions classified elsewhere*
        Code first underlying condition

    **G47.29**   Other **circadian rhythm sleep disorder**

☑5ᵗʰ **G47.3**   Sleep apnea
    Code also any associated underlying condition
    *EXCLUDES 1*   apnea NOS (R06.81)
              Cheyne-Stokes breathing (R06.3)
              pickwickian syndrome (E66.2)
              sleep apnea of newborn (P28.3)

    **G47.30**   Sleep apnea, unspecified
        Sleep apnea NOS

    **G47.31**   Primary central **sleep apnea**
        ► Idiopathic central sleep apnea ◄

    **G47.32**   High altitude periodic breathing

    **G47.33**   Obstructive **sleep apnea** (adult) (pediatric)
        ► Obstructive sleep apnea hypopnea ◄
        *EXCLUDES 1*   obstructive sleep apnea of newborn (P28.3)

    **G47.34**   Idiopathic sleep related nonobstructive alveolar hypoventilation
        Sleep related hypoxia

    **G47.35**   Congenital central alveolar hypoventilation syndrome

    **G47.36**   *Sleep related hypoventilation in conditions classified elsewhere*
        Sleep related hypoxemia in conditions classified
           elsewhere
        Code first underlying condition

    **G47.37**   *Central sleep apnea in conditions classified elsewhere*
        Code first underlying condition

    **G47.39**   Other **sleep apnea**

☑5ᵗʰ **G47.4**   Narcolepsy and cataplexy

  ☑6ᵗʰ **G47.41**   Narcolepsy

        **G47.411**   Narcolepsy with cataplexy

        **G47.419**   Narcolepsy without cataplexy
             Narcolepsy NOS

Ⓝ Newborn: 0   Ⓟ Pediatric: 0-17   Ⓜ Maternity: 12-55   Ⓐ Adult: 15-124   **MCC** Major CC Condition   **PDx MCC** PDx acts as own MCC   `CC` CC Condition   **PDx CC** PDx acts as own CC

**566**                         ICD-10-CM 2018

☑ 6th **G47.42  Narcolepsy in conditions classified elsewhere**
Code first underlying condition

G47.421   *Narcolepsy in conditions classified elsewhere with cataplexy*

G47.429   *Narcolepsy in conditions classified elsewhere without cataplexy*

☑ 5th **G47.5  Parasomnia**
EXCLUDES 1   alcohol induced parasomnia (F10.182, F10.282, F10.982)
drug induced parasomnia (F11.182, F11.282, F11.982, F13.182, F13.282, F13.982, F14.182, F14.282, F14.982, F15.182, F15.282, F15.982, F19.182, F19.282, F19.982)
parasomnia not due to a substance or known physiological condition (F51.8)

**G47.50  Parasomnia, unspecified**
Parasomnia NOS

**G47.51  Confusional arousals**

**G47.52  REM sleep behavior disorder**

**G47.53  Recurrent isolated sleep paralysis**

G47.54   *Parasomnia in conditions classified elsewhere*
Code first underlying condition

**G47.59  Other parasomnia**

☑ 5th **G47.6  Sleep related movement disorders**
EXCLUDES 2   restless legs syndrome (G25.81)

**G47.61  Periodic limb movement disorder**
~~Periodic limb movement disorder~~

**G47.62  Sleep related leg cramps**

**G47.63  Sleep related bruxism**
EXCLUDES 1   psychogenic bruxism (F45.8)

**G47.69  Other sleep related movement disorders**

**G47.8  Other sleep disorders**
▶Other specified sleep-wake disorder◀

**G47.9  Sleep disorder, unspecified**
Sleep disorder NOS
▶Unspecified sleep-wake disorder◀

## Nerve, nerve root and plexus disorders (G50-G59)

EXCLUDES 1   current traumatic nerve, nerve root and plexus disorders—see Injury, nerve by body region
neuralgia NOS (M79.2)
neuritis NOS (M79.2)
peripheral neuritis in pregnancy (O26.82-)
radiculitis NOS (M54.1-)

☑ 4th **G50  Disorders of trigeminal nerve**
INCLUDES   disorders of 5th cranial nerve

**G50.0  Trigeminal neuralgia**
Syndrome of paroxysmal facial pain
Tic douloureux

**G50.1  Atypical facial pain**

**G50.8  Other disorders of trigeminal nerve**

**G50.9  Disorder of trigeminal nerve, unspecified**

### Trigeminal and Facial Nerve Branches

Supratrochlear nerve
Supraorbital nerve
V2 branch
Infraorbital nerve
V1 branch
Trigeminal nerve (CN V) branches in infratemporal fossa
V3 branch
Mental nerve
Mental foramen

☑ 4th **G51  Facial nerve disorders**
INCLUDES   disorders of 7th cranial nerve

**G51.0  Bell's palsy**
Facial palsy

**G51.1  Geniculate ganglionitis**
EXCLUDES 1   postherpetic geniculate ganglionitis (B02.21)

**G51.2  Melkersson's syndrome**
Melkersson-Rosenthal syndrome

**G51.3  Clonic hemifacial spasm**

**G51.4  Facial myokymia**

**G51.8  Other disorders of facial nerve**

**G51.9  Disorder of facial nerve, unspecified**

☑ 4th **G52  Disorders of other cranial nerves**
EXCLUDES 2   disorders of acoustic [8th] nerve (H93.3)
disorders of optic [2nd] nerve (H46, H47.0)
paralytic strabismus due to nerve palsy (H49.0-H49.2)

**G52.0  Disorders of olfactory nerve**
Disorders of 1st cranial nerve

**G52.1  Disorders of glossopharyngeal nerve**
Disorder of 9th cranial nerve
Glossopharyngeal neuralgia

**G52.2  Disorders of vagus nerve**
Disorders of pneumogastric [10th] nerve

**G52.3  Disorders of hypoglossal nerve**
Disorders of 12th cranial nerve

**G52.7  Disorders of multiple cranial nerves**
Polyneuritis cranialis

**G52.8  Disorders of other specified cranial nerves**

**G52.9  Cranial nerve disorder, unspecified**

**G53  *Cranial nerve disorders in diseases classified elsewhere***
Code first underlying disease, such as:
neoplasm (C00-D49)
EXCLUDES 1   multiple cranial nerve palsy in sarcoidosis (D86.82)
multiple cranial nerve palsy in syphilis (A52.15)
postherpetic geniculate ganglionitis (B02.21)
postherpetic trigeminal neuralgia (B02.22)

☑ 4th **G54  Nerve root and plexus disorders**
EXCLUDES 1   current traumatic nerve root and plexus disorders—see nerve injury by body region
intervertebral disc disorders (M50-M51)
neuritis or radiculitis brachial NOS (M54.13)
neuritis or radiculitis lumbar NOS (M54.16)
neuritis or radiculitis lumbosacral NOS (M54.17)
neuritis or radiculitis thoracic NOS (M54.14)
radiculitis NOS (M54.10)
radiculopathy NOS (M54.10)
spondylosis (M47.-)

**G54.0  Brachial plexus disorders**
Thoracic outlet syndrome
**DEF:** Acquired disorder affecting the spinal nerves that send signals to the shoulder, arm, and hand; causes corresponding motor and sensory dysfunction; characterized by regional paresthesia, pain, and muscle weakness, and in severe cases paralysis.

**G54.1  Lumbosacral plexus disorders**

**G54.2  Cervical root disorders, not elsewhere classified**

**G54.3  Thoracic root disorders, not elsewhere classified**

**G54.4  Lumbosacral root disorders, not elsewhere classified**

**G54.5  Neuralgic amyotrophy**
Parsonage-Aldren-Turner syndrome
Shoulder-girdle neuritis
EXCLUDES 1   neuralgic amyotrophy in diabetes mellitus (E08-E13 with .44)

**G54.6  Phantom limb syndrome with pain**     HCC

**G54.7  Phantom limb syndrome without pain**     HCC
Phantom limb syndrome NOS

**G54.8  Other nerve root and plexus disorders**

**G54.9  Nerve root and plexus disorder, unspecified**

**G55  *Nerve root and plexus compressions in diseases classified elsewhere***
Code first underlying disease, such as:
neoplasm (C00-D49)
EXCLUDES 1   nerve root compression (due to) (in) ankylosing spondylitis (M45.-)
nerve root compression (due to) (in) dorsopathies (M53.-, M54.-)
nerve root compression (due to) (in) intervertebral disc disorders (M50.1-, M51.1-)
nerve root compression (due to) (in) spondylopathies (M46.-, M48.-)

**Nerves of Upper Limb**

Radial

Deep branch of radial
Ulnar
Superficial branch of radial
Median

### ✓4ᵗʰ G56  Mononeuropathies of upper limb
> **EXCLUDES 1**  *current traumatic nerve disorder—see nerve injury by body region*

- ✓5ᵗʰ **G56.0  Carpal tunnel syndrome**
  - **G56.00**  Carpal tunnel syndrome, unspecified upper limb
  - **G56.01**  Carpal tunnel syndrome, right upper limb
  - **G56.02**  Carpal tunnel syndrome, left upper limb
  - **G56.03**  Carpal tunnel syndrome, bilateral upper limbs
- ✓5ᵗʰ **G56.1  Other lesions of median nerve**
  - **G56.10**  Other lesions of median nerve, unspecified upper limb
  - **G56.11**  Other lesions of median nerve, right upper limb
  - **G56.12**  Other lesions of median nerve, left upper limb
  - **G56.13**  Other lesions of median nerve, bilateral upper limbs
- ✓5ᵗʰ **G56.2  Lesion of ulnar nerve**
  Tardy ulnar nerve palsy
  - **G56.20**  Lesion of ulnar nerve, unspecified upper limb
  - **G56.21**  Lesion of ulnar nerve, right upper limb
  - **G56.22**  Lesion of ulnar nerve, left upper limb
  - **G56.23**  Lesion of ulnar nerve, bilateral upper limbs
- ✓5ᵗʰ **G56.3  Lesion of radial nerve**
  - **G56.30**  Lesion of radial nerve, unspecified upper limb
  - **G56.31**  Lesion of radial nerve, right upper limb
  - **G56.32**  Lesion of radial nerve, left upper limb
  - **G56.33**  Lesion of radial nerve, bilateral upper limbs
- ✓5ᵗʰ **G56.4  Causalgia of upper limb**
  Complex regional pain syndrome II of upper limb
  > **EXCLUDES 1**  *complex regional pain syndrome I of lower limb (G90.52-)*
  > *complex regional pain syndrome I of upper limb (G90.51-)*
  > *complex regional pain syndrome II of lower limb (G57.7-)*
  > *reflex sympathetic dystrophy of lower limb (G90.52-)*
  > *reflex sympathetic dystrophy of upper limb (G90.51-)*
  - **G56.40**  Causalgia of unspecified upper limb
  - **G56.41**  Causalgia of right upper limb
  - **G56.42**  Causalgia of left upper limb
  - **G56.43**  Causalgia of bilateral upper limbs
- ✓5ᵗʰ **G56.8  Other specified mononeuropathies of upper limb**
  Interdigital neuroma of upper limb
  - **G56.80**  Other specified mononeuropathies of unspecified upper limb
  - **G56.81**  Other specified mononeuropathies of right upper limb
  - **G56.82**  Other specified mononeuropathies of left upper limb

- **G56.83**  Other specified mononeuropathies of bilateral upper limbs
- ✓5ᵗʰ **G56.9  Unspecified mononeuropathy of upper limb**
  - **G56.90**  Unspecified mononeuropathy of unspecified upper limb
  - **G56.91**  Unspecified mononeuropathy of right upper limb
  - **G56.92**  Unspecified mononeuropathy of left upper limb
  - **G56.93**  Unspecified mononeuropathy of bilateral upper limbs

### ✓4ᵗʰ G57  Mononeuropathies of lower limb
> **EXCLUDES 1**  *current traumatic nerve disorder—see nerve injury by body region*

- ✓5ᵗʰ **G57.0  Lesion of sciatic nerve**
  > **EXCLUDES 1**  *sciatica NOS (M54.3-)*
  > **EXCLUDES 2**  *sciatica attributed to intervertebral disc disorder (M51.1-)*
  - **G57.00**  Lesion of sciatic nerve, unspecified lower limb
  - **G57.01**  Lesion of sciatic nerve, right lower limb
  - **G57.02**  Lesion of sciatic nerve, left lower limb
  - **G57.03**  Lesion of sciatic nerve, bilateral lower limbs
- ✓5ᵗʰ **G57.1  Meralgia paresthetica**
  Lateral cutaneous nerve of thigh syndrome
  - **G57.10**  Meralgia paresthetica, unspecified lower limb
  - **G57.11**  Meralgia paresthetica, right lower limb
  - **G57.12**  Meralgia paresthetica, left lower limb
  - **G57.13**  Meralgia paresthetica, bilateral lower limbs
- ✓5ᵗʰ **G57.2  Lesion of femoral nerve**
  - **G57.20**  Lesion of femoral nerve, unspecified lower limb
  - **G57.21**  Lesion of femoral nerve, right lower limb
  - **G57.22**  Lesion of femoral nerve, left lower limb
  - **G57.23**  Lesion of femoral nerve, bilateral lower limbs
- ✓5ᵗʰ **G57.3  Lesion of lateral popliteal nerve**
  Peroneal nerve palsy
  - **G57.30**  Lesion of lateral popliteal nerve, unspecified lower limb
  - **G57.31**  Lesion of lateral popliteal nerve, right lower limb
  - **G57.32**  Lesion of lateral popliteal nerve, left lower limb
  - **G57.33**  Lesion of lateral popliteal nerve, bilateral lower limbs
- ✓5ᵗʰ **G57.4  Lesion of medial popliteal nerve**
  - **G57.40**  Lesion of medial popliteal nerve, unspecified lower limb
  - **G57.41**  Lesion of medial popliteal nerve, right lower limb

**Nerves of Lower Limb**

Obturator nerve

Sciatic nerve

Femoral nerve

Saphenous nerve

Common fibular (peroneal) nerve

Deep fibular (peroneal) nerve

Tibial nerve

Superficial fibular (peroneal) nerve

**N** Newborn: 0   **P** Pediatric: 0-17   **M** Maternity: 12-55   **A** Adult: 15-124   **MCC** Major CC Condition   **PDxMCC** PDx acts as own MCC   **CC** CC Condition   **PDxCC** PDx acts as own CC

568                                                                                                                                           ICD-10-CM 2018

G57.42   **Lesion of medial popliteal nerve, left lower limb**

G57.43   **Lesion of medial popliteal nerve, bilateral lower limbs**

✓5ᵗʰ **G57.5**   **Tarsal tunnel syndrome**

     G57.50   **Tarsal tunnel syndrome, unspecified lower limb**

     G57.51   **Tarsal tunnel syndrome, right lower limb**

     G57.52   **Tarsal tunnel syndrome, left lower limb**

     G57.53   **Tarsal tunnel syndrome, bilateral lower limbs**

✓5ᵗʰ **G57.6**   **Lesion of plantar nerve**
     Morton's metatarsalgia

     G57.60   **Lesion of plantar nerve, unspecified lower limb**

     G57.61   **Lesion of plantar nerve, right lower limb**

     G57.62   **Lesion of plantar nerve, left lower limb**

     G57.63   **Lesion of plantar nerve, bilateral lower limbs**

✓5ᵗʰ **G57.7**   **Causalgia of lower limb**
     Complex regional pain syndrome II of lower limb

     **EXCLUDES 1**   *complex regional pain syndrome I of lower limb (G90.52-)*
         *complex regional pain syndrome I of upper limb (G90.51-)*
         *complex regional pain syndrome II of upper limb (G56.4-)*
         *reflex sympathetic dystrophy of lower limb (G90.52-)*
         *reflex sympathetic dystrophy of upper limb (G90.51-)*

     G57.70   **Causalgia of unspecified lower limb**

     G57.71   **Causalgia of right lower limb**

     G57.72   **Causalgia of left lower limb**

     G57.73   **Causalgia of bilateral lower limbs**

✓5ᵗʰ **G57.8**   **Other specified mononeuropathies of lower limb**
     Interdigital neuroma of lower limb

     G57.80   **Other specified mononeuropathies of unspecified lower limb**

     G57.81   **Other specified mononeuropathies of right lower limb**

     G57.82   **Other specified mononeuropathies of left lower limb**

     G57.83   **Other specified mononeuropathies of bilateral lower limbs**

✓5ᵗʰ **G57.9**   **Unspecified mononeuropathy of lower limb**

     G57.90   **Unspecified mononeuropathy of unspecified lower limb**

     G57.91   **Unspecified mononeuropathy of right lower limb**

     G57.92   **Unspecified mononeuropathy of left lower limb**

     G57.93   **Unspecified mononeuropathy of bilateral lower limbs**

✓4ᵗʰ **G58**   **Other mononeuropathies**

     G58.0   **Intercostal neuropathy**

     G58.7   **Mononeuritis multiplex**

     G58.8   **Other specified mononeuropathies**

     G58.9   **Mononeuropathy, unspecified**

**G59**   *Mononeuropathy in diseases classified elsewhere*
     Code first underlying disease
     **EXCLUDES 1**   *diabetic mononeuropathy (E08-E13 with .41)*
         *syphilitic nerve paralysis (A52.19)*
         *syphilitic neuritis (A52.15)*
         *tuberculous mononeuropathy (A17.83)*

## Polyneuropathies and other disorders of the peripheral nervous system (G60-G65)

     **EXCLUDES 1**   *neuralgia NOS (M79.2)*
         *neuritis NOS (M79.2)*
         *peripheral neuritis in pregnancy (O26.82-)*
         *radiculitis NOS (M54.10)*

✓4ᵗʰ **G60**   **Hereditary and idiopathic neuropathy**

     **G60.0**   **Hereditary motor and sensory neuropathy**
         Charcôt-Marie-Tooth disease
         Déjérine-Sottas disease
         Hereditary motor and sensory neuropathy, types I-IV
         Hypertrophic neuropathy of infancy
         Peroneal muscular atrophy (axonal type) (hypertrophic type)
         Roussy-Levy syndrome

     **G60.1**   **Refsum's disease**   **CC**
         Infantile Refsum disease
         **AHA:** 2014, 2Q, 4
         **DEF:** Genetic disorder of lipid metabolism; characterized by retinitis pigmentosa, degenerative nerve disease, ataxia, and dry, rough, scaly skin.
         **CC Excl:** PDX collection 588

     **G60.2**   **Neuropathy in association with hereditary ataxia**

     **G60.3**   **Idiopathic progressive neuropathy**

     **G60.8**   **Other hereditary and idiopathic neuropathies**
         Dominantly inherited sensory neuropathy
         Morvan's disease
         Nelaton's syndrome
         Recessively inherited sensory neuropathy

     **G60.9**   **Hereditary and idiopathic neuropathy, unspecified**

✓4ᵗʰ **G61**   **Inflammatory polyneuropathy**

     **G61.0**   **Guillain-Barre syndrome**   **CC** **HCC**
         Acute (post-)infective polyneuritis
         Miller Fisher syndrome
         **AHA:** 2014, 2Q, 4
         **CC Excl:** PDX collection 92

     **G61.1**   **Serum neuropathy**   **HCC**
         Use additional code for adverse effect, if applicable, to identify serum (T50.-)

✓5ᵗʰ **G61.8**   **Other inflammatory polyneuropathies**

     G61.81   **Chronic inflammatory demyelinating polyneuritis**   **CC** **HCC**
         **CC Excl:** PDX collection 589

     G61.82   **Multifocal motor neuropathy**   **HCC**
         MMN

     G61.89   **Other inflammatory polyneuropathies**   **HCC**

     **G61.9**   **Inflammatory polyneuropathy, unspecified**   **HCC**

✓4ᵗʰ **G62**   **Other and unspecified polyneuropathies**

     **G62.0**   **Drug-induced polyneuropathy**   **HCC**
         Use additional code for adverse effect, if applicable, to identify drug (T36-T50 with fifth or sixth character 5)

     **G62.1**   **Alcoholic polyneuropathy**   **HCC**

     **G62.2**   **Polyneuropathy due to other toxic agents**   **HCC**
         Code first (T51-T65) to identify toxic agent

✓5ᵗʰ **G62.8**   **Other specified polyneuropathies**

     G62.81   **Critical illness polyneuropathy**   **CC** **HCC**
         Acute motor neuropathy
         **CC Excl:** PDX collection 590

     G62.82   **Radiation-induced polyneuropathy**   **HCC**
         Use additional external cause code (W88-W90, X39.0-) to identify cause

     G62.89   **Other specified polyneuropathies**
         **AHA:** 2016, 2Q, 11

     **G62.9**   **Polyneuropathy, unspecified**
         Neuropathy NOS

**G63**   *Polyneuropathy in diseases classified elsewhere*   **HCC**
     Code first underlying disease, such as:
         amyloidosis (E85.-)
         endocrine disease, except diabetes (E00-E07, E15-E16, E20-E34)
         metabolic diseases (E70-E88)
         neoplasm (C00-D49)
         nutritional deficiency (E40-E64)
     **EXCLUDES 1**   *polyneuropathy (in):*
         *diabetes mellitus (E08-E13 with .42)*
         *diphtheria (A36.83)*
         *infectious mononucleosis (B27.0-B27.9 with 1)*
         *Lyme disease (A69.22)*
         *mumps (B26.84)*
         *postherpetic (B02.23)*
         *rheumatoid arthritis (M05.33)*
         *scleroderma (M34.83)*
         *systemic lupus erythematosus (M32.19)*
     **AHA:** 2012, 4Q, 99

**G64**   **Other disorders of peripheral nervous system**
     Disorder of peripheral nervous system NOS

✓4ᵗʰ **G65**   **Sequelae of inflammatory and toxic polyneuropathies**
     Code first condition resulting from (sequela) of inflammatory and toxic polyneuropathies

     **G65.0**   **Sequelae of Guillain-Barré syndrome**   **HCC**

     **G65.1**   **Sequelae of other inflammatory polyneuropathy**   **HCC**

     **G65.2**   **Sequelae of toxic polyneuropathy**   **HCC**

## Diseases of myoneural junction and muscle (G70-G73)

**☑4ᵗʰ G70 Myasthenia gravis and other myoneural disorders**

> **EXCLUDES 1**   botulism (A05.1, A48.51-A48.52)
> transient neonatal myasthenia gravis (P94.0)

> **CC Excl:** For CC/MCC codes in category G70: PDX collection 591

**☑5ᵗʰ G70.0 Myasthenia gravis**

> **G70.00 Myasthenia gravis without (acute) exacerbation** `HCC`
> Myasthenia gravis NOS

> **G70.01 Myasthenia gravis with (acute) exacerbation** `MCC` `HCC`
> Myasthenia gravis in crisis

**G70.1 Toxic myoneural disorders** `HCC`
> Code first (T51-T65) to identify toxic agent

**G70.2 Congenital and developmental myasthenia** `HCC`

**☑5ᵗʰ G70.8 Other specified myoneural disorders**

> **G70.80 Lambert-Eaton syndrome, unspecified** `CC` `HCC`
> Lambert-Eaton syndrome NOS

> **G70.81 *Lambert-Eaton syndrome in disease classified elsewhere*** `CC` `HCC`
> Code first underlying disease
> > **EXCLUDES 1**   Lambert-Eaton syndrome in neoplastic disease (G73.1)

> **G70.89 Other specified myoneural disorders** `HCC`

**G70.9 Myoneural disorder, unspecified** `HCC`

**☑4ᵗʰ G71 Primary disorders of muscles**

> **EXCLUDES 2**   arthrogryposis multiplex congenita (Q74.3)
> metabolic disorders (E70-E88)
> myositis (M60.-)

**G71.0 Muscular dystrophy** `CC` `HCC`
> Autosomal recessive, childhood type, muscular dystrophy resembling Duchenne or Becker muscular dystrophy
> Benign [Becker] muscular dystrophy
> Benign scapuloperoneal muscular dystrophy with early contractures [Emery-Dreifuss]
> Congenital muscular dystrophy NOS
> Congenital muscular dystrophy with specific morphological abnormalities of the muscle fiber
> Distal muscular dystrophy
> Facioscapulohumeral muscular dystrophy
> Limb-girdle muscular dystrophy
> Ocular muscular dystrophy
> Oculopharyngeal muscular dystrophy
> Scapuloperoneal muscular dystrophy
> Severe [Duchenne] muscular dystrophy
> **CC Excl:** PDX collection 592

**☑5ᵗʰ G71.1 Myotonic disorders**

> **G71.11 Myotonic muscular dystrophy** `HCC`
> Dystrophia myotonica [Steinert]
> Myotonia atrophica
> Myotonic dystrophy
> Proximal myotonic myopathy (PROMM)
> Steinert disease

> **G71.12 Myotonia congenita**
> Acetazolamide responsive myotonia congenita
> Dominant myotonia congenita [Thomsen disease]
> Myotonia levior
> Recessive myotonia congenita [Becker disease]

> **G71.13 Myotonic chondrodystrophy**
> Chondrodystrophic myotonia
> Congenital myotonic chondrodystrophy
> Schwartz-Jampel disease

> **G71.14 Drug induced myotonia**
> Use additional code for adverse effect, if applicable, to identify drug (T36-T50 with fifth or sixth character 5)

> **G71.19 Other specified myotonic disorders**
> Myotonia fluctuans
> Myotonia permanens
> Neuromyotonia [Isaacs]
> Paramyotonia congenita (of von Eulenburg)
> Pseudomyotonia
> Symptomatic myotonia

**G71.2 Congenital myopathies** `CC` `HCC`
> Central core disease
> Fiber-type disproportion
> Minicore disease
> Multicore disease
> Myotubular (centronuclear) myopathy
> Nemaline myopathy
> > **EXCLUDES 1**   arthrogryposis multiplex congenita (Q74.3)
> **CC Excl:** PDX collection 592

**G71.3 Mitochondrial myopathy, not elsewhere classified**
> > **EXCLUDES 1**   Kearns-Sayre syndrome (H49.81)
> > Leber's disease (H47.21)
> > Leigh's encephalopathy (G31.82)
> > mitochondrial metabolism disorders (E88.4-)
> > Reye's syndrome (G93.7)

**G71.8 Other primary disorders of muscles**

**G71.9 Primary disorder of muscle, unspecified**
> Hereditary myopathy NOS

**☑4ᵗʰ G72 Other and unspecified myopathies**

> **EXCLUDES 1**   arthrogryposis multiplex congenita (Q74.3)
> dermatopolymyositis (M33.-)
> ischemic infarction of muscle (M62.2-)
> myositis (M60.-)
> polymyositis (M33.2-)

**G72.0 Drug-induced myopathy** `CC`
> Use additional code for adverse effect, if applicable, to identify drug (T36-T50 with fifth or sixth character 5)
> **CC Excl:** PDX collection 593

**G72.1 Alcoholic myopathy** `CC`
> Use additional code to identify alcoholism (F10.-)
> **CC Excl:** PDX collection 593

**G72.2 Myopathy due to other toxic agents** `CC`
> Code first (T51-T65) to identify toxic agent
> **CC Excl:** PDX collection 593

**G72.3 Periodic paralysis**
> Familial periodic paralysis
> Hyperkalemic periodic paralysis (familial)
> Hypokalemic periodic paralysis (familial)
> Myotonic periodic paralysis (familial)
> Normokalemic paralysis (familial)
> Potassium sensitive periodic paralysis
> > **EXCLUDES 1**   paramyotonia congenita (of von Eulenburg) (G71.19)

**☑5ᵗʰ G72.4 Inflammatory and immune myopathies, not elsewhere classified**

> **G72.41 Inclusion body myositis [IBM]**

> **G72.49 Other inflammatory and immune myopathies, not elsewhere classified**
> Inflammatory myopathy NOS

**☑5ᵗʰ G72.8 Other specified myopathies**

> **G72.81 Critical illness myopathy** `CC`
> Acute necrotizing myopathy
> Acute quadriplegic myopathy
> Intensive care (ICU) myopathy
> Myopathy of critical illness
> **CC Excl:** PDX collection 594

> **G72.89 Other specified myopathies**

**G72.9 Myopathy, unspecified**

**☑4ᵗʰ G73 Disorders of myoneural junction and muscle in diseases classified elsewhere**

> **G73.1 *Lambert-Eaton syndrome in neoplastic disease*** `CC` `HCC`
> Code first underlying neoplasm (C00-D49)
> > **EXCLUDES 1**   Lambert-Eaton syndrome not associated with neoplasm (G70.80-G70.81)
> **CC Excl:** PDX collection 591

> **G73.3 *Myasthenic syndromes in other diseases classified elsewhere*** `CC` `HCC`
> Code first underlying disease, such as:
> neoplasm (C00-D49)
> thyrotoxicosis (E05.-)
> **CC Excl:** PDX collection 591

☑ Newborn: 0   ☑ Pediatric: 0-17   ☑ Maternity: 12-55   ☑ Adult: 15-124   `MCC` Major CC Condition   `PDxMCC` PDx acts as own MCC   `CC` CC Condition   `PDxCC` PDx acts as own CC

570        ICD-10-CM 2018

**G73.7** *Myopathy in diseases classified elsewhere*

Code first underlying disease, such as:
hyperparathyroidism (E21.0, E21.3)
hypoparathyroidism (E20.-)
glycogen storage disease (E74.0)
lipid storage disorders (E75.-)

> EXCLUDES 1    *myopathy in:*
> *rheumatoid arthritis (M05.4-)*
> *sarcoidosis (D86.87)*
> *scleroderma (M34.82)*
> *sicca syndrome [Sjögren] (M35.03)*
> *systemic lupus erythematosus (M32.19)*

## Cerebral palsy and other paralytic syndromes (G80-G83)

### ✓4th **G80** **Cerebral palsy**

> EXCLUDES 1    *hereditary spastic paraplegia (G11.4)*

**G80.0** **Spastic quadriplegic cerebral palsy**   MCC HCC
Congenital spastic paralysis (cerebral)
CC Excl: PDX collection 595

**G80.1** **Spastic diplegic cerebral palsy**   CC HCC
Spastic cerebral palsy NOS
CC Excl: PDX collection 596

**G80.2** **Spastic hemiplegic cerebral palsy**   CC HCC
CC Excl: PDX collection 597

**G80.3** **Athetoid cerebral palsy**   CC HCC
Double athetosis (syndrome)
Dyskinetic cerebral palsy
Dystonic cerebral palsy
Vogt disease
CC Excl: PDX collection 598

**G80.4** **Ataxic cerebral palsy**   HCC

**G80.8** **Other cerebral palsy**   HCC
Mixed cerebral palsy syndromes

**G80.9** **Cerebral palsy, unspecified**   HCC
Cerebral palsy NOS

### ✓4th **G81** **Hemiplegia and hemiparesis**

> NOTE    This category is to be used only when hemiplegia (complete)(incomplete) is reported without further specification, or is stated to be old or longstanding but of unspecified cause. The category is also for use in multiple coding to identify these types of hemiplegia resulting from any cause.

> EXCLUDES 1    *congenital cerebral palsy (G80.-)*
> *hemiplegia and hemiparesis due to sequela of cerebrovascular disease (I69.05-, I69.15-, I69.25-, I69.35-, I69.85-, I69.95-)*

**AHA:** 2015, 1Q, 25

CC Excl: For CC codes in category G81: PDX collection 561

#### ✓5th **G81.0** **Flaccid hemiplegia**

**G81.00** **Flaccid hemiplegia affecting unspecified side**   CC HCC

**G81.01** **Flaccid hemiplegia affecting right dominant side**   CC HCC

**G81.02** **Flaccid hemiplegia affecting left dominant side**   CC HCC

**G81.03** **Flaccid hemiplegia affecting right nondominant side**   CC HCC

**G81.04** **Flaccid hemiplegia affecting left nondominant side**   CC HCC

#### ✓5th **G81.1** **Spastic hemiplegia**

**G81.10** **Spastic hemiplegia affecting unspecified side**   CC HCC

**G81.11** **Spastic hemiplegia affecting right dominant side**   CC HCC

**G81.12** **Spastic hemiplegia affecting left dominant side**   CC HCC

**G81.13** **Spastic hemiplegia affecting right nondominant side**   CC HCC

**G81.14** **Spastic hemiplegia affecting left nondominant side**   CC HCC

#### ✓5th **G81.9** **Hemiplegia, unspecified**
**AHA:** 2014, 1Q, 23

**G81.90** **Hemiplegia, unspecified affecting unspecified side**   CC HCC

**G81.91** **Hemiplegia, unspecified affecting right dominant side**   CC HCC

**G81.92** **Hemiplegia, unspecified affecting left dominant side**   CC HCC

**G81.93** **Hemiplegia, unspecified affecting right nondominant side**   CC HCC

**G81.94** **Hemiplegia, unspecified affecting left nondominant side**   CC HCC

### ✓4th **G82** **Paraplegia (paraparesis) and quadriplegia (quadriparesis)**

> NOTE    This category is to be used only when the listed conditions are reported without further specification, or are stated to be old or longstanding but of unspecified cause. The category is also for use in multiple coding to identify these conditions resulting from any cause

> EXCLUDES 1    *congenital cerebral palsy (G80.-)*
> *functional quadriplegia (R53.2)*
> *hysterical paralysis (F44.4)*

#### ✓5th **G82.2** **Paraplegia**
Paralysis of both lower limbs NOS
Paraparesis (lower) NOS
Paraplegia (lower) NOS

CC Excl: For CC codes in subcategory G82.2:
PDX collection 561

**G82.20** **Paraplegia, unspecified**   CC HCC

**G82.21** **Paraplegia, complete**   CC HCC

**G82.22** **Paraplegia, incomplete**   CC HCC

#### ✓5th **G82.5** **Quadriplegia**

CC Excl: For MCC codes in subcategory G82.5:
PDX collection 595

**G82.50** **Quadriplegia, unspecified**   MCC HCC

**G82.51** **Quadriplegia, C1-C4 complete**   MCC HCC

**G82.52** **Quadriplegia, C1-C4 incomplete**   MCC HCC

**G82.53** **Quadriplegia, C5-C7 complete**   MCC HCC

**G82.54** **Quadriplegia, C5-C7 incomplete**   MCC HCC

### ✓4th **G83** **Other paralytic syndromes**

> NOTE    This category is to be used only when the listed conditions are reported without further specification, or are stated to be old or longstanding but of unspecified cause. The category is also for use in multiple coding to identify these conditions resulting from any cause.

> INCLUDES    paralysis (complete) (incomplete), except as in G80-G82

**G83.0** **Diplegia of upper limbs**   CC HCC
Diplegia (upper)
Paralysis of both upper limbs
CC Excl: PDX collection 599

#### ✓5th **G83.1** **Monoplegia of lower limb**
Paralysis of lower limb

> EXCLUDES 1    *monoplegia of lower limbs due to sequela of cerebrovascular disease (I69.04-, I69.14-, I69.24-, I69.34-, I69.84-, I69.94-)*

**G83.10** **Monoplegia of lower limb affecting unspecified side**   HCC

**G83.11** **Monoplegia of lower limb affecting right dominant side**   HCC

**G83.12** **Monoplegia of lower limb affecting left dominant side**   HCC

**G83.13** **Monoplegia of lower limb affecting right nondominant side**   HCC

**G83.14** **Monoplegia of lower limb affecting left nondominant side**   HCC

#### ✓5th **G83.2** **Monoplegia of upper limb**
Paralysis of upper limb

> EXCLUDES 1    *monoplegia of upper limbs due to sequela of cerebrovascular disease (I69.03-, I69.13-, I69.23-, I69.33-, I69.83-, I69.93-)*

**G83.20** **Monoplegia of upper limb affecting unspecified side**   HCC

**G83.21** **Monoplegia of upper limb affecting right dominant side**   HCC

**G83.22** **Monoplegia of upper limb affecting left dominant side**   HCC

**G83.23** **Monoplegia of upper limb affecting right nondominant side**   HCC

**G83.24** **Monoplegia of upper limb affecting left nondominant side**   HCC

#### ✓5th **G83.3** **Monoplegia, unspecified**

**G83.30** **Monoplegia, unspecified affecting unspecified side**   HCC

**G83.31** **Monoplegia, unspecified affecting right dominant side**   HCC

✓ Additional Character Req   ✓x7th Placeholder Alert   Unacceptable PDx   Manifestation   H1-H14 HAC   HCC CMS-HCC Condition   EXCLUDES1 Not Coded Here   EXCLUDES2 Not Included Here

ICD-10-CM 2018          **571**

**G83.32**   **Monoplegia, unspecified affecting** left **dominant side**    `HCC`

**G83.33**   **Monoplegia, unspecified affecting** right **nondominant side**    `HCC`

**G83.34**   **Monoplegia, unspecified affecting** left **nondominant side**    `HCC`

**G83.4**   **Cauda equina syndrome**    `CC` `HCC`
Neurogenic bladder due to cauda equina syndrome
> *EXCLUDES 1*   cord bladder NOS (G95.89)
>          neurogenic bladder NOS (N31.9)
**CC Excl:** PDX collection 600

**G83.5**   **Locked-in state**    `MCC` `HCC`
**CC Excl:** PDX collection 601

√5ᵗʰ **G83.8**   **Other specified paralytic syndromes**
> *EXCLUDES 1*   paralytic syndromes due to current spinal cord
>          injury—code to spinal cord injury (S14, S24, S34)

**G83.81**   **Brown-Séquard syndrome**    `HCC`

**G83.82**   **Anterior cord syndrome**    `HCC`

**G83.83**   **Posterior cord syndrome**    `HCC`

**G83.84**   **Todd's paralysis (postepileptic)**    `HCC`

**G83.89**   **Other specified paralytic syndromes**    `HCC`

**G83.9**   **Paralytic syndrome, unspecified**    `HCC`

## Other disorders of the nervous system (G89-G99)

√4ᵗʰ **G89**   **Pain, not elsewhere classified**
Code also related psychological factors associated with pain (F45.42)
> *EXCLUDES 1*   generalized pain NOS (R52)
>          pain disorders exclusively related to psychological factors
>            (F45.41)
>          pain NOS (R52)
> *EXCLUDES 2*   atypical face pain (G50.1)
>          headache syndromes (G44.-)
>          localized pain, unspecified type—code to pain by site, such as:
>            abdomen pain (R10.-)
>            back pain (M54.9)
>            breast pain (N64.4)
>            chest pain (R07.1-R07.9)
>            ear pain (H92.0-)
>            eye pain (H57.1)
>            headache (R51)
>            joint pain (M25.5-)
>            limb pain (M79.6-)
>            lumbar region pain (M54.5)
>            painful urination (R30.9)
>            pelvic and perineal pain (R10.2)
>            renal colic (N23)
>            shoulder pain (M25.51-)
>            spine pain (M54.-)
>            throat pain (R07.0)
>            tongue pain (K14.6)
>            tooth pain (K08.8)
>           migraines (G43.-)
>          myalgia (M79.1)
>          pain from prosthetic devices, implants, and grafts (T82.84,
>            T83.84, T84.84, T85.84-)
>          phantom limb syndrome with pain (G54.6)
>          vulvar vestibulitis (N94.810)
>          vulvodynia (N94.81-)

**G89.0**   **Central pain syndrome**
Déjérine-Roussy syndrome
Myelopathic pain syndrome
Thalamic pain syndrome (hyperesthetic)

√5ᵗʰ **G89.1**   **Acute pain, not elsewhere classified**

**G89.11**   **Acute pain due to trauma**

**G89.12**   **Acute post-thoracotomy pain**
Post-thoracotomy pain NOS

**G89.18**   **Other acute postprocedural pain**
Postoperative pain NOS
Postprocedural pain NOS

√5ᵗʰ **G89.2**   **Chronic pain, not elsewhere classified**
> *EXCLUDES 1*   causalgia, lower limb (G57.7-)
>          causalgia, upper limb (G56.4-)
>          central pain syndrome (G89.0)
>          chronic pain syndrome (G89.4)
>          complex regional pain syndrome II, lower limb (G57.7-)
>          complex regional pain syndrome II, upper limb (G56.4-)
>          neoplasm related chronic pain (G89.3)
>          reflex sympathetic dystrophy (G90.5-)

**G89.21**   **Chronic pain due to trauma**

**G89.22**   **Chronic post-thoracotomy pain**

**G89.28**   **Other chronic postprocedural pain**
Other chronic postoperative pain

**G89.29**   **Other chronic pain**

**G89.3**   **Neoplasm related pain (acute) (chronic)**
Cancer associated pain
Pain due to malignancy (primary) (secondary)
Tumor associated pain

**G89.4**   **Chronic pain syndrome**
Chronic pain associated with significant psychosocial dysfunction

√4ᵗʰ **G90**   **Disorders of autonomic nervous system**
> *EXCLUDES 1*   dysfunction of the autonomic nervous system due to alcohol
>          (G31.2)

√5ᵗʰ **G90.0**   **Idiopathic peripheral autonomic neuropathy**

**G90.01**   **Carotid sinus syncope**
Carotid sinus syndrome
**DEF:** Vagal activation caused by pressure on the carotid sinus baroreceptors; sympathetic nerve impulses may cause sinus arrest or AV block.

**G90.09**   **Other idiopathic peripheral autonomic neuropathy**
Idiopathic peripheral autonomic neuropathy NOS

**G90.1**   **Familial dysautonomia [Riley-Day]**    `HCC`

**G90.2**   **Horner's syndrome**
Bernard(-Horner) syndrome
Cervical sympathetic dystrophy or paralysis

**G90.3**   **Multi-system degeneration of the autonomic nervous**    `CC` `HCC`
**system**
Neurogenic orthostatic hypotension [Shy-Drager]
> *EXCLUDES 1*   orthostatic hypotension NOS (I95.1)
**CC Excl:** PDX collection 573

**G90.4**   **Autonomic dysreflexia**
Use additional code to identify the cause, such as:
>    fecal impaction (K56.41)
>    pressure ulcer (pressure area) (L89.-)
>    urinary tract infection (N39.0)

√5ᵗʰ **G90.5**   **Complex regional pain syndrome I (CRPS I)**
Reflex sympathetic dystrophy
> *EXCLUDES 1*   causalgia of lower limb (G57.7-)
>          causalgia of upper limb (G56.4-)
>          complex regional pain syndrome II of lower limb
>            (G57.7-)
>          complex regional pain syndrome II of upper limb
>            (G56.4-)

**CC Excl: For CC codes in subcategory G90.5, unless otherwise noted:** PDX collection 603

**G90.50**   **Complex regional pain syndrome I, unspecified**    `CC`
**CC Excl:** PDX collection 602

√6ᵗʰ **G90.51**   **Complex regional pain syndrome I of upper limb**

**G90.511**   **Complex regional pain syndrome I of right upper limb**    `CC`

**G90.512**   **Complex regional pain syndrome I of left upper limb**    `CC`

**G90.513**   **Complex regional pain syndrome I of upper limb, bilateral**    `CC`

**G90.519**   **Complex regional pain syndrome I of unspecified upper limb**    `CC`

√6ᵗʰ **G90.52**   **Complex regional pain syndrome I of lower limb**

**G90.521**   **Complex regional pain syndrome I of right lower limb**    `CC`

**G90.522**   **Complex regional pain syndrome I of left lower limb**    `CC`

**G90.523**   **Complex regional pain syndrome I of lower limb, bilateral**    `CC`

**G90.529**   **Complex regional pain syndrome I of unspecified lower limb**    `CC`

**G90.59**   **Complex regional pain syndrome I of other specified site**    `CC`

**G90.8**   **Other disorders of autonomic nervous system**

**G90.9**   **Disorder of the autonomic nervous system, unspecified**

---

N Newborn: 0   P Pediatric: 0-17   M Maternity: 12-55   A Adult: 15-124   `MCC` Major CC Condition   `PDxMCC` PDx acts as own MCC   `CC` CC Condition   `PDxCC` PDx acts as own CC

**572**          ICD-10-CM 2018

**Hydrocephalus (Acquired)**

Normal ventricles          Hydrocephalic ventricles

✓4th **G91 Hydrocephalus**
     INCLUDES   acquired hydrocephalus
     EXCLUDES 1   Arnold-Chiari syndrome with hydrocephalus (Q07.-)
          congenital hydrocephalus (Q03.-)
          spina bifida with hydrocephalus (Q05.-)

     **CC Excl: For CC codes in category G91, unless otherwise noted:**
     PDX collection 605

     **G91.0 Communicating hydrocephalus**    CC
         Secondary normal pressure hydrocephalus
         **CC Excl:** PDX collection 604

     **G91.1 Obstructive hydrocephalus**    CC
         **DEF:** Obstruction of cerebrospinal fluid passage from brain into
         spinal canal; characterized by headaches, drowsiness, poor
         coordination, urinary incontinence, nausea, vomiting, and
         papilledema.

     **G91.2 (Idiopathic) normal pressure hydrocephalus**    CC
         Normal pressure hydrocephalus NOS
         **CC Excl:** PDX collection 604

     **G91.3 Post-traumatic hydrocephalus, unspecified**    CC

     *G91.4 Hydrocephalus in diseases classified elsewhere*
         Code first underlying condition, such as:
           congenital syphilis (A50.4-)
           neoplasm (C00-D49)
         EXCLUDES 1   hydrocephalus due to congenital toxoplasmosis
               (P37.1)
         **AHA:** 2014, 3Q, 3

     **G91.8 Other hydrocephalus**    CC

     **G91.9 Hydrocephalus, unspecified**    CC

**G92 Toxic encephalopathy**    MCC
     Toxic encephalitis
     Toxic metabolic encephalopathy
     ▶Code first, if applicable, drug induced (T36-T50)◀
     Code first (T51-T65) to identify toxic agent
     **AHA:** 2017, 1Q, 39-40
     **DEF:** Brain tissue degeneration due to toxic substance.
     **CC Excl:** PDX collection 606

✓4th **G93 Other disorders of brain**

     **G93.0 Cerebral cysts**
         Arachnoid cyst
         Porencephalic cyst, acquired
         EXCLUDES 1   acquired periventricular cysts of newborn (P91.1)
               congenital cerebral cysts (Q04.6)

     **G93.1 Anoxic brain damage, not elsewhere classified**    CC HCC
         EXCLUDES 1   cerebral anoxia due to anesthesia during labor and
               delivery (O74.3)
               cerebral anoxia due to anesthesia during the
               puerperium (O89.2)
               neonatal anoxia (P84)
         **DEF:** Brain injury not resulting from birth trauma that is due to lack
         of oxygen. Brain cells, when deprived of oxygen, begin to expire
         after 4 minutes.
         **CC Excl:** PDX collection 607

     **G93.2 Benign intracranial hypertension**
         EXCLUDES 1   hypertensive encephalopathy (I67.4)

     **G93.3 Postviral fatigue syndrome**
         Benign myalgic encephalomyelitis
         EXCLUDES 1   chronic fatigue syndrome NOS (R53.82)

✓5th    **G93.4 Other and unspecified encephalopathy**
         EXCLUDES 1   alcoholic encephalopathy (G31.2)
               encephalopathy in diseases classified elsewhere (G94)
               hypertensive encephalopathy (I67.4)
               toxic (metabolic) encephalopathy (G92)

         **G93.40 Encephalopathy, unspecified**    HIV MCC
             **AHA:** 2017, 2Q, 8
             **CC Excl:** PDX collection 608

         **G93.41 Metabolic encephalopathy**    HIV MCC
             Septic encephalopathy
             **AHA:** 2017, 2Q, 8; 2016, 3Q, 42; 2015, 3Q, 21
             **CC Excl:** GPDX collection 609

         **G93.49 Other encephalopathy**    HIV MCC
             Encephalopathy NEC
             **AHA:** 2017, 2Q, 9
             **CC Excl:** PDX collection 610

     **G93.5 Compression of brain**    MCC HCC
         Arnold-Chiari type 1 compression of brain
         Compression of brain (stem)
         Herniation of brain (stem)
         EXCLUDES 1   diffuse traumatic compression of brain (S06.2-)
               focal traumatic compression of brain (S06.3-)
         **CC Excl:** PDX collection 611

     **G93.6 Cerebral edema**    MCC HCC
         EXCLUDES 1   cerebral edema due to birth injury (P11.0)
               traumatic cerebral edema (S06.1-)
         **CC Excl:** PDX collection 612

     **G93.7 Reye's syndrome**    MCC P
         ~~Code first (T39.0-), if salicylates-induced~~
         ▶Code first poisoning due to salicylates, if applicable (T39.0-, with
           sixth character 1-4)◀
         ▶Use additional code for adverse effect due to salicylates, if
           applicable (T39.0-, with sixth character 5)◀
         **DEF:** Rare childhood illness often developed after a viral upper
         respiratory infection; characterized by vomiting, elevated serum
         transaminase, brain swelling, disturbances of consciousness,
         seizures, and changes in liver and other viscera; can be fatal.
         **CC Excl:** PDX collection 613

✓5th    **G93.8 Other specified disorders of brain**

         **G93.81 Temporal sclerosis**
             Hippocampal sclerosis
             Mesial temporal sclerosis

         **G93.82 Brain death**    MCC
             **CC Excl:** PDX collection 515

         **G93.89 Other specified disorders of brain**
             Postradiation encephalopathy

     **G93.9 Disorder of brain, unspecified**    HIV

*G94 Other disorders of brain in diseases classified elsewhere*
     Code first underlying disease
     EXCLUDES 1   encephalopathy in congenital syphilis (A50.49)
          encephalopathy in influenza (J09.X9, J10.81, J11.81)
          encephalopathy in syphilis (A52.19)
          hydrocephalus in diseases classified elsewhere (G91.4)

✓4th **G95 Other and unspecified diseases of spinal cord**
     EXCLUDES 2   myelitis (G04.-)

     **G95.0 Syringomyelia and syringobulbia**    CC HCC
         **CC Excl:** PDX collection 614

✓5th    **G95.1 Vascular myelopathies**
         EXCLUDES 2   intraspinal phlebitis and thrombophlebitis, except
               non-pyogenic (G08)

         **G95.11 Acute infarction of spinal cord (embolic)**    MCC HCC
            **(nonembolic)**
             Anoxia of spinal cord
             Arterial thrombosis of spinal cord
             **CC Excl:** PDX collection 603

         **G95.19 Other vascular myelopathies**    MCC HCC
             Edema of spinal cord
             Hematomyelia
             Nonpyogenic intraspinal phlebitis and
               thrombophlebitis
             Subacute necrotic myelopathy
             **CC Excl:** PDX collection 603

☑ Additional Character Req    ✓x7th Placeholder Alert    Unacceptable PDx    Manifestation    H1-H14 HAC    HCC CMS-HCC Condition    EXCLUDES 1 Not Coded Here    EXCLUDES 2 Not Included Here

ICD-10-CM 2018                                                            573

G91–G95.19

✓5th **G95.2 Other and unspecified cord compression**

**G95.20 Unspecified cord compression** `HIV` `CC` `HCC`
CC Excl: PDX collection 615

**G95.29 Other cord compression** `HIV` `CC` `HCC`
CC Excl: PDX collection 615

✓5th **G95.8 Other specified diseases of spinal cord**
EXCLUDES 1   *neurogenic bladder NOS (N31.9)*
*neurogenic bladder due to cauda equina syndrome (G83.4)*
*neuromuscular dysfunction of bladder without spinal cord lesion (N31.-)*

**G95.81 Conus medullaris syndrome** `CC` `HCC`
CC Excl: PDX collection 603

**G95.89 Other specified diseases of spinal cord** `CC` `HCC`
Cord bladder NOS
Drug-induced myelopathy
Radiation-induced myelopathy
EXCLUDES 1   *myelopathy NOS (G95.9)*
CC Excl: PDX collection 603

**G95.9 Disease of spinal cord, unspecified** `HIV` `CC` `HCC`
Myelopathy NOS
CC Excl: PDX collection 615

✓4th **G96 Other disorders of central nervous system**

**G96.0 Cerebrospinal fluid leak** `CC`
EXCLUDES 1   *cerebrospinal fluid leak from spinal puncture (G97.0)*
DEF: Cerebrospinal fluid discharging from the nose or the ear; caused by fracture of frontal bone with tearing of dura mater and arachnoid; characterized by watery drainage usually from only one side of the nose or one ear, headache, vision changes, and hearing loss.
CC Excl: PDX collection 616

✓5th **G96.1 Disorders of meninges, not elsewhere classified**

**G96.11 Dural tear** `CC`
EXCLUDES 1   *accidental puncture or laceration of dura during a procedure (G97.41)*
AHA: 2014, 4Q, 24
CC Excl: PDX collection 509

**G96.12 Meningeal adhesions (cerebral) (spinal)**

**G96.19 Other disorders of meninges, not elsewhere classified**

**G96.8 Other specified disorders of central nervous system**

**G96.9 Disorder of central nervous system, unspecified** `HIV`

✓4th **G97 Intraoperative and postprocedural complications and disorders of nervous system, not elsewhere classified**
EXCLUDES 2   *intraoperative and postprocedural cerebrovascular infarction (I97.81-, I97.82-)*

**G97.0 Cerebrospinal fluid leak from spinal puncture** `CC`
CC Excl: PDX collection 617

**G97.1 Other reaction to spinal and lumbar puncture**
Headache due to lumbar puncture

**G97.2 Intracranial hypotension following ventricular shunting** `CC`
CC Excl: PDX collection 617

✓5th **G97.3 Intraoperative hemorrhage and hematoma of a nervous system organ or structure complicating a procedure**
EXCLUDES 1   *intraoperative hemorrhage and hematoma of a nervous system organ or structure due to accidental puncture and laceration during a procedure (G97.4-)*

**G97.31 Intraoperative hemorrhage and hematoma of a nervous system organ or structure complicating a nervous system procedure** `CC`
CC Excl: PDX collection 618

**G97.32 Intraoperative hemorrhage and hematoma of a nervous system organ or structure complicating other procedure** `CC`
CC Excl: PDX collection 618

✓5th **G97.4 Accidental puncture and laceration of a nervous system organ or structure during a procedure**

CC Excl: For CC codes in subcategory G97.4:
PDX collection 509

**G97.41 Accidental puncture or laceration of dura during a procedure** `CC`
Incidental (inadvertent) durotomy
AHA: 2014, 4Q, 24

**G97.48 Accidental puncture and laceration of other nervous system organ or structure during a nervous system procedure** `CC`

**Spinal Puncture**
- Spinal cord
- Epidural space
- Subarachnoid space
- Vertebra
- Spinal needle
- Lumbar area

**G97.49 Accidental puncture and laceration of other nervous system organ or structure during other procedure** `CC`

✓5th **G97.5 Postprocedural hemorrhage of a nervous system organ or structure following a procedure**

**G97.51 Postprocedural hemorrhage of a nervous system organ or structure following a nervous system procedure** `CC`
CC Excl: PDX collection 619

**G97.52 Postprocedural hemorrhage of a nervous system organ or structure following other procedure** `CC`
CC Excl: PDX collection 619

✓5th **G97.6 Postprocedural hematoma and seroma of a nervous system organ or structure following a procedure**

CC Excl: For CC codes in subcategory G97.6, unless otherwise noted: PDX collection 619

**G97.61 Postprocedural hematoma of a nervous system organ or structure following a nervous system procedure** `CC`

**G97.62 Postprocedural hematoma of a nervous system organ or structure following other procedure** `CC`

**G97.63 Postprocedural seroma of a nervous system organ or structure following a nervous system procedure** `CC`

**G97.64 Postprocedural seroma of a nervous system organ or structure following other procedure** `CC`

✓5th **G97.8 Other intraoperative and postprocedural complications and disorders of nervous system**
Use additional code to further specify disorder

**G97.81 Other intraoperative complications of nervous system** `CC`
CC Excl: PDX collection 617

**G97.82 Other postprocedural complications and disorders of nervous system** `CC`
CC Excl: PDX collection 617

✓4th **G98 Other disorders of nervous system not elsewhere classified**
INCLUDES   nervous system disorder NOS

**G98.0 Neurogenic arthritis, not elsewhere classified**
Nonsyphilitic neurogenic arthropathy NEC
Nonsyphilitic neurogenic spondylopathy NEC
EXCLUDES 1   *spondylopathy (in):*
*syringomyelia and syringobulbia (G95.0)*
*tabes dorsalis (A52.11)*

**G98.8 Other disorders of nervous system** `HIV`
Nervous system disorder NOS

✓4th **G99 Other disorders of nervous system in diseases classified elsewhere**

**G99.0 Autonomic neuropathy in diseases classified elsewhere** `CC`
Code first underlying disease, such as:
amyloidosis (E85.-)
gout ( M1A.-, M10.-)
hyperthyroidism (E05.-)
EXCLUDES 1   *diabetic autonomic neuropathy (E08-E13 with .43)*
CC Excl: PDX collection 620

N Newborn: 0   P Pediatric: 0-17   M Maternity: 12-55   A Adult: 15-124   MCC Major CC Condition   PDxMCC PDx acts as own MCC   CC CC Condition   PDxCC PDx acts as own CC

574      ICD-10-CM 2018

**G99.2** **Myelopathy in diseases classified elsewhere**   CC HCC

    Code first underlying disease, such as:
       neoplasm (C00-D49)

    *EXCLUDES 1*   *myelopathy in:*
           *intervertebral disease (M50.0-, M51.0-)*
           *spondylosis (M47.0-, M47.1-)*

    **CC Excl:** PDX collection 603

**G99.8** **Other specified disorders of nervous system in diseases classified elsewhere**

    Code first underlying disorder, such as:
       amyloidosis (E85.-)
       avitaminosis (E56.9)

    *EXCLUDES 1*   *nervous system involvement in:*
           *cysticercosis (B69.0)*
           *rubella (B06.0-)*
           *syphilis (A52.1-)*

☑Additional Character Req   *√x7ᵗʰ* Placeholder Alert   Unacceptable PDx   Manifestation   H1-H14 HAC   HCC CMS-HCC Condition   *EXCLUDES 1* Not Coded Here   *EXCLUDES 2* Not Included Here

ICD-10-CM 2018                  **575**

**G99.2–G99.8**

# Chapter 7. Diseases of the Eye and Adnexa (H00–H59)

## Chapter Specific Guidelines with Coding Examples

The chapter specific guidelines from the ICD-10-CM Official Guidelines for Coding and Reporting have been provided below. Along with these guidelines are coding examples, contained in the shaded boxes, that have been developed to help illustrate the coding and/or sequencing guidance found in these guidelines.

### a. Glaucoma

#### 1) Assigning glaucoma codes

Assign as many codes from category H40, Glaucoma, as needed to identify the type of glaucoma, the affected eye, and the glaucoma stage.

#### 2) Bilateral glaucoma with same type and stage

When a patient has bilateral glaucoma and both eyes are documented as being the same type and stage, and there is a code for bilateral glaucoma, report only the code for the type of glaucoma, bilateral, with the seventh character for the stage.

> Bilateral severe stage pigmentary glaucoma
>
> **H40.1333    Pigmentary glaucoma, bilateral, severe stage**
>
> *Explanation*: In this scenario, the patient has the same type and stage of glaucoma in both eyes. As this type of glaucoma has a code for bilateral, assign only the code for the bilateral glaucoma with the seventh character for the stage.

When a patient has bilateral glaucoma and both eyes are documented as being the same type and stage, and the classification does not provide a code for bilateral glaucoma (i.e. subcategories H40.10, H40.11 and H40.20) report only one code for the type of glaucoma with the appropriate seventh character for the stage.

> Bilateral open-angle glaucoma; not specified as to type and stage indeterminate in both eyes
>
> **H40.10X4    Unspecified open-angle glaucoma, indeterminate stage**
>
> *Explanation*: In this scenario, the patient has glaucoma of the same type and stage of both eyes, but there is no code specifically for bilateral glaucoma. Only one code is assigned with the appropriate seventh character for the stage.

#### 3) Bilateral glaucoma stage with different types or stages

When a patient has bilateral glaucoma and each eye is documented as having a different type or stage, and the classification distinguishes laterality, assign the appropriate code for each eye rather than the code for bilateral glaucoma.

> Bilateral chronic angle-closure glaucoma; right eye is documented as mild stage and left eye as moderate stage
>
> **H40.2211    Chronic angle-closure glaucoma, right eye, mild stage**
>
> **H40.2222    Chronic angle-closure glaucoma, left eye, moderate stage**
>
> *Explanation*: In this scenario the patient has the same type of glaucoma in both eyes, but each eye is at a different stage. Because the subcategory for this condition identifies laterality, one code is assigned for the right eye and one code is assigned for the left eye, each with the appropriate seventh character for the stage appended.

When a patient has bilateral glaucoma and each eye is documented as having a different type, and the classification does not distinguish laterality (i.e. subcategories H40.10, H40.11 and H40.20), assign one code for each type of glaucoma with the appropriate seventh character for the stage.

> Documentation relates mild, unspecified primary angle-closure glaucoma of the left eye with mild unspecified open-angle glaucoma of the right eye
>
> **H40.20X1    Unspecified primary angle-closure glaucoma, mild stage**
>
> **H40.10X1    Unspecified open-angle glaucoma, mild stage**
>
> *Explanation*: In this scenario the patient has a different type of glaucoma in each eye and the classification does not distinguish laterality. A code for each type of glaucoma is assigned, each with the appropriate seventh character for the stage.

When a patient has bilateral glaucoma and each eye is documented as having the same type, but different stage, and the classification does not distinguish laterality (i.e. subcategories H40.10, H40.11 and H40.20), assign a code for the type of glaucoma for each eye with the seventh character for the specific glaucoma stage documented for each eye.

> Bilateral open-angle glaucoma, not specified as to type; the right eye is documented to be in mild stage and the left eye as being in moderate stage
>
> **H40.10X1    Unspecified open-angle glaucoma, mild stage**
>
> **H40.10X2    Unspecified open-angle glaucoma, moderate stage**
>
> *Explanation*: In this scenario the patient has the same type of glaucoma in each eye but each eye is at a different stage, and the classification does not distinguish laterality at this subcategory level. Two codes are assigned; both codes represent the same type of glaucoma but each has a different seventh character identifying the appropriate stage for each eye.

#### 4) Patient admitted with glaucoma and stage evolves during the admission

If a patient is admitted with glaucoma and the stage progresses during the admission, assign the code for highest stage documented.

> Patient admitted with mild low-tension glaucoma of the right eye, which progresses to moderate stage during the patient's stay
>
> **H40.1212    Low-tension glaucoma, right eye, moderate stage**
>
> *Explanation*: When the glaucoma stage progresses during an admission, assign only the code for the highest stage documented.

#### 5) Indeterminate stage glaucoma

Assignment of the seventh character "4" for "indeterminate stage" should be based on the clinical documentation. The seventh character "4" is used for glaucomas whose stage cannot be clinically determined. This seventh character should not be confused with the seventh character "0", unspecified, which should be assigned when there is no documentation regarding the stage of the glaucoma.

## Chapter 7. Diseases of the Eye and Adnexa (H00-H59)

**NOTE**   Use an external cause code following the code for the eye condition, if applicable, to identify the cause of the eye condition.

**EXCLUDES 2**   certain conditions originating in the perinatal period (P04-P96)
certain infectious and parasitic diseases (A00-B99)
complications of pregnancy, childbirth and the puerperium (O00-O9A)
congenital malformations, deformations, and chromosomal abnormalities (Q00-Q99)
diabetes mellitus related eye conditions (E09.3-, E10.3-, E11.3-, E13.3-)
endocrine, nutritional and metabolic diseases (E00-E88)
injury (trauma) of eye and orbit (S05.-)
injury, poisoning and certain other consequences of external causes (S00-T88)
neoplasms (C00-D49)
symptoms, signs and abnormal clinical and laboratory findings, not elsewhere classified (R00-R94)
syphilis related eye disorders (A50.01, A50.3-, A51.43, A52.71)

This chapter contains the following blocks:

| | |
|---|---|
| H00-H05 | Disorders of eyelid, lacrimal system and orbit |
| H10-H11 | Disorders of conjunctiva |
| H15-H22 | Disorders of sclera, cornea, iris and ciliary body |
| H25-H28 | Disorders of lens |
| H30-H36 | Disorders of choroid and retina |
| H40-H42 | Glaucoma |
| H43-H44 | Disorders of vitreous body and globe |
| H46-H47 | Disorders of optic nerve and visual pathways |
| H49-H52 | Disorders of ocular muscles, binocular movement, accommodation and refraction |
| H53-H54 | Visual disturbances and blindness |
| H55-H57 | Other disorders of eye and adnexa |
| H59 | Intraoperative and postprocedural complications and disorders of eye and adnexa, not elsewhere classified |

### Disorders of eyelid, lacrimal system and orbit (H00-H05)

**EXCLUDES 2**   open wound of eyelid (S01.1-)
superficial injury of eyelid (S00.1-, S00.2-)

**✓4ᵗʰ H00   Hordeolum and chalazion**

   **✓5ᵗʰ H00.0   Hordeolum (externum) (internum) of eyelid**

     **✓6ᵗʰ H00.01   Hordeolum externum**
Hordeolum NOS
Stye
     **H00.011   Hordeolum externum right upper eyelid**
     **H00.012   Hordeolum externum right lower eyelid**
     **H00.013   Hordeolum externum right eye, unspecified eyelid**
     **H00.014   Hordeolum externum left upper eyelid**
     **H00.015   Hordeolum externum left lower eyelid**
     **H00.016   Hordeolum externum left eye, unspecified eyelid**
     **H00.019   Hordeolum externum unspecified eye, unspecified eyelid**

     **✓6ᵗʰ H00.02   Hordeolum internum**
Infection of meibomian gland
     **H00.021   Hordeolum internum right upper eyelid**
     **H00.022   Hordeolum internum right lower eyelid**
     **H00.023   Hordeolum internum right eye, unspecified eyelid**
     **H00.024   Hordeolum internum left upper eyelid**
     **H00.025   Hordeolum internum left lower eyelid**
     **H00.026   Hordeolum internum left eye, unspecified eyelid**
     **H00.029   Hordeolum internum unspecified eye, unspecified eyelid**

     **✓6ᵗʰ H00.03   Abscess of eyelid**
Furuncle of eyelid
     **H00.031   Abscess of right upper eyelid**
     **H00.032   Abscess of right lower eyelid**
     **H00.033   Abscess of eyelid right eye, unspecified eyelid**
     **H00.034   Abscess of left upper eyelid**
     **H00.035   Abscess of left lower eyelid**
     **H00.036   Abscess of eyelid left eye, unspecified eyelid**
     **H00.039   Abscess of eyelid unspecified eye, unspecified eyelid**

   **✓5ᵗʰ H00.1   Chalazion**
Meibomian (gland) cyst
**EXCLUDES 2**   infected meibomian gland (H00.02-)
   **H00.11   Chalazion right upper eyelid**
   **H00.12   Chalazion right lower eyelid**
   **H00.13   Chalazion right eye, unspecified eyelid**
   **H00.14   Chalazion left upper eyelid**
   **H00.15   Chalazion left lower eyelid**
   **H00.16   Chalazion left eye, unspecified eyelid**
   **H00.19   Chalazion unspecified eye, unspecified eyelid**

**✓4ᵗʰ H01   Other inflammation of eyelid**

   **✓5ᵗʰ H01.0   Blepharitis**
**EXCLUDES 1**   blepharoconjunctivitis (H10.5-)

     **✓6ᵗʰ H01.00   Unspecified blepharitis**
     **H01.001   Unspecified blepharitis right upper eyelid**
     **H01.002   Unspecified blepharitis right lower eyelid**
     **H01.003   Unspecified blepharitis right eye, unspecified eyelid**
     **H01.004   Unspecified blepharitis left upper eyelid**
     **H01.005   Unspecified blepharitis left lower eyelid**
     **H01.006   Unspecified blepharitis left eye, unspecified eyelid**
     **H01.009   Unspecified blepharitis unspecified eye, unspecified eyelid**

     **✓6ᵗʰ H01.01   Ulcerative blepharitis**
     **H01.011   Ulcerative blepharitis right upper eyelid**
     **H01.012   Ulcerative blepharitis right lower eyelid**
     **H01.013   Ulcerative blepharitis right eye, unspecified eyelid**
     **H01.014   Ulcerative blepharitis left upper eyelid**
     **H01.015   Ulcerative blepharitis left lower eyelid**
     **H01.016   Ulcerative blepharitis left eye, unspecified eyelid**
     **H01.019   Ulcerative blepharitis unspecified eye, unspecified eyelid**

     **✓6ᵗʰ H01.02   Squamous blepharitis**
     **H01.021   Squamous blepharitis right upper eyelid**
     **H01.022   Squamous blepharitis right lower eyelid**
     **H01.023   Squamous blepharitis right eye, unspecified eyelid**
     **H01.024   Squamous blepharitis left upper eyelid**
     **H01.025   Squamous blepharitis left lower eyelid**
     **H01.026   Squamous blepharitis left eye, unspecified eyelid**
     **H01.029   Squamous blepharitis unspecified eye, unspecified eyelid**

   **✓5ᵗʰ H01.1   Noninfectious dermatoses of eyelid**

     **✓6ᵗʰ H01.11   Allergic dermatitis of eyelid**
Contact dermatitis of eyelid
     **H01.111   Allergic dermatitis of right upper eyelid**
     **H01.112   Allergic dermatitis of right lower eyelid**
     **H01.113   Allergic dermatitis of right eye, unspecified eyelid**
     **H01.114   Allergic dermatitis of left upper eyelid**
     **H01.115   Allergic dermatitis of left lower eyelid**
     **H01.116   Allergic dermatitis of left eye, unspecified eyelid**
     **H01.119   Allergic dermatitis of unspecified eye, unspecified eyelid**

     **✓6ᵗʰ H01.12   Discoid lupus erythematosus of eyelid**
     **H01.121   Discoid lupus erythematosus of right upper eyelid**
     **H01.122   Discoid lupus erythematosus of right lower eyelid**
     **H01.123   Discoid lupus erythematosus of right eye, unspecified eyelid**
     **H01.124   Discoid lupus erythematosus of left upper eyelid**
     **H01.125   Discoid lupus erythematosus of left lower eyelid**
     **H01.126   Discoid lupus erythematosus of left eye, unspecified eyelid**
     **H01.129   Discoid lupus erythematosus of unspecified eye, unspecified eyelid**

**N** Newborn: 0   **P** Pediatric: 0-17   **M** Maternity: 12-55   **A** Adult: 15-124   **MCC** Major CC Condition   **PDxMCC** PDx acts as own MCC   **CC** CC Condition   **PDxCC** PDx acts as own CC

**578**          ICD-10-CM 2018

✓6th **H01.13 Eczematous dermatitis of eyelid**
    **H01.131 Eczematous dermatitis of** right upper eyelid
    **H01.132 Eczematous dermatitis of** right lower eyelid
    **H01.133 Eczematous dermatitis of** right eye, unspecified eyelid
    **H01.134 Eczematous dermatitis of** left upper eyelid
    **H01.135 Eczematous dermatitis of** left lower eyelid
    **H01.136 Eczematous dermatitis of** left eye, unspecified eyelid
    **H01.139 Eczematous dermatitis of** unspecified eye, unspecified eyelid

✓6th **H01.14 Xeroderma of eyelid**
    **H01.141 Xeroderma of** right upper eyelid
    **H01.142 Xeroderma of** right lower eyelid
    **H01.143 Xeroderma of** right eye, unspecified eyelid
    **H01.144 Xeroderma of** left upper eyelid
    **H01.145 Xeroderma of** left lower eyelid
    **H01.146 Xeroderma of** left eye, unspecified eyelid
    **H01.149 Xeroderma of** unspecified eye, unspecified eyelid

**H01.8 Other specified inflammations of eyelid**

**H01.9 Unspecified inflammation of eyelid**
    Inflammation of eyelid NOS

✓4th **H02 Other disorders of eyelid**
    EXCLUDES 1 *congenital malformations of eyelid (Q10.0-Q10.3)*

✓5th **H02.0 Entropion and trichiasis of eyelid**
  ✓6th **H02.00 Unspecified entropion of eyelid**
    **H02.001 Unspecified entropion of** right upper eyelid
    **H02.002 Unspecified entropion of** right lower eyelid
    **H02.003 Unspecified entropion of** right eye, unspecified eyelid
    **H02.004 Unspecified entropion of** left upper eyelid
    **H02.005 Unspecified entropion of** left lower eyelid
    **H02.006 Unspecified entropion of** left eye, unspecified eyelid
    **H02.009 Unspecified entropion of** unspecified eye, unspecified eyelid

  ✓6th **H02.01 Cicatricial entropion of eyelid**
    **H02.011 Cicatricial entropion of** right upper eyelid
    **H02.012 Cicatricial entropion of** right lower eyelid
    **H02.013 Cicatricial entropion of** right eye, unspecified eyelid
    **H02.014 Cicatricial entropion of** left upper eyelid
    **H02.015 Cicatricial entropion of** left lower eyelid
    **H02.016 Cicatricial entropion of** left eye, unspecified eyelid
    **H02.019 Cicatricial entropion of** unspecified eye, unspecified eyelid

  ✓6th **H02.02 Mechanical entropion of eyelid**
    **H02.021 Mechanical entropion of** right upper eyelid
    **H02.022 Mechanical entropion of** right lower eyelid
    **H02.023 Mechanical entropion of** right eye, unspecified eyelid
    **H02.024 Mechanical entropion of** left upper eyelid
    **H02.025 Mechanical entropion of** left lower eyelid
    **H02.026 Mechanical entropion of** left eye, unspecified eyelid
    **H02.029 Mechanical entropion of** unspecified eye, unspecified eyelid

  ✓6th **H02.03 Senile entropion of eyelid**
    **H02.031 Senile entropion of** right upper eyelid Ⓐ
    **H02.032 Senile entropion of** right lower eyelid Ⓐ
    **H02.033 Senile entropion of** right eye, unspecified eyelid Ⓐ
    **H02.034 Senile entropion of** left upper eyelid Ⓐ
    **H02.035 Senile entropion of** left lower eyelid Ⓐ
    **H02.036 Senile entropion of** left eye, unspecified eyelid Ⓐ
    **H02.039 Senile entropion of** unspecified eye, unspecified eyelid Ⓐ

**Entropion and Ectropion**

Normal eyelid    Entropion    Ectropion

✓6th **H02.04 Spastic entropion of eyelid**
    **H02.041 Spastic entropion of** right upper eyelid
    **H02.042 Spastic entropion of** right lower eyelid
    **H02.043 Spastic entropion of** right eye, unspecified eyelid
    **H02.044 Spastic entropion of** left upper eyelid
    **H02.045 Spastic entropion of** left lower eyelid
    **H02.046 Spastic entropion of** left eye, unspecified eyelid
    **H02.049 Spastic entropion of** unspecified eye, unspecified eyelid

▲ ✓6th **H02.05 Trichiasis without entropion**
▲    **H02.051 Trichiasis without entropion** right upper eyelid
▲    **H02.052 Trichiasis without entropion** right lower eyelid
▲    **H02.053 Trichiasis without entropion** right eye, unspecified eyelid
▲    **H02.054 Trichiasis without entropion** left upper eyelid
▲    **H02.055 Trichiasis without entropion** left lower eyelid
▲    **H02.056 Trichiasis without entropion** left eye, unspecified eyelid
▲    **H02.059 Trichiasis without entropion** unspecified eye, unspecified eyelid

✓5th **H02.1 Ectropion of eyelid**
  ✓6th **H02.10 Unspecified ectropion of eyelid**
    **H02.101 Unspecified ectropion of** right upper eyelid
    **H02.102 Unspecified ectropion of** right lower eyelid
    **H02.103 Unspecified ectropion of** right eye, unspecified eyelid
    **H02.104 Unspecified ectropion of** left upper eyelid
    **H02.105 Unspecified ectropion of** left lower eyelid
    **H02.106 Unspecified ectropion of** left eye, unspecified eyelid
    **H02.109 Unspecified ectropion of** unspecified eye, unspecified eyelid

  ✓6th **H02.11 Cicatricial ectropion of eyelid**
    **H02.111 Cicatricial ectropion of** right upper eyelid
    **H02.112 Cicatricial ectropion of** right lower eyelid
    **H02.113 Cicatricial ectropion of** right eye, unspecified eyelid
    **H02.114 Cicatricial ectropion of** left upper eyelid
    **H02.115 Cicatricial ectropion of** left lower eyelid
    **H02.116 Cicatricial ectropion of** left eye, unspecified eyelid
    **H02.119 Cicatricial ectropion of** unspecified eye, unspecified eyelid

  ✓6th **H02.12 Mechanical ectropion of eyelid**
    **H02.121 Mechanical ectropion of** right upper eyelid
    **H02.122 Mechanical ectropion of** right lower eyelid
    **H02.123 Mechanical ectropion of** right eye, unspecified eyelid
    **H02.124 Mechanical ectropion of** left upper eyelid
    **H02.125 Mechanical ectropion of** left lower eyelid
    **H02.126 Mechanical ectropion of** left eye, unspecified eyelid
    **H02.129 Mechanical ectropion of** unspecified eye, unspecified eyelid

**Chapter 7. Diseases of the Eye and Adnexa**

**H02.13–H02.536**

✓6ᵗʰ **H02.13 Senile ectropion of eyelid**
- H02.131 Senile ectropion of right upper eyelid  A
- H02.132 Senile ectropion of right lower eyelid  A
- H02.133 Senile ectropion of right eye, unspecified eyelid  A
- H02.134 Senile ectropion of left upper eyelid  A
- H02.135 Senile ectropion of left lower eyelid  A
- H02.136 Senile ectropion of left eye, unspecified eyelid  A
- H02.139 Senile ectropion of unspecified eye, unspecified eyelid  A

✓6ᵗʰ **H02.14 Spastic ectropion of eyelid**
- H02.141 Spastic ectropion of right upper eyelid
- H02.142 Spastic ectropion of right lower eyelid
- H02.143 Spastic ectropion of right eye, unspecified eyelid
- H02.144 Spastic ectropion of left upper eyelid
- H02.145 Spastic ectropion of left lower eyelid
- H02.146 Spastic ectropion of left eye, unspecified eyelid
- H02.149 Spastic ectropion of unspecified eye, unspecified eyelid

✓5ᵗʰ **H02.2 Lagophthalmos**

✓6ᵗʰ **H02.20 Unspecified lagophthalmos**
- H02.201 Unspecified lagophthalmos right upper eyelid
- H02.202 Unspecified lagophthalmos right lower eyelid
- H02.203 Unspecified lagophthalmos right eye, unspecified eyelid
- H02.204 Unspecified lagophthalmos left upper eyelid
- H02.205 Unspecified lagophthalmos left lower eyelid
- H02.206 Unspecified lagophthalmos left eye, unspecified eyelid
- H02.209 Unspecified lagophthalmos unspecified eye, unspecified eyelid

✓6ᵗʰ **H02.21 Cicatricial lagophthalmos**
- H02.211 Cicatricial lagophthalmos right upper eyelid
- H02.212 Cicatricial lagophthalmos right lower eyelid
- H02.213 Cicatricial lagophthalmos right eye, unspecified eyelid
- H02.214 Cicatricial lagophthalmos left upper eyelid
- H02.215 Cicatricial lagophthalmos left lower eyelid
- H02.216 Cicatricial lagophthalmos left eye, unspecified eyelid
- H02.219 Cicatricial lagophthalmos unspecified eye, unspecified eyelid

✓6ᵗʰ **H02.22 Mechanical lagophthalmos**
- H02.221 Mechanical lagophthalmos right upper eyelid
- H02.222 Mechanical lagophthalmos right lower eyelid
- H02.223 Mechanical lagophthalmos right eye, unspecified eyelid
- H02.224 Mechanical lagophthalmos left upper eyelid
- H02.225 Mechanical lagophthalmos left lower eyelid
- H02.226 Mechanical lagophthalmos left eye, unspecified eyelid
- H02.229 Mechanical lagophthalmos unspecified eye, unspecified eyelid

✓6ᵗʰ **H02.23 Paralytic lagophthalmos**
- H02.231 Paralytic lagophthalmos right upper eyelid
- H02.232 Paralytic lagophthalmos right lower eyelid
- H02.233 Paralytic lagophthalmos right eye, unspecified eyelid
- H02.234 Paralytic lagophthalmos left upper eyelid
- H02.235 Paralytic lagophthalmos left lower eyelid
- H02.236 Paralytic lagophthalmos left eye, unspecified eyelid
- H02.239 Paralytic lagophthalmos unspecified eye, unspecified eyelid

✓5ᵗʰ **H02.3 Blepharochalasis**
    Pseudoptosis
- H02.30 Blepharochalasis unspecified eye, unspecified eyelid
- H02.31 Blepharochalasis right upper eyelid
- H02.32 Blepharochalasis right lower eyelid
- H02.33 Blepharochalasis right eye, unspecified eyelid
- H02.34 Blepharochalasis left upper eyelid
- H02.35 Blepharochalasis left lower eyelid
- H02.36 Blepharochalasis left eye, unspecified eyelid

✓5ᵗʰ **H02.4 Ptosis of eyelid**

✓6ᵗʰ **H02.40 Unspecified ptosis of eyelid**
- H02.401 Unspecified ptosis of right eyelid
- H02.402 Unspecified ptosis of left eyelid
- H02.403 Unspecified ptosis of bilateral eyelids
- H02.409 Unspecified ptosis of unspecified eyelid

✓6ᵗʰ **H02.41 Mechanical ptosis of eyelid**
- H02.411 Mechanical ptosis of right eyelid
- H02.412 Mechanical ptosis of left eyelid
- H02.413 Mechanical ptosis of bilateral eyelids
- H02.419 Mechanical ptosis of unspecified eyelid

✓6ᵗʰ **H02.42 Myogenic ptosis of eyelid**
- H02.421 Myogenic ptosis of right eyelid
- H02.422 Myogenic ptosis of left eyelid
- H02.423 Myogenic ptosis of bilateral eyelids
- H02.429 Myogenic ptosis of unspecified eyelid

✓6ᵗʰ **H02.43 Paralytic ptosis of eyelid**
    Neurogenic ptosis of eyelid
- H02.431 Paralytic ptosis of right eyelid
- H02.432 Paralytic ptosis of left eyelid
- H02.433 Paralytic ptosis of bilateral eyelids
- H02.439 Paralytic ptosis unspecified eyelid

✓5ᵗʰ **H02.5 Other disorders affecting eyelid function**
    *EXCLUDES 2*   blepharospasm (G24.5)
                    organic tic (G25.69)
                    psychogenic tic (F95.-)

✓6ᵗʰ **H02.51 Abnormal innervation syndrome**
- H02.511 Abnormal innervation syndrome right upper eyelid
- H02.512 Abnormal innervation syndrome right lower eyelid
- H02.513 Abnormal innervation syndrome right eye, unspecified eyelid
- H02.514 Abnormal innervation syndrome left upper eyelid
- H02.515 Abnormal innervation syndrome left lower eyelid
- H02.516 Abnormal innervation syndrome left eye, unspecified eyelid
- H02.519 Abnormal innervation syndrome unspecified eye, unspecified eyelid

✓6ᵗʰ **H02.52 Blepharophimosis**
    Ankyloblepharon
- H02.521 Blepharophimosis right upper eyelid
- H02.522 Blepharophimosis right lower eyelid
- H02.523 Blepharophimosis right eye, unspecified eyelid
- H02.524 Blepharophimosis left upper eyelid
- H02.525 Blepharophimosis left lower eyelid
- H02.526 Blepharophimosis left eye, unspecified eyelid
- H02.529 Blepharophimosis unspecified eye, unspecified lid

✓6ᵗʰ **H02.53 Eyelid retraction**
    Eyelid lag
- H02.531 Eyelid retraction right upper eyelid
- H02.532 Eyelid retraction right lower eyelid
- H02.533 Eyelid retraction right eye, unspecified eyelid
- H02.534 Eyelid retraction left upper eyelid
- H02.535 Eyelid retraction left lower eyelid
- H02.536 Eyelid retraction left eye, unspecified eyelid

N Newborn: 0    P Pediatric: 0-17    M Maternity: 12-55    A Adult: 15-124    MCC Major CC Condition    PDx MCC PDx acts as own MCC    CC CC Condition    PDx CC PDx acts as own CC

580                                                ICD-10-CM 2018

    **H02.539**   **Eyelid retraction** unspecified eye, unspecified lid

   **H02.59**   **Other disorders affecting eyelid function**
Deficient blink reflex
Sensory disorders

✓5ᵗʰ **H02.6**   **Xanthelasma of eyelid**

   **H02.60**   **Xanthelasma of** unspecified eye, unspecified eyelid

   **H02.61**   **Xanthelasma of** right upper eyelid

   **H02.62**   **Xanthelasma of** right lower eyelid

   **H02.63**   **Xanthelasma of** right eye, unspecified eyelid

   **H02.64**   **Xanthelasma of** left upper eyelid

   **H02.65**   **Xanthelasma of** left lower eyelid

   **H02.66**   **Xanthelasma of** left eye, unspecified eyelid

✓5ᵗʰ **H02.7**   **Other and unspecified degenerative disorders of eyelid and periocular area**

   **H02.70**   **Unspecified degenerative disorders of eyelid and periocular area**

✓6ᵗʰ  **H02.71**   **Chloasma of eyelid and periocular area**
Dyspigmentation of eyelid
Hyperpigmentation of eyelid

   **H02.711**   **Chloasma of** right upper **eyelid and periocular area**

   **H02.712**   **Chloasma of** right lower **eyelid and periocular area**

   **H02.713**   **Chloasma of** right eye, unspecified **eyelid and periocular area**

   **H02.714**   **Chloasma of** left upper **eyelid and periocular area**

   **H02.715**   **Chloasma of** left lower **eyelid and periocular area**

   **H02.716**   **Chloasma of** left eye, unspecified **eyelid and periocular area**

   **H02.719**   **Chloasma of** unspecified eye, unspecified **eyelid and periocular area**

✓6ᵗʰ  **H02.72**   **Madarosis of eyelid and periocular area**
Hypotrichosis of eyelid

   **H02.721**   **Madarosis of** right upper **eyelid and periocular area**

   **H02.722**   **Madarosis of** right lower **eyelid and periocular area**

   **H02.723**   **Madarosis of** right eye, unspecified **eyelid and periocular area**

   **H02.724**   **Madarosis of** left upper **eyelid and periocular area**

   **H02.725**   **Madarosis of** left lower **eyelid and periocular area**

   **H02.726**   **Madarosis of** left eye, unspecified **eyelid and periocular area**

   **H02.729**   **Madarosis of** unspecified eye, unspecified **eyelid and periocular area**

✓6ᵗʰ  **H02.73**   **Vitiligo of eyelid and periocular area**
Hypopigmentation of eyelid

   **H02.731**   **Vitiligo of** right upper **eyelid and periocular area**

   **H02.732**   **Vitiligo of** right lower **eyelid and periocular area**

   **H02.733**   **Vitiligo of** right eye, unspecified **eyelid and periocular area**

   **H02.734**   **Vitiligo of** left upper **eyelid and periocular area**

   **H02.735**   **Vitiligo of** left lower **eyelid and periocular area**

   **H02.736**   **Vitiligo of** left eye, unspecified **eyelid and periocular area**

   **H02.739**   **Vitiligo of** unspecified eye, unspecified **eyelid and periocular area**

   **H02.79**   **Other degenerative disorders of eyelid and periocular area**

✓5ᵗʰ **H02.8**   **Other specified disorders of eyelid**

✓6ᵗʰ  **H02.81**   **Retained foreign body in eyelid**
Use additional code to identify the type of retained foreign body (Z18.-)

   **EXCLUDES 1**   *laceration of eyelid with foreign body (S01.12-)*
*retained intraocular foreign body (H44.6-, H44.7-)*
*superficial foreign body of eyelid and periocular area (S00.25-)*

   **H02.811**   **Retained foreign body in** right upper eyelid

   **H02.812**   **Retained foreign body in** right lower eyelid

   **H02.813**   **Retained foreign body in** right eye, unspecified eyelid

   **H02.814**   **Retained foreign body in** left upper eyelid

   **H02.815**   **Retained foreign body in** left lower eyelid

   **H02.816**   **Retained foreign body in** left eye, unspecified eyelid

   **H02.819**   **Retained foreign body in** unspecified eye, unspecified eyelid

✓6ᵗʰ  **H02.82**   **Cysts of eyelid**
Sebaceous cyst of eyelid

   **H02.821**   **Cysts of** right upper eyelid

   **H02.822**   **Cysts of** right lower eyelid

   **H02.823**   **Cysts of** right eye, unspecified eyelid

   **H02.824**   **Cysts of** left upper eyelid

   **H02.825**   **Cysts of** left lower eyelid

   **H02.826**   **Cysts of** left eye, unspecified eyelid

   **H02.829**   **Cysts of** unspecified eye, unspecified eyelid

✓6ᵗʰ  **H02.83**   **Dermatochalasis of eyelid**
**DEF:** Acquired form of connective tissue disorder associated with decreased elastic tissue and abnormal elastin formation, resulting in loss of elasticity of the skin of the eyelid; generally associated with aging.

   **H02.831**   **Dermatochalasis of** right upper eyelid

   **H02.832**   **Dermatochalasis of** right lower eyelid

   **H02.833**   **Dermatochalasis of** right eye, unspecified eyelid

   **H02.834**   **Dermatochalasis of** left upper eyelid

   **H02.835**   **Dermatochalasis of** left lower eyelid

   **H02.836**   **Dermatochalasis of** left eye, unspecified eyelid

   **H02.839**   **Dermatochalasis of** unspecified eye, unspecified eyelid

✓6ᵗʰ  **H02.84**   **Edema of eyelid**
Hyperemia of eyelid

   **H02.841**   **Edema of** right upper eyelid

   **H02.842**   **Edema of** right lower eyelid

   **H02.843**   **Edema of** right eye, unspecified eyelid

   **H02.844**   **Edema of** left upper eyelid

   **H02.845**   **Edema of** left lower eyelid

   **H02.846**   **Edema of** left eye, unspecified eyelid

   **H02.849**   **Edema of** unspecified eye, unspecified eyelid

✓6ᵗʰ  **H02.85**   **Elephantiasis of eyelid**

   **H02.851**   **Elephantiasis of** right upper eyelid

   **H02.852**   **Elephantiasis of** right lower eyelid

   **H02.853**   **Elephantiasis of** right eye, unspecified eyelid

   **H02.854**   **Elephantiasis of** left upper eyelid

   **H02.855**   **Elephantiasis of** left lower eyelid

   **H02.856**   **Elephantiasis of** left eye, unspecified eyelid

   **H02.859**   **Elephantiasis of** unspecified eye, unspecified eyelid

✓6ᵗʰ  **H02.86**   **Hypertrichosis of eyelid**

   **H02.861**   **Hypertrichosis of** right upper eyelid

   **H02.862**   **Hypertrichosis of** right lower eyelid

   **H02.863**   **Hypertrichosis of** right eye, unspecified eyelid

   **H02.864**   **Hypertrichosis of** left upper eyelid

   **H02.865**   **Hypertrichosis of** left lower eyelid

   **H02.866**   **Hypertrichosis of** left eye, unspecified eyelid

☑ Additional Character Req   ✓ˣ7ᵗʰ Placeholder Alert   Unacceptable PDx   Manifestation   **H1**-**H14** HAC   **HCC** CMS-HCC Condition   **EXCLUDES 1** Not Coded Here   **EXCLUDES 2** Not Included Here

ICD-10-CM 2018         581

    **H02.869**    Hypertrichosis of unspecified eye, unspecified eyelid

✓6th **H02.87**    Vascular anomalies of eyelid
    **H02.871**    Vascular anomalies of right upper eyelid
    **H02.872**    Vascular anomalies of right lower eyelid
    **H02.873**    Vascular anomalies of right eye, unspecified eyelid
    **H02.874**    Vascular anomalies of left upper eyelid
    **H02.875**    Vascular anomalies of left lower eyelid
    **H02.876**    Vascular anomalies of left eye, unspecified eyelid
    **H02.879**    Vascular anomalies of unspecified eye, unspecified eyelid

    **H02.89**    Other specified disorders of eyelid
         Hemorrhage of eyelid

  **H02.9**    Unspecified disorder of eyelid
       Disorder of eyelid NOS

✓4th **H04**    **Disorders of lacrimal system**
    EXCLUDES 1    *congenital malformations of lacrimal system (Q10.4-Q10.6)*

✓5th **H04.0**    Dacryoadenitis
 ✓6th **H04.00**    Unspecified dacryoadenitis
    **H04.001**    Unspecified dacryoadenitis, right lacrimal gland
    **H04.002**    Unspecified dacryoadenitis, left lacrimal gland
    **H04.003**    Unspecified dacryoadenitis, bilateral lacrimal glands
    **H04.009**    Unspecified dacryoadenitis, unspecified lacrimal gland

 ✓6th **H04.01**    Acute dacryoadenitis
    **H04.011**    Acute dacryoadenitis, right lacrimal gland
    **H04.012**    Acute dacryoadenitis, left lacrimal gland
    **H04.013**    Acute dacryoadenitis, bilateral lacrimal glands
    **H04.019**    Acute dacryoadenitis, unspecified lacrimal gland

 ✓6th **H04.02**    Chronic dacryoadenitis
    **H04.021**    Chronic dacryoadenitis, right lacrimal gland
    **H04.022**    Chronic dacryoadenitis, left lacrimal gland
    **H04.023**    Chronic dacryoadenitis, bilateral lacrimal glands
    **H04.029**    Chronic dacryoadenitis, unspecified lacrimal gland

 ✓6th **H04.03**    Chronic enlargement of lacrimal gland
    **H04.031**    Chronic enlargement of right lacrimal gland
    **H04.032**    Chronic enlargement of left lacrimal gland
    **H04.033**    Chronic enlargement of bilateral lacrimal glands
    **H04.039**    Chronic enlargement of unspecified lacrimal gland

✓5th **H04.1**    Other disorders of lacrimal gland
 ✓6th **H04.11**    Dacryops
    **H04.111**    Dacryops of right lacrimal gland
    **H04.112**    Dacryops of left lacrimal gland
    **H04.113**    Dacryops of bilateral lacrimal glands
    **H04.119**    Dacryops of unspecified lacrimal gland

 ✓6th **H04.12**    Dry eye syndrome
       Tear film insufficiency, NOS
    **H04.121**    Dry eye syndrome of right lacrimal gland
    **H04.122**    Dry eye syndrome of left lacrimal gland
    **H04.123**    Dry eye syndrome of bilateral lacrimal glands
    **H04.129**    Dry eye syndrome of unspecified lacrimal gland

 ✓6th **H04.13**    Lacrimal cyst
       Lacrimal cystic degeneration
    **H04.131**    Lacrimal cyst, right lacrimal gland
    **H04.132**    Lacrimal cyst, left lacrimal gland
    **H04.133**    Lacrimal cyst, bilateral lacrimal glands
    **H04.139**    Lacrimal cyst, unspecified lacrimal gland

 ✓6th **H04.14**    Primary lacrimal gland atrophy
    **H04.141**    Primary lacrimal gland atrophy, right lacrimal gland

    **H04.142**    Primary lacrimal gland atrophy, left lacrimal gland
    **H04.143**    Primary lacrimal gland atrophy, bilateral lacrimal glands
    **H04.149**    Primary lacrimal gland atrophy, unspecified lacrimal gland

 ✓6th **H04.15**    Secondary lacrimal gland atrophy
    **H04.151**    Secondary lacrimal gland atrophy, right lacrimal gland
    **H04.152**    Secondary lacrimal gland atrophy, left lacrimal gland
    **H04.153**    Secondary lacrimal gland atrophy, bilateral lacrimal glands
    **H04.159**    Secondary lacrimal gland atrophy, unspecified lacrimal gland

 ✓6th **H04.16**    Lacrimal gland dislocation
    **H04.161**    Lacrimal gland dislocation, right lacrimal gland
    **H04.162**    Lacrimal gland dislocation, left lacrimal gland
    **H04.163**    Lacrimal gland dislocation, bilateral lacrimal glands
    **H04.169**    Lacrimal gland dislocation, unspecified lacrimal gland

    **H04.19**    Other specified disorders of lacrimal gland

✓5th **H04.2**    Epiphora
 ✓6th **H04.20**    Unspecified epiphora
    **H04.201**    Unspecified epiphora, right lacrimal gland
    **H04.202**    Unspecified epiphora, left lacrimal gland
    **H04.203**    Unspecified epiphora, bilateral lacrimal glands
    **H04.209**    Unspecified epiphora, unspecified lacrimal gland

 ✓6th **H04.21**    Epiphora due to excess lacrimation
    **H04.211**    Epiphora due to excess lacrimation, right lacrimal gland
    **H04.212**    Epiphora due to excess lacrimation, left lacrimal gland
    **H04.213**    Epiphora due to excess lacrimation, bilateral lacrimal glands
    **H04.219**    Epiphora due to excess lacrimation, unspecified lacrimal gland

 ✓6th **H04.22**    Epiphora due to insufficient drainage
    **H04.221**    Epiphora due to insufficient drainage, right lacrimal gland
    **H04.222**    Epiphora due to insufficient drainage, left lacrimal gland
    **H04.223**    Epiphora due to insufficient drainage, bilateral lacrimal glands
    **H04.229**    Epiphora due to insufficient drainage, unspecified lacrimal gland

✓5th **H04.3**    Acute and unspecified inflammation of lacrimal passages
    EXCLUDES 1    *neonatal dacryocystitis (P39.1)*
 ✓6th **H04.30**    Unspecified dacryocystitis
    **H04.301**    Unspecified dacryocystitis of right lacrimal passage
    **H04.302**    Unspecified dacryocystitis of left lacrimal passage
    **H04.303**    Unspecified dacryocystitis of bilateral lacrimal passages
    **H04.309**    Unspecified dacryocystitis of unspecified lacrimal passage

 ✓6th **H04.31**    Phlegmonous dacryocystitis
    **H04.311**    Phlegmonous dacryocystitis of right lacrimal passage
    **H04.312**    Phlegmonous dacryocystitis of left lacrimal passage
    **H04.313**    Phlegmonous dacryocystitis of bilateral lacrimal passages
    **H04.319**    Phlegmonous dacryocystitis of unspecified lacrimal passage

 ✓6th **H04.32**    Acute dacryocystitis
       Acute dacryopericystitis
    **H04.321**    Acute dacryocystitis of right lacrimal passage
    **H04.322**    Acute dacryocystitis of left lacrimal passage

N Newborn: 0    P Pediatric: 0-17    M Maternity: 12-55    A Adult: 15-124    MCC Major CC Condition    PDxMCC PDx acts as own MCC    CC CC Condition    PDxCC PDx acts as own CC

582             ICD-10-CM 2018

**H04.323** Acute dacryocystitis of bilateral lacrimal passages

**H04.329** Acute dacryocystitis of unspecified lacrimal passage

✓6ᵗʰ **H04.33** Acute lacrimal canaliculitis

**H04.331** Acute lacrimal canaliculitis of right lacrimal passage

**H04.332** Acute lacrimal canaliculitis of left lacrimal passage

**H04.333** Acute lacrimal canaliculitis of bilateral lacrimal passages

**H04.339** Acute lacrimal canaliculitis of unspecified lacrimal passage

✓5ᵗʰ **H04.4** Chronic inflammation of lacrimal passages

✓6ᵗʰ **H04.41** Chronic dacryocystitis

**H04.411** Chronic dacryocystitis of right lacrimal passage

**H04.412** Chronic dacryocystitis of left lacrimal passage

**H04.413** Chronic dacryocystitis of bilateral lacrimal passages

**H04.419** Chronic dacryocystitis of unspecified lacrimal passage

✓6ᵗʰ **H04.42** Chronic lacrimal canaliculitis

**H04.421** Chronic lacrimal canaliculitis of right lacrimal passage

**H04.422** Chronic lacrimal canaliculitis of left lacrimal passage

**H04.423** Chronic lacrimal canaliculitis of bilateral lacrimal passages

**H04.429** Chronic lacrimal canaliculitis of unspecified lacrimal passage

✓6ᵗʰ **H04.43** Chronic lacrimal mucocele

**H04.431** Chronic lacrimal mucocele of right lacrimal passage

**H04.432** Chronic lacrimal mucocele of left lacrimal passage

**H04.433** Chronic lacrimal mucocele of bilateral lacrimal passages

**H04.439** Chronic lacrimal mucocele of unspecified lacrimal passage

✓5ᵗʰ **H04.5** Stenosis and insufficiency of lacrimal passages

✓6ᵗʰ **H04.51** Dacryolith

**H04.511** Dacryolith of right lacrimal passage

**H04.512** Dacryolith of left lacrimal passage

**H04.513** Dacryolith of bilateral lacrimal passages

**H04.519** Dacryolith of unspecified lacrimal passage

✓6ᵗʰ **H04.52** Eversion of lacrimal punctum

**H04.521** Eversion of right lacrimal punctum

**H04.522** Eversion of left lacrimal punctum

**H04.523** Eversion of bilateral lacrimal punctum

**H04.529** Eversion of unspecified lacrimal punctum

✓6ᵗʰ **H04.53** Neonatal obstruction of nasolacrimal duct

EXCLUDES 1 *congenital stenosis and stricture of lacrimal duct (Q10.5)*

**H04.531** Neonatal obstruction of right nasolacrimal duct                    [N]

**H04.532** Neonatal obstruction of left nasolacrimal duct                     [N]

**H04.533** Neonatal obstruction of bilateral nasolacrimal duct               [N]

**H04.539** Neonatal obstruction of unspecified nasolacrimal duct            [N]

✓6ᵗʰ **H04.54** Stenosis of lacrimal canaliculi

**H04.541** Stenosis of right lacrimal canaliculi

**H04.542** Stenosis of left lacrimal canaliculi

**H04.543** Stenosis of bilateral lacrimal canaliculi

**H04.549** Stenosis of unspecified lacrimal canaliculi

✓6ᵗʰ **H04.55** Acquired stenosis of nasolacrimal duct

**H04.551** Acquired stenosis of right nasolacrimal duct

**H04.552** Acquired stenosis of left nasolacrimal duct

**H04.553** Acquired stenosis of bilateral nasolacrimal duct

**H04.559** Acquired stenosis of unspecified nasolacrimal duct

✓6ᵗʰ **H04.56** Stenosis of lacrimal punctum

**H04.561** Stenosis of right lacrimal punctum

**H04.562** Stenosis of left lacrimal punctum

**H04.563** Stenosis of bilateral lacrimal punctum

**H04.569** Stenosis of unspecified lacrimal punctum

✓6ᵗʰ **H04.57** Stenosis of lacrimal sac

**H04.571** Stenosis of right lacrimal sac

**H04.572** Stenosis of left lacrimal sac

**H04.573** Stenosis of bilateral lacrimal sac

**H04.579** Stenosis of unspecified lacrimal sac

✓5ᵗʰ **H04.6** Other changes of lacrimal passages

✓6ᵗʰ **H04.61** Lacrimal fistula

**H04.611** Lacrimal fistula right lacrimal passage

**H04.612** Lacrimal fistula left lacrimal passage

**H04.613** Lacrimal fistula bilateral lacrimal passages

**H04.619** Lacrimal fistula unspecified lacrimal passage

**H04.69** Other changes of lacrimal passages

✓5ᵗʰ **H04.8** Other disorders of lacrimal system

✓6ᵗʰ **H04.81** Granuloma of lacrimal passages

**H04.811** Granuloma of right lacrimal passage

**H04.812** Granuloma of left lacrimal passage

**H04.813** Granuloma of bilateral lacrimal passages

**H04.819** Granuloma of unspecified lacrimal passage

**H04.89** Other disorders of lacrimal system

**H04.9** Disorder of lacrimal system, unspecified

✓4ᵗʰ **H05** Disorders of orbit

EXCLUDES 1 *congenital malformation of orbit (Q10.7)*

✓5ᵗʰ **H05.0** Acute inflammation of orbit

**H05.00** Unspecified acute inflammation of orbit

✓6ᵗʰ **H05.01** Cellulitis of orbit

Abscess of orbit

CC Excl: For CC codes in subcategory H05.01: PDX collection 621

**H05.011** Cellulitis of right orbit                    CC

**H05.012** Cellulitis of left orbit                     CC

**H05.013** Cellulitis of bilateral orbits              CC

**H05.019** Cellulitis of unspecified orbit            CC

✓6ᵗʰ **H05.02** Osteomyelitis of orbit

CC Excl: For CC codes in subcategory H05.02: PDX collection 622

**H05.021** Osteomyelitis of right orbit             CC

**H05.022** Osteomyelitis of left orbit              CC

**H05.023** Osteomyelitis of bilateral orbits        CC

**H05.029** Osteomyelitis of unspecified orbit       CC

✓6ᵗʰ **H05.03** Periostitis of orbit

CC Excl: For CC codes in subcategory H05.03: PDX collection 623

**H05.031** Periostitis of right orbit               CC

**H05.032** Periostitis of left orbit                CC

**H05.033** Periostitis of bilateral orbits          CC

**H05.039** Periostitis of unspecified orbit         CC

✓6ᵗʰ **H05.04** Tenonitis of orbit

**H05.041** Tenonitis of right orbit

**H05.042** Tenonitis of left orbit

**H05.043** Tenonitis of bilateral orbits

**H05.049** Tenonitis of unspecified orbit

✓5ᵗʰ **H05.1** Chronic inflammatory disorders of orbit

**H05.10** Unspecified chronic inflammatory disorders of orbit

✓6ᵗʰ **H05.11** Granuloma of orbit

Pseudotumor (inflammatory) of orbit

**H05.111** Granuloma of right orbit

**H05.112** Granuloma of left orbit

**H05.113** Granuloma of bilateral orbits

**H05.119** Granuloma of unspecified orbit

✓6ᵗʰ **H05.12** Orbital myositis

**H05.121** Orbital myositis, right orbit

**H05.122** Orbital myositis, left orbit

**H05.123** Orbital myositis, bilateral

H05.129    Orbital myositis, unspecified orbit

✓5ᵗʰ  **H05.2  Exophthalmic conditions**

    **H05.20  Unspecified exophthalmos**

    ✓6ᵗʰ  **H05.21  Displacement (lateral) of globe**

        H05.211    Displacement (lateral) of globe, right eye

        H05.212    Displacement (lateral) of globe, left eye

        H05.213    Displacement (lateral) of globe, bilateral

        H05.219    Displacement (lateral) of globe, unspecified eye

    ✓6ᵗʰ  **H05.22  Edema of orbit**
        Orbital congestion

        H05.221    Edema of right orbit

        H05.222    Edema of left orbit

        H05.223    Edema of bilateral orbit

        H05.229    Edema of unspecified orbit

    ✓6ᵗʰ  **H05.23  Hemorrhage of orbit**

        H05.231    Hemorrhage of right orbit

        H05.232    Hemorrhage of left orbit

        H05.233    Hemorrhage of bilateral orbit

        H05.239    Hemorrhage of unspecified orbit

    ✓6ᵗʰ  **H05.24  Constant exophthalmos**

        H05.241    Constant exophthalmos, right eye

        H05.242    Constant exophthalmos, left eye

        H05.243    Constant exophthalmos, bilateral

        H05.249    Constant exophthalmos, unspecified eye

    ✓6ᵗʰ  **H05.25  Intermittent exophthalmos**

        H05.251    Intermittent exophthalmos, right eye

        H05.252    Intermittent exophthalmos, left eye

        H05.253    Intermittent exophthalmos, bilateral

        H05.259    Intermittent exophthalmos, unspecified eye

    ✓6ᵗʰ  **H05.26  Pulsating exophthalmos**

        H05.261    Pulsating exophthalmos, right eye

        H05.262    Pulsating exophthalmos, left eye

        H05.263    Pulsating exophthalmos, bilateral

        H05.269    Pulsating exophthalmos, unspecified eye

✓5ᵗʰ  **H05.3  Deformity of orbit**

    *EXCLUDES 1*  congenital deformity of orbit (Q10.7)
        hypertelorism (Q75.2)

    **H05.30  Unspecified deformity of orbit**

    ✓6ᵗʰ  **H05.31  Atrophy of orbit**

        H05.311    Atrophy of right orbit

        H05.312    Atrophy of left orbit

        H05.313    Atrophy of bilateral orbit

        H05.319    Atrophy of unspecified orbit

    ✓6ᵗʰ  **H05.32  Deformity of orbit due to bone disease**
        Code also associated bone disease

        H05.321    Deformity of right orbit due to bone disease

        H05.322    Deformity of left orbit due to bone disease

        H05.323    Deformity of bilateral orbits due to bone disease

        H05.329    Deformity of unspecified orbit due to bone disease

    ✓6ᵗʰ  **H05.33  Deformity of orbit due to trauma or surgery**

        H05.331    Deformity of right orbit due to trauma or surgery

        H05.332    Deformity of left orbit due to trauma or surgery

        H05.333    Deformity of bilateral orbits due to trauma or surgery

        H05.339    Deformity of unspecified orbit due to trauma or surgery

    ✓6ᵗʰ  **H05.34  Enlargement of orbit**

        H05.341    Enlargement of right orbit

        H05.342    Enlargement of left orbit

        H05.343    Enlargement of bilateral orbits

        H05.349    Enlargement of unspecified orbit

    ✓6ᵗʰ  **H05.35  Exostosis of orbit**

        H05.351    Exostosis of right orbit

        H05.352    Exostosis of left orbit

        H05.353    Exostosis of bilateral orbits

        H05.359    Exostosis of unspecified orbit

---

✓5ᵗʰ  **H05.4  Enophthalmos**

    ✓6ᵗʰ  **H05.40  Unspecified enophthalmos**

        H05.401    Unspecified enophthalmos, right eye

        H05.402    Unspecified enophthalmos, left eye

        H05.403    Unspecified enophthalmos, bilateral

        H05.409    Unspecified enophthalmos, unspecified eye

    ✓6ᵗʰ  **H05.41  Enophthalmos due to atrophy of orbital tissue**

        H05.411    Enophthalmos due to atrophy of orbital tissue, right eye

        H05.412    Enophthalmos due to atrophy of orbital tissue, left eye

        H05.413    Enophthalmos due to atrophy of orbital tissue, bilateral

        H05.419    Enophthalmos due to atrophy of orbital tissue, unspecified eye

    ✓6ᵗʰ  **H05.42  Enophthalmos due to trauma or surgery**

        H05.421    Enophthalmos due to trauma or surgery, right eye

        H05.422    Enophthalmos due to trauma or surgery, left eye

        H05.423    Enophthalmos due to trauma or surgery, bilateral

        H05.429    Enophthalmos due to trauma or surgery, unspecified eye

✓5ᵗʰ  **H05.5  Retained (old) foreign body following penetrating wound of orbit**
    Retrobulbar foreign body
    Use additional code to identify the type of retained foreign body (Z18.-)

    *EXCLUDES 1*  current penetrating wound of orbit (S05.4-)

    *EXCLUDES 2*  retained foreign body of eyelid (H02.81-)
        retained intraocular foreign body (H44.6-, H44.7-)

    **H05.50  Retained (old) foreign body following penetrating wound of unspecified orbit**

    **H05.51  Retained (old) foreign body following penetrating wound of right orbit**

    **H05.52  Retained (old) foreign body following penetrating wound of left orbit**

    **H05.53  Retained (old) foreign body following penetrating wound of bilateral orbits**

✓5ᵗʰ  **H05.8  Other disorders of orbit**

    ✓6ᵗʰ  **H05.81  Cyst of orbit**
        Encephalocele of orbit

        H05.811    Cyst of right orbit

        H05.812    Cyst of left orbit

        H05.813    Cyst of bilateral orbits

        H05.819    Cyst of unspecified orbit

    ✓6ᵗʰ  **H05.82  Myopathy of extraocular muscles**

        H05.821    Myopathy of extraocular muscles, right orbit

        H05.822    Myopathy of extraocular muscles, left orbit

        H05.823    Myopathy of extraocular muscles, bilateral

        H05.829    Myopathy of extraocular muscles, unspecified orbit

    **H05.89  Other disorders of orbit**

    **H05.9  Unspecified disorder of orbit**

### Disorders of conjunctiva (H10-H11)

✓4ᵗʰ  **H10  Conjunctivitis**

    *EXCLUDES 1*  keratoconjunctivitis (H16.2-)

    ✓5ᵗʰ  **H10.0  Mucopurulent conjunctivitis**

        ✓6ᵗʰ  **H10.01  Acute follicular conjunctivitis**

            H10.011    Acute follicular conjunctivitis, right eye

            H10.012    Acute follicular conjunctivitis, left eye

            H10.013    Acute follicular conjunctivitis, bilateral

            H10.019    Acute follicular conjunctivitis, unspecified eye

        ✓6ᵗʰ  **H10.02  Other mucopurulent conjunctivitis**

            H10.021    Other mucopurulent conjunctivitis, right eye

            H10.022    Other mucopurulent conjunctivitis, left eye

Ⓝ Newborn: 0   Ⓟ Pediatric: 0-17   Ⓜ Maternity: 12-55   Ⓐ Adult: 15-124   MCC Major CC Condition   PDx MCC PDx acts as own MCC   CC CC Condition   PDx CC PDx acts as own CC

584                                                                                                              ICD-10-CM 2018

H10.023    Other mucopurulent conjunctivitis, bilateral

H10.029    Other mucopurulent conjunctivitis, unspecified eye

✓5ᵗʰ **H10.1**    **Acute atopic conjunctivitis**
Acute papillary conjunctivitis

H10.10    **Acute atopic conjunctivitis, unspecified eye**

H10.11    **Acute atopic conjunctivitis, right eye**

H10.12    **Acute atopic conjunctivitis, left eye**

H10.13    **Acute atopic conjunctivitis, bilateral**

✓5ᵗʰ **H10.2**    **Other acute conjunctivitis**

✓6ᵗʰ **H10.21**    **Acute toxic conjunctivitis**
Acute chemical conjunctivitis
Code first (T51-T65) to identify chemical and intent
EXCLUDES 1    burn and corrosion of eye and adnexa (T26.-)

H10.211    **Acute toxic conjunctivitis, right eye**

H10.212    **Acute toxic conjunctivitis, left eye**

H10.213    **Acute toxic conjunctivitis, bilateral**

H10.219    **Acute toxic conjunctivitis, unspecified eye**

✓6ᵗʰ **H10.22**    **Pseudomembranous conjunctivitis**

H10.221    **Pseudomembranous conjunctivitis, right eye**

H10.222    **Pseudomembranous conjunctivitis, left eye**

H10.223    **Pseudomembranous conjunctivitis, bilateral**

H10.229    **Pseudomembranous conjunctivitis, unspecified eye**

✓6ᵗʰ **H10.23**    **Serous conjunctivitis, except viral**
EXCLUDES 1    viral conjunctivitis (B30.-)

H10.231    **Serous conjunctivitis, except viral, right eye**

H10.232    **Serous conjunctivitis, except viral, left eye**

H10.233    **Serous conjunctivitis, except viral, bilateral**

H10.239    **Serous conjunctivitis, except viral, unspecified eye**

✓5ᵗʰ **H10.3**    **Unspecified acute conjunctivitis**
EXCLUDES 1    ophthalmia neonatorum NOS (P39.1)

H10.30    **Unspecified acute conjunctivitis, unspecified eye**

H10.31    **Unspecified acute conjunctivitis, right eye**

H10.32    **Unspecified acute conjunctivitis, left eye**

H10.33    **Unspecified acute conjunctivitis, bilateral**

✓5ᵗʰ **H10.4**    **Chronic conjunctivitis**

✓6ᵗʰ **H10.40**    **Unspecified chronic conjunctivitis**

H10.401    **Unspecified chronic conjunctivitis, right eye**

H10.402    **Unspecified chronic conjunctivitis, left eye**

H10.403    **Unspecified chronic conjunctivitis, bilateral**

H10.409    **Unspecified chronic conjunctivitis, unspecified eye**

✓6ᵗʰ **H10.41**    **Chronic giant papillary conjunctivitis**

H10.411    **Chronic giant papillary conjunctivitis, right eye**

H10.412    **Chronic giant papillary conjunctivitis, left eye**

H10.413    **Chronic giant papillary conjunctivitis, bilateral**

H10.419    **Chronic giant papillary conjunctivitis, unspecified eye**

✓6ᵗʰ **H10.42**    **Simple chronic conjunctivitis**

H10.421    **Simple chronic conjunctivitis, right eye**

H10.422    **Simple chronic conjunctivitis, left eye**

H10.423    **Simple chronic conjunctivitis, bilateral**

H10.429    **Simple chronic conjunctivitis, unspecified eye**

✓6ᵗʰ **H10.43**    **Chronic follicular conjunctivitis**

H10.431    **Chronic follicular conjunctivitis, right eye**

H10.432    **Chronic follicular conjunctivitis, left eye**

H10.433    **Chronic follicular conjunctivitis, bilateral**

H10.439    **Chronic follicular conjunctivitis, unspecified eye**

H10.44    **Vernal conjunctivitis**
EXCLUDES 1    vernal keratoconjunctivitis with limbar and corneal involvement (H16.26-)

H10.45    **Other chronic allergic conjunctivitis**

✓5ᵗʰ **H10.5**    **Blepharoconjunctivitis**

✓6ᵗʰ **H10.50**    **Unspecified blepharoconjunctivitis**

H10.501    **Unspecified blepharoconjunctivitis, right eye**

H10.502    **Unspecified blepharoconjunctivitis, left eye**

H10.503    **Unspecified blepharoconjunctivitis, bilateral**

H10.509    **Unspecified blepharoconjunctivitis, unspecified eye**

✓6ᵗʰ **H10.51**    **Ligneous conjunctivitis**

H10.511    **Ligneous conjunctivitis, right eye**

H10.512    **Ligneous conjunctivitis, left eye**

H10.513    **Ligneous conjunctivitis, bilateral**

H10.519    **Ligneous conjunctivitis, unspecified eye**

✓6ᵗʰ **H10.52**    **Angular blepharoconjunctivitis**

H10.521    **Angular blepharoconjunctivitis, right eye**

H10.522    **Angular blepharoconjunctivitis, left eye**

H10.523    **Angular blepharoconjunctivitis, bilateral**

H10.529    **Angular blepharoconjunctivitis, unspecified eye**

✓6ᵗʰ **H10.53**    **Contact blepharoconjunctivitis**

H10.531    **Contact blepharoconjunctivitis, right eye**

H10.532    **Contact blepharoconjunctivitis, left eye**

H10.533    **Contact blepharoconjunctivitis, bilateral**

H10.539    **Contact blepharoconjunctivitis, unspecified eye**

✓5ᵗʰ **H10.8**    **Other conjunctivitis**

✓6ᵗʰ **H10.81**    **Pingueculitis**
EXCLUDES 1    pinguecula (H11.15-)

H10.811    **Pingueculitis, right eye**

H10.812    **Pingueculitis, left eye**

H10.813    **Pingueculitis, bilateral**

H10.819    **Pingueculitis, unspecified eye**

H10.89    **Other conjunctivitis**

H10.9    **Unspecified conjunctivitis**

✓4ᵗʰ **H11**    **Other disorders of conjunctiva**
EXCLUDES 1    keratoconjunctivitis (H16.2-)

✓5ᵗʰ **H11.0**    **Pterygium of eye**
EXCLUDES 1    pseudopterygium (H11.81-)

✓6ᵗʰ **H11.00**    **Unspecified pterygium of eye**

H11.001    **Unspecified pterygium of right eye**

H11.002    **Unspecified pterygium of left eye**

H11.003    **Unspecified pterygium of eye, bilateral**

H11.009    **Unspecified pterygium of unspecified eye**

✓6ᵗʰ **H11.01**    **Amyloid pterygium**

H11.011    **Amyloid pterygium of right eye**

H11.012    **Amyloid pterygium of left eye**

H11.013    **Amyloid pterygium of eye, bilateral**

H11.019    **Amyloid pterygium of unspecified eye**

✓6ᵗʰ **H11.02**    **Central pterygium of eye**

H11.021    **Central pterygium of right eye**

H11.022    **Central pterygium of left eye**

H11.023    **Central pterygium of eye, bilateral**

**Pterygium**

Pterygium

☑ Additional Character Req    ✓×7ᵗʰ Placeholder Alert    Unacceptable PDx    Manifestation    H1-H14 HAC    HCC CMS-HCC Condition    EXCLUDES 1 Not Coded Here    EXCLUDES 2 Not Included Here

ICD-10-CM 2018      585

    H11.029   **Central** pterygium of **unspecified** eye

✓6th   **H11.03**   **Double** pterygium of eye
    H11.031   Double pterygium of **right** eye
    H11.032   Double pterygium of **left** eye
    H11.033   Double pterygium of eye, **bilateral**
    H11.039   Double pterygium of **unspecified** eye

✓6th   **H11.04**   **Peripheral** pterygium of eye, **stationary**
    H11.041   Peripheral pterygium, stationary, **right** eye
    H11.042   Peripheral pterygium, stationary, **left** eye
    H11.043   Peripheral pterygium, stationary, **bilateral**
    H11.049   Peripheral pterygium, stationary, **unspecified** eye

✓6th   **H11.05**   **Peripheral** pterygium of eye, **progressive**
    H11.051   Peripheral pterygium, progressive, **right** eye
    H11.052   Peripheral pterygium, progressive, **left** eye
    H11.053   Peripheral pterygium, progressive, **bilateral**
    H11.059   Peripheral pterygium, progressive, **unspecified** eye

✓6th   **H11.06**   **Recurrent** pterygium of eye
    H11.061   Recurrent pterygium of **right** eye
    H11.062   Recurrent pterygium of **left** eye
    H11.063   Recurrent pterygium of eye, **bilateral**
    H11.069   Recurrent pterygium of **unspecified** eye

✓5th   **H11.1**   **Conjunctival degenerations and deposits**
    **EXCLUDES 2**   *pseudopterygium (H11.81)*

    **H11.10**   **Unspecified conjunctival degenerations**

✓6th   **H11.11**   **Conjunctival deposits**
    H11.111   Conjunctival deposits, **right** eye
    H11.112   Conjunctival deposits, **left** eye
    H11.113   Conjunctival deposits, **bilateral**
    H11.119   Conjunctival deposits, **unspecified** eye

✓6th   **H11.12**   **Conjunctival** concretions
    H11.121   Conjunctival concretions, **right** eye
    H11.122   Conjunctival concretions, **left** eye
    H11.123   Conjunctival concretions, **bilateral**
    H11.129   Conjunctival concretions, **unspecified** eye

✓6th   **H11.13**   **Conjunctival** pigmentations
    Conjunctival argyrosis [argyria]
    H11.131   Conjunctival pigmentations, **right** eye
    H11.132   Conjunctival pigmentations, **left** eye
    H11.133   Conjunctival pigmentations, **bilateral**
    H11.139   Conjunctival pigmentations, **unspecified** eye

✓6th   **H11.14**   **Conjunctival xerosis, unspecified**
    **EXCLUDES 1**   *xerosis of conjunctiva due to vitamin A deficiency (E50.0, E50.1)*
    **DEF:** Abnormal dryness of conjunctiva due to lack of insufficient tears or conjunctival secretions.
    H11.141   Conjunctival xerosis, unspecified, **right** eye
    H11.142   Conjunctival xerosis , unspecified, **left** eye
    H11.143   Conjunctival xerosis, unspecified, **bilateral**
    H11.149   Conjunctival xerosis, unspecified, **unspecified** eyed

✓6th   **H11.15**   **Pinguecula**
    **EXCLUDES 1**   *pingueculitis (H10.81-)*
    H11.151   Pinguecula, **right** eye
    H11.152   Pinguecula, **left** eye
    H11.153   Pinguecula, **bilateral**
    H11.159   Pinguecula, **unspecified** eye

✓5th   **H11.2**   **Conjunctival scars**

✓6th   **H11.21**   **Conjunctival** adhesions and strands **(localized)**
    H11.211   Conjunctival adhesions and strands (localized), **right** eye
    H11.212   Conjunctival adhesions and strands (localized), **left** eye
    H11.213   Conjunctival adhesions and strands (localized), **bilateral**
    H11.219   Conjunctival adhesions and strands (localized), **unspecified** eye

**Pinguecula**

Pinguecula

✓6th   **H11.22**   **Conjunctival** granuloma
    H11.221   Conjunctival granuloma, **right** eye
    H11.222   Conjunctival granuloma, **left** eye
    H11.223   Conjunctival granuloma, **bilateral**
    H11.229   Conjunctival granuloma, **unspecified**

✓6th   **H11.23**   **Symblepharon**
    H11.231   Symblepharon, **right** eye
    H11.232   Symblepharon, **left** eye
    H11.233   Symblepharon, **bilateral**
    H11.239   Symblepharon, **unspecified** eye

✓6th   **H11.24**   **Scarring of conjunctiva**
    H11.241   Scarring of conjunctiva, **right** eye
    H11.242   Scarring of conjunctiva, **left** eye
    H11.243   Scarring of conjunctiva, **bilateral**
    H11.249   Scarring of conjunctiva, **unspecified** eye

✓5th   **H11.3**   **Conjunctival hemorrhage**
    Subconjunctival hemorrhage
    H11.30   Conjunctival hemorrhage, **unspecified** eye
    H11.31   Conjunctival hemorrhage, **right** eye
    H11.32   Conjunctival hemorrhage, **left** eye
    H11.33   Conjunctival hemorrhage, **bilateral**

✓5th   **H11.4**   **Other conjunctival vascular disorders and cysts**

✓6th   **H11.41**   **Vascular abnormalities** of conjunctiva
    Conjunctival aneurysm
    H11.411   Vascular abnormalities of conjunctiva, **right** eye
    H11.412   Vascular abnormalities of conjunctiva, **left** eye
    H11.413   Vascular abnormalities of conjunctiva, **bilateral**
    H11.419   Vascular abnormalities of conjunctiva, **unspecified** eye

✓6th   **H11.42**   **Conjunctival edema**
    H11.421   Conjunctival edema, **right** eye
    H11.422   Conjunctival edema, **left** eye
    H11.423   Conjunctival edema, **bilateral**
    H11.429   Conjunctival edema, **unspecified** eye

✓6th   **H11.43**   **Conjunctival** hyperemia
    H11.431   Conjunctival hyperemia, **right** eye
    H11.432   Conjunctival hyperemia, **left** eye
    H11.433   Conjunctival hyperemia, **bilateral**
    H11.439   Conjunctival hyperemia, **unspecified** eye

✓6th   **H11.44**   **Conjunctival cysts**
    H11.441   Conjunctival cysts, **right** eye
    H11.442   Conjunctival cysts, **left** eye
    H11.443   Conjunctival cysts, **bilateral**
    H11.449   Conjunctival cysts, **unspecified** eye

✓5th   **H11.8**   **Other specified disorders of conjunctiva**

✓6th   **H11.81**   **Pseudopterygium of conjunctiva**
    H11.811   Pseudopterygium of conjunctiva, **right** eye
    H11.812   Pseudopterygium of conjunctiva, **left** eye
    H11.813   Pseudopterygium of conjunctiva, **bilateral**
    H11.819   Pseudopterygium of conjunctiva, **unspecified** eye

✓6th   **H11.82**   **Conjunctivochalasis**
    H11.821   Conjunctivochalasis, **right** eye

**N** Newborn: 0    **P** Pediatric: 0-17    **M** Maternity: 12-55    **A** Adult: 15-124    **MCC** Major CC Condition    **PDx MCC** PDx acts as own MCC    **CC** CC Condition    **PDx CC** PDx acts as own CC

**586**          ICD-10-CM 2018

**H11.822**   Conjunctivochalasis, left eye
**H11.823**   Conjunctivochalasis, bilateral
**H11.829**   Conjunctivochalasis, unspecified eye
**H11.89**   Other specified disorders of conjunctiva
**H11.9**   Unspecified disorder of conjunctiva

## Disorders of sclera, cornea, iris and ciliary body (H15-H22)

### ✓4ᵗʰ H15   Disorders of sclera

- ✓5ᵗʰ **H15.0**   Scleritis
  - ✓6ᵗʰ **H15.00**   Unspecified scleritis
    - **H15.001**   Unspecified scleritis, right eye
    - **H15.002**   Unspecified scleritis, left eye
    - **H15.003**   Unspecified scleritis, bilateral
    - **H15.009**   Unspecified scleritis, unspecified eye
  - ✓6ᵗʰ **H15.01**   Anterior scleritis
    - **H15.011**   Anterior scleritis, right eye
    - **H15.012**   Anterior scleritis, left eye
    - **H15.013**   Anterior scleritis, bilateral
    - **H15.019**   Anterior scleritis, unspecified eye
  - ✓6ᵗʰ **H15.02**   Brawny scleritis
    - **H15.021**   Brawny scleritis, right eye
    - **H15.022**   Brawny scleritis, left eye
    - **H15.023**   Brawny scleritis, bilateral
    - **H15.029**   Brawny scleritis, unspecified eye
  - ✓6ᵗʰ **H15.03**   Posterior scleritis
    - Sclerotenonitis
    - **H15.031**   Posterior scleritis, right eye
    - **H15.032**   Posterior scleritis, left eye
    - **H15.033**   Posterior scleritis, bilateral
    - **H15.039**   Posterior scleritis, unspecified eye
  - ✓6ᵗʰ **H15.04**   Scleritis with corneal involvement
    - **H15.041**   Scleritis with corneal involvement, right eye
    - **H15.042**   Scleritis with corneal involvement, left eye
    - **H15.043**   Scleritis with corneal involvement, bilateral
    - **H15.049**   Scleritis with corneal involvement, unspecified eye
  - ✓6ᵗʰ **H15.05**   Scleromalacia perforans
    - **H15.051**   Scleromalacia perforans, right eye
    - **H15.052**   Scleromalacia perforans, left eye
    - **H15.053**   Scleromalacia perforans, bilateral
    - **H15.059**   Scleromalacia perforans, unspecified eye
  - ✓6ᵗʰ **H15.09**   Other scleritis
    - Scleral abscess
    - **H15.091**   Other scleritis, right eye
    - **H15.092**   Other scleritis, left eye
    - **H15.093**   Other scleritis, bilateral
    - **H15.099**   Other scleritis, unspecified eye
- ✓5ᵗʰ **H15.1**   Episcleritis
  - ✓6ᵗʰ **H15.10**   Unspecified episcleritis
    - **H15.101**   Unspecified episcleritis, right eye
    - **H15.102**   Unspecified episcleritis, left eye
    - **H15.103**   Unspecified episcleritis, bilateral
    - **H15.109**   Unspecified episcleritis, unspecified eye
  - ✓6ᵗʰ **H15.11**   Episcleritis periodica fugax
    - **H15.111**   Episcleritis periodica fugax, right eye
    - **H15.112**   Episcleritis periodica fugax, left eye
    - **H15.113**   Episcleritis periodica fugax, bilateral
    - **H15.119**   Episcleritis periodica fugax, unspecified eye
  - ✓6ᵗʰ **H15.12**   Nodular episcleritis
    - **H15.121**   Nodular episcleritis, right eye
    - **H15.122**   Nodular episcleritis, left eye
    - **H15.123**   Nodular episcleritis, bilateral
    - **H15.129**   Nodular episcleritis, unspecified eye
- ✓5ᵗʰ **H15.8**   Other disorders of sclera
  - *EXCLUDES 2*   blue sclera (Q13.5)
    - degenerative myopia (H44.2-)
  - ✓6ᵗʰ **H15.81**   Equatorial staphyloma
    - **H15.811**   Equatorial staphyloma, right eye
    - **H15.812**   Equatorial staphyloma, left eye

**H15.813**   Equatorial staphyloma, bilateral
**H15.819**   Equatorial staphyloma, unspecified eye
- ✓6ᵗʰ **H15.82**   Localized anterior staphyloma
  - **H15.821**   Localized anterior staphyloma, right eye
  - **H15.822**   Localized anterior staphyloma, left eye
  - **H15.823**   Localized anterior staphyloma, bilateral
  - **H15.829**   Localized anterior staphyloma, unspecified eye
- ✓6ᵗʰ **H15.83**   Staphyloma posticum
  - **H15.831**   Staphyloma posticum, right eye
  - **H15.832**   Staphyloma posticum, left eye
  - **H15.833**   Staphyloma posticum, bilateral
  - **H15.839**   Staphyloma posticum, unspecified eye
- ✓6ᵗʰ **H15.84**   Scleral ectasia
  - **H15.841**   Scleral ectasia, right eye
  - **H15.842**   Scleral ectasia, left eye
  - **H15.843**   Scleral ectasia, bilateral
  - **H15.849**   Scleral ectasia, unspecified eye
- ✓6ᵗʰ **H15.85**   Ring staphyloma
  - **H15.851**   Ring staphyloma, right eye
  - **H15.852**   Ring staphyloma, left eye
  - **H15.853**   Ring staphyloma, bilateral
  - **H15.859**   Ring staphyloma, unspecified eye
- **H15.89**   Other disorders of sclera
- **H15.9**   Unspecified disorder of sclera

### ✓4ᵗʰ H16   Keratitis

- ✓5ᵗʰ **H16.0**   Corneal ulcer
  - ✓6ᵗʰ **H16.00**   Unspecified corneal ulcer
    - **H16.001**   Unspecified corneal ulcer, right eye
    - **H16.002**   Unspecified corneal ulcer, left eye
    - **H16.003**   Unspecified corneal ulcer, bilateral
    - **H16.009**   Unspecified corneal ulcer, unspecified eye
  - ✓6ᵗʰ **H16.01**   Central corneal ulcer
    - **H16.011**   Central corneal ulcer, right eye
    - **H16.012**   Central corneal ulcer, left eye
    - **H16.013**   Central corneal ulcer, bilateral
    - **H16.019**   Central corneal ulcer, unspecified eye
  - ✓6ᵗʰ **H16.02**   Ring corneal ulcer
    - **H16.021**   Ring corneal ulcer, right eye
    - **H16.022**   Ring corneal ulcer, left eye
    - **H16.023**   Ring corneal ulcer, bilateral
    - **H16.029**   Ring corneal ulcer, unspecified eye
  - ✓6ᵗʰ **H16.03**   Corneal ulcer with hypopyon
    - **H16.031**   Corneal ulcer with hypopyon, right eye
    - **H16.032**   Corneal ulcer with hypopyon, left eye
    - **H16.033**   Corneal ulcer with hypopyon, bilateral
    - **H16.039**   Corneal ulcer with hypopyon, unspecified eye
  - ✓6ᵗʰ **H16.04**   Marginal corneal ulcer
    - **H16.041**   Marginal corneal ulcer, right eye
    - **H16.042**   Marginal corneal ulcer, left eye
    - **H16.043**   Marginal corneal ulcer, bilateral
    - **H16.049**   Marginal corneal ulcer, unspecified eye
  - ✓6ᵗʰ **H16.05**   Mooren's corneal ulcer
    - **H16.051**   Mooren's corneal ulcer, right eye
    - **H16.052**   Mooren's corneal ulcer, left eye
    - **H16.053**   Mooren's corneal ulcer, bilateral
    - **H16.059**   Mooren's corneal ulcer, unspecified eye
  - ✓6ᵗʰ **H16.06**   Mycotic corneal ulcer
    - **H16.061**   Mycotic corneal ulcer, right eye
    - **H16.062**   Mycotic corneal ulcer, left eye
    - **H16.063**   Mycotic corneal ulcer, bilateral
    - **H16.069**   Mycotic corneal ulcer, unspecified eye
  - ✓6ᵗʰ **H16.07**   Perforated corneal ulcer
    - **H16.071**   Perforated corneal ulcer, right eye
    - **H16.072**   Perforated corneal ulcer, left eye
    - **H16.073**   Perforated corneal ulcer, bilateral
    - **H16.079**   Perforated corneal ulcer, unspecified eye

✓ Additional Character Req    ✓x7ᵗʰ Placeholder Alert    Unacceptable PDx    Manifestation    **H1**-**H14** HAC    **HCC** CMS-HCC Condition    *EXCLUDES 1* Not Coded Here    *EXCLUDES 2* Not Included Here

ICD-10-CM 2018                          587

✓5th **H16.1 Other and unspecified superficial keratitis without conjunctivitis**

  ✓6th **H16.10 Unspecified superficial keratitis**

    **H16.101 Unspecified superficial keratitis, right eye**

    **H16.102 Unspecified superficial keratitis, left eye**

    **H16.103 Unspecified superficial keratitis, bilateral**

    **H16.109 Unspecified superficial keratitis, unspecified eye**

  ✓6th **H16.11 Macular keratitis**
    Areolar keratitis
    Nummular keratitis
    Stellate keratitis
    Striate keratitis

    **H16.111 Macular keratitis, right eye**

    **H16.112 Macular keratitis, left eye**

    **H16.113 Macular keratitis, bilateral**

    **H16.119 Macular keratitis, unspecified eye**

  ✓6th **H16.12 Filamentary keratitis**

    **H16.121 Filamentary keratitis, right eye**

    **H16.122 Filamentary keratitis, left eye**

    **H16.123 Filamentary keratitis, bilateral**

    **H16.129 Filamentary keratitis, unspecified eye**

  ✓6th **H16.13 Photokeratitis**
    Snow blindness
    Welders keratitis

    **H16.131 Photokeratitis, right eye**

    **H16.132 Photokeratitis, left eye**

    **H16.133 Photokeratitis, bilateral**

    **H16.139 Photokeratitis, unspecified eye**

  ✓6th **H16.14 Punctate keratitis**

    **H16.141 Punctate keratitis, right eye**

    **H16.142 Punctate keratitis, left eye**

    **H16.143 Punctate keratitis, bilateral**

    **H16.149 Punctate keratitis, unspecified eye**

✓5th **H16.2 Keratoconjunctivitis**

  ✓6th **H16.20 Unspecified keratoconjunctivitis**
    Superficial keratitis with conjunctivitis NOS

    **H16.201 Unspecified keratoconjunctivitis, right eye**

    **H16.202 Unspecified keratoconjunctivitis, left eye**

    **H16.203 Unspecified keratoconjunctivitis, bilateral**

    **H16.209 Unspecified keratoconjunctivitis, unspecified eye**

  ✓6th **H16.21 Exposure keratoconjunctivitis**

    **H16.211 Exposure keratoconjunctivitis, right eye**

    **H16.212 Exposure keratoconjunctivitis, left eye**

    **H16.213 Exposure keratoconjunctivitis, bilateral**

    **H16.219 Exposure keratoconjunctivitis, unspecified eye**

  ✓6th **H16.22 Keratoconjunctivitis sicca, not specified as Sjögren's**
    **EXCLUDES 1** *Sjögren's syndrome (M35.01)*

    **H16.221 Keratoconjunctivitis sicca, not specified as Sjögren's, right eye**

    **H16.222 Keratoconjunctivitis sicca, not specified as Sjögren's, left eye**

    **H16.223 Keratoconjunctivitis sicca, not specified as Sjögren's, bilateral**

    **H16.229 Keratoconjunctivitis sicca, not specified as Sjögren's, unspecified eye**

  ✓6th **H16.23 Neurotrophic keratoconjunctivitis**

    **H16.231 Neurotrophic keratoconjunctivitis, right eye**

    **H16.232 Neurotrophic keratoconjunctivitis, left eye**

    **H16.233 Neurotrophic keratoconjunctivitis, bilateral**

    **H16.239 Neurotrophic keratoconjunctivitis, unspecified eye**

  ✓6th **H16.24 Ophthalmia nodosa**

    **H16.241 Ophthalmia nodosa, right eye**

    **H16.242 Ophthalmia nodosa, left eye**

    **H16.243 Ophthalmia nodosa, bilateral**

    **H16.249 Ophthalmia nodosa, unspecified eye**

  ✓6th **H16.25 Phlyctenular keratoconjunctivitis**

    **H16.251 Phlyctenular keratoconjunctivitis, right eye**

    **H16.252 Phlyctenular keratoconjunctivitis, left eye**

    **H16.253 Phlyctenular keratoconjunctivitis, bilateral**

    **H16.259 Phlyctenular keratoconjunctivitis, unspecified eye**

  ✓6th **H16.26 Vernal keratoconjunctivitis, with limbar and corneal involvement**
    **EXCLUDES 1** *vernal conjunctivitis without limbar and corneal involvement (H10.44)*

    **H16.261 Vernal keratoconjunctivitis, with limbar and corneal involvement, right eye**

    **H16.262 Vernal keratoconjunctivitis, with limbar and corneal involvement, left eye**

    **H16.263 Vernal keratoconjunctivitis, with limbar and corneal involvement, bilateral**

    **H16.269 Vernal keratoconjunctivitis, with limbar and corneal involvement, unspecified eye**

  ✓6th **H16.29 Other keratoconjunctivitis**

    **H16.291 Other keratoconjunctivitis, right eye**

    **H16.292 Other keratoconjunctivitis, left eye**

    **H16.293 Other keratoconjunctivitis, bilateral**

    **H16.299 Other keratoconjunctivitis, unspecified eye**

✓5th **H16.3 Interstitial and deep keratitis**

  ✓6th **H16.30 Unspecified interstitial keratitis**

    **H16.301 Unspecified interstitial keratitis, right eye**

    **H16.302 Unspecified interstitial keratitis, left eye**

    **H16.303 Unspecified interstitial keratitis, bilateral**

    **H16.309 Unspecified interstitial keratitis, unspecified eye**

  ✓6th **H16.31 Corneal abscess**

    **H16.311 Corneal abscess, right eye**

    **H16.312 Corneal abscess, left eye**

    **H16.313 Corneal abscess, bilateral**

    **H16.319 Corneal abscess, unspecified eye**

  ✓6th **H16.32 Diffuse interstitial keratitis**
    Cogan's syndrome

    **H16.321 Diffuse interstitial keratitis, right eye**

    **H16.322 Diffuse interstitial keratitis, left eye**

    **H16.323 Diffuse interstitial keratitis, bilateral**

    **H16.329 Diffuse interstitial keratitis, unspecified eye**

  ✓6th **H16.33 Sclerosing keratitis**

    **H16.331 Sclerosing keratitis, right eye**

    **H16.332 Sclerosing keratitis, left eye**

    **H16.333 Sclerosing keratitis, bilateral**

    **H16.339 Sclerosing keratitis, unspecified eye**

  ✓6th **H16.39 Other interstitial and deep keratitis**

    **H16.391 Other interstitial and deep keratitis, right eye**

    **H16.392 Other interstitial and deep keratitis, left eye**

    **H16.393 Other interstitial and deep keratitis, bilateral**

    **H16.399 Other interstitial and deep keratitis, unspecified eye**

✓5th **H16.4 Corneal neovascularization**

  ✓6th **H16.40 Unspecified corneal neovascularization**

    **H16.401 Unspecified corneal neovascularization, right eye**

    **H16.402 Unspecified corneal neovascularization, left eye**

    **H16.403 Unspecified corneal neovascularization, bilateral**

    **H16.409 Unspecified corneal neovascularization, unspecified eye**

  ✓6th **H16.41 Ghost vessels (corneal)**

    **H16.411 Ghost vessels (corneal), right eye**

    **H16.412 Ghost vessels (corneal), left eye**

    **H16.413 Ghost vessels (corneal), bilateral**

    **H16.419 Ghost vessels (corneal), unspecified eye**

N Newborn: 0   P Pediatric: 0-17   M Maternity: 12-55   A Adult: 15-124   MCC Major CC Condition   PDx MCC PDx acts as own MCC   CC CC Condition   PDx CC PDx acts as own CC

588           ICD-10-CM 2018

√6th **H16.42 Pannus (corneal)**
     H16.421   **Pannus (corneal), right eye**
     H16.422   **Pannus (corneal), left eye**
     H16.423   **Pannus (corneal), bilateral**
     H16.429   **Pannus (corneal), unspecified eye**

√6th **H16.43 Localized vascularization of cornea**
     H16.431   **Localized vascularization of cornea, right eye**
     H16.432   **Localized vascularization of cornea, left eye**
     H16.433   **Localized vascularization of cornea, bilateral**
     H16.439   **Localized vascularization of cornea, unspecified eye**

√6th **H16.44 Deep vascularization of cornea**
     H16.441   **Deep vascularization of cornea, right eye**
     H16.442   **Deep vascularization of cornea, left eye**
     H16.443   **Deep vascularization of cornea, bilateral**
     H16.449   **Deep vascularization of cornea, unspecified eye**

**H16.8 Other keratitis**
**H16.9 Unspecified keratitis**

√4th **H17 Corneal scars and opacities**

√5th **H17.0 Adherent leukoma**
     H17.00   **Adherent leukoma, unspecified eye**
     H17.01   **Adherent leukoma, right eye**
     H17.02   **Adherent leukoma, left eye**
     H17.03   **Adherent leukoma, bilateral**

√5th **H17.1 Central corneal opacity**
     H17.10   **Central corneal opacity, unspecified eye**
     H17.11   **Central corneal opacity, right eye**
     H17.12   **Central corneal opacity, left eye**
     H17.13   **Central corneal opacity, bilateral**

√5th **H17.8 Other corneal scars and opacities**
   √6th **H17.81 Minor opacity of cornea**
       Corneal nebula
     H17.811   **Minor opacity of cornea, right eye**
     H17.812   **Minor opacity of cornea, left eye**
     H17.813   **Minor opacity of cornea, bilateral**
     H17.819   **Minor opacity of cornea, unspecified eye**
   √6th **H17.82 Peripheral opacity of cornea**
     H17.821   **Peripheral opacity of cornea, right eye**
     H17.822   **Peripheral opacity of cornea, left eye**
     H17.823   **Peripheral opacity of cornea, bilateral**
     H17.829   **Peripheral opacity of cornea, unspecified eye**
     H17.89   **Other corneal scars and opacities**
**H17.9 Unspecified corneal scar and opacity**

√4th **H18 Other disorders of cornea**

√5th **H18.0 Corneal pigmentations and deposits**
   √6th **H18.00 Unspecified corneal deposit**
     H18.001   **Unspecified corneal deposit, right eye**
     H18.002   **Unspecified corneal deposit, left eye**
     H18.003   **Unspecified corneal deposit, bilateral**
     H18.009   **Unspecified corneal deposit, unspecified eye**
   √6th **H18.01 Anterior corneal pigmentations**
       Staehli's line
     H18.011   **Anterior corneal pigmentations, right eye**
     H18.012   **Anterior corneal pigmentations, left eye**
     H18.013   **Anterior corneal pigmentations, bilateral**
     H18.019   **Anterior corneal pigmentations, unspecified eye**
   √6th **H18.02 Argentous corneal deposits**
     H18.021   **Argentous corneal deposits, right eye**
     H18.022   **Argentous corneal deposits, left eye**
     H18.023   **Argentous corneal deposits, bilateral**
     H18.029   **Argentous corneal deposits, unspecified eye**

√6th **H18.03 Corneal deposits in metabolic disorders**
       Code also associated metabolic disorder
     H18.031   **Corneal deposits in metabolic disorders, right eye**
     H18.032   **Corneal deposits in metabolic disorders, left eye**
     H18.033   **Corneal deposits in metabolic disorders, bilateral**
     H18.039   **Corneal deposits in metabolic disorders, unspecified eye**

√6th **H18.04 Kayser-Fleischer ring**
       Code also associated Wilson's disease (E83.01)
     H18.041   **Kayser-Fleischer ring, right eye**
     H18.042   **Kayser-Fleischer ring, left eye**
     H18.043   **Kayser-Fleischer ring, bilateral**
     H18.049   **Kayser-Fleischer ring, unspecified eye**

√6th **H18.05 Posterior corneal pigmentations**
       Krukenberg's spindle
     H18.051   **Posterior corneal pigmentations, right eye**
     H18.052   **Posterior corneal pigmentations, left eye**
     H18.053   **Posterior corneal pigmentations, bilateral**
     H18.059   **Posterior corneal pigmentations, unspecified eye**

√6th **H18.06 Stromal corneal pigmentations**
       Hematocornea
     H18.061   **Stromal corneal pigmentations, right eye**
     H18.062   **Stromal corneal pigmentations, left eye**
     H18.063   **Stromal corneal pigmentations, bilateral**
     H18.069   **Stromal corneal pigmentations, unspecified eye**

√5th **H18.1 Bullous keratopathy**
       **DEF:** Corneal swelling due to damaged corneal endothelium; characterized by recurring, rupturing epithelial "blisters"; occurs in glaucoma, iridocyclitis and Fuchs dystrophy.
     H18.10   **Bullous keratopathy, unspecified eye**
     H18.11   **Bullous keratopathy, right eye**
     H18.12   **Bullous keratopathy, left eye**
     H18.13   **Bullous keratopathy, bilateral**

√5th **H18.2 Other and unspecified corneal edema**
     H18.20   **Unspecified corneal edema**
   √6th **H18.21 Corneal edema secondary to contact lens**
       EXCLUDES 2   *other corneal disorders due to contact lens (H18.82-)*
     H18.211   **Corneal edema secondary to contact lens, right eye**
     H18.212   **Corneal edema secondary to contact lens, left eye**
     H18.213   **Corneal edema secondary to contact lens, bilateral**
     H18.219   **Corneal edema secondary to contact lens, unspecified eye**
   √6th **H18.22 Idiopathic corneal edema**
     H18.221   **Idiopathic corneal edema, right eye**
     H18.222   **Idiopathic corneal edema, left eye**
     H18.223   **Idiopathic corneal edema, bilateral**
     H18.229   **Idiopathic corneal edema, unspecified eye**
   √6th **H18.23 Secondary corneal edema**
     H18.231   **Secondary corneal edema, right eye**
     H18.232   **Secondary corneal edema, left eye**
     H18.233   **Secondary corneal edema, bilateral**
     H18.239   **Secondary corneal edema, unspecified eye**

√5th **H18.3 Changes of corneal membranes**
     H18.30   **Unspecified corneal membrane change**
   √6th **H18.31 Folds and rupture in Bowman's membrane**
     H18.311   **Folds and rupture in Bowman's membrane, right eye**
     H18.312   **Folds and rupture in Bowman's membrane, left eye**
     H18.313   **Folds and rupture in Bowman's membrane, bilateral**
     H18.319   **Folds and rupture in Bowman's membrane, unspecified eye**
   √6th **H18.32 Folds in Descemet's membrane**
     H18.321   **Folds in Descemet's membrane, right eye**
     H18.322   **Folds in Descemet's membrane, left eye**

✔ Additional Character Req    √x7th Placeholder Alert    Unacceptable PDx    Manifestation    **H1**-**H14** HAC    **HCC** CMS-HCC Condition    *EXCLUDES 1* Not Coded Here    *EXCLUDES 2* Not Included Here

ICD-10-CM 2018        **589**

**Chapter 7. Diseases of the Eye and Adnexa**

H18.323    **Folds in Descemet's membrane,** bilateral
H18.329    **Folds in Descemet's membrane,** unspecified eye

√6ᵗʰ   **H18.33**   Rupture in Descemet's membrane
H18.331    **Rupture in Descemet's membrane,** right eye
H18.332    **Rupture in Descemet's membrane,** left eye
H18.333    **Rupture in Descemet's membrane,** bilateral
H18.339    **Rupture in Descemet's membrane,** unspecified eye

√5ᵗʰ   **H18.4**   Corneal degeneration
    *EXCLUDES 1*   Mooren's ulcer (H16.0-)
                 recurrent erosion of cornea (H18.83-)
H18.40    Unspecified **corneal degeneration**

√6ᵗʰ   **H18.41**   Arcus senilis
       Senile corneal changes
H18.411    **Arcus senilis,** right eye
H18.412    **Arcus senilis,** left eye
H18.413    **Arcus senilis,** bilateral
H18.419    **Arcus senilis,** unspecified eye

√6ᵗʰ   **H18.42**   Band keratopathy
H18.421    **Band keratopathy,** right eye
H18.422    **Band keratopathy,** left eye
H18.423    **Band keratopathy,** bilateral
H18.429    **Band keratopathy,** unspecified eye

H18.43    Other **calcerous corneal degeneration**

√6ᵗʰ   **H18.44**   Keratomalacia
    *EXCLUDES 1*   keratomalacia due to vitamin A deficiency (E50.4)
H18.441    **Keratomalacia,** right eye
H18.442    **Keratomalacia,** left eye
H18.443    **Keratomalacia,** bilateral
H18.449    **Keratomalacia,** unspecified eye

√6ᵗʰ   **H18.45**   Nodular corneal degeneration
H18.451    **Nodular corneal degeneration,** right eye
H18.452    **Nodular corneal degeneration,** left eye
H18.453    **Nodular corneal degeneration,** bilateral
H18.459    **Nodular corneal degeneration,** unspecified eye

√6ᵗʰ   **H18.46**   Peripheral corneal degeneration
H18.461    **Peripheral corneal degeneration,** right eye
H18.462    **Peripheral corneal degeneration,** left eye
H18.463    **Peripheral corneal degeneration,** bilateral
H18.469    **Peripheral corneal degeneration,** unspecified eye

H18.49    Other **corneal degeneration**

√5ᵗʰ   **H18.5**   Hereditary corneal dystrophies
H18.50    Unspecified **hereditary corneal dystrophies**
H18.51    Endothelial **corneal dystrophy**
       Fuchs' dystrophy
H18.52    Epithelial **(juvenile) corneal dystrophy**
H18.53    Granular **corneal dystrophy**
H18.54    Lattice **corneal dystrophy**
H18.55    Macular **corneal dystrophy**
H18.59    Other **hereditary corneal dystrophies**

√5ᵗʰ   **H18.6**   Keratoconus

√6ᵗʰ   **H18.60**   Keratoconus, unspecified
H18.601    **Keratoconus, unspecified,** right eye
H18.602    **Keratoconus, unspecified,** left eye
H18.603    **Keratoconus, unspecified,** bilateral
H18.609    **Keratoconus, unspecified,** unspecified eye

√6ᵗʰ   **H18.61**   Keratoconus, stable
H18.611    **Keratoconus, stable,** right eye
H18.612    **Keratoconus, stable,** left eye
H18.613    **Keratoconus, stable,** bilateral
H18.619    **Keratoconus, stable,** unspecified eye

√6ᵗʰ   **H18.62**   Keratoconus, unstable
       Acute hydrops
H18.621    **Keratoconus, unstable,** right eye
H18.622    **Keratoconus, unstable,** left eye
H18.623    **Keratoconus, unstable,** bilateral
H18.629    **Keratoconus, unstable,** unspecified eye

√5ᵗʰ   **H18.7**   Other and unspecified corneal deformities
    *EXCLUDES 1*   congenital malformations of cornea (Q13.3-Q13.4)
H18.70    Unspecified **corneal deformity**

√6ᵗʰ   **H18.71**   Corneal ectasia
H18.711    **Corneal ectasia,** right eye
H18.712    **Corneal ectasia,** left eye
H18.713    **Corneal ectasia,** bilateral
H18.719    **Corneal ectasia,** unspecified eye

√6ᵗʰ   **H18.72**   Corneal staphyloma
H18.721    **Corneal staphyloma,** right eye
H18.722    **Corneal staphyloma,** left eye
H18.723    **Corneal staphyloma,** bilateral
H18.729    **Corneal staphyloma,** unspecified eye

√6ᵗʰ   **H18.73**   Descemetocele
H18.731    **Descemetocele,** right eye
H18.732    **Descemetocele,** left eye
H18.733    **Descemetocele,** bilateral
H18.739    **Descemetocele,** unspecified eye

√6ᵗʰ   **H18.79**   Other corneal deformities
H18.791    **Other corneal deformities,** right eye
H18.792    **Other corneal deformities,** left eye
H18.793    **Other corneal deformities,** bilateral
H18.799    **Other corneal deformities,** unspecified eye

√5ᵗʰ   **H18.8**   Other specified disorders of cornea

√6ᵗʰ   **H18.81**   Anesthesia and hypoesthesia of cornea
H18.811    **Anesthesia and hypoesthesia of cornea,** right eye
H18.812    **Anesthesia and hypoesthesia of cornea,** left eye
H18.813    **Anesthesia and hypoesthesia of cornea,** bilateral
H18.819    **Anesthesia and hypoesthesia of cornea,** unspecified eye

√6ᵗʰ   **H18.82**   Corneal disorder due to contact lens
    *EXCLUDES 2*   corneal edema due to contact lens (H18.21-)
H18.821    **Corneal disorder due to contact lens,** right eye
H18.822    **Corneal disorder due to contact lens,** left eye
H18.823    **Corneal disorder due to contact lens,** bilateral
H18.829    **Corneal disorder due to contact lens,** unspecified eye

√6ᵗʰ   **H18.83**   Recurrent erosion of cornea
H18.831    **Recurrent erosion of cornea,** right eye
H18.832    **Recurrent erosion of cornea,** left eye
H18.833    **Recurrent erosion of cornea,** bilateral
H18.839    **Recurrent erosion of cornea,** unspecified eye

√6ᵗʰ   **H18.89**   Other specified disorders of cornea
H18.891    **Other specified disorders of cornea,** right eye
H18.892    **Other specified disorders of cornea,** left eye
H18.893    **Other specified disorders of cornea,** bilateral
H18.899    **Other specified disorders of cornea,** unspecified eye

**H18.9 Unspecified disorder of cornea**

✓4ᵗʰ **H20** **Iridocyclitis**

**CC Excl: For CC codes in category H20:** PDX collection 624

✓5ᵗʰ **H20.0** **Acute and subacute iridocyclitis**
　　　Acute anterior uveitis
　　　Acute cyclitis
　　　Acute iritis
　　　Subacute anterior uveitis
　　　Subacute cyclitis
　　　Subacute iritis
　　　*EXCLUDES 1*　 *iridocyclitis, iritis, uveitis (due to) (in) diabetes mellitus (E08-E13 with .39)*
　　　　　*iridocyclitis, iritis, uveitis (due to) (in) diphtheria (A36.89)*
　　　　　*iridocyclitis, iritis, uveitis (due to) (in) gonococcal (A54.32)*
　　　　　*iridocyclitis, iritis, uveitis (due to) (in) herpes (simplex) (B00.51)*
　　　　　*iridocyclitis, iritis, uveitis (due to) (in) herpes zoster (B02.32)*
　　　　　*iridocyclitis, iritis, uveitis (due to) (in) late congenital syphilis (A50.39)*
　　　　　*iridocyclitis, iritis, uveitis (due to) (in) late syphilis (A52.71)*
　　　　　*iridocyclitis, iritis, uveitis (due to) (in) sarcoidosis (D86.83)*
　　　　　*iridocyclitis, iritis, uveitis (due to) (in) syphilis (A51.43)*
　　　　　*iridocyclitis, iritis, uveitis (due to) (in) toxoplasmosis (B58.09)*
　　　　　*iridocyclitis, iritis, uveitis (due to) (in) tuberculosis (A18.54)*
　　　**H20.00**　**Unspecified acute and subacute iridocyclitis**　CC
✓6ᵗʰ **H20.01**　**Primary iridocyclitis**
　　　**H20.011**　**Primary iridocyclitis, right eye**　CC
　　　**H20.012**　**Primary iridocyclitis, left eye**　CC
　　　**H20.013**　**Primary iridocyclitis, bilateral**　CC
　　　**H20.019**　**Primary iridocyclitis, unspecified eye**　CC
✓6ᵗʰ **H20.02**　**Recurrent acute iridocyclitis**
　　　**H20.021**　**Recurrent acute iridocyclitis, right eye**　CC
　　　**H20.022**　**Recurrent acute iridocyclitis, left eye**　CC
　　　**H20.023**　**Recurrent acute iridocyclitis, bilateral**　CC
　　　**H20.029**　**Recurrent acute iridocyclitis, unspecified eye**　CC
✓6ᵗʰ **H20.03**　**Secondary infectious iridocyclitis**
　　　**H20.031**　**Secondary infectious iridocyclitis, right eye**　CC
　　　**H20.032**　**Secondary infectious iridocyclitis, left eye**　CC
　　　**H20.033**　**Secondary infectious iridocyclitis, bilateral**　CC
　　　**H20.039**　**Secondary infectious iridocyclitis, unspecified eye**　CC
✓6ᵗʰ **H20.04**　**Secondary noninfectious iridocyclitis**
　　　**H20.041**　**Secondary noninfectious iridocyclitis, right eye**
　　　**H20.042**　**Secondary noninfectious iridocyclitis, left eye**
　　　**H20.043**　**Secondary noninfectious iridocyclitis, bilateral**
　　　**H20.049**　**Secondary noninfectious iridocyclitis, unspecified eye**
✓6ᵗʰ **H20.05**　**Hypopyon**
　　　**H20.051**　**Hypopyon, right eye**
　　　**H20.052**　**Hypopyon, left eye**
　　　**H20.053**　**Hypopyon, bilateral**
　　　**H20.059**　**Hypopyon, unspecified eye**
✓5ᵗʰ **H20.1** **Chronic iridocyclitis**
　　　Use additional code for any associated cataract (H26.21-)
　　　*EXCLUDES 2*　 *posterior cyclitis (H30.2-)*
　　　**H20.10**　**Chronic iridocyclitis, unspecified eye**
　　　**H20.11**　**Chronic iridocyclitis, right eye**
　　　**H20.12**　**Chronic iridocyclitis, left eye**
　　　**H20.13**　**Chronic iridocyclitis, bilateral**
✓5ᵗʰ **H20.2** **Lens-induced iridocyclitis**
　　　**H20.20**　**Lens-induced iridocyclitis, unspecified eye**
　　　**H20.21**　**Lens-induced iridocyclitis, right eye**
　　　**H20.22**　**Lens-induced iridocyclitis, left eye**
　　　**H20.23**　**Lens-induced iridocyclitis, bilateral**

**Hyphema**

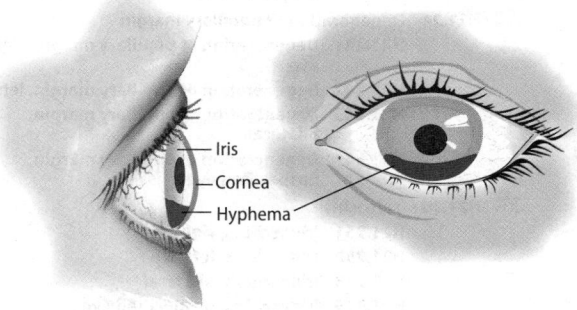

Iris
Cornea
Hyphema

✓5ᵗʰ **H20.8** **Other iridocyclitis**
　　　*EXCLUDES 2*　 *glaucomatocyclitis crises (H40.4-)*
　　　　　*posterior cyclitis (H30.2-)*
　　　　　*sympathetic uveitis (H44.13-)*
✓6ᵗʰ **H20.81**　**Fuchs' heterochromic cyclitis**
　　　**H20.811**　**Fuchs' heterochromic cyclitis, right eye**
　　　**H20.812**　**Fuchs' heterochromic cyclitis, left eye**
　　　**H20.813**　**Fuchs' heterochromic cyclitis, bilateral**
　　　**H20.819**　**Fuchs' heterochromic cyclitis, unspecified eye**
✓6ᵗʰ **H20.82**　**Vogt-Koyanagi syndrome**
　　　**H20.821**　**Vogt-Koyanagi syndrome, right eye**
　　　**H20.822**　**Vogt-Koyanagi syndrome, left eye**
　　　**H20.823**　**Vogt-Koyanagi syndrome, bilateral**
　　　**H20.829**　**Vogt-Koyanagi syndrome, unspecified eye**
**H20.9** **Unspecified iridocyclitis**　CC
　　　Uveitis NOS

✓4ᵗʰ **H21** **Other disorders of iris and ciliary body**
　　　*EXCLUDES 2*　 *sympathetic uveitis (H44.1-)*
✓5ᵗʰ **H21.0** **Hyphema**
　　　*EXCLUDES 1*　 *traumatic hyphema (S05.1-)*
　　　**H21.00**　**Hyphema, unspecified eye**
　　　**H21.01**　**Hyphema, right eye**
　　　**H21.02**　**Hyphema, left eye**
　　　**H21.03**　**Hyphema, bilateral**
✓5ᵗʰ **H21.1** **Other vascular disorders of iris and ciliary body**
　　　Neovascularization of iris or ciliary body
　　　Rubeosis iridis
　　　Rubeosis of iris
✓6ᵗʰ **H21.1X**　**Other vascular disorders of iris and ciliary body**
　　　**H21.1X1**　**Other vascular disorders of iris and ciliary body, right eye**
　　　**H21.1X2**　**Other vascular disorders of iris and ciliary body, left eye**
　　　**H21.1X3**　**Other vascular disorders of iris and ciliary body, bilateral**
　　　**H21.1X9**　**Other vascular disorders of iris and ciliary body, unspecified eye**
✓5ᵗʰ **H21.2** **Degeneration of iris and ciliary body**
✓6ᵗʰ **H21.21**　**Degeneration of chamber angle**
　　　**H21.211**　**Degeneration of chamber angle, right eye**
　　　**H21.212**　**Degeneration of chamber angle, left eye**
　　　**H21.213**　**Degeneration of chamber angle, bilateral**
　　　**H21.219**　**Degeneration of chamber angle, unspecified eye**
✓6ᵗʰ **H21.22**　**Degeneration of ciliary body**
　　　**H21.221**　**Degeneration of ciliary body, right eye**
　　　**H21.222**　**Degeneration of ciliary body, left eye**
　　　**H21.223**　**Degeneration of ciliary body, bilateral**
　　　**H21.229**　**Degeneration of ciliary body, unspecified eye**
✓6ᵗʰ **H21.23**　**Degeneration of iris (pigmentary)**
　　　Translucency of iris
　　　**H21.231**　**Degeneration of iris (pigmentary), right eye**
　　　**H21.232**　**Degeneration of iris (pigmentary), left eye**
　　　**H21.233**　**Degeneration of iris (pigmentary), bilateral**

H21.239   **Degeneration of iris (pigmentary), unspecified eye**

✓6ᵗʰ   **H21.24**   **Degeneration of pupillary margin**

    H21.241   **Degeneration of pupillary margin, right eye**

    H21.242   **Degeneration of pupillary margin, left eye**

    H21.243   **Degeneration of pupillary margin, bilateral**

    H21.249   **Degeneration of pupillary margin, unspecified eye**

✓6ᵗʰ   **H21.25**   **Iridoschisis**

    H21.251   **Iridoschisis, right eye**

    H21.252   **Iridoschisis, left eye**

    H21.253   **Iridoschisis, bilateral**

    H21.259   **Iridoschisis, unspecified eye**

✓6ᵗʰ   **H21.26**   **Iris atrophy (essential) (progressive)**

    H21.261   **Iris atrophy (essential) (progressive), right eye**

    H21.262   **Iris atrophy (essential) (progressive), left eye**

    H21.263   **Iris atrophy (essential) (progressive), bilateral**

    H21.269   **Iris atrophy (essential) (progressive), unspecified eye**

✓6ᵗʰ   **H21.27**   **Miotic pupillary cyst**

    H21.271   **Miotic pupillary cyst, right eye**

    H21.272   **Miotic pupillary cyst, left eye**

    H21.273   **Miotic pupillary cyst, bilateral**

    H21.279   **Miotic pupillary cyst, unspecified eye**

    **H21.29**   **Other iris atrophy**

✓5ᵗʰ   **H21.3**   **Cyst of iris, ciliary body and anterior chamber**

    EXCLUDES 2   *miotic pupillary cyst (H21.27-)*

✓6ᵗʰ   **H21.30**   **Idiopathic cysts of iris, ciliary body or anterior chamber**

     Cyst of iris, ciliary body or anterior chamber NOS

    H21.301   **Idiopathic cysts of iris, ciliary body or anterior chamber, right eye**

    H21.302   **Idiopathic cysts of iris, ciliary body or anterior chamber, left eye**

    H21.303   **Idiopathic cysts of iris, ciliary body or anterior chamber, bilateral**

    H21.309   **Idiopathic cysts of iris, ciliary body or anterior chamber, unspecified eye**

✓6ᵗʰ   **H21.31**   **Exudative cysts of iris or anterior chamber**

    H21.311   **Exudative cysts of iris or anterior chamber, right eye**

    H21.312   **Exudative cysts of iris or anterior chamber, left eye**

    H21.313   **Exudative cysts of iris or anterior chamber, bilateral**

    H21.319   **Exudative cysts of iris or anterior chamber, unspecified eye**

✓6ᵗʰ   **H21.32**   **Implantation cysts of iris, ciliary body or anterior chamber**

    H21.321   **Implantation cysts of iris, ciliary body or anterior chamber, right eye**

    H21.322   **Implantation cysts of iris, ciliary body or anterior chamber, left eye**

    H21.323   **Implantation cysts of iris, ciliary body or anterior chamber, bilateral**

    H21.329   **Implantation cysts of iris, ciliary body or anterior chamber, unspecified eye**

✓6ᵗʰ   **H21.33**   **Parasitic cyst of iris, ciliary body or anterior chamber**

> **CC Excl:** For CC codes in subcategory H21.33: PDX collection 625

    H21.331   **Parasitic cyst of iris, ciliary body or anterior chamber, right eye**   `CC`

    H21.332   **Parasitic cyst of iris, ciliary body or anterior chamber, left eye**   `CC`

    H21.333   **Parasitic cyst of iris, ciliary body or anterior chamber, bilateral**   `CC`

    H21.339   **Parasitic cyst of iris, ciliary body or anterior chamber, unspecified eye**   `CC`

✓6ᵗʰ   **H21.34**   **Primary cyst of pars plana**

    H21.341   **Primary cyst of pars plana, right eye**

    H21.342   **Primary cyst of pars plana, left eye**

    H21.343   **Primary cyst of pars plana, bilateral**

    H21.349   **Primary cyst of pars plana, unspecified eye**

✓6ᵗʰ   **H21.35**   **Exudative cyst of pars plana**

     **DEF:** Protein, fatty-filled bullous elevation of nonpigmented outermost ciliary epithelium of pars plana; due to fluid leak from blood vessels.

    H21.351   **Exudative cyst of pars plana, right eye**

    H21.352   **Exudative cyst of pars plana, left eye**

    H21.353   **Exudative cyst of pars plana, bilateral**

    H21.359   **Exudative cyst of pars plana, unspecified eye**

✓5ᵗʰ   **H21.4**   **Pupillary membranes**

    Iris bombé      Pupillary seclusion

    Pupillary occlusion

    EXCLUDES 1   *congenital pupillary membranes (Q13.8)*

    **H21.40**   **Pupillary membranes, unspecified eye**

    **H21.41**   **Pupillary membranes, right eye**

    **H21.42**   **Pupillary membranes, left eye**

    **H21.43**   **Pupillary membranes, bilateral**

✓5ᵗʰ   **H21.5**   **Other and unspecified adhesions and disruptions of iris and ciliary body**

    EXCLUDES 1   *corectopia (Q13.2)*

✓6ᵗʰ   **H21.50**   **Unspecified adhesions of iris**

     Synechia (iris) NOS

    H21.501   **Unspecified adhesions of iris, right eye**

    H21.502   **Unspecified adhesions of iris, left eye**

    H21.503   **Unspecified adhesions of iris, bilateral**

    H21.509   **Unspecified adhesions of iris and ciliary body, unspecified eye**

✓6ᵗʰ   **H21.51**   **Anterior synechiae (iris)**

    H21.511   **Anterior synechiae (iris), right eye**

    H21.512   **Anterior synechiae (iris), left eye**

    H21.513   **Anterior synechiae (iris), bilateral**

    H21.519   **Anterior synechiae (iris), unspecified eye**

✓6ᵗʰ   **H21.52**   **Goniosynechiae**

    H21.521   **Goniosynechiae, right eye**

    H21.522   **Goniosynechiae, left eye**

    H21.523   **Goniosynechiae, bilateral**

    H21.529   **Goniosynechiae, unspecified eye**

✓6ᵗʰ   **H21.53**   **Iridodialysis**

    H21.531   **Iridodialysis, right eye**

    H21.532   **Iridodialysis, left eye**

    H21.533   **Iridodialysis, bilateral**

    H21.539   **Iridodialysis, unspecified eye**

✓6ᵗʰ   **H21.54**   **Posterior synechiae (iris)**

    H21.541   **Posterior synechiae (iris), right eye**

    H21.542   **Posterior synechiae (iris), left eye**

    H21.543   **Posterior synechiae (iris), bilateral**

    H21.549   **Posterior synechiae (iris), unspecified eye**

✓6ᵗʰ   **H21.55**   **Recession of chamber angle**

    H21.551   **Recession of chamber angle, right eye**

    H21.552   **Recession of chamber angle, left eye**

    H21.553   **Recession of chamber angle, bilateral**

    H21.559   **Recession of chamber angle, unspecified eye**

✓6ᵗʰ   **H21.56**   **Pupillary abnormalities**

    Deformed pupil      Rupture of sphincter, pupil

    Ectopic pupil

    EXCLUDES 1   *congenital deformity of pupil (Q13.2-)*

    H21.561   **Pupillary abnormality, right eye**

    H21.562   **Pupillary abnormality, left eye**

    H21.563   **Pupillary abnormality, bilateral**

    H21.569   **Pupillary abnormality, unspecified eye**

✓5ᵗʰ   **H21.8**   **Other specified disorders of iris and ciliary body**

    **H21.81**   **Floppy iris syndrome**

     Intraoperative floppy iris syndrome (IFIS)

     Use additional code for adverse effect, if applicable, to identify drug (T36-T50 with fifth or sixth character 5)

    **H21.82**   **Plateau iris syndrome (post-iridectomy) (postprocedural)**

**H21.89**   Other specified disorders of iris and ciliary body

**H21.9**   Unspecified disorder of iris and ciliary body

**H22**   *Disorders of iris and ciliary body in diseases classified elsewhere*

Code first underlying disease, such as:
gout (M1A.-, M10.-)
leprosy (A30.-)
parasitic disease (B89)

## Disorders of lens (H25-H28)

✓4ᵗʰ **H25**   **Age-related cataract**
Senile cataract
*EXCLUDES 2*   capsular glaucoma with pseudoexfoliation of lens (H40.1-)

  ✓5ᵗʰ **H25.0**   **Age-related incipient cataract**

    ✓6ᵗʰ **H25.01**   **Cortical age-related cataract**

       **H25.011**   **Cortical age-related cataract, right** eye   Ⓐ

       **H25.012**   **Cortical age-related cataract, left** eye   Ⓐ

       **H25.013**   **Cortical age-related cataract, bilateral**   Ⓐ

       **H25.019**   **Cortical age-related cataract, unspecified** eye   Ⓐ

    ✓6ᵗʰ **H25.03**   **Anterior subcapsular polar age-related cataract**

       **H25.031**   **Anterior subcapsular polar age-related cataract, right** eye   Ⓐ

       **H25.032**   **Anterior subcapsular polar age-related cataract, left** eye   Ⓐ

       **H25.033**   **Anterior subcapsular polar age-related cataract, bilateral**   Ⓐ

       **H25.039**   **Anterior subcapsular polar age-related cataract, unspecified** eye   Ⓐ

    ✓6ᵗʰ **H25.04**   **Posterior subcapsular polar age-related cataract**

       **H25.041**   **Posterior subcapsular polar age-related cataract, right** eye   Ⓐ

       **H25.042**   **Posterior subcapsular polar age-related cataract, left** eye   Ⓐ

       **H25.043**   **Posterior subcapsular polar age-related cataract, bilateral**   Ⓐ

       **H25.049**   **Posterior subcapsular polar age-related cataract, unspecified** eye   Ⓐ

    ✓6ᵗʰ **H25.09**   **Other age-related incipient cataract**
Coronary age-related cataract
Punctate age-related cataract
Water clefts

       **H25.091**   **Other age-related incipient cataract, right** eye   Ⓐ

       **H25.092**   **Other age-related incipient cataract, left** eye   Ⓐ

       **H25.093**   **Other age-related incipient cataract, bilateral**   Ⓐ

       **H25.099**   **Other age-related incipient cataract, unspecified** eye   Ⓐ

  ✓5ᵗʰ **H25.1**   **Age-related nuclear cataract**
Cataracta brunescens
Nuclear sclerosis cataract
**AHA:** 2016, 1Q, 32

     **H25.10**   **Age-related nuclear cataract, unspecified** eye   Ⓐ

     **H25.11**   **Age-related nuclear cataract, right** eye   Ⓐ

### Cataracts

Vitreous
Iris
Cornea
Retina
Pupil
Lens

Normal lens

Clouded lens

Lens affected by cataracts

---

     **H25.12**   **Age-related nuclear cataract, left** eye   Ⓐ

     **H25.13**   **Age-related nuclear cataract, bilateral**   Ⓐ

  ✓5ᵗʰ **H25.2**   **Age-related cataract, morgagnian type**
Age-related hypermature cataract

     **H25.20**   **Age-related cataract, morgagnian type, unspecified** eye   Ⓐ

     **H25.21**   **Age-related cataract, morgagnian type, right** eye   Ⓐ

     **H25.22**   **Age-related cataract, morgagnian type, left** eye   Ⓐ

     **H25.23**   **Age-related cataract, morgagnian type, bilateral**   Ⓐ

  ✓5ᵗʰ **H25.8**   **Other age-related cataract**

    ✓6ᵗʰ **H25.81**   **Combined forms of age-related cataract**

       **H25.811**   **Combined forms of age-related cataract, right** eye   Ⓐ

       **H25.812**   **Combined forms of age-related cataract, left** eye   Ⓐ

       **H25.813**   **Combined forms of age-related cataract, bilateral**   Ⓐ

       **H25.819**   **Combined forms of age-related cataract, unspecified** eye   Ⓐ

     **H25.89**   **Other age-related cataract**   Ⓐ

   **H25.9**   **Unspecified age-related cataract**   Ⓐ

✓4ᵗʰ **H26**   **Other cataract**
*EXCLUDES 1*   congenital cataract (Q12.0)

  ✓5ᵗʰ **H26.0**   **Infantile and juvenile cataract**

    ✓6ᵗʰ **H26.00**   **Unspecified infantile and juvenile cataract**

       **H26.001**   **Unspecified infantile and juvenile cataract, right** eye   Ⓟ

       **H26.002**   **Unspecified infantile and juvenile cataract, left** eye   Ⓟ

       **H26.003**   **Unspecified infantile and juvenile cataract, bilateral**   Ⓟ

       **H26.009**   **Unspecified infantile and juvenile cataract, unspecified** eye   Ⓟ

    ✓6ᵗʰ **H26.01**   **Infantile and juvenile cortical, lamellar, or zonular cataract**

       **H26.011**   **Infantile and juvenile cortical, lamellar, or zonular cataract, right** eye   Ⓟ

       **H26.012**   **Infantile and juvenile cortical, lamellar, or zonular cataract, left** eye   Ⓟ

       **H26.013**   **Infantile and juvenile cortical, lamellar, or zonular cataract, bilateral**   Ⓟ

       **H26.019**   **Infantile and juvenile cortical, lamellar, or zonular cataract, unspecified** eye   Ⓟ

    ✓6ᵗʰ **H26.03**   **Infantile and juvenile nuclear cataract**

       **H26.031**   **Infantile and juvenile nuclear cataract, right** eye   Ⓟ

       **H26.032**   **Infantile and juvenile nuclear cataract, left** eye   Ⓟ

       **H26.033**   **Infantile and juvenile nuclear cataract, bilateral**   Ⓟ

       **H26.039**   **Infantile and juvenile nuclear cataract, unspecified** eye   Ⓟ

    ✓6ᵗʰ **H26.04**   **Anterior subcapsular polar infantile and juvenile cataract**

       **H26.041**   **Anterior subcapsular polar infantile and juvenile cataract, right** eye   Ⓟ

       **H26.042**   **Anterior subcapsular polar infantile and juvenile cataract, left** eye   Ⓟ

       **H26.043**   **Anterior subcapsular polar infantile and juvenile cataract, bilateral**   Ⓟ

       **H26.049**   **Anterior subcapsular polar infantile and juvenile cataract, unspecified** eye   Ⓟ

    ✓6ᵗʰ **H26.05**   **Posterior subcapsular polar infantile and juvenile cataract**

       **H26.051**   **Posterior subcapsular polar infantile and juvenile cataract, right** eye   Ⓟ

       **H26.052**   **Posterior subcapsular polar infantile and juvenile cataract, left** eye   Ⓟ

       **H26.053**   **Posterior subcapsular polar infantile and juvenile cataract, bilateral**   Ⓟ

       **H26.059**   **Posterior subcapsular polar infantile and juvenile cataract, unspecified** eye   Ⓟ

    ✓6ᵗʰ **H26.06**   **Combined forms of infantile and juvenile cataract**

       **H26.061**   **Combined forms of infantile and juvenile cataract, right** eye   Ⓟ

---

✓ Additional Character Req   ✓x7ᵗʰ Placeholder Alert   Unacceptable PDx   Manifestation   H1-H14 HAC   HCC CMS-HCC Condition   *EXCLUDES 1* Not Coded Here   *EXCLUDES 2* Not Included Here

ICD-10-CM 2018          **593**

     H26.062  **Combined forms of infantile and juvenile cataract, left eye** P

     H26.063  **Combined forms of infantile and juvenile cataract, bilateral** P

     H26.069  **Combined forms of infantile and juvenile cataract, unspecified eye** P

   H26.09  **Other infantile and juvenile cataract** P

✓5th **H26.1**  **Traumatic cataract**

     Use additional code (Chapter 20) to identify external cause

   ✓6th **H26.10**  **Unspecified traumatic cataract**

     H26.101  **Unspecified traumatic cataract, right eye**

     H26.102  **Unspecified traumatic cataract, left eye**

     H26.103  **Unspecified traumatic cataract, bilateral**

     H26.109  **Unspecified traumatic cataract, unspecified eye**

   ✓6th **H26.11**  **Localized traumatic opacities**

     H26.111  **Localized traumatic opacities, right eye**

     H26.112  **Localized traumatic opacities, left eye**

     H26.113  **Localized traumatic opacities, bilateral**

     H26.119  **Localized traumatic opacities, unspecified eye**

   ✓6th **H26.12**  **Partially resolved traumatic cataract**

     H26.121  **Partially resolved traumatic cataract, right eye**

     H26.122  **Partially resolved traumatic cataract, left eye**

     H26.123  **Partially resolved traumatic cataract, bilateral**

     H26.129  **Partially resolved traumatic cataract, unspecified eye**

   ✓6th **H26.13**  **Total traumatic cataract**

     H26.131  **Total traumatic cataract, right eye**

     H26.132  **Total traumatic cataract, left eye**

     H26.133  **Total traumatic cataract, bilateral**

     H26.139  **Total traumatic cataract, unspecified eye**

✓5th **H26.2**  **Complicated cataract**

   H26.20  **Unspecified complicated cataract**

     Cataracta complicata NOS

   ✓6th **H26.21**  **Cataract with neovascularization**

     Code also associated condition, such as: chronic iridocyclitis (H20.1-)

     H26.211  **Cataract with neovascularization, right eye**

     H26.212  **Cataract with neovascularization, left eye**

     H26.213  **Cataract with neovascularization, bilateral**

     H26.219  **Cataract with neovascularization, unspecified eye**

   ✓6th **H26.22**  **Cataract secondary to ocular disorders (degenerative) (inflammatory)**

     Code also associated ocular disorder

     H26.221  **Cataract secondary to ocular disorders (degenerative) (inflammatory), right eye**

     H26.222  **Cataract secondary to ocular disorders (degenerative) (inflammatory), left eye**

     H26.223  **Cataract secondary to ocular disorders (degenerative) (inflammatory), bilateral**

     H26.229  **Cataract secondary to ocular disorders (degenerative) (inflammatory), unspecified eye**

   ✓6th **H26.23**  **Glaucomatous flecks (subcapsular)**

     Code first underlying glaucoma (H40-H42)

     H26.231  **Glaucomatous flecks (subcapsular), right eye**

     H26.232  **Glaucomatous flecks (subcapsular), left eye**

     H26.233  **Glaucomatous flecks (subcapsular), bilateral**

     H26.239  **Glaucomatous flecks (subcapsular), unspecified eye**

✓5th **H26.3**  **Drug-induced cataract**

     Toxic cataract

     Use additional code for adverse effect, if applicable, to identify drug (T36-T50 with fifth or sixth character 5)

   H26.30  **Drug-induced cataract, unspecified eye**

   H26.31  **Drug-induced cataract, right eye**

   H26.32  **Drug-induced cataract, left eye**

   H26.33  **Drug-induced cataract, bilateral**

✓5th **H26.4**  **Secondary cataract**

   H26.40  **Unspecified secondary cataract**

   ✓6th **H26.41**  **Soemmering's ring**

     H26.411  **Soemmering's ring, right eye**

     H26.412  **Soemmering's ring, left eye**

     H26.413  **Soemmering's ring, bilateral**

     H26.419  **Soemmering's ring, unspecified eye**

   ✓6th **H26.49**  **Other secondary cataract**

     H26.491  **Other secondary cataract, right eye**

     H26.492  **Other secondary cataract, left eye**

     H26.493  **Other secondary cataract, bilateral**

     H26.499  **Other secondary cataract, unspecified eye**

   H26.8  **Other specified cataract**

   H26.9  **Unspecified cataract**

✓4th **H27**  **Other disorders of lens**

     **EXCLUDES 1**  *congenital lens malformations (Q12.-)*
         *mechanical complications of intraocular lens implant (T85.2)*
         *pseudophakia (Z96.1)*

   ✓5th **H27.0**  **Aphakia**

     Acquired absence of lens
     Acquired aphakia
     Aphakia due to trauma

     **EXCLUDES 1**  *cataract extraction status (Z98.4-)*
         *congenital absence of lens (Q12.3)*
         *congenital aphakia (Q12.3)*

     H27.00  **Aphakia, unspecified eye**

     H27.01  **Aphakia, right eye**

     H27.02  **Aphakia, left eye**

     H27.03  **Aphakia, bilateral**

   ✓5th **H27.1**  **Dislocation of lens**

     H27.10  **Unspecified dislocation of lens**

     ✓6th **H27.11**  **Subluxation of lens**

       H27.111  **Subluxation of lens, right eye**

       H27.112  **Subluxation of lens, left eye**

       H27.113  **Subluxation of lens, bilateral**

       H27.119  **Subluxation of lens, unspecified eye**

     ✓6th **H27.12**  **Anterior dislocation of lens**

       H27.121  **Anterior dislocation of lens, right eye**

       H27.122  **Anterior dislocation of lens, left eye**

       H27.123  **Anterior dislocation of lens, bilateral**

       H27.129  **Anterior dislocation of lens, unspecified eye**

     ✓6th **H27.13**  **Posterior dislocation of lens**

       H27.131  **Posterior dislocation of lens, right eye**

       H27.132  **Posterior dislocation of lens, left eye**

       H27.133  **Posterior dislocation of lens, bilateral**

       H27.139  **Posterior dislocation of lens, unspecified eye**

   H27.8  **Other specified disorders of lens**

   H27.9  **Unspecified disorder of lens**

**H28**  *Cataract in diseases classified elsewhere*

     Code first underlying disease, such as:
       hypoparathyroidism (E20.-)
       myotonia (G71.1-)
       myxedema (E03.-)
       protein-calorie malnutrition (E40-E46)

     **EXCLUDES 1**  *cataract in diabetes mellitus (E08.36, E09.36, E10.36, E11.36, E13.36)*

N Newborn: 0    P Pediatric: 0-17    M Maternity: 12-55    A Adult: 15-124    MCC Major CC Condition    PDx MCC PDx acts as own MCC    CC CC Condition    PDx CC PDx acts as own CC

594      ICD-10-CM 2018

### Disorders of choroid and retina (H30-H36)

✓4ᵗʰ **H30**  **Chorioretinal inflammation**

> **CC Excl: For CC codes in category H30:** PDX collection 626

✓5ᵗʰ **H30.0**  **Focal chorioretinal inflammation**
Focal chorioretinitis
Focal choroiditis
Focal retinitis
Focal retinochoroiditis

  ✓6ᵗʰ **H30.00**  **Unspecified** **focal chorioretinal inflammation**
Focal chorioretinitis NOS
Focal choroiditis NOS
Focal retinitis NOS
Focal retinochoroiditis NOS

    **H30.001**  **Unspecified focal chorioretinal inflammation, right eye**
    **H30.002**  **Unspecified focal chorioretinal inflammation, left eye**
    **H30.003**  **Unspecified focal chorioretinal inflammation, bilateral**
    **H30.009**  **Unspecified focal chorioretinal inflammation, unspecified eye**

  ✓6ᵗʰ **H30.01**  **Focal chorioretinal inflammation, juxtapapillary**
    **H30.011**  **Focal chorioretinal inflammation, juxtapapillary, right eye**
    **H30.012**  **Focal chorioretinal inflammation, juxtapapillary, left eye**
    **H30.013**  **Focal chorioretinal inflammation, juxtapapillary, bilateral**
    **H30.019**  **Focal chorioretinal inflammation, juxtapapillary, unspecified eye**

  ✓6ᵗʰ **H30.02**  **Focal chorioretinal inflammation of posterior pole**
    **H30.021**  **Focal chorioretinal inflammation of posterior pole, right eye**
    **H30.022**  **Focal chorioretinal inflammation of posterior pole, left eye**
    **H30.023**  **Focal chorioretinal inflammation of posterior pole, bilateral**
    **H30.029**  **Focal chorioretinal inflammation of posterior pole, unspecified eye**

  ✓6ᵗʰ **H30.03**  **Focal chorioretinal inflammation, peripheral**
    **H30.031**  **Focal chorioretinal inflammation, peripheral, right eye**
    **H30.032**  **Focal chorioretinal inflammation, peripheral, left eye**
    **H30.033**  **Focal chorioretinal inflammation, peripheral, bilateral**
    **H30.039**  **Focal chorioretinal inflammation, peripheral, unspecified eye**

  ✓6ᵗʰ **H30.04**  **Focal chorioretinal inflammation, macular or paramacular**
    **H30.041**  **Focal chorioretinal inflammation, macular or paramacular, right eye**
    **H30.042**  **Focal chorioretinal inflammation, macular or paramacular, left eye**
    **H30.043**  **Focal chorioretinal inflammation, macular or paramacular, bilateral**
    **H30.049**  **Focal chorioretinal inflammation, macular or paramacular, unspecified eye**

✓5ᵗʰ **H30.1**  **Disseminated chorioretinal inflammation**
Disseminated chorioretinitis
Disseminated choroiditis
Disseminated retinitis
Disseminated retinochoroiditis
> *EXCLUDES 2*  *exudative retinopathy (H35.02-)*

  ✓6ᵗʰ **H30.10**  **Unspecified disseminated chorioretinal inflammation**
Disseminated chorioretinitis NOS
Disseminated choroiditis NOS
Disseminated retinitis NOS
Disseminated retinochoroiditis NOS
    **H30.101**  **Unspecified disseminated chorioretinal inflammation, right eye** CC
    **H30.102**  **Unspecified disseminated chorioretinal inflammation, left eye** CC
    **H30.103**  **Unspecified disseminated chorioretinal inflammation, bilateral** CC
    **H30.109**  **Unspecified disseminated chorioretinal inflammation, unspecified eye** CC

  ✓6ᵗʰ **H30.11**  **Disseminated chorioretinal inflammation of posterior pole**
    **H30.111**  **Disseminated chorioretinal inflammation of posterior pole, right eye** CC
    **H30.112**  **Disseminated chorioretinal inflammation of posterior pole, left eye** CC
    **H30.113**  **Disseminated chorioretinal inflammation of posterior pole, bilateral** CC
    **H30.119**  **Disseminated chorioretinal inflammation of posterior pole, unspecified eye** CC

  ✓6ᵗʰ **H30.12**  **Disseminated chorioretinal inflammation, peripheral**
    **H30.121**  **Disseminated chorioretinal inflammation, peripheral right eye** CC
    **H30.122**  **Disseminated chorioretinal inflammation, peripheral, left eye** CC
    **H30.123**  **Disseminated chorioretinal inflammation, peripheral, bilateral** CC
    **H30.129**  **Disseminated chorioretinal inflammation, peripheral, unspecified eye** CC

  ✓6ᵗʰ **H30.13**  **Disseminated chorioretinal inflammation, generalized**
    **H30.131**  **Disseminated chorioretinal inflammation, generalized, right eye** CC
    **H30.132**  **Disseminated chorioretinal inflammation, generalized, left eye** CC
    **H30.133**  **Disseminated chorioretinal inflammation, generalized, bilateral** CC
    **H30.139**  **Disseminated chorioretinal inflammation, generalized, unspecified eye** CC

  ✓6ᵗʰ **H30.14**  **Acute posterior multifocal placoid pigment epitheliopathy**
    **H30.141**  **Acute posterior multifocal placoid pigment epitheliopathy, right eye** CC
    **H30.142**  **Acute posterior multifocal placoid pigment epitheliopathy, left eye** CC
    **H30.143**  **Acute posterior multifocal placoid pigment epitheliopathy, bilateral** CC
    **H30.149**  **Acute posterior multifocal placoid pigment epitheliopathy, unspecified eye** CC

✓5ᵗʰ **H30.2**  **Posterior cyclitis**
Pars planitis
    **H30.20**  **Posterior cyclitis, unspecified eye**
    **H30.21**  **Posterior cyclitis, right eye**
    **H30.22**  **Posterior cyclitis, left eye**
    **H30.23**  **Posterior cyclitis, bilateral**

✓5ᵗʰ **H30.8**  **Other chorioretinal inflammations**
  ✓6ᵗʰ **H30.81**  **Harada's disease**
    **H30.811**  **Harada's disease, right eye**
    **H30.812**  **Harada's disease, left eye**
    **H30.813**  **Harada's disease, bilateral**
    **H30.819**  **Harada's disease, unspecified eye**

  ✓6ᵗʰ **H30.89**  **Other chorioretinal inflammations**
    **H30.891**  **Other chorioretinal inflammations, right eye** CC
    **H30.892**  **Other chorioretinal inflammations, left eye** CC
    **H30.893**  **Other chorioretinal inflammations, bilateral** CC
    **H30.899**  **Other chorioretinal inflammations, unspecified eye** CC

✓5ᵗʰ **H30.9**  **Unspecified chorioretinal inflammation**
Chorioretinitis NOS
Choroiditis NOS
Neuroretinitis NOS
Retinitis NOS
Retinochoroiditis NOS
    **H30.90**  **Unspecified chorioretinal inflammation, unspecified eye** CC

---

✓ Additional Character Req   ✓x7ᵗʰ Placeholder Alert   Unacceptable PDx   Manifestation   **H1 - H14** HAC   **HCC** CMS-HCC Condition   *EXCLUDES 1* Not Coded Here   *EXCLUDES 2* Not Included Here

**Chapter 7. Diseases of the Eye and Adnexa**

     **H30.91**    Unspecified chorioretinal inflammation, right eye    `CC`

     **H30.92**    Unspecified chorioretinal inflammation, left eye    `CC`

     **H30.93**    Unspecified chorioretinal inflammation, bilateral    `CC`

✓4ᵗʰ **H31**    **Other disorders of choroid**

     **CC Excl: For CC codes in category H31:** PDX collection 627

   ✓5ᵗʰ **H31.0**    **Chorioretinal** scars

       *EXCLUDES 2*    *postsurgical chorioretinal scars (H59.81-)*

     ✓6ᵗʰ **H31.00**    **Unspecified chorioretinal scars**

        **H31.001**    Unspecified chorioretinal scars, right eye

        **H31.002**    Unspecified chorioretinal scars, left eye

        **H31.003**    Unspecified chorioretinal scars, bilateral

        **H31.009**    Unspecified chorioretinal scars, unspecified eye

     ✓6ᵗʰ **H31.01**    **Macula scars of posterior pole (postinflammatory) (post-traumatic)**

        *EXCLUDES 1*    *postprocedural chorioretinal scar (H59.81-)*

        **H31.011**    Macula scars of posterior pole (postinflammatory) (post-traumatic), right eye

        **H31.012**    Macula scars of posterior pole (postinflammatory) (post-traumatic), left eye

        **H31.013**    Macula scars of posterior pole (postinflammatory) (post-traumatic), bilateral

        **H31.019**    Macula scars of posterior pole (postinflammatory) (post-traumatic), unspecified eye

     ✓6ᵗʰ **H31.02**    **Solar retinopathy**

        **H31.021**    Solar retinopathy, right eye

        **H31.022**    Solar retinopathy, left eye

        **H31.023**    Solar retinopathy, bilateral

        **H31.029**    Solar retinopathy, unspecified eye

     ✓6ᵗʰ **H31.09**    **Other chorioretinal scars**

        **H31.091**    Other chorioretinal scars, right eye

        **H31.092**    Other chorioretinal scars, left eye

        **H31.093**    Other chorioretinal scars, bilateral

        **H31.099**    Other chorioretinal scars, unspecified eye

   ✓5ᵗʰ **H31.1**    **Choroidal** degeneration

       *EXCLUDES 2*    *angioid streaks of macula (H35.33)*

     ✓6ᵗʰ **H31.10**    **Unspecified choroidal degeneration**
        Choroidal sclerosis NOS

        **H31.101**    Choroidal degeneration, unspecified, right eye

        **H31.102**    Choroidal degeneration, unspecified, left eye

        **H31.103**    Choroidal degeneration, unspecified, bilateral

        **H31.109**    Choroidal degeneration, unspecified, unspecified eye

     ✓6ᵗʰ **H31.11**    **Age-related** choroidal atrophy

        **H31.111**    Age-related choroidal atrophy, right eye    `A`

        **H31.112**    Age-related choroidal atrophy, left eye    `A`

        **H31.113**    Age-related choroidal atrophy, bilateral    `A`

        **H31.119**    Age-related choroidal atrophy, unspecified eye

     ✓6ᵗʰ **H31.12**    **Diffuse secondary** atrophy of choroid

        **H31.121**    Diffuse secondary atrophy of choroid, right eye

        **H31.122**    Diffuse secondary atrophy of choroid, left eye

        **H31.123**    Diffuse secondary atrophy of choroid, bilateral

        **H31.129**    Diffuse secondary atrophy of choroid, unspecified eye

   ✓5ᵗʰ **H31.2**    **Hereditary choroidal dystrophy**

       *EXCLUDES 2*    *hyperornithinemia (E72.4)*
                        *ornithinemia (E72.4)*

     **H31.20**    **Hereditary choroidal dystrophy, unspecified**

     **H31.21**    **Choroideremia**

     **H31.22**    **Choroidal dystrophy (central areolar) (generalized) (peripapillary)**

     **H31.23**    **Gyrate atrophy, choroid**

     **H31.29**    **Other hereditary choroidal dystrophy**

   ✓5ᵗʰ **H31.3**    **Choroidal** hemorrhage and rupture

     ✓6ᵗʰ **H31.30**    **Unspecified** choroidal hemorrhage

        **H31.301**    Unspecified choroidal hemorrhage, right eye

        **H31.302**    Unspecified choroidal hemorrhage, left eye

        **H31.303**    Unspecified choroidal hemorrhage, bilateral

        **H31.309**    Unspecified choroidal hemorrhage, unspecified eye

     ✓6ᵗʰ **H31.31**    **Expulsive** choroidal hemorrhage

        **H31.311**    Expulsive choroidal hemorrhage, right eye

        **H31.312**    Expulsive choroidal hemorrhage, left eye

        **H31.313**    Expulsive choroidal hemorrhage, bilateral

        **H31.319**    Expulsive choroidal hemorrhage, unspecified eye

     ✓6ᵗʰ **H31.32**    **Choroidal** rupture

        **H31.321**    Choroidal rupture, right eye    `CC`

        **H31.322**    Choroidal rupture, left eye    `CC`

        **H31.323**    Choroidal rupture, bilateral    `CC`

        **H31.329**    Choroidal rupture, unspecified eye    `CC`

   ✓5ᵗʰ **H31.4**    **Choroidal** detachment

     ✓6ᵗʰ **H31.40**    **Unspecified** choroidal detachment

        **H31.401**    Unspecified choroidal detachment, right eye    `CC`

        **H31.402**    Unspecified choroidal detachment, left eye    `CC`

        **H31.403**    Unspecified choroidal detachment, bilateral    `CC`

        **H31.409**    Unspecified choroidal detachment, unspecified eye    `CC`

     ✓6ᵗʰ **H31.41**    **Hemorrhagic** choroidal detachment

        **H31.411**    Hemorrhagic choroidal detachment, right eye    `CC`

        **H31.412**    Hemorrhagic choroidal detachment, left eye    `CC`

        **H31.413**    Hemorrhagic choroidal detachment, bilateral    `CC`

        **H31.419**    Hemorrhagic choroidal detachment, unspecified eye    `CC`

     ✓6ᵗʰ **H31.42**    **Serous** choroidal detachment

        **H31.421**    Serous choroidal detachment, right eye    `CC`

        **H31.422**    Serous choroidal detachment, left eye    `CC`

        **H31.423**    Serous choroidal detachment, bilateral    `CC`

        **H31.429**    Serous choroidal detachment, unspecified eye    `CC`

     **H31.8**    **Other specified disorders of choroid**

     **H31.9**    **Unspecified disorder of choroid**

**H32**    *Chorioretinal disorders in diseases classified elsewhere*

     Code first underlying disease, such as:
       congenital toxoplasmosis (P37.1)
       histoplasmosis (B39.-)
       leprosy (A30.-)

     *EXCLUDES 1*    *chorioretinitis (in):*
                  *toxoplasmosis (acquired) (B58.01)*
                  *tuberculosis (A18.53)*

✓4ᵗʰ **H33**    **Retinal detachments and breaks**

     *EXCLUDES 1*    *detachment of retinal pigment epithelium (H35.72-, H35.73-)*

     **CC Excl: For CC codes in category H33, unless otherwise noted:** PDX collection 628

   ✓5ᵗʰ **H33.0**    **Retinal detachment** with retinal break
       Rhegmatogenous retinal detachment

       *EXCLUDES 1*    *serous retinal detachment (without retinal break) (H33.2-)*

     ✓6ᵗʰ **H33.00**    **Unspecified** retinal detachment with retinal break

        **H33.001**    Unspecified retinal detachment with retinal break, right eye

`N` Newborn: 0    `P` Pediatric: 0-17    `M` Maternity: 12-55    `A` Adult: 15-124    `MCC` Major CC Condition    `PDx MCC` PDx acts as own MCC    `CC` CC Condition    `PDx CC` PDx acts as own CC

**596**                                                   ICD-10-CM 2018

**Retinal Detachment**

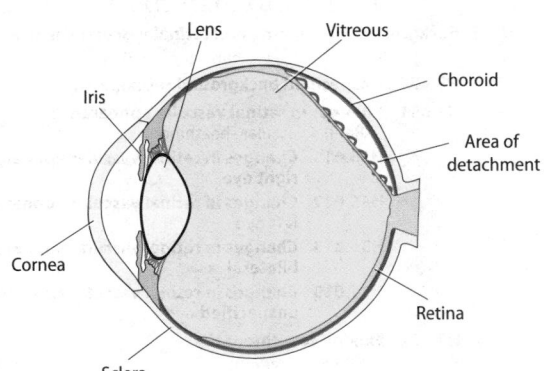

**H33.002**   **Unspecified retinal detachment with retinal break, left eye**

**H33.003**   **Unspecified retinal detachment with retinal break, bilateral**

**H33.009**   **Unspecified retinal detachment with retinal break, unspecified eye**

✓6ᵗʰ **H33.01**   **Retinal detachment with single break**

    **H33.011**   **Retinal detachment with single break, right eye**

    **H33.012**   **Retinal detachment with single break, left eye**

    **H33.013**   **Retinal detachment with single break, bilateral**

    **H33.019**   **Retinal detachment with single break, unspecified eye**

✓6ᵗʰ **H33.02**   **Retinal detachment with multiple breaks**

    **H33.021**   **Retinal detachment with multiple breaks, right eye**

    **H33.022**   **Retinal detachment with multiple breaks, left eye**

    **H33.023**   **Retinal detachment with multiple breaks, bilateral**

    **H33.029**   **Retinal detachment with multiple breaks, unspecified eye**

✓6ᵗʰ **H33.03**   **Retinal detachment with giant retinal tear**

    **H33.031**   **Retinal detachment with giant retinal tear, right eye**

    **H33.032**   **Retinal detachment with giant retinal tear, left eye**

    **H33.033**   **Retinal detachment with giant retinal tear, bilateral**

    **H33.039**   **Retinal detachment with giant retinal tear, unspecified eye**

✓6ᵗʰ **H33.04**   **Retinal detachment with retinal dialysis**

    **H33.041**   **Retinal detachment with retinal dialysis, right eye**

    **H33.042**   **Retinal detachment with retinal dialysis, left eye**

    **H33.043**   **Retinal detachment with retinal dialysis, bilateral**

    **H33.049**   **Retinal detachment with retinal dialysis, unspecified eye**

✓6ᵗʰ **H33.05**   **Total retinal detachment**

    **H33.051**   **Total retinal detachment, right eye**

    **H33.052**   **Total retinal detachment, left eye**

    **H33.053**   **Total retinal detachment, bilateral**

    **H33.059**   **Total retinal detachment, unspecified eye**

✓5ᵗʰ **H33.1**   **Retinoschisis and retinal cysts**

    *EXCLUDES 1*   *congenital retinoschisis (Q14.1)*

             *microcystoid degeneration of retina (H35.42-)*

✓6ᵗʰ **H33.10**   **Unspecified retinoschisis**

    **H33.101**   **Unspecified retinoschisis, right eye**

    **H33.102**   **Unspecified retinoschisis, left eye**

    **H33.103**   **Unspecified retinoschisis, bilateral**

    **H33.109**   **Unspecified retinoschisis, unspecified eye**

✓6ᵗʰ **H33.11**   **Cyst of ora serrata**

    **H33.111**   **Cyst of ora serrata, right eye**

    **H33.112**   **Cyst of ora serrata, left eye**

    **H33.113**   **Cyst of ora serrata, bilateral**

    **H33.119**   **Cyst of ora serrata, unspecified eye**

✓6ᵗʰ **H33.12**   **Parasitic cyst of retina**

> **CC Excl: For CC codes in subcategory H33.12:** PDX collection 625

    **H33.121**   **Parasitic cyst of retina, right eye**   `CC`

    **H33.122**   **Parasitic cyst of retina, left eye**   `CC`

    **H33.123**   **Parasitic cyst of retina, bilateral**   `CC`

    **H33.129**   **Parasitic cyst of retina, unspecified eye**   `CC`

✓6ᵗʰ **H33.19**   **Other retinoschisis and retinal cysts**

    Pseudocyst of retina

    **H33.191**   **Other retinoschisis and retinal cysts, right eye**

    **H33.192**   **Other retinoschisis and retinal cysts, left eye**

    **H33.193**   **Other retinoschisis and retinal cysts, bilateral**

    **H33.199**   **Other retinoschisis and retinal cysts, unspecified eye**

✓5ᵗʰ **H33.2**   **Serous retinal detachment**

    Retinal detachment NOS

    Retinal detachment without retinal break

    *EXCLUDES 1*   *central serous chorioretinopathy (H35.71-)*

    **H33.20**   **Serous retinal detachment, unspecified eye**   `CC`

    **H33.21**   **Serous retinal detachment, right eye**   `CC`

    **H33.22**   **Serous retinal detachment, left eye**   `CC`

    **H33.23**   **Serous retinal detachment, bilateral**   `CC`

✓5ᵗʰ **H33.3**   **Retinal breaks without detachment**

    *EXCLUDES 1*   *chorioretinal scars after surgery for detachment (H59.81-)*

             *peripheral retinal degeneration without break (H35.4-)*

✓6ᵗʰ **H33.30**   **Unspecified retinal break**

    **H33.301**   **Unspecified retinal break, right eye**

    **H33.302**   **Unspecified retinal break, left eye**

    **H33.303**   **Unspecified retinal break, bilateral**

    **H33.309**   **Unspecified retinal break, unspecified eye**

✓6ᵗʰ **H33.31**   **Horseshoe tear of retina without detachment**

    Operculum of retina without detachment

    **H33.311**   **Horseshoe tear of retina without detachment, right eye**

    **H33.312**   **Horseshoe tear of retina without detachment, left eye**

    **H33.313**   **Horseshoe tear of retina without detachment, bilateral**

    **H33.319**   **Horseshoe tear of retina without detachment, unspecified eye**

✓6ᵗʰ **H33.32**   **Round hole of retina without detachment**

    **H33.321**   **Round hole, right eye**

    **H33.322**   **Round hole, left eye**

    **H33.323**   **Round hole, bilateral**

    **H33.329**   **Round hole, unspecified eye**

✓6ᵗʰ **H33.33**   **Multiple defects of retina without detachment**

    **H33.331**   **Multiple defects of retina without detachment, right eye**

    **H33.332**   **Multiple defects of retina without detachment, left eye**

    **H33.333**   **Multiple defects of retina without detachment, bilateral**

    **H33.339**   **Multiple defects of retina without detachment, unspecified eye**

✓5ᵗʰ **H33.4**   **Traction detachment of retina**

    Proliferative vitreo-retinopathy with retinal detachment

    **H33.40**   **Traction detachment of retina, unspecified eye**   `CC`

    **H33.41**   **Traction detachment of retina, right eye**   `CC`

    **H33.42**   **Traction detachment of retina, left eye**   `CC`

    **H33.43**   **Traction detachment of retina, bilateral**   `CC`

**H33.8**   **Other retinal detachments**

✓ Additional Character Req   ✓x7ᵗʰ Placeholder Alert   Unacceptable PDx   **Manifestation**   **H1** - **H14** HAC   **HCC** CMS-HCC Condition   *EXCLUDES 1* Not Coded Here   *EXCLUDES 2* Not Included Here

ICD-10-CM 2018          **597**

✓4ᵗʰ **H34    Retinal vascular occlusions**
*EXCLUDES 1*    amaurosis fugax (G45.3)

**CC Excl: For CC codes in category H34:** PDX collection 587

✓5ᵗʰ **H34.0    Transient** retinal artery occlusion
**H34.00    Transient retinal artery occlusion, unspecified eye**   CC
**H34.01    Transient retinal artery occlusion, right eye**   CC
**H34.02    Transient retinal artery occlusion, left eye**   CC
**H34.03    Transient retinal artery occlusion, bilateral**   CC

✓5ᵗʰ **H34.1    Central** retinal artery occlusion
**H34.10    Central retinal artery occlusion, unspecified eye**   CC
**H34.11    Central retinal artery occlusion, right eye**   CC
**H34.12    Central retinal artery occlusion, left eye**   CC
**H34.13    Central retinal artery occlusion, bilateral**   CC

✓5ᵗʰ **H34.2    Other** retinal artery occlusions
✓6ᵗʰ **H34.21    Partial** retinal artery occlusion
Hollenhorst's plaque
Retinal microembolism
**H34.211    Partial retinal artery occlusion, right eye**   CC
**H34.212    Partial retinal artery occlusion, left eye**   CC
**H34.213    Partial retinal artery occlusion, bilateral**   CC
**H34.219    Partial retinal artery occlusion, unspecified eye**   CC

✓6ᵗʰ **H34.23    Retinal artery branch occlusion**
**H34.231    Retinal artery branch occlusion, right eye**   CC
**H34.232    Retinal artery branch occlusion, left eye**   CC
**H34.233    Retinal artery branch occlusion, bilateral**   CC
**H34.239    Retinal artery branch occlusion, unspecified eye**   CC

✓5ᵗʰ **H34.8    Other retinal vascular occlusions**
✓6ᵗʰ **H34.81    Central retinal vein occlusion**

One of the following 7th characters is to be assigned to codes in subcategory H34.81 to designate the severity of the occlusion:
Ø    with macular edema
1    with retinal neovascularization
2    stable
     old central retinal vein occlusion

✓7ᵗʰ **H34.811    Central retinal vein occlusion, right eye** CC
✓7ᵗʰ **H34.812    Central retinal vein occlusion, left eye**   CC
✓7ᵗʰ **H34.813    Central retinal vein occlusion, bilateral** CC
✓7ᵗʰ **H34.819    Central retinal vein occlusion, unspecified eye**   CC

✓6ᵗʰ **H34.82    Venous engorgement**
Incipient retinal vein occlusion
Partial retinal vein occlusion
**H34.821    Venous engorgement, right eye**
**H34.822    Venous engorgement, left eye**
**H34.823    Venous engorgement, bilateral**
**H34.829    Venous engorgement, unspecified eye**

✓6ᵗʰ **H34.83    Tributary (branch) retinal vein occlusion**

One of the following 7th characters is to be assigned to codes in subcategory H34.83 to designate the severity of the occlusion:
Ø    with macular edema
1    with retinal neovascularization
2    stable
     old tributary (branch) retinal vein occlusion

✓7ᵗʰ **H34.831    Tributary (branch) retinal vein occlusion, right eye**
✓7ᵗʰ **H34.832    Tributary (branch) retinal vein occlusion, left eye**
✓7ᵗʰ **H34.833    Tributary (branch) retinal vein occlusion, bilateral**
✓7ᵗʰ **H34.839    Tributary (branch) retinal vein occlusion, unspecified eye**

**H34.9    Unspecified retinal vascular occlusion**   CC

✓4ᵗʰ **H35    Other retinal disorders**
*EXCLUDES 2*    diabetic retinal disorders (E08.311- E08.359, E09.311- E09.359, E10.311- E10.359, E11.311- E11.359, E13.311- E13.359)

✓5ᵗʰ **H35.0    Background retinopathy and retinal vascular changes**
Code also any associated hypertension (I10.-)
**H35.00    Unspecified background retinopathy**

✓6ᵗʰ **H35.01    Changes in retinal vascular appearance**
Retinal vascular sheathing
**H35.011    Changes in retinal vascular appearance, right eye**
**H35.012    Changes in retinal vascular appearance, left eye**
**H35.013    Changes in retinal vascular appearance, bilateral**
**H35.019    Changes in retinal vascular appearance, unspecified eye**

✓6ᵗʰ **H35.02    Exudative retinopathy**
Coats retinopathy
**H35.021    Exudative retinopathy, right eye**
**H35.022    Exudative retinopathy, left eye**
**H35.023    Exudative retinopathy, bilateral**
**H35.029    Exudative retinopathy, unspecified eye**

✓6ᵗʰ **H35.03    Hypertensive retinopathy**
**H35.031    Hypertensive retinopathy, right eye**
**H35.032    Hypertensive retinopathy, left eye**
**H35.033    Hypertensive retinopathy, bilateral**
**H35.039    Hypertensive retinopathy, unspecified eye**

✓6ᵗʰ **H35.04    Retinal micro-aneurysms, unspecified**
**H35.041    Retinal micro-aneurysms, unspecified, right eye**
**H35.042    Retinal micro-aneurysms, unspecified, left eye**
**H35.043    Retinal micro-aneurysms, unspecified, bilateral**
**H35.049    Retinal micro-aneurysms, unspecified, unspecified eye**

✓6ᵗʰ **H35.05    Retinal neovascularization, unspecified**
**H35.051    Retinal neovascularization, unspecified, right eye**
**H35.052    Retinal neovascularization, unspecified, left eye**
**H35.053    Retinal neovascularization, unspecified, bilateral**
**H35.059    Retinal neovascularization, unspecified, unspecified eye**

✓6ᵗʰ **H35.06    Retinal vasculitis**
Eales disease
Retinal perivasculitis
**DEF:** Sight-threatening intraocular inflammation of the retinal blood vessels; causes minimal, partial, or even complete blindness.
**H35.061    Retinal vasculitis, right eye**
**H35.062    Retinal vasculitis, left eye**
**H35.063    Retinal vasculitis, bilateral**
**H35.069    Retinal vasculitis, unspecified eye**

✓6ᵗʰ **H35.07    Retinal telangiectasis**
**H35.071    Retinal telangiectasis, right eye**
**H35.072    Retinal telangiectasis, left eye**
**H35.073    Retinal telangiectasis, bilateral**
**H35.079    Retinal telangiectasis, unspecified eye**

**H35.09    Other intraretinal microvascular abnormalities**
Retinal varices

✓5ᵗʰ **H35.1    Retinopathy of prematurity**
✓6ᵗʰ **H35.10    Retinopathy of prematurity, unspecified**
Retinopathy of prematurity NOS
**H35.101    Retinopathy of prematurity, unspecified, right eye**
**H35.102    Retinopathy of prematurity, unspecified, left eye**
**H35.103    Retinopathy of prematurity, unspecified, bilateral**
**H35.109    Retinopathy of prematurity, unspecified, unspecified eye**

N Newborn: 0   P Pediatric: 0-17   M Maternity: 12-55   A Adult: 15-124   MCC Major CC Condition   PDx MCC PDx acts as own MCC   CC CC Condition   PDx CC PDx acts as own CC

598
ICD-10-CM 2018

✓6ᵗʰ **H35.11 Retinopathy of prematurity, stage 0**

   **H35.111 Retinopathy of prematurity, stage 0, right eye**

   **H35.112 Retinopathy of prematurity, stage 0, left eye**

   **H35.113 Retinopathy of prematurity, stage 0, bilateral**

   **H35.119 Retinopathy of prematurity, stage 0, unspecified eye**

✓6ᵗʰ **H35.12 Retinopathy of prematurity, stage 1**

   **H35.121 Retinopathy of prematurity, stage 1, right eye**

   **H35.122 Retinopathy of prematurity, stage 1, left eye**

   **H35.123 Retinopathy of prematurity, stage 1, bilateral**

   **H35.129 Retinopathy of prematurity, stage 1, unspecified eye**

✓6ᵗʰ **H35.13 Retinopathy of prematurity, stage 2**

   **H35.131 Retinopathy of prematurity, stage 2, right eye**

   **H35.132 Retinopathy of prematurity, stage 2, left eye**

   **H35.133 Retinopathy of prematurity, stage 2, bilateral**

   **H35.139 Retinopathy of prematurity, stage 2, unspecified eye**

✓6ᵗʰ **H35.14 Retinopathy of prematurity, stage 3**

   **H35.141 Retinopathy of prematurity, stage 3, right eye**

   **H35.142 Retinopathy of prematurity, stage 3, left eye**

   **H35.143 Retinopathy of prematurity, stage 3, bilateral**

   **H35.149 Retinopathy of prematurity, stage 3, unspecified eye**

✓6ᵗʰ **H35.15 Retinopathy of prematurity, stage 4**

   **H35.151 Retinopathy of prematurity, stage 4, right eye**

   **H35.152 Retinopathy of prematurity, stage 4, left eye**

   **H35.153 Retinopathy of prematurity, stage 4, bilateral**

   **H35.159 Retinopathy of prematurity, stage 4, unspecified eye**

✓6ᵗʰ **H35.16 Retinopathy of prematurity, stage 5**

   **H35.161 Retinopathy of prematurity, stage 5, right eye**

   **H35.162 Retinopathy of prematurity, stage 5, left eye**

   **H35.163 Retinopathy of prematurity, stage 5, bilateral**

   **H35.169 Retinopathy of prematurity, stage 5, unspecified eye**

✓6ᵗʰ **H35.17 Retrolental fibroplasia**

   **H35.171 Retrolental fibroplasia, right eye**

   **H35.172 Retrolental fibroplasia, left eye**

   **H35.173 Retrolental fibroplasia, bilateral**

   **H35.179 Retrolental fibroplasia, unspecified eye**

✓5ᵗʰ **H35.2 Other non-diabetic proliferative retinopathy**

Proliferative vitreo-retinopathy

**EXCLUDES 1** *proliferative vitreo-retinopathy with retinal detachment (H33.4-)*

   **H35.20 Other non-diabetic proliferative retinopathy, unspecified eye**

   **H35.21 Other non-diabetic proliferative retinopathy, right eye**

   **H35.22 Other non-diabetic proliferative retinopathy, left eye**

   **H35.23 Other non-diabetic proliferative retinopathy, bilateral**

✓5ᵗʰ **H35.3 Degeneration of macula and posterior pole**

   **H35.30 Unspecified macular degeneration**    Ⓐ

Age-related macular degeneration

✓6ᵗʰ **H35.31 Nonexudative age-related macular degeneration**

Atrophic age-related macular degeneration

Dry age-related macular degeneration

**AHA:** 2016, 4Q, 21

One of the following 7th characters is to be assigned to codes in subcategory H35.31 to designate the stage of the disease:

0   stage unspecified

1   early dry stage

2   intermediate dry stage

3   advanced atrophic without subfoveal involvement

    advanced dry stage

4   advanced atrophic with subfoveal involvement

   ✓7ᵗʰ **H35.311 Nonexudative age-related macular degeneration, right eye**   Ⓐ

   ✓7ᵗʰ **H35.312 Nonexudative age-related macular degeneration, left eye**   Ⓐ

   ✓7ᵗʰ **H35.313 Nonexudative age-related macular degeneration, bilateral**   Ⓐ

   ✓7ᵗʰ **H35.319 Nonexudative age-related macular degeneration, unspecified eye**   Ⓐ

✓6ᵗʰ **H35.32 Exudative age-related macular degeneration**

Wet age-related macular degeneration

One of the following 7th characters is to be assigned to codes in subcategory H35.32 to designate the stage of the disease:

0   stage unspecified

1   with active choroidal neovascularization

2   with inactive choroidal neovascularization

    with involuted or regressed neovascularization

3   with inactive scar

   ✓7ᵗʰ **H35.321 Exudative age-related macular degeneration, right eye**   HCC Ⓐ

   ✓7ᵗʰ **H35.322 Exudative age-related macular degeneration, left eye**   HCC Ⓐ

   ✓7ᵗʰ **H35.323 Exudative age-related macular degeneration, bilateral**   HCC Ⓐ

   ✓7ᵗʰ **H35.329 Exudative age-related macular degeneration, unspecified eye**   HCC Ⓐ

   **H35.33 Angioid streaks of macula**

**DEF:** Degeneration of choroid; characterized by broad, irregular, dark brown streaks radiating from optic disc; occurs with pseudoxanthoma elasticum or Paget's disease.

✓6ᵗʰ **H35.34 Macular cyst, hole, or pseudohole**

   **H35.341 Macular cyst, hole, or pseudohole, right eye**

   **H35.342 Macular cyst, hole, or pseudohole, left eye**

   **H35.343 Macular cyst, hole, or pseudohole, bilateral**

   **H35.349 Macular cyst, hole, or pseudohole, unspecified eye**

✓6ᵗʰ **H35.35 Cystoid macular degeneration**

**EXCLUDES 1** *cystoid macular edema following cataract surgery (H59.03-)*

   **H35.351 Cystoid macular degeneration, right eye**

   **H35.352 Cystoid macular degeneration, left eye**

   **H35.353 Cystoid macular degeneration, bilateral**

   **H35.359 Cystoid macular degeneration, unspecified eye**

✓6ᵗʰ **H35.36 Drusen (degenerative) of macula**

**AHA:** 2017, 1Q, 51; 2016, 4Q, 21

   **H35.361 Drusen (degenerative) of macula, right eye**

   **H35.362 Drusen (degenerative) of macula, left eye**

   **H35.363 Drusen (degenerative) of macula, bilateral**

   **H35.369 Drusen (degenerative) of macula, unspecified eye**

✓6ᵗʰ **H35.37 Puckering of macula**

   **H35.371 Puckering of macula, right eye**

   **H35.372 Puckering of macula, left eye**

   **H35.373 Puckering of macula, bilateral**

   **H35.379 Puckering of macula, unspecified eye**

---

✓ Additional Character Req   ✓x7ᵗʰ Placeholder Alert   Unacceptable PDx   Manifestation   H1-H14 HAC   HCC CMS-HCC Condition   EXCLUDES 1 Not Coded Here   EXCLUDES 2 Not Included Here

ICD-10-CM 2018                                                              599

**Chapter 7. Diseases of the Eye and Adnexa**

✓6ᵗʰ **H35.38 Toxic maculopathy**
Code first poisoning due to drug or toxin, if applicable (T36-T65 with fifth or sixth character 1-4 or 6)
Use additional code for adverse effect, if applicable, to identify drug (T36-T50 with fifth or sixth character 5)

H35.381 **Toxic maculopathy, right eye**
H35.382 **Toxic maculopathy, left eye**
H35.383 **Toxic maculopathy, bilateral**
H35.389 **Toxic maculopathy, unspecified eye**

✓5ᵗʰ **H35.4 Peripheral retinal degeneration**
*EXCLUDES 1*   *hereditary retinal degeneration (dystrophy) (H35.5-)*
*peripheral retinal degeneration with retinal break (H33.3-)*

H35.40 **Unspecified peripheral retinal degeneration**

✓6ᵗʰ **H35.41 Lattice degeneration of retina**
Palisade degeneration of retina
**DEF:** Degeneration of retina; often bilateral, usually benign; characterized by lines intersecting at irregular intervals in peripheral retina; retinal thinning and retinal holes may occur.

H35.411 **Lattice degeneration of retina, right eye**
H35.412 **Lattice degeneration of retina, left eye**
H35.413 **Lattice degeneration of retina, bilateral**
H35.419 **Lattice degeneration of retina, unspecified eye**

✓6ᵗʰ **H35.42 Microcystoid degeneration of retina**
H35.421 **Microcystoid degeneration of retina, right eye**
H35.422 **Microcystoid degeneration of retina, left eye**
H35.423 **Microcystoid degeneration of retina, bilateral**
H35.429 **Microcystoid degeneration of retina, unspecified eye**

✓6ᵗʰ **H35.43 Paving stone degeneration of retina**
H35.431 **Paving stone degeneration of retina, right eye**
H35.432 **Paving stone degeneration of retina, left eye**
H35.433 **Paving stone degeneration of retina, bilateral**
H35.439 **Paving stone degeneration of retina, unspecified eye**

✓6ᵗʰ **H35.44 Age-related reticular degeneration of retina**
H35.441 **Age-related reticular degeneration of retina, right eye** Ⓐ
H35.442 **Age-related reticular degeneration of retina, left eye** Ⓐ
H35.443 **Age-related reticular degeneration of retina, bilateral** Ⓐ
H35.449 **Age-related reticular degeneration of retina, unspecified eye** Ⓐ

✓6ᵗʰ **H35.45 Secondary pigmentary degeneration**
H35.451 **Secondary pigmentary degeneration, right eye**
H35.452 **Secondary pigmentary degeneration, left eye**
H35.453 **Secondary pigmentary degeneration, bilateral**
H35.459 **Secondary pigmentary degeneration, unspecified eye**

✓6ᵗʰ **H35.46 Secondary vitreoretinal degeneration**
H35.461 **Secondary vitreoretinal degeneration, right eye**
H35.462 **Secondary vitreoretinal degeneration, left eye**
H35.463 **Secondary vitreoretinal degeneration, bilateral**
H35.469 **Secondary vitreoretinal degeneration, unspecified eye**

✓5ᵗʰ **H35.5 Hereditary retinal dystrophy**
*EXCLUDES 1*   *dystrophies primarily involving Bruch's membrane (H31.1-)*

H35.50 **Unspecified hereditary retinal dystrophy**
H35.51 **Vitreoretinal dystrophy**

H35.52 **Pigmentary retinal dystrophy**
Albipunctate retinal dystrophy
Retinitis pigmentosa
Tapetoretinal dystrophy

H35.53 **Other dystrophies primarily involving the sensory retina**
Stargardt's disease

H35.54 **Dystrophies primarily involving the retinal pigment epithelium**
Vitelliform retinal dystrophy

✓5ᵗʰ **H35.6 Retinal hemorrhage**
H35.60 **Retinal hemorrhage, unspecified eye**
H35.61 **Retinal hemorrhage, right eye**
H35.62 **Retinal hemorrhage, left eye**
H35.63 **Retinal hemorrhage, bilateral**

✓5ᵗʰ **H35.7 Separation of retinal layers**
*EXCLUDES 1*   *retinal detachment (serous) (H33.2-)*
*rhegmatogenous retinal detachment (H33.0-)*

**CC Excl: For CC codes in subcategory H35.7:**
PDX collection 628

H35.70 **Unspecified separation of retinal layers** CC

✓6ᵗʰ **H35.71 Central serous chorioretinopathy**
H35.711 **Central serous chorioretinopathy, right eye**
H35.712 **Central serous chorioretinopathy, left eye**
H35.713 **Central serous chorioretinopathy, bilateral**
H35.719 **Central serous chorioretinopathy, unspecified eye**

✓6ᵗʰ **H35.72 Serous detachment of retinal pigment epithelium**
H35.721 **Serous detachment of retinal pigment epithelium, right eye** CC
H35.722 **Serous detachment of retinal pigment epithelium, left eye** CC
H35.723 **Serous detachment of retinal pigment epithelium, bilateral** CC
H35.729 **Serous detachment of retinal pigment epithelium, unspecified eye** CC

✓6ᵗʰ **H35.73 Hemorrhagic detachment of retinal pigment epithelium**
H35.731 **Hemorrhagic detachment of retinal pigment epithelium, right eye** CC
H35.732 **Hemorrhagic detachment of retinal pigment epithelium, left eye** CC
H35.733 **Hemorrhagic detachment of retinal pigment epithelium, bilateral** CC
H35.739 **Hemorrhagic detachment of retinal pigment epithelium, unspecified eye** CC

✓5ᵗʰ **H35.8 Other specified retinal disorders**
*EXCLUDES 2*   *retinal hemorrhage (H35.6-)*

H35.81 **Retinal edema**
Retinal cotton wool spots

H35.82 **Retinal ischemia** CC
**CC Excl:** PDX collection 629

H35.89 **Other specified retinal disorders**

H35.9 **Unspecified retinal disorder**

**H36 Retinal disorders in diseases classified elsewhere**
Code first underlying disease, such as:
lipid storage disorders (E75.-)
sickle-cell disorders (D57.-)
*EXCLUDES 1*   *arteriosclerotic retinopathy (H35.0-)*
*diabetic retinopathy (E08.3-, E09.3-, E10.3-, E11.3-, E13.3-)*

## Glaucoma (H40-H42)

✓4ᵗʰ **H40 Glaucoma**
*EXCLUDES 1*   *absolute glaucoma (H44.51-)*
*congenital glaucoma (Q15.0)*
*traumatic glaucoma due to birth injury (P15.3)*

✓5ᵗʰ **H40.0 Glaucoma suspect**
✓6ᵗʰ **H40.00 Preglaucoma, unspecified**
H40.001 **Preglaucoma, unspecified, right eye**
H40.002 **Preglaucoma, unspecified, left eye**
H40.003 **Preglaucoma, unspecified, bilateral**
H40.009 **Preglaucoma, unspecified, unspecified eye**

Ⓝ Newborn: 0   Ⓟ Pediatric: 0-17   Ⓜ Maternity: 12-55   Ⓐ Adult: 15-124   **MCC** Major CC Condition   **PDx MCC** PDx acts as own MCC   **CC** CC Condition   **PDx CC** PDx acts as own CC

600

ICD-10-CM 2018

**✓6ᵗʰ H40.01 Open angle with borderline findings, low risk**
Open angle, low risk

    **H40.011 Open angle with borderline findings, low risk, right eye**

    **H40.012 Open angle with borderline findings, low risk, left eye**

    **H40.013 Open angle with borderline findings, low risk, bilateral**

    **H40.019 Open angle with borderline findings, low risk, unspecified eye**

**✓6ᵗʰ H40.02 Open angle with borderline findings, high risk**
Open angle, high risk

    **H40.021 Open angle with borderline findings, high risk, right eye**

    **H40.022 Open angle with borderline findings, high risk, left eye**

    **H40.023 Open angle with borderline findings, high risk, bilateral**

    **H40.029 Open angle with borderline findings, high risk, unspecified eye**

**✓6ᵗʰ H40.03 Anatomical narrow angle**
Primary angle closure suspect

    **H40.031 Anatomical narrow angle, right eye**

    **H40.032 Anatomical narrow angle, left eye**

    **H40.033 Anatomical narrow angle, bilateral**

    **H40.039 Anatomical narrow angle, unspecified eye**

**✓6ᵗʰ H40.04 Steroid responder**

    **H40.041 Steroid responder, right eye**

    **H40.042 Steroid responder, left eye**

    **H40.043 Steroid responder, bilateral**

    **H40.049 Steroid responder, unspecified eye**

**✓6ᵗʰ H40.05 Ocular hypertension**

    **H40.051 Ocular hypertension, right eye**

    **H40.052 Ocular hypertension, left eye**

    **H40.053 Ocular hypertension, bilateral**

    **H40.059 Ocular hypertension, unspecified eye**

**✓6ᵗʰ H40.06 Primary angle closure without glaucoma damage**

    **H40.061 Primary angle closure without glaucoma damage, right eye**

    **H40.062 Primary angle closure without glaucoma damage, left eye**

    **H40.063 Primary angle closure without glaucoma damage, bilateral**

    **H40.069 Primary angle closure without glaucoma damage, unspecified eye**

**✓5ᵗʰ H40.1 Open-angle glaucoma**

One of the following 7th characters is to be assigned to each code in subcategories H40.10, H40.11-, H40.12-, H40.13-, and H40.14- to designate the stage of glaucoma.
Ø  stage unspecified
1  mild stage
2  moderate stage
3  severe stage
4  indeterminate stage

**✓x7ᵗʰ H40.10 Unspecified open-angle glaucoma**

**✓6ᵗʰ H40.11 Primary open-angle glaucoma**
Chronic simple glaucoma

    **✓7ᵗʰ H40.111 Primary open-angle glaucoma, right eye**

    **✓7ᵗʰ H40.112 Primary open-angle glaucoma, left eye**

    **✓7ᵗʰ H40.113 Primary open-angle glaucoma, bilateral**

    **✓7ᵗʰ H40.119 Primary open-angle glaucoma, unspecified eye**

**✓6ᵗʰ H40.12 Low-tension glaucoma**

    **✓7ᵗʰ H40.121 Low-tension glaucoma, right eye**

    **✓7ᵗʰ H40.122 Low-tension glaucoma, left eye**

    **✓7ᵗʰ H40.123 Low-tension glaucoma, bilateral**

    **✓7ᵗʰ H40.129 Low-tension glaucoma, unspecified eye**

**✓6ᵗʰ H40.13 Pigmentary glaucoma**

    **✓7ᵗʰ H40.131 Pigmentary glaucoma, right eye**

    **✓7ᵗʰ H40.132 Pigmentary glaucoma, left eye**

    **✓7ᵗʰ H40.133 Pigmentary glaucoma, bilateral**

    **✓7ᵗʰ H40.139 Pigmentary glaucoma, unspecified eye**

**Open Angle/Angle Closure Glaucoma**

Open angle — Closed angle — Fluid flow — Lens — Lens — Iris — Cornea — Fluid flow — Drainage canal

**✓6ᵗʰ H40.14 Capsular glaucoma with pseudoexfoliation of lens**

    **✓7ᵗʰ H40.141 Capsular glaucoma with pseudoexfoliation of lens, right eye**

    **✓7ᵗʰ H40.142 Capsular glaucoma with pseudoexfoliation of lens, left eye**

    **✓7ᵗʰ H40.143 Capsular glaucoma with pseudoexfoliation of lens, bilateral**

    **✓7ᵗʰ H40.149 Capsular glaucoma with pseudoexfoliation of lens, unspecified eye**

**✓6ᵗʰ H40.15 Residual stage of open-angle glaucoma**

    **H40.151 Residual stage of open-angle glaucoma, right eye**

    **H40.152 Residual stage of open-angle glaucoma, left eye**

    **H40.153 Residual stage of open-angle glaucoma, bilateral**

    **H40.159 Residual stage of open-angle glaucoma, unspecified eye**

**✓5ᵗʰ H40.2 Primary angle-closure glaucoma**
**EXCLUDES 1**   *aqueous misdirection (H40.83-)*
          *malignant glaucoma (H40.83-)*

One of the following 7th characters is to be assigned to each code in subcategories H40.20 and H40.22- to designate the stage of glaucoma.
Ø  stage unspecified
1  mild stage
2  moderate stage
3  severe stage
4  indeterminate stage

**✓x7ᵗʰ H40.20 Unspecified primary angle-closure glaucoma**

**✓6ᵗʰ H40.21 Acute angle-closure glaucoma**
Acute angle-closure glaucoma attack
Acute angle-closure glaucoma crisis

**CC Excl: For CC codes in subcategory H40.21:**
PDX collection 630

    **H40.211 Acute angle-closure glaucoma, right eye**    `CC`

    **H40.212 Acute angle-closure glaucoma, left eye**    `CC`

    **H40.213 Acute angle-closure glaucoma, bilateral**    `CC`

    **H40.219 Acute angle-closure glaucoma, unspecified eye**    `CC`

**✓6ᵗʰ H40.22 Chronic angle-closure glaucoma**
Chronic primary angle-closure glaucoma

    **✓7ᵗʰ H40.221 Chronic angle-closure glaucoma, right eye**

    **✓7ᵗʰ H40.222 Chronic angle-closure glaucoma, left eye**

    **✓7ᵗʰ H40.223 Chronic angle-closure glaucoma, bilateral**

    **✓7ᵗʰ H40.229 Chronic angle-closure glaucoma, unspecified eye**

**✓6ᵗʰ H40.23 Intermittent angle-closure glaucoma**

    **H40.231 Intermittent angle-closure glaucoma, right eye**

    **H40.232 Intermittent angle-closure glaucoma, left eye**

    **H40.233 Intermittent angle-closure glaucoma, bilateral**

    **H40.239 Intermittent angle-closure glaucoma, unspecified eye**

✓ Additional Character Req   ✓x7ᵗʰ Placeholder Alert   Unacceptable PDx   Manifestation   **H1**-**H14** HAC   **HCC** CMS-HCC Condition   **EXCLUDES 1** Not Coded Here   **EXCLUDES 2** Not Included Here

ICD-10-CM 2018                          **601**

**✓6ᵗʰ H40.24 Residual stage** of angle-closure glaucoma

H40.241 **Residual stage of angle-closure glaucoma, right eye**

H40.242 **Residual stage of angle-closure glaucoma, left eye**

H40.243 **Residual stage of angle-closure glaucoma, bilateral**

H40.249 **Residual stage of angle-closure glaucoma, unspecified eye**

**✓5ᵗʰ H40.3 Glaucoma secondary to eye trauma**
Code also underlying condition

> One of the following 7th characters is to be assigned to each code in subcategory H40.3- to designate the stage of glaucoma.
> Ø   stage unspecified
> 1   mild stage
> 2   moderate stage
> 3   severe stage
> 4   indeterminate stage

**✓x7ᵗʰ H40.30 Glaucoma secondary to eye trauma, unspecified eye**

**✓x7ᵗʰ H40.31 Glaucoma secondary to eye trauma, right eye**

**✓x7ᵗʰ H40.32 Glaucoma secondary to eye trauma, left eye**

**✓x7ᵗʰ H40.33 Glaucoma secondary to eye trauma, bilateral**

**✓5ᵗʰ H40.4 Glaucoma secondary to eye inflammation**
Code also underlying condition

> One of the following 7th characters is to be assigned to each code in subcategory H40.4- to designate the stage of glaucoma.
> Ø   stage unspecified
> 1   mild stage
> 2   moderate stage
> 3   severe stage
> 4   indeterminate stage

**✓x7ᵗʰ H40.40 Glaucoma secondary to eye inflammation, unspecified eye**

**✓x7ᵗʰ H40.41 Glaucoma secondary to eye inflammation, right eye**

**✓x7ᵗʰ H40.42 Glaucoma secondary to eye inflammation, left eye**

**✓x7ᵗʰ H40.43 Glaucoma secondary to eye inflammation, bilateral**

**✓5ᵗʰ H40.5 Glaucoma secondary to other eye disorders**
Code also underlying eye disorder

> One of the following 7th characters is to be assigned to each code in subcategory H40.5- to designate the stage of glaucoma.
> Ø   stage unspecified
> 1   mild stage
> 2   moderate stage
> 3   severe stage
> 4   indeterminate stage

**✓x7ᵗʰ H40.50 Glaucoma secondary to other eye disorders, unspecified eye**

**✓x7ᵗʰ H40.51 Glaucoma secondary to other eye disorders, right eye**

**✓x7ᵗʰ H40.52 Glaucoma secondary to other eye disorders, left eye**

**✓x7ᵗʰ H40.53 Glaucoma secondary to other eye disorders, bilateral**

**✓5ᵗʰ H40.6 Glaucoma secondary to drugs**
Use additional code for adverse effect, if applicable, to identify drug (T36-T50 with fifth or sixth character 5)

> One of the following 7th characters is to be assigned to each code in subcategory H40.6- to designate the stage of glaucoma.
> Ø   stage unspecified
> 1   mild stage
> 2   moderate stage
> 3   severe stage
> 4   indeterminate stage

**✓x7ᵗʰ H40.60 Glaucoma secondary to drugs, unspecified eye**

**✓x7ᵗʰ H40.61 Glaucoma secondary to drugs, right eye**

**✓x7ᵗʰ H40.62 Glaucoma secondary to drugs, left eye**

**✓x7ᵗʰ H40.63 Glaucoma secondary to drugs, bilateral**

**✓5ᵗʰ H40.8 Other glaucoma**

**✓6ᵗʰ H40.81 Glaucoma with increased episcleral venous pressure**

H40.811 **Glaucoma with increased episcleral venous pressure, right eye**

H40.812 **Glaucoma with increased episcleral venous pressure, left eye**

H40.813 **Glaucoma with increased episcleral venous pressure, bilateral**

H40.819 **Glaucoma with increased episcleral venous pressure, unspecified eye**

**✓6ᵗʰ H40.82 Hypersecretion glaucoma**

H40.821 **Hypersecretion glaucoma, right eye**

H40.822 **Hypersecretion glaucoma, left eye**

H40.823 **Hypersecretion glaucoma, bilateral**

H40.829 **Hypersecretion glaucoma, unspecified eye**

**✓6ᵗʰ H40.83 Aqueous misdirection**
Malignant glaucoma

H40.831 **Aqueous misdirection, right eye**

H40.832 **Aqueous misdirection, left eye**

H40.833 **Aqueous misdirection, bilateral**

H40.839 **Aqueous misdirection, unspecified eye**

H40.89 **Other specified glaucoma**

H40.9 **Unspecified glaucoma**

**H42 *Glaucoma in diseases classified elsewhere***
Code first underlying condition, such as:
amyloidosis (E85.-)
aniridia (Q13.1)
▶glaucoma (in) diabetes mellitus (EØ8.39, EØ9.39, E1Ø.39, E11.39, E13.39)◀
Lowe's syndrome (E72.Ø3)
Reiger's anomaly (Q13.81)
specified metabolic disorder (E7Ø-E88)

**EXCLUDES 1**   *glaucoma (in) onchocerciasis (B73.Ø2)*
*glaucoma (in) syphilis (A52.71)*
*glaucoma (in) tuberculous (A18.59)*

**EXCLUDES 2**   *glaucoma (in) diabetes mellitus (EØ8.39, EØ9.39, E1Ø.39, E11.39, E13.39)*

## Disorders of vitreous body and globe (H43-H44)

**✓4ᵗʰ H43 Disorders of vitreous body**

**✓5ᵗʰ H43.0 Vitreous prolapse**

**EXCLUDES 1**   *traumatic vitreous prolapse (SØ5.2-)*
*vitreous syndrome following cataract surgery (H59.Ø-)*

H43.00 **Vitreous prolapse, unspecified eye**

H43.01 **Vitreous prolapse, right eye**

H43.02 **Vitreous prolapse, left eye**

H43.03 **Vitreous prolapse, bilateral**

**✓5ᵗʰ H43.1 Vitreous hemorrhage**

H43.10 **Vitreous hemorrhage, unspecified eye**   `HCC`

H43.11 **Vitreous hemorrhage, right eye**   `HCC`

H43.12 **Vitreous hemorrhage, left eye**   `HCC`

H43.13 **Vitreous hemorrhage, bilateral**   `HCC`

**✓5ᵗʰ H43.2 Crystalline deposits in vitreous body**

H43.20 **Crystalline deposits in vitreous body, unspecified eye**

H43.21 **Crystalline deposits in vitreous body, right eye**

H43.22 **Crystalline deposits in vitreous body, left eye**

H43.23 **Crystalline deposits in vitreous body, bilateral**

**✓5ᵗʰ H43.3 Other vitreous opacities**

**✓6ᵗʰ H43.31 Vitreous membranes and strands**

H43.311 **Vitreous membranes and strands, right eye**

H43.312 **Vitreous membranes and strands, left eye**

H43.313 **Vitreous membranes and strands, bilateral**

H43.319 **Vitreous membranes and strands, unspecified eye**

**✓6ᵗʰ H43.39 Other vitreous opacities**
Vitreous floaters

H43.391 **Other vitreous opacities, right eye**

H43.392 **Other vitreous opacities, left eye**

H43.393 **Other vitreous opacities, bilateral**

H43.399 **Other vitreous opacities, unspecified eye**

N Newborn: 0   P Pediatric: 0-17   M Maternity: 12-55   A Adult: 15-124   MCC Major CC Condition   PDx MCC PDx acts as own MCC   CC CC Condition   PDx CC PDx acts as own CC

602   ICD-10-CM 2018

✓5ᵗʰ **H43.8  Other disorders of vitreous body**
  EXCLUDES 1   *proliferative vitreo-retinopathy with retinal detachment (H33.4-)*
  EXCLUDES 2   *vitreous abscess (H44.02-)*

  ✓6ᵗʰ **H43.81  Vitreous degeneration**
        Vitreous detachment
        **H43.811  Vitreous degeneration, right eye**
        **H43.812  Vitreous degeneration, left eye**
        **H43.813  Vitreous degeneration, bilateral**
        **H43.819  Vitreous degeneration, unspecified eye**
  ✓6ᵗʰ **H43.82  Vitreomacular adhesion**
        Vitreomacular traction
        **H43.821  Vitreomacular adhesion, right eye**  [A]
        **H43.822  Vitreomacular adhesion, left eye**  [A]
        **H43.823  Vitreomacular adhesion, bilateral**  [A]
        **H43.829  Vitreomacular adhesion, unspecified eye**  [A]
        **H43.89  Other disorders of vitreous body**
      **H43.9  Unspecified disorder of vitreous body**

✓4ᵗʰ **H44  Disorders of globe**
  INCLUDES   disorders affecting multiple structures of eye

  ✓5ᵗʰ **H44.0  Purulent endophthalmitis**
        Use additional code to identify organism
      EXCLUDES 1   *bleb associated endophthalmitis (H59.4-)*

  ✓6ᵗʰ **H44.00  Unspecified purulent endophthalmitis**

        CC Excl: For CC codes in subcategory H44.00:
        PDX collection 625

        **H44.001  Unspecified purulent endophthalmitis, right eye**  CC
        **H44.002  Unspecified purulent endophthalmitis, left eye**  CC
        **H44.003  Unspecified purulent endophthalmitis, bilateral**  CC
        **H44.009  Unspecified purulent endophthalmitis, unspecified eye**  CC
  ✓6ᵗʰ **H44.01  Panophthalmitis (acute)**

        CC Excl: For CC codes in subcategory H44.01:
        PDX collection 625

        **H44.011  Panophthalmitis (acute), right eye**  CC
        **H44.012  Panophthalmitis (acute), left eye**  CC
        **H44.013  Panophthalmitis (acute), bilateral**  CC
        **H44.019  Panophthalmitis (acute), unspecified eye**  CC
  ✓6ᵗʰ **H44.02  Vitreous abscess (chronic)**

        CC Excl: For CC codes in subcategory H44.02:
        PDX collection 631

        **H44.021  Vitreous abscess (chronic), right eye**  CC
        **H44.022  Vitreous abscess (chronic), left eye**  CC
        **H44.023  Vitreous abscess (chronic), bilateral**  CC
        **H44.029  Vitreous abscess (chronic), unspecified eye**  CC

  ✓5ᵗʰ **H44.1  Other endophthalmitis**
      EXCLUDES 1   *bleb associated endophthalmitis (H59.4-)*
      EXCLUDES 2   *ophthalmia nodosa (H16.2-)*

  ✓6ᵗʰ **H44.11  Panuveitis**
        DEF: Inflammation of all layers of uvea of eye, including choroid, iris, and ciliary body; also typically involves lens, retina, optic nerve, and vitreous; causes reduced vision or blindness.

        CC Excl: For CC codes in subcategory H44.11:
        PDX collection 632

        **H44.111  Panuveitis, right eye**  CC
        **H44.112  Panuveitis, left eye**  CC
        **H44.113  Panuveitis, bilateral**  CC
        **H44.119  Panuveitis, unspecified eye**  CC
  ✓6ᵗʰ **H44.12  Parasitic endophthalmitis, unspecified**

        CC Excl: For CC codes in subcategory H44.12:
        PDX collection 625

        **H44.121  Parasitic endophthalmitis, unspecified, right eye**  CC
        **H44.122  Parasitic endophthalmitis, unspecified, left eye**  CC

        **H44.123  Parasitic endophthalmitis, unspecified, bilateral**  CC
        **H44.129  Parasitic endophthalmitis, unspecified, unspecified eye**  CC
  ✓6ᵗʰ **H44.13  Sympathetic uveitis**

        CC Excl: For CC codes in subcategory H44.13:
        PDX collection 632

        **H44.131  Sympathetic uveitis, right eye**  CC
        **H44.132  Sympathetic uveitis, left eye**  CC
        **H44.133  Sympathetic uveitis, bilateral**  CC
        **H44.139  Sympathetic uveitis, unspecified eye**  CC
        **H44.19  Other endophthalmitis**  CC
              CC Excl: PDX collection 625

  ✓5ᵗʰ **H44.2  Degenerative myopia**
        Malignant myopia
        **H44.20  Degenerative myopia, unspecified eye**
        **H44.21  Degenerative myopia, right eye**
        **H44.22  Degenerative myopia, left eye**
        **H44.23  Degenerative myopia, bilateral**
  ✓6ᵗʰ **H44.2A  Degenerative myopia with choroidal neovascularization**
        Use additional code for any associated choroid disorders (H31.-)
        **H44.2A1  Degenerative myopia with choroidal neovascularization, right eye**
        **H44.2A2  Degenerative myopia with choroidal neovascularization, left eye**
        **H44.2A3  Degenerative myopia with choroidal neovascularization, bilateral eye**
        **H44.2A9  Degenerative myopia with choroidal neovascularization, unspecified eye**
  ✓6ᵗʰ **H44.2B  Degenerative myopia with macular hole**
        **H44.2B1  Degenerative myopia with macular hole, right eye**
        **H44.2B2  Degenerative myopia with macular hole, left eye**
        **H44.2B3  Degenerative myopia with macular hole, bilateral eye**
        **H44.2B9  Degenerative myopia with macular hole, unspecified eye**
  ✓6ᵗʰ **H44.2C  Degenerative myopia with retinal detachment**
        Use additional code to identify the retinal detachment (H33.-)
        **H44.2C1  Degenerative myopia with retinal detachment, right eye**
        **H44.2C2  Degenerative myopia with retinal detachment, left eye**
        **H44.2C3  Degenerative myopia with retinal detachment, bilateral eye**
        **H44.2C9  Degenerative myopia with retinal detachment, unspecified eye**
  ✓6ᵗʰ **H44.2D  Degenerative myopia with foveoschisis**
        **H44.2D1  Degenerative myopia with foveoschisis, right eye**
        **H44.2D2  Degenerative myopia with foveoschisis, left eye**
        **H44.2D3  Degenerative myopia with foveoschisis, bilateral eye**
        **H44.2D9  Degenerative myopia with foveoschisis, unspecified eye**
  ✓6ᵗʰ **H44.2E  Degenerative myopia with other maculopathy**
        **H44.2E1  Degenerative myopia with other maculopathy, right eye**
        **H44.2E2  Degenerative myopia with other maculopathy, left eye**
        **H44.2E3  Degenerative myopia with other maculopathy, bilateral eye**
        **H44.2E9  Degenerative myopia with other maculopathy, unspecified eye**

✓ Additional Character Req   ✓x7ᵗʰ Placeholder Alert   Unacceptable PDx   Manifestation   H1 - H14 HAC   HCC CMS-HCC Condition   EXCLUDES 1 Not Coded Here   EXCLUDES 2 Not Included Here

ICD-10-CM 2018                                                                        603

✓5ᵗʰ **H44.3** **Other and unspecified degenerative disorders of globe**

    **H44.30** **Unspecified degenerative disorder of globe**

✓6ᵗʰ **H44.31** **Chalcosis**

    **H44.311** **Chalcosis, right eye**

    **H44.312** **Chalcosis, left eye**

    **H44.313** **Chalcosis, bilateral**

    **H44.319** **Chalcosis, unspecified eye**

✓6ᵗʰ **H44.32** **Siderosis of eye**

    **DEF:** Iron pigment deposits within tissue of eyeball; caused by high iron content of blood; characterized by cataract, rust-colored anterior subcapsular deposits, iris heterochromia, pupillary mydriasis, and depressed electroretinogram amplitudes.

    **H44.321** **Siderosis of eye, right eye**

    **H44.322** **Siderosis of eye, left eye**

    **H44.323** **Siderosis of eye, bilateral**

    **H44.329** **Siderosis of eye, unspecified eye**

✓6ᵗʰ **H44.39** **Other degenerative disorders of globe**

    **H44.391** **Other degenerative disorders of globe, right eye**

    **H44.392** **Other degenerative disorders of globe, left eye**

    **H44.393** **Other degenerative disorders of globe, bilateral**

    **H44.399** **Other degenerative disorders of globe, unspecified eye**

✓5ᵗʰ **H44.4** **Hypotony of eye**

    **H44.40** **Unspecified hypotony of eye**

✓6ᵗʰ **H44.41** **Flat anterior chamber hypotony of eye**

    **H44.411** **Flat anterior chamber hypotony of right eye**

    **H44.412** **Flat anterior chamber hypotony of left eye**

    **H44.413** **Flat anterior chamber hypotony of eye, bilateral**

    **H44.419** **Flat anterior chamber hypotony of unspecified eye**

✓6ᵗʰ **H44.42** **Hypotony of eye due to ocular fistula**

    **H44.421** **Hypotony of right eye due to ocular fistula**

    **H44.422** **Hypotony of left eye due to ocular fistula**

    **H44.423** **Hypotony of eye due to ocular fistula, bilateral**

    **H44.429** **Hypotony of unspecified eye due to ocular fistula**

✓6ᵗʰ **H44.43** **Hypotony of eye due to other ocular disorders**

    **H44.431** **Hypotony of eye due to other ocular disorders, right eye**

    **H44.432** **Hypotony of eye due to other ocular disorders, left eye**

    **H44.433** **Hypotony of eye due to other ocular disorders, bilateral**

    **H44.439** **Hypotony of eye due to other ocular disorders, unspecified eye**

✓6ᵗʰ **H44.44** **Primary hypotony of eye**

    **H44.441** **Primary hypotony of right eye**

    **H44.442** **Primary hypotony of left eye**

    **H44.443** **Primary hypotony of eye, bilateral**

    **H44.449** **Primary hypotony of unspecified eye**

✓5ᵗʰ **H44.5** **Degenerated conditions of globe**

    **H44.50** **Unspecified degenerated conditions of globe**

✓6ᵗʰ **H44.51** **Absolute glaucoma**

    **H44.511** **Absolute glaucoma, right eye**

    **H44.512** **Absolute glaucoma, left eye**

    **H44.513** **Absolute glaucoma, bilateral**

    **H44.519** **Absolute glaucoma, unspecified eye**

✓6ᵗʰ **H44.52** **Atrophy of globe**

    Phthisis bulbi

    **H44.521** **Atrophy of globe, right eye**

    **H44.522** **Atrophy of globe, left eye**

    **H44.523** **Atrophy of globe, bilateral**

    **H44.529** **Atrophy of globe, unspecified eye**

✓6ᵗʰ **H44.53** **Leucocoria**

    **H44.531** **Leucocoria, right eye**

    **H44.532** **Leucocoria, left eye**

    **H44.533** **Leucocoria, bilateral**

    **H44.539** **Leucocoria, unspecified eye**

✓5ᵗʰ **H44.6** **Retained (old) intraocular foreign body, magnetic**

    Use additional code to identify magnetic foreign body (Z18.11)

    *EXCLUDES 1* current intraocular foreign body (S05.-)

    *EXCLUDES 2* retained foreign body in eyelid (H02.81-)

        retained (old) foreign body following penetrating wound of orbit (H05.5-)

        retained (old) intraocular foreign body, nonmagnetic (H44.7-)

✓6ᵗʰ **H44.60** **Unspecified retained (old) intraocular foreign body, magnetic**

    **H44.601** **Unspecified retained (old) intraocular foreign body, magnetic, right eye**

    **H44.602** **Unspecified retained (old) intraocular foreign body, magnetic, left eye**

    **H44.603** **Unspecified retained (old) intraocular foreign body, magnetic, bilateral**

    **H44.609** **Unspecified retained (old) intraocular foreign body, magnetic, unspecified eye**

✓6ᵗʰ **H44.61** **Retained (old) magnetic foreign body in anterior chamber**

    **H44.611** **Retained (old) magnetic foreign body in anterior chamber, right eye**

    **H44.612** **Retained (old) magnetic foreign body in anterior chamber, left eye**

    **H44.613** **Retained (old) magnetic foreign body in anterior chamber, bilateral**

    **H44.619** **Retained (old) magnetic foreign body in anterior chamber, unspecified eye**

✓6ᵗʰ **H44.62** **Retained (old) magnetic foreign body in iris or ciliary body**

    **H44.621** **Retained (old) magnetic foreign body in iris or ciliary body, right eye**

    **H44.622** **Retained (old) magnetic foreign body in iris or ciliary body, left eye**

    **H44.623** **Retained (old) magnetic foreign body in iris or ciliary body, bilateral**

    **H44.629** **Retained (old) magnetic foreign body in iris or ciliary body, unspecified eye**

✓6ᵗʰ **H44.63** **Retained (old) magnetic foreign body in lens**

    **H44.631** **Retained (old) magnetic foreign body in lens, right eye**

    **H44.632** **Retained (old) magnetic foreign body in lens, left eye**

    **H44.633** **Retained (old) magnetic foreign body in lens, bilateral**

    **H44.639** **Retained (old) magnetic foreign body in lens, unspecified eye**

✓6ᵗʰ **H44.64** **Retained (old) magnetic foreign body in posterior wall of globe**

    **H44.641** **Retained (old) magnetic foreign body in posterior wall of globe, right eye**

    **H44.642** **Retained (old) magnetic foreign body in posterior wall of globe, left eye**

    **H44.643** **Retained (old) magnetic foreign body in posterior wall of globe, bilateral**

    **H44.649** **Retained (old) magnetic foreign body in posterior wall of globe, unspecified eye**

✓6ᵗʰ **H44.65** **Retained (old) magnetic foreign body in vitreous body**

    **H44.651** **Retained (old) magnetic foreign body in vitreous body, right eye**

    **H44.652** **Retained (old) magnetic foreign body in vitreous body, left eye**

    **H44.653** **Retained (old) magnetic foreign body in vitreous body, bilateral**

    **H44.659** **Retained (old) magnetic foreign body in vitreous body, unspecified eye**

✓6ᵗʰ **H44.69** **Retained (old) intraocular foreign body, magnetic, in other or multiple sites**

    **H44.691** **Retained (old) intraocular foreign body, magnetic, in other or multiple sites, right eye**

    **H44.692** **Retained (old) intraocular foreign body, magnetic, in other or multiple sites, left eye**

    **H44.693** **Retained (old) intraocular foreign body, magnetic, in other or multiple sites, bilateral**

N Newborn: 0    P Pediatric: 0-17    M Maternity: 12-55    A Adult: 15-124    MCC Major CC Condition    PDx MCC PDx acts as own MCC    CC CC Condition    PDx CC PDx acts as own CC

**604**      ICD-10-CM 2018

H44.699   **Retained (old) intraocular foreign body, magnetic, in other or multiple sites, unspecified eye**

✓5ᵗʰ **H44.7**   **Retained (old) intraocular foreign body, nonmagnetic**
Use additional code to identify nonmagnetic foreign body (Z18.01–Z18.10, Z18.12, Z18.2–Z18.9)
    **EXCLUDES 1**   current intraocular foreign body (S05.-)
    **EXCLUDES 2**   retained foreign body in eyelid (H02.81-)
          retained (old) foreign body following penetrating wound of orbit (H05.5-)
          retained (old) intraocular foreign body, magnetic (H44.6-)

✓6ᵗʰ **H44.70**   **Unspecified retained (old) intraocular foreign body, nonmagnetic**
    H44.701   **Unspecified retained (old) intraocular foreign body, nonmagnetic, right eye**
    H44.702   **Unspecified retained (old) intraocular foreign body, nonmagnetic, left eye**
    H44.703   **Unspecified retained (old) intraocular foreign body, nonmagnetic, bilateral**
    H44.709   **Unspecified retained (old) intraocular foreign body, nonmagnetic, unspecified eye**
         Retained (old) intraocular foreign body NOS

✓6ᵗʰ **H44.71**   **Retained (nonmagnetic) (old) foreign body in anterior chamber**
    H44.711   **Retained (nonmagnetic) (old) foreign body in anterior chamber, right eye**
    H44.712   **Retained (nonmagnetic) (old) foreign body in anterior chamber, left eye**
    H44.713   **Retained (nonmagnetic) (old) foreign body in anterior chamber, bilateral**
    H44.719   **Retained (nonmagnetic) (old) foreign body in anterior chamber, unspecified eye**

✓6ᵗʰ **H44.72**   **Retained (nonmagnetic) (old) foreign body in iris or ciliary body**
    H44.721   **Retained (nonmagnetic) (old) foreign body in iris or ciliary body, right eye**
    H44.722   **Retained (nonmagnetic) (old) foreign body in iris or ciliary body, left eye**
    H44.723   **Retained (nonmagnetic) (old) foreign body in iris or ciliary body, bilateral**
    H44.729   **Retained (nonmagnetic) (old) foreign body in iris or ciliary body, unspecified eye**

✓6ᵗʰ **H44.73**   **Retained (nonmagnetic) (old) foreign body in lens**
    H44.731   **Retained (nonmagnetic) (old) foreign body in lens, right eye**
    H44.732   **Retained (nonmagnetic) (old) foreign body in lens, left eye**
    H44.733   **Retained (nonmagnetic) (old) foreign body in lens, bilateral**
    H44.739   **Retained (nonmagnetic) (old) foreign body in lens, unspecified eye**

✓6ᵗʰ **H44.74**   **Retained (nonmagnetic) (old) foreign body in posterior wall of globe**
    H44.741   **Retained (nonmagnetic) (old) foreign body in posterior wall of globe, right eye**
    H44.742   **Retained (nonmagnetic) (old) foreign body in posterior wall of globe, left eye**
    H44.743   **Retained (nonmagnetic) (old) foreign body in posterior wall of globe, bilateral**
    H44.749   **Retained (nonmagnetic) (old) foreign body in posterior wall of globe, unspecified eye**

✓6ᵗʰ **H44.75**   **Retained (nonmagnetic) (old) foreign body in vitreous body**
    H44.751   **Retained (nonmagnetic) (old) foreign body in vitreous body, right eye**
    H44.752   **Retained (nonmagnetic) (old) foreign body in vitreous body, left eye**
    H44.753   **Retained (nonmagnetic) (old) foreign body in vitreous body, bilateral**
    H44.759   **Retained (nonmagnetic) (old) foreign body in vitreous body, unspecified eye**

✓6ᵗʰ **H44.79**   **Retained (old) intraocular foreign body, nonmagnetic, in other or multiple sites**
    H44.791   **Retained (old) intraocular foreign body, nonmagnetic, in other or multiple sites, right eye**
    H44.792   **Retained (old) intraocular foreign body, nonmagnetic, in other or multiple sites, left eye**
    H44.793   **Retained (old) intraocular foreign body, nonmagnetic, in other or multiple sites, bilateral**
    H44.799   **Retained (old) intraocular foreign body, nonmagnetic, in other or multiple sites, unspecified eye**

✓5ᵗʰ **H44.8**   **Other disorders of globe**
   ✓6ᵗʰ **H44.81**   **Hemophthalmos**
      **DEF:** Pool of blood within eyeball, not from current injury.
    H44.811   **Hemophthalmos, right eye**
    H44.812   **Hemophthalmos, left eye**
    H44.813   **Hemophthalmos, bilateral**
    H44.819   **Hemophthalmos, unspecified eye**
   ✓6ᵗʰ **H44.82**   **Luxation of globe**
    H44.821   **Luxation of globe, right eye**
    H44.822   **Luxation of globe, left eye**
    H44.823   **Luxation of globe, bilateral**
    H44.829   **Luxation of globe, unspecified eye**
    **H44.89**   **Other disorders of globe**
  **H44.9**   **Unspecified disorder of globe**

## Disorders of optic nerve and visual pathways (H46-H47)

✓4ᵗʰ **H46**   **Optic neuritis**
    **EXCLUDES 2**   ischemic optic neuropathy (H47.01-)
          neuromyelitis optica [Devic] (G36.0)

    **CC Excl: For CC codes in category H46:** PDX collection 633

✓5ᵗʰ **H46.0**   **Optic papillitis**
    **H46.00**   **Optic papillitis, unspecified eye**   `CC`
    **H46.01**   **Optic papillitis, right eye**   `CC`
    **H46.02**   **Optic papillitis, left eye**   `CC`
    **H46.03**   **Optic papillitis, bilateral**   `CC`
✓5ᵗʰ **H46.1**   **Retrobulbar neuritis**
    Retrobulbar neuritis NOS
    **EXCLUDES 1**   syphilitic retrobulbar neuritis (A52.15)
    **H46.10**   **Retrobulbar neuritis, unspecified eye**   `CC`
    **H46.11**   **Retrobulbar neuritis, right eye**   `CC`
    **H46.12**   **Retrobulbar neuritis, left eye**   `CC`
    **H46.13**   **Retrobulbar neuritis, bilateral**   `CC`
  **H46.2**   **Nutritional optic neuropathy**
  **H46.3**   **Toxic optic neuropathy**
    Code first (T51-T65) to identify cause
  **H46.8**   **Other optic neuritis**   `CC`
  **H46.9**   **Unspecified optic neuritis**   `CC`

✓4ᵗʰ **H47**   **Other disorders of optic [2nd] nerve and visual pathways**
✓5ᵗʰ **H47.0**   **Disorders of optic nerve, not elsewhere classified**
   ✓6ᵗʰ **H47.01**   **Ischemic optic neuropathy**
    H47.011   **Ischemic optic neuropathy, right eye**
    H47.012   **Ischemic optic neuropathy, left eye**
    H47.013   **Ischemic optic neuropathy, bilateral**
    H47.019   **Ischemic optic neuropathy, unspecified eye**
   ✓6ᵗʰ **H47.02**   **Hemorrhage in optic nerve sheath**
    H47.021   **Hemorrhage in optic nerve sheath, right eye**
    H47.022   **Hemorrhage in optic nerve sheath, left eye**
    H47.023   **Hemorrhage in optic nerve sheath, bilateral**
    H47.029   **Hemorrhage in optic nerve sheath, unspecified eye**
   ✓6ᵗʰ **H47.03**   **Optic nerve hypoplasia**
    H47.031   **Optic nerve hypoplasia, right eye**
    H47.032   **Optic nerve hypoplasia, left eye**
    H47.033   **Optic nerve hypoplasia, bilateral**
    H47.039   **Optic nerve hypoplasia, unspecified eye**

☑6ᵗʰ **H47.09** **Other disorders of optic nerve, not elsewhere classified**
　　Compression of optic nerve

　　**H47.091** **Other disorders of optic nerve, not elsewhere classified, right eye**

　　**H47.092** **Other disorders of optic nerve, not elsewhere classified, left eye**

　　**H47.093** **Other disorders of optic nerve, not elsewhere classified, bilateral**

　　**H47.099** **Other disorders of optic nerve, not elsewhere classified, unspecified eye**

☑5ᵗʰ **H47.1** **Papilledema**

　　**H47.10** **Unspecified papilledema** `CC`
　　　CC Excl: PDX collection 634

　　**H47.11** **Papilledema associated with increased intracranial pressure** `CC`
　　　CC Excl: PDX collection 634

　　**H47.12** **Papilledema associated with decreased ocular pressure**

　　**H47.13** **Papilledema associated with retinal disorder**

☑6ᵗʰ **H47.14** **Foster-Kennedy syndrome**

　　**H47.141** **Foster-Kennedy syndrome, right eye**

　　**H47.142** **Foster-Kennedy syndrome, left eye**

　　**H47.143** **Foster-Kennedy syndrome, bilateral**

　　**H47.149** **Foster-Kennedy syndrome, unspecified eye**

☑5ᵗʰ **H47.2** **Optic atrophy**

　　**H47.20** **Unspecified optic atrophy**

☑6ᵗʰ **H47.21** **Primary optic atrophy**

　　**H47.211** **Primary optic atrophy, right eye**

　　**H47.212** **Primary optic atrophy, left eye**

　　**H47.213** **Primary optic atrophy, bilateral**

　　**H47.219** **Primary optic atrophy, unspecified eye**

　　**H47.22** **Hereditary optic atrophy**
　　　Leber's optic atrophy

☑6ᵗʰ **H47.23** **Glaucomatous optic atrophy**

　　**H47.231** **Glaucomatous optic atrophy, right eye**

　　**H47.232** **Glaucomatous optic atrophy, left eye**

　　**H47.233** **Glaucomatous optic atrophy, bilateral**

　　**H47.239** **Glaucomatous optic atrophy, unspecified eye**

☑6ᵗʰ **H47.29** **Other optic atrophy**
　　　Temporal pallor of optic disc

　　**H47.291** **Other optic atrophy, right eye**

　　**H47.292** **Other optic atrophy, left eye**

　　**H47.293** **Other optic atrophy, bilateral**

　　**H47.299** **Other optic atrophy, unspecified eye**

☑5ᵗʰ **H47.3** **Other disorders of optic disc**

☑6ᵗʰ **H47.31** **Coloboma of optic disc**

　　**H47.311** **Coloboma of optic disc, right eye**

　　**H47.312** **Coloboma of optic disc, left eye**

　　**H47.313** **Coloboma of optic disc, bilateral**

　　**H47.319** **Coloboma of optic disc, unspecified eye**

☑6ᵗʰ **H47.32** **Drusen of optic disc**

　　**H47.321** **Drusen of optic disc, right eye**

　　**H47.322** **Drusen of optic disc, left eye**

　　**H47.323** **Drusen of optic disc, bilateral**

　　**H47.329** **Drusen of optic disc, unspecified eye**

☑6ᵗʰ **H47.33** **Pseudopapilledema of optic disc**

　　**H47.331** **Pseudopapilledema of optic disc, right eye**

　　**H47.332** **Pseudopapilledema of optic disc, left eye**

　　**H47.333** **Pseudopapilledema of optic disc, bilateral**

　　**H47.339** **Pseudopapilledema of optic disc, unspecified eye**

☑6ᵗʰ **H47.39** **Other disorders of optic disc**

　　**H47.391** **Other disorders of optic disc, right eye**

　　**H47.392** **Other disorders of optic disc, left eye**

　　**H47.393** **Other disorders of optic disc, bilateral**

　　**H47.399** **Other disorders of optic disc, unspecified eye**

☑5ᵗʰ **H47.4** **Disorders of optic chiasm**
　　　Code also underlying condition

　　CC Excl: For CC codes in subcategory H47.4:
　　PDX collection 635

　　**H47.41** **Disorders of optic chiasm in (due to) inflammatory disorders** `CC`

　　**H47.42** **Disorders of optic chiasm in (due to) neoplasm** `CC`

　　**H47.43** **Disorders of optic chiasm in (due to) vascular disorders** `CC`

　　**H47.49** **Disorders of optic chiasm in (due to) other disorders** `CC`

☑5ᵗʰ **H47.5** **Disorders of other visual pathways**
　　　Disorders of optic tracts, geniculate nuclei and optic radiations
　　　Code also underlying condition

　　CC Excl: For CC codes in subcategory H47.5:
　　PDX collection 635

☑6ᵗʰ **H47.51** **Disorders of visual pathways in (due to) inflammatory disorders**

　　**H47.511** **Disorders of visual pathways in (due to) inflammatory disorders, right side** `CC`

　　**H47.512** **Disorders of visual pathways in (due to) inflammatory disorders, left side** `CC`

　　**H47.519** **Disorders of visual pathways in (due to) inflammatory disorders, unspecified side** `CC`

☑6ᵗʰ **H47.52** **Disorders of visual pathways in (due to) neoplasm**

　　**H47.521** **Disorders of visual pathways in (due to) neoplasm, right side** `CC`

　　**H47.522** **Disorders of visual pathways in (due to) neoplasm, left side** `CC`

　　**H47.529** **Disorders of visual pathways in (due to) neoplasm, unspecified side** `CC`

☑6ᵗʰ **H47.53** **Disorders of visual pathways in (due to) vascular disorders**

　　**H47.531** **Disorders of visual pathways in (due to) vascular disorders, right side** `CC`

　　**H47.532** **Disorders of visual pathways in (due to) vascular disorders, left side** `CC`

　　**H47.539** **Disorders of visual pathways in (due to) vascular disorders, unspecified side** `CC`

☑5ᵗʰ **H47.6** **Disorders of visual cortex**
　　　Code also underlying condition
　　　**EXCLUDES 1** injury to visual cortex S04.04

　　CC Excl: For CC codes in subcategory H47.6:
　　PDX collection 636

☑6ᵗʰ **H47.61** **Cortical blindness**

　　**H47.611** **Cortical blindness, right side of brain**

　　**H47.612** **Cortical blindness, left side of brain**

　　**H47.619** **Cortical blindness, unspecified side of brain**

☑6ᵗʰ **H47.62** **Disorders of visual cortex in (due to) inflammatory disorders**

　　**H47.621** **Disorders of visual cortex in (due to) inflammatory disorders, right side of brain** `CC`

　　**H47.622** **Disorders of visual cortex in (due to) inflammatory disorders, left side of brain** `CC`

　　**H47.629** **Disorders of visual cortex in (due to) inflammatory disorders, unspecified side of brain** `CC`

☑6ᵗʰ **H47.63** **Disorders of visual cortex in (due to) neoplasm**

　　**H47.631** **Disorders of visual cortex in (due to) neoplasm, right side of brain** `CC`

　　**H47.632** **Disorders of visual cortex in (due to) neoplasm, left side of brain** `CC`

　　**H47.639** **Disorders of visual cortex in (due to) neoplasm, unspecified side of brain** `CC`

☑6ᵗʰ **H47.64** **Disorders of visual cortex in (due to) vascular disorders**

　　**H47.641** **Disorders of visual cortex in (due to) vascular disorders, right side of brain** `CC`

H47.642   **Disorders of visual cortex in (due to)** `CC`
**vascular disorders, left side of brain**

H47.649   **Disorders of visual cortex in (due to)** `CC`
**vascular disorders, unspecified side of
brain**

**H47.9   Unspecified disorder of visual pathways**

## Disorders of ocular muscles, binocular movement, accommodation and refraction (H49–H52)

> *EXCLUDES 2*   *nystagmus and other irregular eye movements (H55)*

☑4th **H49   Paralytic strabismus**
> *EXCLUDES 2*   *internal ophthalmoplegia (H52.51-)*
> *internuclear ophthalmoplegia (H51.2-)*
> *progressive supranuclear ophthalmoplegia (G23.1)*

☑5th **H49.0   Third [oculomotor] nerve palsy**
   H49.00   **Third [oculomotor] nerve palsy, unspecified eye**
   H49.01   **Third [oculomotor] nerve palsy, right eye**
   H49.02   **Third [oculomotor] nerve palsy, left eye**
   H49.03   **Third [oculomotor] nerve palsy, bilateral**

☑5th **H49.1   Fourth [trochlear] nerve palsy**
   H49.10   **Fourth [trochlear] nerve palsy, unspecified eye**
   H49.11   **Fourth [trochlear] nerve palsy, right eye**
   H49.12   **Fourth [trochlear] nerve palsy, left eye**
   H49.13   **Fourth [trochlear] nerve palsy, bilateral**

☑5th **H49.2   Sixth [abducent] nerve palsy**
   H49.20   **Sixth [abducent] nerve palsy, unspecified eye**
   H49.21   **Sixth [abducent] nerve palsy, right eye**
   H49.22   **Sixth [abducent] nerve palsy, left eye**
   H49.23   **Sixth [abducent] nerve palsy, bilateral**

☑5th **H49.3   Total (external) ophthalmoplegia**
   H49.30   **Total (external) ophthalmoplegia, unspecified eye**
   H49.31   **Total (external) ophthalmoplegia, right eye**
   H49.32   **Total (external) ophthalmoplegia, left eye**
   H49.33   **Total (external) ophthalmoplegia, bilateral**

☑5th **H49.4   Progressive external ophthalmoplegia**
> *EXCLUDES 1*   *Kearns-Sayre syndrome (H49.81-)*

   H49.40   **Progressive external ophthalmoplegia, unspecified
eye**
   H49.41   **Progressive external ophthalmoplegia, right eye**
   H49.42   **Progressive external ophthalmoplegia, left eye**
   H49.43   **Progressive external ophthalmoplegia, bilateral**

☑5th **H49.8   Other paralytic strabismus**

> **CC Excl: For CC codes in subcategory H49.8:**
> PDX collection 545

☑6th **H49.81   Kearns-Sayre syndrome**
Progressive external ophthalmoplegia with
pigmentary retinopathy
Use additional code for other manifestation, such as:
heart block (I45.9)
   H49.811   **Kearns-Sayre syndrome, right eye** `CC` `HCC`
   H49.812   **Kearns-Sayre syndrome, left eye** `CC` `HCC`
   H49.813   **Kearns-Sayre syndrome, bilateral** `CC` `HCC`
   H49.819   **Kearns-Sayre syndrome,** `CC` `HCC`
**unspecified eye**

☑6th **H49.88   Other paralytic strabismus**
External ophthalmoplegia NOS
   H49.881   **Other paralytic strabismus, right eye**
   H49.882   **Other paralytic strabismus, left eye**
   H49.883   **Other paralytic strabismus, bilateral**
   H49.889   **Other paralytic strabismus, unspecified
eye**

**H49.9   Unspecified paralytic strabismus**

☑4th **H50   Other strabismus**
☑5th **H50.0   Esotropia**
Convergent concomitant strabismus
> *EXCLUDES 1*   *intermittent esotropia (H50.31-, H50.32)*

   H50.00   **Unspecified esotropia**
☑6th **H50.01   Monocular esotropia**
   H50.011   **Monocular esotropia, right eye**
   H50.012   **Monocular esotropia, left eye**

**Eye Muscle Diseases**

R.      L.
Monocular (one eye only) esotropia (inward)

Monocular exotropia (outward)

Monocular hypertropia (upward)

☑6th **H50.02   Monocular esotropia with A pattern**
   H50.021   **Monocular esotropia with A pattern,
right eye**
   H50.022   **Monocular esotropia with A pattern,
left eye**

☑6th **H50.03   Monocular esotropia with V pattern**
   H50.031   **Monocular esotropia with V pattern,
right eye**
   H50.032   **Monocular esotropia with V pattern,
left eye**

☑6th **H50.04   Monocular esotropia with other noncomitancies**
   H50.041   **Monocular esotropia with other
noncomitancies, right eye**
   H50.042   **Monocular esotropia with other
noncomitancies, left eye**

   H50.05   **Alternating esotropia**
   H50.06   **Alternating esotropia with A pattern**
   H50.07   **Alternating esotropia with V pattern**
   H50.08   **Alternating esotropia with other noncomitancies**

☑5th **H50.1   Exotropia**
Divergent concomitant strabismus
> *EXCLUDES 1*   *intermittent exotropia (H50.33-, H50.34)*

   H50.10   **Unspecified exotropia**
☑6th **H50.11   Monocular exotropia**
   H50.111   **Monocular exotropia, right eye**
   H50.112   **Monocular exotropia, left eye**
☑6th **H50.12   Monocular exotropia with A pattern**
   H50.121   **Monocular exotropia with A pattern,
right eye**
   H50.122   **Monocular exotropia with A pattern,
left eye**
☑6th **H50.13   Monocular exotropia with V pattern**
   H50.131   **Monocular exotropia with V pattern,
right eye**
   H50.132   **Monocular exotropia with V pattern,
left eye**
☑6th **H50.14   Monocular exotropia with other noncomitancies**
   H50.141   **Monocular exotropia with other
noncomitancies, right eye**
   H50.142   **Monocular exotropia with other
noncomitancies, left eye**

   H50.15   **Alternating exotropia**
   H50.16   **Alternating exotropia with A pattern**
   H50.17   **Alternating exotropia with V pattern**
   H50.18   **Alternating exotropia with other noncomitancies**

☑5th **H50.2   Vertical strabismus**
Hypertropia
   H50.21   **Vertical strabismus, right eye**
   H50.22   **Vertical strabismus, left eye**

☑5th **H50.3   Intermittent heterotropia**
   H50.30   **Unspecified intermittent heterotropia**

---

☑ Additional Character Req    ☑x7th Placeholder Alert    Unacceptable PDx    Manifestation    `H1`-`H14` HAC    `HCC` CMS-HCC Condition    *EXCLUDES 1* Not Coded Here    *EXCLUDES 2* Not Included Here

ICD-10-CM 2018                                         **607**

✓6th **H50.31** Intermittent monocular esotropia
    **H50.311** Intermittent monocular esotropia, right eye
    **H50.312** Intermittent monocular esotropia, left eye
**H50.32** Intermittent alternating esotropia
✓6th **H50.33** Intermittent monocular exotropia
    **H50.331** Intermittent monocular exotropia, right eye
    **H50.332** Intermittent monocular exotropia, left eye
**H50.34** Intermittent alternating exotropia
✓5th **H50.4** Other and unspecified heterotropia
    **H50.40** Unspecified heterotropia
✓6th **H50.41** Cyclotropia
    **H50.411** Cyclotropia, right eye
    **H50.412** Cyclotropia, left eye
**H50.42** Monofixation syndrome
**H50.43** Accommodative component in esotropia
✓5th **H50.5** Heterophoria
    **H50.50** Unspecified heterophoria
    **H50.51** Esophoria
    **H50.52** Exophoria
    **H50.53** Vertical heterophoria
    **H50.54** Cyclophoria
    **H50.55** Alternating heterophoria
✓5th **H50.6** Mechanical strabismus
    **H50.60** Mechanical strabismus, unspecified
✓6th **H50.61** Brown's sheath syndrome
    **H50.611** Brown's sheath syndrome, right eye
    **H50.612** Brown's sheath syndrome, left eye
**H50.69** Other mechanical strabismus
    Strabismus due to adhesions
    Traumatic limitation of duction of eye muscle
✓5th **H50.8** Other specified strabismus
✓6th **H50.81** Duane's syndrome
    **H50.811** Duane's syndrome, right eye
    **H50.812** Duane's syndrome, left eye
**H50.89** Other specified strabismus
**H50.9** Unspecified strabismus

✓4th **H51** Other disorders of binocular movement
**H51.0** Palsy (spasm) of conjugate gaze
✓5th **H51.1** Convergence insufficiency and excess
    **H51.11** Convergence insufficiency
    **H51.12** Convergence excess
✓5th **H51.2** Internuclear ophthalmoplegia
    **H51.20** Internuclear ophthalmoplegia, unspecified eye
    **H51.21** Internuclear ophthalmoplegia, right eye
    **H51.22** Internuclear ophthalmoplegia, left eye
    **H51.23** Internuclear ophthalmoplegia, bilateral
**H51.8** Other specified disorders of binocular movement
**H51.9** Unspecified disorder of binocular movement

✓4th **H52** Disorders of refraction and accommodation
✓5th **H52.0** Hypermetropia
    **H52.00** Hypermetropia, unspecified eye
    **H52.01** Hypermetropia, right eye
    **H52.02** Hypermetropia, left eye
    **H52.03** Hypermetropia, bilateral
✓5th **H52.1** Myopia
    EXCLUDES 1 *degenerative myopia (H44.2-)*
    **H52.10** Myopia, unspecified eye
    **H52.11** Myopia, right eye
    **H52.12** Myopia, left eye
    **H52.13** Myopia, bilateral
✓5th **H52.2** Astigmatism
✓6th **H52.20** Unspecified astigmatism
    **H52.201** Unspecified astigmatism, right eye
    **H52.202** Unspecified astigmatism, left eye
    **H52.203** Unspecified astigmatism, bilateral
    **H52.209** Unspecified astigmatism, unspecified eye

✓6th **H52.21** Irregular astigmatism
    **H52.211** Irregular astigmatism, right eye
    **H52.212** Irregular astigmatism, left eye
    **H52.213** Irregular astigmatism, bilateral
    **H52.219** Irregular astigmatism, unspecified eye
✓6th **H52.22** Regular astigmatism
    **H52.221** Regular astigmatism, right eye
    **H52.222** Regular astigmatism, left eye
    **H52.223** Regular astigmatism, bilateral
    **H52.229** Regular astigmatism, unspecified eye
✓5th **H52.3** Anisometropia and aniseikonia
    **H52.31** Anisometropia
    **H52.32** Aniseikonia
**H52.4** Presbyopia
✓5th **H52.5** Disorders of accommodation
✓6th **H52.51** Internal ophthalmoplegia (complete) (total)
    **H52.511** Internal ophthalmoplegia (complete) (total), right eye
    **H52.512** Internal ophthalmoplegia (complete) (total), left eye
    **H52.513** Internal ophthalmoplegia (complete) (total), bilateral
    **H52.519** Internal ophthalmoplegia (complete) (total), unspecified eye
✓6th **H52.52** Paresis of accommodation
    **H52.521** Paresis of accommodation, right eye
    **H52.522** Paresis of accommodation, left eye
    **H52.523** Paresis of accommodation, bilateral
    **H52.529** Paresis of accommodation, unspecified eye
✓6th **H52.53** Spasm of accommodation
    **H52.531** Spasm of accommodation, right eye
    **H52.532** Spasm of accommodation, left eye
    **H52.533** Spasm of accommodation, bilateral
    **H52.539** Spasm of accommodation, unspecified eye
**H52.6** Other disorders of refraction
**H52.7** Unspecified disorder of refraction

### Visual disturbances and blindness (H53-H54)

✓4th **H53** Visual disturbances
✓5th **H53.0** Amblyopia ex anopsia
    EXCLUDES 1 *amblyopia due to vitamin A deficiency (E50.5)*
✓6th **H53.00** Unspecified amblyopia
    **H53.001** Unspecified amblyopia, right eye
    **H53.002** Unspecified amblyopia, left eye
    **H53.003** Unspecified amblyopia, bilateral
    **H53.009** Unspecified amblyopia, unspecified eye
✓6th **H53.01** Deprivation amblyopia
    **H53.011** Deprivation amblyopia, right eye
    **H53.012** Deprivation amblyopia, left eye
    **H53.013** Deprivation amblyopia, bilateral
    **H53.019** Deprivation amblyopia, unspecified eye
✓6th **H53.02** Refractive amblyopia
    **H53.021** Refractive amblyopia, right eye
    **H53.022** Refractive amblyopia, left eye
    **H53.023** Refractive amblyopia, bilateral
    **H53.029** Refractive amblyopia, unspecified eye
✓6th **H53.03** Strabismic amblyopia
    EXCLUDES 1 *strabismus (H50.-)*
    **H53.031** Strabismic amblyopia, right eye
    **H53.032** Strabismic amblyopia, left eye
    **H53.033** Strabismic amblyopia, bilateral
    **H53.039** Strabismic amblyopia, unspecified eye
✓6th **H53.04** Amblyopia suspect
    **H53.041** Amblyopia suspect, right eye
    **H53.042** Amblyopia suspect, left eye
    **H53.043** Amblyopia suspect, bilateral
    **H53.049** Amblyopia suspect, unspecified eye

N Newborn: 0  P Pediatric: 0-17  M Maternity: 12-55  A Adult: 15-124  MCC Major CC Condition  PDxMCC PDx acts as own MCC  CC CC Condition  PDxCC PDx acts as own CC

**608**    ICD-10-CM 2018

✓5ᵗʰ **H53.1 Subjective visual disturbances**
> EXCLUDES 1 · *subjective visual disturbances due to vitamin A deficiency (E50.5)*
> *visual hallucinations (R44.1)*

**CC Excl: For CC codes in subcategory H53.1:**
PDX collection 637

**H53.10 Unspecified subjective visual disturbances**

**H53.11 Day blindness**
Hemeralopia

✓6ᵗʰ **H53.12 Transient visual loss**
Scintillating scotoma
> EXCLUDES 1 · *amaurosis fugax (G45.3-)*
> *transient retinal artery occlusion (H34.0-)*

**H53.121 Transient visual loss, right eye** CC
**H53.122 Transient visual loss, left eye** CC
**H53.123 Transient visual loss, bilateral** CC
**H53.129 Transient visual loss, unspecified eye** CC

✓6ᵗʰ **H53.13 Sudden visual loss**

**H53.131 Sudden visual loss, right eye** CC
**H53.132 Sudden visual loss, left eye** CC
**H53.133 Sudden visual loss, bilateral** CC
**H53.139 Sudden visual loss, unspecified eye** CC

✓6ᵗʰ **H53.14 Visual discomfort**
Asthenopia
Photophobia

**H53.141 Visual discomfort, right eye**
**H53.142 Visual discomfort, left eye**
**H53.143 Visual discomfort, bilateral**
**H53.149 Visual discomfort, unspecified**

**H53.15 Visual distortions of shape and size**
Metamorphopsia

**H53.16 Psychophysical visual disturbances**

**H53.19 Other subjective visual disturbances**
Visual halos

**H53.2 Diplopia**
Double vision

✓5ᵗʰ **H53.3 Other and unspecified disorders of binocular vision**

**H53.30 Unspecified disorder of binocular vision**
**H53.31 Abnormal retinal correspondence**
**H53.32 Fusion with defective stereopsis**
**H53.33 Simultaneous visual perception without fusion**
**H53.34 Suppression of binocular vision**

✓5ᵗʰ **H53.4 Visual field defects**

**H53.40 Unspecified visual field defects**

✓6ᵗʰ **H53.41 Scotoma involving central area**
Central scotoma

**H53.411 Scotoma involving central area, right eye**
**H53.412 Scotoma involving central area, left eye**
**H53.413 Scotoma involving central area, bilateral**
**H53.419 Scotoma involving central area, unspecified eye**

✓6ᵗʰ **H53.42 Scotoma of blind spot area**
Enlarged blind spot

**H53.421 Scotoma of blind spot area, right eye**
**H53.422 Scotoma of blind spot area, left eye**
**H53.423 Scotoma of blind spot area, bilateral**
**H53.429 Scotoma of blind spot area, unspecified eye**

✓6ᵗʰ **H53.43 Sector or arcuate defects**
Arcuate scotoma
Bjerrum scotoma

**H53.431 Sector or arcuate defects, right eye**
**H53.432 Sector or arcuate defects, left eye**
**H53.433 Sector or arcuate defects, bilateral**
**H53.439 Sector or arcuate defects, unspecified eye**

✓6ᵗʰ **H53.45 Other localized visual field defect**
Peripheral visual field defect
Ring scotoma NOS
Scotoma NOS

**H53.451 Other localized visual field defect, right eye**
**H53.452 Other localized visual field defect, left eye**
**H53.453 Other localized visual field defect, bilateral**

**H53.459 Other localized visual field defect, unspecified eye**

✓6ᵗʰ **H53.46 Homonymous bilateral field defects**
Homonymous hemianopia
Homonymous hemianopsia
Quadrant anopia
Quadrant anopsia

**H53.461 Homonymous bilateral field defects, right side**
**H53.462 Homonymous bilateral field defects, left side**
**H53.469 Homonymous bilateral field defects, unspecified side**
Homonymous bilateral field defects NOS

**H53.47 Heteronymous bilateral field defects**
Heteronymous hemianop(s)ia

✓6ᵗʰ **H53.48 Generalized contraction of visual field**

**H53.481 Generalized contraction of visual field, right eye**
**H53.482 Generalized contraction of visual field, left eye**
**H53.483 Generalized contraction of visual field, bilateral**
**H53.489 Generalized contraction of visual field, unspecified eye**

✓5ᵗʰ **H53.5 Color vision deficiencies**
Color blindness
> EXCLUDES 2 · *day blindness (H53.11)*

**H53.50 Unspecified color vision deficiencies**
Color blindness NOS

**H53.51 Achromatopsia**
**DEF:** Nonprogressive genetic visual disorder; characterized by complete color blindness, decreased vision, and light sensitivity.

**H53.52 Acquired color vision deficiency**

**H53.53 Deuteranomaly**
Deuteranopia
**DEF:** Male-only genetic disorder; difficulty in distinguishing green and red, no shortened spectrum.

**H53.54 Protanomaly**
Protanopia

**H53.55 Tritanomaly**
Tritanopia

**H53.59 Other color vision deficiencies**

✓5ᵗʰ **H53.6 Night blindness**
> EXCLUDES 1 · *night blindness due to vitamin A deficiency (E50.5)*

**H53.60 Unspecified night blindness**
**H53.61 Abnormal dark adaptation curve**
**H53.62 Acquired night blindness**
**H53.63 Congenital night blindness**
**H53.69 Other night blindness**

✓5ᵗʰ **H53.7 Vision sensitivity deficiencies**

**H53.71 Glare sensitivity**
**H53.72 Impaired contrast sensitivity**

**H53.8 Other visual disturbances**

**H53.9 Unspecified visual disturbance**

✓4ᵗʰ **H54 Blindness and low vision**
> NOTE · For definition of visual impairment categories see table below
>
> Code first any associated underlying cause of the blindness
> EXCLUDES 1 · *amaurosis fugax (G45.3)*

✓5ᵗʰ **H54.0 Blindness, both eyes**
Visual impairment categories 3, 4, 5 in both eyes.

● ✓6ᵗʰ **H54.0X Blindness, both eyes, different category levels**

● ✓7ᵗʰ **H54.0X3 Blindness right eye, category 3**

● **H54.0X33 Blindness right eye category 3, blindness left eye category 3**
● **H54.0X34 Blindness right eye category 3, blindness left eye category 4**
● **H54.0X35 Blindness right eye category 3, blindness left eye category 5**

● ✓7ᵗʰ **H54.0X4 Blindness right eye, category 4**

● **H54.0X43 Blindness right eye category 4, blindness left eye category 3**
● **H54.0X44 Blindness right eye category 4, blindness left eye category 4**

✓ Additional Character Req · ✓x7ᵗʰ Placeholder Alert · Unacceptable PDx · Manifestation · H1–H14 HAC · HCC CMS-HCC Condition · EXCLUDES 1 Not Coded Here · EXCLUDES 2 Not Included Here

ICD-10-CM 2018

609

- ●   H54.0X45   **Blindness right eye category 4, blindness left eye category 5**
- ●   √7ᵗʰ   **H54.0X5**   **Blindness right eye, category 5**
- ●   H54.0X53   **Blindness right eye category 5, blindness left eye category 3**
- ●   H54.0X54   **Blindness right eye category 5, blindness left eye category 4**
- ●   H54.0X55   **Blindness right eye category 5, blindness left eye category 5**

√5ᵗʰ   **H54.1**   **Blindness, one eye, low vision other eye**
Visual impairment categories 3, 4, 5 in one eye, with categories 1 or 2 in the other eye.

     H54.10   **Blindness, one eye, low vision other eye, unspecified eyes**

√6ᵗʰ   **H54.11**   **Blindness, right eye, low vision left eye**

- ●   √7ᵗʰ   **H54.113**   **Blindness right eye category 3, low vision left eye**
- ●   H54.1131   **Blindness right eye category 3, low vision left eye category 1**
- ●   H54.1132   **Blindness right eye category 3, low vision left eye category 2**
- ●   √7ᵗʰ   **H54.114**   **Blindness right eye category 4, low vision left eye**
- ●   H54.1141   **Blindness right eye category 4, low vision left eye category 1**
- ●   H54.1142   **Blindness right eye category 4, low vision left eye category 2**
- ●   √7ᵗʰ   **H54.115**   **Blindness right eye category 5, low vision left eye**
- ●   H54.1151   **Blindness right eye category 5, low vision left eye category 1**
- ●   H54.1152   **Blindness right eye category 5, low vision left eye category 2**

√6ᵗʰ   **H54.12**   **Blindness, left eye, low vision right eye**

- ●   √7ᵗʰ   **H54.121**   **Low vision right eye category 1, blindness left eye**
- ●   H54.1213   **Low vision right eye category 1, blindness left eye category 3**
- ●   H54.1214   **Low vision right eye category 1, blindness left eye category 4**
- ●   H54.1215   **Low vision right eye category 1, blindness left eye category 5**
- ●   √7ᵗʰ   **H54.122**   **Low vision right eye category 2, blindness left eye**
- ●   H54.1223   **Low vision right eye category 2, blindness left eye category 3**
- ●   H54.1224   **Low vision right eye category 2, blindness left eye category 4**
- ●   H54.1225   **Low vision right eye category 2, blindness left eye category 5**

√5ᵗʰ   **H54.2**   **Low vision, both eyes**
Visual impairment categories 1 or 2 in both eyes.

- ●   √6ᵗʰ   **H54.2X**   **Low vision, both eyes, different category levels**
- ●   √7ᵗʰ   **H54.2X1**   **Low vision, right eye, category 1**
- ●   H54.2X11   **Low vision right eye category 1, low vision left eye category 1**
- ●   H54.2X12   **Low vision right eye category 1, low vision left eye category 2**

- ●   √7ᵗʰ   **H54.2X2**   **Low vision, right eye, category 2**
- ●   H54.2X21   **Low vision right eye category 2, low vision left eye category 1**
- ●   H54.2X22   **Low vision right eye category 2, low vision left eye category 2**

   **H54.3**   **Unqualified visual loss, both eyes**
Visual impairment category 9 in both eyes.

√5ᵗʰ   **H54.4**   **Blindness, one eye**
Visual impairment categories 3, 4, 5 in one eye [normal vision in other eye].

     H54.40   **Blindness, one eye, unspecified eye**

√6ᵗʰ   **H54.41**   **Blindness, right eye, normal vision left eye**

- ●   √7ᵗʰ   **H54.413**   **Blindness, right eye, category 3**
- ●   H54.413A   **Blindness right eye category 3, normal vision left eye**
- ●   √7ᵗʰ   **H54.414**   **Blindness, right eye, category 4**
- ●   H54.414A   **Blindness right eye category 4, normal vision left eye**
- ●   √7ᵗʰ   **H54.415**   **Blindness, right eye, category 5**
- ●   H54.415A   **Blindness right eye category 5, normal vision left eye**

√6ᵗʰ   **H54.42**   **Blindness, left eye, normal vision right eye**

- ●   √7ᵗʰ   **H54.42A**   **Blindness, left eye, category 3-5**
- ●   H54.42A3   **Blindness left eye category 3, normal vision right eye**
- ●   H54.42A4   **Blindness left eye category 4, normal vision right eye**
- ●   H54.42A5   **Blindness left eye category 5, normal vision right eye**

√5ᵗʰ   **H54.5**   **Low vision, one eye**
Visual impairment categories 1 or 2 in one eye [normal vision in other eye].

     H54.50   **Low vision, one eye, unspecified eye**

√6ᵗʰ   **H54.51**   **Low vision, right eye, normal vision left eye**

- ●   √7ᵗʰ   **H54.511**   **Low vision, right eye, category 1-2**
- ●   H54.511A   **Low vision right eye category 1, normal vision left eye**
- ●   H54.512A   **Low vision right eye category 2, normal vision left eye**

√6ᵗʰ   **H54.52**   **Low vision, left eye, normal vision right eye**

- ●   √7ᵗʰ   **H54.52A**   **Low vision, left eye, category 1-2**
- ●   H54.52A1   **Low vision left eye category 1, normal vision right eye**
- ●   H54.52A2   **Low vision left eye category 2, normal vision right eye**

√5ᵗʰ   **H54.6**   **Unqualified visual loss, one eye**
Visual impairment category 9 in one eye [normal vision in other eye].

     H54.60   **Unqualified visual loss, one eye, unspecified**

     H54.61   **Unqualified visual loss, right eye, normal vision left eye**

     H54.62   **Unqualified visual loss, left eye, normal vision right eye**

   **H54.7**   **Unspecified visual loss**
Visual impairment category 9 NOS

   **H54.8**   **Legal blindness, as defined in USA**
Blindness NOS according to USA definition

     **EXCLUDES 1**   *legal blindness with specification of impairment level (H54.0–H54.7)*

N Newborn: 0   P Pediatric: 0-17   M Maternity: 12-55   A Adult: 15-124   **MCC** Major CC Condition   **PDxMCC** PDx acts as own MCC   **CC** CC Condition   **PDxCC** PDx acts as own CC

**610**        ICD-10-CM 2018

**NOTE** The table below gives a classification of severity of visual impairment recommended by a WHO Study Group on the Prevention of Blindness, Geneva, 6-10 November l972.

The term "low vision" in category H54 comprises categories 1 and 2 of the table, the term "blindness" categories 3, 4 and 5, and the term "unqualified visual loss" category 9.

If the extent of the visual field is taken into account, patients with a field no greater than 10 but greater than 5 around central fixation should be placed in category 3 and patients with a field no greater than 5 around central fixation should be placed in category 4, even if the central acuity is not impaired.

| Category of visual impairment | Visual acuity with best possible correction | |
| --- | --- | --- |
| | Maximum less than: | Minimum equal to or better than: |
| 1 | 6/18<br>3/10 (0.3)<br>20/70 | 6/60<br>1/10 (0.1)<br>20/200 |
| 2 | 6/60<br>1/10 (0.1)<br>20/200 | 3/60<br>1/20 (0.05)<br>20/400 |
| 3 | 3/60<br><br>1/200 (0.05)<br>20/400 | 1/60 (finger counting at one meter)<br>1/50 (0.02)<br>5/300 (20/1200) |
| 4 | 1/60 (finger counting at one meter)<br>1/50 (0.02)<br>5/300 | Light perception |
| 5 | No light perception | |
| 9 | Undetermined or unspecified | |

## Other disorders of eye and adnexa (H55-H57)

✓4ᵗʰ **H55** **Nystagmus and other** irregular eye movements

  ✓5ᵗʰ **H55.0** **Nystagmus**

    **H55.00** **Unspecified nystagmus**

    **H55.01** **Congenital nystagmus**

    **H55.02** **Latent nystagmus**

    **H55.03** **Visual deprivation nystagmus**

    **H55.04** **Dissociated nystagmus**

    **H55.09** **Other** forms of nystagmus

  ✓5ᵗʰ **H55.8** **Other irregular eye movements**

    **H55.81** **Saccadic eye movements**

    **H55.89** **Other** irregular eye movements

✓4ᵗʰ **H57** **Other disorders of eye and adnexa**

  ✓5ᵗʰ **H57.0** **Anomalies of pupillary function**

    **H57.00** **Unspecified anomaly of pupillary function**

    **H57.01** **Argyll Robertson pupil, atypical**
        *EXCLUDES 1*   syphilitic Argyll Robertson pupil (A52.19)

    **H57.02** **Anisocoria**

    **H57.03** **Miosis**

    **H57.04** **Mydriasis**

    ✓6ᵗʰ **H57.05** **Tonic pupil**

      **H57.051** **Tonic pupil,** right eye

      **H57.052** **Tonic pupil,** left eye

      **H57.053** **Tonic pupil,** bilateral

      **H57.059** **Tonic pupil,** unspecified eye

    **H57.09** **Other** anomalies of pupillary function

  ✓5ᵗʰ **H57.1** **Ocular pain**

    **H57.10** **Ocular pain,** unspecified eye

    **H57.11** **Ocular pain,** right eye

    **H57.12** **Ocular pain,** left eye

    **H57.13** **Ocular pain,** bilateral

  **H57.8** **Other specified disorders of eye and adnexa**

  **H57.9** **Unspecified disorder of eye and adnexa**

## Intraoperative and postprocedural complications and disorders of eye and adnexa, not elsewhere classified (H59)

✓4ᵗʰ **H59** **Intraoperative and postprocedural complications and disorders of eye and adnexa, not elsewhere classified**
    *EXCLUDES 1*   mechanical complication of intraocular lens (T85.2)
        mechanical complication of other ocular prosthetic devices, implants and grafts (T85.3)
        pseudophakia (Z96.1)
        secondary cataracts (H26.4-)

  ✓5ᵗʰ **H59.0** **Disorders of the eye** following cataract surgery

    **CC Excl: For CC codes in subcategory H59.0:**
    PDX collection 638

    ✓6ᵗʰ **H59.01** **Keratopathy (bullous aphakic) following cataract surgery**
      Vitreal corneal syndrome
      Vitreous (touch) syndrome

      **H59.011** **Keratopathy (bullous aphakic) following cataract surgery,** right eye   CC

      **H59.012** **Keratopathy (bullous aphakic) following cataract surgery,** left eye   CC

      **H59.013** **Keratopathy (bullous aphakic) following cataract surgery,** bilateral   CC

      **H59.019** **Keratopathy (bullous aphakic) following cataract surgery,** unspecified eye   CC

    ✓6ᵗʰ **H59.02** **Cataract (lens) fragments in eye following cataract surgery**

      **H59.021** **Cataract (lens) fragments in eye following cataract surgery,** right eye

      **H59.022** **Cataract (lens) fragments in eye following cataract surgery,** left eye

      **H59.023** **Cataract (lens) fragments in eye following cataract surgery,** bilateral

      **H59.029** **Cataract (lens) fragments in eye following cataract surgery,** unspecified eye

    ✓6ᵗʰ **H59.03** **Cystoid macular edema following cataract surgery**

      **H59.031** **Cystoid macular edema following cataract surgery,** right eye   CC

      **H59.032** **Cystoid macular edema following cataract surgery,** left eye   CC

      **H59.033** **Cystoid macular edema following cataract surgery,** bilateral   CC

      **H59.039** **Cystoid macular edema following cataract surgery,** unspecified eye   CC

    ✓6ᵗʰ **H59.09** **Other disorders of the eye following cataract surgery**

      **H59.091** **Other disorders of the** right eye following cataract surgery   CC

      **H59.092** **Other disorders of the** left eye following cataract surgery   CC

      **H59.093** **Other disorders of the eye following cataract surgery,** bilateral   CC

      **H59.099** **Other disorders of** unspecified eye following cataract surgery   CC

  ✓5ᵗʰ **H59.1** **Intraoperative hemorrhage and hematoma of eye and adnexa complicating a procedure**
    *EXCLUDES 1*   intraoperative hemorrhage and hematoma of eye and adnexa due to accidental puncture or laceration during a procedure (H59.2-)

    **CC Excl: For CC codes in subcategory H59.1:**
    PDX collection 639

    ✓6ᵗʰ **H59.11** **Intraoperative hemorrhage and hematoma of eye and adnexa complicating an** ophthalmic procedure

      **H59.111** **Intraoperative hemorrhage and hematoma of** right **eye and adnexa complicating an ophthalmic procedure**   CC

      **H59.112** **Intraoperative hemorrhage and hematoma of** left **eye and adnexa complicating an ophthalmic procedure**   CC

      **H59.113** **Intraoperative hemorrhage and hematoma of eye and adnexa complicating an ophthalmic procedure,** bilateral   CC

      **H59.119** **Intraoperative hemorrhage and hematoma of** unspecified **eye and adnexa complicating an ophthalmic procedure**   CC

✓ Additional Character Req   ✓x7ᵗʰ Placeholder Alert   Unacceptable PDx   Manifestation   **H1**–**H14** HAC   **HCC** CMS-HCC Condition   *EXCLUDES 1* Not Coded Here   *EXCLUDES 2* Not Included Here

ICD-10-CM 2018      **611**

**Chapter 7. Diseases of the Eye and Adnexa**

✓6ᵗʰ **H59.12 Intraoperative hemorrhage and hematoma of eye and adnexa complicating other procedure**

     **H59.121** Intraoperative hemorrhage and hematoma of right eye and adnexa complicating other procedure    CC

     **H59.122** Intraoperative hemorrhage and hematoma of left eye and adnexa complicating other procedure    CC

     **H59.123** Intraoperative hemorrhage and hematoma of eye and adnexa complicating other procedure, bilateral    CC

     **H59.129** Intraoperative hemorrhage and hematoma of unspecified eye and adnexa complicating other procedure    CC

✓5ᵗʰ **H59.2 Accidental puncture and laceration of eye and adnexa during a procedure**

     **CC Excl: For CC codes in subcategory H59.2:**
     PDX collection 509

✓6ᵗʰ **H59.21 Accidental puncture and laceration of eye and adnexa during an ophthalmic procedure**

     **H59.211** Accidental puncture and laceration of right eye and adnexa during an ophthalmic procedure    CC

     **H59.212** Accidental puncture and laceration of left eye and adnexa during an ophthalmic procedure    CC

     **H59.213** Accidental puncture and laceration of eye and adnexa during an ophthalmic procedure, bilateral    CC

     **H59.219** Accidental puncture and laceration of unspecified eye and adnexa during an ophthalmic procedure    CC

✓6ᵗʰ **H59.22 Accidental puncture and laceration of eye and adnexa during other procedure**

     **H59.221** Accidental puncture and laceration of right eye and adnexa during other procedure    CC

     **H59.222** Accidental puncture and laceration of left eye and adnexa during other procedure    CC

     **H59.223** Accidental puncture and laceration of eye and adnexa during other procedure, bilateral    CC

     **H59.229** Accidental puncture and laceration of unspecified eye and adnexa during other procedure    CC

✓5ᵗʰ **H59.3 Postprocedural hemorrhage, hematoma, and seroma of eye and adnexa following a procedure**

     **CC Excl: For CC codes in subcategory H59.3:**
     PDX collection 639

✓6ᵗʰ **H59.31 Postprocedural hemorrhage of eye and adnexa following an ophthalmic procedure**

     **H59.311** Postprocedural hemorrhage of right eye and adnexa following an ophthalmic procedure    CC

     **H59.312** Postprocedural hemorrhage of left eye and adnexa following an ophthalmic procedure    CC

     **H59.313** Postprocedural hemorrhage of eye and adnexa following an ophthalmic procedure, bilateral    CC

     **H59.319** Postprocedural hemorrhage of unspecified eye and adnexa following an ophthalmic procedure    CC

✓6ᵗʰ **H59.32 Postprocedural hemorrhage of eye and adnexa following other procedure**

     **H59.321** Postprocedural hemorrhage of right eye and adnexa following other procedure    CC

     **H59.322** Postprocedural hemorrhage of left eye and adnexa following other procedure    CC

     **H59.323** Postprocedural hemorrhage of eye and adnexa following other procedure, bilateral    CC

     **H59.329** Postprocedural hemorrhage of unspecified eye and adnexa following other procedure    CC

✓6ᵗʰ **H59.33 Postprocedural hematoma of eye and adnexa following an ophthalmic procedure**

     **H59.331** Postprocedural hematoma of right eye and adnexa following an ophthalmic procedure    CC

     **H59.332** Postprocedural hematoma of left eye and adnexa following an ophthalmic procedure    CC

     **H59.333** Postprocedural hematoma of eye and adnexa following an ophthalmic procedure, bilateral    CC

     **H59.339** Postprocedural hematoma of unspecified eye and adnexa following an ophthalmic procedure    CC

✓6ᵗʰ **H59.34 Postprocedural hematoma of eye and adnexa following other procedure**

     **H59.341** Postprocedural hematoma of right eye and adnexa following other procedure    CC

     **H59.342** Postprocedural hematoma of left eye and adnexa following other procedure    CC

     **H59.343** Postprocedural hematoma of eye and adnexa following other procedure, bilateral    CC

     **H59.349** Postprocedural hematoma of unspecified eye and adnexa following other procedure    CC

✓6ᵗʰ **H59.35 Postprocedural seroma of eye and adnexa following an ophthalmic procedure**

     **H59.351** Postprocedural seroma of right eye and adnexa following an ophthalmic procedure    CC

     **H59.352** Postprocedural seroma of left eye and adnexa following an ophthalmic procedure    CC

     **H59.353** Postprocedural seroma of eye and adnexa following an ophthalmic procedure, bilateral    CC

     **H59.359** Postprocedural seroma of unspecified eye and adnexa following an ophthalmic procedure    CC

✓6ᵗʰ **H59.36 Postprocedural seroma of eye and adnexa following other procedure**

     **H59.361** Postprocedural seroma of right eye and adnexa following other procedure    CC

     **H59.362** Postprocedural seroma of left eye and adnexa following other procedure    CC

     **H59.363** Postprocedural seroma of eye and adnexa following other procedure, bilateral    CC

     **H59.369** Postprocedural seroma of unspecified eye and adnexa following other procedurec    CC

✓5ᵗʰ **H59.4 Inflammation (infection) of postprocedural bleb**

     Postprocedural blebitis

     **EXCLUDES 1** *filtering (vitreous) bleb after glaucoma surgery status (Z98.83)*

     **H59.40** Inflammation (infection) of postprocedural bleb, unspecified

     **H59.41** Inflammation (infection) of postprocedural bleb, stage 1

     **H59.42** Inflammation (infection) of postprocedural bleb, stage 2

     **H59.43** Inflammation (infection) of postprocedural bleb, stage 3
       Bleb endophthalmitis

N Newborn: 0    P Pediatric: 0-17    M Maternity: 12-55    A Adult: 15-124    **MCC** Major CC Condition    **PDxMCC** PDx acts as own MCC    **CC** CC Condition    **PDxCC** PDx acts as own CC

612               ICD-10-CM 2018

✓5ᵗʰ **H59.8** **Other intraoperative and postprocedural complications and disorders of eye and adnexa, not elsewhere classified**

> **CC Excl: For CC codes in subcategory H59.8:**
> PDX collection 638

✓6ᵗʰ **H59.81** **Chorioretinal scars after surgery for detachment**

     **H59.811** **Chorioretinal scars after surgery for detachment, right eye**    `CC`

     **H59.812** **Chorioretinal scars after surgery for detachment, left eye**    `CC`

     **H59.813** **Chorioretinal scars after surgery for detachment, bilateral**    `CC`

     **H59.819** **Chorioretinal scars after surgery for detachment, unspecified eye**    `CC`

**H59.88** **Other intraoperative complications of eye and adnexa, not elsewhere classified**    `CC`

**H59.89** **Other postprocedural complications and disorders of eye and adnexa, not elsewhere classified**    `CC`

---

✔ Additional Character Req   ✔x7ᵗʰ Placeholder Alert   Unacceptable PDx   **Manifestation**   **H1**-**H14** HAC   **HCC** CMS-HCC Condition   *EXCLUDES 1* Not Coded Here   *EXCLUDES 2* Not Included Here

# Chapter 8. Diseases of the Ear and Mastoid Process (H60–H95)

**Chapter Specific Coding Guidelines and Examples**
Reserved for future guideline expansion.

# Chapter 8. Diseases of the Ear and Mastoid Process (H60-H95)

**NOTE** Use an external cause code following the code for the ear condition, if applicable, to identify the cause of the ear condition.

**EXCLUDES 2** *certain conditions originating in the perinatal period (P04-P96)*
*certain infectious and parasitic diseases (A00-B99)*
*complications of pregnancy, childbirth and the puerperium (O00-O9A)*
*congenital malformations, deformations and chromosomal abnormalities (Q00-Q99)*
*endocrine, nutritional and metabolic diseases (E00-E88)*
*injury, poisoning and certain other consequences of external causes (S00-T88)*
*neoplasms (C00-D49)*
*symptoms, signs and abnormal clinical and laboratory findings, not elsewhere classified (R00-R94)*

This chapter contains the following blocks:
H60-H62    Diseases of external ear
H65-H75    Diseases of middle ear and mastoid
H80-H83    Diseases of inner ear
H90-H94    Other disorders of ear
H95        Intraoperative and postprocedural complications and disorders of ear and mastoid process, not elsewhere classified

## Diseases of external ear (H60-H62)

✓4ᵗʰ **H60  Otitis externa**

✓5ᵗʰ **H60.0  Abscess of external ear**
    Boil of external ear
    Carbuncle of auricle or external auditory canal
    Furuncle of external ear
    **H60.00  Abscess of external ear, unspecified ear**
    **H60.01  Abscess of right external ear**
    **H60.02  Abscess of left external ear**
    **H60.03  Abscess of external ear, bilateral**

✓5ᵗʰ **H60.1  Cellulitis of external ear**
    Cellulitis of auricle
    Cellulitis of external auditory canal
    **H60.10  Cellulitis of external ear, unspecified ear**
    **H60.11  Cellulitis of right external ear**
    **H60.12  Cellulitis of left external ear**
    **H60.13  Cellulitis of external ear, bilateral**

✓5ᵗʰ **H60.2  Malignant otitis externa**

> **CC Excl: For CC codes in subcategory H60.2:**
> PDX collection 640

    **H60.20  Malignant otitis externa, unspecified ear**    CC
    **H60.21  Malignant otitis externa, right ear**    CC
    **H60.22  Malignant otitis externa, left ear**    CC
    **H60.23  Malignant otitis externa, bilateral**    CC

✓5ᵗʰ **H60.3  Other infective otitis externa**
    ✓6ᵗʰ **H60.31  Diffuse otitis externa**
        **H60.311  Diffuse otitis externa, right ear**
        **H60.312  Diffuse otitis externa, left ear**
        **H60.313  Diffuse otitis externa, bilateral**
        **H60.319  Diffuse otitis externa, unspecified ear**
    ✓6ᵗʰ **H60.32  Hemorrhagic otitis externa**
        **H60.321  Hemorrhagic otitis externa, right ear**
        **H60.322  Hemorrhagic otitis externa, left ear**
        **H60.323  Hemorrhagic otitis externa, bilateral**
        **H60.329  Hemorrhagic otitis externa, unspecified ear**
    ✓6ᵗʰ **H60.33  Swimmer's ear**
        **DEF:** Otitis externa; commonly occurs when water gets trapped in the ear after swimming.
        **H60.331  Swimmer's ear, right ear**
        **H60.332  Swimmer's ear, left ear**
        **H60.333  Swimmer's ear, bilateral**
        **H60.339  Swimmer's ear, unspecified ear**
    ✓6ᵗʰ **H60.39  Other infective otitis externa**
        **H60.391  Other infective otitis externa, right ear**
        **H60.392  Other infective otitis externa, left ear**
        **H60.393  Other infective otitis externa, bilateral**
        **H60.399  Other infective otitis externa, unspecified ear**

✓5ᵗʰ **H60.4  Cholesteatoma of external ear**
    Keratosis obturans of external ear (canal)
    **EXCLUDES 2** *cholesteatoma of middle ear (H71.-)*
        *recurrent cholesteatoma of postmastoidectomy cavity (H95.0-)*
    **H60.40  Cholesteatoma of external ear, unspecified ear**
    **H60.41  Cholesteatoma of right external ear**
    **H60.42  Cholesteatoma of left external ear**
    **H60.43  Cholesteatoma of external ear, bilateral**

✓5ᵗʰ **H60.5  Acute noninfective otitis externa**
    ✓6ᵗʰ **H60.50  Unspecified acute noninfective otitis externa**
        Acute otitis externa NOS
        **H60.501  Unspecified acute noninfective otitis externa, right ear**
        **H60.502  Unspecified acute noninfective otitis externa, left ear**
        **H60.503  Unspecified acute noninfective otitis externa, bilateral**
        **H60.509  Unspecified acute noninfective otitis externa, unspecified ear**
    ✓6ᵗʰ **H60.51  Acute actinic otitis externa**
        **H60.511  Acute actinic otitis externa, right ear**
        **H60.512  Acute actinic otitis externa, left ear**
        **H60.513  Acute actinic otitis externa, bilateral**
        **H60.519  Acute actinic otitis externa, unspecified ear**
    ✓6ᵗʰ **H60.52  Acute chemical otitis externa**
        **H60.521  Acute chemical otitis externa, right ear**
        **H60.522  Acute chemical otitis externa, left ear**
        **H60.523  Acute chemical otitis externa, bilateral**
        **H60.529  Acute chemical otitis externa, unspecified ear**
    ✓6ᵗʰ **H60.53  Acute contact otitis externa**
        **H60.531  Acute contact otitis externa, right ear**
        **H60.532  Acute contact otitis externa, left ear**
        **H60.533  Acute contact otitis externa, bilateral**
        **H60.539  Acute contact otitis externa, unspecified ear**
    ✓6ᵗʰ **H60.54  Acute eczematoid otitis externa**
        **H60.541  Acute eczematoid otitis externa, right ear**
        **H60.542  Acute eczematoid otitis externa, left ear**
        **H60.543  Acute eczematoid otitis externa, bilateral**
        **H60.549  Acute eczematoid otitis externa, unspecified ear**
    ✓6ᵗʰ **H60.55  Acute reactive otitis externa**
        **H60.551  Acute reactive otitis externa, right ear**
        **H60.552  Acute reactive otitis externa, left ear**
        **H60.553  Acute reactive otitis externa, bilateral**
        **H60.559  Acute reactive otitis externa, unspecified ear**
    ✓6ᵗʰ **H60.59  Other noninfective acute otitis externa**
        **H60.591  Other noninfective acute otitis externa, right ear**
        **H60.592  Other noninfective acute otitis externa, left ear**
        **H60.593  Other noninfective acute otitis externa, bilateral**
        **H60.599  Other noninfective acute otitis externa, unspecified ear**

✓5ᵗʰ **H60.6  Unspecified chronic otitis externa**
    **H60.60  Unspecified chronic otitis externa, unspecified ear**
    **H60.61  Unspecified chronic otitis externa, right ear**
    **H60.62  Unspecified chronic otitis externa, left ear**
    **H60.63  Unspecified chronic otitis externa, bilateral**

✓5ᵗʰ **H60.8  Other otitis externa**
    ✓6ᵗʰ **H60.8X  Other otitis externa**
        **H60.8X1  Other otitis externa, right ear**
        **H60.8X2  Other otitis externa, left ear**
        **H60.8X3  Other otitis externa, bilateral**
        **H60.8X9  Other otitis externa, unspecified ear**

---

Ⓝ Newborn: 0    Ⓟ Pediatric: 0-17    Ⓜ Maternity: 12-55    Ⓐ Adult: 15-124    **MCC** Major CC Condition    **PDxMCC** PDx acts as own MCC    **CC** CC Condition    **PDxCC** PDx acts as own CC

✓5ᵗʰ **H60.9** **Unspecified otitis externa**
- **H60.90** **Unspecified otitis externa,** unspecified **ear**
- **H60.91** **Unspecified otitis externa,** right **ear**
- **H60.92** **Unspecified otitis externa,** left **ear**
- **H60.93** **Unspecified otitis externa,** bilateral

✓4ᵗʰ **H61** **Other disorders of external ear**

✓5ᵗʰ **H61.0** **Chondritis and perichondritis of external ear**
Chondrodermatitis nodularis chronica helicis
Perichondritis of auricle
Perichondritis of pinna

✓6ᵗʰ **H61.00** **Unspecified perichondritis of external ear**
- **H61.001** **Unspecified perichondritis of** right **external ear**
- **H61.002** **Unspecified perichondritis of** left **external ear**
- **H61.003** **Unspecified perichondritis of external ear,** bilateral
- **H61.009** **Unspecified perichondritis of external ear,** unspecified **ear**

✓6ᵗʰ **H61.01** **Acute perichondritis of external ear**
- **H61.011** **Acute perichondritis of** right **external ear**
- **H61.012** **Acute perichondritis of** left **external ear**
- **H61.013** **Acute perichondritis of external ear,** bilateral
- **H61.019** **Acute perichondritis of external ear,** unspecified **ear**

✓6ᵗʰ **H61.02** **Chronic perichondritis of external ear**
- **H61.021** **Chronic perichondritis of** right **external ear**
- **H61.022** **Chronic perichondritis of** left **external ear**
- **H61.023** **Chronic perichondritis of external ear,** bilateral
- **H61.029** **Chronic perichondritis of external ear,** unspecified **ear**

✓6ᵗʰ **H61.03** **Chondritis of external ear**
Chondritis of auricle     Chondritis of pinna
**AHA:** 2015, 1Q, 18
**DEF:** Infection that has progressed into the cartilage; presents as indurated and edematous skin over the pinna; vascular compromise occurs with tissue necrosis and deformity.
- **H61.031** **Chondritis of** right **external ear**
- **H61.032** **Chondritis of** left **external ear**
- **H61.033** **Chondritis of external ear,** bilateral
- **H61.039** **Chondritis of external ear,** unspecified **ear**

✓5ᵗʰ **H61.1** **Noninfective disorders of pinna**
EXCLUDES 2   cauliflower ear (M95.1-)
              gouty tophi of ear (M1A.-)

✓6ᵗʰ **H61.10** **Unspecified noninfective disorders of pinna**
Disorder of pinna NOS
- **H61.101** **Unspecified noninfective disorders of pinna,** right **ear**
- **H61.102** **Unspecified noninfective disorders of pinna,** left **ear**
- **H61.103** **Unspecified noninfective disorders of pinna,** bilateral
- **H61.109** **Unspecified noninfective disorders of pinna,** unspecified **ear**

✓6ᵗʰ **H61.11** **Acquired deformity of pinna**
Acquired deformity of auricle
EXCLUDES 2   cauliflower ear (M95.1-)
- **H61.111** **Acquired deformity of pinna,** right **ear**
- **H61.112** **Acquired deformity of pinna,** left **ear**
- **H61.113** **Acquired deformity of pinna,** bilateral
- **H61.119** **Acquired deformity of pinna,** unspecified **ear**

✓6ᵗʰ **H61.12** **Hematoma of pinna**
Hematoma of auricle
- **H61.121** **Hematoma of pinna,** right **ear**
- **H61.122** **Hematoma of pinna,** left **ear**
- **H61.123** **Hematoma of pinna,** bilateral
- **H61.129** **Hematoma of pinna,** unspecified **ear**

✓6ᵗʰ **H61.19** **Other noninfective disorders of pinna**
- **H61.191** **Noninfective disorders of pinna,** right **ear**
- **H61.192** **Noninfective disorders of pinna,** left **ear**
- **H61.193** **Noninfective disorders of pinna,** bilateral
- **H61.199** **Noninfective disorders of pinna,** unspecified **ear**

✓5ᵗʰ **H61.2** **Impacted cerumen**
Wax in ear
- 4 **H61.20** **Impacted cerumen,** unspecified **ear**
- 4 **H61.21** **Impacted cerumen,** right **ear**
- 4 **H61.22** **Impacted cerumen,** left **ear**
- 4 **H61.23** **Impacted cerumen,** bilateral

✓5ᵗʰ **H61.3** **Acquired stenosis of external ear canal**
Collapse of external ear canal
EXCLUDES 1   postprocedural stenosis of external ear canal (H95.81-)

✓6ᵗʰ **H61.30** **Acquired stenosis of external ear canal,** unspecified
- **H61.301** **Acquired stenosis of** right **external ear canal,** unspecified
- **H61.302** **Acquired stenosis of** left **external ear canal,** unspecified
- **H61.303** **Acquired stenosis of external ear canal,** unspecified, bilateral
- **H61.309** **Acquired stenosis of external ear canal,** unspecified, unspecified **ear**

✓6ᵗʰ **H61.31** **Acquired stenosis of external ear canal** secondary to trauma
- **H61.311** **Acquired stenosis of** right **external ear canal secondary to trauma**
- **H61.312** **Acquired stenosis of** left **external ear canal secondary to trauma**
- **H61.313** **Acquired stenosis of external ear canal secondary to trauma,** bilateral
- **H61.319** **Acquired stenosis of external ear canal secondary to trauma,** unspecified **ear**

✓6ᵗʰ **H61.32** **Acquired stenosis of external ear canal** secondary to inflammation and infection
**DEF:** Narrowing of the external ear canal; due to chronic inflammation or infection.
- **H61.321** **Acquired stenosis of** right **external ear canal secondary to inflammation and infection**
- **H61.322** **Acquired stenosis of** left **external ear canal secondary to inflammation and infection**
- **H61.323** **Acquired stenosis of external ear canal secondary to inflammation and infection,** bilateral
- **H61.329** **Acquired stenosis of external ear canal secondary to inflammation and infection,** unspecified **ear**

✓6ᵗʰ **H61.39** **Other** acquired stenosis of external ear canal
- **H61.391** **Other acquired stenosis of** right **external ear canal**
- **H61.392** **Other acquired stenosis of** left **external ear canal**
- **H61.393** **Other acquired stenosis of external ear canal,** bilateral
- **H61.399** **Other acquired stenosis of external ear canal,** unspecified **ear**

✓5ᵗʰ **H61.8** **Other specified disorders of external ear**

✓6ᵗʰ **H61.81** **Exostosis of external canal**
- **H61.811** **Exostosis of** right **external canal**
- **H61.812** **Exostosis of** left **external canal**
- **H61.813** **Exostosis of external canal,** bilateral
- **H61.819** **Exostosis of external canal,** unspecified **ear**

✓6ᵗʰ **H61.89** **Other specified disorders of external ear**
- **H61.891** **Other specified disorders of** right **external ear**
- **H61.892** **Other specified disorders of** left **external ear**
- **H61.893** **Other specified disorders of external ear,** bilateral
- **H61.899** **Other specified disorders of external ear,** unspecified **ear**

---

4   Questionable admission when used as PDx.

✓ Additional Character Req   ✓x 7ᵗʰ Placeholder Alert   Unacceptable PDx   Manifestation   ▆H1▆-▆H14▆ HAC   ▆HCC▆ CMS-HCC Condition   *EXCLUDES 1* Not Coded Here   *EXCLUDES 2* Not Included Here

ICD-10-CM 2018            **617**

**Chapter 8. Diseases of the Ear and Mastoid Process**

✓5ᵗʰ **H61.9 Disorder of external ear, unspecified**

     **H61.90 Disorder of external ear, unspecified, unspecified ear**

     **H61.91 Disorder of right external ear, unspecified**

     **H61.92 Disorder of left external ear, unspecified**

     **H61.93 Disorder of external ear, unspecified, bilateral**

✓4ᵗʰ **H62 Disorders of external ear in diseases classified elsewhere**

✓5ᵗʰ **H62.4 Otitis externa in other diseases classified elsewhere**

     Code first underlying disease, such as:
         erysipelas (A46)
         impetigo (L01.0)

     **EXCLUDES 1**   otitis externa (in):
         candidiasis (B37.84)
         herpes viral [herpes simplex] (B00.1)
         herpes zoster (B02.8)

     *H62.40 Otitis externa in other diseases classified elsewhere, unspecified ear*

     *H62.41 Otitis externa in other diseases classified elsewhere, right ear*

     *H62.42 Otitis externa in other diseases classified elsewhere, left ear*

     *H62.43 Otitis externa in other diseases classified elsewhere, bilateral*

✓5ᵗʰ **H62.8 Other disorders of external ear in diseases classified elsewhere**

     Code first underlying disease, such as:
         gout (M1A.-, M10.-)

✓6ᵗʰ **H62.8X Other disorders of external ear in diseases classified elsewhere**

     *H62.8X1 Other disorders of right external ear in diseases classified elsewhere*

     *H62.8X2 Other disorders of left external ear in diseases classified elsewhere*

     *H62.8X3 Other disorders of external ear in diseases classified elsewhere, bilateral*

     *H62.8X9 Other disorders of external ear in diseases classified elsewhere, unspecified ear*

### Diseases of middle ear and mastoid (H65-H75)

✓4ᵗʰ **H65 Nonsuppurative otitis media**

     **INCLUDES**   nonsuppurative otitis media with myringitis

     Use additional code for any associated perforated tympanic membrane (H72.-)

     Use additional code to identify:
         exposure to environmental tobacco smoke (Z77.22)
         exposure to tobacco smoke in the perinatal period (P96.81)
         history of tobacco dependence (Z87.891)
         occupational exposure to environmental tobacco smoke (Z57.31)
         tobacco dependence (F17.-)
         tobacco use (Z72.0)

✓5ᵗʰ **H65.0 Acute serous otitis media**

     Acute and subacute secretory otitis

     **H65.00 Acute serous otitis media, unspecified ear**

     **H65.01 Acute serous otitis media, right ear**

     **H65.02 Acute serous otitis media, left ear**

     **H65.03 Acute serous otitis media, bilateral**

     **H65.04 Acute serous otitis media, recurrent, right ear**

     **H65.05 Acute serous otitis media, recurrent, left ear**

     **H65.06 Acute serous otitis media, recurrent, bilateral**

     **H65.07 Acute serous otitis media, recurrent, unspecified ear**

✓5ᵗʰ **H65.1 Other acute nonsuppurative otitis media**

     **EXCLUDES 1**   otitic barotrauma (T70.0)
                otitis media (acute) NOS (H66.9)

✓6ᵗʰ **H65.11 Acute and subacute allergic otitis media (mucoid) (sanguinous) (serous)**

     **H65.111 Acute and subacute allergic otitis media (mucoid) (sanguinous) (serous), right ear**

     **H65.112 Acute and subacute allergic otitis media (mucoid) (sanguinous) (serous), left ear**

     **H65.113 Acute and subacute allergic otitis media (mucoid) (sanguinous) (serous), bilateral**

     **H65.114 Acute and subacute allergic otitis media (mucoid) (sanguinous) (serous), recurrent, right ear**

     **H65.115 Acute and subacute allergic otitis media (mucoid) (sanguinous) (serous), recurrent, left ear**

     **H65.116 Acute and subacute allergic otitis media (mucoid) (sanguinous) (serous), recurrent, bilateral**

     **H65.117 Acute and subacute allergic otitis media (mucoid) (sanguinous) (serous), recurrent, unspecified ear**

     **H65.119 Acute and subacute allergic otitis media (mucoid) (sanguinous) (serous), unspecified ear**

✓6ᵗʰ **H65.19 Other acute nonsuppurative otitis media**

     Acute and subacute mucoid otitis media
     Acute and subacute nonsuppurative otitis media NOS
     Acute and subacute sanguinous otitis media
     Acute and subacute seromucinous otitis media

     **H65.191 Other acute nonsuppurative otitis media, right ear**

     **H65.192 Other acute nonsuppurative otitis media, left ear**

     **H65.193 Other acute nonsuppurative otitis media, bilateral**

     **H65.194 Other acute nonsuppurative otitis media, recurrent, right ear**

     **H65.195 Other acute nonsuppurative otitis media, recurrent, left ear**

     **H65.196 Other acute nonsuppurative otitis media, recurrent, bilateral**

     **H65.197 Other acute nonsuppurative otitis media, recurrent, unspecified ear**

     **H65.199 Other acute nonsuppurative otitis media, unspecified ear**

✓5ᵗʰ **H65.2 Chronic serous otitis media**

     Chronic tubotympanal catarrh

     **H65.20 Chronic serous otitis media, unspecified ear**

     **H65.21 Chronic serous otitis media, right ear**

     **H65.22 Chronic serous otitis media, left ear**

     **H65.23 Chronic serous otitis media, bilateral**

✓5ᵗʰ **H65.3 Chronic mucoid otitis media**

     Chronic mucinous otitis media
     Chronic secretory otitis media
     Chronic transudative otitis media
     Glue ear

     **EXCLUDES 1**   *adhesive middle ear disease (H74.1)*

     **H65.30 Chronic mucoid otitis media, unspecified ear**

     **H65.31 Chronic mucoid otitis media, right ear**

     **H65.32 Chronic mucoid otitis media, left ear**

     **H65.33 Chronic mucoid otitis media, bilateral**

✓5ᵗʰ **H65.4 Other chronic nonsuppurative otitis media**

✓6ᵗʰ **H65.41 Chronic allergic otitis media**

     **H65.411 Chronic allergic otitis media, right ear**

     **H65.412 Chronic allergic otitis media, left ear**

     **H65.413 Chronic allergic otitis media, bilateral**

     **H65.419 Chronic allergic otitis media, unspecified ear**

✓6ᵗʰ **H65.49 Other chronic nonsuppurative otitis media**

     Chronic exudative otitis media
     Chronic nonsuppurative otitis media NOS
     Chronic otitis media with effusion (nonpurulent)
     Chronic seromucinous otitis media

     **H65.491 Other chronic nonsuppurative otitis media, right ear**

     **H65.492 Other chronic nonsuppurative otitis media, left ear**

     **H65.493 Other chronic nonsuppurative otitis media, bilateral**

     **H65.499 Other chronic nonsuppurative otitis media, unspecified ear**

**N** Newborn: 0   **P** Pediatric: 0-17   **M** Maternity: 12-55   **A** Adult: 15-124   **MCC** Major CC Condition   **PDx MCC** PDx acts as own MCC   **CC** CC Condition   **PDx CC** PDx acts as own CC

**618**

ICD-10-CM 2018

✓5ᵗʰ **H65.9  Unspecified nonsuppurative otitis media**
Allergic otitis media NOS
Catarrhal otitis media NOS
Exudative otitis media NOS
Mucoid otitis media NOS
Otitis media with effusion (nonpurulent) NOS
Secretory otitis media NOS
Seromucinous otitis media NOS
Serous otitis media NOS
Transudative otitis media NOS

**H65.90  Unspecified nonsuppurative otitis media, unspecified ear**

**H65.91  Unspecified nonsuppurative otitis media, right ear**

**H65.92  Unspecified nonsuppurative otitis media, left ear**

**H65.93  Unspecified nonsuppurative otitis media, bilateral**

✓4ᵗʰ **H66  Suppurative and unspecified otitis media**
INCLUDES  suppurative and unspecified otitis media with myringitis
Use additional code to identify:
exposure to environmental tobacco smoke (Z77.22)
exposure to tobacco smoke in the perinatal period (P96.81)
history of tobacco dependence (Z87.891)
occupational exposure to environmental tobacco smoke (Z57.31)
tobacco dependence (F17.-)
tobacco use (Z72.0)
AHA: 2016, 1Q, 34

✓5ᵗʰ **H66.0  Acute suppurative otitis media**

✓6ᵗʰ **H66.00  Acute suppurative otitis media without spontaneous rupture of ear drum**

**H66.001  Acute suppurative otitis media without spontaneous rupture of ear drum, right ear**

**H66.002  Acute suppurative otitis media without spontaneous rupture of ear drum, left ear**

**H66.003  Acute suppurative otitis media without spontaneous rupture of ear drum, bilateral**

**H66.004  Acute suppurative otitis media without spontaneous rupture of ear drum, recurrent, right ear**

**H66.005  Acute suppurative otitis media without spontaneous rupture of ear drum, recurrent, left ear**

**H66.006  Acute suppurative otitis media without spontaneous rupture of ear drum, recurrent, bilateral**

**H66.007  Acute suppurative otitis media without spontaneous rupture of ear drum, recurrent, unspecified ear**

**H66.009  Acute suppurative otitis media without spontaneous rupture of ear drum, unspecified ear**

✓6ᵗʰ **H66.01  Acute suppurative otitis media with spontaneous rupture of ear drum**
DEF: Sudden, severe inflammation of middle ear, with pressure causing the perforation of ear drum tissue.

**H66.011  Acute suppurative otitis media with spontaneous rupture of ear drum, right ear**

**H66.012  Acute suppurative otitis media with spontaneous rupture of ear drum, left ear**

**H66.013  Acute suppurative otitis media with spontaneous rupture of ear drum, bilateral**

**H66.014  Acute suppurative otitis media with spontaneous rupture of ear drum, recurrent, right ear**

**H66.015  Acute suppurative otitis media with spontaneous rupture of ear drum, recurrent, left ear**

**H66.016  Acute suppurative otitis media with spontaneous rupture of ear drum, recurrent, bilateral**

**H66.017  Acute suppurative otitis media with spontaneous rupture of ear drum, recurrent, unspecified ear**

**H66.019  Acute suppurative otitis media with spontaneous rupture of ear drum, unspecified ear**

✓5ᵗʰ **H66.1  Chronic tubotympanic suppurative otitis media**
Benign chronic suppurative otitis media
Chronic tubotympanic disease
Use additional code for any associated perforated tympanic membrane (H72.-)

**H66.10  Chronic tubotympanic suppurative otitis media, unspecified**

**H66.11  Chronic tubotympanic suppurative otitis media, right ear**

**H66.12  Chronic tubotympanic suppurative otitis media, left ear**

**H66.13  Chronic tubotympanic suppurative otitis media, bilateral**

✓5ᵗʰ **H66.2  Chronic atticoantral suppurative otitis media**
Chronic atticoantral disease
Use additional code for any associated perforated tympanic membrane (H72.-)

**H66.20  Chronic atticoantral suppurative otitis media, unspecified ear**

**H66.21  Chronic atticoantral suppurative otitis media, right ear**

**H66.22  Chronic atticoantral suppurative otitis media, left ear**

**H66.23  Chronic atticoantral suppurative otitis media, bilateral**

✓5ᵗʰ **H66.3  Other chronic suppurative otitis media**
Chronic suppurative otitis media NOS
Use additional code for any associated perforated tympanic membrane (H72.-)
EXCLUDES 1  *tuberculous otitis media (A18.6)*

✓6ᵗʰ **H66.3X  Other chronic suppurative otitis media**

**H66.3X1  Other chronic suppurative otitis media, right ear**

**H66.3X2  Other chronic suppurative otitis media, left ear**

**H66.3X3  Other chronic suppurative otitis media, bilateral**

**H66.3X9  Other chronic suppurative otitis media, unspecified ear**

✓5ᵗʰ **H66.4  Suppurative otitis media, unspecified**
Purulent otitis media NOS
Use additional code for any associated perforated tympanic membrane (H72.-)

**H66.40  Suppurative otitis media, unspecified, unspecified ear**

**H66.41  Suppurative otitis media, unspecified, right ear**

**H66.42  Suppurative otitis media, unspecified, left ear**

**H66.43  Suppurative otitis media, unspecified, bilateral**

✓5ᵗʰ **H66.9  Otitis media, unspecified**
Otitis media NOS
Acute otitis media NOS
Chronic otitis media NOS
Use additional code for any associated perforated tympanic membrane (H72.-)

**H66.90  Otitis media, unspecified, unspecified ear**

**H66.91  Otitis media, unspecified, right ear**

**H66.92  Otitis media, unspecified, left ear**

**H66.93  Otitis media, unspecified, bilateral**

✓4ᵗʰ **H67  Otitis media in diseases classified elsewhere**
Code first underlying disease, such as:
viral disease NEC (B00-B34)
Use additional code for any associated perforated tympanic membrane (H72.-)
EXCLUDES 1  *otitis media in:*
*influenza (J09.X9, J10.83, J11.83)*
*measles (B05.3)*
*scarlet fever (A38.0)*
*tuberculosis (A18.6)*

**H67.1  *Otitis media in diseases classified elsewhere, right ear***

**H67.2  *Otitis media in diseases classified elsewhere, left ear***

**H67.3  *Otitis media in diseases classified elsewhere, bilateral***

**H67.9  *Otitis media in diseases classified elsewhere, unspecified ear***

## ✓4th H68 Eustachian salpingitis and obstruction

### ✓5th H68.0 Eustachian salpingitis

#### ✓6th H68.00 Unspecified Eustachian salpingitis

H68.001 Unspecified Eustachian salpingitis, right ear

H68.002 Unspecified Eustachian salpingitis, left ear

H68.003 Unspecified Eustachian salpingitis, bilateral

H68.009 Unspecified Eustachian salpingitis, unspecified ear

#### ✓6th H68.01 Acute Eustachian salpingitis

H68.011 Acute Eustachian salpingitis, right ear

H68.012 Acute Eustachian salpingitis, left ear

H68.013 Acute Eustachian salpingitis, bilateral

H68.019 Acute Eustachian salpingitis, unspecified ear

#### ✓6th H68.02 Chronic Eustachian salpingitis

H68.021 Chronic Eustachian salpingitis, right ear

H68.022 Chronic Eustachian salpingitis, left ear

H68.023 Chronic Eustachian salpingitis, bilateral

H68.029 Chronic Eustachian salpingitis, unspecified ear

### ✓5th H68.1 Obstruction of Eustachian tube
Stenosis of Eustachian tube
Stricture of Eustachian tube

#### ✓6th H68.10 Unspecified obstruction of Eustachian tube

H68.101 Unspecified obstruction of Eustachian tube, right ear

H68.102 Unspecified obstruction of Eustachian tube, left ear

H68.103 Unspecified obstruction of Eustachian tube, bilateral

H68.109 Unspecified obstruction of Eustachian tube, unspecified ear

#### ✓6th H68.11 Osseous obstruction of Eustachian tube

H68.111 Osseous obstruction of Eustachian tube, right ear

H68.112 Osseous obstruction of Eustachian tube, left ear

H68.113 Osseous obstruction of Eustachian tube, bilateral

H68.119 Osseous obstruction of Eustachian tube, unspecified ear

#### ✓6th H68.12 Intrinsic cartilagenous obstruction of Eustachian tube

H68.121 Intrinsic cartilagenous obstruction of Eustachian tube, right ear

H68.122 Intrinsic cartilagenous obstruction of Eustachian tube, left ear

H68.123 Intrinsic cartilagenous obstruction of Eustachian tube, bilateral

H68.129 Intrinsic cartilagenous obstruction of Eustachian tube, unspecified ear

#### ✓6th H68.13 Extrinsic cartilagenous obstruction of Eustachian tube
Compression of Eustachian tube

H68.131 Extrinsic cartilagenous obstruction of Eustachian tube, right ear

H68.132 Extrinsic cartilagenous obstruction of Eustachian tube, left ear

H68.133 Extrinsic cartilagenous obstruction of Eustachian tube, bilateral

H68.139 Extrinsic cartilagenous obstruction of Eustachian tube, unspecified ear

## ✓4th H69 Other and unspecified disorders of Eustachian tube

### ✓5th H69.0 Patulous Eustachian tube

H69.00 Patulous Eustachian tube, unspecified ear

H69.01 Patulous Eustachian tube, right ear

H69.02 Patulous Eustachian tube, left ear

H69.03 Patulous Eustachian tube, bilateral

### ✓5th H69.8 Other specified disorders of Eustachian tube

H69.80 Other specified disorders of Eustachian tube, unspecified ear

H69.81 Other specified disorders of Eustachian tube, right ear

H69.82 Other specified disorders of Eustachian tube, left ear

H69.83 Other specified disorders of Eustachian tube, bilateral

### ✓5th H69.9 Unspecified Eustachian tube disorder

H69.90 Unspecified Eustachian tube disorder, unspecified ear

H69.91 Unspecified Eustachian tube disorder, right ear

H69.92 Unspecified Eustachian tube disorder, left ear

H69.93 Unspecified Eustachian tube disorder, bilateral

## ✓4th H70 Mastoiditis and related conditions

### ✓5th H70.0 Acute mastoiditis
Abscess of mastoid
Empyema of mastoid

> **CC Excl: For CC codes in subcategory H70.0:**
> PDX collection 641

#### ✓6th H70.00 Acute mastoiditis without complications

H70.001 Acute mastoiditis without complications, right ear `CC`

H70.002 Acute mastoiditis without complications, left ear `CC`

H70.003 Acute mastoiditis without complications, bilateral `CC`

H70.009 Acute mastoiditis without complications, unspecified ear `CC`

#### ✓6th H70.01 Subperiosteal abscess of mastoid

H70.011 Subperiosteal abscess of mastoid, right ear `CC`

H70.012 Subperiosteal abscess of mastoid, left ear `CC`

H70.013 Subperiosteal abscess of mastoid, bilateral `CC`

H70.019 Subperiosteal abscess of mastoid, unspecified ear `CC`

#### ✓6th H70.09 Acute mastoiditis with other complications

H70.091 Acute mastoiditis with other complications, right ear `CC`

H70.092 Acute mastoiditis with other complications, left ear `CC`

H70.093 Acute mastoiditis with other complications, bilateral `CC`

H70.099 Acute mastoiditis with other complications, unspecified ear `CC`

### ✓5th H70.1 Chronic mastoiditis
Caries of mastoid
Fistula of mastoid
**EXCLUDES 1**   *tuberculous mastoiditis (A18.03)*

H70.10 Chronic mastoiditis, unspecified ear

H70.11 Chronic mastoiditis, right ear

H70.12 Chronic mastoiditis, left ear

H70.13 Chronic mastoiditis, bilateral

### ✓5th H70.2 Petrositis
Inflammation of petrous bone

#### ✓6th H70.20 Unspecified petrositis

H70.201 Unspecified petrositis, right ear

H70.202 Unspecified petrositis, left ear

H70.203 Unspecified petrositis, bilateral

H70.209 Unspecified petrositis, unspecified ear

#### ✓6th H70.21 Acute petrositis
**DEF:** Sudden, severe inflammation of petrous temporal bone behind the ear; associated with middle ear infection.

H70.211 Acute petrositis, right ear

H70.212 Acute petrositis, left ear

H70.213 Acute petrositis, bilateral

H70.219 Acute petrositis, unspecified ear

#### ✓6th H70.22 Chronic petrositis

H70.221 Chronic petrositis, right ear

H70.222 Chronic petrositis, left ear

H70.223 Chronic petrositis, bilateral

H70.229 Chronic petrositis, unspecified ear

✓5ᵗʰ **H70.8** **Other mastoiditis and related conditions**
　　　*EXCLUDES 1*　*preauricular sinus and cyst (Q18.1)*
　　　　　　*sinus, fistula, and cyst of branchial cleft (Q18.0)*

　✓6ᵗʰ **H70.81** **Postauricular fistula**
　　　**H70.811** **Postauricular fistula, right ear**
　　　**H70.812** **Postauricular fistula, left ear**
　　　**H70.813** **Postauricular fistula, bilateral**
　　　**H70.819** **Postauricular fistula, unspecified ear**

　✓6ᵗʰ **H70.89** **Other mastoiditis and related conditions**
　　　**H70.891** **Other mastoiditis and related conditions, right ear**
　　　**H70.892** **Other mastoiditis and related conditions, left ear**
　　　**H70.893** **Other mastoiditis and related conditions, bilateral**
　　　**H70.899** **Other mastoiditis and related conditions, unspecified ear**

✓5ᵗʰ **H70.9** **Unspecified mastoiditis**
　　　**H70.90** **Unspecified mastoiditis, unspecified ear**
　　　**H70.91** **Unspecified mastoiditis, right ear**
　　　**H70.92** **Unspecified mastoiditis, left ear**
　　　**H70.93** **Unspecified mastoiditis, bilateral**

✓4ᵗʰ **H71** **Cholesteatoma of middle ear**
　　　*EXCLUDES 2*　*cholesteatoma of external ear (H60.4-)*
　　　　　　*recurrent cholesteatoma of postmastoidectomy cavity (H95.0-)*

✓5ᵗʰ **H71.0** **Cholesteatoma of attic**
　　　**H71.00** **Cholesteatoma of attic, unspecified ear**
　　　**H71.01** **Cholesteatoma of attic, right ear**
　　　**H71.02** **Cholesteatoma of attic, left ear**
　　　**H71.03** **Cholesteatoma of attic, bilateral**

✓5ᵗʰ **H71.1** **Cholesteatoma of tympanum**
　　　**H71.10** **Cholesteatoma of tympanum, unspecified ear**
　　　**H71.11** **Cholesteatoma of tympanum, right ear**
　　　**H71.12** **Cholesteatoma of tympanum, left ear**
　　　**H71.13** **Cholesteatoma of tympanum, bilateral**

✓5ᵗʰ **H71.2** **Cholesteatoma of mastoid**
　　　**H71.20** **Cholesteatoma of mastoid, unspecified ear**
　　　**H71.21** **Cholesteatoma of mastoid, right ear**
　　　**H71.22** **Cholesteatoma of mastoid, left ear**
　　　**H71.23** **Cholesteatoma of mastoid, bilateral**

✓5ᵗʰ **H71.3** **Diffuse cholesteatosis**
　　　**H71.30** **Diffuse cholesteatosis, unspecified ear**
　　　**H71.31** **Diffuse cholesteatosis, right ear**
　　　**H71.32** **Diffuse cholesteatosis, left ear**
　　　**H71.33** **Diffuse cholesteatosis, bilateral**

✓5ᵗʰ **H71.9** **Unspecified cholesteatoma**
　　　**H71.90** **Unspecified cholesteatoma, unspecified ear**
　　　**H71.91** **Unspecified cholesteatoma, right ear**
　　　**H71.92** **Unspecified cholesteatoma, left ear**
　　　**H71.93** **Unspecified cholesteatoma, bilateral**

**Cholesteatoma of Middle Ear**

Middle ear chamber

Ear drum

Cholesteatoma sac

✓4ᵗʰ **H72** **Perforation of tympanic membrane**
　　　[INCLUDES]　persistent post-traumatic perforation of ear drum
　　　　　　postinflammatory perforation of ear drum
　　　Code first any associated otitis media (H65.-, H66.1-, H66.2-, H66.3-, H66.4-, H66.9-, H67.-)
　　　*EXCLUDES 1*　*acute suppurative otitis media with rupture of the tympanic membrane (H66.01-)*
　　　　　　*traumatic rupture of ear drum (S09.2-)*

✓5ᵗʰ **H72.0** **Central perforation of tympanic membrane**
　　　**H72.00** **Central perforation of tympanic membrane, unspecified ear**
　　　**H72.01** **Central perforation of tympanic membrane, right ear**
　　　**H72.02** **Central perforation of tympanic membrane, left ear**
　　　**H72.03** **Central perforation of tympanic membrane, bilateral**

✓5ᵗʰ **H72.1** **Attic perforation of tympanic membrane**
　　　Perforation of pars flaccida
　　　**H72.10** **Attic perforation of tympanic membrane, unspecified ear**
　　　**H72.11** **Attic perforation of tympanic membrane, right ear**
　　　**H72.12** **Attic perforation of tympanic membrane, left ear**
　　　**H72.13** **Attic perforation of tympanic membrane, bilateral**

✓5ᵗʰ **H72.2** **Other marginal perforations of tympanic membrane**
　✓6ᵗʰ **H72.2X** **Other marginal perforations of tympanic membrane**
　　　**H72.2X1** **Other marginal perforations of tympanic membrane, right ear**
　　　**H72.2X2** **Other marginal perforations of tympanic membrane, left ear**
　　　**H72.2X3** **Other marginal perforations of tympanic membrane, bilateral**
　　　**H72.2X9** **Other marginal perforations of tympanic membrane, unspecified ear**

✓5ᵗʰ **H72.8** **Other perforations of tympanic membrane**
　✓6ᵗʰ **H72.81** **Multiple perforations of tympanic membrane**
　　　**H72.811** **Multiple perforations of tympanic membrane, right ear**
　　　**H72.812** **Multiple perforations of tympanic membrane, left ear**
　　　**H72.813** **Multiple perforations of tympanic membrane, bilateral**
　　　**H72.819** **Multiple perforations of tympanic membrane, unspecified ear**
　✓6ᵗʰ **H72.82** **Total perforations of tympanic membrane**
　　　**H72.821** **Total perforations of tympanic membrane, right ear**
　　　**H72.822** **Total perforations of tympanic membrane, left ear**
　　　**H72.823** **Total perforations of tympanic membrane, bilateral**
　　　**H72.829** **Total perforations of tympanic membrane, unspecified ear**

✓5ᵗʰ **H72.9** **Unspecified perforation of tympanic membrane**
　　　**H72.90** **Unspecified perforation of tympanic membrane, unspecified ear**
　　　**H72.91** **Unspecified perforation of tympanic membrane, right ear**
　　　**H72.92** **Unspecified perforation of tympanic membrane, left ear**
　　　**H72.93** **Unspecified perforation of tympanic membrane, bilateral**

✓4ᵗʰ **H73** **Other disorders of tympanic membrane**
✓5ᵗʰ **H73.0** **Acute myringitis**
　　　*EXCLUDES 1*　*acute myringitis with otitis media (H65, H66)*

　✓6ᵗʰ **H73.00** **Unspecified acute myringitis**
　　　Acute tympanitis NOS
　　　**H73.001** **Acute myringitis, right ear**
　　　**H73.002** **Acute myringitis, left ear**
　　　**H73.003** **Acute myringitis, bilateral**
　　　**H73.009** **Acute myringitis, unspecified ear**

　✓6ᵗʰ **H73.01** **Bullous myringitis**
　　　**DEF:** Bacterial or viral otitis media; characterized by the appearance of serous or hemorrhagic blebs on the ear drum and sudden onset of severe pain in ear.
　　　**H73.011** **Bullous myringitis, right ear**
　　　**H73.012** **Bullous myringitis, left ear**

H73.Ø13 **Bullous myringitis**, bilateral

H73.Ø19 **Bullous myringitis**, unspecified ear

✓6ᵗʰ H73.Ø9 **Other acute myringitis**

H73.Ø91 **Other acute myringitis**, right ear

H73.Ø92 **Other acute myringitis**, left ear

H73.Ø93 **Other acute myringitis**, bilateral

H73.Ø99 **Other acute myringitis**, unspecified ear

✓5ᵗʰ **H73.1 Chronic myringitis**

Chronic tympanitis

EXCLUDES 1 *chronic myringitis with otitis media (H65, H66)*

H73.1Ø **Chronic myringitis**, unspecified ear

H73.11 **Chronic myringitis**, right ear

H73.12 **Chronic myringitis**, left ear

H73.13 **Chronic myringitis**, bilateral

✓5ᵗʰ **H73.2 Unspecified myringitis**

H73.2Ø **Unspecified myringitis**, unspecified ear

H73.21 **Unspecified myringitis**, right ear

H73.22 **Unspecified myringitis**, left ear

H73.23 **Unspecified myringitis**, bilateral

✓5ᵗʰ **H73.8 Other specified disorders of tympanic membrane**

✓6ᵗʰ H73.81 **Atrophic flaccid tympanic membrane**

H73.811 **Atrophic flaccid tympanic membrane, right ear**

H73.812 **Atrophic flaccid tympanic membrane, left ear**

H73.813 **Atrophic flaccid tympanic membrane, bilateral**

H73.819 **Atrophic flaccid tympanic membrane, unspecified ear**

✓6ᵗʰ H73.82 **Atrophic nonflaccid tympanic membrane**

H73.821 **Atrophic nonflaccid tympanic membrane, right ear**

H73.822 **Atrophic nonflaccid tympanic membrane, left ear**

H73.823 **Atrophic nonflaccid tympanic membrane, bilateral**

H73.829 **Atrophic nonflaccid tympanic membrane, unspecified ear**

✓6ᵗʰ H73.89 **Other specified disorders of tympanic membrane**

H73.891 **Other specified disorders of tympanic membrane, right ear**

H73.892 **Other specified disorders of tympanic membrane, left ear**

H73.893 **Other specified disorders of tympanic membrane, bilateral**

H73.899 **Other specified disorders of tympanic membrane, unspecified ear**

✓5ᵗʰ **H73.9 Unspecified disorder of tympanic membrane**

H73.9Ø **Unspecified disorder of tympanic membrane, unspecified ear**

H73.91 **Unspecified disorder of tympanic membrane, right ear**

H73.92 **Unspecified disorder of tympanic membrane, left ear**

H73.93 **Unspecified disorder of tympanic membrane, bilateral**

✓4ᵗʰ **H74 Other disorders of middle ear mastoid**

EXCLUDES 2 *mastoiditis (H7Ø.-)*

✓5ᵗʰ **H74.Ø Tympanosclerosis**

**DEF:** Calcification of tissue in the ear drum, middle ear bones, and middle ear canal.

H74.Ø1 **Tympanosclerosis**, right ear

H74.Ø2 **Tympanosclerosis**, left ear

H74.Ø3 **Tympanosclerosis**, bilateral

H74.Ø9 **Tympanosclerosis**, unspecified ear

✓5ᵗʰ **H74.1 Adhesive middle ear disease**

Adhesive otitis

EXCLUDES 1 *glue ear (H65.3-)*

H74.11 **Adhesive right middle ear disease**

H74.12 **Adhesive left middle ear disease**

H74.13 **Adhesive middle ear disease**, bilateral

H74.19 **Adhesive middle ear disease**, unspecified ear

✓5ᵗʰ **H74.2 Discontinuity and dislocation of ear ossicles**

H74.2Ø **Discontinuity and dislocation of ear ossicles, unspecified ear**

H74.21 **Discontinuity and dislocation of right ear ossicles**

H74.22 **Discontinuity and dislocation of left ear ossicles**

H74.23 **Discontinuity and dislocation of ear ossicles, bilateral**

✓5ᵗʰ **H74.3 Other acquired abnormalities of ear ossicles**

✓6ᵗʰ H74.31 **Ankylosis of ear ossicles**

H74.311 **Ankylosis of ear ossicles**, right ear

H74.312 **Ankylosis of ear ossicles**, left ear

H74.313 **Ankylosis of ear ossicles**, bilateral

H74.319 **Ankylosis of ear ossicles**, unspecified ear

✓6ᵗʰ H74.32 **Partial loss of ear ossicles**

H74.321 **Partial loss of ear ossicles**, right ear

H74.322 **Partial loss of ear ossicles**, left ear

H74.323 **Partial loss of ear ossicles**, bilateral

H74.329 **Partial loss of ear ossicles**, unspecified ear

✓6ᵗʰ H74.39 **Other acquired abnormalities of ear ossicles**

H74.391 **Other acquired abnormalities of right ear ossicles**

H74.392 **Other acquired abnormalities of left ear ossicles**

H74.393 **Other acquired abnormalities of ear ossicles, bilateral**

H74.399 **Other acquired abnormalities of ear ossicles, unspecified ear**

✓5ᵗʰ **H74.4 Polyp of middle ear**

H74.4Ø **Polyp of middle ear**, unspecified ear

H74.41 **Polyp of right middle ear**

H74.42 **Polyp of left middle ear**

H74.43 **Polyp of middle ear**, bilateral

✓5ᵗʰ **H74.8 Other specified disorders of middle ear and mastoid**

✓6ᵗʰ H74.8X **Other specified disorders of middle ear and mastoid**

H74.8X1 **Other specified disorders of right middle ear and mastoid**

H74.8X2 **Other specified disorders of left middle ear and mastoid**

H74.8X3 **Other specified disorders of middle ear and mastoid, bilateral**

H74.8X9 **Other specified disorders of middle ear and mastoid, unspecified ear**

✓5ᵗʰ **H74.9 Unspecified disorder of middle ear and mastoid**

H74.9Ø **Unspecified disorder of middle ear and mastoid, unspecified ear**

H74.91 **Unspecified disorder of right middle ear and mastoid**

H74.92 **Unspecified disorder of left middle ear and mastoid**

H74.93 **Unspecified disorder of middle ear and mastoid, bilateral**

✓4ᵗʰ **H75 Other disorders of middle ear and mastoid in diseases classified elsewhere**

Code first underlying disease

✓5ᵗʰ **H75.Ø Mastoiditis in infectious and parasitic diseases classified elsewhere**

EXCLUDES 1 *mastoiditis (in):*
*syphilis (A52.77)*
*tuberculosis (A18.Ø3)*

H75.ØØ *Mastoiditis in infectious and parasitic diseases classified elsewhere, unspecified ear*

H75.Ø1 *Mastoiditis in infectious and parasitic diseases classified elsewhere, right ear*

H75.Ø2 *Mastoiditis in infectious and parasitic diseases classified elsewhere, left ear*

H75.Ø3 *Mastoiditis in infectious and parasitic diseases classified elsewhere, bilateral*

✓5ᵗʰ **H75.8 Other specified disorders of middle ear and mastoid in diseases classified elsewhere**

H75.8Ø *Other specified disorders of middle ear and mastoid in diseases classified elsewhere, unspecified ear*

H75.81 *Other specified disorders of right middle ear and mastoid in diseases classified elsewhere*

H75.82 *Other specified disorders of left middle ear and mastoid in diseases classified elsewhere*

Ⓝ Newborn: 0   Ⓟ Pediatric: 0-17   Ⓜ Maternity: 12-55   Ⓐ Adult: 15-124   **MCC** Major CC Condition   **PDxMCC** PDx acts as own MCC   **CC** CC Condition   **PDxCC** PDx acts as own CC

**622**  ICD-10-CM 2018

**H75.83**  *Other specified disorders of middle ear and mastoid in diseases classified elsewhere, bilateral*

## Diseases of inner ear (H80-H83)

✓4ᵗʰ **H80  Otosclerosis**
INCLUDES  otospongiosis

✓5ᵗʰ **H80.0  Otosclerosis involving oval window, nonobliterative**
- **H80.00  Otosclerosis involving oval window, nonobliterative, unspecified ear**
- **H80.01  Otosclerosis involving oval window, nonobliterative, right ear**
- **H80.02  Otosclerosis involving oval window, nonobliterative, left ear**
- **H80.03  Otosclerosis involving oval window, nonobliterative, bilateral**

✓5ᵗʰ **H80.1  Otosclerosis involving oval window, obliterative**
- **H80.10  Otosclerosis involving oval window, obliterative, unspecified ear**
- **H80.11  Otosclerosis involving oval window, obliterative, right ear**
- **H80.12  Otosclerosis involving oval window, obliterative, left ear**
- **H80.13  Otosclerosis involving oval window, obliterative, bilateral**

✓5ᵗʰ **H80.2  Cochlear otosclerosis**
Otosclerosis involving otic capsule
Otosclerosis involving round window
- **H80.20  Cochlear otosclerosis, unspecified ear**
- **H80.21  Cochlear otosclerosis, right ear**
- **H80.22  Cochlear otosclerosis, left ear**
- **H80.23  Cochlear otosclerosis, bilateral**

✓5ᵗʰ **H80.8  Other otosclerosis**
- **H80.80  Other otosclerosis, unspecified ear**
- **H80.81  Other otosclerosis, right ear**
- **H80.82  Other otosclerosis, left ear**
- **H80.83  Other otosclerosis, bilateral**

✓5ᵗʰ **H80.9  Unspecified otosclerosis**
- **H80.90  Unspecified otosclerosis, unspecified ear**
- **H80.91  Unspecified otosclerosis, right ear**
- **H80.92  Unspecified otosclerosis, left ear**
- **H80.93  Unspecified otosclerosis, bilateral**

✓4ᵗʰ **H81  Disorders of vestibular function**
EXCLUDES 1  epidemic vertigo (A88.1)
vertigo NOS (R42)

✓5ᵗʰ **H81.0  Ménière's disease**
Labyrinthine hydrops
Ménière's syndrome or vertigo
- **H81.01  Ménière's disease, right ear**
- **H81.02  Ménière's disease, left ear**
- **H81.03  Ménière's disease, bilateral**
- **H81.09  Ménière's disease, unspecified ear**

✓5ᵗʰ **H81.1  Benign paroxysmal vertigo**
- **H81.10  Benign paroxysmal vertigo, unspecified ear**
- **H81.11  Benign paroxysmal vertigo, right ear**
- **H81.12  Benign paroxysmal vertigo, left ear**
- **H81.13  Benign paroxysmal vertigo, bilateral**

✓5ᵗʰ **H81.2  Vestibular neuronitis**
**DEF:** Transient benign vertigo, caused by inflammation of the vestibular nerve; characterized by response to caloric stimulation on one side, nystagmus with rhythmic movement of eyes; normal auditory function present.
- **H81.20  Vestibular neuronitis, unspecified ear**
- **H81.21  Vestibular neuronitis, right ear**
- **H81.22  Vestibular neuronitis, left ear**
- **H81.23  Vestibular neuronitis, bilateral**

✓5ᵗʰ **H81.3  Other peripheral vertigo**
✓6ᵗʰ **H81.31  Aural vertigo**
- **H81.311  Aural vertigo, right ear**
- **H81.312  Aural vertigo, left ear**
- **H81.313  Aural vertigo, bilateral**
- **H81.319  Aural vertigo, unspecified ear**

✓6ᵗʰ **H81.39  Other peripheral vertigo**
Lermoyez' syndrome
Otogenic vertigo
Peripheral vertigo NOS
- **H81.391  Other peripheral vertigo, right ear**
- **H81.392  Other peripheral vertigo, left ear**
- **H81.393  Other peripheral vertigo, bilateral**
- **H81.399  Other peripheral vertigo, unspecified ear**

✓5ᵗʰ **H81.4  Vertigo of central origin**
Central positional nystagmus
- **H81.41  Vertigo of central origin, right ear**
- **H81.42  Vertigo of central origin, left ear**
- **H81.43  Vertigo of central origin, bilateral**
- **H81.49  Vertigo of central origin, unspecified ear**

✓5ᵗʰ **H81.8  Other disorders of vestibular function**
✓6ᵗʰ **H81.8X  Other disorders of vestibular function**
- **H81.8X1  Other disorders of vestibular function, right ear**
- **H81.8X2  Other disorders of vestibular function, left ear**
- **H81.8X3  Other disorders of vestibular function, bilateral**
- **H81.8X9  Other disorders of vestibular function, unspecified ear**

✓5ᵗʰ **H81.9  Unspecified disorder of vestibular function**
Vertiginous syndrome NOS
- **H81.90  Unspecified disorder of vestibular function, unspecified ear**
- **H81.91  Unspecified disorder of vestibular function, right ear**
- **H81.92  Unspecified disorder of vestibular function, left ear**
- **H81.93  Unspecified disorder of vestibular function, bilateral**

✓4ᵗʰ **H82  Vertiginous syndromes in diseases classified elsewhere**
Code first underlying disease
EXCLUDES 1  epidemic vertigo (A88.1)

**H82.1**  *Vertiginous syndromes in diseases classified elsewhere, right ear*

**H82.2**  *Vertiginous syndromes in diseases classified elsewhere, left ear*

**H82.3**  *Vertiginous syndromes in diseases classified elsewhere, bilateral*

**H82.9**  *Vertiginous syndromes in diseases classified elsewhere, unspecified ear*

✓4ᵗʰ **H83  Other diseases of inner ear**
✓5ᵗʰ **H83.0  Labyrinthitis**
**DEF:** Inflammation of the inner ear, or labyrinth; characterized by pus, vertigo, dizziness, nausea, and hearing loss.
- **H83.01  Labyrinthitis, right ear**
- **H83.02  Labyrinthitis, left ear**
- **H83.03  Labyrinthitis, bilateral**
- **H83.09  Labyrinthitis, unspecified ear**

✓5ᵗʰ **H83.1  Labyrinthine fistula**
- **H83.11  Labyrinthine fistula, right ear**
- **H83.12  Labyrinthine fistula, left ear**
- **H83.13  Labyrinthine fistula, bilateral**
- **H83.19  Labyrinthine fistula, unspecified ear**

✓5ᵗʰ **H83.2  Labyrinthine dysfunction**
Labyrinthine hypersensitivity
Labyrinthine hypofunction
Labyrinthine loss of function
**DEF:** Decreased function of the labyrinth sensors.
✓6ᵗʰ **H83.2X  Labyrinthine dysfunction**
- **H83.2X1  Labyrinthine dysfunction, right ear**
- **H83.2X2  Labyrinthine dysfunction, left ear**
- **H83.2X3  Labyrinthine dysfunction, bilateral**
- **H83.2X9  Labyrinthine dysfunction, unspecified ear**

✓5ᵗʰ **H83.3  Noise effects on inner ear**
Acoustic trauma of inner ear
Noise-induced hearing loss of inner ear
✓6ᵗʰ **H83.3X  Noise effects on inner ear**
- **H83.3X1  Noise effects on right inner ear**
- **H83.3X2  Noise effects on left inner ear**
- **H83.3X3  Noise effects on inner ear, bilateral**
- **H83.3X9  Noise effects on inner ear, unspecified ear**

✓ Additional Character Req   ✓x7ᵗʰ Placeholder Alert   Unacceptable PDx   Manifestation   **H1**-**H14** HAC   HCC CMS-HCC Condition   EXCLUDES 1 Not Coded Here   EXCLUDES 2 Not Included Here

ICD-10-CM 2018                                                                              **623**

Chapter 8. Diseases of the Ear and Mastoid Process

H75.83–H83.3X9

✓5ᵗʰ **H83.8 Other specified diseases of inner ear**

    ✓6ᵗʰ **H83.8X Other specified diseases of inner ear**

        **H83.8X1 Other specified diseases of right inner ear**

        **H83.8X2 Other specified diseases of left inner ear**

        **H83.8X3 Other specified diseases of inner ear, bilateral**

        **H83.8X9 Other specified diseases of inner ear, unspecified ear**

✓5ᵗʰ **H83.9 Unspecified disease of inner ear**

    **H83.90 Unspecified disease of inner ear, unspecified ear**

    **H83.91 Unspecified disease of right inner ear**

    **H83.92 Unspecified disease of left inner ear**

    **H83.93 Unspecified disease of inner ear, bilateral**

### Other disorders of ear (H90-H94)

✓4ᵗʰ **H90 Conductive and sensorineural hearing loss**

    **EXCLUDES 1**    *deaf nonspeaking NEC (H91.3)*
         *deafness NOS (H91.9-)*
         *hearing loss NOS (H91.9-)*
         *noise-induced hearing loss (H83.3-)*
         *ototoxic hearing loss (H91.0-)*
         *sudden (idiopathic) hearing loss (H91.2-)*

    **AHA:** 2015, 2Q, 7

    **H90.0 Conductive hearing loss, bilateral**

✓5ᵗʰ **H90.1 Conductive hearing loss, unilateral with unrestricted hearing on the contralateral side**

    **H90.11 Conductive hearing loss, unilateral, right ear, with unrestricted hearing on the contralateral side**

    **H90.12 Conductive hearing loss, unilateral, left ear, with unrestricted hearing on the contralateral side**

    **H90.2 Conductive hearing loss, unspecified**
        Conductive deafness NOS

    **H90.3 Sensorineural hearing loss, bilateral**

✓5ᵗʰ **H90.4 Sensorineural hearing loss, unilateral with unrestricted hearing on the contralateral side**

    **H90.41 Sensorineural hearing loss, unilateral, right ear, with unrestricted hearing on the contralateral side**

    **H90.42 Sensorineural hearing loss, unilateral, left ear, with unrestricted hearing on the contralateral side**

    **H90.5 Unspecified sensorineural hearing loss**
        Central hearing loss NOS      Perceptive hearing loss NOS
        Congenital deafness NOS      Sensorineural deafness NOS
        Neural hearing loss NOS      Sensory hearing loss NOS

        **EXCLUDES 1**    *abnormal auditory perception (H93.2-)*
             *psychogenic deafness (F44.6)*

    **H90.6 Mixed conductive and sensorineural hearing loss, bilateral**
        **AHA:** 2015, 2Q, 7

✓5ᵗʰ **H90.7 Mixed conductive and sensorineural hearing loss, unilateral with unrestricted hearing on the contralateral side**

    **H90.71 Mixed conductive and sensorineural hearing loss, unilateral, right ear, with unrestricted hearing on the contralateral side**

    **H90.72 Mixed conductive and sensorineural hearing loss, unilateral, left ear, with unrestricted hearing on the contralateral side**

    **H90.8 Mixed conductive and sensorineural hearing loss, unspecified**

✓5ᵗʰ **H90.A Conductive and sensorineural hearing loss with restricted hearing on the contralateral side**

    ✓6ᵗʰ **H90.A1 Conductive hearing loss, unilateral, with restricted hearing on the contralateral side**

        **H90.A11 Conductive hearing loss, unilateral, right ear with restricted hearing on the contralateral side**

        **H90.A12 Conductive hearing loss, unilateral, left ear with restricted hearing on the contralateral side**

    ✓6ᵗʰ **H90.A2 Sensorineural hearing loss, unilateral, with restricted hearing on the contralateral side**

        **H90.A21 Sensorineural hearing loss, unilateral, right ear, with restricted hearing on the contralateral side**

        **H90.A22 Sensorineural hearing loss, unilateral, left ear, with restricted hearing on the contralateral side**

    ✓6ᵗʰ **H90.A3 Mixed conductive and sensorineural hearing loss, unilateral with restricted hearing on the contralateral side**

        **H90.A31 Mixed conductive and sensorineural hearing loss, unilateral, right ear with restricted hearing on the contralateral side**

        **H90.A32 Mixed conductive and sensorineural hearing loss, unilateral, left ear with restricted hearing on the contralateral side**

✓4ᵗʰ **H91 Other and unspecified hearing loss**

    **EXCLUDES 1**    *abnormal auditory perception (H93.2-)*
         *hearing loss as classified in H90-*
         *impacted cerumen (H61.2-)*
         *noise-induced hearing loss (H83.3-)*
         *psychogenic deafness (F44.6)*
         *transient ischemic deafness (H93.01-)*

✓5ᵗʰ **H91.0 Ototoxic hearing loss**

    Code first poisoning due to drug or toxin, if applicable (T36-T65 with fifth or sixth character 1-4 or 6)

    Use additional code for adverse effect, if applicable, to identify drug (T36-T50 with fifth or sixth character 5)

    **H91.01 Ototoxic hearing loss, right ear**

    **H91.02 Ototoxic hearing loss, left ear**

    **H91.03 Ototoxic hearing loss, bilateral**

    **H91.09 Ototoxic hearing loss, unspecified ear**

✓5ᵗʰ **H91.1 Presbycusis**
    Presbyacusia

    **H91.10 Presbycusis, unspecified ear**

    **H91.11 Presbycusis, right ear**

    **H91.12 Presbycusis, left ear**

    **H91.13 Presbycusis, bilateral**

✓5ᵗʰ **H91.2 Sudden idiopathic hearing loss**
    Sudden hearing loss NOS

    **H91.20 Sudden idiopathic hearing loss, unspecified ear**

    **H91.21 Sudden idiopathic hearing loss, right ear**

    **H91.22 Sudden idiopathic hearing loss, left ear**

    **H91.23 Sudden idiopathic hearing loss, bilateral**

    **H91.3 Deaf nonspeaking, not elsewhere classified**

✓5ᵗʰ **H91.8 Other specified hearing loss**

    ✓6ᵗʰ **H91.8X Other specified hearing loss**

        **H91.8X1 Other specified hearing loss, right ear**

        **H91.8X2 Other specified hearing loss, left ear**

        **H91.8X3 Other specified hearing loss, bilateral**

        **H91.8X9 Other specified hearing loss, unspecified ear**

✓5ᵗʰ **H91.9 Unspecified hearing loss**
    Deafness NOS
    High frequency deafness
    Low frequency deafness

    **H91.90 Unspecified hearing loss, unspecified ear**

    **H91.91 Unspecified hearing loss, right ear**

    **H91.92 Unspecified hearing loss, left ear**

    **H91.93 Unspecified hearing loss, bilateral**

✓4ᵗʰ **H92 Otalgia and effusion of ear**

✓5ᵗʰ **H92.0 Otalgia**

    **H92.01 Otalgia, right ear**

    **H92.02 Otalgia, left ear**

    **H92.03 Otalgia, bilateral**

    **H92.09 Otalgia, unspecified ear**

✓5ᵗʰ **H92.1 Otorrhea**

    **EXCLUDES 1**    *leakage of cerebrospinal fluid through ear (G96.0)*

    **H92.10 Otorrhea, unspecified ear**

    **H92.11 Otorrhea, right ear**

    **H92.12 Otorrhea, left ear**

    **H92.13 Otorrhea, bilateral**

✓5ᵗʰ **H92.2 Otorrhagia**

    **EXCLUDES 1**    *traumatic otorrhagia—code to injury*

    **H92.20 Otorrhagia, unspecified ear**

    **H92.21 Otorrhagia, right ear**

    **H92.22 Otorrhagia, left ear**

    **H92.23 Otorrhagia, bilateral**

Ⓝ Newborn: 0    Ⓟ Pediatric: 0-17    Ⓜ Maternity: 12-55    Ⓐ Adult: 15-124    **MCC** Major CC Condition    **PDxMCC** PDx acts as own MCC    **CC** CC Condition    **PDxCC** PDx acts as own CC

**624**      ICD-10-CM 2018

### ✓4th H93 Other disorders of ear, not elsewhere classified

#### ✓5th H93.0 Degenerative and vascular disorders of ear
EXCLUDES 1   presbycusis (H91.1)

##### ✓6th H93.01 Transient ischemic deafness
- H93.011 Transient ischemic deafness, right ear
- H93.012 Transient ischemic deafness, left ear
- H93.013 Transient ischemic deafness, bilateral
- H93.019 Transient ischemic deafness, unspecified ear

##### ✓6th H93.09 Unspecified degenerative and vascular disorders of ear
- H93.091 Unspecified degenerative and vascular disorders of right ear
- H93.092 Unspecified degenerative and vascular disorders of left ear
- H93.093 Unspecified degenerative and vascular disorders of ear, bilateral
- H93.099 Unspecified degenerative and vascular disorders of unspecified ear

#### ✓5th H93.1 Tinnitus
- H93.11 Tinnitus, right ear
- H93.12 Tinnitus, left ear
- H93.13 Tinnitus, bilateral
- H93.19 Tinnitus, unspecified ear

#### ✓5th H93.A Pulsatile Tinnitus
- H93.A1 Pulsatile tinnitus, right ear
- H93.A2 Pulsatile tinnitus, left ear
- H93.A3 Pulsatile tinnitus, bilateral
- H93.A9 Pulsatile tinnitus, unspecified ear

#### ✓5th H93.2 Other abnormal auditory perceptions
EXCLUDES 2   auditory hallucinations (R44.0)

##### ✓6th H93.21 Auditory recruitment
- H93.211 Auditory recruitment, right ear
- H93.212 Auditory recruitment, left ear
- H93.213 Auditory recruitment, bilateral
- H93.219 Auditory recruitment, unspecified ear

##### ✓6th H93.22 Diplacusis
- H93.221 Diplacusis, right ear
- H93.222 Diplacusis, left ear
- H93.223 Diplacusis, bilateral
- H93.229 Diplacusis, unspecified ear

##### ✓6th H93.23 Hyperacusis
DEF: Exceptionally acute sense of hearing caused by such conditions as Bell's palsy; this term may also refer to painful sensitivity to sounds.
- H93.231 Hyperacusis, right ear
- H93.232 Hyperacusis, left ear
- H93.233 Hyperacusis, bilateral
- H93.239 Hyperacusis, unspecified ear

##### ✓6th H93.24 Temporary auditory threshold shift
- H93.241 Temporary auditory threshold shift, right ear
- H93.242 Temporary auditory threshold shift, left ear
- H93.243 Temporary auditory threshold shift, bilateral
- H93.249 Temporary auditory threshold shift, unspecified ear

##### H93.25 Central auditory processing disorder
Congenital auditory imperception
Word deafness
EXCLUDES 1   mixed receptive-expressive language disorder (F80.2)

##### ✓6th H93.29 Other abnormal auditory perceptions
- H93.291 Other abnormal auditory perceptions, right ear
- H93.292 Other abnormal auditory perceptions, left ear
- H93.293 Other abnormal auditory perceptions, bilateral
- H93.299 Other abnormal auditory perceptions, unspecified ear

#### ✓5th H93.3 Disorders of acoustic nerve
Disorder of 8th cranial nerve
EXCLUDES 1   acoustic neuroma (D33.3)
     syphilitic acoustic neuritis (A52.15)

##### ✓6th H93.3X Disorders of acoustic nerve
- H93.3X1 Disorders of right acoustic nerve
- H93.3X2 Disorders of left acoustic nerve
- H93.3X3 Disorders of bilateral acoustic nerves
- H93.3X9 Disorders of unspecified acoustic nerve

#### ✓5th H93.8 Other specified disorders of ear

##### ✓6th H93.8X Other specified disorders of ear
- H93.8X1 Other specified disorders of right ear
- H93.8X2 Other specified disorders of left ear
- H93.8X3 Other specified disorders of ear, bilateral
- H93.8X9 Other specified disorders of ear, unspecified ear

#### ✓5th H93.9 Unspecified disorder of ear
- H93.90 Unspecified disorder of ear, unspecified ear
- H93.91 Unspecified disorder of right ear
- H93.92 Unspecified disorder of left ear
- H93.93 Unspecified disorder of ear, bilateral

### ✓4th H94 Other disorders of ear in diseases classified elsewhere

#### ✓5th H94.0 Acoustic neuritis in infectious and parasitic diseases classified elsewhere
Code first underlying disease, such as:
parasitic disease (B65-B89)
EXCLUDES 1   acoustic neuritis (in):
     herpes zoster (B02.29)
     syphilis (A52.15)
- H94.00 Acoustic neuritis in infectious and parasitic diseases classified elsewhere, unspecified ear
- H94.01 Acoustic neuritis in infectious and parasitic diseases classified elsewhere, right ear
- H94.02 Acoustic neuritis in infectious and parasitic diseases classified elsewhere, left ear
- H94.03 Acoustic neuritis in infectious and parasitic diseases classified elsewhere, bilateral

#### ✓5th H94.8 Other specified disorders of ear in diseases classified elsewhere
Code first underlying disease, such as:
congenital syphilis (A50.0)
EXCLUDES 1   aural myiasis (B87.4)
     syphilitic labyrinthitis (A52.79)
- H94.80 Other specified disorders of ear in diseases classified elsewhere, unspecified ear
- H94.81 Other specified disorders of right ear in diseases classified elsewhere
- H94.82 Other specified disorders of left ear in diseases classified elsewhere
- H94.83 Other specified disorders of ear in diseases classified elsewhere, bilateral

## Intraoperative and postprocedural complications and disorders of ear and mastoid process, not elsewhere classified (H95)

### ✓4th H95 Intraoperative and postprocedural complications and disorders of ear and mastoid process, not elsewhere classified

#### ✓5th H95.0 Recurrent cholesteatoma of postmastoidectomy cavity
- H95.00 Recurrent cholesteatoma of postmastoidectomy cavity, unspecified ear
- H95.01 Recurrent cholesteatoma of postmastoidectomy cavity, right ear
- H95.02 Recurrent cholesteatoma of postmastoidectomy cavity, left ear
- H95.03 Recurrent cholesteatoma of postmastoidectomy cavity, bilateral ears

#### ✓5th H95.1 Other disorders of ear and mastoid process following mastoidectomy

##### ✓6th H95.11 Chronic inflammation of postmastoidectomy cavity
- H95.111 Chronic inflammation of postmastoidectomy cavity, right ear
- H95.112 Chronic inflammation of postmastoidectomy cavity, left ear
- H95.113 Chronic inflammation of postmastoidectomy cavity, bilateral ears

**Chapter 8. Diseases of the Ear and Mastoid Process**

H95.119    **Chronic inflammation of postmastoidectomy cavity, unspecified ear**

✓6ᵗʰ   **H95.12**    **Granulation of postmastoidectomy cavity**

H95.121    **Granulation of postmastoidectomy cavity, right ear**

H95.122    **Granulation of postmastoidectomy cavity, left ear**

H95.123    **Granulation of postmastoidectomy cavity, bilateral ears**

H95.129    **Granulation of postmastoidectomy cavity, unspecified ear**

✓6ᵗʰ   **H95.13**    **Mucosal cyst of postmastoidectomy cavity**

H95.131    **Mucosal cyst of postmastoidectomy cavity, right ear**

H95.132    **Mucosal cyst of postmastoidectomy cavity, left ear**

H95.133    **Mucosal cyst of postmastoidectomy cavity, bilateral ears**

H95.139    **Mucosal cyst of postmastoidectomy cavity, unspecified ear**

✓6ᵗʰ   **H95.19**    **Other disorders following mastoidectomy**

H95.191    **Other disorders following mastoidectomy, right ear**

H95.192    **Other disorders following mastoidectomy, left ear**

H95.193    **Other disorders following mastoidectomy, bilateral ears**

H95.199    **Other disorders following mastoidectomy, unspecified ear**

✓5ᵗʰ   **H95.2**    **Intraoperative hemorrhage and hematoma of ear and mastoid process complicating a procedure**

*EXCLUDES 1*    *intraoperative hemorrhage and hematoma of ear and mastoid process due to accidental puncture or laceration during a procedure (H95.3-)*

H95.21    **Intraoperative hemorrhage and hematoma of ear and mastoid process complicating a procedure on the ear and mastoid process**    `CC`
**CC Excl:** PDX collection 642

H95.22    **Intraoperative hemorrhage and hematoma of of ear and mastoid process complicating other procedure**    `CC`
**CC Excl:** PDX collection 642

✓5ᵗʰ   **H95.3**    **Accidental puncture and laceration of ear and mastoid process during a procedure**

H95.31    **Accidental puncture and laceration of the ear and mastoid process during a procedure on the ear and mastoid process**    `CC`
**CC Excl:** PDX collection 509

H95.32    **Accidental puncture and laceration of the ear and mastoid process during other procedure**    `CC`
**CC Excl:** PDX collection 509

✓5ᵗʰ   **H95.4**    **Postprocedural hemorrhage of ear and mastoid process following a procedure**

H95.41    **Postprocedural hemorrhage of ear and mastoid process following a procedure on the ear and mastoid process**    `CC`
**CC Excl:** PDX collection 642

H95.42    **Postprocedural hemorrhage of ear and mastoid process following other procedure**    `CC`
**CC Excl:** PDX collection 642

✓5ᵗʰ   **H95.5**    **Postprocedural hematoma and seroma of ear and mastoid process following a procedure**

**CC Excl: For CC codes in subcategory H95.5:**
PDX collection 642

H95.51    **Postprocedural hematoma of ear and mastoid process following a procedure on the ear and mastoid process**    `CC`

H95.52    **Postprocedural hematoma of ear and mastoid process following other procedure**    `CC`

H95.53    **Postprocedural seroma of ear and mastoid process following a procedure on the ear and mastoid process**    `CC`

H95.54    **Postprocedural seroma of ear and mastoid process following other procedure**    `CC`

✓5ᵗʰ   **H95.8**    **Other intraoperative and postprocedural complications and disorders of the ear and mastoid process, not elsewhere classified**

*EXCLUDES 2*    *postprocedural complications and disorders following mastoidectomy (H95.0-, H95.1-)*

**CC Excl: For CC codes in subcategory H95.8:**
PDX collection 643

✓6ᵗʰ   **H95.81**    **Postprocedural stenosis of external ear canal**

H95.811    **Postprocedural stenosis of right external ear canal**    `CC`

H95.812    **Postprocedural stenosis of left external ear canal**    `CC`

H95.813    **Postprocedural stenosis of external ear canal, bilateral**    `CC`

H95.819    **Postprocedural stenosis of unspecified external ear canal**    `CC`

H95.88    **Other intraoperative complications and disorders of the ear and mastoid process, not elsewhere classified**    `CC`
Use additional code, if applicable, to further specify disorder

H95.89    **Other postprocedural complications and disorders of the ear and mastoid process, not elsewhere classified**    `CC`
Use additional code, if applicable, to further specify disorder

N Newborn: 0   P Pediatric: 0-17   M Maternity: 12-55   A Adult: 15-124   **MCC** Major CC Condition   **PDx MCC** PDx acts as own MCC   **CC** CC Condition   **PDx CC** PDx acts as own CC

**626**      ICD-10-CM 2018

# Chapter 9. Diseases of the Circulatory System (I00–I99)

## Chapter Specific Guidelines with Coding Examples

The chapter specific guidelines from the ICD-10-CM Official Guidelines for Coding and Reporting have been provided below. Along with these guidelines are coding examples, contained in the shaded boxes, that have been developed to help illustrate the coding and/or sequencing guidance found in these guidelines.

### a. Hypertension

The classification presumes a causal relationship between hypertension and heart involvement and between hypertension and kidney involvement, as the two conditions are linked by the term "with" in the Alphabetic Index. These conditions should be coded as related even in the absence of provider documentation explicitly linking them, unless the documentation clearly states the conditions are unrelated.

For hypertension and conditions not specifically linked by relational terms such as "with," "associated with" or "due to" in the classification, provider documentation must link the conditions in order to code them as related.

#### 1) Hypertension with heart disease

Hypertension with heart conditions classified to I50.- or I51.4-I51.9, are assigned to a code from category I11, Hypertensive heart disease. Use an additional code from category I50, Heart failure, to identify the type of heart failure in those patients with heart failure.

The same heart conditions (I50.-, I51.4-I51.9) with hypertension are coded separately if the provider has specifically documented a different cause. Sequence according to the circumstances of the admission/encounter.

> Patient is admitted in left heart failure. Patient also has a history of hypertension managed by medication.
>
> **11.0**      **Hypertensive heart disease with heart failure**
>
> **I50.1**      **Left ventricular failure, unspecified**
>
> *Explanation*: Without a diagnostic statement to the contrary, hypertension and heart failure have an assumed causal relationship, and a combination code should be used. An additional code to identify the type of heart failure (I50.-) should also be provided.

#### 2) Hypertensive chronic kidney disease

Assign codes from category I12, Hypertensive chronic kidney disease, when both hypertension and a condition classifiable to category N18, Chronic kidney disease (CKD), are present. CKD should not be coded as hypertensive if the physician has specifically documented a different cause.

The appropriate code from category N18 should be used as a secondary code with a code from category I12 to identify the stage of chronic kidney disease.

*See Section I.C.14. Chronic kidney disease.*

If a patient has hypertensive chronic kidney disease and acute renal failure, an additional code for the acute renal failure is required.

> Patient is admitted with stage IV chronic kidney disease (CKD). The patient also has documented hypertension secondary to primary hyperparathyroidism.
>
> **N18.4**      **Chronic kidney disease, stage 4 (severe)**
>
> **I10**      **Essential (primary) hypertension**
>
> **E21.0**      **Primary hyperparathyroidism**
>
> *Explanation*: A combination code describing a relationship between hypertension and CKD is not used due to the physician documentation identifying the primary hyperparathyroidism as the cause for the hypertension.

#### 3) Hypertensive heart and chronic kidney disease

Assign codes from combination category I13, Hypertensive heart and chronic kidney disease, when there is hypertension with both heart and kidney involvement. If heart failure is present, assign an additional code from category I50 to identify the type of heart failure.

The appropriate code from category N18, Chronic kidney disease, should be used as a secondary code with a code from category I13 to identify the stage of chronic kidney disease.

*See Section I.C.14. Chronic kidney disease.*

The codes in category I13, Hypertensive heart and chronic kidney disease, are combination codes that include hypertension, heart disease and chronic kidney disease. The Includes note at I13 specifies that the conditions included at I11 and I12 are included together in I13. If a patient

has hypertension, heart disease and chronic kidney disease, then a code from I13 should be used, not individual codes for hypertension, heart disease and chronic kidney disease, or codes from I11 or I12.

For patients with both acute renal failure and chronic kidney disease, an additional code for acute renal failure is required.

> Hypertensive heart and kidney disease with congestive heart failure and stage 2 chronic kidney disease
>
> **I13.0**      **Hypertensive heart and chronic kidney disease with heart failure and stage 1 through stage 4 chronic kidney disease, or unspecified chronic kidney disease**
>
> **I50.9**      **Heart failure, unspecified**
>
> **N18.2**      **Chronic kidney disease, stage 2 (mild)**
>
> *Explanation*: Combination codes in category I13 are used to report conditions classifiable to *both* categories I11 and I12. Do not report conditions classifiable to I11 and I12 separately. Use additional codes to report type of heart failure and stage of CKD.

#### 4) Hypertensive cerebrovascular disease

For hypertensive cerebrovascular disease, first assign the appropriate code from categories I60-I69, followed by the appropriate hypertension code.

> Rupture of cerebral aneurysm caused by malignant hypertension
>
> **I60.7**      **Nontraumatic subarachnoid hemorrhage from unspecified intracranial artery**
>
> **I10**      **Essential (primary) hypertension**
>
> *Explanation*: Hypertensive cerebrovascular disease requires two codes: the appropriate I60–I69 code followed by the appropriate hypertension code.

#### 5) Hypertensive retinopathy

Subcategory H35.0, Background retinopathy and retinal vascular changes, should be used with a code from category I10 – I15, Hypertensive disease to include the systemic hypertension. The sequencing is based on the reason for the encounter.

> Hypertensive retinopathy of the right eye
>
> **H35.031**      **Hypertensive retinopathy, right eye**
>
> **I10**      **Essential (primary) hypertension**
>
> *Explanation*: Hypertensive retinopathy requires two codes: the appropriate subcategory H35.0 code and a code for the hypertension.

#### 6) Hypertension, secondary

Secondary hypertension is due to an underlying condition. Two codes are required: one to identify the underlying etiology and one from category I15 to identify the hypertension. Sequencing of codes is determined by the reason for admission/encounter.

> Renovascular hypertension due to renal artery atherosclerosis
>
> **I15.0**      **Renovascular hypertension**
>
> **I70.1**      **Atherosclerosis of renal artery**
>
> *Explanation*: Secondary hypertension requires two codes: a code to identify the etiology and the appropriate I15 code.

#### 7) Hypertension, transient

Assign code R03.0, Elevated blood pressure reading without diagnosis of hypertension, unless patient has an established diagnosis of hypertension. Assign code O13.-, Gestational [pregnancy-induced] hypertension without significant proteinuria, or O14.-, Pre-eclampsia, for transient hypertension of pregnancy.

#### 8) Hypertension, controlled

This diagnostic statement usually refers to an existing state of hypertension under control by therapy. Assign the appropriate code from categories I10-I15, Hypertensive diseases.

#### 9) Hypertension, uncontrolled

Uncontrolled hypertension may refer to untreated hypertension or hypertension not responding to current therapeutic regimen. In either case, assign the appropriate code from categories I10-I15, Hypertensive diseases.

#### 10) Hypertensive Crisis

Assign a code from category I16, Hypertensive crisis, for documented hypertensive urgency, hypertensive emergency or unspecified hypertensive crisis. Code also any identified hypertensive disease (I10–I15). The sequencing is based on the reason for the encounter.

### b. Atherosclerotic coronary artery disease and angina

ICD-10-CM has combination codes for atherosclerotic heart disease with angina pectoris. The subcategories for these codes are I25.11, Atherosclerotic heart disease of native coronary artery with angina pectoris and I25.7, Atherosclerosis of coronary artery bypass graft(s) and coronary artery of transplanted heart with angina pectoris.

When using one of these combination codes it is not necessary to use an additional code for angina pectoris. A causal relationship can be assumed in a patient with both atherosclerosis and angina pectoris, unless the documentation indicates the angina is due to something other than the atherosclerosis.

If a patient with coronary artery disease is admitted due to an acute myocardial infarction (AMI), the AMI should be sequenced before the coronary artery disease.

*See Section I.C.9. Acute myocardial infarction (AMI)*

Patient is being seen for spastic angina pectoris. She also has a documented history of progressive coronary artery disease of the native vessels.

**I25.111**    **Atherosclerotic heart disease of native coronary artery with angina pectoris with documented spasm**

*Explanation*: Report the combination code for atherosclerotic heart disease (coronary artery disease) with angina pectoris. A causal relationship is assumed in a patient with both atherosclerosis and angina pectoris, unless the documentation indicates the angina is due to something other than the atherosclerosis. When using one of these combination codes, it is not necessary to use an additional code for angina pectoris.

### c. Intraoperative and postprocedural cerebrovascular accident

Medical record documentation should clearly specify the cause- and- effect relationship between the medical intervention and the cerebrovascular accident in order to assign a code for intraoperative or postprocedural cerebrovascular accident.

Proper code assignment depends on whether it was an infarction or hemorrhage and whether it occurred intraoperatively or postoperatively. If it was a cerebral hemorrhage, code assignment depends on the type of procedure performed.

Embolic cerebral infarction of the right middle cerebral artery that occurred during hip replacement surgery. The surgeon documented as due to the surgery.

**I97.811**    **Intraoperative cerebrovascular infarction during other surgery**

**I63.411**    **Cerebral infarction due to embolism of right middle cerebral artery**

*Explanation*: Code assignment for intraoperative or postprocedural cerebrovascular accident is based on the provider's documentation of a cause-and-effect relationship between the condition and the procedure. Proper code assignment also depends on whether the cerebrovascular accident was an infarction or hemorrhage, occurred intraoperatively or postoperatively, and the type of procedure performed.

### d. Sequelae of cerebrovascular disease

#### 1) Category I69, Sequelae of cerebrovascular disease

Category I69 is used to indicate conditions classifiable to categories I60-I67 as the causes of sequela (neurologic deficits), themselves classified elsewhere. These "late effects" include neurologic deficits that persist after initial onset of conditions classifiable to categories I60-I67. The neurologic deficits caused by cerebrovascular disease may be present from the onset or may arise at any time after the onset of the condition classifiable to categories I60-I67.

Codes from category I69, Sequelae of cerebrovascular disease, that specify hemiplegia, hemiparesis and monoplegia identify whether the dominant or nondominant side is affected. Should the affected side be documented, but not specified as dominant or nondominant, and the classification system does not indicate a default, code selection is as follows:

- For ambidextrous patients, the default should be dominant.
- If the left side is affected, the default is non-dominant.
- If the right side is affected, the default is dominant.

#### 2) Codes from category I69 with codes from I60–I67

Codes from category I69 may be assigned on a health care record with codes from I60-I67, if the patient has a current cerebrovascular disease and deficits from an old cerebrovascular disease.

#### 3) Codes from category I69 and personal history of transient ischemic attack (TIA) and cerebral infarction (Z86.73)

Codes from category I69 should not be assigned if the patient does not have neurologic deficits.

*See Section I.C.21. 4. History (of) for use of personal history codes*

### e. Acute myocardial infarction (AMI)

#### 1) ST elevation myocardial infarction (STEMI) and non ST elevation myocardial infarction (NSTEMI)

The ICD-10-CM codes for acute myocardial infarction (AMI) identify the site, such as anterolateral wall or true posterior wall. Subcategories I21.0-I21.2 and code I21.3 are used for ST elevation myocardial infarction (STEMI). Code I21.4, Non-ST elevation (NSTEMI) myocardial infarction, is used for non ST elevation myocardial infarction (NSTEMI) and nontransmural MIs.

If NSTEMI evolves to STEMI, assign the STEMI code. If STEMI converts to NSTEMI due to thrombolytic therapy, it is still coded as STEMI.

Acute inferior NSTEMI evolved into STEMI

**I21.19**    **ST elevation (STEMI) myocardial infarction involving other coronary artery of inferior wall**

*Explanation*: If an NSTEMI converts to a STEMI, report only the STEMI code.

For encounters occurring while the myocardial infarction is equal to, or less than, four weeks old, including transfers to another acute setting or a postacute setting, and the myocardial infarction meets the definition for "other diagnoses" (see Section III, Reporting Additional Diagnoses), codes from category I21 may continue to be reported. For encounters after the 4 week time frame and the patient is still receiving care related to the myocardial infarction, the appropriate aftercare code should be assigned, rather than a code from category I21. For old or healed myocardial infarctions not requiring further care, code I25.2, Old myocardial infarction, may be assigned.

#### 2) Acute myocardial infarction, unspecified

Code I21.3, ST elevation (STEMI) myocardial infarction of unspecified site, is the default for unspecified acute myocardial infarction. If only STEMI or transmural MI without the site is documented, assign code I21.3.

#### 3) AMI documented as nontransmural or subendocardial but site provided

If an AMI is documented as nontransmural or subendocardial, but the site is provided, it is still coded as a subendocardial AMI.

*See Section I.C.21.3 for information on coding status post administration of tPA in a different facility within the last 24 hours.*

Acute inferior subendocardial myocardial infarction (NSTEMI)

**I21.4**    **Non-ST elevation (NSTEMI) myocardial infarction**

*Explanation*: An AMI documented as subendocardial or nontransmural is coded as such (I21.4, I22.2), even if the site of infarction is specified.

#### 4) Subsequent acute myocardial infarction

A code from category I22, Subsequent ST elevation (STEMI) and non ST elevation (NSTEMI) myocardial infarction, is to be used when a patient who has suffered an AMI has a new AMI within the 4 week time frame of the initial AMI. A code from category I22 must be used in conjunction with a code from category I21. The sequencing of the I22 and I21 codes depends on the circumstances of the encounter.

Acute inferior STEMI status post acute NSTEMI two weeks ago.

**I22.1**    **Subsequent ST elevation (STEMI) myocardial infarction of inferior wall**

**I21.4**    **Non-ST elevation (NSTEMI) myocardial infarction**

*Explanation*: A code from I22 must be used in conjunction with a code from I21 when a patient who has suffered an AMI has a new AMI within four weeks of the initial one. Category I22 is never reported alone. The guidelines for assigning the correct I22 code are the same as those for reporting the initial MI (I21). Sequencing is determined by the circumstances of the encounter.

# Chapter 9. Diseases of the Circulatory System (I00-I99)

**EXCLUDES 2**   *certain conditions originating in the perinatal period (P04-P96)*
*certain infectious and parasitic diseases (A00-B99)*
*complications of pregnancy, childbirth and the puerperium (O00-O9A)*
*congenital malformations, deformations, and chromosomal abnormalities (Q00-Q99)*
*endocrine, nutritional and metabolic diseases (E00-E88)*
*injury, poisoning and certain other consequences of external causes (S00-T88)*
*neoplasms (C00-D49)*
*symptoms, signs and abnormal clinical and laboratory findings, not elsewhere classified (R00-R94)*
*systemic connective tissue disorders (M30-M36)*
*transient cerebral ischemic attacks and related syndromes (G45.-)*

This chapter contains the following blocks:

| | |
|---|---|
| I00-I02 | Acute rheumatic fever |
| I05-I09 | Chronic rheumatic heart diseases |
| I10-I16 | Hypertensive diseases |
| I20-I25 | Ischemic heart diseases |
| I26-I28 | Pulmonary heart disease and diseases of pulmonary circulation |
| I30-I52 | Other forms of heart disease |
| I60-I69 | Cerebrovascular diseases |
| I70-I79 | Diseases of arteries, arterioles and capillaries |
| I80-I89 | Diseases of veins, lymphatic vessels and lymph nodes, not elsewhere classified |
| I95-I99 | Other and unspecified disorders of the circulatory system |

## Acute rheumatic fever (I00-I02)

**I00**   **Rheumatic fever without heart involvement**
   **INCLUDES**   arthritis, rheumatic, acute or subacute
   **EXCLUDES 1**   *rheumatic fever with heart involvement (I01.0-I01.9)*

√4ᵗʰ **I01**   **Rheumatic fever with heart involvement**
   **EXCLUDES 1**   *chronic diseases of rheumatic origin (I05-I09) unless rheumatic fever is also present or there is evidence of reactivation or activity of the rheumatic process.*

   **I01.0**   **Acute rheumatic pericarditis**    `CC`
     Any condition in I00 with pericarditis
     Rheumatic pericarditis (acute)
     **EXCLUDES 1**   *acute pericarditis not specified as rheumatic (I30.-)*
     **CC Excl:** PDX collection 188

   **I01.1**   **Acute rheumatic endocarditis**    `CC`
     Any condition in I00 with endocarditis or valvulitis
     Acute rheumatic valvulitis
     **CC Excl:** PDX collection 644

   **I01.2**   **Acute rheumatic myocarditis**    `CC`
     Any condition in I00 with myocarditis
     **CC Excl:** PDX collection 186

   **I01.8**   **Other acute rheumatic heart disease**    `CC`
     Any condition in I00 with other or multiple types of heart involvement
     Acute rheumatic pancarditis
     **CC Excl:** PDX collection 645

   **I01.9**   **Acute rheumatic heart disease, unspecified**    `CC`
     Any condition in I00 with unspecified type of heart involvement
     Rheumatic carditis, acute
     Rheumatic heart disease, active or acute
     **CC Excl:** PDX collection 646

√4ᵗʰ **I02**   **Rheumatic chorea**
   **INCLUDES**   Sydenham's chorea
   **EXCLUDES 1**   *chorea NOS (G25.5)*
            *Huntington's chorea (G10)*

   **I02.0**   **Rheumatic chorea with heart involvement**    `CC`
     Chorea NOS with heart involvement
     Rheumatic chorea with heart involvement of any type classifiable under I01-
     **CC Excl:** PDX collection 645

   **I02.9**   **Rheumatic chorea without heart involvement**    `CC`
     Rheumatic chorea NOS
     **CC Excl:** PDX collection 646

## Chronic rheumatic heart diseases (I05-I09)

√4ᵗʰ **I05**   **Rheumatic mitral valve diseases**
   **INCLUDES**   conditions classifiable to both I05.0 and I05.2-I05.9, whether specified as rheumatic or not
   **EXCLUDES 1**   *mitral valve disease specified as nonrheumatic (I34.-)*
            *mitral valve disease with aortic and/or tricuspid valve involvement (I08.-)*

   **I05.0**   **Rheumatic mitral stenosis**
     Mitral (valve) obstruction (rheumatic)
     **DEF:** Narrowing of mitral valve between left atrium and left ventricle; due to rheumatic fever; characterized by shortness of breath during or after exercise, fatigue, palpitations, chest discomfort, and swelling of feet or legs.

   **I05.1**   **Rheumatic mitral insufficiency**
     Rheumatic mitral incompetence
     Rheumatic mitral regurgitation
     **EXCLUDES 1**   *mitral insufficiency not specified as rheumatic (I34.0)*

   **I05.2**   **Rheumatic mitral stenosis with insufficiency**
     Rheumatic mitral stenosis with incompetence or regurgitation

   **I05.8**   **Other rheumatic mitral valve diseases**
     Rheumatic mitral (valve) failure

   **I05.9**   **Rheumatic mitral valve disease, unspecified**
     Rheumatic mitral (valve) disorder (chronic) NOS

√4ᵗʰ **I06**   **Rheumatic aortic valve diseases**
   **EXCLUDES 1**   *aortic valve disease not specified as rheumatic (I35.-)*
            *aortic valve disease with mitral and/or tricuspid valve involvement (I08.-)*

   **I06.0**   **Rheumatic aortic stenosis**
     Rheumatic aortic (valve) obstruction

   **I06.1**   **Rheumatic aortic insufficiency**
     Rheumatic aortic incompetence
     Rheumatic aortic regurgitation

   **I06.2**   **Rheumatic aortic stenosis with insufficiency**
     Rheumatic aortic stenosis with incompetence or regurgitation

   **I06.8**   **Other rheumatic aortic valve diseases**

   **I06.9**   **Rheumatic aortic valve disease, unspecified**
     Rheumatic aortic (valve) disease NOS

√4ᵗʰ **I07**   **Rheumatic tricuspid valve diseases**
   **INCLUDES**   rheumatic tricuspid valve diseases specified as rheumatic or unspecified
   **EXCLUDES 1**   *tricuspid valve disease specified as nonrheumatic (I36.-)*
            *tricuspid valve disease with aortic and/or mitral valve involvement (I08.-)*

   **I07.0**   **Rheumatic tricuspid stenosis**
     Tricuspid (valve) stenosis (rheumatic)

   **I07.1**   **Rheumatic tricuspid insufficiency**
     Tricuspid (valve) insufficiency (rheumatic)

   **I07.2**   **Rheumatic tricuspid stenosis and insufficiency**

   **I07.8**   **Other rheumatic tricuspid valve diseases**

   **I07.9**   **Rheumatic tricuspid valve disease, unspecified**
     Rheumatic tricuspid valve disorder NOS

√4ᵗʰ **I08**   **Multiple valve diseases**
   **INCLUDES**   multiple valve diseases specified as rheumatic or unspecified
   **EXCLUDES 1**   *endocarditis, valve unspecified (I38)*
            *multiple valve disease specified a nonrheumatic (I34.-, I35.-, I36.-, I37.-, I38.-, Q22.-, Q23.-, Q24.8-)*
            *rheumatic valve disease NOS (I09.1)*

   **I08.0**   **Rheumatic disorders of both mitral and aortic valves**
     Involvement of both mitral and aortic valves specified as rheumatic or unspecified

   **I08.1**   **Rheumatic disorders of both mitral and tricuspid valves**

   **I08.2**   **Rheumatic disorders of both aortic and tricuspid valves**

   **I08.3**   **Combined rheumatic disorders of mitral, aortic and tricuspid valves**

   **I08.8**   **Other rheumatic multiple valve diseases**

   **I08.9**   **Rheumatic multiple valve disease, unspecified**

√4ᵗʰ **I09**   **Other rheumatic heart diseases**

   **I09.0**   **Rheumatic myocarditis**    `CC`
     **EXCLUDES 1**   *myocarditis not specified as rheumatic (I51.4)*
     **CC Excl:** PDX collection 647

   **I09.1**   **Rheumatic diseases of endocardium, valve unspecified**
     Rheumatic endocarditis (chronic)
     Rheumatic valvulitis (chronic)
     **EXCLUDES 1**   *endocarditis, valve unspecified (I38)*

---

✔ Additional Character Req    ✔x7ᵗʰ Placeholder Alert    Unacceptable PDx    Manifestation    **H1** - **H14** HAC    **HCC** CMS-HCC Condition    **EXCLUDES 1** Not Coded Here    **EXCLUDES 2** Not Included Here

**I09.2 Chronic rheumatic pericarditis** ⸰CC
Adherent pericardium, rheumatic
Chronic rheumatic mediastinopericarditis
Chronic rheumatic myopericarditis
**EXCLUDES 1** *chronic pericarditis not specified as rheumatic (I31.-)*
CC Excl: PDX collection 188

✓5th **I09.8 Other specified rheumatic heart diseases**

**I09.81 Rheumatic heart failure** CC HCC
Use additional code to identify type of heart failure
(I50.-)
**DEF:** Decreased cardiac output, edema, and
hypertension; due to rheumatic heart disease.
CC Excl: PDX collection 648

**I09.89 Other specified rheumatic heart diseases**
Rheumatic disease of pulmonary valve

**I09.9 Rheumatic heart disease, unspecified**
Rheumatic carditis
**EXCLUDES 1** *rheumatoid carditis (M05.31)*

## Hypertensive diseases (I10-I16)

Use additional code to identify:
exposure to environmental tobacco smoke (Z77.22)
history of tobacco dependence (Z87.891)
occupational exposure to environmental tobacco smoke (Z57.31)
tobacco dependence (F17.-)
tobacco use (Z72.0)
**EXCLUDES 1** *neonatal hypertension (P29.2)*
*primary pulmonary hypertension (I27.0)*
**EXCLUDES 2** *hypertensive disease complicating pregnancy, childbirth and the*
*puerperium (O10-O11, O13-O16)*

⁴ **I10 Essential (primary) hypertension**
**INCLUDES** high blood pressure
hypertension (arterial) (benign) (essential) (malignant)
(primary) (systemic)
**EXCLUDES 1** *hypertensive disease complicating pregnancy, childbirth and*
*the puerperium (O10-O11, O13-O16)*
**EXCLUDES 2** *essential (primary) hypertension involving vessels of brain*
*(I60-I69)*
*essential (primary) hypertension involving vessels of eye*
*(H35.0-)*
**AHA:** 2016, 4Q, 27

✓4th **I11 Hypertensive heart disease**
**INCLUDES** ▶ any condition in I50.-, I51.4-I51.9 due to hypertension ◀

**I11.0 Hypertensive heart disease with heart failure** HCC
Hypertensive heart failure
Use additional code to identify type of heart failure (I50.-)
**AHA:** 2017, 1Q, 47

**I11.9 Hypertensive heart disease without heart failure**
Hypertensive heart disease NOS

✓4th **I12 Hypertensive chronic kidney disease**
**INCLUDES** any condition in N18 and N26- due to hypertension
arteriosclerosis of kidney
arteriosclerotic nephritis (chronic) (interstitial)
hypertensive nephropathy
nephrosclerosis
**EXCLUDES 1** *hypertension due to kidney disease (I15.0, I15.1)*
*renovascular hypertension (I15.0)*
*secondary hypertension (I15.-)*
**EXCLUDES 2** *acute kidney failure (N17.-)*
**AHA:** 2016, 3Q, 22

**I12.0 Hypertensive chronic kidney disease with stage 5** CC HCC
**chronic kidney disease or end stage renal disease**
Use additional code to identify the stage of chronic kidney
disease (N18.5, N18.6)
CC Excl: PDX collection 649

**I12.9 Hypertensive chronic kidney disease with stage 1 through**
**stage 4 chronic kidney disease, or unspecified chronic kidney**
**disease**
Hypertensive chronic kidney disease NOS
Hypertensive renal disease NOS
Use additional code to identify the stage of chronic kidney
disease (N18.1-N18.4, N18.9)

✓4th **I13 Hypertensive heart and chronic kidney disease**
**INCLUDES** any condition in I11.- with any condition in I12.-
cardiorenal disease
cardiovascular renal disease

**CC Excl: For CC codes in category I13:** PDX collection 650

**I13.0 Hypertensive heart and chronic kidney disease with** CC HCC
**heart failure and stage 1 through stage 4 chronic kidney**
**disease, or unspecified chronic kidney disease**
Use additional code to identify type of heart failure (I50.-)
Use additional code to identify stage of chronic kidney disease
(N18.1-N18.4, N18.9)

✓5th **I13.1 Hypertensive heart and chronic kidney disease without heart**
**failure**

**I13.10 Hypertensive heart and chronic kidney disease**
**without heart failure, with stage 1 through stage 4**
**chronic kidney disease, or unspecified chronic**
**kidney disease**
Hypertensive heart disease and hypertensive chronic
kidney disease NOS
Use additional code to identify the stage of chronic
kidney disease (N18.1-N18.4, N18.9)

**I13.11 Hypertensive heart and chronic kidney** CC HCC
**disease without heart failure, with stage 5**
**chronic kidney disease, or end stage renal disease**
Use additional code to identify the stage of chronic
kidney disease (N18.5, N18.6)

**I13.2 Hypertensive heart and chronic kidney disease** CC HCC
**with heart failure and with stage 5 chronic kidney**
**disease, or end stage renal disease**
Use additional code to identify type of heart failure (I50.-)
Use additional code to identify the stage of chronic kidney
disease (N18.5, N18.6)

✓4th **I15 Secondary hypertension**
Code also underlying condition
**EXCLUDES 1** *postprocedural hypertension (I97.3)*
**EXCLUDES 2** *secondary hypertension involving vessels of brain (I60-I69)*
*secondary hypertension involving vessels of eye (H35.0-)*

**I15.0 Renovascular hypertension**

**I15.1 Hypertension secondary to other renal disorders**
**AHA:** 2016, 3Q, 22

**I15.2 Hypertension secondary to endocrine disorders**

**I15.8 Other secondary hypertension**

**I15.9 Secondary hypertension, unspecified**

✓4th **I16 Hypertensive crisis**
Code also any identified hypertensive disease (I10-I15)
**AHA:** 2016, 4Q, 27

**I16.0 Hypertensive urgency**

**I16.1 Hypertensive emergency** CC
CC Excl: No Excl

**I16.9 Hypertensive crisis, unspecified** CC
CC Excl: No Excl

## Ischemic heart diseases (I20-I25)

Use additional code to identify presence of hypertension (I10-I16)

✓4th **I20 Angina pectoris**
Use additional code to identify:
exposure to environmental tobacco smoke (Z77.22)
history of tobacco dependence (Z87.891)
occupational exposure to environmental tobacco smoke (Z57.31)
tobacco dependence (F17.-)
tobacco use (Z72.0)
**EXCLUDES 1** *angina pectoris with atherosclerotic heart disease of native*
*coronary arteries (I25.1-)*
*atherosclerosis of coronary artery bypass graft(s) and coronary*
*artery of transplanted heart with angina pectoris (I25.7-)*
*postinfarction angina (I23.7)*

**I20.0 Unstable angina** CC HCC
Accelerated angina
Crescendo angina
De novo effort angina
Intermediate coronary syndrome
Preinfarction syndrome
Worsening effort angina
**DEF:** A condition representing an intermediate stage between
angina of effort and acute myocardial infarction.
CC Excl: PDX collection 651

---

⁴ Questionable admission when used as PDx.

**N** Newborn: 0  **P** Pediatric: 0-17  **M** Maternity: 12-55  **A** Adult: 15-124  **MCC** Major CC Condition  **PDxMCC** PDx acts as own MCC  **CC** CC Condition  **PDxCC** PDx acts as own CC

**630**
ICD-10-CM 2018

**I20.1**   **Angina pectoris with documented spasm**   `CC` `HCC`
Angiospastic angina
Prinzmetal angina
Spasm-induced angina
Variant angina
**CC Excl:** PDX collection 652

**I20.8**   **Other forms of angina pectoris**   `HCC`
Angina equivalent
Angina of effort
Coronary slow flow syndrome
Stable angina
Stenocardia
Use additional code(s) for symptoms associated with angina equivalent

**I20.9**   **Angina pectoris, unspecified**   `HCC`
Angina NOS
Anginal syndrome
Cardiac angina
Ischemic chest pain

▲ `√4ᵗʰ` **I21 Acute myocardial infarction**
    `INCLUDES`   cardiac infarction
coronary (artery) embolism
coronary (artery) occlusion
coronary (artery) rupture
coronary (artery) thrombosis
infarction of heart, myocardium, or ventricle
myocardial infarction specified as acute or with a stated duration of 4 weeks (28 days) or less from onset
Use additional code, if applicable, to identify:
exposure to environmental tobacco smoke (Z77.22)
history of tobacco dependence (Z87.891)
occupational exposure to environmental tobacco smoke (Z57.31)
status post administration of tPA (rtPA) in a different facility within the last 24 hours prior to admission to current facility (Z92.82)
tobacco dependence (F17.-)
tobacco use (Z72.0)
`EXCLUDES 2`   *old myocardial infarction (I25.2)*
*postmyocardial infarction syndrome (I24.1)*
►*subsequent type 1 myocardial infarction◄ (I22.-)*
**AHA:** 2017, 1Q, 44-45; 2016, 4Q, 140; 2015, 2Q, 16; 2013, 1Q, 25; 2012, 4Q, 96, 102-103

> **CC Excl: For MCC codes in category I21:** PDX collection 653

`√5ᵗʰ` **I21.0**   **ST elevation (STEMI) myocardial infarction of anterior wall**
►Type 1 ST elevation myocardial infarction of anterior wall◄

**I21.01**   **ST elevation (STEMI) myocardial infarction**   `MCC` `HCC`
**involving left main coronary artery**

**I21.02**   **ST elevation (STEMI) myocardial infarction**   `MCC` `HCC`
**involving left anterior descending coronary artery**
ST elevation (STEMI) myocardial infarction involving diagonal coronary artery
**AHA:** 2013, 1Q, 25

**I21.09**   **ST elevation (STEMI) myocardial infarction**   `MCC` `HCC`
**involving other coronary artery of anterior wall**
Acute transmural myocardial infarction of anterior wall
Anteroapical transmural (Q wave) infarction (acute)
Anterolateral transmural (Q wave) infarction (acute)
Anteroseptal transmural (Q wave) infarction (acute)
Transmural (Q wave) infarction (acute) (of) anterior (wall) NOS
**AHA:** 2012, 4Q, 102-103

`√5ᵗʰ` **I21.1**   **ST elevation (STEMI) myocardial infarction of inferior wall**
►Type 1 ST elevation myocardial infarction of inferior wall◄

**I21.11**   **ST elevation (STEMI) myocardial infarction**   `MCC` `HCC`
**involving right coronary artery**
Inferoposterior transmural (Q wave) infarction (acute)

**I21.19**   **ST elevation (STEMI) myocardial infarction**   `MCC` `HCC`
**involving other coronary artery of inferior wall**
Acute transmural myocardial infarction of inferior wall
Inferolateral transmural (Q wave) infarction (acute)
Transmural (Q wave) infarction (acute) (of) diaphragmatic wall
Transmural (Q wave) infarction (acute) (of) inferior (wall) NOS
`EXCLUDES 2`   *ST elevation (STEMI) myocardial infarction involving left circumflex coronary artery (I21.21)*
**AHA:** 2012, 4Q, 96

`√5ᵗʰ` **I21.2**   **ST elevation (STEMI) myocardial infarction of other sites**
►Type 1 ST elevation myocardial infarction of other sites◄

**I21.21**   **ST elevation (STEMI) myocardial infarction**   `MCC` `HCC`
**involving left circumflex coronary artery**
ST elevation (STEMI) myocardial infarction involving oblique marginal coronary artery

**I21.29**   **ST elevation (STEMI) myocardial infarction**   `MCC` `HCC`
**involving other sites**
Acute transmural myocardial infarction of other sites
Apical-lateral transmural (Q wave) infarction (acute)
Basal-lateral transmural (Q wave) infarction (acute)
High lateral transmural (Q wave) infarction (acute)
Lateral (wall) NOS transmural (Q wave) infarction (acute)
Posterior (true) transmural (Q wave) infarction (acute)
Posterobasal transmural (Q wave) infarction (acute)
Posterolateral transmural (Q wave) infarction (acute)
Posteroseptal transmural (Q wave) infarction (acute)
Septal transmural (Q wave) infarction (acute) NOS

**I21.3**   **ST elevation (STEMI) myocardial infarction of**   `MCC` `HCC`
**unspecified site**
Acute transmural myocardial infarction of unspecified site
~~Myocardial infarction (acute) NOS~~
Transmural (Q wave) myocardial infarction NOS
►Type 1 ST elevation myocardial infarction of unspecified site◄

**I21.4**   **Non-ST elevation (NSTEMI) myocardial infarction**   `MCC` `HCC`
Acute subendocardial myocardial infarction
Non-Q wave myocardial infarction NOS
Nontransmural myocardial infarction NOS
►Type 1 non-ST elevation myocardial infarction◄
**AHA:** 2017, 1Q, 44-45

● **I21.9**   **Acute myocardial infarction, unspecified**
Myocardial infarction (acute) NOS

● `√5ᵗʰ` **I21.A**   **Other type of myocardial infarction**

● **I21.A1**   **Myocardial infarction type 2**
Myocardial infarction due to demand ischemia
Myocardial infarction secondary to ischemic imbalance
Code also the underlying cause, if known and applicable, such as:
anemia (D50.0-D64.9)
chronic obstructive pulmonary disease (J44.-)
heart failure (I50.-)
paroxysmal tachycardia (I47.0-I47.9)
renal failure (N17.0-N19)
shock (R57.0-R57.9)

● **I21.A9**   **Other myocardial infarction type**
Myocardial infarction associated with revascularization procedure
Myocardial infarction type 3
Myocardial infarction type 4a
Myocardial infarction type 4b
Myocardial infarction type 4c
Myocardial infarction type 5
Code first, if applicable, postprocedural myocardial infarction following cardiac surgery (I97.190), or postprocedural myocardial infarction during cardiac surgery (I97.790)
Code also complication, if known and applicable, such as:
(acute) stent occlusion (T82.897-)
(acute) stent stenosis (T82.857-)
(acute) stent thrombosis (T82.867-)
cardiac arrest due to underlying cardiac condition (I46.2)
complication of percutaneous coronary intervention (PCI) (I97.89)
occlusion of coronary artery bypass graft (T82.218-)

☑ Additional Character Req   `√x7ᵗʰ` Placeholder Alert   Unacceptable PDx   ■ Manifestation   `H1`-`H14` HAC   `HCC` CMS-HCC Condition   `EXCLUDES 1` Not Coded Here   `EXCLUDES 2` Not Included Here

ICD-10-CM 2018        **631**

✓4ᵗʰ **I22 Subsequent ST elevation (STEMI) and non-ST elevation (NSTEMI) myocardial infarction**

INCLUDES   acute myocardial infarction occurring within four weeks (28 days) of a previous acute myocardial infarction, regardless of site
cardiac infarction
coronary (artery) embolism
coronary (artery) occlusion
coronary (artery) rupture
coronary (artery) thrombosis
infarction of heart, myocardium, or ventricle
recurrent myocardial infarction
reinfarction of myocardium
rupture of heart, myocardium, or ventricle
▶subsequent type 1 myocardial infarction◀

Use additional code, if applicable, to identify:
exposure to environmental tobacco smoke (Z77.22)
history of tobacco dependence (Z87.891)
occupational exposure to environmental tobacco smoke (Z57.31)
status post administration of tPA (rtPA) in a different facility within the last 24 hours prior to admission to current facility (Z92.82)
tobacco dependence (F17.-)
tobacco use (Z72.0)

EXCLUDES 1 ▶ subsequent myocardial infarction, type 2 (I21.A1)
subsequent myocardial infarction of other type (type 3) (type 4) (type 5) (I21.A9)◀

**AHA:** 2017, 2Q, 11; 2013, 1Q, 25; 2012, 4Q, 97, 102-103

CC Excl: For MCC codes in category I22: PDX collection 653

**I22.0 Subsequent ST elevation (STEMI) myocardial infarction of anterior wall**    MCC HCC
Subsequent acute transmural myocardial infarction of anterior wall
Subsequent transmural (Q wave) infarction (acute)(of) anterior (wall) NOS
Subsequent anteroapical transmural (Q wave) infarction (acute)
Subsequent anterolateral transmural (Q wave) infarction (acute)
Subsequent anteroseptal transmural (Q wave) infarction (acute)

**I22.1 Subsequent ST elevation (STEMI) myocardial infarction of inferior wall**    MCC HCC
Subsequent acute transmural myocardial infarction of inferior wall
Subsequent transmural (Q wave) infarction (acute)(of) diaphragmatic wall
Subsequent transmural (Q wave) infarction (acute)(of) inferior (wall) NOS
Subsequent inferolateral transmural (Q wave) infarction (acute)
Subsequent inferoposterior transmural (Q wave) infarction (acute)
**AHA:** 2012, 4Q, 102

**I22.2 Subsequent non-ST elevation (NSTEMI) myocardial infarction**    MCC HCC
Subsequent acute subendocardial myocardial infarction
Subsequent non-Q wave myocardial infarction NOS
Subsequent nontransmural myocardial infarction NOS

**I22.8 Subsequent ST elevation (STEMI) myocardial infarction of other sites**    MCC HCC
Subsequent acute transmural myocardial infarction of other sites
Subsequent apical-lateral transmural (Q wave) myocardial infarction (acute)
Subsequent basal-lateral transmural (Q wave) myocardial infarction (acute)
Subsequent high lateral transmural (Q wave) myocardial infarction (acute)
Subsequent transmural (Q wave) myocardial infarction (acute)(of) lateral (wall) NOS
Subsequent posterior (true)transmural (Q wave) myocardial infarction (acute)
Subsequent posterobasal transmural (Q wave) myocardial infarction (acute)
Subsequent posterolateral transmural (Q wave) myocardial infarction (acute)
Subsequent posteroseptal transmural (Q wave) myocardial infarction (acute)
Subsequent septal NOS transmural (Q wave) myocardial infarction (acute)

**I22.9 Subsequent ST elevation (STEMI) myocardial infarction of unspecified site**    MCC HCC
Subsequent acute myocardial infarction of unspecified site
Subsequent myocardial infarction (acute) NOS

✓4ᵗʰ **I23 Certain current complications following ST elevation (STEMI) and non-ST elevation (NSTEMI) myocardial infarction (within the 28 day period)**
**AHA:** 2017, 2Q, 11

CC Excl: For CC codes in category I23, unless otherwise noted: PDX collection 654

**I23.0 Hemopericardium as current complication following acute myocardial infarction**    CC HCC A
EXCLUDES 1   hemopericardium not specified as current complication following acute myocardial infarction (I31.2)

**I23.1 Atrial septal defect as current complication following acute myocardial infarction**    CC HCC A
EXCLUDES 1   acquired atrial septal defect not specified as current complication following acute myocardial infarction (I51.0)

**I23.2 Ventricular septal defect as current complication following acute myocardial infarction**    CC HCC A
EXCLUDES 1   acquired ventricular septal defect not specified as current complication following acute myocardial infarction (I51.0)

**I23.3 Rupture of cardiac wall without hemopericardium as current complication following acute myocardial infarction**    CC HCC A

**I23.4 Rupture of chordae tendineae as current complication following acute myocardial infarction**    MCC HCC
EXCLUDES 1   rupture of chordae tendineae not specified as current complication following acute myocardial infarction (I51.1)
CC Excl: PDX collection 655

**I23.5 Rupture of papillary muscle as current complication following acute myocardial infarction**    MCC HCC
EXCLUDES 1   rupture of papillary muscle not specified as current complication following acute myocardial infarction (I51.2)
CC Excl: PDX collection 656

**I23.6 Thrombosis of atrium, auricular appendage, and ventricle as current complications following acute myocardial infarction**    CC HCC A
EXCLUDES 1   thrombosis of atrium, auricular appendage, and ventricle not specified as current complication following acute myocardial infarction (I51.3)

**I23.7 Postinfarction angina**    CC HCC A
**AHA:** 2015, 2Q, 16

**I23.8 Other current complications following acute myocardial infarction**    CC HCC A

✓4ᵗʰ **I24 Other acute ischemic heart diseases**
EXCLUDES 1   angina pectoris (I20.-)
transient myocardial ischemia in newborn (P29.4)

CC Excl: For CC codes in category I24, unless otherwise noted: PDX collection 657

**I24.0 Acute coronary thrombosis not resulting in myocardial infarction**    CC HCC
Acute coronary (artery) (vein) embolism not resulting in myocardial infarction
Acute coronary (artery) (vein) occlusion not resulting in myocardial infarction
Acute coronary (artery) (vein) thromboembolism not resulting in myocardial infarction
EXCLUDES 1   atherosclerotic heart disease (I25.1-)
**AHA:** 2013, 1Q, 24

**I24.1 Dressler's syndrome**    CC HCC
Postmyocardial infarction syndrome
EXCLUDES 1   postinfarction angina (I23.7)
CC Excl: PDX collection 658

**I24.8 Other forms of acute ischemic heart disease**    CC HCC
EXCLUDES 1 ▶ myocardial infarction due to demand ischemia (I21.A1)◀

**I24.9 Acute ischemic heart disease, unspecified**    CC HCC
EXCLUDES 1   ischemic heart disease (chronic) NOS (I25.9)

N Newborn: 0   P Pediatric: 0-17   M Maternity: 12-55   A Adult: 15-124   MCC Major CC Condition   PDxMCC PDx acts as own MCC   CC CC Condition   PDxCC PDx acts as own CC

632          ICD-10-CM 2018

**Atheromas**

Atheromas (fatty tissue and/or plaque)

Lumen

✅ 4ᵗʰ **I25**    **Chronic ischemic heart disease**
Use additional code to identify:
chronic total occlusion of coronary artery (I25.82)
exposure to environmental tobacco smoke (Z77.22)
history of tobacco dependence (Z87.891)
occupational exposure to environmental tobacco smoke (Z57.31)
tobacco dependence (F17,-)
tobacco use (Z72.0)

✅ 5ᵗʰ   **I25.1**    **Atherosclerotic heart disease of** native **coronary artery**
Atherosclerotic cardiovascular disease
Coronary (artery) atheroma
Coronary (artery) atherosclerosis
Coronary (artery) disease
Coronary (artery) sclerosis
Use additional code, if applicable, to identify:
coronary atherosclerosis due to calcified coronary lesion (I25.84)
coronary atherosclerosis due to lipid rich plaque (I25.83)
EXCLUDES 2 *atheroembolism (I75.-)*
*atherosclerosis of coronary artery bypass graft(s) and transplanted heart (I25.7-)*

    **I25.10**    **Atherosclerotic heart disease of native coronary** Ⓐ **artery** without **angina pectoris**
Atherosclerotic heart disease NOS
**AHA:** 2015, 2Q, 16; 2012, 4Q, 92

✅ 6ᵗʰ   **I25.11**    **Atherosclerotic heart disease of native coronary artery** with **angina pectoris**

      **I25.110**   **Atherosclerotic heart** PDxCC CC HCC Ⓐ **disease of native coronary artery with** unstable **angina pectoris**
EXCLUDES 1 *unstable angina without atherosclerotic heart disease (I20.0)*
**CC Excl:** PDX collection 651

      **I25.111**   **Atherosclerotic heart disease of** HCC Ⓐ **native coronary artery with angina pectoris with** documented spasm
EXCLUDES 1 *angina pectoris with documented spasm without atherosclerotic heart disease (I20.1)*

      **I25.118**   **Atherosclerotic heart disease of** HCC Ⓐ **native coronary artery with** other **forms of angina pectoris**
EXCLUDES 1 *other forms of angina pectoris without atherosclerotic heart disease (I20.8)*
**AHA:** 2015, 2Q, 16

      **I25.119**   **Atherosclerotic heart disease of** HCC Ⓐ **native coronary artery with** unspecified **angina pectoris**
Atherosclerotic heart disease with angina NOS
Atherosclerotic heart disease with ischemic chest pain
EXCLUDES 1 *unspecified angina pectoris without atherosclerotic heart disease (I20.9)*

    **I25.2**    **Old myocardial infarction**
Healed myocardial infarction
Past myocardial infarction diagnosed by ECG or other investigation, but currently presenting no symptoms

    **I25.3**    **Aneurysm of heart**           CC
Mural aneurysm
Ventricular aneurysm
**CC Excl:** PDX collection 659

✅ 5ᵗʰ   **I25.4**    **Coronary artery aneurysm and dissection**

    **I25.41**    **Coronary artery aneurysm**
Coronary arteriovenous fistula, acquired
EXCLUDES 1 *congenital coronary (artery) aneurysm (Q24.5)*

    **I25.42**    **Coronary artery dissection**       MCC
**DEF:** A tear in the intimal arterial wall of a coronary artery resulting in the sudden intrusion of blood within the layers of the wall.
**CC Excl:** PDX collection 660

    **I25.5**    **Ischemic cardiomyopathy**
EXCLUDES 2 *coronary atherosclerosis (I25.1-, I25.7-)*

    **I25.6**    **Silent myocardial ischemia**

✅ 5ᵗʰ   **I25.7**    **Atherosclerosis of coronary artery** bypass graft(s) **and coronary artery of** transplanted heart **with angina pectoris**
Use additional code, if applicable, to identify:
coronary atherosclerosis due to calcified coronary lesion (I25.84)
coronary atherosclerosis due to lipid rich plaque (I25.83)
EXCLUDES 1 *atherosclerosis of bypass graft(s) of transplanted heart without angina pectoris (I25.812)*
*atherosclerosis of coronary artery bypass graft(s) without angina pectoris (I25.810)*
*atherosclerosis of native coronary artery of transplanted heart without angina pectoris (I25.811)*
*~~embolism or thrombus of coronary artery bypass graft(s) (T82.8-)~~*

✅ 6ᵗʰ   **I25.70**    **Atherosclerosis of coronary artery** bypass graft(s), unspecified, **with angina pectoris**

      **I25.700**   **Atherosclerosis of** PDxCC CC HCC Ⓐ **coronary artery bypass graft(s), unspecified, with** unstable **angina pectoris**
EXCLUDES 1 *unstable angina pectoris without atherosclerosis of coronary artery bypass graft (I20.0)*
**CC Excl:** PDX collection 651

      **I25.701**   **Atherosclerosis of coronary artery** HCC Ⓐ **bypass graft(s), unspecified, with angina pectoris with** documented spasm
EXCLUDES 1 *angina pectoris with documented spasm without atherosclerosis of coronary artery bypass graft (I20.1)*

      **I25.708**   **Atherosclerosis of coronary artery** HCC Ⓐ **bypass graft(s), unspecified, with** other **forms of angina pectoris**
EXCLUDES 1 *other forms of angina pectoris without atherosclerosis of coronary artery bypass graft (I20.8)*

      **I25.709**   **Atherosclerosis of coronary artery** HCC Ⓐ **bypass graft(s), unspecified, with** unspecified **angina pectoris**
EXCLUDES 1 *unspecified angina pectoris without atherosclerosis of coronary artery bypass graft (I20.9)*

✅ 6ᵗʰ   **I25.71**    **Atherosclerosis of** autologous vein **coronary artery bypass graft(s) with angina pectoris**

**CC Excl: For CC codes in subcategory I25.71, unless otherwise noted: PDX collection 662**

      **I25.710**   **Atherosclerosis of** PDxCC CC HCC Ⓐ **autologous vein coronary artery bypass graft(s) with** unstable **angina pectoris**
EXCLUDES 1 *unstable angina without atherosclerosis of autologous vein coronary artery bypass graft(s) (I20.0)*
EXCLUDES 2 ▶*embolism or thrombus of coronary artery bypass graft(s) (T82.8-)*◄
**CC Excl:** PDX collection 661

      **I25.711**   **Atherosclerosis of autologous** CC HCC Ⓐ **vein coronary artery bypass graft(s) with angina pectoris with** documented spasm
EXCLUDES 1 *angina pectoris with documented spasm without atherosclerosis of autologous vein coronary artery bypass graft(s) (I20.1)*

**Chapter 9. Diseases of the Circulatory System**

**I25.718**   Atherosclerosis of autologous `CC` `HCC` `A`
vein coronary artery bypass graft(s) with
other forms of angina pectoris
> *EXCLUDES 1*   other forms of angina pectoris
> without atherosclerosis of
> autologous vein coronary
> artery bypass graft(s) (I20.8)

**I25.719**   Atherosclerosis of autologous `CC` `HCC`
vein coronary artery bypass graft(s) with
unspecified angina pectoris
> *EXCLUDES 1*   unspecified angina pectoris
> without atherosclerosis of
> autologous vein coronary
> artery bypass graft(s) (I20.9)

✓6ᵗʰ **I25.72**   Atherosclerosis of autologous artery coronary artery
bypass graft(s) with angina pectoris
> Atherosclerosis of internal mammary artery graft with
> angina pectoris

> **CC Excl: For CC codes in subcategories I25.72,
> unless otherwise noted: PDX collection 662**

**I25.720**   Atherosclerosis of `PDxCC` `CC` `HCC` `A`
autologous artery coronary artery bypass
graft(s) with unstable angina pectoris
> *EXCLUDES 1*   unstable angina without
> atherosclerosis of
> autologous artery coronary
> artery bypass graft(s) (I20.0)
> **CC Excl:** PDX collection 661

**I25.721**   Atherosclerosis of autologous `CC` `HCC` `A`
artery coronary artery bypass graft(s) with
angina pectoris with documented spasm
> *EXCLUDES 1*   angina pectoris with documented
> spasm without
> atherosclerosis of
> autologous artery coronary
> artery bypass graft(s) (I20.1)

**I25.728**   Atherosclerosis of autologous `CC` `HCC` `A`
artery coronary artery bypass graft(s)
with other forms of angina pectoris
> *EXCLUDES 1*   other forms of angina pectoris
> without atherosclerosis of
> autologous artery coronary
> artery bypass graft(s) (I20.8)

**I25.729**   Atherosclerosis of autologous `CC` `HCC` `A`
artery coronary artery bypass graft(s) with
unspecified angina pectoris
> *EXCLUDES 1*   unspecified angina pectoris
> without atherosclerosis of
> autologous artery coronary
> artery bypass graft(s) (I20.9)

✓6ᵗʰ **I25.73**   Atherosclerosis of nonautologous biological
coronary artery bypass graft(s) with angina pectoris

> **CC Excl: For CC codes in subcategories I25.73,
> unless otherwise noted: PDX collection 662**

**I25.730**   Atherosclerosis of `PDxCC` `CC` `HCC` `A`
nonautologous biological
coronary artery bypass graft(s)
with unstable angina pectoris
> *EXCLUDES 1*   unstable angina without
> atherosclerosis of
> nonautologous biological
> coronary artery bypass
> graft(s) (I20.0)
> **CC Excl:** PDX collection 661

**I25.731**   Atherosclerosis of `CC` `HCC` `A`
nonautologous biological coronary
artery bypass graft(s) with angina
pectoris with documented spasm
> *EXCLUDES 1*   angina pectoris with documented
> spasm without
> atherosclerosis of
> nonautologous biological
> coronary artery bypass
> graft(s) (I20.1)

**I25.738**   Atherosclerosis of `CC` `HCC` `A`
nonautologous biological coronary
artery bypass graft(s) with other forms of
angina pectoris
> *EXCLUDES 1*   other forms of angina pectoris
> without atherosclerosis of
> nonautologous biological
> coronary artery bypass
> graft(s) (I20.8)

**I25.739**   Atherosclerosis of `CC` `HCC` `A`
nonautologous biological coronary
artery bypass graft(s) with unspecified
angina pectoris
> *EXCLUDES 1*   unspecified angina pectoris
> without atherosclerosis of
> nonautologous biological
> coronary artery bypass
> graft(s) (I20.9)

✓6ᵗʰ **I25.75**   Atherosclerosis of native coronary artery of
transplanted heart with angina pectoris
> *EXCLUDES 1*   atherosclerosis of native coronary artery of
> transplanted heart without angina
> pectoris (I25.811)

> **CC Excl: For CC codes in subcategory I25.75,
> unless otherwise noted: PDX collection 664**

**I25.750**   Atherosclerosis of native `PDxCC` `CC` `HCC`
coronary artery of transplanted heart
with unstable angina
> **CC Excl:** PDX collection 663

**I25.751**   Atherosclerosis of native coronary `CC` `HCC`
artery of transplanted heart with angina
pectoris with documented spasm

**I25.758**   Atherosclerosis of native coronary `CC` `HCC`
artery of transplanted heart with other
forms of angina pectoris

**I25.759**   Atherosclerosis of native coronary `CC` `HCC`
artery of transplanted heart with
unspecified angina pectoris

✓6ᵗʰ **I25.76**   Atherosclerosis of bypass graft of coronary artery of
transplanted heart with angina pectoris
> *EXCLUDES 1*   atherosclerosis of bypass graft of coronary
> artery of transplanted heart without
> angina pectoris (I25.812)

> **CC Excl: For CC codes in subcategory I25.76,
> unless otherwise noted: PDX collection 666**

**I25.760**   Atherosclerosis of bypass `PDxCC` `CC` `HCC` `A`
graft of coronary artery of transplanted
heart with unstable angina
> **CC Excl:** PDX collection 665

**I25.761**   Atherosclerosis of bypass graft `CC` `HCC`
of coronary artery of transplanted
heart with angina pectoris with
documented spasm

**I25.768**   Atherosclerosis of bypass graft `CC` `HCC`
of coronary artery of transplanted
heart with other forms of angina
pectoris

**I25.769**   Atherosclerosis of bypass graft `CC` `HCC`
of coronary artery of transplanted
heart with unspecified angina pectoris

✓6ᵗʰ **I25.79**   Atherosclerosis of other coronary artery bypass
graft(s) with angina pectoris

**I25.790**   Atherosclerosis of other `PDxCC` `CC` `HCC` `A`
coronary artery bypass graft(s)
with unstable angina pectoris
> *EXCLUDES 1*   unstable angina without
> atherosclerosis of other
> coronary artery bypass
> graft(s) (I20.0)
> **CC Excl:** PDX collection 651

**I25.791**   Atherosclerosis of other `CC` `HCC` `A`
coronary artery bypass graft(s) with
angina pectoris with documented spasm
> *EXCLUDES 1*   angina pectoris with documented
> spasm without
> atherosclerosis of other
> coronary artery bypass
> graft(s) (I20.1)
> **CC Excl:** No Excl

**I25.798**   Atherosclerosis of other `CC` `HCC` `A`
coronary artery bypass graft(s) with
other forms of angina pectoris
> *EXCLUDES 1*   other forms of angina pectoris
> without atherosclerosis of
> other coronary artery bypass
> graft(s) (I20.8)
> **CC Excl:** No Excl

---

`N` Newborn: 0   `P` Pediatric: 0-17   `M` Maternity: 12-55   `A` Adult: 15-124   `MCC` Major CC Condition   `PDxMCC` PDx acts as own MCC   `CC` CC Condition   `PDxCC` PDx acts as own CC

**I25.799** Atherosclerosis of other `CC` `HCC` `A`
coronary artery bypass graft(s) with
unspecified angina pectoris
> *EXCLUDES 1* *unspecified angina pectoris*
> *without atherosclerosis of*
> *other coronary artery bypass*
> *graft(s) (I20.9)*

**CC Excl:** No Excl

**✓5ᵗʰ I25.8** **Other forms of chronic ischemic heart disease**

**✓6ᵗʰ I25.81** Atherosclerosis of other coronary vessels without
angina pectoris
> Use additional code, if applicable, to identify:
> coronary atherosclerosis due to calcified coronary
> lesion (I25.84)
> coronary atherosclerosis due to lipid rich plaque
> (I25.83)
> *EXCLUDES 1* *atherosclerotic heart disease of native*
> *coronary artery without angina pectoris*
> *(I25.10)*

**I25.810** Atherosclerosis of coronary artery `CC` `A`
bypass graft(s) without angina pectoris
> Atherosclerosis of coronary artery bypass
> graft NOS
> *EXCLUDES 1* *atherosclerosis of coronary*
> *bypass graft(s) with angina*
> *pectoris (I25.70--I25.73-,*
> *I25.79-)*

**CC Excl:** No Excl

**I25.811** Atherosclerosis of native coronary `CC`
artery of transplanted heart without
angina pectoris
> Atherosclerosis of native coronary artery of
> transplanted heart NOS
> *EXCLUDES 1* *atherosclerosis of native coronary*
> *artery of transplanted heart*
> *with angina pectoris*
> *(I25.75-)*

**CC Excl:** PDX collection 664

**I25.812** Atherosclerosis of bypass graft of `CC` `A`
coronary artery of transplanted heart
without angina pectoris
> Atherosclerosis of bypass graft of
> transplanted heart NOS
> *EXCLUDES 1* *atherosclerosis of bypass graft of*
> *transplanted heart with*
> *angina pectoris (I25.76)*

**CC Excl:** PDX collection 666

**I25.82** Chronic total occlusion of coronary artery
> Complete occlusion of coronary artery
> Total occlusion of coronary artery
> Code first coronary atherosclerosis (I25.1-, I25.7-,
> I25.81-)
> *EXCLUDES 1* ▶*acute coronary occlusion with myocardial*
> *infarction (I21.0-I21.9, I22.-)*◄
> ▶*acute coronary occlusion without*
> *myocardial infarction*◄ *(I24.0)*
> **DEF:** Complete blockage of coronary artery due to
> plaque accumulation over an extended period of time;
> results in substantial reduction of blood flow;
> characterized by angina or chest pain.

**I25.83** Coronary atherosclerosis due to lipid rich plaque `A`
> Code first coronary atherosclerosis (I25.1-, I25.7-,
> I25.81-)

**I25.84** Coronary atherosclerosis due to calcified coronary
lesion
> Coronary atherosclerosis due to severely calcified
> coronary lesion
> Code first coronary atherosclerosis (I25.1-, I25.7-,
> I25.81-)

**I25.89** Other forms of chronic ischemic heart disease

**I25.9** Chronic ischemic heart disease, unspecified
> Ischemic heart disease (chronic) NOS

---

## Pulmonary heart disease and diseases of pulmonary circulation (I26-I28)

**✓4ᵗʰ I26** **Pulmonary embolism**
> `INCLUDES` pulmonary (acute) (artery)(vein) infarction
> pulmonary (acute) (artery)(vein) thromboembolism
> pulmonary (acute) (artery)(vein) thrombosis
> *EXCLUDES 2* *chronic pulmonary embolism (I27.82)*
> *personal history of pulmonary embolism (Z86.711)*
> *pulmonary embolism due to trauma (T79.0, T79.1)*
> *pulmonary embolism due to complications of surgical and*
> *medical care (T80.0, T81.7-, T82.8-)*
> *pulmonary embolism complicating abortion, ectopic or molar*
> *pregnancy (O00-O07, O08.2)*
> *pulmonary embolism complicating pregnancy, childbirth and*
> *the puerperium (O88.-)*
> *septic (non-pulmonary) arterial embolism (I76)*

**✓5ᵗʰ I26.0** **Pulmonary embolism with acute cor pulmonale**

> **CC Excl:** For MCC codes in subcategory I26.0, unless
> otherwise noted: PDX collection 667

**I26.01** Septic pulmonary embolism with `PDxMCC` `MCC` `HCC`
acute cor pulmonale
> Code first underlying infection

**I26.02** Saddle embolus of pulmonary `PDxMCC` `MCC` `H10` `HCC`
artery with acute cor pulmonale

**I26.09** Other pulmonary embolism with `PDxMCC` `MCC` `H10` `HCC`
acute cor pulmonale
> Acute cor pulmonale NOS
> **AHA:** 2014, 4Q, 21

**✓5ᵗʰ I26.9** **Pulmonary embolism without acute cor pulmonale**

**I26.90** Septic pulmonary embolism without acute `MCC` `HCC`
cor pulmonale
> Code first underlying infection
> **CC Excl:** PDX collection 668

**I26.92** Saddle embolus of pulmonary artery `MCC` `H10` `HCC`
without acute cor pulmonale
> **CC Excl:** PDX collection 669

**I26.99** Other pulmonary embolism without `MCC` `H10` `HCC`
acute cor pulmonale
> Acute pulmonary embolism NOS
> Pulmonary embolism NOS
> **CC Excl:** PDX collection 670

**✓4ᵗʰ I27** **Other pulmonary heart diseases**

**I27.0** **Primary pulmonary hypertension** `CC` `HCC`
> ▶Heritable pulmonary arterial hypertension
> Idiopathic pulmonary arterial hypertension
> Primary group 1 pulmonary hypertension
> Primary pulmonary arterial hypertension◄
> *EXCLUDES 1* ▶*persistent pulmonary hypertension of newborn*
> *(P29.30)*◄
> *pulmonary hypertension NOS* ▶*(I27.20)*◄
> ▶*secondary pulmonary arterial hypertension (I27.21)*◄
> *secondary pulmonary hypertension* ▶*(I27.29)*◄
> **CC Excl:** PDX collection 671

**I27.1** **Kyphoscoliotic heart disease** `CC` `HCC`
> **CC Excl:** PDX collection 533

**✓5ᵗʰ I27.2** **Other secondary pulmonary hypertension**
> ~~Pulmonary hypertension NOS~~
> Code also associated underlying condition
> *EXCLUDES 1* ▶*Eisenmenger's syndrome (I27.83)*◄
> **AHA:** 2014, 4Q, 21

● **I27.20** **Pulmonary hypertension, unspecified**
> Pulmonary hypertension NOS

● **I27.21** **Secondary pulmonary arterial hypertension**
> (Associated) (drug-induced) (toxin-induced)
> pulmonary arterial hypertension NOS
> (Associated) (drug-induced) (toxin-induced)
> (secondary) group 1 pulmonary hypertension
> Code also associated conditions if applicable, or
> adverse effects of drugs or toxins, such as:
> adverse effect of appetite depressants (T50.5X5)
> congenital heart disease (Q20-Q28)
> human immunodeficiency virus [HIV] disease (B20)
> polymyositis (M33.2-)
> portal hypertension (K76.6)
> rheumatoid arthritis (M05.-)
> schistosomiasis (B65.-)
> Sjögren syndrome (M35.0-)
> systemic sclerosis (M34.-)

---

✓Additional Character Req    `✓x7ᵗʰ` Placeholder Alert    Unacceptable PDx    Manifestation    `H1`-`H14` HAC    `HCC` CMS-HCC Condition    *EXCLUDES 1* Not Coded Here    *EXCLUDES 2* Not Included Here

ICD-10-CM 2018     635

**I27.22**   **Pulmonary hypertension** due to left heart disease
Group 2 pulmonary hypertension
Code also associated left heart disease, if known, such as:
     multiple valve disease (I08.-)
     rheumatic mitral valve diseases (I05.-)
     rheumatic aortic valve diseases (I06.-)

**I27.23**   **Pulmonary hypertension** due to lung diseases and hypoxia
Group 3 pulmonary hypertension
Code also associated lung disease, if known, such as:
     bronchiectasis (J47.-)
     cystic fibrosis with pulmonary manifestations (E84.0)
     interstitial lung disease (J84.-)
     pleural effusion (J90)
     sleep apnea (G47.3-)

**I27.24**   **Chronic thromboembolic pulmonary hypertension**
Group 4 pulmonary hypertension
Code also associated pulmonary embolism, if applicable (I26.-, I27.82)

**I27.29**   **Other secondary pulmonary hypertension**
Group 5 pulmonary hypertension
Pulmonary hypertension with unclear multifactorial mechanisms
Pulmonary hypertension due to hematologic disorders
Pulmonary hypertension due to metabolic disorders
Pulmonary hypertension due to other systemic disorders
Code also other associated disorders, if known, such as:
     chronic myeloid leukemia (C92.10- C92.22)
     essential thrombocythemia (D47.3)
     Gaucher disease (E75.22)
     hypertensive chronic kidney disease with end stage renal disease (I12.0, I12.11, I13.2)
     hyperthyroidism (E05.-)
     hypothyroidism (E00-E03)
     polycythemia vera (D45)
     sarcoidosis (D86.-)
**AHA:** 2016, 2Q, 8

☑5ᵗʰ **I27.8**   **Other specified pulmonary heart diseases**

**I27.81**   **Cor pulmonale (chronic)**   `HCC`
Cor pulmonale NOS
**EXCLUDES 1**   *acute cor pulmonale (I26.0-)*
**AHA:** 2014, 4Q, 21

**I27.82**   **Chronic pulmonary embolism**   `CC` `HCC`
Use additional code, if applicable, for associated long-term (current) use of anticoagulants (Z79.01)
**EXCLUDES 1**   *personal history of pulmonary embolism (Z86.711)*
**DEF:** A long-standing condition commonly associated with pulmonary hypertension in which small blood clots travel to the lungs repeatedly over many weeks, months, or years, requiring continuation of established anticoagulant or thrombolytic therapy.
**CC Excl:** PDX collection 669

**I27.83**   **Eisenmenger's syndrome**
Eisenmenger's complex
(Irreversible) Eisenmenger's disease
Pulmonary hypertension with right to left shunt related to congenital heart disease
Code also underlying heart defect, if known, such as:
     atrial septal defect (Q21.1)
     Eisenmenger's defect (Q21.8)
     patent ductus arteriosus (Q25.0)
     ventricular septal defect (Q21.0)

**I27.89**   **Other specified pulmonary heart diseases**   `HCC`
~~Eisenmenger's complex~~
~~Eisenmenger's syndrome~~
**EXCLUDES 1**   ~~*Eisenmenger's defect (Q21.8)*~~

**I27.9**   **Pulmonary heart disease, unspecified**   `HCC`
Chronic cardiopulmonary disease

☑4ᵗʰ **I28**   **Other diseases of pulmonary vessels**

**I28.0**   **Arteriovenous fistula of pulmonary vessels**   `CC` `HCC`
**EXCLUDES 1**   *congenital arteriovenous fistula (Q25.72)*
**CC Excl:** PDX collection 672

**I28.1**   **Aneurysm of pulmonary artery**   `CC` `HCC`
**EXCLUDES 1**   *congenital aneurysm (Q25.79)*
         *congenital arteriovenous aneurysm (Q25.72)*
**CC Excl:** PDX collection 672

**I28.8**   **Other diseases of pulmonary vessels**   `HCC`
Pulmonary arteritis
Pulmonary endarteritis
Rupture of pulmonary vessels
Stenosis of pulmonary vessels
Stricture of pulmonary vessels

**I28.9**   **Disease of pulmonary vessels, unspecified**   `HCC`

## Other forms of heart disease (I30-I52)

☑4ᵗʰ **I30**   **Acute pericarditis**
**INCLUDES**   acute mediastinopericarditis
     acute myopericarditis
     acute pericardial effusion
     acute pleuropericarditis
     acute pneumopericarditis
**EXCLUDES 1**   *Dressler's syndrome (I24.1)*
     *rheumatic pericarditis (acute) (I01.0)*
     ▶*viral pericarditis due to Coxsakie virus (B33.23)*◀

**CC Excl: For CC codes in category I30:** PDX collection 673

**I30.0**   **Acute nonspecific idiopathic pericarditis**   `CC`

**I30.1**   **Infective pericarditis**   `CC`
Pneumococcal pericarditis
Pneumopyopericardium
Purulent pericarditis
Pyopericarditis
Pyopericardium
Pyopneumopericardium
Staphylococcal pericarditis
Streptococcal pericarditis
Suppurative pericarditis
Viral pericarditis
Use additional code (B95-B97) to identify infectious agent

**I30.8**   **Other forms of acute pericarditis**   `CC`

**I30.9**   **Acute pericarditis, unspecified**   `CC`

☑4ᵗʰ **I31**   **Other diseases of pericardium**
**EXCLUDES 1**   *diseases of pericardium specified as rheumatic (I09.2)*
     *postcardiotomy syndrome (I97.0)*
     *traumatic injury to pericardium (S26.-)*

**I31.0**   **Chronic adhesive pericarditis**   `CC`
Accretio cordis
Adherent pericardium
Adhesive mediastinopericarditis
**CC Excl:** PDX collection 674

**I31.1**   **Chronic constrictive pericarditis**   `CC`
Concretio cordis
Pericardial calcification
**CC Excl:** PDX collection 674

**I31.2**   **Hemopericardium, not elsewhere classified**   `CC`
**EXCLUDES 1**   *hemopericardium as current complication following acute myocardial infarction (I23.0)*
**DEF:** Presence of blood in the pericardial sac (pericardium). It can lead to potentially fatal cardiac tamponade if enough blood enters the pericardial cavity.
**CC Excl:** PDX collection 674

**I31.3**   **Pericardial effusion (noninflammatory)**   `CC`
Chylopericardium
**EXCLUDES 1**   *acute pericardial effusion (I30.9)*
**CC Excl:** PDX collection 188

**I31.4**   **Cardiac tamponade**   `CC`
Code first underlying cause
**CC Excl:** PDX collection 188

**I31.8**   **Other specified diseases of pericardium**   `CC`
Epicardial plaques      Focal pericardial adhesions
**CC Excl:** PDX collection 188

**I31.9**   **Disease of pericardium, unspecified**   `CC`
Pericarditis (chronic) NOS
**CC Excl:** PDX collection 188

**Cardiac Tamponade**

Normal

Acute Pericardial Effusion with Cardiac Tamponade

Excessive fluid in pericardial space

Serous pericardium (visceral layer)

Fibrous pericardium

Pericardial space (potential)

Serous pericardium (parietal layer)

constricted areas

**I32**    *Pericarditis in diseases classified elsewhere*    `CC`

Code first underlying disease

*EXCLUDES 1*    *pericarditis (in):*
*coxsackie (virus) (B33.23)*
*gonococcal (A54.83)*
*meningococcal (A39.53)*
*rheumatoid (arthritis) (M05.31)*
*syphilitic (A52.06)*
*systemic lupus erythematosus (M32.12)*
*tuberculosis (A18.84)*

**CC Excl:** PDX collection 673

**✓4th I33**    **Acute and subacute endocarditis**

*EXCLUDES 1*    *acute rheumatic endocarditis (I01.1)*
*endocarditis NOS (I38)*

**I33.0**    **Acute and subacute infective endocarditis**    `HIV` `MCC`
Bacterial endocarditis (acute) (subacute)
Infective endocarditis (acute) (subacute) NOS
Endocarditis lenta (acute) (subacute)
Malignant endocarditis (acute) (subacute)
Purulent endocarditis (acute) (subacute)
Septic endocarditis (acute) (subacute)
Ulcerative endocarditis (acute) (subacute)
Vegetative endocarditis (acute) (subacute)
Use additional code (B95-B97) to identify infectious agent
**CC Excl:** PDX collection 675

**I33.9**    **Acute and subacute endocarditis, unspecified**    `HIV` `MCC`
Acute endocarditis NOS
Acute myoendocarditis NOS
Acute periendocarditis NOS
Subacute endocarditis NOS
Subacute myoendocarditis NOS
Subacute periendocarditis NOS
**CC Excl:** PDX collection 675

**✓4th I34**    **Nonrheumatic mitral valve disorders**

*EXCLUDES 1*    *mitral valve disease (I05.9)*
*mitral valve failure (I05.8)*
*mitral valve stenosis (I05.0)*
*mitral valve disorder of unspecified cause with diseases of aortic and/or tricuspid valve(s) (I08.-)*
*mitral valve disorder of unspecified cause with mitral stenosis or obstruction (I05.0)*
*mitral valve disorder specified as congenital ▶(Q23.2, Q23.9)◀*
*mitral valve disorder specified as rheumatic (I05.-)*

**I34.0**    **Nonrheumatic mitral (valve) insufficiency**
Nonrheumatic mitral (valve) incompetence NOS
Nonrheumatic mitral (valve) regurgitation NOS

**I34.1**    **Nonrheumatic mitral (valve) prolapse**
Floppy nonrheumatic mitral valve syndrome
*EXCLUDES 1*    *Marfan's syndrome (Q87.4-)*

**I34.2**    **Nonrheumatic mitral (valve) stenosis**

**I34.8**    **Other nonrheumatic mitral valve disorders**

**I34.9**    **Nonrheumatic mitral valve disorder, unspecified**

**✓4th I35**    **Nonrheumatic aortic valve disorders**

*EXCLUDES 1*    *aortic valve disorder of unspecified cause but with diseases of mitral and/or tricuspid valve(s) (I08.-)*
*aortic valve disorder specified as congenital (Q23.0, Q23.1)*
*aortic valve disorder specified as rheumatic (I06.-)*
*hypertrophic subaortic stenosis (I42.1)*

**I35.0**    **Nonrheumatic aortic (valve) stenosis**

**I35.1**    **Nonrheumatic aortic (valve) insufficiency**
Nonrheumatic aortic (valve) incompetence NOS
Nonrheumatic aortic (valve) regurgitation NOS

**I35.2**    **Nonrheumatic aortic (valve) stenosis with insufficiency**

**I35.8**    **Other nonrheumatic aortic valve disorders**

**I35.9**    **Nonrheumatic aortic valve disorder, unspecified**

**✓4th I36**    **Nonrheumatic tricuspid valve disorders**

*EXCLUDES 1*    *tricuspid valve disorders of unspecified cause (I07.-)*
*tricuspid valve disorders specified as congenital (Q22.4, Q22.8, Q22.9)*
*tricuspid valve disorders specified as rheumatic (I07.-)*
*tricuspid valve disorders with aortic and/or mitral valve involvement (I08.-)*

**I36.0**    **Nonrheumatic tricuspid (valve) stenosis**

**I36.1**    **Nonrheumatic tricuspid (valve) insufficiency**
Nonrheumatic tricuspid (valve) incompetence
Nonrheumatic tricuspid (valve) regurgitation

**I36.2**    **Nonrheumatic tricuspid (valve) stenosis with insufficiency**

**I36.8**    **Other nonrheumatic tricuspid valve disorders**

**I36.9**    **Nonrheumatic tricuspid valve disorder, unspecified**

**✓4th I37**    **Nonrheumatic pulmonary valve disorders**

*EXCLUDES 1*    *pulmonary valve disorder specified as congenital (Q22.1, Q22.2, Q22.3)*
*pulmonary valve disorder specified as rheumatic (I09.89)*

**I37.0**    **Nonrheumatic pulmonary valve stenosis**

**I37.1**    **Nonrheumatic pulmonary valve insufficiency**
Nonrheumatic pulmonary valve incompetence
Nonrheumatic pulmonary valve regurgitation

**I37.2**    **Nonrheumatic pulmonary valve stenosis with insufficiency**

**I37.8**    **Other nonrheumatic pulmonary valve disorders**

**I37.9**    **Nonrheumatic pulmonary valve disorder, unspecified**

**I38**    **Endocarditis, valve unspecified**    `CC`

*INCLUDES*    endocarditis (chronic) NOS
valvular incompetence NOS
valvular insufficiency NOS
valvular regurgitation NOS
valvular stenosis NOS
valvulitis (chronic) NOS

*EXCLUDES 1*    *congenital insufficiency of cardiac valve NOS (Q24.8)*
*congenital stenosis of cardiac valve NOS (Q24.8)*
*endocardial fibroelastosis (I42.4)*
*endocarditis specified as rheumatic (I09.1)*

**CC Excl:** PDX collection 676

**I39**    *Endocarditis and heart valve disorders in diseases classified elsewhere*    `CC`

Code first underlying disease, such as:
Q fever (A78)

*EXCLUDES 1*    *endocardial involvement in:*
*candidiasis (B37.6)*
*gonococcal infection (A54.83)*
*Libman-Sacks disease (M32.11)*
*listerosis (A32.82)*
*meningococcal infection (A39.51)*
*rheumatoid arthritis (M05.31)*
*syphilis (A52.03)*
*tuberculosis (A18.84)*
*typhoid fever (A01.02)*

**CC Excl:** PDX collection 676

**✓4th I40**    **Acute myocarditis**

*INCLUDES*    subacute myocarditis
*EXCLUDES 1*    *acute rheumatic myocarditis (I01.2)*

**CC Excl: For MCC codes in category I40:** PDX collection 677

**I40.0**    **Infective myocarditis**    `HIV` `MCC`
Septic myocarditis
Use additional code (B95-B97) to identify infectious agent

**I40.1**    **Isolated myocarditis**    `HIV` `MCC`
Fiedler's myocarditis
Giant cell myocarditis
Idiopathic myocarditis

**I40.8**    **Other acute myocarditis**    `HIV` `MCC`

**I40.9**    **Acute myocarditis, unspecified**    `HIV` `MCC`

Chapter 9. Diseases of the Circulatory System

I32–I40.9

✓ Additional Character Req    ✓x7th Placeholder Alert    Unacceptable PDx    Manifestation    `H1`-`H14` HAC    `HCC` CMS-HCC Condition    *EXCLUDES 1* Not Coded Here    *EXCLUDES 2* Not Included Here

ICD-10-CM 2018              637

**I41**    *Myocarditis in diseases classified elsewhere*    `MCC`

     Code first underlying disease, such as:
         typhus (A75.Ø-A75.9)

     `EXCLUDES 1`   myocarditis (in):
         Chagas' disease (chronic) (B57.2)
           acute (B57.Ø)
         coxsackie (virus) infection (B33.22)
         diphtheritic (A36.81)
         gonococcal (A54.83)
         influenzal (JØ9.X9, J1Ø.82, J11.82)
         meningococcal (A39.52)
         mumps (B26.82)
         rheumatoid arthritis (MØ5.31)
         sarcoid (D86.85)
         syphilis (A52.Ø6)
         toxoplasmosis (B58.81)
         tuberculous (A18.84)

     **CC Excl:** PDX collection 677

**✓4ᵗʰ I42**   **Cardiomyopathy**

     `INCLUDES`   myocardiopathy

     Code first pre-existing cardiomyopathy complicating pregnancy and puerperium (O99.4)

     `EXCLUDES 2`   ischemic cardiomyopathy (I25.5)
         peripartum cardiomyopathy (O9Ø.3)
         ventricular hypertrophy (I51.7)

     **CC Excl: For CC codes in category I42:** PDX collection 678

   **I42.Ø**   **Dilated cardiomyopathy**   `CC` `HCC`
       Congestive cardiomyopathy

   **I42.1**   **Obstructive hypertrophic cardiomyopathy**   `CC` `HCC`
       Hypertrophic subaortic stenosis (idiopathic)
       **DEF:** Cardiomyopathy marked by left ventricle hypertrophy, enlarged septum; results in obstructed blood flow, arrhythmias, mitral regurgitation, and sudden cardiac death.

   **I42.2**   **Other hypertrophic cardiomyopathy**   `CC` `HCC`
       Nonobstructive hypertrophic cardiomyopathy

   **I42.3**   **Endomyocardial (eosinophilic) disease**   `CC` `HCC`
       Endomyocardial (tropical) fibrosis
       Löffler's endocarditis

   **I42.4**   **Endocardial fibroelastosis**   `CC` `HCC`
       Congenital cardiomyopathy
       Elastomyofibrosis

   **I42.5**   **Other restrictive cardiomyopathy**   `CC` `HCC`
       Constrictive cardiomyopathy NOS

   **I42.6**   **Alcoholic cardiomyopathy**   `CC` `HCC`
       Code also presence of alcoholism (F1Ø.-)

   **I42.7**   **Cardiomyopathy due to drug and external agent**   `CC` `HCC`
       Code first poisoning due to drug or toxin, if applicable (T36-T65 with fifth or sixth character 1-4 or 6)
       Use additional code for adverse effect, if applicable, to identify drug (T36-T5Ø with fifth or sixth character 5)

   **I42.8**   **Other cardiomyopathies**   `CC` `HCC`

   **I42.9**   **Cardiomyopathy, unspecified**   `CC` `HCC`
       Cardiomyopathy (primary) (secondary) NOS

**I43**    *Cardiomyopathy in diseases classified elsewhere*   `CC` `HCC`

     Code first underlying disease, such as:
         amyloidosis (E85.-)
         glycogen storage disease (E74.Ø)
         gout (M1Ø.Ø-)
         thyrotoxicosis (EØ5.Ø-EØ5.9-)

     `EXCLUDES 1`   cardiomyopathy (in):
         coxsackie (virus) (B33.24)
         diphtheria (A36.81)
         sarcoidosis (D86.85)
         tuberculosis (A18.84)

     **CC Excl:** PDX collection 678

**✓4ᵗʰ I44**   **Atrioventricular and left bundle-branch block**

   **I44.Ø**   **Atrioventricular block, first degree**

   **I44.1**   **Atrioventricular block, second degree**
       Atrioventricular block, type I and II
       Möbitz block, type I and II
       Second degree block, type I and II
       Wenckebach's block

   **I44.2**   **Atrioventricular block, complete**   `CC` `HCC`
       Complete heart block NOS      Third degree block
       **CC Excl:** PDX collection 679

   **✓5ᵗʰ I44.3**   **Other and unspecified atrioventricular block**
       Atrioventricular block NOS

      **I44.3Ø**   **Unspecified atrioventricular block**

---

      **I44.39**   **Other atrioventricular block**

   4   **I44.4**   **Left anterior fascicular block**

   4   **I44.5**   **Left posterior fascicular block**

   ✓5ᵗʰ   **I44.6**   **Other and unspecified fascicular block**

      4   **I44.6Ø**   **Unspecified fascicular block**
         Left bundle-branch hemiblock NOS

      4   **I44.69**   **Other fascicular block**

   4   **I44.7**   **Left bundle-branch block, unspecified**

**✓4ᵗʰ I45**   **Other conduction disorders**

     **CC Excl: For CC codes in category I45:** PDX collection 679

   4   **I45.Ø**   **Right fascicular block**

   ✓5ᵗʰ   **I45.1**   **Other and unspecified right bundle-branch block**

      4   **I45.1Ø**   **Unspecified right bundle-branch block**
         Right bundle-branch block NOS

      4   **I45.19**   **Other right bundle-branch block**

   **I45.2**   **Bifascicular block**   `CC`

   **I45.3**   **Trifascicular block**   `CC`

   **I45.4**   **Nonspecific intraventricular block**
       Bundle-branch block NOS

   **I45.5**   **Other specified heart block**
       Sinoatrial block      Sinoauricular block
       `EXCLUDES 1`   heart block NOS (I45.9)

   **I45.6**   **Pre-excitation syndrome**
       Accelerated atrioventricular conduction
       Accessory atrioventricular conduction
       Anomalous atrioventricular excitation
       Lown-Ganong-Levine syndrome
       Pre-excitation atrioventricular conduction
       Wolff-Parkinson-White syndrome

   ✓5ᵗʰ   **I45.8**   **Other specified conduction disorders**

      **I45.81**   **Long QT syndrome**
         **DEF:** Condition characterized by recurrent syncope, malignant arrhythmias, and sudden death; characteristic prolonged Q-T interval on electrocardiogram.

      **I45.89**   **Other specified conduction disorders**   `CC`
         Atrioventricular [AV] dissociation
         Interference dissociation
         Isorhythmic dissociation
         Nonparoxysmal AV nodal tachycardia
         **AHA:** 2013, 2Q, 31

   **I45.9**   **Conduction disorder, unspecified**
       Heart block NOS
       Stokes-Adams syndrome

**Conduction Disorders**

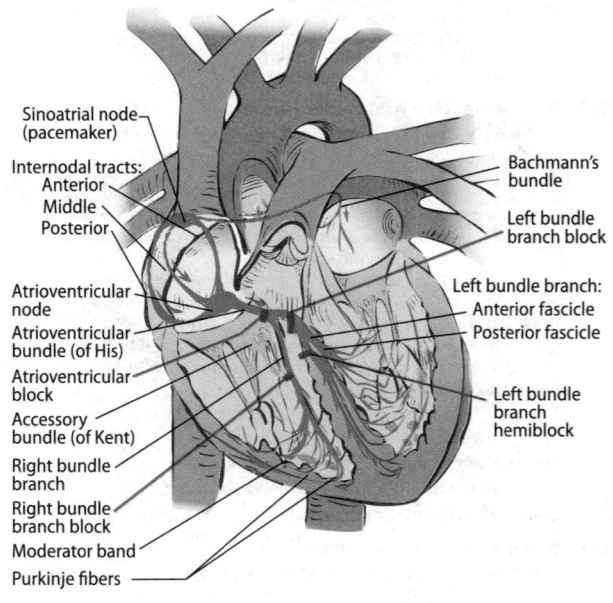

Labels: Sinoatrial node (pacemaker); Internodal tracts: Anterior, Middle, Posterior; Atrioventricular node; Atrioventricular bundle (of His); Atrioventricular block; Accessory bundle (of Kent); Right bundle branch; Right bundle branch block; Moderator band; Purkinje fibers; Bachmann's bundle; Left bundle branch block; Left bundle branch: Anterior fascicle, Posterior fascicle; Left bundle branch hemiblock

---

4   Questionable admission when used as PDx.

`N` Newborn: 0   `P` Pediatric: 0-17   `M` Maternity: 12-55   `A` Adult: 15-124   `MCC` Major CC Condition   `PDxMCC` PDx acts as own MCC   `CC` CC Condition   `PDxCC` PDx acts as own CC

638                                                    ICD-10-CM 2018

✓4ᵗʰ **I46** **Cardiac arrest**

> *EXCLUDES 1*    cardiogenic shock (R57.0)

> **CC Excl: For MCC codes in category I46:** PDX collection 680

[1] **I46.2** **Cardiac arrest due to underlying cardiac condition**   MCC HCC
> Code first underlying cardiac condition

[1] **I46.8** **Cardiac arrest due to other underlying condition**   MCC HCC
> Code first underlying condition

[1] **I46.9** **Cardiac arrest, cause unspecified**   MCC HCC

✓4ᵗʰ **I47** **Paroxysmal tachycardia**

> Code first tachycardia complicating:
> abortion or ectopic or molar pregnancy (O00–O07, O08.8)
> obstetric surgery and procedures (O75.4)

> *EXCLUDES 1*    tachycardia NOS (R00.0)
> sinoauricular tachycardia NOS (R00.0)
> sinus [sinusal] tachycardia NOS (R00.0)

> **CC Excl: For CC codes in category I47:** PDX collection 679

**I47.0** **Re-entry ventricular arrhythmia**   CC HCC

**I47.1** **Supraventricular tachycardia**   CC HCC
> Atrial (paroxysmal) tachycardia
> Atrioventricular [AV] (paroxysmal) tachycardia
> Atrioventricular re-entrant (nodal) tachycardia [AVNRT] [AVRT]
> Junctional (paroxysmal) tachycardia
> Nodal (paroxysmal) tachycardia

**I47.2** **Ventricular tachycardia**   CC HCC
> AHA: 2013, 3Q, 23

**I47.9** **Paroxysmal tachycardia, unspecified**   HCC
> Bouveret (-Hoffman) syndrome

✓4ᵗʰ **I48** **Atrial fibrillation and flutter**

> **CC Excl: For CC codes in category I48:** PDX collection 679

**I48.0** **Paroxysmal atrial fibrillation**   HCC

**I48.1** **Persistent atrial fibrillation**   CC HCC

**I48.2** **Chronic atrial fibrillation**   HCC
> Permanent atrial fibrillation

**I48.3** **Typical atrial flutter**   CC HCC
> Type I atrial flutter

**I48.4** **Atypical atrial flutter**   CC HCC
> Type II atrial flutter

✓5ᵗʰ **I48.9** **Unspecified atrial fibrillation and atrial flutter**

    **I48.91** **Unspecified atrial fibrillation**   HCC

    **I48.92** **Unspecified atrial flutter**   CC HCC

✓4ᵗʰ **I49** **Other cardiac arrhythmias**

> Code first cardiac arrhythmia complicating:
> abortion or ectopic or molar pregnancy (O00–O07, O08.8)
> obstetric surgery and procedures (O75.4)

> *EXCLUDES 1*    bradycardia NOS (R00.1)
> neonatal dysrhythmia (P29.1-)
> sinoatrial bradycardia (R00.1)
> sinus bradycardia (R00.1)
> vagal bradycardia (R00.1)

> *EXCLUDES 2* ▶bradycardia NOS (R00.1)◄

> **CC Excl: For CC/MCC codes in category I49:**
> PDX collection 679

✓5ᵗʰ **I49.0** **Ventricular fibrillation and flutter**

    [1] **I49.01** **Ventricular fibrillation**   MCC HCC

    **I49.02** **Ventricular flutter**   MCC HCC

**I49.1** **Atrial premature depolarization**
> Atrial premature beats

**I49.2** **Junctional premature depolarization**   CC HCC

**I49.3** **Ventricular premature depolarization**

✓5ᵗʰ **I49.4** **Other and unspecified premature depolarization**

    **I49.40** **Unspecified premature depolarization**
> Premature beats NOS

    **I49.49** **Other premature depolarization**
> Ectopic beats
> Extrasystoles
> Extrasystolic arrhythmias
> Premature contractions

**I49.5** **Sick sinus syndrome**   HCC
> Tachycardia-bradycardia syndrome

**I49.8** **Other specified cardiac arrhythmias**
> ▶Brugada syndrome◄
> Coronary sinus rhythm disorder
> Ectopic rhythm disorder
> Nodal rhythm disorder

**I49.9** **Cardiac arrhythmia, unspecified**
> Arrhythmia (cardiac) NOS

✓4ᵗʰ **I50** **Heart failure**

> Code first:
> heart failure complicating abortion or ectopic or molar pregnancy
> (O00–O07, O08.8)
> heart failure following surgery (I97.13-)
> heart failure due to hypertension (I11.0)
> heart failure due to hypertension with chronic kidney disease (I13.-)
> obstetric surgery and procedures (O75.4)
> rheumatic heart failure (I09.81)

> *EXCLUDES 1*    neonatal cardiac failure (P29.0)
> *EXCLUDES 2*    cardiac arrest (I46.-)

> AHA: 2017, 1Q, 47; 2014, 1Q, 25; 2013, 2Q, 33

> **CC Excl: For CC/MCC codes in category I50, unless otherwise noted:** PDX collection 682

▲ **I50.1** **Left ventricular failure, unspecified**   CC HCC
> Cardiac asthma
> Edema of lung with heart disease NOS
> Edema of lung with heart failure
> Left heart failure
> Pulmonary edema with heart disease NOS
> Pulmonary edema with heart failure

> *EXCLUDES 1*    edema of lung without heart disease or heart failure
> (J81.-)
> pulmonary edema without heart disease or failure
> (J81.-)

> **CC Excl:** PDX collection 681

✓5ᵗʰ **I50.2** **Systolic (congestive) heart failure**
> ▶Heart failure with reduced ejection fraction [HFrEF]
> Systolic left ventricular heart failure◄
> ▶Code also end stage heart failure, if applicable (I50.84)◄

> *EXCLUDES 1*    combined systolic (congestive) and diastolic
> (congestive) heart failure (I50.4-)

> AHA: 2017, 1Q, 46; 2016, 1Q, 10

    **I50.20** **Unspecified systolic (congestive) heart**   CC HCC
> **failure**

    **I50.21** **Acute systolic (congestive) heart failure**   MCC HCC

    **I50.22** **Chronic systolic (congestive) heart failure**   CC HCC

    **I50.23** **Acute on chronic systolic (congestive) heart**   MCC HCC
> **failure**

✓5ᵗʰ **I50.3** **Diastolic (congestive) heart failure**
> ▶Diastolic left ventricular heart failure
> Heart failure with normal ejection fraction
> Heart failure with preserved ejection fraction [HFpEF]◄
> ▶Code also end stage heart failure, if applicable (I50.84)◄

> *EXCLUDES 1*    combined systolic (congestive) and diastolic
> (congestive) heart failure (I50.4-)

> AHA: 2017, 1Q, 46; 2016, 1Q, 10

    **I50.30** **Unspecified diastolic (congestive) heart**   CC HCC
> **failure**

    **I50.31** **Acute diastolic (congestive) heart failure**   MCC HCC

    **I50.32** **Chronic diastolic (congestive) heart failure**   CC HCC

    **I50.33** **Acute on chronic diastolic (congestive)**   MCC HCC
> **heart failure**

✓5ᵗʰ **I50.4** **Combined systolic (congestive) and diastolic (congestive) heart failure**
> ▶Combined systolic and diastolic left ventricular heart failure
> Heart failure with reduced ejection fraction and diastolic
> dysfunction◄
> ▶Code also end stage heart failure, if applicable (I50.84)◄
> AHA: 2017, 1Q, 46; 2016, 1Q, 10

    **I50.40** **Unspecified combined systolic (congestive)**   CC HCC
> **and diastolic (congestive) heart failure**

    **I50.41** **Acute combined systolic (congestive) and**   MCC HCC
> **diastolic (congestive) heart failure**

    **I50.42** **Chronic combined systolic (congestive) and**   CC HCC
> **diastolic (congestive) heart failure**

    **I50.43** **Acute on chronic combined systolic**   MCC HCC
> **(congestive) and diastolic (congestive) heart failure**

---

[1]   MCC only if patient is discharged alive.

✓ Additional Character Req    ✓x7ᵗʰ Placeholder Alert    Unacceptable PDx    Manifestation    H1-H14 HAC    HCC CMS-HCC Condition    *EXCLUDES 1* Not Coded Here    *EXCLUDES 2* Not Included Here

**ICD-10-CM 2018**       **639**

**I46–I50.43**

**Chapter 9. Diseases of the Circulatory System**

- ✓5th **I50.8** **Other heart failure**
- ✓6th **I50.81** **Right heart failure**
  Right ventricular failure
  - **I50.810** **Right heart failure, unspecified**
    Right heart failure without mention of left heart failure
    Right ventricular failure NOS
  - **I50.811** **Acute right heart failure**
    Acute isolated right heart failure
    Acute (isolated) right ventricular failure
  - **I50.812** **Chronic right heart failure**
    Chronic isolated right heart failure
    Chronic (isolated) right ventricular failure
  - **I50.813** **Acute on chronic right heart failure**
    Acute on chronic isolated right heart failure
    Acute on chronic (isolated) right ventricular failure
    Acute decompensation of chronic (isolated) right ventricular failure
    Acute exacerbation of chronic (isolated) right ventricular failure
  - **I50.814** **Right heart failure due to left heart failure**
    Right ventricular failure secondary to left ventricular failure
    Code also the type of left ventricular failure, if known (I50.2-I50.43)
    *EXCLUDES 1*   *right heart failure with but not due to left heart failure (I50.82)*
- **I50.82** **Biventricular heart failure**
  Code also the type of left ventricular failure as systolic, diastolic, or combined, if known (I50.2-I50.43)
- **I50.83** **High output heart failure**
- **I50.84** **End stage heart failure**
  Stage D heart failure
  Code also the type of heart failure as systolic, diastolic, or combined, if known (I50.2-I50.43)
- **I50.89** **Other heart failure**
- **I50.9** **Heart failure, unspecified**   HCC
  Biventricular (heart) failure NOS
  Cardiac, heart or myocardial failure NOS
  Congestive heart disease
  Congestive heart failure NOS
  ~~Right ventricular failure (secondary to left heart failure)~~
  *EXCLUDES 2*   *fluid overload (E87.70)*
  **AHA:** 2017, 1Q, 45-46; 2014, 4Q, 21; 2012, 4Q, 92

- ✓4th **I51** **Complications and ill-defined descriptions of heart disease**
  *EXCLUDES 1*   *any condition in I51.4-I51.9 due to hypertension (I11.-)*
       *any condition in I51.4-I51.9 due to hypertension and chronic kidney disease (I13.-)*
       *heart disease specified as rheumatic (I00-I09)*
  - **I51.0** **Cardiac septal defect, acquired**   CC A
    Acquired septal atrial defect (old)
    Acquired septal auricular defect (old)
    Acquired septal ventricular defect (old)
    *EXCLUDES 1*   *cardiac septal defect as current complication following acute myocardial infarction (I23.1, I23.2)*
    **DEF:** Abnormal communication between opposite heart chambers due to defect of septum; not present at birth.
    **CC Excl:** PDX collection 654
  - **I51.1** **Rupture of chordae tendineae, not elsewhere classified**   MCC HCC
    *EXCLUDES 1*   *rupture of chordae tendineae as current complication following acute myocardial infarction (I23.4)*
    **CC Excl:** PDX collection 655
  - **I51.2** **Rupture of papillary muscle, not elsewhere classified**   MCC HCC
    *EXCLUDES 1*   *rupture of papillary muscle as current complication following acute myocardial infarction (I23.5)*
    **CC Excl:** PDX collection 656
  - **I51.3** **Intracardiac thrombosis, not elsewhere classified**
    Apical thrombosis (old)
    Atrial thrombosis (old)
    Auricular thrombosis (old)
    Mural thrombosis (old)
    Ventricular thrombosis (old)
    *EXCLUDES 1*   *intracardiac thrombosis as current complication following acute myocardial infarction (I23.6)*
    **AHA:** 2013, 1Q, 24

- **I51.4** **Myocarditis, unspecified**   HCC
  Chronic (interstitial) myocarditis
  Myocardial fibrosis
  Myocarditis NOS
  *EXCLUDES 1*   *acute or subacute myocarditis (I40.-)*
- **I51.5** **Myocardial degeneration**   HCC
  Fatty degeneration of heart or myocardium
  Myocardial disease
  Senile degeneration of heart or myocardium
- **I51.7** **Cardiomegaly**
  Cardiac dilatation
  Cardiac hypertrophy
  Ventricular dilatation
- ✓5th **I51.8** **Other ill-defined heart diseases**
  - **I51.81** **Takotsubo syndrome**   CC
    Reversible left ventricular dysfunction following sudden emotional stress
    Stress induced cardiomyopathy
    Takotsubo cardiomyopathy
    Transient left ventricular apical ballooning syndrome
    **CC Excl:** PDX collection 683
  - **I51.89** **Other ill-defined heart diseases**
    Carditis (acute)(chronic)
    Pancarditis (acute)(chronic)
- **I51.9** **Heart disease, unspecified**

- **I52** *Other heart disorders in diseases classified elsewhere*
  Code first underlying disease, such as:
  congenital syphilis (A50.5)
  mucopolysaccharidosis (E76.3)
  schistosomiasis (B65.0-B65.9)
  *EXCLUDES 1*   *heart disease (in):*
       *gonococcal infection (A54.83)*
       *meningococcal infection (A39.50)*
       *rheumatoid arthritis (M05.31)*
       *syphilis (A52.06)*

## Cerebrovascular diseases (I60-I69)

Use additional code to identify presence of:
alcohol abuse and dependence (F10.-)
exposure to environmental tobacco smoke (Z77.22)
history of tobacco dependence (Z87.891)
hypertension (I10-I15)
occupational exposure to environmental tobacco smoke (Z57.31)
tobacco dependence (F17.-)
tobacco use (Z72.0)
*EXCLUDES 1*   *transient cerebral ischemic attacks and related syndromes (G45.-)*
     *traumatic intracranial hemorrhage (S06.-)*
**AHA:** 2014, 3Q, 5; 2012, 4Q, 91-92

- ✓4th **I60** **Nontraumatic subarachnoid hemorrhage**
  *INCLUDES*   ruptured cerebral aneurysm
  *EXCLUDES 1*   *syphilitic ruptured cerebral aneurysm (A52.05)*
  *EXCLUDES 2*   *sequelae of subarachnoid hemorrhage (I69.0-)*

  **CC Excl: For MCC codes in category I60:** PDX collection 684

- ✓5th **I60.0** **Nontraumatic subarachnoid hemorrhage from carotid siphon and bifurcation**
  - **I60.00** **Nontraumatic subarachnoid hemorrhage from unspecified carotid siphon and bifurcation**   MCC HCC
  - **I60.01** **Nontraumatic subarachnoid hemorrhage from right carotid siphon and bifurcation**   MCC HCC
  - **I60.02** **Nontraumatic subarachnoid hemorrhage from left carotid siphon and bifurcation**   MCC HCC
- ✓5th **I60.1** **Nontraumatic subarachnoid hemorrhage from middle cerebral artery**
  - **I60.10** **Nontraumatic subarachnoid hemorrhage from unspecified middle cerebral artery**   MCC HCC
  - **I60.11** **Nontraumatic subarachnoid hemorrhage from right middle cerebral artery**   MCC HCC
  - **I60.12** **Nontraumatic subarachnoid hemorrhage from left middle cerebral artery**   MCC HCC
- **I60.2** **Nontraumatic subarachnoid hemorrhage from anterior communicating artery**   MCC HCC
- ✓5th **I60.3** **Nontraumatic subarachnoid hemorrhage from posterior communicating artery**
  - **I60.30** **Nontraumatic subarachnoid hemorrhage from unspecified posterior communicating artery**   MCC HCC
  - **I60.31** **Nontraumatic subarachnoid hemorrhage from right posterior communicating artery**   MCC HCC

N Newborn: 0   P Pediatric: 0-17   M Maternity: 12-55   A Adult: 15-124   MCC Major CC Condition   PDxMCC PDx acts as own MCC   CC CC Condition   PDxCC PDx acts as own CC

**640**        ICD-10-CM 2018

**I60.32**   **Nontraumatic subarachnoid hemorrhage from** left **posterior communicating artery** `MCC` `HCC`

**I60.4**   **Nontraumatic subarachnoid hemorrhage from basilar artery** `MCC` `HCC`

✓5ᵗʰ **I60.5**   **Nontraumatic subarachnoid hemorrhage from** vertebral **artery**

**I60.50**   **Nontraumatic subarachnoid hemorrhage from** unspecified **vertebral artery** `MCC` `HCC`

**I60.51**   **Nontraumatic subarachnoid hemorrhage from** right **vertebral artery** `MCC` `HCC`

**I60.52**   **Nontraumatic subarachnoid hemorrhage from** left **vertebral artery** `MCC` `HCC`

**I60.6**   **Nontraumatic subarachnoid hemorrhage from** other **intracranial arteries** `MCC` `HCC`

**I60.7**   **Nontraumatic subarachnoid hemorrhage from** unspecified **intracranial artery** `MCC` `HCC`
Ruptured (congenital) berry aneurysm
Ruptured (congenital) cerebral aneurysm
Subarachnoid hemorrhage (nontraumatic) from cerebral artery NOS
Subarachnoid hemorrhage (nontraumatic) from communicating artery NOS
*EXCLUDES 1*   berry aneurysm, nonruptured (I67.1)

**I60.8**   Other **nontraumatic subarachnoid hemorrhage** `MCC` `HCC`
Meningeal hemorrhage
Rupture of cerebral arteriovenous malformation

**I60.9**   **Nontraumatic subarachnoid hemorrhage, unspecified** `MCC` `HCC`

✓4ᵗʰ **I61**   **Nontraumatic intracerebral hemorrhage**
*EXCLUDES 2*   sequelae of intracerebral hemorrhage (I69.1-)
**AHA:** 2017, 2Q, 9-10

CC Excl: For MCC codes in category I61: PDX collection 684

**I61.0**   **Nontraumatic intracerebral hemorrhage in** hemisphere, subcortical `MCC` `HCC`
Deep intracerebral hemorrhage (nontraumatic)

**I61.1**   **Nontraumatic intracerebral hemorrhage in** hemisphere, cortical `MCC` `HCC`
Cerebral lobe hemorrhage (nontraumatic)
Superficial intracerebral hemorrhage (nontraumatic)

**I61.2**   **Nontraumatic intracerebral hemorrhage in** hemisphere, unspecified `MCC` `HCC`

**I61.3**   **Nontraumatic intracerebral hemorrhage in** brain **stem** `MCC` `HCC`

**I61.4**   **Nontraumatic intracerebral hemorrhage in** cerebellum `MCC` `HCC`

**I61.5**   **Nontraumatic intracerebral hemorrhage, intraventricular** `MCC` `HCC`

**I61.6**   **Nontraumatic intracerebral hemorrhage,** multiple **localized** `MCC` `HCC`

**I61.8**   Other **nontraumatic intracerebral hemorrhage** `MCC` `HCC`

**I61.9**   **Nontraumatic intracerebral hemorrhage, unspecified** `MCC` `HCC`

✓4ᵗʰ **I62**   **Other and unspecified nontraumatic intracranial hemorrhage**
*EXCLUDES 2*   sequelae of intracranial hemorrhage (I69.2)

CC Excl: For CC/MCC codes in category I62: PDX collection 684

✓5ᵗʰ **I62.0**   **Nontraumatic** subdural **hemorrhage**

**I62.00**   **Nontraumatic subdural hemorrhage, unspecified** `MCC` `HCC`

**I62.01**   **Nontraumatic** acute **subdural hemorrhage** `MCC` `HCC`

**I62.02**   **Nontraumatic** subacute **subdural hemorrhage** `MCC` `HCC`

**I62.03**   **Nontraumatic** chronic **subdural hemorrhage** `MCC` `HCC`

**I62.1**   **Nontraumatic** extradural **hemorrhage** `MCC` `HCC`
Nontraumatic epidural hemorrhage

**I62.9**   **Nontraumatic intracranial hemorrhage,** unspecified `CC` `HCC`

✓4ᵗʰ **I63**   **Cerebral infarction**
`INCLUDES`   occlusion and stenosis of cerebral and precerebral arteries, resulting in cerebral infarction
Use additional code, if applicable, to identify status post administration of tPA (rtPA) in a different facility within the last 24 hours prior to admission to current facility (Z92.82)
Use additional code, if known, to indicate National Institutes of Health Stroke Scale (NIHSS) score (R29.7-)
*EXCLUDES 2*   sequelae of cerebral infarction (I69.3-)
**AHA:** 2017, 2Q, 9-10; 2014, 1Q, 23

✓5ᵗʰ **I63.0**   **Cerebral infarction due to** thrombosis of precerebral **arteries**

**I63.00**   **Cerebral infarction due to thrombosis of** unspecified **precerebral artery** `MCC` `HCC`
CC Excl: PDX collection 685

✓6ᵗʰ **I63.01**   **Cerebral infarction due to thrombosis of** vertebral **artery**

CC Excl: For MCC codes in subcategory I63.01: PDX collection 686

**I63.011**   **Cerebral infarction due to thrombosis of** right **vertebral artery** `MCC` `HCC`

**I63.012**   **Cerebral infarction due to thrombosis of** left **vertebral artery** `MCC` `HCC`

**I63.013**   **Cerebral infarction due to thrombosis of** bilateral **vertebral arteries** `MCC` `HCC`

**I63.019**   **Cerebral infarction due to thrombosis of** unspecified **vertebral artery** `MCC` `HCC`

**I63.02**   **Cerebral infarction due to thrombosis of** basilar **artery** `MCC` `HCC`
CC Excl: PDX collection 685

✓6ᵗʰ **I63.03**   **Cerebral infarction due to thrombosis of** carotid **artery**

CC Excl: For MCC codes in subcategory I63.03: PDX collection 687

**I63.031**   **Cerebral infarction due to thrombosis of** right **carotid artery** `MCC` `HCC`

**I63.032**   **Cerebral infarction due to thrombosis of** left **carotid artery** `MCC` `HCC`

**I63.033**   **Cerebral infarction due to thrombosis of** bilateral **carotid arteries** `MCC` `HCC`

**I63.039**   **Cerebral infarction due to thrombosis of** unspecified **carotid artery** `MCC` `HCC`

**I63.09**   **Cerebral infarction due to thrombosis of** other **precerebral** artery `MCC` `HCC`
CC Excl: PDX collection 685

✓5ᵗʰ **I63.1**   **Cerebral infarction due to** embolism of precerebral **arteries**

**I63.10**   **Cerebral infarction due to embolism of** unspecified **precerebral artery** `MCC` `HCC`
CC Excl: PDX collection 685

✓6ᵗʰ **I63.11**   **Cerebral infarction due to embolism of** vertebral **artery**

CC Excl: For MCC codes in subcategory I63.11: PDX collection 686

**I63.111**   **Cerebral infarction due to embolism of** right **vertebral artery** `MCC` `HCC`

**I63.112**   **Cerebral infarction due to embolism of** left **vertebral artery** `MCC` `HCC`

**I63.113**   **Cerebral infarction due to embolism of** bilateral **vertebral arteries** `MCC` `HCC`

**I63.119**   **Cerebral infarction due to embolism of** unspecified **vertebral artery** `MCC` `HCC`

**I63.12**   **Cerebral infarction due to embolism of** basilar **artery** `MCC` `HCC`
CC Excl: PDX collection 685

✓6ᵗʰ **I63.13**   **Cerebral infarction due to embolism of** carotid **artery**

CC Excl: For MCC codes in subcategory I63.13: PDX collection 687

**I63.131**   **Cerebral infarction due to embolism of** right **carotid artery** `MCC` `HCC`

**I63.132**   **Cerebral infarction due to embolism of** left **carotid artery** `MCC` `HCC`

**I63.133**   **Cerebral infarction due to embolism of** bilateral **carotid arteries** `MCC` `HCC`

**I63.139**   **Cerebral infarction due to embolism of** unspecified **carotid artery** `MCC` `HCC`

Chapter 9. Diseases of the Circulatory System

I63.19–I63.439

I63.19   **Cerebral infarction due to embolism of** `MCC` `HCC`
other **precerebral artery**
CC Excl: PDX collection 685

✓5th   **I63.2**   **Cerebral infarction due to** unspecified occlusion or stenosis of
precerebral **arteries**

     I63.20   **Cerebral infarction due to unspecified** `MCC` `HCC`
**occlusion or stenosis of** unspecified **precerebral
arteries**
CC Excl: PDX collection 685

     ✓6th   I63.21   **Cerebral infarction due to unspecified occlusion or
stenosis of** vertebral **arteries**

         **CC Excl: For MCC codes in subcategory I63.21:**
PDX collection 686

▲      I63.211   **Cerebral infarction due to** `MCC` `HCC`
**unspecified occlusion or stenosis
of** right **vertebral artery**

▲      I63.212   **Cerebral infarction due to** `MCC` `HCC`
**unspecified occlusion or stenosis
of** left **vertebral artery**

     I63.213   **Cerebral infarction due to** `MCC` `HCC`
**unspecified occlusion or stenosis
of** bilateral **vertebral arteries**

     I63.219   **Cerebral infarction due to** `MCC` `HCC`
**unspecified occlusion or stenosis
of** unspecified **vertebral arteries**

▲      I63.22   **Cerebral infarction due to unspecified** `MCC` `HCC`
**occlusion or stenosis of** basilar **artery**
CC Excl: PDX collection 685

▲   ✓6th   I63.23   **Cerebral infarction due to unspecified occlusion or
stenosis of** carotid **arteries**

         **CC Excl: For MCC codes in subcategory I63.23:**
PDX collection 687

     I63.231   **Cerebral infarction due to** `MCC` `HCC`
**unspecified occlusion or stenosis
of** right **carotid arteries**

     I63.232   **Cerebral infarction due to** `MCC` `HCC`
**unspecified occlusion or stenosis
of** left **carotid arteries**

     I63.233   **Cerebral infarction due to** `MCC` `HCC`
**unspecified occlusion or stenosis
of** bilateral **carotid arteries**

     I63.239   **Cerebral infarction due to** `MCC` `HCC`
**unspecified occlusion or stenosis
of** unspecified **carotid arteries**

     I63.29   **Cerebral infarction due to unspecified** `MCC` `HCC`
**occlusion or stenosis of** other **precerebral arteries**
CC Excl: PDX collection 685

✓5th   **I63.3**   **Cerebral infarction due to** thrombosis of cerebral **arteries**

     **CC Excl: For MCC codes in subcategory I63.3:**
PDX collection 688

     I63.30   **Cerebral infarction due to thrombosis of** `MCC` `HCC`
unspecified **cerebral artery**

     ✓6th   I63.31   **Cerebral infarction due to thrombosis of** middle
**cerebral artery**

     I63.311   **Cerebral infarction due to** `MCC` `HCC`
**thrombosis of** right **middle
cerebral artery**

     I63.312   **Cerebral infarction due to** `MCC` `HCC`
**thrombosis of** left **middle
cerebral artery**

     I63.313   **Cerebral infarction due to** `MCC` `HCC`
**thrombosis of** bilateral **middle
cerebral arteries**

     I63.319   **Cerebral infarction due to** `MCC` `HCC`
**thrombosis of** unspecified **middle
cerebral artery**

     ✓6th   I63.32   **Cerebral infarction due to thrombosis of** anterior
**cerebral artery**

     I63.321   **Cerebral infarction due to** `MCC` `HCC`
**thrombosis of** right **anterior
cerebral artery**

     I63.322   **Cerebral infarction due to** `MCC` `HCC`
**thrombosis of** left **anterior
cerebral artery**

▲      I63.323   **Cerebral infarction due to** `MCC` `HCC`
**thrombosis of** bilateral **anterior
cerebral arteries**

     I63.329   **Cerebral infarction due to** `MCC` `HCC`
**thrombosis of** unspecified **anterior
cerebral artery**

✓6th   I63.33   **Cerebral infarction due to thrombosis of** posterior
**cerebral artery**

     I63.331   **Cerebral infarction due to** `MCC` `HCC`
**thrombosis of** right **posterior
cerebral artery**

     I63.332   **Cerebral infarction due to** `MCC` `HCC`
**thrombosis of** left **posterior
cerebral artery**

     I63.333   **Cerebral infarction to thrombosis** `MCC` `HCC`
**of** bilateral **posterior cerebral arteries**

     I63.339   **Cerebral infarction due to** `MCC` `HCC`
**thrombosis of** unspecified **posterior
cerebral artery**

▲   ✓6th   I63.34   **Cerebral infarction due to thrombosis of** cerebellar
**artery**

     I63.341   **Cerebral infarction due to** `MCC` `HCC`
**thrombosis of** right **cerebellar
artery**

     I63.342   **Cerebral infarction due to** `MCC` `HCC`
**thrombosis of** left **cerebellar
artery**

     I63.343   **Cerebral infarction to** `MCC` `HCC`
**thrombosis of** bilateral **cerebellar
arteries**

     I63.349   **Cerebral infarction due to** `MCC` `HCC`
**thrombosis of** unspecified
**cerebellar artery**

     I63.39   **Cerebral infarction due to thrombosis of** `MCC` `HCC`
other **cerebral artery**

✓5th   **I63.4**   **Cerebral infarction due to** embolism of cerebral **arteries**

     **CC Excl: For MCC codes in subcategory I63.4:**
PDX collection 688

     I63.40   **Cerebral infarction due to embolism of** `MCC` `HCC`
unspecified **cerebral artery**

     ✓6th   I63.41   **Cerebral infarction due to embolism of** middle
**cerebral artery**

     I63.411   **Cerebral infarction due to** `MCC` `HCC`
**embolism of** right **middle
cerebral artery**

     I63.412   **Cerebral infarction due to** `MCC` `HCC`
**embolism of** left **middle
cerebral artery**

     I63.413   **Cerebral infarction due to** `MCC` `HCC`
**embolism of** bilateral **middle
cerebral arteries**

     I63.419   **Cerebral infarction due to** `MCC` `HCC`
**embolism of** unspecified **middle
cerebral artery**

     ✓6th   I63.42   **Cerebral infarction due to embolism of** anterior
**cerebral artery**

     I63.421   **Cerebral infarction due to** `MCC` `HCC`
**embolism of** right **anterior
cerebral artery**

     I63.422   **Cerebral infarction due to** `MCC` `HCC`
**embolism of** left **anterior
cerebral artery**

     I63.423   **Cerebral infarction due to** `MCC` `HCC`
**embolism of** bilateral **anterior
cerebral arteries**

     I63.429   **Cerebral infarction due to** `MCC` `HCC`
**embolism of** unspecified **anterior
cerebral artery**

     ✓6th   I63.43   **Cerebral infarction due to embolism of** posterior
**cerebral artery**

     I63.431   **Cerebral infarction due to** `MCC` `HCC`
**embolism of** right **posterior
cerebral artery**

     I63.432   **Cerebral infarction due to** `MCC` `HCC`
**embolism of** left **posterior
cerebral artery**

     I63.433   **Cerebral infarction due to** `MCC` `HCC`
**embolism of** bilateral **posterior
cerebral arteries**

     I63.439   **Cerebral infarction due to** `MCC` `HCC`
**embolism of** unspecified **posterior
cerebral artery**

Ⓝ Newborn: 0   Ⓟ Pediatric: 0-17   Ⓜ Maternity: 12-55   Ⓐ Adult: 15-124   `MCC` Major CC Condition   `PDxMCC` PDx acts as own MCC   `CC` CC Condition   `PDxCC` PDx acts as own CC

**642**

ICD-10-CM 2018

✓6ᵗʰ **I63.44**   **Cerebral infarction due to embolism of** cerebellar artery

    **I63.441**   **Cerebral infarction due to embolism of** right **cerebellar artery**    MCC HCC

    **I63.442**   **Cerebral infarction due to embolism of** left **cerebellar artery**    MCC HCC

    **I63.443**   **Cerebral infarction due to embolism of** bilateral **cerebellar arteries**    MCC HCC

    **I63.449**   **Cerebral infarction due to embolism of** unspecified **cerebellar artery**    MCC HCC

   **I63.49**   **Cerebral infarction due to embolism of** other **cerebral artery**    MCC HCC

✓5ᵗʰ **I63.5**   **Cerebral infarction due to** unspecified occlusion or stenosis of cerebral **arteries**

    **CC Excl: For MCC codes in subcategory I63.5:** PDX collection 688

   **I63.50**   **Cerebral infarction due to unspecified occlusion or stenosis of** unspecified **cerebral artery**    MCC HCC

✓6ᵗʰ **I63.51**   **Cerebral infarction due to unspecified occlusion or stenosis of** middle **cerebral artery**

    **I63.511**   **Cerebral infarction due to unspecified occlusion or stenosis of** right **middle cerebral artery**    MCC HCC

    **I63.512**   **Cerebral infarction due to unspecified occlusion or stenosis of** left **middle cerebral artery**    MCC HCC

    **I63.513**   **Cerebral infarction due to unspecified occlusion or stenosis of** bilateral **middle cerebral arteries**    MCC HCC

    **I63.519**   **Cerebral infarction due to unspecified occlusion or stenosis of** unspecified **middle cerebral artery**    MCC HCC

✓6ᵗʰ **I63.52**   **Cerebral infarction due to unspecified occlusion or stenosis of** anterior **cerebral artery**

    **I63.521**   **Cerebral infarction due to unspecified occlusion or stenosis of** right **anterior cerebral artery**    MCC HCC

    **I63.522**   **Cerebral infarction due to unspecified occlusion or stenosis of** left **anterior cerebral artery**    MCC HCC

    **I63.523**   **Cerebral infarction due to unspecified occlusion or stenosis of** bilateral **anterior cerebral arteries**    MCC HCC

    **I63.529**   **Cerebral infarction due to unspecified occlusion or stenosis of** unspecified **anterior cerebral artery**    MCC HCC

✓6ᵗʰ **I63.53**   **Cerebral infarction due to unspecified occlusion or stenosis of** posterior **cerebral artery**

    **I63.531**   **Cerebral infarction due to unspecified occlusion or stenosis of** right **posterior cerebral artery**    MCC HCC

    **I63.532**   **Cerebral infarction due to unspecified occlusion or stenosis of** left **posterior cerebral artery**    MCC HCC

    **I63.533**   **Cerebral infarction due to unspecified occlusion or stenosis of** bilateral **posterior cerebral arteries**    MCC HCC

    **I63.539**   **Cerebral infarction due to unspecified occlusion or stenosis of** unspecified **posterior cerebral artery**    MCC HCC

✓6ᵗʰ **I63.54**   **Cerebral infarction due to unspecified occlusion or stenosis of** cerebellar **artery**

    **I63.541**   **Cerebral infarction due to unspecified occlusion or stenosis of** right **cerebellar artery**    MCC HCC

    **I63.542**   **Cerebral infarction due to unspecified occlusion or stenosis of** left **cerebellar artery**    MCC HCC

    **I63.543**   **Cerebral infarction due to unspecified occlusion or stenosis of** bilateral **cerebellar arteries**    MCC HCC

    **I63.549**   **Cerebral infarction due to unspecified occlusion or stenosis of** unspecified **cerebellar artery**    MCC HCC

---

   **I63.59**   **Cerebral infarction due to unspecified occlusion or stenosis of** other **cerebral artery**    MCC HCC

   **I63.6**   **Cerebral infarction due to** cerebral venous **thrombosis, nonpyogenic**    MCC HCC
    **CC Excl:** PDX collection 688

   **I63.8**   **Other cerebral infarction**    MCC HCC
    **CC Excl:**.PDX collection 688

   **I63.9**   **Cerebral infarction, unspecified**    MCC HCC
    Stroke NOS
    *EXCLUDES 2* ►*transient cerebral ischemic attacks and related syndromes (G45.-)*◄
    **AHA:** 2015, 1Q, 25
    **CC Excl:** PDX collection 688

✓4ᵗʰ **I65**   **Occlusion and stenosis of** precerebral **arteries, not resulting in cerebral infarction**
    **INCLUDES**   embolism of precerebral artery
          narrowing of precerebral artery
          obstruction (complete) (partial) of precerebral artery
          thrombosis of precerebral artery
    *EXCLUDES 1*   *insufficiency, NOS, of precerebral artery (G45.-)*
          *insufficiency of precerebral arteries causing cerebral infarction (I63.0-I63.2)*

   ✓5ᵗʰ **I65.0**   **Occlusion and stenosis of** vertebral **artery**

    **I65.01**   **Occlusion and stenosis of** right **vertebral artery**

    **I65.02**   **Occlusion and stenosis of** left **vertebral artery**

    **I65.03**   **Occlusion and stenosis of** bilateral **vertebral arteries**

    **I65.09**   **Occlusion and stenosis of** unspecified **vertebral artery**

   **I65.1**   **Occlusion and stenosis of** basilar **artery**

   ✓5ᵗʰ **I65.2**   **Occlusion and stenosis of** carotid **artery**

    **I65.21**   **Occlusion and stenosis of** right **carotid artery**

    **I65.22**   **Occlusion and stenosis of** left **carotid artery**

    **I65.23**   **Occlusion and stenosis of** bilateral **carotid arteries**

    **I65.29**   **Occlusion and stenosis of** unspecified **carotid artery**

   **I65.8**   **Occlusion and stenosis of** other **precerebral arteries**

   **I65.9**   **Occlusion and stenosis of** unspecified **precerebral artery**
    Occlusion and stenosis of precerebral artery NOS

✓4ᵗʰ **I66**   **Occlusion and stenosis of** cerebral **arteries, not resulting in cerebral infarction**
    **INCLUDES**   embolism of cerebral artery
          narrowing of cerebral artery
          obstruction (complete) (partial) of cerebral artery
          thrombosis of cerebral artery
    *EXCLUDES 1*   *occlusion and stenosis of cerebral artery causing cerebral infarction (I63.3-I63.5)*

   ✓5ᵗʰ **I66.0**   **Occlusion and stenosis of** middle **cerebral artery**

    **I66.01**   **Occlusion and stenosis of** right **middle cerebral artery**

    **I66.02**   **Occlusion and stenosis of** left **middle cerebral artery**

    **I66.03**   **Occlusion and stenosis of** bilateral **middle cerebral arteries**

    **I66.09**   **Occlusion and stenosis of** unspecified **middle cerebral artery**

   ✓5ᵗʰ **I66.1**   **Occlusion and stenosis of** anterior **cerebral artery**

    **I66.11**   **Occlusion and stenosis of** right **anterior cerebral artery**

    **I66.12**   **Occlusion and stenosis of** left **anterior cerebral artery**

    **I66.13**   **Occlusion and stenosis of** bilateral **anterior cerebral arteries**

    **I66.19**   **Occlusion and stenosis of** unspecified **anterior cerebral artery**

   ✓5ᵗʰ **I66.2**   **Occlusion and stenosis of** posterior **cerebral artery**

    **I66.21**   **Occlusion and stenosis of** right **posterior cerebral artery**

    **I66.22**   **Occlusion and stenosis of** left **posterior cerebral artery**

    **I66.23**   **Occlusion and stenosis of** bilateral **posterior cerebral arteries**

    **I66.29**   **Occlusion and stenosis of** unspecified **posterior cerebral artery**

   **I66.3**   **Occlusion and stenosis of** cerebellar **arteries**

   **I66.8**   **Occlusion and stenosis of** other **cerebral arteries**
    Occlusion and stenosis of perforating arteries

   **I66.9**   **Occlusion and stenosis of** unspecified **cerebral artery**

---

✓ Additional Character Req    ✓x7ᵗʰ Placeholder Alert    Unacceptable PDx    Manifestation    H1 - H14 HAC    HCC CMS-HCC Condition    *EXCLUDES 1* Not Coded Here    *EXCLUDES 2* Not Included Here

**Berry Aneurysm**

Berry aneurysms form at the site of a weakness in an arterial wall, often at a junction

Berry aneurysm

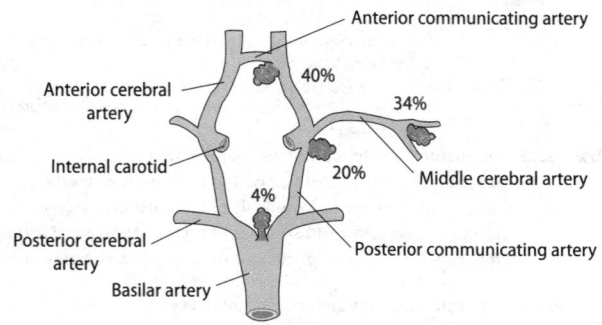

Anterior communicating artery

Anterior cerebral artery

Internal carotid

40%

34%

20%

4%

Middle cerebral artery

Posterior cerebral artery

Posterior communicating artery

Basilar artery

Common sites of berry aneurysms in the circle of Willis arteries

✓4ᵗʰ **I67**    **Other cerebrovascular diseases**
> *EXCLUDES 2*   *sequelae of the listed conditions (I69.8)*

**I67.0**    **Dissection of cerebral arteries, nonruptured**    `MCC` `HCC`
> *EXCLUDES 1*   *ruptured cerebral arteries (I60.7)*
> **CC Excl:** PDX collection 689

**I67.1**    **Cerebral aneurysm, nonruptured**
> Cerebral aneurysm NOS
> Cerebral arteriovenous fistula, acquired
> Internal carotid artery aneurysm, intracranial portion
> Internal carotid artery aneurysm, NOS
> *EXCLUDES 1*   *congenital cerebral aneurysm, nonruptured (Q28.-)*
>                *ruptured cerebral aneurysm (I60.7)*

**I67.2**    **Cerebral atherosclerosis**    `A`
> Atheroma of cerebral and precerebral arteries

**I67.3**    **Progressive vascular leukoencephalopathy**    `HIV` `CC`
> Binswanger's disease
> **CC Excl:** PDX collection 133

**I67.4**    **Hypertensive encephalopathy**    `CC`
> *EXCLUDES 2* ▶*insufficiency, NOS, of precerebral arteries (G45.2)*◀
> **CC Excl:** PDX collection 690

**I67.5**    **Moyamoya disease**    `CC`
> **DEF:** Cerebrovascular ischemia; vessels occlude and rupture, causing tiny hemorrhages at base of brain; affects predominantly Japanese people.
> **CC Excl:** PDX collection 691

**I67.6**    **Nonpyogenic thrombosis of intracranial venous system**    `CC`
> Nonpyogenic thrombosis of cerebral vein
> Nonpyogenic thrombosis of intracranial venous sinus
> *EXCLUDES 1*   *nonpyogenic thrombosis of intracranial venous system causing infarction (I63.6)*
> **CC Excl:** PDX collection 692

**I67.7**    **Cerebral arteritis, not elsewhere classified**    `CC`
> Granulomatous angiitis of the nervous system
> *EXCLUDES 1*   *allergic granulomatous angiitis (M30.1)*
> **CC Excl:** PDX collection 693

✓5ᵗʰ **I67.8**    **Other specified cerebrovascular diseases**

     **I67.81**    **Acute cerebrovascular insufficiency**    `CC`
> Acute cerebrovascular insufficiency unspecified as to location or reversibility
> **CC Excl:** PDX collection 694

     **I67.82**    **Cerebral ischemia**    `CC`
> Chronic cerebral ischemia
> **CC Excl:** PDX collection 694

     **I67.83**    **Posterior reversible encephalopathy syndrome**    `HIV` `MCC`
> PRES
> **CC Excl:** PDX collection 610

---

✓6ᵗʰ **I67.84**    **Cerebral vasospasm and vasoconstriction**

     **I67.841**    **Reversible cerebrovascular vasoconstriction syndrome**    `CC`
> Call-Fleming syndrome
> Code first underlying condition, if applicable, such as eclampsia (O15.00-O15.9)
> **CC Excl:** PDX collection 586

     **I67.848**    **Other cerebrovascular vasospasm and vasoconstriction**    `CC`
> **CC Excl:** PDX collection 586

     **I67.89**    **Other cerebrovascular disease**    `CC`
> **CC Excl:** PDX collection 694

**I67.9**    **Cerebrovascular disease, unspecified**

✓4ᵗʰ **I68**    **Cerebrovascular disorders in diseases classified elsewhere**

**I68.0**    ***Cerebral amyloid angiopathy***
> Code first underlying amyloidosis (E85.-)

**I68.2**    ***Cerebral arteritis in other diseases classified elsewhere***    `CC`
> Code first underlying disease
> *EXCLUDES 1*   *cerebral arteritis (in):*
>             *listerosis (A32.89)*
>             *systemic lupus erythematosus (M32.19)*
>             *syphilis (A52.04)*
>             *tuberculosis (A18.89)*
> **CC Excl:** PDX collection 693

**I68.8**    ***Other cerebrovascular disorders in diseases classified elsewhere***
> Code first underlying disease
> *EXCLUDES 1*   *syphilitic cerebral aneurysm (A52.05)*

✓4ᵗʰ **I69**    **Sequelae of cerebrovascular disease**
> `NOTE`   Category I69 is to be used to indicate conditions in I60-I67 as the cause of sequelae. The "sequelae" include conditions specified as such or as residuals which may occur at any time after the onset of the causal condition
> *EXCLUDES 1*   *personal history of cerebral infarction without residual deficit (Z86.73)*
>             *personal history of prolonged reversible ischemic neurologic deficit (PRIND) (Z86.73)*
>             *personal history of reversible ischemic neurologcial deficit (RIND) (Z86.73)*
>             *sequelae of traumatic intracranial injury (S06.-)*
>             ~~*transient ischemic attack (TIA) (G45.9)*~~
> **AHA:** 2017, 1Q, 47; 2015, 1Q, 25; 2012, 4Q, 106

✓5ᵗʰ **I69.0**    **Sequelae of nontraumatic subarachnoid hemorrhage**

     **I69.00**    **Unspecified sequelae of nontraumatic subarachnoid hemorrhage**

✓6ᵗʰ **I69.01**    **Cognitive deficits following nontraumatic subarachnoid hemorrhage**

     **I69.010**    **Attention and concentration deficit following nontraumatic subarachnoid hemorrhage**

     **I69.011**    **Memory deficit following nontraumatic subarachnoid hemorrhage**

     **I69.012**    **Visuospatial deficit and spatial neglect following nontraumatic subarachnoid hemorrhage**

     **I69.013**    **Psychomotor deficit following nontraumatic subarachnoid hemorrhage**

     **I69.014**    **Frontal lobe and executive function deficit following nontraumatic subarachnoid hemorrhage**

     **I69.015**    **Cognitive social or emotional deficit following nontraumatic subarachnoid hemorrhage**

     **I69.018**    **Other symptoms and signs involving cognitive functions following nontraumatic subarachnoid hemorrhage**

     **I69.019**    **Unspecified symptoms and signs involving cognitive functions following nontraumatic subarachnoid hemorrhage**

✓6ᵗʰ **I69.02**    **Speech and language deficits following nontraumatic subarachnoid hemorrhage**

     **I69.020**    **Aphasia following nontraumatic subarachnoid hemorrhage**

     **I69.021**    **Dysphasia following nontraumatic subarachnoid hemorrhage**

     **I69.022**    **Dysarthria following nontraumatic subarachnoid hemorrhage**

`N` Newborn: 0    `P` Pediatric: 0-17    `M` Maternity: 12-55    `A` Adult: 15-124    `MCC` Major CC Condition    `PDxMCC` PDx acts as own MCC    `CC` CC Condition    `PDxCC` PDx acts as own CC

**644**                                                               ICD-10-CM 2018

**I69.023**   **Fluency disorder** following **nontraumatic subarachnoid hemorrhage**
Stuttering following nontraumatic subarachnoid hemorrhage

**I69.028**   **Other speech and language deficits following nontraumatic subarachnoid hemorrhage**

✓6th **I69.03**   Monoplegia of upper limb following nontraumatic subarachnoid hemorrhage
AHA: 2017, 1Q, 47

**I69.031**   Monoplegia of upper limb following `HCC` nontraumatic subarachnoid hemorrhage affecting **right dominant** side

**I69.032**   Monoplegia of upper limb following `HCC` nontraumatic subarachnoid hemorrhage affecting **left dominant** side

**I69.033**   Monoplegia of upper limb following `HCC` nontraumatic subarachnoid hemorrhage affecting **right non-dominant** side

**I69.034**   Monoplegia of upper limb following `HCC` nontraumatic subarachnoid hemorrhage affecting **left non-dominant** side

**I69.039**   Monoplegia of upper limb following `HCC` nontraumatic subarachnoid hemorrhage affecting **unspecified** side

✓6th **I69.04**   Monoplegia of lower limb following nontraumatic subarachnoid hemorrhage
AHA: 2017, 1Q, 47

**I69.041**   Monoplegia of lower limb following `HCC` nontraumatic subarachnoid hemorrhage affecting **right dominant** side

**I69.042**   Monoplegia of lower limb following `HCC` nontraumatic subarachnoid hemorrhage affecting **left dominant** side

**I69.043**   Monoplegia of lower limb following `HCC` nontraumatic subarachnoid hemorrhage affecting **right non-dominant** side

**I69.044**   Monoplegia of lower limb following `HCC` nontraumatic subarachnoid hemorrhage affecting **left non-dominant** side

**I69.049**   Monoplegia of lower limb following `HCC` nontraumatic subarachnoid hemorrhage affecting **unspecified** side

✓6th **I69.05**   Hemiplegia and hemiparesis following nontraumatic subarachnoid hemorrhage
AHA: 2015, 1Q, 25

**I69.051**   Hemiplegia and hemiparesis `CC` `HCC` following nontraumatic subarachnoid hemorrhage affecting **right dominant** side
CC Excl: PDX collection 695

**I69.052**   Hemiplegia and hemiparesis `CC` `HCC` following nontraumatic subarachnoid hemorrhage affecting **left dominant** side
CC Excl: PDX collection 695

**I69.053**   Hemiplegia and hemiparesis `CC` `HCC` following nontraumatic subarachnoid hemorrhage affecting **right non-dominant** side
CC Excl: PDX collection 696

**I69.054**   Hemiplegia and hemiparesis `CC` `HCC` following nontraumatic subarachnoid hemorrhage affecting **left non-dominant** side
CC Excl: PDX collection 696

**I69.059**   Hemiplegia and hemiparesis `CC` `HCC` following nontraumatic subarachnoid hemorrhage affecting **unspecified** side
CC Excl: PDX collection 697

✓6th **I69.06**   Other paralytic syndrome following nontraumatic subarachnoid hemorrhage
Use additional code to identify type of paralytic syndrome, such as:
locked-in state (G83.5)
quadriplegia (G82.5-)
*EXCLUDES 1*   *hemiplegia/hemiparesis following nontraumatic subarachnoid hemorrhage (I69.05-)*
*monoplegia of lower limb following nontraumatic subarachnoid hemorrhage (I69.04-)*
*monoplegia of upper limb following nontraumatic subarachnoid hemorrhage (I69.03-)*

**I69.061**   Other paralytic syndrome following `HCC` nontraumatic subarachnoid hemorrhage affecting **right dominant** side

**I69.062**   Other paralytic syndrome following `HCC` nontraumatic subarachnoid hemorrhage affecting **left dominant** side

**I69.063**   Other paralytic syndrome following `HCC` nontraumatic subarachnoid hemorrhage affecting **right non-dominant** side

**I69.064**   Other paralytic syndrome following `HCC` nontraumatic subarachnoid hemorrhage affecting **left non-dominant** side

**I69.065**   Other paralytic syndrome following `HCC` nontraumatic subarachnoid hemorrhage, **bilateral**

**I69.069**   Other paralytic syndrome following `HCC` nontraumatic subarachnoid hemorrhage affecting **unspecified** side

✓6th **I69.09**   Other sequelae of nontraumatic subarachnoid hemorrhage

**I69.090**   **Apraxia** following nontraumatic subarachnoid hemorrhage

**I69.091**   **Dysphagia** following nontraumatic subarachnoid hemorrhage
Use additional code to identify the type of dysphagia, if known (R13.1-)

**I69.092**   **Facial weakness** following nontraumatic subarachnoid hemorrhage
Facial droop following nontraumatic subarachnoid hemorrhage

**I69.093**   **Ataxia** following nontraumatic subarachnoid hemorrhage

**I69.098**   **Other sequelae** following nontraumatic subarachnoid hemorrhage
Alterations of sensation following nontraumatic subarachnoid hemorrhage
Disturbance of vision following nontraumatic subarachnoid hemorrhage
Use additional code to identify the sequelae

✓5th **I69.1**   Sequelae of nontraumatic intracerebral hemorrhage

**I69.10**   Unspecified sequelae of nontraumatic intracerebral hemorrhage

✓6th **I69.11**   Cognitive deficits following nontraumatic intracerebral hemorrhage

**I69.110**   **Attention and concentration deficit** following nontraumatic intracerebral hemorrhage

**I69.111**   **Memory deficit** following nontraumatic intracerebral hemorrhage

**I69.112**   **Visuospatial deficit and spatial neglect** following nontraumatic intracerebral hemorrhage

**I69.113**   **Psychomotor deficit** following nontraumatic intracerebral hemorrhage

**I69.114**   **Frontal lobe and executive function deficit** following nontraumatic intracerebral hemorrhage

**I69.115**   **Cognitive social or emotional deficit** following nontraumatic intracerebral hemorrhage

**I69.118**   **Other symptoms and signs involving cognitive functions** following nontraumatic intracerebral hemorrhage

**I69.119**   **Unspecified symptoms and signs involving cognitive functions** following nontraumatic intracerebral hemorrhage

✓6th **I69.12**   Speech and language deficits following nontraumatic intracerebral hemorrhage

**I69.120**   **Aphasia** following nontraumatic intracerebral hemorrhage

**I69.121**   **Dysphasia** following nontraumatic intracerebral hemorrhage

**I69.122**   **Dysarthria** following nontraumatic intracerebral hemorrhage

**I69.123**   **Fluency disorder** following nontraumatic intracerebral hemorrhage
Stuttering following nontraumatic intracerebral hemorrhage

**I69.128**   Other speech and language deficits following nontraumatic intracerebral hemorrhage

✓6ᵗʰ **I69.13**   Monoplegia of upper limb following nontraumatic intracerebral hemorrhage
AHA: 2017, 1Q, 47

**I69.131**   Monoplegia of upper limb following nontraumatic intracerebral hemorrhage affecting right dominant side   HCC

**I69.132**   Monoplegia of upper limb following nontraumatic intracerebral hemorrhage affecting left dominant side   HCC

**I69.133**   Monoplegia of upper limb following nontraumatic intracerebral hemorrhage affecting right non-dominant side   HCC

**I69.134**   Monoplegia of upper limb following nontraumatic intracerebral hemorrhage affecting left non-dominant side   HCC

**I69.139**   Monoplegia of upper limb following nontraumatic intracerebral hemorrhage affecting unspecified side   HCC

✓6ᵗʰ **I69.14**   Monoplegia of lower limb following nontraumatic intracerebral hemorrhage
AHA: 2017, 1Q, 47

**I69.141**   Monoplegia of lower limb following nontraumatic intracerebral hemorrhage affecting right dominant side   HCC

**I69.142**   Monoplegia of lower limb following nontraumatic intracerebral hemorrhage affecting left dominant side   HCC

**I69.143**   Monoplegia of lower limb following nontraumatic intracerebral hemorrhage affecting right non-dominant side   HCC

**I69.144**   Monoplegia of lower limb following nontraumatic intracerebral hemorrhage affecting left non-dominant side   HCC

**I69.149**   Monoplegia of lower limb following nontraumatic intracerebral hemorrhage affecting unspecified side   HCC

✓6ᵗʰ **I69.15**   Hemiplegia and hemiparesis following nontraumatic intracerebral hemorrhage
AHA: 2015, 1Q, 25

**I69.151**   Hemiplegia and hemiparesis following nontraumatic intracerebral hemorrhage affecting right dominant side   CC HCC
CC Excl: PDX collection 695

**I69.152**   Hemiplegia and hemiparesis following nontraumatic intracerebral hemorrhage affecting left dominant side   CC HCC
CC Excl: PDX collection 695

**I69.153**   Hemiplegia and hemiparesis following nontraumatic intracerebral hemorrhage affecting right non-dominant side   CC HCC
CC Excl: PDX collection 696

**I69.154**   Hemiplegia and hemiparesis following nontraumatic intracerebral hemorrhage affecting left non-dominant side   CC HCC
CC Excl: PDX collection 696

**I69.159**   Hemiplegia and hemiparesis following nontraumatic intracerebral hemorrhage affecting unspecified side   CC HCC
CC Excl: PDX collection 697

✓6ᵗʰ **I69.16**   Other paralytic syndrome following nontraumatic intracerebral hemorrhage
Use additional code to identify type of paralytic syndrome, such as:
locked-in state (G83.5)
quadriplegia (G82.5-)
*EXCLUDES 1*   hemiplegia/hemiparesis following nontraumatic intracerebral hemorrhage (I69.15-)
monoplegia of lower limb following nontraumatic intracerebral hemorrhage (I69.14-)
monoplegia of upper limb following nontraumatic intracerebral hemorrhage (I69.13-)

**I69.161**   Other paralytic syndrome following nontraumatic intracerebral hemorrhage affecting right dominant side   HCC

**I69.162**   Other paralytic syndrome following nontraumatic intracerebral hemorrhage affecting left dominant side   HCC

**I69.163**   Other paralytic syndrome following nontraumatic intracerebral hemorrhage affecting right non-dominant side   HCC

**I69.164**   Other paralytic syndrome following nontraumatic intracerebral hemorrhage affecting left non-dominant side   HCC

**I69.165**   Other paralytic syndrome following nontraumatic intracerebral hemorrhage, bilateral   HCC

**I69.169**   Other paralytic syndrome following nontraumatic intracerebral hemorrhage affecting unspecified side   HCC

✓6ᵗʰ **I69.19**   Other sequelae of nontraumatic intracerebral hemorrhage

**I69.190**   Apraxia following nontraumatic intracerebral hemorrhage

**I69.191**   Dysphagia following nontraumatic intracerebral hemorrhage
Use additional code to identify the type of dysphagia, if known (R13.1-)

**I69.192**   Facial weakness following nontraumatic intracerebral hemorrhage
Facial droop following nontraumatic intracerebral hemorrhage

**I69.193**   Ataxia following nontraumatic intracerebral hemorrhage

**I69.198**   Other sequelae of nontraumatic intracerebral hemorrhage
Alteration of sensations following nontraumatic intracerebral hemorrhage
Disturbance of vision following nontraumatic intracerebral hemorrhage
Use additional code to identify the sequelae

✓5ᵗʰ **I69.2**   Sequelae of other nontraumatic intracranial hemorrhage

**I69.20**   Unspecified sequelae of other nontraumatic intracranial hemorrhage

✓6ᵗʰ **I69.21**   Cognitive deficits following other nontraumatic intracranial hemorrhage

**I69.210**   Attention and concentration deficit following other nontraumatic intracranial hemorrhage

**I69.211**   Memory deficit following other nontraumatic intracranial hemorrhage

**I69.212**   Visuospatial deficit and spatial neglect following other nontraumatic intracranial hemorrhage

**I69.213**   Psychomotor deficit following other nontraumatic intracranial hemorrhage

**I69.214**   Frontal lobe and executive function deficit following other nontraumatic intracranial hemorrhage

**I69.215**   Cognitive social or emotional deficit following other nontraumatic intracranial hemorrhage

**I69.218**   Other symptoms and signs involving cognitive functions following other nontraumatic intracranial hemorrhage

**I69.219**   Unspecified symptoms and signs involving cognitive functions following other nontraumatic intracranial hemorrhage

✓6ᵗʰ **I69.22**   Speech and language deficits following other nontraumatic intracranial hemorrhage

**I69.220**   Aphasia following other nontraumatic intracranial hemorrhage

**I69.221**   Dysphasia following other nontraumatic intracranial hemorrhage

**I69.222**   Dysarthria following other nontraumatic intracranial hemorrhage

**I69.223**   Fluency disorder following other nontraumatic intracranial hemorrhage
Stuttering following other nontraumatic intracranial hemorrhage

I69.228 **Other** speech and language deficits following other nontraumatic intracranial hemorrhage

☑6ᵗʰ I69.23 Monoplegia of upper limb following other nontraumatic intracranial hemorrhage
**AHA:** 2017, 1Q, 47

I69.231 **Monoplegia of upper limb following other nontraumatic intracranial hemorrhage affecting right dominant side** `HCC`

I69.232 **Monoplegia of upper limb following other nontraumatic intracranial hemorrhage affecting left dominant side** `HCC`

I69.233 **Monoplegia of upper limb following other nontraumatic intracranial hemorrhage affecting right non-dominant side** `HCC`

I69.234 **Monoplegia of upper limb following other nontraumatic intracranial hemorrhage affecting left non-dominant side** `HCC`

I69.239 **Monoplegia of upper limb following other nontraumatic intracranial hemorrhage affecting unspecified side** `HCC`

☑6ᵗʰ I69.24 Monoplegia of lower limb following other nontraumatic intracranial hemorrhage
**AHA:** 2017, 1Q, 47

I69.241 **Monoplegia of lower limb following other nontraumatic intracranial hemorrhage affecting right dominant side** `HCC`

I69.242 **Monoplegia of lower limb following other nontraumatic intracranial hemorrhage affecting left dominant side** `HCC`

I69.243 **Monoplegia of lower limb following other nontraumatic intracranial hemorrhage affecting right non-dominant side** `HCC`

I69.244 **Monoplegia of lower limb following other nontraumatic intracranial hemorrhage affecting left non-dominant side** `HCC`

I69.249 **Monoplegia of lower limb following other nontraumatic intracranial hemorrhage affecting unspecified side** `HCC`

☑6ᵗʰ I69.25 Hemiplegia and hemiparesis following other nontraumatic intracranial hemorrhage
**AHA:** 2015, 1Q, 25

I69.251 **Hemiplegia and hemiparesis following other nontraumatic intracranial hemorrhage affecting right dominant side** `CC` `HCC`
**CC Excl:** PDX collection 695

I69.252 **Hemiplegia and hemiparesis following other nontraumatic intracranial hemorrhage affecting left dominant side** `CC` `HCC`
**CC Excl:** PDX collection 695

I69.253 **Hemiplegia and hemiparesis following other nontraumatic intracranial hemorrhage affecting right non-dominant side** `CC` `HCC`
**CC Excl:** PDX collection 696

I69.254 **Hemiplegia and hemiparesis following other nontraumatic intracranial hemorrhage affecting left non-dominant side** `CC` `HCC`
**CC Excl:** PDX collection 696

I69.259 **Hemiplegia and hemiparesis following other nontraumatic intracranial hemorrhage affecting unspecified side** `CC` `HCC`
**CC Excl:** PDX collection 697

☑6ᵗʰ I69.26 **Other paralytic syndrome following other nontraumatic intracranial hemorrhage**
Use additional code to identify type of paralytic syndrome, such as:
locked-in state (G83.5)
quadriplegia (G82.5-)
*EXCLUDES 1* hemiplegia/hemiparesis following other nontraumatic intracranial hemorrhage (I69.25-)
monoplegia of lower limb following other nontraumatic intracranial hemorrhage (I69.24-)
monoplegia of upper limb following other nontraumatic intracranial hemorrhage (I69.23-)

I69.261 **Other paralytic syndrome following other nontraumatic intracranial hemorrhage affecting right dominant side** `HCC`

I69.262 **Other paralytic syndrome following other nontraumatic intracranial hemorrhage affecting left dominant side** `HCC`

I69.263 **Other paralytic syndrome following other nontraumatic intracranial hemorrhage affecting right non-dominant side** `HCC`

I69.264 **Other paralytic syndrome following other nontraumatic intracranial hemorrhage affecting left non-dominant side** `HCC`

I69.265 **Other paralytic syndrome following other nontraumatic intracranial hemorrhage, bilateral** `HCC`

I69.269 **Other paralytic syndrome following other nontraumatic intracranial hemorrhage affecting unspecified side** `HCC`

☑6ᵗʰ I69.29 **Other sequelae of other nontraumatic intracranial hemorrhage**

I69.290 **Apraxia following other nontraumatic intracranial hemorrhage**

I69.291 **Dysphagia following other nontraumatic intracranial hemorrhage**
Use additional code to identify the type of dysphagia, if known (R13.1-)

I69.292 **Facial weakness following other nontraumatic intracranial hemorrhage**
Facial droop following other nontraumatic intracranial hemorrhage

I69.293 **Ataxia following other nontraumatic intracranial hemorrhage**

I69.298 **Other sequelae of other nontraumatic intracranial hemorrhage**
Alteration of sensation following other nontraumatic intracranial hemorrhage
Disturbance of vision following other nontraumatic intracranial hemorrhage
Use additional code to identify the sequelae

☑5ᵗʰ I69.3 **Sequelae of cerebral infarction**
Sequelae of stroke NOS
**AHA:** 2013, 4Q, 127-128; 2012, 4Q, 92, 94

I69.30 **Unspecified sequelae of cerebral infarction**

☑6ᵗʰ I69.31 **Cognitive deficits following cerebral infarction**

I69.310 **Attention and concentration deficit following cerebral infarction**

I69.311 **Memory deficit following cerebral infarction**

I69.312 **Visuospatial deficit and spatial neglect following cerebral infarction**

I69.313 **Psychomotor deficit following cerebral infarction**

I69.314 **Frontal lobe and executive function deficit following cerebral infarction**

I69.315 **Cognitive social or emotional deficit following cerebral infarction**

I69.318 **Other symptoms and signs involving cognitive functions following cerebral infarction**

I69.319 **Unspecified symptoms and signs involving cognitive functions following cerebral infarction**

✓6ᵗʰ **I69.32** **Speech and language deficits following cerebral infarction**

    **I69.320** **Aphasia following cerebral infarction**

    **I69.321** **Dysphasia following cerebral infarction**
        **AHA:** 2012, 4Q, 91

    **I69.322** **Dysarthria following cerebral infarction**
        *EXCLUDES 2* ▶*transient ischemic attack (TIA) (G45.9)*◀

    **I69.323** **Fluency disorder following cerebral infarction**
        Stuttering following cerebral infarction

    **I69.328** **Other speech and language deficits following cerebral infarction**

✓6ᵗʰ **I69.33** **Monoplegia of upper limb following cerebral infarction**
    **AHA:** 2017, 1Q, 47

    **I69.331** **Monoplegia of upper limb following cerebral infarction affecting right dominant side** HCC

    **I69.332** **Monoplegia of upper limb following cerebral infarction affecting left dominant side** HCC

    **I69.333** **Monoplegia of upper limb following cerebral infarction affecting right non-dominant side** HCC

    **I69.334** **Monoplegia of upper limb following cerebral infarction affecting left non-dominant side** HCC

    **I69.339** **Monoplegia of upper limb following cerebral infarction affecting unspecified side** HCC

✓6ᵗʰ **I69.34** **Monoplegia of lower limb following cerebral infarction**
    **AHA:** 2017, 1Q, 47

    **I69.341** **Monoplegia of lower limb following cerebral infarction affecting right dominant side** HCC

    **I69.342** **Monoplegia of lower limb following cerebral infarction affecting left dominant side** HCC

    **I69.343** **Monoplegia of lower limb following cerebral infarction affecting right non-dominant side** HCC

    **I69.344** **Monoplegia of lower limb following cerebral infarction affecting left non-dominant side** HCC

    **I69.349** **Monoplegia of lower limb following cerebral infarction affecting unspecified side** HCC

✓6ᵗʰ **I69.35** **Hemiplegia and hemiparesis following cerebral infarction**
    **AHA:** 2015, 1Q, 25

    **I69.351** **Hemiplegia and hemiparesis following cerebral infarction affecting right dominant side** CC HCC
        *EXCLUDES 2* ▶*transient ischemic attack (TIA) (G45.9)*◀
        **CC Excl:** PDX collection 695

    **I69.352** **Hemiplegia and hemiparesis following cerebral infarction affecting left dominant side** CC HCC
        **CC Excl:** PDX collection 695

    **I69.353** **Hemiplegia and hemiparesis following cerebral infarction affecting right non-dominant side** CC HCC
        **CC Excl:** PDX collection 696

    **I69.354** **Hemiplegia and hemiparesis following cerebral infarction affecting left non-dominant side** CC HCC
        **AHA:** 2012, 4Q, 91
        **CC Excl:** PDX collection 696

    **I69.359** **Hemiplegia and hemiparesis following cerebral infarction affecting unspecified side** CC HCC
        **CC Excl:** PDX collection 697

✓6ᵗʰ **I69.36** **Other paralytic syndrome following cerebral infarction**
    Use additional code to identify type of paralytic syndrome, such as:
        locked-in state (G83.5)
        quadriplegia (G82.5-)
    *EXCLUDES 1* *hemiplegia/hemiparesis following cerebral infarction (I69.35-)*
        *monoplegia of lower limb following cerebral infarction (I69.34-)*
        *monoplegia of upper limb following cerebral infarction (I69.33-)*

    **I69.361** **Other paralytic syndrome following cerebral infarction affecting right dominant side** HCC

    **I69.362** **Other paralytic syndrome following cerebral infarction affecting left dominant side** HCC

    **I69.363** **Other paralytic syndrome following cerebral infarction affecting right non-dominant side** HCC

    **I69.364** **Other paralytic syndrome following cerebral infarction affecting left non-dominant side** HCC

    **I69.365** **Other paralytic syndrome following cerebral infarction, bilateral** HCC

    **I69.369** **Other paralytic syndrome following cerebral infarction affecting unspecified side** HCC

✓6ᵗʰ **I69.39** **Other sequelae of cerebral infarction**

    **I69.390** **Apraxia following cerebral infarction**

    **I69.391** **Dysphagia following cerebral infarction**
        Use additional code to identify the type of dysphagia, if known (R13.1-)

    **I69.392** **Facial weakness following cerebral infarction**
        Facial droop following cerebral infarction

    **I69.393** **Ataxia following cerebral infarction**

    **I69.398** **Other sequelae of cerebral infarction**
        Alteration of sensation following cerebral infarction
        Disturbance of vision following cerebral infarction
        Use additional code to identify the sequelae

✓5ᵗʰ **I69.8** **Sequelae of other cerebrovascular diseases**
    *EXCLUDES 1* *sequelae of traumatic intracranial injury (S06.-)*

    **I69.80** **Unspecified sequelae of other cerebrovascular disease**

✓6ᵗʰ **I69.81** **Cognitive deficits following other cerebrovascular disease**

    **I69.810** **Attention and concentration deficit following other cerebrovascular disease**

    **I69.811** **Memory deficit following other cerebrovascular disease**

    **I69.812** **Visuospatial deficit and spatial neglect following other cerebrovascular disease**

    **I69.813** **Psychomotor deficit following other cerebrovascular disease**

    **I69.814** **Frontal lobe and executive function deficit following other cerebrovascular disease**

    **I69.815** **Cognitive social or emotional deficit following other cerebrovascular disease**

    **I69.818** **Other symptoms and signs involving cognitive functions following other cerebrovascular disease**

    **I69.819** **Unspecified symptoms and signs involving cognitive functions following other cerebrovascular disease**

✓6ᵗʰ **I69.82** **Speech and language deficits following other cerebrovascular disease**

    **I69.820** **Aphasia following other cerebrovascular disease**

    **I69.821** **Dysphasia following other cerebrovascular disease**

    **I69.822** **Dysarthria following other cerebrovascular disease**

**N** Newborn: 0    **P** Pediatric: 0-17    **M** Maternity: 12-55    **A** Adult: 15-124    **MCC** Major CC Condition    **PDxMCC** PDx acts as own MCC    **CC** CC Condition    **PDxCC** PDx acts as own CC

648      ICD-10-CM 2018

**I69.823** **Fluency disorder following other cerebrovascular disease**
Stuttering following other cerebrovascular disease

**I69.828** **Other speech and language deficits following other cerebrovascular disease**

✓6th **I69.83** **Monoplegia of upper limb following other cerebrovascular disease**
AHA: 2017, 1Q, 47

**I69.831** **Monoplegia of upper limb following other cerebrovascular disease affecting right dominant side** HCC

**I69.832** **Monoplegia of upper limb following other cerebrovascular disease affecting left dominant side** HCC

**I69.833** **Monoplegia of upper limb following other cerebrovascular disease affecting right non-dominant side** HCC

**I69.834** **Monoplegia of upper limb following other cerebrovascular disease affecting left non-dominant side** HCC

**I69.839** **Monoplegia of upper limb following other cerebrovascular disease affecting unspecified side** HCC

✓6th **I69.84** **Monoplegia of lower limb following other cerebrovascular disease**
AHA: 2017, 1Q, 47

**I69.841** **Monoplegia of lower limb following other cerebrovascular disease affecting right dominant side** HCC

**I69.842** **Monoplegia of lower limb following other cerebrovascular disease affecting left dominant side** HCC

**I69.843** **Monoplegia of lower limb following other cerebrovascular disease affecting right non-dominant side** HCC

**I69.844** **Monoplegia of lower limb following other cerebrovascular disease affecting left non-dominant side** HCC

**I69.849** **Monoplegia of lower limb following other cerebrovascular disease affecting unspecified side** HCC

✓6th **I69.85** **Hemiplegia and hemiparesis following other cerebrovascular disease**
AHA: 2015, 1Q, 25

**I69.851** **Hemiplegia and hemiparesis following other cerebrovascular disease affecting right dominant side** CC HCC
CC Excl: PDX collection 695

**I69.852** **Hemiplegia and hemiparesis following other cerebrovascular disease affecting left dominant side** CC HCC
CC Excl: PDX collection 695

**I69.853** **Hemiplegia and hemiparesis following other cerebrovascular disease affecting right non-dominant side** CC HCC
CC Excl: PDX collection 696

**I69.854** **Hemiplegia and hemiparesis following other cerebrovascular disease affecting left non-dominant side** CC HCC
CC Excl: PDX collection 696

**I69.859** **Hemiplegia and hemiparesis following other cerebrovascular disease affecting unspecified side** CC HCC
CC Excl: PDX collection 697

✓6th **I69.86** **Other paralytic syndrome following other cerebrovascular disease**
Use additional code to identify type of paralytic syndrome, such as:
locked-in state (G83.5)
quadriplegia (G82.5-)
*EXCLUDES 1* *hemiplegia/hemiparesis following other cerebrovascular disease (I69.85-)*
*monoplegia of lower limb following other cerebrovascular disease (I69.84-)*
*monoplegia of upper limb following other cerebrovascular disease (I69.83-)*

**I69.861** **Other paralytic syndrome following other cerebrovascular disease affecting right dominant side** HCC

**I69.862** **Other paralytic syndrome following other cerebrovascular disease affecting left dominant side** HCC

**I69.863** **Other paralytic syndrome following other cerebrovascular disease affecting right non-dominant side** HCC

**I69.864** **Other paralytic syndrome following other cerebrovascular disease affecting left non-dominant side** HCC

**I69.865** **Other paralytic syndrome following other cerebrovascular disease, bilateral** HCC

**I69.869** **Other paralytic syndrome following other cerebrovascular disease affecting unspecified side** HCC

✓6th **I69.89** **Other sequelae of other cerebrovascular disease**

**I69.890** **Apraxia following other cerebrovascular disease**

**I69.891** **Dysphagia following other cerebrovascular disease**
Use additional code to identify the type of dysphagia, if known (R13.1-)

**I69.892** **Facial weakness following other cerebrovascular disease**
Facial droop following other cerebrovascular disease

**I69.893** **Ataxia following other cerebrovascular disease**

**I69.898** **Other sequelae of other cerebrovascular disease**
Alteration of sensation following other cerebrovascular disease
Disturbance of vision following other cerebrovascular disease
Use additional code to identify the sequelae

✓5th **I69.9** **Sequelae of unspecified cerebrovascular diseases**
*EXCLUDES 1* *sequelae of stroke (I69.3)*
*sequelae of traumatic intracranial injury (S06.-)*

**I69.90** **Unspecified sequelae of unspecified cerebrovascular disease**

✓6th **I69.91** **Cognitive deficits following unspecified cerebrovascular disease**

**I69.910** **Attention and concentration deficit following unspecified cerebrovascular disease**

**I69.911** **Memory deficit following unspecified cerebrovascular disease**

**I69.912** **Visuospatial deficit and spatial neglect following unspecified cerebrovascular disease**

**I69.913** **Psychomotor deficit following unspecified cerebrovascular disease**

**I69.914** **Frontal lobe and executive function deficit following unspecified cerebrovascular disease**

**I69.915** **Cognitive social or emotional deficit following unspecified cerebrovascular disease**

**I69.918** **Other symptoms and signs involving cognitive functions following unspecified cerebrovascular disease**

**I69.919** **Unspecified symptoms and signs involving cognitive functions following unspecified cerebrovascular disease**

✓6th **I69.92** **Speech and language deficits following unspecified cerebrovascular disease**

**I69.920** **Aphasia following unspecified cerebrovascular disease**

**I69.921** **Dysphasia following unspecified cerebrovascular disease**

**I69.922** **Dysarthria following unspecified cerebrovascular disease**

**I69.923** **Fluency disorder following unspecified cerebrovascular disease**
Stuttering following unspecified cerebrovascular disease

**I69.928** **Other speech and language deficits following unspecified cerebrovascular disease**

✓ Additional Character Req   ✓x7th Placeholder Alert   Unacceptable PDx   Manifestation   H1 - H14 HAC   HCC CMS-HCC Condition   *EXCLUDES 1* Not Coded Here   *EXCLUDES 2* Not Included Here

ICD-10-CM 2018                  **649**

**Chapter 9. Diseases of the Circulatory System**

✓6th **I69.93** Monoplegia of upper limb following unspecified cerebrovascular disease
AHA: 2017, 1Q, 47

**I69.931** Monoplegia of upper limb following unspecified cerebrovascular disease affecting right dominant side `HCC`

**I69.932** Monoplegia of upper limb following unspecified cerebrovascular disease affecting left dominant side `HCC`

**I69.933** Monoplegia of upper limb following unspecified cerebrovascular disease affecting right non-dominant side `HCC`

**I69.934** Monoplegia of upper limb following unspecified cerebrovascular disease affecting left non-dominant side `HCC`

**I69.939** Monoplegia of upper limb following unspecified cerebrovascular disease affecting unspecified side `HCC`

✓6th **I69.94** Monoplegia of lower limb following unspecified cerebrovascular disease
AHA: 2017, 1Q, 47

**I69.941** Monoplegia of lower limb following unspecified cerebrovascular disease affecting right dominant side `HCC`

**I69.942** Monoplegia of lower limb following unspecified cerebrovascular disease affecting left dominant side `HCC`

**I69.943** Monoplegia of lower limb following unspecified cerebrovascular disease affecting right non-dominant side `HCC`

**I69.944** Monoplegia of lower limb following unspecified cerebrovascular disease affecting left non-dominant side `HCC`

**I69.949** Monoplegia of lower limb following unspecified cerebrovascular disease affecting unspecified side `HCC`

✓6th **I69.95** Hemiplegia and hemiparesis following unspecified cerebrovascular disease
AHA: 2015, 1Q, 25

**I69.951** Hemiplegia and hemiparesis following unspecified cerebrovascular disease affecting right dominant side `CC` `HCC`
CC Excl: PDX collection 695

**I69.952** Hemiplegia and hemiparesis following unspecified cerebrovascular disease affecting left dominant side `CC` `HCC`
CC Excl: PDX collection 695

**I69.953** Hemiplegia and hemiparesis following unspecified cerebrovascular disease affecting right non-dominant side `CC` `HCC`
CC Excl: PDX collection 696

**I69.954** Hemiplegia and hemiparesis following unspecified cerebrovascular disease affecting left non-dominant side `CC` `HCC`
CC Excl: PDX collection 696

**I69.959** Hemiplegia and hemiparesis following unspecified cerebrovascular disease affecting unspecified side `CC` `HCC`
CC Excl: PDX collection 697

✓6th **I69.96** Other paralytic syndrome following unspecified cerebrovascular disease
Use additional code to identify type of paralytic syndrome, such as:
locked-in state (G83.5)
quadriplegia (G82.5-)
EXCLUDES 1 hemiplegia/hemiparesis following unspecified cerebrovascular disease (I69.95-)
monoplegia of lower limb following unspecified cerebrovascular disease (I69.94-)
monoplegia of upper limb following unspecified cerebrovascular disease (I69.93-)

**I69.961** Other paralytic syndrome following unspecified cerebrovascular disease affecting right dominant side `HCC`

**I69.962** Other paralytic syndrome following unspecified cerebrovascular disease affecting left dominant side `HCC`

**I69.963** Other paralytic syndrome following unspecified cerebrovascular disease affecting right non-dominant side `HCC`

**I69.964** Other paralytic syndrome following unspecified cerebrovascular disease affecting left non-dominant side `HCC`

**I69.965** Other paralytic syndrome following unspecified cerebrovascular disease, bilateral `HCC`

**I69.969** Other paralytic syndrome following unspecified cerebrovascular disease affecting unspecified side `HCC`

✓6th **I69.99** Other sequelae of unspecified cerebrovascular disease

**I69.990** Apraxia following unspecified cerebrovascular disease

**I69.991** Dysphagia following unspecified cerebrovascular disease
Use additional code to identify the type of dysphagia, if known (R13.1-)

**I69.992** Facial weakness following unspecified cerebrovascular disease
Facial droop following unspecified cerebrovascular disease

**I69.993** Ataxia following unspecified cerebrovascular disease

**I69.998** Other sequelae following unspecified cerebrovascular disease
Alteration in sensation following unspecified cerebrovascular disease
Disturbance of vision following unspecified cerebrovascular disease
Use additional code to identify the sequelae

## Diseases of arteries, arterioles and capillaries (I70-I79)

✓4th **I70** **Atherosclerosis**
INCLUDES  arteriolosclerosis
arterial degeneration
arteriosclerosis
arteriosclerotic vascular disease
arteriovascular degeneration
atheroma
endarteritis deformans or obliterans
senile arteritis
senile endarteritis
vascular degeneration
Use additional code to identify:
exposure to environmental tobacco smoke (Z77.22)
history of tobacco dependence (Z87.891)
occupational exposure to environmental tobacco smoke (Z57.31)
tobacco dependence (F17.-)
tobacco use (Z72.0)
EXCLUDES 2 arteriosclerotic cardiovascular disease (I25.1-)
arteriosclerotic heart disease (I25.1-)
atheroembolism (I75.-)
cerebral atherosclerosis (I67.2)
coronary atherosclerosis (I25.1-)
mesenteric atherosclerosis (K55.1)
precerebral atherosclerosis (I67.2)
primary pulmonary atherosclerosis (I27.0)

**I70.0** Atherosclerosis of aorta `HCC` `A`

**I70.1** Atherosclerosis of renal artery `HCC` `A`
Goldblatt's kidney
EXCLUDES 2 atherosclerosis of renal arterioles (I12.-)

✓5th **I70.2** Atherosclerosis of native arteries of the extremities
Mönckeberg's (medial) sclerosis
Use additional code, if applicable, to identify chronic total occlusion of artery of extremity (I70.92)
EXCLUDES 2 atherosclerosis of bypass graft of extremities (I70.30-I70.79)

✓6th **I70.20** Unspecified atherosclerosis of native arteries of extremities

**I70.201** Unspecified atherosclerosis of native arteries of extremities, right leg `HCC` `A`

**I70.202** Unspecified atherosclerosis of native arteries of extremities, left leg `HCC` `A`

**I70.203** Unspecified atherosclerosis of native arteries of extremities, bilateral legs `HCC` `A`

**I70.208** Unspecified atherosclerosis of native arteries of extremities, other extremity `HCC` `A`

Ⓝ Newborn: 0   Ⓟ Pediatric: 0-17   Ⓜ Maternity: 12-55   Ⓐ Adult: 15-124   `MCC` Major CC Condition   `PDxMCC` PDx acts as own MCC   `CC` CC Condition   `PDxCC` PDx acts as own CC

**650**                                                                                                                    ICD-10-CM 2018

**I70.209**   **Unspecified atherosclerosis of** HCC A
**native arteries of extremities, unspecified**
**extremity**

✓6ᵗʰ **I70.21**   **Atherosclerosis of native arteries of extremities with**
**intermittent claudication**

**I70.211**   **Atherosclerosis of native arteries of** HCC A
**extremities with intermittent**
**claudication, right leg**

**I70.212**   **Atherosclerosis of native arteries of** HCC A
**extremities with intermittent**
**claudication, left leg**

**I70.213**   **Atherosclerosis of native arteries of** HCC A
**extremities with intermittent**
**claudication, bilateral legs**

**I70.218**   **Atherosclerosis of native arteries of** HCC A
**extremities with intermittent**
**claudication, other extremity**

**I70.219**   **Atherosclerosis of native arteries of** HCC A
**extremities with intermittent**
**claudication, unspecified extremity**

✓6ᵗʰ **I70.22**   **Atherosclerosis of native arteries of extremities with**
**rest pain**
INCLUDES   any condition classifiable to I70.21-

**I70.221**   **Atherosclerosis of native arteries of** HCC A
**extremities with rest pain, right leg**

**I70.222**   **Atherosclerosis of native arteries of** HCC A
**extremities with rest pain, left leg**

**I70.223**   **Atherosclerosis of native arteries of** HCC A
**extremities with rest pain, bilateral legs**

**I70.228**   **Atherosclerosis of native arteries of** HCC A
**extremities with rest pain, other**
**extremity**

**I70.229**   **Atherosclerosis of native arteries of** HCC A
**extremities with rest pain, unspecified**
**extremity**

✓6ᵗʰ **I70.23**   **Atherosclerosis of native arteries of right leg with**
**ulceration**
INCLUDES   any condition classifiable to I70.211 and
I70.221
Use additional code to identify severity of ulcer (L97.-)

**I70.231**   **Atherosclerosis of native arteries of** HCC A
**right leg with ulceration of thigh**

**I70.232**   **Atherosclerosis of native arteries of** HCC A
**right leg with ulceration of calf**

**I70.233**   **Atherosclerosis of native arteries of** HCC A
**right leg with ulceration of ankle**

**I70.234**   **Atherosclerosis of native arteries of** HCC A
**right leg with ulceration of heel and**
**midfoot**
Atherosclerosis of native arteries of right
leg with ulceration of plantar surface
of midfoot

**I70.235**   **Atherosclerosis of native arteries of** HCC A
**right leg with ulceration of other part of**
**foot**
Atherosclerosis of native arteries of right
leg extremities with ulceration of toe

**I70.238**   **Atherosclerosis of native arteries of** HCC A
**right leg with ulceration of other part of**
**lower right leg**

**I70.239**   **Atherosclerosis of native arteries of** HCC A
**right leg with ulceration of**
**unspecified site**

✓6ᵗʰ **I70.24**   **Atherosclerosis of native arteries of left leg with**
**ulceration**
INCLUDES   any condition classifiable to I70.212 and
I70.222
Use additional code to identify severity of ulcer (L97.-)

**I70.241**   **Atherosclerosis of native arteries of** HCC A
**left leg with ulceration of thigh**

**I70.242**   **Atherosclerosis of native arteries of** HCC A
**left leg with ulceration of calf**

**I70.243**   **Atherosclerosis of native arteries of** HCC A
**left leg with ulceration of ankle**

**I70.244**   **Atherosclerosis of native arteries of** HCC A
**left leg with ulceration of heel and**
**midfoot**
Atherosclerosis of native arteries of left leg
with ulceration of plantar surface of
midfoot

**I70.245**   **Atherosclerosis of native arteries** HCC A
**of left leg with ulceration of other**
**part of foot**
Atherosclerosis of native arteries of left leg
extremities with ulceration of toe

**I70.248**   **Atherosclerosis of native arteries of** HCC A
**left leg with ulceration of other part**
**of lower left leg**

**I70.249**   **Atherosclerosis of native arteries of** HCC A
**left leg with ulceration of**
**unspecified site**

**I70.25**   **Atherosclerosis of native arteries of other** HCC A
**extremities with ulceration**
INCLUDES   any condition classifiable to I70.218 and
I70.228
Use additional code to identify the severity of the ulcer
(L98.49-)

✓6ᵗʰ **I70.26**   **Atherosclerosis of native arteries of extremities with**
**gangrene**
INCLUDES   any condition classifiable to I70.21-, I70.22-,
I70.23-, I70.24-, and I70.25-
Use additional code to identify the severity of any
ulcer (L97.-, L98.49-), if applicable

**CC Excl: For CC codes in subcategory I70.26:**
PDX collection 519

**I70.261**   **Atherosclerosis of native** CC HCC A
**arteries of extremities with**
**gangrene, right leg**

**I70.262**   **Atherosclerosis of native** CC HCC A
**arteries of extremities with**
**gangrene, left leg**

**I70.263**   **Atherosclerosis of native** CC HCC A
**arteries of extremities with**
**gangrene, bilateral legs**

**I70.268**   **Atherosclerosis of native** CC HCC A
**arteries of extremities with**
**gangrene, other extremity**

**I70.269**   **Atherosclerosis of native** CC HCC A
**arteries of extremities with**
**gangrene, unspecified extremity**

✓6ᵗʰ **I70.29**   **Other atherosclerosis of native arteries of**
**extremities**

**I70.291**   **Other atherosclerosis of native** HCC A
**arteries of extremities, right leg**

**I70.292**   **Other atherosclerosis of native** HCC A
**arteries of extremities, left leg**

**I70.293**   **Other atherosclerosis of native** HCC A
**arteries of extremities, bilateral legs**

**I70.298**   **Other atherosclerosis of native** HCC A
**arteries of extremities, other extremity**

**I70.299**   **Other atherosclerosis of native** HCC A
**arteries of extremities, unspecified**
**extremity**

✓5ᵗʰ **I70.3**   **Atherosclerosis of unspecified type of bypass graft(s) of the**
**extremities**
Use additional code, if applicable, to identify chronic total
occlusion of artery of extremity (I70.92)
EXCLUDES 1   embolism or thrombus of bypass graft(s) of extremities
(T82.8-)

✓6ᵗʰ **I70.30**   **Unspecified atherosclerosis of unspecified type of**
**bypass graft(s) of the extremities**

**I70.301**   **Unspecified atherosclerosis of** HCC A
**unspecified type of bypass graft(s)**
**of the extremities, right leg**

**I70.302**   **Unspecified atherosclerosis of** HCC A
**unspecified type of bypass graft(s)**
**of the extremities, left leg**

**I70.303**   **Unspecified atherosclerosis of** HCC A
**unspecified type of bypass graft(s)**
**of the extremities, bilateral legs**

**I70.308**   **Unspecified atherosclerosis of** HCC A
**unspecified type of bypass graft(s)**
**of the extremities, other extremity**

**I70.309**   **Unspecified atherosclerosis of** HCC A
**unspecified type of bypass graft(s)**
**of the extremities, unspecified**
**extremity**

✓Additional Character Req   ✓x7ᵗʰ Placeholder Alert   Unacceptable PDx   Manifestation   H1-H14 HAC   HCC CMS-HCC Condition   EXCLUDES 1 Not Coded Here   EXCLUDES 2 Not Included Here

ICD-10-CM 2018       651

**Chapter 9. Diseases of the Circulatory System**

✓6ᵗʰ **I70.31** **Atherosclerosis of unspecified type of bypass graft(s) of the extremities with intermittent claudication**

     **I70.311** **Atherosclerosis of unspecified type** HCC A **of bypass graft(s) of the extremities with intermittent claudication, right leg**

     **I70.312** **Atherosclerosis of unspecified type** HCC A **of bypass graft(s) of the extremities with intermittent claudication, left leg**

     **I70.313** **Atherosclerosis of unspecified type** HCC A **of bypass graft(s) of the extremities with intermittent claudication, bilateral legs**

     **I70.318** **Atherosclerosis of unspecified type** HCC A **of bypass graft(s) of the extremities with intermittent claudication, other extremity**

     **I70.319** **Atherosclerosis of unspecified type** HCC A **of bypass graft(s) of the extremities with intermittent claudication, unspecified extremity**

✓6ᵗʰ **I70.32** **Atherosclerosis of unspecified type of bypass graft(s) of the extremities with rest pain**
     INCLUDES any condition classifiable to I70.31-

     **I70.321** **Atherosclerosis of unspecified type** HCC A **of bypass graft(s) of the extremities with rest pain, right leg**

     **I70.322** **Atherosclerosis of unspecified type** HCC A **of bypass graft(s) of the extremities with rest pain, left leg**

     **I70.323** **Atherosclerosis of unspecified type** HCC A **of bypass graft(s) of the extremities with rest pain, bilateral legs**

     **I70.328** **Atherosclerosis of unspecified type** HCC A **of bypass graft(s) of the extremities with rest pain, other extremity**

     **I70.329** **Atherosclerosis of unspecified type** HCC A **of bypass graft(s) of the extremities with rest pain, unspecified extremity**

✓6ᵗʰ **I70.33** **Atherosclerosis of unspecified type of bypass graft(s) of the right leg with ulceration**
     INCLUDES any condition classifiable to I70.311 and I70.321
     Use additional code to identify severity of ulcer (L97.-)

     **CC Excl: For CC codes in subcategory I70.33:** PDX collection 698

     **I70.331** **Atherosclerosis of** PDxCC CC HCC A **unspecified type of bypass graft(s) of the right leg with ulceration of thigh**

     **I70.332** **Atherosclerosis of** PDxCC CC HCC A **unspecified type of bypass graft(s) of the right leg with ulceration of calf**

     **I70.333** **Atherosclerosis of** PDxCC CC HCC A **type of bypass graft(s) of the unspecified right leg with ulceration of ankle**

     **I70.334** **Atherosclerosis of** PDxCC CC HCC A **unspecified type of bypass graft(s) of the right leg with ulceration of heel and midfoot**
         Atherosclerosis of unspecified type of bypass graft(s) of right leg with ulceration of plantar surface of midfoot

     **I70.335** **Atherosclerosis of unspecified type** HCC A **of bypass graft(s) of the right leg with ulceration of other part of foot**
         Atherosclerosis of unspecified type of bypass graft(s) of the right leg with ulceration of toe

     **I70.338** **Atherosclerosis of** PDxCC CC HCC A **unspecified type of bypass graft(s) of the right leg with ulceration of other part of lower leg**

     **I70.339** **Atherosclerosis of** PDxCC CC HCC A **unspecified type of bypass graft(s) of the right leg with ulceration of unspecified site**

✓6ᵗʰ **I70.34** **Atherosclerosis of unspecified type of bypass graft(s) of the left leg with ulceration**
     INCLUDES any condition classifiable to I70.312 and I70.322
     Use additional code to identify severity of ulcer (L97.-)

     **CC Excl: For CC codes in subcategory I70.34:** PDX collection 698

     **I70.341** **Atherosclerosis of** PDxCC CC HCC A **unspecified type of bypass graft(s) of the left leg with ulceration of thigh**

     **I70.342** **Atherosclerosis of** PDxCC CC HCC A **unspecified type of bypass graft(s) of the left leg with ulceration of calf**

     **I70.343** **Atherosclerosis of** PDxCC CC HCC A **unspecified type of bypass graft(s) of the left leg with ulceration of ankle**

     **I70.344** **Atherosclerosis of** PDxCC CC HCC A **unspecified type of bypass graft(s) of the left leg with ulceration of heel and midfoot**
         Atherosclerosis of unspecified type of bypass graft(s) of left leg with ulceration of plantar surface of midfoot

     **I70.345** **Atherosclerosis of unspecified** HCC A **type of bypass graft(s) of the left leg with ulceration of other part of foot**
         Atherosclerosis of unspecified type of bypass graft(s) of the left leg with ulceration of toe

     **I70.348** **Atherosclerosis of** PDxCC CC HCC A **unspecified type of bypass graft(s) of the left leg with ulceration of other part of lower leg**

     **I70.349** **Atherosclerosis of** PDxCC CC HCC A **unspecified type of bypass graft(s) of the left leg with ulceration of unspecified site**

**I70.35** **Atherosclerosis of unspecified type of bypass** HCC A **graft(s) of other extremity with ulceration**
     INCLUDES any condition classifiable to I70.318 and I70.328
     Use additional code to identify severity of ulcer (L98.49-)

✓6ᵗʰ **I70.36** **Atherosclerosis of unspecified type of bypass graft(s) of the extremities with gangrene**
     INCLUDES any condition classifiable to I70.31-, I70.32-, I70.33-, I70.34-, I70.35
     Use additional code to identify the severity of any ulcer (L97.-, L98.49-), if applicable

     **CC Excl: For CC codes in subcategory I70.36, unless otherwise noted:** PDX collection 519

     **I70.361** **Atherosclerosis of** PDxCC CC HCC A **unspecified type of bypass graft(s) of the extremities with gangrene, right leg**

     **I70.362** **Atherosclerosis of** PDxCC CC HCC A **unspecified type of bypass graft(s) of the extremities with gangrene, left leg**

     **I70.363** **Atherosclerosis of** PDxCC CC HCC A **unspecified type of bypass graft(s) of the extremities with gangrene, bilateral legs**

     **I70.368** **Atherosclerosis of** PDxCC CC HCC A **unspecified type of bypass graft(s) of the extremities with gangrene, other extremity**

     **I70.369** **Atherosclerosis of** PDxCC CC HCC A **unspecified type of bypass graft(s) of the extremities with gangrene, unspecified extremity**

✓6ᵗʰ **I70.39** **Other atherosclerosis of unspecified type of bypass graft(s) of the extremities**

     **I70.391** **Other atherosclerosis of** HCC A **unspecified type of bypass graft(s) of the extremities, right leg**

N Newborn: 0   P Pediatric: 0-17   M Maternity: 12-55   A Adult: 15-124   MCC Major CC Condition   PDxMCC PDx acts as own MCC   CC CC Condition   PDxCC PDx acts as own CC

**652**          ICD-10-CM 2018

**I70.392**    Other atherosclerosis of unspecified type of bypass graft(s) of the extremities, left leg   HCC A

**I70.393**    Other atherosclerosis of unspecified type of bypass graft(s) of the extremities, bilateral legs   HCC A

**I70.398**    Other atherosclerosis of unspecified type of bypass graft(s) of the extremities, other extremity   HCC A

**I70.399**    Other atherosclerosis of unspecified type of bypass graft(s) of the extremities, unspecified extremity   HCC A

✓5th **I70.4**    Atherosclerosis of autologous vein bypass graft(s) of the extremities

    Use additional code, if applicable, to identify chronic total occlusion of artery of extremity (I70.92)

✓6th **I70.40**    Unspecified atherosclerosis of autologous vein bypass graft(s) of the extremities

**I70.401**    Unspecified atherosclerosis of autologous vein bypass graft(s) of the extremities, right leg   HCC A

**I70.402**    Unspecified atherosclerosis of autologous vein bypass graft(s) of the extremities, left leg   HCC A

**I70.403**    Unspecified atherosclerosis of autologous vein bypass graft(s) of the extremities, bilateral legs   HCC A

**I70.408**    Unspecified atherosclerosis of autologous vein bypass graft(s) of the extremities, other extremity   HCC A

**I70.409**    Unspecified atherosclerosis of autologous vein bypass graft(s) of the extremities, unspecified extremity   HCC A

✓6th **I70.41**    Atherosclerosis of autologous vein bypass graft(s) of the extremities with intermittent claudication

**I70.411**    Atherosclerosis of autologous vein bypass graft(s) of the extremities with intermittent claudication, right leg   HCC A

**I70.412**    Atherosclerosis of autologous vein bypass graft(s) of the extremities with intermittent claudication, left leg   HCC A

**I70.413**    Atherosclerosis of autologous vein bypass graft(s) of the extremities with intermittent claudication, bilateral legs   HCC A

**I70.418**    Atherosclerosis of autologous vein bypass graft(s) of the extremities with intermittent claudication, other extremity   HCC A

**I70.419**    Atherosclerosis of autologous vein bypass graft(s) of the extremities with intermittent claudication, unspecified extremity   HCC A

✓6th **I70.42**    Atherosclerosis of autologous vein bypass graft(s) of the extremities with rest pain

    INCLUDES   any condition classifiable to I70.41-

**I70.421**    Atherosclerosis of autologous vein bypass graft(s) of the extremities with rest pain, right leg   HCC A

**I70.422**    Atherosclerosis of autologous vein bypass graft(s) of the extremities with rest pain, left leg   HCC A

**I70.423**    Atherosclerosis of autologous vein bypass graft(s) of the extremities with rest pain, bilateral legs   HCC A

**I70.428**    Atherosclerosis of autologous vein bypass graft(s) of the extremities with rest pain, other extremity   HCC A

**I70.429**    Atherosclerosis of autologous vein bypass graft(s) of the extremities with rest pain, unspecified extremity   HCC A

✓6th **I70.43**    Atherosclerosis of autologous vein bypass graft(s) of the right leg with ulceration

    INCLUDES   any condition classifiable to I70.411 and I70.421

    Use additional code to identify severity of ulcer (L97.-)

    **CC Excl: For CC codes in subcategory I70.43:** PDX collection 698

**I70.431**    Atherosclerosis of autologous vein bypass graft(s) of the right leg with ulceration of thigh   PDxCC CC HCC A

**I70.432**    Atherosclerosis of autologous vein bypass graft(s) of the right leg with ulceration of calf   PDxCC CC HCC A

**I70.433**    Atherosclerosis of autologous vein bypass graft(s) of the right leg with ulceration of ankle   PDxCC CC HCC A

**I70.434**    Atherosclerosis of autologous vein bypass graft(s) of the right leg with ulceration of heel and midfoot   PDxCC CC HCC A

    Atherosclerosis of autologous vein bypass graft(s) of right leg with ulceration of plantar surface of midfoot

**I70.435**    Atherosclerosis of autologous vein bypass graft(s) of the right leg with ulceration of other part of foot   HCC A

    Atherosclerosis of autologous vein bypass graft(s) of right leg with ulceration of toe

**I70.438**    Atherosclerosis of autologous vein bypass graft(s) of the right leg with ulceration of other part of lower leg   PDxCC CC HCC A

**I70.439**    Atherosclerosis of autologous vein bypass graft(s) of the right leg with ulceration of unspecified site   PDxCC CC HCC A

✓6th **I70.44**    Atherosclerosis of autologous vein bypass graft(s) of the left leg with ulceration

    INCLUDES   any condition classifiable to I70.412 and I70.422

    Use additional code to identify severity of ulcer (L97.-)

    **CC Excl: For CC codes in subcategory I70.44:** PDX collection 698

**I70.441**    Atherosclerosis of autologous vein bypass graft(s) of the left leg with ulceration of thigh   PDxCC CC HCC A

**I70.442**    Atherosclerosis of autologous vein bypass graft(s) of the left leg with ulceration of calf   PDxCC CC HCC A

**I70.443**    Atherosclerosis of autologous vein bypass graft(s) of the left leg with ulceration of ankle   PDxCC CC HCC A

**I70.444**    Atherosclerosis of autologous vein bypass graft(s) of the left leg with ulceration of heel and midfoot   PDxCC CC HCC A

    Atherosclerosis of autologous vein bypass graft(s) of left leg with ulceration of plantar surface of midfoot

**I70.445**    Atherosclerosis of autologous vein bypass graft(s) of the left leg with ulceration of other part of foot   HCC A

    Atherosclerosis of autologous vein bypass graft(s) of left leg with ulceration of toe

**I70.448**    Atherosclerosis of autologous vein bypass graft(s) of the left leg with ulceration of other part of lower leg   PDxCC CC HCC A

**I70.449**    Atherosclerosis of autologous vein bypass graft(s) of the left leg with ulceration of unspecified site   PDxCC CC HCC A

**I70.45**    Atherosclerosis of autologous vein bypass graft(s) of other extremity with ulceration   HCC A

    INCLUDES   any condition classifiable to I70.418, I70.428, and I70.438

    Use additional code to identify severity of ulcer (L98.49)

✓6th **I70.46**    Atherosclerosis of autologous vein bypass graft(s) of the extremities with gangrene

    INCLUDES   any condition classifiable to I70.41-, I70.42-, and I70.43-, I70.44-, I70.45

    Use additional code to identify the severity of any ulcer (L97.-, L98.49-), if applicable

    **CC Excl: For CC codes in subcategory I70.46:** PDX collection 519

**I70.461**    Atherosclerosis of autologous vein bypass graft(s) of the extremities with gangrene, right leg   PDxCC CC HCC A

✓ Additional Character Req   ✓x7th Placeholder Alert   Unacceptable PDx   Manifestation   H1 - H14 HAC   HCC CMS-HCC Condition   EXCLUDES 1 Not Coded Here   EXCLUDES 2 Not Included Here

ICD-10-CM 2018         653

**I70.462**   Atherosclerosis of `PDxCC` `CC` `HCC` `A`
autologous vein bypass graft(s)
of the extremities with gangrene,
left leg

**I70.463**   Atherosclerosis of `PDxCC` `CC` `HCC` `A`
autologous vein bypass graft(s)
of the extremities with gangrene,
bilateral legs

**I70.468**   Atherosclerosis of `PDxCC` `CC` `HCC` `A`
autologous vein bypass graft(s)
of the extremities with gangrene,
other extremity

**I70.469**   Atherosclerosis of `PDxCC` `CC` `HCC` `A`
autologous vein bypass graft(s)
of the extremities with gangrene,
unspecified extremity

√6th **I70.49**   Other atherosclerosis of autologous vein bypass
graft(s) of the extremities

**I70.491**   Other atherosclerosis of `HCC` `A`
autologous vein bypass graft(s)
of the extremities, right leg

**I70.492**   Other atherosclerosis of `HCC` `A`
autologous vein bypass graft(s)
of the extremities, left leg

**I70.493**   Other atherosclerosis of `HCC` `A`
autologous vein bypass graft(s)
of the extremities, bilateral legs

**I70.498**   Other atherosclerosis of `HCC` `A`
autologous vein bypass graft(s)
of the extremities, other extremity

**I70.499**   Other atherosclerosis of `HCC` `A`
autologous vein bypass graft(s) of the
extremities, unspecified extremity

√5th **I70.5**   Atherosclerosis of nonautologous biological bypass graft(s)
of the extremities
Use additional code, if applicable, to identify chronic total
occlusion of artery of extremity (I70.92)

√6th **I70.50**   Unspecified atherosclerosis of nonautologous
biological bypass graft(s) of the extremities

**I70.501**   Unspecified atherosclerosis of `HCC` `A`
nonautologous biological bypass
graft(s) of the extremities, right leg

**I70.502**   Unspecified atherosclerosis of `HCC` `A`
nonautologous biological bypass
graft(s) of the extremities, left leg

**I70.503**   Unspecified atherosclerosis of `HCC` `A`
nonautologous biological bypass
graft(s) of the extremities, bilateral legs

**I70.508**   Unspecified atherosclerosis of `HCC` `A`
nonautologous biological bypass
graft(s) of the extremities, other extremity

**I70.509**   Unspecified atherosclerosis of `HCC` `A`
nonautologous biological bypass
graft(s) of the extremities, unspecified
extremity

√6th **I70.51**   Atherosclerosis of nonautologous biological bypass
graft(s) of the extremities with intermittent
claudication

**I70.511**   Atherosclerosis of nonautologous `HCC` `A`
biological bypass graft(s) of the
extremities with intermittent
claudication, right leg

**I70.512**   Atherosclerosis of nonautologous `HCC` `A`
biological bypass graft(s) of the
extremities with intermittent
claudication, left leg

**I70.513**   Atherosclerosis of nonautologous `HCC` `A`
biological bypass graft(s) of the
extremities with intermittent
claudication, bilateral legs

**I70.518**   Atherosclerosis of nonautologous `HCC` `A`
biological bypass graft(s) of the
extremities with intermittent
claudication, other extremity

**I70.519**   Atherosclerosis of nonautologous `HCC` `A`
biological bypass graft(s) of the
extremities with intermittent
claudication, unspecified extremity

√6th **I70.52**   Atherosclerosis of nonautologous biological bypass
graft(s) of the extremities with rest pain
`INCLUDES`   any condition classifiable to I70.51-

**I70.521**   Atherosclerosis of nonautologous `HCC` `A`
biological bypass graft(s) of the
extremities with rest pain, right leg

**I70.522**   Atherosclerosis of nonautologous `HCC` `A`
biological bypass graft(s) of the
extremities with rest pain, left leg

**I70.523**   Atherosclerosis of nonautologous `HCC` `A`
biological bypass graft(s) of the
extremities with rest pain, bilateral legs

**I70.528**   Atherosclerosis of nonautologous `HCC` `A`
biological bypass graft(s) of the
extremities with rest pain, other extremity

**I70.529**   Atherosclerosis of nonautologous `HCC` `A`
biological bypass graft(s) of the
extremities with rest pain, unspecified
extremity

√6th **I70.53**   Atherosclerosis of nonautologous biological bypass
graft(s) of the right leg with ulceration
`INCLUDES`   any condition classifiable to I70.511 and
I70.521
Use additional code to identify severity of ulcer (L97.-)

> **CC Excl: For CC codes in subcategory I70.53:**
> PDX collection 698

**I70.531**   Atherosclerosis of `PDxCC` `CC` `HCC` `A`
biological nonautologous bypass graft(s)
of the right leg with ulceration of thigh

**I70.532**   Atherosclerosis of `PDxCC` `CC` `HCC` `A`
bilological nonautologous bypass graft(s)
of the right leg with ulceration of calf

**I70.533**   Atherosclerosis of `PDxCC` `CC` `HCC` `A`
nonautologous biological bypass graft(s)
of the right leg with ulceration of ankle

**I70.534**   Atherosclerosis of `PDxCC` `CC` `HCC` `A`
nonautologous biological bypass graft(s)
of the right leg with ulceration of heel and
midfoot
Atherosclerosis of nonautologous
biological bypass graft(s) of right leg
with ulceration of plantar surface of
midfoot

**I70.535**   Atherosclerosis of nonautologous `HCC` `A`
biological bypass graft(s) of the right leg
with ulceration of other part of foot
Atherosclerosis of nonautologous
biological bypass graft(s) of the right
leg with ulceration of toe

**I70.538**   Atherosclerosis of `PDxCC` `CC` `HCC` `A`
nonautologous biological bypass graft(s)
of the right leg with ulceration of other
part of lower leg

**I70.539**   Atherosclerosis of `PDxCC` `CC` `HCC` `A`
nonautologous biological bypass graft(s)
of the right leg with ulceration of
unspecified site

√6th **I70.54**   Atherosclerosis of nonautologous biological bypass
graft(s) of the left leg with ulceration
`INCLUDES`   any condition classifiable to I70.512 and
I70.522
Use additional code to identify severity of ulcer (L97.-)

> **CC Excl: For CC codes in subcategory I70.54:**
> PDX collection 698

**I70.541**   Atherosclerosis of `PDxCC` `CC` `HCC` `A`
nonautologous biological bypass graft(s)
of the left leg with ulceration of thigh

**I70.542**   Atherosclerosis of `PDxCC` `CC` `HCC` `A`
nonautologous biological bypass graft(s)
of the left leg with ulceration of calf

**I70.543**   Atherosclerosis of `PDxCC` `CC` `HCC` `A`
nonautologous biological bypass graft(s)
of the left leg with ulceration of ankle

**I70.544**   Atherosclerosis of `PDxCC` `CC` `HCC` `A`
nonautologous biological bypass graft(s)
of the left leg with ulceration of heel and
midfoot
Atherosclerosis of nonautologous
biological bypass graft(s) of left leg
with ulceration of plantar surface of
midfoot

**I70.545** **Atherosclerosis of nonautologous** `HCC` `A`
**biological bypass graft(s) of the left leg**
**with ulceration of** other part of foot
> Atherosclerosis of nonautologous
> biological bypass graft(s) of the left leg
> with ulceration of toe

**I70.548** **Atherosclerosis of** `PDxCC` `CC` `HCC` `A`
**nonautologous biological bypass**
**graft(s) of the left leg with ulceration**
**of** other part of lower leg

**I70.549** **Atherosclerosis of** `PDxCC` `CC` `HCC` `A`
**nonautologous biological bypass**
**graft(s) of the left leg with ulceration**
**of** unspecified site

**I70.55** **Atherosclerosis of nonautologous biological** `HCC` `A`
**bypass graft(s) of** other extremity with ulceration
> `INCLUDES` any condition classifiable to I70.518,
> I70.528, and I70.538
> Use additional code to identify severity of ulcer
> (L98.49)

✓6ᵗʰ **I70.56** **Atherosclerosis of nonautologous biological bypass**
**graft(s) of the extremities with** gangrene
> `INCLUDES` any condition classifiable to I70.51-, I70.52-,
> and I70.53-, I70.54-, I70.55
> Use additional code to identify the severity of any
> ulcer (L97.-, L98.49-), if applicable

> **CC Excl: For CC codes in subcategory I70.56:**
> PDX collection 519

**I70.561** **Atherosclerosis of** `PDxCC` `CC` `HCC` `A`
**nonautologous biological bypass graft(s)**
**of the extremities with gangrene,** right leg

**I70.562** **Atherosclerosis of** `PDxCC` `CC` `HCC` `A`
**nonautologous biological bypass graft(s)**
**of the extremities with gangrene,** left leg

**I70.563** **Atherosclerosis of** `PDxCC` `CC` `HCC` `A`
**nonautologous biological bypass graft(s)**
**of the extremities with gangrene,**
**bilateral legs**

**I70.568** **Atherosclerosis of** `PDxCC` `CC` `HCC` `A`
**nonautologous biological bypass graft(s)**
**of the extremities with gangrene,** other
**extremity**

**I70.569** **Atherosclerosis of** `PDxCC` `CC` `HCC` `A`
**nonautologous biological bypass graft(s)**
**of the extremities with gangrene,**
**unspecified extremity**

✓6ᵗʰ **I70.59** **Other atherosclerosis of nonautologous biological**
**bypass graft(s) of the extremities**

**I70.591** **Other atherosclerosis of** `HCC` `A`
**biological nonautologous bypass**
**graft(s) of the extremities,** right leg

**I70.592** **Other atherosclerosis of** `HCC` `A`
**nonautologous biological bypass**
**graft(s) of the extremities,** left leg

**I70.593** **Other atherosclerosis of** `HCC` `A`
**nonautologous biological bypass**
**graft(s) of the extremities,**
**bilateral legs**

**I70.598** **Other atherosclerosis of** `HCC` `A`
**nonautologous biological bypass**
**graft(s) of the extremities,**
**other extremity**

**I70.599** **Other atherosclerosis of** `HCC` `A`
**nonautologous biological bypass**
**graft(s) of the extremities,**
**unspecified extremity**

✓5ᵗʰ **I70.6** **Atherosclerosis of** nonbiological bypass graft(s) of the
**extremities**
> Use additional code, if applicable, to identify chronic total
> occlusion of artery of extremity (I70.92)

✓6ᵗʰ **I70.60** **Unspecified atherosclerosis of nonbiological bypass**
**graft(s) of the extremities**

**I70.601** **Unspecified atherosclerosis of** `HCC` `A`
**nonbiological bypass graft(s) of the**
**extremities,** right leg

**I70.602** **Unspecified atherosclerosis of** `HCC` `A`
**nonbiological bypass graft(s) of the**
**extremities,** left leg

**I70.603** **Unspecified atherosclerosis of** `HCC` `A`
**nonbiological bypass graft(s) of the**
**extremities,** bilateral legs

**I70.608** **Unspecified atherosclerosis of** `HCC` `A`
**nonbiological bypass graft(s) of the**
**extremities,** other extremity

**I70.609** **Unspecified atherosclerosis of** `HCC` `A`
**nonbiological bypass graft(s) of the**
**extremities,** unspecified extremity

✓6ᵗʰ **I70.61** **Atherosclerosis of nonbiological bypass graft(s) of**
**the extremities with** intermittent claudication

**I70.611** **Atherosclerosis of nonbiological** `HCC` `A`
**bypass graft(s) of the extremities with**
**intermittent claudication,** right leg

**I70.612** **Atherosclerosis of nonbiological** `HCC` `A`
**bypass graft(s) of the extremities with**
**intermittent claudication,** left leg

**I70.613** **Atherosclerosis of nonbiological** `HCC` `A`
**bypass graft(s) of the extremities with**
**intermittent claudication,** bilateral legs

**I70.618** **Atherosclerosis of nonbiological** `HCC` `A`
**bypass graft(s) of the extremities with**
**intermittent claudication,**
**other extremity**

**I70.619** **Atherosclerosis of nonbiological** `HCC` `A`
**bypass graft(s) of the extremities with**
**intermittent claudication,** unspecified
**extremity**

✓6ᵗʰ **I70.62** **Atherosclerosis of nonbiological bypass graft(s) of**
**the extremities with** rest pain
> `INCLUDES` any condition classifiable to I70.61-

**I70.621** **Atherosclerosis of nonbiological** `HCC` `A`
**bypass graft(s) of the extremities with**
**rest pain,** right leg

**I70.622** **Atherosclerosis of nonbiological** `HCC` `A`
**bypass graft(s) of the extremities**
**with rest pain,** left leg

**I70.623** **Atherosclerosis of nonbiological** `HCC` `A`
**bypass graft(s) of the extremities with rest**
**pain,** bilateral legs

**I70.628** **Atherosclerosis of nonbiological** `HCC` `A`
**bypass graft(s) of the extremities**
**with rest pain,** other extremity

**I70.629** **Atherosclerosis of nonbiological** `HCC` `A`
**bypass graft(s) of the extremities**
**with rest pain,** unspecified extremity

✓6ᵗʰ **I70.63** **Atherosclerosis of nonbiological bypass graft(s) of**
**the** right leg with ulceration
> `INCLUDES` any condition classifiable to I70.611 and
> I70.621
> Use additional code to identify severity of ulcer (L97.-)

> **CC Excl: For CC codes in subcategory I70.63:**
> PDX collection 698

**I70.631** **Atherosclerosis of** `PDxCC` `CC` `HCC` `A`
**nonbiological bypass graft(s) of the**
**right leg with ulceration of** thigh

**I70.632** **Atherosclerosis of** `PDxCC` `CC` `HCC` `A`
**nonbiological bypass graft(s) of the**
**right leg with ulceration of** calf

**I70.633** **Atherosclerosis of** `PDxCC` `CC` `HCC` `A`
**nonbiological bypass graft(s) of the**
**right leg with ulceration of** ankle

**I70.634** **Atherosclerosis of** `PDxCC` `CC` `HCC` `A`
**nonbiological bypass graft(s) of the**
**right leg with ulceration of** heel and
**midfoot**
> Atherosclerosis of nonbiological bypass
> graft(s) of right leg with ulceration of
> plantar surface of midfoot

**I70.635** **Atherosclerosis of nonbiological** `HCC` `A`
**bypass graft(s) of the right leg with**
**ulceration of** other part of foot
> Atherosclerosis of nonbiological bypass
> graft(s) of the right leg with ulceration
> of toe

**I70.638** **Atherosclerosis of** `PDxCC` `CC` `HCC` `A`
**nonbiological bypass graft(s) of the**
**right leg with ulceration of** other part
**of lower leg**

**I70.639** **Atherosclerosis of** `PDxCC` `CC` `HCC` `A`
**nonbiological bypass graft(s) of the**
**right leg with ulceration of** unspecified
**site**

---

✓ Additional Character Req   ✓x7ᵗʰ Placeholder Alert   Unacceptable PDx   Manifestation   `H1`-`H14` HAC   `HCC` CMS-HCC Condition   *EXCLUDES 1* Not Coded Here   *EXCLUDES 2* Not Included Here

**✓6th I70.64 Atherosclerosis of nonbiological bypass graft(s) of the left leg with ulceration**

INCLUDES any condition classifiable to I70.612 and I70.622

Use additional code to identify severity of ulcer (L97.-)

CC Excl: For CC codes in subcategory I70.64:
PDX collection 698

**I70.641 Atherosclerosis of** PDxCC CC HCC A
**nonbiological bypass graft(s) of the left leg with ulceration of thigh**

**I70.642 Atherosclerosis of** PDxCC CC HCC A
**nonbiological bypass graft(s) of the left leg with ulceration of calf**

**I70.643 Atherosclerosis of** PDxCC CC HCC A
**nonbiological bypass graft(s) of the left leg with ulceration of ankle**

**I70.644 Atherosclerosis of** PDxCC CC HCC A
**nonbiological bypass graft(s) of the left leg with ulceration of heel and midfoot**

Atherosclerosis of nonbiological bypass graft(s) of left leg with ulceration of plantar surface of midfoot

**I70.645 Atherosclerosis of nonbiological** HCC A
**bypass graft(s) of the left leg with ulceration of other part of foot**

Atherosclerosis of nonbiological bypass graft(s) of the left leg with ulceration of toe

**I70.648 Atherosclerosis of** PDxCC CC HCC A
**nonbiological bypass graft(s) of the left leg with ulceration of other part of lower leg**

**I70.649 Atherosclerosis of** PDxCC CC HCC A
**nonbiological bypass graft(s) of the left leg with ulceration of unspecified site**

**I70.65 Atherosclerosis of nonbiological bypass** HCC A
**graft(s) of other extremity with ulceration**

INCLUDES any condition classifiable to I70.618 and I70.628

Use additional code to identify severity of ulcer (L98.49)

**✓6th I70.66 Atherosclerosis of nonbiological bypass graft(s) of the extremities with gangrene**

INCLUDES any condition classifiable to I70.61-, I70.62-, I70.63-, I70.64-, I70.65

Use additional code to identify the severity of any ulcer (L97.-, L98.49-), if applicable

CC Excl: For CC codes in subcategory I70.66:
PDX collection 519

**I70.661 Atherosclerosis of** PDxCC CC HCC A
**nonbiological bypass graft(s) of the extremities with gangrene, right leg**

**I70.662 Atherosclerosis of** PDxCC CC HCC A
**nonbiological bypass graft(s) of the extremities with gangrene, left leg**

**I70.663 Atherosclerosis of** PDxCC CC HCC A
**nonbiological bypass graft(s) of the extremities with gangrene, bilateral legs**

**I70.668 Atherosclerosis of** PDxCC CC HCC A
**nonbiological bypass graft(s) of the extremities with gangrene, other extremity**

**I70.669 Atherosclerosis of** PDxCC CC HCC A
**nonbiological bypass graft(s) of the extremities with gangrene, unspecified extremity**

**✓6th I70.69 Other atherosclerosis of nonbiological bypass graft(s) of the extremities**

**I70.691 Other atherosclerosis of** HCC A
**nonbiological bypass graft(s) of the extremities, right leg**

**I70.692 Other atherosclerosis of** HCC A
**nonbiological bypass graft(s) of the extremities, left leg**

**I70.693 Other atherosclerosis of** HCC A
**nonbiological bypass graft(s) of the extremities, bilateral legs**

**I70.698 Other atherosclerosis of** HCC A
**nonbiological bypass graft(s) of the extremities, other extremity**

**I70.699 Other atherosclerosis of** HCC A
**nonbiological bypass graft(s) of the extremities, unspecified extremity**

**✓5th I70.7 Atherosclerosis of other type of bypass graft(s) of the extremities**

Use additional code, if applicable, to identify chronic total occlusion of artery of extremity (I70.92)

**✓6th I70.70 Unspecified atherosclerosis of other type of bypass graft(s) of the extremities**

**I70.701 Unspecified atherosclerosis of** HCC A
**other type of bypass graft(s) of the extremities, right leg**

**I70.702 Unspecified atherosclerosis of** HCC A
**other type of bypass graft(s) of the extremities, left leg**

**I70.703 Unspecified atherosclerosis of** HCC A
**other type of bypass graft(s) of the extremities, bilateral legs**

**I70.708 Unspecified atherosclerosis of** HCC A
**other type of bypass graft(s) of the extremities, other extremity**

**I70.709 Unspecified atherosclerosis of** HCC A
**other type of bypass graft(s) of the extremities, unspecified extremity**

**✓6th I70.71 Atherosclerosis of other type of bypass graft(s) of the extremities with intermittent claudication**

**I70.711 Atherosclerosis of other type of** HCC A
**bypass graft(s) of the extremities with intermittent claudication, right leg**

**I70.712 Atherosclerosis of other type of** HCC A
**bypass graft(s) of the extremities with intermittent claudication, left leg**

**I70.713 Atherosclerosis of other type of** HCC A
**bypass graft(s) of the extremities with intermittent claudication, bilateral legs**

**I70.718 Atherosclerosis of other type of** HCC A
**bypass graft(s) of the extremities with intermittent claudication, other extremity**

**I70.719 Atherosclerosis of other type of** HCC A
**bypass graft(s) of the extremities with intermittent claudication, unspecified extremity**

**✓6th I70.72 Atherosclerosis of other type of bypass graft(s) of the extremities with rest pain**

INCLUDES any condition classifiable to I70.71-

**I70.721 Atherosclerosis of other type of** HCC A
**bypass graft(s) of the extremities with rest pain, right leg**

**I70.722 Atherosclerosis of other type of** HCC A
**bypass graft(s) of the extremities with rest pain, left leg**

**I70.723 Atherosclerosis of other type of** HCC A
**bypass graft(s) of the extremities with rest pain, bilateral legs**

**I70.728 Atherosclerosis of other type of** HCC A
**bypass graft(s) of the extremities with rest pain, other extremity**

**I70.729 Atherosclerosis of other type of** HCC A
**bypass graft(s) of the extremities with rest pain, unspecified extremity**

**✓6th I70.73 Atherosclerosis of other type of bypass graft(s) of the right leg with ulceration**

INCLUDES any condition classifiable to I70.711 and I70.721

Use additional code to identify severity of ulcer (L97.-)

CC Excl: For CC codes in subcategory I70.73:
PDX collection 698

**I70.731 Atherosclerosis of other** PDxCC CC HCC A
**type of bypass graft(s) of the right leg with ulceration of thigh**

**I70.732 Atherosclerosis of other** PDxCC CC HCC A
**type of bypass graft(s) of the right leg with ulceration of calf**

**I70.733 Atherosclerosis of other** PDxCC CC HCC A
**type of bypass graft(s) of the right leg with ulceration of ankle**

N Newborn: 0   P Pediatric: 0-17   M Maternity: 12-55   A Adult: 15-124   MCC Major CC Condition   PDxMCC PDx acts as own MCC   CC CC Condition   PDxCC PDx acts as own CC

656   ICD-10-CM 2018

**I70.734** **Atherosclerosis of other type of bypass graft(s) of the right leg with ulceration of heel and midfoot** `PDxCC` `CC` `HCC` `A`
Atherosclerosis of other type of bypass graft(s) of right leg with ulceration of plantar surface of midfoot

**I70.735** **Atherosclerosis of other type of bypass graft(s) of the right leg with ulceration of other part of foot** `HCC` `A`
Atherosclerosis of other type of bypass graft(s) of right leg with ulceration of toe

**I70.738** **Atherosclerosis of other type of bypass graft(s) of the right leg with ulceration of other part of lower leg** `PDxCC` `CC` `HCC` `A`

**I70.739** **Atherosclerosis of other type of bypass graft(s) of the right leg with ulceration of unspecified site** `PDxCC` `CC` `HCC` `A`

√6th **I70.74** **Atherosclerosis of other type of bypass graft(s) of the left leg with ulceration**
**INCLUDES** any condition classifiable to I70.712 and I70.722
Use additional code to identify severity of ulcer (L97.-)

> **CC Excl: For CC codes in subcategory I70.74:** PDX collection 698

**I70.741** **Atherosclerosis of other type of bypass graft(s) of the left leg with ulceration of thigh** `PDxCC` `CC` `HCC` `A`

**I70.742** **Atherosclerosis of other type of bypass graft(s) of the left leg with ulceration of calf** `PDxCC` `CC` `HCC` `A`

**I70.743** **Atherosclerosis of other type of bypass graft(s) of the left leg with ulceration of ankle** `PDxCC` `CC` `HCC` `A`

**I70.744** **Atherosclerosis of other type of bypass raft(s) of the left leg with ulceration of heel and midfoot** `PDxCC` `CC` `HCC` `A`
Atherosclerosis of other type of bypass graft(s) of left leg with ulceration of plantar surface of midfoot

**I70.745** **Atherosclerosis of other type of bypass graft(s) of the left leg with ulceration of other part of foot** `HCC` `A`
Atherosclerosis of other type of bypass graft(s) of left leg with ulceration of toe

**I70.748** **Atherosclerosis of other type of bypass graft(s) of the left leg with ulceration of other part of lower leg** `PDxCC` `CC` `HCC` `A`

**I70.749** **Atherosclerosis of other type of bypass graft(s) of the left leg with ulceration of unspecified site** `PDxCC` `CC` `HCC` `A`

**I70.75** **Atherosclerosis of other type of bypass graft(s) of other extremity with ulceration** `HCC` `A`
**INCLUDES** any condition classifiable to I70.718 and I70.728
Use additional code to identify severity of ulcer (L98.49)

√6th **I70.76** **Atherosclerosis of other type of bypass graft(s) of the extremities with gangrene**
**INCLUDES** any condition classifiable to I70.71-, I70.72-, I70.73-, I70.74-, I70.75
Use additional code to identify the severity of any ulcer (L97.-, L98.49-), if applicable

> **CC Excl: For CC codes in subcategory I70.76:** PDX collection 519

**I70.761** **Atherosclerosis of other type of bypass graft(s) of the extremities with gangrene, right leg** `PDxCC` `CC` `HCC` `A`

**I70.762** **Atherosclerosis of other type of bypass graft(s) of the extremities with gangrene, left leg** `PDxCC` `CC` `HCC` `A`

**I70.763** **Atherosclerosis of other type of bypass graft(s) of the extremities with gangrene, bilateral legs** `PDxCC` `CC` `HCC` `A`

**I70.768** **Atherosclerosis of other type of bypass graft(s) of the extremities with gangrene, other extremity** `PDxCC` `CC` `HCC` `A`

**I70.769** **Atherosclerosis of other type of bypass graft(s) of the extremities with gangrene, unspecified extremity** `PDxCC` `CC` `HCC` `A`

√6th **I70.79** **Other atherosclerosis of other type of bypass graft(s) of the extremities**

**I70.791** **Other atherosclerosis of other type of bypass graft(s) of the extremities, right leg** `HCC` `A`

**I70.792** **Other atherosclerosis of other type of bypass graft(s) of the extremities, left leg** `HCC` `A`

**I70.793** **Other atherosclerosis of other type of bypass graft(s) of the extremities, bilateral legs** `HCC` `A`

**I70.798** **Other atherosclerosis of other type of bypass graft(s) of the extremities, other extremity** `HCC` `A`

**I70.799** **Other atherosclerosis of other type of bypass graft(s) of the extremities, unspecified extremity** `HCC` `A`

**I70.8** **Atherosclerosis of other arteries** `A`
**TIP:** Arteriosclerosis of the iliac arteries is coded here.

√5th **I70.9** **Other and unspecified atherosclerosis**

**I70.90** **Unspecified atherosclerosis** `A`

**I70.91** **Generalized atherosclerosis** `A`

**I70.92** **Chronic total occlusion of artery of the extremities** `CC` `HCC` `A`
Complete occlusion of artery of the extremities
Total occlusion of artery of the extremities
Code first atherosclerosis of arteries of the extremities (I70.2-, I70.3-, I70.4-, I70.5-, I70.6-, I70.7-)
**CC Excl:** PDX collection 699

√4th **I71** **Aortic aneurysm and dissection**
**EXCLUDES 1** aortic ectasia (I77.81-)
syphilitic aortic aneurysm (A52.01)
traumatic aortic aneurysm (S25.09, S35.09)

> **CC Excl: For MCC codes in category I71:** PDX collection 700

√5th **I71.0** **Dissection of aorta**

**I71.00** **Dissection of unspecified site of aorta** `MCC` `HCC`

**I71.01** **Dissection of thoracic aorta** `MCC` `HCC`

**I71.02** **Dissection of abdominal aorta** `MCC` `HCC`

**I71.03** **Dissection of thoracoabdominal aorta** `MCC` `HCC`

**I71.1** **Thoracic aortic aneurysm, ruptured** `MCC` `HCC`

**I71.2** **Thoracic aortic aneurysm, without rupture** `HCC`

**I71.3** **Abdominal aortic aneurysm, ruptured** `MCC` `HCC`

**I71.4** **Abdominal aortic aneurysm, without rupture** `HCC`

**I71.5** **Thoracoabdominal aortic aneurysm, ruptured** `MCC` `HCC`

**I71.6** **Thoracoabdominal aortic aneurysm, without rupture** `HCC`

**I71.8** **Aortic aneurysm of unspecified site, ruptured** `MCC` `HCC`
Rupture of aorta NOS

**I71.9** **Aortic aneurysm of unspecified site, without rupture** `HCC`
Aneurysm of aorta     Hyaline necrosis of aorta
Dilatation of aorta

√4th **I72** **Other aneurysm**
**INCLUDES** aneurysm (cirsoid) (false) (ruptured)
**EXCLUDES 2** acquired aneurysm (I77.0)
aneurysm (of) aorta (I71.-)
aneurysm (of) arteriovenous NOS (Q27.3-)
carotid artery dissection (I77.71)
cerebral (nonruptured) aneurysm (I67.1)
coronary aneurysm (I25.4)
coronary artery dissection (I25.42)
dissection of artery NEC (I77.79)
dissection of precerebral artery, congenital (nonruptured) (Q28.1)
heart aneurysm (I25.3)
iliac artery dissection (I77.72)
▶precerebral artery, congenital (nonruptured) (Q28.1)◀
pulmonary artery aneurysm (I28.1)
renal artery dissection (I77.73)
retinal aneurysm (H35.0)
ruptured cerebral aneurysm (I60.7)
varicose aneurysm (I77.0)
vertebral artery dissection (I77.74)

**I72.0** **Aneurysm of carotid artery** `HCC`
Aneurysm of common carotid artery
Aneurysm of external carotid artery
Aneurysm of internal carotid artery, extracranial portion
**EXCLUDES 1** aneurysm of internal carotid artery, intracranial portion (I67.1)
aneurysm of internal carotid artery NOS (I67.1)

**Aneurysm**

Outer layer

Layers of muscular
and elastic tissue

Inner layer

Aneurysm

**I72.1**  **Aneurysm of artery of upper extremity**  `HCC`

**I72.2**  **Aneurysm of renal artery**  `HCC`

**I72.3**  **Aneurysm of iliac artery**  `HCC`

**I72.4**  **Aneurysm of artery of lower extremity**  `HCC`

**I72.5**  **Aneurysm of other precerebral arteries**  `HCC`
Aneurysm of basilar artery (trunk)
`EXCLUDES 2`  *aneurysm of carotid artery (I72.Ø)*
*aneurysm of vertebral artery (I72.6)*
*dissection of carotid artery (I77.71)*
*dissection of other precerebral arteries (I77.75)*
*dissection of vertebral artery (I77.74)*

**I72.6**  **Aneurysm of vertebral artery**  `HCC`
`EXCLUDES 2`  *dissection of vertebral artery (I77.74)*

**I72.8**  **Aneurysm of other specified arteries**  `HCC`

**I72.9**  **Aneurysm of unspecified site**  `HCC`

`✓4ᵗʰ` **I73**  **Other peripheral vascular diseases**
`EXCLUDES 2`  *chilblains (T69.1)*
*frostbite (T33- T34)*
*immersion hand or foot (T69.Ø-)*
*spasm of cerebral artery (G45.9)*

`✓5ᵗʰ` **I73.Ø**  **Raynaud's syndrome**
Raynaud's disease
Raynaud's phenomenon (secondary)

**I73.ØØ**  **Raynaud's syndrome without gangrene**

**I73.Ø1**  **Raynaud's syndrome with gangrene**  `PDxCC` `CC` `HCC`
**CC Excl:** PDX collection 519

**I73.1**  **Thromboangiitis obliterans [Buerger's disease]**  `HCC`
**DEF:** Inflammatory disease of extremity blood vessels, mainly the
lower; associated with heavy tobacco use; arteries are more
affected than veins; occurs primarily in young men and leads to
tissue ischemia and gangrene.

`✓5ᵗʰ` **I73.8**  **Other specified peripheral vascular diseases**
`EXCLUDES 1`  *diabetic (peripheral) angiopathy (EØ8-E13 with .51-*
*.52)*

**I73.81**  **Erythromelalgia**  `HCC`

**I73.89**  **Other specified peripheral vascular diseases**  `HCC`
Acrocyanosis
Erythrocyanosis
Simple acroparesthesia [Schultze's type]
Vasomotor acroparesthesia [Nothnagel's type]

**I73.9**  **Peripheral vascular disease, unspecified**  `HCC`
Intermittent claudication
Peripheral angiopathy NOS
Spasm of artery
`EXCLUDES 1`  *atherosclerosis of the extremities (I70.2--I70.7-)*

`✓4ᵗʰ` **I74**  **Arterial embolism and thrombosis**
`INCLUDES`  embolic infarction
embolic occlusion
thrombotic infarction
thrombotic occlusion
Code first:
embolism and thrombosis complicating abortion or ectopic or molar
pregnancy (OØØ-OØ7, OØ8.2)
embolism and thrombosis complicating pregnancy, childbirth and
the puerperium (O88.-)
`EXCLUDES 2`  *atheroembolism (I75.-)*
*basilar embolism and thrombosis (I63.Ø-I63.2, I65.1)*
*carotid embolism and thrombosis (I63.Ø-I63.2, I65.2)*
*cerebral embolism and thrombosis (I63.3-I63.5, I66-)*
*coronary embolism and thrombosis (I21-I25)*
*mesenteric embolism and thrombosis (K55.Ø-)*
*ophthalmic embolism and thrombosis (H34.-)*
*precerebral embolism and thrombosis NOS (I63.Ø-I63.2, I65.9)*
*pulmonary embolism and thrombosis (I26.-)*
*renal embolism and thrombosis (N28.Ø)*
*retinal embolism and thrombosis (H34.-)*
*septic embolism and thrombosis (I76)*
*vertebral embolism and thrombosis (I63.Ø-I63.2, I65.Ø)*

`✓5ᵗʰ` **I74.Ø**  **Embolism and thrombosis of abdominal aorta**

**I74.Ø1**  **Saddle embolus of abdominal aorta**  `MCC` `HCC`
**CC Excl:** PDX collection 669

**I74.Ø9**  **Other arterial embolism and thrombosis of**  `CC` `HCC`
**abdominal aorta**
Aortic bifurcation syndrome       Leriche's syndrome
Aortoiliac obstruction
**CC Excl:** PDX collection 669

`✓5ᵗʰ` **I74.1**  **Embolism and thrombosis of other and unspecified parts of**
**aorta**

**I74.10**  **Embolism and thrombosis of unspecified**  `CC` `HCC`
**parts of aorta**
**CC Excl:** PDX collection 669

**I74.11**  **Embolism and thrombosis of thoracic aorta**  `CC` `HCC`
**CC Excl:** PDX collection 701

**I74.19**  **Embolism and thrombosis of other parts of**  `CC` `HCC`
**aorta**
**CC Excl:** PDX collection 669

**I74.2**  **Embolism and thrombosis of arteries of the upper**  `CC` `HCC`
**extremities**
**CC Excl:** PDX collection 702

**I74.3**  **Embolism and thrombosis of arteries of the lower**  `CC` `HCC`
**extremities**
**CC Excl:** PDX collection 703

**I74.4**  **Embolism and thrombosis of arteries of extremities,**  `CC` `HCC`
**unspecified**
Peripheral arterial embolism NOS
**CC Excl:** PDX collection 703

**I74.5**  **Embolism and thrombosis of iliac artery**  `CC` `HCC`
**CC Excl:** PDX collection 704

**I74.8**  **Embolism and thrombosis of other arteries**  `CC` `HCC`
**CC Excl:** PDX collection 705

**I74.9**  **Embolism and thrombosis of unspecified artery**  `CC` `HCC`
**CC Excl:** PDX collection 705

`✓4ᵗʰ` **I75**  **Atheroembolism**
`INCLUDES`  atherothrombotic microembolism
cholesterol embolism

`✓5ᵗʰ` **I75.Ø**  **Atheroembolism of extremities**

`✓6ᵗʰ` **I75.Ø1**  **Atheroembolism of upper extremity**

**CC Excl: For CC codes in subcategory I75.Ø1:**
PDX collection 706

**I75.Ø11**  **Atheroembolism of right upper**  `CC` `HCC`
**extremity**

**I75.Ø12**  **Atheroembolism of left upper**  `CC` `HCC`
**extremity**

**I75.Ø13**  **Atheroembolism of bilateral**  `CC` `HCC`
**upper extremities**

**I75.Ø19**  **Atheroembolism of unspecified**  `CC` `HCC`
**upper extremity**

`✓6ᵗʰ` **I75.Ø2**  **Atheroembolism of lower extremity**

**CC Excl: For CC codes in subcategory I75.Ø2:**
PDX collection 707

**I75.Ø21**  **Atheroembolism of right lower**  `CC` `HCC`
**extremity**

**I75.Ø22**  **Atheroembolism of left lower**  `CC` `HCC`
**extremity**

`N` Newborn: 0   `P` Pediatric: 0-17   `M` Maternity: 12-55   `A` Adult: 15-124   `MCC` Major CC Condition   `PDxMCC` PDx acts as own MCC   `CC` CC Condition   `PDxCC` PDx acts as own CC

658                                                                                                                ICD-10-CM 2018

    **I75.Ø23** **Atheroembolism of bilateral lower** `CC` `HCC`
                **extremities**

    **I75.Ø29** **Atheroembolism of unspecified** `CC` `HCC`
                **lower extremity**

✓5ᵗʰ **I75.8** **Atheroembolism of other sites**

    **I75.81** **Atheroembolism of kidney** `CC` `HCC`
            Use additional code for any associated acute kidney
            failure and chronic kidney disease (N17.-, N18.-)
            **CC Excl:** PDX collection 7Ø8

    **I75.89** **Atheroembolism of other site** `CC` `HCC`
            **CC Excl:** PDX collection 7Ø9

**I76** **Septic arterial embolism** `CC` `HCC`
     Code first underlying infection, such as:
       infective endocarditis (I33.Ø)
       lung abscess (J85.-)
     Use additional code to identify the site of the embolism (I74.-)
     *EXCLUDES 2*   *septic pulmonary embolism (I26.Ø1, I26.9Ø)*
     **CC Excl:** PDX collection 7Ø5

✓4ᵗʰ **I77** **Other disorders of arteries and arterioles**
     *EXCLUDES 2*   *collagen (vascular) diseases (M3Ø-M36)*
                   *hypersensitivity angiitis (M31.Ø)*
                   *pulmonary artery (I28.-)*

    **I77.Ø** **Arteriovenous fistula, acquired** `HCC`
         Aneurysmal varix
         Arteriovenous aneurysm, acquired
         *EXCLUDES 1*   *arteriovenous aneurysm NOS (Q27.3-)*
                   *presence of arteriovenous shunt (fistula) for dialysis*
                     *(Z99.2)*
                   *traumatic—see injury of blood vessel by body region*
         *EXCLUDES 2*   *cerebral (I67.1)*
                   *coronary (I25.4)*
         **DEF:** Communication between an artery and vein; caused by
         trauma or invasive procedures.

    **I77.1** **Stricture of artery** `HCC`
         Narrowing of artery

    **I77.2** **Rupture of artery** `CC` `HCC`
         Erosion of artery
         Fistula of artery
         Ulcer of artery
         *EXCLUDES 1*   *traumatic rupture of artery—see injury of blood vessel*
                   *by body region*
         **CC Excl:** PDX collection 71Ø

    **I77.3** **Arterial fibromuscular dysplasia** `HCC`
         Fibromuscular hyperplasia (of) carotid artery
         Fibromuscular hyperplasia (of) renal artery

    **I77.4** **Celiac artery compression syndrome** `CC` `HCC`
         **CC Excl:** PDX collection 711

    **I77.5** **Necrosis of artery** `CC` `HCC`
         **CC Excl:** PDX collection 712

    **I77.6** **Arteritis, unspecified** `HCC`
         Aortitis NOS
         Endarteritis NOS
         *EXCLUDES 1*   *arteritis or endarteritis:*
                   *aortic arch (M31.4)*
                   *cerebral NEC (I67.7)*
                   *coronary (I25.89)*
                   *deformans (I7Ø.-)*
                   *giant cell (M31.5., M31.6)*
                   *obliterans (I7Ø.-)*
                   *senile (I7Ø.-)*

✓5ᵗʰ **I77.7** **Other arterial dissection**
         *EXCLUDES 2*   *dissection of aorta (I71.Ø-)*
                   *dissection of coronary artery (I25.42)*

    **CC Excl: For MCC codes in subcategory I77.7:**
    PDX collection 689

    **I77.7Ø** **Dissection of unspecified artery** `MCC` `HCC`

    **I77.71** **Dissection of carotid artery** `MCC` `HCC`

    **I77.72** **Dissection of iliac artery** `MCC` `HCC`

    **I77.73** **Dissection of renal artery** `MCC` `HCC`

    **I77.74** **Dissection of vertebral artery** `MCC` `HCC`
         *EXCLUDES 2*   *aneurysm of vertebral artery (I72.6)*

    **I77.75** **Dissection of other precerebral arteries** `MCC` `HCC`
         Dissection of basilar artery (trunk)
         *EXCLUDES 2*   *aneurysm of carotid artery (I72.Ø)*
                   *aneurysm of other precerebral arteries (I72.5)*
                   *aneurysm of vertebral artery (I72.6)*
                   *dissection of carotid artery (I77.71)*
                   *dissection of vertebral artery (I77.74)*

    **I77.76** **Dissection of artery of upper extremity** `MCC` `HCC`

    **I77.77** **Dissection of artery of lower extremity** `MCC` `HCC`

    **I77.79** **Dissection of other specified artery** `MCC` `HCC`

✓5ᵗʰ **I77.8** **Other specified disorders of arteries and arterioles**

    ✓6ᵗʰ **I77.81** **Aortic ectasia**
         Ectasis aorta
         *EXCLUDES 1*   *aortic aneurysm and dissection (I71.Ø-)*

        **I77.81Ø** **Thoracic aortic ectasia** `HCC`

        **I77.811** **Abdominal aortic ectasia** `HCC`

        **I77.812** **Thoracoabdominal aortic ectasia** `HCC`

        **I77.819** **Aortic ectasia, unspecified site** `HCC`

    **I77.89** **Other specified disorders of arteries and** `HCC`
                **arterioles**

    **I77.9** **Disorder of arteries and arterioles, unspecified** `HCC`

✓4ᵗʰ **I78** **Diseases of capillaries**

    **I78.Ø** **Hereditary hemorrhagic telangiectasia** `HCC`
         Rendu-Osler-Weber disease

    **I78.1** **Nevus, non-neoplastic**
         Araneus nevus        Spider nevus
         Senile nevus          Stellar nevus
         *EXCLUDES 1*   *nevus NOS (D22.-)*
                   *vascular NOS (Q82.5)*
         *EXCLUDES 2*   *blue nevus (D22.-)*
                   *flammeus nevus (Q82.5)*
                   *hairy nevus (D22.-)*
                   *melanocytic nevus (D22.-)*
                   *pigmented nevus (D22.-)*
                   *portwine nevus (Q82.5)*
                   *sanguineous nevus (Q82.5)*
                   *strawberry nevus (Q82.5)*
                   *verrucous nevus (Q82.5)*

    **I78.8** **Other diseases of capillaries**

    **I78.9** **Disease of capillaries, unspecified**

✓4ᵗʰ **I79** **Disorders of arteries, arterioles and capillaries in diseases classified elsewhere**

    ***I79.Ø*** ***Aneurysm of aorta in diseases classified elsewhere*** `HCC`
         Code first underlying disease
         *EXCLUDES 1*   *syphilitic aneurysm (A52.Ø1)*

    ***I79.1*** ***Aortitis in diseases classified elsewhere*** `HCC`
         Code first underlying disease
         *EXCLUDES 1*   *syphilitic aortitis (A52.Ø2)*

    ***I79.8*** ***Other disorders of arteries, arterioles and capillaries*** `HCC`
    ***in diseases classified elsewhere***
         Code first underlying disease, such as:
           amyloidosis (E85.-)
         *EXCLUDES 1*   *diabetic (peripheral) angiopathy (EØ8-E13 with .51-*
                   *.52)*
                   *syphilitic endarteritis (A52.Ø9)*
                   *tuberculous endarteritis (A18.89)*

## Diseases of veins, lymphatic vessels and lymph nodes, not elsewhere classified (I8Ø-I89)

✓4ᵗʰ **I8Ø** **Phlebitis and thrombophlebitis**
     `INCLUDES`   endophlebitis
                inflammation, vein
                periphlebitis
                suppurative phlebitis
     Code first:
       phlebitis and thrombophlebitis complicating abortion, ectopic or
         molar pregnancy (OØØ-OØ7, OØ8.7)
       phlebitis and thrombophlebitis complicating pregnancy, childbirth
         and the puerperium (O22.-, O87.-)
     *EXCLUDES 1*   *venous embolism and thrombosis of lower extremities (I82.4-,*
                   *I82.5-, I82.81-)*

    **CC Excl: For CC codes in category I8Ø:** PDX collection 713

✓5ᵗʰ **I8Ø.Ø** **Phlebitis and thrombophlebitis of superficial vessels of lower extremities**
         Phlebitis and thrombophlebitis of femoropopliteal vein

    **I8Ø.ØØ** **Phlebitis and thrombophlebitis of superficial vessels of unspecified lower extremity**

    **I8Ø.Ø1** **Phlebitis and thrombophlebitis of superficial vessels of right lower extremity**

    **I8Ø.Ø2** **Phlebitis and thrombophlebitis of superficial vessels of left lower extremity**

    **I8Ø.Ø3** **Phlebitis and thrombophlebitis of superficial vessels of lower extremities, bilateral**

**✓5th I80.1 Phlebitis and thrombophlebitis of femoral vein**

**I80.10** Phlebitis and thrombophlebitis of unspecified femoral vein `CC HCC`

**I80.11** Phlebitis and thrombophlebitis of right femoral vein `CC HCC`

**I80.12** Phlebitis and thrombophlebitis of left femoral vein `CC HCC`

**I80.13** Phlebitis and thrombophlebitis of femoral vein, bilateral `CC HCC`

**✓5th I80.2 Phlebitis and thrombophlebitis of other and unspecified deep vessels of lower extremities**

**✓6th I80.20** Phlebitis and thrombophlebitis of unspecified deep vessels of lower extremities

**I80.201** Phlebitis and thrombophlebitis of unspecified deep vessels of right lower extremity `CC HCC`

**I80.202** Phlebitis and thrombophlebitis of unspecified deep vessels of left lower extremity `CC HCC`

**I80.203** Phlebitis and thrombophlebitis of unspecified deep vessels of lower extremities, bilateral `CC HCC`

**I80.209** Phlebitis and thrombophlebitis of unspecified deep vessels of unspecified lower extremity `CC HCC`

**✓6th I80.21** Phlebitis and thrombophlebitis of iliac vein

**I80.211** Phlebitis and thrombophlebitis of right iliac vein `CC HCC`

**I80.212** Phlebitis and thrombophlebitis of left iliac vein `CC HCC`

**I80.213** Phlebitis and thrombophlebitis of iliac vein, bilateral `CC HCC`

**I80.219** Phlebitis and thrombophlebitis of unspecified iliac vein `CC HCC`

**✓6th I80.22** Phlebitis and thrombophlebitis of popliteal vein

**I80.221** Phlebitis and thrombophlebitis of right popliteal vein `CC HCC`

**I80.222** Phlebitis and thrombophlebitis of left popliteal vein `CC HCC`

**I80.223** Phlebitis and thrombophlebitis of popliteal vein, bilateral `CC HCC`

**I80.229** Phlebitis and thrombophlebitis of unspecified popliteal vein `CC HCC`

**✓6th I80.23** Phlebitis and thrombophlebitis of tibial vein

**I80.231** Phlebitis and thrombophlebitis of right tibial vein `CC HCC`

**I80.232** Phlebitis and thrombophlebitis of left tibial vein `CC HCC`

**I80.233** Phlebitis and thrombophlebitis of tibial vein, bilateral `CC HCC`

**I80.239** Phlebitis and thrombophlebitis of unspecified tibial vein `CC HCC`

**✓6th I80.29** Phlebitis and thrombophlebitis of other deep vessels of lower extremities

**I80.291** Phlebitis and thrombophlebitis of other deep vessels of right lower extremity `CC HCC`

**I80.292** Phlebitis and thrombophlebitis of other deep vessels of left lower extremity `CC HCC`

**I80.293** Phlebitis and thrombophlebitis of other deep vessels of lower extremity, bilateral `CC HCC`

**I80.299** Phlebitis and thrombophlebitis of other deep vessels of unspecified lower extremity `CC HCC`

**I80.3 Phlebitis and thrombophlebitis of lower extremities, unspecified**

**I80.8 Phlebitis and thrombophlebitis of other sites**

**I80.9 Phlebitis and thrombophlebitis of unspecified site**

**I81 Portal vein thrombosis** `MCC`
Portal (vein) obstruction

*EXCLUDES 2*   hepatic vein thrombosis (I82.0)
     phlebitis of portal vein (K75.1)

**CC Excl:** PDX collection 714

**✓4th I82 Other venous embolism and thrombosis**
Code first venous embolism and thrombosis complicating:
   abortion, ectopic or molar pregnancy (O00-O07, O08.7)
   pregnancy, childbirth and the puerperium (O22.-, O87.-)

*EXCLUDES 2*   venous embolism and thrombosis (of):
     cerebral (I63.6, I67.6)
     coronary (I21-I25)
     intracranial and intraspinal, septic or NOS (G08)
     intracranial, nonpyogenic (I67.6)
     intraspinal, nonpyogenic (G95.1)
     mesenteric (K55.0-)
     portal (I81)
     pulmonary (I26.-)

**I82.0 Budd-Chiari syndrome** `MCC HCC`
Hepatic vein thrombosis
**DEF:** Thrombosis or other obstruction of hepatic veins; symptoms include enlarged liver, extensive collateral vessels, intractable ascites, and severe portal hypertension.
**CC Excl:** PDX collection 715

**I82.1 Thrombophlebitis migrans** `CC`
**CC Excl:** PDX collection 716

**✓5th I82.2 Embolism and thrombosis of vena cava and other thoracic veins**

**CC Excl: For CC codes in subcategory I82.2, unless otherwise noted:** PDX collection 717

**✓6th I82.21** Embolism and thrombosis of superior vena cava

**I82.210** Acute embolism and thrombosis of superior vena cava `CC HCC`
Embolism and thrombosis of superior vena cava NOS

**I82.211** Chronic embolism and thrombosis of superior vena cava `CC HCC`

**✓6th I82.22** Embolism and thrombosis of inferior vena cava

**I82.220** Acute embolism and thrombosis of inferior vena cava `MCC HCC`
Embolism and thrombosis of inferior vena cava NOS
**CC Excl:** PDX collection 718

**I82.221** Chronic embolism and thrombosis of inferior vena cava `MCC HCC`
**CC Excl:** PDX collection 718

**✓6th I82.29** Embolism and thrombosis of other thoracic veins
Embolism and thrombosis of brachiocephalic (innominate) vein

**I82.290** Acute embolism and thrombosis of other thoracic veins `CC HCC`

**I82.291** Chronic embolism and thrombosis of other thoracic veins `CC HCC`

**I82.3 Embolism and thrombosis of renal vein** `CC HCC`
**CC Excl:** PDX collection 719

**✓5th I82.4 Acute embolism and thrombosis of deep veins of lower extremity**

**CC Excl: For CC codes in subcategory I82.4:** PDX collection 717

**✓6th I82.40** Acute embolism and thrombosis of unspecified deep veins of lower extremity
Deep vein thrombosis NOS
DVT NOS

*EXCLUDES 1*   acute embolism and thrombosis of unspecified deep veins of distal lower extremity (I82.4Z-)
     acute embolism and thrombosis of unspecified deep veins of proximal lower extremity (I82.4Y-)

**I82.401** Acute embolism and thrombosis of unspecified deep veins of right lower extremity `CC H10 HCC`

**I82.402** Acute embolism and thrombosis of unspecified deep veins of left lower extremity `CC H10 HCC`

**I82.403** Acute embolism and thrombosis of unspecified deep veins of lower extremity, bilateral `CC H10 HCC`

**I82.409** Acute embolism and thrombosis of unspecified deep veins of unspecified lower extremity `CC H10 HCC`

**✓6th I82.41** Acute embolism and thrombosis of femoral vein

**I82.411** Acute embolism and thrombosis of right femoral vein `CC H10 HCC`

**I82.412** Acute embolism and thrombosis of left femoral vein `CC H10 HCC`

---

N Newborn: 0   P Pediatric: 0-17   M Maternity: 12-55   A Adult: 15-124   **MCC** Major CC Condition   **PDxMCC** PDx acts as own MCC   **CC** CC Condition   **PDxCC** PDx acts as own CC

660          ICD-10-CM 2018

**I82.413** Acute embolism and thrombosis of femoral vein, bilateral `CC` `H10` `HCC`

**I82.419** Acute embolism and thrombosis of unspecified femoral vein `CC` `H10` `HCC`

✓6ᵗʰ **I82.42** Acute embolism and thrombosis of iliac vein

**I82.421** Acute embolism and thrombosis of right iliac vein `CC` `H10` `HCC`

**I82.422** Acute embolism and thrombosis of left iliac vein `CC` `H10` `HCC`

**I82.423** Acute embolism and thrombosis of iliac vein, bilateral `CC` `H10` `HCC`

**I82.429** Acute embolism and thrombosis of unspecified iliac vein `CC` `H10` `HCC`

✓6ᵗʰ **I82.43** Acute embolism and thrombosis of popliteal vein

**I82.431** Acute embolism and thrombosis of right popliteal vein `CC` `H10` `HCC`

**I82.432** Acute embolism and thrombosis of left popliteal vein `CC` `H10` `HCC`

**I82.433** Acute embolism and thrombosis of popliteal vein, bilateral `CC` `H10` `HCC`

**I82.439** Acute embolism and thrombosis of unspecified popliteal vein `CC` `H10` `HCC`

✓6ᵗʰ **I82.44** Acute embolism and thrombosis of tibial vein

**I82.441** Acute embolism and thrombosis of right tibial vein `CC` `H10` `HCC`

**I82.442** Acute embolism and thrombosis of left tibial vein `CC` `H10` `HCC`

**I82.443** Acute embolism and thrombosis of tibial vein, bilateral `CC` `H10` `HCC`

**I82.449** Acute embolism and unspecified tibial vein `CC` `H10` `HCC`

✓6ᵗʰ **I82.49** Acute embolism and thrombosis of other specified deep vein of lower extremity

**I82.491** Acute embolism and thrombosis of other specified deep vein of right lower extremity `CC` `H10` `HCC`

**I82.492** Acute embolism and thrombosis of other specified deep vein of left lower extremity `CC` `H10` `HCC`

**I82.493** Acute embolism and thrombosis of other specified deep vein of lower extremity, bilateral `CC` `H10` `HCC`

**I82.499** Acute embolism and thrombosis of other specified deep vein of unspecified lower extremity `CC` `H10` `HCC`

✓6ᵗʰ **I82.4Y** Acute embolism and thrombosis of unspecified deep veins of proximal lower extremity
Acute embolism and thrombosis of deep vein of thigh NOS
Acute embolism and thrombosis of deep vein of upper leg NOS

**I82.4Y1** Acute embolism and thrombosis of unspecified deep veins of right proximal lower extremity `CC` `H10` `HCC`

**I82.4Y2** Acute embolism and thrombosis of unspecified deep veins of left proximal lower extremity `CC` `H10` `HCC`

**I82.4Y3** Acute embolism and thrombosis of unspecified deep veins of proximal lower extremity, bilateral `CC` `H10` `HCC`

**I82.4Y9** Acute embolism and thrombosis of unspecified deep veins of unspecified proximal lower extremity `CC` `H10` `HCC`

✓6ᵗʰ **I82.4Z** Acute embolism and thrombosis of unspecified deep veins of distal lower extremity
Acute embolism and thrombosis of deep vein of calf NOS
Acute embolism and thrombosis of deep vein of lower leg NOS

**I82.4Z1** Acute embolism and thrombosis of unspecified deep veins of right distal lower extremity `CC` `H10` `HCC`

**I82.4Z2** Acute embolism and thrombosis of unspecified deep veins of left distal lower extremity `CC` `H10` `HCC`

**I82.4Z3** Acute embolism and thrombosis of unspecified deep veins of distal lower extremity, bilateral `CC` `H10` `HCC`

**I82.4Z9** Acute embolism and thrombosis of unspecified deep veins of unspecified distal lower extremity `CC` `H10` `HCC`

✓5ᵗʰ **I82.5** Chronic embolism and thrombosis of deep veins of lower extremity
Use additional code, if applicable, for associated long-term (current) use of anticoagulants (Z79.01)
*EXCLUDES 1*    personal history of venous embolism and thrombosis (Z86.718)

**CC Excl: For CC codes in subcategory I82.5:**
PDX collection 717

✓6ᵗʰ **I82.50** Chronic embolism and thrombosis of unspecified deep veins of lower extremity
*EXCLUDES 1*    chronic embolism and thrombosis of unspecified deep veins of distal lower extremity (I82.5Z-)
chronic embolism and thrombosis of unspecified deep veins of proximal lower extremity (I82.5Y-)

**I82.501** Chronic embolism and thrombosis of unspecified deep veins of right lower extremity `CC` `HCC`

**I82.502** Chronic embolism and thrombosis of unspecified deep veins of left lower extremity `CC` `HCC`

**I82.503** Chronic embolism and thrombosis of unspecified deep veins of lower extremity, bilateral `CC` `HCC`

**I82.509** Chronic embolism and thrombosis of unspecified deep veins of unspecified lower extremity `CC` `HCC`

✓6ᵗʰ **I82.51** Chronic embolism and thrombosis of femoral vein

**I82.511** Chronic embolism and thrombosis of right femoral vein `CC` `HCC`

**I82.512** Chronic embolism and thrombosis of left femoral vein `CC` `HCC`

**I82.513** Chronic embolism and thrombosis of femoral vein, bilateral `CC` `HCC`

**I82.519** Chronic embolism and thrombosis of unspecified femoral vein `CC` `HCC`

✓6ᵗʰ **I82.52** Chronic embolism and thrombosis of iliac vein

**I82.521** Chronic embolism and thrombosis of right iliac vein `CC` `HCC`

**I82.522** Chronic embolism and thrombosis of left iliac vein `CC` `HCC`

**I82.523** Chronic embolism and thrombosis of iliac vein, bilateral `CC` `HCC`

**I82.529** Chronic embolism and thrombosis of unspecified iliac vein `CC` `HCC`

✓6ᵗʰ **I82.53** Chronic embolism and thrombosis of popliteal vein

**I82.531** Chronic embolism and thrombosis of right popliteal vein `CC` `HCC`

**I82.532** Chronic embolism and thrombosis of left popliteal vein `CC` `HCC`

**I82.533** Chronic embolism and thrombosis of popliteal vein, bilateral `CC` `HCC`

**I82.539** Chronic embolism and thrombosis of unspecified popliteal vein `CC` `HCC`

✓6ᵗʰ **I82.54** Chronic embolism and thrombosis of tibial vein

**I82.541** Chronic embolism and thrombosis of right tibial vein `CC` `HCC`

**I82.542** Chronic embolism and thrombosis of left tibial vein `CC` `HCC`

**I82.543** Chronic embolism and thrombosis of tibial vein, bilateral `CC` `HCC`

**I82.549** Chronic embolism and thrombosis of unspecified tibial vein `CC` `HCC`

✓6ᵗʰ **I82.59** Chronic embolism and thrombosis of other specified deep vein of lower extremity

**I82.591** Chronic embolism and thrombosis of other specified deep vein of right lower extremity `CC` `HCC`

**I82.592** Chronic embolism and thrombosis of other specified deep vein of left lower extremity `CC` `HCC`

✓ Additional Character Req    ✓x7ᵗʰ Placeholder Alert    Unacceptable PDx    Manifestation    `H1`–`H14` HAC    `HCC` CMS-HCC Condition    *EXCLUDES 1* Not Coded Here    *EXCLUDES 2* Not Included Here

**ICD-10-CM 2018**                                                                                                                **661**

**I82.593** Chronic embolism and thrombosis `CC` `HCC` of other specified deep vein of lower extremity, **bilateral**

**I82.599** Chronic embolism and thrombosis `CC` `HCC` of other specified deep vein of **unspecified lower extremity**

✓6ᵗʰ **I82.5Y** Chronic embolism and thrombosis of **unspecified deep veins of proximal lower extremity**
Chronic embolism and thrombosis of deep veins of thigh NOS
Chronic embolism and thrombosis of deep veins of upper leg NOS

**I82.5Y1** Chronic embolism and thrombosis `CC` `HCC` of unspecified deep veins of **right proximal lower extremity**

**I82.5Y2** Chronic embolism and thrombosis `CC` `HCC` of unspecified deep veins of **left** proximal lower extremity

**I82.5Y3** Chronic embolism and thrombosis `CC` `HCC` of unspecified deep veins of proximal lower extremity, **bilateral**

**I82.5Y9** Chronic embolism and thrombosis `CC` `HCC` of unspecified deep veins of **unspecified proximal lower extremity**

✓6ᵗʰ **I82.5Z** Chronic embolism and thrombosis of **unspecified deep veins of distal lower extremity**
Chronic embolism and thrombosis of deep veins of calf NOS
Chronic embolism and thrombosis of deep veins of lower leg NOS

**I82.5Z1** Chronic embolism and thrombosis `CC` `HCC` of unspecified deep veins of **right** distal lower extremity

**I82.5Z2** Chronic embolism and thrombosis `CC` `HCC` of unspecified deep veins of **left** distal lower extremity

**I82.5Z3** Chronic embolism and thrombosis `CC` `HCC` of unspecified deep veins of distal lower extremity, **bilateral**

**I82.5Z9** Chronic embolism and thrombosis `CC` `HCC` of unspecified deep veins of **unspecified distal lower extremity**

✓5ᵗʰ **I82.6** Acute **embolism and thrombosis of veins of** upper extremity

**CC Excl: For CC codes in subcategory I82.6:**
PDX collection 717

✓6ᵗʰ **I82.60** Acute embolism and thrombosis of **unspecified veins of upper extremity**

**I82.601** Acute embolism and thrombosis of `CC` unspecified veins of **right** upper extremity

**I82.602** Acute embolism and thrombosis of `CC` unspecified veins of **left** upper extremity

**I82.603** Acute embolism and thrombosis of `CC` unspecified veins of upper extremity, **bilateral**

**I82.609** Acute embolism and thrombosis of `CC` unspecified veins of **unspecified** upper extremity

✓6ᵗʰ **I82.61** Acute embolism and thrombosis of **superficial veins of upper extremity**
Acute embolism and thrombosis of antecubital vein
Acute embolism and thrombosis of basilic vein
Acute embolism and thrombosis of cephalic vein

**I82.611** Acute embolism and thrombosis of `CC` superficial veins of **right** upper extremity

**I82.612** Acute embolism and thrombosis of `CC` superficial veins of **left** upper extremity

**I82.613** Acute embolism and thrombosis of `CC` superficial veins of upper extremity, **bilateral**

**I82.619** Acute embolism and thrombosis of `CC` superficial veins of unspecified upper extremity

✓6ᵗʰ **I82.62** Acute embolism and thrombosis of **deep veins** of upper extremity
Acute embolism and thrombosis of brachial vein
Acute embolism and thrombosis of radial vein
Acute embolism and thrombosis of ulnar vein

**I82.621** Acute embolism and thrombosis of `CC` `HCC` deep veins of **right** upper extremity

**I82.622** Acute embolism and thrombosis of `CC` `HCC` deep veins of **left** upper extremity

**I82.623** Acute embolism and thrombosis of `CC` `HCC` deep veins of upper extremity, **bilateral**

**I82.629** Acute embolism and thrombosis of `CC` `HCC` deep veins of **unspecified** upper extremity

✓5ᵗʰ **I82.7** Chronic **embolism and thrombosis of veins of** upper extremity
Use additional code, if applicable, for associated long-term (current) use of anticoagulants (Z79.01)
**EXCLUDES 1** *personal history of venous embolism and thrombosis (Z86.718)*

**CC Excl: For CC codes in subcategory I82.7:**
PDX collection 717

✓6ᵗʰ **I82.70** Chronic embolism and thrombosis of **unspecified veins of upper extremity**

**I82.701** Chronic embolism and thrombosis of `CC` unspecified veins of **right** upper extremity

**I82.702** Chronic embolism and thrombosis of `CC` unspecified veins of **left** upper extremity

**I82.703** Chronic embolism and thrombosis of `CC` unspecified veins of upper extremity, **bilateral**

**I82.709** Chronic embolism and thrombosis of `CC` unspecified veins of **unspecified** upper extremity

✓6ᵗʰ **I82.71** Chronic embolism and thrombosis of **superficial veins of upper extremity**
Chronic embolism and thrombosis of antecubital vein
Chronic embolism and thrombosis of basilic vein
Chronic embolism and thrombosis of cephalic vein

**I82.711** Chronic embolism and thrombosis of `CC` superficial veins of **right** upper extremity

**I82.712** Chronic embolism and thrombosis of `CC` superficial veins of **left** upper extremity

**I82.713** Chronic embolism and thrombosis of `CC` superficial veins of upper extremity, **bilateral**

**I82.719** Chronic embolism and thrombosis of `CC` superficial veins of **unspecified** upper extremity

✓6ᵗʰ **I82.72** Chronic embolism and thrombosis of **deep veins** of upper extremity
Chronic embolism and thrombosis of brachial vein
Chronic embolism and thrombosis of radial vein
Chronic embolism and thrombosis of ulnar vein

**I82.721** Chronic embolism and thrombosis `CC` `HCC` of deep veins of **right** upper extremity

**I82.722** Chronic embolism and thrombosis `CC` `HCC` of deep veins of **left** upper extremity

**I82.723** Chronic embolism and thrombosis `CC` `HCC` of deep veins of **upper** extremity, **bilateral**

**I82.729** Chronic embolism and thrombosis `CC` `HCC` of deep veins of **unspecified** upper extremity

✓5ᵗʰ **I82.A** Embolism and thrombosis of **axillary vein**

**CC Excl: For CC codes in subcategory I82.A:**
PDX collection 717

✓6ᵗʰ **I82.A1** Acute **embolism and thrombosis of axillary vein**

**I82.A11** Acute embolism and thrombosis `CC` `HCC` of **right** axillary vein

**I82.A12** Acute embolism and thrombosis `CC` `HCC` of **left** axillary vein

**I82.A13** Acute embolism and thrombosis `CC` `HCC` of axillary vein, **bilateral**

Ⓝ Newborn: 0   Ⓟ Pediatric: 0-17   Ⓜ Maternity: 12-55   Ⓐ Adult: 15-124   `MCC` Major CC Condition   `PDxMCC` PDx acts as own MCC   `CC` CC Condition   `PDxCC` PDx acts as own CC

**662**                                                       ICD-10-CM 2018

I82.A19    **Acute embolism and thrombosis** `CC` `HCC`
of **unspecified axillary** vein

✓6ᵗʰ I82.A2    Chronic **embolism and thrombosis of axillary vein**

I82.A21    **Chronic embolism and thrombosis** `CC` `HCC`
of **right axillary** vein

I82.A22    **Chronic embolism and thrombosis** `CC` `HCC`
of **left axillary** vein

I82.A23    **Chronic embolism and thrombosis** `CC` `HCC`
of axillary vein, **bilateral**

I82.A29    **Chronic embolism and thrombosis** `CC` `HCC`
of **unspecified axillary** vein

✓5ᵗʰ I82.B    **Embolism and thrombosis of subclavian vein**

**CC Excl: For CC codes in subcategory I82.B:**
PDX collection 717

✓6ᵗʰ I82.B1    Acute **embolism and thrombosis of subclavian vein**

I82.B11    **Acute embolism and thrombosis** `CC` `HCC`
of **right subclavian** vein

I82.B12    **Acute embolism and thrombosis** `CC` `HCC`
of **left subclavian** vein

I82.B13    **Acute embolism and thrombosis** `CC` `HCC`
of subclavian vein, **bilateral**

I82.B19    **Acute embolism and thrombosis** `CC` `HCC`
of **unspecified subclavian** vein

✓6ᵗʰ I82.B2    Chronic **embolism and thrombosis of subclavian
vein**

I82.B21    **Chronic embolism and thrombosis** `CC` `HCC`
of **right subclavian** vein

I82.B22    **Chronic embolism and thrombosis** `CC` `HCC`
of **left subclavian** vein

I82.B23    **Chronic embolism and thrombosis** `CC` `HCC`
of subclavian vein, **bilateral**

I82.B29    **Chronic embolism and thrombosis** `CC` `HCC`
of **unspecified subclavian** vein

✓5ᵗʰ I82.C    **Embolism and thrombosis of internal jugular vein**

**CC Excl: For CC codes in subcategory I82.C:**
PDX collection 717

✓6ᵗʰ I82.C1    Acute **embolism and thrombosis of internal jugular
vein**

I82.C11    **Acute embolism and thrombosis** `CC` `HCC`
of **right internal jugular** vein

I82.C12    **Acute embolism and thrombosis** `CC` `HCC`
of **left internal jugular** vein

I82.C13    **Acute embolism and thrombosis** `CC` `HCC`
of internal jugular vein, **bilateral**

I82.C19    **Acute embolism and thrombosis** `CC` `HCC`
of **unspecified internal jugular** vein

✓6ᵗʰ I82.C2    Chronic **embolism and thrombosis of internal
jugular vein**

I82.C21    **Chronic embolism and thrombosis** `CC` `HCC`
of **right internal jugular** vein

I82.C22    **Chronic embolism and thrombosis** `CC` `HCC`
of **left internal jugular** vein

I82.C23    **Chronic embolism and thrombosis** `CC` `HCC`
of internal jugular vein, **bilateral**

I82.C29    **Chronic embolism and thrombosis** `CC` `HCC`
of **unspecified internal jugular** vein

✓5ᵗʰ I82.8    **Embolism and thrombosis of other specified veins**
Use additional code, if applicable, for associated long-term
(current) use of anticoagulants (Z79.01)

**CC Excl: For CC codes in subcategory I82.8:**
PDX collection 717

✓6ᵗʰ I82.81    **Embolism and thrombosis of superficial veins of
lower extremities**
Embolism and thrombosis of saphenous vein (greater)
(lesser)

▲    I82.811    **Embolism and thrombosis of** `CC`
**superficial veins of right lower
extremity**

▲    I82.812    **Embolism and thrombosis of** `CC`
**superficial veins of left lower
extremity**

I82.813    **Embolism and thrombosis of** `CC`
**superficial veins of lower
extremities, bilateral**

▲    I82.819    **Embolism and thrombosis of** `CC`
**superficial veins of unspecified
lower extremity**

✓6ᵗʰ I82.89    **Embolism and thrombosis of other specified veins**

I82.890    **Acute embolism and thrombosis of** `CC`
**other specified veins**

I82.891    **Chronic embolism and thrombosis of** `CC`
**other specified veins**

✓5ᵗʰ I82.9    **Embolism and thrombosis of unspecified vein**

**CC Excl: For CC codes in subcategory I82.9:**
PDX collection 717

I82.90    **Acute embolism and thrombosis of unspecified** `CC`
**vein**
Embolism of vein NOS
Thrombosis (vein) NOS

I82.91    **Chronic embolism and thrombosis of** `CC`
**unspecified vein**

✓4ᵗʰ **I83**    **Varicose veins of lower extremities**
EXCLUDES 1    varicose veins complicating pregnancy (O22.0-)
varicose veins complicating the puerperium (O87.4)

✓5ᵗʰ I83.0    **Varicose veins of lower extremities with ulcer**
Use additional code to identify severity of ulcer (L97.-)

✓6ᵗʰ I83.00    **Varicose veins of unspecified lower extremity with
ulcer**

I83.001    **Varicose veins of unspecified lower** `HCC` `A`
**extremity with ulcer of thigh**

I83.002    **Varicose veins of unspecified lower** `HCC` `A`
**extremity with ulcer of calf**

I83.003    **Varicose veins of unspecified lower** `HCC` `A`
**extremity with ulcer of ankle**

I83.004    **Varicose veins of unspecified lower** `HCC` `A`
**extremity with ulcer of heel and midfoot**
Varicose veins of unspecified lower
extremity with ulcer of plantar surface
of midfoot

I83.005    **Varicose veins of unspecified lower** `HCC` `A`
**extremity with ulcer other part of foot**
Varicose veins of unspecified lower
extremity with ulcer of toe

I83.008    **Varicose veins of unspecified lower** `HCC` `A`
**extremity with ulcer other part of
lower leg**

I83.009    **Varicose veins of unspecified lower** `HCC` `A`
**extremity with ulcer of unspecified site**

✓6ᵗʰ I83.01    **Varicose veins of right lower extremity with ulcer**

I83.011    **Varicose veins of right lower** `HCC` `A`
**extremity with ulcer of thigh**

I83.012    **Varicose veins of right lower** `HCC` `A`
**extremity with ulcer of calf**

I83.013    **Varicose veins of right lower** `HCC` `A`
**extremity with ulcer of ankle**

I83.014    **Varicose veins of right lower** `HCC` `A`
**extremity with ulcer of heel and midfoot**
Varicose veins of right lower extremity with
ulcer of plantar surface of midfoot

I83.015    **Varicose veins of right lower** `HCC` `A`
**extremity with ulcer other part of foot**
Varicose veins of right lower extremity with
ulcer of toe

I83.018    **Varicose veins of right lower** `HCC` `A`
**extremity with ulcer other part of lower
leg**

I83.019    **Varicose veins of right lower** `HCC` `A`
**extremity with ulcer of unspecified site**

✓6ᵗʰ I83.02    **Varicose veins of left lower extremity with ulcer**

I83.021    **Varicose veins of left lower** `HCC` `A`
**extremity with ulcer of thigh**

I83.022    **Varicose veins of left lower** `HCC` `A`
**extremity with ulcer of calf**

I83.023    **Varicose veins of left lower** `HCC` `A`
**extremity with ulcer of ankle**

I83.024    **Varicose veins of left lower** `HCC` `A`
**extremity with ulcer of heel and midfoot**
Varicose veins of left lower extremity with
ulcer of plantar surface of midfoot

**183.025**    Varicose veins of left lower    HCC A
extremity with ulcer other part of foot
     Varicose veins of left lower extremity with
ulcer of toe

**183.028**    Varicose veins of left lower    HCC A
extremity with ulcer other part of lower
leg

**183.029**    Varicose veins of left lower    HCC A
extremity with ulcer of unspecified site

✓5ᵗʰ **183.1**    Varicose veins of lower extremities with inflammation

**183.10**    Varicose veins of unspecified lower extremity    A
with inflammation

**183.11**    Varicose veins of right lower extremity with    A
inflammation

**183.12**    Varicose veins of left lower extremity with    A
inflammation

✓5ᵗʰ **183.2**    Varicose veins of lower extremities with both ulcer and
inflammation
     Use additional code to identify severity of ulcer (L97.-)

> **CC Excl: For CC codes in subcategory 183.2:**
> PDX collection 720

✓6ᵗʰ **183.20**    Varicose veins of unspecified lower extremity with
both ulcer and inflammation

**183.201**    Varicose veins of unspecified    CC HCC A
lower extremity with both ulcer of thigh
and inflammation

**183.202**    Varicose veins of unspecified    CC HCC A
lower extremity with both ulcer of calf and
inflammation

**183.203**    Varicose veins of unspecified    CC HCC A
lower extremity with both ulcer of ankle
and inflammation

**183.204**    Varicose veins of unspecified    CC HCC A
lower extremity with both ulcer of heel
and midfoot and inflammation
     Varicose veins of unspecified lower
extremity with both ulcer of plantar
surface of midfoot and inflammation

**183.205**    Varicose veins of unspecified    CC HCC A
lower extremity with both ulcer of other
part of foot and inflammation
     Varicose veins of unspecified lower
extremity with both ulcer of toe and
inflammation

**183.208**    Varicose veins of unspecified    CC HCC A
lower extremity with both ulcer
of other part of lower extremity and
inflammation

**183.209**    Varicose veins of unspecified    CC HCC A
lower extremity with both ulcer of
unspecified site and inflammation

✓6ᵗʰ **183.21**    Varicose veins of right lower extremity with both
ulcer and inflammation

**183.211**    Varicose veins of right lower    CC HCC A
extremity with both ulcer of thigh
and inflammation

**183.212**    Varicose veins of right lower    CC HCC A
extremity with both ulcer of calf
and inflammation

**183.213**    Varicose veins of right lower    CC HCC A
extremity with both ulcer of ankle
and inflammation

**183.214**    Varicose veins of right lower    CC HCC A
extremity with both ulcer of heel
and midfoot and inflammation
     Varicose veins of right lower extremity with
both ulcer of plantar surface of
midfoot and inflammation

**183.215**    Varicose veins of right lower    CC HCC A
extremity with both ulcer other
part of foot and inflammation
     Varicose veins of right lower extremity with
both ulcer of toe and inflammation

**183.218**    Varicose veins of right lower    CC HCC A
extremity with both ulcer of other
part of lower extremity and
inflammation

**183.219**    Varicose veins of right lower    CC HCC A
extremity with both ulcer of
unspecified site and inflammation

✓6ᵗʰ **183.22**    Varicose veins of left lower extremity with both ulcer
and inflammation

**183.221**    Varicose veins of left lower    CC HCC A
extremity with both ulcer of thigh
and inflammation

**183.222**    Varicose veins of left lower    CC HCC A
extremity with both ulcer of calf
and inflammation

**183.223**    Varicose veins of left lower    CC HCC A
extremity with both ulcer of ankle
and inflammation

**183.224**    Varicose veins of left lower    CC HCC A
extremity with both ulcer of heel and
midfoot and inflammation
     Varicose veins of left lower extremity with
both ulcer of plantar surface of
midfoot and inflammation

**183.225**    Varicose veins of left lower    CC HCC A
extremity with both ulcer other
part of foot and inflammation
     Varicose veins of left lower extremity with
both ulcer of toe and inflammation

**183.228**    Varicose veins of left lower    CC HCC A
extremity with both ulcer of other
part of lower extremity and
inflammation

**183.229**    Varicose veins of left lower    CC HCC A
extremity with both ulcer of
unspecified site and inflammation

✓5ᵗʰ **183.8**    Varicose veins of lower extremities with other complications

✓6ᵗʰ **183.81**    Varicose veins of lower extremities with pain

▲ **183.811**    Varicose veins of right lower    A
extremity with pain

▲ **183.812**    Varicose veins of left lower extremity    A
with pain

**183.813**    Varicose veins of bilateral lower    A
extremities with pain

▲ **183.819**    Varicose veins of unspecified lower    A
extremity with pain

✓6ᵗʰ **183.89**    Varicose veins of lower extremities with other
complications
     Varicose veins of lower extremities with edema
     Varicose veins of lower extremities with swelling

▲ **183.891**    Varicose veins of right lower    A
extremity with other complications

▲ **183.892**    Varicose veins of left lower extremity    A
with other complications

**183.893**    Varicose veins of bilateral lower    A
extremities with other complications

▲ **183.899**    Varicose veins of unspecified lower    A
extremity with other complications

✓5ᵗʰ **183.9**    Asymptomatic varicose veins of lower extremities
     Phlebectasia of lower extremities
     Varicose veins of lower extremities
     Varix of lower extremities

**183.90**    Asymptomatic varicose veins of unspecified    A
lower extremity
     Varicose veins NOS

**183.91**    Asymptomatic varicose veins of right lower    A
extremity

**183.92**    Asymptomatic varicose veins of left lower    A
extremity

**183.93**    Asymptomatic varicose veins of bilateral lower    A
extremities

✓4ᵗʰ **185**    **Esophageal varices**
     Use additional code to identify:
       alcohol abuse and dependence (F10.-)

✓5ᵗʰ **185.0**    **Esophageal varices**
     Idiopathic esophageal varices
     Primary esophageal varices

**185.00**    Esophageal varices without bleeding    CC HCC
     Esophageal varices NOS
     **CC Excl:** PDX collection 721

**185.01**    Esophageal varices with bleeding    MCC HCC
     **CC Excl:** PDX collection 722

N Newborn: 0    P Pediatric: 0-17    M Maternity: 12-55    A Adult: 15-124    MCC Major CC Condition    PDxMCC PDx acts as own MCC    CC CC Condition    PDxCC PDx acts as own CC

**664**          ICD-10-CM 2018

✓5ᵗʰ **I85.1 Secondary esophageal varices**
Esophageal varices secondary to alcoholic liver disease
Esophageal varices secondary to cirrhosis of liver
Esophageal varices secondary to schistosomiasis
Esophageal varices secondary to toxic liver disease
Code first underlying disease

     **I85.10 Secondary esophageal varices without bleeding** `CC` `HCC`
         CC Excl: PDX collection 723

     **I85.11 Secondary esophageal varices with bleeding** `MCC` `HCC`
         CC Excl: PDX collection 724

✓4ᵗʰ **I86 Varicose veins of other sites**
   **EXCLUDES 1**   varicose veins of unspecified site (I83.9-)
   **EXCLUDES 2**   retinal varices (H35.0-)

   **I86.0 Sublingual varices**
     DEF: Distended, tortuous veins beneath tongue.

   **I86.1 Scrotal varices**      ♂
     Varicocele

   **I86.2 Pelvic varices**

   **I86.3 Vulval varices**      ♀
     **EXCLUDES 1**   vulval varices complicating childbirth and the puerperium (O87.8)
         vulval varices complicating pregnancy (O22.1-)

   **I86.4 Gastric varices**

   **I86.8 Varicose veins of other specified sites**    `A`
     Varicose ulcer of nasal septum

✓4ᵗʰ **I87 Other disorders of veins**

✓5ᵗʰ **I87.0 Postthrombotic syndrome**
Chronic venous hypertension due to deep vein thrombosis
Postphlebitic syndrome
   **EXCLUDES 1**   chronic venous hypertension without deep vein thrombosis (I87.3-)

**CC Excl: For CC codes in subcategory I87.0:**
PDX collection 725

✓6ᵗʰ **I87.00 Postthrombotic syndrome without complications**
Asymptomatic postthrombotic syndrome
   **I87.001 Postthrombotic syndrome without complications of right lower extremity**
   **I87.002 Postthrombotic syndrome without complications of left lower extremity**
   **I87.003 Postthrombotic syndrome without complications of bilateral lower extremity**
   **I87.009 Postthrombotic syndrome without complications of unspecified extremity**
     Postthrombotic syndrome NOS

✓6ᵗʰ **I87.01 Postthrombotic syndrome with ulcer**
Use additional code to specify site and severity of ulcer (L97.-)
   **I87.011 Postthrombotic syndrome with ulcer of right lower extremity** `CC` `HCC`
   **I87.012 Postthrombotic syndrome with ulcer of left lower extremity** `CC` `HCC`
   **I87.013 Postthrombotic syndrome with ulcer of bilateral lower extremity** `CC` `HCC`
   **I87.019 Postthrombotic syndrome with ulcer of unspecified lower extremity** `CC` `HCC`

✓6ᵗʰ **I87.02 Postthrombotic syndrome with inflammation**
   **I87.021 Postthrombotic syndrome with inflammation of right lower extremity**
   **I87.022 Postthrombotic syndrome with inflammation of left lower extremity**
   **I87.023 Postthrombotic syndrome with inflammation of bilateral lower extremity**
   **I87.029 Postthrombotic syndrome with inflammation of unspecified lower extremity**

✓6ᵗʰ **I87.03 Postthrombotic syndrome with ulcer and inflammation**
Use additional code to specify site and severity of ulcer (L97.-)
   **I87.031 Postthrombotic syndrome with ulcer and inflammation of right lower extremity** `CC` `HCC`
   **I87.032 Postthrombotic syndrome with ulcer and inflammation of left lower extremity** `CC` `HCC`

   **I87.033 Postthrombotic syndrome with ulcer and inflammation of bilateral lower extremity** `CC` `HCC`
   **I87.039 Postthrombotic syndrome with ulcer and inflammation of unspecified lower extremity** `CC` `HCC`

✓6ᵗʰ **I87.09 Postthrombotic syndrome with other complications**
   **I87.091 Postthrombotic syndrome with other complications of right lower extremity**
   **I87.092 Postthrombotic syndrome with other complications of left lower extremity**
   **I87.093 Postthrombotic syndrome with other complications of bilateral lower extremity**
   **I87.099 Postthrombotic syndrome with other complications of unspecified lower extremity**

**I87.1 Compression of vein**    `CC`
Stricture of vein
Vena cava syndrome (inferior) (superior)
   **EXCLUDES 2**   compression of pulmonary vein (I28.8)
CC Excl: PDX collection 726

**I87.2 Venous insufficiency (chronic) (peripheral)**
Stasis dermatitis
   **EXCLUDES 1**   stasis dermatitis with varicose veins of lower extremities (I83.1-, I83.2-)
DEF: Insufficient drainage of venous blood in any part of body; results in edema or dermatosis.

✓5ᵗʰ **I87.3 Chronic venous hypertension (idiopathic)**
Stasis edema
   **EXCLUDES 1**   chronic venous hypertension due to deep vein thrombosis (I87.0-)
         varicose veins of lower extremities (I83.-)

**CC Excl: For CC codes in subcategory I87.3:**
PDX collection 727

✓6ᵗʰ **I87.30 Chronic venous hypertension (idiopathic) without complications**
Asymptomatic chronic venous hypertension (idiopathic)
   **I87.301 Chronic venous hypertension (idiopathic) without complications of right lower extremity**
   **I87.302 Chronic venous hypertension (idiopathic) without complications of left lower extremity**
   **I87.303 Chronic venous hypertension (idiopathic) without complications of bilateral lower extremity**
   **I87.309 Chronic venous hypertension (idiopathic) without complications of unspecified lower extremity**
     Chronic venous hypertension NOS

✓6ᵗʰ **I87.31 Chronic venous hypertension (idiopathic) with ulcer**
Use additional code to specify site and severity of ulcer (L97.-)
   **I87.311 Chronic venous hypertension (idiopathic) with ulcer of right lower extremity** `CC` `HCC`
   **I87.312 Chronic venous hypertension (idiopathic) with ulcer of left lower extremity** `CC` `HCC`
   **I87.313 Chronic venous hypertension (idiopathic) with ulcer of bilateral lower extremity** `CC` `HCC`
   **I87.319 Chronic venous hypertension (idiopathic) with ulcer of unspecified lower extremity** `CC` `HCC`

✓6ᵗʰ **I87.32 Chronic venous hypertension (idiopathic) with inflammation**
   **I87.321 Chronic venous hypertension (idiopathic) with inflammation of right lower extremity**
   **I87.322 Chronic venous hypertension (idiopathic) with inflammation of left lower extremity**
   **I87.323 Chronic venous hypertension (idiopathic) with inflammation of bilateral lower extremity**
   **I87.329 Chronic venous hypertension (idiopathic) with inflammation of unspecified lower extremity**

✓ Additional Character Req   ✓x7ᵗʰ Placeholder Alert   Unacceptable PDx   Manifestation   **H1**-**H14** HAC   **HCC** CMS-HCC Condition   **EXCLUDES 1** Not Coded Here   **EXCLUDES 2** Not Included Here
ICD-10-CM 2018      665
I85.1–I87.329

**Chapter 9. Diseases of the Circulatory System**

**I87.33–I97.191**

✓6ᵗʰ **I87.33   Chronic venous hypertension (idiopathic) with ulcer and inflammation**
> Use additional code to specify site and severity of ulcer (L97.-)

    **I87.331   Chronic venous hypertension (idiopathic) with ulcer and inflammation of right lower extremity**   CC HCC

    **I87.332   Chronic venous hypertension (idiopathic) with ulcer and inflammation of left lower extremity**   CC HCC

    **I87.333   Chronic venous hypertension (idiopathic) with ulcer and inflammation of bilateral lower extremity**   CC HCC

    **I87.339   Chronic venous hypertension (idiopathic) with ulcer and inflammation of unspecified lower extremity**   CC HCC

✓6ᵗʰ **I87.39   Chronic venous hypertension (idiopathic) with other complications**

    **I87.391   Chronic venous hypertension (idiopathic) with other complications of right lower extremity**

    **I87.392   Chronic venous hypertension (idiopathic) with other complications of left lower extremity**

    **I87.393   Chronic venous hypertension (idiopathic) with other complications of bilateral lower extremity**

    **I87.399   Chronic venous hypertension (idiopathic) with other complications of unspecified lower extremity**

**I87.8   Other specified disorders of veins**
> Phlebosclerosis
> Venofibrosis

**I87.9   Disorder of vein, unspecified**

✓4ᵗʰ **I88   Nonspecific lymphadenitis**
> *EXCLUDES 1*   *acute lymphadenitis, except mesenteric (L04.-)*
> *enlarged lymph nodes NOS (R59.-)*
> *human immunodeficiency virus [HIV] disease resulting in generalized lymphadenopathy (B20)*

**I88.0   Nonspecific mesenteric lymphadenitis**
> Mesenteric lymphadenitis (acute)(chronic)

**I88.1   Chronic lymphadenitis, except mesenteric**
> Adenitis
> Lymphadenitis

**I88.8   Other nonspecific lymphadenitis**

**I88.9   Nonspecific lymphadenitis, unspecified**
> Lymphadenitis NOS

✓4ᵗʰ **I89   Other noninfective disorders of lymphatic vessels and lymph nodes**
> *EXCLUDES 1*   *chylocele, tunica vaginalis (nonfilarial) NOS (N50.89)*
> *enlarged lymph nodes NOS (R59.-)*
> *filarial chylocele (B74.-)*
> *hereditary lymphedema (Q82.0)*

**I89.0   Lymphedema, not elsewhere classified**
> Elephantiasis (nonfilarial) NOS
> Lymphangiectasis
> Obliteration, lymphatic vessel
> Praecox lymphedema
> Secondary lymphedema
> *EXCLUDES 1*   *postmastectomy lymphedema (I97.2)*

**I89.1   Lymphangitis**
> Chronic lymphangitis
> Lymphangitis NOS
> Subacute lymphangitis
> *EXCLUDES 1*   *acute lymphangitis (L03.-)*

**I89.8   Other specified noninfective disorders of lymphatic vessels and lymph nodes**
> Chylocele (nonfilarial)
> Chylous ascites
> Chylous cyst
> Lipomelanotic reticulosis
> Lymph node or vessel fistula
> Lymph node or vessel infarction
> Lymph node or vessel rupture

**I89.9   Noninfective disorder of lymphatic vessels and lymph nodes, unspecified**
> Disease of lymphatic vessels NOS

## Other and unspecified disorders of the circulatory system (I95-I99)

✓4ᵗʰ **I95   Hypotension**
> *EXCLUDES 1*   *cardiovascular collapse (R57.9)*
> *maternal hypotension syndrome (O26.5-)*
> *nonspecific low blood pressure reading NOS (R03.1)*

**I95.0   Idiopathic hypotension**

**I95.1   Orthostatic hypotension**
> Hypotension, postural
> *EXCLUDES 1*   *neurogenic orthostatic hypotension [Shy-Drager] (G90.3)*
> *orthostatic hypotension due to drugs (I95.2)*

**I95.2   Hypotension due to drugs**
> Orthostatic hypotension due to drugs
> Use additional code for adverse effect, if applicable, to identify drug (T36-T50 with fifth or sixth character 5)

**I95.3   Hypotension of hemodialysis**
> Intra-dialytic hypotension

✓5ᵗʰ **I95.8   Other hypotension**

    **I95.81   Postprocedural hypotension**

    **I95.89   Other hypotension**
> Chronic hypotension

**I95.9   Hypotension, unspecified**

**I96   Gangrene, not elsewhere classified**   CC HCC
> Gangrenous cellulitis
> *EXCLUDES 1*   *gangrene in atherosclerosis of native arteries of the extremities (I70.26)*
> *gangrene in diabetes mellitus (E08-E13 with .52)*
> *gangrene in hernia (K40.1, K40.4, K41.1, K41.4, K42.1, K43.1-, K44.1, K45.1, K46.1)*
> *gangrene in other peripheral vascular diseases (I73.-)*
> *gangrene of certain specified sites—see Alphabetical Index*
> *gas gangrene (A48.0)*
> *pyoderma gangrenosum (L88)*
> *EXCLUDES 2*   ►*gangrene in diabetes mellitus (E08-E13 with .52)*◄
> **AHA:** 2013, 2Q, 34
> **CC Excl:** PDX collection 519

✓4ᵗʰ **I97   Intraoperative and postprocedural complications and disorders of circulatory system, not elsewhere classified**
> *EXCLUDES 2*   *postprocedural shock (T81.1-)*

**I97.0   Postcardiotomy syndrome**

✓5ᵗʰ **I97.1   Other postprocedural cardiac functional disturbances**
> *EXCLUDES 2*   *acute pulmonary insufficiency following thoracic surgery (J95.1)*
> *intraoperative cardiac functional disturbances (I97.7-)*

> **CC Excl: For CC codes in subcategory I97.1:**
> PDX collection 728

✓6ᵗʰ **I97.11   Postprocedural cardiac insufficiency**

    **I97.110   Postprocedural cardiac insufficiency following cardiac surgery**   CC

    **I97.111   Postprocedural cardiac insufficiency following other surgery**   CC

✓6ᵗʰ **I97.12   Postprocedural cardiac arrest**

    **I97.120   Postprocedural cardiac arrest following cardiac surgery**   CC

    **I97.121   Postprocedural cardiac arrest following other surgery**   CC

✓6ᵗʰ **I97.13   Postprocedural heart failure**
> Use additional code to identify the heart failure (I50.-)

    **I97.130   Postprocedural heart failure following cardiac surgery**   CC

    **I97.131   Postprocedural heart failure following other surgery**   CC

✓6ᵗʰ **I97.19   Other postprocedural cardiac functional disturbances**
> Use additional code, if applicable, to further specify disorder

    **I97.190   Other postprocedural cardiac functional disturbances following cardiac surgery**   CC
> ►Use additional code, if applicable, for type 4 or type 5 myocardial infarction, to further specify disorder◄

    **I97.191   Other postprocedural cardiac functional disturbances following other surgery**   CC

N Newborn: 0    P Pediatric: 0-17    M Maternity: 12-55    A Adult: 15-124    MCC Major CC Condition    PDxMCC PDx acts as own MCC    CC CC Condition    PDxCC PDx acts as own CC

666          ICD-10-CM 2018

**I97.2** **Postmastectomy lymphedema syndrome** A
Elephantiasis due to mastectomy
Obliteration of lymphatic vessels

**I97.3** **Postprocedural hypertension**

✓5th **I97.4** **Intraoperative hemorrhage and hematoma of a circulatory system organ or structure complicating a procedure**
EXCLUDES 1   *intraoperative hemorrhage and hematoma of a circulatory system organ or structure due to accidental puncture and laceration during a procedure (I97.5-)*
EXCLUDES 2   *intraoperative cerebrovascular hemorrhage complicating a procedure (G97.3-)*

CC Excl: For CC codes in subcategory I97.4:
PDX collection 729

✓6th **I97.41** **Intraoperative hemorrhage and hematoma of a circulatory system organ or structure complicating a circulatory system procedure**
**I97.410** **Intraoperative hemorrhage and hematoma of a circulatory system organ or structure complicating a cardiac catheterization** CC
**I97.411** **Intraoperative hemorrhage and hematoma of a circulatory system organ or structure complicating a cardiac bypass** CC
**I97.418** **Intraoperative hemorrhage and hematoma of a circulatory system organ or structure complicating** other circulatory system procedure CC

**I97.42** **Intraoperative hemorrhage and hematoma of a circulatory system organ or structure complicating other procedure** CC

✓5th **I97.5** **Accidental puncture and laceration of a circulatory system organ or structure during a procedure**
EXCLUDES 2   *accidental puncture and laceration of brain during a procedure (G97.4-)*
**I97.51** **Accidental puncture and laceration of a circulatory system organ or structure during a circulatory system procedure** CC
CC Excl: PDX collection 509
**I97.52** **Accidental puncture and laceration of a circulatory system organ or structure during** other procedure CC
CC Excl: PDX collection 509

✓5th **I97.6** **Postprocedural hemorrhage, hematoma and seroma of a circulatory system organ or structure following a procedure**
EXCLUDES 2   *postprocedural cerebrovascular hemorrhage complicating a procedure (G97.5-)*

CC Excl: For CC codes in subcategory I97.6:
PDX collection 729

✓6th **I97.61** **Postprocedural** hemorrhage **of a circulatory system organ or structure following a** circulatory system procedure
**I97.610** **Postprocedural hemorrhage of a circulatory system organ or structure following a** cardiac catheterization CC
**I97.611** **Postprocedural hemorrhage of a circulatory system organ or structure following** cardiac bypass CC
**I97.618** **Postprocedural hemorrhage of a circulatory system organ or structure following** other circulatory system procedure CC

✓6th **I97.62** **Postprocedural hemorrhage, hematoma and seroma of a circulatory system organ or structure following** other procedure
**I97.620** **Postprocedural** hemorrhage **of a circulatory system organ or structure following other procedure** CC
**I97.621** **Postprocedural** hematoma **of a circulatory system organ or structure following other procedure** CC
**I97.622** **Postprocedural** seroma **of a circulatory system organ or structure following procedure** CC

✓6th **I97.63** **Postprocedural hematoma of a circulatory system organ or structure following a** circulatory system procedure
**I97.630** **Postprocedural hematoma of a circulatory system organ or structure following a** cardiac catheterization CC
**I97.631** **Postprocedural hematoma of a circulatory system organ or structure following** cardiac bypass CC
**I97.638** **Postprocedural hematoma of a circulatory system organ or structure following** other circulatory system procedure CC

✓6th **I97.64** **Postprocedural seroma of a circulatory system organ or structure following a circulatory system procedure**
**I97.640** **Postprocedural seroma of a circulatory system organ or structure following a** cardiac catheterization CC
**I97.641** **Postprocedural seroma of a circulatory system organ or structure following** cardiac bypass CC
**I97.648** **Postprocedural seroma of a circulatory system organ or structure following** other circulatory system procedure CC

✓5th **I97.7** **Intraoperative** cardiac **functional disturbances**
EXCLUDES 2   *acute pulmonary insufficiency following thoracic surgery (J95.1)*
*postprocedural cardiac functional disturbances (I97.1-)*

CC Excl: For CC codes in subcategory I97.7:
PDX collection 728

✓6th **I97.71** **Intraoperative** cardiac arrest
**I97.710** **Intraoperative cardiac arrest during cardiac surgery** CC
**I97.711** **Intraoperative cardiac arrest during other surgery** CC

✓6th **I97.79** **Other** intraoperative cardiac functional disturbances
Use additional code, if applicable, to further specify disorder
**I97.790** **Other intraoperative cardiac functional disturbances during cardiac surgery** CC
**I97.791** **Other intraoperative cardiac functional disturbances during** other surgery CC

✓5th **I97.8** **Other intraoperative and postprocedural complications and disorders of the circulatory system, not elsewhere classified**
Use additional code, if applicable, to further specify disorder

CC Excl: For CC codes in subcategory I97.8, unless otherwise noted: PDX collection 617

✓6th **I97.81** **Intraoperative** cerebrovascular infarction
**I97.810** **Intraoperative cerebrovascular infarction during** cardiac surgery CC HCC
**I97.811** **Intraoperative cerebrovascular infarction during** other surgery CC HCC

✓6th **I97.82** **Postprocedural** cerebrovascular infarction
**I97.820** **Postprocedural cerebrovascular infarction following** cardiac surgery CC HCC
**I97.821** **Postprocedural cerebrovascular infarction following** other surgery CC HCC

**I97.88** **Other intraoperative complications of the circulatory system, not elsewhere classified** CC
CC Excl: PDX collection 728

**I97.89** **Other postprocedural complications and disorders of the circulatory system, not elsewhere classified** CC
CC Excl: PDX collection 728

✓4th **I99** **Other and unspecified disorders of circulatory system**
**I99.8** **Other disorder of circulatory system**
**I99.9** **Unspecified disorder of circulatory system**

# Chapter 10. Diseases of the Respiratory System (J00–J99)

## Chapter Specific Guidelines with Coding Examples

The chapter specific guidelines from the ICD-10-CM Official Guidelines for Coding and Reporting have been provided below. Along with these guidelines are coding examples, contained in the shaded boxes, that have been developed to help illustrate the coding and/or sequencing guidance found in these guidelines.

### a. Chronic obstructive pulmonary disease [COPD] and asthma

#### 1) Acute exacerbation of chronic obstructive bronchitis and asthma

The codes in categories J44 and J45 distinguish between uncomplicated cases and those in acute exacerbation. An acute exacerbation is a worsening or a decompensation of a chronic condition. An acute exacerbation is not equivalent to an infection superimposed on a chronic condition, though an exacerbation may be triggered by an infection.

---

Vancomycin IV was started to treat a patient with acute pneumonia due to *Streptococcus pneumoniae*. Patient also with acute exacerbation of COPD continued on home meds.

| J13 | Pneumonia due to Streptococcus pneumoniae |
|---|---|
| J44.0 | Chronic obstructive pulmonary disease with acute lower respiratory infection |
| J44.1 | Chronic obstructive pulmonary disease with (acute) exacerbation |

*Explanation*: ICD-10-CM uses combination codes to create organism-specific classifications for acute pneumonia. Category J44 codes include combination codes with severity components, which differentiate between COPD with acute lower respiratory infection (acute pneumonia), COPD with acute exacerbation, and COPD without mention of a complication (unspecified).

An acute exacerbation is a worsening or a decompensation of a chronic condition. An acute exacerbation is not equivalent to an infection superimposed on a chronic condition, though an exacerbation may be triggered by an infection, as in this example. Treatment of the pneumonia necessitated the inpatient admission. Instructional notes at J44.0 say to "code also to identify the infection," which informs the coder that another code must be assigned if applicable. Sequencing of the pneumonia and COPD exacerbation are governed by the Section II, "Selection of Principal Diagnosis," guidelines. In this case it was the pneumonia that was "chiefly responsible for occasioning the admission" with the IV vancomycin treatment.

---

Exacerbation of moderate persistent asthma with status asthmaticus

| J45.42 | Moderate persistent asthma with status asthmaticus |
|---|---|

*Explanation*: Category J45 Asthma includes severity-specific subcategories and fifth-character codes to distinguish between uncomplicated cases, those in acute exacerbation, and those with status asthmaticus.

---

### b. Acute respiratory failure

#### 1) Acute respiratory failure as principal diagnosis

A code from subcategory J96.0, Acute respiratory failure, or subcategory J96.2, Acute and chronic respiratory failure, may be assigned as a principal diagnosis when it is the condition established after study to be chiefly responsible for occasioning the admission to the hospital, and the selection is supported by the Alphabetic Index and Tabular List. However, chapter-specific coding guidelines (such as obstetrics, poisoning, HIV, newborn) that provide sequencing direction take precedence.

---

Acute hypoxic respiratory failure due to COPD exacerbation

| J96.01 | Acute respiratory failure with hypoxia |
|---|---|
| J44.1 | Chronic obstructive pulmonary disease with (acute) exacerbation |

*Explanation*: Category J96 classifies respiratory failure with combination codes that designate the severity and the presence of hypoxia and hypercapnia. Code J96.01 is sequenced as the first-listed diagnosis, as the reason for the admission. Respiratory failure may be assigned as a principal diagnosis when it is the condition established after study to be chiefly responsible for occasioning the admission to the hospital and the selection is supported by the Alphabetic Index and Tabular List.

---

#### 2) Acute respiratory failure as secondary diagnosis

Respiratory failure may be listed as a secondary diagnosis if it occurs after admission, or if it is present on admission, but does not meet the definition of principal diagnosis.

---

Acute respiratory failure due to accidental oxycodone overdose

| T40.2X1A | Poisoning by other opioids, accidental (unintentional), initial encounter |
|---|---|
| J96.00 | Acute respiratory failure, unspecified whether with hypoxia or hypercapnia |

*Explanation*: Respiratory failure may be assigned as a principal diagnosis when it is the condition established after study to be chiefly responsible for occasioning the admission to the hospital, and the selection is supported by the Alphabetic Index and Tabular List. However, chapter-specific coding guidelines, such as poisoning, that provide sequencing direction take precedence. When coding a poisoning or reaction to the improper use of a medication (e.g. overdose, wrong substance given or taken in error, wrong route of administration), first assign the appropriate code from categories T36–T50. Use additional code(s) for all manifestations of the poisoning. In this instance, the respiratory failure is a manifestation of the poisoning and is sequenced as a secondary diagnosis.

---

Acute pneumococcal pneumonia with subsequent development of acute respiratory failure

| J13 | Pneumonia due to Streptococcus pneumoniae |
|---|---|
| J96.00 | Acute respiratory failure, unspecified whether with hypoxia or hypercapnia |

*Explanation*: Acute respiratory failure may be listed as a secondary diagnosis if it occurs after admission, or if it is present on admission but does not meet the definition of principal diagnosis.

---

#### 3) Sequencing of acute respiratory failure and another acute condition

When a patient is admitted with respiratory failure and another acute condition, (e.g., myocardial infarction, cerebrovascular accident, aspiration pneumonia), the principal diagnosis will not be the same in every situation. This applies whether the other acute condition is a respiratory or nonrespiratory condition. Selection of the principal diagnosis will be dependent on the circumstances of admission. If both the respiratory failure and the other acute condition are equally responsible for occasioning the admission to the hospital, and there are no chapter-specific sequencing rules, the guideline regarding two or more diagnoses that equally meet the definition for principal diagnosis (Section II, C.) may be applied in these situations.

If the documentation is not clear as to whether acute respiratory failure and another condition are equally responsible for occasioning the admission, query the provider for clarification.

---

Acute pneumococcal pneumonia and acute respiratory failure, both present on admission

| J96.00 | Acute respiratory failure, unspecified whether with hypoxia or hypercapnia |
|---|---|
| J13 | Pneumonia due to Streptococcus pneumoniae |

*Explanation*: When a patient is admitted with respiratory failure and another acute condition, such as a bacterial pneumonia, the principal diagnosis is not the same in every situation. This applies whether the other acute condition is a respiratory or nonrespiratory condition. The principal diagnosis depends on the circumstances of admission.

---

### c. Influenza due to certain identified influenza viruses

Code only confirmed cases of influenza due to certain identified influenza viruses (category J09), and due to other identified influenza virus (category J10). This is an exception to the hospital inpatient guideline Section II, H. (Uncertain Diagnosis).

In this context, "confirmation" does not require documentation of positive laboratory testing specific for avian or other novel influenza A or other identified influenza virus. However, coding should be based on the provider's diagnostic statement that the patient has avian influenza, or other novel influenza A, for category J09, or has another particular identified strain of influenza, such as H1N1 or H3N2, but not identified as novel or variant, for category J10.

If the provider records "suspected" or "possible" or "probable" avian influenza, or novel influenza, or other identified influenza, then the appropriate influenza code from category J11, Influenza due to unidentified influenza virus, should be assigned. A code from category J09, Influenza due to certain identified influenza viruses, should not be assigned nor should a code from category J10, Influenza due to other identified influenza virus.

---

Influenza due to avian influenza virus with pneumonia

**J09.X1**      **Influenza due to identified novel influenza A virus with pneumonia**

*Explanation*: Codes in category J09 Influenza due to certain identified influenza viruses should be assigned only for confirmed cases. "Confirmation" does not require positive laboratory testing of a specific influenza virus but does need to be based on the provider's diagnostic statement, which should not include terms such as "possible," "probable," or "suspected."

---

### d. Ventilator associated pneumonia

#### 1) Documentation of ventilator associated pneumonia

As with all procedural or postprocedural complications, code assignment is based on the provider's documentation of the relationship between the condition and the procedure.

Code J95.851, Ventilator associated pneumonia, should be assigned only when the provider has documented ventilator associated pneumonia (VAP). An additional code to identify the organism (e.g., Pseudomonas aeruginosa, code B96.5) should also be assigned. Do not assign an additional code from categories J12-J18 to identify the type of pneumonia.

Code J95.851 should not be assigned for cases where the patient has pneumonia and is on a mechanical ventilator and the provider has not specifically stated that the pneumonia is ventilator-associated pneumonia. If the documentation is unclear as to whether the patient has a pneumonia that is a complication attributable to the mechanical ventilator, query the provider.

#### 2) Ventilator associated pneumonia develops after admission

A patient may be admitted with one type of pneumonia (e.g., code J13, Pneumonia due to Streptococcus pneumonia) and subsequently develop VAP. In this instance, the principal diagnosis would be the appropriate code from categories J12-J18 for the pneumonia diagnosed at the time of admission. Code J95.851, Ventilator associated pneumonia, would be assigned as an additional diagnosis when the provider has also documented the presence of ventilator associated pneumonia.

---

Patient with pneumonia due to *Klebsiella pneumoniae* develops superimposed MRSA ventilator-associated pneumonia

**J15.0**      **Pneumonia due to Klebsiella pneumoniae**

**J95.851**      **Ventilator associated pneumonia**

**B95.62**      **Methicillin resistant Staphylococcus aureus infection as the cause of diseases classified elsewhere**

*Explanation*: Code assignment for ventilator-associated pneumonia is based on the provider's documentation of the relationship between the condition and the procedure and is reported only when the provider has documented ventilator-associated pneumonia (VAP).

A patient may be admitted with one type of pneumonia and subsequently develop VAP. In this example, the principal diagnosis code describes the pneumonia diagnosed at the time of admission, with code J95.851 Ventilator associated pneumonia, assigned as secondary.

---

# Chapter 10. Diseases of the Respiratory System (J00-J99)

**NOTE** When a respiratory condition is described as occurring in more than one site and is not specifically indexed, it should be classified to the lower anatomic site (e.g. tracheobronchitis to bronchitis in J40).

Use additional code, where applicable, to identify:
exposure to environmental tobacco smoke (Z77.22)
exposure to tobacco smoke in the perinatal period (P96.81)
history of tobacco dependence (Z87.891)
occupational exposure to environmental tobacco smoke (Z57.31)
tobacco dependence (F17.-)
tobacco use (Z72.0)

*EXCLUDES 2*   *certain conditions originating in the perinatal period (P04-P96)*
*certain infectious and parasitic diseases (A00-B99)*
*complications of pregnancy, childbirth and the puerperium (O00-O9A)*
*congenital malformations, deformations and chromosomal abnormalities (Q00-Q99)*
*endocrine, nutritional and metabolic diseases (E00-E88)*
*injury, poisoning and certain other consequences of external causes (S00-T88)*
*neoplasms (C00-D49)*
*smoke inhalation (T59.81-)*
*symptoms, signs and abnormal clinical and laboratory findings, not elsewhere classified (R00-R94)*

This chapter contains the following blocks:
J00-J06    Acute upper respiratory infections
J09-J18    Influenza and pneumonia
J20-J22    Other acute lower respiratory infections
J30-J39    Other diseases of upper respiratory tract
J40-J47    Chronic lower respiratory diseases
J60-J70    Lung diseases due to external agents
J80-J84    Other respiratory diseases principally affecting the interstitium
J85-J86    Suppurative and necrotic conditions of the lower respiratory tract
J90-J94    Other diseases of the pleura
J95    Intraoperative and postprocedural complications and disorders of respiratory system, not elsewhere classified
J96-J99    Other diseases of the respiratory system

### Acute upper respiratory infections (J00-J06)

*EXCLUDES 1*   *chronic obstructive pulmonary disease with acute lower respiratory infection (J44.0)*
*influenza virus with other respiratory manifestations (J09.X2, J10.1, J11.1)*

**J00   Acute nasopharyngitis (common cold)**
Acute rhinitis      Infective rhinitis
Coryza (acute)      Nasal catarrh, acute
Infective nasopharyngitis NOS    Nasopharyngitis NOS

*EXCLUDES 1*   *acute pharyngitis (J02.-)*
*acute sore throat NOS (J02.9)*
*pharyngitis NOS (J02.9)*
*rhinitis NOS (J31.0)*
*sore throat NOS (J02.9)*

*EXCLUDES 2*   *allergic rhinitis (J30.1-J30.9)*
*chronic pharyngitis (J31.2)*
*chronic rhinitis (J31.0)*
*chronic sore throat (J31.2)*
*nasopharyngitis, chronic (J31.1)*
*vasomotor rhinitis (J30.0)*

**DEF:** Acute inflammation of mucous membranes; extends from nares to pharynx; characterized by nasal obstruction, sneezing, runny nose, and sore throat.

**✓4ᵗʰ J01   Acute sinusitis**
**INCLUDES**   acute abscess of sinus
acute empyema of sinus
acute infection of sinus
acute inflammation of sinus
acute suppuration of sinus

Use additional code (B95-B97) to identify infectious agent
*EXCLUDES 1*   *sinusitis NOS (J32.9)*
*EXCLUDES 2*   *chronic sinusitis (J32.0-J32.8)*

**✓5ᵗʰ J01.0   Acute maxillary sinusitis**
Acute antritis
   **J01.00   Acute maxillary sinusitis, unspecified**
   **J01.01   Acute recurrent maxillary sinusitis**

**✓5ᵗʰ J01.1   Acute frontal sinusitis**
   **J01.10   Acute frontal sinusitis, unspecified**
   **J01.11   Acute recurrent frontal sinusitis**

**✓5ᵗʰ J01.2   Acute ethmoidal sinusitis**
   **J01.20   Acute ethmoidal sinusitis, unspecified**
   **J01.21   Acute recurrent ethmoidal sinusitis**

**✓5ᵗʰ J01.3   Acute sphenoidal sinusitis**
   **J01.30   Acute sphenoidal sinusitis, unspecified**
   **J01.31   Acute recurrent sphenoidal sinusitis**

**✓5ᵗʰ J01.4   Acute pansinusitis**
   **J01.40   Acute pansinusitis, unspecified**
   **J01.41   Acute recurrent pansinusitis**

**✓5ᵗʰ J01.8   Other acute sinusitis**
   **J01.80   Other acute sinusitis**
     Acute sinusitis involving more than one sinus but not pansinusitis
   **J01.81   Other acute recurrent sinusitis**
     Acute recurrent sinusitis involving more than one sinus but not pansinusitis

**✓5ᵗʰ J01.9   Acute sinusitis, unspecified**
   **J01.90   Acute sinusitis, unspecified**
   **J01.91   Acute recurrent sinusitis, unspecified**

**✓4ᵗʰ J02   Acute pharyngitis**
**INCLUDES**   acute sore throat
*EXCLUDES 1*   *acute laryngopharyngitis (J06.0)*
*peritonsillar abscess (J36)*
*pharyngeal abscess (J39.1)*
*retropharyngeal abscess (J39.0)*
*EXCLUDES 2*   *chronic pharyngitis (J31.2)*

**J02.0   Streptococcal pharyngitis**
Septic pharyngitis
Streptococcal sore throat
*EXCLUDES 2*   *scarlet fever (A38.-)*

**J02.8   Acute pharyngitis due to other specified organisms**
Use additional code (B95-B97) to identify infectious agent
*EXCLUDES 1*   *acute pharyngitis due to coxsackie virus (B08.5)*
*acute pharyngitis due to gonococcus (A54.5)*
*acute pharyngitis due to herpes [simplex] virus (B00.2)*
*acute pharyngitis due to infectious mononucleosis (B27.-)*
*enteroviral vesicular pharyngitis (B08.5)*

**J02.9   Acute pharyngitis, unspecified**
Gangrenous pharyngitis (acute)
Infective pharyngitis (acute) NOS
Pharyngitis (acute) NOS
Sore throat (acute) NOS
Suppurative pharyngitis (acute)
Ulcerative pharyngitis (acute)

**✓4ᵗʰ J03   Acute tonsillitis**
*EXCLUDES 1*   *acute sore throat (J02.-)*
*hypertrophy of tonsils (J35.1)*
*peritonsillar abscess (J36)*
*sore throat NOS (J02.9)*
*streptococcal sore throat (J02.0)*
*EXCLUDES 2*   *chronic tonsillitis (J35.0)*

**✓5ᵗʰ J03.0   Streptococcal tonsillitis**
   **J03.00   Acute streptococcal tonsillitis, unspecified**
   **J03.01   Acute recurrent streptococcal tonsillitis**

**✓5ᵗʰ J03.8   Acute tonsillitis due to other specified organisms**
Use additional code (B95-B97) to identify infectious agent
*EXCLUDES 1*   *diphtheritic tonsillitis (A36.0)*
*herpesviral pharyngotonsillitis (B00.2)*
*streptococcal tonsillitis (J03.0)*
*tuberculous tonsillitis (A15.8)*
*Vincent's tonsillitis (A69.1)*
   **J03.80   Acute tonsillitis due to other specified organisms**
   **J03.81   Acute recurrent tonsillitis due to other specified organisms**

**✓5ᵗʰ J03.9   Acute tonsillitis, unspecified**
Follicular tonsillitis (acute)
Gangrenous tonsillitis (acute)
Infective tonsillitis (acute)
Tonsillitis (acute) NOS
Ulcerative tonsillitis (acute)
   **J03.90   Acute tonsillitis, unspecified**
   **J03.91   Acute recurrent tonsillitis, unspecified**

## ✓4th J04 Acute laryngitis and tracheitis

Use additional code (B95-B97) to identify infectious agent

EXCLUDES 1   *acute obstructive laryngitis [croup] and epiglottitis (J05.-)*

EXCLUDES 2   *laryngismus (stridulus) (J38.5)*

### J04.0 Acute laryngitis

Edematous laryngitis (acute)
Laryngitis (acute) NOS
Subglottic laryngitis (acute)
Suppurative laryngitis (acute)
Ulcerative laryngitis (acute)

EXCLUDES 1   *acute obstructive laryngitis (J05.0)*

EXCLUDES 2   *chronic laryngitis (J37.0)*

### ✓5th J04.1 Acute tracheitis

Acute viral tracheitis
Catarrhal tracheitis (acute)
Tracheitis (acute) NOS

EXCLUDES 2   *chronic tracheitis (J42)*

#### J04.10 Acute tracheitis without obstruction

#### J04.11 Acute tracheitis with obstruction   `MCC`
CC Excl: PDX collection 730

### J04.2 Acute laryngotracheitis

Laryngotracheitis NOS
Tracheitis (acute) with laryngitis (acute)

EXCLUDES 1   *acute obstructive laryngotracheitis (J05.0)*

EXCLUDES 2   *chronic laryngotracheitis (J37.1)*

### ✓5th J04.3 Supraglottitis, unspecified

#### J04.30 Supraglottitis, unspecified, without obstruction

#### J04.31 Supraglottitis, unspecified, with obstruction   `MCC`
CC Excl: PDX collection 731

## ✓4th J05 Acute obstructive laryngitis [croup] and epiglottitis

Use additional code (B95-B97) to identify infectious agent

### J05.0 Acute obstructive laryngitis [croup]

Obstructive laryngitis (acute) NOS
Obstructive laryngotracheitis NOS

**DEF:** Acute laryngeal obstruction due to allergy, foreign body, or in the majority of cases a viral infection; symptoms include harsh, barking cough, hoarseness, and persistent high-pitched respiratory sound (stridor).

### ✓5th J05.1 Acute epiglottitis

EXCLUDES 2   *epiglottitis, chronic (J37.0)*

#### J05.10 Acute epiglottitis without obstruction   `CC`
Epiglottitis NOS
CC Excl: PDX collection 732

#### J05.11 Acute epiglottitis with obstruction   `MCC`
CC Excl: PDX collection 730

## ✓4th J06 Acute upper respiratory infections of multiple and unspecified sites

EXCLUDES 1   *acute respiratory infection NOS (J22)*
*streptococcal pharyngitis (J02.0)*

### J06.0 Acute laryngopharyngitis

### J06.9 Acute upper respiratory infection, unspecified

Upper respiratory disease, acute
Upper respiratory infection NOS

## Influenza and pneumonia (J09-J18)

EXCLUDES 2   *allergic or eosinophilic pneumonia (J82)*
*aspiration pneumonia NOS (J69.0)*
*congenital pneumonia (P23.9)*
*lipid pneumonia (J69.1)*
*meconium pneumonia (P24.01)*
*neonatal aspiration pneumonia (P24.-)*
*pneumonia due to solids and liquids (J69.-)*
*rheumatic pneumonia (I00)*
*ventilator associated pneumonia (J95.851)*

## ✓4th J09 Influenza due to certain identified influenza viruses

EXCLUDES 1   ▶*influenza A/H1N1 (J10.-)*◀
*influenza due to other identified influenza virus (J10.-)*
*influenza due to unidentified influenza virus (J11.-)*
*seasonal influenza due to other identified influenza virus (J10.-)*
*seasonal influenza due to unidentified influenza virus (J11.-)*

### ✓5th J09.X Influenza due to identified novel influenza A virus

Avian influenza
Bird influenza
Influenza A/H5N1
Influenza of other animal origin, not bird or swine
Swine influenza virus (viruses that normally cause infections in pigs)

**AHA:** 2016, 3Q, 10

#### J09.X1 Influenza due to identified novel influenza A virus with pneumonia   `HIV` `MCC`

Code also, if applicable, associated:
lung abscess (J85.1)
other specified type of pneumonia
CC Excl: PDX collection 110

#### J09.X2 Influenza due to identified novel influenza A virus with other respiratory manifestations

Influenza due to identified novel influenza A virus NOS
Influenza due to identified novel influenza A virus with laryngitis
Influenza due to identified novel influenza A virus with pharyngitis
Influenza due to identified novel influenza A virus with upper respiratory symptoms

Use additional code, if applicable, for associated:
pleural effusion (J91.8)
sinusitis (J01.-)

#### J09.X3 Influenza due to identified novel influenza A virus with gastrointestinal manifestations

Influenza due to identified novel influenza A virus gastroenteritis

EXCLUDES 1   *'intestinal flu' [viral gastroenteritis] (A08.-)*

#### J09.X9 Influenza due to identified novel influenza A virus with other manifestations

Influenza due to identified novel influenza A virus with encephalopathy
Influenza due to identified novel influenza A virus with myocarditis
Influenza due to identified novel influenza A virus with otitis media

Use additional code to identify manifestation

## ✓4th J10 Influenza due to other identified influenza virus

EXCLUDES 1   *influenza due to avian influenza virus (J09.X-)*
*influenza due to swine flu (J09.X-)*
*influenza due to unidentifed influenza virus (J11.-)*

### ✓5th J10.0 Influenza due to other identified influenza virus with pneumonia

Code also associated lung abscess, if applicable (J85.1)

#### J10.00 Influenza due to other identified influenza virus with unspecified type of pneumonia   `MCC`
CC Excl: PDX collection 110

#### J10.01 Influenza due to other identified influenza virus with the same other identified influenza virus pneumonia   `MCC`
CC Excl: PDX collection 110

#### J10.08 Influenza due to other identified influenza virus with other specified pneumonia   `HIV` `MCC`
Code also other specified type of pneumonia
CC Excl: PDX collection 733

N Newborn: 0   P Pediatric: 0-17   M Maternity: 12-55   A Adult: 15-124   `MCC` Major CC Condition   `PDxMCC` PDx acts as own MCC   `CC` CC Condition   `PDxCC` PDx acts as own CC

672          ICD-10-CM 2018

**J10.1**   **Influenza due to other identified influenza virus with other respiratory manifestations**
Influenza due to other identified influenza virus NOS
Influenza due to other identified influenza virus with laryngitis
Influenza due to other identified influenza virus with pharyngitis
Influenza due to other identified influenza virus with upper respiratory symptoms
Use additional code for associated pleural effusion, if applicable (J91.8)
Use additional code for associated sinusitis, if applicable (J01.-)
**AHA:** 2016, 3Q, 10-11

**J10.2**   **Influenza due to other identified influenza virus with gastrointestinal manifestations**
Influenza due to other identified influenza virus gastroenteritis
   EXCLUDES 1   *'intestinal flu' [viral gastroenteritis] (A08.-)*

✓5th **J10.8**   **Influenza due to other identified influenza virus with other manifestations**

    **J10.81**   **Influenza due to other identified influenza virus with encephalopathy**

    **J10.82**   **Influenza due to other identified influenza virus with myocarditis**

    **J10.83**   **Influenza due to other identified influenza virus with otitis media**
      Use additional code for any associated perforated tympanic membrane (H72.-)

    **J10.89**   **Influenza due to other identified influenza virus with other manifestations**
      Use additional codes to identify the manifestations

✓4th **J11**   **Influenza due to unidentified influenza virus**

✓5th **J11.0**   **Influenza due to unidentified influenza virus with pneumonia**
Code also associated lung abscess, if applicable (J85.1)
**AHA:** 2016, 3Q, 11

    **J11.00**   **Influenza due to unidentified influenza virus with unspecified type of pneumonia**   MCC
Influenza with pneumonia NOS
**CC Excl:** PDX collection 110

    **J11.08**   **Influenza due to unidentified influenza virus with specified pneumonia**   MCC
Code also other specified type of pneumonia
**CC Excl:** PDX collection 110

**J11.1**   **Influenza due to unidentified influenza virus with other respiratory manifestations**
Influenza NOS
Influenzal laryngitis NOS
Influenzal pharyngitis NOS
Influenza with upper respiratory symptoms NOS
Use additional code for associated pleural effusion, if applicable (J91.8)
Use additional code for associated sinusitis, if applicable (J01.-)

**J11.2**   **Influenza due to unidentified influenza virus with gastrointestinal manifestations**
Influenza gastroenteritis NOS
   EXCLUDES 1   *'intestinal flu' [viral gastroenteritis] (A08.-)*

✓5th **J11.8**   **Influenza due to unidentified influenza virus with other manifestations**

    **J11.81**   **Influenza due to unidentified influenza virus with encephalopathy**
Influenzal encephalopathy NOS

    **J11.82**   **Influenza due to unidentified influenza virus with myocarditis**
Influenzal myocarditis NOS

    **J11.83**   **Influenza due to unidentified influenza virus with otitis media**
Influenzal otitis media NOS
Use additional code for any associated perforated tympanic membrane (H72.-)

    **J11.89**   **Influenza due to unidentified influenza virus with other manifestations**
Use additional codes to identify the manifestations

✓4th **J12**   **Viral pneumonia, not elsewhere classified**
   INCLUDES   bronchopneumonia due to viruses other than influenza viruses
Code first associated influenza, if applicable (J09.X1, J10.0-, J11.0-)
Code also associated abscess, if applicable (J85.1)
   EXCLUDES 1   *aspiration pneumonia due to anesthesia during labor and delivery (O74.0)*
*aspiration pneumonia due to anesthesia during pregnancy (O29)*
*aspiration pneumonia due to anesthesia during puerperium (O89.0)*
*aspiration pneumonia due to solids and liquids (J69.-)*
*aspiration pneumonia NOS (J69.0)*
*congenital pneumonia (P23.0)*
*congenital rubella pneumonitis (P35.0)*
*interstitial pneumonia NOS (J84.9)*
*lipid pneumonia (J69.1)*
*neonatal aspiration pneumonia (P24.-)*
**AHA:** 2016, 3Q, 15; 2013, 4Q, 118

> **CC Excl: For MCC codes in category J12, unless otherwise noted:** PDX collection 734

**J12.0**   **Adenoviral pneumonia**   MCC

**J12.1**   **Respiratory syncytial virus pneumonia**   MCC

**J12.2**   **Parainfluenza virus pneumonia**   MCC

**J12.3**   **Human metapneumovirus pneumonia**   HIV MCC

✓5th **J12.8**   **Other viral pneumonia**

    **J12.81**   **Pneumonia due to SARS-associated coronavirus**   HIV MCC
Severe acute respiratory syndrome NOS
**DEF:** A severe adult respiratory syndrome caused by the coronavirus, specified as inflammation of the lungs with consolidation.
**CC Excl:** PDX collection 735

    **J12.89**   **Other viral pneumonia**   HIV MCC

**J12.9**   **Viral pneumonia, unspecified**   HIV MCC

**J13**   **Pneumonia due to Streptococcus pneumoniae**   HIV MCC HCC
Bronchopneumonia due to S. pneumoniae
Code first associated influenza, if applicable (J09.X1, J10.0-, J11.0-)
Code also associated lung abscess, if applicable (J85.1)
   EXCLUDES 1   *congenital pneumonia due to S. pneumoniae (P23.6)*
*lobar pneumonia, unspecified organism (J18.1)*
*pneumonia due to other streptococci (J15.3-J15.4)*
**AHA:** 2016, 3Q, 15; 2013, 4Q, 118
**CC Excl:** PDX collection 110

**J14**   **Pneumonia due to Hemophilus influenzae**   HIV MCC HCC
Bronchopneumonia due to H. influenzae
Code first associated influenza, if applicable (J09.X1, J10.0-, J11.0-)
Code also associated lung abscess, if applicable (J85.1)
   EXCLUDES 1   *congenital pneumonia due to H. influenzae (P23.6)*
**AHA:** 2016, 3Q, 15; 2013, 4Q, 118
**CC Excl:** PDX collection 110

✓4th **J15**   **Bacterial pneumonia, not elsewhere classified**
   INCLUDES   bronchopneumonia due to bacteria other than S. pneumoniae and H. influenzae
Code first associated influenza, if applicable (J09.X1, J10.0-, J11.0-)
Code also associated lung abscess, if applicable (J85.1)
   EXCLUDES 1   *chlamydial pneumonia (J16.0)*
*congenital pneumonia (P23.-)*
*Legionnaires' disease (A48.1)*
*spirochetal pneumonia (A69.8)*
**AHA:** 2016, 3Q, 15; 2013, 4Q, 118

> **CC Excl: For MCC codes in category J15:** PDX collection 110

**J15.0**   **Pneumonia due to Klebsiella pneumoniae**   HIV MCC HCC

**J15.1**   **Pneumonia due to Pseudomonas**   HIV MCC HCC

✓5th **J15.2**   **Pneumonia due to staphylococcus**

    **J15.20**   **Pneumonia due to staphylococcus, unspecified**   HIV MCC HCC

   ✓6th **J15.21**   **Pneumonia due to Staphylococcus aureus**

      **J15.211**   **Pneumonia due to Methicillin susceptible Staphylococcus aureus**   HIV MCC HCC
MSSA pneumonia
Pneumonia due to Staphylococcus aureus NOS

      **J15.212**   **Pneumonia due to Methicillin resistant Staphylococcus aureus**   HIV MCC HCC

    **J15.29**   **Pneumonia due to other staphylococcus**   HIV MCC HCC

**J15.3**   **Pneumonia due to streptococcus, group B**   HIV MCC HCC

✓ Additional Character Req   ✓x7th Placeholder Alert   Unacceptable PDx   Manifestation   H1-H14 HAC   HCC CMS-HCC Condition   EXCLUDES 1 Not Coded Here   EXCLUDES 2 Not Included Here

ICD-10-CM 2018                                        **673**

**Chapter 10. Diseases of the Respiratory System**

**J15.4 Pneumonia due to other streptococci** `HIV` `MCC` `HCC`
> *EXCLUDES 1*   pneumonia due to streptococcus, group B (J15.3)
> pneumonia due to Streptococcus pneumoniae (J13)

**J15.5 Pneumonia due to Escherichia coli** `HIV` `MCC` `HCC`

▲ **J15.6 Pneumonia due to other Gram-negative bacteria** `HIV` `MCC` `HCC`
> ►Pneumonia due to other aerobic Gram-negative bacteria◄
> Pneumonia due to Serratia marcescens

**J15.7 Pneumonia due to Mycoplasma pneumoniae** `MCC`

**J15.8 Pneumonia due to other specified bacteria** `HIV` `MCC` `HCC`

**J15.9 Unspecified bacterial pneumonia** `HIV` `MCC`
> Pneumonia due to gram-positive bacteria

✓4th **J16 Pneumonia due to other infectious organisms, not elsewhere classified**
> Code first associated influenza, if applicable (J09.X1, J10.0-, J11.0-)
> Code also associated lung abscess, if applicable (J85.1)
> *EXCLUDES 1*   congenital pneumonia (P23.-)
> ornithosis (A70)
> pneumocystosis (B59)
> pneumonia NOS (J18.9)
> **AHA:** 2016, 3Q, 15; 2013, 4Q, 118

**J16.0 Chlamydial pneumonia** `MCC`
> **CC Excl:** PDX collection 110

**J16.8 Pneumonia due to other specified infectious organisms** `MCC`
> **CC Excl:** PDX collection 110

**J17 *Pneumonia in diseases classified elsewhere*** `MCC`
> Code first underlying disease, such as:
> Q fever (A78)
> rheumatic fever (I00)
> schistosomiasis (B65.0-B65.9)
> *EXCLUDES 1*   candidial pneumonia (B37.1)
> chlamydial pneumonia (J16.0)
> gonorrheal pneumonia (A54.84)
> histoplasmosis pneumonia (B39.0-B39.2)
> measles pneumonia (B05.2)
> nocardiosis pneumonia (A43.0)
> pneumocystosis (B59)
> pneumonia due to Pneumocystis carinii (B59)
> pneumonia due to Pneumocystis jiroveci (B59)
> pneumonia in actinomycosis (A42.0)
> pneumonia in anthrax (A22.1)
> pneumonia in ascariasis (B77.81)
> pneumonia in aspergillosis (B44.0-B44.1)
> pneumonia in coccidioidomycosis (B38.0-B38.2)
> pneumonia in cytomegalovirus disease (B25.0)
> pneumonia in toxoplasmosis (B58.3)
> rubella pneumonia (B06.81)
> salmonella pneumonia (A02.22)
> spirochetal infection NEC with pneumonia (A69.8)
> tularemia pneumonia (A21.2)
> typhoid fever with pneumonia (A01.03)
> varicella pneumonia (B01.2)
> whooping cough with pneumonia (A37 with fifth-character 1)
> **AHA:** 2016, 3Q, 15; 2013, 4Q, 118
> **CC Excl:** PDX collection 110

✓4th **J18 Pneumonia, unspecified organism**
> Code first associated influenza, if applicable (J09.X1, J10.0-, J11.0-)
> *EXCLUDES 1*   abscess of lung with pneumonia (J85.1)
> aspiration pneumonia due to anesthesia during labor and delivery (O74.0)
> aspiration pneumonia due to anesthesia during pregnancy (O29)
> aspiration pneumonia due to anesthesia during puerperium (O89.0)
> aspiration pneumonia due to solids and liquids (J69.-)
> aspiration pneumonia NOS (J69.0)
> congenital pneumonia (P23.0)
> drug-induced interstitial lung disorder (J70.2-J70.4)
> interstitial pneumonia NOS (J84.9)
> lipid pneumonia (J69.1)
> neonatal aspiration pneumonia (P24.-)
> pneumonitis due to external agents (J67-J70)
> pneumonitis due to fumes and vapors (J68.0)
> usual interstitial pneumonia (J84.17)
> **AHA:** 2016, 3Q, 15; 2013, 4Q, 118

> **CC Excl: For MCC codes in category J18, unless otherwise noted:** PDX collection 110

**J18.0 Bronchopneumonia, unspecified organism** `MCC`
> *EXCLUDES 1*   hypostatic bronchopneumonia (J18.2)
> lipid pneumonia (J69.1)
> *EXCLUDES 2*   acute bronchiolitis (J21.-)
> chronic bronchiolitis (J44.9)

**J18.1 Lobar pneumonia, unspecified organism** `HIV` `MCC` `HCC`

**J18.2 Hypostatic pneumonia, unspecified organism** `CC`
> Hypostatic bronchopneumonia
> Passive pneumonia
> **CC Excl:** PDX collection 736

**J18.8 Other pneumonia, unspecified organism** `HIV` `MCC`

**J18.9 Pneumonia, unspecified organism** `HIV` `MCC`
> **AHA:** 2014, 3Q, 4; 2013, 4Q, 119; 2012, 4Q, 94

## Other acute lower respiratory infections (J20-J22)

> *EXCLUDES 2*   chronic obstructive pulmonary disease with acute lower respiratory infection (J44.0)

✓4th **J20 Acute bronchitis**
> *INCLUDES*   acute and subacute bronchitis (with) bronchospasm
> acute and subacute bronchitis (with) tracheitis
> acute and subacute bronchitis (with) tracheobronchitis, acute
> acute and subacute fibrinous bronchitis
> acute and subacute membranous bronchitis
> acute and subacute purulent bronchitis
> acute and subacute septic bronchitis
> *EXCLUDES 1*   bronchitis NOS (J40)
> tracheobronchitis NOS (J40)
> *EXCLUDES 2*   acute bronchitis with bronchiectasis (J47.0)
> acute bronchitis with chronic obstructive asthma (J44.0)
> acute bronchitis with chronic obstructive pulmonary disease (J44.0)
> allergic bronchitis NOS (J45.909)
> bronchitis due to chemicals, fumes and vapors (J68.0)
> chronic bronchitis NOS (J42)
> chronic mucopurulent bronchitis (J41.1)
> chronic obstructive bronchitis (J44.-)
> chronic obstructive tracheobronchitis (J44.-)
> chronic simple bronchitis (J41.0)
> chronic tracheobronchitis (J42)
> **AHA:** 2016, 3Q, 10, 16
> **DEF:** Acute inflammation of main branches of bronchial tree due to infectious or irritant agents; symptoms include cough with a varied production of sputum, fever, substernal soreness, and lung rales; usually last for three to 10 days.

**J20.0 Acute bronchitis due to Mycoplasma pneumoniae**

**J20.1 Acute bronchitis due to Hemophilus influenzae**

**J20.2 Acute bronchitis due to streptococcus**

**J20.3 Acute bronchitis due to coxsackievirus**

**J20.4 Acute bronchitis due to parainfluenza virus**

**J20.5 Acute bronchitis due to respiratory syncytial virus**

**J20.6 Acute bronchitis due to rhinovirus**

**J20.7 Acute bronchitis due to echovirus**

**J20.8 Acute bronchitis due to other specified organisms**

**J20.9 Acute bronchitis, unspecified**

✓4th **J21 Acute bronchiolitis**
> *INCLUDES*   acute bronchiolitis with bronchospasm
> *EXCLUDES 2*   respiratory bronchiolitis interstitial lung disease (J84.115)

> **CC Excl: For CC codes in category J21, unless otherwise noted:** PDX collection 738

**J21.0 Acute bronchiolitis due to respiratory syncytial virus** `CC`
> **CC Excl:** PDX collection 737

**J21.1 Acute bronchiolitis due to human metapneumovirus** `CC`

**J21.8 Acute bronchiolitis due to other specified organisms** `CC`

**J21.9 Acute bronchiolitis, unspecified** `CC`
> Bronchiolitis (acute)
> *EXCLUDES 1*   chronic bronchiolitis (J44.-)

**J22 Unspecified acute lower respiratory infection**
> Acute (lower) respiratory (tract) infection NOS
> *EXCLUDES 1*   upper respiratory infection (acute) (J06.9)

## Other diseases of upper respiratory tract (J30-J39)

✓4th **J30 Vasomotor and allergic rhinitis**
> *INCLUDES*   spasmodic rhinorrhea
> *EXCLUDES 1*   allergic rhinitis with asthma (bronchial) (J45.909)
> rhinitis NOS (J31.0)

**J30.0 Vasomotor rhinitis**

**J30.1 Allergic rhinitis due to pollen**
> Allergy NOS due to pollen
> Hay fever
> Pollinosis

**J30.2 Other seasonal allergic rhinitis**

`N` Newborn: 0   `P` Pediatric: 0-17   `M` Maternity: 12-55   `A` Adult: 15-124   `MCC` Major CC Condition   `PDxMCC` PDx acts as own MCC   `CC` CC Condition   `PDxCC` PDx acts as own CC

**674**        ICD-10-CM 2018

J30.5　**Allergic rhinitis due to food**

✓5ᵗʰ J30.8　**Other allergic rhinitis**

　　J30.81　**Allergic rhinitis due to animal (cat) (dog) hair and dander**

　　J30.89　**Other allergic rhinitis**
　　　　　　Perennial allergic rhinitis

J30.9　**Allergic rhinitis, unspecified**

✓4ᵗʰ **J31　Chronic rhinitis, nasopharyngitis and pharyngitis**

　　Use additional code to identify:
　　　exposure to environmental tobacco smoke (Z77.22)
　　　exposure to tobacco smoke in the perinatal period (P96.81)
　　　history of tobacco dependence (Z87.891)
　　　occupational exposure to environmental tobacco smoke (Z57.31)
　　　tobacco dependence (F17.-)
　　　tobacco use (Z72.0)

J31.0　**Chronic rhinitis**
　　　Atrophic rhinitis (chronic)
　　　Granulomatous rhinitis (chronic)
　　　Hypertrophic rhinitis (chronic)
　　　Obstructive rhinitis (chronic)
　　　Ozena
　　　Purulent rhinitis (chronic)
　　　Rhinitis (chronic) NOS
　　　Ulcerative rhinitis (chronic)
　　　**EXCLUDES 1**　*allergic rhinitis (J30.1-J30.9)*
　　　　　　　　　*vasomotor rhinitis (J30.0)*
　　　**DEF:** Persistent inflammation of mucous membranes of nose; characterized by postnasal drip.

J31.1　**Chronic nasopharyngitis**
　　　**EXCLUDES 2**　*acute nasopharyngitis (J00)*
　　　**DEF:** Persistent inflammation of mucous membranes extending from nares to pharynx; characterized by constant irritation in nasopharynx and postnasal drip.

J31.2　**Chronic pharyngitis**
　　　Atrophic pharyngitis (chronic)
　　　Chronic sore throat
　　　Granular pharyngitis (chronic)
　　　Hypertrophic pharyngitis (chronic)
　　　**EXCLUDES 2**　*acute pharyngitis (J02.9)*

✓4ᵗʰ **J32　Chronic sinusitis**
　　　**INCLUDES**　sinus abscess
　　　　　　　　sinus empyema
　　　　　　　　sinus infection
　　　　　　　　sinus suppuration
　　Use additional code to identify:
　　　exposure to environmental tobacco smoke (Z77.22)
　　　exposure to tobacco smoke in the perinatal period (P96.81)
　　　history of tobacco dependence (Z87.891)
　　　infectious agent (B95-B97)
　　　occupational exposure to environmental tobacco smoke (Z57.31)
　　　tobacco dependence (F17.-)
　　　tobacco use (Z72.0)
　　　**EXCLUDES 2**　*acute sinusitis (J01.-)*

J32.0　**Chronic maxillary sinusitis**
　　　Antritis (chronic)
　　　Maxillary sinusitis NOS

J32.1　**Chronic frontal sinusitis**
　　　Frontal sinusitis NOS

J32.2　**Chronic ethmoidal sinusitis**
　　　Ethmoidal sinusitis NOS
　　　**EXCLUDES 1**　*Woakes' ethmoiditis (J33.1)*

J32.3　**Chronic sphenoidal sinusitis**
　　　Sphenoidal sinusitis NOS

J32.4　**Chronic pansinusitis**
　　　Pansinusitis NOS

J32.8　**Other chronic sinusitis**
　　　Sinusitis (chronic) involving more than one sinus but not pansinusitis

J32.9　**Chronic sinusitis, unspecified**
　　　Sinusitis (chronic) NOS

✓4ᵗʰ **J33　Nasal polyp**
　　Use additional code to identify:
　　　exposure to environmental tobacco smoke (Z77.22)
　　　exposure to tobacco smoke in the perinatal period (P96.81)
　　　history of tobacco dependence (Z87.891)
　　　occupational exposure to environmental tobacco smoke (Z57.31)
　　　tobacco dependence (F17.-)
　　　tobacco use (Z72.0)
　　　**EXCLUDES 1**　*adenomatous polyps (D14.0)*

J33.0　**Polyp of nasal cavity**
　　　Choanal polyp
　　　Nasopharyngeal polyp

J33.1　**Polypoid sinus degeneration**
　　　Woakes' syndrome or ethmoiditis

J33.8　**Other polyp of sinus**
　　　Accessory polyp of sinus
　　　Ethmoidal polyp of sinus
　　　Maxillary polyp of sinus
　　　Sphenoidal polyp of sinus

J33.9　**Nasal polyp, unspecified**

✓4ᵗʰ **J34　Other and unspecified disorders of nose and nasal sinuses**
　　　**EXCLUDES 2**　*varicose ulcer of nasal septum (I86.8)*

J34.0　**Abscess, furuncle and carbuncle of nose**
　　　Cellulitis of nose　　　Ulceration of nose
　　　Necrosis of nose

J34.1　**Cyst and mucocele of nose and nasal sinus**

J34.2　**Deviated nasal septum**
　　　Deflection or deviation of septum (nasal) (acquired)
　　　**EXCLUDES 1**　*congenital deviated nasal septum (Q67.4)*

J34.3　**Hypertrophy of nasal turbinates**

✓5ᵗʰ J34.8　**Other specified disorders of nose and nasal sinuses**

　　J34.81　**Nasal mucositis (ulcerative)**
　　　　　　Code also type of associated therapy, such as:
　　　　　　　antineoplastic and immunosuppressive drugs (T45.1X-)
　　　　　　　radiological procedure and radiotherapy (Y84.2)
　　　　　　**EXCLUDES 2**　*gastrointestinal mucositis (ulcerative) (K92.81)*
　　　　　　　　　　　　*mucositis (ulcerative) of vagina and vulva (N76.81)*
　　　　　　　　　　　　*oral mucositis (ulcerative) (K12.3-)*

　　J34.89　**Other specified disorders of nose and nasal sinuses**
　　　　　　Perforation of nasal septum NOS
　　　　　　Rhinolith

J34.9　**Unspecified disorder of nose and nasal sinuses**

✓4ᵗʰ **J35　Chronic diseases of tonsils and adenoids**
　　Use additional code to identify:
　　　exposure to environmental tobacco smoke (Z77.22)
　　　exposure to tobacco smoke in the perinatal period (P96.81)
　　　history of tobacco dependence (Z87.891)
　　　occupational exposure to environmental tobacco smoke (Z57.31)
　　　tobacco dependence (F17.-)
　　　tobacco use (Z72.0)

✓5ᵗʰ J35.0　**Chronic tonsillitis and adenoiditis**
　　　**EXCLUDES 2**　*acute tonsillitis (J03.-)*

　　J35.01　**Chronic tonsillitis**

　　J35.02　**Chronic adenoiditis**

　　J35.03　**Chronic tonsillitis and adenoiditis**

J35.1　**Hypertrophy of tonsils**
　　　Enlargement of tonsils
　　　**EXCLUDES 1**　*hypertrophy of tonsils with tonsillitis (J35.0-)*

J35.2　**Hypertrophy of adenoids**
　　　Enlargement of adenoids
　　　**EXCLUDES 1**　*hypertrophy of adenoids with adenoiditis (J35.0-)*

J35.3　**Hypertrophy of tonsils with hypertrophy of adenoids**
　　　**EXCLUDES 1**　*hypertrophy of tonsils and adenoids with tonsillitis and adenoiditis (J35.03)*

J35.8　**Other chronic diseases of tonsils and adenoids**
　　　Adenoid vegetations　　　　Tonsillar tag
　　　Amygdalolith　　　　　　　Ulcer of tonsil
　　　Calculus, tonsil
　　　Cicatrix of tonsil (and adenoid)

J35.9　**Chronic disease of tonsils and adenoids, unspecified**
　　　Disease (chronic) of tonsils and adenoids NOS

✓ Additional Character Req　　✓x7ᵗʰ Placeholder Alert　　Unacceptable PDx　　Manifestation　　**H1**-**H14** HAC　　**HCC** CMS-HCC Condition　　**EXCLUDES 1** Not Coded Here　　**EXCLUDES 2** Not Included Here

ICD-10-CM 2018　　　　　　　　　　　　　　　　　　　　　　　　　　　　　　　　　　**675**

**Chapter 10. Diseases of the Respiratory System**

**J36    Peritonsillar abscess**    `CC`
    `INCLUDES`   abscess of tonsil
                peritonsillar cellulitis
                quinsy
    Use additional code (B95-B97) to identify infectious agent
    `EXCLUDES 1`   *acute tonsillitis (J03.-)*
                *chronic tonsillitis (J35.0)*
                *retropharyngeal abscess (J39.0)*
                *tonsillitis NOS (J03.9-)*
    **CC Excl:** PDX collection 739

**✓4ᵗʰ J37    Chronic laryngitis and laryngotracheitis**
    Use additional code to identify:
      exposure to environmental tobacco smoke (Z77.22)
      exposure to tobacco smoke in the perinatal period (P96.81)
      history of tobacco dependence (Z87.891)
      infectious agent (B95-B97)
      occupational exposure to environmental tobacco smoke (Z57.31)
      tobacco dependence (F17.-)
      tobacco use (Z72.0)

    **J37.0    Chronic laryngitis**
       Catarrhal laryngitis
       Hypertrophic laryngitis
       Sicca laryngitis
       `EXCLUDES 2`   *acute laryngitis (J04.0)*
                  *obstructive (acute) laryngitis (J05.0)*

    **J37.1    Chronic laryngotracheitis**
       Laryngitis, chronic, with tracheitis (chronic)
       Tracheitis, chronic, with laryngitis
       `EXCLUDES 1`   *chronic tracheitis (J42)*
       `EXCLUDES 2`   *acute laryngotracheitis (J04.2)*
                  *acute tracheitis (J04.1)*

**✓4ᵗʰ J38    Diseases of vocal cords and larynx, not elsewhere classified**
    Use additional code to identify:
      exposure to environmental tobacco smoke (Z77.22)
      exposure to tobacco smoke in the perinatal period (P96.81)
      history of tobacco dependence (Z87.891)
      occupational exposure to environmental tobacco smoke (Z57.31)
      tobacco dependence (F17.-)
      tobacco use (Z72.0)
    `EXCLUDES 1`   *congenital laryngeal stridor (P28.89)*
               *obstructive laryngitis (acute) (J05.0)*
               *postprocedural subglottic stenosis (J95.5)*
               *stridor (R06.1)*
               *ulcerative laryngitis (J04.0)*

    **✓5ᵗʰ J38.0    Paralysis of vocal cords and larynx**
       Laryngoplegia
       Paralysis of glottis

       **J38.00    Paralysis of vocal cords and larynx, unspecified**
       **J38.01    Paralysis of vocal cords and larynx, unilateral**
       **J38.02    Paralysis of vocal cords and larynx, bilateral**

    **J38.1    Polyp of vocal cord and larynx**
       `EXCLUDES 1`   *adenomatous polyps (D14.1)*

    **J38.2    Nodules of vocal cords**
       Chorditis (fibrinous)(nodosa)(tuberosa)
       Singer's nodes
       Teacher's nodes

    **J38.3    Other diseases of vocal cords**
       Abscess of vocal cords
       Cellulitis of vocal cords
       Granuloma of vocal cords
       Leukokeratosis of vocal cords
       Leukoplakia of vocal cords

    **J38.4    Edema of larynx**
       Edema (of) glottis
       Subglottic edema
       Supraglottic edema
       `EXCLUDES 1`   *acute obstructive laryngitis [croup] (J05.0)*
                  *edematous laryngitis (J04.0)*

    **J38.5    Laryngeal spasm**
       Laryngismus (stridulus)

    **J38.6    Stenosis of larynx**

    **J38.7    Other diseases of larynx**
       Abscess of larynx
       Cellulitis of larynx
       Disease of larynx NOS
       Necrosis of larynx
       Pachyderma of larynx
       Perichondritis of larynx
       Ulcer of larynx

**✓4ᵗʰ J39    Other diseases of upper respiratory tract**
    `EXCLUDES 1`   *acute respiratory infection NOS (J22)*
               *acute upper respiratory infection (J06.9)*
               *upper respiratory inflammation due to chemicals, gases, fumes*
                   *or vapors (J68.2)*

    **J39.0    Retropharyngeal and parapharyngeal abscess**    `CC`
       Peripharyngeal abscess
       `EXCLUDES 1`   *peritonsillar abscess (J36)*
       **DEF:** Purulent infection behind pharynx and front of precerebral
       fascia; characterized by neck stiffness, cervical lymphadenopathy,
       sore throat, fever, and stridor.
       **CC Excl:** PDX collection 740

    **J39.1    Other abscess of pharynx**    `CC`
       Cellulitis of pharynx
       Nasopharyngeal abscess
       **CC Excl:** PDX collection 740

    **J39.2    Other diseases of pharynx**
       Cyst of pharynx
       Edema of pharynx
       `EXCLUDES 2`   *chronic pharyngitis (J31.2)*
                  *ulcerative pharyngitis (J02.9)*

    **J39.3    Upper respiratory tract hypersensitivity reaction, site unspecified**
       `EXCLUDES 1`   *hypersensitivity reaction of upper respiratory tract,*
                   *such as:*
                     *extrinsic allergic alveolitis (J67.9)*
                     *pneumoconiosis (J60-J67.9)*

    **J39.8    Other specified diseases of upper respiratory tract**

    **J39.9    Disease of upper respiratory tract, unspecified**

### Chronic lower respiratory diseases (J40-J47)

    `EXCLUDES 1`   *bronchitis due to chemicals, gases, fumes and vapors (J68.0)*
    `EXCLUDES 2`   *cystic fibrosis (E84.-)*

**J40    Bronchitis, not specified as acute or chronic**
    Bronchitis NOS
    Bronchitis with tracheitis NOS
    Catarrhal bronchitis
    Tracheobronchitis NOS
    Use additional code to identify:
      exposure to environmental tobacco smoke (Z77.22)
      exposure to tobacco smoke in the perinatal period (P96.81)
      history of tobacco dependence (Z87.891)
      occupational exposure to environmental tobacco smoke (Z57.31)
      tobacco dependence (F17.-)
      tobacco use (Z72.0)
    `EXCLUDES 1`   *acute bronchitis (J20.-)*
               *allergic bronchitis NOS (J45.909)*
               *asthmatic bronchitis NOS (J45.9-)*
               *bronchitis due to chemicals, gases, fumes and vapors (J68.0)*

**✓4ᵗʰ J41    Simple and mucopurulent chronic bronchitis**
    Use additional code to identify:
      exposure to environmental tobacco smoke (Z77.22)
      exposure to tobacco smoke in the perinatal period (P96.81)
      history of tobacco dependence (Z87.891)
      occupational exposure to environmental tobacco smoke (Z57.31)
      tobacco dependence (F17.-)
      tobacco use (Z72.0)
    `EXCLUDES 1`   *chronic bronchitis NOS (J42)*
               *chronic obstructive bronchitis (J44.-)*

    **J41.0    Simple chronic bronchitis**    `HCC`
    **J41.1    Mucopurulent chronic bronchitis**    `HCC`
    **J41.8    Mixed simple and mucopurulent chronic bronchitis**    `HCC`

**J42    Unspecified chronic bronchitis**    `HCC`
    Chronic bronchitis NOS
    Chronic tracheitis
    Chronic tracheobronchitis
    Use additional code to identify:
      exposure to environmental tobacco smoke (Z77.22)
      exposure to tobacco smoke in the perinatal period (P96.81)
      history of tobacco dependence (Z87.891)
      occupational exposure to environmental tobacco smoke (Z57.31)
      tobacco dependence (F17.-)
      tobacco use (Z72.0)
    `EXCLUDES 1`   *chronic asthmatic bronchitis (J44.-)*
               *chronic bronchitis with airways obstruction (J44.-)*
               *chronic emphysematous bronchitis (J44.-)*
               *chronic obstructive pulmonary disease NOS (J44.9)*
               *simple and mucopurulent chronic bronchitis (J41.-)*

`N` Newborn: 0    `P` Pediatric: 0-17    `M` Maternity: 12-55    `A` Adult: 15-124    `MCC` Major CC Condition    `PDxMCC` PDx acts as own MCC    `CC` CC Condition    `PDxCC` PDx acts as own CC

**676**            ICD-10-CM 2018

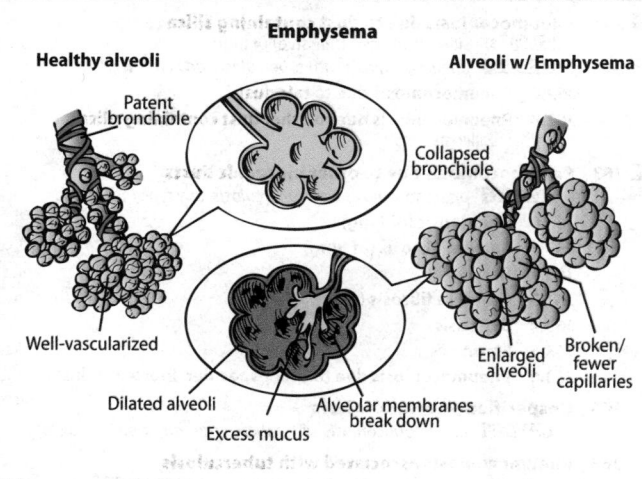

**Emphysema**

Healthy alveoli                    Alveoli w/ Emphysema

Patent bronchiole

Collapsed bronchiole

Well-vascularized

Dilated alveoli

Enlarged alveoli

Broken/ fewer capillaries

Alveolar membranes break down

Excess mucus

### ✓4th J43   Emphysema

Use additional code to identify:
exposure to environmental tobacco smoke (Z77.22)
history of tobacco dependence (Z87.891)
occupational exposure to environmental tobacco smoke (Z57.31)
tobacco dependence (F17.-)
tobacco use (Z72.0)

**EXCLUDES 1**   *compensatory emphysema (J98.3)*
*emphysema due to inhalation of chemicals, gases, fumes or vapors (J68.4)*
*emphysema with chronic (obstructive) bronchitis (J44.-)*
*emphysematous (obstructive) bronchitis (J44.-)*
*interstitial emphysema (J98.2)*
*mediastinal emphysema (J98.2)*
*neonatal interstitial emphysema (P25.0)*
*surgical (subcutaneous) emphysema (T81.82)*
*traumatic subcutaneous emphysema (T79.7)*

**J43.0**   **Unilateral pulmonary emphysema [MacLeod's syndrome]** HCC
Swyer-James syndrome
Unilateral emphysema
Unilateral hyperlucent lung
Unilateral pulmonary artery functional hypoplasia
Unilateral transparency of lung

**J43.1**   **Panlobular emphysema**                                    HCC
Panacinar emphysema

**J43.2**   **Centrilobular emphysema**                               HCC

**J43.8**   **Other emphysema**                                       HCC

**J43.9**   **Emphysema, unspecified**                                HCC
Bullous emphysema (lung)(pulmonary)
Emphysema (lung)(pulmonary) NOS
Emphysematous bleb
Vesicular emphysema (lung)(pulmonary)

### ✓4th J44   Other chronic obstructive pulmonary disease

**INCLUDES**   asthma with chronic obstructive pulmonary disease
chronic asthmatic (obstructive) bronchitis
chronic bronchitis with airways obstruction
chronic bronchitis with emphysema
chronic emphysematous bronchitis
chronic obstructive asthma
chronic obstructive bronchitis
chronic obstructive tracheobronchitis

Code also type of asthma, if applicable (J45.-)
Use additional code to identify:
exposure to environmental tobacco smoke (Z77.22)
history of tobacco dependence (Z87.891)
occupational exposure to environmental tobacco smoke (Z57.31)
tobacco dependence (F17.-)
tobacco use (Z72.0)

**EXCLUDES 1**   *bronchiectasis (J47.-)*
*chronic bronchitis NOS (J42)*
*chronic simple and mucopurulent bronchitis (J41.-)*
*chronic tracheitis (J42)*
*chronic tracheobronchitis (J42)*
*emphysema without chronic bronchitis (J43.-)*

**EXCLUDES 2**   ~~*lung diseases due to external agents (J60-J70)*~~

**AHA:** 2017, 1Q, 25-26; 2016, 3Q, 15-16; 2013, 4Q, 109

**J44.0**   **Chronic obstructive pulmonary disease with acute** CC HCC
**lower respiratory infection**
▶Code also to identify the infection◀
~~Use additional code to identify the infection~~
**AHA:** 2017, 1Q, 24-25
**CC Excl:** PDX collection 741

**J44.1**   **Chronic obstructive pulmonary disease with (acute)** CC HCC
**exacerbation**
Decompensated COPD
Decompensated COPD with (acute) exacerbation
**EXCLUDES 2**   *chronic obstructive pulmonary disease [COPD] with acute bronchitis (J44.0)*
▶*lung diseases due to external agents (J60-J70)*◀
**AHA:** 2017, 1Q, 26; 2016, 1Q, 36
**CC Excl:** PDX collection 741

**J44.9**   **Chronic obstructive pulmonary disease, unspecified** HCC
Chronic obstructive airway disease NOS
Chronic obstructive lung disease NOS
**EXCLUDES 2**▶*lung diseases due to external agents (J60-J70)*◀
**AHA:** 2016, 1Q, 36; 2014, 4Q, 21; 2013, 4Q, 109

### ✓4th J45   Asthma

**INCLUDES**   allergic (predominantly) asthma
allergic bronchitis NOS
allergic rhinitis with asthma
atopic asthma
extrinsic allergic asthma
hay fever with asthma
idiosyncratic asthma
intrinsic nonallergic asthma
nonallergic asthma

Use additional code to identify:
exposure to environmental tobacco smoke (Z77.22)
exposure to tobacco smoke in the perinatal period (P96.81)
history of tobacco dependence (Z87.891)
occupational exposure to environmental tobacco smoke (Z57.31)
tobacco dependence (F17.-)
tobacco use (Z72.0)

**EXCLUDES 1**   *detergent asthma (J69.8)*
*eosinophilic asthma (J82)*
~~*lung diseases due to external agents (J60-J70)*~~
*miner's asthma (J60)*
*wheezing NOS (R06.2)*
*wood asthma (J67.8)*

**EXCLUDES 2**   *asthma with chronic obstructive pulmonary disease (J44.9)*
*chronic asthmatic (obstructive) bronchitis (J44.9)*
*chronic obstructive asthma (J44.9)*

**AHA:** 2017, 1Q, 25-26; 2012, 4Q, 99
**DEF:** Status asthmaticus: Severe, intractable episode of asthma that is unresponsive to normal therapeutic measures.

**CC Excl: For CC codes in category J45:** PDX collection 742

### ✓5th J45.2   Mild intermittent asthma

**J45.20**   **Mild intermittent asthma, uncomplicated**
Mild intermittent asthma NOS

**J45.21**   **Mild intermittent asthma with (acute)** CC
**exacerbation**

**J45.22**   **Mild intermittent asthma with status** CC
**asthmaticus**

### ✓5th J45.3   Mild persistent asthma

**J45.30**   **Mild persistent asthma, uncomplicated**
Mild persistent asthma NOS

**J45.31**   **Mild persistent asthma with (acute) exacerbation** CC
**AHA:** 2016, 1Q, 35

**J45.32**   **Mild persistent asthma with status asthmaticus** CC

### ✓5th J45.4   Moderate persistent asthma

**J45.40**   **Moderate persistent asthma, uncomplicated**
Moderate persistent asthma NOS

**J45.41**   **Moderate persistent asthma with (acute)** CC
**exacerbation**
**AHA:** 2017, 1Q, 26

**J45.42**   **Moderate persistent asthma with status** CC
**asthmaticus**

### ✓5th J45.5   Severe persistent asthma

**J45.50**   **Severe persistent asthma, uncomplicated**
Severe persistent asthma NOS

**J45.51**   **Severe persistent asthma with (acute)** CC
**exacerbation**

**J45.52**   **Severe persistent asthma with status** CC
**asthmaticus**

---

✓Additional Character Req   ✓x7th Placeholder Alert   Unacceptable PDx   Manifestation   H1 - H14 HAC   HCC CMS-HCC Condition   EXCLUDES 1 Not Coded Here   EXCLUDES 2 Not Included Here

### Asthma

Smooth muscle fibres

Contraction of smooth muscle fibres

Respiratory bronchiole

Mucus lining bronchial tubes

Extra mucus secretion in inflamed bronchial tubes

Air trapped within alveoli

Alveoli

Normal alveoli          Asthmatic alveoli

✓5th **J45.9**  **Other and unspecified asthma**

✓6th  **J45.90**  **Unspecified asthma**
Asthmatic bronchitis NOS
Childhood asthma NOS
Late onset asthma

**J45.901**  **Unspecified asthma with (acute)**  CC
**exacerbation**

**J45.902**  **Unspecified asthma with status**  CC
**asthmaticus**

**J45.909**  **Unspecified asthma, uncomplicated**
Asthma NOS
**EXCLUDES 2** ▶lung diseases due to external
agents (J60-J70)◀
**AHA:** 2017, 1Q, 25

✓6th  **J45.99**  **Other asthma**

**J45.990**  **Exercise induced bronchospasm**

**J45.991**  **Cough variant asthma**

**J45.998**  **Other asthma**

✓4th **J47**  **Bronchiectasis**
**INCLUDES** bronchiolectasis
Use additional code to identify:
exposure to environmental tobacco smoke (Z77.22)
exposure to tobacco smoke in the perinatal period (P96.81)
history of tobacco dependence (Z87.891)
occupational exposure to environmental tobacco smoke (Z57.31)
tobacco dependence (F17.-)
tobacco use (Z72.0)
**EXCLUDES 1** congenital bronchiectasis (Q33.4)
tuberculous bronchiectasis (current disease) (A15.0)

**J47.0**  **Bronchiectasis with acute lower respiratory infection**  CC HCC
Bronchiectasis with acute bronchitis
Use additional code to identify the infection
**CC Excl:** PDX collection 743

**J47.1**  **Bronchiectasis with (acute) exacerbation**  CC HCC
**CC Excl:** PDX collection 743

**J47.9**  **Bronchiectasis, uncomplicated**  HCC
Bronchiectasis NOS

### Lung diseases due to external agents (J60-J70)

**EXCLUDES 2** asthma (J45.-)
malignant neoplasm of bronchus and lung (C34.-)

**J60**  **Coalworker's pneumoconiosis**  A HCC
Anthracosilicosis
Anthracosis
Black lung disease
Coalworker's lung
**EXCLUDES 1** coalworker pneumoconiosis with tuberculosis, any type in A15 (J65)

**J61**  **Pneumoconiosis due to asbestos and other mineral fibers**  A HCC
Asbestosis
**EXCLUDES 1** pleural plaque with asbestosis (J92.0)
pneumoconiosis with tuberculosis, any type in A15 (J65)

✓4th **J62**  **Pneumoconiosis due to dust containing silica**
**INCLUDES** silicotic fibrosis (massive) of lung
**EXCLUDES 1** pneumoconiosis with tuberculosis, any type in A15 (J65)

**J62.0**  **Pneumoconiosis due to talc dust**  HCC

**J62.8**  **Pneumoconiosis due to other dust containing silica**  HCC
Silicosis NOS

✓4th **J63**  **Pneumoconiosis due to other inorganic dusts**
**EXCLUDES 1** pneumoconiosis with tuberculosis, any type in A15 (J65)

**J63.0**  **Aluminosis (of lung)**  HCC

**J63.1**  **Bauxite fibrosis (of lung)**  HCC

**J63.2**  **Berylliosis**  HCC

**J63.3**  **Graphite fibrosis (of lung)**  HCC

**J63.4**  **Siderosis**  HCC

**J63.5**  **Stannosis**  HCC

**J63.6**  **Pneumoconiosis due to other specified inorganic dusts**  HCC

**J64**  **Unspecified pneumoconiosis**  HCC
**EXCLUDES 1** pneumonoconiosis with tuberculosis, any type in A15 (J65)

**J65**  **Pneumoconiosis associated with tuberculosis**  HCC
Any condition in J60-J64 with tuberculosis, any type in A15
Silicotuberculosis

✓4th **J66**  **Airway disease due to specific organic dust**
**EXCLUDES 2** allergic alveolitis (J67.-)
asbestosis (J61)
bagassosis (J67.1)
farmer's lung (J67.0)
hypersensitivity pneumonitis due to organic dust (J67.-)
reactive airways dysfunction syndrome (J68.3)

**J66.0**  **Byssinosis**  HCC
Airway disease due to cotton dust

**J66.1**  **Flax-dressers' disease**  HCC

**J66.2**  **Cannabinosis**  HCC

**J66.8**  **Airway disease due to other specific organic dusts**  HCC

✓4th **J67**  **Hypersensitivity pneumonitis due to organic dust**
**INCLUDES** allergic alveolitis and pneumonitis due to inhaled organic
dust and particles of fungal, actinomycetic or other
origin
**EXCLUDES 1** pneumonitis due to inhalation of chemicals, gases, fumes or
vapors (J68.0)

**CC Excl: For CC codes in category J67, unless otherwise noted:**
PDX collection 110

**J67.0**  **Farmer's lung**  HCC
Harvester's lung
Haymaker's lung
Moldy hay disease

**J67.1**  **Bagassosis**  HCC
Bagasse disease
Bagasse pneumonitis

**J67.2**  **Bird fancier's lung**  HCC
Budgerigar fancier's disease or lung
Pigeon fancier's disease or lung

**J67.3**  **Suberosis**  HCC
Corkhandler's disease or lung
Corkworker's disease or lung

**J67.4**  **Maltworker's lung**  HCC
Alveolitis due to Aspergillus clavatus

**J67.5**  **Mushroom-worker's lung**  HCC

**J67.6**  **Maple-bark-stripper's lung**  HCC
Alveolitis due to Cryptostroma corticale
Cryptostromosis

**J67.7**  **Air conditioner and humidifier lung**  CC HCC
Allergic alveolitis due to fungal, thermophilic actinomycetes and
other organisms growing in ventilation [air conditioning]
systems

**J67.8**  **Hypersensitivity pneumonitis due to other**  CC HCC
**organic dusts**
Cheese-washer's lung
Coffee-worker's lung
Fish-meal worker's lung
Furrier's lung
Sequoiosis

**J67.9**  **Hypersensitivity pneumonitis due to unspecified**  CC HCC
**organic dust**
Allergic alveolitis (extrinsic) NOS
Hypersensitivity pneumonitis NOS

Chapter 10. Diseases of the Respiratory System

**✓4ᵗʰ J68   Respiratory conditions due to inhalation of chemicals, gases, fumes and vapors**

Code first (T51-T65) to identify cause
Use additional code to identify associated respiratory conditions, such as:
   acute respiratory failure (J96.0-)

> **CC Excl: For CC/MCC codes in category J68:** PDX collection 110

**J68.0   Bronchitis and pneumonitis due to chemicals, gases, fumes and vapors**   `CC` `HCC`
   Chemical bronchitis (acute)

**J68.1   Pulmonary edema due to chemicals, gases, fumes and vapors**   `MCC` `HCC`
   Chemical pulmonary edema (acute) (chronic)
   *EXCLUDES 1*   *pulmonary edema (acute) (chronic) NOS (J81.-)*

**J68.2   Upper respiratory inflammation due to chemicals, gases, fumes and vapors, not elsewhere classified**   `HCC`

**J68.3   Other acute and subacute respiratory conditions due to chemicals, gases, fumes and vapors**   `HCC`
   Reactive airways dysfunction syndrome

**J68.4   Chronic respiratory conditions due to chemicals, gases, fumes and vapors**   `HCC`
   Emphysema (diffuse) (chronic) due to inhalation of chemicals, gases, fumes and vapors
   Obliterative bronchiolitis (chronic) (subacute) due to inhalation of chemicals, gases, fumes and vapors
   Pulmonary fibrosis (chronic) due to inhalation of chemicals, gases, fumes and vapors
   *EXCLUDES 1*   *chronic pulmonary edema due to chemicals, gases, fumes and vapors (J68.1)*

**J68.8   Other respiratory conditions due to chemicals, gases, fumes and vapors**   `HCC`

**J68.9   Unspecified respiratory condition due to chemicals, gases, fumes and vapors**   `HCC`

**✓4ᵗʰ J69   Pneumonitis due to solids and liquids**
   *EXCLUDES 1*   *neonatal aspiration syndromes (P24.-)*
           *postprocedural pneumonitis (J95.4)*
   AHA: 2017, 1Q, 24

> **CC Excl: For MCC codes in category J69:** PDX collection 110

**J69.0   Pneumonitis due to inhalation of food and vomit**   `MCC` `HCC`
   Aspiration pneumonia NOS
   Aspiration pneumonia (due to) food (regurgitated)
   Aspiration pneumonia (due to) gastric secretions
   Aspiration pneumonia (due to) milk
   Aspiration pneumonia (due to) vomit
   Code also any associated foreign body in respiratory tract (T17.-)
   *EXCLUDES 1*   *chemical pneumonitis due to anesthesia (J95.4)*
           *obstetric aspiration pneumonitis (O74.0)*

**J69.1   Pneumonitis due to inhalation of oils and essences**   `MCC` `HCC`
   Exogenous lipoid pneumonia
   Lipid pneumonia NOS
   Code first (T51-T65) to identify substance
   *EXCLUDES 1*   *endogenous lipoid pneumonia (J84.89)*

**J69.8   Pneumonitis due to inhalation of other solids and liquids**   `MCC` `HCC`
   Pneumonitis due to aspiration of blood
   Pneumonitis due to aspiration of detergent
   Code first (T51-T65) to identify substance

**✓4ᵗʰ J70   Respiratory conditions due to other external agents**

> **CC Excl: For CC codes in category J70:** PDX collection 110

**J70.0   Acute pulmonary manifestations due to radiation**   `CC` `HCC`
   Radiation pneumonitis
   Use additional code (W88-W90, X39.0-) to identify the external cause

**J70.1   Chronic and other pulmonary manifestations due to radiation**   `CC` `HCC`
   Fibrosis of lung following radiation
   Use additional code (W88-W90, X39.0-) to identify the external cause

**J70.2   Acute drug-induced interstitial lung disorders**   `HCC`
   Use additional code for adverse effect, if applicable, to identify drug (T36-T50 with fifth or sixth character 5)
   *EXCLUDES 1*   *interstitial pneumonia NOS (J84.9)*
           *lymphoid interstitial pneumonia (J84.2)*

**J70.3   Chronic drug-induced interstitial lung disorders**   `HCC`
   Use additional code for adverse effect, if applicable, to identify drug (T36-T50 with fifth or sixth character 5)
   *EXCLUDES 1*   *interstitial pneumonia NOS (J84.9)*
           *lymphoid interstitial pneumonia (J84.2)*

**J70.4   Drug-induced interstitial lung disorders, unspecified**   `HCC`
   Use additional code for adverse effect, if applicable, to identify drug (T36-T50 with fifth or sixth character 5)
   *EXCLUDES 1*   *interstitial pneumonia NOS (J84.9)*
           *lymphoid interstitial pneumonia (J84.2)*

**J70.5   Respiratory conditions due to smoke inhalation**   `HCC`
   Smoke inhalation NOS
   *EXCLUDES 1*   *smoke inhalation due to chemicals, gases, fumes and vapors (J68.9)*
   AHA: 2013, 4Q, 121

**J70.8   Respiratory conditions due to other specified external agents**   `HCC`
   Code first (T51-T65) to identify the external agent

**J70.9   Respiratory conditions due to unspecified external agent**   `HCC`
   Code first (T51-T65) to identify the external agent

## Other respiratory diseases principally affecting the interstitium (J80-J84)

**J80   Acute respiratory distress syndrome**   `CC` `HCC`
   Acute respiratory distress syndrome in adult or child
   Adult hyaline membrane disease
   *EXCLUDES 1*   *respiratory distress syndrome in newborn (perinatal) (P22.0)*
   AHA: 2017, 1Q, 26
   **CC Excl:** PDX collection 744

**✓4ᵗʰ J81   Pulmonary edema**
   Use additional code to identify:
      exposure to environmental tobacco smoke (Z77.22)
      history of tobacco dependence (Z87.891)
      occupational exposure to environmental tobacco smoke (Z57.31)
      tobacco dependence (F17.-)
      tobacco use (Z72.0)
   *EXCLUDES 1*   *chemical (acute) pulmonary edema (J68.1)*
           *hypostatic pneumonia (J18.2)*
           *passive pneumonia (J18.2)*
           *pulmonary edema due to external agents (J60-J70)*
           *pulmonary edema with heart disease NOS (I50.1)*
           *pulmonary edema with heart failure (I50.1)*

**J81.0   Acute pulmonary edema**   `MCC` `HCC`
   Acute edema of lung
   **CC Excl:** PDX collection 745

**J81.1   Chronic pulmonary edema**   `CC`
   Pulmonary congestion (chronic) (passive)
   Pulmonary edema NOS
   **CC Excl:** PDX collection 736

**J82   Pulmonary eosinophilia, not elsewhere classified**   `CC` `HCC`
   Allergic pneumonia
   Eosinophilic asthma
   Eosinophilic pneumonia
   Löffler's pneumonia
   Tropical (pulmonary) eosinophilia NOS
   *EXCLUDES 1*   *pulmonary eosinophilia due to aspergillosis (B44.-)*
           *pulmonary eosinophilia due to drugs (J70.2-J70.4)*
           *pulmonary eosinophilia due to specified parasitic infection (B50-B83)*
           *pulmonary eosinophilia due to systemic connective tissue disorders (M30-M36)*
           *pulmonary infiltrate NOS (R91.8)*
   **CC Excl:** PDX collection 746

**✓4ᵗʰ J84   Other interstitial pulmonary diseases**
   *EXCLUDES 1*   *drug-induced interstitial lung disorders (J70.2-J70.4)*
           *interstitial emphysema (J98.2)*
           ~~*lung diseases due to external agents (J60-J70)*~~
   *EXCLUDES 2*   ▶*lung diseases due to external agents (J60-J70)*◀

**✓5ᵗʰ J84.0   Alveolar and parieto-alveolar conditions**

> **CC Excl: For CC codes in subcategory J84.0:** PDX collection 747

   **J84.01   Alveolar proteinosis**   `CC` `HCC`
      **DEF:** Reduced ventilation due to proteinaceous deposits on alveoli; symptoms include dyspnea, cough, chest pain, weakness, weight loss, and hemoptysis.

   **J84.02   Pulmonary alveolar microlithiasis**   `CC` `HCC`

---

✓ Additional Character Req   ✓×7ᵗʰ Placeholder Alert   Unacceptable PDx   Manifestation   `H1`-`H14` HAC   `HCC` CMS-HCC Condition   *EXCLUDES 1* Not Coded Here   *EXCLUDES 2* Not Included Here

**J84.03**   *Idiopathic pulmonary hemosiderosis*   CC HCC
Essential brown induration of lung
Code first underlying disease, such as:
   disorders of iron metabolism (E83.1-)
EXCLUDES 1   *acute idiopathic pulmonary hemorrhage in infants [AIPHI] (R04.81)*
**DEF:** Fibrosis of alveolar walls; marked by abnormal accumulation of iron as hemosiderin in lungs; primarily affects children; symptoms include anemia, fluid in lungs, and blood in sputum; etiology unknown.

**J84.09**   **Other alveolar and parieto-alveolar conditions**   CC HCC

√5th **J84.1**   **Other interstitial pulmonary diseases with fibrosis**
EXCLUDES 1   *pulmonary fibrosis (chronic) due to inhalation of chemicals, gases, fumes or vapors (J68.4)*
*pulmonary fibrosis (chronic) following radiation (J70.1)*

CC Excl: For CC codes in subcategory J84.1:
PDX collection 747

**J84.10**   **Pulmonary fibrosis, unspecified**   HCC
Capillary fibrosis of lung
Cirrhosis of lung (chronic) NOS
Fibrosis of lung (atrophic) (chronic) (confluent) (massive) (perialveolar) (peribronchial) NOS
Induration of lung (chronic) NOS
Postinflammatory pulmonary fibrosis

√6th **J84.11**   **Idiopathic interstitial pneumonia**
EXCLUDES 1   *lymphoid interstitial pneumonia (J84.2)*
*pneumocystis pneumonia (B59)*

**J84.111**   **Idiopathic interstitial pneumonia, not otherwise specified**   HCC

**J84.112**   **Idiopathic pulmonary fibrosis**   HCC
Cryptogenic fibrosing alveolitis
Idiopathic fibrosing alveolitis

**J84.113**   **Idiopathic non-specific interstitial pneumonitis**   HCC
EXCLUDES 1   *non-specific interstitial pneumonia NOS, or due to known underlying cause (J84.89)*

**J84.114**   **Acute interstitial pneumonitis**   CC HCC
Hamman-Rich syndrome
EXCLUDES 1   *pneumocystis pneumonia (B59)*

**J84.115**   **Respiratory bronchiolitis interstitial lung disease**   HCC

**J84.116**   **Cryptogenic organizing pneumonia**   CC HCC
EXCLUDES 1   *organizing pneumonia NOS, or due to known underlying cause (J84.89)*

**J84.117**   **Desquamative interstitial pneumonia**   CC HCC

**J84.17**   *Other interstitial pulmonary diseases with fibrosis in diseases classified elsewhere*   HCC
Interstitial pneumonia (nonspecific) (usual) due to collagen vascular disease
Interstitial pneumonia (nonspecific) (usual) in diseases classified elsewhere
Organizing pneumonia due to collagen vascular disease
Organizing pneumonia in diseases classified elsewhere
Code first underlying disease, such as:
   progressive systemic sclerosis (M34.0)
   rheumatoid arthritis (M05.00-M06.9)
   systemic lupus erythematosis (M32.0-M32.9)

**J84.2**   **Lymphoid interstitial pneumonia**   CC HCC
Lymphoid interstitial pneumonitis
CC Excl: PDX collection 747

√5th **J84.8**   **Other specified interstitial pulmonary diseases**
EXCLUDES 1   *exogenous lipoid pneumonia (J69.1)*
*unspecified lipoid pneumonia (J69.1)*

**J84.81**   **Lymphangioleiomyomatosis**   MCC HCC
Lymphangiomyomatosis
CC Excl: PDX collection 747

**J84.82**   **Adult pulmonary Langerhans cell histiocytosis**   CC HCC A
Adult PLCH
CC Excl: PDX collection 747

**J84.83**   **Surfactant mutations of the lung**   MCC HCC
**DEF:** Genetic disorder resulting in insufficient secretion of a complex mixture of phospholipids and proteins that reduce surface tension in the alveoli following the onset of breathing to facilitate lung expansion in the newborn; leading indication for pediatric lung transplantation.
CC Excl: PDX collection 748

√6th **J84.84**   **Other interstitial lung diseases of childhood**

CC Excl: For MCC codes in subcategory J84.84, unless otherwise noted: PDX collection 748

**J84.841**   **Neuroendocrine cell hyperplasia of infancy**   MCC HCC

**J84.842**   **Pulmonary interstitial glycogenosis**   MCC HCC

**J84.843**   **Alveolar capillary dysplasia with vein misalignment**   MCC HCC

**J84.848**   **Other interstitial lung diseases of childhood**   MCC HCC

**J84.89**   **Other specified interstitial pulmonary diseases**   HCC
Endogenous lipoid pneumonia
Interstitial pneumonitis
Non-specific interstitial pneumonitis NOS
Organizing pneumonia NOS
Code first, if applicable:
   poisoning due to drug or toxin (T51-T65 with fifth or sixth character to indicate intent), for toxic pneumonopathy
   underlying cause of pneumonopathy, if known
Use additional code, for adverse effect, to identify drug (T36-T50 with fifth or sixth character 5), if drug-induced
EXCLUDES 1   *cryptogenic organizing pneumonia (J84.116)*
*idiopathic non-specific interstitial pneumonitis (J84.113)*
*lipoid pneumonia, exogenous or unspecified (J69.1)*
*lymphoid interstitial pneumonia (J84.2)*

**J84.9**   **Interstitial pulmonary disease, unspecified**   CC HCC
Interstitial pneumonia NOS
CC Excl: PDX collection 747

## Suppurative and necrotic conditions of the lower respiratory tract (J85-J86)

√4th **J85**   **Abscess of lung and mediastinum**
Use additional code (B95-B97) to identify infectious agent

CC Excl: For MCC codes in category J85, unless otherwise noted: PDX collection 749

**J85.0**   **Gangrene and necrosis of lung**   MCC HCC

**J85.1**   **Abscess of lung with pneumonia**   MCC HCC
Code also the type of pneumonia

**J85.2**   **Abscess of lung without pneumonia**   MCC HCC
Abscess of lung NOS

**J85.3**   **Abscess of mediastinum**   MCC HCC
CC Excl: PDX collection 750

√4th **J86**   **Pyothorax**
Use additional code (B95-B97) to identify infectious agent
EXCLUDES 1   *abscess of lung (J85.-)*
*pyothorax due to tuberculosis (A15.6)*

**J86.0**   **Pyothorax with fistula**   MCC HCC
Bronchocutaneous fistula
Bronchopleural fistula
Hepatopleural fistula
Mediastinal fistula
Pleural fistula
Thoracic fistula
Any condition classifiable to J86.9 with fistula
**DEF:** Purulent infection of respiratory cavity, with communication from cavity to another structure.
CC Excl: PDX collection 751

**J86.9**   **Pyothorax without fistula**   MCC HCC
Abscess of pleura
Abscess of thorax
Empyema (chest) (lung) (pleura)
Fibrinopurulent pleurisy
Purulent pleurisy
Pyopneumothorax
Septic pleurisy
Seropurulent pleurisy
Suppurative pleurisy
CC Excl: PDX collection 751

N Newborn: 0   P Pediatric: 0-17   M Maternity: 12-55   A Adult: 15-124   MCC Major CC Condition   PDxMCC PDx acts as own MCC   CC CC Condition   PDxCC PDx acts as own CC

680      ICD-10-CM 2018

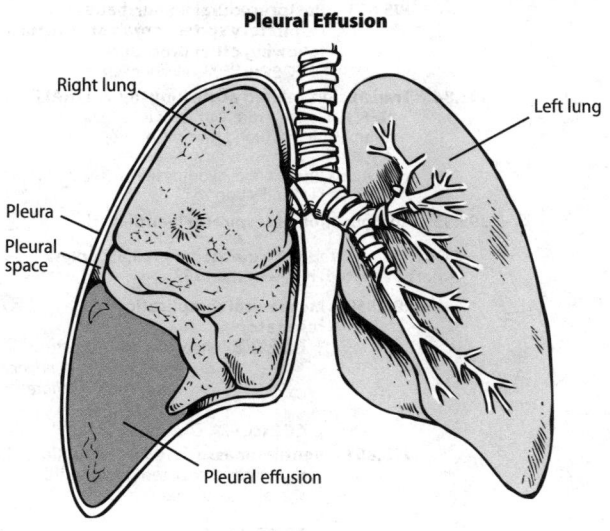

**Pleural Effusion**

Right lung

Left lung

Pleura

Pleural space

Pleural effusion

## Other diseases of the pleura (J90-J94)

**J90**   **Pleural effusion, not elsewhere classified**    `CC`
Encysted pleurisy
Pleural effusion NOS
Pleurisy with effusion (exudative) (serous)
    **EXCLUDES 1**   *chylous (pleural) effusion (J94.0)*
         *malignant pleural effusion (J91.0))*
         *pleurisy NOS (R09.1)*
         *tuberculous pleural effusion (A15.6)*
    **CC Excl:** PDX collection 752

✓4ᵗʰ **J91**   **Pleural effusion in conditions classified elsewhere**
    **EXCLUDES 2**   *pleural effusion in heart failure (I50.-)*
         *pleural effusion in systemic lupus erythematosus (M32.13)*

    **J91.0**   *Malignant pleural effusion*    `CC`
       Code first underlying neoplasm
       **CC Excl:** PDX collection 753

    **J91.8**   *Pleural effusion in other conditions classified elsewhere*    `CC`
       Code first underlying disease, such as:
         filariasis (B74.0-B74.9)
         influenza (J09.X2, J10.1, J11.1)
       **AHA:** 2015, 2Q, 15
       **CC Excl:** PDX collection 752

✓4ᵗʰ **J92**   **Pleural plaque**
    **INCLUDES**   pleural thickening

    **J92.0**   **Pleural plaque with presence of asbestos**

    **J92.9**   **Pleural plaque without asbestos**
       Pleural plaque NOS

✓4ᵗʰ **J93**   **Pneumothorax and air leak**
    **EXCLUDES 1**   *congenital or perinatal pneumothorax (P25.1)*
         *postprocedural air leak (J95.812)*
         *postprocedural pneumothorax (J95.811)*
         *traumatic pneumothorax (S27.0)*
         *tuberculous (current disease) pneumothorax (A15.-)*
         *pyopneumothorax (J86.-)*

    **CC Excl: For CC/MCC codes in category J93:** PDX collection 754

    **J93.0**   **Spontaneous tension pneumothorax**    `MCC`
       **DEF:** Leaking air from lung into lining, causing collapse.

✓5ᵗʰ   **J93.1**   **Other spontaneous pneumothorax**

       **J93.11**   **Primary spontaneous pneumothorax**    `CC`

       **J93.12**   **Secondary spontaneous pneumothorax**    `CC`
          Code first underlying condition, such as:
            catamenial pneumothorax due to endometriosis (N80.8)
            cystic fibrosis (E84.-)
            eosinophilic pneumonia (J82)
            lymphangioleiomyomatosis (J84.81)
            malignant neoplasm of bronchus and lung (C34.-)
            Marfan's syndrome (Q87.4)
            pneumonia due to Pneumocystis carinii (B59)
            secondary malignant neoplasm of lung (C78.0-)
            spontaneous rupture of the esophagus (K22.3)

✓5ᵗʰ   **J93.8**   **Other pneumothorax and air leak**

       **J93.81**   **Chronic pneumothorax**    `CC`

---

       **J93.82**   **Other air leak**    `CC`
          Persistent air leak

       **J93.83**   **Other pneumothorax**    `CC`
          Acute pneumothorax
          Spontaneous pneumothorax NOS

    **J93.9**   **Pneumothorax, unspecified**    `CC`
       Pneumothorax NOS

✓4ᵗʰ **J94**   **Other pleural conditions**
    **EXCLUDES 1**   *pleurisy NOS (R09.1)*
         *traumatic hemopneumothorax (S27.2)*
         *traumatic hemothorax (S27.1)*
         *tuberculous pleural conditions (current disease) (A15.-)*

    **J94.0**   **Chylous effusion**    `CC`
       Chyliform effusion
       **CC Excl:** PDX collection 752

    **J94.1**   **Fibrothorax**

    **J94.2**   **Hemothorax**    `CC`
       Hemopneumothorax
       **CC Excl:** PDX collection 752

    **J94.8**   **Other specified pleural conditions**    `CC`
       Hydropneumothorax
       Hydrothorax
       **CC Excl:** No excl

    **J94.9**   **Pleural condition, unspecified**

## Intraoperative and postprocedural complications and disorders of respiratory system, not elsewhere classified (J95)

✓4ᵗʰ **J95**   **Intraoperative and postprocedural complications and disorders of respiratory system, not elsewhere classified**
    **EXCLUDES 2**   *aspiration pneumonia (J69.-)*
         *emphysema (subcutaneous) resulting from a procedure (T81.82)*
         *hypostatic pneumonia (J18.2)*
         *pulmonary manifestations due to radiation (J70.0- J70.1)*

✓5ᵗʰ   **J95.0**   **Tracheostomy complications**

    **CC Excl: For CC codes in subcategory J95.0, unless otherwise noted:** PDX collection 755

       **J95.00**   **Unspecified tracheostomy complication**    `CC` `HCC`

       **J95.01**   **Hemorrhage from tracheostomy stoma**    `CC` `HCC`

       **J95.02**   **Infection of tracheostomy stoma**    `CC` `HCC`
          Use additional code to identify type of infection, such as:
            cellulitis of neck ▶(L03.221)◄
            sepsis (A40, A41-)

       **J95.03**   **Malfunction of tracheostomy stoma**    `CC` `HCC`
          Mechanical complication of tracheostomy stoma
          Obstruction of tracheostomy airway
          Tracheal stenosis due to tracheostomy

**Tracheostomy**

Tracheostomy in place

Incision in trachea

Trachea

Tracheostomy tube

---

✓ Additional Character Req    ✓x7ᵗʰ Placeholder Alert    Unacceptable PDx    Manifestation    **H1**–**H14** HAC    `HCC` CMS-HCC Condition    **EXCLUDES 1** Not Coded Here    **EXCLUDES 2** Not Included Here

**J95.04**   Tracheo-esophageal fistula **following tracheostomy**    `CC` `HCC`

**J95.09**   Other **tracheostomy complication**    `CC` `HCC`

**J95.1**   Acute pulmonary insufficiency **following** thoracic surgery    `MCC` `HCC`
> *EXCLUDES 2*   *functional disturbances following cardiac surgery (I97.0, I97.1-)*
> **CC Excl:** PDX collection 756

**J95.2**   Acute pulmonary insufficiency **following nonthoracic surgery**    `MCC` `HCC`
> *EXCLUDES 2*   *functional disturbances following cardiac surgery (I97.0, I97.1-)*
> **CC Excl:** PDX collection 756

**J95.3**   Chronic pulmonary insufficiency **following surgery**    `MCC` `HCC`
> *EXCLUDES 2*   *functional disturbances following cardiac surgery (I97.0, I97.1-)*
> **CC Excl:** PDX collection 756

**J95.4**   Chemical pneumonitis **due to anesthesia**    `CC`
> Mendelson's syndrome
> Postprocedural aspiration pneumonia
> Use additional code for adverse effect, if applicable, to identify drug (T41.- with fifth or sixth character 5)
> *EXCLUDES 1*   *aspiration pneumonitis due to anesthesia complicating labor and delivery (O74.0)*
> *aspiration pneumonitis due to anesthesia complicating pregnancy (O29)*
> *aspiration pneumonitis due to anesthesia complicating the puerperium (O89.01)*
> **CC Excl:** PDX collection 757

**J95.5**   Postprocedural subglottic stenosis    `CC`
> **CC Excl:** PDX collection 757

√5th **J95.6**   Intraoperative hemorrhage and hematoma **of a respiratory system organ or structure complicating a procedure**
> *EXCLUDES 1*   *intraoperative hemorrhage and hematoma of a respiratory system organ or structure due to accidental puncture and laceration during procedure (J95.7-)*

**J95.61**   Intraoperative hemorrhage and hematoma of a respiratory system organ or structure complicating a respiratory system procedure    `CC`
> **CC Excl:** PDX collection 758

**J95.62**   Intraoperative hemorrhage and hematoma of a respiratory system organ or structure complicating other procedure    `CC`
> **CC Excl:** PDX collection 758

√5th **J95.7**   Accidental puncture and laceration **of a respiratory system organ or structure during a procedure**
> *EXCLUDES 2*   *postprocedural pneumothorax (J95.811)*

**J95.71**   Accidental puncture and laceration of a respiratory system organ or structure during a respiratory system procedure    `CC`
> **CC Excl:** PDX collection 509

**J95.72**   Accidental puncture and laceration of a respiratory system organ or structure during other procedure    `CC`
> **CC Excl:** PDX collection 509

√5th **J95.8**   Other **intraoperative and postprocedural complications and disorders of respiratory system, not elsewhere classified**

√6th **J95.81**   Postprocedural **pneumothorax and air leak**

**J95.811**   Postprocedural **pneumothorax**    `CC` `H14`
> **CC Excl:** PDX collection 754

**J95.812**   Postprocedural **air leak**    `CC`
> **CC Excl:** PDX collection 754

√6th **J95.82**   Postprocedural **respiratory failure**
> *EXCLUDES 1*   *respiratory failure in other conditions (J96.-)*

**J95.821**   Acute **postprocedural respiratory failure**    `MCC` `HCC`
> Postprocedural respiratory failure NOS
> **CC Excl:** PDX collection 756

**J95.822**   Acute and chronic **postprocedural respiratory failure**    `MCC` `HCC`
> **CC Excl:** PDX collection 756

√6th **J95.83**   Postprocedural **hemorrhage of a respiratory system organ or structure following a procedure**

**J95.830**   Postprocedural **hemorrhage of a respiratory system organ or structure following a respiratory system procedure**    `CC`
> **CC Excl:** PDX collection 758

**J95.831**   Postprocedural **hemorrhage of a respiratory system organ or structure following other procedure**    `CC`
> **CC Excl:** PDX collection 758

**J95.84**   Transfusion-related acute lung injury **(TRALI)**    `CC`
> **DEF:** A relatively rare, but serious, pulmonary complication of blood transfusion, with acute respiratory distress, noncardiogenic pulmonary edema, cyanosis, hypoxemia, hypotension, fever, and chills.
> **CC Excl:** PDX collection 757

√6th **J95.85**   **Complication of respirator [ventilator]**

> **CC Excl: For CC codes in subcategory J95.85, unless otherwise noted:** PDX collection 757

**J95.850**   Mechanical **complication of respirator**    `CC` `HCC`
> *EXCLUDES 1*   *encounter for respirator [ventilator] dependence during power failure (Z99.12)*
> **CC Excl:** PDX collection 759

**J95.851**   Ventilator **associated pneumonia**    `HCC`
> Ventilator associated pneumonitis
> Use additional code to identify the organism, if known (B95.-, B96.-, B97.-)
> *EXCLUDES 1*   *ventilator lung in newborn (P27.8)*
> **AHA:** 2017, 1Q, 25

**J95.859**   Other **complication of respirator [ventilator]**    `CC` `HCC`

√6th **J95.86**   Postprocedural **hematoma and seroma of a respiratory system organ or structure following a procedure**

> **CC Excl: For CC codes in subcategory J95.86:** PDX collection 758

**J95.860**   Postprocedural **hematoma of a respiratory system organ or structure following a respiratory system procedure**    `CC`

**J95.861**   Postprocedural **hematoma of a respiratory system organ or structure following other procedure**    `CC`

**J95.862**   Postprocedural **seroma of a respiratory system organ or structure following a respiratory system procedure**    `CC`

**J95.863**   Postprocedural **seroma of a respiratory system organ or structure following other procedure**    `CC`

**J95.88**   Other intraoperative **complications of respiratory system, not elsewhere classified**    `CC`
> **CC Excl:** PDX collection 757

**J95.89**   Other postprocedural **complications and disorders of respiratory system, not elsewhere classified**    `CC`
> Use additional code to identify disorder, such as:
> aspiration pneumonia (J69.-)
> bacterial or viral pneumonia (J12-J18)
> *EXCLUDES 2*   *acute pulmonary insufficiency following thoracic surgery (J95.1)*
> *postprocedural subglottic stenosis (J95.5)*
> **CC Excl:** PDX collection 757

## Other diseases of the respiratory system (J96-J99)

√4th **J96**   **Respiratory failure, not elsewhere classified**
> *EXCLUDES 1*   *acute respiratory distress syndrome (J80)*
> *cardiorespiratory failure (R09.2)*
> *newborn respiratory distress syndrome (P22.0)*
> *postprocedural respiratory failure (J95.82-)*
> *respiratory arrest (R09.2)*
> *respiratory arrest of newborn (P28.81)*
> *respiratory failure of newborn (P28.5)*

> **CC Excl: For CC/MCC codes in category J96:** PDX collection 744

√5th **J96.0**   **Acute respiratory failure**

**J96.00**   Acute respiratory failure, unspecified **whether with hypoxia or hypercapnia**    `MCC` `HCC`
> **AHA:** 2016, 3Q, 14; 2013, 4Q, 121

**J96.01**   Acute respiratory failure with **hypoxia**    `MCC` `HCC`

**J96.02**   Acute respiratory failure with **hypercapnia**    `MCC` `HCC`

`N` Newborn: 0   `P` Pediatric: 0-17   `M` Maternity: 12-55   `A` Adult: 15-124   `MCC` Major CC Condition   `PDxMCC` PDx acts as own MCC   `CC` CC Condition   `PDxCC` PDx acts as own CC

682        ICD-10-CM 2018

☑5ᵗʰ **J96.1** **Chronic** respiratory failure

    **J96.10** **Chronic respiratory failure, unspecified** `CC` `HCC`
           **whether with hypoxia or hypercapnia**
           **AHA:** 2016, 1Q, 38; 2015, 1Q, 21

    **J96.11** **Chronic respiratory failure with** hypoxia `CC` `HCC`
           **AHA:** 2013, 4Q, 129

    **J96.12** **Chronic respiratory failure with** hypercapnia `CC` `HCC`

☑5ᵗʰ **J96.2** **Acute and chronic** respiratory failure
    Acute on chronic respiratory failure

    **J96.20** **Acute and chronic respiratory failure,** `MCC` `HCC`
           **unspecified whether with hypoxia or**
           **hypercapnia**

    **J96.21** **Acute and chronic respiratory failure with** `MCC` `HCC`
           **hypoxia**

    **J96.22** **Acute and chronic respiratory failure with** `MCC` `HCC`
           **hypercapnia**

☑5ᵗʰ **J96.9** **Respiratory failure,** unspecified

    **J96.90** **Respiratory failure, unspecified,** `MCC` `HCC`
           **unspecified whether with hypoxia**
           **or hypercapnia**

    **J96.91** **Respiratory failure, unspecified with** `MCC` `HCC`
           **hypoxia**

    **J96.92** **Respiratory failure, unspecified with** `MCC` `HCC`
           **hypercapnia**

☑4ᵗʰ **J98** **Other respiratory disorders**
    Use additional code to identify:
      exposure to environmental tobacco smoke (Z77.22)
      exposure to tobacco smoke in the perinatal period (P96.81)
      history of tobacco dependence (Z87.891)
      occupational exposure to environmental tobacco smoke (Z57.31)
      tobacco dependence (F17.-)
      tobacco use (Z72.0)
    *EXCLUDES 1*　newborn apnea (P28.4)
             newborn sleep apnea (P28.3)
    *EXCLUDES 2*　apnea NOS (R06.81)
             sleep apnea (G47.3-)

☑5ᵗʰ **J98.0** **Diseases of bronchus, not elsewhere classified**

    **J98.01** **Acute bronchospasm**
        *EXCLUDES 1*　acute bronchiolitis with bronchospasm
                (J21.-)
               acute bronchitis with bronchospasm (J20.-)
               asthma (J45.-)
               exercise induced bronchospasm (J45.990)

    **J98.09** **Other diseases of bronchus, not elsewhere classified**
        Broncholithiasis
        Calcification of bronchus
        Stenosis of bronchus
        Tracheobronchial collapse
        Tracheobronchial dyskinesia
        Ulcer of bronchus

☑5ᵗʰ **J98.1** **Pulmonary collapse**
    *EXCLUDES 1*　therapeutic collapse of lung status (Z98.3)

    **J98.11** **Atelectasis** `CC`
        *EXCLUDES 1*　newborn atelectasis
                tuberculous atelectasis (current disease)
                   (A15)
        **CC Excl:** PDX collection 760

    **J98.19** **Other pulmonary collapse** `CC`
        **CC Excl:** PDX collection 760

    **J98.2** **Interstitial emphysema** `HCC`
        Mediastinal emphysema
        *EXCLUDES 1*　emphysema NOS (J43.9)
               emphysema in newborn (P25.0)
               surgical emphysema (subcutaneous) (T81.82)
               traumatic subcutaneous emphysema (T79.7)

**J98.3** **Compensatory emphysema** `HCC`
    **DEF:** Distention of all or part of the lung caused by disease
    processes or surgical intervention that decreased volume in
    another part of the lung; overcompensation reaction to the loss of
    capacity in another part of the lung; occurs in association with
    pneumonias, pleural effusions, atelectasis, empyema, and
    pneumothorax.

**J98.4** **Other disorders of lung**
    Calcification of lung
    Cystic lung disease (acquired)
    Lung disease NOS
    Pulmolithiasis
    *EXCLUDES 1*　acute interstitial pneumonitis (J84.114)
             pulmonary insufficiency following surgery (J95.1-
               J95.2)

☑5ᵗʰ **J98.5** **Diseases of mediastinum, not elsewhere classified**
    *EXCLUDES 2*　abscess of mediastinum (J85.3)

    **J98.51** **Mediastinitis** `MCC` `H8`
        Code first:
          underlying condition, if applicable, such as
              postoperative mediastinitis (T81.-)
        **CC Excl:** No Excl

    **J98.59** **Other diseases of mediastinum, not** `MCC` `H8`
        **elsewhere classified**
        Fibrosis of mediastinum
        Hernia of mediastinum
        Retraction of mediastinum
        **CC Excl:** No Excl

**J98.6** **Disorders of diaphragm**
    Diaphragmatitis
    Paralysis of diaphragm
    Relaxation of diaphragm
    *EXCLUDES 1*　congenital malformation of diaphragm NEC (Q79.1)
             congenital diaphragmatic hernia (Q79.0)
    *EXCLUDES 2*　diaphragmatic hernia (K44.-)

**J98.8** **Other specified respiratory disorders**

**J98.9** **Respiratory disorder, unspecified**
    Respiratory disease (chronic) NOS

**J99** ***Respiratory disorders in diseases classified elsewhere*** `HCC`
    Code first underlying disease, such as:
      amyloidosis (E85.-)
      ankylosing spondylitis (M45)
      congenital syphilis (A50.5)
      cryoglobulinemia (D89.1)
      early congenital syphilis (A50.0)
      schistosomiasis (B65.0-B65.9)
    *EXCLUDES 1*　respiratory disorders in:
             amebiasis (A06.5)
             blastomycosis (B40.0-B40.2)
             candidiasis (B37.1)
             coccidioidomycosis (B38.0-B38.2)
             cystic fibrosis with pulmonary manifestations (E84.0)
             dermatomyositis (M33.01, M33.11)
             histoplasmosis (B39.0-B39.2)
             late syphilis (A52.72, A52.73)
             polymyositis (M33.21)
             sicca syndrome (M35.02)
             systemic lupus erythematosus (M32.13)
             systemic sclerosis (M34.81)
             Wegener's granulomatosis (M31.30-M31.31)

☑Additional Character Req　☑x7ᵗʰ Placeholder Alert　Unacceptable PDx　Manifestation　`H1`-`H14` HAC　`HCC` CMS-HCC Condition　*EXCLUDES 1* Not Coded Here　*EXCLUDES 2* Not Included Here

ICD-10-CM 2018　　　　　683

# Chapter 11. Diseases of the Digestive System (KØØ–K95)

**Chapter Specific Coding Guidelines and Examples**
Reserved for future guideline expansion.

**Chapter 11. Diseases of the Digestive System**
*(continued in left margin: Chapter 11. Diseases of the Digestive System)*

# Chapter 11. Diseases of the Digestive System (K00-K95)

**EXCLUDES 2** *certain conditions originating in the perinatal period (P04-P96)*
*certain infectious and parasitic diseases (A00-B99)*
*complications of pregnancy, childbirth and the puerperium (O00-O9A)*
*congenital malformations, deformations and chromosomal abnormalities (Q00-Q99)*
*endocrine, nutritional and metabolic diseases (E00-E88)*
*injury, poisoning and certain other consequences of external causes (S00-T88)*
*neoplasms (C00-D49)*
*symptoms, signs and abnormal clinical and laboratory findings, not elsewhere classified (R00-R94)*

This chapter contains the following blocks:

| | |
|---|---|
| K00-K14 | Diseases of oral cavity and salivary glands |
| K20-K31 | Diseases of esophagus, stomach and duodenum |
| K35-K38 | Diseases of appendix |
| K40-K46 | Hernia |
| K50-K52 | Noninfective enteritis and colitis |
| K55-K64 | Other diseases of intestines |
| K65-K68 | Diseases of peritoneum and retroperitoneum |
| K70-K77 | Diseases of liver |
| K80-K87 | Disorders of gallbladder, biliary tract and pancreas |
| K90-K95 | Other diseases of the digestive system |

## Diseases of oral cavity and salivary glands (K00-K14)

**✓4ᵗʰ K00 Disorders of tooth development and eruption**
    **EXCLUDES 2** *embedded and impacted teeth (K01.-)*

**K00.0 Anodontia**
    Hypodontia
    Oligodontia
    **EXCLUDES 1** *acquired absence of teeth (K08.1-)*

**K00.1 Supernumerary teeth**
    Distomolar
    Fourth molar
    Mesiodens
    Paramolar
    Supplementary teeth
    **EXCLUDES 2** *supernumerary roots (K00.2)*

**K00.2 Abnormalities of size and form of teeth**
    Concrescence of teeth
    Dens evaginatus
    Dens in dente
    Dens invaginatus
    Enamel pearls
    Fusion of teeth
    Gemination of teeth
    Macrodontia
    Microdontia
    Peg-shaped [conical] teeth
    Supernumerary roots
    Taurodontism
    Tuberculum paramolare
    **EXCLUDES 1** *abnormalities of teeth due to congenital syphilis (A50.5)*
    *tuberculum Carabelli, which is regarded as a normal variation and should not be coded*

**K00.3 Mottled teeth**
    Dental fluorosis
    Mottling of enamel
    Nonfluoride enamel opacities
    **EXCLUDES 2** *deposits [accretions] on teeth (K03.6)*

**K00.4 Disturbances in tooth formation**
    Aplasia and hypoplasia of cementum
    Dilaceration of tooth
    Enamel hypoplasia (neonatal) (postnatal) (prenatal)
    Regional odontodysplasia
    Turner's tooth
    **EXCLUDES 1** *Hutchinson's teeth and mulberry molars in congenital syphilis (A50.5)*
    **EXCLUDES 2** *mottled teeth (K00.3)*

**K00.5 Hereditary disturbances in tooth structure, not elsewhere classified**
    Amelogenesis imperfecta
    Dentinogenesis imperfecta
    Odontogenesis imperfecta
    Dentinal dysplasia
    Shell teeth

**Tooth Anatomy**

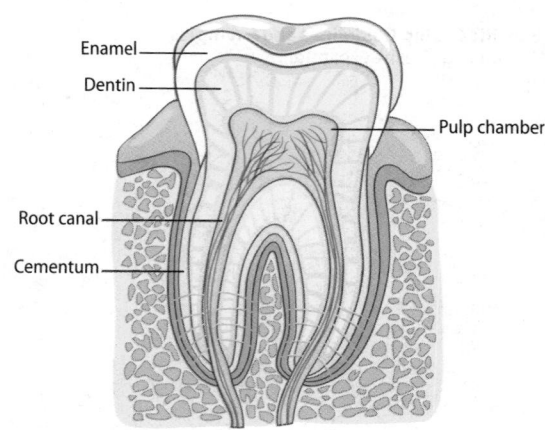

Enamel
Dentin
Pulp chamber
Root canal
Cementum

**K00.6 Disturbances in tooth eruption**
    Dentia praecox
    Natal tooth
    Neonatal tooth
    Premature eruption of tooth
    Premature shedding of primary [deciduous] tooth
    Prenatal teeth
    Retained [persistent] primary tooth
    **EXCLUDES 2** *embedded and impacted teeth (K01.-)*

**K00.7 Teething syndrome**

**K00.8 Other disorders of tooth development**
    Color changes during tooth formation
    Intrinsic staining of teeth NOS
    **EXCLUDES 2** *posteruptive color changes (K03.7)*

**K00.9 Disorder of tooth development, unspecified**
    Disorder of odontogenesis NOS

**✓4ᵗʰ K01 Embedded and impacted teeth**
    **EXCLUDES 1** *abnormal position of fully erupted teeth (M26.3-)*

**K01.0 Embedded teeth**

**K01.1 Impacted teeth**

**✓4ᵗʰ K02 Dental caries**
    **INCLUDES** caries of dentine
    dental cavities
    early childhood caries
    pre-eruptive caries
    recurrent caries (dentino enamel junction) (enamel) (to the pulp)
    tooth decay

**K02.3 Arrested dental caries**
    Arrested coronal and root caries

**✓5ᵗʰ K02.5 Dental caries on pit and fissure surface**
    Dental caries on chewing surface of tooth

    **K02.51 Dental caries on pit and fissure surface limited to enamel**
        White spot lesions [initial caries] on pit and fissure surface of tooth

    **K02.52 Dental caries on pit and fissure surface penetrating into dentin**
        Primary dental caries, cervical origin

    **K02.53 Dental caries on pit and fissure surface penetrating into pulp**

**✓5ᵗʰ K02.6 Dental caries on smooth surface**

    **K02.61 Dental caries on smooth surface limited to enamel**
        White spot lesions [initial caries] on smooth surface of tooth

    **K02.62 Dental caries on smooth surface penetrating into dentin**

    **K02.63 Dental caries on smooth surface penetrating into pulp**

**K02.7 Dental root caries**

**K02.9 Dental caries, unspecified**

N Newborn: 0    P Pediatric: 0-17    M Maternity: 12-55    A Adult: 15-124    MCC Major CC Condition    PDxMCC PDx acts as own MCC    CC CC Condition    PDxCC PDx acts as own CC

686      ICD-10-CM 2018

✓4ᵗʰ **K03** **Other diseases of hard tissues of teeth**
> EXCLUDES 2   *bruxism (F45.8)*
> *dental caries (K02.-)*
> *teeth-grinding NOS (F45.8)*

**K03.0** **Excessive attrition of teeth**
Approximal wear of teeth
Occlusal wear of teeth

**K03.1** **Abrasion of teeth**
Dentifrice abrasion of teeth
Habitual abrasion of teeth
Occupational abrasion of teeth
Ritual abrasion of teeth
Traditional abrasion of teeth
Wedge defect NOS

**K03.2** **Erosion of teeth**
Erosion of teeth due to diet
Erosion of teeth due to drugs and medicaments
Erosion of teeth due to persistent vomiting
Erosion of teeth NOS
Idiopathic erosion of teeth
Occupational erosion of teeth

**K03.3** **Pathological resorption of teeth**
Internal granuloma of pulp
Resorption of teeth (external)

**K03.4** **Hypercementosis**
Cementation hyperplasia

**K03.5** **Ankylosis of teeth**

**K03.6** **Deposits [accretions] on teeth**
Betel deposits [accretions] on teeth
Black deposits [accretions] on teeth
Extrinsic staining of teeth NOS
Green deposits [accretions] on teeth
Materia alba deposits [accretions] on teeth
Orange deposits [accretions] on teeth
Staining of teeth NOS
Subgingival dental calculus
Supragingival dental calculus
Tobacco deposits [accretions] on teeth

**K03.7** **Posteruptive color changes of dental hard tissues**
> EXCLUDES 2   *deposits [accretions] on teeth (K03.6)*

✓5ᵗʰ **K03.8** **Other specified diseases of hard tissues of teeth**
**K03.81** **Cracked tooth**
> EXCLUDES 1   *asymptomatic craze lines in enamel—omit code*
> *broken or fractured tooth due to trauma (S02.5)*

**K03.89** **Other specified diseases of hard tissues of teeth**

**K03.9** **Disease of hard tissues of teeth, unspecified**

✓4ᵗʰ **K04** **Diseases of pulp and periapical tissues**

> **CC Excl: For CC codes in category K04:** PDX collection 761

✓5ᵗʰ **K04.0** **Pulpitis**
Acute pulpitis
Chronic (hyperplastic) (ulcerative) pulpitis

**K04.01** **Reversible pulpitis**    CC

**K04.02** **Irreversible pulpitis**    CC

**K04.1** **Necrosis of pulp**
Pulpal gangrene

**K04.2** **Pulp degeneration**
Denticles
Pulpal calcifications
Pulpal stones

**K04.3** **Abnormal hard tissue formation in pulp**
Secondary or irregular dentine

**K04.4** **Acute apical periodontitis of pulpal origin**    CC
Acute apical periodontitis NOS
> EXCLUDES 1   *acute periodontitis (K05.2)*

> **DEF:** Severe inflammation of the area surrounding the tip of a tooth's root; often secondary to infection or trauma.
> **CC Excl:** PDX collection 761

**K04.5** **Chronic apical periodontitis**
Apical or periapical granuloma
Apical periodontitis NOS
> EXCLUDES 1   *chronic periodontitis (K05.3-)*

**K04.6** **Periapical abscess with sinus**
Dental abscess with sinus
Dentoalveolar abscess with sinus

**K04.7** **Periapical abscess without sinus**
Dental abscess without sinus
Dentoalveolar abscess without sinus
~~Periapical abscess without sinus~~

**K04.8** **Radicular cyst**
Apical (periodontal) cyst
Periapical cyst
Residual radicular cyst
> EXCLUDES 2   *lateral periodontal cyst (K09.0)*

> **DEF:** Most common odontogenic cyst in tissue around tooth apex due to chronic inflammation of dental pulp.

✓5ᵗʰ **K04.9** **Other and unspecified diseases of pulp and periapical tissues**
**K04.90** **Unspecified diseases of pulp and periapical tissues**

**K04.99** **Other diseases of pulp and periapical tissues**

✓4ᵗʰ **K05** **Gingivitis and periodontal diseases**
Use additional code to identify:
alcohol abuse and dependence (F10.-)
exposure to environmental tobacco smoke (Z77.22)
exposure to tobacco smoke in the perinatal period (P96.81)
history of tobacco dependence (Z87.891)
occupational exposure to environmental tobacco smoke (Z57.31)
tobacco dependence (F17.-)
tobacco use (Z72.0)

✓5ᵗʰ **K05.0** **Acute gingivitis**
> EXCLUDES 1   *acute necrotizing ulcerative gingivitis (A69.1)*
> *herpesviral [herpes simplex] gingivostomatitis (B00.2)*

**K05.00** **Acute gingivitis, plaque induced**
Acute gingivitis NOS
Plaque induced gingival disease

**K05.01** **Acute gingivitis, non-plaque induced**

✓5ᵗʰ **K05.1** **Chronic gingivitis**
Desquamative gingivitis (chronic)
Gingivitis (chronic) NOS
Hyperplastic gingivitis (chronic)
Pregnancy associated gingivitis
Simple marginal gingivitis (chronic)
Ulcerative gingivitis (chronic)
Code first, if applicable, diseases of the digestive system complicating pregnancy (O99.61-)

**K05.10** **Chronic gingivitis, plaque induced**
Chronic gingivitis NOS
Gingivitis NOS

**K05.11** **Chronic gingivitis, non-plaque induced**

✓5ᵗʰ **K05.2** **Aggressive periodontitis**
Acute pericoronitis
> EXCLUDES 1   *acute apical periodontitis (K04.4)*
> *periapical abscess (K04.7)*
> *periapical abscess with sinus (K04.6)*

**K05.20** **Aggressive periodontitis, unspecified**

✓6ᵗʰ **K05.21** **Aggressive periodontitis, localized**
Periodontal abscess
**K05.211** **Aggressive periodontitis, localized, slight**

**K05.212** **Aggressive periodontitis, localized, moderate**

**K05.213** **Aggressive periodontitis, localized, severe**

**K05.219** **Aggressive periodontitis, localized, unspecified severity**

✓6ᵗʰ **K05.22** **Aggressive periodontitis, generalized**
**K05.221** **Aggressive periodontitis, generalized, slight**

**K05.222** **Aggressive periodontitis, generalized, moderate**

**K05.223** **Aggressive periodontitis, generalized, severe**

**K05.229** **Aggressive periodontitis, generalized, unspecified severity**

✓5ᵗʰ **K05.3** **Chronic periodontitis**
Chronic pericoronitis      Periodontitis NOS
Complex periodontitis      Simplex periodontitis
> EXCLUDES 1   *chronic apical periodontitis (K04.5)*

**K05.30** **Chronic periodontitis, unspecified**

✓6ᵗʰ **K05.31** **Chronic periodontitis, localized**
**K05.311** **Chronic periodontitis, localized, slight**

**K05.312** **Chronic periodontitis, localized, moderate**

        **K05.313**   **Chronic periodontitis, localized, severe**

        **K05.319**   **Chronic periodontitis, localized, unspecified severity**

   ✓6th **K05.32**   **Chronic periodontitis, generalized**

        **K05.321**   **Chronic periodontitis, generalized, slight**

        **K05.322**   **Chronic periodontitis, generalized, moderate**

        **K05.323**   **Chronic periodontitis, generalized, severe**

        **K05.329**   **Chronic periodontitis, generalized, unspecified severity**

  **K05.4**   **Periodontosis**
      Juvenile periodontosis

  **K05.5**   **Other periodontal diseases**
      Combined periodontic-endodontic lesion
      Narrow gingival width (of periodontal soft tissue)
      EXCLUDES 2   *leukoplakia of gingiva (K13.21)*

  **K05.6**   **Periodontal disease, unspecified**

✓4th **K06**   **Other disorders of gingiva and edentulous alveolar ridge**
    EXCLUDES 2   *acute gingivitis (K05.0)*
            *atrophy of edentulous alveolar ridge (K08.2)*
            *chronic gingivitis (K05.1)*
            *gingivitis NOS (K05.1)*

  ✓5th **K06.0**   **Gingival recession**
      ▶Gingival recession (postinfective) (postprocedural)◀

    ✓6th **K06.01**   **Gingival recession, localized**

      **K06.010**   **Localized gingival recession, unspecified**
           Localized gingival recession, NOS

      **K06.011**   **Localized gingival recession, minimal**

      **K06.012**   **Localized gingival recession, moderate**

      **K06.013**   **Localized gingival recession, severe**

    ✓6th **K06.02**   **Gingival recession, generalized**

      **K06.020**   **Generalized gingival recession, unspecified**
           Generalized gingival recession, NOS

      **K06.021**   **Generalized gingival recession, minimal**

      **K06.022**   **Generalized gingival recession, moderate**

      **K06.023**   **Generalized gingival recession, severe**

  **K06.1**   **Gingival enlargement**
      Gingival fibromatosis

  **K06.2**   **Gingival and edentulous alveolar ridge lesions associated with trauma**
      Irritative hyperplasia of edentulous ridge [denture hyperplasia]
      Use additional code (Chapter 20) to identify external cause or denture status (Z97.2)

  **K06.3**   **Horizontal alveolar bone loss**

  **K06.8**   **Other specified disorders of gingiva and edentulous alveolar ridge**
      Fibrous epulis
      Flabby alveolar ridge
      Giant cell epulis
      Peripheral giant cell granuloma of gingiva
      Pyogenic granuloma of gingiva
      Vertical ridge deficiency
      EXCLUDES 2   *gingival cyst (K09.0)*

  **K06.9**   **Disorder of gingiva and edentulous alveolar ridge, unspecified**

✓4th **K08**   **Other disorders of teeth and supporting structures**
    EXCLUDES 2   *dentofacial anomalies [including malocclusion] (M26.-)*
            *disorders of jaw (M27.-)*

  **K08.0**   **Exfoliation of teeth due to systemic causes**
      Code also underlying systemic condition

  ✓5th **K08.1**   **Complete loss of teeth**
      Acquired loss of teeth, complete
      EXCLUDES 1   *congenital absence of teeth (K00.0)*
            *exfoliation of teeth due to systemic causes (K08.0)*
            *partial loss of teeth (K08.4-)*

    ✓6th **K08.10**   **Complete loss of teeth, unspecified cause**

      **K08.101**   **Complete loss of teeth, unspecified cause, class I**

      **K08.102**   **Complete loss of teeth, unspecified cause, class II**

      **K08.103**   **Complete loss of teeth, unspecified cause, class III**

      **K08.104**   **Complete loss of teeth, unspecified cause, class IV**

      **K08.109**   **Complete loss of teeth, unspecified cause, unspecified class**
           Edentulism NOS

    ✓6th **K08.11**   **Complete loss of teeth due to trauma**

      **K08.111**   **Complete loss of teeth due to trauma, class I**

      **K08.112**   **Complete loss of teeth due to trauma, class II**

      **K08.113**   **Complete loss of teeth due to trauma, class III**

      **K08.114**   **Complete loss of teeth due to trauma, class IV**

      **K08.119**   **Complete loss of teeth due to trauma, unspecified class**

    ✓6th **K08.12**   **Complete loss of teeth due to periodontal diseases**

      **K08.121**   **Complete loss of teeth due to periodontal diseases, class I**

      **K08.122**   **Complete loss of teeth due to periodontal diseases, class II**

      **K08.123**   **Complete loss of teeth due to periodontal diseases, class III**

      **K08.124**   **Complete loss of teeth due to periodontal diseases, class IV**

      **K08.129**   **Complete loss of teeth due to periodontal diseases, unspecified class**

    ✓6th **K08.13**   **Complete loss of teeth due to caries**

      **K08.131**   **Complete loss of teeth due to caries, class I**

      **K08.132**   **Complete loss of teeth due to caries, class II**

      **K08.133**   **Complete loss of teeth due to caries, class III**

      **K08.134**   **Complete loss of teeth due to caries, class IV**

      **K08.139**   **Complete loss of teeth due to caries, unspecified class**

    ✓6th **K08.19**   **Complete loss of teeth due to other specified cause**

      **K08.191**   **Complete loss of teeth due to other specified cause, class I**

      **K08.192**   **Complete loss of teeth due to other specified cause, class II**

      **K08.193**   **Complete loss of teeth due to other specified cause, class III**

      **K08.194**   **Complete loss of teeth due to other specified cause, class IV**

      **K08.199**   **Complete loss of teeth due to other specified cause, unspecified class**

  ✓5th **K08.2**   **Atrophy of edentulous alveolar ridge**

      **K08.20**   **Unspecified atrophy of edentulous alveolar ridge**
           Atrophy of the mandible NOS
           Atrophy of the maxilla NOS

      **K08.21**   **Minimal atrophy of the mandible**
           Minimal atrophy of the edentulous mandible

      **K08.22**   **Moderate atrophy of the mandible**
           Moderate atrophy of the edentulous mandible

      **K08.23**   **Severe atrophy of the mandible**
           Severe atrophy of the edentulous mandible

      **K08.24**   **Minimal atrophy of maxilla**
           Minimal atrophy of the edentulous maxilla

      **K08.25**   **Moderate atrophy of the maxilla**
           Moderate atrophy of the edentulous maxilla

      **K08.26**   **Severe atrophy of the maxilla**
           Severe atrophy of the edentulous maxilla

  **K08.3**   **Retained dental root**

  ✓5th **K08.4**   **Partial loss of teeth**
      Acquired loss of teeth, partial
      EXCLUDES 1   *complete loss of teeth (K08.1-)*
            *congenital absence of teeth (K00.0)*
      EXCLUDES 2   *exfoliation of teeth due to systemic causes (K08.0)*

    ✓6th **K08.40**   **Partial loss of teeth, unspecified cause**

      **K08.401**   **Partial loss of teeth, unspecified cause, class I**

      **K08.402**   **Partial loss of teeth, unspecified cause, class II**

      **K08.403**   **Partial loss of teeth, unspecified cause, class III**

N Newborn: 0   P Pediatric: 0-17   M Maternity: 12-55   A Adult: 15-124   MCC Major CC Condition   PDxMCC PDx acts as own MCC   CC CC Condition   PDxCC PDx acts as own CC

688                  ICD-10-CM 2018

    **K08.404**    **Partial loss of teeth, unspecified cause, class IV**

    **K08.409**    **Partial loss of teeth, unspecified cause, unspecified class**
         Tooth extraction status NOS

✓6th **K08.41**   **Partial loss of teeth due to trauma**

    **K08.411**    **Partial loss of teeth due to trauma, class I**

    **K08.412**    **Partial loss of teeth due to trauma, class II**

    **K08.413**    **Partial loss of teeth due to trauma, class III**

    **K08.414**    **Partial loss of teeth due to trauma, class IV**

    **K08.419**    **Partial loss of teeth due to trauma, unspecified class**

✓6th **K08.42**   **Partial loss of teeth due to periodontal diseases**

    **K08.421**    **Partial loss of teeth due to periodontal diseases, class I**

    **K08.422**    **Partial loss of teeth due to periodontal diseases, class II**

    **K08.423**    **Partial loss of teeth due to periodontal diseases, class III**

    **K08.424**    **Partial loss of teeth due to periodontal diseases, class IV**

    **K08.429**    **Partial loss of teeth due to periodontal diseases, unspecified class**

✓6th **K08.43**   **Partial loss of teeth due to caries**

    **K08.431**    **Partial loss of teeth due to caries, class I**

    **K08.432**    **Partial loss of teeth due to caries, class II**

    **K08.433**    **Partial loss of teeth due to caries, class III**

    **K08.434**    **Partial loss of teeth due to caries, class IV**

    **K08.439**    **Partial loss of teeth due to caries, unspecified class**

✓6th **K08.49**   **Partial loss of teeth due to other specified cause**

    **K08.491**    **Partial loss of teeth due to other specified cause, class I**

    **K08.492**    **Partial loss of teeth due to other specified cause, class II**

    **K08.493**    **Partial loss of teeth due to other specified cause, class III**

    **K08.494**    **Partial loss of teeth due to other specified cause, class IV**

    **K08.499**    **Partial loss of teeth due to other specified cause, unspecified class**

✓5th **K08.5**   **Unsatisfactory restoration of tooth**
     Defective bridge, crown, filling
     Defective dental restoration
     *EXCLUDES 1*   *dental restoration status (Z98.811)*
     *EXCLUDES 2*   *endosseous dental implant failure (M27.6-)*
         *unsatisfactory endodontic treatment (M27.5-)*

    **K08.50**    **Unsatisfactory restoration of tooth, unspecified**
         Defective dental restoration NOS

    **K08.51**    **Open restoration margins of tooth**
         Dental restoration failure of marginal integrity
         Open margin on tooth restoration
         Poor gingival margin to tooth restoration

    **K08.52**    **Unrepairable overhanging of dental restorative materials**
         Overhanging of tooth restoration

✓6th     **K08.53**    **Fractured dental restorative material**
         *EXCLUDES 1*   *cracked tooth (K03.81)*
            *traumatic fracture of tooth (S02.5)*

        **K08.530**    **Fractured dental restorative material without loss of material**

        **K08.531**    **Fractured dental restorative material with loss of material**

        **K08.539**    **Fractured dental restorative material, unspecified**

    **K08.54**    **Contour of existing restoration of tooth biologically incompatible with oral health**
         Dental restoration failure of periodontal anatomical integrity
         Unacceptable contours of existing restoration of tooth
         Unacceptable morphology of existing restoration of tooth

    **K08.55**    **Allergy to existing dental restorative material**
         Use additional code to identify the specific type of allergy

    **K08.56**    **Poor aesthetic of existing restoration of tooth**
         Dental restoration aesthetically inadequate or displeasing

    **K08.59**    **Other unsatisfactory restoration of tooth**
         Other defective dental restoration

✓5th **K08.8**   **Other specified disorders of teeth and supporting structures**

    **K08.81**    **Primary occlusal trauma**

    **K08.82**    **Secondary occlusal trauma**

    **K08.89**    **Other specified disorders of teeth and supporting structures**
         Enlargement of alveolar ridge NOS
         Insufficient anatomic crown height
         Insufficient clinical crown length
         Irregular alveolar process
         Toothache NOS

**K08.9**   **Disorder of teeth and supporting structures, unspecified**

✓4th **K09**   **Cysts of oral region, not elsewhere classified**
     *INCLUDES*   lesions showing histological features both of aneurysmal cyst and of another fibro-osseous lesion
     *EXCLUDES 2*   *cysts of jaw (M27.0-, M27.4-)*
         *radicular cyst (K04.8)*

**K09.0**   **Developmental odontogenic cysts**
     Dentigerous cyst
     Eruption cyst
     Follicular cyst
     Gingival cyst
     Lateral periodontal cyst
     Primordial cyst
     *EXCLUDES 2*   *keratocysts (D16.4, D16.5)*
         *odontogenic keratocystic tumors (D16.4, D16.5)*

**K09.1**   **Developmental (nonodontogenic) cysts of oral region**
     Cyst (of) incisive canal
     Cyst (of) palatine of papilla
     Globulomaxillary cyst
     Median palatal cyst
     Nasoalveolar cyst
     Nasolabial cyst
     Nasopalatine duct cyst

**K09.8**   **Other cysts of oral region, not elsewhere classified**
     Dermoid cyst
     Epidermoid cyst
     Lymphoepithelial cyst
     Epstein's pearl

**K09.9**   **Cyst of oral region, unspecified**

✓4th **K11**   **Diseases of salivary glands**
     Use additional code to identify:
     alcohol abuse and dependence (F10.-)
     exposure to environmental tobacco smoke (Z77.22)
     exposure to tobacco smoke in the perinatal period (P96.81)
     history of tobacco dependence (Z87.891)
     occupational exposure to environmental tobacco smoke (Z57.31)
     tobacco dependence (F17.-)
     tobacco use (Z72.0)

**K11.0**   **Atrophy of salivary gland**

**K11.1**   **Hypertrophy of salivary gland**
     **DEF:** Overgrowth of or enlarged salivary gland tissue; caused by infection, salivary duct blockage, autoimmune diseases, and benign and malignant tumors.

✓5th **K11.2**   **Sialoadenitis**
     Parotitis
     *EXCLUDES 1*   *epidemic parotitis (B26.-)*
         *mumps (B26.-)*
         *uveoparotid fever [Heerfordt] (D86.89)*

    **K11.20**    **Sialoadenitis, unspecified**

    **K11.21**    **Acute sialoadenitis**
         *EXCLUDES 1*   *acute recurrent sialoadenitis (K11.22)*

    **K11.22**    **Acute recurrent sialoadenitis**

    **K11.23**    **Chronic sialoadenitis**

**K11.3**   **Abscess of salivary gland**    `CC`
     **CC Excl:** PDX collection 762

**K11.4**   **Fistula of salivary gland**    `CC`
     *EXCLUDES 1*   *congenital fistula of salivary gland (Q38.4)*
     **CC Excl:** PDX collection 762

**K11.5**   **Sialolithiasis**
     Calculus of salivary gland or duct
     Stone of salivary gland or duct

✓ Additional Character Req    ✓x7th Placeholder Alert    Unacceptable PDx    Manifestation    H1-H14 HAC    HCC CMS-HCC Condition    *EXCLUDES 1* Not Coded Here    *EXCLUDES 2* Not Included Here

ICD-10-CM 2018          **689**

**K11.6 Mucocele** of salivary gland
Mucous extravasation cyst of salivary gland
Mucous retention cyst of salivary gland
Ranula

**K11.7 Disturbances of salivary secretion**
Hypoptyalism
Ptyalism
Xerostomia
EXCLUDES 2   *dry mouth NOS (R68.2)*

**K11.8 Other diseases of salivary glands**
Benign lymphoepithelial lesion of salivary gland
Mikulicz' disease
Necrotizing sialometaplasia
Sialectasia
Stenosis of salivary duct
Stricture of salivary duct
EXCLUDES 1   *sicca syndrome [Sjögren] (M35.0-)*

**K11.9 Disease of salivary gland, unspecified**
Sialoadenopathy NOS

✓4ᵗʰ **K12 Stomatitis and related lesions**
Use additional code to identify:
alcohol abuse and dependence (F10.-)
exposure to environmental tobacco smoke (Z77.22)
exposure to tobacco smoke in the perinatal period (P96.81)
history of tobacco dependence (Z87.891)
occupational exposure to environmental tobacco smoke (Z57.31)
tobacco dependence (F17.-)
tobacco use (Z72.0)
EXCLUDES 1   *cancrum oris (A69.0)*
     *cheilitis (K13.0)*
     *gangrenous stomatitis (A69.0)*
     *herpesviral [herpes simplex] gingivostomatitis (B00.2)*
     *noma (A69.0)*

**K12.0 Recurrent oral aphthae**
Aphthous stomatitis (major) (minor)
Bednar's aphthae
Periadenitis mucosa necrotica recurrens
Recurrent aphthous ulcer
Stomatitis herpetiformis
**DEF:** Disorder of unknown etiology with small oval or round painful ulcers of the mouth marked by a grayish exudate and a red halo effect.

**K12.1 Other forms of stomatitis**
Stomatitis NOS
Denture stomatitis
Ulcerative stomatitis
Vesicular stomatitis
EXCLUDES 1   *acute necrotizing ulcerative stomatitis (A69.1)*
     *Vincent's stomatitis (A69.1)*

**K12.2 Cellulitis and abscess of mouth**    CC
Cellulitis of mouth (floor)
Submandibular abscess
EXCLUDES 2   *abscess of salivary gland (K11.3)*
     *abscess of tongue (K14.0)*
     *periapical abscess (K04.6-K04.7)*
     *periodontal abscess (K05.21)*
     *peritonsillar abscess (J36)*
**CC Excl:** PDX collection 763

✓5ᵗʰ **K12.3 Oral mucositis (ulcerative)**
Mucositis (oral) (oropharyneal)
EXCLUDES 2   *gastrointestinal mucositis (ulcerative) (K92.81)*
     *mucositis (ulcerative) of vagina and vulva (N76.81)*
     *nasal mucositis (ulcerative) (J34.81)*

**K12.30 Oral mucositis (ulcerative), unspecified**

**K12.31 Oral mucositis (ulcerative) due to antineoplastic therapy**
Use additional code for adverse effect, if applicable, to identify antineoplastic and immunosuppressive drugs (T45.1X5)
Use additional code for other antineoplastic therapy, such as:
radiological procedure and radiotherapy (Y84.2)

**K12.32 Oral mucositis (ulcerative) due to other drugs**
Use additional code for adverse effect, if applicable, to identify drug (T36-T50 with fifth or sixth character 5)

**K12.33 Oral mucositis (ulcerative) due to radiation**
Use additional external cause code (W88-W90, X39.0-) to identify cause

**K12.39 Other oral mucositis (ulcerative)**
Viral oral mucositis (ulcerative)

✓4ᵗʰ **K13 Other diseases of lip and oral mucosa**
INCLUDES   epithelial disturbances of tongue
Use additional code to identify:
alcohol abuse and dependence (F10.-)
exposure to environmental tobacco smoke (Z77.22)
exposure to tobacco smoke in the perinatal period (P96.81)
history of tobacco dependence (Z87.891)
occupational exposure to environmental tobacco smoke (Z57.31)
tobacco dependence (F17.-)
tobacco use (Z72.0)
EXCLUDES 2   *certain disorders of gingiva and edentulous alveolar ridge (K05-K06)*
     *cysts of oral region (K09.-)*
     *diseases of tongue (K14.-)*
     *stomatitis and related lesions (K12.-)*

**K13.0 Diseases of lips**
Abscess of lips
Angular cheilitis
Cellulitis of lips
Cheilitis NOS
Cheilodynia
Cheilosis
Exfoliative cheilitis
Fistula of lips
Glandular cheilitis
Hypertrophy of lips
Perlèche NEC
EXCLUDES 1   *ariboflavinosis (E53.0)*
     *cheilitis due to radiation-related disorders (L55-L59)*
     *congenital fistula of lips (Q38.0)*
     *congenital hypertrophy of lips (Q18.6)*
     *Perlèche due to candidiasis (B37.83)*
     *Perlèche due to riboflavin deficiency (E53.0)*

**K13.1 Cheek and lip biting**

✓5ᵗʰ **K13.2 Leukoplakia and other disturbances of oral epithelium, including tongue**
EXCLUDES 1   *carcinoma in situ of oral epithelium (D00.0-)*
     *hairy leukoplakia (K13.3)*

**K13.21 Leukoplakia of oral mucosa, including tongue**
Leukokeratosis of oral mucosa
Leukoplakia of gingiva, lips, tongue
EXCLUDES 1   *hairy leukoplakia (K13.3)*
     *leukokeratosis nicotina palati (K13.24)*

**K13.22 Minimal keratinized residual ridge mucosa**
Minimal keratinization of alveolar ridge mucosa

**K13.23 Excessive keratinized residual ridge mucosa**
Excessive keratinization of alveolar ridge mucosa

**K13.24 Leukokeratosis nicotina palati**
Smoker's palate

**K13.29 Other disturbances of oral epithelium, including tongue**
Erythroplakia of mouth or tongue
Focal epithelial hyperplasia of mouth or tongue
Leukoedema of mouth or tongue
Other oral epithelium disturbances

**K13.3 Hairy leukoplakia**

**K13.4 Granuloma and granuloma-like lesions of oral mucosa**
Eosinophilic granuloma
Granuloma pyogenicum
Verrucous xanthoma

**K13.5 Oral submucous fibrosis**
Submucous fibrosis of tongue

**K13.6 Irritative hyperplasia of oral mucosa**
EXCLUDES 2   *irritative hyperplasia of edentulous ridge [denture hyperplasia] (K06.2)*

✓5ᵗʰ **K13.7 Other and unspecified lesions of oral mucosa**
**K13.70 Unspecified lesions of oral mucosa**
**K13.79 Other lesions of oral mucosa**
Focal oral mucinosis

---

N Newborn: 0   P Pediatric: 0-17   M Maternity: 12-55   A Adult: 15-124   MCC Major CC Condition   PDxMCC PDx acts as own MCC   CC CC Condition   PDxCC PDx acts as own CC

## ✓4th K14 Diseases of tongue

Use additional code to identify:
alcohol abuse and dependence (F10.-)
exposure to environmental tobacco smoke (Z77.22)
history of tobacco dependence (Z87.891)
occupational exposure to environmental tobacco smoke (Z57.31)
tobacco dependence (F17.-)
tobacco use (Z72.0)

*EXCLUDES 2*    *erythroplakia (K13.29)*
*focal epithelial hyperplasia (K13.29)*
*leukedema of tongue (K13.29)*
*leukoplakia of tongue (K13.21)*
*hairy leukoplakia (K13.3)*
*macroglossia (congenital) (Q38.2)*
*submucous fibrosis of tongue (K13.5)*

### K14.0 Glossitis
Abscess of tongue
Ulceration (traumatic) of tongue
*EXCLUDES 1*   *atrophic glossitis (K14.4)*

### K14.1 Geographic tongue
Benign migratory glossitis
Glossitis areata exfoliativa

### K14.2 Median rhomboid glossitis

### K14.3 Hypertrophy of tongue papillae
Black hairy tongue
Coated tongue
Hypertrophy of foliate papillae
Lingua villosa nigra

### K14.4 Atrophy of tongue papillae
Atrophic glossitis

### K14.5 Plicated tongue
Fissured tongue
Furrowed tongue
Scrotal tongue
*EXCLUDES 1*   *fissured tongue, congenital (Q38.3)*

### K14.6 Glossodynia
Glossopyrosis
Painful tongue

### K14.8 Other diseases of tongue
Atrophy of tongue
Crenated tongue
Enlargement of tongue
Glossocele
Glossoptosis
Hypertrophy of tongue

### K14.9 Disease of tongue, unspecified
Glossopathy NOS

## Diseases of esophagus, stomach and duodenum (K20-K31)

*EXCLUDES 2*   *hiatus hernia (K44.-)*

## ✓4th K20 Esophagitis

Use additional code to identify:
alcohol abuse and dependence (F10.-)
*EXCLUDES 1*   *erosion of esophagus (K22.1-)*
*esophagitis with gastro-esophageal reflux disease (K21.0)*
*reflux esophagitis (K21.0)*
*ulcerative esophagitis (K22.1-)*
*EXCLUDES 2*   *eosinophilic gastritis or gastroenteritis (K52.81)*

### K20.0 Eosinophilic esophagitis

### K20.8 Other esophagitis
Abscess of esophagus

### K20.9 Esophagitis, unspecified
Esophagitis NOS

## ✓4th K21 Gastro-esophageal reflux disease

*EXCLUDES 1*   *newborn esophageal reflux (P78.83)*

### K21.0 Gastro-esophageal reflux disease with esophagitis
Reflux esophagitis

### K21.9 Gastro-esophageal reflux disease without esophagitis
Esophageal reflux NOS
**AHA:** 2016, 1Q, 18

## ✓4th K22 Other diseases of esophagus

*EXCLUDES 2*   *esophageal varices (I85.-)*

### K22.0 Achalasia of cardia
Achalasia NOS
Cardiospasm
*EXCLUDES 1*   *congenital cardiospasm (Q39.5)*
**DEF:** Esophageal motility disorder; caused by absence of esophageal peristalsis and impaired relaxation of lower esophageal sphincter; characterized by dysphagia, regurgitation, and heartburn.

### ✓5th K22.1 Ulcer of esophagus
Barrett's ulcer
Erosion of esophagus
Fungal ulcer of esophagus
Peptic ulcer of esophagus
Ulcer of esophagus due to ingestion of chemicals
Ulcer of esophagus due to ingestion of drugs and medicaments
Ulcerative esophagitis

Code first poisoning due to drug or toxin, if applicable (T36-T65 with fifth or sixth character 1-4 or 6)

Use additional code for adverse effect, if applicable, to identify drug (T36-T50 with fifth or sixth character 5)

*EXCLUDES 1*   *Barrett's esophagus (K22.7-)*

#### K22.10 Ulcer of esophagus without bleeding   `CC`
Ulcer of esophagus NOS
**CC Excl:** PDX collection 764

#### K22.11 Ulcer of esophagus with bleeding   `MCC`
*EXCLUDES 2*   *bleeding esophageal varices (I85.01, I85.11)*
**CC Excl:** PDX collection 765

### K22.2 Esophageal obstruction
Compression of esophagus
Constriction of esophagus
Stenosis of esophagus
Stricture of esophagus
*EXCLUDES 1*   *congenital stenosis or stricture of esophagus (Q39.3)*

### K22.3 Perforation of esophagus   `MCC`
Rupture of esophagus
*EXCLUDES 1*   *traumatic perforation of (thoracic) esophagus (S27.8-)*
**CC Excl:** PDX collection 766

### K22.4 Dyskinesia of esophagus
Corkscrew esophagus
Diffuse esophageal spasm
Spasm of esophagus
*EXCLUDES 1*   *cardiospasm (K22.0)*

### K22.5 Diverticulum of esophagus, acquired
Esophageal pouch, acquired
*EXCLUDES 1*   *diverticulum of esophagus (congenital) (Q39.6)*

### K22.6 Gastro-esophageal laceration-hemorrhage syndrome   `MCC`
Mallory-Weiss syndrome
**CC Excl:** PDX collection 767

### ✓5th K22.7 Barrett's esophagus
Barrett's disease
Barrett's syndrome
*EXCLUDES 1*   *Barrett's ulcer (K22.1)*
*malignant neoplasm of esophagus (C15.)*
**DEF:** A metaplastic disorder in which specialized columnar epithelial cells replace the normal squamous epithelial cells; secondary to chronic gastroesophageal reflux damage to the mucosa; increases risk of developing adenocarcinoma.

#### K22.70 Barrett's esophagus without dysplasia
Barrett's esophagus NOS

#### ✓6th K22.71 Barrett's esophagus with dysplasia

##### K22.710 Barrett's esophagus with low grade dysplasia

##### K22.711 Barrett's esophagus with high grade dysplasia

##### K22.719 Barrett's esophagus with dysplasia, unspecified

### K22.8 Other specified diseases of esophagus
Hemorrhage of esophagus NOS
*EXCLUDES 2*   *esophageal varices (I85.-)*
*Paterson-Kelly syndrome (D50.1)*

### K22.9 Disease of esophagus, unspecified

---

**Chapter 11. Diseases of the Digestive System**

**K23–K29.41**

## Gastrointestinal Ulcers

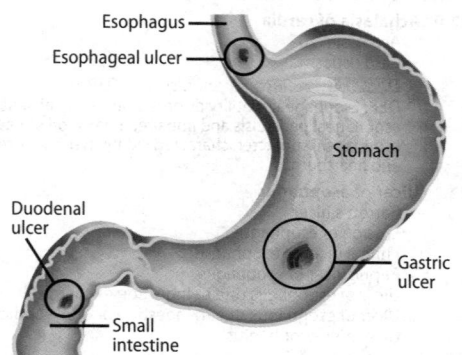

Esophagus

Esophageal ulcer

Stomach

Duodenal ulcer

Gastric ulcer

Small intestine

### K23   *Disorders of esophagus in diseases classified elsewhere*

Code first underlying disease, such as:
    congenital syphilis (A50.5)
> **EXCLUDES 1**   *late syphilis (A52.79)*
>     *megaesophagus due to Chagas' disease (B57.31)*
>     *tuberculosis (A18.83)*

### ✓4ᵗʰ K25   Gastric **ulcer**

> **INCLUDES**   erosion (acute) of stomach
>     pylorus ulcer (peptic)
>     stomach ulcer (peptic)

Use additional code to identify:
    alcohol abuse and dependence (F10.-)
> **EXCLUDES 1**   *acute gastritis (K29.0-)*
>     *peptic ulcer NOS (K27.-)*

**CC Excl: For CC/MCC codes in category K25:** PDX collection 765

| | | |
|---|---|---|
| **K25.0** | Acute **gastric ulcer** with hemorrhage | MCC |
| **K25.1** | Acute **gastric ulcer** with perforation | MCC HCC |
| **K25.2** | Acute **gastric ulcer** with both hemorrhage and perforation | MCC HCC |
| **K25.3** | Acute **gastric ulcer** without hemorrhage or perforation | CC |
| **K25.4** | Chronic or unspecified **gastric ulcer** with hemorrhage | MCC |
| **K25.5** | Chronic or unspecified **gastric ulcer** with perforation | MCC HCC |
| **K25.6** | Chronic or unspecified **gastric ulcer** with both hemorrhage and perforation | MCC HCC |
| **K25.7** | Chronic **gastric ulcer** without hemorrhage or perforation | |
| **K25.9** | **Gastric ulcer, unspecified** as acute or chronic, without hemorrhage or perforation | |

### ✓4ᵗʰ K26   Duodenal **ulcer**

> **INCLUDES**   erosion (acute) of duodenum
>     duodenum ulcer (peptic)
>     postpyloric ulcer (peptic)

Use additional code to identify:
    alcohol abuse and dependence (F10.-)
> **EXCLUDES 1**   *peptic ulcer NOS (K27.-)*

**CC Excl: For MCC codes in category K26, unless otherwise noted:** PDX collection 768

| | | |
|---|---|---|
| **K26.0** | Acute **duodenal ulcer** with hemorrhage | MCC |
| **K26.1** | Acute **duodenal ulcer** with perforation | MCC HCC |
| **K26.2** | Acute **duodenal ulcer** with both hemorrhage and perforation | MCC HCC |
| **K26.3** | Acute **duodenal ulcer** without hemorrhage or perforation | CC |
| |     **CC Excl:** PDX collection 769 | |
| **K26.4** | Chronic or unspecified **duodenal ulcer** with hemorrhage | MCC |
| |     **AHA:** 2016, 1Q, 14 | |
| **K26.5** | Chronic or unspecified **duodenal ulcer** with perforation | MCC HCC |
| **K26.6** | Chronic or unspecified **duodenal ulcer** with both hemorrhage and perforation | MCC HCC |
| **K26.7** | Chronic **duodenal ulcer** without hemorrhage or perforation | |
| **K26.9** | **Duodenal ulcer, unspecified** as acute or chronic, without hemorrhage or perforation | |

### ✓4ᵗʰ K27   Peptic **ulcer, site unspecified**

> **INCLUDES**   gastroduodenal ulcer NOS
>     peptic ulcer NOS

Use additional code to identify:
    alcohol abuse and dependence (F10.-)
> **EXCLUDES 1**   *peptic ulcer of newborn (P78.82)*

**CC Excl: For CC/MCC codes in category K27:** PDX collection 768

| | | |
|---|---|---|
| **K27.0** | Acute **peptic ulcer, site unspecified, with** hemorrhage | MCC |
| **K27.1** | Acute **peptic ulcer, site unspecified, with** perforation | MCC HCC |
| **K27.2** | Acute **peptic ulcer, site unspecified, with both** hemorrhage and perforation | MCC HCC |
| **K27.3** | Acute **peptic ulcer, site unspecified, without** hemorrhage or perforation | CC |
| **K27.4** | Chronic or unspecified **peptic ulcer, site unspecified, with** hemorrhage | MCC |
| **K27.5** | Chronic or unspecified **peptic ulcer, site unspecified, with** perforation | HCC |
| **K27.6** | Chronic or unspecified **peptic ulcer, site unspecified, with both** hemorrhage and perforation | MCC HCC |
| **K27.7** | Chronic **peptic ulcer, site unspecified, without** hemorrhage or perforation | |
| **K27.9** | **Peptic ulcer, site unspecified, unspecified as acute or chronic,** without hemorrhage or perforation | |

### ✓4ᵗʰ K28   Gastrojejunal **ulcer**

> **INCLUDES**   anastomotic ulcer (peptic) or erosion
>     gastrocolic ulcer (peptic) or erosion
>     gastrointestinal ulcer (peptic) or erosion
>     gastrojejunal ulcer (peptic) or erosion
>     jejunal ulcer (peptic) or erosion
>     marginal ulcer (peptic) or erosion
>     stomal ulcer (peptic) or erosion

Use additional code to identify:
    alcohol abuse and dependence (F10.-)
> **EXCLUDES 1**   *primary ulcer of small intestine (K63.3)*

**CC Excl: For CC/MCC codes in category K28:** PDX collection 765

| | | |
|---|---|---|
| **K28.0** | Acute **gastrojejunal ulcer** with hemorrhage | MCC |
| **K28.1** | Acute **gastrojejunal ulcer** with perforation | MCC HCC |
| **K28.2** | Acute **gastrojejunal ulcer** with both hemorrhage and perforation | MCC HCC |
| **K28.3** | Acute **gastrojejunal ulcer** without hemorrhage or perforation | CC |
| **K28.4** | Chronic or unspecified **gastrojejunal ulcer** with hemorrhage | MCC |
| **K28.5** | Chronic or unspecified **gastrojejunal ulcer** with perforation | MCC HCC |
| **K28.6** | Chronic or unspecified **gastrojejunal ulcer** with both hemorrhage and perforation | MCC HCC |
| **K28.7** | Chronic **gastrojejunal ulcer** without hemorrhage or perforation | |
| **K28.9** | **Gastrojejunal ulcer, unspecified as acute or chronic,** without hemorrhage or perforation | |

### ✓4ᵗʰ K29   Gastritis and duodenitis

> **EXCLUDES 1**   *eosinophilic gastritis or gastroenteritis (K52.81)*
>     *Zollinger-Ellison syndrome (E16.4)*

**CC Excl: For MCC codes in category K29:** PDX collection 770

#### ✓5ᵗʰ K29.0   Acute **gastritis**

Use additional code to identify:
    alcohol abuse and dependence (F10.-)
> **EXCLUDES 1**   *erosion (acute) of stomach (K25.-)*

| | | |
|---|---|---|
| **K29.00** | Acute **gastritis** without bleeding | |
| **K29.01** | Acute **gastritis** with bleeding | MCC |

#### ✓5ᵗʰ K29.2   Alcoholic **gastritis**

Use additional code to identify:
    alcohol abuse and dependence (F10.-)

| | | |
|---|---|---|
| **K29.20** | Alcoholic **gastritis** without bleeding | |
| **K29.21** | Alcoholic **gastritis** with bleeding | MCC |

#### ✓5ᵗʰ K29.3   Chronic superficial **gastritis**

| | | |
|---|---|---|
| **K29.30** | Chronic superficial **gastritis** without bleeding | |
| **K29.31** | Chronic superficial **gastritis** with bleeding | MCC |

#### ✓5ᵗʰ K29.4   Chronic atrophic **gastritis**

Gastric atrophy

| | | |
|---|---|---|
| **K29.40** | Chronic atrophic **gastritis** without bleeding | |
| **K29.41** | Chronic atrophic **gastritis** with bleeding | MCC |

**N** Newborn: 0    **P** Pediatric: 0-17    **M** Maternity: 12-55    **A** Adult: 15-124    **MCC** Major CC Condition    **PDxMCC** PDx acts as own MCC    **CC** CC Condition    **PDxCC** PDx acts as own CC

**692**

ICD-10-CM 2018

✓5ᵗʰ **K29.5 Unspecified chronic gastritis**
Chronic antral gastritis
Chronic fundal gastritis

**K29.50 Unspecified chronic gastritis without bleeding**

**K29.51 Unspecified chronic gastritis with bleeding** MCC

✓5ᵗʰ **K29.6 Other gastritis**
Giant hypertrophic gastritis
Granulomatous gastritis
Ménétrier's disease

**K29.60 Other gastritis without bleeding**

**K29.61 Other gastritis with bleeding** MCC

✓5ᵗʰ **K29.7 Gastritis, unspecified**

**K29.70 Gastritis, unspecified, without bleeding**

**K29.71 Gastritis, unspecified, with bleeding** MCC

✓5ᵗʰ **K29.8 Duodenitis**

**K29.80 Duodenitis without bleeding**

**K29.81 Duodenitis with bleeding** MCC

✓5ᵗʰ **K29.9 Gastroduodenitis, unspecified**

**K29.90 Gastroduodenitis, unspecified, without bleeding**

**K29.91 Gastroduodenitis, unspecified, with bleeding** MCC

**K30 Functional dyspepsia**
Indigestion
*EXCLUDES 1*   dyspepsia NOS (R10.13)
heartburn (R12)
nervous dyspepsia (F45.8)
neurotic dyspepsia (F45.8)
psychogenic dyspepsia (F45.8)

✓4ᵗʰ **K31 Other diseases of stomach and duodenum**
*INCLUDES*   functional disorders of stomach
*EXCLUDES 2*   diabetic gastroparesis (E08.43, E09.43, E10.43, E11.43, E13.43)
diverticulum of duodenum (K57.00-K57.13)

**K31.0 Acute dilatation of stomach** CC
Acute distention of stomach
**CC Excl:** PDX collection 771

**K31.1 Adult hypertrophic pyloric stenosis** CC A
Pyloric stenosis NOS
*EXCLUDES 1*   congenital or infantile pyloric stenosis (Q40.0)
**CC Excl:** PDX collection 772

**K31.2 Hourglass stricture and stenosis of stomach**
*EXCLUDES 1*   congenital hourglass stomach (Q40.2)
hourglass contraction of stomach (K31.89)

**K31.3 Pylorospasm, not elsewhere classified**
*EXCLUDES 1*   congenital or infantile pylorospasm (Q40.0)
neurotic pylorospasm (F45.8)
psychogenic pylorospasm (F45.8)

**K31.4 Gastric diverticulum**
*EXCLUDES 1*   congenital diverticulum of stomach (Q40.2)

**K31.5 Obstruction of duodenum** CC
Constriction of duodenum
Duodenal ileus (chronic)
Stenosis of duodenum
Stricture of duodenum
Volvulus of duodenum
*EXCLUDES 1*   congenital stenosis of duodenum (Q41.0)
**CC Excl:** PDX collection 773

**K31.6 Fistula of stomach and duodenum** CC
Gastrocolic fistula
Gastrojejunocolic fistula
**CC Excl:** PDX collection 774

**K31.7 Polyp of stomach and duodenum**
*EXCLUDES 1*   adenomatous polyp of stomach (D13.1)

✓5ᵗʰ **K31.8 Other specified diseases of stomach and duodenum**

✓6ᵗʰ **K31.81 Angiodysplasia of stomach and duodenum**

**K31.811 Angiodysplasia of stomach and duodenum with bleeding** MCC
**CC Excl:** PDX collection 770

**K31.819 Angiodysplasia of stomach and duodenum without bleeding**
Angiodysplasia of stomach and duodenum NOS

**K31.82 Dieulafoy lesion (hemorrhagic) of stomach and duodenum** MCC
*EXCLUDES 2*   Dieulafoy lesion of intestine (K63.81)
**CC Excl:** PDX collection 775

**K31.83 Achlorhydria**
**DEF:** Absence of hydrochloric acid in gastric secretions due to gastric mucosa atrophy; unresponsive to histamines; also known as gastric anacidity.

**K31.84 Gastroparesis**
Gastroparalysis
Code first underlying disease, if known, such as:
anorexia nervosa (F50.0-)
diabetes mellitus (E08.43, E09.43, E10.43, E11.43, E13.43)
scleroderma (M34.-)
**AHA:** 2013, 4Q, 114

**K31.89 Other diseases of stomach and duodenum**
**AHA:** 2017, 1Q, 28

**K31.9 Disease of stomach and duodenum, unspecified**

## Diseases of appendix (K35-K38)

✓4ᵗʰ **K35 Acute appendicitis**

**CC Excl: For CC/MCC codes in category K35:** PDX collection 776

**K35.2 Acute appendicitis with generalized peritonitis** MCC
Appendicitis (acute) with generalized (diffuse) peritonitis following rupture or perforation of appendix
Perforated appendix NOS
Ruptured appendix NOS

**K35.3 Acute appendicitis with localized peritonitis** MCC
Acute appendicitis with or without perforation or rupture with peritonitis NOS
Acute appendicitis with or without perforation or rupture with localized peritonitis
Acute appendicitis with peritoneal abscess

✓5ᵗʰ **K35.8 Other and unspecified acute appendicitis**

**K35.80 Unspecified acute appendicitis** CC
Acute appendicitis NOS
Acute appendicitis without (localized) (generalized) peritonitis

**K35.89 Other acute appendicitis** CC

**K36 Other appendicitis**
Chronic appendicitis
Recurrent appendicitis

**K37 Unspecified appendicitis**
*EXCLUDES 1*   unspecified appendicitis with peritonitis (K35.2-K35.3)

✓4ᵗʰ **K38 Other diseases of appendix**

**K38.0 Hyperplasia of appendix**

**K38.1 Appendicular concretions**
Fecalith of appendix
Stercolith of appendix

**K38.2 Diverticulum of appendix**

**K38.3 Fistula of appendix**

**K38.8 Other specified diseases of appendix**
Intussusception of appendix

**K38.9 Disease of appendix, unspecified**

## Hernia (K40-K46)

*NOTE*   Hernia with both gangrene and obstruction is classified to hernia with gangrene.

*INCLUDES*   acquired hernia
congenital [except diaphragmatic or hiatus] hernia
recurrent hernia

✓4ᵗʰ **K40 Inguinal hernia**
*INCLUDES*   bubonocele
direct inguinal hernia
double inguinal hernia
indirect inguinal hernia
inguinal hernia NOS
oblique inguinal hernia
scrotal hernia

**CC Excl: For CC/MCC codes in category K40:** PDX collection 777

✓5ᵗʰ **K40.0 Bilateral inguinal hernia, with obstruction, without gangrene**
Inguinal hernia (bilateral) causing obstruction without gangrene
Incarcerated inguinal hernia (bilateral) without gangrene
Irreducible inguinal hernia (bilateral) without gangrene
Strangulated inguinal hernia (bilateral) without gangrene

**K40.00 Bilateral inguinal hernia, with obstruction, without gangrene, not specified as recurrent**
Bilateral inguinal hernia, with obstruction, without gangrene NOS

✓ Additional Character Req   ✓x7ᵗʰ Placeholder Alert   Unacceptable PDx   Manifestation   H1-H14 HAC   HCC CMS-HCC Condition   *EXCLUDES 1* Not Coded Here   *EXCLUDES 2* Not Included Here

ICD-10-CM 2018

**693**

**Chapter 11. Diseases of the Digestive System**

**Hernia Sites**

Abdominal ring
Indirect inguinal hernia
Anterior inguinal wall
Direct inguinal hernia
Spermatic cord
Femoral hernia
Inguinal ligament
Femoral sheath
Epigastric hernia
Paraumbilical hernia
Inguinal hernias
Femoral hernia

**K40.01**   **Bilateral inguinal hernia, with obstruction, without gangrene, recurrent**   `CC`

✓5ᵗʰ **K40.1**   Bilateral **inguinal hernia, with gangrene**

    **K40.10**   **Bilateral inguinal hernia, with gangrene,** not **specified as recurrent**   `MCC`
       Bilateral inguinal hernia, with gangrene NOS

    **K40.11**   **Bilateral inguinal hernia, with gangrene, recurrent**   `MCC`

✓5ᵗʰ **K40.2**   Bilateral **inguinal hernia, without obstruction or gangrene**

    **K40.20**   **Bilateral inguinal hernia, without obstruction or gangrene, not specified as recurrent**
       Bilateral inguinal hernia NOS

    **K40.21**   **Bilateral inguinal hernia, without obstruction or gangrene, recurrent**

✓5ᵗʰ **K40.3**   Unilateral **inguinal hernia, with obstruction, without gangrene**
       Inguinal hernia (unilateral) causing obstruction without gangrene
       Incarcerated inguinal hernia (unilateral) without gangrene
       Irreducible inguinal hernia (unilateral) without gangrene
       Strangulated inguinal hernia (unilateral) without gangrene

    **K40.30**   **Unilateral inguinal hernia, with obstruction, without gangrene,** not specified as recurrent   `CC`
       Inguinal hernia, with obstruction NOS
       Unilateral inguinal hernia, with obstruction, without gangrene NOS

    **K40.31**   **Unilateral inguinal hernia, with obstruction, without gangrene, recurrent**   `CC`

✓5ᵗʰ **K40.4**   Unilateral **inguinal hernia, with gangrene**

    **K40.40**   **Unilateral inguinal hernia, with gangrene,** not **specified as recurrent**   `MCC`
       Inguinal hernia with gangrene NOS
       Unilateral inguinal hernia with gangrene NOS

    **K40.41**   **Unilateral inguinal hernia, with gangrene, recurrent**   `MCC`

✓5ᵗʰ **K40.9**   Unilateral **inguinal hernia, without obstruction or gangrene**

    **K40.90**   **Unilateral inguinal hernia, without obstruction or gangrene,** not specified as recurrent
       Inguinal hernia NOS
       Unilateral inguinal hernia NOS

    **K40.91**   **Unilateral inguinal hernia, without obstruction or gangrene, recurrent**

✓4ᵗʰ **K41**   **Femoral hernia**

> **CC Excl: For CC/MCC codes in category K41, unless otherwise noted:** PDX collection 778

✓5ᵗʰ **K41.0**   Bilateral **femoral hernia, with obstruction, without gangrene**
       Femoral hernia (bilateral) causing obstruction, without gangrene
       Incarcerated femoral hernia (bilateral), without gangrene
       Irreducible femoral hernia (bilateral), without gangrene
       Strangulated femoral hernia (bilateral), without gangrene

    **K41.00**   **Bilateral femoral hernia, with obstruction, without gangrene,** not specified as recurrent   `CC`
       Bilateral femoral hernia, with obstruction, without gangrene NOS

    **K41.01**   **Bilateral femoral hernia, with obstruction, without gangrene, recurrent**   `CC`

✓5ᵗʰ **K41.1**   Bilateral **femoral hernia, with gangrene**

    **K41.10**   **Bilateral femoral hernia, with gangrene,** not **specified as recurrent**   `MCC`
       Bilateral femoral hernia, with gangrene NOS
       **CC Excl:** PDX collection 779

    **K41.11**   **Bilateral femoral hernia, with gangrene, recurrent**   `MCC`
       **CC Excl:** PDX collection 779

✓5ᵗʰ **K41.2**   Bilateral **femoral hernia, without obstruction or gangrene**

    **K41.20**   **Bilateral femoral hernia, without obstruction or gangrene, not specified as recurrent**
       Bilateral femoral hernia NOS

    **K41.21**   **Bilateral femoral hernia, without obstruction or gangrene, recurrent**

✓5ᵗʰ **K41.3**   Unilateral **femoral hernia, with obstruction, without gangrene**
       Femoral hernia (unilateral) causing obstruction, without gangrene
       Incarcerated femoral hernia (unilateral), without gangrene
       Irreducible femoral hernia (unilateral), without gangrene
       Strangulated femoral hernia (unilateral), without gangrene

    **K41.30**   **Unilateral femoral hernia, with obstruction, without gangrene,** not specified as recurrent   `CC`
       Femoral hernia, with obstruction NOS
       Unilateral femoral hernia, with obstruction NOS

    **K41.31**   **Unilateral femoral hernia, with obstruction, without gangrene, recurrent**   `CC`

✓5ᵗʰ **K41.4**   Unilateral **femoral hernia, with gangrene**

    **K41.40**   **Unilateral femoral hernia, with gangrene,** not **specified as recurrent**   `MCC`
       Femoral hernia, with gangrene NOS
       Unilateral femoral hernia, with gangrene NOS
       **CC Excl:** PDX collection 779

    **K41.41**   **Unilateral femoral hernia, with gangrene, recurrent**   `MCC`
       **CC Excl:** PDX collection 779

✓5ᵗʰ **K41.9**   Unilateral **femoral hernia, without obstruction or gangrene**

    **K41.90**   **Unilateral femoral hernia, without obstruction or gangrene, not specified as recurrent**
       Femoral hernia NOS
       Unilateral femoral hernia NOS

    **K41.91**   **Unilateral femoral hernia, without obstruction or gangrene, recurrent**

✓4ᵗʰ **K42**   **Umbilical hernia**
    **INCLUDES**   paraumbilical hernia
    **EXCLUDES 1**   *omphalocele (Q79.2)*

    **K42.0**   **Umbilical hernia with obstruction, without gangrene**   `CC`
       Umbilical hernia causing obstruction, without gangrene
       Incarcerated umbilical hernia, without gangrene
       Irreducible umbilical hernia, without gangrene
       Strangulated umbilical hernia, without gangrene
       **CC Excl:** PDX collection 780

    **K42.1**   **Umbilical hernia with gangrene**   `MCC`
       Gangrenous umbilical hernia
       **CC Excl:** PDX collection 781

    **K42.9**   **Umbilical hernia without obstruction or gangrene**
       Umbilical hernia NOS

✓4ᵗʰ **K43**   **Ventral hernia**

    **K43.0**   **Incisional hernia with obstruction, without gangrene**   `CC`
       Incisional hernia causing obstruction, without gangrene
       Incarcerated incisional hernia, without gangrene
       Irreducible incisional hernia, without gangrene
       Strangulated incisional hernia, without gangrene
       **CC Excl:** PDX collection 780

    **K43.1**   **Incisional hernia with gangrene**   `MCC`
       Gangrenous incisional hernia
       **CC Excl:** PDX collection 781

    **K43.2**   **Incisional hernia without obstruction or gangrene**
       Incisional NOS

    **K43.3**   **Parastomal hernia with obstruction, without gangrene**   `CC`
       Incarcerated parastomal hernia, without gangrene
       Irreducible parastomal hernia, without gangrene
       Parastomal hernia causing obstruction, without gangrene
       Strangulated parastomal hernia, without gangrene
       **CC Excl:** PDX collection 780

    **K43.4**   **Parastomal hernia with gangrene**   `MCC`
       Gangrenous parastomal hernia
       **CC Excl:** PDX collection 781

    **K43.5**   **Parastomal hernia without obstruction or gangrene**
       Parastomal hernia NOS

**N** Newborn: 0   **P** Pediatric: 0-17   **M** Maternity: 12-55   **A** Adult: 15-124   **MCC** Major CC Condition   **PDx MCC** PDx acts as own MCC   **CC** CC Condition   **PDx CC** PDx acts as own CC

694        ICD-10-CM 2018

K40.01–K43.5

**K43.6**   **Other and unspecified ventral hernia with obstruction, without gangrene**    `CC`
  Epigastric hernia causing obstruction, without gangrene
  Hypogastric hernia causing obstruction, without gangrene
  Incarcerated epigastric hernia without gangrene
  Incarcerated hypogastric hernia without gangrene
  Incarcerated midline hernia without gangrene
  Incarcerated spigelian hernia without gangrene
  Incarcerated subxiphoid hernia without gangrene
  Irreducible epigastric hernia without gangrene
  Irreducible hypogastric hernia without gangrene
  Irreducible midline hernia without gangrene
  Irreducible spigelian hernia without gangrene
  Irreducible subxiphoid hernia without gangrene
  Midline hernia causing obstruction, without gangrene
  Spigelian hernia causing obstruction, without gangrene
  Strangulated epigastric hernia without gangrene
  Strangulated hypogastric hernia without gangrene
  Strangulated midline hernia without gangrene
  Strangulated spigelian hernia without gangrene
  Strangulated subxiphoid hernia without gangrene
  Subxiphoid hernia causing obstruction, without gangrene
  **CC Excl:** PDX collection 780

**K43.7**   **Other and unspecified ventral hernia with gangrene**    `MCC`
  Any condition listed under K43.6 specified as gangrenous
  **CC Excl:** PDX collection 781

**K43.9**   **Ventral hernia without obstruction or gangrene**
  Epigastric hernia
  Ventral hernia NOS

`✓4ᵗʰ` **K44**   **Diaphragmatic hernia**
  `INCLUDES`   hiatus hernia (esophageal) (sliding)
    paraesophageal hernia
  `EXCLUDES 1`   *congenital diaphragmatic hernia (Q79.0)*
    *congenital hiatus hernia (Q40.1)*

**K44.0**   **Diaphragmatic hernia with obstruction, without gangrene**    `CC`
  Diaphragmatic hernia causing obstruction
  Incarcerated diaphragmatic hernia
  Irreducible diaphragmatic hernia
  Strangulated diaphragmatic hernia
  **CC Excl:** PDX collection 782

**K44.1**   **Diaphragmatic hernia with gangrene**    `MCC`
  Gangrenous diaphragmatic hernia
  **CC Excl:** PDX collection 782

**K44.9**   **Diaphragmatic hernia without obstruction or gangrene**
  Diaphragmatic hernia NOS

### Hiatal Hernia

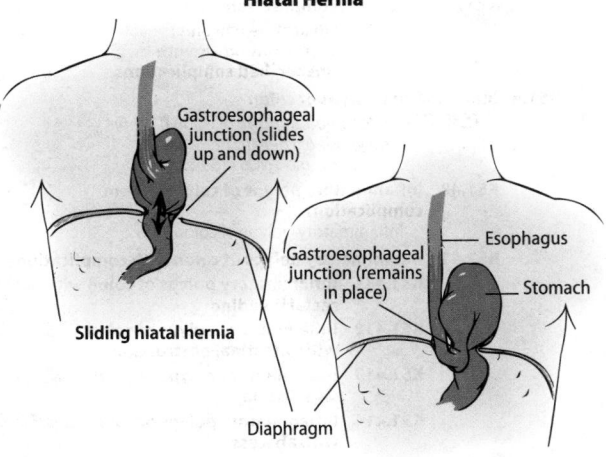

Gastroesophageal junction (slides up and down)

**Sliding hiatal hernia**

Gastroesophageal junction (remains in place)

Esophagus

Stomach

Diaphragm

**Paraesophageal hiatal hernia**

---

`✓4ᵗʰ` **K45**   **Other abdominal hernia**
  `INCLUDES`   abdominal hernia, specified site NEC
    lumbar hernia
    obturator hernia
    pudendal hernia
    retroperitoneal hernia
    sciatic hernia

**K45.0**   **Other specified abdominal hernia with obstruction, without gangrene**    `CC`
  Other specified abdominal hernia causing obstruction
  Other specified incarcerated abdominal hernia
  Other specified irreducible abdominal hernia
  Other specified strangulated abdominal hernia
  **CC Excl:** PDX collection 783

**K45.1**   **Other specified abdominal hernia with gangrene**    `MCC`
  Any condition listed under K45 specified as gangrenous
  **CC Excl:** PDX collection 784

**K45.8**   **Other specified abdominal hernia without obstruction or gangrene**

`✓4ᵗʰ` **K46**   **Unspecified abdominal hernia**
  `INCLUDES`   enterocele
    epiplocele
    hernia NOS
    interstitial hernia
    intestinal hernia
    intra-abdominal hernia
  `EXCLUDES 1`   *vaginal enterocele (N81.5)*

**K46.0**   **Unspecified abdominal hernia with obstruction, without gangrene**    `CC`
  Unspecified abdominal hernia causing obstruction
  Unspecified incarcerated abdominal hernia
  Unspecified irreducible abdominal hernia
  Unspecified strangulated abdominal hernia
  **CC Excl:** PDX collection 783

**K46.1**   **Unspecified abdominal hernia with gangrene**    `MCC`
  Any condition listed under K46 specified as gangrenous
  **CC Excl:** PDX collection 784

**K46.9**   **Unspecified abdominal hernia without obstruction or gangrene**
  Abdominal hernia NOS

## Noninfective enteritis and colitis (K50-K52)

`INCLUDES`   noninfective inflammatory bowel disease
`EXCLUDES 1`   *irritable bowel syndrome (K58.-)*
  *megacolon (K59.3-)*

`✓4ᵗʰ` **K50**   **Crohn's disease [regional enteritis]**
  `INCLUDES`   granulomatous enteritis
  Use additional code to identify manifestations, such as:
    pyoderma gangrenosum (L88)
  `EXCLUDES 1`   *ulcerative colitis (K51.-)*
  **AHA:** 2012, 4Q, 104

  **CC Excl: For CC codes in category K50, unless otherwise noted:** PDX collection 785

`✓5ᵗʰ` **K50.0**   **Crohn's disease of small intestine**
  Crohn's disease [regional enteritis] of duodenum
  Crohn's disease [regional enteritis] of ileum
  Crohn's disease [regional enteritis] of jejunum
  Regional ileitis
  Terminal ileitis
  `EXCLUDES 1`   *Crohn's disease of both small and large intestine (K50.8-)*

  **K50.00**   **Crohn's disease of small intestine without complications**    `CC` `HCC`

  `✓6ᵗʰ` **K50.01**   **Crohn's disease of small intestine with complications**

    **K50.011**   **Crohn's disease of small intestine with rectal bleeding**    `CC` `HCC`

    **K50.012**   **Crohn's disease of small intestine with intestinal obstruction**    `PDx CC` `CC` `HCC`

    **K50.013**   **Crohn's disease of small intestine with fistula**    `PDx CC` `CC` `HCC`

    **K50.014**   **Crohn's disease of small intestine with abscess**    `PDx CC` `CC` `HCC`
      **AHA:** 2012, 4Q, 104

    **K50.018**   **Crohn's disease of small intestine with other complication**    `CC` `HCC`

    **K50.019**   **Crohn's disease of small intestine with unspecified complications**    `CC` `HCC`

---

`✓` Additional Character Req   `✓x7ᵗʰ` Placeholder Alert   Unacceptable PDx   **Manifestation**   `H1`-`H14` HAC   `HCC` CMS-HCC Condition   `EXCLUDES 1` Not Coded Here   `EXCLUDES 2` Not Included Here

✓5ᵗʰ **K50.1** **Crohn's disease of large intestine**
Crohn's disease [regional enteritis] of colon
Crohn's disease [regional enteritis] of large bowel
Crohn's disease [regional enteritis] of rectum
Granulomatous colitis
Regional colitis
EXCLUDES 1 Crohn's disease of both small and large intestine (K50.8)

**K50.10** **Crohn's disease of large intestine** without complications `CC` `HCC`

✓6ᵗʰ **K50.11** **Crohn's disease of large intestine** with complications

**K50.111** **Crohn's disease of large intestine** with rectal bleeding `CC` `HCC`

**K50.112** **Crohn's disease of large intestine with intestinal obstruction** `PDxCC` `CC` `HCC`

**K50.113** **Crohn's disease of large intestine with fistula** `PDxCC` `CC` `HCC`

**K50.114** **Crohn's disease of large intestine with abscess** `PDxCC` `CC` `HCC`

**K50.118** **Crohn's disease of large intestine with other complication** `CC` `HCC`

**K50.119** **Crohn's disease of large intestine with unspecified complications** `CC` `HCC`

✓5ᵗʰ **K50.8** **Crohn's disease of both small and large intestine**

**K50.80** **Crohn's disease of both small and large intestine** without complications `CC` `HCC`

✓6ᵗʰ **K50.81** **Crohn's disease of both small and large intestine with complications**

**K50.811** **Crohn's disease of both small and large intestine with rectal bleeding** `CC` `HCC`

**K50.812** **Crohn's disease of both small and large intestine with intestinal obstruction** `PDxCC` `CC` `HCC`

**K50.813** **Crohn's disease of both small and large intestine with fistula** `PDxCC` `CC` `HCC`

**K50.814** **Crohn's disease of both small and large intestine with abscess** `PDxCC` `CC` `HCC`

**K50.818** **Crohn's disease of both small and large intestine with other complication** `CC` `HCC`

**K50.819** **Crohn's disease of both small and large intestine with unspecified complications** `CC` `HCC`

✓5ᵗʰ **K50.9** **Crohn's disease, unspecified**

CC Excl: For CC codes in subcategory K50.9:
PDX collection 786

**K50.90** **Crohn's disease, unspecified, without complications** `CC` `HCC`
Crohn's disease NOS
Regional enteritis NOS

✓6ᵗʰ **K50.91** **Crohn's disease, unspecified, with complications**

**K50.911** **Crohn's disease, unspecified, with rectal bleeding** `CC` `HCC`

**K50.912** **Crohn's disease, unspecified, with intestinal obstruction** `PDxCC` `CC` `HCC`

**K50.913** **Crohn's disease, unspecified, with fistula** `PDxCC` `CC` `HCC`

**K50.914** **Crohn's disease, unspecified, with abscess** `PDxCC` `CC` `HCC`

**K50.918** **Crohn's disease, unspecified, with other complication** `CC` `HCC`

**K50.919** **Crohn's disease, unspecified, with unspecified complications** `CC` `HCC`

✓4ᵗʰ **K51** **Ulcerative colitis**
Use additional code to identify manifestations, such as:
pyoderma gangrenosum (L88)
EXCLUDES 1 Crohn's disease [regional enteritis] (K50.-)

CC Excl: For CC codes in category K51, unless otherwise noted:
PDX collection 785

✓5ᵗʰ **K51.0** **Ulcerative (chronic) pancolitis**
Backwash ileitis

**K51.00** **Ulcerative (chronic) pancolitis** without complications `CC` `HCC`
Ulcerative (chronic) pancolitis NOS

✓6ᵗʰ **K51.01** **Ulcerative (chronic) pancolitis** with complications

**K51.011** **Ulcerative (chronic) pancolitis with** rectal bleeding `CC` `HCC`

**K51.012** **Ulcerative (chronic) pancolitis** `PDxCC` `CC` `HCC`
with **intestinal obstruction**

**K51.013** **Ulcerative (chronic) pancolitis** `PDxCC` `CC` `HCC`
with **fistula**

**K51.014** **Ulcerative (chronic) pancolitis** `PDxCC` `CC` `HCC`
with **abscess**

**K51.018** **Ulcerative (chronic) pancolitis with** `CC` `HCC`
other complication

**K51.019** **Ulcerative (chronic) pancolitis with** `CC` `HCC`
unspecified complications

✓5ᵗʰ **K51.2** **Ulcerative (chronic) proctitis**

**K51.20** **Ulcerative (chronic) proctitis** without `CC` `HCC`
complications
Ulcerative (chronic) proctitis NOS

✓6ᵗʰ **K51.21** **Ulcerative (chronic) proctitis** with complications

**K51.211** **Ulcerative (chronic) proctitis with** `CC` `HCC`
rectal bleeding

**K51.212** **Ulcerative (chronic) proctitis** `PDxCC` `CC` `HCC`
with intestinal obstruction

**K51.213** **Ulcerative (chronic) proctitis** `PDxCC` `CC` `HCC`
with fistula

**K51.214** **Ulcerative (chronic) proctitis** `PDxCC` `CC` `HCC`
with abscess

**K51.218** **Ulcerative (chronic) proctitis with** `CC` `HCC`
other complication

**K51.219** **Ulcerative (chronic) proctitis with** `CC` `HCC`
unspecified complications

✓5ᵗʰ **K51.3** **Ulcerative (chronic) rectosigmoiditis**

**K51.30** **Ulcerative (chronic) rectosigmoiditis** without `CC` `HCC`
complications
Ulcerative (chronic) rectosigmoiditis NOS

✓6ᵗʰ **K51.31** **Ulcerative (chronic) rectosigmoiditis** with
complications

**K51.311** **Ulcerative (chronic)** `CC` `HCC`
**rectosigmoiditis** with rectal
bleeding

**K51.312** **Ulcerative (chronic)** `PDxCC` `CC` `HCC`
**rectosigmoiditis** with intestinal
obstruction

**K51.313** **Ulcerative (chronic)** `PDxCC` `CC` `HCC`
**rectosigmoiditis** with fistula

**K51.314** **Ulcerative (chronic)** `PDxCC` `CC` `HCC`
**rectosigmoiditis** with abscess

**K51.318** **Ulcerative (chronic) r** `CC` `HCC`
**ectosigmoiditis** with other
complication

**K51.319** **Ulcerative (chronic)** `CC` `HCC`
**rectosigmoiditis** with
unspecified complications

✓5ᵗʰ **K51.4** **Inflammatory polyps of colon**
EXCLUDES 1 adenomatous polyp of colon (D12.6)
polyposis of colon (D12.6)
polyps of colon NOS (K63.5)

**K51.40** **Inflammatory polyps of colon** without `CC` `HCC`
complications
Inflammatory polyps of colon NOS

✓6ᵗʰ **K51.41** **Inflammatory polyps of colon** with complications

**K51.411** **Inflammatory polyps of colon with** `CC` `HCC`
rectal bleeding

**K51.412** **Inflammatory polyps of colon** `PDxCC` `CC` `HCC`
with intestinal obstruction

**K51.413** **Inflammatory polyps of colon** `PDxCC` `CC` `HCC`
with fistula

**K51.414** **Inflammatory polyps of colon** `PDxCC` `CC` `HCC`
with abscess

**K51.418** **Inflammatory polyps of colon with** `CC` `HCC`
other complication

**K51.419** **Inflammatory polyps of colon with** `CC` `HCC`
unspecified complications

✓5ᵗʰ **K51.5** **Left sided colitis**
Left hemicolitis

**K51.50** **Left sided colitis** without complications `CC` `HCC`
Left sided colitis NOS

✓6ᵗʰ **K51.51** **Left sided colitis** with complications

**K51.511** **Left sided colitis with** rectal `CC` `HCC`
bleeding

**K51.512** **Left sided colitis with** `PDxCC` `CC` `HCC`
intestinal obstruction

---

`N` Newborn: 0　`P` Pediatric: 0-17　`M` Maternity: 12-55　`A` Adult: 15-124　`MCC` Major CC Condition　`PDxMCC` PDx acts as own MCC　`CC` CC Condition　`PDxCC` PDx acts as own CC

**K51.513** Left sided colitis with fistula `PDxCC` `CC` `HCC`
**K51.514** Left sided colitis with abscess `PDxCC` `CC` `HCC`
**K51.518** Left sided colitis with other complication `CC` `HCC`
**K51.519** Left sided colitis with unspecified complications `CC` `HCC`

✓5ᵗʰ **K51.8** **Other ulcerative colitis**
**K51.80** Other ulcerative colitis without complications `CC` `HCC`
✓6ᵗʰ **K51.81** **Other ulcerative colitis with complications**
**K51.811** Other ulcerative colitis with rectal bleeding `CC` `HCC`
**K51.812** Other ulcerative colitis with intestinal obstruction `PDxCC` `CC` `HCC`
**K51.813** Other ulcerative colitis with fistula `PDxCC` `CC` `HCC`
**K51.814** Other ulcerative colitis with abscess `PDxCC` `CC` `HCC`
**K51.818** Other ulcerative colitis with other complication `CC` `HCC`
**K51.819** Other ulcerative colitis with unspecified complications `CC` `HCC`

✓5ᵗʰ **K51.9** **Ulcerative colitis, unspecified**

> **CC Excl: For CC codes in subcategory K51.9:**
> PDX collection 787

**K51.90** Ulcerative colitis, unspecified, without complications `CC` `HCC`
✓6ᵗʰ **K51.91** **Ulcerative colitis, unspecified, with complications**
**K51.911** Ulcerative colitis, unspecified with rectal bleeding `CC` `HCC`
**K51.912** Ulcerative colitis, unspecified with intestinal obstruction `PDxCC` `CC` `HCC`
**K51.913** Ulcerative colitis, unspecified with fistula `PDxCC` `CC` `HCC`
**K51.914** Ulcerative colitis, unspecified with abscess `PDxCC` `CC` `HCC`
**K51.918** Ulcerative colitis, unspecified with other complication `CC` `HCC`
**K51.919** Ulcerative colitis, unspecified with unspecified complications `CC` `HCC`

✓4ᵗʰ **K52** **Other and unspecified noninfective gastroenteritis and colitis**
**K52.0** **Gastroenteritis and colitis due to radiation** `CC`
**CC Excl:** PDX collection 788
**K52.1** **Toxic gastroenteritis and colitis** `CC`
Drug-induced gastroenteritis and colitis
Code first (T51-T65) to identify toxic agent
Use additional code for adverse effect, if applicable, to identify drug (T36-T50 with fifth or sixth character 5)
**CC Excl:** PDX collection 789
✓5ᵗʰ **K52.2** **Allergic and dietetic gastroenteritis and colitis**
Use additional code to identify type of food allergy (Z91.01-, Z91.02-)
*EXCLUDES 2* allergic eosinophilic colitis (K52.82)
allergic eosinophilic esophagitis (K20.0)
allergic eosinophilic gastritis (K52.81)
allergic eosinophilic gastroenteritis (K52.81)
food protein-induced proctocolitis (K52.82)
**DEF:** True immunoglobulin E (IgE)-mediated allergic reaction of the lining of the stomach, intestines, or colon to food proteins; causes nausea, vomiting, diarrhea, and abdominal cramping.
**K52.21** **Food protein-induced enterocolitis syndrome**
Use additional code for hypovolemic shock, if present (R57.1)
**K52.22** **Food protein-induced enteropathy**
**K52.29** **Other allergic and dietetic gastroenteritis and colitis**
Food hypersensitivity gastroenteritis or colitis
Immediate gastrointestinal hypersensitivity
**K52.3** **Indeterminate colitis**
Colonic inflammatory bowel disease unclassified (IBDU)
*EXCLUDES 1* unspecified colitis (K52.9)
✓5ᵗʰ **K52.8** **Other specified noninfective gastroenteritis and colitis**
**K52.81** **Eosinophilic gastritis or gastroenteritis**
Eosinophilic enteritis
*EXCLUDES 2* eosinophilic esophagitis (K20.0)

**K52.82** **Eosinophilic colitis**
Allergic proctocolitis
Food-induced eosinophilic proctocolitis
Food protein-induced proctocolitis
Milk protein-induced proctocolitis
✓6ᵗʰ **K52.83** **Microscopic colitis**
**K52.831** **Collagenous colitis**
**K52.832** **Lymphocytic colitis**
**K52.838** **Other microscopic colitis**
**K52.839** **Microscopic colitis, unspecified**
**K52.89** **Other specified noninfective gastroenteritis and colitis**
**K52.9** **Noninfective gastroenteritis and colitis, unspecified**
Colitis NOS                   Ileitis NOS
Enteritis NOS                 Jejunitis NOS
Gastroenteritis NOS           Sigmoiditis NOS
*EXCLUDES 1* diarrhea NOS (R19.7)
functional diarrhea (K59.1)
infectious gastroenteritis and colitis NOS (A09)
neonatal diarrhea (noninfective) (P78.3)
psychogenic diarrhea (F45.8)

### Other diseases of intestines (K55-K64)

✓4ᵗʰ **K55** **Vascular disorders of intestine**
*EXCLUDES 1* necrotizing enterocolitis of newborn (P77.-)

> **CC Excl: For MCC codes in category K55, unless otherwise noted:**
> PDX collection 790

✓5ᵗʰ **K55.0** **Acute vascular disorders of intestine**
Infarction of appendices epiploicae
Mesenteric (artery) (vein) embolism
Mesenteric (artery) (vein) infarction
Mesenteric (artery) (vein) thrombosis
✓6ᵗʰ **K55.01** **Acute (reversible) ischemia of small intestine**
**K55.011** Focal (segmental) acute (reversible) ischemia of small intestine `MCC` `HCC`
**K55.012** Diffuse acute (reversible) ischemia of small intestine `MCC` `HCC`
**K55.019** Acute (reversible) ischemia of small intestine, extent unspecified `MCC` `HCC`
✓6ᵗʰ **K55.02** **Acute infarction of small intestine**
Gangrene of small intestine
Necrosis of small intestine
**K55.021** Focal (segmental) acute infarction of small intestine `MCC` `HCC`
**K55.022** Diffuse acute infarction of small intestine `MCC` `HCC`
**K55.029** Acute infarction of small intestine, extent unspecified `MCC` `HCC`
✓6ᵗʰ **K55.03** **Acute (reversible) ischemia of large intestine**
Acute fulminant ischemic colitis
Subacute ischemic colitis
**K55.031** Focal (segmental) acute (reversible) ischemia of large intestine `MCC` `HCC`
**K55.032** Diffuse acute (reversible) ischemia of large intestine `MCC` `HCC`
**K55.039** Acute (reversible) ischemia of large intestine, extent unspecified `MCC` `HCC`
✓6ᵗʰ **K55.04** **Acute infarction of large intestine**
Gangrene of large intestine
Necrosis of large intestine
**K55.041** Focal (segmental) acute infarction of large intestine `MCC` `HCC`
**K55.042** Diffuse acute infarction of large intestine `MCC` `HCC`
**K55.049** Acute infarction of large intestine, extent unspecified `MCC` `HCC`
✓6ᵗʰ **K55.05** **Acute (reversible) ischemia of intestine, part unspecified**
**K55.051** Focal (segmental) acute (reversible) ischemia of intestine, part unspecified `MCC` `HCC`
**K55.052** Diffuse acute (reversible) ischemia of intestine, part unspecified `MCC` `HCC`
**K55.059** Acute (reversible) ischemia of intestine, part and extent unspecified `MCC` `HCC`

---

✓ Additional Character Req   ✓x7ᵗʰ Placeholder Alert   Unacceptable PDx   Manifestation   `H1`-`H14` HAC   `HCC` CMS-HCC Condition   *EXCLUDES 1* Not Coded Here   *EXCLUDES 2* Not Included Here

✓6ᵗʰ **K55.06** **Acute infarction of intestine, part unspecified**
Acute intestinal infarction
Gangrene of intestine
Necrosis of intestine

     **K55.061** **Focal (segmental) acute infarction** MCC HCC
**of intestine, part unspecified**

     **K55.062** **Diffuse acute infarction of** MCC HCC
**intestine, part unspecified**

     **K55.069** **Acute infarction of intestine, part** MCC HCC
**and extent unspecified**

**K55.1** **Chronic vascular disorders of intestine** CC HCC
Chronic ischemic colitis
Chronic ischemic enteritis
Chronic ischemic enterocolitis
Ischemic stricture of intestine
Mesenteric atherosclerosis
Mesenteric vascular insufficiency
**CC Excl:** PDX collection 791

✓5ᵗʰ **K55.2** **Angiodysplasia of colon**

     **K55.20** **Angiodysplasia of colon without hemorrhage**

     **K55.21** **Angiodysplasia of colon with hemorrhage** MCC
**DEF:** Small vascular abnormalities due to fragile blood
vessels in the colon; results in blood loss from the
gastrointestinal (GI) tract.
**CC Excl:** PDX collection 770

✓5ᵗʰ **K55.3** **Necrotizing enterocolitis**
EXCLUDES 1    *necrotizing enterocolitis of newborn (P77.-)*
EXCLUDES 2    *necrotizing enterocolitis due to Clostridium difficile*
▶*(A04.7-)*◀

     **K55.30** **Necrotizing enterocolitis, unspecified** MCC HCC
Necrotizing enterocolitis, NOS

     **K55.31** **Stage 1 necrotizing enterocolitis** MCC HCC
Necrotizing enterocolitis without pneumatosis,
without perforation

     **K55.32** **Stage 2 necrotizing enterocolitis** MCC HCC
Necrotizing enterocolitis with pneumatosis, without
perforation

     **K55.33** **Stage 3 necrotizing enterocolitis** MCC HCC
Necrotizing enterocolitis with perforation
Necrotizing enterocolitis with pneumatosis and
perforation

**K55.8** **Other vascular disorders of intestine** CC HCC
**CC Excl:** PDX collection 791

**K55.9** **Vascular disorder of intestine, unspecified** CC HCC
Ischemic colitis
Ischemic enteritis
Ischemic enterocolitis
**CC Excl:** PDX collection 791

✓4ᵗʰ **K56** **Paralytic ileus and intestinal obstruction without hernia**
EXCLUDES 1    *congenital stricture or stenosis of intestine (Q41-Q42)*
*cystic fibrosis with meconium ileus (E84.11)*
*intestinal obstruction with hernia (K40-K46)*
*ischemic stricture of intestine (K55.1)*
*meconium ileus NOS (P76.0)*
*neonatal intestinal obstructions classifiable to P76-*
*obstruction of duodenum (K31.5)*
*postprocedural intestinal obstruction* ▶*(K91.3-)*◀
*stenosis of anus or rectum (K62.4)*

**CC Excl: For CC/MCC codes in category K56:** PDX collection 792

**K56.0** **Paralytic ileus** CC HCC
Paralysis of bowel    Paralysis of intestine    Paralysis of colon
EXCLUDES 1    *gallstone ileus (K56.3)*
*ileus NOS (K56.7)*
*obstructive ileus NOS* ▶*(K56.69-)*◀

**K56.1** **Intussusception** CC HCC
Intussusception or invagination of bowel
Intussusception or invagination of colon
Intussusception or invagination of intestine
Intussusception or invagination of rectum
EXCLUDES 2    *intussusception of appendix (K38.8)*
**DEF:** Intestinal obstruction due to prolapse of a bowel section into
adjacent section; occurs primarily in children; symptoms include
acute abdominal pain, vomiting, and passage of blood and mucus
from rectum.

**K56.2** **Volvulus** MCC HCC
Strangulation of colon or intestine
Torsion of colon or intestine
Twist of colon or intestine
EXCLUDES 2    *volvulus of duodenum (K31.5)*

**Volvulus**

Knotted
intestine
(volvulus)

**K56.3** **Gallstone ileus** CC HCC
Obstruction of intestine by gallstone

✓5ᵗʰ **K56.4** **Other impaction of intestine**

     **K56.41** **Fecal impaction** HCC
EXCLUDES 1    *constipation (K59.0-)*
*incomplete defecation (R15.0)*

     **K56.49** **Other impaction of intestine** CC HCC

▲ ✓5ᵗʰ **K56.5** **Intestinal adhesions [bands] with obstruction**
**(postinfection)**
Abdominal hernia due to adhesions with obstruction
▶Peritoneal adhesions [bands] with intestinal obstruction
(postinfection)◀

●      **K56.50** **Intestinal adhesions [bands], unspecified as** CC
**to partial versus complete obstruction**
Intestinal adhesions with obstruction NOS

●      **K56.51** **Intestinal adhesions [bands], with partial** CC
**obstruction**
Intestinal adhesions with incomplete obstruction

●      **K56.52** **Intestinal adhesions [bands] with complete** CC
**obstruction**

✓5ᵗʰ **K56.6** **Other and unspecified intestinal obstruction**
**AHA:** 2017, 2Q, 12

     ✓6ᵗʰ **K56.60** **Unspecified intestinal obstruction**
~~Intestinal obstruction NOS~~
EXCLUDES 1    *intestinal obstruction due to specified*
*condition—code to condition*

●        **K56.600** **Partial intestinal obstruction,** CC
**unspecified as to cause**
Incomplete intestinal obstruction, NOS

●        **K56.601** **Complete intestinal obstruction,** CC
**unspecified as to cause**

●        **K56.609** **Unspecified intestinal obstruction,** CC
**unspecified as to partial versus**
**complete obstruction**
Intestinal obstruction NOS

     ✓6ᵗʰ **K56.69** **Other intestinal obstruction**
Enterostenosis NOS
Obstructive ileus NOS
Occlusion of colon or intestine NOS
Stenosis of colon or intestine NOS
Stricture of colon or intestine NOS
EXCLUDES 1    *intestinal obstruction due to specified*
*condition—code to condition*

●        **K56.690** **Other partial intestinal obstruction** CC
Other incomplete intestinal obstruction

●        **K56.691** **Other complete intestinal obstruction** CC

●        **K56.699** **Other intestinal obstruction** CC
**unspecified as to partial versus**
**complete obstruction**
Other intestinal obstruction, NEC

**K56.7** **Ileus, unspecified** CC HCC
EXCLUDES 1    *obstructive ileus* ▶*(K56.69-)*◀
EXCLUDES 2    ▶*intestinal obstruction with hernia (K40-K46)*◀
**AHA:** 2017, 1Q, 40

N Newborn: 0    P Pediatric: 0-17    M Maternity: 12-55    A Adult: 15-124    MCC Major CC Condition    PDxMCC PDx acts as own MCC    CC CC Condition    PDxCC PDx acts as own CC

**698**      ICD-10-CM 2018

☑4ᵗʰ **K57  Diverticular disease of intestine**
> *EXCLUDES 1*  congenital diverticulum of intestine (Q43.8)
> Meckel's diverticulum (Q43.0)
> *EXCLUDES 2*  diverticulum of appendix (K38.2)

**CC Excl: For MCC codes in category K57, unless otherwise noted:**
PDX collection 770

☑5ᵗʰ **K57.0  Diverticulitis of small intestine with perforation and abscess**
> Diverticulitis of small intestine with peritonitis
> *EXCLUDES 1*  diverticulitis of both small and large intestine with perforation and abscess (K57.4-)

**K57.00  Diverticulitis of small intestine with perforation and abscess without bleeding**  `PDxCC` `CC`
> **CC Excl:** PDX collection 793

**K57.01  Diverticulitis of small intestine with perforation and abscess with bleeding**  `PDxCC` `MCC`

☑5ᵗʰ **K57.1  Diverticular disease of small intestine without perforation or abscess**
> *EXCLUDES 1*  diverticular disease of both small and large intestine without perforation or abscess (K57.5-)

**K57.10  Diverticulosis of small intestine without perforation or abscess without bleeding**
> Diverticular disease of small intestine NOS

**K57.11  Diverticulosis of small intestine without perforation or abscess with bleeding**  `MCC`

**K57.12  Diverticulitis of small intestine without perforation or abscess without bleeding**  `CC`
> **CC Excl:** PDX collection 793

**K57.13  Diverticulitis of small intestine without perforation or abscess with bleeding**  `MCC`

☑5ᵗʰ **K57.2  Diverticulitis of large intestine with perforation and abscess**
> Diverticulitis of colon with peritonitis
> *EXCLUDES 1*  diverticulitis of both small and large intestine with perforation and abscess (K57.4-)

**K57.20  Diverticulitis of large intestine with perforation and abscess without bleeding**  `PDxCC` `CC`
> **CC Excl:** PDX collection 794

**K57.21  Diverticulitis of large intestine with perforation and abscess with bleeding**  `PDxCC` `MCC`

☑5ᵗʰ **K57.3  Diverticular disease of large intestine without perforation or abscess**
> *EXCLUDES 1*  diverticular disease of both small and large intestine without perforation or abscess (K57.5-)

**K57.30  Diverticulosis of large intestine without perforation or abscess without bleeding**
> Diverticular disease of colon NOS

**K57.31  Diverticulosis of large intestine without perforation or abscess with bleeding**  `MCC`

**K57.32  Diverticulitis of large intestine without perforation or abscess without bleeding**  `CC`
> **CC Excl:** PDX collection 794

**K57.33  Diverticulitis of large intestine without perforation or abscess with bleeding**  `MCC`

☑5ᵗʰ **K57.4  Diverticulitis of both small and large intestine with perforation and abscess**
> Diverticulitis of both small and large intestine with peritonitis

**K57.40  Diverticulitis of both small and large intestine with perforation and abscess without bleeding**  `PDxCC` `CC`
> **CC Excl:** PDX collection 794

**K57.41  Diverticulitis of both small and large intestine with perforation and abscess with bleeding**  `PDxCC` `MCC`

☑5ᵗʰ **K57.5  Diverticular disease of both small and large intestine without perforation or abscess**

**K57.50  Diverticulosis of both small and large intestine without perforation or abscess without bleeding**
> Diverticular disease of both small and large intestine NOS

**K57.51  Diverticulitis of both small and large intestine without perforation or abscess with bleeding**  `MCC`

**K57.52  Diverticulitis of both small and large intestine without perforation or abscess without bleeding**  `PDxCC` `CC`
> **CC Excl:** PDX collection 794

**K57.53  Diverticulitis of both small and large intestine without perforation or abscess with bleeding**  `MCC`

☑5ᵗʰ **K57.8  Diverticulitis of intestine, part unspecified, with perforation and abscess**
> Diverticulitis of intestine NOS with peritonitis

**K57.80  Diverticulitis of intestine, part unspecified, with perforation and abscess without bleeding**  `PDxCC` `CC`
> **CC Excl:** PDX collection 794

**K57.81  Diverticulitis of intestine, part unspecified, with perforation and abscess with bleeding**  `PDxCC` `MCC`

☑5ᵗʰ **K57.9  Diverticular disease of intestine, part unspecified, without perforation or abscess**

**K57.90  Diverticulosis of intestine, part unspecified, without perforation or abscess without bleeding**
> Diverticular disease of intestine NOS

**K57.91  Diverticulosis of intestine, part unspecified, without perforation or abscess with bleeding**  `MCC`

**K57.92  Diverticulitis of intestine, part unspecified, without perforation or abscess without bleeding**  `CC`
> **CC Excl:** PDX collection 794

**K57.93  Diverticulitis of intestine, part unspecified, without perforation or abscess with bleeding**  `MCC`

☑4ᵗʰ **K58  Irritable bowel syndrome**
> *INCLUDES*  irritable colon
> spastic colon

**K58.0  Irritable bowel syndrome with diarrhea**

**K58.1  Irritable bowel syndrome with constipation**

**K58.2  Mixed irritable bowel syndrome**

**K58.8  Other irritable bowel syndrome**

**K58.9  Irritable bowel syndrome without diarrhea**
> Irritable bowel syndrome NOS

☑4ᵗʰ **K59  Other functional intestinal disorders**
> *EXCLUDES 1*  change in bowel habit NOS (R19.4)
> intestinal malabsorption (K90.-)
> psychogenic intestinal disorders (F45.8)
> *EXCLUDES 2*  functional disorders of stomach (K31.-)

☑5ᵗʰ **K59.0  Constipation**
> Use additional code for adverse effect, if applicable, to identify drug (T36-T50 with fifth or sixth character 5)
> *EXCLUDES 1*  fecal impaction (K56.41)
> incomplete defecation (R15.0)

**K59.00  Constipation, unspecified**

**K59.01  Slow transit constipation**
> **DEF:** Delay in the transit of fecal material through the colon secondary to smooth muscle dysfunction or decreased peristaltic contractions along the colon: also called colonic inertia or delayed transit.

**K59.02  Outlet dysfunction constipation**

**K59.03  Drug induced constipation**
> Use additional code for adverse effect, if applicable, to identify drug (T36-T50 with fifth or sixth character 5)

**K59.04  Chronic idiopathic constipation**
> Functional constipation

**K59.09  Other constipation**
> Chronic constipation

**K59.1  Functional diarrhea**
> *EXCLUDES 1*  diarrhea NOS (R19.7)
> irritable bowel syndrome with diarrhea (K58.0)

**K59.2  Neurogenic bowel, not elsewhere classified**  `CC`
> **DEF:** Disorder of bowel due to spinal cord lesion due to injury or as a complication of conditions such as multiple sclerosis (MS) or spina bifida; loss of bowel control is the primary symptom, manifested as constipation or bowel incontinence.
> **CC Excl:** PDX collection 795

☑5ᵗʰ **K59.3  Megacolon, not elsewhere classified**
> Dilatation of colon
> Code first, if applicable (T51-T65) to identify toxic agent
> *EXCLUDES 1*  congenital megacolon (aganglionic) (Q43.1)
> megacolon (due to) (in) Chagas' disease (B57.32)
> megacolon (due to) (in) Clostridium difficile
> ►(A04.7-)◄
> megacolon (due to) (in) Hirschsprung's disease (Q43.1)

**CC Excl: For CC codes in subcategory K59.3:**
PDX collection 795

**K59.31  Toxic megacolon**  `CC` `HCC`

**K59.39  Other megacolon**  `CC`
> Megacolon NOS

---

☑ Additional Character Req   ☑x7ᵗʰ Placeholder Alert   Unacceptable PDx   Manifestation   `H1`-`H14` HAC   `HCC` CMS-HCC Condition   *EXCLUDES 1* Not Coded Here   *EXCLUDES 2* Not Included Here

**Chapter 11. Diseases of the Digestive System**

**K59.4**   **Anal spasm**
Proctalgia fugax

**K59.8**   **Other specified functional intestinal disorders**
Atony of colon
Pseudo-obstruction (acute) (chronic) of intestine

**K59.9**   **Functional intestinal disorder, unspecified**

✓4ᵗʰ **K60**   **Fissure and fistula of anal and rectal regions**
EXCLUDES 1   *fissure and fistula of anal and rectal regions with abscess or cellulitis (K61.-)*
EXCLUDES 2   *anal sphincter tear (healed) (nontraumatic) (old) (K62.81)*

**K60.0**   **Acute anal fissure**

**K60.1**   **Chronic anal fissure**

**K60.2**   **Anal fissure, unspecified**

**K60.3**   **Anal fistula**

**K60.4**   **Rectal fistula**
Fistula of rectum to skin
EXCLUDES 1   *rectovaginal fistula (N82.3)*
     *vesicorectal fistual (N32.1)*

**K60.5**   **Anorectal fistula**

✓4ᵗʰ **K61**   **Abscess of anal and rectal regions**
INCLUDES   abscess of anal and rectal regions
     cellulitis of anal and rectal regions

CC Excl: For CC codes in category K61: PDX collection 796

**K61.0**   **Anal abscess**    CC
Perianal abscess
EXCLUDES 1   *intrasphincteric abscess (K61.4)*

**K61.1**   **Rectal abscess**    CC
Perirectal abscess
EXCLUDES 1   *ischiorectal abscess (K61.3)*
AHA: 2012, 4Q, 104

**K61.2**   **Anorectal abscess**    CC

**K61.3**   **Ischiorectal abscess**    CC
Abscess of ischiorectal fossa

**K61.4**   **Intrasphincteric abscess**    CC

✓4ᵗʰ **K62**   **Other diseases of anus and rectum**
INCLUDES   anal canal
EXCLUDES 2   *colostomy and enterostomy malfunction (K94.0-, K94.1-)*
     *fecal incontinence (R15.-)*
     *hemorrhoids (K64.-)*

**K62.0**   **Anal polyp**

**K62.1**   **Rectal polyp**
EXCLUDES 1   *adenomatous polyp (D12.8)*

**K62.2**   **Anal prolapse**
Prolapse of anal canal

**K62.3**   **Rectal prolapse**
Prolapse of rectal mucosa

**K62.4**   **Stenosis of anus and rectum**
Stricture of anus (sphincter)

**K62.5**   **Hemorrhage of anus and rectum**    CC
EXCLUDES 1   *gastrointestinal bleeding NOS (K92.2)*
     *melena (K92.1)*
     *neonatal rectal hemorrhage (P54.2)*
CC Excl: PDX collection 770

**K62.6**   **Ulcer of anus and rectum**    CC
Solitary ulcer of anus and rectum
Stercoral ulcer of anus and rectum
EXCLUDES 1   *fissure and fistula of anus and rectum (K60.-)*
     *ulcerative colitis (K51.-)*
CC Excl: PDX collection 797

**K62.7**   **Radiation proctitis**
Use additional code to identify the type of radiation (W90.-)

✓5ᵗʰ **K62.8**   **Other specified diseases of anus and rectum**
EXCLUDES 2   *ulcerative proctitis (K51.2)*

**K62.81**   **Anal sphincter tear (healed) (nontraumatic) (old)**
Tear of anus, nontraumatic
Use additional code for any associated fecal incontinence (R15.-)
EXCLUDES 2   *anal fissure (K60.-)*
     *anal sphincter tear (healed) (old) complicating delivery (O34.7-)*
     *traumatic tear of anal sphincter (S31.831)*

**K62.82**   **Dysplasia of anus**
Anal intraepithelial neoplasia I and II (AIN I and II) (histologically confirmed)
Dysplasia of anus NOS
Mild and moderate dysplasia of anus (histologically confirmed)
EXCLUDES 1   *abnormal results from anal cytologic examination without histologic confirmation (R85.61-)*
     *anal intraepithelial neoplasia III (D01.3)*
     *carcinoma in situ of anus (D01.3)*
     *HGSIL of anus (R85.613)*
     *severe dysplasia of anus (D01.3)*

**K62.89**   **Other specified diseases of anus and rectum**
Proctitis NOS
Use additional code for any associated fecal incontinence (R15.-)

**K62.9**   **Disease of anus and rectum, unspecified**

✓4ᵗʰ **K63**   **Other diseases of intestine**

**K63.0**   **Abscess of intestine**    CC
EXCLUDES 1   *abscess of intestine with Crohn's disease (K50.014, K50.114, K50.814, K50.914)*
     *abscess of intestine with diverticular disease (K57.0, K57.2, K57.4, K57.8)*
     *abscess of intestine with ulcerative colitis (K51.014, K51.214, K51.314, K51.414, K51.514, K51.814, K51.914)*
EXCLUDES 2   *abscess of anal and rectal regions (K61.-)*
     *abscess of appendix (K35.3)*
CC Excl: PDX collection 798

**K63.1**   **Perforation of intestine (nontraumatic)**    MCC HCC
Perforation (nontraumatic) of rectum
EXCLUDES 1   *perforation (nontraumatic) of duodenum (K26.-)*
     *perforation (nontraumatic) of intestine with diverticular disease (K57.0, K57.2, K57.4, K57.8)*
EXCLUDES 2   *perforation (nontraumatic) of appendix (K35.2, K35.3)*
CC Excl: PDX collection 799

**K63.2**   **Fistula of intestine**    CC
EXCLUDES 1   *fistula of duodenum (K31.6)*
     *fistula of intestine with Crohn's disease (K50.013, K50.113, K50.813, K50.913)*
     *fistula of intestine with ulcerative colitis (K51.013, K51.213, K51.313, K51.413, K51.513, K51.813, K51.913)*
EXCLUDES 2   *fistula of anal and rectal regions (K60.-)*
     *fistula of appendix (K38.3)*
     *intestinal-genital fistula, female (N82.2-N82.4)*
     *vesicointestinal fistula (N32.1)*
CC Excl: PDX collection 800

**K63.3**   **Ulcer of intestine**    CC
Primary ulcer of small intestine
EXCLUDES 1   *duodenal ulcer (K26.-)*
     *gastrointestinal ulcer (K28.-)*
     *gastrojejunal ulcer (K28.-)*
     *jejunal ulcer (K28.-)*
     *peptic ulcer, site unspecified (K27.-)*
     *ulcer of intestine with perforation (K63.1)*
     *ulcer of anus or rectum (K62.6)*
     *ulcerative colitis (K51.-)*
CC Excl: PDX collection 801

**K63.4**   **Enteroptosis**

**K63.5**   **Polyp of colon**
EXCLUDES 1   *adenomatous polyp of colon (D12.6)*
     *inflammatory polyp of colon (K51.4-)*
     *polyposis of colon (D12.6)*
AHA: 2017, 1Q, 15; 2015, 2Q, 14

✓5ᵗʰ **K63.8**   **Other specified diseases of intestine**

**K63.81**   **Dieulafoy lesion of intestine**    MCC
EXCLUDES 2   *Dieulafoy lesion of stomach and duodenum (K31.82)*
CC Excl: PDX collection 802

**K63.89**   **Other specified diseases of intestine**
AHA: 2013, 2Q, 31

**K63.9**   **Disease of intestine, unspecified**

✓4ᵗʰ **K64**   **Hemorrhoids and perianal venous thrombosis**
INCLUDES   piles
EXCLUDES 1   *hemorrhoids complicating childbirth and the puerperium (O87.2)*
     *hemorrhoids complicating pregnancy (O22.4)*

**K64.0**   **First degree hemorrhoids**
Grade/stage I hemorrhoids
Hemorrhoids (bleeding) without prolapse outside of anal canal

N Newborn: 0   P Pediatric: 0-17   M Maternity: 12-55   A Adult: 15-124   MCC Major CC Condition   PDx MCC PDx acts as own MCC   CC CC Condition   PDx CC PDx acts as own CC

700       ICD-10-CM 2018

### Hemorrhoids

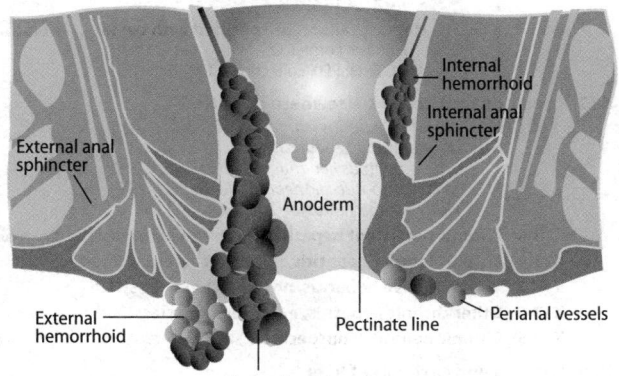

**K64.1** **Second degree hemorrhoids**
Grade/stage II hemorrhoids
Hemorrhoids (bleeding) that prolapse with straining, but retract spontaneously

**K64.2** **Third degree hemorrhoids**
Grade/stage III hemorrhoids
Hemorrhoids (bleeding) that prolapse with straining and require manual replacement back inside anal canal

**K64.3** **Fourth degree hemorrhoids**
Grade/stage IV hemorrhoids
Hemorrhoids (bleeding) with prolapsed tissue that cannot be manually replaced

**K64.4** **Residual hemorrhoidal skin tags**
External hemorrhoids, NOS
Skin tags of anus

**K64.5** **Perianal venous thrombosis**
External hemorrhoids with thrombosis
Perianal hematoma
Thrombosed hemorrhoids NOS

**K64.8** **Other hemorrhoids**
Internal hemorrhoids, without mention of degree
Prolapsed hemorrhoids, degree not specified

**K64.9** **Unspecified hemorrhoids**
Hemorrhoids (bleeding) NOS
Hemorrhoids (bleeding) without mention of degree

## Diseases of peritoneum and retroperitoneum (K65-K68)

**✓4ᵗʰ K65** **Peritonitis**
Use additional code (B95-B97), to identify infectious agent
*EXCLUDES 1*   *acute appendicitis with generalized peritonitis (K35.2)*
*aseptic peritonitis (T81.6)*
*benign paroxysmal peritonitis (E85.0)*
*chemical peritonitis (T81.6)*
*diverticulitis of both small and large intestine with peritonitis (K57.4-)*
*diverticulitis of colon with peritonitis (K57.2-)*
*diverticulitis of intestine, NOS, with peritonitis (K57.8-)*
*diverticulitis of small intestine with peritonitis (K57.0-)*
*gonococcal peritonitis (A54.85)*
*neonatal peritonitis (P78.0-P78.1)*
*pelvic peritonitis, female (N73.3-N73.5)*
*periodic familial peritonitis (E85.0)*
*peritonitis due to talc or other foreign substance (T81.6)*
*peritonitis in chlamydia (A74.81)*
*peritonitis in diphtheria (A36.89)*
*peritonitis in syphilis (late) (A52.74)*
*peritonitis in tuberculosis (A18.31)*
*peritonitis with or following abortion or ectopic or molar pregnancy (O00-O07, O08.0)*
*peritonitis with or following appendicitis (K35.-)*
*peritonitis with or following diverticular disease of intestine (K57.-)*
*puerperal peritonitis (O85)*
*retroperitoneal infections (K68.-)*

**CC Excl: For CC/MCC codes in category K65:** PDX collection 803

**K65.0** **Generalized (acute) peritonitis** `MCC` `HCC`
Pelvic peritonitis (acute), male
Subphrenic peritonitis (acute)
Suppurative peritonitis (acute)

**K65.1** **Peritoneal abscess** `MCC` `HCC`
Abdominopelvic abscess    Subdiaphragmatic abscess
Abscess (of) omentum    Subhepatic abscess
Abscess (of) peritoneum    Subphrenic abscess
Mesenteric abscess
Retrocecal abscess

**K65.2** **Spontaneous bacterial peritonitis** `MCC` `HCC`
*EXCLUDES 1*   *bacterial peritonitis NOS (K65.9)*

**K65.3** **Choleperitonitis** `MCC` `HCC`
Peritonitis due to bile
**DEF:** Inflammation of the peritoneum due to leakage of bile into the peritoneal cavity resulting from rupture of the bile passages or gallbladder.

**K65.4** **Sclerosing mesenteritis** `CC` `HCC`
Fat necrosis of peritoneum
(Idiopathic) sclerosing mesenteric fibrosis
Mesenteric lipodystrophy
Mesenteric panniculitis
Retractile mesenteritis

**K65.8** **Other peritonitis** `MCC` `HCC`
Chronic proliferative peritonitis    Peritonitis due to urine

**K65.9** **Peritonitis, unspecified** `MCC` `HCC`
Bacterial peritonitis NOS
**AHA:** 2013, 2Q, 31

**✓4ᵗʰ K66** **Other disorders of peritoneum**
*EXCLUDES 2*   *ascites (R18.-)*
*peritoneal effusion (chronic) (R18.8)*

**K66.0** **Peritoneal adhesions (postprocedural) (postinfection)**
Adhesions (of) abdominal (wall)    Adhesions (of) omentum
Adhesions (of) diaphragm    Adhesions (of) stomach
Adhesions (of) intestine    Adhesive bands
Adhesions (of) male pelvis    Mesenteric adhesions
*EXCLUDES 1*   *female pelvic adhesions [bands] (N73.6)*
*peritoneal adhesions with intestinal obstruction* ▶*(K56.5-)*◀

**K66.1** **Hemoperitoneum** `MCC`
*EXCLUDES 1*   *traumatic hemoperitoneum (S36.8-)*
**CC Excl:** PDX collection 804

**K66.8** **Other specified disorders of peritoneum**

**K66.9** **Disorder of peritoneum, unspecified**

**K67** *Disorders of peritoneum in infectious diseases classified elsewhere* `MCC` `HCC`
Code first underlying disease, such as:
congenital syphilis (A50.0)
helminthiasis (B65.0-B83.9)
*EXCLUDES 1*   *peritonitis in chlamydia (A74.81)*
*peritonitis in diphtheria (A36.89)*
*peritonitis in gonococcal (A54.85)*
*peritonitis in syphilis (late) (A52.74)*
*peritonitis in tuberculosis (A18.31)*
**CC Excl:** PDX collection 803

**✓4ᵗʰ K68** **Disorders of retroperitoneum**

**✓5ᵗʰ K68.1** **Retroperitoneal abscess**

**K68.11** **Postprocedural retroperitoneal abscess** `CC` `H11` `H12` `H13`
**CC Excl:** PDX collection 805

**K68.12** **Psoas muscle abscess** `MCC` `HCC`
**CC Excl:** PDX collection 806

**K68.19** **Other retroperitoneal abscess** `MCC` `HCC`
**CC Excl:** PDX collection 803

**K68.9** **Other disorders of retroperitoneum** `MCC`
**CC Excl:** PDX collection 803

## Diseases of liver (K70-K77)

*EXCLUDES 1*   *jaundice NOS (R17)*
*EXCLUDES 2*   *hemochromatosis (E83.11-)*
*Reye's syndrome (G93.7)*
*viral hepatitis (B15-B19)*
*Wilson's disease (E83.0)*

**✓4ᵗʰ K70** **Alcoholic liver disease**
Use additional code to identify:
alcohol abuse and dependence (F10.-)

**K70.0** **Alcoholic fatty liver** `A`

**✓5ᵗʰ K70.1** **Alcoholic hepatitis** `A`
**K70.10** **Alcoholic hepatitis without ascites** `A`
**K70.11** **Alcoholic hepatitis with ascites** `A`

**K70.2** **Alcoholic fibrosis and sclerosis of liver** `A`

✓ Additional Character Req    ✓x7ᵗʰ Placeholder Alert    Unacceptable PDx    Manifestation    `H1`-`H14` HAC    `HCC` CMS-HCC Condition    *EXCLUDES 1* Not Coded Here    *EXCLUDES 2* Not Included Here

ICD-10-CM 2018      701

K64.1–K70.2

**Chapter 11. Diseases of the Digestive System**

**K70.3-K75.89**

√5ᵗʰ **K70.3 Alcoholic cirrhosis of liver**
Alcoholic cirrhosis NOS

    **K70.30 Alcoholic cirrhosis of liver without ascites** `HCC` `A`
    **K70.31 Alcoholic cirrhosis of liver with ascites** `HCC` `A`

√5ᵗʰ **K70.4 Alcoholic hepatic failure**
Acute alcoholic hepatic failure
Alcoholic hepatic failure NOS
Chronic alcoholic hepatic failure
Subacute alcoholic hepatic failure

    **K70.40 Alcoholic hepatic failure without coma** `HCC` `A`
    **K70.41 Alcoholic hepatic failure with coma** `PDxMCC` `MCC` `HCC` `A`
        **CC Excl:** PDX collection 807

**K70.9 Alcoholic liver disease, unspecified** `HCC` `A`

√4ᵗʰ **K71 Toxic liver disease**
    **INCLUDES** drug-induced idiosyncratic (unpredictable) liver disease
        drug-induced toxic (predictable) liver disease
    Code first poisoning due to drug or toxin, if applicable (T36-T65 with fifth or sixth character 1-4 or 6)
    Use additional code for adverse effect, if applicable, to identify drug (T36-T50 with fifth or sixth character 5)
    **EXCLUDES 2** *alcoholic liver disease (K70.-)*
        *Budd-Chiari syndrome (I82.0)*

**K71.0 Toxic liver disease with cholestasis**
Cholestasis with hepatocyte injury
"Pure" cholestasis

√5ᵗʰ **K71.1 Toxic liver disease with hepatic necrosis**
Hepatic failure (acute) (chronic) due to drugs

    **K71.10 Toxic liver disease with hepatic necrosis, without coma**
    **K71.11 Toxic liver disease with hepatic necrosis, with coma** `PDxMCC` `MCC` `HCC`
        **CC Excl:** PDX collection 807

**K71.2 Toxic liver disease with acute hepatitis**

**K71.3 Toxic liver disease with chronic persistent hepatitis**

**K71.4 Toxic liver disease with chronic lobular hepatitis**

√5ᵗʰ **K71.5 Toxic liver disease with chronic active hepatitis**
Toxic liver disease with lupoid hepatitis

    **K71.50 Toxic liver disease with chronic active hepatitis without ascites**
    **K71.51 Toxic liver disease with chronic active hepatitis with ascites**

**K71.6 Toxic liver disease with hepatitis, not elsewhere classified**

**K71.7 Toxic liver disease with fibrosis and cirrhosis of liver**

**K71.8 Toxic liver disease with other disorders of liver**
Toxic liver disease with focal nodular hyperplasia
Toxic liver disease with hepatic granulomas
Toxic liver disease with peliosis hepatis
Toxic liver disease with veno-occlusive disease of liver

**K71.9 Toxic liver disease, unspecified**

√4ᵗʰ **K72 Hepatic failure, not elsewhere classified**
    **INCLUDES** fulminant hepatitis NEC, with hepatic failure
        hepatic encephalopathy NOS
        liver (cell) necrosis with hepatic failure
        malignant hepatitis NEC, with hepatic failure
        yellow liver atrophy or dystrophy
    **EXCLUDES 1** *alcoholic hepatic failure (K70.4)*
        *hepatic failure with toxic liver disease (K71.1-)*
        *icterus of newborn (P55-P59)*
        *postprocedural hepatic failure (K91.82)*
    **EXCLUDES 2** *hepatic failure complicating abortion or ectopic or molar pregnancy (O00-O07, O08.8)*
        *hepatic failure complicating pregnancy, childbirth and the puerperium (O26.6-)*
        *viral hepatitis with hepatic coma (B15-B19)*
    **AHA:** 2017, 1Q, 41

√5ᵗʰ **K72.0 Acute and subacute hepatic failure**
Acute non-viral hepatitis NOS
**AHA:** 2015, 2Q, 17; 2014, 2Q, 13

    **K72.00 Acute and subacute hepatic failure without coma** `MCC`
        **CC Excl:** PDX collection 808
    **K72.01 Acute and subacute hepatic failure with coma** `PDxMCC` `MCC` `HCC`
        **CC Excl:** PDX collection 808

√5ᵗʰ **K72.1 Chronic hepatic failure**
    **K72.10 Chronic hepatic failure without coma** `HCC`
    **K72.11 Chronic hepatic failure with coma** `PDxMCC` `MCC` `HCC`
        **CC Excl:** PDX collection 807

√5ᵗʰ **K72.9 Hepatic failure, unspecified**
    **K72.90 Hepatic failure, unspecified without coma** `HCC`
        **AHA:** 2016, 2Q, 35
    **K72.91 Hepatic failure, unspecified with coma** `MCC` `HCC`
        Hepatic coma NOS
        **CC Excl:** PDX collection 807

√4ᵗʰ **K73 Chronic hepatitis, not elsewhere classified**
    **EXCLUDES 1** *alcoholic hepatitis (chronic) (K70.1-)*
        *drug-induced hepatitis (chronic) (K71.-)*
        *granulomatous hepatitis (chronic) NEC (K75.3)*
        *reactive, nonspecific hepatitis (chronic) (K75.2)*
        *viral hepatitis (chronic) (B15-B19)*

**K73.0 Chronic persistent hepatitis, not elsewhere classified** `HCC`

**K73.1 Chronic lobular hepatitis, not elsewhere classified** `HCC`

**K73.2 Chronic active hepatitis, not elsewhere classified** `HCC`

**K73.8 Other chronic hepatitis, not elsewhere classified** `HCC`

**K73.9 Chronic hepatitis, unspecified** `HCC`

√4ᵗʰ **K74 Fibrosis and cirrhosis of liver**
    Code also, if applicable, viral hepatitis (acute) (chronic) (B15-B19)
    **EXCLUDES 1** *alcoholic cirrhosis (of liver) (K70.3)*
        *alcoholic fibrosis of liver (K70.2)*
        *cardiac sclerosis of liver (K76.1)*
        *cirrhosis (of liver) with toxic liver disease (K71.7)*
        *congenital cirrhosis (of liver) (P78.81)*
        *pigmentary cirrhosis (of liver) (E83.110)*

**K74.0 Hepatic fibrosis**

**K74.1 Hepatic sclerosis**

**K74.2 Hepatic fibrosis with hepatic sclerosis**

**K74.3 Primary biliary cirrhosis** `HCC`
Chronic nonsuppurative destructive cholangitis

**K74.4 Secondary biliary cirrhosis** `HCC`

**K74.5 Biliary cirrhosis, unspecified** `HCC`

√5ᵗʰ **K74.6 Other and unspecified cirrhosis of liver**
    **K74.60 Unspecified cirrhosis of liver** `HCC`
        Cirrhosis (of liver) NOS
    **K74.69 Other cirrhosis of liver** `HCC`
        Cryptogenic cirrhosis (of liver)
        Macronodular cirrhosis (of liver)
        Micronodular cirrhosis (of liver)
        Mixed type cirrhosis (of liver)
        Portal cirrhosis (of liver)
        Postnecrotic cirrhosis (of liver)

√4ᵗʰ **K75 Other inflammatory liver diseases**
    **EXCLUDES 2** *toxic liver disease (K71.-)*

**K75.0 Abscess of liver** `MCC`
Cholangitic hepatic abscess
Hematogenic hepatic abscess
Hepatic abscess NOS
Lymphogenic hepatic abscess
Pylephlebitic hepatic abscess
    **EXCLUDES 2** *acute or subacute hepatitis NOS (B17.9)*
        *acute or subacute non-viral hepatitis (K72.0)*
        *chronic hepatitis NEC (K73.8)*
    **CC Excl:** PDX collection 809

**K75.1 Phlebitis of portal vein** `MCC`
Pylephlebitis
    **EXCLUDES 1** *pylephlebitic liver abscess (K75.0)*
    **DEF:** Inflammation of portal vein or branches; may be due to diverticulitis, perforated appendicitis, or peritonitis; symptoms include fever, chills, jaundice, sweating, and abscess in various body parts.
    **CC Excl:** PDX collection 809

**K75.2 Nonspecific reactive hepatitis**
    **EXCLUDES 1** *acute or subacute hepatitis (K72.0-)*
        *chronic hepatitis NEC (K73.-)*
        *viral hepatitis (B15-B19)*

**K75.3 Granulomatous hepatitis, not elsewhere classified**
    **EXCLUDES 1** *acute or subacute hepatitis (K72.0-)*
        *chronic hepatitis NEC (K73.-)*
        *viral hepatitis (B15-B19)*

**K75.4 Autoimmune hepatitis** `HCC`
Lupoid hepatitis NEC

√5ᵗʰ **K75.8 Other specified inflammatory liver diseases**
    **K75.81 Nonalcoholic steatohepatitis (NASH)**
    **K75.89 Other specified inflammatory liver diseases**

`N` Newborn: 0   `P` Pediatric: 0-17   `M` Maternity: 12-55   `A` Adult: 15-124   `MCC` Major CC Condition   `PDxMCC` PDx acts as own MCC   `CC` CC Condition   `PDxCC` PDx acts as own CC

702          ICD-10-CM 2018

### K75.9 Inflammatory liver disease, unspecified
Hepatitis NOS

**EXCLUDES 1** *acute or subacute hepatitis (K72.0-)*
*chronic hepatitis NEC (K73.-)*
*viral hepatitis (B15-B19)*

**AHA:** 2015, 2Q, 17

### ✓4th K76 Other diseases of liver
**EXCLUDES 2** *alcoholic liver disease (K70.-)*
*amyloid degeneration of liver (E85.-)*
*cystic disease of liver (congenital) (Q44.6)*
*hepatic vein thrombosis (I82.0)*
*hepatomegaly NOS (R16.0)*
*pigmentary cirrhosis (of liver) (E83.110)*
*portal vein thrombosis (I81)*
*toxic liver disease (K71.-)*

### K76.0 Fatty (change of) liver, not elsewhere classified
Nonalcoholic fatty liver disease (NAFLD)

**EXCLUDES 1** *nonalcoholic steatohepatitis (NASH) (K75.81)*

### K76.1 Chronic passive congestion of liver
Cardiac cirrhosis
Cardiac sclerosis

### K76.2 Central hemorrhagic necrosis of liver  MCC
**EXCLUDES 1** *liver necrosis with hepatic failure (K72.-)*
**CC Excl:** PDX collection 808

### K76.3 Infarction of liver  MCC
**CC Excl:** PDX collection 808

### K76.4 Peliosis hepatis
Hepatic angiomatosis

### K76.5 Hepatic veno-occlusive disease
**EXCLUDES 1** *Budd-Chiari syndrome (I82.0)*

### K76.6 Portal hypertension  CC  HCC
Use additional code for any associated complications, such as:
portal hypertensive gastropathy (K31.89)
**CC Excl:** PDX collection 810

### K76.7 Hepatorenal syndrome  MCC  HCC
**EXCLUDES 1** *hepatorenal syndrome following labor and delivery (O90.4)*
*postprocedural hepatorenal syndrome (K91.83)*
**CC Excl:** PDX collection 811

### ✓5th K76.8 Other specified diseases of liver
#### K76.81 Hepatopulmonary syndrome  HCC
Code first underlying liver disease, such as:
alcoholic cirrhosis of liver (K70.3-)
cirrhosis of liver without mention of alcohol (K74.6-)

#### K76.89 Other specified diseases of liver
Cyst (simple) of liver
Focal nodular hyperplasia of liver
Hepatoptosis

### K76.9 Liver disease, unspecified

### *K77 Liver disorders in diseases classified elsewhere*  CC
Code first underlying disease, such as:
amyloidosis (E85.-)
congenital syphilis (A50.0, A50.5)
congenital toxoplasmosis (P37.1)
schistosomiasis (B65.0-B65.9)

**EXCLUDES 1** *alcoholic hepatitis (K70.1-)*
*alcoholic liver disease (K70-.)*
*cytomegaloviral hepatitis (B25.1)*
*herpesviral [herpes simplex] hepatitis (B00.81)*
*infectious mononucleosis with liver disease (B27.0-B27.9 with .9)*
*mumps hepatitis (B26.81)*
*sarcoidosis with liver disease (D86.89)*
*secondary syphilis with liver disease (A51.45)*
*syphilis (late) with liver disease (A52.74)*
*toxoplasmosis (acquired) hepatitis (B58.1)*
*tuberculosis with liver disease (A18.83)*
**CC Excl:** No Excl

## Disorders of gallbladder, biliary tract and pancreas (K80-K87)

### ✓4th K80 Cholelithiasis
**EXCLUDES 1** *retained cholelithiasis following cholecystectomy (K91.86)*

#### ✓5th K80.0 Calculus of gallbladder with acute cholecystitis
Any condition listed in K80.2 with acute cholecystitis

##### K80.00 Calculus of gallbladder with acute cholecystitis  CC
without obstruction
**CC Excl:** PDX collection 812

**Cholelithiasis**

### K80.01 Calculus of gallbladder with acute cholecystitis  CC
with obstruction
**CC Excl:** PDX collection 813

#### ✓5th K80.1 Calculus of gallbladder with other cholecystitis

**CC Excl: For CC codes in subcategory K80.1, unless otherwise noted:** PDX collection 813

##### K80.10 Calculus of gallbladder with chronic  CC
cholecystitis without obstruction
Cholelithiasis with cholecystitis NOS

##### K80.11 Calculus of gallbladder with chronic  CC
cholecystitis with obstruction

##### K80.12 Calculus of gallbladder with acute and chronic  CC
cholecystitis without obstruction
**CC Excl:** PDX collection 812

##### K80.13 Calculus of gallbladder with acute and chronic  CC
cholecystitis with obstruction

##### K80.18 Calculus of gallbladder with other cholecystitis  CC
without obstruction

##### K80.19 Calculus of gallbladder with other cholecystitis  CC
with obstruction

#### ✓5th K80.2 Calculus of gallbladder without cholecystitis
Cholecystolithiasis without cholecystitis
Cholelithiasis (without cholecystitis)
Colic (recurrent) of gallbladder (without cholecystitis)
Gallstone (impacted) of cystic duct (without cholecystitis)
Gallstone (impacted) of gallbladder (without cholecystitis)

##### K80.20 Calculus of gallbladder without cholecystitis without
obstruction

##### K80.21 Calculus of gallbladder without cholecystitis  CC
with obstruction
**CC Excl:** PDX collection 813

#### ✓5th K80.3 Calculus of bile duct with cholangitis
Any condition listed in K80.5 with cholangitis

**CC Excl: For CC codes in subcategory K80.3, unless otherwise noted:** PDX collection 814

##### K80.30 Calculus of bile duct with cholangitis,  PDxCC CC
unspecified, without obstruction

##### K80.31 Calculus of bile duct with cholangitis,  PDxCC CC
unspecified, with obstruction
**CC Excl:** PDX collection 815

##### K80.32 Calculus of bile duct with acute cholangitis  PDxCC CC
without obstruction

##### K80.33 Calculus of bile duct with acute cholangitis  PDxCC CC
with obstruction
**CC Excl:** PDX collection 815

##### K80.34 Calculus of bile duct with chronic  PDxCC CC
cholangitis without obstruction

##### K80.35 Calculus of bile duct with chronic  PDxCC CC
cholangitis with obstruction
**CC Excl:** PDX collection 815

##### K80.36 Calculus of bile duct with acute and chronic  PDxCC CC
cholangitis without obstruction

##### K80.37 Calculus of bile duct with acute and chronic  PDxCC CC
cholangitis with obstruction
**CC Excl:** PDX collection 815

---

✓ Additional Character Req  ✓x7th Placeholder Alert  Unacceptable PDx  Manifestation  **H1**-**H14** HAC  **HCC** CMS-HCC Condition  **EXCLUDES 1** Not Coded Here  **EXCLUDES 2** Not Included Here

**Chapter 11. Diseases of the Digestive System**

**K80.4–K83.9**

✓5ᵗʰ **K80.4 Calculus of bile duct with cholecystitis**
Any condition listed in K80.5 with cholecystitis (with cholangitis)

> **CC Excl: For CC codes in subcategory K80.4:** PDX collection 815

     **K80.40 Calculus of bile duct with cholecystitis, unspecified, without obstruction** `CC`

     **K80.41 Calculus of bile duct with cholecystitis, unspecified, with obstruction** `CC`

     **K80.42 Calculus of bile duct with acute cholecystitis without obstruction** `CC`

     **K80.43 Calculus of bile duct with acute cholecystitis with obstruction** `CC`

     **K80.44 Calculus of bile duct with chronic cholecystitis without obstruction** `CC`

     **K80.45 Calculus of bile duct with chronic cholecystitis with obstruction** `CC`

     **K80.46 Calculus of bile duct with acute and chronic cholecystitis without obstruction** `CC`

     **K80.47 Calculus of bile duct with acute and chronic cholecystitis with obstruction** `CC`

✓5ᵗʰ **K80.5 Calculus of bile duct without cholangitis or cholecystitis**
Choledocholithiasis (without cholangitis or cholecystitis)
Gallstone (impacted) of bile duct NOS (without cholangitis or cholecystitis)
Gallstone (impacted) of common duct (without cholangitis or cholecystitis)
Gallstone (impacted) of hepatic duct (without cholangitis or cholecystitis)
Hepatic cholelithiasis (without cholangitis or cholecystitis)
Hepatic colic (recurrent) (without cholangitis or cholecystitis)

     **K80.50 Calculus of bile duct without cholangitis or cholecystitis without obstruction**

     **K80.51 Calculus of bile duct without cholangitis or cholecystitis with obstruction** `CC`
       **CC Excl:** PDX collection 815

✓5ᵗʰ **K80.6 Calculus of gallbladder and bile duct with cholecystitis**

> **CC Excl: For CC codes in subcategory K80.6, unless otherwise noted:** PDX collection 815

     **K80.60 Calculus of gallbladder and bile duct with cholecystitis, unspecified, without obstruction** `CC`

     **K80.61 Calculus of gallbladder and bile duct with cholecystitis, unspecified, with obstruction** `CC`

     **K80.62 Calculus of gallbladder and bile duct with acute cholecystitis without obstruction** `CC`
       **CC Excl:** PDX collection 816

     **K80.63 Calculus of gallbladder and bile duct with acute cholecystitis with obstruction** `CC`
       **CC Excl:** PDX collection 816

     **K80.64 Calculus of gallbladder and bile duct with chronic cholecystitis without obstruction** `CC`

     **K80.65 Calculus of gallbladder and bile duct with chronic cholecystitis with obstruction** `CC`

     **K80.66 Calculus of gallbladder and bile duct with acute and chronic cholecystitis without obstruction** `CC`
       **CC Excl:** PDX collection 817

     **K80.67 Calculus of gallbladder and bile duct with acute and chronic cholecystitis with obstruction** `MCC`
       **CC Excl:** PDX collection 817

✓5ᵗʰ **K80.7 Calculus of gallbladder and bile duct without cholecystitis**

     **K80.70 Calculus of gallbladder and bile duct without cholecystitis without obstruction**

     **K80.71 Calculus of gallbladder and bile duct without cholecystitis with obstruction** `CC`
       **CC Excl:** PDX collection 815

✓5ᵗʰ **K80.8 Other cholelithiasis**

     **K80.80 Other cholelithiasis without obstruction**

     **K80.81 Other cholelithiasis with obstruction** `CC`
       **CC Excl:** PDX collection 815

---

✓4ᵗʰ **K81 Cholecystitis**
   *EXCLUDES 1*   cholecystitis with cholelithiasis (K80.-)

     **K81.0 Acute cholecystitis** `CC`
Abscess of gallbladder
Angiocholecystitis
Emphysematous (acute) cholecystitis
Empyema of gallbladder
Gangrene of gallbladder
Gangrenous cholecystitis
Suppurative cholecystitis
**CC Excl:** PDX collection 818

     **K81.1 Chronic cholecystitis**

     **K81.2 Acute cholecystitis with chronic cholecystitis** `CC`
**CC Excl:** PDX collection 819

     **K81.9 Cholecystitis, unspecified**

✓4ᵗʰ **K82 Other diseases of gallbladder**
   *EXCLUDES 1*   nonvisualization of gallbladder (R93.2)
             postcholecystectomy syndrome (K91.5)

> **CC Excl: For CC/MCC codes in category K82:** PDX collection 820

     **K82.0 Obstruction of gallbladder** `CC`
Occlusion of cystic duct or gallbladder without cholelithiasis
Stenosis of cystic duct or gallbladder without cholelithiasis
Stricture of cystic duct or gallbladder without cholelithiasis
   *EXCLUDES 1*   obstruction of gallbladder with cholelithiasis (K80.-)

     **K82.1 Hydrops of gallbladder** `CC`
Mucocele of gallbladder

     **K82.2 Perforation of gallbladder** `MCC`
Rupture of cystic duct or gallbladder

     **K82.3 Fistula of gallbladder** `CC`
Cholecystocolic fistula
Cholecystoduodenal fistula

     **K82.4 Cholesterolosis of gallbladder**
Strawberry gallbladder
   *EXCLUDES 1*   cholesterolosis of gallbladder with cholecystitis (K81.-)
             cholesterolosis of gallbladder with cholelithiasis (K80.-)

     **K82.8 Other specified diseases of gallbladder**
Adhesions of cystic duct or gallbladder
Atrophy of cystic duct or gallbladder
Cyst of cystic duct or gallbladder
Dyskinesia of cystic duct or gallbladder
Hypertrophy of cystic duct or gallbladder
Nonfunctioning of cystic duct or gallbladder
Ulcer of cystic duct or gallbladder

     **K82.9 Disease of gallbladder, unspecified**

✓4ᵗʰ **K83 Other diseases of biliary tract**
   *EXCLUDES 1*   postcholecystectomy syndrome (K91.5)
   *EXCLUDES 2*   conditions involving the gallbladder (K81-K82)
             conditions involving the cystic duct (K81-K82)

     **K83.0 Cholangitis** `CC`
Ascending cholangitis      Sclerosing cholangitis
Cholangitis NOS      Secondary cholangitis
Primary cholangitis      Stenosing cholangitis
Recurrent cholangitis      Suppurative cholangitis
   *EXCLUDES 1*   cholangitic liver abscess (K75.0)
             cholangitis with choledocholithiasis (K80.3-, K80.4-)
             chronic nonsuppurative destructive cholangitis (K74.3)
**CC Excl:** PDX collection 814

     **K83.1 Obstruction of bile duct** `MCC`
Occlusion of bile duct without cholelithiasis
Stenosis of bile duct without cholelithiasis
Stricture of bile duct without cholelithiasis
   *EXCLUDES 1*   congenital obstruction of bile duct (Q44.3)
             obstruction of bile duct with cholelithiasis (K80.-)
**AHA:** 2016, 1Q, 18
**CC Excl:** PDX collection 821

     **K83.2 Perforation of bile duct** `MCC`
Rupture of bile duct
**CC Excl:** PDX collection 822

     **K83.3 Fistula of bile duct** `CC`
Choledochoduodenal fistula
**CC Excl:** PDX collection 822

     **K83.4 Spasm of sphincter of Oddi**

     **K83.5 Biliary cyst**

     **K83.8 Other specified diseases of biliary tract**
Adhesions of biliary tract      Hypertrophy of biliary tract
Atrophy of biliary tract      Ulcer of biliary tract

     **K83.9 Disease of biliary tract, unspecified**

---

**N** Newborn: 0   **P** Pediatric: 0-17   **M** Maternity: 12-55   **A** Adult: 15-124   **MCC** Major CC Condition   **PDxMCC** PDx acts as own MCC   **CC** CC Condition   **PDxCC** PDx acts as own CC

704          ICD-10-CM 2018

## ✓4th K85  Acute pancreatitis

INCLUDES   acute (recurrent) pancreatitis
subacute pancreatitis

**CC Excl: For MCC codes in category K85:** PDX collection 177

### ✓5th K85.0  Idiopathic acute pancreatitis

**K85.00   Idiopathic acute pancreatitis without necrosis or infection**   MCC

**K85.01   Idiopathic acute pancreatitis with uninfected necrosis**   MCC

**K85.02   Idiopathic acute pancreatitis with infected necrosis**   MCC

### ✓5th K85.1  Biliary acute pancreatitis
Gallstone pancreatitis

**K85.10   Biliary acute pancreatitis without necrosis or infection**   MCC

**K85.11   Biliary acute pancreatitis with uninfected necrosis**   MCC

**K85.12   Biliary acute pancreatitis with infected necrosis**   MCC

### ✓5th K85.2  Alcohol induced acute pancreatitis
EXCLUDES 2   *alcohol induced chronic pancreatitis (K86.0)*

**K85.20   Alcohol induced acute pancreatitis without necrosis or infection**   MCC

**K85.21   Alcohol induced acute pancreatitis with uninfected necrosis**   MCC

**K85.22   Alcohol induced acute pancreatitis with infected necrosis**   MCC

### ✓5th K85.3  Drug induced acute pancreatitis
Use additional code for adverse effect, if applicable, to identify drug (T36-T50 with fifth or sixth character 5)
Use additional code to identify drug abuse and dependence (F11. – F17.-)

**K85.30   Drug induced acute pancreatitis without necrosis or infection**   MCC

**K85.31   Drug induced acute pancreatitis with uninfected necrosis**   MCC

**K85.32   Drug induced acute pancreatitis with infected necrosis**   MCC

### ✓5th K85.8  Other acute pancreatitis

**K85.80   Other acute pancreatitis without necrosis or infection**   MCC

**K85.81   Other acute pancreatitis with uninfected necrosis**   MCC

**K85.82   Other acute pancreatitis with infected necrosis**   MCC

### ✓5th K85.9  Acute pancreatitis, unspecified
Pancreatitis NOS

**K85.90   Acute pancreatitis without necrosis or infection, unspecified**   MCC

**K85.91   Acute pancreatitis with uninfected necrosis, unspecified**   MCC

**K85.92   Acute pancreatitis with infected necrosis, unspecified**   MCC

## ✓4th K86  Other diseases of pancreas

EXCLUDES 2   *fibrocystic disease of pancreas (E84.-)*
*islet cell tumor (of pancreas) (D13.7)*
*pancreatic steatorrhea (K90.3)*

### K86.0  Alcohol-induced chronic pancreatitis   CC HCC
Code also exocrine pancreatic insufficiency (K86.81)
Use additional code to identify:
alcohol abuse and dependence (F10.-)
EXCLUDES 2   *alcohol induced acute pancreatitis (K85.2-)*
**CC Excl:** PDX collection 823

### K86.1  Other chronic pancreatitis   CC HCC
Chronic pancreatitis NOS
Infectious chronic pancreatitis
Recurrent chronic pancreatitis
Relapsing chronic pancreatitis
Code also exocrine pancreatic insufficiency (K86.81)
**CC Excl:** PDX collection 823

### K86.2  Cyst of pancreas   CC
**CC Excl:** PDX collection 824

### K86.3  Pseudocyst of pancreas   CC
**CC Excl:** PDX collection 824

### ✓5th K86.8  Other specified diseases of pancreas

**K86.81   Exocrine pancreatic insufficiency**

---

**K86.89   Other specified diseases of pancreas**
Aseptic pancreatic necrosis, unrelated to acute pancreatitis
Atrophy of pancreas
Calculus of pancreas
Cirrhosis of pancreas
Fibrosis of pancreas
Pancreatic fat necrosis, unrelated to acute pancreatitis
Pancreatic infantilism
Pancreatic necrosis NOS, unrelated to acute pancreatitis

### K86.9  Disease of pancreas, unspecified

## K87  Disorders of gallbladder, biliary tract and pancreas in diseases classified elsewhere
Code first underlying disease
EXCLUDES 1   *cytomegaloviral pancreatitis (B25.2)*
*mumps pancreatitis (B26.3)*
*syphilitic gallbladder (A52.74)*
*syphilitic pancreas (A52.74)*
*tuberculosis of gallbladder (A18.83)*
*tuberculosis of pancreas (A18.83)*

# Other diseases of the digestive system (K90-K95)

## ✓4th K90  Intestinal malabsorption
EXCLUDES 1   *intestinal malabsorption following gastrointestinal surgery (K91.2)*

**CC Excl: For CC codes in category K90, unless otherwise noted:** PDX collection 825

### K90.0  Celiac disease
Celiac disease with steatorrhea
►Celiac gluten-sensitive enteropathy◄
Nontropical sprue
Use additional code for associated disorders including:
dermatitis herpetiformis (L13.0)
gluten ataxia (G32.81)
Code also exocrine pancreatic insufficiency (K86.81)
**DEF:** Malabsorption syndrome due to gluten consumption; symptoms include fetid, bulky, frothy, oily stools, distended abdomen, gas, asthenia, electrolyte depletion, and vitamin B, D, and K deficiency.

### K90.1  Tropical sprue   CC
Sprue NOS
Tropical steatorrhea

### K90.2  Blind loop syndrome, not elsewhere classified   CC
Blind loop syndrome NOS
EXCLUDES 1   *congenital blind loop syndrome (Q43.8)*
*postsurgical blind loop syndrome (K91.2)*

### K90.3  Pancreatic steatorrhea   CC

### ✓5th K90.4  Other malabsorption due to intolerance   
EXCLUDES 2   ►*celiac gluten-sensitive enteropathy◄ (K90.0)*
*lactose intolerance (E73.-)*

**K90.41   Non-celiac gluten sensitivity**   CC
Gluten sensitivity NOS
Non-celiac gluten sensitive enteropathy

**K90.49   Malabsorption due to intolerance, not elsewhere classified**   CC
Malabsorption due to intolerance to carbohydrate
Malabsorption due to intolerance to fat
Malabsorption due to intolerance to protein
Malabsorption due to intolerance to starch

### ✓5th K90.8  Other intestinal malabsorption

**K90.81   Whipple's disease**   CC
**CC Excl:** PDX collection 826

**K90.89   Other intestinal malabsorption**   CC

### K90.9  Intestinal malabsorption, unspecified   CC

## ✓4th K91  Intraoperative and postprocedural complications and disorders of digestive system, not elsewhere classified
EXCLUDES 2   *complications of artificial opening of digestive system (K94.-)*
*complications of bariatric procedures (K95.-)*
*gastrojejunal ulcer (K28.-)*
*postprocedural (radiation) retroperitoneal abscess (K68.11)*
*radiation colitis (K52.0)*
*radiation gastroenteritis (K52.0)*
*radiation proctitis (K62.7)*

### K91.0  Vomiting following gastrointestinal surgery

### K91.1  Postgastric surgery syndromes
Dumping syndrome
Postgastrectomy syndrome
Postvagotomy syndrome

---

**K91.2 Postsurgical malabsorption, not elsewhere classified** `CC`
Postsurgical blind loop syndrome
*EXCLUDES 1*    *malabsorption osteomalacia in adults (M83.2)*
*malabsorption osteoporosis, postsurgical (M80.8-, M81.8)*
**CC Excl:** PDX collection 827

✓5ᵗʰ **K91.3 Postprocedural intestinal obstruction**
**AHA:** 2017, 1Q, 40

●    **K91.30 Postprocedural intestinal obstruction, unspecified as to partial versus complete** `CC`
Postprocedural intestinal obstruction NOS

●    **K91.31 Postprocedural partial intestinal obstruction** `CC`
Postprocedural incomplete intestinal obstruction

●    **K91.32 Postprocedural complete intestinal obstruction** `CC`

**K91.5 Postcholecystectomy syndrome**

✓5ᵗʰ **K91.6 Intraoperative hemorrhage and hematoma of a digestive system organ or structure complicating a procedure**
*EXCLUDES 1*    *intraoperative hemorrhage and hematoma of a digestive system organ or structure due to accidental puncture and laceration during a procedure (K91.7-)*

   **K91.61 Intraoperative hemorrhage and hematoma of a digestive system organ or structure complicating a digestive system procedure** `CC`
**CC Excl:** PDX collection 829

   **K91.62 Intraoperative hemorrhage and hematoma of a digestive system organ or structure complicating other procedure** `CC`
**CC Excl:** PDX collection 829

✓5ᵗʰ **K91.7 Accidental puncture and laceration of a digestive system organ or structure during a procedure**

   **K91.71 Accidental puncture and laceration of a digestive system organ or structure during a digestive system procedure** `CC`
**CC Excl:** PDX collection 509

   **K91.72 Accidental puncture and laceration of a digestive system organ or structure during other procedure** `CC`
**CC Excl:** PDX collection 509

✓5ᵗʰ **K91.8 Other intraoperative and postprocedural complications and disorders of digestive system**

**CC Excl: For CC codes in subcategory K91.8, unless otherwise noted:** PDX collection 828

   **K91.81 Other intraoperative complications of digestive system** `CC`

   **K91.82 Postprocedural hepatic failure** `CC`

   **K91.83 Postprocedural hepatorenal syndrome** `CC`

✓6ᵗʰ **K91.84 Postprocedural hemorrhage of a digestive system organ or structure following a procedure**

   **K91.840 Postprocedural hemorrhage of a digestive system organ or structure following a digestive system procedure** `CC`
**AHA:** 2016, 1Q, 15
**CC Excl:** PDX collection 829

   **K91.841 Postprocedural hemorrhage of a digestive system organ or structure following other procedure** `CC`
**CC Excl:** PDX collection 829

✓6ᵗʰ **K91.85 Complications of intestinal pouch**

   **K91.850 Pouchitis** `CC` `HCC`
Inflammation of internal ileoanal pouch
**DEF:** Inflammatory complication of an existing surgically created ileoanal pouch, resulting in multiple GI complaints, including diarrhea, abdominal pain, rectal bleeding, fecal urgency, or incontinence.

   **K91.858 Other complications of intestinal pouch** `CC` `HCC`

   **K91.86 Retained cholelithiasis following cholecystectomy** `CC`

✓6ᵗʰ **K91.87 Postprocedural hematoma and seroma of a digestive system organ or structure following a procedure**

**CC Excl: For CC codes in subcategory K91.87:** PDX collection 829

   **K91.870 Postprocedural hematoma of a digestive system organ or structure following a digestive system procedure** `CC`

   **K91.871 Postprocedural hematoma of a digestive system organ or structure following other procedure** `CC`

   **K91.872 Postprocedural seroma of a digestive system organ or structure following a digestive system procedure** `CC`

   **K91.873 Postprocedural seroma of a digestive system organ or structure following other procedure** `CC`

   **K91.89 Other postprocedural complications and disorders of digestive system** `CC`
Use additional code, if applicable, to further specify disorder
*EXCLUDES 2*    *postprocedural retroperitoneal abscess (K68.11)*
**AHA:** 2017, 1Q, 40
**CC Excl:** PDX collection 828

✓4ᵗʰ **K92 Other diseases of digestive system**
*EXCLUDES 1*    *neonatal gastrointestinal hemorrhage (P54.0-P54.3)*

**CC Excl: For CC codes in category K92, unless otherwise noted:** PDX collection 770

**K92.0 Hematemesis** `CC`

**K92.1 Melena** `CC`
*EXCLUDES 1*    *occult blood in feces (R19.5)*

**K92.2 Gastrointestinal hemorrhage, unspecified** `CC`
Gastric hemorrhage NOS
Intestinal hemorrhage NOS
*EXCLUDES 1*    *acute hemorrhagic gastritis (K29.01)*
*hemorrhage of anus and rectum (K62.5)*
*angiodysplasia of stomach with hemorrhage (K31.811)*
*diverticular disease with hemorrhage (K57.-)*
*gastritis and duodenitis with hemorrhage (K29.-)*
*peptic ulcer with hemorrhage (K25-K28)*

✓5ᵗʰ **K92.8 Other specified diseases of the digestive system**

   **K92.81 Gastrointestinal mucositis (ulcerative)** `CC`
Code also type of associated therapy, such as:
antineoplastic and immunosuppressive drugs (T45.1X-)
radiological procedure and radiotherapy (Y84.2)
*EXCLUDES 2*    *mucositis (ulcerative) of vagina and vulva (N76.81)*
*nasal mucositis (ulcerative) (J34.81)*
*oral mucositis (ulcerative) (K12.3-)*
**CC Excl:** PDX collection 765

   **K92.89 Other specified diseases of the digestive system**

**K92.9 Disease of digestive system, unspecified**

✓4ᵗʰ **K94 Complications of artificial openings of the digestive system**

✓5ᵗʰ **K94.0 Colostomy complications**

**CC Excl: For CC codes in subcategory K94.0, unless otherwise noted:** PDX collection 830

   **K94.00 Colostomy complication, unspecified** `HCC`

   **K94.01 Colostomy hemorrhage** `CC` `HCC`

   **K94.02 Colostomy infection** `CC` `HCC`
Use additional code to specify type of infection, such as:
cellulitis of abdominal wall (L03.311)
sepsis (A40-, A41-)

   **K94.03 Colostomy malfunction** `CC` `HCC`
Mechanical complication of colostomy
**CC Excl:** PDX collection 831

   **K94.09 Other complications of colostomy** `CC` `HCC`

✓5ᵗʰ **K94.1 Enterostomy complicatiCC Excl: PDX collection 831ons**

**CC Excl: For CC codes in subcategory K94.1, unless otherwise noted:** PDX collection 830

   **K94.10 Enterostomy complication, unspecified** `HCC`

   **K94.11 Enterostomy hemorrhage** `CC` `HCC`

   **K94.12 Enterostomy infection** `CC` `HCC`
Use additional code to specify type of infection, such as:
cellulitis of abdominal wall (L03.311)
sepsis (A40-, A41-)

   **K94.13 Enterostomy malfunction** `CC` `HCC`
Mechanical complication of enterostomy
**CC Excl:** PDX collection 831

   **K94.19 Other complications of enterostomy** `CC` `HCC`

Ⓝ Newborn: 0   Ⓟ Pediatric: 0-17   Ⓜ Maternity: 12-55   Ⓐ Adult: 15-124   **MCC** Major CC Condition   **PDxMCC** PDx acts as own MCC   **CC** CC Condition   **PDxCC** PDx acts as own CC

706          ICD-10-CM 2018

**✓5ᵗʰ K94.2**   **Gastrostomy** complications

     **K94.20**   **Gastrostomy complication, unspecified**    `HCC`

     **K94.21**   **Gastrostomy** hemorrhage    `HCC`

     **K94.22**   **Gastrostomy** infection    `CC` `HCC`

           Use additional code to specify type of infection, such as:

             cellulitis of abdominal wall (LØ3.311)

             sepsis (A4Ø-, A41-)

           **CC Excl:** PDX collection 828

     **K94.23**   **Gastrostomy** malfunction    `CC` `HCC`

           Mechanical complication of gastrostomy

           **CC Excl:** PDX collection 828

     **K94.29**   **Other** complications of gastrostomy    `HCC`

**✓5ᵗʰ K94.3**   **Esophagostomy** complications

> **CC Excl: For CC codes in subcategory K94.3:** PDX collection 828

     **K94.30**   **Esophagostomy complications, unspecified**    `CC` `HCC`

     **K94.31**   **Esophagostomy** hemorrhage    `CC` `HCC`

     **K94.32**   **Esophagostomy** infection    `CC` `HCC`

           Use additional code to identify the infection

     **K94.33**   **Esophagostomy** malfunction    `CC` `HCC`

           Mechanical complication of esophagostomy

     **K94.39**   **Other** complications of esophagostomy    `CC` `HCC`

**✓4ᵗʰ K95**   **Complications of bariatric procedures**

> **CC Excl: For CC codes in category K95:** PDX collection 828

**✓5ᵗʰ K95.Ø**   **Complications of** gastric band procedure

     **K95.Ø1**   **Infection** due to gastric band procedure    `CC` `H11`

           Use additional code to specify type of infection or organism, such as:

             bacterial and viral infectious agents (B95.-, B96.-)

             cellulitis of abdominal wall (LØ3.311)

             sepsis (A4Ø.-, A41.-)

     **K95.Ø9**   **Other** complications of gastric band procedure    `CC`

           Use additional code, if applicable, to further specify complication

**✓5ᵗʰ K95.8**   **Complications of** other bariatric procedure

        *EXCLUDES 1*   complications of gastric band surgery (K95.Ø-)

     **K95.81**   **Infection** due to other bariatric procedure    `CC` `H11`

           Use additional code to specify type of infection or organism, such as:

             bacterial and viral infectious agents (B95.-, B96.-)

             cellulitis of abdominal wall (LØ3.311)

             sepsis (A4Ø.-, A41.-)

     **K95.89**   **Other** complications of other bariatric procedure    `CC`

           Use additional code, if applicable, to further specify complication

---

✓ Additional Character Req    ✓x7ᵗʰ Placeholder Alert    Unacceptable PDx    Manifestation    `H1`-`H14` HAC    `HCC` CMS-HCC Condition    *EXCLUDES 1* Not Coded Here    *EXCLUDES 2* Not Included Here

ICD-10-CM 2018                                                     **707**

# Chapter 12. Diseases of the Skin and Subcutaneous Tissue (L00–L99)

## Chapter Specific Guidelines with Coding Examples

The chapter specific guidelines from the ICD-10-CM Official Guidelines for Coding and Reporting have been provided below. Along with these guidelines are coding examples, contained in the shaded boxes, that have been developed to help illustrate the coding and/or sequencing guidance found in these guidelines.

### a. Pressure ulcer stage codes

#### 1) Pressure ulcer stages

Codes from category L89, Pressure ulcer, identify the site of the pressure ulcer as well as the stage of the ulcer.

The ICD-10-CM classifies pressure ulcer stages based on severity, which is designated by stages 1-4, unspecified stage and unstageable.

Assign as many codes from category L89 as needed to identify all the pressure ulcers the patient has, if applicable.

---

Stage 4 pressure ulcer right heel, 9 x 10 cm that invades the muscle and fascia; stage 2 pressure ulcer of left elbow

**L89.614     Pressure ulcer of right heel, stage 4**

**L89.022     Pressure ulcer of left elbow, stage 2**

*Explanation:* Patient has a right heel pressure ulcer documented as stage 4 and a left elbow pressure ulcer documented as stage 2. Combination codes from category L89 Pressure ulcer, identify the site of the pressure ulcer as well as the stage. Assign as many codes from category L89 as needed to identify all the pressure ulcers the patient has.

---

#### 2) Unstageable pressure ulcers

Assignment of the code for unstageable pressure ulcer (L89.--0) should be based on the clinical documentation. These codes are used for pressure ulcers whose stage cannot be clinically determined (e.g., the ulcer is covered by eschar or has been treated with a skin or muscle graft) and pressure ulcers that are documented as deep tissue injury but not documented as due to trauma. This code should not be confused with the codes for unspecified stage (L89.--9). When there is no documentation regarding the stage of the pressure ulcer, assign the appropriate code for unspecified stage (L89.--9).

---

Pressure ulcer of the right lower back documented as unstageable due to the presence of thick eschar covering the ulcer

**L89.130     Pressure ulcer of right lower back, unstageable**

*Explanation:* Codes for unstageable pressure ulcers are assigned when the stage cannot be clinically determined (e.g., the ulcer is covered by eschar or has been treated with a skin or muscle graft).

---

#### 3) Documented pressure ulcer stage

Assignment of the pressure ulcer stage code should be guided by clinical documentation of the stage or documentation of the terms found in the Alphabetic Index. For clinical terms describing the stage that are not found in the Alphabetic Index, and there is no documentation of the stage, the provider should be queried.

---

Left heel pressure ulcer with partial thickness skin loss involving the dermis

**L89.622     Pressure ulcer of left heel, stage 2**

*Explanation:* Code assignment for the pressure ulcer stage should be guided by either the clinical documentation of the stage or the documentation of terms found in the Alphabetic Index. The clinical documentation describing the left heel pressure ulcer "partial thickness skin loss involving the dermis" matches the ICD-10-CM index parenthetical description for stage 2 "(abrasion, blister, partial thickness skin loss involving epidermis and/or dermis)."

---

#### 4) Patients admitted with pressure ulcers documented as healed

No code is assigned if the documentation states that the pressure ulcer is completely healed.

---

Admission orders noted to watch closely for evolving pressure ulcers as patient history noted a healed pressure ulcer of the foot.

**Z87.2     Personal history of diseases of the skin and subcutaneous tissue**

*Explanation:* A code is assigned only for the personal history of the pressure ulcer. Personal history code Z87.2 includes conditions classifiable to L00–L99 such as pressure ulcer. No code is assigned for a pressure ulcer documented as completely healed.

---

#### 5) Patients admitted with pressure ulcers documented as healing

Pressure ulcers described as healing should be assigned the appropriate pressure ulcer stage code based on the documentation in the medical record. If the documentation does not provide information about the stage of the healing pressure ulcer, assign the appropriate code for unspecified stage.

If the documentation is unclear as to whether the patient has a current (new) pressure ulcer or if the patient is being treated for a healing pressure ulcer, query the provider.

For ulcers that were present on admission but healed at the time of discharge, assign the code for the site and stage of the pressure ulcer at the time of admission.

---

H & P noted healing stage 2 sacral pressure ulcer. Resolved at time of discharge summary.

**L89.152     Pressure ulcer of sacral region, stage 2**

*Explanation:* Although completely healed upon discharge, the pressure ulcer required observation and/or treatment and should be coded based on the site and stage upon admission.

---

#### 6) Patient admitted with pressure ulcer evolving into another stage during the admission

If a patient is admitted with a pressure ulcer at one stage and it progresses to a higher stage, two separate codes should be assigned: one code for the site and stage of the ulcer on admission and a second code for the same ulcer site and the highest stage reported during the stay.

---

Stage 3 right hip pressure ulcer worsened during admission to a stage 4

**L89.213     Pressure ulcer of right hip, stage 3**

**L89.214     Pressure ulcer of right hip, stage 4**

*Explanation:* A pressure ulcer that progresses from a lower stage to a higher stage is assigned two codes, one for the documented stage upon admission and one for the documented stage at discharge.

---

# Chapter 12. Diseases of the Skin and Subcutaneous Tissue (L00-L99)

EXCLUDES 2   *certain conditions originating in the perinatal period (P04-P96)*
*certain infectious and parasitic diseases (A00-B99)*
*complications of pregnancy, childbirth and the puerperium (O00-O9A)*
*congenital malformations, deformations, and chromosomal abnormalities (Q00-Q99)*
*endocrine, nutritional and metabolic diseases (E00-E88)*
*lipomelanotic reticulosis (I89.8)*
*neoplasms (C00-D49)*
*symptoms, signs and abnormal clinical and laboratory findings, not elsewhere classified (R00-R94)*
*systemic connective tissue disorders (M30-M36)*
*viral warts (B07.-)*

This chapter contains the following blocks:

| | |
|---|---|
| L00-L08 | Infections of the skin and subcutaneous tissue |
| L10-L14 | Bullous disorders |
| L20-L30 | Dermatitis and eczema |
| L40-L45 | Papulosquamous disorders |
| L49-L54 | Urticaria and erythema |
| L55-L59 | Radiation-related disorders of the skin and subcutaneous tissue |
| L60-L75 | Disorders of skin appendages |
| L76 | Intraoperative and postprocedural complications of skin and subcutaneous tissue |
| L80-L99 | Other disorders of the skin and subcutaneous tissue |

## Infections of the skin and subcutaneous tissue (L00-L08)

Use additional code (B95-B97) to identify infectious agent

EXCLUDES 2   *hordeolum (H00.0)*
*infective dermatitis (L30.3)*
*local infections of skin classified in Chapter 1*
*lupus panniculitis (L93.2)*
*panniculitis NOS (M79.3)*
*panniculitis of neck and back (M54.0-)*
*Perlèche NOS (K13.0)*
*Perlèche due to candidiasis (B37.0)*
*Perlèche due to riboflavin deficiency (E53.0)*
*pyogenic granuloma (L98.0)*
*relapsing panniculitis [Weber-Christian] (M35.6)*
*viral warts (B07.-)*
*zoster (B02.-)*

**L00    Staphylococcal scalded skin syndrome**
Ritter's disease
Use additional code to identify percentage of skin exfoliation (L49.-)

EXCLUDES 1   *bullous impetigo (L01.03)*
*pemphigus neonatorum (L01.03)*
*toxic epidermal necrolysis [Lyell] (L51.2)*

**DEF:** Infectious skin disease of children younger than 5 years marked by eruptions ranging from a few localized blisters to widespread, easily ruptured, fine vesicles and bullae affecting almost the entire body; results in exfoliation of large planes of skin and leaves raw areas.

✓4ᵗʰ **L01    Impetigo**

EXCLUDES 1   *impetigo herpetiformis (L40.1)*

✓5ᵗʰ **L01.0    Impetigo**
Impetigo contagiosa
Impetigo vulgaris

**L01.00    Impetigo, unspecified**
Impetigo NOS

**L01.01    Non-bullous impetigo**

**L01.02    Bockhart's impetigo**
Impetigo folliculitis
Perifolliculitis NOS
Superficial pustular perifolliculitis

**L01.03    Bullous impetigo**
Impetigo neonatorum
Pemphigus neonatorum

**L01.09    Other impetigo**
Ulcerative impetigo

**L01.1    Impetiginization of other dermatoses**

✓4ᵗʰ **L02    Cutaneous abscess, furuncle and carbuncle**
Use additional code to identify organism (B95-B96)

EXCLUDES 2   *abscess of anus and rectal regions (K61.-)*
*abscess of female genital organs (external) (N76.4)*
*abscess of male genital organs (external) (N48.2, N49-)*

✓5ᵗʰ **L02.0    Cutaneous abscess, furuncle and carbuncle of face**

EXCLUDES 2   *abscess of ear, external (H60.0)*
*abscess of eyelid (H00.0)*
*abscess of head [any part, except face] (L02.8)*
*abscess of lacrimal gland (H04.0)*
*abscess of lacrimal passages (H04.3)*
*abscess of mouth (K12.2)*
*abscess of nose (J34.0)*
*abscess of orbit (H05.0)*
*submandibular abscess (K12.2)*

**L02.01    Cutaneous abscess of face**            **CC**
CC Excl: No Excl

**L02.02    Furuncle of face**
Boil of face
Folliculitis of face

**L02.03    Carbuncle of face**

✓5ᵗʰ **L02.1    Cutaneous abscess, furuncle and carbuncle of neck**

**L02.11    Cutaneous abscess of neck**            **CC**
CC Excl: PDX collection 832

**L02.12    Furuncle of neck**
Boil of neck
Folliculitis of neck

**L02.13    Carbuncle of neck**

✓5ᵗʰ **L02.2    Cutaneous abscess, furuncle and carbuncle of trunk**

EXCLUDES 1   *non-newborn omphalitis (L08.82)*
*omphalitis of newborn (P38.-)*

EXCLUDES 2   *abscess of breast (N61.1)*
*abscess of buttocks (L02.3)*
*abscess of female external genital organs (N76.4)*
*abscess of hip (L02.4)*
*abscess of male external genital organs (N48.2, N49.-)*

**CC Excl: For CC codes in subcategory L02.2:**
PDX collection 833

✓6ᵗʰ **L02.21    Cutaneous abscess of trunk**
**L02.211    Cutaneous abscess of abdominal wall**   **CC**
**L02.212    Cutaneous abscess of back [any part, except buttock]**   **CC**
**L02.213    Cutaneous abscess of chest wall**   **CC**
**L02.214    Cutaneous abscess of groin**   **CC**
**L02.215    Cutaneous abscess of perineum**   **CC**
**L02.216    Cutaneous abscess of umbilicus**   **CC**
**L02.219    Cutaneous abscess of trunk, unspecified**   **CC**

✓6ᵗʰ **L02.22    Furuncle of trunk**
Boil of trunk       Folliculitis of trunk
**L02.221    Furuncle of abdominal wall**
**L02.222    Furuncle of back [any part, except buttock]**
**L02.223    Furuncle of chest wall**
**L02.224    Furuncle of groin**
**L02.225    Furuncle of perineum**
**L02.226    Furuncle of umbilicus**
**L02.229    Furuncle of trunk, unspecified**

✓6ᵗʰ **L02.23    Carbuncle of trunk**
**L02.231    Carbuncle of abdominal wall**
**L02.232    Carbuncle of back [any part, except buttock]**
**L02.233    Carbuncle of chest wall**
**L02.234    Carbuncle of groin**
**L02.235    Carbuncle of perineum**
**L02.236    Carbuncle of umbilicus**
**L02.239    Carbuncle of trunk, unspecified**

✓5ᵗʰ **L02.3    Cutaneous abscess, furuncle and carbuncle of buttock**

EXCLUDES 1   *pilonidal cyst with abscess (L05.01)*

**L02.31    Cutaneous abscess of buttock**            **CC**
Cutaneous abscess of gluteal region
CC Excl: PDX collection 834

**L02.32    Furuncle of buttock**
Boil of buttock
Folliculitis of buttock
Furuncle of gluteal region

Ⓝ Newborn: 0    Ⓟ Pediatric: 0-17    Ⓜ Maternity: 12-55    Ⓐ Adult: 15-124    ᴹᶜᶜ Major CC Condition    ᴾᴰˣᴹᶜᶜ PDx acts as own MCC    ᶜᶜ CC Condition    ᴾᴰˣᶜᶜ PDx acts as own CC

710                                                                                                                    ICD-10-CM 2018

**L02.33**   **Carbuncle of buttock**
Carbuncle of gluteal region

☑5ᵗʰ **L02.4**   **Cutaneous abscess, furuncle and carbuncle of limb**
*EXCLUDES 2*   *cutaneous abscess, furuncle and carbuncle of groin (L02.214, L02.224, L02.234)*
*cutaneous abscess, furuncle and carbuncle of hand (L02.5-)*
*cutaneous abscess, furuncle and carbuncle of foot (L02.6-)*

**CC Excl: For CC codes in subcategory L02.4, unless otherwise noted:** PDX collection 835

☑6ᵗʰ **L02.41**   **Cutaneous abscess of limb**
**L02.411**   **Cutaneous abscess of right axilla**   CC
**L02.412**   **Cutaneous abscess of left axilla**   CC
**L02.413**   **Cutaneous abscess of right upper limb**   CC
**L02.414**   **Cutaneous abscess of left upper limb**   CC
**L02.415**   **Cutaneous abscess of right lower limb**   CC
     **CC Excl:** PDX collection 836
**L02.416**   **Cutaneous abscess of left lower limb**   CC
     **CC Excl:** PDX collection 836
**L02.419**   **Cutaneous abscess of limb, unspecified**   CC
     **CC Excl:** PDX collection 836

☑6ᵗʰ **L02.42**   **Furuncle of limb**
Boil of limb
Folliculitis of limb
**L02.421**   **Furuncle of right axilla**
**L02.422**   **Furuncle of left axilla**
**L02.423**   **Furuncle of right upper limb**
**L02.424**   **Furuncle of left upper limb**
**L02.425**   **Furuncle of right lower limb**
**L02.426**   **Furuncle of left lower limb**
**L02.429**   **Furuncle of limb, unspecified**

☑6ᵗʰ **L02.43**   **Carbuncle of limb**
**L02.431**   **Carbuncle of right axilla**
**L02.432**   **Carbuncle of left axilla**
**L02.433**   **Carbuncle of right upper limb**
**L02.434**   **Carbuncle of left upper limb**
**L02.435**   **Carbuncle of right lower limb**
**L02.436**   **Carbuncle of left lower limb**
**L02.439**   **Carbuncle of limb, unspecified**

☑5ᵗʰ **L02.5**   **Cutaneous abscess, furuncle and carbuncle of hand**

**CC Excl: For CC codes in subcategory L02.5:** PDX collection 837

☑6ᵗʰ **L02.51**   **Cutaneous abscess of hand**
**L02.511**   **Cutaneous abscess of right hand**   CC
**L02.512**   **Cutaneous abscess of left hand**   CC
**L02.519**   **Cutaneous abscess of unspecified hand**   CC

☑6ᵗʰ **L02.52**   **Furuncle hand**
Boil of hand
Folliculitis of hand
**L02.521**   **Furuncle right hand**
**L02.522**   **Furuncle left hand**
**L02.529**   **Furuncle unspecified hand**

☑6ᵗʰ **L02.53**   **Carbuncle of hand**
**L02.531**   **Carbuncle of right hand**
**L02.532**   **Carbuncle of left hand**
**L02.539**   **Carbuncle of unspecified hand**

☑5ᵗʰ **L02.6**   **Cutaneous abscess, furuncle and carbuncle of foot**

**CC Excl: For CC codes in subcategory L02.6:** PDX collection 838

☑6ᵗʰ **L02.61**   **Cutaneous abscess of foot**
**L02.611**   **Cutaneous abscess of right foot**   CC
**L02.612**   **Cutaneous abscess of left foot**   CC
**L02.619**   **Cutaneous abscess of unspecified foot**   CC

☑6ᵗʰ **L02.62**   **Furuncle of foot**
Boil of foot      Folliculitis of foot
**L02.621**   **Furuncle of right foot**
**L02.622**   **Furuncle of left foot**
**L02.629**   **Furuncle of unspecified foot**

☑6ᵗʰ **L02.63**   **Carbuncle of foot**
**L02.631**   **Carbuncle of right foot**
**L02.632**   **Carbuncle of left foot**
**L02.639**   **Carbuncle of unspecified foot**

☑5ᵗʰ **L02.8**   **Cutaneous abscess, furuncle and carbuncle of other sites**
☑6ᵗʰ **L02.81**   **Cutaneous abscess of other sites**
**L02.811**   **Cutaneous abscess of head [any part, except face]**   CC
     **CC Excl:** PDX collection 839
**L02.818**   **Cutaneous abscess of other sites**   CC
     **CC Excl:** PDX collection 839

☑6ᵗʰ **L02.82**   **Furuncle of other sites**
Boil of other sites      Folliculitis of other sites
**L02.821**   **Furuncle of head [any part, except face]**
**L02.828**   **Furuncle of other sites**

☑6ᵗʰ **L02.83**   **Carbuncle of other sites**
**L02.831**   **Carbuncle of head [any part, except face]**
**L02.838**   **Carbuncle of other sites**

☑5ᵗʰ **L02.9**   **Cutaneous abscess, furuncle and carbuncle, unspecified**
**L02.91**   **Cutaneous abscess, unspecified**   CC
     **CC Excl:** PDX collection 839
**L02.92**   **Furuncle, unspecified**
Boil NOS      Furunculosis NOS
**L02.93**   **Carbuncle, unspecified**

☑4ᵗʰ **L03**   **Cellulitis and acute lymphangitis**
*EXCLUDES 2*   *cellulitis of anal and rectal region (K61.-)*
*cellulitis of external auditory canal (H60.1)*
*cellulitis of eyelid (H00.03-)*
*cellulitis of female external genital organs (N76.4)*
*cellulitis of lacrimal apparatus (H04.3)*
*cellulitis of male external genital organs (N48.2, N49-)*
*cellulitis of mouth (K12.2)*
*cellulitis of nose (J34.0)*
*eosinophilic cellulitis [Wells] (L98.3)*
*febrile neutrophilic dermatosis [Sweet] (L98.2)*
*lymphangitis (chronic) (subacute) (I89.1)*

☑5ᵗʰ **L03.0**   **Cellulitis and acute lymphangitis of finger and toe**
Infection of nail
Onychia
Paronychia
Perionychia

☑6ᵗʰ **L03.01**   **Cellulitis of finger**
Felon
Whitlow
*EXCLUDES 1*   *herpetic whitlow (B00.89)*
**DEF:** Felon: Superficial bacterial skin infection at the tip of the finger.
**L03.011**   **Cellulitis of right finger**
**L03.012**   **Cellulitis of left finger**
**L03.019**   **Cellulitis of unspecified finger**

☑6ᵗʰ **L03.02**   **Acute lymphangitis of finger**
Hangnail with lymphangitis of finger
**L03.021**   **Acute lymphangitis of right finger**
**L03.022**   **Acute lymphangitis of left finger**
**L03.029**   **Acute lymphangitis of unspecified finger**

☑6ᵗʰ **L03.03**   **Cellulitis of toe**
**L03.031**   **Cellulitis of right toe**
**L03.032**   **Cellulitis of left toe**
**L03.039**   **Cellulitis of unspecified toe**

☑6ᵗʰ **L03.04**   **Acute lymphangitis of toe**
Hangnail with lymphangitis of toe
**L03.041**   **Acute lymphangitis of right toe**
**L03.042**   **Acute lymphangitis of left toe**
**L03.049**   **Acute lymphangitis of unspecified toe**

☑5ᵗʰ **L03.1**   **Cellulitis and acute lymphangitis of other parts of limb**

**CC Excl: For CC codes in subcategory L03.1, unless otherwise noted:** PDX collection 835

☑6ᵗʰ **L03.11**   **Cellulitis of other parts of limb**
*EXCLUDES 2*   *cellulitis of fingers (L03.01-)*
*cellulitis of toes (L03.03-)*
*groin (L03.314)*
**L03.111**   **Cellulitis of right axilla**   CC
**L03.112**   **Cellulitis of left axilla**   CC
**L03.113**   **Cellulitis of right upper limb**   CC
**L03.114**   **Cellulitis of left upper limb**   CC

☑Additional Character Req   ☑7ᵗʰ Placeholder Alert   Unacceptable PDx   **Manifestation**   **H1**-**H14** HAC   **HCC** CMS-HCC Condition   *EXCLUDES 1* Not Coded Here   *EXCLUDES 2* Not Included Here

ICD-10-CM 2018      **711**

**L03.115**   **Cellulitis of right lower limb**   `CC`
     **CC Excl:** PDX collection 836

**L03.116**   **Cellulitis of left lower limb**   `CC`
     **CC Excl:** PDX collection 836

**L03.119**   **Cellulitis of unspecified part of limb**   `CC`
     **CC Excl:** PDX collection 836

✓6ᵗʰ **L03.12**   **Acute lymphangitis of other parts of limb**
     *EXCLUDES 2*   *acute lymphangitis of fingers (L03.02-)*
                *acute lymphangitis of groin (L03.324)*
                *acute lymphangitis of toes (L03.04-)*

**L03.121**   **Acute lymphangitis of right axilla**   `CC`

**L03.122**   **Acute lymphangitis of left axilla**   `CC`

**L03.123**   **Acute lymphangitis of right upper limb**   `CC`

**L03.124**   **Acute lymphangitis of left upper limb**   `CC`

**L03.125**   **Acute lymphangitis of right lower limb**   `CC`
     **CC Excl:** PDX collection 836

**L03.126**   **Acute lymphangitis of left lower limb**   `CC`
     **CC Excl:** PDX collection 836

**L03.129**   **Acute lymphangitis of unspecified part of limb**   `CC`
     **CC Excl:** PDX collection 836

✓5ᵗʰ **L03.2**   **Cellulitis and acute lymphangitis of face and neck**

   ✓6ᵗʰ **L03.21**   **Cellulitis and acute lymphangitis of face**

**L03.211**   **Cellulitis of face**   `CC`
     *EXCLUDES 2*   *abscess of orbit (H05.01-)*
                *cellulitis of ear (H60.1-)*
                *cellulitis of eyelid (H00.03-)*
                *cellulitis of head (L03.811)*
                *cellulitis of lacrimal apparatus*
                   *(H04.3)*
                *cellulitis of lip (K13.0)*
                *cellulitis of mouth (K12.2)*
                *cellulitis of nose (internal) (J34.0)*
                *cellulitis of orbit (H05.01-)*
                *cellulitis of scalp (L03.811)*
     **AHA:** 2013, 4Q, 123
     **CC Excl:** PDX collection 840

**L03.212**   **Acute lymphangitis of face**   `CC`
     **CC Excl:** No Excl

**L03.213**   **Periorbital cellulitis**   `CC`
     Preseptal cellulitis
     **CC Excl:** PDX collection 840

   ✓6ᵗʰ **L03.22**   **Cellulitis and acute lymphangitis of neck**

**L03.221**   **Cellulitis of neck**   `CC`
     **CC Excl:** PDX collection 832

**L03.222**   **Acute lymphangitis of neck**   `CC`
     **CC Excl:** PDX collection 832

✓5ᵗʰ **L03.3**   **Cellulitis and acute lymphangitis of trunk**

> **CC Excl: For CC codes in subcategory L03.3, unless otherwise noted:** PDX collection 833

   ✓6ᵗʰ **L03.31**   **Cellulitis of trunk**
     *EXCLUDES 2*   *cellulitis of anal and rectal regions (K61.-)*
                *cellulitis of breast NOS (N61.0)*
                *cellulitis of female external genital organs*
                   *(N76.4)*
                *cellulitis of male external genital organs*
                   *(N48.2, N49-)*
                *omphalitis of newborn (P38.-)*
                *puerperal cellulitis of breast (O91.2)*

**L03.311**   **Cellulitis of abdominal wall**   `CC`
     *EXCLUDES 2*   *cellulitis of umbilicus (L03.316)*
                *cellulitis of groin (L03.314)*

**L03.312**   **Cellulitis of back [any part except buttock]**   `CC`

**L03.313**   **Cellulitis of chest wall**   `CC`

**L03.314**   **Cellulitis of groin**   `CC`

**L03.315**   **Cellulitis of perineum**   `CC`

**L03.316**   **Cellulitis of umbilicus**   `CC`

**L03.317**   **Cellulitis of buttock**   `CC`
     **CC Excl:** PDX collection 834

**L03.319**   **Cellulitis of trunk, unspecified**   `CC`

   ✓6ᵗʰ **L03.32**   **Acute lymphangitis of trunk**

**L03.321**   **Acute lymphangitis of abdominal wall**   `CC`

**L03.322**   **Acute lymphangitis of back [any part except buttock]**   `CC`

**L03.323**   **Acute lymphangitis of chest wall**   `CC`

**L03.324**   **Acute lymphangitis of groin**   `CC`

**L03.325**   **Acute lymphangitis of perineum**   `CC`

---

**L03.326**   **Acute lymphangitis of umbilicus**   `CC`

**L03.327**   **Acute lymphangitis of buttock**   `CC`
     **CC Excl:** PDX collection 834

**L03.329**   **Acute lymphangitis of trunk, unspecified**   `CC`

✓5ᵗʰ **L03.8**   **Cellulitis and acute lymphangitis of other sites**

> **CC Excl: For CC codes in subcategory L03.8:** PDX collection 839

   ✓6ᵗʰ **L03.81**   **Cellulitis of other sites**

**L03.811**   **Cellulitis of head [any part, except face]**   `CC`
     Cellulitis of scalp
     *EXCLUDES 2*   *cellulitis of face (L03.211)*

**L03.818**   **Cellulitis of other sites**   `CC`

   ✓6ᵗʰ **L03.89**   **Acute lymphangitis of other sites**

**L03.891**   **Acute lymphangitis of head [any part, except face]**   `CC`

**L03.898**   **Acute lymphangitis of other sites**   `CC`

✓5ᵗʰ **L03.9**   **Cellulitis and acute lymphangitis, unspecified**

> **CC Excl: For CC codes in subcategory L03.9:** PDX collection 839

**L03.90**   **Cellulitis, unspecified**   `CC`

**L03.91**   **Acute lymphangitis, unspecified**   `CC`
     *EXCLUDES 1*   *lymphangitis NOS (I89.1)*

✓4ᵗʰ **L04**   **Acute lymphadenitis**
     *INCLUDES*   abscess (acute) of lymph nodes, except mesenteric
                 acute lymphadenitis, except mesenteric
     *EXCLUDES 1*   *chronic or subacute lymphadenitis, except mesenteric (I88.1)*
                *enlarged lymph nodes (R59.-)*
                *human immunodeficiency virus [HIV] disease resulting in*
                   *generalized lymphadenopathy (B20)*
                *lymphadenitis NOS (I88.9)*
                *nonspecific mesenteric lymphadenitis (I88.0)*

**L04.0**   **Acute lymphadenitis of face, head and neck**

**L04.1**   **Acute lymphadenitis of trunk**

**L04.2**   **Acute lymphadenitis of upper limb**
     Acute lymphadenitis of axilla      Acute lymphadenitis of shoulder

**L04.3**   **Acute lymphadenitis of lower limb**
     Acute lymphadenitis of hip
     *EXCLUDES 2*   *acute lymphadenitis of groin (L04.1)*

**L04.8**   **Acute lymphadenitis of other sites**

**L04.9**   **Acute lymphadenitis, unspecified**

✓4ᵗʰ **L05**   **Pilonidal cyst and sinus**

   ✓5ᵗʰ **L05.0**   **Pilonidal cyst and sinus with abscess**

**L05.01**   **Pilonidal cyst with abscess**   `CC`
     Pilonidal abscess
     Pilonidal dimple with abscess
     Postanal dimple with abscess
     *EXCLUDES 2*   *congenital sacral dimple (Q82.6)*
                *parasacral dimple (Q82.6)*
     **CC Excl:** PDX collection 841

**L05.02**   **Pilonidal sinus with abscess**   `CC`
     Coccygeal fistula with abscess
     Coccygeal sinus with abscess
     Pilonidal fistula with abscess
     **CC Excl:** PDX collection 841

**Pilonidal Cyst**

Skin

Fistula

Pilonidal cyst

Fat

Bone

---

`N` Newborn: 0    `P` Pediatric: 0-17    `M` Maternity: 12-55    `A` Adult: 15-124    `MCC` Major CC Condition    `PDxMCC` PDx acts as own MCC    `CC` CC Condition    `PDxCC` PDx acts as own CC

**712**                                                  ICD-10-CM 2018

√5ᵗʰ **L05.9** **Pilonidal cyst and sinus** without abscess

     **L05.91** **Pilonidal cyst** without abscess
         Pilonidal dimple
         Postanal dimple
         Pilonidal cyst NOS
         *EXCLUDES 2*   *congenital sacral dimple (Q82.6)*
                 *parasacral dimple (Q82.6)*

     **L05.92** **Pilonidal sinus** without abscess
         Coccygeal fistula
         Coccygeal sinus without abscess
         Pilonidal fistula

√4ᵗʰ **L08** **Other local infections of skin and subcutaneous tissue**

     **L08.0** **Pyoderma**
         Dermatitis gangrenosa
         Purulent dermatitis
         Septic dermatitis
         Suppurative dermatitis
         *EXCLUDES 1*   *pyoderma gangrenosum (L88)*
                 *pyoderma vegetans (L08.81)*

     **L08.1** **Erythrasma**      HIV CC
         **CC Excl:** PDX collection 107

√5ᵗʰ **L08.8** **Other specified local infections of the skin and subcutaneous tissue**

     **L08.81** **Pyoderma vegetans**
         *EXCLUDES 1*   *pyoderma gangrenosum (L88)*
                 *pyoderma NOS (L08.0)*

     **L08.82** **Omphalitis** not of newborn
         *EXCLUDES 1*   *omphalitis of newborn (P38.-)*

     **L08.89** **Other specified local infections of the skin and subcutaneous tissue**

     **L08.9** **Local infection of the skin and subcutaneous tissue, unspecified**

### Bullous disorders (L10-L14)

*EXCLUDES 1*   *benign familial pemphigus [Hailey-Hailey] (Q82.8)*
            *staphylococcal scalded skin syndrome (L00)*
            *toxic epidermal necrolysis [Lyell] (L51.2)*

√4ᵗʰ **L10** **Pemphigus**
     *EXCLUDES 1*   *pemphigus neonatorum (L01.03)*

     **CC Excl: For CC codes in category L10:** PDX collection 842

     **L10.0** **Pemphigus vulgaris**      CC
     **L10.1** **Pemphigus vegetans**      CC
     **L10.2** **Pemphigus foliaceous**      CC
     **L10.3** **Brazilian pemphigus [fogo selvagem]**      CC
     **L10.4** **Pemphigus erythematosus**      CC
         Senear-Usher syndrome
     **L10.5** **Drug-induced pemphigus**      CC
         Use additional code for adverse effect, if applicable, to identify drug (T36-T50 with fifth or sixth character 5)

√5ᵗʰ **L10.8** **Other pemphigus**
     **L10.81** **Paraneoplastic pemphigus**      CC
     **L10.89** **Other pemphigus**      CC
     **L10.9** **Pemphigus, unspecified**      CC

√4ᵗʰ **L11** **Other acantholytic disorders**

     **L11.0** **Acquired keratosis follicularis**
         *EXCLUDES 1*   *keratosis follicularis (congenital) [Darier-White] (Q82.8)*

     **L11.1** **Transient acantholytic dermatosis [Grover]**
     **L11.8** **Other specified acantholytic disorders**
     **L11.9** **Acantholytic disorder, unspecified**

√4ᵗʰ **L12** **Pemphigoid**
     *EXCLUDES 1*   *herpes gestationis (O26.4-)*
            *impetigo herpetiformis (L40.1)*

     **CC Excl: For CC codes in category L12, unless otherwise noted:** PDX collection 842

     **L12.0** **Bullous pemphigoid**      CC
     **L12.1** **Cicatricial pemphigoid**
         Benign mucous membrane pemphigoid
         **DEF:** Chronic autoimmune disease characterized by subepidermal blistering lesions of mucosa, including the conjunctiva; seen predominantly in the elderly; produces adhesions and scarring.
     **L12.2** **Chronic bullous disease of childhood**      P
         Juvenile dermatitis herpetiformis

√5ᵗʰ **L12.3** **Acquired epidermolysis bullosa**
     *EXCLUDES 1*   *epidermolysis bullosa (congenital) (Q81.-)*

     **L12.30** **Acquired epidermolysis bullosa, unspecified**      CC HCC
         **CC Excl:** PDX collection 843
     **L12.31** **Epidermolysis bullosa due to drug**      CC HCC
         Use additional code for adverse effect, if applicable, to identify drug (T36-T50 with fifth or sixth character 5)
         **CC Excl:** PDX collection 843
     **L12.35** **Other acquired epidermolysis bullosa**      CC HCC
         **CC Excl:** PDX collection 843

     **L12.8** **Other pemphigoid**      CC
     **L12.9** **Pemphigoid, unspecified**      CC

√4ᵗʰ **L13** **Other bullous disorders**

     **L13.0** **Dermatitis herpetiformis**
         Duhring's disease
         Hydroa herpetiformis
         *EXCLUDES 1*   *juvenile dermatitis herpetiformis (L12.2)*
                 *senile dermatitis herpetiformis (L12.0)*
         **DEF:** Skin disease to which people are genetically predisposed resulting from an immunological response to gluten; seen as an extremely pruritic eruption of various lesions that frequently heal, leaving hyperpigmentation or hypopigmentation and occasionally scarring; usually associated with an asymptomatic gluten-sensitive enteropathy.

     **L13.1** **Subcorneal pustular dermatitis**
         Sneddon-Wilkinson disease
     **L13.8** **Other specified bullous disorders**
     **L13.9** **Bullous disorder, unspecified**

*L14*   *Bullous disorders in diseases classified elsewhere*
     Code first underlying disease

### Dermatitis and eczema (L20-L30)

**NOTE**   In this block the terms dermatitis and eczema are used synonymously and interchangeably.

*EXCLUDES 2*   *chronic (childhood) granulomatous disease (D71)*
            *dermatitis gangrenosa (L08.0)*
            *dermatitis herpetiformis (L13.0)*
            *dry skin dermatitis (L85.3)*
            *factitial dermatitis (L98.1)*
            *perioral dermatitis (L71.0)*
            *radiation-related disorders of the skin and subcutaneous tissue (L55-L59)*
            *stasis dermatitis (I87.2)*

√4ᵗʰ **L20** **Atopic dermatitis**
     **L20.0** **Besnier's prurigo**
√5ᵗʰ **L20.8** **Other atopic dermatitis**
     *EXCLUDES 2*   *circumscribed neurodermatitis (L28.0)*

     **L20.81** **Atopic neurodermatitis**
         Diffuse neurodermatitis
     **L20.82** **Flexural eczema**
     **L20.83** **Infantile (acute) (chronic) eczema**      P
     **L20.84** **Intrinsic (allergic) eczema**
     **L20.89** **Other atopic dermatitis**
     **L20.9** **Atopic dermatitis, unspecified**

√4ᵗʰ **L21** **Seborrheic dermatitis**
     *EXCLUDES 2*   *infective dermatitis (L30.3)*
            *seborrheic keratosis (L82.-)*

     **L21.0** **Seborrhea capitis**
         Cradle cap
     **L21.1** **Seborrheic infantile dermatitis**      P
     **L21.8** **Other seborrheic dermatitis**
     **L21.9** **Seborrheic dermatitis, unspecified**
         Seborrhea NOS

     **L22** **Diaper dermatitis**
         Diaper erythema
         Diaper rash
         Psoriasiform diaper rash

✔ Additional Character Req   ✔x7ᵗʰ Placeholder Alert   Unacceptable PDx   **Manifestation**   H1 - H14 HAC   HCC CMS-HCC Condition   *EXCLUDES 1* Not Coded Here   *EXCLUDES 2* Not Included Here

ICD-10-CM 2018          **713**

**Chapter 12. Diseases of the Skin and Subcutaneous Tissue**

**L23–L29.8**

✓4ᵗʰ **L23**   **Allergic contact dermatitis**

> **EXCLUDES 1**   allergy NOS (T78.40)
> contact dermatitis NOS (L25.9)
> dermatitis NOS (L30.9)
>
> **EXCLUDES 2**   dermatitis due to substances taken internally (L27.-)
> dermatitis of eyelid (H01.1-)
> diaper dermatitis (L22)
> eczema of external ear (H60.5-)
> irritant contact dermatitis (L24.-)
> perioral dermatitis (L71.0)
> radiation-related disorders of the skin and subcutaneous tissue (L55-L59)

**L23.0**   **Allergic contact dermatitis due to metals**
> Allergic contact dermatitis due to chromium
> Allergic contact dermatitis due to nickel

**L23.1**   **Allergic contact dermatitis due to adhesives**

**L23.2**   **Allergic contact dermatitis due to cosmetics**

**L23.3**   **Allergic contact dermatitis due to drugs in contact with skin**
> Use additional code for adverse effect, if applicable, to identify drug (T36-T50 with fifth or sixth character 5)
>
> **EXCLUDES 2**   dermatitis due to ingested drugs and medicaments (L27.0-L27.1)

**L23.4**   **Allergic contact dermatitis due to dyes**

**L23.5**   **Allergic contact dermatitis due to other chemical products**
> Allergic contact dermatitis due to cement
> Allergic contact dermatitis due to insecticide
> Allergic contact dermatitis due to plastic
> Allergic contact dermatitis due to rubber

**L23.6**   **Allergic contact dermatitis due to food in contact with the skin**
> **EXCLUDES 2**   dermatitis due to ingested food (L27.2)

**L23.7**   **Allergic contact dermatitis due to plants, except food**
> **EXCLUDES 2**   allergy NOS due to pollen (J30.1)

✓5ᵗʰ **L23.8**   **Allergic contact dermatitis due to other agents**

> **L23.81**   **Allergic contact dermatitis due to animal (cat) (dog) dander**
> > Allergic contact dermatitis due to animal (cat) (dog) hair
>
> **L23.89**   **Allergic contact dermatitis due to other agents**

**L23.9**   **Allergic contact dermatitis, unspecified cause**
> Allergic contact eczema NOS

✓4ᵗʰ **L24**   **Irritant contact dermatitis**

> **EXCLUDES 1**   allergy NOS (T78.40)
> contact dermatitis NOS (L25.9)
> dermatitis NOS (L30.9)
>
> **EXCLUDES 2**   allergic contact dermatitis (L23.-)
> dermatitis due to substances taken internally (L27.-)
> dermatitis of eyelid (H01.1-)
> diaper dermatitis (L22)
> eczema of external ear (H60.5-)
> perioral dermatitis (L71.0)
> radiation-related disorders of the skin and subcutaneous tissue (L55-L59)

**L24.0**   **Irritant contact dermatitis due to detergents**

**L24.1**   **Irritant contact dermatitis due to oils and greases**

**L24.2**   **Irritant contact dermatitis due to solvents**
> Irritant contact dermatitis due to chlorocompound
> Irritant contact dermatitis due to cyclohexane
> Irritant contact dermatitis due to ester
> Irritant contact dermatitis due to glycol
> Irritant contact dermatitis due to hydrocarbon
> Irritant contact dermatitis due to ketone

**L24.3**   **Irritant contact dermatitis due to cosmetics**

**L24.4**   **Irritant contact dermatitis due to drugs in contact with skin**
> Use additional code for adverse effect, if applicable, to identify drug (T36-T50 with fifth or sixth character 5)

**L24.5**   **Irritant contact dermatitis due to other chemical products**
> Irritant contact dermatitis due to cement
> Irritant contact dermatitis due to insecticide
> Irritant contact dermatitis due to plastic
> Irritant contact dermatitis due to rubber

**L24.6**   **Irritant contact dermatitis due to food in contact with skin**
> **EXCLUDES 2**   dermatitis due to ingested food (L27.2)

**L24.7**   **Irritant contact dermatitis due to plants, except food**
> **EXCLUDES 2**   allergy NOS to pollen (J30.1)

✓5ᵗʰ **L24.8**   **Irritant contact dermatitis due to other agents**

> **L24.81**   **Irritant contact dermatitis due to metals**
> > Irritant contact dermatitis due to chromium
> > Irritant contact dermatitis due to nickel

> **L24.89**   **Irritant contact dermatitis due to other agents**
> > Irritant contact dermatitis due to dyes

**L24.9**   **Irritant contact dermatitis, unspecified cause**
> Irritant contact eczema NOS

✓4ᵗʰ **L25**   **Unspecified contact dermatitis**

> **EXCLUDES 1**   allergic contact dermatitis (L23.-)
> allergy NOS (T78.40)
> dermatitis NOS (L30.9)
> irritant contact dermatitis (L24.-)
>
> **EXCLUDES 2**   dermatitis due to ingested substances (L27.-)
> dermatitis of eyelid (H01.1-)
> eczema of external ear (H60.5-)
> perioral dermatitis (L71.0)
> radiation-related disorders of the skin and subcutaneous tissue (L55-L59)

**L25.0**   **Unspecified contact dermatitis due to cosmetics**

**L25.1**   **Unspecified contact dermatitis due to drugs in contact with skin**
> Use additional code for adverse effect, if applicable, to identify drug (T36-T50 with fifth or sixth character 5)
>
> **EXCLUDES 2**   dermatitis due to ingested drugs and medicaments (L27.0-L27.1)

**L25.2**   **Unspecified contact dermatitis due to dyes**

**L25.3**   **Unspecified contact dermatitis due to other chemical products**
> Unspecified contact dermatitis due to cement
> Unspecified contact dermatitis due to insecticide

**L25.4**   **Unspecified contact dermatitis due to food in contact with skin**
> **EXCLUDES 2**   dermatitis due to ingested food (L27.2)

**L25.5**   **Unspecified contact dermatitis due to plants, except food**
> **EXCLUDES 1**   nettle rash (L50.9)
>
> **EXCLUDES 2**   allergy NOS due to pollen (J30.1)

**L25.8**   **Unspecified contact dermatitis due to other agents**

**L25.9**   **Unspecified contact dermatitis, unspecified cause**
> Contact dermatitis (occupational) NOS
> Contact eczema (occupational) NOS

**L26**   **Exfoliative dermatitis**
> Hebra's pityriasis
>
> **EXCLUDES 1**   Ritter's disease (L00)

✓4ᵗʰ **L27**   **Dermatitis due to substances taken internally**

> **EXCLUDES 1**   allergy NOS (T78.40)
>
> **EXCLUDES 2**   adverse food reaction, except dermatitis (T78.0-T78.1)
> contact dermatitis (L23-L25)
> drug photoallergic response (L56.1)
> drug phototoxic response (L56.0)
> urticaria (L50.-)

**L27.0**   **Generalized skin eruption due to drugs and medicaments taken internally**
> Use additional code for adverse effect, if applicable, to identify drug (T36-T50 with fifth or sixth character 5)

**L27.1**   **Localized skin eruption due to drugs and medicaments taken internally**
> Use additional code for adverse effect, if applicable, to identify drug (T36-T50 with fifth or sixth character 5)

**L27.2**   **Dermatitis due to ingested food**
> **EXCLUDES 2**   dermatitis due to food in contact with skin (L23.6, L24.6, L25.4)

**L27.8**   **Dermatitis due to other substances taken internally**

**L27.9**   **Dermatitis due to unspecified substance taken internally**

✓4ᵗʰ **L28**   **Lichen simplex chronicus and prurigo**

**L28.0**   **Lichen simplex chronicus**
> Circumscribed neurodermatitis
> Lichen NOS

**L28.1**   **Prurigo nodularis**

**L28.2**   **Other prurigo**
> Prurigo NOS      Prurigo mitis
> Prurigo Hebra      Urticaria papulosa

✓4ᵗʰ **L29**   **Pruritus**

> **EXCLUDES 1**   neurotic excoriation (L98.1)
> psychogenic pruritus (F45.8)

**L29.0**   **Pruritus ani**

**L29.1**   **Pruritus scroti**          ♂

**L29.2**   **Pruritus vulvae**          ♀

**L29.3**   **Anogenital pruritus, unspecified**

**L29.8**   **Other pruritus**

Ⓝ Newborn: 0   Ⓟ Pediatric: 0-17   Ⓜ Maternity: 12-55   Ⓐ Adult: 15-124   **MCC** Major CC Condition   **PDxMCC** PDx acts as own MCC   **CC** CC Condition   **PDxCC** PDx acts as own CC

714        ICD-10-CM 2018

**L29.9**   **Pruritus, unspecified**
Itch NOS

✓4th **L30**   **Other and unspecified dermatitis**
> *EXCLUDES 2*   *contact dermatitis (L23-L25)*
> *dry skin dermatitis (L85.3)*
> *small plaque parapsoriasis (L41.3)*
> *stasis dermatitis (I87.2)*

**L30.0**   **Nummular dermatitis**

**L30.1**   **Dyshidrosis [pompholyx]**

**L30.2**   **Cutaneous autosensitization**
Candidid [levurid]
Dermatophytid
Eczematid

**L30.3**   **Infective dermatitis**
Infectious eczematoid dermatitis

**L30.4**   **Erythema intertrigo**

**L30.5**   **Pityriasis alba**

**L30.8**   **Other specified dermatitis**

**L30.9**   **Dermatitis, unspecified**
Eczema NOS

## Papulosquamous disorders (L40-L45)

✓4th **L40**   **Psoriasis**

**L40.0**   **Psoriasis vulgaris**
Nummular psoriasis
Plaque psoriasis

**L40.1**   **Generalized pustular psoriasis**
Impetigo herpetiformis
Von Zumbusch's disease

**L40.2**   **Acrodermatitis continua**

**L40.3**   **Pustulosis palmaris et plantaris**

**L40.4**   **Guttate psoriasis**

✓5th **L40.5**   **Arthropathic psoriasis**

     **L40.50**   **Arthropathic psoriasis, unspecified**   `HCC`

     **L40.51**   **Distal interphalangeal psoriatic arthropathy**   `HCC`

     **L40.52**   **Psoriatic arthritis mutilans**   `HCC`

     **L40.53**   **Psoriatic spondylitis**   `HCC`

     **L40.54**   **Psoriatic juvenile arthropathy**   `HCC`

     **L40.59**   **Other psoriatic arthropathy**   `HCC`

**L40.8**   **Other psoriasis**
Flexural psoriasis

**L40.9**   **Psoriasis, unspecified**

✓4th **L41**   **Parapsoriasis**
> *EXCLUDES 1*   *poikiloderma vasculare atrophicans (L94.5)*

**L41.0**   **Pityriasis lichenoides et varioliformis acuta**
Mucha-Habermann disease

**L41.1**   **Pityriasis lichenoides chronica**

**L41.3**   **Small plaque parapsoriasis**

**L41.4**   **Large plaque parapsoriasis**

**L41.5**   **Retiform parapsoriasis**

**L41.8**   **Other parapsoriasis**

**L41.9**   **Parapsoriasis, unspecified**

**L42**   **Pityriasis rosea**

✓4th **L43**   **Lichen planus**
> *EXCLUDES 1*   *lichen planopilaris (L66.1)*

**L43.0**   **Hypertrophic lichen planus**

**L43.1**   **Bullous lichen planus**

**L43.2**   **Lichenoid drug reaction**
Use additional code for adverse effect, if applicable, to identify drug (T36-T50 with fifth or sixth character 5)

**L43.3**   **Subacute (active) lichen planus**
Lichen planus tropicus

**L43.8**   **Other lichen planus**

**L43.9**   **Lichen planus, unspecified**

✓4th **L44**   **Other papulosquamous disorders**

**L44.0**   **Pityriasis rubra pilaris**

**L44.1**   **Lichen nitidus**
**DEF:** Chronic, inflammatory, asymptomatic skin disorder, characterized by numerous glistening, flat-topped, discrete, skin-colored micropapules, most often on the penis, lower abdomen, inner thighs, wrists, forearms, breasts and buttocks.

**L44.2**   **Lichen striatus**

**L44.3**   **Lichen ruber moniliformis**

**L44.4**   **Infantile papular acrodermatitis [Gianotti-Crosti]**   `P`

**L44.8**   **Other specified papulosquamous disorders**

**L44.9**   **Papulosquamous disorder, unspecified**

**L45**   ***Papulosquamous disorders in diseases classified elsewhere***
Code first underlying disease

## Urticaria and erythema (L49-L54)

> *EXCLUDES 1*   *Lyme disease (A69.2-)*
> *rosacea (L71.-)*

✓4th **L49**   **Exfoliation due to erythematous conditions according to extent of body surface involved**
Code first erythematous condition causing exfoliation, such as:
Ritter's disease (L00)
(Staphylococcal) scalded skin syndrom (L00)
Stevens-Johnson syndrome (L51.1)
Stevens-Johnson syndrome-toxic epidermal necrolysis overlap syndrome (L51.3)
toxic epidermal necrolysis (L51.2)

**L49.0**   **Exfoliation due to erythematous condition involving less than 10 percent of body surface**
Exfoliation due to erythematous condition NOS

**L49.1**   **Exfoliation due to erythematous condition involving 10-19 percent of body surface**

**L49.2**   **Exfoliation due to erythematous condition involving 20-29 percent of body surface**

**L49.3**   **Exfoliation due to erythematous condition involving 30-39 percent of body surface**   `CC`
CC Excl: PDX collection 844

**L49.4**   **Exfoliation due to erythematous condition involving 40-49 percent of body surface**   `CC`
CC Excl: PDX collection 845

**L49.5**   **Exfoliation due to erythematous condition involving 50-59 percent of body surface**   `CC`
CC Excl: PDX collection 846

**L49.6**   **Exfoliation due to erythematous condition involving 60-69 percent of body surface**   `CC`
CC Excl: PDX collection 847

**L49.7**   **Exfoliation due to erythematous condition involving 70-79 percent of body surface**   `CC`
CC Excl: PDX collection 848

**L49.8**   **Exfoliation due to erythematous condition involving 80-89 percent of body surface**   `CC`
CC Excl: PDX collection 849

**L49.9**   **Exfoliation due to erythematous condition involving 90 or more percent of body surface**   `CC`
CC Excl: PDX collection 850

✓4th **L50**   **Urticaria**
> *EXCLUDES 1*   *allergic contact dermatitis (L23.-)*
> *angioneurotic edema (T78.3)*
> *giant urticaria (T78.3)*
> *hereditary angio-edema (D84.1)*
> *Quincke's edema (T78.3)*
> *serum urticaria (T80.6-)*
> *solar urticaria (L56.3)*
> *urticaria neonatorum (P83.8)*
> *urticaria papulosa (L28.2)*
> *urticaria pigmentosa (Q82.2)*

**L50.0**   **Allergic urticaria**

**L50.1**   **Idiopathic urticaria**

**L50.2**   **Urticaria due to cold and heat**
> *EXCLUDES 2* *familial cold urticaria (M04.2)*

**L50.3**   **Dermatographic urticaria**

**L50.4**   **Vibratory urticaria**

**L50.5**   **Cholinergic urticaria**

**L50.6**   **Contact urticaria**

**L50.8**   **Other urticaria**
Chronic urticaria
Recurrent periodic urticaria

**L50.9**   **Urticaria, unspecified**

---

✓ Additional Character Req    ✓x7th Placeholder Alert    Unacceptable PDx    Manifestation    **H1**-**H14** HAC    `HCC` CMS-HCC Condition    *EXCLUDES 1* Not Coded Here    *EXCLUDES 2* Not Included Here

☑4ᵗʰ **L51** **Erythema multiforme**
Use additional code for adverse effect, if applicable, to identify drug (T36-T50 with fifth or sixth character 5)
Use additional code to identify associated manifestations, such as:
arthropathy associated with dermatological disorders (M14.8-)
conjunctival edema (H11.42)
conjunctivitis (H10.22-)
corneal scars and opacities (H17.-)
corneal ulcer (H16.0-)
edema of eyelid (H02.84)
inflammation of eyelid (H01.8)
keratoconjunctivitis sicca (H16.22-)
mechanical lagophthalmos (H02.22-)
stomatitis (K12.-)
symblepharon (H11.23-)
Use additional code to identify percentage of skin exfoliation (L49.-)
**EXCLUDES 1**  *staphylococcal scalded skin syndrome (L00)*
*Ritter's disease (L00)*

**L51.0** **Nonbullous erythema multiforme**

**L51.1** **Stevens-Johnson syndrome**    `CC` `HCC`
CC Excl: PDX collection 843

**L51.2** **Toxic epidermal necrolysis [Lyell]**    `CC` `HCC`
CC Excl: PDX collection 843

**L51.3** **Stevens-Johnson syndrome-toxic epidermal**    `CC` `HCC`
**necrolysis overlap syndrome**
SJS-TEN overlap syndrome
CC Excl: PDX collection 843

**L51.8** **Other erythema multiforme**

**L51.9** **Erythema multiforme, unspecified**
Erythema iris
Erythema multiforme major NOS
Erythema multiforme minor NOS
Herpes iris

**L52** **Erythema nodosum**
**EXCLUDES 1**  *tuberculous erythema nodosum (A18.4)*
**DEF:** A form of panniculitis (inflammation of the fat layer beneath the skin) of particularly women, usually seen as a hypersensitivity reaction to infections, drugs, sarcoidosis, and specific enteropathies; the acute stage is associated with fever, malaise, and arthralgia; the lesions are pink to blue in color as tender nodules and are found on the front of the legs below the knees.

☑4ᵗʰ **L53** **Other erythematous conditions**
**EXCLUDES 1**  *erythema ab igne (L59.0)*
*erythema due to external agents in contact with skin (L23-L25)*
*erythema intertrigo (L30.4)*

CC Excl: For CC codes in category L53: PDX collection 851

**L53.0** **Toxic erythema**    `CC`
Code first poisoning due to drug or toxin, if applicable (T36-T65 with fifth or sixth character 1-4 or 6)
Use additional code for adverse effect, if applicable, to identify drug (T36-T50 with fifth or sixth character 5)
**EXCLUDES 1**  *neonatal erythema toxicum (P83.1)*

**L53.1** **Erythema annulare centrifugum**    `CC`

**L53.2** **Erythema marginatum**    `CC`

**L53.3** **Other chronic figurate erythema**    `CC`

**L53.8** **Other specified erythematous conditions**

**L53.9** **Erythematous condition, unspecified**
Erythema NOS
Erythroderma NOS

**L54** *Erythema in diseases classified elsewhere*
Code first underlying disease

### Radiation-related disorders of the skin and subcutaneous tissue (L55-L59)

☑4ᵗʰ **L55** **Sunburn**
**L55.0** **Sunburn of first degree**
**L55.1** **Sunburn of second degree**
**L55.2** **Sunburn of third degree**
**L55.9** **Sunburn, unspecified**

☑4ᵗʰ **L56** **Other acute skin changes due to ultraviolet radiation**
Use additional code to identify the source of the ultraviolet radiation (W89, X32)

**L56.0** **Drug phototoxic response**
Use additional code for adverse effect, if applicable, to identify drug (T36-T50 with fifth or sixth character 5)

**L56.1** **Drug photoallergic response**
Use additional code for adverse effect, if applicable, to identify drug (T36-T50 with fifth or sixth character 5)

**L56.2** **Photocontact dermatitis [berloque dermatitis]**

**L56.3** **Solar urticaria**

**L56.4** **Polymorphous light eruption**

**L56.5** **Disseminated superficial actinic porokeratosis (DSAP)**
**DEF:** Autosomal dominant skin condition occurring in sun-exposed areas of the skin (particularly the arms and legs); characterized by superficial annular, keratotic, brownish-red spots or thickenings with depressed centers and sharp, ridged borders; may evolve into squamous cell carcinoma.

**L56.8** **Other specified acute skin changes due to ultraviolet radiation**

**L56.9** **Acute skin change due to ultraviolet radiation, unspecified**

☑4ᵗʰ **L57** **Skin changes due to chronic exposure to nonionizing radiation**
Use additional code to identify the source of the ultraviolet radiation ▶(W89)◀

**L57.0** **Actinic keratosis**
Keratosis NOS
Senile keratosis
Solar keratosis

**L57.1** **Actinic reticuloid**

**L57.2** **Cutis rhomboidalis nuchae**

**L57.3** **Poikiloderma of Civatte**

**L57.4** **Cutis laxa senilis**
Elastosis senilis

**L57.5** **Actinic granuloma**

**L57.8** **Other skin changes due to chronic exposure to nonionizing radiation**
Farmer's skin
Sailor's skin
Solar dermatitis

**L57.9** **Skin changes due to chronic exposure to nonionizing radiation, unspecified**

☑4ᵗʰ **L58** **Radiodermatitis**
Use additional code to identify the source of the radiation (W88, W90)

**L58.0** **Acute radiodermatitis**

**L58.1** **Chronic radiodermatitis**

**L58.9** **Radiodermatitis, unspecified**

☑4ᵗʰ **L59** **Other disorders of skin and subcutaneous tissue related to radiation**

**L59.0** **Erythema ab igne [dermatitis ab igne]**

**L59.8** **Other specified disorders of the skin and subcutaneous tissue related to radiation**
AHA: 2017, 1Q, 33

**L59.9** **Disorder of the skin and subcutaneous tissue related to radiation, unspecified**

### Disorders of skin appendages (L60-L75)
**EXCLUDES 1**  *congenital malformations of integument (Q84.-)*

☑4ᵗʰ **L60** **Nail disorders**
**EXCLUDES 2**  *clubbing of nails (R68.3)*
*onychia and paronychia (L03.0-)*

**L60.0** **Ingrowing nail**

**Nail Disorders**

Normal

Koilonychia

Beau's Lines

Ⓝ Newborn: 0    Ⓟ Pediatric: 0-17    Ⓜ Maternity: 12-55    Ⓐ Adult: 15-124    `MCC` Major CC Condition    `PDxMCC` PDx acts as own MCC    `CC` CC Condition    `PDxCC` PDx acts as own CC

716    ICD-10-CM 2018

L60.1   **Onycholysis**

L60.2   **Onychogryphosis**

L60.3   **Nail dystrophy**

L60.4   **Beau's lines**

L60.5   **Yellow nail syndrome**

L60.8   **Other nail disorders**

L60.9   **Nail disorder, unspecified**

### L62   *Nail disorders in diseases classified elsewhere*

Code first underlying disease, such as:
pachydermoperiostosis (M89.4-)

### ✓4ᵗʰ L63   Alopecia areata

L63.0   **Alopecia (capitis) totalis**

L63.1   **Alopecia universalis**

L63.2   **Ophiasis**

L63.8   **Other alopecia areata**

L63.9   **Alopecia areata, unspecified**

### ✓4ᵗʰ L64   Androgenic alopecia

**INCLUDES**   male-pattern baldness

L64.0   **Drug-induced androgenic alopecia**

Use additional code for adverse effect, if applicable, to identify drug (T36-T50 with fifth or sixth character 5)

L64.8   **Other androgenic alopecia**

L64.9   **Androgenic alopecia, unspecified**

### ✓4ᵗʰ L65   Other nonscarring hair loss

Use additional code for adverse effect, if applicable, to identify drug (T36-T50 with fifth or sixth character 5)

**EXCLUDES 1**   *trichotillomania (F63.3)*

L65.0   **Telogen effluvium**

**DEF:** A form of nonscarring alopecia characterized by shedding of hair from premature telogen development in follicles due to stress, including shock, childbirth, surgery, drugs, or weight loss.

L65.1   **Anagen effluvium**

L65.2   **Alopecia mucinosa**

L65.8   **Other specified nonscarring hair loss**

L65.9   **Nonscarring hair loss, unspecified**

Alopecia NOS

### ✓4ᵗʰ L66   Cicatricial alopecia [scarring hair loss]

L66.0   **Pseudopelade**

L66.1   **Lichen planopilaris**

Follicular lichen planus

L66.2   **Folliculitis decalvans**

L66.3   **Perifolliculitis capitis abscedens**

L66.4   **Folliculitis ulerythematosa reticulata**

L66.8   **Other cicatricial alopecia**

**AHA:** 2015, 1Q, 19

L66.9   **Cicatricial alopecia, unspecified**

### ✓4ᵗʰ L67   Hair color and hair shaft abnormalities

**EXCLUDES 1**   *monilethrix (Q84.1)*
*pili annulati (Q84.1)*
*telogen effluvium (L65.0)*

L67.0   **Trichorrhexis nodosa**

L67.1   **Variations in hair color**

Canities
Greyness, hair (premature)
Heterochromia of hair
Poliosis circumscripta, acquired
Poliosis NOS

L67.8   **Other hair color and hair shaft abnormalities**

Fragilitas crinium

L67.9   **Hair color and hair shaft abnormality, unspecified**

### ✓4ᵗʰ L68   Hypertrichosis

**INCLUDES**   excess hair
**EXCLUDES 1**   *congenital hypertrichosis (Q84.2)*
*persistent lanugo (Q84.2)*

L68.0   **Hirsutism**

L68.1   **Acquired hypertrichosis lanuginosa**

L68.2   **Localized hypertrichosis**

L68.3   **Polytrichia**

L68.8   **Other hypertrichosis**

L68.9   **Hypertrichosis, unspecified**

### ✓4ᵗʰ L70   Acne

**EXCLUDES 2**   *acne keloid (L73.0)*

L70.0   **Acne vulgaris**

L70.1   **Acne conglobata**

L70.2   **Acne varioliformis**

Acne necrotica miliaris

**DEF:** Rare form of acne characterized by development of persistent brown papulo-pustules followed by scar formation; usually on the brow and temporoparietal part of the scalp.

L70.3   **Acne tropica**

L70.4   **Infantile acne**     P

L70.5   **Acné excoriée**

Acné excoriée des jeunes filles
Picker's acne

L70.8   **Other acne**

L70.9   **Acne, unspecified**

### ✓4ᵗʰ L71   Rosacea

Use additional code for adverse effect, if applicable, to identify drug (T36-T50 with fifth or sixth character 5)

L71.0   **Perioral dermatitis**

L71.1   **Rhinophyma**

L71.8   **Other rosacea**

L71.9   **Rosacea, unspecified**

### ✓4ᵗʰ L72   Follicular cysts of skin and subcutaneous tissue

L72.0   **Epidermal cyst**

✓5ᵗʰ L72.1   **Pilar and trichodermal cyst**

L72.11   **Pilar cyst**

L72.12   **Trichodermal cyst**

Trichilemmal (proliferating) cyst

L72.2   **Steatocystoma multiplex**

L72.3   **Sebaceous cyst**

**EXCLUDES 2**   *pilar cyst (L72.11)*
*trichilemmal (proliferating) cyst (L72.12)*

L72.8   **Other follicular cysts of the skin and subcutaneous tissue**

L72.9   **Follicular cyst of the skin and subcutaneous tissue, unspecified**

### ✓4ᵗʰ L73   Other follicular disorders

L73.0   **Acne keloid**

L73.1   **Pseudofolliculitis barbae**

L73.2   **Hidradenitis suppurativa**

L73.8   **Other specified follicular disorders**

Sycosis barbae

L73.9   **Follicular disorder, unspecified**

### ✓4ᵗʰ L74   Eccrine sweat disorders

**EXCLUDES 2**   *generalized hyperhidrosis (R61)*

L74.0   **Miliaria rubra**

L74.1   **Miliaria crystallina**

L74.2   **Miliaria profunda**

Miliaria tropicalis

L74.3   **Miliaria, unspecified**

L74.4   **Anhidrosis**

Hypohidrosis

✓5ᵗʰ L74.5   **Focal hyperhidrosis**

✓6ᵗʰ L74.51   **Primary focal hyperhidrosis**

L74.510   **Primary focal hyperhidrosis, axilla**

L74.511   **Primary focal hyperhidrosis, face**

L74.512   **Primary focal hyperhidrosis, palms**

L74.513   **Primary focal hyperhidrosis, soles**

L74.519   **Primary focal hyperhidrosis, unspecified**

L74.52   **Secondary focal hyperhidrosis**

Frey's syndrome

L74.8   **Other eccrine sweat disorders**

L74.9   **Eccrine sweat disorder, unspecified**

Sweat gland disorder NOS

### ✓4ᵗʰ L75   Apocrine sweat disorders

**EXCLUDES 1**   *dyshidrosis (L30.1)*
*hidradenitis suppurativa (L73.2)*

L75.0   **Bromhidrosis**

L75.1   **Chromhidrosis**

✓ Additional Character Req   ✓x7ᵗʰ Placeholder Alert   Unacceptable PDx   Manifestation   **H1 - H14** HAC   **HCC** CMS-HCC Condition   **EXCLUDES 1** Not Coded Here   **EXCLUDES 2** Not Included Here

ICD-10-CM 2018                                                       **717**

**L75.2** **Apocrine miliaria**
Fox-Fordyce disease
**DEF:** Chronic, usually pruritic disease evidenced by small follicular papular eruptions, especially in the axillary and pubic areas; develops from the closure and rupture of the affected apocrine glands' intraepidermal portion of the ducts.

**L75.8** **Other apocrine sweat disorders**

**L75.9** **Apocrine sweat disorder, unspecified**

## Intraoperative and postprocedural complications of skin and subcutaneous tissue (L76)

☑4th **L76** **Intraoperative and postprocedural complications of skin and subcutaneous tissue**

> **CC Excl:** For CC codes in category L76, unless otherwise noted: PDX collection 852

☑5th **L76.0** **Intraoperative hemorrhage and hematoma of skin and subcutaneous tissue complicating a procedure**
> **EXCLUDES 1** *intraoperative hemorrhage and hematoma of skin and subcutaneous tissue due to accidental puncture and laceration during a procedure (L76.1-)*

**L76.01** **Intraoperative hemorrhage and hematoma of skin and subcutaneous tissue complicating a dermatologic procedure** `CC`

**L76.02** **Intraoperative hemorrhage and hematoma of skin and subcutaneous tissue complicating other procedure** `CC`

☑5th **L76.1** **Accidental puncture and laceration of skin and subcutaneous tissue during a procedure**

**L76.11** **Accidental puncture and laceration of skin and subcutaneous tissue during a dermatologic procedure** `CC`
**CC Excl:** PDX collection 509

**L76.12** **Accidental puncture and laceration of skin and subcutaneous tissue during other procedure** `CC`
**CC Excl:** PDX collection 509

☑5th **L76.2** **Postprocedural hemorrhage of skin and subcutaneous tissue following a procedure**

**L76.21** **Postprocedural hemorrhage of skin and subcutaneous tissue following a dermatologic procedure** `CC`

**L76.22** **Postprocedural hemorrhage of skin and subcutaneous tissue following other procedure** `CC`

☑5th **L76.3** **Postprocedural hematoma and seroma of skin and subcutaneous tissue following a procedure**

**L76.31** **Postprocedural hematoma of skin and subcutaneous tissue following a dermatologic procedure** `CC`

**L76.32** **Postprocedural hematoma of skin and subcutaneous tissue following other procedure** `CC`

**L76.33** **Postprocedural seroma of skin and subcutaneous tissue following a dermatologic procedure** `CC`

**L76.34** **Postprocedural seroma of skin and subcutaneous tissue following other procedure** `CC`

☑5th **L76.8** **Other intraoperative and postprocedural complications of skin and subcutaneous tissue**
> Use additional code, if applicable, to further specify disorder

**L76.81** **Other intraoperative complications of skin and subcutaneous tissue**

**L76.82** **Other postprocedural complications of skin and subcutaneous tissue**

## Other disorders of the skin and subcutaneous tissue (L80-L99)

**L80** **Vitiligo**
> **EXCLUDES 2** *vitiligo of eyelids (H02.73-)*
> *vitiligo of vulva (N90.89)*
**DEF:** Persistent, progressive development of nonpigmented white patches on otherwise normal skin.

☑4th **L81** **Other disorders of pigmentation**
> **EXCLUDES 1** *birthmark NOS (Q82.5)*
> *Peutz-Jeghers syndrome (Q85.8)*
> **EXCLUDES 2** *nevus—see Alphabetical Index*

**L81.0** **Postinflammatory hyperpigmentation**

**L81.1** **Chloasma**

**L81.2** **Freckles**

**L81.3** **Café au lait spots**

**L81.4** **Other melanin hyperpigmentation**
Lentigo

**L81.5** **Leukoderma, not elsewhere classified**

**L81.6** **Other disorders of diminished melanin formation**

**L81.7** **Pigmented purpuric dermatosis**
Angioma serpiginosum

**L81.8** **Other specified disorders of pigmentation**
Iron pigmentation
Tattoo pigmentation

**L81.9** **Disorder of pigmentation, unspecified**

☑4th **L82** **Seborrheic keratosis**
> **INCLUDES** basal cell papilloma
> dermatosis papulosa nigra
> Leser-Trélat disease
> **EXCLUDES 2** *seborrheic dermatitis (L21.-)*

**L82.0** **Inflamed seborrheic keratosis**

**L82.1** **Other seborrheic keratosis**
Seborrheic keratosis NOS

**L83** **Acanthosis nigricans**
Confluent and reticulated papillomatosis
**DEF:** Diffuse, velvety hyperplasia of the spinous skin layer of the axilla and other body folds marked by gray, brown, or black pigmentation; in adult form often associated with malignant acanthosis nigricans in a benign, nevoid form relatively generalized.

**L84** **Corns and callosities**
Callus     Clavus

☑4th **L85** **Other epidermal thickening**
> **EXCLUDES 2** *hypertrophic disorders of the skin (L91.-)*

**L85.0** **Acquired ichthyosis**
> **EXCLUDES 1** *congenital ichthyosis (Q80.-)*

**L85.1** **Acquired keratosis [keratoderma] palmaris et plantaris**
> **EXCLUDES 1** *inherited keratosis palmaris et plantaris (Q82.8)*

**L85.2** **Keratosis punctata (palmaris et plantaris)**

**L85.3** **Xerosis cutis**
Dry skin dermatitis

**L85.8** **Other specified epidermal thickening**
Cutaneous horn

**L85.9** **Epidermal thickening, unspecified**

*L86* *Keratoderma in diseases classified elsewhere*
> Code first underlying disease, such as:
> Reiter's disease (M02.3-)
> **EXCLUDES 1** *gonococcal keratoderma (A54.89)*
> *gonococcal keratosis (A54.89)*
> *keratoderma due to vitamin A deficiency (E50.8)*
> *keratosis due to vitamin A deficiency (E50.8)*
> *xeroderma due to vitamin A deficiency (E50.8)*

☑4th **L87** **Transepidermal elimination disorders**
> **EXCLUDES 1** *granuloma annulare (perforating) (L92.0)*

**L87.0** **Keratosis follicularis et parafollicularis in cutem penetrans**
Hyperkeratosis follicularis penetrans
Kyrle disease

**L87.1** **Reactive perforating collagenosis**

**L87.2** **Elastosis perforans serpiginosa**

**L87.8** **Other transepidermal elimination disorders**

**L87.9** **Transepidermal elimination disorder, unspecified**

**L88** **Pyoderma gangrenosum** `CC`
Phagedenic pyoderma
> **EXCLUDES 1** *dermatitis gangrenosa (L08.0)*
**DEF:** Persistent debilitating skin disease characterized by irregular, boggy, blue-red ulcerations, with central healing and undermined edges.
**CC Excl:** PDX collection 853

---

**N** Newborn: 0  **P** Pediatric: 0-17  **M** Maternity: 12-55  **A** Adult: 15-124  **MCC** Major CC Condition  **PDxMCC** PDx acts as own MCC  **CC** CC Condition  **PDxCC** PDx acts as own CC

**718**                                                                                                        ICD-10-CM 2018

## Four Stages of Pressure Ulcer

Epidermis
Dermis

**Stage 1**
Persistent focal erythema

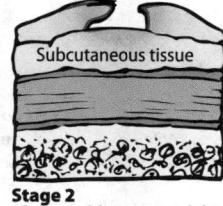

Subcutaneous tissue

**Stage 2**
Abrasion, blister, partial thickness skin loss involving epidermis and/or dermis

Superficial fascia
Muscle

**Stage 3**
Full thickness skin loss involving damage or necrosis of subcutaneous tissue

Deep fascia
Bone

**Stage 4**
Necrosis of soft tissues through to underlying muscle, tendon, or bone

### ✓4th L89  Pressure ulcer

INCLUDES
bed sore
decubitus ulcer
plaster ulcer
pressure area
pressure sore

Code first any associated gangrene (I96)

EXCLUDES 2 *decubitus (trophic) ulcer of cervix (uteri) (N86)*
*diabetic ulcers (E08.621, E08.622, E09.621, E09.622, E10.621, E10.622, E11.621, E11.622, E13.621, E13.622)*
*non-pressure chronic ulcer of skin (L97.-)*
*skin infections (L00-L08)*
*varicose ulcer (I83.0, I83.2)*

**AHA:** 2017, 1Q, 49; 2016, 4Q, 143

**CC Excl: For MCC codes in category L89:** PDX collection 854

### ✓5th L89.0  Pressure ulcer of elbow

#### ✓6th L89.00  Pressure ulcer of unspecified elbow

**L89.000  Pressure ulcer of unspecified elbow, unstageable**  HCC

**L89.001  Pressure ulcer of unspecified elbow, stage 1**
Healing pressure ulcer of unspecified elbow, stage 1
Pressure pre-ulcer skin changes limited to persistent focal edema, unspecified elbow

**L89.002  Pressure ulcer of unspecified elbow, stage 2**
Healing pressure ulcer of unspecified elbow, stage 2
Pressure ulcer with abrasion, blister, partial thickness skin loss involving epidermis and/or dermis, unspecified elbow

**L89.003  Pressure ulcer of unspecified elbow, stage 3**  PDx MCC  MCC  H4  HCC
Healing pressure ulcer of unspecified elbow, stage 3
Pressure ulcer with full thickness skin loss involving damage or necrosis of subcutaneous tissue, unspecified elbow

**L89.004  Pressure ulcer of unspecified elbow, stage 4**  PDx MCC  MCC  H4  HCC
Healing pressure ulcer of unspecified elbow, stage 4
Pressure ulcer with necrosis of soft tissues through to underlying muscle, tendon, or bone, unspecified elbow

**L89.009  Pressure ulcer of unspecified elbow, unspecified stage**
Healing pressure ulcer of elbow NOS
Healing pressure ulcer of unspecified elbow, unspecified stage

#### ✓6th L89.01  Pressure ulcer of right elbow

**L89.010  Pressure ulcer of right elbow, unstageable**  HCC

**L89.011  Pressure ulcer of right elbow, stage 1**
Healing pressure ulcer of right elbow, stage 1
Pressure pre-ulcer skin changes limited to persistent focal edema, right elbow

**L89.012  Pressure ulcer of right elbow, stage 2**
Healing pressure ulcer of right elbow, stage 2
Pressure ulcer with abrasion, blister, partial thickness skin loss involving epidermis and/or dermis, right elbow

**L89.013  Pressure ulcer of right elbow, stage 3**  PDx MCC  MCC  H4  HCC
Healing pressure ulcer of right elbow, stage 3
Pressure ulcer with full thickness skin loss involving damage or necrosis of subcutaneous tissue, right elbow

**L89.014  Pressure ulcer of right elbow, stage 4**  PDx MCC  MCC  H4  HCC
Healing pressure ulcer of right elbow, stage 4
Pressure ulcer with necrosis of soft tissues through to underlying muscle, tendon, or bone, right elbow

**L89.019  Pressure ulcer of right elbow, unspecified stage**
Healing pressure right of elbow NOS
▶Healing pressure ulcer of right elbow, unspecified stage◀

#### ✓6th L89.02  Pressure ulcer of left elbow

**L89.020  Pressure ulcer of left elbow, unstageable**  HCC

**L89.021  Pressure ulcer of left elbow, stage 1**
Healing pressure ulcer of left elbow, stage 1
Pressure pre-ulcer skin changes limited to persistent focal edema, left elbow

**L89.022  Pressure ulcer of left elbow, stage 2**
Healing pressure ulcer of left elbow, stage 2
Pressure ulcer with abrasion, blister, partial thickness skin loss involving epidermis and/or dermis, left elbow

**L89.023  Pressure ulcer of left elbow, stage 3**  PDx MCC  MCC  H4  HCC
Healing pressure ulcer of left elbow, stage 3
Pressure ulcer with full thickness skin loss involving damage or necrosis of subcutaneous tissue, left elbow

**L89.024  Pressure ulcer of left elbow, stage 4**  PDx MCC  MCC  H4  HCC
Healing pressure ulcer of left elbow, stage 4
Pressure ulcer with necrosis of soft tissues through to underlying muscle, tendon, or bone, left elbow

**L89.029  Pressure ulcer of left elbow, unspecified stage**
Healing pressure ulcer of left of elbow NOS
▶Healing pressure ulcer of left elbow, unspecified stage◀

### ✓5th L89.1  Pressure ulcer of back

#### ✓6th L89.10  Pressure ulcer of unspecified part of back

**L89.100  Pressure ulcer of unspecified part of back, unstageable**  HCC

**L89.101  Pressure ulcer of unspecified part of back, stage 1**
Healing pressure ulcer of unspecified part of back, stage 1
Pressure pre-ulcer skin changes limited to persistent focal edema, unspecified part of back

**L89.102  Pressure ulcer of unspecified part of back, stage 2**
Healing pressure ulcer of unspecified part of back, stage 2
Pressure ulcer with abrasion, blister, partial thickness skin loss involving epidermis and/or dermis, unspecified part of back

✓ Additional Character Req  √x 7th Placeholder Alert  Unacceptable PDx  Manifestation  H1 - H14 HAC  HCC CMS-HCC Condition  EXCLUDES 1 Not Coded Here  EXCLUDES 2 Not Included Here

ICD-10-CM 2018  719

**Chapter 12. Diseases of the Skin and Subcutaneous Tissue**

**L89.1Ø3** **Pressure ulcer of unspecified part of back, stage 3** `PDxMCC` `MCC` `H4` `HCC`
　　Healing pressure ulcer of unspecified part of back, stage 3
　　Pressure ulcer with full thickness skin loss involving damage or necrosis of subcutaneous tissue, unspecified part of back

**L89.1Ø4** **Pressure ulcer of unspecified part of back, stage 4** `PDxMCC` `MCC` `H4` `HCC`
　　Healing pressure ulcer of unspecified part of back, stage 4
　　Pressure ulcer with necrosis of soft tissues through to underlying muscle, tendon, or bone, unspecified part of back

**L89.1Ø9** **Pressure ulcer of unspecified part of back, unspecified stage**
　　Healing pressure ulcer of unspecified part of back NOS
　　Healing pressure ulcer of unspecified part of back, unspecified stage

✓6ᵗʰ **L89.11** **Pressure ulcer of right upper back**
　Pressure ulcer of right shoulder blade

**L89.11Ø** **Pressure ulcer of right upper back, unstageable** `HCC`

**L89.111** **Pressure ulcer of right upper back, stage 1**
　　Healing pressure ulcer of right upper back, stage 1
　　Pressure pre-ulcer skin changes limited to persistent focal edema, right upper back

**L89.112** **Pressure ulcer of right upper back, stage 2**
　　Healing pressure ulcer of right upper back, stage 2
　　Pressure ulcer with abrasion, blister, partial thickness skin loss involving epidermis and/or dermis, right upper back

**L89.113** **Pressure ulcer of right upper back, stage 3** `PDxMCC` `MCC` `H4` `HCC`
　　Healing pressure ulcer of right upper back, stage 3
　　Pressure ulcer with full thickness skin loss involving damage or necrosis of subcutaneous tissue, right upper back

**L89.114** **Pressure ulcer of right upper back, stage 4** `PDxMCC` `MCC` `H4` `HCC`
　　Healing pressure ulcer of right upper back, stage 4
　　Pressure ulcer with necrosis of soft tissues through to underlying muscle, tendon, or bone, right upper back

**L89.119** **Pressure ulcer of right upper back, unspecified stage**
　　Healing pressure ulcer of right upper back NOS
　　Healing pressure ulcer of right upper back, unspecified stage

✓6ᵗʰ **L89.12** **Pressure ulcer of left upper back**
　Pressure ulcer of left shoulder blade

**L89.12Ø** **Pressure ulcer of left upper back, unstageable** `HCC`

**L89.121** **Pressure ulcer of left upper back, stage 1**
　　Healing pressure ulcer of left upper back, stage 1
　　Pressure pre-ulcer skin changes limited to persistent focal edema, left upper back

**L89.122** **Pressure ulcer of left upper back, stage 2**
　　Healing pressure ulcer of left upper back, stage 2
　　Pressure ulcer with abrasion, blister, partial thickness skin loss involving epidermis and/or dermis, left upper back

**L89.123** **Pressure ulcer of left upper back, stage 3** `PDxMCC` `MCC` `H4` `HCC`
　　Healing pressure ulcer of left upper back, stage 3
　　Pressure ulcer with full thickness skin loss involving damage or necrosis of subcutaneous tissue, left upper back

**L89.124** **Pressure ulcer of left upper back, stage 4** `PDxMCC` `MCC` `H4` `HCC`
　　Healing pressure ulcer of left upper back, stage 4
　　Pressure ulcer with necrosis of soft tissues through to underlying muscle, tendon, or bone, left upper back

**L89.129** **Pressure ulcer of left upper back, unspecified stage**
　　Healing pressure ulcer of left upper back NOS
　　Healing pressure ulcer of left upper back, unspecified stage

✓6ᵗʰ **L89.13** **Pressure ulcer of right lower back**

**L89.13Ø** **Pressure ulcer of right lower back, unstageable** `HCC`

**L89.131** **Pressure ulcer of right lower back, stage 1**
　　Healing pressure ulcer of right lower back, stage 1
　　Pressure pre-ulcer skin changes limited to persistent focal edema, right lower back

**L89.132** **Pressure ulcer of right lower back, stage 2**
　　Healing pressure ulcer of right lower back, stage 2
　　Pressure ulcer with abrasion, blister, partial thickness skin loss involving epidermis and/or dermis, right lower back

**L89.133** **Pressure ulcer of right lower back, stage 3** `PDxMCC` `MCC` `H4` `HCC`
　　Healing pressure ulcer of right lower back, stage 3
　　Pressure ulcer with full thickness skin loss involving damage or necrosis of subcutaneous tissue, right lower back

**L89.134** **Pressure ulcer of right lower back, stage 4** `PDxMCC` `MCC` `H4` `HCC`
　　Healing pressure ulcer of right lower back, stage 4
　　Pressure ulcer with necrosis of soft tissues through to underlying muscle, tendon, or bone, right lower back

**L89.139** **Pressure ulcer of right lower back, unspecified stage**
　　Healing pressure ulcer of right lower back NOS
　　Healing pressure ulcer of right lower back, unspecified stage

✓6ᵗʰ **L89.14** **Pressure ulcer of left lower back**

**L89.14Ø** **Pressure ulcer of left lower back, unstageable** `HCC`

**L89.141** **Pressure ulcer of left lower back, stage 1**
　　Healing pressure ulcer of left lower back, stage 1
　　Pressure pre-ulcer skin changes limited to persistent focal edema, left lower back

**L89.142** **Pressure ulcer of left lower back, stage 2**
　　Healing pressure ulcer of left lower back, stage 2
　　Pressure ulcer with abrasion, blister, partial thickness skin loss involving epidermis and/or dermis, left lower back

**L89.143** **Pressure ulcer of left lower back, stage 3** `PDxMCC` `MCC` `H4` `HCC`
　　Healing pressure ulcer of left lower back, stage 3
　　Pressure ulcer with full thickness skin loss involving damage or necrosis of subcutaneous tissue, left lower back

**L89.144** **Pressure ulcer of left lower back, stage 4** `PDxMCC` `MCC` `H4` `HCC`
　　Healing pressure ulcer of left lower back, stage 4
　　Pressure ulcer with necrosis of soft tissues through to underlying muscle, tendon, or bone, left lower back

**L89.149** **Pressure ulcer of left lower back, unspecified stage**
　　Healing pressure ulcer of left lower back NOS
　　Healing pressure ulcer of left lower back, unspecified stage

Ⓝ Newborn: 0　Ⓟ Pediatric: 0-17　Ⓜ Maternity: 12-55　Ⓐ Adult: 15-124　`MCC` Major CC Condition　`PDxMCC` PDx acts as own MCC　`CC` CC Condition　`PDxCC` PDx acts as own CC

**720**
ICD-10-CM 2018

✓6ᵗʰ **L89.15** **Pressure ulcer of** sacral region
     Pressure ulcer of coccyx
     Pressure ulcer of tailbone

**L89.150** **Pressure ulcer of sacral region,** HCC
     **unstageable**

**L89.151** **Pressure ulcer of sacral region,** stage 1
     Healing pressure ulcer of sacral region,
       stage 1
     Pressure pre-ulcer skin changes limited to
       persistent focal edema, sacral region

**L89.152** **Pressure ulcer of sacral region,** stage 2
     Healing pressure ulcer of sacral region,
       stage 2
     Pressure ulcer with abrasion, blister, partial
       thickness skin loss involving epidermis
       and/or dermis, sacral region

**L89.153** **Pressure ulcer of sacral** PDxMCC MCC H4 HCC
     **region, stage 3**
     Healing pressure ulcer of sacral region,
       stage 3
     Pressure ulcer with full thickness skin loss
       involving damage or necrosis of
       subcutaneous tissue, sacral region

**L89.154** **Pressure ulcer of sacral** PDxMCC MCC H4 HCC
     **region, stage 4**
     Healing pressure ulcer of sacral region,
       stage 4
     Pressure ulcer with necrosis of soft tissues
       through to underlying muscle,
       tendon, or bone, sacral region

**L89.159** **Pressure ulcer of sacral region,**
     **unspecified stage**
     Healing pressure ulcer of sacral region NOS
     Healing pressure ulcer of sacral region,
       unspecified stage

✓5ᵗʰ **L89.2** **Pressure ulcer of** hip

✓6ᵗʰ **L89.20** **Pressure ulcer of** unspecified hip

**L89.200** **Pressure ulcer of unspecified hip,** HCC
     **unstageable**

**L89.201** **Pressure ulcer of unspecified hip,** stage 1
     Healing pressure ulcer of unspecified hip
       back, stage 1
     Pressure pre-ulcer skin changes limited to
       persistent focal edema, unspecified hip

**L89.202** **Pressure ulcer of unspecified hip,** stage 2
     Healing pressure ulcer of unspecified hip,
       stage 2
     Pressure ulcer with abrasion, blister, partial
       thickness skin loss involving epidermis
       and/or dermis, unspecified hip

**L89.203** **Pressure ulcer of** PDxMCC MCC H4 HCC
     **unspecified hip, stage 3**
     Healing pressure ulcer of unspecified hip,
       stage 3
     Pressure ulcer with full thickness skin loss
       involving damage or necrosis of
       subcutaneous tissue, unspecified hip

**L89.204** **Pressure ulcer of** PDxMCC MCC H4 HCC
     **unspecified hip, stage 4**
     Healing pressure ulcer of unspecified hip,
       stage 4
     Pressure ulcer with necrosis of soft tissues
       through to underlying muscle,
       tendon, or bone, unspecified hip

**L89.209** **Pressure ulcer of unspecified hip,**
     **unspecified stage**
     Healing pressure ulcer of unspecified hip
       NOS
     Healing pressure ulcer of unspecified hip,
       unspecified stage

✓6ᵗʰ **L89.21** **Pressure ulcer of** right hip

**L89.210** **Pressure ulcer of right hip,** HCC
     **unstageable**

**L89.211** **Pressure ulcer of right hip,** stage 1
     Healing pressure ulcer of right hip back,
       stage 1
     Pressure pre-ulcer skin changes limited to
       persistent focal edema, right hip

**L89.212** **Pressure ulcer of right hip,** stage 2
     Healing pressure ulcer of right hip, stage 2
     Pressure ulcer with abrasion, blister, partial
       thickness skin loss involving epidermis
       and/or dermis, right hip

**L89.213** **Pressure ulcer of right** PDxMCC MCC H4 HCC
     **hip, stage 3**
     Healing pressure ulcer of right hip, stage 3
     Pressure ulcer with full thickness skin loss
       involving damage or necrosis of
       subcutaneous tissue, right hip

**L89.214** **Pressure ulcer of right** PDxMCC MCC H4 HCC
     **hip, stage 4**
     Healing pressure ulcer of right hip, stage 4
     Pressure ulcer with necrosis of soft tissues
       through to underlying muscle,
       tendon, or bone, right hip

**L89.219** **Pressure ulcer of right hip,** unspecified
     stage
     Healing pressure ulcer of right hip NOS
     Healing pressure ulcer of right hip,
       unspecified stage

✓6ᵗʰ **L89.22** **Pressure ulcer of** left hip

**L89.220** **Pressure ulcer of left hip,** unstageable HCC

**L89.221** **Pressure ulcer of left hip,** stage 1
     Healing pressure ulcer of left hip back,
       stage 1
     Pressure pre-ulcer skin changes limited to
       persistent focal edema, left hip

**L89.222** **Pressure ulcer of left hip,** stage 2
     Healing pressure ulcer of left hip, stage 2
     Pressure ulcer with abrasion, blister, partial
       thickness skin loss involving epidermis
       and/or dermis, left hip

**L89.223** **Pressure ulcer of left** PDxMCC MCC H4 HCC
     **hip, stage 3**
     Healing pressure ulcer of left hip, stage 3
     Pressure ulcer with full thickness skin loss
       involving damage or necrosis of
       subcutaneous tissue, left hip

**L89.224** **Pressure ulcer of left** PDxMCC MCC H4 HCC
     **hip, stage 4**
     Healing pressure ulcer of left hip, stage 4
     Pressure ulcer with necrosis of soft tissues
       through to underlying muscle,
       tendon, or bone, left hip

**L89.229** **Pressure ulcer of left hip,** unspecified
     stage
     Healing pressure ulcer of left hip NOS
     Healing pressure ulcer of left hip,
       unspecified stage

✓5ᵗʰ **L89.3** **Pressure ulcer of** buttock

✓6ᵗʰ **L89.30** **Pressure ulcer of** unspecified buttock

**L89.300** **Pressure ulcer of unspecified buttock,** HCC
     **unstageable**

**L89.301** **Pressure ulcer of unspecified buttock,**
     **stage 1**
     Healing pressure ulcer of unspecified
       buttock, stage 1
     Pressure pre-ulcer skin changes limited to
       persistent focal edema, unspecified
       buttock

**L89.302** **Pressure ulcer of unspecified buttock,**
     **stage 2**
     Healing pressure ulcer of unspecified
       buttock, stage 2
     Pressure ulcer with abrasion, blister, partial
       thickness skin loss involving epidermis
       and/or dermis, unspecified buttock

**L89.303** **Pressure ulcer of** PDxMCC MCC H4 HCC
     **unspecified buttock, stage 3**
     Healing pressure ulcer of unspecified
       buttock, stage 3
     Pressure ulcer with full thickness skin loss
       involving damage or necrosis of
       subcutaneous tissue, unspecified
       buttock

**L89.304** **Pressure ulcer of** PDxMCC MCC H4 HCC
     **unspecified buttock, stage 4**
     Healing pressure ulcer of unspecified
       buttock, stage 4
     Pressure ulcer with necrosis of soft tissues
       through to underlying muscle,
       tendon, or bone, unspecified buttock

---

✔ Additional Character Req    ✔x7ᵗʰ Placeholder Alert    Unacceptable PDx    Manifestation    **H1**-**H14** HAC    HCC CMS-HCC Condition    *EXCLUDES 1* Not Coded Here    *EXCLUDES 2* Not Included Here

**Chapter 12. Diseases of the Skin and Subcutaneous Tissue**

    **L89.3Ø9**   **Pressure ulcer of unspecified buttock, unspecified stage**
         Healing pressure ulcer of unspecified buttock NOS
         Healing pressure ulcer of unspecified buttock, unspecified stage

✓6ᵗʰ  **L89.31**   **Pressure ulcer of** right buttock
    **L89.31Ø**   **Pressure ulcer of right buttock,**   HCC
         **unstageable**
    **L89.311**   **Pressure ulcer of right buttock,** stage 1
         Healing pressure ulcer of right buttock, stage 1
         Pressure pre-ulcer skin changes limited to persistent focal edema, right buttock
    **L89.312**   **Pressure ulcer of right buttock,** stage 2
         Healing pressure ulcer of right buttock, stage 2
         Pressure ulcer with abrasion, blister, partial thickness skin loss involving epidermis and/or dermis, right buttock
    **L89.313**   **Pressure ulcer of right buttock, unspecified** stage 3   PDxMCC MCC H4 HCC
         Healing pressure ulcer of right buttock, stage 3
         Pressure ulcer with full thickness skin loss involving damage or necrosis of subcutaneous tissue, right buttock
    **L89.314**   **Pressure ulcer of right buttock, unspecified** stage 4   PDxMCC MCC H4 HCC
         Healing pressure ulcer of right buttock, stage 4
         Pressure ulcer with necrosis of soft tissues through to underlying muscle, tendon, or bone, right buttock
    **L89.319**   **Pressure ulcer of right buttock, unspecified stage**
         Healing pressure ulcer of right buttock NOS
         Healing pressure ulcer of right buttock, unspecified stage

✓6ᵗʰ  **L89.32**   **Pressure ulcer of** left buttock
    **L89.32Ø**   **Pressure ulcer of left buttock,**   HCC
         **unstageable**
    **L89.321**   **Pressure ulcer of left buttock,** stage 1
         Healing pressure ulcer of left buttock, stage 1
         Pressure pre-ulcer skin changes limited to persistent focal edema, left buttock
    **L89.322**   **Pressure ulcer of left buttock,** stage 2
         Healing pressure ulcer of left buttock, stage 2
         Pressure ulcer with abrasion, blister, partial thickness skin loss involving epidermis and/or dermis, left buttock
    **L89.323**   **Pressure ulcer of left buttock, stage 3**   PDxMCC MCC H4 HCC
         Healing pressure ulcer of left buttock, stage 3
         Pressure ulcer with full thickness skin loss involving damage or necrosis of subcutaneous tissue, left buttock
    **L89.324**   **Pressure ulcer of left buttock, stage 4**   PDxMCC MCC H4 HCC
         Healing pressure ulcer of left buttock, stage 4
         Pressure ulcer with necrosis of soft tissues through to underlying muscle, tendon, or bone, left buttock
    **L89.329**   **Pressure ulcer of left buttock, unspecified stage**
         Healing pressure ulcer of left buttock NOS
         Healing pressure ulcer of left buttock, unspecified stage

✓5ᵗʰ  **L89.4**   **Pressure ulcer of contiguous site of** back, buttock and hip
    **L89.4Ø**   **Pressure ulcer of contiguous site of back, buttock and hip, unspecified stage**
         Healing pressure ulcer of contiguous site of back, buttock and hip NOS
         Healing pressure ulcer of contiguous site of back, buttock and hip, unspecified stage

**L89.41**   **Pressure ulcer of contiguous site of back, buttock and hip, stage 1**
     Healing pressure ulcer of contiguous site of back, buttock and hip, stage 1
     Pressure pre-ulcer skin changes limited to persistent focal edema, contiguous site of back, buttock and hip

**L89.42**   **Pressure ulcer of contiguous site of back, buttock and hip, stage 2**
     Healing pressure ulcer of contiguous site of back, buttock and hip, stage 2
     Pressure ulcer with abrasion, blister, partial thickness skin loss involving epidermis and/or dermis, contiguous site of back, buttock and hip

**L89.43**   **Pressure ulcer of contiguous site of back, buttock and hip, stage 3**   PDxMCC MCC H4 HCC
     Healing pressure ulcer of contiguous site of back, buttock and hip, stage 3
     Pressure ulcer with full thickness skin loss involving damage or necrosis of subcutaneous tissue, contiguous site of back, buttock and hip

**L89.44**   **Pressure ulcer of contiguous site of back, buttock and hip, stage 4**   PDxMCC MCC H4 HCC
     Healing pressure ulcer of contiguous site of back, buttock and hip, stage 4
     Pressure ulcer with necrosis of soft tissues through to underlying muscle, tendon, or bone, contiguous site of back, buttock and hip

**L89.45**   **Pressure ulcer of contiguous site of back, buttock and hip, unstageable**   HCC

✓5ᵗʰ  **L89.5**   **Pressure ulcer of** ankle
✓6ᵗʰ  **L89.5Ø**   **Pressure ulcer of** unspecified ankle
    **L89.5ØØ**   **Pressure ulcer of unspecified ankle, unstageable**   HCC
    **L89.5Ø1**   **Pressure ulcer of unspecified ankle, stage 1**
         Healing pressure ulcer of unspecified ankle, stage 1
         Pressure pre-ulcer skin changes limited to persistent focal edema, unspecified ankle
    **L89.5Ø2**   **Pressure ulcer of unspecified ankle, stage 2**
         Healing pressure ulcer of unspecified ankle, stage 2
         Pressure ulcer with abrasion, blister, partial thickness skin loss involving epidermis and/or dermis, unspecified ankle
    **L89.5Ø3**   **Pressure ulcer of unspecified ankle, stage 3**   PDxMCC MCC H4 HCC
         Healing pressure ulcer of unspecified ankle, stage 3
         Pressure ulcer with full thickness skin loss involving damage or necrosis of subcutaneous tissue, unspecified ankle
    **L89.5Ø4**   **Pressure ulcer of unspecified ankle, stage 4**   PDxMCC MCC H4 HCC
         Healing pressure ulcer of unspecified ankle, stage 4
         Pressure ulcer with necrosis of soft tissues through to underlying muscle, tendon, or bone, unspecified ankle
    **L89.5Ø9**   **Pressure ulcer of unspecified ankle, unspecified stage**
         Healing pressure ulcer of unspecified ankle NOS
         Healing pressure ulcer of unspecified ankle, unspecified stage

✓6ᵗʰ  **L89.51**   **Pressure ulcer of** right ankle
    **L89.51Ø**   **Pressure ulcer of right ankle, unstageable**   HCC
    **L89.511**   **Pressure ulcer of right ankle,** stage 1
         Healing pressure ulcer of right ankle, stage 1
         Pressure pre-ulcer skin changes limited to persistent focal edema, right ankle
    **L89.512**   **Pressure ulcer of right ankle,** stage 2
         Healing pressure ulcer of right ankle, stage 2
         Pressure pre-ulcer skin changes limited to persistent focal edema, right ankle

N Newborn: 0   P Pediatric: 0-17   M Maternity: 12-55   A Adult: 15-124   MCC Major CC Condition   PDxMCC PDx acts as own MCC   CC CC Condition   PDxCC PDx acts as own CC

722                                                     ICD-10-CM 2018

**L89.513  Pressure ulcer of right** `PDx MCC` `MCC` `H4` `HCC`
**ankle, stage 3**
Healing pressure ulcer of right ankle, stage 3
Pressure ulcer with full thickness skin loss involving damage or necrosis of subcutaneous tissue, right ankle

**L89.514  Pressure ulcer of right** `PDx MCC` `MCC` `H4` `HCC`
**ankle, stage 4**
Healing pressure ulcer of right ankle, stage 4
Pressure ulcer with necrosis of soft tissues through to underlying muscle, tendon, or bone, right ankle

**L89.519  Pressure ulcer of right ankle, unspecified stage**
Healing pressure ulcer of right ankle NOS
Healing pressure ulcer of right ankle, unspecified stage

`✓6ᵗʰ` **L89.52  Pressure ulcer of left ankle**

**L89.520  Pressure ulcer of left ankle,** `HCC`
**unstageable**

**L89.521  Pressure ulcer of left ankle, stage 1**
Healing pressure ulcer of left ankle, stage 1
Pressure pre-ulcer skin changes limited to persistent focal edema, left ankle

**L89.522  Pressure ulcer of left ankle, stage 2**
Healing pressure ulcer of left ankle, stage 2
Pressure ulcer with abrasion, blister, partial thickness skin loss involving epidermis and/or dermis, left ankle

**L89.523  Pressure ulcer of left** `PDx MCC` `MCC` `H4` `HCC`
**ankle, stage 3**
Healing pressure ulcer of left ankle, stage 3
Pressure ulcer with full thickness skin loss involving damage or necrosis of subcutaneous tissue, left ankle

**L89.524  Pressure ulcer of left** `PDx MCC` `MCC` `H4` `HCC`
**ankle, stage 4**
Healing pressure ulcer of left ankle, stage 4
Pressure ulcer with necrosis of soft tissues through to underlying muscle, tendon, or bone, left ankle

**L89.529  Pressure ulcer of left ankle, unspecified stage**
Healing pressure ulcer of left ankle NOS
Healing pressure ulcer of left ankle, unspecified stage

`✓5ᵗʰ` **L89.6  Pressure ulcer of heel**

`✓6ᵗʰ` **L89.60  Pressure ulcer of unspecified heel**

**L89.600  Pressure ulcer of unspecified heel,** `HCC`
**unstageable**

**L89.601  Pressure ulcer of unspecified heel, stage 1**
Healing pressure ulcer of unspecified heel, stage 1
Pressure pre-ulcer skin changes limited to persistent focal edema, unspecified heel

**L89.602  Pressure ulcer of unspecified heel, stage 2**
Healing pressure ulcer of unspecified heel, stage 2
Pressure ulcer with abrasion, blister, partial thickness skin loss involving epidermis and/or dermis, unspecified heel

**L89.603  Pressure ulcer of** `PDx MCC` `MCC` `H4` `HCC`
**unspecified heel, stage 3**
Healing pressure ulcer of unspecified heel, stage 3
Pressure ulcer with full thickness skin loss involving damage or necrosis of subcutaneous tissue, unspecified heel

**L89.604  Pressure ulcer of** `PDx MCC` `MCC` `H4` `HCC`
**unspecified heel, stage 4**
Healing pressure ulcer of unspecified heel, stage 4
Pressure ulcer with necrosis of soft tissues through to underlying muscle, tendon, or bone, unspecified heel

**L89.609  Pressure ulcer of unspecified heel, unspecified stage**
Healing pressure ulcer of unspecified heel NOS
Healing pressure ulcer of unspecified heel, unspecified stage

`✓6ᵗʰ` **L89.61  Pressure ulcer of right heel**

**L89.610  Pressure ulcer of right heel,** `HCC`
**unstageable**

**L89.611  Pressure ulcer of right heel, stage 1**
Healing pressure ulcer of right heel, stage 1
Pressure pre-ulcer skin changes limited to persistent focal edema, right heel

**L89.612  Pressure ulcer of right heel, stage 2**
Healing pressure ulcer of right heel, stage 2
Pressure ulcer with abrasion, blister, partial thickness skin loss involving epidermis and/or dermis, right heel

**L89.613  Pressure ulcer of right** `PDx MCC` `MCC` `H4` `HCC`
**heel, stage 3**
Healing pressure ulcer of right heel, stage 3
Pressure ulcer with full thickness skin loss involving damage or necrosis of subcutaneous tissue, right heel

**L89.614  Pressure ulcer of right** `PDx MCC` `MCC` `H4` `HCC`
**heel, stage 4**
Healing pressure ulcer of right heel, stage 4
Pressure ulcer with necrosis of soft tissues through to underlying muscle, tendon, or bone, right heel

**L89.619  Pressure ulcer of right heel, unspecified stage**
Healing pressure ulcer of right heel NOS
►Healing pressure ulcer of right heel, unspecified stage◄

`✓6ᵗʰ` **L89.62  Pressure ulcer of left heel**

**L89.620  Pressure ulcer of left heel,** `HCC`
**unstageable**

**L89.621  Pressure ulcer of left heel, stage 1**
Healing pressure ulcer of left heel, stage 1
Pressure pre-ulcer skin changes limited to persistent focal edema, left heel

**L89.622  Pressure ulcer of left heel, stage 2**
Healing pressure ulcer of left heel, stage 2
Pressure ulcer with abrasion, blister, partial thickness skin loss involving epidermis and/or dermis, left heel

**L89.623  Pressure ulcer of left** `PDx MCC` `MCC` `H4` `HCC`
**heel, stage 3**
Healing pressure ulcer of left heel, stage 3
Pressure ulcer with full thickness skin loss involving damage or necrosis of subcutaneous tissue, left heel

**L89.624  Pressure ulcer of left** `PDx MCC` `MCC` `H4` `HCC`
**heel, stage 4**
Healing pressure ulcer of left heel, stage 4
Pressure ulcer with necrosis of soft tissues through to underlying muscle, tendon, or bone, left heel

**L89.629  Pressure ulcer of left heel, unspecified stage**
Healing pressure ulcer of left heel NOS
Healing pressure ulcer of left heel, unspecified stage

`✓5ᵗʰ` **L89.8  Pressure ulcer of other site**

`✓6ᵗʰ` **L89.81  Pressure ulcer of head**
Pressure ulcer of face

**L89.810  Pressure ulcer of head, unstageable** `HCC`

**L89.811  Pressure ulcer of head, stage 1**
Healing pressure ulcer of head, stage 1
Pressure pre-ulcer skin changes limited to persistent focal edema, head

**L89.812  Pressure ulcer of head, stage 2**
Healing pressure ulcer of head, stage 2
Pressure ulcer with abrasion, blister, partial thickness skin loss involving epidermis and/or dermis, head

*Chapter 12. Diseases of the Skin and Subcutaneous Tissue*

**L89.513–L89.812**

---

**Chapter 12. Diseases of the Skin and Subcutaneous Tissue**

**L89.813**   **Pressure ulcer of head,** `PDxMCC` `MCC` `H4` `HCC`
**stage 3**
    Healing pressure ulcer of head, stage 3
    Pressure ulcer with full thickness skin loss
      involving damage or necrosis of
      subcutaneous tissue, head

**L89.814**   **Pressure ulcer of head,** `PDxMCC` `MCC` `H4` `HCC`
**stage 4**
    Healing pressure ulcer of head, stage 4
    Pressure ulcer with necrosis of soft tissues
      through to underlying muscle,
      tendon, or bone, head

**L89.819**   **Pressure ulcer of head, unspecified stage**
    Healing pressure ulcer of head NOS
    Healing pressure ulcer of head, unspecified
      stage

✓6th **L89.89**   **Pressure ulcer of other site**

**L89.890**   **Pressure ulcer of other site,** `HCC`
**unstageable**

**L89.891**   **Pressure ulcer of other site, stage 1**
    Healing pressure ulcer of other site, stage 1
    Pressure pre-ulcer skin changes limited to
      persistent focal edema, other site

**L89.892**   **Pressure ulcer of other site, stage 2**
    Healing pressure ulcer of other site, stage 2
    Pressure ulcer with abrasion, blister, partial
      thickness skin loss involving epidermis
      and/or dermis, other site

**L89.893**   **Pressure ulcer of other** `PDxMCC` `MCC` `H4` `HCC`
**site, stage 3**
    Healing pressure ulcer of other site, stage 3
    Pressure ulcer with full thickness skin loss
      involving damage or necrosis of
      subcutaneous tissue, other site

**L89.894**   **Pressure ulcer of other** `PDxMCC` `MCC` `H4` `HCC`
**site, stage 4**
    Healing pressure ulcer of other site, stage 4
    Pressure ulcer with necrosis of soft tissues
      through to underlying muscle,
      tendon, or bone, other site

**L89.899**   **Pressure ulcer of other site, unspecified
stage**
    Healing pressure ulcer of other site NOS
    Healing pressure ulcer of other site,
      unspecified stage

✓5th **L89.9**   **Pressure ulcer of unspecified site**

**L89.90**   **Pressure ulcer of unspecified site, unspecified stage**
    Healing pressure ulcer of unspecified site NOS
    Healing pressure ulcer of unspecified site, unspecified
      stage

**L89.91**   **Pressure ulcer of unspecified site, stage 1**
    Healing pressure ulcer of unspecified site, stage 1
    Pressure pre-ulcer skin changes limited to persistent
      focal edema, unspecified site

**L89.92**   **Pressure ulcer of unspecified site, stage 2**
    Healing pressure ulcer of unspecified site, stage 2
    Pressure ulcer with abrasion, blister, partial thickness
      skin loss involving epidermis and/or dermis,
      unspecified site

**L89.93**   **Pressure ulcer of unspecified site,** `PDxMCC` `MCC` `H4` `HCC`
**stage 3**
    Healing pressure ulcer of unspecified site, stage 3
    Pressure ulcer with full thickness skin loss involving
      damage or necrosis of subcutaneous tissue,
      unspecified site

**L89.94**   **Pressure ulcer of unspecified site,** `PDxMCC` `MCC` `H4` `HCC`
**stage 4**
    Healing pressure ulcer of unspecified site, stage 4
    Pressure ulcer with necrosis of soft tissues through to
      underlying muscle, tendon, or bone, unspecified
      site

**L89.95**   **Pressure ulcer of unspecified site, unstageable** `HCC`

✓4th **L90**   **Atrophic disorders of skin**

**L90.0**   **Lichen sclerosus et atrophicus**
    `EXCLUDES 2` *lichen sclerosus of external female genital organs
      (N90.4)*
      *lichen sclerosus of external male genital organs (N48.0)*

**L90.1**   **Anetoderma of Schweninger-Buzzi**

**L90.2**   **Anetoderma of Jadassohn-Pellizzari**

**L90.3**   **Atrophoderma of Pasini and Pierini**

**L90.4**   **Acrodermatitis chronica atrophicans**

**L90.5**   **Scar conditions and fibrosis of skin**
    Adherent scar (skin)
    Cicatrix
    Disfigurement of skin due to scar
    Fibrosis of skin NOS
    Scar NOS
    `EXCLUDES 2` *hypertrophic scar (L91.0)*
      *keloid scar (L91.0)*
    **AHA:** 2016, 2Q, 5; 2015, 1Q, 19

**L90.6**   **Striae atrophicae**

**L90.8**   **Other atrophic disorders of skin**

**L90.9**   **Atrophic disorder of skin, unspecified**

✓4th **L91**   **Hypertrophic disorders of skin**

**L91.0**   **Hypertrophic scar**
    Keloid
    Keloid scar
    `EXCLUDES 2` *acne keloid (L73.0)*
      *scar NOS (L90.5)*
    **DEF:** Overgrowth of scar tissue due to excess amounts of collagen
    during connective tissue repair; occurs mainly on upper trunk,
    face.

**L91.8**   **Other hypertrophic disorders of the skin**

**L91.9**   **Hypertrophic disorder of the skin, unspecified**

✓4th **L92**   **Granulomatous disorders of skin and subcutaneous tissue**
    `EXCLUDES 2` *actinic granuloma (L57.5)*

**L92.0**   **Granuloma annulare**
    Perforating granuloma annulare

**L92.1**   **Necrobiosis lipoidica, not elsewhere classified**
    `EXCLUDES 1` *necrobiosis lipoidica associated with diabetes mellitus
      (E08-E13 with .620)*

**L92.2**   **Granuloma faciale [eosinophilic granuloma of skin]**

**L92.3**   **Foreign body granuloma of the skin and subcutaneous tissue**
    Use additional code to identify the type of retained foreign body
      (Z18.-)

**L92.8**   **Other granulomatous disorders of the skin and subcutaneous
tissue**

**L92.9**   **Granulomatous disorder of the skin and subcutaneous tissue,
unspecified**
    `EXCLUDES 2` ▶*umbilical granuloma (P83.81)*◀

✓4th **L93**   **Lupus erythematosus**
    Use additional code for adverse effect, if applicable, to identify drug
      (T36-T50 with fifth or sixth character 5)
    `EXCLUDES 1` *lupus exedens (A18.4)*
      *lupus vulgaris (A18.4)*
      *scleroderma (M34.-)*
      *systemic lupus erythematosus (M32.-)*

**L93.0**   **Discoid lupus erythematosus**
    Lupus erythematosus NOS

**L93.1**   **Subacute cutaneous lupus erythematosus**

**L93.2**   **Other local lupus erythematosus**
    Lupus erythematosus profundus
    Lupus panniculitis

✓4th **L94**   **Other localized connective tissue disorders**
    `EXCLUDES 1` *systemic connective tissue disorders (M30-M36)*

**L94.0**   **Localized scleroderma [morphea]**
    Circumscribed scleroderma

**L94.1**   **Linear scleroderma**
    En coup de sabre lesion

**L94.2**   **Calcinosis cutis**

**L94.3**   **Sclerodactyly**

**L94.4**   **Gottron's papules**

**L94.5**   **Poikiloderma vasculare atrophicans**

**L94.6**   **Ainhum**

**L94.8**   **Other specified localized connective tissue disorders**

**L94.9**   **Localized connective tissue disorder, unspecified**

`N` Newborn: 0   `P` Pediatric: 0-17   `M` Maternity: 12-55   `A` Adult: 15-124   `MCC` Major CC Condition   `PDxMCC` PDx acts as own MCC   `CC` CC Condition   `PDxCC` PDx acts as own CC

724       ICD-10-CM 2018

✓4ᵗʰ **L95**   **Vasculitis limited to skin, not elsewhere classified**

    EXCLUDES 1    angioma serpiginosum (L81.7)
                  Henoch(-Schönlein) purpura (D69.0)
                  hypersensitivity angiitis (M31.0)
                  lupus panniculitis (L93.2)
                  panniculitis NOS (M79.3)
                  panniculitis of neck and back (M54.0-)
                  polyarteritis nodosa (M30.0)
                  relapsing panniculitis (M35.6)
                  rheumatoid vasculitis (M05.2)
                  serum sickness (T80.6-)
                  urticaria (L50.-)
                  Wegener's granulomatosis (M31.3-)

    **L95.0**   **Livedoid vasculitis**
         Atrophie blanche (en plaque)

    **L95.1**   **Erythema elevatum diutinum**

    **L95.8**   **Other vasculitis limited to the skin**

    **L95.9**   **Vasculitis limited to the skin, unspecified**

✓4ᵗʰ **L97**   **Non-pressure chronic ulcer of lower limb, not elsewhere classified**

    INCLUDES    chronic ulcer of skin of lower limb NOS
                  non-healing ulcer of skin
                  non-infected sinus of skin
                  trophic ulcer NOS
                  tropical ulcer NOS
                  ulcer of skin of lower limb NOS

    Code first any associated underlying condition, such as:
       any associated gangrene (I96)
       atherosclerosis of the lower extremities (I70.23-, I70.24-, I70.33-, I70.34-, I70.43-, I70.44-, I70.53-, I70.54-, I70.63-, I70.64-, I70.73-, I70.74-)
       chronic venous hypertension (I87.31-, I87.33-)
       diabetic ulcers (E08.621, E08.622, E09.621, E09.622, E10.621, E10.622, E11.621, E11.622, E13.621, E13.622)
       postphlebitic syndrome (I87.01-, I87.03-)
       postthrombotic syndrome (I87.01-, I87.03-)
       varicose ulcer (I83.0-, I83.2-)

    EXCLUDES 2    pressure ulcer (pressure area) (L89.-)
                  skin infections (L00-L08)
                  specific infections classified to A00-B99

    **CC Excl: For CC codes in category L97:** PDX collection 698

✓5ᵗʰ **L97.1**   **Non-pressure chronic ulcer of thigh**

    ✓6ᵗʰ **L97.10**   **Non-pressure chronic ulcer of unspecified thigh**

       **L97.101**   **Non-pressure chronic ulcer of** CC HCC **unspecified thigh limited to breakdown of skin**

       **L97.102**   **Non-pressure chronic ulcer of** CC HCC **unspecified thigh with fat layer exposed**

       **L97.103**   **Non-pressure chronic ulcer of** CC HCC **unspecified thigh with necrosis of muscle**

       **L97.104**   **Non-pressure chronic ulcer of** CC HCC **unspecified thigh with necrosis of bone**

●    **L97.105**   **Non-pressure chronic ulcer of** CC **unspecified thigh with muscle involvement without evidence of necrosis**

●    **L97.106**   **Non-pressure chronic ulcer of** CC **unspecified thigh with bone involvement without evidence of necrosis**

●    **L97.108**   **Non-pressure chronic ulcer of** CC **unspecified thigh with other specified severity**

       **L97.109**   **Non-pressure chronic ulcer of** CC HCC **unspecified thigh with unspecified severity**

    ✓6ᵗʰ **L97.11**   **Non-pressure chronic ulcer of right thigh**

       **L97.111**   **Non-pressure chronic ulcer of right** CC HCC **thigh limited to breakdown of skin**

       **L97.112**   **Non-pressure chronic ulcer of right** CC HCC **thigh with fat layer exposed**

       **L97.113**   **Non-pressure chronic ulcer of right** CC HCC **thigh with necrosis of muscle**

       **L97.114**   **Non-pressure chronic ulcer of right** CC HCC **thigh with necrosis of bone**

●    **L97.115**   **Non-pressure chronic ulcer of right** CC **thigh with muscle involvement without evidence of necrosis**

       **L97.116**   **Non-pressure chronic ulcer of right** CC **thigh with bone involvement without evidence of necrosis**

       **L97.118**   **Non-pressure chronic ulcer of right** CC **thigh with other specified severity**

       **L97.119**   **Non-pressure chronic ulcer of right** CC HCC **thigh with unspecified severity**

    ✓6ᵗʰ **L97.12**   **Non-pressure chronic ulcer of left thigh**

       **L97.121**   **Non-pressure chronic ulcer of left** CC HCC **thigh limited to breakdown of skin**

       **L97.122**   **Non-pressure chronic ulcer of left** CC HCC **thigh with fat layer exposed**

       **L97.123**   **Non-pressure chronic ulcer of left** CC HCC **thigh with necrosis of muscle**

       **L97.124**   **Non-pressure chronic ulcer of left** CC HCC **thigh with necrosis of bone**

●    **L97.125**   **Non-pressure chronic ulcer of left** CC **thigh with muscle involvement without evidence of necrosis**

●    **L97.126**   **Non-pressure chronic ulcer of left** CC **thigh with bone involvement without evidence of necrosis**

●    **L97.128**   **Non-pressure chronic ulcer of left** CC **thigh with other specified severity**

       **L97.129**   **Non-pressure chronic ulcer of left** CC HCC **thigh with unspecified severity**

✓5ᵗʰ **L97.2**   **Non-pressure chronic ulcer of calf**

    ✓6ᵗʰ **L97.20**   **Non-pressure chronic ulcer of unspecified calf**

       **L97.201**   **Non-pressure chronic ulcer of** CC HCC **unspecified calf limited to breakdown of skin**

       **L97.202**   **Non-pressure chronic ulcer of** CC HCC **unspecified calf with fat layer exposed**

       **L97.203**   **Non-pressure chronic ulcer of** CC HCC **unspecified calf with necrosis of muscle**

       **L97.204**   **Non-pressure chronic ulcer of** CC HCC **unspecified calf with necrosis of bone**

●    **L97.205**   **Non-pressure chronic ulcer of** CC **unspecified calf with muscle involvement without evidence of necrosis**

●    **L97.206**   **Non-pressure chronic ulcer of** CC **unspecified calf with bone involvement without evidence of necrosis**

●    **L97.208**   **Non-pressure chronic ulcer of** CC **unspecified calf with other specified severity**

       **L97.209**   **Non-pressure chronic ulcer of** CC HCC **unspecified calf with unspecified severity**

    ✓6ᵗʰ **L97.21**   **Non-pressure chronic ulcer of right calf**

       **L97.211**   **Non-pressure chronic ulcer of right** CC HCC **calf limited to breakdown of skin**

       **L97.212**   **Non-pressure chronic ulcer of right** CC HCC **calf with fat layer exposed**

       **L97.213**   **Non-pressure chronic ulcer of right** CC HCC **calf with necrosis of muscle**

       **L97.214**   **Non-pressure chronic ulcer of right** CC HCC **calf with necrosis of bone**

●    **L97.215**   **Non-pressure chronic ulcer of right** CC **calf with muscle involvement without evidence of necrosis**

●    **L97.216**   **Non-pressure chronic ulcer of right** CC **calf with bone involvement without evidence of necrosis**

●    **L97.218**   **Non-pressure chronic ulcer of right** CC **calf with other specified severity**

       **L97.219**   **Non-pressure chronic ulcer of right** CC HCC **calf with unspecified severity**

    ✓6ᵗʰ **L97.22**   **Non-pressure chronic ulcer of left calf**

       **L97.221**   **Non-pressure chronic ulcer of left** CC HCC **calf limited to breakdown of skin**

       **L97.222**   **Non-pressure chronic ulcer of left** CC HCC **calf with fat layer exposed**

       **L97.223**   **Non-pressure chronic ulcer of left** CC HCC **calf with necrosis of muscle**

       **L97.224**   **Non-pressure chronic ulcer of left** CC HCC **calf with necrosis of bone**

- L97.225 **Non-pressure chronic ulcer of left calf** with muscle involvement without evidence of necrosis `CC`
- L97.226 **Non-pressure chronic ulcer of left calf** with bone involvement without evidence of necrosis `CC`
- L97.228 **Non-pressure chronic ulcer of left calf** with other specified severity `CC`
  L97.229 **Non-pressure chronic ulcer of left calf** with unspecified severity `CC` `HCC`

✓5ᵗʰ **L97.3 Non-pressure chronic ulcer of ankle**

  ✓6ᵗʰ **L97.30 Non-pressure chronic ulcer of** unspecified ankle

    L97.301 **Non-pressure chronic ulcer of unspecified ankle** limited to breakdown of skin `CC` `HCC`

    L97.302 **Non-pressure chronic ulcer of unspecified ankle** with fat layer exposed `CC` `HCC`

    L97.303 **Non-pressure chronic ulcer of unspecified ankle** with necrosis of muscle `CC` `HCC`

    L97.304 **Non-pressure chronic ulcer of unspecified ankle** with necrosis of bone `CC` `HCC`

-     L97.305 **Non-pressure chronic ulcer of unspecified ankle** with muscle involvement without evidence of necrosis `CC`

-     L97.306 **Non-pressure chronic ulcer of unspecified ankle** with bone involvement without evidence of necrosis `CC`

-     L97.308 **Non-pressure chronic ulcer of unspecified ankle** with other specified severity `CC`

    L97.309 **Non-pressure chronic ulcer of unspecified ankle** with unspecified severity `CC` `HCC`

  ✓6ᵗʰ **L97.31 Non-pressure chronic ulcer of** right ankle

    L97.311 **Non-pressure chronic ulcer of right ankle** limited to breakdown of skin `CC` `HCC`

    L97.312 **Non-pressure chronic ulcer of right ankle** with fat layer exposed `CC` `HCC`

    L97.313 **Non-pressure chronic ulcer of right ankle** with necrosis of muscle `CC` `HCC`

    L97.314 **Non-pressure chronic ulcer of right ankle** with necrosis of bone `CC` `HCC`

-     L97.315 **Non-pressure chronic ulcer of right ankle** with muscle involvement without evidence of necrosis `CC`

-     L97.316 **Non-pressure chronic ulcer of right ankle** with bone involvement without evidence of necrosis `CC`

    L97.318 **Non-pressure chronic ulcer of right ankle** with other specified severity `CC`

    L97.319 **Non-pressure chronic ulcer of right ankle** with unspecified severity `CC` `HCC`

  ✓6ᵗʰ **L97.32 Non-pressure chronic ulcer of** left ankle

    L97.321 **Non-pressure chronic ulcer of left ankle** limited to breakdown of skin `CC` `HCC`

    L97.322 **Non-pressure chronic ulcer of left ankle** with fat layer exposed `CC` `HCC`

    L97.323 **Non-pressure chronic ulcer of left ankle** with necrosis of muscle `CC` `HCC`

    L97.324 **Non-pressure chronic ulcer of left ankle** with necrosis of bone `CC` `HCC`

-     L97.325 **Non-pressure chronic ulcer of left ankle** with muscle involvement without evidence of necrosis `CC`

-     L97.326 **Non-pressure chronic ulcer of left ankle** with bone involvement without evidence of necrosis `CC`

-     L97.328 **Non-pressure chronic ulcer of left ankle** with other specified severity `CC`

    L97.329 **Non-pressure chronic ulcer of left ankle** with unspecified severity `CC` `HCC`

✓5ᵗʰ **L97.4 Non-pressure chronic ulcer of** heel and midfoot
  Non-pressure chronic ulcer of plantar surface of midfoot

  ✓6ᵗʰ **L97.40 Non-pressure chronic ulcer of** unspecified heel and midfoot

    L97.401 **Non-pressure chronic ulcer of unspecified heel and midfoot** limited to breakdown of skin `CC` `HCC`

L97.402 **Non-pressure chronic ulcer of unspecified heel and midfoot** with fat layer exposed `CC` `HCC`

L97.403 **Non-pressure chronic ulcer of unspecified heel and midfoot** with necrosis of muscle `CC` `HCC`

L97.404 **Non-pressure chronic ulcer of unspecified heel and midfoot** with necrosis of bone `CC` `HCC`

- L97.405 **Non-pressure chronic ulcer of unspecified heel and midfoot** with muscle involvement without evidence of necrosis `CC`

- L97.406 **Non-pressure chronic ulcer of unspecified heel and midfoot** with bone involvement without evidence of necrosis `CC`

- L97.408 **Non-pressure chronic ulcer of unspecified heel and midfoot with** other specified severity `CC`

L97.409 **Non-pressure chronic ulcer of unspecified heel and midfoot** with unspecified severity `CC` `HCC`

  ✓6ᵗʰ **L97.41 Non-pressure chronic ulcer of** right heel and midfoot

    L97.411 **Non-pressure chronic ulcer of right heel and midfoot** limited to breakdown of skin `CC` `HCC`

    L97.412 **Non-pressure chronic ulcer of right heel and midfoot** with fat layer exposed `CC` `HCC`

    L97.413 **Non-pressure chronic ulcer of right heel and midfoot** with necrosis of muscle `CC` `HCC`

    L97.414 **Non-pressure chronic ulcer of right heel and midfoot** with necrosis of bone `CC` `HCC`

-     L97.415 **Non-pressure chronic ulcer of right heel and midfoot** with muscle involvement without evidence of necrosis `CC`

-     L97.416 **Non-pressure chronic ulcer of right heel and midfoot** with bone involvement without evidence of necrosis `CC`

-     L97.418 **Non-pressure chronic ulcer of right heel and midfoot with other specified severity** `CC`

    L97.419 **Non-pressure chronic ulcer of right heel and midfoot** with unspecified severity `CC` `HCC`

  ✓6ᵗʰ **L97.42 Non-pressure chronic ulcer of** left heel and midfoot

    L97.421 **Non-pressure chronic ulcer of left heel and midfoot** limited to breakdown of skin `CC` `HCC`
      **AHA:** 2016, 1Q, 12

    L97.422 **Non-pressure chronic ulcer of left heel and midfoot** with fat layer exposed `CC` `HCC`

    L97.423 **Non-pressure chronic ulcer of left heel and midfoot** with necrosis of muscle `CC` `HCC`

    L97.424 **Non-pressure chronic ulcer of left heel and midfoot** with necrosis of bone `CC` `HCC`

-     L97.425 **Non-pressure chronic ulcer of left heel and midfoot** with muscle involvement without evidence of necrosis `CC`

-     L97.426 **Non-pressure chronic ulcer of left heel and midfoot** with bone involvement without evidence of necrosis `CC`

-     L97.428 **Non-pressure chronic ulcer of left heel and midfoot with other specified severity** `CC`

    L97.429 **Non-pressure chronic ulcer of left heel and midfoot** with unspecified severity `CC` `HCC`

✓5ᵗʰ **L97.5 Non-pressure chronic ulcer of** other part of foot
  Non-pressure chronic ulcer of toe

  ✓6ᵗʰ **L97.50 Non-pressure chronic ulcer of** other part of unspecified foot

    L97.501 **Non-pressure chronic ulcer of other part of unspecified foot** limited to breakdown of skin `HCC`

N Newborn: 0   P Pediatric: 0-17   M Maternity: 12-55   A Adult: 15-124   MCC Major CC Condition   PDxMCC PDx acts as own MCC   CC CC Condition   PDxCC PDx acts as own CC

726     ICD-10-CM 2018

L97.502 **Non-pressure chronic ulcer of other** `HCC`
**part of unspecified foot with fat layer
exposed**

L97.503 **Non-pressure chronic ulcer of other** `HCC`
**part of unspecified foot with necrosis of
muscle**

L97.504 **Non-pressure chronic ulcer of other** `HCC`
**part of unspecified foot with necrosis of
bone**

● L97.505 **Non-pressure chronic ulcer of other** `CC`
**part of unspecified foot with muscle
involvement without evidence of
necrosis**

● L97.506 **Non-pressure chronic ulcer of other** `CC`
**part of unspecified foot with bone
involvement without evidence of
necrosis**

● L97.508 **Non-pressure chronic ulcer of other** `CC`
**part of unspecified foot with other
specified severity**

L97.509 **Non-pressure chronic ulcer of other** `HCC`
**part of unspecified foot with unspecified
severity**

`✓6ᵗʰ` **L97.51 Non-pressure chronic ulcer of** other part of right foot

L97.511 **Non-pressure chronic ulcer of other** `HCC`
**part of right foot limited to breakdown of
skin**

L97.512 **Non-pressure chronic ulcer of other** `HCC`
**part of right foot with fat layer exposed**

L97.513 **Non-pressure chronic ulcer of other** `HCC`
**part of right foot with necrosis of muscle**

L97.514 **Non-pressure chronic ulcer of other** `HCC`
**part of right foot with necrosis of bone**

● L97.515 **Non-pressure chronic ulcer of other** `CC`
**part of right foot with muscle
involvement without evidence
of necrosis**

● L97.516 **Non-pressure chronic ulcer of other** `CC`
**part of right foot with bone
involvement without evidence
of necrosis**

● L97.518 **Non-pressure chronic ulcer of other** `CC`
**part of right foot with other specified
severity**

L97.519 **Non-pressure chronic ulcer of other** `HCC`
**part of right foot with unspecified severity**

`✓6ᵗʰ` **L97.52 Non-pressure chronic ulcer of** other part of left foot

L97.521 **Non-pressure chronic ulcer of other** `HCC`
**part of left foot limited to breakdown of
skin**

L97.522 **Non-pressure chronic ulcer of other** `HCC`
**part of left foot with fat layer exposed**

L97.523 **Non-pressure chronic ulcer of other** `HCC`
**part of left foot with necrosis of muscle**

L97.524 **Non-pressure chronic ulcer of other** `HCC`
**part of left foot with necrosis of bone**

● L97.525 **Non-pressure chronic ulcer of other** `CC`
**part of left foot with muscle involvement
without evidence of necrosis**

● L97.526 **Non-pressure chronic ulcer of other** `CC`
**part of left foot with bone involvement
without evidence of necrosis**

● L97.528 **Non-pressure chronic ulcer of other** `CC`
**part of left foot with other specified
severity**

L97.529 **Non-pressure chronic ulcer of other** `HCC`
**part of left foot with unspecified severity**

`✓5ᵗʰ` **L97.8 Non-pressure chronic ulcer of** other part of lower leg

`✓6ᵗʰ` **L97.80 Non-pressure chronic ulcer of** other part of
unspecified lower leg

L97.801 **Non-pressure chronic ulcer of other** `CC` `HCC`
**part of unspecified lower leg limited to
breakdown of skin**

L97.802 **Non-pressure chronic ulcer of other** `CC` `HCC`
**part of unspecified lower leg with fat
layer exposed**

L97.803 **Non-pressure chronic ulcer of other** `CC` `HCC`
**part of unspecified lower leg with
necrosis of muscle**

L97.804 **Non-pressure chronic ulcer of other** `CC` `HCC`
**part of unspecified lower leg with
necrosis of bone**

● L97.805 **Non-pressure chronic ulcer of other** `CC`
**part of unspecified lower leg with
muscle involvement without evidence
of necrosis**

● L97.806 **Non-pressure chronic ulcer of other** `CC`
**part of unspecified lower leg with
bone involvement without evidence
of necrosis**

● L97.808 **Non-pressure chronic ulcer of other** `CC`
**part of unspecified lower leg with
other specified severity**

L97.809 **Non-pressure chronic ulcer of other** `CC` `HCC`
**part of unspecified lower leg with
unspecified severity**

`✓6ᵗʰ` **L97.81 Non-pressure chronic ulcer of** other part of right
lower leg

L97.811 **Non-pressure chronic ulcer of other** `CC` `HCC`
**part of right lower leg limited to
breakdown of skin**

L97.812 **Non-pressure chronic ulcer of other** `CC` `HCC`
**part of right lower leg with fat layer
exposed**

L97.813 **Non-pressure chronic ulcer of other** `CC` `HCC`
**part of right lower leg with necrosis of
muscle**

L97.814 **Non-pressure chronic ulcer of other** `CC` `HCC`
**part of right lower leg with necrosis of
bone**

● L97.815 **Non-pressure chronic ulcer of other** `CC`
**part of right lower leg with muscle
involvement without evidence
of necrosis**

● L97.816 **Non-pressure chronic ulcer of other** `CC`
**part of right lower leg with bone
involvement without evidence
of necrosis**

● L97.818 **Non-pressure chronic ulcer of other** `CC`
**part of right lower leg with other
specified severity**

L97.819 **Non-pressure chronic ulcer of other** `CC` `HCC`
**part of right lower leg with unspecified
severity**

`✓6ᵗʰ` **L97.82 Non-pressure chronic ulcer of** other part of left
lower leg

L97.821 **Non-pressure chronic ulcer of other** `CC` `HCC`
**part of left lower leg limited to
breakdown of skin**

L97.822 **Non-pressure chronic ulcer of other** `CC` `HCC`
**part of left lower leg with fat layer
exposed**

L97.823 **Non-pressure chronic ulcer of other** `CC` `HCC`
**part of left lower leg with necrosis of
muscle**

L97.824 **Non-pressure chronic ulcer of other** `CC` `HCC`
**part of left lower leg with necrosis
of bone**

● L97.825 **Non-pressure chronic ulcer of other** `CC`
**part of left lower leg with muscle
involvement without evidence
of necrosis**

● L97.826 **Non-pressure chronic ulcer of other** `CC`
**part of left lower leg with bone
involvement without evidence
of necrosis**

● L97.828 **Non-pressure chronic ulcer of other** `CC`
**part of left lower leg with other
specified severity**

L97.829 **Non-pressure chronic ulcer of other** `CC` `HCC`
**part of left lower leg with unspecified
severity**

`✓5ᵗʰ` **L97.9 Non-pressure chronic ulcer of** unspecified part of lower leg

`✓6ᵗʰ` **L97.90 Non-pressure chronic ulcer of** unspecified part of
unspecified lower leg

L97.901 **Non-pressure chronic ulcer of** `CC` `HCC`
**unspecified part of unspecified lower
leg limited to breakdown of skin**

---

☑Additional Character Req    `✓x7ᵗʰ` Placeholder Alert    Unacceptable PDx    Manifestation    `H1`-`H14` HAC    `HCC`CMS-HCC Condition    *EXCLUDES 1* Not Coded Here    *EXCLUDES 2* Not Included Here

**Chapter 12. Diseases of the Skin and Subcutaneous Tissue**

**L97.902** Non-pressure chronic ulcer of unspecified part of unspecified lower leg with fat layer exposed   `CC` `HCC`

**L97.903** Non-pressure chronic ulcer of unspecified part of unspecified lower leg with necrosis of muscle   `CC` `HCC`

**L97.904** Non-pressure chronic ulcer of unspecified part of unspecified lower leg with necrosis of bone   `CC` `HCC`

● **L97.905** Non-pressure chronic ulcer of unspecified part of unspecified lower leg with muscle involvement without evidence of necrosis   `CC`

● **L97.906** Non-pressure chronic ulcer of unspecified part of unspecified lower leg with bone involvement without evidence of necrosis   `CC`

● **L97.908** Non-pressure chronic ulcer of unspecified part of unspecified lower leg with other specified severity   `CC`

**L97.909** Non-pressure chronic ulcer of unspecified part of unspecified lower leg with unspecified severity   `CC` `HCC`

✓6th **L97.91** Non-pressure chronic ulcer of unspecified part of right lower leg

**L97.911** Non-pressure chronic ulcer of unspecified part of right lower leg limited to breakdown of skin   `CC` `HCC`

**L97.912** Non-pressure chronic ulcer of unspecified part of right lower leg with fat layer exposed   `CC` `HCC`

**L97.913** Non-pressure chronic ulcer of unspecified part of right lower leg with necrosis of muscle   `CC` `HCC`

**L97.914** Non-pressure chronic ulcer of unspecified part of right lower leg with necrosis of bone   `CC` `HCC`

● **L97.915** Non-pressure chronic ulcer of unspecified part of right lower leg with muscle involvement without evidence of necrosis   `CC`

● **L97.916** Non-pressure chronic ulcer of unspecified part of right lower leg with bone involvement without evidence of necrosis   `CC`

● **L97.918** Non-pressure chronic ulcer of unspecified part of right lower leg with other specified severity   `CC`

**L97.919** Non-pressure chronic ulcer of unspecified part of right lower leg with unspecified severity   `CC` `HCC`

✓6th **L97.92** Non-pressure chronic ulcer of unspecified part of left lower leg

**L97.921** Non-pressure chronic ulcer of unspecified part of left lower leg limited to breakdown of skin   `CC` `HCC`

**L97.922** Non-pressure chronic ulcer of unspecified part of left lower leg with fat layer exposed   `CC` `HCC`

**L97.923** Non-pressure chronic ulcer of unspecified part of left lower leg with necrosis of muscle   `CC` `HCC`

**L97.924** Non-pressure chronic ulcer of unspecified part of left lower leg with necrosis of bone   `CC` `HCC`

● **L97.925** Non-pressure chronic ulcer of unspecified part of left lower leg with muscle involvement without evidence of necrosis   `CC`

● **L97.926** Non-pressure chronic ulcer of unspecified part of left lower leg with bone involvement without evidence of necrosis   `CC`

● **L97.928** Non-pressure chronic ulcer of unspecified part of left lower leg with other specified severity   `CC`

**L97.929** Non-pressure chronic ulcer of unspecified part of left lower leg with unspecified severity   `CC` `HCC`

✓4th **L98** Other disorders of skin and subcutaneous tissue, not elsewhere classified

**L98.0** Pyogenic granuloma

*EXCLUDES 2*   *pyogenic granuloma of gingiva (K06.8)*
*pyogenic granuloma of maxillary alveolar ridge (K04.5)*
*pyogenic granuloma of oral mucosa (K13.4)*

**DEF:** Solitary polypoid capillary hemangioma often associated with local irritation, trauma, and superimposed inflammation; located on the skin and gingival or oral mucosa; they bleed easily and may ulcerate and form crusted sores.

**L98.1** Factitial dermatitis
Neurotic excoriation

*EXCLUDES 1*   *excoriation (skin-picking) disorder (F42.4)*

**DEF:** Self-inflicted skin lesions to satisfy an unconscious psychological or emotional need; methods used to injure the skin include deep excoriations with a sharp instrument, scarification with a knife, or the application of caustic chemicals and burning, sometimes with a cigarette.

**L98.2** Febrile neutrophilic dermatosis [Sweet]

**L98.3** Eosinophilic cellulitis [Wells]   `CC`
**CC Excl:** PDX collection 839

✓5th **L98.4** Non-pressure chronic ulcer of skin, not elsewhere classified
Chronic ulcer of skin NOS
Tropical ulcer NOS
Ulcer of skin NOS

*EXCLUDES 2*   *pressure ulcer (pressure area) (L89.-)*
*gangrene (I96)*
*skin infections (L00-L08)*
*specific infections classified to A00-B99*
*ulcer of lower limb NEC (L97.-)*
*varicose ulcer (I83.0-I82.2)*

**CC Excl: For CC codes in subcategory L98.4:** PDX collection 698

✓6th **L98.41** Non-pressure chronic ulcer of buttock

**L98.411** Non-pressure chronic ulcer of buttock limited to breakdown of skin   `HCC`

**L98.412** Non-pressure chronic ulcer of buttock with fat layer exposed   `HCC`

**L98.413** Non-pressure chronic ulcer of buttock with necrosis of muscle   `HCC`

**L98.414** Non-pressure chronic ulcer of buttock with necrosis of bone   `HCC`

● **L98.415** Non-pressure chronic ulcer of buttock with muscle involvement without evidence of necrosis   `CC`

● **L98.416** Non-pressure chronic ulcer of buttock with bone involvement without evidence of necrosis   `CC`

● **L98.418** Non-pressure chronic ulcer of buttock with other specified severity   `CC`

**L98.419** Non-pressure chronic ulcer of buttock with unspecified severity   `HCC`

✓6th **L98.42** Non-pressure chronic ulcer of back

**L98.421** Non-pressure chronic ulcer of back limited to breakdown of skin   `HCC`

**L98.422** Non-pressure chronic ulcer of back with fat layer exposed   `HCC`

**L98.423** Non-pressure chronic ulcer of back with necrosis of muscle   `HCC`

**L98.424** Non-pressure chronic ulcer of back with necrosis of bone   `HCC`

● **L98.425** Non-pressure chronic ulcer of back with muscle involvement without evidence of necrosis   `CC`

● **L98.426** Non-pressure chronic ulcer of back with bone involvement without evidence of necrosis   `CC`

● **L98.428** Non-pressure chronic ulcer of back with other specified severity   `CC`

**L98.429** Non-pressure chronic ulcer of back with unspecified severity   `HCC`

✓6th **L98.49** Non-pressure chronic ulcer of skin of other sites
Non-pressure chronic ulcer of skin NOS

**L98.491** Non-pressure chronic ulcer of skin of other sites limited to breakdown of skin   `HCC`

**L98.492** Non-pressure chronic ulcer of skin of other sites with fat layer exposed   `HCC`

`N` Newborn: 0   `P` Pediatric: 0-17   `M` Maternity: 12-55   `A` Adult: 15-124   `MCC` Major CC Condition   `PDxMCC` PDx acts as own MCC   `CC` CC Condition   `PDxCC` PDx acts as own CC

**728**      ICD-10-CM 2018

Chapter 12. Diseases of the Skin and Subcutaneous Tissue

L97.902–L98.492

**L98.493**   **Non-pressure chronic ulcer of skin of other sites** with necrosis of muscle   `HCC`

**L98.494**   **Non-pressure chronic ulcer of skin of other sites** with necrosis of bone   `HCC`

●    **L98.495**   **Non-pressure chronic ulcer of other sites** with muscle involvement without evidence of necrosis   `CC`

●    **L98.496**   **Non-pressure chronic ulcer of other sites** with bone involvement without evidence of necrosis   `CC`

●    **L98.498**   **Non-pressure chronic ulcer of other sites with other specified severity**   `CC`

**L98.499**   **Non-pressure chronic ulcer of skin of other sites** with unspecified severity   `HCC`

**L98.5**   **Mucinosis of the skin**
Focal mucinosis
Lichen myxedematosus
Reticular erythematous mucinosis
> *EXCLUDES 1*   *focal oral mucinosis (K13.79)*
> *myxedema (E03.9)*

**L98.6**   **Other infiltrative disorders of the skin and subcutaneous tissue**
> *EXCLUDES 1*   *hyalinosis cutis et mucosae (E78.89)*

**L98.7**   **Excessive and redundant skin and subcutaneous tissue**
Loose or sagging skin following bariatric surgery weight loss
Loose or sagging skin following dietary weight loss
Loose or sagging skin, NOS
> *EXCLUDES 2*   *acquired excess or redundant skin of eyelid (H02.3-)*
> *congenital excess or redundant skin of eyelid (Q10.3)*
> *skin changes due to chronic exposure to nonionizing radiation (L57.-)*

**L98.8**   **Other specified disorders of the skin and subcutaneous tissue**
**AHA:** 2013, 2Q, 32

**L98.9**   **Disorder of the skin and subcutaneous tissue, unspecified**

**L99**   *Other disorders of skin and subcutaneous tissue in diseases classified elsewhere*
Code first underlying disease, such as:
amyloidosis (E85.-)
> *EXCLUDES 1*   *skin disorders in diabetes (E08-E13 with .62)*
> *skin disorders in gonorrhea (A54.89)*
> *skin disorders in syphilis (A51.31, A52.79)*

☑ Additional Character Req   ✓x7ᵗʰ Placeholder Alert   Unacceptable PDx   Manifestation   `H1`-`H14` HAC   `HCC` CMS-HCC Condition   *EXCLUDES 1* Not Coded Here   *EXCLUDES 2* Not Included Here

ICD-10-CM 2018      **729**

# Chapter 13. Diseases of the Musculoskeletal System and Connective Tissue (M00–M99)

## Chapter Specific Guidelines with Coding Examples

The chapter specific guidelines from the ICD-10-CM Official Guidelines for Coding and Reporting have been provided below. Along with these guidelines are coding examples, contained in the shaded boxes, that have been developed to help illustrate the coding and/or sequencing guidance found in these guidelines.

### a. Site and laterality

Most of the codes within Chapter 13 have site and laterality designations. The site represents the bone, joint or the muscle involved. For some conditions where more than one bone, joint or muscle is usually involved, such as osteoarthritis, there is a "multiple sites" code available. For categories where no multiple site code is provided and more than one bone, joint or muscle is involved, multiple codes should be used to indicate the different sites involved.

> Rheumatoid arthritis of multiple sites without rheumatoid factor
>
> **M06.09**    **Rheumatoid arthritis without rheumatoid factor, multiple sites**
>
> *Explanation:* For some conditions where more than one bone, joint or muscle is usually involved, such as osteoarthritis, there is a "multiple sites" code available.

> Osteomyelitis of the fourth thoracic and second lumbar vertebrae
>
> **M46.24**    **Osteomyelitis of vertebra, thoracic region**
>
> **M46.26**    **Osteomyelitis of vertebra, lumbar region**
>
> *Explanation:* For categories without a multiple site code and more than one bone, joint, or muscle is involved, multiple codes should be used to indicate the different sites involved.

#### 1) Bone versus joint

For certain conditions, the bone may be affected at the upper or lower end, (e.g., avascular necrosis of bone, M87, Osteoporosis, M80, M81). Though the portion of the bone affected may be at the joint, the site designation will be the bone, not the joint.

> Idiopathic avascular necrosis of the femoral head of the left hip joint
>
> **M87.052**    **Idiopathic aseptic necrosis of left femur**
>
> *Explanation:* For certain conditions such as avascular necrosis, the bone may be affected at the joint, but the site designation is the bone, not the joint.

### b. Acute traumatic versus chronic or recurrent musculoskeletal conditions

Many musculoskeletal conditions are a result of previous injury or trauma to a site, or are recurrent conditions. Bone, joint or muscle conditions that are the result of a healed injury are usually found in chapter 13. Recurrent bone, joint or muscle conditions are also usually found in chapter 13. Any current, acute injury should be coded to the appropriate injury code from chapter 19. Chronic or recurrent conditions should generally be coded with a code from chapter 13. If it is difficult to determine from the documentation in the record which code is best to describe a condition, query the provider.

> Acute traumatic bucket handle tear of right medial meniscus
>
> **S83.211A**    **Bucket-handle tear of medial meniscus, current injury, right knee, initial encounter**
>
> *Explanation:* Any current, acute injury is not coded in chapter 13. It should instead be coded to the appropriate injury code from chapter 19.

> Old bucket handle tear of right medial meniscus
>
> **M23.203**    **Derangement of unspecified medial meniscus due to old tear or injury, right knee**
>
> *Explanation:* Chronic or recurrent conditions should generally be coded with a code from chapter 13.

### c. Coding of Pathologic Fractures

7th character A is for use as long as the patient is receiving active treatment for the fracture. Examples of active treatment are: surgical treatment, emergency department encounter, evaluation and continuing treatment by the same or a different physician. While the patient may be seen by a new or different provider over the course of treatment for a pathological fracture, assignment of the 7th character is based on whether the patient is

undergoing active treatment and not whether the provider is seeing the patient for the first time.

> Patient admitted for repair of pathologic fracture of left foot, unknown cause. The surgery will be performed by his orthopedic specialist who he has been seeing for this fracture for the past month.
>
> **M84.475A**    **Pathological fracture, left foot, initial encounter for fracture**
>
> *Explanation:* Seventh character A is for use as long as the patient is receiving active treatment for a pathologic fracture. Examples of active treatment are surgical treatment, emergency department encounter, evaluation, and continuing treatment by the same or a different physician.
>
> The seventh character is based on whether the patient is undergoing active treatment such as surgery, and not whether the provider is seeing the patient for the first time.

7th character, D is to be used for encounters after the patient has completed active treatment. The other 7th characters, listed under each subcategory in the Tabular List, are to be used for subsequent encounters for treatment of problems associated with the healing, such as malunions, nonunions, and sequelae.

Care for complications of surgical treatment for fracture repairs during the healing or recovery phase should be coded with the appropriate complication codes.

*See Section I.C.19. Coding of traumatic fractures.*

### d. Osteoporosis

Osteoporosis is a systemic condition, meaning that all bones of the musculoskeletal system are affected. Therefore, site is not a component of the codes under category M81, Osteoporosis without current pathological fracture. The site codes under category M80, Osteoporosis with current pathological fracture, identify the site of the fracture, not the osteoporosis.

#### 1) Osteoporosis without pathological fracture

Category M81, Osteoporosis without current pathological fracture, is for use for patients with osteoporosis who do not currently have a pathologic fracture due to the osteoporosis, even if they have had a fracture in the past. For patients with a history of osteoporosis fractures, status code Z87.310, Personal history of (healed) osteoporosis fracture, should follow the code from M81.

> Age-related osteoporosis with healed osteoporotic fracture of the lumbar vertebra
>
> **M81.0**    **Age-related osteoporosis without current pathological fracture**
>
> **Z87.310**    **Personal history of (healed) osteoporosis fracture**
>
> *Explanation:* Category M81 is used for patients with osteoporosis who do not currently have a pathologic fracture due to the osteoporosis. To report a previous (healed) fracture, status code Z87.310 Personal history of (healed) osteoporosis fracture, should follow the code from M81.

#### 2) Osteoporosis with current pathological fracture

Category M80, Osteoporosis with current pathological fracture, is for patients who have a current pathologic fracture at the time of an encounter. The codes under M80 identify the site of the fracture. A code from category M80, not a traumatic fracture code, should be used for any patient with known osteoporosis who suffers a fracture, even if the patient had a minor fall or trauma, if that fall or trauma would not usually break a normal, healthy bone.

> Disuse osteoporosis with current fracture of right shoulder sustained lifting a grocery bag, initial encounter
>
> **M80.811A**    **Other osteoporosis with current pathological fracture, right shoulder, initial encounter for fracture**
>
> *Explanation:* A code from category M80, not a traumatic fracture code, should be used for any patient with known osteoporosis who suffers a fracture, even if the patient had a minor fall or trauma, if that fall or trauma would not usually break a normal, healthy bone.

# Muscle/Tendon Table

ICD-10-CM categorizes certain muscles and tendons in the upper and lower extremities by their action (e.g., extension, flexion), their anatomical location (e.g., posterior, anterior), and/or whether they are intrinsic or extrinsic to a certain anatomical area. The Muscle/Tendon Table is provided at the beginning of chapters 13 and 19 as a resource to help users when code selection depends on one or more of these characteristics. Please note that this table is not all-inclusive, and proper code assignment should be based on the provider's documentation.

| Body Region | Muscle | Extensor Tendon | Flexor Tendon | Other Tendon |
|---|---|---|---|---|
| **Shoulder** | | | | |
| | Deltoid | Posterior deltoid | Anterior deltoid | |
| | Rotator cuff | | | |
| |   Infraspinatus | | | Infraspinatus |
| |   Subscapularis | | | Subscapularis |
| |   Supraspinatus | | | Supraspinatus |
| |   Teres minor | | | Teres minor |
| | Teres major | Teres major | | |
| **Upper arm** | | | | |
| | Anterior muscles | | | |
| |   Biceps brachii — long head | | Biceps brachii — long head | |
| |   Biceps brachii — short head | | Biceps brachii — short head | |
| |   Brachialis | | Brachialis | |
| |   Coracobrachialis | | Coracobrachialis | |
| | Posterior muscles | | | |
| |   Triceps brachii | Triceps brachii | | |
| **Forearm** | | | | |
| | Anterior muscles | | | |
| | Flexors | | | |
| |   Deep | | | |
| |     Flexor digitorum profundus | | Flexor digitorum profundus | |
| |     Flexor pollicis longus | | Flexor pollicis longus | |
| |   Intermediate | | | |
| |     Flexor digitorum superficialis | | Flexor digitorum superficialis | |
| |   Superficial | | | |
| |     Flexor carpi radialis | | Flexor carpi radialis | |
| |     Flexor carpi ulnaris | | Flexor carpi ulnaris | |
| |     Palmaris longus | | Palmaris longus | |
| | Pronators | | | |
| |   Pronator quadratus | | | Pronator quadratus |
| |   Pronator teres | | | Pronator teres |
| | Posterior muscles | | | |
| | Extensors | | | |
| |   Deep | | | |
| |     Abductor pollicis longus | | | Abductor pollicis longus |
| |     Extensor indicis | Extensor indicis | | |
| |     Extensor pollicis brevis | Extensor pollicis brevis | | |
| |     Extensor pollicis longus | Extensor pollicis longus | | |
| |   Superficial | | | |
| |     Brachioradialis | | | Brachioradialis |
| |     Extensor carpi radialis brevis | Extensor carpi radialis brevis | | |
| |     Extensor carpi radialis longus | Extensor carpi radialis longus | | |
| |     Extensor carpi ulnaris | Extensor carpi ulnaris | | |
| |     Extensor digiti minimi | Extensor digiti minimi | | |
| |     Extensor digitorum | Extensor digitorum | | |
| |     Anconeus | Anconeus | | |
| | Supinator | | | Supinator |

| Body Region | Muscle | Extensor Tendon | Flexor Tendon | Other Tendon |
|---|---|---|---|---|
| **Hand** | | | | |
| Extrinsic — attach to a site in the forearm as well as a site in the hand with action related to hand movement at the wrist | | | | |
| | Extensor carpi radialis brevis | Extensor carpi radialis brevis | | |
| | Extensor carpi radialis longus | Extensor carpie radialis longus | | |
| | Extensor carpi ulnaris | Extensor carpi ulnaris | | |
| | Flexor carpi radialis | | Flexor carpi radialis | |
| | Flexor carpi ulnaris | | Flexor carpi ulnaris | |
| | Flexor digitorum superficialis | | Flexor digitorum superficialis | |
| | Palmaris longus | | Palmaris longus | |
| Extrinsic — attach to a site in the forearm as well as a site in the hand with action in the hand related to finger movement | | | | |
| | Adductor pollicis longus | | | Adductor pollicis longus |
| | Extensor digiti minimi | Extensor digiti minimi | | |
| | Extensor digitorum | Extensor digitorum | | |
| | Extensor indicis | Extensor indicis | | |
| | Flexor digitorum profundus | | Flexor digitorum profundus | |
| | Flexor digitorum superficialis | | Flexor digitorum superficialis | |
| Extrinsic — attach to a site in the forearm as well as a site in the hand with action in the hand related to thumb movement | | | | |
| | Extensor pollicis brevis | Extensor pollicis brevis | | |
| | Extensor pollicis longus | Extensor pollicis longus | | |
| | Flexor pollicis longus | | Flexor pollicis longus | |
| Intrinsic — found within the hand only | | | | |
| | Adductor pollicis | | | Adductor pollicis |
| | Dorsal interossei | Dorsal interossei | Dorsal interossei | |
| | Lumbricals | Lumbricals | Lumbricals | |
| | Palmaris brevis | | | Palmaris brevis |
| | Palmar interossei | Palmar interossei | Palmar interossei | |
| | Hypothenar muscles | | | |
| |   Abductor digiti minimi | | | Abductor digiti minimi |
| |   Flexor digiti minimi brevis | | Flexor digiti minimi brevis | |
| |   Oppenens digiti minimi | | Oppenens digiti minimi | |
| | Thenar muscles | | | |
| |   Abductor pollicis brevis | | | Abductor pollicis brevis |
| |   Flexor pollicis brevis | | Flexor pollicis brevis | |
| |   Oppenens pollicis | | Oppenens pollicis | |
| **Thigh** | | | | |
| | Anterior muscles | | | |
| |   Iliopsoas | | Iliopsoas | |
| |   Pectineus | | Pectineus | |
| |   Quadriceps | Quadriceps | | |
| |     Rectus femoris | Rectus femoris — Extends knee | Rectus femoris — Flexes hip | |
| |     Vastus intermedius | Vastus intermedius | | |
| |     Vastus lateralis | Vastus lateralis | | |
| |     Vastus medialis | Vastus medialis | | |
| |   Sartorius | | Sartorius | |
| | Medial muscles | | | |
| |   Adductor brevis | | | Adductor brevis |
| |   Adductor longus | | | Adductor longus |
| |   Adductor magnus | | | Adductor magnus |
| |   Gracilis | | | Gracilis |
| |   Obturator externus | | | Obturator externus |
| | Posterior muscles | | | |
| |   Hamstring | Hamstring — Extends hip | Hamstring — Flexes knee | |
| |     Biceps femoris | Biceps femoris | Biceps femoris | |
| |     Semimembranosus | Semimembranosus | Semimembranosus | |
| |     Semitendinosus | Semitendinosus | Semitendinosus | |

Chapter 13. Diseases of the Musculoskeletal System and Connective Tissue

Chapter 13. Diseases of the Musculoskeletal System and Connective Tissue

| Body Region | Muscle | Extensor Tendon | Flexor Tendon | Other Tendon |
|---|---|---|---|---|
| **Lower leg** | | | | |
| | Anterior muscles | | | |
| | Extensor digitorum longus | Extensor digitorum longus | | |
| | Extensor hallucis longus | Extensor hallucis longus | | |
| | Fibularis (peroneus) tertius | Fibularis (peroneus) tertius | | |
| | Tibialis anterior | Tibialis anterior | | Tibialis anterior |
| | Lateral muscles | | | |
| | Fibularis (peroneus) brevis | | Fibularis (peroneus) brevis | |
| | Fibularis (peroneus) longus | | Fibularis (peroneus) longus | |
| | Posterior muscles | | | |
| | Deep | | | |
| | Flexor digitorum longus | | Flexor digitorum longus | |
| | Flexor hallucis longus | | Flexor hallucis longus | |
| | Popliteus | | Popliteus | |
| | Tibialis posterior | | Tibialis posterior | |
| | Superficial | | | |
| | Gastrocnemius | | Gastrocnemius | |
| | Plantaris | | Plantaris | |
| | Soleus | | Soleus | |
| | | | | Calcaneal (Achilles) |
| **Ankle/Foot** | | | | |
| **Extrinsic — attach to a site in the lower leg as well as a site in the foot with action related to foot movement at the ankle** | | | | |
| | Plantaris | | Plantaris | |
| | Soleus | | Soleus | |
| | Tibialis anterior | Tibialis anterior | | |
| | Tibialis posterior | | Tibialis posterior | |
| **Extrinsic — attach to a site in the lower leg as well as a site in the foot with action in the foot related to toe movement** | | | | |
| | Extensor digitorum longus | Extensor digitorum longus | | |
| | Extensor hallicus longus | Extensor hallicus longus | | |
| | Flexor digitorum longus | | Flexor digitorum longus | |
| | Flexor hallucis longus | | Flexor hallucis longus | |
| **Intrinsic — found within the ankle/foot only** | | | | |
| | Dorsal muscles | | | |
| | Extensor digitorum brevis | Extensor digitorum brevis | | |
| | Extensor hallucis brevis | Extensor hallucis brevis | | |
| | Plantar muscles | | | |
| | Abductor digiti minimi | | Abductor digiti minimi | |
| | Abductor hallucis | | Abductor hallucis | |
| | Dorsal interossei | Dorsal interossei | Dorsal interossei | |
| | Flexor digiti minimi brevis | | Flexor digiti minimi brevis | |
| | Flexor digitorum brevis | | Flexor digitorum brevis | |
| | Flexor hallucis brevis | | Flexor hallucis brevis | |
| | Lumbricals | Lumbricals | Lumbricals | |
| | Quadratus plantae | | Quadratus plantae | |
| | Plantar interossei | Plantar interossei | Plantar interossei | |

# Chapter 13. Diseases of the Musculoskeletal System and Connective Tissue (M00-M99)

**NOTE** Use an external cause code following the code for the musculoskeletal condition, if applicable, to identify the cause of the musculoskeletal condition.

**EXCLUDES 2** arthropathic psoriasis (L40.5-)
certain conditions originating in the perinatal period (P04-P96)
certain infectious and parasitic diseases (A00-B99)
compartment syndrome (traumatic) (T79.A-)
complications of pregnancy, childbirth and the puerperium (O00-O9A)
congenital malformations, deformations, and chromosomal abnormalities (Q00-Q99)
endocrine, nutritional and metabolic diseases (E00-E88)
injury, poisoning and certain other consequences of external causes (S00-T88)
neoplasms (C00-D49)
symptoms, signs and abnormal clinical and laboratory findings, not elsewhere classified (R00-R94)

This chapter contains the following blocks:

| | |
|---|---|
| M00-M02 | Infectious arthropathies |
| ~~M04~~ | ~~Autoinflammatory syndromes~~ |
| M05-M14 | Inflammatory polyarthropathies |
| M15-M19 | Osteoarthritis |
| M20-M25 | Other joint disorders |
| M26-M27 | Dentofacial anomalies [including malocclusion] and other disorders of jaw |
| M30-M36 | Systemic connective tissue disorders |
| M40-M43 | Deforming dorsopathies |
| M45-M49 | Spondylopathies |
| M50-M54 | Other dorsopathies |
| M60-M63 | Disorders of muscles |
| M65-M67 | Disorders of synovium and tendon |
| M70-M79 | Other soft tissue disorders |
| M80-M85 | Disorders of bone density and structure |
| M86-M90 | Other osteopathies |
| M91-M94 | Chondropathies |
| M95 | Other disorders of the musculoskeletal system and connective tissue |
| M96 | Intraoperative and postprocedural complications and disorders of musculoskeletal system, not elsewhere classified |
| ~~M97~~ | ~~Periprosthetic fracture around internal prosthetic joint~~ |
| M99 | Biomechanical lesions, not elsewhere classified |

## ARTHROPATHIES (M00-M25)

**INCLUDES** disorders affecting predominantly peripheral (limb) joints

### Infectious arthropathies (M00-M02)

**NOTE** This block comprises arthropathies due to microbiological agents. Distinction is made between the following types of etiological relationship:
a) direct infection of joint, where organisms invade synovial tissue and microbial antigen is present in the joint;
b) indirect infection, which may be of two types: a reactive arthropathy, where microbial infection of the body is established but neither organisms nor antigens can be identified in the joint, and a postinfective arthropathy, where microbial antigen is present but recovery of an organism is inconstant and evidence of local multiplication is lacking.

√4ᵗʰ **M00 Pyogenic arthritis**

√5ᵗʰ **M00.0 Staphylococcal arthritis and polyarthritis**
Use additional code (B95.61-B95.8) to identify bacterial agent
**EXCLUDES 2** infection and inflammatory reaction due to internal joint prosthesis (T84.5-)

**M00.00 Staphylococcal arthritis, unspecified joint** CC HCC
CC Excl: PDX collection 855

√6ᵗʰ **M00.01 Staphylococcal arthritis, shoulder**

> **CC Excl: For all CC codes in subcategory M00.01:** PDX collection 856

**M00.011 Staphylococcal arthritis, right shoulder** CC HCC

**M00.012 Staphylococcal arthritis, left shoulder** CC HCC

**M00.019 Staphylococcal arthritis, unspecified shoulder** CC HCC

**M00.02 Staphylococcal arthritis, elbow**

> **CC Excl: For all CC codes in subcategory M00.02:** PDX collection 857

**M00.021 Staphylococcal arthritis, right elbow** CC HCC

**M00.022 Staphylococcal arthritis, left elbow** CC HCC

**M00.029 Staphylococcal arthritis, unspecified elbow** CC HCC

√6ᵗʰ **M00.03 Staphylococcal arthritis, wrist**
Staphylococcal arthritis of carpal bones

> **CC Excl: For all CC codes in subcategory M00.03:** PDX collection 858

**M00.031 Staphylococcal arthritis, right wrist** CC HCC

**M00.032 Staphylococcal arthritis, left wrist** CC HCC

**M00.039 Staphylococcal arthritis, unspecified wrist** CC HCC

√6ᵗʰ **M00.04 Staphylococcal arthritis, hand**
Staphylococcal arthritis of metacarpus and phalanges

> **CC Excl: For all CC codes in subcategory M00.04:** PDX collection 859

**M00.041 Staphylococcal arthritis, right hand** CC HCC

**M00.042 Staphylococcal arthritis, left hand** CC HCC

**M00.049 Staphylococcal arthritis, unspecified hand** CC HCC

√6ᵗʰ **M00.05 Staphylococcal arthritis, hip**

> **CC Excl: For all CC codes in subcategory M00.05:** PDX collection 860

**M00.051 Staphylococcal arthritis, right hip** CC HCC
**M00.052 Staphylococcal arthritis, left hip** CC HCC
**M00.059 Staphylococcal arthritis, unspecified hip** CC HCC

√6ᵗʰ **M00.06 Staphylococcal arthritis, knee**

> **CC Excl: For all CC codes in subcategory M00.06:** PDX collection 861

**M00.061 Staphylococcal arthritis, right knee** CC HCC
**M00.062 Staphylococcal arthritis, left knee** CC HCC
**M00.069 Staphylococcal arthritis, unspecified knee** CC HCC

√6ᵗʰ **M00.07 Staphylococcal arthritis, ankle and foot**
Staphylococcal arthritis, tarsus, metatarsus and phalanges

> **CC Excl: For all CC codes in subcategory M00.07:** PDX collection 862

**M00.071 Staphylococcal arthritis, right ankle and foot** CC HCC

**M00.072 Staphylococcal arthritis, left ankle and foot** CC HCC

**M00.079 Staphylococcal arthritis, unspecified ankle and foot** CC HCC

**M00.08 Staphylococcal arthritis, vertebrae** CC HCC
CC Excl: PDX collection 855

**M00.09 Staphylococcal polyarthritis** CC HCC
CC Excl: PDX collection 855

√5ᵗʰ **M00.1 Pneumococcal arthritis and polyarthritis**
**M00.10 Pneumococcal arthritis, unspecified joint** CC HCC
CC Excl: PDX collection 855

√6ᵗʰ **M00.11 Pneumococcal arthritis, shoulder**

> **CC Excl: For CC codes in subcategory M00.11:** PDX collection 856

**M00.111 Pneumococcal arthritis, right shoulder** CC HCC

**M00.112 Pneumococcal arthritis, left shoulder** CC HCC

**M00.119 Pneumococcal arthritis, unspecified shoulder** CC HCC

☑ Additional Character Req   √x7ᵗʰ Placeholder Alert   Unacceptable PDx   Manifestation   **H1**-**H14** HAC   HCC CMS-HCC Condition   EXCLUDES 1 Not Coded Here   EXCLUDES 2 Not Included Here

ICD-10-CM 2018   735

M00–M00.119

**Chapter 13. Diseases of the Musculoskeletal System and Connective Tissue**

✓6ᵗʰ **M00.12 Pneumococcal arthritis,** elbow

> **CC Excl: For CC codes in subcategory M00.12:**
> PDX collection 857

  **M00.121 Pneumococcal arthritis, right elbow** `CC` `HCC`

  **M00.122 Pneumococcal arthritis, left elbow** `CC` `HCC`

  **M00.129 Pneumococcal arthritis, unspecified elbow** `CC` `HCC`

✓6ᵗʰ **M00.13 Pneumococcal arthritis,** wrist
Pneumococcal arthritis of carpal bones

> **CC Excl: For CC codes in subcategory M00.13:**
> PDX collection 858

  **M00.131 Pneumococcal arthritis, right wrist** `CC` `HCC`

  **M00.132 Pneumococcal arthritis, left wrist** `CC` `HCC`

  **M00.139 Pneumococcal arthritis, unspecified wrist** `CC` `HCC`

✓6ᵗʰ **M00.14 Pneumococcal arthritis,** hand
Pneumococcal arthritis of metacarpus and phalanges

> **CC Excl: For CC codes in subcategory M00.14:**
> PDX collection 859

  **M00.141 Pneumococcal arthritis, right hand** `CC` `HCC`

  **M00.142 Pneumococcal arthritis, left hand** `CC` `HCC`

  **M00.149 Pneumococcal arthritis, unspecified hand** `CC` `HCC`

✓6ᵗʰ **M00.15 Pneumococcal arthritis,** hip

> **CC Excl: For CC codes in subcategory M00.15:**
> PDX collection 860

  **M00.151 Pneumococcal arthritis, right hip** `CC` `HCC`

  **M00.152 Pneumococcal arthritis, left hip** `CC` `HCC`

  **M00.159 Pneumococcal arthritis, unspecified hip** `CC` `HCC`

✓6ᵗʰ **M00.16 Pneumococcal arthritis,** knee

> **CC Excl: For CC codes in subcategory M00.16:**
> PDX collection 861

  **M00.161 Pneumococcal arthritis, right knee** `CC` `HCC`

  **M00.162 Pneumococcal arthritis, left knee** `CC` `HCC`

  **M00.169 Pneumococcal arthritis, unspecified knee** `CC` `HCC`

✓6ᵗʰ **M00.17 Pneumococcal arthritis,** ankle and foot
Pneumococcal arthritis, tarsus, metatarsus and phalanges

> **CC Excl: For CC codes in subcategory M00.17:**
> PDX collection 862

  **M00.171 Pneumococcal arthritis, right ankle and foot** `CC` `HCC`

  **M00.172 Pneumococcal arthritis, left ankle and foot** `CC` `HCC`

  **M00.179 Pneumococcal arthritis, unspecified ankle and foot** `CC` `HCC`

**M00.18 Pneumococcal arthritis,** vertebrae `CC` `HCC`
**CC Excl:** PDX collection 855

**M00.19 Pneumococcal polyarthritis** `CC` `HCC`
**CC Excl:** PDX collection 855

✓5ᵗʰ **M00.2 Other streptococcal arthritis and polyarthritis**
Use additional code (B95.0-B95.2, B95.4-B95.5) to identify bacterial agent

**M00.20 Other streptococcal arthritis,** unspecified joint `CC` `HCC`
**CC Excl:** PDX collection 855

✓6ᵗʰ **M00.21 Other streptococcal arthritis,** shoulder

> **CC Excl: For CC codes in subcategory M00.21:**
> PDX collection 856

  **M00.211 Other streptococcal arthritis, right shoulder** `CC` `HCC`

  **M00.212 Other streptococcal arthritis, left shoulder** `CC` `HCC`

  **M00.219 Other streptococcal arthritis, unspecified shoulder** `CC` `HCC`

✓6ᵗʰ **M00.22 Other streptococcal arthritis,** elbow

> **CC Excl: For CC codes in subcategory M00.22:**
> PDX collection 857

  **M00.221 Other streptococcal arthritis, right elbow** `CC` `HCC`

  **M00.222 Other streptococcal arthritis, left elbow** `CC` `HCC`

  **M00.229 Other streptococcal arthritis, unspecified elbow** `CC` `HCC`

✓6ᵗʰ **M00.23 Other streptococcal arthritis,** wrist
Other streptococcal arthritis of carpal bones

> **CC Excl: For CC codes in subcategory M00.23:**
> PDX collection 858

  **M00.231 Other streptococcal arthritis, right wrist** `CC` `HCC`

  **M00.232 Other streptococcal arthritis, left wrist** `CC` `HCC`

  **M00.239 Other streptococcal arthritis, unspecified wrist** `CC` `HCC`

✓6ᵗʰ **M00.24 Other streptococcal arthritis,** hand
Other streptococcal arthritis metacarpus and phalanges

> **CC Excl: For CC codes in subcategory M00.24:**
> PDX collection 859

  **M00.241 Other streptococcal arthritis, right hand** `CC` `HCC`

  **M00.242 Other streptococcal arthritis, left hand** `CC` `HCC`

  **M00.249 Other streptococcal arthritis, unspecified hand** `CC` `HCC`

✓6ᵗʰ **M00.25 Other streptococcal arthritis,** hip

> **CC Excl: For CC codes in subcategory M00.25:**
> PDX collection 860

  **M00.251 Other streptococcal arthritis, right hip** `CC` `HCC`

  **M00.252 Other streptococcal arthritis, left hip** `CC` `HCC`

  **M00.259 Other streptococcal arthritis, unspecified hip** `CC` `HCC`

✓6ᵗʰ **M00.26 Other streptococcal arthritis,** knee

> **CC Excl: For CC codes in subcategory M00.26:**
> PDX collection 861

  **M00.261 Other streptococcal arthritis, right knee** `CC` `HCC`

  **M00.262 Other streptococcal arthritis, left knee** `CC` `HCC`

  **M00.269 Other streptococcal arthritis, unspecified knee** `CC` `HCC`

✓6ᵗʰ **M00.27 Other streptococcal arthritis,** ankle and foot
Other streptococcal arthritis, tarsus, metatarsus and phalanges

> **CC Excl: For CC codes in subcategory M00.27:**
> PDX collection 862

  **M00.271 Other streptococcal arthritis, right ankle and foot** `CC` `HCC`

  **M00.272 Other streptococcal arthritis, left ankle and foot** `CC` `HCC`

  **M00.279 Other streptococcal arthritis, unspecified ankle and foot** `CC` `HCC`

**M00.28 Other streptococcal arthritis,** vertebrae `CC` `HCC`
**CC Excl:** PDX collection 855

**M00.29 Other streptococcal polyarthritis** `CC` `HCC`
**CC Excl:** PDX collection 855

✓5ᵗʰ **M00.8 Arthritis and polyarthritis due to other bacteria**
Use additional code (B96) to identify bacteria

**M00.80 Arthritis due to other bacteria,** unspecified joint `CC` `HCC`
**CC Excl:** PDX collection 855

Ⓝ Newborn: 0   Ⓟ Pediatric: 0-17   Ⓜ Maternity: 12-55   Ⓐ Adult: 15-124   `MCC` Major CC Condition   `PDxMCC` PDx acts as own MCC   `CC` CC Condition   `PDxCC` PDx acts as own CC

**736**      ICD-10-CM 2018

✓6ᵗʰ **M00.81** **Arthritis due to other bacteria, shoulder**

> **CC Excl: For CC codes in subcategory M00.81:**
> PDX collection 856

**M00.811** **Arthritis due to other bacteria,** `CC` `HCC`
**right shoulder**

**M00.812** **Arthritis due to other bacteria,** `CC` `HCC`
**left shoulder**

**M00.819** **Arthritis due to other bacteria,** `CC` `HCC`
**unspecified shoulder**

✓6ᵗʰ **M00.82** **Arthritis due to other bacteria, elbow**

> **CC Excl: For CC codes in subcategory M00.82:**
> PDX collection 857

**M00.821** **Arthritis due to other bacteria,** `CC` `HCC`
**right elbow**

**M00.822** **Arthritis due to other bacteria,** `CC` `HCC`
**left elbow**

**M00.829** **Arthritis due to other bacteria,** `CC` `HCC`
**unspecified elbow**

✓6ᵗʰ **M00.83** **Arthritis due to other bacteria, wrist**
Arthritis due to other bacteria, carpal bones

> **CC Excl: For CC codes in subcategory M00.83:**
> PDX collection 858

**M00.831** **Arthritis due to other bacteria,** `CC` `HCC`
**right wrist**

**M00.832** **Arthritis due to other bacteria,** `CC` `HCC`
**left wrist**

**M00.839** **Arthritis due to other bacteria,** `CC` `HCC`
**unspecified wrist**

✓6ᵗʰ **M00.84** **Arthritis due to other bacteria, hand**
Arthritis due to other bacteria, metacarpus and
phalanges

> **CC Excl: For CC codes in subcategory M00.84:**
> PDX collection 859

**M00.841** **Arthritis due to other bacteria,** `CC` `HCC`
**right hand**

**M00.842** **Arthritis due to other bacteria,** `CC` `HCC`
**left hand**

**M00.849** **Arthritis due to other bacteria,** `CC` `HCC`
**unspecified hand**

✓6ᵗʰ **M00.85** **Arthritis due to other bacteria, hip**

> **CC Excl: For CC codes in subcategory M00.85:**
> PDX collection 860

**M00.851** **Arthritis due to other bacteria,** `CC` `HCC`
**right hip**

**M00.852** **Arthritis due to other bacteria,** `CC` `HCC`
**left hip**

**M00.859** **Arthritis due to other bacteria,** `CC` `HCC`
**unspecified hip**

✓6ᵗʰ **M00.86** **Arthritis due to other bacteria, knee**

> **CC Excl: For CC codes in subcategory M00.86:**
> PDX collection 861

**M00.861** **Arthritis due to other bacteria,** `CC` `HCC`
**right knee**

**M00.862** **Arthritis due to other bacteria,** `CC` `HCC`
**left knee**

**M00.869** **Arthritis due to other bacteria,** `CC` `HCC`
**unspecified knee**

✓6ᵗʰ **M00.87** **Arthritis due to other bacteria, ankle and foot**
Arthritis due to other bacteria, tarsus, metatarsus,
and phalanges

> **CC Excl: For CC codes in subcategory M00.87:**
> PDX collection 862

**M00.871** **Arthritis due to other bacteria,** `CC` `HCC`
**right ankle and foot**

**M00.872** **Arthritis due to other bacteria,** `CC` `HCC`
**left ankle and foot**

**M00.879** **Arthritis due to other bacteria,** `CC` `HCC`
**unspecified ankle and foot**

**M00.88** **Arthritis due to other bacteria, vertebrae** `CC` `HCC`
**CC Excl:** PDX collection 855

**M00.89** **Polyarthritis due to other bacteria** `CC` `HCC`
**CC Excl:** PDX collection 855

**M00.9** **Pyogenic arthritis, unspecified** `CC` `HCC`
Infective arthritis NOS
**CC Excl:** PDX collection 855

✓4ᵗʰ **M01** **Direct infections of joint in infectious and parasitic diseases classified elsewhere**

Code first underlying disease, such as:
leprosy [Hansen's disease] (A30.-)
mycoses (B35-B49)
O'nyong-nyong fever (A92.1)
paratyphoid fever (A01.1-A01.4)

> *EXCLUDES 1*   arthropathy in Lyme disease (A69.23)
> gonococcal arthritis (A54.42)
> meningococcal arthritis (A39.83)
> mumps arthritis (B26.85)
> postinfective arthropathy (M02.-)
> postmeningococcal arthritis (A39.84)
> reactive arthritis (M02.3)
> rubella arthritis (B06.82)
> sarcoidosis arthritis (D86.86)
> typhoid fever arthritis (A01.04)
> tuberculosis arthritis (A18.01-A18.02)

> **CC Excl: For CC codes in category M01, unless otherwise noted:** PDX collection 863

✓5ᵗʰ **M01.X** **Direct infection of joint in infectious and parasitic diseases classified elsewhere**

**M01.X0** *Direct infection of unspecified joint in* `CC` `HCC`
*infectious and parasitic diseases classified elsewhere*

✓6ᵗʰ **M01.X1** **Direct infection of shoulder joint in infectious and parasitic diseases classified elsewhere**

> **CC Excl: For CC codes in subcategory M01.X1, unless otherwise noted:** PDX collection 864

**M01.X11** *Direct infection of right shoulder in* `CC` `HCC`
*infectious and parasitic diseases classified elsewhere*

**M01.X12** *Direct infection of left shoulder in* `CC` `HCC`
*infectious and parasitic diseases classified elsewhere*

**M01.X19** *Direct infection of unspecified* `CC` `HCC`
*shoulder in infectious and parasitic diseases classified elsewhere*

✓6ᵗʰ **M01.X2** **Direct infection of elbow in infectious and parasitic diseases classified elsewhere**

**M01.X21** *Direct infection of right elbow in* `CC` `HCC`
*infectious and parasitic diseases classified elsewhere*

**M01.X22** *Direct infection of left elbow in* `CC` `HCC`
*infectious and parasitic diseases classified elsewhere*

**M01.X29** *Direct infection of unspecified elbow* `CC` `HCC`
*in infectious and parasitic diseases classified elsewhere*

✓6ᵗʰ **M01.X3** **Direct infection of wrist in infectious and parasitic diseases classified elsewhere**
Direct infection of carpal bones in infectious and
parasitic diseases classified elsewhere

**M01.X31** *Direct infection of right wrist in* `CC` `HCC`
*infectious and parasitic diseases classified elsewhere*

**M01.X32** *Direct infection of left wrist in* `CC` `HCC`
*infectious and parasitic diseases classified elsewhere*

**M01.X39** *Direct infection of unspecified wrist* `CC` `HCC`
*in infectious and parasitic diseases classified elsewhere*

✓6ᵗʰ **M01.X4** **Direct infection of hand in infectious and parasitic diseases classified elsewhere**
Direct infection of metacarpus and phalanges in
infectious and parasitic diseases classified
elsewhere

**M01.X41** *Direct infection of right hand in* `CC` `HCC`
*infectious and parasitic diseases classified elsewhere*

**M01.X42** *Direct infection of left hand in* `CC` `HCC`
*infectious and parasitic diseases classified elsewhere*

**M01.X49** *Direct infection of unspecified hand* `CC` `HCC`
*in infectious and parasitic diseases classified elsewhere*

✓6ᵗʰ **M01.X5** Direct infection of hip in infectious and parasitic diseases classified elsewhere

    *M01.X51*   *Direct infection of right hip in infectious and parasitic diseases classified elsewhere*   CC HCC

    *M01.X52*   *Direct infection of left hip in infectious and parasitic diseases classified elsewhere*   CC HCC

    *M01.X59*   *Direct infection of unspecified hip in infectious and parasitic diseases classified elsewhere*   CC HCC

✓6ᵗʰ **M01.X6** Direct infection of knee in infectious and parasitic diseases classified elsewhere

    *M01.X61*   *Direct infection of right knee in infectious and parasitic diseases classified elsewhere*   CC HCC

    *M01.X62*   *Direct infection of left knee in infectious and parasitic diseases classified elsewhere*   CC HCC

    *M01.X69*   *Direct infection of unspecified knee in infectious and parasitic diseases classified elsewhere*   CC HCC

✓6ᵗʰ **M01.X7** Direct infection of ankle and foot in infectious and parasitic diseases classified elsewhere

    Direct infection of tarsus, metatarsus and phalanges in infectious and parasitic diseases classified elsewhere

    *M01.X71*   *Direct infection of right ankle and foot in infectious and parasitic diseases classified elsewhere*   CC HCC

    *M01.X72*   *Direct infection of left ankle and foot in infectious and parasitic diseases classified elsewhere*   CC HCC

    *M01.X79*   *Direct infection of unspecified ankle and foot in infectious and parasitic diseases classified elsewhere*   CC HCC

    *M01.X8*   *Direct infection of vertebrae in infectious and parasitic diseases classified elsewhere*   CC HCC

    *M01.X9*   *Direct infection of multiple joints in infectious and parasitic diseases classified elsewhere*   CC HCC

✓4ᵗʰ **M02 Postinfective and reactive arthropathies**

    Code first underlying disease, such as:
      congenital syphilis [Clutton's joints] (A50.5)
      enteritis due to Yersinia enterocolitica (A04.6)
      infective endocarditis (I33.0)
      viral hepatitis (B15-B19)

    **EXCLUDES 1**   *Behçet's disease (M35.2)*
        *direct infections of joint in infectious and parasitic diseases classified elsewhere (M01.-)*
        *mumps arthritis (B26.85)*
        *postmeningococcal arthritis (A39.84)*
        *rheumatic fever (I00)*
        *rubella arthritis (B06.82)*
        *syphilis arthritis (late) (A52.77)*
        *tabetic arthropathy [Charcôt's] (A52.16)*

✓5ᵗʰ **M02.0 Arthropathy following intestinal bypass**

    **M02.00**   Arthropathy following intestinal bypass, unspecified site

    ✓6ᵗʰ **M02.01**   Arthropathy following intestinal bypass, shoulder

        **M02.011**   Arthropathy following intestinal bypass, right shoulder

        **M02.012**   Arthropathy following intestinal bypass, left shoulder

        **M02.019**   Arthropathy following intestinal bypass, unspecified shoulder

    ✓6ᵗʰ **M02.02**   Arthropathy following intestinal bypass, elbow

        **M02.021**   Arthropathy following intestinal bypass, right elbow

        **M02.022**   Arthropathy following intestinal bypass, left elbow

        **M02.029**   Arthropathy following intestinal bypass, unspecified elbow

    ✓6ᵗʰ **M02.03**   Arthropathy following intestinal bypass, wrist
        Arthropathy following intestinal bypass, carpal bones

        **M02.031**   Arthropathy following intestinal bypass, right wrist

        **M02.032**   Arthropathy following intestinal bypass, left wrist

        **M02.039**   Arthropathy following intestinal bypass, unspecified wrist

    ✓6ᵗʰ **M02.04**   Arthropathy following intestinal bypass, hand
        Arthropathy following intestinal bypass, metacarpals and phalanges

        **M02.041**   Arthropathy following intestinal bypass, right hand

        **M02.042**   Arthropathy following intestinal bypass, left hand

        **M02.049**   Arthropathy following intestinal bypass, unspecified hand

    ✓6ᵗʰ **M02.05**   Arthropathy following intestinal bypass, hip

        **M02.051**   Arthropathy following intestinal bypass, right hip

        **M02.052**   Arthropathy following intestinal bypass, left hip

        **M02.059**   Arthropathy following intestinal bypass, unspecified hip

    ✓6ᵗʰ **M02.06**   Arthropathy following intestinal bypass, knee

        **M02.061**   Arthropathy following intestinal bypass, right knee

        **M02.062**   Arthropathy following intestinal bypass, left knee

        **M02.069**   Arthropathy following intestinal bypass, unspecified knee

    ✓6ᵗʰ **M02.07**   Arthropathy following intestinal bypass, ankle and foot

        Arthropathy following intestinal bypass, tarsus, metatarsus and phalanges

        **M02.071**   Arthropathy following intestinal bypass, right ankle and foot

        **M02.072**   Arthropathy following intestinal bypass, left ankle and foot

        **M02.079**   Arthropathy following intestinal bypass, unspecified ankle and foot

    **M02.08**   Arthropathy following intestinal bypass, vertebrae

    **M02.09**   Arthropathy following intestinal bypass, multiple sites

✓5ᵗʰ **M02.1 Postdysenteric arthropathy**

    **CC Excl: For CC codes in subcategory M02.1, unless otherwise noted:** PDX collection 863

    **M02.10**   Postdysenteric arthropathy, unspecified site   CC HCC

    ✓6ᵗʰ **M02.11**   Postdysenteric arthropathy, shoulder

        **M02.111**   Postdysenteric arthropathy, right shoulder   CC HCC

        **M02.112**   Postdysenteric arthropathy, left shoulder   CC HCC

        **M02.119**   Postdysenteric arthropathy, unspecified shoulder   CC HCC

    ✓6ᵗʰ **M02.12**   Postdysenteric arthropathy, elbow

        **M02.121**   Postdysenteric arthropathy, right elbow   CC HCC

        **M02.122**   Postdysenteric arthropathy, left elbow   CC HCC

        **M02.129**   Postdysenteric arthropathy, unspecified elbow   CC HCC

    ✓6ᵗʰ **M02.13**   Postdysenteric arthropathy, wrist
        Postdysenteric arthropathy, carpal bones

        **M02.131**   Postdysenteric arthropathy, right wrist   CC HCC

        **M02.132**   Postdysenteric arthropathy, left wrist   CC HCC

        **M02.139**   Postdysenteric arthropathy, unspecified wrist   CC HCC

    ✓6ᵗʰ **M02.14**   Postdysenteric arthropathy, hand
        Postdysenteric arthropathy, metacarpus and phalanges

        **M02.141**   Postdysenteric arthropathy, right hand   CC HCC

        **M02.142**   Postdysenteric arthropathy, left hand   CC HCC

        **M02.149**   Postdysenteric arthropathy, unspecified hand   CC HCC

    ✓6ᵗʰ **M02.15**   Postdysenteric arthropathy, hip

        **M02.151**   Postdysenteric arthropathy, right hip   CC HCC

        **M02.152**   Postdysenteric arthropathy, left hip   CC HCC

Ⓝ Newborn: 0   Ⓟ Pediatric: 0-17   Ⓜ Maternity: 12-55   Ⓐ Adult: 15-124   **MCC** Major CC Condition   **PDxMCC** PDx acts as own MCC   **CC** CC Condition   **PDxCC** PDx acts as own CC

**738**      ICD-10-CM 2018

M02.159 **Postdysenteric arthropathy, unspecified hip** `CC` `HCC`

✓6ᵗʰ **M02.16 Postdysenteric arthropathy, knee**

> **CC Excl: For CC codes in subcategory M02.16:** PDX collection 865

M02.161 **Postdysenteric arthropathy, right knee** `CC` `HCC`

M02.162 **Postdysenteric arthropathy, left knee** `CC` `HCC`

M02.169 **Postdysenteric arthropathy, unspecified knee** `CC` `HCC`

✓6ᵗʰ **M02.17 Postdysenteric arthropathy, ankle and foot**
Postdysenteric arthropathy, tarsus, metatarsus and phalanges

M02.171 **Postdysenteric arthropathy, right ankle and foot** `CC` `HCC`

M02.172 **Postdysenteric arthropathy, left ankle and foot** `CC` `HCC`

M02.179 **Postdysenteric arthropathy, unspecified ankle and foot** `CC` `HCC`

M02.18 **Postdysenteric arthropathy, vertebrae** `CC` `HCC`
**CC Excl:** PDX collection 866

M02.19 **Postdysenteric arthropathy, multiple sites** `CC` `HCC`

✓5ᵗʰ **M02.2 Postimmunization arthropathy**

M02.20 **Postimmunization arthropathy, unspecified site**

✓6ᵗʰ **M02.21 Postimmunization arthropathy, shoulder**

M02.211 **Postimmunization arthropathy, right shoulder**

M02.212 **Postimmunization arthropathy, left shoulder**

M02.219 **Postimmunization arthropathy, unspecified shoulder**

✓6ᵗʰ **M02.22 Postimmunization arthropathy, elbow**

M02.221 **Postimmunization arthropathy, right elbow**

M02.222 **Postimmunization arthropathy, left elbow**

M02.229 **Postimmunization arthropathy, unspecified elbow**

✓6ᵗʰ **M02.23 Postimmunization arthropathy, wrist**
Postimmunization arthropathy, carpal bones

M02.231 **Postimmunization arthropathy, right wrist**

M02.232 **Postimmunization arthropathy, left wrist**

M02.239 **Postimmunization arthropathy, unspecified wrist**

✓6ᵗʰ **M02.24 Postimmunization arthropathy, hand**
Postimmunization arthropathy, metacarpus and phalanges

M02.241 **Postimmunization arthropathy, right hand**

M02.242 **Postimmunization arthropathy, left hand**

M02.249 **Postimmunization arthropathy, unspecified hand**

✓6ᵗʰ **M02.25 Postimmunization arthropathy, hip**

M02.251 **Postimmunization arthropathy, right hip**

M02.252 **Postimmunization arthropathy, left hip**

M02.259 **Postimmunization arthropathy, unspecified hip**

✓6ᵗʰ **M02.26 Postimmunization arthropathy, knee**

M02.261 **Postimmunization arthropathy, right knee**

M02.262 **Postimmunization arthropathy, left knee**

M02.269 **Postimmunization arthropathy, unspecified knee**

✓6ᵗʰ **M02.27 Postimmunization arthropathy, ankle and foot**
Postimmunization arthropathy, tarsus, metatarsus and phalanges

M02.271 **Postimmunization arthropathy, right ankle and foot**

M02.272 **Postimmunization arthropathy, left ankle and foot**

M02.279 **Postimmunization arthropathy, unspecified ankle and foot**

M02.28 **Postimmunization arthropathy, vertebrae**

M02.29 **Postimmunization arthropathy, multiple sites**

✓5ᵗʰ **M02.3 Reiter's disease**
Reactive arthritis

> **CC Excl: For CC codes in subcategory M02.3:** PDX collection 863

M02.30 **Reiter's disease, unspecified site** `PDx CC` `CC` `HCC`

✓6ᵗʰ **M02.31 Reiter's disease, shoulder**

M02.311 **Reiter's disease, right shoulder** `PDx CC` `CC` `HCC`

M02.312 **Reiter's disease, left shoulder** `PDx CC` `CC` `HCC`

M02.319 **Reiter's disease, unspecified shoulder** `PDx CC` `CC` `HCC`

✓6ᵗʰ **M02.32 Reiter's disease, elbow**

M02.321 **Reiter's disease, right elbow** `PDx CC` `CC` `HCC`

M02.322 **Reiter's disease, left elbow** `PDx CC` `CC` `HCC`

M02.329 **Reiter's disease, unspecified elbow** `PDx CC` `CC` `HCC`

✓6ᵗʰ **M02.33 Reiter's disease, wrist**
Reiter's disease, carpal bones

M02.331 **Reiter's disease, right wrist** `PDx CC` `CC` `HCC`

M02.332 **Reiter's disease, left wrist** `PDx CC` `CC` `HCC`

M02.339 **Reiter's disease, unspecified wrist** `PDx CC` `CC` `HCC`

✓6ᵗʰ **M02.34 Reiter's disease, hand**
Reiter's disease, metacarpus and phalanges

M02.341 **Reiter's disease, right hand** `PDx CC` `CC` `HCC`

M02.342 **Reiter's disease, left hand** `PDx CC` `CC` `HCC`

M02.349 **Reiter's disease, unspecified hand** `PDx CC` `CC` `HCC`

✓6ᵗʰ **M02.35 Reiter's disease, hip**

M02.351 **Reiter's disease, right hip** `PDx CC` `CC` `HCC`

M02.352 **Reiter's disease, left hip** `PDx CC` `CC` `HCC`

M02.359 **Reiter's disease, unspecified hip** `PDx CC` `CC` `HCC`

✓6ᵗʰ **M02.36 Reiter's disease, knee**

M02.361 **Reiter's disease, right knee** `PDx CC` `CC` `HCC`

M02.362 **Reiter's disease, left knee** `PDx CC` `CC` `HCC`

M02.369 **Reiter's disease, unspecified knee** `PDx CC` `CC` `HCC`

✓6ᵗʰ **M02.37 Reiter's disease, ankle and foot**
Reiter's disease, tarsus, metatarsus and phalanges

M02.371 **Reiter's disease, right ankle and foot** `PDx CC` `CC` `HCC`

M02.372 **Reiter's disease, left ankle and foot** `PDx CC` `CC` `HCC`

M02.379 **Reiter's disease, unspecified ankle and foot** `PDx CC` `CC` `HCC`

M02.38 **Reiter's disease, vertebrae** `PDx CC` `CC` `HCC`

M02.39 **Reiter's disease, multiple sites** `PDx CC` `CC` `HCC`

✓5ᵗʰ **M02.8 Other reactive arthropathies**

> **CC Excl: For CC codes in subcategory M02.8, unless otherwise noted:** PDX collection 863

*M02.80* *Other reactive arthropathies, unspecified site* `CC` `HCC`

✓6ᵗʰ **M02.81 Other reactive arthropathies, shoulder**

> **CC Excl: For CC codes in subcategory M02.81:** PDX collection 864

*M02.811* *Other reactive arthropathies, right shoulder* `CC` `HCC`

*M02.812* *Other reactive arthropathies, left shoulder* `CC` `HCC`

*M02.819* *Other reactive arthropathies, unspecified shoulder* `CC` `HCC`

✓6ᵗʰ **M02.82 Other reactive arthropathies, elbow**

*M02.821* *Other reactive arthropathies, right elbow* `CC` `HCC`

*M02.822* *Other reactive arthropathies, left elbow* `CC` `HCC`

*M02.829* *Other reactive arthropathies, unspecified elbow* `CC` `HCC`

✓6th **M02.83** **Other reactive arthropathies, wrist**
Other reactive arthropathies, carpal bones

**M02.831** *Other reactive arthropathies, right wrist* `CC` `HCC`

**M02.832** *Other reactive arthropathies, left wrist* `CC` `HCC`

**M02.839** *Other reactive arthropathies, unspecified wrist* `CC` `HCC`

✓6th **M02.84** **Other reactive arthropathies, hand**
Other reactive arthropathies, metacarpus and phalanges

**M02.841** *Other reactive arthropathies, right hand* `CC` `HCC`

**M02.842** *Other reactive arthropathies, left hand* `CC` `HCC`

**M02.849** *Other reactive arthropathies, unspecified hand* `CC` `HCC`

✓6th **M02.85** **Other reactive arthropathies, hip**

**M02.851** *Other reactive arthropathies, right hip* `CC` `HCC`

**M02.852** *Other reactive arthropathies, left hip* `CC` `HCC`

**M02.859** *Other reactive arthropathies, unspecified hip* `CC` `HCC`

✓6th **M02.86** **Other reactive arthropathies, knee**

**M02.861** *Other reactive arthropathies, right knee* `CC` `HCC`

**M02.862** *Other reactive arthropathies, left knee* `CC` `HCC`

**M02.869** *Other reactive arthropathies, unspecified knee* `CC` `HCC`

✓6th **M02.87** **Other reactive arthropathies, ankle and foot**
Other reactive arthropathies, tarsus, metatarsus and phalanges

**M02.871** *Other reactive arthropathies, right ankle and foot* `CC` `HCC`

**M02.872** *Other reactive arthropathies, left ankle and foot* `CC` `HCC`

**M02.879** *Other reactive arthropathies, unspecified ankle and foot* `CC` `HCC`

**M02.88** *Other reactive arthropathies, vertebrae* `CC` `HCC`

**M02.89** *Other reactive arthropathies, multiple sites* `CC` `HCC`

**M02.9** *Reactive arthropathy, unspecified* `HCC`

## Autoinflammatory syndromes (M04)

✓4th **M04** **Autoinflammatory syndromes**
EXCLUDES 2 *Crohn's disease (K50.-)*

**M04.1** **Periodic fever syndromes** `HCC`
Familial Mediterranean fever
Hyperimmunoglobin D syndrome
Mevalonate kinase deficiency
Tumor necrosis factor receptor associated periodic syndrome [TRAPS]

**M04.2** **Cryopyrin-associated periodic syndromes** `HCC`
Chronic infantile neurological, cutaneous and articular syndrome [CINCA]
Familial cold autoinflammatory syndrome
Familial cold urticaria
Muckle-Wells syndrome
Neonatal onset multisystemic inflammatory disorder [NOMID]

**M04.8** **Other autoinflammatory syndromes** `HCC`
Blau syndrome
Deficiency of interleukin 1 receptor antagonist [DIRA]
Majeed syndrome
Periodic fever, aphthous stomatitis, pharyngitis, and adenopathy syndrome [PFAPA]
Pyogenic arthritis, pyoderma gangrenosum, and acne syndrome [PAPA]

**M04.9** **Autoinflammatory syndrome, unspecified** `HCC`

## Inflammatory polyarthropathies (M05-M14)

✓4th **M05** **Rheumatoid arthritis with rheumatoid factor**
EXCLUDES 1 *rheumatic fever (I00)*
*juvenile rheumatoid arthritis (M08.-)*
*rheumatoid arthritis of spine (M45.-)*
**DEF:** Rheumatoid arthritis: Autoimmune systemic disease that causes chronic inflammation of joints and other areas of the body, manifested by inflammatory changes in articular structures and synovial membranes, atrophy, and loss in bone density.

✓5th **M05.0** **Felty's syndrome**
Rheumatoid arthritis with splenoadenomegaly and leukopenia

**M05.00** **Felty's syndrome, unspecified site** `HCC`

✓6th **M05.01** **Felty's syndrome, shoulder**

**M05.011** **Felty's syndrome, right shoulder** `HCC`

**M05.012** **Felty's syndrome, left shoulder** `HCC`

**M05.019** **Felty's syndrome, unspecified shoulder** `HCC`

✓6th **M05.02** **Felty's syndrome, elbow**

**M05.021** **Felty's syndrome, right elbow** `HCC`

**M05.022** **Felty's syndrome, left elbow** `HCC`

**M05.029** **Felty's syndrome, unspecified elbow** `HCC`

✓6th **M05.03** **Felty's syndrome, wrist**
Felty's syndrome, carpal bones

**M05.031** **Felty's syndrome, right wrist** `HCC`

**M05.032** **Felty's syndrome, left wrist** `HCC`

**M05.039** **Felty's syndrome, unspecified wrist** `HCC`

✓6th **M05.04** **Felty's syndrome, hand**
Felty's syndrome, metacarpus and phalanges

**M05.041** **Felty's syndrome, right hand** `HCC`

**M05.042** **Felty's syndrome, left hand** `HCC`

**M05.049** **Felty's syndrome, unspecified hand** `HCC`

✓6th **M05.05** **Felty's syndrome, hip**

**M05.051** **Felty's syndrome, right hip** `HCC`

**M05.052** **Felty's syndrome, left hip** `HCC`

**M05.059** **Felty's syndrome, unspecified hip** `HCC`

✓6th **M05.06** **Felty's syndrome, knee**

**M05.061** **Felty's syndrome, right knee** `HCC`

**M05.062** **Felty's syndrome, left knee** `HCC`

**M05.069** **Felty's syndrome, unspecified knee** `HCC`

✓6th **M05.07** **Felty's syndrome, ankle and foot**
Felty's syndrome, tarsus, metatarsus and phalanges

**M05.071** **Felty's syndrome, right ankle and foot** `HCC`

**M05.072** **Felty's syndrome, left ankle and foot** `HCC`

**M05.079** **Felty's syndrome, unspecified ankle and foot** `HCC`

**M05.09** **Felty's syndrome, multiple sites** `HCC`

✓5th **M05.1** **Rheumatoid lung disease with rheumatoid arthritis**
**DEF:** Lung disorders associated with rheumatoid arthritis.

**M05.10** **Rheumatoid lung disease with rheumatoid arthritis of unspecified site** `HCC`

✓6th **M05.11** **Rheumatoid lung disease with rheumatoid arthritis of shoulder**

**M05.111** **Rheumatoid lung disease with rheumatoid arthritis of right shoulder** `HCC`

**M05.112** **Rheumatoid lung disease with rheumatoid arthritis of left shoulder** `HCC`

**M05.119** **Rheumatoid lung disease with rheumatoid arthritis of unspecified shoulder** `HCC`

✓6th **M05.12** **Rheumatoid lung disease with rheumatoid arthritis of elbow**

**M05.121** **Rheumatoid lung disease with rheumatoid arthritis of right elbow** `HCC`

**M05.122** **Rheumatoid lung disease with rheumatoid arthritis of left elbow** `HCC`

**M05.129** **Rheumatoid lung disease with rheumatoid arthritis of unspecified elbow** `HCC`

N Newborn: 0  P Pediatric: 0-17  M Maternity: 12-55  A Adult: 15-124  MCC Major CC Condition  PDxMCC PDx acts as own MCC  CC CC Condition  PDxCC PDx acts as own CC

740

ICD-10-CM 2018

✔6ᵗʰ **M05.13** **Rheumatoid lung disease with rheumatoid arthritis of** wrist
     Rheumatoid lung disease with rheumatoid arthritis, carpal bones

     **M05.131** **Rheumatoid lung disease with rheumatoid arthritis of** right **wrist** `HCC`

     **M05.132** **Rheumatoid lung disease with rheumatoid arthritis of** left **wrist** `HCC`

     **M05.139** **Rheumatoid lung disease with rheumatoid arthritis of** unspecified **wrist** `HCC`

✔6ᵗʰ **M05.14** **Rheumatoid lung disease with rheumatoid arthritis of** hand
     Rheumatoid lung disease with rheumatoid arthritis, metacarpus and phalanges

     **M05.141** **Rheumatoid lung disease with rheumatoid arthritis of** right **hand** `HCC`

     **M05.142** **Rheumatoid lung disease with rheumatoid arthritis of** left **hand** `HCC`

     **M05.149** **Rheumatoid lung disease with rheumatoid arthritis of** unspecified **hand** `HCC`

✔6ᵗʰ **M05.15** **Rheumatoid lung disease with rheumatoid arthritis of** hip

     **M05.151** **Rheumatoid lung disease with rheumatoid arthritis of** right **hip** `HCC`

     **M05.152** **Rheumatoid lung disease with rheumatoid arthritis of** left **hip** `HCC`

     **M05.159** **Rheumatoid lung disease with rheumatoid arthritis of** unspecified **hip** `HCC`

✔6ᵗʰ **M05.16** **Rheumatoid lung disease with rheumatoid arthritis of** knee

     **M05.161** **Rheumatoid lung disease with rheumatoid arthritis of** right **knee** `HCC`

     **M05.162** **Rheumatoid lung disease with rheumatoid arthritis of** left **knee** `HCC`

     **M05.169** **Rheumatoid lung disease with rheumatoid arthritis of** unspecified **knee** `HCC`

✔6ᵗʰ **M05.17** **Rheumatoid lung disease with rheumatoid arthritis of** ankle and foot
     Rheumatoid lung disease with rheumatoid arthritis, tarsus, metatarsus and phalanges

     **M05.171** **Rheumatoid lung disease with rheumatoid arthritis of** right **ankle and foot** `HCC`

     **M05.172** **Rheumatoid lung disease with rheumatoid arthritis of** left **ankle and foot** `HCC`

     **M05.179** **Rheumatoid lung disease with rheumatoid arthritis of** unspecified **ankle and foot** `HCC`

     **M05.19** **Rheumatoid lung disease with rheumatoid arthritis of** multiple sites `HCC`

✔5ᵗʰ **M05.2** **Rheumatoid** vasculitis with rheumatoid arthritis

     **M05.20** **Rheumatoid vasculitis with rheumatoid arthritis of** unspecified site `HCC`

✔6ᵗʰ **M05.21** **Rheumatoid vasculitis with rheumatoid arthritis of** shoulder

     **M05.211** **Rheumatoid vasculitis with rheumatoid arthritis of** right **shoulder** `HCC`

     **M05.212** **Rheumatoid vasculitis with rheumatoid arthritis of** left **shoulder** `HCC`

     **M05.219** **Rheumatoid vasculitis with rheumatoid arthritis of** unspecified **shoulder** `HCC`

✔6ᵗʰ **M05.22** **Rheumatoid vasculitis with rheumatoid arthritis of** elbow

     **M05.221** **Rheumatoid vasculitis with rheumatoid arthritis of** right **elbow** `HCC`

     **M05.222** **Rheumatoid vasculitis with rheumatoid arthritis of** left **elbow** `HCC`

     **M05.229** **Rheumatoid vasculitis with rheumatoid arthritis of** unspecified **elbow** `HCC`

✔6ᵗʰ **M05.23** **Rheumatoid vasculitis with rheumatoid arthritis of** wrist
     Rheumatoid vasculitis with rheumatoid arthritis, carpal bones

     **M05.231** **Rheumatoid vasculitis with rheumatoid arthritis of** right **wrist** `HCC`

     **M05.232** **Rheumatoid vasculitis with rheumatoid arthritis of** left **wrist** `HCC`

     **M05.239** **Rheumatoid vasculitis with rheumatoid arthritis of** unspecified **wrist** `HCC`

✔6ᵗʰ **M05.24** **Rheumatoid vasculitis with rheumatoid arthritis of** hand
     Rheumatoid vasculitis with rheumatoid arthritis, metacarpus and phalanges

     **M05.241** **Rheumatoid vasculitis with rheumatoid arthritis of** right **hand** `HCC`

     **M05.242** **Rheumatoid vasculitis with rheumatoid arthritis of** left **hand** `HCC`

     **M05.249** **Rheumatoid vasculitis with rheumatoid arthritis of** unspecified **hand** `HCC`

✔6ᵗʰ **M05.25** **Rheumatoid vasculitis with rheumatoid arthritis of** hip

     **M05.251** **Rheumatoid vasculitis with rheumatoid arthritis of** right **hip** `HCC`

     **M05.252** **Rheumatoid vasculitis with rheumatoid arthritis of** left **hip** `HCC`

     **M05.259** **Rheumatoid vasculitis with rheumatoid arthritis of** unspecified **hip** `HCC`

✔6ᵗʰ **M05.26** **Rheumatoid vasculitis with rheumatoid arthritis of** knee

     **M05.261** **Rheumatoid vasculitis with rheumatoid arthritis of** right **knee** `HCC`

     **M05.262** **Rheumatoid vasculitis with rheumatoid arthritis of** left **knee** `HCC`

     **M05.269** **Rheumatoid vasculitis with rheumatoid arthritis of** unspecified **knee** `HCC`

✔6ᵗʰ **M05.27** **Rheumatoid vasculitis with rheumatoid arthritis of** ankle and foot
     Rheumatoid vasculitis with rheumatoid arthritis, tarsus, metatarsus and phalanges

     **M05.271** **Rheumatoid vasculitis with rheumatoid arthritis of** right **ankle and foot** `HCC`

     **M05.272** **Rheumatoid vasculitis with rheumatoid arthritis of** left **ankle and foot** `HCC`

     **M05.279** **Rheumatoid vasculitis with rheumatoid arthritis of** unspecified **ankle and foot** `HCC`

     **M05.29** **Rheumatoid vasculitis with rheumatoid arthritis of** multiple sites `HCC`

✔5ᵗʰ **M05.3** **Rheumatoid** heart disease with rheumatoid arthritis
     Rheumatoid carditis      Rheumatoid myocarditis
     Rheumatoid endocarditis      Rheumatoid pericarditis

     **M05.30** **Rheumatoid heart disease with rheumatoid arthritis of** unspecified site `HCC`

✔6ᵗʰ **M05.31** **Rheumatoid heart disease with rheumatoid arthritis of** shoulder

     **M05.311** **Rheumatoid heart disease with rheumatoid arthritis of** right **shoulder** `HCC`

     **M05.312** **Rheumatoid heart disease with rheumatoid arthritis of** left **shoulder** `HCC`

     **M05.319** **Rheumatoid heart disease with rheumatoid arthritis of** unspecified **shoulder** `HCC`

✔6ᵗʰ **M05.32** **Rheumatoid heart disease with rheumatoid arthritis of** elbow

     **M05.321** **Rheumatoid heart disease with rheumatoid arthritis of** right **elbow** `HCC`

     **M05.322** **Rheumatoid heart disease with rheumatoid arthritis of** left **elbow** `HCC`

     **M05.329** **Rheumatoid heart disease with rheumatoid arthritis of** unspecified **elbow** `HCC`

✔6ᵗʰ **M05.33** **Rheumatoid heart disease with rheumatoid arthritis of** wrist
     Rheumatoid heart disease with rheumatoid arthritis, carpal bones

     **M05.331** **Rheumatoid heart disease with rheumatoid arthritis of** right **wrist** `HCC`

     **M05.332** **Rheumatoid heart disease with rheumatoid arthritis of** left **wrist** `HCC`

     **M05.339** **Rheumatoid heart disease with rheumatoid arthritis of** unspecified **wrist** `HCC`

---

✔ Additional Character Req    ✔x7ᵗʰ Placeholder Alert    Unacceptable PDx    Manifestation    `H1`-`H14` HAC    `HCC` CMS-HCC Condition    *EXCLUDES 1* Not Coded Here    *EXCLUDES 2* Not Included Here

✓6ᵗʰ **M05.34 Rheumatoid heart disease with rheumatoid arthritis of** hand
Rheumatoid heart disease with rheumatoid arthritis, metacarpus and phalanges

M05.341 **Rheumatoid heart disease with rheumatoid arthritis of** right **hand** `HCC`

M05.342 **Rheumatoid heart disease with rheumatoid arthritis of** left **hand** `HCC`

M05.349 **Rheumatoid heart disease with rheumatoid arthritis of** unspecified **hand** `HCC`

✓6ᵗʰ **M05.35 Rheumatoid heart disease with rheumatoid arthritis of** hip

M05.351 **Rheumatoid heart disease with rheumatoid arthritis of** right **hip** `HCC`

M05.352 **Rheumatoid heart disease with rheumatoid arthritis of** left **hip** `HCC`

M05.359 **Rheumatoid heart disease with rheumatoid arthritis of** unspecified **hip** `HCC`

✓6ᵗʰ **M05.36 Rheumatoid heart disease with rheumatoid arthritis of** knee

M05.361 **Rheumatoid heart disease with rheumatoid arthritis of** right **knee** `HCC`

M05.362 **Rheumatoid heart disease with rheumatoid arthritis of** left **knee** `HCC`

M05.369 **Rheumatoid heart disease with rheumatoid arthritis of** unspecified **knee** `HCC`

✓6ᵗʰ **M05.37 Rheumatoid heart disease with rheumatoid arthritis of** ankle and foot
Rheumatoid heart disease with rheumatoid arthritis, tarsus, metatarsus and phalanges

M05.371 **Rheumatoid heart disease with rheumatoid arthritis of** right **ankle and foot** `HCC`

M05.372 **Rheumatoid heart disease with rheumatoid arthritis of** left **ankle and foot** `HCC`

M05.379 **Rheumatoid heart disease with rheumatoid arthritis of** unspecified **ankle and foot** `HCC`

M05.39 **Rheumatoid heart disease with rheumatoid arthritis of** multiple sites `HCC`

✓5ᵗʰ **M05.4 Rheumatoid** myopathy with rheumatoid arthritis

**CC Excl: For CC codes in subcategory M05.4:**
PDX collection 867

M05.40 **Rheumatoid myopathy with rheumatoid arthritis of** unspecified **site** `PDxCC` `CC` `HCC`

✓6ᵗʰ **M05.41 Rheumatoid myopathy with rheumatoid arthritis of** shoulder

M05.411 **Rheumatoid myopathy with rheumatoid arthritis of** right **shoulder** `PDxCC` `CC` `HCC`

M05.412 **Rheumatoid myopathy with rheumatoid arthritis of** left **shoulder** `PDxCC` `CC` `HCC`

M05.419 **Rheumatoid myopathy with rheumatoid arthritis of** unspecified **shoulder** `PDxCC` `CC` `HCC`

✓6ᵗʰ **M05.42 Rheumatoid myopathy with rheumatoid arthritis of** elbow

M05.421 **Rheumatoid myopathy with rheumatoid arthritis of** right **elbow** `PDxCC` `CC` `HCC`

M05.422 **Rheumatoid myopathy with rheumatoid arthritis of** left **elbow** `PDxCC` `CC` `HCC`

M05.429 **Rheumatoid myopathy with rheumatoid arthritis of** unspecified **elbow** `PDxCC` `CC` `HCC`

✓6ᵗʰ **M05.43 Rheumatoid myopathy with rheumatoid arthritis of** wrist
Rheumatoid myopathy with rheumatoid arthritis, carpal bones

M05.431 **Rheumatoid myopathy with rheumatoid arthritis of** right **wrist** `PDxCC` `CC` `HCC`

M05.432 **Rheumatoid myopathy with rheumatoid arthritis of** left **wrist** `PDxCC` `CC` `HCC`

M05.439 **Rheumatoid myopathy with rheumatoid arthritis of** unspecified **wrist** `PDxCC` `CC` `HCC`

✓6ᵗʰ **M05.44 Rheumatoid myopathy with rheumatoid arthritis of** hand
Rheumatoid myopathy with rheumatoid arthritis, metacarpus and phalanges

M05.441 **Rheumatoid myopathy with rheumatoid arthritis of** right **hand** `PDxCC` `CC` `HCC`

M05.442 **Rheumatoid myopathy with rheumatoid arthritis of** left **hand** `PDxCC` `CC` `HCC`

M05.449 **Rheumatoid myopathy with rheumatoid arthritis of** unspecified **hand** `PDxCC` `CC` `HCC`

✓6ᵗʰ **M05.45 Rheumatoid myopathy with rheumatoid arthritis of** hip

M05.451 **Rheumatoid myopathy with rheumatoid arthritis of** right **hip** `PDxCC` `CC` `HCC`

M05.452 **Rheumatoid myopathy with rheumatoid arthritis of** left **hip** `PDxCC` `CC` `HCC`

M05.459 **Rheumatoid myopathy with rheumatoid arthritis of** unspecified **hip** `PDxCC` `CC` `HCC`

✓6ᵗʰ **M05.46 Rheumatoid myopathy with rheumatoid arthritis of** knee

M05.461 **Rheumatoid myopathy with rheumatoid arthritis of** right **knee** `PDxCC` `CC` `HCC`

M05.462 **Rheumatoid myopathy with rheumatoid arthritis of** left **knee** `PDxCC` `CC` `HCC`

M05.469 **Rheumatoid myopathy with rheumatoid arthritis of** unspecified **knee** `PDxCC` `CC` `HCC`

✓6ᵗʰ **M05.47 Rheumatoid myopathy with rheumatoid arthritis of** ankle and foot
Rheumatoid myopathy with rheumatoid arthritis, tarsus, metatarsus and phalanges

M05.471 **Rheumatoid myopathy with rheumatoid arthritis of** right **ankle and foot** `PDxCC` `CC` `HCC`

M05.472 **Rheumatoid myopathy with rheumatoid arthritis of** left **ankle and foot** `PDxCC` `CC` `HCC`

M05.479 **Rheumatoid myopathy with rheumatoid arthritis of** unspecified **ankle and foot** `PDxCC` `CC` `HCC`

M05.49 **Rheumatoid myopathy with rheumatoid arthritis of** multiple sites `PDxCC` `CC` `HCC`

✓5ᵗʰ **M05.5 Rheumatoid** polyneuropathy with rheumatoid arthritis

M05.50 **Rheumatoid polyneuropathy with rheumatoid arthritis of** unspecified **site** `HCC`

✓6ᵗʰ **M05.51 Rheumatoid polyneuropathy with rheumatoid arthritis of** shoulder

M05.511 **Rheumatoid polyneuropathy with rheumatoid arthritis of** right **shoulder** `HCC`

M05.512 **Rheumatoid polyneuropathy with rheumatoid arthritis of** left **shoulder** `HCC`

M05.519 **Rheumatoid polyneuropathy with rheumatoid arthritis of** unspecified **shoulder** `HCC`

✓6ᵗʰ **M05.52 Rheumatoid polyneuropathy with rheumatoid arthritis of** elbow

M05.521 **Rheumatoid polyneuropathy with rheumatoid arthritis of** right **elbow** `HCC`

M05.522 **Rheumatoid polyneuropathy with rheumatoid arthritis of** left **elbow** `HCC`

M05.529 **Rheumatoid polyneuropathy with rheumatoid arthritis of** unspecified **elbow** `HCC`

✓6ᵗʰ **M05.53 Rheumatoid polyneuropathy with rheumatoid arthritis of** wrist
Rheumatoid polyneuropathy with rheumatoid arthritis, carpal bones

M05.531 **Rheumatoid polyneuropathy with rheumatoid arthritis of** right **wrist** `HCC`

M05.532 **Rheumatoid polyneuropathy with rheumatoid arthritis of** left **wrist** `HCC`

M05.539 **Rheumatoid polyneuropathy with rheumatoid arthritis of** unspecified **wrist** `HCC`

Ⓝ Newborn: 0 Ⓟ Pediatric: 0-17 Ⓜ Maternity: 12-55 Ⓐ Adult: 15-124 `MCC` Major CC Condition `PDxMCC` PDx acts as own MCC `CC` CC Condition `PDxCC` PDx acts as own CC

742

ICD-10-CM 2018

✓6ᵗʰ **M05.54** **Rheumatoid polyneuropathy with rheumatoid arthritis of hand**
Rheumatoid polyneuropathy with rheumatoid arthritis, metacarpus and phalanges

**M05.541** **Rheumatoid polyneuropathy with rheumatoid arthritis of right hand** ᴴᶜᶜ

**M05.542** **Rheumatoid polyneuropathy with rheumatoid arthritis of left hand** ᴴᶜᶜ

**M05.549** **Rheumatoid polyneuropathy with rheumatoid arthritis of unspecified hand** ᴴᶜᶜ

✓6ᵗʰ **M05.55** **Rheumatoid polyneuropathy with rheumatoid arthritis of hip**

**M05.551** **Rheumatoid polyneuropathy with rheumatoid arthritis of right hip** ᴴᶜᶜ

**M05.552** **Rheumatoid polyneuropathy with rheumatoid arthritis of left hip** ᴴᶜᶜ

**M05.559** **Rheumatoid polyneuropathy with rheumatoid arthritis of unspecified hip** ᴴᶜᶜ

✓6ᵗʰ **M05.56** **Rheumatoid polyneuropathy with rheumatoid arthritis of knee**

**M05.561** **Rheumatoid polyneuropathy with rheumatoid arthritis of right knee** ᴴᶜᶜ

**M05.562** **Rheumatoid polyneuropathy with rheumatoid arthritis of left knee** ᴴᶜᶜ

**M05.569** **Rheumatoid polyneuropathy with rheumatoid arthritis of unspecified knee** ᴴᶜᶜ

✓6ᵗʰ **M05.57** **Rheumatoid polyneuropathy with rheumatoid arthritis of ankle and foot**
Rheumatoid polyneuropathy with rheumatoid arthritis, tarsus, metatarsus and phalanges

**M05.571** **Rheumatoid polyneuropathy with rheumatoid arthritis of right ankle and foot** ᴴᶜᶜ

**M05.572** **Rheumatoid polyneuropathy with rheumatoid arthritis of left ankle and foot** ᴴᶜᶜ

**M05.579** **Rheumatoid polyneuropathy with rheumatoid arthritis of unspecified ankle and foot** ᴴᶜᶜ

**M05.59** **Rheumatoid polyneuropathy with rheumatoid arthritis of multiple sites** ᴴᶜᶜ

✓5ᵗʰ **M05.6** **Rheumatoid arthritis with involvement of other organs and systems**

**M05.60** **Rheumatoid arthritis of unspecified site with involvement of other organs and systems** ᴴᶜᶜ

✓6ᵗʰ **M05.61** **Rheumatoid arthritis of shoulder with involvement of other organs and systems**

**M05.611** **Rheumatoid arthritis of right shoulder with involvement of other organs and systems** ᴴᶜᶜ

**M05.612** **Rheumatoid arthritis of left shoulder with involvement of other organs and systems** ᴴᶜᶜ

**M05.619** **Rheumatoid arthritis of unspecified shoulder with involvement of other organs and systems** ᴴᶜᶜ

✓6ᵗʰ **M05.62** **Rheumatoid arthritis of elbow with involvement of other organs and systems**

**M05.621** **Rheumatoid arthritis of right elbow with involvement of other organs and systems** ᴴᶜᶜ

**M05.622** **Rheumatoid arthritis of left elbow with involvement of other organs and systems** ᴴᶜᶜ

**M05.629** **Rheumatoid arthritis of unspecified elbow with involvement of other organs and systems** ᴴᶜᶜ

✓6ᵗʰ **M05.63** **Rheumatoid arthritis of wrist with involvement of other organs and systems**
Rheumatoid arthritis of carpal bones with involvement of other organs and systems

**M05.631** **Rheumatoid arthritis of right wrist with involvement of other organs and systems** ᴴᶜᶜ

**M05.632** **Rheumatoid arthritis of left wrist with involvement of other organs and systems** ᴴᶜᶜ

**M05.639** **Rheumatoid arthritis of unspecified wrist with involvement of other organs and systems** ᴴᶜᶜ

✓6ᵗʰ **M05.64** **Rheumatoid arthritis of hand with involvement of other organs and systems**
Rheumatoid arthritis of metacarpus and phalanges with involvement of other organs and systems

**M05.641** **Rheumatoid arthritis of right hand with involvement of other organs and systems** ᴴᶜᶜ

**M05.642** **Rheumatoid arthritis of left hand with involvement of other organs and systems** ᴴᶜᶜ

**M05.649** **Rheumatoid arthritis of unspecified hand with involvement of other organs and systems** ᴴᶜᶜ

✓6ᵗʰ **M05.65** **Rheumatoid arthritis of hip with involvement of other organs and systems**

**M05.651** **Rheumatoid arthritis of right hip with involvement of other organs and systems** ᴴᶜᶜ

**M05.652** **Rheumatoid arthritis of left hip with involvement of other organs and systems** ᴴᶜᶜ

**M05.659** **Rheumatoid arthritis of unspecified hip with involvement of other organs and systems** ᴴᶜᶜ

✓6ᵗʰ **M05.66** **Rheumatoid arthritis of knee with involvement of other organs and systems**

**M05.661** **Rheumatoid arthritis of right knee with involvement of other organs and systems** ᴴᶜᶜ

**M05.662** **Rheumatoid arthritis of left knee with involvement of other organs and systems** ᴴᶜᶜ

**M05.669** **Rheumatoid arthritis of unspecified knee with involvement of other organs and systems** ᴴᶜᶜ

✓6ᵗʰ **M05.67** **Rheumatoid arthritis of ankle and foot with involvement of other organs and systems**
Rheumatoid arthritis of tarsus, metatarsus and phalanges with involvement of other organs and systems

**M05.671** **Rheumatoid arthritis of right ankle and foot with involvement of other organs and systems** ᴴᶜᶜ

**M05.672** **Rheumatoid arthritis of left ankle and foot with involvement of other organs and systems** ᴴᶜᶜ

**M05.679** **Rheumatoid arthritis of unspecified ankle and foot with involvement of other organs and systems** ᴴᶜᶜ

**M05.69** **Rheumatoid arthritis of multiple sites with involvement of other organs and systems** ᴴᶜᶜ

✓5ᵗʰ **M05.7** **Rheumatoid arthritis with rheumatoid factor without organ or systems involvement**

**M05.70** **Rheumatoid arthritis with rheumatoid factor of unspecified site without organ or systems involvement** ᴴᶜᶜ

✓6ᵗʰ **M05.71** **Rheumatoid arthritis with rheumatoid factor of shoulder without organ or systems involvement**

**M05.711** **Rheumatoid arthritis with rheumatoid factor of right shoulder without organ or systems involvement** ᴴᶜᶜ

**M05.712** **Rheumatoid arthritis with rheumatoid factor of left shoulder without organ or systems involvement** ᴴᶜᶜ

**M05.719** **Rheumatoid arthritis with rheumatoid factor of unspecified shoulder without organ or systems involvement** ᴴᶜᶜ

✓6ᵗʰ **M05.72** **Rheumatoid arthritis with rheumatoid factor of elbow without organ or systems involvement**

**M05.721** **Rheumatoid arthritis with rheumatoid factor of right elbow without organ or systems involvement** ᴴᶜᶜ

**M05.722** **Rheumatoid arthritis with rheumatoid factor of left elbow without organ or systems involvement** ᴴᶜᶜ

✔ Additional Character Req  ✔x7ᵗʰ Placeholder Alert  Unacceptable PDx  Manifestation  H1 - H14 HAC  ᴴᶜᶜ CMS-HCC Condition  *EXCLUDES 1* Not Coded Here  *EXCLUDES 2* Not Included Here

ICD-10-CM 2018  **743**

**M05.729** Rheumatoid arthritis with rheumatoid factor of unspecified elbow without organ or systems involvement

✓6ᵗʰ **M05.73** Rheumatoid arthritis with rheumatoid factor of wrist without organ or systems involvement

**M05.731** Rheumatoid arthritis with rheumatoid factor of right wrist without organ or systems involvement  `HCC`

**M05.732** Rheumatoid arthritis with rheumatoid factor of left wrist without organ or systems involvement  `HCC`

**M05.739** Rheumatoid arthritis with rheumatoid factor of unspecified wrist without organ or systems involvement  `HCC`

✓6ᵗʰ **M05.74** Rheumatoid arthritis with rheumatoid factor of hand without organ or systems involvement

**M05.741** Rheumatoid arthritis with rheumatoid factor of right hand without organ or systems involvement  `HCC`

**M05.742** Rheumatoid arthritis with rheumatoid factor of left hand without organ or systems involvement  `HCC`

**M05.749** Rheumatoid arthritis with rheumatoid factor of unspecified hand without organ or systems involvement  `HCC`

✓6ᵗʰ **M05.75** Rheumatoid arthritis with rheumatoid factor of hip without organ or systems involvement

**M05.751** Rheumatoid arthritis with rheumatoid factor of right hip without organ or systems involvement  `HCC`

**M05.752** Rheumatoid arthritis with rheumatoid factor of left hip without organ or systems involvement  `HCC`

**M05.759** Rheumatoid arthritis with rheumatoid factor of unspecified hip without organ or systems involvement  `HCC`

✓6ᵗʰ **M05.76** Rheumatoid arthritis with rheumatoid factor of knee without organ or systems involvement

**M05.761** Rheumatoid arthritis with rheumatoid factor of right knee without organ or systems involvement  `HCC`

**M05.762** Rheumatoid arthritis with rheumatoid factor of left knee without organ or systems involvement  `HCC`

**M05.769** Rheumatoid arthritis with rheumatoid factor of unspecified knee without organ or systems involvement  `HCC`

✓6ᵗʰ **M05.77** Rheumatoid arthritis with rheumatoid factor of ankle and foot without organ or systems involvement

**M05.771** Rheumatoid arthritis with rheumatoid factor of right ankle and foot without organ or systems involvement  `HCC`

**M05.772** Rheumatoid arthritis with rheumatoid factor of left ankle and foot without organ or systems involvement  `HCC`

**M05.779** Rheumatoid arthritis with heumatoid factor of unspecified ankle and foot without organ or systems involvement  `HCC`

**M05.79** Rheumatoid arthritis with rheumatoid factor of multiple sites without organ or systems involvement  `HCC`

✓5ᵗʰ **M05.8** Other rheumatoid arthritis with rheumatoid factor

**M05.80** Other rheumatoid arthritis with rheumatoid actor of unspecified site  `HCC`

✓6ᵗʰ **M05.81** Other rheumatoid arthritis with rheumatoid factor of shoulder

**M05.811** Other rheumatoid arthritis with rheumatoid factor of right shoulder  `HCC`

**M05.812** Other rheumatoid arthritis with rheumatoid factor of left shoulder  `HCC`

**M05.819** Other rheumatoid arthritis with rheumatoid factor of unspecified shoulder  `HCC`

✓6ᵗʰ **M05.82** Other rheumatoid arthritis with rheumatoid factor of elbow

**M05.821** Other rheumatoid arthritis with rheumatoid factor of right elbow  `HCC`

**M05.822** Other rheumatoid arthritis with rheumatoid factor of left elbow  `HCC`

**M05.829** Other rheumatoid arthritis with rheumatoid factor of unspecified elbow  `HCC`

✓6ᵗʰ **M05.83** Other rheumatoid arthritis with rheumatoid factor of wrist

**M05.831** Other rheumatoid arthritis with rheumatoid factor of right wrist  `HCC`

**M05.832** Other rheumatoid arthritis with rheumatoid factor of left wrist  `HCC`

**M05.839** Other rheumatoid arthritis with rheumatoid factor of unspecified wrist  `HCC`

✓6ᵗʰ **M05.84** Other rheumatoid arthritis with rheumatoid factor of hand

**M05.841** Other rheumatoid arthritis with rheumatoid factor of right hand  `HCC`

**M05.842** Other rheumatoid arthritis with rheumatoid factor of left hand  `HCC`

**M05.849** Other rheumatoid arthritis with rheumatoid factor of unspecified hand  `HCC`

✓6ᵗʰ **M05.85** Other rheumatoid arthritis with rheumatoid factor of hip

**M05.851** Other rheumatoid arthritis with rheumatoid factor of right hip  `HCC`

**M05.852** Other rheumatoid arthritis with rheumatoid factor of left hip  `HCC`

**M05.859** Other rheumatoid arthritis with rheumatoid factor of unspecified hip  `HCC`

✓6ᵗʰ **M05.86** Other rheumatoid arthritis with rheumatoid factor of knee

**M05.861** Other rheumatoid arthritis with rheumatoid factor of right knee  `HCC`

**M05.862** Other rheumatoid arthritis with rheumatoid factor of left knee  `HCC`

**M05.869** Other rheumatoid arthritis with rheumatoid factor of unspecified knee  `HCC`

✓6ᵗʰ **M05.87** Other rheumatoid arthritis with rheumatoid factor of ankle and foot

**M05.871** Other rheumatoid arthritis with rheumatoid factor of right ankle and foot  `HCC`

**M05.872** Other rheumatoid arthritis with rheumatoid factor of left ankle and foot  `HCC`

**M05.879** Other rheumatoid arthritis with rheumatoid factor of unspecified ankle and foot  `HCC`

**M05.89** Other rheumatoid arthritis with rheumatoid factor of multiple sites  `HCC`

**M05.9** Rheumatoid arthritis with rheumatoid factor, unspecified  `HCC`

✓4ᵗʰ **M06** **Other rheumatoid arthritis**

**DEF:** Rheumatoid arthritis: Autoimmune systemic disease that causes chronic inflammation of joints and other areas of the body, manifested by inflammatory changes in articular structures and synovial membranes, atrophy, and loss in bone density.

✓5ᵗʰ **M06.0** Rheumatoid arthritis without rheumatoid factor

**M06.00** Rheumatoid arthritis without rheumatoid factor, unspecified site  `HCC`

✓6ᵗʰ **M06.01** Rheumatoid arthritis without rheumatoid factor, shoulder

**M06.011** Rheumatoid arthritis without rheumatoid factor, right shoulder  `HCC`

**M06.012** Rheumatoid arthritis without rheumatoid factor, left shoulder  `HCC`

**M06.019** Rheumatoid arthritis without rheumatoid factor, unspecified shoulder  `HCC`

✓6ᵗʰ **M06.02** Rheumatoid arthritis without rheumatoid factor, elbow

**M06.021** Rheumatoid arthritis without rheumatoid factor, right elbow  `HCC`

**M06.022** Rheumatoid arthritis without rheumatoid factor, left elbow  `HCC`

**M06.029** Rheumatoid arthritis without rheumatoid factor, unspecified elbow  `HCC`

**N** Newborn: 0   **P** Pediatric: 0-17   **M** Maternity: 12-55   **A** Adult: 15-124   **MCC** Major CC Condition   **PDxMCC** PDx acts as own MCC   **CC** CC Condition   **PDxCC** PDx acts as own CC

**744**                                                      ICD-10-CM 2018

✓6th **M06.03 Rheumatoid arthritis without rheumatoid factor, wrist**
- M06.031 Rheumatoid arthritis without rheumatoid factor, **right wrist** `HCC`
- M06.032 Rheumatoid arthritis without rheumatoid factor, **left wrist** `HCC`
- M06.039 Rheumatoid arthritis without rheumatoid factor, **unspecified** wrist `HCC`

✓6th **M06.04 Rheumatoid arthritis without rheumatoid factor, hand**
- M06.041 Rheumatoid arthritis without rheumatoid factor, **right hand** `HCC`
- M06.042 Rheumatoid arthritis without rheumatoid factor, **left hand** `HCC`
- M06.049 Rheumatoid arthritis without rheumatoid factor, **unspecified hand** `HCC`

✓6th **M06.05 Rheumatoid arthritis without rheumatoid factor, hip**
- M06.051 Rheumatoid arthritis without rheumatoid factor, **right hip** `HCC`
- M06.052 Rheumatoid arthritis without rheumatoid factor, **left hip** `HCC`
- M06.059 Rheumatoid arthritis without rheumatoid factor, **unspecified hip** `HCC`

✓6th **M06.06 Rheumatoid arthritis without rheumatoid factor, knee**
- M06.061 Rheumatoid arthritis without rheumatoid factor, **right knee** `HCC`
- M06.062 Rheumatoid arthritis without rheumatoid factor, **left knee** `HCC`
- M06.069 Rheumatoid arthritis without rheumatoid factor, **unspecified knee** `HCC`

✓6th **M06.07 Rheumatoid arthritis without rheumatoid factor, ankle and foot**
- M06.071 Rheumatoid arthritis without rheumatoid factor, **right ankle and foot** `HCC`
- M06.072 Rheumatoid arthritis without rheumatoid factor, **left ankle and foot** `HCC`
- M06.079 Rheumatoid arthritis without rheumatoid factor, **unspecified ankle and foot** `HCC`

M06.08 Rheumatoid arthritis without rheumatoid factor, **vertebrae** `HCC`

M06.09 Rheumatoid arthritis without rheumatoid factor, **multiple sites** `HCC`

**M06.1 Adult-onset Still's disease** `HCC` `A`
> *EXCLUDES 1*   Still's disease NOS (M08.2-)

✓5th **M06.2 Rheumatoid bursitis**

M06.20 Rheumatoid bursitis, **unspecified site** `HCC`

✓6th **M06.21 Rheumatoid bursitis, shoulder**
- M06.211 Rheumatoid bursitis, **right shoulder** `HCC`
- M06.212 Rheumatoid bursitis, **left shoulder** `HCC`
- M06.219 Rheumatoid bursitis, **unspecified shoulder** `HCC`

✓6th **M06.22 Rheumatoid bursitis, elbow**
- M06.221 Rheumatoid bursitis, **right elbow** `HCC`
- M06.222 Rheumatoid bursitis, **left elbow** `HCC`
- M06.229 Rheumatoid bursitis, **unspecified elbow** `HCC`

✓6th **M06.23 Rheumatoid bursitis, wrist**
- M06.231 Rheumatoid bursitis, **right wrist** `HCC`
- M06.232 Rheumatoid bursitis, **left wrist** `HCC`
- M06.239 Rheumatoid bursitis, **unspecified wrist** `HCC`

✓6th **M06.24 Rheumatoid bursitis, hand**
- M06.241 Rheumatoid bursitis, **right hand** `HCC`
- M06.242 Rheumatoid bursitis, **left hand** `HCC`
- M06.249 Rheumatoid bursitis, **unspecified hand** `HCC`

✓6th **M06.25 Rheumatoid bursitis, hip**
- M06.251 Rheumatoid bursitis, **right hip** `HCC`
- M06.252 Rheumatoid bursitis, **left hip** `HCC`
- M06.259 Rheumatoid bursitis, **unspecified hip** `HCC`

✓6th **M06.26 Rheumatoid bursitis, knee**
- M06.261 Rheumatoid bursitis, **right knee** `HCC`
- M06.262 Rheumatoid bursitis, **left knee** `HCC`
- M06.269 Rheumatoid bursitis, **unspecified knee** `HCC`

✓6th **M06.27 Rheumatoid bursitis, ankle and foot**
- M06.271 Rheumatoid bursitis, **right ankle and foot** `HCC`
- M06.272 Rheumatoid bursitis, **left ankle and foot** `HCC`
- M06.279 Rheumatoid bursitis, **unspecified ankle and foot** `HCC`

M06.28 Rheumatoid bursitis, **vertebrae** `HCC`

M06.29 Rheumatoid bursitis, **multiple sites** `HCC`

✓5th **M06.3 Rheumatoid nodule**

M06.30 Rheumatoid nodule, **unspecified site** `HCC`

✓6th **M06.31 Rheumatoid nodule, shoulder**
- M06.311 Rheumatoid nodule, **right shoulder** `HCC`
- M06.312 Rheumatoid nodule, **left shoulder** `HCC`
- M06.319 Rheumatoid nodule, **unspecified shoulder** `HCC`

✓6th **M06.32 Rheumatoid nodule, elbow**
- M06.321 Rheumatoid nodule, **right elbow** `HCC`
- M06.322 Rheumatoid nodule, **left elbow** `HCC`
- M06.329 Rheumatoid nodule, **unspecified elbow** `HCC`

✓6th **M06.33 Rheumatoid nodule, wrist**
- M06.331 Rheumatoid nodule, **right wrist** `HCC`
- M06.332 Rheumatoid nodule, **left wrist** `HCC`
- M06.339 Rheumatoid nodule, **unspecified wrist** `HCC`

✓6th **M06.34 Rheumatoid nodule, hand**
- M06.341 Rheumatoid nodule, **right hand** `HCC`
- M06.342 Rheumatoid nodule, **left hand** `HCC`
- M06.349 Rheumatoid nodule, **unspecified hand** `HCC`

✓6th **M06.35 Rheumatoid nodule, hip**
- M06.351 Rheumatoid nodule, **right hip** `HCC`
- M06.352 Rheumatoid nodule, **left hip** `HCC`
- M06.359 Rheumatoid nodule, **unspecified hip** `HCC`

✓6th **M06.36 Rheumatoid nodule, knee**
- M06.361 Rheumatoid nodule, **right knee** `HCC`
- M06.362 Rheumatoid nodule, **left knee** `HCC`
- M06.369 Rheumatoid nodule, **unspecified knee** `HCC`

✓6th **M06.37 Rheumatoid nodule, ankle and foot**
- M06.371 Rheumatoid nodule, **right ankle and foot** `HCC`
- M06.372 Rheumatoid nodule, **left ankle and foot** `HCC`
- M06.379 Rheumatoid nodule, **unspecified ankle and foot** `HCC`

M06.38 Rheumatoid nodule, **vertebrae** `HCC`

M06.39 Rheumatoid nodule, **multiple sites** `HCC`

**M06.4 Inflammatory polyarthropathy** `HCC`
> *EXCLUDES 1*   polyarthritis NOS (M13.0)

✓5th **M06.8 Other specified rheumatoid arthritis**

M06.80 Other specified rheumatoid arthritis, **unspecified site** `HCC`

✓6th **M06.81 Other specified rheumatoid arthritis, shoulder**
- M06.811 Other specified rheumatoid arthritis, **right shoulder** `HCC`
- M06.812 Other specified rheumatoid arthritis, **left shoulder** `HCC`
- M06.819 Other specified rheumatoid arthritis, **unspecified shoulder** `HCC`

✓6th **M06.82 Other specified rheumatoid arthritis, elbow**
- M06.821 Other specified rheumatoid arthritis, **right elbow** `HCC`
- M06.822 Other specified rheumatoid arthritis, **left elbow** `HCC`
- M06.829 Other specified rheumatoid arthritis, **unspecified elbow** `HCC`

✓6th **M06.83 Other specified rheumatoid arthritis, wrist**
- M06.831 Other specified rheumatoid arthritis, **right wrist** `HCC`

        **M06.832** Other specified rheumatoid arthritis, **HCC**
left wrist

        **M06.839** Other specified rheumatoid arthritis, **HCC**
unspecified wrist

✓6ᵗʰ **M06.84** Other specified rheumatoid arthritis, hand

        **M06.841** Other specified rheumatoid arthritis, **HCC**
right hand

        **M06.842** Other specified rheumatoid arthritis, **HCC**
left hand

        **M06.849** Other specified rheumatoid arthritis, **HCC**
unspecified hand

✓6ᵗʰ **M06.85** Other specified rheumatoid arthritis, hip

        **M06.851** Other specified rheumatoid arthritis, **HCC**
right hip

        **M06.852** Other specified rheumatoid arthritis, **HCC**
left hip

        **M06.859** Other specified rheumatoid arthritis, **HCC**
unspecified hip

✓6ᵗʰ **M06.86** Other specified rheumatoid arthritis, knee

        **M06.861** Other specified rheumatoid arthritis, **HCC**
right knee

        **M06.862** Other specified rheumatoid arthritis, **HCC**
left knee

        **M06.869** Other specified rheumatoid arthritis, **HCC**
unspecified knee

✓6ᵗʰ **M06.87** Other specified rheumatoid arthritis, ankle and foot

        **M06.871** Other specified rheumatoid arthritis, **HCC**
right ankle and foot

        **M06.872** Other specified rheumatoid arthritis, **HCC**
left ankle and foot

        **M06.879** Other specified rheumatoid arthritis, **HCC**
unspecified ankle and foot

    **M06.88** Other specified rheumatoid arthritis, vertebrae **HCC**

    **M06.89** Other specified rheumatoid arthritis, multiple **HCC**
sites

  **M06.9** Rheumatoid arthritis, unspecified **HCC**

✓4ᵗʰ **M07** Enteropathic arthropathies

    Code also associated enteropathy, such as:
      regional enteritis [Crohn's disease] (K50.-)
      ulcerative colitis (K51.-)
      **EXCLUDES 1** *psoriatic arthropathies (L40.5-)*

✓5ᵗʰ **M07.6** Enteropathic arthropathies

    **M07.60** Enteropathic arthropathies, unspecified site

  ✓6ᵗʰ **M07.61** Enteropathic arthropathies, shoulder

        **M07.611** Enteropathic arthropathies, right
shoulder

        **M07.612** Enteropathic arthropathies, left shoulder

        **M07.619** Enteropathic arthropathies, unspecified
shoulder

  ✓6ᵗʰ **M07.62** Enteropathic arthropathies, elbow

        **M07.621** Enteropathic arthropathies, right elbow

        **M07.622** Enteropathic arthropathies, left elbow

        **M07.629** Enteropathic arthropathies, unspecified
elbow

  ✓6ᵗʰ **M07.63** Enteropathic arthropathies, wrist

        **M07.631** Enteropathic arthropathies, right wrist

        **M07.632** Enteropathic arthropathies, left wrist

        **M07.639** Enteropathic arthropathies, unspecified
wrist

  ✓6ᵗʰ **M07.64** Enteropathic arthropathies, hand

        **M07.641** Enteropathic arthropathies, right hand

        **M07.642** Enteropathic arthropathies, left hand

        **M07.649** Enteropathic arthropathies, unspecified
hand

  ✓6ᵗʰ **M07.65** Enteropathic arthropathies, hip

        **M07.651** Enteropathic arthropathies, right hip

        **M07.652** Enteropathic arthropathies, left hip

        **M07.659** Enteropathic arthropathies, unspecified
hip

  ✓6ᵗʰ **M07.66** Enteropathic arthropathies, knee

        **M07.661** Enteropathic arthropathies, right knee

        **M07.662** Enteropathic arthropathies, left knee

        **M07.669** Enteropathic arthropathies, unspecified
knee

  ✓6ᵗʰ **M07.67** Enteropathic arthropathies, ankle and foot

        **M07.671** Enteropathic arthropathies, right ankle
and foot

        **M07.672** Enteropathic arthropathies, left ankle and
foot

        **M07.679** Enteropathic arthropathies, unspecified
ankle and foot

    **M07.68** Enteropathic arthropathies, vertebrae

    **M07.69** Enteropathic arthropathies, multiple sites

✓4ᵗʰ **M08** Juvenile arthritis

    Code also any associated underlying condition, such as:
      regional enteritis [Crohn's disease] (K50.-)
      ulcerative colitis (K51.-)
      **EXCLUDES 1** *arthropathy in Whipple's disease (M14.8)*
          *Felty's syndrome (M05.0)*
          *juvenile dermatomyositis (M33.0-)*
          *psoriatic juvenile arthropathy (L40.54)*

  ✓5ᵗʰ **M08.0** Unspecified juvenile rheumatoid arthritis

    Juvenile rheumatoid arthritis with or without rheumatoid factor

    **M08.00** Unspecified juvenile rheumatoid arthritis of **HCC**
unspecified site

  ✓6ᵗʰ **M08.01** Unspecified juvenile rheumatoid arthritis, shoulder

        **M08.011** Unspecified juvenile rheumatoid **HCC**
arthritis, right shoulder

        **M08.012** Unspecified juvenile rheumatoid **HCC**
arthritis, left shoulder

        **M08.019** Unspecified juvenile rheumatoid **HCC**
arthritis, unspecified shoulder

  ✓6ᵗʰ **M08.02** Unspecified juvenile rheumatoid arthritis of elbow

        **M08.021** Unspecified juvenile rheumatoid **HCC**
arthritis, right elbow

        **M08.022** Unspecified juvenile rheumatoid **HCC**
arthritis, left elbow

        **M08.029** Unspecified juvenile rheumatoid **HCC**
arthritis, unspecified elbow

  ✓6ᵗʰ **M08.03** Unspecified juvenile rheumatoid arthritis, wrist

        **M08.031** Unspecified juvenile rheumatoid **HCC**
arthritis, right wrist

        **M08.032** Unspecified juvenile rheumatoid **HCC**
arthritis, left wrist

        **M08.039** Unspecified juvenile rheumatoid **HCC**
arthritis, unspecified wrist

  ✓6ᵗʰ **M08.04** Unspecified juvenile rheumatoid arthritis, hand

        **M08.041** Unspecified juvenile rheumatoid **HCC**
arthritis, right hand

        **M08.042** Unspecified juvenile rheumatoid **HCC**
arthritis, left hand

        **M08.049** Unspecified juvenile rheumatoid **HCC**
arthritis, unspecified hand

  ✓6ᵗʰ **M08.05** Unspecified juvenile rheumatoid arthritis, hip

        **M08.051** Unspecified juvenile rheumatoid **HCC**
arthritis, right hip

        **M08.052** Unspecified juvenile rheumatoid **HCC**
arthritis, left hip

        **M08.059** Unspecified juvenile rheumatoid **HCC**
arthritis, unspecified hip

  ✓6ᵗʰ **M08.06** Unspecified juvenile rheumatoid arthritis, knee

        **M08.061** Unspecified juvenile rheumatoid **HCC**
arthritis, right knee

        **M08.062** Unspecified juvenile rheumatoid **HCC**
arthritis, left knee

        **M08.069** Unspecified juvenile rheumatoid **HCC**
arthritis, unspecified knee

  ✓6ᵗʰ **M08.07** Unspecified juvenile rheumatoid arthritis, ankle and
foot

        **M08.071** Unspecified juvenile rheumatoid **HCC**
arthritis, right ankle and foot

        **M08.072** Unspecified juvenile rheumatoid **HCC**
arthritis, left ankle and foot

        **M08.079** Unspecified juvenile rheumatoid **HCC**
arthritis, unspecified ankle and foot

    **M08.08** Unspecified juvenile rheumatoid arthritis, **HCC**
vertebrae

    **M08.09** Unspecified juvenile rheumatoid arthritis, **HCC**
multiple sites

---

**N** Newborn: 0   **P** Pediatric: 0-17   **M** Maternity: 12-55   **A** Adult: 15-124   **MCC** Major CC Condition   **PDx MCC** PDx acts as own MCC   **CC** CC Condition   **PDx CC** PDx acts as own CC

746                                                        ICD-10-CM 2018

**M08.1**   **Juvenile** ankylosing spondylitis   `HCC`
> *EXCLUDES 1*   *ankylosing spondylitis in adults (M45.0-)*

✓5ᵗʰ **M08.2**   **Juvenile rheumatoid arthritis** with systemic onset
> Still's disease NOS
>> *EXCLUDES 1*   *adult-onset Still's disease (M06.1-)*

    **M08.20**   **Juvenile rheumatoid arthritis with systemic**   `HCC`
      **onset, unspecified site**

   ✓6ᵗʰ **M08.21**   **Juvenile rheumatoid arthritis with systemic onset, shoulder**
      **M08.211**   **Juvenile rheumatoid arthritis with**   `HCC`
       **systemic onset, right shoulder**
      **M08.212**   **Juvenile rheumatoid arthritis with**   `HCC`
       **systemic onset, left shoulder**
      **M08.219**   **Juvenile rheumatoid arthritis with**   `HCC`
       **systemic onset, unspecified shoulder**

   ✓6ᵗʰ **M08.22**   **Juvenile rheumatoid arthritis with systemic onset, elbow**
      **M08.221**   **Juvenile rheumatoid arthritis with**   `HCC`
       **systemic onset, right elbow**
      **M08.222**   **Juvenile rheumatoid arthritis with**   `HCC`
       **systemic onset, left elbow**
      **M08.229**   **Juvenile rheumatoid arthritis with**   `HCC`
       **systemic onset, unspecified elbow**

   ✓6ᵗʰ **M08.23**   **Juvenile rheumatoid arthritis with systemic onset, wrist**
      **M08.231**   **Juvenile rheumatoid arthritis with**   `HCC`
       **systemic onset, right wrist**
      **M08.232**   **Juvenile rheumatoid arthritis with**   `HCC`
       **systemic onset, left wrist**
      **M08.239**   **Juvenile rheumatoid arthritis with**   `HCC`
       **systemic onset, unspecified wrist**

   ✓6ᵗʰ **M08.24**   **Juvenile rheumatoid arthritis with systemic onset, hand**
      **M08.241**   **Juvenile rheumatoid arthritis with**   `HCC`
       **systemic onset, right hand**
      **M08.242**   **Juvenile rheumatoid arthritis with**   `HCC`
       **systemic onset, left hand**
      **M08.249**   **Juvenile rheumatoid arthritis with**   `HCC`
       **systemic onset, unspecified hand**

   ✓6ᵗʰ **M08.25**   **Juvenile rheumatoid arthritis with systemic onset, hip**
      **M08.251**   **Juvenile rheumatoid arthritis with**   `HCC`
       **systemic onset, right hip**
      **M08.252**   **Juvenile rheumatoid arthritis with**   `HCC`
       **systemic onset, left hip**
      **M08.259**   **Juvenile rheumatoid arthritis with**   `HCC`
       **systemic onset, unspecified hip**

   ✓6ᵗʰ **M08.26**   **Juvenile rheumatoid arthritis with systemic onset, knee**
      **M08.261**   **Juvenile rheumatoid arthritis with**   `HCC`
       **systemic onset, right knee**
      **M08.262**   **Juvenile rheumatoid arthritis with**   `HCC`
       **systemic onset, left knee**
      **M08.269**   **Juvenile rheumatoid arthritis with**   `HCC`
       **systemic onset, unspecified knee**

   ✓6ᵗʰ **M08.27**   **Juvenile rheumatoid arthritis with systemic onset, ankle and foot**
      **M08.271**   **Juvenile rheumatoid arthritis with**   `HCC`
       **systemic onset, right ankle and foot**
      **M08.272**   **Juvenile rheumatoid arthritis with**   `HCC`
       **systemic onset, left ankle and foot**
      **M08.279**   **Juvenile rheumatoid arthritis with**   `HCC`
       **systemic onset, unspecified ankle and foot**

    **M08.28**   **Juvenile rheumatoid arthritis with systemic**   `HCC`
      **onset, vertebrae**
    **M08.29**   **Juvenile rheumatoid arthritis with systemic**   `HCC`
      **onset, multiple sites**

**M08.3**   **Juvenile rheumatoid** polyarthritis (seronegative)   `HCC`

✓5ᵗʰ **M08.4**   **Pauciarticular** juvenile rheumatoid arthritis
    **M08.40**   **Pauciarticular juvenile rheumatoid arthritis,**   `HCC`
      **unspecified site**
   ✓6ᵗʰ **M08.41**   **Pauciarticular juvenile rheumatoid arthritis, shoulder**
      **M08.411**   **Pauciarticular juvenile rheumatoid**   `HCC`
       **arthritis, right shoulder**

      **M08.412**   **Pauciarticular juvenile rheumatoid**   `HCC`
       **arthritis, left shoulder**
      **M08.419**   **Pauciarticular juvenile rheumatoid**   `HCC`
       **arthritis, unspecified shoulder**

   ✓6ᵗʰ **M08.42**   **Pauciarticular juvenile rheumatoid arthritis, elbow**
      **M08.421**   **Pauciarticular juvenile rheumatoid**   `HCC`
       **arthritis, right elbow**
      **M08.422**   **Pauciarticular juvenile rheumatoid**   `HCC`
       **arthritis, left elbow**
      **M08.429**   **Pauciarticular juvenile rheumatoid**   `HCC`
       **arthritis, unspecified elbow**

   ✓6ᵗʰ **M08.43**   **Pauciarticular juvenile rheumatoid arthritis, wrist**
      **M08.431**   **Pauciarticular juvenile rheumatoid**   `HCC`
       **arthritis, right wrist**
      **M08.432**   **Pauciarticular juvenile rheumatoid**   `HCC`
       **arthritis, left wrist**
      **M08.439**   **Pauciarticular juvenile rheumatoid**   `HCC`
       **arthritis, unspecified wrist**

   ✓6ᵗʰ **M08.44**   **Pauciarticular juvenile rheumatoid arthritis, hand**
      **M08.441**   **Pauciarticular juvenile rheumatoid**   `HCC`
       **arthritis, right hand**
      **M08.442**   **Pauciarticular juvenile rheumatoid**   `HCC`
       **arthritis, left hand**
      **M08.449**   **Pauciarticular juvenile rheumatoid**   `HCC`
       **arthritis, unspecified hand**

   ✓6ᵗʰ **M08.45**   **Pauciarticular juvenile rheumatoid arthritis, hip**
      **M08.451**   **Pauciarticular juvenile rheumatoid**   `HCC`
       **arthritis, right hip**
      **M08.452**   **Pauciarticular juvenile rheumatoid**   `HCC`
       **arthritis, left hip**
      **M08.459**   **Pauciarticular juvenile rheumatoid**   `HCC`
       **arthritis, unspecified hip**

   ✓6ᵗʰ **M08.46**   **Pauciarticular juvenile rheumatoid arthritis, knee**
      **M08.461**   **Pauciarticular juvenile rheumatoid**   `HCC`
       **arthritis, right knee**
      **M08.462**   **Pauciarticular juvenile rheumatoid**   `HCC`
       **arthritis, left knee**
      **M08.469**   **Pauciarticular juvenile rheumatoid**   `HCC`
       **arthritis, unspecified knee**

   ✓6ᵗʰ **M08.47**   **Pauciarticular juvenile rheumatoid arthritis, ankle and foot**
      **M08.471**   **Pauciarticular juvenile rheumatoid**   `HCC`
       **arthritis, right ankle and foot**
      **M08.472**   **Pauciarticular juvenile rheumatoid**   `HCC`
       **arthritis, left ankle and foot**
      **M08.479**   **Pauciarticular juvenile rheumatoid**   `HCC`
       **arthritis, unspecified ankle and foot**

    **M08.48**   **Pauciarticular juvenile rheumatoid arthritis,**   `HCC`
      **vertebrae**

✓5ᵗʰ **M08.8**   **Other** juvenile arthritis
    **M08.80**   **Other juvenile arthritis, unspecified site**   `HCC`
   ✓6ᵗʰ **M08.81**   **Other juvenile arthritis, shoulder**
      **M08.811**   **Other juvenile arthritis, right**   `HCC`
       **shoulder**
      **M08.812**   **Other juvenile arthritis, left shoulder**   `HCC`
      **M08.819**   **Other juvenile arthritis, unspecified**   `HCC`
       **shoulder**

   ✓6ᵗʰ **M08.82**   **Other juvenile arthritis, elbow**
      **M08.821**   **Other juvenile arthritis, right elbow**   `HCC`
      **M08.822**   **Other juvenile arthritis, left elbow**   `HCC`
      **M08.829**   **Other juvenile arthritis, unspecified**   `HCC`
       **elbow**

   ✓6ᵗʰ **M08.83**   **Other juvenile arthritis, wrist**
      **M08.831**   **Other juvenile arthritis, right wrist**   `HCC`
      **M08.832**   **Other juvenile arthritis, left wrist**   `HCC`
      **M08.839**   **Other juvenile arthritis, unspecified**   `HCC`
       **wrist**

   ✓6ᵗʰ **M08.84**   **Other juvenile arthritis, hand**
      **M08.841**   **Other juvenile arthritis, right hand**   `HCC`
      **M08.842**   **Other juvenile arthritis, left hand**   `HCC`
      **M08.849**   **Other juvenile arthritis, unspecified**   `HCC`
       **hand**

   ✓6ᵗʰ **M08.85**   **Other juvenile arthritis, hip**
      **M08.851**   **Other juvenile arthritis, right hip**   `HCC`
      **M08.852**   **Other juvenile arthritis, left hip**   `HCC`

☑ Additional Character Req   ✓x7ᵗʰ Placeholder Alert   Unacceptable PDx   Manifestation   `H1`-`H14` HAC   `HCC` CMS-HCC Condition   *EXCLUDES 1* Not Coded Here   *EXCLUDES 2* Not Included Here

ICD-10-CM 2018                      **747**

**Chapter 13. Diseases of the Musculoskeletal System and Connective Tissue**

**M08.859–M1A.132**

          **M08.859** Other juvenile arthritis, unspecified hip — HCC

✓6ᵗʰ **M08.86** Other juvenile arthritis, knee
      **M08.861** Other juvenile arthritis, right knee — HCC
      **M08.862** Other juvenile arthritis, left knee — HCC
      **M08.869** Other juvenile arthritis, unspecified knee — HCC

✓6ᵗʰ **M08.87** Other juvenile arthritis, ankle and foot
      **M08.871** Other juvenile arthritis, right ankle and foot — HCC
      **M08.872** Other juvenile arthritis, left ankle and foot — HCC
      **M08.879** Other juvenile arthritis, unspecified ankle and foot — HCC

   **M08.88** Other juvenile arthritis, other specified site — HCC
      Other juvenile arthritis, vertebrae

   **M08.89** Other juvenile arthritis, multiple sites — HCC

✓5ᵗʰ **M08.9** Juvenile arthritis, unspecified
     *EXCLUDES 1*   juvenile rheumatoid arthritis, unspecified (M08.0-)

   **M08.90** Juvenile arthritis, unspecified, unspecified site — HCC

✓6ᵗʰ **M08.91** Juvenile arthritis, unspecified, shoulder
      **M08.911** Juvenile arthritis, unspecified, right shoulder — HCC
      **M08.912** Juvenile arthritis, unspecified, left shoulder — HCC
      **M08.919** Juvenile arthritis, unspecified, unspecified shoulder — HCC

✓6ᵗʰ **M08.92** Juvenile arthritis, unspecified, elbow
      **M08.921** Juvenile arthritis, unspecified, right elbow — HCC
      **M08.922** Juvenile arthritis, unspecified, left elbow — HCC
      **M08.929** Juvenile arthritis, unspecified, unspecified elbow — HCC

✓6ᵗʰ **M08.93** Juvenile arthritis, unspecified, wrist
      **M08.931** Juvenile arthritis, unspecified, right wrist — HCC
      **M08.932** Juvenile arthritis, unspecified, left wrist — HCC
      **M08.939** Juvenile arthritis, unspecified, unspecified wrist — HCC

✓6ᵗʰ **M08.94** Juvenile arthritis, unspecified, hand
      **M08.941** Juvenile arthritis, unspecified, right hand — HCC
      **M08.942** Juvenile arthritis, unspecified, left hand — HCC
      **M08.949** Juvenile arthritis, unspecified, unspecified hand — HCC

✓6ᵗʰ **M08.95** Juvenile arthritis, unspecified, hip
      **M08.951** Juvenile arthritis, unspecified, right hip — HCC
      **M08.952** Juvenile arthritis, unspecified, left hip — HCC
      **M08.959** Juvenile arthritis, unspecified, unspecified hip — HCC

✓6ᵗʰ **M08.96** Juvenile arthritis, unspecified, knee
      **M08.961** Juvenile arthritis, unspecified, right knee — HCC
      **M08.962** Juvenile arthritis, unspecified, left knee — HCC
      **M08.969** Juvenile arthritis, unspecified, unspecified knee — HCC

✓6ᵗʰ **M08.97** Juvenile arthritis, unspecified, ankle and foot
      **M08.971** Juvenile arthritis, unspecified, right ankle and foot — HCC
      **M08.972** Juvenile arthritis, unspecified, left ankle and foot — HCC
      **M08.979** Juvenile arthritis, unspecified, unspecified ankle and foot — HCC

   **M08.98** Juvenile arthritis, unspecified, vertebrae — HCC
   **M08.99** Juvenile arthritis, unspecified, multiple sites — HCC

---

✓4ᵗʰ **M1A Chronic gout**

Use additional code to identify:
  autonomic neuropathy in diseases classified elsewhere (G99.0)
  calculus of urinary tract in diseases classified elsewhere (N22)
  cardiomyopathy in diseases classified elsewhere (I43)
  disorders of external ear in diseases classified elsewhere (H61.1-, H62.8-)
  disorders of iris and ciliary body in diseases classified elsewhere (H22)
  glomerular disorders in diseases classified elsewhere (N08)

*EXCLUDES 1*   gout NOS (M10.-)
*EXCLUDES 2*   acute gout (M10.-)

The appropriate 7th character is to be added to each code from category M1A.
Ø     without tophus (tophi)
1     with tophus (tophi)

✓5ᵗʰ **M1A.0** Idiopathic chronic gout
     Chronic gouty bursitis
     Primary chronic gout

✓x7ᵗʰ **M1A.00** Idiopathic chronic gout, unspecified site

✓6ᵗʰ **M1A.01** Idiopathic chronic gout, shoulder
    ✓7ᵗʰ **M1A.011** Idiopathic chronic gout, right shoulder
    ✓7ᵗʰ **M1A.012** Idiopathic chronic gout, left shoulder
    ✓7ᵗʰ **M1A.019** Idiopathic chronic gout, unspecified shoulder

✓6ᵗʰ **M1A.02** Idiopathic chronic gout, elbow
    ✓7ᵗʰ **M1A.021** Idiopathic chronic gout, right elbow
    ✓7ᵗʰ **M1A.022** Idiopathic chronic gout, left elbow
    ✓7ᵗʰ **M1A.029** Idiopathic chronic gout, unspecified elbow

✓6ᵗʰ **M1A.03** Idiopathic chronic gout, wrist
    ✓7ᵗʰ **M1A.031** Idiopathic chronic gout, right wrist
    ✓7ᵗʰ **M1A.032** Idiopathic chronic gout, left wrist
    ✓7ᵗʰ **M1A.039** Idiopathic chronic gout, unspecified wrist

✓6ᵗʰ **M1A.04** Idiopathic chronic gout, hand
    ✓7ᵗʰ **M1A.041** Idiopathic chronic gout, right hand
    ✓7ᵗʰ **M1A.042** Idiopathic chronic gout, left hand
    ✓7ᵗʰ **M1A.049** Idiopathic chronic gout, unspecified hand

✓6ᵗʰ **M1A.05** Idiopathic chronic gout, hip
    ✓7ᵗʰ **M1A.051** Idiopathic chronic gout, right hip
    ✓7ᵗʰ **M1A.052** Idiopathic chronic gout, left hip
    ✓7ᵗʰ **M1A.059** Idiopathic chronic gout, unspecified hip

✓6ᵗʰ **M1A.06** Idiopathic chronic gout, knee
    ✓7ᵗʰ **M1A.061** Idiopathic chronic gout, right knee
    ✓7ᵗʰ **M1A.062** Idiopathic chronic gout, left knee
    ✓7ᵗʰ **M1A.069** Idiopathic chronic gout, unspecified knee

✓6ᵗʰ **M1A.07** Idiopathic chronic gout, ankle and foot
    ✓7ᵗʰ **M1A.071** Idiopathic chronic gout, right ankle and foot
    ✓7ᵗʰ **M1A.072** Idiopathic chronic gout, left ankle and foot
    ✓7ᵗʰ **M1A.079** Idiopathic chronic gout, unspecified ankle and foot

✓x7ᵗʰ **M1A.08** Idiopathic chronic gout, vertebrae
✓x7ᵗʰ **M1A.09** Idiopathic chronic gout, multiple sites

✓5ᵗʰ **M1A.1** Lead-induced chronic gout
     Code first toxic effects of lead and its compounds (T56.0-)

✓x7ᵗʰ **M1A.10** Lead-induced chronic gout, unspecified site

✓6ᵗʰ **M1A.11** Lead-induced chronic gout, shoulder
    ✓7ᵗʰ **M1A.111** Lead-induced chronic gout, right shoulder
    ✓7ᵗʰ **M1A.112** Lead-induced chronic gout, left shoulder
    ✓7ᵗʰ **M1A.119** Lead-induced chronic gout, unspecified shoulder

✓6ᵗʰ **M1A.12** Lead-induced chronic gout, elbow
    ✓7ᵗʰ **M1A.121** Lead-induced chronic gout, right elbow
    ✓7ᵗʰ **M1A.122** Lead-induced chronic gout, left elbow
    ✓7ᵗʰ **M1A.129** Lead-induced chronic gout, unspecified elbow

✓6ᵗʰ **M1A.13** Lead-induced chronic gout, wrist
    ✓7ᵗʰ **M1A.131** Lead-induced chronic gout, right wrist
    ✓7ᵗʰ **M1A.132** Lead-induced chronic gout, left wrist

N Newborn: 0   P Pediatric: 0-17   M Maternity: 12-55   A Adult: 15-124   MCC Major CC Condition   PDx MCC PDx acts as own MCC   CC CC Condition   PDx CC PDx acts as own CC

748                                                            ICD-10-CM 2018

☑7ᵗʰ **M1A.139** Lead-induced chronic gout, unspecified wrist

☑6ᵗʰ **M1A.14** Lead-induced chronic gout, hand
- ☑7ᵗʰ **M1A.141** Lead-induced chronic gout, right hand
- ☑7ᵗʰ **M1A.142** Lead-induced chronic gout, left hand
- ☑7ᵗʰ **M1A.149** Lead-induced chronic gout, unspecified hand

☑6ᵗʰ **M1A.15** Lead-induced chronic gout, hip
- ☑7ᵗʰ **M1A.151** Lead-induced chronic gout, right hip
- ☑7ᵗʰ **M1A.152** Lead-induced chronic gout, left hip
- ☑7ᵗʰ **M1A.159** Lead-induced chronic gout, unspecified hip

☑6ᵗʰ **M1A.16** Lead-induced chronic gout, knee
- ☑7ᵗʰ **M1A.161** Lead-induced chronic gout, right knee
- ☑7ᵗʰ **M1A.162** Lead-induced chronic gout, left knee
- ☑7ᵗʰ **M1A.169** Lead-induced chronic gout, unspecified knee

☑6ᵗʰ **M1A.17** Lead-induced chronic gout, ankle and foot
- ☑7ᵗʰ **M1A.171** Lead-induced chronic gout, right ankle and foot
- ☑7ᵗʰ **M1A.172** Lead-induced chronic gout, left ankle and foot
- ☑7ᵗʰ **M1A.179** Lead-induced chronic gout, unspecified ankle and foot

☑x7ᵗʰ **M1A.18** Lead-induced chronic gout, vertebrae

☑x7ᵗʰ **M1A.19** Lead-induced chronic gout, multiple sites

☑5ᵗʰ **M1A.2** Drug-induced chronic gout

Use additional code for adverse effect, if applicable, to identify drug (T36-T50 with fifth or sixth character 5)

☑x7ᵗʰ **M1A.20** Drug-induced chronic gout, unspecified site

☑6ᵗʰ **M1A.21** Drug-induced chronic gout, shoulder
- ☑7ᵗʰ **M1A.211** Drug-induced chronic gout, right shoulder
- ☑7ᵗʰ **M1A.212** Drug-induced chronic gout, left shoulder
- ☑7ᵗʰ **M1A.219** Drug-induced chronic gout, unspecified shoulder

☑6ᵗʰ **M1A.22** Drug-induced chronic gout, elbow
- ☑7ᵗʰ **M1A.221** Drug-induced chronic gout, right elbow
- ☑7ᵗʰ **M1A.222** Drug-induced chronic gout, left elbow
- ☑7ᵗʰ **M1A.229** Drug-induced chronic gout, unspecified elbow

☑6ᵗʰ **M1A.23** Drug-induced chronic gout, wrist
- ☑7ᵗʰ **M1A.231** Drug-induced chronic gout, right wrist
- ☑7ᵗʰ **M1A.232** Drug-induced chronic gout, left wrist
- ☑7ᵗʰ **M1A.239** Drug-induced chronic gout, unspecified wrist

☑6ᵗʰ **M1A.24** Drug-induced chronic gout, hand
- ☑7ᵗʰ **M1A.241** Drug-induced chronic gout, right hand
- ☑7ᵗʰ **M1A.242** Drug-induced chronic gout, left hand
- ☑7ᵗʰ **M1A.249** Drug-induced chronic gout, unspecified hand

☑6ᵗʰ **M1A.25** Drug-induced chronic gout, hip
- ☑7ᵗʰ **M1A.251** Drug-induced chronic gout, right hip
- ☑7ᵗʰ **M1A.252** Drug-induced chronic gout, left hip
- ☑7ᵗʰ **M1A.259** Drug-induced chronic gout, unspecified hip

☑6ᵗʰ **M1A.26** Drug-induced chronic gout, knee
- ☑7ᵗʰ **M1A.261** Drug-induced chronic gout, right knee
- ☑7ᵗʰ **M1A.262** Drug-induced chronic gout, left knee
- ☑7ᵗʰ **M1A.269** Drug-induced chronic gout, unspecified knee

☑6ᵗʰ **M1A.27** Drug-induced chronic gout, ankle and foot
- ☑7ᵗʰ **M1A.271** Drug-induced chronic gout, right ankle and foot
- ☑7ᵗʰ **M1A.272** Drug-induced chronic gout, left ankle and foot
- ☑7ᵗʰ **M1A.279** Drug-induced chronic gout, unspecified ankle and foot

☑x7ᵗʰ **M1A.28** Drug-induced chronic gout, vertebrae

☑x7ᵗʰ **M1A.29** Drug-induced chronic gout, multiple sites

☑5ᵗʰ **M1A.3** Chronic gout due to renal impairment

Code first associated renal disease

☑7ᵗʰ **M1A.30** Chronic gout due to renal impairment, unspecified site

☑6ᵗʰ **M1A.31** Chronic gout due to renal impairment, shoulder
- ☑7ᵗʰ **M1A.311** Chronic gout due to renal impairment, right shoulder
- ☑7ᵗʰ **M1A.312** Chronic gout due to renal impairment, left shoulder
- ☑7ᵗʰ **M1A.319** Chronic gout due to renal impairment, unspecified shoulder

☑6ᵗʰ **M1A.32** Chronic gout due to renal impairment, elbow
- ☑7ᵗʰ **M1A.321** Chronic gout due to renal impairment, right elbow
- ☑7ᵗʰ **M1A.322** Chronic gout due to renal impairment, left elbow
- ☑7ᵗʰ **M1A.329** Chronic gout due to renal impairment, unspecified elbow

☑6ᵗʰ **M1A.33** Chronic gout due to renal impairment, wrist
- ☑7ᵗʰ **M1A.331** Chronic gout due to renal impairment, right wrist
- ☑7ᵗʰ **M1A.332** Chronic gout due to renal impairment, left wrist
- ☑7ᵗʰ **M1A.339** Chronic gout due to renal impairment, unspecified wrist

☑6ᵗʰ **M1A.34** Chronic gout due to renal impairment, hand
- ☑7ᵗʰ **M1A.341** Chronic gout due to renal impairment, right hand
- ☑7ᵗʰ **M1A.342** Chronic gout due to renal impairment, left hand
- ☑7ᵗʰ **M1A.349** Chronic gout due to renal impairment, unspecified hand

☑6ᵗʰ **M1A.35** Chronic gout due to renal impairment, hip
- ☑7ᵗʰ **M1A.351** Chronic gout due to renal impairment, right hip
- ☑7ᵗʰ **M1A.352** Chronic gout due to renal impairment, left hip
- ☑7ᵗʰ **M1A.359** Chronic gout due to renal impairment, unspecified hip

☑6ᵗʰ **M1A.36** Chronic gout due to renal impairment, knee
- ☑7ᵗʰ **M1A.361** Chronic gout due to renal impairment, right knee
- ☑7ᵗʰ **M1A.362** Chronic gout due to renal impairment, left knee
- ☑7ᵗʰ **M1A.369** Chronic gout due to renal impairment, unspecified knee

☑6ᵗʰ **M1A.37** Chronic gout due to renal impairment, ankle and foot
- ☑7ᵗʰ **M1A.371** Chronic gout due to renal impairment, right ankle and foot
- ☑7ᵗʰ **M1A.372** Chronic gout due to renal impairment, left ankle and foot
- ☑7ᵗʰ **M1A.379** Chronic gout due to renal impairment, unspecified ankle and foot

☑x7ᵗʰ **M1A.38** Chronic gout due to renal impairment, vertebrae

☑x7ᵗʰ **M1A.39** Chronic gout due to renal impairment, multiple sites

☑5ᵗʰ **M1A.4** Other secondary chronic gout

Code first associated condition

☑x7ᵗʰ **M1A.40** Other secondary chronic gout, unspecified site

☑6ᵗʰ **M1A.41** Other secondary chronic gout, shoulder
- ☑7ᵗʰ **M1A.411** Other secondary chronic gout, right shoulder
- ☑7ᵗʰ **M1A.412** Other secondary chronic gout, left shoulder
- ☑7ᵗʰ **M1A.419** Other secondary chronic gout, unspecified shoulder

☑6ᵗʰ **M1A.42** Other secondary chronic gout, elbow
- ☑7ᵗʰ **M1A.421** Other secondary chronic gout, right elbow
- ☑7ᵗʰ **M1A.422** Other secondary chronic gout, left elbow
- ☑7ᵗʰ **M1A.429** Other secondary chronic gout, unspecified elbow

☑ Additional Character Req    ☑x7ᵗʰ Placeholder Alert    Unacceptable PDx    Manifestation    **H1**-**H14** HAC    **HCC** CMS-HCC Condition    *EXCLUDES 1* Not Coded Here    *EXCLUDES 2* Not Included Here

ICD-10-CM 2018        749

**✓6ᵗʰ M1A.43 Other secondary chronic gout, wrist**
- ✓7ᵗʰ M1A.431 Other secondary chronic gout, right wrist
- ✓7ᵗʰ M1A.432 Other secondary chronic gout, left wrist
- ✓7ᵗʰ M1A.439 Other secondary chronic gout, unspecified wrist

**✓6ᵗʰ M1A.44 Other secondary chronic gout, hand**
- ✓7ᵗʰ M1A.441 Other secondary chronic gout, right hand
- ✓7ᵗʰ M1A.442 Other secondary chronic gout, left hand
- ✓7ᵗʰ M1A.449 Other secondary chronic gout, unspecified hand

**✓6ᵗʰ M1A.45 Other secondary chronic gout, hip**
- ✓7ᵗʰ M1A.451 Other secondary chronic gout, right hip
- ✓7ᵗʰ M1A.452 Other secondary chronic gout, left hip
- ✓7ᵗʰ M1A.459 Other secondary chronic gout, unspecified hip

**✓6ᵗʰ M1A.46 Other secondary chronic gout, knee**
- ✓7ᵗʰ M1A.461 Other secondary chronic gout, right knee
- ✓7ᵗʰ M1A.462 Other secondary chronic gout, left knee
- ✓7ᵗʰ M1A.469 Other secondary chronic gout, unspecified knee

**✓6ᵗʰ M1A.47 Other secondary chronic gout, ankle and foot**
- ✓7ᵗʰ M1A.471 Other secondary chronic gout, right ankle and foot
- ✓7ᵗʰ M1A.472 Other secondary chronic gout, left ankle and foot
- ✓7ᵗʰ M1A.479 Other secondary chronic gout, unspecified ankle and foot

**✓x 7ᵗʰ M1A.48 Other secondary chronic gout, vertebrae**

**✓x 7ᵗʰ M1A.49 Other secondary chronic gout, multiple sites**

**✓x 7ᵗʰ M1A.9 Chronic gout, unspecified**

**✓4ᵗʰ M10 Gout**

Acute gout
Gout attack
Gout flare
Podagra

Use additional code to identify:
- autonomic neuropathy in diseases classified elsewhere (G99.0)
- calculus of urinary tract in diseases classified elsewhere (N22)
- cardiomyopathy in diseases classified elsewhere (I43)
- disorders of external ear in diseases classified elsewhere (H61.1-, H62.8-)
- disorders of iris and ciliary body in diseases classified elsewhere (H22)
- glomerular disorders in diseases classified elsewhere (N08)

EXCLUDES 2   chronic gout (M1A.-)

**DEF:** Purine and pyrimidine metabolic disorders; manifested by hyperuricemia and recurrent acute inflammatory arthritis; monosodium urate or monohydrate crystals may be deposited in and around the joints, leading to joint destruction and severe crippling.

**✓5ᵗʰ M10.0 Idiopathic gout**

Gouty bursitis
Primary gout

**M10.00 Idiopathic gout, unspecified site**

**✓6ᵗʰ M10.01 Idiopathic gout, shoulder**
- M10.011 Idiopathic gout, right shoulder
- M10.012 Idiopathic gout, left shoulder
- M10.019 Idiopathic gout, unspecified shoulder

**✓6ᵗʰ M10.02 Idiopathic gout, elbow**
- M10.021 Idiopathic gout, right elbow
- M10.022 Idiopathic gout, left elbow
- M10.029 Idiopathic gout, unspecified elbow

**✓6ᵗʰ M10.03 Idiopathic gout, wrist**
- M10.031 Idiopathic gout, right wrist
- M10.032 Idiopathic gout, left wrist
- M10.039 Idiopathic gout, unspecified wrist

**✓6ᵗʰ M10.04 Idiopathic gout, hand**
- M10.041 Idiopathic gout, right hand
- M10.042 Idiopathic gout, left hand
- M10.049 Idiopathic gout, unspecified hand

**✓6ᵗʰ M10.05 Idiopathic gout, hip**
- M10.051 Idiopathic gout, right hip
- M10.052 Idiopathic gout, left hip
- M10.059 Idiopathic gout, unspecified hip

**✓6ᵗʰ M10.06 Idiopathic gout, knee**
- M10.061 Idiopathic gout, right knee
- M10.062 Idiopathic gout, left knee
- M10.069 Idiopathic gout, unspecified knee

**✓6ᵗʰ M10.07 Idiopathic gout, ankle and foot**
- M10.071 Idiopathic gout, right ankle and foot
- M10.072 Idiopathic gout, left ankle and foot
- M10.079 Idiopathic gout, unspecified ankle and foot

**M10.08 Idiopathic gout, vertebrae**

**M10.09 Idiopathic gout, multiple sites**

**✓5ᵗʰ M10.1 Lead-induced gout**

Code first toxic effects of lead and its compounds (T56.0-)

**M10.10 Lead-induced gout, unspecified site**

**✓6ᵗʰ M10.11 Lead-induced gout, shoulder**
- M10.111 Lead-induced gout, right shoulder
- M10.112 Lead-induced gout, left shoulder
- M10.119 Lead-induced gout, unspecified shoulder

**✓6ᵗʰ M10.12 Lead-induced gout, elbow**
- M10.121 Lead-induced gout, right elbow
- M10.122 Lead-induced gout, left elbow
- M10.129 Lead-induced gout, unspecified elbow

**✓6ᵗʰ M10.13 Lead-induced gout, wrist**
- M10.131 Lead-induced gout, right wrist
- M10.132 Lead-induced gout, left wrist
- M10.139 Lead-induced gout, unspecified wrist

**✓6ᵗʰ M10.14 Lead-induced gout, hand**
- M10.141 Lead-induced gout, right hand
- M10.142 Lead-induced gout, left hand
- M10.149 Lead-induced gout, unspecified hand

**✓6ᵗʰ M10.15 Lead-induced gout, hip**
- M10.151 Lead-induced gout, right hip
- M10.152 Lead-induced gout, left hip
- M10.159 Lead-induced gout, unspecified hip

**✓6ᵗʰ M10.16 Lead-induced gout, knee**
- M10.161 Lead-induced gout, right knee
- M10.162 Lead-induced gout, left knee
- M10.169 Lead-induced gout, unspecified knee

**✓6ᵗʰ M10.17 Lead-induced gout, ankle and foot**
- M10.171 Lead-induced gout, right ankle and foot
- M10.172 Lead-induced gout, left ankle and foot
- M10.179 Lead-induced gout, unspecified ankle and foot

**M10.18 Lead-induced gout, vertebrae**

**M10.19 Lead-induced gout, multiple sites**

**✓5ᵗʰ M10.2 Drug-induced gout**

Use additional code for adverse effect, if applicable, to identify drug (T36-T50 with fifth or sixth character 5)

**M10.20 Drug-induced gout, unspecified site**

**✓6ᵗʰ M10.21 Drug-induced gout, shoulder**
- M10.211 Drug-induced gout, right shoulder
- M10.212 Drug-induced gout, left shoulder
- M10.219 Drug-induced gout, unspecified shoulder

**✓6ᵗʰ M10.22 Drug-induced gout, elbow**
- M10.221 Drug-induced gout, right elbow
- M10.222 Drug-induced gout, left elbow
- M10.229 Drug-induced gout, unspecified elbow

**✓6ᵗʰ M10.23 Drug-induced gout, wrist**
- M10.231 Drug-induced gout, right wrist
- M10.232 Drug-induced gout, left wrist
- M10.239 Drug-induced gout, unspecified wrist

**✓6ᵗʰ M10.24 Drug-induced gout, hand**
- M10.241 Drug-induced gout, right hand
- M10.242 Drug-induced gout, left hand
- M10.249 Drug-induced gout, unspecified hand

**✓6ᵗʰ M10.25 Drug-induced gout, hip**
- M10.251 Drug-induced gout, right hip
- M10.252 Drug-induced gout, left hip
- M10.259 Drug-induced gout, unspecified hip

N Newborn: 0   P Pediatric: 0-17   M Maternity: 12-55   A Adult: 15-124   MCC Major CC Condition   PDx MCC PDx acts as own MCC   CC CC Condition   PDx CC PDx acts as own CC

750      ICD-10-CM 2018

√6ᵗʰ **M10.26 Drug-induced gout,** knee
     **M10.261 Drug-induced gout,** right **knee**
     **M10.262 Drug-induced gout,** left **knee**
     **M10.269 Drug-induced gout,** unspecified **knee**

√6ᵗʰ **M10.27 Drug-induced gout,** ankle and foot
     **M10.271 Drug-induced gout,** right **ankle and foot**
     **M10.272 Drug-induced gout,** left **ankle and foot**
     **M10.279 Drug-induced gout,** unspecified **ankle and foot**

   **M10.28 Drug-induced gout,** vertebrae
   **M10.29 Drug-induced gout,** multiple sites

√5ᵗʰ **M10.3 Gout due to** renal impairment
     Code first associated renal disease

   **M10.30 Gout due to renal impairment,** unspecified site

√6ᵗʰ **M10.31 Gout due to renal impairment,** shoulder
     **M10.311 Gout due to renal impairment,** right **shoulder**
     **M10.312 Gout due to renal impairment,** left **shoulder**
     **M10.319 Gout due to renal impairment,** unspecified **shoulder**

√6ᵗʰ **M10.32 Gout due to renal impairment,** elbow
     **M10.321 Gout due to renal impairment,** right **elbow**
     **M10.322 Gout due to renal impairment,** left **elbow**
     **M10.329 Gout due to renal impairment,** unspecified **elbow**

√6ᵗʰ **M10.33 Gout due to renal impairment,** wrist
     **M10.331 Gout due to renal impairment,** right **wrist**
     **M10.332 Gout due to renal impairment,** left **wrist**
     **M10.339 Gout due to renal impairment,** unspecified **wrist**

√6ᵗʰ **M10.34 Gout due to renal impairment,** hand
     **M10.341 Gout due to renal impairment,** right **hand**
     **M10.342 Gout due to renal impairment,** left **hand**
     **M10.349 Gout due to renal impairment,** unspecified **hand**

√6ᵗʰ **M10.35 Gout due to renal impairment,** hip
     **M10.351 Gout due to renal impairment,** right **hip**
     **M10.352 Gout due to renal impairment,** left **hip**
     **M10.359 Gout due to renal impairment,** unspecified **hip**

√6ᵗʰ **M10.36 Gout due to renal impairment,** knee
     **M10.361 Gout due to renal impairment,** right **knee**
     **M10.362 Gout due to renal impairment,** left **knee**
     **M10.369 Gout due to renal impairment,** unspecified **knee**

√6ᵗʰ **M10.37 Gout due to renal impairment,** ankle and foot
     **M10.371 Gout due to renal impairment,** right **ankle and foot**
     **M10.372 Gout due to renal impairment,** left **ankle and foot**
     **M10.379 Gout due to renal impairment,** unspecified **ankle and foot**

   **M10.38 Gout due to renal impairment,** vertebrae
   **M10.39 Gout due to renal impairment,** multiple sites

√5ᵗʰ **M10.4 Other secondary gout**
     Code first associated condition

   **M10.40 Other secondary gout,** unspecified site

√6ᵗʰ **M10.41 Other secondary gout,** shoulder
     **M10.411 Other secondary gout,** right **shoulder**
     **M10.412 Other secondary gout,** left **shoulder**
     **M10.419 Other secondary gout,** unspecified **shoulder**

√6ᵗʰ **M10.42 Other secondary gout,** elbow
     **M10.421 Other secondary gout,** right **elbow**
     **M10.422 Other secondary gout,** left **elbow**
     **M10.429 Other secondary gout,** unspecified **elbow**

√6ᵗʰ **M10.43 Other secondary gout,** wrist
     **M10.431 Other secondary gout,** right **wrist**
     **M10.432 Other secondary gout,** left **wrist**
     **M10.439 Other secondary gout,** unspecified **wrist**

√6ᵗʰ **M10.44 Other secondary gout,** hand
     **M10.441 Other secondary gout,** right **hand**
     **M10.442 Other secondary gout,** left **hand**
     **M10.449 Other secondary gout,** unspecified **hand**

√6ᵗʰ **M10.45 Other secondary gout,** hip
     **M10.451 Other secondary gout,** right **hip**
     **M10.452 Other secondary gout,** left **hip**
     **M10.459 Other secondary gout,** unspecified **hip**

√6ᵗʰ **M10.46 Other secondary gout,** knee
     **M10.461 Other secondary gout,** right **knee**
     **M10.462 Other secondary gout,** left **knee**
     **M10.469 Other secondary gout,** unspecified **knee**

√6ᵗʰ **M10.47 Other secondary gout,** ankle and foot
     **M10.471 Other secondary gout,** right **ankle and foot**
     **M10.472 Other secondary gout,** left **ankle and foot**
     **M10.479 Other secondary gout,** unspecified **ankle and foot**

   **M10.48 Other secondary gout,** vertebrae
   **M10.49 Other secondary gout,** multiple sites

 **M10.9 Gout,** unspecified
     Gout NOS

√4ᵗʰ **M11 Other crystal arthropathies**

√5ᵗʰ **M11.0 Hydroxyapatite deposition disease**

   **M11.00 Hydroxyapatite deposition disease,** unspecified site

√6ᵗʰ **M11.01 Hydroxyapatite deposition disease,** shoulder
     **M11.011 Hydroxyapatite deposition disease,** right **shoulder**
     **M11.012 Hydroxyapatite deposition disease,** left **shoulder**
     **M11.019 Hydroxyapatite deposition disease,** unspecified **shoulder**

√6ᵗʰ **M11.02 Hydroxyapatite deposition disease,** elbow
     **M11.021 Hydroxyapatite deposition disease,** right **elbow**
     **M11.022 Hydroxyapatite deposition disease,** left **elbow**
     **M11.029 Hydroxyapatite deposition disease,** unspecified **elbow**

√6ᵗʰ **M11.03 Hydroxyapatite deposition disease,** wrist
     **M11.031 Hydroxyapatite deposition disease,** right **wrist**
     **M11.032 Hydroxyapatite deposition disease,** left **wrist**
     **M11.039 Hydroxyapatite deposition disease,** unspecified **wrist**

√6ᵗʰ **M11.04 Hydroxyapatite deposition disease,** hand
     **M11.041 Hydroxyapatite deposition disease,** right **hand**
     **M11.042 Hydroxyapatite deposition disease,** left **hand**
     **M11.049 Hydroxyapatite deposition disease,** unspecified **hand**

√6ᵗʰ **M11.05 Hydroxyapatite deposition disease,** hip
     **M11.051 Hydroxyapatite deposition disease,** right **hip**
     **M11.052 Hydroxyapatite deposition disease,** left **hip**
     **M11.059 Hydroxyapatite deposition disease,** unspecified **hip**

√6ᵗʰ **M11.06 Hydroxyapatite deposition disease,** knee
     **M11.061 Hydroxyapatite deposition disease,** right **knee**
     **M11.062 Hydroxyapatite deposition disease,** left **knee**
     **M11.069 Hydroxyapatite deposition disease,** unspecified **knee**

√6ᵗʰ **M11.07 Hydroxyapatite deposition disease,** ankle and foot
     **M11.071 Hydroxyapatite deposition disease,** right **ankle and foot**
     **M11.072 Hydroxyapatite deposition disease,** left **ankle and foot**
     **M11.079 Hydroxyapatite deposition disease,** unspecified **ankle and foot**

---

M11.Ø8    **Hydroxyapatite deposition disease, vertebrae**

M11.Ø9    **Hydroxyapatite deposition disease, multiple sites**

✓5ᵗʰ   **M11.1   Familial chondrocalcinosis**

     M11.1Ø   **Familial chondrocalcinosis, unspecified site**

   ✓6ᵗʰ   **M11.11   Familial chondrocalcinosis, shoulder**

       M11.111   **Familial chondrocalcinosis, right shoulder**

       M11.112   **Familial chondrocalcinosis, left shoulder**

       M11.119   **Familial chondrocalcinosis, unspecified shoulder**

   ✓6ᵗʰ   **M11.12   Familial chondrocalcinosis, elbow**

       M11.121   **Familial chondrocalcinosis, right elbow**

       M11.122   **Familial chondrocalcinosis, left elbow**

       M11.129   **Familial chondrocalcinosis, unspecified elbow**

   ✓6ᵗʰ   **M11.13   Familial chondrocalcinosis, wrist**

       M11.131   **Familial chondrocalcinosis, right wrist**

       M11.132   **Familial chondrocalcinosis, left wrist**

       M11.139   **Familial chondrocalcinosis, unspecified wrist**

   ✓6ᵗʰ   **M11.14   Familial chondrocalcinosis, hand**

       M11.141   **Familial chondrocalcinosis, right hand**

       M11.142   **Familial chondrocalcinosis, left hand**

       M11.149   **Familial chondrocalcinosis, unspecified hand**

   ✓6ᵗʰ   **M11.15   Familial chondrocalcinosis, hip**

       M11.151   **Familial chondrocalcinosis, right hip**

       M11.152   **Familial chondrocalcinosis, left hip**

       M11.159   **Familial chondrocalcinosis, unspecified hip**

   ✓6ᵗʰ   **M11.16   Familial chondrocalcinosis, knee**

       M11.161   **Familial chondrocalcinosis, right knee**

       M11.162   **Familial chondrocalcinosis, left knee**

       M11.169   **Familial chondrocalcinosis, unspecified knee**

   ✓6ᵗʰ   **M11.17   Familial chondrocalcinosis, ankle and foot**

       M11.171   **Familial chondrocalcinosis, right ankle and foot**

       M11.172   **Familial chondrocalcinosis, left ankle and foot**

       M11.179   **Familial chondrocalcinosis, unspecified ankle and foot**

     M11.18   **Familial chondrocalcinosis, vertebrae**

     M11.19   **Familial chondrocalcinosis, multiple sites**

✓5ᵗʰ   **M11.2   Other chondrocalcinosis**

     Chondrocalcinosis NOS

     M11.2Ø   **Other chondrocalcinosis, unspecified site**

   ✓6ᵗʰ   **M11.21   Other chondrocalcinosis, shoulder**

       M11.211   **Other chondrocalcinosis, right shoulder**

       M11.212   **Other chondrocalcinosis, left shoulder**

       M11.219   **Other chondrocalcinosis, unspecified shoulder**

   ✓6ᵗʰ   **M11.22   Other chondrocalcinosis, elbow**

       M11.221   **Other chondrocalcinosis, right elbow**

       M11.222   **Other chondrocalcinosis, left elbow**

       M11.229   **Other chondrocalcinosis, unspecified elbow**

   ✓6ᵗʰ   **M11.23   Other chondrocalcinosis, wrist**

       M11.231   **Other chondrocalcinosis, right wrist**

       M11.232   **Other chondrocalcinosis, left wrist**

       M11.239   **Other chondrocalcinosis, unspecified wrist**

   ✓6ᵗʰ   **M11.24   Other chondrocalcinosis, hand**

       M11.241   **Other chondrocalcinosis, right hand**

       M11.242   **Other chondrocalcinosis, left hand**

       M11.249   **Other chondrocalcinosis, unspecified hand**

   ✓6ᵗʰ   **M11.25   Other chondrocalcinosis, hip**

       M11.251   **Other chondrocalcinosis, right hip**

       M11.252   **Other chondrocalcinosis, left hip**

       M11.259   **Other chondrocalcinosis, unspecified hip**

   ✓6ᵗʰ   **M11.26   Other chondrocalcinosis, knee**

       M11.261   **Other chondrocalcinosis, right knee**

       M11.262   **Other chondrocalcinosis, left knee**

       M11.269   **Other chondrocalcinosis, unspecified knee**

   ✓6ᵗʰ   **M11.27   Other chondrocalcinosis, ankle and foot**

       M11.271   **Other chondrocalcinosis, right ankle and foot**

       M11.272   **Other chondrocalcinosis, left ankle and foot**

       M11.279   **Other chondrocalcinosis, unspecified ankle and foot**

     M11.28   **Other chondrocalcinosis, vertebrae**

     M11.29   **Other chondrocalcinosis, multiple sites**

✓5ᵗʰ   **M11.8   Other specified crystal arthropathies**

     M11.8Ø   **Other specified crystal arthropathies, unspecified site**

   ✓6ᵗʰ   **M11.81   Other specified crystal arthropathies, shoulder**

       M11.811   **Other specified crystal arthropathies, right shoulder**

       M11.812   **Other specified crystal arthropathies, left shoulder**

       M11.819   **Other specified crystal arthropathies, unspecified shoulder**

   ✓6ᵗʰ   **M11.82   Other specified crystal arthropathies, elbow**

       M11.821   **Other specified crystal arthropathies, right elbow**

       M11.822   **Other specified crystal arthropathies, left elbow**

       M11.829   **Other specified crystal arthropathies, unspecified elbow**

   ✓6ᵗʰ   **M11.83   Other specified crystal arthropathies, wrist**

       M11.831   **Other specified crystal arthropathies, right wrist**

       M11.832   **Other specified crystal arthropathies, left wrist**

       M11.839   **Other specified crystal arthropathies, unspecified wrist**

   ✓6ᵗʰ   **M11.84   Other specified crystal arthropathies, hand**

       M11.841   **Other specified crystal arthropathies, right hand**

       M11.842   **Other specified crystal arthropathies, left hand**

       M11.849   **Other specified crystal arthropathies, unspecified hand**

   ✓6ᵗʰ   **M11.85   Other specified crystal arthropathies, hip**

       M11.851   **Other specified crystal arthropathies, right hip**

       M11.852   **Other specified crystal arthropathies, left hip**

       M11.859   **Other specified crystal arthropathies, unspecified hip**

   ✓6ᵗʰ   **M11.86   Other specified crystal arthropathies, knee**

       M11.861   **Other specified crystal arthropathies, right knee**

       M11.862   **Other specified crystal arthropathies, left knee**

       M11.869   **Other specified crystal arthropathies, unspecified knee**

   ✓6ᵗʰ   **M11.87   Other specified crystal arthropathies, ankle and foot**

       M11.871   **Other specified crystal arthropathies, right ankle and foot**

       M11.872   **Other specified crystal arthropathies, left ankle and foot**

       M11.879   **Other specified crystal arthropathies, unspecified ankle and foot**

     M11.88   **Other specified crystal arthropathies, vertebrae**

     M11.89   **Other specified crystal arthropathies, multiple sites**

     M11.9   **Crystal arthropathy, unspecified**

✓4ᵗʰ   **M12   Other and unspecified arthropathy**

     *EXCLUDES 1*   *arthrosis (M15-M19)*

               *cricoarytenoid arthropathy (J38.7)*

   ✓5ᵗʰ   **M12.Ø   Chronic postrheumatic arthropathy [Jaccoud]**

       M12.ØØ   **Chronic postrheumatic arthropathy [Jaccoud], unspecified site**   HCC

     ✓6ᵗʰ   **M12.Ø1   Chronic postrheumatic arthropathy [Jaccoud], shoulder**

         M12.Ø11   **Chronic postrheumatic arthropathy [Jaccoud], right shoulder**   HCC

         M12.Ø12   **Chronic postrheumatic arthropathy [Jaccoud], left shoulder**   HCC

N Newborn: 0   P Pediatric: 0-17   M Maternity: 12-55   A Adult: 15-124   **MCC** Major CC Condition   **PDxMCC** PDx acts as own MCC   **CC** CC Condition   **PDxCC** PDx acts as own CC

**752**                                                      ICD-10-CM 2018

M12.019 **Chronic postrheumatic arthropathy** [Jaccoud], **unspecified shoulder** `HCC`

✅6th M12.02 **Chronic postrheumatic arthropathy [Jaccoud], elbow**

M12.021 **Chronic postrheumatic arthropathy [Jaccoud], right elbow** `HCC`

M12.022 **Chronic postrheumatic arthropathy [Jaccoud], left elbow** `HCC`

M12.029 **Chronic postrheumatic arthropathy [Jaccoud], unspecified elbow** `HCC`

✅6th M12.03 **Chronic postrheumatic arthropathy [Jaccoud], wrist**

M12.031 **Chronic postrheumatic arthropathy [Jaccoud], right wrist** `HCC`

M12.032 **Chronic postrheumatic arthropathy [Jaccoud], left wrist** `HCC`

M12.039 **Chronic postrheumatic arthropathy [Jaccoud], unspecified wrist** `HCC`

✅6th M12.04 **Chronic postrheumatic arthropathy [Jaccoud], hand**

M12.041 **Chronic postrheumatic arthropathy [Jaccoud], right hand** `HCC`

M12.042 **Chronic postrheumatic arthropathy [Jaccoud], left hand** `HCC`

M12.049 **Chronic postrheumatic arthropathy [Jaccoud], unspecified hand** `HCC`

✅6th M12.05 **Chronic postrheumatic arthropathy [Jaccoud], hip**

M12.051 **Chronic postrheumatic arthropathy [Jaccoud], right hip** `HCC`

M12.052 **Chronic postrheumatic arthropathy [Jaccoud], left hip** `HCC`

M12.059 **Chronic postrheumatic arthropathy [Jaccoud], unspecified hip** `HCC`

✅6th M12.06 **Chronic postrheumatic arthropathy [Jaccoud], knee**

M12.061 **Chronic postrheumatic arthropathy [Jaccoud], right knee** `HCC`

M12.062 **Chronic postrheumatic arthropathy [Jaccoud], left knee** `HCC`

M12.069 **Chronic postrheumatic arthropathy [Jaccoud], unspecified knee** `HCC`

✅6th M12.07 **Chronic postrheumatic arthropathy [Jaccoud], ankle and foot**

M12.071 **Chronic postrheumatic arthropathy [Jaccoud], right ankle and foot** `HCC`

M12.072 **Chronic postrheumatic arthropathy [Jaccoud], left ankle and foot** `HCC`

M12.079 **Chronic postrheumatic arthropathy [Jaccoud], unspecified ankle and foot** `HCC`

M12.08 **Chronic postrheumatic arthropathy [Jaccoud], other specified site** `HCC`
Chronic postrheumatic arthropathy [Jaccoud], vertebrae

M12.09 **Chronic postrheumatic arthropathy [Jaccoud], multiple sites** `HCC`

✅5th M12.1 **Kaschin-Beck disease**
Osteochondroarthrosis deformans endemica

M12.10 **Kaschin-Beck disease, unspecified site**

✅6th M12.11 **Kaschin-Beck disease, shoulder**

M12.111 **Kaschin-Beck disease, right shoulder**
M12.112 **Kaschin-Beck disease, left shoulder**
M12.119 **Kaschin-Beck disease, unspecified shoulder**

✅6th M12.12 **Kaschin-Beck disease, elbow**

M12.121 **Kaschin-Beck disease, right elbow**
M12.122 **Kaschin-Beck disease, left elbow**
M12.129 **Kaschin-Beck disease, unspecified elbow**

✅6th M12.13 **Kaschin-Beck disease, wrist**

M12.131 **Kaschin-Beck disease, right wrist**
M12.132 **Kaschin-Beck disease, left wrist**
M12.139 **Kaschin-Beck disease, unspecified wrist**

✅6th M12.14 **Kaschin-Beck disease, hand**

M12.141 **Kaschin-Beck disease, right hand**
M12.142 **Kaschin-Beck disease, left hand**
M12.149 **Kaschin-Beck disease, unspecified hand**

✅6th M12.15 **Kaschin-Beck disease, hip**

M12.151 **Kaschin-Beck disease, right hip**
M12.152 **Kaschin-Beck disease, left hip**
M12.159 **Kaschin-Beck disease, unspecified hip**

✅6th M12.16 **Kaschin-Beck disease, knee**

M12.161 **Kaschin-Beck disease, right knee**
M12.162 **Kaschin-Beck disease, left knee**
M12.169 **Kaschin-Beck disease, unspecified knee**

✅6th M12.17 **Kaschin-Beck disease, ankle and foot**

M12.171 **Kaschin-Beck disease, right ankle and foot**
M12.172 **Kaschin-Beck disease, left ankle and foot**
M12.179 **Kaschin-Beck disease, unspecified ankle and foot**

M12.18 **Kaschin-Beck disease, vertebrae**

M12.19 **Kaschin-Beck disease, multiple sites**

✅5th M12.2 **Villonodular synovitis (pigmented)**

M12.20 **Villonodular synovitis (pigmented), unspecified site**

✅6th M12.21 **Villonodular synovitis (pigmented), shoulder**

M12.211 **Villonodular synovitis (pigmented), right shoulder**
M12.212 **Villonodular synovitis (pigmented), left shoulder**
M12.219 **Villonodular synovitis (pigmented), unspecified shoulder**

✅6th M12.22 **Villonodular synovitis (pigmented), elbow**

M12.221 **Villonodular synovitis (pigmented), right elbow**
M12.222 **Villonodular synovitis (pigmented), left elbow**
M12.229 **Villonodular synovitis (pigmented), unspecified elbow**

✅6th M12.23 **Villonodular synovitis (pigmented), wrist**

M12.231 **Villonodular synovitis (pigmented), right wrist**
M12.232 **Villonodular synovitis (pigmented), left wrist**
M12.239 **Villonodular synovitis (pigmented), unspecified wrist**

✅6th M12.24 **Villonodular synovitis (pigmented), hand**

M12.241 **Villonodular synovitis (pigmented), right hand**
M12.242 **Villonodular synovitis (pigmented), left hand**
M12.249 **Villonodular synovitis (pigmented), unspecified hand**

✅6th M12.25 **Villonodular synovitis (pigmented), hip**

M12.251 **Villonodular synovitis (pigmented), right hip**
M12.252 **Villonodular synovitis (pigmented), left hip**
M12.259 **Villonodular synovitis (pigmented), unspecified hip**

✅6th M12.26 **Villonodular synovitis (pigmented), knee**

M12.261 **Villonodular synovitis (pigmented), right knee**
M12.262 **Villonodular synovitis (pigmented), left knee**
M12.269 **Villonodular synovitis (pigmented), unspecified knee**

✅6th M12.27 **Villonodular synovitis (pigmented), ankle and foot**

M12.271 **Villonodular synovitis (pigmented), right ankle and foot**
M12.272 **Villonodular synovitis (pigmented), left ankle and foot**
M12.279 **Villonodular synovitis (pigmented), unspecified ankle and foot**

M12.28 **Villonodular synovitis (pigmented), other specified site**
Villonodular synovitis (pigmented), vertebrae

M12.29 **Villonodular synovitis (pigmented), multiple sites**

✅5th M12.3 **Palindromic rheumatism**

M12.30 **Palindromic rheumatism, unspecified site**

✅6th M12.31 **Palindromic rheumatism, shoulder**

M12.311 **Palindromic rheumatism, right shoulder**
M12.312 **Palindromic rheumatism, left shoulder**
M12.319 **Palindromic rheumatism, unspecified shoulder**

---

✅ Additional Character Req   ✅x7th Placeholder Alert   Unacceptable PDx   Manifestation   `H1`-`H14` HAC   `HCC` CMS-HCC Condition   *EXCLUDES 1* Not Coded Here   *EXCLUDES 2* Not Included Here

ICD-10-CM 2018   753

✓6ᵗʰ **M12.32** **Palindromic rheumatism,** elbow
　　**M12.321** **Palindromic rheumatism, right elbow**
　　**M12.322** **Palindromic rheumatism, left elbow**
　　**M12.329** **Palindromic rheumatism, unspecified elbow**

✓6ᵗʰ **M12.33** **Palindromic rheumatism,** wrist
　　**M12.331** **Palindromic rheumatism, right wrist**
　　**M12.332** **Palindromic rheumatism, left wrist**
　　**M12.339** **Palindromic rheumatism, unspecified wrist**

✓6ᵗʰ **M12.34** **Palindromic rheumatism,** hand
　　**M12.341** **Palindromic rheumatism, right hand**
　　**M12.342** **Palindromic rheumatism, left hand**
　　**M12.349** **Palindromic rheumatism, unspecified hand**

✓6ᵗʰ **M12.35** **Palindromic rheumatism,** hip
　　**M12.351** **Palindromic rheumatism, right hip**
　　**M12.352** **Palindromic rheumatism, left hip**
　　**M12.359** **Palindromic rheumatism, unspecified hip**

✓6ᵗʰ **M12.36** **Palindromic rheumatism,** knee
　　**M12.361** **Palindromic rheumatism, right knee**
　　**M12.362** **Palindromic rheumatism, left knee**
　　**M12.369** **Palindromic rheumatism, unspecified knee**

✓6ᵗʰ **M12.37** **Palindromic rheumatism,** ankle and foot
　　**M12.371** **Palindromic rheumatism, right ankle and foot**
　　**M12.372** **Palindromic rheumatism, left ankle and foot**
　　**M12.379** **Palindromic rheumatism, unspecified ankle and foot**

　　**M12.38** **Palindromic rheumatism,** other specified site
　　　　Palindromic rheumatism, vertebrae

　　**M12.39** **Palindromic rheumatism,** multiple sites

✓5ᵗʰ **M12.4** **Intermittent hydrarthrosis**
　　**M12.40** **Intermittent hydrarthrosis,** unspecified site

✓6ᵗʰ **M12.41** **Intermittent hydrarthrosis,** shoulder
　　**M12.411** **Intermittent hydrarthrosis, right shoulder**
　　**M12.412** **Intermittent hydrarthrosis, left shoulder**
　　**M12.419** **Intermittent hydrarthrosis, unspecified shoulder**

✓6ᵗʰ **M12.42** **Intermittent hydrarthrosis,** elbow
　　**M12.421** **Intermittent hydrarthrosis, right elbow**
　　**M12.422** **Intermittent hydrarthrosis, left elbow**
　　**M12.429** **Intermittent hydrarthrosis, unspecified elbow**

✓6ᵗʰ **M12.43** **Intermittent hydrarthrosis,** wrist
　　**M12.431** **Intermittent hydrarthrosis, right wrist**
　　**M12.432** **Intermittent hydrarthrosis, left wrist**
　　**M12.439** **Intermittent hydrarthrosis, unspecified wrist**

✓6ᵗʰ **M12.44** **Intermittent hydrarthrosis,** hand
　　**M12.441** **Intermittent hydrarthrosis, right hand**
　　**M12.442** **Intermittent hydrarthrosis, left hand**
　　**M12.449** **Intermittent hydrarthrosis, unspecified hand**

✓6ᵗʰ **M12.45** **Intermittent hydrarthrosis,** hip
　　**M12.451** **Intermittent hydrarthrosis, right hip**
　　**M12.452** **Intermittent hydrarthrosis, left hip**
　　**M12.459** **Intermittent hydrarthrosis, unspecified hip**

✓6ᵗʰ **M12.46** **Intermittent hydrarthrosis,** knee
　　**M12.461** **Intermittent hydrarthrosis, right knee**
　　**M12.462** **Intermittent hydrarthrosis, left knee**
　　**M12.469** **Intermittent hydrarthrosis, unspecified knee**

✓6ᵗʰ **M12.47** **Intermittent hydrarthrosis,** ankle and foot
　　**M12.471** **Intermittent hydrarthrosis, right ankle and foot**
　　**M12.472** **Intermittent hydrarthrosis, left ankle and foot**
　　**M12.479** **Intermittent hydrarthrosis, unspecified ankle and foot**

　　**M12.48** **Intermittent hydrarthrosis,** other site

　　**M12.49** **Intermittent hydrarthrosis,** multiple sites

✓5ᵗʰ **M12.5** **Traumatic arthropathy**
　　EXCLUDES 1　current injury—see Alphabetic Index
　　　　post-traumatic osteoarthritis NOS (M19.1-)
　　　　post-traumatic osteoarthritis of first carpometacarpal joint (M18.2-M18.3)
　　　　post-traumatic osteoarthritis of hip (M16.4-M16.5)
　　　　post-traumatic osteoarthritis of knee (M17.2-M17.3)
　　　　post-traumatic osteoarthritis of other single joints (M19.1-)
　　**AHA:** 2015, 1Q, 17

　　**M12.50** **Traumatic arthropathy,** unspecified site

✓6ᵗʰ **M12.51** **Traumatic arthropathy,** shoulder
　　**M12.511** **Traumatic arthropathy, right shoulder**
　　**M12.512** **Traumatic arthropathy, left shoulder**
　　**M12.519** **Traumatic arthropathy, unspecified shoulder**

✓6ᵗʰ **M12.52** **Traumatic arthropathy,** elbow
　　**M12.521** **Traumatic arthropathy, right elbow**
　　**M12.522** **Traumatic arthropathy, left elbow**
　　**M12.529** **Traumatic arthropathy, unspecified elbow**

✓6ᵗʰ **M12.53** **Traumatic arthropathy,** wrist
　　**M12.531** **Traumatic arthropathy, right wrist**
　　**M12.532** **Traumatic arthropathy, left wrist**
　　**M12.539** **Traumatic arthropathy, unspecified wrist**

✓6ᵗʰ **M12.54** **Traumatic arthropathy,** hand
　　**M12.541** **Traumatic arthropathy, right hand**
　　**M12.542** **Traumatic arthropathy, left hand**
　　**M12.549** **Traumatic arthropathy, unspecified hand**

✓6ᵗʰ **M12.55** **Traumatic arthropathy,** hip
　　**M12.551** **Traumatic arthropathy, right hip**
　　**M12.552** **Traumatic arthropathy, left hip**
　　**M12.559** **Traumatic arthropathy, unspecified hip**

✓6ᵗʰ **M12.56** **Traumatic arthropathy,** knee
　　**M12.561** **Traumatic arthropathy, right knee**
　　**M12.562** **Traumatic arthropathy, left knee**
　　**M12.569** **Traumatic arthropathy, unspecified knee**

✓6ᵗʰ **M12.57** **Traumatic arthropathy,** ankle and foot
　　**M12.571** **Traumatic arthropathy, right ankle and foot**
　　**M12.572** **Traumatic arthropathy, left ankle and foot**
　　**M12.579** **Traumatic arthropathy, unspecified ankle and foot**

　　**M12.58** **Traumatic arthropathy,** other specified site
　　　　Traumatic arthropathy, vertebrae

　　**M12.59** **Traumatic arthropathy,** multiple sites

✓5ᵗʰ **M12.8** **Other specific arthropathies, not elsewhere classified**
　　Transient arthropathy

　　**M12.80** **Other specific arthropathies, not elsewhere classified,** unspecified site

✓6ᵗʰ **M12.81** **Other specific arthropathies, not elsewhere classified,** shoulder
　　**M12.811** **Other specific arthropathies, not elsewhere classified, right shoulder**
　　**M12.812** **Other specific arthropathies, not elsewhere classified, left shoulder**
　　**M12.819** **Other specific arthropathies, not elsewhere classified, unspecified shoulder**

✓6ᵗʰ **M12.82** **Other specific arthropathies, not elsewhere classified,** elbow
　　**M12.821** **Other specific arthropathies, not elsewhere classified, right elbow**
　　**M12.822** **Other specific arthropathies, not elsewhere classified, left elbow**
　　**M12.829** **Other specific arthropathies, not elsewhere classified, unspecified elbow**

✓6ᵗʰ **M12.83** **Other specific arthropathies, not elsewhere classified,** wrist
　　**M12.831** **Other specific arthropathies, not elsewhere classified, right wrist**
　　**M12.832** **Other specific arthropathies, not elsewhere classified, left wrist**
　　**M12.839** **Other specific arthropathies, not elsewhere classified, unspecified wrist**

N Newborn: 0　P Pediatric: 0-17　M Maternity: 12-55　A Adult: 15-124　MCC Major CC Condition　PDxMCC PDx acts as own MCC　CC CC Condition　PDxCC PDx acts as own CC

754

ICD-10-CM 2018

✓6ᵗʰ **M12.84** **Other specific arthropathies, not elsewhere classified,** hand

    **M12.841** **Other specific arthropathies, not elsewhere classified,** right **hand**

    **M12.842** **Other specific arthropathies, not elsewhere classified,** left **hand**

    **M12.849** **Other specific arthropathies, not elsewhere classified,** unspecified **hand**

✓6ᵗʰ **M12.85** **Other specific arthropathies, not elsewhere classified,** hip

    **M12.851** **Other specific arthropathies, not elsewhere classified,** right **hip**

    **M12.852** **Other specific arthropathies, not elsewhere classified,** left **hip**

    **M12.859** **Other specific arthropathies, not elsewhere classified,** unspecified **hip**

✓6ᵗʰ **M12.86** **Other specific arthropathies, not elsewhere classified,** knee

    **M12.861** **Other specific arthropathies, not elsewhere classified,** right **knee**

    **M12.862** **Other specific arthropathies, not elsewhere classified,** left **knee**

    **M12.869** **Other specific arthropathies, not elsewhere classified,** unspecified **knee**

✓6ᵗʰ **M12.87** **Other specific arthropathies, not elsewhere classified,** ankle and foot

    **M12.871** **Other specific arthropathies, not elsewhere classified,** right **ankle and foot**

    **M12.872** **Other specific arthropathies, not elsewhere classified,** left **ankle and foot**

    **M12.879** **Other specific arthropathies, not elsewhere classified,** unspecified **ankle and foot**

    **M12.88** **Other specific arthropathies, not elsewhere classified,** other specified site

        Other specific arthropathies, not elsewhere classified, vertebrae

    **M12.89** **Other specific arthropathies, not elsewhere classified,** multiple sites

**M12.9** **Arthropathy,** unspecified

✓4ᵗʰ **M13** **Other arthritis**

    *EXCLUDES 1*    arthrosis (M15-M19)

                osteoarthritis (M15-M19)

**M13.0** **Polyarthritis,** unspecified

✓5ᵗʰ **M13.1** **Monoarthritis, not elsewhere classified**

    **M13.10** **Monoarthritis, not elsewhere classified,** unspecified site

✓6ᵗʰ **M13.11** **Monoarthritis, not elsewhere classified,** shoulder

    **M13.111** **Monoarthritis, not elsewhere classified,** right **shoulder**

    **M13.112** **Monoarthritis, not elsewhere classified,** left **shoulder**

    **M13.119** **Monoarthritis, not elsewhere classified,** unspecified **shoulder**

✓6ᵗʰ **M13.12** **Monoarthritis, not elsewhere classified,** elbow

    **M13.121** **Monoarthritis, not elsewhere classified,** right **elbow**

    **M13.122** **Monoarthritis, not elsewhere classified,** left **elbow**

    **M13.129** **Monoarthritis, not elsewhere classified,** unspecified **elbow**

✓6ᵗʰ **M13.13** **Monoarthritis, not elsewhere classified,** wrist

    **M13.131** **Monoarthritis, not elsewhere classified,** right **wrist**

    **M13.132** **Monoarthritis, not elsewhere classified,** left **wrist**

    **M13.139** **Monoarthritis, not elsewhere classified,** unspecified **wrist**

✓6ᵗʰ **M13.14** **Monoarthritis, not elsewhere classified,** hand

    **M13.141** **Monoarthritis, not elsewhere classified,** right **hand**

    **M13.142** **Monoarthritis, not elsewhere classified,** left **hand**

    **M13.149** **Monoarthritis, not elsewhere classified,** unspecified **hand**

✓6ᵗʰ **M13.15** **Monoarthritis, not elsewhere classified,** hip

    **M13.151** **Monoarthritis, not elsewhere classified,** right **hip**

    **M13.152** **Monoarthritis, not elsewhere classified,** left **hip**

    **M13.159** **Monoarthritis, not elsewhere classified,** unspecified **hip**

✓6ᵗʰ **M13.16** **Monoarthritis, not elsewhere classified,** knee

    **M13.161** **Monoarthritis, not elsewhere classified,** right **knee**

    **M13.162** **Monoarthritis, not elsewhere classified,** left **knee**

    **M13.169** **Monoarthritis, not elsewhere classified,** unspecified **knee**

✓6ᵗʰ **M13.17** **Monoarthritis, not elsewhere classified,** ankle and foot

    **M13.171** **Monoarthritis, not elsewhere classified,** right **ankle and foot**

    **M13.172** **Monoarthritis, not elsewhere classified,** left **ankle and foot**

    **M13.179** **Monoarthritis, not elsewhere classified,** unspecified **ankle and foot**

✓5ᵗʰ **M13.8** **Other specified arthritis**

    Allergic arthritis

    *EXCLUDES 1*    osteoarthritis (M15-M19)

    **M13.80** **Other specified arthritis,** unspecified site

✓6ᵗʰ **M13.81** **Other specified arthritis,** shoulder

    **M13.811** **Other specified arthritis,** right **shoulder**

    **M13.812** **Other specified arthritis,** left **shoulder**

    **M13.819** **Other specified arthritis,** unspecified **shoulder**

✓6ᵗʰ **M13.82** **Other specified arthritis,** elbow

    **M13.821** **Other specified arthritis,** right **elbow**

    **M13.822** **Other specified arthritis,** left **elbow**

    **M13.829** **Other specified arthritis,** unspecified **elbow**

✓6ᵗʰ **M13.83** **Other specified arthritis,** wrist

    **M13.831** **Other specified arthritis,** right **wrist**

    **M13.832** **Other specified arthritis,** left **wrist**

    **M13.839** **Other specified arthritis,** unspecified **wrist**

✓6ᵗʰ **M13.84** **Other specified arthritis,** hand

    **M13.841** **Other specified arthritis,** right **hand**

    **M13.842** **Other specified arthritis,** left **hand**

    **M13.849** **Other specified arthritis,** unspecified **hand**

✓6ᵗʰ **M13.85** **Other specified arthritis,** hip

    **M13.851** **Other specified arthritis,** right **hip**

    **M13.852** **Other specified arthritis,** left **hip**

    **M13.859** **Other specified arthritis,** unspecified **hip**

✓6ᵗʰ **M13.86** **Other specified arthritis,** knee

    **M13.861** **Other specified arthritis,** right **knee**

    **M13.862** **Other specified arthritis,** left **knee**

    **M13.869** **Other specified arthritis,** unspecified **knee**

✓6ᵗʰ **M13.87** **Other specified arthritis,** ankle and foot

    **M13.871** **Other specified arthritis,** right **ankle and foot**

    **M13.872** **Other specified arthritis,** left **ankle and foot**

    **M13.879** **Other specified arthritis,** unspecified **ankle and foot**

    **M13.88** **Other specified arthritis,** other site

    **M13.89** **Other specified arthritis,** multiple sites

✓ Additional Character Req    ✓×7ᵗʰ Placeholder Alert    Unacceptable PDx    Manifestation    H1 - H14 HAC    HCC CMS-HCC Condition    *EXCLUDES 1* Not Coded Here    *EXCLUDES 2* Not Included Here

ICD-10-CM 2018      755

✓4th **M14 Arthropathies in other diseases classified elsewhere**
> EXCLUDES 1 *arthropathy in:*
>> *diabetes mellitus (E08-E13 with .61-)*
>> *hematological disorders (M36.2-M36.3)*
>> *hypersensitivity reactions (M36.4)*
>> *neoplastic disease (M36.1)*
>> *neurosyphillis (A52.16)*
>> *sarcoidosis (D86.86)*
>> *enteropathic arthropathies (M07.-)*
>> *juvenile psoriatic arthropathy (L40.54)*
>> *lipoid dermatoarthritis (E78.81)*

✓5th **M14.6 Charcôt's joint**
> Neuropathic arthropathy
>> EXCLUDES 1 *Charcôt's joint in diabetes mellitus (E08-E13 with .610-)*
>> *Charcôt's joint in tabes dorsalis (A52.16)*

> **M14.60 Charcôt's joint, unspecified site**

> ✓6th **M14.61 Charcôt's joint, shoulder**
>> **M14.611 Charcôt's joint, right shoulder**
>> **M14.612 Charcôt's joint, left shoulder**
>> **M14.619 Charcôt's joint, unspecified shoulder**

> ✓6th **M14.62 Charcôt's joint, elbow**
>> **M14.621 Charcôt's joint, right elbow**
>> **M14.622 Charcôt's joint, left elbow**
>> **M14.629 Charcôt's joint, unspecified elbow**

> ✓6th **M14.63 Charcôt's joint, wrist**
>> **M14.631 Charcôt's joint, right wrist**
>> **M14.632 Charcôt's joint, left wrist**
>> **M14.639 Charcôt's joint, unspecified wrist**

> ✓6th **M14.64 Charcôt's joint, hand**
>> **M14.641 Charcôt's joint, right hand**
>> **M14.642 Charcôt's joint, left hand**
>> **M14.649 Charcôt's joint, unspecified hand**

> ✓6th **M14.65 Charcôt's joint, hip**
>> **M14.651 Charcôt's joint, right hip**
>> **M14.652 Charcôt's joint, left hip**
>> **M14.659 Charcôt's joint, unspecified hip**

> ✓6th **M14.66 Charcôt's joint, knee**
>> **M14.661 Charcôt's joint, right knee**
>> **M14.662 Charcôt's joint, left knee**
>> **M14.669 Charcôt's joint, unspecified knee**

> ✓6th **M14.67 Charcôt's joint, ankle and foot**
>> **M14.671 Charcôt's joint, right ankle and foot**
>> **M14.672 Charcôt's joint, left ankle and foot**
>> **M14.679 Charcôt's joint, unspecified ankle and foot**

> **M14.68 Charcôt's joint, vertebrae**
> **M14.69 Charcôt's joint, multiple sites**

✓5th **M14.8 Arthropathies in other specified diseases classified elsewhere**
> Code first underlying disease, such as:
>> amyloidosis (E85.-)
>> erythema multiforme (L51.-)
>> erythema nodosum (L52)
>> hemochromatosis (E83.11-)
>> hyperparathyroidism (E21.-)
>> hypothyroidism (E00-E03)
>> sickle-cell disorders (D57.-)
>> thyrotoxicosis [hyperthyroidism] (E05.-)
>> Whipple's disease (K90.81)

> *M14.80 Arthropathies in other specified diseases classified elsewhere, unspecified site*

> ✓6th **M14.81 Arthropathies in other specified diseases classified elsewhere, shoulder**
>> *M14.811 Arthropathies in other specified diseases classified elsewhere, right shoulder*
>> *M14.812 Arthropathies in other specified diseases classified elsewhere, left shoulder*
>> *M14.819 Arthropathies in other specified diseases classified elsewhere, unspecified shoulder*

> ✓6th **M14.82 Arthropathies in other specified diseases classified elsewhere, elbow**
>> *M14.821 Arthropathies in other specified diseases classified elsewhere, right elbow*
>> *M14.822 Arthropathies in other specified diseases classified elsewhere, left elbow*
>> *M14.829 Arthropathies in other specified diseases classified elsewhere, unspecified elbow*

✓6th **M14.83 Arthropathies in other specified diseases classified elsewhere, wrist**
> *M14.831 Arthropathies in other specified diseases classified elsewhere, right wrist*
> *M14.832 Arthropathies in other specified diseases classified elsewhere, left wrist*
> *M14.839 Arthropathies in other specified diseases classified elsewhere, unspecified wrist*

✓6th **M14.84 Arthropathies in other specified diseases classified elsewhere, hand**
> *M14.841 Arthropathies in other specified diseases classified elsewhere, right hand*
> *M14.842 Arthropathies in other specified diseases classified elsewhere, left hand*
> *M14.849 Arthropathies in other specified diseases classified elsewhere, unspecified hand*

✓6th **M14.85 Arthropathies in other specified diseases classified elsewhere, hip**
> *M14.851 Arthropathies in other specified diseases classified elsewhere, right hip*
> *M14.852 Arthropathies in other specified diseases classified elsewhere, left hip*
> *M14.859 Arthropathies in other specified diseases classified elsewhere, unspecified hip*

✓6th **M14.86 Arthropathies in other specified diseases classified elsewhere, knee**
> *M14.861 Arthropathies in other specified diseases classified elsewhere, right knee*
> *M14.862 Arthropathies in other specified diseases classified elsewhere, left knee*
> *M14.869 Arthropathies in other specified diseases classified elsewhere, unspecified knee*

✓6th **M14.87 Arthropathies in other specified diseases classified elsewhere, ankle and foot**
> *M14.871 Arthropathies in other specified diseases classified elsewhere, right ankle and foot*
> *M14.872 Arthropathies in other specified diseases classified elsewhere, left ankle and foot*
> *M14.879 Arthropathies in other specified diseases classified elsewhere, unspecified ankle and foot*

> *M14.88 Arthropathies in other specified diseases classified elsewhere, vertebrae*
> *M14.89 Arthropathies in other specified diseases classified elsewhere, multiple sites*

## Osteoarthritis (M15-M19)
> EXCLUDES 2 *osteoarthritis of spine (M47.-)*

✓4th **M15 Polyosteoarthritis**
> INCLUDES arthritis of multiple sites
> EXCLUDES 1 *bilateral involvement of single joint (M16-M19)*

> **M15.0 Primary generalized (osteo)arthritis**

> **M15.1 Heberden's nodes (with arthropathy)**
>> Interphalangeal distal osteoarthritis

> **M15.2 Bouchard's nodes (with arthropathy)**
>> Juxtaphalangeal distal osteoarthritis

> **M15.3 Secondary multiple arthritis**
>> Post-traumatic polyosteoarthritis

> **M15.4 Erosive (osteo)arthritis**

> **M15.8 Other polyosteoarthritis**

> **M15.9 Polyosteoarthritis, unspecified**
>> Generalized osteoarthritis NOS

✓4th **M16 Osteoarthritis of hip**
> AHA: 2016, 4Q, 146

> **M16.0 Bilateral primary osteoarthritis of hip**

> ✓5th **M16.1 Unilateral primary osteoarthritis of hip**
>> Primary osteoarthritis of hip NOS
>>> **M16.10 Unilateral primary osteoarthritis, unspecified hip**
>>> **M16.11 Unilateral primary osteoarthritis, right hip**
>>> **M16.12 Unilateral primary osteoarthritis, left hip**

> **M16.2 Bilateral osteoarthritis resulting from hip dysplasia**

> ✓5th **M16.3 Unilateral osteoarthritis resulting from hip dysplasia**
>> Dysplastic osteoarthritis of hip NOS
>>> **M16.30 Unilateral osteoarthritis resulting from hip dysplasia, unspecified hip**

     **M16.31**   Unilateral osteoarthritis resulting from hip dysplasia, right hip

     **M16.32**   Unilateral osteoarthritis resulting from hip dysplasia, left hip

   **M16.4**   Bilateral post-traumatic osteoarthritis of hip

✓5ᵗʰ **M16.5**   Unilateral post-traumatic osteoarthritis of hip
     Post-traumatic osteoarthritis of hip NOS

     **M16.50**   Unilateral post-traumatic osteoarthritis, unspecified hip

     **M16.51**   Unilateral post-traumatic osteoarthritis, right hip

     **M16.52**   Unilateral post-traumatic osteoarthritis, left hip

   **M16.6**   Other bilateral secondary osteoarthritis of hip

   **M16.7**   Other unilateral secondary osteoarthritis of hip
     Secondary osteoarthritis of hip NOS

   **M16.9**   Osteoarthritis of hip, unspecified

✓4ᵗʰ **M17**   **Osteoarthritis of knee**
     AHA: 2016, 4Q, 146-147

   **M17.0**   Bilateral primary osteoarthritis of knee

✓5ᵗʰ **M17.1**   Unilateral primary osteoarthritis of knee
     Primary osteoarthritis of knee NOS

     **M17.10**   Unilateral primary osteoarthritis, unspecified knee

     **M17.11**   Unilateral primary osteoarthritis, right knee

     **M17.12**   Unilateral primary osteoarthritis, left knee

   **M17.2**   Bilateral post-traumatic osteoarthritis of knee

✓5ᵗʰ **M17.3**   Unilateral post-traumatic osteoarthritis of knee
     Post-traumatic osteoarthritis of knee NOS

     **M17.30**   Unilateral post-traumatic osteoarthritis, unspecified knee

     **M17.31**   Unilateral post-traumatic osteoarthritis, right knee

     **M17.32**   Unilateral post-traumatic osteoarthritis, left knee

   **M17.4**   Other bilateral secondary osteoarthritis of knee

   **M17.5**   Other unilateral secondary osteoarthritis of knee
     Secondary osteoarthritis of knee NOS

   **M17.9**   Osteoarthritis of knee, unspecified

✓4ᵗʰ **M18**   **Osteoarthritis of first carpometacarpal joint**

   **M18.0**   Bilateral primary osteoarthritis of first carpometacarpal joints

✓5ᵗʰ **M18.1**   Unilateral primary osteoarthritis of first carpometacarpal joint
     Primary osteoarthritis of first carpometacarpal joint NOS

     **M18.10**   Unilateral primary osteoarthritis of first carpometacarpal joint, unspecified hand

     **M18.11**   Unilateral primary osteoarthritis of first carpometacarpal joint, right hand

     **M18.12**   Unilateral primary osteoarthritis of first carpometacarpal joint, left hand

   **M18.2**   Bilateral post-traumatic osteoarthritis of first carpometacarpal joints

✓5ᵗʰ **M18.3**   Unilateral post-traumatic osteoarthritis of first carpometacarpal joint
     Post-traumatic osteoarthritis of first carpometacarpal joint NOS

     **M18.30**   Unilateral post-traumatic osteoarthritis of first carpometacarpal joint, unspecified hand

     **M18.31**   Unilateral post-traumatic osteoarthritis of first carpometacarpal joint, right hand

     **M18.32**   Unilateral post-traumatic osteoarthritis of first carpometacarpal joint, left hand

   **M18.4**   Other bilateral secondary osteoarthritis of first carpometacarpal joints

✓5ᵗʰ **M18.5**   Other unilateral secondary osteoarthritis of first carpometacarpal joint
     Secondary osteoarthritis of first carpometacarpal joint NOS

     **M18.50**   Other unilateral secondary osteoarthritis of first carpometacarpal joint, unspecified hand

     **M18.51**   Other unilateral secondary osteoarthritis of first carpometacarpal joint, right hand

     **M18.52**   Other unilateral secondary osteoarthritis of first carpometacarpal joint, left hand

   **M18.9**   Osteoarthritis of first carpometacarpal joint, unspecified

✓4ᵗʰ **M19**   **Other and unspecified osteoarthritis**
     EXCLUDES 1   polyarthritis (M15.-)
     EXCLUDES 2   arthrosis of spine (M47.-)
             hallux rigidus (M20.2)
             osteoarthritis of spine (M47.-)

✓5ᵗʰ **M19.0**   Primary osteoarthritis of other joints
     AHA: 2016, 4Q, 145

   ✓6ᵗʰ **M19.01**   Primary osteoarthritis, shoulder

     **M19.011**   Primary osteoarthritis, right shoulder

     **M19.012**   Primary osteoarthritis, left shoulder

     **M19.019**   Primary osteoarthritis, unspecified shoulder

   ✓6ᵗʰ **M19.02**   Primary osteoarthritis, elbow

     **M19.021**   Primary osteoarthritis, right elbow

     **M19.022**   Primary osteoarthritis, left elbow

     **M19.029**   Primary osteoarthritis, unspecified elbow

   ✓6ᵗʰ **M19.03**   Primary osteoarthritis, wrist

     **M19.031**   Primary osteoarthritis, right wrist

     **M19.032**   Primary osteoarthritis, left wrist

     **M19.039**   Primary osteoarthritis, unspecified wrist

   ✓6ᵗʰ **M19.04**   Primary osteoarthritis, hand
     EXCLUDES 2   primary osteoarthritis of first carpometacarpal joint (M18.0-, M18.1-)

     **M19.041**   Primary osteoarthritis, right hand

     **M19.042**   Primary osteoarthritis, left hand

     **M19.049**   Primary osteoarthritis, unspecified hand

   ✓6ᵗʰ **M19.07**   Primary osteoarthritis ankle and foot

     **M19.071**   Primary osteoarthritis, right ankle and foot

     **M19.072**   Primary osteoarthritis, left ankle and foot

     **M19.079**   Primary osteoarthritis, unspecified ankle and foot

✓5ᵗʰ **M19.1**   Post-traumatic osteoarthritis of other joints

   ✓6ᵗʰ **M19.11**   Post-traumatic osteoarthritis, shoulder

     **M19.111**   Post-traumatic osteoarthritis, right shoulder

     **M19.112**   Post-traumatic osteoarthritis, left shoulder

     **M19.119**   Post-traumatic osteoarthritis, unspecified shoulder

   ✓6ᵗʰ **M19.12**   Post-traumatic osteoarthritis, elbow

     **M19.121**   Post-traumatic osteoarthritis, right elbow

     **M19.122**   Post-traumatic osteoarthritis, left elbow

     **M19.129**   Post-traumatic osteoarthritis, unspecified elbow

   ✓6ᵗʰ **M19.13**   Post-traumatic osteoarthritis, wrist

     **M19.131**   Post-traumatic osteoarthritis, right wrist

     **M19.132**   Post-traumatic osteoarthritis, left wrist

     **M19.139**   Post-traumatic osteoarthritis, unspecified wrist

   ✓6ᵗʰ **M19.14**   Post-traumatic osteoarthritis, hand
     EXCLUDES 2   post-traumatic osteoarthritis of first carpometacarpal joint (M18.2-, M18.3-)

     **M19.141**   Post-traumatic osteoarthritis, right hand

     **M19.142**   Post-traumatic osteoarthritis, left hand

     **M19.149**   Post-traumatic osteoarthritis, unspecified hand

   ✓6ᵗʰ **M19.17**   Post-traumatic osteoarthritis, ankle and foot

     **M19.171**   Post-traumatic osteoarthritis, right ankle and foot

     **M19.172**   Post-traumatic osteoarthritis, left ankle and foot

     **M19.179**   Post-traumatic osteoarthritis, unspecified ankle and foot

✓5ᵗʰ **M19.2**   Secondary osteoarthritis of other joints

   ✓6ᵗʰ **M19.21**   Secondary osteoarthritis, shoulder

     **M19.211**   Secondary osteoarthritis, right shoulder

     **M19.212**   Secondary osteoarthritis, left shoulder

     **M19.219**   Secondary osteoarthritis, unspecified shoulder

   ✓6ᵗʰ **M19.22**   Secondary osteoarthritis, elbow

     **M19.221**   Secondary osteoarthritis, right elbow

     **M19.222**   Secondary osteoarthritis, left elbow

✓ Additional Character Req   ✓x7ᵗʰ Placeholder Alert   Unacceptable PDx   Manifestation   H1 - H14 HAC   HCC CMS-HCC Condition   EXCLUDES 1 Not Coded Here   EXCLUDES 2 Not Included Here

ICD-10-CM 2018      757

M16.31–M19.222

M19.229   Secondary osteoarthritis, unspecified elbow

✓6ᵗʰ   **M19.23**   Secondary osteoarthritis, wrist

M19.231   Secondary osteoarthritis, right wrist

M19.232   Secondary osteoarthritis, left wrist

M19.239   Secondary osteoarthritis, unspecified wrist

✓6ᵗʰ   **M19.24**   Secondary osteoarthritis, hand

M19.241   Secondary osteoarthritis, right hand

M19.242   Secondary osteoarthritis, left hand

M19.249   Secondary osteoarthritis, unspecified hand

✓6ᵗʰ   **M19.27**   Secondary osteoarthritis, ankle and foot

M19.271   Secondary osteoarthritis, right ankle and foot

M19.272   Secondary osteoarthritis, left ankle and foot

M19.279   Secondary osteoarthritis, unspecified ankle and foot

✓5ᵗʰ   **M19.9**   Osteoarthritis, unspecified site

**M19.90**   Unspecified osteoarthritis, unspecified site
Arthrosis NOS
Arthritis NOS
Osteoarthritis NOS
**AHA:** 2016, 4Q, 147

**M19.91**   Primary osteoarthritis, unspecified site
Primary osteoarthritis NOS

**M19.92**   Post-traumatic osteoarthritis, unspecified site
Post-traumatic osteoarthritis NOS

**M19.93**   Secondary osteoarthritis, unspecified site
Secondary osteoarthritis NOS

### Other joint disorders (M20-M25)

EXCLUDES 2   *joints of the spine (M40-M54)*

✓4ᵗʰ   **M20**   **Acquired deformities of fingers and toes**

EXCLUDES 1   *acquired absence of fingers and toes (Z89.-)*
*congenital absence of fingers and toes (Q71.3-, Q72.3-)*
*congenital deformities and malformations of fingers and toes (Q66-, Q68-Q70, Q74-)*

✓5ᵗʰ   **M20.0**   **Deformity of finger(s)**

EXCLUDES 1   *clubbing of fingers (R68.3)*
*palmar fascial fibromatosis [Dupuytren] (M72.0)*
*trigger finger (M65.3)*

✓6ᵗʰ   **M20.00**   Unspecified deformity of finger(s)

M20.001   Unspecified deformity of right finger(s)

M20.002   Unspecified deformity of left finger(s)

M20.009   Unspecified deformity of unspecified finger(s)

✓6ᵗʰ   **M20.01**   Mallet finger

M20.011   Mallet finger of right finger(s)

M20.012   Mallet finger of left finger(s)

M20.019   Mallet finger of unspecified finger(s)d

✓6ᵗʰ   **M20.02**   Boutonnière deformity
**DEF:** A deformity of the finger caused by flexion of the proximal interphalangeal joint and hyperextension of the distal joint; results from rheumatoid arthritis, osteoarthritis, or injury; also called buttonhole deformity.

M20.021   Boutonnière deformity of right finger(s)

M20.022   Boutonnière deformity of left finger(s)

M20.029   Boutonnière deformity of unspecified finger(s)

✓6ᵗʰ   **M20.03**   Swan-neck deformity
**DEF:** Flexed distal and hyperextended proximal interphalangeal joint; most commonly caused by rheumatoid arthritis.

M20.031   Swan-neck deformity of right finger(s)

M20.032   Swan-neck deformity of left finger(s)

M20.039   Swan-neck deformity of unspecified finger(s)

✓6ᵗʰ   **M20.09**   Other deformity of finger(s)

M20.091   Other deformity of right finger(s)

M20.092   Other deformity of left finger(s)

M20.099   Other deformity of finger(s), unspecified finger(s)

**Hallux Valgus**

Hallux valgus

Medial eminence of metatarsal bone

Right foot

✓5ᵗʰ   **M20.1**   Hallux valgus (acquired)

EXCLUDES 2   *bunion (M21.6-)*

M20.10   Hallux valgus (acquired), unspecified foot

M20.11   Hallux valgus (acquired), right foot

M20.12   Hallux valgus (acquired), left foot

✓5ᵗʰ   **M20.2**   Hallux rigidus

M20.20   Hallux rigidus, unspecified foot

M20.21   Hallux rigidus, right foot

M20.22   Hallux rigidus, left foot

✓5ᵗʰ   **M20.3**   Hallux varus (acquired)

M20.30   Hallux varus (acquired), unspecified foot

M20.31   Hallux varus (acquired), right foot

M20.32   Hallux varus (acquired), left foot

✓5ᵗʰ   **M20.4**   Other hammer toe(s) (acquired)

M20.40   Other hammer toe(s) (acquired), unspecified foot

M20.41   Other hammer toe(s) (acquired), right foot

M20.42   Other hammer toe(s) (acquired), left foot

✓5ᵗʰ   **M20.5**   Other deformities of toe(s) (acquired)

✓6ᵗʰ   **M20.5X**   Other deformities of toe(s) (acquired)

M20.5X1   Other deformities of toe(s) (acquired), right foot

M20.5X2   Other deformities of toe(s) (acquired), left foot

M20.5X9   Other deformities of toe(s) (acquired), unspecified foot

✓5ᵗʰ   **M20.6**   Acquired deformities of toe(s), unspecified

M20.60   Acquired deformities of toe(s), unspecified, unspecified foot

M20.61   Acquired deformities of toe(s), unspecified, right foot

M20.62   Acquired deformities of toe(s), unspecified, left foot

✓4ᵗʰ   **M21**   **Other acquired deformities of limbs**

EXCLUDES 1   *acquired absence of limb (Z89.-)*
*congenital absence of limbs (Q71-Q73)*
*congenital deformities and malformations of limbs (Q65-Q66, Q68-Q74)*

EXCLUDES 2   *acquired deformities of fingers or toes (M20.-)*
*coxa plana (M91.2)*

✓5ᵗʰ   **M21.0**   Valgus deformity, not elsewhere classified

EXCLUDES 1   *metatarsus valgus (Q66.6)*
*talipes calcaneovalgus (Q66.4)*

M21.00   Valgus deformity, not elsewhere classified, unspecified site

✓6ᵗʰ   **M21.02**   Valgus deformity, not elsewhere classified, elbow
Cubitus valgus

M21.021   Valgus deformity, not elsewhere classified, right elbow

M21.022   Valgus deformity, not elsewhere classified, left elbow

M21.029   Valgus deformity, not elsewhere classified, unspecified elbow

N Newborn: 0   P Pediatric: 0-17   M Maternity: 12-55   A Adult: 15-124   MCC Major CC Condition   PDxMCC PDx acts as own MCC   CC CC Condition   PDxCC PDx acts as own CC

**758**        ICD-10-CM 2018

**Genu Valga (knock-knee)**

**Genu Varus (bowleg)**

✓6ᵗʰ **M21.05** Valgus deformity, not elsewhere classified, hip
- **M21.051** Valgus deformity, not elsewhere classified, **right** hip
- **M21.052** Valgus deformity, not elsewhere classified, **left** hip
- **M21.059** Valgus deformity, not elsewhere classified, **unspecified** hip

✓6ᵗʰ **M21.06** Valgus deformity, not elsewhere classified, knee
Genu valgum
Knock knee
- **M21.061** Valgus deformity, not elsewhere classified, **right** knee
- **M21.062** Valgus deformity, not elsewhere classified, **left** knee
- **M21.069** Valgus deformity, not elsewhere classified, **unspecified** knee

✓6ᵗʰ **M21.07** Valgus deformity, not elsewhere classified, ankle
- **M21.071** Valgus deformity, not elsewhere classified, **right** ankle
- **M21.072** Valgus deformity, not elsewhere classified, **left** ankle
- **M21.079** Valgus deformity, not elsewhere classified, **unspecified** ankle

✓5ᵗʰ **M21.1** Varus deformity, not elsewhere classified
> **EXCLUDES 1**   *metatarsus varus (Q66.22)*
> *tibia vara (M92.5)*

- **M21.10** Varus deformity, not elsewhere classified, **unspecified site**

✓6ᵗʰ **M21.12** Varus deformity, not elsewhere classified, elbow
Cubitus varus, elbow
- **M21.121** Varus deformity, not elsewhere classified, **right** elbow
- **M21.122** Varus deformity, not elsewhere classified, **left** elbow
- **M21.129** Varus deformity, not elsewhere classified, **unspecified** elbow

✓6ᵗʰ **M21.15** Varus deformity, not elsewhere classified, hip
- **M21.151** Varus deformity, not elsewhere classified, **right** hip
- **M21.152** Varus deformity, not elsewhere classified, **left** hip
- **M21.159** Varus deformity, not elsewhere classified, **unspecified**

✓6ᵗʰ **M21.16** Varus deformity, not elsewhere classified, knee
Bow leg
Genu varum
- **M21.161** Varus deformity, not elsewhere classified, **right** knee
- **M21.162** Varus deformity, not elsewhere classified, **left** knee
- **M21.169** Varus deformity, not elsewhere classified, **unspecified** knee

✓6ᵗʰ **M21.17** Varus deformity, not elsewhere classified, ankle
- **M21.171** Varus deformity, not elsewhere classified, **right** ankle
- **M21.172** Varus deformity, not elsewhere classified, **left** ankle
- **M21.179** Varus deformity, not elsewhere classified, **unspecified** ankle

✓5ᵗʰ **M21.2** Flexion deformity
- **M21.20** Flexion deformity, **unspecified site**

✓6ᵗʰ **M21.21** Flexion deformity, shoulder
- **M21.211** Flexion deformity, **right** shoulder
- **M21.212** Flexion deformity, **left** shoulder
- **M21.219** Flexion deformity, **unspecified** shoulder

✓6ᵗʰ **M21.22** Flexion deformity, elbow
- **M21.221** Flexion deformity, **right** elbow
- **M21.222** Flexion deformity, **left** elbow
- **M21.229** Flexion deformity, **unspecified** elbow

✓6ᵗʰ **M21.23** Flexion deformity, wrist
- **M21.231** Flexion deformity, **right** wrist
- **M21.232** Flexion deformity, **left** wrist
- **M21.239** Flexion deformity, **unspecified** wrist

✓6ᵗʰ **M21.24** Flexion deformity, finger joints
- **M21.241** Flexion deformity, **right** finger joints
- **M21.242** Flexion deformity, **left** finger joints
- **M21.249** Flexion deformity, **unspecified** finger joints

✓6ᵗʰ **M21.25** Flexion deformity, hip
- **M21.251** Flexion deformity, **right** hip
- **M21.252** Flexion deformity, **left** hip
- **M21.259** Flexion deformity, **unspecified** hip

✓6ᵗʰ **M21.26** Flexion deformity, knee
- **M21.261** Flexion deformity, **right** knee
- **M21.262** Flexion deformity, **left** knee
- **M21.269** Flexion deformity, **unspecified** knee

✓6ᵗʰ **M21.27** Flexion deformity, ankle and toes
- **M21.271** Flexion deformity, **right** ankle and toes
- **M21.272** Flexion deformity, **left** ankle and toes
- **M21.279** Flexion deformity, **unspecified** ankle and toes

✓5ᵗʰ **M21.3** Wrist or foot drop (acquired)

✓6ᵗʰ **M21.33** Wrist drop (acquired)
- **M21.331** Wrist drop, **right** wrist
- **M21.332** Wrist drop, **left** wrist
- **M21.339** Wrist drop, **unspecified** wrist

✓6ᵗʰ **M21.37** Foot drop (acquired)
- **M21.371** Foot drop, **right** foot
- **M21.372** Foot drop, **left** foot
- **M21.379** Foot drop, **unspecified** foot

---

✓ Additional Character Req   ✓x7ᵗʰ Placeholder Alert   Unacceptable PDx   Manifestation   H1-H14 HAC   HCC CMS-HCC Condition   EXCLUDES 1 Not Coded Here   EXCLUDES 2 Not Included Here

ICD-10-CM 2018      759

✓5ᵗʰ **M21.4** Flat foot [pes planus] (acquired)
     EXCLUDES 1   *congenital pes planus (Q66.5-)*
     **M21.40** Flat foot [pes planus] (acquired), unspecified foot
     **M21.41** Flat foot [pes planus] (acquired), right foot
     **M21.42** Flat foot [pes planus] (acquired), left foot

✓5ᵗʰ **M21.5** Acquired clawhand, clubhand, clawfoot and clubfoot
     EXCLUDES 1   *clubfoot, not specified as acquired (Q66.89)*
     ✓6ᵗʰ **M21.51** Acquired clawhand
         **M21.511** Acquired clawhand, right hand
         **M21.512** Acquired clawhand, left hand
         **M21.519** Acquired clawhand, unspecified hand
     ✓6ᵗʰ **M21.52** Acquired clubhand
         **M21.521** Acquired clubhand, right hand
         **M21.522** Acquired clubhand, left hand
         **M21.529** Acquired clubhand, unspecified hand
     ✓6ᵗʰ **M21.53** Acquired clawfoot
         **DEF:** High foot arch with hyperextended toes at metatarsophalangeal joint and flexed toes at distal joints.
         **M21.531** Acquired clawfoot, right foot
         **M21.532** Acquired clawfoot, left foot
         **M21.539** Acquired clawfoot, unspecified foot
     ✓6ᵗʰ **M21.54** Acquired clubfoot
         **M21.541** Acquired clubfoot, right foot
         **M21.542** Acquired clubfoot, left foot
         **M21.549** Acquired clubfoot, unspecified foot

✓5ᵗʰ **M21.6** Other acquired deformities of foot
     EXCLUDES 2   *deformities of toe (acquired) (M20.1-M20.6-)*
     ✓6ᵗʰ **M21.61** Bunion
         **M21.611** Bunion of right foot
         **M21.612** Bunion of left foot
         **M21.619** Bunion of unspecified foot
     ✓6ᵗʰ **M21.62** Bunionette
         **M21.621** Bunionette of right foot
         **M21.622** Bunionette of left foot
         **M21.629** Bunionette of unspecified foot
     ✓6ᵗʰ **M21.6X** Other acquired deformities of foot
         **M21.6X1** Other acquired deformities of right foot
         **M21.6X2** Other acquired deformities of left foot
         **M21.6X9** Other acquired deformities of unspecified foot

✓5ᵗʰ **M21.7** Unequal limb length (acquired)
     NOTE   The site used should correspond to the shorter limb.
     **M21.70** Unequal limb length (acquired), unspecified site
     ✓6ᵗʰ **M21.72** Unequal limb length (acquired), humerus
         **M21.721** Unequal limb length (acquired), right humerus
         **M21.722** Unequal limb length (acquired), left humerus
         **M21.729** Unequal limb length (acquired), unspecified humerus
     ✓6ᵗʰ **M21.73** Unequal limb length (acquired), ulna and radius
         **M21.731** Unequal limb length (acquired), right ulna
         **M21.732** Unequal limb length (acquired), left ulna
         **M21.733** Unequal limb length (acquired), right radius
         **M21.734** Unequal limb length (acquired), left radius
         **M21.739** Unequal limb length (acquired), unspecified ulna and radius
     ✓6ᵗʰ **M21.75** Unequal limb length (acquired), femur
         **M21.751** Unequal limb length (acquired), right femur
         **M21.752** Unequal limb length (acquired), left femur
         **M21.759** Unequal limb length (acquired), unspecified femur
     ✓6ᵗʰ **M21.76** Unequal limb length (acquired), tibia and fibula
         **M21.761** Unequal limb length (acquired), right tibia
         **M21.762** Unequal limb length (acquired), left tibia
         **M21.763** Unequal limb length (acquired), right fibula
         **M21.764** Unequal limb length (acquired), left fibula
         **M21.769** Unequal limb length (acquired), unspecified tibia and fibula

✓5ᵗʰ **M21.8** Other specified acquired deformities of limbs
     EXCLUDES 2   *coxa plana (M91.2)*
     **M21.80** Other specified acquired deformities of unspecified limb
     ✓6ᵗʰ **M21.82** Other specified acquired deformities of upper arm
         **M21.821** Other specified acquired deformities of right upper arm
         **M21.822** Other specified acquired deformities of left upper arm
         **M21.829** Other specified acquired deformities of unspecified upper arm
     ✓6ᵗʰ **M21.83** Other specified acquired deformities of forearm
         **M21.831** Other specified acquired deformities of right forearm
         **M21.832** Other specified acquired deformities of left forearm
         **M21.839** Other specified acquired deformities of unspecified forearm
     ✓6ᵗʰ **M21.85** Other specified acquired deformities of thigh
         **M21.851** Other specified acquired deformities of right thigh
         **M21.852** Other specified acquired deformities of left thigh
         **M21.859** Other specified acquired deformities of unspecified thigh
     ✓6ᵗʰ **M21.86** Other specified acquired deformities of lower leg
         **M21.861** Other specified acquired deformities of right lower leg
         **M21.862** Other specified acquired deformities of left lower leg
         **M21.869** Other specified acquired deformities of unspecified lower leg

✓5ᵗʰ **M21.9** Unspecified acquired deformity of limb and hand
     **M21.90** Unspecified acquired deformity of unspecified limb
     ✓6ᵗʰ **M21.92** Unspecified acquired deformity of upper arm
         **M21.921** Unspecified acquired deformity of right upper arm
         **M21.922** Unspecified acquired deformity of left upper arm
         **M21.929** Unspecified acquired deformity of unspecified upper arm
     ✓6ᵗʰ **M21.93** Unspecified acquired deformity of forearm
         **M21.931** Unspecified acquired deformity of right forearm
         **M21.932** Unspecified acquired deformity of left forearm
         **M21.939** Unspecified acquired deformity of unspecified forearm
     ✓6ᵗʰ **M21.94** Unspecified acquired deformity of hand
         **M21.941** Unspecified acquired deformity of hand, right hand
         **M21.942** Unspecified acquired deformity of hand, left hand
         **M21.949** Unspecified acquired deformity of hand, unspecified hand
     ✓6ᵗʰ **M21.95** Unspecified acquired deformity of thigh
         **M21.951** Unspecified acquired deformity of right thigh
         **M21.952** Unspecified acquired deformity of left thigh
         **M21.959** Unspecified acquired deformity of unspecified thigh
     ✓6ᵗʰ **M21.96** Unspecified acquired deformity of lower leg
         **M21.961** Unspecified acquired deformity of right lower leg
         **M21.962** Unspecified acquired deformity of left lower leg
         **M21.969** Unspecified acquired deformity of unspecified lower leg

☑️⁴ᵗʰ **M22 Disorder of patella**
> *EXCLUDES 1*    *traumatic dislocation of patella (S83.0-)*

☑️⁵ᵗʰ **M22.0 Recurrent dislocation of patella**
- **M22.00** Recurrent dislocation of patella, unspecified knee
- **M22.01** Recurrent dislocation of patella, right knee
- **M22.02** Recurrent dislocation of patella, left knee

☑️⁵ᵗʰ **M22.1 Recurrent subluxation of patella**
> Incomplete dislocation of patella
- **M22.10** Recurrent subluxation of patella, unspecified knee
- **M22.11** Recurrent subluxation of patella, right knee
- **M22.12** Recurrent subluxation of patella, left knee

☑️⁵ᵗʰ **M22.2 Patellofemoral disorders**
- ☑️⁶ᵗʰ **M22.2X Patellofemoral disorders**
  - **M22.2X1** Patellofemoral disorders, right knee
  - **M22.2X2** Patellofemoral disorders, left knee
  - **M22.2X9** Patellofemoral disorders, unspecified knee

☑️⁵ᵗʰ **M22.3 Other derangements of patella**
- ☑️⁶ᵗʰ **M22.3X Other derangements of patella**
  - **M22.3X1** Other derangements of patella, right knee
  - **M22.3X2** Other derangements of patella, left knee
  - **M22.3X9** Other derangements of patella, unspecified knee

☑️⁵ᵗʰ **M22.4 Chondromalacia patellae**
- **M22.40** Chondromalacia patellae, unspecified knee
- **M22.41** Chondromalacia patellae, right knee
- **M22.42** Chondromalacia patellae, left knee

☑️⁵ᵗʰ **M22.8 Other disorders of patella**
- ☑️⁶ᵗʰ **M22.8X Other disorders of patella**
  - **M22.8X1** Other disorders of patella, right knee
  - **M22.8X2** Other disorders of patella, left knee
  - **M22.8X9** Other disorders of patella, unspecified knee

☑️⁵ᵗʰ **M22.9 Unspecified disorder of patella**
- **M22.90** Unspecified disorder of patella, unspecified knee
- **M22.91** Unspecified disorder of patella, right knee
- **M22.92** Unspecified disorder of patella, left knee

☑️⁴ᵗʰ **M23 Internal derangement of knee**
> *EXCLUDES 1*    *ankylosis (M24.66)*
> *current injury—see injury of knee and lower leg (S80-S89)*
> *deformity of knee (M21.-)*
> *osteochondritis dissecans (M93.2)*
> *recurrent dislocation or subluxation of joints (M24.4)*
> *recurrent dislocation or subluxation of patella (M22.0-M22.1)*

☑️⁵ᵗʰ **M23.0 Cystic meniscus**
- ☑️⁶ᵗʰ **M23.00 Cystic meniscus, unspecified meniscus**
  > Cystic meniscus, unspecified lateral meniscus
  > Cystic meniscus, unspecified medial meniscus
  - **M23.000** Cystic meniscus, unspecified lateral meniscus, right knee
  - **M23.001** Cystic meniscus, unspecified lateral meniscus, left knee
  - **M23.002** Cystic meniscus, unspecified lateral meniscus, unspecified knee
  - **M23.003** Cystic meniscus, unspecified medial meniscus, right knee
  - **M23.004** Cystic meniscus, unspecified medial meniscus, left knee
  - **M23.005** Cystic meniscus, unspecified medial meniscus, unspecified knee
  - **M23.006** Cystic meniscus, unspecified meniscus, right knee
  - **M23.007** Cystic meniscus, unspecified meniscus, left knee
  - **M23.009** Cystic meniscus, unspecified meniscus, unspecified knee
- ☑️⁶ᵗʰ **M23.01 Cystic meniscus, anterior horn of medial meniscus**
  - **M23.011** Cystic meniscus, anterior horn of medial meniscus, right knee
  - **M23.012** Cystic meniscus, anterior horn of medial meniscus, left knee
  - **M23.019** Cystic meniscus, anterior horn of medial meniscus, unspecified knee

- ☑️⁶ᵗʰ **M23.02 Cystic meniscus, posterior horn of medial meniscus**
  - **M23.021** Cystic meniscus, posterior horn of medial meniscus, right knee
  - **M23.022** Cystic meniscus, posterior horn of medial meniscus, left knee
  - **M23.029** Cystic meniscus, posterior horn of medial meniscus, unspecified knee
- ☑️⁶ᵗʰ **M23.03 Cystic meniscus, other medial meniscus**
  - **M23.031** Cystic meniscus, other medial meniscus, right knee
  - **M23.032** Cystic meniscus, other medial meniscus, left knee
  - **M23.039** Cystic meniscus, other medial meniscus, unspecified knee
- ☑️⁶ᵗʰ **M23.04 Cystic meniscus, anterior horn of lateral meniscus**
  - **M23.041** Cystic meniscus, anterior horn of lateral meniscus, right knee
  - **M23.042** Cystic meniscus, anterior horn of lateral meniscus, left knee
  - **M23.049** Cystic meniscus, anterior horn of lateral meniscus, unspecified knee
- ☑️⁶ᵗʰ **M23.05 Cystic meniscus, posterior horn of lateral meniscus**
  - **M23.051** Cystic meniscus, posterior horn of lateral meniscus, right knee
  - **M23.052** Cystic meniscus, posterior horn of lateral meniscus, left knee
  - **M23.059** Cystic meniscus, posterior horn of lateral meniscus, unspecified knee
- ☑️⁶ᵗʰ **M23.06 Cystic meniscus, other lateral meniscus**
  - **M23.061** Cystic meniscus, other lateral meniscus, right knee
  - **M23.062** Cystic meniscus, other lateral meniscus, left knee
  - **M23.069** Cystic meniscus, other lateral meniscus, unspecified knee

☑️⁵ᵗʰ **M23.2 Derangement of meniscus due to old tear or injury**
> Old bucket-handle tear
- ☑️⁶ᵗʰ **M23.20 Derangement of unspecified meniscus due to old tear or injury**
  > Derangement of unspecified lateral meniscus due to old tear or injury
  > Derangement of unspecified medial meniscus due to old tear or injury
  - **M23.200** Derangement of unspecified lateral meniscus due to old tear or injury, right knee
  - **M23.201** Derangement of unspecified lateral meniscus due to old tear or injury, left knee

**Derangement of Meniscus**

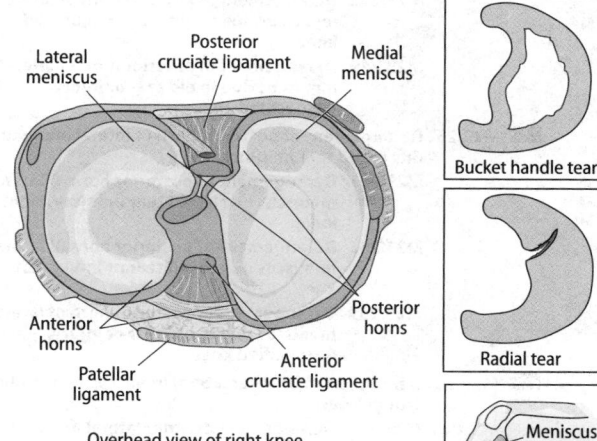

Overhead view of right knee

☑️Additional Character Req   ✓ˣ⁷ᵗʰ Placeholder Alert   Unacceptable PDx   Manifestation   **H1**-**H14** HAC   **HCC** CMS-HCC Condition   *EXCLUDES 1* Not Coded Here   *EXCLUDES 2* Not Included Here

ICD-10-CM 2018      761

**Chapter 13. Diseases of the Musculoskeletal System and Connective Tissue**

**M23.202**   Derangement of unspecified lateral meniscus due to old tear or injury, unspecified knee

**M23.203**   Derangement of unspecified medial meniscus due to old tear or injury, right knee

**M23.204**   Derangement of unspecified medial meniscus due to old tear or injury, left knee

**M23.205**   Derangement of unspecified medial meniscus due to old tear or injury, unspecified knee

**M23.206**   Derangement of unspecified meniscus due to old tear or injury, right knee

**M23.207**   Derangement of unspecified meniscus due to old tear or injury, left knee

**M23.209**   Derangement of unspecified meniscus due to old tear or injury, unspecified knee

✓6ᵗʰ **M23.21**   Derangement of anterior horn of medial meniscus due to old tear or injury

**M23.211**   Derangement of anterior horn of medial meniscus due to old tear or injury, right knee

**M23.212**   Derangement of anterior horn of medial meniscus due to old tear or injury, left knee

**M23.219**   Derangement of anterior horn of medial meniscus due to old tear or injury, unspecified knee

✓6ᵗʰ **M23.22**   Derangement of posterior horn of medial meniscus due to old tear or injury

**M23.221**   Derangement of posterior horn of medial meniscus due to old tear or injury, right knee

**M23.222**   Derangement of posterior horn of medial meniscus due to old tear or injury, left knee

**M23.229**   Derangement of posterior horn of medial meniscus due to old tear or injury, unspecified knee

✓6ᵗʰ **M23.23**   Derangement of other medial meniscus due to old tear or injury

**M23.231**   Derangement of other medial meniscus due to old tear or injury, right knee

**M23.232**   Derangement of other medial meniscus due to old tear or injury, left knee

**M23.239**   Derangement of other medial meniscus due to old tear or injury, unspecified knee

✓6ᵗʰ **M23.24**   Derangement of anterior horn of lateral meniscus due to old tear or injury

**M23.241**   Derangement of anterior horn of lateral meniscus due to old tear or injury, right knee

**M23.242**   Derangement of anterior horn of lateral meniscus due to old tear or injury, left knee

**M23.249**   Derangement of anterior horn of lateral meniscus due to old tear or injury, unspecified knee

✓6ᵗʰ **M23.25**   Derangement of posterior horn of lateral meniscus due to old tear or injury

**M23.251**   Derangement of posterior horn of lateral meniscus due to old tear or injury, right knee

**M23.252**   Derangement of posterior horn of lateral meniscus due to old tear or injury, left knee

**M23.259**   Derangement of posterior horn of lateral meniscus due to old tear or injury, unspecified knee

✓6ᵗʰ **M23.26**   Derangement of other lateral meniscus due to old tear or injury

**M23.261**   Derangement of other lateral meniscus due to old tear or injury, right knee

**M23.262**   Derangement of other lateral meniscus due to old tear or injury, left knee

**M23.269**   Derangement of other lateral meniscus due to old tear or injury, unspecified knee

✓5ᵗʰ **M23.3**   **Other meniscus derangements**
Degenerate meniscus
Detached meniscus
Retained meniscus

✓6ᵗʰ **M23.30**   Other meniscus derangements, unspecified meniscus
Other meniscus derangements, unspecified lateral meniscus
Other meniscus derangements, unspecified medial meniscus

**M23.300**   Other meniscus derangements, unspecified lateral meniscus, right knee

**M23.301**   Other meniscus derangements, unspecified lateral meniscus, left knee

**M23.302**   Other meniscus derangements, unspecified lateral meniscus, unspecified knee

**M23.303**   Other meniscus derangements, unspecified medial meniscus, right knee

**M23.304**   Other meniscus derangements, unspecified medial meniscus, left knee

**M23.305**   Other meniscus derangements, unspecified medial meniscus, unspecified knee

**M23.306**   Other meniscus derangements, unspecified meniscus, right knee

**M23.307**   Other meniscus derangements, unspecified meniscus, left knee

**M23.309**   Other meniscus derangements, unspecified meniscus, unspecified knee

✓6ᵗʰ **M23.31**   Other meniscus derangements, anterior horn of medial meniscus

**M23.311**   Other meniscus derangements, anterior horn of medial meniscus, right knee

**M23.312**   Other meniscus derangements, anterior horn of medial meniscus, left knee

**M23.319**   Other meniscus derangements, anterior horn of medial meniscus, unspecified knee

✓6ᵗʰ **M23.32**   Other meniscus derangements, posterior horn of medial meniscus

**M23.321**   Other meniscus derangements, posterior horn of medial meniscus, right knee

**M23.322**   Other meniscus derangements, posterior horn of medial meniscus, left knee

**M23.329**   Other meniscus derangements, posterior horn of medial meniscus, unspecified knee

✓6ᵗʰ **M23.33**   Other meniscus derangements, other medial meniscus

**M23.331**   Other meniscus derangements, other medial meniscus, right knee

**M23.332**   Other meniscus derangements, other medial meniscus, left knee

**M23.339**   Other meniscus derangements, other medial meniscus, unspecified knee

✓6ᵗʰ **M23.34**   Other meniscus derangements, anterior horn of lateral meniscus

**M23.341**   Other meniscus derangements, anterior horn of lateral meniscus, right knee

**M23.342**   Other meniscus derangements, anterior horn of lateral meniscus, left knee

**M23.349**   Other meniscus derangements, anterior horn of lateral meniscus, unspecified knee

✓6ᵗʰ **M23.35**   Other meniscus derangements, posterior horn of lateral meniscus

**M23.351**   Other meniscus derangements, posterior horn of lateral meniscus, right knee

**M23.352**   Other meniscus derangements, posterior horn of lateral meniscus, left knee

**M23.359**   Other meniscus derangements, posterior horn of lateral meniscus, unspecified knee

✓6ᵗʰ **M23.36**   Other meniscus derangements, other lateral meniscus

**M23.361**   Other meniscus derangements, other lateral meniscus, right knee

**M23.362**   Other meniscus derangements, other lateral meniscus, left knee

**M23.369**   Other meniscus derangements, other lateral meniscus, unspecified knee

Ⓝ Newborn: 0   Ⓟ Pediatric: 0-17   Ⓜ Maternity: 12-55   Ⓐ Adult: 15-124   **MCC** Major CC Condition   **PDxMCC** PDx acts as own MCC   **CC** CC Condition   **PDxCC** PDx acts as own CC

762       ICD-10-CM 2018

✓5ᵗʰ **M23.4 Loose body in knee**

    **M23.40**   Loose body in knee, unspecified knee

    **M23.41**   Loose body in knee, right knee

    **M23.42**   Loose body in knee, left knee

✓5ᵗʰ **M23.5 Chronic instability of knee**

    **M23.50**   Chronic instability of knee, unspecified knee

    **M23.51**   Chronic instability of knee, right knee

    **M23.52**   Chronic instability of knee, left knee

✓5ᵗʰ **M23.6 Other spontaneous disruption of ligament(s) of knee**

  ✓6ᵗʰ **M23.60**   Other spontaneous disruption of unspecified ligament of knee

    **M23.601**   Other spontaneous disruption of unspecified ligament of right knee

    **M23.602**   Other spontaneous disruption of unspecified ligament of left knee

    **M23.609**   Other spontaneous disruption of unspecified ligament of unspecified knee

  ✓6ᵗʰ **M23.61**   Other spontaneous disruption of anterior cruciate ligament of knee

    **M23.611**   Other spontaneous disruption of anterior cruciate ligament of right knee

    **M23.612**   Other spontaneous disruption of anterior cruciate ligament of left knee

    **M23.619**   Other spontaneous disruption of anterior cruciate ligament of unspecified knee

  ✓6ᵗʰ **M23.62**   Other spontaneous disruption of posterior cruciate ligament of knee

    **M23.621**   Other spontaneous disruption of posterior cruciate ligament of right knee

    **M23.622**   Other spontaneous disruption of posterior cruciate ligament of left knee

    **M23.629**   Other spontaneous disruption of posterior cruciate ligament of unspecified knee

  ✓6ᵗʰ **M23.63**   Other spontaneous disruption of medial collateral ligament of knee

    **M23.631**   Other spontaneous disruption of medial collateral ligament of right knee

    **M23.632**   Other spontaneous disruption of medial collateral ligament of left knee

    **M23.639**   Other spontaneous disruption of medial collateral ligament of unspecified knee

  ✓6ᵗʰ **M23.64**   Other spontaneous disruption of lateral collateral ligament of knee

    **M23.641**   Other spontaneous disruption of lateral collateral ligament of right knee

    **M23.642**   Other spontaneous disruption of lateral collateral ligament of left knee

    **M23.649**   Other spontaneous disruption of lateral collateral ligament of unspecified knee

  ✓6ᵗʰ **M23.67**   Other spontaneous disruption of capsular ligament of knee

    **M23.671**   Other spontaneous disruption of capsular ligament of right knee

    **M23.672**   Other spontaneous disruption of capsular ligament of left knee

    **M23.679**   Other spontaneous disruption of capsular ligament of unspecified knee

✓5ᵗʰ **M23.8 Other internal derangements of knee**

    Laxity of ligament of knee

    Snapping knee

  ✓6ᵗʰ **M23.8X**   Other internal derangements of knee

    **M23.8X1**   Other internal derangements of right knee

    **M23.8X2**   Other internal derangements of left knee

    **M23.8X9**   Other internal derangements of unspecified knee

✓5ᵗʰ **M23.9 Unspecified internal derangement of knee**

    **M23.90**   Unspecified internal derangement of unspecified knee

    **M23.91**   Unspecified internal derangement of right knee

    **M23.92**   Unspecified internal derangement of left knee

✓4ᵗʰ **M24 Other specific joint derangements**

    *EXCLUDES 1*   current injury—see injury of joint by body region

    *EXCLUDES 2*   ganglion (M67.4)

              snapping knee (M23.8-)

              temporomandibular joint disorders (M26.6-)

  ✓5ᵗʰ **M24.0 Loose body in joint**

    *EXCLUDES 2*   loose body in knee (M23.4)

    **M24.00**   Loose body in unspecified joint

  ✓6ᵗʰ **M24.01**   Loose body in shoulder

    **M24.011**   Loose body in right shoulder

    **M24.012**   Loose body in left shoulder

    **M24.019**   Loose body in unspecified shoulder

  ✓6ᵗʰ **M24.02**   Loose body in elbow

    **M24.021**   Loose body in right elbow

    **M24.022**   Loose body in left elbow

    **M24.029**   Loose body in unspecified elbow

  ✓6ᵗʰ **M24.03**   Loose body in wrist

    **M24.031**   Loose body in right wrist

    **M24.032**   Loose body in left wrist

    **M24.039**   Loose body in unspecified wrist

  ✓6ᵗʰ **M24.04**   Loose body in finger joints

    **M24.041**   Loose body in right finger joint(s)

    **M24.042**   Loose body in left finger joint(s)

    **M24.049**   Loose body in unspecified finger joint(s)

  ✓6ᵗʰ **M24.05**   Loose body in hip

    **M24.051**   Loose body in right hip

    **M24.052**   Loose body in left hip

    **M24.059**   Loose body in unspecified hip

  ✓6ᵗʰ **M24.07**   Loose body in ankle and toe joints

    **M24.071**   Loose body in right ankle

    **M24.072**   Loose body in left ankle

    **M24.073**   Loose body in unspecified ankle

    **M24.074**   Loose body in right toe joint(s)

    **M24.075**   Loose body in left toe joint(s)

    **M24.076**   Loose body in unspecified toe joints

    **M24.08**   Loose body, other site

  ✓5ᵗʰ **M24.1 Other articular cartilage disorders**

    *EXCLUDES 2*   chondrocalcinosis (M11.1, M11.2-)

              internal derangement of knee (M23.-)

              metastatic calcification (E83.5)

              ochronosis (E70.2)

    **M24.10**   Other articular cartilage disorders, unspecified site

  ✓6ᵗʰ **M24.11**   Other articular cartilage disorders, shoulder

    **M24.111**   Other articular cartilage disorders, right shoulder

    **M24.112**   Other articular cartilage disorders, left shoulder

    **M24.119**   Other articular cartilage disorders, unspecified shoulder

  ✓6ᵗʰ **M24.12**   Other articular cartilage disorders, elbow

    **M24.121**   Other articular cartilage disorders, right elbow

    **M24.122**   Other articular cartilage disorders, left elbow

    **M24.129**   Other articular cartilage disorders, unspecified elbow

  ✓6ᵗʰ **M24.13**   Other articular cartilage disorders, wrist

    **M24.131**   Other articular cartilage disorders, right wrist

    **M24.132**   Other articular cartilage disorders, left wrist

    **M24.139**   Other articular cartilage disorders, unspecified wrist

  ✓6ᵗʰ **M24.14**   Other articular cartilage disorders, hand

    **M24.141**   Other articular cartilage disorders, right hand

    **M24.142**   Other articular cartilage disorders, left hand

    **M24.149**   Other articular cartilage disorders, unspecified hand

✓ Additional Character Req   ✓ x7ᵗʰ Placeholder Alert   Unacceptable PDx   Manifestation   H1 - H14 HAC   HCC CMS-HCC Condition   *EXCLUDES 1* Not Coded Here   *EXCLUDES 2* Not Included Here

ICD-10-CM 2018                                                            **763**

✓6ᵗʰ **M24.15 Other articular cartilage disorders, hip**
- **M24.151 Other articular cartilage disorders, right hip**
- **M24.152 Other articular cartilage disorders, left hip**
- **M24.159 Other articular cartilage disorders, unspecified hip**

✓6ᵗʰ **M24.17 Other articular cartilage disorders, ankle and foot**
- **M24.171 Other articular cartilage disorders, right ankle**
- **M24.172 Other articular cartilage disorders, left ankle**
- **M24.173 Other articular cartilage disorders, unspecified ankle**
- **M24.174 Other articular cartilage disorders, right foot**
- **M24.175 Other articular cartilage disorders, left foot**
- **M24.176 Other articular cartilage disorders, unspecified foot**

✓5ᵗʰ **M24.2 Disorder of ligament**
Instability secondary to old ligament injury
Ligamentous laxity NOS
EXCLUDES 1    *familial ligamentous laxity (M35.7)*
EXCLUDES 2    *internal derangement of knee (M23.5-M23.89)*

**M24.20 Disorder of ligament, unspecified site**

✓6ᵗʰ **M24.21 Disorder of ligament, shoulder**
- **M24.211 Disorder of ligament, right shoulder**
- **M24.212 Disorder of ligament, left shoulder**
- **M24.219 Disorder of ligament, unspecified shoulder**

✓6ᵗʰ **M24.22 Disorder of ligament, elbow**
- **M24.221 Disorder of ligament, right elbow**
- **M24.222 Disorder of ligament, left elbow**
- **M24.229 Disorder of ligament, unspecified elbow**

✓6ᵗʰ **M24.23 Disorder of ligament, wrist**
- **M24.231 Disorder of ligament, right wrist**
- **M24.232 Disorder of ligament, left wrist**
- **M24.239 Disorder of ligament, unspecified wrist**

✓6ᵗʰ **M24.24 Disorder of ligament, hand**
- **M24.241 Disorder of ligament, right hand**
- **M24.242 Disorder of ligament, left hand**
- **M24.249 Disorder of ligament, unspecified hand**

✓6ᵗʰ **M24.25 Disorder of ligament, hip**
- **M24.251 Disorder of ligament, right hip**
- **M24.252 Disorder of ligament, left hip**
- **M24.259 Disorder of ligament, unspecified hip**

✓6ᵗʰ **M24.27 Disorder of ligament, ankle and foot**
- **M24.271 Disorder of ligament, right ankle**
- **M24.272 Disorder of ligament, left ankle**
- **M24.273 Disorder of ligament, unspecified ankle**
- **M24.274 Disorder of ligament, right foot**
- **M24.275 Disorder of ligament, left foot**
- **M24.276 Disorder of ligament, unspecified foot**

**M24.28 Disorder of ligament, vertebrae**

✓5ᵗʰ **M24.3 Pathological dislocation of joint, not elsewhere classified**
EXCLUDES 1    *congenital dislocation or displacement of joint—see congenital malformations and deformations of the musculoskeletal system (Q65-Q79)*
*current injury—see injury of joints and ligaments by body region*
*recurrent dislocation of joint (M24.4-)*

**M24.30 Pathological dislocation of unspecified joint, not elsewhere classified**

✓6ᵗʰ **M24.31 Pathological dislocation of shoulder, not elsewhere classified**
- **M24.311 Pathological dislocation of right shoulder, not elsewhere classified**
- **M24.312 Pathological dislocation of left shoulder, not elsewhere classified**
- **M24.319 Pathological dislocation of unspecified shoulder, not elsewhere classified**

✓6ᵗʰ **M24.32 Pathological dislocation of elbow, not elsewhere classified**
- **M24.321 Pathological dislocation of right elbow, not elsewhere classified**
- **M24.322 Pathological dislocation of left elbow, not elsewhere classified**
- **M24.329 Pathological dislocation of unspecified elbow, not elsewhere classified**

✓6ᵗʰ **M24.33 Pathological dislocation of wrist, not elsewhere classified**
- **M24.331 Pathological dislocation of right wrist, not elsewhere classified**
- **M24.332 Pathological dislocation of left wrist, not elsewhere classified**
- **M24.339 Pathological dislocation of unspecified wrist, not elsewhere classified**

✓6ᵗʰ **M24.34 Pathological dislocation of hand, not elsewhere classified**
- **M24.341 Pathological dislocation of right hand, not elsewhere classified**
- **M24.342 Pathological dislocation of left hand, not elsewhere classified**
- **M24.349 Pathological dislocation of unspecified hand, not elsewhere classified**

✓6ᵗʰ **M24.35 Pathological dislocation of hip, not elsewhere classified**
- **M24.351 Pathological dislocation of right hip, not elsewhere classified**
- **M24.352 Pathological dislocation of left hip, not elsewhere classified**
- **M24.359 Pathological dislocation of unspecified hip, not elsewhere classified**

✓6ᵗʰ **M24.36 Pathological dislocation of knee, not elsewhere classified**
- **M24.361 Pathological dislocation of right knee, not elsewhere classified**
- **M24.362 Pathological dislocation of left knee, not elsewhere classified**
- **M24.369 Pathological dislocation of unspecified knee, not elsewhere classified**

✓6ᵗʰ **M24.37 Pathological dislocation of ankle and foot, not elsewhere classified**
- **M24.371 Pathological dislocation of right ankle, not elsewhere classified**
- **M24.372 Pathological dislocation of left ankle, not elsewhere classified**
- **M24.373 Pathological dislocation of unspecified ankle, not elsewhere classified**
- **M24.374 Pathological dislocation of right foot, not elsewhere classified**
- **M24.375 Pathological dislocation of left foot, not elsewhere classified**
- **M24.376 Pathological dislocation of unspecified foot, not elsewhere classified**

✓5ᵗʰ **M24.4 Recurrent dislocation of joint**
Recurrent subluxation of joint
EXCLUDES 2    *recurrent dislocation of patella (M22.0-M22.1)*
*recurrent vertebral dislocation (M43.3-, M43.4, M43.5-)*

**M24.40 Recurrent dislocation, unspecified joint**

✓6ᵗʰ **M24.41 Recurrent dislocation, shoulder**
- **M24.411 Recurrent dislocation, right shoulder**
- **M24.412 Recurrent dislocation, left shoulder**
- **M24.419 Recurrent dislocation, unspecified shoulder**

✓6ᵗʰ **M24.42 Recurrent dislocation, elbow**
- **M24.421 Recurrent dislocation, right elbow**
- **M24.422 Recurrent dislocation, left elbow**
- **M24.429 Recurrent dislocation, unspecified elbow**

✓6ᵗʰ **M24.43 Recurrent dislocation, wrist**
- **M24.431 Recurrent dislocation, right wrist**
- **M24.432 Recurrent dislocation, left wrist**
- **M24.439 Recurrent dislocation, unspecified wrist**

✓6ᵗʰ **M24.44 Recurrent dislocation, hand and finger(s)**
- **M24.441 Recurrent dislocation, right hand**
- **M24.442 Recurrent dislocation, left hand**
- **M24.443 Recurrent dislocation, unspecified hand**
- **M24.444 Recurrent dislocation, right finger**
- **M24.445 Recurrent dislocation, left finger**
- **M24.446 Recurrent dislocation, unspecified finger**

N Newborn: 0   P Pediatric: 0-17   M Maternity: 12-55   A Adult: 15-124   MCC Major CC Condition   PDx MCC PDx acts as own MCC   CC CC Condition   PDx CC PDx acts as own CC

764          ICD-10-CM 2018

✓6ᵗʰ **M24.45** **Recurrent dislocation,** hip
    **M24.451** **Recurrent dislocation,** right **hip**
    **M24.452** **Recurrent dislocation,** left **hip**
    **M24.459** **Recurrent dislocation,** unspecified **hip**

✓6ᵗʰ **M24.46** **Recurrent dislocation,** knee
    **M24.461** **Recurrent dislocation,** right **knee**
    **M24.462** **Recurrent dislocation,** left **knee**
    **M24.469** **Recurrent dislocation,** unspecified **knee**

✓6ᵗʰ **M24.47** **Recurrent dislocation,** ankle, foot and toes
    **M24.471** **Recurrent dislocation,** right **ankle**
    **M24.472** **Recurrent dislocation,** left **ankle**
    **M24.473** **Recurrent dislocation,** unspecified **ankle**
    **M24.474** **Recurrent dislocation,** right **foot**
    **M24.475** **Recurrent dislocation,** left **foot**
    **M24.476** **Recurrent dislocation,** unspecified **foot**
    **M24.477** **Recurrent dislocation,** right **toe(s)**
    **M24.478** **Recurrent dislocation,** left **toe(s)**
    **M24.479** **Recurrent dislocation,** unspecified **toe(s)**

✓5ᵗʰ **M24.5** **Contracture of joint**
    **EXCLUDES 1** *contracture of muscle without contracture of joint (M62.4-)*
    *contracture of tendon (sheath) without contracture of joint (M62.4-)*
    *Dupuytren's contracture (M72.0)*
    **EXCLUDES 2** *acquired deformities of limbs (M20-M21)*
    **AHA:** 2016, 2Q, 6

    **M24.50** **Contracture,** unspecified joint

✓6ᵗʰ **M24.51** **Contracture,** shoulder
    **M24.511** **Contracture,** right **shoulder**
    **M24.512** **Contracture,** left **shoulder**
    **M24.519** **Contracture,** unspecified **shoulder**

✓6ᵗʰ **M24.52** **Contracture,** elbow
    **M24.521** **Contracture,** right **elbow**
    **M24.522** **Contracture,** left **elbow**
    **M24.529** **Contracture,** unspecified **elbow**

✓6ᵗʰ **M24.53** **Contracture,** wrist
    **M24.531** **Contracture,** right **wrist**
    **M24.532** **Contracture,** left **wrist**
    **M24.539** **Contracture,** unspecified **wrist**

✓6ᵗʰ **M24.54** **Contracture,** hand
    **M24.541** **Contracture,** right **hand**
    **M24.542** **Contracture,** left **hand**
    **M24.549** **Contracture,** unspecified **hand**

✓6ᵗʰ **M24.55** **Contracture,** hip
    **M24.551** **Contracture,** right **hip**
    **M24.552** **Contracture,** left **hip**
    **M24.559** **Contracture,** unspecified **hip**

✓6ᵗʰ **M24.56** **Contracture,** knee
    **M24.561** **Contracture,** right **knee**
    **M24.562** **Contracture,** left **knee**
    **M24.569** **Contracture,** unspecified **knee**

✓6ᵗʰ **M24.57** **Contracture,** ankle and foot
    **M24.571** **Contracture,** right **ankle**
    **M24.572** **Contracture,** left **ankle**
    **M24.573** **Contracture,** unspecified **ankle**
    **M24.574** **Contracture,** right **foot**
    **M24.575** **Contracture,** left **foot**
    **M24.576** **Contracture,** unspecified **foot**

✓5ᵗʰ **M24.6** **Ankylosis of joint**
    **EXCLUDES 1** *stiffness of joint without ankylosis (M25.6-)*
    **EXCLUDES 2** *spine (M43.2-)*

    **M24.60** **Ankylosis,** unspecified joint

✓6ᵗʰ **M24.61** **Ankylosis,** shoulder
    **M24.611** **Ankylosis,** right **shoulder**
    **M24.612** **Ankylosis,** left **shoulder**
    **M24.619** **Ankylosis,** unspecified **shoulder**

✓6ᵗʰ **M24.62** **Ankylosis,** elbow
    **M24.621** **Ankylosis,** right **elbow**
    **M24.622** **Ankylosis,** left **elbow**
    **M24.629** **Ankylosis,** unspecified **elbow**

✓6ᵗʰ **M24.63** **Ankylosis,** wrist
    **M24.631** **Ankylosis,** right **wrist**

    **M24.632** **Ankylosis,** left **wrist**
    **M24.639** **Ankylosis,** unspecified **wrist**

✓6ᵗʰ **M24.64** **Ankylosis,** hand
    **M24.641** **Ankylosis,** right **hand**
    **M24.642** **Ankylosis,** left **hand**
    **M24.649** **Ankylosis,** unspecified **hand**

✓6ᵗʰ **M24.65** **Ankylosis,** hip
    **M24.651** **Ankylosis,** right **hip**
    **M24.652** **Ankylosis,** left **hip**
    **M24.659** **Ankylosis,** unspecified **hip**

✓6ᵗʰ **M24.66** **Ankylosis,** knee
    **M24.661** **Ankylosis,** right **knee**
    **M24.662** **Ankylosis,** left **knee**
    **M24.669** **Ankylosis,** unspecified **knee**

✓6ᵗʰ **M24.67** **Ankylosis,** ankle and foot
    **M24.671** **Ankylosis,** right **ankle**
    **M24.672** **Ankylosis,** left **ankle**
    **M24.673** **Ankylosis,** unspecified **ankle**
    **M24.674** **Ankylosis,** right **foot**
    **M24.675** **Ankylosis,** left **foot**
    **M24.676** **Ankylosis,** unspecified **foot**

**M24.7** **Protrusio acetabuli**

✓5ᵗʰ **M24.8** **Other specific joint derangements, not elsewhere classified**
    **EXCLUDES 2** *iliotibial band syndrome (M76.3)*

    **M24.80** **Other specific joint derangements of** unspecified joint, not elsewhere classified

✓6ᵗʰ **M24.81** **Other specific joint derangements of** shoulder, not elsewhere classified
    **M24.811** **Other specific joint derangements of** right shoulder, not elsewhere classified
    **M24.812** **Other specific joint derangements of** left shoulder, not elsewhere classified
    **M24.819** **Other specific joint derangements of** unspecified shoulder, not elsewhere classified

✓6ᵗʰ **M24.82** **Other specific joint derangements of** elbow, not elsewhere classified
    **M24.821** **Other specific joint derangements of** right elbow, not elsewhere classified
    **M24.822** **Other specific joint derangements of** left elbow, not elsewhere classified
    **M24.829** **Other specific joint derangements of** unspecified elbow, not elsewhere classified

✓6ᵗʰ **M24.83** **Other specific joint derangements of** wrist, not elsewhere classified
    **M24.831** **Other specific joint derangements of** right wrist, not elsewhere classified
    **M24.832** **Other specific joint derangements of** left wrist, not elsewhere classified
    **M24.839** **Other specific joint derangements of** unspecified wrist, not elsewhere classified

✓6ᵗʰ **M24.84** **Other specific joint derangements of** hand, not elsewhere classified
    **M24.841** **Other specific joint derangements of** right hand, not elsewhere classified
    **M24.842** **Other specific joint derangements of** left hand, not elsewhere classified
    **M24.849** **Other specific joint derangements of** unspecified hand, not elsewhere classified

✓6ᵗʰ **M24.85** **Other specific joint derangements of** hip, not elsewhere classified
    Irritable hip
    **M24.851** **Other specific joint derangements of** right hip, not elsewhere classified
    **M24.852** **Other specific joint derangements of** left hip, not elsewhere classified
    **M24.859** **Other specific joint derangements of** unspecified hip, not elsewhere classified

✓6ᵗʰ **M24.87** **Other specific joint derangements of** ankle and foot, not elsewhere classified
    **M24.871** **Other specific joint derangements of** right ankle, not elsewhere classified
    **M24.872** **Other specific joint derangements of** left ankle, not elsewhere classified

✓ Additional Character Req   ✓x7ᵗʰ Placeholder Alert   Unacceptable PDx   Manifestation   H1 - H14 HAC   HCC CMS-HCC Condition   EXCLUDES 1 Not Coded Here   EXCLUDES 2 Not Included Here

ICD-10-CM 2018      765

**Chapter 13. Diseases of the Musculoskeletal System and Connective Tissue**

M24.873–M25.28

        M24.873   **Other specific joint derangements of unspecified ankle, not elsewhere classified**

        M24.874   **Other specific joint derangements of** right **foot, not elsewhere classified**

        M24.875   **Other specific joint derangements** left **foot, not elsewhere classified**

        M24.876   **Other specific joint derangements of unspecified foot, not elsewhere classified**

    M24.9   **Joint derangement, unspecified**

✓4ᵗʰ **M25   Other joint disorder, not elsewhere classified**

EXCLUDES 2   *abnormality of gait and mobility (R26.-)*
*acquired deformities of limb (M20-M21)*
*calcification of bursa (M71.4-)*
*calcification of shoulder (joint) (M75.3)*
*calcification of tendon (M65.2-)*
*difficulty in walking (R26.2)*
*temporomandibular joint disorder (M26.6-)*

✓5ᵗʰ **M25.0   Hemarthrosis**

EXCLUDES 1   *current injury—see injury of joint by body region*
*hemophilic arthropathy (M36.2)*

    M25.00   **Hemarthrosis, unspecified joint**   CC
        CC Excl: PDX collection 868

✓6ᵗʰ   M25.01   **Hemarthrosis, shoulder**

        **CC Excl: For CC codes in subcategory M25.01:** PDX collection 869

        M25.011   **Hemarthrosis, right shoulder**   CC
        M25.012   **Hemarthrosis, left shoulder**   CC
        M25.019   **Hemarthrosis, unspecified shoulder**   CC

✓6ᵗʰ   M25.02   **Hemarthrosis, elbow**

        **CC Excl: For CC codes in subcategory M25.02:** PDX collection 870

        M25.021   **Hemarthrosis, right elbow**   CC
        M25.022   **Hemarthrosis, left elbow**   CC
        M25.029   **Hemarthrosis, unspecified elbow**   CC

✓6ᵗʰ   M25.03   **Hemarthrosis, wrist**

        **CC Excl: For CC codes in subcategory M25.03:** PDX collection 871

        M25.031   **Hemarthrosis, right wrist**   CC
        M25.032   **Hemarthrosis, left wrist**   CC
        M25.039   **Hemarthrosis, unspecified wrist**   CC

✓6ᵗʰ   M25.04   **Hemarthrosis, hand**

        **CC Excl: For CC codes in subcategory M25.04:** PDX collection 872

        M25.041   **Hemarthrosis, right hand**   CC
        M25.042   **Hemarthrosis, left hand**   CC
        M25.049   **Hemarthrosis, unspecified hand**   CC

✓6ᵗʰ   M25.05   **Hemarthrosis, hip**

        **CC Excl: For CC codes in subcategory M25.05:** PDX collection 868

        M25.051   **Hemarthrosis, right hip**   CC
        M25.052   **Hemarthrosis, left hip**   CC
        M25.059   **Hemarthrosis, unspecified hip**   CC

✓6ᵗʰ   M25.06   **Hemarthrosis, knee**

        **CC Excl: For CC codes in subcategory M25.06:** PDX collection 873

        M25.061   **Hemarthrosis, right knee**   CC
        M25.062   **Hemarthrosis, left knee**   CC
        M25.069   **Hemarthrosis, unspecified knee**   CC

✓6ᵗʰ   M25.07   **Hemarthrosis, ankle and foot**

        **CC Excl: For CC codes in subcategory M25.07:** PDX collection 873

        M25.071   **Hemarthrosis, right ankle**   CC
        M25.072   **Hemarthrosis, left ankle**   CC
        M25.073   **Hemarthrosis, unspecified ankle**   CC
        M25.074   **Hemarthrosis, right foot**   CC
        M25.075   **Hemarthrosis, left foot**   CC
        M25.076   **Hemarthrosis, unspecified foot**   CC

    M25.08   **Hemarthrosis, other specified site**   CC
        Hemarthrosis, vertebrae
        **CC Excl:** PDX collection 868

✓5ᵗʰ **M25.1   Fistula of joint**

    M25.10   **Fistula, unspecified joint**

✓6ᵗʰ   M25.11   **Fistula, shoulder**

        M25.111   **Fistula, right shoulder**
        M25.112   **Fistula, left shoulder**
        M25.119   **Fistula, unspecified shoulder**

✓6ᵗʰ   M25.12   **Fistula, elbow**

        M25.121   **Fistula, right elbow**
        M25.122   **Fistula, left elbow**
        M25.129   **Fistula, unspecified elbow**

✓6ᵗʰ   M25.13   **Fistula, wrist**

        M25.131   **Fistula, right wrist**
        M25.132   **Fistula, left wrist**
        M25.139   **Fistula, unspecified wrist**

✓6ᵗʰ   M25.14   **Fistula, hand**

        M25.141   **Fistula, right hand**
        M25.142   **Fistula, left hand**
        M25.149   **Fistula, unspecified hand**

✓6ᵗʰ   M25.15   **Fistula, hip**

        M25.151   **Fistula, right hip**
        M25.152   **Fistula, left hip**
        M25.159   **Fistula, unspecified hip**

✓6ᵗʰ   M25.16   **Fistula, knee**

        M25.161   **Fistula, right knee**
        M25.162   **Fistula, left knee**
        M25.169   **Fistula, unspecified knee**

✓6ᵗʰ   M25.17   **Fistula, ankle and foot**

        M25.171   **Fistula, right ankle**
        M25.172   **Fistula, left ankle**
        M25.173   **Fistula, unspecified ankle**
        M25.174   **Fistula, right foot**
        M25.175   **Fistula, left foot**
        M25.176   **Fistula, unspecified foot**

    M25.18   **Fistula, other specified site**
        Fistula, vertebrae

✓5ᵗʰ **M25.2   Flail joint**

    M25.20   **Flail joint, unspecified joint**

✓6ᵗʰ   M25.21   **Flail joint, shoulder**

        M25.211   **Flail joint, right shoulder**
        M25.212   **Flail joint, left shoulder**
        M25.219   **Flail joint, unspecified shoulder**

✓6ᵗʰ   M25.22   **Flail joint, elbow**

        M25.221   **Flail joint, right elbow**
        M25.222   **Flail joint, left elbow**
        M25.229   **Flail joint, unspecified elbow**

✓6ᵗʰ   M25.23   **Flail joint, wrist**

        M25.231   **Flail joint, right wrist**
        M25.232   **Flail joint, left wrist**
        M25.239   **Flail joint, unspecified wrist**

✓6ᵗʰ   M25.24   **Flail joint, hand**

        M25.241   **Flail joint, right hand**
        M25.242   **Flail joint, left hand**
        M25.249   **Flail joint, unspecified hand**

✓6ᵗʰ   M25.25   **Flail joint, hip**

        M25.251   **Flail joint, right hip**
        M25.252   **Flail joint, left hip**
        M25.259   **Flail joint, unspecified hip**

✓6ᵗʰ   M25.26   **Flail joint, knee**

        M25.261   **Flail joint, right knee**
        M25.262   **Flail joint, left knee**
        M25.269   **Flail joint, unspecified knee**

✓6ᵗʰ   M25.27   **Flail joint, ankle and foot**

        M25.271   **Flail joint, right ankle and foot**
        M25.272   **Flail joint, left ankle and foot**
        M25.279   **Flail joint, unspecified ankle and foot**

    M25.28   **Flail joint, other site**

N Newborn: 0   P Pediatric: 0-17   M Maternity: 12-55   A Adult: 15-124   MCC Major CC Condition   PDx MCC PDx acts as own MCC   CC CC Condition   PDx CC PDx acts as own CC

**766**      ICD-10-CM 2018

✓5ᵗʰ **M25.3 Other instability of joint**

     *EXCLUDES 1*    instability of joint secondary to old ligament injury (M24.2-)
            instability of joint secondary to removal of joint prosthesis (M96.8-)
     *EXCLUDES 2*    spinal instabilities (M53.2-)

     **M25.30 Other instability, unspecified joint**

✓6ᵗʰ   **M25.31 Other instability, shoulder**
       **M25.311 Other instability, right shoulder**
       **M25.312 Other instability, left shoulder**
       **M25.319 Other instability, unspecified shoulder**

✓6ᵗʰ   **M25.32 Other instability, elbow**
       **M25.321 Other instability, right elbow**
       **M25.322 Other instability, left elbow**
       **M25.329 Other instability, unspecified elbow**

✓6ᵗʰ   **M25.33 Other instability, wrist**
       **M25.331 Other instability, right wrist**
       **M25.332 Other instability, left wrist**
       **M25.339 Other instability, unspecified wrist**

✓6ᵗʰ   **M25.34 Other instability, hand**
       **M25.341 Other instability, right hand**
       **M25.342 Other instability, left hand**
       **M25.349 Other instability, unspecified hand**

✓6ᵗʰ   **M25.35 Other instability, hip**
       **M25.351 Other instability, right hip**
       **M25.352 Other instability, left hip**
       **M25.359 Other instability, unspecified hip**

✓6ᵗʰ   **M25.36 Other instability, knee**
       **M25.361 Other instability, right knee**
       **M25.362 Other instability, left knee**
       **M25.369 Other instability, unspecified knee**

✓6ᵗʰ   **M25.37 Other instability, ankle and foot**
       **M25.371 Other instability, right ankle**
       **M25.372 Other instability, left ankle**
       **M25.373 Other instability, unspecified ankle**
       **M25.374 Other instability, right foot**
       **M25.375 Other instability, left foot**
       **M25.376 Other instability, unspecified foot**

✓5ᵗʰ **M25.4 Effusion of joint**

     *EXCLUDES 1*    hydrarthrosis in yaws (A66.6)
            intermittent hydrarthrosis (M12.4-)
            other infective (teno)synovitis (M65.1-)

     **M25.40 Effusion, unspecified joint**

✓6ᵗʰ   **M25.41 Effusion, shoulder**
       **M25.411 Effusion, right shoulder**
       **M25.412 Effusion, left shoulder**
       **M25.419 Effusion, unspecified shoulder**

✓6ᵗʰ   **M25.42 Effusion, elbow**
       **M25.421 Effusion, right elbow**
       **M25.422 Effusion, left elbow**
       **M25.429 Effusion, unspecified elbow**

✓6ᵗʰ   **M25.43 Effusion, wrist**
       **M25.431 Effusion, right wrist**
       **M25.432 Effusion, left wrist**
       **M25.439 Effusion, unspecified wrist**

✓6ᵗʰ   **M25.44 Effusion, hand**
       **M25.441 Effusion, right hand**
       **M25.442 Effusion, left hand**
       **M25.449 Effusion, unspecified hand**

✓6ᵗʰ   **M25.45 Effusion, hip**
       **M25.451 Effusion, right hip**
       **M25.452 Effusion, left hip**
       **M25.459 Effusion, unspecified hip**

✓6ᵗʰ   **M25.46 Effusion, knee**
       **M25.461 Effusion, right knee**
       **M25.462 Effusion, left knee**
       **M25.469 Effusion, unspecified knee**

✓6ᵗʰ   **M25.47 Effusion, ankle and foot**
       **M25.471 Effusion, right ankle**
       **M25.472 Effusion, left ankle**
       **M25.473 Effusion, unspecified ankle**
       **M25.474 Effusion, right foot**
       **M25.475 Effusion, left foot**
       **M25.476 Effusion, unspecified foot**

     **M25.48 Effusion, other site**

✓5ᵗʰ **M25.5 Pain in joint**

     *EXCLUDES 2*    pain in hand (M79.64-)
            pain in fingers (M79.64-)
            pain in foot (M79.67-)
            pain in limb (M79.6-)
            pain in toes (M79.67-)

     **M25.50 Pain in unspecified joint**

✓6ᵗʰ   **M25.51 Pain in shoulder**
       **M25.511 Pain in right shoulder**
       **M25.512 Pain in left shoulder**
       **M25.519 Pain in unspecified shoulder**

✓6ᵗʰ   **M25.52 Pain in elbow**
       **M25.521 Pain in right elbow**
       **M25.522 Pain in left elbow**
       **M25.529 Pain in unspecified elbow**

✓6ᵗʰ   **M25.53 Pain in wrist**
       **M25.531 Pain in right wrist**
       **M25.532 Pain in left wrist**
       **M25.539 Pain in unspecified wrist**

✓6ᵗʰ   **M25.54 Pain in joints of hand**
       **M25.541 Pain in joints of right hand**
       **M25.542 Pain in joints of left hand**
       **M25.549 Pain in joints of unspecified hand**
            Pain in joints of hand NOS

✓6ᵗʰ   **M25.55 Pain in hip**
       **M25.551 Pain in right hip**
       **M25.552 Pain in left hip**
       **M25.559 Pain in unspecified hip**

✓6ᵗʰ   **M25.56 Pain in knee**
       **M25.561 Pain in right knee**
       **M25.562 Pain in left knee**
       **M25.569 Pain in unspecified knee**

✓6ᵗʰ   **M25.57 Pain in ankle and joints of foot**
       **M25.571 Pain in right ankle and joints of right foot**
       **M25.572 Pain in left ankle and joints of left foot**
       **M25.579 Pain in unspecified ankle and joints of unspecified foot**

✓5ᵗʰ **M25.6 Stiffness of joint, not elsewhere classified**

     *EXCLUDES 1*    ankylosis of joint (M24.6-)
            contracture of joint (M24.5-)

     **M25.60 Stiffness of unspecified joint, not elsewhere classified**

✓6ᵗʰ   **M25.61 Stiffness of shoulder, not elsewhere classified**
       **M25.611 Stiffness of right shoulder, not elsewhere classified**
       **M25.612 Stiffness of left shoulder, not elsewhere classified**
       **M25.619 Stiffness of unspecified shoulder, not elsewhere classified**

✓6ᵗʰ   **M25.62 Stiffness of elbow, not elsewhere classified**
       **M25.621 Stiffness of right elbow, not elsewhere classified**
       **M25.622 Stiffness of left elbow, not elsewhere classified**
       **M25.629 Stiffness of unspecified elbow, not elsewhere classified**

✓6ᵗʰ   **M25.63 Stiffness of wrist, not elsewhere classified**
       **M25.631 Stiffness of right wrist, not elsewhere classified**
       **M25.632 Stiffness of left wrist, not elsewhere classified**
       **M25.639 Stiffness of unspecified wrist, not elsewhere classified**

✓6ᵗʰ   **M25.64 Stiffness of hand, not elsewhere classified**
       **M25.641 Stiffness of right hand, not elsewhere classified**
       **M25.642 Stiffness of left hand, not elsewhere classified**
       **M25.649 Stiffness of unspecified hand, not elsewhere classified**

✅ Additional Character Req    ✓x7ᵗʰ Placeholder Alert    Unacceptable PDx    Manifestation    H1 - H14 HAC    HCC CMS-HCC Condition    *EXCLUDES 1* Not Coded Here    *EXCLUDES 2* Not Included Here

ICD-10-CM 2018          767

M25.3–M25.649

✓6th **M25.65 Stiffness of hip, not elsewhere classified**
   **M25.651** Stiffness of right hip, not elsewhere classified
   **M25.652** Stiffness of left hip, not elsewhere classified
   **M25.659** Stiffness of unspecified hip, not elsewhere classified

✓6th **M25.66 Stiffness of knee, not elsewhere classified**
   **M25.661** Stiffness of right knee, not elsewhere classified
   **M25.662** Stiffness of left knee, not elsewhere classified
   **M25.669** Stiffness of unspecified knee, not elsewhere classified

✓6th **M25.67 Stiffness of ankle and foot, not elsewhere classified**
   **M25.671** Stiffness of right ankle, not elsewhere classified
   **M25.672** Stiffness of left ankle, not elsewhere classified
   **M25.673** Stiffness of unspecified ankle, not elsewhere classified
   **M25.674** Stiffness of right foot, not elsewhere classified
   **M25.675** Stiffness of left foot, not elsewhere classified
   **M25.676** Stiffness of unspecified foot, not elsewhere classified

✓5th **M25.7 Osteophyte**
   **M25.70** Osteophyte, unspecified joint

✓6th **M25.71 Osteophyte, shoulder**
   **M25.711** Osteophyte, right shoulder
   **M25.712** Osteophyte, left shoulder
   **M25.719** Osteophyte, unspecified shoulder

✓6th **M25.72 Osteophyte, elbow**
   **M25.721** Osteophyte, right elbow
   **M25.722** Osteophyte, left elbow
   **M25.729** Osteophyte, unspecified elbow

✓6th **M25.73 Osteophyte, wrist**
   **M25.731** Osteophyte, right wrist
   **M25.732** Osteophyte, left wrist
   **M25.739** Osteophyte, unspecified wrist

✓6th **M25.74 Osteophyte, hand**
   **M25.741** Osteophyte, right hand
   **M25.742** Osteophyte, left hand
   **M25.749** Osteophyte, unspecified hand

✓6th **M25.75 Osteophyte, hip**
   **M25.751** Osteophyte, right hip
   **M25.752** Osteophyte, left hip
   **M25.759** Osteophyte, unspecified hip

✓6th **M25.76 Osteophyte, knee**
   **M25.761** Osteophyte, right knee
   **M25.762** Osteophyte, left knee
   **M25.769** Osteophyte, unspecified knee

✓6th **M25.77 Osteophyte, ankle and foot**
   **M25.771** Osteophyte, right ankle
   **M25.772** Osteophyte, left ankle
   **M25.773** Osteophyte, unspecified ankle
   **M25.774** Osteophyte, right foot
   **M25.775** Osteophyte, left foot
   **M25.776** Osteophyte, unspecified foot

   **M25.78** Osteophyte, vertebrae

✓5th **M25.8 Other specified joint disorders**
   **M25.80** Other specified joint disorders, unspecified joint

✓6th **M25.81 Other specified joint disorders, shoulder**
   **M25.811** Other specified joint disorders, right shoulder
   **M25.812** Other specified joint disorders, left shoulder
   **M25.819** Other specified joint disorders, unspecified shoulder

✓6th **M25.82 Other specified joint disorders, elbow**
   **M25.821** Other specified joint disorders, right elbow
   **M25.822** Other specified joint disorders, left elbow

   **M25.829** Other specified joint disorders, unspecified elbow

✓6th **M25.83 Other specified joint disorders, wrist**
   **M25.831** Other specified joint disorders, right wrist
   **M25.832** Other specified joint disorders, left wrist
   **M25.839** Other specified joint disorders, unspecified wrist

✓6th **M25.84 Other specified joint disorders, hand**
   **M25.841** Other specified joint disorders, right hand
   **M25.842** Other specified joint disorders, left hand
   **M25.849** Other specified joint disorders, unspecified hand

✓6th **M25.85 Other specified joint disorders, hip**
   **AHA:** 2014, 4Q, 25
   **M25.851** Other specified joint disorders, right hip
   **M25.852** Other specified joint disorders, left hip
   **M25.859** Other specified joint disorders, unspecified hip

✓6th **M25.86 Other specified joint disorders, knee**
   **M25.861** Other specified joint disorders, right knee
   **M25.862** Other specified joint disorders, left knee
   **M25.869** Other specified joint disorders, unspecified knee

✓6th **M25.87 Other specified joint disorders, ankle and foot**
   **M25.871** Other specified joint disorders, right ankle and foot
   **M25.872** Other specified joint disorders, left ankle and foot
   **M25.879** Other specified joint disorders, unspecified ankle and foot

   **M25.9 Joint disorder, unspecified**

## Dentofacial anomalies [including malocclusion] and other disorders of jaw (M26-M27)

**EXCLUDES 1** *hemifacial atrophy or hypertrophy (Q67.4)*
*unilateral condylar hyperplasia or hypoplasia (M27.8)*

✓4th **M26 Dentofacial anomalies [including malocclusion]**

✓5th **M26.0 Major anomalies of jaw size**
   **EXCLUDES 1** *acromegaly (E22.0)*
   *Robin's syndrome (Q87.0)*
   **M26.00** Unspecified anomaly of jaw size
   **M26.01** Maxillary hyperplasia
   **M26.02** Maxillary hypoplasia
      **AHA:** 2014, 3Q, 23
   **M26.03** Mandibular hyperplasia
   **M26.04** Mandibular hypoplasia
   **M26.05** Macrogenia
   **M26.06** Microgenia
   **M26.07** Excessive tuberosity of jaw
      Entire maxillary tuberosity
   **M26.09** Other specified anomalies of jaw size

✓5th **M26.1 Anomalies of jaw-cranial base relationship**
   **M26.10** Unspecified anomaly of jaw-cranial base relationship
   **M26.11** Maxillary asymmetry
   **M26.12** Other jaw asymmetry
   **M26.19** Other specified anomalies of jaw-cranial base relationship

✓5th **M26.2 Anomalies of dental arch relationship**
   **M26.20** Unspecified anomaly of dental arch relationship

✓6th **M26.21 Malocclusion, Angle's class**
   **M26.211** Malocclusion, Angle's class I
      Neutro-occlusion
   **M26.212** Malocclusion, Angle's class II
      Disto-occlusion Division I
      Disto-occlusion Division II
   **M26.213** Malocclusion, Angle's class III
      Mesio-occlusion
   **M26.219** Malocclusion, Angle's class, unspecified

✓6th **M26.22 Open occlusal relationship**
   **M26.220** Open anterior occlusal relationship
      Anterior openbite
   **M26.221** Open posterior occlusal relationship
      Posterior openbite

Ⓝ Newborn: 0   Ⓟ Pediatric: 0-17   Ⓜ Maternity: 12-55   Ⓐ Adult: 15-124   MCC Major CC Condition   PDxMCC PDx acts as own MCC   CC CC Condition   PDxCC PDx acts as own CC

768   ICD-10-CM 2018

**M26.23**   **Excessive horizontal overlap**
Excessive horizontal overjet

**M26.24**   **Reverse articulation**
Crossbite (anterior) (posterior)

**M26.25**   **Anomalies of interarch distance**

**M26.29**   **Other anomalies of dental arch relationship**
Midline deviation of dental arch
Overbite (excessive) deep
Overbite (excessive) horizontal
Overbite (excessive) vertical
Posterior lingual occlusion of mandibular teeth

✓5ᵗʰ   **M26.3**   **Anomalies of tooth position of fully erupted tooth or teeth**
     *EXCLUDES 2*   *embedded and impacted teeth (KØ1.-)*

**M26.30**   **Unspecified anomaly of tooth position of fully erupted tooth or teeth**
Abnormal spacing of fully erupted tooth or teeth NOS
Displacement of fully erupted tooth or teeth NOS
Transposition of fully erupted tooth or teeth NOS

**M26.31**   **Crowding of fully erupted teeth**

**M26.32**   **Excessive spacing of fully erupted teeth**
Diastema of fully erupted tooth or teeth NOS

**M26.33**   **Horizontal displacement of fully erupted tooth or teeth**
Tipped tooth or teeth
Tipping of fully erupted tooth

**M26.34**   **Vertical displacement of fully erupted tooth or teeth**
Extruded tooth
Infraeruption of tooth or teeth
Supraeruption of tooth or teeth

**M26.35**   **Rotation of fully erupted tooth or teeth**

**M26.36**   **Insufficient interocclusal distance of fully erupted teeth (ridge)**
Lack of adequate intermaxillary vertical dimension of fully erupted teeth

**M26.37**   **Excessive interocclusal distance of fully erupted teeth**
Excessive intermaxillary vertical dimension of fully erupted teeth
Loss of occlusal vertical dimension of fully erupted teeth

**M26.39**   **Other anomalies of tooth position of fully erupted tooth or teeth**

**M26.4**   **Malocclusion, unspecified**

✓5ᵗʰ   **M26.5**   **Dentofacial functional abnormalities**
     *EXCLUDES 1*   *bruxism (F45.8)*
          *teeth-grinding NOS (F45.8)*

**M26.50**   **Dentofacial functional abnormalities, unspecified**

**M26.51**   **Abnormal jaw closure**

**M26.52**   **Limited mandibular range of motion**

**M26.53**   **Deviation in opening and closing of the mandible**

**M26.54**   **Insufficient anterior guidance**
Insufficient anterior occlusal guidance

**M26.55**   **Centric occlusion maximum intercuspation discrepancy**
     *EXCLUDES 1*   *centric occlusion NOS (M26.59)*

**M26.56**   **Non-working side interference**
Balancing side interference

**M26.57**   **Lack of posterior occlusal support**

**M26.59**   **Other dentofacial functional abnormalities**
Centric occlusion (of teeth) NOS
Malocclusion due to abnormal swallowing
Malocclusion due to mouth breathing
Malocclusion due to tongue, lip or finger habits

✓5ᵗʰ   **M26.6**   **Temporomandibular joint disorders**
     *EXCLUDES 2*   *current temporomandibular joint dislocation (SØ3.Ø)*
          *current temporomandibular joint sprain (SØ3.4)*

✓6ᵗʰ   **M26.60**   **Temporomandibular joint disorder, unspecified**

**M26.601**   **Right temporomandibular joint disorder, unspecified**

**M26.602**   **Left temporomandibular joint disorder, unspecified**

**M26.603**   **Bilateral temporomandibular joint disorder, unspecified**

**M26.609**   **Unspecified temporomandibular joint disorder, unspecified side**
Temporomandibular joint disorder NOS

**Temporomandibular Joint**

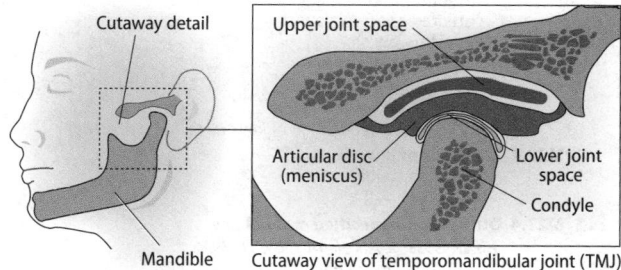

Cutaway view of temporomandibular joint (TMJ)

✓6ᵗʰ   **M26.61**   **Adhesions and ankylosis of temporomandibular joint**

**M26.611**   **Adhesions and ankylosis of right temporomandibular joint**

**M26.612**   **Adhesions and ankylosis of left temporomandibular joint**

**M26.613**   **Adhesions and ankylosis of bilateral temporomandibular joint**

**M26.619**   **Adhesions and ankylosis of temporomandibular joint, unspecified side**

✓6ᵗʰ   **M26.62**   **Arthralgia of temporomandibular joint**

**M26.621**   **Arthralgia of right temporomandibular joint**

**M26.622**   **Arthralgia of left temporomandibular joint**

**M26.623**   **Arthralgia of bilateral temporomandibular joint**

**M26.629**   **Arthralgia of temporomandibular joint, unspecified side**

✓6ᵗʰ   **M26.63**   **Articular disc disorder of temporomandibular joint**

**M26.631**   **Articular disc disorder of right temporomandibular joint**

**M26.632**   **Articular disc disorder of left temporomandibular joint**

**M26.633**   **Articular disc disorder of bilateral temporomandibular joint**

**M26.639**   **Articular disc disorder of temporomandibular joint, unspecified side**

**M26.69**   **Other specified disorders of temporomandibular joint**

✓5ᵗʰ   **M26.7**   **Dental alveolar anomalies**

**M26.70**   **Unspecified alveolar anomaly**

**M26.71**   **Alveolar maxillary hyperplasia**

**M26.72**   **Alveolar mandibular hyperplasia**

**M26.73**   **Alveolar maxillary hypoplasia**

**M26.74**   **Alveolar mandibular hypoplasia**

**M26.79**   **Other specified alveolar anomalies**

✓5ᵗʰ   **M26.8**   **Other dentofacial anomalies**

**M26.81**   **Anterior soft tissue impingement**
Anterior soft tissue impingement on teeth

**M26.82**   **Posterior soft tissue impingement**
Posterior soft tissue impingement on teeth

**M26.89**   **Other dentofacial anomalies**

**M26.9**   **Dentofacial anomaly, unspecified**

✓4ᵗʰ   **M27**   **Other diseases of jaws**

**M27.0**   **Developmental disorders of jaws**
Latent bone cyst of jaw
Stafne's cyst
Torus mandibularis
Torus palatinus

**M27.1**   **Giant cell granuloma, central**
Giant cell granuloma NOS
     *EXCLUDES 1*   *peripheral giant cell granuloma (KØ6.8)*

✓ Additional Character Req    ✓x7ᵗʰ Placeholder Alert    Unacceptable PDx    Manifestation    H1-H14 HAC    HCC CMS-HCC Condition    *EXCLUDES 1* Not Coded Here    *EXCLUDES 2* Not Included Here

ICD-10-CM 2018      769

**Chapter 13. Diseases of the Musculoskeletal System and Connective Tissue**

### M27.2 Inflammatory conditions of jaws
Osteitis of jaw(s)
Osteomyelitis (neonatal) jaw(s)
Osteoradionecrosis jaw(s)
Periostitis jaw(s)
Sequestrum of jaw bone
Use additional code (W88-W90, X39.0) to identify radiation, if radiation-induced
*EXCLUDES 2*   osteonecrosis of jaw due to drug (M87.180)

### M27.3 Alveolitis of jaws
Alveolar osteitis
Dry socket

### ✓5ᵗʰ M27.4 Other and unspecified cysts of jaw
*EXCLUDES 1*   cysts of oral region (K09.-)
latent bone cyst of jaw (M27.0)
Stafne's cyst (M27.0)

#### M27.40 Unspecified cyst of jaw
Cyst of jaw NOS

#### M27.49 Other cysts of jaw
Aneurysmal cyst of jaw
Hemorrhagic cyst of jaw
Traumatic cyst of jaw

### ✓5ᵗʰ M27.5 Periradicular pathology associated with previous endodontic treatment

#### M27.51 Perforation of root canal space due to endodontic treatment

#### M27.52 Endodontic overfill

#### M27.53 Endodontic underfill

#### M27.59 Other periradicular pathology associated with previous endodontic treatment

### ✓5ᵗʰ M27.6 Endosseous dental implant failure

#### M27.61 Osseointegration failure of dental implant
Hemorrhagic complications of dental implant placement
Iatrogenic osseointegration failure of dental implant
Osseointegration failure of dental implant due to complications of systemic disease
Osseointegration failure of dental implant due to poor bone quality
Pre-integration failure of dental implant NOS
Pre-osseointegration failure of dental implant

#### M27.62 Post-osseointegration biological failure of dental implant
Failure of dental implant due to lack of attached gingiva
Failure of dental implant due to occlusal trauma (caused by poor prosthetic design)
Failure of dental implant due to parafunctional habits
Failure of dental implant due to periodontal infection (peri-implantitis)
Failure of dental implant due to poor oral hygiene
Iatrogenic post-osseointegration failure of dental implant
Post-osseointegration failure of dental implant due to complications of systemic disease

#### M27.63 Post-osseointegration mechanical failure of dental implant
Failure of dental prosthesis causing loss of dental implant
Fracture of dental implant
*EXCLUDES 2*   cracked tooth (K03.81)
fractured dental restorative material with loss of material (K08.531)
fractured dental restorative material without loss of material (K08.530)
fractured tooth (S02.5)

#### M27.69 Other endosseous dental implant failure
Dental implant failure NOS

### M27.8 Other specified diseases of jaws
Cherubism
Exostosis
Fibrous dysplasia
Unilateral condylar hyperplasia
Unilateral condylar hypoplasia
*EXCLUDES 1*   jaw pain (R68.84)

### M27.9 Disease of jaws, unspecified

## Systemic connective tissue disorders (M30-M36)
**INCLUDES**   autoimmune disease NOS
collagen (vascular) disease NOS
systemic autoimmune disease
systemic collagen (vascular) disease
*EXCLUDES 1*   autoimmune disease, single organ or single cell-type—code to relevant condition category

### ✓4ᵗʰ M30 Polyarteritis nodosa and related conditions
*EXCLUDES 1*   microscopic polyarteritis (M31.7)

**CC Excl: For CC codes in category M30, unless otherwise noted:** PDX collection 874

#### M30.0 Polyarteritis nodosa   `CC` `HCC`

#### M30.1 Polyarteritis with lung involvement [Churg-Strauss]   `CC` `HCC`
Allergic granulomatous angiitis

#### M30.2 Juvenile polyarteritis   `CC` `HCC`

#### M30.3 Mucocutaneous lymph node syndrome [Kawasaki]   `CC` `HCC`
**CC Excl:** PDX collection 875

#### M30.8 Other conditions related to polyarteritis nodosa   `CC` `HCC`
Polyangiitis overlap syndrome

### ✓4ᵗʰ M31 Other necrotizing vasculopathies

**CC Excl: For CC/MCC codes in category M31, unless otherwise noted:** PDX collection 874

#### M31.0 Hypersensitivity angiitis   `CC` `HCC`
Goodpasture's syndrome

#### M31.1 Thrombotic microangiopathy   `MCC` `HCC`
Thrombotic thrombocytopenic purpura

#### M31.2 Lethal midline granuloma   `CC` `HCC`

### ✓5ᵗʰ M31.3 Wegener's granulomatosis
Necrotizing respiratory granulomatosis

#### M31.30 Wegener's granulomatosis without renal involvement   `CC` `HCC`
Wegener's granulomatosis NOS

#### M31.31 Wegener's granulomatosis with renal involvement   `CC` `HCC`

#### M31.4 Aortic arch syndrome [Takayasu]   `CC` `HCC`

#### M31.5 Giant cell arteritis with polymyalgia rheumatica   `HCC`

#### M31.6 Other giant cell arteritis   `HCC`

#### M31.7 Microscopic polyangiitis   `CC` `HCC`
Microscopic polyarteritis
*EXCLUDES 1*   polyarteritis nodosa (M30.0)

#### M31.8 Other specified necrotizing vasculopathies   `CC` `HCC`
Hypocomplementemic vasculitis
Septic vasculitis
**CC Excl:** PDX collection 712

#### M31.9 Necrotizing vasculopathy, unspecified   `CC` `HCC`
**CC Excl:** PDX collection 712

### ✓4ᵗʰ M32 Systemic lupus erythematosus (SLE)
*EXCLUDES 1*   lupus erythematosus (discoid) (NOS) (L93.0)

#### M32.0 Drug-induced systemic lupus erythematosus   `HCC`
Use additional code for adverse effect, if applicable, to identify drug (T36-T50 with fifth or sixth character 5)

### ✓5ᵗʰ M32.1 Systemic lupus erythematosus with organ or system involvement

#### M32.10 Systemic lupus erythematosus, organ or system involvement unspecified   `HCC`

#### M32.11 Endocarditis in systemic lupus erythematosus   `PDxCC` `CC` `HCC`
Libman-Sacks disease
**CC Excl:** PDX collection 676

#### M32.12 Pericarditis in systemic lupus erythematosus   `PDxCC` `CC` `HCC`
Lupus pericarditis
**CC Excl:** PDX collection 673

#### M32.13 Lung involvement in systemic lupus erythematosus   `HCC`
Pleural effusion due to systemic lupus erythematosus

#### M32.14 Glomerular disease in systemic lupus erythematosus   `HCC`
Lupus renal disease NOS
**AHA:** 2013, 4Q, 125

#### M32.15 Tubulo-interstitial nephropathy in systemic lupus erythematosus   `HCC`

#### M32.19 Other organ or system involvement in systemic lupus erythematosus   `HCC`

#### M32.8 Other forms of systemic lupus erythematosus   `HCC`

---

`N` Newborn: 0   `P` Pediatric: 0-17   `M` Maternity: 12-55   `A` Adult: 15-124   `MCC` Major CC Condition   `PDxMCC` PDx acts as own MCC   `CC` CC Condition   `PDxCC` PDx acts as own CC

770      ICD-10-CM 2018

**M32.9 Systemic lupus erythematosus,** unspecified `HCC`
SLE NOS
Systemic lupus erythematosus NOS
Systemic lupus erythematosus without organ involvement

✓4ᵗʰ **M33 Dermatopolymyositis**

**CC Excl: For CC codes in category M33, unless otherwise noted:**
PDX collection 876

▲ ✓5ᵗʰ **M33.0 Juvenile dermatomyositis**

▲ **M33.00 Juvenile dermatomyositis, organ** `CC` `HCC`
**involvement** unspecified

▲ **M33.01 Juvenile dermatomyositis with** respiratory `CC` `HCC`
**involvement**

▲ **M33.02 Juvenile dermatomyositis with** `PDxCC` `CC` `HCC`
myopathy
CC Excl: PDX collection 877

● **M33.03 Juvenile dermatomyositis without myopathy** `CC`

▲ **M33.09 Juvenile dermatomyositis with** other organ `CC` `HCC`
involvement

▲ ✓5ᵗʰ **M33.1 Other dermatomyositis** ◄
▶Adult dermatomyositis◄

▲ **M33.10 Other dermatomyositis, organ involvement** `CC` `HCC`
**unspecified**

▲ **M33.11 Other dermatomyositis with** respiratory `CC` `HCC`
**involvement**

▲ **M33.12 Other dermatomyositis with** myopathy `PDxCC` `CC` `HCC`
CC Excl: PDX collection 877

● **M33.13 Other dermatomyositis without myopathy** `CC`
Dermatomyositis NOS

▲ **M33.19 Other dermatomyositis with** other organ `CC` `HCC`
involvement

✓5ᵗʰ **M33.2 Polymyositis**

**M33.20 Polymyositis, organ involvement** unspecified `CC` `HCC`
CC Excl: PDX collection 878

**M33.21 Polymyositis with** respiratory involvement `CC` `HCC`
CC Excl: PDX collection 878

**M33.22 Polymyositis with** myopathy `PDxCC` `CC` `HCC`
CC Excl: PDX collection 879

**M33.29 Polymyositis with** other organ involvement `CC` `HCC`
CC Excl: PDX collection 878

✓5ᵗʰ **M33.9 Dermatopolymyositis,** unspecified

**M33.90 Dermatopolymyositis, unspecified, organ** `CC` `HCC`
**involvement** unspecified

**M33.91 Dermatopolymyositis, unspecified with** `CC` `HCC`
respiratory **involvement**

**M33.92 Dermatopolymyositis, unspecified with** `PDxCC` `CC` `HCC`
myopathy
CC Excl: PDX collection 877

● **M33.93 Dermatopolymyositis, unspecified without** `CC`
myopathy

**M33.99 Dermatopolymyositis, unspecified with** `CC` `HCC`
other organ involvement

✓4ᵗʰ **M34 Systemic sclerosis [scleroderma]**
*EXCLUDES 1* *circumscribed scleroderma (L94.0)*
*neonatal scleroderma (P83.8)*

**M34.0 Progressive** systemic sclerosis `HCC`

**M34.1 CR(E)ST syndrome** `HCC`
Combination of calcinosis, Raynaud's phenomenon, esophageal
dysfunction, sclerodactyly, telangiectasia

**M34.2 Systemic sclerosis** induced by drug and chemical `HCC`
Code first poisoning due to drug or toxin, if applicable (T36-T65
with fifth or sixth character 1-4 or 6)
Use additional code for adverse effect, if applicable, to identify
drug (T36-T50 with fifth or sixth character 5)

✓5ᵗʰ **M34.8 Other forms of systemic sclerosis**

**M34.81 Systemic sclerosis with** lung `PDxCC` `CC` `HCC`
**involvement**
CC Excl: No excl

**M34.82 Systemic sclerosis with** myopathy `PDxCC` `CC` `HCC`
CC Excl: PDX collection 867

**M34.83 Systemic sclerosis with** polyneuropathy `HCC`

**M34.89 Other** systemic sclerosis `HCC`

**M34.9 Systemic sclerosis,** unspecified `HCC`

✓4ᵗʰ **M35 Other systemic involvement of connective tissue**
*EXCLUDES 1* *reactive perforating collagenosis (L87.1)*

✓5ᵗʰ **M35.0 Sicca syndrome [Sjögren]**
**DEF:** Autoimmune disease; associated with keratoconjunctivitis,
laryngopharyngitis, rhinitis, dry mouth, enlarged parotid gland,
and chronic polyarthritis.

**M35.00 Sicca syndrome,** unspecified `HCC`

**M35.01 Sicca syndrome with** keratoconjunctivitis `HCC`

**M35.02 Sicca syndrome with** lung involvement `HCC`

**M35.03 Sicca syndrome with** myopathy `PDxCC` `CC` `HCC`
CC Excl: PDX collection 867

**M35.04 Sicca syndrome with** tubulo-interstitial `HCC`
**nephropathy**
Renal tubular acidosis in sicca syndrome

**M35.09 Sicca syndrome with** other organ **involvement** `HCC`

**M35.1 Other overlap syndromes** `CC` `HCC`
Mixed connective tissue disease
*EXCLUDES 1* *polyangiitis overlap syndrome (M30.8)*
CC Excl: PDX collection 880

**M35.2 Behçet's disease** `CC` `HCC`
CC Excl: PDX collection 863

**M35.3 Polymyalgia rheumatica** `HCC`
*EXCLUDES 1* *polymyalgia rheumatica with giant cell arteritis*
*(M31.5)*

**M35.4 Diffuse (eosinophilic) fasciitis**

**M35.5 Multifocal fibrosclerosis** `CC` `HCC`
CC Excl: PDX collection 880

**M35.6 Relapsing panniculitis [Weber-Christian]**
*EXCLUDES 1* *lupus panniculitis (L93.2)*
*panniculitis NOS (M79.3-)*

**M35.7 Hypermobility syndrome**
Familial ligamentous laxity
*EXCLUDES 1* *Ehlers-Danlos syndrome (Q79.6)*
*ligamentous laxity, NOS (M24.2-)*

**M35.8 Other specified systemic involvement of connective** `CC` `HCC`
**tissue**
CC Excl: PDX collection 880

**M35.9 Systemic involvement of connective tissue, unspecified** `HCC`
Autoimmune disease (systemic) NOS
Collagen (vascular) disease NOS

✓4ᵗʰ **M36 Systemic disorders of connective tissue in diseases classified**
**elsewhere**
*EXCLUDES 2* *arthropathies in diseases classified elsewhere (M14.-)*

**M36.0 Dermato(poly)myositis in neoplastic disease** `CC` `HCC`
Code first underlying neoplasm (C00-D49)
CC Excl: PDX collection 876

**M36.1 Arthropathy in neoplastic disease**
Code first underlying neoplasm, such as:
leukemia (C91-C95)
malignant histiocytosis (C96.A)
multiple myeloma (C90.0)

**M36.2 Hemophilic arthropathy**
Hemarthrosis in hemophilic arthropathy
Code first underlying disease, such as:
factor VIII deficiency (D66)
with vascular defect (D68.0)
factor IX deficiency (D67)
hemophilia (classical) (D66)
hemophilia B (D67)
hemophilia C (D68.1)

**M36.3 Arthropathy in other blood disorders**

**M36.4 Arthropathy in hypersensitivity reactions classified elsewhere**
Code first underlying disease, such as:
Henoch (-Schönlein) purpura (D69.0)
serum sickness (T80.6-)

**M36.8 Systemic disorders of connective tissue in other diseases** `HCC`
**classified elsewhere**
Code first underlying disease, such as:
alkaptonuria (E70.2)
hypogammaglobulinemia (D80.-)
ochronosis (E70.2)

# DORSOPATHIES (M40–M54)

## Deforming dorsopathies (M40-M43)

### ✓4th M40 Kyphosis and lordosis

**EXCLUDES 1** *congenital kyphosis and lordosis (Q76.4)*
*kyphoscoliosis (M41.-)*
*postprocedural kyphosis and lordosis (M96.-)*

**✓5th M40.0 Postural kyphosis**

**EXCLUDES 1** *osteochondrosis of spine (M42.-)*

- **M40.00** Postural kyphosis, site unspecified
- **M40.03** Postural kyphosis, cervicothoracic **region**
- **M40.04** Postural kyphosis, thoracic **region**
- **M40.05** Postural kyphosis, thoracolumbar **region**

**✓5th M40.1 Other secondary kyphosis**

- **M40.10** Other secondary kyphosis, site unspecified
- **M40.12** Other secondary kyphosis, cervical **region**
- **M40.13** Other secondary kyphosis, cervicothoracic **region**
- **M40.14** Other secondary kyphosis, thoracic **region**
- **M40.15** Other secondary kyphosis, thoracolumbar **region**

**✓5th M40.2 Other and unspecified kyphosis**

**✓6th M40.20 Unspecified kyphosis**

- **M40.202** Unspecified kyphosis, cervical region
- **M40.203** Unspecified kyphosis, cervicothoracic region
- **M40.204** Unspecified kyphosis, thoracic region
- **M40.205** Unspecified kyphosis, thoracolumbar region
- **M40.209** Unspecified kyphosis, site unspecified

**✓6th M40.29 Other kyphosis**

- **M40.292** Other kyphosis, cervical **region**
- **M40.293** Other kyphosis, cervicothoracic **region**
- **M40.294** Other kyphosis, thoracic **region**
- **M40.295** Other kyphosis, thoracolumbar **region**
- **M40.299** Other kyphosis, site unspecified

**✓5th M40.3 Flatback syndrome**

- **M40.30** Flatback syndrome, site unspecified
- **M40.35** Flatback syndrome, thoracolumbar **region**
- **M40.36** Flatback syndrome, lumbar **region**
- **M40.37** Flatback syndrome, lumbosacral **region**

**✓5th M40.4 Postural lordosis**
Acquired lordosis

- **M40.40** Postural lordosis, site unspecified
- **M40.45** Postural lordosis, thoracolumbar **region**
- **M40.46** Postural lordosis, lumbar **region**
- **M40.47** Postural lordosis, lumbosacral **region**

**✓5th M40.5 Lordosis, unspecified**

- **M40.50** Lordosis, unspecified, site unspecified
- **M40.55** Lordosis, unspecified, thoracolumbar **region**
- **M40.56** Lordosis, unspecified, lumbar **region**
- **M40.57** Lordosis, unspecified, lumbosacral **region**

### ✓4th M41 Scoliosis

**INCLUDES** kyphoscoliosis

**EXCLUDES 1** *congenital scoliosis due to bony malformation (Q76.3)*
*congenital scoliosis NOS (Q67.5)*
*kyphoscoliotic heart disease (I27.1)*
*postprocedural scoliosis (M96.-)*
*postural congenital scoliosis (Q67.5)*

**✓5th M41.0 Infantile idiopathic scoliosis**
**AHA:** 2014, 4Q, 26

- **M41.00** Infantile idiopathic scoliosis, site unspecified
- **M41.02** Infantile idiopathic scoliosis, cervical **region**
- **M41.03** Infantile idiopathic scoliosis, cervicothoracic **region**
- **M41.04** Infantile idiopathic scoliosis, thoracic **region**
- **M41.05** Infantile idiopathic scoliosis, thoracolumbar **region**
- **M41.06** Infantile idiopathic scoliosis, lumbar **region**
- **M41.07** Infantile idiopathic scoliosis, lumbosacral **region**
- **M41.08** Infantile idiopathic scoliosis, sacral and sacrococcygeal **region**

**✓5th M41.1 Juvenile and adolescent idiopathic scoliosis**

**✓6th M41.11 Juvenile idiopathic scoliosis**
**AHA:** 2014, 4Q, 28

- **M41.112** Juvenile idiopathic scoliosis, cervical **region**
- **M41.113** Juvenile idiopathic scoliosis, cervicothoracic **region**
- **M41.114** Juvenile idiopathic scoliosis, thoracic **region**
- **M41.115** Juvenile idiopathic scoliosis, thoracolumbar **region**
- **M41.116** Juvenile idiopathic scoliosis, lumbar **region**
- **M41.117** Juvenile idiopathic scoliosis, lumbosacral **region**
- **M41.119** Juvenile idiopathic scoliosis, site unspecified

**✓6th M41.12 Adolescent scoliosis**

- **M41.122** Adolescent idiopathic scoliosis, cervical **region**
- **M41.123** Adolescent idiopathic scoliosis, cervicothoracic **region**
- **M41.124** Adolescent idiopathic scoliosis, thoracic **region**
- **M41.125** Adolescent idiopathic scoliosis, thoracolumbar **region**
- **M41.126** Adolescent idiopathic scoliosis, lumbar **region**
- **M41.127** Adolescent idiopathic scoliosis, lumbosacral **region**
- **M41.129** Adolescent idiopathic scoliosis, site unspecified

**✓5th M41.2 Other idiopathic scoliosis**

- **M41.20** Other idiopathic scoliosis, site unspecified
- **M41.22** Other idiopathic scoliosis, cervical **region**

### Kyphosis and Lordosis

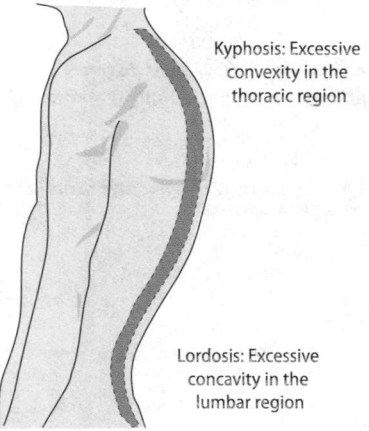

Kyphosis: Excessive convexity in the thoracic region

Lordosis: Excessive concavity in the lumbar region

### Scoliosis

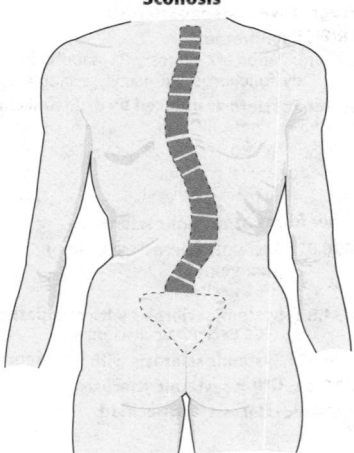

Lateral curvature of spine

**N** Newborn: 0   **P** Pediatric: 0-17   **M** Maternity: 12-55   **A** Adult: 15-124   **MCC** Major CC Condition   **PDx MCC** PDx acts as own MCC   **CC** CC Condition   **PDx CC** PDx acts as own CC

772          ICD-10-CM 2018

M41.23   **Other idiopathic scoliosis, cervicothoracic region**
M41.24   **Other idiopathic scoliosis, thoracic region**
M41.25   **Other idiopathic scoliosis, thoracolumbar region**
M41.26   **Other idiopathic scoliosis, lumbar region**
M41.27   **Other idiopathic scoliosis, lumbosacral region**

✓5ᵗʰ **M41.3   Thoracogenic scoliosis**
M41.30   **Thoracogenic scoliosis, site unspecified**
M41.34   **Thoracogenic scoliosis, thoracic region**
M41.35   **Thoracogenic scoliosis, thoracolumbar region**

✓5ᵗʰ **M41.4   Neuromuscular scoliosis**
Scoliosis secondary to cerebral palsy, Friedreich's ataxia, poliomyelitis and other neuromuscular disorders
Code also underlying condition
**AHA:** 2014, 4Q, 27
M41.40   **Neuromuscular scoliosis, site unspecified**
M41.41   **Neuromuscular scoliosis, occipito-atlanto-axial region**
M41.42   **Neuromuscular scoliosis, cervical region**
M41.43   **Neuromuscular scoliosis, cervicothoracic region**
M41.44   **Neuromuscular scoliosis, thoracic region**
M41.45   **Neuromuscular scoliosis, thoracolumbar region**
M41.46   **Neuromuscular scoliosis, lumbar region**
M41.47   **Neuromuscular scoliosis, lumbosacral region**

✓5ᵗʰ **M41.5   Other secondary scoliosis**
M41.50   **Other secondary scoliosis, site unspecified**
M41.52   **Other secondary scoliosis, cervical region**
M41.53   **Other secondary scoliosis, cervicothoracic region**
M41.54   **Other secondary scoliosis, thoracic region**
M41.55   **Other secondary scoliosis, thoracolumbar region**
M41.56   **Other secondary scoliosis, lumbar region**
M41.57   **Other secondary scoliosis, lumbosacral region**

✓5ᵗʰ **M41.8   Other forms of scoliosis**
M41.80   **Other forms of scoliosis, site unspecified**
M41.82   **Other forms of scoliosis, cervical region**
M41.83   **Other forms of scoliosis, cervicothoracic region**
M41.84   **Other forms of scoliosis, thoracic region**
M41.85   **Other forms of scoliosis, thoracolumbar region**
M41.86   **Other forms of scoliosis, lumbar region**
M41.87   **Other forms of scoliosis, lumbosacral region**

M41.9   **Scoliosis, unspecified**

✓4ᵗʰ **M42   Spinal osteochondrosis**

✓5ᵗʰ **M42.0   Juvenile osteochondrosis of spine**
Calvé's disease
Scheuermann's disease
*EXCLUDES 1*   postural kyphosis (M40.0)
M42.00   **Juvenile osteochondrosis of spine, site unspecified**
M42.01   **Juvenile osteochondrosis of spine, occipito-atlanto-axial region**
M42.02   **Juvenile osteochondrosis of spine, cervical region**
M42.03   **Juvenile osteochondrosis of spine, cervicothoracic region**
M42.04   **Juvenile osteochondrosis of spine, thoracic region**
M42.05   **Juvenile osteochondrosis of spine, thoracolumbar region**
M42.06   **Juvenile osteochondrosis of spine, lumbar region**
M42.07   **Juvenile osteochondrosis of spine, lumbosacral region**
M42.08   **Juvenile osteochondrosis of spine, sacral and sacrococcygeal region**
M42.09   **Juvenile osteochondrosis of spine, multiple sites in spine**

✓5ᵗʰ **M42.1   Adult osteochondrosis of spine**
M42.10   **Adult osteochondrosis of spine, site unspecified**   Ⓐ
M42.11   **Adult osteochondrosis of spine, occipito-atlanto-axial region**   Ⓐ
M42.12   **Adult osteochondrosis of spine, cervical region**   Ⓐ
M42.13   **Adult osteochondrosis of spine, cervicothoracic region**   Ⓐ
M42.14   **Adult osteochondrosis of spine, thoracic region**   Ⓐ
M42.15   **Adult osteochondrosis of spine, thoracolumbar region**   Ⓐ
M42.16   **Adult osteochondrosis of spine, lumbar region**   Ⓐ
M42.17   **Adult osteochondrosis of spine, lumbosacral region**   Ⓐ
M42.18   **Adult osteochondrosis of spine, sacral and sacrococcygeal region**   Ⓐ
M42.19   **Adult osteochondrosis of spine, multiple sites in spine**   Ⓐ
M42.9   **Spinal osteochondrosis, unspecified**

✓4ᵗʰ **M43   Other deforming dorsopathies**
*EXCLUDES 1*   congenital spondylolysis and spondylolisthesis (Q76.2)
hemivertebra (Q76.3-Q76.4)
Klippel-Feil syndrome (Q76.1)
lumbarization and sacralization (Q76.4)
platyspondylisis (Q76.4)
spina bifida occulta (Q76.0)
spinal curvature in osteoporosis (M80.-)
spinal curvature in Paget's disease of bone [osteitis deformans] (M88.-)

✓5ᵗʰ **M43.0   Spondylolysis**
*EXCLUDES 1*   congenital spondylolysis (Q76.2)
spondylolisthesis (M43.1)
M43.00   **Spondylolysis, site unspecified**
M43.01   **Spondylolysis, occipito-atlanto-axial region**
M43.02   **Spondylolysis, cervical region**
M43.03   **Spondylolysis, cervicothoracic region**
M43.04   **Spondylolysis, thoracic region**
M43.05   **Spondylolysis, thoracolumbar region**
M43.06   **Spondylolysis, lumbar region**
M43.07   **Spondylolysis, lumbosacral region**
M43.08   **Spondylolysis, sacral and sacrococcygeal region**
M43.09   **Spondylolysis, multiple sites in spine**

✓5ᵗʰ **M43.1   Spondylolisthesis**
*EXCLUDES 1*   acute traumatic of lumbosacral region (S33.1)
acute traumatic of sites other than lumbosacral— code to Fracture, vertebra, by region
congenital spondylolisthesis (Q76.2)
M43.10   **Spondylolisthesis, site unspecified**
M43.11   **Spondylolisthesis, occipito-atlanto-axial region**
M43.12   **Spondylolisthesis, cervical region**
M43.13   **Spondylolisthesis, cervicothoracic region**
M43.14   **Spondylolisthesis, thoracic region**
M43.15   **Spondylolisthesis, thoracolumbar region**
M43.16   **Spondylolisthesis, lumbar region**
M43.17   **Spondylolisthesis, lumbosacral region**
M43.18   **Spondylolisthesis, sacral and sacrococcygeal region**
M43.19   **Spondylolisthesis, multiple sites in spine**

✓5ᵗʰ **M43.2   Fusion of spine**
Ankylosis of spinal joint
*EXCLUDES 1*   ankylosing spondylitis (M45.0-)
congenital fusion of spine (Q76.4)
*EXCLUDES 2*   arthrodesis status (Z98.1)
pseudoarthrosis after fusion or arthrodesis (M96.0)
M43.20   **Fusion of spine, site unspecified**
M43.21   **Fusion of spine, occipito-atlanto-axial region**
M43.22   **Fusion of spine, cervical region**
M43.23   **Fusion of spine, cervicothoracic region**
M43.24   **Fusion of spine, thoracic region**
M43.25   **Fusion of spine, thoracolumbar region**
M43.26   **Fusion of spine, lumbar region**
M43.27   **Fusion of spine, lumbosacral region**
M43.28   **Fusion of spine, sacral and sacrococcygeal region**

M43.3   **Recurrent atlantoaxial dislocation with myelopathy**
M43.4   **Other recurrent atlantoaxial dislocation**

✓5ᵗʰ **M43.5   Other recurrent vertebral dislocation**
*EXCLUDES 1*   biomechanical lesions NEC (M99.-)
✓6ᵗʰ **M43.5X   Other recurrent vertebral dislocation**
M43.5X2   **Other recurrent vertebral dislocation, cervical region**
M43.5X3   **Other recurrent vertebral dislocation, cervicothoracic region**
M43.5X4   **Other recurrent vertebral dislocation, thoracic region**
M43.5X5   **Other recurrent vertebral dislocation, thoracolumbar region**

✓ Additional Character Req   ✓x7ᵗʰ Placeholder Alert   Unacceptable PDx   **Manifestation**   H1 - H14 HAC   HCC CMS-HCC Condition   *EXCLUDES 1* Not Coded Here   *EXCLUDES 2* Not Included Here

ICD-10-CM 2018      773

Chapter 13. Diseases of the Musculoskeletal System and Connective Tissue

M41.23–M43.5X5

**M43.5X6**   **Other recurrent vertebral dislocation, lumbar region**

**M43.5X7**   **Other recurrent vertebral dislocation, lumbosacral region**

**M43.5X8**   **Other recurrent vertebral dislocation, sacral and sacrococcygeal region**

**M43.5X9**   **Other recurrent vertebral dislocation, site unspecified**

**M43.6 Torticollis**
> *EXCLUDES 1*   congenital (sternomastoid) torticollis (Q68.0)
> current injury—see Injury, of spine, by body region
> ocular torticollis (R29.891)
> psychogenic torticollis (F45.8)
> spasmodic torticollis (G24.3)
> torticollis due to birth injury (P15.2)

✓5ᵗʰ **M43.8 Other specified deforming dorsopathies**
> *EXCLUDES 2*   kyphosis and lordosis (M40.-)
> scoliosis (M41.-)

   ✓6ᵗʰ **M43.8X**   **Other specified deforming dorsopathies**

**M43.8X1**   **Other specified deforming dorsopathies, occipito-atlanto-axial region**

**M43.8X2**   **Other specified deforming dorsopathies, cervical region**

**M43.8X3**   **Other specified deforming dorsopathies, cervicothoracic region**

**M43.8X4**   **Other specified deforming dorsopathies, thoracic region**

**M43.8X5**   **Other specified deforming dorsopathies, thoracolumbar region**

**M43.8X6**   **Other specified deforming dorsopathies, lumbar region**

**M43.8X7**   **Other specified deforming dorsopathies, lumbosacral region**

**M43.8X8**   **Other specified deforming dorsopathies, sacral and sacrococcygeal region**

**M43.8X9**   **Other specified deforming dorsopathies, site unspecified**

**M43.9 Deforming dorsopathy, unspecified**
> Curvature of spine NOS

## Spondylopathies (M45-M49)

✓4ᵗʰ **M45 Ankylosing spondylitis**
> Rheumatoid arthritis of spine
> *EXCLUDES 1*   arthropathy in Reiter's disease (M02.3-)
> juvenile (ankylosing) spondylitis (M08.1)
> *EXCLUDES 2*   Behçet's disease (M35.2)

**M45.0 Ankylosing spondylitis of multiple sites in spine**   `HCC`

**M45.1 Ankylosing spondylitis of occipito-atlanto-axial region**   `HCC`

**M45.2 Ankylosing spondylitis of cervical region**   `HCC`

**M45.3 Ankylosing spondylitis of cervicothoracic region**   `HCC`

**M45.4 Ankylosing spondylitis of thoracic region**   `HCC`

**M45.5 Ankylosing spondylitis of thoracolumbar region**   `HCC`

**M45.6 Ankylosing spondylitis lumbar region**   `HCC`

**M45.7 Ankylosing spondylitis of lumbosacral region**   `HCC`

**M45.8 Ankylosing spondylitis sacral and sacrococcygeal region**   `HCC`

**M45.9 Ankylosing spondylitis of unspecified sites in spine**   `HCC`

✓4ᵗʰ **M46 Other inflammatory spondylopathies**

   ✓5ᵗʰ **M46.0 Spinal enthesopathy**
> Disorder of ligamentous or muscular attachments of spine

**M46.00**   **Spinal enthesopathy, site unspecified**   `HCC`

**M46.01**   **Spinal enthesopathy, occipito-atlanto-axial region**   `HCC`

**M46.02**   **Spinal enthesopathy, cervical region**   `HCC`

**M46.03**   **Spinal enthesopathy, cervicothoracic region**   `HCC`

**M46.04**   **Spinal enthesopathy, thoracic region**   `HCC`

**M46.05**   **Spinal enthesopathy, thoracolumbar region**   `HCC`

**M46.06**   **Spinal enthesopathy, lumbar region**   `HCC`

**M46.07**   **Spinal enthesopathy, lumbosacral region**   `HCC`

**M46.08**   **Spinal enthesopathy, sacral and sacrococcygeal region**   `HCC`

**M46.09**   **Spinal enthesopathy, multiple sites in spine**   `HCC`

**M46.1 Sacroiliitis, not elsewhere classified**   `HCC`
> **DEF:** Inflammation of sacroiliac joint (situated at juncture of sacrum and hip); characterized by pain in buttocks or lower back that can extend down one or both legs.

---

✓5ᵗʰ **M46.2 Osteomyelitis of vertebra**

> **CC Excl: For CC codes in subcategory M46.2:**
> PDX collection 881

**M46.20**   **Osteomyelitis of vertebra, site unspecified**   `CC` `HCC`

**M46.21**   **Osteomyelitis of vertebra, occipito-atlanto-axial region**   `HCC`

**M46.22**   **Osteomyelitis of vertebra, cervical region**   `CC` `HCC`

**M46.23**   **Osteomyelitis of vertebra, cervicothoracic region**   `CC` `HCC`

**M46.24**   **Osteomyelitis of vertebra, thoracic region**   `CC` `HCC`

**M46.25**   **Osteomyelitis of vertebra, thoracolumbar region**   `CC` `HCC`

**M46.26**   **Osteomyelitis of vertebra, lumbar region**   `CC` `HCC`

**M46.27**   **Osteomyelitis of vertebra, lumbosacral region**   `CC` `HCC`

**M46.28**   **Osteomyelitis of vertebra, sacral and sacrococcygeal region**   `CC` `HCC`

✓5ᵗʰ **M46.3 Infection of intervertebral disc (pyogenic)**
> Use additional code (B95-B97) to identify infectious agent

> **CC Excl: For CC codes in subcategory M46.3:**
> PDX collection 882

**M46.30**   **Infection of intervertebral disc (pyogenic), site unspecified**   `CC` `HCC`

**M46.31**   **Infection of intervertebral disc (pyogenic), occipito-atlanto-axial region**   `CC` `HCC`

**M46.32**   **Infection of intervertebral disc (pyogenic), cervical region**   `CC` `HCC`

**M46.33**   **Infection of intervertebral disc (pyogenic), cervicothoracic region**   `CC` `HCC`

**M46.34**   **Infection of intervertebral disc (pyogenic), thoracic region**   `CC` `HCC`

**M46.35**   **Infection of intervertebral disc (pyogenic), thoracolumbar region**   `CC` `HCC`

**M46.36**   **Infection of intervertebral disc (pyogenic), lumbar region**   `CC` `HCC`

**M46.37**   **Infection of intervertebral disc (pyogenic), lumbosacral region**   `CC` `HCC`

**M46.38**   **Infection of intervertebral disc (pyogenic), sacral and sacrococcygeal region**   `CC` `HCC`

**M46.39**   **Infection of intervertebral disc (pyogenic), multiple sites in spine**   `CC` `HCC`

✓5ᵗʰ **M46.4 Discitis, unspecified**

**M46.40**   **Discitis, unspecified, site unspecified**

**M46.41**   **Discitis, unspecified, occipito-atlanto-axial region**

**M46.42**   **Discitis, unspecified, cervical region**

**M46.43**   **Discitis, unspecified, cervicothoracic region**

**M46.44**   **Discitis, unspecified, thoracic region**

**M46.45**   **Discitis, unspecified, thoracolumbar region**

**M46.46**   **Discitis, unspecified, lumbar region**

**M46.47**   **Discitis, unspecified, lumbosacral region**

**M46.48**   **Discitis, unspecified, sacral and sacrococcygeal region**

**M46.49**   **Discitis, unspecified, multiple sites in spine**

✓5ᵗʰ **M46.5 Other infective spondylopathies**

**M46.50**   **Other infective spondylopathies, site unspecified**   `HCC`

**M46.51**   **Other infective spondylopathies, occipito-atlanto-axial region**   `HCC`

**M46.52**   **Other infective spondylopathies, cervical region**   `HCC`

**M46.53**   **Other infective spondylopathies, cervicothoracic region**   `HCC`

**M46.54**   **Other infective spondylopathies, thoracic region**   `HCC`

**M46.55**   **Other infective spondylopathies, thoracolumbar region**   `HCC`

**M46.56**   **Other infective spondylopathies, lumbar region**   `HCC`

**M46.57**   **Other infective spondylopathies, lumbosacral region**   `HCC`

**M46.58**   **Other infective spondylopathies, sacral and sacrococcygeal region**   `HCC`

**M46.59**   **Other infective spondylopathies, multiple sites in spine**   `HCC`

---

Ⓝ Newborn: 0   Ⓟ Pediatric: 0-17   Ⓜ Maternity: 12-55   Ⓐ Adult: 15-124   `MCC` Major CC Condition   `PDxMCC` PDx acts as own MCC   `CC` CC Condition   `PDxCC` PDx acts as own CC

774        ICD-10-CM 2018

✓5ᵗʰ **M46.8 Other specified inflammatory spondylopathies**

**M46.80** Other specified inflammatory spondylopathies, HCC
site unspecified

**M46.81** Other specified inflammatory spondylopathies, HCC
occipito-atlanto-axial region

**M46.82** Other specified inflammatory spondylopathies, HCC
cervical region

**M46.83** Other specified inflammatory spondylopathies, HCC
cervicothoracic region

**M46.84** Other specified inflammatory spondylopathies, HCC
thoracic region

**M46.85** Other specified inflammatory spondylopathies, HCC
thoracolumbar region

**M46.86** Other specified inflammatory spondylopathies, HCC
lumbar region

**M46.87** Other specified inflammatory spondylopathies, HCC
lumbosacral region

**M46.88** Other specified inflammatory spondylopathies, HCC
sacral and sacrococcygeal region

**M46.89** Other specified inflammatory spondylopathies, HCC
multiple sites in spine

✓5ᵗʰ **M46.9 Unspecified inflammatory spondylopathy**

**M46.90** Unspecified inflammatory spondylopathy, HCC
site unspecified

**M46.91** Unspecified inflammatory spondylopathy, HCC
occipito-atlanto-axial region

**M46.92** Unspecified inflammatory spondylopathy, HCC
cervical region

**M46.93** Unspecified inflammatory spondylopathy, HCC
cervicothoracic region

**M46.94** Unspecified inflammatory spondylopathy, HCC
thoracic region

**M46.95** Unspecified inflammatory spondylopathy, HCC
thoracolumbar region

**M46.96** Unspecified inflammatory spondylopathy, HCC
lumbar region

**M46.97** Unspecified inflammatory spondylopathy, HCC
lumbosacral region

**M46.98** Unspecified inflammatory spondylopathy, HCC
sacral and sacrococcygeal region

**M46.99** Unspecified inflammatory spondylopathy, HCC
multiple sites in spine

✓4ᵗʰ **M47 Spondylosis**

INCLUDES   arthrosis or osteoarthritis of spine
degeneration of facet joints

✓5ᵗʰ **M47.0 Anterior spinal and vertebral artery compression syndromes**

> **CC Excl: For CC codes in subcategory M47.0:**
> PDX collection 883

✓6ᵗʰ **M47.01 Anterior spinal artery compression syndromes**

**M47.011** Anterior spinal artery compression CC
syndromes, occipito-atlanto-axial
region

**M47.012** Anterior spinal artery compression CC
syndromes, cervical region

**M47.013** Anterior spinal artery compression CC
syndromes, cervicothoracic region

**M47.014** Anterior spinal artery compression CC
syndromes, thoracic region

**M47.015** Anterior spinal artery compression CC
syndromes, thoracolumbar region

**M47.016** Anterior spinal artery compression CC
syndromes, lumbar region

**M47.019** Anterior spinal artery compression CC
syndromes, site unspecified

✓6ᵗʰ **M47.02 Vertebral artery compression syndromes**

**M47.021** Vertebral artery compression CC
syndromes, occipito-atlanto-axial
region

**M47.022** Vertebral artery compression CC
syndromes, cervical region

**M47.029** Vertebral artery compression CC
syndromes, site unspecified

✓5ᵗʰ **M47.1 Other spondylosis with myelopathy**
Spondylogenic compression of spinal cord
EXCLUDES 1   vertebral subluxation (M43.3-M43.5X9)

**M47.10** Other spondylosis with myelopathy, site CC
unspecified
CC Excl: PDX collection 884

**M47.11** Other spondylosis with myelopathy, CC
occipito-atlanto-axial region
CC Excl: PDX collection 883

**M47.12** Other spondylosis with myelopathy, cervical CC
region
CC Excl: PDX collection 883

**M47.13** Other spondylosis with myelopathy, CC
cervicothoracic region
CC Excl: PDX collection 883

**M47.14** Other spondylosis with myelopathy, thoracic CC
region
CC Excl: PDX collection 885

**M47.15** Other spondylosis with myelopathy, CC
thoracolumbar region
CC Excl: PDX collection 885

**M47.16** Other spondylosis with myelopathy, lumbar CC
region
CC Excl: PDX collection 886

✓5ᵗʰ **M47.2 Other spondylosis with radiculopathy**

**M47.20** Other spondylosis with radiculopathy, site
unspecified

**M47.21** Other spondylosis with radiculopathy, occipito-
atlanto-axial region

**M47.22** Other spondylosis with radiculopathy, cervical
region

**M47.23** Other spondylosis with radiculopathy,
cervicothoracic region

**M47.24** Other spondylosis with radiculopathy, thoracic
region

**M47.25** Other spondylosis with radiculopathy,
thoracolumbar region

**M47.26** Other spondylosis with radiculopathy, lumbar
region

**M47.27** Other spondylosis with radiculopathy, lumbosacral
region

**M47.28** Other spondylosis with radiculopathy, sacral and
sacrococcygeal region

✓5ᵗʰ **M47.8 Other spondylosis**

✓6ᵗʰ **M47.81 Spondylosis without myelopathy or radiculopathy**

**M47.811** Spondylosis without myelopathy or
radiculopathy, occipito-atlanto-axial
region

**M47.812** Spondylosis without myelopathy or
radiculopathy, cervical region

**M47.813** Spondylosis without myelopathy or
radiculopathy, cervicothoracic region

**M47.814** Spondylosis without myelopathy or
radiculopathy, thoracic region

**M47.815** Spondylosis without myelopathy or
radiculopathy, thoracolumbar region

**M47.816** Spondylosis without myelopathy or
radiculopathy, lumbar region

**M47.817** Spondylosis without myelopathy or
radiculopathy, lumbosacral region

**M47.818** Spondylosis without myelopathy or
radiculopathy, sacral and sacrococcygeal
region

**M47.819** Spondylosis without myelopathy or
radiculopathy, site unspecified

✓6ᵗʰ **M47.89 Other spondylosis**

**M47.891** Other spondylosis, occipito-atlanto-axial
region

**M47.892** Other spondylosis, cervical region

**M47.893** Other spondylosis, cervicothoracic region

**M47.894** Other spondylosis, thoracic region

**M47.895** Other spondylosis, thoracolumbar region

**M47.896** Other spondylosis, lumbar region

**M47.897** Other spondylosis, lumbosacral region

**M47.898** Other spondylosis, sacral and
sacrococcygeal region

**M47.899** Other spondylosis, site unspecified

☑ Additional Character Req   ✓x7ᵗʰ Placeholder Alert   Unacceptable PDx   Manifestation   H1-H14 HAC   HCC CMS-HCC Condition   EXCLUDES 1 Not Coded Here   EXCLUDES 2 Not Included Here

ICD-10-CM 2018      **775**

M47.9    **Spondylosis,** unspecified

✓4th **M48 Other spondylopathies**

✓5th   **M48.0 Spinal stenosis**
Caudal stenosis

     **M48.00 Spinal stenosis, site unspecified**

     **M48.01 Spinal stenosis, occipito-atlanto-axial region**

     **M48.02 Spinal stenosis, cervical region**

     **M48.03 Spinal stenosis, cervicothoracic region**

     **M48.04 Spinal stenosis, thoracic region**

     **M48.05 Spinal stenosis, thoracolumbar region**

✓6th     **M48.06 Spinal stenosis, lumbar region**
**DEF:** Spinal canal narrowing in the lumbar area with nerve root compression, causing muscle pain, fatigue, and weakness during extension of the lumbar spine; pain is relieved by sitting or bending.

●      **M48.061 Spinal stenosis, lumbar region without neurogenic claudication**
Spinal stenosis, lumbar region NOS

●      **M48.062 Spinal stenosis, lumbar region with neurogenic claudication**

     **M48.07 Spinal stenosis, lumbosacral region**

     **M48.08 Spinal stenosis, sacral and sacrococcygeal region**

✓5th   **M48.1 Ankylosing hyperostosis [Forestier]**
Diffuse idiopathic skeletal hyperostosis [DISH]

     **M48.10 Ankylosing hyperostosis [Forestier], site unspecified**

     **M48.11 Ankylosing hyperostosis [Forestier], occipito-atlanto-axial region**

     **M48.12 Ankylosing hyperostosis [Forestier], cervical region**

     **M48.13 Ankylosing hyperostosis [Forestier], cervicothoracic region**

     **M48.14 Ankylosing hyperostosis [Forestier], thoracic region**

     **M48.15 Ankylosing hyperostosis [Forestier], thoracolumbar region**

     **M48.16 Ankylosing hyperostosis [Forestier], lumbar region**

     **M48.17 Ankylosing hyperostosis [Forestier], lumbosacral region**

     **M48.18 Ankylosing hyperostosis [Forestier], sacral and sacrococcygeal region**

     **M48.19 Ankylosing hyperostosis [Forestier], multiple sites in spine**

✓5th   **M48.2 Kissing spine**

     **M48.20 Kissing spine, site unspecified**

     **M48.21 Kissing spine, occipito-atlanto-axial region**

     **M48.22 Kissing spine, cervical region**

     **M48.23 Kissing spine, cervicothoracic region**

     **M48.24 Kissing spine, thoracic region**

     **M48.25 Kissing spine, thoracolumbar region**

     **M48.26 Kissing spine, lumbar region**

     **M48.27 Kissing spine, lumbosacral region**

✓5th   **M48.3 Traumatic spondylopathy**

**CC Excl: For CC codes in subcategory M48.3:**
PDX collection 887

     **M48.30 Traumatic spondylopathy, site unspecified**   CC

     **M48.31 Traumatic spondylopathy, occipito-atlanto-axial region**   CC

     **M48.32 Traumatic spondylopathy, cervical region**   CC

     **M48.33 Traumatic spondylopathy, cervicothoracic region**   CC

     **M48.34 Traumatic spondylopathy, thoracic region**   CC

     **M48.35 Traumatic spondylopathy, thoracolumbar region**   CC

     **M48.36 Traumatic spondylopathy, lumbar region**   CC

     **M48.37 Traumatic spondylopathy, lumbosacral region**   CC

     **M48.38 Traumatic spondylopathy, sacral and sacrococcygeal region**   CC

---

✓5th   **M48.4 Fatigue fracture of vertebra**
Stress fracture of vertebra
**EXCLUDES 1**   *pathological fracture NOS (M84.4-)*
*pathological fracture of vertebra due to neoplasm (M84.58)*
*pathological fracture of vertebra due to other diagnosis (M84.68)*
*pathological fracture of vertebra due to osteoporosis (M80.-)*
*traumatic fracture of vertebrae (S12.0-S12.3-, S22.0-, S32.0-)*

The appropriate 7th character is to be added to each code from subcategory M48.4.
A   initial encounter for fracture
D   subsequent encounter for fracture with routine healing
G   subsequent encounter for fracture with delayed healing
S   sequela of fracture

✓x7th   **M48.40 Fatigue fracture of vertebra, site unspecified**

✓x7th   **M48.41 Fatigue fracture of vertebra, occipito-atlanto-axial region**

✓x7th   **M48.42 Fatigue fracture of vertebra, cervical region**

✓x7th   **M48.43 Fatigue fracture of vertebra, cervicothoracic region**

✓x7th   **M48.44 Fatigue fracture of vertebra, thoracic region**

✓x7th   **M48.45 Fatigue fracture of vertebra, thoracolumbar region**

✓x7th   **M48.46 Fatigue fracture of vertebra, lumbar region**

✓x7th   **M48.47 Fatigue fracture of vertebra, lumbosacral region**

✓x7th   **M48.48 Fatigue fracture of vertebra, sacral and sacrococcygeal region**

✓5th   **M48.5 Collapsed vertebra, not elsewhere classified**
Collapsed vertebra NOS
Compression fracture of vertebra NOS
Wedging of vertebra NOS
**EXCLUDES 1**   *current injury—see Injury of spine, by body region*
*fatigue fracture of vertebra (M48.4)*
*pathological fracture of vertebra due to neoplasm (M84.58)*
*pathological fracture of vertebra due to other diagnosis (M84.68)*
*pathological fracture of vertebra due to osteoporosis (M80.-)*
*pathological fracture NOS (M84.4-)*
*stress fracture of vertebra (M48.4-)*
*traumatic fracture of vertebra (S12-, S22-, S32-)*

The appropriate 7th character is to be added to each code from subcategory M48.5.
A   initial encounter for fracture
D   subsequent encounter for fracture with routine healing
G   subsequent encounter for fracture with delayed healing
S   sequela of fracture

**CC Excl: For CC codes in subcategory M48.5:**
PDX collection 888

10 ✓x7th   **M48.50 Collapsed vertebra, not elsewhere classified, site unspecified**   CC HCC

10 ✓x7th   **M48.51 Collapsed vertebra, not elsewhere classified, occipito-atlanto-axial region**   CC HCC

10 ✓x7th   **M48.52 Collapsed vertebra, not elsewhere classified, cervical region**   CC HCC

10 ✓x7th   **M48.53 Collapsed vertebra, not elsewhere classified, cervicothoracic region**   CC HCC

10 ✓x7th   **M48.54 Collapsed vertebra, not elsewhere classified, thoracic region**   CC HCC

10 ✓x7th   **M48.55 Collapsed vertebra, not elsewhere classified, thoracolumbar region**   CC HCC

10 ✓x7th   **M48.56 Collapsed vertebra, not elsewhere classified, lumbar region**   CC HCC

10 ✓x7th   **M48.57 Collapsed vertebra, not elsewhere classified, lumbosacral region**   CC HCC

10 ✓x7th   **M48.58 Collapsed vertebra, not elsewhere classified, sacral and sacrococcygeal region**   CC HCC

---

10   HCC with 7th character indicating initial encounter (A, B or C - specific to category).

N Newborn: 0   P Pediatric: 0-17   M Maternity: 12-55   A Adult: 15-124   MCC Major CC Condition   PDxMCC PDx acts as own MCC   CC CC Condition   PDxCC PDx acts as own CC

**776**      ICD-10-CM 2018

☑5ᵗʰ **M48.8  Other specified spondylopathies**
Ossification of posterior longitudinal ligament

☑6ᵗʰ **M48.8X  Other specified spondylopathies**

**M48.8X1  Other specified spondylopathies, occipito-atlanto-axial region**  `HCC`

**M48.8X2  Other specified spondylopathies, cervical region**  `HCC`

**M48.8X3  Other specified spondylopathies, cervicothoracic region**  `HCC`

**M48.8X4  Other specified spondylopathies, thoracic region**  `HCC`

**M48.8X5  Other specified spondylopathies, thoracolumbar region**  `HCC`

**M48.8X6  Other specified spondylopathies, lumbar region**  `HCC`

**M48.8X7  Other specified spondylopathies, lumbosacral region**  `HCC`

**M48.8X8  Other specified spondylopathies, sacral and sacrococcygeal region**  `HCC`

**M48.8X9  Other specified spondylopathies, site unspecified**  `HCC`

**M48.9  Spondylopathy, unspecified**

☑4ᵗʰ **M49  Spondylopathies in diseases classified elsewhere**
**INCLUDES**   curvature of spine in diseases classified elsewhere
deformity of spine in diseases classified elsewhere
kyphosis in diseases classified elsewhere
scoliosis in diseases classified elsewhere
spondylopathy in diseases classified elsewhere
Code first underlying disease, such as:
brucellosis (A23.-)
Charcôt-Marie-Tooth disease (G60.0)
enterobacterial infections (A01-A04)
osteitis fibrosa cystica (E21.0)
**EXCLUDES 1**   *curvature of spine in tuberculosis [Pott's] (A18.01)*
*enteropathic arthropathies (M07.-)*
*gonococcal spondylitis (A54.41)*
*neuropathic [tabes dorsalis] spondylitis (A52.11)*
*neuropathic spondylopathy in syringomyelia (G95.0)*
*neuropathic spondylopathy in tabes dorsalis (A52.11)*
*nonsyphilitic neuropathic spondylopathy NEC (G98.0)*
*spondylitis in syphilis (acquired) (A52.77)*
*tuberculous spondylitis (A18.01)*
*typhoid fever spondylitis (A01.05)*

☑5ᵗʰ **M49.8  Spondylopathy in diseases classified elsewhere**

*M49.80  Spondylopathy in diseases classified elsewhere, site unspecified*  `HCC`

*M49.81  Spondylopathy in diseases classified elsewhere, occipito-atlanto-axial region*  `HCC`

*M49.82  Spondylopathy in diseases classified elsewhere, cervical region*  `HCC`

*M49.83  Spondylopathy in diseases classified elsewhere, cervicothoracic region*  `HCC`

*M49.84  Spondylopathy in diseases classified elsewhere, thoracic region*  `HCC`

*M49.85  Spondylopathy in diseases classified elsewhere, thoracolumbar region*  `HCC`

*M49.86  Spondylopathy in diseases classified elsewhere, lumbar region*  `HCC`

*M49.87  Spondylopathy in diseases classified elsewhere, lumbosacral region*  `HCC`

*M49.88  Spondylopathy in diseases classified elsewhere, sacral and sacrococcygeal region*  `HCC`

*M49.89  Spondylopathy in diseases classified elsewhere, multiple sites in spine*  `HCC`

## Other dorsopathies (M50-M54)

**EXCLUDES 1**   *current injury—see injury of spine by body region*
*discitis NOS (M46.4-)*

☑4ᵗʰ **M50  Cervical disc disorders**
**NOTE**   Code to the most superior level of disorder.
**INCLUDES**   cervicothoracic disc disorders with cervicalgia
cervicothoracic disc disorders
**AHA:** 2016, 1Q, 17

☑5ᵗʰ **M50.0  Cervical disc disorder with myelopathy**

**CC Excl: For CC codes in subcategory M50.0:**
PDX collection 889

**M50.00  Cervical disc disorder with myelopathy, unspecified cervical region**  `CC`

**M50.01  Cervical disc disorder with myelopathy, high cervical region**  `CC`
C2-C3 disc disorder with myelopathy
C3-C4 disc disorder with myelopathy

☑6ᵗʰ **M50.02  Cervical disc disorder with myelopathy, mid-cervical region**

**M50.020  Cervical disc disorder with myelopathy, mid-cervical region, unspecified level**  `CC`

**M50.021  Cervical disc disorder at C4-C5 level with myelopathy**  `CC`
C4-C5 disc disorder with myelopathy

**M50.022  Cervical disc disorder at C5-C6 level with myelopathy**  `CC`
C5-C6 disc disorder with myelopathy

**M50.023  Cervical disc disorder at C6-C7 level with myelopathy**  `CC`
C6-C7 disc disorder with myelopathy

**M50.03  Cervical disc disorder with myelopathy, cervicothoracic region**  `CC`
C7-T1 disc disorder with myelopathy

☑5ᵗʰ **M50.1  Cervical disc disorder with radiculopathy**
**EXCLUDES 2**   *brachial radiculitis NOS (M54.13)*

**M50.10  Cervical disc disorder with radiculopathy, unspecified cervical region**

**M50.11  Cervical disc disorder with radiculopathy, high cervical region**
C2-C3 disc disorder with radiculopathy
C3 radiculopathy due to disc disorder
C3-C4 disc disorder with radiculopathy
C4 radiculopathy due to disc disorder

☑6ᵗʰ **M50.12  Cervical disc disorder with radiculopathy, mid-cervical region**

**M50.120  Mid-cervical disc disorder, unspecified**

**M50.121  Cervical disc disorder at C4-C5 level with radiculopathy**
C4-C5 disc disorder with radiculopathy
C5 radiculopathy due to disc disorder

**M50.122  Cervical disc disorder at C5-C6 level with radiculopathy**
C5-C6 disc disorder with radiculopathy
C6 radiculopathy due to disc disorder

**M50.123  Cervical disc disorder at C6-C7 level with radiculopathy**
C6-C7 disc disorder with radiculopathy
C7 radiculopathy due to disc disorder

**M50.13  Cervical disc disorder with radiculopathy, cervicothoracic region**
C7-T1 disc disorder with radiculopathy
C8 radiculopathy due to disc disorder

☑5ᵗʰ **M50.2  Other cervical disc displacement**

**M50.20  Other cervical disc displacement, unspecified cervical region**

**M50.21  Other cervical disc displacement, high cervical region**
Other C2-C3 cervical disc displacement
Other C3-C4 cervical disc displacement

☑6ᵗʰ **M50.22  Other cervical disc displacement, mid-cervical region**

**M50.220  Other cervical disc displacement, mid-cervical region, unspecified level**

**M50.221  Other cervical disc displacement at C4-C5 level**
Other C4-C5 cervical disc displacement

**M50.222  Other cervical disc displacement at C5-C6 level**
Other C5-C6 cervical disc displacement

**M50.223  Other cervical disc displacement at C6-C7 level**
Other C6-C7 cervical disc displacement

**M50.23  Other cervical disc displacement, cervicothoracic region**
Other C7-T1 cervical disc displacement

☑5ᵗʰ **M50.3  Other cervical disc degeneration**

**M50.30  Other cervical disc degeneration, unspecified cervical region**

**M50.31  Other cervical disc degeneration, high cervical region**
Other C2-C3 cervical disc degeneration
Other C3-C4 cervical disc degeneration

✓6th **M50.32  Other cervical disc degeneration, mid-cervical region**
- **M50.320  Other cervical disc degeneration, mid-cervical region, unspecified level**
- **M50.321  Other cervical disc degeneration at C4-C5 level**
  Other C4-C5 cervical disc degeneration
- **M50.322  Other cervical disc degeneration at C5-C6 level**
  Other C5-C6 cervical disc degeneration
- **M50.323  Other cervical disc degeneration at C6-C7 level**
  Other C6-C7 cervical disc degeneration

**M50.33  Other cervical disc degeneration, cervicothoracic region**
Other C7-T1 cervical disc degeneration

✓5th **M50.8  Other cervical disc disorders**
- **M50.80  Other cervical disc disorders, unspecified cervical region**
- **M50.81  Other cervical disc disorders, high cervical region**
  Other C2-C3 cervical disc disorders
  Other C3-C4 cervical disc disorders
- ✓6th **M50.82  Other cervical disc disorders, mid-cervical region**
  - **M50.820  Other cervical disc disorders, mid-cervical region, unspecified level**
  - **M50.821  Other cervical disc disorders at C4-C5 level**
    Other C4-C5 cervical disc disorders
  - **M50.822  Other cervical disc disorders at C5-C6 level**
    Other C5-C6 cervical disc disorders
  - **M50.823  Other cervical disc disorders at C6-C7 level**
    Other C6-C7 cervical disc disorders
- **M50.83  Other cervical disc disorders, cervicothoracic region**
  Other C7-T1 cervical disc disorders

✓5th **M50.9  Cervical disc disorder, unspecified**
- **M50.90  Cervical disc disorder, unspecified, unspecified cervical region**
- **M50.91  Cervical disc disorder, unspecified, high cervical region**
  C2-C3 cervical disc disorder, unspecified
  C3-C4 cervical disc disorder, unspecified
- ✓6th **M50.92  Cervical disc disorder, unspecified, mid-cervical region**
  - **M50.920  Unspecified cervical disc disorder, mid-cervical region, unspecified level**
  - **M50.921  Unspecified cervical disc disorder at C4-C5 level**
    Unspecified C4-C5 cervical disc disorder
  - **M50.922  Unspecified cervical disc disorder at C5-C6 level**
    Unspecified C5-C6 cervical disc disorder
  - **M50.923  Unspecified cervical disc disorder at C6-C7 level**
    Unspecified C6-C7 cervical disc disorder
- **M50.93  Cervical disc disorder, unspecified, cervicothoracic region**
  C7-T1 cervical disc disorder, unspecified

✓4th **M51  Thoracic, thoracolumbar, and lumbosacral intervertebral disc disorders**
- EXCLUDES 2 *cervical and cervicothoracic disc disorders (M50.-)*
  *sacral and sacrococcygeal disorders (M53.3)*

✓5th **M51.0  Thoracic, thoracolumbar and lumbosacral intervertebral disc disorders with myelopathy**
- **M51.04  Intervertebral disc disorders with myelopathy, thoracic region**  CC
  **CC Excl:** PDX collection 890
- **M51.05  Intervertebral disc disorders with myelopathy, thoracolumbar region**  CC
  **CC Excl:** PDX collection 890
- **M51.06  Intervertebral disc disorders with myelopathy, lumbar region**  CC
  **CC Excl:** PDX collection 891

✓5th **M51.1  Thoracic, thoracolumbar and lumbosacral intervertebral disc disorders with radiculopathy**
Sciatica due to intervertebral disc disorder
- EXCLUDES 1 *lumbar radiculitis NOS (M54.16)*
  *sciatica NOS (M54.3)*
- **M51.14  Intervertebral disc disorders with radiculopathy, thoracic region**

### Displacement Intervertebral Disc

Normal Top View — Herniated Top View

Labels: Lamina, Ligamentum flavum, Disc annulus, Nucleus pulposus, Nucleus pulposus, Herniates through annulus, Spinal cord, Spinal nerve

- **M51.15  Intervertebral disc disorders with radiculopathy, thoracolumbar region**
- **M51.16  Intervertebral disc disorders with radiculopathy, lumbar region**
- **M51.17  Intervertebral disc disorders with radiculopathy, lumbosacral region**

✓5th **M51.2  Other thoracic, thoracolumbar and lumbosacral intervertebral disc displacement**
Lumbago due to displacement of intervertebral disc
- **M51.24  Other intervertebral disc displacement, thoracic region**
- **M51.25  Other intervertebral disc displacement, thoracolumbar region**
- **M51.26  Other intervertebral disc displacement, lumbar region**
- **M51.27  Other intervertebral disc displacement, lumbosacral region**

✓5th **M51.3  Other thoracic, thoracolumbar and lumbosacral intervertebral disc degeneration**
**AHA:** 2013, 3Q, 22
- **M51.34  Other intervertebral disc degeneration, thoracic region**
- **M51.35  Other intervertebral disc degeneration, thoracolumbar region**
- **M51.36  Other intervertebral disc degeneration, lumbar region**
- **M51.37  Other intervertebral disc degeneration, lumbosacral region**

✓5th **M51.4  Schmorl's nodes**
**DEF:** Irregular bone defect in the margin of the vertebral body; causes herniation into end plate of vertebral body.
- **M51.44  Schmorl's nodes, thoracic region**
- **M51.45  Schmorl's nodes, thoracolumbar region**
- **M51.46  Schmorl's nodes, lumbar region**
- **M51.47  Schmorl's nodes, lumbosacral region**

✓5th **M51.8  Other thoracic, thoracolumbar and lumbosacral intervertebral disc disorders**
- **M51.84  Other intervertebral disc disorders, thoracic region**
- **M51.85  Other intervertebral disc disorders, thoracolumbar region**
- **M51.86  Other intervertebral disc disorders, lumbar region**
- **M51.87  Other intervertebral disc disorders, lumbosacral region**

**M51.9  Unspecified thoracic, thoracolumbar and lumbosacral intervertebral disc disorder**

✓4th **M53  Other and unspecified dorsopathies, not elsewhere classified**
**M53.0  Cervicocranial syndrome**
Posterior cervical sympathetic syndrome

**M53.1  Cervicobrachial syndrome**
- EXCLUDES 2 *cervical disc disorder (M50.-)*
  *thoracic outlet syndrome (G54.0)*

✓5th **M53.2  Spinal instabilities**
- ✓6th **M53.2X  Spinal instabilities**
  - **M53.2X1  Spinal instabilities, occipito-atlanto-axial region**
  - **M53.2X2  Spinal instabilities, cervical region**
  - **M53.2X3  Spinal instabilities, cervicothoracic region**
  - **M53.2X4  Spinal instabilities, thoracic region**

---

Ⓝ Newborn: 0  Ⓟ Pediatric: 0-17  Ⓜ Maternity: 12-55  Ⓐ Adult: 15-124  **MCC** Major CC Condition  **PDxMCC** PDx acts as own MCC  **CC** CC Condition  **PDxCC** PDx acts as own CC

M53.2X5   **Spinal instabilities, thoracolumbar region**
M53.2X6   **Spinal instabilities, lumbar region**
M53.2X7   **Spinal instabilities, lumbosacral region**
M53.2X8   **Spinal instabilities, sacral and sacrococcygeal region**
M53.2X9   **Spinal instabilities, site unspecified**

**M53.3   Sacrococcygeal disorders, not elsewhere classified**
Coccygodynia

✓5ᵗʰ **M53.8   Other specified dorsopathies**
M53.80   **Other specified dorsopathies, site unspecified**
M53.81   **Other specified dorsopathies, occipito-atlanto-axial region**
M53.82   **Other specified dorsopathies, cervical region**
M53.83   **Other specified dorsopathies, cervicothoracic region**
M53.84   **Other specified dorsopathies, thoracic region**
M53.85   **Other specified dorsopathies, thoracolumbar region**
M53.86   **Other specified dorsopathies, lumbar region**
M53.87   **Other specified dorsopathies, lumbosacral region**
M53.88   **Other specified dorsopathies, sacral and sacrococcygeal region**

**M53.9   Dorsopathy, unspecified**

✓4ᵗʰ **M54   Dorsalgia**
*EXCLUDES 1*   psychogenic dorsalgia (F45.41)

✓5ᵗʰ **M54.0   Panniculitis affecting regions of neck and back**
*EXCLUDES 1*   lupus panniculitis (L93.2)
panniculitis NOS (M79.3)
relapsing [Weber-Christian] panniculitis (M35.6)
M54.00   **Panniculitis affecting regions of neck and back, site unspecified**
M54.01   **Panniculitis affecting regions of neck and back, occipito-atlanto-axial region**
M54.02   **Panniculitis affecting regions of neck and back, cervical region**
M54.03   **Panniculitis affecting regions of neck and back, cervicothoracic region**
M54.04   **Panniculitis affecting regions of neck and back, thoracic region**
M54.05   **Panniculitis affecting regions of neck and back, thoracolumbar region**
M54.06   **Panniculitis affecting regions of neck and back, lumbar region**
M54.07   **Panniculitis affecting regions of neck and back, lumbosacral region**
M54.08   **Panniculitis affecting regions of neck and back, sacral and sacrococcygeal region**
M54.09   **Panniculitis affecting regions, neck and back, multiple sites in spine**

✓5ᵗʰ **M54.1   Radiculopathy**
Brachial neuritis or radiculitis NOS
Lumbar neuritis or radiculitis NOS
Lumbosacral neuritis or radiculitis NOS
Thoracic neuritis or radiculitis NOS
Radiculitis NOS
*EXCLUDES 1*   neuralgia and neuritis NOS (M79.2)
radiculopathy with cervical disc disorder (M50.1)
radiculopathy with lumbar and other intervertebral disc disorder (M51.1-)
radiculopathy with spondylosis (M47.2-)
M54.10   **Radiculopathy, site unspecified**
M54.11   **Radiculopathy, occipito-atlanto-axial region**
M54.12   **Radiculopathy, cervical region**
M54.13   **Radiculopathy, cervicothoracic region**
M54.14   **Radiculopathy, thoracic region**
M54.15   **Radiculopathy, thoracolumbar region**
M54.16   **Radiculopathy, lumbar region**
M54.17   **Radiculopathy, lumbosacral region**
M54.18   **Radiculopathy, sacral and sacrococcygeal region**

**M54.2   Cervicalgia**
*EXCLUDES 1*   cervicalgia due to intervertebral cervical disc disorder (M50.-)

✓5ᵗʰ **M54.3   Sciatica**
*EXCLUDES 1*   lesion of sciatic nerve (G57.0)
sciatica due to intervertebral disc disorder (M51.1-)
sciatica with lumbago (M54.4-)
M54.30   **Sciatica, unspecified side**
M54.31   **Sciatica, right side**
M54.32   **Sciatica, left side**

✓5ᵗʰ **M54.4   Lumbago with sciatica**
*EXCLUDES 1*   lumbago with sciatica due to intervertebral disc disorder (M51.1-)
**AHA:** 2016, 2Q, 7
M54.40   **Lumbago with sciatica, unspecified side**
M54.41   **Lumbago with sciatica, right side**
M54.42   **Lumbago with sciatica, left side**

**M54.5   Low back pain**
Loin pain
Lumbago NOS
*EXCLUDES 1*   low back strain (S39.012)
lumbago due to intervertebral disc displacement (M51.2-)
lumbago with sciatica (M54.4-)

**M54.6   Pain in thoracic spine**
*EXCLUDES 1*   pain in thoracic spine due to intervertebral disc disorder (M51.-)

✓5ᵗʰ **M54.8   Other dorsalgia**
*EXCLUDES 1*   dorsalgia in thoracic region (M54.6)
low back pain (M54.5)
M54.81   **Occipital neuralgia**
M54.89   **Other dorsalgia**

**M54.9   Dorsalgia, unspecified**
Backache NOS
Back pain NOS

## SOFT TISSUE DISORDERS (M60-M79)

### Disorders of muscles (M60-M63)

*EXCLUDES 1*   dermatopolymyositis (M33.-)
muscular dystrophies and myopathies (G71-G72)
myopathy in amyloidosis (E85.-)
myopathy in polyarteritis nodosa (M30.0)
myopathy in rheumatoid arthritis (M05.32)
myopathy in scleroderma (M34.-)
myopathy in Sjögren's syndrome (M35.03)
myopathy in systemic lupus erythematosus (M32.-)

✓4ᵗʰ **M60   Myositis**
*EXCLUDES 2*   inclusion body myositis [IBM] (G72.41)

✓5ᵗʰ **M60.0   Infective myositis**
Tropical pyomyositis
Use additional code (B95-B97) to identify infectious agent

> **CC Excl: For CC codes in subcategory M60.0:**
> PDX collection 806

✓6ᵗʰ **M60.00   Infective myositis, unspecified site**
M60.000   **Infective myositis, unspecified right arm**   `CC`
Infective myositis, right upper limb NOS
M60.001   **Infective myositis, unspecified left arm**   `CC`
Infective myositis, left upper limb NOS
M60.002   **Infective myositis, unspecified arm**   `CC`
Infective myositis, upper limb NOS
M60.003   **Infective myositis, unspecified right leg**   `CC`
Infective myositis, right lower limb NOS
M60.004   **Infective myositis, unspecified left leg**   `CC`
Infective myositis, left lower limb NOS
M60.005   **Infective myositis, unspecified leg**   `CC`
Infective myositis, lower limb NOS
M60.009   **Infective myositis, unspecified site**   `CC`

✓6ᵗʰ **M60.01   Infective myositis, shoulder**
M60.011   **Infective myositis, right shoulder**   `CC`
M60.012   **Infective myositis, left shoulder**   `CC`
M60.019   **Infective myositis, unspecified shoulder**   `CC`

✓6ᵗʰ **M60.02   Infective myositis, upper arm**
M60.021   **Infective myositis, right upper arm**   `CC`
M60.022   **Infective myositis, left upper arm**   `CC`

✓ Additional Character Req   ✓7ᵗʰ Placeholder Alert   Unacceptable PDx   Manifestation   **H1**-**H14** HAC   **HCC** CMS-HCC Condition   *EXCLUDES 1* Not Coded Here   *EXCLUDES 2* Not Included Here

ICD-10-CM 2018       **779**

M53.2X5–M60.022

M60.029   Infective myositis, unspecified **upper arm**   `CC`

✓6th   **M60.03**   Infective myositis, **forearm**
    M60.031   Infective myositis, right **forearm**   `CC`
    M60.032   Infective myositis, left **forearm**   `CC`
    M60.039   Infective myositis, unspecified **forearm**   `CC`

✓6th   **M60.04**   Infective myositis, **hand and fingers**
    M60.041   Infective myositis, right **hand**   `CC`
    M60.042   Infective myositis, left **hand**   `CC`
    M60.043   Infective myositis, unspecified **hand**   `CC`
    M60.044   Infective myositis, right **finger(s)**   `CC`
    M60.045   Infective myositis, left **finger(s)**   `CC`
    M60.046   Infective myositis, unspecified **finger(s)**   `CC`

✓6th   **M60.05**   Infective myositis, **thigh**
    M60.051   Infective myositis, right **thigh**   `CC`
    M60.052   Infective myositis, left **thigh**   `CC`
    M60.059   Infective myositis, unspecified **thigh**   `CC`

✓6th   **M60.06**   Infective myositis, **lower leg**
    M60.061   Infective myositis, right **lower leg**   `CC`
    M60.062   Infective myositis, left **lower leg**   `CC`
    M60.069   Infective myositis, unspecified **lower leg**   `CC`

✓6th   **M60.07**   Infective myositis, **ankle, foot and toes**
    M60.070   Infective myositis, right **ankle**   `CC`
    M60.071   Infective myositis, left **ankle**   `CC`
    M60.072   Infective myositis, unspecified **ankle**   `CC`
    M60.073   Infective myositis, right **foot**   `CC`
    M60.074   Infective myositis, left **foot**   `CC`
    M60.075   Infective myositis, unspecified **foot**   `CC`
    M60.076   Infective myositis, right **toe(s)**   `CC`
    M60.077   Infective myositis, left **toe(s)**   `CC`
    M60.078   Infective myositis, unspecified **toe(s)**   `CC`

  M60.08   Infective myositis, **other site**   `CC`
  M60.09   Infective myositis, **multiple sites**   `CC`

**M60.1   Interstitial myositis**
  M60.10   Interstitial myositis of **unspecified site**

✓6th   **M60.11**   Interstitial myositis, **shoulder**
    M60.111   Interstitial myositis, right **shoulder**
    M60.112   Interstitial myositis, left **shoulder**
    M60.119   Interstitial myositis, unspecified **shoulder**

✓6th   **M60.12**   Interstitial myositis, **upper arm**
    M60.121   Interstitial myositis, right **upper arm**
    M60.122   Interstitial myositis, left **upper arm**
    M60.129   Interstitial myositis, unspecified **upper arm**

✓6th   **M60.13**   Interstitial myositis, **forearm**
    M60.131   Interstitial myositis, right **forearm**
    M60.132   Interstitial myositis, left **forearm**
    M60.139   Interstitial myositis, unspecified **forearm**

✓6th   **M60.14**   Interstitial myositis, **hand**
    M60.141   Interstitial myositis, right **hand**
    M60.142   Interstitial myositis, left **hand**
    M60.149   Interstitial myositis, unspecified **hand**

✓6th   **M60.15**   Interstitial myositis, **thigh**
    M60.151   Interstitial myositis, right **thigh**
    M60.152   Interstitial myositis, left **thigh**
    M60.159   Interstitial myositis, unspecified **thigh**

✓6th   **M60.16**   Interstitial myositis, **lower leg**
    M60.161   Interstitial myositis, right **lower leg**
    M60.162   Interstitial myositis, left **lower leg**
    M60.169   Interstitial myositis, unspecified **lower leg**

✓6th   **M60.17**   Interstitial myositis, **ankle and foot**
    M60.171   Interstitial myositis, right **ankle and foot**
    M60.172   Interstitial myositis, left **ankle and foot**
    M60.179   Interstitial myositis, unspecified **ankle and foot**

  M60.18   Interstitial myositis, **other site**
  M60.19   Interstitial myositis, **multiple sites**

✓5th   **M60.2   Foreign body granuloma of soft tissue, not elsewhere classified**
   Use additional code to identify the type of retained foreign body (Z18.-)
   **EXCLUDES 1**   *foreign body granuloma of skin and subcutaneous tissue (L92.3)*

  M60.20   Foreign body granuloma of soft tissue, not elsewhere classified, **unspecified site**

✓6th   **M60.21**   Foreign body granuloma of soft tissue, not elsewhere classified, **shoulder**
    M60.211   Foreign body granuloma of soft tissue, not elsewhere classified, right **shoulder**
    M60.212   Foreign body granuloma of soft tissue, not elsewhere classified, left **shoulder**
    M60.219   Foreign body granuloma of soft tissue, not elsewhere classified, unspecified **shoulder**

✓6th   **M60.22**   Foreign body granuloma of soft tissue, not elsewhere classified, **upper arm**
    M60.221   Foreign body granuloma of soft tissue, not elsewhere classified, right **upper arm**
    M60.222   Foreign body granuloma of soft tissue, not elsewhere classified, left **upper arm**
    M60.229   Foreign body granuloma of soft tissue, not elsewhere classified, unspecified **upper arm**

✓6th   **M60.23**   Foreign body granuloma of soft tissue, not elsewhere classified, **forearm**
    M60.231   Foreign body granuloma of soft tissue, not elsewhere classified, right **forearm**
    M60.232   Foreign body granuloma of soft tissue, not elsewhere classified, left **forearm**
    M60.239   Foreign body granuloma of soft tissue, not elsewhere classified, unspecified **forearm**

✓6th   **M60.24**   Foreign body granuloma of soft tissue, not elsewhere classified, **hand**
    M60.241   Foreign body granuloma of soft tissue, not elsewhere classified, right **hand**
    M60.242   Foreign body granuloma of soft tissue, not elsewhere classified, left **hand**
    M60.249   Foreign body granuloma of soft tissue, not elsewhere classified, unspecified **hand**

✓6th   **M60.25**   Foreign body granuloma of soft tissue, not elsewhere classified, **thigh**
    M60.251   Foreign body granuloma of soft tissue, not elsewhere classified, right **thigh**
    M60.252   Foreign body granuloma of soft tissue, not elsewhere classified, left **thigh**
    M60.259   Foreign body granuloma of soft tissue, not elsewhere classified, unspecified **thigh**

✓6th   **M60.26**   Foreign body granuloma of soft tissue, not elsewhere classified, **lower leg**
    M60.261   Foreign body granuloma of soft tissue, not elsewhere classified, right **lower leg**
    M60.262   Foreign body granuloma of soft tissue, not elsewhere classified, left **lower leg**
    M60.269   Foreign body granuloma of soft tissue, not elsewhere classified, unspecified **lower leg**

✓6th   **M60.27**   Foreign body granuloma of soft tissue, not elsewhere classified, **ankle and foot**
    M60.271   Foreign body granuloma of soft tissue, not elsewhere classified, right **ankle and foot**
    M60.272   Foreign body granuloma of soft tissue, not elsewhere classified, left **ankle and foot**
    M60.279   Foreign body granuloma of soft tissue, not elsewhere classified, unspecified **ankle and foot**

  M60.28   Foreign body granuloma of soft tissue, not elsewhere classified, **other site**

✓5th   **M60.8   Other myositis**
  M60.80   Other myositis, **unspecified site**

✓6th   **M60.81**   Other myositis **shoulder**
    M60.811   Other myositis, right **shoulder**
    M60.812   Other myositis, left **shoulder**
    M60.819   Other myositis, unspecified **shoulder**

✓6th   **M60.82**   Other myositis, **upper arm**
    M60.821   Other myositis, right **upper arm**
    M60.822   Other myositis, left **upper arm**

M60.829   Other myositis, unspecified upper arm

✓6ᵗʰ **M60.83 Other myositis, forearm**
     M60.831   Other myositis, right forearm
     M60.832   Other myositis, left forearm
     M60.839   Other myositis, unspecified forearm

✓6ᵗʰ **M60.84 Other myositis, hand**
     M60.841   Other myositis, right hand
     M60.842   Other myositis, left hand
     M60.849   Other myositis, unspecified hand

✓6ᵗʰ **M60.85 Other myositis, thigh**
     M60.851   Other myositis, right thigh
     M60.852   Other myositis, left thigh
     M60.859   Other myositis, unspecified thigh

✓6ᵗʰ **M60.86 Other myositis, lower leg**
     M60.861   Other myositis, right lower leg
     M60.862   Other myositis, left lower leg
     M60.869   Other myositis, unspecified lower leg

✓6ᵗʰ **M60.87 Other myositis, ankle and foot**
     M60.871   Other myositis, right ankle and foot
     M60.872   Other myositis, left ankle and foot
     M60.879   Other myositis, unspecified ankle and foot

M60.88   Other myositis, other site
M60.89   Other myositis, multiple sites

M60.9   Myositis, unspecified

✓4ᵗʰ **M61 Calcification and ossification of muscle**

✓5ᵗʰ **M61.0 Myositis ossificans traumatica**
     M61.00   Myositis ossificans traumatica, unspecified site

✓6ᵗʰ **M61.01 Myositis ossificans traumatica, shoulder**
     M61.011   Myositis ossificans traumatica, right shoulder
     M61.012   Myositis ossificans traumatica, left shoulder
     M61.019   Myositis ossificans traumatica, unspecified shoulder

✓6ᵗʰ **M61.02 Myositis ossificans traumatica, upper arm**
     M61.021   Myositis ossificans traumatica, right upper arm
     M61.022   Myositis ossificans traumatica, left upper arm
     M61.029   Myositis ossificans traumatica, unspecified upper arm

✓6ᵗʰ **M61.03 Myositis ossificans traumatica, forearm**
     M61.031   Myositis ossificans traumatica, right forearm
     M61.032   Myositis ossificans traumatica, left forearm
     M61.039   Myositis ossificans traumatica, unspecified forearm

✓6ᵗʰ **M61.04 Myositis ossificans traumatica, hand**
     M61.041   Myositis ossificans traumatica, right hand
     M61.042   Myositis ossificans traumatica, left hand
     M61.049   Myositis ossificans traumatica, unspecified hand

✓6ᵗʰ **M61.05 Myositis ossificans traumatica, thigh**
     M61.051   Myositis ossificans traumatica, right thigh
     M61.052   Myositis ossificans traumatica, left thigh
     M61.059   Myositis ossificans traumatica, unspecified thigh

✓6ᵗʰ **M61.06 Myositis ossificans traumatica, lower leg**
     M61.061   Myositis ossificans traumatica, right lower leg
     M61.062   Myositis ossificans traumatica, left lower leg
     M61.069   Myositis ossificans traumatica, unspecified lower leg

✓6ᵗʰ **M61.07 Myositis ossificans traumatica, ankle and foot**
     M61.071   Myositis ossificans traumatica, right ankle and foot
     M61.072   Myositis ossificans traumatica, left ankle and foot
     M61.079   Myositis ossificans traumatica, unspecified ankle and foot

M61.08   Myositis ossificans traumatica, other site

M61.09   Myositis ossificans traumatica, multiple sites

✓5ᵗʰ **M61.1 Myositis ossificans progressiva**
     Fibrodysplasia ossificans progressiva
     M61.10   Myositis ossificans progressiva, unspecified site

✓6ᵗʰ **M61.11 Myositis ossificans progressiva, shoulder**
     M61.111   Myositis ossificans progressiva, right shoulder
     M61.112   Myositis ossificans progressiva, left shoulder
     M61.119   Myositis ossificans progressiva, unspecified shoulder

✓6ᵗʰ **M61.12 Myositis ossificans progressiva, upper arm**
     M61.121   Myositis ossificans progressiva, right upper arm
     M61.122   Myositis ossificans progressiva, left upper arm
     M61.129   Myositis ossificans progressiva, unspecified arm

✓6ᵗʰ **M61.13 Myositis ossificans progressiva, forearm**
     M61.131   Myositis ossificans progressiva, right forearm
     M61.132   Myositis ossificans progressiva, left forearm
     M61.139   Myositis ossificans progressiva, unspecified forearm

✓6ᵗʰ **M61.14 Myositis ossificans progressiva, hand and finger(s)**
     M61.141   Myositis ossificans progressiva, right hand
     M61.142   Myositis ossificans progressiva, left hand
     M61.143   Myositis ossificans progressiva, unspecified hand
     M61.144   Myositis ossificans progressiva, right finger(s)
     M61.145   Myositis ossificans progressiva, left finger(s)
     M61.146   Myositis ossificans progressiva, unspecified finger(s)

✓6ᵗʰ **M61.15 Myositis ossificans progressiva, thigh**
     M61.151   Myositis ossificans progressiva, right thigh
     M61.152   Myositis ossificans progressiva, left thigh
     M61.159   Myositis ossificans progressiva, unspecified thigh

✓6ᵗʰ **M61.16 Myositis ossificans progressiva, lower leg**
     M61.161   Myositis ossificans progressiva, right lower leg
     M61.162   Myositis ossificans progressiva, left lower leg
     M61.169   Myositis ossificans progressiva, unspecified lower leg

✓6ᵗʰ **M61.17 Myositis ossificans progressiva, ankle, foot and toe(s)**
     M61.171   Myositis ossificans progressiva, right ankle
     M61.172   Myositis ossificans progressiva, left ankle
     M61.173   Myositis ossificans progressiva, unspecified ankle
     M61.174   Myositis ossificans progressiva, right foot
     M61.175   Myositis ossificans progressiva, left foot
     M61.176   Myositis ossificans progressiva, unspecified foot
     M61.177   Myositis ossificans progressiva, right toe(s)
     M61.178   Myositis ossificans progressiva, left toe(s)
     M61.179   Myositis ossificans progressiva, unspecified toe(s)

M61.18   Myositis ossificans progressiva, other site

M61.19   Myositis ossificans progressiva, multiple sites

✓5ᵗʰ **M61.2 Paralytic calcification and ossification of muscle**
     Myositis ossificans associated with quadriplegia or paraplegia
     M61.20   Paralytic calcification and ossification of muscle, unspecified site

✓6ᵗʰ **M61.21 Paralytic calcification and ossification of muscle, shoulder**
     M61.211   Paralytic calcification and ossification of muscle, right shoulder

✓ Additional Character Req    ✓x7ᵗʰ Placeholder Alert    Unacceptable PDx    Manifestation    **H1–H14** HAC    **HCC** CMS-HCC Condition    **EXCLUDES 1** Not Coded Here    **EXCLUDES 2** Not Included Here

ICD-10-CM 2018      781

**M61.212** Paralytic calcification and ossification of muscle, left shoulder

**M61.219** Paralytic calcification and ossification of muscle, unspecified shoulder

✓6ᵗʰ **M61.22** Paralytic calcification and ossification of muscle, upper arm

**M61.221** Paralytic calcification and ossification of muscle, right upper arm

**M61.222** Paralytic calcification and ossification of muscle, left upper arm

**M61.229** Paralytic calcification and ossification of muscle, unspecified upper arm

✓6ᵗʰ **M61.23** Paralytic calcification and ossification of muscle, forearm

**M61.231** Paralytic calcification and ossification of muscle, right forearm

**M61.232** Paralytic calcification and ossification of muscle, left forearm

**M61.239** Paralytic calcification and ossification of muscle, unspecified forearm

✓6ᵗʰ **M61.24** Paralytic calcification and ossification of muscle, hand

**M61.241** Paralytic calcification and ossification of muscle, right hand

**M61.242** Paralytic calcification and ossification of muscle, left hand

**M61.249** Paralytic calcification and ossification of muscle, unspecified hand

✓6ᵗʰ **M61.25** Paralytic calcification and ossification of muscle, thigh

**M61.251** Paralytic calcification and ossification of muscle, right thigh

**M61.252** Paralytic calcification and ossification of muscle, left thigh

**M61.259** Paralytic calcification and ossification of muscle, unspecified thigh

✓6ᵗʰ **M61.26** Paralytic calcification and ossification of muscle, lower leg

**M61.261** Paralytic calcification and ossification of muscle, right lower leg

**M61.262** Paralytic calcification and ossification of muscle, left lower leg

**M61.269** Paralytic calcification and ossification of muscle, unspecified lower leg

✓6ᵗʰ **M61.27** Paralytic calcification and ossification of muscle, ankle and foot

**M61.271** Paralytic calcification and ossification of muscle, right ankle and foot

**M61.272** Paralytic calcification and ossification of muscle, left ankle and foot

**M61.279** Paralytic calcification and ossification of muscle, unspecified ankle and foot

**M61.28** Paralytic calcification and ossification of muscle, other site

**M61.29** Paralytic calcification and ossification of muscle, multiple sites

✓5ᵗʰ **M61.3** Calcification and ossification of muscles associated with burns

    Myositis ossificans associated with burns

**M61.30** Calcification and ossification of muscles associated with burns, unspecified site

✓6ᵗʰ **M61.31** Calcification and ossification of muscles associated with burns, shoulder

**M61.311** Calcification and ossification of muscles associated with burns, right shoulder

**M61.312** Calcification and ossification of muscles associated with burns, left shoulder

**M61.319** Calcification and ossification of muscles associated with burns, unspecified shoulder

✓6ᵗʰ **M61.32** Calcification and ossification of muscles associated with burns, upper arm

**M61.321** Calcification and ossification of muscles associated with burns, right upper arm

**M61.322** Calcification and ossification of muscles associated with burns, left upper arm

**M61.329** Calcification and ossification of muscles associated with burns, unspecified upper arm

✓6ᵗʰ **M61.33** Calcification and ossification of muscles associated with burns, forearm

**M61.331** Calcification and ossification of muscles associated with burns, right forearm

**M61.332** Calcification and ossification of muscles associated with burns, left forearm

**M61.339** Calcification and ossification of muscles associated with burns, unspecified forearm

✓6ᵗʰ **M61.34** Calcification and ossification of muscles associated with burns, hand

**M61.341** Calcification and ossification of muscles associated with burns, right hand

**M61.342** Calcification and ossification of muscles associated with burns, left hand

**M61.349** Calcification and ossification of muscles associated with burns, unspecified hand

✓6ᵗʰ **M61.35** Calcification and ossification of muscles associated with burns, thigh

**M61.351** Calcification and ossification of muscles associated with burns, right thigh

**M61.352** Calcification and ossification of muscles associated with burns, left thigh

**M61.359** Calcification and ossification of muscles associated with burns, unspecified thigh

✓6ᵗʰ **M61.36** Calcification and ossification of muscles associated with burns, lower leg

**M61.361** Calcification and ossification of muscles associated with burns, right lower leg

**M61.362** Calcification and ossification of muscles associated with burns, left lower leg

**M61.369** Calcification and ossification of muscles associated with burns, unspecified lower leg

✓6ᵗʰ **M61.37** Calcification and ossification of muscles associated with burns, ankle and foot

**M61.371** Calcification and ossification of muscles associated with burns, right ankle and foot

**M61.372** Calcification and ossification of muscles associated with burns, left ankle and foot

**M61.379** Calcification and ossification of muscles associated with burns, unspecified ankle and foot

**M61.38** Calcification and ossification of muscles associated with burns, other site

**M61.39** Calcification and ossification of muscles associated with burns, multiple sites

✓5ᵗʰ **M61.4** Other calcification of muscle

    **EXCLUDES 1**   calcific tendinitis NOS (M65.2-)
                  calcific tendinitis of shoulder (M75.3)

**M61.40** Other calcification of muscle, unspecified site

✓6ᵗʰ **M61.41** Other calcification of muscle, shoulder

**M61.411** Other calcification of muscle, right shoulder

**M61.412** Other calcification of muscle, left shoulder

**M61.419** Other calcification of muscle, unspecified shoulder

✓6ᵗʰ **M61.42** Other calcification of muscle, upper arm

**M61.421** Other calcification of muscle, right upper arm

**M61.422** Other calcification of muscle, left upper arm

**M61.429** Other calcification of muscle, unspecified upper arm

✓6ᵗʰ **M61.43** Other calcification of muscle, forearm

**M61.431** Other calcification of muscle, right forearm

**M61.432** Other calcification of muscle, left forearm

**M61.439** Other calcification of muscle, unspecified forearm

Ⓝ Newborn: 0   Ⓟ Pediatric: 0-17   Ⓜ Maternity: 12-55   Ⓐ Adult: 15-124   **MCC** Major CC Condition   **PDx MCC** PDx acts as own MCC   **CC** CC Condition   **PDx CC** PDx acts as own CC

**782**     ICD-10-CM 2018

✓6ᵗʰ **M61.44** **Other calcification of muscle, hand**
     M61.441 **Other calcification of muscle, right hand**
     M61.442 **Other calcification of muscle, left hand**
     M61.449 **Other calcification of muscle, unspecified hand**

✓6ᵗʰ **M61.45** **Other calcification of muscle, thigh**
     M61.451 **Other calcification of muscle, right thigh**
     M61.452 **Other calcification of muscle, left thigh**
     M61.459 **Other calcification of muscle, unspecified thigh**

✓6ᵗʰ **M61.46** **Other calcification of muscle, lower leg**
     M61.461 **Other calcification of muscle, right lower leg**
     M61.462 **Other calcification of muscle, left lower leg**
     M61.469 **Other calcification of muscle, unspecified lower leg**

✓6ᵗʰ **M61.47** **Other calcification of muscle, ankle and foot**
     M61.471 **Other calcification of muscle, right ankle and foot**
     M61.472 **Other calcification of muscle, left ankle and foot**
     M61.479 **Other calcification of muscle, unspecified ankle and foot**

     **M61.48** **Other calcification of muscle, other site**
     **M61.49** **Other calcification of muscle, multiple sites**

✓5ᵗʰ **M61.5** Other ossification of muscle
     **M61.50** **Other ossification of muscle, unspecified site**

✓6ᵗʰ **M61.51** **Other ossification of muscle, shoulder**
     M61.511 **Other ossification of muscle, right shoulder**
     M61.512 **Other ossification of muscle, left shoulder**
     M61.519 **Other ossification of muscle, unspecified shoulder**

✓6ᵗʰ **M61.52** **Other ossification of muscle, upper arm**
     M61.521 **Other ossification of muscle, right upper arm**
     M61.522 **Other ossification of muscle, left upper arm**
     M61.529 **Other ossification of muscle, unspecified upper arm**

✓6ᵗʰ **M61.53** **Other ossification of muscle, forearm**
     M61.531 **Other ossification of muscle, right forearm**
     M61.532 **Other ossification of muscle, left forearm**
     M61.539 **Other ossification of muscle, unspecified forearm**

✓6ᵗʰ **M61.54** **Other ossification of muscle, hand**
     M61.541 **Other ossification of muscle, right hand**
     M61.542 **Other ossification of muscle, left hand**
     M61.549 **Other ossification of muscle, unspecified hand**

✓6ᵗʰ **M61.55** **Other ossification of muscle, thigh**
     M61.551 **Other ossification of muscle, right thigh**
     M61.552 **Other ossification of muscle, left thigh**
     M61.559 **Other ossification of muscle, unspecified thigh**

✓6ᵗʰ **M61.56** **Other ossification of muscle, lower leg**
     M61.561 **Other ossification of muscle, right lower leg**
     M61.562 **Other ossification of muscle, left lower leg**
     M61.569 **Other ossification of muscle, unspecified lower leg**

✓6ᵗʰ **M61.57** **Other ossification of muscle, ankle and foot**
     M61.571 **Other ossification of muscle, right ankle and foot**
     M61.572 **Other ossification of muscle, left ankle and foot**
     M61.579 **Other ossification of muscle, unspecified ankle and foot**

     **M61.58** **Other ossification of muscle, other site**
     **M61.59** **Other ossification of muscle, multiple sites**
     **M61.9** **Calcification and ossification of muscle, unspecified**

✓4ᵗʰ **M62** **Other disorders of muscle**
     *EXCLUDES 1*    *alcoholic myopathy (G72.1)*
           *cramp and spasm (R25.2)*
           *drug-induced myopathy (G72.0)*
           *myalgia (M79.1)*
           *stiff-man syndrome (G25.82)*
     *EXCLUDES 2*    *nontraumatic hematoma of muscle (M79.81)*

✓5ᵗʰ **M62.0** **Separation of muscle (nontraumatic)**
     Diastasis of muscle
     *EXCLUDES 1*    *diastasis recti complicating pregnancy, labor and delivery (O71.8)*
           *traumatic separation of muscle—see strain of muscle by body region*

     **M62.00** **Separation of muscle (nontraumatic), unspecified site**

✓6ᵗʰ **M62.01** **Separation of muscle (nontraumatic), shoulder**
     M62.011 **Separation of muscle (nontraumatic), right shoulder**
     M62.012 **Separation of muscle (nontraumatic), left shoulder**
     M62.019 **Separation of muscle (nontraumatic), unspecified shoulder**

✓6ᵗʰ **M62.02** **Separation of muscle (nontraumatic), upper arm**
     M62.021 **Separation of muscle (nontraumatic), right upper arm**
     M62.022 **Separation of muscle (nontraumatic), left upper arm**
     M62.029 **Separation of muscle (nontraumatic), unspecified upper arm**

✓6ᵗʰ **M62.03** **Separation of muscle (nontraumatic), forearm**
     M62.031 **Separation of muscle (nontraumatic), right forearm**
     M62.032 **Separation of muscle (nontraumatic), left forearm**
     M62.039 **Separation of muscle (nontraumatic), unspecified forearm**

✓6ᵗʰ **M62.04** **Separation of muscle (nontraumatic), hand**
     M62.041 **Separation of muscle (nontraumatic), right hand**
     M62.042 **Separation of muscle (nontraumatic), left hand**
     M62.049 **Separation of muscle (nontraumatic), unspecified hand**

✓6ᵗʰ **M62.05** **Separation of muscle (nontraumatic), thigh**
     M62.051 **Separation of muscle (nontraumatic), right thigh**
     M62.052 **Separation of muscle (nontraumatic), left thigh**
     M62.059 **Separation of muscle (nontraumatic), unspecified thigh**

✓6ᵗʰ **M62.06** **Separation of muscle (nontraumatic), lower leg**
     M62.061 **Separation of muscle (nontraumatic), right lower leg**
     M62.062 **Separation of muscle (nontraumatic), left lower leg**
     M62.069 **Separation of muscle (nontraumatic), unspecified lower leg**

✓6ᵗʰ **M62.07** **Separation of muscle (nontraumatic), ankle and foot**
     M62.071 **Separation of muscle (nontraumatic), right ankle and foot**
     M62.072 **Separation of muscle (nontraumatic), left ankle and foot**
     M62.079 **Separation of muscle (nontraumatic), unspecified ankle and foot**

     **M62.08** **Separation of muscle (nontraumatic), other site**

✓5ᵗʰ **M62.1** **Other rupture of muscle (nontraumatic)**
     *EXCLUDES 1*    *traumatic rupture of muscle—see strain of muscle by body region*
     *EXCLUDES 2*    *rupture of tendon (M66.-)*

     **M62.10** **Other rupture of muscle (nontraumatic), unspecified site**

✓6ᵗʰ **M62.11** **Other rupture of muscle (nontraumatic), shoulder**
     M62.111 **Other rupture of muscle (nontraumatic), right shoulder**
     M62.112 **Other rupture of muscle (nontraumatic), left shoulder**

**M62.119** Other rupture of muscle (nontraumatic), unspecified **shoulder**

✓6ᵗʰ **M62.12** Other rupture of muscle (nontraumatic), **upper arm**

**M62.121** Other rupture of muscle (nontraumatic), **right upper arm**

**M62.122** Other rupture of muscle (nontraumatic), **left upper arm**

**M62.129** Other rupture of muscle (nontraumatic), unspecified **upper arm**

✓6ᵗʰ **M62.13** Other rupture of muscle (nontraumatic), **forearm**

**M62.131** Other rupture of muscle (nontraumatic), **right forearm**

**M62.132** Other rupture of muscle (nontraumatic), **left forearm**

**M62.139** Other rupture of muscle (nontraumatic), unspecified **forearm**

✓6ᵗʰ **M62.14** Other rupture of muscle (nontraumatic), **hand**

**M62.141** Other rupture of muscle (nontraumatic), **right hand**

**M62.142** Other rupture of muscle (nontraumatic), **left hand**

**M62.149** Other rupture of muscle (nontraumatic), unspecified **hand**

✓6ᵗʰ **M62.15** Other rupture of muscle (nontraumatic), **thigh**

**M62.151** Other rupture of muscle (nontraumatic), **right thigh**

**M62.152** Other rupture of muscle (nontraumatic), **left thigh**

**M62.159** Other rupture of muscle (nontraumatic), unspecified **thigh**

✓6ᵗʰ **M62.16** Other rupture of muscle (nontraumatic), **lower leg**

**M62.161** Other rupture of muscle (nontraumatic), **right lower leg**

**M62.162** Other rupture of muscle (nontraumatic), **left lower leg**

**M62.169** Other rupture of muscle (nontraumatic), unspecified **lower leg**

✓6ᵗʰ **M62.17** Other rupture of muscle (nontraumatic), **ankle and foot**

**M62.171** Other rupture of muscle (nontraumatic), **right ankle and foot**

**M62.172** Other rupture of muscle (nontraumatic), **left ankle and foot**

**M62.179** Other rupture of muscle (nontraumatic), unspecified **ankle and foot**

**M62.18** Other rupture of muscle (nontraumatic), **other site**

✓5ᵗʰ **M62.2 Nontraumatic ischemic infarction of muscle**

EXCLUDES 1    compartment syndrome (traumatic) (T79.A-)
nontraumatic compartment syndrome (M79.A-)
rhabdomyolysis (M62.82)
traumatic ischemia of muscle (T79.6)
Volkmann's ischemic contracture (T79.6)

**M62.20** Nontraumatic ischemic infarction of muscle, unspecified site

✓6ᵗʰ **M62.21** Nontraumatic ischemic infarction of muscle, shoulder

**M62.211** Nontraumatic ischemic infarction of muscle, **right shoulder**

**M62.212** Nontraumatic ischemic infarction of muscle, **left shoulder**

**M62.219** Nontraumatic ischemic infarction of muscle, unspecified **shoulder**

✓6ᵗʰ **M62.22** Nontraumatic ischemic infarction of muscle, upper arm

**M62.221** Nontraumatic ischemic infarction of muscle, **right upper arm**

**M62.222** Nontraumatic ischemic infarction of muscle, **left upper arm**

**M62.229** Nontraumatic ischemic infarction of muscle, unspecified **upper arm**

✓6ᵗʰ **M62.23** Nontraumatic ischemic infarction of muscle, **forearm**

**M62.231** Nontraumatic ischemic infarction of muscle, **right forearm**

**M62.232** Nontraumatic ischemic infarction of muscle, **left forearm**

**M62.239** Nontraumatic ischemic infarction of muscle, unspecified **forearm**

✓6ᵗʰ **M62.24** Nontraumatic ischemic infarction of muscle, **hand**

**M62.241** Nontraumatic ischemic infarction of muscle, **right hand**

**M62.242** Nontraumatic ischemic infarction of muscle, **left hand**

**M62.249** Nontraumatic ischemic infarction of muscle, unspecified **hand**

✓6ᵗʰ **M62.25** Nontraumatic ischemic infarction of muscle, **thigh**

**M62.251** Nontraumatic ischemic infarction of muscle, **right thigh**

**M62.252** Nontraumatic ischemic infarction of muscle, **left thigh**

**M62.259** Nontraumatic ischemic infarction of muscle, unspecified **thigh**

✓6ᵗʰ **M62.26** Nontraumatic ischemic infarction of muscle, **lower leg**

**M62.261** Nontraumatic ischemic infarction of muscle, **right lower leg**

**M62.262** Nontraumatic ischemic infarction of muscle, **left lower leg**

**M62.269** Nontraumatic ischemic infarction of muscle, unspecified **lower leg**

✓6ᵗʰ **M62.27** Nontraumatic ischemic infarction of muscle, **ankle and foot**

**M62.271** Nontraumatic ischemic infarction of muscle, **right ankle and foot**

**M62.272** Nontraumatic ischemic infarction of muscle, **left ankle and foot**

**M62.279** Nontraumatic ischemic infarction of muscle, unspecified **ankle and foot**

**M62.28** Nontraumatic ischemic infarction of muscle, **other site**

**M62.3 Immobility syndrome (paraplegic)**

✓5ᵗʰ **M62.4 Contracture of muscle**

Contracture of tendon (sheath)

EXCLUDES 1    contracture of joint (M24.5-)

**M62.40** Contracture of muscle, **unspecified site**

✓6ᵗʰ **M62.41** Contracture of muscle, **shoulder**

**M62.411** Contracture of muscle, **right shoulder**

**M62.412** Contracture of muscle, **left shoulder**

**M62.419** Contracture of muscle, unspecified **shoulder**

✓6ᵗʰ **M62.42** Contracture of muscle, **upper arm**

**M62.421** Contracture of muscle, **right upper arm**

**M62.422** Contracture of muscle, **left upper arm**

**M62.429** Contracture of muscle, unspecified **upper arm**

✓6ᵗʰ **M62.43** Contracture of muscle, **forearm**

**M62.431** Contracture of muscle, **right forearm**

**M62.432** Contracture of muscle, **left forearm**

**M62.439** Contracture of muscle, unspecified **forearm**

✓6ᵗʰ **M62.44** Contracture of muscle, **hand**

**M62.441** Contracture of muscle, **right hand**

**M62.442** Contracture of muscle, **left hand**

**M62.449** Contracture of muscle, unspecified **hand**

✓6ᵗʰ **M62.45** Contracture of muscle, **thigh**

**M62.451** Contracture of muscle, **right thigh**

**M62.452** Contracture of muscle, **left thigh**

**M62.459** Contracture of muscle, unspecified **thigh**

✓6ᵗʰ **M62.46** Contracture of muscle, **lower leg**

**M62.461** Contracture of muscle, **right lower leg**

**M62.462** Contracture of muscle, **left lower leg**

**M62.469** Contracture of muscle, unspecified **lower leg**

✓6ᵗʰ **M62.47** Contracture of muscle, **ankle and foot**

**M62.471** Contracture of muscle, **right ankle and foot**

**M62.472** Contracture of muscle, **left ankle and foot**

**M62.479** Contracture of muscle, unspecified **ankle and foot**

**M62.48** Contracture of muscle, **other site**

**M62.49** Contracture of muscle, **multiple sites**

N Newborn: 0    P Pediatric: 0-17    M Maternity: 12-55    A Adult: 15-124    MCC Major CC Condition    PDx MCC PDx acts as own MCC    CC CC Condition    PDx CC PDx acts as own CC

784    ICD-10-CM 2018

☑5ᵗʰ **M62.5** **Muscle wasting and atrophy, not elsewhere classified**
Disuse atrophy NEC
*EXCLUDES 1*   *neuralgic amyotrophy (G54.5)*
        *progressive muscular atrophy ▶(G12.21)◀*
        *sarcopenia (M62.84)*
*EXCLUDES 2*   *pelvic muscle wasting (N81.84)*

    **M62.50** **Muscle wasting and atrophy, not elsewhere classified, unspecified site**

☑6ᵗʰ **M62.51** **Muscle wasting and atrophy, not elsewhere classified, shoulder**
      **M62.511** Muscle wasting and atrophy, not elsewhere classified, right shoulder
      **M62.512** Muscle wasting and atrophy, not elsewhere classified, left shoulder
      **M62.519** Muscle wasting and atrophy, not elsewhere classified, unspecified shoulder

☑6ᵗʰ **M62.52** **Muscle wasting and atrophy, not elsewhere classified, upper arm**
      **M62.521** Muscle wasting and atrophy, not elsewhere classified, right upper arm
      **M62.522** Muscle wasting and atrophy, not elsewhere classified, left upper arm
      **M62.529** Muscle wasting and atrophy, not elsewhere classified, unspecified upper arm

☑6ᵗʰ **M62.53** **Muscle wasting and atrophy, not elsewhere classified, forearm**
      **M62.531** Muscle wasting and atrophy, not elsewhere classified, right forearm
      **M62.532** Muscle wasting and atrophy, not elsewhere classified, left forearm
      **M62.539** Muscle wasting and atrophy, not elsewhere classified, unspecified forearm

☑6ᵗʰ **M62.54** **Muscle wasting and atrophy, not elsewhere classified, hand**
      **M62.541** Muscle wasting and atrophy, not elsewhere classified, right hand
      **M62.542** Muscle wasting and atrophy, not elsewhere classified, left hand
      **M62.549** Muscle wasting and atrophy, not elsewhere classified, unspecified hand

☑6ᵗʰ **M62.55** **Muscle wasting and atrophy, not elsewhere classified, thigh**
      **M62.551** Muscle wasting and atrophy, not elsewhere classified, right thigh
      **M62.552** Muscle wasting and atrophy, not elsewhere classified, left thigh
      **M62.559** Muscle wasting and atrophy, not elsewhere classified, unspecified thigh

☑6ᵗʰ **M62.56** **Muscle wasting and atrophy, not elsewhere classified, lower leg**
      **M62.561** Muscle wasting and atrophy, not elsewhere classified, right lower leg
      **M62.562** Muscle wasting and atrophy, not elsewhere classified, left lower leg
      **M62.569** Muscle wasting and atrophy, not elsewhere classified, unspecified lower leg

☑6ᵗʰ **M62.57** **Muscle wasting and atrophy, not elsewhere classified, ankle and foot**
      **M62.571** Muscle wasting and atrophy, not elsewhere classified, right ankle and foot
      **M62.572** Muscle wasting and atrophy, not elsewhere classified, left ankle and foot
      **M62.579** Muscle wasting and atrophy, not elsewhere classified, unspecified ankle and foot

    **M62.58** **Muscle wasting and atrophy, not elsewhere classified, other site**

    **M62.59** **Muscle wasting and atrophy, not elsewhere classified, multiple sites**

☑5ᵗʰ **M62.8** **Other specified disorders of muscle**
*EXCLUDES 2*   *nontraumatic hematoma of muscle (M79.81)*

    **M62.81** **Muscle weakness (generalized)**
      *EXCLUDES 1*   *muscle weakness in sarcopenia (M62.84)*

    **M62.82** **Rhabdomyolysis**      CC
      *EXCLUDES 1*   *traumatic rhabdomyolysis (T79.6)*
      **DEF:** Rapid disintegration or destruction of skeletal muscle caused by direct or indirect injury; resulting in the excretion of muscle protein myoglobin into the urine.
      **CC Excl:** PDX collection 892

☑6ᵗʰ **M62.83** **Muscle spasm**
      **M62.830** Muscle spasm of back
      **M62.831** Muscle spasm of calf
        Charley-horse
      **M62.838** Other muscle spasm

    **M62.84** **Sarcopenia**
      Age-related sarcopenia
      Code first underlying disease, if applicable, such as:
        disorders of myoneural junction and muscle disease in diseases classified elsewhere (G73.-)
        other and unspecified myopathies (G72.-)
        primary disorders of muscles (G71.-)

    **M62.89** **Other specified disorders of muscle**
      Muscle (sheath) hernia

  **M62.9** **Disorder of muscle, unspecified**

☑4ᵗʰ **M63** **Disorders of muscle in diseases classified elsewhere**
Code first underlying disease, such as:
   leprosy (A30.-)
   neoplasm (C49-, C79.89, D21-, D48.1)
   schistosomiasis (B65.-)
   trichinellosis (B75)
*EXCLUDES 1*   *myopathy in cysticercosis (B69.81)*
        *myopathy in endocrine diseases (G73.7)*
        *myopathy in metabolic diseases (G73.7)*
        *myopathy in sarcoidosis (D86.87)*
        *myopathy in secondary syphilis (A51.49)*
        *myopathy in syphilis (late) (A52.78)*
        *myopathy in toxoplasmosis (B58.82)*
        *myopathy in tuberculosis (A18.09)*

☑5ᵗʰ **M63.8** **Disorders of muscle in diseases classified elsewhere**
    *M63.80*   *Disorders of muscle in diseases classified elsewhere, unspecified site*

☑6ᵗʰ **M63.81** **Disorders of muscle in diseases classified elsewhere, shoulder**
      *M63.811*   *Disorders of muscle in diseases classified elsewhere, right shoulder*
      *M63.812*   *Disorders of muscle in diseases classified elsewhere, left shoulder*
      *M63.819*   *Disorders of muscle in diseases classified elsewhere, unspecified shoulder*

☑6ᵗʰ **M63.82** **Disorders of muscle in diseases classified elsewhere, upper arm**
      *M63.821*   *Disorders of muscle in diseases classified elsewhere, right upper arm*
      *M63.822*   *Disorders of muscle in diseases classified elsewhere, left upper arm*
      *M63.829*   *Disorders of muscle in diseases classified elsewhere, unspecified upper arm*

☑6ᵗʰ **M63.83** **Disorders of muscle in diseases classified elsewhere, forearm**
      *M63.831*   *Disorders of muscle in diseases classified elsewhere, right forearm*
      *M63.832*   *Disorders of muscle in diseases classified elsewhere, left forearm*
      *M63.839*   *Disorders of muscle in diseases classified elsewhere, unspecified forearm*

☑6ᵗʰ **M63.84** **Disorders of muscle in diseases classified elsewhere, hand**
      *M63.841*   *Disorders of muscle in diseases classified elsewhere, right hand*
      *M63.842*   *Disorders of muscle in diseases classified elsewhere, left hand*
      *M63.849*   *Disorders of muscle in diseases classified elsewhere, unspecified hand*

---

☑Additional Character Req    ☑x7ᵗʰ Placeholder Alert    Unacceptable PDx    **Manifestation**    **H1 - H14** HAC    **HCC** CMS-HCC Condition    *EXCLUDES 1* Not Coded Here    *EXCLUDES 2* Not Included Here

**ICD-10-CM 2018**                                                      **785**

√6ᵗʰ **M63.85** Disorders of muscle in diseases classified elsewhere, thigh

**M63.851** *Disorders of muscle in diseases classified elsewhere, right thigh*

**M63.852** *Disorders of muscle in diseases classified elsewhere, left thigh*

**M63.859** *Disorders of muscle in diseases classified elsewhere, unspecified thigh*

√6ᵗʰ **M63.86** Disorders of muscle in diseases classified elsewhere, lower leg

**M63.861** *Disorders of muscle in diseases classified elsewhere, right lower leg*

**M63.862** *Disorders of muscle in diseases classified elsewhere, left lower leg*

**M63.869** *Disorders of muscle in diseases classified elsewhere, unspecified lower leg*

√6ᵗʰ **M63.87** Disorders of muscle in diseases classified elsewhere, ankle and foot

**M63.871** *Disorders of muscle in diseases classified elsewhere, right ankle and foot*

**M63.872** *Disorders of muscle in diseases classified elsewhere, left ankle and foot*

**M63.879** *Disorders of muscle in diseases classified elsewhere, unspecified ankle and foot*

**M63.88** *Disorders of muscle in diseases classified elsewhere, other site*

**M63.89** *Disorders of muscle in diseases classified elsewhere, multiple sites*

## Disorders of synovium and tendon (M65-M67)

√4ᵗʰ **M65 Synovitis and tenosynovitis**

**EXCLUDES 1** *chronic creptant synovitis of hand and wrist (M70.0-)*
*current injury—see injury of ligament or tendon by body region*
*soft tissue disorders related to use, overuse and pressure (M70.-)*

√5ᵗʰ **M65.0 Abscess of tendon sheath**

Use additional code (B95-B96) to identify bacterial agent.

**M65.00** Abscess of tendon sheath, unspecified site

√6ᵗʰ **M65.01** Abscess of tendon sheath, shoulder

**M65.011** Abscess of tendon sheath, right shoulder
**M65.012** Abscess of tendon sheath, left shoulder
**M65.019** Abscess of tendon sheath, unspecified shoulder

√6ᵗʰ **M65.02** Abscess of tendon sheath, upper arm

**M65.021** Abscess of tendon sheath, right upper arm
**M65.022** Abscess of tendon sheath, left upper arm
**M65.029** Abscess of tendon sheath, unspecified upper arm

√6ᵗʰ **M65.03** Abscess of tendon sheath, forearm

**M65.031** Abscess of tendon sheath, right forearm
**M65.032** Abscess of tendon sheath, left forearm
**M65.039** Abscess of tendon sheath, unspecified forearm

√6ᵗʰ **M65.04** Abscess of tendon sheath, hand

**M65.041** Abscess of tendon sheath, right hand
**M65.042** Abscess of tendon sheath, left hand
**M65.049** Abscess of tendon sheath, unspecified hand

√6ᵗʰ **M65.05** Abscess of tendon sheath, thigh

**M65.051** Abscess of tendon sheath, right thigh
**M65.052** Abscess of tendon sheath, left thigh
**M65.059** Abscess of tendon sheath, unspecified thigh

√6ᵗʰ **M65.06** Abscess of tendon sheath, lower leg

**M65.061** Abscess of tendon sheath, right lower leg
**M65.062** Abscess of tendon sheath, left lower leg
**M65.069** Abscess of tendon sheath, unspecified lower leg

√6ᵗʰ **M65.07** Abscess of tendon sheath, ankle and foot

**M65.071** Abscess of tendon sheath, right ankle and foot
**M65.072** Abscess of tendon sheath, left ankle and foot
**M65.079** Abscess of tendon sheath, unspecified ankle and foot

**M65.08** Abscess of tendon sheath, other site

√5ᵗʰ **M65.1 Other infective (teno)synovitis**

**M65.10** Other infective (teno)synovitis, unspecified site

√6ᵗʰ **M65.11** Other infective (teno)synovitis, shoulder

**M65.111** Other infective (teno)synovitis, right shoulder
**M65.112** Other infective (teno)synovitis, left shoulder
**M65.119** Other infective (teno)synovitis, unspecified shoulder

√6ᵗʰ **M65.12** Other infective (teno)synovitis, elbow

**M65.121** Other infective (teno)synovitis, right elbow
**M65.122** Other infective (teno)synovitis, left elbow
**M65.129** Other infective (teno)synovitis, unspecified elbow

√6ᵗʰ **M65.13** Other infective (teno)synovitis, wrist

**M65.131** Other infective (teno)synovitis, right wrist
**M65.132** Other infective (teno)synovitis, left wrist
**M65.139** Other infective (teno)synovitis, unspecified wrist

√6ᵗʰ **M65.14** Other infective (teno)synovitis, hand

**M65.141** Other infective (teno)synovitis, right hand
**M65.142** Other infective (teno)synovitis, left hand
**M65.149** Other infective (teno)synovitis, unspecified hand

√6ᵗʰ **M65.15** Other infective (teno)synovitis, hip

**M65.151** Other infective (teno)synovitis, right hip
**M65.152** Other infective (teno)synovitis, left hip
**M65.159** Other infective (teno)synovitis, unspecified hip

√6ᵗʰ **M65.16** Other infective (teno)synovitis, knee

**M65.161** Other infective (teno)synovitis, right knee
**M65.162** Other infective (teno)synovitis, left knee
**M65.169** Other infective (teno)synovitis, unspecified knee

√6ᵗʰ **M65.17** Other infective (teno)synovitis, ankle and foot

**M65.171** Other infective (teno)synovitis, right ankle and foot
**M65.172** Other infective (teno)synovitis, left ankle and foot
**M65.179** Other infective (teno)synovitis, unspecified ankle and foot

**M65.18** Other infective (teno)synovitis, other site

**M65.19** Other infective (teno)synovitis, multiple sites

√5ᵗʰ **M65.2 Calcific tendinitis**

**EXCLUDES 1** *tendinitis as classified in M75-M77*
*calcified tendinitis of shoulder (M75.3)*

**M65.20** Calcific tendinitis, unspecified site

√6ᵗʰ **M65.22** Calcific tendinitis, upper arm

**M65.221** Calcific tendinitis, right upper arm
**M65.222** Calcific tendinitis, left upper arm
**M65.229** Calcific tendinitis, unspecified upper arm

√6ᵗʰ **M65.23** Calcific tendinitis, forearm

**M65.231** Calcific tendinitis, right forearm
**M65.232** Calcific tendinitis, left forearm
**M65.239** Calcific tendinitis, unspecified forearm

√6ᵗʰ **M65.24** Calcific tendinitis, hand

**M65.241** Calcific tendinitis, right hand
**M65.242** Calcific tendinitis, left hand
**M65.249** Calcific tendinitis, unspecified hand

√6ᵗʰ **M65.25** Calcific tendinitis, thigh

**M65.251** Calcific tendinitis, right thigh
**M65.252** Calcific tendinitis, left thigh
**M65.259** Calcific tendinitis, unspecified thigh

√6ᵗʰ **M65.26** Calcific tendinitis, lower leg

**M65.261** Calcific tendinitis, right lower leg
**M65.262** Calcific tendinitis, left lower leg
**M65.269** Calcific tendinitis, unspecified lower leg

√6ᵗʰ **M65.27** Calcific tendinitis, ankle and foot

**M65.271** Calcific tendinitis, right ankle and foot
**M65.272** Calcific tendinitis, left ankle and foot
**M65.279** Calcific tendinitis, unspecified ankle and foot

N Newborn: 0   P Pediatric: 0-17   M Maternity: 12-55   A Adult: 15-124   MCC Major CC Condition   PDx MCC PDx acts as own MCC   CC CC Condition   PDx CC PDx acts as own CC

786
ICD-10-CM 2018

M65.28   Calcific tendinitis, **other site**

M65.29   Calcific tendinitis, **multiple sites**

√5ᵗʰ **M65.3**   **Trigger finger**
     Nodular tendinous disease

    M65.30   Trigger finger, **unspecified finger**

    √6ᵗʰ **M65.31**   **Trigger thumb**

       M65.311   Trigger thumb, **right thumb**

       M65.312   Trigger thumb, **left thumb**

       M65.319   Trigger thumb, **unspecified thumb**

    √6ᵗʰ **M65.32**   **Trigger finger, index finger**

       M65.321   Trigger finger, **right index finger**

       M65.322   Trigger finger, **left index finger**

       M65.329   Trigger finger, **unspecified index finger**

    √6ᵗʰ **M65.33**   **Trigger finger, middle finger**

       M65.331   Trigger finger, **right middle finger**

       M65.332   Trigger finger, **left middle finger**

       M65.339   Trigger finger, **unspecified middle finger**

    √6ᵗʰ **M65.34**   **Trigger finger, ring finger**

       M65.341   Trigger finger, **right ring finger**

       M65.342   Trigger finger, **left ring finger**

       M65.349   Trigger finger, **unspecified ring finger**

    √6ᵗʰ **M65.35**   **Trigger finger, little finger**

       M65.351   Trigger finger, **right little finger**

       M65.352   Trigger finger, **left little finger**

       M65.359   Trigger finger, **unspecified little finger**

**M65.4**   Radial styloid tenosynovitis [de Quervain]

√5ᵗʰ **M65.8**   **Other synovitis and tenosynovitis**

    M65.80   Other synovitis and tenosynovitis, **unspecified site**

    √6ᵗʰ **M65.81**   **Other synovitis and tenosynovitis, shoulder**

       M65.811   Other synovitis and tenosynovitis, **right shoulder**

       M65.812   Other synovitis and tenosynovitis, **left shoulder**

       M65.819   Other synovitis and tenosynovitis, **unspecified shoulder**

    √6ᵗʰ **M65.82**   **Other synovitis and tenosynovitis, upper arm**

       M65.821   Other synovitis and tenosynovitis, **right upper arm**

       M65.822   Other synovitis and tenosynovitis, **left upper arm**

       M65.829   Other synovitis and tenosynovitis, **unspecified upper arm**

    √6ᵗʰ **M65.83**   **Other synovitis and tenosynovitis, forearm**

       M65.831   Other synovitis and tenosynovitis, **right forearm**

       M65.832   Other synovitis and tenosynovitis, **left forearm**

       M65.839   Other synovitis and tenosynovitis, **unspecified forearm**

    √6ᵗʰ **M65.84**   **Other synovitis and tenosynovitis, hand**

       M65.841   Other synovitis and tenosynovitis, **right hand**

       M65.842   Other synovitis and tenosynovitis, **left hand**

       M65.849   Other synovitis and tenosynovitis, **unspecified hand**

    √6ᵗʰ **M65.85**   **Other synovitis and tenosynovitis, thigh**

       M65.851   Other synovitis and tenosynovitis, **right thigh**

       M65.852   Other synovitis and tenosynovitis, **left thigh**

       M65.859   Other synovitis and tenosynovitis, **unspecified thigh**

    √6ᵗʰ **M65.86**   **Other synovitis and tenosynovitis, lower leg**

       M65.861   Other synovitis and tenosynovitis, **right lower leg**

       M65.862   Other synovitis and tenosynovitis, **left lower leg**

       M65.869   Other synovitis and tenosynovitis, **unspecified lower leg**

    √6ᵗʰ **M65.87**   **Other synovitis and tenosynovitis, ankle and foot**

       M65.871   Other synovitis and tenosynovitis, **right ankle and foot**

       M65.872   Other synovitis and tenosynovitis, **left ankle and foot**

       M65.879   Other synovitis and tenosynovitis, **unspecified ankle and foot**

    M65.88   Other synovitis and tenosynovitis, **other site**

    M65.89   Other synovitis and tenosynovitis, **multiple sites**

**M65.9**   Synovitis and tenosynovitis, **unspecified**

√4ᵗʰ **M66**   **Spontaneous rupture of synovium and tendon**

    **INCLUDES**   rupture that occurs when a normal force is applied to tissues that are inferred to have less than normal strength

    *EXCLUDES 2*   *rotator cuff syndrome (M75.1-)*
       *rupture where an abnormal force is applied to normal tissue—see injury of tendon by body region*

**M66.0**   **Rupture of popliteal cyst**

√5ᵗʰ **M66.1**   **Rupture of synovium**
     Rupture of synovial cyst
     *EXCLUDES 2*   *rupture of popliteal cyst (M66.0)*

    M66.10   Rupture of synovium, **unspecified joint**

    √6ᵗʰ **M66.11**   **Rupture of synovium, shoulder**

       M66.111   Rupture of synovium, **right shoulder**

       M66.112   Rupture of synovium, **left shoulder**

       M66.119   Rupture of synovium, **unspecified shoulder**

    √6ᵗʰ **M66.12**   **Rupture of synovium, elbow**

       M66.121   Rupture of synovium, **right elbow**

       M66.122   Rupture of synovium, **left elbow**

       M66.129   Rupture of synovium, **unspecified elbow**

    √6ᵗʰ **M66.13**   **Rupture of synovium, wrist**

       M66.131   Rupture of synovium, **right wrist**

       M66.132   Rupture of synovium, **left wrist**

       M66.139   Rupture of synovium, **unspecified wrist**

    √6ᵗʰ **M66.14**   **Rupture of synovium, hand and fingers**

       M66.141   Rupture of synovium, **right hand**

       M66.142   Rupture of synovium, **left hand**

       M66.143   Rupture of synovium, **unspecified hand**

       M66.144   Rupture of synovium, **right finger(s)**

       M66.145   Rupture of synovium, **left finger(s)**

       M66.146   Rupture of synovium, **unspecified finger(s)**

    √6ᵗʰ **M66.15**   **Rupture of synovium, hip**

       M66.151   Rupture of synovium, **right hip**

       M66.152   Rupture of synovium, **left hip**

       M66.159   Rupture of synovium, **unspecified hip**

    √6ᵗʰ **M66.17**   **Rupture of synovium, ankle, foot and toes**

       M66.171   Rupture of synovium, **right ankle**

       M66.172   Rupture of synovium, **left ankle**

       M66.173   Rupture of synovium, **unspecified ankle**

       M66.174   Rupture of synovium, **right foot**

       M66.175   Rupture of synovium, **left foot**

       M66.176   Rupture of synovium, **unspecified foot**

       M66.177   Rupture of synovium, **right toe(s)**

       M66.178   Rupture of synovium, **left toe(s)**

       M66.179   Rupture of synovium, **unspecified toe(s)**

    M66.18   Rupture of synovium, **other site**

√5ᵗʰ **M66.2**   **Spontaneous rupture of extensor tendons**
     **TIP:** Refer to the Muscle/Tendon table at the beginning of this chapter.

    M66.20   Spontaneous rupture of extensor tendons, **unspecified site**

    √6ᵗʰ **M66.21**   **Spontaneous rupture of extensor tendons, shoulder**

       M66.211   Spontaneous rupture of extensor tendons, **right shoulder**

       M66.212   Spontaneous rupture of extensor tendons, **left shoulder**

       M66.219   Spontaneous rupture of extensor tendons, **unspecified shoulder**

    √6ᵗʰ **M66.22**   **Spontaneous rupture of extensor tendons, upper arm**

       M66.221   Spontaneous rupture of extensor tendons, **right upper arm**

       M66.222   Spontaneous rupture of extensor tendons, **left upper arm**

       M66.229   Spontaneous rupture of extensor tendons, **unspecified upper arm**

√ Additional Character Req   √x7ᵗʰ Placeholder Alert   Unacceptable PDx   Manifestation   **H1** - **H14** HAC   **HCC** CMS-HCC Condition   *EXCLUDES 1* Not Coded Here   *EXCLUDES 2* Not Included Here

ICD-10-CM 2018      787

✓6ᵗʰ **M66.23** **Spontaneous rupture of extensor tendons,** forearm

**M66.231** **Spontaneous rupture of extensor tendons, right forearm**

**M66.232** **Spontaneous rupture of extensor tendons, left forearm**

**M66.239** **Spontaneous rupture of extensor tendons, unspecified forearm**

✓6ᵗʰ **M66.24** **Spontaneous rupture of extensor tendons,** hand

**M66.241** **Spontaneous rupture of extensor tendons, right hand**

**M66.242** **Spontaneous rupture of extensor tendons, left hand**

**M66.249** **Spontaneous rupture of extensor tendons, unspecified hand**

✓6ᵗʰ **M66.25** **Spontaneous rupture of extensor tendons,** thigh

**M66.251** **Spontaneous rupture of extensor tendons, right thigh**

**M66.252** **Spontaneous rupture of extensor tendons, left thigh**

**M66.259** **Spontaneous rupture of extensor tendons, unspecified thigh**

✓6ᵗʰ **M66.26** **Spontaneous rupture of extensor tendons,** lower leg

**M66.261** **Spontaneous rupture of extensor tendons, right lower leg**

**M66.262** **Spontaneous rupture of extensor tendons, left lower leg**

**M66.269** **Spontaneous rupture of extensor tendons, unspecified lower leg**

✓6ᵗʰ **M66.27** **Spontaneous rupture of extensor tendons, ankle and foot**

**M66.271** **Spontaneous rupture of extensor tendons, right ankle and foot**

**M66.272** **Spontaneous rupture of extensor tendons, left ankle and foot**

**M66.279** **Spontaneous rupture of extensor tendons, unspecified ankle and foot**

**M66.28** **Spontaneous rupture of extensor tendons,** other site

**M66.29** **Spontaneous rupture of extensor tendons,** multiple sites

✓5ᵗʰ **M66.3** **Spontaneous rupture of** flexor tendons

**TIP:** Refer to the Muscle/Tendon table at the beginning of this chapter.

**M66.30** **Spontaneous rupture of flexor tendons, unspecified site**

✓6ᵗʰ **M66.31** **Spontaneous rupture of flexor tendons,** shoulder

**M66.311** **Spontaneous rupture of flexor tendons, right shoulder**

**M66.312** **Spontaneous rupture of flexor tendons, left shoulder**

**M66.319** **Spontaneous rupture of flexor tendons, unspecified shoulder**

✓6ᵗʰ **M66.32** **Spontaneous rupture of flexor tendons,** upper arm

**M66.321** **Spontaneous rupture of flexor tendons, right upper arm**

**M66.322** **Spontaneous rupture of flexor tendons, left upper arm**

**M66.329** **Spontaneous rupture of flexor tendons, unspecified upper arm**

✓6ᵗʰ **M66.33** **Spontaneous rupture of flexor tendons,** forearm

**M66.331** **Spontaneous rupture of flexor tendons, right forearm**

**M66.332** **Spontaneous rupture of flexor tendons, left forearm**

**M66.339** **Spontaneous rupture of flexor tendons, unspecified forearm**

✓6ᵗʰ **M66.34** **Spontaneous rupture of flexor tendons,** hand

**M66.341** **Spontaneous rupture of flexor tendons, right hand**

**M66.342** **Spontaneous rupture of flexor tendons, left hand**

**M66.349** **Spontaneous rupture of flexor tendons, unspecified hand**

✓6ᵗʰ **M66.35** **Spontaneous rupture of flexor tendons,** thigh

**M66.351** **Spontaneous rupture of flexor tendons, right thigh**

**M66.352** **Spontaneous rupture of flexor tendons, left thigh**

**M66.359** **Spontaneous rupture of flexor tendons, unspecified thigh**

✓6ᵗʰ **M66.36** **Spontaneous rupture of flexor tendons,** lower leg

**M66.361** **Spontaneous rupture of flexor tendons, right lower leg**

**M66.362** **Spontaneous rupture of flexor tendons, left lower leg**

**M66.369** **Spontaneous rupture of flexor tendons, unspecified lower leg**

✓6ᵗʰ **M66.37** **Spontaneous rupture of flexor tendons, ankle and foot**

**M66.371** **Spontaneous rupture of flexor tendons, right ankle and foot**

**M66.372** **Spontaneous rupture of flexor tendons, left ankle and foot**

**M66.379** **Spontaneous rupture of flexor tendons, unspecified ankle and foot**

**M66.38** **Spontaneous rupture of flexor tendons,** other site

**M66.39** **Spontaneous rupture of flexor tendons,** multiple sites

✓5ᵗʰ **M66.8** **Spontaneous rupture of** other tendons

**TIP:** Refer to the Muscle/Tendon table at the beginning of this chapter.

**M66.80** **Spontaneous rupture of other tendons, unspecified site**

✓6ᵗʰ **M66.81** **Spontaneous rupture of other tendons,** shoulder

**M66.811** **Spontaneous rupture of other tendons, right shoulder**

**M66.812** **Spontaneous rupture of other tendons, left shoulder**

**M66.819** **Spontaneous rupture of other tendons, unspecified shoulder**

✓6ᵗʰ **M66.82** **Spontaneous rupture of other tendons,** upper arm

**M66.821** **Spontaneous rupture of other tendons, right upper arm**

**M66.822** **Spontaneous rupture of other tendons, left upper arm**

**M66.829** **Spontaneous rupture of other tendons, unspecified upper arm**

✓6ᵗʰ **M66.83** **Spontaneous rupture of other tendons,** forearm

**M66.831** **Spontaneous rupture of other tendons, right forearm**

**M66.832** **Spontaneous rupture of other tendons, left forearm**

**M66.839** **Spontaneous rupture of other tendons, unspecified forearm**

✓6ᵗʰ **M66.84** **Spontaneous rupture of other tendons,** hand

**M66.841** **Spontaneous rupture of other tendons, right hand**

**M66.842** **Spontaneous rupture of other tendons, left hand**

**M66.849** **Spontaneous rupture of other tendons, unspecified hand**

✓6ᵗʰ **M66.85** **Spontaneous rupture of other tendons,** thigh

**M66.851** **Spontaneous rupture of other tendons, right thigh**

**M66.852** **Spontaneous rupture of other tendons, left thigh**

**M66.859** **Spontaneous rupture of other tendons, unspecified thigh**

✓6ᵗʰ **M66.86** **Spontaneous rupture of other tendons,** lower leg

**M66.861** **Spontaneous rupture of other tendons, right lower leg**

**M66.862** **Spontaneous rupture of other tendons, left lower leg**

**M66.869** **Spontaneous rupture of other tendons, unspecified lower leg**

✓6ᵗʰ **M66.87** **Spontaneous rupture of other tendons, ankle and foot**

**M66.871** **Spontaneous rupture of other tendons, right ankle and foot**

**M66.872** **Spontaneous rupture of other tendons, left ankle and foot**

**M66.879** **Spontaneous rupture of other tendons, unspecified ankle and foot**

**M66.88** **Spontaneous rupture of other tendons,** other

N Newborn: 0    P Pediatric: 0-17    M Maternity: 12-55    A Adult: 15-124    MCC Major CC Condition    PDx MCC PDx acts as own MCC    CC CC Condition    PDx CC PDx acts as own CC

788

ICD-10-CM 2018

    **M66.89**    Spontaneous rupture of other tendons, **multiple sites**

  **M66.9**   Spontaneous rupture of **unspecified tendon**
       Rupture at musculotendinous junction, nontraumatic

**☑4ᵗʰ M67 Other disorders of synovium and tendon**
     *EXCLUDES 1*    palmar fascial fibromatosis [Dupuytren] (M72.0)
              tendinitis NOS (M77.9-)
              xanthomatosis localized to tendons (E78.2)

  **☑5ᵗʰ M67.0 Short Achilles tendon (acquired)**
    **M67.00**    Short Achilles tendon (acquired), **unspecified ankle**
    **M67.01**    Short Achilles tendon (acquired), **right ankle**
    **M67.02**    Short Achilles tendon (acquired), **left ankle**

  **☑5ᵗʰ M67.2 Synovial hypertrophy, not elsewhere classified**
       *EXCLUDES 1*    villonodular synovitis (pigmented) (M12.2-)
    **M67.20**    Synovial hypertrophy, not elsewhere classified, **unspecified site**
  **☑6ᵗʰ M67.21**    Synovial hypertrophy, not elsewhere classified, **shoulder**
      **M67.211**    Synovial hypertrophy, not elsewhere classified, **right shoulder**
      **M67.212**    Synovial hypertrophy, not elsewhere classified, **left shoulder**
      **M67.219**    Synovial hypertrophy, not elsewhere classified, **unspecified shoulder**
  **☑6ᵗʰ M67.22**    Synovial hypertrophy, not elsewhere classified, **upper arm**
      **M67.221**    Synovial hypertrophy, not elsewhere classified, **right upper arm**
      **M67.222**    Synovial hypertrophy, not elsewhere classified, **left upper arm**
      **M67.229**    Synovial hypertrophy, not elsewhere classified, **unspecified upper arm**
  **☑6ᵗʰ M67.23**    Synovial hypertrophy, not elsewhere classified, **forearm**
      **M67.231**    Synovial hypertrophy, not elsewhere classified, **right forearm**
      **M67.232**    Synovial hypertrophy, not elsewhere classified, **left forearm**
      **M67.239**    Synovial hypertrophy, not elsewhere classified, **unspecified forearm**
  **☑6ᵗʰ M67.24**    Synovial hypertrophy, not elsewhere classified, **hand**
      **M67.241**    Synovial hypertrophy, not elsewhere classified, **right hand**
      **M67.242**    Synovial hypertrophy, not elsewhere classified, **left hand**
      **M67.249**    Synovial hypertrophy, not elsewhere classified, **unspecified hand**
  **☑6ᵗʰ M67.25**    Synovial hypertrophy, not elsewhere classified, **thigh**
      **M67.251**    Synovial hypertrophy, not elsewhere classified, **right thigh**
      **M67.252**    Synovial hypertrophy, not elsewhere classified, **left thigh**
      **M67.259**    Synovial hypertrophy, not elsewhere classified, **unspecified thigh**
  **☑6ᵗʰ M67.26**    Synovial hypertrophy, not elsewhere classified, **lower leg**
      **M67.261**    Synovial hypertrophy, not elsewhere classified, **right lower leg**
      **M67.262**    Synovial hypertrophy, not elsewhere classified, **left lower leg**
      **M67.269**    Synovial hypertrophy, not elsewhere classified, **unspecified lower leg**
  **☑6ᵗʰ M67.27**    Synovial hypertrophy, not elsewhere classified, **ankle and foot**
      **M67.271**    Synovial hypertrophy, not elsewhere classified, **right ankle and foot**
      **M67.272**    Synovial hypertrophy, not elsewhere classified, **left ankle and foot**
      **M67.279**    Synovial hypertrophy, not elsewhere classified, **unspecified ankle and foot**
    **M67.28**    Synovial hypertrophy, not elsewhere classified, **other site**
    **M67.29**    Synovial hypertrophy, not elsewhere classified, **multiple sites**

  **☑5ᵗʰ M67.3 Transient synovitis**
     Toxic synovitis
       *EXCLUDES 1*    palindromic rheumatism (M12.3-)
    **M67.30**    Transient synovitis, **unspecified site**
  **☑6ᵗʰ M67.31**    Transient synovitis, **shoulder**
      **M67.311**    Transient synovitis, **right shoulder**
      **M67.312**    Transient synovitis, **left shoulder**
      **M67.319**    Transient synovitis, **unspecified shoulder**
  **☑6ᵗʰ M67.32**    Transient synovitis, **elbow**
      **M67.321**    Transient synovitis, **right elbow**
      **M67.322**    Transient synovitis, **left elbow**
      **M67.329**    Transient synovitis, **unspecified elbow**
  **☑6ᵗʰ M67.33**    Transient synovitis, **wrist**
      **M67.331**    Transient synovitis, **right wrist**
      **M67.332**    Transient synovitis, **left wrist**
      **M67.339**    Transient synovitis, **unspecified wrist**
  **☑6ᵗʰ M67.34**    Transient synovitis, **hand**
      **M67.341**    Transient synovitis, **right hand**
      **M67.342**    Transient synovitis, **left hand**
      **M67.349**    Transient synovitis, **unspecified hand**
  **☑6ᵗʰ M67.35**    Transient synovitis, **hip**
      **M67.351**    Transient synovitis, **right hip**
      **M67.352**    Transient synovitis, **left hip**
      **M67.359**    Transient synovitis, **unspecified hip**
  **☑6ᵗʰ M67.36**    Transient synovitis, **knee**
      **M67.361**    Transient synovitis, **right knee**
      **M67.362**    Transient synovitis, **left knee**
      **M67.369**    Transient synovitis, **unspecified knee**
  **☑6ᵗʰ M67.37**    Transient synovitis, **ankle and foot**
      **M67.371**    Transient synovitis, **right ankle and foot**
      **M67.372**    Transient synovitis, **left ankle and foot**
      **M67.379**    Transient synovitis, **unspecified ankle and foot**
    **M67.38**    Transient synovitis, **other site**
    **M67.39**    Transient synovitis, **multiple sites**

  **☑5ᵗʰ M67.4 Ganglion**
     Ganglion of joint or tendon (sheath)
       *EXCLUDES 1*    ganglion in yaws (A66.6)
       *EXCLUDES 2*    cyst of bursa (M71.2-M71.3)
              cyst of synovium (M71.2-M71.3)
    **M67.40**    Ganglion, **unspecified site**
  **☑6ᵗʰ M67.41**    Ganglion, **shoulder**
      **M67.411**    Ganglion, **right shoulder**
      **M67.412**    Ganglion, **left shoulder**
      **M67.419**    Ganglion, **unspecified shoulder**
  **☑6ᵗʰ M67.42**    Ganglion, **elbow**
      **M67.421**    Ganglion, **right elbow**
      **M67.422**    Ganglion, **left elbow**
      **M67.429**    Ganglion, **unspecified elbow**
  **☑6ᵗʰ M67.43**    Ganglion, **wrist**
      **M67.431**    Ganglion, **right wrist**

**Ganglion of Wrist**

Extensor tendon sheaths

Ganglion of wrist (fluid-filled sac)

☑ Additional Character Req   ☑x7ᵗʰ Placeholder Alert   Unacceptable PDx   Manifestation   **H1**-**H14** HAC   **HCC** CMS-HCC Condition   *EXCLUDES 1* Not Coded Here   *EXCLUDES 2* Not Included Here

ICD-10-CM 2018          **789**

        M67.432   Ganglion, left wrist
        M67.439   Ganglion, unspecified wrist

✓6th   M67.44   Ganglion, hand
        M67.441   Ganglion, right hand
        M67.442   Ganglion, left hand
        M67.449   Ganglion, unspecified hand

✓6th   M67.45   Ganglion, hip
        M67.451   Ganglion, right hip
        M67.452   Ganglion, left hip
        M67.459   Ganglion, unspecified hip

✓6th   M67.46   Ganglion, knee
        M67.461   Ganglion, right knee
        M67.462   Ganglion, left knee
        M67.469   Ganglion, unspecified knee

✓6th   M67.47   Ganglion, ankle and foot
        M67.471   Ganglion, right ankle and foot
        M67.472   Ganglion, left ankle and foot
        M67.479   Ganglion, unspecified ankle and foot

    M67.48   Ganglion, other site
    M67.49   Ganglion, multiple sites

✓5th   **M67.5   Plica syndrome**
       Plica knee
    M67.50   Plica syndrome, unspecified knee
    M67.51   Plica syndrome, right knee
    M67.52   Plica syndrome, left knee

✓5th   **M67.8   Other specified disorders of synovium and tendon**
    M67.80   Other specified disorders of synovium and tendon, unspecified site

✓6th   M67.81   Other specified disorders of synovium and tendon, shoulder
        M67.811   Other specified disorders of synovium, right shoulder
        M67.812   Other specified disorders of synovium, left shoulder
        M67.813   Other specified disorders of tendon, right shoulder
        M67.814   Other specified disorders of tendon, left shoulder
        M67.819   Other specified disorders of synovium and tendon, unspecified shoulder

✓6th   M67.82   Other specified disorders of synovium and tendon, elbow
        M67.821   Other specified disorders of synovium, right elbow
        M67.822   Other specified disorders of synovium, left elbow
        M67.823   Other specified disorders of tendon, right elbow
        M67.824   Other specified disorders of tendon, left elbow
        M67.829   Other specified disorders of synovium and tendon, unspecified elbow

✓6th   M67.83   Other specified disorders of synovium and tendon, wrist
        M67.831   Other specified disorders of synovium, right wrist
        M67.832   Other specified disorders of synovium, left wrist
        M67.833   Other specified disorders of tendon, right wrist
        M67.834   Other specified disorders of tendon, left wrist
        M67.839   Other specified disorders of synovium and tendon, unspecified forearm

✓6th   M67.84   Other specified disorders of synovium and tendon, hand
        M67.841   Other specified disorders of synovium, right hand
        M67.842   Other specified disorders of synovium, left hand
        M67.843   Other specified disorders of tendon, right hand
        M67.844   Other specified disorders of tendon, left hand
        M67.849   Other specified disorders of synovium and tendon, unspecified hand

✓6th   M67.85   Other specified disorders of synovium and tendon, hip
        M67.851   Other specified disorders of synovium, right hip
        M67.852   Other specified disorders of synovium, left hip
        M67.853   Other specified disorders of tendon, right hip
        M67.854   Other specified disorders of tendon, left hip
        M67.859   Other specified disorders of synovium and tendon, unspecified hip

✓6th   M67.86   Other specified disorders of synovium and tendon, knee
        M67.861   Other specified disorders of synovium, right knee
        M67.862   Other specified disorders of synovium, left knee
        M67.863   Other specified disorders of tendon, right knee
        M67.864   Other specified disorders of tendon, left knee
        M67.869   Other specified disorders of synovium and tendon, unspecified knee

✓6th   M67.87   Other specified disorders of synovium and tendon, ankle and foot
        M67.871   Other specified disorders of synovium, right ankle and foot
        M67.872   Other specified disorders of synovium, left ankle and foot
        M67.873   Other specified disorders of tendon, right ankle and foot
        M67.874   Other specified disorders of tendon, left ankle and foot
        M67.879   Other specified disorders of synovium and tendon, unspecified ankle and foot

    M67.88   Other specified disorders of synovium and tendon, other site
    M67.89   Other specified disorders of synovium and tendon, multiple sites

✓5th   **M67.9   Unspecified disorder of synovium and tendon**
    M67.90   Unspecified disorder of synovium and tendon, unspecified site

✓6th   M67.91   Unspecified disorder of synovium and tendon, shoulder
        M67.911   Unspecified disorder of synovium and tendon, right shoulder
        M67.912   Unspecified disorder of synovium and tendon, left shoulder
        M67.919   Unspecified disorder of synovium and tendon, unspecified shoulder

✓6th   M67.92   Unspecified disorder of synovium and tendon, upper arm
        M67.921   Unspecified disorder of synovium and tendon, right upper arm
        M67.922   Unspecified disorder of synovium and tendon, left upper arm
        M67.929   Unspecified disorder of synovium and tendon, unspecified upper arm

✓6th   M67.93   Unspecified disorder of synovium and tendon, forearm
        M67.931   Unspecified disorder of synovium and tendon, right forearm
        M67.932   Unspecified disorder of synovium and tendon, left forearm
        M67.939   Unspecified disorder of synovium and tendon, unspecified forearm

✓6th   M67.94   Unspecified disorder of synovium and tendon, hand
        M67.941   Unspecified disorder of synovium and tendon, right hand
        M67.942   Unspecified disorder of synovium and tendon, left hand
        M67.949   Unspecified disorder of synovium and tendon, unspecified hand

✓6ᵗʰ **M67.95** Unspecified disorder of synovium and tendon, **thigh**

    **M67.951** Unspecified disorder of synovium and tendon, **right thigh**

    **M67.952** Unspecified disorder of synovium and tendon, **left thigh**

    **M67.959** Unspecified disorder of synovium and tendon, **unspecified thigh**

✓6ᵗʰ **M67.96** Unspecified disorder of synovium and tendon, **lower leg**

    **M67.961** Unspecified disorder of synovium and tendon, **right lower leg**

    **M67.962** Unspecified disorder of synovium and tendon, **left lower leg**

    **M67.969** Unspecified disorder of synovium and tendon, **unspecified lower leg**

✓6ᵗʰ **M67.97** Unspecified disorder of synovium and tendon, **ankle and foot**

    **M67.971** Unspecified disorder of synovium and tendon, **right ankle and foot**

    **M67.972** Unspecified disorder of synovium and tendon, **left ankle and foot**

    **M67.979** Unspecified disorder of synovium and tendon, **unspecified ankle and foot**

**M67.98** Unspecified disorder of synovium and tendon, **other site**

**M67.99** Unspecified disorder of synovium and tendon, **multiple sites**

### Other soft tissue disorders (M70-M79)

✓4ᵗʰ **M70 Soft tissue disorders related to use, overuse and pressure**

    **INCLUDES** soft tissue disorders of occupational origin

    Use additional external cause code to identify activity causing disorder (Y93.-)

    **EXCLUDES 1** bursitis NOS (M71.9-)

    **EXCLUDES 2** bursitis of shoulder (M75.5)
       enthesopathies (M76-M77)
       pressure ulcer (pressure area) (L89.-)

✓5ᵗʰ **M70.0 Crepitant synovitis (acute) (chronic) of hand and wrist**

    ✓6ᵗʰ **M70.03 Crepitant synovitis (acute) (chronic), wrist**

       **M70.031** Crepitant synovitis (acute) (chronic), **right wrist**

       **M70.032** Crepitant synovitis (acute) (chronic), **left wrist**

       **M70.039** Crepitant synovitis (acute) (chronic), **unspecified wrist**

    ✓6ᵗʰ **M70.04 Crepitant synovitis (acute) (chronic), hand**

       **M70.041** Crepitant synovitis (acute) (chronic), **right hand**

       **M70.042** Crepitant synovitis (acute) (chronic), **left hand**

       **M70.049** Crepitant synovitis (acute) (chronic), **unspecified hand**

✓5ᵗʰ **M70.1 Bursitis of hand**

    **M70.10** Bursitis, **unspecified hand**

    **M70.11** Bursitis, **right hand**

    **M70.12** Bursitis, **left hand**

✓5ᵗʰ **M70.2 Olecranon bursitis**

    **M70.20** Olecranon bursitis, **unspecified elbow**

    **M70.21** Olecranon bursitis, **right elbow**

    **M70.22** Olecranon bursitis, **left elbow**

✓5ᵗʰ **M70.3 Other bursitis of elbow**

    **M70.30** Other bursitis of elbow, **unspecified elbow**

    **M70.31** Other bursitis of elbow, **right elbow**

    **M70.32** Other bursitis of elbow, **left elbow**

✓5ᵗʰ **M70.4 Prepatellar bursitis**

    **M70.40** Prepatellar bursitis, **unspecified knee**

    **M70.41** Prepatellar bursitis, **right knee**

    **M70.42** Prepatellar bursitis, **left knee**

✓5ᵗʰ **M70.5 Other bursitis of knee**

    **M70.50** Other bursitis of knee, **unspecified knee**

    **M70.51** Other bursitis of knee, **right knee**

    **M70.52** Other bursitis of knee, **left knee**

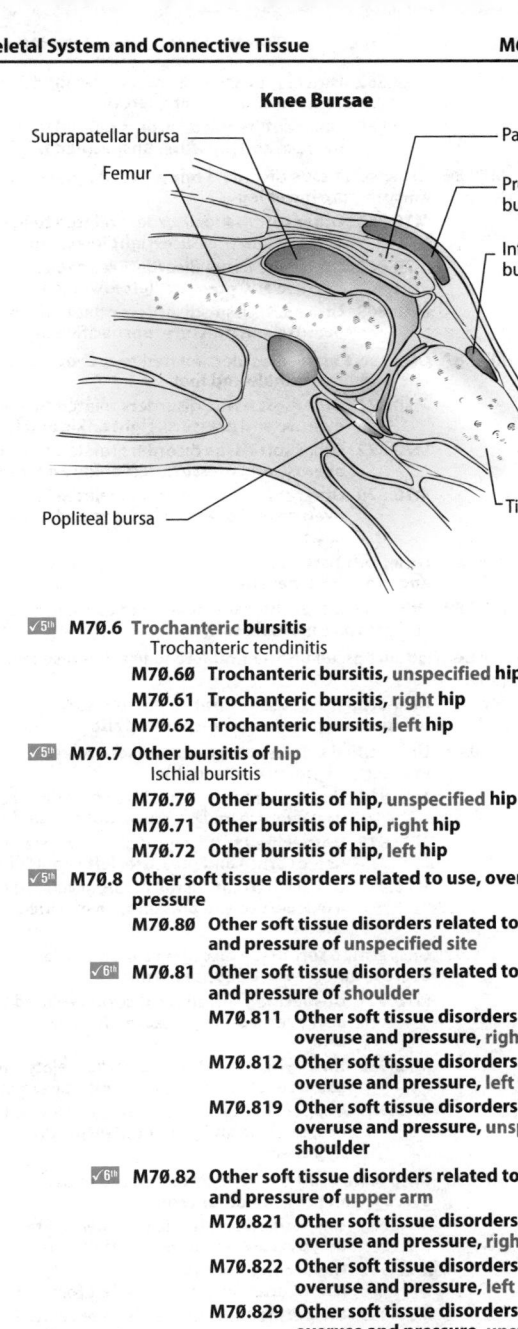

**Knee Bursae**

Suprapatellar bursa — Femur — Patella — Prepatellar bursa — Infrapatellar bursa — Popliteal bursa — Tibia

✓5ᵗʰ **M70.6 Trochanteric bursitis**

    Trochanteric tendinitis

    **M70.60** Trochanteric bursitis, **unspecified hip**

    **M70.61** Trochanteric bursitis, **right hip**

    **M70.62** Trochanteric bursitis, **left hip**

✓5ᵗʰ **M70.7 Other bursitis of hip**

    Ischial bursitis

    **M70.70** Other bursitis of hip, **unspecified hip**

    **M70.71** Other bursitis of hip, **right hip**

    **M70.72** Other bursitis of hip, **left hip**

✓5ᵗʰ **M70.8 Other soft tissue disorders related to use, overuse and pressure**

    **M70.80** Other soft tissue disorders related to use, overuse and pressure of **unspecified site**

    ✓6ᵗʰ **M70.81** Other soft tissue disorders related to use, overuse and pressure of **shoulder**

       **M70.811** Other soft tissue disorders related to use, overuse and pressure, **right shoulder**

       **M70.812** Other soft tissue disorders related to use, overuse and pressure, **left shoulder**

       **M70.819** Other soft tissue disorders related to use, overuse and pressure, **unspecified shoulder**

    ✓6ᵗʰ **M70.82** Other soft tissue disorders related to use, overuse and pressure of **upper arm**

       **M70.821** Other soft tissue disorders related to use, overuse and pressure, **right upper arm**

       **M70.822** Other soft tissue disorders related to use, overuse and pressure, **left upper arm**

       **M70.829** Other soft tissue disorders related to use, overuse and pressure, **unspecified upper arms**

    ✓6ᵗʰ **M70.83** Other soft tissue disorders related to use, overuse and pressure of **forearm**

       **M70.831** Other soft tissue disorders related to use, overuse and pressure, **right forearm**

       **M70.832** Other soft tissue disorders related to use, overuse and pressure, **left forearm**

       **M70.839** Other soft tissue disorders related to use, overuse and pressure, **unspecified forearm**

    ✓6ᵗʰ **M70.84** Other soft tissue disorders related to use, overuse and pressure of **hand**

       **M70.841** Other soft tissue disorders related to use, overuse and pressure, **right hand**

       **M70.842** Other soft tissue disorders related to use, overuse and pressure, **left hand**

       **M70.849** Other soft tissue disorders related to use, overuse and pressure, **unspecified hand**

    ✓6ᵗʰ **M70.85** Other soft tissue disorders related to use, overuse and pressure of **thigh**

       **M70.851** Other soft tissue disorders related to use, overuse and pressure, **right thigh**

✓ Additional Character Req    ✓x7ᵗʰ Placeholder Alert    Unacceptable PDx    Manifestation    **H1** - **H14** HAC    **HCC** CMS-HCC Condition    **EXCLUDES 1** Not Coded Here    **EXCLUDES 2** Not Included Here

ICD-10-CM 2018        791

M70.852　Other soft tissue disorders related to use, overuse and pressure, left thigh

M70.859　Other soft tissue disorders related to use, overuse and pressure, unspecified thigh

✓6th M70.86　Other soft tissue disorders related to use, overuse and pressure lower leg

M70.861　Other soft tissue disorders related to use, overuse and pressure, right lower leg

M70.862　Other soft tissue disorders related to use, overuse and pressure, left lower leg

M70.869　Other soft tissue disorders related to use, overuse and pressure, unspecified leg

✓6th M70.87　Other soft tissue disorders related to use, overuse and pressure of ankle and foot

M70.871　Other soft tissue disorders related to use, overuse and pressure, right ankle and foot

M70.872　Other soft tissue disorders related to use, overuse and pressure, left ankle and foot

M70.879　Other soft tissue disorders related to use, overuse and pressure, unspecified ankle and foot

M70.88　Other soft tissue disorders related to use, overuse and pressure other site

M70.89　Other soft tissue disorders related to use, overuse and pressure multiple sites

✓5th M70.9　Unspecified soft tissue disorder related to use, overuse and pressure

M70.90　Unspecified soft tissue disorder related to use, overuse and pressure of unspecified site

✓6th M70.91　Unspecified soft tissue disorder related to use, overuse and pressure of shoulder

M70.911　Unspecified soft tissue disorder related to use, overuse and pressure, right shoulder

M70.912　Unspecified soft tissue disorder related to use, overuse and pressure, left shoulder

M70.919　Unspecified soft tissue disorder related to use, overuse and pressure, unspecified shoulder

✓6th M70.92　Unspecified soft tissue disorder related to use, overuse and pressure of upper arm

M70.921　Unspecified soft tissue disorder related to use, overuse and pressure, right upper arm

M70.922　Unspecified soft tissue disorder related to use, overuse and pressure, left upper arm

M70.929　Unspecified soft tissue disorder related to use, overuse and pressure, unspecified upper arm

✓6th M70.93　Unspecified soft tissue disorder related to use, overuse and pressure of forearm

M70.931　Unspecified soft tissue disorder related to use, overuse and pressure, right forearm

M70.932　Unspecified soft tissue disorder related to use, overuse and pressure, left forearm

M70.939　Unspecified soft tissue disorder related to use, overuse and pressure, unspecified forearm

✓6th M70.94　Unspecified soft tissue disorder related to use, overuse and pressure of hand

M70.941　Unspecified soft tissue disorder related to use, overuse and pressure, right hand

M70.942　Unspecified soft tissue disorder related to use, overuse and pressure, left hand

M70.949　Unspecified soft tissue disorder related to use, overuse and pressure, unspecified hand

✓6th M70.95　Unspecified soft tissue disorder related to use, overuse and pressure of thigh

M70.951　Unspecified soft tissue disorder related to use, overuse and pressure, right thigh

M70.952　Unspecified soft tissue disorder related to use, overuse and pressure, left thigh

M70.959　Unspecified soft tissue disorder related to use, overuse and pressure, unspecified thigh

✓6th M70.96　Unspecified soft tissue disorder related to use, overuse and pressure lower leg

M70.961　Unspecified soft tissue disorder related to use, overuse and pressure, right lower leg

M70.962　Unspecified soft tissue disorder related to use, overuse and pressure, left lower leg

M70.969　Unspecified soft tissue disorder related to use, overuse and pressure, unspecified lower leg

✓6th M70.97　Unspecified soft tissue disorder related to use, overuse and pressure of ankle and foot

M70.971　Unspecified soft tissue disorder related to use, overuse and pressure, right ankle and foot

M70.972　Unspecified soft tissue disorder related to use, overuse and pressure, left ankle and foot

M70.979　Unspecified soft tissue disorder related to use, overuse and pressure, unspecified ankle and foot

M70.98　Unspecified soft tissue disorder related to use, overuse and pressure other

M70.99　Unspecified soft tissue disorder related to use, overuse and pressure multiple sites

✓4th M71　Other bursopathies

EXCLUDES 1　bunion (M20.1)
bursitis related to use, overuse or pressure (M70.-)
enthesopathies (M76-M77)

✓5th M71.0　Abscess of bursa

Use additional code (B95.-, B96.-) to identify causative organism

M71.00　Abscess of bursa, unspecified site

✓6th M71.01　Abscess of bursa, shoulder

M71.011　Abscess of bursa, right shoulder

M71.012　Abscess of bursa, left shoulder

M71.019　Abscess of bursa, unspecified shoulder

✓6th M71.02　Abscess of bursa, elbow

M71.021　Abscess of bursa, right elbow

M71.022　Abscess of bursa, left elbow

M71.029　Abscess of bursa, unspecified elbow

✓6th M71.03　Abscess of bursa, wrist

M71.031　Abscess of bursa, right wrist

M71.032　Abscess of bursa, left wrist

M71.039　Abscess of bursa, unspecified wrist

✓6th M71.04　Abscess of bursa, hand

M71.041　Abscess of bursa, right hand

M71.042　Abscess of bursa, left hand

M71.049　Abscess of bursa, unspecified hand

✓6th M71.05　Abscess of bursa, hip

M71.051　Abscess of bursa, right hip

M71.052　Abscess of bursa, left hip

M71.059　Abscess of bursa, unspecified hip

✓6th M71.06　Abscess of bursa, knee

M71.061　Abscess of bursa, right knee

M71.062　Abscess of bursa, left knee

M71.069　Abscess of bursa, unspecified knee

✓6th M71.07　Abscess of bursa, ankle and foot

M71.071　Abscess of bursa, right ankle and foot

M71.072　Abscess of bursa, left ankle and foot

M71.079　Abscess of bursa, unspecified ankle and foot

M71.08　Abscess of bursa, other site

M71.09　Abscess of bursa, multiple sites

✓5th M71.1　Other infective bursitis

Use additional code (B95.-, B96.-) to identify causative organism

M71.10　Other infective bursitis, unspecified site

✓6th M71.11　Other infective bursitis, shoulder

M71.111　Other infective bursitis, right shoulder

M71.112　Other infective bursitis, left shoulder

M71.119　Other infective bursitis, unspecified shoulder

✓6th M71.12　Other infective bursitis, elbow

M71.121　Other infective bursitis, right elbow

M71.122　Other infective bursitis, left elbow

M71.129　Other infective bursitis, unspecified elbow

✓6th M71.13　Other infective bursitis, wrist

M71.131　Other infective bursitis, right wrist

M71.132　Other infective bursitis, left wrist

N Newborn: 0　P Pediatric: 0-17　M Maternity: 12-55　A Adult: 15-124　MCC Major CC Condition　PDxMCC PDx acts as own MCC　CC CC Condition　PDxCC PDx acts as own CC

792　　ICD-10-CM 2018

M71.139  Other infective bursitis, unspecified wrist

✔6ᵗʰ M71.14  **Other infective bursitis, hand**
- M71.141  Other infective bursitis, right hand
- M71.142  Other infective bursitis, left hand
- M71.149  Other infective bursitis, unspecified hand

✔6ᵗʰ M71.15  **Other infective bursitis, hip**
- M71.151  Other infective bursitis, right hip
- M71.152  Other infective bursitis, left hip
- M71.159  Other infective bursitis, unspecified hip

✔6ᵗʰ M71.16  **Other infective bursitis, knee**
- M71.161  Other infective bursitis, right knee
- M71.162  Other infective bursitis, left knee
- M71.169  Other infective bursitis, unspecified knee

✔6ᵗʰ M71.17  **Other infective bursitis, ankle and foot**
- M71.171  Other infective bursitis, right ankle and foot
- M71.172  Other infective bursitis, left ankle and foot
- M71.179  Other infective bursitis, unspecified ankle and foot

M71.18  **Other infective bursitis, other site**

M71.19  **Other infective bursitis, multiple sites**

✔5ᵗʰ M71.2  **Synovial cyst of popliteal space [Baker]**
> EXCLUDES 1  *synovial cyst of popliteal space with rupture (M66.0)*
- M71.20  Synovial cyst of popliteal space [Baker], unspecified knee
- M71.21  Synovial cyst of popliteal space [Baker], right knee
- M71.22  Synovial cyst of popliteal space [Baker], left knee

✔5ᵗʰ M71.3  **Other bursal cyst**
Synovial cyst NOS
> EXCLUDES 1  *synovial cyst with rupture (M66.1-)*
- M71.30  Other bursal cyst, unspecified site

✔6ᵗʰ M71.31  **Other bursal cyst, shoulder**
- M71.311  Other bursal cyst, right shoulder
- M71.312  Other bursal cyst, left shoulder
- M71.319  Other bursal cyst, unspecified shoulder

✔6ᵗʰ M71.32  **Other bursal cyst, elbow**
- M71.321  Other bursal cyst, right elbow
- M71.322  Other bursal cyst, left elbow
- M71.329  Other bursal cyst, unspecified elbow

✔6ᵗʰ M71.33  **Other bursal cyst, wrist**
- M71.331  Other bursal cyst, right wrist
- M71.332  Other bursal cyst, left wrist
- M71.339  Other bursal cyst, unspecified wrist

✔6ᵗʰ M71.34  **Other bursal cyst, hand**
- M71.341  Other bursal cyst, right hand
- M71.342  Other bursal cyst, left hand
- M71.349  Other bursal cyst, unspecified hand

**Baker's Cyst**

Baker's cyst connected to knee joint synovial cavity

✔6ᵗʰ M71.35  **Other bursal cyst, hip**
- M71.351  Other bursal cyst, right hip
- M71.352  Other bursal cyst, left hip
- M71.359  Other bursal cyst, unspecified hip

✔6ᵗʰ M71.37  **Other bursal cyst, ankle and foot**
- M71.371  Other bursal cyst, right ankle and foot
- M71.372  Other bursal cyst, left ankle and foot
- M71.379  Other bursal cyst, unspecified ankle and foot

M71.38  **Other bursal cyst, other site**

M71.39  **Other bursal cyst, multiple sites**

✔5ᵗʰ M71.4  **Calcium deposit in bursa**
> EXCLUDES 2  *calcium deposit in bursa of shoulder (M75.3)*
- M71.40  Calcium deposit in bursa, unspecified site

✔6ᵗʰ M71.42  **Calcium deposit in bursa, elbow**
- M71.421  Calcium deposit in bursa, right elbow
- M71.422  Calcium deposit in bursa, left elbow
- M71.429  Calcium deposit in bursa, unspecified elbow

✔6ᵗʰ M71.43  **Calcium deposit in bursa, wrist**
- M71.431  Calcium deposit in bursa, right wrist
- M71.432  Calcium deposit in bursa, left wrist
- M71.439  Calcium deposit in bursa, unspecified wrist

✔6ᵗʰ M71.44  **Calcium deposit in bursa, hand**
- M71.441  Calcium deposit in bursa, right hand
- M71.442  Calcium deposit in bursa, left hand
- M71.449  Calcium deposit in bursa, unspecified hand

✔6ᵗʰ M71.45  **Calcium deposit in bursa, hip**
- M71.451  Calcium deposit in bursa, right hip
- M71.452  Calcium deposit in bursa, left hip
- M71.459  Calcium deposit in bursa, unspecified hip

✔6ᵗʰ M71.46  **Calcium deposit in bursa, knee**
- M71.461  Calcium deposit in bursa, right knee
- M71.462  Calcium deposit in bursa, left knee
- M71.469  Calcium deposit in bursa, unspecified knee

✔6ᵗʰ M71.47  **Calcium deposit in bursa, ankle and foot**
- M71.471  Calcium deposit in bursa, right ankle and foot
- M71.472  Calcium deposit in bursa, left ankle and foot
- M71.479  Calcium deposit in bursa, unspecified ankle and foot

M71.48  **Calcium deposit in bursa, other site**

M71.49  **Calcium deposit in bursa, multiple sites**

✔5ᵗʰ M71.5  **Other bursitis, not elsewhere classified**
> EXCLUDES 1  *bursitis NOS (M71.9-)*
> EXCLUDES 2  *bursitis of shoulder (M75.5)*
> *bursitis of tibial collateral [Pellegrini-Stieda] (M76.4-)*
- M71.50  Other bursitis, not elsewhere classified, unspecified site

✔6ᵗʰ M71.52  **Other bursitis, not elsewhere classified, elbow**
- M71.521  Other bursitis, not elsewhere classified, right elbow
- M71.522  Other bursitis, not elsewhere classified, left elbow
- M71.529  Other bursitis, not elsewhere classified, unspecified elbow

✔6ᵗʰ M71.53  **Other bursitis, not elsewhere classified, wrist**
- M71.531  Other bursitis, not elsewhere classified, right wrist
- M71.532  Other bursitis, not elsewhere classified, left wrist
- M71.539  Other bursitis, not elsewhere classified, unspecified wrist

✔6ᵗʰ M71.54  **Other bursitis, not elsewhere classified, hand**
- M71.541  Other bursitis, not elsewhere classified, right hand
- M71.542  Other bursitis, not elsewhere classified, left hand

M71.549   **Other bursitis, not elsewhere classified, unspecified hand**

✓6ᵗʰ **M71.55 Other bursitis, not elsewhere classified, hip**

M71.551   **Other bursitis, not elsewhere classified, right hip**

M71.552   **Other bursitis, not elsewhere classified, left hip**

M71.559   **Other bursitis, not elsewhere classified, unspecified hip**

✓6ᵗʰ **M71.56 Other bursitis, not elsewhere classified, knee**

M71.561   **Other bursitis, not elsewhere classified, right knee**

M71.562   **Other bursitis, not elsewhere classified, left knee**

M71.569   **Other bursitis, not elsewhere classified, unspecified knee**

✓6ᵗʰ **M71.57 Other bursitis, not elsewhere classified, ankle and foot**

M71.571   **Other bursitis, not elsewhere classified, right ankle and foot**

M71.572   **Other bursitis, not elsewhere classified, left ankle and foot**

M71.579   **Other bursitis, not elsewhere classified, unspecified ankle and foot**

M71.58   **Other bursitis, not elsewhere classified,** other site

✓5ᵗʰ **M71.8 Other specified bursopathies**

M71.80   **Other specified bursopathies,** unspecified site

✓6ᵗʰ **M71.81 Other specified bursopathies,** shoulder

M71.811   **Other specified bursopathies,** right **shoulder**

M71.812   **Other specified bursopathies,** left **shoulder**

M71.819   **Other specified bursopathies,** unspecified **shoulder**

✓6ᵗʰ **M71.82 Other specified bursopathies,** elbow

M71.821   **Other specified bursopathies,** right **elbow**

M71.822   **Other specified bursopathies,** left **elbow**

M71.829   **Other specified bursopathies,** unspecified **elbow**

✓6ᵗʰ **M71.83 Other specified bursopathies,** wrist

M71.831   **Other specified bursopathies,** right **wrist**

M71.832   **Other specified bursopathies,** left **wrist**

M71.839   **Other specified bursopathies,** unspecified **wrist**

✓6ᵗʰ **M71.84 Other specified bursopathies,** hand

M71.841   **Other specified bursopathies,** right **hand**

M71.842   **Other specified bursopathies,** left **hand**

M71.849   **Other specified bursopathies,** unspecified **hand**

✓6ᵗʰ **M71.85 Other specified bursopathies,** hip

M71.851   **Other specified bursopathies,** right **hip**

M71.852   **Other specified bursopathies,** left **hip**

M71.859   **Other specified bursopathies,** unspecified **hip**

✓6ᵗʰ **M71.86 Other specified bursopathies,** knee

M71.861   **Other specified bursopathies,** right **knee**

M71.862   **Other specified bursopathies,** left **knee**

M71.869   **Other specified bursopathies,** unspecified **knee**

✓6ᵗʰ **M71.87 Other specified bursopathies,** ankle and foot

M71.871   **Other specified bursopathies,** right **ankle and foot**

M71.872   **Other specified bursopathies,** left **ankle and foot**

M71.879   **Other specified bursopathies,** unspecified **ankle and foot**

M71.88   **Other specified bursopathies,** other site

M71.89   **Other specified bursopathies,** multiple sites

**M71.9 Bursopathy, unspecified**
Bursitis NOS

✓4ᵗʰ **M72 Fibroblastic disorders**

*EXCLUDES 2*   *retroperitoneal fibromatosis (D48.3)*

**M72.0 Palmar fascial fibromatosis [Dupuytren]**   A
**DEF:** Dupuytren's contracture: Flexion deformity of finger, due to shortened, thickened fibrosing of palmar fascia; cause unknown; associated with long-standing epilepsy.

**M72.1 Knuckle pads**

**M72.2 Plantar fascial fibromatosis**
Plantar fasciitis
**DEF:** Rapid-growing and multiplanar nodular swellings and pain in the foot; not associated with contractures.

**M72.4 Pseudosarcomatous fibromatosis**
Nodular fasciitis

**M72.6 Necrotizing fasciitis**   MCC HCC
Use additional code (B95.-, B96.-) to identify causative organism
**CC Excl:** PDX collection 806

**M72.8 Other fibroblastic disorders**
Abscess of fascia
Fasciitis NEC
Other infective fasciitis
Use additional code to (B95.-, B96.-) identify causative organism
*EXCLUDES 1*   *diffuse (eosinophilic) fasciitis (M35.4)*
*necrotizing fasciitis (M72.6)*
*nodular fasciitis (M72.4)*
*perirenal fasciitis NOS (N13.5)*
*perirenal fasciitis with infection (N13.6)*
*plantar fasciitis (M72.2)*

**M72.9 Fibroblastic disorder, unspecified**
Fasciitis NOS
Fibromatosis NOS

✓4ᵗʰ **M75 Shoulder lesions**

*EXCLUDES 2*   *shoulder-hand syndrome (M89.0-)*

✓5ᵗʰ **M75.0 Adhesive capsulitis of shoulder**
Frozen shoulder
Periarthritis of shoulder
**AHA:** 2015, 2Q, 23

M75.00   **Adhesive capsulitis of** unspecified **shoulder**

M75.01   **Adhesive capsulitis of** right **shoulder**

M75.02   **Adhesive capsulitis of** left **shoulder**

✓5ᵗʰ **M75.1 Rotator cuff tear or rupture, not specified as traumatic**
Rotator cuff syndrome
Supraspinatus syndrome
Supraspinatus tear or rupture, not specified as traumatic
*EXCLUDES 1*   *tear of rotator cuff, traumatic (S46.01-)*

✓6ᵗʰ **M75.10 Unspecified rotator cuff tear or rupture, not specified as traumatic**

M75.100   **Unspecified rotator cuff tear or rupture of** unspecified **shoulder, not specified as traumatic**

M75.101   **Unspecified rotator cuff tear or rupture of** right **shoulder, not specified as traumatic**

M75.102   **Unspecified rotator cuff tear or rupture of** left **shoulder, not specified as traumatic**

✓6ᵗʰ **M75.11 Incomplete rotator cuff tear or rupture not specified as traumatic**

M75.110   **Incomplete rotator cuff tear or rupture of** unspecified **shoulder, not specified as traumatic**

M75.111   **Incomplete rotator cuff tear or rupture of** right **shoulder, not specified as traumatic**

M75.112   **Incomplete rotator cuff tear or rupture of** left **shoulder, not specified as traumatic**

✓6ᵗʰ **M75.12 Complete rotator cuff tear or rupture not specified as traumatic**

M75.120   **Complete rotator cuff tear or rupture of** unspecified **shoulder, not specified as traumatic**

M75.121   **Complete rotator cuff tear or rupture of** right **shoulder, not specified as traumatic**

M75.122   **Complete rotator cuff tear or rupture of** left **shoulder, not specified as traumatic**

✓5ᵗʰ **M75.2 Bicipital tendinitis**

M75.20   **Bicipital tendinitis,** unspecified **shoulder**

M75.21   **Bicipital tendinitis,** right **shoulder**

M75.22   **Bicipital tendinitis,** left **shoulder**

✓5ᵗʰ **M75.3 Calcific tendinitis of shoulder**
Calcified bursa of shoulder

     **M75.30 Calcific tendinitis of** unspecified **shoulder**
     **M75.31 Calcific tendinitis of** right **shoulder**
     **M75.32 Calcific tendinitis of** left **shoulder**

✓5ᵗʰ **M75.4 Impingement syndrome of shoulder**

     **M75.40 Impingement syndrome of** unspecified **shoulder**
     **M75.41 Impingement syndrome of** right **shoulder**
     **M75.42 Impingement syndrome of** left **shoulder**

✓5ᵗʰ **M75.5 Bursitis of shoulder**

     **M75.50 Bursitis of** unspecified **shoulder**
     **M75.51 Bursitis of** right **shoulder**
     **M75.52 Bursitis of** left **shoulder**

✓5ᵗʰ **M75.8 Other shoulder lesions**

     **M75.80 Other shoulder lesions,** unspecified **shoulder**
     **M75.81 Other shoulder lesions,** right **shoulder**
     **M75.82 Other shoulder lesions,** left **shoulder**

✓5ᵗʰ **M75.9 Shoulder lesion,** unspecified

     **M75.90 Shoulder lesion, unspecified,** unspecified **shoulder**
     **M75.91 Shoulder lesion, unspecified,** right **shoulder**
     **M75.92 Shoulder lesion, unspecified,** left **shoulder**

✓4ᵗʰ **M76 Enthesopathies, lower limb, excluding foot**
     *EXCLUDES 2*   bursitis due to use, overuse and pressure (M70.-)
                 enthesopathies of ankle and foot (M77.5-)

✓5ᵗʰ **M76.0 Gluteal tendinitis**

     **M76.00 Gluteal tendinitis,** unspecified **hip**
     **M76.01 Gluteal tendinitis,** right **hip**
     **M76.02 Gluteal tendinitis,** left **hip**

✓5ᵗʰ **M76.1 Psoas tendinitis**

     **M76.10 Psoas tendinitis,** unspecified **hip**
     **M76.11 Psoas tendinitis,** right **hip**
     **M76.12 Psoas tendinitis,** left **hip**

✓5ᵗʰ **M76.2 Iliac crest spur**

     **M76.20 Iliac crest spur,** unspecified **hip**
     **M76.21 Iliac crest spur,** right **hip**
     **M76.22 Iliac crest spur,** left **hip**

✓5ᵗʰ **M76.3 Iliotibial band syndrome**

     **M76.30 Iliotibial band syndrome,** unspecified **leg**
     **M76.31 Iliotibial band syndrome,** right **leg**
     **M76.32 Iliotibial band syndrome,** left **leg**

✓5ᵗʰ **M76.4 Tibial collateral bursitis [Pellegrini-Stieda]**

     **M76.40 Tibial collateral bursitis [Pellegrini-Stieda],** unspecified **leg**
     **M76.41 Tibial collateral bursitis [Pellegrini-Stieda],** right **leg**
     **M76.42 Tibial collateral bursitis [Pellegrini-Stieda],** left **leg**

✓5ᵗʰ **M76.5 Patellar tendinitis**

     **M76.50 Patellar tendinitis,** unspecified **knee**
     **M76.51 Patellar tendinitis,** right **knee**
     **M76.52 Patellar tendinitis,** left **knee**

✓5ᵗʰ **M76.6 Achilles tendinitis**
Achilles bursitis

     **M76.60 Achilles tendinitis,** unspecified **leg**
     **M76.61 Achilles tendinitis,** right **leg**
     **M76.62 Achilles tendinitis,** left **leg**

✓5ᵗʰ **M76.7 Peroneal tendinitis**

     **M76.70 Peroneal tendinitis,** unspecified **leg**
     **M76.71 Peroneal tendinitis,** right **leg**
     **M76.72 Peroneal tendinitis,** left **leg**

✓5ᵗʰ **M76.8 Other specified enthesopathies of lower limb, excluding foot**

     ✓6ᵗʰ **M76.81 Anterior tibial syndrome**
         **M76.811 Anterior tibial syndrome,** right **leg**
         **M76.812 Anterior tibial syndrome,** left **leg**
         **M76.819 Anterior tibial syndrome,** unspecified **leg**

     ✓6ᵗʰ **M76.82 Posterior tibial tendinitis**
         **M76.821 Posterior tibial tendinitis,** right **leg**
         **M76.822 Posterior tibial tendinitis,** left **leg**
         **M76.829 Posterior tibial tendinitis,** unspecified **leg**

     ✓6ᵗʰ **M76.89 Other specified enthesopathies of lower limb, excluding foot**
         **M76.891 Other specified enthesopathies of** right **lower limb, excluding foot**
         **M76.892 Other specified enthesopathies of** left **lower limb, excluding foot**
         **M76.899 Other specified enthesopathies of** unspecified **lower limb, excluding foot**

     **M76.9 Unspecified enthesopathy, lower limb, excluding foot**

✓4ᵗʰ **M77 Other enthesopathies**
     *EXCLUDES 1*   bursitis NOS (M71.9-)
     *EXCLUDES 2*   bursitis due to use, overuse and pressure (M70.-)
                 osteophyte (M25.7)
                 spinal enthesopathy (M46.0-)

✓5ᵗʰ **M77.0 Medial epicondylitis**

     **M77.00 Medial epicondylitis,** unspecified **elbow**
     **M77.01 Medial epicondylitis,** right **elbow**
     **M77.02 Medial epicondylitis,** left **elbow**

✓5ᵗʰ **M77.1 Lateral epicondylitis**
Tennis elbow

     **M77.10 Lateral epicondylitis,** unspecified **elbow**
     **M77.11 Lateral epicondylitis,** right **elbow**
     **M77.12 Lateral epicondylitis,** left **elbow**

✓5ᵗʰ **M77.2 Periarthritis of wrist**

     **M77.20 Periarthritis,** unspecified **wrist**
     **M77.21 Periarthritis,** right **wrist**
     **M77.22 Periarthritis,** left **wrist**

✓5ᵗʰ **M77.3 Calcaneal spur**
**DEF:** Overgrowth of calcaneus bone on underside of the heel; causes pain on walking; due to chronic avulsion injury of plantar fascia from calcaneus.

     **M77.30 Calcaneal spur,** unspecified **foot**
     **M77.31 Calcaneal spur,** right **foot**
     **M77.32 Calcaneal spur,** left **foot**

✓5ᵗʰ **M77.4 Metatarsalgia**
     *EXCLUDES 1*   Morton's metatarsalgia (G57.6)

     **M77.40 Metatarsalgia,** unspecified **foot**
     **M77.41 Metatarsalgia,** right **foot**
     **M77.42 Metatarsalgia,** left **foot**

✓5ᵗʰ **M77.5 Other enthesopathy of foot**

     **M77.50 Other enthesopathy of** unspecified **foot**
     **M77.51 Other enthesopathy of** right **foot**
     **M77.52 Other enthesopathy of** left **foot**

     **M77.8 Other enthesopathies, not elsewhere classified**

     **M77.9 Enthesopathy,** unspecified
     Bone spur NOS      Periarthritis NOS
     Capsulitis NOS      Tendinitis NOS

✓4ᵗʰ **M79 Other and unspecified soft tissue disorders, not elsewhere classified**
     *EXCLUDES 1*   psychogenic rheumatism (F45.8)
                 soft tissue pain, psychogenic (F45.41)

     **M79.0 Rheumatism, unspecified**
         *EXCLUDES 1*   fibromyalgia (M79.7)
                     palindromic rheumatism (M12.3-)

     **M79.1 Myalgia**
     Myofascial pain syndrome
         *EXCLUDES 1*   fibromyalgia (M79.7)
                     myositis (M60.-)

     **M79.2 Neuralgia and neuritis, unspecified**
         *EXCLUDES 1*   brachial radiculitis NOS (M54.1)
                     lumbosacral radiculitis NOS (M54.1)
                     mononeuropathies (G56-G58)
                     radiculitis NOS (M54.1)
                     sciatica (M54.3-M54.4)

     **M79.3 Panniculitis, unspecified**
         *EXCLUDES 1*   lupus panniculitis (L93.2)
                     neck and back panniculitis (M54.0-)
                     relapsing [Weber-Christian] panniculitis (M35.6)

     **M79.4 Hypertrophy of (infrapatellar) fat pad**

     **M79.5 Residual foreign body in soft tissue**
         *EXCLUDES 1*   foreign body granuloma of skin and subcutaneous tissue (L92.3)
                     foreign body granuloma of soft tissue (M60.2-)

✓ Additional Character Req    ✓x7ᵗʰ Placeholder Alert    Unacceptable PDx    Manifestation    H1-H14 HAC    HCC CMS-HCC Condition    *EXCLUDES 1* Not Coded Here    *EXCLUDES 2* Not Included Here

ICD-10-CM 2018          **795**

✓5th **M79.6 Pain in limb, hand, foot, fingers and toes**
> EXCLUDES 2   *pain in joint (M25.5-)*

✓6th **M79.60 Pain in limb, unspecified**
    **M79.601 Pain in right arm**
      Pain in right upper limb NOS
    **M79.602 Pain in left arm**
      Pain in left upper limb NOS
    **M79.603 Pain in arm, unspecified**
      Pain in upper limb NOS
    **M79.604 Pain in right leg**
      Pain in right lower limb NOS
    **M79.605 Pain in left leg**
      Pain in left lower limb NOS
    **M79.606 Pain in leg, unspecified**
      Pain in lower limb NOS
    **M79.609 Pain in unspecified limb**
      Pain in limb NOS

✓6th **M79.62 Pain in upper arm**
    Pain in axillary region
    **M79.621 Pain in right upper arm**
    **M79.622 Pain in left upper arm**
    **M79.629 Pain in unspecified upper arm**

✓6th **M79.63 Pain in forearm**
    **M79.631 Pain in right forearm**
    **M79.632 Pain in left forearm**
    **M79.639 Pain in unspecified forearm**

✓6th **M79.64 Pain in hand and fingers**
    **M79.641 Pain in right hand**
    **M79.642 Pain in left hand**
    **M79.643 Pain in unspecified hand**
    **M79.644 Pain in right finger(s)**
    **M79.645 Pain in left finger(s)**
    **M79.646 Pain in unspecified finger(s)**

✓6th **M79.65 Pain in thigh**
    **M79.651 Pain in right thigh**
    **M79.652 Pain in left thigh**
    **M79.659 Pain in unspecified thigh**

✓6th **M79.66 Pain in lower leg**
    **M79.661 Pain in right lower leg**
    **M79.662 Pain in left lower leg**
    **M79.669 Pain in unspecified lower leg**

✓6th **M79.67 Pain in foot and toes**
    **M79.671 Pain in right foot**
    **M79.672 Pain in left foot**
    **M79.673 Pain in unspecified foot**
    **M79.674 Pain in right toe(s)**
    **M79.675 Pain in left toe(s)**
    **M79.676 Pain in unspecified toe(s)**

**M79.7 Fibromyalgia**
    Fibromyositis
    Fibrositis
    Myofibrositis

✓5th **M79.A Nontraumatic compartment syndrome**
    Code first, if applicable, associated postprocedural complication
> EXCLUDES 1   *compartment syndrome NOS (T79.A-)*
> *fibromyalgia (M79.7)*
> *nontraumatic ischemic infarction of muscle (M62.2-)*
> *traumatic compartment syndrome (T79.A-)*

✓6th **M79.A1 Nontraumatic compartment syndrome of upper extremity**
    Nontraumatic compartment syndrome of shoulder, arm, forearm, wrist, hand, and fingers

> **CC Excl: For CC codes in subcategory M79.A1:**
> PDX collection 893

    **M79.A11 Nontraumatic compartment syndrome** CC **of right upper extremity**
    **M79.A12 Nontraumatic compartment syndrome** CC **of left upper extremity**
    **M79.A19 Nontraumatic compartment syndrome** CC **of unspecified upper extremity**

✓6th **M79.A2 Nontraumatic compartment syndrome of lower extremity**
    Nontraumatic compartment syndrome of hip, buttock, thigh, leg, foot, and toes

> **CC Excl: For CC codes in subcategory M79.A2:**
> PDX collection 894

    **M79.A21 Nontraumatic compartment syndrome** CC **of right lower extremity**
    **M79.A22 Nontraumatic compartment syndrome** CC **of left lower extremity**
    **M79.A29 Nontraumatic compartment syndrome** CC **of unspecified lower extremity**

    **M79.A3 Nontraumatic compartment syndrome of abdomen** CC
      **CC Excl:** PDX collection 895

    **M79.A9 Nontraumatic compartment syndrome of other sites** CC
      **CC Excl:** PDX collection 896

✓5th **M79.8 Other specified soft tissue disorders**
    **M79.81 Nontraumatic hematoma of soft tissue**
      Nontraumatic hematoma of muscle
      Nontraumatic seroma of muscle and soft tissue

    **M79.89 Other specified soft tissue disorders**
      Polyalgia

**M79.9 Soft tissue disorder, unspecified**

## OSTEOPATHIES AND CHONDROPATHIES (M80-M94)

### Disorders of bone density and structure (M80-M85)

✓4th **M80 Osteoporosis with current pathological fracture**
> INCLUDES   osteoporosis with current fragility fracture

Use additional code to identify major osseous defect, if applicable (M89.7-)
> EXCLUDES 1   *collapsed vertebra NOS (M48.5)*
> *pathological fracture NOS (M84.4)*
> *wedging of vertebra NOS (M48.5)*
> EXCLUDES 2   *personal history of (healed) osteoporosis fracture (Z87.310)*

> The appropriate 7th character is to be added to each code from category M80.
> A   initial encounter for fracture
> D   subsequent encounter for fracture with routine healing
> G   subsequent encounter for fracture with delayed healing
> K   subsequent encounter for fracture with nonunion
> P   subsequent encounter for fracture with malunion
> S   sequela

> **CC Excl: For codes in category M80, unless otherwise noted:**
> **CC with 7th character A:** PDX collection 888
> **CC with 7th character K or P:** PDX collection 897

✓5th **M80.0 Age-related osteoporosis with current pathological fracture**
    Involutional osteoporosis with current pathological fracture
    Osteoporosis NOS with current pathological fracture
    Postmenopausal osteoporosis with current pathological fracture
    Senile osteoporosis with current pathological fracture

[7] ✓x7th **M80.00 Age-related osteoporosis with current pathological fracture, unspecified site** CC A

✓6th **M80.01 Age-related osteoporosis with current pathological fracture, shoulder**
    [7] ✓7th **M80.011 Age-related osteoporosis with current pathological fracture, right shoulder** CC A
    [7] ✓7th **M80.012 Age-related osteoporosis with current pathological fracture, left shoulder** CC A
    [7] ✓7th **M80.019 Age-related osteoporosis with current pathological fracture, unspecified shoulder** CC A

✓6th **M80.02 Age-related osteoporosis with current pathological fracture, humerus**
    [7] ✓7th **M80.021 Age-related osteoporosis with current pathological fracture, right humerus** CC A
    [7] ✓7th **M80.022 Age-related osteoporosis with current pathological fracture, left humerus** CC A

---

[7]   CC when reported as an initial encounter (7th character A, B, or C – specific to category) OR a subsequent encounter for nonunion or malunion (7th character K, M, N, P, Q, or R – specific to category).

N Newborn: 0   P Pediatric: 0-17   M Maternity: 12-55   A Adult: 15-124   MCC Major CC Condition   PDxMCC PDx acts as own MCC   CC CC Condition   PDxCC PDx acts as own CC

796     ICD-10-CM 2018

**Chapter 13. Diseases of the Musculoskeletal System and Connective Tissue**

7 ✓7ᵗʰ **M80.029** Age-related osteoporosis with current pathological fracture, unspecified humerus `CC` `A`

✓6ᵗʰ **M80.03** Age-related osteoporosis with current pathological fracture, forearm
Age-related osteoporosis with current pathological fracture of wrist

7 ✓7ᵗʰ **M80.031** Age-related osteoporosis with current pathological fracture, right forearm `CC` `A`

7 ✓7ᵗʰ **M80.032** Age-related osteoporosis with current pathological fracture, left forearm `CC` `A`

7 ✓7ᵗʰ **M80.039** Age-related osteoporosis with current pathological fracture, unspecified forearm `CC` `A`

✓6ᵗʰ **M80.04** Age-related osteoporosis with current pathological fracture, hand

7 ✓7ᵗʰ **M80.041** Age-related osteoporosis with current pathological fracture, right hand `CC` `A`

7 ✓7ᵗʰ **M80.042** Age-related osteoporosis with current pathological fracture, left hand `CC` `A`

7 ✓7ᵗʰ **M80.049** Age-related osteoporosis with current pathological fracture, unspecified hand `CC` `A`

✓6ᵗʰ **M80.05** Age-related osteoporosis with current pathological fracture, femur
Age-related osteoporosis with current pathological fracture of hip

7, 10 ✓7ᵗʰ **M80.051** Age-related osteoporosis with current pathological fracture, right femur `CC` `HCC` `A`

7, 10 ✓7ᵗʰ **M80.052** Age-related osteoporosis with current pathological fracture, left femur `CC` `HCC` `A`

7, 10 ✓7ᵗʰ **M80.059** Age-related osteoporosis with current pathological fracture, unspecified femur `CC` `HCC` `A`

✓6ᵗʰ **M80.06** Age-related osteoporosis with current pathological fracture, lower leg

7 ✓7ᵗʰ **M80.061** Age-related osteoporosis with current pathological fracture, right lower leg `CC` `A`

7 ✓7ᵗʰ **M80.062** Age-related osteoporosis with current pathological fracture, left lower leg `CC` `A`

7 ✓7ᵗʰ **M80.069** Age-related osteoporosis with current pathological fracture, unspecified lower leg `CC` `A`

✓6ᵗʰ **M80.07** Age-related osteoporosis with current pathological fracture, ankle and foot

7 ✓7ᵗʰ **M80.071** Age-related osteoporosis with current pathological fracture, right ankle and foot `CC` `A`

7 ✓7ᵗʰ **M80.072** Age-related osteoporosis with current pathological fracture, left ankle and foot `CC` `A`

7 ✓7ᵗʰ **M80.079** Age-related osteoporosis with current pathological fracture, unspecified ankle and foot `CC` `A`

7, 10 ✓x7ᵗʰ **M80.08** Age-related osteoporosis with current pathological fracture, vertebra(e) `CC` `HCC` `A`

✓5ᵗʰ **M80.8** Other osteoporosis with current pathological fracture
Drug-induced osteoporosis with current pathological fracture
Idiopathic osteoporosis with current pathological fracture
Osteoporosis of disuse with current pathological fracture
Postoophorectomy osteoporosis with current pathological fracture
Postsurgical malabsorption osteoporosis with current pathological fracture
Post-traumatic osteoporosis with current pathological fracture
Use additional code for adverse effect, if applicable, to identify drug (T36-T50 with fifth or sixth character 5)

7 ✓x7ᵗʰ **M80.80** Other osteoporosis with current pathological fracture, unspecified site `CC`

✓6ᵗʰ **M80.81** Other osteoporosis with pathological fracture, shoulder

7 ✓7ᵗʰ **M80.811** Other osteoporosis with current pathological fracture, right shoulder `CC`

7 ✓7ᵗʰ **M80.812** Other osteoporosis with current pathological fracture, left shoulder `CC`

7 ✓7ᵗʰ **M80.819** Other osteoporosis with current pathological fracture, unspecified shoulder `CC`

✓6ᵗʰ **M80.82** Other osteoporosis with current pathological fracture, humerus

7 ✓7ᵗʰ **M80.821** Other osteoporosis with current pathological fracture, right humerus `CC`

7 ✓7ᵗʰ **M80.822** Other osteoporosis with current pathological fracture, left humerus `CC`

7 ✓7ᵗʰ **M80.829** Other osteoporosis with current pathological fracture, unspecified humerus `CC`

✓6ᵗʰ **M80.83** Other osteoporosis with current pathological fracture, forearm
Other osteoporosis with current pathological fracture of wrist

7 ✓7ᵗʰ **M80.831** Other osteoporosis with current pathological fracture, right forearm `CC`

7 ✓7ᵗʰ **M80.832** Other osteoporosis with current pathological fracture, left forearm `CC`

7 ✓7ᵗʰ **M80.839** Other osteoporosis with current pathological fracture, unspecified forearm `CC`

✓6ᵗʰ **M80.84** Other osteoporosis with current pathological fracture, hand

7 ✓7ᵗʰ **M80.841** Other osteoporosis with current pathological fracture, right hand `CC`

7 ✓7ᵗʰ **M80.842** Other osteoporosis with current pathological fracture, left hand `CC`

7 ✓7ᵗʰ **M80.849** Other osteoporosis with current pathological fracture, unspecified hand `CC`

✓6ᵗʰ **M80.85** Other osteoporosis with current pathological fracture, femur
Other osteoporosis with current pathological fracture of hip

7, 10 ✓7ᵗʰ **M80.851** Other osteoporosis with current pathological fracture, right femur `CC` `HCC`

7, 10 ✓7ᵗʰ **M80.852** Other osteoporosis with current pathological fracture, left femur `CC` `HCC`

7, 10 ✓7ᵗʰ **M80.859** Other osteoporosis with current pathological fracture, unspecified femur `CC` `HCC`

✓6ᵗʰ **M80.86** Other osteoporosis with current pathological fracture, lower leg

7 ✓7ᵗʰ **M80.861** Other osteoporosis with current pathological fracture, right lower leg `CC`

7 ✓7ᵗʰ **M80.862** Other osteoporosis with current pathological fracture, left lower leg `CC`

7 ✓7ᵗʰ **M80.869** Other osteoporosis with current pathological fracture, unspecified lower leg `CC`

✓6ᵗʰ **M80.87** Other osteoporosis with current pathological fracture, ankle and foot

7 ✓7ᵗʰ **M80.871** Other osteoporosis with current pathological fracture, right ankle and foot `CC`

7 ✓7ᵗʰ **M80.872** Other osteoporosis with current pathological fracture, left ankle and foot `CC`

7 ✓7ᵗʰ **M80.879** Other osteoporosis with current pathological fracture, unspecified ankle and foot `CC`

7, 10 ✓x7ᵗʰ **M80.88** Other osteoporosis with current pathological fracture, vertebra(e) `CC` `HCC`

---

7 CC when reported as an initial encounter (7th character A, B, or C – specific to category) OR a subsequent encounter for nonunion or malunion (7th character K, M, N, P, Q, or R – specific to category).
10 HCC with 7th character indicating initial encounter (A, B or C - specific to category).

✓ Additional Character Req   ✓x7ᵗʰ Placeholder Alert   Unacceptable PDx   Manifestation   `H1`-`H14` HAC   `HCC` CMS-HCC Condition   *EXCLUDES 1* Not Coded Here   *EXCLUDES 2* Not Included Here

**✓4ᵗʰ M81 Osteoporosis without current pathological fracture**

Use additional code to identify:
  major osseous defect, if applicable (M89.7-)
  personal history of (healed) osteoporosis fracture, if applicable (Z87.310)
    **EXCLUDES 1**   *osteoporosis with current pathological fracture (M80.-)*
          *Sudeck's atrophy (M89.0)*

**M81.0 Age-related osteoporosis without current pathological fracture**   Ⓐ
  Involutional osteoporosis without current pathological fracture
  Osteoporosis NOS
  Postmenopausal osteoporosis without current pathological fracture
  Senile osteoporosis without current pathological fracture

**M81.6 Localized osteoporosis [Lequesne]**
    **EXCLUDES 1**   *Sudeck's atrophy (M89.0)*

**M81.8 Other osteoporosis without current pathological fracture**
  Drug-induced osteoporosis without current pathological fracture
  Idiopathic osteoporosis without current pathological fracture
  Osteoporosis of disuse without current pathological fracture
  Postoophorectomy osteoporosis without current pathological fracture
  Postsurgical malabsorption osteoporosis without current pathological fracture
  Post-traumatic osteoporosis without current pathological fracture
  Use additional code for adverse effect, if applicable, to identify drug (T36-T50 with fifth or sixth character 5)

**✓4ᵗʰ M83 Adult osteomalacia**
    **EXCLUDES 1**   *infantile and juvenile osteomalacia (E55.0)*
          *renal osteodystrophy (N25.0)*
          *rickets (active) (E55.0)*
          *rickets (active) sequelae (E64.3)*
          *vitamin D-resistant osteomalacia (E83.3)*
          *vitamin D-resistant rickets (active) (E83.3)*

**M83.0 Puerperal osteomalacia**   Ⓜ ♀

**M83.1 Senile osteomalacia**   Ⓐ

**M83.2 Adult osteomalacia due to malabsorption**   Ⓐ
  Postsurgical malabsorption osteomalacia in adults

**M83.3 Adult osteomalacia due to malnutrition**   Ⓐ

**M83.4 Aluminum bone disease**

**M83.5 Other drug-induced osteomalacia in adults**   Ⓐ
  Use additional code for adverse effect, if applicable, to identify drug (T36-T50 with fifth or sixth character 5)

**M83.8 Other adult osteomalacia**   Ⓐ

**M83.9 Adult osteomalacia, unspecified**   Ⓐ

**✓4ᵗʰ M84 Disorder of continuity of bone**
    **EXCLUDES 2**   *traumatic fracture of bone-see fracture, by site*

**✓5ᵗʰ M84.3 Stress fracture**
  Fatigue fracture      Stress fracture NOS
  March fracture       Stress reaction
  Use additional external cause code(s) to identify the cause of the stress fracture
    **EXCLUDES 1**   *pathological fracture NOS (M84.4-)*
          *pathological fracture due to osteoporosis (M80.-)*
          *traumatic fracture (S12-, S22-, S32-, S42-, S52-, S62-, S72-, S82-, S92-)*
    **EXCLUDES 2**   *personal history of (healed) stress (fatigue) fracture (Z87.312)*
          *stress fracture of vertebra (M48.4-)*

The appropriate 7th character is to be added to each code from subcategory M84.3.
  A      initial encounter for fracture
  D      subsequent encounter for fracture with routine healing
  G      subsequent encounter for fracture with delayed healing
  K      subsequent encounter for fracture with nonunion
  P      subsequent encounter for fracture with malunion
  S      sequela

**CC Excl: For codes in subcategory M84.3:**
**CC with 7th character K or P:** PDX collection 897

8   **✓x7ᵗʰ M84.30 Stress fracture, unspecified site**    CC

---

**✓6ᵗʰ M84.31 Stress fracture, shoulder**
  8   ✓7ᵗʰ   **M84.311 Stress fracture, right shoulder**   CC
  8   ✓7ᵗʰ   **M84.312 Stress fracture, left shoulder**   CC
  8   ✓7ᵗʰ   **M84.319 Stress fracture, unspecified shoulder**   CC

**✓6ᵗʰ M84.32 Stress fracture, humerus**
  8   ✓7ᵗʰ   **M84.321 Stress fracture, right humerus**   CC
  8   ✓7ᵗʰ   **M84.322 Stress fracture, left humerus**   CC
  8   ✓7ᵗʰ   **M84.329 Stress fracture, unspecified humerus**   CC

**✓6ᵗʰ M84.33 Stress fracture, ulna and radius**
  8   ✓7ᵗʰ   **M84.331 Stress fracture, right ulna**   CC
  8   ✓7ᵗʰ   **M84.332 Stress fracture, left ulna**   CC
  8   ✓7ᵗʰ   **M84.333 Stress fracture, right radius**   CC
  8   ✓7ᵗʰ   **M84.334 Stress fracture, left radius**   CC
  8   ✓7ᵗʰ   **M84.339 Stress fracture, unspecified ulna and radius**   CC

**✓6ᵗʰ M84.34 Stress fracture, hand and fingers**
  8   ✓7ᵗʰ   **M84.341 Stress fracture, right hand**   CC
  8   ✓7ᵗʰ   **M84.342 Stress fracture, left hand**   CC
  8   ✓7ᵗʰ   **M84.343 Stress fracture, unspecified hand**   CC
  8   ✓7ᵗʰ   **M84.344 Stress fracture, right finger(s)**   CC
  8   ✓7ᵗʰ   **M84.345 Stress fracture, left finger(s)**   CC
  8   ✓7ᵗʰ   **M84.346 Stress fracture, unspecified finger(s)**   CC

**✓6ᵗʰ M84.35 Stress fracture, pelvis and femur**
  Stress fracture, hip
  8   ✓7ᵗʰ   **M84.350 Stress fracture, pelvis**   CC
  8   ✓7ᵗʰ   **M84.351 Stress fracture, right femur**   CC
  8   ✓7ᵗʰ   **M84.352 Stress fracture, left femur**   CC
  8   ✓7ᵗʰ   **M84.353 Stress fracture, unspecified femur**   CC
  8   ✓7ᵗʰ   **M84.359 Stress fracture, hip, unspecified**   CC

**✓6ᵗʰ M84.36 Stress fracture, tibia and fibula**
  8   ✓7ᵗʰ   **M84.361 Stress fracture, right tibia**   CC
  8   ✓7ᵗʰ   **M84.362 Stress fracture, left tibia**   CC
  8   ✓7ᵗʰ   **M84.363 Stress fracture, right fibula**   CC
  8   ✓7ᵗʰ   **M84.364 Stress fracture, left fibula**   CC
  8   ✓7ᵗʰ   **M84.369 Stress fracture, unspecified tibia and fibula**   CC

**✓6ᵗʰ M84.37 Stress fracture, ankle, foot and toes**
  8   ✓7ᵗʰ   **M84.371 Stress fracture, right ankle**   CC
  8   ✓7ᵗʰ   **M84.372 Stress fracture, left ankle**   CC
  8   ✓7ᵗʰ   **M84.373 Stress fracture, unspecified ankle**   CC
  8   ✓7ᵗʰ   **M84.374 Stress fracture, right foot**   CC
  8   ✓7ᵗʰ   **M84.375 Stress fracture, left foot**   CC
  8   ✓7ᵗʰ   **M84.376 Stress fracture, unspecified foot**   CC
  8   ✓7ᵗʰ   **M84.377 Stress fracture, right toe(s)**   CC
  8   ✓7ᵗʰ   **M84.378 Stress fracture, left toe(s)**   CC
  8   ✓7ᵗʰ   **M84.379 Stress fracture, unspecified toe(s)**   CC

8   **✓x7ᵗʰ M84.38 Stress fracture, other site**   CC
    **EXCLUDES 2**   *stress fracture of vertebra (M48.4-)*

---

8   CC when reported as a subsequent encounter for nonunion or malunion (7th character K, M, N, P, Q, or R – specific to category).

Ⓝ Newborn: 0    Ⓟ Pediatric: 0-17    Ⓜ Maternity: 12-55    Ⓐ Adult: 15-124    **MCC** Major CC Condition    **PDxMCC** PDx acts as own MCC    **CC** CC Condition    **PDxCC** PDx acts as own CC

798      ICD-10-CM 2018

✓5th **M84.4 Pathological fracture, not elsewhere classified**
Chronic fracture
Pathological fracture NOS

> EXCLUDES 1   *collapsed vertebra NEC (M48.5)*
> *pathological fracture in neoplastic disease (M84.5-)*
> *pathological fracture in osteoporosis (M80.-)*
> *pathological fracture in other disease (M84.6-)*
> *stress fracture (M84.3-)*
> *traumatic fracture (S12.-, S22.-, S32.-, S42.-, S52.-,*
> *S62.-, S72.-, S82.-, S92.-)*

> EXCLUDES 2   *personal history of (healed) pathological fracture*
> *(Z87.311)*

The appropriate 7th character is to be added to each code
from subcategory M84.4.
A   initial encounter for fracture
D   subsequent encounter for fracture with routine healing
G   subsequent encounter for fracture with delayed healing
K   subsequent encounter for fracture with nonunion
P   subsequent encounter for fracture with malunion
S   sequela

**CC Excl: For codes in subcategory M84.4:**
**CC with 7th character A:** PDX collection 888
**CC with 7th character K or P:** PDX collection 897

7   ✓x7th   **M84.40 Pathological fracture, unspecified site**   CC
    ✓6th   **M84.41 Pathological fracture, shoulder**
       7   ✓7th   **M84.411 Pathological fracture, right shoulder**   CC
       7   ✓7th   **M84.412 Pathological fracture, left shoulder**   CC
       7   ✓7th   **M84.419 Pathological fracture, unspecified shoulder**   CC
    ✓6th   **M84.42 Pathological fracture, humerus**
       7   ✓7th   **M84.421 Pathological fracture, right humerus**   CC
       7   ✓7th   **M84.422 Pathological fracture, left humerus**   CC
       7   ✓7th   **M84.429 Pathological fracture, unspecified humerus**   CC
    ✓6th   **M84.43 Pathological fracture, ulna and radius**
       7   ✓7th   **M84.431 Pathological fracture, right ulna**   CC
       7   ✓7th   **M84.432 Pathological fracture, left ulna**   CC
       7   ✓7th   **M84.433 Pathological fracture, right radius**   CC
       7   ✓7th   **M84.434 Pathological fracture, left radius**   CC
       7   ✓7th   **M84.439 Pathological fracture, unspecified ulna and radius**   CC
    ✓6th   **M84.44 Pathological fracture, hand and fingers**
       7   ✓7th   **M84.441 Pathological fracture, right hand**   CC
       7   ✓7th   **M84.442 Pathological fracture, left hand**   CC
       7   ✓7th   **M84.443 Pathological fracture, unspecified hand**   CC
       7   ✓7th   **M84.444 Pathological fracture, right finger(s)**   CC
       7   ✓7th   **M84.445 Pathological fracture, left finger(s)**   CC
       7   ✓7th   **M84.446 Pathological fracture, unspecified finger(s)**   CC
    ✓6th   **M84.45 Pathological fracture, femur and pelvis**
       7, 10   ✓7th   **M84.451 Pathological fracture, right femur**   CC HCC
       7, 10   ✓7th   **M84.452 Pathological fracture, left femur**   CC HCC
       7, 10   ✓7th   **M84.453 Pathological fracture, unspecified femur**   CC HCC
       7   ✓7th   **M84.454 Pathological fracture, pelvis**   CC
       7, 10   ✓7th   **M84.459 Pathological fracture, hip, unspecified**   CC HCC
    ✓6th   **M84.46 Pathological fracture, tibia and fibula**
       7   ✓7th   **M84.461 Pathological fracture, right tibia**   CC
       7   ✓7th   **M84.462 Pathological fracture, left tibia**   CC
       7   ✓7th   **M84.463 Pathological fracture, right fibula**   CC
       7   ✓7th   **M84.464 Pathological fracture, left fibula**   CC
       7   ✓7th   **M84.469 Pathological fracture, unspecified tibia and fibula**   CC
    ✓6th   **M84.47 Pathological fracture, ankle, foot and toes**
       7   ✓7th   **M84.471 Pathological fracture, right ankle**   CC
       7   ✓7th   **M84.472 Pathological fracture, left ankle**   CC
       7   ✓7th   **M84.473 Pathological fracture, unspecified ankle**   CC

       7   ✓7th   **M84.474 Pathological fracture, right foot**   CC
       7   ✓7th   **M84.475 Pathological fracture, left foot**   CC
       7   ✓7th   **M84.476 Pathological fracture, unspecified foot**   CC
       7   ✓7th   **M84.477 Pathological fracture, right toe(s)**   CC
       7   ✓7th   **M84.478 Pathological fracture, left toe(s)**   CC
       7   ✓7th   **M84.479 Pathological fracture, unspecified toe(s)**   CC
7   ✓x7th   **M84.48 Pathological fracture, other site**   CC

✓5th **M84.5 Pathological fracture in neoplastic disease**
Code also underlying neoplasm

The appropriate 7th character is to be added to each code
from subcategory M84.5.
A   initial encounter for fracture
D   subsequent encounter for fracture with routine healing
G   subsequent encounter for fracture with delayed healing
K   subsequent encounter for fracture with nonunion
P   subsequent encounter for fracture with malunion
S   sequela

**CC Excl: For codes in subcategory M84.5:**
**CC with 7th character A:** PDX collection 888
**CC with 7th character K or P:** PDX collection 897

7   ✓x7th   **M84.50 Pathological fracture in neoplastic disease, unspecified site**   CC
    ✓6th   **M84.51 Pathological fracture in neoplastic disease, shoulder**
       7   ✓7th   **M84.511 Pathological fracture in neoplastic disease, right shoulder**   CC
       7   ✓7th   **M84.512 Pathological fracture in neoplastic disease, left shoulder**   CC
       7   ✓7th   **M84.519 Pathological fracture in neoplastic disease, unspecified shoulder**   CC
    ✓6th   **M84.52 Pathological fracture in neoplastic disease, humerus**
       7   ✓7th   **M84.521 Pathological fracture in neoplastic disease, right humerus**   CC
       7   ✓7th   **M84.522 Pathological fracture in neoplastic disease, left humerus**   CC
       7   ✓7th   **M84.529 Pathological fracture in neoplastic disease, unspecified humerus**   CC
    ✓6th   **M84.53 Pathological fracture in neoplastic disease, ulna and radius**
       7   ✓7th   **M84.531 Pathological fracture in neoplastic disease, right ulna**   CC
       7   ✓7th   **M84.532 Pathological fracture in neoplastic disease, left ulna**   CC
       7   ✓7th   **M84.533 Pathological fracture in neoplastic disease, right radius**   CC
       7   ✓7th   **M84.534 Pathological fracture in neoplastic disease, left radius**   CC
       7   ✓7th   **M84.539 Pathological fracture in neoplastic disease, unspecified ulna and radius**   CC
    ✓6th   **M84.54 Pathological fracture in neoplastic disease, hand**
       7   ✓7th   **M84.541 Pathological fracture in neoplastic disease, right hand**   CC
       7   ✓7th   **M84.542 Pathological fracture in neoplastic disease, left hand**   CC
       7   ✓7th   **M84.549 Pathological fracture in neoplastic disease, unspecified hand**   CC
    ✓6th   **M84.55 Pathological fracture in neoplastic disease, pelvis and femur**
       7   ✓7th   **M84.550 Pathological fracture in neoplastic disease, pelvis**   CC
       7, 10   ✓7th   **M84.551 Pathological fracture in neoplastic disease, right femur**   CC HCC
       7, 10   ✓7th   **M84.552 Pathological fracture in neoplastic disease, left femur**   CC HCC
       7, 10   ✓7th   **M84.553 Pathological fracture in neoplastic disease, unspecified femur**   CC HCC
       7, 10   ✓7th   **M84.559 Pathological fracture in neoplastic disease, hip, unspecified**   CC HCC

---

7   CC when reported as an initial encounter (7th character A, B, or C – specific to category) OR a subsequent encounter for nonunion or malunion
    (7th character K, M, N, P, Q, or R – specific to category).
10   HCC with 7th character indicating initial encounter (A, B or C - specific to category).

**Chapter 13. Diseases of the Musculoskeletal System and Connective Tissue**

✓6th **M84.56 Pathological fracture in neoplastic disease, tibia and fibula**

    7 ✓7th **M84.561 Pathological fracture in neoplastic disease, right tibia** CC

    7 ✓7th **M84.562 Pathological fracture in neoplastic disease, left tibia** CC

    7 ✓7th **M84.563 Pathological fracture in neoplastic disease, right fibula** CC

    7 ✓7th **M84.564 Pathological fracture in neoplastic disease, left fibula** CC

    7 ✓7th **M84.569 Pathological fracture in neoplastic disease, unspecified tibia and fibula** CC

✓6th **M84.57 Pathological fracture in neoplastic disease, ankle and foot**

    7 ✓7th **M84.571 Pathological fracture in neoplastic disease, right ankle** CC

    7 ✓7th **M84.572 Pathological fracture in neoplastic disease, left ankle** CC

    7 ✓7th **M84.573 Pathological fracture in neoplastic disease, unspecified ankle** CC

    7 ✓7th **M84.574 Pathological fracture in neoplastic disease, right foot** CC

    7 ✓7th **M84.575 Pathological fracture in neoplastic disease, left foot** CC

    7 ✓7th **M84.576 Pathological fracture in neoplastic disease, unspecified foot** CC

✓x7th **M84.58 Pathological fracture in neoplastic disease, other specified site** CC

      Pathological fracture in neoplastic disease, vertebrae

✓5th **M84.6 Pathological fracture in other disease**

   Code also underlying condition

   **EXCLUDES 1**   *pathological fracture in osteoporosis (M80.-)*

> The appropriate 7th character is to be added to each code from subcategory M84.6.
> A   initial encounter for fracture
> D   subsequent encounter for fracture with routine healing
> G   subsequent encounter for fracture with delayed healing
> K   subsequent encounter for fracture with nonunion
> P   subsequent encounter for fracture with malunion
> S   sequela

> **CC Excl: For codes in subcategory M84.6:**
> **CC with 7th character A:** PDX collection 888
> **CC with 7th character K or P:** PDX collection 897

  7 ✓x7th **M84.60 Pathological fracture in other disease, unspecified site** CC

✓6th **M84.61 Pathological fracture in other disease, shoulder**

    7 ✓7th **M84.611 Pathological fracture in other disease, right shoulder** CC

    7 ✓7th **M84.612 Pathological fracture in other disease, left shoulder** CC

    7 ✓7th **M84.619 Pathological fracture in other disease, unspecified shoulder** CC

✓6th **M84.62 Pathological fracture in other disease, humerus**

    7 ✓7th **M84.621 Pathological fracture in other disease, right humerus** CC

    7 ✓7th **M84.622 Pathological fracture in other disease, left humerus** CC

    7 ✓7th **M84.629 Pathological fracture in other disease, unspecified humerus** CC

✓6th **M84.63 Pathological fracture in other disease, ulna and radius**

    7 ✓7th **M84.631 Pathological fracture in other disease, right ulna** CC

    7 ✓7th **M84.632 Pathological fracture in other disease, left ulna** CC

    7 ✓7th **M84.633 Pathological fracture in other disease, right radius** CC

    7 ✓7th **M84.634 Pathological fracture in other disease, left radius** CC

    7 ✓7th **M84.639 Pathological fracture in other disease, unspecified ulna and radius** CC

✓6th **M84.64 Pathological fracture in other disease, hand**

    7 ✓7th **M84.641 Pathological fracture in other disease, right hand** CC

    7 ✓7th **M84.642 Pathological fracture in other disease, left hand** CC

    7 ✓7th **M84.649 Pathological fracture in other disease, unspecified hand** CC

✓6th **M84.65 Pathological fracture in other disease, pelvis and femur**

    7 ✓7th **M84.650 Pathological fracture in other disease, pelvis** CC

    7, 10 ✓7th **M84.651 Pathological fracture in other disease, right femur** CC HCC

    7, 10 ✓7th **M84.652 Pathological fracture in other disease, left femur** CC HCC

    7, 10 ✓7th **M84.653 Pathological fracture in other disease, unspecified femur** CC HCC

    7, 10 ✓7th **M84.659 Pathological fracture in other disease, hip, unspecified** CC HCC

✓6th **M84.66 Pathological fracture in other disease, tibia and fibula**

    7 ✓7th **M84.661 Pathological fracture in other disease, right tibia** CC

    7 ✓7th **M84.662 Pathological fracture in other disease, left tibia** CC

    7 ✓7th **M84.663 Pathological fracture in other disease, right fibula** CC

    7 ✓7th **M84.664 Pathological fracture in other disease, left fibula** CC

    7 ✓7th **M84.669 Pathological fracture in other disease, unspecified tibia and fibula** CC

✓6th **M84.67 Pathological fracture in other disease, ankle and foot**

    7 ✓7th **M84.671 Pathological fracture in other disease, right ankle** CC

    7 ✓7th **M84.672 Pathological fracture in other disease, left ankle** CC

    7 ✓7th **M84.673 Pathological fracture in other disease, unspecified ankle** CC

    7 ✓7th **M84.674 Pathological fracture in other disease, right foot** CC

    7 ✓7th **M84.675 Pathological fracture in other disease, left foot** CC

    7 ✓7th **M84.676 Pathological fracture in other disease, unspecified foot** CC

  7 ✓x7th **M84.68 Pathological fracture in other disease, other site** CC

✓5th **M84.7 Nontraumatic fracture, not elsewhere classified**

✓6th **M84.75 Atypical femoral fracture**

> The appropriate 7th character is to be added to each code from subcategory M84.75.
> A   initial encounter for fracture
> D   subsequent encounter for fracture with routine healing
> G   subsequent encounter for fracture with delayed healing
> K   subsequent encounter for fracture with nonunion
> P   subsequent encounter for fracture with malunion
> S   sequela

> **CC Excl: For CC codes in subcategory M84.75:**
> **CC with 7th character A:** PDX collection 888
> **CC with 7th character K or P:** PDX collection 897

    7 ✓7th **M84.750 Atypical femoral fracture, unspecified** CC

    7 ✓7th **M84.751 Incomplete atypical femoral fracture, right leg** CC

    7 ✓7th **M84.752 Incomplete atypical femoral fracture, left leg** CC

    7 ✓7th **M84.753 Incomplete atypical femoral fracture, unspecified leg** CC

---

7   CC when reported as an initial encounter (7th character A, B, or C – specific to category) OR a subsequent encounter for nonunion or malunion (7th character K, M, N, P, Q, or R – specific to category).

10   HCC with 7th character indicating initial encounter (A, B or C - specific to category).

N Newborn: 0   P Pediatric: 0-17   M Maternity: 12-55   A Adult: 15-124   **MCC** Major CC Condition   **PDx MCC** PDx acts as own MCC   **CC** CC Condition   **PDx CC** PDx acts as own CC

800                                     ICD-10-CM 2018

7, 10 ✓7th **M84.754** Complete transverse **atypical femoral fracture, right leg** `CC` `HCC`

7, 10 ✓7th **M84.755** Complete transverse **atypical femoral fracture, left leg** `CC` `HCC`

7, 10 ✓7th **M84.756** Complete transverse **atypical femoral fracture, unspecified leg** `CC` `HCC`

7, 10 ✓7th **M84.757** Complete oblique **atypical femoral fracture, right leg** `CC` `HCC`

7, 10 ✓7th **M84.758** Complete oblique **atypical femoral fracture, left leg** `CC` `HCC`

7, 10 ✓7th **M84.759** Complete oblique **atypical femoral fracture, unspecified leg** `CC` `HCC`

✓5th **M84.8** Other disorders of continuity of bone

    **M84.80** Other disorders of continuity of bone, unspecified site

    ✓6th **M84.81** Other disorders of continuity of bone, **shoulder**

       **M84.811** Other disorders of continuity of bone, right **shoulder**

       **M84.812** Other disorders of continuity of bone, left **shoulder**

       **M84.819** Other disorders of continuity of bone, unspecified **shoulder**

    ✓6th **M84.82** Other disorders of continuity of bone, **humerus**

       **M84.821** Other disorders of continuity of bone, right **humerus**

       **M84.822** Other disorders of continuity of bone, left **humerus**

       **M84.829** Other disorders of continuity of bone, unspecified **humerus**

    ✓6th **M84.83** Other disorders of continuity of bone, **ulna and radius**

       **M84.831** Other disorders of continuity of bone, right **ulna**

       **M84.832** Other disorders of continuity of bone, left **ulna**

       **M84.833** Other disorders of continuity of bone, right **radius**

       **M84.834** Other disorders of continuity of bone, left **radius**

       **M84.839** Other disorders of continuity of bone, unspecified **ulna and radius**

    ✓6th **M84.84** Other disorders of continuity of bone, **hand**

       **M84.841** Other disorders of continuity of bone, right **hand**

       **M84.842** Other disorders of continuity of bone, left **hand**

       **M84.849** Other disorders of continuity of bone, unspecified **hand**

    ✓6th **M84.85** Other disorders of continuity of bone, **pelvic region and thigh**

       **M84.851** Other disorders of continuity of bone, right **pelvic region and thigh**

       **M84.852** Other disorders of continuity of bone, left **pelvic region and thigh**

       **M84.859** Other disorders of continuity of bone, unspecified **pelvic region and thigh**

    ✓6th **M84.86** Other disorders of continuity of bone, **tibia and fibula**

       **M84.861** Other disorders of continuity of bone, right **tibia**

       **M84.862** Other disorders of continuity of bone, left **tibia**

       **M84.863** Other disorders of continuity of bone, right **fibula**

       **M84.864** Other disorders of continuity of bone, left **fibula**

       **M84.869** Other disorders of continuity of bone, unspecified **tibia and fibula**

    ✓6th **M84.87** Other disorders of continuity of bone, **ankle and foot**

       **M84.871** Other disorders of continuity of bone, right **ankle and foot**

       **M84.872** Other disorders of continuity of bone, left **ankle and foot**

**M84.879** Other disorders of continuity of bone, unspecified **ankle and foot**

**M84.88** Other disorders of continuity of bone, other site

**M84.9** Disorder of continuity of bone, unspecified

✓4th **M85** Other disorders of bone density and structure

    EXCLUDES 1   osteogenesis imperfecta (Q78.0)
                osteopetrosis (Q78.2)
                osteopoikilosis (Q78.8)
                polyostotic fibrous dysplasia (Q78.1)

✓5th **M85.0** Fibrous dysplasia (monostotic)

    EXCLUDES 2   fibrous dysplasia of jaw (M27.8)

    **M85.00** Fibrous dysplasia (monostotic), unspecified site

    ✓6th **M85.01** Fibrous dysplasia (monostotic), shoulder

       **M85.011** Fibrous dysplasia (monostotic), right shoulder

       **M85.012** Fibrous dysplasia (monostotic), left shoulder

       **M85.019** Fibrous dysplasia (monostotic), unspecified shoulder

    ✓6th **M85.02** Fibrous dysplasia (monostotic), upper arm

       **M85.021** Fibrous dysplasia (monostotic), right upper arm

       **M85.022** Fibrous dysplasia (monostotic), left upper arm

       **M85.029** Fibrous dysplasia (monostotic), unspecified upper arm

    ✓6th **M85.03** Fibrous dysplasia (monostotic), forearm

       **M85.031** Fibrous dysplasia (monostotic), right forearm

       **M85.032** Fibrous dysplasia (monostotic), left forearm

       **M85.039** Fibrous dysplasia (monostotic), unspecified forearm

    ✓6th **M85.04** Fibrous dysplasia (monostotic), hand

       **M85.041** Fibrous dysplasia (monostotic), right hand

       **M85.042** Fibrous dysplasia (monostotic), left hand

       **M85.049** Fibrous dysplasia (monostotic), unspecified hand

    ✓6th **M85.05** Fibrous dysplasia (monostotic), thigh

       **M85.051** Fibrous dysplasia (monostotic), right thigh

       **M85.052** Fibrous dysplasia (monostotic), left thigh

       **M85.059** Fibrous dysplasia (monostotic), unspecified thigh

    ✓6th **M85.06** Fibrous dysplasia (monostotic), lower leg

       **M85.061** Fibrous dysplasia (monostotic), right lower leg

       **M85.062** Fibrous dysplasia (monostotic), left lower leg

       **M85.069** Fibrous dysplasia (monostotic), unspecified lower leg

    ✓6th **M85.07** Fibrous dysplasia (monostotic), ankle and foot

       **M85.071** Fibrous dysplasia (monostotic), right ankle and foot

       **M85.072** Fibrous dysplasia (monostotic), left ankle and foot

       **M85.079** Fibrous dysplasia (monostotic), unspecified ankle and foot

    **M85.08** Fibrous dysplasia (monostotic), other site

    **M85.09** Fibrous dysplasia (monostotic), multiple sites

✓5th **M85.1** Skeletal fluorosis

    **M85.10** Skeletal fluorosis, unspecified site

    ✓6th **M85.11** Skeletal fluorosis, shoulder

       **M85.111** Skeletal fluorosis, right shoulder

       **M85.112** Skeletal fluorosis, left shoulder

       **M85.119** Skeletal fluorosis, unspecified shoulder

    ✓6th **M85.12** Skeletal fluorosis, upper arm

       **M85.121** Skeletal fluorosis, right upper arm

       **M85.122** Skeletal fluorosis, left upper arm

       **M85.129** Skeletal fluorosis, unspecified upper arm

    ✓6th **M85.13** Skeletal fluorosis, forearm

       **M85.131** Skeletal fluorosis, right forearm

---

7   CC when reported as an initial encounter (7th character A, B, or C – specific to category) OR a subsequent encounter for nonunion or malunion (7th character K, M, N, P, Q, or R – specific to category).

10   HCC with 7th character indicating initial encounter (A, B or C - specific to category).

✓ Additional Character Req   vx 7th Placeholder Alert   Unacceptable PDx   Manifestation   H1 - H14 HAC   HCC CMS-HCC Condition   EXCLUDES 1 Not Coded Here   EXCLUDES 2 Not Included Here

ICD-10-CM 2018                                                            **801**

          M85.132   Skeletal fluorosis, left forearm
          M85.139   Skeletal fluorosis, unspecified forearm

√6th   **M85.14**   **Skeletal fluorosis, hand**
          M85.141   Skeletal fluorosis, right hand
          M85.142   Skeletal fluorosis, left hand
          M85.149   Skeletal fluorosis, unspecified hand

√6th   **M85.15**   **Skeletal fluorosis, thigh**
          M85.151   Skeletal fluorosis, right thigh
          M85.152   Skeletal fluorosis, left thigh
          M85.159   Skeletal fluorosis, unspecified thigh

√6th   **M85.16**   **Skeletal fluorosis, lower leg**
          M85.161   Skeletal fluorosis, right lower leg
          M85.162   Skeletal fluorosis, left lower leg
          M85.169   Skeletal fluorosis, unspecified lower leg

√6th   **M85.17**   **Skeletal fluorosis, ankle and foot**
          M85.171   Skeletal fluorosis, right ankle and foot
          M85.172   Skeletal fluorosis, left ankle and foot
          M85.179   Skeletal fluorosis, unspecified ankle and foot

      **M85.18**   **Skeletal fluorosis, other site**
      **M85.19**   **Skeletal fluorosis, multiple sites**

**M85.2**   **Hyperostosis of skull**
      **DEF:** Abnormal bone growth on inner aspect of cranial bones.

√5th   **M85.3**   **Osteitis condensans**
      **M85.30**   **Osteitis condensans, unspecified site**

√6th   **M85.31**   **Osteitis condensans, shoulder**
          M85.311   Osteitis condensans, right shoulder
          M85.312   Osteitis condensans, left shoulder
          M85.319   Osteitis condensans, unspecified shoulder

√6th   **M85.32**   **Osteitis condensans, upper arm**
          M85.321   Osteitis condensans, right upper arm
          M85.322   Osteitis condensans, left upper arm
          M85.329   Osteitis condensans, unspecified upper arm

√6th   **M85.33**   **Osteitis condensans, forearm**
          M85.331   Osteitis condensans, right forearm
          M85.332   Osteitis condensans, left forearm
          M85.339   Osteitis condensans, unspecified forearm

√6th   **M85.34**   **Osteitis condensans, hand**
          M85.341   Osteitis condensans, right hand
          M85.342   Osteitis condensans, left hand
          M85.349   Osteitis condensans, unspecified hand

√6th   **M85.35**   **Osteitis condensans, thigh**
          M85.351   Osteitis condensans, right thigh
          M85.352   Osteitis condensans, left thigh
          M85.359   Osteitis condensans, unspecified thigh

√6th   **M85.36**   **Osteitis condensans, lower leg**
          M85.361   Osteitis condensans, right lower leg
          M85.362   Osteitis condensans, left lower leg
          M85.369   Osteitis condensans, unspecified lower leg

√6th   **M85.37**   **Osteitis condensans, ankle and foot**
          M85.371   Osteitis condensans, right ankle and foot
          M85.372   Osteitis condensans, left ankle and foot
          M85.379   Osteitis condensans, unspecified ankle and foot

      **M85.38**   **Osteitis condensans, other site**
      **M85.39**   **Osteitis condensans, multiple sites**

√5th   **M85.4**   **Solitary bone cyst**
      EXCLUDES 2   *solitary cyst of jaw (M27.4)*
      **M85.40**   **Solitary bone cyst, unspecified site**

√6th   **M85.41**   **Solitary bone cyst, shoulder**
          M85.411   Solitary bone cyst, right shoulder
          M85.412   Solitary bone cyst, left shoulder
          M85.419   Solitary bone cyst, unspecified shoulder

√6th   **M85.42**   **Solitary bone cyst, humerus**
          M85.421   Solitary bone cyst, right humerus
          M85.422   Solitary bone cyst, left humerus
          M85.429   Solitary bone cyst, unspecified humerus

√6th   **M85.43**   **Solitary bone cyst, ulna and radius**
          M85.431   Solitary bone cyst, right ulna and radius
          M85.432   Solitary bone cyst, left ulna and radius

          M85.439   Solitary bone cyst, unspecified ulna and radius

√6th   **M85.44**   **Solitary bone cyst, hand**
          M85.441   Solitary bone cyst, right hand
          M85.442   Solitary bone cyst, left hand
          M85.449   Solitary bone cyst, unspecified hand

√6th   **M85.45**   **Solitary bone cyst, pelvis**
          M85.451   Solitary bone cyst, right pelvis
          M85.452   Solitary bone cyst, left pelvis
          M85.459   Solitary bone cyst, unspecified pelvis

√6th   **M85.46**   **Solitary bone cyst, tibia and fibula**
          M85.461   Solitary bone cyst, right tibia and fibula
          M85.462   Solitary bone cyst, left tibia and fibula
          M85.469   Solitary bone cyst, unspecified tibia and fibula

√6th   **M85.47**   **Solitary bone cyst, ankle and foot**
          M85.471   Solitary bone cyst, right ankle and foot
          M85.472   Solitary bone cyst, left ankle and foot
          M85.479   Solitary bone cyst, unspecified ankle and foot

      **M85.48**   **Solitary bone cyst, other site**

√5th   **M85.5**   **Aneurysmal bone cyst**
      EXCLUDES 2   *aneurysmal cyst of jaw (M27.4)*
      **DEF:** Solitary bone lesion, bulges into periosteum; marked by calcified rim.
      **M85.50**   **Aneurysmal bone cyst, unspecified site**

√6th   **M85.51**   **Aneurysmal bone cyst, shoulder**
          M85.511   Aneurysmal bone cyst, right shoulder
          M85.512   Aneurysmal bone cyst, left shoulder
          M85.519   Aneurysmal bone cyst, unspecified shoulder

√6th   **M85.52**   **Aneurysmal bone cyst, upper arm**
          M85.521   Aneurysmal bone cyst, right upper arm
          M85.522   Aneurysmal bone cyst, left upper arm
          M85.529   Aneurysmal bone cyst, unspecified upper arm

√6th   **M85.53**   **Aneurysmal bone cyst, forearm**
          M85.531   Aneurysmal bone cyst, right forearm
          M85.532   Aneurysmal bone cyst, left forearm
          M85.539   Aneurysmal bone cyst, unspecified forearm

√6th   **M85.54**   **Aneurysmal bone cyst, hand**
          M85.541   Aneurysmal bone cyst, right hand
          M85.542   Aneurysmal bone cyst, left hand
          M85.549   Aneurysmal bone cyst, unspecified hand

√6th   **M85.55**   **Aneurysmal bone cyst, thigh**
          M85.551   Aneurysmal bone cyst, right thigh
          M85.552   Aneurysmal bone cyst, left thigh
          M85.559   Aneurysmal bone cyst, unspecified thigh

√6th   **M85.56**   **Aneurysmal bone cyst, lower leg**
          M85.561   Aneurysmal bone cyst, right lower leg
          M85.562   Aneurysmal bone cyst, left lower leg
          M85.569   Aneurysmal bone cyst, unspecified lower leg

√6th   **M85.57**   **Aneurysmal bone cyst, ankle and foot**
          M85.571   Aneurysmal bone cyst, right ankle and foot
          M85.572   Aneurysmal bone cyst, left ankle and foot
          M85.579   Aneurysmal bone cyst, unspecified ankle and foot

      **M85.58**   **Aneurysmal bone cyst, other site**
      **M85.59**   **Aneurysmal bone cyst, multiple sites**

√5th   **M85.6**   **Other cyst of bone**
      EXCLUDES 1   *cyst of jaw NEC (M27.4)*
              *osteitis fibrosa cystica generalisata [von Recklinghausen's disease of bone] (E21.0)*
      **M85.60**   **Other cyst of bone, unspecified site**

√6th   **M85.61**   **Other cyst of bone, shoulder**
          M85.611   Other cyst of bone, right shoulder
          M85.612   Other cyst of bone, left shoulder
          M85.619   Other cyst of bone, unspecified shoulder

√6th   **M85.62**   **Other cyst of bone, upper arm**
          M85.621   Other cyst of bone, right upper arm

M85.622  Other cyst of bone, left upper arm

M85.629  Other cyst of bone, unspecified upper arm

✓6ᵗʰ **M85.63**  Other cyst of bone, forearm

M85.631  Other cyst of bone, right forearm

M85.632  Other cyst of bone, left forearm

M85.639  Other cyst of bone, unspecified forearm

✓6ᵗʰ **M85.64**  Other cyst of bone, hand

M85.641  Other cyst of bone, right hand

M85.642  Other cyst of bone, left hand

M85.649  Other cyst of bone, unspecified hand

✓6ᵗʰ **M85.65**  Other cyst of bone, thigh

M85.651  Other cyst of bone, right thigh

M85.652  Other cyst of bone, left thigh

M85.659  Other cyst of bone, unspecified thigh

✓6ᵗʰ **M85.66**  Other cyst of bone, lower leg

M85.661  Other cyst of bone, right lower leg

M85.662  Other cyst of bone, left lower leg

M85.669  Other cyst of bone, unspecified lower leg

✓6ᵗʰ **M85.67**  Other cyst of bone, ankle and foot

M85.671  Other cyst of bone, right ankle and foot

M85.672  Other cyst of bone, left ankle and foot

M85.679  Other cyst of bone, unspecified ankle and foot

**M85.68**  Other cyst of bone, other site

**M85.69**  Other cyst of bone, multiple sites

✓5ᵗʰ **M85.8**  Other specified disorders of bone density and structure

Hyperostosis of bones, except skull

Osteosclerosis, acquired

*EXCLUDES 1*  diffuse idiopathic skeletal hyperostosis [DISH] (M48.1)
osteosclerosis congenita (Q77.4)
osteosclerosis fragilitas (generalista) (Q78.2)
osteosclerosis myelofibrosis (D75.81)

**M85.80**  Other specified disorders of bone density and structure, unspecified site

✓6ᵗʰ **M85.81**  Other specified disorders of bone density and structure, shoulder

M85.811  Other specified disorders of bone density and structure, right shoulder

M85.812  Other specified disorders of bone density and structure, left shoulder

M85.819  Other specified disorders of bone density and structure, unspecified shoulder

✓6ᵗʰ **M85.82**  Other specified disorders of bone density and structure, upper arm

M85.821  Other specified disorders of bone density and structure, right upper arm

M85.822  Other specified disorders of bone density and structure, left upper arm

M85.829  Other specified disorders of bone density and structure, unspecified upper arm

✓6ᵗʰ **M85.83**  Other specified disorders of bone density and structure, forearm

M85.831  Other specified disorders of bone density and structure, right forearm

M85.832  Other specified disorders of bone density and structure, left forearm

M85.839  Other specified disorders of bone density and structure, unspecified forearm

✓6ᵗʰ **M85.84**  Other specified disorders of bone density and structure, hand

M85.841  Other specified disorders of bone density and structure, right hand

M85.842  Other specified disorders of bone density and structure, left hand

M85.849  Other specified disorders of bone density and structure, unspecified hand

✓6ᵗʰ **M85.85**  Other specified disorders of bone density and structure, thigh

M85.851  Other specified disorders of bone density and structure, right thigh

M85.852  Other specified disorders of bone density and structure, left thigh

M85.859  Other specified disorders of bone density and structure, unspecified thigh

✓6ᵗʰ **M85.86**  Other specified disorders of bone density and structure, lower leg

M85.861  Other specified disorders of bone density and structure, right lower leg

M85.862  Other specified disorders of bone density and structure, left lower leg

M85.869  Other specified disorders of bone density and structure, unspecified lower leg

✓6ᵗʰ **M85.87**  Other specified disorders of bone density and structure, ankle and foot

M85.871  Other specified disorders of bone density and structure, right ankle and foot

M85.872  Other specified disorders of bone density and structure, left ankle and foot

M85.879  Other specified disorders of bone density and structure, unspecified ankle and foot

**M85.88**  Other specified disorders of bone density and structure, other site

**M85.89**  Other specified disorders of bone density and structure, multiple sites

**M85.9**  Disorder of bone density and structure, unspecified

## Other osteopathies (M86-M90)

*EXCLUDES 1*  postprocedural osteopathies (M96.-)

✓4ᵗʰ **M86**  **Osteomyelitis**

Use additional code (B95-B97) to identify infectious agent

Use additional code to identify major osseous defect, if applicable (M89.7-)

*EXCLUDES 1*  osteomyelitis due to:
echinococcus (B67.2)
gonococcus (A54.43)
salmonella (A02.24)

*EXCLUDES 2*  ostemyelitis of:
orbit (H05.0-)
petrous bone (H70.2-)
vertebra (M46.2-)

✓5ᵗʰ **M86.0**  Acute hematogenous osteomyelitis

**M86.00**  Acute hematogenous osteomyelitis, unspecified site  `CC` `HCC`

CC Excl: PDX collection 898

✓6ᵗʰ **M86.01**  Acute hematogenous osteomyelitis, shoulder

CC Excl: For CC codes in subcategory M86.01: PDX collection 899

M86.011  Acute hematogenous osteomyelitis, right shoulder  `CC` `HCC`

M86.012  Acute hematogenous osteomyelitis, left shoulder  `CC` `HCC`

M86.019  Acute hematogenous osteomyelitis, unspecified shoulder  `CC` `HCC`

✓6ᵗʰ **M86.02**  Acute hematogenous osteomyelitis, humerus

CC Excl: For CC codes in subcategory M86.02: PDX collection 900

M86.021  Acute hematogenous osteomyelitis, right humerus  `CC` `HCC`

M86.022  Acute hematogenous osteomyelitis, left humerus  `CC` `HCC`

M86.029  Acute hematogenous osteomyelitis, unspecified humerus  `CC` `HCC`

✓6ᵗʰ **M86.03**  Acute hematogenous osteomyelitis, radius and ulna

CC Excl: For CC codes in subcategory M86.03: PDX collection 901

M86.031  Acute hematogenous osteomyelitis, right radius and ulna  `CC` `HCC`

M86.032  Acute hematogenous osteomyelitis, left radius and ulna  `CC` `HCC`

M86.039  Acute hematogenous osteomyelitis, unspecified radius and ulna  `CC` `HCC`

✓6ᵗʰ **M86.04**  Acute hematogenous osteomyelitis, hand

CC Excl: For CC codes in subcategory M86.04: PDX collection 902

M86.041  Acute hematogenous osteomyelitis, right hand  `CC` `HCC`

M86.042  Acute hematogenous osteomyelitis, left hand  `CC` `HCC`

✓ Additional Character Req  ✓x7ᵗʰ Placeholder Alert  Unacceptable PDx  Manifestation  H1-H14 HAC  HCC CMS-HCC Condition  *EXCLUDES 1* Not Coded Here  *EXCLUDES 2* Not Included Here

ICD-10-CM 2018  **803**

M86.049   **Acute hematogenous osteomyelitis, unspecified hand** `CC` `HCC`

☑6ᵗʰ   M86.05   **Acute hematogenous osteomyelitis, femur**

> **CC Excl: For CC codes in subcategory M86.05:**
> PDX collection 903

M86.051   **Acute hematogenous osteomyelitis, right femur** `CC` `HCC`

M86.052   **Acute hematogenous osteomyelitis, left femur** `CC` `HCC`

M86.059   **Acute hematogenous osteomyelitis, femur** `CC` `HCC`

☑6ᵗʰ   M86.06   **Acute hematogenous osteomyelitis, tibia and fibula**

> **CC Excl: For CC codes in subcategory M86.06:**
> PDX collection 904

M86.061   **Acute hematogenous osteomyelitis, right tibia and fibula** `CC` `HCC`

M86.062   **Acute hematogenous osteomyelitis, left tibia and fibula** `CC` `HCC`

M86.069   **Acute hematogenous osteomyelitis, unspecified tibia and fibula** `CC` `HCC`

☑6ᵗʰ   M86.07   **Acute hematogenous osteomyelitis, ankle and foot**

> **CC Excl: For CC codes in subcategory M86.07:**
> PDX collection 905

M86.071   **Acute hematogenous osteomyelitis, right ankle and foot** `CC` `HCC`

M86.072   **Acute hematogenous osteomyelitis, left ankle and foot** `CC` `HCC`

M86.079   **Acute hematogenous osteomyelitis, unspecified ankle and foot** `CC` `HCC`

M86.08   **Acute hematogenous osteomyelitis, other sites** `CC` `HCC`
CC Excl: PDX collection 882

M86.09   **Acute hematogenous osteomyelitis, multiple sites** `CC` `HCC`
CC Excl: PDX collection 898

☑5ᵗʰ   M86.1   **Other acute osteomyelitis**

M86.10   **Other acute osteomyelitis, unspecified site** `CC` `HCC`
CC Excl: PDX collection 898

☑6ᵗʰ   M86.11   **Other acute osteomyelitis, shoulder**

> **CC Excl: For CC codes in subcategory M86.11:**
> PDX collection 899

M86.111   **Other acute osteomyelitis, right shoulder** `CC` `HCC`

M86.112   **Other acute osteomyelitis, left shoulder** `CC` `HCC`

M86.119   **Other acute osteomyelitis, unspecified shoulder** `CC` `HCC`

☑6ᵗʰ   M86.12   **Other acute osteomyelitis, humerus**

> **CC Excl: For CC codes in subcategory M86.12:**
> PDX collection 900

M86.121   **Other acute osteomyelitis, right humerus** `CC` `HCC`

M86.122   **Other acute osteomyelitis, left humerus** `CC` `HCC`

M86.129   **Other acute osteomyelitis, unspecified humerus** `CC` `HCC`

☑6ᵗʰ   M86.13   **Other acute osteomyelitis, radius and ulna**

> **CC Excl: For CC codes in subcategory M86.13:**
> PDX collection 901

M86.131   **Other acute osteomyelitis, right radius and ulna** `CC` `HCC`

M86.132   **Other acute osteomyelitis, left radius and ulna** `CC` `HCC`

M86.139   **Other acute osteomyelitis, unspecified radius and ulna** `CC` `HCC`

☑6ᵗʰ   M86.14   **Other acute osteomyelitis, hand**

> **CC Excl: For CC codes in subcategory M86.14:**
> PDX collection 902

M86.141   **Other acute osteomyelitis, right hand** `CC` `HCC`

M86.142   **Other acute osteomyelitis, left hand** `CC` `HCC`

M86.149   **Other acute osteomyelitis, unspecified hand** `CC` `HCC`

☑6ᵗʰ   M86.15   **Other acute osteomyelitis, femur**

> **CC Excl: For CC codes in subcategory M86.15:**
> PDX collection 903

M86.151   **Other acute osteomyelitis, right femur** `CC` `HCC`

M86.152   **Other acute osteomyelitis, left femur** `CC` `HCC`

M86.159   **Other acute osteomyelitis, unspecified femur** `CC` `HCC`

☑6ᵗʰ   M86.16   **Other acute osteomyelitis, tibia and fibula**

> **CC Excl: For CC codes in subcategory M86.16:**
> PDX collection 904

M86.161   **Other acute osteomyelitis, right tibia and fibula** `CC` `HCC`

M86.162   **Other acute osteomyelitis, left tibia and fibula** `CC` `HCC`

M86.169   **Other acute osteomyelitis, unspecified tibia and fibula** `CC` `HCC`

☑6ᵗʰ   M86.17   **Other acute osteomyelitis, ankle and foot**

> **CC Excl: For CC codes in subcategory M86.17:**
> PDX collection 905

M86.171   **Other acute osteomyelitis, right ankle and foot** `CC` `HCC`

M86.172   **Other acute osteomyelitis, left ankle and foot** `CC` `HCC`

M86.179   **Other acute osteomyelitis, unspecified ankle and foot** `CC` `HCC`

M86.18   **Other acute osteomyelitis, other site** `CC` `HCC`
CC Excl: PDX collection 882

M86.19   **Other acute osteomyelitis, multiple sites** `CC` `HCC`
CC Excl: PDX collection 898

☑5ᵗʰ   M86.2   **Subacute osteomyelitis**

M86.20   **Subacute osteomyelitis, unspecified site** `CC` `HCC`
CC Excl: PDX collection 898

☑6ᵗʰ   M86.21   **Subacute osteomyelitis, shoulder**

> **CC Excl: For CC codes in subcategory M86.21:**
> PDX collection 899

M86.211   **Subacute osteomyelitis, right shoulder** `CC` `HCC`

M86.212   **Subacute osteomyelitis, left shoulder** `CC` `HCC`

M86.219   **Subacute osteomyelitis, unspecified shoulder** `CC` `HCC`

☑6ᵗʰ   M86.22   **Subacute osteomyelitis, humerus**

> **CC Excl: For CC codes in subcategory M86.22:**
> PDX collection 900

M86.221   **Subacute osteomyelitis, right humerus** `CC` `HCC`

M86.222   **Subacute osteomyelitis, left humerus** `CC` `HCC`

M86.229   **Subacute osteomyelitis, unspecified humerus** `CC` `HCC`

☑6ᵗʰ   M86.23   **Subacute osteomyelitis, radius and ulna**

> **CC Excl: For CC codes in subcategory M86.23:**
> PDX collection 901

M86.231   **Subacute osteomyelitis, right radius and ulna** `CC` `HCC`

M86.232   **Subacute osteomyelitis, left radius and ulna** `CC` `HCC`

M86.239   **Subacute osteomyelitis, unspecified radius and ulna** `CC` `HCC`

☑6ᵗʰ   M86.24   **Subacute osteomyelitis, hand**

> **CC Excl: For CC codes in subcategory M86.24:**
> PDX collection 902

M86.241   **Subacute osteomyelitis, right hand** `CC` `HCC`

M86.242   **Subacute osteomyelitis, left hand** `CC` `HCC`

M86.249   **Subacute osteomyelitis, unspecified hand** `CC` `HCC`

Ⓝ Newborn: 0   Ⓟ Pediatric: 0-17   Ⓜ Maternity: 12-55   Ⓐ Adult: 15-124   **MCC** Major CC Condition   **PDxMCC** PDx acts as own MCC   **CC** CC Condition   **PDxCC** PDx acts as own CC

**804**        ICD-10-CM 2018

√6ᵗʰ **M86.25** **Subacute osteomyelitis, femur**

> **CC Excl: For CC codes in subcategory M86.25:**
> PDX collection 903

     **M86.251** **Subacute osteomyelitis, right** `CC` `HCC`
                **femur**

     **M86.252** **Subacute osteomyelitis, left** `CC` `HCC`
                **femur**

     **M86.259** **Subacute osteomyelitis,** `CC` `HCC`
                **unspecified femur**

√6ᵗʰ **M86.26** **Subacute osteomyelitis, tibia and fibula**

> **CC Excl: For CC codes in subcategory M86.26:**
> PDX collection 904

     **M86.261** **Subacute osteomyelitis, right tibia** `CC` `HCC`
                **and fibula**

     **M86.262** **Subacute osteomyelitis, left tibia** `CC` `HCC`
                **and fibula**

     **M86.269** **Subacute osteomyelitis,** `CC` `HCC`
                **unspecified tibia and fibula**

√6ᵗʰ **M86.27** **Subacute osteomyelitis, ankle and foot**

> **CC Excl: For CC codes in subcategory M86.27:**
> PDX collection 905

     **M86.271** **Subacute osteomyelitis, right** `CC` `HCC`
                **ankle and foot**

     **M86.272** **Subacute osteomyelitis, left** `CC` `HCC`
                **ankle and foot**

     **M86.279** **Subacute osteomyelitis,** `CC` `HCC`
                **unspecified ankle and foot**

**M86.28** **Subacute osteomyelitis, other site** `CC` `HCC`
        **CC Excl:** PDX collection 882

**M86.29** **Subacute osteomyelitis, multiple sites** `CC` `HCC`
        **CC Excl:** PDX collection 898

√5ᵗʰ **M86.3** **Chronic multifocal osteomyelitis**

> **CC Excl: For CC codes in subcategory M86.3, unless**
> **otherwise noted:** PDX collection 881

**M86.30** **Chronic multifocal osteomyelitis,** `CC` `HCC`
**unspecified site**
        **CC Excl:** PDX collection 906

√6ᵗʰ **M86.31** **Chronic multifocal osteomyelitis, shoulder**

     **M86.311** **Chronic multifocal osteomyelitis,** `CC` `HCC`
                **right shoulder**

     **M86.312** **Chronic multifocal osteomyelitis,** `CC` `HCC`
                **left shoulder**

     **M86.319** **Chronic multifocal osteomyelitis,** `CC` `HCC`
                **unspecified shoulder**

√6ᵗʰ **M86.32** **Chronic multifocal osteomyelitis, humerus**

     **M86.321** **Chronic multifocal osteomyelitis,** `CC` `HCC`
                **right humerus**

     **M86.322** **Chronic multifocal osteomyelitis,** `CC` `HCC`
                **left humerus**

     **M86.329** **Chronic multifocal osteomyelitis,** `CC` `HCC`
                **unspecified humerus**

√6ᵗʰ **M86.33** **Chronic multifocal osteomyelitis, radius and ulna**

     **M86.331** **Chronic multifocal osteomyelitis,** `CC` `HCC`
                **right radius and ulna**

     **M86.332** **Chronic multifocal osteomyelitis,** `CC` `HCC`
                **left radius and ulna**

     **M86.339** **Chronic multifocal osteomyelitis,** `CC` `HCC`
                **unspecified radius and ulna**

√6ᵗʰ **M86.34** **Chronic multifocal osteomyelitis, hand**

     **M86.341** **Chronic multifocal osteomyelitis,** `CC` `HCC`
                **right hand**

     **M86.342** **Chronic multifocal osteomyelitis,** `CC` `HCC`
                **left hand**

     **M86.349** **Chronic multifocal osteomyelitis,** `CC` `HCC`
                **unspecified hand**

√6ᵗʰ **M86.35** **Chronic multifocal osteomyelitis, femur**

     **M86.351** **Chronic multifocal osteomyelitis,** `CC` `HCC`
                **right femur**

     **M86.352** **Chronic multifocal osteomyelitis,** `CC` `HCC`
                **left femur**

     **M86.359** **Chronic multifocal osteomyelitis,** `CC` `HCC`
                **unspecified femur**

√6ᵗʰ **M86.36** **Chronic multifocal osteomyelitis, tibia and fibula**

     **M86.361** **Chronic multifocal osteomyelitis,** `CC` `HCC`
                **right tibia and fibula**

     **M86.362** **Chronic multifocal osteomyelitis,** `CC` `HCC`
                **left tibia and fibula**

     **M86.369** **Chronic multifocal osteomyelitis,** `CC` `HCC`
                **unspecified tibia and fibula**

√6ᵗʰ **M86.37** **Chronic multifocal osteomyelitis, ankle and foot**

     **M86.371** **Chronic multifocal osteomyelitis,** `CC` `HCC`
                **right ankle and foot**

     **M86.372** **Chronic multifocal osteomyelitis,** `CC` `HCC`
                **left ankle and foot**

     **M86.379** **Chronic multifocal osteomyelitis,** `CC` `HCC`
                **unspecified ankle and foot**

**M86.38** **Chronic multifocal osteomyelitis, other site** `CC` `HCC`

**M86.39** **Chronic multifocal osteomyelitis, multiple** `CC` `HCC`
**sites**

√5ᵗʰ **M86.4** **Chronic osteomyelitis with draining sinus**

> **CC Excl: For CC codes in subcategory M86.4, unless**
> **otherwise noted:** PDX collection 881

**M86.40** **Chronic osteomyelitis with draining sinus,** `CC` `HCC`
**unspecified site**
        **CC Excl:** PDX collection 906

√6ᵗʰ **M86.41** **Chronic osteomyelitis with draining sinus, shoulder**

     **M86.411** **Chronic osteomyelitis with** `CC` `HCC`
                **draining sinus, right shoulder**

     **M86.412** **Chronic osteomyelitis with** `CC` `HCC`
                **draining sinus, left shoulder**

     **M86.419** **Chronic osteomyelitis with** `CC` `HCC`
                **draining sinus, unspecified shoulder**

√6ᵗʰ **M86.42** **Chronic osteomyelitis with draining sinus, humerus**

     **M86.421** **Chronic osteomyelitis with** `CC` `HCC`
                **draining sinus, right humerus**

     **M86.422** **Chronic osteomyelitis with** `CC` `HCC`
                **draining sinus, left humerus**

     **M86.429** **Chronic osteomyelitis with** `CC` `HCC`
                **draining sinus, unspecified humerus**

√6ᵗʰ **M86.43** **Chronic osteomyelitis with draining sinus, radius and ulna**

     **M86.431** **Chronic osteomyelitis with** `CC` `HCC`
                **draining sinus, right radius and ulna**

     **M86.432** **Chronic osteomyelitis with** `CC` `HCC`
                **draining sinus, left radius and ulna**

     **M86.439** **Chronic osteomyelitis with** `CC` `HCC`
                **draining sinus, unspecified radius and ulna**

√6ᵗʰ **M86.44** **Chronic osteomyelitis with draining sinus, hand**

     **M86.441** **Chronic osteomyelitis with** `CC` `HCC`
                **draining sinus, right hand**

     **M86.442** **Chronic osteomyelitis with** `CC` `HCC`
                **draining sinus, left hand**

     **M86.449** **Chronic osteomyelitis with** `CC` `HCC`
                **draining sinus, unspecified hand**

√6ᵗʰ **M86.45** **Chronic osteomyelitis with draining sinus, femur**

     **M86.451** **Chronic osteomyelitis with** `CC` `HCC`
                **draining sinus, right femur**

     **M86.452** **Chronic osteomyelitis with** `CC` `HCC`
                **draining sinus, left femur**

     **M86.459** **Chronic osteomyelitis with** `CC` `HCC`
                **draining sinus, unspecified femur**

√6ᵗʰ **M86.46** **Chronic osteomyelitis with draining sinus, tibia and fibula**

     **M86.461** **Chronic osteomyelitis with** `CC` `HCC`
                **draining sinus, right tibia and fibula**

     **M86.462** **Chronic osteomyelitis with** `CC` `HCC`
                **draining sinus, left tibia and fibula**

     **M86.469** **Chronic osteomyelitis with** `CC` `HCC`
                **draining sinus, unspecified tibia and fibula**

√6ᵗʰ **M86.47** **Chronic osteomyelitis with draining sinus, ankle and foot**

     **M86.471** **Chronic osteomyelitis with** `CC` `HCC`
                **draining sinus, right ankle and foot**

     **M86.472** **Chronic osteomyelitis with** `CC` `HCC`
                **draining sinus, left ankle and foot**

✓ Additional Character Req   √ₓ7ᵗʰ Placeholder Alert   Unacceptable PDx   Manifestation   **H1–H14** HAC   `HCC` CMS-HCC Condition   *EXCLUDES 1* Not Coded Here   *EXCLUDES 2* Not Included Here

ICD-10-CM 2018                          **805**

**M86.479** Chronic osteomyelitis with draining sinus, **unspecified** ankle and foot `CC` `HCC`

**M86.48** Chronic osteomyelitis with draining sinus, other site `CC` `HCC`

**M86.49** Chronic osteomyelitis with draining sinus, multiple sites `CC` `HCC`

✓5ᵗʰ **M86.5** Other chronic hematogenous **osteomyelitis**

> **CC Excl: For CC codes in subcategory M86.5, unless otherwise noted:** PDX collection 881

**M86.50** Other chronic hematogenous osteomyelitis, **unspecified site** `CC` `HCC`
> **CC Excl:** PDX collection 906

✓6ᵗʰ **M86.51** Other chronic hematogenous osteomyelitis, **shoulder**

    **M86.511** Other chronic hematogenous osteomyelitis, **right** shoulder `CC` `HCC`

    **M86.512** Other chronic hematogenous osteomyelitis, **left** shoulder `CC` `HCC`

    **M86.519** Other chronic hematogenous osteomyelitis, **unspecified** shoulder `CC` `HCC`

✓6ᵗʰ **M86.52** Other chronic hematogenous osteomyelitis, **humerus**

    **M86.521** Other chronic hematogenous osteomyelitis, **right** humerus `CC` `HCC`

    **M86.522** Other chronic hematogenous osteomyelitis, **left** humerus `CC` `HCC`

    **M86.529** Other chronic hematogenous osteomyelitis, **unspecified** humerus `CC` `HCC`

✓6ᵗʰ **M86.53** Other chronic hematogenous osteomyelitis, **radius and ulna**

    **M86.531** Other chronic hematogenous osteomyelitis, **right** radius and ulna `CC` `HCC`

    **M86.532** Other chronic hematogenous osteomyelitis, **left** radius and ulna `CC` `HCC`

    **M86.539** Other chronic hematogenous osteomyelitis, **unspecified** radius and ulna `CC` `HCC`

✓6ᵗʰ **M86.54** Other chronic hematogenous osteomyelitis, **hand**

    **M86.541** Other chronic hematogenous osteomyelitis, **right** hand `CC` `HCC`

    **M86.542** Other chronic hematogenous osteomyelitis, **left** hand `CC` `HCC`

    **M86.549** Other chronic hematogenous osteomyelitis, **unspecified** hand `CC` `HCC`

✓6ᵗʰ **M86.55** Other chronic hematogenous osteomyelitis, **femur**

    **M86.551** Other chronic hematogenous osteomyelitis, **right** femur `CC` `HCC`

    **M86.552** Other chronic hematogenous osteomyelitis, **left** femur `CC` `HCC`

    **M86.559** Other chronic hematogenous osteomyelitis, **unspecified** femur `CC` `HCC`

✓6ᵗʰ **M86.56** Other chronic hematogenous osteomyelitis, **tibia and fibula**

    **M86.561** Other chronic hematogenous osteomyelitis, **right** tibia and fibula `CC` `HCC`

    **M86.562** Other chronic hematogenous osteomyelitis, **left** tibia and fibula `CC` `HCC`

    **M86.569** Other chronic hematogenous osteomyelitis, **unspecified** tibia and fibula `CC` `HCC`

✓6ᵗʰ **M86.57** Other chronic hematogenous osteomyelitis, **ankle and foot**

    **M86.571** Other chronic hematogenous osteomyelitis, **right** ankle and foot `CC` `HCC`

    **M86.572** Other chronic hematogenous osteomyelitis, **left** ankle and foot `CC` `HCC`

    **M86.579** Other chronic hematogenous osteomyelitis, **unspecified** ankle and foot `CC` `HCC`

**M86.58** Other chronic hematogenous osteomyelitis, **other site** `CC` `HCC`

**M86.59** Other chronic hematogenous osteomyelitis, **multiple sites** `CC` `HCC`

✓5ᵗʰ **M86.6** Other chronic **osteomyelitis**

> **CC Excl: For CC codes in subcategory M86.6, unless otherwise noted:** PDX collection 881

**M86.60** Other chronic osteomyelitis, **unspecified site** `CC` `HCC`
> **CC Excl:** PDX collection 906

✓6ᵗʰ **M86.61** Other chronic osteomyelitis, **shoulder**

    **M86.611** Other chronic osteomyelitis, **right** shoulder `CC` `HCC`

    **M86.612** Other chronic osteomyelitis, **left** shoulder `CC` `HCC`

    **M86.619** Other chronic osteomyelitis, **unspecified** shoulder `CC` `HCC`

✓6ᵗʰ **M86.62** Other chronic osteomyelitis, **humerus**

    **M86.621** Other chronic osteomyelitis, **right** humerus `CC` `HCC`

    **M86.622** Other chronic osteomyelitis, **left** humerus `CC` `HCC`

    **M86.629** Other chronic osteomyelitis, **unspecified** humerus `CC` `HCC`

✓6ᵗʰ **M86.63** Other chronic osteomyelitis, **radius and ulna**

    **M86.631** Other chronic osteomyelitis, **right** radius and ulna `CC` `HCC`

    **M86.632** Other chronic osteomyelitis, **left** radius and ulna `CC` `HCC`

    **M86.639** Other chronic osteomyelitis, **unspecified** radius and ulna `CC` `HCC`

✓6ᵗʰ **M86.64** Other chronic osteomyelitis, **hand**

    **M86.641** Other chronic osteomyelitis, **right** hand `CC` `HCC`

    **M86.642** Other chronic osteomyelitis, **left** hand `CC` `HCC`

    **M86.649** Other chronic osteomyelitis, **unspecified** hand `CC` `HCC`

✓6ᵗʰ **M86.65** Other chronic osteomyelitis, **thigh**

    **M86.651** Other chronic osteomyelitis, **right** thigh `CC` `HCC`

    **M86.652** Other chronic osteomyelitis, **left** thigh `CC` `HCC`

    **M86.659** Other chronic osteomyelitis, **unspecified** thigh `CC` `HCC`

✓6ᵗʰ **M86.66** Other chronic osteomyelitis, **tibia and fibula**

    **M86.661** Other chronic osteomyelitis, **right** tibia and fibula `CC` `HCC`

    **M86.662** Other chronic osteomyelitis, **left** tibia and fibula `CC` `HCC`

    **M86.669** Other chronic osteomyelitis, **unspecified** tibia and fibula `CC` `HCC`

✓6ᵗʰ **M86.67** Other chronic osteomyelitis, **ankle and foot**

    **M86.671** Other chronic osteomyelitis, **right** ankle and foot `CC` `HCC`
> **AHA:** 2016, 1Q, 13

    **M86.672** Other chronic osteomyelitis, **left** ankle and foot `CC` `HCC`

    **M86.679** Other chronic osteomyelitis, **unspecified** ankle and foot `CC` `HCC`

**M86.68** Other chronic osteomyelitis, **other site** `CC` `HCC`

**M86.69** Other chronic osteomyelitis, **multiple sites** `CC` `HCC`

✓5ᵗʰ **M86.8** Other **osteomyelitis**
Brodie's abscess

> **CC Excl: For CC codes in subcategory M86.8, unless otherwise noted:** PDX collection 881

✓6ᵗʰ **M86.8X** Other **osteomyelitis**

    **M86.8X0** Other osteomyelitis, **multiple sites** `CC` `HCC`

    **M86.8X1** Other osteomyelitis, **shoulder** `CC` `HCC`

    **M86.8X2** Other osteomyelitis, **upper arm** `CC` `HCC`

    **M86.8X3** Other osteomyelitis, **forearm** `CC` `HCC`

    **M86.8X4** Other osteomyelitis, **hand** `CC` `HCC`

    **M86.8X5** Other osteomyelitis, **thigh** `CC` `HCC`

    **M86.8X6** Other osteomyelitis, **lower leg** `CC` `HCC`

    **M86.8X7** Other osteomyelitis, **ankle and foot** `CC` `HCC`

    **M86.8X8** Other osteomyelitis, **other site** `CC` `HCC`

    **M86.8X9** Other osteomyelitis, **unspecified sites** `CC` `HCC`
> **CC Excl:** PDX collection 906

**M86.9 Osteomyelitis, unspecified**
Infection of bone NOS
Periostitis without osteomyelitis
**CC Excl:** PDX collection 906

**✓4th M87 Osteonecrosis**
**INCLUDES**   avascular necrosis of bone
Use additional code to identify major osseous defect, if applicable
(M89.7-)
**EXCLUDES 1**   juvenile osteonecrosis (M91-M92)
            osteochondropathies (M90-M93)

**CC Excl: For CC codes in category M87, unless otherwise noted:** PDX collection 907

**✓5th M87.0 Idiopathic aseptic necrosis of bone**
     **M87.00 Idiopathic aseptic necrosis of unspecified** CC HCC
               **bone**
    **✓6th M87.01 Idiopathic aseptic necrosis of shoulder**
               Idiopathic aseptic necrosis of clavicle and scapula

**CC Excl: For CC codes in subcategory M87.01:**
PDX collection 908

       **M87.011 Idiopathic aseptic necrosis of right** CC HCC
                   **shoulder**
       **M87.012 Idiopathic aseptic necrosis of left** CC HCC
                   **shoulder**
       **M87.019 Idiopathic aseptic necrosis of** CC HCC
                   **unspecified shoulder**
    **✓6th M87.02 Idiopathic aseptic necrosis of humerus**

**CC Excl: For CC codes in subcategory M87.02:**
PDX collection 908

       **M87.021 Idiopathic aseptic necrosis of right** CC HCC
                   **humerus**
       **M87.022 Idiopathic aseptic necrosis of left** CC HCC
                   **humerus**
       **M87.029 Idiopathic aseptic necrosis of** CC HCC
                   **unspecified humerus**
    **✓6th M87.03 Idiopathic aseptic necrosis of radius, ulna and carpus**
       **M87.031 Idiopathic aseptic necrosis of right** CC HCC
                   **radius**
       **M87.032 Idiopathic aseptic necrosis of left** CC HCC
                   **radius**
       **M87.033 Idiopathic aseptic necrosis of** CC HCC
                   **unspecified radius**
       **M87.034 Idiopathic aseptic necrosis of** CC HCC
                   **right ulna**
       **M87.035 Idiopathic aseptic necrosis of** CC HCC
                   **left ulna**
       **M87.036 Idiopathic aseptic necrosis of** CC HCC
                   **unspecified ulna**
       **M87.037 Idiopathic aseptic necrosis of right** CC HCC
                   **carpus**
       **M87.038 Idiopathic aseptic necrosis of left** CC HCC
                   **carpus**
       **M87.039 Idiopathic aseptic necrosis of** CC HCC
                   **unspecified carpus**
    **✓6th M87.04 Idiopathic aseptic necrosis of hand and fingers**
               Idiopathic aseptic necrosis of metacarpals and
               phalanges of hands
       **M87.041 Idiopathic aseptic necrosis of right** CC HCC
                   **hand**
       **M87.042 Idiopathic aseptic necrosis of left** CC HCC
                   **hand**
       **M87.043 Idiopathic aseptic necrosis of** CC HCC
                   **unspecified hand**
       **M87.044 Idiopathic aseptic necrosis of right** CC HCC
                   **finger(s)**
       **M87.045 Idiopathic aseptic necrosis of left** CC HCC
                   **finger(s)**
       **M87.046 Idiopathic aseptic necrosis of** CC HCC
                   **unspecified finger(s)**
    **✓6th M87.05 Idiopathic aseptic necrosis of pelvis and femur**
       **M87.050 Idiopathic aseptic necrosis of** CC HCC
                   **pelvis**
       **M87.051 Idiopathic aseptic necrosis of** CC HCC
                   **right femur**
            **CC Excl:** PDX collection 909

**M87.052 Idiopathic aseptic necrosis of** CC HCC
            **left femur**
               **CC Excl:** PDX collection 909
**M87.059 Idiopathic aseptic necrosis of** CC HCC
            **unspecified femur**
               Idiopathic aseptic necrosis of hip NOS
               **CC Excl:** PDX collection 909
**✓6th M87.06 Idiopathic aseptic necrosis of tibia and fibula**
       **M87.061 Idiopathic aseptic necrosis of** CC HCC
            **right tibia**
       **M87.062 Idiopathic aseptic necrosis of** CC HCC
            **left tibia**
       **M87.063 Idiopathic aseptic necrosis of** CC HCC
            **unspecified tibia**
       **M87.064 Idiopathic aseptic necrosis of** CC HCC
            **right fibula**
       **M87.065 Idiopathic aseptic necrosis of** CC HCC
            **left fibula**
       **M87.066 Idiopathic aseptic necrosis of** CC HCC
            **unspecified fibula**
**✓6th M87.07 Idiopathic aseptic necrosis of ankle, foot and toes**
               Idiopathic aseptic necrosis of metatarsus, tarsus, and
               phalanges of toes
       **M87.071 Idiopathic aseptic necrosis of right** CC HCC
            **ankle**
       **M87.072 Idiopathic aseptic necrosis of left** CC HCC
            **ankle**
       **M87.073 Idiopathic aseptic necrosis of** CC HCC
            **unspecified ankle**
       **M87.074 Idiopathic aseptic necrosis of** CC HCC
            **right foot**
               **CC Excl:** PDX collection 910
       **M87.075 Idiopathic aseptic necrosis of** CC HCC
            **left foot**
               **CC Excl:** PDX collection 910
       **M87.076 Idiopathic aseptic necrosis of** CC HCC
            **unspecified foot**
               **CC Excl:** PDX collection 910
       **M87.077 Idiopathic aseptic necrosis of** CC HCC
            **right toe(s)**
       **M87.078 Idiopathic aseptic necrosis of** CC HCC
            **left toe(s)**
       **M87.079 Idiopathic aseptic necrosis of** CC HCC
            **unspecified toe(s)**
    **M87.08 Idiopathic aseptic necrosis of bone, other** CC HCC
           **site**
    **M87.09 Idiopathic aseptic necrosis of bone,** CC HCC
           **multiple sites**
**✓5th M87.1 Osteonecrosis due to drugs**
       Use additional code for adverse effect, if applicable, to identify
       drug (T36-T50 with fifth or sixth character 5)
    **M87.10 Osteonecrosis due to drugs, unspecified** CC HCC
           **bone**
    **✓6th M87.11 Osteonecrosis due to drugs, shoulder**
       **M87.111 Osteonecrosis due to drugs, right** CC HCC
            **shoulder**
       **M87.112 Osteonecrosis due to drugs, left** CC HCC
            **shoulder**
       **M87.119 Osteonecrosis due to drugs,** CC HCC
            **unspecified shoulder**
    **✓6th M87.12 Osteonecrosis due to drugs, humerus**

**CC Excl: For CC codes in subcategory M87.12:**
PDX collection 908

       **M87.121 Osteonecrosis due to drugs, right** CC HCC
            **humerus**
       **M87.122 Osteonecrosis due to drugs, left** CC HCC
            **humerus**
       **M87.129 Osteonecrosis due to drugs,** CC HCC
            **unspecified humerus**
    **✓6th M87.13 Osteonecrosis due to drugs of radius, ulna and**
           **carpus**
       **M87.131 Osteonecrosis due to drugs of right** CC HCC
            **radius**
       **M87.132 Osteonecrosis due to drugs of left** CC HCC
            **radius**
       **M87.133 Osteonecrosis due to drugs of** CC HCC
            **unspecified radius**

M87.134 **Osteonecrosis due to drugs of right ulna** `CC` `HCC`

M87.135 **Osteonecrosis due to drugs of left ulna** `CC` `HCC`

M87.136 **Osteonecrosis due to drugs of unspecified ulna** `CC` `HCC`

M87.137 **Osteonecrosis due to drugs of** right **carpus** `CC` `HCC`

M87.138 **Osteonecrosis due to drugs of** left **carpus** `CC` `HCC`

M87.139 **Osteonecrosis due to drugs of unspecified carpus** `CC` `HCC`

✓6ᵗʰ M87.14 **Osteonecrosis due to drugs, hand and fingers**

M87.141 **Osteonecrosis due to drugs, right hand** `CC` `HCC`

M87.142 **Osteonecrosis due to drugs,** left **hand** `CC` `HCC`

M87.143 **Osteonecrosis due to drugs, unspecified hand** `CC` `HCC`

M87.144 **Osteonecrosis due to drugs, right finger(s)** `CC` `HCC`

M87.145 **Osteonecrosis due to drugs,** left **finger(s)** `CC` `HCC`

M87.146 **Osteonecrosis due to drugs, unspecified finger(s)** `CC` `HCC`

✓6ᵗʰ M87.15 **Osteonecrosis due to drugs, pelvis and femur**

> **CC Excl: For CC codes in subcategory M87.15:** PDX collection 909

M87.150 **Osteonecrosis due to drugs, pelvis** `CC` `HCC`

M87.151 **Osteonecrosis due to drugs, right femur** `CC` `HCC`

M87.152 **Osteonecrosis due to drugs,** left **femur** `CC` `HCC`

M87.159 **Osteonecrosis due to drugs, unspecified femur** `CC` `HCC`

✓6ᵗʰ M87.16 **Osteonecrosis due to drugs, tibia and fibula**

M87.161 **Osteonecrosis due to drugs, right tibia** `CC` `HCC`

M87.162 **Osteonecrosis due to drugs, left tibia** `CC` `HCC`

M87.163 **Osteonecrosis due to drugs, unspecified tibia** `CC` `HCC`

M87.164 **Osteonecrosis due to drugs, right fibula** `CC` `HCC`

M87.165 **Osteonecrosis due to drugs, left fibula** `CC` `HCC`

M87.166 **Osteonecrosis due to drugs, unspecified fibula** `CC` `HCC`

✓6ᵗʰ M87.17 **Osteonecrosis due to drugs, ankle, foot and toes**

M87.171 **Osteonecrosis due to drugs, right ankle** `CC` `HCC`

M87.172 **Osteonecrosis due to drugs, left ankle** `CC` `HCC`

M87.173 **Osteonecrosis due to drugs, unspecified ankle** `CC` `HCC`

M87.174 **Osteonecrosis due to drugs, right foot** `CC` `HCC`
> **CC Excl:** PDX collection 910

M87.175 **Osteonecrosis due to drugs, left foot** `CC` `HCC`
> **CC Excl:** PDX collection 910

M87.176 **Osteonecrosis due to drugs, unspecified foot** `CC` `HCC`
> **CC Excl:** PDX collection 910

M87.177 **Osteonecrosis due to drugs, right toe(s)** `CC` `HCC`

M87.178 **Osteonecrosis due to drugs, left toe(s)** `CC` `HCC`

M87.179 **Osteonecrosis due to drugs, unspecified toe(s)** `CC` `HCC`

✓6ᵗʰ M87.18 **Osteonecrosis due to drugs, other site**

M87.180 **Osteonecrosis due to drugs, jaw** `CC` `HCC`

M87.188 **Osteonecrosis due to drugs, other site** `CC` `HCC`

M87.19 **Osteonecrosis due to drugs, multiple sites** `CC` `HCC`

✓5ᵗʰ M87.2 **Osteonecrosis** due to previous trauma

M87.20 **Osteonecrosis due to previous trauma, unspecified bone** `CC` `HCC`

✓6ᵗʰ M87.21 **Osteonecrosis due to previous trauma, shoulder**

M87.211 **Osteonecrosis due to previous trauma, right shoulder** `CC` `HCC`

M87.212 **Osteonecrosis due to previous trauma, left shoulder** `CC` `HCC`

M87.219 **Osteonecrosis due to previous trauma, unspecified shoulder** `CC` `HCC`

✓6ᵗʰ M87.22 **Osteonecrosis due to previous trauma, humerus**

> **CC Excl: For CC codes in subcategory M87.22:** PDX collection 908

M87.221 **Osteonecrosis due to previous trauma, right humerus** `CC` `HCC`

M87.222 **Osteonecrosis due to previous trauma, left humerus** `CC` `HCC`

M87.229 **Osteonecrosis due to previous trauma, unspecified humerus** `CC` `HCC`

✓6ᵗʰ M87.23 **Osteonecrosis due to previous trauma of radius, ulna and carpus**

M87.231 **Osteonecrosis due to previous trauma of right radius** `CC` `HCC`

M87.232 **Osteonecrosis due to previous trauma of left radius** `CC` `HCC`

M87.233 **Osteonecrosis due to previous trauma of unspecified radius** `CC` `HCC`

M87.234 **Osteonecrosis due to previous trauma of right ulna** `CC` `HCC`

M87.235 **Osteonecrosis due to previous trauma of left ulna** `CC` `HCC`

M87.236 **Osteonecrosis due to previous trauma of unspecified ulna** `CC` `HCC`

M87.237 **Osteonecrosis due to previous trauma of right carpus** `CC` `HCC`

M87.238 **Osteonecrosis due to previous trauma of left carpus** `CC` `HCC`

M87.239 **Osteonecrosis due to previous trauma of unspecified carpus** `CC` `HCC`

✓6ᵗʰ M87.24 **Osteonecrosis due to previous trauma, hand and fingers**

M87.241 **Osteonecrosis due to previous trauma, right hand** `CC` `HCC`

M87.242 **Osteonecrosis due to previous trauma, left hand** `CC` `HCC`

M87.243 **Osteonecrosis due to previous trauma, unspecified hand** `CC` `HCC`

M87.244 **Osteonecrosis due to previous trauma, right finger(s)** `CC` `HCC`

M87.245 **Osteonecrosis due to previous trauma, left finger(s)** `CC` `HCC`

M87.246 **Osteonecrosis due to previous trauma, unspecified finger(s)** `CC` `HCC`

✓6ᵗʰ M87.25 **Osteonecrosis due to previous trauma, pelvis and femur**

M87.250 **Osteonecrosis due to previous trauma, pelvis** `CC` `HCC`

M87.251 **Osteonecrosis due to previous trauma, right femur** `CC` `HCC`
> **CC Excl:** PDX collection 909

M87.252 **Osteonecrosis due to previous trauma, left femur** `CC` `HCC`
> **CC Excl:** PDX collection 909

M87.256 **Osteonecrosis due to previous trauma, unspecified femur** `CC` `HCC`
> **CC Excl:** PDX collection 909

✓6ᵗʰ M87.26 **Osteonecrosis due to previous trauma, tibia and fibula**

M87.261 **Osteonecrosis due to previous trauma, right tibia** `CC` `HCC`

M87.262 **Osteonecrosis due to previous trauma, left tibia** `CC` `HCC`

M87.263 **Osteonecrosis due to previous trauma, unspecified tibia** `CC` `HCC`

M87.264 **Osteonecrosis due to previous trauma, right fibula** `CC` `HCC`

M87.265 **Osteonecrosis due to previous trauma, left fibula** `CC` `HCC`

---

`N` Newborn: 0    `P` Pediatric: 0-17    `M` Maternity: 12-55    `A` Adult: 15-124    `MCC` Major CC Condition    `PDxMCC` PDx acts as own MCC    `CC` CC Condition    `PDxCC` PDx acts as own CC

M87.266 **Osteonecrosis due to previous** `CC` `HCC`
**trauma, unspecified fibula**

✓6ᵗʰ M87.27 **Osteonecrosis due to previous trauma, ankle, foot and toes**

　　M87.271 **Osteonecrosis due to previous** `CC` `HCC`
**trauma, right ankle**

　　M87.272 **Osteonecrosis due to previous** `CC` `HCC`
**trauma, left ankle**

　　M87.273 **Osteonecrosis due to previous** `CC` `HCC`
**trauma, unspecified ankle**

　　M87.274 **Osteonecrosis due to previous** `CC` `HCC`
**trauma, right foot**
　　　　**CC Excl:** PDX collection 91Ø

　　M87.275 **Osteonecrosis due to previous** `CC` `HCC`
**trauma, left foot**
　　　　**CC Excl:** PDX collection 91Ø

　　M87.276 **Osteonecrosis due to previous** `CC` `HCC`
**trauma, unspecified foot**
　　　　**CC Excl:** PDX collection 91Ø

　　M87.277 **Osteonecrosis due to previous** `CC` `HCC`
**trauma, right toe(s)**

　　M87.278 **Osteonecrosis due to previous** `CC` `HCC`
**trauma, left toe(s)**

　　M87.279 **Osteonecrosis due to previous** `CC` `HCC`
**trauma, unspecified toe(s)**

M87.28 **Osteonecrosis due to previous trauma,** `CC` `HCC`
**other site**

M87.29 **Osteonecrosis due to previous trauma,** `CC` `HCC`
**multiple sites**

✓5ᵗʰ M87.3 **Other secondary osteonecrosis**

M87.30 **Other secondary osteonecrosis,** `CC` `HCC`
**unspecified bone**

✓6ᵗʰ M87.31 **Other secondary osteonecrosis, shoulder**

　　M87.311 **Other secondary osteonecrosis,** `CC` `HCC`
**right shoulder**

　　M87.312 **Other secondary osteonecrosis,** `CC` `HCC`
**left shoulder**

　　M87.319 **Other secondary osteonecrosis,** `CC` `HCC`
**unspecified shoulder**

✓6ᵗʰ M87.32 **Other secondary osteonecrosis, humerus**

> **CC Excl: For CC codes in subcategory M87.32:** PDX collection 9Ø8

　　M87.321 **Other secondary osteonecrosis,** `CC` `HCC`
**right humerus**

　　M87.322 **Other secondary osteonecrosis,** `CC` `HCC`
**left humerus**

　　M87.329 **Other secondary osteonecrosis,** `CC` `HCC`
**unspecified humerus**

✓6ᵗʰ M87.33 **Other secondary osteonecrosis of radius, ulna and carpus**

　　M87.331 **Other secondary osteonecrosis** `CC` `HCC`
**of right radius**

　　M87.332 **Other secondary osteonecrosis** `CC` `HCC`
**of left radius**

　　M87.333 **Other secondary osteonecrosis** `CC` `HCC`
**of unspecified radius**

　　M87.334 **Other secondary osteonecrosis** `CC` `HCC`
**of right ulna**

　　M87.335 **Other secondary osteonecrosis** `CC` `HCC`
**of left ulna**

　　M87.336 **Other secondary osteonecrosis** `CC` `HCC`
**of unspecified ulna**

　　M87.337 **Other secondary osteonecrosis** `CC` `HCC`
**of right carpus**

　　M87.338 **Other secondary osteonecrosis** `CC` `HCC`
**of left carpus**

　　M87.339 **Other secondary osteonecrosis** `CC` `HCC`
**of unspecified carpus**

✓6ᵗʰ M87.34 **Other secondary osteonecrosis, hand and fingers**

　　M87.341 **Other secondary osteonecrosis,** `CC` `HCC`
**right hand**

　　M87.342 **Other secondary osteonecrosis,** `CC` `HCC`
**left hand**

　　M87.343 **Other secondary osteonecrosis,** `CC` `HCC`
**unspecified hand**

　　M87.344 **Other secondary osteonecrosis,** `CC` `HCC`
**right finger(s)**

　　M87.345 **Other secondary osteonecrosis,** `CC` `HCC`
**left finger(s)**

　　M87.346 **Other secondary osteonecrosis,** `CC` `HCC`
**unspecified finger(s)**

✓6ᵗʰ M87.35 **Other secondary osteonecrosis, pelvis and femur**

> **CC Excl: For CC codes in subcategory M87.35:** PDX collection 9Ø9

　　M87.35Ø **Other secondary osteonecrosis,** `CC` `HCC`
**pelvis**

　　M87.351 **Other secondary osteonecrosis,** `CC` `HCC`
**right femur**

　　M87.352 **Other secondary osteonecrosis,** `CC` `HCC`
**left femur**

　　M87.353 **Other secondary osteonecrosis,** `CC` `HCC`
**unspecified femur**

✓6ᵗʰ M87.36 **Other secondary osteonecrosis, tibia and fibula**

　　M87.361 **Other secondary osteonecrosis,** `CC` `HCC`
**right tibia**

　　M87.362 **Other secondary osteonecrosis,** `CC` `HCC`
**left tibia**

　　M87.363 **Other secondary osteonecrosis,** `CC` `HCC`
**unspecified tibia**

　　M87.364 **Other secondary osteonecrosis,** `CC` `HCC`
**right fibula**

　　M87.365 **Other secondary osteonecrosis,** `CC` `HCC`
**left fibula**

　　M87.366 **Other secondary osteonecrosis,** `CC` `HCC`
**unspecified fibula**

✓6ᵗʰ M87.37 **Other secondary osteonecrosis, ankle and foot**

　　M87.371 **Other secondary osteonecrosis,** `CC` `HCC`
**right ankle**

　　M87.372 **Other secondary osteonecrosis,** `CC` `HCC`
**left ankle**

　　M87.373 **Other secondary osteonecrosis,** `CC` `HCC`
**unspecified ankle**

　　M87.374 **Other secondary osteonecrosis,** `CC` `HCC`
**right foot**
　　　　**CC Excl:** PDX collection 91Ø

　　M87.375 **Other secondary osteonecrosis,** `CC` `HCC`
**left foot**
　　　　**CC Excl:** PDX collection 91Ø

　　M87.376 **Other secondary osteonecrosis,** `CC` `HCC`
**unspecified foot**
　　　　**CC Excl:** PDX collection 91Ø

　　M87.377 **Other secondary osteonecrosis,** `CC` `HCC`
**right toe(s)**

　　M87.378 **Other secondary osteonecrosis,** `CC` `HCC`
**left toe(s)**

　　M87.379 **Other secondary osteonecrosis,** `CC` `HCC`
**unspecified toe(s)**

M87.38 **Other secondary osteonecrosis, other site** `CC` `HCC`

M87.39 **Other secondary osteonecrosis, multiple** `CC` `HCC`
**sites**

✓5ᵗʰ M87.8 **Other osteonecrosis**

M87.8Ø **Other osteonecrosis, unspecified bone** `CC` `HCC`

✓6ᵗʰ M87.81 **Other osteonecrosis, shoulder**

　　M87.811 **Other osteonecrosis, right** `CC` `HCC`
**shoulder**

　　M87.812 **Other osteonecrosis, left** `CC` `HCC`
**shoulder**

　　M87.819 **Other osteonecrosis, unspecified** `CC` `HCC`
**shoulder**

✓6ᵗʰ M87.82 **Other osteonecrosis, humerus**

> **CC Excl: For CC codes in subcategory M87.82:** PDX collection 9Ø8

　　M87.821 **Other osteonecrosis, right** `CC` `HCC`
**humerus**

　　M87.822 **Other osteonecrosis, left** `CC` `HCC`
**humerus**

　　M87.829 **Other osteonecrosis, unspecified** `CC` `HCC`
**humerus**

✓6ᵗʰ M87.83 **Other osteonecrosis of radius, ulna and carpus**

　　M87.831 **Other osteonecrosis of right radius** `CC` `HCC`

　　M87.832 **Other osteonecrosis of left radius** `CC` `HCC`

　　M87.833 **Other osteonecrosis of unspecified** `CC` `HCC`
**radius**

✓ Additional Character Req　✓7ᵗʰ Placeholder Alert　Unacceptable PDx　Manifestation　H1-H14 HAC　HCC CMS-HCC Condition　EXCLUDES1 Not Coded Here　EXCLUDES2 Not Included Here

ICD-10-CM 2018　　809

M87.834   Other osteonecrosis of right ulna   `CC` `HCC`
M87.835   Other osteonecrosis of left ulna   `CC` `HCC`
M87.836   Other osteonecrosis of unspecified ulna   `CC` `HCC`
M87.837   Other osteonecrosis of right carpus   `CC` `HCC`
M87.838   Other osteonecrosis of left carpus   `CC` `HCC`
M87.839   Other osteonecrosis of unspecified carpus   `CC` `HCC`

✓6th **M87.84 Other osteonecrosis, hand and fingers**
M87.841   Other osteonecrosis, right hand   `CC` `HCC`
M87.842   Other osteonecrosis, left hand   `CC` `HCC`
M87.843   Other osteonecrosis, unspecified hand   `CC` `HCC`
M87.844   Other osteonecrosis, right finger(s)   `CC` `HCC`
M87.845   Other osteonecrosis, left finger(s)   `CC` `HCC`
M87.849   Other osteonecrosis, unspecified finger(s)   `CC` `HCC`

✓6th **M87.85 Other osteonecrosis, pelvis and femur**

> **CC Excl:** For CC codes in subcategory M87.85: PDX collection 909

M87.850   Other osteonecrosis, pelvis   `CC` `HCC`
M87.851   Other osteonecrosis, right femur   `CC` `HCC`
M87.852   Other osteonecrosis, left femur   `CC` `HCC`
M87.859   Other osteonecrosis, unspecified femur   `CC` `HCC`

✓6th **M87.86 Other osteonecrosis, tibia and fibula**
M87.861   Other osteonecrosis, right tibia   `CC` `HCC`
M87.862   Other osteonecrosis, left tibia   `CC` `HCC`
M87.863   Other osteonecrosis, unspecified tibia   `CC` `HCC`
M87.864   Other osteonecrosis, right fibula   `CC` `HCC`
M87.865   Other osteonecrosis, left fibula   `CC` `HCC`
M87.869   Other osteonecrosis, unspecified fibula   `CC` `HCC`

✓6th **M87.87 Other osteonecrosis, ankle, foot and toes**
M87.871   Other osteonecrosis, right ankle   `CC` `HCC`
M87.872   Other osteonecrosis, left ankle   `CC` `HCC`
M87.873   Other osteonecrosis, unspecified ankle   `CC` `HCC`
M87.874   Other osteonecrosis, right foot   `CC` `HCC`
     **CC Excl:** PDX collection 910
M87.875   Other osteonecrosis, left foot   `CC` `HCC`
     **CC Excl:** PDX collection 910
M87.876   Other osteonecrosis, unspecified foot   `CC` `HCC`
     **CC Excl:** PDX collection 910
M87.877   Other osteonecrosis, right toe(s)   `CC` `HCC`
M87.878   Other osteonecrosis, left toe(s)   `CC` `HCC`
M87.879   Other osteonecrosis, unspecified toe(s)   `CC` `HCC`

M87.88   Other osteonecrosis, other site   `CC` `HCC`
M87.89   Other osteonecrosis, multiple sites   `CC` `HCC`

**M87.9 Osteonecrosis, unspecified**   `CC` `HCC`
     Necrosis of bone NOS

✓4th **M88 Osteitis deformans [Paget's disease of bone]**
     **EXCLUDES 1**   osteitis deformans in neoplastic disease (M90.6)

**M88.0 Osteitis deformans of skull**

**M88.1 Osteitis deformans of vertebrae**

✓5th **M88.8 Osteitis deformans of other bones**

✓6th **M88.81 Osteitis deformans of shoulder**
M88.811   Osteitis deformans of right shoulder
M88.812   Osteitis deformans of left shoulder
M88.819   Osteitis deformans of unspecified shoulder

✓6th **M88.82 Osteitis deformans of upper arm**
M88.821   Osteitis deformans of right upper arm
M88.822   Osteitis deformans of left upper arm
M88.829   Osteitis deformans of unspecified upper arm

✓6th **M88.83 Osteitis deformans of forearm**
M88.831   Osteitis deformans of right forearm
M88.832   Osteitis deformans of left forearm
M88.839   Osteitis deformans of unspecified forearm

✓6th **M88.84 Osteitis deformans of hand**
M88.841   Osteitis deformans of right hand
M88.842   Osteitis deformans of left hand
M88.849   Osteitis deformans of unspecified hand

✓6th **M88.85 Osteitis deformans of thigh**
M88.851   Osteitis deformans of right thigh
M88.852   Osteitis deformans of left thigh
M88.859   Osteitis deformans of unspecified thigh

✓6th **M88.86 Osteitis deformans of lower leg**
M88.861   Osteitis deformans of right lower leg
M88.862   Osteitis deformans of left lower leg
M88.869   Osteitis deformans of unspecified lower leg

✓6th **M88.87 Osteitis deformans of ankle and foot**
M88.871   Osteitis deformans of right ankle and foot
M88.872   Osteitis deformans of left ankle and foot
M88.879   Osteitis deformans of unspecified ankle and foot

M88.88   Osteitis deformans of other bones
     **EXCLUDES 2**   osteitis deformans of skull (M88.0)
         osteitis deformans of vertebrae (M88.1)

M88.89   Osteitis deformans of multiple sites

**M88.9 Osteitis deformans of unspecified bone**

✓4th **M89 Other disorders of bone**

✓5th **M89.0 Algoneurodystrophy**
     Shoulder-hand syndrome
     Sudeck's atrophy
     **EXCLUDES 1**   causalgia, lower limb (G57.7-)
         causalgia, upper limb (G56.4-)
         complex regional pain syndrome II, lower limb (G57.7-)
         complex regional pain syndrome II, upper limb (G56.4-)
         reflex sympathetic dystrophy (G90.5-)

M89.00   Algoneurodystrophy, unspecified site

✓6th **M89.01 Algoneurodystrophy, shoulder**
M89.011   Algoneurodystrophy, right shoulder
M89.012   Algoneurodystrophy, left shoulder
M89.019   Algoneurodystrophy, unspecified shoulder

✓6th **M89.02 Algoneurodystrophy, upper arm**
M89.021   Algoneurodystrophy, right upper arm
M89.022   Algoneurodystrophy, left upper arm
M89.029   Algoneurodystrophy, unspecified upper arm

✓6th **M89.03 Algoneurodystrophy, forearm**
M89.031   Algoneurodystrophy, right forearm
M89.032   Algoneurodystrophy, left forearm
M89.039   Algoneurodystrophy, unspecified forearm

✓6th **M89.04 Algoneurodystrophy, hand**
M89.041   Algoneurodystrophy, right hand
M89.042   Algoneurodystrophy, left hand
M89.049   Algoneurodystrophy, unspecified hand

✓6th **M89.05 Algoneurodystrophy, thigh**
M89.051   Algoneurodystrophy, right thigh
M89.052   Algoneurodystrophy, left thigh
M89.059   Algoneurodystrophy, unspecified thigh

✓6th **M89.06 Algoneurodystrophy, lower leg**
M89.061   Algoneurodystrophy, right lower leg
M89.062   Algoneurodystrophy, left lower leg
M89.069   Algoneurodystrophy, unspecified lower leg

✓6th **M89.07 Algoneurodystrophy, ankle and foot**
M89.071   Algoneurodystrophy, right ankle and foot
M89.072   Algoneurodystrophy, left ankle and foot
M89.079   Algoneurodystrophy, unspecified ankle and foot

M89.08   Algoneurodystrophy, other site
M89.09   Algoneurodystrophy, multiple sites

`N` Newborn: 0   `P` Pediatric: 0-17   `M` Maternity: 12-55   `A` Adult: 15-124   `MCC` Major CC Condition   `PDxMCC` PDx acts as own MCC   `CC` CC Condition   `PDxCC` PDx acts as own CC

810      ICD-10-CM 2018

✓5ᵗʰ **M89.1 Physeal arrest**
Arrest of growth plate
Epiphyseal arrest
Growth plate arrest

✓6ᵗʰ **M89.12 Physeal arrest, humerus**
- **M89.121 Complete physeal arrest, right proximal humerus**
- **M89.122 Complete physeal arrest, left proximal humerus**
- **M89.123 Partial physeal arrest, right proximal humerus**
- **M89.124 Partial physeal arrest, left proximal humerus**
- **M89.125 Complete physeal arrest, right distal humerus**
- **M89.126 Complete physeal arrest, left distal humerus**
- **M89.127 Partial physeal arrest, right distal humerus**
- **M89.128 Partial physeal arrest, left distal humerus**
- **M89.129 Physeal arrest, humerus, unspecified**

✓6ᵗʰ **M89.13 Physeal arrest, forearm**
- **M89.131 Complete physeal arrest, right distal radius**
- **M89.132 Complete physeal arrest, left distal radius**
- **M89.133 Partial physeal arrest, right distal radius**
- **M89.134 Partial physeal arrest, left distal radius**
- **M89.138 Other physeal arrest of forearm**
- **M89.139 Physeal arrest, forearm, unspecified**

✓6ᵗʰ **M89.15 Physeal arrest, femur**
- **M89.151 Complete physeal arrest, right proximal femur**
- **M89.152 Complete physeal arrest, left proximal femur**
- **M89.153 Partial physeal arrest, right proximal femur**
- **M89.154 Partial physeal arrest, left proximal femur**
- **M89.155 Complete physeal arrest, right distal femur**
- **M89.156 Complete physeal arrest, left distal femur**
- **M89.157 Partial physeal arrest, right distal femur**
- **M89.158 Partial physeal arrest, left distal femur**
- **M89.159 Physeal arrest, femur, unspecified**

✓6ᵗʰ **M89.16 Physeal arrest, lower leg**
- **M89.160 Complete physeal arrest, right proximal tibia**
- **M89.161 Complete physeal arrest, left proximal tibia**
- **M89.162 Partial physeal arrest, right proximal tibia**
- **M89.163 Partial physeal arrest, left proximal tibia**
- **M89.164 Complete physeal arrest, right distal tibia**
- **M89.165 Complete physeal arrest, left distal tibia**
- **M89.166 Partial physeal arrest, right distal tibia**
- **M89.167 Partial physeal arrest, left distal tibia**
- **M89.168 Other physeal arrest of lower leg**
- **M89.169 Physeal arrest, lower leg, unspecified**

**M89.18 Physeal arrest, other site**

✓5ᵗʰ **M89.2 Other disorders of bone development and growth**
**M89.20 Other disorders of bone development and growth, unspecified site**

✓6ᵗʰ **M89.21 Other disorders of bone development and growth, shoulder**
- **M89.211 Other disorders of bone development and growth, right shoulder**
- **M89.212 Other disorders of bone development and growth, left shoulder**
- **M89.219 Other disorders of bone development and growth, unspecified shoulder**

✓6ᵗʰ **M89.22 Other disorders of bone development and growth, humerus**
- **M89.221 Other disorders of bone development and growth, right humerus**
- **M89.222 Other disorders of bone development and growth, left humerus**
- **M89.229 Other disorders of bone development and growth, unspecified humerus**

✓6ᵗʰ **M89.23 Other disorders of bone development and growth, ulna and radius**
- **M89.231 Other disorders of bone development and growth, right ulna**
- **M89.232 Other disorders of bone development and growth, left ulna**
- **M89.233 Other disorders of bone development and growth, right radius**
- **M89.234 Other disorders of bone development and growth, left radius**
- **M89.239 Other disorders of bone development and growth, unspecified ulna and radius**

✓6ᵗʰ **M89.24 Other disorders of bone development and growth, hand**
- **M89.241 Other disorders of bone development and growth, right hand**
- **M89.242 Other disorders of bone development and growth, left hand**
- **M89.249 Other disorders of bone development and growth, unspecified hand**

✓6ᵗʰ **M89.25 Other disorders of bone development and growth, femur**
- **M89.251 Other disorders of bone development and growth, right femur**
- **M89.252 Other disorders of bone development and growth, left femur**
- **M89.259 Other disorders of bone development and growth, unspecified femur**

✓6ᵗʰ **M89.26 Other disorders of bone development and growth, tibia and fibula**
- **M89.261 Other disorders of bone development and growth, right tibia**
- **M89.262 Other disorders of bone development and growth, left tibia**
- **M89.263 Other disorders of bone development and growth, right fibula**
- **M89.264 Other disorders of bone development and growth, left fibula**
- **M89.269 Other disorders of bone development and growth, unspecified lower leg**

✓6ᵗʰ **M89.27 Other disorders of bone development and growth, ankle and foot**
- **M89.271 Other disorders of bone development and growth, right ankle and foot**
- **M89.272 Other disorders of bone development and growth, left ankle and foot**
- **M89.279 Other disorders of bone development and growth, unspecified ankle and foot**

**M89.28 Other disorders of bone development and growth, other site**

**M89.29 Other disorders of bone development and growth, multiple sites**

✓5ᵗʰ **M89.3 Hypertrophy of bone**
**M89.30 Hypertrophy of bone, unspecified site**

✓6ᵗʰ **M89.31 Hypertrophy of bone, shoulder**
- **M89.311 Hypertrophy of bone, right shoulder**
- **M89.312 Hypertrophy of bone, left shoulder**
- **M89.319 Hypertrophy of bone, unspecified shoulder**

✓6ᵗʰ **M89.32 Hypertrophy of bone, humerus**
- **M89.321 Hypertrophy of bone, right humerus**
- **M89.322 Hypertrophy of bone, left humerus**
- **M89.329 Hypertrophy of bone, unspecified humerus**

✓6ᵗʰ **M89.33 Hypertrophy of bone, ulna and radius**
- **M89.331 Hypertrophy of bone, right ulna**
- **M89.332 Hypertrophy of bone, left ulna**
- **M89.333 Hypertrophy of bone, right radius**
- **M89.334 Hypertrophy of bone, left radius**
- **M89.339 Hypertrophy of bone, unspecified ulna and radius**

✓6ᵗʰ **M89.34 Hypertrophy of bone, hand**
- **M89.341 Hypertrophy of bone, right hand**
- **M89.342 Hypertrophy of bone, left hand**
- **M89.349 Hypertrophy of bone, unspecified hand**

---

✓ Additional Character Req  ✓x7ᵗʰ Placeholder Alert  Unacceptable PDx  Manifestation  **H1**-**H14** HAC  **HCC** CMS-HCC Condition  *EXCLUDES 1* Not Coded Here  *EXCLUDES 2* Not Included Here

✓6ᵗʰ **M89.35  Hypertrophy of bone, femur**
    **M89.351  Hypertrophy of bone, right femur**
    **M89.352  Hypertrophy of bone, left femur**
    **M89.359  Hypertrophy of bone, unspecified femur**

✓6ᵗʰ **M89.36  Hypertrophy of bone, tibia and fibula**
    **M89.361  Hypertrophy of bone, right tibia**
    **M89.362  Hypertrophy of bone, left tibia**
    **M89.363  Hypertrophy of bone, right fibula**
    **M89.364  Hypertrophy of bone, left fibula**
    **M89.369  Hypertrophy of bone, unspecified tibia and fibula**

✓6ᵗʰ **M89.37  Hypertrophy of bone, ankle and foot**
    **M89.371  Hypertrophy of bone, right ankle and foot**
    **M89.372  Hypertrophy of bone, left ankle and foot**
    **M89.379  Hypertrophy of bone, unspecified ankle and foot**

    **M89.38  Hypertrophy of bone, other site**
    **M89.39  Hypertrophy of bone, multiple sites**

✓5ᵗʰ **M89.4  Other hypertrophic osteoarthropathy**
    Marie-Bamberger disease
    Pachydermoperiostosis
    **M89.40  Other hypertrophic osteoarthropathy, unspecified site**

✓6ᵗʰ **M89.41  Other hypertrophic osteoarthropathy, shoulder**
    **M89.411  Other hypertrophic osteoarthropathy, right shoulder**
    **M89.412  Other hypertrophic osteoarthropathy, left shoulder**
    **M89.419  Other hypertrophic osteoarthropathy, unspecified shoulder**

✓6ᵗʰ **M89.42  Other hypertrophic osteoarthropathy, upper arm**
    **M89.421  Other hypertrophic osteoarthropathy, right upper arm**
    **M89.422  Other hypertrophic osteoarthropathy, left upper arm**
    **M89.429  Other hypertrophic osteoarthropathy, unspecified upper arm**

✓6ᵗʰ **M89.43  Other hypertrophic osteoarthropathy, forearm**
    **M89.431  Other hypertrophic osteoarthropathy, right forearm**
    **M89.432  Other hypertrophic osteoarthropathy, left forearm**
    **M89.439  Other hypertrophic osteoarthropathy, unspecified forearm**

✓6ᵗʰ **M89.44  Other hypertrophic osteoarthropathy, hand**
    **M89.441  Other hypertrophic osteoarthropathy, right hand**
    **M89.442  Other hypertrophic osteoarthropathy, left hand**
    **M89.449  Other hypertrophic osteoarthropathy, unspecified hand**

✓6ᵗʰ **M89.45  Other hypertrophic osteoarthropathy, thigh**
    **M89.451  Other hypertrophic osteoarthropathy, right thigh**
    **M89.452  Other hypertrophic osteoarthropathy, left thigh**
    **M89.459  Other hypertrophic osteoarthropathy, unspecified thigh**

✓6ᵗʰ **M89.46  Other hypertrophic osteoarthropathy, lower leg**
    **M89.461  Other hypertrophic osteoarthropathy, right lower leg**
    **M89.462  Other hypertrophic osteoarthropathy, left lower leg**
    **M89.469  Other hypertrophic osteoarthropathy, unspecified lower leg**

✓6ᵗʰ **M89.47  Other hypertrophic osteoarthropathy, ankle and foot**
    **M89.471  Other hypertrophic osteoarthropathy, right ankle and foot**
    **M89.472  Other hypertrophic osteoarthropathy, left ankle and foot**
    **M89.479  Other hypertrophic osteoarthropathy, unspecified ankle and foot**

    **M89.48  Other hypertrophic osteoarthropathy, other site**
    **M89.49  Other hypertrophic osteoarthropathy, multiple sites**

✓5ᵗʰ **M89.5  Osteolysis**
    Use additional code to identify major osseous defect, if applicable (M89.7-)
    **EXCLUDES 2**  *periprosthetic osteolysis of internal prosthetic joint (T84.05-)*
    **M89.50  Osteolysis, unspecified site**

✓6ᵗʰ **M89.51  Osteolysis, shoulder**
    **M89.511  Osteolysis, right shoulder**
    **M89.512  Osteolysis, left shoulder**
    **M89.519  Osteolysis, unspecified shoulder**

✓6ᵗʰ **M89.52  Osteolysis, upper arm**
    **M89.521  Osteolysis, right upper arm**
    **M89.522  Osteolysis, left upper arm**
    **M89.529  Osteolysis, unspecified upper arm**

✓6ᵗʰ **M89.53  Osteolysis, forearm**
    **M89.531  Osteolysis, right forearm**
    **M89.532  Osteolysis, left forearm**
    **M89.539  Osteolysis, unspecified forearm**

✓6ᵗʰ **M89.54  Osteolysis, hand**
    **M89.541  Osteolysis, right hand**
    **M89.542  Osteolysis, left hand**
    **M89.549  Osteolysis, unspecified hand**

✓6ᵗʰ **M89.55  Osteolysis, thigh**
    **M89.551  Osteolysis, right thigh**
    **M89.552  Osteolysis, left thigh**
    **M89.559  Osteolysis, unspecified thigh**

✓6ᵗʰ **M89.56  Osteolysis, lower leg**
    **M89.561  Osteolysis, right lower leg**
    **M89.562  Osteolysis, left lower leg**
    **M89.569  Osteolysis, unspecified lower leg**

✓6ᵗʰ **M89.57  Osteolysis, ankle and foot**
    **M89.571  Osteolysis, right ankle and foot**
    **M89.572  Osteolysis, left ankle and foot**
    **M89.579  Osteolysis, unspecified ankle and foot**

    **M89.58  Osteolysis, other site**
    **M89.59  Osteolysis, multiple sites**

✓5ᵗʰ **M89.6  Osteopathy after poliomyelitis**
    Use additional code (B91) to identify previous poliomyelitis
    **EXCLUDES 1**  *postpolio syndrome (G14)*
    **M89.60  Osteopathy after poliomyelitis, unspecified site** ᴴᶜᶜ

✓6ᵗʰ **M89.61  Osteopathy after poliomyelitis, shoulder**
    **M89.611  Osteopathy after poliomyelitis, right shoulder** ᴴᶜᶜ
    **M89.612  Osteopathy after poliomyelitis, left shoulder** ᴴᶜᶜ
    **M89.619  Osteopathy after poliomyelitis, unspecified shoulder** ᴴᶜᶜ

✓6ᵗʰ **M89.62  Osteopathy after poliomyelitis, upper arm**
    **M89.621  Osteopathy after poliomyelitis, right upper arm** ᴴᶜᶜ
    **M89.622  Osteopathy after poliomyelitis, left upper arm** ᴴᶜᶜ
    **M89.629  Osteopathy after poliomyelitis, unspecified upper arm** ᴴᶜᶜ

✓6ᵗʰ **M89.63  Osteopathy after poliomyelitis, forearm**
    **M89.631  Osteopathy after poliomyelitis, right forearm** ᴴᶜᶜ
    **M89.632  Osteopathy after poliomyelitis, left forearm** ᴴᶜᶜ
    **M89.639  Osteopathy after poliomyelitis, unspecified forearm** ᴴᶜᶜ

✓6ᵗʰ **M89.64  Osteopathy after poliomyelitis, hand**
    **M89.641  Osteopathy after poliomyelitis, right hand** ᴴᶜᶜ
    **M89.642  Osteopathy after poliomyelitis, left hand** ᴴᶜᶜ
    **M89.649  Osteopathy after poliomyelitis, unspecified hand** ᴴᶜᶜ

✓6ᵗʰ **M89.65  Osteopathy after poliomyelitis, thigh**
    **M89.651  Osteopathy after poliomyelitis, right thigh** ᴴᶜᶜ
    **M89.652  Osteopathy after poliomyelitis, left thigh** ᴴᶜᶜ

Ⓝ Newborn: 0   Ⓟ Pediatric: 0-17   Ⓜ Maternity: 12-55   Ⓐ Adult: 15-124   **MCC** Major CC Condition   **PDxMCC** PDx acts as own MCC   **CC** CC Condition   **PDxCC** PDx acts as own CC

**812**                                                                                      ICD-10-CM 2018

M89.659 Osteopathy after poliomyelitis, unspecified **thigh** `HCC`

✓6ᵗʰ **M89.66** **Osteopathy after poliomyelitis, lower leg**

M89.661 Osteopathy after poliomyelitis, right lower leg `HCC`

M89.662 Osteopathy after poliomyelitis, left lower leg `HCC`

M89.669 Osteopathy after poliomyelitis, unspecified **lower leg** `HCC`

✓6ᵗʰ **M89.67** **Osteopathy after poliomyelitis, ankle and foot**

M89.671 Osteopathy after poliomyelitis, right ankle and foot `HCC`

M89.672 Osteopathy after poliomyelitis, left ankle and foot `HCC`

M89.679 Osteopathy after poliomyelitis, unspecified **ankle and foot** `HCC`

**M89.68** Osteopathy after poliomyelitis, **other site** `HCC`

**M89.69** Osteopathy after poliomyelitis, **multiple sites** `HCC`

✓5ᵗʰ **M89.7** **Major osseous defect**

Code first underlying disease, if known, such as:
aseptic necrosis of bone (M87.-)
malignant neoplasm of bone (C40.-)
osteolysis (M89.5)
osteomyelitis (M86.-)
osteonecrosis (M87.-)
osteoporosis (M80.-, M81.-)
periprosthetic osteolysis (T84.05-)

**M89.70** Major osseous defect, unspecified site

✓6ᵗʰ **M89.71** **Major osseous defect, shoulder region**
Major osseous defect clavicle or scapula

M89.711 Major osseous defect, right shoulder region

M89.712 Major osseous defect, left shoulder region

M89.719 Major osseous defect, unspecified shoulder region

✓6ᵗʰ **M89.72** **Major osseous defect, humerus**

M89.721 Major osseous defect, right humerus

M89.722 Major osseous defect, left humerus

M89.729 Major osseous defect, unspecified humerus

✓6ᵗʰ **M89.73** **Major osseous defect, forearm**
Major osseous defect of radius and ulna

M89.731 Major osseous defect, right forearm

M89.732 Major osseous defect, left forearm

M89.739 Major osseous defect, unspecified forearm

✓6ᵗʰ **M89.74** **Major osseous defect, hand**
Major osseous defect of carpus, fingers, metacarpus

M89.741 Major osseous defect, right hand

M89.742 Major osseous defect, left hand

M89.749 Major osseous defect, unspecified hand

✓6ᵗʰ **M89.75** **Major osseous defect, pelvic region and thigh**
Major osseous defect of femur and pelvis

M89.751 Major osseous defect, right pelvic region and thigh

M89.752 Major osseous defect, left pelvic region and thigh

M89.759 Major osseous defect, unspecified pelvic region and thigh

✓6ᵗʰ **M89.76** **Major osseous defect, lower leg**
Major osseous defect of fibula and tibia

M89.761 Major osseous defect, right lower leg

M89.762 Major osseous defect, left lower leg

M89.769 Major osseous defect, unspecified lower leg

✓6ᵗʰ **M89.77** **Major osseous defect, ankle and foot**
Major osseous defect of metatarsus, tarsus, toes

M89.771 Major osseous defect, right ankle and foot

M89.772 Major osseous defect, left ankle and foot

M89.779 Major osseous defect, unspecified ankle and foot

**M89.78** Major osseous defect, other site

**M89.79** Major osseous defect, multiple sites

✓5ᵗʰ **M89.8** **Other specified disorders of bone**
Infantile cortical hyperostoses
Post-traumatic subperiosteal ossification

✓6ᵗʰ **M89.8X** **Other specified disorders of bone**

M89.8X0 Other specified disorders of bone, multiple sites

M89.8X1 Other specified disorders of bone, shoulder

M89.8X2 Other specified disorders of bone, upper arm

M89.8X3 Other specified disorders of bone, forearm

M89.8X4 Other specified disorders of bone, hand

M89.8X5 Other specified disorders of bone, thigh

M89.8X6 Other specified disorders of bone, lower leg

M89.8X7 Other specified disorders of bone, ankle and foot

M89.8X8 Other specified disorders of bone, other site

M89.8X9 Other specified disorders of bone, unspecified site

**M89.9** **Disorder of bone, unspecified**

✓4ᵗʰ **M90** **Osteopathies in diseases classified elsewhere**
**EXCLUDES 1** *osteochondritis, osteomyelitis, and osteopathy (in):*
*cryptococcosis (B45.3)*
*diabetes mellitus (E08-E13 with .69-)*
*gonococcal (A54.43)*
*neurogenic syphilis (A52.11)*
*renal osteodystrophy (N25.0)*
*salmonellosis (A02.24)*
*secondary syphilis (A51.46)*
*syphilis (late) (A52.77)*

✓5ᵗʰ **M90.5** **Osteonecrosis in diseases classified elsewhere**
Code first underlying disease, such as:
caisson disease (T70.3)
hemoglobinopathy (D50-D64)

**CC Excl: For CC codes in subcategory M90.5, unless otherwise noted:** PDX collection 907

*M90.50* *Osteonecrosis in diseases classified elsewhere, unspecified site* `PDxCC` `CC` `HCC`

✓6ᵗʰ **M90.51** **Osteonecrosis in diseases classified elsewhere, shoulder**

**CC Excl: For CC codes in subcategory M90.51:** PDX collection 908

*M90.511* *Osteonecrosis in diseases classified elsewhere, right shoulder* `PDxCC` `CC` `HCC`

*M90.512* *Osteonecrosis in diseases classified elsewhere, left shoulder* `PDxCC` `CC` `HCC`

*M90.519* *Osteonecrosis in diseases classified elsewhere, unspecified shoulder* `PDxCC` `CC` `HCC`

✓6ᵗʰ **M90.52** **Osteonecrosis in diseases classified elsewhere, upper arm**

*M90.521* *Osteonecrosis in diseases classified elsewhere, right upper arm* `PDxCC` `CC` `HCC`

*M90.522* *Osteonecrosis in diseases classified elsewhere, left upper arm* `PDxCC` `CC` `HCC`

*M90.529* *Osteonecrosis in diseases classified elsewhere, unspecified upper arm* `PDxCC` `CC` `HCC`

✓6ᵗʰ **M90.53** **Osteonecrosis in diseases classified elsewhere, forearm**

*M90.531* *Osteonecrosis in diseases classified elsewhere, right forearm* `PDxCC` `CC` `HCC`

*M90.532* *Osteonecrosis in diseases classified elsewhere, left forearm* `PDxCC` `CC` `HCC`

*M90.539* *Osteonecrosis in diseases classified elsewhere, unspecified forearm* `PDxCC` `CC` `HCC`

✓6ᵗʰ **M90.54** **Osteonecrosis in diseases classified elsewhere, hand**

*M90.541* *Osteonecrosis in diseases classified elsewhere, right hand* `PDxCC` `CC` `HCC`

*M90.542* *Osteonecrosis in diseases classified elsewhere, left hand* `PDxCC` `CC` `HCC`

*M90.549* *Osteonecrosis in diseases classified elsewhere, unspecified hand* `PDxCC` `CC` `HCC`

✓ Additional Character Req   ✓x7ᵗʰ Placeholder Alert   Unacceptable PDx   Manifestation   **H1**-**H14** HAC   `HCC` CMS-HCC Condition   **EXCLUDES 1** Not Coded Here   **EXCLUDES 2** Not Included Here

**ICD-10-CM 2018**                                                                                                                **813**

✓6th **M90.55 Osteonecrosis in diseases classified elsewhere, thigh**

> **CC Excl: For CC codes in subcategory M90.55:**
> PDX collection 909

     *M90.551*   **Osteonecrosis in diseases classified elsewhere, *right* thigh** `PDxCC` `CC` `HCC`

     *M90.552*   **Osteonecrosis in diseases classified elsewhere, *left* thigh** `PDxCC` `CC` `HCC`

     *M90.559*   **Osteonecrosis in diseases classified elsewhere, *unspecified* thigh**

✓6th **M90.56 Osteonecrosis in diseases classified elsewhere, lower leg**

     *M90.561*   **Osteonecrosis in diseases classified elsewhere, *right* lower leg** `PDxCC` `CC` `HCC`

     *M90.562*   **Osteonecrosis in diseases classified elsewhere, *left* lower leg** `PDxCC` `CC` `HCC`

     *M90.569*   **Osteonecrosis in diseases classified elsewhere, *unspecified* lower leg** `PDxCC` `CC` `HCC`

✓6th **M90.57 Osteonecrosis in diseases classified elsewhere, ankle and foot**

     *M90.571*   **Osteonecrosis in diseases classified elsewhere, *right* ankle and foot** `PDxCC` `CC` `HCC`

     *M90.572*   **Osteonecrosis in diseases classified elsewhere, *left* ankle and foot** `PDxCC` `CC` `HCC`

     *M90.579*   **Osteonecrosis in diseases classified elsewhere, *unspecified* ankle and foot** `PDxCC` `CC` `HCC`

   *M90.58*   **Osteonecrosis in diseases classified elsewhere, *other site*** `PDxCC` `CC` `HCC`

   *M90.59*   **Osteonecrosis in diseases classified elsewhere, *multiple sites*** `PDxCC` `CC` `HCC`

✓5th **M90.6 Osteitis deformans in neoplastic diseases**
     Osteitis deformans in malignant neoplasm of bone
     Code first the neoplasm (C40-, C41-)
     **EXCLUDES 1**   osteitis deformans [Paget's disease of bone] (M88.-)

   *M90.60*   **Osteitis deformans in neoplastic diseases, *unspecified site***

✓6th **M90.61 Osteitis deformans in neoplastic diseases, shoulder**

     *M90.611*   **Osteitis deformans in neoplastic diseases, *right* shoulder**

     *M90.612*   **Osteitis deformans in neoplastic diseases, *left* shoulder**

     *M90.619*   **Osteitis deformans in neoplastic diseases, *unspecified* shoulder**

✓6th **M90.62 Osteitis deformans in neoplastic diseases, upper arm**

     *M90.621*   **Osteitis deformans in neoplastic diseases, *right* upper arm**

     *M90.622*   **Osteitis deformans in neoplastic diseases, *left* upper arm**

     *M90.629*   **Osteitis deformans in neoplastic diseases, *unspecified* upper arm**

✓6th **M90.63 Osteitis deformans in neoplastic diseases, forearm**

     *M90.631*   **Osteitis deformans in neoplastic diseases, *right* forearm**

     *M90.632*   **Osteitis deformans in neoplastic diseases, *left* forearm**

     *M90.639*   **Osteitis deformans in neoplastic diseases, *unspecified* forearm**

✓6th **M90.64 Osteitis deformans in neoplastic diseases, hand**

     *M90.641*   **Osteitis deformans in neoplastic diseases, *right* hand**

     *M90.642*   **Osteitis deformans in neoplastic diseases, *left* hand**

     *M90.649*   **Osteitis deformans in neoplastic diseases, *unspecified* hand**

✓6th **M90.65 Osteitis deformans in neoplastic diseases, thigh**

     *M90.651*   **Osteitis deformans in neoplastic diseases, *right* thigh**

     *M90.652*   **Osteitis deformans in neoplastic diseases, *left* thigh**

     *M90.659*   **Osteitis deformans in neoplastic diseases, *unspecified* thigh**

✓6th **M90.66 Osteitis deformans in neoplastic diseases, lower leg**

     *M90.661*   **Osteitis deformans in neoplastic diseases, *right* lower leg**

     *M90.662*   **Osteitis deformans in neoplastic diseases, *left* lower leg**

     *M90.669*   **Osteitis deformans in neoplastic diseases, *unspecified* lower leg**

✓6th **M90.67 Osteitis deformans in neoplastic diseases, ankle and foot**

     *M90.671*   **Osteitis deformans in neoplastic diseases, *right* ankle and foot**

     *M90.672*   **Osteitis deformans in neoplastic diseases, *left* ankle and foot**

     *M90.679*   **Osteitis deformans in neoplastic diseases, *unspecified* ankle and foot**

   *M90.68*   **Osteitis deformans in neoplastic diseases, *other site***

   *M90.69*   **Osteitis deformans in neoplastic diseases, *multiple sites***

✓5th **M90.8 Osteopathy in diseases classified elsewhere**
     Code first underlying disease, such as:
       rickets (E55.0)
       vitamin-D-resistant rickets (E83.3)

   *M90.80*   **Osteopathy in diseases classified elsewhere, *unspecified site***

✓6th **M90.81 Osteopathy in diseases classified elsewhere, shoulder**

     *M90.811*   **Osteopathy in diseases classified elsewhere, *right* shoulder**

     *M90.812*   **Osteopathy in diseases classified elsewhere, *left* shoulder**

     *M90.819*   **Osteopathy in diseases classified elsewhere, *unspecified* shoulder**

✓6th **M90.82 Osteopathy in diseases classified elsewhere, upper arm**

     *M90.821*   **Osteopathy in diseases classified elsewhere, *right* upper arm**

     *M90.822*   **Osteopathy in diseases classified elsewhere, *left* upper arm**

     *M90.829*   **Osteopathy in diseases classified elsewhere, *unspecified* upper arm**

✓6th **M90.83 Osteopathy in diseases classified elsewhere, forearm**

     *M90.831*   **Osteopathy in diseases classified elsewhere, *right* forearm**

     *M90.832*   **Osteopathy in diseases classified elsewhere, *left* forearm**

     *M90.839*   **Osteopathy in diseases classified elsewhere, *unspecified* forearm**

✓6th **M90.84 Osteopathy in diseases classified elsewhere, hand**

     *M90.841*   **Osteopathy in diseases classified elsewhere, *right* hand**

     *M90.842*   **Osteopathy in diseases classified elsewhere, *left* hand**

     *M90.849*   **Osteopathy in diseases classified elsewhere, *unspecified* hand**

✓6th **M90.85 Osteopathy in diseases classified elsewhere, thigh**

     *M90.851*   **Osteopathy in diseases classified elsewhere, *right* thigh**

     *M90.852*   **Osteopathy in diseases classified elsewhere, *left* thigh**

     *M90.859*   **Osteopathy in diseases classified elsewhere, *unspecified* thigh**

✓6th **M90.86 Osteopathy in diseases classified elsewhere, lower leg**

     *M90.861*   **Osteopathy in diseases classified elsewhere, *right* lower leg**

     *M90.862*   **Osteopathy in diseases classified elsewhere, *left* lower leg**

     *M90.869*   **Osteopathy in diseases classified elsewhere, *unspecified* lower leg**

✓6th **M90.87 Osteopathy in diseases classified elsewhere, ankle and foot**

     *M90.871*   **Osteopathy in diseases classified elsewhere, *right* ankle and foot**

     *M90.872*   **Osteopathy in diseases classified elsewhere, *left* ankle and foot**

     *M90.879*   **Osteopathy in diseases classified elsewhere, *unspecified* ankle and foot**

N Newborn: 0   P Pediatric: 0-17   M Maternity: 12-55   A Adult: 15-124   **MCC** Major CC Condition   **PDxMCC** PDx acts as own MCC   **CC** CC Condition   **PDxCC** PDx acts as own CC

814          ICD-10-CM 2018

M90.88　***Osteopathy in diseases classified elsewhere,*** *other site*

M90.89　***Osteopathy in diseases classified elsewhere,*** *multiple sites*

### Chondropathies (M91-M94)

EXCLUDES 1　*postprocedural chondropathies (M96.-)*

✔4ᵗʰ **M91　Juvenile osteochondrosis of** hip and pelvis

　　　　EXCLUDES 1　*slipped upper femoral epiphysis (nontraumatic) (M93.0)*

　**M91.0　Juvenile osteochondrosis of** pelvis
　　　Osteochondrosis (juvenile) of acetabulum
　　　Osteochondrosis (juvenile) of iliac crest [Buchanan]
　　　Osteochondrosis (juvenile) of ischiopubic synchondrosis [van Neck]
　　　Osteochondrosis (juvenile) of symphysis pubis [Pierson]

✔5ᵗʰ **M91.1　Juvenile osteochondrosis of** head of femur **[Legg-Calvé-Perthes]**

　　**M91.10　Juvenile osteochondrosis of head of femur [Legg-Calvé-Perthes],** unspecified **leg**

　　**M91.11　Juvenile osteochondrosis of head of femur [Legg-Calvé-Perthes],** right **leg**

　　**M91.12　Juvenile osteochondrosis of head of femur [Legg-Calvé-Perthes],** left **leg**

✔5ᵗʰ **M91.2　Coxa plana**
　　　Hip deformity due to previous juvenile osteochondrosis

　　**M91.20　Coxa plana,** unspecified **hip**

　　**M91.21　Coxa plana,** right **hip**

　　**M91.22　Coxa plana,** left **hip**

✔5ᵗʰ **M91.3　Pseudocoxalgia**

　　**M91.30　Pseudocoxalgia,** unspecified **hip**

　　**M91.31　Pseudocoxalgia,** right **hip**

　　**M91.32　Pseudocoxalgia,** left **hip**

✔5ᵗʰ **M91.4　Coxa magna**

　　**M91.40　Coxa magna,** unspecified **hip**

　　**M91.41　Coxa magna,** right **hip**

　　**M91.42　Coxa magna,** left **hip**

✔5ᵗʰ **M91.8　Other juvenile osteochondrosis of hip and pelvis**
　　　Juvenile osteochondrosis after reduction of congenital dislocation of hip

　　**M91.80　Other juvenile osteochondrosis of hip and pelvis,** unspecified **leg**

　　**M91.81　Other juvenile osteochondrosis of hip and pelvis,** right **leg**

　　**M91.82　Other juvenile osteochondrosis of hip and pelvis,** left **leg**

✔5ᵗʰ **M91.9　Juvenile osteochondrosis of hip and pelvis,** unspecified

　　**M91.90　Juvenile osteochondrosis of hip and pelvis, unspecified,** unspecified **leg**

　　**M91.91　Juvenile osteochondrosis of hip and pelvis, unspecified,** right **leg**

　　**M91.92　Juvenile osteochondrosis of hip and pelvis, unspecified,** left **leg**

✔4ᵗʰ **M92　Other juvenile osteochondrosis**

✔5ᵗʰ **M92.0　Juvenile osteochondrosis of** humerus
　　　Osteochondrosis (juvenile) of capitulum of humerus [Panner]
　　　Osteochondrosis (juvenile) of head of humerus [Haas]

　　**M92.00　Juvenile osteochondrosis of humerus,** unspecified **arm**

　　**M92.01　Juvenile osteochondrosis of humerus,** right **arm**

　　**M92.02　Juvenile osteochondrosis of humerus,** left **arm**

✔5ᵗʰ **M92.1　Juvenile osteochondrosis of** radius and ulna
　　　Osteochondrosis (juvenile) of lower ulna [Burns]
　　　Osteochondrosis (juvenile) of radial head [Brailsford]

　　**M92.10　Juvenile osteochondrosis of radius and ulna,** unspecified **arm**

　　**M92.11　Juvenile osteochondrosis of radius and ulna,** right **arm**

　　**M92.12　Juvenile osteochondrosis of radius and ulna,** left **arm**

✔5ᵗʰ **M92.2　Juvenile osteochondrosis,** hand

　✔6ᵗʰ **M92.20　Unspecified juvenile osteochondrosis,** hand

　　　**M92.201　Unspecified juvenile osteochondrosis,** right **hand**

　　　**M92.202　Unspecified juvenile osteochondrosis,** left **hand**

　　　**M92.209　Unspecified juvenile osteochondrosis,** unspecified **hand**

　✔6ᵗʰ **M92.21　Osteochondrosis (juvenile) of** carpal lunate **[Kienböck]**

　　　**M92.211　Osteochondrosis (juvenile) of carpal lunate [Kienböck],** right **hand**

　　　**M92.212　Osteochondrosis (juvenile) of carpal lunate [Kienböck],** left **hand**

　　　**M92.219　Osteochondrosis (juvenile) of carpal lunate [Kienböck],** unspecified **hand**

　✔6ᵗʰ **M92.22　Osteochondrosis (juvenile) of** metacarpal heads **[Mauclaire]**

　　　**M92.221　Osteochondrosis (juvenile) of metacarpal heads [Mauclaire],** right **hand**

　　　**M92.222　Osteochondrosis (juvenile) of metacarpal heads [Mauclaire],** left **hand**

　　　**M92.229　Osteochondrosis (juvenile) of metacarpal heads [Mauclaire],** unspecified **hand**

　✔6ᵗʰ **M92.29　Other** juvenile osteochondrosis, hand

　　　**M92.291　Other juvenile osteochondrosis,** right **hand**

　　　**M92.292　Other juvenile osteochondrosis,** left **hand**

　　　**M92.299　Other juvenile osteochondrosis,** unspecified **hand**

✔5ᵗʰ **M92.3　Other juvenile osteochondrosis, upper limb**

　　**M92.30　Other juvenile osteochondrosis, unspecified upper limb**

　　**M92.31　Other juvenile osteochondrosis, right upper limb**

　　**M92.32　Other juvenile osteochondrosis, left upper limb**

✔5ᵗʰ **M92.4　Juvenile osteochondrosis of** patella
　　　Osteochondrosis (juvenile) of primary patellar center [Köhler]
　　　Osteochondrosis (juvenile) of secondary patellar centre [Sinding Larsen]

　　**M92.40　Juvenile osteochondrosis of patella,** unspecified **knee**

　　**M92.41　Juvenile osteochondrosis of patella,** right **knee**

　　**M92.42　Juvenile osteochondrosis of patella,** left **knee**

✔5ᵗʰ **M92.5　Juvenile osteochondrosis of** tibia and fibula
　　　Osteochondrosis (juvenile) of proximal tibia [Blount]
　　　Osteochondrosis (juvenile) of tibial tubercle [Osgood-Schlatter]
　　　Tibia vara

　　**M92.50　Juvenile osteochondrosis of tibia and fibula,** unspecified **leg**

　　**M92.51　Juvenile osteochondrosis of tibia and fibula,** right **leg**

　　**M92.52　Juvenile osteochondrosis of tibia and fibula,** left **leg**

✔5ᵗʰ **M92.6　Juvenile osteochondrosis of** tarsus
　　　Osteochondrosis (juvenile) of calcaneum [Sever]
　　　Osteochondrosis (juvenile) of os tibiale externum [Haglund]
　　　Osteochondrosis (juvenile) of talus [Diaz]
　　　Osteochondrosis (juvenile) of tarsal navicular [Köhler]

　　**M92.60　Juvenile osteochondrosis of tarsus,** unspecified **ankle**

　　**M92.61　Juvenile osteochondrosis of tarsus,** right **ankle**

　　**M92.62　Juvenile osteochondrosis of tarsus,** left **ankle**

✔5ᵗʰ **M92.7　Juvenile osteochondrosis of** metatarsus
　　　Osteochondrosis (juvenile) of fifth metatarsus [Iselin]
　　　Osteochondrosis (juvenile) of second metatarsus [Freiberg]

　　**M92.70　Juvenile osteochondrosis of metatarsus,** unspecified **foot**

　　**M92.71　Juvenile osteochondrosis of metatarsus,** right **foot**

　　**M92.72　Juvenile osteochondrosis of metatarsus,** left **foot**

　**M92.8　Other specified juvenile osteochondrosis**
　　　Calcaneal apophysitis

　**M92.9　Juvenile osteochondrosis,** unspecified
　　　Juvenile apophysitis NOS
　　　Juvenile epiphysitis NOS
　　　Juvenile osteochondritis NOS
　　　Juvenile osteochondrosis NOS

---

✔ Additional Character Req　✔7ᵗʰ Placeholder Alert　Unacceptable PDx　Manifestation　H1 -H14 HAC　HCC CMS-HCC Condition　EXCLUDES 1 Not Coded Here　EXCLUDES 2 Not Included Here

✓4ᵗʰ **M93 Other osteochondropathies**

> EXCLUDES 2   *osteochondrosis of spine (M42.-)*

✓5ᵗʰ **M93.0 Slipped upper femoral epiphysis (nontraumatic)**

> Use additional code for associated chondrolysis (M94.3)

  ✓6ᵗʰ **M93.00 Unspecified slipped upper femoral epiphysis (nontraumatic)**

    **M93.001 Unspecified slipped upper femoral epiphysis (nontraumatic), right hip**

    **M93.002 Unspecified slipped upper femoral epiphysis (nontraumatic), left hip**

    **M93.003 Unspecified slipped upper femoral epiphysis (nontraumatic), unspecified hip**

  ✓6ᵗʰ **M93.01 Acute slipped upper femoral epiphysis (nontraumatic)**

    **M93.011 Acute slipped upper femoral epiphysis (nontraumatic), right hip**

    **M93.012 Acute slipped upper femoral epiphysis (nontraumatic), left hip**

    **M93.013 Acute slipped upper femoral epiphysis (nontraumatic), unspecified hip**

  ✓6ᵗʰ **M93.02 Chronic slipped upper femoral epiphysis (nontraumatic)**

    **M93.021 Chronic slipped upper femoral epiphysis (nontraumatic), right hip**

    **M93.022 Chronic slipped upper femoral epiphysis (nontraumatic), left hip**

    **M93.023 Chronic slipped upper femoral epiphysis (nontraumatic), unspecified hip**

  ✓6ᵗʰ **M93.03 Acute on chronic slipped upper femoral epiphysis (nontraumatic)**

    **M93.031 Acute on chronic slipped upper femoral epiphysis (nontraumatic), right hip**

    **M93.032 Acute on chronic slipped upper femoral epiphysis (nontraumatic), left hip**

    **M93.033 Acute on chronic slipped upper femoral epiphysis (nontraumatic), unspecified hip**

**M93.1 Kienböck's disease of adults**    🅰

> Adult osteochondrosis of carpal lunates

✓5ᵗʰ **M93.2 Osteochondritis dissecans**

  **M93.20 Osteochondritis dissecans of unspecified site**

  ✓6ᵗʰ **M93.21 Osteochondritis dissecans of shoulder**

    **M93.211 Osteochondritis dissecans, right shoulder**

    **M93.212 Osteochondritis dissecans, left shoulder**

    **M93.219 Osteochondritis dissecans, unspecified shoulder**

  ✓6ᵗʰ **M93.22 Osteochondritis dissecans of elbow**

    **M93.221 Osteochondritis dissecans, right elbow**

    **M93.222 Osteochondritis dissecans, left elbow**

    **M93.229 Osteochondritis dissecans, unspecified elbow**

  ✓6ᵗʰ **M93.23 Osteochondritis dissecans of wrist**

    **M93.231 Osteochondritis dissecans, right wrist**

    **M93.232 Osteochondritis dissecans, left wrist**

    **M93.239 Osteochondritis dissecans, unspecified wrist**

  ✓6ᵗʰ **M93.24 Osteochondritis dissecans of joints of hand**

    **M93.241 Osteochondritis dissecans, joints of right hand**

    **M93.242 Osteochondritis dissecans, joints of left hand**

    **M93.249 Osteochondritis dissecans, joints of unspecified hand**

  ✓6ᵗʰ **M93.25 Osteochondritis dissecans of hip**

    **M93.251 Osteochondritis dissecans, right hip**

    **M93.252 Osteochondritis dissecans, left hip**

    **M93.259 Osteochondritis dissecans, unspecified hip**

  ✓6ᵗʰ **M93.26 Osteochondritis dissecans knee**

    **M93.261 Osteochondritis dissecans, right knee**

    **M93.262 Osteochondritis dissecans, left knee**

    **M93.269 Osteochondritis dissecans, unspecified knee**

  ✓6ᵗʰ **M93.27 Osteochondritis dissecans of ankle and joints of foot**

    **M93.271 Osteochondritis dissecans, right ankle and joints of right foot**

    **M93.272 Osteochondritis dissecans, left ankle and joints of left foot**

    **M93.279 Osteochondritis dissecans, unspecified ankle and joints of foot**

  **M93.28 Osteochondritis dissecans other site**

  **M93.29 Osteochondritis dissecans multiple sites**

✓5ᵗʰ **M93.8 Other specified osteochondropathies**

  **M93.80 Other specified osteochondropathies of unspecified site**

  ✓6ᵗʰ **M93.81 Other specified osteochondropathies of shoulder**

    **M93.811 Other specified osteochondropathies, right shoulder**

    **M93.812 Other specified osteochondropathies, left shoulder**

    **M93.819 Other specified osteochondropathies, unspecified shoulder**

  ✓6ᵗʰ **M93.82 Other specified osteochondropathies of upper arm**

    **M93.821 Other specified osteochondropathies, right upper arm**

    **M93.822 Other specified osteochondropathies, left upper arm**

    **M93.829 Other specified osteochondropathies, unspecified upper arm**

  ✓6ᵗʰ **M93.83 Other specified osteochondropathies of forearm**

    **M93.831 Other specified osteochondropathies, right forearm**

    **M93.832 Other specified osteochondropathies, left forearm**

    **M93.839 Other specified osteochondropathies, unspecified forearm**

  ✓6ᵗʰ **M93.84 Other specified osteochondropathies of hand**

    **M93.841 Other specified osteochondropathies, right hand**

    **M93.842 Other specified osteochondropathies, left hand**

    **M93.849 Other specified osteochondropathies, unspecified hand**

  ✓6ᵗʰ **M93.85 Other specified osteochondropathies of thigh**

    **M93.851 Other specified osteochondropathies, right thigh**

    **M93.852 Other specified osteochondropathies, left thigh**

    **M93.859 Other specified osteochondropathies, unspecified thigh**

  ✓6ᵗʰ **M93.86 Other specified osteochondropathies lower leg**

    **M93.861 Other specified osteochondropathies, right lower leg**

    **M93.862 Other specified osteochondropathies, left lower leg**

    **M93.869 Other specified osteochondropathies, unspecified lower leg**

  ✓6ᵗʰ **M93.87 Other specified osteochondropathies of ankle and foot**

    **M93.871 Other specified osteochondropathies, right ankle and foot**

    **M93.872 Other specified osteochondropathies, left ankle and foot**

    **M93.879 Other specified osteochondropathies, unspecified ankle and foot**

  **M93.88 Other specified osteochondropathies other site**

  **M93.89 Other specified osteochondropathies multiple sites**

✓5ᵗʰ **M93.9 Osteochondropathy, unspecified**

> Apophysitis NOS      Osteochondritis NOS
> Epiphysitis NOS      Osteochondrosis NOS

  **M93.90 Osteochondropathy, unspecified of unspecified site**

  ✓6ᵗʰ **M93.91 Osteochondropathy, unspecified of shoulder**

    **M93.911 Osteochondropathy, unspecified, right shoulder**

    **M93.912 Osteochondropathy, unspecified, left shoulder**

    **M93.919 Osteochondropathy, unspecified, unspecified shoulder**

  ✓6ᵗʰ **M93.92 Osteochondropathy, unspecified of upper arm**

    **M93.921 Osteochondropathy, unspecified, right upper arm**

🅝 Newborn: 0   🅟 Pediatric: 0-17   🅜 Maternity: 12-55   🅐 Adult: 15-124   **MCC** Major CC Condition   **PDxMCC** PDx acts as own MCC   **CC** CC Condition   **PDxCC** PDx acts as own CC

816      ICD-10-CM 2018

      **M93.922** Osteochondropathy, unspecified, left upper arm

      **M93.929** Osteochondropathy, unspecified, unspecified upper arm

    ✓6ᵗʰ **M93.93** Osteochondropathy, unspecified of forearm

      **M93.931** Osteochondropathy, unspecified, right forearm

      **M93.932** Osteochondropathy, unspecified, left forearm

      **M93.939** Osteochondropathy, unspecified, unspecified forearm

    ✓6ᵗʰ **M93.94** Osteochondropathy, unspecified of hand

      **M93.941** Osteochondropathy, unspecified, right hand

      **M93.942** Osteochondropathy, unspecified, left hand

      **M93.949** Osteochondropathy, unspecified, unspecified hand

    ✓6ᵗʰ **M93.95** Osteochondropathy, unspecified of thigh

      **M93.951** Osteochondropathy, unspecified, right thigh

      **M93.952** Osteochondropathy, unspecified, left thigh

      **M93.959** Osteochondropathy, unspecified, unspecified thigh

    ✓6ᵗʰ **M93.96** Osteochondropathy, unspecified lower leg

      **M93.961** Osteochondropathy, unspecified, right lower leg

      **M93.962** Osteochondropathy, unspecified, left lower leg

      **M93.969** Osteochondropathy, unspecified, unspecified lower leg

    ✓6ᵗʰ **M93.97** Osteochondropathy, unspecified of ankle and foot

      **M93.971** Osteochondropathy, unspecified, right ankle and foot

      **M93.972** Osteochondropathy, unspecified, left ankle and foot

      **M93.979** Osteochondropathy, unspecified, unspecified ankle and foot

      **M93.98** Osteochondropathy, unspecified other site

      **M93.99** Osteochondropathy, unspecified multiple sites

✓4ᵗʰ **M94** **Other disorders of cartilage**

    **M94.0** **Chondrocostal junction syndrome [Tietze]**
      Costochondritis

    **M94.1** **Relapsing polychondritis**

  ✓5ᵗʰ **M94.2** **Chondromalacia**
      *EXCLUDES 1*    chondromalacia patellae (M22.4)

    **M94.20** Chondromalacia, unspecified site

  ✓6ᵗʰ **M94.21** Chondromalacia, shoulder

    **M94.211** Chondromalacia, right shoulder

    **M94.212** Chondromalacia, left shoulder

    **M94.219** Chondromalacia, unspecified shoulder

  ✓6ᵗʰ **M94.22** Chondromalacia, elbow

    **M94.221** Chondromalacia, right elbow

    **M94.222** Chondromalacia, left elbow

    **M94.229** Chondromalacia, unspecified elbow

  ✓6ᵗʰ **M94.23** Chondromalacia, wrist

    **M94.231** Chondromalacia, right wrist

    **M94.232** Chondromalacia, left wrist

    **M94.239** Chondromalacia, unspecified wrist

  ✓6ᵗʰ **M94.24** Chondromalacia, joints of hand

    **M94.241** Chondromalacia, joints of right hand

    **M94.242** Chondromalacia, joints of left hand

    **M94.249** Chondromalacia, joints of unspecified hand

  ✓6ᵗʰ **M94.25** Chondromalacia, hip

    **M94.251** Chondromalacia, right hip

    **M94.252** Chondromalacia, left hip

    **M94.259** Chondromalacia, unspecified hip

  ✓6ᵗʰ **M94.26** Chondromalacia, knee

    **M94.261** Chondromalacia, right knee

    **M94.262** Chondromalacia, left knee

    **M94.269** Chondromalacia, unspecified knee

  ✓6ᵗʰ **M94.27** Chondromalacia, ankle and joints of foot

    **M94.271** Chondromalacia, right ankle and joints of right foot

    **M94.272** Chondromalacia, left ankle and joints of left foot

    **M94.279** Chondromalacia, unspecified ankle and joints of foot

    **M94.28** Chondromalacia, other site

    **M94.29** Chondromalacia, multiple sites

  ✓5ᵗʰ **M94.3** **Chondrolysis**
    Code first any associated slipped upper femoral epiphysis (nontraumatic) (M93.0-)

  ✓6ᵗʰ **M94.35** Chondrolysis, hip

    **M94.351** Chondrolysis, right hip

    **M94.352** Chondrolysis, left hip

    **M94.359** Chondrolysis, unspecified hip

  ✓5ᵗʰ **M94.8** **Other specified disorders of cartilage**

  ✓6ᵗʰ **M94.8X** Other specified disorders of cartilage

    **M94.8X0** Other specified disorders of cartilage, multiple sites

    **M94.8X1** Other specified disorders of cartilage, shoulder

    **M94.8X2** Other specified disorders of cartilage, upper arm

    **M94.8X3** Other specified disorders of cartilage, forearm

    **M94.8X4** Other specified disorders of cartilage, hand

    **M94.8X5** Other specified disorders of cartilage, thigh

    **M94.8X6** Other specified disorders of cartilage, lower leg

    **M94.8X7** Other specified disorders of cartilage, ankle and foot

    **M94.8X8** Other specified disorders of cartilage, other site

    **M94.8X9** Other specified disorders of cartilage, unspecified sites

    **M94.9** **Disorder of cartilage, unspecified**

## Other disorders of the musculoskeletal system and connective tissue (M95)

✓4ᵗʰ **M95** **Other acquired deformities of musculoskeletal system and connective tissue**
    *EXCLUDES 2*   acquired absence of limbs and organs (Z89-Z90)
         acquired deformities of limbs (M20-M21)
         congenital malformations and deformations of the musculoskeletal system (Q65-Q79)
         deforming dorsopathies (M40-M43)
         dentofacial anomalies [including malocclusion] (M26.-)
         postprocedural musculoskeletal disorders (M96.-)

    **M95.0** **Acquired deformity of nose**
      *EXCLUDES 2*   deviated nasal septum (J34.2)

  ✓5ᵗʰ **M95.1** **Cauliflower ear**
      *EXCLUDES 2*   other acquired deformities of ear (H61.1)
      **DEF:** Acquired deformity of the external ear; due to injury, subsequent perichondritis.

    **M95.10** Cauliflower ear, unspecified ear

    **M95.11** Cauliflower ear, right ear

    **M95.12** Cauliflower ear, left ear

    **M95.2** **Other acquired deformity of head**

    **M95.3** **Acquired deformity of neck**

    **M95.4** **Acquired deformity of chest and rib**
      **AHA:** 2014, 4Q, 26-27

    **M95.5** **Acquired deformity of pelvis**
      *EXCLUDES 1*   maternal care for known or suspected disproportion (O33.-)

    **M95.8** **Other specified acquired deformities of musculoskeletal system**

    **M95.9** **Acquired deformity of musculoskeletal system, unspecified**

✔ Additional Character Req    ✔x7ᵗʰ Placeholder Alert    Unacceptable PDx    **Manifestation**    **H1**-**H14** HAC    **HCC** CMS-HCC Condition    *EXCLUDES 1* Not Coded Here    *EXCLUDES 2* Not Included Here

**ICD-10-CM 2018**          817

## Intraoperative and postprocedural complications and disorders of musculoskeletal system, not elsewhere classified (M96)

**√4ᵗʰ M96 Intraoperative and postprocedural complications and disorders of musculoskeletal system, not elsewhere classified**

> *EXCLUDES 2*   arthropathy following intestinal bypass (M02.0-)
> complications of internal orthopedic prosthetic devices, implants and grafts (T84.-)
> disorders associated with osteoporosis (M80)
> periprosthetic fracture around internal prosthetic joint (M97.-)
> presence of functional implants and other devices (Z96-Z97)

**M96.0 Pseudarthrosis after fusion or arthrodesis**   CC
> **CC Excl:** No Excl

**M96.1 Postlaminectomy syndrome, not elsewhere classified**

**M96.2 Postradiation kyphosis**

**M96.3 Postlaminectomy kyphosis**

**M96.4 Postsurgical lordosis**

**M96.5 Postradiation scoliosis**

**√5ᵗʰ M96.6 Fracture of bone following insertion of orthopedic implant, joint prosthesis, or bone plate**
> Intraoperative fracture of bone during insertion of orthopedic implant, joint prosthesis, or bone plate
> *EXCLUDES 2*   complication of internal orthopedic devices, implants or grafts (T84.-)

> **CC Excl: For CC codes in subcategory M96.6:** PDX collection 911

    **√6ᵗʰ M96.62 Fracture of humerus following insertion of orthopedic implant, joint prosthesis, or bone plate**
       **M96.621 Fracture of humerus following insertion of orthopedic implant, joint prosthesis, or bone plate, right arm**   CC HCC
       **M96.622 Fracture of humerus following insertion of orthopedic implant, joint prosthesis, or bone plate, left arm**   CC HCC
       **M96.629 Fracture of humerus following insertion of orthopedic implant, joint prosthesis, or bone plate, unspecified arm**   CC HCC

    **√6ᵗʰ M96.63 Fracture of radius or ulna following insertion of orthopedic implant, joint prosthesis, or bone plate**
       **M96.631 Fracture of radius or ulna following nsertion of orthopedic implant, joint prosthesis, or bone plate, right arm**   CC HCC
       **M96.632 Fracture of radius or ulna following insertion of orthopedic implant, joint prosthesis, or bone plate, left arm**   CC HCC
       **M96.639 Fracture of radius or ulna following insertion of orthopedic implant, joint prosthesis, or bone plate, unspecified arm**   CC HCC

    **M96.65 Fracture of pelvis following insertion of orthopedic implant, joint prosthesis, or bone plate**   CC HCC

    **√6ᵗʰ M96.66 Fracture of femur following insertion of orthopedic implant, joint prosthesis, or bone plate**
       **M96.661 Fracture of femur following insertion of orthopedic implant, joint prosthesis, or bone plate, right leg**   CC HCC
       **M96.662 Fracture of femur following insertion of orthopedic implant, joint prosthesis, or bone plate, left leg**   CC HCC
       **M96.669 Fracture of femur following insertion of orthopedic implant, joint prosthesis, or bone plate, unspecified leg**   CC HCC

    **√6ᵗʰ M96.67 Fracture of tibia or fibula following insertion of orthopedic implant, joint prosthesis, or bone plate**
       **M96.671 Fracture of tibia or fibula following insertion of orthopedic implant, joint prosthesis, or bone plate, right leg**   CC HCC
       **M96.672 Fracture of tibia or fibula following insertion of orthopedic implant, joint prosthesis, or bone plate, left leg**   CC HCC
       **M96.679 Fracture of tibia or fibula following insertion of orthopedic implant, joint prosthesis, or bone plate, unspecified leg**   CC HCC

    **M96.69 Fracture of other bone following insertion of orthopedic implant, joint prosthesis, or bone plate**   CC HCC

**√5ᵗʰ M96.8 Other intraoperative and postprocedural complications and disorders of musculoskeletal system, not elsewhere classified**

> **CC Excl: For CC codes in subcategory M96.8, unless otherwise noted:** PDX collection 912

    **√6ᵗʰ M96.81 Intraoperative hemorrhage and hematoma of a musculoskeletal structure complicating a procedure**
> *EXCLUDES 1*   intraoperative hemorrhage and hematoma of a musculoskeletal structure due to accidental puncture and laceration during a procedure (M96.82-)

       **M96.810 Intraoperative hemorrhage and hematoma of a musculoskeletal structure complicating a musculoskeletal system procedure**   CC
       **M96.811 Intraoperative hemorrhage and hematoma of a musculoskeletal structure complicating other procedure**   CC

    **√6ᵗʰ M96.82 Accidental puncture and laceration of a musculoskeletal structure during a procedure**
       **M96.820 Accidental puncture and laceration of a musculoskeletal structure during a musculoskeletal system procedure**   CC
>         **CC Excl:** PDX collection 509
       **M96.821 Accidental puncture and laceration of a musculoskeletal structure during other procedure**   CC
>         **CC Excl:** PDX collection 509

    **√6ᵗʰ M96.83 Postprocedural hemorrhage of a musculoskeletal structure following a procedure**
       **M96.830 Postprocedural hemorrhage of a musculoskeletal structure following a musculoskeletal system procedure**   CC
       **M96.831 Postprocedural hemorrhage of a musculoskeletal structure following other procedure**   CC

    **√6ᵗʰ M96.84 Postprocedural hematoma and seroma of a musculoskeletal structure following a procedure**
       **M96.840 Postprocedural hematoma of a musculoskeletal structure following a musculoskeletal system procedure**   CC
       **M96.841 Postprocedural hematoma of a musculoskeletal structure following other procedure**   CC
       **M96.842 Postprocedural seroma of a musculoskeletal structure following a musculoskeletal system procedure**   CC
       **M96.843 Postprocedural seroma of a musculoskeletal structure following other procedure**   CC

    **M96.89 Other intraoperative and postprocedural complications and disorders of the musculoskeletal system**   CC
> Instability of joint secondary to removal of joint prosthesis
> Use additional code, if applicable, to further specify disorder
> **CC Excl:** PDX collection 643

## Periprosthetic fracture around internal prosthetic joint (M97)

**√4ᵗʰ M97 Periprosthetic fracture around internal prosthetic joint**
> *EXCLUDES 2*   breakage (fracture) of prosthetic joint (T84.01-)
> fracture of bone following insertion of orthopedic implant, joint prosthesis or bone plate (M96.6-)

> The appropriate 7th character is to be added to each code from category M97.
> A   initial encounter
> D   subsequent encounter
> S   sequela

> **CC Excl: For CC codes in category M97:** PDX collection 911

**√5ᵗʰ M97.0 Periprosthetic fracture around internal prosthetic hip joint**
    7, 10  √x7ᵗʰ **M97.01 Periprosthetic fracture around internal prosthetic right hip joint**   CC HCC
    7, 10  √x7ᵗʰ **M97.02 Periprosthetic fracture around internal prosthetic left hip joint**   CC HCC

---

[7]   CC when reported as an initial encounter (7th character A, B, or C – specific to category) OR a subsequent encounter for nonunion or malunion (7th character K, M, N, P, Q, or R – specific to category).

[10]   HCC with 7th character indicating initial encounter (A, B or C - specific to category).

---

N Newborn: 0   P Pediatric: 0-17   M Maternity: 12-55   A Adult: 15-124   MCC Major CC Condition   PDx MCC PDx acts as own MCC   CC CC Condition   PDx CC PDx acts as own CC

818              ICD-10-CM 2018

☑5ᵗʰ **M97.1** Periprosthetic fracture around internal prosthetic knee joint

   ☑x7ᵗʰ **M97.11** Periprosthetic fracture around internal prosthetic right knee joint `CC`

   ☑x7ᵗʰ **M97.12** Periprosthetic fracture around internal prosthetic left knee joint `CC`

☑5ᵗʰ **M97.2** Periprosthetic fracture around internal prosthetic ankle joint

   ☑x7ᵗʰ **M97.21** Periprosthetic fracture around internal prosthetic right ankle joint `CC`

   ☑x7ᵗʰ **M97.22** Periprosthetic fracture around internal prosthetic left ankle joint `CC`

☑5ᵗʰ **M97.3** Periprosthetic fracture around internal prosthetic shoulder joint

   ☑x7ᵗʰ **M97.31** Periprosthetic fracture around internal prosthetic right shoulder joint `CC`

   ☑x7ᵗʰ **M97.32** Periprosthetic fracture around internal prosthetic left shoulder joint `CC`

☑5ᵗʰ **M97.4** Periprosthetic fracture around internal prosthetic elbow joint

   ☑x7ᵗʰ **M97.41** Periprosthetic fracture around internal prosthetic right elbow joint `CC`

   ☑x7ᵗʰ **M97.42** Periprosthetic fracture around internal prosthetic left elbow joint `CC`

☑x7ᵗʰ **M97.8** Periprosthetic fracture around other internal prosthetic joint `CC`
Periprosthetic fracture around internal prosthetic finger joint
Periprosthetic fracture around internal prosthetic spinal joint
Periprosthetic fracture around internal prosthetic toe joint
Periprosthetic fracture around internal prosthetic wrist joint
Use additional code to identify the joint (Z96.6-)

☑x7ᵗʰ **M97.9** Periprosthetic fracture around unspecified internal prosthetic joint `CC`

## Biomechanical lesions, not elsewhere classified (M99)

☑4ᵗʰ **M99 Biomechanical lesions, not elsewhere classified**
   **NOTE**    This category should not be used if the condition can be classified elsewhere.

☑5ᵗʰ **M99.0** Segmental and somatic dysfunction

   **M99.00** Segmental and somatic dysfunction of head region

   **M99.01** Segmental and somatic dysfunction of cervical region

   **M99.02** Segmental and somatic dysfunction of thoracic region

   **M99.03** Segmental and somatic dysfunction of lumbar region

   **M99.04** Segmental and somatic dysfunction of sacral region

   **M99.05** Segmental and somatic dysfunction of pelvic region

   **M99.06** Segmental and somatic dysfunction of lower extremity

   **M99.07** Segmental and somatic dysfunction of upper extremity

   **M99.08** Segmental and somatic dysfunction of rib cage

   **M99.09** Segmental and somatic dysfunction of abdomen and other regions

☑5ᵗʰ **M99.1** Subluxation complex (vertebral)

   **CC Excl:** For CC codes in subcategory M99.1, unless otherwise noted: PDX collection 913

   **M99.10** Subluxation complex (vertebral) of head region `CC` `H5`

   **M99.11** Subluxation complex (vertebral) of cervical region `CC` `H5`

   **M99.12** Subluxation complex (vertebral) of thoracic region

   **M99.13** Subluxation complex (vertebral) of lumbar region

   **M99.14** Subluxation complex (vertebral) of sacral region

   **M99.15** Subluxation complex (vertebral) of pelvic region

   **M99.16** Subluxation complex (vertebral) of lower extremity

   **M99.17** Subluxation complex (vertebral) of upper extremity

   **M99.18** Subluxation complex (vertebral) of rib cage `CC` `H5`
      **CC Excl:** PDX collection 914

   **M99.19** Subluxation complex (vertebral) of abdomen and other regions

☑5ᵗʰ **M99.2** Subluxation stenosis of neural canal

   **M99.20** Subluxation stenosis of neural canal of head region

   **M99.21** Subluxation stenosis of neural canal of cervical region

   **M99.22** Subluxation stenosis of neural canal of thoracic region

   **M99.23** Subluxation stenosis of neural canal of lumbar region

   **M99.24** Subluxation stenosis of neural canal of sacral region

   **M99.25** Subluxation stenosis of neural canal of pelvic region

   **M99.26** Subluxation stenosis of neural canal of lower extremity

   **M99.27** Subluxation stenosis of neural canal of upper extremity

   **M99.28** Subluxation stenosis of neural canal of rib cage

   **M99.29** Subluxation stenosis of neural canal of abdomen and other regions

☑5ᵗʰ **M99.3** Osseous stenosis of neural canal

   **M99.30** Osseous stenosis of neural canal of head region

   **M99.31** Osseous stenosis of neural canal of cervical region

   **M99.32** Osseous stenosis of neural canal of thoracic region

   **M99.33** Osseous stenosis of neural canal of lumbar region

   **M99.34** Osseous stenosis of neural canal of sacral region

   **M99.35** Osseous stenosis of neural canal of pelvic region

   **M99.36** Osseous stenosis of neural canal of lower extremity

   **M99.37** Osseous stenosis of neural canal of upper extremity

   **M99.38** Osseous stenosis of neural canal of rib cage

   **M99.39** Osseous stenosis of neural canal of abdomen and other regions

☑5ᵗʰ **M99.4** Connective tissue stenosis of neural canal

   **M99.40** Connective tissue stenosis of neural canal of head region

   **M99.41** Connective tissue stenosis of neural canal of cervical region

   **M99.42** Connective tissue stenosis of neural canal of thoracic region

   **M99.43** Connective tissue stenosis of neural canal of lumbar region

   **M99.44** Connective tissue stenosis of neural canal of sacral region

   **M99.45** Connective tissue stenosis of neural canal of pelvic region

   **M99.46** Connective tissue stenosis of neural canal of lower extremity

   **M99.47** Connective tissue stenosis of neural canal of upper extremity

   **M99.48** Connective tissue stenosis of neural canal of rib cage

   **M99.49** Connective tissue stenosis of neural canal of abdomen and other regions

☑5ᵗʰ **M99.5** Intervertebral disc stenosis of neural canal

   **M99.50** Intervertebral disc stenosis of neural canal of head region

   **M99.51** Intervertebral disc stenosis of neural canal of cervical region

   **M99.52** Intervertebral disc stenosis of neural canal of thoracic region

   **M99.53** Intervertebral disc stenosis of neural canal of lumbar region

   **M99.54** Intervertebral disc stenosis of neural canal of sacral region

   **M99.55** Intervertebral disc stenosis of neural canal of pelvic region

   **M99.56** Intervertebral disc stenosis of neural canal of lower extremity

   **M99.57** Intervertebral disc stenosis of neural canal of upper extremity

   **M99.58** Intervertebral disc stenosis of neural canal of rib cage

   **M99.59** Intervertebral disc stenosis of neural canal of abdomen and other regions

☑5ᵗʰ **M99.6** Osseous and subluxation stenosis of intervertebral foramina

   **M99.60** Osseous and subluxation stenosis of intervertebral foramina of head region

   **M99.61** Osseous and subluxation stenosis of intervertebral foramina of cervical region

   **M99.62** Osseous and subluxation stenosis of intervertebral foramina of thoracic region

   **M99.63** Osseous and subluxation stenosis of intervertebral foramina of lumbar region

☑Additional Character Req   ☑x7ᵗʰ Placeholder Alert   Unacceptable PDx   Manifestation   `H1`-`H14` HAC   `HCC` CMS-HCC Condition   *EXCLUDES 1* Not Coded Here   *EXCLUDES 2* Not Included Here

ICD-10-CM 2018      **819**

M99.64   **Osseous and subluxation stenosis of intervertebral foramina of** sacral **region**

M99.65   **Osseous and subluxation stenosis of intervertebral foramina of** pelvic **region**

M99.66   **Osseous and subluxation stenosis of intervertebral foramina of** lower extremity

M99.67   **Osseous and subluxation stenosis of intervertebral foramina of** upper extremity

M99.68   **Osseous and subluxation stenosis of intervertebral foramina of** rib cage

M99.69   **Osseous and subluxation stenosis of intervertebral foramina of** abdomen and other **regions**

✓5ᵗʰ **M99.7   Connective tissue and disc stenosis of intervertebral foramina**

M99.70   **Connective tissue and disc stenosis of intervertebral foramina of** head **region**

M99.71   **Connective tissue and disc stenosis of intervertebral foramina of** cervical **region**

M99.72   **Connective tissue and disc stenosis of intervertebral foramina of** thoracic **region**

M99.73   **Connective tissue and disc stenosis of intervertebral foramina of** lumbar **region**

M99.74   **Connective tissue and disc stenosis of intervertebral foramina of** sacral **region**

M99.75   **Connective tissue and disc stenosis of intervertebral foramina of** pelvic **region**

M99.76   **Connective tissue and disc stenosis of intervertebral foramina of** lower extremity

M99.77   **Connective tissue and disc stenosis of intervertebral foramina of** upper extremity

M99.78   **Connective tissue and disc stenosis of intervertebral foramina of** rib cage

M99.79   **Connective tissue and disc stenosis of intervertebral foramina of** abdomen and other **regions**

✓5ᵗʰ **M99.8   Other biomechanical lesions**

M99.80   **Other biomechanical lesions of** head **region**

M99.81   **Other biomechanical lesions of** cervical **region**

M99.82   **Other biomechanical lesions of** thoracic **region**

M99.83   **Other biomechanical lesions of** lumbar **region**

M99.84   **Other biomechanical lesions of** sacral **region**

M99.85   **Other biomechanical lesions of** pelvic **region**

M99.86   **Other biomechanical lesions of** lower extremity

M99.87   **Other biomechanical lesions of** upper extremity

M99.88   **Other biomechanical lesions of** rib cage

M99.89   **Other biomechanical lesions of** abdomen and other **regions**

**M99.9   Biomechanical lesion,** unspecified

N Newborn: 0   P Pediatric: 0-17   M Maternity: 12-55   A Adult: 15-124   MCC Major CC Condition   PDxMCC PDx acts as own MCC   CC CC Condition   PDxCC PDx acts as own CC

820           ICD-10-CM 2018

# Chapter 14. Diseases of Genitourinary System (NØØ–N99)

## Chapter Specific Guidelines with Coding Examples

The chapter specific guidelines from the ICD-10-CM Official Guidelines for Coding and Reporting have been provided below. Along with these guidelines are coding examples, contained in the shaded boxes, that have been developed to help illustrate the coding and/or sequencing guidance found in these guidelines.

### a. Chronic kidney disease

#### 1) Stages of chronic kidney disease (CKD)

The ICD-10-CM classifies CKD based on severity. The severity of CKD is designated by stages 1-5. Stage 2, code N18.2, equates to mild CKD; stage 3, code N18.3, equates to moderate CKD; and stage 4, code N18.4, equates to severe CKD. Code N18.6, End stage renal disease (ESRD), is assigned when the provider has documented end-stage-renal disease (ESRD).

If both a stage of CKD and ESRD are documented, assign code N18.6 only.

---

Stage 5 chronic kidney disease with ESRD requiring chronic dialysis

**N18.6**      **End stage renal disease**

**Z99.2**      **Dependence on renal dialysis**

*Explanation:* The diagnostic statement indicates the patient has chronic kidney disease, documented both as stage 5 and as ESRD requiring chronic dialysis. Code N18.6 End stage renal disease (ESRD), is assigned when the provider has documented end-stage-renal disease (ESRD). If both a stage of CKD and ESRD are documented, assign code N18.6 only.

---

#### 2) Chronic kidney disease and kidney transplant status

Patients who have undergone kidney transplant may still have some form of chronic kidney disease (CKD) because the kidney transplant may not fully restore kidney function. Therefore, the presence of CKD alone does not constitute a transplant complication. Assign the appropriate N18 code for the patient's stage of CKD and code Z94.Ø, Kidney transplant status. If a transplant complication such as failure or rejection or other transplant complication is documented, see section I.C.19.g for information on coding complications of a kidney transplant. If the documentation is unclear as to whether the patient has a complication of the transplant, query the provider.

---

Patient with residual chronic kidney disease stage 1 after kidney transplant

**N18.1**      **Chronic kidney disease, stage 1**

**Z94.Ø**      **Kidney transplant status**

*Explanation:* Patients who have undergone kidney transplant may still have some form of chronic kidney disease (CKD) because the kidney transplant may not fully restore kidney function. The presence of CKD alone does not constitute a transplant complication. Assign the appropriate N18 code for the patient's stage of CKD and code Z94.0 Kidney transplant status.

---

#### 3) Chronic kidney disease with other conditions

Patients with CKD may also suffer from other serious conditions, most commonly diabetes mellitus and hypertension. The sequencing of the CKD code in relationship to codes for other contributing conditions is based on the conventions in the Tabular List.

*See I.C.9. Hypertensive chronic kidney disease.*

*See I.C.19. Chronic kidney disease and kidney transplant complications.*

---

Type 1 diabetic chronic kidney disease, stage 2

**E1Ø.22**      **Type 1 diabetes mellitus with diabetic chronic kidney disease**

**N18.2**      **Chronic kidney disease, stage 2 (mild)**

*Explanation:* Patients with CKD may also suffer from other serious conditions such as diabetes mellitus. The sequencing of the CKD code in relationship to codes for other contributing conditions is based on the conventions in the Tabular List. Diabetic CKD code E10.22 includes an instructional note to "Use additional code to identify stage of chronic kidney disease (N18.1–N18.6)," thus providing sequencing direction.

---

# Chapter 14. Diseases of the Genitourinary System (N00-N99)

*EXCLUDES 2*   *certain conditions originating in the perinatal period (P04-P96)*
*certain infectious and parasitic diseases (A00-B99)*
*complications of pregnancy, childbirth and the puerperium (O00-O9A)*
*congenital malformations, deformations and chromosomal abnormalities (Q00-Q99)*
*endocrine, nutritional and metabolic diseases (E00-E88)*
*injury, poisoning and certain other consequences of external causes (S00-T88)*
*neoplasms (C00-D49)*
*symptoms, signs and abnormal clinical and laboratory findings, not elsewhere classified (R00-R94)*

This chapter contains the following blocks:

## Glomerular diseases (N00-N08)

Code also any associated kidney failure (N17-N19).
*EXCLUDES 1*   *hypertensive chronic kidney disease (I12.-)*

### ✓4ᵗʰ N00   Acute nephritic syndrome
INCLUDES   acute glomerular disease
acute glomerulonephritis
acute nephritis
*EXCLUDES 1*   *acute tubulo-interstitial nephritis (N10)*
*nephritic syndrome NOS (N05.-)*

**CC Excl: For MCC codes in category N00, unless otherwise noted:** PDX collection 915

**N00.0   Acute nephritic syndrome with minor glomerular abnormality**   `MCC`
Acute nephritic syndrome with minimal change lesion

**N00.1   Acute nephritic syndrome with focal and segmental glomerular lesions**   `MCC`
Acute nephritic syndrome with focal and segmental hyalinosis
Acute nephritic syndrome with focal and segmental sclerosis
Acute nephritic syndrome with focal glomerulonephritis

**N00.2   Acute nephritic syndrome with diffuse membranous glomerulonephritis**   `MCC`

**N00.3   Acute nephritic syndrome with diffuse mesangial proliferative glomerulonephritis**   `MCC`

**N00.4   Acute nephritic syndrome with diffuse endocapillary proliferative glomerulonephritis**   `MCC`

**N00.5   Acute nephritic syndrome with diffuse mesangiocapillary glomerulonephritis**   `MCC`
Acute nephritic syndrome with membranoproliferative glomerulonephritis, types 1 and 3, or NOS

**N00.6   Acute nephritic syndrome with dense deposit disease**   `MCC`
Acute nephritic syndrome with membranoproliferative glomerulonephritis, type 2

**N00.7   Acute nephritic syndrome with diffuse crescentic glomerulonephritis**   `MCC`
Acute nephritic syndrome with extracapillary glomerulonephritis

**N00.8   Acute nephritic syndrome with other morphologic changes**   `MCC`
Acute nephritic syndrome with proliferative glomerulonephritis NOS
**CC Excl:** PDX collection 916

**N00.9   Acute nephritic syndrome with unspecified morphologic changes**   `MCC`

### ✓4ᵗʰ N01   Rapidly progressive nephritic syndrome
INCLUDES   rapidly progressive glomerular disease
rapidly progressive glomerulonephritis
rapidly progressive nephritis
*EXCLUDES 1*   *nephritic syndrome NOS (N05.-)*

**CC Excl: For MCC codes in category N01:** PDX collection 915

**N01.0   Rapidly progressive nephritic syndrome with minor glomerular abnormality**   `MCC`
Rapidly progressive nephritic syndrome with minimal change lesion

**N01.1   Rapidly progressive nephritic syndrome with focal and segmental glomerular lesions**   `MCC`
Rapidly progressive nephritic syndrome with focal and segmental hyalinosis
Rapidly progressive nephritic syndrome with focal and segmental sclerosis
Rapidly progressive nephritic syndrome with focal glomerulonephritis

**N01.2   Rapidly progressive nephritic syndrome with diffuse membranous glomerulonephritis**   `MCC`

**N01.3   Rapidly progressive nephritic syndrome with diffuse mesangial proliferative glomerulonephritis**   `MCC`

**N01.4   Rapidly progressive nephritic syndrome with diffuse endocapillary proliferative glomerulonephritis**   `MCC`

**N01.5   Rapidly progressive nephritic syndrome with diffuse mesangiocapillary glomerulonephritis**   `MCC`
Rapidly progressive nephritic syndrome with membranoproliferative glomerulonephritis, types 1 and 3, or NOS

**N01.6   Rapidly progressive nephritic syndrome with dense deposit disease**   `MCC`
Rapidly progressive nephritic syndrome with membranoproliferative glomerulonephritis, type 2

**N01.7   Rapidly progressive nephritic syndrome with diffuse crescentic glomerulonephritis**   `MCC`
Rapidly progressive nephritic syndrome with extracapillary glomerulonephritis

**N01.8   Rapidly progressive nephritic syndrome with other morphologic changes**   `MCC`
Rapidly progressive nephritic syndrome with proliferative glomerulonephritis NOS

**N01.9   Rapidly progressive nephritic syndrome with unspecified morphologic changes**   `MCC`

### ✓4ᵗʰ N02   Recurrent and persistent hematuria
*EXCLUDES 1*   *acute cystitis with hematuria (N30.01)*
*hematuria NOS (R31.9)*
*hematuria not associated with specified morphologic lesions (R31.-)*

**CC Excl: For CC codes in category N02, unless otherwise noted:** PDX collection 917

**N02.0   Recurrent and persistent hematuria with minor glomerular abnormality**   `CC`
Recurrent and persistent hematuria with minimal change lesion

**N02.1   Recurrent and persistent hematuria with focal and segmental glomerular lesions**   `CC`
Recurrent and persistent hematuria with focal and segmental hyalinosis
Recurrent and persistent hematuria with focal and segmental sclerosis
Recurrent and persistent hematuria with focal glomerulonephritis

**N02.2   Recurrent and persistent hematuria with diffuse membranous glomerulonephritis**   `CC`

**N02.3   Recurrent and persistent hematuria with diffuse mesangial proliferative glomerulonephritis**   `CC`

**N02.4   Recurrent and persistent hematuria with diffuse endocapillary proliferative glomerulonephritis**   `CC`

**N02.5   Recurrent and persistent hematuria with diffuse mesangiocapillary glomerulonephritis**   `CC`
Recurrent and persistent hematuria with membranoproliferative glomerulonephritis, types 1 and 3, or NOS

**N02.6   Recurrent and persistent hematuria with dense deposit disease**   `CC`
Recurrent and persistent hematuria with membranoproliferative glomerulonephritis, type 2

Ⓝ Newborn: 0   🅿 Pediatric: 0-17   Ⓜ Maternity: 12-55   🅰 Adult: 15-124   `MCC` Major CC Condition   `PDxMCC` PDx acts as own MCC   `CC` CC Condition   `PDxCC` PDx acts as own CC

822                                                                                         ICD-10-CM 2018

**N02.7**  **Recurrent and persistent hematuria with** diffuse crescentic glomerulonephritis   `CC`
    Recurrent and persistent hematuria with extracapillary glomerulonephritis

**N02.8**  **Recurrent and persistent hematuria with** other morphologic changes   `CC`
    Recurrent and persistent hematuria with proliferative glomerulonephritis NOS
    **CC Excl:** PDX collection 915

**N02.9**  **Recurrent and persistent hematuria with** unspecified morphologic changes   `CC`
    **AHA:** 2017, 2Q, 5
    **CC Excl:** PDX collection 915

✓4ᵗʰ  **N03**  **Chronic nephritic syndrome**
    `INCLUDES`  chronic glomerular disease
             chronic glomerulonephritis
             chronic nephritis
    *EXCLUDES 1*  *chronic tubulo-interstitial nephritis (N11.-)*
             *diffuse sclerosing glomerulonephritis (N05.8-)*
             *nephritic syndrome NOS (N05.-)*
    **DEF:** Slow, progressive type of nephritis characterized by inflammation of the capillary loops in the glomeruli of the kidney, which leads to renal failure.

    **CC Excl: For CC codes in catagory N03:** PDX collection 918

**N03.0**  **Chronic nephritic syndrome with** minor glomerular abnormality   `CC`
    Chronic nephritic syndrome with minimal change lesion

**N03.1**  **Chronic nephritic syndrome with** focal and segmental glomerular lesions   `CC`
    Chronic nephritic syndrome with focal and segmental hyalinosis
    Chronic nephritic syndrome with focal and segmental sclerosis
    Chronic nephritic syndrome with focal glomerulonephritis

**N03.2**  **Chronic nephritic syndrome with** diffuse membranous glomerulonephritis   `CC`

**N03.3**  **Chronic nephritic syndrome with** diffuse mesangial proliferative glomerulonephritis   `CC`

**N03.4**  **Chronic nephritic syndrome with** diffuse endocapillary proliferative glomerulonephritis   `CC`

**N03.5**  **Chronic nephritic syndrome with** diffuse mesangiocapillary glomerulonephritis   `CC`
    Chronic nephritic syndrome with membranoproliferative glomerulonephritis, types 1 and 3, or NOS

**N03.6**  **Chronic nephritic syndrome with** dense deposit disease   `CC`
    Chronic nephritic syndrome with membranoproliferative glomerulonephritis, type 2

**N03.7**  **Chronic nephritic syndrome with** diffuse crescentic glomerulonephritis   `CC`
    Chronic nephritic syndrome with extracapillary glomerulonephritis

**N03.8**  **Chronic nephritic syndrome with** other morphologic changes   `CC`
    Chronic nephritic syndrome with proliferative glomerulonephritis NOS

**N03.9**  **Chronic nephritic syndrome with** unspecified morphologic changes   `CC`

✓4ᵗʰ  **N04**  **Nephrotic syndrome**
    `INCLUDES`  congenital nephrotic syndrome
             lipoid nephrosis

    **CC Excl: For CC codes in category N04, unless otherwise noted:** PDX collection 917

**N04.0**  **Nephrotic syndrome with** minor glomerular abnormality   `CC`
    Nephrotic syndrome with minimal change lesion

**N04.1**  **Nephrotic syndrome with** focal and segmental glomerular lesions   `CC`
    Nephrotic syndrome with focal and segmental hyalinosis
    Nephrotic syndrome with focal and segmental sclerosis
    Nephrotic syndrome with focal glomerulonephritis

**N04.2**  **Nephrotic syndrome with** diffuse membranous glomerulonephritis   `CC`

**N04.3**  **Nephrotic syndrome with** diffuse mesangial proliferative glomerulonephritis   `CC`

**N04.4**  **Nephrotic syndrome with** diffuse endocapillary proliferative glomerulonephritis   `CC`

**N04.5**  **Nephrotic syndrome with** diffuse mesangiocapillary glomerulonephritis   `CC`
    Nephrotic syndrome with membranoproliferative glomerulonephritis, types 1 and 3, or NOS

**N04.6**  **Nephrotic syndrome with** dense deposit disease   `CC`
    Nephrotic syndrome with membranoproliferative glomerulonephritis, type 2

**N04.7**  **Nephrotic syndrome with** diffuse crescentic glomerulonephritis   `CC`
    Nephrotic syndrome with extracapillary glomerulonephritis
    **CC Excl:** PDX collection 915

**N04.8**  **Nephrotic syndrome with** other morphologic changes   `CC`
    Nephrotic syndrome with proliferative glomerulonephritis NOS
    **CC Excl:** PDX collection 915

**N04.9**  **Nephrotic syndrome with** unspecified morphologic changes   `CC`
    **CC Excl:** PDX collection 915

✓4ᵗʰ  **N05**  **Unspecified nephritic syndrome**
    `INCLUDES`  glomerular disease NOS
             glomerulonephritis NOS
             nephritis NOS
             nephropathy NOS and renal disease NOS with morphological lesion specified in .0-.8
    *EXCLUDES 1*  *nephropathy NOS with no stated morphological lesion (N28.9)*
             *renal disease NOS with no stated morphological lesion (N28.9)*
             *tubulo-interstitial nephritis NOS (N12)*

    **CC Excl: For CC codes in category N05:** PDX collection 918

**N05.0**  **Unspecified nephritic syndrome with** minor glomerular abnormality
    Unspecified nephritic syndrome with minimal change lesion

**N05.1**  **Unspecified nephritic syndrome with** focal and segmental glomerular lesions
    Unspecified nephritic syndrome with focal and segmental hyalinosis
    Unspecified nephritic syndrome with focal and segmental sclerosis
    Unspecified nephritic syndrome with focal glomerulonephritis

**N05.2**  **Unspecified nephritic syndrome with** diffuse membranous glomerulonephritis   `CC`

**N05.3**  **Unspecified nephritic syndrome with** diffuse mesangial proliferative glomerulonephritis   `CC`

**N05.4**  **Unspecified nephritic syndrome with** diffuse endocapillary proliferative glomerulonephritis   `CC`

**N05.5**  **Unspecified nephritic syndrome with** diffuse mesangiocapillary glomerulonephritis   `CC`
    Unspecified nephritic syndrome with membranoproliferative glomerulonephritis, types 1 and 3, or NOS

**N05.6**  **Unspecified nephritic syndrome with** dense deposit disease
    Unspecified nephritic syndrome with membranoproliferative glomerulonephritis, type 2

**N05.7**  **Unspecified nephritic syndrome with** diffuse crescentic glomerulonephritis
    Unspecified nephritic syndrome with extracapillary glomerulonephritis

**N05.8**  **Unspecified nephritic syndrome with** other morphologic changes
    Unspecified nephritic syndrome with proliferative glomerulonephritis NOS

**N05.9**  **Unspecified nephritic syndrome with** unspecified morphologic changes

✓4ᵗʰ  **N06**  **Isolated proteinuria with specified morphological lesion**
    *EXCLUDES 1*  *proteinuria not associated with specific morphologic lesions (R80.0)*

    **CC Excl: For CC codes in category N06:** PDX collection 918

**N06.0**  **Isolated proteinuria with** minor glomerular abnormality
    Isolated proteinuria with minimal change lesion

**N06.1**  **Isolated proteinuria with** focal and segmental glomerular lesions
    Isolated proteinuria with focal and segmental hyalinosis
    Isolated proteinuria with focal and segmental sclerosis
    Isolated proteinuria with focal glomerulonephritis

**N06.2**  **Isolated proteinuria with** diffuse membranous glomerulonephritis   `CC`

**N06.3**  **Isolated proteinuria with** diffuse mesangial proliferative glomerulonephritis   `CC`

**N06.4**  **Isolated proteinuria with** diffuse endocapillary proliferative glomerulonephritis   `CC`

**N06.5**  **Isolated proteinuria with** diffuse mesangiocapillary glomerulonephritis   `CC`
    Isolated proteinuria with membranoproliferative glomerulonephritis, types 1 and 3, or NOS

✔Additional Character Req   ✓x7ᵗʰ Placeholder Alert   Unacceptable PDx   Manifestation   **H1**–**H14** HAC   `HCC` CMS-HCC Condition   *EXCLUDES 1* Not Coded Here   *EXCLUDES 2* Not Included Here

ICD-10-CM 2018                                                                   **823**

**N06.6 Isolated proteinuria with dense deposit disease**
Isolated proteinuria with membranoproliferative glomerulonephritis, type 2

**N06.7 Isolated proteinuria with diffuse crescentic glomerulonephritis**
Isolated proteinuria with extracapillary glomerulonephritis

**N06.8 Isolated proteinuria with other morphologic lesion**
Isolated proteinuria with proliferative glomerulonephritis NOS

**N06.9 Isolated proteinuria with unspecified morphologic lesion**

✓4ᵗʰ **N07 Hereditary nephropathy, not elsewhere classified**
EXCLUDES 2   Alport's syndrome (Q87.81-)
hereditary amyloid nephropathy (E85.-)
nail patella syndrome (Q87.2)
non-neuropathic heredofamilial amyloidosis (E85.-)

CC Excl: For CC codes in category N07: PDX collection 918

**N07.0 Hereditary nephropathy, not elsewhere classified with minor glomerular abnormality**
Hereditary nephropathy, not elsewhere classified with minimal change lesion

**N07.1 Hereditary nephropathy, not elsewhere classified with focal and segmental glomerular lesions**
Hereditary nephropathy, not elsewhere classified with focal and segmental hyalinosis
Hereditary nephropathy, not elsewhere classified with focal and segmental sclerosis
Hereditary nephropathy, not elsewhere classified with focal glomerulonephritis

**N07.2 Hereditary nephropathy, not elsewhere classified with diffuse membranous glomerulonephritis**   CC

**N07.3 Hereditary nephropathy, not elsewhere classified with diffuse mesangial proliferative glomerulonephritis**   CC

**N07.4 Hereditary nephropathy, not elsewhere classified with diffuse endocapillary proliferative glomerulonephritis**   CC

**N07.5 Hereditary nephropathy, not elsewhere classified with diffuse mesangiocapillary glomerulonephritis**   CC
Hereditary nephropathy, not elsewhere classified with membranoproliferative glomerulonephritis, types 1 and 3, or NOS

**N07.6 Hereditary nephropathy, not elsewhere classified with dense deposit disease**
Hereditary nephropathy, not elsewhere classified with membranoproliferative glomerulonephritis, type 2

**N07.7 Hereditary nephropathy, not elsewhere classified with diffuse crescentic glomerulonephritis**
Hereditary nephropathy, not elsewhere classified with extracapillary glomerulonephritis

**N07.8 Hereditary nephropathy, not elsewhere classified with other morphologic lesions**
Hereditary nephropathy, not elsewhere classified with proliferative glomerulonephritis NOS

**N07.9 Hereditary nephropathy, not elsewhere classified with unspecified morphologic lesions**

**N08 *Glomerular disorders in diseases classified elsewhere***
Glomerulonephritis
Nephritis
Nephropathy
Code first underlying disease, such as:
amyloidosis (E85.-)
congenital syphilis (A50.5)
cryoglobulinemia (D89.1)
disseminated intravascular coagulation (D65)
gout (M1A.-, M10.-)
microscopic polyangiitis (M31.7)
multiple myeloma (C90.0-)
sepsis (A40.0-A41.9)
sickle-cell disease (D57.0-D57.8)
EXCLUDES 1   glomerulonephritis, nephritis and nephropathy (in):
antiglomerular basement membrane disease (M31.0)
diabetes (E08-E13 with .21)
gonococcal (A54.21)
Goodpasture's syndrome (M31.0)
hemolytic-uremic syndrome (D59.3)
lupus (M32.14)
mumps (B26.83)
syphilis (A52.75)
systemic lupus erythematosus (M32.14)
Wegener's granulomatosis (M31.31)
pyelonephritis in diseases classified elsewhere (N16)
renal tubulo-interstitial disorders classified elsewhere (N16)

## Renal tubulo-interstitial diseases (N10-N16)

INCLUDES   pyelonephritis
EXCLUDES 1   pyeloureteritis cystica (N28.85)

**N10 Acute pyelonephritis**   CC  H6
Acute infectious interstitial nephritis
Acute pyelitis
Acute tubulo-interstitial nephritis
Hemoglobin nephrosis
Myoglobin nephrosis
Use additional code (B95-B97), to identify infectious agent
CC Excl: PDX collection 919

✓4ᵗʰ **N11 Chronic tubulo-interstitial nephritis**
INCLUDES   chronic infectious interstitial nephritis
chronic pyelitis
chronic pyelonephritis
Use additional code (B95-B97), to identify infectious agent

**N11.0 Nonobstructive reflux-associated chronic pyelonephritis**
Pyelonephritis (chronic) associated with (vesicoureteral) reflux
EXCLUDES 1   vesicoureteral reflux NOS (N13.70)

**N11.1 Chronic obstructive pyelonephritis**   PDx CC  CC
Pyelonephritis (chronic) associated with anomaly of pelviureteric junction
Pyelonephritis (chronic) associated with anomaly of pyeloureteric junction
Pyelonephritis (chronic) associated with crossing of vessel
Pyelonephritis (chronic) associated with kinking of ureter
Pyelonephritis (chronic) associated with obstruction of ureter
Pyelonephritis (chronic) associated with stricture of pelviureteric junction
Pyelonephritis (chronic) associated with stricture of ureter
EXCLUDES 1   calculous pyelonephritis (N20.9)
obstructive uropathy (N13.-)
CC Excl: PDX collection 920

**N11.8 Other chronic tubulo-interstitial nephritis**   CC
Nonobstructive chronic pyelonephritis NOS
CC Excl: PDX collection 921

**N11.9 Chronic tubulo-interstitial nephritis, unspecified**   CC  H6
Chronic interstitial nephritis NOS
Chronic pyelitis NOS
Chronic pyelonephritis NOS
CC Excl: PDX collection 922

**N12 Tubulo-interstitial nephritis, not specified as acute or chronic**   CC  H6
Interstitial nephritis NOS
Pyelitis NOS
Pyelonephritis NOS
EXCLUDES 1   calculous pyelonephritis (N20.9)
CC Excl: PDX collection 922

✓4ᵗʰ **N13 Obstructive and reflux uropathy**
EXCLUDES 2   calculus of kidney and ureter without hydronephrosis (N20.-)
congenital obstructive defects of renal pelvis and ureter (Q62.0-Q62.3)
hydronephrosis with ureteropelvic junction obstruction ▶(Q62.11)◀
obstructive pyelonephritis (N11.1)

CC Excl: For CC codes in category N13, unless otherwise noted: PDX collection 922

**N13.0 Hydronephrosis with ureteropelvic junction obstruction**   PDx CC  CC
Hydronephrosis due to acquired occlusion of ureteropelvic junction
EXCLUDES 2   hydronephrosis with ureteropelvic junction obstruction due to calculus (N13.2)

**N13.1 Hydronephrosis with ureteral stricture, not elsewhere classified**   PDx CC  CC
EXCLUDES 1   hydronephrosis with ureteral stricture with infection (N13.6)

**N13.2 Hydronephrosis with renal and ureteral calculous obstruction**   PDx CC  CC
EXCLUDES 1   hydronephrosis with renal and ureteral calculous obstruction with infection (N13.6)

✓5ᵗʰ **N13.3 Other and unspecified hydronephrosis**
EXCLUDES 1   hydronephrosis with infection (N13.6)
**N13.30 Unspecified hydronephrosis**   CC
**N13.39 Other hydronephrosis**   CC

N Newborn: 0   P Pediatric: 0-17   M Maternity: 12-55   A Adult: 15-124   MCC Major CC Condition   PDx MCC PDx acts as own MCC   CC CC Condition   PDx CC PDx acts as own CC

824   ICD-10-CM 2018

**Hydronephrosis/UPJ Obstruction**

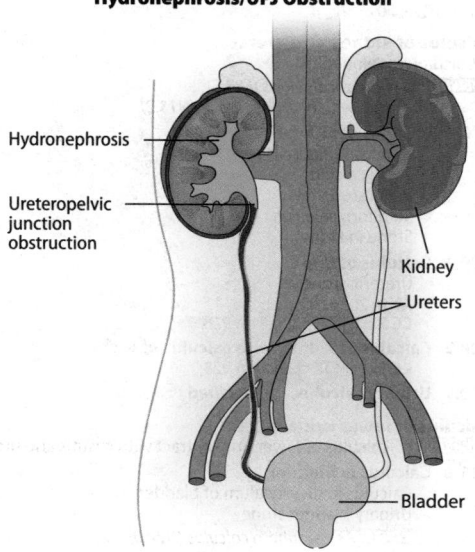

Hydronephrosis

Ureteropelvic junction obstruction

Kidney

Ureters

Bladder

**N13.4  Hydroureter**                                                            **CC**
> *EXCLUDES 1*  *congenital hydroureter (Q62.3-)*
>                  *hydroureter with infection (N13.6)*
>                  *vesicoureteral-reflux with hydroureter (N13.73-)*
> **CC Excl:** PDX collection 923

**N13.5  Crossing vessel and stricture of ureter without hydronephrosis**
> Kinking and stricture of ureter without hydronephrosis
> *EXCLUDES 1*  *crossing vessel and stricture of ureter without
>                  hydronephrosis with infection (N13.6)*

**N13.6  Pyonephrosis**                                                      **CC  H6**
> Conditions in N13.Ø-N13.5 with infection
> Obstructive uropathy with infection
> Use additional code (B95-B97), to identify infectious agent

**√5ᵗʰ N13.7  Vesicoureteral-reflux**
> *EXCLUDES 1*  *reflux-associated pyelonephritis (N11.Ø)*

> **N13.7Ø  Vesicoureteral-reflux, unspecified**
>            Vesicoureteral-reflux NOS

> **N13.71  Vesicoureteral-reflux without reflux nephropathy**

> **√6ᵗʰ N13.72  Vesicoureteral-reflux with reflux nephropathy without hydroureter**

>> **N13.721  Vesicoureteral-reflux with reflux
>>             nephropathy without hydroureter,
>>             unilateral**

>> **N13.722  Vesicoureteral-reflux with reflux
>>             nephropathy without hydroureter,
>>             bilateral**

>> **N13.729  Vesicoureteral-reflux with reflux
>>             nephropathy without hydroureter,
>>             unspecified**

**Vesicoureteral Reflux**

Kidneys

Ureters

Bladder

Normal flow of urine          Urine flowing the wrong way (VUR)

**√6ᵗʰ N13.73  Vesicoureteral-reflux with reflux nephropathy with hydroureter**

> **N13.731  Vesicoureteral-reflux with reflux
>             nephropathy with hydroureter, unilateral**

> **N13.732  Vesicoureteral-reflux with reflux
>             nephropathy with hydroureter, bilateral**

> **N13.739  Vesicoureteral-reflux with reflux
>             nephropathy with hydroureter,
>             unspecified**

**N13.8  Other obstructive and reflux uropathy**                      **CC**
> Urinary tract obstruction due to specified cause
> Code first, if applicable, any causal condition, such as:
>     enlarged prostate (N4Ø.1)
> **CC Excl:** PDX collection 920

**N13.9  Obstructive and reflux uropathy, unspecified**
> Urinary tract obstruction NOS

**√4ᵗʰ N14  Drug- and heavy-metal-induced tubulo-interstitial and tubular conditions**
> Code first poisoning due to drug or toxin, if applicable (T36-T65 with
>     fifth or sixth character 1-4 or 6)
> Use additional code for adverse effect, if applicable, to identify drug
>     (T36-T5Ø with fifth or sixth character 5)

**N14.Ø  Analgesic nephropathy**

**N14.1  Nephropathy induced by other drugs, medicaments and
        biological substances**

**N14.2  Nephropathy induced by unspecified drug, medicament or
        biological substance**

**N14.3  Nephropathy induced by heavy metals**

**N14.4  Toxic nephropathy, not elsewhere classified**

**√4ᵗʰ N15  Other renal tubulo-interstitial diseases**

**N15.Ø  Balkan nephropathy**
> Balkan endemic nephropathy

**N15.1  Renal and perinephric abscess**                           **MCC  H6**
> **CC Excl:** PDX collection 919

**N15.8  Other specified renal tubulo-interstitial diseases**

**N15.9  Renal tubulo-interstitial disease, unspecified**
> Infection of kidney NOS
> *EXCLUDES 1*  *urinary tract infection NOS (N39.Ø)*

**N16  *Renal tubulo-interstitial disorders in diseases classified elsewhere***
> Pyelonephritis
> Tubulo-interstitial nephritis
> Code first underlying disease, such as:
>     brucellosis (A23.Ø-A23.9)
>     cryoglobulinemia (D89.1)
>     glycogen storage disease (E74.Ø)
>     leukemia (C91-C95)
>     lymphoma (C81.Ø-C85.9, C96.Ø-C96.9)
>     multiple myeloma (C9Ø.Ø-)
>     sepsis (A4Ø.Ø-A41.9)
>     Wilson's disease (E83.Ø)
> *EXCLUDES 1*  *diphtheritic pyelonephritis and tubulo-interstitial nephritis
>                  (A36.84)*
>                  *pyelonephritis and tubulo-interstitial nephritis in candidiasis
>                  (B37.49)*
>                  *pyelonephritis and tubulo-interstitial nephritis in cystinosis
>                  (E72.Ø4)*
>                  *pyelonephritis and tubulo-interstitial nephritis in salmonella
>                  infection (AØ2.25)*
>                  *pyelonephritis and tubulo-interstitial nephritis in sarcoidosis
>                  (D86.84)*
>                  *pyelonephritis and tubulo-interstitial nephritis in sicca
>                  syndrome [Sjogren's] (M35.Ø4)*
>                  *pyelonephritis and tubulo-interstitial nephritis in systemic lupus
>                  erythematosus (M32.15)*
>                  *pyelonephritis and tubulo-interstitial nephritis in toxoplasmosis
>                  (B58.83)*
>                  *renal tubular degeneration in diabetes (EØ8-E13 with .29)*
>                  *syphilitic pyelonephritis and tubulo-interstitial nephritis
>                  (A52.75)*

---

✓Additional Character Req   ✓x7ᵗʰ Placeholder Alert   Unacceptable PDx   Manifestation   **H1**-**H14** HAC   **HCC** CMS-HCC Condition   *EXCLUDES 1* Not Coded Here   *EXCLUDES 2* Not Included Here

Chapter 14. Diseases of Genitourinary System

## Acute kidney failure and chronic kidney disease (N17-N19)

EXCLUDES 2   congenital renal failure (P96.0)
     drug- and heavy-metal-induced tubulo-interstitial and tubular
       conditions (N14.-)
     extrarenal uremia (R39.2)
     hemolytic-uremic syndrome (D59.3)
     hepatorenal syndrome (K76.7)
     postpartum hepatorenal syndrome (O90.4)
     posttraumatic renal failure (T79.5)
     prerenal uremia (R39.2)
     renal failure complicating abortion or ectopic or molar pregnancy (O00-
       O07, O08.4)
     renal failure following labor and delivery (O90.4)
     renal failure postprocedural (N99.0)

✓4ᵗʰ **N17 Acute kidney failure**
     Code also associated underlying condition
     EXCLUDES 1   posttraumatic renal failure (T79.5)
     **AHA:** 2013, 4Q, 124

     CC Excl: For CC/MCC codes in category N17: PDX collection 924

   **N17.0 Acute kidney failure with tubular necrosis**    MCC HCC
     Acute tubular necrosis
     Renal tubular necrosis
     Tubular necrosis NOS

   **N17.1 Acute kidney failure with acute cortical necrosis**    MCC HCC
     Acute cortical necrosis
     Cortical necrosis NOS
     Renal cortical necrosis

   **N17.2 Acute kidney failure with medullary necrosis**    MCC HCC
     Medullary [papillary] necrosis NOS
     Acute medullary [papillary] necrosis
     Renal medullary [papillary] necrosis

   **N17.8 Other acute kidney failure**    CC HCC
     CC Excl: PDX collection 925

   **N17.9 Acute kidney failure, unspecified**    CC HCC
     Acute kidney injury (nontraumatic)
     EXCLUDES 2   traumatic kidney injury (S37.0-)

✓4ᵗʰ **N18 Chronic kidney disease (CKD)**
     Code first any associated:
       diabetic chronic kidney disease (E08.22, E09.22, E10.22, E11.22,
         E13.22)
       hypertensive chronic kidney disease (I12-, I13-)
     Use additional code to identify kidney transplant status, if applicable,
       (Z94.0)
     **AHA:** 2013, 1Q, 24

   **N18.1 Chronic kidney disease, stage 1**

   **N18.2 Chronic kidney disease, stage 2 (mild)**

   **N18.3 Chronic kidney disease, stage 3 (moderate)**

   **N18.4 Chronic kidney disease, stage 4 (severe)**    CC HCC
     CC Excl: PDX collection 926

   **N18.5 Chronic kidney disease, stage 5**    CC HCC
     EXCLUDES 1   chronic kidney disease, stage 5 requiring chronic
         dialysis (N18.6)
     **DEF:** End-stage renal disease (ESRD) with GFR value of 15 ml/min
     or less not yet requiring chronic dialysis.
     CC Excl: PDX collection 926

   **N18.6 End stage renal disease**    MCC HCC
     Chronic kidney disease requiring chronic dialysis
     Use additional code to identify dialysis status (Z99.2)
     **AHA:** 2016, 3Q, 22; 2016, 1Q, 12; 2013, 4Q, 124-125
     CC Excl: PDX collection 927

   **N18.9 Chronic kidney disease, unspecified**
     Chronic renal disease
     Chronic renal failure NOS
     Chronic renal insufficiency
     ▶Chronic uremia NOS
     Diffuse sclerosing glomerulonephritis NOS◄

**N19 Unspecified kidney failure**
     Uremia NOS
     EXCLUDES 1   acute kidney failure (N17.-)
       chronic kidney disease (N18.-)
       chronic uremia (N18.9)
       extrarenal uremia (R39.2)
       prerenal uremia (R39.2)
       renal insufficiency (acute) (N28.9)
       uremia of newborn (P96.0)

## Urolithiasis (N20-N23)

   **AHA:** 2017, 1Q, 5; 2015, 2Q, 8

✓4ᵗʰ **N20 Calculus of kidney and ureter**
     Calculous pyelonephritis
     EXCLUDES 1   nephrocalcinosis (E83.5)
       that with hydronephrosis (N13.2)

   **N20.0 Calculus of kidney**
     Nephrolithiasis NOS
     Renal calculus
     Renal stone
     Staghorn calculus
     Stone in kidney

   **N20.1 Calculus of ureter**    CC
     Ureteric stone
     **AHA:** 2016, 3Q, 22
     CC Excl: PDX collection 928

   **N20.2 Calculus of kidney with calculus of ureter**    CC
     CC Excl: PDX collection 928

   **N20.9 Urinary calculus, unspecified**

✓4ᵗʰ **N21 Calculus of lower urinary tract**
     INCLUDES   calculus of lower urinary tract with cystitis and urethritis

   **N21.0 Calculus in bladder**
     Calculus in diverticulum of bladder
     Urinary bladder stone
     EXCLUDES 2   staghorn calculus (N20.0)

   **N21.1 Calculus in urethra**
     EXCLUDES 2   calculus of prostate (N42.0)

   **N21.8 Other lower urinary tract calculus**

   **N21.9 Calculus of lower urinary tract, unspecified**
     EXCLUDES 1   calculus of urinary tract NOS (N20.9)

***N22 Calculus of urinary tract in diseases classified elsewhere***
     Code first underlying disease, such as:
       gout (M1A.-, M10.-)
       schistosomiasis (B65.0-B65.9)

**N23 Unspecified renal colic**

## Other disorders of kidney and ureter (N25-N29)

   EXCLUDES 2   disorders of kidney and ureter with urolithiasis (N20-N23)

✓4ᵗʰ **N25 Disorders resulting from impaired renal tubular function**
     EXCLUDES 1   ~~metabolic disorders classifiable to E70-E88~~

   **N25.0 Renal osteodystrophy**
     Azotemic osteodystrophy
     Phosphate-losing tubular disorders
     Renal rickets
     Renal short stature
     EXCLUDES 2   ▶metabolic disorders classifiable to E70-E88◄

   **N25.1 Nephrogenic diabetes insipidus**    CC HCC
     EXCLUDES 1   diabetes insipidus NOS (E23.2)
     **DEF:** Type of diabetes due to inability of renal tubules to reabsorb
     water back into the body; not responsive to vasopressin
     (antidiuretic hormone); characterized by excessive thirst and
     excessive urine production; may develop into chronic renal
     insufficiency.
     CC Excl: PDX collection 929

✓5ᵗʰ **N25.8 Other disorders resulting from impaired renal tubular
     function**

     **N25.81 Secondary hyperparathyroidism of renal**    CC HCC
       **origin**
       EXCLUDES 1   secondary hyperparathyroidism, non-renal
         (E21.1)
       EXCLUDES 2   ▶metabolic disorders classifiable to
         E70-E88◄
       **DEF:** Parathyroid dysfunction caused by chronic renal
       failure; phosphate clearance is impaired, phosphate is
       released from bone, vitamin D is not produced,
       intestinal calcium absorption is low, and blood levels of
       calcium are lowered, causing excessive production of
       parathyroid hormone.
       CC Excl: PDX collection 930

     **N25.89 Other disorders resulting from impaired renal
       tubular function**
       Hypokalemic nephropathy
       Lightwood-Albright syndrome
       Renal tubular acidosis NOS

   **N25.9 Disorder resulting from impaired renal tubular function,
     unspecified**

Ⓝ Newborn: 0   Ⓟ Pediatric: 0-17   Ⓜ Maternity: 12-55   Ⓐ Adult: 15-124   MCC Major CC Condition   PDxMCC PDx acts as own MCC   CC CC Condition   PDxCC PDx acts as own CC

826                                                  ICD-10-CM 2018

☑4ᵗʰ **N26**   **Unspecified contracted kidney**
> *EXCLUDES 1*   *contracted kidney due to hypertension (I12.-)*
> *diffuse sclerosing glomerulonephritis (N05.8-)*
> *hypertensive nephrosclerosis (arteriolar) (arteriosclerotic) (I12.-)*
> *small kidney of unknown cause (N27.-)*

   **N26.1**   **Atrophy of kidney (terminal)**
   **N26.2**   **Page kidney**
   **N26.9**   **Renal sclerosis, unspecified**

☑4ᵗʰ **N27**   **Small kidney of unknown cause**
> **INCLUDES**   oligonephronia

   **N27.0**   **Small kidney, unilateral**
   **N27.1**   **Small kidney, bilateral**
   **N27.9**   **Small kidney, unspecified**

☑4ᵗʰ **N28**   **Other disorders of kidney and ureter, not elsewhere classified**
   **N28.0**   **Ischemia and infarction of kidney**    `CC` `HCC`
       Renal artery embolism
       Renal artery obstruction
       Renal artery occlusion
       Renal artery thrombosis
       Renal infarct
> *EXCLUDES 1*   *atherosclerosis of renal artery (extrarenal part) (I70.1)*
> *congenital stenosis of renal artery (Q27.1)*
> *Goldblatt's kidney (I70.1)*

       **CC Excl:** PDX collection 931

   **N28.1**   **Cyst of kidney, acquired**
       ►Cyst (multiple) (solitary) of kidney (acquired)◄
> *EXCLUDES 1*   *cystic kidney disease (congenital) (Q61.-)*

☑5ᵗʰ   **N28.8**   **Other specified disorders of kidney and ureter**
> *EXCLUDES 1*   *hydroureter (N13.4)*
> *ureteric stricture with hydronephrosis (N13.1)*
> *ureteric stricture without hydronephrosis (N13.5)*

       **CC Excl: For CC codes in subcategory N28.8:**
       PDX collection 922

     **N28.81**   **Hypertrophy of kidney**
     **N28.82**   **Megaloureter**
     **N28.83**   **Nephroptosis**
     **N28.84**   **Pyelitis cystica**    `CC` `H6`
     **N28.85**   **Pyeloureteritis cystica**    `CC` `H6`
     **N28.86**   **Ureteritis cystica**    `CC` `H6`
     **N28.89**   **Other specified disorders of kidney and ureter**

   **N28.9**   **Disorder of kidney and ureter, unspecified**
       Nephropathy NOS
       Renal disease (acute) NOS
       Renal insufficiency (acute)
> *EXCLUDES 1*   *chronic renal insufficiency (N18.9)*
> *unspecified nephritic syndrome (N05.-)*

       **AHA:** 2016, 1Q, 13

*N29*   *Other disorders of kidney and ureter in diseases classified elsewhere*
       Code first underlying disease, such as:
       amyloidosis (E85.-)
       nephrocalcinosis (E83.5)
       schistosomiasis (B65.0-B65.9)
> *EXCLUDES 1*   *disorders of kidney and ureter in:*
> *cystinosis (E72.0)*
> *gonorrhea (A54.21)*
> *syphilis (A52.75)*
> *tuberculosis (A18.11)*

### Other diseases of the urinary system (N30-N39)
> *EXCLUDES 1*   *urinary infection (complicating):*
> *abortion or ectopic or molar pregnancy (O00-O07, O08.8)*
> *pregnancy, childbirth and the puerperium (O23-, O75.3, O86.2-)*

☑4ᵗʰ **N30**   **Cystitis**
       Use additional code to identify infectious agent (B95-B97)
> *EXCLUDES 1*   *prostatocystitis (N41.3)*

       **AHA:** 2017, 1Q, 6

       **CC Excl: For CC codes in category N30:** PDX collection 932

☑5ᵗʰ   **N30.0**   **Acute cystitis**
> *EXCLUDES 1*   *irradiation cystitis (N30.4-)*
> *trigonitis (N30.3-)*

     **N30.00**   **Acute cystitis without hematuria**    `CC` `H6`
     **N30.01**   **Acute cystitis with hematuria**    `CC` `H6`

☑5ᵗʰ   **N30.1**   **Interstitial cystitis (chronic)**
     **N30.10**   **Interstitial cystitis (chronic) without hematuria**
     **N30.11**   **Interstitial cystitis (chronic) with hematuria**

☑5ᵗʰ   **N30.2**   **Other chronic cystitis**
     **N30.20**   **Other chronic cystitis without hematuria**
     **N30.21**   **Other chronic cystitis with hematuria**

☑5ᵗʰ   **N30.3**   **Trigonitis**
       Urethrotrigonitis
     **N30.30**   **Trigonitis without hematuria**
     **N30.31**   **Trigonitis with hematuria**

☑5ᵗʰ   **N30.4**   **Irradiation cystitis**
     **N30.40**   **Irradiation cystitis without hematuria**    `CC`
     **N30.41**   **Irradiation cystitis with hematuria**    `CC`

☑5ᵗʰ   **N30.8**   **Other cystitis**
       Abscess of bladder
     **N30.80**   **Other cystitis without hematuria**
     **N30.81**   **Other cystitis with hematuria**

☑5ᵗʰ   **N30.9**   **Cystitis, unspecified**
     **N30.90**   **Cystitis, unspecified without hematuria**
     **N30.91**   **Cystitis, unspecified with hematuria**

☑4ᵗʰ **N31**   **Neuromuscular dysfunction of bladder, not elsewhere classified**
       Use additional code to identify any associated urinary incontinence (N39.3-N39.4-)
> *EXCLUDES 1*   *cord bladder NOS (G95.89)*
> *neurogenic bladder due to cauda equina syndrome (G83.4)*
> *neuromuscular dysfunction due to spinal cord lesion (G95.89)*

   **N31.0**   **Uninhibited neuropathic bladder, not elsewhere classified**
   **N31.1**   **Reflex neuropathic bladder, not elsewhere classified**
   **N31.2**   **Flaccid neuropathic bladder, not elsewhere classified**
       Atonic (motor) (sensory) neuropathic bladder
       Autonomous neuropathic bladder
       Nonreflex neuropathic bladder
   **N31.8**   **Other neuromuscular dysfunction of bladder**
   **N31.9**   **Neuromuscular dysfunction of bladder, unspecified**
       Neurogenic bladder dysfunction NOS

☑4ᵗʰ **N32**   **Other disorders of bladder**
> *EXCLUDES 2*   *calculus of bladder (N21.0)*
> *cystocele (N81.1-)*
> *hernia or prolapse of bladder, female (N81.1-)*

   **N32.0**   **Bladder-neck obstruction**
       Bladder-neck stenosis (acquired)
> *EXCLUDES 1*   *congenital bladder-neck obstruction (Q64.3-)*

       **DEF:** Bladder outlet and vesicourethral obstruction; occurs as a consequence of benign prostatic hypertrophy or prostatic cancer; may also occur in either sex due to strictures, radiation, cystoscopy, catheterization, injury, infection, blood clots, bladder cancer, impaction, or other disease that compresses the bladder neck.

   **N32.1**   **Vesicointestinal fistula**    `CC`
       Vesicorectal fistula
       **CC Excl:** PDX collection 933

   **N32.2**   **Vesical fistula, not elsewhere classified**    `CC`
> *EXCLUDES 1*   *fistula between bladder and female genital tract (N82.0-N82.1)*

       **CC Excl:** PDX collection 933

   **N32.3**   **Diverticulum of bladder**
> *EXCLUDES 1*   *congenital diverticulum of bladder (Q64.6)*
> *diverticulitis of bladder (N30.8-)*

☑5ᵗʰ   **N32.8**   **Other specified disorders of bladder**
     **N32.81**   **Overactive bladder**
       Detrusor muscle hyperactivity
> *EXCLUDES 1*   *frequent urination due to specified bladder condition—code to condition*

       **DEF:** Sudden involuntary contractions of the muscular wall of bladder; results in sudden, strong urge to urinate.

     **N32.89**   **Other specified disorders of bladder**
       Bladder hemorrhage
       Bladder hypertrophy
       Calcified bladder
       Contracted bladder

   **N32.9**   **Bladder disorder, unspecified**

☑ Additional Character Req   ☑x7ᵗʰ Placeholder Alert   Unacceptable PDx   Manifestation   `H1`-`H14` HAC   `HCC` CMS-HCC Condition   *EXCLUDES 1* Not Coded Here   *EXCLUDES 2* Not Included Here

ICD-10-CM 2018                              **827**

**N26–N32.9**

**Chapter 14. Diseases of Genitourinary System**

**N33** *Bladder disorders in diseases classified elsewhere*
Code first underlying disease, such as:
schistosomiasis (B65.0-B65.9)
*EXCLUDES 1*    *bladder disorder in syphilis (A52.76)*
*bladder disorder in tuberculosis (A18.12)*
*candidal cystitis (B37.41)*
*chlamydial cystitis (A56.01)*
*cystitis in gonorrhea (A54.01)*
*cystitis in neurogenic bladder (N31.-)*
*diphtheritic cystitis (A36.85)*
*neurogenic bladder (N31.-)*
*syphilitic cystitis (A52.76)*
*trichomonal cystitis (A59.03)*

**√4ᵗʰ N34** **Urethritis and urethral syndrome**
Use additional code (B95-B97), to identify infectious agent
*EXCLUDES 2*    *Reiter's disease (M02.3-)*
*urethritis in diseases with a predominantly sexual mode of*
*transmission (A50-A64)*
*urethrotrigonitis (N30.3-)*
**AHA:** 2017, 1Q, 6

**N34.0** **Urethral abscess**      CC H6
Abscess (of) Cowper's gland
Abscess (of) Littrés gland
Abscess (of) urethral (gland)
Periurethral abscess
*EXCLUDES 1*    *urethral caruncle (N36.2)*
**CC Excl:** PDX collection 934

**N34.1** **Nonspecific urethritis**
Nongonococcal urethritis
Nonvenereal urethritis

**N34.2** **Other urethritis**
Meatitis, urethral
Postmenopausal urethritis
Ulcer of urethra (meatus)
Urethritis NOS

**N34.3** **Urethral syndrome, unspecified**

**√4ᵗʰ N35** **Urethral stricture**
*EXCLUDES 1*    *congenital urethral stricture (Q64.3-)*
*postprocedural urethral stricture (N99.1-)*

**√5ᵗʰ N35.0** **Post-traumatic urethral stricture**
Urethral stricture due to injury
*EXCLUDES 1*    *postprocedural urethral stricture (N99.1-)*

   **√6ᵗʰ N35.01** **Post-traumatic urethral stricture, male**
     **N35.010** **Post-traumatic urethral stricture,**    ♂
**male, meatal**
     **N35.011** **Post-traumatic bulbous urethral**    ♂
**stricture**
     **N35.012** **Post-traumatic membranous urethral**    ♂
**stricture**
     **N35.013** **Post-traumatic anterior urethral**    ♂
**stricture**
     **N35.014** **Post-traumatic urethral stricture,**    ♂
**male, unspecified**

   **√6ᵗʰ N35.02** **Post-traumatic urethral stricture, female**
     **N35.021** **Urethral stricture due to childbirth**    ♀
     **N35.028** **Other post-traumatic urethral stricture,**    ♀
**female**

**√5ᵗʰ N35.1** **Postinfective urethral stricture, not elsewhere classified**
*EXCLUDES 1*    *urethral stricture associated with schistosomiasis*
*(B65-, N29)*
*gonococcal urethral stricture (A54.01)*
*syphilitic urethral stricture (A52.76)*

   **√6ᵗʰ N35.11** **Postinfective urethral stricture, not elsewhere**
**classified, male**
     **N35.111** **Postinfective urethral stricture, not**    ♂
**elsewhere classified, male, meatal**
▲      **N35.112** **Postinfective bulbous urethral**    ♂
**stricture, not elsewhere classified, male**
▲      **N35.113** **Postinfective membranous urethral**    ♂
**stricture, not elsewhere classified, male**
▲      **N35.114** **Postinfective anterior urethral**    ♂
**stricture, not elsewhere classified, male**
     **N35.119** **Postinfective urethral stricture, not**    ♂
**elsewhere classified, male, unspecified**
   **N35.12** **Postinfective urethral stricture, not elsewhere**    ♀
**classified, female**

**N35.8** **Other urethral stricture**
*EXCLUDES 1*    *postprocedural urethral stricture (N99.1-)*

**N35.9** **Urethral stricture, unspecified**

**√4ᵗʰ N36** **Other disorders of urethra**
**N36.0** **Urethral fistula**      CC
Urethroperineal fistula
Urethrorectal fistula
Urinary fistula NOS
*EXCLUDES 1*    *urethroscrotal fistula (N50.89)*
*urethrovaginal fistula (N82.1)*
*urethrovesicovaginal fistula (N82.1)*
**CC Excl:** PDX collection 935

**N36.1** **Urethral diverticulum**
**N36.2** **Urethral caruncle**

**√5ᵗʰ N36.4** **Urethral functional and muscular disorders**
Use additional code to identify associated urinary stress
incontinence (N39.3)

**N36.41** **Hypermobility of urethra**
**N36.42** **Intrinsic sphincter deficiency (ISD)**
**N36.43** **Combined hypermobility of urethra and intrinsic**
**sphincter deficiency**
**N36.44** **Muscular disorders of urethra**
Bladder sphincter dyssynergy

**N36.5** **Urethral false passage**
**N36.8** **Other specified disorders of urethra**
*EXCLUDES 1*    *congenital urethrocele (Q64.7)*
*female urethrocele (N81.0)*

**N36.9** **Urethral disorder, unspecified**

**N37** *Urethral disorders in diseases classified elsewhere*
Code first underlying disease
*EXCLUDES 1*    *urethritis (in):*
*candidal infection (B37.41)*
*chlamydial (A56.01)*
*gonorrhea (A54.01)*
*syphilis (A52.76)*
*trichomonal infection (A59.03)*
*tuberculosis (A18.13)*

**√4ᵗʰ N39** **Other disorders of urinary system**
*EXCLUDES 2*    *hematuria NOS (R31.-)*
*recurrent or persistent hematuria (N02.-)*
*recurrent or persistent hematuria with specified morphological*
*lesion (N02.-)*
*proteinuria NOS (R80.-)*

**N39.0** **Urinary tract infection, site not specified**      CC H6
Use additional code (B95-B97), to identify infectious agent
*EXCLUDES 1*    *candidiasis of urinary tract (B37.4-)*
*neonatal urinary tract infection (P39.3)*
*urinary tract infection of specified site, such as:*
*cystitis (N30.-)*
*urethritis (N34.-)*
**AHA:** 2017, 1Q, 6; 2012, 4Q, 94
**CC Excl:** PDX collection 936

**N39.3** **Stress incontinence (female) (male)**
Code also any associated overactive bladder (N32.81)
*EXCLUDES 1*    *mixed incontinence (N39.46)*

**√5ᵗʰ N39.4** **Other specified urinary incontinence**
Code also any associated overactive bladder (N32.81)
*EXCLUDES 1*    *enuresis NOS (R32)*
*functional urinary incontinence (R39.81)*
*urinary incontinence associated with cognitive*
*impairment (R39.81)*
*urinary incontinence NOS (R32)*
*urinary incontinence of nonorganic origin (F98.0)*

**N39.41** **Urge incontinence**
*EXCLUDES 1*    *mixed incontinence (N39.46)*
**N39.42** **Incontinence without sensory awareness**
Insensible (urinary) incontinence
**N39.43** **Post-void dribbling**
**N39.44** **Nocturnal enuresis**
**N39.45** **Continuous leakage**
**N39.46** **Mixed incontinence**
Urge and stress incontinence

   **√6ᵗʰ N39.49** **Other specified urinary incontinence**
     **N39.490** **Overflow incontinence**
     **N39.491** **Coital incontinence**
     **N39.492** **Postural (urinary) incontinence**

N Newborn: 0   P Pediatric: 0-17   M Maternity: 12-55   A Adult: 15-124   MCC Major CC Condition   PDxMCC PDx acts as own MCC   CC CC Condition   PDxCC PDx acts as own CC

828          ICD-10-CM 2018

**N39.498**   **Other specified urinary incontinence**
Reflex incontinence
Total incontinence

**N39.8**   **Other specified disorders of urinary system**

**N39.9**   **Disorder of urinary system, unspecified**

### Diseases of male genital organs (N40-N53)

✓4ᵗʰ **N40**   **Benign prostatic hyperplasia**
   INCLUDES   adenofibromatous hypertrophy of prostate
          benign hypertrophy of the prostate
          benign prostatic hypertrophy
          BPH
          enlarged prostate
          nodular prostate
          polyp of prostate
   EXCLUDES 1   benign neoplasms of prostate (adenoma, benign)
          (fibroadenoma) (fibroma) (myoma) (D29.1)
   EXCLUDES 2   malignant neoplasm of prostate (C61)

**N40.0**   **Benign prostatic hyperplasia** without lower    A♂
**urinary tract symptoms**
Enlarged prostate NOS
Enlarged prostate without LUTS

**N40.1**   **Benign prostatic hyperplasia** with lower urinary tract   A♂
**symptoms**
Enlarged prostate with LUTS
Use additional code for associated symptoms, when specified:
    incomplete bladder emptying (R39.14)
    nocturia (R35.1)
    straining on urination (R39.16)
    urinary frequency (R35.0)
    urinary hesitancy (R39.11)
    urinary incontinence (N39.4-)
    urinary obstruction (N13.8)
    urinary retention (R33.8)
    urinary urgency (R39.15)
    weak urinary stream (R39.12)

**N40.2**   **Nodular** prostate without lower urinary tract symptoms   A♂
Nodular prostate without LUTS

**N40.3**   **Nodular** prostate with lower urinary tract symptoms   A♂
Use additional code for associated symptoms, when specified:
    incomplete bladder emptying (R39.14)
    nocturia (R35.1)
    straining on urination (R39.16)
    urinary frequency (R35.0)
    urinary hesitancy (R39.11)
    urinary incontinence (N39.4-)
    urinary obstruction (N13.8)
    urinary retention (R33.8)
    urinary urgency (R39.15)
    weak urinary stream (R39.12)

✓4ᵗʰ **N41**   **Inflammatory diseases of prostate**
Use additional code (B95-B97), to identify infectious agent

**N41.0**   **Acute prostatitis**    CC A♂
    **CC Excl:** PDX collection 937

**N41.1**   **Chronic prostatitis**    A♂

**N41.2**   **Abscess of prostate**    CC A♂
    **CC Excl:** PDX collection 937

**N41.3**   **Prostatocystitis**    A♂

**N41.4**   **Granulomatous prostatitis**    A♂

**N41.8**   **Other inflammatory diseases of prostate**    A♂

**N41.9**   **Inflammatory disease of prostate, unspecified**    A♂
Prostatitis NOS

✓4ᵗʰ **N42**   **Other and unspecified disorders of prostate**

**N42.0**   **Calculus of prostate**    A♂
Prostatic stone
**DEF:** Formation of small, solid stone often composed of calcium
carbonate or calcium phosphate in the prostate gland.

**N42.1**   **Congestion and hemorrhage of prostate**    A♂
   EXCLUDES 1   enlarged prostate (N40.-)
          hematuria (R31.-)
          hyperplasia of prostate (N40.-)
          inflammatory diseases of prostate (N41.-)

✓5ᵗʰ **N42.3**   **Dysplasia of prostate**

**N42.30**   **Unspecified dysplasia of prostate**    ♂

---

**N42.31**   **Prostatic intraepithelial neoplasia**    ♂
PIN
Prostatic intraepithelial neoplasia I (PIN I)
Prostatic intraepithelial neoplasia II (PIN II)
   EXCLUDES 1   prostatic intraepithelial neoplasia III (PIN III)
          (D07.5)
**DEF:** Abnormality of shape and size of the intraepithelial
tissues of the prostate; premalignant condition
characterized by stalks and absence of a basilar cell
layer; synonyms are intraductal dysplasia, large acinar
atypical hyperplasia, atypical primary hyperplasia,
hyperplasia with malignant changes, marked atypia, or
duct-acinar dysplasia.

**N42.32**   **Atypical small acinar proliferation of prostate**   ♂

**N42.39**   **Other dysplasia of prostate**    ♂

✓5ᵗʰ **N42.8**   **Other specified disorders of prostate**

**N42.81**   **Prostatodynia syndrome**    A♂
Painful prostate syndrome

**N42.82**   **Prostatosis syndrome**    A♂

**N42.83**   **Cyst of prostate**    A♂

**N42.89**   **Other specified disorders of prostate**    A♂

**N42.9**   **Disorder of prostate, unspecified**    A♂

✓4ᵗʰ **N43**   **Hydrocele and spermatocele**
   INCLUDES   hydrocele of spermatic cord, testis or tunica vaginalis
   EXCLUDES 1   congenital hydrocele (P83.5)

**N43.0**   **Encysted hydrocele**    ♂

**N43.1**   **Infected hydrocele**    CC ♂
    Use additional code (B95-B97), to identify infectious agent
    **CC Excl:** PDX collection 938

**N43.2**   **Other hydrocele**    ♂

**N43.3**   **Hydrocele, unspecified**    ♂

✓5ᵗʰ **N43.4**   **Spermatocele of epididymis**
Spermatic cyst

**N43.40**   **Spermatocele of epididymis, unspecified**   ♂

**N43.41**   **Spermatocele of epididymis, single**    ♂

**N43.42**   **Spermatocele of epididymis, multiple**    ♂

✓4ᵗʰ **N44**   **Noninflammatory disorders of testis**

    **CC Excl: For CC codes in category N44:** PDX collection 939

✓5ᵗʰ **N44.0**   **Torsion of testis**

**N44.00**   **Torsion of testis, unspecified**    CC ♂

**N44.01**   **Extravaginal torsion of spermatic cord**    CC ♂
**DEF:** Torsion of the spermatic cord just below the tunica
vaginalis attachments.

**N44.02**   **Intravaginal torsion of spermatic cord**    CC ♂
Torsion of spermatic cord NOS

**N44.03**   **Torsion of appendix testis**    CC ♂

**N44.04**   **Torsion of appendix epididymis**    CC ♂

**N44.1**   **Cyst of tunica albuginea testis**    ♂

**N44.2**   **Benign cyst of testis**    ♂

**N44.8**   **Other noninflammatory disorders of the testis**    ♂

✓4ᵗʰ **N45**   **Orchitis and epididymitis**
Use additional code (B95-B97), to identify infectious agent

**N45.1**   **Epididymitis**    ♂

**N45.2**   **Orchitis**    ♂

**N45.3**   **Epididymo-orchitis**    ♂

**N45.4**   **Abscess of epididymis or testis**    CC ♂
    **CC Excl:** PDX collection 940

**Hydrocele**

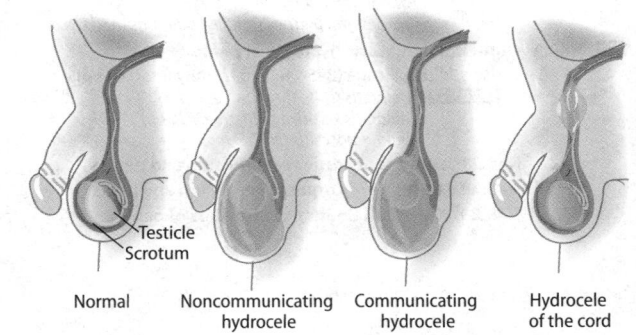

Normal     Noncommunicating hydrocele     Communicating hydrocele     Hydrocele of the cord

Testicle
Scrotum

---

☑ Additional Character Req   ✓x7ᵗʰ Placeholder Alert   Unacceptable PDx   Manifestation   H1-H14 HAC   HCC CMS-HCC Condition   EXCLUDES 1 Not Coded Here   EXCLUDES 2 Not Included Here

**ICD-10-CM 2018**          **829**

**☑4ᵗʰ N46 Male infertility**
> EXCLUDES 1   vasectomy status (Z98.52)

**☑5ᵗʰ N46.0 Azoospermia**
Absolute male infertility
Male infertility due to germinal (cell) aplasia
Male infertility due to spermatogenic arrest (complete)

    **N46.01 Organic azoospermia**    A ♂
        Azoospermia NOS

    **☑6ᵗʰ N46.02 Azoospermia due to extratesticular causes**
        Code also associated cause
        **N46.021 Azoospermia due to drug therapy**   A ♂
        **N46.022 Azoospermia due to infection**   A ♂
        **N46.023 Azoospermia due to obstruction of**   A ♂
           **efferent ducts**
        **N46.024 Azoospermia due to radiation**   A ♂
        **N46.025 Azoospermia due to systemic disease**   A ♂
        **N46.029 Azoospermia due to other**   A ♂
           **extratesticular causes**

**☑5ᵗʰ N46.1 Oligospermia**
Male infertility due to germinal cell desquamation
Male infertility due to hypospermatogenesis
Male infertility due to incomplete spermatogenic arrest

    **N46.11 Organic oligospermia**   A ♂
        Oligospermia NOS

    **☑6ᵗʰ N46.12 Oligospermia due to extratesticular causes**
        Code also associated cause
        **N46.121 Oligospermia due to drug therapy**   A ♂
        **N46.122 Oligospermia due to infection**   A ♂
        **N46.123 Oligospermia due to obstruction of**   A ♂
           **efferent ducts**
        **N46.124 Oligospermia due to radiation**   A ♂
        **N46.125 Oligospermia due to systemic disease**   A ♂
        **N46.129 Oligospermia due to other**   A ♂
           **extratesticular causes**

**N46.8 Other male infertility**   A ♂
**N46.9 Male infertility, unspecified**   A ♂

**☑4ᵗʰ N47 Disorders of prepuce**
**N47.0 Adherent prepuce, newborn**   N ♂
**N47.1 Phimosis**   ♂
**N47.2 Paraphimosis**   ♂
**N47.3 Deficient foreskin**   ♂
**N47.4 Benign cyst of prepuce**   ♂
**N47.5 Adhesions of prepuce and glans penis**   ♂
**N47.6 Balanoposthitis**   ♂
> Use additional code (B95-B97), to identify infectious agent
> EXCLUDES 1   balanitis (N48.1)

**N47.7 Other inflammatory diseases of prepuce**   ♂
> Use additional code (B95-B97), to identify infectious agent

**N47.8 Other disorders of prepuce**   ♂

**☑4ᵗʰ N48 Other disorders of penis**
**N48.0 Leukoplakia of penis**   ♂
Balanitis xerotica obliterans
Kraurosis of penis
Lichen sclerosus of external male genital organs
> EXCLUDES 1   carcinoma in situ of penis (D07.4)

**N48.1 Balanitis**   ♂
> Use additional code (B95-B97), to identify infectious agent
> EXCLUDES 1   amebic balanitis (A06.8)
>           balanitis xerotica obliterans (N48.0)
>           candidal balanitis (B37.42)
>           gonococcal balanitis (A54.23)
>           herpesviral [herpes simplex] balanitis (A60.01)

**☑5ᵗʰ N48.2 Other inflammatory disorders of penis**
> Use additional code (B95-B97), to identify infectious agent
> EXCLUDES 1   balanitis (N48.1)
>           balanitis xerotica obliterans (N48.0)
>           balanoposthitis (N47.6)

    **N48.21 Abscess of corpus cavernosum and penis**   ♂
    **N48.22 Cellulitis of corpus cavernosum and penis**   ♂
    **N48.29 Other inflammatory disorders of penis**   ♂

**☑5ᵗʰ N48.3 Priapism**
Painful erection
Code first underlying cause

> **CC Excl: For CC codes in subcategory N48.3:**
> PDX collection 941

    **N48.30 Priapism, unspecified**   CC ♂
    **N48.31 Priapism due to trauma**   CC ♂
    *N48.32 Priapism due to disease classified elsewhere*   CC ♂
    **N48.33 Priapism, drug-induced**   CC ♂
    **N48.39 Other priapism**   CC ♂

**N48.5 Ulcer of penis**   ♂
**N48.6 Induration penis plastica**   ♂
Peyronie's disease
Plastic induration of penis

**☑5ᵗʰ N48.8 Other specified disorders of penis**
    **N48.81 Thrombosis of superficial vein of penis**   ♂
    **N48.82 Acquired torsion of penis**   ♂
        Acquired torsion of penis NOS
        > EXCLUDES 1   congenital torsion of penis (Q55.63)
    **N48.83 Acquired buried penis**   ♂
        > EXCLUDES 1   congenital hidden penis (Q55.64)
    **N48.89 Other specified disorders of penis**   ♂

**N48.9 Disorder of penis, unspecified**   ♂

**☑4ᵗʰ N49 Inflammatory disorders of male genital organs, not elsewhere classified**
> Use additional code (B95-B97), to identify infectious agent
> EXCLUDES 1   inflammation of penis (N48.1, N48.2-)
>           orchitis and epididymitis (N45.-)

**N49.0 Inflammatory disorders of seminal vesicle**   ♂
Vesiculitis NOS
**N49.1 Inflammatory disorders of spermatic cord, tunica**   ♂
**vaginalis and vas deferens**
Vasitis
**N49.2 Inflammatory disorders of scrotum**   ♂
**N49.3 Fournier gangrene**   ♂
**N49.8 Inflammatory disorders of other specified male genital**   ♂
**organs**
Inflammation of multiple sites in male genital organs
**N49.9 Inflammatory disorder of unspecified male genital**   ♂
**organ**
Abscess of unspecified male genital organ
Boil of unspecified male genital organ
Carbuncle of unspecified male genital organ
Cellulitis of unspecified male genital organ

**☑4ᵗʰ N50 Other and unspecified disorders of male genital organs**
> EXCLUDES 2   torsion of testis (N44.0-)

**N50.0 Atrophy of testis**   ♂
**N50.1 Vascular disorders of male genital organs**   ♂
Hematocele, NOS, of male genital organs
Hemorrhage of male genital organs
Thrombosis of male genital organs
**N50.3 Cyst of epididymis**   ♂

**☑5ᵗʰ N50.8 Other specified disorders of male genital organs**
    **☑6ᵗʰ N50.81 Testicular pain**
        **N50.811 Right testicular pain**   ♂
        **N50.812 Left testicular pain**   ♂
        **N50.819 Testicular pain, unspecified**   ♂
    **N50.82 Scrotal pain**   ♂
    **N50.89 Other specified disorders of the male genital**   ♂
        **organs**
        Atrophy of scrotum, seminal vesicle, spermatic cord, tunica vaginalis and vas deferens
        Chylocele, tunica vaginalis (nonfilarial) NOS
        Edema of scrotum, seminal vesicle, spermatic cord, tunica vaginalis and vas deferens
        Hypertrophy of scrotum, seminal vesicle, spermatic cord, tunica vaginalis and vas deferens
        Stricture of spermatic cord, tunica vaginalis, and vas deferens
        Ulcer of scrotum, seminal vesicle, spermatic cord, testis, tunica vaginalis and vas deferens
        Urethroscrotal fistula

**N50.9 Disorder of male genital organs, unspecified**   ♂

N Newborn: 0   P Pediatric: 0-17   M Maternity: 12-55   A Adult: 15-124   MCC Major CC Condition   PDxMCC PDx acts as own MCC   CC CC Condition   PDxCC PDx acts as own CC

830                                     ICD-10-CM 2018

**N51  Disorders of male genital organs in diseases classified elsewhere**                                                        ♂
    Code first underlying disease, such as:
      filariasis (B74.0-B74.9)
    *EXCLUDES 1*  amebic balanitis (A06.8)
          candidal balanitis (B37.42)
          gonococcal balanitis (A54.23)
          gonococcal prostatitis (A54.22)
          herpesviral [herpes simplex] balanitis (A60.01)
          trichomonal prostatitis (A59.02)
          tuberculous prostatitis (A18.14)

**✓4th N52  Male erectile dysfunction**
    *EXCLUDES 1*  psychogenic impotence (F52.21)

   **✓5th N52.0  Vasculogenic erectile dysfunction**
      **N52.01  Erectile dysfunction due to arterial insufficiency**  A ♂
      **N52.02  Corporo-venous occlusive erectile dysfunction**  A ♂
      **N52.03  Combined arterial insufficiency and corporo-venous occlusive erectile dysfunction**  A ♂

   **N52.1  Erectile dysfunction due to diseases classified elsewhere**
      Code first underlying disease

   **N52.2  Drug-induced erectile dysfunction**  A ♂

   **✓5th N52.3  Postprocedural erectile dysfunction**
      **N52.31  Erectile dysfunction following radical prostatectomy**  A ♂
      **N52.32  Erectile dysfunction following radical cystectomy**  A ♂
      **N52.33  Erectile dysfunction following urethral surgery**  A ♂
      **N52.34  Erectile dysfunction following simple prostatectomy**  A ♂
      **N52.35  Erectile dysfunction following radiation therapy**  A ♂
      **N52.36  Erectile dysfunction following interstitial seed therapy**  A ♂
      **N52.37  Erectile dysfunction following prostate ablative therapy**  A ♂
         Erectile dysfunction following cryotherapy
         Erectile dysfunction following other prostate ablative therapies
         Erectile dysfunction following ultrasound ablative therapies
      **N52.39  Other and unspecified postprocedural erectile dysfunction**  A ♂

   **N52.8  Other male erectile dysfunction**  A ♂
   **N52.9  Male erectile dysfunction, unspecified**  A ♂
      Impotence NOS

**✓4th N53  Other male sexual dysfunction**
    *EXCLUDES 1*  psychogenic sexual dysfunction (F52.-)

   **✓5th N53.1  Ejaculatory dysfunction**
    *EXCLUDES 1*  premature ejaculation (F52.4)
      **N53.11  Retarded ejaculation**  ♂
      **N53.12  Painful ejaculation**  ♂
      **N53.13  Anejaculatory orgasm**  ♂
      **N53.14  Retrograde ejaculation**  ♂
         **DEF:** A form of male sexual dysfunction in which the semen enters the bladder instead of going out through the urethra during ejaculation.
      **N53.19  Other ejaculatory dysfunction**  ♂
         Ejaculatory dysfunction NOS

   **N53.8  Other male sexual dysfunction**  ♂
   **N53.9  Unspecified male sexual dysfunction**  ♂

### Disorders of breast (N60-N65)

*EXCLUDES 1*  disorders of breast associated with childbirth (O91-O92)

**✓4th N60  Benign mammary dysplasia**
    *INCLUDES*  fibrocystic mastopathy

   **✓5th N60.0  Solitary cyst of breast**
      Cyst of breast
      **N60.01  Solitary cyst of right breast**
      **N60.02  Solitary cyst of left breast**
      **N60.09  Solitary cyst of unspecified breast**

   **✓5th N60.1  Diffuse cystic mastopathy**
      Cystic breast
      Fibrocystic disease of breast
    *EXCLUDES 1*  diffuse cystic mastopathy with epithelial proliferation (N60.3-)
      **N60.11  Diffuse cystic mastopathy of right breast**  A
      **N60.12  Diffuse cystic mastopathy of left breast**  A
      **N60.19  Diffuse cystic mastopathy of unspecified breast**  A

   **✓5th N60.2  Fibroadenosis of breast**
      Adenofibrosis of breast
    *EXCLUDES 2*  fibroadenoma of breast (D24.-)
      **N60.21  Fibroadenosis of right breast**
      **N60.22  Fibroadenosis of left breast**
      **N60.29  Fibroadenosis of unspecified breast**

   **✓5th N60.3  Fibrosclerosis of breast**
      Cystic mastopathy with epithelial proliferation
      **N60.31  Fibrosclerosis of right breast**
      **N60.32  Fibrosclerosis of left breast**
      **N60.39  Fibrosclerosis of unspecified breast**

   **✓5th N60.4  Mammary duct ectasia**
      **N60.41  Mammary duct ectasia of right breast**
      **N60.42  Mammary duct ectasia of left breast**
      **N60.49  Mammary duct ectasia of unspecified breast**

   **✓5th N60.8  Other benign mammary dysplasias**
      **N60.81  Other benign mammary dysplasias of right breast**
      **N60.82  Other benign mammary dysplasias of left breast**
      **N60.89  Other benign mammary dysplasias of unspecified breast**

   **✓5th N60.9  Unspecified benign mammary dysplasia**
      **N60.91  Unspecified benign mammary dysplasia of right breast**
      **N60.92  Unspecified benign mammary dysplasia of left breast**
      **N60.99  Unspecified benign mammary dysplasia of unspecified breast**

**✓4th N61  Inflammatory disorders of breast**
    *EXCLUDES 1*  inflammatory carcinoma of breast (C50.9)
          inflammatory disorder of breast associated with childbirth (O91.-)
          neonatal infective mastitis (P39.0)
          thrombophlebitis of breast [Mondor's disease] (I80.8)

   **N61.0  Mastitis without abscess**
      Infective mastitis (acute) (nonpuerperal) (subacute)
      Mastitis (acute) (nonpuerperal) (subacute) NOS
      Cellulitis (acute) (nonpuerperal) (subacute) of breast NOS
      Cellulitis (acute) (nonpuerperal) (subacute) of nipple NOS

   **N61.1  Abscess of the breast and nipple**
      Abscess (acute) (chronic) (nonpuerperal) of areola
      Abscess (acute) (chronic) (nonpuerperal) of breast
      Carbuncle of breast
      Mastitis with abscess

**N62  Hypertrophy of breast**
    Gynecomastia
    Hypertrophy of breast NOS
    Massive pubertal hypertrophy of breast
    *EXCLUDES 1*  breast engorgement of newborn (P83.4)
          disproportion of reconstructed breast (N65.1)

**✓4th N63  Unspecified lump in breast**
    Nodule(s) NOS in breast

   ● **N63.0  Unspecified lump in unspecified breast**

   ● **✓5th N63.1  Unspecified lump in the right breast**
      ● **N63.10  Unspecified lump in the right breast, unspecified quadrant**
      ● **N63.11  Unspecified lump in the right breast, upper outer quadrant**
      ● **N63.12  Unspecified lump in the right breast, upper inner quadrant**
      ● **N63.13  Unspecified lump in the right breast, lower outer quadrant**
      ● **N63.14  Unspecified lump in the right breast, lower inner quadrant**

   ● **✓5th N63.2  Unspecified lump in the left breast**
      ● **N63.20  Unspecified lump in the left breast, unspecified quadrant**
      ● **N63.21  Unspecified lump in the left breast, upper outer quadrant**

✓ Additional Character Req  ✓x7th Placeholder Alert  Unacceptable PDx  Manifestation  H1-H14 HAC  HCC CMS-HCC Condition  *EXCLUDES 1* Not Coded Here  *EXCLUDES 2* Not Included Here

ICD-10-CM 2018        831

**Chapter 14. Diseases of Genitourinary System**

-     **N63.22**   Unspecified lump in the left breast, upper inner quadrant
-     **N63.23**   Unspecified lump in the left breast, lower outer quadrant
-     **N63.24**   Unspecified lump in the left breast, lower inner quadrant
- ✓5ᵗʰ **N63.3**   Unspecified lump in axillary tail
-     **N63.31**   Unspecified lump in axillary tail of the right breast
-     **N63.32**   Unspecified lump in axillary tail of the left breast
- ✓5ᵗʰ **N63.4**   Unspecified lump in breast, subareolar
-     **N63.41**   Unspecified lump in right breast, subareolar
-     **N63.42**   Unspecified lump in left breast, subareolar

✓4ᵗʰ **N64**   **Other disorders of breast**
     *EXCLUDES 2*   *mechanical complication of breast prosthesis and implant (T85.4-)*

    **N64.0**   **Fissure and fistula of nipple**

    **N64.1**   **Fat necrosis of breast**
        Fat necrosis (segmental) of breast
        Code first breast necrosis due to breast graft (T85.898)

    **N64.2**   **Atrophy of breast**

    **N64.3**   **Galactorrhea not associated with childbirth**

    **N64.4**   **Mastodynia**

✓5ᵗʰ **N64.5**   **Other signs and symptoms in breast**
        *EXCLUDES 2*   *abnormal findings on diagnostic imaging of breast (R92.-)*

    **N64.51**   **Induration of breast**

    **N64.52**   **Nipple discharge**
        *EXCLUDES 1*   *abnormal findings in nipple discharge (R89.-)*

    **N64.53**   **Retraction of nipple**

    **N64.59**   **Other signs and symptoms in breast**

✓5ᵗʰ **N64.8**   **Other specified disorders of breast**

    **N64.81**   **Ptosis of breast**   Ⓐ
        *EXCLUDES 1*   *ptosis of native breast in relation to reconstructed breast (N65.1)*

    **N64.82**   **Hypoplasia of breast**   Ⓐ
        Micromastia
        *EXCLUDES 1*   *congenital absence of breast (Q83.0)*
                  *hypoplasia of native breast in relation to reconstructed breast (N65.1)*

    **N64.89**   **Other specified disorders of breast**
        Galactocele
        Subinvolution of breast (postlactational)

    **N64.9**   **Disorder of breast, unspecified**

✓4ᵗʰ **N65**   **Deformity and disproportion of reconstructed breast**

    **N65.0**   **Deformity of reconstructed breast**   Ⓐ
        Contour irregularity in reconstructed breast
        Excess tissue in reconstructed breast
        Misshapen reconstructed breast

    **N65.1**   **Disproportion of reconstructed breast**   Ⓐ
        Breast asymmetry between native breast and reconstructed breast
        Disproportion between native breast and reconstructed breast

## Inflammatory diseases of female pelvic organs (N70-N77)

     *EXCLUDES 1*   *inflammatory diseases of female pelvic organs complicating:*
        *abortion or ectopic or molar pregnancy (O00-O07, O08.0)*
        *pregnancy, childbirth and the puerperium (O23-, O75.3, O85, O86-)*

✓4ᵗʰ **N70**   **Salpingitis and oophoritis**
     *INCLUDES*   abscess (of) fallopian tube
              abscess (of) ovary
              pyosalpinx
              salpingo-oophoritis
              tubo-ovarian abscess
              tubo-ovarian inflammatory disease
     Use additional code (B95-B97), to identify infectious agent
     *EXCLUDES 1*   *gonococcal infection (A54.24)*
                *tuberculous infection (A18.17)*

     **CC Excl: For CC codes in category N70: PDX collection 942**

✓5ᵗʰ **N70.0**   **Acute salpingitis and oophoritis**
    **N70.01**   **Acute salpingitis**   CC ♀
    **N70.02**   **Acute oophoritis**   CC ♀
    **N70.03**   **Acute salpingitis and oophoritis**   CC ♀

✓5ᵗʰ **N70.1**   **Chronic salpingitis and oophoritis**
        Hydrosalpinx
    **N70.11**   **Chronic salpingitis**   ♀
    **N70.12**   **Chronic oophoritis**   ♀
    **N70.13**   **Chronic salpingitis and oophoritis**   ♀

✓5ᵗʰ **N70.9**   **Salpingitis and oophoritis, unspecified**
    **N70.91**   **Salpingitis, unspecified**   ♀
    **N70.92**   **Oophoritis, unspecified**   ♀
    **N70.93**   **Salpingitis and oophoritis, unspecified**   ♀

✓4ᵗʰ **N71**   **Inflammatory disease of uterus, except cervix**
     *INCLUDES*   endo (myo) metritis
              metritis
              myometritis
              pyometra
              uterine abscess
     Use additional code (B95-B97), to identify infectious agent
     *EXCLUDES 1*   *hyperplastic endometritis (N85.0-)*
                *infection of uterus following delivery (O85, O86.-)*

    **N71.0**   **Acute inflammatory disease of uterus**   CC ♀
        **CC Excl: PDX collection 943**

    **N71.1**   **Chronic inflammatory disease of uterus**   ♀

    **N71.9**   **Inflammatory disease of uterus, unspecified**   ♀

**N72**   **Inflammatory disease of cervix uteri**   ♀
     *INCLUDES*   cervicitis (with or without erosion or ectropion)
              endocervicitis (with or without erosion or ectropion)
              exocervicitis (with or without erosion or ectropion)
     Use additional code (B95-B97), to identify infectious agent
     *EXCLUDES 1*   *erosion and ectropion of cervix without cervicitis (N86)*

✓4ᵗʰ **N73**   **Other female pelvic inflammatory diseases**
     Use additional code (B95-B97), to identify infectious agent

     **CC Excl: For CC/MCC codes in category N73: PDX collection 942**

    **N73.0**   **Acute parametritis and pelvic cellulitis**   CC ♀
        Abscess of broad ligament
        Abscess of parametrium
        Pelvic cellulitis, female
        **DEF:** Parametritis: Inflammation of the parametrium; pelvic cellulitis is a synonym for parametritis.

    **N73.1**   **Chronic parametritis and pelvic cellulitis**   ♀
        Any condition in N73.0 specified as chronic
        *EXCLUDES 1*   *tuberculous parametritis and pelvic cellutis (A18.17)*

    **N73.2**   **Unspecified parametritis and pelvic cellulitis**   ♀
        Any condition in N73.0 unspecified whether acute or chronic

    **N73.3**   **Female acute pelvic peritonitis**   MCC ♀

    **N73.4**   **Female chronic pelvic peritonitis**   CC ♀
        *EXCLUDES 1*   *tuberculous pelvic (female) peritonitis (A18.17)*

    **N73.5**   **Female pelvic peritonitis, unspecified**   ♀

    **N73.6**   **Female pelvic peritoneal adhesions (postinfective)**   ♀
        *EXCLUDES 2*   *postprocedural pelvic peritoneal adhesions (N99.4)*
        **AHA: 2014, 1Q, 6**

    **N73.8**   **Other specified female pelvic inflammatory diseases**   ♀

    **N73.9**   **Female pelvic inflammatory disease, unspecified**   ♀
        Female pelvic infection or inflammation NOS

**N74**   *Female pelvic inflammatory disorders in diseases classified elsewhere*   ♀
     Code first underlying disease
     *EXCLUDES 1*   *chlamydial cervicitis (A56.02)*
                *chlamydial pelvic inflammatory disease (A56.11)*
                *gonococcal cervicitis (A54.03)*
                *gonococcal pelvic inflammatory disease (A54.24)*
                *herpesviral [herpes simplex] cervicitis (A60.03)*
                *herpesviral [herpes simplex] pelvic inflammatory disease (A60.09)*
                *syphilitic cervicitis (A52.76)*
                *syphilitic pelvic inflammatory disease (A52.76)*
                *trichomonal cervicitis (A59.09)*
                *tuberculous cervicitis (A18.16)*
                *tuberculous pelvic inflammatory disease (A18.17)*

✓4ᵗʰ **N75**   **Diseases of Bartholin's gland**

    **N75.0**   **Cyst of Bartholin's gland**   ♀

    **N75.1**   **Abscess of Bartholin's gland**   CC ♀
        **CC Excl: PDX collection 944**

    **N75.8**   **Other diseases of Bartholin's gland**   ♀
        Bartholinitis

    **N75.9**   **Disease of Bartholin's gland, unspecified**   ♀

Ⓝ Newborn: 0   Ⓟ Pediatric: 0-17   Ⓜ Maternity: 12-55   Ⓐ Adult: 15-124   MCC Major CC Condition   PDx MCC PDx acts as own MCC   CC CC Condition   PDx CC PDx acts as own CC

832                                                          ICD-10-CM 2018

**Chapter 14. Diseases of Genitourinary System**

**✓4ᵗʰ N76 Other inflammation of vagina and vulva**
    Use additional code (B95-B97), to identify infectious agent
    *EXCLUDES 2*    *senile (atrophic) vaginitis (N95.2)*
               *vulvar vestibulitis (N94.810)*

  **N76.0 Acute vaginitis**       ♀
      Acute vulvovaginitis      Vulvovaginitis NOS
      Vaginitis NOS

  **N76.1 Subacute and chronic vaginitis**       ♀
      Chronic vulvovaginitis
      Subacute vulvovaginitis

  **N76.2 Acute vulvitis**       ♀
      Vulvitis NOS

  **N76.3 Subacute and chronic vulvitis**       ♀

  **N76.4 Abscess of vulva**       `CC` ♀
      Furuncle of vulva
      **CC Excl:** PDX collection 944

  **N76.5 Ulceration of vagina**       ♀

  **N76.6 Ulceration of vulva**       ♀

  **✓5ᵗʰ N76.8 Other specified inflammation of vagina and vulva**
    **N76.81 Mucositis (ulcerative) of vagina and vulva**    `CC` ♀
        Code also type of associated therapy, such as:
          antineoplastic and immunosuppressive drugs
            (T45.1X-)
          radiological procedure and radiotherapy (Y84.2)
        *EXCLUDES 2*   *gastrointestinal mucositis (ulcerative)*
               *(K92.81)*
              *nasal mucositis (ulcerative) (J34.81)*
              *oral mucositis (ulcerative) (K12.3-)*
        **CC Excl:** PDX collection 945

    **N76.89 Other specified inflammation of vagina and vulva** ♀

**✓4ᵗʰ N77 Vulvovaginal ulceration and inflammation in diseases classified elsewhere**

  **N77.0 *Ulceration of vulva in diseases classified elsewhere***     ♀
      Code first underlying disease, such as:
        Behçet's disease (M35.2)
      *EXCLUDES 1*   *ulceration of vulva in gonococcal infection (A54.02)*
              *ulceration of vulva in herpesviral [herpes simplex]*
                 *infection (A60.04)*
              *ulceration of vulva in syphilis (A51.0)*
              *ulceration of vulva in tuberculosis (A18.18)*

  **N77.1 *Vaginitis, vulvitis and vulvovaginitis in diseases classified elsewhere***     ♀
      Code first underlying disease, such as:
        pinworm (B80)
      *EXCLUDES 1*   *candidal vulvovaginitis (B37.3)*
              *chlamydial vulvovaginitis (A56.02)*
              *gonococcal vulvovaginitis (A54.02)*
              *herpesviral [herpes simplex] vulvovaginitis (A60.04)*
              *trichomonal vulvovaginitis (A59.01)*
              *tuberculous vulvovaginitis (A18.18)*
              *vulvovaginitis in early syphilis (A51.0)*
              *vulvovaginitis in late syphilis (A52.76)*

## Noninflammatory disorders of female genital tract (N80-N98)

**✓4ᵗʰ N80 Endometriosis**

  **N80.0 Endometriosis of uterus**       ♀
      Adenomyosis
      *EXCLUDES 1*   *stromal endometriosis (D39.0)*

  **N80.1 Endometriosis of ovary**       ♀

  **N80.2 Endometriosis of fallopian tube**       ♀

  **N80.3 Endometriosis of pelvic peritoneum**       ♀

  **N80.4 Endometriosis of rectovaginal septum and vagina**       ♀

  **N80.5 Endometriosis of intestine**       ♀

  **N80.6 Endometriosis in cutaneous scar**       ♀

  **N80.8 Other endometriosis**       ♀
      ▶Endometriosis of thorax◀

  **N80.9 Endometriosis, unspecified**       ♀

**✓4ᵗʰ N81 Female genital prolapse**
    *EXCLUDES 1*   *genital prolapse complicating pregnancy, labor or delivery*
             *(O34.5-)*
             *prolapse and hernia of ovary and fallopian tube (N83.4-)*
             *prolapse of vaginal vault after hysterectomy (N99.3)*

  **N81.0 Urethrocele**       ♀
      *EXCLUDES 1*   *urethrocele with cystocele (N81.1-)*
              *urethrocele with prolapse of uterus (N81.2-N81.4)*

### Types of Pelvic Organ Prolapse

Urethrocele · Cystocele · Rectocele · Enterocele

  **✓5ᵗʰ N81.1 Cystocele**
      Cystocele with urethrocele
      Cystourethrocele
      *EXCLUDES 1*   *cystocele with prolapse of uterus (N81.2-N81.4)*

    **N81.10 Cystocele, unspecified**       ♀
        Prolapse of (anterior) vaginal wall NOS

    **N81.11 Cystocele, midline**       ♀

    **N81.12 Cystocele, lateral**       ♀
        Paravaginal cystocele
        **DEF:** Detachment of the lateral support connections of
        the vagina at the arcus tendineus fasciae pelvis (ATFP)
        results in bladder drop; bladder herniates into the
        vagina laterally.

  **N81.2 Incomplete uterovaginal prolapse**       ♀
      First degree uterine prolapse
      Prolapse of cervix NOS
      Second degree uterine prolapse
      *EXCLUDES 1* ▶*cervical stump prolapse*◀ *(N81.85)*

  **N81.3 Complete uterovaginal prolapse**       ♀
      Procidentia (uteri) NOS
      Third degree uterine prolapse

  **N81.4 Uterovaginal prolapse, unspecified**       ♀
      Prolapse of uterus NOS

  **N81.5 Vaginal enterocele**       ♀
      *EXCLUDES 1*   *enterocele with prolapse of uterus (N81.2-N81.4)*

  **N81.6 Rectocele**       ♀
      Prolapse of posterior vaginal wall
      Use additional code for any associated fecal incontinence, if
        applicable (R15.-)
      *EXCLUDES 2*   *perineocele (N81.81)*
              *rectal prolapse (K62.3)*
              *rectocele with prolapse of uterus (N81.2-N81.4)*

  **✓5ᵗʰ N81.8 Other female genital prolapse**
    **N81.81 Perineocele**       ♀

    **N81.82 Incompetence or weakening of pubocervical tissue**       ♀

    **N81.83 Incompetence or weakening of rectovaginal tissue**       ♀

    **N81.84 Pelvic muscle wasting**       ♀
        Disuse atrophy of pelvic muscles and anal sphincter

    **N81.85 Cervical stump prolapse**       ♀

    **N81.89 Other female genital prolapse**       ♀
        Deficient perineum
        Old laceration of muscles of pelvic floor

  **N81.9 Female genital prolapse, unspecified**       ♀

**✓4ᵗʰ N82 Fistulae involving female genital tract**
    *EXCLUDES 1*   *vesicointestinal fistulae (N32.1)*

  **CC Excl: For CC codes in category N82:** PDX collection 946

  **N82.0 Vesicovaginal fistula**       `CC`

  **N82.1 Other female urinary-genital tract fistulae**       `CC` ♀
      Cervicovesical fistula      Uteroureteric fistula
      Ureterovaginal fistula      Uterovesical fistula
      Urethrovaginal fistula

✓ Additional Character Req    ✓x7ᵗʰ Placeholder Alert    Unacceptable PDx    Manifestation    `H1`-`H14` HAC    `HCC` CMS-HCC Condition    *EXCLUDES 1* Not Coded Here    *EXCLUDES 2* Not Included Here

ICD-10-CM 2018                                    **833**

**N82.2** **Fistula of vagina to** small **intestine** CC ♀

**N82.3** **Fistula of vagina to** large **intestine** CC ♀
Rectovaginal fistula

**N82.4** **Other female** intestinal-genital tract **fistulae** CC ♀
Intestinouterine fistula

**N82.5** **Female** genital tract-skin **fistulae** CC ♀
Uterus to abdominal wall fistula
Vaginoperineal fistula

**N82.8** **Other** female genital tract fistulae CC ♀

**N82.9** **Female genital tract fistula,** unspecified CC ♀

✓4th **N83** **Noninflammatory disorders of ovary, fallopian tube and broad ligament**
EXCLUDES 2  hydrosalpinx (N70.1-)

✓5th **N83.0** **Follicular cyst of ovary**
Cyst of graafian follicle
Hemorrhagic follicular cyst (of ovary)

**N83.00** **Follicular cyst of ovary,** unspecified **side** ♀

**N83.01** **Follicular cyst of** right **ovary** ♀

**N83.02** **Follicular cyst of** left **ovary** ♀

✓5th **N83.1** **Corpus luteum cyst**
Hemorrhagic corpus luteum cyst

**N83.10** **Corpus luteum cyst of ovary,** unspecified **side** ♀

**N83.11** **Corpus luteum cyst of** right **ovary** ♀

**N83.12** **Corpus luteum cyst of** left **ovary** ♀

✓5th **N83.2** **Other and unspecified ovarian cysts**
EXCLUDES 1  developmental ovarian cyst (Q50.1)
neoplastic ovarian cyst (D27.-)
polycystic ovarian syndrome (E28.2)
Stein-Leventhal syndrome (E28.2)

✓6th **N83.20** **Unspecified ovarian cysts**

**N83.201** **Unspecified ovarian cyst,** right **side** ♀

**N83.202** **Unspecified ovarian cyst,** left **side** ♀

**N83.209** **Unspecified ovarian cyst,** unspecified **side** ♀
Ovarian cyst, NOS

✓6th **N83.29** **Other ovarian cysts**
Retention cyst of ovary
Simple cyst of ovary

**N83.291** **Other ovarian cyst,** right **side** ♀

**N83.292** **Other ovarian cyst,** left **side** ♀

**N83.299** **Other ovarian cyst,** unspecified **side** ♀

✓5th **N83.3** **Acquired atrophy of ovary and fallopian tube**

✓6th **N83.31** **Acquired atrophy of** ovary

**N83.311** **Acquired atrophy of** right **ovary** ♀

**N83.312** **Acquired atrophy of** left **ovary** ♀

**N83.319** **Acquired atrophy of ovary,** unspecified **side** ♀
Acquired atrophy of ovary, NOS

✓6th **N83.32** **Acquired atrophy of** fallopian tube

**N83.321** **Acquired atrophy of** right **fallopian tube** ♀

**N83.322** **Acquired atrophy of** left **fallopian tube** ♀

**N83.329** **Acquired atrophy of fallopian tube,** unspecified **side** ♀
Acquired atrophy of fallopian tube, NOS

✓6th **N83.33** **Acquired atrophy of** ovary and fallopian tube

**N83.331** **Acquired atrophy of** right **ovary and fallopian tube** ♀

**N83.332** **Acquired atrophy of** left **ovary and fallopian tube** ♀

**N83.339** **Acquired atrophy of ovary and fallopian tube,** unspecified **side** ♀
Acquired atrophy of ovary and fallopian tube, NOS

✓5th **N83.4** **Prolapse and hernia of ovary and fallopian tube**

**N83.40** **Prolapse and hernia of ovary and fallopian tube,** unspecified **side** ♀
Prolapse and hernia of ovary and fallopian tube, NOS

**N83.41** **Prolapse and hernia of** right **ovary and fallopian tube** ♀

**N83.42** **Prolapse and hernia of** left **ovary and fallopian tube** ♀

✓5th **N83.5** **Torsion of ovary, ovarian pedicle and fallopian tube**
Torsion of accessory tube

**CC Excl: For CC codes in subcategory N83.5:**
PDX collection 947

✓6th **N83.51** **Torsion of** ovary and ovarian pedicle

**N83.511** **Torsion of** right **ovary and ovarian pedicle** CC ♀

**N83.512** **Torsion of** left **ovary and ovarian pedicle** CC ♀

**N83.519** **Torsion of ovary and ovarian pedicle,** unspecified **side** CC ♀
Torsion of ovary and ovarian pedicle, NOS

✓6th **N83.52** **Torsion of** fallopian tube
Torsion of hydatid of Morgagni

**N83.521** **Torsion of** right **fallopian tube** CC ♀

**N83.522** **Torsion of** left **fallopian tube** CC ♀

**N83.529** **Torsion of fallopian tube,** unspecified **side** CC ♀
Torsion of fallopian tube, NOS

**N83.53** **Torsion of** ovary, ovarian pedicle and fallopian tube CC ♀

**N83.6** **Hematosalpinx** ♀
EXCLUDES 1  hematosalpinx (with) (in):
hematocolpos (N89.7)
hematometra (N85.7)
tubal pregnancy (O00.1-)

**N83.7** **Hematoma of broad ligament** ♀

**N83.8** **Other noninflammatory disorders of ovary, fallopian tube and broad ligament** ♀
Broad ligament laceration syndrome [Allen-Masters]

**N83.9** **Noninflammatory disorder of ovary, fallopian tube and broad ligament, unspecified**

✓4th **N84** **Polyp of female genital tract**
EXCLUDES 1  adenomatous polyp (D28.-)
placental polyp (O90.89)

**N84.0** **Polyp of** corpus uteri ♀
Polyp of endometrium      Polyp of uterus NOS
EXCLUDES 1  polypoid endometrial hyperplasia (N85.0-)

**N84.1** **Polyp of** cervix uteri ♀
Mucous polyp of cervix

**N84.2** **Polyp of** vagina ♀

**N84.3** **Polyp of** vulva ♀
Polyp of labia

**N84.8** **Polyp of** other parts of female genital tract ♀

**N84.9** **Polyp of female genital tract,** unspecified ♀

✓4th **N85** **Other noninflammatory disorders of uterus, except cervix**
EXCLUDES 1  endometriosis (N80.-)
inflammatory diseases of uterus (N71.-)
noninflammatory disorders of cervix, except malposition (N86-N88)
polyp of corpus uteri (N84.0)
uterine prolapse (N81.-)

✓5th **N85.0** **Endometrial hyperplasia**

**N85.00** **Endometrial hyperplasia,** unspecified ♀
Hyperplasia (adenomatous) (cystic) (glandular) of endometrium
Hyperplastic endometritis

**N85.01** **Benign** endometrial hyperplasia ♀
Endometrial hyperplasia (complex) (simple) without atypia

**N85.02** **Endometrial intraepithelial neoplasia [EIN]** ♀
Endometrial hyperplasia with atypia
EXCLUDES 1  malignant neoplasm of endometrium (with endometrial intraepithelial neoplasia [EIN]) (C54.1)

**N85.2** **Hypertrophy of uterus** ♀
Bulky or enlarged uterus
EXCLUDES 1  puerperal hypertrophy of uterus (O90.89)

**N85.3** **Subinvolution of uterus** ♀
EXCLUDES 1  puerperal subinvolution of uterus (O90.89)

**N85.4** **Malposition of uterus** ♀
Anteversion of uterus
Retroflexion of uterus
Retroversion of uterus
EXCLUDES 1  malposition of uterus complicating pregnancy, labor or delivery (O34.5-, O65.5)

N Newborn: 0   P Pediatric: 0-17   M Maternity: 12-55   A Adult. 15-124   MCC Major CC Condition   PDxMCC PDx acts as own MCC   CC CC Condition   PDxCC PDx acts as own CC

834

ICD-10-CM 2018

**Inversion of Uterus**

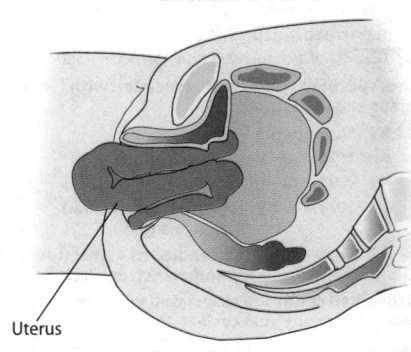

Uterus

**N85.5 Inversion of uterus** ♀
> **EXCLUDES 1**   current obstetric trauma (O71.2)
>      postpartum inversion of uterus (O71.2)

**N85.6 Intrauterine synechiae** ♀

**N85.7 Hematometra** ♀
> Hematosalpinx with hematometra
> **EXCLUDES 1**   hematometra with hematocolpos (N89.7)
> **DEF:** Accumulation of blood within the uterus.

**N85.8 Other specified noninflammatory disorders of uterus** ♀
> Atrophy of uterus, acquired
> Fibrosis of uterus NOS

**N85.9 Noninflammatory disorder of uterus, unspecified** ♀
> Disorder of uterus NOS

**N86 Erosion and ectropion of cervix uteri** ♀
> Decubitus (trophic) ulcer of cervix
> Eversion of cervix
> **EXCLUDES 1**   erosion and ectropion of cervix with cervicitis (N72)

✓4th **N87 Dysplasia of cervix uteri**
> **EXCLUDES 1**   abnormal results from cervical cytologic examination without
>      histologic confirmation (R87.61-)
>      carcinoma in situ of cervix uteri (D06.-)
>      cervical intraepithelial neoplasia III [CIN III] (D06.-)
>      HGSIL of cervix (R87.613)
>      severe dysplasia of cervix uteri (D06.-)

**N87.0 Mild cervical dysplasia** ♀
> Cervical intraepithelial neoplasia I [CIN I]

**N87.1 Moderate cervical dysplasia** ♀
> Cervical intraepithelial neoplasia II [CIN II]

**N87.9 Dysplasia of cervix uteri, unspecified** ♀
> Anaplasia of cervix
> Cervical atypism
> Cervical dysplasia NOS

✓4th **N88 Other noninflammatory disorders of cervix uteri**
> **EXCLUDES 2**   inflammatory disease of cervix (N72)
>      polyp of cervix (N84.1)

**N88.0 Leukoplakia of cervix uteri** ♀

**N88.1 Old laceration of cervix uteri** ♀
> Adhesions of cervix
> **EXCLUDES 1**   current obstetric trauma (O71.3)

**N88.2 Stricture and stenosis of cervix uteri** ♀
> **EXCLUDES 1**   stricture and stenosis of cervix uteri complicating labor
>      (O65.5)

**N88.3 Incompetence of cervix uteri** ♀
> Investigation and management of (suspected) cervical
> incompetence in a nonpregnant woman
> **EXCLUDES 1**   cervical incompetence complicating pregnancy
>      (O34.3-)

**N88.4 Hypertrophic elongation of cervix uteri** ♀

**N88.8 Other specified noninflammatory disorders of cervix uteri** ♀
> **EXCLUDES 1**   current obstetric trauma (O71.3)

**N88.9 Noninflammatory disorder of cervix uteri, unspecified** ♀

✓4th **N89 Other noninflammatory disorders of vagina**
> **EXCLUDES 1**   abnormal results from vaginal cytologic examination without
>      histologic confirmation (R87.62-)
>      carcinoma in situ of vagina (D07.2)
>      HGSIL of vagina (R87.623)
>      inflammation of vagina (N76.-)
>      senile (atrophic) vaginitis (N95.2)
>      severe dysplasia of vagina (D07.2)
>      trichomonal leukorrhea (A59.00)
>      vaginal intraepithelial neoplasia [VAIN], grade III (D07.2)

**N89.0 Mild vaginal dysplasia** ♀
> Vaginal intraepithelial neoplasia [VAIN], grade I

**N89.1 Moderate vaginal dysplasia** ♀
> Vaginal intraepithelial neoplasia [VAIN], grade II

**N89.3 Dysplasia of vagina, unspecified** ♀

**N89.4 Leukoplakia of vagina** ♀

**N89.5 Stricture and atresia of vagina** ♀
> Vaginal adhesions    Vaginal stenosis
> **EXCLUDES 1**   congenital atresia or stricture (Q52.4)
>      postprocedural adhesions of vagina (N99.2)

**N89.6 Tight hymenal ring** ♀
> Rigid hymen
> Tight introitus
> **EXCLUDES 1**   imperforate hymen (Q52.3)

**N89.7 Hematocolpos** ♀
> Hematocolpos with hematometra or hematosalpinx

**N89.8 Other specified noninflammatory disorders of vagina** ♀
> Leukorrhea NOS
> Old vaginal laceration
> Pessary ulcer of vagina
> **EXCLUDES 1**   current obstetric trauma (O70-, O71.4, O71.7-O71.8)
>      old laceration involving muscles of pelvic floor (N81.8)

**N89.9 Noninflammatory disorder of vagina, unspecified** ♀

✓4th **N90 Other noninflammatory disorders of vulva and perineum**
> **EXCLUDES 1**   anogenital (venereal) warts (A63.0)
>      carcinoma in situ of vulva (D07.1)
>      condyloma acuminatum (A63.0)
>      current obstetric trauma (O70-, O71.7-O71.8)
>      inflammation of vulva (N76.-)
>      severe dysplasia of vulva (D07.1)
>      vulvar intraepithelial neoplasm III [VIN III] (D07.1)

**N90.0 Mild vulvar dysplasia** ♀
> Vulvar intraepithelial neoplasia [VIN], grade I

**N90.1 Moderate vulvar dysplasia** ♀
> Vulvar intraepithelial neoplasia [VIN], grade II

**N90.3 Dysplasia of vulva, unspecified** ♀

**N90.4 Leukoplakia of vulva** ♀
> Dystrophy of vulva
> Kraurosis of vulva
> Lichen sclerosus of external female genital organs

**N90.5 Atrophy of vulva** ♀
> Stenosis of vulva

✓5th **N90.6 Hypertrophy of vulva**
> **N90.60 Unspecified hypertrophy of vulva** ♀
>      Unspecified hypertrophy of labia
>
> **N90.61 Childhood asymmetric labium majus enlargement** ♀
>      CALME
>
> **N90.69 Other specified hypertrophy of vulva** ♀
>      Other specified hypertrophy of labia

**N90.7 Vulvar cyst** ♀

✓5th **N90.8 Other specified noninflammatory disorders of vulva and perineum**
> ✓6th **N90.81 Female genital mutilation status**
>      Female genital cutting status
>      **N90.810 Female genital mutilation status,** ♀
>          **unspecified**
>          Female genital cutting status, unspecified
>          Female genital mutilation status NOS
>      **N90.811 Female genital mutilation Type I status** ♀
>          Clitorectomy status
>          Female genital cutting Type I status
>      **N90.812 Female genital mutilation Type II status** ♀
>          Clitorectomy with excision of labia minora
>          status
>          Female genital cutting Type II status
>      **N90.813 Female genital mutilation Type III status** ♀
>          Female genital cutting Type III status
>          Infibulation status

**N90.818** **Other** female genital mutilation status ♀
Female genital cutting Type IV status
Female genital mutilation Type IV status
Other female genital cutting status

**N90.89** **Other specified noninflammatory disorders of vulva and perineum** ♀
Adhesions of vulva
Hypertrophy of clitoris

**N90.9** **Noninflammatory disorder of vulva and perineum, unspecified** ♀

✓4ᵗʰ **N91** **Absent, scanty and rare menstruation**
*EXCLUDES 1*   *ovarian dysfunction (E28.-)*

**N91.0** **Primary amenorrhea** ♀
**N91.1** **Secondary amenorrhea** ♀
**N91.2** **Amenorrhea, unspecified** ♀
**N91.3** **Primary oligomenorrhea** ♀
**N91.4** **Secondary oligomenorrhea** ♀
**N91.5** **Oligomenorrhea, unspecified** ♀
Hypomenorrhea NOS

✓4ᵗʰ **N92** **Excessive, frequent and irregular menstruation**
*EXCLUDES 1*   *postmenopausal bleeding (N95.0)*
*precocious puberty (menstruation) (E30.1)*

**N92.0** **Excessive and frequent menstruation** with regular cycle ♀
Heavy periods NOS
Menorrhagia NOS
Polymenorrhea

**N92.1** **Excessive and frequent menstruation** with irregular cycle ♀
Irregular intermenstrual bleeding
Irregular, shortened intervals between menstrual bleeding
Menometrorrhagia
Metrorrhagia

**N92.2** **Excessive menstruation at puberty** P♀
Excessive bleeding associated with onset of menstrual periods
Pubertal menorrhagia
Puberty bleeding

**N92.3** **Ovulation bleeding** ♀
Regular intermenstrual bleeding

**N92.4** **Excessive bleeding in the premenopausal period** ♀
Climacteric menorrhagia or metrorrhagia
Menopausal menorrhagia or metrorrhagia
Preclimacteric menorrhagia or metrorrhagia
Premenopausal menorrhagia or metrorrhagia

**N92.5** **Other specified irregular menstruation** ♀
**N92.6** **Irregular menstruation, unspecified** ♀
Irregular bleeding NOS
Irregular periods NOS
*EXCLUDES 1*   *irregular menstruation with:*
*lengthened intervals or scanty bleeding (N91.3-N91.5)*
*shortened intervals or excessive bleeding (N92.1)*

✓4ᵗʰ **N93** **Other abnormal uterine and vaginal bleeding**
*EXCLUDES 1*   *neonatal vaginal hemorrhage (P54.6)*
*precocious puberty (menstruation) (E30.1)*
*pseudomenses (P54.6)*

**N93.0** **Postcoital and contact bleeding** ♀
**N93.1** **Pre-pubertal vaginal bleeding** ♀
**N93.8** **Other specified abnormal uterine and vaginal bleeding** ♀
Dysfunctional or functional uterine or vaginal bleeding NOS

**N93.9** **Abnormal uterine and vaginal bleeding, unspecified** ♀

✓4ᵗʰ **N94** **Pain and other conditions associated with female genital organs and menstrual cycle**

**N94.0** **Mittelschmerz** ♀
**DEF:** One-sided, lower abdominal pain occurring between menstrual periods; associated with ovulation.

✓5ᵗʰ **N94.1** **Dyspareunia**
*EXCLUDES 1*   *psychogenic dyspareunia (F52.6)*
**N94.10** **Unspecified dyspareunia** ♀
**N94.11** **Superficial (introital) dyspareunia** ♀
**N94.12** **Deep dyspareunia** ♀
**N94.19** **Other specified dyspareunia** ♀

**N94.2** **Vaginismus** ♀
*EXCLUDES 1*   *psychogenic vaginismus (F52.5)*

**N94.3** **Premenstrual tension syndrome** ♀
~~Premenstrual dysphoric disorder~~
Code also associated menstrual migraine (G43.82-, G43.83-)
*EXCLUDES 1*   *premenstrual dysphoric disorder (F32.81)*

**N94.4** **Primary dysmenorrhea** ♀
**N94.5** **Secondary dysmenorrhea** ♀
**N94.6** **Dysmenorrhea, unspecified** ♀
*EXCLUDES 1*   *psychogenic dysmenorrhea (F45.8)*

✓5ᵗʰ **N94.8** **Other specified conditions associated with female genital organs and menstrual cycle**

✓6ᵗʰ **N94.81** **Vulvodynia**
**N94.810** **Vulvar vestibulitis** ♀
**N94.818** **Other vulvodynia** ♀
**N94.819** **Vulvodynia, unspecified** ♀
Vulvodynia NOS

**N94.89** **Other specified conditions associated with female genital organs and menstrual cycle** ♀

**N94.9** **Unspecified condition associated with female genital organs and menstrual cycle** ♀

✓4ᵗʰ **N95** **Menopausal and other perimenopausal disorders**
Menopausal and other perimenopausal disorders due to naturally occurring (age-related) menopause and perimenopause
*EXCLUDES 1*   *excessive bleeding in the premenopausal period (N92.4)*
*menopausal and perimenopausal disorders due to artificial or premature menopause (E89.4-, E28.31-)*
*premature menopause (E28.31-)*
*EXCLUDES 2*   *postmenopausal osteoporosis (M81.0-)*
*postmenopausal osteoporosis with current pathological fracture (M80.0-)*
*postmenopausal urethritis (N34.2)*

**N95.0** **Postmenopausal bleeding** ♀
**N95.1** **Menopausal and female climacteric states** ♀
Symptoms such as flushing, sleeplessness, headache, lack of concentration, associated with natural (age-related) menopause
Use additional code for associated symptoms
*EXCLUDES 1*   *asymptomatic menopausal state (Z78.0)*
*symptoms associated with artificial menopause (E89.41)*
*symptoms associated with premature menopause (E28.310)*

**N95.2** **Postmenopausal atrophic vaginitis** ♀
Senile (atrophic) vaginitis

**N95.8** **Other specified menopausal and perimenopausal disorders** ♀
**N95.9** **Unspecified menopausal and perimenopausal disorder** ♀

**N96** **Recurrent pregnancy loss** ♀
Investigation or care in a nonpregnant woman with history of recurrent pregnancy loss
*EXCLUDES 1*   *recurrent pregnancy loss with current pregnancy (O26.2-)*

✓4ᵗʰ **N97** **Female infertility**
**INCLUDES**   inability to achieve a pregnancy
sterility, female NOS
*EXCLUDES 1*   *female infertility associated with:*
*hypopituitarism (E23.0)*
*Stein-Leventhal syndrome (E28.2)*
*EXCLUDES 2*   *incompetence of cervix uteri (N88.3)*
**DEF:** Infertility: Inability to conceive for at least one year with regular intercourse.
**DEF:** Primary infertility: Infertility occurring in patients who have never conceived.
**DEF:** Secondary infertility: Infertility occurring in patients who have previously conceived.

**N97.0** **Female infertility** associated with anovulation ♀
**N97.1** **Female infertility of** tubal origin ♀
Female infertility associated with congenital anomaly of tube
Female infertility due to tubal block
Female infertility due to tubal occlusion
Female infertility due to tubal stenosis

**N97.2** **Female infertility of** uterine origin ♀
Female infertility associated with congenital anomaly of uterus
Female infertility due to nonimplantation of ovum

**N97.8** **Female infertility of** other origin ♀
**N97.9** **Female infertility,** unspecified ♀

✓4ᵗʰ **N98** **Complications associated with artificial fertilization**

CC Excl: For CC codes in category N98, unless otherwise noted:
PDX collection 643

**N98.0** **Infection associated with artificial insemination** cc♀
**CC Excl:** PDX collection 948

**N98.1** **Hyperstimulation of** ovaries cc♀
Hyperstimulation of ovaries NOS
Hyperstimulation of ovaries associated with induced ovulation

---

N Newborn: 0   P Pediatric: 0-17   M Maternity: 12-55   A Adult: 15-124   MCC Major CC Condition   PDxMCC PDx acts as own MCC   CC CC Condition   PDxCC PDx acts as own CC

**N98.2**   **Complications of attempted** introduction of fertilized ovum **following in vitro fertilization**   `CC` ♀

**N98.3**   **Complications of attempted** introduction of embryo **in embryo transfer**   `CC` ♀

**N98.8**   Other **complications associated with artificial fertilization**   `CC` ♀

**N98.9**   **Complication associated with artificial fertilization,** unspecified   `CC` ♀

## Intraoperative and postprocedural complications and disorders of genitourinary system, not elsewhere classified (N99)

✔4ᵗʰ **N99**   **Intraoperative and postprocedural complications and disorders of genitourinary system, not elsewhere classified**
> *EXCLUDES 2*   irradiation cystitis (N30.4-)
> postoophorectomy osteoporosis with current pathological fracture (M80.8-)
> postoophorectomy osteoporosis without current pathological fracture (M81.8)

**N99.0**   **Postprocedural (acute) (chronic)** kidney failure
> Use additional code for type of kidney disease

✔5ᵗʰ **N99.1**   **Postprocedural** urethral stricture
> Postcatheterization urethral stricture

   ✔6ᵗʰ **N99.11**   **Postprocedural urethral stricture,** male

     **N99.110**   **Postprocedural urethral stricture, male,** meatal   ♂

▲      **N99.111**   **Postprocedural** bulbous **urethral stricture, male**   ♂

▲      **N99.112**   **Postprocedural** membranous **urethral stricture, male**   ♂

▲      **N99.113**   **Postprocedural** anterior bulbous **urethral stricture, male**   ♂

     **N99.114**   **Postprocedural urethral stricture, male,** unspecified   ♂

     **N99.115**   **Postprocedural** fossa navicularis **urethral stricture**   ♂

   **N99.12**   **Postprocedural urethral stricture,** female   ♀

**N99.2**   **Postprocedural** adhesions of vagina   ♀

**N99.3**   **Prolapse of vaginal vault** after hysterectomy   ♀

**N99.4**   **Postprocedural** pelvic peritoneal adhesions
> *EXCLUDES 2*   pelvic peritoneal adhesions NOS (N73.6)
> postinfective pelvic peritoneal adhesions (N73.6)

✔5ᵗʰ **N99.5**   **Complications of stoma of urinary tract**
> *EXCLUDES 2*   mechanical complication of urinary catheter (T83.0-)

   ✔6ᵗʰ **N99.51**   **Complication of** cystostomy

     **N99.510**   **Cystostomy** hemorrhage   `CC` `HCC`
>        **CC Excl:** PDX collection 949

     **N99.511**   **Cystostomy** infection   `CC` `HCC`
>        **CC Excl:** PDX collection 950

     **N99.512**   **Cystostomy** malfunction   `CC` `HCC`
>        **CC Excl:** PDX collection 951

     **N99.518**   **Other cystostomy complication**   `CC` `HCC`
>        **CC Excl:** PDX collection 949

   ✔6ᵗʰ **N99.52**   **Complication of** incontinent external stoma of urinary tract

     **N99.520**   Hemorrhage of incontinent external stoma of urinary tract   `HCC`

     **N99.521**   Infection of incontinent external stoma of urinary tract   `HCC`

     **N99.522**   Malfunction of incontinent external stoma of urinary tract   `HCC`

     **N99.523**   Herniation of incontinent stoma of urinary tract   `HCC`

     **N99.524**   Stenosis of incontinent stoma of urinary tract   `HCC`

     **N99.528**   Other complication of incontinent external stoma of urinary tract   `HCC`

   ✔6ᵗʰ **N99.53**   **Complication of** continent stoma of urinary tract

     **N99.530**   Hemorrhage of continent stoma of urinary tract   `HCC`

     **N99.531**   Infection of continent stoma of urinary tract   `HCC`

     **N99.532**   Malfunction of continent stoma of urinary tract   `HCC`

     **N99.533**   Herniation of continent stoma of urinary tract   `HCC`

     **N99.534**   Stenosis of continent stoma of urinary tract   `HCC`

     **N99.538**   Other complication of continent stoma of urinary tract   `HCC`

✔5ᵗʰ **N99.6**   Intraoperative hemorrhage and hematoma of a genitourinary system organ or structure complicating a procedure
> *EXCLUDES 1*   intraoperative hemorrhage and hematoma of a genitourinary system organ or structure due to accidental puncture or laceration during a procedure (N99.7-)

   **N99.61**   Intraoperative hemorrhage and hematoma of a genitourinary system organ or structure complicating a genitourinary system procedure   `CC`
>        **CC Excl:** PDX collection 952

   **N99.62**   Intraoperative hemorrhage and hematoma of a genitourinary system organ or structure complicating other procedure   `CC`
>        **CC Excl:** PDX collection 952

✔5ᵗʰ **N99.7**   Accidental puncture and laceration of a genitourinary system organ or structure during a procedure

   **N99.71**   Accidental puncture and laceration of a genitourinary system organ or structure during a genitourinary system procedure   `CC`
>        **CC Excl:** PDX collection 509

   **N99.72**   Accidental puncture and laceration of a genitourinary system organ or structure during other procedure   `CC`
>        **CC Excl:** PDX collection 509

✔5ᵗʰ **N99.8**   Other intraoperative and postprocedural complications and disorders of genitourinary system

> **CC Excl:** For CC codes in subcategory N99.8, unless otherwise noted: PDX collection 952

   **N99.81**   Other intraoperative complications of genitourinary system

   ✔6ᵗʰ **N99.82**   Postprocedural hemorrhage of a genitourinary system organ or structure following a procedure

     **N99.820**   Postprocedural hemorrhage of a genitourinary system organ or structure following a genitourinary system procedure   `CC`

     **N99.821**   Postprocedural hemorrhage of a genitourinary system organ or structure following other procedure   `CC`

   **N99.83**   Residual ovary syndrome   ♀

   ✔6ᵗʰ **N99.84**   Postprocedural hematoma and seroma of a genitourinary system organ or structure following a procedure

     **N99.840**   Postprocedural hematoma of a genitourinary system organ or structure following a genitourinary system procedure   `CC`

     **N99.841**   Postprocedural hematoma of a genitourinary system organ or structure following other procedure   `CC`

     **N99.842**   Postprocedural seroma of a genitourinary system organ or structure following a genitourinary system procedure   `CC`

     **N99.843**   Postprocedural seroma of a genitourinary system organ or structure following other procedure   `CC`

   **N99.89**   Other postprocedural complications and disorders of genitourinary system

---

✔ Additional Character Req    ✔x7ᵗʰ Placeholder Alert    Unacceptable PDx    Manifestation    `H1`-`H14` HAC    `HCC` CMS-HCC Condition    *EXCLUDES 1* Not Coded Here    *EXCLUDES 2* Not Included Here

# Chapter 15. Pregnancy, Childbirth and the Puerperium (O00–O9A)

## Chapter Specific Guidelines with Coding Examples

The chapter specific guidelines from the ICD-10-CM Official Guidelines for Coding and Reporting have been provided below. Along with these guidelines are coding examples, contained in the shaded boxes, that have been developed to help illustrate the coding and/or sequencing guidance found in these guidelines.

### a. General rules for obstetric cases

#### 1) Codes from Chapter 15 and sequencing priority

Obstetric cases require codes from chapter 15, codes in the range O00-O9A, Pregnancy, Childbirth, and the Puerperium. Chapter 15 codes have sequencing priority over codes from other chapters. Additional codes from other chapters may be used in conjunction with chapter 15 codes to further specify conditions. Should the provider document that the pregnancy is incidental to the encounter, then code Z33.1, Pregnant state, incidental, should be used in place of any chapter 15 codes. It is the provider's responsibility to state that the condition being treated is not affecting the pregnancy.

> Pregnant patient at 25 weeks' gestation admitted for bladder abscess.
>
> **O23.12**    **Infections of bladder in pregnancy, second trimester**
>
> **N30.80**    **Other cystitis without hematuria**
>
> **Z3A.25**    **25 weeks gestation of pregnancy**
>
> *Explanation:* The documentation does not indicate that the pregnancy is incidental or in any way unaffected by the bladder abscess; therefore, an obstetrics code should be sequenced first. An additional code was provided to identify the specific bladder condition as this information is not called out specifically in the obstetrics code.

#### 2) Chapter 15 codes used only on the maternal record

Chapter 15 codes are to be used only on the maternal record, never on the record of the newborn.

#### 3) Final character for trimester

The majority of codes in Chapter 15 have a final character indicating the trimester of pregnancy. The timeframes for the trimesters are indicated at the beginning of the chapter. If trimester is not a component of a code, it is because the condition always occurs in a specific trimester, or the concept of trimester of pregnancy is not applicable. Certain codes have characters for only certain trimesters because the condition does not occur in all trimesters, but it may occur in more than just one. Assignment of the final character for trimester should be based on the provider's documentation of the trimester (or number of weeks) for the current admission/encounter. This applies to the assignment of trimester for pre-existing conditions as well as those that develop during or are due to the pregnancy. The provider's documentation of the number of weeks may be used to assign the appropriate code identifying the trimester.

Whenever delivery occurs during the current admission, and there is an "in childbirth" option for the obstetric complication being coded, the "in childbirth" code should be assigned.

> Pregnant patient at 21 weeks' gestation admitted with excessive vomiting
>
> **O21.2**    **Late vomiting of pregnancy**
>
> **Z3A.21**    **21 weeks gestation of pregnancy**
>
> *Explanation:* Category O21 classifies vomiting in pregnancy. Although code selection is based on whether the vomiting is before or after 20 completed weeks, these codes are not further classified by trimester. If vomiting only in the second trimester was documented, the provider should be queried for the specific week of gestation, as this will affect code selection.

#### 4) Selection of trimester for inpatient admissions that encompass more than one trimester

In instances when a patient is admitted to a hospital for complications of pregnancy during one trimester and remains in the hospital into a subsequent trimester, the trimester character for the antepartum complication code should be assigned on the basis of the trimester when the complication developed, not the trimester of the discharge. If the condition developed prior to the current admission/encounter or represents a pre-existing condition, the trimester character for the trimester at the time of the admission/encounter should be assigned.

> Patient admitted at 27 6/7 weeks' gestation for hemorrhaging from partial placenta previa; three days after admission at 28 1/7 weeks' gestation, she developed gestational hypertension
>
> **O44.32**    **Partial placenta previa with hemorrhage, second trimester**
>
> **O13.3**    **Gestational [pregnancy-induced] hypertension without significant proteinuria, third trimester**
>
> **Z3A.27**    **27 weeks gestation of pregnancy**
>
> *Explanation:* The patient presented with hemorrhaging from partial placenta previa while still in her 27th week, which falls within the second trimester. The gestational hypertension did not occur until three days after admission, putting the patient in her 28th week of pregnancy or what is considered to be the third trimester. The weeks of gestation captured by a code from category Z3A should represent only the gestational weeks upon admission.

#### 5) Unspecified trimester

Each category that includes codes for trimester has a code for "unspecified trimester." The "unspecified trimester" code should rarely be used, such as when the documentation in the record is insufficient to determine the trimester and it is not possible to obtain clarification.

#### 6) 7th character for fetus identification

Where applicable, a 7th character is to be assigned for certain categories (O31, O32, O33.3 - O33.6, O35, O36, O40, O41, O60.1, O60.2, O64, and O69) to identify the fetus for which the complication code applies.

Assign 7th character "0":

- For single gestations
- When the documentation in the record is insufficient to determine the fetus affected and it is not possible to obtain clarification.
- When it is not possible to clinically determine which fetus is affected.

> Maternal patient with twin gestations is seen after ultrasound identifies fetus B to be in breech presentation
>
> **O32.1XX2**    **Maternal care for breech presentation, fetus 2**
>
> *Explanation:* The documentation indicates that although there are two fetuses, only one fetus is determined to be in breech presentation. Whether fetus 2 or fetus B is used, the coder can assign the seventh character of 2 to identify the second fetus as the one in breech.

### b. Selection of OB principal or first-listed diagnosis

#### 1) Routine outpatient prenatal visits

For routine outpatient prenatal visits when no complications are present, a code from category Z34, Encounter for supervision of normal pregnancy, should be used as the first-listed diagnosis. These codes should not be used in conjunction with chapter 15 codes.

#### 2) *Supervision of high-risk pregnancy*

Codes from category O09, Supervision of high-risk pregnancy, are intended for use only during the prenatal period. For complications during the labor or delivery episode as a result of a high-risk pregnancy, assign the applicable complication codes from Chapter 15. If there are no complications during the labor or delivery episode, assign code O80, Encounter for full-term uncomplicated delivery.

For routine prenatal outpatient visits for patients with high-risk pregnancies, a code from category O09, Supervision of high-risk pregnancy, should be used as the first-listed diagnosis. Secondary chapter 15 codes may be used in conjunction with these codes if appropriate.

> 36-year-old admitted in labor with second child at 39 weeks' gestation, delivered a healthy baby, delivery complicated by tear of fourchette that was repaired
>
> **O70.0**    **First degree perineal laceration during delivery**
>
> **Z3A.39**    **39 weeks gestation of pregnancy**
>
> **Z37.0**    **Single live birth**
>
> Explanation: Although this patient is over 35 and having her second child (elderly multigravida), do not append a code from subcategory O09.52-. A code describing the tear of the fourchette, which complicated the delivery, should be used in addition to the applicable Z codes.

### 3) Episodes when no delivery occurs

In episodes when no delivery occurs, the principal diagnosis should correspond to the principal complication of the pregnancy which necessitated the encounter. Should more than one complication exist, all of which are treated or monitored, any of the complications codes may be sequenced first.

### 4) When a delivery occurs

When an obstetric patient is admitted and delivers during that admission, the condition that prompted the admission should be sequenced as the principal diagnosis. If multiple conditions prompted the admission, sequence the one most related to the delivery as the principal diagnosis. A code for any complication of the delivery should be assigned as an additional diagnosis. In cases of cesarean delivery, if the patient was admitted with a condition that resulted in the performance of a cesarean procedure, that condition should be selected as the principal diagnosis. If the reason for the admission was unrelated to the condition resulting in the cesarean delivery, the condition related to the reason for the admission should be selected as the principal diagnosis.

Maternal patient with diet-controlled gestational diabetes was admitted at 38 weeks' gestation in obstructed labor due to footling presentation; cesarean performed for the malpresentation

| | |
|---|---|
| O64.8XX0 | Obstructed labor due to other malposition and malpresentation, not applicable or unspecified |
| O24.420 | Gestational diabetes mellitus in childbirth, diet controlled |
| Z3A.38 | 38 weeks gestation of pregnancy |
| Z37.0 | Single live birth |

*Explanation:* The obstructed labor necessitated the cesarean procedure.

At 39 weeks' gestation, a maternal patient presents with hemorrhage with coagulation defect; the next day the patient goes into labor and eventually delivers via cesarean section due to arrested active phase of labor

| | |
|---|---|
| O46.003 | Antepartum hemorrhage with coagulation defect, unspecified, third trimester |
| O62.1 | Secondary uterine inertia |
| Z3A.39 | 39 weeks gestation of pregnancy |
| Z37.0 | Single live birth |

*Explanation:* The patient was admitted because of the antepartum hemorrhage with coagulation defect. The arrested active phase, although the reason for the cesarean delivery, did not develop until later into the stay.

### 5) Outcome of delivery

A code from category Z37, Outcome of delivery, should be included on every maternal record when a delivery has occurred. These codes are not to be used on subsequent records or on the newborn record.

### c. Pre-existing conditions versus conditions due to the pregnancy

Certain categories in Chapter 15 distinguish between conditions of the mother that existed prior to pregnancy (pre-existing) and those that are a direct result of pregnancy. When assigning codes from Chapter 15, it is important to assess if a condition was pre-existing prior to pregnancy or developed during or due to the pregnancy in order to assign the correct code.

Categories that do not distinguish between pre-existing and pregnancy-related conditions may be used for either. It is acceptable to use codes specifically for the puerperium with codes complicating pregnancy and childbirth if a condition arises postpartum during the delivery encounter.

### d. Pre-existing hypertension in pregnancy

Category O10, Pre-existing hypertension complicating pregnancy, childbirth and the puerperium, includes codes for hypertensive heart and hypertensive chronic kidney disease. When assigning one of the O10 codes that includes hypertensive heart disease or hypertensive chronic kidney disease, it is necessary to add a secondary code from the appropriate hypertension category to specify the type of heart failure or chronic kidney disease.

*See Section I.C.9. Hypertension.*

### e. Fetal conditions affecting the management of the mother

#### 1) Codes from categories O35 and O36

Codes from categories O35, Maternal care for known or suspected fetal abnormality and damage, and O36, Maternal care for other fetal problems, are assigned only when the fetal condition is actually responsible for modifying the management of the mother, i.e., by requiring diagnostic studies, additional observation, special care, or termination of pregnancy. The fact that the fetal condition exists does not justify assigning a code from this series to the mother's record.

A patient is seen in ED for spotting 15 weeks into her pregnancy; the doctors also suspect fetal hydrocephalus.

| | |
|---|---|
| O26.852 | Spotting complicating pregnancy, second trimester |
| Z3A.15 | 15 weeks gestation of pregnancy |

*Explanation:* Whether the fetal hydrocephalus was suspected or confirmed, an additional code is not warranted for this condition as the documentation does not indicate that this fetal condition is in any way altering the management of the mother or complicating her pregnancy.

#### 2) In utero surgery

In cases when surgery is performed on the fetus, a diagnosis code from category O35, Maternal care for known or suspected fetal abnormality and damage, should be assigned identifying the fetal condition. Assign the appropriate procedure code for the procedure performed.

No code from Chapter 16, the perinatal codes, should be used on the mother's record to identify fetal conditions. Surgery performed in utero on a fetus is still to be coded as an obstetric encounter.

### f. HIV infection in pregnancy, childbirth and the puerperium

During pregnancy, childbirth or the puerperium, a patient admitted because of an HIV-related illness should receive a principal diagnosis from subcategory O98.7-, Human immunodeficiency [HIV] disease complicating pregnancy, childbirth and the puerperium, followed by the code(s) for the HIV-related illness(es).

Patients with asymptomatic HIV infection status admitted during pregnancy, childbirth, or the puerperium should receive codes of O98.7- and Z21, Asymptomatic human immunodeficiency virus [HIV] infection status.

A previously asymptomatic HIV patient who is 13 weeks pregnant is admitted with oral thrush.

| | |
|---|---|
| O98.711 | Human immunodeficiency virus [HIV] disease complicating pregnancy, first trimester |
| B20 | Human immunodeficiency virus [HIV] disease |
| B37.0 | Candidal stomatitis |
| Z3A.13 | 13 weeks gestation of pregnancy |

*Explanation:* Because oral thrush is an HIV-related condition, this patient is now considered to have HIV disease. An obstetrics code indicating that HIV is complicating the pregnancy is coded first, followed by B20 for HIV disease as well as a code for the oral thrush.

### g. Diabetes mellitus in pregnancy

Diabetes mellitus is a significant complicating factor in pregnancy. Pregnant women who are diabetic should be assigned a code from category O24, Diabetes mellitus in pregnancy, childbirth, and the puerperium, first, followed by the appropriate diabetes code(s) (E08-E13) from Chapter 4.

### h. Long term use of insulin and oral hypoglycemics

Code Z79.4, Long-term (current) use of insulin, or code Z79.84, Long-term (current) use of oral hypoglycemic drugs, should also be assigned if the diabetes mellitus is being treated with insulin or oral medications. If the patient is treated with both oral medications and insulin, only the code for insulin-controlled should be assigned.

### i. Gestational (pregnancy induced) diabetes

Gestational (pregnancy induced) diabetes can occur during the second and third trimester of pregnancy in women who were not diabetic prior to pregnancy. Gestational diabetes can cause complications in the pregnancy similar to those of pre-existing diabetes mellitus. It also puts the woman at greater risk of developing diabetes after the pregnancy. Codes for gestational diabetes are in subcategory O24.4, Gestational diabetes mellitus. No other code from category O24, Diabetes mellitus in pregnancy, childbirth, and the puerperium, should be used with a code from O24.4.

The codes under subcategory O24.4 include diet controlled, insulin controlled, and controlled by oral hypoglycemic drugs. If a patient with gestational diabetes is treated with both diet and insulin, only the code for insulin-controlled is required. If a patient with gestational diabetes is treated with both diet and oral hypoglycemic medications, only the code for "controlled by oral hypoglycemic drugs" is required. Code Z79.4, Long-term (current) use of insulin or code Z79.84, Long-term (current) use of oral hypoglycemic drugs, should not be assigned with codes from subcategory O24.4.

An abnormal glucose tolerance in pregnancy is assigned a code from subcategory O99.81, Abnormal glucose complicating pregnancy, childbirth, and the puerperium.

> Patient at 39 weeks term pregnancy with gestational diabetes was admitted in labor and delivered a healthy newborn. Patient is on diabetes diet with daily metformin.
>
> | **O24.425** | **Gestational diabetes mellitus in childbirth, controlled by oral hypoglycemic drugs** |
> |---|---|
> | **Z3A.39** | **39 weeks gestation of pregnancy** |
> | **Z37.0** | **Single live birth** |
>
> *Explanation:* When the patient is admitted for delivery and the patient's gestational diabetes is controlled by both diet and oral hypoglycemic medications, only the combination code in subcategory O24.4-Gestational diabetes mellitus, is reported. No code is added for diet controlled diabetes, and no Z code for long-term use of oral hypoglycemics is reported with the O24.4 combination codes.

### j. Sepsis and septic shock complicating abortion, pregnancy, childbirth and the puerperium

When assigning a chapter 15 code for sepsis complicating abortion, pregnancy, childbirth, and the puerperium, a code for the specific type of infection should be assigned as an additional diagnosis. If severe sepsis is present, a code from subcategory R65.2, Severe sepsis, and code(s) for associated organ dysfunction(s) should also be assigned as additional diagnoses.

> Patient is seen several days after a miscarriage with sepsis; cultures return MSSA
>
> | **O03.87** | **Sepsis following complete or unspecified spontaneous abortion** |
> |---|---|
> | **B95.61** | **Methicillin susceptible Staphylococcus aureus infection as the cause of diseases classified elsewhere** |
>
> *Explanation:* The type of infection that caused this patient to become septic was methicillin susceptible *Staphylococcus aureus* (MSSA), which as a secondary code helps capture all aspects related to this patient's septic condition.

### k. Puerperal sepsis

Code O85, Puerperal sepsis, should be assigned with a secondary code to identify the causal organism (e.g., for a bacterial infection, assign a code from category B95-B96, Bacterial infections in conditions classified elsewhere). A code from category A40, Streptococcal sepsis, or A41, Other sepsis, should not be used for puerperal sepsis. If applicable, use additional codes to identify severe sepsis (R65.2-) and any associated acute organ dysfunction.

### l. Alcohol and tobacco use during pregnancy, childbirth and the puerperium

#### 1) Alcohol use during pregnancy, childbirth and the puerperium

Codes under subcategory O99.31, Alcohol use complicating pregnancy, childbirth, and the puerperium, should be assigned for any pregnancy case when a mother uses alcohol during the pregnancy or postpartum. A secondary code from category F10, Alcohol related disorders, should also be assigned to identify manifestations of the alcohol use.

#### 2) Tobacco use during pregnancy, childbirth and the puerperium

Codes under subcategory O99.33, Smoking (tobacco) complicating pregnancy, childbirth, and the puerperium, should be assigned for any pregnancy case when a mother uses any type of tobacco product during the pregnancy or postpartum. A secondary code from category F17, Nicotine dependence, should also be assigned to identify the type of nicotine dependence.

### m. Poisoning, toxic effects, adverse effects and underdosing in a pregnant patient

A code from subcategory O9A.2, Injury, poisoning and certain other consequences of external causes complicating pregnancy, childbirth, and the puerperium, should be sequenced first, followed by the appropriate injury, poisoning, toxic effect, adverse effect or underdosing code, and

then the additional code(s) that specifies the condition caused by the poisoning, toxic effect, adverse effect or underdosing.

*See Section I.C.19. Adverse effects, poisoning, underdosing and toxic effects.*

> Patient admitted with accidental carbon monoxide poisoning from a gas heating implement; the patient is 18 weeks' pregnant
>
> | **O9A.212** | **Injury, poisoning and certain other consequences of external causes complicating pregnancy, second trimester** |
> |---|---|
> | **T58.11XA** | **Toxic effect of carbon monoxide from utility gas, accidental (unintentional), initial encounter** |
> | **Z3A.18** | **18 weeks gestation of pregnancy** |
>
> *Explanation:* Although the carbon monoxide poisoning is the reason the patient was admitted, a code from the obstetrics chapter must be sequenced first. Chapter 15 codes have sequencing priority over codes from other chapters.

### n. Normal delivery, code O80

#### 1) Encounter for full term uncomplicated delivery

Code O80 should be assigned when a woman is admitted for a full-term normal delivery and delivers a single, healthy infant without any complications antepartum, during the delivery, or postpartum during the delivery episode. Code O80 is always a principal diagnosis. It is not to be used if any other code from chapter 15 is needed to describe a current complication of the antenatal, delivery, or perinatal period. Additional codes from other chapters may be used with code O80 if they are not related to or are in any way complicating the pregnancy.

#### 2) Uncomplicated delivery with resolved antepartum complication

Code O80 may be used if the patient had a complication at some point during the pregnancy, but the complication is not present at the time of the admission for delivery.

> Patient presents in labor at 39 weeks' gestation and delivers a healthy newborn; patient had abnormal glucose levels in her first trimester, which have since resolved
>
> | **O80** | **Encounter for full-term uncomplicated delivery** |
> |---|---|
> | **Z37.0** | **Single live birth** |
>
> *Explanation:* The abnormal glucose levels during the first trimester cannot be coded if they are not affecting the patient's current trimester. Without additional complications associated with the pregnancy, fetus, or mother, code O80 is appropriate.

#### 3) Outcome of delivery for O80

Z37.0, Single live birth, is the only outcome of delivery code appropriate for use with O80.

### o. The peripartum and postpartum periods

#### 1) Peripartum and postpartum periods

The postpartum period begins immediately after delivery and continues for six weeks following delivery. The peripartum period is defined as the last month of pregnancy to five months postpartum.

#### 2) Peripartum and postpartum complication

A postpartum complication is any complication occurring within the six-week period.

#### 3) Pregnancy-related complications after 6 week period

Chapter 15 codes may also be used to describe pregnancy-related complications after the peripartum or postpartum period if the provider documents that a condition is pregnancy related.

> Patient admitted for varicose veins. She had a baby boy three months ago; the varicose veins started to appear one month ago. The doctor attributes the patient's pregnancy as the cause of the varicose veins, which continue to be painful and bother the patient. She is seeking surgical relief.
>
> | **O87.4** | **Varicose veins of the lower extremity in the puerperium** |
> |---|---|
>
> *Explanation:* Although the varicose veins occurred several months after the delivery of the newborn, the doctor attributed the varicose veins to pregnancy and therefore a code from chapter 15 is appropriate.

#### 4) Admission for routine postpartum care following delivery outside hospital

When the mother delivers outside the hospital prior to admission and is admitted for routine postpartum care and no complications are noted, code Z39.0, Encounter for care and examination of mother immediately after delivery, should be assigned as the principal diagnosis.

**5) Pregnancy associated cardiomyopathy**

Pregnancy associated cardiomyopathy, code O90.3, is unique in that it may be diagnosed in the third trimester of pregnancy but may continue to progress months after delivery. For this reason, it is referred to as peripartum cardiomyopathy. Code O90.3 is only for use when the cardiomyopathy develops as a result of pregnancy in a woman who did not have pre-existing heart disease.

**p. Code O94, Sequelae of complication of pregnancy, childbirth, and the puerperium**

**1) Code O94**

Code O94, Sequelae of complication of pregnancy, childbirth, and the puerperium, is for use in those cases when an initial complication of a pregnancy develops a sequelae requiring care or treatment at a future date.

**2) After the initial postpartum period**

This code may be used at any time after the initial postpartum period.

**3) Sequencing of code O94**

This code, like all sequela codes, is to be sequenced following the code describing the sequelae of the complication.

**q. Termination of pregnancy and spontaneous abortions**

**1) Abortion with liveborn fetus**

When an attempted termination of pregnancy results in a liveborn fetus, assign code Z33.2, Encounter for elective termination of pregnancy and a code from category Z37, Outcome of Delivery.

**2) Retained products of conception following an abortion**

Subsequent encounters for retained products of conception following a spontaneous abortion or elective termination of pregnancy are assigned the appropriate code from category O03, Spontaneous abortion, or codes O07.4, Failed attempted termination of pregnancy without complication and Z33.2, Encounter for elective termination of pregnancy. This advice is appropriate even when the patient was discharged previously with a discharge diagnosis of complete abortion.

> Patient was seen two days ago for complete spontaneous abortion but returns today for urinary tract infection (UTI) with ultrasound showing retained products of conception
>
> **O03.38　　Urinary tract infection following incomplete spontaneous abortion**
>
> *Explanation:* Although the diagnosis from the patient's previous stay indicated that the patient had a complete abortion, it is now determined that there were actually retained products of conception (POC). An abortion with retained POC is considered incomplete and in this case resulted in the patient developing a UTI.

**3) Complications leading to abortion**

Codes from Chapter 15 may be used as additional codes to identify any documented complications of the pregnancy in conjunction with codes in categories in O07 and O08.

**r. Abuse in a pregnant patient**

For suspected or confirmed cases of abuse of a pregnant patient, a code(s) from subcategories O9A.3, Physical abuse complicating pregnancy, childbirth, and the puerperium, O9A.4, Sexual abuse complicating pregnancy, childbirth, and the puerperium, and O9A.5, Psychological abuse complicating pregnancy, childbirth, and the puerperium, should be sequenced first, followed by the appropriate codes (if applicable) to identify any associated current injury due to physical abuse, sexual abuse, and the perpetrator of abuse.

*See Section I.C.19. Adult and child abuse, neglect and other maltreatment.*

# Chapter 15. Pregnancy, Childbirth and the Puerperium (O00-O9A)

**NOTE**　CODES FROM THIS CHAPTER ARE FOR USE ONLY ON MATERNAL RECORDS, NEVER ON NEWBORN RECORDS.

Codes from this chapter are for use for conditions related to or aggravated by the pregnancy, childbirth, or by the puerperium (maternal causes or obstetric causes).

**NOTE**　Trimesters are counted from the first day of the last menstrual period. They are defined as follows:

　1st trimester- less than 14 weeks 0 days
　2nd trimester- 14 weeks 0 days to less than 28 weeks 0 days
　3rd trimester- 28 weeks 0 days until delivery

Use additional code from category Z3A, Weeks of gestation, to identify the specific week of the pregnancy, if known

**EXCLUDES 1**　*supervision of normal pregnancy (Z34.-)*
**EXCLUDES 2**　*mental and behavioral disorders associated with the puerperium (F53)*
　　*dobstetrical tetanus (A34)*
　　*postpartum necrosis of pituitary gland (E23.0)*
　　*puerperal osteomalacia (M83.0)*

**AHA:** 2016, 1Q, 3-5; 2014, 3Q, 17

This chapter contains the following blocks:
O00-O08　Pregnancy with abortive outcome
O09　Supervision of high risk pregnancy
O10-O16　Edema, proteinuria and hypertensive disorders in pregnancy, childbirth and the puerperium
O20-O29　Other maternal disorders predominantly related to pregnancy
O30-O48　Maternal care related to the fetus and amniotic cavity and possible delivery problems
O60-O77　Complications of labor and delivery
O80, O82　Encounter for delivery
O85-O92　Complications predominantly related to the puerperium
O94-O9A　Other obstetric conditions, not elsewhere classified

## Pregnancy with abortive outcome (O00-O08)

**EXCLUDES 1**　*continuing pregnancy in multiple gestation after abortion of one fetus or more (O31.1-, O31.3-)*

**✓4ᵗʰ O00　Ectopic pregnancy**
　**INCLUDES**　ruptured ectopic pregnancy
　Use additional code from category O08 to identify any associated complication
　**AHA:** 2014, 3Q, 17
　**DEF:** Implantation of fertilized egg outside the uterus, usually in fallopian tube or abdomen; requires emergency treatment.

　**CC Excl: For CC codes in category O00:** PDX collection 953

　**✓5ᵗʰ O00.0　Abdominal pregnancy**
　　**EXCLUDES 1**　*maternal care for viable fetus in abdominal pregnancy (O36.7-)*

　　**O00.00　Abdominal pregnancy without intrauterine pregnancy**　CC M ♀
　　　Abdominal pregnancy NOS

　　**O00.01　Abdominal pregnancy with intrauterine pregnancy**　CC M ♀

　**✓5ᵗʰ O00.1　Tubal pregnancy**
　　Fallopian pregnancy
　　Rupture of (fallopian) tube due to pregnancy
　　Tubal abortion

　　**✓6ᵗʰ O00.10　Tubal pregnancy without intrauterine pregnancy**
　　　Tubal pregnancy NOS

　　　● **O00.101　Right tubal pregnancy without intrauterine pregnancy**　CC M

　　　● **O00.102　Left tubal pregnancy without intrauterine pregnancy**　CC M

　　　● **O00.109　Unspecified tubal pregnancy without intrauterine pregnancy**　CC M

　　**✓6ᵗʰ O00.11　Tubal pregnancy with intrauterine pregnancy**
　　　● **O00.111　Right tubal pregnancy with intrauterine pregnancy**　CC M

　　　● **O00.112　Left tubal pregnancy with intrauterine pregnancy**　CC M

　　　● **O00.119　Unspecified tubal pregnancy with intrauterine pregnancy**　CC M

　**✓5ᵗʰ O00.2　Ovarian pregnancy**
　　**✓6ᵗʰ O00.20　Ovarian pregnancy without intrauterine pregnancy**
　　　Ovarian pregnancy NOS

　　　● **O00.201　Right ovarian pregnancy without intrauterine pregnancy**　CC M

　　　● **O00.202　Left ovarian pregnancy without intrauterine pregnancy**　CC M

　　　● **O00.209　Unspecified ovarian pregnancy without intrauterine pregnancy**　CC M

　　**✓6ᵗʰ O00.21　Ovarian pregnancy with intrauterine pregnancy**
　　　● **O00.211　Right ovarian pregnancy with intrauterine pregnancy**　CC M

　　　● **O00.212　Left ovarian pregnancy with intrauterine pregnancy**　CC M

　　　● **O00.219　Unspecified ovarian pregnancy with intrauterine pregnancy**　CC M

　**✓5ᵗʰ O00.8　Other ectopic pregnancy**
　　Cervical pregnancy
　　Cornual pregnancy
　　Intraligamentous pregnancy
　　Mural pregnancy

　　**O00.80　Other ectopic pregnancy without intrauterine pregnancy**　CC M ♀
　　　Other ectopic pregnancy NOS

　　**O00.81　Other ectopic pregnancy with intrauterine pregnancy**　CC M ♀

　**✓5ᵗʰ O00.9　Ectopic pregnancy, unspecified**
　　**O00.90　Unspecified ectopic pregnancy without intrauterine pregnancy**　CC M ♀
　　　Ectopic pregnancy NOS

　　**O00.91　Unspecified ectopic pregnancy with intrauterine pregnancy**　CC M ♀

**✓4ᵗʰ O01　Hydatidiform mole**
　Use additional code from category O08 to identify any associated complication
　**EXCLUDES 1**　*chorioadenoma (destruens) (D39.2)*
　　*malignant hydatidiform mole (D39.2)*
　**AHA:** 2014, 3Q, 17
　**DEF:** Abnormal product of pregnancy; marked by mass of cysts resembling bunch of grapes due to chorionic villi proliferation and dissolution; must be surgically removed.

　**O01.0　Classical hydatidiform mole**　M ♀
　　Complete hydatidiform mole

　**O01.1　Incomplete and partial hydatidiform mole**　M ♀

　**O01.9　Hydatidiform mole, unspecified**　M ♀
　　Trophoblastic disease NOS
　　Vesicular mole NOS

**✓4ᵗʰ O02　Other abnormal products of conception**
　Use additional code from category O08 to identify any associated complication
　**EXCLUDES 1**　*papyraceous fetus (O31.0-)*
　**AHA:** 2014, 3Q, 17

　**O02.0　Blighted ovum and nonhydatidiform mole**　M ♀
　　Carneous mole
　　Fleshy mole
　　Intrauterine mole NOS
　　Molar pregnancy NEC
　　Pathological ovum

**Ectopic Pregnancy**

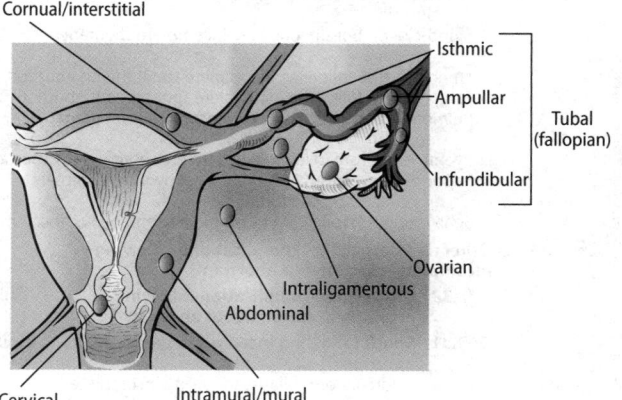

Cornual/interstitial — Isthmic — Ampullar — Tubal (fallopian) — Infundibular — Ovarian — Intraligamentous — Abdominal — Cervical — Intramural/mural

**O02.1 Missed abortion**   Ⓜ♀

Early fetal death, before completion of 20 weeks of gestation, with retention of dead fetus

> EXCLUDES 1   *failed induced abortion (O07.-)*
> *fetal death (intrauterine) (late) (O36.4)*
> *missed abortion with blighted ovum (O02.0)*
> *missed abortion with hydatidiform mole (O01.-)*
> *missed abortion with nonhydatidiform (O02.0)*
> *missed abortion with other abnormal products of conception (O02.8-)*
> *missed delivery (O36.4)*
> *stillbirth (P95)*

✓5ᵗʰ **O02.8 Other specified abnormal products of conception**

> EXCLUDES 1   *abnormal products of conception with blighted ovum (O02.0)*
> *abnormal products of conception with hydatidiform mole (O01.-)*
> *abnormal products of conception with nonhydatidiform mole (O02.0)*

**O02.81 Inappropriate change in quantitative human chorionic gonadotropin (hCG) in early pregnancy**   Ⓜ♀

Biochemical pregnancy

Chemical pregnancy

Inappropriate level of quantitative human chorionic gonadotropin (hCG) for gestational age in early pregnancy

**O02.89 Other abnormal products of conception**   Ⓜ♀

**O02.9 Abnormal product of conception, unspecified**   Ⓜ♀

✓4ᵗʰ **O03 Spontaneous abortion**

> NOTE   Incomplete abortion includes retained products of conception following spontaneous abortion
> INCLUDES   miscarriage

> CC Excl: For CC/MCC codes in category O03: PDX collection 954

**O03.0 Genital tract and pelvic infection following incomplete spontaneous abortion**   cc Ⓜ♀

Endometritis following incomplete spontaneous abortion

Oophoritis following incomplete spontaneous abortion

Parametritis following incomplete spontaneous abortion

Pelvic peritonitis following incomplete spontaneous abortion

Salpingitis following incomplete spontaneous abortion

Salpingo-oophoritis following incomplete spontaneous abortion

> EXCLUDES 1   *sepsis following incomplete spontaneous abortion (O03.37)*
> *urinary tract infection following incomplete spontaneous abortion (O03.38)*

**O03.1 Delayed or excessive hemorrhage following incomplete spontaneous abortion**   Ⓜ♀

Afibrinogenemia following incomplete spontaneous abortion

Defibrination syndrome following incomplete spontaneous abortion

Hemolysis following incomplete spontaneous abortion

Intravascular coagulation following incomplete spontaneous abortion

**O03.2 Embolism following incomplete spontaneous abortion**   mcc Ⓜ♀

Air embolism following incomplete spontaneous abortion

Amniotic fluid embolism following incomplete spontaneous abortion

Blood-clot embolism following incomplete spontaneous abortion

Embolism NOS following incomplete spontaneous abortion

Fat embolism following incomplete spontaneous abortion

Pulmonary embolism following incomplete spontaneous abortion

Pyemic embolism following incomplete spontaneous abortion

Septic or septicopyemic embolism following incomplete spontaneous abortion

Soap embolism following incomplete spontaneous abortion

✓5ᵗʰ **O03.3 Other and unspecified complications following incomplete spontaneous abortion**

**O03.30 Unspecified complication following incomplete spontaneous abortion**   cc Ⓜ♀

**O03.31 Shock following incomplete spontaneous abortion**   mcc Ⓜ♀

Circulatory collapse following incomplete spontaneous abortion

Shock (postprocedural) following incomplete spontaneous abortion

> EXCLUDES 1   *shock due to infection following incomplete spontaneous abortion (O03.37)*

**O03.32 Renal failure following incomplete spontaneous abortion**   mcc Ⓜ♀

Kidney failure (acute) following incomplete spontaneous abortion

Oliguria following incomplete spontaneous abortion

Renal shutdown following incomplete spontaneous abortion

Renal tubular necrosis following incomplete spontaneous abortion

Uremia following incomplete spontaneous abortion

**O03.33 Metabolic disorder following incomplete spontaneous abortion**   cc Ⓜ♀

**O03.34 Damage to pelvic organs following incomplete spontaneous abortion**   cc Ⓜ♀

Laceration, perforation, tear or chemical damage of bladder following incomplete spontaneous abortion

Laceration, perforation, tear or chemical damage of bowel following incomplete spontaneous abortion

Laceration, perforation, tear or chemical damage of broad ligament following incomplete spontaneous abortion

Laceration, perforation, tear or chemical damage of cervix following incomplete spontaneous abortion

Laceration, perforation, tear or chemical damage of periurethral tissue following incomplete spontaneous abortion

Laceration, perforation, tear or chemical damage of uterus following incomplete spontaneous abortion

Laceration, perforation, tear or chemical damage of vagina following incomplete spontaneous abortion

**O03.35 Other venous complications following incomplete spontaneous abortion**   cc Ⓜ♀

**O03.36 Cardiac arrest following incomplete spontaneous abortion**   cc Ⓜ♀

**O03.37 Sepsis following incomplete spontaneous abortion**   cc Ⓜ♀

Use additional code to identify infectious agent (B95-B97)

Use additional code to identify severe sepsis, if applicable (R65.2-)

> EXCLUDES 1   *septic or septicopyemic embolism following incomplete spontaneous abortion (O03.2)*

**O03.38 Urinary tract infection following incomplete spontaneous abortion**   cc Ⓜ♀

Cystitis following incomplete spontaneous abortion

**O03.39 Incomplete spontaneous abortion with other complications**   cc Ⓜ♀

**O03.4 Incomplete spontaneous abortion without complication**   Ⓜ♀

**O03.5 Genital tract and pelvic infection following complete or unspecified spontaneous abortion**   cc Ⓜ♀

Endometritis following complete or unspecified spontaneous abortion

Oophoritis following complete or unspecified spontaneous abortion

Parametritis following complete or unspecified spontaneous abortion

Pelvic peritonitis following complete or unspecified spontaneous abortion

Salpingitis following complete or unspecified spontaneous abortion

Salpingo-oophoritis following complete or unspecified spontaneous abortion

> EXCLUDES 1   *sepsis following complete or unspecified spontaneous abortion (O03.87)*
> *urinary tract infection following complete or unspecified spontaneous abortion (O03.88)*

**O03.6 Delayed or excessive hemorrhage following complete or unspecified spontaneous abortion**   Ⓜ♀

Afibrinogenemia following complete or unspecified spontaneous abortion

Defibrination syndrome following complete or unspecified spontaneous abortion

Hemolysis following complete or unspecified spontaneous abortion

Intravascular coagulation following complete or unspecified spontaneous abortion

Ⓝ Newborn: 0    Ⓟ Pediatric: 0-17    Ⓜ Maternity: 12-55    Ⓐ Adult: 15-124    mcc Major CC Condition    PDxMCC PDx acts as own MCC    cc CC Condition    PDxCC PDx acts as own CC

844          ICD-10-CM 2018

**O03.7**   **Embolism following complete or unspecified** `CC` `M` ♀
**spontaneous abortion**
     Air embolism following complete or unspecified spontaneous abortion
     Amniotic fluid embolism following complete or unspecified spontaneous abortion
     Blood-clot embolism following complete or unspecified spontaneous abortion
     Embolism NOS following complete or unspecified spontaneous abortion
     Fat embolism following complete or unspecified spontaneous abortion
     Pulmonary embolism following complete or unspecified spontaneous abortion
     Pyemic embolism following complete or unspecified spontaneous abortion
     Septic or septicopyemic embolism following complete or unspecified spontaneous abortion
     Soap embolism following complete or unspecified spontaneous abortion

✓5th **O03.8**   **Other and unspecified complications following complete or unspecified spontaneous abortion**

   **O03.80**   **Unspecified complication following complete** `CC` `M` ♀
         **or unspecified spontaneous abortion**

   **O03.81**   **Shock following complete or unspecified** `MCC` `M` ♀
         **spontaneous abortion**
         Circulatory collapse following complete or unspecified spontaneous abortion
         Shock (postprocedural) following complete or unspecified spontaneous abortion
         `EXCLUDES 1` *shock due to infection following complete or unspecified spontaneous abortion (O03.87)*

   **O03.82**   **Renal failure following complete or** `MCC` `M` ♀
         **unspecified spontaneous abortion**
         Kidney failure (acute) following complete or unspecified spontaneous abortion
         Oliguria following complete or unspecified spontaneous abortion
         Renal shutdown following complete or unspecified spontaneous abortion
         Renal tubular necrosis following complete or unspecified spontaneous abortion
         Uremia following complete or unspecified spontaneous abortion

   **O03.83**   **Metabolic disorder following complete or** `CC` `M` ♀
         **unspecified spontaneous abortion**

   **O03.84**   **Damage to pelvic organs following complete** `CC` `M` ♀
         **or unspecified spontaneous abortion**
         Laceration, perforation, tear or chemical damage of bladder following complete or unspecified spontaneous abortion
         Laceration, perforation, tear or chemical damage of bowel following complete or unspecified spontaneous abortion
         Laceration, perforation, tear or chemical damage of broad ligament following complete or unspecified spontaneous abortion
         Laceration, perforation, tear or chemical damage of cervix following complete or unspecified spontaneous abortion
         Laceration, perforation, tear or chemical damage of periurethral tissue following complete or unspecified spontaneous abortion
         Laceration, perforation, tear or chemical damage of uterus following complete or unspecified spontaneous abortion
         Laceration, perforation, tear or chemical damage of vagina following complete or unspecified spontaneous abortion

   **O03.85**   **Other venous complications following** `CC` `M` ♀
         **complete or unspecified spontaneous abortion**

   **O03.86**   **Cardiac arrest following complete or** `CC` `M` ♀
         **unspecified spontaneous abortion**

   **O03.87**   **Sepsis following complete or unspecified** `CC` `M` ♀
         **spontaneous abortion**
         Use additional code to identify infectious agent (B95-B97)
         Use additional code to identify severe sepsis, if applicable (R65.2-)
         `EXCLUDES 1` *septic or septicopyemic embolism following complete or unspecified spontaneous abortion (O03.7)*

**O03.88**   **Urinary tract infection following complete or** `CC` `M` ♀
         **unspecified spontaneous abortion**
         Cystitis following complete or unspecified spontaneous abortion

**O03.89**   **Complete or unspecified spontaneous** `CC` `M` ♀
         **abortion with other complications**

**O03.9**   **Complete or unspecified spontaneous abortion without** `M` ♀
**complication**
     Miscarriage NOS
     Spontaneous abortion NOS

✓4th **O04**   **Complications following (induced) termination of pregnancy**
     `INCLUDES`   complications following (induced) termination of pregnancy
     `EXCLUDES 1`   *encounter for elective termination of pregnancy, uncomplicated (Z33.2)*
              *failed attempted termination of pregnancy (O07.-)*

> **CC Excl: For CC/MCC codes in category O04, unless otherwise noted:** PDX collection 954

**O04.5**   **Genital tract and pelvic infection following (induced)** `CC` `M` ♀
**termination of pregnancy**
     Endometritis following (induced) termination of pregnancy
     Oophoritis following (induced) termination of pregnancy
     Parametritis following (induced) termination of pregnancy
     Pelvic peritonitis following (induced) termination of pregnancy
     Salpingitis following (induced) termination of pregnancy
     Salpingo-oophoritis following (induced) termination of pregnancy
     `EXCLUDES 1`   *sepsis following (induced) termination of pregnancy (O04.87)*
              *urinary tract infection following (induced) termination of pregnancy (O04.88)*

**O04.6**   **Delayed or excessive hemorrhage following (induced)** `M` ♀
**termination of pregnancy**
     Afibrinogenemia following (induced) termination of pregnancy
     Defibrination syndrome following (induced) termination of pregnancy
     Hemolysis following (induced) termination of pregnancy
     Intravascular coagulation following (induced) termination of pregnancy

**O04.7**   **Embolism following (induced) termination of** `MCC` `M` ♀
**pregnancy**
     Air embolism following (induced) termination of pregnancy
     Amniotic fluid embolism following (induced) termination of pregnancy
     Blood-clot embolism following (induced) termination of pregnancy
     Embolism NOS following (induced) termination of pregnancy
     Fat embolism following (induced) termination of pregnancy
     Pulmonary embolism following (induced) termination of pregnancy
     Pyemic embolism following (induced) termination of pregnancy
     Septic or septicopyemic embolism following (induced) termination of pregnancy
     Soap embolism following (induced) termination of pregnancy

✓5th **O04.8**   **(Induced) termination of pregnancy with other and unspecified complications**

   **O04.80**   **(Induced) termination of pregnancy with** `CC` `M` ♀
         **unspecified complications**

   **O04.81**   **Shock following (induced) termination of** `MCC` `M` ♀
         **pregnancy**
         Circulatory collapse following (induced) termination of pregnancy
         Shock (postprocedural) following (induced) termination of pregnancy
         `EXCLUDES 1` *shock due to infection following (induced) termination of pregnancy (O04.87)*

   **O04.82**   **Renal failure following (induced)** `MCC` `M` ♀
         **termination of pregnancy**
         Kidney failure (acute) following (induced) termination of pregnancy
         Oliguria following (induced) termination of pregnancy
         Renal shutdown following (induced) termination of pregnancy
         Renal tubular necrosis following (induced) termination of pregnancy
         Uremia following (induced) termination of pregnancy

   **O04.83**   **Metabolic disorder following (induced)** `CC` `M` ♀
         **termination of pregnancy**

---

✓ Additional Character Req    ✓x7th Placeholder Alert    Unacceptable PDx    Manifestation    `H1`-`H14` HAC    `HCC` CMS-HCC Condition    `EXCLUDES 1` Not Coded Here    `EXCLUDES 2` Not Included Here

**Chapter 15. Pregnancy, Childbirth and the Puerperium**

**O04.84**   **Damage to pelvic organs following (induced)** CC M♀
**termination of pregnancy**
Laceration, perforation, tear or chemical damage of
bladder following (induced) termination of
pregnancy
Laceration, perforation, tear or chemical damage of
bowel following (induced) termination of
pregnancy
Laceration, perforation, tear or chemical damage of
broad ligament following (induced) termination
of pregnancy
Laceration, perforation, tear or chemical damage of
cervix following (induced) termination of
pregnancy
Laceration, perforation, tear or chemical damage of
periurethral tissue following (induced)
termination of pregnancy
Laceration, perforation, tear or chemical damage of
uterus following (induced) termination of
pregnancy
Laceration, perforation, tear or chemical damage of
vagina following (induced) termination of
pregnancy

**O04.85**   **Other venous complications following**   CC M♀
**(induced) termination of pregnancy**

**O04.86**   **Cardiac arrest following (induced)**   CC M♀
**termination of pregnancy**

**O04.87**   **Sepsis following (induced) termination of**   CC M♀
**pregnancy**
Use additional code to identify infectious agent
(B95-B97)
Use additional code to identify severe sepsis, if
applicable (R65.2-)
**EXCLUDES 1**   *septic or septicopyemic embolism following
(induced) termination of pregnancy
(O04.7)*
**CC Excl:** PDX collection 955

**O04.88**   **Urinary tract infection following (induced)**   CC M♀
**termination of pregnancy**
Cystitis following (induced) termination of pregnancy

**O04.89**   **(Induced) termination of pregnancy with**   CC M♀
**other complications**

✓4th **O07**   **Failed attempted termination of pregnancy**
**INCLUDES**   failure of attempted induction of termination of pregnancy
incomplete elective abortion
**EXCLUDES 1**   *incomplete spontaneous abortion (O03.0-)*

**O07.0**   **Genital tract and pelvic infection following failed**   CC M♀
**attempted termination of pregnancy**
Endometritis following failed attempted termination of
pregnancy
Oophoritis following failed attempted termination of pregnancy
Parametritis following failed attempted termination of
pregnancy
Pelvic peritonitis following failed attempted termination of
pregnancy
Salpingitis following failed attempted termination of pregnancy
Salpingo-oophoritis following failed attempted termination of
pregnancy
**EXCLUDES 1**   *sepsis following failed attempted termination of
pregnancy (O07.37)
urinary tract infection following failed attempted
termination of pregnancy (O07.38)*
**CC Excl:** PDX collection 956

**O07.1**   **Delayed or excessive hemorrhage following failed**   CC M♀
**attempted termination of pregnancy**
Afibrinogenemia following failed attempted termination of
pregnancy
Defibrination syndrome following failed attempted termination
of pregnancy
Hemolysis following failed attempted termination of pregnancy
Intravascular coagulation following failed attempted
termination of pregnancy
**CC Excl:** PDX collection 957

**O07.2**   **Embolism following failed attempted termination of**   MCC M♀
**pregnancy**
Air embolism following failed attempted termination of
pregnancy
Amniotic fluid embolism following failed attempted termination
of pregnancy
Blood-clot embolism following failed attempted termination of
pregnancy
Embolism NOS following failed attempted termination of
pregnancy
Fat embolism following failed attempted termination of
pregnancy
Pulmonary embolism following failed attempted termination of
pregnancy
Pyemic embolism following failed attempted termination of
pregnancy
Septic or septicopyemic embolism following failed attempted
termination of pregnancy
Soap embolism following failed attempted termination of
pregnancy
**CC Excl:** PDX collection 958

✓5th **O07.3**   **Failed attempted termination of pregnancy with other and**
**unspecified complications**

**O07.30**   **Failed attempted termination of pregnancy**   CC M♀
**with unspecified complications**
**CC Excl:** PDX collection 954

**O07.31**   **Shock following failed attempted**   MCC M♀
**termination of pregnancy**
Circulatory collapse following failed attempted
termination of pregnancy
Shock (postprocedural) following failed attempted
termination of pregnancy
**EXCLUDES 1**   *shock due to infection following failed
attempted termination of pregnancy
(O07.37)*
**CC Excl:** PDX collection 959

**O07.32**   **Renal failure following failed attempted**   MCC M♀
**termination of pregnancy**
Kidney failure (acute) following failed attempted
termination of pregnancy
Oliguria following failed attempted termination of
pregnancy
Renal shutdown following failed attempted
termination of pregnancy
Renal tubular necrosis following failed attempted
termination of pregnancy
Uremia following failed attempted termination of
pregnancy
**CC Excl:** PDX collection 960

**O07.33**   **Metabolic disorder following failed**   CC M♀
**attempted termination of pregnancy**
**CC Excl:** PDX collection 954

**O07.34**   **Damage to pelvic organs following failed**   CC M♀
**attempted termination of pregnancy**
Laceration, perforation, tear or chemical damage of
bladder following failed attempted termination
of pregnancy
Laceration, perforation, tear or chemical damage of
bowel following failed attempted termination of
pregnancy
Laceration, perforation, tear or chemical damage of
broad ligament following failed attempted
termination of pregnancy
Laceration, perforation, tear or chemical damage of
cervix following failed attempted termination of
pregnancy
Laceration, perforation, tear or chemical damage of
periurethral tissue following failed attempted
termination of pregnancy
Laceration, perforation, tear or chemical damage of
uterus following failed attempted termination of
pregnancy
Laceration, perforation, tear or chemical damage of
vagina following failed attempted termination of
pregnancy
**CC Excl:** PDX collection 961

**O07.35**   **Other venous complications following failed**   CC M♀
**attempted termination of pregnancy**
**CC Excl:** PDX collection 954

**O07.36**   **Cardiac arrest following failed attempted**   CC M♀
**termination of pregnancy**
**CC Excl:** PDX collection 954

---

N Newborn: 0   P Pediatric: 0-17   M Maternity: 12-55   A Adult: 15-124   MCC Major CC Condition   PDxMCC PDx acts as own MCC   CC CC Condition   PDxCC PDx acts as own CC

**846**      ICD-10-CM 2018

**O07.37** **Sepsis following failed attempted termination of pregnancy**   `CC` `M` ♀
Use additional code to identify infectious agent (B95-B97)
Use additional code to identify severe sepsis, if applicable (R65.2-)
   *EXCLUDES 1*   *septic or septicopyemic embolism following failed attempted termination of pregnancy (O07.2)*
**CC Excl:** PDX collection 956

**O07.38** **Urinary tract infection following failed attempted termination of pregnancy**   `CC` `M` ♀
Cystitis following failed attempted termination of pregnancy
**CC Excl:** PDX collection 954

**O07.39** **Failed attempted termination of pregnancy with other complications**   `CC` `M` ♀
**CC Excl:** PDX collection 954

**O07.4** **Failed attempted termination of pregnancy** without complication   `M` ♀

✅4th **O08** **Complications following ectopic and molar pregnancy**
This category is for use with categories O00-O02 to identify any associated complications

> **CC Excl:** For CC/MCC codes in category O08, unless otherwise noted: PDX collection 963

**O08.0** **Genital tract and pelvic infection following ectopic and molar pregnancy**   `CC` `M` ♀
Endometritis following ectopic and molar pregnancy
Oophoritis following ectopic and molar pregnancy
Parametritis following ectopic and molar pregnancy
Pelvic peritonitis following ectopic and molar pregnancy
Salpingitis following ectopic and molar pregnancy
Salpingo-oophoritis following ectopic and molar pregnancy
   *EXCLUDES 1*   *sepsis following ectopic and molar pregnancy (O08.82)*
*urinary tract infection (O08.83)*
**CC Excl:** PDX collection 85

**O08.1** **Delayed or excessive hemorrhage following ectopic and molar pregnancy**   `CC` ♀
Afibrinogenemia following ectopic and molar pregnancy
Defibrination syndrome following ectopic and molar pregnancy
Hemolysis following ectopic and molar pregnancy
Intravascular coagulation following ectopic and molar pregnancy
   *EXCLUDES 1*   *delayed or excessive hemorrhage due to incomplete abortion (O03.1)*
**CC Excl:** PDX collection 962

**O08.2** **Embolism following ectopic and molar pregnancy**   `MCC` `M` ♀
Air embolism following ectopic and molar pregnancy
Amniotic fluid embolism following ectopic and molar pregnancy
Blood-clot embolism following ectopic and molar pregnancy
Embolism NOS following ectopic and molar pregnancy
Fat embolism following ectopic and molar pregnancy
Pulmonary embolism following ectopic and molar pregnancy
Pyemic embolism following ectopic and molar pregnancy
Septic or septicopyemic embolism following ectopic and molar pregnancy
Soap embolism following ectopic and molar pregnancy

**O08.3** **Shock following ectopic and molar pregnancy**   `MCC` ♀
Circulatory collapse following ectopic and molar pregnancy
Shock (postprocedural) following ectopic and molar pregnancy
   *EXCLUDES 1*   *shock due to infection following ectopic and molar pregnancy (O08.82)*

**O08.4** **Renal failure following ectopic and molar pregnancy**   `MCC` ♀
Kidney failure (acute) following ectopic and molar pregnancy
Oliguria following ectopic and molar pregnancy
Renal shutdown following ectopic and molar pregnancy
Renal tubular necrosis following ectopic and molar pregnancy
Uremia following ectopic and molar pregnancy

**O08.5** **Metabolic disorders following an ectopic and molar pregnancy**   `CC` `M` ♀

**O08.6** **Damage to pelvic organs and tissues following an ectopic and molar pregnancy**   `CC` `M` ♀
Laceration, perforation, tear or chemical damage of bladder following an ectopic and molar pregnancy
Laceration, perforation, tear or chemical damage of bowel following an ectopic and molar pregnancy
Laceration, perforation, tear or chemical damage of broad ligament following an ectopic and molar pregnancy
Laceration, perforation, tear or chemical damage of cervix following an ectopic and molar pregnancy
Laceration, perforation, tear or chemical damage of periurethral tissue following an ectopic and molar pregnancy
Laceration, perforation, tear or chemical damage of uterus following an ectopic and molar pregnancy
Laceration, perforation, tear or chemical damage of vagina following an ectopic and molar pregnancy

**O08.7** **Other venous complications following an ectopic and molar pregnancy**   `CC` `M` ♀

✅5th **O08.8** **Other complications following an ectopic and molar pregnancy**

**O08.81** **Cardiac arrest following an ectopic and molar pregnancy**   `CC` `M` ♀

**O08.82** **Sepsis following ectopic and molar pregnancy**   `CC` `M` ♀
Use additional code to identify infectious agent (B95-B97)
Use additional code to identify severe sepsis, if applicable (R65.2-)
   *EXCLUDES 1*   *septic or septicopyemic embolism following ectopic and molar pregnancy (O08.2)*
**CC Excl:** PDX collection 85

**O08.83** **Urinary tract infection following an ectopic and molar pregnancy**   `CC` `M` ♀
Cystitis following an ectopic and molar pregnancy

**O08.89** **Other complications following an ectopic and molar pregnancy**   `CC` `M` ♀

**O08.9** **Unspecified complication following an ectopic and molar pregnancy**   `CC` `M` ♀

### Supervision of high risk pregnancy (O09)

✅4th **O09** **Supervision of high risk pregnancy**
**AHA:** 2016, 4Q, 150

✅5th **O09.0** **Supervision of pregnancy with history of infertility**

**O09.00** **Supervision of pregnancy with history of infertility, unspecified trimester**   `M` ♀

**O09.01** **Supervision of pregnancy with history of infertility, first trimester**   `M` ♀

**O09.02** **Supervision of pregnancy with history of infertility, second trimester**   `M` ♀

**O09.03** **Supervision of pregnancy with history of infertility, third trimester**   `M` ♀

✅5th **O09.1** **Supervision of pregnancy with history of ectopic pregnancy**

**O09.10** **Supervision of pregnancy with history of ectopic pregnancy, unspecified trimester**   `M` ♀

**O09.11** **Supervision of pregnancy with history of ectopic pregnancy, first trimester**   `M` ♀

**O09.12** **Supervision of pregnancy with history of ectopic pregnancy, second trimester**   `M` ♀

**O09.13** **Supervision of pregnancy with history of ectopic pregnancy, third trimester**   `M` ♀

✅5th **O09.A** **Supervision of pregnancy with history of molar pregnancy**

**O09.A0** **Supervision of pregnancy with history of molar pregnancy, unspecified trimester**   `M` ♀

**O09.A1** **Supervision of pregnancy with history of molar pregnancy, first trimester**   `M` ♀

**O09.A2** **Supervision of pregnancy with history of molar pregnancy, second trimester**   `M` ♀

**O09.A3** **Supervision of pregnancy with history of molar pregnancy, third trimester**   `M` ♀

✅5th **O09.2** **Supervision of pregnancy with other poor reproductive or obstetric history**
   *EXCLUDES 2*   *pregnancy care for patient with history of recurrent pregnancy loss (O26.2-)*

✅6th **O09.21** **Supervision of pregnancy with history of pre-term labor**

**O09.211** **Supervision of pregnancy with history of pre-term labor, first trimester**   `M` ♀

**O09.212** **Supervision of pregnancy with history of pre-term labor, second trimester**   `M` ♀

O09.213 **Supervision of pregnancy with history** Ⓜ♀
**of pre-term labor, third trimester**

O09.219 **Supervision of pregnancy with history** Ⓜ♀
**of pre-term labor, unspecified trimester**

√6ᵗʰ O09.29 **Supervision of pregnancy with other poor**
**reproductive or obstetric history**
Supervision of pregnancy with history of neonatal
death
Supervision of pregnancy with history of stillbirth

O09.291 **Supervision of pregnancy with other** Ⓜ♀
**poor reproductive or obstetric**
**history, first trimester**

O09.292 **Supervision of pregnancy with other** Ⓜ♀
**poor reproductive or obstetric**
**history, second trimester**

O09.293 **Supervision of pregnancy with other** Ⓜ♀
**poor reproductive or obstetric**
**history, third trimester**

O09.299 **Supervision of pregnancy with other** Ⓜ♀
**poor reproductive or obstetric**
**history, unspecified trimester**

√5ᵗʰ O09.3 **Supervision of pregnancy with insufficient antenatal care**
Supervision of concealed pregnancy
Supervision of hidden pregnancy

O09.30 **Supervision of pregnancy with insufficient** Ⓜ♀
**antenatal care, unspecified trimester**

O09.31 **Supervision of pregnancy with insufficient** Ⓜ♀
**antenatal care, first trimester**

O09.32 **Supervision of pregnancy with insufficient** Ⓜ♀
**antenatal care, second trimester**

O09.33 **Supervision of pregnancy with insufficient** Ⓜ♀
**antenatal care, third trimester**

√5ᵗʰ O09.4 **Supervision of pregnancy with grand multiparity**

O09.40 **Supervision of pregnancy with grand** Ⓜ♀
**multiparity, unspecified trimester**

O09.41 **Supervision of pregnancy with grand** Ⓜ♀
**multiparity, first trimester**

O09.42 **Supervision of pregnancy with grand** Ⓜ♀
**multiparity, second trimester**

O09.43 **Supervision of pregnancy with grand** Ⓜ♀
**multiparity, third trimester**

√5ᵗʰ O09.5 **Supervision of elderly primigravida and multigravida**
Pregnancy for a female 35 years and older at expected date of
delivery

√6ᵗʰ O09.51 **Supervision of elderly primigravida**

O09.511 **Supervision of elderly primigravida,** Ⓜ♀
**first trimester**

O09.512 **Supervision of elderly primigravida,** Ⓜ♀
**second trimester**

O09.513 **Supervision of elderly primigravida,** Ⓜ♀
**third trimester**

O09.519 **Supervision of elderly primigravida,** Ⓜ♀
**unspecified trimester**

√6ᵗʰ O09.52 **Supervision of elderly multigravida**

O09.521 **Supervision of elderly multigravida,** Ⓜ♀
**first trimester**

O09.522 **Supervision of elderly multigravida,** Ⓜ♀
**second trimester**

O09.523 **Supervision of elderly multigravida,** Ⓜ♀
**third trimester**

O09.529 **Supervision of elderly multigravida,** Ⓜ♀
**unspecified trimester**

√5ᵗʰ O09.6 **Supervision of young primigravida and multigravida**
Supervision of pregnancy for a female less than 16 years old at
expected date of delivery

√6ᵗʰ O09.61 **Supervision of young primigravida**

O09.611 **Supervision of young primigravida,** Ⓜ♀
**first trimester**

O09.612 **Supervision of young primigravida,** Ⓜ♀
**second trimester**

O09.613 **Supervision of young primigravida,** Ⓜ♀
**third trimester**

O09.619 **Supervision of young primigravida,** Ⓜ♀
**unspecified trimester**

√6ᵗʰ O09.62 **Supervision of young multigravida**

O09.621 **Supervision of young multigravida,** Ⓜ♀
**first trimester**

O09.622 **Supervision of young multigravida,** Ⓜ♀
**second trimester**

O09.623 **Supervision of young multigravida,** Ⓜ♀
**third trimester**

O09.629 **Supervision of young multigravida,** Ⓜ♀
**unspecified trimester**

√5ᵗʰ O09.7 **Supervision of high risk pregnancy due to social problems**

O09.70 **Supervision of high risk pregnancy due to** Ⓜ♀
**social problems, unspecified trimester**

O09.71 **Supervision of high risk pregnancy due to** Ⓜ♀
**social problems, first trimester**

O09.72 **Supervision of high risk pregnancy due to** Ⓜ♀
**social problems, second trimester**

O09.73 **Supervision of high risk pregnancy due to** Ⓜ♀
**social problems, third trimester**

√5ᵗʰ O09.8 **Supervision of other high risk pregnancies**

√6ᵗʰ O09.81 **Supervision of pregnancy resulting from assisted**
**reproductive technology**
Supervision of pregnancy resulting from in-vitro
fertilization

EXCLUDES 2    *gestational carrier status (Z33.3)*

O09.811 **Supervision of pregnancy resulting** Ⓜ♀
**from assisted reproductive**
**technology, first trimester**

O09.812 **Supervision of pregnancy resulting** Ⓜ♀
**from assisted reproductive**
**technology, second trimester**

O09.813 **Supervision of pregnancy resulting** Ⓜ♀
**from assisted reproductive**
**technology, third trimester**

O09.819 **Supervision of pregnancy resulting** Ⓜ♀
**from assisted reproductive**
**technology, unspecified trimester**

√6ᵗʰ O09.82 **Supervision of pregnancy with history of in utero**
**procedure during previous pregnancy**

O09.821 **Supervision of pregnancy with history** Ⓜ♀
**of in utero procedure during previous**
**pregnancy, first trimester**

O09.822 **Supervision of pregnancy with history** Ⓜ♀
**of in utero procedure during previous**
**pregnancy, second trimester**

O09.823 **Supervision of pregnancy with history** Ⓜ♀
**of in utero procedure during previous**
**pregnancy, third trimester**

O09.829 **Supervision of pregnancy with history** Ⓜ♀
**of in utero procedure during previous**
**pregnancy, unspecified trimester**

EXCLUDES 1    *supervision of pregnancy affected*
*by in utero procedure during*
*current pregnancy (O35.7)*

√6ᵗʰ O09.89 **Supervision of other high risk pregnancies**

O09.891 **Supervision of other high risk** Ⓜ♀
**pregnancies, first trimester**

O09.892 **Supervision of other high risk** Ⓜ♀
**pregnancies, second trimester**

O09.893 **Supervision of other high risk** Ⓜ♀
**pregnancies, third trimester**

O09.899 **Supervision of other high risk** Ⓜ♀
**pregnancies, unspecified trimester**

√5ᵗʰ O09.9 **Supervision of high risk pregnancy, unspecified**

O09.90 **Supervision of high risk pregnancy,** Ⓜ♀
**unspecified, unspecified trimester**

O09.91 **Supervision of high risk pregnancy,** Ⓜ♀
**unspecified, first trimester**

O09.92 **Supervision of high risk pregnancy,** Ⓜ♀
**unspecified, second trimester**

O09.93 **Supervision of high risk pregnancy,** Ⓜ♀
**unspecified, third trimester**

Ⓝ Newborn: 0   Ⓟ Pediatric: 0-17   Ⓜ Maternity: 12-55   Ⓐ Adult: 15-124   MCC Major CC Condition   PDx MCC PDx acts as own MCC   CC CC Condition   PDx CC PDx acts as own CC

848      ICD-10-CM 2018

## Edema, proteinuria and hypertensive disorders in pregnancy, childbirth and the puerperium (O10-O16)

☑4ᵗʰ **O10** Pre-existing **hypertension complicating pregnancy, childbirth and the puerperium**

> **INCLUDES**   pre-existing hypertension with pre-existing proteinuria complicating pregnancy, childbirth and the puerperium
>
> *EXCLUDES 2*   *pre-existing hypertension with superimposed pre-eclampsia complicating pregnancy, childbirth and the puerperium (O11.-)*

**CC Excl: For CC/MCC codes in category O10:** PDX collection 964

☑5ᵗʰ **O10.0** **Pre-existing** essential **hypertension complicating pregnancy, childbirth and the puerperium**
> Any condition in I10 specified as a reason for obstetric care during pregnancy, childbirth or the puerperium

> ☑6ᵗʰ **O10.01** Pre-existing essential hypertension complicating pregnancy
>> **O10.011** **Pre-existing essential hypertension** CC M ♀ **complicating pregnancy, first trimester**
>>
>> **O10.012** **Pre-existing essential hypertension** CC M ♀ **complicating pregnancy, second trimester**
>>
>> **O10.013** **Pre-existing essential hypertension** CC M ♀ **complicating pregnancy, third trimester**
>>
>> **O10.019** **Pre-existing essential hypertension** M ♀ **complicating pregnancy, unspecified trimester**
>
> **O10.02** **Pre-existing essential hypertension** CC M ♀ **complicating childbirth**
>
> **O10.03** **Pre-existing essential hypertension** M ♀ **complicating the puerperium**

☑5ᵗʰ **O10.1** **Pre-existing hypertensive** heart disease **complicating pregnancy, childbirth and the puerperium**
> Any condition in I11 specified as a reason for obstetric care during pregnancy, childbirth or the puerperium
> Use additional code from I11 to identify the type of hypertensive heart disease

> ☑6ᵗʰ **O10.11** Pre-existing hypertensive heart disease complicating pregnancy
>> **O10.111** **Pre-existing hypertensive heart** M ♀ **disease complicating pregnancy, first trimester**
>>
>> **O10.112** **Pre-existing hypertensive heart** M ♀ **disease complicating pregnancy, second trimester**
>>
>> **O10.113** **Pre-existing hypertensive heart** M ♀ **disease complicating pregnancy, third trimester**
>>
>> **O10.119** **Pre-existing hypertensive heart** M ♀ **disease complicating pregnancy, unspecified trimester**
>
> **O10.12** **Pre-existing hypertensive heart disease** M ♀ **complicating childbirth**
>
> **O10.13** **Pre-existing hypertensive heart disease** M ♀ **complicating the puerperium**

☑5ᵗʰ **O10.2** **Pre-existing hypertensive** chronic kidney disease **complicating pregnancy, childbirth and the puerperium**
> Any condition in I12 specified as a reason for obstetric care during pregnancy, childbirth or the puerperium
> Use additional code from I12 to identify the type of hypertensive chronic kidney disease

> ☑6ᵗʰ **O10.21** Pre-existing hypertensive chronic kidney disease complicating pregnancy
>> **O10.211** **Pre-existing hypertensive chronic** M ♀ **kidney disease complicating pregnancy, first trimester**
>>
>> **O10.212** **Pre-existing hypertensive chronic** M ♀ **kidney disease complicating pregnancy, second trimester**
>>
>> **O10.213** **Pre-existing hypertensive chronic** M ♀ **kidney disease complicating pregnancy, third trimester**
>>
>> **O10.219** **Pre-existing hypertensive chronic** M ♀ **kidney disease complicating pregnancy, unspecified trimester**
>
> **O10.22** **Pre-existing hypertensive chronic kidney** M ♀ **disease complicating** childbirth

> **O10.23** **Pre-existing hypertensive chronic kidney** M ♀ **disease complicating the** puerperium

☑5ᵗʰ **O10.3** **Pre-existing hypertensive** heart and chronic kidney disease **complicating pregnancy, childbirth and the puerperium**
> Any condition in I13 specified as a reason for obstetric care during pregnancy, childbirth or the puerperium
> Use additional code from I13 to identify the type of hypertensive heart and chronic kidney disease

> ☑6ᵗʰ **O10.31** Pre-existing hypertensive heart and chronic kidney disease complicating pregnancy
>> **O10.311** **Pre-existing hypertensive heart and** M ♀ **chronic kidney disease complicating pregnancy, first trimester**
>>
>> **O10.312** **Pre-existing hypertensive heart and** M ♀ **chronic kidney disease complicating pregnancy, second trimester**
>>
>> **O10.313** **Pre-existing hypertensive heart and** M ♀ **chronic kidney disease complicating pregnancy, third trimester**
>>
>> **O10.319** **Pre-existing hypertensive heart and** M ♀ **chronic kidney disease complicating pregnancy, unspecified trimester**
>
> **O10.32** **Pre-existing hypertensive heart and chronic** M ♀ **kidney disease complicating** childbirth
>
> **O10.33** **Pre-existing hypertensive heart and chronic** M ♀ **kidney disease complicating the** puerperium

☑5ᵗʰ **O10.4** **Pre-existing** secondary **hypertension complicating pregnancy, childbirth and the puerperium**
> Any condition in I15 specified as a reason for obstetric care during pregnancy, childbirth or the puerperium
> Use additional code from I15 to identify the type of secondary hypertension

> ☑6ᵗʰ **O10.41** Pre-existing secondary hypertension complicating pregnancy
>> **O10.411** **Pre-existing secondary** CC M ♀ **hypertension complicating pregnancy, first trimester**
>>
>> **O10.412** **Pre-existing secondary** CC M ♀ **hypertension complicating pregnancy, second trimester**
>>
>> **O10.413** **Pre-existing secondary** CC M ♀ **hypertension complicating pregnancy, third trimester**
>>
>> **O10.419** **Pre-existing secondary hypertension** M ♀ **complicating pregnancy, unspecified trimester**
>
> **O10.42** **Pre-existing secondary hypertension** MCC M ♀ **complicating** childbirth
>
> **O10.43** **Pre-existing secondary hypertension** CC M ♀ **complicating the** puerperium

☑5ᵗʰ **O10.9** Unspecified **pre-existing hypertension complicating pregnancy, childbirth and the puerperium**

> ☑6ᵗʰ **O10.91** Unspecified pre-existing hypertension complicating pregnancy
>> **O10.911** **Unspecified pre-existing** CC M ♀ **hypertension complicating pregnancy, first trimester**
>>
>> **O10.912** **Unspecified pre-existing** CC M ♀ **hypertension complicating pregnancy, second trimester**
>>
>> **O10.913** **Unspecified pre-existing** CC M ♀ **hypertension complicating pregnancy, third trimester**
>>
>> **O10.919** **Unspecified pre-existing** M ♀ **hypertension complicating pregnancy, unspecified trimester**
>
> **O10.92** **Unspecified pre-existing hypertension** CC M ♀ **complicating** childbirth
>
> **O10.93** **Unspecified pre-existing hypertension** M ♀ **complicating the** puerperium

☑4ᵗʰ **O11** Pre-existing **hypertension** with pre-eclampsia
> **INCLUDES**   conditions in O10 complicated by pre-eclampsia
> pre-eclampsia superimposed pre-existing hypertension
> Use additional code from O10 to identify the type of hypertension

**CC Excl: For MCC codes in category O11:** PDX collection 964

> **O11.1** **Pre-existing hypertension with pre-eclampsia,** MCC M ♀ **first trimester**

☑ Additional Character Req   ☑·7ᵗʰ Placeholder Alert   Unacceptable PDx   Manifestation   **H1 - H14** HAC   **HCC** CMS-HCC Condition   *EXCLUDES 1* Not Coded Here   *EXCLUDES 2* Not Included Here

ICD-10-CM 2018     **849**

Chapter 15. Pregnancy, Childbirth and the Puerperium

O10–O11.1

**Chapter 15. Pregnancy, Childbirth and the Puerperium**

**O11.2**   **Pre-existing hypertension with pre-eclampsia, second trimester**   MCC M♀

**O11.3**   **Pre-existing hypertension with pre-eclampsia, third trimester**   MCC M♀

**O11.4**   **Pre-existing hypertension with pre-eclampsia, complicating childbirth**   M♀

**O11.5**   **Pre-existing hypertension with pre-eclampsia, complicating the puerperium**   M♀

**O11.9**   **Pre-existing hypertension with pre-eclampsia, unspecified trimester**   M♀

✓4th **O12**   **Gestational [pregnancy-induced] edema and proteinuria without hypertension**

> **CC Excl: For CC codes in category O12:** PDX collection 965

  ✓5th **O12.0**   **Gestational edema**

     **O12.00**   **Gestational edema, unspecified trimester**   M♀

     **O12.01**   **Gestational edema, first trimester**   M♀

     **O12.02**   **Gestational edema, second trimester**   M♀

     **O12.03**   **Gestational edema, third trimester**   M♀

     **O12.04**   **Gestational edema, complicating childbirth**   M♀

     **O12.05**   **Gestational edema, complicating the puerperium**   M♀

  ✓5th **O12.1**   **Gestational proteinuria**

     **O12.10**   **Gestational proteinuria, unspecified trimester**   M♀

     **O12.11**   **Gestational proteinuria, first trimester**   CC M♀

     **O12.12**   **Gestational proteinuria, second trimester**   CC M♀

     **O12.13**   **Gestational proteinuria, third trimester**   CC M♀

     **O12.14**   **Gestational proteinuria, complicating childbirth**   M♀

     **O12.15**   **Gestational proteinuria, complicating the puerperium**   M♀

  ✓5th **O12.2**   **Gestational edema with proteinuria**

     **O12.20**   **Gestational edema with proteinuria, unspecified trimester**   M♀

     **O12.21**   **Gestational edema with proteinuria, first trimester**   PDxCC CC M♀

     **O12.22**   **Gestational edema with proteinuria, second trimester**   PDxCC CC M♀

     **O12.23**   **Gestational edema with proteinuria, third trimester**   PDxCC CC M♀

     **O12.24**   **Gestational edema with proteinuria, complicating childbirth**   M♀

     **O12.25**   **Gestational edema with proteinuria, complicating the puerperium**   M♀

✓4th **O13**   **Gestational [pregnancy-induced] hypertension without significant proteinuria**

> **INCLUDES** gestational hypertension NOS
> transient hypertension of pregnancy

**AHA:** 2016, 1Q, 5

   **O13.1**   **Gestational [pregnancy-induced] hypertension without significant proteinuria, first trimester**   M♀

   **O13.2**   **Gestational [pregnancy-induced] hypertension without significant proteinuria, second trimester**   M♀

   **O13.3**   **Gestational [pregnancy-induced] hypertension without significant proteinuria, third trimester**   M♀

   **O13.4**   **Gestational [pregnancy-induced] hypertension without significant proteinuria, complicating childbirth**   M♀

   **O13.5**   **Gestational [pregnancy-induced] hypertension without significant proteinuria, complicating the puerperium**   M♀

   **O13.9**   **Gestational [pregnancy-induced] hypertension without significant proteinuria, unspecified trimester**   M♀

✓4th **O14**   **Pre-eclampsia**

> **EXCLUDES 1** pre-existing hypertension with pre-eclampsia (O11)

> **CC Excl: For CC /MCC codes in category O14:** PDX collection 964

  ✓5th **O14.0**   **Mild to moderate pre-eclampsia**

     **O14.00**   **Mild to moderate pre-eclampsia, unspecified trimester**   M♀

     **O14.02**   **Mild to moderate pre-eclampsia, second trimester**   CC M♀

     **O14.03**   **Mild to moderate pre-eclampsia, third trimester**   CC M♀

     **O14.04**   **Mild to moderate pre-eclampsia, complicating childbirth**   M♀

     **O14.05**   **Mild to moderate pre-eclampsia, complicating the puerperium**   M♀

  ✓5th **O14.1**   **Severe pre-eclampsia**

> **EXCLUDES 1** HELLP syndrome (O14.2-)

     **O14.10**   **Severe pre-eclampsia, unspecified trimester**   M♀

     **O14.12**   **Severe pre-eclampsia, second trimester**   MCC M♀

     **O14.13**   **Severe pre-eclampsia, third trimester**   MCC M♀

     **O14.14**   **Severe pre-eclampsia complicating childbirth**   M♀

     **O14.15**   **Severe pre-eclampsia, complicating the puerperium**   M♀

  ✓5th **O14.2**   **HELLP syndrome**

> Severe pre-eclampsia with hemolysis, elevated liver enzymes and low platelet count (HELLP)

     **O14.20**   **HELLP syndrome (HELLP), unspecified trimester**   M♀

     **O14.22**   **HELLP syndrome (HELLP), second trimester**   MCC M♀

     **O14.23**   **HELLP syndrome (HELLP), third trimester**   MCC M♀

     **O14.24**   **HELLP syndrome, complicating childbirth**   M♀

     **O14.25**   **HELLP syndrome, complicating the puerperium**   M♀

  ✓5th **O14.9**   **Unspecified pre-eclampsia**

     **O14.90**   **Unspecified pre-eclampsia, unspecified trimester**   M♀

     **O14.92**   **Unspecified pre-eclampsia, second trimester**   CC M♀

     **O14.93**   **Unspecified pre-eclampsia, third trimester**   CC M♀

     **O14.94**   **Unspecified pre-eclampsia, complicating childbirth**   M♀

     **O14.95**   **Unspecified pre-eclampsia, complicating the puerperium**   M♀

✓4th **O15**   **Eclampsia**

> **INCLUDES** convulsions following conditions in O10-O14 and O16

> **CC Excl: For MCC codes in category O15:** PDX collection 964

  ✓5th **O15.0**   **Eclampsia complicating pregnancy**

     **O15.00**   **Eclampsia complicating pregnancy, unspecified trimester**   M♀

     **O15.02**   **Eclampsia complicating pregnancy, second trimester**   MCC M♀

     **O15.03**   **Eclampsia complicating pregnancy, third trimester**   MCC M♀

   **O15.1**   **Eclampsia complicating labor**   MCC M♀

   **O15.2**   **Eclampsia complicating the puerperium**   MCC M♀

   **O15.9**   **Eclampsia, unspecified as to time period**  
Eclampsia NOS

✓4th **O16**   **Unspecified maternal hypertension**

> **CC Excl: For CC codes in category O16:** PDX collection 964

   **O16.1**   **Unspecified maternal hypertension, first trimester**   CC M♀

   **O16.2**   **Unspecified maternal hypertension, second trimester**   CC M♀

   **O16.3**   **Unspecified maternal hypertension, third trimester**   CC M♀

   **O16.4**   **Unspecified maternal hypertension, complicating childbirth**   M♀

   **O16.5**   **Unspecified maternal hypertension, complicating the puerperium**   M♀

   **O16.9**   **Unspecified maternal hypertension, unspecified trimester**   M♀

## Other maternal disorders predominantly related to pregnancy (O20-O29)

> **EXCLUDES 2** maternal care related to the fetus and amniotic cavity and possible delivery problems (O30-O48)
> maternal diseases classifiable elsewhere but complicating pregnancy, labor and delivery, and the puerperium (O98-O99)

✓4th **O20**   **Hemorrhage in early pregnancy**

> Hemorrhage before completion of 20 weeks gestation
> **EXCLUDES 1** pregnancy with abortive outcome (O00-O08)

   **O20.0**   **Threatened abortion**   CC M♀

> Hemorrhage specified as due to threatened abortion
> **DEF:** Bloody discharge during pregnancy; cervix may be dilated and pregnancy threatened, but the pregnancy is not terminated.
> **CC Excl:** PDX collection 966

   **O20.8**   **Other hemorrhage in early pregnancy**   M♀

   **O20.9**   **Hemorrhage in early pregnancy, unspecified**   CC M♀
> **CC Excl:** PDX collection 966

N Newborn: 0   P Pediatric: 0-17   M Maternity: 12-55   A Adult: 15-124   MCC Major CC Condition   PDxMCC PDx acts as own MCC   CC CC Condition   PDxCC PDx acts as own CC

850      ICD-10-CM 2018

**✓4th O21 Excessive vomiting in pregnancy**

**O21.0**   Mild **hyperemesis gravidarum**   M♀
     Hyperemesis gravidarum, mild or unspecified, starting before the end of the 20th week of gestation

**O21.1**   **Hyperemesis gravidarum with** metabolic disturbance   M♀
     Hyperemesis gravidarum, starting before the end of the 20th week of gestation, with metabolic disturbance such as carbohydrate depletion
     Hyperemesis gravidarum, starting before the end of the 20th week of gestation, with metabolic disturbance such as dehydration
     Hyperemesis gravidarum, starting before the end of the 20th week of gestation, with metabolic disturbance such as electrolyte imbalance

**O21.2**   Late **vomiting of pregnancy**   M♀
     Excessive vomiting starting after 20 completed weeks of gestation

**O21.8**   Other **vomiting complicating pregnancy**   M♀
     Vomiting due to diseases classified elsewhere, complicating pregnancy
     Use additional code to identify cause

**O21.9**   **Vomiting of pregnancy,** unspecified   M♀

**✓4th O22 Venous complications and hemorrhoids in pregnancy**

   *EXCLUDES 1*   venous complications of:
      abortion NOS (O03.9)
      ectopic or molar pregnancy (O08.7)
      failed attempted abortion (O07.35)
      induced abortion (O04.85)
      spontaneous abortion (O03.89)

   *EXCLUDES 2*   obstetric pulmonary embolism (O88.-)
      venous complications and hemorrhoids of childbirth and the puerperium (O87.-)

---

**CC Excl: For CC/MCC codes in category O22:** PDX collection 967

---

**✓5th O22.0**   Varicose veins of lower extremity **in pregnancy**
     Varicose veins NOS in pregnancy
     **DEF:** Distended, tortuous veins of lower extremities associated with pregnancy.

**O22.00**   **Varicose veins of lower extremity in pregnancy,** unspecified trimester   M♀

**O22.01**   **Varicose veins of lower extremity in pregnancy,** first trimester   M♀

**O22.02**   **Varicose veins of lower extremity in pregnancy,** second trimester   M♀

**O22.03**   **Varicose veins of lower extremity in pregnancy,** third trimester   M♀

**✓5th O22.1**   Genital varices **in pregnancy**
     Perineal varices in pregnancy
     Vaginal varices in pregnancy
     Vulval varices in pregnancy

**O22.10**   **Genital varices in pregnancy,** unspecified trimester   M♀

**O22.11**   **Genital varices in pregnancy,** first trimester   M♀

**O22.12**   **Genital varices in pregnancy,** second trimester   M♀

**O22.13**   **Genital varices in pregnancy,** third trimester   M♀

**✓5th O22.2**   Superficial thrombophlebitis **in pregnancy**
     Phlebitis in pregnancy NOS
     Thrombophlebitis of legs in pregnancy
     Thrombosis in pregnancy NOS
     Use additional code to identify the superficial thrombophlebitis (I80.0-)

**O22.20**   **Superficial thrombophlebitis in pregnancy,** unspecified trimester   CC M♀

**O22.21**   **Superficial thrombophlebitis in pregnancy,** first trimester   CC M♀

**O22.22**   **Superficial thrombophlebitis in pregnancy,** second trimester   CC M♀

**O22.23**   **Superficial thrombophlebitis in pregnancy,** third trimester   CC M♀

**✓5th O22.3**   Deep phlebothrombosis **in pregnancy**
     Deep vein thrombosis, antepartum
     Use additional code to identify the deep vein thrombosis (I82.4-, I82.5-, I82.62-. I82.72-)
     Use additional code, if applicable, for associated long-term (current) use of anticoagulants (Z79.01)

**O22.30**   **Deep phlebothrombosis in pregnancy,** unspecified trimester   CC M♀

**O22.31**   **Deep phlebothrombosis in pregnancy,** first trimester   MCC M♀

**O22.32**   **Deep phlebothrombosis in pregnancy,** second trimester   MCC M♀

**O22.33**   **Deep phlebothrombosis in pregnancy,** third trimester   MCC M♀

**✓5th O22.4**   Hemorrhoids **in pregnancy**

**O22.40**   **Hemorrhoids in pregnancy,** unspecified trimester   CC M♀

**O22.41**   **Hemorrhoids in pregnancy,** first trimester   CC M♀

**O22.42**   **Hemorrhoids in pregnancy,** second trimester   CC M♀

**O22.43**   **Hemorrhoids in pregnancy,** third trimester   CC M♀

**✓5th O22.5**   Cerebral venous thrombosis **in pregnancy**
     Cerebrovenous sinus thrombosis in pregnancy

**O22.50**   **Cerebral venous thrombosis in pregnancy,** unspecified trimester   CC M♀

**O22.51**   **Cerebral venous thrombosis in pregnancy,** first trimester   CC M♀

**O22.52**   **Cerebral venous thrombosis in pregnancy,** second trimester   CC M♀

**O22.53**   **Cerebral venous thrombosis in pregnancy,** third trimester   CC M♀

**✓5th O22.8**   Other venous complications **in pregnancy**

**✓6th O22.8X**   Other **venous complications in pregnancy**

**O22.8X1**   **Other venous complications in pregnancy,** first trimester   CC M♀

**O22.8X2**   **Other venous complications in pregnancy,** second trimester   CC M♀

**O22.8X3**   **Other venous complications in pregnancy,** third trimester   CC M♀

**O22.8X9**   **Other venous complications in pregnancy,** unspecified trimester   CC M♀

**✓5th O22.9**   Venous complication **in pregnancy,** unspecified
     Gestational phlebitis NOS
     Gestational phlebopathy NOS
     Gestational thrombosis NOS

**O22.90**   **Venous complication in pregnancy, unspecified,** unspecified trimester   CC M♀

**O22.91**   **Venous complication in pregnancy, unspecified,** first trimester   M♀

**O22.92**   **Venous complication in pregnancy, unspecified,** second trimester   M♀

**O22.93**   **Venous complication in pregnancy, unspecified,** third trimester   M♀

**✓4th O23 Infections of genitourinary tract in pregnancy**

     Use additional code to identify organism (B95.-, B96.-)

   *EXCLUDES 2*   gonococcal infections complicating pregnancy, childbirth and the puerperium (O98.2)
      infections with a predominantly sexual mode of transmission NOS complicating pregnancy, childbirth and the puerperium (O98.3)
      syphilis complicating pregnancy, childbirth and the puerperium (O98.1)
      tuberculosis of genitourinary system complicating pregnancy, childbirth and the puerperium (O98.0)
      venereal disease NOS complicating pregnancy, childbirth and the puerperium (O98.3)

---

**CC Excl: For CC codes in category O23:** PDX collection 968

---

**✓5th O23.0**   Infections of kidney **in pregnancy**
     Pyelonephritis in pregnancy

**O23.00**   **Infections of kidney in pregnancy,** unspecified trimester   M♀

**O23.01**   **Infections of kidney in pregnancy,** first trimester   CC M♀

**O23.02**   **Infections of kidney in pregnancy,** second trimester   CC M♀

**O23.03**   **Infections of kidney in pregnancy,** third trimester   CC M♀

**✓5th O23.1**   Infections of bladder **in pregnancy**

**O23.10**   **Infections of bladder in pregnancy,** unspecified trimester   M♀

**O23.11**   **Infections of bladder in pregnancy,** first trimester   CC M♀

**O23.12**   **Infections of bladder in pregnancy,** second trimester   CC M♀

**O23.13**   **Infections of bladder in pregnancy,** third trimester   CC M♀

---

✓ Additional Character Req   ✓x7th Placeholder Alert   Unacceptable PDx   Manifestation   H1 - H14 HAC   HCC CMS-HCC Condition   *EXCLUDES 1* Not Coded Here   *EXCLUDES 2* Not Included Here

ICD-10-CM 2018      **851**

✓5ᵗʰ **O23.2** **Infections of** urethra **in pregnancy**

    **O23.20** **Infections of urethra in pregnancy,** **unspecified trimester**   M♀

    **O23.21** **Infections of urethra in pregnancy,** **first trimester**   CC M♀

    **O23.22** **Infections of urethra in pregnancy,** **second trimester**   CC M♀

    **O23.23** **Infections of urethra in pregnancy,** **third trimester**   CC M♀

✓5ᵗʰ **O23.3** **Infections of** other parts **of urinary tract in pregnancy**

    **O23.30** **Infections of other parts of urinary tract in** **pregnancy,** unspecified trimester   M♀

    **O23.31** **Infections of other parts of urinary tract in** **pregnancy,** first trimester   CC M♀

    **O23.32** **Infections of other parts of urinary tract in** **pregnancy,** second trimester   CC M♀

    **O23.33** **Infections of other parts of urinary tract in** **pregnancy,** third trimester   CC M♀

✓5ᵗʰ **O23.4** **Unspecified infection of urinary tract in pregnancy**

    **O23.40** **Unspecified infection of urinary tract in** **pregnancy,** unspecified trimester   M♀

    **O23.41** **Unspecified infection of urinary tract in** **pregnancy,** first trimester   CC M♀

    **O23.42** **Unspecified infection of urinary tract in** **pregnancy,** second trimester   CC M♀

    **O23.43** **Unspecified infection of urinary tract in** **pregnancy,** third trimester   CC M♀

✓5ᵗʰ **O23.5** **Infections of the** genital tract **in pregnancy**

  ✓6ᵗʰ **O23.51** **Infection of** cervix **in pregnancy**

    **O23.511** **Infections of cervix in pregnancy,** **first trimester**   CC M♀

    **O23.512** **Infections of cervix in pregnancy,** **second trimester**   CC M♀

    **O23.513** **Infections of cervix in pregnancy,** **third trimester**   CC M♀

    **O23.519** **Infections of cervix in pregnancy,** **unspecified trimester**   M♀

  ✓6ᵗʰ **O23.52** **Salpingo-oophoritis** **in pregnancy**
    Oophoritis in pregnancy
    Salpingitis in pregnancy

    **O23.521** **Salpingo-oophoritis in pregnancy,** **first trimester**   CC M♀

    **O23.522** **Salpingo-oophoritis in pregnancy,** **second trimester**   CC M♀

    **O23.523** **Salpingo-oophoritis in pregnancy,** **third trimester**   CC M♀

    **O23.529** **Salpingo-oophoritis in pregnancy,** **unspecified trimester**   M♀

  ✓6ᵗʰ **O23.59** **Infection of** other part **of genital tract in pregnancy**

    **O23.591** **Infection of other part of genital** **tract in pregnancy,** first trimester   CC M♀

    **O23.592** **Infection of other part of genital** **tract in pregnancy,** second trimester   CC M♀

    **O23.593** **Infection of other part of genital** **tract in pregnancy,** third trimester   CC M♀

    **O23.599** **Infection of other part of genital tract** **in pregnancy,** unspecified trimester   M♀

✓5ᵗʰ **O23.9** **Unspecified** genitourinary tract infection in pregnancy
    Genitourinary tract infection in pregnancy NOS

    **O23.90** **Unspecified genitourinary tract infection in** **pregnancy,** unspecified trimester   M♀

    **O23.91** **Unspecified genitourinary tract infection in** **pregnancy,** first trimester   CC M♀

    **O23.92** **Unspecified genitourinary tract infection in** **pregnancy,** second trimester   CC M♀

    **O23.93** **Unspecified genitourinary tract infection in** **pregnancy,** third trimester   CC M♀

---

✓4ᵗʰ **O24** **Diabetes mellitus** in pregnancy, childbirth, and the puerperium

    **CC Excl: For CC/MCC codes in category O24:** PDX collection 969

✓5ᵗʰ **O24.0** **Pre-existing type 1** diabetes mellitus, in pregnancy, childbirth and the puerperium
    Juvenile onset diabetes mellitus, in pregnancy, childbirth and the puerperium
    Ketosis-prone diabetes mellitus in pregnancy, childbirth and the puerperium
    Use additional code from category E10 to further identify any manifestations

  ✓6ᵗʰ **O24.01** **Pre-existing type 1 diabetes mellitus, in** pregnancy

    **O24.011** **Pre-existing type 1diabetes** **mellitus, in pregnancy,** **first trimester**   CC M♀

    **O24.012** **Pre-existing type 1diabetes** **mellitus, in pregnancy,** **second trimester**   CC M♀

    **O24.013** **Pre-existing type 1diabetes** **mellitus, in pregnancy,** **third trimester**   CC M♀

    **O24.019** **Pre-existing type 1diabetes** **mellitus, in pregnancy,** **unspecified trimester**   CC M♀

    **O24.02** **Pre-existing type 1diabetes mellitus, in** childbirth   MCC M♀

    **O24.03** **Pre-existing type 1 diabetes mellitus, in** the puerperium   CC M♀

✓5ᵗʰ **O24.1** **Pre-existing type 2** diabetes mellitus, in pregnancy, childbirth and the puerperium
    Insulin-resistant diabetes mellitus in pregnancy, childbirth and the puerperium
    Use additional code (for):
      from category E11 to further identify any manifestations
      long-term (current) use of insulin (Z79.4)

  ✓6ᵗʰ **O24.11** **Pre-existing type 2 diabetes mellitus, in** pregnancy

    **O24.111** **Pre-existing type 2 diabetes** **mellitus, in pregnancy,** **first trimester**   CC M♀

    **O24.112** **Pre-existing type 2 diabetes** **mellitus, in pregnancy,** **second trimester**   CC ♀

    **O24.113** **Pre-existing type 2 diabetes** **mellitus, in pregnancy,** **third trimester**   CC M♀

    **O24.119** **Pre-existing type 2 diabetes** **mellitus, in pregnancy,** **unspecified trimester**   CC M♀

    **O24.12** **Pre-existing type 2 diabetes mellitus, in** childbirth   MCC M♀

    **O24.13** **Pre-existing type 2 diabetes mellitus, in the** puerperium   CC M♀

✓5ᵗʰ **O24.3** **Unspecified pre-existing** diabetes mellitus in pregnancy, childbirth and the puerperium
    Use additional code (for):
      from category E11 to further identify any manifestation
      long-term (current) use of insulin (Z79.4)

  ✓6ᵗʰ **O24.31** **Unspecified** pre-existing diabetes mellitus in **pregnancy**

    **O24.311** **Unspecified pre-existing diabetes** **mellitus in pregnancy,** first trimester   CC M♀

    **O24.312** **Unspecified pre-existing diabetes** **mellitus in pregnancy,** second trimester   CC M♀

    **O24.313** **Unspecified pre-existing diabetes** **mellitus in pregnancy,** third trimester   CC M♀

    **O24.319** **Unspecified pre-existing diabetes** **mellitus in pregnancy,** unspecified **trimester**   CC M♀

    **O24.32** **Unspecified pre-existing diabetes mellitus** **in** childbirth   MCC M♀

    **O24.33** **Unspecified pre-existing diabetes mellitus** **in the** puerperium   CC M♀

✓5ᵗʰ **O24.4** **Gestational** diabetes mellitus
    Diabetes mellitus arising in pregnancy
    Gestational diabetes mellitus NOS

  ✓6ᵗʰ **O24.41** **Gestational diabetes mellitus in** pregnancy

    **O24.410** **Gestational diabetes mellitus in** **pregnancy,** diet controlled   M♀

---

N Newborn: 0   P Pediatric: 0-17   M Maternity: 12-55   A Adult: 15-124   MCC Major CC Condition   PDxMCC PDx acts as own MCC   CC CC Condition   PDxCC PDx acts as own CC

852      ICD-10-CM 2018

**O24.414** **Gestational diabetes mellitus in pregnancy, insulin controlled** Ⓜ♀

**O24.415** **Gestational diabetes mellitus in pregnancy, controlled by oral hypoglycemic drugs** Ⓜ♀
Gestational diabetes mellitus in pregnancy, controlled by oral antidiabetic drugs

**O24.419** **Gestational diabetes mellitus in pregnancy, unspecified control** Ⓜ♀
**AHA:** 2015, 4Q, 34

✓6ᵗʰ **O24.42** **Gestational diabetes mellitus in childbirth**
**AHA:** 2016, 1Q, 5

**O24.420** **Gestational diabetes mellitus in childbirth, diet controlled** Ⓜ♀

**O24.424** **Gestational diabetes mellitus in childbirth, insulin controlled** Ⓜ♀

**O24.425** **Gestational diabetes mellitus in childbirth, controlled by oral hypoglycemic drugs** Ⓜ♀
Gestational diabetes mellitus in childbirth, controlled by oral antidiabetic drugs

**O24.429** **Gestational diabetes mellitus in childbirth, unspecified control** Ⓜ♀
**AHA:** 2015, 4Q, 34

✓6ᵗʰ **O24.43** **Gestational diabetes mellitus in the puerperium**

**O24.430** **Gestational diabetes mellitus in the puerperium, diet controlled** Ⓜ♀

**O24.434** **Gestational diabetes mellitus in the puerperium, insulin controlled** Ⓜ♀

**O24.435** **Gestational diabetes mellitus in puerperium, controlled by oral hypoglycemic drugs** Ⓜ♀
Gestational diabetes mellitus in puerperium, controlled by oral antidiabetic drugs

**O24.439** **Gestational diabetes mellitus in the puerperium, unspecified control** Ⓜ♀
**AHA:** 2015, 4Q, 34

✓5ᵗʰ **O24.8** **Other pre-existing diabetes mellitus in pregnancy, childbirth, and the puerperium**
Use additional code (for):
from categories E08, E09 and E13 to further identify any manifestation
long-term (current) use of insulin (Z79.4)

✓6ᵗʰ **O24.81** **Other pre-existing diabetes mellitus in pregnancy**

**O24.811** **Other pre-existing diabetes mellitus in pregnancy, first trimester** CC Ⓜ♀

**O24.812** **Other pre-existing diabetes mellitus in pregnancy, second trimester** CC Ⓜ♀

**O24.813** **Other pre-existing diabetes mellitus in pregnancy, third trimester** CC Ⓜ♀

**O24.819** **Other pre-existing diabetes mellitus in pregnancy, unspecified trimester** CC Ⓜ♀

**O24.82** **Other pre-existing diabetes mellitus in childbirth** MCC Ⓜ♀

**O24.83** **Other pre-existing diabetes mellitus in the puerperium** CC Ⓜ♀

✓5ᵗʰ **O24.9** **Unspecified diabetes mellitus in pregnancy, childbirth and the puerperium**
Use additional code for long-term (current) use of insulin (Z79.4)

✓6ᵗʰ **O24.91** **Unspecified diabetes mellitus in pregnancy**

**O24.911** **Unspecified diabetes mellitus in pregnancy, first trimester** CC Ⓜ♀

**O24.912** **Unspecified diabetes mellitus in pregnancy, second trimester** CC Ⓜ♀

**O24.913** **Unspecified diabetes mellitus in pregnancy, third trimester** CC Ⓜ♀

**O24.919** **Unspecified diabetes mellitus in pregnancy, unspecified trimester** CC Ⓜ♀

**O24.92** **Unspecified diabetes mellitus in childbirth** Ⓜ♀

**O24.93** **Unspecified diabetes mellitus in the puerperium** CC Ⓜ♀

✓4ᵗʰ **O25** **Malnutrition in pregnancy, childbirth and the puerperium**

✓5ᵗʰ **O25.1** **Malnutrition in pregnancy**

**O25.10** **Malnutrition in pregnancy, unspecified trimester** Ⓜ♀

**O25.11** **Malnutrition in pregnancy, first trimester** Ⓜ♀

**O25.12** **Malnutrition in pregnancy, second trimester** Ⓜ♀

**O25.13** **Malnutrition in pregnancy, third trimester** Ⓜ♀

**O25.2** **Malnutrition in childbirth** Ⓜ♀

**O25.3** **Malnutrition in the puerperium** Ⓜ♀

✓4ᵗʰ **O26** **Maternal care for other conditions predominantly related to pregnancy**

✓5ᵗʰ **O26.0** **Excessive weight gain in pregnancy**
*EXCLUDES 2* gestational edema (O12.0, O12.2)

**O26.00** **Excessive weight gain in pregnancy, unspecified trimester** Ⓜ♀

**O26.01** **Excessive weight gain in pregnancy, first trimester** Ⓜ♀

**O26.02** **Excessive weight gain in pregnancy, second trimester** Ⓜ♀

**O26.03** **Excessive weight gain in pregnancy, third trimester** Ⓜ♀

✓5ᵗʰ **O26.1** **Low weight gain in pregnancy**

**O26.10** **Low weight gain in pregnancy, unspecified trimester** Ⓜ♀

**O26.11** **Low weight gain in pregnancy, first trimester** Ⓜ♀

**O26.12** **Low weight gain in pregnancy, second trimester** Ⓜ♀

**O26.13** **Low weight gain in pregnancy, third trimester** Ⓜ♀

✓5ᵗʰ **O26.2** **Pregnancy care for patient with recurrent pregnancy loss**

**O26.20** **Pregnancy care for patient with recurrent pregnancy loss, unspecified trimester** Ⓜ♀

**O26.21** **Pregnancy care for patient with recurrent pregnancy loss, first trimester** Ⓜ♀

**O26.22** **Pregnancy care for patient with recurrent pregnancy loss, second trimester** Ⓜ♀

**O26.23** **Pregnancy care for patient with recurrent pregnancy loss, third trimester** Ⓜ♀

✓5ᵗʰ **O26.3** **Retained intrauterine contraceptive device in pregnancy**

**O26.30** **Retained intrauterine contraceptive device in pregnancy, unspecified trimester** Ⓜ♀

**O26.31** **Retained intrauterine contraceptive device in pregnancy, first trimester** Ⓜ♀

**O26.32** **Retained intrauterine contraceptive device in pregnancy, second trimester** Ⓜ♀

**O26.33** **Retained intrauterine contraceptive device in pregnancy, third trimester** Ⓜ♀

✓5ᵗʰ **O26.4** **Herpes gestationis**

**O26.40** **Herpes gestationis, unspecified trimester** Ⓜ♀

**O26.41** **Herpes gestationis, first trimester** Ⓜ♀

**O26.42** **Herpes gestationis, second trimester** Ⓜ♀

**O26.43** **Herpes gestationis, third trimester** Ⓜ♀

✓5ᵗʰ **O26.5** **Maternal hypotension syndrome**
Supine hypotensive syndrome

**O26.50** **Maternal hypotension syndrome, unspecified trimester** Ⓜ♀

**O26.51** **Maternal hypotension syndrome, first trimester** Ⓜ♀

**O26.52** **Maternal hypotension syndrome, second trimester** Ⓜ♀

**O26.53** **Maternal hypotension syndrome, third trimester** Ⓜ♀

✓5ᵗʰ **O26.6** **Liver and biliary tract disorders in pregnancy, childbirth and the puerperium**
Use additional code to identify the specific disorder
*EXCLUDES 2* hepatorenal syndrome following labor and delivery (O90.4)

**CC Excl: For CC codes in subcategory O26.6:**
PDX collection 972

✓6ᵗʰ **O26.61** **Liver and biliary tract disorders in pregnancy**

**O26.611** **Liver and biliary tract disorders in pregnancy, first trimester** CC Ⓜ♀

**O26.612** **Liver and biliary tract disorders in pregnancy, second trimester** CC Ⓜ♀

**O26.613** **Liver and biliary tract disorders in pregnancy, third trimester** CC Ⓜ♀

**O26.619** **Liver and biliary tract disorders in pregnancy, unspecified trimester** Ⓜ♀

**O26.62** **Liver and biliary tract disorders in childbirth** CC Ⓜ♀

**O26.63** **Liver and biliary tract disorders in the puerperium** Ⓜ♀

**Chapter 15. Pregnancy, Childbirth and the Puerperium**

**O26.7-O29.Ø19**

√5ᵗʰ **O26.7 Subluxation of symphysis (pubis) in pregnancy, childbirth and the puerperium**
> EXCLUDES 1   traumatic separation of symphysis (pubis) during childbirth (O71.6)

√6ᵗʰ **O26.71 Subluxation of symphysis (pubis) in pregnancy**
- **O26.711 Subluxation of symphysis (pubis) in pregnancy, first trimester** Ⓜ♀
- **O26.712 Subluxation of symphysis (pubis) in pregnancy, second trimester** Ⓜ♀
- **O26.713 Subluxation of symphysis (pubis) in pregnancy, third trimester** Ⓜ♀
- **O26.719 Subluxation of symphysis (pubis) in pregnancy, unspecified trimester** Ⓜ♀

**O26.72 Subluxation of symphysis (pubis) in childbirth** Ⓜ♀
**O26.73 Subluxation of symphysis (pubis) in the puerperium** Ⓜ♀

√5ᵗʰ **O26.8 Other specified pregnancy related conditions**

√6ᵗʰ **O26.81 Pregnancy related exhaustion and fatigue**
- **O26.811 Pregnancy related exhaustion and fatigue, first trimester** Ⓜ♀
- **O26.812 Pregnancy related exhaustion and fatigue, second trimester** Ⓜ♀
- **O26.813 Pregnancy related exhaustion and fatigue, third trimester** Ⓜ♀
- **O26.819 Pregnancy related exhaustion and fatigue, unspecified trimester** Ⓜ♀

√6ᵗʰ **O26.82 Pregnancy related peripheral neuritis**
- **O26.821 Pregnancy related peripheral neuritis, first trimester** Ⓜ♀
- **O26.822 Pregnancy related peripheral neuritis, second trimester** Ⓜ♀
- **O26.823 Pregnancy related peripheral neuritis, third trimester** Ⓜ♀
- **O26.829 Pregnancy related peripheral neuritis, unspecified trimester** Ⓜ♀

√6ᵗʰ **O26.83 Pregnancy related renal disease**
> Use additional code to identify the specific disorder

> **CC Excl: For CC codes in subcategory O26.83:** PDX collection 965

- **O26.831 Pregnancy related renal disease, first trimester** CC Ⓜ♀
- **O26.832 Pregnancy related renal disease, second trimester** CC Ⓜ♀
- **O26.833 Pregnancy related renal disease, third trimester** CC Ⓜ♀
- **O26.839 Pregnancy related renal disease, unspecified trimester** Ⓜ♀

√6ᵗʰ **O26.84 Uterine size-date discrepancy complicating pregnancy**
> EXCLUDES 1   encounter for suspected problem with fetal growth ruled out (Z03.74)

- **O26.841 Uterine size-date discrepancy, first trimester** Ⓜ♀
- **O26.842 Uterine size-date discrepancy, second trimester** Ⓜ♀
- **O26.843 Uterine size-date discrepancy, third trimester** Ⓜ♀
- **O26.849 Uterine size-date discrepancy, unspecified trimester** Ⓜ♀

√6ᵗʰ **O26.85 Spotting complicating pregnancy**
- **O26.851 Spotting complicating pregnancy, first trimester** Ⓜ♀
- **O26.852 Spotting complicating pregnancy, second trimester** Ⓜ♀
- **O26.853 Spotting complicating pregnancy, third trimester** Ⓜ♀
- **O26.859 Spotting complicating pregnancy, unspecified trimester** Ⓜ♀

**O26.86 Pruritic urticarial papules and plaques of pregnancy (PUPPP)** Ⓜ♀
> Polymorphic eruption of pregnancy

√6ᵗʰ **O26.87 Cervical shortening**
> EXCLUDES 1   encounter for suspected cervical shortening ruled out (Z03.75)

> **DEF:** A cervix that has shortened to < 25 mm before the 24th week of pregnancy; warning sign for impending premature delivery; treated by cervical cerclage placement or progesterone.

> **CC Excl: For CC codes in subcategory O26.87:** PDX collection 973

- **O26.872 Cervical shortening, second trimester** CC Ⓜ♀
- **O26.873 Cervical shortening, third trimester** CC Ⓜ♀
- **O26.879 Cervical shortening, unspecified trimester** CC Ⓜ♀

√6ᵗʰ **O26.89 Other specified pregnancy related conditions**
> **AHA:** 2015, 3Q, 40

- **O26.891 Other specified pregnancy related conditions, first trimester** Ⓜ♀
- **O26.892 Other specified pregnancy related conditions, second trimester** Ⓜ♀
- **O26.893 Other specified pregnancy related conditions, third trimester** Ⓜ♀
- **O26.899 Other specified pregnancy related conditions, unspecified trimester** Ⓜ♀

√5ᵗʰ **O26.9 Pregnancy related conditions, unspecified**
- **O26.90 Pregnancy related conditions, unspecified, unspecified trimester** Ⓜ♀
- **O26.91 Pregnancy related conditions, unspecified, first trimester** Ⓜ♀
- **O26.92 Pregnancy related conditions, unspecified, second trimester** Ⓜ♀
- **O26.93 Pregnancy related conditions, unspecified, third trimester** Ⓜ♀

√4ᵗʰ **O28 Abnormal findings on antenatal screening of mother**
> EXCLUDES 1   diagnostic findings classified elsewhere—see Alphabetical Index

**O28.0 Abnormal hematological finding on antenatal screening of mother** Ⓜ♀
**O28.1 Abnormal biochemical finding on antenatal screening of mother** Ⓜ♀
**O28.2 Abnormal cytological finding on antenatal screening of mother** Ⓜ♀
**O28.3 Abnormal ultrasonic finding on antenatal screening of mother** Ⓜ♀
**O28.4 Abnormal radiological finding on antenatal screening of mother** Ⓜ♀
**O28.5 Abnormal chromosomal and genetic finding on antenatal screening of mother** Ⓜ♀
**O28.8 Other abnormal findings on antenatal screening of mother** Ⓜ♀
**O28.9 Unspecified abnormal findings on antenatal screening of mother** Ⓜ♀

√4ᵗʰ **O29 Complications of anesthesia during pregnancy**
> INCLUDES   maternal complications arising from the administration of a general, regional or local anesthetic, analgesic or other sedation during pregnancy
> Use additional code, if necessary, to identify the complication
> EXCLUDES 2   complications of anesthesia during labor and delivery (O74.-)
> complications of anesthesia during the puerperium (O89.-)

√5ᵗʰ **O29.Ø Pulmonary complications of anesthesia during pregnancy**

√6ᵗʰ **O29.Ø1 Aspiration pneumonitis due to anesthesia during pregnancy**
> Inhalation of stomach contents or secretions NOS due to anesthesia during pregnancy
> Mendelson's syndrome due to anesthesia during pregnancy

- **O29.Ø11 Aspiration pneumonitis due to anesthesia during pregnancy, first trimester** Ⓜ♀
- **O29.Ø12 Aspiration pneumonitis due to anesthesia during pregnancy, second trimester** Ⓜ♀
- **O29.Ø13 Aspiration pneumonitis due to anesthesia during pregnancy, third trimester** Ⓜ♀
- **O29.Ø19 Aspiration pneumonitis due to anesthesia during pregnancy, unspecified trimester** Ⓜ♀

---

Ⓝ Newborn: 0   Ⓟ Pediatric: 0-17   Ⓜ Maternity: 12-55   Ⓐ Adult: 15-124   MCC Major CC Condition   PDxMCC PDx acts as own MCC   CC CC Condition   PDxCC PDx acts as own CC

**854**      ICD-10-CM 2018

✓6ᵗʰ **O29.02** **Pressure collapse of lung** due to anesthesia during pregnancy

    **O29.021** **Pressure collapse of lung due to anesthesia during pregnancy,** first trimester  Ⓜ♀

    **O29.022** **Pressure collapse of lung due to anesthesia during pregnancy,** second trimester  Ⓜ♀

    **O29.023** **Pressure collapse of lung due to anesthesia during pregnancy,** third trimester  Ⓜ♀

    **O29.029** **Pressure collapse of lung due to anesthesia during pregnancy,** unspecified trimester  Ⓜ♀

✓6ᵗʰ **O29.09** **Other pulmonary complications** of anesthesia during pregnancy

    **O29.091** **Other pulmonary complications of anesthesia during pregnancy,** first trimester  Ⓜ♀

    **O29.092** **Other pulmonary complications of anesthesia during pregnancy,** second trimester  Ⓜ♀

    **O29.093** **Other pulmonary complications of anesthesia during pregnancy,** third trimester  Ⓜ♀

    **O29.099** **Other pulmonary complications of anesthesia during pregnancy,** unspecified trimester  Ⓜ♀

✓5ᵗʰ **O29.1** **Cardiac** complications of anesthesia during pregnancy

  ✓6ᵗʰ **O29.11** **Cardiac arrest** due to anesthesia during pregnancy

    **O29.111** **Cardiac arrest due to anesthesia during pregnancy,** first trimester  Ⓜ♀

    **O29.112** **Cardiac arrest due to anesthesia during pregnancy,** second trimester  Ⓜ♀

    **O29.113** **Cardiac arrest due to anesthesia during pregnancy,** third trimester  Ⓜ♀

    **O29.119** **Cardiac arrest due to anesthesia during pregnancy,** unspecified trimester  Ⓜ♀

  ✓6ᵗʰ **O29.12** **Cardiac failure** due to anesthesia during pregnancy

    **O29.121** **Cardiac failure due to anesthesia during pregnancy,** first trimester  Ⓜ♀

    **O29.122** **Cardiac failure due to anesthesia during pregnancy,** second trimester  Ⓜ♀

    **O29.123** **Cardiac failure due to anesthesia during pregnancy,** third trimester  Ⓜ♀

    **O29.129** **Cardiac failure due to anesthesia during pregnancy,** unspecified trimester  Ⓜ♀

  ✓6ᵗʰ **O29.19** **Other cardiac complications** of anesthesia during pregnancy

    **O29.191** **Other cardiac complications of anesthesia during pregnancy,** first trimester  Ⓜ♀

    **O29.192** **Other cardiac complications of anesthesia during pregnancy,** second trimester  Ⓜ♀

    **O29.193** **Other cardiac complications of anesthesia during pregnancy,** third trimester  Ⓜ♀

    **O29.199** **Other cardiac complications of anesthesia during pregnancy,** unspecified trimester  Ⓜ♀

✓5ᵗʰ **O29.2** **Central nervous system** complications of anesthesia during pregnancy

  ✓6ᵗʰ **O29.21** **Cerebral anoxia** due to anesthesia during pregnancy

    **O29.211** **Cerebral anoxia due to anesthesia during pregnancy,** first trimester  Ⓜ♀

    **O29.212** **Cerebral anoxia due to anesthesia during pregnancy,** second trimester  Ⓜ♀

    **O29.213** **Cerebral anoxia due to anesthesia during pregnancy,** third trimester  Ⓜ♀

    **O29.219** **Cerebral anoxia due to anesthesia during pregnancy,** unspecified trimester  Ⓜ♀

  ✓6ᵗʰ **O29.29** **Other central nervous system complications** of anesthesia during pregnancy

    **O29.291** **Other central nervous system complications of anesthesia during pregnancy,** first trimester  ♀

    **O29.292** **Other central nervous system complications of anesthesia during pregnancy,** second trimester  Ⓜ♀

    **O29.293** **Other central nervous system complications of anesthesia during pregnancy,** third trimester  Ⓜ♀

    **O29.299** **Other central nervous system complications of anesthesia during pregnancy,** unspecified trimester  Ⓜ♀

✓5ᵗʰ **O29.3** **Toxic reaction** to local anesthesia during pregnancy

  ✓6ᵗʰ **O29.3X** **Toxic reaction to local anesthesia during pregnancy**

    **O29.3X1** **Toxic reaction to local anesthesia during pregnancy,** first trimester  Ⓜ♀

    **O29.3X2** **Toxic reaction to local anesthesia during pregnancy,** second trimester  Ⓜ♀

    **O29.3X3** **Toxic reaction to local anesthesia during pregnancy,** third trimester  Ⓜ♀

    **O29.3X9** **Toxic reaction to local anesthesia during pregnancy,** unspecified trimester  Ⓜ♀

✓5ᵗʰ **O29.4** **Spinal and epidural anesthesia induced headache** during pregnancy

    **O29.40** **Spinal and epidural anesthesia induced headache during pregnancy,** unspecified trimester  Ⓜ♀

    **O29.41** **Spinal and epidural anesthesia induced headache during pregnancy,** first trimester  Ⓜ♀

    **O29.42** **Spinal and epidural anesthesia induced headache during pregnancy,** second trimester  Ⓜ♀

    **O29.43** **Spinal and epidural anesthesia induced headache during pregnancy,** third trimester  Ⓜ♀

✓5ᵗʰ **O29.5** **Other complications** of spinal and epidural anesthesia during pregnancy

  ✓6ᵗʰ **O29.5X** **Other complications of spinal and epidural anesthesia during pregnancy**

    **O29.5X1** **Other complications of spinal and epidural anesthesia during pregnancy,** first trimester  Ⓜ♀

    **O29.5X2** **Other complications of spinal and epidural anesthesia during pregnancy,** second trimester  Ⓜ♀

    **O29.5X3** **Other complications of spinal and epidural anesthesia during pregnancy,** third trimester  Ⓜ♀

    **O29.5X9** **Other complications of spinal and epidural anesthesia during pregnancy,** unspecified trimester  Ⓜ♀

✓5ᵗʰ **O29.6** **Failed or difficult intubation** for anesthesia during pregnancy

    **O29.60** **Failed or difficult intubation for anesthesia during pregnancy,** unspecified trimester  Ⓜ♀

    **O29.61** **Failed or difficult intubation for anesthesia during pregnancy,** first trimester  Ⓜ♀

    **O29.62** **Failed or difficult intubation for anesthesia during pregnancy,** second trimester  Ⓜ♀

    **O29.63** **Failed or difficult intubation for anesthesia during pregnancy,** third trimester  Ⓜ♀

✓5ᵗʰ **O29.8** **Other complications** of anesthesia during pregnancy

  ✓6ᵗʰ **O29.8X** **Other complications of anesthesia during pregnancy**

    **O29.8X1** **Other complications of anesthesia during pregnancy,** first trimester  Ⓜ♀

    **O29.8X2** **Other complications of anesthesia during pregnancy,** second trimester  Ⓜ♀

    **O29.8X3** **Other complications of anesthesia during pregnancy,** third trimester  Ⓜ♀

    **O29.8X9** **Other complications of anesthesia during pregnancy,** unspecified trimester  Ⓜ♀

✓5ᵗʰ **O29.9** **Unspecified complication** of anesthesia during pregnancy

    **O29.90** **Unspecified complication of anesthesia during pregnancy,** unspecified trimester  Ⓜ♀

    **O29.91** **Unspecified complication of anesthesia during pregnancy,** first trimester  Ⓜ♀

    **O29.92** **Unspecified complication of anesthesia during pregnancy,** second trimester  Ⓜ♀

    **O29.93** **Unspecified complication of anesthesia during pregnancy,** third trimester  Ⓜ♀

---

✔ Additional Character Req    ✔x7ᵗʰ Placeholder Alert    Unacceptable PDx    Manifestation    **H1**-**H14** HAC    **HCC** CMS-HCC Condition    *EXCLUDES 1* Not Coded Here    *EXCLUDES 2* Not Included Here

### Twin Gestation – Monochorionic/Monoamniotic

- 1 Chorionic sac
- 1 Amniotic sac
- 2 Fetuses
- 2 Umbilical cords
- 1 Placenta

### Maternal care related to the fetus and amniotic cavity and possible delivery problems (O30-O48)

**✓4ᵗʰ O30 Multiple gestation**

Code also any complications specific to multiple gestation

**CC Excl: For CC codes in category O30:** PDX collection 976

**✓5ᵗʰ O30.0 Twin pregnancy**

**✓6ᵗʰ O30.00 Twin pregnancy, unspecified number of placenta and unspecified number of amniotic sacs**

- O30.001   Twin pregnancy, unspecified number of placenta and unspecified number of amniotic sacs, **first trimester**   Ⓜ♀
- O30.002   Twin pregnancy, unspecified number of placenta and unspecified number of amniotic sacs, **second trimester**   Ⓜ♀
- O30.003   Twin pregnancy, unspecified number of placenta and unspecified number of amniotic sacs, **third trimester**   Ⓜ♀
- O30.009   Twin pregnancy, unspecified number of placenta and unspecified number of amniotic sacs, **unspecified trimester**   Ⓜ♀

**✓6ᵗʰ O30.01 Twin pregnancy, monochorionic/monoamniotic**
Twin pregnancy, one placenta, one amniotic sac
**EXCLUDES 1** conjoined twins (O30.02-)

- O30.011   Twin pregnancy, monochorionic/monoamniotic, **first trimester**   Ⓜ♀
- O30.012   Twin pregnancy, monochorionic/monoamniotic, **second trimester**   Ⓜ♀
- O30.013   Twin pregnancy, monochorionic/monoamniotic, **third trimester**   Ⓜ♀
- O30.019   Twin pregnancy, monochorionic/monoamniotic, **unspecified trimester**   Ⓜ♀

**✓6ᵗʰ O30.02 Conjoined twin pregnancy**

- O30.021   Conjoined twin pregnancy, **first trimester**   Ⓜ♀
- O30.022   Conjoined twin pregnancy, **second trimester**   Ⓜ♀
- O30.023   Conjoined twin pregnancy, **third trimester**   Ⓜ♀
- O30.029   Conjoined twin pregnancy, **unspecified trimester**   Ⓜ♀

### Twin Gestation – Dichorionic/Diamniotic

- 2 Chorionic sacs
- 2 Amniotic sacs
- 2 Fetuses
- 2 Umbilical cords
- 2 Placentas

### Twin Gestation – Monochorionic/Diamniotic

- 1 Chorionic sac
- 2 Amniotic sacs
- 2 Fetuses
- 2 Umbilical cords
- 1 Placenta

**✓6ᵗʰ O30.03 Twin pregnancy, monochorionic/diamniotic**
Twin pregnancy, one placenta, two amniotic sacs

- O30.031   Twin pregnancy, monochorionic/diamniotic, **first trimester**   Ⓜ♀
- O30.032   Twin pregnancy, monochorionic/diamniotic, **second trimester**   Ⓜ♀
- O30.033   Twin pregnancy, monochorionic/diamniotic, **third trimester**   Ⓜ♀
- O30.039   Twin pregnancy, monochorionic/diamniotic, **unspecified trimester**   Ⓜ♀

**✓6ᵗʰ O30.04 Twin pregnancy, dichorionic/diamniotic**
Twin pregnancy, two placentae, two amniotic sacs

- O30.041   Twin pregnancy, dichorionic/diamniotic, **first trimester**   Ⓜ♀
- O30.042   Twin pregnancy, dichorionic/diamniotic, **second trimester**   Ⓜ♀
- O30.043   Twin pregnancy, dichorionic/diamniotic, **third trimester**   Ⓜ♀
- O30.049   Twin pregnancy, dichorionic/diamniotic, **unspecified trimester**   Ⓜ♀

**✓6ᵗʰ O30.09 Twin pregnancy, unable to determine number of placenta and number of amniotic sacs**

- O30.091   Twin pregnancy, unable to determine number of placenta and number of amniotic sacs, **first trimester**   Ⓜ♀
- O30.092   Twin pregnancy, unable to determine number of placenta and number of amniotic sacs, **second trimester**   Ⓜ♀
- O30.093   Twin pregnancy, unable to determine number of placenta and number of amniotic sacs, **third trimester**   Ⓜ♀
- O30.099   Twin pregnancy, unable to determine number of placenta and number of amniotic sacs, **unspecified trimester**   Ⓜ♀

**✓5ᵗʰ O30.1 Triplet pregnancy**

**✓6ᵗʰ O30.10 Triplet pregnancy, unspecified number of placenta and unspecified number of amniotic sacs**
**AHA:** 2016, 2Q, 8

- O30.101   Triplet pregnancy, unspecified number of placenta and unspecified number of amniotic sacs, **first trimester**   Ⓒ Ⓜ♀
- O30.102   Triplet pregnancy, unspecified number of placenta and unspecified number of amniotic sacs, **second trimester**   Ⓒ Ⓜ♀
- O30.103   Triplet pregnancy, unspecified number of placenta and unspecified number of amniotic sacs, **third trimester**   Ⓒ Ⓜ♀
- O30.109   Triplet pregnancy, unspecified number of placenta and unspecified number of amniotic sacs, **unspecified trimester**   Ⓜ♀

**✓6ᵗʰ O30.11 Triplet pregnancy with two or more monochorionic fetuses**

- O30.111   Triplet pregnancy with two or more monochorionic fetuses, **first trimester**   Ⓒ Ⓜ♀

Ⓝ Newborn: 0    Ⓟ Pediatric: 0-17    Ⓜ Maternity: 12-55    Ⓐ Adult: 15-124    **MCC** Major CC Condition    **PDxMCC** PDx acts as own MCC    **CC** CC Condition    **PDxCC** PDx acts as own CC

856          ICD-10-CM 2018

O3Ø.112 **Triplet pregnancy with two or more** [cc] [M] ♀ **monochorionic fetuses, second trimester**

O3Ø.113 **Triplet pregnancy with two or more** [cc] [M] ♀ **monochorionic fetuses, third trimester**

O3Ø.119 **Triplet pregnancy with two or more** [M] ♀ **monochorionic fetuses, unspecified trimester**

✓6th **O3Ø.12 Triplet pregnancy with** two or more monoamniotic fetuses

O3Ø.121 **Triplet pregnancy with two or more** [cc] [M] ♀ **monoamniotic fetuses, first trimester**

O3Ø.122 **Triplet pregnancy with two or more** [cc] [M] ♀ **monoamniotic fetuses, second trimester**

O3Ø.123 **Triplet pregnancy with two or more** [cc] [M] ♀ **monoamniotic fetuses, third trimester**

O3Ø.129 **Triplet pregnancy with two or more** [M] ♀ **monoamniotic fetuses, unspecified trimester**

✓6th **O3Ø.19 Triplet pregnancy,** unable to determine number of placenta and number of amniotic sacs

O3Ø.191 **Triplet pregnancy, unable to** [cc] [M] ♀ **determine number of placenta and number of amniotic sacs, first trimester**

O3Ø.192 **Triplet pregnancy, unable to** [cc] [M] ♀ **determine number of placenta and number of amniotic sacs, second trimester**

O3Ø.193 **Triplet pregnancy, unable to** [cc] [M] ♀ **determine number of placenta and number of amniotic sacs, third trimester**

O3Ø.199 **Triplet pregnancy, unable to** [M] ♀ **determine number of placenta and number of amniotic sacs, unspecified trimester**

✓5th **O3Ø.2 Quadruplet pregnancy**

✓6th **O3Ø.20 Quadruplet pregnancy,** unspecified number of placenta and unspecified number of amniotic sacs

O3Ø.201 **Quadruplet pregnancy, unspecified** [cc] [M] ♀ **number of placenta and unspecified number of amniotic sacs, first trimester**

O3Ø.202 **Quadruplet pregnancy, unspecified** [cc] [M] ♀ **number of placenta and unspecified number of amniotic sacs, second trimester**

O3Ø.203 **Quadruplet pregnancy, unspecified** [cc] [M] ♀ **number of placenta and unspecified number of amniotic sacs, third trimester**

O3Ø.209 **Quadruplet pregnancy, unspecified** [M] ♀ **number of placenta and unspecified number of amniotic sacs, unspecified trimester**

✓6th **O3Ø.21 Quadruplet pregnancy with** two or more monochorionic fetuses

O3Ø.211 **Quadruplet pregnancy with two or** [cc] [M] ♀ **more monochorionic fetuses, first trimester**

O3Ø.212 **Quadruplet pregnancy with two or** [cc] [M] ♀ **more monochorionic fetuses, second trimester**

O3Ø.213 **Quadruplet pregnancy with two or** [cc] [M] ♀ **more monochorionic fetuses, third trimester**

O3Ø.219 **Quadruplet pregnancy with two or** [M] ♀ **more monochorionic fetuses, unspecified trimester**

✓6th **O3Ø.22 Quadruplet pregnancy with** two or more monoamniotic fetuses

O3Ø.221 **Quadruplet pregnancy with two or** [cc] [M] ♀ **more monoamniotic fetuses, first trimester**

O3Ø.222 **Quadruplet pregnancy with two or** [cc] [M] ♀ **more monoamniotic fetuses, second trimester**

O3Ø.223 **Quadruplet pregnancy with two or** [cc] [M] ♀ **more monoamniotic fetuses, third trimester**

O3Ø.229 **Quadruplet pregnancy with two or** [M] ♀ **more monoamniotic fetuses, unspecified trimester**

✓6th **O3Ø.29 Quadruplet pregnancy,** unable to determine number of placenta and number of amniotic sacs

O3Ø.291 **Quadruplet pregnancy, unable to** [cc] [M] ♀ **determine number of placenta and number of amniotic sacs, first trimester**

O3Ø.292 **Quadruplet pregnancy, unable to** [cc] [M] ♀ **determine number of placenta and number of amniotic sacs, second trimester**

O3Ø.293 **Quadruplet pregnancy, unable to** [cc] [M] ♀ **determine number of placenta and number of amniotic sacs, third trimester**

O3Ø.299 **Quadruplet pregnancy, unable to** [M] ♀ **determine number of placenta and number of amniotic sacs, unspecified trimester**

✓5th **O3Ø.8 Other specified multiple gestation**
Multiple gestation pregnancy greater than quadruplets

✓6th **O3Ø.80 Other specified multiple gestation,** unspecified number of placenta and unspecified number of amniotic sacs

O3Ø.801 **Other specified multiple gestation,** [cc] [M] ♀ **unspecified number of placenta and unspecified number of amniotic sacs, first trimester**

O3Ø.802 **Other specified multiple gestation,** [cc] [M] ♀ **unspecified number of placenta and unspecified number of amniotic sacs, second trimester**

O3Ø.803 **Other specified multiple gestation,** [cc] [M] ♀ **unspecified number of placenta and unspecified number of amniotic sacs, third trimester**

O3Ø.809 **Other specified multiple gestation,** [M] ♀ **unspecified number of placenta and unspecified number of amniotic sacs, unspecified trimester**

✓6th **O3Ø.81 Other specified multiple gestation with** two or more monochorionic fetuses

O3Ø.811 **Other specified multiple gestation** [cc] [M] ♀ **with two or more monochorionic fetuses, first trimester**

O3Ø.812 **Other specified multiple gestation** [cc] [M] ♀ **with two or more monochorionic fetuses, second trimester**

O3Ø.813 **Other specified multiple gestation** [cc] [M] ♀ **with two or more monochorionic fetuses, third trimester**

O3Ø.819 **Other specified multiple gestation** [M] ♀ **with two or more monochorionic fetuses, unspecified trimester**

✓6th **O3Ø.82 Other specified multiple gestation with** two or more monoamniotic fetuses

O3Ø.821 **Other specified multiple gestation** [cc] [M] ♀ **with two or more monoamniotic fetuses, first trimester**

O3Ø.822 **Other specified multiple gestation** [cc] [M] ♀ **with two or more monoamniotic fetuses, second trimester**

O3Ø.823 **Other specified multiple gestation** [cc] [M] ♀ **with two or more monoamniotic fetuses, third trimester**

O3Ø.829 **Other specified multiple gestation** [M] ♀ **with two or more monoamniotic fetuses, unspecified trimester**

☑ Additional Character Req   ✓x7th Placeholder Alert   Unacceptable PDx   ■ Manifestation   H1 - H14 HAC   HCC CMS-HCC Condition   EXCLUDES 1 Not Coded Here   EXCLUDES 2 Not Included Here

ICD-10-CM 2018   857

O3Ø.112–O3Ø.829

**Chapter 15. Pregnancy, Childbirth and the Puerperium**

✓6th **O30.89** **Other** specified multiple gestation, unable to determine number of placenta and number of amniotic sacs

    **O30.891** Other specified multiple gestation, CC M♀ unable to determine number of placenta and number of amniotic sacs, first trimester

    **O30.892** Other specified multiple gestation, CC M♀ unable to determine number of placenta and number of amniotic sacs, second trimester

    **O30.893** Other specified multiple gestation, CC M♀ unable to determine number of placenta and number of amniotic sacs, third trimester

    **O30.899** Other specified multiple gestation, M♀ unable to determine number of placenta and number of amniotic sacs, unspecified trimester

✓5th **O30.9** Multiple gestation, unspecified
    Multiple pregnancy NOS

    **O30.90** Multiple gestation, unspecified, unspecified M♀ trimester

    **O30.91** Multiple gestation, unspecified, first trimester M♀

    **O30.92** Multiple gestation, unspecified, second M♀ trimester

    **O30.93** Multiple gestation, unspecified, third trimester M♀

✓4th **O31** **Complications specific to multiple gestation**
    EXCLUDES 2   *delayed delivery of second twin, triplet, etc. (O63.2)*
          *malpresentation of one fetus or more (O32.9)*
          *placental transfusion syndromes (O43.0-)*
    AHA: 2012, 4Q, 107

> One of the following 7th characters is to be assigned to each code under category O31. 7th character Ø is for single gestations and multiple gestations where the fetus is unspecified. 7th characters 1 through 9 are for cases of multiple gestations to identify the fetus for which the code applies. The appropriate code from category O30, Multiple gestation, must also be assigned when assigning a code from category O31 that has a 7th character of 1 through 9.
>
> | Ø | not applicable or unspecified | 3 | fetus 3 |
> |---|---|---|---|
> |   |   | 4 | fetus 4 |
> | 1 | fetus 1 | 5 | fetus 5 |
> | 2 | fetus 2 | 9 | other fetus |

✓5th **O31.0** **Papyraceous fetus**
    Fetus compressus

    ✓x7th **O31.00** **Papyraceous fetus,** unspecified trimester M♀

    ✓x7th **O31.01** **Papyraceous fetus,** first trimester M♀

    ✓x7th **O31.02** **Papyraceous fetus,** second trimester M♀

    ✓x7th **O31.03** **Papyraceous fetus,** third trimester M♀

✓5th **O31.1** **Continuing pregnancy** after spontaneous abortion of one fetus or more

    ✓x7th **O31.10** **Continuing pregnancy after spontaneous** M♀ abortion of one fetus or more, unspecified trimester

    ✓x7th **O31.11** **Continuing pregnancy after spontaneous** M♀ abortion of one fetus or more, first trimester

    ✓x7th **O31.12** **Continuing pregnancy after spontaneous** M♀ abortion of one fetus or more, second trimester

    ✓x7th **O31.13** **Continuing pregnancy after spontaneous** M♀ abortion of one fetus or more, third trimester

✓5th **O31.2** **Continuing pregnancy** after intrauterine death of one fetus or more

    ✓x7th **O31.20** **Continuing pregnancy after intrauterine death** M♀ of one fetus or more, unspecified trimester

    ✓x7th **O31.21** **Continuing pregnancy after intrauterine death** M♀ of one fetus or more, first trimester

    ✓x7th **O31.22** **Continuing pregnancy after intrauterine death** M♀ of one fetus or more, second trimester

    ✓x7th **O31.23** **Continuing pregnancy after intrauterine death** M♀ of one fetus or more, third trimester

✓5th **O31.3** **Continuing pregnancy after** elective fetal reduction of one fetus or more
    Continuing pregnancy after selective termination of one fetus or more

    ✓x7th **O31.30** **Continuing pregnancy after elective fetal** M♀ reduction of one fetus or more, unspecified trimester

---

✓x7th **O31.31** **Continuing pregnancy after elective fetal** M♀ reduction of one fetus or more, first trimester

✓x7th **O31.32** **Continuing pregnancy after elective fetal** M♀ reduction of one fetus or more, second trimester

✓x7th **O31.33** **Continuing pregnancy after elective fetal** M♀ reduction of one fetus or more, third trimester

✓5th **O31.8** Other complications specific to multiple gestation

    ✓6th **O31.8X** Other complications specific to multiple gestation

> **CC Excl: For CC codes in subcategory O31.8X:**
> PDX collection 976

    ✓7th **O31.8X1** Other complications specific to CC M♀ multiple gestation, first trimester

    ✓7th **O31.8X2** Other complications specific to CC M♀ multiple gestation, second trimester

    ✓7th **O31.8X3** Other complications specific to CC M♀ multiple gestation, third trimester

    ✓7th **O31.8X9** Other complications specific to M♀ multiple gestation, unspecified trimester

✓4th **O32** **Maternal care for malpresentation of fetus**
    INCLUDES   the listed conditions as a reason for observation, hospitalization or other obstetric care of the mother, or for cesarean delivery before onset of labor
    EXCLUDES 1   *malpresentation of fetus with obstructed labor (O64.-)*
    AHA: 2012, 4Q, 107

> One of the following 7th characters is to be assigned to each code under category O32. 7th character Ø is for single gestations and multiple gestations where the fetus is unspecified. 7th characters 1 through 9 are for cases of multiple gestations to identify the fetus for which the code applies. The appropriate code from category O30, Multiple gestation, must also be assigned when assigning a code from category O32 that has a 7th character of 1 through 9.
>
> | Ø | not applicable or unspecified | 3 | fetus 3 |
> |---|---|---|---|
> |   |   | 4 | fetus 4 |
> | 1 | fetus 1 | 5 | fetus 5 |
> | 2 | fetus 2 | 9 | other fetus |

✓x7th **O32.0** **Maternal care for** unstable lie M♀

✓x7th **O32.1** **Maternal care for** breech presentation M♀
    Maternal care for buttocks presentation
    Maternal care for complete breech
    Maternal care for frank breech
    EXCLUDES 1   *footling presentation (O32.8)*
          *incomplete breech (O32.8)*
    **DEF:** Fetus presentation in a longitudinal lie with the buttocks or feet closest to birth canal; may require external cephalic version or cesarean delivery.

✓x7th **O32.2** **Maternal care for** transverse and oblique lie M♀
    Maternal care for oblique presentation
    Maternal care for transverse presentation

✓x7th **O32.3** **Maternal care for** face, brow and chin presentation M♀

✓x7th **O32.4** **Maternal care for** high head at term M♀
    Maternal care for failure of head to enter pelvic brim

✓x7th **O32.6** **Maternal care for** compound presentation M♀

✓x7th **O32.8** **Maternal care for** other malpresentation of fetus M♀
    Maternal care for footling presentation
    Maternal care for incomplete breech

✓x7th **O32.9** **Maternal care for malpresentation of fetus,** unspecified M♀

**Fetal Malpresentation**

Breech
Mother's pelvis

Face (mentum)

Shoulder (arm prolapse)

Compound (extremity together with head)

Oblique

N Newborn: 0   P Pediatric: 0-17   M Maternity: 12-55   A Adult: 15-124   MCC Major CC Condition   PDx MCC PDx acts as own MCC   CC CC Condition   PDx CC PDx acts as own CC

858         ICD-10-CM 2018

✓4ᵗʰ **O33 Maternal care for disproportion**

> INCLUDES   the listed conditions as a reason for observation, hospitalization or other obstetric care of the mother, or for cesarean delivery before onset of labor
>
> EXCLUDES 1   *disproportion with obstructed labor (O65-O66)*

**O33.0 Maternal care for disproportion due to deformity of maternal pelvic bones**   CC M♀

> Maternal care for disproportion due to pelvic deformity causing disproportion NOS
>
> **CC Excl:** PDX collection 977

**O33.1 Maternal care for disproportion due to generally contracted pelvis**   M♀

> Maternal care for disproportion due to contracted pelvis NOS causing disproportion

**O33.2 Maternal care for disproportion due to inlet contraction of pelvis**   M♀

> Maternal care for disproportion due to inlet contraction (pelvis) causing disproportion

✓x7ᵗʰ **O33.3 Maternal care for disproportion due to outlet contraction of pelvis**   M♀

> Maternal care for disproportion due to mid-cavity contraction (pelvis)
>
> Maternal care for disproportion due to outlet contraction (pelvis)
>
> One of the following 7th characters is to be assigned to code O33.3. 7th character Ø is for single gestations and multiple gestations where the fetus is unspecified. 7th characters 1 through 9 are for cases of multiple gestations to identify the fetus for which the code applies. The appropriate code from category O3Ø, Multiple gestation, must also be assigned when assigning code O33.3 with a 7th character of 1 through 9.

| | | | |
|---|---|---|---|
| Ø | not applicable or unspecified | 3 | fetus 3 |
| | | 4 | fetus 4 |
| 1 | fetus 1 | 5 | fetus 5 |
| 2 | fetus 2 | 9 | other fetus |

✓x7ᵗʰ **O33.4 Maternal care for disproportion of mixed maternal and fetal origin**   M♀

> One of the following 7th characters is to be assigned to code O33.4. 7th character Ø is for single gestations and multiple gestations where the fetus is unspecified. 7th characters 1 through 9 are for cases of multiple gestations to identify the fetus for which the code applies. The appropriate code from category O3Ø, Multiple gestation, must also be assigned when assigning code O33.4 with a 7th character of 1 through 9.

| | | | |
|---|---|---|---|
| Ø | not applicable or unspecified | 3 | fetus 3 |
| | | 4 | fetus 4 |
| 1 | fetus 1 | 5 | fetus 5 |
| 2 | fetus 2 | 9 | other fetus |

✓x7ᵗʰ **O33.5 Maternal care for disproportion due to unusually large fetus**   M♀

> Maternal care for disproportion due to disproportion of fetal origin with normally formed fetus
>
> Maternal care for disproportion due to fetal disproportion NOS
>
> One of the following 7th characters is to be assigned to code O33.5. 7th character Ø is for single gestations and multiple gestations where the fetus is unspecified. 7th characters 1 through 9 are for cases of multiple gestations to identify the fetus for which the code applies. The appropriate code from category O3Ø, Multiple gestation, must also be assigned when assigning code O33.5 with a 7th character of 1 through 9.

| | | | |
|---|---|---|---|
| Ø | not applicable or unspecified | 3 | fetus 3 |
| | | 4 | fetus 4 |
| 1 | fetus 1 | 5 | fetus 5 |
| 2 | fetus 2 | 9 | other fetus |

✓x7ᵗʰ **O33.6 Maternal care for disproportion due to hydrocephalic fetus**   M♀

> One of the following 7th characters is to be assigned to code O33.6. 7th character Ø is for single gestations and multiple gestations where the fetus is unspecified. 7th characters 1 through 9 are for cases of multiple gestations to identify the fetus for which the code applies. The appropriate code from category O3Ø, Multiple gestation, must also be assigned when assigning code O33.6 with a 7th character of 1 through 9.

| | | | |
|---|---|---|---|
| Ø | not applicable or unspecified | 3 | fetus 3 |
| | | 4 | fetus 4 |
| 1 | fetus 1 | 5 | fetus 5 |
| 2 | fetus 2 | 9 | other fetus |

✓x7ᵗʰ **O33.7 Maternal care for disproportion due to other fetal deformities**   M♀

> Maternal care for disproportion due to fetal ascites
>
> Maternal care for disproportion due to fetal hydrops
>
> Maternal care for disproportion due to fetal meningomyelocele
>
> Maternal care for disproportion due to fetal sacral teratoma
>
> Maternal care for disproportion due to fetal tumor
>
> EXCLUDES 1   *obstructed labor due to other fetal deformities (O66.3)*
>
> One of the following 7th characters is to be assigned to code O33.7. 7th character Ø is for single gestations and multiple gestations where the fetus is unspecified. 7th characters 1 through 9 are for cases of multiple gestations to identify the fetus for which the code applies. The appropriate code from category O3Ø, Multiple gestation, must also be assigned when assigning code O33.7 with a 7th character of 1 through 9.

| | | | |
|---|---|---|---|
| Ø | not applicable or unspecified | 3 | fetus 3 |
| | | 4 | fetus 4 |
| 1 | fetus 1 | 5 | fetus 5 |
| 2 | fetus 2 | 9 | other fetus |

**O33.8 Maternal care for disproportion of other origin**   M♀

**O33.9 Maternal care for disproportion, unspecified**   M♀

> Maternal care for disproportion due to cephalopelvic disproportion NOS
>
> Maternal care for disproportion due to fetopelvic disproportion NOS

✓4ᵗʰ **O34 Maternal care for abnormality of pelvic organs**

> INCLUDES   the listed conditions as a reason for hospitalization or other obstetric care of the mother, or for cesarean delivery before onset of labor
>
> Code first any associated obstructed labor (O65.5)
>
> Use additional code for specific condition

✓5ᵗʰ **O34.0 Maternal care for congenital malformation of uterus**

> Maternal care for double uterus
>
> Maternal care for uterus bicornis

    **O34.00 Maternal care for unspecified congenital malformation of uterus, unspecified trimester**   M♀

    **O34.01 Maternal care for unspecified congenital malformation of uterus, first trimester**   M♀

    **O34.02 Maternal care for unspecified congenital malformation of uterus, second trimester**   M♀

    **O34.03 Maternal care for unspecified congenital malformation of uterus, third trimester**   M♀

✓5ᵗʰ **O34.1 Maternal care for benign tumor of corpus uteri**

> EXCLUDES 2   *maternal care for benign tumor of cervix (O34.4-)*
> *maternal care for malignant neoplasm of uterus (O9A.1-)*

    **O34.10 Maternal care for benign tumor of corpus uteri, unspecified trimester**   M♀

    **O34.11 Maternal care for benign tumor of corpus uteri, first trimester**   M♀

    **O34.12 Maternal care for benign tumor of corpus uteri, second trimester**   M♀

    **O34.13 Maternal care for benign tumor of corpus uteri, third trimester**   M♀

✓5ᵗʰ **O34.2 Maternal care due to uterine scar from previous surgery**

    ✓6ᵗʰ **O34.21 Maternal care for scar from previous cesarean delivery**

       **O34.211 Maternal care for low transverse scar from previous cesarean delivery**   M♀

       **O34.212 Maternal care for vertical scar from previous cesarean delivery**   M♀

> Maternal care for classical scar from previous cesarean delivery

       **O34.219 Maternal care for unspecified type scar from previous cesarean delivery**   M♀

    **O34.29 Maternal care due to uterine scar from other previous surgery**   M♀

> Maternal care due to uterine scar from other transmural uterine incision

---

✓ Additional Character Req    ✓x7ᵗʰ Placeholder Alert    Unacceptable PDx    **Manifestation**    H1 -H14 HAC    HCC CMS-HCC Condition    EXCLUDES 1 Not Coded Here    EXCLUDES 2 Not Included Here

ICD-10-CM 2018            **859**

**Chapter 15. Pregnancy, Childbirth and the Puerperium**

✓5th **O34.3 Maternal care for** cervical incompetence
Maternal care for cerclage with or without cervical incompetence
Maternal care for Shirodkar suture with or without cervical incompetence
**DEF:** Inadequate functioning of cervix marked by abnormal widening during pregnancy that may cause premature birth or miscarriage.

**CC Excl: For MCC codes in subcategory O34.3:**
PDX collection 973

O34.30   **Maternal care for cervical incompetence,** unspecified trimester    M♀

O34.31   **Maternal care for cervical incompetence,** first trimester    MCC M♀

O34.32   **Maternal care for cervical incompetence,** second trimester    MCC M♀

O34.33   **Maternal care for cervical incompetence,** third trimester    MCC M♀

✓5th **O34.4 Maternal care for** other abnormalities of cervix

O34.40   **Maternal care for other abnormalities of cervix,** unspecified trimester    M♀

O34.41   **Maternal care for other abnormalities of cervix,** first trimester    M♀

O34.42   **Maternal care for other abnormalities of cervix,** second trimester    M♀

O34.43   **Maternal care for other abnormalities of cervix,** third trimester    M♀

✓5th **O34.5 Maternal care for** other abnormalities of gravid uterus

✓6th **O34.51 Maternal care for** incarceration of gravid uterus

O34.511   **Maternal care for incarceration of gravid uterus,** first trimester    M♀

O34.512   **Maternal care for incarceration of gravid uterus,** second trimester    M♀

O34.513   **Maternal care for incarceration of gravid uterus,** third trimester    M♀

O34.519   **Maternal care for incarceration of gravid uterus,** unspecified trimester    M♀

✓6th **O34.52 Maternal care for** prolapse of gravid uterus

O34.521   **Maternal care for prolapse of gravid uterus,** first trimester    M♀

O34.522   **Maternal care for prolapse of gravid uterus,** second trimester    M♀

O34.523   **Maternal care for prolapse of gravid uterus,** third trimester    M♀

O34.529   **Maternal care for prolapse of gravid uterus,** unspecified trimester    M♀

✓6th **O34.53 Maternal care for** retroversion of gravid uterus

O34.531   **Maternal care for retroversion of gravid uterus,** first trimester    M♀

O34.532   **Maternal care for retroversion of gravid uterus,** second trimester    M♀

O34.533   **Maternal care for retroversion of gravid uterus,** third trimester    M♀

O34.539   **Maternal care for retroversion of gravid uterus,** unspecified trimester    M♀

✓6th **O34.59 Maternal care for** other abnormalities of gravid uterus

O34.591   **Maternal care for other abnormalities of gravid uterus,** first trimester    M♀

O34.592   **Maternal care for other abnormalities of gravid uterus,** second trimester    M♀

O34.593   **Maternal care for other abnormalities of gravid uterus,** third trimester    M♀

O34.599   **Maternal care for other abnormalities of gravid uterus,** unspecified trimester    M♀

✓5th **O34.6 Maternal care for** abnormality of vagina
EXCLUDES 2   maternal care for vaginal varices in pregnancy (O22.1-)

O34.60   **Maternal care for abnormality of vagina,** unspecified trimester    M♀

O34.61   **Maternal care for abnormality of vagina,** first trimester    M♀

O34.62   **Maternal care for abnormality of vagina,** second trimester    M♀

O34.63   **Maternal care for abnormality of vagina,** third trimester    M♀

✓5th **O34.7 Maternal care for** abnormality of vulva and perineum
EXCLUDES 2   maternal care for perineal and vulval varices in pregnancy (O22.1-)

O34.70   **Maternal care for abnormality of vulva and perineum,** unspecified trimester    M♀

O34.71   **Maternal care for abnormality of vulva and perineum,** first trimester    M♀

O34.72   **Maternal care for abnormality of vulva and perineum,** second trimester    M♀

O34.73   **Maternal care for abnormality of vulva and perineum,** third trimester    M♀

✓5th **O34.8 Maternal care for** other abnormalities of pelvic organs

O34.80   **Maternal care for other abnormalities of pelvic organs,** unspecified trimester    M♀

O34.81   **Maternal care for other abnormalities of pelvic organs,** first trimester    M♀

O34.82   **Maternal care for other abnormalities of pelvic organs,** second trimester    M♀

O34.83   **Maternal care for other abnormalities of pelvic organs,** third trimester    M♀

✓5th **O34.9 Maternal care for abnormality of pelvic organ,** unspecified

O34.90   **Maternal care for abnormality of pelvic organ, unspecified,** unspecified trimester    M♀

O34.91   **Maternal care for abnormality of pelvic organ, unspecified,** first trimester    M♀

O34.92   **Maternal care for abnormality of pelvic organ, unspecified,** second trimester    M♀

O34.93   **Maternal care for abnormality of pelvic organ, unspecified,** third trimester    M♀

✓4th **O35 Maternal care for known or suspected fetal abnormality and damage**
INCLUDES   the listed conditions in the fetus as a reason for hospitalization or other obstetric care to the mother, or for termination of pregnancy
Code also any associated maternal condition
EXCLUDES 1   encounter for suspected maternal and fetal conditions ruled out (Z03.7-)

One of the following 7th characters is to be assigned to each code under category O35. 7th character 0 is for single gestations and multiple gestations where the fetus is unspecified. 7th characters 1 through 9 are for cases of multiple gestations to identify the fetus for which the code applies. The appropriate code from category O30, Multiple gestation, must also be assigned when assigning a code from category O35 that has a 7th character of 1 through 9.
0   not applicable or     3   fetus 3
     unspecified         4   fetus 4
1   fetus 1             5   fetus 5
2   fetus 2             9   other fetus

✓x7th **O35.0 Maternal care for (suspected)** central nervous system malformation in fetus    M♀
Maternal care for fetal anencephaly
Maternal care for fetal hydrocephalus
Maternal care for fetal spina bifida
EXCLUDES 2   chromosomal abnormality in fetus (O35.1)

✓x7th **O35.1 Maternal care for (suspected)** chromosomal abnormality in fetus    M♀

✓x7th **O35.2 Maternal care for (suspected)** hereditary disease in fetus    M♀
EXCLUDES 2   chromosomal abnormality in fetus (O35.1)

✓x7th **O35.3 Maternal care for (suspected)** damage to fetus from viral disease in mother    M♀
Maternal care for damage to fetus from maternal cytomegalovirus infection
Maternal care for damage to fetus from maternal rubella

✓x7th **O35.4 Maternal care for (suspected)** damage to fetus from alcohol    M♀

✓x7th **O35.5 Maternal care for (suspected)** damage to fetus by drugs    M♀
Maternal care for damage to fetus from drug addiction

✓x7th **O35.6 Maternal care for (suspected)** damage to fetus by radiation    M♀

✓x7th **O35.7 Maternal care for (suspected)** damage to fetus by other medical procedures    M♀
Maternal care for damage to fetus by amniocentesis
Maternal care for damage to fetus by biopsy procedures
Maternal care for damage to fetus by hematological investigation
Maternal care for damage to fetus by intrauterine contraceptive device
Maternal care for damage to fetus by intrauterine surgery

**✔x7ᵗʰ O35.8 Maternal care for other (suspected) fetal abnormality and damage** Ⓜ♀
     Maternal care for damage to fetus from maternal listeriosis
     Maternal care for damage to fetus from maternal toxoplasmosis

**✔x7ᵗʰ O35.9 Maternal care for (suspected) fetal abnormality and damage, unspecified** Ⓜ♀

**✔4ᵗʰ O36 Maternal care for other fetal problems**
   **INCLUDES** the listed conditions in the fetus as a reason for hospitalization or other obstetric care of the mother, or for termination of pregnancy
   **EXCLUDES 1** encounter for suspected maternal and fetal conditions ruled out (Z03.7-)
         placental transfusion syndromes (O43.0-)
   **EXCLUDES 2** labor and delivery complicated by fetal stress (O77.-)
   **AHA:** 2015, 3Q, 40

> One of the following 7th characters is to be assigned to each code under category O36. 7th character 0 is for single gestations and multiple gestations where the fetus is unspecified. 7th characters 1 through 9 are for cases of multiple gestations to identify the fetus for which the code applies. The appropriate code from category O30, Multiple gestation, must also be assigned when assigning a code from category O36 that has a 7th character of 1 through 9.
> | | | | |
> |---|---|---|---|
> | 0 | not applicable or unspecified | 3 | fetus 3 |
> | | | 4 | fetus 4 |
> | 1 | fetus 1 | 5 | fetus 5 |
> | 2 | fetus 2 | 9 | other fetus |

**✔5ᵗʰ O36.0 Maternal care for rhesus isoimmunization**
     Maternal care for Rh incompatibility (with hydrops fetalis)

> **CC Excl: For CC codes in subcategory O36.0:**
> PDX collection 978

   **✔6ᵗʰ O36.01 Maternal care for anti-D [Rh] antibodies**
         **AHA:** 2014, 4Q, 17
     **✔7ᵗʰ O36.011 Maternal care for anti-D [Rh] antibodies, first trimester** CC Ⓜ♀
     **✔7ᵗʰ O36.012 Maternal care for anti-D [Rh] antibodies, second trimester** CC Ⓜ♀
     **✔7ᵗʰ O36.013 Maternal care for anti-D [Rh] antibodies, third trimester** CC Ⓜ♀
     **✔7ᵗʰ O36.019 Maternal care for anti-D [Rh] antibodies, unspecified trimester** Ⓜ♀

   **✔6ᵗʰ O36.09 Maternal care for other rhesus isoimmunization**
     **✔7ᵗʰ O36.091 Maternal care for other rhesus isoimmunization, first trimester** CC Ⓜ♀
     **✔7ᵗʰ O36.092 Maternal care for other rhesus isoimmunization, second trimester** CC Ⓜ♀
     **✔7ᵗʰ O36.093 Maternal care for other rhesus isoimmunization, third trimester** CC Ⓜ♀
     **✔7ᵗʰ O36.099 Maternal care for other rhesus isoimmunization, unspecified trimester** Ⓜ♀

**✔5ᵗʰ O36.1 Maternal care for other isoimmunization**
     Maternal care for ABO isoimmunization

   **✔6ᵗʰ O36.11 Maternal care for Anti-A sensitization**
     Maternal care for isoimmunization NOS (with hydrops fetalis)
     **✔7ᵗʰ O36.111 Maternal care for Anti-A sensitization, first trimester** Ⓜ♀
     **✔7ᵗʰ O36.112 Maternal care for Anti-A sensitization, second trimester** Ⓜ♀
     **✔7ᵗʰ O36.113 Maternal care for Anti-A sensitization, third trimester** Ⓜ♀
     **✔7ᵗʰ O36.119 Maternal care for Anti-A sensitization, unspecified trimester** Ⓜ♀

   **✔6ᵗʰ O36.19 Maternal care for other isoimmunization**
     Maternal care for Anti-B sensitization
     **✔7ᵗʰ O36.191 Maternal care for other isoimmunization, first trimester** Ⓜ♀
     **✔7ᵗʰ O36.192 Maternal care for other isoimmunization, second trimester** Ⓜ♀
     **✔7ᵗʰ O36.193 Maternal care for other isoimmunization, third trimester** Ⓜ♀
     **✔7ᵗʰ O36.199 Maternal care for other isoimmunization, unspecified trimester** Ⓜ♀

**✔5ᵗʰ O36.2 Maternal care for hydrops fetalis**
     Maternal care for hydrops fetalis NOS
     Maternal care for hydrops fetalis not associated with isoimmunization
   **EXCLUDES 1** hydrops fetalis associated with ABO isoimmunization (O36.1-)
         hydrops fetalis associated with rhesus isoimmunization (O36.0-)
   **✔x7ᵗʰ O36.20 Maternal care for hydrops fetalis, unspecified trimester** Ⓜ♀
   **✔x7ᵗʰ O36.21 Maternal care for hydrops fetalis, first trimester** Ⓜ♀
   **✔x7ᵗʰ O36.22 Maternal care for hydrops fetalis, second trimester** Ⓜ♀
   **✔x7ᵗʰ O36.23 Maternal care for hydrops fetalis, third trimester** Ⓜ♀

**✔x7ᵗʰ O36.4 Maternal care for intrauterine death** CC Ⓜ♀
     Maternal care for intrauterine fetal death NOS
     Maternal care for intrauterine fetal death after completion of 20 weeks of gestation
     Maternal care for late fetal death
     Maternal care for missed delivery
   **EXCLUDES 1** missed abortion (O02.1)
         stillbirth (P95)
   **CC Excl:** PDX collection 979

**✔5ᵗʰ O36.5 Maternal care for known or suspected poor fetal growth**
   **✔6ᵗʰ O36.51 Maternal care for known or suspected placental insufficiency**
     **✔7ᵗʰ O36.511 Maternal care for known or suspected placental insufficiency, first trimester** Ⓜ♀
     **✔7ᵗʰ O36.512 Maternal care for known or suspected placental insufficiency, second trimester** Ⓜ♀
     **✔7ᵗʰ O36.513 Maternal care for known or suspected placental insufficiency, third trimester** Ⓜ♀
     **✔7ᵗʰ O36.519 Maternal care for known or suspected placental insufficiency, unspecified trimester** Ⓜ♀

   **✔6ᵗʰ O36.59 Maternal care for other known or suspected poor fetal growth**
     Maternal care for known or suspected light-for-dates NOS
     Maternal care for known or suspected small-for-dates NOS
     **✔7ᵗʰ O36.591 Maternal care for other known or suspected poor fetal growth, first trimester** Ⓜ♀
     **✔7ᵗʰ O36.592 Maternal care for other known or suspected poor fetal growth, second trimester** Ⓜ♀
     **✔7ᵗʰ O36.593 Maternal care for other known or suspected poor fetal growth, third trimester** Ⓜ♀
     **✔7ᵗʰ O36.599 Maternal care for other known or suspected poor fetal growth, unspecified trimester** Ⓜ♀

**✔5ᵗʰ O36.6 Maternal care for excessive fetal growth**
     Maternal care for known or suspected large-for-dates
   **✔x7ᵗʰ O36.60 Maternal care for excessive fetal growth, unspecified trimester** Ⓜ♀
   **✔x7ᵗʰ O36.61 Maternal care for excessive fetal growth, first trimester** Ⓜ♀
   **✔x7ᵗʰ O36.62 Maternal care for excessive fetal growth, second trimester** Ⓜ♀
   **✔x7ᵗʰ O36.63 Maternal care for excessive fetal growth, third trimester** Ⓜ♀

**✔5ᵗʰ O36.7 Maternal care for viable fetus in abdominal pregnancy**
   **✔x7ᵗʰ O36.70 Maternal care for viable fetus in abdominal pregnancy, unspecified trimester** Ⓜ♀
   **✔x7ᵗʰ O36.71 Maternal care for viable fetus in abdominal pregnancy, first trimester** Ⓜ♀
   **✔x7ᵗʰ O36.72 Maternal care for viable fetus in abdominal pregnancy, second trimester** Ⓜ♀
   **✔x7ᵗʰ O36.73 Maternal care for viable fetus in abdominal pregnancy, third trimester** Ⓜ♀

✔ Additional Character Req   ✔x7ᵗʰ Placeholder Alert   Unacceptable PDx   Manifestation   H1-H14 HAC   HCC CMS-HCC Condition   EXCLUDES 1 Not Coded Here   EXCLUDES 2 Not Included Here

ICD-10-CM 2018      **861**

**Chapter 15. Pregnancy, Childbirth and the Puerperium** (side margin)

√5ᵗʰ **O36.8　Maternal care for other specified fetal problems**

√7ᵗʰ **O36.80　Pregnancy with inconclusive fetal viability**　Ⓜ♀
Encounter to determine fetal viability of pregnancy

√6ᵗʰ **O36.81　Decreased fetal movements**

√7ᵗʰ **O36.812　Decreased fetal movements, second trimester**　Ⓜ♀

√7ᵗʰ **O36.813　Decreased fetal movements, third trimester**　Ⓜ♀

√7ᵗʰ **O36.819　Decreased fetal movements, unspecified trimester**　Ⓜ♀

√6ᵗʰ **O36.82　Fetal anemia and thrombocytopenia**

√7ᵗʰ **O36.821　Fetal anemia and thrombocytopenia, first trimester**　Ⓜ♀

√7ᵗʰ **O36.822　Fetal anemia and thrombocytopenia, second trimester**　Ⓜ♀

√7ᵗʰ **O36.823　Fetal anemia and thrombocytopenia, third trimester**　Ⓜ♀

√7ᵗʰ **O36.829　Fetal anemia and thrombocytopenia, unspecified trimester**　Ⓜ♀

● √6ᵗʰ **O36.83　Maternal care for abnormalities of the fetal heart rate or rhythm**

● √7ᵗʰ **O36.831　Maternal care for abnormalities of the fetal heart rate or rhythm, first trimester**　Ⓜ

● √7ᵗʰ **O36.832　Maternal care for abnormalities of the fetal heart rate or rhythm, second trimester**　Ⓜ

● √7ᵗʰ **O36.833　Maternal care for abnormalities of the fetal heart rate or rhythm, third trimester**　Ⓜ

● √7ᵗʰ **O36.839　Maternal care for abnormalities of the fetal heart rate or rhythm, unspecified trimester**　Ⓜ

√6ᵗʰ **O36.89　Maternal care for other specified fetal problems**

√7ᵗʰ **O36.891　Maternal care for other specified fetal problems, first trimester**　Ⓜ♀

√7ᵗʰ **O36.892　Maternal care for other specified fetal problems, second trimester**　Ⓜ♀

√7ᵗʰ **O36.893　Maternal care for other specified fetal problems, third trimester**　Ⓜ♀

√7ᵗʰ **O36.899　Maternal care for other specified fetal problems, unspecified trimester**　Ⓜ♀

√5ᵗʰ **O36.9　Maternal care for fetal problem, unspecified**

√x7ᵗʰ **O36.90　Maternal care for fetal problem, unspecified, unspecified trimester**　Ⓜ♀

√x7ᵗʰ **O36.91　Maternal care for fetal problem, unspecified, first trimester**　Ⓜ♀

√x7ᵗʰ **O36.92　Maternal care for fetal problem, unspecified, second trimester**　Ⓜ♀

√x7ᵗʰ **O36.93　Maternal care for fetal problem, unspecified, third trimester**　Ⓜ♀

√4ᵗʰ **O40　Polyhydramnios**

**INCLUDES**　hydramnios

**EXCLUDES 1**　encounter for suspected maternal and fetal conditions ruled out (Z03.7-)

**AHA:** 2016, 1Q, 4

One of the following 7th characters is to be assigned to each code under category O40. 7th character 0 is for single gestations and multiple gestations where the fetus is unspecified. 7th characters 1 through 9 are for cases of multiple gestations to identify the fetus for which the code applies. The appropriate code from category O30, Multiple gestation, must also be assigned when assigning a code from category O40 that has a 7th character of 1 through 9.

| | | | |
|---|---|---|---|
| 0 | not applicable or unspecified | 3 | fetus 3 |
| | | 4 | fetus 4 |
| 1 | fetus 1 | 5 | fetus 5 |
| 2 | fetus 2 | 9 | other fetus |

√x7ᵗʰ **O40.1　Polyhydramnios, first trimester**　Ⓜ♀

√x7ᵗʰ **O40.2　Polyhydramnios, second trimester**　Ⓜ♀

√x7ᵗʰ **O40.3　Polyhydramnios, third trimester**　Ⓜ♀

√x7ᵗʰ **O40.9　Polyhydramnios, unspecified trimester**　Ⓜ♀

√4ᵗʰ **O41　Other disorders of amniotic fluid and membranes**

**EXCLUDES 1**　encounter for suspected maternal and fetal conditions ruled out (Z03.7-)

One of the following 7th characters is to be assigned to each code under category O41. 7th character 0 is for single gestations and multiple gestations where the fetus is unspecified. 7th characters 1 through 9 are for cases of multiple gestations to identify the fetus for which the code applies. The appropriate code from category O30, Multiple gestation, must also be assigned when assigning a code from category O41 that has a 7th character of 1 through 9.

| | | | |
|---|---|---|---|
| 0 | not applicable or unspecified | 3 | fetus 3 |
| | | 4 | fetus 4 |
| 1 | fetus 1 | 5 | fetus 5 |
| 2 | fetus 2 | 9 | other fetus |

√5ᵗʰ **O41.0　Oligohydramnios**
Oligohydramnios without rupture of membranes

**CC Excl: For CC codes in subcategory O41.0:**
PDX collection 982

√x7ᵗʰ **O41.00　Oligohydramnios, unspecified trimester**　Ⓜ♀

√x7ᵗʰ **O41.01　Oligohydramnios, first trimester**　CC Ⓜ♀

√x7ᵗʰ **O41.02　Oligohydramnios, second trimester**　CC Ⓜ♀

√x7ᵗʰ **O41.03　Oligohydramnios, third trimester**　CC Ⓜ♀

√5ᵗʰ **O41.1　Infection of amniotic sac and membranes**

**CC Excl: For MCC codes in subcategory O41.1:**
PDX collection 983

√6ᵗʰ **O41.10　Infection of amniotic sac and membranes, unspecified**

√7ᵗʰ **O41.101　Infection of amniotic sac and membranes, unspecified, first trimester**　MCC Ⓜ♀

√7ᵗʰ **O41.102　Infection of amniotic sac and membranes, unspecified, second trimester**　MCC Ⓜ♀

√7ᵗʰ **O41.103　Infection of amniotic sac and membranes, unspecified, third trimester**　MCC Ⓜ♀

√7ᵗʰ **O41.109　Infection of amniotic sac and membranes, unspecified, unspecified trimester**　Ⓜ♀

√6ᵗʰ **O41.12　Chorioamnionitis**

√7ᵗʰ **O41.121　Chorioamnionitis, first trimester**　MCC Ⓜ♀

√7ᵗʰ **O41.122　Chorioamnionitis, second trimester**　MCC Ⓜ♀

√7ᵗʰ **O41.123　Chorioamnionitis, third trimester**　MCC Ⓜ♀

√7ᵗʰ **O41.129　Chorioamnionitis, unspecified trimester**　Ⓜ♀

√6ᵗʰ **O41.14　Placentitis**

√7ᵗʰ **O41.141　Placentitis, first trimester**　MCC Ⓜ♀

√7ᵗʰ **O41.142　Placentitis, second trimester**　MCC Ⓜ♀

√7ᵗʰ **O41.143　Placentitis, third trimester**　MCC Ⓜ♀

√7ᵗʰ **O41.149　Placentitis, unspecified trimester**　Ⓜ♀

√5ᵗʰ **O41.8　Other specified disorders of amniotic fluid and membranes**

√6ᵗʰ **O41.8X　Other specified disorders of amniotic fluid and membranes**

√7ᵗʰ **O41.8X1　Other specified disorders of amniotic fluid and membranes, first trimester**　Ⓜ♀

√7ᵗʰ **O41.8X2　Other specified disorders of amniotic fluid and membranes, second trimester**　Ⓜ♀

√7ᵗʰ **O41.8X3　Other specified disorders of amniotic fluid and membranes, third trimester**　Ⓜ♀

√7ᵗʰ **O41.8X9　Other specified disorders of amniotic fluid and membranes, unspecified trimester**　Ⓜ♀

√5ᵗʰ **O41.9　Disorder of amniotic fluid and membranes, unspecified**

√x7ᵗʰ **O41.90　Disorder of amniotic fluid and membranes, unspecified, unspecified trimester**　Ⓜ♀

√x7ᵗʰ **O41.91　Disorder of amniotic fluid and membranes, unspecified, first trimester**　Ⓜ♀

√x7ᵗʰ **O41.92　Disorder of amniotic fluid and membranes, unspecified, second trimester**　Ⓜ♀

Ⓝ Newborn: 0　Ⓟ Pediatric: 0-17　Ⓜ Maternity: 12-55　Ⓐ Adult: 15-124　**MCC** Major CC Condition　**PDxMCC** PDx acts as own MCC　**CC** CC Condition　**PDxCC** PDx acts as own CC

862　　　　　　　　　　ICD-10-CM 2018

√x7ᵗʰ **O41.93 Disorder of amniotic fluid and membranes, unspecified, third trimester** Ⓜ♀

√4ᵗʰ **O42 Premature rupture of membranes**
AHA: 2016, 1Q, 3

√5ᵗʰ **O42.0 Premature rupture of membranes, onset of labor within 24 hours of rupture**

**O42.00 Premature rupture of membranes, onset of labor within 24 hours of rupture, unspecified weeks of gestation** Ⓜ♀

√6ᵗʰ **O42.01 Preterm premature rupture of membranes, onset of labor within 24 hours of rupture**
Premature rupture of membranes before 37 completed weeks of gestation

**O42.011 Preterm premature rupture of membranes, onset of labor within 24 hours of rupture, first trimester** Ⓜ♀

**O42.012 Preterm premature rupture of membranes, onset of labor within 24 hours of rupture, second trimester** Ⓜ♀

**O42.013 Preterm premature rupture of membranes, onset of labor within 24 hours of rupture, third trimester** Ⓜ♀

**O42.019 Preterm premature rupture of membranes, onset of labor within 24 hours of rupture, unspecified trimester** Ⓜ♀

**O42.02 Full-term premature rupture of membranes, onset of labor within 24 hours of rupture** Ⓜ♀
Premature rupture of membranes at or after 37 completed weeks of gestation, onset of labor within 24 hours of rupture

√5ᵗʰ **O42.1 Premature rupture of membranes, onset of labor more than 24 hours following rupture**
AHA: 2016, 1Q, 5

**O42.10 Premature rupture of membranes, onset of labor more than 24 hours following rupture, unspecified weeks of gestation** Ⓜ♀

√6ᵗʰ **O42.11 Preterm premature rupture of membranes, onset of labor more than 24 hours following rupture**
Premature rupture of membranes before 37 completed weeks of gestation

**O42.111 Preterm premature rupture of membranes, onset of labor more than 24 hours following rupture, first trimester** Ⓜ♀

**O42.112 Preterm premature rupture of membranes, onset of labor more than 24 hours following rupture, second trimester** Ⓜ♀

**O42.113 Preterm premature rupture of membranes, onset of labor more than 24 hours following rupture, third trimester** Ⓜ♀

**O42.119 Preterm premature rupture of membranes, onset of labor more than 24 hours following rupture, unspecified trimester** ♀

**O42.12 Full-term premature rupture of membranes, onset of labor more than 24 hours following rupture** Ⓜ♀
Premature rupture of membranes at or after 37 completed weeks of gestation, onset of labor more than 24 hours following rupture

√5ᵗʰ **O42.9 Premature rupture of membranes, unspecified as to length of time between rupture and onset of labor**

**O42.90 Premature rupture of membranes, unspecified as to length of time between rupture and onset of labor, unspecified weeks of gestation** Ⓜ♀

√6ᵗʰ **O42.91 Preterm premature rupture of membranes, unspecified as to length of time between rupture and onset of labor**
Premature rupture of membranes before 37 completed weeks of gestation

**O42.911 Preterm premature rupture of membranes, unspecified as to length of time between rupture and onset of labor, first trimester** Ⓜ♀

**O42.912 Preterm premature rupture of membranes, unspecified as to length of time between rupture and onset of labor, second trimester** Ⓜ♀

**O42.913 Preterm premature rupture of membranes, unspecified as to length of time between rupture and onset of labor, third trimester** Ⓜ♀

**O42.919 Preterm premature rupture of membranes, unspecified as to length of time between rupture and onset of labor, unspecified trimester** Ⓜ♀

**O42.92 Full-term premature rupture of membranes, unspecified as to length of time between rupture and onset of labor** Ⓜ♀
Premature rupture of membranes at or after 37 completed weeks of gestation, unspecified as to length of time between rupture and onset of labor

√4ᵗʰ **O43 Placental disorders**
EXCLUDES 2    maternal care for poor fetal growth due to placental insufficiency (O36.5-)
placenta previa (O44.-)
placental polyp (O90.89)
placentitis (O41.14-)
premature separation of placenta [abruptio placentae] (O45.-)

√5ᵗʰ **O43.0 Placental transfusion syndromes**

√6ᵗʰ **O43.01 Fetomaternal placental transfusion syndrome**
Maternofetal placental transfusion syndrome

**O43.011 Fetomaternal placental transfusion syndrome, first trimester** Ⓜ♀

**O43.012 Fetomaternal placental transfusion syndrome, second trimester** Ⓜ♀

**O43.013 Fetomaternal placental transfusion syndrome, third trimester** Ⓜ♀

**O43.019 Fetomaternal placental transfusion syndrome, unspecified trimester** Ⓜ♀

√6ᵗʰ **O43.02 Fetus-to-fetus placental transfusion syndrome**

**O43.021 Fetus-to-fetus placental transfusion syndrome, first trimester** Ⓜ♀

**O43.022 Fetus-to-fetus placental transfusion syndrome, second trimester** Ⓜ♀

**O43.023 Fetus-to-fetus placental transfusion syndrome, third trimester** Ⓜ♀

**O43.029 Fetus-to-fetus placental transfusion syndrome, unspecified trimester** Ⓜ♀

√5ᵗʰ **O43.1 Malformation of placenta**

√6ᵗʰ **O43.10 Malformation of placenta, unspecified**
Abnormal placenta NOS

**O43.101 Malformation of placenta, unspecified, first trimester** Ⓜ♀

**O43.102 Malformation of placenta, unspecified, second trimester** Ⓜ♀

**O43.103 Malformation of placenta, unspecified, third trimester** Ⓜ♀

**O43.109 Malformation of placenta, unspecified, unspecified trimester** Ⓜ♀

√6ᵗʰ **O43.11 Circumvallate placenta**

**O43.111 Circumvallate placenta, first trimester** Ⓜ♀

**O43.112 Circumvallate placenta, second trimester** Ⓜ♀

**O43.113 Circumvallate placenta, third trimester** Ⓜ♀

**Twin to Twin Transfusion Syndrome (TTTS)**

Healthy twins      Twins with TTTS

**O43.119**   Circumvallate placenta, unspecified trimester   M♀

✓6ᵗʰ **O43.12**   Velamentous insertion of umbilical cord

     **O43.121**   Velamentous insertion of umbilical cord, first trimester   M♀

     **O43.122**   Velamentous insertion of umbilical cord, second trimester   M♀

     **O43.123**   Velamentous insertion of umbilical cord, third trimester   M♀

     **O43.129**   Velamentous insertion of umbilical cord, unspecified trimester   M♀

✓6ᵗʰ **O43.19**   Other malformation of placenta

     **O43.191**   Other malformation of placenta, first trimester   M♀

     **O43.192**   Other malformation of placenta, second trimester   M♀

     **O43.193**   Other malformation of placenta, third trimester   M♀

     **O43.199**   Other malformation of placenta, unspecified trimester   M♀

✓5ᵗʰ **O43.2**   Morbidly adherent placenta

Code also associated third stage postpartum hemorrhage, if applicable (O72.0)

EXCLUDES 1   retained placenta (O73.-)

✓6ᵗʰ **O43.21**   Placenta accreta

     **O43.211**   Placenta accreta, first trimester   M♀
     **O43.212**   Placenta accreta, second trimester   M♀
     **O43.213**   Placenta accreta, third trimester   M♀
     **O43.219**   Placenta accreta, unspecified trimester   M♀

✓6ᵗʰ **O43.22**   Placenta increta

     **O43.221**   Placenta increta, first trimester   M♀
     **O43.222**   Placenta increta, second trimester   M♀
     **O43.223**   Placenta increta, third trimester   M♀
     **O43.229**   Placenta increta, unspecified trimester   M♀

✓6ᵗʰ **O43.23**   Placenta percreta

     **O43.231**   Placenta percreta, first trimester   M♀
     **O43.232**   Placenta percreta, second trimester   M♀
     **O43.233**   Placenta percreta, third trimester   M♀
     **O43.239**   Placenta percreta, unspecified trimester   M♀

✓5ᵗʰ **O43.8**   Other placental disorders

✓6ᵗʰ **O43.81**   Placental infarction

     **O43.811**   Placental infarction, first trimester   M♀
     **O43.812**   Placental infarction, second trimester   M♀
     **O43.813**   Placental infarction, third trimester   M♀
     **O43.819**   Placental infarction, unspecified trimester   M♀

✓6ᵗʰ **O43.89**   Other placental disorders

Placental dysfunction

     **O43.891**   Other placental disorders, first trimester   M♀
     **O43.892**   Other placental disorders, second trimester   M♀
     **O43.893**   Other placental disorders, third trimester   M♀
     **O43.899**   Other placental disorders, unspecified trimester   M♀

✓5ᵗʰ **O43.9**   Unspecified placental disorder

     **O43.90**   Unspecified placental disorder, unspecified trimester   M♀
     **O43.91**   Unspecified placental disorder, first trimester   M♀
     **O43.92**   Unspecified placental disorder, second trimester   M♀
     **O43.93**   Unspecified placental disorder, third trimester   M♀

✓4ᵗʰ **O44**   Placenta previa

**DEF:** Placenta implanted in lower segment of uterus; commonly causes hemorrhage in the last trimester of pregnancy.

CC Excl: For CC/MCC codes in category O44: PDX collection 966

✓5ᵗʰ **O44.0**   Complete placenta previa NOS or without hemorrhage

Placenta previa NOS

     **O44.00**   Complete placenta previa NOS or without hemorrhage, unspecified trimester   M♀

     **O44.01**   Complete placenta previa NOS or without hemorrhage, first trimester   CC M♀

     **O44.02**   Complete placenta previa NOS or without hemorrhage, second trimester   CC M♀

     **O44.03**   Complete placenta previa NOS or without hemorrhage, third trimester   CC M♀

✓5ᵗʰ **O44.1**   Complete placenta previa with hemorrhage

EXCLUDES 1   labor and delivery complicated by hemorrhage from vasa previa (O69.4)

     **O44.10**   Complete placenta previa with hemorrhage, unspecified trimester   M♀

     **O44.11**   Complete placenta previa with hemorrhage, first trimester   MCC M♀

     **O44.12**   Complete placenta previa with hemorrhage, second trimester   MCC M♀

     **O44.13**   Complete placenta previa with hemorrhage, third trimester   MCC M♀

✓5ᵗʰ **O44.2**   Partial placenta previa without hemorrhage

Marginal placenta previa, NOS or without hemorrhage

     **O44.20**   Partial placenta previa NOS or without hemorrhage, unspecified trimester   M♀

     **O44.21**   Partial placenta previa NOS or without hemorrhage, first trimester   CC M♀

     **O44.22**   Partial placenta previa NOS or without hemorrhage, second trimester   CC M♀

     **O44.23**   Partial placenta previa NOS or without hemorrhage, third trimester   CC M♀

✓5ᵗʰ **O44.3**   Partial placenta previa with hemorrhage

Marginal placenta previa with hemorrhage

     **O44.30**   Partial placenta previa with hemorrhage, unspecified trimester   M♀

     **O44.31**   Partial placenta previa with hemorrhage, first trimester   MCC M♀

     **O44.32**   Partial placenta previa with hemorrhage, second trimester   MCC M♀

     **O44.33**   Partial placenta previa with hemorrhage, third trimester   MCC ♀

✓5ᵗʰ **O44.4**   Low lying placenta NOS or without hemorrhage

Low implantation of placenta NOS or without hemorrhage

     **O44.40**   Low lying placenta NOS or without hemorrhage, unspecified trimester   M♀

     **O44.41**   Low lying placenta NOS or without hemorrhage, first trimester   CC ♀

     **O44.42**   Low lying placenta NOS or without hemorrhage, second trimester   CC M♀

     **O44.43**   Low lying placenta NOS or without hemorrhage, third trimester   CC M♀

✓5ᵗʰ **O44.5**   Low lying placenta with hemorrhage

Low implantation of placenta with hemorrhage

     **O44.50**   Low lying placenta with hemorrhage, unspecified trimester   M♀

     **O44.51**   Low lying placenta with hemorrhage, first trimester   MCC M♀

     **O44.52**   Low lying placenta with hemorrhage, second trimester   MCC M♀

     **O44.53**   Low lying placenta with hemorrhage, third trimester   MCC M♀

✓4ᵗʰ **O45**   Premature separation of placenta [abruptio placentae]

✓5ᵗʰ **O45.0**   Premature separation of placenta with coagulation defect

CC Excl: For MCC codes in subcategory O45.0: PDX collection 985

✓6ᵗʰ **O45.00**   Premature separation of placenta with coagulation defect, unspecified

     **O45.001**   Premature separation of placenta with coagulation defect, unspecified, first trimester   MCC M♀

     **O45.002**   Premature separation of placenta with coagulation defect, unspecified, second trimester   MCC M♀

     **O45.003**   Premature separation of placenta with coagulation defect, unspecified, third trimester   MCC M♀

     **O45.009**   Premature separation of placenta with coagulation defect, unspecified, unspecified trimester   M♀

N Newborn: 0   P Pediatric: 0-17   M Maternity: 12-55   A Adult: 15-124   MCC Major CC Condition   PDx MCC PDx acts as own MCC   CC CC Condition   PDx CC PDx acts as own CC

**864**      ICD-10-CM 2018

√6ᵗʰ **O45.01** **Premature separation of placenta with afibrinogenemia**
Premature separation of placenta with hypofibrinogenemia

**O45.011** **Premature separation of placenta with afibrinogenemia, first trimester** MCC M ♀

**O45.012** **Premature separation of placenta with afibrinogenemia, second trimester** MCC M ♀

**O45.013** **Premature separation of placenta with afibrinogenemia, third trimester** MCC M ♀

**O45.019** **Premature separation of placenta with afibrinogenemia, unspecified trimester** M ♀

√6ᵗʰ **O45.02** **Premature separation of placenta with disseminated intravascular coagulation**

**O45.021** **Premature separation of placenta with disseminated intravascular coagulation, first trimester** MCC M ♀

**O45.022** **Premature separation of placenta with disseminated intravascular coagulation, second trimester** MCC M ♀

**O45.023** **Premature separation of placenta with disseminated intravascular coagulation, third trimester** MCC M ♀

**O45.029** **Premature separation of placenta with disseminated intravascular coagulation, unspecified trimester** M ♀

√6ᵗʰ **O45.09** **Premature separation of placenta with other coagulation defect**

**O45.091** **Premature separation of placenta with other coagulation defect, first trimester** MCC M ♀

**O45.092** **Premature separation of placenta with other coagulation defect, second trimester** MCC M ♀

**O45.093** **Premature separation of placenta with other coagulation defect, third trimester** MCC M ♀

**O45.099** **Premature separation of placenta with other coagulation defect, unspecified trimester** M ♀

√5ᵗʰ **O45.8** **Other premature separation of placenta**

**CC Excl: For MCC codes in subcategory O45.8:** PDX collection 986

√6ᵗʰ **O45.8X** **Other premature separation of placenta**

**O45.8X1** **Other premature separation of placenta, first trimester** MCC M ♀

**O45.8X2** **Other premature separation of placenta, second trimester** MCC M ♀

**O45.8X3** **Other premature separation of placenta, third trimester** MCC M ♀

**O45.8X9** **Other premature separation of placenta, unspecified trimester** M ♀

√5ᵗʰ **O45.9** **Premature separation of placenta, unspecified**
Abruptio placentae NOS

**CC Excl: For MCC codes in subcategory O45.9:** PDX collection 986

**O45.90** **Premature separation of placenta, unspecified, unspecified trimester** M ♀

**O45.91** **Premature separation of placenta, unspecified, first trimester** MCC M ♀

**O45.92** **Premature separation of placenta, unspecified, second trimester** MCC M ♀

**O45.93** **Premature separation of placenta, unspecified, third trimester** MCC M ♀

√4ᵗʰ **O46** **Antepartum hemorrhage, not elsewhere classified**

**EXCLUDES 1**   *hemorrhage in early pregnancy (O20.-)*
*intrapartum hemorrhage NEC (O67.-)*
*placenta previa (O44.-)*
*premature separation of placenta [abruptio placentae] (O45.-)*

**DEF:** Uterine hemorrhage prior to delivery; not related to placenta previa or abruptio placentae.

√5ᵗʰ **O46.0** **Antepartum hemorrhage with coagulation defect**

**CC Excl: For MCC codes in subcategory O46.0:** PDX collection 985

√6ᵗʰ **O46.00** **Antepartum hemorrhage with coagulation defect, unspecified**

**O46.001** **Antepartum hemorrhage with coagulation defect, unspecified, first trimester** MCC M ♀

**O46.002** **Antepartum hemorrhage with coagulation defect, unspecified, second trimester** MCC M ♀

**O46.003** **Antepartum hemorrhage with coagulation defect, unspecified, third trimester** MCC M ♀

**O46.009** **Antepartum hemorrhage with coagulation defect, unspecified, unspecified trimester** M ♀

√6ᵗʰ **O46.01** **Antepartum hemorrhage with afibrinogenemia**
Antepartum hemorrhage with hypofibrinogenemia

**O46.011** **Antepartum hemorrhage with afibrinogenemia, first trimester** MCC M ♀

**O46.012** **Antepartum hemorrhage with afibrinogenemia, second trimester** MCC M ♀

**O46.013** **Antepartum hemorrhage with afibrinogenemia, third trimester** MCC M ♀

**O46.019** **Antepartum hemorrhage with afibrinogenemia, unspecified trimester** M ♀

√6ᵗʰ **O46.02** **Antepartum hemorrhage with disseminated intravascular coagulation**

**O46.021** **Antepartum hemorrhage with disseminated intravascular coagulation, first trimester** MCC M ♀

**O46.022** **Antepartum hemorrhage with disseminated intravascular coagulation, second trimester** MCC M ♀

**O46.023** **Antepartum hemorrhage with disseminated intravascular coagulation, third trimester** MCC M ♀

**O46.029** **Antepartum hemorrhage with disseminated intravascular coagulation, unspecified trimester** M ♀

√6ᵗʰ **O46.09** **Antepartum hemorrhage with other coagulation defect**

**O46.091** **Antepartum hemorrhage with other coagulation defect, first trimester** MCC M ♀

**O46.092** **Antepartum hemorrhage with other coagulation defect, second trimester** MCC M ♀

**O46.093** **Antepartum hemorrhage with other coagulation defect, third trimester** MCC M ♀

**O46.099** **Antepartum hemorrhage with other coagulation defect, unspecified trimester** M ♀

√5ᵗʰ **O46.8** **Other antepartum hemorrhage**

√6ᵗʰ **O46.8X** **Other antepartum hemorrhage**

**O46.8X1** **Other antepartum hemorrhage, first trimester** M ♀

**O46.8X2** **Other antepartum hemorrhage, second trimester** M ♀

**O46.8X3** **Other antepartum hemorrhage, third trimester** M ♀

**O46.8X9** **Other antepartum hemorrhage, unspecified trimester** M ♀

√5ᵗʰ **O46.9** **Antepartum hemorrhage, unspecified**

**O46.90** **Antepartum hemorrhage, unspecified, unspecified trimester** M ♀

**O46.91** **Antepartum hemorrhage, unspecified, first trimester** M ♀

☑ Additional Character Req   √x7ᵗʰ Placeholder Alert   Unacceptable PDx   Manifestation   H1 - H14 HAC   MCC CMS-HCC Condition   EXCLUDES 1 Not Coded Here   EXCLUDES 2 Not Included Here

ICD-10-CM 2018      **865**

**O46.92**    **Antepartum hemorrhage, unspecified, second trimester**    M ♀

**O46.93**    **Antepartum hemorrhage, unspecified, third trimester**    M ♀

### ✓4ᵗʰ O47 False labor

INCLUDES   Braxton Hicks contractions
      threatened labor

EXCLUDES 1   *preterm labor (O60.-)*

**CC Excl: For CC codes in catagory O47:** PDX collection 987

#### ✓5ᵗʰ O47.0 False labor before 37 completed weeks of gestation

**O47.00**   **False labor before 37 completed weeks of gestation, unspecified trimester**    M ♀

**O47.02**   **False labor before 37 completed weeks of gestation, second trimester**    CC M ♀

**O47.03**   **False labor before 37 completed weeks of gestation, third trimester**    CC M ♀

**O47.1**   **False labor at or after 37 completed weeks of gestation**    CC M ♀

**O47.9**   **False labor, unspecified**    M ♀

### ✓4ᵗʰ O48 Late pregnancy

**O48.0**   **Post-term pregnancy**    M ♀
     Pregnancy over 40 completed weeks to 42 completed weeks gestation

**O48.1**   **Prolonged pregnancy**    M ♀
     Pregnancy which has advanced beyond 42 completed weeks gestation
     **AHA:** 2016, 1Q, 5

## Complications of labor and delivery (O60-O77)

### ✓4ᵗʰ O60 Preterm labor

INCLUDES   onset (spontaneous) of labor before 37 completed weeks of gestation

EXCLUDES 1   *false labor (O47.0-)*
          *threatened labor NOS (O47.0-)*

**CC Excl: For CC/MCC codes in category O60:** PDX collection 987

#### ✓5ᵗʰ O60.0 Preterm labor without delivery

**O60.00**   **Preterm labor without delivery, unspecified trimester**    M ♀

**O60.02**   **Preterm labor without delivery, second trimester**    MCC M ♀

**O60.03**   **Preterm labor without delivery, third trimester**    MCC M ♀

#### ✓5ᵗʰ O60.1 Preterm labor with preterm delivery
**AHA:** 2016, 2Q, 10

One of the following 7th characters is to be assigned to each code under subcategory O60.1. 7th character 0 is for single gestations and multiple gestations where the fetus is unspecified. 7th characters 1 through 9 are for cases of multiple gestations to identify the fetus for which the code applies. The appropriate code from category O30, Multiple gestation, must also be assigned when assigning a code from subcategory O60.1 that has a 7th character of 1 through 9.

| 0 | not applicable or unspecified | 3 | fetus 3 |
|---|---|---|---|
| 1 | fetus 1 | 4 | fetus 4 |
| 2 | fetus 2 | 5 | fetus 5 |
| | | 9 | other fetus |

**✓x7ᵗʰ O60.10**   **Preterm labor with preterm delivery, unspecified trimester**    CC M ♀
     Preterm labor with delivery NOS

**✓x7ᵗʰ O60.12**   **Preterm labor second trimester with preterm delivery second trimester**    MCC M ♀

**✓x7ᵗʰ O60.13**   **Preterm labor second trimester with preterm delivery third trimester**    MCC M ♀

**✓x7ᵗʰ O60.14**   **Preterm labor third trimester with preterm delivery third trimester**    MCC M ♀

#### ✓5ᵗʰ O60.2 Term delivery with preterm labor

One of the following 7th characters is to be assigned to each code under subcategory O60.2. 7th character 0 is for single gestations and multiple gestations where the fetus is unspecified. 7th characters 1 through 9 are for cases of multiple gestations to identify the fetus for which the code applies. The appropriate code from category O30, Multiple gestation, must also be assigned when assigning a code from subcategory O60.2 that has a 7th character of 1 through 9.

| 0 | not applicable or unspecified | 3 | fetus 3 |
|---|---|---|---|
| 1 | fetus 1 | 4 | fetus 4 |
| 2 | fetus 2 | 5 | fetus 5 |
| | | 9 | other fetus |

**✓x7ᵗʰ O60.20**   **Term delivery with preterm labor, unspecified trimester**    CC M ♀

**✓x7ᵗʰ O60.22**   **Term delivery with preterm labor, second trimester**    MCC M ♀

**✓x7ᵗʰ O60.23**   **Term delivery with preterm labor, third trimester**    MCC M ♀

### ✓4ᵗʰ O61 Failed induction of labor

**O61.0**   **Failed medical induction of labor**    M ♀
     Failed induction (of labor) by oxytocin
     Failed induction (of labor) by prostaglandins

**O61.1**   **Failed instrumental induction of labor**    M ♀
     Failed mechanical induction (of labor)
     Failed surgical induction (of labor)

**O61.8**   **Other failed induction of labor**    M ♀

**O61.9**   **Failed induction of labor, unspecified**    M ♀

### ✓4ᵗʰ O62 Abnormalities of forces of labor

**O62.0**   **Primary inadequate contractions**    M ♀
     Failure of cervical dilatation
     Primary hypotonic uterine dysfunction
     Uterine inertia during latent phase of labor

**O62.1**   **Secondary uterine inertia**    M ♀
     Arrested active phase of labor
     Secondary hypotonic uterine dysfunction

**O62.2**   **Other uterine inertia**    M ♀
     Atony of uterus without hemorrhage
     Atony of uterus NOS
     Desultory labor
     Hypotonic uterine dysfunction NOS
     Irregular labor
     Poor contractions
     Slow slope active phase of labor
     Uterine inertia NOS

     EXCLUDES 1   *atony of uterus with hemorrhage (postpartum) (O72.1)*
                *postpartum atony of uterus without hemorrhage (O75.89)*

**O62.3**   **Precipitate labor**    M ♀

**O62.4**   **Hypertonic, incoordinate, and prolonged uterine contractions**    M ♀
     Cervical spasm
     Contraction ring dystocia
     Dyscoordinate labor
     Hour-glass contraction of uterus
     Hypertonic uterine dysfunction
     Incoordinate uterine action
     Tetanic contractions
     Uterine dystocia NOS
     Uterine spasm

     EXCLUDES 1   *dystocia (fetal) (maternal) NOS (O66.9)*

**O62.8**   **Other abnormalities of forces of labor**    M ♀

**O62.9**   **Abnormality of forces of labor, unspecified**    M ♀

### ✓4ᵗʰ O63 Long labor

**O63.0**   **Prolonged first stage (of labor)**    M ♀

**O63.1**   **Prolonged second stage (of labor)**    M ♀

**O63.2**   **Delayed delivery of second twin, triplet, etc.**    M ♀

**O63.9**   **Long labor, unspecified**    CC M ♀
     Prolonged labor NOS
     **CC Excl:** PDX collection 988

N Newborn: 0    P Pediatric: 0-17    M Maternity: 12-55    A Adult: 15-124    MCC Major CC Condition    PDx MCC PDx acts as own MCC    CC CC Condition    PDx CC PDx acts as own CC

866                         ICD-10-CM 2018

**Fetal Malposition**

Breech

Shoulder
(arm prolapse)

Mother's pelvis

Face
(mentum)

Compound
(extremity
together
with head)

Oblique

✓4th **O64 Obstructed labor due to malposition and malpresentation of fetus**

> One of the following 7th characters is to be assigned to each code under category O64. 7th character Ø is for single gestations and multiple gestations where the fetus is unspecified. 7th characters 1 through 9 are for cases of multiple gestations to identify the fetus for which the code applies. The appropriate code from category O3Ø, Multiple gestation, must also be assigned when assigning a code from category O64 that has a 7th character of 1 through 9.
>
> | | | | |
> |---|---|---|---|
> | Ø | not applicable or | 3 | fetus 3 |
> | | unspecified | 4 | fetus 4 |
> | 1 | fetus 1 | 5 | fetus 5 |
> | 2 | fetus 2 | 9 | other fetus |

✓x7th **O64.Ø Obstructed labor due to incomplete rotation of fetal head**   Ⓜ♀
Deep transverse arrest
Obstructed labor due to persistent occipitoiliac (position)
Obstructed labor due to persistent occipitoposterior (position)
Obstructed labor due to persistent occipitosacral (position)
Obstructed labor due to persistent occipitotransverse (position)

✓x7th **O64.1 Obstructed labor due to breech presentation**   Ⓜ♀
Obstructed labor due to buttocks presentation
Obstructed labor due to complete breech presentation
Obstructed labor due to frank breech presentation

✓x7th **O64.2 Obstructed labor due to face presentation**   Ⓜ♀
Obstructed labor due to chin presentation

✓x7th **O64.3 Obstructed labor due to brow presentation**   Ⓜ♀

✓x7th **O64.4 Obstructed labor due to shoulder presentation**   Ⓜ♀
Prolapsed arm
> EXCLUDES 1   impacted shoulders (O66.Ø)
>          shoulder dystocia (O66.Ø)

✓x7th **O64.5 Obstructed labor due to compound presentation**   Ⓜ♀

✓x7th **O64.8 Obstructed labor due to other malposition and malpresentation**   Ⓜ♀
Obstructed labor due to footling presentation
Obstructed labor due to incomplete breech presentation

✓x7th **O64.9 Obstructed labor due to malposition and malpresentation, unspecified**   Ⓜ♀

✓4th **O65 Obstructed labor due to maternal pelvic abnormality**

**O65.Ø Obstructed labor due to deformed pelvis**   Ⓜ♀

**O65.1 Obstructed labor due to generally contracted pelvis**   Ⓜ♀

**O65.2 Obstructed labor due to pelvic inlet contraction**   Ⓜ♀

**O65.3 Obstructed labor due to pelvic outlet and mid-cavity contraction**   Ⓜ♀

**O65.4 Obstructed labor due to fetopelvic disproportion, unspecified**   Ⓜ♀
> EXCLUDES 1   dystocia due to abnormality of fetus (O66.2-O66.3)

**O65.5 Obstructed labor due to abnormality of maternal pelvic organs**   Ⓜ♀
Obstructed labor due to conditions listed in O34-
Use additional code to identify abnormality of pelvic organs (O34.-)

**O65.8 Obstructed labor due to other maternal pelvic abnormalities**   Ⓜ♀

**O65.9 Obstructed labor due to maternal pelvic abnormality, unspecified**   Ⓜ♀

✓4th **O66 Other obstructed labor**

**O66.Ø Obstructed labor due to shoulder dystocia**   Ⓜ♀
Impacted shoulders
**DEF:** Obstructed labor due to impacted fetal shoulders; emergency condition that may require cesarean section, forceps delivery, vacuum extraction, or simphysiotomy.

**O66.1 Obstructed labor due to locked twins**   Ⓜ♀

**O66.2 Obstructed labor due to unusually large fetus**   Ⓜ♀

**O66.3 Obstructed labor due to other abnormalities of fetus**   Ⓜ♀
Dystocia due to fetal ascites
Dystocia due to fetal hydrops
Dystocia due to fetal meningomyelocele
Dystocia due to fetal sacral teratoma
Dystocia due to fetal tumor
Dystocia due to hydrocephalic fetus
Use additional code to identify cause of obstruction

✓5th **O66.4 Failed trial of labor**

**O66.4Ø Failed trial of labor, unspecified**   Ⓜ♀

**O66.41 Failed attempted vaginal birth after previous cesarean delivery**   Ⓜ♀
Code first rupture of uterus, if applicable (O71.Ø-, O71.1)

**O66.5 Attempted application of vacuum extractor and forceps**   Ⓜ♀
Attempted application of vacuum or forceps, with subsequent delivery by forceps or cesarean delivery

**O66.6 Obstructed labor due to other multiple fetuses**   Ⓜ♀

**O66.8 Other specified obstructed labor**   Ⓜ♀
Use additional code to identify cause of obstruction

**O66.9 Obstructed labor, unspecified**   Ⓜ♀
Dystocia NOS
Fetal dystocia NOS
Maternal dystocia NOS

✓4th **O67 Labor and delivery complicated by intrapartum hemorrhage, not elsewhere classified**
> EXCLUDES 1   antepartum hemorrhage NEC (O46.-)
>          placenta previa (O44.-)
>          premature separation of placenta [abruptio placentae] (O45.-)
> EXCLUDES 2   postpartum hemorrhage (O72.-)

**O67.Ø Intrapartum hemorrhage with coagulation defect**   MCC Ⓜ♀
Intrapartum hemorrhage (excessive) associated with afibrinogenemia
Intrapartum hemorrhage (excessive) associated with disseminated intravascular coagulation
Intrapartum hemorrhage (excessive) associated with hyperfibrinolysis
Intrapartum hemorrhage (excessive) associated with hypofibrinogenemia
**CC Excl:** PDX collection 985

**O67.8 Other intrapartum hemorrhage**   Ⓜ♀
Excessive intrapartum hemorrhage

**O67.9 Intrapartum hemorrhage, unspecified**   Ⓜ♀

**O68 Labor and delivery complicated by abnormality of fetal acid-base balance**   CC Ⓜ♀
Fetal acidemia complicating labor and delivery
Fetal acidosis complicating labor and delivery
Fetal alkalosis complicating labor and delivery
Fetal metabolic acidemia complicating labor and delivery
> EXCLUDES 1   fetal stress NOS (O77.9)
>          labor and delivery complicated by electrocardiographic evidence of fetal stress (O77.8)
>          labor and delivery complicated by ultrasonic evidence of fetal stress (O77.8)
> EXCLUDES 2   abnormality in fetal heart rate or rhythm (O76)
>          labor and delivery complicated by meconium in amniotic fluid (O77.Ø)
**CC Excl:** PDX collection 989

✓ Additional Character Req   ✓x7th Placeholder Alert   Unacceptable PDx   Manifestation   H1 - H14 HAC   HCC CMS-HCC Condition   EXCLUDES 1 Not Coded Here   EXCLUDES 2 Not Included Here

ICD-10-CM 2018             867

**Chapter 15. Pregnancy, Childbirth and the Puerperium**

✓4ᵗʰ **O69   Labor and delivery complicated by umbilical cord complications**
AHA: 2016, 1Q, 5

One of the following 7th characters is to be assigned to each code under category O69. 7th character Ø is for single gestations and multiple gestations where the fetus is unspecified. 7th characters 1 through 9 are for cases of multiple gestations to identify the fetus for which the code applies. The appropriate code from category O30, Multiple gestation, must also be assigned when assigning a code from category O69 that has a 7th character of 1 through 9.

| Ø | not applicable or unspecified | 3 | fetus 3 |
|---|---|---|---|
| | | 4 | fetus 4 |
| 1 | fetus 1 | 5 | fetus 5 |
| 2 | fetus 2 | 9 | other fetus |

✓x7ᵗʰ **O69.Ø   Labor and delivery complicated by prolapse of cord** Ⓜ♀
DEF: Abnormal presentation of fetus; marked by protruding umbilical cord during labor; can cause fetal death.

✓x7ᵗʰ **O69.1   Labor and delivery complicated by cord around neck, with compression** Ⓜ♀
EXCLUDES 1   *labor and delivery complicated by cord around neck, without compression (O69.81)*

✓x7ᵗʰ **O69.2   Labor and delivery complicated by other cord entanglement, with compression** Ⓜ♀
Labor and delivery complicated by compression of cord NOS
Labor and delivery complicated by entanglement of cords of twins in monoamniotic sac
Labor and delivery complicated by knot in cord
EXCLUDES 1   *labor and delivery complicated by other cord entanglement, without compression (O69.82)*

✓x7ᵗʰ **O69.3   Labor and delivery complicated by short cord** Ⓜ♀

✓x7ᵗʰ **O69.4   Labor and delivery complicated by vasa previa** Ⓜ♀
Labor and delivery complicated by hemorrhage from vasa previa

✓x7ᵗʰ **O69.5   Labor and delivery complicated by vascular lesion of cord** Ⓜ♀
Labor and delivery complicated by cord bruising
Labor and delivery complicated by cord hematoma
Labor and delivery complicated by thrombosis of umbilical vessels

✓5ᵗʰ **O69.8   Labor and delivery complicated by other cord complications**

✓x7ᵗʰ **O69.81   Labor and delivery complicated by cord around neck, without compression** Ⓜ♀
AHA: 2016, 1Q, 5

✓x7ᵗʰ **O69.82   Labor and delivery complicated by other cord entanglement, without compression** Ⓜ♀

✓x7ᵗʰ **O69.89   Labor and delivery complicated by other cord complications** Ⓜ♀

✓x7ᵗʰ **O69.9   Labor and delivery complicated by cord complication, unspecified** Ⓜ♀

✓4ᵗʰ **O7Ø   Perineal laceration during delivery**
INCLUDES   episiotomy extended by laceration
EXCLUDES 1   *obstetric high vaginal laceration alone (O71.4)*
AHA: 2016, 2Q, 34; 2016, 1Q, 3-4, 5

**O7Ø.Ø   First degree perineal laceration during delivery** Ⓜ♀
Perineal laceration, rupture or tear involving fourchette during delivery
Perineal laceration, rupture or tear involving labia during delivery
Perineal laceration, rupture or tear involving skin during delivery
Perineal laceration, rupture or tear involving vagina during delivery
Perineal laceration, rupture or tear involving vulva during delivery
Slight perineal laceration, rupture or tear during delivery

**O7Ø.1   Second degree perineal laceration during delivery** Ⓜ♀
Perineal laceration, rupture or tear during delivery as in O70.0, also involving pelvic floor
Perineal laceration, rupture or tear during delivery as in O70.0, also involving perineal muscles
Perineal laceration, rupture or tear during delivery as in O70.0, also involving vaginal muscles
EXCLUDES 1   *perineal laceration involving anal sphincter (O70.2)*

✓5ᵗʰ **O7Ø.2   Third degree perineal laceration during delivery**
Perineal laceration, rupture or tear during delivery as in O70.1, also involving anal sphincter
Perineal laceration, rupture or tear during delivery as in O70.1, also involving rectovaginal septum
Perineal laceration, rupture or tear during delivery as in O70.1, also involving sphincter NOS
EXCLUDES 1   *anal sphincter tear during delivery without third degree perineal laceration (O70.4)*
     *perineal laceration involving anal or rectal mucosa (O70.3)*

CC Excl: For CC codes in subcategory O7Ø.2:
PDX collection 99Ø

**O7Ø.20   Third degree perineal laceration during delivery, unspecified** CC Ⓜ♀

**O7Ø.21   Third degree perineal laceration during delivery, IIIa** CC Ⓜ♀
Third degree perineal laceration during delivery with less than 50% of external anal sphincter (EAS) thickness torn

**O7Ø.22   Third degree perineal laceration during delivery, IIIb** CC Ⓜ♀
Third degree perineal laceration during delivery with more than 50% external anal sphincter (EAS) thickness torn

**O7Ø.23   Third degree perineal laceration during delivery, IIIc** CC Ⓜ♀
Third degree perineal laceration during delivery with both external anal sphincter (EAS) and internal anal sphincter (IAS) torn

**O7Ø.3   Fourth degree perineal laceration during delivery** CC Ⓜ♀
Perineal laceration, rupture or tear during delivery as in O70.2, also involving anal mucosa
Perineal laceration, rupture or tear during delivery as in O70.2, also involving rectal mucosa
CC Excl: PDX collection 991

**O7Ø.4   Anal sphincter tear complicating delivery, not associated with third degree laceration** CC Ⓜ♀
EXCLUDES 1   *anal sphincter tear with third degree perineal laceration (O70.2)*
CC Excl: PDX collection 992

**O7Ø.9   Perineal laceration during delivery, unspecified** Ⓜ♀

✓4ᵗʰ **O71   Other obstetric trauma**
Obstetric damage from instruments

✓5ᵗʰ **O71.Ø   Rupture of uterus (spontaneous) before onset of labor**
EXCLUDES 1   *disruption of (current) cesarean delivery wound (O90.0)*
     *laceration of uterus, NEC (O71.81)*

**O71.ØØ   Rupture of uterus before onset of labor, unspecified trimester** Ⓜ♀

**O71.Ø2   Rupture of uterus before onset of labor, second trimester** MCC Ⓜ♀
CC Excl: PDX collection 993

**O71.Ø3   Rupture of uterus before onset of labor, third trimester** MCC Ⓜ♀
CC Excl: PDX collection 993

**O71.1   Rupture of uterus during labor** MCC Ⓜ♀
Rupture of uterus not stated as occurring before onset of labor
EXCLUDES 1   *disruption of cesarean delivery wound (O90.0)*
     *laceration of uterus, NEC (O71.81)*
CC Excl: PDX collection 993

**O71.2   Postpartum inversion of uterus** CC Ⓜ♀
CC Excl: PDX collection 994

**O71.3   Obstetric laceration of cervix** CC Ⓜ♀
Annular detachment of cervix
CC Excl: PDX collection 995

**O71.4   Obstetric high vaginal laceration alone** CC Ⓜ♀
Laceration of vaginal wall without perineal laceration
EXCLUDES 1   *obstetric high vaginal laceration with perineal laceration (O70.-)*
AHA: 2016, 1Q, 5
CC Excl: PDX collection 996

**O71.5   Other obstetric injury to pelvic organs** CC Ⓜ♀
Obstetric injury to bladder
Obstetric injury to urethra
EXCLUDES 2   *obstetric periurethral trauma (O71.82)*
AHA: 2014, 4Q, 18
CC Excl: PDX collection 993

Ⓝ Newborn: 0   Ⓟ Pediatric: 0-17   Ⓜ Maternity: 12-55   Ⓐ Adult: 15-124   MCC Major CC Condition   PDx MCC PDx acts as own MCC   CC CC Condition   PDx CC PDx acts as own CC

**868**      ICD-10-CM 2018

**O71.6 Obstetric damage to pelvic joints and ligaments** `cc` `M♀`
Obstetric avulsion of inner symphyseal cartilage
Obstetric damage to coccyx
Obstetric traumatic separation of symphysis (pubis)
**CC Excl:** PDX collection 997

**O71.7 Obstetric hematoma of pelvis** `cc` `M♀`
Obstetric hematoma of perineum
Obstetric hematoma of vagina
Obstetric hematoma of vulva
**CC Excl:** PDX collection 998

✓5ᵗʰ **O71.8 Other specified obstetric trauma**

    **O71.81 Laceration of uterus, not elsewhere classified** `M♀`

    **O71.82 Other specified trauma to perineum and vulva** `M♀`
      Obstetric periurethral trauma
      **AHA:** 2016, 1Q, 4; 2014, 4Q, 18

    **O71.89 Other specified obstetric trauma** `M♀`

**O71.9 Obstetric trauma, unspecified** `M♀`

✓4ᵗʰ **O72 Postpartum hemorrhage**
**INCLUDES** hemorrhage after delivery of fetus or infant

**O72.0 Third-stage hemorrhage** `cc` `M♀`
Hemorrhage associated with retained, trapped or adherent placenta
Retained placenta NOS
Code also type of adherent placenta (O43.2-)
**CC Excl:** PDX collection 999

**O72.1 Other immediate postpartum hemorrhage** `cc` `M♀`
Hemorrhage following delivery of placenta
Postpartum hemorrhage (atonic) NOS
Uterine atony with hemorrhage
**EXCLUDES 1** uterine atony NOS (O62.2)
uterine atony without hemorrhage (O62.2)
postpartum atony of uterus without hemorrhage (O75.89)
**AHA:** 2016, 1Q, 4
**CC Excl:** PDX collection 1000

**O72.2 Delayed and secondary postpartum hemorrhage** `cc` `M♀`
Hemorrhage associated with retained portions of placenta or membranes after the first 24 hours following delivery of placenta
Retained products of conception NOS, following delivery
**CC Excl:** PDX collection 1001

**O72.3 Postpartum coagulation defects** `M♀`
Postpartum afibrinogenemia
Postpartum fibrinolysis

✓4ᵗʰ **O73 Retained placenta and membranes, without hemorrhage**
**EXCLUDES 1** placenta accreta (O43.21-)
placenta increta (O43.22-)
placenta percreta (O43.23-)
**DEF:** Postpartum condition resulting from failure to expel placental membrane tissues due to failed contractions of uterine wall.

**O73.0 Retained placenta without hemorrhage** `M♀`
Adherent placenta, without hemorrhage
Trapped placenta without hemorrhage

**O73.1 Retained portions of placenta and membranes, without hemorrhage** `M♀`
Retained products of conception following delivery, without hemorrhage

✓4ᵗʰ **O74 Complications of anesthesia during labor and delivery**
**INCLUDES** maternal complications arising from the administration of a general, regional or local anesthetic, analgesic or other sedation during labor and delivery
Use additional code, if applicable, to identify specific complication

**O74.0 Aspiration pneumonitis due to anesthesia during labor and delivery** `M♀`
Inhalation of stomach contents or secretions NOS due to anesthesia during labor and delivery
Mendelson's syndrome due to anesthesia during labor and delivery

**O74.1 Other pulmonary complications of anesthesia during labor and delivery** `M♀`

**O74.2 Cardiac complications of anesthesia during labor and delivery** `M♀`

**O74.3 Central nervous system complications of anesthesia during labor and delivery** `M♀`

**O74.4 Toxic reaction to local anesthesia during labor and delivery** `M♀`

**O74.5 Spinal and epidural anesthesia-induced headache during labor and delivery** `M♀`

**O74.6 Other complications of spinal and epidural anesthesia during labor and delivery** `M♀`

**O74.7 Failed or difficult intubation for anesthesia during labor and delivery** `M♀`

**O74.8 Other complications of anesthesia during labor and delivery** `M♀`

**O74.9 Complication of anesthesia during labor and delivery, unspecified** `M♀`

✓4ᵗʰ **O75 Other complications of labor and delivery, not elsewhere classified**
**EXCLUDES 2** puerperal (postpartum) infection (O86.-)
puerperal (postpartum) sepsis (O85)

**O75.0 Maternal distress during labor and delivery** `M♀`

**O75.1 Shock during or following labor and delivery** `MCC` `M♀`
Obstetric shock following labor and delivery
**CC Excl:** PDX collection 1002

**O75.2 Pyrexia during labor, not elsewhere classified** `cc` `M♀`
**CC Excl:** PDX collection 1003

**O75.3 Other infection during labor** `MCC` `M♀`
Sepsis during labor
Use additional code (B95-B97), to identify infectious agent
**CC Excl:** PDX collection 1004

**O75.4 Other complications of obstetric surgery and procedures** `M♀`
Cardiac arrest following obstetric surgery or procedures
Cardiac failure following obstetric surgery or procedures
Cerebral anoxia following obstetric surgery or procedures
Pulmonary edema following obstetric surgery or procedures
Use additional code to identify specific complication
**EXCLUDES 2** complications of anesthesia during labor and delivery (O74.-)
disruption of obstetrical (surgical) wound (O90.0-O90.1)
hematoma of obstetrical (surgical) wound (O90.2)
infection of obstetrical (surgical) wound (O86.0)

**O75.5 Delayed delivery after artificial rupture of membranes** `M♀`

✓5ᵗʰ **O75.8 Other specified complications of labor and delivery**

    **O75.81 Maternal exhaustion complicating labor and delivery** `M♀`

    **O75.82 Onset (spontaneous) of labor after 37 completed weeks of gestation but before 39 completed weeks gestation, with delivery by (planned) cesarean section** `M♀`
      Delivery by (planned) cesarean section occurring after 37 completed weeks of gestation but before 39 completed weeks gestation due to (spontaneous) onset of labor
      Code first to specify reason for planned cesarean section such as:
        cephalopelvic disproportion (normally formed fetus) (O33.9)
        previous cesarean delivery (O34.21)

    **O75.89 Other specified complications of labor and delivery** `M♀`

**O75.9 Complication of labor and delivery, unspecified** `M♀`

**O76 Abnormality in fetal heart rate and rhythm complicating labor and delivery** `M♀`
Depressed fetal heart rate tones complicating labor and delivery
Fetal bradycardia complicating labor and delivery
Fetal heart rate abnormal variability complicating labor and delivery
Fetal heart rate decelerations complicating labor and delivery
Fetal heart rate irregularity complicating labor and delivery
Fetal tachycardia complicating labor and delivery
Non-reassuring fetal heart rate or rhythm complicating labor and delivery
**EXCLUDES 1** fetal stress NOS (O77.9)
labor and delivery complicated by electrocardiographic evidence of fetal stress (O77.8)
labor and delivery complicated by ultrasonic evidence of fetal stress (O77.8)
**EXCLUDES 2** fetal metabolic acidemia (O68)
other fetal stress (O77.0-O77.1)
**AHA:** 2013, 4Q, 118

✓4ᵗʰ **O77 Other fetal stress complicating labor and delivery**

**O77.0 Labor and delivery complicated by meconium in amniotic fluid** `M♀`
**AHA:** 2013, 4Q, 117-118

**O77.1 Fetal stress in labor or delivery due to drug administration** `M♀`

---

✓ Additional Character Req   ✓ₓ7ᵗʰ Placeholder Alert   Unacceptable PDx   Manifestation   H1 - H14 HAC   HCC CMS-HCC Condition   EXCLUDES 1 Not Coded Here   EXCLUDES 2 Not Included Here

ICD-10-CM 2018                                                        869

O71.6–O77.1

**O77.8 Labor and delivery complicated by other evidence of fetal stress**   M♀

Labor and delivery complicated by electrocardiographic evidence of fetal stress

Labor and delivery complicated by ultrasonic evidence of fetal stress

EXCLUDES 1   *abnormality in fetal heart rate or rhythm (O76)*
*abnormality of fetal acid-base balance (O68)*
*fetal metabolic acidemia (O68)*

**O77.9 Labor and delivery complicated by fetal stress, unspecified**   M♀

EXCLUDES 1   *abnormality in fetal heart rate or rhythm (O76)*
*abnormality of fetal acid-base balance (O68)*
*fetal metabolic acidemia (O68)*

## Encounter for delivery (O80-O82)

**O80 Encounter for full-term uncomplicated delivery**   M♀

NOTE   Delivery requiring minimal or no assistance, with or without episiotomy, without fetal manipulation [e.g., rotation version] or instrumentation [forceps] of a spontaneous, cephalic, vaginal, full-term, single, live-born infant. This code is for use as a single diagnosis code and is not to be used with any other code from chapter 15.

Use additional code to indicate outcome of delivery (Z37.0)

AHA: 2016, 4Q, 150; 2014, 2Q, 9

**O82 Encounter for cesarean delivery without indication**   M♀

Use additional code to indicate outcome of delivery (Z37.0)

## Complications predominantly related to the puerperium (O85-O92)

EXCLUDES 2   *mental and behavioral disorders associated with the puerperium (F53)*
*obstetrical tetanus (A34)*
*puerperal osteomalacia (M83.0)*

**O85 Puerperal sepsis**   MCC M♀

Postpartum sepsis
Puerperal peritonitis
Puerperal pyemia

Use additional code (B95-B97), to identify infectious agent
Use additional code (R65.2-) to identify severe sepsis, if applicable

EXCLUDES 1   *fever of unknown origin following delivery (O86.4)*
*genital tract infection following delivery (O86.1-)*
*obstetric pyemic and septic embolism (O88.3-)*
*puerperal septic thrombophlebitis (O86.81)*
*urinary tract infection following delivery (O86.2-)*

EXCLUDES 2   *sepsis during labor (O75.3)*
CC Excl: PDX collection 1005

**✓4ᵗʰ O86 Other puerperal infections**

Use additional code (B95-B97), to identify infectious agent
EXCLUDES 2   *infection during labor (O75.3)*
*obstetrical tetanus (A34)*

CC Excl: For CC codes in category O86, unless otherwise noted: PDX collection 968

**O86.0 Infection of obstetric surgical wound**   M♀

Infected cesarean delivery wound following delivery
Infected perineal repair following delivery

**✓5ᵗʰ O86.1 Other infection of genital tract following delivery**

**O86.11 Cervicitis following delivery**   CC M♀

**O86.12 Endometritis following delivery**   CC M♀
CC Excl: PDX collection 1005

**O86.13 Vaginitis following delivery**   CC M♀

**O86.19 Other infection of genital tract following delivery**   CC M♀

**✓5ᵗʰ O86.2 Urinary tract infection following delivery**

**O86.20 Urinary tract infection following delivery, unspecified**   CC M♀
Puerperal urinary tract infection NOS

**O86.21 Infection of kidney following delivery**   CC M♀

**O86.22 Infection of bladder following delivery**   CC M♀
Infection of urethra following delivery

**O86.29 Other urinary tract infection following delivery**   CC M♀

**O86.4 Pyrexia of unknown origin following delivery**   CC M♀

Puerperal infection NOS following delivery
Puerperal pyrexia NOS following delivery

EXCLUDES 2   *pyrexia during labor (O75.2)*

DEF: Fever of unknown origin experienced by the mother after childbirth.
CC Excl: PDX collection 1006

**✓5ᵗʰ O86.8 Other specified puerperal infections**

**O86.81 Puerperal septic thrombophlebitis**   MCC M♀
CC Excl: PDX collection 1005

**O86.89 Other specified puerperal infections**   MCC M♀
CC Excl: PDX collection 1005

**✓4ᵗʰ O87 Venous complications and hemorrhoids in the puerperium**

INCLUDES   venous complications in labor, delivery and the puerperium
EXCLUDES 2   *obstetric embolism (O88.-)*
*puerperal septic thrombophlebitis (O86.81)*
*venous complications in pregnancy (O22.-)*

CC Excl: For CC/MCC codes in category O87: PDX collection 967

**O87.0 Superficial thrombophlebitis in the puerperium**   CC M♀
Puerperal phlebitis NOS
Puerperal thrombosis NOS

**O87.1 Deep phlebothrombosis in the puerperium**   MCC M♀
Deep vein thrombosis, postpartum
Pelvic thrombophlebitis, postpartum

Use additional code to identify the deep vein thrombosis (I82.4-, I82.5-, I82.62-. I82.72-)
Use additional code, if applicable, for associated long-term (current) use of anticoagulants (Z79.01)

**O87.2 Hemorrhoids in the puerperium**   CC M♀

**O87.3 Cerebral venous thrombosis in the puerperium**   CC M♀
Cerebrovenous sinus thrombosis in the puerperium

**O87.4 Varicose veins of lower extremity in the puerperium**   M♀

**O87.8 Other venous complications in the puerperium**   CC M♀
Genital varices in the puerperium

**O87.9 Venous complication in the puerperium, unspecified**   M♀
Puerperal phlebopathy NOS

**✓4ᵗʰ O88 Obstetric embolism**

EXCLUDES 1   *embolism complicating abortion NOS (O03.2)*
*embolism complicating ectopic or molar pregnancy (O08.2)*
*embolism complicating failed attempted abortion (O07.2)*
*embolism complicating induced abortion (O04.7)*
*embolism complicating spontaneous abortion (O03.2, O03.7)*

CC Excl: For CC/MCC codes in category O88: PDX collection 1007

**✓5ᵗʰ O88.0 Obstetric air embolism**
DEF: Sudden blocking of pulmonary artery or right ventricle with air or nitrogen bubbles.

**✓6ᵗʰ O88.01 Obstetric air embolism in pregnancy**

**O88.011 Air embolism in pregnancy, first trimester**   MCC M♀

**O88.012 Air embolism in pregnancy, second trimester**   MCC M♀

**O88.013 Air embolism in pregnancy, third trimester**   MCC M♀

**O88.019 Air embolism in pregnancy, unspecified trimester**   M♀

**O88.02 Air embolism in childbirth**   MCC M♀

**O88.03 Air embolism in the puerperium**   MCC M♀

**✓5ᵗʰ O88.1 Amniotic fluid embolism**
Anaphylactoid syndrome in pregnancy

**✓6ᵗʰ O88.11 Amniotic fluid embolism in pregnancy**

**O88.111 Amniotic fluid embolism in pregnancy, first trimester**   MCC M♀

**O88.112 Amniotic fluid embolism in pregnancy, second trimester**   MCC M♀

**O88.113 Amniotic fluid embolism in pregnancy, third trimester**   MCC M♀

**O88.119 Amniotic fluid embolism in pregnancy, unspecified trimester**   M♀

**O88.12 Amniotic fluid embolism in childbirth**   MCC M♀

**O88.13 Amniotic fluid embolism in the puerperium**   MCC M♀

**✓5ᵗʰ O88.2 Obstetric thromboembolism**

**✓6ᵗʰ O88.21 Thromboembolism in pregnancy**
Obstetric (pulmonary) embolism NOS

**O88.211 Thromboembolism in pregnancy, first trimester**   MCC M♀

**O88.212 Thromboembolism in pregnancy, second trimester**   MCC M♀

**O88.213 Thromboembolism in pregnancy, third trimester**   MCC M♀

**O88.219 Thromboembolism in pregnancy, unspecified trimester**   M♀

**O88.22 Thromboembolism in childbirth**   MCC M♀

N Newborn: 0   P Pediatric: 0-17   M Maternity: 12-55   A Adult: 15-124   MCC Major CC Condition   PDxMCC PDx acts as own MCC   CC CC Condition   PDxCC PDx acts as own CC

870      ICD-10-CM 2018

**O88.23** **Thromboembolism in the puerperium** `MCC` `M♀`
Puerperal (pulmonary) embolism NOS

√5ᵗʰ **O88.3** **Obstetric pyemic and septic embolism**

√6ᵗʰ **O88.31** **Pyemic and septic embolism in pregnancy**

**O88.311** **Pyemic and septic embolism in** `MCC` `M♀`
**pregnancy, first trimester**

**O88.312** **Pyemic and septic embolism in** `MCC` `M♀`
**pregnancy, second trimester**

**O88.313** **Pyemic and septic embolism in** `MCC` `M♀`
**pregnancy, third trimester**

**O88.319** **Pyemic and septic embolism in** `CC` `M♀`
**pregnancy, unspecified trimester**

**O88.32** **Pyemic and septic embolism in childbirth** `MCC` `M♀`

**O88.33** **Pyemic and septic embolism in the** `MCC` `M♀`
**puerperium**

√5ᵗʰ **O88.8** **Other obstetric embolism**
Obstetric fat embolism

√6ᵗʰ **O88.81** **Other embolism in pregnancy**

**O88.811** **Other embolism in pregnancy,** `MCC` `M♀`
**first trimester**

**O88.812** **Other embolism in pregnancy,** `MCC` `M♀`
**second trimester**

**O88.813** **Other embolism in pregnancy,** `MCC` `M♀`
**third trimester**

**O88.819** **Other embolism in pregnancy,** `M♀`
**unspecified trimester**

**O88.82** **Other embolism in childbirth** `MCC` `M♀`

**O88.83** **Other embolism in the puerperium** `MCC` `M♀`

√4ᵗʰ **O89** **Complications of anesthesia during the puerperium**
`INCLUDES` maternal complications arising from the administration of a
general, regional or local anesthetic, analgesic or other
sedation during the puerperium
Use additional code, if applicable, to identify specific complication

√5ᵗʰ **O89.0** **Pulmonary complications of anesthesia during the**
**puerperium**

**O89.01** **Aspiration pneumonitis due to anesthesia** `M♀`
**during the puerperium**
Inhalation of stomach contents or secretions NOS due
to anesthesia during the puerperium
Mendelson's syndrome due to anesthesia during the
puerperium

**O89.09** **Other pulmonary complications of anesthesia** `M♀`
**during the puerperium**

**O89.1** **Cardiac complications of anesthesia during the** `M♀`
**puerperium**

**O89.2** **Central nervous system complications of anesthesia** `M♀`
**during the puerperium**

**O89.3** **Toxic reaction to local anesthesia during the puerperium** `M♀`

**O89.4** **Spinal and epidural anesthesia-induced headache** `M♀`
**during the puerperium**

**O89.5** **Other complications of spinal and epidural anesthesia** `M♀`
**during the puerperium**

**O89.6** **Failed or difficult intubation for anesthesia during the** `M♀`
**puerperium**

**O89.8** **Other complications of anesthesia during the puerperium** `M♀`

**O89.9** **Complication of anesthesia during the puerperium,** `M♀`
**unspecified**

√4ᵗʰ **O90** **Complications of the puerperium, not elsewhere classified**

**O90.0** **Disruption of cesarean delivery wound** `M♀`
Dehiscence of cesarean delivery wound
`EXCLUDES 1` rupture of uterus (spontaneous) before onset of labor
(O71.0-)
rupture of uterus during labor (O71.1)

**O90.1** **Disruption of perineal obstetric wound** `M♀`
Disruption of wound of episiotomy
Disruption of wound of perineal laceration
Secondary perineal tear

**O90.2** **Hematoma of obstetric wound** `M♀`

**O90.3** **Peripartum cardiomyopathy** `MCC` `M♀`
Conditions in I42- arising during pregnancy and the puerperium
`EXCLUDES 1` pre-existing heart disease complicating pregnancy and
the puerperium (O99.4-)
**DEF:** Any structural or functional abnormality of the ventricular
myocardium, noninflammatory disease of obscure or unknown
etiology with onset during the postpartum period.
**CC Excl:** PDX collection 1008

**O90.4** **Postpartum acute kidney failure** `MCC` `M♀`
Hepatorenal syndrome following labor and delivery
**CC Excl:** PDX collection 1009

**O90.5** **Postpartum thyroiditis** `M♀`

**O90.6** **Postpartum mood disturbance** `M♀`
Postpartum blues
Postpartum dysphoria
Postpartum sadness
`EXCLUDES 1` postpartum depression (F53)
puerperal psychosis (F53)

√5ᵗʰ **O90.8** **Other complications of the puerperium, not elsewhere**
**classified**

**O90.81** **Anemia of the puerperium** `M♀`
Postpartum anemia NOS
`EXCLUDES 1` pre-existing anemia complicating the
puerperium (O99.03)

**O90.89** **Other complications of the puerperium, not** `M♀`
**elsewhere classified**
Placental polyp

**O90.9** **Complication of the puerperium, unspecified** `M♀`

√4ᵗʰ **O91** **Infections of breast associated with pregnancy, the puerperium**
**and lactation**
Use additional code to identify infection

√5ᵗʰ **O91.0** **Infection of nipple associated with pregnancy, the**
**puerperium and lactation**

√6ᵗʰ **O91.01** **Infection of nipple associated with pregnancy**
Gestational abscess of nipple

**O91.011** **Infection of nipple associated with** `M♀`
**pregnancy, first trimester**

**O91.012** **Infection of nipple associated with** `M♀`
**pregnancy, second trimester**

**O91.013** **Infection of nipple associated with** `M♀`
**pregnancy, third trimester**

**O91.019** **Infection of nipple associated with** `M♀`
**pregnancy, unspecified trimester**

**O91.02** **Infection of nipple associated with the** `M♀`
**puerperium**
Puerperal abscess of nipple

**O91.03** **Infection of nipple associated with lactation** `M♀`
Abscess of nipple associated with lactation

√5ᵗʰ **O91.1** **Abscess of breast associated with pregnancy, the puerperium**
**and lactation**

√6ᵗʰ **O91.11** **Abscess of breast associated with pregnancy**
Gestational mammary abscess
Gestational purulent mastitis
Gestational subareolar abscess

**O91.111** **Abscess of breast associated with** `M♀`
**pregnancy, first trimester**

**O91.112** **Abscess of breast associated with** `M♀`
**pregnancy, second trimester**

**O91.113** **Abscess of breast associated with** `M♀`
**pregnancy, third trimester**

**O91.119** **Abscess of breast associated with** `M♀`
**pregnancy, unspecified trimester**

**O91.12** **Abscess of breast associated with the** `M♀`
**puerperium**
Puerperal mammary abscess
Puerperal purulent mastitis
Puerperal subareolar abscess

**O91.13** **Abscess of breast associated with lactation** `M♀`
Mammary abscess associated with lactation
Purulent mastitis associated with lactation
Subareolar abscess associated with lactation

√5ᵗʰ **O91.2** **Nonpurulent mastitis associated with pregnancy, the**
**puerperium and lactation**

√6ᵗʰ **O91.21** **Nonpurulent mastitis associated with pregnancy**
Gestational interstitial mastitis
Gestational lymphangitis of breast
Gestational mastitis NOS
Gestational parenchymatous mastitis

**O91.211** **Nonpurulent mastitis associated with** `M♀`
**pregnancy, first trimester**

**O91.212** **Nonpurulent mastitis associated with** `M♀`
**pregnancy, second trimester**

**O91.213** **Nonpurulent mastitis associated with** `M♀`
**pregnancy, third trimester**

**O91.219** **Nonpurulent mastitis associated with** `M♀`
**pregnancy, unspecified trimester**

O91.22 **Nonpurulent mastitis associated with the puerperium** Ⓜ♀
    Puerperal interstitial mastitis
    Puerperal lymphangitis of breast
    Puerperal mastitis NOS
    Puerperal parenchymatous mastitis

O91.23 **Nonpurulent mastitis associated with lactation** Ⓜ♀
    Interstitial mastitis associated with lactation
    Lymphangitis of breast associated with lactation
    Mastitis NOS associated with lactation
    Parenchymatous mastitis associated with lactation

✓4ᵗʰ **O92 Other disorders of breast and disorders of lactation associated with pregnancy and the puerperium**

  ✓5ᵗʰ **O92.0 Retracted nipple associated with pregnancy, the puerperium, and lactation**

    ✓6ᵗʰ **O92.01 Retracted nipple associated with pregnancy**

      O92.011 **Retracted nipple associated with pregnancy, first trimester** Ⓜ♀

      O92.012 **Retracted nipple associated with pregnancy, second trimester** Ⓜ♀

      O92.013 **Retracted nipple associated with pregnancy, third trimester** Ⓜ♀

      O92.019 **Retracted nipple associated with pregnancy, unspecified trimester** Ⓜ♀

    O92.02 **Retracted nipple associated with the puerperium** Ⓜ♀

    O92.03 **Retracted nipple associated with lactation** Ⓜ♀

  ✓5ᵗʰ **O92.1 Cracked nipple associated with pregnancy, the puerperium, and lactation**
    Fissure of nipple, gestational or puerperal

    ✓6ᵗʰ **O92.11 Cracked nipple associated with pregnancy**

      O92.111 **Cracked nipple associated with pregnancy, first trimester** Ⓜ♀

      O92.112 **Cracked nipple associated with pregnancy, second trimester** Ⓜ♀

      O92.113 **Cracked nipple associated with pregnancy, third trimester** Ⓜ♀

      O92.119 **Cracked nipple associated with pregnancy, unspecified trimester** Ⓜ♀

    O92.12 **Cracked nipple associated with the puerperium** Ⓜ♀

    O92.13 **Cracked nipple associated with lactation** Ⓜ♀

  ✓5ᵗʰ **O92.2 Other and unspecified disorders of breast associated with pregnancy and the puerperium**

    O92.20 **Unspecified disorder of breast associated with pregnancy and the puerperium** Ⓜ♀

    O92.29 **Other disorders of breast associated with pregnancy and the puerperium** Ⓜ♀

  **O92.3 Agalactia** Ⓜ♀
    Primary agalactia
    EXCLUDES 1   *elective agalactia (O92.5)*
              *secondary agalactia (O92.5)*
              *therapeutic agalactia (O92.5)*
    **DEF:** Absence of milk secretion in a female after delivery.

  **O92.4 Hypogalactia** Ⓜ♀

  **O92.5 Suppressed lactation** Ⓜ♀
    Elective agalactia
    Secondary agalactia
    Therapeutic agalactia
    EXCLUDES 1   *primary agalactia (O92.3)*

  **O92.6 Galactorrhea** Ⓜ♀
    **DEF:** Excessive or persistent milk secretion by breast; may occur in absence of nursing.

  ✓5ᵗʰ **O92.7 Other and unspecified disorders of lactation**

    O92.70 **Unspecified disorders of lactation** Ⓜ♀

    O92.79 **Other disorders of lactation** Ⓜ♀
      Puerperal galactocele

## Other obstetric conditions, not elsewhere classified (O94-O9A)

**O94 Sequelae of complication of pregnancy, childbirth, and the puerperium** Ⓜ♀
    NOTE   This category is to be used to indicate conditions in O00-O77.-, O85-O94 and O98-O9A.- as the cause of late effects. The sequelae include conditions specified as such, or as late effects, which may occur at any time after the puerperium.
    Code first condition resulting from (sequela) of complication of pregnancy, childbirth, and the puerperium

✓4ᵗʰ **O98 Maternal infectious and parasitic diseases classifiable elsewhere but complicating pregnancy, childbirth and the puerperium**
    INCLUDES   the listed conditions when complicating the pregnant state, when aggravated by the pregnancy, or as a reason for obstetric care
    Use additional code (Chapter 1), to identify specific infectious or parasitic disease
    EXCLUDES 2   *herpes gestationis (O26.4-)*
              *infectious carrier state (O99.82-, O99.83-)*
              *obstetrical tetanus (A34)*
              *puerperal infection (O86.-)*
              *puerperal sepsis (O85)*
              *when the reason for maternal care is that the disease is known or suspected to have affected the fetus (O35-O36)*

  ✓5ᵗʰ **O98.0 Tuberculosis complicating pregnancy, childbirth and the puerperium**
    Conditions in A15-A19

    **CC Excl: For CC codes in subcategory O98.0:**
    PDX collection 1011

    ✓6ᵗʰ **O98.01 Tuberculosis complicating pregnancy**

      O98.011 **Tuberculosis complicating pregnancy, first trimester** cc Ⓜ♀

      O98.012 **Tuberculosis complicating pregnancy, second trimester** cc Ⓜ♀

      O98.013 **Tuberculosis complicating pregnancy, third trimester** cc Ⓜ♀

      O98.019 **Tuberculosis complicating pregnancy, unspecified trimester** Ⓜ♀

    O98.02 **Tuberculosis complicating childbirth** cc Ⓜ♀

    O98.03 **Tuberculosis complicating the puerperium** cc Ⓜ♀

  ✓5ᵗʰ **O98.1 Syphilis complicating pregnancy, childbirth and the puerperium**
    Conditions in A50-A53

    **CC Excl: For CC codes in subcategory O98.1:**
    PDX collection 1012

    ✓6ᵗʰ **O98.11 Syphilis complicating pregnancy**

      O98.111 **Syphilis complicating pregnancy, first trimester** cc Ⓜ♀

      O98.112 **Syphilis complicating pregnancy, second trimester** cc Ⓜ♀

      O98.113 **Syphilis complicating pregnancy, third trimester** cc Ⓜ♀

      O98.119 **Syphilis complicating pregnancy, unspecified trimester** Ⓜ♀

    O98.12 **Syphilis complicating childbirth** cc Ⓜ♀

    O98.13 **Syphilis complicating the puerperium** cc Ⓜ♀

  ✓5ᵗʰ **O98.2 Gonorrhea complicating pregnancy, childbirth and the puerperium**
    Conditions in A54-

    **CC Excl: For CC codes in subcategory O98.2:**
    PDX collection 1012

    ✓6ᵗʰ **O98.21 Gonorrhea complicating pregnancy**

      O98.211 **Gonorrhea complicating pregnancy, first trimester** cc Ⓜ♀

      O98.212 **Gonorrhea complicating pregnancy, second trimester** cc Ⓜ♀

      O98.213 **Gonorrhea complicating pregnancy, third trimester** cc Ⓜ♀

      O98.219 **Gonorrhea complicating pregnancy, unspecified trimester** Ⓜ♀

    O98.22 **Gonorrhea complicating childbirth** cc Ⓜ♀

    O98.23 **Gonorrhea complicating the puerperium** cc Ⓜ♀

  ✓5ᵗʰ **O98.3 Other infections with a predominantly sexual mode of transmission complicating pregnancy, childbirth and the puerperium**
    Conditions in A55-A64

    **CC Excl: For CC codes in subcategory O98.3:**
    PDX collection 1012

    ✓6ᵗʰ **O98.31 Other infections with a predominantly sexual mode of transmission complicating pregnancy**

      O98.311 **Other infections with a predominantly sexual mode of transmission complicating pregnancy, first trimester** cc Ⓜ♀

Ⓝ Newborn: 0   Ⓟ Pediatric: 0-17   Ⓜ Maternity: 12-55   Ⓐ Adult: 15-124   MCC Major CC Condition   PDxMCC PDx acts as own MCC   cc CC Condition   PDxCC PDx acts as own CC

872        ICD-10-CM 2018

**O98.312** Other infections with a predominantly sexual mode of transmission complicating pregnancy, **second trimester** `CC` `M` ♀

**O98.313** Other infections with a predominantly sexual mode of transmission complicating pregnancy, **third trimester** `CC` `M` ♀

**O98.319** Other infections with a predominantly sexual mode of transmission complicating pregnancy, **unspecified trimester** `M` ♀

**O98.32** Other infections with a predominantly sexual mode of transmission complicating **childbirth** `CC` `M` ♀

**O98.33** Other infections with a predominantly sexual mode of transmission complicating the **puerperium** `CC` `M` ♀

✓5th **O98.4** **Viral hepatitis complicating pregnancy, childbirth and the puerperium**
Conditions in B15-B19

> **CC Excl: For CC codes in subcategory O98.4:**
> PDX collection 1013

✓6th **O98.41** **Viral hepatitis complicating pregnancy**

**O98.411** Viral hepatitis complicating pregnancy, **first trimester** `CC` `M` ♀

**O98.412** Viral hepatitis complicating pregnancy, **second trimester** `CC` `M` ♀

**O98.413** Viral hepatitis complicating pregnancy, **third trimester** `CC` `M` ♀

**O98.419** Viral hepatitis complicating pregnancy, **unspecified trimester** `M` ♀

**O98.42** Viral hepatitis complicating **childbirth** `CC` `M` ♀

**O98.43** Viral hepatitis complicating the **puerperium** `CC` `M` ♀

✓5th **O98.5** **Other viral diseases complicating pregnancy, childbirth and the puerperium**
Conditions in A80-B09, B25-B34, R87.81-, R87.82-
> `EXCLUDES 1` human immunodeficiency virus [HIV] disease complicating pregnancy, childbirth and the puerperium (O98.7-)

> **CC Excl: For CC codes in subcategory O98.5:**
> PDX collection 1013

✓6th **O98.51** **Other viral diseases complicating pregnancy**

**O98.511** Other viral diseases complicating pregnancy, **first trimester** `CC` `M` ♀

**O98.512** Other viral diseases complicating pregnancy, **second trimester** `CC` `M` ♀

**O98.513** Other viral diseases complicating pregnancy, **third trimester** `CC` `M` ♀

**O98.519** Other viral diseases complicating pregnancy, **unspecified trimester** `M` ♀

**O98.52** Other viral diseases complicating **childbirth** `CC` `M` ♀

**O98.53** Other viral diseases complicating the **puerperium** `CC` `M` ♀

✓5th **O98.6** **Protozoal diseases complicating pregnancy, childbirth and the puerperium**
Conditions in B50-B64

> **CC Excl: For CC codes in subcategory O98.6, unless otherwise noted:** PDX collection 1014

✓6th **O98.61** **Protozoal diseases complicating pregnancy**

**O98.611** Protozoal diseases complicating pregnancy, **first trimester** `CC` `M` ♀

**O98.612** Protozoal diseases complicating pregnancy, **second trimester** `CC` `M` ♀

**O98.613** Protozoal diseases complicating pregnancy, **third trimester** `CC` `M` ♀

**O98.619** Protozoal diseases complicating pregnancy, **unspecified trimester** `M` ♀

**O98.62** Protozoal diseases complicating **childbirth** `CC` `M` ♀
CC Excl: PDX collection 1015

**O98.63** Protozoal diseases complicating the **puerperium** `CC` `M` ♀
CC Excl: PDX collection 1015

✓5th **O98.7** **Human immunodeficiency virus [HIV] disease complicating pregnancy, childbirth and the puerperium**
Use additional code to identify the type of HIV disease:
acquired immune deficiency syndrome (AIDS) (B20)
asymptomatic HIV status (Z21)
HIV positive NOS (Z21)
symptomatic HIV disease (B20)

> **CC Excl: For CC codes in subcategory O98.7:**
> PDX collection 1013

✓6th **O98.71** **Human immunodeficiency virus [HIV] disease complicating pregnancy**

**O98.711** Human immunodeficiency virus [HIV] disease complicating pregnancy, **first trimester** `CC` `M` ♀

**O98.712** Human immunodeficiency virus [HIV] disease complicating pregnancy, **second trimester** `CC` `M` ♀

**O98.713** Human immunodeficiency virus [HIV] disease complicating pregnancy, **third trimester** `CC` `M` ♀

**O98.719** Human immunodeficiency virus [HIV] disease complicating pregnancy, **unspecified trimester** `M` ♀

**O98.72** Human immunodeficiency virus [HIV] disease complicating **childbirth** `CC` `M` ♀

**O98.73** Human immunodeficiency virus [HIV] disease complicating the **puerperium** `CC` `M` ♀

✓5th **O98.8** **Other maternal infectious and parasitic diseases complicating pregnancy, childbirth and the puerperium**

> **CC Excl: For CC codes in subcategory O98.8:**
> PDX collection 1013

✓6th **O98.81** **Other maternal infectious and parasitic diseases complicating pregnancy**

**O98.811** Other maternal infectious and parasitic diseases complicating pregnancy, **first trimester** `CC` `M` ♀

**O98.812** Other maternal infectious and parasitic diseases complicating pregnancy, **second trimester** `CC` `M` ♀

**O98.813** Other maternal infectious and parasitic diseases complicating pregnancy, **third trimester** `CC` `M` ♀

**O98.819** Other maternal infectious and parasitic diseases complicating pregnancy, **unspecified trimester** `M` ♀

**O98.82** Other maternal infectious and parasitic diseases complicating **childbirth** `CC` `M` ♀

**O98.83** Other maternal infectious and parasitic diseases complicating the **puerperium** `CC` `M` ♀

✓5th **O98.9** **Unspecified maternal infectious and parasitic disease complicating pregnancy, childbirth and the puerperium**

> **CC Excl: For CC codes in subcategory O98.9:**
> PDX collection 1013

✓6th **O98.91** **Unspecified maternal infectious and parasitic disease complicating pregnancy**

**O98.911** Unspecified maternal infectious and parasitic disease complicating pregnancy, **first trimester** `CC` `M` ♀

**O98.912** Unspecified maternal infectious and parasitic disease complicating pregnancy, **second trimester** `CC` `M` ♀

**O98.913** Unspecified maternal infectious and parasitic disease complicating pregnancy, **third trimester** `CC` `M` ♀

**O98.919** Unspecified maternal infectious and parasitic disease complicating pregnancy, **unspecified trimester** `M` ♀

**O98.92** Unspecified maternal infectious and parasitic disease complicating **childbirth** `CC` `M` ♀

**O98.93** Unspecified maternal infectious and parasitic disease complicating the **puerperium** `CC` `M` ♀

---

✓ Additional Character Req   ✓7th Placeholder Alert   Unacceptable PDx   Manifestation   `H1`-`H14` HAC   `HCC` CMS-HCC Condition   `EXCLUDES 1` Not Coded Here   `EXCLUDES 2` Not Included Here

**Chapter 15. Pregnancy, Childbirth and the Puerperium**

☑4ᵗʰ **O99** **Other maternal diseases classifiable elsewhere but complicating pregnancy, childbirth and the puerperium**

INCLUDES   conditions which complicate the pregnant state, are aggravated by the pregnancy or are a main reason for obstetric care

Use additional code to identify specific condition

EXCLUDES 2   *when the reason for maternal care is that the condition is known or suspected to have affected the fetus (O35-O36)*

☑5ᵗʰ **O99.0** **Anemia complicating pregnancy, childbirth and the puerperium**

Conditions in D50-D64

EXCLUDES 1   *anemia arising in the puerperium (O90.81)*
*postpartum anemia NOS (O90.81)*

☑6ᵗʰ **O99.01** **Anemia complicating pregnancy**
AHA: 2016, 1Q, 4

    **O99.011** **Anemia complicating pregnancy, first trimester**    Ⓜ♀

    **O99.012** **Anemia complicating pregnancy, second trimester**    Ⓜ♀

    **O99.013** **Anemia complicating pregnancy, third trimester**    Ⓜ♀

    **O99.019** **Anemia complicating pregnancy, unspecified trimester**    Ⓜ♀

   **O99.02** **Anemia complicating childbirth**    Ⓜ♀

   **O99.03** **Anemia complicating the puerperium**    Ⓜ♀

EXCLUDES 1   *postpartum anemia not pre-existing prior to delivery (O90.81)*

☑5ᵗʰ **O99.1** **Other diseases of the blood and blood-forming organs and certain disorders involving the immune mechanism complicating pregnancy, childbirth and the puerperium**

Conditions in D65-D89

EXCLUDES 1 ▶*hemorrhage with coagulation defects (O45.-, O46.0-, O67.0, O72.3)*◀

EXCLUDES 2 *hemorrhage with coagulation defects (O45.-, O46.0-, O67.0, O72.3)*

**CC Excl: For CC codes in subcategory O99.1, unless otherwise noted: PDX collection 1016**

☑6ᵗʰ **O99.11** **Other diseases of the blood and blood-forming organs and certain disorders involving the immune mechanism complicating pregnancy**

    **O99.111** **Other diseases of the blood and blood-forming organs and certain disorders involving the immune mechanism complicating pregnancy, first trimester**    CC Ⓜ♀

    **O99.112** **Other diseases of the blood and blood-forming organs and certain disorders involving the immune mechanism complicating pregnancy, second trimester**    CC Ⓜ♀

    **O99.113** **Other diseases of the blood and blood-forming organs and certain disorders involving the immune mechanism complicating pregnancy, third trimester**    CC Ⓜ♀

    **O99.119** **Other diseases of the blood and blood-forming organs and certain disorders involving the immune mechanism complicating pregnancy, unspecified trimester**    CC Ⓜ♀
**CC Excl: PDX collection 1017**

   **O99.12** **Other diseases of the blood and blood-forming organs and certain disorders involving the immune mechanism complicating childbirth**    CC Ⓜ♀

   **O99.13** **Other diseases of the blood and blood-forming organs and certain disorders involving the immune mechanism complicating the puerperium**    CC Ⓜ♀

☑5ᵗʰ **O99.2** **Endocrine, nutritional and metabolic diseases complicating pregnancy, childbirth, and the puerperium**

Conditions in E00-E88

EXCLUDES 2   *diabetes mellitus (O24.-)*
*malnutrition (O25.-)*
*postpartum thyroiditis (O90.5)*

☑6ᵗʰ **O99.21** **Obesity complicating pregnancy, childbirth, and the puerperium**

Use additional code to identify the type of obesity (E66.-)

    **O99.210** **Obesity complicating pregnancy, unspecified trimester**    Ⓜ♀

    **O99.211** **Obesity complicating pregnancy, first trimester**    Ⓜ♀

    **O99.212** **Obesity complicating pregnancy, second trimester**    Ⓜ♀

    **O99.213** **Obesity complicating pregnancy, third trimester**    Ⓜ♀

    **O99.214** **Obesity complicating childbirth**    Ⓜ♀

    **O99.215** **Obesity complicating the puerperium**    Ⓜ♀

☑6ᵗʰ **O99.28** **Other endocrine, nutritional and metabolic diseases complicating pregnancy, childbirth and the puerperium**

    **O99.280** **Endocrine, nutritional and metabolic diseases complicating pregnancy, unspecified trimester**    Ⓜ♀

    **O99.281** **Endocrine, nutritional and metabolic diseases complicating pregnancy, first trimester**    Ⓜ♀

    **O99.282** **Endocrine, nutritional and metabolic diseases complicating pregnancy, second trimester**    Ⓜ♀

    **O99.283** **Endocrine, nutritional and metabolic diseases complicating pregnancy, third trimester**    Ⓜ♀

    **O99.284** **Endocrine, nutritional and metabolic diseases complicating childbirth**    Ⓜ♀

    **O99.285** **Endocrine, nutritional and metabolic diseases complicating the puerperium**    Ⓜ♀

☑5ᵗʰ **O99.3** **Mental disorders and diseases of the nervous system complicating pregnancy, childbirth and the puerperium**

**CC Excl: For CC codes in subcategory O99.3, unless otherwise noted: PDX collection 1018**

☑6ᵗʰ **O99.31** **Alcohol use complicating pregnancy, childbirth, and the puerperium**

Use additional code(s) from F10 to identify manifestations of the alcohol use

    **O99.310** **Alcohol use complicating pregnancy, unspecified trimester**    Ⓜ♀

    **O99.311** **Alcohol use complicating pregnancy, first trimester**    Ⓜ♀

    **O99.312** **Alcohol use complicating pregnancy, second trimester**    Ⓜ♀

    **O99.313** **Alcohol use complicating pregnancy, third trimester**    Ⓜ♀

    **O99.314** **Alcohol use complicating childbirth**    Ⓜ♀

    **O99.315** **Alcohol use complicating the puerperium**    Ⓜ♀

☑6ᵗʰ **O99.32** **Drug use complicating pregnancy, childbirth, and the puerperium**

Use additional code(s) from F11-F16 and F18-F19 to identify manifestations of the drug use

    **O99.320** **Drug use complicating pregnancy, unspecified trimester**    Ⓜ♀

    **O99.321** **Drug use complicating pregnancy, first trimester**    CC Ⓜ♀

    **O99.322** **Drug use complicating pregnancy, second trimester**    CC Ⓜ♀

    **O99.323** **Drug use complicating pregnancy, third trimester**    CC Ⓜ♀

    **O99.324** **Drug use complicating childbirth**    CC Ⓜ♀

    **O99.325** **Drug use complicating the puerperium**    CC Ⓜ♀

Ⓝ Newborn: 0   Ⓟ Pediatric: 0-17   Ⓜ Maternity: 12-55   Ⓐ Adult: 15-124   MCC Major CC Condition   PDxMCC PDx acts as own MCC   CC CC Condition   PDxCC PDx acts as own CC

**874**      ICD-10-CM 2018

✓6th **O99.33** **Tobacco use disorder complicating pregnancy, childbirth, and the puerperium**
Smoking complicating pregnancy, childbirth, and the puerperium
Use additional code from category F17 to identify type of tobacco nicotine dependence

**O99.330** **Smoking (tobacco) complicating pregnancy, unspecified trimester** Ⓜ♀

**O99.331** **Smoking (tobacco) complicating pregnancy, first trimester** Ⓜ♀

**O99.332** **Smoking (tobacco) complicating pregnancy, second trimester** Ⓜ♀

**O99.333** **Smoking (tobacco) complicating pregnancy, third trimester** Ⓜ♀

**O99.334** **Smoking (tobacco) complicating childbirth** Ⓜ♀

**O99.335** **Smoking (tobacco) complicating the puerperium** Ⓜ♀

✓6th **O99.34** **Other mental disorders complicating pregnancy, childbirth, and the puerperium**
Conditions in F01-F09 and F20-F99
EXCLUDES 2 *postpartum mood disturbance (O90.6)*
*postnatal psychosis (F53)*
*puerperal psychosis (F53)*

**O99.340** **Other mental disorders complicating pregnancy, unspecified trimester** Ⓜ♀

**O99.341** **Other mental disorders complicating pregnancy, first trimester** Ⓜ♀

**O99.342** **Other mental disorders complicating pregnancy, second trimester** Ⓜ♀

**O99.343** **Other mental disorders complicating pregnancy, third trimester** Ⓜ♀

**O99.344** **Other mental disorders complicating childbirth** Ⓜ♀

**O99.345** **Other mental disorders complicating the puerperium** Ⓜ♀

✓6th **O99.35** **Diseases of the nervous system complicating pregnancy, childbirth, and the puerperium**
Conditions in G00-G99
EXCLUDES 2 *pregnancy related peripheral neuritis (O26.8-)*

**O99.350** **Diseases of the nervous system complicating pregnancy, unspecified trimester** Ⓜ♀

**O99.351** **Diseases of the nervous system complicating pregnancy, first trimester** Ⓜ♀

**O99.352** **Diseases of the nervous system complicating pregnancy, second trimester** Ⓜ♀

**O99.353** **Diseases of the nervous system complicating pregnancy, third trimester** Ⓜ♀

**O99.354** **Diseases of the nervous system complicating childbirth** cc Ⓜ♀
**CC Excl:** PDX collection 1016

**O99.355** **Diseases of the nervous system complicating the puerperium** cc Ⓜ♀
**CC Excl:** PDX collection 1016

✓5th **O99.4** **Diseases of the circulatory system complicating pregnancy, childbirth and the puerperium**
Conditions in I00-I99
EXCLUDES 1 *peripartum cardiomyopathy (O90.3)*
EXCLUDES 2 *hypertensive disorders (O10-O16)*
*obstetric embolism (O88.-)*
*venous complications and cerebrovenous sinus thrombosis in labor, childbirth and the puerperium (O87.-)*
*venous complications and cerebrovenous sinus thrombosis in pregnancy (O22.-)*

**AHA:** 2016, 2Q, 8

**CC Excl: For CC codes in subcategory O99.4, unless otherwise noted:** PDX collection 1019

✓6th **O99.41** **Diseases of the circulatory system complicating pregnancy**

**O99.411** **Diseases of the circulatory system complicating pregnancy, first trimester** cc Ⓜ♀

**O99.412** **Diseases of the circulatory system complicating pregnancy, second trimester** cc Ⓜ♀

**O99.413** **Diseases of the circulatory system complicating pregnancy, third trimester** cc Ⓜ♀

**O99.419** **Diseases of the circulatory system complicating pregnancy, unspecified trimester** Ⓜ♀

**O99.42** **Diseases of the circulatory system complicating childbirth** MCC Ⓜ♀
**CC Excl:** PDX collection 1008

**O99.43** **Diseases of the circulatory system complicating the puerperium** cc Ⓜ♀

✓5th **O99.5** **Diseases of the respiratory system complicating pregnancy, childbirth and the puerperium**
Conditions in J00-J99

✓6th **O99.51** **Diseases of the respiratory system complicating pregnancy**

**O99.511** **Diseases of the respiratory system complicating pregnancy, first trimester** Ⓜ♀

**O99.512** **Diseases of the respiratory system complicating pregnancy, second trimester** Ⓜ♀

**O99.513** **Diseases of the respiratory system complicating pregnancy, third trimester** Ⓜ♀

**O99.519** **Diseases of the respiratory system complicating pregnancy, unspecified trimester** Ⓜ♀

**O99.52** **Diseases of the respiratory system complicating childbirth** Ⓜ♀

**O99.53** **Diseases of the respiratory system complicating the puerperium** Ⓜ♀

✓5th **O99.6** **Diseases of the digestive system complicating pregnancy, childbirth and the puerperium**
Conditions in K00-K93
EXCLUDES 2 *hemorrhoids in pregnancy (O22.4-)*
*liver and biliary tract disorders in pregnancy, childbirth and the puerperium (O26.6-)*

✓6th **O99.61** **Diseases of the digestive system complicating pregnancy**
**AHA:** 2016, 1Q, 4

**O99.611** **Diseases of the digestive system complicating pregnancy, first trimester** Ⓜ♀

**O99.612** **Diseases of the digestive system complicating pregnancy, second trimester** Ⓜ♀

**O99.613** **Diseases of the digestive system complicating pregnancy, third trimester** Ⓜ♀

**O99.619** **Diseases of the digestive system complicating pregnancy, unspecified trimester** Ⓜ♀

**O99.62** **Diseases of the digestive system complicating childbirth** Ⓜ♀

**O99.63** **Diseases of the digestive system complicating the puerperium** Ⓜ♀

✓5th **O99.7** **Diseases of the skin and subcutaneous tissue complicating pregnancy, childbirth and the puerperium**
Conditions in L00-L99
EXCLUDES 2 *herpes gestationis (O26.4)*
*pruritic urticarial papules and plaques of pregnancy (PUPPP) (O26.86)*

✓6th **O99.71** **Diseases of the skin and subcutaneous tissue complicating pregnancy**

**O99.711** **Diseases of the skin and subcutaneous tissue complicating pregnancy, first trimester** Ⓜ♀

**O99.712** **Diseases of the skin and subcutaneous tissue complicating pregnancy, second trimester** Ⓜ♀

**O99.713** **Diseases of the skin and subcutaneous tissue complicating pregnancy, third trimester** Ⓜ♀

**O99.719** **Diseases of the skin and subcutaneous tissue complicating pregnancy, unspecified trimester** Ⓜ♀

**O99.72** **Diseases of the skin and subcutaneous tissue complicating childbirth** Ⓜ♀

**O99.73** **Diseases of the skin and subcutaneous tissue complicating the puerperium** Ⓜ♀

**Chapter 15. Pregnancy, Childbirth and the Puerperium**

✓5ᵗʰ **O99.8** **Other specified diseases and conditions complicating pregnancy, childbirth and the puerperium**
Conditions in D00-D48, H00-H95, M00-N99, and Q00-Q99
Use additional code to identify condition

> EXCLUDES 2 *genitourinary infections in pregnancy (O23.-)*
> *infection of genitourinary tract following delivery (O86.1-O86.3)*
> *malignant neoplasm complicating pregnancy, childbirth and the puerperium (O9A.1-)*
> *maternal care for known or suspected abnormality of maternal pelvic organs (O34.-)*
> *postpartum acute kidney failure (O90.4)*
> *traumatic injuries in pregnancy (O9A.2)*

**CC Excl: For CC codes in subcategory O99.8:**
**PDX collection 1013**

✓6ᵗʰ **O99.81** **Abnormal glucose complicating pregnancy, childbirth and the puerperium**
> EXCLUDES 1 *gestational diabetes (O24.4-)*

   **O99.810** **Abnormal glucose complicating pregnancy** Ⓜ♀
   **O99.814** **Abnormal glucose complicating childbirth** Ⓜ♀
   **O99.815** **Abnormal glucose complicating the puerperium** Ⓜ♀

✓6ᵗʰ **O99.82** **Streptococcus B carrier state complicating pregnancy, childbirth and the puerperium**
> EXCLUDES 1 *carrier of streptococcus group B (GBS) in a nonpregnant woman (Z22.330)*

   **O99.820** **Streptococcus B carrier state complicating pregnancy** Ⓜ♀
   **O99.824** **Streptococcus B carrier state complicating childbirth** Ⓜ♀
   **O99.825** **Streptococcus B carrier state complicating the puerperium** Ⓜ♀

✓6ᵗʰ **O99.83** **Other infection carrier state complicating pregnancy, childbirth and the puerperium**
Use additional code to identify the carrier state (Z22.-)

   **O99.830** **Other infection carrier state complicating pregnancy** CC Ⓜ♀
   **O99.834** **Other infection carrier state complicating childbirth** CC Ⓜ♀
   **O99.835** **Other infection carrier state complicating the puerperium** CC Ⓜ♀

✓6ᵗʰ **O99.84** **Bariatric surgery status complicating pregnancy, childbirth and the puerperium**
Gastric banding status complicating pregnancy, childbirth and the puerperium
Gastric bypass status for obesity complicating pregnancy, childbirth and the puerperium
Obesity surgery status complicating pregnancy, childbirth and the puerperium

   **O99.840** **Bariatric surgery status complicating pregnancy, unspecified trimester** Ⓜ♀
   **O99.841** **Bariatric surgery status complicating pregnancy, first trimester** Ⓜ♀
   **O99.842** **Bariatric surgery status complicating pregnancy, second trimester** Ⓜ♀
   **O99.843** **Bariatric surgery status complicating pregnancy, third trimester** Ⓜ♀
   **O99.844** **Bariatric surgery status complicating childbirth** Ⓜ♀
   **O99.845** **Bariatric surgery status complicating the puerperium** Ⓜ♀

   **O99.89** **Other specified diseases and conditions complicating pregnancy, childbirth and the puerperium** Ⓜ♀

✓4ᵗʰ **O9A** **Maternal malignant neoplasms, traumatic injuries and abuse classifiable elsewhere but complicating pregnancy, childbirth and the puerperium**

✓5ᵗʰ **O9A.1** **Malignant neoplasm complicating pregnancy, childbirth and the puerperium**
Conditions in C00-C96
Use additional code to identify neoplasm
> EXCLUDES 2 *maternal care for benign tumor of corpus uteri (O34.1-)*
> *maternal care for benign tumor of cervix (O34.4-)*

**AHA:** 2015, 3Q, 19

✓6ᵗʰ **O9A.11** **Malignant neoplasm complicating pregnancy**
   **O9A.111** **Malignant neoplasm complicating pregnancy, first trimester** Ⓜ♀

   **O9A.112** **Malignant neoplasm complicating pregnancy, second trimester** Ⓜ♀
   **O9A.113** **Malignant neoplasm complicating pregnancy, third trimester** Ⓜ♀
   **O9A.119** **Malignant neoplasm complicating pregnancy, unspecified trimester** Ⓜ♀

   **O9A.12** **Malignant neoplasm complicating childbirth** Ⓜ♀
   **O9A.13** **Malignant neoplasm complicating the puerperium** Ⓜ♀

✓5ᵗʰ **O9A.2** **Injury, poisoning and certain other consequences of external causes complicating pregnancy, childbirth and the puerperium**
Conditions in S00-T88, except T74 and T76
Use additional code(s) to identify the injury or poisoning
> EXCLUDES 2 *physical, sexual and psychological abuse complicating pregnancy, childbirth and the puerperium (O9A.3-, O9A.4-, O9A.5-)*

✓6ᵗʰ **O9A.21** **Injury, poisoning and certain other consequences of external causes complicating pregnancy**
   **O9A.211** **Injury, poisoning and certain other consequences of external causes complicating pregnancy, first trimester** Ⓜ♀
   **O9A.212** **Injury, poisoning and certain other consequences of external causes complicating pregnancy, second trimester** Ⓜ♀
   **O9A.213** **Injury, poisoning and certain other consequences of external causes complicating pregnancy, third trimester** Ⓜ♀
   **O9A.219** **Injury, poisoning and certain other consequences of external causes complicating pregnancy, unspecified trimester** Ⓜ♀

   **O9A.22** **Injury, poisoning and certain other consequences of external causes complicating childbirth** Ⓜ♀
   **O9A.23** **Injury, poisoning and certain other consequences of external causes complicating the puerperium** Ⓜ♀

✓5ᵗʰ **O9A.3** **Physical abuse complicating pregnancy, childbirth and the puerperium**
Conditions in T74.11 or T76.11
Use additional code (if applicable):
   to identify any associated current injury due to physical abuse
   to identify the perpetrator of abuse (Y07.-)
> EXCLUDES 2 *sexual abuse complicating pregnancy, childbirth and the puerperium (O9A.4)*

✓6ᵗʰ **O9A.31** **Physical abuse complicating pregnancy**
   **O9A.311** **Physical abuse complicating pregnancy, first trimester** Ⓜ♀
   **O9A.312** **Physical abuse complicating pregnancy, second trimester** Ⓜ♀
   **O9A.313** **Physical abuse complicating pregnancy, third trimester** Ⓜ♀
   **O9A.319** **Physical abuse complicating pregnancy, unspecified trimester** Ⓜ♀

   **O9A.32** **Physical abuse complicating childbirth** Ⓜ♀
   **O9A.33** **Physical abuse complicating the puerperium** Ⓜ♀

✓5ᵗʰ **O9A.4** **Sexual abuse complicating pregnancy, childbirth and the puerperium**
Conditions in T74.21 or T76.21
Use additional code (if applicable):
   to identify any associated current injury due to sexual abuse
   to identify the perpetrator of abuse (Y07.-)

✓6ᵗʰ **O9A.41** **Sexual abuse complicating pregnancy**
   **O9A.411** **Sexual abuse complicating pregnancy, first trimester** Ⓜ♀
   **O9A.412** **Sexual abuse complicating pregnancy, second trimester** Ⓜ♀
   **O9A.413** **Sexual abuse complicating pregnancy, third trimester** Ⓜ♀
   **O9A.419** **Sexual abuse complicating pregnancy, unspecified trimester** Ⓜ♀

   **O9A.42** **Sexual abuse complicating childbirth** Ⓜ♀
   **O9A.43** **Sexual abuse complicating the puerperium** Ⓜ♀

Ⓝ Newborn: 0   Ⓟ Pediatric: 0-17   Ⓜ Maternity: 12-55   Ⓐ Adult: 15-124   MCC Major CC Condition   PDxMCC PDx acts as own MCC   CC CC Condition   PDxCC PDx acts as own CC

876    ICD-10-CM 2018

☑5ᵗʰ **O9A.5** Psychological abuse **complicating pregnancy, childbirth and the puerperium**
Conditions in T74.31 or T76.31
Use additional code to identify the perpetrator of abuse (YØ7.-)

☑6ᵗʰ **O9A.51** **Psychological abuse complicating** pregnancy

**O9A.511** **Psychological abuse complicating pregnancy,** first trimester    Ⓜ♀

**O9A.512** **Psychological abuse complicating pregnancy,** second trimester    Ⓜ♀

**O9A.513** **Psychological abuse complicating pregnancy,** third trimester    Ⓜ♀

**O9A.519** **Psychological abuse complicating pregnancy,** unspecified trimester    Ⓜ♀

**O9A.52** **Psychological abuse complicating** childbirth    Ⓜ♀

**O9A.53** **Psychological abuse complicating the** puerperium    Ⓜ♀

☑Additional Character Req   ☑x7ᵗʰ Placeholder Alert   Unacceptable PDx   Manifestation   H1-H14 HAC   HCC CMS-HCC Condition   *EXCLUDES 1* Not Coded Here   *EXCLUDES 2* Not Included Here

ICD-10-CM 2018      877

# Chapter 16. Certain Conditions Originating in the Perinatal Period (P00–P96)

## Chapter Specific Guidelines with Coding Examples

The chapter specific guidelines from the ICD-10-CM Official Guidelines for Coding and Reporting have been provided below. Along with these guidelines are coding examples, contained in the shaded boxes, that have been developed to help illustrate the coding and/or sequencing guidance found in these guidelines.

For coding and reporting purposes the perinatal period is defined as before birth through the 28th day following birth. The following guidelines are provided for reporting purposes

### a. General perinatal rules

#### 1) Use of Chapter 16 codes

Codes in this chapter are <u>never</u> for use on the maternal record. Codes from Chapter 15, the obstetric chapter, are never permitted on the newborn record. Chapter 16 codes may be used throughout the life of the patient if the condition is still present.

#### 2) Principal diagnosis for birth record

When coding the birth episode in a newborn record, assign a code from category Z38, Liveborn infants according to place of birth and type of delivery, as the principal diagnosis. A code from category Z38 is assigned only once, to a newborn at the time of birth. If a newborn is transferred to another institution, a code from category Z38 should not be used at the receiving hospital.

A code from category Z38 is used only on the newborn record, not on the mother's record.

> Newborn delivered via vaginal delivery in Rural Hospital A, experienced meconium aspiration resulting in pneumonia. Rural Hospital A is not equipped to handle the extensive respiratory therapy this baby needs and transfers the patient to Metropolis Hospital B, where the pneumonia resolves and the newborn is eventually discharged.
>
> *Rural Hospital A*
>
> **Z38.00    Single liveborn infant, delivered vaginally**
>
> **P24.01    Meconium aspiration with respiratory symptoms**
>
> *Metropolis Hospital B*
>
> **P24.01    Meconium aspiration with respiratory symptoms**
>
> *Explanation:* A code from category Z38 is a one-time use only code. The hospital that actually delivered the newborn, in this case Rural Hospital A, can append a code from category Z38 but for the delivery admission only. Once the patient is transferred or discharged, the Z38 category no longer applies for that patient.
>
> The reason for the transfer to Metropolis Hospital B was for the respiratory symptoms (pneumonia) the newborn was exhibiting secondary to aspirating meconium.

#### 3) Use of codes from other chapters with codes from Chapter 16

Codes from other chapters may be used with codes from chapter 16 if the codes from the other chapters provide more specific detail. Codes for signs and symptoms may be assigned when a definitive diagnosis has not been established. If the reason for the encounter is a perinatal condition, the code from chapter 16 should be sequenced first.

#### 4) Use of Chapter 16 codes after the perinatal period

Should a condition originate in the perinatal period, and continue throughout the life of the patient, the perinatal code should continue to be used regardless of the patient's age.

> A 7-year-old patient with history of birth injury that resulted in Erb's palsy is seen for subscapularis release
>
> **P14.0    Erb's paralysis due to birth injury**
>
> *Explanation:* Although in this instance Erb's palsy is specifically related to a birth injury, it has not resolved and continues to be a health concern. A perinatal code is appropriate even though this patient is beyond the perinatal period.

#### 5) Birth process or community acquired conditions

If a newborn has a condition that may be either due to the birth process or community acquired and the documentation does not indicate which it is, the default is due to the birth process and the code from Chapter 16 should be used. If the condition is community-acquired, a code from Chapter 16 should not be assigned.

#### 6) Code all clinically significant conditions

All clinically significant conditions noted on routine newborn examination should be coded. A condition is clinically significant if it requires:

clinical evaluation; or

therapeutic treatment; or

diagnostic procedures; or

extended length of hospital stay; or

increased nursing care and/or monitoring; or

has implications for future health care needs

**Note:** The perinatal guidelines listed above are the same as the general coding guidelines for "additional diagnoses", except for the final point regarding implications for future health care needs. Codes should be assigned for conditions that have been specified by the provider as having implications for future health care needs.

### b. Observation and evaluation of newborns for suspected conditions not found

#### 1) Assign a code from category Z05, Observation and evaluation of newborns and infants for suspected conditions ruled out, to identify those instances when a healthy newborn is evaluated for a suspected condition that is determined after study not to be present. Do not use a code from category Z05 when the patient has identified signs or symptoms of a suspected problem; in such cases code the sign or symptom.

#### 2) A code from category Z05 may also be assigned as a principal or first-listed code for readmissions or encounters when the code from category Z38 code no longer applies. Codes from category Z05 are for use only for healthy newborns and infants for which no condition after study is found to be present.

#### 3) Z05 on a birth record

A code from category Z05 is to be used as a secondary code after the code from category Z38, Liveborn infants according to place of birth and type of delivery.

> Newborn delivered via vaginal delivery; previous ultrasounds showed what appeared to be an abnormality of the right kidney. Kidney function tests were performed and ultrasounds taken and any genitourinary conditions ruled out.
>
> **Z38.00    Single liveborn infant, delivered vaginally**
>
> **Z05.6    Observation and evaluation of newborn for suspected genitourinary condition ruled out**
>
> Explanation: The newborn had no signs or symptoms of kidney or other genitourinary condition but was evaluated after delivery due to the abnormal prenatal ultrasound findings. A Z code describing the type and place of birth should be coded first, followed by a Z05 category code for the work performed to rule out a suspected genitourinary condition.

### c. Coding additional perinatal diagnoses

#### 1) Assigning codes for conditions that require treatment

Assign codes for conditions that require treatment or further investigation, prolong the length of stay, or require resource utilization.

**2) Codes for conditions specified as having implications for future health care needs**

Assign codes for conditions that have been specified by the provider as having implications for future health care needs.

**Note:** This guideline should not be used for adult patients.

> An abnormal noise was heard in the left hip of a post-term newborn during a physical examination. The pediatrician would like to follow the patient after discharge as a hip click can be an early sign of hip dysplasia. The newborn was delivered via cesarean at 41 weeks.
>
> **Z38.01**    **Single liveborn infant, delivered by cesarean**
>
> **P08.21**    **Post-term newborn**
>
> **R29.4**    **Clicking hip**
>
> *Explanation:* The abnormal hip noise or click is appended as a secondary diagnosis not only because it is an abnormal finding upon examination, but also due to its potential to be part of a bigger health issue. The hip dysplasia has not yet been diagnosed and does not warrant a code at this time.

**d. Prematurity and fetal growth retardation**

Providers utilize different criteria in determining prematurity. A code for prematurity should not be assigned unless it is documented. Assignment of codes in categories P05, Disorders of newborn related to slow fetal growth and fetal malnutrition, and P07, Disorders of newborn related to short gestation and low birth weight, not elsewhere classified, should be based on the recorded birth weight and estimated gestational age. Codes from category P05 should not be assigned with codes from category P07.

When both birth weight and gestational age are available, two codes from category P07 should be assigned, with the code for birth weight sequenced before the code for gestational age.

**e. Low birth weight and immaturity status**

Codes from category P07, Disorders of newborn related to short gestation and low birth weight, not elsewhere classified, are for use for a child or adult who was premature or had a low birth weight as a newborn and this is affecting the patient's current health status.

*See Section I.C.21. Factors influencing health status and contact with health services, Status.*

> A 35-year-old patient, who weighed 659 grams at birth, is seen for heart disease documented as being a consequence of the low birth weight
>
> **I51.9**    **Heart disease, unspecified**
>
> **P07.02**    **Extremely low birth weight newborn, 500–749 grams**
>
> *Explanation:* A code from subcategories P07.0- and P07.1- is appropriate, regardless of the age of the patient, as long as the documentation provides a clear link between the patient's current illness and the low birth weight.

**f. Bacterial sepsis of newborn**

Category P36, Bacterial sepsis of newborn, includes congenital sepsis. If a perinate is documented as having sepsis without documentation of congenital or community acquired, the default is congenital and a code from category P36 should be assigned. If the P36 code includes the causal organism, an additional code from category B95, Streptococcus, Staphylococcus, and Enterococcus as the cause of diseases classified elsewhere, or B96, Other bacterial agents as the cause of diseases classified elsewhere, should not be assigned. If the P36 code does not include the causal organism, assign an additional code from category B96. If applicable, use additional codes to identify severe sepsis (R65.2-) and any associated acute organ dysfunction.

> A full-term infant develops severe sepsis 24 hours after discharge from the hospital and is readmitted; cultures identified *E. coli* as the infective agent
>
> **P36.4**    **Sepsis of newborn due to Escherichia coli**
>
> **R65.20**    **Severe sepsis without septic shock**
>
> *Explanation:* Even though this newborn was discharged and could have acquired *E. coli* from his/her external environment, due to the lack of documentation specifying specifically how this pathogen was acquired, the default is to code the *E. coli* sepsis as congenital. A code from chapter 1, "Certain Infectious and Parasitic Diseases," is not required because the perinatal sepsis code identifies both the sepsis and the bacteria causing the sepsis.

**g. Stillbirth**

Code P95, Stillbirth, is only for use in institutions that maintain separate records for stillbirths. No other code should be used with P95. Code P95 should not be used on the mother's record.

# Chapter 16. Certain Conditions Originating in the Perinatal Period (P00-P96)

**NOTE** Codes from this chapter are for use on newborn records only, never on maternal records.

**INCLUDES** conditions that have their origin in the fetal or perinatal period (before birth through the first 28 days after birth) even if morbidity occurs later

**EXCLUDES 2** *congenital malformations, deformations and chromosomal abnormalities (Q00-Q99)*
*endocrine, nutritional and metabolic diseases (E00-E88)*
*injury, poisoning and certain other consequences of external causes (S00-T88)*
*neoplasms (C00-D49)*
*tetanus neonatorum (A33)*

This chapter contains the following blocks:

P00-P04   Newborn affected by maternal factors and by complications of pregnancy, labor, and delivery
P05-P08   Disorders of newborn related to length of gestation and fetal growth
P09   Abnormal findings on neonatal screening
P10-P15   Birth trauma
P19-P29   Respiratory and cardiovascular disorders specific to the perinatal period
P35-P39   Infections specific to the perinatal period
P50-P61   Hemorrhagic and hematological disorders of newborn
P70-P74   Transitory endocrine and metabolic disorders specific to newborn
P76-P78   Digestive system disorders of newborn
P80-P83   Conditions involving the integument and temperature regulation of newborn
P84   Other problems with newborn
P90-P96   Other disorders originating in the perinatal period

## Newborn affected by maternal factors and by complications of pregnancy, labor, and delivery (P00-P04)

**NOTE** These codes are for use when the listed maternal conditions are specified as the cause of confirmed morbidity or potential morbidity which have their origin in the perinatal period (before birth through the first 28 days after birth).

**✓4ᵗʰ P00 Newborn affected by maternal conditions that may be unrelated to present pregnancy**

Code first any current condition in newborn

**EXCLUDES 2** *encounter for observation of newborn for suspected diseases and conditions ruled out (Z05.-)*
*newborn affected by maternal complications of pregnancy (P01.-)*
*newborn affected by maternal endocrine and metabolic disorders (P70-P74)*
*newborn affected by noxious substances transmitted via placenta or breast milk (P04.-)*

**P00.0 Newborn affected by maternal hypertensive disorders**
Newborn affected by maternal conditions classifiable to O10-O11, O13-O16

**P00.1 Newborn affected by maternal renal and urinary tract diseases**
Newborn affected by maternal conditions classifiable to N00-N39

**P00.2 Newborn affected by maternal infectious and parasitic diseases**
Newborn affected by maternal infectious disease classifiable to A00-B99, J09 and J10
**EXCLUDES 1** *infections specific to the perinatal period (P35-P39)*
*maternal genital tract or other localized infections (P00.8)*
**EXCLUDES 2** ▶*infections specific to the perinatal period (P35-P39)*◀
**AHA:** 2015, 3Q, 20

**P00.3 Newborn affected by other maternal circulatory and respiratory diseases**
Newborn affected by maternal conditions classifiable to I00-I99, J00-J99, Q20-Q34 and not included in P00.0, P00.2

**P00.4 Newborn affected by maternal nutritional disorders**
Newborn affected by maternal disorders classifiable to E40-E64
Maternal malnutrition NOS

**P00.5 Newborn affected by maternal injury**
Newborn affected by maternal conditions classifiable to O9A.2-

**P00.6 Newborn affected by surgical procedure on mother**
Newborn affected by amniocentesis
**EXCLUDES 1** *Cesarean delivery for present delivery (P03.4)*
*damage to placenta from amniocentesis, Cesarean delivery or surgical induction (P02.1)*
*previous surgery to uterus or pelvic organs (P03.89)*
**EXCLUDES 2** *newborn affected by complication of (fetal) intrauterine procedure (P96.5)*

**P00.7 Newborn affected by other medical procedures on mother, not elsewhere classified**
Newborn affected by radiation to mother
**EXCLUDES 1** *damage to placenta from amniocentesis, cesarean delivery or surgical induction (P02.1)*
*newborn affected by other complications of labor and delivery (P03.-)*

**✓5ᵗʰ P00.8 Newborn affected by other maternal conditions**
**P00.81 Newborn affected by periodontal disease in mother**
**P00.89 Newborn affected by other maternal conditions**
Newborn affected by conditions classifiable to T80-T88
Newborn affected by maternal genital tract or other localized infections
Newborn affected by maternal systemic lupus erythematosus

**P00.9 Newborn affected by unspecified maternal condition**

**✓4ᵗʰ P01 Newborn affected by maternal complications of pregnancy**

Code first any current condition in newborn
**EXCLUDES 2** *encounter for observation of newborn for suspected diseases and conditions ruled out (Z05.-)*

**P01.0 Newborn affected by incompetent cervix**

**P01.1 Newborn affected by premature rupture of membranes**

**P01.2 Newborn affected by oligohydramnios**
**EXCLUDES 1** *oligohydramnios due to premature rupture of membranes (P01.1)*
**DEF:** Low amniotic fluid level, resulting in underdeveloped organs in the fetus.

**P01.3 Newborn affected by polyhydramnios**
Newborn affected by hydramnios

**P01.4 Newborn affected by ectopic pregnancy**
Newborn affected by abdominal pregnancy

**P01.5 Newborn affected by multiple pregnancy**
Newborn affected by triplet (pregnancy)
Newborn affected by twin (pregnancy)

**P01.6 Newborn affected by maternal death**

**P01.7 Newborn affected by malpresentation before labor**
Newborn affected by breech presentation before labor
Newborn affected by external version before labor
Newborn affected by face presentation before labor
Newborn affected by transverse lie before labor
Newborn affected by unstable lie before labor

**P01.8 Newborn affected by other maternal complications of pregnancy**

**P01.9 Newborn affected by maternal complication of pregnancy, unspecified**

**✓4ᵗʰ P02 Newborn affected by complications of placenta, cord and membranes**

Code first any current condition in newborn
**EXCLUDES 2** *encounter for observation of newborn for suspected diseases and conditions ruled out (Z05.-)*

**P02.0 Newborn affected by placenta previa**
**DEF:** Placenta developed in lower segment of uterus; can cause hemorrhaging leading to preterm delivery.

**P02.1 Newborn affected by other forms of placental separation and hemorrhage**
Newborn affected by abruptio placenta
Newborn affected by accidental hemorrhage
Newborn affected by antepartum hemorrhage
Newborn affected by damage to placenta from amniocentesis, cesarean delivery or surgical induction
Newborn affected by maternal blood loss
Newborn affected by premature separation of placenta

**✓5ᵗʰ P02.2 Newborn affected by other and unspecified morphological and functional abnormalities of placenta**
**P02.20 Newborn affected by unspecified morphological and functional abnormalities of placenta**

✓ Additional Character Req   ✓x7ᵗʰ Placeholder Alert   Unacceptable PDx   Manifestation   H1-H14 HAC   HCC CMS-HCC Condition   EXCLUDES 1 Not Coded Here   EXCLUDES 2 Not Included Here

ICD-10-CM 2018      881

**P02.29 Newborn affected by other morphological and functional abnormalities of placenta**
Newborn affected by placental dysfunction
Newborn affected by placental infarction
Newborn affected by placental insufficiency

**P02.3 Newborn affected by placental transfusion syndromes**
Newborn affected by placental and cord abnormalities resulting in twin-to-twin or other transplacental transfusion

**P02.4 Newborn affected by prolapsed cord**

**P02.5 Newborn affected by other compression of umbilical cord**
Newborn affected by umbilical cord (tightly) around neck
Newborn affected by entanglement of umbilical cord
Newborn affected by knot in umbilical cord

✓5ᵗʰ **P02.6 Newborn affected by other and unspecified conditions of umbilical cord**

    **P02.60 Newborn affected by unspecified conditions of umbilical cord**

    **P02.69 Newborn affected by other conditions of umbilical cord**
    Newborn affected by short umbilical cord
    Newborn affected by vasa previa
    **EXCLUDES 1** *newborn affected by single umbilical artery (Q27.0)*

**P02.7 Newborn affected by chorioamnionitis**
Newborn affected by amnionitis
Newborn affected by membranitis
Newborn affected by placentitis
**DEF:** Inflammation of the fetal membranes due to maternal infection; characterized by fetal tachycardia, respiratory distress, apnea, weak cries, and poor sucking.

**P02.8 Newborn affected by other abnormalities of membranes**

**P02.9 Newborn affected by abnormality of membranes, unspecified**

✓4ᵗʰ **P03 Newborn affected by other complications of labor and delivery**
Code first any current condition in newborn
**EXCLUDES 2** *encounter for observation of newborn for suspected diseases and conditions ruled out (Z05.-)*

**P03.0 Newborn affected by breech delivery and extraction**

**P03.1 Newborn affected by other malpresentation, malposition and disproportion during labor and delivery**
Newborn affected by contracted pelvis
Newborn affected by conditions classifiable to O64-O66
Newborn affected by persistent occipitoposterior
Newborn affected by transverse lie

**P03.2 Newborn affected by forceps delivery**

### Forceps Assisted Birth

Forceps extractor

### Vacuum Assisted Birth

Vacuum extractor

**P03.3 Newborn affected by delivery by vacuum extractor [ventouse]**

**P03.4 Newborn affected by Cesarean delivery**

**P03.5 Newborn affected by precipitate delivery**
Newborn affected by rapid second stage

**P03.6 Newborn affected by abnormal uterine contractions**
Newborn affected by conditions classifiable to O62.-, except O62.3
Newborn affected by hypertonic labor
Newborn affected by uterine inertia

✓5ᵗʰ **P03.8 Newborn affected by other specified complications of labor and delivery**

    ✓6ᵗʰ **P03.81 Newborn affected by abnormality in fetal (intrauterine) heart rate or rhythm**
    **EXCLUDES 1** *neonatal cardiac dysrhythmia (P29.1-)*

        **P03.810 Newborn affected by abnormality in fetal (intrauterine) heart rate or rhythm before the onset of labor**

        **P03.811 Newborn affected by abnormality in fetal (intrauterine) heart rate or rhythm during labor**

        **P03.819 Newborn affected by abnormality in fetal (intrauterine) heart rate or rhythm, unspecified as to time of onset**

    **P03.82 Meconium passage during delivery**
    **EXCLUDES 1** *meconium aspiration (P24.00, P24.01)*
    *meconium staining (P96.83)*
    **DEF:** Fetal intestinal activity that increases in response to a fetomaternal distressed state during delivery; the anal sphincter relaxes, and meconium is passed into the amniotic fluid.

    **P03.89 Newborn affected by other specified complications of labor and delivery**
    Newborn affected by abnormality of maternal soft tissues
    Newborn affected by conditions classifiable to O60-O75 and by procedures used in labor and delivery not included in P02.- and P03.0-P03.6
    Newborn affected by induction of labor

**P03.9 Newborn affected by complication of labor and delivery, unspecified**

✓4ᵗʰ **P04 Newborn affected by noxious substances transmitted via placenta or breast milk**
**INCLUDES** nonteratogenic effects of substances transmitted via placenta
**EXCLUDES 2** *congenital malformations (Q00-Q99)*
*encounter for observation of newborn for suspected diseases and conditions ruled out (Z05.-)*
*neonatal jaundice from excessive hemolysis due to drugs or toxins transmitted from mother (P58.4)*
*newborn in contact with and (suspected) exposures hazardous to health not transmitted via placenta or breast milk (Z77.-)*

**P04.0 Newborn affected by maternal anesthesia and analgesia in pregnancy, labor and delivery**
Newborn affected by reactions and intoxications from maternal opiates and tranquilizers administered during labor and delivery

**P04.1 Newborn affected by other maternal medication**
Newborn affected by cancer chemotherapy
Newborn affected by cytotoxic drugs
**EXCLUDES 1** *dysmorphism due to warfarin (Q86.2)*
*fetal hydantoin syndrome (Q86.1)*
*maternal use of drugs of addiction (P04.4-)*

**P04.2 Newborn affected by maternal use of tobacco**
Newborn affected by exposure in utero to tobacco smoke
**EXCLUDES 2** *newborn exposure to environmental tobacco smoke (P96.81)*

**P04.3 Newborn affected by maternal use of alcohol**
**EXCLUDES 1** *fetal alcohol syndrome (Q86.0)*

✓5ᵗʰ **P04.4 Newborn affected by maternal use of drugs of addiction**

    **P04.41 Newborn affected by maternal use of cocaine**
    "Crack baby"

    **P04.49 Newborn affected by maternal use of other drugs of addiction**
    **EXCLUDES 2** *newborn affected by maternal anesthesia and analgesia (P04.0)*
    *withdrawal symptoms from maternal use of drugs of addiction (P96.1)*

**P04.5 Newborn affected by maternal use of nutritional chemical substances**

P04.6 **Newborn affected by maternal exposure to** environmental chemical substances

P04.8 **Newborn affected by other maternal** noxious substances

P04.9 **Newborn affected by maternal noxious substance,** unspecified

## Disorders of newborn related to length of gestation and fetal growth (P05-P08)

✓4ᵗʰ **P05** **Disorders of newborn related to slow fetal growth and fetal malnutrition**

✓5ᵗʰ **P05.0** **Newborn light for gestational age**
Newborn light-for-dates
Weight below but length above 10th percentile for gestational age

**P05.00** **Newborn light for gestational age,** unspecified weight

**P05.01** **Newborn light for gestational age,** less than 500 grams

**P05.02** **Newborn light for gestational age,** 500-749 grams

**P05.03** **Newborn light for gestational age,** 750-999 grams

**P05.04** **Newborn light for gestational age,** 1000-1249 grams

**P05.05** **Newborn light for gestational age,** 1250-1499 grams

**P05.06** **Newborn light for gestational age,** 1500-1749 grams

**P05.07** **Newborn light for gestational age,** 1750-1999 grams

**P05.08** **Newborn light for gestational age,** 2000-2499 grams

**P05.09** **Newborn light for gestational age,** 2500 grams and over
Newborn light for gestational age, other

✓5ᵗʰ **P05.1** **Newborn small for gestational age**
Newborn small-and-light-for-dates
Newborn small-for-dates
Weight and length below 10th percentile for gestational age

**P05.10** **Newborn small for gestational age,** unspecified weight

**P05.11** **Newborn small for gestational age,** less than 500 grams

**P05.12** **Newborn small for gestational age,** 500-749 grams

**P05.13** **Newborn small for gestational age,** 750-999 grams

**P05.14** **Newborn small for gestational age,** 1000-1249 grams

**P05.15** **Newborn small for gestational age,** 1250-1499 grams

**P05.16** **Newborn small for gestational age,** 1500-1749 grams

**P05.17** **Newborn small for gestational age,** 1750-1999 grams

**P05.18** **Newborn small for gestational age,** 2000-2499 grams

**P05.19** **Newborn small for gestational age,** other
Newborn small for gestational age, 2500 grams and over

**P05.2** **Newborn affected by** fetal (intrauterine) malnutrition **not light or small for gestational age**
Infant, not light or small for gestational age, showing signs of fetal malnutrition, such as dry, peeling skin and loss of subcutaneous tissue
*EXCLUDES 1* *newborn affected by fetal malnutrition with light for gestational age (P05.0-)*
*newborn affected by fetal malnutrition with small for gestational age (P05.1-)*

**P05.9** **Newborn affected by** slow intrauterine growth**, unspecified**
Newborn affected by fetal growth retardation NOS

✓4ᵗʰ **P07** **Disorders of newborn related to short gestation and low birth weight, not elsewhere classified**
**NOTE** When both birth weight and gestational age of the newborn are available, both should be coded with birth weight sequenced before gestational age
**INCLUDES** the listed conditions, without further specification, as the cause of morbidity or additional care, in newborn

✓5ᵗʰ **P07.0** **Extremely low** birth weight newborn
Newborn birth weight 999 g. or less
*EXCLUDES 1* *low birth weight due to slow fetal growth and fetal malnutrition (P05.-)*

**P07.00** **Extremely low birth weight newborn,** unspecified weight

**P07.01** **Extremely low birth weight newborn,** less than 500 grams

**P07.02** **Extremely low birth weight newborn,** 500-749 grams

**P07.03** **Extremely low birth weight newborn,** 750-999 grams

✓5ᵗʰ **P07.1** **Other low** birth weight newborn
Newborn birth weight 1000-2499 g.
*EXCLUDES 1* *low birth weight due to slow fetal growth and fetal malnutrition (P05.-)*

**P07.10** **Other low birth weight newborn,** unspecified weight

**P07.14** **Other low birth weight newborn,** 1000-1249 grams

**P07.15** **Other low birth weight newborn,** 1250-1499 grams

**P07.16** **Other low birth weight newborn,** 1500-1749 grams

**P07.17** **Other low birth weight newborn,** 1750-1999 grams

**P07.18** **Other low birth weight newborn,** 2000-2499 grams

✓5ᵗʰ **P07.2** **Extreme immaturity of** newborn
Less than 28 completed weeks (less than 196 completed days) of gestation.

**P07.20** **Extreme immaturity of newborn,** unspecified weeks of gestation
Gestational age less than 28 completed weeks NOS

**P07.21** **Extreme immaturity of newborn, gestational age less than 23 completed weeks**
Extreme immaturity of newborn, gestational age less than 23 weeks, 0 days

**P07.22** **Extreme immaturity of newborn, gestational age 23 completed weeks**
Extreme immaturity of newborn, gestational age 23 weeks, 0 days through 23 weeks, 6 days

**P07.23** **Extreme immaturity of newborn, gestational age 24 completed weeks**
Extreme immaturity of newborn, gestational age 24 weeks, 0 days through 24 weeks, 6 days

**P07.24** **Extreme immaturity of newborn, gestational age 25 completed weeks**
Extreme immaturity of newborn, gestational age 25 weeks, 0 days through 25 weeks, 6 days

**P07.25** **Extreme immaturity of newborn, gestational age 26 completed weeks**
Extreme immaturity of newborn, gestational age 26 weeks, 0 days through 26 weeks, 6 days

**P07.26** **Extreme immaturity of newborn, gestational age 27 completed weeks**
Extreme immaturity of newborn, gestational age 27 weeks, 0 days through 27 weeks, 6 days

✓5ᵗʰ **P07.3** **Preterm [premature] newborn [other]**
28 completed weeks or more but less than 37 completed weeks (196 completed days but less than 259 completed days) of gestation
Prematurity NOS

**P07.30** **Preterm newborn,** unspecified weeks of gestation

**P07.31** **Preterm newborn, gestational age 28 completed weeks**
Preterm newborn, gestational age 28 weeks, 0 days through 28 weeks, 6 days

**P07.32** **Preterm newborn, gestational age 29 completed weeks**
Preterm newborn, gestational age 29 weeks, 0 days through 29 weeks, 6 days

**P07.33** **Preterm newborn, gestational age 30 completed weeks**
Preterm newborn, gestational age 30 weeks, 0 days through 30 weeks, 6 days

**P07.34** **Preterm newborn, gestational age 31 completed weeks**
Preterm newborn, gestational age 31 weeks, 0 days through 31 weeks, 6 days

**P07.35** **Preterm newborn, gestational age 32 completed weeks**
Preterm newborn, gestational age 32 weeks, 0 days through 32 weeks, 6 days

**P07.36** **Preterm newborn, gestational age 33 completed weeks**
Preterm newborn, gestational age 33 weeks, 0 days through 33 weeks, 6 days

**P07.37** **Preterm newborn, gestational age 34 completed weeks**
Preterm newborn, gestational age 34 weeks, 0 days through 34 weeks, 6 days

✓ Additional Character Req   ✓x7ᵗʰ Placeholder Alert   Unacceptable PDx   Manifestation   **H1**-**H14** HAC   **HCC** CMS-HCC Condition   *EXCLUDES 1* Not Coded Here   *EXCLUDES 2* Not Included Here

**P07.38**   **Preterm newborn, gestational age 35 completed weeks**
Preterm newborn, gestational age 35 weeks, 0 days through 35 weeks, 6 days

**P07.39**   **Preterm newborn, gestational age 36 completed weeks**
Preterm newborn, gestational age 36 weeks, 0 days through 36 weeks, 6 days

✅4ᵗʰ **P08**   **Disorders of newborn related to long gestation and high birth weight**

NOTE   When both birth weight and gestational age of the newborn are available, priority of assignment should be given to birth weight

INCLUDES   the listed conditions, without further specification, as causes of morbidity or additional care, in newborn

**P08.0**   **Exceptionally large newborn baby**
Usually implies a birth weight of 4500 g. or more
EXCLUDES 1   *syndrome of infant of diabetic mother (P70.1)*
*syndrome of infant of mother with gestational diabetes (P70.0)*

**P08.1**   **Other heavy for gestational age newborn**
Other newborn heavy- or large-for-dates regardless of period of gestation
Usually implies a birth weight of 4000 g. to 4499 g.
EXCLUDES 1   *newborn with a birth weight of 4500 or more (P08.0)*
*syndrome of infant of diabetic mother (P70.1)*
*syndrome of infant of mother with gestational diabetes (P70.0).*

✅5ᵗʰ **P08.2**   **Late newborn, not heavy for gestational age**
AHA: 2014, 1Q, 14

**P08.21**   **Post-term newborn**
Newborn with gestation period over 40 completed weeks to 42 completed weeks

**P08.22**   **Prolonged gestation of newborn**
Newborn with gestation period over 42 completed weeks (294 days or more), not heavy- or large-for-dates.
Postmaturity NOS

## Abnormal findings on neonatal screening (P09)

**P09**   **Abnormal findings on neonatal screening**
Use additional code to identify signs, symptoms and conditions associated with the screening
EXCLUDES 2   *nonspecific serologic evidence of human immunodeficiency virus [HIV] (R75)*

## Birth trauma (P10-P15)

✅4ᵗʰ **P10**   **Intracranial laceration and hemorrhage due to birth injury**
EXCLUDES 1   *intracranial hemorrhage of newborn NOS (P52.9)*
*intracranial hemorrhage of newborn due to anoxia or hypoxia (P52.-)*
*nontraumatic intracranial hemorrhage of newborn (P52.-)*

CC Excl: For MCC codes in category P10, unless otherwise noted:
PDX collection 1020

**P10.0**   **Subdural hemorrhage due to birth injury**   MCC
Subdural hematoma (localized) due to birth injury
EXCLUDES 1   *subdural hemorrhage accompanying tentorial tear (P10.4)*

**P10.1**   **Cerebral hemorrhage due to birth injury**   MCC

**P10.2**   **Intraventricular hemorrhage due to birth injury**   CC
CC Excl: PDX collection 1021

**P10.3**   **Subarachnoid hemorrhage due to birth injury**   MCC
CC Excl: PDX collection 1022

**P10.4**   **Tentorial tear due to birth injury**   MCC

**P10.8**   **Other intracranial lacerations and hemorrhages due to birth injury**   MCC

**P10.9**   **Unspecified intracranial laceration and hemorrhage due to birth injury**   MCC

✅4ᵗʰ **P11**   **Other birth injuries to central nervous system**

CC Excl: For MCC codes in category P11, unless otherwise noted:
PDX collection 1020

**P11.0**   **Cerebral edema due to birth injury**   MCC

**P11.1**   **Other specified brain damage due to birth injury**

**P11.2**   **Unspecified brain damage due to birth injury**   MCC

**P11.3**   **Birth injury to facial nerve**
Facial palsy due to birth injury

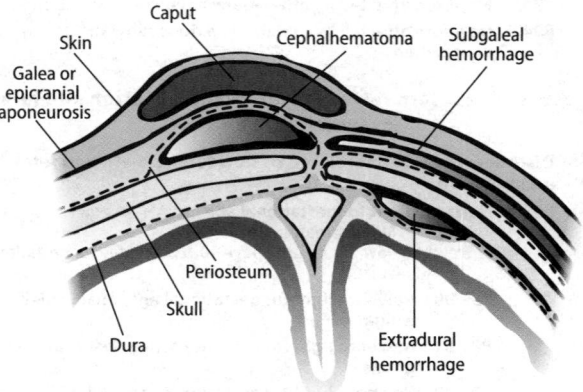

**Birth Injuries to Scalp**

**P11.4**   **Birth injury to other cranial nerves**

**P11.5**   **Birth injury to spine and spinal cord**
Fracture of spine due to birth injury

**P11.9**   **Birth injury to central nervous system, unspecified**   MCC

✅4ᵗʰ **P12**   **Birth injury to scalp**

**P12.0**   **Cephalhematoma due to birth injury**

**P12.1**   **Chignon (from vacuum extraction) due to birth injury**

**P12.2**   **Epicranial subaponeurotic hemorrhage due to birth injury**   CC
Subgaleal hemorrhage
CC Excl: PDX collection 1023

**P12.3**   **Bruising of scalp due to birth injury**

**P12.4**   **Injury of scalp of newborn due to monitoring equipment**
Sampling incision of scalp of newborn
Scalp clip (electrode) injury of newborn

✅5ᵗʰ **P12.8**   **Other birth injuries to scalp**

**P12.81**   **Caput succedaneum**

**P12.89**   **Other birth injuries to scalp**

**P12.9**   **Birth injury to scalp, unspecified**

✅4ᵗʰ **P13**   **Birth injury to skeleton**
EXCLUDES 2   *birth injury to spine (P11.5)*

**P13.0**   **Fracture of skull due to birth injury**

**P13.1**   **Other birth injuries to skull**
EXCLUDES 1   *cephalhematoma (P12.0)*

**P13.2**   **Birth injury to femur**

**P13.3**   **Birth injury to other long bones**

**P13.4**   **Fracture of clavicle due to birth injury**

**P13.8**   **Birth injuries to other parts of skeleton**

**P13.9**   **Birth injury to skeleton, unspecified**

✅4ᵗʰ **P14**   **Birth injury to peripheral nervous system**

**P14.0**   **Erb's paralysis due to birth injury**

**P14.1**   **Klumpke's paralysis due to birth injury**

**P14.2**   **Phrenic nerve paralysis due to birth injury**

**P14.3**   **Other brachial plexus birth injuries**

**P14.8**   **Birth injuries to other parts of peripheral nervous system**

**P14.9**   **Birth injury to peripheral nervous system, unspecified**

✅4ᵗʰ **P15**   **Other birth injuries**

**P15.0**   **Birth injury to liver**
Rupture of liver due to birth injury

**P15.1**   **Birth injury to spleen**
Rupture of spleen due to birth injury

**P15.2**   **Sternomastoid injury due to birth injury**

**P15.3**   **Birth injury to eye**
Subconjunctival hemorrhage due to birth injury
Traumatic glaucoma due to birth injury

**P15.4**   **Birth injury to face**
Facial congestion due to birth injury

**P15.5**   **Birth injury to external genitalia**

**P15.6**   **Subcutaneous fat necrosis due to birth injury**

**P15.8**   **Other specified birth injuries**
TIP: Use for any injury of newborn from scalpel.

**P15.9**   **Birth injury, unspecified**

Ⓝ Newborn: 0   Ⓟ Pediatric: 0-17   Ⓜ Maternity: 12-55   Ⓐ Adult: 15-124   MCC Major CC Condition   PDxMCC PDx acts as own MCC   CC CC Condition   PDxCC PDx acts as own CC

884      ICD-10-CM 2018

## Respiratory and cardiovascular disorders specific to the perinatal period (P19-P29)

**✓4ᵗʰ P19 Metabolic acidemia in newborn**
> INCLUDES metabolic acidemia in newborn

**P19.0 Metabolic acidemia in newborn first noted before onset of labor**

**P19.1 Metabolic acidemia in newborn first noted during labor**

**P19.2 Metabolic acidemia noted at birth**

**P19.9 Metabolic acidemia, unspecified**

**✓4ᵗʰ P22 Respiratory distress of newborn**
> EXCLUDES 1 respiratory arrest of newborn (P28.81)
> respiratory failure of newborn NOS (P28.5)

**P22.0 Respiratory distress syndrome of newborn**   MCC
> Cardiorespiratory distress syndrome of newborn
> Hyaline membrane disease
> Idiopathic respiratory distress syndrome [IRDS or RDS] of newborn
> Pulmonary hypoperfusion syndrome
> Respiratory distress syndrome, type I
> **DEF:** Severe chest contractions upon air intake and expiratory grunting; infant appears blue due to oxygen deficiency and has rapid respiratory rate; formerly called hyaline membrane disease.
> **CC Excl:** PDX collection 748

**P22.1 Transient tachypnea of newborn**
> Idiopathic tachypnea of newborn
> Respiratory distress syndrome, type II
> Wet lung syndrome
> **DEF:** Rapid, labored breathing of newborn; short-term problem that begins after birth and lasts about three days.

**P22.8 Other respiratory distress of newborn**

**P22.9 Respiratory distress of newborn, unspecified**

**✓4ᵗʰ P23 Congenital pneumonia**
> INCLUDES infective pneumonia acquired in utero or during birth
> EXCLUDES 1 neonatal pneumonia resulting from aspiration (P24.-)

> **CC Excl: For MCC codes in subcategory P23:** PDX collection 748

**P23.0 Congenital pneumonia due to viral agent**   MCC
> Use additional code (B97) to identify organism
> EXCLUDES 1 congenital rubella pneumonitis (P35.0)

**P23.1 Congenital pneumonia due to Chlamydia**   MCC

**P23.2 Congenital pneumonia due to staphylococcus**   MCC

**P23.3 Congenital pneumonia due to streptococcus, group B**   MCC

**P23.4 Congenital pneumonia due to Escherichia coli**   MCC

**P23.5 Congenital pneumonia due to Pseudomonas**   MCC

**P23.6 Congenital pneumonia due to other bacterial agents**   MCC
> Congenital pneumonia due to Hemophilus influenzae
> Congenital pneumonia due to Klebsiella pneumoniae
> Congenital pneumonia due to Mycoplasma
> Congenital pneumonia due to Streptococcus, except group B
> Use additional code (B95-B96) to identify organism

**P23.8 Congenital pneumonia due to other organisms**   MCC

**P23.9 Congenital pneumonia, unspecified**   MCC

**✓4ᵗʰ P24 Neonatal aspiration**
> INCLUDES aspiration in utero and during delivery

> **CC Excl: For MCC codes in category P24:** PDX collection 748

**✓5ᵗʰ P24.0 Meconium aspiration**
> EXCLUDES 1 meconium passage (without aspiration) during delivery (P03.82)
> meconium staining (P96.83)

**P24.00 Meconium aspiration without respiratory symptoms**
> Meconium aspiration NOS

**P24.01 Meconium aspiration with respiratory symptoms**   MCC
> Meconium aspiration pneumonia
> Meconium aspiration pneumonitis
> Meconium aspiration syndrome NOS
> Use additional code to identify any secondary pulmonary hypertension, if applicable ▶(I27.2-)◀
> **DEF:** Aspiration of fetal intestinal material during or prior to delivery; usually a complication of placental insufficiency, causing pneumonitis and bronchial obstruction (inflammatory reaction of lungs).
> **CC Excl:** PDX collection 748

**✓5ᵗʰ P24.1 Neonatal aspiration of (clear) amniotic fluid and mucus**
> Neonatal aspiration of liquor (amnii)

**P24.10 Neonatal aspiration of (clear) amniotic fluid and mucus without respiratory symptoms**
> Neonatal aspiration of amniotic fluid and mucus NOS

**P24.11 Neonatal aspiration of (clear) amniotic fluid and mucus with respiratory symptoms**   MCC
> Neonatal aspiration of amniotic fluid and mucus with pneumonia
> Neonatal aspiration of amniotic fluid and mucus with pneumonitis
> Use additional code to identify any secondary pulmonary hypertension, if applicable ▶(I27.2-)◀
> **CC Excl:** PDX collection 748

**✓5ᵗʰ P24.2 Neonatal aspiration of blood**

**P24.20 Neonatal aspiration of blood without respiratory symptoms**
> Neonatal aspiration of blood NOS

**P24.21 Neonatal aspiration of blood with respiratory symptoms**   MCC
> Neonatal aspiration of blood with pneumonia
> Neonatal aspiration of blood with pneumonitis
> Use additional code to identify any secondary pulmonary hypertension, if applicable ▶(I27.2-)◀
> **CC Excl:** PDX collection 748

**✓5ᵗʰ P24.3 Neonatal aspiration of milk and regurgitated food**
> Neonatal aspiration of stomach contents

**P24.30 Neonatal aspiration of milk and regurgitated food without respiratory symptoms**
> Neonatal aspiration of milk and regurgitated food NOS

**P24.31 Neonatal aspiration of milk and regurgitated food with respiratory symptoms**   MCC
> Neonatal aspiration of milk and regurgitated food with pneumonia
> Neonatal aspiration of milk and regurgitated food with pneumonitis
> Use additional code to identify any secondary pulmonary hypertension, if applicable ▶(I27.2-)◀
> **CC Excl:** PDX collection 748

**✓5ᵗʰ P24.8 Other neonatal aspiration**

**P24.80 Other neonatal aspiration without respiratory symptoms**
> Neonatal aspiration NEC

**P24.81 Other neonatal aspiration with respiratory symptoms**   MCC
> Neonatal aspiration pneumonia NEC
> Neonatal aspiration with pneumonitis NEC
> Neonatal aspiration with pneumonia NOS
> Neonatal aspiration with pneumonitis NOS
> Use additional code to identify any secondary pulmonary hypertension, if applicable ▶(I27.2-)◀
> **CC Excl:** PDX collection 748

**P24.9 Neonatal aspiration, unspecified**

**✓4ᵗʰ P25 Interstitial emphysema and related conditions originating in the perinatal period**

> **CC Excl: For MCC codes in subcategory P25:** PDX collection 748

**P25.0 Interstitial emphysema originating in the perinatal period**   MCC

**P25.1 Pneumothorax originating in the perinatal period**   MCC

**P25.2 Pneumomediastinum originating in the perinatal period**   MCC

**P25.3 Pneumopericardium originating in the perinatal period**   MCC

**P25.8 Other conditions related to interstitial emphysema originating in the perinatal period**   MCC

**✓4ᵗʰ P26 Pulmonary hemorrhage originating in the perinatal period**
> EXCLUDES 1 acute idiopathic hemorrhage in infants over 28 days old (R04.81)

> **CC Excl: For MCC codes in subcategory P26:** PDX collection 748

**P26.0 Tracheobronchial hemorrhage originating in the perinatal period**   MCC

**P26.1 Massive pulmonary hemorrhage originating in the perinatal period**   MCC

**P26.8 Other pulmonary hemorrhages originating in the perinatal period**   MCC

**P26.9 Unspecified pulmonary hemorrhage originating in the perinatal period**   MCC

**Chapter 16. Certain Conditions Originating in the Perinatal Period**

P27–P37.1

✓4ᵗʰ **P27** **Chronic respiratory disease originating in the perinatal period**
> *EXCLUDES 1*   *respiratory distress of newborn (P22.0–P22.9)*
> *EXCLUDES 2* ▶*respiratory distress of newborn (P22.0-P22.9)*◀

    **P27.0**   **Wilson-Mikity syndrome**    `MCC`
       Pulmonary dysmaturity

    **P27.1**   **Bronchopulmonary dysplasia originating in the**   `MCC`
       **perinatal period**

    **P27.8**   **Other chronic respiratory diseases originating in the**   `MCC`
       **perinatal period**
       Congenital pulmonary fibrosis     Ventilator lung in newborn

    **P27.9**   **Unspecified chronic respiratory disease originating in**   `MCC`
       **the perinatal period**

✓4ᵗʰ **P28** **Other respiratory conditions originating in the perinatal period**
> *EXCLUDES 1*   *congenital malformations of the respiratory system (Q30-Q34)*

> **CC Excl: For CC/MCC codes in subcategory P28, unless otherwise noted:** PDX collection 748

    **P28.0**   **Primary atelectasis of newborn**    `CC`
       Primary failure to expand terminal respiratory units
       Pulmonary hypoplasia associated with short gestation
       Pulmonary immaturity NOS

    ✓5ᵗʰ **P28.1**   **Other and unspecified atelectasis of newborn**

       **P28.10**   **Unspecified atelectasis of newborn**    `CC`
          Atelectasis of newborn NOS

       **P28.11**   **Resorption atelectasis without respiratory**    `CC`
          **distress syndrome**
> *EXCLUDES 1*   *resorption atelectasis with respiratory distress syndrome (P22.0)*

       **P28.19**   **Other atelectasis of newborn**    `CC`
          Partial atelectasis of newborn
          Secondary atelectasis of newborn

    **P28.2**   **Cyanotic attacks of newborn**    `CC`
> *EXCLUDES 1*   *apnea of newborn (P28.3-P28.4)*
       **CC Excl:** PDX collection 1024

    **P28.3**   **Primary sleep apnea of newborn**    `CC`
       Central sleep apnea of newborn
       Obstructive sleep apnea of newborn
       Sleep apnea of newborn NOS
       **DEF:** Unexplained cessation of breathing when a neonate makes no respiratory effort for 20 seconds or longer, or when neonate's breathing cessation is accompanied by cyanosis, bradycardia, or hypotonia.
       **CC Excl:** PDX collection 1025

    **P28.4**   **Other apnea of newborn**    `CC`
       Apnea of prematurity
       Obstructive apnea of newborn
> *EXCLUDES 1*   *obstructive sleep apnea of newborn (P28.3)*
       **CC Excl:** PDX collection 1026

    **P28.5**   **Respiratory failure of newborn**    `MCC`
> *EXCLUDES 1*   *respiratory arrest of newborn (P28.81)*
>           *respiratory distress of newborn (P22.0-)*

    ✓5ᵗʰ **P28.8**   **Other specified respiratory conditions of newborn**

       **P28.81**   **Respiratory arrest of newborn**    `MCC`
          **CC Excl:** PDX collection 1027

       **P28.89**   **Other specified respiratory conditions of newborn**
          Congenital laryngeal stridor
          Sniffles in newborn
          Snuffles in newborn
> *EXCLUDES 1*   *early congenital syphilitic rhinitis (A50.05)*

    **P28.9**   **Respiratory condition of newborn, unspecified**
       Respiratory depression in newborn

✓4ᵗʰ **P29** **Cardiovascular disorders originating in the perinatal period**
> *EXCLUDES 1*   *congenital malformations of the circulatory system (Q20-Q28)*

    **P29.0**   **Neonatal cardiac failure**

    ✓5ᵗʰ **P29.1**   **Neonatal cardiac dysrhythmia**

       **P29.11**   **Neonatal tachycardia**

       **P29.12**   **Neonatal bradycardia**

    **P29.2**   **Neonatal hypertension**

    ✓5ᵗʰ **P29.3**   **Persistent fetal circulation**
       ~~Delayed closure of ductus arteriosus~~
       ~~(Persistent) pulmonary hypertension of newborn~~

> **CC Excl: For codes in subcategory P29.3:** PDX collection 1028

●      **P29.30**   **Pulmonary hypertension of newborn**    `MCC`
          Persistent pulmonary hypertension of newborn

●      **P29.38**   **Other persistent fetal circulation**    `MCC`
          Delayed closure of ductus arteriosus

    **P29.4**   **Transient myocardial ischemia in newborn**

    ✓5ᵗʰ **P29.8**   **Other cardiovascular disorders originating in the perinatal period**

       **P29.81**   **Cardiac arrest of newborn**    `MCC`
          **CC Excl:** PDX collection 1029

       **P29.89**   **Other cardiovascular disorders originating in the perinatal period**
          **AHA:** 2014, 4Q, 23

    **P29.9**   **Cardiovascular disorder originating in the perinatal period, unspecified**

## Infections specific to the perinatal period (P35-P39)

Infections acquired in utero, during birth via the umbilicus, or during the first 28 days after birth
> *EXCLUDES 2*   *asymptomatic human immunodeficiency virus [HIV] infection status (Z21)*
>           *congenital gonococcal infection (A54.-)*
>           *congenital pneumonia (P23.-)*
>           *congenital syphilis (A50.-)*
>           *human immunodeficiency virus [HIV] disease (B20)*
>           *infant botulism (A48.51)*
>           *infectious diseases not specific to the perinatal period (A00-B99, J09, J10-)*
>           *intestinal infectious disease (A00-A09)*
>           *laboratory evidence of human immunodeficiency virus [HIV] (R75)*
>           *tetanus neonatorum (A33)*

✓4ᵗʰ **P35** **Congenital viral diseases**
> *INCLUDES*   infections acquired in utero or during birth

> **CC Excl: For MCC codes in category P35, unless otherwise noted:** PDX collection 562

    **P35.0**   **Congenital rubella syndrome**    `CC`
       Congenital rubella pneumonitis
       **CC Excl:** PDX collection 1030

    **P35.1**   **Congenital cytomegalovirus infection**    `MCC`
       **CC Excl:** PDX collection 1030

    **P35.2**   **Congenital herpesviral [herpes simplex] infection**    `MCC`

    **P35.3**   **Congenital viral hepatitis**    `MCC`

    **P35.8**   **Other congenital viral diseases**    `MCC`
       Congenital varicella [chickenpox]

    **P35.9**   **Congenital viral disease, unspecified**    `MCC`

✓4ᵗʰ **P36** **Bacterial sepsis of newborn**
> *INCLUDES*   congenital sepsis

Use additional code(s), if applicable, to identify severe sepsis (R65.2-) and associated acute organ dysfunction(s)

> **CC Excl: For MCC codes in subcategory P36:** PDX collection 1031

    **P36.0**   **Sepsis of newborn due to streptococcus, group B**    `MCC` `HCC`

    ✓5ᵗʰ **P36.1**   **Sepsis of newborn due to other and unspecified streptococci**

       **P36.10**   **Sepsis of newborn due to unspecified streptococci**    `MCC` `HCC`

       **P36.19**   **Sepsis of newborn due to other streptococci**    `MCC` `HCC`

    **P36.2**   **Sepsis of newborn due to Staphylococcus aureus**    `MCC` `HCC`

    ✓5ᵗʰ **P36.3**   **Sepsis of newborn due to other and unspecified staphylococci**

       **P36.30**   **Sepsis of newborn due to unspecified staphylococci**    `MCC` `HCC`

       **P36.39**   **Sepsis of newborn due to other staphylococci**    `MCC` `HCC`

    **P36.4**   **Sepsis of newborn due to Escherichia coli**    `MCC` `HCC`

    **P36.5**   **Sepsis of newborn due to anaerobes**    `MCC` `HCC`

    **P36.8**   **Other bacterial sepsis of newborn**    `MCC` `HCC`
       Use additional code from category B96 to identify organism

    **P36.9**   **Bacterial sepsis of newborn, unspecified**    `MCC` `HCC`

✓4ᵗʰ **P37** **Other congenital infectious and parasitic diseases**
> *EXCLUDES 2*   *congenital syphilis (A50.-)*
>           *infectious neonatal diarrhea (A00-A09)*
>           *necrotizing enterocolitis in newborn (P77.-)*
>           *noninfectious neonatal diarrhea (P78.3)*
>           *ophthalmia neonatorum due to gonococcus (A54.31)*
>           *tetanus neonatorum (A33)*

> **CC Excl: For MCC codes in subcategory P37:** PDX collection 562

    **P37.0**   **Congenital tuberculosis**    `MCC`

    **P37.1**   **Congenital toxoplasmosis**    `MCC`
       Hydrocephalus due to congenital toxoplasmosis

---

Ⓝ Newborn: 0   Ⓟ Pediatric: 0-17   Ⓜ Maternity: 12-55   Ⓐ Adult: 15-124   `MCC` Major CC Condition   `PDxMCC` PDx acts as own MCC   `CC` CC Condition   `PDxCC` PDx acts as own CC

P37.2 **Neonatal (disseminated)** listeriosis    `MCC`

P37.3 **Congenital** falciparum malaria    `MCC`

P37.4 **Other congenital** malaria    `MCC`

P37.5 **Neonatal** candidiasis

P37.8 **Other** specified congenital infectious and parasitic diseases    `MCC`

P37.9 **Congenital infectious or parasitic disease,** unspecified    `MCC`

☑4ᵗʰ **P38 Omphalitis of newborn**
  *EXCLUDES 1*  omphalitis not of newborn (L08.82)
         tetanus omphalitis (A33)
         umbilical hemorrhage of newborn (P51.-)

P38.1 **Omphalitis with mild hemorrhage**    `CC`
    **CC Excl:** PDX collection 1032

P38.9 **Omphalitis without hemorrhage**    `CC`
    Omphalitis of newborn NOS
    **CC Excl:** PDX collection 1032

☑4ᵗʰ **P39 Other infections specific to the perinatal period**
  Use additional code to identify organism or specific infection

  **CC Excl: For CC codes in category P39, unless otherwise noted:** PDX collection 1033

P39.0 **Neonatal infective** mastitis    `CC`
    *EXCLUDES 1*  breast engorgement of newborn (P83.4)
           noninfective mastitis of newborn (P83.4)
    **CC Excl:** PDX collection 1032

P39.1 **Neonatal** conjunctivitis and dacryocystitis
    Neonatal chlamydial conjunctivitis
    Ophthalmia neonatorum NOS
    *EXCLUDES 1*  gonococcal conjunctivitis (A54.31)

P39.2 **Intra-amniotic infection affecting newborn, not elsewhere classified**    `CC`

P39.3 **Neonatal** urinary tract infection    `CC`
    **CC Excl:** PDX collection 1034

P39.4 **Neonatal** skin infection    `CC`
    Neonatal pyoderma
    *EXCLUDES 1*  pemphigus neonatorum (L00)
           staphylococcal scalded skin syndrome (L00)

P39.8 **Other** specified infections specific to the perinatal period    `CC`

P39.9 **Infection specific to the perinatal period,** unspecified    `CC`

## Hemorrhagic and hematological disorders of newborn (P50-P61)

*EXCLUDES 1*  congenital stenosis and stricture of bile ducts (Q44.3)
       Crigler-Najjar syndrome (E80.5)
       Dubin-Johnson syndrome (E80.6)
       Gilbert syndrome (E80.4)
       hereditary hemolytic anemias (D55-D58)

☑4ᵗʰ **P50 Newborn affected by intrauterine (fetal) blood loss**
  *EXCLUDES 1*  congenital anemia from intrauterine (fetal) blood loss (P61.3)

P50.0 **Newborn affected by intrauterine (fetal) blood loss from vasa previa**

P50.1 **Newborn affected by intrauterine (fetal) blood loss from ruptured cord**

P50.2 **Newborn affected by intrauterine (fetal) blood loss from placenta**

P50.3 **Newborn affected by hemorrhage into** co-twin

P50.4 **Newborn affected by hemorrhage into** maternal circulation

P50.5 **Newborn affected by intrauterine (fetal) blood loss from cut end of co-twin's cord**

P50.8 **Newborn affected by other intrauterine (fetal) blood loss**

P50.9 **Newborn affected by intrauterine (fetal) blood loss, unspecified**
    Newborn affected by fetal hemorrhage NOS

☑4ᵗʰ **P51 Umbilical hemorrhage of newborn**
  *EXCLUDES 1*  omphalitis with mild hemorrhage (P38.1)
         umbilical hemorrhage from cut end of co-twins cord (P50.5)

P51.0 **Massive umbilical hemorrhage of newborn**

P51.8 **Other umbilical hemorrhages of newborn**
    Slipped umbilical ligature NOS

P51.9 **Umbilical hemorrhage of newborn,** unspecified

☑4ᵗʰ **P52 Intracranial nontraumatic hemorrhage of newborn**
  `INCLUDES`  intracranial hemorrhage due to anoxia or hypoxia
  *EXCLUDES 1*  intracranial hemorrhage due to birth injury (P10.-)
         intracranial hemorrhage due to other injury (S06.-)

P52.0 **Intraventricular (nontraumatic) hemorrhage, grade 1, of newborn**    `CC`
    Subependymal hemorrhage (without intraventricular extension)
    Bleeding into germinal matrix
    **CC Excl:** PDX collection 1021

P52.1 **Intraventricular (nontraumatic) hemorrhage, grade 2, of newborn**    `CC`
    Subependymal hemorrhage with intraventricular extension
    Bleeding into ventricle
    **CC Excl:** PDX collection 1021

☑5ᵗʰ **P52.2 Intraventricular (nontraumatic) hemorrhage, grade 3 and grade 4, of newborn**

P52.21 **Intraventricular (nontraumatic) hemorrhage, grade 3, of newborn**    `MCC`
    Subependymal hemorrhage with intraventricular extension with enlargement of ventricle
    **CC Excl:** PDX collection 1021

P52.22 **Intraventricular (nontraumatic) hemorrhage, grade 4, of newborn**    `MCC`
    Bleeding into cerebral cortex
    Subependymal hemorrhage with intracerebral extension
    **CC Excl:** PDX collection 1021

P52.3 **Unspecified intraventricular (nontraumatic) hemorrhage of newborn**    `CC`
    **CC Excl:** PDX collection 1021

P52.4 **Intracerebral (nontraumatic) hemorrhage of newborn**    `MCC`
    **CC Excl:** PDX collection 1020

P52.5 **Subarachnoid (nontraumatic) hemorrhage of newborn**    `MCC`
    **CC Excl:** PDX collection 1022

P52.6 **Cerebellar (nontraumatic) and posterior fossa hemorrhage of newborn**    `MCC`
    **CC Excl:** PDX collection 1020

P52.8 **Other intracranial (nontraumatic) hemorrhages of newborn**    `MCC`
    **CC Excl:** PDX collection 1020

P52.9 **Intracranial (nontraumatic) hemorrhage of newborn, unspecified**    `MCC`
    **CC Excl:** PDX collection 1020

P53 **Hemorrhagic disease of newborn**    `CC`
    Vitamin K deficiency of newborn
    **CC Excl:** PDX collection 1035

☑4ᵗʰ **P54 Other neonatal hemorrhages**
  *EXCLUDES 1*  newborn affected by (intrauterine) blood loss (P50.-)
         pulmonary hemorrhage originating in the perinatal period (P26.-)

  **CC Excl: For CC/MCC codes in category P54:** PDX collection 1036

P54.0 **Neonatal hematemesis**
    *EXCLUDES 1*  neonatal hematemesis due to swallowed maternal blood (P78.2)

P54.1 **Neonatal melena**    `MCC`
    *EXCLUDES 1*  neonatal melena due to swallowed maternal blood (P78.2)

P54.2 **Neonatal rectal hemorrhage**    `MCC`

P54.3 **Other neonatal gastrointestinal hemorrhage**    `MCC`

P54.4 **Neonatal adrenal hemorrhage**    `CC`

P54.5 **Neonatal cutaneous hemorrhage**
    Neonatal bruising
    Neonatal ecchymoses
    Neonatal petechiae
    Neonatal superficial hematomata
    *EXCLUDES 2*  bruising of scalp due to birth injury (P12.3)
           cephalhematoma due to birth injury (P12.0)

P54.6 **Neonatal vaginal hemorrhage**    ♀
    Neonatal pseudomenses

P54.8 **Other specified neonatal hemorrhages**

P54.9 **Neonatal hemorrhage, unspecified**

**Chapter 16. Certain Conditions Originating in the Perinatal Period**

**P55-P71.8**

### ✓4th P55 Hemolytic disease of newborn

**P55.0 Rh isoimmunization of newborn**
DEF: Incompatible Rh fetal-maternal blood grouping; prematurely destroys red blood cells; characterized by jaundice, asphyxia, pulmonary hypertension, edema, respiratory distress, kernicterus, and coagulopathies; detected by Coombs test.

**P55.1 ABO isoimmunization of newborn**
AHA: 2015, 3Q, 20

**P55.8 Other hemolytic diseases of newborn**

**P55.9 Hemolytic disease of newborn, unspecified**

### ✓4th P56 Hydrops fetalis due to hemolytic disease

EXCLUDES 1   hydrops fetalis NOS (P83.2)

**CC Excl: For MCC codes in subcategory P56: PDX collection 1037**

**P56.0 Hydrops fetalis due to isoimmunization**   MCC

✓5th **P56.9 Hydrops fetalis due to other and unspecified hemolytic disease**

**P56.90 Hydrops fetalis due to unspecified hemolytic disease**   MCC

**P56.99 Hydrops fetalis due to other hemolytic disease**   MCC

### ✓4th P57 Kernicterus

**P57.0 Kernicterus due to isoimmunization**   MCC
DEF: Complication of erythroblastosis fetalis associated with severe neural symptoms, high blood bilirubin levels and nerve cell destruction; results in bilirubin-pigmented gray matter of central nervous system.
CC Excl: PDX collection 1037

**P57.8 Other specified kernicterus**   MCC
EXCLUDES 1   Crigler-Najjar syndrome (E80.5)
CC Excl: PDX collection 1038

**P57.9 Kernicterus, unspecified**   MCC
CC Excl: PDX collection 1038

### ✓4th P58 Neonatal jaundice due to other excessive hemolysis

EXCLUDES 1   jaundice due to isoimmunization (P55-P57)

**P58.0 Neonatal jaundice due to bruising**

**P58.1 Neonatal jaundice due to bleeding**

**P58.2 Neonatal jaundice due to infection**

**P58.3 Neonatal jaundice due to polycythemia**

✓5th **P58.4 Neonatal jaundice due to drugs or toxins transmitted from mother or given to newborn**
Code first poisoning due to drug or toxin, if applicable (T36-T65 with fifth or sixth character 1-4 or 6)
Use additional code for adverse effect, if applicable, to identify drug (T36-T50 with fifth or sixth character 5)

**P58.41 Neonatal jaundice due to drugs or toxins transmitted from mother**

**P58.42 Neonatal jaundice due to drugs or toxins given to newborn**

**P58.5 Neonatal jaundice due to swallowed maternal blood**

**P58.8 Neonatal jaundice due to other specified excessive hemolysis**

**P58.9 Neonatal jaundice due to excessive hemolysis, unspecified**

### ✓4th P59 Neonatal jaundice from other and unspecified causes

EXCLUDES 1   jaundice due to inborn errors of metabolism (E70-E88)
kernicterus (P57.-)

**CC Excl: For MCC codes in category P59: PDX collection 1038**

**P59.0 Neonatal jaundice associated with preterm delivery**
Hyperbilirubinemia of prematurity
Jaundice due to delayed conjugation associated with preterm delivery

**P59.1 Inspissated bile syndrome**   MCC

✓5th **P59.2 Neonatal jaundice from other and unspecified hepatocellular damage**
EXCLUDES 1   congenital viral hepatitis (P35.3)

**P59.20 Neonatal jaundice from unspecified hepatocellular damage**   MCC

**P59.29 Neonatal jaundice from other hepatocellular damage**   MCC
Neonatal giant cell hepatitis
Neonatal (idiopathic) hepatitis

**P59.3 Neonatal jaundice from breast milk inhibitor**

**P59.8 Neonatal jaundice from other specified causes**

**P59.9 Neonatal jaundice, unspecified**
Neonatal physiological jaundice (intense)(prolonged) NOS
AHA: 2015, 3Q, 20

---

### P60 Disseminated intravascular coagulation of newborn   MCC
Defibrination syndrome of newborn
CC Excl: PDX collection 1035

### ✓4th P61 Other perinatal hematological disorders

EXCLUDES 1   transient hypogammaglobulinemia of infancy (D80.7)

**P61.0 Transient neonatal thrombocytopenia**   MCC
Neonatal thrombocytopenia due to exchange transfusion
Neonatal thrombocytopenia due to idiopathic maternal thrombocytopenia
Neonatal thrombocytopenia due to isoimmunization
DEF: Temporary decrease in blood platelets of newborn; secondary to placental insufficiency.
CC Excl: PDX collection 1035

**P61.1 Polycythemia neonatorum**
DEF: Abnormal increase of total red blood cells of newborn; results in hyperviscosity, which slows the flow of blood through small blood vessels.

**P61.2 Anemia of prematurity**   CC
CC Excl: PDX collection 1039

**P61.3 Congenital anemia from fetal blood loss**   CC
CC Excl: PDX collection 1039

**P61.4 Other congenital anemias, not elsewhere classified**   CC
Congenital anemia NOS
CC Excl: PDX collection 1039

**P61.5 Transient neonatal neutropenia**   MCC
EXCLUDES 1   congenital neutropenia (nontransient) (D70.0)
DEF: Low blood neutrophil counts of newborn; occurs due to maternal hypertension, sepsis, twin-twin transfusion, alloimmunization, and hemolytic disease.
CC Excl: PDX collection 1040

**P61.6 Other transient neonatal disorders of coagulation**   CC
CC Excl: PDX collection 1035

**P61.8 Other specified perinatal hematological disorders**

**P61.9 Perinatal hematological disorder, unspecified**

## Transitory endocrine and metabolic disorders specific to newborn (P70-P74)

INCLUDES   transitory endocrine and metabolic disturbances caused by the infant's response to maternal endocrine and metabolic factors, or its adjustment to extrauterine environment

### ✓4th P70 Transitory disorders of carbohydrate metabolism specific to newborn

**P70.0 Syndrome of infant of mother with gestational diabetes**
Newborn (with hypoglycemia) affected by maternal gestational diabetes
EXCLUDES 1   newborn (with hypoglycemia) affected by maternal (pre-existing) diabetes mellitus (P70.1)
syndrome of infant of a diabetic mother (P70.1)

**P70.1 Syndrome of infant of a diabetic mother**
Newborn (with hypoglycemia) affected by maternal (pre-existing) diabetes mellitus
EXCLUDES 1   newborn (with hypoglycemia) affected by maternal gestational diabetes (P70.0)
syndrome of infant of mother with gestational diabetes (P70.0)

**P70.2 Neonatal diabetes mellitus**   CC
CC Excl: PDX collection 1041

**P70.3 Iatrogenic neonatal hypoglycemia**

**P70.4 Other neonatal hypoglycemia**
Transitory neonatal hypoglycemia

**P70.8 Other transitory disorders of carbohydrate metabolism of newborn**   CC
CC Excl: PDX collection 1042

**P70.9 Transitory disorder of carbohydrate metabolism of newborn, unspecified**

### ✓4th P71 Transitory neonatal disorders of calcium and magnesium metabolism

**CC Excl: For CC codes in category P71: PDX collection 1041**

**P71.0 Cow's milk hypocalcemia in newborn**   CC

**P71.1 Other neonatal hypocalcemia**   CC
EXCLUDES 1   neonatal hypoparathyroidism (P71.4)

**P71.2 Neonatal hypomagnesemia**   CC

**P71.3 Neonatal tetany without calcium or magnesium deficiency**   CC
Neonatal tetany NOS

**P71.4 Transitory neonatal hypoparathyroidism**   CC

**P71.8 Other transitory neonatal disorders of calcium and magnesium metabolism**   CC

---

N Newborn: 0    P Pediatric: 0-17    M Maternity: 12-55    A Adult: 15-124    MCC Major CC Condition    PDx MCC PDx acts as own MCC    CC CC Condition    PDx CC PDx acts as own CC

**P71.9**   **Transitory neonatal disorder of calcium and magnesium metabolism, unspecified**   CC

☑4th **P72**   **Other transitory neonatal endocrine disorders**
> EXCLUDES 1   congenital hypothyroidism with or without goiter (E03.0-E03.1)
> dyshormogenetic goiter (E07.1)
> Pendred's syndrome (E07.1)

> **CC Excl: For CC codes in category P72:** PDX collection 1042

**P72.0**   **Neonatal goiter, not elsewhere classified**   CC
> Transitory congenital goiter with normal functioning

**P72.1**   **Transitory neonatal hyperthyroidism**   CC
> Neonatal thyrotoxicosis
> **CC Excl:** PDX collection 1041

**P72.2**   **Other transitory neonatal disorders of thyroid function, not elsewhere classified**   CC
> Transitory neonatal hypothyroidism

**P72.8**   **Other specified transitory neonatal endocrine disorders**   CC

**P72.9**   **Transitory neonatal endocrine disorder, unspecified**

☑4th **P74**   **Other transitory neonatal electrolyte and metabolic disturbances**

> **CC Excl: For CC codes in category P74:** PDX collection 1042

**P74.0**   **Late metabolic acidosis of newborn**   MCC
> EXCLUDES 1   (fetal) metabolic acidosis of newborn (P19)
> **CC Excl:** PDX collection 1041

**P74.1**   **Dehydration of newborn**

**P74.2**   **Disturbances of sodium balance of newborn**

**P74.3**   **Disturbances of potassium balance of newborn**

**P74.4**   **Other transitory electrolyte disturbances of newborn**

**P74.5**   **Transitory tyrosinemia of newborn**   CC

**P74.6**   **Transitory hyperammonemia of newborn**   CC

**P74.8**   **Other transitory metabolic disturbances of newborn**   CC
> Amino-acid metabolic disorders described as transitory

**P74.9**   **Transitory metabolic disturbance of newborn, unspecified**

### Digestive system disorders of newborn (P76-P78)

☑4th **P76**   **Other intestinal obstruction of newborn**

**P76.0**   **Meconium plug syndrome**
> Meconium ileus NOS
> EXCLUDES 1   meconium ileus in cystic fibrosis (E84.11)

**P76.1**   **Transitory ileus of newborn**   CC
> EXCLUDES 1   Hirschsprung's disease (Q43.1)
> **CC Excl:** PDX collection 1043

**P76.2**   **Intestinal obstruction due to inspissated milk**

**P76.8**   **Other specified intestinal obstruction of newborn**
> EXCLUDES 1   intestinal obstruction classifiable to K56-.

**P76.9**   **Intestinal obstruction of newborn, unspecified**

☑4th **P77**   **Necrotizing enterocolitis of newborn**
> **DEF:** Serious intestinal infection and inflammation in preterm infants; severity is measured by stages and may progress to life-threatening perforation or peritonitis; resection surgical treatment may be necessary.

> **CC Excl: For MCC codes in category P77:** PDX collection 1044

**P77.1**   **Stage 1 necrotizing enterocolitis in newborn**   MCC
> Necrotizing enterocolitis without pneumatosis, without perforation
> **DEF:** Broad-spectrum symptoms with nonspecific signs, including feeding intolerance, abdominal distention, bradycardia, and metabolic abnormalities.

**P77.2**   **Stage 2 necrotizing enterocolitis in newborn**   MCC
> Necrotizing enterocolitis with pneumatosis, without perforation
> **DEF:** Radiographic confirmation of necrotizing enterocolitis showing intestinal dilatation, fixed loops of bowels, pneumatosis intestinalis, metabolic acidosis, and thrombocytopenia.

**P77.3**   **Stage 3 necrotizing enterocolitis in newborn**   MCC
> Necrotizing enterocolitis with perforation
> Necrotizing enterocolitis with pneumatosis and perforation
> **DEF:** Advanced stage in which infant demonstrates signs of bowel perforation, septic shock, metabolic acidosis, ascites, disseminated intravascular coagulopathy, neutropenia.

**P77.9**   **Necrotizing enterocolitis in newborn, unspecified**   MCC
> Necrotizing enterocolitis in newborn, NOS

☑4th **P78**   **Other perinatal digestive system disorders**
> EXCLUDES 1   cystic fibrosis (E84.0-E84.9)
> neonatal gastrointestinal hemorrhages (P54.0-P54.3)

**P78.0**   **Perinatal intestinal perforation**   MCC
> Meconium peritonitis
> **CC Excl:** PDX collection 1044

**P78.1**   **Other neonatal peritonitis**
> Neonatal peritonitis NOS

**P78.2**   **Neonatal hematemesis and melena due to swallowed maternal blood**

**P78.3**   **Noninfective neonatal diarrhea**
> Neonatal diarrhea NOS

☑5th **P78.8**   **Other specified perinatal digestive system disorders**

**P78.81**   **Congenital cirrhosis (of liver)**

**P78.82**   **Peptic ulcer of newborn**

**P78.83**   **Newborn esophageal reflux**
> Neonatal esophageal reflux

● **P78.84**   **Gestational alloimmune liver disease**
> GALD
> Neonatal hemochromatosis
> EXCLUDES 1   hemochromatosis (E83.11-)

**P78.89**   **Other specified perinatal digestive system disorders**

**P78.9**   **Perinatal digestive system disorder, unspecified**

### Conditions involving the integument and temperature regulation of newborn (P80-P83)

☑4th **P80**   **Hypothermia of newborn**

**P80.0**   **Cold injury syndrome**
> Severe and usually chronic hypothermia associated with a pink flushed appearance, edema and neurological and biochemical abnormalities.
> EXCLUDES 1   mild hypothermia of newborn (P80.8)

**P80.8**   **Other hypothermia of newborn**
> Mild hypothermia of newborn

**P80.9**   **Hypothermia of newborn, unspecified**

☑4th **P81**   **Other disturbances of temperature regulation of newborn**

**P81.0**   **Environmental hyperthermia of newborn**

**P81.8**   **Other specified disturbances of temperature regulation of newborn**

**P81.9**   **Disturbance of temperature regulation of newborn, unspecified**
> Fever of newborn NOS

☑4th **P83**   **Other conditions of integument specific to newborn**
> EXCLUDES 1   congenital malformations of skin and integument (Q80-Q84)
> hydrops fetalis due to hemolytic disease (P56.-)
> neonatal skin infection (P39.4)
> staphylococcal scalded skin syndrome (L00)
> EXCLUDES 2   cradle cap (L21.0)
> diaper [napkin] dermatitis (L22)

**P83.0**   **Sclerema neonatorum**   CC
> **DEF:** Diffuse, rapidly progressing white, waxy, nonpitting hardening of tissue, usually of legs and feet that is life-threatening; found in preterm or debilitated infants; unknown etiology.
> **CC Excl:** PDX collection 1045

**P83.1**   **Neonatal erythema toxicum**

**P83.2**   **Hydrops fetalis not due to hemolytic disease**   MCC
> Hydrops fetalis NOS
> **DEF:** Severe, life-threatening problem of newborn characterized by severe edema of entire body; unrelated to immune response.
> **CC Excl:** PDX collection 1046

☑5th **P83.3**   **Other and unspecified edema specific to newborn**

**P83.30**   **Unspecified edema specific to newborn**   CC
> **CC Excl:** PDX collection 1047

**P83.39**   **Other edema specific to newborn**   CC
> **CC Excl:** PDX collection 1047

**P83.4**   **Breast engorgement of newborn**
> Noninfective mastitis of newborn

**P83.5**   **Congenital hydrocele**   ♂

**P83.6**   **Umbilical polyp of newborn**

☑ Additional Character Req   ☑x7th Placeholder Alert   Unacceptable PDx   Manifestation   H1-H14 HAC   HCC CMS-HCC Condition   EXCLUDES 1 Not Coded Here   EXCLUDES 2 Not Included Here

**ICD-10-CM 2018**      **889**

√5ᵗʰ **P83.8** **Other specified conditions of integument specific to newborn**
~~Bronze baby syndrome~~
~~Neonatal scleroderma~~
~~Urticaria neonatorum~~

●    **P83.81** **Umbilical granuloma**
*EXCLUDES 2*   *granulomatous disorder of the skin and subcutaneous tissue, unspecified (L92.9)*

●    **P83.88** **Other specified conditions of integument specific to newborn**
Bronze baby syndrome
Neonatal scleroderma
Urticaria neonatorum

**P83.9** **Condition of the integument specific to newborn, unspecified**

### Other problems with newborn (P84)

**P84** **Other problems with newborn**
Acidemia of newborn     Hypoxemia of newborn
Acidosis of newborn     Hypoxia of newborn NOS
Anoxia of newborn NOS     Mixed metabolic and respiratory
Asphyxia of newborn NOS     acidosis of newborn
Hypercapnia of newborn
*EXCLUDES 1*   *intracranial hemorrhage due to anoxia or hypoxia (P52.-)*
*hypoxic ischemic encephalopathy [HIE] (P91.6-)*
*late metabolic acidosis of newborn (P74.0)*

### Other disorders originating in the perinatal period (P90-P96)

**P90** **Convulsions of newborn**     MCC
*EXCLUDES 1*   *benign myoclonic epilepsy in infancy (G40.3-)*
*benign neonatal convulsions (familial) (G40.3-)*
**CC Excl:** PDX collection 1048

√4ᵗʰ **P91** **Other disturbances of cerebral status of newborn**

**CC Excl: For CC/MCC codes in category P91, unless otherwise noted:** PDX collection 1049

**P91.0** **Neonatal cerebral ischemia**     MCC
**P91.1** **Acquired periventricular cysts of newborn**     MCC
**P91.2** **Neonatal cerebral leukomalacia**     MCC
Periventricular leukomalacia
**CC Excl:** PDX collection 1022
**P91.3** **Neonatal cerebral irritability**     MCC
**P91.4** **Neonatal cerebral depression**     MCC
**P91.5** **Neonatal coma**     MCC

√5ᵗʰ **P91.6** **Hypoxic ischemic encephalopathy [HIE]**
*EXCLUDES 1* ▶*neonatal cerebral depression (P91.4)*
*neonatal cerebral irritability (P91.3)*
*neonatal coma (P91.5)*◀

**CC Excl: For CC/MCC codes in subcategory P91.6:** PDX collection 1050

**P91.60** **Hypoxic ischemic encephalopathy [HIE], unspecified**     CC
**P91.61** **Mild hypoxic ischemic encephalopathy [HIE]**     CC
**P91.62** **Moderate hypoxic ischemic encephalopathy [HIE]**     CC
**P91.63** **Severe hypoxic ischemic encephalopathy [HIE]**     MCC

√5ᵗʰ **P91.8** **Other specified disturbances of cerebral status of newborn**
●    √6ᵗʰ **P91.81** **Neonatal encephalopathy**
●      **P91.811** **Neonatal encephalopathy in diseases classified elsewhere**
Code first underlying condition, if known, such as:
congenital cirrhosis (of liver) (P78.71)
intracranial nontraumatic hemorrhage of newborn (P52.-)
kernicterus (P57.-)
●      **P91.819** **Neonatal encephalopathy, unspecified**
●    **P91.88** **Other specified disturbances of cerebral status of newborn**
**P91.9** **Disturbance of cerebral status of newborn, unspecified**

√4ᵗʰ **P92** **Feeding problems of newborn**
*EXCLUDES 1* ▶*eating disorders (F50.-)*◀
*feeding problems in child over 28 days old (R63.3)*
**AHA:** 2016, 3Q, 19

√5ᵗʰ **P92.0** **Vomiting of newborn**
*EXCLUDES 1*   *vomiting of child over 28 days old (R11.-)*
**P92.01** **Bilious vomiting of newborn**     MCC
*EXCLUDES 1*   *bilious vomiting in child over 28 days old (R11.14)*
**CC Excl:** PDX collection 1051
**P92.09** **Other vomiting of newborn**
*EXCLUDES 1*   *regurgitation of food in newborn (P92.1)*

**P92.1** **Regurgitation and rumination of newborn**
**P92.2** **Slow feeding of newborn**
**P92.3** **Underfeeding of newborn**
**P92.4** **Overfeeding of newborn**
**P92.5** **Neonatal difficulty in feeding at breast**
**AHA:** 2017, 1Q, 28
**P92.6** **Failure to thrive in newborn**
*EXCLUDES 1*   *failure to thrive in child over 28 days old (R62.51)*
**P92.8** **Other feeding problems of newborn**
**P92.9** **Feeding problem of newborn, unspecified**

√4ᵗʰ **P93** **Reactions and intoxications due to drugs administered to newborn**
*INCLUDES*   reactions and intoxications due to drugs administered to fetus affecting newborn
*EXCLUDES 1*   *jaundice due to drugs or toxins transmitted from mother or given to newborn (P58.4-)*
*reactions and intoxications from maternal opiates, tranquilizers and other medication (P04.0-P04.1, P04.4)*
*withdrawal symptoms from maternal use of drugs of addiction (P96.1)*
*withdrawal symptoms from therapeutic use of drugs in newborn (P96.2)*

**P93.0** **Grey baby syndrome**     CC
Grey syndrome from chloramphenicol administration in newborn
**CC Excl:** PDX collection 1052
**P93.8** **Other reactions and intoxications due to drugs administered to newborn**     CC
Use additional code for adverse effect, if applicable, to identify drug (T36-T50 with fifth or sixth character 5)
**CC Excl:** PDX collection 1052

√4ᵗʰ **P94** **Disorders of muscle tone of newborn**
**P94.0** **Transient neonatal myasthenia gravis**     CC
*EXCLUDES 1*   *myasthenia gravis (G70.0)*
**CC Excl:** PDX collection 1041
**P94.1** **Congenital hypertonia**
**P94.2** **Congenital hypotonia**
Floppy baby syndrome, unspecified
**P94.8** **Other disorders of muscle tone of newborn**
**P94.9** **Disorder of muscle tone of newborn, unspecified**

**P95** **Stillbirth**
Deadborn fetus NOS
Fetal death of unspecified cause
Stillbirth NOS
*EXCLUDES 1*   *maternal care for intrauterine death (O36.4)*
*missed abortion (O02.1)*
*outcome of delivery, stillbirth (Z37.1, Z37.3, Z37.4, Z37.7)*

√4ᵗʰ **P96** **Other conditions originating in the perinatal period**
**P96.0** **Congenital renal failure**
Uremia of newborn
**P96.1** **Neonatal withdrawal symptoms from maternal use of drugs of addiction**     CC
Drug withdrawal syndrome in infant of dependent mother
Neonatal abstinence syndrome
*EXCLUDES 1*   *reactions and intoxications from maternal opiates and tranquilizers administered during labor and delivery (P04.0)*
**CC Excl:** PDX collection 1052
**P96.2** **Withdrawal symptoms from therapeutic use of drugs in newborn**     CC
**CC Excl:** PDX collection 1052
**P96.3** **Wide cranial sutures of newborn**
Neonatal craniotabes

N Newborn: 0   P Pediatric: 0-17   M Maternity: 12-55   A Adult: 15-124   MCC Major CC Condition   PDx MCC PDx acts as own MCC   CC CC Condition   PDx CC PDx acts as own CC

P83.8–P96.3

890      ICD-10-CM 2018

**P96.5**    **Complication to newborn due to (fetal) intrauterine procedure**

> EXCLUDES 2    *newborn affected by amniocentesis (P00.6)*

✓5ᵗʰ **P96.8**    **Other specified conditions originating in the perinatal period**

     **P96.81**    **Exposure to (parental) (environmental) tobacco smoke in the perinatal period**

> EXCLUDES 2    *newborn affected by in utero exposure to tobacco (P04.2)*
> *exposure to environmental tobacco smoke after the perinatal period (Z77.22)*

     **P96.82**    **Delayed separation of umbilical cord**

     **P96.83**    **Meconium staining**

> EXCLUDES 1    *meconium aspiration (P24.00, P24.01)*
> *meconium passage during delivery (P03.82)*

     **P96.89**    **Other specified conditions originating in the perinatal period**

        Use additional code to specify condition

**P96.9**    **Condition originating in the perinatal period, unspecified**

     Congenital debility NOS

✓ Additional Character Req    ✓x7ᵗʰ Placeholder Alert    Unacceptable PDx    Manifestation    H1-H14 HAC    HCC CMS-HCC Condition    EXCLUDES 1 Not Coded Here    EXCLUDES 2 Not Included Here

ICD-10-CM 2018            **891**

# Chapter 17. Congenital Malformations, Deformations and Chromosomal Abnormalities (Q00–Q99)

## Chapter Specific Guidelines with Coding Examples

The chapter specific guidelines from the ICD-10-CM Official Guidelines for Coding and Reporting have been provided below. Along with these guidelines are coding examples, contained in the shaded boxes, that have been developed to help illustrate the coding and/or sequencing guidance found in these guidelines.

Assign an appropriate code(s) from categories Q00-Q99, Congenital malformations, deformations, and chromosomal abnormalities when a malformation/deformation or chromosomal abnormality is documented. A malformation/deformation/or chromosomal abnormality may be the principal/first-listed diagnosis on a record or a secondary diagnosis.

When a malformation/deformation/or chromosomal abnormality does not have a unique code assignment, assign additional code(s) for any manifestations that may be present.

When the code assignment specifically identifies the malformation/deformation/or chromosomal abnormality, manifestations that are an inherent component of the anomaly should not be coded separately. Additional codes should be assigned for manifestations that are not an inherent component.

---

8-day-old infant with tetralogy of Fallot and pulmonary stenosis

**Q21.3**    **Tetralogy of Fallot**

*Explanation:* Pulmonary stenosis is inherent in the disease process of tetralogy of Fallot. When the code assignment specifically identifies the malformation/deformation/or chromosomal abnormality, manifestations that are inherent components of the anomaly should not be coded separately.

---

7-month-old infant with Down syndrome and common atrioventricular canal

**Q90.9**    **Down syndrome, unspecified**

**Q21.2**    **Atrioventricular septal defect**

*Explanation:* While a common atrioventricular canal is often associated with patients with Down syndrome, this manifestation is not an inherent component and may be reported separately. When the code assignment specifically identifies the anomaly, manifestations that are inherent components of the condition should not be coded separately. Additional codes should be assigned for manifestations that are not inherent components.

---

Codes from Chapter 17 may be used throughout the life of the patient. If a congenital malformation or deformity has been corrected, a personal history code should be used to identify the history of the malformation or deformity. Although present at birth, malformation/deformation/or chromosomal abnormality may not be identified until later in life. Whenever the condition is diagnosed by the physician, it is appropriate to assign a code from codes Q00-Q99. For the birth admission, the appropriate code from category Z38, Liveborn infants, according to place of birth and type of delivery, should be sequenced as the principal diagnosis, followed by any congenital anomaly codes, Q00- Q99.

---

Three-year-old with history of corrected ventricular septal defect

**Z87.74**    **Personal history of (corrected) congenital malformations of heart and circulatory system**

*Explanation:* If a congenital malformation or deformity has been corrected, a personal history code should be used to identify the history of the malformation or deformity.

---

Forty-year-old man with headaches diagnosed with congenital arteriovenous malformation by brain scan

**Q28.2**    **Arteriovenous malformation of cerebral vessels**

*Explanation:* Although present at birth, malformations may not be identified until later in life. Whenever the condition is diagnosed by the physician, it is appropriate to assign a code from the range Q00–Q99.

---

Newborn with anencephaly delivered vaginally in hospital

**Z38.00**    **Single liveborn infant, delivered vaginally**

**Q00.0**    **Anencephaly**

*Explanation:* For the birth admission, the appropriate code from category Z38 Liveborn infants, according to place of birth and type of delivery, should be sequenced as the principal diagnosis, followed by any congenital anomaly codes, Q00–Q99.

# Chapter 17. Congenital Malformations, Deformations and Chromosomal Abnormalities(Q00-Q99)

**NOTE** Codes from this chapter are not for use on maternal or fetal records.

**EXCLUDES 2** *inborn errors of metabolism (E70-E88)*

This chapter contains the following blocks:

Q00-Q07   Congenital malformations of the nervous system
Q10-Q18   Congenital malformations of eye, ear, face and neck
Q20-Q28   Congenital malformations of the circulatory system
Q30-Q34   Congenital malformations of the respiratory system
Q35-Q37   Cleft lip and cleft palate
Q38-Q45   Other congenital malformations of the digestive system
Q50-Q56   Congenital malformations of genital organs
Q60-Q64   Congenital malformations of the urinary system
Q65-Q79   Congenital malformations and deformations of the musculoskeletal system
Q80-Q89   Other congenital malformations
Q90-Q99   Chromosomal abnormalities, not elsewhere classified

## Congenital malformations of the nervous system (Q00-Q07)

**✓4ᵗʰ Q00 Anencephaly and similar malformations**

**CC Excl: For MCC codes in category Q00:** PDX collection 1053

**Q00.0 Anencephaly** MCC HCC
Acephaly
Acrania
Amyelencephaly
Hemianencephaly
Hemicephaly

**Q00.1 Craniorachischisis** MCC HCC

**Q00.2 Iniencephaly** MCC HCC

**✓4ᵗʰ Q01 Encephalocele**
**INCLUDES** Arnold-Chiari syndrome, type III
encephalocystocele
encephalomyelocele
hydroencephalocele
hydromeningocele, cranial
meningocele, cerebral
meningoencephalocele
**EXCLUDES 1** *Meckel-Gruber syndrome (Q61.9)*

**CC Excl: For CC codes in category Q01:** PDX collection 1054

**Q01.0 Frontal encephalocele** CC HCC
**Q01.1 Nasofrontal encephalocele** CC HCC
**Q01.2 Occipital encephalocele** CC HCC
**Q01.8 Encephalocele of other sites** CC HCC
**Q01.9 Encephalocele, unspecified** CC HCC

**Q02 Microcephaly** HCC
**INCLUDES** hydromicrocephaly
micrencephalon
**EXCLUDES 1** *Meckel-Gruber syndrome (Q61.9)*

**✓4ᵗʰ Q03 Congenital hydrocephalus**
**INCLUDES** hydrocephalus in newborn
**EXCLUDES 1** *Arnold-Chiari syndrome, type II (Q07.0-)*
*acquired hydrocephalus (G91.-)*
*hydrocephalus due to congenital toxoplasmosis (P37.1)*
*hydrocephalus with spina bifida (Q05.0-Q05.4)*

**Q03.0 Malformations of aqueduct of Sylvius** HCC
Anomaly of aqueduct of Sylvius
Obstruction of aqueduct of Sylvius, congenital
Stenosis of aqueduct of Sylvius

**Q03.1 Atresia of foramina of Magendie and Luschka** HCC
Dandy-Walker syndrome

**Q03.8 Other congenital hydrocephalus** HCC
**Q03.9 Congenital hydrocephalus, unspecified** HCC

**✓4ᵗʰ Q04 Other congenital malformations of brain**
**EXCLUDES 1** *cyclopia (Q87.0)*
*macrocephaly (Q75.3)*

**CC Excl: For MCC codes in category Q04, unless otherwise noted:** PDX collection 1054

**Q04.0 Congenital malformations of corpus callosum** MCC HCC
Agenesis of corpus callosum

**Q04.1 Arhinencephaly** MCC HCC

**Q04.2 Holoprosencephaly** MCC HCC

**Congenital Hydrocephalus**

Pressure

Normal ventricles      Hydrocephalic ventricles

**Q04.3 Other reduction deformities of brain** MCC HCC
Absence of part of brain
Agenesis of part of brain
Agyria
Aplasia of part of brain
Hydranencephaly
Hypoplasia of part of brain
Lissencephaly
Microgyria
Pachygyria
**EXCLUDES 1** *congenital malformations of corpus callosum (Q04.0)*

**Q04.4 Septo-optic dysplasia of brain** CC HCC
**CC Excl:** PDX collection 1055

**Q04.5 Megalencephaly** CC HCC
**CC Excl:** PDX collection 1055

**Q04.6 Congenital cerebral cysts** CC HCC
Porencephaly
Schizencephaly
**EXCLUDES 1** *acquired porencephalic cyst (G93.0)*
**CC Excl:** PDX collection 1055

**Q04.8 Other specified congenital malformations of brain** CC HCC
Arnold-Chiari syndrome, type IV
Macrogyria
**CC Excl:** PDX collection 1055

**Q04.9 Congenital malformation of brain, unspecified** HCC
Congenital anomaly NOS of brain
Congenital deformity NOS of brain
Congenital disease or lesion NOS of brain
Multiple anomalies NOS of brain, congenital

**✓4ᵗʰ Q05 Spina bifida**
Hydromeningocele (spinal)
Meningocele (spinal)
Meningomyelocele
Myelocele
Myelomeningocele
Rachischisis
Spina bifida (aperta)(cystica)
Syringomyelocele
Use additional code for any associated paraplegia (paraparesis) (G82.2-)
**EXCLUDES 1** *Arnold-Chiari syndrome, type II (Q07.0-)*
*spina bifida occulta (Q76.0)*

**CC Excl: For CC codes in category Q05:** PDX collection 1056

**Q05.0 Cervical spina bifida with hydrocephalus** CC HCC
**Q05.1 Thoracic spina bifida with hydrocephalus** CC HCC
Dorsal spina bifida with hydrocephalus
Thoracolumbar spina bifida with hydrocephalus

**Q05.2 Lumbar spina bifida with hydrocephalus** CC HCC
Lumbosacral spina bifida with hydrocephalus

**Q05.3 Sacral spina bifida with hydrocephalus** CC HCC
**Q05.4 Unspecified spina bifida with hydrocephalus** CC HCC
**Q05.5 Cervical spina bifida without hydrocephalus** HCC
**Q05.6 Thoracic spina bifida without hydrocephalus** HCC
Dorsal spina bifida NOS
Thoracolumbar spina bifida NOS

**Q05.7 Lumbar spina bifida without hydrocephalus** HCC
Lumbosacral spina bifida NOS

**Q05.8 Sacral spina bifida without hydrocephalus** HCC
**Q05.9 Spina bifida, unspecified** HCC

N Newborn: 0   P Pediatric: 0-17   M Maternity: 12-55   A Adult: 15-124   MCC Major CC Condition   PDx MCC PDx acts as own MCC   CC CC Condition   PDx CC PDx acts as own CC

894      ICD-10-CM 2018

## Spina Bifida

**Spina bifida occulta**    **Meningocele**    **Myelomeningocele**

✓4ᵗʰ **Q06 Other congenital malformations of spinal cord**

**Q06.0 Amyelia**   HCC

**Q06.1 Hypoplasia and dysplasia of spinal cord**   HCC
Atelomyelia
Myelatelia
Myelodysplasia of spinal cord

**Q06.2 Diastematomyelia**   HCC
**DEF:** Rare congenital anomaly often associated with spina bifida; the spinal cord is separated into longitudinal halves by a bony, cartilaginous or fibrous septum, each half surrounded by a dural sac.

**Q06.3 Other congenital cauda equina malformations**   HCC

**Q06.4 Hydromyelia**   HCC
Hydrorachis

**Q06.8 Other specified congenital malformations of spinal cord**   HCC

**Q06.9 Congenital malformation of spinal cord, unspecified**   HCC
Congenital anomaly NOS of spinal cord
Congenital deformity NOS of spinal cord
Congenital disease or lesion NOS of spinal cord

✓4ᵗʰ **Q07 Other congenital malformations of nervous system**
*EXCLUDES 2*   *congenital central alveolar hypoventilation syndrome (G47.35)*
*familial dysautonomia [Riley-Day] (G90.1)*
*neurofibromatosis (nonmalignant) (Q85.0-)*

**CC Excl: For CC codes in category Q007:** PDX collection 1056

✓5ᵗʰ **Q07.0 Arnold-Chiari syndrome**
Arnold-Chiari syndrome, type II
*EXCLUDES 1*   *Arnold-Chiari syndrome, type III (Q01.-)*
*Arnold-Chiari syndrome, type IV (Q04.8)*

**Q07.00 Arnold-Chiari syndrome without spina bifida or hydrocephalus**   HCC

**Q07.01 Arnold-Chiari syndrome with spina bifida**   HCC

**Q07.02 Arnold-Chiari syndrome with hydrocephalus**   CC HCC

**Q07.03 Arnold-Chiari syndrome with spina bifida and hydrocephalus**   CC HCC

**Q07.8 Other specified congenital malformations of nervous system**   HCC
Agenesis of nerve
Displacement of brachial plexus
Jaw-winking syndrome
Marcus Gunn's syndrome

**Q07.9 Congenital malformation of nervous system, unspecified**   HCC
Congenital anomaly NOS of nervous system
Congenital deformity NOS of nervous system
Congenital disease or lesion NOS of nervous system

### Congenital malformations of eye, ear, face and neck (Q10-Q18)
*EXCLUDES 2*   *cleft lip and cleft palate (Q35-Q37)*
*congenital malformation of cervical spine (Q05.0, Q05.5, Q67.5, Q76.0-Q76.4)*
*congenital malformation of larynx (Q31.-)*
*congenital malformation of lip NEC (Q38.0)*
*congenital malformation of nose (Q30.-)*
*congenital malformation of parathyroid gland (Q89.2)*
*congenital malformation of thyroid gland (Q89.2)*

✓4ᵗʰ **Q10 Congenital malformations of eyelid, lacrimal apparatus and orbit**
*EXCLUDES 1*   *cryptophthalmos NOS (Q11.2)*
*cryptophthalmos syndrome (Q87.0)*

**Q10.0 Congenital ptosis**
**DEF:** Congenital drooping of eyelid; mostly idiopathic, but may occur genetically.

**Q10.1 Congenital ectropion**

**Q10.2 Congenital entropion**

**Q10.3 Other congenital malformations of eyelid**
Ablepharon
Blepharophimosis, congenital
Coloboma of eyelid
Congenital absence or agenesis of cilia
Congenital absence or agenesis of eyelid
Congenital accessory eyelid
Congenital accessory eye muscle
Congenital malformation of eyelid NOS

**Q10.4 Absence and agenesis of lacrimal apparatus**
Congenital absence of punctum lacrimale

**Q10.5 Congenital stenosis and stricture of lacrimal duct**

**Q10.6 Other congenital malformations of lacrimal apparatus**
Congenital malformation of lacrimal apparatus NOS

**Q10.7 Congenital malformation of orbit**

✓4ᵗʰ **Q11 Anophthalmos, microphthalmos and macrophthalmos**

**Q11.0 Cystic eyeball**

**Q11.1 Other anophthalmos**
Anophthalmos NOS
Agenesis of eye
Aplasia of eye

**Q11.2 Microphthalmos**
Cryptophthalmos NOS
Dysplasia of eye
Hypoplasia of eye
Rudimentary eye
*EXCLUDES 1*   *cryptophthalmos syndrome (Q87.0)*

**Q11.3 Macrophthalmos**
*EXCLUDES 1*   *macrophthalmos in congenital glaucoma (Q15.0)*

✓4ᵗʰ **Q12 Congenital lens malformations**

**Q12.0 Congenital cataract**

**Q12.1 Congenital displaced lens**

**Q12.2 Coloboma of lens**

**Q12.3 Congenital aphakia**

**Q12.4 Spherophakia**

**Q12.8 Other congenital lens malformations**
Microphakia

**Q12.9 Congenital lens malformation, unspecified**

✓4ᵗʰ **Q13 Congenital malformations of anterior segment of eye**

**Q13.0 Coloboma of iris**
Coloboma NOS

**Q13.1 Absence of iris**
Aniridia
Use additional code for associated glaucoma (H42)
**DEF:** Incompletely formed or absent iris; affects both eyes; dominant trait.

**Q13.2 Other congenital malformations of iris**
Anisocoria, congenital
Atresia of pupil
Congenital malformation of iris NOS
Corectopia

**Q13.3 Congenital corneal opacity**

**Q13.4 Other congenital corneal malformations**
Congenital malformation of cornea NOS
Microcornea
Peter's anomaly

**Q13.5 Blue sclera**

### Coloboma of Lens

Coloboma

☑ Additional Character Req   ✓x 7ᵗʰ Placeholder Alert   Unacceptable PDx   Manifestation   **H1** - **H14** HAC   HCC CMS-HCC Condition   *EXCLUDES 1* Not Coded Here   *EXCLUDES 2* Not Included Here

ICD-10-CM 2018      **895**

**Chapter 17. Congenital Malformations, Deformations and Chromosomal Abnormalities**

✓5ᵗʰ **Q13.8 Other congenital malformations of anterior segment of eye**

**Q13.81 Rieger's anomaly**
Use additional code for associated glaucoma (H42)

**Q13.89 Other congenital malformations of anterior segment of eye**

**Q13.9 Congenital malformation of anterior segment of eye, unspecified**

✓4ᵗʰ **Q14 Congenital malformations of posterior segment of eye**
EXCLUDES 2   optic nerve hypoplasia (H47.03-)

**Q14.0 Congenital malformation of vitreous humor**
Congenital vitreous opacity

**Q14.1 Congenital malformation of retina**
Congenital retinal aneurysm

**Q14.2 Congenital malformation of optic disc**
Coloboma of optic disc

**Q14.3 Congenital malformation of choroid**

**Q14.8 Other congenital malformations of posterior segment of eye**
Coloboma of the fundus

**Q14.9 Congenital malformation of posterior segment of eye, unspecified**

✓4ᵗʰ **Q15 Other congenital malformations of eye**
EXCLUDES 1   congenital nystagmus (H55.01)
ocular albinism (E70.31-)
optic nerve hypoplasia (H47.03-)
retinitis pigmentosa (H35.52)

**Q15.0 Congenital glaucoma**
Axenfeld's anomaly
Buphthalmos
Glaucoma of childhood
Glaucoma of newborn
Hydrophthalmos
Keratoglobus, congenital, with glaucoma
Macrocornea with glaucoma
Macrophthalmos in congenital glaucoma
Megalocornea with glaucoma

**Q15.8 Other specified congenital malformations of eye**

**Q15.9 Congenital malformation of eye, unspecified**
Congenital anomaly of eye
Congenital deformity of eye

✓4ᵗʰ **Q16 Congenital malformations of ear causing impairment of hearing**
EXCLUDES 1   congenital deafness (H90.-)

**Q16.0 Congenital absence of (ear) auricle**

**Q16.1 Congenital absence, atresia and stricture of auditory canal (external)**
Congenital atresia or stricture of osseous meatus

**Q16.2 Absence of eustachian tube**

**Q16.3 Congenital malformation of ear ossicles**
Congenital fusion of ear ossicles

**Q16.4 Other congenital malformations of middle ear**
Congenital malformation of middle ear NOS

**Q16.5 Congenital malformation of inner ear**
Congenital anomaly of membranous labyrinth
Congenital anomaly of organ of Corti

**Q16.9 Congenital malformation of ear causing impairment of hearing, unspecified**
Congenital absence of ear NOS

✓4ᵗʰ **Q17 Other congenital malformations of ear**
EXCLUDES 1   congenital malformations of ear with impairment of hearing (Q16.0- Q16.9)
preauricular sinus (Q18.1)

**Q17.0 Accessory auricle**
Accessory tragus
Polyotia
Preauricular appendage or tag
Supernumerary ear
Supernumerary lobule

**Q17.1 Macrotia**
DEF: Birth defect characterized by abnormal enlargement of the pinna of the ear.

**Q17.2 Microtia**

**Q17.3 Other misshapen ear**
Pointed ear

**Q17.4 Misplaced ear**
Low-set ears
EXCLUDES 1   cervical auricle (Q18.2)

**Q17.5 Prominent ear**
Bat ear

**Q17.8 Other specified congenital malformations of ear**
Congenital absence of lobe of ear

**Q17.9 Congenital malformation of ear, unspecified**
Congenital anomaly of ear NOS

✓4ᵗʰ **Q18 Other congenital malformations of face and neck**
EXCLUDES 1   cleft lip and cleft palate (Q35-Q37)
conditions classified to Q67.0-Q67.4
congenital malformations of skull and face bones (Q75.-)
cyclopia (Q87.0)
dentofacial anomalies [including malocclusion] (M26.-)
malformation syndromes affecting facial appearance (Q87.0)
persistent thyroglossal duct (Q89.2)

**Q18.0 Sinus, fistula and cyst of branchial cleft**
Branchial vestige

**Q18.1 Preauricular sinus and cyst**
Fistula of auricle, congenital
Cervicoaural fistula

**Q18.2 Other branchial cleft malformations**
Branchial cleft malformation NOS
Cervical auricle
Otocephaly

**Q18.3 Webbing of neck**
Pterygium colli
DEF: Congenital malformation characterized by thick, triangular skinfold that stretches from the lateral side of the neck across the shoulder; associated with genetic conditions Turner's and Noonan's syndromes.

**Q18.4 Macrostomia**
DEF: Rare congenital craniofacial bilateral or unilateral anomaly of mouth due to malformed maxillary and mandibular processes; results in abnormally large mouth extending towards ear.

**Q18.5 Microstomia**

**Q18.6 Macrocheilia**
Hypertrophy of lip, congenital

**Q18.7 Microcheilia**

**Q18.8 Other specified congenital malformations of face and neck**
Medial cyst of face and neck
Medial fistula of face and neck
Medial sinus of face and neck

**Q18.9 Congenital malformation of face and neck, unspecified**
Congenital anomaly NOS of face and neck

## Congenital malformations of the circulatory system (Q20-Q28)

✓4ᵗʰ **Q20 Congenital malformations of cardiac chambers and connections**
EXCLUDES 1   dextrocardia with situs inversus (Q89.3)
mirror-image atrial arrangement with situs inversus (Q89.3)

**CC Excl: For CC/MCC codes in category Q20: PDX collection 1057**

**Q20.0 Common arterial trunk**    `MCC`
Persistent truncus arteriosus
EXCLUDES 1   aortic septal defect (Q21.4)

**Q20.1 Double outlet right ventricle**    `MCC`
Taussig-Bing syndrome

**Q20.2 Double outlet left ventricle**    `MCC`

**Q20.3 Discordant ventriculoarterial connection**    `MCC`
Dextrotransposition of aorta
Transposition of great vessels (complete)

**Q20.4 Double inlet ventricle**    `MCC`
Common ventricle
Cor triloculare biatriatum
Single ventricle

**Q20.5 Discordant atrioventricular connection**    `CC`
Corrected transposition
Levotransposition
Ventricular inversion

**Q20.6 Isomerism of atrial appendages**
Isomerism of atrial appendages with asplenia or polysplenia

**Q20.8 Other congenital malformations of cardiac chambers and connections**
Cor binoculare

**Q20.9 Congenital malformation of cardiac chambers and connections, unspecified**

N Newborn: 0   P Pediatric: 0-17   M Maternity: 12-55   A Adult: 15-124   MCC Major CC Condition   PDxMCC PDx acts as own MCC   CC CC Condition   PDxCC PDx acts as own CC

896          ICD-10-CM 2018

## Ventricular Septal Defect

✓4ᵗʰ **Q21 Congenital malformations of cardiac septa**
    *EXCLUDES 1*   acquired cardiac septal defect (I51.0)

**CC Excl: For CC/MCC codes in category Q21, unless otherwise noted:** PDX collection 1057

**Q21.0 Ventricular septal defect**    CC
    Roger's disease

**Q21.1 Atrial septal defect**    CC
    Coronary sinus defect
    Patent or persistent foramen ovale
    Patent or persistent ostium secundum defect (type II)
    Patent or persistent sinus venosus defect
    **CC Excl:** PDX collection 1058

**Q21.2 Atrioventricular septal defect**    CC
    Common atrioventricular canal
    Endocardial cushion defect
    Ostium primum atrial septal defect (type I)

**Q21.3 Tetralogy of Fallot**    MCC
    Ventricular septal defect with pulmonary stenosis or atresia,
      dextroposition of aorta and hypertrophy of right ventricle.
    **AHA:** 2014, 3Q, 16

**Q21.4 Aortopulmonary septal defect**
    Aortic septal defect
    Aortopulmonary window

**Q21.8 Other congenital malformations of cardiac septa**
    Eisenmenger's defect
    Pentalogy of Fallot
    ▶Code also if applicable:
      Eisenmenger's complex (I27.83)
      Eisenmenger's syndrome (I27.83)◀
    *EXCLUDES 1*   *Eisenmenger's complex (I27.8)*
            *Eisenmenger's syndrome (I27.8)*

**Q21.9 Congenital malformation of cardiac septum, unspecified**
    Septal (heart) defect NOS

## Atrial Septal Defect

## Atrioventricular Septal Defect

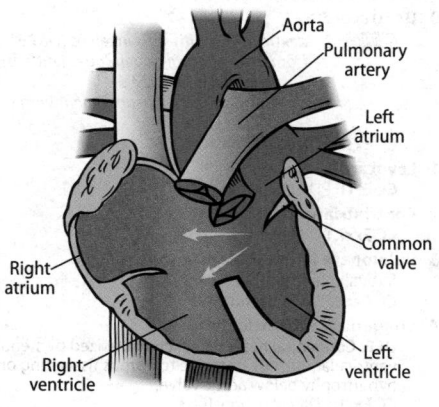

✓4ᵗʰ **Q22 Congenital malformations of pulmonary and tricuspid valves**

**CC Excl: For MCC codes in category Q22, unless otherwise noted:** PDX collection 1061

**Q22.0 Pulmonary valve atresia**    MCC
    **CC Excl:** PDX collection 1059

**Q22.1 Congenital pulmonary valve stenosis**    CC
    **DEF:** Stenosis of opening between pulmonary artery and right
    ventricle; causes obstructed blood outflow from right ventricle.
    **CC Excl:** PDX collection 1059

**Q22.2 Congenital pulmonary valve insufficiency**    CC
    Congenital pulmonary valve regurgitation
    **CC Excl:** PDX collection 1060

**Q22.3 Other congenital malformations of pulmonary valve**    CC
    Congenital malformation of pulmonary valve NOS
    Supernumerary cusps of pulmonary valve
    **CC Excl:** PDX collection 1060

**Q22.4 Congenital tricuspid stenosis**    MCC
    Congenital tricuspid atresia

**Q22.5 Ebstein's anomaly**    MCC
    **DEF:** Malformation of the tricuspid valve characterized by septal
    and posterior leaflets attaching to the wall of the right ventricle;
    causes the right ventricle to fuse with the atrium into a large right
    atrium and a small ventricle; leads to heart failure and abnormal
    cardiac rhythm.

**Q22.6 Hypoplastic right heart syndrome**    MCC

**Q22.8 Other congenital malformations of tricuspid valve**    MCC

**Q22.9 Congenital malformation of tricuspid valve, unspecified**    MCC

✓4ᵗʰ **Q23 Congenital malformations of aortic and mitral valves**

**CC Excl: For CC/MCC codes in category Q23:** PDX collection 1061

**Q23.0 Congenital stenosis of aortic valve**    CC
    Congenital aortic atresia
    Congenital aortic stenosis NOS
    *EXCLUDES 1*   *congenital stenosis of aortic valve in hypoplastic left*
            *heart syndrome (Q23.4)*
            *congenital subaortic stenosis (Q24.4)*
            *supravalvular aortic stenosis (congenital) (Q25.3)*

**Q23.1 Congenital insufficiency of aortic valve**    CC
    Bicuspid aortic valve
    Congenital aortic insufficiency

**Q23.2 Congenital mitral stenosis**    CC
    Congenital mitral atresia
    **DEF:** Congenital stenosis of mitral valve orifice between left
    atrium and ventricle; at the supravalvular, valvular, or subvalvular
    levels; causes obstruction to left ventricular filling.

**Q23.3 Congenital mitral insufficiency**    CC

**Q23.4 Hypoplastic left heart syndrome**    MCC

**Q23.8 Other congenital malformations of aortic and mitral valves**

**Q23.9 Congenital malformation of aortic and mitral valves, unspecified**

✓ Additional Character Req   ✓x7ᵗʰ Placeholder Alert   Unacceptable PDx   Manifestation   H1 - H14 HAC   HCG CMS-HCC Condition   *EXCLUDES 1* Not Coded Here   *EXCLUDES 2* Not Included Here

ICD-10-CM 2018                                         **897**

✓4ᵗʰ **Q24  Other congenital malformations of heart**
**EXCLUDES 1** *endocardial fibroelastosis (I42.4)*

**Q24.Ø  Dextrocardia**  CC
**EXCLUDES 1** *dextrocardia with situs inversus (Q89.3)*
*isomerism of atrial appendages (with asplenia or polysplenia) (Q2Ø.6)*
*mirror-image atrial arrangement with situs inversus (Q89.3)*
**CC Excl:** PDX collection 1Ø62

**Q24.1  Levocardia**  CC
**CC Excl:** PDX collection 1Ø62

**Q24.2  Cor triatriatum**  MCC
**CC Excl:** PDX collection 1Ø63

**Q24.3  Pulmonary infundibular stenosis**  CC
Subvalvular pulmonic stenosis
**CC Excl:** PDX collection 1Ø63

**Q24.4  Congenital subaortic stenosis**  MCC
**DEF:** Congenital heart defect characterized by stenosis of left ventricular outflow tract due to fibrous tissue ring or septal hypertrophy below aortic valve.
**CC Excl:** PDX collection 1Ø63

**Q24.5  Malformation of coronary vessels**  CC
Congenital coronary (artery) aneurysm
**CC Excl:** PDX collection 1Ø64

**Q24.6  Congenital heart block**  MCC
**CC Excl:** PDX collection 1Ø65

**Q24.8  Other specified congenital malformations of heart**
Congenital diverticulum of left ventricle
Congenital malformation of myocardium
Congenital malformation of pericardium
Malposition of heart
Uhl's disease

**Q24.9  Congenital malformation of heart, unspecified**
Congenital anomaly of heart
Congenital disease of heart

✓4ᵗʰ **Q25  Congenital malformations of great arteries**

**Q25.Ø  Patent ductus arteriosus**  CC
Patent ductus Botallo
Persistent ductus arteriosus
**CC Excl:** PDX collection 1Ø66

**Q25.1  Coarctation of aorta**  CC
Coarctation of aorta (preductal) (postductal)
Stenosis of aorta
**CC Excl:** PDX collection 1Ø67

✓5ᵗʰ **Q25.2  Atresia of aorta**

**Q25.21  Interruption of aortic arch**  CC
Atresia of aortic arch
**CC Excl:** PDX collection 1Ø68

**Q25.29  Other atresia of aorta**  CC
Atresia of aorta
**CC Excl:** PDX collection 1Ø68

**Q25.3  Supravalvular aortic stenosis**  CC
**EXCLUDES 1** *congenital aortic stenosis NOS (Q23.Ø)*
*congenital stenosis of aortic valve (Q23.Ø)*
**CC Excl:** PDX collection 1Ø68

**Aortic Arch Anomalies**

Esophagus
Trachea
Aortic arch

Normal aortic arch

Double aortic arch          Right aortic arch

✓5ᵗʰ **Q25.4  Other congenital malformations of aorta**
**EXCLUDES 1** *hypoplasia of aorta in hypoplastic left heart syndrome (Q23.4)*

**CC Excl: For CC codes in subcategory Q25.4:**
PDX collection 1Ø69

**Q25.4Ø  Congenital malformation of aorta unspecified**  CC

**Q25.41  Absence and aplasia of aorta**  CC

**Q25.42  Hypoplasia of aorta**  CC

**Q25.43  Congenital aneurysm of aorta**  CC
Congenital aneurysm of aortic root
Congenital aneurysm of aortic sinus

**Q25.44  Congenital dilation of aorta**  CC

**Q25.45  Double aortic arch**  CC
Vascular ring of aorta

**Q25.46  Tortuous aortic arch**  CC
Persistent convolutions of aortic arch

**Q25.47  Right aortic arch**  CC
Persistent right aortic arch

**Q25.48  Anomalous origin of subclavian artery**  CC

**Q25.49  Other congenital malformations of aorta**  CC
▶Aortic arch
Bovine arch◀

**Q25.5  Atresia of pulmonary artery**  MCC
**CC Excl:** PDX collection 1Ø7Ø

**Q25.6  Stenosis of pulmonary artery**  MCC
Supravalvular pulmonary stenosis
**CC Excl:** PDX collection 1Ø7Ø

✓5ᵗʰ **Q25.7  Other congenital malformations of pulmonary artery**

**CC Excl: For MCC codes in subcategory Q25.7:**
PDX collection 1Ø7Ø

**Q25.71  Coarctation of pulmonary artery**  MCC

**Q25.72  Congenital pulmonary arteriovenous malformation**  MCC
Congenital pulmonary arteriovenous aneurysm

**Q25.79  Other congenital malformations of pulmonary artery**  MCC
Aberrant pulmonary artery
Agenesis of pulmonary artery
Congenital aneurysm of pulmonary artery
Congenital anomaly of pulmonary artery
Hypoplasia of pulmonary artery

**Q25.8  Other congenital malformations of other great arteries**  CC
**CC Excl:** PDX collection 1Ø69

**Q25.9  Congenital malformation of great arteries, unspecified**  CC
**CC Excl:** PDX collection 1Ø69

✓4ᵗʰ **Q26  Congenital malformations of great veins**

**Q26.Ø  Congenital stenosis of vena cava**  CC
Congenital stenosis of vena cava (inferior)(superior)
**CC Excl:** PDX collection 1Ø71

**Patent Ductus Arteriosus**

Patent ductus arteriosus
Pulmonary artery
Aorta
Atria
Superior vena cava
Septum
Patent foramen ovale
Right atrium
Left atrium
Schematic showing foramen ovale

**N** Newborn: 0   **P** Pediatric: 0-17   **M** Maternity: 12-55   **A** Adult: 15-124   **MCC** Major CC Condition   **PDxMCC** PDx acts as own MCC   **CC** CC Condition   **PDxCC** PDx acts as own CC

**898**          ICD-10-CM 2018

**Q26.1** **Persistent left superior vena cava**  `CC`
    **CC Excl:** PDX collection 1071

**Q26.2** **Total anomalous pulmonary venous connection**  `CC`
    Total anomalous pulmonary venous return [TAPVR],
        subdiaphragmatic
    Total anomalous pulmonary venous return [TAPVR],
        supradiaphragmatic
    **CC Excl:** PDX collection 1072

**Q26.3** **Partial anomalous pulmonary venous connection**  `CC`
    Partial anomalous pulmonary venous return
    **CC Excl:** PDX collection 1073

**Q26.4** **Anomalous pulmonary venous connection, unspecified**  `CC`
    **CC Excl:** PDX collection 1073

**Q26.5** **Anomalous portal venous connection**

**Q26.6** **Portal vein-hepatic artery fistula**

**Q26.8** **Other congenital malformations of great veins**  `CC`
    Absence of vena cava (inferior) (superior)
    Azygos continuation of inferior vena cava
    Persistent left posterior cardinal vein
    Scimitar syndrome
    **CC Excl:** PDX collection 1071

**Q26.9** **Congenital malformation of great vein, unspecified**  `CC`
    Congenital anomaly of vena cava (inferior) (superior) NOS
    **CC Excl:** PDX collection 1074

✓4ᵗʰ **Q27** **Other congenital malformations of peripheral vascular system**
    *EXCLUDES 2* *anomalies of cerebral and precerebral vessels (Q28.0-Q28.3)*
        *anomalies of coronary vessels (Q24.5)*
        *anomalies of pulmonary artery (Q25.5-Q25.7)*
        *congenital retinal aneurysm (Q14.1)*
        *hemangioma and lymphangioma (D18.-)*

**Q27.0** **Congenital absence and hypoplasia of umbilical artery**
    Single umbilical artery

**Q27.1** **Congenital renal artery stenosis**

**Q27.2** **Other congenital malformations of renal artery**
    Congenital malformation of renal artery NOS
    Multiple renal arteries

✓5ᵗʰ **Q27.3** **Arteriovenous malformation (peripheral)**
    Arteriovenous aneurysm
    *EXCLUDES 1* *acquired arteriovenous aneurysm (I77.0)*
    *EXCLUDES 2* *arteriovenous malformation of cerebral vessels (Q28.2)*
        *arteriovenous malformation of precerebral vessels*
        *(Q28.0)*

    **Q27.30** **Arteriovenous malformation, site unspecified**  `CC`
        **CC Excl:** PDX collection 1075

    **Q27.31** **Arteriovenous malformation of vessel of upper limb**

    **Q27.32** **Arteriovenous malformation of vessel of lower limb**

    **Q27.33** **Arteriovenous malformation of digestive system vessel**

    **Q27.34** **Arteriovenous malformation of renal vessel**

    **Q27.39** **Arteriovenous malformation, other site**

**Q27.4** **Congenital phlebectasia**  `CC`
    **CC Excl:** PDX collection 1075

**Q27.8** **Other specified congenital malformations of peripheral vascular system**
    Absence of peripheral vascular system
    Atresia of peripheral vascular system
    Congenital aneurysm (peripheral)
    Congenital stricture, artery
    Congenital varix
    *EXCLUDES 1* *arteriovenous malformation (Q27.3-)*

**Q27.9** **Congenital malformation of peripheral vascular system, unspecified**
    Anomaly of artery or vein NOS

✓4ᵗʰ **Q28** **Other congenital malformations of circulatory system**
    *EXCLUDES 1* *congenital aneurysm NOS (Q27.8)*
        *congenital coronary aneurysm (Q24.5)*
        *ruptured cerebral arteriovenous malformation (I60.8)*
        *ruptured malformation of precerebral vessels (I72.0)*
    *EXCLUDES 2* *congenital peripheral aneurysm (Q27.8)*
        *congenital pulmonary aneurysm (Q25.79)*
        *congenital retinal aneurysm (Q14.1)*

    **CC Excl: For CC codes in category Q28, unless otherwise noted:**
    PDX collection 1075

**Q28.0** **Arteriovenous malformation of precerebral vessels**  `CC`
    Congenital arteriovenous precerebral aneurysm (nonruptured)

**Q28.1** **Other malformations of precerebral vessels**  `CC`
    Congenital malformation of precerebral vessels NOS
    Congenital precerebral aneurysm (nonruptured)

**Q28.2** **Arteriovenous malformation of cerebral vessels**  `MCC`
    Arteriovenous malformation of brain NOS
    Congenital arteriovenous cerebral aneurysm (nonruptured)
    **CC Excl:** PDX collection 1076

**Q28.3** **Other malformations of cerebral vessels**  `MCC`
    Congenital cerebral aneurysm (nonruptured)
    Congenital malformation of cerebral vessels NOS
    Developmental venous anomaly
    **CC Excl:** PDX collection 1076

**Q28.8** **Other specified congenital malformations of circulatory system**  `CC`
    Congenital aneurysm, specified site NEC
    Spinal vessel anomaly

**Q28.9** **Congenital malformation of circulatory system, unspecified**  `CC`
    **CC Excl:** PDX collection 1077

## Congenital malformations of the respiratory system (Q30-Q34)

✓4ᵗʰ **Q30** **Congenital malformations of nose**
    *EXCLUDES 1* *congenital deviation of nasal septum (Q67.4)*

**Q30.0** **Choanal atresia**
    Atresia of nares (anterior) (posterior)
    Congenital stenosis of nares (anterior) (posterior)

**Q30.1** **Agenesis and underdevelopment of nose**
    Congenital absent of nose

**Q30.2** **Fissured, notched and cleft nose**

**Q30.3** **Congenital perforated nasal septum**

**Q30.8** **Other congenital malformations of nose**
    Accessory nose
    Congenital anomaly of nasal sinus wall

**Q30.9** **Congenital malformation of nose, unspecified**

✓4ᵗʰ **Q31** **Congenital malformations of larynx**
    *EXCLUDES 1* *congenital laryngeal stridor NOS (P28.89)*

    **CC Excl: For CC codes in category Q31:** PDX collection 1078

**Q31.0** **Web of larynx**
    Glottic web of larynx
    Subglottic web of larynx
    Web of larynx NOS
    **DEF:** Congenital malformation of larynx; marked by thin,
    translucent, or thick, fibrotic membrane-like structure between
    vocal folds; characterized by shortness of breath, and stridor.

**Q31.1** **Congenital subglottic stenosis**  `CC`

**Q31.2** **Laryngeal hypoplasia**  `CC`

**Q31.3** **Laryngocele**  `CC`

**Q31.5** **Congenital laryngomalacia**  `CC`

**Q31.8** **Other congenital malformations of larynx**  `CC`
    Absence of larynx
    Agenesis of larynx
    Atresia of larynx
    Congenital cleft thyroid cartilage
    Congenital fissure of epiglottis
    Congenital stenosis of larynx NEC
    Posterior cleft of cricoid cartilage

**Q31.9** **Congenital malformation of larynx, unspecified**  `CC`

✓4ᵗʰ **Q32** **Congenital malformations of trachea and bronchus**
    *EXCLUDES 1* *congenital bronchiectasis (Q33.4)*

    **CC Excl: For CC codes in category Q32:** PDX collection 1078

**Q32.0** **Congenital tracheomalacia**  `CC`

**Q32.1** **Other congenital malformations of trachea**  `CC`
    Atresia of trachea
    Congenital anomaly of tracheal cartilage
    Congenital dilatation of trachea
    Congenital malformation of trachea
    Congenital stenosis of trachea
    Congenital tracheocele

**Q32.2** **Congenital bronchomalacia**  `CC`

**Q32.3** **Congenital stenosis of bronchus**  `CC`

**Q32.4** **Other congenital malformations of bronchus**  `CC`
    Absence of bronchus
    Agenesis of bronchus
    Atresia of bronchus
    Congenital diverticulum of bronchus
    Congenital malformation of bronchus NOS

✓ Additional Character Req  ✓ₓ7ᵗʰ Placeholder Alert  Unacceptable PDx  Manifestation  **H1**-**H14** HAC  **HCC** CMS-HCC Condition  *EXCLUDES 1* Not Coded Here  *EXCLUDES 2* Not Included Here

ICD-10-CM 2018  **899**

### ✓4ᵗʰ Q33　Congenital malformations of lung

**CC Excl: For CC/MCC codes in category Q33, unless otherwise noted:** PDX collection 1079

**Q33.0　Congenital cystic lung**　CC
Congenital cystic lung disease
Congenital honeycomb lung
Congenital polycystic lung disease
*EXCLUDES 1　cystic fibrosis (E84.0)*
*cystic lung disease, acquired or unspecified (J98.4)*

**Q33.1　Accessory lobe of lung**
Azygos lobe (fissured), lung

**Q33.2　Sequestration of lung**　MCC

**Q33.3　Agenesis of lung**　MCC
Congenital absence of lung (lobe)

**Q33.4　Congenital bronchiectasis**　CC
CC Excl: PDX collection 1080

**Q33.5　Ectopic tissue in lung**

**Q33.6　Congenital hypoplasia and dysplasia of lung**　MCC
*EXCLUDES 1　pulmonary hypoplasia associated with short gestation (P28.0)*

**Q33.8　Other congenital malformations of lung**

**Q33.9　Congenital malformation of lung, unspecified**

### ✓4ᵗʰ Q34　Other congenital malformations of respiratory system
*EXCLUDES 2　congenital central alveolar hypoventilation syndrome (G47.35)*

**Q34.0　Anomaly of pleura**

**Q34.1　Congenital cyst of mediastinum**

**Q34.8　Other specified congenital malformations of respiratory system**
Atresia of nasopharynx

**Q34.9　Congenital malformation of respiratory system, unspecified**
Congenital absence of respiratory system
Congenital anomaly of respiratory system NOS

## Cleft lip and cleft palate (Q35-Q37)

Use additional code to identify associated malformation of the nose (Q30.2)
*EXCLUDES 1　Robin's syndrome (Q87.0)*

### ✓4ᵗʰ Q35　Cleft palate
*INCLUDES　fissure of palate*
*palatoschisis*
*EXCLUDES 1　cleft palate with cleft lip (Q37.-)*

**Q35.1　Cleft hard palate**

**Q35.3　Cleft soft palate**

**Q35.5　Cleft hard palate with cleft soft palate**

**Q35.7　Cleft uvula**

**Q35.9　Cleft palate, unspecified**
Cleft palate NOS

### ✓4ᵗʰ Q36　Cleft lip
*INCLUDES　cheiloschisis*
*congenital fissure of lip*
*harelip*
*labium leporinum*
*EXCLUDES 1　cleft lip with cleft palate (Q37.-)*

**Q36.0　Cleft lip, bilateral**

**Q36.1　Cleft lip, median**

**Q36.9　Cleft lip, unilateral**
Cleft lip NOS

## Cleft Lip

Unilateral incomplete　　Unilateral complete　　Bilateral complete

### ✓4ᵗʰ Q37　Cleft palate with cleft lip
*INCLUDES　cheilopalatoschisis*

**Q37.0　Cleft hard palate with bilateral cleft lip**

**Q37.1　Cleft hard palate with unilateral cleft lip**
Cleft hard palate with cleft lip NOS

**Q37.2　Cleft soft palate with bilateral cleft lip**

**Q37.3　Cleft soft palate with unilateral cleft lip**
Cleft soft palate with cleft lip NOS

**Q37.4　Cleft hard and soft palate with bilateral cleft lip**

**Q37.5　Cleft hard and soft palate with unilateral cleft lip**
Cleft hard and soft palate with cleft lip NOS

**Q37.8　Unspecified cleft palate with bilateral cleft lip**

**Q37.9　Unspecified cleft palate with unilateral cleft lip**
Cleft palate with cleft lip NOS

## Other congenital malformations of the digestive system (Q38-Q45)

### ✓4ᵗʰ Q38　Other congenital malformations of tongue, mouth and pharynx
*EXCLUDES 1　dentofacial anomalies (M26.-)*
*macrostomia (Q18.4)*
*microstomia (Q18.5)*

**Q38.0　Congenital malformations of lips, not elsewhere classified**
Congenital fistula of lip
Congenital malformation of lip NOS
Van der Woude's syndrome
*EXCLUDES 1　cleft lip (Q36.-)*
*cleft lip with cleft palate (Q37.-)*
*macrocheilia (Q18.6)*
*microcheilia (Q18.7)*

**Q38.1　Ankyloglossia**
Tongue tie

**Q38.2　Macroglossia**
Congenital hypertrophy of tongue

**Q38.3　Other congenital malformations of tongue**
Aglossia
Bifid tongue
Congenital adhesion of tongue
Congenital fissure of tongue
Congenital malformation of tongue NOS
Double tongue
Hypoglossia
Hypoplasia of tongue
Microglossia

**Q38.4　Congenital malformations of salivary glands and ducts**
Atresia of salivary glands and ducts
Congenital absence of salivary glands and ducts
Congenital accessory salivary glands and ducts
Congenital fistula of salivary gland

**Q38.5　Congenital malformations of palate, not elsewhere classified**
Congenital absence of uvula
Congenital malformation of palate NOS
Congenital high arched palate
*EXCLUDES 1　cleft palate (Q35.-)*
*cleft palate with cleft lip (Q37.-)*

**Q38.6　Other congenital malformations of mouth**
Congenital malformation of mouth NOS

**Q38.7　Congenital pharyngeal pouch**
Congenital diverticulum of pharynx
*EXCLUDES 1　pharyngeal pouch syndrome (D82.1)*

**Q38.8　Other congenital malformations of pharynx**
Congenital malformation of pharynx NOS
Imperforate pharynx

## Cleft Palate

Cleft in soft palate　　　　　　　　Cleft in hard and soft palate

Hard palate

Soft palate

Cleft　　　　　　　Cleft

N Newborn: 0　P Pediatric: 0-17　M Maternity: 12-55　A Adult: 15-124　MCC Major CC Condition　PDx MCC PDx acts as own MCC　CC CC Condition　PDx CC PDx acts as own CC

900　　　　　　　　　　　　　　　　　　　　　　　　　　　　　　　　　　　　　　ICD-10-CM 2018

✓4th **Q39  Congenital malformations of esophagus**

> **CC Excl: For MCC codes in category Q39:** PDX collection 1081
> **For CC codes in category Q39:** PDX collection 1082

**Q39.0  Atresia of esophagus without fistula**    `MCC`
  Atresia of esophagus NOS

**Q39.1  Atresia of esophagus with tracheo-esophageal fistula**    `MCC`
  Atresia of esophagus with broncho-esophageal fistula

**Q39.2  Congenital tracheo-esophageal fistula without atresia**    `MCC`
  Congenital tracheo-esophageal fistula NOS

**Q39.3  Congenital stenosis and stricture of esophagus**    `MCC`

**Q39.4  Esophageal web**    `MCC`

**Q39.5  Congenital dilatation of esophagus**    `CC`
  Congenital cardiospasm

**Q39.6  Congenital diverticulum of esophagus**    `CC`
  Congenital esophageal pouch

**Q39.8  Other congenital malformations of esophagus**    `CC`
  Congenital absence of esophagus
  Congenital displacement of esophagus
  Congenital duplication of esophagus

**Q39.9  Congenital malformation of esophagus, unspecified**    `CC`

✓4th **Q40  Other congenital malformations of upper alimentary tract**

**Q40.0  Congenital hypertrophic pyloric stenosis**
  Congenital or infantile constriction
  Congenital or infantile hypertrophy
  Congenital or infantile spasm
  Congenital or infantile stenosis
  Congenital or infantile stricture

**Q40.1  Congenital hiatus hernia**
  Congenital displacement of cardia through esophageal hiatus
  *EXCLUDES 1*  *congenital diaphragmatic hernia (Q79.0)*

**Q40.2  Other specified congenital malformations of stomach**
  Congenital displacement of stomach
  Congenital diverticulum of stomach
  Congenital hourglass stomach
  Congenital duplication of stomach
  Megalogastria
  Microgastria

**Q40.3  Congenital malformation of stomach, unspecified**

**Q40.8  Other specified congenital malformations of upper alimentary tract**

**Q40.9  Congenital malformation of upper alimentary tract, unspecified**
  Congenital anomaly of upper alimentary tract
  Congenital deformity of upper alimentary tract

✓4th **Q41  Congenital absence, atresia and stenosis of small intestine**
  *INCLUDES*  congenital obstruction, occlusion or stricture of small intestine or intestine NOS
  *EXCLUDES 1*  *cystic fibrosis with intestinal manifestation (E84.11)*
        *meconium ileus NOS (without cystic fibrosis) (P76.0)*

> **CC Excl: For CC codes in category Q41:** PDX collection 1083

**Q41.0  Congenital absence, atresia and stenosis of duodenum**    `CC`

**Q41.1  Congenital absence, atresia and stenosis of jejunum**    `CC`
  Apple peel syndrome
  Imperforate jejunum

**Q41.2  Congenital absence, atresia and stenosis of ileum**    `CC`

**Q41.8  Congenital absence, atresia and stenosis of other specified parts of small intestine**    `CC`

**Q41.9  Congenital absence, atresia and stenosis of small intestine, part unspecified**    `CC`
  Congenital absence, atresia and stenosis of intestine NOS

✓4th **Q42  Congenital absence, atresia and stenosis of large intestine**
  *INCLUDES*  congenital obstruction, occlusion and stricture of large intestine

> **CC Excl: For CC codes in category Q42:** PDX collection 1084

**Q42.0  Congenital absence, atresia and stenosis of rectum with fistula**    `CC`

**Q42.1  Congenital absence, atresia and stenosis of rectum without fistula**    `CC`
  Imperforate rectum

**Q42.2  Congenital absence, atresia and stenosis of anus with fistula**    `CC`

**Q42.3  Congenital absence, atresia and stenosis of anus without fistula**    `CC`
  Imperforate anus

**Q42.8  Congenital absence, atresia and stenosis of other parts of large intestine**    `CC`

**Q42.9  Congenital absence, atresia and stenosis of large intestine, part unspecified**    `CC`

✓4th **Q43  Other congenital malformations of intestine**

> **CC Excl: For CC codes in category Q43, unless otherwise noted:** PDX collection 1087

**Q43.0  Meckel's diverticulum (displaced) (hypertrophic)**
  Persistent omphalomesenteric duct
  Persistent vitelline duct

**Q43.1  Hirschsprung's disease**    `CC`
  Aganglionosis
  Congenital (aganglionic) megacolon
  **CC Excl:** PDX collection 1085

**Q43.2  Other congenital functional disorders of colon**    `CC`
  Congenital dilatation of colon
  **CC Excl:** PDX collection 1085

**Q43.3  Congenital malformations of intestinal fixation**    `CC`
  Congenital omental, anomalous adhesions [bands]
  Congenital peritoneal adhesions [bands]
  Incomplete rotation of cecum and colon
  Insufficient rotation of cecum and colon
  Jackson's membrane
  Malrotation of colon
  Rotation failure of cecum and colon
  Universal mesentery
  **CC Excl:** DX collection 1086

**Q43.4  Duplication of intestine**    `CC`

**Q43.5  Ectopic anus**    `CC`

**Q43.6  Congenital fistula of rectum and anus**    `CC`
  *EXCLUDES 1*  *congenital fistula of anus with absence, atresia and stenosis (Q42.2)*
        *congenital fistula of rectum with absence, atresia and stenosis (Q42.0)*
        *congenital rectovaginal fistula (Q52.2)*
        *congenital urethrorectal fistula (Q64.73)*
        *pilonidal fistula or sinus (L05.-)*

**Q43.7  Persistent cloaca**    `CC`
  Cloaca NOS

**Q43.8  Other specified congenital malformations of intestine**    `CC`
  Congenital blind loop syndrome
  Congenital diverticulitis, colon
  Congenital diverticulum, intestine
  Dolichocolon
  Megaloappendix
  Megaloduodenum
  Microcolon
  Transposition of appendix
  Transposition of colon
  Transposition of intestine
  **AHA:** 2013, 2Q, 31

**Q43.9  Congenital malformation of intestine, unspecified**    `CC`

✓4th **Q44  Congenital malformations of gallbladder, bile ducts and liver**

> **CC Excl: For CC codes in category Q44, unless otherwise noted:** PDX collection 1088

**Q44.0  Agenesis, aplasia and hypoplasia of gallbladder**    `CC`
  Congenital absence of gallbladder

**Q44.1  Other congenital malformations of gallbladder**    `CC`
  Congenital malformation of gallbladder NOS
  Intrahepatic gallbladder

**Q44.2  Atresia of bile ducts**    `MCC`
  **CC Excl:** PDX collection 1089

**Q44.3  Congenital stenosis and stricture of bile ducts**    `MCC`
  **CC Excl:** PDX collection 1089

**Q44.4  Choledochal cyst**    `CC`

**Q44.5  Other congenital malformations of bile ducts**    `CC`
  Accessory hepatic duct
  Biliary duct duplication
  Congenital malformation of bile duct NOS
  Cystic duct duplication

**Q44.6  Cystic disease of liver**    `CC`
  Fibrocystic disease of liver
  **CC Excl:** PDX collection 1090

**Q44.7  Other congenital malformations of liver**    `CC`
  Accessory liver
  Alagille's syndrome
  Congenital absence of liver
  Congenital hepatomegaly
  Congenital malformation of liver NOS

---

✓ Additional Character Req    ✓7th Placeholder Alert    Unacceptable PDx    Manifestation    `H1`-`H14` HAC    `HCC` CMS-HCC Condition    *EXCLUDES 1* Not Coded Here    *EXCLUDES 2* Not Included Here

✓4ᵗʰ **Q45**   **Other congenital malformations of digestive system**
> EXCLUDES 2   *congenital diaphragmatic hernia (Q79.0)*
> *congenital hiatus hernia (Q40.1)*

> CC Excl: For CC codes in category Q45: PDX collection 1091

**Q45.0**   **Agenesis, aplasia and hypoplasia of pancreas**    CC
Congenital absence of pancreas

**Q45.1**   **Annular pancreas**    CC

**Q45.2**   **Congenital pancreatic cyst**    CC

**Q45.3**   **Other congenital malformations of pancreas and pancreatic duct**    CC
Accessory pancreas
Congenital malformation of pancreas or pancreatic duct NOS
> EXCLUDES 1   *congenital diabetes mellitus (E10.-)*
> *cystic fibrosis (E84.0-E84.9)*
> *fibrocystic disease of pancreas (E84.-)*
> *neonatal diabetes mellitus (P70.2)*

**Q45.8**   **Other specified congenital malformations of digestive system**
Absence (complete) (partial) of alimentary tract NOS
Duplication of digestive system
Malposition, congenital of digestive system

**Q45.9**   **Congenital malformation of digestive system, unspecified**
Congenital anomaly of digestive system
Congenital deformity of digestive system

## Congenital malformations of genital organs (Q50–Q56)

> EXCLUDES 1   *androgen insensitivity syndrome (E34.5-)*
> *syndromes associated with anomalies in the number and form of chromosomes (Q90-Q99)*

✓4ᵗʰ **Q50**   **Congenital malformations of ovaries, fallopian tubes and broad ligaments**

✓5ᵗʰ **Q50.0**   **Congenital absence of ovary**
> EXCLUDES 1   *Turner's syndrome (Q96.-)*

    **Q50.01**   **Congenital absence of ovary, unilateral**    ♀

    **Q50.02**   **Congenital absence of ovary, bilateral**    ♀

**Q50.1**   **Developmental ovarian cyst**    ♀

**Q50.2**   **Congenital torsion of ovary**    ♀

✓5ᵗʰ **Q50.3**   **Other congenital malformations of ovary**

    **Q50.31**   **Accessory ovary**    ♀

    **Q50.32**   **Ovarian streak**    ♀
46, XX with streak gonads

    **Q50.39**   **Other congenital malformation of ovary**    ♀
Congenital malformation of ovary NOS

**Q50.4**   **Embryonic cyst of fallopian tube**    ♀
Fimbrial cyst

**Q50.5**   **Embryonic cyst of broad ligament**    ♀
Epoophoron cyst
Parovarian cyst

**Q50.6**   **Other congenital malformations of fallopian tube and broad ligament**    ♀
Absence of fallopian tube and broad ligament
Accessory fallopian tube and broad ligament
Atresia of fallopian tube and broad ligament
Congenital malformation of fallopian tube or broad ligament NOS

✓4ᵗʰ **Q51**   **Congenital malformations of uterus and cervix**

**Q51.0**   **Agenesis and aplasia of uterus**    ♀
Congenital absence of uterus

✓5ᵗʰ **Q51.1**   **Doubling of uterus with doubling of cervix and vagina**

    **Q51.10**   **Doubling of uterus with doubling of cervix and vagina without obstruction**    ♀
Doubling of uterus with doubling of cervix and vagina NOS

    **Q51.11**   **Doubling of uterus with doubling of cervix and vagina with obstruction**    ♀

**Q51.2**   **Other doubling of uterus**    ♀
Doubling of uterus NOS
Septate uterus, complete or partial

**Q51.3**   **Bicornate uterus**    ♀
Bicornate uterus, complete or partial

**Q51.4**   **Unicornate uterus**    ♀
Unicornate uterus with or without a separate uterine horn
Uterus with only one functioning horn

**Q51.5**   **Agenesis and aplasia of cervix**    ♀
Congenital absence of cervix

**Q51.6**   **Embryonic cyst of cervix**    ♀

**Q51.7**   **Congenital fistulae between uterus and digestive and urinary tracts**    ♀

✓5ᵗʰ **Q51.8**   **Other congenital malformations of uterus and cervix**

   ✓6ᵗʰ **Q51.81**   **Other congenital malformations of uterus**

       **Q51.810**   **Arcuate uterus**    ♀
Arcuatus uterus

       **Q51.811**   **Hypoplasia of uterus**    ♀

       **Q51.818**   **Other congenital malformations of uterus**    ♀
Müllerian anomaly of uterus NEC

   ✓6ᵗʰ **Q51.82**   **Other congenital malformations of cervix**

       **Q51.820**   **Cervical duplication**    ♀

       **Q51.821**   **Hypoplasia of cervix**    ♀

       **Q51.828**   **Other congenital malformations of cervix**    ♀

**Q51.9**   **Congenital malformation of uterus and cervix, unspecified**    ♀

✓4ᵗʰ **Q52**   **Other congenital malformations of female genitalia**

**Q52.0**   **Congenital absence of vagina**    ♀
Vaginal agenesis, total or partial

✓5ᵗʰ **Q52.1**   **Doubling of vagina**
> EXCLUDES 1   *doubling of vagina with doubling of uterus and cervix (Q51.1-)*

    **Q52.10**   **Doubling of vagina, unspecified**    ♀
Septate vagina NOS

    **Q52.11**   **Transverse vaginal septum**    ♀

   ✓6ᵗʰ **Q52.12**   **Longitudinal vaginal septum**

       **Q52.120**   **Longitudinal vaginal septum, nonobstructing**    ♀

       **Q52.121**   **Longitudinal vaginal septum, obstructing, right side**    ♀

       **Q52.122**   **Longitudinal vaginal septum, obstructing, left side**    ♀

       **Q52.123**   **Longitudinal vaginal septum, microperforate, right side**    ♀

       **Q52.124**   **Longitudinal vaginal septum, microperforate, left side**    ♀

       **Q52.129**   **Other and unspecified longitudinal vaginal septum**    ♀

**Q52.2**   **Congenital rectovaginal fistula**    ♀
> EXCLUDES 1   *cloaca (Q43.7)*

**Q52.3**   **Imperforate hymen**    ♀
**DEF:** Obstructive anomaly of vagina, characterized by complete closure of membranous fold around external opening of vagina, obstructing the vaginal introitus.

**Q52.4**   **Other congenital malformations of vagina**    ♀
Canal of Nuck cyst, congenital
Congenital malformation of vagina NOS
Embryonic vaginal cyst
Gartner's duct cyst

**Q52.5**   **Fusion of labia**    ♀

**Q52.6**   **Congenital malformation of clitoris**    ♀

✓5ᵗʰ **Q52.7**   **Other and unspecified congenital malformations of vulva**

    **Q52.70**   **Unspecified congenital malformations of vulva**    ♀
Congenital malformation of vulva NOS

    **Q52.71**   **Congenital absence of vulva**    ♀

    **Q52.79**   **Other congenital malformations of vulva**    ♀
Congenital cyst of vulva

**Q52.8**   **Other specified congenital malformations of female genitalia**    ♀

**Q52.9**   **Congenital malformation of female genitalia, unspecified**    ♀

✓4ᵗʰ **Q53**   **Undescended and ectopic testicle**

✓5ᵗʰ **Q53.0**   **Ectopic testis**

    **Q53.00**   **Ectopic testis, unspecified**    ♂

    **Q53.01**   **Ectopic testis, unilateral**    ♂

    **Q53.02**   **Ectopic testes, bilateral**    ♂

✓5ᵗʰ **Q53.1**   **Undescended testicle, unilateral**

    **Q53.10**   **Unspecified undescended testicle, unilateral**    ♂

   ✓6ᵗʰ **Q53.11**   **Abdominal testis, unilateral**

       ● **Q53.111**   **Unilateral intraabdominal testis**    ♂

       ● **Q53.112**   **Unilateral inguinal testis**    ♂

    **Q53.12**   **Ectopic perineal testis, unilateral**    ♂

    ● **Q53.13**   **Unilateral high scrotal testis**    ♂

Ⓝ Newborn: 0    Ⓟ Pediatric: 0-17    Ⓜ Maternity: 12-55    Ⓐ Adult: 15-124    MCC Major CC Condition    PDxMCC PDx acts as own MCC    CC CC Condition    PDxCC PDx acts as own CC

902                     ICD-10-CM 2018

### Hypospadias and Epispadias

Balanic (glanular, coronal) hypospadias
Subcoronal hypospadias
Penile hypospadias
Penile raphe
Penoscrotal hypospadius
Scrotal hypospadias
Scrotum
Scrotal raphe
Perineal hypospadias

**Hypospadias (ventral view)**

Normal external urethral orifice
Glans penis
Foreskin (retracted)
Epispadias

**Epispadias (dorsal view)**

✓5ᵗʰ **Q53.2 Undescended testicle, bilateral**

     **Q53.20 Undescended testicle, unspecified, bilateral** ♂

     ✓6ᵗʰ **Q53.21 Abdominal testis, bilateral**

-        **Q53.211 Bilateral intraabdominal testes** ♂
-        **Q53.212 Bilateral inguinal testes** ♂

     **Q53.22 Ectopic perineal testis, bilateral** ♂

-      **Q53.23 Bilateral high scrotal testes** ♂

**Q53.9 Undescended testicle, unspecified** ♂
     Cryptorchism NOS

✓4ᵗʰ **Q54 Hypospadias**
     **EXCLUDES 1**   epispadias (Q64.0)
     **DEF:** Abnormal opening of urethra on the ventral (underside) surface of the penis.

     **Q54.0 Hypospadias, balanic** ♂
       Hypospadias, coronal
       Hypospadias, glandular

     **Q54.1 Hypospadias, penile** ♂

     **Q54.2 Hypospadias, penoscrotal** ♂

     **Q54.3 Hypospadias, perineal** ♂

     **Q54.4 Congenital chordee** ♂
       Chordee without hypospadias

     **Q54.8 Other hypospadias** ♂
       Hypospadias with intersex state

     **Q54.9 Hypospadias, unspecified** ♂

✓4ᵗʰ **Q55 Other congenital malformations of male genital organs**
     **EXCLUDES 1**   congenital hydrocele (P83.5)
         hypospadias (Q54.-)

     **Q55.0 Absence and aplasia of testis** ♂
       Monorchism

     **Q55.1 Hypoplasia of testis and scrotum** ♂
       Fusion of testes

     ✓5ᵗʰ **Q55.2 Other and unspecified congenital malformations of testis and scrotum**

       **Q55.20 Unspecified congenital malformations of testis and scrotum** ♂
         Congenital malformation of testis or scrotum NOS

       **Q55.21 Polyorchism** ♂

       **Q55.22 Retractile testis** ♂

       **Q55.23 Scrotal transposition** ♂

       **Q55.29 Other congenital malformations of testis and scrotum** ♂

     **Q55.3 Atresia of vas deferens** ♂
       Code first any associated cystic fibrosis (E84.-)

     **Q55.4 Other congenital malformations of vas deferens, epididymis, seminal vesicles and prostate** ♂
       Absence or aplasia of prostate
       Absence or aplasia of spermatic cord
       Congenital malformation of vas deferens, epididymis, seminal vesicles or prostate NOS

     **Q55.5 Congenital absence and aplasia of penis** ♂

     ✓5ᵗʰ **Q55.6 Other congenital malformations of penis**

       **Q55.61 Curvature of penis (lateral)** ♂

       **Q55.62 Hypoplasia of penis** ♂
         Micropenis

       **Q55.63 Congenital torsion of penis** ♂
         **EXCLUDES 1**   acquired torsion of penis (N48.82)

       **Q55.64 Hidden penis** ♂
         Buried penis
         Concealed penis
         **EXCLUDES 1**   acquired buried penis (N48.83)

       **Q55.69 Other congenital malformation of penis** ♂
         Congenital malformation of penis NOS

     **Q55.7 Congenital vasocutaneous fistula** ♂

     **Q55.8 Other specified congenital malformations of male genital organs** ♂

     **Q55.9 Congenital malformation of male genital organ, unspecified** ♂
       Congenital anomaly of male genital organ
       Congenital deformity of male genital organ

✓4ᵗʰ **Q56 Indeterminate sex and pseudohermaphroditism**
     **EXCLUDES 1**   46, XX true hermaphrodite (Q99.1)
         androgen insensitivity syndrome (E34.5-)
         chimera 46, XX/46, XY true hermaphrodite (Q99.0)
         female pseudohermaphroditism with adrenocortical disorder (E25.-)
         pseudohermaphroditism with specified chromosomal anomaly (Q96-Q99)
         pure gonadal dysgenesis (Q99.1)

     **Q56.0 Hermaphroditism, not elsewhere classified**
       Ovotestis

     **Q56.1 Male pseudohermaphroditism, not elsewhere classified** ♂
       46, XY with streak gonads
       Male pseudohermaphroditism NOS

     **Q56.2 Female pseudohermaphroditism, not elsewhere classified** ♀
       Female pseudohermaphroditism NOS

     **Q56.3 Pseudohermaphroditism, unspecified**

     **Q56.4 Indeterminate sex, unspecified**
       Ambiguous genitalia

## Congenital malformations of the urinary system (Q60-Q64)

✓4ᵗʰ **Q60 Renal agenesis and other reduction defects of kidney**
     **INCLUDES**   congenital absence of kidney
         congenital atrophy of kidney
         infantile atrophy of kidney

     **CC Excl: For CC codes in category Q60:** PDX collection 1092

     **Q60.0 Renal agenesis, unilateral** CC

     **Q60.1 Renal agenesis, bilateral** CC

     **Q60.2 Renal agenesis, unspecified** CC

     **Q60.3 Renal hypoplasia, unilateral** CC

     **Q60.4 Renal hypoplasia, bilateral** CC

     **Q60.5 Renal hypoplasia, unspecified** CC

     **Q60.6 Potter's syndrome** CC

✓4ᵗʰ **Q61 Cystic kidney disease**
     **EXCLUDES 1**   acquired cyst of kidney (N28.1)
         Potter's syndrome (Q60.6)

     ✓5ᵗʰ **Q61.0 Congenital renal cyst**

       **Q61.00 Congenital renal cyst, unspecified** CC
         Cyst of kidney NOS (congenital)
         **CC Excl:** PDX collection 1093

       **Q61.01 Congenital single renal cyst** CC
         **CC Excl:** PDX collection 1094

       **Q61.02 Congenital multiple renal cysts** CC
         **CC Excl:** PDX collection 1095

     ✓5ᵗʰ **Q61.1 Polycystic kidney, infantile type**
       Polycystic kidney, autosomal recessive

       **Q61.11 Cystic dilatation of collecting ducts** CC
         **CC Excl:** PDX collection 1096

       **Q61.19 Other polycystic kidney, infantile type** CC
         **CC Excl:** PDX collection 1096

     **Q61.2 Polycystic kidney, adult type** CC
       Polycystic kidney, autosomal dominant
       **CC Excl:** PDX collection 1096

     **Q61.3 Polycystic kidney, unspecified** CC
       **AHA:** 2016, 3Q, 22
       **CC Excl:** PDX collection 1096

     **Q61.4 Renal dysplasia** CC
       Multicystic dysplastic kidney
       Multicystic kidney (development)
       Multicystic kidney disease
       Multicystic renal dysplasia
       **EXCLUDES 1**   polycystic kidney disease (Q61.11-Q61.3)
       **CC Excl:** PDX collection 1097

✓ Additional Character Req    ✓x7ᵗʰ Placeholder Alert    Unacceptable PDx    Manifestation    **H1**-**H14** HAC    **HCC** CMS-HCC Condition    **EXCLUDES 1** Not Coded Here    **EXCLUDES 2** Not Included Here

ICD-10-CM 2018        **903**

**Chapter 17. Congenital Malformations, Deformations and Chromosomal Abnormalities**     **Q53.2–Q61.4**

**Chapter 17. Congenital Malformations, Deformations and Chromosomal Abnormalities**

**Q61.5 Medullary cystic kidney** `CC`
Nephronopthisis
Sponge kidney NOS
**DEF:** Sponge kidney: Dilated collecting tubules; usually asymptomatic but calcinosis in tubules may cause renal insufficiency.
**CC Excl:** PDX collection 1095

**Q61.8 Other cystic kidney diseases** `CC`
Fibrocystic kidney
Fibrocystic renal degeneration or disease
**CC Excl:** PDX collection 1095

**Q61.9 Cystic kidney disease, unspecified** `CC`
Meckel-Gruber syndrome
**CC Excl:** PDX collection 1093

✓4th **Q62 Congenital obstructive defects of renal pelvis and congenital malformations of ureter**

**CC Excl: For CC codes in category Q62:** PDX collection 1098

**Q62.0 Congenital hydronephrosis** `CC`

✓5th **Q62.1 Congenital occlusion of ureter**
Atresia and stenosis of ureter

    **Q62.10 Congenital occlusion of ureter, unspecified** `CC`

    **Q62.11 Congenital occlusion of ureteropelvic junction** `CC`

    **Q62.12 Congenital occlusion of ureterovesical orifice** `CC`

**Q62.2 Congenital megaureter** `CC`
Congenital dilatation of ureter

✓5th **Q62.3 Other obstructive defects of renal pelvis and ureter**

    **Q62.31 Congenital ureterocele, orthotopic** `CC`

    **Q62.32 Cecoureterocele** `CC`
Ectopic ureterocele

    **Q62.39 Other obstructive defects of renal pelvis and ureter** `CC`
Ureteropelvic junction obstruction NOS

**Q62.4 Agenesis of ureter**
Congenital absence ureter

**Q62.5 Duplication of ureter**
Accessory ureter
Double ureter

✓5th **Q62.6 Malposition of ureter**

    **Q62.60 Malposition of ureter, unspecified**

    **Q62.61 Deviation of ureter**

    **Q62.62 Displacement of ureter**

    **Q62.63 Anomalous implantation of ureter**
Ectopia of ureter
Ectopic ureter

    **Q62.69 Other malposition of ureter**

**Q62.7 Congenital vesico-uretero-renal reflux**

**Q62.8 Other congenital malformations of ureter**
Anomaly of ureter NOS

✓4th **Q63 Other congenital malformations of kidney**
*EXCLUDES 1* congenital nephrotic syndrome (N04.-)

**Q63.0 Accessory kidney**

**Q63.1 Lobulated, fused and horseshoe kidney**

**Q63.2 Ectopic kidney**
Congenital displaced kidney
Malrotation of kidney

**Q63.3 Hyperplastic and giant kidney**
Compensatory hypertrophy of kidney

**Q63.8 Other specified congenital malformations of kidney**
Congenital renal calculi

**Q63.9 Congenital malformation of kidney, unspecified**

✓4th **Q64 Other congenital malformations of urinary system**

**Q64.0 Epispadias**
*EXCLUDES 1* hypospadias (Q54.-)

✓5th **Q64.1 Exstrophy of urinary bladder**

**CC Excl: For CC codes in subcategory Q64.1:**
PDX collection 1099

    **Q64.10 Exstrophy of urinary bladder, unspecified** `CC`
Ectopia vesicae

    **Q64.11 Supravesical fissure of urinary bladder** `CC`

    **Q64.12 Cloacal exstrophy of urinary bladder** `CC`

    **Q64.19 Other exstrophy of urinary bladder** `CC`
Extroversion of bladder

**Q64.2 Congenital posterior urethral valves** `CC`
**CC Excl:** PDX collection 1100

✓5th **Q64.3 Other atresia and stenosis of urethra and bladder neck**

**CC Excl: For CC codes in subcategory Q64.3:**
PDX collection 1100

    **Q64.31 Congenital bladder neck obstruction** `CC`
Congenital obstruction of vesicourethral orifice

    **Q64.32 Congenital stricture of urethra** `CC`

    **Q64.33 Congenital stricture of urinary meatus** `CC`

    **Q64.39 Other atresia and stenosis of urethra and bladder neck** `CC`
Atresia and stenosis of urethra and bladder neck NOS

**Q64.4 Malformation of urachus**
Cyst of urachus
Patent urachus
Prolapse of urachus

**Q64.5 Congenital absence of bladder and urethra**

**Q64.6 Congenital diverticulum of bladder**

✓5th **Q64.7 Other and unspecified congenital malformations of bladder and urethra**
*EXCLUDES 1* congenital prolapse of bladder (mucosa) (Q79.4)

    **Q64.70 Unspecified congenital malformation of bladder and urethra**
Malformation of bladder or urethra NOS

    **Q64.71 Congenital prolapse of urethra**

    **Q64.72 Congenital prolapse of urinary meatus**

    **Q64.73 Congenital urethrorectal fistula**

    **Q64.74 Double urethra**

    **Q64.75 Double urinary meatus**

    **Q64.79 Other congenital malformations of bladder and urethra**

**Q64.8 Other specified congenital malformations of urinary system**

**Q64.9 Congenital malformation of urinary system, unspecified**
Congenital anomaly NOS of urinary system
Congenital deformity NOS of urinary system

## Congenital malformations and deformations of the musculoskeletal system (Q65-Q79)

✓4th **Q65 Congenital deformities of hip**
*EXCLUDES 1* clicking hip (R29.4)

✓5th **Q65.0 Congenital dislocation of hip, unilateral**

    **Q65.00 Congenital dislocation of unspecified hip, unilateral**

    **Q65.01 Congenital dislocation of right hip, unilateral**

    **Q65.02 Congenital dislocation of left hip, unilateral**

**Q65.1 Congenital dislocation of hip, bilateral**

**Q65.2 Congenital dislocation of hip, unspecified**

✓5th **Q65.3 Congenital partial dislocation of hip, unilateral**

    **Q65.30 Congenital partial dislocation of unspecified hip, unilateral**

    **Q65.31 Congenital partial dislocation of right hip, unilateral**

    **Q65.32 Congenital partial dislocation of left hip, unilateral**

**Q65.4 Congenital partial dislocation of hip, bilateral**

**Q65.5 Congenital partial dislocation of hip, unspecified**

**Q65.6 Congenital unstable hip**
Congenital dislocatable hip

✓5th **Q65.8 Other congenital deformities of hip**

    **Q65.81 Congenital coxa valga**

    **Q65.82 Congenital coxa vara**

    **Q65.89 Other specified congenital deformities of hip**
Anteversion of femoral neck
Congenital acetabular dysplasia

**Q65.9 Congenital deformity of hip, unspecified**

✓4th **Q66 Congenital deformities of feet**
*EXCLUDES 1* reduction defects of feet (Q72.-)
valgus deformities (acquired) (M21.0-)
varus deformities (acquired) (M21.1-)

**Q66.0 Congenital talipes equinovarus**

**Q66.1 Congenital talipes calcaneovarus**

✓5th **Q66.2 Congenital metatarsus (primus) varus**

    **Q66.21 Congenital metatarsus primus varus**

    **Q66.22 Congenital metatarsus adductus**
Congenital metatarsus varus

**Q66.3 Other congenital varus deformities of feet**
Hallux varus, congenital

N Newborn: 0   P Pediatric: 0-17   M Maternity: 12-55   A Adult: 15-124   MCC Major CC Condition   PDxMCC PDx acts as own MCC   CC CC Condition   PDxCC PDx acts as own CC

904             ICD-10-CM 2018

**Q66.4  Congenital** talipes calcaneovalgus

✓5ᵗʰ **Q66.5  Congenital** pes planus
Congenital flat foot
Congenital rigid flat foot
Congenital spastic (everted) flat foot
EXCLUDES 1  pes planus, acquired (M21.4)

**Q66.50  Congenital pes planus, unspecified foot**

**Q66.51  Congenital pes planus, right foot**

**Q66.52  Congenital pes planus, left foot**

**Q66.6  Other congenital valgus deformities of feet**
Congenital metatarsus valgus

**Q66.7  Congenital pes cavus**

✓5ᵗʰ **Q66.8  Other congenital deformities of feet**

**Q66.80  Congenital vertical talus deformity, unspecified foot**

**Q66.81  Congenital vertical talus deformity, right foot**

**Q66.82  Congenital vertical talus deformity, left foot**

**Q66.89  Other specified congenital deformities of feet**
Congenital asymmetric talipes
Congenital clubfoot NOS
Congenital talipes NOS
Congenital tarsal coalition
Hammer toe, congenital

**Q66.9  Congenital deformity of feet, unspecified**

✓4ᵗʰ **Q67  Congenital musculoskeletal deformities of head, face, spine and chest**
EXCLUDES 1  congenital malformation syndromes classified to Q87-
Potter's syndrome (Q60.6)

**Q67.0  Congenital facial asymmetry**

**Q67.1  Congenital compression facies**

**Q67.2  Dolichocephaly**

**Q67.3  Plagiocephaly**

**Q67.4  Other congenital deformities of skull, face and jaw**
Congenital depressions in skull
Congenital hemifacial atrophy or hypertrophy
Deviation of nasal septum, congenital
Squashed or bent nose, congenital
EXCLUDES 1  dentofacial anomalies [including malocclusion]
(M26.-)
syphilitic saddle nose (A50.5)

**Q67.5  Congenital deformity of spine**  CC
Congenital postural scoliosis
Congenital scoliosis NOS
EXCLUDES 1  infantile idiopathic scoliosis (M41.0)
scoliosis due to congenital bony malformation (Q76.3)
**AHA:** 2014, 4Q, 26
**CC Excl:** PDX collection 1101

**Q67.6  Pectus excavatum**
Congenital funnel chest

**Q67.7  Pectus carinatum**
Congenital pigeon chest

**Q67.8  Other congenital deformities of chest**  CC
Congenital deformity of chest wall NOS
**CC Excl:** PDX collection 1102

✓4ᵗʰ **Q68  Other congenital musculoskeletal deformities**
EXCLUDES 1  reduction defects of limb(s) (Q71-Q73)
EXCLUDES 2  congenital myotonic chondrodystrophy (G71.13)

**Q68.0  Congenital deformity of sternocleidomastoid muscle**
Congenital contracture of sternocleidomastoid (muscle)
Congenital (sternomastoid) torticollis
Sternomastoid tumor (congenital)

**Q68.1  Congenital deformity of finger(s) and hand**  CC
Congenital clubfinger
Spade-like hand (congenital)
**CC Excl:** PDX collection 1102

**Q68.2  Congenital deformity of knee**
Congenital dislocation of knee
Congenital genu recurvatum

**Q68.3  Congenital bowing of femur**
EXCLUDES 1  anteversion of femur (neck) (Q65.89)

**Q68.4  Congenital bowing of tibia and fibula**

**Q68.5  Congenital bowing of long bones of leg, unspecified**

**Q68.6  Discoid meniscus**

**Q68.8  Other specified congenital musculoskeletal deformities**
Congenital deformity of clavicle
Congenital deformity of elbow
Congenital deformity of forearm
Congenital deformity of scapula
Congenital deformity of wrist
Congenital dislocation of elbow
Congenital dislocation of shoulder
Congenital dislocation of wrist

✓4ᵗʰ **Q69  Polydactyly**

**Q69.0  Accessory finger(s)**

**Q69.1  Accessory thumb(s)**

**Q69.2  Accessory toe(s)**
Accessory hallux

**Q69.9  Polydactyly, unspecified**
Supernumerary digit(s) NOS

✓4ᵗʰ **Q70  Syndactyly**

✓5ᵗʰ **Q70.0  Fused fingers**
Complex syndactyly of fingers with synostosis

**Q70.00  Fused fingers, unspecified hand**

**Q70.01  Fused fingers, right hand**

**Q70.02  Fused fingers, left hand**

**Q70.03  Fused fingers, bilateral**

✓5ᵗʰ **Q70.1  Webbed fingers**
Simple syndactyly of fingers without synostosis

**Q70.10  Webbed fingers, unspecified hand**

**Q70.11  Webbed fingers, right hand**

**Q70.12  Webbed fingers, left hand**

**Q70.13  Webbed fingers, bilateral**

✓5ᵗʰ **Q70.2  Fused toes**
Complex syndactyly of toes with synostosis

**Q70.20  Fused toes, unspecified foot**

**Q70.21  Fused toes, right foot**

**Q70.22  Fused toes, left foot**

**Q70.23  Fused toes, bilateral**

✓5ᵗʰ **Q70.3  Webbed toes**
Simple syndactyly of toes without synostosis

**Q70.30  Webbed toes, unspecified foot**

**Q70.31  Webbed toes, right foot**

**Q70.32  Webbed toes, left foot**

**Q70.33  Webbed toes, bilateral**

**Q70.4  Polysyndactyly, unspecified**
EXCLUDES 1  specified syndactyly of hand and feet—code to
specified conditions (Q70.0-Q70.3-)

**Q70.9  Syndactyly, unspecified**
Symphalangy NOS

✓4ᵗʰ **Q71  Reduction defects of upper limb**

✓5ᵗʰ **Q71.0  Congenital complete absence of upper limb**

**Q71.00  Congenital complete absence of unspecified upper limb**

**Q71.01  Congenital complete absence of right upper limb**

**Q71.02  Congenital complete absence of left upper limb**

**Q71.03  Congenital complete absence of upper limb, bilateral**

✓5ᵗʰ **Q71.1  Congenital absence of upper arm and forearm with hand present**

**Q71.10  Congenital absence of unspecified upper arm and forearm with hand present**

**Q71.11  Congenital absence of right upper arm and forearm with hand present**

**Q71.12  Congenital absence of left upper arm and forearm with hand present**

**Q71.13  Congenital absence of upper arm and forearm with hand present, bilateral**

✓5ᵗʰ **Q71.2  Congenital absence of both forearm and hand**

**Q71.20  Congenital absence of both forearm and hand, unspecified upper limb**

**Q71.21  Congenital absence of both forearm and hand, right upper limb**

**Q71.22  Congenital absence of both forearm and hand, left upper limb**

**Q71.23  Congenital absence of both forearm and hand, bilateral**

✓5th **Q71.3 Congenital absence of hand and finger**
   **Q71.30 Congenital absence of unspecified hand and finger**
   **Q71.31 Congenital absence of right hand and finger**
   **Q71.32 Congenital absence of left hand and finger**
   **Q71.33 Congenital absence of hand and finger, bilateral**

✓5th **Q71.4 Longitudinal reduction defect of radius**
   Clubhand (congenital)
   Radial clubhand
   **Q71.40 Longitudinal reduction defect of unspecified radius**
   **Q71.41 Longitudinal reduction defect of right radius**
   **Q71.42 Longitudinal reduction defect of left radius**
   **Q71.43 Longitudinal reduction defect of radius, bilateral**

✓5th **Q71.5 Longitudinal reduction defect of ulna**
   **Q71.50 Longitudinal reduction defect of unspecified ulna**
   **Q71.51 Longitudinal reduction defect of right ulna**
   **Q71.52 Longitudinal reduction defect of left ulna**
   **Q71.53 Longitudinal reduction defect of ulna, bilateral**

✓5th **Q71.6 Lobster-claw hand**
   **Q71.60 Lobster-claw hand, unspecified hand**
   **Q71.61 Lobster-claw right hand**
   **Q71.62 Lobster-claw left hand**
   **Q71.63 Lobster-claw hand, bilateral**

✓5th **Q71.8 Other reduction defects of upper limb**
  ✓6th **Q71.81 Congenital shortening of upper limb**
    **Q71.811 Congenital shortening of right upper limb**
    **Q71.812 Congenital shortening of left upper limb**
    **Q71.813 Congenital shortening of upper limb, bilateral**
    **Q71.819 Congenital shortening of unspecified upper limb**
  ✓6th **Q71.89 Other reduction defects of upper limb**
    **Q71.891 Other reduction defects of right upper limb**
    **Q71.892 Other reduction defects of left upper limb**
    **Q71.893 Other reduction defects of upper limb, bilateral**
    **Q71.899 Other reduction defects of unspecified upper limb**

✓5th **Q71.9 Unspecified reduction defect of upper limb**
   **Q71.90 Unspecified reduction defect of unspecified upper limb**
   **Q71.91 Unspecified reduction defect of right upper limb**
   **Q71.92 Unspecified reduction defect of left upper limb**
   **Q71.93 Unspecified reduction defect of upper limb, bilateral**

✓4th **Q72 Reduction defects of lower limb**
 ✓5th **Q72.0 Congenital complete absence of lower limb**
   **Q72.00 Congenital complete absence of unspecified lower limb**
   **Q72.01 Congenital complete absence of right lower limb**
   **Q72.02 Congenital complete absence of left lower limb**
   **Q72.03 Congenital complete absence of lower limb, bilateral**

 ✓5th **Q72.1 Congenital absence of thigh and lower leg with foot present**
   **Q72.10 Congenital absence of unspecified thigh and lower leg with foot present**
   **Q72.11 Congenital absence of right thigh and lower leg with foot present**
   **Q72.12 Congenital absence of left thigh and lower leg with foot present**
   **Q72.13 Congenital absence of thigh and lower leg with foot present, bilateral**

 ✓5th **Q72.2 Congenital absence of both lower leg and foot**
   **Q72.20 Congenital absence of both lower leg and foot, unspecified lower limb**
   **Q72.21 Congenital absence of both lower leg and foot, right lower limb**
   **Q72.22 Congenital absence of both lower leg and foot, left lower limb**
   **Q72.23 Congenital absence of both lower leg and foot, bilateral**

 ✓5th **Q72.3 Congenital absence of foot and toe(s)**
   **Q72.30 Congenital absence of unspecified foot and toe(s)**
   **Q72.31 Congenital absence of right foot and toe(s)**

   **Q72.32 Congenital absence of left foot and toe(s)**
   **Q72.33 Congenital absence of foot and toe(s), bilateral**

✓5th **Q72.4 Longitudinal reduction defect of femur**
   Proximal femoral focal deficiency
   **Q72.40 Longitudinal reduction defect of unspecified femur**
   **Q72.41 Longitudinal reduction defect of right femur**
   **Q72.42 Longitudinal reduction defect of left femur**
   **Q72.43 Longitudinal reduction defect of femur, bilateral**

✓5th **Q72.5 Longitudinal reduction defect of tibia**
   **Q72.50 Longitudinal reduction defect of unspecified tibia**
   **Q72.51 Longitudinal reduction defect of right tibia**
   **Q72.52 Longitudinal reduction defect of left tibia**
   **Q72.53 Longitudinal reduction defect of tibia, bilateral**

✓5th **Q72.6 Longitudinal reduction defect of fibula**
   **Q72.60 Longitudinal reduction defect of unspecified fibula**
   **Q72.61 Longitudinal reduction defect of right fibula**
   **Q72.62 Longitudinal reduction defect of left fibula**
   **Q72.63 Longitudinal reduction defect of fibula, bilateral**

✓5th **Q72.7 Split foot**
   **Q72.70 Split foot, unspecified lower limb**
   **Q72.71 Split foot, right lower limb**
   **Q72.72 Split foot, left lower limb**
   **Q72.73 Split foot, bilateral**

✓5th **Q72.8 Other reduction defects of lower limb**
  ✓6th **Q72.81 Congenital shortening of lower limb**
    **Q72.811 Congenital shortening of right lower limb**
    **Q72.812 Congenital shortening of left lower limb**
    **Q72.813 Congenital shortening of lower limb, bilateral**
    **Q72.819 Congenital shortening of unspecified lower limb**
  ✓6th **Q72.89 Other reduction defects of lower limb**
    **Q72.891 Other reduction defects of right lower limb**
    **Q72.892 Other reduction defects of left lower limb**
    **Q72.893 Other reduction defects of lower limb, bilateral**
    **Q72.899 Other reduction defects of unspecified lower limb**

✓5th **Q72.9 Unspecified reduction defect of lower limb**
   **Q72.90 Unspecified reduction defect of unspecified lower limb**
   **Q72.91 Unspecified reduction defect of right lower limb**
   **Q72.92 Unspecified reduction defect of left lower limb**
   **Q72.93 Unspecified reduction defect of lower limb, bilateral**

✓4th **Q73 Reduction defects of unspecified limb**
 **Q73.0 Congenital absence of unspecified limb(s)**
   Amelia NOS
 **Q73.1 Phocomelia, unspecified limb(s)**
   Phocomelia NOS
 **Q73.8 Other reduction defects of unspecified limb(s)**
   Longitudinal reduction deformity of unspecified limb(s)
   Ectromelia of limb NOS
   Hemimelia of limb NOS
   Reduction defect of limb NOS

✓4th **Q74 Other congenital malformations of limb(s)**
  **EXCLUDES1** *polydactyly (Q69.-)*
   *reduction defect of limb (Q71-Q73)*
   *syndactyly (Q70.-)*
 **Q74.0 Other congenital malformations of upper limb(s), including shoulder girdle**
   Accessory carpal bones
   Cleidocranial dysostosis
   Congenital pseudarthrosis of clavicle
   Macrodactylia (fingers)
   Madelung's deformity
   Radioulnar synostosis
   Sprengel's deformity
   Triphalangeal thumb

**Q74.1 Congenital malformation of** knee
    Congenital absence of patella
    Congenital dislocation of patella
    Congenital genu valgum
    Congenital genu varum
    Rudimentary patella
    **EXCLUDES 1**    *congenital dislocation of knee (Q68.2)*
        *congenital genu recurvatum (Q68.2)*
        *nail patella syndrome (Q87.2)*

**Q74.2 Other congenital malformations of** lower limb(s), **including pelvic girdle**
    Congenital fusion of sacroiliac joint
    Congenital malformation of ankle joint
    Congenital malformation of sacroiliac joint
    **EXCLUDES 1**    *anteversion of femur (neck) (Q65.89)*

**Q74.3 Arthrogryposis multiplex congenita**    `CC`
    **CC Excl:** PDX collection 1102

**Q74.8 Other** specified congenital malformations of limb(s)

**Q74.9 Unspecified** congenital malformation of limb(s)
    Congenital anomaly of limb(s) NOS

✓4th **Q75 Other congenital malformations of** skull and face bones
    **EXCLUDES 1**    *congenital malformation of face NOS (Q18.-)*
        *congenital malformation syndromes classified to Q87.-*
        *dentofacial anomalies [including malocclusion] (M26.-)*
        *musculoskeletal deformities of head and face (Q67.0-Q67.4)*
        *skull defects associated with congenital anomalies of brain*
            *such as:*
                *anencephaly (Q00.0)*
                *encephalocele (Q01.-)*
                *hydrocephalus (Q03.-)*
                *microcephaly (Q02)*

**Q75.0 Craniosynostosis**
    Acrocephaly
    Imperfect fusion of skull
    Oxycephaly
    Trigonocephaly

**Q75.1 Craniofacial dysostosis**
    Crouzon's disease

**Q75.2 Hypertelorism**

**Q75.3 Macrocephaly**

**Q75.4 Mandibulofacial dysostosis**
    Franceschetti syndrome
    Treacher Collins syndrome

**Q75.5 Oculomandibular dysostosis**

**Q75.8 Other specified congenital malformations of skull and face bones**
    Absence of skull bone, congenital
    Congenital deformity of forehead
    Platybasia

**Q75.9 Congenital malformation of skull and face bones, unspecified**
    Congenital anomaly of face bones NOS
    Congenital anomaly of skull NOS

✓4th **Q76 Congenital malformations of** spine and bony thorax
    **EXCLUDES 1**    *congenital musculoskeletal deformities of spine and chest (Q67.5-Q67.8)*

**Q76.0 Spina bifida occulta**
    **EXCLUDES 1**    *meningocele (spinal) (Q05.-)*
        *spina bifida (aperta) (cystica) (Q05.-)*

**Q76.1 Klippel-Feil syndrome**
    Cervical fusion syndrome

**Q76.2 Congenital spondylolisthesis**
    Congenital spondylolysis
    **EXCLUDES 1**    *spondylolisthesis (acquired) (M43.1-)*
        *spondylolysis (acquired) (M43.0-)*

**Q76.3 Congenital scoliosis due to congenital bony malformation**    `CC`
    Hemivertebra fusion or failure of segmentation with scoliosis
    **CC Excl:** PDX collection 1101

✓5th **Q76.4 Other congenital malformations of spine, not associated with scoliosis**

    **CC Excl: For CC codes in subcategory Q76.4:**
    PDX collection 1101

    ✓6th **Q76.41 Congenital** kyphosis
        **Q76.411 Congenital kyphosis, occipito-atlanto-axial region**
        **Q76.412 Congenital kyphosis, cervical region**
        **Q76.413 Congenital kyphosis, cervicothoracic region**
        **Q76.414 Congenital kyphosis, thoracic region**

        **Q76.415 Congenital kyphosis, thoracolumbar region**
        **Q76.419 Congenital kyphosis, unspecified region**

    ✓6th **Q76.42 Congenital** lordosis
        **Q76.425 Congenital lordosis, thoracolumbar region**    `CC`
        **Q76.426 Congenital lordosis, lumbar region**    `CC`
        **Q76.427 Congenital lordosis, lumbosacral region**    `CC`
        **Q76.428 Congenital lordosis, sacral and sacrococcygeal region**    `CC`
        **Q76.429 Congenital lordosis, unspecified region**    `CC`

    **Q76.49 Other congenital malformations of spine, not associated with scoliosis**
        Congenital absence of vertebra NOS
        Congenital fusion of spine NOS
        Congenital malformation of lumbosacral (joint) (region) NOS
        Congenital malformation of spine NOS
        Hemivertebra NOS
        Malformation of spine NOS
        Platyspondylisis NOS
        Supernumerary vertebra NOS

**Q76.5 Cervical rib**
    Supernumerary rib in cervical region

**Q76.6 Other congenital malformations of** ribs    `CC`
    Accessory rib
    Congenital absence of rib
    Congenital fusion of ribs
    Congenital malformation of ribs NOS
    **EXCLUDES 1**    *short rib syndrome (Q77.2)*
    **CC Excl:** PDX collection 1103

**Q76.7 Congenital malformation of** sternum    `CC`
    Congenital absence of sternum
    Sternum bifidum
    **CC Excl:** PDX collection 1103

**Q76.8 Other congenital malformations of** bony thorax    `CC`
    **CC Excl:** PDX collection 1103

**Q76.9 Congenital malformation of** bony thorax, unspecified    `CC`
    **CC Excl:** PDX collection 1103

✓4th **Q77 Osteochondrodysplasia with defects of growth of tubular bones and spine**
    **EXCLUDES 1**    *mucopolysaccharidosis (E76.0-E76.3)*
    **EXCLUDES 2**    *congenital myotonic chondrodystrophy (G71.13)*

**Q77.0 Achondrogenesis**
    Hypochondrogenesis

**Q77.1 Thanatophoric short stature**

**Q77.2 Short rib syndrome**    `CC`
    Asphyxiating thoracic dysplasia [Jeune]
    **CC Excl:** PDX collection 1103

**Q77.3 Chondrodysplasia punctata**
    **EXCLUDES 1**    *Rhizomelic chondrodysplasia punctata (E71.43)*

**Q77.4 Achondroplasia**
    Hypochondroplasia
    Osteosclerosis congenita

**Q77.5 Diastrophic dysplasia**

**Q77.6 Chondroectodermal dysplasia**
    Ellis-van Creveld syndrome

**Q77.7 Spondyloepiphyseal dysplasia**

**Q77.8 Other osteochondrodysplasia with defects of growth of tubular bones and spine**

**Q77.9 Osteochondrodysplasia with defects of growth of tubular bones and spine, unspecified**

✓4th **Q78 Other osteochondrodysplasias**
    **EXCLUDES 2**    *congenital myotonic chondrodystrophy (G71.13)*

**Q78.0 Osteogenesis imperfecta**    `CC`
    Fragilitas ossium
    Osteopsathyrosis
    **CC Excl:** PDX collection 1104

**Q78.1 Polyostotic fibrous dysplasia**
    Albright(-McCune)(-Sternberg) syndrome

**Q78.2 Osteopetrosis**    `CC`
    Albers-Schönberg syndrome
    Osteosclerosis NOS
    **CC Excl:** PDX collection 1104

**Q78.3 Progressive diaphyseal dysplasia**
    Camurati-Engelmann syndrome

---

**Chapter 17. Congenital Malformations, Deformations and Chromosomal Abnormalities**

**Gastroschisis**

Herniated small bowel (gastroschisis)

Rectus abdominus m.

Umbilicus

distal

skin

proximal

**Defect**

Q78.4 **Enchondromatosis**
     Maffucci's syndrome
     Ollier's disease

Q78.5 **Metaphyseal dysplasia**
     Pyle's syndrome

Q78.6 **Multiple congenital exostoses**
     Diaphyseal aclasis

Q78.8 **Other specified osteochondrodysplasias**
     Osteopoikilosis

Q78.9 **Osteochondrodysplasia, unspecified**
     Chondrodystrophy NOS
     Osteodystrophy NOS

✓4ᵗʰ **Q79 Congenital malformations of musculoskeletal system, not elsewhere classified**
     *EXCLUDES 2*   congenital (sternomastoid) torticollis (Q68.0)

> **CC Excl: For MCC codes in category Q79, unless otherwise noted:** PDX collection 1106

Q79.0 **Congenital diaphragmatic hernia**   MCC
     *EXCLUDES 1*   congenital hiatus hernia (Q40.1)
     **CC Excl:** PDX collection 1105

Q79.1 **Other congenital malformations of diaphragm**   MCC
     Absence of diaphragm
     Congenital malformation of diaphragm NOS
     Eventration of diaphragm
     **CC Excl:** PDX collection 1105

Q79.2 **Exomphalos**   MCC
     Omphalocele
     *EXCLUDES 1*   umbilical hernia (K42.-)

Q79.3 **Gastroschisis**   MCC

Q79.4 **Prune belly syndrome**   MCC
     Congenital prolapse of bladder mucosa
     Eagle-Barrett syndrome

✓5ᵗʰ Q79.5 **Other congenital malformations of abdominal wall**
     *EXCLUDES 1*   umbilical hernia (K42.-)

     Q79.51 **Congenital hernia of bladder**   MCC

     Q79.59 **Other congenital malformations of abdominal wall**   MCC

Q79.6 **Ehlers-Danlos syndrome**   CC
     **DEF:** Connective tissue disorder that causes hyperextended skin and joints; results in fragile blood vessels with bleeding, poor wound healing, and subcutaneous pseudotumors.
     **CC Excl:** PDX collection 1107

Q79.8 **Other congenital malformations of musculoskeletal system**
     Absence of muscle
     Absence of tendon
     Accessory muscle
     Amyotrophia congenita
     Congenital constricting bands
     Congenital shortening of tendon
     Poland syndrome

Q79.9 **Congenital malformation of musculoskeletal system, unspecified**
     Congenital anomaly of musculoskeletal system NOS
     Congenital deformity of musculoskeletal system NOS

**Other congenital malformations (Q80-Q89)**

✓4ᵗʰ **Q80 Congenital ichthyosis**
     *EXCLUDES 1*   Refsum's disease (G60.1)

Q80.0 **Ichthyosis vulgaris**

Q80.1 **X-linked ichthyosis**

Q80.2 **Lamellar ichthyosis**
     Collodion baby

Q80.3 **Congenital bullous ichthyosiform erythroderma**

Q80.4 **Harlequin fetus**

Q80.8 **Other congenital ichthyosis**

Q80.9 **Congenital ichthyosis, unspecified**

✓4ᵗʰ **Q81 Epidermolysis bullosa**

Q81.0 **Epidermolysis bullosa simplex**
     *EXCLUDES 1*   Cockayne's syndrome (Q87.1)

Q81.1 **Epidermolysis bullosa letalis**
     Herlitz' syndrome

Q81.2 **Epidermolysis bullosa dystrophica**

Q81.8 **Other epidermolysis bullosa**

Q81.9 **Epidermolysis bullosa, unspecified**

✓4ᵗʰ **Q82 Other congenital malformations of skin**
     *EXCLUDES 1*   acrodermatitis enteropathica (E83.2)
         congenital erythropoietic porphyria (E80.0)
         pilonidal cyst or sinus (L05.-)
         Sturge-Weber (-Dimitri) syndrome (Q85.8)

Q82.0 **Hereditary lymphedema**

Q82.1 **Xeroderma pigmentosum**

▲ Q82.2 **Congenital cutaneous mastocytosis**
     ▶Congenital diffuse cutaneous mastocytosis
     Congenital maculopapular cutaneous mastocytosis
     Congenital urticaria pigmentosa◀
     ~~Urticaria pigmentosa~~
     *EXCLUDES 1* ▶cutaneous mastocytosis NOS (D47.01)
         diffuse cutaneous mastocytosis (with onset after newborn period) (D47.01)◀
         malignant mastocytosis ▶(C96.2-)◀
         ▶systemic mastocytosis (D47.02)
         urticaria pigmentosa (non-congenital) (with onset after newborn period) (D47.01)◀

Q82.3 **Incontinentia pigmenti**

Q82.4 **Ectodermal dysplasia (anhidrotic)**
     *EXCLUDES 1*   Ellis-van Creveld syndrome (Q77.6)

Q82.5 **Congenital non-neoplastic nevus**
     Birthmark NOS
     Flammeus Nevus
     Portwine Nevus
     Sanguineous Nevus
     Strawberry Nevus
     Vascular Nevus NOS
     Verrucous Nevus
     *EXCLUDES 2*   araneus nevus (I78.1)
         café au lait spots (L81.3)
         lentigo (L81.4)
         melanocytic nevus (D22.-)
         nevus NOS (D22.-)
         pigmented nevus (D22.-)
         spider nevus (I78.1)
         stellar nevus (I78.1)

Q82.6 **Congenital sacral dimple**
     Parasacral dimple
     *EXCLUDES 2*   pilonidal cyst with abscess (L05.01)
         pilonidal cyst without abscess (L05.91)

Q82.8 **Other specified congenital malformations of skin**
     Abnormal palmar creases
     Accessory skin tags
     Benign familial pemphigus [Hailey-Hailey]
     Congenital poikiloderma
     Cutis laxa (hyperelastica)
     Dermatoglyphic anomalies
     Inherited keratosis palmaris et plantaris
     Keratosis follicularis [Darier-White]
     *EXCLUDES 1*   Ehlers-Danlos syndrome (Q79.6)
     **AHA:** 2016, 1Q, 17

Q82.9 **Congenital malformation of skin, unspecified**

✓4ᵗʰ **Q83 Congenital malformations of breast**
     *EXCLUDES 2*   absence of pectoral muscle (Q79.8)
         hypoplasia of breast (N64.82)
         micromastia (N64.82)

**N** Newborn: 0   **P** Pediatric: 0-17   **M** Maternity: 12-55   **A** Adult: 15-124   **MCC** Major CC Condition   **PDxMCC** PDx acts as own MCC   **CC** CC Condition   **PDxCC** PDx acts as own CC   ICD-10-CM 2018

**908**      ICD-10-CM 2018

**Q83.0**   **Congenital absence of breast with absent nipple**

**Q83.1**   **Accessory breast**
> Supernumerary breast

**Q83.2**   **Absent nipple**

**Q83.3**   **Accessory nipple**
> Supernumerary nipple

**Q83.8**   **Other congenital malformations of breast**

**Q83.9**   **Congenital malformation of breast, unspecified**

☑4ᵗʰ **Q84**   **Other congenital malformations of integument**

**Q84.0**   **Congenital alopecia**
> Congenital atrichosis

**Q84.1**   **Congenital morphological disturbances of hair, not elsewhere classified**
> Beaded hair
> Monilethrix
> Pili annulati
> **EXCLUDES 1**   *Menkes' kinky hair syndrome (E83.0)*

**Q84.2**   **Other congenital malformations of hair**
> Congenital hypertrichosis
> Congenital malformation of hair NOS
> Persistent lanugo

**Q84.3**   **Anonychia**
> **EXCLUDES 1**   *nail patella syndrome (Q87.2)*

**Q84.4**   **Congenital leukonychia**

**Q84.5**   **Enlarged and hypertrophic nails**
> Congenital onychauxis
> Pachyonychia

**Q84.6**   **Other congenital malformations of nails**
> Congenital clubnail
> Congenital koilonychia
> Congenital malformation of nail NOS

**Q84.8**   **Other specified congenital malformations of integument**
> Aplasia cutis congenita

**Q84.9**   **Congenital malformation of integument, unspecified**
> Congenital anomaly of integument NOS
> Congenital deformity of integument NOS

☑4ᵗʰ **Q85**   **Phakomatoses, not elsewhere classified**
> **EXCLUDES 1**   *ataxia telangiectasia [Louis-Bar] (G11.3)*
> *familial dysautonomia [Riley-Day] (G90.1)*

☑5ᵗʰ **Q85.0**   **Neurofibromatosis (nonmalignant)**

**Q85.00**   **Neurofibromatosis, unspecified**   HCC

**Q85.01**   **Neurofibromatosis, type 1**   HCC
> Von Recklinghausen disease

**Q85.02**   **Neurofibromatosis, type 2**   HCC
> Acoustic neurofibromatosis
> **DEF:** Inherited condition with cutaneous lesions, benign tumors of peripheral nerves, and bilateral 8th nerve masses.

**Q85.03**   **Schwannomatosis**   HCC
> **DEF:** A genetic mutation (SMARCB1/INI1) causing multiple benign tumors along nerve pathways; characterized by the exception of 8th cranial nerve involvement.

**Q85.09**   **Other neurofibromatosis**   HCC

**Q85.1**   **Tuberous sclerosis**   CC HCC
> Bourneville's disease
> Epiloia
> **CC Excl:** PDX collection 1108

**Q85.8**   **Other phakomatoses, not elsewhere classified**   CC HCC
> Peutz-Jeghers Syndrome
> Sturge-Weber(-Dimitri) syndrome
> von Hippel-Lindau syndrome
> **EXCLUDES 1**   *Meckel-Gruber syndrome (Q61.9)*
> **CC Excl:** PDX collection 1109

**Q85.9**   **Phakomatosis, unspecified**   CC HCC
> Hamartosis NOS
> **CC Excl:** PDX collection 1109

☑4ᵗʰ **Q86**   **Congenital malformation syndromes due to known exogenous causes, not elsewhere classified**
> **EXCLUDES 2**   *iodine-deficiency-related hypothyroidism (E00-E02)*
> *nonteratogenic effects of substances transmitted via placenta or breast milk (P04.-)*

**Q86.0**   **Fetal alcohol syndrome (dysmorphic)**

**Q86.1**   **Fetal hydantoin syndrome**
> Meadow's syndrome

**Q86.2**   **Dysmorphism due to warfarin**

**Q86.8**   **Other congenital malformation syndromes due to known exogenous causes**

☑4ᵗʰ **Q87**   **Other specified congenital malformation syndromes affecting multiple systems**
> Use additional code(s) to identify all associated manifestations

> **CC Excl: For CC codes in category Q87, unless otherwise noted:**
> PDX collection 540

**Q87.0**   **Congenital malformation syndromes predominantly affecting facial appearance**
> Acrocephalopolysyndactyly
> Acrocephalosyndactyly [Apert]
> Cryptophthalmos syndrome
> Cyclopia
> Goldenhar syndrome
> Moebius syndrome
> Oro-facial-digital syndrome
> Robin syndrome
> Whistling face

**Q87.1**   **Congenital malformation syndromes predominantly associated with short stature**   CC
> Aarskog syndrome
> Cockayne syndrome
> De Lange syndrome
> Dubowitz syndrome
> Noonan syndrome
> Prader-Willi syndrome
> Robinow-Silverman-Smith syndrome
> Russell-Silver syndrome
> Seckel syndrome
> **EXCLUDES 1**   *Ellis-van Creveld syndrome (Q77.6)*
> *Smith-Lemli-Opitz syndrome (E78.72)*
> **CC Excl:** PDX collection 1110

**Q87.2**   **Congenital malformation syndromes predominantly involving limbs**   CC
> Holt-Oram syndrome
> Klippel-Trenaunay-Weber syndrome
> Nail patella syndrome
> Rubinstein-Taybi syndrome
> Sirenomelia syndrome
> Thrombocytopenia with absent radius [TAR] syndrome
> VATER syndrome

**Q87.3**   **Congenital malformation syndromes involving early overgrowth**   CC
> Beckwith-Wiedemann syndrome
> Sotos syndrome
> Weaver syndrome

☑5ᵗʰ **Q87.4**   **Marfan's syndrome**

> **CC Excl: For CC codes in subcategory Q87.4:**
> PDX collection 1110

**Q87.40**   **Marfan's syndrome, unspecified**   CC

☑6ᵗʰ **Q87.41**   **Marfan's syndrome with cardiovascular manifestations**

**Q87.410**   **Marfan's syndrome with aortic dilation**   CC

**Q87.418**   **Marfan's syndrome with other cardiovascular manifestations**   CC

**Q87.42**   **Marfan's syndrome with ocular manifestations**   CC

**Q87.43**   **Marfan's syndrome with skeletal manifestation**   CC

**Q87.5**   **Other congenital malformation syndromes with other skeletal changes**

☑5ᵗʰ **Q87.8**   **Other specified congenital malformation syndromes, not elsewhere classified**
> **EXCLUDES 1**   *Zellweger syndrome (E71.510)*

**Q87.81**   **Alport syndrome**   CC
> Use additional code to identify stage of chronic kidney disease (N18.1-N18.6)

**Q87.82**   **Arterial tortuosity syndrome**   CC

**Q87.89**   **Other specified congenital malformation syndromes, not elsewhere classified**   CC
> Laurence-Moon (-Bardet)-Biedl syndrome

☑4ᵗʰ **Q89**   **Other congenital malformations, not elsewhere classified**

☑5ᵗʰ **Q89.0**   **Congenital absence and malformations of spleen**
> **EXCLUDES 1**   *isomerism of atrial appendages (with asplenia or polysplenia) (Q20.6)*

**Q89.01**   **Asplenia (congenital)**   CC
> **CC Excl:** PDX collection 1111

**Q89.09**   **Congenital malformations of spleen**   CC
> Congenital splenomegaly
> **CC Excl:** PDX collection 1111

☑ Additional Character Req   ☑x7ᵗʰ Placeholder Alert   Unacceptable PDx   Manifestation   **H1-H14** HAC   HCC CMS-HCC Condition   **EXCLUDES 1** Not Coded Here   **EXCLUDES 2** Not Included Here

ICD-10-CM 2018      **909**

**Q89.1　Congenital malformations of adrenal gland**
　　EXCLUDES 1　adrenogenital disorders (E25.-)
　　　　congenital adrenal hyperplasia (E25.0)

**Q89.2　Congenital malformations of other endocrine glands**
　　Congenital malformation of parathyroid or thyroid gland
　　Persistent thyroglossal duct
　　Thyroglossal cyst
　　EXCLUDES 1　congenital goiter (E03.0)
　　　　congenital hypothyroidism (E03.1)

**Q89.3　Situs inversus**　　　　　CC
　　Dextrocardia with situs inversus
　　Mirror-image atrial arrangement with situs inversus
　　Situs inversus or transversus abdominalis
　　Situs inversus or transversus thoracis
　　Transposition of abdominal viscera
　　Transposition of thoracic viscera
　　EXCLUDES 1　dextrocardia NOS (Q24.0)
　　CC Excl: PDX collection 1112

**Q89.4　Conjoined twins**　　　　　MCC
　　Craniopagus
　　Dicephaly
　　Pygopagus
　　Thoracopagus
　　CC Excl: PDX collection 1113

**Q89.7　Multiple congenital malformations, not elsewhere classified**　　　　　CC
　　Multiple congenital anomalies NOS
　　Multiple congenital deformities NOS
　　EXCLUDES 1　congenital malformation syndromes affecting multiple systems (Q87.-)
　　CC Excl: PDX collection 1112

**Q89.8　Other specified congenital malformations**　　　　　CC
　　Use additional code(s) to identify all associated manifestations
　　CC Excl: PDX collection 540

**Q89.9　Congenital malformation, unspecified**
　　Congenital anomaly NOS
　　Congenital deformity NOS

## Chromosomal abnormalities, not elsewhere classified (Q90-Q99)
　　EXCLUDES 2　mitochondrial metabolic disorders (E88.4-)

✓4th **Q90　Down syndrome**
　　Use additional code(s) to identify any associated physical conditions and degree of intellectual disabilities (F70-F79)

**Q90.0　Trisomy 21, nonmosaicism (meiotic nondisjunction)**

**Q90.1　Trisomy 21, mosaicism (mitotic nondisjunction)**

**Q90.2　Trisomy 21, translocation**

**Q90.9　Down syndrome, unspecified**
　　Trisomy 21 NOS

✓4th **Q91　Trisomy 18 and Trisomy 13**

　　CC Excl: For CC codes in category Q91: PDX collection 1114

**Q91.0　Trisomy 18, nonmosaicism (meiotic nondisjunction)**　　CC

**Q91.1　Trisomy 18, mosaicism (mitotic nondisjunction)**　　CC

**Q91.2　Trisomy 18, translocation**　　CC

**Q91.3　Trisomy 18, unspecified**　　CC

**Q91.4　Trisomy 13, nonmosaicism (meiotic nondisjunction)**　　CC

**Q91.5　Trisomy 13, mosaicism (mitotic nondisjunction)**　　CC

**Q91.6　Trisomy 13, translocation**　　CC

**Q91.7　Trisomy 13, unspecified**　　CC

✓4th **Q92　Other trisomies and partial trisomies of the autosomes, not elsewhere classified**
　　INCLUDES　unbalanced translocations and insertions
　　EXCLUDES 1　trisomies of chromosomes 13, 18, 21 (Q90-Q91)

**Q92.0　Whole chromosome trisomy, nonmosaicism (meiotic nondisjunction)**

**Q92.1　Whole chromosome trisomy, mosaicism (mitotic nondisjunction)**

**Q92.2　Partial trisomy**
　　Less than whole arm duplicated
　　Whole arm or more duplicated
　　EXCLUDES 1　partial trisomy due to unbalanced translocation (Q92.5)

**Q92.5　Duplications with other complex rearrangements**
　　Partial trisomy due to unbalanced translocations
　　Code also any associated deletions due to unbalanced translocations, inversions and insertions (Q93.7)

✓5th **Q92.6　Marker chromosomes**
　　Trisomies due to dicentrics
　　Trisomies due to extra rings
　　Trisomies due to isochromosomes
　　Individual with marker heterochromatin

**Q92.61　Marker chromosomes in normal individual**

**Q92.62　Marker chromosomes in abnormal individual**

**Q92.7　Triploidy and polyploidy**

**Q92.8　Other specified trisomies and partial trisomies of autosomes**
　　Duplications identified by fluorescence in situ hybridization (FISH)
　　Duplications identified by in situ hybridization (ISH)
　　Duplications seen only at prometaphase

**Q92.9　Trisomy and partial trisomy of autosomes, unspecified**

✓4th **Q93　Monosomies and deletions from the autosomes, not elsewhere classified**

　　CC Excl: For CC codes in category Q93, unless otherwise noted: PDX collection 1115

**Q93.0　Whole chromosome monosomy, nonmosaicism (meiotic nondisjunction)**

**Q93.1　Whole chromosome monosomy, mosaicism (mitotic nondisjunction)**

**Q93.2　Chromosome replaced with ring, dicentric or isochromosome**

**Q93.3　Deletion of short arm of chromosome 4**　　CC
　　Wolff-Hirschorn syndrome

**Q93.4　Deletion of short arm of chromosome 5**　　CC
　　Cri-du-chat syndrome
　　CC Excl: PDX collection 1116

**Q93.5　Other deletions of part of a chromosome**　　CC
　　Angelman syndrome

**Q93.7　Deletions with other complex rearrangements**　　CC
　　Deletions due to unbalanced translocations, inversions and insertions
　　Code also any associated duplications due to unbalanced translocations, inversions and insertions (Q92.5)

✓5th **Q93.8　Other deletions from the autosomes**

**Q93.81　Velo-cardio-facial syndrome**　　MCC
　　Deletion 22q11.2
　　DEF: Microdeletion syndrome affecting multiple organs; characteristic cleft palate, heart defects, elongated face with almond-shaped eyes, wide nose, small ears, weak immune system, weak musculature, hypothyroidism, short stature, and scoliosis; deletion at q11.2 on the long arm of the chromosome 22.
　　CC Excl: PDX collection 1117

**Q93.88　Other microdeletions**　　CC
　　Miller-Dieker syndrome
　　Smith-Magenis syndrome
　　CC Excl: PDX collection 1118

**Q93.89　Other deletions from the autosomes**　　CC
　　Deletions identified by fluorescence in situ hybridization (FISH)
　　Deletions identified by in situ hybridization (ISH)
　　Deletions seen only at prometaphase

**Q93.9　Deletion from autosomes, unspecified**　　CC

✓4th **Q95　Balanced rearrangements and structural markers, not elsewhere classified**
　　INCLUDES　Robertsonian and balanced reciprocal translocations and insertions

**Q95.0　Balanced translocation and insertion in normal individual**

**Q95.1　Chromosome inversion in normal individual**

**Q95.2　Balanced autosomal rearrangement in abnormal individual**

**Q95.3　Balanced sex/autosomal rearrangement in abnormal individual**

**Q95.5　Individual with autosomal fragile site**

**Q95.8　Other balanced rearrangements and structural markers**

**Q95.9　Balanced rearrangement and structural marker, unspecified**

✓4th **Q96　Turner's syndrome**
　　EXCLUDES 1　Noonan syndrome (Q87.1)

**Q96.0　Karyotype 45, X**　　♀

**Q96.1　Karyotype 46, X iso (Xq)**　　♀
　　Karyotype 46, isochromosome Xq

**Q96.2　Karyotype 46, X with abnormal sex chromosome, except iso (Xq)**　　♀
　　Karyotype 46, X with abnormal sex chromosome, except isochromosome Xq

**Q96.3　Mosaicism, 45, X/46, XX or XY**　　♀

---

N Newborn: 0　　P Pediatric: 0-17　　M Maternity: 12-55　　A Adult: 15-124　　MCC Major CC Condition　　PDxMCC PDx acts as own MCC　　CC CC Condition　　PDxCC PDx acts as own CC

Q96.4  **Mosaicism, 45, X/other cell line(s) with abnormal sex chromosome**   ♀

Q96.8  **Other variants of Turner's syndrome**   ♀

Q96.9  **Turner's syndrome, unspecified**   ♀

✓4ᵗʰ  **Q97**  **Other sex chromosome abnormalities, female phenotype, not elsewhere classified**

      *EXCLUDES 1*   Turner's syndrome (Q96.-)

Q97.0  **Karyotype 47, XXX**   ♀

Q97.1  **Female with more than three X chromosomes**   ♀

Q97.2  **Mosaicism, lines with various numbers of X chromosomes**   ♀

Q97.3  **Female with 46, XY karyotype**   ♀

Q97.8  **Other specified sex chromosome abnormalities, female phenotype**   ♀

Q97.9  **Sex chromosome abnormality, female phenotype, unspecified**   ♀

✓4ᵗʰ  **Q98**  **Other sex chromosome abnormalities, male phenotype, not elsewhere classified**

Q98.0  **Klinefelter syndrome karyotype 47, XXY**   ♂

Q98.1  **Klinefelter syndrome, male with more than two X chromosomes**   ♂

Q98.3  **Other male with 46, XX karyotype**   ♂

Q98.4  **Klinefelter syndrome, unspecified**   ♂

Q98.5  **Karyotype 47, XYY**

Q98.6  **Male with structurally abnormal sex chromosome**   ♂

Q98.7  **Male with sex chromosome mosaicism**   ♂

Q98.8  **Other specified sex chromosome abnormalities, male phenotype**   ♂

Q98.9  **Sex chromosome abnormality, male phenotype, unspecified**   ♂

✓4ᵗʰ  **Q99**  **Other chromosome abnormalities, not elsewhere classified**

Q99.0  **Chimera 46, XX/46, XY**
      Chimera 46, XX/46, XY true hermaphrodite

Q99.1  **46, XX true hermaphrodite**
      46, XX with streak gonads
      46, XY with streak gonads
      Pure gonadal dysgenesis

Q99.2  **Fragile X chromosome**
      Fragile X syndrome

Q99.8  **Other specified chromosome abnormalities**

Q99.9  **Chromosomal abnormality, unspecified**

✓ Additional Character Req  ✓x7ᵗʰ Placeholder Alert  Unacceptable PDx  Manifestation  **H1**-**H14** HAC  **HCC** CMS-HCC Condition  *EXCLUDES 1* Not Coded Here  *EXCLUDES 2* Not Included Here

ICD-10-CM 2018      **911**

# Chapter 18. Symptoms, Signs and Abnormal Clinical and Laboratory Findings, Not Elsewhere Classified (R00–R99)

## Chapter Specific Guidelines with Coding Examples

The chapter specific guidelines from the ICD-10-CM Official Guidelines for Coding and Reporting have been provided below. Along with these guidelines are coding examples, contained in the shaded boxes, that have been developed to help illustrate the coding and/or sequencing guidance found in these guidelines.

Chapter 18 includes symptoms, signs, abnormal results of clinical or other investigative procedures, and ill-defined conditions regarding which no diagnosis classifiable elsewhere is recorded. Signs and symptoms that point to a specific diagnosis have been assigned to a category in other chapters of the classification.

### a. Use of symptom codes

Codes that describe symptoms and signs are acceptable for reporting purposes when a related definitive diagnosis has not been established (confirmed) by the provider.

Chest pain of unknown origin

**R07.9        Chest pain, unspecified**

*Explanation:* Codes that describe symptoms such as chest pain are acceptable for reporting purposes when the provider has not established (confirmed) a related definitive diagnosis.

### b. Use of a symptom code with a definitive diagnosis code

Codes for signs and symptoms may be reported in addition to a related definitive diagnosis when the sign or symptom is not routinely associated with that diagnosis, such as the various signs and symptoms associated with complex syndromes. The definitive diagnosis code should be sequenced before the symptom code.

Signs or symptoms that are associated routinely with a disease process should not be assigned as additional codes, unless otherwise instructed by the classification.

Pneumonia with hemoptysis

**J18.9        Pneumonia, unspecified organism**

**R04.2        Hemoptysis**

*Explanation:* Codes for signs and symptoms may be reported in addition to a related definitive diagnosis when the sign or symptom is not routinely associated with that diagnosis.

Abdominal pain due to acute appendicitis

**K35.80        Unspecified acute appendicitis**

*Explanation:* Codes for signs or symptoms routinely associated with a disease process should not be assigned unless the classification instructs otherwise.

### c. Combination codes that include symptoms

ICD-10-CM contains a number of combination codes that identify both the definitive diagnosis and common symptoms of that diagnosis. When using one of these combination codes, an additional code should not be assigned for the symptom.

Acute gastritis with hemorrhage

**K29.01        Acute gastritis with bleeding**

*Explanation:* When a combination code identifies both the definitive diagnosis and the symptom, an additional code should not be assigned for the symptom.

### d. Repeated falls

Code R29.6, Repeated falls, is for use for encounters when a patient has recently fallen and the reason for the fall is being investigated.

Code Z91.81, History of falling, is for use when a patient has fallen in the past and is at risk for future falls. When appropriate, both codes R29.6 and Z91.81 may be assigned together.

### e. Coma scale

The coma scale codes (R40.2-) can be used in conjunction with traumatic brain injury codes, acute cerebrovascular disease or sequelae of cerebrovascular disease codes. These codes are primarily for use by trauma registries, but they may be used in any setting where this information is collected. The coma scale may also be used to assess the status of the central nervous system for other non-trauma conditions, such as monitoring patients in the intensive care unit regardless of medical condition. The coma scale codes should be sequenced after the diagnosis code(s).

These codes, one from each subcategory, are needed to complete the scale. The 7th character indicates when the scale was recorded. The 7th character should match for all three codes.

At a minimum, report the initial score documented on presentation at your facility. This may be a score from the emergency medicine technician (EMT) or in the emergency department. If desired, a facility may choose to capture multiple coma scale scores.

Assign code R40.24, Glasgow coma scale, total score, when only the total score is documented in the medical record and not the individual score(s).

23-year-old man found down after unknown injury with skull fracture and with concussion and loss of consciousness of unknown duration. EMS evaluated the patient in the field and reported the individual Glasgow coma scores:

Eye opening response—3: eyes open to speech

Verbal response—4: confused but coherent speech

Motor response—6: obeys commands fully

**S02.0XXA        Fracture of vault of skull, initial encounter for closed fracture**

**S06.0X9A        Concussion with loss of consciousness of unspecified duration, initial encounter**

**R40.2131        Coma scale, eyes open, to sound, in the field [EMT or ambulance]**

**R40.2241        Coma scale, best verbal response, confused conversation, in the field [EMT or ambulance]**

**R40.2361        Coma scale, best motor response, obeys commands, in the field [EMT or ambulance]**

*Explanation:* When individual scores for the Glasgow coma scale are documented, one code from each category is needed to complete the scale. The seventh character indicates when the scale was recorded and should match for all three codes. Assign a code from subcategory R40.24-Glasgow coma scale, total score, when only the total and not the individual score(s) is documented.

Patient with intractable epilepsy with status epilepticus arrives to ED with alteration of consciousness. Coma scale performed en route by EMT documented total coma score as 11. Another coma score was performed upon hospital admission that was documented as 14.

**G40.911        Epilepsy, unspecified, intractable, with status epilepticus**

**R40.2421        Iasgow coma scale score 9-12, in the field [EMT or ambulance]**

**R40.2413        Glasgow coma scale score 13-15, at hospital admission**

*Explanation:* Coma scores may be used to assess mental status in non-trauma conditions. Use only code R40.24- Glasgow coma scale, total scores when individual scores are unavailable. Multiple scores may be reported with the seventh character representing where or when the assessment was made.

### f. Functional quadriplegia

Functional quadriplegia (code R53.2) is the lack of ability to use one's limbs or to ambulate due to extreme debility. It is not associated with neurologic deficit or injury, and code R53.2 should not be used for cases of neurologic quadriplegia. It should only be assigned if functional quadriplegia is specifically documented in the medical record.

**g. SIRS due to non-infectious process**

The systemic inflammatory response syndrome (SIRS) can develop as a result of certain non-infectious disease processes, such as trauma, malignant neoplasm, or pancreatitis. When SIRS is documented with a noninfectious condition, and no subsequent infection is documented, the code for the underlying condition, such as an injury, should be assigned, followed by code R65.10, Systemic inflammatory response syndrome (SIRS) of non-infectious origin without acute organ dysfunction, or code R65.11, Systemic inflammatory response syndrome (SIRS) of non-infectious origin with acute organ dysfunction. If an associated acute organ dysfunction is documented, the appropriate code(s) for the specific type of organ dysfunction(s) should be assigned in addition to code R65.11. If acute organ dysfunction is documented, but it cannot be determined if the acute organ dysfunction is associated with SIRS or due to another condition (e.g., directly due to the trauma), the provider should be queried.

Systemic inflammatory response syndrome (SIRS) due to acute gallstone pancreatitis

| K85.10 | Biliary acute pancreatitis without necrosis or infection |
| R65.10 | Systemic inflammatory response syndrome (SIRS) of noninfectious origin without acute organ dysfunction |

*Explanation:* When SIRS is documented with a noninfectious condition without subsequent infection documented, the code for the underlying condition such as pancreatitis should be assigned followed by the appropriate code for SIRS of noninfectious origin, either with or without associated organ dysfunction.

**h. Death NOS**

Code R99, Ill-defined and unknown cause of mortality, is only for use in the very limited circumstance when a patient who has already died is brought into an emergency department or other healthcare facility and is pronounced dead upon arrival. It does not represent the discharge disposition of death.

**i. NIHSS stroke scale**

The NIH stroke scale (NIHSS) codes (R29.7- -) can be used in conjunction with acute stroke codes (I63) to identify the patient's neurological status and the severity of the stroke. The stroke scale codes should be sequenced after the acute stroke diagnosis code(s).

At a minimum, report the initial score documented. If desired, a facility may choose to capture multiple stroke scale scores.

*See Section I.B.14. for information concerning the medical record documentation that may be used for assignment of the NIHSS codes.*

Patient admitted with CVA seen by neurology consult who documents moderate to severe stroke, 17 on NIHSS stroke scale.

| I63.9 | Cerebral infarction, unspecified |
| R29.717 | NIHSS score 17 |

*Explanation:* Unspecified cerebral vascular accident (CVA) is sequenced before the NIHSS stroke scale score code. The stroke scale is an assessment tool to help measure stroke-related neurological deficits. Fifteen items are evaluated by trained observers and include such conditions as levels of consciousness, language, dysarthria, ataxia, and sensory loss. A facility may report multiple stroke scale scores if it wants to.

# Chapter 18. Symptoms, Signs and Abnormal Clinical and Laboratory Findings, Not Elsewhere Classified (R00-R99)

**NOTE**   This chapter includes symptoms, signs, abnormal results of clinical or other investigative procedures, and ill-defined conditions regarding which no diagnosis classifiable elsewhere is recorded.

Signs and symptoms that point rather definitely to a given diagnosis have been assigned to a category in other chapters of the classification. In general, categories in this chapter include the less well-defined conditions and symptoms that, without the necessary study of the case to establish a final diagnosis, point perhaps equally to two or more diseases or to two or more systems of the body. Practically all categories in the chapter could be designated "not otherwise specified", "unknown etiology" or "transient". The Alphabetical Index should be consulted to determine which symptoms and signs are to be allocated here and which to other chapters. The residual subcategories, numbered .8, are generally provided for other relevant symptoms that cannot be allocated elsewhere in the classification.

The conditions and signs or symptoms included in categories R00-R94 consist of:

(a)    cases for which no more specific diagnosis can be made even after all the facts bearing on the case have been investigated;

(b)    signs or symptoms existing at the time of initial encounter that proved to be transient and whose causes could not be determined;

(c)    provisional diagnosis in a patient who failed to return for further investigation or care;

(d)    cases referred elsewhere for investigation or treatment before the diagnosis was made;

(e)    cases in which a more precise diagnosis was not available for any other reason;

(f)    certain symptoms, for which supplementary information is provided, that represent important problems in medical care in their own right.

**EXCLUDES 2**   *abnormal findings on antenatal screening of mother (O28.-)*
*certain conditions originating in the perinatal period (P04-P96)*
*signs and symptoms classified in the body system chapters*
*signs and symptoms of breast (N63, N64.5)*

**AHA:** 2017, 1Q, 6, 7

This chapter contains the following blocks:

R00-R09    Symptoms and signs involving the circulatory and respiratory systems
R10-R19    Symptoms and signs involving the digestive system and abdomen
R20-R23    Symptoms and signs involving the skin and subcutaneous tissue
R25-R29    Symptoms and signs involving the nervous and musculoskeletal systems
R30-R39    Symptoms and signs involving the genitourinary system
R40-R46    Symptoms and signs involving cognition, perception, emotional state and behavior
R47-R49    Symptoms and signs involving speech and voice
R50-R69    General symptoms and signs
R70-R79    Abnormal findings on examination of blood, without diagnosis
R80-R82    Abnormal findings on examination of urine, without diagnosis
R83-R89    Abnormal findings on examination of other body fluids, substances and tissues, without diagnosis
R90-R94    Abnormal findings on diagnostic imaging and in function studies, without diagnosis
R97    Abnormal tumor markers
R99    Ill-defined and unknown cause of mortality

## Symptoms and signs involving the circulatory and respiratory systems (R00-R09)

**✓4ᵗʰ R00**   **Abnormalities of heart beat**
    **EXCLUDES 1**   *abnormalities originating in the perinatal period (P29.1-)*
    **EXCLUDES 2**   *specified arrhythmias (I47-I49)*

   **R00.0**   **Tachycardia,** unspecified
     Rapid heart beat
     Sinoauricular tachycardia NOS
     Sinus [sinusal] tachycardia NOS
     **EXCLUDES 1**   *neonatal tachycardia (P29.11)*
           *paroxysmal tachycardia (I47.-)*
     **DEF:** Excessively rapid heart rate of more than 100 beats per minute.

**R00.1**   **Bradycardia,** unspecified
    Sinoatrial bradycardia
    Sinus bradycardia
    Slow heart beat
    Vagal bradycardia
    Use additional code for adverse effect, if applicable, to identify drug (T36-T50 with fifth or sixth character 5)
    **EXCLUDES 1**   *neonatal bradycardia (P29.12)*

**R00.2**   **Palpitations**
    Awareness of heart beat

**R00.8**   **Other** abnormalities of heart beat

**R00.9**   **Unspecified** abnormalities of heart beat

**✓4ᵗʰ R01**   **Cardiac murmurs and other cardiac sounds**
    **EXCLUDES 1**   *cardiac murmurs and sounds originating in the perinatal period (P29.8)*

   **R01.0**   **Benign and innocent** cardiac murmurs
     Functional cardiac murmur

   **R01.1**   **Cardiac murmur,** unspecified
     Cardiac bruit NOS
     Heart murmur NOS
     Systolic murmur NOS

   **R01.2**   **Other** cardiac sounds
     Cardiac dullness, increased or decreased
     Precordial friction

**✓4ᵗʰ R03**   **Abnormal blood-pressure reading,** without diagnosis

   **4**   **R03.0**   **Elevated blood**-pressure reading, without diagnosis of hypertension
     **NOTE**   This category is to be used to record an episode of elevated blood pressure in a patient in whom no formal diagnosis of hypertension has been made, or as an isolated incidental finding.

   **R03.1**   **Nonspecific low blood**-pressure reading
     **EXCLUDES 1**   *hypotension (I95.-)*
           *maternal hypotension syndrome (O26.5-)*
           *neurogenic orthostatic hypotension (G90.3)*

**✓4ᵗʰ R04**   **Hemorrhage from respiratory passages**

   **CC Excl: For CC codes in category R04:** PDX collection 1119

   **R04.0**   **Epistaxis**
     Hemorrhage from nose
     Nosebleed

   **R04.1**   **Hemorrhage** from throat
     **EXCLUDES 2**   *hemoptysis (R04.2)*

   **R04.2**   **Hemoptysis**            **CC**
     Blood-stained sputum
     Cough with hemorrhage
     **AHA:** 2013, 4Q, 118

**✓5ᵗʰ R04.8**   **Hemorrhage from** other sites **in respiratory passages**

    **R04.81**   **Acute idiopathic pulmonary hemorrhage in**   **CC P**
       **infants**
       AIPHI
       Acute idiopathic hemorrhage in infants over 28 days old
       **EXCLUDES 1**   *perinatal pulmonary hemorrhage (P26.-)*
           *von Willebrand's disease (D68.0)*

    **R04.89**   **Hemorrhage from** other sites **in respiratory**   **CC**
       **passages**
       Pulmonary hemorrhage NOS

   **R04.9**   **Hemorrhage from respiratory passages,** unspecified   **CC**

**R05**   **Cough**
    **EXCLUDES 1**   *cough with hemorrhage (R04.2)*
           *smoker's cough (J41.0)*
    **AHA:** 2016, 2Q, 33

**✓4ᵗʰ R06**   **Abnormalities of breathing**
    **EXCLUDES 1**   *acute respiratory distress syndrome (J80)*
           *respiratory arrest (R09.2)*
           *respiratory arrest of newborn (P28.81)*
           *respiratory distress syndrome of newborn (P22.-)*
           *respiratory failure (J96.-)*
           *respiratory failure of newborn (P28.5)*

**✓5ᵗʰ R06.0**   **Dyspnea**
    **EXCLUDES 1**   *tachypnea NOS (R06.82)*
           *transient tachypnea of newborn (P22.1)*

    **R06.00**   **Dyspnea,** unspecified
       **AHA:** 2017, 1Q, 26

    **R06.01**   **Orthopnea**

---

**4**   Questionable admission when used as PDx.

☑ Additional Character Req   ✓x7ᵗʰ Placeholder Alert   Unacceptable PDx   Manifestation   H1-H14 HAC   HCC CMS-HCC Condition   **EXCLUDES 1** Not Coded Here   **EXCLUDES 2** Not Included Here

ICD-10-CM 2018                                                  **915**

**R06.02**   **Shortness** of breath

**R06.03**   **Acute respiratory distress**

**R06.09**   **Other forms** of dyspnea

**R06.1**   **Stridor**
- *EXCLUDES 1*     *congenital laryngeal stridor (P28.89)*
- *laryngismus (stridulus) (J38.5)*

**R06.2**   **Wheezing**
- *EXCLUDES 1*     *asthma (J45.-)*
- **AHA:** 2016, 2Q, 33
- **DEF:** High-pitched whistling sound during breathing due to stenosis of respiratory passageway; associated with asthma, sleep apnea, bronchiectasis, bronchiolitis, COPD, and pleural effusion.

**R06.3**   **Periodic breathing**     `CC`
- Cheyne-Stokes breathing
- **CC Excl:** PDX collection 1120

**R06.4**   **Hyperventilation**
- *EXCLUDES 1*     *psychogenic hyperventilation (F45.8)*

**R06.5**   **Mouth breathing**
- *EXCLUDES 2*     *dry mouth NOS (R68.2)*

**R06.6**   **Hiccough**
- *EXCLUDES 1*     *psychogenic hiccough (F45.8)*

**R06.7**   **Sneezing**

✓5th   **R06.8**   **Other abnormalities** of breathing

    **R06.81**   **Apnea,** not elsewhere classified
- Apnea NOS
- *EXCLUDES 1*     *apnea (of) newborn (P28.4)*
- *sleep apnea (G47.3-)*
- *sleep apnea of newborn (primary) (P28.3)*

    **R06.82**   **Tachypnea,** not elsewhere classified
- Tachypnea NOS
- *EXCLUDES 1*     *transitory tachypnea of newborn (P22.1)*

    **R06.83**   **Snoring**

    **R06.89**   **Other abnormalities** of breathing
- Breath-holding (spells)
- Sighing

**R06.9**   **Unspecified abnormalities** of breathing

✓4th   **R07**   **Pain in throat and chest**
- *EXCLUDES 1*     *epidemic myalgia (B33.0)*
- *EXCLUDES 2*     *jaw pain (R68.84)*
- *pain in breast (N64.4)*

**R07.0**   **Pain in throat**
- *EXCLUDES 1*     *chronic sore throat (J31.2)*
- *sore throat (acute) NOS (J02.9)*
- *EXCLUDES 2*     *dysphagia (R13.1-)*
- *pain in neck (M54.2)*

**R07.1**   **Chest pain on breathing**
- Painful respiration

**R07.2**   **Precordial pain**

✓5th   **R07.8**   **Other chest pain**

    **R07.81**   **Pleurodynia**
- Pleurodynia NOS
- *EXCLUDES 1*     *epidemic pleurodynia (B33.0)*

    **R07.82**   **Intercostal pain**

    **R07.89**   **Other chest pain**
- Anterior chest-wall pain NOS

**R07.9**   **Chest pain, unspecified**

✓4th   **R09**   **Other symptoms and signs involving the circulatory and respiratory system**
- *EXCLUDES 1*     *acute respiratory distress syndrome (J80)*
- *respiratory arrest of newborn (P28.81)*
- *respiratory distress syndrome of newborn (P22.0)*
- *respiratory failure (J96.-)*
- *respiratory failure of newborn (P28.5)*

✓5th   **R09.0**   **Asphyxia and hypoxemia**
- *EXCLUDES 1*     *asphyxia due to carbon monoxide (T58.-)*
- *asphyxia due to foreign body in respiratory tract (T17.-)*
- *birth (intrauterine) asphyxia (P84)*
- ~~*hypercapnia (R06.4)*~~
- *hyperventilation (R06.4)*
- *traumatic asphyxia (T71.-)*
- *EXCLUDES 2* ▶*hypercapnia (R06.89)*◀

    **R09.01**   **Asphyxia**     `CC`
- **CC Excl:** PDX collection 1121

    **R09.02**   **Hypoxemia**

---

**R09.1**   **Pleurisy**
- *EXCLUDES 1*     *pleurisy with effusion (J90)*

[1] **R09.2**   **Respiratory arrest**     `MCC` `HCC`
- Cardiorespiratory failure
- *EXCLUDES 1*     *cardiac arrest (I46.-)*
- *respiratory arrest of newborn (P28.81)*
- *respiratory distress of newborn (P22.0)*
- *respiratory failure (J96.-)*
- *respiratory failure of newborn (P28.5)*
- *respiratory insufficiency (R06.89)*
- *respiratory insufficiency of newborn (P28.5)*
- **CC Excl:** PDX collection 1121

**R09.3**   **Abnormal sputum**
- Abnormal amount of sputum
- Abnormal color of sputum
- Abnormal odor of sputum
- Excessive sputum
- *EXCLUDES 1*     *blood-stained sputum (R04.2)*

✓5th   **R09.8**   **Other specified symptoms and signs involving the circulatory and respiratory systems**

    **R09.81**   **Nasal congestion**

    **R09.82**   **Postnasal drip**

    **R09.89**   **Other specified symptoms and signs involving the circulatory and respiratory systems**
- Abnormal chest percussion
- Bruit (arterial)
- Chest tympany
- Choking sensation
- Feeling of foreign body in throat
- Friction sounds in chest
- Rales
- Weak pulse
- *EXCLUDES 2*     *foreign body in throat (T17.2-)*
- *wheezing (R06.2)*

## Symptoms and signs involving the digestive system and abdomen (R10-R19)

- *EXCLUDES 2*     *congenital or infantile pylorospasm (Q40.0)*
- *gastrointestinal hemorrhage (K92.0-K92.2)*
- *intestinal obstruction (K56.-)*
- *newborn gastrointestinal hemorrhage (P54.0-P54.3)*
- *newborn intestinal obstruction (P76.-)*
- *pylorospasm (K31.3)*
- *signs and symptoms involving the urinary system (R30-R39)*
- *symptoms referable to female genital organs (N94.-)*
- *symptoms referable to male genital organs (N48-N50)*

✓4th   **R10**   **Abdominal and pelvic pain**
- *EXCLUDES 1*     *renal colic (N23)*
- *EXCLUDES 2*     *dorsalgia (M54.-)*
- *flatulence and related conditions (R14.-)*

**R10.0**   **Acute abdomen**
- Severe abdominal pain (generalized) (with abdominal rigidity)
- *EXCLUDES 1*     *abdominal rigidity NOS (R19.3)*
- *generalized abdominal pain NOS (R10.84)*
- *localized abdominal pain (R10.1-R10.3-)*

**Abdominal Pain**

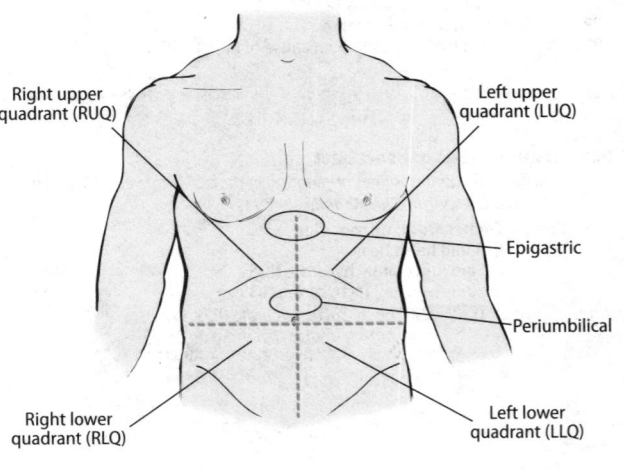

Right upper quadrant (RUQ)     Left upper quadrant (LUQ)     Epigastric     Periumbilical     Right lower quadrant (RLQ)     Left lower quadrant (LLQ)

---

[1]   MCC only if patient is discharged alive.

`N` Newborn: 0   `P` Pediatric: 0-17   `M` Maternity: 12-55   `A` Adult: 15-124   `MCC` Major CC Condition   `PDxMCC` PDx acts as own MCC   `CC` CC Condition   `PDxCC` PDx acts as own CC

**916**      ICD-10-CM 2018

✓5ᵗʰ **R10.1**   **Pain localized to upper abdomen**

     **R10.10**   **Upper abdominal pain, unspecified**

     **R10.11**   **Right upper quadrant pain**

     **R10.12**   **Left upper quadrant pain**

     **R10.13**   **Epigastric pain**
         Dyspepsia
         EXCLUDES 1   *functional dyspepsia (K30)*

**R10.2**   **Pelvic and perineal pain**
     EXCLUDES 1   *vulvodynia (N94.81)*

✓5ᵗʰ **R10.3**   **Pain localized to other parts of lower abdomen**

     **R10.30**   **Lower abdominal pain, unspecified**

     **R10.31**   **Right lower quadrant pain**

     **R10.32**   **Left lower quadrant pain**

     **R10.33**   **Periumbilical pain**

✓5ᵗʰ **R10.8**   **Other abdominal pain**

     ✓6ᵗʰ **R10.81**   **Abdominal tenderness**
         Abdominal tenderness NOS

         **R10.811**   **Right upper quadrant abdominal tenderness**

         **R10.812**   **Left upper quadrant abdominal tenderness**

         **R10.813**   **Right lower quadrant abdominal tenderness**

         **R10.814**   **Left lower quadrant abdominal tenderness**

         **R10.815**   **Periumbilic abdominal tenderness**

         **R10.816**   **Epigastric abdominal tenderness**

         **R10.817**   **Generalized abdominal tenderness**

         **R10.819**   **Abdominal tenderness, unspecified site**

     ✓6ᵗʰ **R10.82**   **Rebound abdominal tenderness**

         **R10.821**   **Right upper quadrant rebound abdominal tenderness**

         **R10.822**   **Left upper quadrant rebound abdominal tenderness**

         **R10.823**   **Right lower quadrant rebound abdominal tenderness**

         **R10.824**   **Left lower quadrant rebound abdominal tenderness**

         **R10.825**   **Periumbilic rebound abdominal tenderness**

         **R10.826**   **Epigastric rebound abdominal tenderness**

         **R10.827**   **Generalized rebound abdominal tenderness**

         **R10.829**   **Rebound abdominal tenderness, unspecified site**

     **R10.83**   **Colic**      P
         Colic NOS
         Infantile colic
         EXCLUDES 1   *colic in adult and child over 12 months old (R10.84)*
         **DEF:** Inconsolable crying in an otherwise well-fed and healthy infant for more than three hours a day, three days a week, for more than three weeks.

     **R10.84**   **Generalized abdominal pain**
         EXCLUDES 1   *generalized abdominal pain associated with acute abdomen (R10.0)*

**R10.9**   **Unspecified abdominal pain**

✓4ᵗʰ **R11**   **Nausea and vomiting**
     EXCLUDES 1   *cyclical vomiting associated with migraine (G43.A-)*
                 *excessive vomiting in pregnancy (O21.-)*
                 *hematemesis (K92.0)*
                 *neonatal hematemesis (P54.0)*
                 *newborn vomiting (P92.0-)*
                 *psychogenic vomiting (F50.89)*
                 *vomiting associated with bulimia nervosa (F50.2)*
                 *vomiting following gastrointestinal surgery (K91.0)*
     **AHA:** 2017, 1Q, 28

     **R11.0**   **Nausea**
         Nausea NOS
         Nausea without vomiting

     ✓5ᵗʰ **R11.1**   **Vomiting**

         **R11.10**   **Vomiting, unspecified**
             Vomiting NOS

         **R11.11**   **Vomiting without nausea**

         **R11.12**   **Projectile vomiting**

         **R11.13**   **Vomiting of fecal matter**

---

**Swallowing Function**

**Oral phase**

**Oropharyngeal phase**

**Pharyngeal phase**

**Pharyngoesophageal phase**

         **R11.14**   **Bilious vomiting**
             Bilious emesis

     **R11.2**   **Nausea with vomiting, unspecified**
         Persistent nausea with vomiting NOS

**R12**   **Heartburn**
     EXCLUDES 1   *dyspepsia NOS (R10.13)*
                 *functional dyspepsia (K30)*

✓4ᵗʰ **R13**   **Aphagia and dysphagia**

     **R13.0**   **Aphagia**
         Inability to swallow
         EXCLUDES 1   *psychogenic aphagia (F50.9)*

     ✓5ᵗʰ **R13.1**   **Dysphagia**
         Code first, if applicable, dysphagia following cerebrovascular disease (I69. with final characters -91)
         EXCLUDES 1   *psychogenic dysphagia (F45.8)*

         **R13.10**   **Dysphagia, unspecified**
             Difficulty in swallowing NOS

         **R13.11**   **Dysphagia, oral phase**

         **R13.12**   **Dysphagia, oropharyngeal phase**

         **R13.13**   **Dysphagia, pharyngeal phase**

         **R13.14**   **Dysphagia, pharyngoesophageal phase**

         **R13.19**   **Other dysphagia**
             Cervical dysphagia
             Neurogenic dysphagia

✓4ᵗʰ **R14**   **Flatulence and related conditions**
     EXCLUDES 1   *psychogenic aerophagy (F45.8)*

     **R14.0**   **Abdominal distension (gaseous)**
         Bloating
         Tympanites (abdominal) (intestinal)

     **R14.1**   **Gas pain**

     **R14.2**   **Eructation**

     **R14.3**   **Flatulence**

✓4ᵗʰ **R15**   **Fecal incontinence**
     INCLUDES   encopresis NOS
     EXCLUDES 1   *fecal incontinence of nonorganic origin (F98.1)*

     **R15.0**   **Incomplete defecation**
         EXCLUDES 1   *constipation (K59.0-)*
                 *fecal impaction (K56.41)*

     **R15.1**   **Fecal smearing**
         Fecal soiling

     **R15.2**   **Fecal urgency**

     **R15.9**   **Full incontinence of feces**
         Fecal incontinence NOS

✓4ᵗʰ **R16**   **Hepatomegaly and splenomegaly, not elsewhere classified**

     **R16.0**   **Hepatomegaly, not elsewhere classified**
         Hepatomegaly NOS

     **R16.1**   **Splenomegaly, not elsewhere classified**
         Splenomegaly NOS

     **R16.2**   **Hepatomegaly with splenomegaly, not elsewhere classified**
         Hepatosplenomegaly NOS

---

✔ Additional Character Req    ✔x7ᵗʰ Placeholder Alert    Unacceptable PDx    Manifestation    H1 - H14 HAC    HCC CMS-HCC Condition    EXCLUDES 1 Not Coded Here    EXCLUDES 2 Not Included Here

**Chapter 18. Symptoms, Signs and Abnormal Clinical and Laboratory Findings, Not Elsewhere Classified**

**R17-R23.3**

**R17**    **Unspecified jaundice**      `CC`
     **EXCLUDES 1**   *neonatal jaundice (P55, P57-P59)*
     **CC Excl:** PDX collection 1122

✓4th **R18**    **Ascites**
     **INCLUDES**   fluid in peritoneal cavity
     **EXCLUDES 1**   *ascites in alcoholic cirrhosis (K70.31)*
           *ascites in alcoholic hepatitis (K70.11)*
           *ascites in toxic liver disease with chronic active hepatitis*
              *(K71.51)*

     **R18.0**   **Malignant ascites**      `CC`
           Code first malignancy, such as:
              malignant neoplasm of ovary (C56.-)
              secondary malignant neoplasm of retroperitoneum and
                peritoneum (C78.6)
           **CC Excl:** PDX collection 1123

     **R18.8**   **Other ascites**      `CC`
           Ascites NOS
           Peritoneal effusion (chronic)
           **CC Excl:** PDX collection 1123

✓4th **R19**    **Other symptoms and signs involving the digestive system and abdomen**
     **EXCLUDES 1**   *acute abdomen (R10.0)*

     ✓5th **R19.0**   **Intra-abdominal and pelvic swelling, mass and lump**
         **EXCLUDES 1**   *abdominal distension (gaseous) (R14.-)*
             *ascites (R18.-)*

         **R19.00**   **Intra-abdominal and pelvic swelling, mass and lump, unspecified site**

         **R19.01**   **Right upper quadrant abdominal swelling, mass and lump**

         **R19.02**   **Left upper quadrant abdominal swelling, mass and lump**

         **R19.03**   **Right lower quadrant abdominal swelling, mass and lump**

         **R19.04**   **Left lower quadrant abdominal swelling, mass and lump**

         **R19.05**   **Periumbilic swelling, mass or lump**
             Diffuse or generalized umbilical swelling or mass

         **R19.06**   **Epigastric swelling, mass or lump**

         **R19.07**   **Generalized intra-abdominal and pelvic swelling, mass and lump**
             Diffuse or generalized intra-abdominal swelling or
               mass NOS
             Diffuse or generalized pelvic swelling or mass NOS

         **R19.09**   **Other intra-abdominal and pelvic swelling, mass and lump**

     ✓5th **R19.1**   **Abnormal bowel sounds**
         **R19.11**   **Absent bowel sounds**
         **R19.12**   **Hyperactive bowel sounds**
         **R19.15**   **Other abnormal bowel sounds**
             Abnormal bowel sounds NOS

     **R19.2**   **Visible peristalsis**
         Hyperperistalsis
         **DEF:** Visible movements of muscular attempts to move food
         through the digestive tract; due to pyloric obstruction, stomach
         obstruction, or intestinal obstruction.

     ✓5th **R19.3**   **Abdominal rigidity**
         **EXCLUDES 1**   *abdominal rigidity with severe abdominal pain (R10.0)*
         **R19.30**   **Abdominal rigidity, unspecified site**
         **R19.31**   **Right upper quadrant abdominal rigidity**
         **R19.32**   **Left upper quadrant abdominal rigidity**
         **R19.33**   **Right lower quadrant abdominal rigidity**
         **R19.34**   **Left lower quadrant abdominal rigidity**
         **R19.35**   **Periumbilic abdominal rigidity**
         **R19.36**   **Epigastric abdominal rigidity**
         **R19.37**   **Generalized abdominal rigidity**

     **R19.4**   **Change in bowel habit**
         **EXCLUDES 1**   *constipation (K59.0-)*
             *functional diarrhea (K59.1)*

     **R19.5**   **Other fecal abnormalities**
         Abnormal stool color
         Bulky stools
         Mucus in stools
         Occult blood in feces
         Occult blood in stools
         **EXCLUDES 1**   *melena (K92.1)*
             *neonatal melena (P54.1)*

**R19.6**    **Halitosis**

**R19.7**    **Diarrhea, unspecified**
     Diarrhea NOS
     **EXCLUDES 1**   *functional diarrhea (K59.1)*
           *neonatal diarrhea (P78.3)*
           *psychogenic diarrhea (F45.8)*

**R19.8**    **Other specified symptoms and signs involving the digestive system and abdomen**

## Symptoms and signs involving the skin and subcutaneous tissue (R20-R23)

**EXCLUDES 2**   *symptoms relating to breast (N64.4-N64.5)*

✓4th **R20**    **Disturbances of skin sensation**
     **EXCLUDES 1**   *dissociative anesthesia and sensory loss (F44.6)*
           *psychogenic disturbances (F45.8)*

     **R20.0**   **Anesthesia of skin**
     **R20.1**   **Hypoesthesia of skin**
     **R20.2**   **Paresthesia of skin**
         Formication
         Pins and needles
         Tingling skin
         **EXCLUDES 1**   *acroparesthesia (I73.8)*

     **R20.3**   **Hyperesthesia**
     **R20.8**   **Other disturbances of skin sensation**
     **R20.9**   **Unspecified disturbances of skin sensation**

**R21**    **Rash and other nonspecific skin eruption**
     **INCLUDES**   rash NOS
     **EXCLUDES 1**   *specified type of rash—code to condition*
           *vesicular eruption (R23.8)*

✓4th **R22**    **Localized swelling, mass and lump of skin and subcutaneous tissue**
     **INCLUDES**   subcutaneous nodules (localized)(superficial)
     **EXCLUDES 1**   *abnormal findings on diagnostic imaging (R90-R93)*
           *edema (R60.-)*
           *enlarged lymph nodes (R59.-)*
           *localized adiposity (E65)*
           *swelling of joint (M25.4-)*

     **R22.0**   **Localized swelling, mass and lump, head**
     **R22.1**   **Localized swelling, mass and lump, neck**
     **R22.2**   **Localized swelling, mass and lump, trunk**
         **EXCLUDES 1**   *intra-abdominal or pelvic mass and lump (R19.0-)*
             *intra-abdominal or pelvic swelling (R19.0-)*
         **EXCLUDES 2**   *breast mass and lump (N63)*

     ✓5th **R22.3**   **Localized swelling, mass and lump, upper limb**
         **R22.30**   **Localized swelling, mass and lump, unspecified upper limb**
         **R22.31**   **Localized swelling, mass and lump, right upper limb**
         **R22.32**   **Localized swelling, mass and lump, left upper limb**
         **R22.33**   **Localized swelling, mass and lump, upper limb, bilateral**

     ✓5th **R22.4**   **Localized swelling, mass and lump, lower limb**
         **R22.40**   **Localized swelling, mass and lump, unspecified lower limb**
         **R22.41**   **Localized swelling, mass and lump, right lower limb**
         **R22.42**   **Localized swelling, mass and lump, left lower limb**
         **R22.43**   **Localized swelling, mass and lump, lower limb, bilateral**

     **R22.9**   **Localized swelling, mass and lump, unspecified**

✓4th **R23**    **Other skin changes**
     **R23.0**   **Cyanosis**
         **EXCLUDES 1**   *acrocyanosis (I73.8)*
             *cyanotic attacks of newborn (P28.2)*
         **DEF:** Bluish or purplish discoloration of the skin due to inadequate
         oxygen level of blood.

     **R23.1**   **Pallor**
         Clammy skin

     **R23.2**   **Flushing**
         Excessive blushing
         Code first, if applicable, menopausal and female climacteric
           states (N95.1)

     **R23.3**   **Spontaneous ecchymoses**
         Petechiae
         **EXCLUDES 1**   *ecchymoses of newborn (P54.5)*
           *purpura (D69.-)*

N Newborn: 0    P Pediatric: 0-17    M Maternity: 12-55    A Adult: 15-124    **MCC** Major CC Condition    **PDxMCC** PDx acts as own MCC    **CC** CC Condition    **PDxCC** PDx acts as own CC

**918**      ICD-10-CM 2018

**R23.4** **Changes in skin texture**
Desquamation of skin
Induration of skin
Scaling of skin
*EXCLUDES 1*  *epidermal thickening NOS (L85.9)*

**R23.8** **Other skin changes**

**R23.9** **Unspecified skin changes**

### Symptoms and signs involving the nervous and musculoskeletal systems (R25-R29)

✓4ᵗʰ **R25** **Abnormal involuntary movements**
*EXCLUDES 1*  *specific movement disorders (G20-G26)*
*stereotyped movement disorders (F98.4)*
*tic disorders (F95.-)*

**R25.0** **Abnormal head movements**

**R25.1** **Tremor, unspecified**
*EXCLUDES 1*  *chorea NOS (G25.5)*
*essential tremor (G25.0)*
*hysterical tremor (F44.4)*
*intention tremor (G25.2)*

**R25.2** **Cramp and spasm**
*EXCLUDES 2*  *carpopedal spasm (R29.0)*
*charley-horse (M62.831)*
*infantile spasms (G40.4-)*
*muscle spasm of back (M62.830)*
*muscle spasm of calf (M62.831)*

**R25.3** **Fasciculation**
Twitching NOS

**R25.8** **Other abnormal involuntary movements**

**R25.9** **Unspecified abnormal involuntary movements**

✓4ᵗʰ **R26** **Abnormalities of gait and mobility**
*EXCLUDES 1*  *ataxia NOS (R27.0)*
*hereditary ataxia (G11.-)*
*locomotor (syphilitic) ataxia (A52.11)*
*immobility syndrome (paraplegic) (M62.3)*

**R26.0** **Ataxic gait**
Staggering gait

**R26.1** **Paralytic gait**
Spastic gait

**R26.2** **Difficulty in walking, not elsewhere classified**
*EXCLUDES 1*  *falling (R29.6)*
*unsteadiness on feet (R26.81)*
**AHA:** 2016, 2Q, 7

✓5ᵗʰ **R26.8** **Other abnormalities of gait and mobility**
**R26.81** **Unsteadiness on feet**
**R26.89** **Other abnormalities of gait and mobility**

**R26.9** **Unspecified abnormalities of gait and mobility**

✓4ᵗʰ **R27** **Other lack of coordination**
*EXCLUDES 1*  *ataxic gait (R26.0)*
*hereditary ataxia (G11.-)*
*vertigo NOS (R42)*

**R27.0** **Ataxia, unspecified**
*EXCLUDES 1*  *ataxia following cerebrovascular disease (I69. with final characters -93)*

**R27.8** **Other lack of coordination**

**R27.9** **Unspecified lack of coordination**

✓4ᵗʰ **R29** **Other symptoms and signs involving the nervous and musculoskeletal systems**

**R29.0** **Tetany**  CC
Carpopedal spasm
*EXCLUDES 1*  *hysterical tetany (F44.5)*
*neonatal tetany (P71.3)*
*parathyroid tetany (E20.9)*
*post-thyroidectomy tetany (E89.2)*
**CC Excl:** PDX collection 1124

**R29.1** **Meningismus**  CC
**CC Excl:** PDX collection 1125

**R29.2** **Abnormal reflex**
*EXCLUDES 2*  *abnormal pupillary reflex (H57.0)*
*hyperactive gag reflex (J39.2)*
*vasovagal reaction or syncope (R55)*

**R29.3** **Abnormal posture**

**R29.4** **Clicking hip**
*EXCLUDES 1*  *congenital deformities of hip (Q65.-)*

**R29.5** **Transient paralysis**  CC
Code first any associated spinal cord injury (S14.0, S14.1-, S24.0, S24.1-, S34.0-, S34.1-)
*EXCLUDES 1*  *transient ischemic attack (G45.9)*
**CC Excl:** PDX collection 1126

**R29.6** **Repeated falls**
Falling
Tendency to fall
*EXCLUDES 2*  *at risk for falling (Z91.81)*
*history of falling (Z91.81)*
**AHA:** 2016, 2Q, 6

✓5ᵗʰ **R29.7** **National Institutes of Health Stroke Scale (NIHSS) score**
Code first the type of cerebral infarction (I63.-)

✓6ᵗʰ **R29.70** **NIHSS score 0-9**
**R29.700** **NIHSS score 0**
**R29.701** **NIHSS score 1**
**R29.702** **NIHSS score 2**
**R29.703** **NIHSS score 3**
**R29.704** **NIHSS score 4**
**R29.705** **NIHSS score 5**
**R29.706** **NIHSS score 6**
**R29.707** **NIHSS score 7**
**R29.708** **NIHSS score 8**
**R29.709** **NIHSS score 9**

✓6ᵗʰ **R29.71** **NIHSS score 10-19**
**R29.710** **NIHSS score 10**
**R29.711** **NIHSS score 11**
**R29.712** **NIHSS score 12**
**R29.713** **NIHSS score 13**
**R29.714** **NIHSS score 14**
**R29.715** **NIHSS score 15**
**R29.716** **NIHSS score 16**
**R29.717** **NIHSS score 17**
**R29.718** **NIHSS score 18**
**R29.719** **NIHSS score 19**

✓6ᵗʰ **R29.72** **NIHSS score 20-29**
**R29.720** **NIHSS score 20**
**R29.721** **NIHSS score 21**
**R29.722** **NIHSS score 22**
**R29.723** **NIHSS score 23**
**R29.724** **NIHSS score 24**
**R29.725** **NIHSS score 25**
**R29.726** **NIHSS score 26**
**R29.727** **NIHSS score 27**
**R29.728** **NIHSS score 28**
**R29.729** **NIHSS score 29**

✓6ᵗʰ **R29.73** **NIHSS score 30-39**
**R29.730** **NIHSS score 30**
**R29.731** **NIHSS score 31**
**R29.732** **NIHSS score 32**
**R29.733** **NIHSS score 33**
**R29.734** **NIHSS score 34**
**R29.735** **NIHSS score 35**
**R29.736** **NIHSS score 36**
**R29.737** **NIHSS score 37**
**R29.738** **NIHSS score 38**
**R29.739** **NIHSS score 39**

✓6ᵗʰ **R29.74** **NIHSS score 40-42**
**R29.740** **NIHSS score 40**
**R29.741** **NIHSS score 41**
**R29.742** **NIHSS score 42**

✓5ᵗʰ **R29.8** **Other symptoms and signs involving the nervous and musculoskeletal systems**

✓6ᵗʰ **R29.81** **Other symptoms and signs involving the nervous system**
**R29.810** **Facial weakness**
Facial droop
*EXCLUDES 1*  *Bell's palsy (G51.0)*
*facial weakness following cerebrovascular disease (I69. with final characters -92)*
**R29.818** **Other symptoms and signs involving the nervous system**

☑6ᵗʰ **R29.89** **Other symptoms and signs involving the musculoskeletal system**
     EXCLUDES 2 *pain in limb (M79.6-)*

     **R29.890** **Loss of height**
         EXCLUDES 1 *osteoporosis (M80-M81)*

     **R29.891** **Ocular torticollis**
         EXCLUDES 1 *congenital (sternomastoid) torticollis Q68.0*
             *psychogenic torticollis (F45.8)*
             *spasmodic torticollis (G24.3)*
             *torticollis due to birth injury (P15.8)*
             *torticollis NOS M43.6*
         **DEF:** Abnormal head posture as a result of a contracted state of cervical muscles to correct a visual disturbance, either double vision or a visual field defect.

     **R29.898** **Other symptoms and signs involving the musculoskeletal system**

☑5ᵗʰ **R29.9** **Unspecified symptoms and signs involving the nervous and musculoskeletal systems**

     **R29.90** **Unspecified symptoms and signs involving the nervous system**

     **R29.91** **Unspecified symptoms and signs involving the musculoskeletal system**

## Symptoms and signs involving the genitourinary system (R30-R39)

☑4ᵗʰ **R30** **Pain associated with micturition**
     EXCLUDES 1 *psychogenic pain associated with micturition (F45.8)*

     **R30.0** **Dysuria**
         Strangury

     **R30.1** **Vesical tenesmus**

     **R30.9** **Painful micturition, unspecified**
         Painful urination NOS

☑4ᵗʰ **R31** **Hematuria**
     EXCLUDES 1 *hematuria included with underlying conditions, such as:*
         *acute cystitis with hematuria (N30.01)*
         *recurrent and persistent hematuria in glomerular diseases (N02.-)*
     **AHA:** 2017, 1Q, 17

     **R31.0** **Gross hematuria**

     **R31.1** **Benign essential microscopic hematuria**

☑5ᵗʰ   **R31.2** **Other microscopic hematuria**

     **R31.21** **Asymptomatic microscopic hematuria**
         AMH

     **R31.29** **Other microscopic hematuria**

     **R31.9** **Hematuria, unspecified**

**R32** **Unspecified urinary incontinence**
     Enuresis NOS
     EXCLUDES 1 *functional urinary incontinence (R39.81)*
         *nonorganic enuresis (F98.0)*
         *stress incontinence and other specified urinary incontinence (N39.3-N39.4-)*
         *urinary incontinence associated with cognitive impairment (R39.81)*

☑4ᵗʰ **R33** **Retention of urine**
     EXCLUDES 1 *psychogenic retention of urine (F45.8)*

     **R33.0** **Drug induced retention of urine**
         Use additional code for adverse effect, if applicable, to identify drug (T36-T50 with fifth or sixth character 5)

     **R33.8** **Other retention of urine**
         Code first, if applicable, any causal condition, such as:
         enlarged prostate (N40.1)

     **R33.9** **Retention of urine, unspecified**

**R34** **Anuria and oliguria**
     EXCLUDES 1 *anuria and oliguria complicating abortion or ectopic or molar pregnancy (O00-O07, O08.4)*
         *anuria and oliguria complicating pregnancy (O26.83-)*
         *anuria and oliguria complicating the puerperium (O90.4)*

☑4ᵗʰ **R35** **Polyuria**
     Code first, if applicable, any causal condition, such as:
     enlarged prostate (N40.1)
     EXCLUDES 1 *psychogenic polyuria (F45.8)*

     **R35.0** **Frequency of micturition**

     **R35.1** **Nocturia**

     **R35.8** **Other polyuria**
         Polyuria NOS

☑4ᵗʰ **R36** **Urethral discharge**

     **R36.0** **Urethral discharge without blood**

     **R36.1** **Hematospermia**      ♂

     **R36.9** **Urethral discharge, unspecified**
         Penile discharge NOS
         Urethrorrhea

**R37** **Sexual dysfunction, unspecified**

☑4ᵗʰ **R39** **Other and unspecified symptoms and signs involving the genitourinary system**

     **R39.0** **Extravasation of urine**      CC
         **CC Excl:** PDX collection 1127

☑5ᵗʰ   **R39.1** **Other difficulties with micturition**
     Code first, if applicable, any causal condition, such as:
     enlarged prostate (N40.1)

     **R39.11** **Hesitancy of micturition**

     **R39.12** **Poor urinary stream**
         Weak urinary steam

     **R39.13** **Splitting of urinary stream**

     **R39.14** **Feeling of incomplete bladder emptying**

     **R39.15** **Urgency of urination**
         EXCLUDES 1 *urge incontinence (N39.41, N39.46)*

     **R39.16** **Straining to void**

☑6ᵗʰ   **R39.19** **Other difficulties with micturition**

     **R39.191** **Need to immediately re-void**

     **R39.192** **Position dependent micturition**

     **R39.198** **Other difficulties with micturition**

     **R39.2** **Extrarenal uremia**
         Prerenal uremia
         EXCLUDES 1 *uremia NOS (N19)*

☑5ᵗʰ   **R39.8** **Other symptoms and signs involving the genitourinary system**

     **R39.81** **Functional urinary incontinence**
         Urinary incontinence due to cognitive impairment, or severe physical disability or immobility
         EXCLUDES 1 *stress incontinence and other specified urinary incontinence (N39.3-N39.4-)*
             *urinary incontinence NOS (R32)*

     **R39.82** **Chronic bladder pain**

     ● **R39.83** **Unilateral non-palpable testicle**      ♂

     ● **R39.84** **Bilateral non-palpable testicles**      ♂

     **R39.89** **Other symptoms and signs involving the genitourinary system**

     **R39.9** **Unspecified symptoms and signs involving the genitourinary system**

## Symptoms and signs involving cognition, perception, emotional state and behavior (R40-R46)

     EXCLUDES 2 *symptoms and signs constituting part of a pattern of mental disorder (F01-F99)*

☑4ᵗʰ **R40** **Somnolence, stupor and coma**
     EXCLUDES 1 *neonatal coma (P91.5)*
         *somnolence, stupor and coma in diabetes (E08-E13)*
         *somnolence, stupor and coma in hepatic failure (K72.-)*
         *somnolence, stupor and coma in hypoglycemia (nondiabetic) (E15)*

     **R40.0** **Somnolence**
         Drowsiness
         EXCLUDES 1 *coma (R40.2-)*

     **R40.1** **Stupor**
         Catatonic stupor
         Semicoma
         EXCLUDES 1 *catatonic schizophrenia (F20.2)*
             *coma (R40.2-)*
             *depressive stupor (F31-F33)*
             *dissociative stupor (F44.2)*
             *manic stupor (F30.2)*

N Newborn: 0   P Pediatric: 0-17   M Maternity: 12-55   A Adult: 15-124   MCC Major CC Condition   PDxMCC PDx acts as own MCC   CC CC Condition   PDxCC PDx acts as own CC

920          ICD-10-CM 2018

√5th **R40.2  Coma**

Code first any associated:
fracture of skull (S02.-)
intracranial injury (S06.-)

NOTE  One code from each subcategory, R40.21-R40.23, is required to complete the coma scale

AHA: 2015, 2Q, 17; 2014, 1Q, 19

CC Excl: For MCC codes in subcategory R40.2:
PDX collection 515

**R40.20  Unspecified coma**  MCC HCC
Coma NOS
Unconsciousness NOS

√6th **R40.21  Coma scale, eyes open**

The following appropriate 7th character is to be added to subcategories R40.21-, R40.22-, R40.23-, and R40.24-.
0  unspecified time
1  in the field [EMT or ambulance]
2  at arrival to emergency department
3  at hospital admission
4  24 hours or more after hospital admission

√7th **R40.211  Coma scale, eyes open, never**  MCC HCC
√7th **R40.212  Coma scale, eyes open, to pain**  MCC HCC
√7th **R40.213  Coma scale, eyes open, to sound**
√7th **R40.214  Coma scale, eyes open, spontaneous**

√6th **R40.22  Coma scale, best verbal response**

√7th **R40.221  Coma scale, best verbal response, none**  MCC HCC

√7th **R40.222  Coma scale, best verbal response, incomprehensible words**  MCC HCC
▶Incomprehensible sounds (2-5 years of age) Moans/grunts to pain; restless (< 2 years old)◀

√7th **R40.223  Coma scale, best verbal response, inappropriate words**
▶Inappropriate crying or screaming (< 2 years of age) Screaming (2-5 years of age)◀

√7th **R40.224  Coma scale, best verbal response, confused conversation**
▶Inappropriate words (2-5 years of age) Irritable cries (< 2 years of age)◀

√7th **R40.225  Coma scale, best verbal response, oriented**
▶Cooing or babbling or crying appropriately (< 2 years of age) Uses appropriate words (2- 5 years of age)◀

√6th **R40.23  Coma scale, best motor response**

√7th **R40.231  Coma scale, best motor response, none**  MCC HCC

√7th **R40.232  Coma scale, best motor response, extension**  MCC HCC
▶Abnormal extensor posturing to pain or noxious stimuli (< 2 years of age) Extensor posturing to pain or noxious stimuli (2-5 years of age)◀

√7th **R40.233  Coma scale, best motor response, abnormal**
▶Abnormal flexure posturing to pain or noxious stimuli (0-5 years of age) Flexion/decorticate posturing (< 2 years of age)◀

√7th **R40.234  Coma scale, best motor response, flexion withdrawal**  MCC HCC
▶Withdraws from pain or noxious stimuli (0-5 years of age)◀

√7th **R40.235  Coma scale, best motor response, localizes pain**
▶Localizes pain (2-5 years of age) Withdraws to touch (< 2 years of age)◀

√7th **R40.236  Coma scale, best motor response, obeys commands**
▶Normal or spontaneous movement (< 2 years of age) Obeys commands (2-5 years of age)◀

√6th **R40.24  Glasgow coma scale, total score**
NOTE  Assign a code from subcategory R40.24, when only the total coma score is documented

√7th **R40.241  Glasgow coma scale score 13-15**
√7th **R40.242  Glasgow coma scale score 9-12**
√7th **R40.243  Glasgow coma scale score 3-8**  HCC
√7th **R40.244  Other coma, without documented Glasgow coma scale score, or with partial score reported**  HCC

**R40.3  Persistent vegetative state**  CC HCC
DEF: Persistent wakefulness without consciousness due to nonfunctioning cerebral cortex.
CC Excl: PDX collection 515

**R40.4  Transient alteration of awareness**

√4th **R41  Other symptoms and signs involving cognitive functions and awareness**
EXCLUDES 1  dissociative [conversion] disorders (F44.-)
mild cognitive impairment, so stated (G31.84)

**R41.0  Disorientation, unspecified**
Confusion NOS
Delirium NOS

**R41.1  Anterograde amnesia**

**R41.2  Retrograde amnesia**

**R41.3  Other amnesia**
Amnesia NOS
Memory loss NOS
EXCLUDES 1  amnestic disorder due to known physiologic condition (F04)
amnestic syndrome due to psychoactive substance use (F10-F19 with 5th character .6)
mild memory disturbance due to known physiological condition (F06.8)
transient global amnesia (G45.4)

**R41.4  Neurologic neglect syndrome**  CC
Asomatognosia
Hemi-akinesia
Hemi-inattention
Hemispatial neglect
Left-sided neglect
Sensory neglect
Visuospatial neglect
EXCLUDES 1  visuospatial deficit (R41.842)
CC Excl: PDX collection 1128

√5th **R41.8  Other symptoms and signs involving cognitive functions and awareness**
**R41.81  Age-related cognitive decline**  A
Senility NOS

**R41.82  Altered mental status, unspecified**
Change in mental status NOS
EXCLUDES 1  altered level of consciousness (R40.-)
altered mental status due to known condition—code to condition
delirium NOS (R41.0)
AHA: 2012, 4Q, 97

**R41.83  Borderline intellectual functioning**
IQ level 71 to 84
EXCLUDES 1  intellectual disabilities (F70-F79)

√6th **R41.84  Other specified cognitive deficit**
EXCLUDES 1  cognitive deficits as sequelae of cerebrovascular disease (I69.01-, I69.11-, I69.21-, I69.31-, I69.81-, I69.91-)

**R41.840  Attention and concentration deficit**
EXCLUDES 1  attention-deficit hyperactivity disorders (F90.-)

**R41.841  Cognitive communication deficit**

**R41.842  Visuospatial deficit**

**R41.843  Psychomotor deficit**

**R41.844  Frontal lobe and executive function deficit**

**R41.89  Other symptoms and signs involving cognitive functions and awareness**
Anosognosia

**R41.9  Unspecified symptoms and signs involving cognitive functions and awareness**
▶Unspecified neurocognitive disorder◀

Chapter 18. Symptoms, Signs and Abnormal Clinical and Laboratory Findings, Not Elsewhere Classified

R40.2–R41.9

**R42 Dizziness and giddiness**
Light-headedness
Vertigo NOS
> **EXCLUDES 1**   vertiginous syndromes (H81.-)
> vertigo from infrasound (T75.23)

**✓4ᵗʰ R43 Disturbances of smell and taste**

**R43.0 Anosmia**

**R43.1 Parosmia**

**R43.2 Parageusia**

**R43.8 Other disturbances of smell and taste**
Mixed disturbance of smell and taste

**R43.9 Unspecified disturbances of smell and taste**

**✓4ᵗʰ R44 Other symptoms and signs involving general sensations and perceptions**
> **EXCLUDES 1**   alcoholic hallucinations (F1.5)
> hallucinations in drug psychosis (F11-F19 with .5)
> hallucinations in mood disorders with psychotic symptoms (F30.2, F31.5, F32.3, F33.3)
> hallucinations in schizophrenia, schizotypal and delusional disorders (F20-F29)
>
> **EXCLUDES 2**   disturbances of skin sensation (R20.-)

> **CC Excl:** For CC codes in category R44: PDX collection 1129

**R44.0 Auditory hallucinations**    `CC`

**R44.1 Visual hallucinations**

**R44.2 Other hallucinations**    `CC`

**R44.3 Hallucinations, unspecified**    `CC`

**R44.8 Other symptoms and signs involving general sensations and perceptions**

**R44.9 Unspecified symptoms and signs involving general sensations and perceptions**

**✓4ᵗʰ R45 Symptoms and signs involving emotional state**

**R45.0 Nervousness**
Nervous tension

**R45.1 Restlessness and agitation**

**R45.2 Unhappiness**

**R45.3 Demoralization and apathy**
> **EXCLUDES 1**   anhedonia (R45.84)

**R45.4 Irritability and anger**

**R45.5 Hostility**

**R45.6 Violent behavior**

**R45.7 State of emotional shock and stress, unspecified**

**✓5ᵗʰ R45.8 Other symptoms and signs involving emotional state**

**R45.81 Low self-esteem**

**R45.82 Worries**

**R45.83 Excessive crying of child, adolescent or adult**
> **EXCLUDES 1**   excessive crying of infant (baby) R68.11

**R45.84 Anhedonia**

**✓6ᵗʰ R45.85 Homicidal and suicidal ideations**
> **EXCLUDES 1**   suicide attempt (T14.91)

**R45.850 Homicidal ideations**

**R45.851 Suicidal ideations**    `CC`
**DEF:** Thoughts of committing suicide; no actual attempt of suicide has been made.
**CC Excl:** PDX collection 1130

**R45.86 Emotional lability**

**R45.87 Impulsiveness**

**R45.89 Other symptoms and signs involving emotional state**

**✓4ᵗʰ R46 Symptoms and signs involving appearance and behavior**
> **EXCLUDES 1**   appearance and behavior in schizophrenia, schizotypal and delusional disorders (F20-F29)
> mental and behavioral disorders (F01-F99)

**R46.0 Very low level of personal hygiene**

**R46.1 Bizarre personal appearance**

**R46.2 Strange and inexplicable behavior**

**R46.3 Overactivity**

**R46.4 Slowness and poor responsiveness**
> **EXCLUDES 1**   stupor (R40.1)

**R46.5 Suspiciousness and marked evasiveness**

**R46.6 Undue concern and preoccupation with stressful events**

**R46.7 Verbosity and circumstantial detail obscuring reason for contact**

**✓5ᵗʰ R46.8 Other symptoms and signs involving appearance and behavior**

**R46.81 Obsessive-compulsive behavior**
> **EXCLUDES 1**   obsessive-compulsive disorder (F42-)

**R46.89 Other symptoms and signs involving appearance and behavior**

## Symptoms and signs involving speech and voice (R47-R49)

**✓4ᵗʰ R47 Speech disturbances, not elsewhere classified**
> **EXCLUDES 1**   autism (F84.0)
> cluttering (F80.81)
> specific developmental disorders of speech and language (F80.-)
> stuttering (F80.81)

**✓5ᵗʰ R47.0 Dysphasia and aphasia**

**R47.01 Aphasia**    `CC`
> **EXCLUDES 1**   aphasia following cerebrovascular disease (I69. with final characters -20)
> progressive isolated aphasia (G31.01)
> **CC Excl:** PDX collection 1131

**R47.02 Dysphasia**
> **EXCLUDES 1**   dysphasia following cerebrovascular disease (I69. with final characters -21)

**R47.1 Dysarthria and anarthria**
> **EXCLUDES 1**   dysarthria following cerebrovascular disease (I69. with final characters -22)

**✓5ᵗʰ R47.8 Other speech disturbances**
> **EXCLUDES 1**   dysarthria following cerebrovascular disease (I69. with final characters -28)

**R47.81 Slurred speech**

**R47.82 _Fluency disorder in conditions classified elsewhere_**
Stuttering in conditions classified elsewhere
Code first underlying disease or condition, such as:
Parkinson's disease (G20)
> **EXCLUDES 1**   adult onset fluency disorder (F98.5)
> childhood onset fluency disorder (F80.81)
> fluency disorder (stuttering) following cerebrovascular disease (I69. with final characters-23)

**R47.89 Other speech disturbances**

**R47.9 Unspecified speech disturbances**

**✓4ᵗʰ R48 Dyslexia and other symbolic dysfunctions, not elsewhere classified**
> **EXCLUDES 1**   specific developmental disorders of scholastic skills (F81.-)

**R48.0 Dyslexia and alexia**

**R48.1 Agnosia**
Astereognosia (astereognosis)
Autotopagnosia
> **EXCLUDES 1**   visual object agnosia (R48.3)

**R48.2 Apraxia**
> **EXCLUDES 1**   apraxia following cerebrovascular disease (I69. with final characters -90)

**R48.3 Visual agnosia**
Prosopagnosia
Simultanagnosia (asimultagnosia)

**R48.8 Other symbolic dysfunctions**
Acalculia
Agraphia
**AHA:** 2017, 1Q, 27

**R48.9 Unspecified symbolic dysfunctions**

**✓4ᵗʰ R49 Voice and resonance disorders**
> **EXCLUDES 1**   psychogenic voice and resonance disorders (F44.4)

**R49.0 Dysphonia**
Hoarseness

**R49.1 Aphonia**
Loss of voice

**✓5ᵗʰ R49.2 Hypernasality and hyponasality**

**R49.21 Hypernasality**

**R49.22 Hyponasality**

**R49.8 Other voice and resonance disorders**

**R49.9 Unspecified voice and resonance disorder**
Change in voice NOS
Resonance disorder NOS

---

**N** Newborn: 0    **P** Pediatric: 0-17    **M** Maternity: 12-55    **A** Adult: 15-124    **MCC** Major CC Condition    **PDxMCC** PDx acts as own MCC    **CC** CC Condition    **PDxCC** PDx acts as own CC

922        ICD-10-CM 2018

R42–R49.9

## General symptoms and signs (R50-R69)

✓4th **R50   Fever of other and unknown origin**

EXCLUDES 1   chills without fever (R68.83)
febrile convulsions (R56.0-)
fever of unknown origin during labor (O75.2)
fever of unknown origin in newborn (P81.9)
hypothermia due to illness (R68.0)
malignant hyperthermia due to anesthesia (T88.3)
puerperal pyrexia NOS (O86.4)

**R50.2   Drug induced fever**

Use additional code for adverse effect, if applicable, to identify drug (T36-T50 with fifth or sixth character 5)

EXCLUDES 1   postvaccination (postimmunization) fever (R50.83)

✓5th **R50.8   Other specified fever**

*R50.81   Fever presenting with conditions classified elsewhere*
Code first underlying condition when associated fever is present, such as with:
leukemia (C91-C95)
neutropenia (D70.-)
sickle-cell disease (D57.-)
**AHA:** 2014, 4Q, 22

**R50.82   Postprocedural fever**

EXCLUDES 1   postprocedural infection (T81.4-)
posttransfusion fever (R50.84)
postvaccination (postimmunization) fever (R50.83)

**R50.83   Postvaccination fever**
Postimmunization fever

**R50.84   Febrile nonhemolytic transfusion reaction**
FNHTR
Posttransfusion fever

**R50.9   Fever, unspecified**
Fever NOS
Fever of unknown origin [FUO]
Fever with chills
Fever with rigors
Hyperpyrexia NOS
Persistent fever
Pyrexia NOS

**R51   Headache**
Facial pain NOS

EXCLUDES 1   atypical face pain (G50.1)
migraine and other headache syndromes (G43-G44)
trigeminal neuralgia (G50.0)

**R52   Pain, unspecified**
Acute pain NOS
Generalized pain NOS
Pain NOS

EXCLUDES 1   acute and chronic pain, not elsewhere classified (G89.-)
localized pain, unspecified type—code to pain by site, such as:
abdomen pain (R10.-)
back pain (M54.9)
breast pain (N64.4)
chest pain (R07.1-R07.9)
ear pain (H92.0-)
eye pain (H57.1)
headache (R51)
joint pain (M25.5-)
limb pain (M79.6-)
lumbar region pain (M54.5)
pelvic and perineal pain (R10.2)
renal colic (N23)
shoulder pain (M25.51-)
spine pain (M54.-)
throat pain (R07.0)
tongue pain (K14.6)
tooth pain (K08.8)
pain disorders exclusively related to psychological factors (F45.41)

✓4th **R53   Malaise and fatigue**

**R53.0   Neoplastic (malignant) related fatigue**
Code first associated neoplasm

**R53.1   Weakness**
Asthenia NOS

EXCLUDES 1   age-related weakness (R54)
muscle weakness (M62.8-)
sarcopenia (M62.84)
senile asthenia (R54)
**AHA:** 2017, 1Q, 7; 2015, 1Q, 25

**R53.2   Functional quadriplegia**   MCC  HCC
Complete immobility due to severe physical disability or frailty

EXCLUDES 1   frailty NOS (R54)
hysterical paralysis (F44.4)
immobility syndrome (M62.3)
neurologic quadriplegia (G82.5-)
quadriplegia (G82.50)
**AHA:** 2016, 2Q, 6
**DEF:** Inability to move due to a nonphysiological condition, such as dementia; no mental ability to move independently; typically found in severely demented patients.
**CC Excl:** PDX collection 595

✓5th **R53.8   Other malaise and fatigue**

EXCLUDES 1   combat exhaustion and fatigue (F43.0)
congenital debility (P96.9)
~~exhaustion and fatigue due to depressive episode (F32.-)~~
exhaustion and fatigue due to excessive exertion (T73.3)
exhaustion and fatigue due to exposure (T73.2)
exhaustion and fatigue due to heat (T67.-)
exhaustion and fatigue due to pregnancy (O26.8-)
exhaustion and fatigue due to recurrent depressive episode (F33)
exhaustion and fatigue due to senile debility (R54)

**R53.81   Other malaise**
Chronic debility          Malaise NOS
Debility NOS              Nervous debility
General physical deterioration
EXCLUDES 1   age-related physical debility (R54)

**R53.82   Chronic fatigue, unspecified**
Chronic fatigue syndrome NOS
EXCLUDES 1   postviral fatigue syndrome (G93.3)

**R53.83   Other fatigue**
Fatigue NOS
Lack of energy
Lethargy
Tiredness
EXCLUDES 2 ▶exhaustion and fatigue due to depressive episode (F32.-)◀

**R54   Age-related physical debility**   A
Frailty          Senile asthenia
Old age          Senile debility
Senescence

EXCLUDES 1   age-related cognitive decline (R41.81)
sarcopenia (M62.84)
senile psychosis (F03)
senility NOS (R41.81)

**R55   Syncope and collapse**
Blackout          Vasovagal attack
Fainting

EXCLUDES 1   cardiogenic shock (R57.0)
carotid sinus syncope (G90.01)
heat syncope (T67.1)
neurocirculatory asthenia (F45.8)
neurogenic orthostatic hypotension (G90.3)
orthostatic hypotension (I95.1)
postprocedural shock (T81.1-)
psychogenic syncope (F48.8)
shock NOS (R57.9)
shock complicating or following abortion or ectopic or molar pregnancy (O00-O07, O08.3)
shock complicating or following labor and delivery (O75.1)
Stokes-Adams attack (I45.9)
unconsciousness NOS (R40.2-)

✓4th **R56   Convulsions, not elsewhere classified**

EXCLUDES 1   dissociative convulsions and seizures (F44.5)
epileptic convulsions and seizures (G40.-)
newborn convulsions and seizures (P90)

✓5th **R56.0   Febrile convulsions**

**R56.00   Simple febrile convulsions**   CC  HCC
Febrile convulsion NOS
Febrile seizure NOS
**CC Excl:** PDX collection 1132

**R56.01   Complex febrile convulsions**   CC  HCC
Atypical febrile seizure
Complex febrile seizure
Complicated febrile seizure
EXCLUDES 1   status epilepticus (G40.901)
**CC Excl:** PDX collection 1132

**R56.1 Post traumatic seizures** `CC` `HCC`

> EXCLUDES 1    *post traumatic epilepsy (G40.-)*
>
> **CC Excl:** PDX collection 582

**R56.9 Unspecified convulsions** `HCC`

> Convulsion disorder
> Fit NOS
> Recurrent convulsions
> Seizure(s) (convulsive) NOS

✓4ᵗʰ **R57 Shock, not elsewhere classified**

> EXCLUDES 1    *anaphylactic shock NOS (T78.2)*
> *anaphylactic reaction or shock due to adverse food reaction (T78.0-)*
> *anaphylactic shock due to adverse effect of correct drug or medicament properly administered (T88.6)*
> *anaphylactic shock due to serum (T80.5-)*
> *anesthetic shock (T88.3)*
> *electric shock (T75.4)*
> *obstetric shock (O75.1)*
> *postprocedural shock (T81.1-)*
> *psychic shock (F43.0)*
> *~~septic shock (R65.21)~~*
> *shock complicating or following ectopic or molar pregnancy (O00-O07, O08.3)*
> *shock due to lightning (T75.01)*
> *traumatic shock (T79.4)*
> *toxic shock syndrome (A48.3)*

> **CC Excl: For CC/MCC codes in category R57:** PDX collection 1133

[1] **R57.0 Cardiogenic shock** `MCC` `HCC`

> EXCLUDES 2    ▶*septic shock (R65.21)*◀
>
> **DEF:** Associated with myocardial infarction, cardiac tamponade, and massive pulmonary embolism; symptoms include mental confusion, reduced blood pressure, tachycardia, pallor, and cold, clammy skin.

[1] **R57.1 Hypovolemic shock** `MCC` `HCC`

[1] **R57.8 Other shock** `MCC` `HCC`

**R57.9 Shock, unspecified** `CC` `HCC`

> Failure of peripheral circulation NOS

**R58 Hemorrhage, not elsewhere classified**

> Hemorrhage NOS
>
> EXCLUDES 1    *hemorrhage included with underlying conditions, such as:*
> *acute duodenal ulcer with hemorrhage (K26.0)*
> *acute gastritis with bleeding (K29.01)*
> *ulcerative enterocolitis with rectal bleeding (K51.01)*

✓4ᵗʰ **R59 Enlarged lymph nodes**

> INCLUDES    swollen glands
>
> EXCLUDES 1    *acute lymphadenitis (L04.-)*
> *chronic lymphadenitis (I88.1)*
> *lymphadenitis NOS (I88.9)*
> *mesenteric (acute) (chronic) lymphadenitis (I88.0)*

**R59.0 Localized enlarged lymph nodes**

**R59.1 Generalized enlarged lymph nodes**

> Lymphadenopathy NOS

**R59.9 Enlarged lymph nodes, unspecified**

✓4ᵗʰ **R60 Edema, not elsewhere classified**

> EXCLUDES 1    *angioneurotic edema (T78.3)*
> *ascites (R18.-)*
> *cerebral edema (G93.6)*
> *cerebral edema due to birth injury (P11.0)*
> *edema of larynx (J38.4)*
> *edema of nasopharynx (J39.2)*
> *edema of pharynx (J39.2)*
> *gestational edema (O12.0-)*
> *hereditary edema (Q82.0)*
> *hydrops fetalis NOS (P83.2)*
> *hydrothorax (J94.8)*
> *~~nutritional edema (E40-E46)~~*
> *hydrops fetalis NOS (P83.2)*
> *newborn edema (P83.3)*
> *pulmonary edema (J81.-)*

**R60.0 Localized edema**

**R60.1 Generalized edema**

> EXCLUDES 2    ▶*nutritional edema (E40-E46)*◀

**R60.9 Edema, unspecified**

> Fluid retention NOS

**R61 Generalized hyperhidrosis**

> Excessive sweating
> Night sweats
> Secondary hyperhidrosis
> Code first, if applicable, menopausal and female climacteric states (N95.1)
>
> EXCLUDES 1    *focal (primary) (secondary) hyperhidrosis (L74.5-)*
> *Frey's syndrome (L74.52)*
> *localized (primary) (secondary) hyperhidrosis (L74.5-)*

✓4ᵗʰ **R62 Lack of expected normal physiological development in childhood and adults**

> EXCLUDES 1    *delayed puberty (E30.0)*
> *gonadal dysgenesis (Q99.1)*
> *hypopituitarism (E23.0)*

**R62.0 Delayed milestone in childhood** `P`

> Delayed attainment of expected physiological developmental stage
> Late talker
> Late walker

✓5ᵗʰ **R62.5 Other and unspecified lack of expected normal physiological development in childhood**

> EXCLUDES 1    *HIV disease resulting in failure to thrive (B20)*
> *physical retardation due to malnutrition (E45)*

**R62.50 Unspecified lack of expected normal physiological development in childhood**

> Infantilism NOS

**R62.51 Failure to thrive (child)** `P`

> Failure to gain weight
>
> EXCLUDES 1    *failure to thrive in child under 28 days old (P92.6)*
>
> **DEF:** Organic failure to thrive (FTT): Acute or chronic illness that interferes with nutritional intake, absorption, metabolism excretion, and energy requirements; nonorganic FTT is a symptom of neglect or abuse.

**R62.52 Short stature (child)**

> Lack of growth
> Physical retardation
> Short stature NOS
>
> EXCLUDES 1    *short stature due to endocrine disorder (E34.3)*

**R62.59 Other lack of expected normal physiological development in childhood**

**R62.7 Adult failure to thrive** `A`

✓4ᵗʰ **R63 Symptoms and signs concerning food and fluid intake**

> EXCLUDES 1    *bulimia NOS (F50.2)*
> *eating disorders of nonorganic origin (F50.-)*
> *malnutrition (E40-E46)*

**R63.0 Anorexia**

> Loss of appetite
>
> EXCLUDES 1    *anorexia nervosa (F50.0-)*
> *loss of appetite of nonorganic origin (F50.89)*

**R63.1 Polydipsia**

> Excessive thirst

**R63.2 Polyphagia**

> Excessive eating
> Hyperalimentation NOS

**R63.3 Feeding difficulties**

> Feeding problem (elderly) (infant) NOS
> ▶Picky eater◀
>
> EXCLUDES 1    ▶*eating disorders (F50.-)*◀
> *feeding problems of newborn (P92.-)*
> *infant feeding disorder of nonorganic origin (F98.2-)*
>
> **AHA:** 2017, 1Q, 28; 2016, 3Q, 19

**R63.4 Abnormal weight loss**

**R63.5 Abnormal weight gain**

> EXCLUDES 1    *excessive weight gain in pregnancy (O26.0-)*
> *obesity (E66.-)*

**R63.6 Underweight**

> Use additional code to identify body mass index (BMI), if known (Z68.-)
>
> EXCLUDES 1    *abnormal weight loss (R63.4)*
> *anorexia nervosa (F50.0-)*
> *malnutrition (E40-E46)*

**R63.8 Other symptoms and signs concerning food and fluid intake**

---

[1]   MCC only if patient is discharged alive.

`N` Newborn: 0   `P` Pediatric: 0-17   `M` Maternity: 12-55   `A` Adult: 15-124   `MCC` Major CC Condition   `PDxMCC` PDx acts as own MCC   `CC` CC Condition   `PDxCC` PDx acts as own CC

**924**      **ICD-10-CM 2018**

**R64   Cachexia**   `CC` `HCC`
Wasting syndrome
Code first underlying condition, if known
*EXCLUDES 1*   *abnormal weight loss (R63.4)*
*nutritional marasmus (E41)*
**CC Excl:** PDX collection 1134

✓4th **R65   Symptoms and signs specifically associated with systemic inflammation and infection**

**CC Excl: For CC/MCC codes in category R65, unless otherwise noted:** PDX collection 71

✓5th **R65.1   Systemic inflammatory response syndrome [SIRS] of non-infectious origin**
Code first underlying condition, such as:
heatstroke (T67.0)
injury and trauma (S00-T88)
*EXCLUDES 1*   *sepsis—code to infection*
*severe sepsis (R65.2)*

**R65.10   Systemic inflammatory response syndrome [SIRS] of non-infectious origin without acute organ dysfunction**   `CC` `HCC`
Systemic inflammatory response syndrome (SIRS) NOS

**R65.11   Systemic inflammatory response syndrome [SIRS] of non-infectious origin with acute organ dysfunction**   `MCC` `HCC`
Use additional code to identify specific acute organ dysfunction, such as:
acute kidney failure (N17.-)
acute respiratory failure (J96.0-)
critical illness myopathy (G72.81)
critical illness polyneuropathy (G62.81)
disseminated intravascular coagulopathy [DIC] (D65)
encephalopathy (metabolic) (septic) (G93.41)
hepatic failure (K72.0-)

✓5th **R65.2   Severe sepsis**
Infection with associated acute organ dysfunction
Sepsis with acute organ dysfunction
Sepsis with multiple organ dysfunction
Systemic inflammatory response syndrome due to infectious process with acute organ dysfunction
Code first underlying infection, such as:
infection following a procedure (T81.4-)
infections following infusion, transfusion and therapeutic injection (T80.2-)
puerperal sepsis (O85)
sepsis following complete or unspecified spontaneous abortion (O03.87)
sepsis following ectopic and molar pregnancy (O08.82)
sepsis following incomplete spontaneous abortion (O03.37)
sepsis following (induced) termination of pregnancy (O04.87)
sepsis NOS (A41.9)
Use additional code to identify specific acute organ dysfunction, such as:
acute kidney failure (N17.-)
acute respiratory failure (J96.0-)
critical illness myopathy (G72.81)
critical illness polyneuropathy (G62.81)
disseminated intravascular coagulopathy [DIC] (D65)
encephalopathy (metabolic) (septic) (G93.41)
hepatic failure (K72.0-)
**AHA:** 2016, 3Q, 8

**R65.20   Severe sepsis without septic shock**   `MCC` `HCC`
Severe sepsis NOS
**AHA:** 2016, 3Q, 14; 2013, 4Q, 119

**R65.21   Severe sepsis with septic shock**   `PDx MCC` `MCC` `HCC`
**CC Excl:** PDX collection 1133

✓4th **R68   Other general symptoms and signs**
**R68.0   Hypothermia, not associated with low environmental temperature**
*EXCLUDES 1*   *hypothermia due to anesthesia (T88.51)*
*hypothermia due to low environmental temperature (T68)*
*hypothermia NOS (accidental) (T68)*
*newborn hypothermia (P80.-)*

✓5th **R68.1   Nonspecific symptoms peculiar to infancy**
*EXCLUDES 1*   *colic, infantile (R10.83)*
*neonatal cerebral irritability (P91.3)*
*teething syndrome (K00.7)*

**R68.11   Excessive crying of infant (baby)**   `P`
*EXCLUDES 1*   *excessive crying of child, adolescent, or adult (R45.83)*

**R68.12   Fussy infant (baby)**   `P`
Irritable infant

**R68.13   Apparent life threatening event in infant (ALTE)**   `P`
Apparent life threatening event in newborn
▶Brief resolved unexplained event (BRUE)◀
Code first confirmed diagnosis, if known
Use additional code(s) for associated signs and symptoms if no confirmed diagnosis established, or if signs and symptoms are not associated routinely with confirmed diagnosis, or provide additional information for cause of ALTE

**R68.19   Other nonspecific symptoms peculiar to infancy**   `P`

**R68.2   Dry mouth, unspecified**
*EXCLUDES 1*   *dry mouth due to dehydration (E86.0)*
*dry mouth due to sicca syndrome [Sjögren] (M35.0-)*
*salivary gland hyposecretion (K11.7)*

**R68.3   Clubbing of fingers**
Clubbing of nails
*EXCLUDES 1*   *congenital clubfinger (Q68.1)*
**DEF:** Enlarged soft tissue of distal fingers; usually occurs in heart and lung diseases.

✓5th **R68.8   Other general symptoms and signs**
**R68.81   Early satiety**
**DEF:** The premature feeling of being full after eating only a small amount of food; mechanism of satiety is multifactorial.

**R68.82   Decreased libido**   `A`
Decreased sexual desire

**R68.83   Chills (without fever)**
Chills NOS
*EXCLUDES 1*   *chills with fever (R50.9)*

**R68.84   Jaw pain**
Mandibular pain
Maxilla pain
*EXCLUDES 1*   *temporomandibular joint arthralgia (M26.62-)*

**R68.89   Other general symptoms and signs**

**R69   Illness, unspecified**
Unknown and unspecified cases of morbidity

## Abnormal findings on examination of blood, without diagnosis (R70-R79)

*EXCLUDES 2*   *abnormal findings on antenatal screening of mother (O28.-)*
*abnormalities of lipids (E78.-)*
*abnormalities of platelets and thrombocytes (D69.-)*
*abnormalities of white blood cells classified elsewhere (D70-D72)*
*coagulation hemorrhagic disorders (D65-D68)*
*diagnostic abnormal findings classified elsewhere—see Alphabetical Index*
*hemorrhagic and hematological disorders of newborn (P50-P61)*

✓4th **R70   Elevated erythrocyte sedimentation rate and abnormality of plasma viscosity**
**R70.0   Elevated erythrocyte sedimentation rate**
**R70.1   Abnormal plasma viscosity**

✓4th **R71   Abnormality of red blood cells**
*EXCLUDES 1*   *anemias (D50-D64)*
*anemia of premature infant (P61.2)*
*benign (familial) polycythemia (D75.0)*
*congenital anemias (P61.2-P61.4)*
*newborn anemia due to isoimmunization (P55.-)*
*polycythemia neonatorum (P61.1)*
*polycythemia NOS (D75.1)*
*polycythemia vera (D45)*
*secondary polycythemia (D75.1)*

**R71.0   Precipitous drop in hematocrit**   `CC`
Drop (precipitous) in hemoglobin
Drop in hematocrit
**CC Excl:** PDX collection 1135

**R71.8   Other abnormality of red blood cells**
Abnormal red-cell morphology NOS        Anisocytosis
Abnormal red-cell volume NOS        Poikilocytosis

**✓4ᵗʰ R73 Elevated blood glucose level**
> EXCLUDES 1   *diabetes mellitus (E08-E13)*
> *diabetes mellitus in pregnancy, childbirth and the puerperium (O24.-)*
> *neonatal disorders (P70.0-P70.2)*
> *postsurgical hypoinsulinemia (E89.1)*

**✓5ᵗʰ R73.0 Abnormal glucose**
> EXCLUDES 1   *abnormal glucose in pregnancy (O99.81-)*
> *diabetes mellitus (E08-E13)*
> *dysmetabolic syndrome X (E88.81)*
> *gestational diabetes (O24.4-)*
> *glycosuria (R81)*
> *hypoglycemia (E16.2)*

    **R73.01 Impaired fasting glucose**
       Elevated fasting glucose

    **R73.02 Impaired glucose tolerance (oral)**
       Elevated glucose tolerance

    **R73.03 Prediabetes**
       Latent diabetes

    **R73.09 Other abnormal glucose**
       Abnormal glucose NOS
       Abnormal non-fasting glucose tolerance

    **R73.9 Hyperglycemia, unspecified**

**✓4ᵗʰ R74 Abnormal serum enzyme levels**
    **R74.0 Nonspecific elevation of levels of transaminase and lactic acid dehydrogenase [LDH]**
    **R74.8 Abnormal levels of other serum enzymes**
       Abnormal level of acid phosphatase
       Abnormal level of alkaline phosphatase
       Abnormal level of amylase
       Abnormal level of lipase [triacylglycerol lipase]
    **R74.9 Abnormal serum enzyme level, unspecified**

**R75 Inconclusive laboratory evidence of human immunodeficiency virus [HIV]**
    Nonconclusive HIV-test finding in infants
> EXCLUDES 1   *asymptomatic human immunodeficiency virus [HIV] infection status (Z21)*
> *human immunodeficiency virus [HIV] disease (B20)*

**✓4ᵗʰ R76 Other abnormal immunological findings in serum**
    **R76.0 Raised antibody titer**
> EXCLUDES 1   *isoimmunization in pregnancy (O36.0-O36.1)*
> *isoimmunization affecting newborn (P55.-)*

**✓5ᵗʰ R76.1 Nonspecific reaction to test for tuberculosis**
    **R76.11 Nonspecific reaction to tuberculin skin test without active tuberculosis**
       Abnormal result of Mantoux test
       PPD positive
       Tuberculin (skin test) positive
       Tuberculin (skin test) reactor
> EXCLUDES 1   *nonspecific reaction to cell mediated immunity measurement of gamma interferon antigen response without active tuberculosis (R76.12)*

    **R76.12 Nonspecific reaction to cell mediated immunity measurement of gamma interferon antigen response without active tuberculosis**
       Nonspecific reaction to QuantiFERON-TB test (QFT) without active tuberculosis
> EXCLUDES 1   *nonspecific reaction to tuberculin skin test without active tuberculosis (R76.11)*
> *positive tuberculin skin test (R76.11)*

    **R76.8 Other specified abnormal immunological findings in serum**
       Raised level of immunoglobulins NOS

    **R76.9 Abnormal immunological finding in serum, unspecified**

**✓4ᵗʰ R77 Other abnormalities of plasma proteins**
> EXCLUDES 1   *disorders of plasma-protein metabolism (E88.0)*

    **R77.0 Abnormality of albumin**
    **R77.1 Abnormality of globulin**
       Hyperglobulinemia NOS
    **R77.2 Abnormality of alphafetoprotein**
    **R77.8 Other specified abnormalities of plasma proteins**
    **R77.9 Abnormality of plasma protein, unspecified**

**✓4ᵗʰ R78 Findings of drugs and other substances, not normally found in blood**
    Use additional code to identify any retained foreign body, if applicable (Z18.-)
> EXCLUDES 1   *mental or behavioral disorders due to psychoactive substance use (F10-F19)*

    **R78.0 Finding of alcohol in blood**
       Use additional external cause code (Y90.-), for detail regarding alcohol level

    **R78.1 Finding of opiate drug in blood**
    **R78.2 Finding of cocaine in blood**
    **R78.3 Finding of hallucinogen in blood**
    **R78.4 Finding of other drugs of addictive potential in blood**
    **R78.5 Finding of other psychotropic drug in blood**
    **R78.6 Finding of steroid agent in blood**

**✓5ᵗʰ R78.7 Finding of abnormal level of heavy metals in blood**
    **R78.71 Abnormal lead level in blood**
> EXCLUDES 1   *lead poisoning (T56.0-)*

    **R78.79 Finding of abnormal level of heavy metals in blood**

**✓5ᵗʰ R78.8 Finding of other specified substances, not normally found in blood**
    **R78.81 Bacteremia**    `CC`
> EXCLUDES 1   *sepsis—code to specified infection*
       **DEF:** Laboratory finding of bacteria in the blood in the absence of two or more signs of sepsis; transient in nature, it progresses to septicemia with severe infectious process.
       **CC Excl:** PDX collection 1136

    **R78.89 Finding of other specified substances, not normally found in blood**
       Finding of abnormal level of lithium in blood

    **R78.9 Finding of unspecified substance, not normally found in blood**

**✓4ᵗʰ R79 Other abnormal findings of blood chemistry**
    Use additional code to identify any retained foreign body, if applicable (Z18.-)
> EXCLUDES 1   *abnormality of fluid, electrolyte or acid-base balance (E86-E87)*
> *asymptomatic hyperuricemia (E79.0)*
> *hyperglycemia NOS (R73.9)*
> *hypoglycemia NOS (E16.2)*
> *neonatal hypoglycemia (P70.3-P70.4)*
> *specific findings indicating disorder of amino-acid metabolism (E70-E72)*
> *specific findings indicating disorder of carbohydrate metabolism (E73-E74)*
> *specific findings indicating disorder of lipid metabolism (E75.-)*

    **R79.0 Abnormal level of blood mineral**
       Abnormal blood level of cobalt
       Abnormal blood level of copper
       Abnormal blood level of iron
       Abnormal blood level of magnesium
       Abnormal blood level of mineral NEC
       Abnormal blood level of zinc
> EXCLUDES 1   *abnormal level of lithium (R78.89)*
> *disorders of mineral metabolism (E83.-)*
> *neonatal hypomagnesemia (P71.2)*
> *nutritional mineral deficiency (E58-E61)*

    **R79.1 Abnormal coagulation profile**
       Abnormal or prolonged bleeding time
       Abnormal or prolonged coagulation time
       Abnormal or prolonged partial thromboplastin time [PTT]
       Abnormal or prolonged prothrombin time [PT]
> EXCLUDES 1   *coagulation defects (D68.-)*
> EXCLUDES 2   ▶*abnormality of fluid, electrolyte or acid-base balance (E86-E87)*◄

**✓5ᵗʰ R79.8 Other specified abnormal findings of blood chemistry**
    **R79.81 Abnormal blood-gas level**
    **R79.82 Elevated C-reactive protein [CRP]**
    **R79.89 Other specified abnormal findings of blood chemistry**

    **R79.9 Abnormal finding of blood chemistry, unspecified**

**N** Newborn: 0   **P** Pediatric: 0-17   **M** Maternity: 12-55   **A** Adult: 15-124   **MCC** Major CC Condition   **PDxMCC** PDx acts as own MCC   **CC** CC Condition   **PDxCC** PDx acts as own CC

926      ICD-10-CM 2018

## Abnormal findings on examination of urine, without diagnosis (R80-R82)

> EXCLUDES 1　abnormal findings on antenatal screening of mother (O28.-)
> diagnostic abnormal findings classified elsewhere—see Alphabetical Index
> specific findings indicating disorder of amino-acid metabolism (E70-E72)

✓4ᵗʰ **R80　Proteinuria**
> EXCLUDES 1　gestational proteinuria (O12.1-)

**R80.0　Isolated proteinuria**
Idiopathic proteinuria
> EXCLUDES 1　isolated proteinuria with specific morphological lesion (N06.-)

**R80.1　Persistent proteinuria, unspecified**

**R80.2　Orthostatic proteinuria, unspecified**
Postural proteinuria

**R80.3　Bence Jones proteinuria**

**R80.8　Other proteinuria**

**R80.9　Proteinuria, unspecified**
Albuminuria NOS

**R81　Glycosuria**
> EXCLUDES 1　renal glycosuria (E74.8)

✓4ᵗʰ **R82　Other and unspecified abnormal findings in urine**
> INCLUDES　chromoabnormalities in urine
> Use additional code to identify any retained foreign body, if applicable (Z18.-)
> EXCLUDES 2　hematuria (R31.-)

**R82.0　Chyluria**　　CC
> EXCLUDES 1　filarial chyluria (B74.-)
**CC Excl:** PDX collection 1137

**R82.1　Myoglobinuria**　　CC
**CC Excl:** PDX collection 1138

**R82.2　Biliuria**

**R82.3　Hemoglobinuria**
> EXCLUDES 1　hemoglobinuria due to hemolysis from external causes NEC (D59.6)
> hemoglobinuria due to paroxysmal nocturnal [Marchiafava-Micheli] (D59.5)
**DEF:** Free hemoglobin in blood due to rapid hemolysis of red blood cells; causes include burns, crushed injury, sickle cell anemia, thalassemia, parasitic infections, or kidney infections.

**R82.4　Acetonuria**
Ketonuria
**DEF:** Excessive excretion of acetone in urine; commonly occurs in diabetic acidosis.

**R82.5　Elevated urine levels of drugs, medicaments and biological substances**
Elevated urine levels of catecholamines
Elevated urine levels of indoleacetic acid
Elevated urine levels of 17-ketosteroids
Elevated urine levels of steroids

**R82.6　Abnormal urine levels of substances chiefly nonmedicinal as to source**
Abnormal urine level of heavy metals

✓5ᵗʰ **R82.7　Abnormal findings on microbiological examination of urine**
> EXCLUDES 1　colonization status (Z22.-)

**R82.71　Bacteriuria**

**R82.79　Other abnormal findings on microbiological examination of urine**
Positive culture findings of urine

**R82.8　Abnormal findings on cytological and histological examination of urine**

✓5ᵗʰ **R82.9　Other and unspecified abnormal findings in urine**

**R82.90　Unspecified abnormal findings in urine**

**R82.91　Other chromoabnormalities of urine**
Chromoconversion (dipstick)
Idiopathic dipstick converts positive for blood with no cellular forms in sediment
> EXCLUDES 1　hemoglobinuria (R82.3)
> myoglobinuria (R82.1)

**R82.99　Other abnormal findings in urine**
Cells and casts in urine
Crystalluria
Melanuria

## Abnormal findings on examination of other body fluids, substances and tissues, without diagnosis (R83-R89)

> EXCLUDES 1　abnormal findings on antenatal screening of mother (O28.-)
> diagnostic abnormal findings classified elsewhere—see Alphabetical Index
> EXCLUDES 2　abnormal findings on examination of blood, without diagnosis (R70-R79)
> abnormal findings on examination of urine, without diagnosis (R80-R82)
> abnormal tumor markers (R97.-)

✓4ᵗʰ **R83　Abnormal findings in cerebrospinal fluid**

**R83.0　Abnormal level of enzymes in cerebrospinal fluid**

**R83.1　Abnormal level of hormones in cerebrospinal fluid**

**R83.2　Abnormal level of other drugs, medicaments and biological substances in cerebrospinal fluid**

**R83.3　Abnormal level of substances chiefly nonmedicinal as to source in cerebrospinal fluid**

**R83.4　Abnormal immunological findings in cerebrospinal fluid**

**R83.5　Abnormal microbiological findings in cerebrospinal fluid**
Positive culture findings in cerebrospinal fluid
> EXCLUDES 1　colonization status (Z22.-)

**R83.6　Abnormal cytological findings in cerebrospinal fluid**

**R83.8　Other abnormal findings in cerebrospinal fluid**
Abnormal chromosomal findings in cerebrospinal fluid

**R83.9　Unspecified abnormal finding in cerebrospinal fluid**

✓4ᵗʰ **R84　Abnormal findings in specimens from respiratory organs and thorax**
> INCLUDES　abnormal findings in bronchial washings
> abnormal findings in nasal secretions
> abnormal findings in pleural fluid
> abnormal findings in sputum
> abnormal findings in throat scrapings
> EXCLUDES 1　blood-stained sputum (R04.2)

**R84.0　Abnormal level of enzymes in specimens from respiratory organs and thorax**

**R84.1　Abnormal level of hormones in specimens from respiratory organs and thorax**

**R84.2　Abnormal level of other drugs, medicaments and biological substances in specimens from respiratory organs and thorax**

**R84.3　Abnormal level of substances chiefly nonmedicinal as to source in specimens from respiratory organs and thorax**

**R84.4　Abnormal immunological findings in specimens from respiratory organs and thorax**

**Cerebrospinal Fluid**

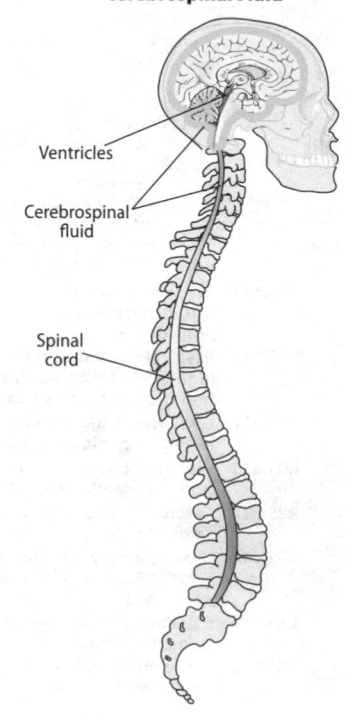

Ventricles

Cerebrospinal fluid

Spinal cord

✓ Additional Character Req　✓x7ᵗʰ Placeholder Alert　Unacceptable PDx　Manifestation　H1-H14 HAC　HCC CMS-HCC Condition　EXCLUDES 1 Not Coded Here　EXCLUDES 2 Not Included Here

**ICD-10-CM 2018**　　　　　　　　　　　　　　　　　　　　　　　　　　**927**

**R84.5**   **Abnormal microbiological findings in specimens from respiratory organs and thorax**
Positive culture findings in specimens from respiratory organs and thorax
*EXCLUDES 1*   *colonization status (Z22.-)*

**R84.6**   **Abnormal cytological findings in specimens from respiratory organs and thorax**

**R84.7**   **Abnormal histological findings in specimens from respiratory organs and thorax**

**R84.8**   **Other abnormal findings in specimens from respiratory organs and thorax**
Abnormal chromosomal findings in specimens from respiratory organs and thorax

**R84.9**   **Unspecified abnormal finding in specimens from respiratory organs and thorax**

✓4ᵗʰ **R85**   **Abnormal findings in specimens from digestive organs and abdominal cavity**
*INCLUDES*   abnormal findings in peritoneal fluid
abnormal findings in saliva
*EXCLUDES 1*   *cloudy peritoneal dialysis effluent (R88.0)*
*fecal abnormalities (R19.5)*

**R85.0**   **Abnormal level of enzymes in specimens from digestive organs and abdominal cavity**

**R85.1**   **Abnormal level of hormones in specimens from digestive organs and abdominal cavity**

**R85.2**   **Abnormal level of other drugs, medicaments and biological substances in specimens from digestive organs and abdominal cavity**

**R85.3**   **Abnormal level of substances chiefly nonmedicinal as to source in specimens from digestive organs and abdominal cavity**

**R85.4**   **Abnormal immunological findings in specimens from digestive organs and abdominal cavity**

**R85.5**   **Abnormal microbiological findings in specimens from digestive organs and abdominal cavity**
Positive culture findings in specimens from digestive organs and abdominal cavity
*EXCLUDES 1*   *colonization status (Z22.-)*

✓5ᵗʰ **R85.6**   **Abnormal cytological findings in specimens from digestive organs and abdominal cavity**

✓6ᵗʰ **R85.61**   **Abnormal cytologic smear of anus**
*EXCLUDES 1*   *abnormal cytological findings in specimens from other digestive organs and abdominal cavity (R85.69)*
*anal intraepithelial neoplasia I [AIN I] (K62.82)*
*anal intraepithelial neoplasia II [AIN II] (K62.82)*
*anal intraepithelial neoplasia III [AIN III] (D01.3)*
*carcinoma in situ of anus (histologically confirmed) (D01.3)*
*dysplasia (mild) (moderate) of anus (histologically confirmed) (K62.82)*
*severe dysplasia of anus (histologically confirmed) (D01.3)*
*EXCLUDES 2*   *anal high risk human papillomavirus (HPV) DNA test positive (R85.81)*
*anal low risk human papillomavirus (HPV) DNA test positive (R85.82)*

**R85.610**   **Atypical squamous cells of undetermined significance on cytologic smear of anus [ASC-US]**

**R85.611**   **Atypical squamous cells cannot exclude high grade squamous intraepithelial lesion on cytologic smear of anus [ASC-H]**

**R85.612**   **Low grade squamous intraepithelial lesion on cytologic smear of anus [LGSIL]**

**R85.613**   **High grade squamous intraepithelial lesion on cytologic smear of anus [HGSIL]**

**R85.614**   **Cytologic evidence of malignancy on smear of anus**

**R85.615**   **Unsatisfactory cytologic smear of anus**
Inadequate sample of cytologic smear of anus

**R85.616**   **Satisfactory anal smear but lacking transformation zone**

**R85.618**   **Other abnormal cytological findings on specimens from anus**

**R85.619**   **Unspecified abnormal cytological findings in specimens from anus**
Abnormal anal cytology NOS
Atypical glandular cells of anus NOS

**R85.69**   **Abnormal cytological findings in specimens from other digestive organs and abdominal cavity**

**R85.7**   **Abnormal histological findings in specimens from digestive organs and abdominal cavity**

✓5ᵗʰ **R85.8**   **Other abnormal findings in specimens from digestive organs and abdominal cavity**

**R85.81**   **Anal high risk human papillomavirus [HPV] DNA test positive**
*EXCLUDES 1*   *anogenital warts due to human papillomavirus (HPV) (A63.0)*
*condyloma acuminatum (A63.0)*

**R85.82**   **Anal low risk human papillomavirus [HPV] DNA test positive**
Use additional code for associated human papillomavirus (B97.7)

**R85.89**   **Other abnormal findings in specimens from digestive organs and abdominal cavity**
Abnormal chromosomal findings in specimens from digestive organs and abdominal cavity

**R85.9**   **Unspecified abnormal finding in specimens from digestive organs and abdominal cavity**

✓4ᵗʰ **R86**   **Abnormal findings in specimens from male genital organs**
*INCLUDES*   abnormal findings in prostatic secretions
abnormal findings in semen, seminal fluid
abnormal spermatozoa
*EXCLUDES 1*   *azoospermia (N46.0-)*
*oligospermia (N46.1-)*

**R86.0**   **Abnormal level of enzymes in specimens from male genital organs**   ♂

**R86.1**   **Abnormal level of hormones in specimens from male genital organs**   ♂

**R86.2**   **Abnormal level of other drugs, medicaments and biological substances in specimens from male genital organs**   ♂

**R86.3**   **Abnormal level of substances chiefly nonmedicinal as to source in specimens from male genital organs**   ♂

**R86.4**   **Abnormal immunological findings in specimens from male genital organs**   ♂

**R86.5**   **Abnormal microbiological findings in specimens from male genital organs**   ♂
Positive culture findings in specimens from male genital organs
*EXCLUDES 1*   *colonization status (Z22.-)*

**R86.6**   **Abnormal cytological findings in specimens from male genital organs**   ♂

**R86.7**   **Abnormal histological findings in specimens from male genital organs**   ♂

**R86.8**   **Other abnormal findings in specimens from male genital organs**   ♂
Abnormal chromosomal findings in specimens from male genital organs

**R86.9**   **Unspecified abnormal finding in specimens from male genital organs**   ♂

✓4ᵗʰ **R87**   **Abnormal findings in specimens from female genital organs**
*INCLUDES*   abnormal findings in secretion and smears from cervix uteri
abnormal findings in secretion and smears from vagina
abnormal findings in secretion and smears from vulva

**R87.0**   **Abnormal level of enzymes in specimens from female genital organs**   ♀

**R87.1**   **Abnormal level of hormones in specimens from female genital organs**   ♀

**R87.2**   **Abnormal level of other drugs, medicaments and biological substances in specimens from female genital organs**   ♀

**R87.3**   **Abnormal level of substances chiefly nonmedicinal as to source in specimens from female genital organs**   ♀

**R87.4**   **Abnormal immunological findings in specimens from female genital organs**   ♀

**R87.5**   **Abnormal microbiological findings in specimens from female genital organs**   ♀
Positive culture findings in specimens from female genital organs
*EXCLUDES 1*   *colonization status (Z22.-)*

N Newborn: 0    P Pediatric: 0-17    M Maternity: 12-55    A Adult: 15-124    MCC Major CC Condition    PDxMCC PDx acts as own MCC    CC CC Condition    PDxCC PDx acts as own CC

**928**      ICD-10-CM 2018

☑5ᵗʰ **R87.6 Abnormal** cytological **findings in specimens from female genital organs**

  ☑6ᵗʰ **R87.61 Abnormal cytological findings in specimens from** cervix uteri

      **EXCLUDES 1** *abnormal cytological findings in specimens from other female genital organs (R87.69)*

                *abnormal cytological findings in specimens from vagina (R87.62-)*

                *carcinoma in situ of cervix uteri (histologically confirmed) (D06.-)*

                *cervical intraepithelial neoplasia I [CIN I] (N87.0)*

                *cervical intraepithelial neoplasia II [CIN II] (N87.1)*

                *cervical intraepithelial neoplasia III [CIN III] (D06.-)*

                *dysplasia (mild) (moderate) of cervix uteri (histologically confirmed) (N87.-)*

                *severe dysplasia of cervix uteri (histologically confirmed) (D06.-)*

      **EXCLUDES 2** *cervical high risk human papillomavirus (HPV) DNA test positive (R87.810)*

                *cervical low risk human papillomavirus (HPV) DNA test positive (R87.820)*

    **R87.610 Atypical squamous cells of** undetermined significance **on cytologic smear of cervix [ASC-US]** ♀

    **R87.611 Atypical squamous cells cannot exclude** high grade **squamous intraepithelial lesion on cytologic smear of cervix [ASC-H]** ♀

    **R87.612** Low grade **squamous intraepithelial lesion on cytologic smear of cervix [LGSIL]** ♀

    **R87.613** High grade **squamous intraepithelial lesion on cytologic smear of cervix [HGSIL]** ♀

    **R87.614 Cytologic evidence of** malignancy **on smear of cervix** ♀

    **R87.615 Unsatisfactory cytologic smear of cervix** ♀

        Inadequate sample of cytologic smear of cervix

    **R87.616 Satisfactory cervical smear but** lacking transformation zone ♀

    **R87.618 Other abnormal cytological findings on specimens from cervix uteri** ♀

    **R87.619 Unspecified abnormal cytological findings in specimens from cervix uteri** ♀

        Abnormal cervical cytology NOS

        Abnormal Papanicolaou smear of cervix NOS

        Abnormal thin preparation smear of cervix NOS

        Atypical endocervical cells of cervix NOS

        Atypical endometrial cells of cervix NOS

        Atypical glandular cells of cervix NOS

  ☑6ᵗʰ **R87.62 Abnormal cytological findings in specimens from** vagina

      Use additional code to identify acquired absence of uterus and cervix, if applicable (Z90.71-)

      **EXCLUDES 1** *abnormal cytological findings in specimens from cervix uteri (R87.61-)*

                *abnormal cytological findings in specimens from other female genital organs (R87.69)*

                *carcinoma in situ of vagina (histologically confirmed) (D07.2)*

                *dysplasia (mild) (moderate) of vagina (histologically confirmed) (N89.-)*

                *severe dysplasia of vagina (histologically confirmed) (D07.2)*

                *vaginal intraepithelial neoplasia I [VAIN I] (N89.0)*

                *vaginal intraepithelial neoplasia II [VAIN II] (N89.1)*

                *vaginal intraepithelial neoplasia III [VAIN III] (D07.2)*

      **EXCLUDES 2** *vaginal high risk human papillomavirus (HPV) DNA test positive (R87.811)*

                *vaginal low risk human papillomavirus (HPV) DNA test positive (R87.821)*

    **R87.620 Atypical squamous cells of** undetermined significance **on cytologic smear of vagina [ASC-US]** ♀

    **R87.621 Atypical squamous cells cannot exclude** high grade **squamous intraepithelial lesion on cytologic smear of vagina [ASC-H]** ♀

    **R87.622** Low grade **squamous intraepithelial lesion on cytologic smear of vagina [LGSIL]** ♀

    **R87.623** High grade **squamous intraepithelial lesion on cytologic smear of vagina [HGSIL]** ♀

    **R87.624 Cytologic evidence of** malignancy **on smear of vagina** ♀

    **R87.625 Unsatisfactory cytologic smear of vagina** ♀

        Inadequate sample of cytologic smear of vagina

    **R87.628 Other abnormal cytological findings on specimens from vagina** ♀

    **R87.629 Unspecified abnormal cytological findings in specimens from vagina** ♀

        Abnormal Papanicolaou smear of vagina NOS

        Abnormal thin preparation smear of vagina NOS

        Abnormal vaginal cytology NOS

        Atypical endocervical cells of vagina NOS

        Atypical endometrial cells of vagina NOS

        Atypical glandular cells of vagina NOS

**R87.69 Abnormal cytological findings in specimens from** other female genital organs ♀

    Abnormal cytological findings in specimens from female genital organs NOS

    **EXCLUDES 1** *dysplasia of vulva (histologically confirmed) (N90.0-N90.3)*

**R87.7 Abnormal histological findings in specimens from female genital organs** ♀

    **EXCLUDES 1** *carcinoma in situ (histologically confirmed) of female genital organs (D06-D07.3)*

                *cervical intraepithelial neoplasia I [CIN I] (N87.0)*

                *cervical intraepithelial neoplasia II [CIN II] (N87.1)*

                *cervical intraepithelial neoplasia III [CIN III] (D06.-)*

                *dysplasia (mild) (moderate) of cervix uteri (histologically confirmed) (N87.-)*

                *dysplasia (mild) (moderate) of vagina (histologically confirmed) (N89.-)*

                *severe dysplasia of cervix uteri (histologically confirmed) (D06.-)*

                *severe dysplasia of vagina (histologically confirmed) (D07.2)*

                *vaginal intraepithelial neoplasia I [VAIN I] (N89.0)*

                *vaginal intraepithelial neoplasia II [VAIN II] (N89.1)*

                *vaginal intraepithelial neoplasia III [VAIN III] (D07.2)*

☑5ᵗʰ **R87.8 Other abnormal findings in specimens from female genital organs**

  ☑6ᵗʰ **R87.81 High risk human papillomavirus [HPV] DNA test positive from female genital organs**

      **EXCLUDES 1** *anogenital warts due to human papillomavirus (HPV) (A63.0)*

                *condyloma acuminatum (A63.0)*

    **R87.810 Cervical high risk human papillomavirus [HPV] DNA test positive** ♀

    **R87.811 Vaginal high risk human papillomavirus [HPV] DNA test positive** ♀

  ☑6ᵗʰ **R87.82 Low risk human papillomavirus [HPV] DNA test positive from female genital organs**

      Use additional code for associated human papillomavirus (B97.7)

    **R87.820 Cervical low risk human papillomavirus [HPV] DNA test positive** ♀

    **R87.821 Vaginal low risk human papillomavirus [HPV] DNA test positive** ♀

  **R87.89 Other abnormal findings in specimens from female genital organs** ♀

    Abnormal chromosomal findings in specimens from female genital organs

☑ Additional Character Req  ☑x7ᵗʰ Placeholder Alert  Unacceptable PDx  Manifestation  H1 - H14 HAC  HCC CMS-HCC Condition  EXCLUDES 1 Not Coded Here  EXCLUDES 2 Not Included Here

ICD-10-CM 2018                **929**

**Chapter 18. Symptoms, Signs and Abnormal Clinical and Laboratory Findings, Not Elsewhere Classified**

**R87.9–R94.02**

R87.9   Unspecified abnormal finding in specimens from female ♀ genital organs

✓4ᵗʰ **R88**   **Abnormal findings in other body fluids and substances**

R88.0   Cloudy (hemodialysis) (peritoneal) dialysis effluent

R88.8   Abnormal findings in other body fluids and substances

✓4ᵗʰ **R89**   **Abnormal findings in specimens from other organs, systems and tissues**

INCLUDES   abnormal findings in nipple discharge
abnormal findings in synovial fluid
abnormal findings in wound secretions

R89.0   **Abnormal level of enzymes in specimens from other organs, systems and tissues**

R89.1   **Abnormal level of hormones in specimens from other organs, systems and tissues**

R89.2   **Abnormal level of other drugs, medicaments and biological substances in specimens from other organs, systems and tissues**

R89.3   **Abnormal level of substances chiefly nonmedicinal as to source in specimens from other organs, systems and tissues**

R89.4   **Abnormal immunological findings in specimens from other organs, systems and tissues**

R89.5   **Abnormal microbiological findings in specimens from other organs, systems and tissues**
Positive culture findings in specimens from other organs, systems and tissues
EXCLUDES 1   colonization status (Z22.-)

R89.6   **Abnormal cytological findings in specimens from other organs, systems and tissues**

R89.7   **Abnormal histological findings in specimens from other organs, systems and tissues**

R89.8   **Other abnormal findings in specimens from other organs, systems and tissues**
Abnormal chromosomal findings in specimens from other organs, systems and tissues

R89.9   **Unspecified abnormal finding in specimens from other organs, systems and tissues**

### Abnormal findings on diagnostic imaging and in function studies, without diagnosis (R90-R94)

INCLUDES   nonspecific abnormal findings on diagnostic imaging by computerized axial tomography [CAT scan]
nonspecific abnormal findings on diagnostic imaging by magnetic resonance imaging [MRI][NMR]
nonspecific abnormal findings on diagnostic imaging by positron emission tomography [PET scan]
nonspecific abnormal findings on diagnostic imaging by thermography
nonspecific abnormal findings on diagnostic imaging by ultrasound [echogram]
nonspecific abnormal findings on diagnostic imaging by X-ray examination

EXCLUDES 1   abnormal findings on antenatal screening of mother (O28.-)
diagnostic abnormal findings classified elsewhere—see Alphabetical Index

✓4ᵗʰ **R90**   **Abnormal findings on diagnostic imaging of central nervous system**

R90.0   **Intracranial space-occupying lesion found on diagnostic imaging of central nervous system**

✓5ᵗʰ R90.8   **Other abnormal findings on diagnostic imaging of central nervous system**

R90.81   Abnormal echoencephalogram

R90.82   White matter disease, unspecified

R90.89   Other abnormal findings on diagnostic imaging of central nervous system
Other cerebrovascular abnormality found on diagnostic imaging of central nervous system

✓4ᵗʰ **R91**   **Abnormal findings on diagnostic imaging of lung**

R91.1   **Solitary pulmonary nodule**
Coin lesion lung
Solitary pulmonary nodule, subsegmental branch of the bronchial tree

R91.8   **Other nonspecific abnormal finding of lung field**
Lung mass NOS found on diagnostic imaging of lung
Pulmonary infiltrate NOS
Shadow, lung

✓4ᵗʰ **R92**   **Abnormal and inconclusive findings on diagnostic imaging of breast**

R92.0   **Mammographic microcalcification found on diagnostic imaging of breast**
EXCLUDES 2   mammographic calcification (calculus) found on diagnostic imaging of breast (R92.1)
DEF: Calcium and cellular debris deposits in the breast that cannot be felt but can be detected on a mammogram; can be a sign of cancer, benign conditions, or changes in the breast tissue as a result of inflammation, injury, or obstructed duct.

R92.1   **Mammographic calcification found on diagnostic imaging of breast**
Mammographic calculus found on diagnostic imaging of breast

R92.2   **Inconclusive mammogram**
Dense breasts NOS
Inconclusive mammogram NEC
Inconclusive mammography due to dense breasts
Inconclusive mammography NEC
AHA: 2015, 1Q, 24

R92.8   **Other abnormal and inconclusive findings on diagnostic imaging of breast**

✓4ᵗʰ **R93**   **Abnormal findings on diagnostic imaging of other body structures**

R93.0   **Abnormal findings on diagnostic imaging of skull and head, not elsewhere classified**
EXCLUDES 1   intracranial space-occupying lesion found on diagnostic imaging (R90.0)

R93.1   **Abnormal findings on diagnostic imaging of heart and coronary circulation**
Abnormal echocardiogram NOS
Abnormal heart shadow

R93.2   **Abnormal findings on diagnostic imaging of liver and biliary tract**
Nonvisualization of gallbladder

R93.3   **Abnormal findings on diagnostic imaging of other parts of digestive tract**

✓5ᵗʰ R93.4   **Abnormal findings on diagnostic imaging of urinary organs**
EXCLUDES 2   hypertrophy of kidney (N28.81)

R93.41   **Abnormal radiological findings on diagnostic imaging of renal pelvis, ureter, or bladder**
Filling defect of bladder found on diagnostic imaging
Filling defect of renal pelvis found on diagnostic imaging
Filling defect of ureter found on diagnostic imaging

✓6ᵗʰ R93.42   **Abnormal radiologic findings on diagnostic imaging of kidney**

R93.421   Abnormal radiologic findings on diagnostic imaging of right kidney

R93.422   Abnormal radiologic findings on diagnostic imaging of left kidney

R93.429   Abnormal radiologic findings on diagnostic imaging of unspecified kidney

R93.49   **Abnormal radiologic findings on diagnostic imaging of other urinary organs**

R93.5   **Abnormal findings on diagnostic imaging of other abdominal regions, including retroperitoneum**

R93.6   **Abnormal findings on diagnostic imaging of limbs**
EXCLUDES 2   abnormal finding in skin and subcutaneous tissue (R93.8)

R93.7   **Abnormal findings on diagnostic imaging of other parts of musculoskeletal system**
EXCLUDES 2   abnormal findings on diagnostic imaging of skull (R93.0)

R93.8   **Abnormal findings on diagnostic imaging of other specified body structures**
Abnormal finding by radioisotope localization of placenta
Abnormal radiological finding in skin and subcutaneous tissue
Mediastinal shift

R93.9   **Diagnostic imaging inconclusive due to excess body fat of patient**

✓4ᵗʰ **R94**   **Abnormal results of function studies**
INCLUDES   abnormal results of radionuclide [radioisotope] uptake studies
abnormal results of scintigraphy

✓5ᵗʰ R94.0   **Abnormal results of function studies of central nervous system**

R94.01   Abnormal electroencephalogram [EEG]

R94.02   Abnormal brain scan

---

Ⓝ Newborn: 0   Ⓟ Pediatric: 0-17   Ⓜ Maternity: 12-55   Ⓐ Adult: 15-124   MCC Major CC Condition   PDxMCC PDx acts as own MCC   CC CC Condition   PDxCC PDx acts as own CC

930     ICD-10-CM 2018

**R94.09** **Abnormal results of** other function studies **of central nervous system**

✓5ᵗʰ **R94.1** **Abnormal results of function studies of** peripheral nervous system and special senses

   ✓6ᵗʰ **R94.11** **Abnormal results of function studies of** eye

      **R94.110** **Abnormal** electro-oculogram [EOG]

      **R94.111** **Abnormal** electroretinogram [ERG]
         Abnormal retinal function study

      **R94.112** **Abnormal** visually evoked potential [VEP]

      **R94.113** **Abnormal** oculomotor **study**

      **R94.118** **Abnormal results of** other **function studies of eye**

   ✓6ᵗʰ **R94.12** **Abnormal results of function studies of** ear and other special senses
      AHA: 2016, 3Q, 17

      **R94.120** **Abnormal** auditory **function study**

      **R94.121** **Abnormal** vestibular **function study**

      **R94.128** **Abnormal results of** other **function studies of ear and other special senses**

   ✓6ᵗʰ **R94.13** **Abnormal results of function studies of** peripheral nervous system

      **R94.130** **Abnormal response to** nerve stimulation, **unspecified**

      **R94.131** Abnormal electromyogram [EMG]
         EXCLUDES 1  *electromyogram of eye (R94.113)*

      **R94.138** **Abnormal results of** other **function studies of peripheral nervous system**

**R94.2** **Abnormal results of** pulmonary function **studies**
   Reduced ventilatory capacity
   Reduced vital capacity

✓5ᵗʰ **R94.3** **Abnormal results of** cardiovascular function **studies**

   **R94.30** **Abnormal result of cardiovascular function study, unspecified**

   **R94.31** **Abnormal** electrocardiogram [ECG] [EKG]
      EXCLUDES 1  *long QT syndrome (I45.81)*

   **R94.39** **Abnormal result of** other **cardiovascular function study**
      Abnormal electrophysiological intracardiac studies
      Abnormal phonocardiogram
      Abnormal vectorcardiogram

**R94.4** **Abnormal results of** kidney function **studies**
   Abnormal renal function test

**R94.5** **Abnormal results of** liver function **studies**

**R94.6** **Abnormal results of** thyroid function **studies**

**R94.7** **Abnormal results of** other endocrine function **studies**
   EXCLUDES 2  *abnormal glucose (R73.0-)*

**R94.8** **Abnormal results of function studies of** other organs and systems
   Abnormal basal metabolic rate [BMR]
   Abnormal bladder function test
   Abnormal splenic function test

## Abnormal tumor markers (R97)

✓4ᵗʰ **R97** **Abnormal tumor markers**
   Elevated tumor associated antigens [TAA]
   Elevated tumor specific antigens [TSA]

**R97.0** **Elevated carcinoembryonic antigen [CEA]**

**R97.1** **Elevated cancer antigen 125 [CA 125]**

✓5ᵗʰ **R97.2** **Elevated prostate specific antigen [PSA]**

   ⁴ **R97.20** **Elevated prostate specific antigen [PSA]**     A♂

   ⁴ **R97.21** **Rising PSA following treatment for malignant neoplasm of prostate**     A♂

**R97.8** **Other abnormal tumor markers**

## Ill-defined and unknown cause of mortality (R99)

**R99** **Ill-defined and unknown cause of mortality**
   Death (unexplained) NOS
   Unspecified cause of mortality

---

⁴ Questionable admission when used as PDx.

# Chapter 19. Injury, Poisoning and Certain Other Consequences of External Causes (S00–T88)

## Chapter Specific Guidelines with Coding Examples

The chapter specific guidelines from the ICD-10-CM Official Guidelines for Coding and Reporting have been provided below. Along with these guidelines are coding examples, contained in the shaded boxes, that have been developed to help illustrate the coding and/or sequencing guidance found in these guidelines.

### a. Application of 7th characters in Chapter 19

Most categories in chapter 19 have a 7th character requirement for each applicable code. Most categories in this chapter have three 7th character values (with the exception of fractures): A, initial encounter, D, subsequent encounter and S, sequela. Categories for traumatic fractures have additional 7th character values. While the patient may be seen by a new or different provider over the course of treatment for an injury, assignment of the 7th character is based on whether the patient is undergoing active treatment and not whether the provider is seeing the patient for the first time.

For complication codes, active treatment refers to treatment for the condition described by the code, even though it may be related to an earlier precipitating problem. For example, code T84.50XA, Infection and inflammatory reaction due to unspecified internal joint prosthesis, initial encounter, is used when active treatment is provided for the infection, even though the condition relates to the prosthetic device, implant or graft that was placed at a previous encounter.

7th character "A", initial encounter is used for each encounter where the patient is receiving active treatment for the condition.

| | |
|---|---|
| Patient admitted after fall from a skateboard onto the sidewalk, x-rays identify a nondisplaced fracture to the distal pole of the right scaphoid bone. The patient is placed in a cast. | |
| **S62.014A** | **Nondisplaced fracture of distal pole of navicular [scaphoid] bone of right wrist, initial encounter for closed fracture** |
| **V00.131A** | **Fall from skateboard, initial encounter** |
| **Y92.480** | **Sidewalk as the place of occurrence of the external cause** |
| **Y93.51** | **Activity, roller skating (inline) and skateboarding** |
| **Y99.8** | **Other external cause status** |

*Explanation:* This fracture would be coded with a seventh character A for initial encounter because the patient received x-rays to identify the site of the fracture and treatment was rendered; this would be considered active treatment.

7th character "D" subsequent encounter is used for encounters after the patient has completed active treatment of the condition and is receiving routine care for the condition during the healing or recovery phase.

| | |
|---|---|
| Patient admitted after fall from a skateboard onto the sidewalk resulted in casting of the right arm. X-rays are taken to evaluate how well the nondisplaced fracture to the distal pole of the right scaphoid bone is healing. The physician feels the fracture is healing appropriately; no adjustments to the cast are made. | |
| **S62.014D** | **Nondisplaced fracture of distal pole of navicular [scaphoid] bone of right wrist, subsequent encounter for fracture with routine healing** |
| **V00.131D** | **Fall from skateboard, subsequent encounter** |

*Explanation:* This fracture would be coded with a seventh character D for subsequent encounter, whether the same physician who provided the initial cast application or a different physician is now seeing the patient. Although the patient received x-rays, the intent of the x-rays was to assess how the fracture was healing. There was no active treatment rendered and the visit is therefore considered a subsequent encounter.

The aftercare Z codes should not be used for aftercare for conditions such as injuries or poisonings, where 7th characters are provided to identify subsequent care. For example, for aftercare of an injury, assign the acute injury code with the 7th character "D" (subsequent encounter).

7th character "S", sequela, is for use for complications or conditions that arise as a direct result of a condition, such as scar formation after a burn. The scars are sequelae of the burn. When using 7th character "S", it is necessary to use both the injury code that precipitated the sequela and the code for the sequela itself. The "S" is added only to the injury code, not the sequela code. The 7th character "S" identifies the injury responsible for the sequela. The specific type of sequela (e.g. scar) is sequenced first, followed by the injury code.

*See Section I.B.10 Sequelae, (Late Effects)*

| | |
|---|---|
| Patient with a history of a nondisplaced fracture to the distal pole of the right scaphoid bone due to a fall from a skateboard is admitted for evaluation of arthritis to the right wrist that has developed as a consequence of the traumatic fracture. | |
| **M12.531** | **Traumatic arthropathy, right wrist** |
| **S62.014S** | **Nondisplaced fracture of distal pole of navicular [scaphoid] bone of right wrist, sequela** |
| **V00.131S** | **Fall from skateboard, sequela** |

*Explanation:* The code identifying the specific sequela condition (traumatic arthritis) should be coded first followed by the injury that instigated the development of the sequela (fracture). The scaphoid fracture injury code is given a 7th character S for sequela to represent its role as the inciting injury. The fracture has healed and is not being managed or treated on this admit and therefore is not applicable as a first listed or principal diagnosis. However, it is directly related to the development of the arthritis and should be appended as a secondary code to signify this cause and effect relationship.

### b. Coding of injuries

When coding injuries, assign separate codes for each injury unless a combination code is provided, in which case the combination code is assigned. Code T07, Unspecified multiple injuries should not be assigned in the inpatient setting unless information for a more specific code is not available. Traumatic injury codes (S00-T14.9) are not to be used for normal, healing surgical wounds or to identify complications of surgical wounds.

| | |
|---|---|
| 11-year-old girl fell from her horse, resulting in a laceration to her right forearm with several large pieces of wooden fragments embedded in the wound as well as abrasions to her right ear; in addition, her right shoulder was dislocated | |
| **S43.004A** | **Unspecified dislocation of right shoulder joint, initial encounter** |
| **S51.821A** | **Laceration with foreign body of right forearm, initial encounter** |
| **S00.411A** | **Abrasion of right ear, initial encounter** |
| **V80.010A** | **Animal-rider injured by fall from or being thrown from horse in noncollision accident, initial encounter** |
| **Y93.52** | **Activity, horseback riding** |

*Explanation:* Each separate injury should be reported. The patient's injury to the forearm is reported with one combination code that captures both the laceration and the foreign body.

The code for the most serious injury, as determined by the provider and the focus of treatment, is sequenced first.

#### 1) Superficial injuries

Superficial injuries such as abrasions or contusions are not coded when associated with more severe injuries of the same site.

#### 2) Primary injury with damage to nerves/blood vessels

When a primary injury results in minor damage to peripheral nerves or blood vessels, the primary injury is sequenced first with additional code(s) for injuries to nerves and spinal cord (such as category S04), and/or injury to blood vessels (such as category S15). When the primary injury is to the blood vessels or nerves, that injury should be sequenced first.

### c. Coding of traumatic fractures

The principles of multiple coding of injuries should be followed in coding fractures. Fractures of specified sites are coded individually by site in accordance with both the provisions within categories S02, S12, S22, S32, S42, S49, S52, S59, S62, S72, S79, S82, S89, S92 and the level of detail furnished by medical record content.

A fracture not indicated as open or closed should be coded to closed. A fracture not indicated whether displaced or not displaced should be coded to displaced.

More specific guidelines are as follows:

### 1) Initial vs. subsequent encounter for fractures

Traumatic fractures are coded using the appropriate 7th character for initial encounter (A, B, C) for each encounter where the patient is receiving active treatment for the fracture. The appropriate 7th character for initial encounter should also be assigned for a patient who delayed seeking treatment for the fracture or nonunion.

Fractures are coded using the appropriate 7th character for subsequent care for encounters after the patient has completed active treatment of the fracture and is receiving routine care for the fracture during the healing or recovery phase.

Care for complications of surgical treatment for fracture repairs during the healing or recovery phase should be coded with the appropriate complication codes.

Care of complications of fractures, such as malunion and nonunion, should be reported with the appropriate 7th character for subsequent care with nonunion (K, M, N,) or subsequent care with malunion (P, Q, R).

Malunion/nonunion: The appropriate 7th character for initial encounter should also be assigned for a patient who delayed seeking treatment for the fracture or nonunion.

---

Female patient fell during a forest hiking excursion almost six months ago and until recently did not feel she needed to seek medical attention for her left ankle pain; x-rays show nonunion of lateral malleolus and surgery has been scheduled

| | |
|---|---|
| **S82.62XA** | **Displaced fracture of lateral malleolus of left fibula, initial encounter for closed fracture** |
| **W01.0XXA** | **Fall on same level from slipping, tripping and stumbling without subsequent striking against object, initial encounter** |
| **Y92.821** | **Forest as place of occurrence of the external cause** |
| **Y93.01** | **Activity, walking, marching and hiking** |
| **Y99.8** | **Other external cause status** |

*Explanation:* A seventh character of A is used for the lateral malleolus nonunion fracture to signify that the fracture is receiving active treatment. The delayed care for the fracture has resulted in a nonunion, but capturing the nonunion in the seventh character is trumped by the provision of active care.

---

The open fracture designations in the assignment of the 7th character for fractures of the forearm, femur and lower leg, including ankle are based on the Gustilo open fracture classification. When the Gustilo classification type is not specified for an open fracture, the 7th character for open fracture type I or II should be assigned (B, E, H, M, Q).

---

A 17-year-old arrives at the trauma center with open, displaced right forearm fracture with extensive soft tissue damage. He fell while being tackled playing football for his high school team. On-call orthopaedic specialist documents segmental type IIIA fracture of shaft radius with no need for plastic consult.

| | |
|---|---|
| **S52.361C** | **Displaced segmental fracture of shaft of radius, right arm, initial encounter for open fracture type IIIA, IIIB, or IIIC** |
| **W03XXXA** | **Other fall on same level due to collision with another person, initial encounter** |
| **Y92.321** | **Football field as the place of occurrence of the external cause** |
| **Y93.61** | **Activity, American tackle football** |

*Explanation:* The seventh character for forearm fractures capture the type of encounter and whether the fracture is open or closed; open fractures are broken down further by the type of fracture based on the Gustilo classification. The Gustilo classification describes the severity of open fracture and soft tissue injury. Type IIIA describes an open fracture with extensive soft tissue injury but adequate soft tissue remaining for wound coverage. A segmental fracture means that the bone is broken in two places, leaving at least one segment unattached to the bone. There is no need to report an additional code for the soft tissue injury as it is captured in the fracture code.

---

A code from category M80, not a traumatic fracture code, should be used for any patient with known osteoporosis who suffers a fracture, even if the patient had a minor fall or trauma, if that fall or trauma would not usually break a normal, healthy bone.

*See Section I.C.13. Osteoporosis.*

The aftercare Z codes should not be used for aftercare for traumatic fractures. For aftercare of a traumatic fracture, assign the acute fracture code with the appropriate 7th character.

### 2) Multiple fractures sequencing

Multiple fractures are sequenced in accordance with the severity of the fracture.

## d. Coding of burns and corrosions

The ICD-10-CM makes a distinction between burns and corrosions. The burn codes are for thermal burns, except sunburns, that come from a heat source, such as a fire or hot appliance. The burn codes are also for burns resulting from electricity and radiation. Corrosions are burns due to chemicals. The guidelines are the same for burns and corrosions.

Current burns (T20-T25) are classified by depth, extent and by agent (X code). Burns are classified by depth as first degree (erythema), second degree (blistering), and third degree (full-thickness involvement). Burns of the eye and internal organs (T26-T28) are classified by site, but not by degree.

### 1) Sequencing of burn and related condition codes

Sequence first the code that reflects the highest degree of burn when more than one burn is present.

   a.   When the reason for the admission or encounter is for treatment of external multiple burns, sequence first the code that reflects the burn of the highest degree.

   b.   When a patient has both internal and external burns, the circumstances of admission govern the selection of the principal diagnosis or first-listed diagnosis.

   c.   When a patient is admitted for burn injuries and other related conditions such as smoke inhalation and/or respiratory failure, the circumstances of admission govern the selection of the principal or first-listed diagnosis.

---

Patient admitted with minor first-degree burns to multiple sites of her right and left hands as well as severe smoke inhalation. While she was sleeping at home, a candle on her dresser lit the bedroom curtains on fire.

| | |
|---|---|
| **T59.811A** | **Toxic effect of smoke, accidental (unintentional), initial encounter** |
| **J70.5** | **Respiratory conditions due to smoke inhalation** |
| **T23.191A** | **Burn of first degree of multiple sites of right wrist and hand, initial encounter** |
| **T23.192A** | **Burn of first degree of multiple sites of left wrist and hand, initial encounter** |
| **X08.8XXA** | **Exposure to other specified smoke, fire and flames, initial encounter** |
| **Y92.003** | **Bedroom of unspecified non-institutional (private) residence as the place of occurrence of the external cause** |
| **Y93.84** | **Activity, sleeping** |

*Explanation:* Based on the documentation, the inhalation injury is more severe than the first-degree burns and is sequenced first. The burns to the hands are appended as secondary diagnoses.

### 2) Burns of the same local site

Classify burns of the same local site (three-character category level, T20-T28) but of different degrees to the subcategory identifying the highest degree recorded in the diagnosis.

---

10-year-old male patient is admitted for third-degree burns of his right palm and second-degree burns of multiple right fingers; right thumb not affected

| | |
|---|---|
| **T23.351A** | **Burn of third degree of right palm, initial encounter** |

*Explanation:* Although there is a code for second-degree burns of multiple fingers, not including the thumb (T23.131-), this code falls in the same three-digit category that the third-degree burn of the right palm falls under, category T23. Only the subcategory identifying the highest degree is captured when different burn degrees are classified to a single category.

Patient is admitted with third-degree burns of the scalp as well as second-degree burns to the back of the right hand

| T20.35XA | Burn of third degree of scalp [any part], initial encounter |
|---|---|
| T23.261A | Burn of second degree of back of right hand, initial encounter |

*Explanation:* Since burns to the hand and scalp are classified to two different three-digit categories, both burns may be reported as they represent distinct sites.

**3) Non-healing burns**

Non-healing burns are coded as acute burns.

Necrosis of burned skin should be coded as a non-healed burn.

**4) Infected burn**

For any documented infected burn site, use an additional code for the infection.

**5) Assign separate codes for each burn site**

When coding burns, assign separate codes for each burn site. Category T30, Burn and corrosion, body region unspecified is extremely vague and should rarely be used.

**6) Burns and corrosions classified according to extent of body surface involved**

Assign codes from category T31, Burns classified according to extent of body surface involved, or T32, Corrosions classified according to extent of body surface involved, when the site of the burn is not specified or when there is a need for additional data. It is advisable to use category T31 as additional coding when needed to provide data for evaluating burn mortality, such as that needed by burn units. It is also advisable to use category T31 as an additional code for reporting purposes when there is mention of a third-degree burn involving 20 percent or more of the body surface.

Categories T31 and T32 are based on the classic "rule of nines" in estimating body surface involved: head and neck are assigned nine percent, each arm nine percent, each leg 18 percent, the anterior trunk 18 percent, posterior trunk 18 percent, and genitalia one percent. Providers may change these percentage assignments where necessary to accommodate infants and children who have proportionately larger heads than adults, and patients who have large buttocks, thighs, or abdomen that involve burns.

Patient seen in burn unit for dressing change after he accidentally spilled acetic acid on himself two days ago. The second-degree burns to his right thigh, covering about 3 percent of his body surface, are healing appropriately.

| T54.2X1D | Toxic effect of corrosive acids and acid-like substances, accidental (unintentional), subsequent encounter |
|---|---|
| T24.611D | Corrosion of second degree of right thigh, subsequent encounter |
| T32.0 | Corrosions involving less than 10% of body surface |

*Explanation:* Code T32.0 provides additional information as to how much of the patient's body was affected by the corrosive substance.

**7) Encounters for treatment of sequela of burns**

Encounters for the treatment of the late effects of burns or corrosions (i.e., scars or joint contractures) should be coded with a burn or corrosion code with the 7th character "S" for sequela.

**8) Sequelae with a late effect code and current burn**

When appropriate, both a code for a current burn or corrosion with 7th character "A" or "D" and a burn or corrosion code with 7th character "S" may be assigned on the same record (when both a current burn and sequelae of an old burn exist). Burns and corrosions do not heal at the same rate and a current healing wound may still exist with sequela of a healed burn or corrosion.

*See Section I.B.10 Sequela (Late Effects)*

Female patient seen in ED for second-degree burn to the left ear; she also has significant scarring on her left elbow from a third-degree burn from childhood

| T20.212A | Burn of second degree of left ear [any part, except ear drum], initial encounter |
|---|---|
| L90.5 | Scar conditions and fibrosis of skin |
| T22.322S | Burn of third degree of left elbow, sequela |

*Explanation:* The patient is being seen for management of a current second-degree burn, which is reflected in the code by appending the seventh character of A, indicating active treatment or management of this burn. The elbow scarring is a sequela of a previous third-degree burn. The sequela condition precedes the original burn injury, which is appended with a seventh character of S.

**9) Use of an external cause code with burns and corrosions**

An external cause code should be used with burns and corrosions to identify the source and intent of the burn, as well as the place where it occurred.

**e. Adverse effects, poisoning, underdosing and toxic effects**

Codes in categories T36-T65 are combination codes that include the substance that was taken as well as the intent. No additional external cause code is required for poisonings, toxic effects, adverse effects and underdosing codes.

**1) Do not code directly from the Table of Drugs**

Do not code directly from the Table of Drugs and Chemicals. Always refer back to the Tabular List.

**2) Use as many codes as necessary to describe**

Use as many codes as necessary to describe completely all drugs, medicinal or biological substances.

**3) If the same code would describe the causative agent**

If the same code would describe the causative agent for more than one adverse reaction, poisoning, toxic effect or underdosing, assign the code only once.

**4) If two or more drugs, medicinal or biological substances**

If two or more drugs, medicinal or biological substances are reported, code each individually unless a combination code is listed in the Table of Drugs and Chemicals.

**5) The occurrence of drug toxicity is classified in ICD-10-CM as follows:**
**(a) Adverse effect**

When coding an adverse effect of a drug that has been correctly prescribed and properly administered, assign the appropriate code for the nature of the adverse effect followed by the appropriate code for the adverse effect of the drug (T36-T50). The code for the drug should have a 5th or 6th character "5" (for example T36.0X5-) Examples of the nature of an adverse effect are tachycardia, delirium, gastrointestinal hemorrhaging, vomiting, hypokalemia, hepatitis, renal failure, or respiratory failure.

Patient admitted for stomach pain and jaundice, indicated by physician as possible side-effects of Inderal, recently started for hypertension. Inderal was discontinued and the patient switched to Atenolol instead.

| R10.9 | Unspecified abdominal pain |
|---|---|
| R17 | Unspecified jaundice |
| T44.7X5A | Adverse effect of beta-adrenoreceptor antagonists, initial encounter |
| I10 | Essential (primary) hypertension |

*Explanation:* The side-effects caused by the drug are listed first, followed by the code for the adverse effect of the drug to capture the specific drug that was used.

**Chapter 19. Injury, Poisoning and Certain Other Consequences of External Causes**

### (b) Poisoning

When coding a poisoning or reaction to the improper use of a medication (e.g., overdose, wrong substance given or taken in error, wrong route of administration), first assign the appropriate code from categories T36-T50. The poisoning codes have an associated intent as their 5th or 6th character (accidental, intentional self-harm, assault and undetermined). If the intent of the poisoning is unknown or unspecified, code the intent as accidental intent. The undetermined intent is only for use if the documentation in the record specifies that the intent cannot be determined. Use additional code(s) for all manifestations of poisonings.

A 55-year-old female status post recent left knee replacement is admitted due to confusion, dizziness, and nausea. Her spouse brought in her prescribed Xanax, Ambien, and Percocet bottles but has no idea how many she took. It is suspected that her symptoms are due to an overdose of these medications.

**T42.4X1A**    **Poisoning by benzodiazepines, accidental (unintentional), initial encounter**

**T42.6X1A**    **Poisoning by other antiepileptic and sedative-hypnotic drugs, accidental (unintentional), initial encounter**

**T40.2X1A**    **Poisoning by other opioids, accidental (unintentional), initial encounter**

**R41.0**    **Disorientation, unspecified**

**R42**    **Dizziness and giddiness**

**R11.0**    **Nausea**

*Explanation:* It was not documented whether the overdose of the drugs was accidental or intentional; therefore the correct reporting of the poisoning codes is accidental intent. The poisoning codes are sequenced first, followed by manifestations of the poisoning.

If there is also a diagnosis of abuse or dependence of the substance, the abuse or dependence is assigned as an additional code.

Examples of poisoning include:

(i) Error was made in drug prescription

Errors made in drug prescription or in the administration of the drug by provider, nurse, patient, or other person.

(ii) Overdose of a drug intentionally taken

If an overdose of a drug was intentionally taken or administered and resulted in drug toxicity, it would be coded as a poisoning.

(iii) Nonprescribed drug taken with correctly prescribed and properly administered drug

If a nonprescribed drug or medicinal agent was taken in combination with a correctly prescribed and properly administered drug, any drug toxicity or other reaction resulting from the interaction of the two drugs would be classified as a poisoning.

(iv) Interaction of drug(s) and alcohol

When a reaction results from the interaction of a drug(s) and alcohol, this would be classified as poisoning.

*See Section I.C.4. if poisoning is the result of insulin pump malfunctions.*

### (c) Underdosing

Underdosing refers to taking less of a medication than is prescribed by a provider or a manufacturer's instruction. For underdosing, assign the code from categories T36-T50 (fifth or sixth character "6").

Codes for underdosing should never be assigned as principal or first-listed codes. If a patient has a relapse or exacerbation of the medical condition for which the drug is prescribed because of the reduction in dose, then the medical condition itself should be coded.

Noncompliance (Z91.12-, Z91.13-) or complication of care (Y63.6-Y63.9) codes are to be used with an underdosing code to indicate intent, if known.

Patient admitted for atrial fibrillation with history of chronic atrial fibrillation for which she is prescribed amiodarone. Financial concerns have left the patient unable to pay for her prescriptions and she has been skipping her amiodarone dose every other day to offset the cost.

**I48.2**    **Chronic atrial fibrillation**

**T46.2X6A**    **Underdosing of other antidysrhythmic drugs, initial encounter**

**Z91.120**    **Patient's intentional underdosing of medication regimen due to financial hardship**

*Explanation:* By skipping her amiodarone pill every other day, the patient's atrial fibrillation returned. The condition for which the drug was being taken is reported first, followed by an underdosing code to show that the patient was not adhering to her prescription regiment. The Z code helps elaborate on the patient's social and/or economic circumstances that led to the patient taking less then what she was prescribed.

### (d) Toxic effects

When a harmful substance is ingested or comes in contact with a person, this is classified as a toxic effect. The toxic effect codes are in categories T51-T65.

Toxic effect codes have an associated intent: accidental, intentional self-harm, assault and undetermined.

## f. Adult and child abuse, neglect and other maltreatment

Sequence first the appropriate code from categories T74.- (Adult and child abuse, neglect and other maltreatment, confirmed) or T76.- (Adult and child abuse, neglect and other maltreatment, suspected) for abuse, neglect and other maltreatment, followed by any accompanying mental health or injury code(s).

If the documentation in the medical record states abuse or neglect it is coded as confirmed (T74.-). It is coded as suspected if it is documented as suspected (T76.-).

For cases of confirmed abuse or neglect an external cause code from the assault section (X92-Y09) should be added to identify the cause of any physical injuries. A perpetrator code (Y07) should be added when the perpetrator of the abuse is known. For suspected cases of abuse or neglect, do not report external cause or perpetrator code.

If a suspected case of abuse, neglect or mistreatment is ruled out during an encounter code Z04.71, Encounter for examination and observation following alleged physical adult abuse, ruled out, or code Z04.72, Encounter for examination and observation following alleged child physical abuse, ruled out, should be used, not a code from T76.

If a suspected case of alleged rape or sexual abuse is ruled out during an encounter code Z04.41, Encounter for examination and observation following alleged adult rape or code Z04.42, Encounter for examination and observation following alleged child rape, should be used, not a code from T76.

*See Section I.C.15. Abuse in a pregnant patient.*

## g. Complications of care

### 1) General guidelines for complications of care

#### (a) Documentation of complications of care

*See Section I.B.16. for information on documentation of complications of care.*

### 2) Pain due to medical devices

Pain associated with devices, implants or grafts left in a surgical site (for example painful hip prosthesis) is assigned to the appropriate code(s) found in Chapter 19, Injury, poisoning, and certain other consequences of external causes. Specific codes for pain due to medical devices are found in the T code section of the ICD-10-CM. Use additional code(s) from category G89 to identify acute or chronic pain due to presence of the device, implant or graft (G89.18 or G89.28).

Chronic left breast pain secondary to breast implant

| **T85.848A** | **Pain due to other internal prosthetic devices, implants and grafts, initial encounter** |
|---|---|
| **N64.4** | **Mastodynia** |
| **G89.28** | **Other chronic postprocedural pain** |

*Explanation:* As the pain is a complication related to the breast implant, the complication code is sequenced first. The T code does not describe the site or type of pain, so additional codes may be appended to indicate that the patient is experiencing chronic pain in the breast.

### 3) Transplant complications

#### (a) Transplant complications other than kidney

Codes under category T86, Complications of transplanted organs and tissues, are for use for both complications and rejection of transplanted organs. A transplant complication code is only assigned if the complication affects the function of the transplanted organ. Two codes are required to fully describe a transplant complication: the appropriate code from category T86 and a secondary code that identifies the complication.

Pre-existing conditions or conditions that develop after the transplant are not coded as complications unless they affect the function of the transplanted organs.

*See I.C.21. for transplant organ removal status*

*See I.C.2. for malignant neoplasm associated with transplanted organ.*

#### (b) Kidney transplant complications

Patients who have undergone kidney transplant may still have some form of chronic kidney disease (CKD) because the kidney transplant may not fully restore kidney function. Code T86.1- should be assigned for documented complications of a kidney transplant, such as transplant failure or rejection or other transplant complication. Code T86.1- should not be assigned for post kidney transplant patients who have chronic kidney (CKD) unless a transplant complication such as transplant failure or rejection is documented. If the documentation is unclear as to whether the patient has a complication of the transplant, query the provider.

Conditions that affect the function of the transplanted kidney, other than CKD, should be assigned a code from subcategory T86.1, Complications of transplanted organ, Kidney, and a secondary code that identifies the complication.

For patients with CKD following a kidney transplant, but who do not have a complication such as failure or rejection, *see section I.C.14. Chronic kidney disease and kidney transplant status*.

Patient with chronic kidney disease stage 2; history of successful kidney transplant with no complications identified

| **N18.2** | **Chronic kidney disease, stage 2 (mild)** |
|---|---|
| **Z94.0** | **Kidney transplant status** |

*Explanation:* This patient's stage 2 CKD is not indicated as being due to the transplanted kidney but instead is just the residual disease the patient had prior to the transplant.

### 4) Complication codes that include the external cause

As with certain other T codes, some of the complications of care codes have the external cause included in the code. The code includes the nature of the complication as well as the type of procedure that caused the complication. No external cause code indicating the type of procedure is necessary for these codes.

### 5) Complications of care codes within the body system chapters

Intraoperative and postprocedural complication codes are found within the body system chapters with codes specific to the organs and structures of that body system. These codes should be sequenced first, followed by a code(s) for the specific complication, if applicable.

During a spinal fusion procedure, the surgeon inadvertently punctured the dura. The midline durotomy was repaired, and the fusion procedure was completed.

| **G97.41** | **Accidental puncture or laceration of dura during a procedure** |
|---|---|

*Explanation:* The accidental durotomy is not coded to an injury code in chapter 19 but instead is categorized to the nervous system chapter.

# Muscle/Tendon Table

ICD-10-CM categorizes certain muscles and tendons in the upper and lower extremities by their action (e.g., extension, flexion), their anatomical location (e.g., posterior, anterior), and/or whether they are intrinsic or extrinsic to a certain anatomical area. The Muscle/Tendon Table is provided at the beginning of chapters 13 and 19 as a resource to help users when code selection depends on one or more of these characteristics. Please note that this table is not all-inclusive, and proper code assignment should be based on the provider's documentation.

| Body Region | Muscle | Extensor Tendon | Flexor Tendon | Other Tendon |
|---|---|---|---|---|
| **Shoulder** | | | | |
| | Deltoid | Posterior deltoid | Anterior deltoid | |
| | Rotator cuff | | | |
| | Infraspinatus | | | Infraspinatus |
| | Subscapularis | | | Subscapularis |
| | Supraspinatus | | | Supraspinatus |
| | Teres minor | | | Teres minor |
| | Teres major | Teres major | | |
| **Upper arm** | | | | |
| | Anterior muscles | | | |
| | Biceps brachii — long head | | Biceps brachii — long head | |
| | Biceps brachii — short head | | Biceps brachii — short head | |
| | Brachialis | | Brachialis | |
| | Coracobrachialis | | Coracobrachialis | |
| | Posterior muscles | | | |
| | Triceps brachii | Triceps brachii | | |
| **Forearm** | | | | |
| | Anterior muscles | | | |
| | Flexors | | | |
| | Deep | | | |
| | Flexor digitorum profundus | | Flexor digitorum profundus | |
| | Flexor pollicis longus | | Flexor pollicis longus | |
| | Intermediate | | | |
| | Flexor digitorum superficialis | | Flexor digitorum superficialis | |
| | Superficial | | | |
| | Flexor carpi radialis | | Flexor carpi radialis | |
| | Flexor carpi ulnaris | | Flexor carpi ulnaris | |
| | Palmaris longus | | Palmaris longus | |
| | Pronators | | | |
| | Pronator quadratus | | | Pronator quadratus |
| | Pronator teres | | | Pronator teres |
| | Posterior muscles | | | |
| | Extensors | | | |
| | Deep | | | |
| | Abductor pollicis longus | | | Abductor pollicis longus |
| | Extensor indicis | Extensor indicis | | |
| | Extensor pollicis brevis | Extensor pollicis brevis | | |
| | Extensor pollicis longus | Extensor pollicis longus | | |
| | Superficial | | | |
| | Brachioradialis | | | Brachioradialis |
| | Extensor carpi radialis brevis | Extensor carpi radialis brevis | | |
| | Extensor carpi radialis longus | Extensor carpi radialis longus | | |
| | Extensor carpi ulnaris | Extensor carpi ulnaris | | |
| | Extensor digiti minimi | Extensor digiti minimi | | |
| | Extensor digitorum | Extensor digitorum | | |
| | Anconeus | Anconeus | | |
| | Supinator | | | Supinator |

| Body Region | Muscle | Extensor Tendon | Flexor Tendon | Other Tendon |
|---|---|---|---|---|
| **Hand** | | | | |
| *Extrinsic — attach to a site in the forearm as well as a site in the hand with action related to hand movement at the wrist* | | | | |
| | Extensor carpi radialis brevis | Extensor carpi radialis brevis | | |
| | Extensor carpi radialis longus | Extensor carpie radialis longus | | |
| | Extensor carpi ulnaris | Extensor carpi ulnaris | | |
| | Flexor carpi radialis | | Flexor carpi radialis | |
| | Flexor carpi ulnaris | | Flexor carpi ulnaris | |
| | Flexor digitorum superficialis | | Flexor digitorum superficialis | |
| | Palmaris longus | | Palmaris longus | |
| *Extrinsic — attach to a site in the forearm as well as a site in the hand with action in the hand related to finger movement* | | | | |
| | Adductor pollicis longus | | | Adductor pollicis longus |
| | Extensor digiti minimi | Extensor digiti minimi | | |
| | Extensor digitorum | Extensor digitorum | | |
| | Extensor indicis | Extensor indicis | | |
| | Flexor digitorum profundus | | Flexor digitorum profundus | |
| | Flexor digitorum superficialis | | Flexor digitorum superficialis | |
| *Extrinsic — attach to a site in the forearm as well as a site in the hand with action in the hand related to thumb movement* | | | | |
| | Extensor pollicis brevis | Extensor pollicis brevis | | |
| | Extensor pollicis longus | Extensor pollicis longus | | |
| | Flexor pollicis longus | | Flexor pollicis longus | |
| *Intrinsic — found within the hand only* | | | | |
| | Adductor pollicis | | | Adductor pollicis |
| | Dorsal interossei | Dorsal interossei | Dorsal interossei | |
| | Lumbricals | Lumbricals | Lumbricals | |
| | Palmaris brevis | | | Palmaris brevis |
| | Palmar interossei | Palmar interossei | Palmar interossei | |
| | Hypothenar muscles | | | |
| |   Abductor digiti minimi | | | Abductor digiti minimi |
| |   Flexor digiti minimi brevis | | Flexor digiti minimi brevis | |
| |   Oppenens digiti minimi | | Oppenens digiti minimi | |
| | Thenar muscles | | | |
| |   Abductor pollicis brevis | | | Abductor pollicis brevis |
| |   Flexor pollicis brevis | | Flexor pollicis brevis | |
| |   Oppenens pollicis | | Oppenens pollicis | |
| **Thigh** | | | | |
| | Anterior muscles | | | |
| |   Iliopsoas | | Iliopsoas | |
| |   Pectineus | | Pectineus | |
| |   Quadriceps | Quadriceps | | |
| |     Rectus femoris | Rectus femoris — Extends knee | Rectus femoris — Flexes hip | |
| |     Vastus intermedius | Vastus intermedius | | |
| |     Vastus lateralis | Vastus lateralis | | |
| |     Vastus medialis | Vastus medialis | | |
| |   Sartorius | | Sartorius | |
| | Medial muscles | | | |
| |   Adductor brevis | | | Adductor brevis |
| |   Adductor longus | | | Adductor longus |
| |   Adductor magnus | | | Adductor magnus |
| |   Gracilis | | | Gracilis |
| |   Obturator externus | | | Obturator externus |
| | Posterior muscles | | | |
| |   Hamstring | Hamstring — Extends hip | Hamstring — Flexes knee | |
| |     Biceps femoris | Biceps femoris | Biceps femoris | |
| |     Semimembranosus | Semimembranosus | Semimembranosus | |
| |     Semitendinosus | Semitendinosus | Semitendinosus | |

| Body Region | Muscle | Extensor Tendon | Flexor Tendon | Other Tendon |
|---|---|---|---|---|
| **Lower leg** | | | | |
| | Anterior muscles | | | |
| | Extensor digitorum longus | Extensor digitorum longus | | |
| | Extensor hallucis longus | Extensor hallucis longus | | |
| | Fibularis (peroneus) tertius | Fibularis (peroneus) tertius | | |
| | Tibialis anterior | Tibialis anterior | | Tibialis anterior |
| | Lateral muscles | | | |
| | Fibularis (peroneus) brevis | | Fibularis (peroneus) brevis | |
| | Fibularis (peroneus) longus | | Fibularis (peroneus) longus | |
| | Posterior muscles | | | |
| | Deep | | | |
| | Flexor digitorum longus | | Flexor digitorum longus | |
| | Flexor hallucis longus | | Flexor hallucis longus | |
| | Popliteus | | Popliteus | |
| | Tibialis posterior | | Tibialis posterior | |
| | Superficial | | | |
| | Gastrocnemius | | Gastrocnemius | |
| | Plantaris | | Plantaris | |
| | Soleus | | Soleus | |
| | | | | Calcaneal (Achilles) |
| **Ankle/Foot** | | | | |
| Extrinsic — attach to a site in the lower leg as well as a site in the foot with action related to foot movement at the ankle | | | | |
| | Plantaris | | Plantaris | |
| | Soleus | | Soleus | |
| | Tibialis anterior | Tibialis anterior | | |
| | Tibialis posterior | | Tibialis posterior | |
| Extrinsic — attach to a site in the lower leg as well as a site in the foot with action in the foot related to toe movement | | | | |
| | Extensor digitorum longus | Extensor digitorum longus | | |
| | Extensor hallicus longus | Extensor hallicus longus | | |
| | Flexor digitorum longus | | Flexor digitorum longus | |
| | Flexor hallucis longus | | Flexor hallucis longus | |
| Intrinsic — found within the ankle/foot only | | | | |
| | Dorsal muscles | | | |
| | Extensor digitorum brevis | Extensor digitorum brevis | | |
| | Extensor hallucis brevis | Extensor hallucis brevis | | |
| | Plantar muscles | | | |
| | Abductor digiti minimi | | Abductor digiti minimi | |
| | Abductor hallucis | | Abductor hallucis | |
| | Dorsal interossei | Dorsal interossei | Dorsal interossei | |
| | Flexor digiti minimi brevis | | Flexor digiti minimi brevis | |
| | Flexor digitorum brevis | | Flexor digitorum brevis | |
| | Flexor hallucis brevis | | Flexor hallucis brevis | |
| | Lumbricals | Lumbricals | Lumbricals | |
| | Quadratus plantae | | Quadratus plantae | |
| | Plantar interossei | Plantar interossei | Plantar interossei | |

# Chapter 19. Injury, Poisoning and Certain Other Consequences of External Causes (S00-T88)

**NOTE**   Use secondary code(s) from Chapter 20, External causes of morbidity, to indicate cause of injury. Codes within the T section that include the external cause do not require an additional external cause code.

Use additional code to identify any retained foreign body, if applicable (Z18.-)

**EXCLUDES 1**   birth trauma (P10-P15)
            obstetric trauma (O70-O71)

**NOTE**   The chapter uses the S-section for coding different types of injuries related to single body regions and the T-section to cover injuries to unspecified body regions as well as poisoning and certain other consequences of external causes.

**AHA:** 2016, 2Q, 3-7; 2015, 4Q, 35-38; 2015, 3Q, 37-39, 40; 2015, 2Q, 6; 2015, 1Q, 3-21

This chapter contains the following blocks:

| | |
|---|---|
| S00-S09 | Injuries to the head |
| S10-S19 | Injuries to the neck |
| S20-S29 | Injuries to the thorax |
| S30-S39 | Injuries to the abdomen, lower back, lumbar spine, pelvis and external genitals |
| S40-S49 | Injuries to the shoulder and upper arm |
| S50-S59 | Injuries to the elbow and forearm |
| S60-S69 | Injuries to the wrist, hand and fingers |
| S70-S79 | Injuries to the hip and thigh |
| S80-S89 | Injuries to the knee and lower leg |
| S90-S99 | Injuries to the ankle and foot |
| T07 | Injuries involving multiple body regions |
| T14 | Injury of unspecified body region |
| T15-T19 | Effects of foreign body entering through natural orifice |
| T20-T25 | Burns and corrosions of external body surface, specified by site |
| T26-T28 | Burns and corrosions confined to eye and internal organs |
| T30-T32 | Burns and corrosions of multiple and unspecified body regions |
| T33-T34 | Frostbite |
| T36-T50 | Poisoning by, adverse effect of and underdosing of drugs, medicaments and biological substances |
| T51-T65 | Toxic effects of substances chiefly nonmedicinal as to source |
| T66-T78 | Other and unspecified effects of external causes |
| T79 | Certain early complications of trauma |
| T80-T88 | Complications of surgical and medical care, not elsewhere classified |

## Injuries to the head (S00-S09)

**INCLUDES**   injuries of ear
            injuries of eye
            injuries of face [any part]
            injuries of gum
            injuries of jaw
            injuries of oral cavity
            injuries of palate
            injuries of periocular area
            injuries of scalp
            injuries of temporomandibular joint area
            injuries of tongue
            injuries of tooth

Code also for any associated infection

**EXCLUDES 2**   burns and corrosions (T20-T32)
            effects of foreign body in ear (T16)
            effects of foreign body in larynx (T17.3)
            effects of foreign body in mouth NOS (T18.0)
            effects of foreign body in nose (T17.0-T17.1)
            effects of foreign body in pharynx (T17.2)
            effects of foreign body on external eye (T15.-)
            frostbite (T33-T34)
            insect bite or sting, venomous (T63.4)

**✓4th S00**   **Superficial injury of head**

**EXCLUDES 1**   diffuse cerebral contusion (S06.2-)
            focal cerebral contusion (S06.3-)
            injury of eye and orbit (S05.-)
            open wound of head (S01.-)

The appropriate 7th character is to be added to each code from category S00.
A    initial encounter
D    subsequent encounter
S    sequela

**✓5th S00.0**   **Superficial injury of** scalp

    **✓x7th S00.00**   Unspecified **superficial injury of scalp**

    **✓x7th S00.01**   Abrasion **of scalp**

    **✓x7th S00.02**   Blister **(nonthermal) of scalp**

    **✓x7th S00.03**   Contusion **of scalp**
            Bruise of scalp
            Hematoma of scalp

    **✓x7th S00.04**   External constriction **of part of scalp**

    **✓x7th S00.05**   Superficial foreign body **of scalp**
            Splinter in the scalp

    **✓x7th S00.06**   Insect bite **(nonvenomous) of scalp**

    **✓x7th S00.07**   Other **superficial bite of scalp**
        **EXCLUDES 1**   open bite of scalp (S01.05)

**✓5th S00.1**   **Contusion of** eyelid and periocular area
          Black eye
        **EXCLUDES 2**   contusion of eyeball and orbital tissues (S05.1)

    **✓x7th S00.10**   Contusion of unspecified **eyelid and periocular area**

    **✓x7th S00.11**   Contusion of right **eyelid and periocular area**

    **✓x7th S00.12**   Contusion of left **eyelid and periocular area**

**✓5th S00.2**   **Other and unspecified superficial injuries of eyelid and periocular area**
        **EXCLUDES 2**   superficial injury of conjunctiva and cornea (S05.0-)

    **✓6th S00.20**   Unspecified **superficial injury of eyelid and periocular area**

       **✓7th S00.201**   **Unspecified superficial injury of** right **eyelid and periocular area**

       **✓7th S00.202**   **Unspecified superficial injury of** left **eyelid and periocular area**

       **✓7th S00.209**   **Unspecified superficial injury of** unspecified **eyelid and periocular area**

    **✓6th S00.21**   Abrasion **of eyelid and periocular area**

       **✓7th S00.211**   **Abrasion of** right **eyelid and periocular area**

       **✓7th S00.212**   **Abrasion of** left **eyelid and periocular area**

       **✓7th S00.219**   **Abrasion of** unspecified **eyelid and periocular area**

    **✓6th S00.22**   Blister **(nonthermal) of eyelid and periocular area**

       **✓7th S00.221**   **Blister (nonthermal) of** right **eyelid and periocular area**

       **✓7th S00.222**   **Blister (nonthermal) of** left **eyelid and periocular area**

       **✓7th S00.229**   **Blister (nonthermal) of** unspecified **eyelid and periocular area**

    **✓6th S00.24**   External constriction **of eyelid and periocular area**

       **✓7th S00.241**   **External constriction of** right **eyelid and periocular area**

       **✓7th S00.242**   **External constriction of** left **eyelid and periocular area**

       **✓7th S00.249**   **External constriction of** unspecified **eyelid and periocular area**

    **✓6th S00.25**   Superficial foreign body **of eyelid and periocular area**
           Splinter of eyelid and periocular area
         **EXCLUDES 2**   retained foreign body in eyelid (H02.81-)

       **✓7th S00.251**   **Superficial foreign body of** right **eyelid and periocular area**

       **✓7th S00.252**   **Superficial foreign body of** left **eyelid and periocular area**

       **✓7th S00.259**   **Superficial foreign body of** unspecified **eyelid and periocular area**

    **✓6th S00.26**   Insect bite **(nonvenomous) of eyelid and periocular area**

       **✓7th S00.261**   **Insect bite (nonvenomous) of** right **eyelid and periocular area**

       **✓7th S00.262**   **Insect bite (nonvenomous) of** left **eyelid and periocular area**

       **✓7th S00.269**   **Insect bite (nonvenomous) of** unspecified **eyelid and periocular area**

    **✓6th S00.27**   Other **superficial bite of eyelid and periocular area**
         **EXCLUDES 1**   open bite of eyelid and periocular area (S01.15)

       **✓7th S00.271**   **Other superficial bite of** right **eyelid and periocular area**

       **✓7th S00.272**   **Other superficial bite of** left **eyelid and periocular area**

       **✓7th S00.279**   **Other superficial bite of** unspecified **eyelid and periocular area**

✓ Additional Character Req   ✓x7th Placeholder Alert   Unacceptable PDx   Manifestation   **H1 - H14** HAC   **HCC** CMS-HCC Condition   **EXCLUDES 1** Not Coded Here   **EXCLUDES 2** Not Included Here

ICD-10-CM 2018                                       941

✓5ᵗʰ **S00.3** **Superficial injury of nose**

    ✓x7ᵗʰ **S00.30** **Unspecified superficial injury of nose**

    ✓x7ᵗʰ **S00.31** **Abrasion of nose**

    ✓x7ᵗʰ **S00.32** **Blister (nonthermal) of nose**

    ✓x7ᵗʰ **S00.33** **Contusion of nose**
        Bruise of nose
        Hematoma of nose

    ✓x7ᵗʰ **S00.34** **External constriction of nose**

    ✓x7ᵗʰ **S00.35** **Superficial foreign body of nose**
        Splinter in the nose

    ✓x7ᵗʰ **S00.36** **Insect bite (nonvenomous) of nose**

    ✓x7ᵗʰ **S00.37** **Other superficial bite of nose**
        **EXCLUDES 1**   open bite of nose (S01.25)

✓5ᵗʰ **S00.4** **Superficial injury of ear**

    ✓6ᵗʰ **S00.40** **Unspecified superficial injury of ear**

        ✓7ᵗʰ **S00.401** **Unspecified superficial injury of right ear**

        ✓7ᵗʰ **S00.402** **Unspecified superficial injury of left ear**

        ✓7ᵗʰ **S00.409** **Unspecified superficial injury of unspecified ear**

    ✓6ᵗʰ **S00.41** **Abrasion of ear**

        ✓7ᵗʰ **S00.411** **Abrasion of right ear**

        ✓7ᵗʰ **S00.412** **Abrasion of left ear**

        ✓7ᵗʰ **S00.419** **Abrasion of unspecified ear**

    ✓6ᵗʰ **S00.42** **Blister (nonthermal) of ear**

        ✓7ᵗʰ **S00.421** **Blister (nonthermal) of right ear**

        ✓7ᵗʰ **S00.422** **Blister (nonthermal) of left ear**

        ✓7ᵗʰ **S00.429** **Blister (nonthermal) of unspecified ear**

    ✓6ᵗʰ **S00.43** **Contusion of ear**
        Bruise of ear
        Hematoma of ear

        ✓7ᵗʰ **S00.431** **Contusion of right ear**

        ✓7ᵗʰ **S00.432** **Contusion of left ear**

        ✓7ᵗʰ **S00.439** **Contusion of unspecified ear**

    ✓6ᵗʰ **S00.44** **External constriction of ear**

        ✓7ᵗʰ **S00.441** **External constriction of right ear**

        ✓7ᵗʰ **S00.442** **External constriction of left ear**

        ✓7ᵗʰ **S00.449** **External constriction of unspecified ear**

    ✓6ᵗʰ **S00.45** **Superficial foreign body of ear**
        Splinter in the ear

        ✓7ᵗʰ **S00.451** **Superficial foreign body of right ear**

        ✓7ᵗʰ **S00.452** **Superficial foreign body of left ear**

        ✓7ᵗʰ **S00.459** **Superficial foreign body of unspecified ear**

    ✓6ᵗʰ **S00.46** **Insect bite (nonvenomous) of ear**

        ✓7ᵗʰ **S00.461** **Insect bite (nonvenomous) of right ear**

        ✓7ᵗʰ **S00.462** **Insect bite (nonvenomous) of left ear**

        ✓7ᵗʰ **S00.469** **Insect bite (nonvenomous) of unspecified ear**

    ✓6ᵗʰ **S00.47** **Other superficial bite of ear**
        **EXCLUDES 1**   open bite of ear (S01.35)

        ✓7ᵗʰ **S00.471** **Other superficial bite of right ear**

        ✓7ᵗʰ **S00.472** **Other superficial bite of left ear**

        ✓7ᵗʰ **S00.479** **Other superficial bite of unspecified ear**

✓5ᵗʰ **S00.5** **Superficial injury of lip and oral cavity**

    ✓6ᵗʰ **S00.50** **Unspecified superficial injury of lip and oral cavity**

        ✓7ᵗʰ **S00.501** **Unspecified superficial injury of lip**

        ✓7ᵗʰ **S00.502** **Unspecified superficial injury of oral cavity**

    ✓6ᵗʰ **S00.51** **Abrasion of lip and oral cavity**

        ✓7ᵗʰ **S00.511** **Abrasion of lip**

        ✓7ᵗʰ **S00.512** **Abrasion of oral cavity**

    ✓6ᵗʰ **S00.52** **Blister (nonthermal) of lip and oral cavity**

        ✓7ᵗʰ **S00.521** **Blister (nonthermal) of lip**

        ✓7ᵗʰ **S00.522** **Blister (nonthermal) of oral cavity**

    ✓6ᵗʰ **S00.53** **Contusion of lip and oral cavity**

        ✓7ᵗʰ **S00.531** **Contusion of lip**
            Bruise of lip
            ►Hematoma of lip◄

        ✓7ᵗʰ **S00.532** **Contusion of oral cavity**
            ►Bruise of oral cavity◄
            Hematoma of oral cavity

    ✓6ᵗʰ **S00.54** **External constriction of lip and oral cavity**

        ✓7ᵗʰ **S00.541** **External constriction of lip**

        ✓7ᵗʰ **S00.542** **External constriction of oral cavity**

    ✓6ᵗʰ **S00.55** **Superficial foreign body of lip and oral cavity**

        ✓7ᵗʰ **S00.551** **Superficial foreign body of lip**
            Splinter of lip and oral cavity

        ✓7ᵗʰ **S00.552** **Superficial foreign body of oral cavity**
            Splinter of lip and oral cavity

    ✓6ᵗʰ **S00.56** **Insect bite (nonvenomous) of lip and oral cavity**

        ✓7ᵗʰ **S00.561** **Insect bite (nonvenomous) of lip**

        ✓7ᵗʰ **S00.562** **Insect bite (nonvenomous) of oral cavity**

    ✓6ᵗʰ **S00.57** **Other superficial bite of lip and oral cavity**

        ✓7ᵗʰ **S00.571** **Other superficial bite of lip**
            **EXCLUDES 1**   open bite of lip (S01.551)

        ✓7ᵗʰ **S00.572** **Other superficial bite of oral cavity**
            **EXCLUDES 1**   open bite of oral cavity (S01.552)

✓5ᵗʰ **S00.8** **Superficial injury of other parts of head**
    Superfical injuries of face [any part]

    ✓x7ᵗʰ **S00.80** **Unspecified superficial injury of other part of head**

    ✓x7ᵗʰ **S00.81** **Abrasion of other part of head**

    ✓x7ᵗʰ **S00.82** **Blister (nonthermal) of other part of head**

    ✓x7ᵗʰ **S00.83** **Contusion of other part of head**
        Bruise of other part of head
        Hematoma of other part of head

    ✓x7ᵗʰ **S00.84** **External constriction of other part of head**

    ✓x7ᵗʰ **S00.85** **Superficial foreign body of other part of head**
        Splinter in other part of head

    ✓x7ᵗʰ **S00.86** **Insect bite (nonvenomous) of other part of head**

    ✓x7ᵗʰ **S00.87** **Other superficial bite of other part of head**
        **EXCLUDES 1**   open bite of other part of head (S01.85)

✓5ᵗʰ **S00.9** **Superficial injury of unspecified part of head**

    ✓x7ᵗʰ **S00.90** **Unspecified superficial injury of unspecified part of head**

    ✓x7ᵗʰ **S00.91** **Abrasion of unspecified part of head**

    ✓x7ᵗʰ **S00.92** **Blister (nonthermal) of unspecified part of head**

    ✓x7ᵗʰ **S00.93** **Contusion of unspecified part of head**
        Bruise of head
        Hematoma of head

    ✓x7ᵗʰ **S00.94** **External constriction of unspecified part of head**

    ✓x7ᵗʰ **S00.95** **Superficial foreign body of unspecified part of head**
        Splinter of head

    ✓x7ᵗʰ **S00.96** **Insect bite (nonvenomous) of unspecified part of head**

    ✓x7ᵗʰ **S00.97** **Other superficial bite of unspecified part of head**
        **EXCLUDES 1**   open bite of head (S01.95)

✓4ᵗʰ **S01** **Open wound of head**
    Code also any associated:
        injury of cranial nerve (S04.-)
        injury of muscle and tendon of head (S09.1-)
        intracranial injury (S06.-)
        wound infection
    **EXCLUDES 1**   open skull fracture (S02- with 7th B)
    **EXCLUDES 2**   injury of eye and orbit (S05.-)
                traumatic amputation of part of head (S08.-)

    The appropriate 7th character is to be added to each code from category S01.
    A    initial encounter
    D    subsequent encounter
    S    sequela

    ✓5ᵗʰ **S01.0** **Open wound of scalp**
        **EXCLUDES 1**   avulsion of scalp (S08.0)

        ✓x7ᵗʰ **S01.00** **Unspecified open wound of scalp**

        ✓x7ᵗʰ **S01.01** **Laceration without foreign body of scalp**

        ✓x7ᵗʰ **S01.02** **Laceration with foreign body of scalp**

        ✓x7ᵗʰ **S01.03** **Puncture wound without foreign body of scalp**

        ✓x7ᵗʰ **S01.04** **Puncture wound with foreign body of scalp**

        ✓x7ᵗʰ **S01.05** **Open bite of scalp**
            Bite of scalp NOS
            **EXCLUDES 1**   superficial bite of scalp (S00.06, S00.07-)

Ⓝ Newborn: 0    Ⓟ Pediatric: 0-17    Ⓜ Maternity: 12-55    Ⓐ Adult: 15-124    **MCC** Major CC Condition    **PDxMCC** PDx acts as own MCC    **CC** CC Condition    **PDxCC** PDx acts as own CC

**942**      ICD-10-CM 2018

✓5th **S01.1** **Open wound of** eyelid and periocular area
Open wound of eyelid and periocular area with or without involvement of lacrimal passages

**CC Excl: For codes in subcategory S01.1:**
PDX collection 1139

✓6th **S01.10** **Unspecified open wound of eyelid and periocular area**

✓7th **S01.101** Unspecified open wound of right eyelid and periocular area   **CC**

✓7th **S01.102** Unspecified open wound of left eyelid and periocular area   **CC**

✓7th **S01.109** Unspecified open wound of unspecified eyelid and periocular area   **CC**

✓6th **S01.11** **Laceration without foreign body of eyelid and periocular area**

✓7th **S01.111** Laceration without foreign body of right eyelid and periocular area

✓7th **S01.112** Laceration without foreign body of left eyelid and periocular area

✓7th **S01.119** Laceration without foreign body of unspecified eyelid and periocular area

✓6th **S01.12** **Laceration with foreign body of eyelid and periocular area**

✓7th **S01.121** Laceration with foreign body of right eyelid and periocular area

✓7th **S01.122** Laceration with foreign body of left eyelid and periocular area

✓7th **S01.129** Laceration with foreign body of unspecified eyelid and periocular area

✓6th **S01.13** **Puncture wound without foreign body of eyelid and periocular area**

✓7th **S01.131** Puncture wound without foreign body of right eyelid and periocular area

✓7th **S01.132** Puncture wound without foreign body of left eyelid and periocular area

✓7th **S01.139** Puncture wound without foreign body of unspecified eyelid and periocular area

✓6th **S01.14** **Puncture wound with foreign body of eyelid and periocular area**

✓7th **S01.141** Puncture wound with foreign body of right eyelid and periocular area

✓7th **S01.142** Puncture wound with foreign body of left eyelid and periocular area

✓7th **S01.149** Puncture wound with foreign body of unspecified eyelid and periocular area

✓6th **S01.15** **Open bite of eyelid and periocular area**
Bite of eyelid and periocular area NOS
*EXCLUDES 1*   superficial bite of eyelid and periocular area (S00.26, S00.27)

✓7th **S01.151** Open bite of right eyelid and periocular area

✓7th **S01.152** Open bite of left eyelid and periocular area

✓7th **S01.159** Open bite of unspecified eyelid and periocular area

✓5th **S01.2** **Open wound of** nose

✓x7th **S01.20** Unspecified open wound of nose

✓x7th **S01.21** Laceration without foreign body of nose

✓x7th **S01.22** Laceration with foreign body of nose

✓x7th **S01.23** Puncture wound without foreign body of nose

✓x7th **S01.24** Puncture wound with foreign body of nose

✓x7th **S01.25** Open bite of nose
Bite of nose NOS
*EXCLUDES 1*   superficial bite of nose (S00.36, S00.37)

✓5th **S01.3** **Open wound of** ear

✓6th **S01.30** **Unspecified open wound of ear**

✓7th **S01.301** Unspecified open wound of right ear

✓7th **S01.302** Unspecified open wound of left ear

✓7th **S01.309** Unspecified open wound of unspecified ear

✓6th **S01.31** **Laceration without foreign body of ear**

✓7th **S01.311** Laceration without foreign body of right ear

✓7th **S01.312** Laceration without foreign body of left ear

✓7th **S01.319** Laceration without foreign body of unspecified ear

✓6th **S01.32** **Laceration with foreign body of ear**

✓7th **S01.321** Laceration with foreign body of right ear

✓7th **S01.322** Laceration with foreign body of left ear

✓7th **S01.329** Laceration with foreign body of unspecified ear

✓6th **S01.33** **Puncture wound without foreign body of ear**

✓7th **S01.331** Puncture wound without foreign body of right ear

✓7th **S01.332** Puncture wound without foreign body of left ear

✓7th **S01.339** Puncture wound without foreign body of unspecified ear

✓6th **S01.34** **Puncture wound with foreign body of ear**

✓7th **S01.341** Puncture wound with foreign body of right ear

✓7th **S01.342** Puncture wound with foreign body of left ear

✓7th **S01.349** Puncture wound with foreign body of unspecified ear

✓6th **S01.35** **Open bite of ear**
Bite of ear NOS
*EXCLUDES 1*   superficial bite of ear (S00.46, S00.47)

✓7th **S01.351** Open bite of right ear

✓7th **S01.352** Open bite of left ear

✓7th **S01.359** Open bite of unspecified ear

✓5th **S01.4** **Open wound of cheek and temporomandibular area**

✓6th **S01.40** **Unspecified open wound of cheek and temporomandibular area**

✓7th **S01.401** Unspecified open wound of right cheek and temporomandibular area

✓7th **S01.402** Unspecified open wound of left cheek and temporomandibular area

✓7th **S01.409** Unspecified open wound of unspecified cheek and temporomandibular area

✓6th **S01.41** **Laceration without foreign body of cheek and temporomandibular area**

✓7th **S01.411** Laceration without foreign body of right cheek and temporomandibular area

✓7th **S01.412** Laceration without foreign body of left cheek and temporomandibular area

✓7th **S01.419** Laceration without foreign body of unspecified cheek and temporomandibular area

✓6th **S01.42** **Laceration with foreign body of cheek and temporomandibular area**

✓7th **S01.421** Laceration with foreign body of right cheek and temporomandibular area

✓7th **S01.422** Laceration with foreign body of left cheek and temporomandibular area

✓7th **S01.429** Laceration with foreign body of unspecified cheek and temporomandibular area

✓6th **S01.43** **Puncture wound without foreign body of cheek and temporomandibular area**

✓7th **S01.431** Puncture wound without foreign body of right cheek and temporomandibular area

✓7th **S01.432** Puncture wound without foreign body of left cheek and temporomandibular area

✓7th **S01.439** Puncture wound without foreign body of unspecified cheek and temporomandibular area

✓6th **S01.44** **Puncture wound with foreign body of cheek and temporomandibular area**

✓7th **S01.441** Puncture wound with foreign body of right cheek and temporomandibular area

✓7th **S01.442** Puncture wound with foreign body of left cheek and temporomandibular area

✓7th **S01.449** Puncture wound with foreign body of unspecified cheek and temporomandibular area

---

✓Additional Character Req   ✓x7th Placeholder Alert   Unacceptable PDx   Manifestation   **H1**-**H14** HAC   **HCC** CMS-HCC Condition   *EXCLUDES 1* Not Coded Here   *EXCLUDES 2* Not Included Here

☑6ᵗʰ **S01.45** **Open bite** of cheek and temporomandibular area
Bite of cheek and temporomandibular area NOS
EXCLUDES 2 *superficial bite of cheek and temporomandibular area (S00.86, S00.87)*

☑7ᵗʰ **S01.451** **Open bite of right cheek and temporomandibular area**

☑7ᵗʰ **S01.452** **Open bite of left cheek and temporomandibular area**

☑7ᵗʰ **S01.459** **Open bite of unspecified cheek and temporomandibular area**

☑5ᵗʰ **S01.5** **Open wound of lip and oral cavity**
EXCLUDES 2 *tooth dislocation (S03.2)*
*tooth fracture (S02.5)*

☑6ᵗʰ **S01.50** **Unspecified open wound of lip and oral cavity**

☑7ᵗʰ **S01.501** **Unspecified open wound of lip**

☑7ᵗʰ **S01.502** **Unspecified open wound of oral cavity**

☑6ᵗʰ **S01.51** **Laceration of lip and oral cavity without foreign body**

☑7ᵗʰ **S01.511** **Laceration without foreign body of lip**

☑7ᵗʰ **S01.512** **Laceration without foreign body of oral cavity**

☑6ᵗʰ **S01.52** **Laceration of lip and oral cavity with foreign body**

☑7ᵗʰ **S01.521** **Laceration with foreign body of lip**

☑7ᵗʰ **S01.522** **Laceration with foreign body of oral cavity**

☑6ᵗʰ **S01.53** **Puncture wound of lip and oral cavity without foreign body**

☑7ᵗʰ **S01.531** **Puncture wound without foreign body of lip**

☑7ᵗʰ **S01.532** **Puncture wound without foreign body of oral cavity**

☑6ᵗʰ **S01.54** **Puncture wound of lip and oral cavity with foreign body**

☑7ᵗʰ **S01.541** **Puncture wound with foreign body of lip**

☑7ᵗʰ **S01.542** **Puncture wound with foreign body of oral cavity**

☑6ᵗʰ **S01.55** **Open bite of lip and oral cavity**

☑7ᵗʰ **S01.551** **Open bite of lip**
Bite of lip NOS
EXCLUDES 1 *superficial bite of lip (S00.571)*

☑7ᵗʰ **S01.552** **Open bite of oral cavity**
Bite of oral cavity NOS
EXCLUDES 1 *superficial bite of oral cavity (S00.572)*

☑5ᵗʰ **S01.8** **Open wound of other parts of head**

☑x7ᵗʰ **S01.80** **Unspecified open wound of other part of head**

☑x7ᵗʰ **S01.81** **Laceration without foreign body of other part of head**

☑x7ᵗʰ **S01.82** **Laceration with foreign body of other part of head**

☑x7ᵗʰ **S01.83** **Puncture wound without foreign body of other part of head**

☑x7ᵗʰ **S01.84** **Puncture wound with foreign body of other part of head**

☑x7ᵗʰ **S01.85** **Open bite of other part of head**
Bite of other part of head NOS
EXCLUDES 1 *superficial bite of other part of head ►(S00.87)◄*

☑5ᵗʰ **S01.9** **Open wound of unspecified part of head**

☑x7ᵗʰ **S01.90** **Unspecified open wound of unspecified part of head**

☑x7ᵗʰ **S01.91** **Laceration without foreign body of unspecified part of head**

☑x7ᵗʰ **S01.92** **Laceration with foreign body of unspecified part of head**

☑x7ᵗʰ **S01.93** **Puncture wound without foreign body of unspecified part of head**

☑x7ᵗʰ **S01.94** **Puncture wound with foreign body of unspecified part of head**

☑x7ᵗʰ **S01.95** **Open bite of unspecified part of head**
Bite of head NOS
EXCLUDES 1 *superficial bite of head NOS (S00.97)*

☑4ᵗʰ **S02** **Fracture of skull and facial bones**
NOTE A fracture not indicated as open or closed should be coded to closed.
Code also any associated intracranial injury (S06.-)
AHA: 2017, 1Q, 42.

The appropriate 7th character is to be added to each code from category S02.
A    initial encounter for closed fracture
B    initial encounter for open fracture
D    subsequent encounter for fracture with routine healing
G    subsequent encounter for fracture with delayed healing
K    subsequent encounter for fracture with nonunion
S    sequela

6, 7,11 ☑x7ᵗʰ **S02.0** **Fracture of vault of skull**    MCC CC H5 HCC
Fracture of frontal bone
Fracture of parietal bone

CC Excl: For codes in subcategory S02.0: CC with 7th character A or MCC with 7th character B:
PDX collection 1140
CC with 7th character K: PDX collection 897

☑5ᵗʰ **S02.1** **Fracture of base of skull**
EXCLUDES 1 *orbit NOS (S02.8)*
EXCLUDES 2 *orbital floor (S02.3-)*

CC Excl: For codes in subcategory S02.1:
CC with 7th character A or MCC with 7th character B:
PDX collection 1140
CC with 7th character K: PDX collection 897

☑6ᵗʰ **S02.10** **Unspecified fracture of base of skull**

6, 7,11 ☑7ᵗʰ **S02.101** **Fracture of base of skull, right side**    MCC CC H5 HCC

6, 7,11 ☑7ᵗʰ **S02.102** **Fracture of base of skull, left side**    MCC CC H5 HCC

6, 7,11 ☑7ᵗʰ **S02.109** **Fracture of base of skull, unspecified side**    MCC CC H5 HCC

☑6ᵗʰ **S02.11** **Fracture of occiput**

6, 7,11 ☑7ᵗʰ **S02.110** **Type I occipital condyle fracture, unspecified side**    MCC CC H5 HCC

6, 7,11 ☑7ᵗʰ **S02.111** **Type II occipital condyle fracture, unspecified side**    MCC CC H5 HCC

6, 7,11 ☑7ᵗʰ **S02.112** **Type III occipital condyle fracture, unspecified side**    MCC CC H5 HCC

6, 7,11 ☑7ᵗʰ **S02.113** **Unspecified occipital condyle fracture**    MCC CC H5 HCC

6, 7,11 ☑7ᵗʰ **S02.118** **Other fracture of occiput, unspecified side**    MCC CC H5 HCC

6, 7,11 ☑7ᵗʰ **S02.119** **Unspecified fracture of occiput**    MCC CC H5 HCC

6, 7,11 ☑7ᵗʰ **S02.11A** **Type I occipital condyle fracture, right side**    MCC CC H5 HCC

6, 7,11 ☑7ᵗʰ **S02.11B** **Type I occipital condyle fracture, left side**    MCC CC H5 HCC

6, 7,11 ☑7ᵗʰ **S02.11C** **Type II occipital condyle fracture, right side**    MCC CC H5 HCC

6, 7,11 ☑7ᵗʰ **S02.11D** **Type II occipital condyle fracture, left side**    MCC CC H5 HCC

6, 7,11 ☑7ᵗʰ **S02.11E** **Type III occipital condyle fracture, right side**    MCC CC H5 HCC

6, 7,11 ☑7ᵗʰ **S02.11F** **Type III occipital condyle fracture, left side**    MCC CC H5 HCC

6, 7,11 ☑7ᵗʰ **S02.11G** **Other fracture of occiput, right side**    MCC CC H5 HCC

6, 7,11 ☑7ᵗʰ **S02.11H** **Other fracture of occiput, left side**    MCC CC H5 HCC

6,7,11 ☑x7ᵗʰ **S02.19** **Other fracture of base of skull**    MCC CC H5 HCC
Fracture of anterior fossa of base of skull
Fracture of ethmoid sinus
Fracture of frontal sinus
Fracture of middle fossa of base of skull
Fracture of orbital roof
Fracture of posterior fossa of base of skull
Fracture of sphenoid
Fracture of temporal bone

---

6   MCC when reported as an open fracture (7th character B or C – specific to category).
7   CC when reported as an initial encounter (7th character A, B, or C – specific to category) OR a subsequent encounter for nonunion or malunion (7th character K, M, N, P, Q, or R – specific to category).
11   HCC with 7th character indicating initial encounter (A or B - specific to category) OR sequela.

**7** ✓x7th **S02.2** **Fracture of** nasal bones    CC H5
       **CC Excl: CC with 7th character B:** PDX collection 1141
       **CC Excl: CC with 7th character K:** PDX collection 897

✓5th **S02.3** **Fracture of** orbital floor
       *EXCLUDES 1*   orbit NOS (S02.8)
       *EXCLUDES 2*   orbital roof (S02.1-)

       **CC Excl: For codes in subcategory S02.3:**
       **CC with 7th character A or B:** PDX collection 1142
       **CC with 7th character K:** PDX collection 897

   **7,11** ✓x7th **S02.30**   **Fracture of orbital floor, unspecified** side   CC H5 HCC
   **7,11** ✓x7th **S02.31**   **Fracture of orbital floor, right** side   CC H5 HCC
   **7,11** ✓x7th **S02.32**   **Fracture of orbital floor, left** side   CC H5 HCC

✓5th **S02.4** **Fracture of** malar, maxillary and zygoma bones
       Fracture of superior maxilla
       Fracture of upper jaw (bone)
       Fracture of zygomatic process of temporal bone

       **CC Excl: For codes in subcategory S02.4, unless otherwise noted:**
       **CC with 7th character A or B:** PDX collection 1143
       **CC with 7th character K:** PDX collection 897

   ✓6th **S02.40**   **Fracture of malar, maxillary and zygoma bones, unspecified**
     **7,11** ✓7th **S02.400**   **Malar fracture, unspecified side**   CC H5 HCC
     **7,11** ✓7th **S02.401**   **Maxillary fracture, unspecified side**   CC H5 HCC
     **7,11** ✓7th **S02.402**   **Zygomatic fracture, unspecified side**   CC H5 HCC
     **7,11** ✓7th **S02.40A**   **Malar fracture, right side**   CC H5 HCC
     **7,11** ✓7th **S02.40B**   **Malar fracture, left side**   CC H5 HCC
     **7,11** ✓7th **S02.40C**   **Maxillary fracture, right side**   CC H5 HCC
     **7,11** ✓7th **S02.40D**   **Maxillary fracture, left side**   CC H5 HCC
     **7,11** ✓7th **S02.40E**   **Zygomatic fracture, right side**   CC H5 HCC
     **7,11** ✓7th **S02.40F**   **Zygomatic fracture, left side**   CC H5 HCC

   ✓6th **S02.41**   **LeFort fracture**
     **7,11** ✓7th **S02.411**   **LeFort I fracture**   CC H5 HCC
     **7,11** ✓7th **S02.412**   **LeFort II fracture**   CC H5 HCC
     **7,11** ✓7th **S02.413**   **LeFort III fracture**   CC H5 HCC

   **7,11** ✓x7th **S02.42**   **Fracture of alveolus of maxilla**   CC H5 HCC
        **CC Excl: CC with 7th character B:** PDX collection 1141
        **CC Excl: CC with 7th character K:** PDX collection 897

**8** ✓x7th **S02.5** **Fracture of** tooth (traumatic)   CC
       Broken tooth
       *EXCLUDES 1*   cracked tooth (nontraumatic) (K03.81)
       **CC Excl: CC with 7th character K:** PDX collection 897

**LeFort Fracture Types**

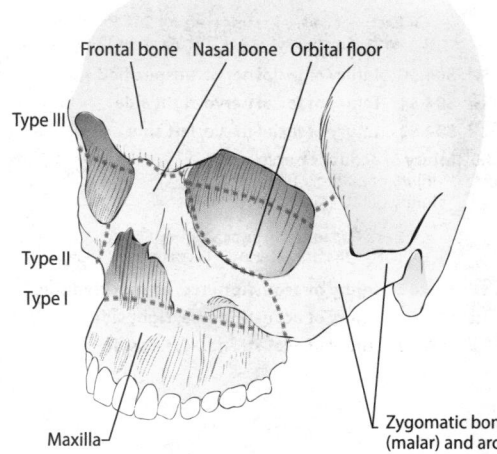

Frontal bone   Nasal bone   Orbital floor
Type III
Type II
Type I
Maxilla
Zygomatic bone (malar) and arch

✓5th **S02.6** **Fracture of** mandible
       Fracture of lower jaw (bone)

       **CC Excl: For codes in subcategory S02.6:**
       **CC with 7th character A or B:** PDX collection 1143
       **CC with 7th character K:** PDX collection 897

   ✓6th **S02.60**   **Fracture of mandible, unspecified**
     **7,11** ✓7th **S02.600**   **Fracture of unspecified part of body of mandible, unspecified side**   CC H5 HCC
     **7,11** ✓7th **S02.601**   **Fracture of unspecified part of body of right mandible**   CC H5 HCC
     **7,11** ✓7th **S02.602**   **Fracture of unspecified part of body of left mandible**   CC H5 HCC
     **7,11** ✓7th **S02.609**   **Fracture of mandible, unspecified**   CC H5 HCC

   ✓6th **S02.61**   **Fracture of condylar process of mandible**
     **7,11** ✓7th **S02.610**   **Fracture of condylar process of mandible, unspecified side**   CC H5 HCC
     **7,11** ✓7th **S02.611**   **Fracture of condylar process of right mandible**   CC H5 HCC
     **7,11** ✓7th **S02.612**   **Fracture of condylar process of left mandible**   CC H5 HCC

   ✓6th **S02.62**   **Fracture of subcondylar process of mandible**
     **7,11** ✓7th **S02.620**   **Fracture of subcondylar process of mandible, unspecified side**   CC H5 HCC
     **7,11** ✓7th **S02.621**   **Fracture of subcondylar process of right mandible**   CC H5 HCC
     **7,11** ✓7th **S02.622**   **Fracture of subcondylar process of left mandible**   CC H5 HCC

   ✓6th **S02.63**   **Fracture of coronoid process of mandible**
     **7,11** ✓7th **S02.630**   **Fracture of coronoid process of mandible, unspecified side**   CC H5 HCC
     **7,11** ✓7th **S02.631**   **Fracture of coronoid process of right mandible**   CC H5 HCC
     **7,11** ✓7th **S02.632**   **Fracture of coronoid process of left mandible**   CC H5 HCC

   ✓6th **S02.64**   **Fracture of ramus of mandible**
     **7,11** ✓7th **S02.640**   **Fracture of ramus of mandible, unspecified side**   CC H5 HCC
     **7,11** ✓7th **S02.641**   **Fracture of ramus of right mandible**   CC H5 HCC
     **7,11** ✓7th **S02.642**   **Fracture of ramus of left mandible**   CC H5 HCC

   ✓6th **S02.65**   **Fracture of angle of mandible**
     **7,11** ✓7th **S02.650**   **Fracture of angle of mandible, unspecified side**   CC H5 HCC
     **7,11** ✓7th **S02.651**   **Fracture of angle of right mandible**   CC H5 HCC
     **7,11** ✓7th **S02.652**   **Fracture of angle of left mandible**   CC H5 HCC

   **7,11** ✓x7th **S02.66**   **Fracture of symphysis of mandible**   CC H5 HCC
   ✓6th **S02.67**   **Fracture of alveolus of mandible**
     **7,11** ✓7th **S02.670**   **Fracture of alveolus of mandible, unspecified side**   CC H5 HCC
     **7,11** ✓7th **S02.671**   **Fracture of alveolus of right mandible**   CC H5 HCC
     **7,11** ✓7th **S02.672**   **Fracture of alveolus of left mandible**   CC H5 HCC

   **7,11** ✓x7th **S02.69**   **Fracture of mandible of other specified site**   CC H5 HCC

✓5th **S02.8** **Fractures of other specified skull and facial bones**
       Fracture of orbit NOS
       Fracture of palate
       *EXCLUDES 1*   fracture of orbital floor (S02.3-)
               fracture of orbital roof (S02.1-)

       **CC Excl: For CC codes in subcategory S02.8:**
       **CC with 7th character A or B:** PDX collection 1142
       **CC with 7th character K:** PDX collection 897

   **7,11** ✓x7th **S02.80**   **Fracture of other specified skull and facial bones, unspecified side**   CC H5 HCC

---

**7**   CC when reported as an initial encounter (7th character A, B, or C – specific to category) OR a subsequent encounter for nonunion or malunion (7th character K, M, N, P, Q, or R – specific to category).

**8**   CC when reported as a subsequent encounter for nonunion or malunion (7th character K, M, N, P, Q, or R – specific to category).

**11**   HCC with 7th character indicating initial encounter (A or B - specific to category) OR sequela.

✓ Additional Character Req   ✓x7th Placeholder Alert   Unacceptable PDx   ■ Manifestation   H1 - H14 HAC   HCC CMS-HCC Condition   *EXCLUDES 1* Not Coded Here   *EXCLUDES 2* Not Included Here

ICD-10-CM 2018                                     **945**

7,11 ✓x7ᵗʰ **S02.81 Fracture of other specified skull and facial** CC H5 HCC
**bones, right side**

7,11 ✓x7ᵗʰ **S02.82 Fracture of other specified skull and facial** CC H5 HCC
**bones, left side**

✓5ᵗʰ **S02.9 Fracture of unspecified skull and facial bones**

6,7,11 ✓x7ᵗʰ **S02.91 Unspecified fracture of skull** MCC CC H5 HCC
CC Excl: CC with 7th character A or MCC with 7th
character B: PDX collection 1140
CC with 7th character K: PDX collection 897

7,11 ✓x7ᵗʰ **S02.92 Unspecified fracture of facial bones** CC H5 HCC
CC Excl: CC with 7th character A or B:
PDX collection 1142
CC with 7th character K: PDX collection 897

✓4ᵗʰ **S03 Dislocation and sprain of joints and ligaments of head**
**INCLUDES** avulsion of joint (capsule) or ligament of head
laceration of cartilage, joint (capsule) or ligament of
head
sprain of cartilage, joint (capsule) or ligament of head
traumatic hemarthrosis of joint or ligament of head
traumatic rupture of joint or ligament of head
traumatic subluxation of joint or ligament of head
traumatic tear of joint or ligament of head
Code also any associated open wound
**EXCLUDES 2** strain of muscle or tendon of head (S09.1)

The appropriate 7th character is to be added to each code from
category S03.
A    initial encounter
D    subsequent encounter
S    sequela

✓5ᵗʰ **S03.0 Dislocation of jaw**
Dislocation of jaw (cartilage) (meniscus)
Dislocation of mandible
Dislocation of temporomandibular (joint)

✓x7ᵗʰ **S03.00 Dislocation of jaw, unspecified side**

✓x7ᵗʰ **S03.01 Dislocation of jaw, right side**

✓x7ᵗʰ **S03.02 Dislocation of jaw, left side**

✓x7ᵗʰ **S03.03 Dislocation of jaw, bilateral**

✓x7ᵗʰ **S03.1 Dislocation of septal cartilage of nose**

✓x7ᵗʰ **S03.2 Dislocation of tooth**

✓5ᵗʰ **S03.4 Sprain of jaw**
Sprain of temporomandibular (joint) (ligament)

✓x7ᵗʰ **S03.40 Sprain of jaw, unspecified side**

✓x7ᵗʰ **S03.41 Sprain of jaw, right side**

✓x7ᵗʰ **S03.42 Sprain of jaw, left side**

✓x7ᵗʰ **S03.43 Sprain of jaw, bilateral**

✓x7ᵗʰ **S03.8 Sprain of joints and ligaments of other parts of head**

✓x7ᵗʰ **S03.9 Sprain of joints and ligaments of unspecified parts of head**

✓4ᵗʰ **S04 Injury of cranial nerve**
The selection of side should be based on the side of the body being
affected
Code first any associated intracranial injury (S06.-)
Code also any associated:
open wound of head (S01.-)
skull fracture (S02.-)

The appropriate 7th character is to be added to each code from
category S04.
A    initial encounter
D    subsequent encounter
S    sequela

✓5ᵗʰ **S04.0 Injury of optic nerve and pathways**
Use additional code to identify any visual field defect or
blindness ▶(H53.4-, H54.-)◀

CC Excl: For codes in subcategory S04.0:
CC with 7th character A: PDX collection 1144

✓6ᵗʰ **S04.01 Injury of optic nerve**
Injury of 2nd cranial nerve

✓7ᵗʰ **S04.011 Injury of optic nerve, right eye** CC

✓7ᵗʰ **S04.012 Injury of optic nerve, left eye** CC

✓7ᵗʰ **S04.019 Injury of optic nerve, unspecified eye** CC
Injury of optic nerve NOS

✓x7ᵗʰ **S04.02 Injury of optic chiasm** CC

✓6ᵗʰ **S04.03 Injury of optic tract and pathways** CC
Injury of optic radiation

▲ ✓7ᵗʰ **S04.031 Injury of optic tract and pathways,** CC
**right side**

▲ ✓7ᵗʰ **S04.032 Injury of optic tract and pathways,** CC
**left side**

▲ ✓7ᵗʰ **S04.039 Injury of optic tract and pathways,** CC
**unspecified side**
Injury of optic tract and pathways NOS

✓6ᵗʰ **S04.04 Injury of visual cortex**

▲ ✓7ᵗʰ **S04.041 Injury of visual cortex, right side** CC

▲ ✓7ᵗʰ **S04.042 Injury of visual cortex, left side** CC

▲ ✓7ᵗʰ **S04.049 Injury of visual cortex, unspecified** CC
**side**
Injury of visual cortex NOS

✓5ᵗʰ **S04.1 Injury of oculomotor nerve**
Injury of 3rd cranial nerve

CC Excl: For codes in subcategory S04.1:
CC with 7th character A: PDX collection 1145

✓x7ᵗʰ **S04.10 Injury of oculomotor nerve, unspecified side** CC

✓x7ᵗʰ **S04.11 Injury of oculomotor nerve, right side** CC

✓x7ᵗʰ **S04.12 Injury of oculomotor nerve, left side** CC

✓5ᵗʰ **S04.2 Injury of trochlear nerve**
Injury of 4th cranial nerve

CC Excl: For codes in subcategory S04.2:
CC with 7th character A: PDX collection 1146

✓x7ᵗʰ **S04.20 Injury of trochlear nerve, unspecified side** CC

✓x7ᵗʰ **S04.21 Injury of trochlear nerve, right side** CC

✓x7ᵗʰ **S04.22 Injury of trochlear nerve, left side** CC

✓5ᵗʰ **S04.3 Injury of trigeminal nerve**
Injury of 5th cranial nerve

CC Excl: For codes in subcategory S04.3:
CC with 7th character A: PDX collection 1147

✓x7ᵗʰ **S04.30 Injury of trigeminal nerve, unspecified side** CC

✓x7ᵗʰ **S04.31 Injury of trigeminal nerve, right side** CC

✓x7ᵗʰ **S04.32 Injury of trigeminal nerve, left side** CC

✓5ᵗʰ **S04.4 Injury of abducent nerve**
Injury of 6th cranial nerve

CC Excl: For codes in subcategory S04.4:
CC with 7th character A: PDX collection 1148

✓x7ᵗʰ **S04.40 Injury of abducent nerve, unspecified side** CC

✓x7ᵗʰ **S04.41 Injury of abducent nerve, right side** CC

✓x7ᵗʰ **S04.42 Injury of abducent nerve, left side** CC

✓5ᵗʰ **S04.5 Injury of facial nerve**
Injury of 7th cranial nerve

CC Excl: For codes in subcategory S04.5:
CC with 7th character A: PDX collection 1149

✓x7ᵗʰ **S04.50 Injury of facial nerve, unspecified side** CC

✓x7ᵗʰ **S04.51 Injury of facial nerve, right side** CC

✓x7ᵗʰ **S04.52 Injury of facial nerve, left side** CC

✓5ᵗʰ **S04.6 Injury of acoustic nerve**
Injury of auditory nerve
Injury of 8th cranial nerve

CC Excl: For codes in subcategory S04.6:
CC with 7th character A: PDX collection 1150

✓x7ᵗʰ **S04.60 Injury of acoustic nerve, unspecified side** CC

✓x7ᵗʰ **S04.61 Injury of acoustic nerve, right side** CC

✓x7ᵗʰ **S04.62 Injury of acoustic nerve, left side** CC

---

6   MCC when reported as an open fracture (7th character B or C – specific to category).

7   CC when reported as an initial encounter (7th character A, B, or C – specific to category) OR a subsequent encounter for nonunion or malunion
(7th character K, M, N, P, Q, or R – specific to category).

11   HCC with 7th character indicating initial encounter (A or B - specific to category) OR sequela.

---

N Newborn: 0   P Pediatric: 0-17   M Maternity: 12-55   A Adult: 15-124   MCC Major CC Condition   PDxMCC PDx acts as own MCC   CC CC Condition   PDxCC PDx acts as own CC

✓5ᵗʰ **S04.7** **Injury of** accessory nerve
Injury of 11th cranial nerve

> CC Excl: For codes in subcategory S04.7:
> CC with 7th character A: PDX collection 1151

   ✓x7ᵗʰ **S04.70** **Injury of accessory nerve,** unspecified **side**   CC
   ✓x7ᵗʰ **S04.71** **Injury of accessory nerve,** right **side**   CC
   ✓x7ᵗʰ **S04.72** **Injury of accessory nerve,** left **side**   CC

✓5ᵗʰ **S04.8** **Injury of** other cranial nerves

> CC Excl: For codes in subcategory S04.8: CC with 7th
> character A: PDX collection 1152

   ✓6ᵗʰ **S04.81** **Injury of** olfactory [1st] nerve
     ✓7ᵗʰ **S04.811** **Injury of olfactory [1st ] nerve,** right **side**   CC
     ✓7ᵗʰ **S04.812** **Injury of olfactory [1st ] nerve,** left **side**   CC
     ✓7ᵗʰ **S04.819** **Injury of olfactory [1st ] nerve,** unspecified **side**   CC

   ✓6ᵗʰ **S04.89** **Injury of** other cranial nerves
Injury of vagus [10th] nerve
     ✓7ᵗʰ **S04.891** **Injury of other cranial nerves,** right **side**   CC
     ✓7ᵗʰ **S04.892** **Injury of other cranial nerves,** left **side**   CC
     ✓7ᵗʰ **S04.899** **Injury of other cranial nerves,** unspecified **side**   CC

✓x7ᵗʰ **S04.9** **Injury of** unspecified **cranial nerve**   CC
     CC Excl: CC with 7th character A: PDX collection 1152

✓4ᵗʰ **S05** **Injury of eye and orbit**
   **INCLUDES** open wound of eye and orbit
   **EXCLUDES 2** 2nd cranial [optic] nerve injury (S04.0-)
     3rd cranial [oculomotor] nerve injury (S04.1-)
     open wound of eyelid and periocular area (S01.1-)
     orbital bone fracture (S02.1-, S02.3-, S02.8-)
     superficial injury of eyelid (S00.1-S00.2)

> The appropriate 7th character is to be added to each code from
> category S05.
> A     initial encounter
> D     subsequent encounter
> S     sequela

> CC Excl: For codes in category S05, unless otherwise noted:
> CC with 7th character A: PDX collection 1139

✓5ᵗʰ **S05.0** **Injury of conjunctiva and corneal abrasion** without foreign body
     **EXCLUDES 1** foreign body in conjunctival sac (T15.1)
       foreign body in cornea (T15.0)

   ✓x7ᵗʰ **S05.00** **Injury of conjunctiva and corneal abrasion without foreign body,** unspecified **eye**
   ✓x7ᵗʰ **S05.01** **Injury of conjunctiva and corneal abrasion without foreign body,** right **eye**
   ✓x7ᵗʰ **S05.02** **Injury of conjunctiva and corneal abrasion without foreign body,** left **eye**

✓5ᵗʰ **S05.1** **Contusion of eyeball and orbital tissues**
Traumatic hyphema
     **EXCLUDES 2** black eye NOS (S00.1)
       contusion of eyelid and periocular area (S00.1)

   ✓x7ᵗʰ **S05.10** **Contusion of eyeball and orbital tissues,** unspecified **eye**
   ✓x7ᵗʰ **S05.11** **Contusion of eyeball and orbital tissues,** right **eye**
   ✓x7ᵗʰ **S05.12** **Contusion of eyeball and orbital tissues,** left **eye**

✓5ᵗʰ **S05.2** **Ocular laceration and rupture** with prolapse or loss of intraocular tissue
   ✓x7ᵗʰ **S05.20** **Ocular laceration and rupture with prolapse or loss of intraocular tissue,** unspecified **eye**   CC
   ✓x7ᵗʰ **S05.21** **Ocular laceration and rupture with prolapse or loss of intraocular tissue,** right **eye**   CC
   ✓x7ᵗʰ **S05.22** **Ocular laceration and rupture with prolapse or loss of intraocular tissue,** left **eye**   CC

✓5ᵗʰ **S05.3** **Ocular laceration** without prolapse or loss of intraocular tissue
Laceration of eye NOS
**DEF:** Tear in ocular tissue without displacing structures; due to blunt trauma; characterized by pain, redness, and decreased vision.

   ✓x7ᵗʰ **S05.30** **Ocular laceration without prolapse or loss of intraocular tissue,** unspecified **eye**   CC
   ✓x7ᵗʰ **S05.31** **Ocular laceration without prolapse or loss of intraocular tissue,** right **eye**   CC
   ✓x7ᵗʰ **S05.32** **Ocular laceration without prolapse or loss of intraocular tissue,** left **eye**   CC

✓5ᵗʰ **S05.4** **Penetrating wound** of orbit with or without foreign body
     **EXCLUDES 2** retained (old) foreign body following penetrating wound in orbit (H05.5-)

   ✓x7ᵗʰ **S05.40** **Penetrating wound of orbit with or without foreign body,** unspecified **eye**   CC
   ✓x7ᵗʰ **S05.41** **Penetrating wound of orbit with or without foreign body,** right **eye**   CC
   ✓x7ᵗʰ **S05.42** **Penetrating wound of orbit with or without foreign body,** left **eye**   CC

✓5ᵗʰ **S05.5** **Penetrating wound with foreign body** of eyeball
     **EXCLUDES 2** retained (old) intraocular foreign body (H44.6-, H44.7)

> CC Excl: For codes in subcategory S05.5:
> CC with 7th character A: PDX collection 1153

   ✓x7ᵗʰ **S05.50** **Penetrating wound with foreign body of** unspecified **eyeball**   CC
   ✓x7ᵗʰ **S05.51** **Penetrating wound with foreign body of** right **eyeball**   CC
   ✓x7ᵗʰ **S05.52** **Penetrating wound with foreign body of** left **eyeball**   CC

✓5ᵗʰ **S05.6** **Penetrating wound without foreign body** of eyeball
Ocular penetration NOS
   ✓x7ᵗʰ **S05.60** **Penetrating wound without foreign body of** unspecified **eyeball**
   ✓x7ᵗʰ **S05.61** **Penetrating wound without foreign body of** right **eyeball**
   ✓x7ᵗʰ **S05.62** **Penetrating wound without foreign body of** left **eyeball**

✓5ᵗʰ **S05.7** **Avulsion of eye**
Traumatic enucleation
   ✓x7ᵗʰ **S05.70** **Avulsion of** unspecified **eye**   CC
   ✓x7ᵗʰ **S05.71** **Avulsion of** right **eye**   CC
   ✓x7ᵗʰ **S05.72** **Avulsion of** left **eye**   CC

✓5ᵗʰ **S05.8** **Other injuries of eye and orbit**
Lacrimal duct injury
   ✓6ᵗʰ **S05.8X** **Other** injuries of eye and orbit
     ✓7ᵗʰ **S05.8X1** **Other injuries of** right **eye and orbit**   CC
     ✓7ᵗʰ **S05.8X2** **Other injuries of** left **eye and orbit**   CC
     ✓7ᵗʰ **S05.8X9** **Other injuries of** unspecified **eye and orbit**   CC

✓5ᵗʰ **S05.9** **Unspecified injury of eye and orbit**
Injury of eye NOS
   ✓x7ᵗʰ **S05.90** **Unspecified injury of** unspecified **eye and orbit**
   ✓x7ᵗʰ **S05.91** **Unspecified injury of** right **eye and orbit**   CC
   ✓x7ᵗʰ **S05.92** **Unspecified injury of** left **eye and orbit**   CC

---

## ✓4th S06  Intracranial injury

**NOTE**  ▶7th characters D and S do not apply to codes in category S06 with 6th character 7 – death due to brain injury prior to regaining consciousness, or 8 – death due to other cause prior to regaining consciousness◄

**INCLUDES**  traumatic brain injury

Code also any associated:
open wound of head (S01.-)
skull fracture (S02.-)

**EXCLUDES 1**  head injury NOS (S09.90)

**AHA:** 2017, 1Q, 42; 2015, 3Q, 37

The appropriate 7th character is to be added to each code from category S06.
A    initial encounter
D    subsequent encounter
S    sequela

CC Excl: For codes in category S06, unless otherwise noted:
CC or MCC with 7th character A: PDX collection 1154

### ✓5th S06.0  Concussion
Commotio cerebri

**EXCLUDES 1**  concussion with other intracranial injuries classified in subcategories S06.1- to S06.6-, S06.81 and S06.82- code to specified intracranial injury

#### ✓6th S06.0X  Concussion

12 ✓7th **S06.0X0  Concussion** without loss of consciousness  `HCC`

12 ✓7th **S06.0X1  Concussion with loss of consciousness of** 30 minutes or less  `CC H5 HCC`

12 ✓7th **S06.0X9  Concussion with loss of consciousness of** unspecified duration  `CC H5 HCC`
Concussion NOS

### ✓5th S06.1  Traumatic cerebral edema
Diffuse traumatic cerebral edema
Focal traumatic cerebral edema

CC Excl: For codes in subcategory S06.1, unless otherwise noted:
MCC with 7th character A: PDX collection 1155

#### ✓6th S06.1X  Traumatic cerebral edema

11 ✓7th **S06.1X0  Traumatic cerebral edema** without loss of consciousness  `PDxMCC MCC HCC`
CC Excl: MCC with 7th character A: PDX collection 612

11 ✓7th **S06.1X1  Traumatic cerebral edema with loss of consciousness of** 30 minutes or less  `PDxMCC MCC H5 HCC`

11 ✓7th **S06.1X2  Traumatic cerebral edema with loss of consciousness of** 31 minutes to 59 minutes  `PDxMCC MCC H5 HCC`

11 ✓7th **S06.1X3  Traumatic cerebral edema with loss of consciousness of** 1 hour to 5 hours 59 minutes  `PDxMCC MCC H5 HCC`

11 ✓7th **S06.1X4  Traumatic cerebral edema with loss of consciousness of** 6 hours to 24 hours  `PDxMCC MCC H5 HCC`

11 ✓7th **S06.1X5  Traumatic cerebral edema with loss of consciousness** greater than 24 hours with return to pre-existing conscious level  `PDxMCC MCC H5 HCC`

11 ✓7th **S06.1X6  Traumatic cerebral edema with loss of consciousness** greater than 24 hours without return to pre-existing conscious level with patient surviving  `PDxMCC MCC H5 HCC`
CC Excl: MCC with 7th character A: PDX collection 1154

✓7th **S06.1X7  Traumatic cerebral edema with loss of consciousness of** any duration with death due to brain injury prior to regaining consciousness  `PDxMCC MCC H5`
CC Excl: MCC with 7th character A: PDX collection 1154

11 ✓7th **S06.1X8  Traumatic cerebral edema with loss of consciousness of** any duration with death due to other cause prior to regaining consciousness  `PDxMCC MCC H5`
CC Excl: MCC with 7th character A: PDX collection 1154

11 ✓7th **S06.1X9  Traumatic cerebral edema with loss of consciousness of** unspecified duration  `PDxMCC MCC H5 HCC`
Traumatic cerebral edema NOS

### ✓5th S06.2  Diffuse traumatic brain injury
Diffuse axonal brain injury

**EXCLUDES 1**  traumatic diffuse cerebral edema (S06.1X-)

#### ✓6th S06.2X  Diffuse traumatic brain injury

11 ✓7th **S06.2X0  Diffuse traumatic brain injury** without loss of consciousness  `HCC`

11 ✓7th **S06.2X1  Diffuse traumatic brain injury with loss of consciousness of** 30 minutes or less  `CC H5 HCC`

11 ✓7th **S06.2X2  Diffuse traumatic brain injury with loss of consciousness of** 31 minutes to 59 minutes  `CC H5 HCC`

11 ✓7th **S06.2X3  Diffuse traumatic brain injury with loss of consciousness of** 1 hour to 5 hours 59 minutes  `CC H5 HCC`

11 ✓7th **S06.2X4  Diffuse traumatic brain injury with loss of consciousness of** 6 hours to 24 hours  `CC H5 HCC`

11 ✓7th **S06.2X5  Diffuse traumatic brain injury with loss of consciousness** greater than 24 hours with return to pre-existing conscious levels  `CC H5 HCC`

11 ✓7th **S06.2X6  Diffuse traumatic brain injury with loss of consciousness** greater than 24 hours without return to pre-existing conscious level with patient surviving  `MCC H5 HCC`

✓7th **S06.2X7  Diffuse traumatic brain injury with loss of consciousness of** any duration with death due to brain injury prior to regaining consciousness  `MCC H5`

✓7th **S06.2X8  Diffuse traumatic brain injury with loss of consciousness of** any duration with death due to other cause prior to regaining consciousness  `MCC H5`

11 ✓7th **S06.2X9  Diffuse traumatic brain injury with loss of consciousness of** unspecified duration  `CC H5 HCC`
Diffuse traumatic brain injury NOS

### ✓5th S06.3  Focal traumatic brain injury

**EXCLUDES 1**  any condition classifiable to S06.4-S06.6
focal cerebral edema (S06.1)

#### ✓6th S06.30  Unspecified focal traumatic brain injury

11 ✓7th **S06.300  Unspecified focal traumatic brain injury** without loss of consciousness  `HCC`

11 ✓7th **S06.301  Unspecified focal traumatic brain injury with loss of consciousness of** 30 minutes or less  `CC H5 HCC`

11 ✓7th **S06.302  Unspecified focal traumatic brain injury with loss of consciousness of** 31 minutes to 59 minutes  `CC H5 HCC`

11 ✓7th **S06.303  Unspecified focal traumatic brain injury with loss of consciousness of** 1 hour to 5 hours 59 minutes  `CC H5 HCC`

11 ✓7th **S06.304  Unspecified focal traumatic brain injury with loss of consciousness of** 6 hours to 24 hours  `CC H5 HCC`

11 ✓7th **S06.305  Unspecified focal traumatic brain injury with loss of consciousness** greater than 24 hours with return to pre-existing conscious level  `CC H5 HCC`

11 ✓7th **S06.306  Unspecified focal traumatic brain injury with loss of consciousness** greater than 24 hours without return to pre-existing conscious level with patient surviving  `MCC H5 HCC`

---

11 HCC with 7th character indicating initial encounter (A or B - specific to category) OR sequela.
12 HCC with 7th character indicating sequela.

---

N Newborn: 0    P Pediatric: 0-17    M Maternity: 12-55    A Adult: 15-124    MCC Major CC Condition    PDxMCC PDx acts as own MCC    CC CC Condition    PDxCC PDx acts as own CC

✓7th **S06.307** **Unspecified focal traumatic brain injury with loss of consciousness of any duration with death due to brain injury prior to regaining consciousness**  `MCC` `H5`

✓7th **S06.308** **Unspecified focal traumatic brain injury with loss of consciousness of any duration with death due to other cause prior to regaining consciousness**  `MCC` `H5`

11 ✓7th **S06.309** **Unspecified focal traumatic brain injury with loss of consciousness of** unspecified duration  `CC` `H5` `HCC`
    Unspecified focal traumatic brain injury NOS

✓6th **S06.31** **Contusion and laceration of** right cerebrum

11 ✓7th **S06.310** **Contusion and laceration of** rightcerebrum **without loss of consciousness**  `MCC` `H5` `HCC`

11 ✓7th **S06.311** **Contusion and laceration of right cerebrum with loss of consciousness of** 30 minutes or less  `MCC` `H5` `HCC`

11 ✓7th **S06.312** **Contusion and laceration of right cerebrum with loss of consciousness of** 31 minutes to 59 minutes  `MCC` `H5` `HCC`

11 ✓7th **S06.313** **Contusion and laceration of right cerebrum with loss of consciousness of** 1 hour to 5 hours 59 minutes  `MCC` `H5` `HCC`

11 ✓7th **S06.314** **Contusion and laceration of right cerebrum with loss of consciousness of** 6 hours to 24 hours  `MCC` `H5` `HCC`

11 ✓7th **S06.315** **Contusion and laceration of right cerebrum with loss of consciousness** greater than 24 hours with return to pre-existing conscious level  `MCC` `H5` `HCC`

11 ✓7th **S06.316** **Contusion and laceration of right cerebrum with loss of consciousness** greater than 24 hours without return to pre-existing conscious level with patient surviving  `MCC` `H5` `HCC`

✓7th **S06.317** **Contusion and laceration of right cerebrum with loss of consciousness of** any duration with death due to brain injury prior to regaining consciousness  `MCC` `H5`

✓7th **S06.318** **Contusion and laceration of right cerebrum with loss of consciousness of** any duration with death due to other cause prior to regaining consciousness  `MCC` `H5`

11 ✓7th **S06.319** **Contusion and laceration of right cerebrum with loss of consciousness of** unspecified duration  `MCC` `H5` `HCC`
    Contusion and laceration of right cerebrum NOS

✓6th **S06.32** **Contusion and laceration of** left cerebrum

11 ✓7th **S06.320** **Contusion and laceration of left cerebrum** without loss of consciousness  `MCC` `H5` `HCC`

11 ✓7th **S06.321** **Contusion and laceration of left cerebrum with loss of consciousness of** 30 minutes or less  `MCC` `H5` `HCC`

11 ✓7th **S06.322** **Contusion and laceration of left cerebrum with loss of consciousness of** 31 minutes to 59 minutes  `MCC` `H5` `HCC`

11 ✓7th **S06.323** **Contusion and laceration of left cerebrum with loss of consciousness of** 1 hour to 5 hours 59 minutes  `MCC` `H5` `HCC`

11 ✓7th **S06.324** **Contusion and laceration of left cerebrum with loss of consciousness of** 6 hours to 24 hours  `MCC` `H5` `HCC`

11 ✓7th **S06.325** **Contusion and laceration of left cerebrum with loss of consciousness** greater than 24 hours with return to pre-existing conscious level  `MCC` `H5` `HCC`

11 ✓7th **S06.326** **Contusion and laceration of left cerebrum with loss of consciousness** greater than 24 hours without return to pre-existing conscious level with patient surviving  `MCC` `H5` `HCC`

✓7th **S06.327** **Contusion and laceration of left cerebrum with loss of consciousness of** any duration with death due to brain injury prior to regaining consciousness  `MCC` `H5`

✓7th **S06.328** **Contusion and laceration of left cerebrum with loss of consciousness of** any duration with death due to other cause prior to regaining consciousness  `MCC` `H5`

11 ✓7th **S06.329** **Contusion and laceration of left cerebrum with loss of consciousness of** unspecified duration  `MCC` `H5` `HCC`
    Contusion and laceration of left cerebrum NOS

✓6th **S06.33** **Contusion and laceration of** cerebrum, unspecified

11 ✓7th **S06.330** **Contusion and laceration of cerebrum, unspecified,** without loss of consciousness  `MCC` `H5` `HCC`

11 ✓7th **S06.331** **Contusion and laceration of cerebrum, unspecified, with loss of consciousness of** 30 minutes or less  `MCC` `H5` `HCC`

11 ✓7th **S06.332** **Contusion and laceration of cerebrum, unspecified, with loss of consciousness of** 31 minutes to 59 minutes  `MCC` `H5` `HCC`

11 ✓7th **S06.333** **Contusion and laceration of cerebrum, unspecified, with loss of consciousness of** 1 hour to 5 hours 59 minutes  `MCC` `H5` `HCC`

11 ✓7th **S06.334** **Contusion and laceration of cerebrum, unspecified, with loss of consciousness of** 6 hours to 24 hours  `MCC` `H5` `HCC`

11 ✓7th **S06.335** **Contusion and laceration of cerebrum, unspecified, with loss of consciousness** greater than 24 hours with return to pre-existing conscious level  `MCC` `H5` `HCC`

11 ✓7th **S06.336** **Contusion and laceration of cerebrum, unspecified, with loss of consciousness** greater than 24 hours without return to pre-existing conscious level with patient surviving  `MCC` `H5` `HCC`

✓7th **S06.337** **Contusion and laceration of cerebrum, unspecified, with loss of consciousness of** any duration with death due to brain injury prior to regaining consciousness  `MCC` `H5`

✓7th **S06.338** **Contusion and laceration of cerebrum, unspecified, with loss of consciousness of** any duration with death due to other cause prior to regaining consciousness  `MCC` `H5`

11 ✓7th **S06.339** **Contusion and laceration of cerebrum, unspecified, with loss of consciousness of** unspecified duration  `MCC` `H5` `HCC`
    Contusion and laceration of cerebrum NOS

✓6th **S06.34** **Traumatic hemorrhage of** right cerebrum
    Traumatic intracerebral hemorrhage and hematoma of right cerebrum

11 ✓7th **S06.340** **Traumatic hemorrhage of right cerebrum** without loss of consciousness  `MCC` `H5` `HCC`

11 ✓7th **S06.341** **Traumatic hemorrhage of right cerebrum with loss of consciousness of** 30 minutes or less  `MCC` `H5` `HCC`

11 ✓7th **S06.342** **Traumatic hemorrhage of right cerebrum with loss of c onsciousness of** 31 minutes to 59 minutes  `MCC` `H5` `HCC`

11 ✓7th **S06.343** **Traumatic hemorrhage of right cerebrum with loss of consciousness of** 1 hours to 5 hours 59 minutes  `MCC` `H5` `HCC`

11 ✓7th **S06.344** **Traumatic hemorrhage of right cerebrum with loss of consciousness of** 6 hours to 24 hours  `MCC` `H5` `HCC`

---

11 HCC with 7th character indicating initial encounter (A or B - specific to category) OR sequela.

✓ Additional Character Req    ✓×7th Placeholder Alert    Unacceptable PDx    Manifestation    `H1`-`H14` HAC    `HCC` CMS-HCC Condition    *EXCLUDES 1* Not Coded Here    *EXCLUDES 2* Not Included Here

ICD-10-CM 2018    **949**

11 ✓7th **S06.345 Traumatic hemorrhage of right cerebrum with loss of consciousness** greater than 24 hours with return to pre-existing conscious level   MCC H5 HCC

11 ✓7th **S06.346 Traumatic hemorrhage of right cerebrum with loss of consciousness** greater than 24 hours without return to pre-existing conscious level with patient surviving   MCC H5 HCC

✓7th **S06.347 Traumatic hemorrhage of right cerebrum with loss of consciousness** of any duration with death due to brain injury prior to regaining consciousness   MCC H5

✓7th **S06.348 Traumatic hemorrhage of right cerebrum with loss of consciousness** of any duration with death due to other cause prior to regaining consciousness   MCC H5

11 ✓7th **S06.349 Traumatic hemorrhage of right cerebrum with loss of consciousness** of unspecified duration   MCC H5 HCC
Traumatic hemorrhage of right cerebrum NOS

✓6th **S06.35 Traumatic hemorrhage of left cerebrum**
Traumatic intracerebral hemorrhage and hematoma of left cerebrum

11 ✓7th **S06.350 Traumatic hemorrhage of left cerebrum** without loss of consciousness   MCC H5 HCC

11 ✓7th **S06.351 Traumatic hemorrhage of left cerebrum with loss of consciousness** of 30 minutes or less   MCC H5 HCC

11 ✓7th **S06.352 Traumatic hemorrhage of left cerebrum with loss of consciousness** of 31 minutes to 59 minutes   MCC H5 HCC

11 ✓7th **S06.353 Traumatic hemorrhage of left cerebrum with loss of consciousness** of 1 hours to 5 hours 59 minutes   MCC H5 HCC

11 ✓7th **S06.354 Traumatic hemorrhage of left cerebrum with loss of consciousness** of 6 hours to 24 hours   MCC H5 HCC

11 ✓7th **S06.355 Traumatic hemorrhage of left cerebrum with loss of consciousness** greater than 24 hours with return to pre-existing conscious level   MCC H5 HCC

11 ✓7th **S06.356 Traumatic hemorrhage of left cerebrum with loss of consciousness** greater than 24 hours without return to pre-existing conscious level with patient surviving   MCC H5 HCC

✓7th **S06.357 Traumatic hemorrhage of left cerebrum with loss of consciousness** of any duration with death due to brain injury prior to regaining consciousness   MCC H5

✓7th **S06.358 Traumatic hemorrhage of left cerebrum with loss of consciousness** of any duration with death due to other cause prior to regaining consciousness   MCC H5

11 ✓7th **S06.359 Traumatic hemorrhage of left cerebrum with loss of consciousness** of unspecified duration   MCC H5 HCC
Traumatic hemorrhage of left cerebrum NOS

✓6th **S06.36 Traumatic hemorrhage of cerebrum, unspecified**
Traumatic intracerebral hemorrhage and hematoma, unspecified

11 ✓7th **S06.360 Traumatic hemorrhage of cerebrum, unspecified,** without loss of consciousness   MCC H5 HCC

11 ✓7th **S06.361 Traumatic hemorrhage of cerebrum, unspecified, with loss of consciousness** of 30 minutes or less   MCC H5 HCC

11 ✓7th **S06.362 Traumatic hemorrhage of cerebrum, unspecified, with loss of consciousness** of 31 minutes to 59 minutes   MCC H5 HCC

11 ✓7th **S06.363 Traumatic hemorrhage of cerebrum, unspecified, with loss of consciousness** of 1 hours to 5 hours 59 minutes   MCC H5 HCC

11 ✓7th **S06.364 Traumatic hemorrhage of cerebrum, unspecified, with loss of consciousness** of 6 hours to 24 hours   MCC H5 HCC

11 ✓7th **S06.365 Traumatic hemorrhage of cerebrum, unspecified, with loss of consciousness** greater than 24 hours with return to pre-existing conscious level   MCC H5 HCC

11 ✓7th **S06.366 Traumatic hemorrhage of cerebrum, unspecified, with loss of consciousness** greater than 24 hours without return to pre-existing conscious level with patient surviving   MCC H5 HCC

✓7th **S06.367 Traumatic hemorrhage of cerebrum, unspecified, with loss of consciousness** of any duration with death due to brain injury prior to regaining consciousness   MCC H5

✓7th **S06.368 Traumatic hemorrhage of cerebrum, unspecified, with loss of consciousness** of any duration with death due to other cause prior to regaining consciousness   MCC H5

11 ✓7th **S06.369 Traumatic hemorrhage of cerebrum, unspecified, with loss of consciousness** of unspecified duration   MCC H5 HCC
Traumatic hemorrhage of cerebrum NOS

✓6th **S06.37 Contusion, laceration, and hemorrhage of cerebellum**

11 ✓7th **S06.370 Contusion, laceration, and hemorrhage of cerebellum** without loss of consciousness   MCC H5 HCC
CC Excl: No Excl

11 ✓7th **S06.371 Contusion, laceration, and hemorrhage of cerebellum with loss of consciousness** of 30 minutes or less   CC H5 HCC

11 ✓7th **S06.372 Contusion, laceration, and hemorrhage of cerebellum with loss of consciousness** of 31 minutes to 59 minutes   CC H5 HCC

11 ✓7th **S06.373 Contusion, laceration, and hemorrhage of cerebellum with loss of consciousness** of 1 hour to 5 hours 59 minutes   CC H5 HCC

11 ✓7th **S06.374 Contusion, laceration, and hemorrhage of cerebellum with loss of consciousness** of 6 hours to 24 hours   CC H5 HCC

11 ✓7th **S06.375 Contusion, laceration, and hemorrhage of cerebellum with loss of consciousness** greater than 24 hours with return to pre-existing conscious level   CC H5 HCC

11 ✓7th **S06.376 Contusion, laceration, and hemorrhage of cerebellum with loss of consciousness** greater than 24 hours without return to pre-existing conscious level with patient surviving   MCC H5 HCC

✓7th **S06.377 Contusion, laceration, and hemorrhage of cerebellum with loss of consciousness** of any duration with death due to brain injury prior to regaining consciousness   MCC H5

✓7th **S06.378 Contusion, laceration, and hemorrhage of cerebellum with loss of consciousness** of any duration with death due to other cause prior to regaining consciousness   MCC H5

11 ✓7th **S06.379 Contusion, laceration, and hemorrhage of cerebellum with loss of consciousness** of unspecified duration   CC H5 HCC
Contusion, laceration, and hemorrhage of cerebellum NOS

✓6th **S06.38 Contusion, laceration, and hemorrhage of brainstem**

11 ✓7th **S06.380 Contusion, laceration, and hemorrhage of brainstem** without loss of consciousness   MCC H5 HCC
CC Excl: No Excl

---

**11** HCC with 7th character indicating initial encounter (A or B - specific to category) OR sequela.

N Newborn: 0   P Pediatric: 0-17   M Maternity: 12-55   A Adult: 15-124   MCC Major CC Condition   PDxMCC PDx acts as own MCC   CC CC Condition   PDxCC PDx acts as own CC

**950**        ICD-10-CM 2018

11 ✓7th **S06.381** **Contusion, laceration, and hemorrhage of brainstem with loss of consciousness of 30 minutes or less** `CC` `H5` `HCC`

11 ✓7th **S06.382** **Contusion, laceration, and hemorrhage of brainstem with loss of consciousness of 31 minutes to 59 minutes** `CC` `H5` `HCC`

11 ✓7th **S06.383** **Contusion, laceration, and hemorrhage of brainstem with loss of consciousness of 1 hour to 5 hours 59 minutes** `CC` `H5` `HCC`

11 ✓7th **S06.384** **Contusion, laceration, and hemorrhage of brainstem with loss of consciousness of 6 hours to 24 hours** `CC` `H5` `HCC`

11 ✓7th **S06.385** **Contusion, laceration, and hemorrhage of brainstem with loss of consciousness greater than 24 hours with return to pre-existing conscious level** `CC` `H5` `HCC`

11 ✓7th **S06.386** **Contusion, laceration, and hemorrhage of brainstem with loss of consciousness greater than 24 hours without return to pre-existing conscious level with patient surviving** `MCC` `H5` `HCC`

✓7th **S06.387** **Contusion, laceration, and hemorrhage of brainstem with loss of consciousness of any duration with death due to brain injury prior to regaining consciousness** `MCC` `H5`

✓7th **S06.388** **Contusion, laceration, and hemorrhage of brainstem with loss of consciousness of any duration with death due to other cause prior to regaining consciousness** `MCC` `H5`

11 ✓7th **S06.389** **Contusion, laceration, and hemorrhage of brainstem with loss of consciousness of unspecified duration** `CC` `H5` `HCC`
Contusion, laceration, and hemorrhage of brainstem NOS

✓5th **S06.4** **Epidural hemorrhage**
Extradural hemorrhage NOS
Extradural hemorrhage (traumatic)

✓6th **S06.4X** **Epidural hemorrhage**

11 ✓7th **S06.4X0** **Epidural hemorrhage without loss of consciousness** `MCC` `H5` `HCC`

11 ✓7th **S06.4X1** **Epidural hemorrhage with loss of consciousness of 30 minutes or less** `MCC` `H5` `HCC`

11 ✓7th **S06.4X2** **Epidural hemorrhage with loss of consciousness of 31 minutes to 59 minutes** `MCC` `H5` `HCC`

11 ✓7th **S06.4X3** **Epidural hemorrhage with loss of consciousness of 1 hour to 5 hours 59 minutes** `MCC` `H5` `HCC`

11 ✓7th **S06.4X4** **Epidural hemorrhage with loss of consciousness of 6 hours to 24 hours** `MCC` `H5` `HCC`

11 ✓7th **S06.4X5** **Epidural hemorrhage with loss of consciousness greater than 24 hours with return to pre-existing conscious level** `MCC` `H5` `HCC`

11 ✓7th **S06.4X6** **Epidural hemorrhage with loss of consciousness greater than 24 hours without return to pre-existing conscious level with patient surviving** `MCC` `H5` `HCC`

✓7th **S06.4X7** **Epidural hemorrhage with loss of consciousness of any duration with death due to brain injury prior to regaining consciousness** `MCC` `H5`

✓7th **S06.4X8** **Epidural hemorrhage with loss of consciousness of any duration with death due to other causes prior to regaining consciousness** `MCC` `H5`

11 ✓7th **S06.4X9** **Epidural hemorrhage with loss of consciousness of unspecified duration** `MCC` `H5` `HCC`
Epidural hemorrhage NOS

✓5th **S06.5** **Traumatic subdural hemorrhage**

✓6th **S06.5X** **Traumatic subdural hemorrhage**

11 ✓7th **S06.5X0** **Traumatic subdural hemorrhage without loss of consciousness** `MCC` `H5` `HCC`

11 ✓7th **S06.5X1** **Traumatic subdural hemorrhage with loss of consciousness of 30 minutes or less** `MCC` `H5` `HCC`

11 ✓7th **S06.5X2** **Traumatic subdural hemorrhage with loss of consciousness of 31 minutes to 59 minutes** `MCC` `H5` `HCC`

11 ✓7th **S06.5X3** **Traumatic subdural hemorrhage with loss of consciousness of 1 hour to 5 hours 59 minutes** `MCC` `H5` `HCC`

11 ✓7th **S06.5X4** **Traumatic subdural hemorrhage with loss of consciousness of 6 hours to 24 hours** `MCC` `H5` `HCC`

11 ✓7th **S06.5X5** **Traumatic subdural hemorrhage with loss of consciousness greater than 24 hours with return to pre-existing conscious level** `MCC` `H5` `HCC`

11 ✓7th **S06.5X6** **Traumatic subdural hemorrhage with loss of consciousness greater than 24 hours without return to pre-existing conscious level with patient surviving** `MCC` `H5` `HCC`

✓7th **S06.5X7** **Traumatic subdural hemorrhage with loss of consciousness of any duration with death due to brain injury before regaining consciousness** `MCC` `H5`

✓7th **S06.5X8** **Traumatic subdural hemorrhage with loss of consciousness of any duration with death due to other cause before regaining consciousness** `MCC` `H5`

11 ✓7th **S06.5X9** **Traumatic subdural hemorrhage with loss of consciousness of unspecified duration** `MCC` `H5` `HCC`
Traumatic subdural hemorrhage NOS

✓5th **S06.6** **Traumatic subarachnoid hemorrhage**

✓6th **S06.6X** **Traumatic subarachnoid hemorrhage**

11 ✓7th **S06.6X0** **Traumatic subarachnoid hemorrhage without loss of consciousness** `MCC` `H5` `HCC`

11 ✓7th **S06.6X1** **Traumatic subarachnoid hemorrhage with loss of consciousness of 30 minutes or less** `MCC` `H5` `HCC`

11 ✓7th **S06.6X2** **Traumatic subarachnoid hemorrhage with loss of consciousness of 31 minutes to 59 minutes** `MCC` `H5` `HCC`

11 ✓7th **S06.6X3** **Traumatic subarachnoid hemorrhage with loss of consciousness of 1 hour to 5 hours 59 minutes** `MCC` `H5` `HCC`

11 ✓7th **S06.6X4** **Traumatic subarachnoid hemorrhage with loss of consciousness of 6 hours to 24 hours** `MCC` `H5` `HCC`

11 ✓7th **S06.6X5** **Traumatic subarachnoid hemorrhage with loss of consciousness greater than 24 hours with return to pre-existing conscious level** `MCC` `H5` `HCC`

11 ✓7th **S06.6X6** **Traumatic subarachnoid hemorrhage with loss of consciousness greater than 24 hours without return to pre-existing conscious level with patient surviving** `MCC` `H5` `HCC`

✓7th **S06.6X7** **Traumatic subarachnoid hemorrhage with loss of consciousness of any duration with death due to brain injury prior to regaining consciousness** `MCC` `H5`

✓7th **S06.6X8** **Traumatic subarachnoid hemorrhage with loss of consciousness of any duration with death due to other cause prior to regaining consciousness** `MCC` `H5`

11 ✓7th **S06.6X9** **Traumatic subarachnoid hemorrhage with loss of consciousness of unspecified duration** `MCC` `H5` `HCC`
Traumatic subarachnoid hemorrhage NOS

---

11 HCC with 7th character indicating initial encounter (A or B - specific to category) OR sequela.

✓Additional Character Req   ✓x7th Placeholder Alert   Unacceptable PDx   Manifestation   `H1`-`H14` HAC   `HCC` CMS-HCC Condition   `EXCLUDES 1` Not Coded Here   `EXCLUDES 2` Not Included Here

☑5ᵗʰ **S06.8** **Other specified intracranial injuries**

  ☑6ᵗʰ **S06.81** **Injury of** right internal carotid artery, intracranial portion, not elsewhere classified

    11 ☑7ᵗʰ **S06.810** **Injury of right internal carotid artery,** HCC **intracranial portion, not elsewhere classified** without loss of consciousness

    11 ☑7ᵗʰ **S06.811** **Injury of right internal carotid** CC H5 HCC **artery, intracranial portion, not elsewhere classified with loss of consciousness of 30 minutes or less**

    11 ☑7ᵗʰ **S06.812** **Injury of right internal carotid** CC H5 HCC **artery, intracranial portion, not elsewhere classified with loss of consciousness of 31 minutes to 59 minutes**

    11 ☑7ᵗʰ **S06.813** **Injury of right internal carotid** CC H5 HCC **artery, intracranial portion, not elsewhere classified with loss of consciousness of 1 hour to 5 hours 59 minutes**

    11 ☑7ᵗʰ **S06.814** **Injury of right internal carotid** CC H5 HCC **artery, intracranial portion, not elsewhere classified with loss of consciousness of 6 hours to 24 hours**

    11 ☑7ᵗʰ **S06.815** **Injury of right internal carotid** CC H5 HCC **artery, intracranial portion, not elsewhere classified with loss of consciousness greater than 24 hours with return to pre-existing conscious level**

    11 ☑7ᵗʰ **S06.816** **Injury of right internal carotid** MCC H5 HCC **artery, intracranial portion, not elsewhere classified with loss of consciousness greater than 24 hours without return to pre-existing conscious level with patient surviving**

    ☑7ᵗʰ **S06.817** **Injury of right internal carotid** MCC H5 **artery, intracranial portion, not elsewhere classified with loss of consciousness of any duration with death due to brain injury prior to regaining consciousness**

    ☑7ᵗʰ **S06.818** **Injury of right internal carotid** MCC H5 **artery, intracranial portion, not elsewhere classified with loss of consciousness of any duration with death due to other cause prior to regaining consciousness**

    11 ☑7ᵗʰ **S06.819** **Injury of right internal carotid** CC H5 HCC **artery, intracranial portion, not elsewhere classified with loss of consciousness of unspecified duration**
         Injury of right internal carotid artery, intracranial portion, not elsewhere classified NOS

  ☑6ᵗʰ **S06.82** **Injury of** left internal carotid artery, intracranial portion, not elsewhere classified

    11 ☑7ᵗʰ **S06.820** **Injury of left internal carotid artery,** HCC **intracranial portion, not elsewhere classified** without loss of consciousness

    11 ☑7ᵗʰ **S06.821** **Injury of left internal carotid** CC H5 HCC **artery, intracranial portion, not elsewhere classified with loss of consciousness of 30 minutes or less**

    11 ☑7ᵗʰ **S06.822** **Injury of left internal carotid** CC H5 HCC **artery, intracranial portion, not elsewhere classified with loss of consciousness of 31 minutes to 59 minutes**

    11 ☑7ᵗʰ **S06.823** **Injury of left internal carotid** CC H5 HCC **artery, intracranial portion, not elsewhere classified with loss of consciousness of 1 hour to 5 hours 59 minutes**

    11 ☑7ᵗʰ **S06.824** **Injury of left internal carotid** CC H5 HCC **artery, intracranial portion, not elsewhere classified with loss of consciousness of 6 hours to 24 hours**

    11 ☑7ᵗʰ **S06.825** **Injury of left internal carotid** CC H5 HCC **artery, intracranial portion, not elsewhere classified with loss of consciousness greater than 24 hours with return to pre-existing conscious level**

    11 ☑7ᵗʰ **S06.826** **Injury of left internal carotid** MCC H5 HCC **artery, intracranial portion, not elsewhere classified with loss of consciousness greater than 24 hours without return to pre-existing conscious level with patient surviving**

    ☑7ᵗʰ **S06.827** **Injury of left internal carotid** MCC H5 **artery, intracranial portion, not elsewhere classified with loss of consciousness of any duration with death due to brain injury prior to regaining consciousness**

    ☑7ᵗʰ **S06.828** **Injury of left internal carotid** MCC H5 **artery, intracranial portion, not elsewhere classified with loss of consciousness of any duration with death due to other cause prior to regaining consciousness**

    11 ☑7ᵗʰ **S06.829** **Injury of left internal carotid** CC H5 HCC **artery, intracranial portion, not elsewhere classified with loss of consciousness of unspecified duration**
         Injury of left internal carotid artery, intracranial portion, not elsewhere classified NOS

  ☑6ᵗʰ **S06.89** **Other specified intracranial injury**
     **EXCLUDES 1** concussion (S06.0X-)

    11 ☑7ᵗʰ **S06.890** **Other specified intracranial injury** HCC **without loss of consciousness**

    11 ☑7ᵗʰ **S06.891** **Other specified intracranial** CC H5 HCC **injury with loss of consciousness of 30 minutes or less**

    11 ☑7ᵗʰ **S06.892** **Other specified intracranial** CC H5 HCC **injury with loss of consciousness of 31 minutes to 59 minutes**

    11 ☑7ᵗʰ **S06.893** **Other specified intracranial** CC H5 HCC **injury with loss of consciousness of 1 hour to 5 hours 59 minutes**

    11 ☑7ᵗʰ **S06.894** **Other specified intracranial** CC H5 HCC **injury with loss of consciousness of 6 hours to 24 hours**

    11 ☑7ᵗʰ **S06.895** **Other specified intracranial** CC H5 HCC **injury with loss of consciousness greater than 24 hours with return to pre-existing conscious level**

    11 ☑7ᵗʰ **S06.896** **Other specified intracranial** MCC H5 HCC **injury with loss of consciousness greater than 24 hours without return to pre-existing conscious level with patient surviving**

    ☑7ᵗʰ **S06.897** **Other specified intracranial injury** MCC H5 **with loss of consciousness of any duration with death due to brain injury prior to regaining consciousness**

    ☑7ᵗʰ **S06.898** **Other specified intracranial injury** MCC H5 **with loss of consciousness of any duration with death due to other cause prior to regaining consciousness**

    11 ☑7ᵗʰ **S06.899** **Other specified intracranial** CC H5 HCC **injury with loss of consciousness of unspecified duration**

☑5ᵗʰ **S06.9** **Unspecified intracranial injury**
     Brain injury NOS
     Head injury NOS with loss of consciousness
     Traumatic brain injury NOS
     **EXCLUDES 1** conditions classifiable to S06.0- to S06.8- code to specified intracranial injury
         head injury NOS (S09.90)

  ☑6ᵗʰ **S06.9X** **Unspecified intracranial injury**

    11 ☑7ᵗʰ **S06.9X0** **Unspecified intracranial injury** HCC **without loss of consciousness**

    11 ☑7ᵗʰ **S06.9X1** **Unspecified intracranial injury** CC H5 HCC **with loss of consciousness of 30 minutes or less**

    11 ☑7ᵗʰ **S06.9X2** **Unspecified intracranial injury** CC H5 HCC **with loss of consciousness of 31 minutes to 59 minutes**

    11 ☑7ᵗʰ **S06.9X3** **Unspecified intracranial injury** CC H5 HCC **with loss of consciousness of 1 hour to 5 hours 59 minutes**

---

11 HCC with 7th character indicating initial encounter (A or B - specific to category) OR sequela.

N Newborn: 0   P Pediatric: 0-17   M Maternity: 12-55   A Adult: 15-124   MCC Major CC Condition   PDxMCC PDx acts as own MCC   CC CC Condition   PDxCC PDx acts as own CC

952             ICD-10-CM 2018

**11** ✓7ᵗʰ **S06.9X4** **Unspecified intracranial injury** CC H5 HCC
**with loss of consciousness of
6 hours to 24 hours**

**11** ✓7ᵗʰ **S06.9X5** **Unspecified intracranial injury** CC H5 HCC
**with loss of consciousness greater
than 24 hours with return to
pre-existing conscious level**

**11** ✓7ᵗʰ **S06.9X6** **Unspecified intracranial injury** MCC H5 HCC
**with loss of consciousness greater
than 24 hours without return to
pre-existing conscious level with
patient surviving**

✓7ᵗʰ **S06.9X7** **Unspecified intracranial injury** MCC H5
**with loss of consciousness of any duration
with death due to brain injury prior
to regaining consciousness**

✓7ᵗʰ **S06.9X8** **Unspecified intracranial injury** MCC H5
**with loss of consciousness of any duration
with death due to other cause prior
to regaining consciousness**

**11** ✓7ᵗʰ **S06.9X9** **Unspecified intracranial injury** CC H5 HCC
**with loss of consciousness of
unspecified duration**

✓4ᵗʰ **S07** **Crushing injury of head**
Use additional code for all associated injuries, such as:
intracranial injuries (S06.-)
skull fractures (S02.-)

The appropriate 7th character is to be added to each code from
category S07.
A     initial encounter
D     subsequent encounter
S     sequela

**CC Excl: For codes in category S07:
CC with 7th character A:** PDX collection 1156

✓x7ᵗʰ **S07.0** **Crushing injury of face** CC H5
✓x7ᵗʰ **S07.1** **Crushing injury of skull** CC H5
✓x7ᵗʰ **S07.8** **Crushing injury of other parts of head** CC H5
✓x7ᵗʰ **S07.9** **Crushing injury of head, part unspecified** CC H5

✓4ᵗʰ **S08** **Avulsion and traumatic amputation of part of head**
An amputation not identified as partial or complete should be coded to
complete

The appropriate 7th character is to be added to each code from
category S08.
A     initial encounter
D     subsequent encounter
S     sequela

✓x7ᵗʰ **S08.0** **Avulsion of scalp**
✓5ᵗʰ **S08.1** **Traumatic amputation of ear**
✓6ᵗʰ **S08.11** **Complete traumatic amputation of ear**
✓7ᵗʰ **S08.111** **Complete traumatic amputation of right
ear**
✓7ᵗʰ **S08.112** **Complete traumatic amputation of left ear**
✓7ᵗʰ **S08.119** **Complete traumatic amputation of
unspecified ear**
✓6ᵗʰ **S08.12** **Partial traumatic amputation of ear**
✓7ᵗʰ **S08.121** **Partial traumatic amputation of right ear**
✓7ᵗʰ **S08.122** **Partial traumatic amputation of left ear**
✓7ᵗʰ **S08.129** **Partial traumatic amputation of
unspecified ear**
✓5ᵗʰ **S08.8** **Traumatic amputation of other parts of head**
✓6ᵗʰ **S08.81** **Traumatic amputation of nose**
✓7ᵗʰ **S08.811** **Complete traumatic amputation of nose**
✓7ᵗʰ **S08.812** **Partial traumatic amputation of nose**
✓x7ᵗʰ **S08.89** **Traumatic amputation of other parts of head**

✓4ᵗʰ **S09** **Other and unspecified injuries of head**

The appropriate 7th character is to be added to each code from
category S09.
A     initial encounter
D     subsequent encounter
S     sequela

**CC Excl: For codes in category S09, unless otherwise noted:
CC with 7th character A:** PDX collection 1158

✓x7ᵗʰ **S09.0** **Injury of blood vessels of head, not elsewhere classified** CC
EXCLUDES 1     injury of cerebral blood vessels (S06.-)
injury of precerebral blood vessels (S15.-)
**CC Excl: CC with 7th character A:** PDX collection 1157

✓5ᵗʰ **S09.1** **Injury of muscle and tendon of head**
Code also any associated open wound (S01.-)
EXCLUDES 2     sprain to joints and ligament of head (S03.9)
✓x7ᵗʰ **S09.10** **Unspecified injury of muscle and tendon of head**
Injury of muscle and tendon of head NOS
✓x7ᵗʰ **S09.11** **Strain of muscle and tendon of head**
✓x7ᵗʰ **S09.12** **Laceration of muscle and tendon of head**
✓x7ᵗʰ **S09.19** **Other specified injury of muscle and tendon of head**

✓5ᵗʰ **S09.2** **Traumatic rupture of ear drum**
EXCLUDES 1     traumatic rupture of ear drum due to blast injury
(S09.31-)
✓x7ᵗʰ **S09.20** **Traumatic rupture of unspecified ear drum** CC
✓x7ᵗʰ **S09.21** **Traumatic rupture of right ear drum** CC
✓x7ᵗʰ **S09.22** **Traumatic rupture of left ear drum** CC

✓5ᵗʰ **S09.3** **Other specified and unspecified injury of middle and inner
ear**
EXCLUDES 1     injury to ear NOS (S09.91-)
EXCLUDES 2     injury to external ear (S00.4-, S01.3-, S08.1-)
✓6ᵗʰ **S09.30** **Unspecified injury of middle and inner ear**
✓7ᵗʰ **S09.301** **Unspecified injury of right middle and** CC
**inner ear**
✓7ᵗʰ **S09.302** **Unspecified injury of left middle and** CC
**inner ear**
✓7ᵗʰ **S09.309** **Unspecified injury of unspecified
middle and inner ear**
✓6ᵗʰ **S09.31** **Primary blast injury of ear**
Blast injury of ear NOS
✓7ᵗʰ **S09.311** **Primary blast injury of right ear** CC
✓7ᵗʰ **S09.312** **Primary blast injury of left ear** CC
✓7ᵗʰ **S09.313** **Primary blast injury of ear, bilateral** CC
✓7ᵗʰ **S09.319** **Primary blast injury of unspecified ear** CC
✓6ᵗʰ **S09.39** **Other specified injury of middle and inner ear**
Secondary blast injury to ear
✓7ᵗʰ **S09.391** **Other specified injury of right middle** CC
**and inner ear**
✓7ᵗʰ **S09.392** **Other specified injury of left middle** CC
**and inner ear**
✓7ᵗʰ **S09.399** **Other specified injury of unspecified** CC
**middle and inner ear**

✓x7ᵗʰ **S09.8** **Other specified injuries of head**
✓5ᵗʰ **S09.9** **Unspecified injury of face and head**
✓x7ᵗʰ **S09.90** **Unspecified injury of head**
Head injury NOS
EXCLUDES 1     brain injury NOS (S06.9-)
head injury NOS with loss of consciousness
(S06.9-)
intracranial injury NOS (S06.9-)
✓x7ᵗʰ **S09.91** **Unspecified injury of ear**
Injury of ear NOS
✓x7ᵗʰ **S09.92** **Unspecified injury of nose**
Injury of nose NOS
✓x7ᵗʰ **S09.93** **Unspecified injury of face**
Injury of face NOS

**11** HCC with 7th character indicating initial encounter (A or B - specific to category) OR sequela.

## Injuries to the neck (S10-S19)

| INCLUDES | injuries of nape |
| | injuries of supraclavicular region |
| | injuries of throat |
| EXCLUDES 2 | burns and corrosions (T20-T32) |
| | effects of foreign body in esophagus (T18.1) |
| | effects of foreign body in larynx (T17.3) |
| | effects of foreign body in pharynx (T17.2) |
| | effects of foreign body in trachea (T17.4) |
| | frostbite (T33-T34) |
| | insect bite or sting, venomous (T63.4) |

### ✓4th S10   Superficial injury of neck

The appropriate 7th character is to be added to each code from category S10.
- A   initial encounter
- D   subsequent encounter
- S   sequela

✓x7th **S10.0**   **Contusion of throat**
Contusion of cervical esophagus
Contusion of larynx
Contusion of pharynx
Contusion of trachea

✓5th **S10.1**   **Other and unspecified superficial injuries of throat**

- ✓x7th **S10.10**   Unspecified superficial injuries of throat
- ✓x7th **S10.11**   Abrasion of throat
- ✓x7th **S10.12**   Blister (nonthermal) of throat
- ✓x7th **S10.14**   External constriction of part of throat
- ✓x7th **S10.15**   Superficial foreign body of throat
  Splinter in the throat
- ✓x7th **S10.16**   Insect bite (nonvenomous) of throat
- ✓x7th **S10.17**   Other superficial bite of throat
  EXCLUDES 1   open bite of throat (S11.85)

✓5th **S10.8**   **Superficial injury of other specified parts of neck**

- ✓x7th **S10.80**   Unspecified superficial injury of other specified part of neck
- ✓x7th **S10.81**   Abrasion of other specified part of neck
- ✓x7th **S10.82**   Blister (nonthermal) of other specified part of neck
- ✓x7th **S10.83**   Contusion of other specified part of neck
- ✓x7th **S10.84**   External constriction of other specified part of neck
- ✓x7th **S10.85**   Superficial foreign body of other specified part of neck
  Splinter in other specified part of neck
- ✓x7th **S10.86**   Insect bite of other specified part of neck
- ✓x7th **S10.87**   Other superficial bite of other specified part of neck
  EXCLUDES 1   open bite of other specified parts of neck (S11.85)

✓5th **S10.9**   **Superficial injury of unspecified part of neck**

- ✓x7th **S10.90**   Unspecified superficial injury of unspecified part of neck
- ✓x7th **S10.91**   Abrasion of unspecified part of neck
- ✓x7th **S10.92**   Blister (nonthermal) of unspecified part of neck
- ✓x7th **S10.93**   Contusion of unspecified part of neck
- ✓x7th **S10.94**   External constriction of unspecified part of neck
- ✓x7th **S10.95**   Superficial foreign body of unspecified part of neck
- ✓x7th **S10.96**   Insect bite of unspecified part of neck
- ✓x7th **S10.97**   Other superficial bite of unspecified part of neck

### ✓4th S11   Open wound of neck

Code also any associated:
   spinal cord injury (S14.0, S14.1-)
   wound infection
EXCLUDES 2   open fracture of vertebra (S12- with 7th B)

The appropriate 7th character is to be added to each code from category S11.
- A   initial encounter
- D   subsequent encounter
- S   sequela

✓5th **S11.0**   **Open wound of larynx and trachea**

CC Excl: For codes in subcategory S11.0, unless otherwise noted:
MCC with 7th character A: PDX collection 1159

✓6th **S11.01**   **Open wound of larynx**
EXCLUDES 2   open wound of vocal cord (S11.03)

- ✓7th **S11.011**   Laceration without foreign body of larynx   MCC
- ✓7th **S11.012**   Laceration with foreign body of larynx   MCC
- ✓7th **S11.013**   Puncture wound without foreign body of larynx   MCC
- ✓7th **S11.014**   Puncture wound with foreign body of larynx   MCC
- ✓7th **S11.015**   Open bite of larynx   MCC
  Bite of larynx NOS
- ✓7th **S11.019**   Unspecified open wound of larynx   MCC

✓6th **S11.02**   **Open wound of trachea**
Open wound of cervical trachea
Open wound of trachea NOS
EXCLUDES 2   open wound of thoracic trachea (S27.5-)

- ✓7th **S11.021**   Laceration without foreign body of trachea   MCC
- ✓7th **S11.022**   Laceration with foreign body of trachea   MCC
- ✓7th **S11.023**   Puncture wound without foreign body of trachea   MCC
- ✓7th **S11.024**   Puncture wound with foreign body of trachea   MCC
- ✓7th **S11.025**   Open bite of trachea   MCC
  Bite of trachea NOS
- ✓7th **S11.029**   Unspecified open wound of trachea   MCC

✓6th **S11.03**   **Open wound of vocal cord**

- ✓7th **S11.031**   Laceration without foreign body of vocal cord   MCC
- ✓7th **S11.032**   Laceration with foreign body of vocal cord   MCC
- ✓7th **S11.033**   Puncture wound without foreign body of vocal cord   MCC
- ✓7th **S11.034**   Puncture wound with foreign body of vocal cord   MCC
- ✓7th **S11.035**   Open bite of vocal cord   MCC
  Bite of vocal cord NOS
- ✓7th **S11.039**   Unspecified open wound of vocal cord   MCC

✓5th **S11.1**   **Open wound of thyroid gland**

CC Excl: For codes in subcategory S11.1, unless otherwise noted:
CC with 7th character A: PDX collection 1160

- ✓x7th **S11.10**   Unspecified open wound of thyroid gland   CC
- ✓x7th **S11.11**   Laceration without foreign body of thyroid gland   CC
- ✓x7th **S11.12**   Laceration with foreign body of thyroid gland   CC
  CC Excl: CC with 7th character A: PDX collection 1161
- ✓x7th **S11.13**   Puncture wound without foreign body of thyroid gland   CC
- ✓x7th **S11.14**   Puncture wound with foreign body of thyroid gland   CC
  CC Excl: CC with 7th character A: PDX collection 1161
- ✓x7th **S11.15**   Open bite of thyroid gland   CC
  Bite of thyroid gland NOS

✓5th **S11.2**   **Open wound of pharynx and cervical esophagus**
EXCLUDES 1   open wound of esophagus NOS (S27.8-)

CC Excl: For codes in subcategory S11.2, unless otherwise noted:
CC with 7th character A: PDX collection 1162

- ✓x7th **S11.20**   Unspecified open wound of pharynx and cervical esophagus   CC
- ✓x7th **S11.21**   Laceration without foreign body of pharynx and cervical esophagus   CC
- ✓x7th **S11.22**   Laceration with foreign body of pharynx and cervical esophagus   CC
  CC Excl: CC with 7th character A: PDX collection 1163
- ✓x7th **S11.23**   Puncture wound without foreign body of pharynx and cervical esophagus   CC

√x7ᵗʰ **S11.24** Puncture wound with foreign body of pharynx and cervical esophagus    `CC`
CC Excl: CC with 7th character A:
PDX collection 1163

√x7ᵗʰ **S11.25** Open bite of pharynx and cervical esophagus    `CC`
Bite of pharynx and cervical esophagus NOS

√5ᵗʰ **S11.8** Open wound of other specified parts of neck

√x7ᵗʰ **S11.80** Unspecified open wound of other specified part of neck

√x7ᵗʰ **S11.81** Laceration without foreign body of other specified part of neck

√x7ᵗʰ **S11.82** Laceration with foreign body of other specified part of neck

√x7ᵗʰ **S11.83** Puncture wound without foreign body of other specified part of neck

√x7ᵗʰ **S11.84** Puncture wound with foreign body of other specified part of neck

√x7ᵗʰ **S11.85** Open bite of other specified part of neck
Bite of other specified part of neck NOS
**EXCLUDES1** *superficial bite of other specified part of neck (S10.87)*

√x7ᵗʰ **S11.89** Other open wound of other specified part of neck

√5ᵗʰ **S11.9** Open wound of unspecified part of neck

√x7ᵗʰ **S11.90** Unspecified open wound of unspecified part of neck

√x7ᵗʰ **S11.91** Laceration without foreign body of unspecified part of neck

√x7ᵗʰ **S11.92** Laceration with foreign body of unspecified part of neck

√x7ᵗʰ **S11.93** Puncture wound without foreign body of unspecified part of neck

√x7ᵗʰ **S11.94** Puncture wound with foreign body of unspecified part of neck

√x7ᵗʰ **S11.95** Open bite of unspecified part of neck
Bite of neck NOS
**EXCLUDES1** *superficial bite of neck (S10.97)*

√4ᵗʰ **S12** Fracture of cervical vertebra and other parts of neck
`NOTE` A fracture not indicated as nondisplaced or displaced should be classified to displaced.
A fracture not indicated as open or closed should be coded to closed.
`INCLUDES` fracture of cervical neural arch
fracture of cervical spine
fracture of cervical spinous process
fracture of cervical transverse process
fracture of cervical vertebral arch
fracture of neck

Code first any associated cervical spinal cord injury (S14.0, S14.1-)
**AHA:** 2015, 3Q, 37-39

The appropriate 7th character is to be added to all codes from subcategories S12.0-S12.6.
A   initial encounter for closed fracture
B   initial encounter for open fracture
D   subsequent encounter for fracture with routine healing
G   subsequent encounter for fracture with delayed healing
K   subsequent encounter for fracture with nonunion
S   sequela

CC Excl: For codes in category S12, unless otherwise noted:
CC with 7th character A or MCC with 7th character B:
PDX collection 1164
CC with 7th character K: PDX collection 897

√5ᵗʰ **S12.0** Fracture of first cervical vertebra
Atlas

√6ᵗʰ **S12.00** Unspecified fracture of first cervical vertebra

6,7,10 √7ᵗʰ **S12.000** Unspecified displaced fracture of first cervical vertebra   `MCC` `CC` `H5` `HCC`

6,7,10 √7ᵗʰ **S12.001** Unspecified nondisplaced fracture of first cervical vertebra   `MCC` `CC` `H5` `HCC`

6,7,10 √x7ᵗʰ **S12.01** Stable burst fracture of first cervical vertebra   `MCC` `CC` `H5` `HCC`

6,7,10 √x7ᵗʰ **S12.02** Unstable burst fracture of first cervical vertebra   `MCC` `CC` `H5` `HCC`

√6ᵗʰ **S12.03** Posterior arch fracture of first cervical vertebra

6,7,10 √7ᵗʰ **S12.030** Displaced posterior arch fracture of first cervical vertebra   `MCC` `CC` `H5` `HCC`

6,7,10 √7ᵗʰ **S12.031** Nondisplaced posterior arch fracture of first cervical vertebra   `MCC` `CC` `H5` `HCC`

√6ᵗʰ **S12.04** Lateral mass fracture of first cervical vertebra

6,7,10 √7ᵗʰ **S12.040** Displaced lateral mass fracture of first cervical vertebra   `MCC` `CC` `H5` `HCC`

6,7,10 √7ᵗʰ **S12.041** Nondisplaced lateral mass fracture of first cervical vertebra   `MCC` `CC` `H5` `HCC`

√6ᵗʰ **S12.09** Other fracture of first cervical vertebra

6,7,10 √7ᵗʰ **S12.090** Other displaced fracture of first cervical vertebra   `MCC` `CC` `H5` `HCC`

6,7,10 √7ᵗʰ **S12.091** Other nondisplaced fracture of first cervical vertebra   `MCC` `CC` `H5` `HCC`

√5ᵗʰ **S12.1** Fracture of second cervical vertebra
Axis

√6ᵗʰ **S12.10** Unspecified fracture of second cervical vertebra

6,7,10 √7ᵗʰ **S12.100** Unspecified displaced fracture of second cervical vertebra   `MCC` `CC` `H5` `HCC`

6,7,10 √7ᵗʰ **S12.101** Unspecified nondisplaced fracture of second cervical vertebra   `MCC` `CC` `H5` `HCC`

√6ᵗʰ **S12.11** Type II dens fracture

6,7,10 √7ᵗʰ **S12.110** Anterior displaced Type II dens fracture   `MCC` `CC` `H5` `HCC`

6,7,10 √7ᵗʰ **S12.111** Posterior displaced Type II dens fracture   `MCC` `CC` `H5` `HCC`

6,7,10 √7ᵗʰ **S12.112** Nondisplaced Type II dens fracture   `MCC` `CC` `H5` `HCC`

√6ᵗʰ **S12.12** Other dens fracture

6,7,10 √7ᵗʰ **S12.120** Other displaced dens fracture   `MCC` `CC` `H5` `HCC`

6,7,10 √7ᵗʰ **S12.121** Other nondisplaced dens fracture   `MCC` `CC` `H5` `HCC`

√6ᵗʰ **S12.13** Unspecified traumatic spondylolisthesis of second cervical vertebra

6,7,10 √7ᵗʰ **S12.130** Unspecified traumatic displaced spondylolisthesis of second cervical vertebra   `MCC` `CC` `H5` `HCC`

6,7,10 √7ᵗʰ **S12.131** Unspecified traumatic nondisplaced spondylolisthesis of second cervical vertebra   `MCC` `CC` `H5` `HCC`

6,7,10 √x7ᵗʰ **S12.14** Type III traumatic spondylolisthesis of second cervical vertebra   `MCC` `CC` `H5` `HCC`

√6ᵗʰ **S12.15** Other traumatic spondylolisthesis of second cervical vertebra

6,7,10 √7ᵗʰ **S12.150** Other traumatic displaced spondylolisthesis of second cervical vertebra   `MCC` `CC` `H5` `HCC`

6,7,10 √7ᵗʰ **S12.151** Other traumatic nondisplaced spondylolisthesis of second cervical vertebra   `MCC` `CC` `H5` `HCC`

√6ᵗʰ **S12.19** Other fracture of second cervical vertebra

6,7,10 √7ᵗʰ **S12.190** Other displaced fracture of second cervical vertebra   `MCC` `CC` `H5` `HCC`

6,7,10 √7ᵗʰ **S12.191** Other nondisplaced fracture of second cervical vertebra   `MCC` `CC` `H5` `HCC`

√5ᵗʰ **S12.2** Fracture of third cervical vertebra

√6ᵗʰ **S12.20** Unspecified fracture of third cervical vertebra

6,7,10 √7ᵗʰ **S12.200** Unspecified displaced fracture of third cervical vertebra   `MCC` `CC` `H5` `HCC`

6,7,10 √7ᵗʰ **S12.201** Unspecified nondisplaced fracture of third cervical vertebra   `MCC` `CC` `H5` `HCC`

√6ᵗʰ **S12.23** Unspecified traumatic spondylolisthesis of third cervical vertebra

6,7,10 √7ᵗʰ **S12.230** Unspecified traumatic displaced spondylolisthesis of third cervical vertebra   `MCC` `CC` `H5` `HCC`

6,7,10 √7ᵗʰ **S12.231** Unspecified traumatic nondisplaced spondylolisthesis of third cervical vertebra   `MCC` `CC` `H5` `HCC`

---

6   MCC when reported as an open fracture (7th character B or C – specific to category).
7   CC when reported as an initial encounter (7th character A, B, or C – specific to category) OR a subsequent encounter for nonunion or malunion (7th character K, M, N, P, Q or R – specific to category).
10   HCC with 7th character indicating initial encounter (A, B or C - specific to category).

√ Additional Character Req    √x7ᵗʰ Placeholder Alert    Unacceptable PDx    Manifestation    `H1`-`H14` HAC    `HCC` CMS-HCC Condition    **EXCLUDES1** Not Coded Here    **EXCLUDES2** Not Included Here

**Chapter 19. Injury, Poisoning and Certain Other Consequences of External Causes**

6,7,10 √x7ᵗʰ **S12.24** Type III traumatic spondylolisthesis of third cervical vertebra `MCC` `CC` `H5` `HCC`

√6ᵗʰ **S12.25** Other traumatic spondylolisthesis of third cervical vertebra

    6,7,10 √7ᵗʰ **S12.250** Other traumatic displaced spondylolisthesis of third cervical vertebra `MCC` `CC` `H5` `HCC`

    6,7,10 √7ᵗʰ **S12.251** Other traumatic nondisplaced spondylolisthesis of third cervical vertebra `MCC` `CC` `H5` `HCC`

√6ᵗʰ **S12.29** Other fracture of third cervical vertebra

    6,7,10 √7ᵗʰ **S12.290** Other displaced fracture of third cervical vertebra `MCC` `CC` `H5` `HCC`

    6,7,10 √7ᵗʰ **S12.291** Other nondisplaced fracture of third cervical vertebra `MCC` `CC` `H5` `HCC`

√5ᵗʰ **S12.3 Fracture of fourth cervical vertebra**

√6ᵗʰ **S12.30** Unspecified fracture of fourth cervical vertebra

    6,7,10 √7ᵗʰ **S12.300** Unspecified displaced fracture of fourth cervical vertebra `MCC` `CC` `H5` `HCC`

    6,7,10 √7ᵗʰ **S12.301** Unspecified nondisplaced fracture of fourth cervical vertebra `MCC` `CC` `H5` `HCC`

√6ᵗʰ **S12.33** Unspecified traumatic spondylolisthesis of fourth cervical vertebra

    6,7,10 √7ᵗʰ **S12.330** Unspecified traumatic displaced spondylolisthesis of fourth cervical vertebra `MCC` `CC` `H5` `HCC`

    6,7,10 √7ᵗʰ **S12.331** Unspecified traumatic nondisplaced spondylolisthesis of fourth cervical vertebra `MCC` `CC` `H5` `HCC`

6,7,10 √x7ᵗʰ **S12.34** Type III traumatic spondylolisthesis of fourth cervical vertebra `MCC` `CC` `H5` `HCC`

√6ᵗʰ **S12.35** Other traumatic spondylolisthesis of fourth cervical vertebra

    6,7,10 √7ᵗʰ **S12.350** Other traumatic displaced spondylolisthesis of fourth cervical vertebra `MCC` `CC` `H5` `HCC`

    6,7,10 √7ᵗʰ **S12.351** Other traumatic nondisplaced spondylolisthesis of fourth cervical vertebra `MCC` `CC` `H5` `HCC`

√6ᵗʰ **S12.39** Other fracture of fourth cervical vertebra

    6,7,10 √7ᵗʰ **S12.390** Other displaced fracture of fourth cervical vertebra `MCC` `CC` `H5` `HCC`

    6,7,10 √7ᵗʰ **S12.391** Other nondisplaced fracture of fourth cervical vertebra `MCC` `CC` `H5` `HCC`

√5ᵗʰ **S12.4 Fracture of fifth cervical vertebra**

√6ᵗʰ **S12.40** Unspecified fracture of fifth cervical vertebra

    6,7,10 √7ᵗʰ **S12.400** Unspecified displaced fracture of fifth cervical vertebra `MCC` `CC` `H5` `HCC`

    6,7,10 √7ᵗʰ **S12.401** Unspecified nondisplaced fracture of fifth cervical vertebra `MCC` `CC` `H5` `HCC`

√6ᵗʰ **S12.43** Unspecified traumatic spondylolisthesis of fifth cervical vertebra

    6,7,10 √7ᵗʰ **S12.430** Unspecified traumatic displaced spondylolisthesis of fifth cervical vertebra `MCC` `CC` `H5` `HCC`

    6,7,10 √7ᵗʰ **S12.431** Unspecified traumatic nondisplaced spondylolisthesis of fifth cervical vertebra `MCC` `CC` `H5` `HCC`

6,7,10 √x7ᵗʰ **S12.44** Type III traumatic spondylolisthesis of fifth cervical vertebra `MCC` `CC` `H5` `HCC`

√6ᵗʰ **S12.45** Other traumatic spondylolisthesis of fifth cervical vertebra

    6,7,10 √7ᵗʰ **S12.450** Other traumatic displaced spondylolisthesis of fifth cervical vertebra `MCC` `CC` `H5` `HCC`

    6,7,10 √7ᵗʰ **S12.451** Other traumatic nondisplaced spondylolisthesis of fifth cervical vertebra `MCC` `CC` `H5` `HCC`

√6ᵗʰ **S12.49** Other fracture of fifth cervical vertebra

    6,7,10 √7ᵗʰ **S12.490** Other displaced fracture of fifth cervical vertebra `MCC` `CC` `H5` `HCC`

6,7,10 √7ᵗʰ **S12.491** Other nondisplaced fracture of fifth cervical vertebra `MCC` `CC` `H5` `HCC`

√5ᵗʰ **S12.5 Fracture of sixth cervical vertebra**

√6ᵗʰ **S12.50** Unspecified fracture of sixth cervical vertebra

    6,7,10 √7ᵗʰ **S12.500** Unspecified displaced fracture of sixth cervical vertebra `MCC` `CC` `H5` `HCC`

    6,7,10 √7ᵗʰ **S12.501** Unspecified nondisplaced fracture of sixth cervical vertebra `MCC` `CC` `H5` `HCC`

√6ᵗʰ **S12.53** Unspecified traumatic spondylolisthesis of sixth cervical vertebra

    6,7,10 √7ᵗʰ **S12.530** Unspecified traumatic displaced spondylolisthesis of sixth cervical vertebra `MCC` `CC` `H5` `HCC`

    6,7,10 √7ᵗʰ **S12.531** Unspecified traumatic nondisplaced spondylolisthesis of sixth cervical vertebra `MCC` `CC` `H5` `HCC`

6,7,10 √x7ᵗʰ **S12.54** Type III traumatic spondylolisthesis of sixth cervical vertebra `MCC` `CC` `H5` `HCC`

√6ᵗʰ **S12.55** Other traumatic spondylolisthesis of sixth cervical vertebra

    6,7,10 √7ᵗʰ **S12.550** Other traumatic displaced spondylolisthesis of sixth cervical vertebra `MCC` `CC` `H5` `HCC`

    6,7,10 √7ᵗʰ **S12.551** Other traumatic nondisplaced spondylolisthesis of sixth cervicalvertebra `MCC` `CC` `H5` `HCC`

√6ᵗʰ **S12.59** Other fracture of sixth cervical vertebra

    6,7,10 √7ᵗʰ **S12.590** Other displaced fracture of sixth cervical vertebra `MCC` `CC` `H5` `HCC`

    6,7,10 √7ᵗʰ **S12.591** Other nondisplaced fracture of sixth cervical vertebra `MCC` `CC` `H5` `HCC`

√5ᵗʰ **S12.6 Fracture of seventh cervical vertebra**

√6ᵗʰ **S12.60** Unspecified fracture of seventh cervical vertebra

    6,7,10 √7ᵗʰ **S12.600** Unspecified displaced fracture of seventh cervical vertebra `MCC` `CC` `H5` `HCC`

    6,7,10 √7ᵗʰ **S12.601** Unspecified nondisplaced fracture of seventh cervical vertebra `MCC` `CC` `H5` `HCC`

√6ᵗʰ **S12.63** Unspecified traumatic spondylolisthesis of seventh cervical vertebra

    6,7,10 √7ᵗʰ **S12.630** Unspecified traumatic displaced spondylolisthesis of seventh cervical vertebra `MCC` `CC` `H5` `HCC`

    6,7,10 √7ᵗʰ **S12.631** Unspecified traumatic nondisplaced spondylolisthesis of seventh cervical vertebra `MCC` `CC` `H5` `HCC`

6,7,10 √x7ᵗʰ **S12.64** Type III traumatic spondylolisthesis of seventh cervical vertebra `MCC` `CC` `H5` `HCC`

√6ᵗʰ **S12.65** Other traumatic spondylolisthesis of seventh cervical vertebra

    6,7,10 √7ᵗʰ **S12.650** Other traumatic displaced spondylolisthesis of seventh cervical vertebra `MCC` `CC` `H5` `HCC`

    6,7,10 √7ᵗʰ **S12.651** Other traumatic nondisplaced spondylolisthesis of seventh cervical vertebra `MCC` `CC` `H5` `HCC`

√6ᵗʰ **S12.69** Other fracture of seventh cervical vertebra

    6,7,10 √7ᵗʰ **S12.690** Other displaced fracture of seventh cervical vertebra `MCC` `CC` `H5` `HCC`

    6,7,10 √7ᵗʰ **S12.691** Other nondisplaced fracture of seventh cervical vertebra `MCC` `CC` `H5` `HCC`

10 √x7ᵗʰ **S12.8 Fracture of other parts of neck** `MCC` `H5` `HCC`

    Hyoid bone       Thyroid cartilage
    Larynx           Trachea

    The appropriate 7th character is to be added to code S12.8.
    A     initial encounter
    D     subsequent encounter
    S     sequela

    **CC Excl: MCC with 7th character A:** PDX collection 1165

---

6   MCC when reported as an open fracture (7th character B or C – specific to category).

7   CC when reported as an initial encounter (7th character A, B, or C – specific to category) OR a subsequent encounter for nonunion or malunion (7th character K, M, N, P, Q, or R – specific to category).

10   HCC with 7th character indicating initial encounter (A, B or C - specific to category).

Ⓝ Newborn: 0   Ⓟ Pediatric: 0-17   Ⓜ Maternity: 12-55   Ⓐ Adult: 15-124   `MCC` Major CC Condition   `PDxMCC` PDx acts as own MCC   `CC` CC Condition   `PDxCC` PDx acts as own CC

**956**                 ICD-10-CM 2018

**10** ✓x7ᵗʰ **S12.9 Fracture of neck, unspecified**   CC H5 HCC
> Fracture of cervical spine NOS
> Fracture of cervical vertebra NOS
> Fracture of neck NOS

> The appropriate 7th character is to be added to code S12.9.
> A    initial encounter
> D    subsequent encounter
> S    sequela

> **CC Excl: CC with 7th character A:** PDX collection 1164

✓4ᵗʰ **S13 Dislocation and sprain of joints and ligaments at neck level**
> INCLUDES   avulsion of joint or ligament at neck level
> laceration of cartilage, joint or ligament at neck level
> sprain of cartilage, joint or ligament at neck level
> traumatic hemarthrosis of joint or ligament at neck level
> traumatic rupture of joint or ligament at neck level
> traumatic subluxation of joint or ligament at neck level
> traumatic tear of joint or ligament at neck level

Code also any associated open wound
> EXCLUDES 2   strain of muscle or tendon at neck level (S16.1)

> The appropriate 7th character is to be added to each code from category S13.
> A    initial encounter
> D    subsequent encounter
> S    sequela

> **CC Excl: For codes in category S13:**
> **CC with 7th character A:** PDX collection 913

✓x7ᵗʰ **S13.0 Traumatic rupture of cervical intervertebral disc**   CC H5
> EXCLUDES 1   rupture or displacement (nontraumatic) of cervical intervertebral disc NOS (M50.-)

✓5ᵗʰ **S13.1 Subluxation and dislocation of cervical vertebrae**
> Code also any associated:
> open wound of neck (S11.-)
> spinal cord injury (S14.1-)
> EXCLUDES 2   fracture of cervical vertebrae (S12.0--S12.3-)

✓6ᵗʰ **S13.10 Subluxation and dislocation of unspecified cervical vertebrae**

✓7ᵗʰ **S13.100 Subluxation of unspecified cervical vertebrae**   CC H5

✓7ᵗʰ **S13.101 Dislocation of unspecified cervical vertebrae**   CC H5

✓6ᵗʰ **S13.11 Subluxation and dislocation of C0/C1 cervical vertebrae**
> Subluxation and dislocation of atlantooccipital joint
> Subluxation and dislocation of atloidooccipital joint
> Subluxation and dislocation of occipitoatloid joint

✓7ᵗʰ **S13.110 Subluxation of C0/C1 cervical vertebrae**   CC H5

✓7ᵗʰ **S13.111 Dislocation of C0/C1 cervical vertebrae**   CC H5

✓6ᵗʰ **S13.12 Subluxation and dislocation of C1/C2 cervical vertebrae**
> Subluxation and dislocation of atlantoaxial joint

✓7ᵗʰ **S13.120 Subluxation of C1/C2 cervical vertebrae**   CC H5

✓7ᵗʰ **S13.121 Dislocation of C1/C2 cervical vertebrae**   CC H5

✓6ᵗʰ **S13.13 Subluxation and dislocation of C2/C3 cervical vertebrae**

✓7ᵗʰ **S13.130 Subluxation of C2/C3 cervical vertebrae**   CC H5

✓7ᵗʰ **S13.131 Dislocation of C2/C3 cervical vertebrae**   CC H5

✓6ᵗʰ **S13.14 Subluxation and dislocation of C3/C4 cervical vertebrae**

✓7ᵗʰ **S13.140 Subluxation of C3/C4 cervical vertebrae**   CC H5

✓7ᵗʰ **S13.141 Dislocation of C3/C4 cervical vertebrae**   CC H5

✓6ᵗʰ **S13.15 Subluxation and dislocation of C4/C5 cervical vertebrae**

✓7ᵗʰ **S13.150 Subluxation of C4/C5 cervical vertebrae**   CC H5

✓7ᵗʰ **S13.151 Dislocation of C4/C5 cervical vertebrae**   CC H5

✓6ᵗʰ **S13.16 Subluxation and dislocation of C5/C6 cervical vertebrae**

✓7ᵗʰ **S13.160 Subluxation of C5/C6 cervical vertebrae**   CC H5

✓7ᵗʰ **S13.161 Dislocation of C5/C6 cervical vertebrae**   CC H5

✓6ᵗʰ **S13.17 Subluxation and dislocation of C6/C7 cervical vertebrae**

✓7ᵗʰ **S13.170 Subluxation of C6/C7 cervical vertebrae**   CC H5

✓7ᵗʰ **S13.171 Dislocation of C6/C7 cervical vertebrae**   CC H5

✓6ᵗʰ **S13.18 Subluxation and dislocation of C7/T1 cervical vertebrae**

✓7ᵗʰ **S13.180 Subluxation of C7/T1 cervical vertebrae**   CC H5

✓7ᵗʰ **S13.181 Dislocation of C7/T1 cervical vertebrae**   CC H5

✓5ᵗʰ **S13.2 Dislocation of other and unspecified parts of neck**

**S13.20 Dislocation of unspecified parts of neck**   CC H5

**S13.29 Dislocation of other parts of neck**   CC H5

✓x7ᵗʰ **S13.4 Sprain of ligaments of cervical spine**
> Sprain of anterior longitudinal (ligament), cervical
> Sprain of atlanto-axial (joints)
> Sprain of atlanto-occipital (joints)
> Whiplash injury of cervical spine

✓x7ᵗʰ **S13.5 Sprain of thyroid region**
> Sprain of cricoarytenoid (joint) (ligament)
> Sprain of cricothyroid (joint) (ligament)
> Sprain of thyroid cartilage

✓x7ᵗʰ **S13.8 Sprain of joints and ligaments of other parts of neck**

✓x7ᵗʰ **S13.9 Sprain of joints and ligaments of unspecified parts of neck**

✓4ᵗʰ **S14 Injury of nerves and spinal cord at neck level**
> NOTE   Code to highest level of cervical cord injury.
> Code also any associated:
> fracture of cervical vertebra (S12.0- – S12.6-)
> open wound of neck (S11.-)
> transient paralysis (R29.5)

> The appropriate 7th character is to be added to each code from category S14.
> A    initial encounter
> D    subsequent encounter
> S    sequela

> **CC Excl: For codes in category S14:**
> **MCC with 7th character A:** PDX collection 1166

✓x7ᵗʰ **S14.0 Concussion and edema of cervical spinal cord**   MCC HCC

✓5ᵗʰ **S14.1 Other and unspecified injuries of cervical spinal cord**

✓6ᵗʰ **S14.10 Unspecified injury of cervical spinal cord**

✓7ᵗʰ **S14.101 Unspecified injury at C1 level of cervical spinal cord**   MCC H5 HCC

✓7ᵗʰ **S14.102 Unspecified injury at C2 level of cervical spinal cord**   MCC H5 HCC

✓7ᵗʰ **S14.103 Unspecified injury at C3 level of cervical spinal cord**   MCC H5 HCC

✓7ᵗʰ **S14.104 Unspecified injury at C4 level of cervical spinal cord**   MCC H5 HCC

✓7ᵗʰ **S14.105 Unspecified injury at C5 level of cervical spinal cord**   MCC H5 HCC

✓7ᵗʰ **S14.106 Unspecified injury at C6 level of cervical spinal cord**   MCC H5 HCC

✓7ᵗʰ **S14.107 Unspecified injury at C7 level of cervical spinal cord**   MCC H5 HCC

✓7ᵗʰ **S14.108 Unspecified injury at C8 level of cervical spinal cord**   MCC HCC

✓7ᵗʰ **S14.109 Unspecified injury at unspecified level of cervical spinal cord**   H5 HCC
> Injury of cervical spinal cord NOS

✓6ᵗʰ **S14.11 Complete lesion of cervical spinal cord**

✓7ᵗʰ **S14.111 Complete lesion at C1 level of cervical spinal cord**   MCC H5 HCC

✓7ᵗʰ **S14.112 Complete lesion at C2 level of cervical spinal cord**   MCC H5 HCC

---

**10** HCC with 7th character indicating initial encounter (A, B or C - specific to category).

✓ Additional Character Req   ✓x7ᵗʰ Placeholder Alert   Unacceptable PDx   Manifestation   H1-H14 HAC   HCC CMS-HCC Condition   EXCLUDES 1 Not Coded Here   EXCLUDES 2 Not Included Here

√7ᵗʰ **S14.113** **Complete lesion at C3 level of cervical spinal cord** MCC H5 HCC

√7ᵗʰ **S14.114** **Complete lesion at C4 level of cervical spinal cord** MCC H5 HCC

√7ᵗʰ **S14.115** **Complete lesion at C5 level of cervical spinal cord** MCC H5 HCC

√7ᵗʰ **S14.116** **Complete lesion at C6 level of cervical spinal cord** MCC H5 HCC

√7ᵗʰ **S14.117** **Complete lesion at C7 level of cervical spinal cord** MCC H5 HCC

√7ᵗʰ **S14.118** **Complete lesion at C8 level of cervical spinal cord** MCC HCC

√7ᵗʰ **S14.119** **Complete lesion at unspecified level of cervical spinal cord** HCC

√6ᵗʰ **S14.12** **Central cord syndrome of cervical spinal cord**

√7ᵗʰ **S14.121** **Central cord syndrome at C1 level of cervical spinal cord** MCC H5 HCC

√7ᵗʰ **S14.122** **Central cord syndrome at C2 level of cervical spinal cord** MCC H5 HCC

√7ᵗʰ **S14.123** **Central cord syndrome at C3 level of cervical spinal cord** MCC H5 HCC

√7ᵗʰ **S14.124** **Central cord syndrome at C4 level of cervical spinal cord** MCC H5 HCC

√7ᵗʰ **S14.125** **Central cord syndrome at C5 level of cervical spinal cord** MCC H5 HCC

√7ᵗʰ **S14.126** **Central cord syndrome at C6 level of cervical spinal cord** MCC H5 HCC

√7ᵗʰ **S14.127** **Central cord syndrome at C7 level of cervical spinal cord** MCC H5 HCC

√7ᵗʰ **S14.128** **Central cord syndrome at C8 level of cervical spinal cord** MCC HCC

√7ᵗʰ **S14.129** **Central cord syndrome at unspecified level of cervical spinal cord** HCC

√6ᵗʰ **S14.13** **Anterior cord syndrome of cervical spinal cord**

√7ᵗʰ **S14.131** **Anterior cord syndrome at C1 level of cervical spinal cord** MCC H5 HCC

√7ᵗʰ **S14.132** **Anterior cord syndrome at C2 level of cervical spinal cord** MCC H5 HCC

√7ᵗʰ **S14.133** **Anterior cord syndrome at C3 level of cervical spinal cord** MCC H5 HCC

√7ᵗʰ **S14.134** **Anterior cord syndrome at C4 level of cervical spinal cord** MCC H5 HCC

√7ᵗʰ **S14.135** **Anterior cord syndrome at C5 level of cervical spinal cord** MCC H5 HCC

√7ᵗʰ **S14.136** **Anterior cord syndrome at C6 level of cervical spinal cord** MCC H5 HCC

√7ᵗʰ **S14.137** **Anterior cord syndrome at C7 level of cervical spinal cord** MCC H5 HCC

√7ᵗʰ **S14.138** **Anterior cord syndrome at C8 level of cervical spinal cord** MCC HCC

√7ᵗʰ **S14.139** **Anterior cord syndrome at unspecified level of cervical spinal cord** HCC

√6ᵗʰ **S14.14** **Brown-Séquard syndrome of cervical spinal cord**

√7ᵗʰ **S14.141** **Brown-Séquard syndrome at C1 level of cervical spinal cord** MCC HCC

√7ᵗʰ **S14.142** **Brown-Séquard syndrome at C2 level of cervical spinal cord** MCC HCC

√7ᵗʰ **S14.143** **Brown-Séquard syndrome at C3 level of cervical spinal cord** MCC HCC

√7ᵗʰ **S14.144** **Brown-Séquard syndrome at C4 level of cervical spinal cord** MCC HCC

√7ᵗʰ **S14.145** **Brown-Séquard syndrome at C5 level of cervical spinal cord** MCC HCC

√7ᵗʰ **S14.146** **Brown-Séquard syndrome at C6 level of cervical spinal cord** MCC HCC

√7ᵗʰ **S14.147** **Brown-Séquard syndrome at C7 level of cervical spinal cord** MCC HCC

√7ᵗʰ **S14.148** **Brown-Séquard syndrome at C8 level of cervical spinal cord** MCC HCC

√7ᵗʰ **S14.149** **Brown-Séquard syndrome at unspecified level of cervical spinal cord** HCC

√6ᵗʰ **S14.15** **Other incomplete lesions of cervical spinal cord**
Incomplete lesion of cervical spinal cord NOS
Posterior cord syndrome of cervical spinal cord

√7ᵗʰ **S14.151** **Other incomplete lesion at C1 level of cervical spinal cord** MCC H5 HCC

√7ᵗʰ **S14.152** **Other incomplete lesion at C2 level of cervical spinal cord** MCC H5 HCC

√7ᵗʰ **S14.153** **Other incomplete lesion at C3 level of cervical spinal cord** MCC H5 HCC

√7ᵗʰ **S14.154** **Other incomplete lesion at C4 level of cervical spinal cord** MCC H5 HCC

√7ᵗʰ **S14.155** **Other incomplete lesion at C5 level of cervical spinal cord** MCC H5 HCC

√7ᵗʰ **S14.156** **Other incomplete lesion at C6 level of cervical spinal cord** MCC H5 HCC

√7ᵗʰ **S14.157** **Other incomplete lesion at C7 level of cervical spinal cord** MCC H5 HCC

√7ᵗʰ **S14.158** **Other incomplete lesion at C8 level of cervical spinal cord** MCC HCC

√7ᵗʰ **S14.159** **Other incomplete lesion at unspecified level of cervical spinal cord** HCC

√x7ᵗʰ **S14.2** **Injury of nerve root of cervical spine**

√x7ᵗʰ **S14.3** **Injury of brachial plexus**

√x7ᵗʰ **S14.4** **Injury of peripheral nerves of neck**

√x7ᵗʰ **S14.5** **Injury of cervical sympathetic nerves**

√x7ᵗʰ **S14.8** **Injury of other specified nerves of neck**

√x7ᵗʰ **S14.9** **Injury of unspecified nerves of neck**

√4ᵗʰ **S15** **Injury of blood vessels at neck level**
Code also any associated open wound (S11.-)

The appropriate 7th character is to be added to each code from category S15.
A    initial encounter
D    subsequent encounter
S    sequela

**CC Excl: For codes in category S15, unless otherwise noted:
CC with 7th character A:** PDX collection 1157

√5ᵗʰ **S15.0** **Injury of carotid artery of neck**
Injury of carotid artery (common) (external) (internal, extracranial portion)
Injury of carotid artery NOS
*EXCLUDES 1*   injury of internal carotid artery, intracranial portion (S06.8)

**CC Excl: For codes in subcategory S15.0:
CC with 7th character A:** PDX collection 1167

√6ᵗʰ **S15.00** **Unspecified injury of carotid artery**

√7ᵗʰ **S15.001** **Unspecified injury of right carotid artery** CC

√7ᵗʰ **S15.002** **Unspecified injury of left carotid artery** CC

√7ᵗʰ **S15.009** **Unspecified injury of unspecified carotid artery** CC

√6ᵗʰ **S15.01** **Minor laceration of carotid artery**
Incomplete transection of carotid artery
Laceration of carotid artery NOS
Superficial laceration of carotid artery

√7ᵗʰ **S15.011** **Minor laceration of right carotid artery** CC

√7ᵗʰ **S15.012** **Minor laceration of left carotid artery** CC

√7ᵗʰ **S15.019** **Minor laceration of unspecified carotid artery** CC

√6ᵗʰ **S15.02** **Major laceration of carotid artery**
Complete transection of carotid artery
Traumatic rupture of carotid artery

√7ᵗʰ **S15.021** **Major laceration of right carotid artery** CC

√7ᵗʰ **S15.022** **Major laceration of left carotid artery** CC

√7ᵗʰ **S15.029** **Major laceration of unspecified carotid artery** CC

√6ᵗʰ **S15.09** **Other specified injury of carotid artery**

√7ᵗʰ **S15.091** **Other specified injury of right carotid artery** CC

√7ᵗʰ **S15.092** **Other specified injury of left carotid artery** CC

N Newborn: 0   P Pediatric: 0-17   M Maternity: 12-55   A Adult: 15-124   MCC Major CC Condition   PDxMCC PDx acts as own MCC   CC CC Condition   PDxCC PDx acts as own CC

958        ICD-10-CM 2018

☑7th **S15.099** Other specified injury of unspecified carotid artery **CC**

☑5th **S15.1** Injury of vertebral artery

  ☑6th **S15.10** Unspecified injury of vertebral artery

    ☑7th **S15.101** Unspecified injury of right vertebral artery **CC**

    ☑7th **S15.102** Unspecified injury of left vertebral artery **CC**

    ☑7th **S15.109** Unspecified injury of unspecified vertebral artery **CC**

  ☑6th **S15.11** Minor laceration of vertebral artery
    Incomplete transection of vertebral artery
    Laceration of vertebral artery NOS
    Superficial laceration of vertebral artery

    ☑7th **S15.111** Minor laceration of right vertebral artery **CC**

    ☑7th **S15.112** Minor laceration of left vertebral artery **CC**

    ☑7th **S15.119** Minor laceration of unspecified vertebral artery **CC**

  ☑6th **S15.12** Major laceration of vertebral artery
    Complete transection of vertebral artery
    Traumatic rupture of vertebral artery

    ☑7th **S15.121** Major laceration of right vertebral artery **CC**

    ☑7th **S15.122** Major laceration of left vertebral artery **CC**

    ☑7th **S15.129** Major laceration of unspecified vertebral artery **CC**

  ☑6th **S15.19** Other specified injury of vertebral artery

    ☑7th **S15.191** Other specified injury of right vertebral artery **CC**

    ☑7th **S15.192** Other specified injury of left vertebral artery **CC**

    ☑7th **S15.199** Other specified injury of unspecified vertebral artery **CC**

☑5th **S15.2** Injury of external jugular vein

  ☑6th **S15.20** Unspecified injury of external jugular vein

    ☑7th **S15.201** Unspecified injury of right external jugular vein **CC**

    ☑7th **S15.202** Unspecified injury of left external jugular vein **CC**

    ☑7th **S15.209** Unspecified injury of unspecified external jugular vein **CC**

  ☑6th **S15.21** Minor laceration of external jugular vein
    Incomplete transection of external jugular vein
    Laceration of external jugular vein NOS
    Superficial laceration of external jugular vein

    ☑7th **S15.211** Minor laceration of right external jugular vein **CC**

    ☑7th **S15.212** Minor laceration of left external jugular vein **CC**

    ☑7th **S15.219** Minor laceration of unspecified external jugular vein **CC**

  ☑6th **S15.22** Major laceration of external jugular vein
    Complete transection of external jugular vein
    Traumatic rupture of external jugular vein

    ☑7th **S15.221** Major laceration of right external jugular vein **CC**

    ☑7th **S15.222** Major laceration of left external jugular vein **CC**

    ☑7th **S15.229** Major laceration of unspecified external jugular vein **CC**

  ☑6th **S15.29** Other specified injury of external jugular vein

    ☑7th **S15.291** Other specified injury of right external jugular vein **CC**

    ☑7th **S15.292** Other specified injury of left external jugular vein **CC**

    ☑7th **S15.299** Other specified injury of unspecified external jugular vein **CC**

☑5th **S15.3** Injury of internal jugular vein

  ☑6th **S15.30** Unspecified injury of internal jugular vein

    ☑7th **S15.301** Unspecified injury of right internal jugular vein **CC**

    ☑7th **S15.302** Unspecified injury of left internal jugular vein **CC**

    ☑7th **S15.309** Unspecified injury of unspecified internal jugular vein **CC**

  ☑6th **S15.31** Minor laceration of internal jugular vein
    Incomplete transection of internal jugular vein
    Laceration of internal jugular vein NOS
    Superficial laceration of internal jugular vein

    ☑7th **S15.311** Minor laceration of right internal jugular vein **CC**

    ☑7th **S15.312** Minor laceration of left internal jugular vein **CC**

    ☑7th **S15.319** Minor laceration of unspecified internal jugular vein **CC**

  ☑6th **S15.32** Major laceration of internal jugular vein
    Complete transection of internal jugular vein
    Traumatic rupture of internal jugular vein

    ☑7th **S15.321** Major laceration of right internal jugular vein **CC**

    ☑7th **S15.322** Major laceration of left internal jugular vein **CC**

    ☑7th **S15.329** Major laceration of unspecified internal jugular vein **CC**

  ☑6th **S15.39** Other specified injury of internal jugular vein

    ☑7th **S15.391** Other specified injury of right internal jugular vein **CC**

    ☑7th **S15.392** Other specified injury of left internal jugular vein **CC**

    ☑7th **S15.399** Other specified injury of unspecified internal jugular vein **CC**

☑x7th **S15.8** Injury of other specified blood vessels at neck level **CC**

☑x7th **S15.9** Injury of unspecified blood vessel at neck level **CC**

☑4th **S16** **Injury of muscle, fascia and tendon at neck level**
    Code also any associated open wound (S11.-)
    *EXCLUDES 2*   sprain of joint or ligament at neck level (S13.9)

    The appropriate 7th character is to be added to each code from category S16.
    A    initial encounter
    D    subsequent encounter
    S    sequela

☑x7th **S16.1** Strain of muscle, fascia and tendon at neck level

☑x7th **S16.2** Laceration of muscle, fascia and tendon at neck level

☑x7th **S16.8** Other specified injury of muscle, fascia and tendon at neck level

☑x7th **S16.9** Unspecified injury of muscle, fascia and tendon at neck level

☑4th **S17** **Crushing injury of neck**
    Use additional code for all associated injuries, such as:
      injury of blood vessels (S15.-)
      open wound of neck (S11.-)
      spinal cord injury (S14.0, S14.1-)
      vertebral fracture (S12.0- – S12.3-)

    The appropriate 7th character is to be added to each code from category S17.
    A    initial encounter
    D    subsequent encounter
    S    sequela

    **CC Excl: For codes in category S17:**
    **CC with 7th character A:** PDX collection 1156

☑x7th **S17.0** Crushing injury of larynx and trachea **CC** **H5**

☑x7th **S17.8** Crushing injury of other specified parts of neck **CC** **H5**

☑x7th **S17.9** Crushing injury of neck, part unspecified **CC** **H5**

☑4th **S19** **Other specified and unspecified injuries of neck**

    The appropriate 7th character is to be added to each code from category S19.
    A    initial encounter
    D    subsequent encounter
    S    sequela

☑5th **S19.8** Other specified injuries of neck

  ☑x7th **S19.80** Other specified injuries of unspecified part of neck

  ☑x7th **S19.81** Other specified injuries of larynx

√x7ᵗʰ **S19.82** **Other specified injuries of cervical** trachea
> EXCLUDES 2   *other specified injury of thoracic trachea (S27.5-)*

√x7ᵗʰ **S19.83** **Other specified injuries of** vocal cord

√x7ᵗʰ **S19.84** **Other specified injuries of** thyroid gland

√x7ᵗʰ **S19.85** **Other specified injuries of** pharynx and cervical esophagus

√x7ᵗʰ **S19.89** **Other specified injuries of** other specified part of neck

√x7ᵗʰ **S19.9** **Unspecified injury of neck**

### Injuries to the thorax (S20-S29)

INCLUDES   injuries of breast
injuries of chest (wall)
injuries of interscapular area
EXCLUDES 2   *burns and corrosions (T20-T32)*
*effects of foreign body in bronchus (T17.5)*
*effects of foreign body in esophagus (T18.1)*
*effects of foreign body in lung (T17.8)*
*effects of foreign body in trachea (T17.4)*
*frostbite (T33-T34)*
*injuries of axilla*
*injuries of clavicle*
*injuries of scapular region*
*injuries of shoulder*
*insect bite or sting, venomous (T63.4)*

√4ᵗʰ **S20** **Superficial injury of thorax**

> The appropriate 7th character is to be added to each code from category S20.
> A    initial encounter
> D    subsequent encounter
> S    sequela

√5ᵗʰ **S20.0** **Contusion** of breast

√x7ᵗʰ **S20.00** **Contusion of breast,** unspecified breast

√x7ᵗʰ **S20.01** **Contusion of** right breast

√x7ᵗʰ **S20.02** **Contusion of** left breast

√5ᵗʰ **S20.1** **Other and unspecified superficial injuries of breast**

√6ᵗʰ **S20.10** Unspecified **superficial injuries of breast**

√7ᵗʰ **S20.101** **Unspecified superficial injuries of breast,** right breast

√7ᵗʰ **S20.102** **Unspecified superficial injuries of breast,** left breast

√7ᵗʰ **S20.109** **Unspecified superficial injuries of breast,** unspecified breast

√6ᵗʰ **S20.11** Abrasion **of breast**

√7ᵗʰ **S20.111** **Abrasion of breast,** right breast

√7ᵗʰ **S20.112** **Abrasion of breast,** left breast

√7ᵗʰ **S20.119** **Abrasion of breast,** unspecified breast

√6ᵗʰ **S20.12** Blister (nonthermal) **of breast**

√7ᵗʰ **S20.121** **Blister (nonthermal) of breast,** right breast

√7ᵗʰ **S20.122** **Blister (nonthermal) of breast,** left breast

√7ᵗʰ **S20.129** **Blister (nonthermal) of breast,** unspecified breast

√6ᵗʰ **S20.14** External constriction **of part of breast**

√7ᵗʰ **S20.141** **External constriction of part of breast,** right breast

√7ᵗʰ **S20.142** **External constriction of part of breast,** left breast

√7ᵗʰ **S20.149** **External constriction of part of breast,** unspecified breast

√6ᵗʰ **S20.15** **Superficial** foreign body **of breast**
Splinter in the breast

√7ᵗʰ **S20.151** **Superficial foreign body of breast,** right breast

√7ᵗʰ **S20.152** **Superficial foreign body of breast,** left breast

√7ᵗʰ **S20.159** **Superficial foreign body of breast,** unspecified breast

√6ᵗʰ **S20.16** Insect bite (nonvenomous) **of breast**

√7ᵗʰ **S20.161** **Insect bite (nonvenomous) of breast,** right breast

√7ᵗʰ **S20.162** **Insect bite (nonvenomous) of breast,** left breast

√7ᵗʰ **S20.169** **Insect bite (nonvenomous) of breast,** unspecified breast

√6ᵗʰ **S20.17** Other **superficial** bite **of breast**
> EXCLUDES 1   *open bite of breast (S21.05-)*

√7ᵗʰ **S20.171** **Other superficial bite of breast,** right breast

√7ᵗʰ **S20.172** **Other superficial bite of breast,** left breast

√7ᵗʰ **S20.179** **Other superficial bite of breast,** unspecified breast

√5ᵗʰ **S20.2** **Contusion of thorax**

√x7ᵗʰ **S20.20** **Contusion of thorax,** unspecified

√6ᵗʰ **S20.21** **Contusion of** front wall **of thorax**

√7ᵗʰ **S20.211** **Contusion of** right **front wall of thorax**

√7ᵗʰ **S20.212** **Contusion of** left **front wall of thorax**

√7ᵗʰ **S20.219** **Contusion of** unspecified **front wall of thorax**

√6ᵗʰ **S20.22** **Contusion of** back wall **of thorax**

√7ᵗʰ **S20.221** **Contusion of** right **back wall of thorax**

√7ᵗʰ **S20.222** **Contusion of** left **back wall of thorax**

√7ᵗʰ **S20.229** **Contusion of** unspecified **back wall of thorax**

√5ᵗʰ **S20.3** **Other and unspecified superficial injuries of** front wall **of thorax**

√6ᵗʰ **S20.30** Unspecified **superficial injuries of front wall of thorax**

√7ᵗʰ **S20.301** **Unspecified superficial injuries of** right **front wall of thorax**

√7ᵗʰ **S20.302** **Unspecified superficial injuries of** left **front wall of thorax**

√7ᵗʰ **S20.309** **Unspecified superficial injuries of** unspecified **front wall of thorax**

√6ᵗʰ **S20.31** Abrasion **of front wall of thorax**

√7ᵗʰ **S20.311** **Abrasion of** right **front wall of thorax**

√7ᵗʰ **S20.312** **Abrasion of** left **front wall of thorax**

√7ᵗʰ **S20.319** **Abrasion of** unspecified **front wall of thorax**

√6ᵗʰ **S20.32** Blister (nonthermal) **of front wall of thorax**

√7ᵗʰ **S20.321** **Blister (nonthermal) of** right **front wall of thorax**

√7ᵗʰ **S20.322** **Blister (nonthermal) of** left **front wall of thorax**

√7ᵗʰ **S20.329** **Blister (nonthermal) of** unspecified **front wall of thorax**

√6ᵗʰ **S20.34** External constriction **of front wall of thorax**

√7ᵗʰ **S20.341** **External constriction of** right **front wall of thorax**

√7ᵗʰ **S20.342** **External constriction of** left **front wall of thorax**

√7ᵗʰ **S20.349** **External constriction of** unspecified **front wall of thorax**

√6ᵗʰ **S20.35** Superficial foreign body **of front wall of thorax**
Splinter in front wall of thorax

√7ᵗʰ **S20.351** **Superficial foreign body of** right **front wall of thorax**

√7ᵗʰ **S20.352** **Superficial foreign body of** left **front wall of thorax**

√7ᵗʰ **S20.359** **Superficial foreign body of** unspecified **front wall of thorax**

√6ᵗʰ **S20.36** Insect bite (nonvenomous) **of front wall of thorax**

√7ᵗʰ **S20.361** **Insect bite (nonvenomous) of** right **front wall of thorax**

√7ᵗʰ **S20.362** **Insect bite (nonvenomous) of** left **front wall of thorax**

√7ᵗʰ **S20.369** **Insect bite (nonvenomous) of** unspecified **front wall of thorax**

√6ᵗʰ **S20.37** Other superficial bite **of front wall of thorax**
> EXCLUDES 1   *open bite of front wall of thorax (S21.14)*

√7ᵗʰ **S20.371** **Other superficial bite of** right **front wall of thorax**

√7ᵗʰ **S20.372** **Other superficial bite of** left **front wall of thorax**

√7ᵗʰ **S20.379** **Other superficial bite of** unspecified **front wall of thorax**

√5th **S20.4** **Other and unspecified superficial injuries of** back wall of thorax

  √6th **S20.40** **Unspecified superficial injuries of back wall of thorax**

    √7th **S20.401** **Unspecified superficial injuries of** right **back wall of thorax**

    √7th **S20.402** **Unspecified superficial injuries of** left **back wall of thorax**

    √7th **S20.409** **Unspecified superficial injuries of** unspecified **back wall of thorax**

  √6th **S20.41** **Abrasion of back wall of thorax**

    √7th **S20.411** **Abrasion of** right **back wall of thorax**

    √7th **S20.412** **Abrasion of** left **back wall of thorax**

    √7th **S20.419** **Abrasion of** unspecified **back wall of thorax**

  √6th **S20.42** **Blister (nonthermal) of back wall of thorax**

    √7th **S20.421** **Blister (nonthermal) of** right **back wall of thorax**

    √7th **S20.422** **Blister (nonthermal) of** left **back wall of thorax**

    √7th **S20.429** **Blister (nonthermal) of** unspecified **back wall of thorax**

  √6th **S20.44** **External constriction of back wall of thorax**

    √7th **S20.441** **External constriction of** right **back wall of thorax**

    √7th **S20.442** **External constriction of** left **back wall of thorax**

    √7th **S20.449** **External constriction of** unspecified **back wall of thorax**

  √6th **S20.45** **Superficial** foreign body **of back wall of thorax**
    Splinter of back wall of thorax

    √7th **S20.451** **Superficial foreign body of** right **back wall of thorax**

    √7th **S20.452** **Superficial foreign body of** left **back wall of thorax**

    √7th **S20.459** **Superficial foreign body of** unspecified **back wall of thorax**

  √6th **S20.46** **Insect bite (nonvenomous) of back wall of thorax**

    √7th **S20.461** **Insect bite (nonvenomous) of** right **back wall of thorax**

    √7th **S20.462** **Insect bite (nonvenomous) of** left **back wall of thorax**

    √7th **S20.469** **Insect bite (nonvenomous) of** unspecified **back wall of thorax**

  √6th **S20.47** **Other superficial** bite **of back wall of thorax**
    *EXCLUDES 1*   *open bite of back wall of thorax (S21.24)*

    √7th **S20.471** **Other superficial bite of** right **back wall of thorax**

    √7th **S20.472** **Other superficial bite of** left **back wall of thorax**

    √7th **S20.479** **Other superficial bite of** unspecified **back wall of thorax**

√5th **S20.9** **Superficial injury of unspecified parts of thorax**
    *EXCLUDES 1*   *contusion of thorax NOS (S20.20)*

  √x7th **S20.90** **Unspecified superficial injury of** unspecified **parts of thorax**
    Superficial injury of thoracic wall NOS

  √x7th **S20.91** **Abrasion of unspecified parts of thorax**

  √x7th **S20.92** **Blister (nonthermal) of unspecified parts of thorax**

  √x7th **S20.94** **External constriction of unspecified parts of thorax**

  √x7th **S20.95** **Superficial** foreign body **of unspecified parts of thorax**
    Splinter in thorax NOS

  √x7th **S20.96** **Insect bite (nonvenomous) of unspecified parts of thorax**

  √x7th **S20.97** **Other superficial** bite **of unspecified parts of thorax**
    *EXCLUDES 1*   *open bite of thorax NOS (S21.95)*

√4th **S21** **Open wound of thorax**
    Code also any associated injury, such as:
    injury of heart (S26.-)
    injury of intrathoracic organs (S27.-)
    rib fracture (S22.3-, S22.4-)
    spinal cord injury (S24.0-, S24.1-)
    traumatic hemopneumothorax (S27.3)
    traumatic hemothorax (S27.1)
    traumatic pneumothorax (S27.0)
    wound infection
    *EXCLUDES 1*   *traumatic amputation (partial) of thorax (S28.1)*

> The appropriate 7th character is to be added to each code from category S21.
> A     initial encounter
> D     subsequent encounter
> S     sequela

√5th **S21.0** **Open wound of** breast

  √6th **S21.00** **Unspecified** open wound of breast

    √7th **S21.001** **Unspecified open wound of** right **breast**

    √7th **S21.002** **Unspecified open wound of** left **breast**

    √7th **S21.009** **Unspecified open wound of** unspecified **breast**

  √6th **S21.01** **Laceration without foreign body of breast**

    √7th **S21.011** **Laceration without foreign body of** right **breast**

    √7th **S21.012** **Laceration without foreign body of** left **breast**

    √7th **S21.019** **Laceration without foreign body of** unspecified **breast**

  √6th **S21.02** **Laceration with foreign body of breast**

    √7th **S21.021** **Laceration with foreign body of** right **breast**

    √7th **S21.022** **Laceration with foreign body of** left **breast**

    √7th **S21.029** **Laceration with foreign body of** unspecified **breast**

  √6th **S21.03** **Puncture wound without foreign body of breast**

    √7th **S21.031** **Puncture wound without foreign body of** right **breast**

    √7th **S21.032** **Puncture wound without foreign body of** left **breast**

    √7th **S21.039** **Puncture wound without foreign body of** unspecified **breast**

  √6th **S21.04** **Puncture wound with foreign body of breast**

    √7th **S21.041** **Puncture wound with foreign body of** right **breast**

    √7th **S21.042** **Puncture wound with foreign body of** left **breast**

    √7th **S21.049** **Puncture wound with foreign body of** unspecified **breast**

  √6th **S21.05** **Open bite of breast**
    Bite of breast NOS
    *EXCLUDES 1*   *superficial bite of breast (S20.17)*

    √7th **S21.051** **Open bite of** right **breast**

    √7th **S21.052** **Open bite of** left **breast**

    √7th **S21.059** **Open bite of** unspecified **breast**

√5th **S21.1** **Open wound of** front wall of thorax without penetration into thoracic cavity
    Open wound of chest without penetration into thoracic cavity

> **CC Excl: For codes in subcategory S21.1:**
> **CC with 7th character A:** PDX collection 1168

  √6th **S21.10** **Unspecified** open wound of front wall of thorax without penetration into thoracic cavity

    √7th **S21.101** **Unspecified open wound of** right **front** `CC` **wall of thorax without penetration into thoracic cavity**

    √7th **S21.102** **Unspecified open wound of** left **front** `CC` **wall of thorax without penetration into thoracic cavity**

    √7th **S21.109** **Unspecified open wound of** `CC` unspecified **front wall of thorax without penetration into thoracic cavity**

√ Additional Character Req   √x7th Placeholder Alert   Unacceptable PDx   Manifestation   **H1**-**H14** HAC   **HCC** CMS-HCC Condition   *EXCLUDES 1* Not Coded Here   *EXCLUDES 2* Not Included Here

ICD-10-CM 2018        **961**

✓6ᵗʰ **S21.11** Laceration without foreign body of front wall of thorax without penetration into thoracic cavity

     ✓7ᵗʰ **S21.111** **Laceration without foreign body of** CC **right front wall of thorax without penetration into thoracic cavity**

     ✓7ᵗʰ **S21.112** **Laceration without foreign body of** CC **left front wall of thorax without penetration into thoracic cavity**

     ✓7ᵗʰ **S21.119** **Laceration without foreign body of** CC **unspecified front wall of thorax without penetration into thoracic cavity**

✓6ᵗʰ **S21.12** Laceration with foreign body of front wall of thorax without penetration into thoracic cavity

     ✓7ᵗʰ **S21.121** **Laceration with foreign body of right** CC **front wall of thorax without penetration into thoracic cavity**

     ✓7ᵗʰ **S21.122** **Laceration with foreign body of left** CC **front wall of thorax without penetration into thoracic cavity**

     ✓7ᵗʰ **S21.129** **Laceration with foreign body of** CC **unspecified front wall of thorax without penetration into thoracic cavity**

✓6ᵗʰ **S21.13** Puncture wound without foreign body of front wall of thorax without penetration into thoracic cavity

     ✓7ᵗʰ **S21.131** **Puncture wound without foreign body** CC **of right front wall of thorax without penetration into thoracic cavity**

     ✓7ᵗʰ **S21.132** **Puncture wound without foreign body** CC **of left front wall of thorax without penetration into thoracic cavity**

     ✓7ᵗʰ **S21.139** **Puncture wound without foreign body** CC **of unspecified front wall of thorax without penetration into thoracic cavity**

✓6ᵗʰ **S21.14** Puncture wound with foreign body of front wall of thorax without penetration into thoracic cavity

     ✓7ᵗʰ **S21.141** **Puncture wound with foreign body of** CC **right front wall of thorax without penetration into thoracic cavity**

     ✓7ᵗʰ **S21.142** **Puncture wound with foreign body of** CC **left front wall of thorax without penetration into thoracic cavity**

     ✓7ᵗʰ **S21.149** **Puncture wound with foreign body of** CC **unspecified front wall of thorax without penetration into thoracic cavity**

✓6ᵗʰ **S21.15** Open bite of front wall of thorax without penetration into thoracic cavity

     Bite of front wall of thorax NOS

     *EXCLUDES 1*   *superficial bite of front wall of thorax (S20.37)*

     ✓7ᵗʰ **S21.151** **Open bite of right front wall of thorax** **without penetration into thoracic cavity**

     ✓7ᵗʰ **S21.152** **Open bite of left front wall of thorax** CC **without penetration into thoracic cavity**

     ✓7ᵗʰ **S21.159** **Open bite of unspecified front wall of** CC **thorax without penetration into thoracic cavity**

✓5ᵗʰ **S21.2** Open wound of back wall of thorax without penetration into thoracic cavity

     ✓6ᵗʰ **S21.20** Unspecified open wound of back wall of thorax without penetration into thoracic cavity

         ✓7ᵗʰ **S21.201** **Unspecified open wound of right back** **wall of thorax without penetration into thoracic cavity**

         ✓7ᵗʰ **S21.202** **Unspecified open wound of left back wall** **of thorax without penetration into thoracic cavity**

         ✓7ᵗʰ **S21.209** **Unspecified open wound of unspecified** **back wall of thorax without penetration into thoracic cavity**

     ✓6ᵗʰ **S21.21** Laceration without foreign body of back wall of thorax without penetration into thoracic cavity

         ✓7ᵗʰ **S21.211** **Laceration without foreign body of right** **back wall of thorax without penetration into thoracic cavity**

         ✓7ᵗʰ **S21.212** **Laceration without foreign body of left** **back wall of thorax without penetration into thoracic cavity**

✓7ᵗʰ **S21.219** **Laceration without foreign body of** **unspecified back wall of thorax without penetration into thoracic cavity**

✓6ᵗʰ **S21.22** Laceration with foreign body of back wall of thorax without penetration into thoracic cavity

     ✓7ᵗʰ **S21.221** **Laceration with foreign body of right back** **wall of thorax without penetration into thoracic cavity**

     ✓7ᵗʰ **S21.222** **Laceration with foreign body of left back** **wall of thorax without penetration into thoracic cavity**

     ✓7ᵗʰ **S21.229** **Laceration with foreign body of** **unspecified back wall of thorax without penetration into thoracic cavity**

✓6ᵗʰ **S21.23** Puncture wound without foreign body of back wall of thorax without penetration into thoracic cavity

     ✓7ᵗʰ **S21.231** **Puncture wound without foreign body of** **right back wall of thorax without penetration into thoracic cavity**

     ✓7ᵗʰ **S21.232** **Puncture wound without foreign body of** **left back wall of thorax without penetration into thoracic cavity**

     ✓7ᵗʰ **S21.239** **Puncture wound without foreign body of** **unspecified back wall of thorax without penetration into thoracic cavity**

✓6ᵗʰ **S21.24** Puncture wound with foreign body of back wall of thorax without penetration into thoracic cavity

     ✓7ᵗʰ **S21.241** **Puncture wound with foreign body of** **right back wall of thorax without penetration into thoracic cavity**

     ✓7ᵗʰ **S21.242** **Puncture wound with foreign body of left** **back wall of thorax without penetration into thoracic cavity**

     ✓7ᵗʰ **S21.249** **Puncture wound with foreign body of** **unspecified back wall of thorax without penetration into thoracic cavity**

✓6ᵗʰ **S21.25** Open bite of back wall of thorax without penetration into thoracic cavity

     Bite of back wall of thorax NOS

     *EXCLUDES 1*   *superficial bite of back wall of thorax (S20.47)*

     ✓7ᵗʰ **S21.251** **Open bite of right back wall of thorax** **without penetration into thoracic cavity**

     ✓7ᵗʰ **S21.252** **Open bite of left back wall of thorax** **without penetration into thoracic cavity**

     ✓7ᵗʰ **S21.259** **Open bite of unspecified back wall of** **thorax without penetration into thoracic cavity**

✓5ᵗʰ **S21.3** Open wound of front wall of thorax with penetration into thoracic cavity

     Open wound of chest with penetration into thoracic cavity

     **CC Excl: For codes in subcategory S21.3, unless otherwise noted:**
     **MCC with 7th character A:** PDX collection 1169

     ✓6ᵗʰ **S21.30** Unspecified open wound of front wall of thorax with penetration into thoracic cavity

         ✓7ᵗʰ **S21.301** **Unspecified open wound of right** MCC **front wall of thorax with penetration into thoracic cavity**

         ✓7ᵗʰ **S21.302** **Unspecified open wound of left front** MCC **wall of thorax with penetration into thoracic cavity**

         ✓7ᵗʰ **S21.309** **Unspecified open wound of** MCC **unspecified front wall of thorax with penetration into thoracic cavity**
             **CC Excl: MCC with 7th character A:** PDX collection 1170

     ✓6ᵗʰ **S21.31** Laceration without foreign body of front wall of thorax with penetration into thoracic cavity

         ✓7ᵗʰ **S21.311** **Laceration without foreign body of** MCC **right front wall of thorax with penetration into thoracic cavity**

         ✓7ᵗʰ **S21.312** **Laceration without foreign body of** MCC **left front wall of thorax with penetration into thoracic cavity**

         ✓7ᵗʰ **S21.319** **Laceration without foreign body of** MCC **unspecified front wall of thorax with penetration into thoracic cavity**

Ⓝ Newborn: 0   Ⓟ Pediatric: 0-17   Ⓜ Maternity: 12-55   Ⓐ Adult: 15-124   MCC Major CC Condition   PDxMCC PDx acts as own MCC   CC CC Condition   PDxCC PDx acts as own CC

**962**      ICD-10-CM 2018

✓6th **S21.32** Laceration with foreign body of front wall of thorax with penetration into thoracic cavity

  ✓7th **S21.321** Laceration with foreign body of right front wall of thorax with penetration into thoracic cavity   MCC

  ✓7th **S21.322** Laceration with foreign body of left front wall of thorax with penetration into thoracic cavity   MCC

  ✓7th **S21.329** Laceration with foreign body of unspecified front wall of thorax with penetration into thoracic cavity   MCC

✓6th **S21.33** Puncture wound without foreign body of front wall of thorax with penetration into thoracic cavity

  ✓7th **S21.331** Puncture wound without foreign body of right front wall of thorax with penetration into thoracic cavity   MCC

  ✓7th **S21.332** Puncture wound without foreign body of left front wall of thorax with penetration into thoracic cavity   MCC

  ✓7th **S21.339** Puncture wound without foreign body of unspecified front wall of thorax with penetration into thoracic cavity   MCC

✓6th **S21.34** Puncture wound with foreign body of front wall of thorax with penetration into thoracic cavity

  ✓7th **S21.341** Puncture wound with foreign body of right front wall of thorax with penetration into thoracic cavity   MCC

  ✓7th **S21.342** Puncture wound with foreign body of left front wall of thorax with penetration into thoracic cavity   MCC

  ✓7th **S21.349** Puncture wound with foreign body of unspecified front wall of thorax with penetration into thoracic cavity   MCC

✓6th **S21.35** Open bite of front wall of thorax with penetration into thoracic cavity

  **EXCLUDES 1** *superficial bite of front wall of thorax (S20.37)*

  ✓7th **S21.351** Open bite of right front wall of thorax with penetration into thoracic cavity   MCC

  ✓7th **S21.352** Open bite of left front wall of thorax with penetration into thoracic cavity   MCC

  ✓7th **S21.359** Open bite of unspecified front wall of thorax with penetration into thoracic cavity   MCC

✓5th **S21.4** Open wound of back wall of thorax with penetration into thoracic cavity

  **CC Excl:** For codes in subcategory S21.4:
  **MCC with 7th character A:** PDX collection 1169

  ✓6th **S21.40** Unspecified open wound of back wall of thorax with penetration into thoracic cavity

    ✓7th **S21.401** Unspecified open wound of right back wall of thorax with penetration into thoracic cavity   MCC

    ✓7th **S21.402** Unspecified open wound of left back wall of thorax with penetration into thoracic cavity   MCC

    ✓7th **S21.409** Unspecified open wound of unspecified back wall of thorax with penetration into thoracic cavity   MCC

  ✓6th **S21.41** Laceration without foreign body of back wall of thorax with penetration into thoracic cavity

    ✓7th **S21.411** Laceration without foreign body of right back wall of thorax with penetration into thoracic cavity   MCC

    ✓7th **S21.412** Laceration without foreign body of left back wall of thorax with penetration into thoracic cavity   MCC

    ✓7th **S21.419** Laceration without foreign body of unspecified back wall of thorax with penetration into thoracic cavity   MCC

✓6th **S21.42** Laceration with foreign body of back wall of thorax with penetration into thoracic cavity

  ✓7th **S21.421** Laceration with foreign body of right back wall of thorax with penetration into thoracic cavity   MCC

  ✓7th **S21.422** Laceration with foreign body of left back wall of thorax with penetration into thoracic cavity   MCC

  ✓7th **S21.429** Laceration with foreign body of unspecified back wall of thorax with penetration into thoracic cavity   MCC

✓6th **S21.43** Puncture wound without foreign body of back wall of thorax with penetration into thoracic cavity

  ✓7th **S21.431** Puncture wound without foreign body of right back wall of thorax with penetration into thoracic cavity   MCC

  ✓7th **S21.432** Puncture wound without foreign body of left back wall of thorax with penetration into thoracic cavity   MCC

  ✓7th **S21.439** Puncture wound without foreign body of unspecified back wall of thorax with penetration into thoracic cavity   MCC

✓6th **S21.44** Puncture wound with foreign body of back wall of thorax with penetration into thoracic cavity

  ✓7th **S21.441** Puncture wound with foreign body of right back wall of thorax with penetration into thoracic cavity   MCC

  ✓7th **S21.442** Puncture wound with foreign body of left back wall of thorax with penetration into thoracic cavity   MCC

  ✓7th **S21.449** Puncture wound with foreign body of unspecified back wall of thorax with penetration into thoracic cavity   MCC

✓6th **S21.45** Open bite of back wall of thorax with penetration into thoracic cavity

  Bite of back wall of thorax NOS
  **EXCLUDES 1** *superficial bite of back wall of thorax (S20.47)*

  ✓7th **S21.451** Open bite of right back wall of thorax with penetration into thoracic cavity   MCC

  ✓7th **S21.452** Open bite of left back wall of thorax with penetration into thoracic cavity   MCC

  ✓7th **S21.459** Open bite of unspecified back wall of thorax with penetration into thoracic cavity   MCC

✓5th **S21.9** Open wound of unspecified part of thorax

  Open wound of thoracic wall NOS

  **CC Excl:** For codes in subcategory S21.9:
  **CC with 7th character A:** PDX collection 1168

  ✓x7th **S21.90** Unspecified open wound of unspecified part of thorax   CC

  ✓x7th **S21.91** Laceration without foreign body of unspecified part of thorax   CC

  ✓x7th **S21.92** Laceration with foreign body of unspecified part of thorax   CC

  ✓x7th **S21.93** Puncture wound without foreign body of unspecified part of thorax   CC

  ✓x7th **S21.94** Puncture wound with foreign body of unspecified part of thorax   CC

  ✓x7th **S21.95** Open bite of unspecified part of thorax   CC

    **EXCLUDES 1** *superficial bite of thorax (S20.97)*

---

✓ Additional Character Req   ✓x7th Placeholder Alert   Unacceptable PDx   Manifestation   H1 - H14 HAC   HCC CMS-HCC Condition   **EXCLUDES 1** Not Coded Here   **EXCLUDES 2** Not Included Here

ICD-10-CM 2018     **963**

☑4th **S22** **Fracture of rib(s), sternum and thoracic spine**

**NOTE** A fracture not indicated as nondisplaced or displaced should be coded to displaced.
A fracture not indicated as open or closed should be coded to closed.

**INCLUDES** fracture of thoracic neural arch
fracture of thoracic spinous process
fracture of thoracic transverse process
fracture of thoracic vertebra
fracture of thoracic vertebral arch

Code first any associated:
injury of intrathoracic organ (S27.-)
spinal cord injury (S24.0-, S24.1-)

**EXCLUDES 1** transection of thorax (S28.1)
**EXCLUDES 2** fracture of clavicle (S42.0-)
fracture of scapula (S42.1-)

**AHA:** 2015, 3Q, 37-39

The appropriate 7th character is to be added to each code from category S22.
A    initial encounter for closed fracture
B    initial encounter for open fracture
D    subsequent encounter for fracture with routine healing
G    subsequent encounter for fracture with delayed healing
K    subsequent encounter for fracture with nonunion
S    sequela

☑5th **S22.0** **Fracture of thoracic vertebra**

**CC Excl: For codes in subcategory S22.0:**
**CC with 7th character A or MCC with 7th character B:** PDX collection 1171
**CC with 7th character K:** PDX collection 897

☑6th **S22.00** **Fracture of unspecified thoracic vertebra**

6, 7, 10 ☑7th **S22.000** Wedge compression fracture of unspecified thoracic vertebra | MCC CC H5 HCC

6,7,10 ☑7th **S22.001** Stable burst fracture of unspecified thoracic vertebra | MCC CC H5 HCC

6,7,10 ☑7th **S22.002** Unstable burst fracture of unspecified thoracic vertebra | MCC CC H5 HCC

6,7,10 ☑7th **S22.008** Other fracture of unspecified thoracic vertebra | MCC CC H5 HCC

6,7,10 ☑7th **S22.009** Unspecified fracture of unspecified thoracic vertebra | MCC CC H5 HCC

☑6th **S22.01** **Fracture of first thoracic vertebra**

6,7,10 ☑7th **S22.010** Wedge compression fracture of first thoracic vertebra | MCC CC H5 HCC

6,7,10 ☑7th **S22.011** Stable burst fracture of first thoracic vertebra | MCC CC H5 HCC

6,7,10 ☑7th **S22.012** Unstable burst fracture of first thoracic vertebra | MCC CC H5 HCC

6,7,10 ☑7th **S22.018** Other fracture of first thoracic vertebra | MCC CC H5 HCC

6,7,10 ☑7th **S22.019** Unspecified fracture of first thoracic vertebra | MCC CC H5 HCC

☑6th **S22.02** **Fracture of second thoracic vertebra**

6,7,10 ☑7th **S22.020** Wedge compression fracture of second thoracic vertebra | MCC CC H5 HCC

6,7,10 ☑7th **S22.021** Stable burst fracture of second thoracic vertebra | MCC CC H5 HCC

6,7,10 ☑7th **S22.022** Unstable burst fracture of second thoracic vertebra | MCC CC H5 HCC

6,7,10 ☑7th **S22.028** Other fracture of second thoracic vertebra | MCC CC H5 HCC

6,7,10 ☑7th **S22.029** Unspecified fracture of second thoracic vertebra | MCC CC H5 HCC

☑6th **S22.03** **Fracture of third thoracic vertebra**

6,7,10 ☑7th **S22.030** Wedge compression fracture of third thoracic vertebra | MCC CC H5 HCC

6,7,10 ☑7th **S22.031** Stable burst fracture of third thoracic vertebra | MCC CC H5 HCC

6,7,10 ☑7th **S22.032** Unstable burst fracture of third thoracic vertebra | MCC CC H5 HCC

6,7,10 ☑7th **S22.038** Other fracture of third thoracic vertebra | MCC CC H5 HCC

6,7,10 ☑7th **S22.039** Unspecified fracture of third thoracic vertebra | MCC CC H5 HCC

☑6th **S22.04** **Fracture of fourth thoracic vertebra**

6,7,10 ☑7th **S22.040** Wedge compression fracture of fourth thoracic vertebra | MCC CC H5 HCC

6,7,10 ☑7th **S22.041** Stable burst fracture of fourth thoracic vertebra | MCC CC H5 HCC

6,7,10 ☑7th **S22.042** Unstable burst fracture of fourth thoracic vertebra | MCC CC H5 HCC

6,7,10 ☑7th **S22.048** Other fracture of fourth thoracic vertebra | MCC CC H5 HCC

6,7,10 ☑7th **S22.049** Unspecified fracture of fourth thoracic vertebra | MCC CC H5 HCC

☑6th **S22.05** **Fracture of T5-T6 vertebra**

6,7,10 ☑7th **S22.050** Wedge compression fracture of T5-T6 vertebra | MCC CC H5 HCC

6,7,10 ☑7th **S22.051** Stable burst fracture of T5-T6 vertebra | MCC CC H5 HCC

6,7,10 ☑7th **S22.052** Unstable burst fracture of T5-T6 vertebra | MCC CC H5 HCC

6,7,10 ☑7th **S22.058** Other fracture of T5-T6 vertebra | MCC CC H5 HCC

6,7,10 ☑7th **S22.059** Unspecified fracture of T5-T6 vertebra | MCC CC H5 HCC

☑6th **S22.06** **Fracture of T7-T8 vertebra**

6,7,10 ☑7th **S22.060** Wedge compression fracture of T7-T8 vertebra | MCC CC H5 HCC

6,7,10 ☑7th **S22.061** Stable burst fracture of T7-T8 vertebra | MCC CC H5 HCC

6,7,10 ☑7th **S22.062** Unstable burst fracture of T7-T8 vertebra | MCC CC H5 HCC

6,7,10 ☑7th **S22.068** Other fracture of T7-T8 thoracic vertebra | MCC CC H5 HCC

6,7,10 ☑7th **S22.069** Unspecified fracture of T7-T8 vertebra | MCC CC H5 HCC

☑6th **S22.07** **Fracture of T9-T10 vertebra**

6,7,10 ☑7th **S22.070** Wedge compression fracture of T9-T10 vertebra | MCC CC H5 HCC

6,7,10 ☑7th **S22.071** Stable burst fracture of T9-T10 vertebra | MCC CC H5 HCC

6,7,10 ☑7th **S22.072** Unstable burst fracture of T9-T10 vertebra | MCC CC H5 HCC

6,7,10 ☑7th **S22.078** Other fracture of T9-T10 vertebra | MCC CC H5 HCC

6,7,10 ☑7th **S22.079** Unspecified fracture of T9-T10 vertebra | MCC CC H5 HCC

☑6th **S22.08** **Fracture of T11-T12 vertebra**

6,7,10 ☑7th **S22.080** Wedge compression fracture of T11-T12 vertebra | MCC CC H5 HCC

6,7,10 ☑7th **S22.081** Stable burst fracture of T11-T12 vertebra | MCC CC H5 HCC

6,7,10 ☑7th **S22.082** Unstable burst fracture of T11-T12 vertebra | MCC CC H5 HCC

6,7,10 ☑7th **S22.088** Other fracture of T11-T12 vertebra | MCC CC H5 HCC

6,7,10 ☑7th **S22.089** Unspecified fracture of T11-T12 vertebra | MCC CC H5 HCC

☑5th **S22.2** **Fracture of sternum**

**DEF:** Break in flat bone (breast bone) in anterior thorax; caused by blunt trauma to anterior chest.

**CC Excl: For codes in subcategory S22.2:**
**CC with 7th character A or MCC with 7th character B:** PDX collection 1172
**CC with 7th character K:** PDX collection 897

6,7 ☑x7th **S22.20** Unspecified fracture of sternum | MCC CC H5

6,7 ☑x7th **S22.21** Fracture of manubrium | MCC CC H5

6,7 ☑x7th **S22.22** Fracture of body of sternum | MCC CC H5

6,7 ☑x7th **S22.23** Sternal manubrial dissociation | MCC CC H5

---

6 MCC when reported as an open fracture (7th character B or C – specific to category).
7 CC when reported as an initial encounter (7th character A, B, or C – specific to category) OR a subsequent encounter for nonunion or malunion (7th character K, M, N, P, Q, or R – specific to category).
10 HCC with 7th character indicating initial encounter (A, B or C - specific to category).

6,7   √x7ᵗʰ   **S22.24**   **Fracture of** xiphoid process    MCC CC H5

√5ᵗʰ   **S22.3**   **Fracture of** one rib

> CC Excl: For codes in subcategory S22.3:
> CC with 7th character A: PDX collection 1173
> MCC with 7th character B: PDX collection 1174
> CC with 7th character K: PDX collection 897

6,7   √x7ᵗʰ   **S22.31**   **Fracture of one rib,** right **side**   MCC CC H5

6,7   √x7ᵗʰ   **S22.32**   **Fracture of one rib,** left **side**   MCC CC H5

6,7   √x7ᵗʰ   **S22.39**   **Fracture of one rib,** unspecified **side**   MCC CC H5

√5ᵗʰ   **S22.4**   **Multiple fractures of ribs**
    Fractures of two or more ribs
    EXCLUDES 1   flail chest (S22.5-)

> CC Excl: For codes in subcategory S22.4, unless
> otherwise noted: CC with 7th character A or MCC with
> 7th character B: PDX collection 1174
> CC with 7th character K: PDX collection 897

6,7   √x7ᵗʰ   **S22.41**   **Multiple fractures of ribs,** right **side**   MCC CC H5

6,7   √x7ᵗʰ   **S22.42**   **Multiple fractures of ribs,** left **side**   MCC CC H5

6,7   √x7ᵗʰ   **S22.43**   **Multiple fractures of ribs,** bilateral   MCC CC H5

6,7   √x7ᵗʰ   **S22.49**   **Multiple fractures of ribs,** unspecified **side**   MCC CC H5
    CC Excl: CC with 7th character A: PDX collection 1174
    MCC with 7th character B: No Excl
    CC with 7th character K: PDX collection 897

8   √x7ᵗʰ   **S22.5**   **Flail chest**   MCC CC H5
    CC Excl: CC with 7th character A or
    MCC with 7th character B: PDX collection 1175
    CC with 7th character K: PDX collection 897

6,7   √x7ᵗʰ   **S22.9**   **Fracture of bony thorax, part unspecified**   MCC CC H5
    CC Excl: CC with 7th character A or
    MCC with 7th character B: PDX collection 1176
    CC with 7th character K: PDX collection 897

√4ᵗʰ   **S23**   **Dislocation and sprain of joints and ligaments of thorax**
    INCLUDES   avulsion of joint or ligament of thorax
      laceration of cartilage, joint or ligament of thorax
      sprain of cartilage, joint or ligament of thorax
      traumatic hemarthrosis of joint or ligament of thorax
      traumatic rupture of joint or ligament of thorax
      traumatic subluxation of joint or ligament of thorax
      traumatic tear of joint or ligament of thorax

Code also any associated open wound
    EXCLUDES 2   dislocation, sprain of sternoclavicular joint (S43.2, S43.6)
       strain of muscle or tendon of thorax (S29.01-)

> The appropriate 7th character is to be added to each code from
> category S23.
> A   initial encounter
> D   subsequent encounter
> S   sequela

√x7ᵗʰ   **S23.0**   **Traumatic rupture of thoracic intervertebral disc**
    EXCLUDES 1   rupture or displacement (nontraumatic) of thoracic
      intervertebral disc NOS (M51- with fifth
      character 4)

√5ᵗʰ   **S23.1**   **Subluxation and dislocation of thoracic vertebra**
    Code also any associated
      open wound of thorax (S21.-)
      spinal cord injury (S24.0-, S24.1-)
    EXCLUDES 2   fracture of thoracic vertebrae (S22.0-)

   √6ᵗʰ   **S23.10**   **Subluxation and dislocation of** unspecified **thoracic vertebra**

     √7ᵗʰ   **S23.100**   **Subluxation of** unspecified thoracic **vertebra**

     √7ᵗʰ   **S23.101**   **Dislocation of** unspecified thoracic **vertebra**

   √6ᵗʰ   **S23.11**   **Subluxation and dislocation of** T1/T2 **thoracic vertebra**

     √7ᵗʰ   **S23.110**   **Subluxation of** T1/T2 thoracic vertebra

     √7ᵗʰ   **S23.111**   **Dislocation of** T1/T2 thoracic vertebra

   √6ᵗʰ   **S23.12**   **Subluxation and dislocation of** T2/T3-T3/T4 **thoracic vertebra**

     √7ᵗʰ   **S23.120**   **Subluxation of** T2/T3 thoracic vertebra

     √7ᵗʰ   **S23.121**   **Dislocation of** T2/T3 thoracic vertebra

     √7ᵗʰ   **S23.122**   **Subluxation of** T3/T4 thoracic vertebra

     √7ᵗʰ   **S23.123**   **Dislocation of** T3/T4 thoracic vertebra

   √6ᵗʰ   **S23.13**   **Subluxation and dislocation of T4/T5-T5/T6 thoracic vertebra**

     √7ᵗʰ   **S23.130**   **Subluxation of T4/T5 thoracic vertebra**

     √7ᵗʰ   **S23.131**   **Dislocation of T4/T5 thoracic vertebra**

     √7ᵗʰ   **S23.132**   **Subluxation of T5/T6 thoracic vertebra**

     √7ᵗʰ   **S23.133**   **Dislocation of T5/T6 thoracic vertebra**

   √6ᵗʰ   **S23.14**   **Subluxation and dislocation of T6/T7-T7/T8 thoracic vertebra**

     √7ᵗʰ   **S23.140**   **Subluxation of T6/T7 thoracic vertebra**

     √7ᵗʰ   **S23.141**   **Dislocation of T6/T7 thoracic vertebra**

     √7ᵗʰ   **S23.142**   **Subluxation of T7/T8 thoracic vertebra**

     √7ᵗʰ   **S23.143**   **Dislocation of T7/T8 thoracic vertebra**

   √6ᵗʰ   **S23.15**   **Subluxation and dislocation of T8/T9-T9/T10 thoracic vertebra**

     √7ᵗʰ   **S23.150**   **Subluxation of T8/T9 thoracic vertebra**

     √7ᵗʰ   **S23.151**   **Dislocation of T8/T9 thoracic vertebra**

     √7ᵗʰ   **S23.152**   **Subluxation of T9/T10 thoracic vertebra**

     √7ᵗʰ   **S23.153**   **Dislocation of T9/T10 thoracic vertebra**

   √6ᵗʰ   **S23.16**   **Subluxation and dislocation of T10/T11-T11/T12 thoracic vertebra**

     √7ᵗʰ   **S23.160**   **Subluxation of T10/T11 thoracic vertebra**

     √7ᵗʰ   **S23.161**   **Dislocation of T10/T11 thoracic vertebra**

     √7ᵗʰ   **S23.162**   **Subluxation of T11/T12 thoracic vertebra**

     √7ᵗʰ   **S23.163**   **Dislocation of T11/T12 thoracic vertebra**

   √6ᵗʰ   **S23.17**   **Subluxation and dislocation of T12/L1 thoracic vertebra**

     √7ᵗʰ   **S23.170**   **Subluxation of T12/L1 thoracic vertebra**

     √7ᵗʰ   **S23.171**   **Dislocation of T12/L1 thoracic vertebra**

√5ᵗʰ   **S23.2**   **Dislocation of other and unspecified parts of thorax**

   √x7ᵗʰ   **S23.20**   **Dislocation of unspecified part of thorax**

   √x7ᵗʰ   **S23.29**   **Dislocation of other parts of thorax**

√x7ᵗʰ   **S23.3**   **Sprain of ligaments of thoracic spine**

√5ᵗʰ   **S23.4**   **Sprain of ribs and sternum**

   √x7ᵗʰ   **S23.41**   **Sprain of ribs**

   √6ᵗʰ   **S23.42**   **Sprain of sternum**

     √7ᵗʰ   **S23.420**   **Sprain of sternoclavicular (joint) (ligament)**

     √7ᵗʰ   **S23.421**   **Sprain of chondrosternal joint**

     √7ᵗʰ   **S23.428**   **Other sprain of sternum**

     √7ᵗʰ   **S23.429**   **Unspecified sprain of sternum**

√x7ᵗʰ   **S23.8**   **Sprain of other specified parts of thorax**

√x7ᵗʰ   **S23.9**   **Sprain of unspecified parts of thorax**

√4ᵗʰ   **S24**   **Injury of nerves and spinal cord at thorax level**
    NOTE   Code to highest level of thoracic spinal cord injury.
      Injuries to the spinal cord (S24.0 and S24.1) refer to the cord
      level and not bone level injury, and can affect nerve roots at
      and below the level given.
    Code also any associated:
      fracture of thoracic vertebra (S22.0-)
      open wound of thorax (S21.-)
      transient paralysis (R29.5)
    EXCLUDES 2   injury of brachial plexus (S14.3)

> The appropriate 7th character is to be added to each code from
> category S24.
> A   initial encounter
> D   subsequent encounter
> S   sequela

> CC Excl: For codes in category S24:
> MCC with 7th character A: PDX collection 1177

√x7ᵗʰ   **S24.0**   **Concussion and edema of thoracic spinal cord**   MCC HCC

√5ᵗʰ   **S24.1**   **Other and unspecified injuries of thoracic spinal cord**

   √6ᵗʰ   **S24.10**   **Unspecified injury of thoracic spinal cord**

     √7ᵗʰ   **S24.101**   **Unspecified injury at T1 level of thoracic spinal cord**   MCC H5 HCC

---

6   MCC when reported as an open fracture (7th character B or C – specific to category).

7   CC when reported as an initial encounter (7th character A, B, or C – specific to category) OR a subsequent encounter for nonunion or malunion
    (7th character K, M, N, P, Q, or R – specific to category).

8   CC when reported as a subsequent encounter for nonunion or malunion (7th character K, M, N, P, Q, or R – specific to category).

---

√ Additional Character Req    √x7ᵗʰ Placeholder Alert    Unacceptable PDx    Manifestation    H1-H14 HAC    HCC CMS-HCC Condition    EXCLUDES 1 Not Coded Here    EXCLUDES 2 Not Included Here

√7ᵗʰ **S24.102** **Unspecified injury at T2-T6 level of thoracic spinal cord** `MCC` `H5` `HCC`

√7ᵗʰ **S24.103** **Unspecified injury at T7-T10 level of thoracic spinal cord** `MCC` `H5` `HCC`

√7ᵗʰ **S24.104** **Unspecified injury at T11-T12 level thoracic spinal cord** `MCC` `H5` `HCC`

√7ᵗʰ **S24.109** **Unspecified injury at unspecified level of thoracic spinal cord** `H5` `HCC`
Injury of thoracic spinal cord NOS

√6ᵗʰ **S24.11** **Complete lesion of thoracic spinal cord**

√7ᵗʰ **S24.111** **Complete lesion at T1 level of thoracic spinal cord** `MCC` `H5` `HCC`

√7ᵗʰ **S24.112** **Complete lesion at T2-T6 level of thoracic spinal cord** `MCC` `H5` `HCC`

√7ᵗʰ **S24.113** **Complete lesion at T7-T10 level of thoracic spinal cord** `MCC` `H5` `HCC`

√7ᵗʰ **S24.114** **Complete lesion at T11-T12 level of thoracic spinal cord** `MCC` `H5` `HCC`

√7ᵗʰ **S24.119** **Complete lesion at unspecified level of thoracic spinal cord** `HCC`

√6ᵗʰ **S24.13** **Anterior cord syndrome of thoracic spinal cord**

√7ᵗʰ **S24.131** **Anterior cord syndrome at T1 level of thoracic spinal cord** `MCC` `H5` `HCC`

√7ᵗʰ **S24.132** **Anterior cord syndrome at T2-T6 level of thoracic spinal cord** `MCC` `H5` `HCC`

√7ᵗʰ **S24.133** **Anterior cord syndrome at T7-T10 level of thoracic spinal cord** `MCC` `H5` `HCC`

√7ᵗʰ **S24.134** **Anterior cord syndrome at T11-T12 level of thoracic spinal cord** `MCC` `H5` `HCC`

√7ᵗʰ **S24.139** **Anterior cord syndrome at unspecified level of thoracic spinal cord** `HCC`

√6ᵗʰ **S24.14** **Brown-Séquard syndrome of thoracic spinal cord**

√7ᵗʰ **S24.141** **Brown-Séquard syndrome at T1 level of thoracic spinal cord** `MCC` `HCC`

√7ᵗʰ **S24.142** **Brown-Séquard syndrome at T2-T6 level of thoracic spinal cord** `MCC` `HCC`

√7ᵗʰ **S24.143** **Brown-Séquard syndrome at T7-T10 level of thoracic spinal cord** `MCC` `HCC`

√7ᵗʰ **S24.144** **Brown-Séquard syndrome at T11-T12 level of thoracic spinal cord** `MCC` `HCC`

√7ᵗʰ **S24.149** **Brown-Séquard syndrome at unspecified level of thoracic spinal cord** `HCC`

√6ᵗʰ **S24.15** **Other incomplete lesions of thoracic spinal cord**
Incomplete lesion of thoracic spinal cord NOS
Posterior cord syndrome of thoracic spinal cord

√7ᵗʰ **S24.151** **Other incomplete lesion at T1 level of thoracic spinal cord** `MCC` `H5` `HCC`

√7ᵗʰ **S24.152** **Other incomplete lesion at T2-T6 level of thoracic spinal cord** `MCC` `H5` `HCC`

√7ᵗʰ **S24.153** **Other incomplete lesion at T7-T10 level of thoracic spinal cord** `MCC` `H5` `HCC`

√7ᵗʰ **S24.154** **Other incomplete lesion at T11-T12 level of thoracic spinal cord** `MCC` `H5` `HCC`

√7ᵗʰ **S24.159** **Other incomplete lesion at unspecified level of thoracic spinal cord** `HCC`

√x7ᵗʰ **S24.2** **Injury of nerve root of thoracic spine**

√x7ᵗʰ **S24.3** **Injury of peripheral nerves of thorax**

√x7ᵗʰ **S24.4** **Injury of thoracic sympathetic nervous system**
Injury of cardiac plexus
Injury of esophageal plexus
Injury of pulmonary plexus
Injury of stellate ganglion
Injury of thoracic sympathetic ganglion

√x7ᵗʰ **S24.8** **Injury of other specified nerves of thorax**

√x7ᵗʰ **S24.9** **Injury of unspecified nerve of thorax**

√4ᵗʰ **S25** **Injury of blood vessels of thorax**
Code also any associated open wound (S21.-)

The appropriate 7th character is to be added to each code from category S25.
A  initial encounter
D  subsequent encounter
S  sequela

√5ᵗʰ **S25.0** **Injury of thoracic aorta**
Injury of aorta NOS

**CC Excl: For codes in subcategory S25.0:**
**MCC with 7th character A:** PDX collection 1178

√x7ᵗʰ **S25.00** **Unspecified injury of thoracic aorta** `MCC`

√x7ᵗʰ **S25.01** **Minor laceration of thoracic aorta** `MCC`
Incomplete transection of thoracic aorta
Laceration of thoracic aorta NOS
Superficial laceration of thoracic aorta

√x7ᵗʰ **S25.02** **Major laceration of thoracic aorta** `MCC`
Complete transection of thoracic aorta
Traumatic rupture of thoracic aorta

√x7ᵗʰ **S25.09** **Other specified injury of thoracic aorta** `MCC`

√5ᵗʰ **S25.1** **Injury of innominate or subclavian artery**

**CC Excl: For codes in subcategory S25.1:**
**MCC with 7th character A:** PDX collection 1179

√6ᵗʰ **S25.10** **Unspecified injury of innominate or subclavian artery**

√7ᵗʰ **S25.101** **Unspecified injury of right innominate or subclavian artery** `MCC`

√7ᵗʰ **S25.102** **Unspecified injury of left innominate or subclavian artery** `MCC`

√7ᵗʰ **S25.109** **Unspecified injury of unspecified innominate or subclavian artery** `MCC`

√6ᵗʰ **S25.11** **Minor laceration of innominate or subclavian artery**
Incomplete transection of innominate or subclavian artery
Laceration of innominate or subclavian artery NOS
Superficial laceration of innominate or subclavian artery

√7ᵗʰ **S25.111** **Minor laceration of right innominate or subclavian artery** `MCC`

√7ᵗʰ **S25.112** **Minor laceration of left innominate or subclavian artery** `MCC`

√7ᵗʰ **S25.119** **Minor laceration of unspecified innominate or subclavian artery** `MCC`

√6ᵗʰ **S25.12** **Major laceration of innominate or subclavian artery**
Complete transection of innominate or subclavian artery
Traumatic rupture of innominate or subclavian artery

√7ᵗʰ **S25.121** **Major laceration of right innominate or subclavian artery** `MCC`

√7ᵗʰ **S25.122** **Major laceration of left innominate or subclavian artery** `MCC`

√7ᵗʰ **S25.129** **Major laceration of unspecified innominate or subclavian artery** `MCC`

√6ᵗʰ **S25.19** **Other specified injury of innominate or subclavian artery**

√7ᵗʰ **S25.191** **Other specified injury of right innominate or subclavian artery** `MCC`

√7ᵗʰ **S25.192** **Other specified injury of left innominate or subclavian artery** `MCC`

√7ᵗʰ **S25.199** **Other specified injury of unspecified innominate or subclavian artery** `MCC`

√5ᵗʰ **S25.2** **Injury of superior vena cava**
Injury of vena cava NOS

**CC Excl: For codes in subcategory S25.2:**
**MCC with 7th character A:** PDX collection 1180

√x7ᵗʰ **S25.20** **Unspecified injury of superior vena cava** `MCC`

√x7ᵗʰ **S25.21** **Minor laceration of superior vena cava** `MCC`
Incomplete transection of superior vena cava
Laceration of superior vena cava NOS
Superficial laceration of superior vena cava

√x7ᵗʰ **S25.22** **Major laceration of superior vena cava** `MCC`
Complete transection of superior vena cava
Traumatic rupture of superior vena cava

√x7ᵗʰ **S25.29** **Other specified injury of superior vena cava** `MCC`

✓5ᵗʰ **S25.3** **Injury of** innominate or subclavian vein

> **CC Excl: For codes in subcategory S25.3:**
> **MCC with 7th character A:** PDX collection 1181

    ✓6ᵗʰ **S25.30** **Unspecified injury of innominate or subclavian vein**

       ✓7ᵗʰ **S25.301** **Unspecified injury of** right **innominate or subclavian vein** `MCC`

       ✓7ᵗʰ **S25.302** **Unspecified injury of** left **innominate or subclavian vein** `MCC`

       ✓7ᵗʰ **S25.309** **Unspecified injury of** unspecified **innominate or subclavian vein** `MCC`

    ✓6ᵗʰ **S25.31** **Minor laceration of innominate or subclavian vein**
> Incomplete transection of innominate or subclavian vein
> Laceration of innominate or subclavian vein NOS
> Superficial laceration of innominate or subclavian vein

       ✓7ᵗʰ **S25.311** **Minor laceration of** right **innominate or subclavian vein** `MCC`

       ✓7ᵗʰ **S25.312** **Minor laceration of** left **innominate or subclavian vein** `MCC`

       ✓7ᵗʰ **S25.319** **Minor laceration of** unspecified **innominate or subclavian vein** `MCC`

    ✓6ᵗʰ **S25.32** **Major laceration of innominate or subclavian vein**
> Complete transection of innominate or subclavian vein
> Traumatic rupture of innominate or subclavian vein

       ✓7ᵗʰ **S25.321** **Major laceration of** right **innominate or subclavian vein** `MCC`

       ✓7ᵗʰ **S25.322** **Major laceration of** left **innominate or subclavian vein** `MCC`

       ✓7ᵗʰ **S25.329** **Major laceration of** unspecified **innominate or subclavian vein** `MCC`

    ✓6ᵗʰ **S25.39** **Other** specified injury of innominate or subclavian **vein**

       ✓7ᵗʰ **S25.391** **Other specified injury of** right **innominate or subclavian vein** `MCC`

       ✓7ᵗʰ **S25.392** **Other specified injury of** left **innominate or subclavian vein** `MCC`

       ✓7ᵗʰ **S25.399** **Other specified injury of** unspecified **innominate or subclavian vein** `MCC`

✓5ᵗʰ **S25.4** **Injury of** pulmonary blood vessels

> **CC Excl: For codes in subcategory S25.4, unless otherwise noted:**
> **MCC with 7th character A:** PDX collection 1182

    ✓6ᵗʰ **S25.40** **Unspecified injury of pulmonary blood vessels**

       ✓7ᵗʰ **S25.401** **Unspecified injury of** right **pulmonary blood vessels** `MCC`

       ✓7ᵗʰ **S25.402** **Unspecified injury of** left **pulmonary blood vessels** `MCC`

       ✓7ᵗʰ **S25.409** **Unspecified injury of** unspecified **pulmonary blood vessels** `MCC`

    ✓6ᵗʰ **S25.41** **Minor laceration of pulmonary blood vessels**
> Incomplete transection of pulmonary blood vessels
> Laceration of pulmonary blood vessels NOS
> Superficial laceration of pulmonary blood vessels

       ✓7ᵗʰ **S25.411** **Minor laceration of** right **pulmonary blood vessels** `MCC`

       ✓7ᵗʰ **S25.412** **Minor laceration of** left **pulmonary blood vessels** `MCC`

       ✓7ᵗʰ **S25.419** **Minor laceration of** unspecified **pulmonary blood vessels** `MCC`

    ✓6ᵗʰ **S25.42** **Major laceration of pulmonary blood vessels**
> Complete transection of pulmonary blood vessels
> Traumatic rupture of pulmonary blood vessels

       ✓7ᵗʰ **S25.421** **Major laceration of** right **pulmonary blood vessels** `MCC`
> > **CC Excl: MCC with 7th character A:**
> > PDX collection 1183

       ✓7ᵗʰ **S25.422** **Major laceration of** left **pulmonary blood vessels** `MCC`

       ✓7ᵗʰ **S25.429** **Major laceration of** unspecified **pulmonary blood vessels** `MCC`

    ✓6ᵗʰ **S25.49** **Other specified injury of pulmonary blood vessels**

       ✓7ᵗʰ **S25.491** **Other specified injury of** right **pulmonary blood vessels** `MCC`

       ✓7ᵗʰ **S25.492** **Other specified injury of** left **pulmonary blood vessels** `MCC`

       ✓7ᵗʰ **S25.499** **Other specified injury of** unspecified **pulmonary blood vessels** `MCC`

✓5ᵗʰ **S25.5** **Injury of** intercostal blood vessels

> **CC Excl: For codes in subcategory S25.5:**
> **CC with 7th character A:** PDX collection 1184

    ✓6ᵗʰ **S25.50** **Unspecified injury of intercostal blood vessels**

       ✓7ᵗʰ **S25.501** **Unspecified injury of intercostal blood vessels,** right **side** `CC`

       ✓7ᵗʰ **S25.502** **Unspecified injury of intercostal blood vessels,** left **side** `CC`

       ✓7ᵗʰ **S25.509** **Unspecified injury of intercostal blood vessels,** unspecified **side** `CC`

    ✓6ᵗʰ **S25.51** **Laceration of intercostal blood vessels**

       ✓7ᵗʰ **S25.511** **Laceration of intercostal blood vessels,** right **side** `CC`

       ✓7ᵗʰ **S25.512** **Laceration of intercostal blood vessels,** left **side** `CC`

       ✓7ᵗʰ **S25.519** **Laceration of intercostal blood vessels,** unspecified **side** `CC`

    ✓6ᵗʰ **S25.59** **Other** specified injury of intercostal **blood vessels**

       ✓7ᵗʰ **S25.591** **Other specified injury of intercostal blood vessels,** right **side** `CC`

       ✓7ᵗʰ **S25.592** **Other specified injury of intercostal blood vessels,** left **side** `CC`

       ✓7ᵗʰ **S25.599** **Other specified injury of intercostal blood vessels,** unspecified **side** `CC`

✓5ᵗʰ **S25.8** **Injury of** other blood vessels **of thorax**
> Injury of azygos vein
> Injury of mammary artery or vein

> **CC Excl: For codes in subcategory S25.8:**
> **CC with 7th character A:** PDX collection 1185

    ✓6ᵗʰ **S25.80** **Unspecified injury of other blood vessels of thorax**

       ✓7ᵗʰ **S25.801** **Unspecified injury of other blood vessels of thorax,** right **side** `CC`

       ✓7ᵗʰ **S25.802** **Unspecified injury of other blood vessels of thorax,** left **side** `CC`

       ✓7ᵗʰ **S25.809** **Unspecified injury of other blood vessels of thorax,** unspecified **side** `CC`

    ✓6ᵗʰ **S25.81** **Laceration of other blood vessels of thorax**

       ✓7ᵗʰ **S25.811** **Laceration of other blood vessels of thorax,** right **side** `CC`

       ✓7ᵗʰ **S25.812** **Laceration of other blood vessels of thorax,** left **side** `CC`

       ✓7ᵗʰ **S25.819** **Laceration of other blood vessels of thorax,** unspecified **side** `CC`

    ✓6ᵗʰ **S25.89** **Other** specified injury of other blood vessels of **thorax**

       ✓7ᵗʰ **S25.891** **Other specified injury of other blood vessels of thorax,** right **side** `CC`

       ✓7ᵗʰ **S25.892** **Other specified injury of other blood vessels of thorax,** left **side** `CC`

       ✓7ᵗʰ **S25.899** **Other specified injury of other blood vessels of thorax,** unspecified **side** `CC`

✓5ᵗʰ **S25.9** **Injury of** unspecified blood vessel **of thorax**

> **CC Excl: For codes in subcategory S25.9:**
> **CC with 7th character A:** PDX collection 1185

    ✓x7ᵗʰ **S25.90** **Unspecified injury of unspecified blood vessel of thorax** `CC`

    ✓x7ᵗʰ **S25.91** **Laceration of unspecified blood vessel of thorax** `CC`

    ✓x7ᵗʰ **S25.99** **Other** specified injury of unspecified **blood vessel of thorax** `CC`

---

**✓4th S26 Injury of heart**

Code also any associated:
open wound of thorax (S21.-)
traumatic hemopneumothorax (S27.2)
traumatic hemothorax (S27.1)
traumatic pneumothorax (S27.0)

The appropriate 7th character is to be added to each code from category S26.
A    initial encounter
D    subsequent encounter
S    sequela

**CC Excl:** For codes in category S26 unless otherwise noted:
**CC or MCC with 7th character A:** PDX collection 1187

**✓5th S26.0 Injury of heart with hemopericardium**

**✓x7th S26.00 Unspecified injury of heart with hemopericardium** `CC`
     **CC Excl:** CC with 7th character A: PDX collection 1186

**✓x7th S26.01 Contusion of heart with hemopericardium** `CC`

**✓6th S26.02 Laceration of heart with hemopericardium**

     **✓7th S26.020 Mild laceration of heart with hemopericardium** `MCC`
         Laceration of heart without penetration of heart chamber

     **✓7th S26.021 Moderate laceration of heart with hemopericardium** `MCC`
         Laceration of heart with penetration of heart chamber

     **✓7th S26.022 Major laceration of heart with hemopericardium** `MCC`
         Laceration of heart with penetration of multiple heart chambers

**✓x7th S26.09 Other injury of heart with hemopericardium** `CC`
     **CC Excl:** CC with 7th character A: PDX collection 1186

**✓5th S26.1 Injury of heart without hemopericardium**

**✓x7th S26.10 Unspecified injury of heart without hemopericardium** `CC`
     **CC Excl:** CC with 7th character A: PDX collection 1186

**✓x7th S26.11 Contusion of heart without hemopericardium** `CC`

**✓x7th S26.12 Laceration of heart without hemopericardium** `MCC`

**✓x7th S26.19 Other injury of heart without hemopericardium** `CC`
     **CC Excl:** CC with 7th character A: PDX collection 1186

**✓5th S26.9 Injury of heart, unspecified with or without hemopericardium**

**✓x7th S26.90 Unspecified injury of heart, unspecified with or without hemopericardium** `CC`
     **CC Excl:** CC with 7th character A: PDX collection 1186

**✓x7th S26.91 Contusion of heart, unspecified with or without hemopericardium** `CC`
     **DEF:** Bruising within the heart muscle with no mention of open wound; usually caused by blunt chest trauma in motor vehicle accidents, falling from great heights, or receiving CPR.

**✓x7th S26.92 Laceration of heart, unspecified with or without hemopericardium** `MCC`
     Laceration of heart NOS

**✓x7th S26.99 Other injury of heart, unspecified with or without hemopericardium** `CC`
     **CC Excl:** CC with 7th character A: PDX collection 1186

**✓4th S27 Injury of other and unspecified intrathoracic organs**

Code also any associated open wound of thorax (S21.-)
*EXCLUDES 2* injury of cervical esophagus (S10-S19)
injury of trachea (cervical) (S10-S19)

The appropriate 7th character is to be added to each code from category S27.
A    initial encounter
D    subsequent encounter
S    sequela

**✓x7th S27.0 Traumatic pneumothorax** `CC`
     *EXCLUDES 1* spontaneous pneumothorax (J93.-)
     **CC Excl:** CC with 7th character A: PDX collection 1188

**✓x7th S27.1 Traumatic hemothorax** `MCC`
     **CC Excl:** MCC with 7th character A: PDX collection 1188

**✓x7th S27.2 Traumatic hemopneumothorax** `MCC`
     **CC Excl:** MCC with 7th character A: PDX collection 1188

**✓5th S27.3 Other and unspecified injuries of lung**

**CC Excl:** For codes in subcategory S27.3, unless otherwise noted:
**CC with 7th character A:** PDX collection 1189

**✓6th S27.30 Unspecified injury of lung**
     **✓7th S27.301 Unspecified injury of lung, unilateral** `CC`
     **✓7th S27.302 Unspecified injury of lung, bilateral** `CC`
     **✓7th S27.309 Unspecified injury of lung, unspecified** `CC`

**✓6th S27.31 Primary blast injury of lung**
     Blast injury of lung NOS
     **✓7th S27.311 Primary blast injury of lung, unilateral** `CC`
     **✓7th S27.312 Primary blast injury of lung, bilateral** `CC`
     **✓7th S27.319 Primary blast injury of lung, unspecified** `CC`

**✓6th S27.32 Contusion of lung**
     **DEF:** Bruising of lung without mention of open wound.
     **✓7th S27.321 Contusion of lung, unilateral** `CC`
     **✓7th S27.322 Contusion of lung, bilateral** `CC`
     **✓7th S27.329 Contusion of lung, unspecified** `CC`

**✓6th S27.33 Laceration of lung**
     **CC Excl:** For codes in subcategory S27.33:
     **MCC with 7th character A:** PDX collection 1190
     **✓7th S27.331 Laceration of lung, unilateral** `MCC`
     **✓7th S27.332 Laceration of lung, bilateral** `MCC`
     **✓7th S27.339 Laceration of lung, unspecified** `MCC`

**✓6th S27.39 Other injuries of lung**
     Secondary blast injury of lung
     **✓7th S27.391 Other injuries of lung, unilateral** `CC`
     **✓7th S27.392 Other injuries of lung, bilateral** `CC`
     **✓7th S27.399 Other injuries of lung, unspecified** `CC`

**✓5th S27.4 Injury of bronchus**

**CC Excl:** For codes in subcategory S27.4:
**MCC with 7th character A:** PDX collection 1191

**✓6th S27.40 Unspecified injury of bronchus**
     **✓7th S27.401 Unspecified injury of bronchus, unilateral** `MCC`
     **✓7th S27.402 Unspecified injury of bronchus, bilateral** `MCC`
     **✓7th S27.409 Unspecified injury of bronchus, unspecified** `MCC`

**✓6th S27.41 Primary blast injury of bronchus**
     Blast injury of bronchus NOS
     **✓7th S27.411 Primary blast injury of bronchus, unilateral** `MCC`
     **✓7th S27.412 Primary blast injury of bronchus, bilateral** `MCC`
     **✓7th S27.419 Primary blast injury of bronchus, unspecified** `MCC`

**✓6th S27.42 Contusion of bronchus**
     **✓7th S27.421 Contusion of bronchus, unilateral** `MCC`
     **✓7th S27.422 Contusion of bronchus, bilateral** `MCC`
     **✓7th S27.429 Contusion of bronchus, unspecified** `MCC`

**✓6th S27.43 Laceration of bronchus**
     **✓7th S27.431 Laceration of bronchus, unilateral** `MCC`
     **✓7th S27.432 Laceration of bronchus, bilateral** `MCC`
     **✓7th S27.439 Laceration of bronchus, unspecified** `MCC`

**✓6th S27.49 Other injury of bronchus**
     Secondary blast injury of bronchus
     **✓7th S27.491 Other injury of bronchus, unilateral** `MCC`
     **✓7th S27.492 Other injury of bronchus, bilateral** `MCC`
     **✓7th S27.499 Other injury of bronchus, unspecified** `MCC`

**✓5th S27.5 Injury of thoracic trachea**

**CC Excl:** For codes in subcategory S27.5:
**CC with 7th character A:** PDX collection 1169

**✓x7th S27.50 Unspecified injury of thoracic trachea** `CC`

**✓x7th S27.51 Primary blast injury of thoracic trachea** `CC`
     Blast injury of thoracic trachea NOS

**✓x7th S27.52 Contusion of thoracic trachea** `CC`

**✓x7th S27.53 Laceration of thoracic trachea** `CC`

√x7ᵗʰ **S27.59**   Other injury of thoracic trachea   CC
     Secondary blast injury of thoracic trachea

√5ᵗʰ **S27.6**   Injury of pleura

> **CC Excl: For codes in subcategory S27.6:**
> **CC with 7th character A:** PDX collection 1169

√x7ᵗʰ **S27.60**   Unspecified injury of pleura   CC

√x7ᵗʰ **S27.63**   Laceration of pleura   CC

√x7ᵗʰ **S27.69**   Other injury of pleura   CC

√5ᵗʰ **S27.8**   Injury of other specified intrathoracic organs

√6ᵗʰ **S27.80**   Injury of diaphragm

> **CC Excl: For codes in subcategory S27.80:**
> **CC with 7th character A:** PDX collection 1192

√7ᵗʰ **S27.802**   Contusion of diaphragm   CC

√7ᵗʰ **S27.803**   Laceration of diaphragm   CC

√7ᵗʰ **S27.808**   Other injury of diaphragm   CC

√7ᵗʰ **S27.809**   Unspecified injury of diaphragm   CC

√6ᵗʰ **S27.81**   Injury of esophagus (thoracic part)

> **CC Excl: For codes in subcategory S27.81:**
> **MCC with 7th character A:** PDX collection 1193

√7ᵗʰ **S27.812**   Contusion of esophagus   MCC
     (thoracic part)

√7ᵗʰ **S27.813**   Laceration of esophagus   MCC
     (thoracic part)

√7ᵗʰ **S27.818**   Other injury of esophagus   MCC
     (thoracic part)

√7ᵗʰ **S27.819**   Unspecified injury of esophagus   MCC
     (thoracic part)

√6ᵗʰ **S27.89**   Injury of other specified intrathoracic organs
     Injury of lymphatic thoracic duct
     Injury of thymus gland

> **CC Excl: For codes in subcategory S27.89:**
> **CC with 7th character A:** PDX collection 1169

√7ᵗʰ **S27.892**   Contusion of other specified   CC
     intrathoracic organs

√7ᵗʰ **S27.893**   Laceration of other specified   CC
     intrathoracic organs

√7ᵗʰ **S27.898**   Other injury of other specified   CC
     intrathoracic organs

√7ᵗʰ **S27.899**   Unspecified injury of other specified   CC
     intrathoracic organs

√x7ᵗʰ **S27.9**   Injury of unspecified intrathoracic organ   CC
     **CC Excl: CC with 7th character A:** PDX collection 1194

√4ᵗʰ **S28**   **Crushing injury of thorax, and traumatic amputation of part of thorax**

> The appropriate 7th character is to be added to each code from category S28.
> A   initial encounter
> D   subsequent encounter
> S   sequela

√x7ᵗʰ **S28.0**   Crushed chest
     Use additional code for all associated injuries
     *EXCLUDES 1*   flail chest (S22.5)

√x7ᵗʰ **S28.1**   Traumatic amputation (partial) of part of thorax,   CC
   except breast
     **CC Excl: CC with 7th character A:** PDX collection 1168

√5ᵗʰ **S28.2**   Traumatic amputation of breast

√6ᵗʰ **S28.21**   Complete traumatic amputation of breast
     Traumatic amputation of breast NOS

√7ᵗʰ **S28.211**   Complete traumatic amputation of right breast

√7ᵗʰ **S28.212**   Complete traumatic amputation of left breast

√7ᵗʰ **S28.219**   Complete traumatic amputation of unspecified breast

√6ᵗʰ **S28.22**   Partial traumatic amputation of breast

√7ᵗʰ **S28.221**   Partial traumatic amputation of right breast

√7ᵗʰ **S28.222**   Partial traumatic amputation of left breast

√7ᵗʰ **S28.229**   Partial traumatic amputation of unspecified breast

√4ᵗʰ **S29**   **Other and unspecified injuries of thorax**
     Code also any associated open wound (S21.-)

> The appropriate 7th character is to be added to each code from category S29.
> A   initial encounter
> D   subsequent encounter
> S   sequela

√5ᵗʰ **S29.0**   Injury of muscle and tendon at thorax level

√6ᵗʰ **S29.00**   Unspecified injury of muscle and tendon of thorax

√7ᵗʰ **S29.001**   Unspecified injury of muscle and tendon of front wall of thorax

√7ᵗʰ **S29.002**   Unspecified injury of muscle and tendon of back wall of thorax

√7ᵗʰ **S29.009**   Unspecified injury of muscle and tendon of unspecified wall of thorax

√6ᵗʰ **S29.01**   Strain of muscle and tendon of thorax

√7ᵗʰ **S29.011**   Strain of muscle and tendon of front wall of thorax

√7ᵗʰ **S29.012**   Strain of muscle and tendon of back wall of thorax

√7ᵗʰ **S29.019**   Strain of muscle and tendon of unspecified wall of thorax

√6ᵗʰ **S29.02**   Laceration of muscle and tendon of thorax

√7ᵗʰ **S29.021**   Laceration of muscle and tendon of   CC
     front wall of thorax
     **CC Excl: CC with 7th character A:**
     PDX collection 1168

√7ᵗʰ **S29.022**   Laceration of muscle and tendon of back wall of thorax

√7ᵗʰ **S29.029**   Laceration of muscle and tendon of   CC
     unspecified wall of thorax
     **CC Excl: CC with 7th character A:**
     PDX collection 1168

√6ᵗʰ **S29.09**   Other injury of muscle and tendon of thorax

√7ᵗʰ **S29.091**   Other injury of muscle and tendon of front wall of thorax

√7ᵗʰ **S29.092**   Other injury of muscle and tendon of back wall of thorax

√7ᵗʰ **S29.099**   Other injury of muscle and tendon of unspecified wall of thorax

√x7ᵗʰ **S29.8**   Other specified injuries of thorax

√x7ᵗʰ **S29.9**   Unspecified injury of thorax

## Injuries to the abdomen, lower back, lumbar spine, pelvis and external genitals (S30-S39)

**INCLUDES**   injuries to the abdominal wall
     injuries to the anus
     injuries to the buttock
     injuries to the external genitalia
     injuries to the flank
     injuries to the groin

*EXCLUDES 2*   *burns and corrosions (T20-T32)*
     *effects of foreign body in anus and rectum (T18.5)*
     *effects of foreign body in genitourinary tract (T19.-)*
     *effects of foreign body in stomach, small intestine and colon (T18.2-T18.4)*
     *frostbite (T33-T34)*
     *insect bite or sting, venomous (T63.4)*

√4ᵗʰ **S30**   **Superficial injury of abdomen, lower back, pelvis and external genitals**
     *EXCLUDES 2*   *superficial injury of hip (S70.-)*

> The appropriate 7th character is to be added to each code from category S30.
> A   initial encounter
> D   subsequent encounter
> S   sequela

√x7ᵗʰ **S30.0**   Contusion of lower back and pelvis
     Contusion of buttock

√x7ᵗʰ **S30.1**   Contusion of abdominal wall
     Contusion of flank
     Contusion of groin

√5ᵗʰ **S30.2**   Contusion of external genital organs

√6ᵗʰ **S30.20**   Contusion of unspecified external genital organ

√7ᵗʰ **S30.201**   Contusion of unspecified external   ♂
     genital organ, male

---

☑ Additional Character Req   √x7ᵗʰ Placeholder Alert   Unacceptable PDx   Manifestation   **H1** – **H14** HAC   **HCC** CMS-HCC Condition   *EXCLUDES 1* Not Coded Here   *EXCLUDES 2* Not Included Here

√7ᵗʰ **S30.202** **Contusion of unspecified external genital organ,** female ♀

√x7ᵗʰ **S30.21** **Contusion of penis** ♂

√x7ᵗʰ **S30.22** **Contusion of scrotum and testes** ♂

√x7ᵗʰ **S30.23** **Contusion of vagina and vulva** ♀

√x7ᵗʰ **S30.3** **Contusion of anus**

√5ᵗʰ **S30.8** **Other superficial injuries of abdomen, lower back, pelvis and external genitals**

√6ᵗʰ **S30.81** **Abrasion of abdomen, lower back, pelvis and external genitals**

√7ᵗʰ **S30.810** **Abrasion of lower back and pelvis**

√7ᵗʰ **S30.811** **Abrasion of abdominal wall**

√7ᵗʰ **S30.812** **Abrasion of penis** ♂

√7ᵗʰ **S30.813** **Abrasion of scrotum and testes** ♂

√7ᵗʰ **S30.814** **Abrasion of vagina and vulva** ♀

√7ᵗʰ **S30.815** **Abrasion of unspecified external genital organs, male** ♂

√7ᵗʰ **S30.816** **Abrasion of unspecified external genital organs, female** ♀

√7ᵗʰ **S30.817** **Abrasion of anus**

√6ᵗʰ **S30.82** **Blister (nonthermal) of abdomen, lower back, pelvis and external genitals**

√7ᵗʰ **S30.820** **Blister (nonthermal) of lower back and pelvis**

√7ᵗʰ **S30.821** **Blister (nonthermal) of abdominal wall**

√7ᵗʰ **S30.822** **Blister (nonthermal) of penis** ♂

√7ᵗʰ **S30.823** **Blister (nonthermal) of scrotum and testes** ♂

√7ᵗʰ **S30.824** **Blister (nonthermal) of vagina and vulva** ♀

√7ᵗʰ **S30.825** **Blister (nonthermal) of unspecified external genital organs, male** ♂

√7ᵗʰ **S30.826** **Blister (nonthermal) of unspecified external genital organs, female** ♀

√7ᵗʰ **S30.827** **Blister (nonthermal) of anus**

√6ᵗʰ **S30.84** **External constriction of abdomen, lower back, pelvis and external genitals**

√7ᵗʰ **S30.840** **External constriction of lower back and pelvis**

√7ᵗʰ **S30.841** **External constriction of abdominal wall**

√7ᵗʰ **S30.842** **External constriction of penis** ♂
Hair tourniquet syndrome of penis
Use additional cause code to identify the constricting item (W49.0-)

√7ᵗʰ **S30.843** **External constriction of scrotum and testes** ♂

√7ᵗʰ **S30.844** **External constriction of vagina and vulva** ♀

√7ᵗʰ **S30.845** **External constriction of unspecified external genital organs, male** ♂

√7ᵗʰ **S30.846** **External constriction of unspecified external genital organs, female** ♀

√6ᵗʰ **S30.85** **Superficial foreign body of abdomen, lower back, pelvis and external genitals**
Splinter in the abdomen, lower back, pelvis and external genitals

√7ᵗʰ **S30.850** **Superficial foreign body of lower back and pelvis**

√7ᵗʰ **S30.851** **Superficial foreign body of abdominal wall**

√7ᵗʰ **S30.852** **Superficial foreign body of penis** ♂

√7ᵗʰ **S30.853** **Superficial foreign body of scrotum and testes** ♂

√7ᵗʰ **S30.854** **Superficial foreign body of vagina and vulva** ♀

√7ᵗʰ **S30.855** **Superficial foreign body of unspecified external genital organs, male** ♂

√7ᵗʰ **S30.856** **Superficial foreign body of unspecified external genital organs, female** ♀

√7ᵗʰ **S30.857** **Superficial foreign body of anus**

√6ᵗʰ **S30.86** **Insect bite (nonvenomous) of abdomen, lower back, pelvis and external genitals**

√7ᵗʰ **S30.860** **Insect bite (nonvenomous) of lower back and pelvis**

√7ᵗʰ **S30.861** **Insect bite (nonvenomous) of abdominal wall**

√7ᵗʰ **S30.862** **Insect bite (nonvenomous) of penis** ♂

√7ᵗʰ **S30.863** **Insect bite (nonvenomous) of scrotum and testes** ♂

√7ᵗʰ **S30.864** **Insect bite (nonvenomous) of vagina and vulva** ♀

√7ᵗʰ **S30.865** **Insect bite (nonvenomous) of unspecified external genital organs, male** ♂

√7ᵗʰ **S30.866** **Insect bite (nonvenomous) of unspecified external genital organs, female** ♀

√7ᵗʰ **S30.867** **Insect bite (nonvenomous) of anus**

√6ᵗʰ **S30.87** **Other superficial bite of abdomen, lower back, pelvis and external genitals**
**EXCLUDES 1** *open bite of abdomen, lower back, pelvis and external genitals (S31.05, S31.15, S31.25, S31.35, S31.45, S31.55)*

√7ᵗʰ **S30.870** **Other superficial bite of lower back and pelvis**

√7ᵗʰ **S30.871** **Other superficial bite of abdominal wall**

√7ᵗʰ **S30.872** **Other superficial bite of penis** ♂

√7ᵗʰ **S30.873** **Other superficial bite of scrotum and testes** ♂

√7ᵗʰ **S30.874** **Other superficial bite of vagina and vulva** ♀

√7ᵗʰ **S30.875** **Other superficial bite of unspecified external genital organs, male** ♂

√7ᵗʰ **S30.876** **Other superficial bite of unspecified external genital organs, female** ♀

√7ᵗʰ **S30.877** **Other superficial bite of anus**

√5ᵗʰ **S30.9** **Unspecified superficial injury of abdomen, lower back, pelvis and external genitals**

√x7ᵗʰ **S30.91** **Unspecified superficial injury of lower back and pelvis**

√x7ᵗʰ **S30.92** **Unspecified superficial injury of abdominal wall**

√x7ᵗʰ **S30.93** **Unspecified superficial injury of penis** ♂

√x7ᵗʰ **S30.94** **Unspecified superficial injury of scrotum and testes** ♂

√x7ᵗʰ **S30.95** **Unspecified superficial injury of vagina and vulva** ♀

√x7ᵗʰ **S30.96** **Unspecified superficial injury of unspecified external genital organs, male** ♂

√x7ᵗʰ **S30.97** **Unspecified superficial injury of unspecified external genital organs, female** ♀

√x7ᵗʰ **S30.98** **Unspecified superficial injury of anus**

√4ᵗʰ **S31** **Open wound of abdomen, lower back, pelvis and external genitals**
Code also any associated:
spinal cord injury (S24.0, S24.1-, S34.0-, S34.1-)
wound infection
**EXCLUDES 1** *traumatic amputation of part of abdomen, lower back and pelvis (S38.2-, S38.3)*
**EXCLUDES 2** *open wound of hip (S71.00-S71.02)*
*open fracture of pelvis (S32.1- – S32.9 with 7th B)*

The appropriate 7th character is to be added to each code from category S31.
A    initial encounter
D    subsequent encounter
S    sequela

**CC Excl: For codes in category S31:**
**MCC with 7th character A:** PDX collection 1195

√5ᵗʰ **S31.0** **Open wound of lower back and pelvis**

√6ᵗʰ **S31.00** **Unspecified open wound of lower back and pelvis**

√7ᵗʰ **S31.000** **Unspecified open wound of lower back and pelvis without penetration into retroperitoneum**
Unspecified open wound of lower back and pelvis NOS

√7ᵗʰ **S31.001** **Unspecified open wound of lower back and pelvis with penetration into retroperitoneum** MCC

Ⓝ Newborn: 0    Ⓟ Pediatric: 0-17    Ⓜ Maternity: 12-55    Ⓐ Adult: 15-124    **MCC** Major CC Condition    **PDxMCC** PDx acts as own MCC    **CC** CC Condition    **PDxCC** PDx acts as own CC

**970**        ICD-10-CM 2018

√6ᵗʰ **S31.01** Laceration without foreign body **of lower back and pelvis**

   √7ᵗʰ **S31.010** **Laceration without foreign body of lower back and pelvis** without penetration into retroperitoneum
     Laceration without foreign body of lower back and pelvis NOS

   √7ᵗʰ **S31.011** **Laceration without foreign body of lower back and pelvis** with penetration into retroperitoneum    `MCC`

√6ᵗʰ **S31.02** Laceration with foreign body **of lower back and pelvis**

   √7ᵗʰ **S31.020** **Laceration with foreign body of lower back and pelvis** without penetration into retroperitoneum
     Laceration with foreign body of lower back and pelvis NOS

   √7ᵗʰ **S31.021** **Laceration with foreign body of lower back and pelvis** with penetration into retroperitoneum    `MCC`

√6ᵗʰ **S31.03** Puncture wound without foreign body **of lower back and pelvis**

   √7ᵗʰ **S31.030** **Puncture wound without foreign body of lower back and pelvis** without penetration into retroperitoneum
     Puncture wound without foreign body of lower back and pelvis NOS

   √7ᵗʰ **S31.031** **Puncture wound without foreign body of lower back and pelvis** with penetration into retroperitoneum    `MCC`

√6ᵗʰ **S31.04** Puncture wound with foreign body **of lower back and pelvis**

   √7ᵗʰ **S31.040** **Puncture wound with foreign body of lower back and pelvis** without penetration into retroperitoneum
     Puncture wound with foreign body of lower back and pelvis NOS

   √7ᵗʰ **S31.041** **Puncture wound with foreign body of lower back and pelvis** with penetration into retroperitoneum    `MCC`

√6ᵗʰ **S31.05** Open bite **of lower back and pelvis**
   Bite of lower back and pelvis NOS
   `EXCLUDES 1` *superficial bite of lower back and pelvis (S30.860, S30.870)*

   √7ᵗʰ **S31.050** **Open bite of lower back and pelvis** without penetration into retroperitoneum
     Open bite of lower back and pelvis NOS

   √7ᵗʰ **S31.051** **Open bite of lower back and pelvis** with penetration into retroperitoneum    `MCC`

√5ᵗʰ **S31.1** Open wound of abdominal wall without penetration into peritoneal cavity
   Open wound of abdominal wall NOS
   `EXCLUDES 2` *open wound of abdominal wall with penetration into peritoneal cavity (S31.6-)*

√6ᵗʰ **S31.10** Unspecified **open wound of abdominal wall without penetration into peritoneal cavity**

   √7ᵗʰ **S31.100** **Unspecified open wound of abdominal wall,** right upper quadrant **without penetration into peritoneal cavity**

   √7ᵗʰ **S31.101** **Unspecified open wound of abdominal wall,** left upper quadrant **without penetration into peritoneal cavity**

   √7ᵗʰ **S31.102** **Unspecified open wound of abdominal wall,** epigastric region **without penetration into peritoneal cavity**

   √7ᵗʰ **S31.103** **Unspecified open wound of abdominal wall,** right lower quadrant **without penetration into peritoneal cavity**

   √7ᵗʰ **S31.104** **Unspecified open wound of abdominal wall,** left lower quadrant **without penetration into peritoneal cavity**

   √7ᵗʰ **S31.105** **Unspecified open wound of abdominal wall,** periumbilic region **without penetration into peritoneal cavity**

   √7ᵗʰ **S31.109** **Unspecified open wound of abdominal wall,** unspecified quadrant **without penetration into peritoneal cavity**
     Unspecified open wound of abdominal wall NOS

√6ᵗʰ **S31.11** Laceration without foreign body **of abdominal wall without penetration into peritoneal cavity**

   √7ᵗʰ **S31.110** **Laceration without foreign body of abdominal wall,** right upper quadrant **without penetration into peritoneal cavity**

   √7ᵗʰ **S31.111** **Laceration without foreign body of abdominal wall,** left upper quadrant **without penetration into peritoneal cavity**

   √7ᵗʰ **S31.112** **Laceration without foreign body of abdominal wall,** epigastric region **without penetration into peritoneal cavity**

   √7ᵗʰ **S31.113** **Laceration without foreign body of abdominal wall,** right lower quadrant **without penetration into peritoneal cavity**

   √7ᵗʰ **S31.114** **Laceration without foreign body of abdominal wall,** left lower quadrant **without penetration into peritoneal cavity**

   √7ᵗʰ **S31.115** **Laceration without foreign body of abdominal wall,** periumbilic region **without penetration into peritoneal cavity**

   √7ᵗʰ **S31.119** **Laceration without foreign body of abdominal wall,** unspecified quadrant **without penetration into peritoneal cavity**

√6ᵗʰ **S31.12** Laceration with foreign body **of abdominal wall without penetration into peritoneal cavity**

   √7ᵗʰ **S31.120** **Laceration of abdominal wall with foreign body,** right upper quadrant **without penetration into peritoneal cavity**

   √7ᵗʰ **S31.121** **Laceration of abdominal wall with foreign body,** left upper quadrant **without penetration into peritoneal cavity**

   √7ᵗʰ **S31.122** **Laceration of abdominal wall with foreign body,** epigastric region **without penetration into peritoneal cavity**

   √7ᵗʰ **S31.123** **Laceration of abdominal wall with foreign body,** right lower quadrant **without penetration into peritoneal cavity**

   √7ᵗʰ **S31.124** **Laceration of abdominal wall with foreign body,** left lower quadrant **without penetration into peritoneal cavity**

   √7ᵗʰ **S31.125** **Laceration of abdominal wall with foreign body,** periumbilic region **without penetration into peritoneal cavity**

   √7ᵗʰ **S31.129** **Laceration of abdominal wall with foreign body,** unspecified quadrant **without penetration into peritoneal cavity**

√6ᵗʰ **S31.13** Puncture wound **of abdominal wall without foreign body without penetration into peritoneal cavity**

   √7ᵗʰ **S31.130** **Puncture wound of abdominal wall without foreign body,** right upper quadrant **without penetration into peritoneal cavity**

   √7ᵗʰ **S31.131** **Puncture wound of abdominal wall without foreign body,** left upper quadrant **without penetration into peritoneal cavity**

   √7ᵗʰ **S31.132** **Puncture wound of abdominal wall without foreign body,** epigastric region **without penetration into peritoneal cavity**

   √7ᵗʰ **S31.133** **Puncture wound of abdominal wall without foreign body,** right lower quadrant **without penetration into peritoneal cavity**

   √7ᵗʰ **S31.134** **Puncture wound of abdominal wall without foreign body,** left lower quadrant **without penetration into peritoneal cavity**

   √7ᵗʰ **S31.135** **Puncture wound of abdominal wall without foreign body,** periumbilic region **without penetration into peritoneal cavity**

   √7ᵗʰ **S31.139** **Puncture wound of abdominal wall without foreign body,** unspecified quadrant **without penetration into peritoneal cavity**

√6ᵗʰ **S31.14** Puncture wound **of abdominal wall with foreign body without penetration into peritoneal cavity**

   √7ᵗʰ **S31.140** **Puncture wound of abdominal wall with foreign body,** right upper quadrant **without penetration into peritoneal cavity**

---

√ Additional Character Req   √x7ᵗʰ Placeholder Alert   Unacceptable PDx   Manifestation   `H1`-`H14` HAC   `HCC` CMS-HCC Condition   `EXCLUDES 1` Not Coded Here   `EXCLUDES 2` Not Included Here

√7ᵗʰ **S31.141** **Puncture wound of abdominal wall with foreign body, left upper quadrant without penetration into peritoneal cavity**

√7ᵗʰ **S31.142** **Puncture wound of abdominal wall with foreign body, epigastric region without penetration into peritoneal cavity**

√7ᵗʰ **S31.143** **Puncture wound of abdominal wall with foreign body, right lower quadrant without penetration into peritoneal cavity**

√7ᵗʰ **S31.144** **Puncture wound of abdominal wall with foreign body, left lower quadrant without penetration into peritoneal cavity**

√7ᵗʰ **S31.145** **Puncture wound of abdominal wall with foreign body, periumbilic region without penetration into peritoneal cavity**

√7ᵗʰ **S31.149** **Puncture wound of abdominal wall with foreign body, unspecified quadrant without penetration into peritoneal cavity**

√6ᵗʰ **S31.15** **Open bite of abdominal wall without penetration into peritoneal cavity**
Bite of abdominal wall NOS
*EXCLUDES 1*   *superficial bite of abdominal wall (S30.871)*

√7ᵗʰ **S31.150** **Open bite of abdominal wall, right upper quadrant without penetration into peritoneal cavity**

√7ᵗʰ **S31.151** **Open bite of abdominal wall, left upper quadrant without penetration into peritoneal cavity**

√7ᵗʰ **S31.152** **Open bite of abdominal wall, epigastric region without penetration into peritoneal cavity**

√7ᵗʰ **S31.153** **Open bite of abdominal wall, right lower quadrant without penetration into peritoneal cavity**

√7ᵗʰ **S31.154** **Open bite of abdominal wall, left lower quadrant without penetration into peritoneal cavity**

√7ᵗʰ **S31.155** **Open bite of abdominal wall, periumbilic region without penetration into peritoneal cavity**

√7ᵗʰ **S31.159** **Open bite of abdominal wall, unspecified quadrant without penetration into peritoneal cavity**

√5ᵗʰ **S31.2** **Open wound of penis**

√x7ᵗʰ **S31.20** **Unspecified open wound of penis**    ♂

√x7ᵗʰ **S31.21** **Laceration without foreign body of penis**    ♂

√x7ᵗʰ **S31.22** **Laceration with foreign body of penis**    ♂

√x7ᵗʰ **S31.23** **Puncture wound without foreign body of penis**    ♂

√x7ᵗʰ **S31.24** **Puncture wound with foreign body of penis**    ♂

√x7ᵗʰ **S31.25** **Open bite of penis**    ♂
Bite of penis NOS
*EXCLUDES 1*   *superficial bite of penis (S30.862, S30.872)*

√5ᵗʰ **S31.3** **Open wound of scrotum and testes**

√x7ᵗʰ **S31.30** **Unspecified open wound of scrotum and testes**    ♂

√x7ᵗʰ **S31.31** **Laceration without foreign body of scrotum and testes**    ♂

√x7ᵗʰ **S31.32** **Laceration with foreign body of scrotum and testes**    ♂

√x7ᵗʰ **S31.33** **Puncture wound without foreign body of scrotum and testes**    ♂

√x7ᵗʰ **S31.34** **Puncture wound with foreign body of scrotum and testes**    ♂

√x7ᵗʰ **S31.35** **Open bite of scrotum and testes**    ♂
Bite of scrotum and testes NOS
*EXCLUDES 1*   *superficial bite of scrotum and testes (S30.863, S30.873)*

√5ᵗʰ **S31.4** **Open wound of vagina and vulva**
*EXCLUDES 1*   *injury to vagina and vulva during delivery (O70-, O71.4)*

√x7ᵗʰ **S31.40** **Unspecified open wound of vagina and vulva**    ♀

√x7ᵗʰ **S31.41** **Laceration without foreign body of vagina and vulva**    ♀

√x7ᵗʰ **S31.42** **Laceration with foreign body of vagina and vulva**    ♀

√x7ᵗʰ **S31.43** **Puncture wound without foreign body of vagina and vulva**    ♀

√x7ᵗʰ **S31.44** **Puncture wound with foreign body of vagina and vulva**    ♀

√x7ᵗʰ **S31.45** **Open bite of vagina and vulva**    ♀
Bite of vagina and vulva NOS
*EXCLUDES 1*   *superficial bite of vagina and vulva (S30.864, S30.874)*

√5ᵗʰ **S31.5** **Open wound of unspecified external genital organs**
*EXCLUDES 1*   *traumatic amputation of external genital organs (S38.21, S38.22)*

√6ᵗʰ **S31.50** **Unspecified open wound of unspecified external genital organs**

√7ᵗʰ **S31.501** **Unspecified open wound of unspecified external genital organs, male**    ♂

√7ᵗʰ **S31.502** **Unspecified open wound of unspecified external genital organs, female**    ♀

√6ᵗʰ **S31.51** **Laceration without foreign body of unspecified external genital organs**

√7ᵗʰ **S31.511** **Laceration without foreign body of unspecified external genital organs, male**    ♂

√7ᵗʰ **S31.512** **Laceration without foreign body of unspecified external genital organs, female**    ♀

√6ᵗʰ **S31.52** **Laceration with foreign body of unspecified external genital organs**

√7ᵗʰ **S31.521** **Laceration with foreign body of unspecified external genital organs, male**    ♂

√7ᵗʰ **S31.522** **Laceration with foreign body of unspecified external genital organs, female**    ♀

√6ᵗʰ **S31.53** **Puncture wound without foreign body of unspecified external genital organs**

√7ᵗʰ **S31.531** **Puncture wound without foreign body of unspecified external genital organs, male**    ♂

√7ᵗʰ **S31.532** **Puncture wound without foreign body of unspecified external genital organs, female**    ♀

√6ᵗʰ **S31.54** **Puncture wound with foreign body of unspecified external genital organs**

√7ᵗʰ **S31.541** **Puncture wound with foreign body of unspecified external genital organs, male**    ♂

√7ᵗʰ **S31.542** **Puncture wound with foreign body of unspecified external genital organs, female**    ♀

√6ᵗʰ **S31.55** **Open bite of unspecified external genital organs**
Bite of unspecified external genital organs NOS
*EXCLUDES 1*   *superficial bite of unspecified external genital organs (S30.865, S30.866, S30.875, S30.876)*

√7ᵗʰ **S31.551** **Open bite of unspecified external genital organs, male**    ♂

√7ᵗʰ **S31.552** **Open bite of unspecified external genital organs, female**    ♀

√5ᵗʰ **S31.6** **Open wound of abdominal wall with penetration into peritoneal cavity**

√6ᵗʰ **S31.60** **Unspecified open wound of abdominal wall with penetration into peritoneal cavity**

√7ᵗʰ **S31.600** **Unspecified open wound of abdominal wall, right upper quadrant with penetration into peritoneal cavity**    MCC

√7ᵗʰ **S31.601** **Unspecified open wound of abdominal wall, left upper quadrant with penetration into peritoneal cavity**    MCC

√7ᵗʰ **S31.602** **Unspecified open wound of abdominal wall, epigastric region with penetration into peritoneal cavity**    MCC

√7ᵗʰ **S31.603** **Unspecified open wound of abdominal wall, right lower quadrant with penetration into peritoneal cavity**    MCC

√7ᵗʰ **S31.604** **Unspecified open wound of abdominal wall, left lower quadrant with penetration into peritoneal cavity**    MCC

√7ᵗʰ **S31.605** **Unspecified open wound of abdominal wall, periumbilic region with penetration into peritoneal cavity**    MCC

Ⓝ Newborn: 0   Ⓟ Pediatric: 0-17   Ⓜ Maternity: 12-55   Ⓐ Adult: 15-124   **MCC** Major CC Condition   **PDxMCC** PDx acts as own MCC   **CC** CC Condition   **PDxCC** PDx acts as own CC

**972**      ICD-10-CM 2018

☑7ᵗʰ **S31.609** Unspecified open wound of abdominal wall, unspecified quadrant with penetration into peritoneal cavity   MCC

☑6ᵗʰ **S31.61** Laceration without foreign body of abdominal wall with penetration into peritoneal cavity

  ☑7ᵗʰ **S31.610** Laceration without foreign body of abdominal wall, right upper quadrant with penetration into peritoneal cavity   MCC

  ☑7ᵗʰ **S31.611** Laceration without foreign body of abdominal wall, left upper quadrant with penetration into peritoneal cavity   MCC

  ☑7ᵗʰ **S31.612** Laceration without foreign body of abdominal wall, epigastric region with penetration into peritoneal cavity   MCC

  ☑7ᵗʰ **S31.613** Laceration without foreign body of abdominal wall, right lower quadrant with penetration into peritoneal cavity   MCC

  ☑7ᵗʰ **S31.614** Laceration without foreign body of abdominal wall, left lower quadrant with penetration into peritoneal cavity   MCC

  ☑7ᵗʰ **S31.615** Laceration without foreign body of abdominal wall, periumbilic region with penetration into peritoneal cavity   MCC

  ☑7ᵗʰ **S31.619** Laceration without foreign body of abdominal wall, unspecified quadrant with penetration into peritoneal cavity   MCC

☑6ᵗʰ **S31.62** Laceration with foreign body of abdominal wall with penetration into peritoneal cavity

  ☑7ᵗʰ **S31.620** Laceration with foreign body of abdominal wall, right upper quadrant with penetration into peritoneal cavity   MCC

  ☑7ᵗʰ **S31.621** Laceration with foreign body of abdominal wall, left upper quadrant with penetration into peritoneal cavity   MCC

  ☑7ᵗʰ **S31.622** Laceration with foreign body of abdominal wall, epigastric region with penetration into peritoneal cavity   MCC

  ☑7ᵗʰ **S31.623** Laceration with foreign body of abdominal wall, right lower quadrant with penetration into peritoneal cavity   MCC

  ☑7ᵗʰ **S31.624** Laceration with foreign body of abdominal wall, left lower quadrant with penetration into peritoneal cavity   MCC

  ☑7ᵗʰ **S31.625** Laceration with foreign body of abdominal wall, periumbilic region with penetration into peritoneal cavity   MCC

  ☑7ᵗʰ **S31.629** Laceration with foreign body of abdominal wall, unspecified quadrant with penetration into peritoneal cavity   MCC

☑6ᵗʰ **S31.63** Puncture wound without foreign body of abdominal wall with penetration into peritoneal cavity

  ☑7ᵗʰ **S31.630** Puncture wound without foreign body of abdominal wall, right upper quadrant with penetration into peritoneal cavity   MCC

  ☑7ᵗʰ **S31.631** Puncture wound without foreign body of abdominal wall, left upper quadrant with penetration into peritoneal cavity   MCC

  ☑7ᵗʰ **S31.632** Puncture wound without foreign body of abdominal wall, epigastric region with penetration into peritoneal cavity   MCC

  ☑7ᵗʰ **S31.633** Puncture wound without foreign body of abdominal wall, right lower quadrant with penetration into peritoneal cavity   MCC

  ☑7ᵗʰ **S31.634** Puncture wound without foreign body of abdominal wall, left lower quadrant with penetration into peritoneal cavity   MCC

  ☑7ᵗʰ **S31.635** Puncture wound without foreign body of abdominal wall, periumbilic region with penetration into peritoneal cavity   MCC

  ☑7ᵗʰ **S31.639** Puncture wound without foreign body of abdominal wall, unspecified quadrant with penetration into peritoneal cavity   MCC

☑6ᵗʰ **S31.64** Puncture wound with foreign body of abdominal wall with penetration into peritoneal cavity

  ☑7ᵗʰ **S31.640** Puncture wound with foreign body of abdominal wall, right upper quadrant with penetration into peritoneal cavity   MCC

  ☑7ᵗʰ **S31.641** Puncture wound with foreign body of abdominal wall, left upper quadrant with penetration into peritoneal cavity   MCC

  ☑7ᵗʰ **S31.642** Puncture wound with foreign body of abdominal wall, epigastric region with penetration into peritoneal cavity   MCC

  ☑7ᵗʰ **S31.643** Puncture wound with foreign body of abdominal wall, right lower quadrant with penetration into peritoneal cavity   MCC

  ☑7ᵗʰ **S31.644** Puncture wound with foreign body of abdominal wall, left lower quadrant with penetration into peritoneal cavity   MCC

  ☑7ᵗʰ **S31.645** Puncture wound with foreign body of abdominal wall, periumbilic region with penetration into peritoneal cavity   MCC

  ☑7ᵗʰ **S31.649** Puncture wound with foreign body of abdominal wall, unspecified quadrant with penetration into peritoneal cavity   MCC

☑6ᵗʰ **S31.65** Open bite of abdominal wall with penetration into peritoneal cavity

     *EXCLUDES 1*   superficial bite of abdominal wall (S30.861, S30.871)

  ☑7ᵗʰ **S31.650** Open bite of abdominal wall, right upper quadrant with penetration into peritoneal cavity   MCC

  ☑7ᵗʰ **S31.651** Open bite of abdominal wall, left upper quadrant with penetration into peritoneal cavity   MCC

  ☑7ᵗʰ **S31.652** Open bite of abdominal wall, epigastric region with penetration into peritoneal cavity   MCC

  ☑7ᵗʰ **S31.653** Open bite of abdominal wall, right lower quadrant with penetration into peritoneal cavity   MCC

  ☑7ᵗʰ **S31.654** Open bite of abdominal wall, left lower quadrant with penetration into peritoneal cavity   MCC

  ☑7ᵗʰ **S31.655** Open bite of abdominal wall, periumbilic region with penetration into peritoneal cavity   MCC

  ☑7ᵗʰ **S31.659** Open bite of abdominal wall, unspecified quadrant with penetration into peritoneal cavity   MCC

☑5ᵗʰ **S31.8** Open wound of other parts of abdomen, lower back and pelvis

☑6ᵗʰ **S31.80** Open wound of unspecified buttock

  ☑7ᵗʰ **S31.801** Laceration without foreign body of unspecified buttock

  ☑7ᵗʰ **S31.802** Laceration with foreign body of unspecified buttock

  ☑7ᵗʰ **S31.803** Puncture wound without foreign body of unspecified buttock

  ☑7ᵗʰ **S31.804** Puncture wound with foreign body of unspecified buttock

  ☑7ᵗʰ **S31.805** Open bite of unspecified buttock
     Bite of buttock NOS
     *EXCLUDES 1*   superficial bite of buttock (S30.870)

  ☑7ᵗʰ **S31.809** Unspecified open wound of unspecified buttock

☑6ᵗʰ **S31.81** Open wound of right buttock

  ☑7ᵗʰ **S31.811** Laceration without foreign body of right buttock

  ☑7ᵗʰ **S31.812** Laceration with foreign body of right buttock

  ☑7ᵗʰ **S31.813** Puncture wound without foreign body of right buttock

  ☑7ᵗʰ **S31.814** Puncture wound with foreign body of right buttock

  ☑7ᵗʰ **S31.815** Open bite of right buttock
     Bite of right buttock NOS
     *EXCLUDES 1*   superficial bite of buttock (S30.870)

☑ Additional Character Req   ☑✗7ᵗʰ Placeholder Alert   Unacceptable PDx   Manifestation   H1–H14 HAC   HCC CMS-HCC Condition   *EXCLUDES 1* Not Coded Here   *EXCLUDES 2* Not Included Here

ICD-10-CM 2018      973

      ✓7ᵗʰ **S31.819**   **Unspecified open wound of right buttock**

   ✓6ᵗʰ **S31.82**   **Open wound of left buttock**

      ✓7ᵗʰ **S31.821**   **Laceration without foreign body of left buttock**

      ✓7ᵗʰ **S31.822**   **Laceration with foreign body of left buttock**

      ✓7ᵗʰ **S31.823**   **Puncture wound without foreign body of left buttock**

      ✓7ᵗʰ **S31.824**   **Puncture wound with foreign body of left buttock**

      ✓7ᵗʰ **S31.825**   **Open bite of left buttock**
          Bite of left buttock NOS
          **EXCLUDES 1**   *superficial bite of buttock (S30.870)*

      ✓7ᵗʰ **S31.829**   **Unspecified open wound of left buttock**

   ✓6ᵗʰ **S31.83**   **Open wound of anus**

      ✓7ᵗʰ **S31.831**   **Laceration without foreign body of anus**

      ✓7ᵗʰ **S31.832**   **Laceration with foreign body of anus**

      ✓7ᵗʰ **S31.833**   **Puncture wound without foreign body of anus**

      ✓7ᵗʰ **S31.834**   **Puncture wound with foreign body of anus**

      ✓7ᵗʰ **S31.835**   **Open bite of anus**
          Bite of anus NOS
          **EXCLUDES 1**   *superficial bite of anus (S30.877)*

      ✓7ᵗʰ **S31.839**   **Unspecified open wound of anus**

✓4ᵗʰ **S32**   **Fracture of lumbar spine and pelvis**

     **NOTE**   A fracture not indicated as displaced or nondisplaced should be coded to displaced.
         A fracture not indicated as opened or closed should be coded to closed.

     **INCLUDES**   fracture of lumbosacral neural arch
         fracture of lumbosacral spinous process
         fracture of lumbosacral transverse process
         fracture of lumbosacral vertebra
         fracture of lumbosacral vertebral arch

     Code first any associated spinal cord and spinal nerve injury (S34.-)
     **EXCLUDES 1**   *transection of abdomen (S38.3)*
     **EXCLUDES 2**   *fracture of hip NOS (S72.0-)*
     AHA: 2015, 3Q, 37-39; 2012, 4Q, 93

     The appropriate 7th character is to be added to each code from category S32.
     A     initial encounter for closed fracture
     B     initial encounter for open fracture
     D     subsequent encounter for fracture with routine healing
     G     subsequent encounter for fracture with delayed healing
     K     subsequent encounter for fracture with nonunion
     S     sequela

  ✓5ᵗʰ **S32.0**   **Fracture of lumbar vertebra**
     Fracture of lumbar spine NOS

     **CC Excl: For codes in subcategory S32.0:**
     **CC with 7th character A or MCC with 7th character B:** PDX collection 1196
     **CC with 7th character K:** PDX collection 897

   ✓6ᵗʰ **S32.00**   **Fracture of unspecified lumbar vertebra**

6,7,10   ✓7ᵗʰ **S32.000**   **Wedge compression fracture of unspecified lumbar vertebra**   MCC CC H5 HCC

6,7,10   ✓7ᵗʰ **S32.001**   **Stable burst fracture of unspecified lumbar vertebra**   MCC CC H5 HCC

6,7,10   ✓7ᵗʰ **S32.002**   **Unstable burst fracture of unspecified lumbar vertebra**   MCC CC H5 HCC

6,7,10   ✓7ᵗʰ **S32.008**   **Other fracture of unspecified lumbar vertebra**   MCC CC H5 HCC

6,7,10   ✓7ᵗʰ **S32.009**   **Unspecified fracture of unspecified lumbar vertebra**   MCC CC H5 HCC

   ✓6ᵗʰ **S32.01**   **Fracture of first lumbar vertebra**

6,7,10   ✓7ᵗʰ **S32.010**   **Wedge compression fracture of first lumbar vertebra**   MCC CC H5 HCC

6,7,10   ✓7ᵗʰ **S32.011**   **Stable burst fracture of first lumbar vertebra**   MCC CC H5 HCC

6,7,10   ✓7ᵗʰ **S32.012**   **Unstable burst fracture of first lumbar vertebra**   MCC CC H5 HCC

6,7,10   ✓7ᵗʰ **S32.018**   **Other fracture of first lumbar vertebra**   MCC CC H5 HCC

6,7,10   ✓7ᵗʰ **S32.019**   **Unspecified fracture of first lumbar vertebra**   MCC CC H5 HCC

   ✓6ᵗʰ **S32.02**   **Fracture of second lumbar vertebra**

6,7,10   ✓7ᵗʰ **S32.020**   **Wedge compression fracture of second lumbar vertebra**   MCC CC H5 HCC

6,7,10   ✓7ᵗʰ **S32.021**   **Stable burst fracture of second lumbar vertebra**   MCC CC H5 HCC

6,7,10   ✓7ᵗʰ **S32.022**   **Unstable burst fracture of second lumbar vertebra**   MCC CC H5 HCC

6,7,10   ✓7ᵗʰ **S32.028**   **Other fracture of second lumbar vertebra**   MCC CC H5 HCC

6,7,10   ✓7ᵗʰ **S32.029**   **Unspecified fracture of second lumbar vertebra**   MCC CC H5 HCC

   ✓6ᵗʰ **S32.03**   **Fracture of third lumbar vertebra**

6,7,10   ✓7ᵗʰ **S32.030**   **Wedge compression fracture of third lumbar vertebra**   MCC CC H5 HCC

6,7,10   ✓7ᵗʰ **S32.031**   **Stable burst fracture of third lumbar vertebra**   MCC CC H5 HCC

6,7,10   ✓7ᵗʰ **S32.032**   **Unstable burst fracture of third lumbar vertebra**   MCC CC H5 HCC

6,7,10   ✓7ᵗʰ **S32.038**   **Other fracture of third lumbar vertebra**   MCC CC H5 HCC

6,7,10   ✓7ᵗʰ **S32.039**   **Unspecified fracture of third lumbar vertebra**   MCC CC H5 HCC

   ✓6ᵗʰ **S32.04**   **Fracture of fourth lumbar vertebra**

6,7,10   ✓7ᵗʰ **S32.040**   **Wedge compression fracture of fourth lumbar vertebra**   MCC CC H5 HCC

6,7,10   ✓7ᵗʰ **S32.041**   **Stable burst fracture of fourth lumbar vertebra**   MCC CC H5 HCC

6,7,10   ✓7ᵗʰ **S32.042**   **Unstable burst fracture of fourth lumbar vertebra**   MCC CC H5 HCC

6,7,10   ✓7ᵗʰ **S32.048**   **Other fracture of fourth lumbar vertebra**   MCC CC H5 HCC

6,7,10   ✓7ᵗʰ **S32.049**   **Unspecified fracture of fourth lumbar vertebra**   MCC CC H5 HCC

   ✓6ᵗʰ **S32.05**   **Fracture of fifth lumbar vertebra**

6,7,10   ✓7ᵗʰ **S32.050**   **Wedge compression fracture of fifth lumbar vertebra**   MCC CC H5 HCC

6,7,10   ✓7ᵗʰ **S32.051**   **Stable burst fracture of fifth lumbar vertebra**   MCC CC H5 HCC

6,7,10   ✓7ᵗʰ **S32.052**   **Unstable burst fracture of fifth lumbar vertebra**   MCC CC H5 HCC

6,7,10   ✓7ᵗʰ **S32.058**   **Other fracture of fifth lumbar vertebra**   MCC CC H5 HCC

6,7,10   ✓7ᵗʰ **S32.059**   **Unspecified fracture of fifth lumbar vertebra**   MCC CC H5 HCC

  ✓5ᵗʰ **S32.1**   **Fracture of sacrum**

     **NOTE**   For vertical fractures, code to most medial fracture extension.
         Use two codes if both a vertical and transverse fracture are present.

     Code also any associated fracture of pelvic ring (S32.8-)

     **CC Excl: For codes in subcategory S32.1:**
     **CC with 7th character A or MCC with 7th character B:** PDX collection 1197
     **CC with 7th character K:** PDX collection 897

6,7,10   ✓x7ᵗʰ **S32.10**   **Unspecified fracture of sacrum**   MCC CC H5 HCC

   ✓6ᵗʰ **S32.11**   **Zone I fracture of sacrum**
     Vertical sacral ala fracture of sacrum

6,7,10   ✓7ᵗʰ **S32.110**   **Nondisplaced Zone I fracture of sacrum**   MCC CC H5 HCC

6,7,10   ✓7ᵗʰ **S32.111**   **Minimally displaced Zone I fracture of sacrum**   MCC CC H5 HCC

6,7,10   ✓7ᵗʰ **S32.112**   **Severely displaced Zone I fracture of sacrum**   MCC CC H5 HCC

---

⁶   MCC when reported as an open fracture (7th character B or C – specific to category).
⁷   CC when reported as an initial encounter (7th character A, B, or C – specific to category) OR a subsequent encounter for nonunion or malunion (7th character K, M, N, P, Q, or R – specific to category).
¹⁰   HCC with 7th character indicating initial encounter (A, B or C - specific to category).

Ⓝ Newborn: 0   Ⓟ Pediatric: 0-17   Ⓜ Maternity: 12-55   Ⓐ Adult: 15-124   **MCC** Major CC Condition   **PDxMCC** PDx acts as own MCC   **CC** CC Condition   **PDxCC** PDx acts as own CC

**974**        ICD-10-CM 2018

**Vertical Sacral Fracture Zones**

Zones: ① ② ③

**Transverse Sacral Fracture Types**

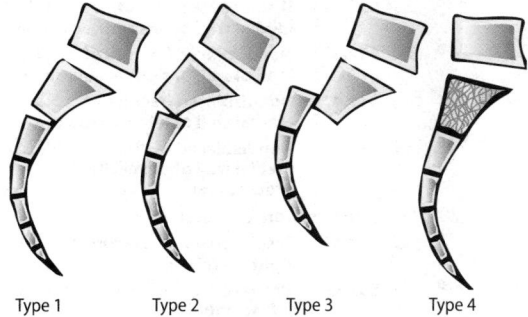

Type 1     Type 2     Type 3     Type 4

6,7,10 ✓7ᵗʰ **S32.119** **Unspecified Zone I fracture of sacrum** `MCC` `CC` `H5` `HCC`

✓6ᵗʰ **S32.12** **Zone II fracture of sacrum**
Vertical foraminal region fracture of sacrum

6,7,10 ✓7ᵗʰ **S32.120** **Nondisplaced Zone II fracture of sacrum** `MCC` `CC` `H5` `HCC`

6,7,10 ✓7ᵗʰ **S32.121** **Minimally displaced Zone II fracture of sacrum** `MCC` `CC` `H5` `HCC`

6,7,10 ✓7ᵗʰ **S32.122** **Severely displaced Zone II fracture of sacrum** `MCC` `CC` `H5` `HCC`

6,7,10 ✓7ᵗʰ **S32.129** **Unspecified Zone II fracture of sacrum** `MCC` `CC` `H5` `HCC`

✓6ᵗʰ **S32.13** **Zone III fracture of sacrum**
Vertical fracture into spinal canal region of sacrum

6,7,10 ✓7ᵗʰ **S32.130** **Nondisplaced Zone III fracture of sacrum** `MCC` `CC` `H5` `HCC`

6,7,10 ✓7ᵗʰ **S32.131** **Minimally displaced Zone III fracture of sacrum** `MCC` `CC` `H5` `HCC`

6,7,10 ✓7ᵗʰ **S32.132** **Severely displaced Zone III fracture of sacrum** `MCC` `CC` `H5` `HCC`

6,7,10 ✓7ᵗʰ **S32.139** **Unspecified Zone III fracture of sacrum** `MCC` `CC` `H5` `HCC`

6,7,10 ✓x7ᵗʰ **S32.14** **Type 1 fracture of sacrum** `MCC` `CC` `H5` `HCC`
Transverse flexion fracture of sacrum without displacement

6,7,10 ✓x7ᵗʰ **S32.15** **Type 2 fracture of sacrum** `MCC` `CC` `H5` `HCC`
Transverse flexion fracture of sacrum with posterior displacement

6,7,10 ✓x7ᵗʰ **S32.16** **Type 3 fracture of sacrum** `MCC` `CC` `H5` `HCC`
Transverse extension fracture of sacrum with anterior displacement

6,7,10 ✓x7ᵗʰ **S32.17** **Type 4 fracture of sacrum** `MCC` `CC` `H5` `HCC`
Transverse segmental comminution of upper sacrum

6,7,10 ✓x7ᵗʰ **S32.19** **Other fracture of sacrum** `MCC` `CC` `H5` `HCC`

6,7,10 ✓x7ᵗʰ **S32.2** **Fracture of coccyx** `MCC` `CC` `H5` `HCC`
**CC Excl:** See code S32.1

---

✓5ᵗʰ **S32.3** **Fracture of ilium**
*EXCLUDES 1*   fracture of ilium with associated disruption of pelvic ring (S32.8-)

> **CC Excl: For codes in subcategory S32.3:**
> **CC with 7th character A:** PDX collection 1176
> **MCC with 7th character B:** PDX collection 1198
> **CC with 7th character K:** PDX collection 897

✓6ᵗʰ **S32.30** **Unspecified fracture of ilium**

6,7,10 ✓7ᵗʰ **S32.301** **Unspecified fracture of right ilium** `MCC` `CC` `H5` `HCC`

6,7,10 ✓7ᵗʰ **S32.302** **Unspecified fracture of left ilium** `MCC` `CC` `H5` `HCC`

6,7,10 ✓7ᵗʰ **S32.309** **Unspecified fracture of unspecified ilium** `MCC` `CC` `H5` `HCC`

✓6ᵗʰ **S32.31** **Avulsion fracture of ilium**

6,7,10 ✓7ᵗʰ **S32.311** **Displaced avulsion fracture of right ilium** `MCC` `CC` `H5` `HCC`

6,7,10 ✓7ᵗʰ **S32.312** **Displaced avulsion fracture of left ilium** `MCC` `CC` `H5` `HCC`

6,7,10 ✓7ᵗʰ **S32.313** **Displaced avulsion fracture of unspecified ilium** `MCC` `CC` `H5` `HCC`

6,7,10 ✓7ᵗʰ **S32.314** **Nondisplaced avulsion fracture of right ilium** `MCC` `CC` `H5` `HCC`

6,7,10 ✓7ᵗʰ **S32.315** **Nondisplaced avulsion fracture of left ilium** `MCC` `CC` `H5` `HCC`

6,7,10 ✓7ᵗʰ **S32.316** **Nondisplaced avulsion fracture of unspecified ilium** `MCC` `CC` `H5` `HCC`

✓6ᵗʰ **S32.39** **Other fracture of ilium**

6,7,10 ✓7ᵗʰ **S32.391** **Other fracture of right ilium** `MCC` `CC` `H5` `HCC`

6,7,10 ✓7ᵗʰ **S32.392** **Other fracture of left ilium** `MCC` `CC` `H5` `HCC`

6,7,10 ✓7ᵗʰ **S32.399** **Other fracture of unspecified ilium** `MCC` `CC` `H5` `HCC`

✓5ᵗʰ **S32.4** **Fracture of acetabulum**
Code also any associated fracture of pelvic ring (S32.8-)
**AHA:** 2016, 3Q, 16

> **CC Excl: For codes in subcategory S32.4:**
> **MCC with 7th character A:** PDX collection 1199
> **MCC with 7th character B:** PDX collection 1200
> **CC with 7th character K:** PDX collection 897

✓6ᵗʰ **S32.40** **Unspecified fracture of acetabulum**

8,10 ✓7ᵗʰ **S32.401** **Unspecified fracture of right acetabulum** `MCC` `CC` `H5` `HCC`

8,10 ✓7ᵗʰ **S32.402** **Unspecified fracture of left acetabulum** `MCC` `CC` `H5` `HCC`

8,10 ✓7ᵗʰ **S32.409** **Unspecified fracture of unspecified acetabulum** `MCC` `CC` `H5` `HCC`

✓6ᵗʰ **S32.41** **Fracture of anterior wall of acetabulum**

8,10 ✓7ᵗʰ **S32.411** **Displaced fracture of anterior wall of right acetabulum** `MCC` `CC` `H5` `HCC`

8,10 ✓7ᵗʰ **S32.412** **Displaced fracture of anterior wall of left acetabulum** `MCC` `CC` `H5` `HCC`

8,10 ✓7ᵗʰ **S32.413** **Displaced fracture of anterior wall of unspecified acetabulum** `MCC` `CC` `H5` `HCC`

8,10 ✓7ᵗʰ **S32.414** **Nondisplaced fracture of anterior wall of right acetabulum** `MCC` `CC` `H5` `HCC`

8,10 ✓7ᵗʰ **S32.415** **Nondisplaced fracture of anterior wall of left acetabulum** `MCC` `CC` `H5` `HCC`

8,10 ✓7ᵗʰ **S32.416** **Nondisplaced fracture of anterior wall of unspecified acetabulum** `MCC` `CC` `H5` `HCC`

✓6ᵗʰ **S32.42** **Fracture of posterior wall of acetabulum**

8,10 ✓7ᵗʰ **S32.421** **Displaced fracture of posterior wall of right acetabulum** `MCC` `CC` `H5` `HCC`

---

**6**   MCC when reported as an open fracture (7th character B or C – specific to category).
**7**   CC when reported as an initial encounter (7th character A, B, or C – specific to category) OR a subsequent encounter for nonunion or malunion (7th character K, M, N, P, Q, or R – specific to category).
**8**   CC when reported as a subsequent encounter for nonunion or malunion (7th character K, M, N, P, Q, or R – specific to category).
**10**   HCC with 7th character indicating initial encounter (A, B or C - specific to category).

---

☑ Additional Character Req    ✓x7ᵗʰ Placeholder Alert    Unacceptable PDx    ■ Manifestation    `H1`-`H14` HAC    `HCC` CMS-HCC Condition    *EXCLUDES 1* Not Coded Here    *EXCLUDES 2* Not Included Here

ICD-10-CM 2018          **975**

8,10 ✓7ᵗʰ **S32.422** Displaced **fracture** of **posteriorwall** of **left** **acetabulum**   `MCC CC H5 HCC`

8,10 ✓7ᵗʰ **S32.423** Displaced **fracture** of **posterior wall** of **unspecified** **acetabulum**   `MCC CC H5 HCC`

8,10 ✓7ᵗʰ **S32.424** Nondisplaced **fracture** of **posterior wall** of **right acetabulum**   `MCC CC H5 HCC`

8,10 ✓7ᵗʰ **S32.425** Nondisplaced **fracture** of **posterior wall** of **left acetabulum**   `MCC CC H5 HCC`

8,10 ✓7ᵗʰ **S32.426** Nondisplaced **fracture** of **posterior wall** of **unspecified acetabulum**   `MCC CC H5 HCC`

✓6ᵗʰ **S32.43** **Fracture** of **anterior column [iliopubic]** of **acetabulum**

8,10 ✓7ᵗʰ **S32.431** Displaced **fracture** of **anterior column [iliopubic]** of **right acetabulum**   `MCC CC H5 HCC`

8,10 ✓7ᵗʰ **S32.432** Displaced **fracture** of **anterior column [iliopubic]** of **left acetabulum**   `MCC CC H5 HCC`

8,10 ✓7ᵗʰ **S32.433** Displaced **fracture** of **anterior column [iliopubic]** of **unspecified acetabulum**   `MCC CC H5 HCC`

8,10 ✓7ᵗʰ **S32.434** Nondisplaced **fracture** of **anterior column [iliopubic]** of **right** **acetabulum**   `MCC CC H5 HCC`

8,10 ✓7ᵗʰ **S32.435** Nondisplaced **fracture** of **anterior column [iliopubic]** of **left** **acetabulum**   `MCC CC H5 HCC`

8,10 ✓7ᵗʰ **S32.436** Nondisplaced **fracture** of **anterior column [iliopubic]** of **unspecified acetabulum**   `MCC CC H5 HCC`

✓6ᵗʰ **S32.44** **Fracture** of **posterior column [ilioischial]** of **acetabulum**

8,10 ✓7ᵗʰ **S32.441** Displaced **fracture** of **posterior column [ilioischial]** of **right acetabulum**   `MCC CC H5 HCC`

8,10 ✓7ᵗʰ **S32.442** Displaced **fracture** of **posteriorcolumn [ilioischial]** of **left acetabulum**   `MCC CC H5 HCC`

8,10 ✓7ᵗʰ **S32.443** Displaced **fracture** of **posterior column [ilioischial]** of **unspecified acetabulum**   `MCC CC H5 HCC`

8,10 ✓7ᵗʰ **S32.444** Nondisplaced **fracture** of **posterior column [ilioischial]** of **right acetabulum**   `MCC CC H5 HCC`

8,10 ✓7ᵗʰ **S32.445** Nondisplaced **fracture** of **posterior column [ilioischial]** of **left** **acetabulum**   `MCC CC H5 HCC`

8,10 ✓7ᵗʰ **S32.446** Nondisplaced **fracture** of **posterior column [ilioischial]** of **unspecified acetabulum**   `MCC CC H5 HCC`

✓6ᵗʰ **S32.45** **Transverse** **fracture of acetabulum**

8,10 ✓7ᵗʰ **S32.451** Displaced **transverse** **fracture** of **right acetabulum**   `MCC CC H5 HCC`

8,10 ✓7ᵗʰ **S32.452** Displaced **transverse** **fractureof** **left acetabulum**   `MCC CC H5 HCC`

8,10 ✓7ᵗʰ **S32.453** Displaced **transverse** **fracture** of **unspecified** **acetabulum**   `MCC CC H5 HCC`

8,10 ✓7ᵗʰ **S32.454** Nondisplaced **transverse** **fracture** of **right acetabulum**   `MCC CC H5 HCC`

8,10 ✓7ᵗʰ **S32.455** Nondisplaced **transverse** **fracture** of **left acetabulum**   `MCC CC H5 HCC`

8,10 ✓7ᵗʰ **S32.456** Nondisplaced **transverse** **fracture** of **unspecified acetabulum**   `MCC CC H5 HCC`

✓6ᵗʰ **S32.46** **Associated transverse-posterior** **fracture** of **acetabulum**

8,10 ✓7ᵗʰ **S32.461** Displaced **associated** **transverse-posterior fracture** of **right acetabulum**   `MCC CC H5 HCC`

8,10 ✓7ᵗʰ **S32.462** Displaced **associated** **transverse-posterior fracture** of **left acetabulum**   `MCC CC H5 HCC`

8,10 ✓7ᵗʰ **S32.463** Displaced **associated** **transverse-posterior fracture** of **unspecified acetabulum**   `MCC CC H5 HCC`

8,10 ✓7ᵗʰ **S32.464** Nondisplaced **associated** **transverse-posterior fracture** of **right acetabulum**   `MCC CC H5 HCC`

8,10 ✓7ᵗʰ **S32.465** Nondisplaced **associated** **transverse-posterior fracture** of **left acetabulum**   `MCC CC H5 HCC`

8,10 ✓7ᵗʰ **S32.466** Nondisplaced **associated** **transverse-posterior fracture** of **unspecified acetabulum**   `MCC CC H5 HCC`

✓6ᵗʰ **S32.47** **Fracture** of **medial wall** of **acetabulum**

8,10 ✓7ᵗʰ **S32.471** Displaced **fracture** of **medial wall** of **right acetabulum**   `MCC CC H5 HCC`

8,10 ✓7ᵗʰ **S32.472** Displaced **fracture** of **medial wall** of **left acetabulum**   `MCC CC H5 HCC`

8,10 ✓7ᵗʰ **S32.473** Displaced **fracture** of **medial wall** of **unspecified acetabulum**   `MCC CC H5 HCC`

8,10 ✓7ᵗʰ **S32.474** Nondisplaced **fracture** of **medial wall** of **right acetabulum**   `MCC CC H5 HCC`

8,10 ✓7ᵗʰ **S32.475** Nondisplaced **fracture** of **medial wall** of **left acetabulum**   `MCC CC H5 HCC`

8,10 ✓7ᵗʰ **S32.476** Nondisplaced **fracture** of **medial wall** of **unspecified** **acetabulum**   `MCC CC H5 HCC`

✓6ᵗʰ **S32.48** **Dome fracture of acetabulum**

8,10 ✓7ᵗʰ **S32.481** Displaced **dome fracture of** **right acetabulum**   `MCC CC H5 HCC`

8,10 ✓7ᵗʰ **S32.482** Displaced **dome fracture of** **left acetabulum**   `MCC CC H5 HCC`

8,10 ✓7ᵗʰ **S32.483** Displaced **dome fracture of** **unspecified acetabulum**   `MCC CC H5 HCC`

8,10 ✓7ᵗʰ **S32.484** Nondisplaced **dome** **fracture of right acetabulum**   `MCC CC H5 HCC`

8,10 ✓7ᵗʰ **S32.485** Nondisplaced **dome** **fracture of left acetabulum**   `MCC CC H5 HCC`

8,10 ✓7ᵗʰ **S32.486** Nondisplaced **dome** **fracture of unspecified acetabulum**   `MCC CC H5 HCC`

✓6ᵗʰ **S32.49** **Other specified fracture of acetabulum**

8,10 ✓7ᵗʰ **S32.491** **Other specified fracture of** **right acetabulum**   `MCC CC H5 HCC`

8,10 ✓7ᵗʰ **S32.492** **Other specified fracture of** **left acetabulum**   `MCC CC H5 HCC`

8,10 ✓7ᵗʰ **S32.499** **Other specified fracture of** **unspecified acetabulum**   `MCC CC H5 HCC`

✓5ᵗʰ **S32.5** **Fracture of pubis**

    `EXCLUDES 1` *fracture of pubis with associated disruption of pelvic ring (S32.8-)*

> **CC Excl: For codes in subcategory S32.5:**
> **CC with 7th character A or MCC with 7th character B:** PDX collection 1201
> **CC with 7th character K:** PDX collection 897

✓6ᵗʰ **S32.50** **Unspecified fracture of pubis**

6,7,10 ✓7ᵗʰ **S32.501** **Unspecified fracture of right** **pubis**   `MCC CC HCC`

6,7,10 ✓7ᵗʰ **S32.502** **Unspecified fracture of left** **pubis**   `MCC CC H5 HCC`

6,7,10 ✓7ᵗʰ **S32.509** **Unspecified fracture of** **unspecified pubis**   `MCC CC H5 HCC`

✓6ᵗʰ **S32.51** **Fracture of superior rim of pubis**

6,7,10 ✓7ᵗʰ **S32.511** **Fracture of superior rim of** **right pubis**   `MCC CC H5 HCC`

6,7,10 ✓7ᵗʰ **S32.512** **Fracture of superior rim of** **left pubis**   `MCC CC H5 HCC`

6,7,10 ✓7ᵗʰ **S32.519** **Fracture of superior rim of** **unspecified pubis**   `MCC CC H5 HCC`

---

**6**   MCC when reported as an open fracture (7th character B or C – specific to category).

**7**   CC when reported as an initial encounter (7th character A, B, or C – specific to category) OR a subsequent encounter for nonunion or malunion (7th character K, M, N, P, Q, or R – specific to category).

**8**   CC when reported as a subsequent encounter for nonunion or malunion (7th character K, M, N, P, Q, or R – specific to category).

**10**   HCC with 7th character indicating initial encounter (A, B or C - specific to category).

Ⓝ Newborn: 0   Ⓟ Pediatric: 0-17   Ⓜ Maternity: 12-55   Ⓐ Adult: 15-124   `MCC` Major CC Condition   `PDxMCC` PDx acts as own MCC   `CC` CC Condition   `PDxCC` PDx acts as own CC

976     ICD-10-CM 2018

✓6th **S32.59**   Other **specified fracture of pubis**

6,7,10   ✓7th **S32.591**   Other **specified fracture of right pubis**   MCC CC H5 HCC

6,7,10   ✓7th **S32.592**   Other **specified fracture of left pubis**   MCC CC H5 HCC

6,7,10   ✓7th **S32.599**   Other **specified fracture of unspecified pubis**   MCC CC H5 HCC

✓5th **S32.6**   **Fracture of ischium**

> EXCLUDES 1   fracture of ischium with associated disruption of pelvic ring (S32.8-)

> **CC Excl: For codes in subcategory S32.6:**
> **CC with 7th character A: PDX collection 1202**
> **MCC with 7th character B: PDX collection 1203**
> **CC with 7th character K: PDX collection 897**

✓6th **S32.60**   **Unspecified fracture of ischium**

6,7,10   ✓7th **S32.601**   **Unspecified fracture of right ischium**   MCC CC H5 HCC

6,7,10   ✓7th **S32.602**   **Unspecified fracture of left ischium**   MCC CC H5 HCC

6,7,10   ✓7th **S32.609**   **Unspecified fracture of unspecified ischium**   MCC CC H5 HCC

✓6th **S32.61**   **Avulsion fracture of ischium**

6,7,10   ✓7th **S32.611**   **Displaced avulsion fracture of right ischium**   MCC CC H5 HCC

6,7,10   ✓7th **S32.612**   **Displaced avulsion fracture of left ischium**   MCC CC H5 HCC

6,7,10   ✓7th **S32.613**   **Displaced avulsion fracture of unspecified ischium**   MCC CC H5 HCC

6,7,10   ✓7th **S32.614**   **Nondisplaced avulsion fracture of right ischium**   MCC CC H5 HCC

6,7,10   ✓7th **S32.615**   **Nondisplaced avulsion fracture of left ischium**   MCC CC H5 HCC

6,7,10   ✓7th **S32.616**   **Nondisplaced avulsion fracture of unspecified ischium**   MCC CC H5 HCC

✓6th **S32.69**   Other **specified fracture of ischium**

6,7,10   ✓7th **S32.691**   Other **specified fracture of right ischium**   MCC CC H5 HCC

6,7,10   ✓7th **S32.692**   Other **specified fracture of left ischium**   MCC CC H5 HCC

6,7,10   ✓7th **S32.699**   Other **specified fracture of unspecified ischium**   MCC CC H5 HCC

✓5th **S32.8**   **Fracture of other parts of pelvis**

> Code also any associated:
> fracture of acetabulum (S32.4-)
> sacral fracture (S32.1-)

✓6th **S32.81**   **Multiple fractures of pelvis with disruption of pelvic ring**

> Multiple pelvic fractures with disruption of pelvic circle

> **CC Excl: For codes in subcategory S32.81:**
> **CC with 7th character A or MCC with 7th character B: PDX collection 1204**
> **CC with 7th character K: PDX collection 897**

6,7,10   ✓7th **S32.810**   **Multiple fractures of pelvis with stable disruption of pelvic ring**   MCC CC H5 HCC

**Fractures Disrupting Pelvic Circle**

6,7,10   ✓7th **S32.811**   **Multiple fractures of pelvis with unstable disruption of pelvic ring**   MCC CC H5 HCC

6,7,10   ✓x7th **S32.82**   **Multiple fractures of pelvis without disruption of pelvic ring**   MCC CC H5 HCC

> Multiple pelvic fractures without disruption of pelvic circle
> **CC Excl: CC with 7th character A or MCC with 7th character B: PDX collection 1205**
> **CC with 7th character K: PDX collection 897**

6,7,10   ✓x7th **S32.89**   **Fracture of other parts of pelvis**   MCC CC H5 HCC

> **CC Excl: CC with 7th character A or MCC with 7th character B: PDX collection 1206**
> **CC with 7th character K: PDX collection 897**

6,7,10 ✓x7th **S32.9**   **Fracture of unspecified parts of lumbosacral spine and pelvis**   MCC CC H5 HCC

> Fracture of lumbosacral spine NOS
> Fracture of pelvis NOS
> **AHA:** 2012, 4Q, 93
> **CC Excl: CC with 7th character A or MCC with 7th character B:** PDX collection 1204
> **CC with 7th character K:** PDX collection 897

✓4th **S33**   **Dislocation and sprain of joints and ligaments of lumbar spine and pelvis**

> INCLUDES   avulsion of joint or ligament of lumbar spine and pelvis
> laceration of cartilage, joint or ligament of lumbar spine and pelvis
> sprain of cartilage, joint or ligament of lumbar spine and pelvis
> traumatic hemarthrosis of joint or ligament of lumbar spine and pelvis
> traumatic rupture of joint or ligament of lumbar spine and pelvis
> traumatic subluxation of joint or ligament of lumbar spine and pelvis
> traumatic tear of joint or ligament of lumbar spine and pelvis

> Code also any associated open wound
> EXCLUDES 1   nontraumatic rupture or displacement of lumbar intervertebral disc NOS (M51.-)
> obstetric damage to pelvic joints and ligaments (O71.6)
> EXCLUDES 2   dislocation and sprain of joints and ligaments of hip (S73.-)
> strain of muscle of lower back and pelvis (S39.01-)

> The appropriate 7th character is to be added to each code from category S33.
> A   initial encounter
> D   subsequent encounter
> S   sequela

✓x7th **S33.0**   **Traumatic rupture of lumbar intervertebral disc**

> EXCLUDES 1   rupture or displacement (nontraumatic) of lumbar intervertebral disc NOS (M51- with fifth character 6)

✓5th **S33.1**   **Subluxation and dislocation of lumbar vertebra**

> Code also any associated:
> open wound of abdomen, lower back and pelvis (S31)
> spinal cord injury (S24.0, S24.1-, S34.0-, S34.1-)
> EXCLUDES 2   fracture of lumbar vertebrae (S32.0-)

✓6th **S33.10**   **Subluxation and dislocation of unspecified lumbar vertebra**

✓7th **S33.100**   **Subluxation of unspecified lumbar vertebra**

✓7th **S33.101**   **Dislocation of unspecified lumbar vertebra**

✓6th **S33.11**   **Subluxation and dislocation of L1/L2 lumbar vertebra**

✓7th **S33.110**   **Subluxation of L1/L2 lumbar vertebra**

✓7th **S33.111**   **Dislocation of L1/L2 lumbar vertebra**

✓6th **S33.12**   **Subluxation and dislocation of L2/L3 lumbar vertebra**

✓7th **S33.120**   **Subluxation of L2/L3 lumbar vertebra**

✓7th **S33.121**   **Dislocation of L2/L3 lumbar vertebra**

✓6th **S33.13**   **Subluxation and dislocation of L3/L4 lumbar vertebra**

✓7th **S33.130**   **Subluxation of L3/L4 lumbar vertebra**

✓7th **S33.131**   **Dislocation of L3/L4 lumbar vertebra**

---

6   MCC when reported as an open fracture (7th character B or C – specific to category).

7   CC when reported as an initial encounter (7th character A, B, or C – specific to category) OR a subsequent encounter for nonunion or malunion (7th character K, M, N, P, Q, or R – specific to category).

10   HCC with 7th character indicating initial encounter (A, B, or C - specific to category).

✓ Additional Character Req   ✓x7th Placeholder Alert   Unacceptable PDx   Manifestation   H1 - H14 HAC   HCC CMS-HCC Condition   EXCLUDES 1 Not Coded Here   EXCLUDES 2 Not Included Here

ICD-10-CM 2018      **977**

S32.59-S33.131

**√6ᵗʰ S33.14 Subluxation and dislocation of L4/L5 lumbar vertebra**

    √7ᵗʰ **S33.140** Subluxation of L4/L5 lumbar vertebra

    √7ᵗʰ **S33.141** Dislocation of L4/L5 lumbar vertebra

√x7ᵗʰ **S33.2 Dislocation of** sacroiliac **and** sacrococcygeal **joint**

√5ᵗʰ **S33.3 Dislocation of** other and unspecified parts **of lumbar spine and pelvis**

    √x7ᵗʰ **S33.30 Dislocation of** unspecified **parts of lumbar spine and pelvis**

    √x7ᵗʰ **S33.39 Dislocation of** other **parts of lumbar spine and pelvis**

√x7ᵗʰ **S33.4 Traumatic rupture of** symphysis pubis

√x7ᵗʰ **S33.5 Sprain of ligaments of** lumbar spine

√x7ᵗʰ **S33.6 Sprain of** sacroiliac joint

√x7ᵗʰ **S33.8 Sprain of** other **parts of lumbar spine and pelvis**

√x7ᵗʰ **S33.9 Sprain of** unspecified **parts of lumbar spine and pelvis**

√4ᵗʰ **S34 Injury of lumbar and sacral spinal cord and nerves at abdomen, lower back and pelvis level**

    **NOTE**   Code to highest level of lumbar cord injury.
    Injuries to the spinal cord (S34.0 and S34.1) refer to the cord level and not bone level injury, and can affect nerve roots at and below the level given.

    Code also any associated:
        fracture of vertebra (S22.0-, S32.0-)
        open wound of abdomen, lower back and pelvis (S31.-)
        transient paralysis (R29.5)

    The appropriate 7th character is to be added to each code from category S34.
    A    initial encounter
    D    subsequent encounter
    S    sequela

    **CC Excl: For codes in category S34 unless otherwise noted: MCC with 7th character A:** PDX collection 1207

√5ᵗʰ **S34.0 Concussion and edema of lumbar and sacral spinal cord**

    √x7ᵗʰ **S34.01 Concussion and edema of** lumbar **spinal cord** `MCC` `HCC`

    √x7ᵗʰ **S34.02 Concussion and edema of** sacral **spinal cord** `MCC` `HCC`
        Concussion and edema of conus medullaris
        **CC Excl: MCC with 7th character A:** PDX collection 1208

√5ᵗʰ **S34.1 Other and unspecified injury of lumbar and sacral spinal cord**

    √6ᵗʰ **S34.10 Unspecified injury to lumbar spinal cord**

        √7ᵗʰ **S34.101 Unspecified injury to L1 level of lumbar spinal cord** `MCC` `H5` `HCC`
            Unspecified injury to lumbar spinal cord level 1

        √7ᵗʰ **S34.102 Unspecified injury to L2 level of lumbar spinal cord** `MCC` `H5` `HCC`
            Unspecified injury to lumbar spinal cord level 2

        √7ᵗʰ **S34.103 Unspecified injury to L3 level of lumbar spinal cord** `MCC` `H5` `HCC`
            Unspecified injury to lumbar spinal cord level 3

        √7ᵗʰ **S34.104 Unspecified injury to L4 level of lumbar spinal cord** `MCC` `H5` `HCC`
            Unspecified injury to lumbar spinal cord level 4

        √7ᵗʰ **S34.105 Unspecified injury to L5 level of lumbar spinal cord** `MCC` `H5` `HCC`
            Unspecified injury to lumbar spinal cord level 5

        √7ᵗʰ **S34.109 Unspecified injury to unspecified level of lumbar spinal cord** `MCC` `H5` `HCC`

    √6ᵗʰ **S34.11 Complete lesion of lumbar spinal cord**

        √7ᵗʰ **S34.111 Complete lesion of L1 level of lumbar spinal cord** `MCC` `H5` `HCC`
            Complete lesion of lumbar spinal cord level 1

        √7ᵗʰ **S34.112 Complete lesion of L2 level of lumbar spinal cord** `MCC` `H5` `HCC`
            Complete lesion of lumbar spinal cord level 2

        √7ᵗʰ **S34.113 Complete lesion of L3 level of lumbar spinal cord** `MCC` `H5` `HCC`
            Complete lesion of lumbar spinal cord level 3

        √7ᵗʰ **S34.114 Complete lesion of L4 level of lumbar spinal cord** `MCC` `H5` `HCC`
            Complete lesion of lumbar spinal cord level 4

        √7ᵗʰ **S34.115 Complete lesion of L5 level of lumbar spinal cord** `MCC` `H5` `HCC`
            Complete lesion of lumbar spinal cord level 5

        √7ᵗʰ **S34.119 Complete lesion of unspecified level of lumbar spinal cord** `MCC` `H5` `HCC`

    √6ᵗʰ **S34.12 Incomplete lesion of lumbar spinal cord**

        √7ᵗʰ **S34.121 Incomplete lesion of L1 level of** `MCC` `H5` `HCC` **lumbar spinal cord**
            Incomplete lesion of lumbar spinal cord level 1

        √7ᵗʰ **S34.122 Incomplete lesion of L2 level of lumbar spinal cord** `MCC` `H5` `HCC`
            Incomplete lesion of lumbar spinal cord level 2

        √7ᵗʰ **S34.123 Incomplete lesion of L3 level of lumbar spinal cord** `MCC` `H5` `HCC`
            Incomplete lesion of lumbar spinal cord level 3

        √7ᵗʰ **S34.124 Incomplete lesion of L4 level of lumbar spinal cord** `MCC` `H5` `HCC`
            Incomplete lesion of lumbar spinal cord level 4

        √7ᵗʰ **S34.125 Incomplete lesion of L5 level of lumbar spinal cord** `MCC` `H5` `HCC`
            Incomplete lesion of lumbar spinal cord level 5

        √7ᵗʰ **S34.129 Incomplete lesion of unspecified level of lumbar spinal cord** `MCC` `H5` `HCC`

    √6ᵗʰ **S34.13 Other and unspecified injury to** sacral **spinal cord**
        Other injury to conus medullaris

        **CC Excl: For codes in subcategory S34.13: MCC with 7th character A:** PDX collection 1208

        √7ᵗʰ **S34.131 Complete lesion of sacral spinal cord** `MCC` `H5` `HCC`
            Complete lesion of conus medullaris

        √7ᵗʰ **S34.132 Incomplete lesion of sacral spinal cord** `MCC` `H5` `HCC`
            Incomplete lesion of conus medullaris

        √7ᵗʰ **S34.139 Unspecified injury to sacral spinal cord** `MCC` `H5` `HCC`
            Unspecified injury of conus medullaris

√5ᵗʰ **S34.2 Injury of nerve root of lumbar and sacral spine**

    √x7ᵗʰ **S34.21 Injury of nerve root of** lumbar spine

    √x7ᵗʰ **S34.22 Injury of nerve root of** sacral spine

10 √x7ᵗʰ **S34.3 Injury of cauda equina** `MCC` `H5` `HCC`
    **CC Excl: MCC with 7th character A:** PDX collection 1208

√x7ᵗʰ **S34.4 Injury of lumbosacral plexus**

√x7ᵗʰ **S34.5 Injury of lumbar, sacral and pelvic sympathetic nerves**
    Injury of celiac ganglion or plexus
    Injury of hypogastric plexus
    Injury of mesenteric plexus (inferior) (superior)
    Injury of splanchnic nerve

√x7ᵗʰ **S34.6 Injury of peripheral nerve(s) at abdomen, lower back and pelvis level**

√x7ᵗʰ **S34.8 Injury of other nerves at abdomen, lower back and pelvis level**

√x7ᵗʰ **S34.9 Injury of unspecified nerves at abdomen, lower back and pelvis level**

---

10 HCC with 7th character indicating initial encounter (A, B or C - specific to category).

N Newborn: 0   P Pediatric: 0-17   M Maternity: 12-55   A Adult: 15-124   `MCC` Major CC Condition   `PDxMCC` PDx acts as own MCC   `CC` CC Condition   `PDxCC` PDx acts as own CC

**978**

**ICD-10-CM 2018**

✓4ᵗʰ **S35   Injury of blood vessels at abdomen, lower back and pelvis level**
Code also any associated open wound (S31.-)

The appropriate 7th character is to be added to each code from category S35.
A     initial encounter
D     subsequent encounter
S     sequela

✓5ᵗʰ **S35.0   Injury of abdominal aorta**
> *EXCLUDES 1*   injury of aorta NOS (S25.0)

> **CC Excl: For codes in subcategory S35.0:**
> **MCC with 7th character A:** PDX collection 1209

   ✓x7ᵗʰ **S35.00   Unspecified injury of abdominal aorta**   `MCC`

   ✓x7ᵗʰ **S35.01   Minor laceration of abdominal aorta**   `MCC`
         Incomplete transection of abdominal aorta
         Laceration of abdominal aorta NOS
         Superficial laceration of abdominal aorta

   ✓x7ᵗʰ **S35.02   Major laceration of abdominal aorta**   `MCC`
         Complete transection of abdominal aorta
         Traumatic rupture of abdominal aorta

   ✓x7ᵗʰ **S35.09   Other injury of abdominal aorta**   `MCC`

✓5ᵗʰ **S35.1   Injury of inferior vena cava**
Injury of hepatic vein
> *EXCLUDES 1*   injury of vena cava NOS (S25.2)

> **CC Excl: For codes in subcategory S35.1:**
> **MCC with 7th character A:** PDX collection 1210

   ✓x7ᵗʰ **S35.10   Unspecified injury of inferior vena cava**   `MCC`

   ✓x7ᵗʰ **S35.11   Minor laceration of inferior vena cava**   `MCC`
         Incomplete transection of inferior vena cava
         Laceration of inferior vena cava NOS
         Superficial laceration of inferior vena cava

   ✓x7ᵗʰ **S35.12   Major laceration of inferior vena cava**   `MCC`
         Complete transection of inferior vena cava
         Traumatic rupture of inferior vena cava

   ✓x7ᵗʰ **S35.19   Other injury of inferior vena cava**   `MCC`

✓5ᵗʰ **S35.2   Injury of celiac or mesenteric artery and branches**
   ✓6ᵗʰ **S35.21   Injury of celiac artery**

> **CC Excl: For codes in subcategory S35.21:**
> **MCC with 7th character A:** PDX collection 1211

     ✓7ᵗʰ **S35.211   Minor laceration of celiac artery**   `MCC`
           Incomplete transection of celiac artery
           Laceration of celiac artery NOS
           Superficial laceration of celiac artery

     ✓7ᵗʰ **S35.212   Major laceration of celiac artery**   `MCC`
           Complete transection of celiac artery
           Traumatic rupture of celiac artery

     ✓7ᵗʰ **S35.218   Other injury of celiac artery**   `MCC`

     ✓7ᵗʰ **S35.219   Unspecified injury of celiac artery**   `MCC`

   ✓6ᵗʰ **S35.22   Injury of superior mesenteric artery**

> **CC Excl: For codes in subcategory S35.22:**
> **MCC with 7th character A:** PDX collection 1212

     ✓7ᵗʰ **S35.221   Minor laceration of superior mesenteric artery**   `MCC`
           Incomplete transection of superior mesenteric artery
           Laceration of superior mesenteric artery NOS
           Superficial laceration of superior mesenteric artery

     ✓7ᵗʰ **S35.222   Major laceration of superior mesenteric artery**   `MCC`
           Complete transection of superior mesenteric artery
           Traumatic rupture of superior mesenteric artery

     ✓7ᵗʰ **S35.228   Other injury of superior mesenteric artery**   `MCC`

     ✓7ᵗʰ **S35.229   Unspecified injury of superior mesenteric artery**   `MCC`

   ✓6ᵗʰ **S35.23   Injury of inferior mesenteric artery**

> **CC Excl: For codes in subcategory S35.23:**
> **MCC with 7th character A:** PDX collection 1213

     ✓7ᵗʰ **S35.231   Minor laceration of inferior mesenteric artery**   `MCC`
           Incomplete transection of inferior mesenteric artery
           Laceration of inferior mesenteric artery NOS
           Superficial laceration of inferior mesenteric artery

     ✓7ᵗʰ **S35.232   Major laceration of inferior mesenteric artery**   `MCC`
           Complete transection of inferior mesenteric artery
           Traumatic rupture of inferior mesenteric artery

     ✓7ᵗʰ **S35.238   Other injury of inferior mesenteric artery**   `MCC`

     ✓7ᵗʰ **S35.239   Unspecified injury of inferior mesenteric artery**   `MCC`

   ✓6ᵗʰ **S35.29   Injury of branches of celiac and mesenteric artery**
       Injury of gastric artery
       Injury of gastroduodenal artery
       Injury of hepatic artery
       Injury of splenic artery

     ✓7ᵗʰ **S35.291   Minor laceration of branches of celiac and mesenteric artery**   `MCC`
           Incomplete transection of branches of celiac and mesenteric artery
           Laceration of branches of celiac and mesenteric artery NOS
           Superficial laceration of branches of celiac and mesenteric artery
>            **CC Excl: MCC with 7th character A:**
>            PDX collection 1214

     ✓7ᵗʰ **S35.292   Major laceration of branches of celiac and mesenteric artery**   `MCC`
           Complete transection of branches of celiac and mesenteric artery
           Traumatic rupture of branches of celiac and mesenteric artery
>            **CC Excl: MCC with 7th character A:**
>            PDX collection 1215

     ✓7ᵗʰ **S35.298   Other injury of branches of celiac and mesenteric artery**   `MCC`
>            **CC Excl: MCC with 7th character A:**
>            PDX collection 1215

     ✓7ᵗʰ **S35.299   Unspecified injury of branches of celiac and mesenteric artery**   `MCC`
>            **CC Excl: MCC with 7th character A:**
>            PDX collection 1216

✓5ᵗʰ **S35.3   Injury of portal or splenic vein and branches**
   ✓6ᵗʰ **S35.31   Injury of portal vein**

> **CC Excl: For codes in subcategory S35.31:**
> **MCC with 7th character A:** PDX collection 1217

     ✓7ᵗʰ **S35.311   Laceration of portal vein**   `MCC`
     ✓7ᵗʰ **S35.318   Other specified injury of portal vein**   `MCC`
     ✓7ᵗʰ **S35.319   Unspecified injury of portal vein**   `MCC`

   ✓6ᵗʰ **S35.32   Injury of splenic vein**

> **CC Excl: For codes in subcategory S35.32:**
> **MCC with 7th character A:** PDX collection 1218

     ✓7ᵗʰ **S35.321   Laceration of splenic vein**   `MCC`
     ✓7ᵗʰ **S35.328   Other specified injury of splenic vein**   `MCC`
     ✓7ᵗʰ **S35.329   Unspecified injury of splenic vein**   `MCC`

   ✓6ᵗʰ **S35.33   Injury of superior mesenteric vein**

> **CC Excl: For codes in subcategory S35.33:**
> **MCC with 7th character A:** PDX collection 1219

     ✓7ᵗʰ **S35.331   Laceration of superior mesenteric vein**   `MCC`
     ✓7ᵗʰ **S35.338   Other specified injury of superior mesenteric vein**   `MCC`
     ✓7ᵗʰ **S35.339   Unspecified injury of superior mesenteric vein**   `MCC`

---

√6ᵗʰ **S35.34** Injury of inferior mesenteric vein

> **CC Excl: For codes in subcategory S35.34:**
> **MCC with 7th character A:** PDX collection 1220

√7ᵗʰ **S35.341** Laceration of inferior mesenteric vein `MCC`

√7ᵗʰ **S35.348** Other specified injury of inferior mesenteric vein `MCC`

√7ᵗʰ **S35.349** Unspecified injury of inferior mesenteric vein `MCC`

√5ᵗʰ **S35.4** Injury of renal blood vessels

> **CC Excl: For codes in subcategory S35.4, unless**
> **otherwise noted: MCC with 7th character A:**
> PDX collection 1221

√6ᵗʰ **S35.40** Unspecified injury of renal blood vessel

√7ᵗʰ **S35.401** Unspecified injury of right renal artery `MCC`

√7ᵗʰ **S35.402** Unspecified injury of left renal artery `MCC`

√7ᵗʰ **S35.403** Unspecified injury of unspecified renal artery `MCC`

√7ᵗʰ **S35.404** Unspecified injury of right renal vein `MCC`
> **CC Excl: MCC with 7th character A:**
> PDX collection 1222

√7ᵗʰ **S35.405** Unspecified injury of left renal vein `MCC`
> **CC Excl: MCC with 7th character A:**
> PDX collection 1222

√7ᵗʰ **S35.406** Unspecified injury of unspecified renal vein `MCC`
> **CC Excl: MCC with 7th character A:**
> PDX collection 1222

√6ᵗʰ **S35.41** Laceration of renal blood vessel

√7ᵗʰ **S35.411** Laceration of right renal artery `MCC`

√7ᵗʰ **S35.412** Laceration of left renal artery `MCC`

√7ᵗʰ **S35.413** Laceration of unspecified renal artery `MCC`

√7ᵗʰ **S35.414** Laceration of right renal vein `MCC`
> **CC Excl: MCC with 7th character A:**
> PDX collection 1222

√7ᵗʰ **S35.415** Laceration of left renal vein `MCC`
> **CC Excl: MCC with 7th character A:**
> PDX collection 1222

√7ᵗʰ **S35.416** Laceration of unspecified renal vein `MCC`
> **CC Excl: MCC with 7th character A:**
> PDX collection 1222

√6ᵗʰ **S35.49** Other specified injury of renal blood vessel

√7ᵗʰ **S35.491** Other specified injury of right renal artery `MCC`

√7ᵗʰ **S35.492** Other specified injury of left renal artery `MCC`

√7ᵗʰ **S35.493** Other specified injury of unspecified renal artery `MCC`

√7ᵗʰ **S35.494** Other specified injury of right renal vein `MCC`
> **CC Excl: MCC with 7th character A:**
> PDX collection 1222

√7ᵗʰ **S35.495** Other specified injury of left renal vein `MCC`
> **CC Excl: MCC with 7th character A:**
> PDX collection 1222

√7ᵗʰ **S35.496** Other specified injury of unspecified renal vein `MCC`
> **CC Excl: MCC with 7th character A:**
> PDX collection 1222

√5ᵗʰ **S35.5** Injury of iliac blood vessels

√x7ᵗʰ **S35.50** Injury of unspecified iliac blood vessel(s) `MCC`
> **CC Excl: MCC with 7th character A:** PDX collection
> 1223

√6ᵗʰ **S35.51** Injury of iliac artery or vein
Injury of hypogastric artery or vein

√7ᵗʰ **S35.511** Injury of right iliac artery `MCC`
> **CC Excl: MCC with 7th character A:**
> PDX collection 1224

√7ᵗʰ **S35.512** Injury of left iliac artery `MCC`
> **CC Excl: MCC with 7th character A:**
> PDX collection 1224

√7ᵗʰ **S35.513** Injury of unspecified iliac artery `MCC`
> **CCC Excl: MCC with 7th character A:**
> PDX collection 1224

√7ᵗʰ **S35.514** Injury of right iliac vein `MCC`
> **CC Excl: MCC with 7th character A:**
> PDX collection 1225

√7ᵗʰ **S35.515** Injury of left iliac vein `MCC`
> **CC Excl: MCC with 7th character A:**
> PDX collection 1225

√7ᵗʰ **S35.516** Injury of unspecified iliac vein `MCC`
> **CC Excl: MCC with 7th character A:**
> PDX collection 1225

√6ᵗʰ **S35.53** Injury of uterine artery or vein

√7ᵗʰ **S35.531** Injury of right uterine artery `CC`♀
> **CC Excl: CC with 7th character A:**
> PDX collection 1226

√7ᵗʰ **S35.532** Injury of left uterine artery `CC`♀
> **CC Excl: CC with 7th character A:**
> PDX collection 1226

√7ᵗʰ **S35.533** Injury of unspecified uterine artery `CC`♀
> **CC Excl: CC with 7th character A:**
> PDX collection 1226

√7ᵗʰ **S35.534** Injury of right uterine vein `CC`♀
> **CC Excl: CC with 7th character A:**
> PDX collection 1227

√7ᵗʰ **S35.535** Injury of left uterine vein `CC`♀
> **CC Excl: CC with 7th character A:**
> PDX collection 1227

√7ᵗʰ **S35.536** Injury of unspecified uterine vein `CC`♀
> **CC Excl: CC with 7th character A:**
> PDX collection 1227

√x7ᵗʰ **S35.59** Injury of other iliac blood vessels `MCC`
> **CC Excl: MCC with 7th character A:**
> PDX collection 1223

√5ᵗʰ **S35.8** Injury of other blood vessels at abdomen, lower back and pelvis level
Injury of ovarian artery or vein

√6ᵗʰ **S35.8X** Injury of other blood vessels at abdomen, lower back and pelvis level

> **CC Excl: For codes in subcategory S35.8X:**
> **CC with 7th character A:** PDX collection 1228

√7ᵗʰ **S35.8X1** Laceration of other blood vessels at abdomen, lower back and pelvis level `CC`

√7ᵗʰ **S35.8X8** Other specified injury of other blood vessels at abdomen, lower back and pelvis level `CC`

√7ᵗʰ **S35.8X9** Unspecified injury of other blood vessels at abdomen, lower back and pelvis level `CC`

√5ᵗʰ **S35.9** Injury of unspecified blood vessel at abdomen, lower back and pelvis level

> **CC Excl: For codes in subcategory S35.9:**
> **CC with 7th character A:** PDX collection 1229

√x7ᵗʰ **S35.90** Unspecified injury of unspecified blood vessel at abdomen, lower back and pelvis level `CC`

√x7ᵗʰ **S35.91** Laceration of unspecified blood vessel at abdomen, lower back and pelvis level `CC`

√x7ᵗʰ **S35.99** Other specified injury of unspecified blood vessel at abdomen, lower back and pelvis level `CC`

√4ᵗʰ **S36** Injury of intra-abdominal organs
Code also any associated open wound (S31.-)

> The appropriate 7th character is to be added to each code from
> category S36.
> A    initial encounter
> D    subsequent encounter
> S    sequela

√5ᵗʰ **S36.0** Injury of spleen
**AHA:** 2015, 2Q, 36; 2015, 1Q, 10

> **CC Excl: For codes in subcategory S36.0:**
> **CC or MCC with 7th character A:** PDX collection 1230

√x7ᵗʰ **S36.00** Unspecified injury of spleen `CC`

√6ᵗʰ **S36.02** Contusion of spleen

√7ᵗʰ **S36.020** Minor contusion of spleen `CC`
Contusion of spleen less than 2 cm

√7ᵗʰ **S36.021** Major contusion of spleen `CC`
Contusion of spleen greater than 2 cm

√7ᵗʰ **S36.029** Unspecified contusion of spleen `CC`

---

N Newborn: 0   P Pediatric: 0-17   M Maternity: 12-55   A Adult: 15-124   `MCC` Major CC Condition   `PDxMCC` PDx acts as own MCC   `CC` CC Condition   `PDxCC` PDx acts as own CC

**980**                                                           ICD-10-CM 2018

✓6ᵗʰ **S36.03** Laceration of spleen

     ✓7ᵗʰ **S36.030** **Superficial (capsular) laceration of spleen**    `CC`
         Laceration of spleen less than 1cm
         Minor laceration of spleen

     ✓7ᵗʰ **S36.031** **Moderate laceration of spleen**    `MCC`
         Laceration of spleen 1 to 3 cm

     ✓7ᵗʰ **S36.032** **Major laceration of spleen**    `MCC`
         Avulsion of spleen
         Laceration of spleen greater than 3 cm
         Massive laceration of spleen
         Multiple moderate lacerations of spleen
         Stellate laceration of spleen

     ✓7ᵗʰ **S36.039** **Unspecified laceration of spleen**    `CC`

✓x7ᵗʰ **S36.09** **Other injury of spleen**    `CC`

✓5ᵗʰ **S36.1** **Injury of liver and gallbladder and bile duct**

     ✓6ᵗʰ **S36.11** **Injury of liver**

         **CC Excl: For codes in subcategory S36.11:**
         **CC or MCC with 7th character A:**
         PDX collection 1231

     ✓7ᵗʰ **S36.112** **Contusion of liver**    `CC`

     ✓7ᵗʰ **S36.113** **Laceration of liver, unspecified degree**    `CC`

     ✓7ᵗʰ **S36.114** **Minor laceration of liver**    `CC`
         Laceration involving capsule only, or,
            without significant involvement of
            hepatic parenchyma [i.e., less than
            1cm deep]

     ✓7ᵗʰ **S36.115** **Moderate laceration of liver**    `MCC`
         Laceration involving parenchyma but
            without major disruption of
            parenchyma [i.e., less than 10 cm long
            and less than 3 cm deep]

     ✓7ᵗʰ **S36.116** **Major laceration of liver**    `MCC`
         Laceration with significant disruption of
            hepatic parenchyma [i.e., greater than
            10 cm long and 3 cm deep]
         Multiple moderate lacerations, with or
            without hematoma
         Stellate laceration of liver

     ✓7ᵗʰ **S36.118** **Other injury of liver**    `CC`

     ✓7ᵗʰ **S36.119** **Unspecified injury of liver**    `CC`

     ✓6ᵗʰ **S36.12** **Injury of gallbladder**

         **CC Excl: For codes in subcategory S36.12:**
         **CC with 7th character A:** PDX collection 1232

     ✓7ᵗʰ **S36.122** **Contusion of gallbladder**    `CC`

     ✓7ᵗʰ **S36.123** **Laceration of gallbladder**    `CC`

     ✓7ᵗʰ **S36.128** **Other injury of gallbladder**    `CC`

     ✓7ᵗʰ **S36.129** **Unspecified injury of gallbladder**    `CC`

     ✓x7ᵗʰ **S36.13** **Injury of bile duct**    `CC`
         **CC Excl: CC with 7th character A:** PDX collection 1232

✓5ᵗʰ **S36.2** **Injury of pancreas**

         **CC Excl: For codes in subcategory S36.2:**
         **CC with 7th character A:** PDX collection 1233

     ✓6ᵗʰ **S36.20** **Unspecified injury of pancreas**

     ✓7ᵗʰ **S36.200** **Unspecified injury of head of pancreas**    `CC`

     ✓7ᵗʰ **S36.201** **Unspecified injury of body of pancreas**    `CC`

     ✓7ᵗʰ **S36.202** **Unspecified injury of tail of pancreas**    `CC`

     ✓7ᵗʰ **S36.209** **Unspecified injury of unspecified part of pancreas**    `CC`

     ✓6ᵗʰ **S36.22** **Contusion of pancreas**

     ✓7ᵗʰ **S36.220** **Contusion of head of pancreas**    `CC`

     ✓7ᵗʰ **S36.221** **Contusion of body of pancreas**    `CC`

     ✓7ᵗʰ **S36.222** **Contusion of tail of pancreas**    `CC`

     ✓7ᵗʰ **S36.229** **Contusion of unspecified part of pancreas**    `CC`

     ✓6ᵗʰ **S36.23** **Laceration of pancreas, unspecified degree**

     ✓7ᵗʰ **S36.230** **Laceration of head of pancreas, unspecified degree**    `CC`

     ✓7ᵗʰ **S36.231** **Laceration of body of pancreas, unspecified degree**    `CC`

     ✓7ᵗʰ **S36.232** **Laceration of tail of pancreas, unspecified degree**    `CC`

     ✓7ᵗʰ **S36.239** **Laceration of unspecified part of pancreas, unspecified degree**    `CC`

     ✓6ᵗʰ **S36.24** **Minor laceration of pancreas**

     ✓7ᵗʰ **S36.240** **Minor laceration of head of pancreas**    `CC`

     ✓7ᵗʰ **S36.241** **Minor laceration of body of pancreas**    `CC`

     ✓7ᵗʰ **S36.242** **Minor laceration of tail of pancreas**    `CC`

     ✓7ᵗʰ **S36.249** **Minor laceration of unspecified part of pancreas**    `CC`

     ✓6ᵗʰ **S36.25** **Moderate laceration of pancreas**

     ✓7ᵗʰ **S36.250** **Moderate laceration of head of pancreas**    `CC`

     ✓7ᵗʰ **S36.251** **Moderate laceration of body of pancreas**    `CC`

     ✓7ᵗʰ **S36.252** **Moderate laceration of tail of pancreas**    `CC`

     ✓7ᵗʰ **S36.259** **Moderate laceration of unspecified part of pancreas**    `CC`

     ✓6ᵗʰ **S36.26** **Major laceration of pancreas**

     ✓7ᵗʰ **S36.260** **Major laceration of head of pancreas**    `CC`

     ✓7ᵗʰ **S36.261** **Major laceration of body of pancreas**    `CC`

     ✓7ᵗʰ **S36.262** **Major laceration of tail of pancreas**    `CC`

     ✓7ᵗʰ **S36.269** **Major laceration of unspecified part of pancreas**    `CC`

     ✓6ᵗʰ **S36.29** **Other injury of pancreas**

     ✓7ᵗʰ **S36.290** **Other injury of head of pancreas**    `CC`

     ✓7ᵗʰ **S36.291** **Other injury of body of pancreas**    `CC`

     ✓7ᵗʰ **S36.292** **Other injury of tail of pancreas**    `CC`

     ✓7ᵗʰ **S36.299** **Other injury of unspecified part of pancreas**    `CC`

✓5ᵗʰ **S36.3** **Injury of stomach**

         **CC Excl: For codes in subcategory S36.3:**
         **CC with 7th character A:** PDX collection 1234

     ✓x7ᵗʰ **S36.30** **Unspecified injury of stomach**    `CC`

     ✓x7ᵗʰ **S36.32** **Contusion of stomach**    `CC`

     ✓x7ᵗʰ **S36.33** **Laceration of stomach**    `CC`

     ✓x7ᵗʰ **S36.39** **Other injury of stomach**    `CC`

✓5ᵗʰ **S36.4** **Injury of small intestine**

         **CC Excl: For codes in subcategory S36.4:**
         **CC with 7th character A:** PDX collection 1235

     ✓6ᵗʰ **S36.40** **Unspecified injury of small intestine**

     ✓7ᵗʰ **S36.400** **Unspecified injury of duodenum**    `CC`

     ✓7ᵗʰ **S36.408** **Unspecified injury of other part of small intestine**    `CC`

     ✓7ᵗʰ **S36.409** **Unspecified injury of unspecified part of small intestine**    `CC`

     ✓6ᵗʰ **S36.41** **Primary blast injury of small intestine**
         Blast injury of small intestine NOS

     ✓7ᵗʰ **S36.410** **Primary blast injury of duodenum**    `CC`

     ✓7ᵗʰ **S36.418** **Primary blast injury of other part of small intestine**    `CC`

     ✓7ᵗʰ **S36.419** **Primary blast injury of unspecified part of small intestine**    `CC`

     ✓6ᵗʰ **S36.42** **Contusion of small intestine**

     ✓7ᵗʰ **S36.420** **Contusion of duodenum**    `CC`

     ✓7ᵗʰ **S36.428** **Contusion of other part of small intestine**    `CC`

     ✓7ᵗʰ **S36.429** **Contusion of unspecified part of small intestine**    `CC`

     ✓6ᵗʰ **S36.43** **Laceration of small intestine**

     ✓7ᵗʰ **S36.430** **Laceration of duodenum**    `CC`

     ✓7ᵗʰ **S36.438** **Laceration of other part of small intestine**    `CC`

     ✓7ᵗʰ **S36.439** **Laceration of unspecified part of small intestine**    `CC`

     ✓6ᵗʰ **S36.49** **Other injury of small intestine**

     ✓7ᵗʰ **S36.490** **Other injury of duodenum**    `CC`

     ✓7ᵗʰ **S36.498** **Other injury of other part of small intestine**    `CC`

     ✓7ᵗʰ **S36.499** **Other injury of unspecified part of small intestine**    `CC`

---

☑ Additional Character Req    ✓x7ᵗʰ Placeholder Alert    Unacceptable PDx    Manifestation    `H1`-`H14` HAC    `HCC` CMS-HCC Condition    *EXCLUDES1* Not Coded Here    *EXCLUDES2* Not Included Here

√5ᵗʰ **S36.5　Injury of colon**
　　EXCLUDES 2　injury of rectum (S36.6-)

> **CC Excl: For codes in subcategory S36.5:**
> **CC with 7th character A:** PDX collection 1236

√6ᵗʰ **S36.50　Unspecified injury of colon**
- √7ᵗʰ **S36.500　Unspecified injury of** ascending [right] colon `CC`
- √7ᵗʰ **S36.501　Unspecified injury of** transverse colon `CC`
- √7ᵗʰ **S36.502　Unspecified injury of** descending [left] colon `CC`
- √7ᵗʰ **S36.503　Unspecified injury of** sigmoid colon `CC`
- √7ᵗʰ **S36.508　Unspecified injury of** other part of colon `CC`
- √7ᵗʰ **S36.509　Unspecified injury of** unspecified part of colon `CC`

√6ᵗʰ **S36.51　Primary blast injury of colon**
　　Blast injury of colon NOS
- √7ᵗʰ **S36.510　Primary blast injury of** ascending [right] colon `CC`
- √7ᵗʰ **S36.511　Primary blast injury of** transverse colon `CC`
- √7ᵗʰ **S36.512　Primary blast injury of** descending [left] colon `CC`
- √7ᵗʰ **S36.513　Primary blast injury of** sigmoid colon `CC`
- √7ᵗʰ **S36.518　Primary blast injury of** other part of colon `CC`
- √7ᵗʰ **S36.519　Primary blast injury of** unspecified part of colon `CC`

√6ᵗʰ **S36.52　Contusion of colon**
- √7ᵗʰ **S36.520　Contusion of** ascending [right] colon `CC`
- √7ᵗʰ **S36.521　Contusion of** transverse colon `CC`
- √7ᵗʰ **S36.522　Contusion of** descending [left] colon `CC`
- √7ᵗʰ **S36.523　Contusion of** sigmoid colon `CC`
- √7ᵗʰ **S36.528　Contusion of** other part of colon `CC`
- √7ᵗʰ **S36.529　Contusion of** unspecified part of colon `CC`

√6ᵗʰ **S36.53　Laceration of colon**
- √7ᵗʰ **S36.530　Laceration of** ascending [right] colon `CC`
- √7ᵗʰ **S36.531　Laceration of** transverse colon `CC`
- √7ᵗʰ **S36.532　Laceration of** descending [left] colon `CC`
- √7ᵗʰ **S36.533　Laceration of** sigmoid colon `CC`
- √7ᵗʰ **S36.538　Laceration of** other part of colon `CC`
- √7ᵗʰ **S36.539　Laceration of** unspecified part of colon `CC`

√6ᵗʰ **S36.59　Other injury of colon**
　　Secondary blast injury of colon
- √7ᵗʰ **S36.590　Other injury of** ascending [right] colon `CC`
- √7ᵗʰ **S36.591　Other injury of** transverse colon `CC`
- √7ᵗʰ **S36.592　Other injury of** descending [left] colon `CC`
- √7ᵗʰ **S36.593　Other injury of** sigmoid colon `CC`
- √7ᵗʰ **S36.598　Other injury of** other part of colon `CC`
- √7ᵗʰ **S36.599　Other injury of** unspecified part of colon `CC`

√5ᵗʰ **S36.6　Injury of rectum**

> **CC Excl: For codes in subcategory S36.6:**
> **CC with 7th character A:** PDX collection 1236

- √x7ᵗʰ **S36.60　Unspecified injury of rectum** `CC`
- √x7ᵗʰ **S36.61　Primary blast injury of rectum** `CC`
　　Blast injury of rectum NOS
- √x7ᵗʰ **S36.62　Contusion of rectum** `CC`
- √x7ᵗʰ **S36.63　Laceration of rectum** `CC`
- √x7ᵗʰ **S36.69　Other injury of rectum** `CC`
　　Secondary blast injury of rectum

√5ᵗʰ **S36.8　Injury of other intra-abdominal organs**

> **CC Excl: For codes in subcategory S36.8:**
> **CC with 7th character A:** PDX collection 1195

- √x7ᵗʰ **S36.81　Injury of peritoneum** `CC`
- √6ᵗʰ **S36.89　Injury of** other **intra-abdominal organs**
　　Injury of retroperitoneum
  - √7ᵗʰ **S36.892　Contusion of other intra-abdominal organs** `CC`

- √7ᵗʰ **S36.893　Laceration of other intra-abdominal organs** `CC`
- √7ᵗʰ **S36.898　Other injury of other intra-abdominal organs** `CC`
- √7ᵗʰ **S36.899　Unspecified injury of other intra-abdominal organs** `CC`

√5ᵗʰ **S36.9　Injury of unspecified intra-abdominal organ**

> **CC Excl: For codes in subcategory S36.9:**
> **CC with 7th character A:** PDX collection 1195

- √x7ᵗʰ **S36.90　Unspecified injury of unspecified intra-abdominal organ** `CC`
- √x7ᵗʰ **S36.92　Contusion of unspecified intra-abdominal organ** `CC`
- √x7ᵗʰ **S36.93　Laceration of unspecified intra-abdominal organ** `CC`
- √x7ᵗʰ **S36.99　Other injury of unspecified intra-abdominal organ** `CC`

√4ᵗʰ **S37　Injury of urinary and pelvic organs**
　　Code also any associated open wound (S31.-)
　　EXCLUDES 1　obstetric trauma to pelvic organs (O71.-)
　　EXCLUDES 2　injury of peritoneum (S36.81)
　　　　　　　　injury of retroperitoneum (S36.89-)

> The appropriate 7th character is to be added to each code from category S37.
> A　initial encounter
> D　subsequent encounter
> S　sequela

√5ᵗʰ **S37.0　Injury of kidney**
　　EXCLUDES 2　acute kidney injury (nontraumatic) (N17.9)

> **CC Excl: For codes in subcategory S37.0:**
> **CC or MCC with 7th character A:** PDX collection 1237

√6ᵗʰ **S37.00　Unspecified injury of kidney**
- √7ᵗʰ **S37.001　Unspecified injury of** right kidney `CC`
- √7ᵗʰ **S37.002　Unspecified injury of** left kidney `CC`
- √7ᵗʰ **S37.009　Unspecified injury of** unspecified kidney `CC`

√6ᵗʰ **S37.01　Minor contusion of kidney**
　　Contusion of kidney less than 2 cm
　　Contusion of kidney NOS
- √7ᵗʰ **S37.011　Minor contusion of** right kidney `CC`
- √7ᵗʰ **S37.012　Minor contusion of** left kidney `CC`
- √7ᵗʰ **S37.019　Minor contusion of** unspecified kidney `CC`

√6ᵗʰ **S37.02　Major contusion of kidney**
　　Contusion of kidney greater than 2 cm
- √7ᵗʰ **S37.021　Major contusion of** right kidney `CC`
- √7ᵗʰ **S37.022　Major contusion of** left kidney `CC`
- √7ᵗʰ **S37.029　Major contusion of** unspecified kidney `CC`

√6ᵗʰ **S37.03　Laceration of kidney, unspecified degree**
- √7ᵗʰ **S37.031　Laceration of** right **kidney, unspecified degree** `CC`
- √7ᵗʰ **S37.032　Laceration of** left **kidney, unspecified degree** `CC`
- √7ᵗʰ **S37.039　Laceration of** unspecified **kidney, unspecified degree** `CC`

√6ᵗʰ **S37.04　Minor laceration of kidney**
　　Laceration of kidney less than 1 cm
- √7ᵗʰ **S37.041　Minor laceration of** right kidney `CC`
- √7ᵗʰ **S37.042　Minor laceration of** left kidney `CC`
- √7ᵗʰ **S37.049　Minor laceration of** unspecified kidney `CC`

√6ᵗʰ **S37.05　Moderate laceration of kidney**
　　Laceration of kidney 1 to 3 cm
- √7ᵗʰ **S37.051　Moderate laceration of** right kidney `CC`
- √7ᵗʰ **S37.052　Moderate laceration of** left kidney `CC`
- √7ᵗʰ **S37.059　Moderate laceration of** unspecified kidney `CC`

√6ᵗʰ **S37.06　Major laceration of kidney**
　　Avulsion of kidney
　　Laceration of kidney greater than 3 cm
　　Massive laceration of kidney
　　Multiple moderate lacerations of kidney
　　Stellate laceration of kidney
- √7ᵗʰ **S37.061　Major laceration of** right kidney `MCC`
- √7ᵗʰ **S37.062　Major laceration of** left kidney `MCC`

Ⓝ Newborn: 0　Ⓟ Pediatric: 0-17　Ⓜ Maternity: 12-55　Ⓐ Adult: 15-124　`MCC` Major CC Condition　`PDxMCC` PDx acts as own MCC　`CC` CC Condition　`PDxCC` PDx acts as own CC

982

ICD-10-CM 2018

√7th **S37.069**   **Major laceration of** unspecified **kidney**   `MCC`

√6th **S37.09**   **Other injury of kidney**

√7th **S37.091**   **Other injury of** right **kidney**   `MCC`

√7th **S37.092**   **Other injury of** left **kidney**   `MCC`

√7th **S37.099**   **Other injury of** unspecified **kidney**   `MCC`

√5th **S37.1**   **Injury of** ureter

> **CC Excl: For codes in subcategory S37.1:**
> **CC with 7th character A:** PDX collection 1238

√x7th **S37.10**   **Unspecified injury of ureter**   `CC`

√x7th **S37.12**   **Contusion of ureter**   `CC`

√x7th **S37.13**   **Laceration of ureter**   `CC`

√x7th **S37.19**   **Other injury of ureter**   `CC`

√5th **S37.2**   **Injury of** bladder

> **CC Excl: For codes in subcategory S37.2:**
> **CC with 7th character A:** PDX collection 1239

√x7th **S37.20**   **Unspecified injury of bladder**   `CC`

√x7th **S37.22**   **Contusion of bladder**   `CC`

√x7th **S37.23**   **Laceration of bladder**   `CC`

√x7th **S37.29**   **Other injury of bladder**   `CC`

√5th **S37.3**   **Injury of** urethra

> **CC Excl: For codes in subcategory S37.3:**
> **CC with 7th character A:** PDX collection 1239

√x7th **S37.30**   **Unspecified injury of urethra**   `CC`

√x7th **S37.32**   **Contusion of urethra**   `CC`

√x7th **S37.33**   **Laceration of urethra**   `CC`

√x7th **S37.39**   **Other injury of urethra**   `CC`

√5th **S37.4**   **Injury of** ovary

√6th **S37.40**   **Unspecified injury of ovary**

√7th **S37.401**   **Unspecified injury of ovary,** unilateral   ♀

√7th **S37.402**   **Unspecified injury of ovary,** bilateral   ♀

√7th **S37.409**   **Unspecified injury of ovary,** unspecified   ♀

√6th **S37.42**   **Contusion of ovary**

√7th **S37.421**   **Contusion of ovary,** unilateral   ♀

√7th **S37.422**   **Contusion of ovary,** bilateral   ♀

√7th **S37.429**   **Contusion of ovary,** unspecified   ♀

√6th **S37.43**   **Laceration of ovary**

√7th **S37.431**   **Laceration of ovary,** unilateral   ♀

√7th **S37.432**   **Laceration of ovary,** bilateral   ♀

√7th **S37.439**   **Laceration of ovary,** unspecified   ♀

√6th **S37.49**   **Other injury of ovary**

√7th **S37.491**   **Other injury of ovary,** unilateral   ♀

√7th **S37.492**   **Other injury of ovary,** bilateral   ♀

√7th **S37.499**   **Other injury of ovary,** unspecified   ♀

√5th **S37.5**   **Injury of** fallopian tube

√6th **S37.50**   **Unspecified injury of fallopian tube**

√7th **S37.501**   **Unspecified injury of fallopian tube,** unilateral   ♀

√7th **S37.502**   **Unspecified injury of fallopian tube,** bilateral   ♀

√7th **S37.509**   **Unspecified injury of fallopian tube,** unspecified   ♀

√6th **S37.51**   **Primary blast injury of fallopian tube**
Blast injury of fallopian tube NOS

√7th **S37.511**   **Primary blast injury of fallopian tube,** unilateral   ♀

√7th **S37.512**   **Primary blast injury of fallopian tube,** bilateral   ♀

√7th **S37.519**   **Primary blast injury of fallopian tube,** unspecified   ♀

√6th **S37.52**   **Contusion of fallopian tube**

√7th **S37.521**   **Contusion of fallopian tube,** unilateral   ♀

√7th **S37.522**   **Contusion of fallopian tube,** bilateral   ♀

√7th **S37.529**   **Contusion of fallopian tube,** unspecified   ♀

√6th **S37.53**   **Laceration of fallopian tube**

√7th **S37.531**   **Laceration of fallopian tube,** unilateral   ♀

√7th **S37.532**   **Laceration of fallopian tube,** bilateral   ♀

√7th **S37.539**   **Laceration of fallopian tube,** unspecified   ♀

√6th **S37.59**   **Other injury of fallopian tube**
Secondary blast injury of fallopian tube

√7th **S37.591**   **Other injury of fallopian tube,** unilateral   ♀

√7th **S37.592**   **Other injury of fallopian tube,** bilateral   ♀

√7th **S37.599**   **Other injury of fallopian tube,** unspecified   ♀

√5th **S37.6**   **Injury of** uterus

> *EXCLUDES 1*   injury to gravid uterus (O9A.2-)
> injury to uterus during delivery (O71.-)

> **CC Excl: For codes in subcategory S37.6:**
> **CC with 7th character A:** PDX collection 1240

√x7th **S37.60**   **Unspecified injury of uterus**   `CC` ♀

√x7th **S37.62**   **Contusion of uterus**   `CC` ♀

√x7th **S37.63**   **Laceration of uterus**   `CC` ♀

√x7th **S37.69**   **Other injury of uterus**   `CC` ♀

√5th **S37.8**   **Injury of other urinary and pelvic organs**

√6th **S37.81**   **Injury of adrenal gland**

> **CC Excl: For codes in subcategory S37.81:**
> **CC with 7th character A:** PDX collection 1241

√7th **S37.812**   **Contusion of adrenal gland**   `CC`

√7th **S37.813**   **Laceration of adrenal gland**   `CC`

√7th **S37.818**   **Other injury of adrenal gland**   `CC`

√7th **S37.819**   **Unspecified injury of adrenal gland**   `CC`

√6th **S37.82**   **Injury of prostate**

√7th **S37.822**   **Contusion of prostate**   ♂

√7th **S37.823**   **Laceration of prostate**   ♂

√7th **S37.828**   **Other injury of prostate**   ♂

√7th **S37.829**   **Unspecified injury of prostate**   ♂

√6th **S37.89**   **Injury of other urinary and pelvic organ**

> **CC Excl: For codes in subcategory S37.89:**
> **CC with 7th character A:** PDX collection 1242

√7th **S37.892**   **Contusion of other urinary and pelvic organ**   `CC`

√7th **S37.893**   **Laceration of other urinary and pelvic organ**   `CC`

√7th **S37.898**   **Other injury of other urinary and pelvic organ**

√7th **S37.899**   **Unspecified injury of other urinary and pelvic organ**   `CC`

√5th **S37.9**   **Injury of unspecified urinary and pelvic organ**

> **CC Excl: For codes in subcategory S37.9:**
> **CC with 7th character A:** PDX collection 1242

√x7th **S37.90**   **Unspecified injury of unspecified urinary and pelvic organ**   `CC`

√x7th **S37.92**   **Contusion of unspecified urinary and pelvic organ**   `CC`

√x7th **S37.93**   **Laceration of unspecified urinary and pelvic organ**   `CC`

√x7th **S37.99**   **Other injury of unspecified urinary and pelvic organ**   `CC`

√4th **S38**   **Crushing injury and traumatic amputation of abdomen, lower back, pelvis and external genitals**
An amputation not identified as partial or complete should be coded to complete.

> The appropriate 7th character is to be added to each code from category S38.
> A   initial encounter
> D   subsequent encounter
> S   sequela

√5th **S38.0**   **Crushing injury of external genital organs**
Use additional code for any associated injuries

√6th **S38.00**   **Crushing injury of unspecified external genital organs**

√7th **S38.001**   **Crushing injury of unspecified external genital organs, male**   ♂

✓7ᵗʰ   **S38.002**   **Crushing injury of unspecified external genital organs, female** ♀

✓x7ᵗʰ   **S38.01**   **Crushing injury of** penis ♂

✓x7ᵗʰ   **S38.02**   **Crushing injury of** scrotum and testis ♂

✓x7ᵗʰ   **S38.03**   **Crushing injury of** vulva ♀

✓x7ᵗʰ   **S38.1**   **Crushing injury of abdomen, lower back, and pelvis**

Use additional code for all associated injuries, such as:
fracture of thoracic or lumbar spine and pelvis (S22.0-, S32-)
injury to intra-abdominal organs (S36.-)
injury to urinary and pelvic organs (S37.-)
open wound of abdominal wall (S31.-)
spinal cord injury (S34.0, S34.1-)

EXCLUDES 2   crushing injury of external genital organs (S38.0-)

✓5ᵗʰ   **S38.2**   **Traumatic amputation of external genital organs**

✓6ᵗʰ   **S38.21**   **Traumatic amputation of** female **external genital organs**

Traumatic amputation of clitoris
Traumatic amputation of labium (majus) (minus)
Traumatic amputation of vulva

✓7ᵗʰ   **S38.211**   **Complete traumatic amputation of female external genital organs** ♀

✓7ᵗʰ   **S38.212**   **Partial traumatic amputation of female external genital organs** ♀

✓6ᵗʰ   **S38.22**   **Traumatic amputation of** penis

✓7ᵗʰ   **S38.221**   **Complete traumatic amputation of penis** ♂

✓7ᵗʰ   **S38.222**   **Partial traumatic amputation of penis** ♂

✓6ᵗʰ   **S38.23**   **Traumatic amputation of** scrotum and testis

✓7ᵗʰ   **S38.231**   **Complete traumatic amputation of scrotum and testis** ♂

✓7ᵗʰ   **S38.232**   **Partial traumatic amputation of scrotum and testis** ♂

✓x7ᵗʰ   **S38.3**   **Transection (partial) of abdomen**

✓4ᵗʰ   **S39**   **Other and unspecified injuries of abdomen, lower back, pelvis and external genitals**

Code also any associated open wound (S31.-)
EXCLUDES 2   sprain of joints and ligaments of lumbar spine and pelvis (S33.-)

The appropriate 7th character is to be added to each code from category S39.
A   initial encounter
D   subsequent encounter
S   sequela

✓5ᵗʰ   **S39.0**   **Injury of muscle, fascia and tendon of abdomen, lower back and pelvis**

✓6ᵗʰ   **S39.00**   **Unspecified injury of muscle, fascia and tendon of abdomen, lower back and pelvis**

✓7ᵗʰ   **S39.001**   **Unspecified injury of muscle, fascia and tendon of** abdomen

✓7ᵗʰ   **S39.002**   **Unspecified injury of muscle, fascia and tendon of** lower back

✓7ᵗʰ   **S39.003**   **Unspecified injury of muscle, fascia and tendon of** pelvis

✓6ᵗʰ   **S39.01**   **Strain of muscle, fascia and tendon of abdomen, lower back and pelvis**

✓7ᵗʰ   **S39.011**   **Strain of muscle, fascia and tendon of** abdomen

✓7ᵗʰ   **S39.012**   **Strain of muscle, fascia and tendon of** lower back

✓7ᵗʰ   **S39.013**   **Strain of muscle, fascia and tendon of** pelvis

✓6ᵗʰ   **S39.02**   **Laceration of muscle, fascia and tendon of abdomen, lower back and pelvis**

✓7ᵗʰ   **S39.021**   **Laceration of muscle, fascia and tendon of** abdomen

✓7ᵗʰ   **S39.022**   **Laceration of muscle, fascia and tendon of** lower back

✓7ᵗʰ   **S39.023**   **Laceration of muscle, fascia and tendon of** pelvis

✓6ᵗʰ   **S39.09**   **Other injury of muscle, fascia and tendon of abdomen, lower back and pelvis**

✓7ᵗʰ   **S39.091**   **Other injury of muscle, fascia and tendon of** abdomen

✓7ᵗʰ   **S39.092**   **Other injury of muscle, fascia and tendon of** lower back

✓7ᵗʰ   **S39.093**   **Other injury of muscle, fascia and tendon of** pelvis

✓5ᵗʰ   **S39.8**   **Other** specified **injuries of abdomen, lower back, pelvis and external genitals**

✓x7ᵗʰ   **S39.81**   **Other specified injuries of** abdomen

✓x7ᵗʰ   **S39.82**   **Other specified injuries of** lower back

✓x7ᵗʰ   **S39.83**   **Other specified injuries of** pelvis

✓6ᵗʰ   **S39.84**   **Other specified injuries of** external genitals

✓7ᵗʰ   **S39.840**   **Fracture of corpus cavernosum penis** ♂

✓7ᵗʰ   **S39.848**   **Other specified injuries of external genitals**

✓5ᵗʰ   **S39.9**   **Unspecified injury of abdomen, lower back, pelvis and external genitals**

✓x7ᵗʰ   **S39.91**   **Unspecified injury of** abdomen

✓x7ᵗʰ   **S39.92**   **Unspecified injury of** lower back

✓x7ᵗʰ   **S39.93**   **Unspecified injury of** pelvis

✓x7ᵗʰ   **S39.94**   **Unspecified injury of** external genitals

## Injuries to the shoulder and upper arm (S40-S49)

INCLUDES   injuries of axilla
injuries of scapular region
EXCLUDES 2   burns and corrosions (T20-T32)
frostbite (T33-T34)
injuries of elbow (S50-S59)
insect bite or sting, venomous (T63.4)

✓4ᵗʰ   **S40**   **Superficial injury of shoulder and upper arm**

The appropriate 7th character is to be added to each code from category S40.
A   initial encounter
D   subsequent encounter
S   sequela

✓5ᵗʰ   **S40.0**   **Contusion of shoulder and upper arm**

✓6ᵗʰ   **S40.01**   **Contusion of** shoulder

✓7ᵗʰ   **S40.011**   **Contusion of right shoulder**

✓7ᵗʰ   **S40.012**   **Contusion of left shoulder**

✓7ᵗʰ   **S40.019**   **Contusion of unspecified shoulder**

✓6ᵗʰ   **S40.02**   **Contusion of** upper arm

✓7ᵗʰ   **S40.021**   **Contusion of right upper arm**

✓7ᵗʰ   **S40.022**   **Contusion of left upper arm**

✓7ᵗʰ   **S40.029**   **Contusion of unspecified upper arm**

✓5ᵗʰ   **S40.2**   **Other superficial injuries of shoulder**

✓6ᵗʰ   **S40.21**   **Abrasion of** shoulder

✓7ᵗʰ   **S40.211**   **Abrasion of right shoulder**

✓7ᵗʰ   **S40.212**   **Abrasion of left shoulder**

✓7ᵗʰ   **S40.219**   **Abrasion of unspecified shoulder**

✓6ᵗʰ   **S40.22**   **Blister (nonthermal) of shoulder**

✓7ᵗʰ   **S40.221**   **Blister (nonthermal) of right shoulder**

✓7ᵗʰ   **S40.222**   **Blister (nonthermal) of left shoulder**

✓7ᵗʰ   **S40.229**   **Blister (nonthermal) of unspecified shoulder**

✓6ᵗʰ   **S40.24**   **External constriction of shoulder**

✓7ᵗʰ   **S40.241**   **External constriction of right shoulder**

✓7ᵗʰ   **S40.242**   **External constriction of left shoulder**

✓7ᵗʰ   **S40.249**   **External constriction of unspecified shoulder**

✓6ᵗʰ   **S40.25**   **Superficial foreign body of shoulder**

Splinter in the shoulder

✓7ᵗʰ   **S40.251**   **Superficial foreign body of right shoulder**

✓7ᵗʰ   **S40.252**   **Superficial foreign body of left shoulder**

✓7ᵗʰ   **S40.259**   **Superficial foreign body of unspecified shoulder**

✓6ᵗʰ   **S40.26**   **Insect bite (nonvenomous) of shoulder**

✓7ᵗʰ   **S40.261**   **Insect bite (nonvenomous) of right shoulder**

✓7ᵗʰ   **S40.262**   **Insect bite (nonvenomous) of left shoulder**

✓7ᵗʰ   **S40.269**   **Insect bite (nonvenomous) of unspecified shoulder**

✓6ᵗʰ   **S40.27**   **Other superficial bite of shoulder**

EXCLUDES 1   open bite of shoulder (S41.05)

✓7ᵗʰ   **S40.271**   **Other superficial bite of right shoulder**

N Newborn: 0   P Pediatric: 0-17   M Maternity: 12-55   A Adult: 15-124   MCC Major CC Condition   PDx MCC PDx acts as own MCC   CC CC Condition   PDx CC PDx acts as own CC

984

ICD-10-CM 2018

√7ᵗʰ **S40.272** Other superficial bite of left shoulder

√7ᵗʰ **S40.279** Other superficial bite of unspecified shoulder

√5ᵗʰ **S40.8** Other superficial injuries of upper arm

√6ᵗʰ **S40.81** Abrasion of upper arm

√7ᵗʰ **S40.811** Abrasion of right upper arm

√7ᵗʰ **S40.812** Abrasion of left upper arm

√7ᵗʰ **S40.819** Abrasion of unspecified upper arm

√6ᵗʰ **S40.82** Blister (nonthermal) of upper arm

√7ᵗʰ **S40.821** Blister (nonthermal) of right upper arm

√7ᵗʰ **S40.822** Blister (nonthermal) of left upper arm

√7ᵗʰ **S40.829** Blister (nonthermal) of unspecified arm

√6ᵗʰ **S40.84** External constriction of upper arm

√7ᵗʰ **S40.841** External constriction of right upper arm

√7ᵗʰ **S40.842** External constriction of left upper arm

√7ᵗʰ **S40.849** External constriction of unspecified upper arm

√6ᵗʰ **S40.85** Superficial foreign body of upper arm
Splinter in the upper arm

√7ᵗʰ **S40.851** Superficial foreign body of right upper arm

√7ᵗʰ **S40.852** Superficial foreign body of left upper arm

√7ᵗʰ **S40.859** Superficial foreign body of unspecified upper arm

√6ᵗʰ **S40.86** Insect bite (nonvenomous) of upper arm

√7ᵗʰ **S40.861** Insect bite (nonvenomous) of right upper arm

√7ᵗʰ **S40.862** Insect bite (nonvenomous) of left upper arm

√7ᵗʰ **S40.869** Insect bite (nonvenomous) of unspecified upper arm

√6ᵗʰ **S40.87** Other superficial bite of upper arm
EXCLUDES 1   open bite of upper arm (S41.14)
EXCLUDES 2   other superficial bite of shoulder (S40.27-)

√7ᵗʰ **S40.871** Other superficial bite of right upper arm

√7ᵗʰ **S40.872** Other superficial bite of left upper arm

√7ᵗʰ **S40.879** Other superficial bite of unspecified upper arm

√5ᵗʰ **S40.9** Unspecified superficial injury of shoulder and upper arm

√6ᵗʰ **S40.91** Unspecified superficial injury of shoulder

√7ᵗʰ **S40.911** Unspecified superficial injury of right shoulder

√7ᵗʰ **S40.912** Unspecified superficial injury of left shoulder

√7ᵗʰ **S40.919** Unspecified superficial injury of unspecified shoulder

√6ᵗʰ **S40.92** Unspecified superficial injury of upper arm

√7ᵗʰ **S40.921** Unspecified superficial injury of right upper arm

√7ᵗʰ **S40.922** Unspecified superficial injury of left upper arm

√7ᵗʰ **S40.929** Unspecified superficial injury of unspecified upper arm

√4ᵗʰ **S41** **Open wound of shoulder and upper arm**
Code also any associated wound infection
EXCLUDES 1   traumatic amputation of shoulder and upper arm (S48.-)
EXCLUDES 2   open fracture of shoulder and upper arm (S42.- with 7th character B or C)

The appropriate 7th character is to be added to each code from category S41.
A    initial encounter
D    subsequent encounter
S    sequela

√5ᵗʰ **S41.0** Open wound of shoulder

√6ᵗʰ **S41.00** Unspecified open wound of shoulder

√7ᵗʰ **S41.001** Unspecified open wound of right shoulder

√7ᵗʰ **S41.002** Unspecified open wound of left shoulder

√7ᵗʰ **S41.009** Unspecified open wound of unspecified shoulder

√6ᵗʰ **S41.01** Laceration without foreign body of shoulder

√7ᵗʰ **S41.011** Laceration without foreign body of right shoulder

√7ᵗʰ **S41.012** Laceration without foreign body of left shoulder

√7ᵗʰ **S41.019** Laceration without foreign body of unspecified shoulder

√6ᵗʰ **S41.02** Laceration with foreign body of shoulder

√7ᵗʰ **S41.021** Laceration with foreign body of right shoulder

√7ᵗʰ **S41.022** Laceration with foreign body of left shoulder

√7ᵗʰ **S41.029** Laceration with foreign body of unspecified shoulder

√6ᵗʰ **S41.03** Puncture wound without foreign body of shoulder

√7ᵗʰ **S41.031** Puncture wound without foreign body of right shoulder

√7ᵗʰ **S41.032** Puncture wound without foreign body of left shoulder

√7ᵗʰ **S41.039** Puncture wound without foreign body of unspecified shoulder

√6ᵗʰ **S41.04** Puncture wound with foreign body of shoulder

√7ᵗʰ **S41.041** Puncture wound with foreign body of right shoulder

√7ᵗʰ **S41.042** Puncture wound with foreign body of left shoulder

√7ᵗʰ **S41.049** Puncture wound with foreign body of unspecified shoulder

√6ᵗʰ **S41.05** Open bite of shoulder
Bite of shoulder NOS
EXCLUDES 1   superficial bite of shoulder (S40.27)

√7ᵗʰ **S41.051** Open bite of right shoulder

√7ᵗʰ **S41.052** Open bite of left shoulder

√7ᵗʰ **S41.059** Open bite of unspecified shoulder

√5ᵗʰ **S41.1** Open wound of upper arm

√6ᵗʰ **S41.10** Unspecified open wound of upper arm
AHA: 2016, 3Q, 24

√7ᵗʰ **S41.101** Unspecified open wound of right upper arm

√7ᵗʰ **S41.102** Unspecified open wound of left upper arm

√7ᵗʰ **S41.109** Unspecified open wound of unspecified upper arm

√6ᵗʰ **S41.11** Laceration without foreign body of upper arm

√7ᵗʰ **S41.111** Laceration without foreign body of right upper arm

√7ᵗʰ **S41.112** Laceration without foreign body of left upper arm

√7ᵗʰ **S41.119** Laceration without foreign body of unspecified upper arm

√6ᵗʰ **S41.12** Laceration with foreign body of upper arm

√7ᵗʰ **S41.121** Laceration with foreign body of right upper arm

√7ᵗʰ **S41.122** Laceration with foreign body of left upper arm

√7ᵗʰ **S41.129** Laceration with foreign body of unspecified upper arm

√6ᵗʰ **S41.13** Puncture wound without foreign body of upper arm
AHA: 2016, 3Q, 24

√7ᵗʰ **S41.131** Puncture wound without foreign body of right upper arm

√7ᵗʰ **S41.132** Puncture wound without foreign body of left upper arm

√7ᵗʰ **S41.139** Puncture wound without foreign body of unspecified upper arm

√6ᵗʰ **S41.14** Puncture wound with foreign body of upper arm
AHA: 2016, 3Q, 24

√7ᵗʰ **S41.141** Puncture wound with foreign body of right upper arm

√7ᵗʰ **S41.142** Puncture wound with foreign body of left upper arm

√7ᵗʰ **S41.149** Puncture wound with foreign body of unspecified upper arm

✔ Additional Character Req   √x7ᵗʰ Placeholder Alert   Unacceptable PDx   Manifestation   H1-H14 HAC   HCC CMS-HCC Condition   EXCLUDES 1 Not Coded Here   EXCLUDES 2 Not Included Here

ICD-10-CM 2018      985

**Chapter 19. Injury, Poisoning and Certain Other Consequences of External Causes** *(left margin, vertical)*

**S41.15–S42.146** *(left margin, vertical)*

✓6th **S41.15** **Open bite** of upper arm
Bite of upper arm NOS
*EXCLUDES 1* *superficial bite of upper arm (S40.87)*

✓7th **S41.151** **Open bite** of **right upper arm**

✓7th **S41.152** **Open bite** of **left upper arm**

✓7th **S41.159** **Open bite** of **unspecified upper arm**

✓4th **S42** **Fracture of shoulder and upper arm**

**NOTE** A fracture not indicated as displaced or nondisplaced should be coded to displaced.
A fracture not indicated as open or closed should be coded to closed.

*EXCLUDES 1* *traumatic amputation of shoulder and upper arm (S48.-)*
**AHA:** 2015, 3Q, 37-39

The appropriate 7th character is to be added to all codes from category S42 [unless otherwise indicated].
A    initial encounter for closed fracture
B    initial encounter for open fracture
D    subsequent encounter for fracture with routine healing
G    subsequent encounter for fracture with delayed healing
K    subsequent encounter for fracture with nonunion
P    subsequent encounter for fracture with malunion
S    sequela

✓5th **S42.0** **Fracture of clavicle**

**CC Excl: For codes in subcategory S42.0:**
**CC with 7th character B:** PDX collection 1243
**CC with 7th character K or P:** PDX collection 897

✓6th **S42.00** **Fracture of unspecified part of clavicle**

7 ✓7th **S42.001** **Fracture of unspecified part of right clavicle** CC H5

7 ✓7th **S42.002** **Fracture of unspecified part of left clavicle** CC H5

7 ✓7th **S42.009** **Fracture of unspecified part of unspecified clavicle** CC H5
**AHA:** 2012, 4Q, 93

✓6th **S42.01** **Fracture of sternal end of clavicle**

7 ✓7th **S42.011** **Anterior displaced fracture of sternal end of right clavicle** CC H5

7 ✓7th **S42.012** **Anterior displaced fracture of sternal end of left clavicle** CC H5

7 ✓7th **S42.013** **Anterior displaced fracture of sternal end of unspecified clavicle** CC H5
Displaced fracture of sternal end of clavicle NOS

7 ✓7th **S42.014** **Posterior displaced fracture of sternal end of right clavicle** CC H5

7 ✓7th **S42.015** **Posterior displaced fracture of sternal end of left clavicle** CC H5

7 ✓7th **S42.016** **Posterior displaced fracture of sternal end of unspecified clavicle** CC H5

7 ✓7th **S42.017** **Nondisplaced fracture of sternal end of right clavicle** CC H5

7 ✓7th **S42.018** **Nondisplaced fracture of sternal end of left clavicle** CC H5

7 ✓7th **S42.019** **Nondisplaced fracture of sternal end of unspecified clavicle** CC H5

✓6th **S42.02** **Fracture of shaft of clavicle**

7 ✓7th **S42.021** **Displaced fracture of shaft of right clavicle** CC H5

7 ✓7th **S42.022** **Displaced fracture of shaft of left clavicle** CC H5

7 ✓7th **S42.023** **Displaced fracture of shaft of unspecified clavicle** CC H5

7 ✓7th **S42.024** **Nondisplaced fracture of shaft of right clavicle** CC H5

7 ✓7th **S42.025** **Nondisplaced fracture of shaft of left clavicle** CC H5

7 ✓7th **S42.026** **Nondisplaced fracture of shaft of unspecified clavicle** CC H5

✓6th **S42.03** **Fracture of lateral end of clavicle**
Fracture of acromial end of clavicle

7 ✓7th **S42.031** **Displaced fracture of lateral end of right clavicle** CC H5

7 ✓7th **S42.032** **Displaced fracture of lateral end of left clavicle** CC H5

7 ✓7th **S42.033** **Displaced fracture of lateral end of unspecified clavicle** CC H5

7 ✓7th **S42.034** **Nondisplaced fracture of lateral end of right clavicle** CC H5

7 ✓7th **S42.035** **Nondisplaced fracture of lateral end of left clavicle** CC H5

7 ✓7th **S42.036** **Nondisplaced fracture of lateral end of unspecified clavicle** CC H5

✓5th **S42.1** **Fracture of scapula**

**CC Excl: For codes in subcatagory S42.1:**
**CC with 7th character B:** PDX collection 1244
**CC with 7th character K or P:** PDX collection 897

✓6th **S42.10** **Fracture of unspecified part of scapula**

7 ✓7th **S42.101** **Fracture of unspecified part of scapula, right shoulder** CC H5

7 ✓7th **S42.102** **Fracture of unspecified part of scapula, left shoulder** CC H5

7 ✓7th **S42.109** **Fracture of unspecified part of scapula, unspecified shoulder** CC H5

✓6th **S42.11** **Fracture of body of scapula**

7 ✓7th **S42.111** **Displaced fracture of body of scapula, right shoulder** CC H5

7 ✓7th **S42.112** **Displaced fracture of body of scapula, left shoulder** CC H5

7 ✓7th **S42.113** **Displaced fracture of body of scapula, unspecified shoulder** CC H5

7 ✓7th **S42.114** **Nondisplaced fracture of body of scapula, right shoulder** CC H5

7 ✓7th **S42.115** **Nondisplaced fracture of body of scapula, left shoulder** CC H5

7 ✓7th **S42.116** **Nondisplaced fracture of body of scapula, unspecified shoulder** CC H5

✓6th **S42.12** **Fracture of acromial process**

7 ✓7th **S42.121** **Displaced fracture of acromial process, right shoulder** CC H5

7 ✓7th **S42.122** **Displaced fracture of acromial process, left shoulder** CC H5

7 ✓7th **S42.123** **Displaced fracture of acromial process, unspecified shoulder** CC H5

7 ✓7th **S42.124** **Nondisplaced fracture of acromial process, right shoulder** CC H5

7 ✓7th **S42.125** **Nondisplaced fracture of acromial process, left shoulder** CC H5

7 ✓7th **S42.126** **Nondisplaced fracture of acromial process, unspecified shoulder** CC H5

✓6th **S42.13** **Fracture of coracoid process**

7 ✓7th **S42.131** **Displaced fracture of coracoid process, right shoulder** CC H5

7 ✓7th **S42.132** **Displaced fracture of coracoid process, left shoulder** CC H5

7 ✓7th **S42.133** **Displaced fracture of coracoid process, unspecified shoulder** CC H5

7 ✓7th **S42.134** **Nondisplaced fracture of coracoid process, right shoulder** CC H5

7 ✓7th **S42.135** **Nondisplaced fracture of coracoid process, left shoulder** CC H5

7 ✓7th **S42.136** **Nondisplaced fracture of coracoid process, unspecified shoulder** CC H5

✓6th **S42.14** **Fracture of glenoid cavity of scapula**

7 ✓7th **S42.141** **Displaced fracture of glenoid cavity of scapula, right shoulder** CC H5

7 ✓7th **S42.142** **Displaced fracture of glenoid cavity of scapula, left shoulder** CC H5

7 ✓7th **S42.143** **Displaced fracture of glenoid cavity of scapula, unspecified shoulder** CC H5

7 ✓7th **S42.144** **Nondisplaced fracture of glenoid cavity of scapula, right shoulder** CC H5

7 ✓7th **S42.145** **Nondisplaced fracture of glenoid cavity of scapula, left shoulder** CC H5

7 ✓7th **S42.146** **Nondisplaced fracture of glenoid cavity of scapula, unspecified shoulder** CC H5

---

**7**   CC when reported as an initial encounter (7th character A, B, or C – specific to category) OR a subsequent encounter for nonunion or malunion (7th character K, M, N, P, Q, or R – specific to category).

**N** Newborn: 0    **P** Pediatric: 0-17    **M** Maternity: 12-55    **A** Adult: 15-124    **MCC** Major CC Condition    **PDx MCC** PDx acts as own MCC    **CC** CC Condition    **PDx CC** PDx acts as own CC

√6ᵗʰ **S42.15** **Fracture of neck of scapula**

   7   √7ᵗʰ **S42.151** **Displaced fracture of neck of scapula, right shoulder**   `CC` `H5`

   7   √7ᵗʰ **S42.152** **Displaced fracture of neck of scapula, left shoulder**   `CC` `H5`

   7   √7ᵗʰ **S42.153** **Displaced fracture of neck of scapula, unspecified shoulder**   `CC` `H5`

   7   √7ᵗʰ **S42.154** **Nondisplaced fracture of neck of scapula, right shoulder**   `CC` `H5`

   7   √7ᵗʰ **S42.155** **Nondisplaced fracture of neck of scapula, left shoulder**   `CC` `H5`

   7   √7ᵗʰ **S42.156** **Nondisplaced fracture of neck of scapula, unspecified shoulder**   `CC` `H5`

√6ᵗʰ **S42.19** **Fracture of other part of scapula**

   7   √7ᵗʰ **S42.191** **Fracture of other part of scapula, right shoulder**   `CC` `H5`

   7   √7ᵗʰ **S42.192** **Fracture of other part of scapula, left shoulder**   `CC` `H5`

   7   √7ᵗʰ **S42.199** **Fracture of other part of scapula, unspecified shoulder**   `CC` `H5`

√5ᵗʰ **S42.2** **Fracture of upper end of humerus**
Fracture of proximal end of humerus

    *EXCLUDES 2*   fracture of shaft of humerus (S42.3-)
                 physeal fracture of upper end of humerus (S49.0-)

> **CC Excl: For CC/MCC codes in subcategory S42.2, unless otherwise noted:**
> **Right side:** See code S42.201
> **Left side:** See code S42.202
> **Unspecified side:** See code S42.209

√6ᵗʰ **S42.20** **Unspecified fracture of upper end of humerus**

  6,7   √7ᵗʰ **S42.201** **Unspecified fracture of upper end of right humerus**   `MCC` `CC` `H5`
         **CC Excl: CC with 7th character A:**
         PDX collection 1245
         **MCC with 7th character B:**
         PDX collection 1246
         **CC with 7th character K or P:**
         PDX collection 897

  6,7   √7ᵗʰ **S42.202** **Unspecified fracture of upper end of left humerus**   `MCC` `CC` `H5`
         **CC Excl: CC with 7th character A:**
         PDX collection 1247
         **MCC with 7th character B:**
         PDX collection 1246
         **CC with 7th character K or P:**
         PDX collection 897

  6,7   √7ᵗʰ **S42.209** **Unspecified fracture of upper end of unspecified humerus**   `MCC` `CC` `H5`
         **CC Excl: CC with 7th character A:**
         PDX collection 1248
         **MCC with 7th character B:**
         PDX collection 1246
         **CC with 7th character K or P:**
         PDX collection 897

√6ᵗʰ **S42.21** **Unspecified fracture of surgical neck of humerus**
Fracture of neck of humerus NOS

  6,7   √7ᵗʰ **S42.211** **Unspecified displaced fracture of surgical neck of right humerus**   `MCC` `CC` `H5`

  6,7   √7ᵗʰ **S42.212** **Unspecified displaced fracture of surgical neck of left humerus**   `MCC` `CC` `H5`

  6,7   √7ᵗʰ **S42.213** **Unspecified displaced fracture of surgical neck of unspecified humerus**   `MCC` `CC` `H5`

  6,7   √7ᵗʰ **S42.214** **Unspecified nondisplaced fracture of surgical neck of right humerus**   `MCC` `CC` `H5`

  6,7   √7ᵗʰ **S42.215** **Unspecified nondisplaced fracture of surgical neck of left humerus**   `MCC` `CC` `H5`

  6,7   √7ᵗʰ **S42.216** **Unspecified nondisplaced fracture of surgical neck of unspecified humerus**   `MCC` `CC` `H5`

√6ᵗʰ **S42.22** **2-part fracture of surgical neck of humerus**

  6,7   √7ᵗʰ **S42.221** **2-part displaced fracture of surgical neck of right humerus**   `MCC` `CC` `H5`

  6,7   √7ᵗʰ **S42.222** **2-part displaced fracture of surgical neck of left humerus**   `MCC` `CC` `H5`

  6,7   √7ᵗʰ **S42.223** **2-part displaced fracture of surgical neck of unspecified humerus**   `MCC` `CC` `H5`

  6,7   √7ᵗʰ **S42.224** **2-part nondisplaced fracture of surgical neck of right humerus**   `MCC` `CC` `H5`

  6,7   √7ᵗʰ **S42.225** **2-part nondisplaced fracture of surgical neck of left humerus**   `MCC` `CC` `H5`

  6,7   √7ᵗʰ **S42.226** **2-part nondisplaced fracture of surgical neck of unspecified humerus**   `MCC` `CC` `H5`

√6ᵗʰ **S42.23** **3-part fracture of surgical neck of humerus**

  6,7   √7ᵗʰ **S42.231** **3-part fracture of surgical neck of right humerus**   `MCC` `CC` `H5`

  6,7   √7ᵗʰ **S42.232** **3-part fracture of surgical neck of left humerus**   `MCC` `CC` `H5`

  6,7   √7ᵗʰ **S42.239** **3-part fracture of surgical neck of unspecified humerus**   `MCC` `CC` `H5`

√6ᵗʰ **S42.24** **4-part fracture of surgical neck of humerus**

  6,7   √7ᵗʰ **S42.241** **4-part fracture of surgical neck of right humerus**   `MCC` `CC` `H5`

  6,7   √7ᵗʰ **S42.242** **4-part fracture of surgical neck of left humerus**   `MCC` `CC` `H5`

  6,7   √7ᵗʰ **S42.249** **4-part fracture of surgical neck of unspecified humerus**   `MCC` `CC` `H5`

√6ᵗʰ **S42.25** **Fracture of greater tuberosity of humerus**

  6,7   √7ᵗʰ **S42.251** **Displaced fracture of greater tuberosity of right humerus**   `MCC` `CC` `H5`

  6,7   √7ᵗʰ **S42.252** **Displaced fracture of greater tuberosity of left humerus**   `MCC` `CC` `H5`

  6,7   √7ᵗʰ **S42.253** **Displaced fracture of greater tuberosity of unspecified humerus**   `MCC` `CC` `H5`

  6,7   √7ᵗʰ **S42.254** **Nondisplaced fracture of greater tuberosity of right humerus**   `MCC` `CC` `H5`

  6,7   √7ᵗʰ **S42.255** **Nondisplaced fracture of greater tuberosity of left humerus**   `MCC` `CC` `H5`

  6,7   √7ᵗʰ **S42.256** **Nondisplaced fracture of greater tuberosity of unspecified humerus**   `MCC` `CC` `H5`

√6ᵗʰ **S42.26** **Fracture of lesser tuberosity of humerus**

  6,7   √7ᵗʰ **S42.261** **Displaced fracture of lesser tuberosity of right humerus**   `MCC` `CC` `H5`

  6,7   √7ᵗʰ **S42.262** **Displaced fracture of lesser tuberosity of left humerus**   `MCC` `CC` `H5`

  6,7   √7ᵗʰ **S42.263** **Displaced fracture of lesser tuberosity of unspecified humerus**   `MCC` `CC` `H5`

  6,7   √7ᵗʰ **S42.264** **Nondisplaced fracture of lesser tuberosity of right humerus**   `MCC` `CC` `H5`

  6,7   √7ᵗʰ **S42.265** **Nondisplaced fracture of lesser tuberosity of left humerus**   `MCC` `CC` `H5`

  6,7   √7ᵗʰ **S42.266** **Nondisplaced fracture of lesser tuberosity of unspecified humerus**   `MCC` `CC` `H5`

√6ᵗʰ **S42.27** **Torus fracture of upper end of humerus**

> The appropriate 7th character is to be added to all codes in subcategory S42.27.
> A   initial encounter for closed fracture
> D   subsequent encounter for fracture with routine healing
> G   subsequent encounter for fracture with delayed healing
> K   subsequent encounter for fracture with nonunion
> P   subsequent encounter for fracture with malunion
> S   sequela

   7   √7ᵗʰ **S42.271** **Torus fracture of upper end of right humerus**   `CC` `H5`
         **CC Excl: CC with 7th character A:**
         PDX collection 1245
         **CC with 7th character K or P:**
         PDX collection 897

   7   √7ᵗʰ **S42.272** **Torus fracture of upper end of left humerus**   `CC` `H5`
         **CC Excl: CC with 7th character A:**
         PDX collection 1247
         **CC with 7th character K or P:**
         PDX collection 897

---

6   MCC when reported as an open fracture (7th character B or C – specific to category).

7   CC when reported as an initial encounter (7th character A, B, or C – specific to category) OR a subsequent encounter for nonunion or malunion (7th character K, M, N, P, Q, or R – specific to category).

---

✔Additional Character Req   ✔x7ᵗʰ Placeholder Alert   Unacceptable PDx   Manifestation   `H1`-`H14` HAC   `HCC` CMS-HCC Condition   *EXCLUDES 1* Not Coded Here   *EXCLUDES 2* Not Included Here

ICD-10-CM 2018      987

*Chapter 19. Injury, Poisoning and Certain Other Consequences of External Causes*

*S42.15–S42.272*

**7** ✓7th **S42.279** **Torus fracture of upper end of unspecified humerus** `CC` `H5`
     CC Excl: CC with 7th character A:
     PDX collection 1248
     CC with 7th character K or P:
     PDX collection 897

✓6th **S42.29** **Other fracture of upper end of humerus**
     Fracture of anatomical neck of humerus
     Fracture of articular head of humerus

**6, 7** ✓7th **S42.291** **Other displaced fracture of upper end of right humerus** `MCC` `CC` `H5`

**6, 7** ✓7th **S42.292** **Other displaced fracture of upper end of left humerus** `MCC` `CC` `H5`

**6, 7** ✓7th **S42.293** **Other displaced fracture of upper end of unspecified humerus** `MCC` `CC` `H5`

**6, 7** ✓7th **S42.294** **Other nondisplaced fracture of upper end of right humerus** `MCC` `CC` `H5`

**6, 7** ✓7th **S42.295** **Other nondisplaced fracture of upper end of left humerus** `MCC` `CC` `H5`

**6, 7** ✓7th **S42.296** **Other nondisplaced fracture of upper end of unspecified humerus** `MCC` `CC` `H5`

✓5th **S42.3** **Fracture of shaft of humerus**
     Fracture of humerus NOS
     Fracture of upper arm NOS
     *EXCLUDES 2*    physeal fractures of upper end of humerus (S49.0-)
              physeal fractures of lower end of humerus (S49.1-)

> **CC Excl: For CC/MCC codes in subcategory S42.3, unless otherwise noted:**
> **Right side:** See code S42.321
> **Left side:** See code S42.322
> **Unspecified side:** See code S42.323

✓6th **S42.30** **Unspecified fracture of shaft of humerus**

**6, 7** ✓7th **S42.301** **Unspecified fracture of shaft of humerus, right arm** `MCC` `CC` `H5`

**6, 7** ✓7th **S42.302** **Unspecified fracture of shaft of humerus, left arm** `MCC` `CC` `H5`

**6, 7** ✓7th **S42.309** **Unspecified fracture of shaft of humerus, unspecified arm** `MCC` `CC` `H5`

✓6th **S42.31** **Greenstick fracture of shaft of humerus**

> The appropriate 7th character is to be added to all codes in subcategory S42.31.
> A    initial encounter for closed fracture
> D    subsequent encounter for fracture with routine healing
> G    subsequent encounter for fracture with delayed healing
> K    subsequent encounter for fracture with nonunion
> P    subsequent encounter for fracture with malunion
> S    sequela

**7** ✓7th **S42.311** **Greenstick fracture of shaft of humerus, right arm** `CC` `H5`
     CC Excl: CC with 7th character A:
     PDX collection 1249
     CC with 7th character K or P:
     PDX collection 897

**7** ✓7th **S42.312** **Greenstick fracture of shaft of humerus, left arm** `CC` `H5`
     CC Excl: CC with 7th character A:
     PDX collection 1250
     CC with 7th character K or P:
     PDX collection 897

**7** ✓7th **S42.319** **Greenstick fracture of shaft of humerus, unspecified arm** `CC` `H5`
     CC Excl: CC with 7th character A:
     PDX collection 1251
     CC with 7th character K or P:
     PDX collection 897

✓6th **S42.32** **Transverse fracture of shaft of humerus**

**6, 7** ✓7th **S42.321** **Displaced transverse fracture of shaft of humerus, right arm** `MCC` `CC` `H5`
     CC Excl: CC with 7th character A:
     PDX collection 1249
     MCC with 7th character B:
     PDX collection 1246
     CC with 7th character K or P:
     PDX collection 897

**6, 7** ✓7th **S42.322** **Displaced transverse fracture of shaft of humerus, left arm** `MCC` `CC` `H5`
     CC Excl: CC with 7th character A:
     PDX collection 1250
     MCC with 7th character B:
     PDX collection 1246
     CC with 7th character K or P:
     PDX collection 897

**6, 7** ✓7th **S42.323** **Displaced transverse fracture of shaft of humerus, unspecified arm** `MCC` `CC` `H5`
     CC Excl: CC with 7th character A:
     PDX collection 1251
     MCC with 7th character B:
     PDX collection 1246
     CC with 7th character K or P:
     PDX collection 897

**6, 7** ✓7th **S42.324** **Nondisplaced transverse fracture of shaft of humerus, right arm** `MCC` `CC` `H5`

**6, 7** ✓7th **S42.325** **Nondisplaced transverse fracture of shaft of humerus, left arm** `MCC` `CC` `H5`

**6, 7** ✓7th **S42.326** **Nondisplaced transverse fracture of shaft of humerus, unspecified arm** `MCC` `CC` `H5`

✓6th **S42.33** **Oblique fracture of shaft of humerus**

**6, 7** ✓7th **S42.331** **Displaced oblique fracture of shaft of humerus, right arm** `MCC` `CC` `H5`

**6, 7** ✓7th **S42.332** **Displaced oblique fracture of shaft of humerus, left arm** `MCC` `CC` `H5`

**6, 7** ✓7th **S42.333** **Displaced oblique fracture of shaft of humerus, unspecified arm** `MCC` `CC` `H5`

**6, 7** ✓7th **S42.334** **Nondisplaced oblique fracture of shaft of humerus, right arm** `MCC` `CC` `H5`

**6, 7** ✓7th **S42.335** **Nondisplaced oblique fracture of shaft of humerus, left arm** `MCC` `CC` `H5`

**6, 7** ✓7th **S42.336** **Nondisplaced oblique fracture of shaft of humerus, unspecified arm** `MCC` `CC` `H5`

✓6th **S42.34** **Spiral fracture of shaft of humerus**

**6, 7** ✓7th **S42.341** **Displaced spiral fracture of shaft of humerus, right arm** `MCC` `CC` `H5`

**6, 7** ✓7th **S42.342** **Displaced spiral fracture of sharft of humerus, left arm** `MCC` `CC` `H5`

**6, 7** ✓7th **S42.343** **Displaced spiral fracture of shaft of humerus, unspecified arm** `MCC` `CC` `H5`

**6, 7** ✓7th **S42.344** **Nondisplaced spiral fracture of shaft of humerus, right arm** `MCC` `CC` `H5`

**6, 7** ✓7th **S42.345** **Nondisplaced spiral fracture of shaft of humerus, left arm** `MCC` `CC` `H5`

**6, 7** ✓7th **S42.346** **Nondisplaced spiral fracture of shaft of humerus, unspecified arm** `MCC` `CC` `H5`

✓6th **S42.35** **Comminuted fracture of shaft of humerus**

**6, 7** ✓7th **S42.351** **Displaced comminuted fracture of shaft of humerus, right arm** `MCC` `CC` `H5`

**6, 7** ✓7th **S42.352** **Displaced comminuted fracture of shaft of humerus, left arm** `MCC` `CC` `H5`

**6, 7** ✓7th **S42.353** **Displaced comminuted fracture of shaft of humerus, unspecified arm** `MCC` `CC` `H5`

**6, 7** ✓7th **S42.354** **Nondisplaced comminuted fracture of shaft of humerus, right arm** `MCC` `CC` `H5`

**6, 7** ✓7th **S42.355** **Nondisplaced comminuted fracture of shaft of humerus, left arm** `MCC` `CC` `H5`

**6, 7** ✓7th **S42.356** **Nondisplaced comminuted fracture of shaft of humerus, unspecified arm** `MCC` `CC` `H5`

✓6th **S42.36** **Segmental fracture of shaft of humerus**

**6, 7** ✓7th **S42.361** **Displaced segmental fracture of shaft of humerus, right arm** `MCC` `CC` `H5`

---

**6**   MCC when reported as an open fracture (7th character B or C – specific to category).
**7**   CC when reported as an initial encounter (7th character A, B, or C – specific to category) OR a subsequent encounter for nonunion or malunion (7th character K, M, N, P, Q, or R – specific to category).

---

`N` Newborn: 0   `P` Pediatric: 0-17   `M` Maternity: 12-55   `A` Adult: 15-124   `MCC` Major CC Condition   `PDxMCC` PDx acts as own MCC   `CC` CC Condition   `PDxCC` PDx acts as own CC

**988**      ICD-10-CM 2018

6, 7 ✓7ᵗʰ **S42.362** Displaced **segmental fracture** of shaft of humerus, **left arm** `MCC` `CC` `H5`

6, 7 ✓7ᵗʰ **S42.363** Displaced **segmental fracture** of shaft of humerus, **unspecified arm** `MCC` `CC` `H5`

6, 7 ✓7ᵗʰ **S42.364** Nondisplaced **segmental fracture of shaft of humerus, right arm** `MCC` `CC` `H5`

6, 7 ✓7ᵗʰ **S42.365** Nondisplaced **segmental fracture of shaft of humerus, left arm** `MCC` `CC` `H5`

6, 7 ✓7ᵗʰ **S42.366** Nondisplaced **segmental fracture of shaft of humerus, unspecified arm** `MCC` `CC` `H5`

✓6ᵗʰ **S42.39** Other **fracture of shaft of humerus**

6, 7 ✓7ᵗʰ **S42.391** Other fracture of shaft of **right** humerus `MCC` `CC` `H5`

6, 7 ✓7ᵗʰ **S42.392** Other fracture of shaft of **left** humerus `MCC` `CC` `H5`

6, 7 ✓7ᵗʰ **S42.399** Other fracture of shaft of **unspecified** humerus `MCC` `CC` `H5`

✓5ᵗʰ **S42.4** Fracture of **lower end of humerus**
Fracture of distal end of humerus

*EXCLUDES 2*   fracture of shaft of humerus (S42.3-)
physeal fracture of lower end of humerus (S49.1-)

> **CC Excl: For CC/MCC codes in subcategory S42.4, unless otherwise noted:**
> **Right side:** See code S42.201
> **Left side:** See code S42.202
> **Unspecified side:** See code S42.209

✓6ᵗʰ **S42.40** Unspecified **fracture of lower end of humerus**
Fracture of elbow NOS

6, 7 ✓7ᵗʰ **S42.401** Unspecified fracture of lower end of **right** humerus `MCC` `CC` `H5`

6, 7 ✓7ᵗʰ **S42.402** Unspecified fracture of lower end of **left** humerus `MCC` `CC` `H5`

6, 7 ✓7ᵗʰ **S42.409** Unspecified fracture of lower end of **unspecified** humerus `MCC` `CC` `H5`

✓6ᵗʰ **S42.41** Simple supracondylar **fracture without** intercondylar **fracture of humerus**

6, 7 ✓7ᵗʰ **S42.411** Displaced **simple supracondylar fracture without intercondylar fracture of right humerus** `MCC` `CC` `H5`

6, 7 ✓7ᵗʰ **S42.412** Displaced **simple supracondylar fracture without intercondylar fracture of left humerus** `MCC` `CC` `H5`

6, 7 ✓7ᵗʰ **S42.413** Displaced **simple supracondylar fracture without intercondylar fracture of unspecified humerus** `MCC` `CC` `H5`

6, 7 ✓7ᵗʰ **S42.414** Nondisplaced **simple supracondylar fracture without intercondylar fracture of right humerus** `MCC` `CC` `H5`

6, 7 ✓7ᵗʰ **S42.415** Nondisplaced **simple supracondylar fracture without intercondylar fracture of left humerus** `MCC` `CC` `H5`

6, 7 ✓7ᵗʰ **S42.416** Nondisplaced **simple supracondylar fracture without intercondylar fracture of unspecified humerus** `MCC` `CC` `H5`

✓6ᵗʰ **S42.42** Comminuted supracondylar **fracture without** intercondylar **fracture of humerus**

6, 7 ✓7ᵗʰ **S42.421** Displaced **comminuted supracondylar fracture without intercondylar fracture of right humerus** `MCC` `CC` `H5`

6, 7 ✓7ᵗʰ **S42.422** Displaced **comminuted supracondylar fracture without intercondylar fracture of left humerus** `MCC` `CC` `H5`

6, 7 ✓7ᵗʰ **S42.423** Displaced **comminuted supracondylar fracture without intercondylar fracture of unspecified humerus** `MCC` `CC` `H5`

6, 7 ✓7ᵗʰ **S42.424** Nondisplaced **comminuted supracondylar fracture without intercondylar fracture of right humerus** `MCC` `CC` `H5`

6, 7 ✓7ᵗʰ **S42.425** Nondisplaced **comminuted supracondylar fracture without intercondylar fracture of left humerus** `MCC` `CC` `H5`

6, 7 ✓7ᵗʰ **S42.426** Nondisplaced **comminuted supracondylar fracture without intercondylar fracture of unspecified humerus** `MCC` `CC` `H5`

✓6ᵗʰ **S42.43** Fracture (avulsion) of **lateral epicondyle of humerus**

6, 7 ✓7ᵗʰ **S42.431** Displaced **fracture (avulsion) of lateral epicondyle of right humerus** `MCC` `CC` `H5`

6, 7 ✓7ᵗʰ **S42.432** Displaced **fracture (avulsion) of lateral epicondyle of left humerus** `MCC` `CC` `H5`

6, 7 ✓7ᵗʰ **S42.433** Displaced **fracture (avulsion) of lateral epicondyle of unspecified humerus** `MCC` `CC` `H5`

6, 7 ✓7ᵗʰ **S42.434** Nondisplaced **fracture (avulsion) of lateral epicondyle of right humerus** `MCC` `CC` `H5`

6, 7 ✓7ᵗʰ **S42.435** Nondisplaced **fracture (avulsion) of lateral epicondyle of left humerus** `MCC` `CC` `H5`

6, 7 ✓7ᵗʰ **S42.436** Nondisplaced **fracture (avulsion) of lateral epicondyle of unspecified humerus** `MCC` `CC` `H5`

✓6ᵗʰ **S42.44** Fracture (avulsion) of **medial epicondyle of humerus**

6, 7 ✓7ᵗʰ **S42.441** Displaced **fracture (avulsion) of medial epicondyle of right humerus** `MCC` `CC` `H5`

6, 7 ✓7ᵗʰ **S42.442** Displaced **fracture (avulsion) of medial epicondyle of left humerus** `MCC` `CC` `H5`

6, 7 ✓7ᵗʰ **S42.443** Displaced **fracture (avulsion) of medial epicondyle of unspecified humerus** `MCC` `CC` `H5`

6, 7 ✓7ᵗʰ **S42.444** Nondisplaced **fracture (avulsion) of medial epicondyle of right humerus** `MCC` `CC` `H5`

6, 7 ✓7ᵗʰ **S42.445** Nondisplaced **fracture (avulsion) of medial epicondyle of left humerus** `MCC` `CC` `H5`

6, 7 ✓7ᵗʰ **S42.446** Nondisplaced **fracture (avulsion) of medial epicondyle of unspecified of humerus** `MCC` `CC` `H5`

6, 7 ✓7ᵗʰ **S42.447** Incarcerated **fracture (avulsion) of medial epicondyle of right humerus** `MCC` `CC` `H5`

6, 7 ✓7ᵗʰ **S42.448** Incarcerated **fracture (avulsion) of medial epicondyle of left humerus** `MCC` `CC` `H5`

6, 7 ✓7ᵗʰ **S42.449** Incarcerated **fracture (avulsion) of medial epicondyle of unspecified humerus** `MCC` `CC` `H5`

✓6ᵗʰ **S42.45** Fracture of **lateral condyle of humerus**
Fracture of capitellum of humerus

6, 7 ✓7ᵗʰ **S42.451** Displaced **fracture of lateral condyle of right humerus** `MCC` `CC` `H5`

6, 7 ✓7ᵗʰ **S42.452** Displaced **fracture of lateral condyle of left humerus** `MCC` `CC` `H5`

6, 7 ✓7ᵗʰ **S42.453** Displaced **fracture of lateral condyle of unspecified humerus** `MCC` `CC` `H5`

6, 7 ✓7ᵗʰ **S42.454** Nondisplaced **fracture of lateral condyle of right humerus** `MCC` `CC` `H5`

6, 7 ✓7ᵗʰ **S42.455** Nondisplaced **fracture of lateral condyle of left humerus** `MCC` `CC` `H5`

6, 7 ✓7ᵗʰ **S42.456** Nondisplaced **fracture of lateral condyle of unspecified humerus** `MCC` `CC` `H5`

✓6ᵗʰ **S42.46** Fracture of **medial condyle of humerus**
Trochlea fracture of humerus

6, 7 ✓7ᵗʰ **S42.461** Displaced **fracture of medial condyle of right humerus** `MCC` `CC` `H5`

6, 7 ✓7ᵗʰ **S42.462** Displaced **fracture of medial condyle of left humerus** `MCC` `CC` `H5`

6, 7 ✓7ᵗʰ **S42.463** Displaced **fracture of medial condyle of unspecified humerus** `MCC` `CC` `H5`

6, 7 ✓7ᵗʰ **S42.464** Nondisplaced **fracture of medial condyle of right humerus** `MCC` `CC` `H5`

---

**6**   MCC when reported as an open fracture (7th character B or C – specific to category).

**7**   CC when reported as an initial encounter (7th character A, B, or C – specific to category) OR a subsequent encounter for nonunion or malunion (7th character K, M, N, P, Q, or R – specific to category).

---

✓ Additional Character Req    ✓ˣ7ᵗʰ Placeholder Alert    Unacceptable PDx    Manifestation    `H1`-`H14` HAC    `HCC` CMS-HCC Condition    *EXCLUDES 1* Not Coded Here    *EXCLUDES 2* Not Included Here

**6,7** ✓7th **S42.465** **Nondisplaced** fracture of medial condyle of **left** humerus `MCC` `CC` `H5`

**6,7** ✓7th **S42.466** **Nondisplaced** fracture of medial condyle of **unspecified** humerus `MCC` `CC` `H5`

✓6th **S42.47** **Transcondylar** fracture of humerus

**6,7** ✓7th **S42.471** **Displaced transcondylar** fracture of **right** humerus `MCC` `CC` `H5`

**6,7** ✓7th **S42.472** **Displaced transcondylar** fracture of **left** humerus `MCC` `CC` `H5`

**6,7** ✓7th **S42.473** **Displaced transcondylar** fracture of **unspecified** humerus `MCC` `CC` `H5`

**6,7** ✓7th **S42.474** **Nondisplaced transcondylar** fracture of **right** humerus `MCC` `CC` `H5`

**6,7** ✓7th **S42.475** **Nondisplaced transcondylar** fracture of **left** humerus `MCC` `CC` `H5`

**6,7** ✓7th **S42.476** **Nondisplaced transcondylar** fracture of **unspecified** humerus `MCC` `CC` `H5`

✓6th **S42.48** **Torus** fracture of lower end of humerus

The appropriate 7th character is to be added to all codes in subcategory S42.48.
A   initial encounter for closed fracture
D   subsequent encounter for fracture with routine healing
G   subsequent encounter for fracture with delayed healing
K   subsequent encounter for fracture with nonunion
P   subsequent encounter for fracture with malunion
S   sequela

**7** ✓7th **S42.481** **Torus** fracture of lower end of **right** humerus `CC` `H5`
     **CC Excl: CC with 7th character A:**
     PDX collection 1245
     **CC with 7th character K or P:**
     PDX collection 897

**7** ✓7th **S42.482** **Torus** fracture of lower end of **left** humerus `CC` `H5`
     **CC Excl: CC with 7th character A:**
     PDX collection 1247
     **CC with 7th character K or P:**
     PDX collection 897

**7** ✓7th **S42.489** **Torus** fracture of lower end of **unspecified** humerus `CC` `H5`
     **CC Excl: CC with 7th character A:**
     PDX collection 1248
     **CC with 7th character K or P:**
     PDX collection 897

✓6th **S42.49** **Other** fracture of lower end of humerus

**6,7** ✓7th **S42.491** **Other displaced** fracture of lower end of **right** humerus `MCC` `CC` `H5`

**6,7** ✓7th **S42.492** **Other displaced** fracture of lower end of **left** humerus `MCC` `CC` `H5`

**6,7** ✓7th **S42.493** **Other displaced** fracture of lower end of **unspecified** humerus `MCC` `CC` `H5`

**6,7** ✓7th **S42.494** **Other nondisplaced** fracture of lower end of **right** humerus `MCC` `CC` `H5`

**6,7** ✓7th **S42.495** **Other nondisplaced** fracture of lower end of **left** humerus `MCC` `CC` `H5`

**6,7** ✓7th **S42.496** **Other nondisplaced** fracture of lower end of **unspecified** humerus `MCC` `CC` `H5`

✓5th **S42.9** **Fracture of shoulder girdle, part unspecified**
Fracture of shoulder NOS

**CC Excl: For CC/MCC codes in subcategory S42.9:**
See code S42.209

**6,7** ✓x7th **S42.90** **Fracture of unspecified shoulder girdle, part unspecified** `MCC` `CC` `H5`

**6,7** ✓x7th **S42.91** **Fracture of right shoulder girdle, part unspecified** `MCC` `CC` `H5`

**6,7** ✓x7th **S42.92** **Fracture of left shoulder girdle, part unspecified** `MCC` `CC` `H5`

✓4th **S43** **Dislocation and sprain of joints and ligaments of shoulder girdle**
`INCLUDES` avulsion of joint or ligament of shoulder girdle
laceration of cartilage, joint or ligament of shoulder girdle
sprain of cartilage, joint or ligament of shoulder girdle
traumatic hemarthrosis of joint or ligament of shoulder girdle
traumatic rupture of joint or ligament of shoulder girdle
traumatic subluxation of joint or ligament of shoulder girdle
traumatic tear of joint or ligament of shoulder girdle

Code also any associated open wound

`EXCLUDES 2` *strain of muscle, fascia and tendon of shoulder and upper arm (S46.-)*

The appropriate 7th character is to be added to each code from category S43.
A   initial encounter
D   subsequent encounter
S   sequela

✓5th **S43.0** **Subluxation and dislocation of shoulder joint**
Dislocation of glenohumeral joint
Subluxation of glenohumeral joint

✓6th **S43.00** **Unspecified subluxation and dislocation of shoulder joint**
Dislocation of humerus NOS
Subluxation of humerus NOS

     ✓7th **S43.001** **Unspecified subluxation of right shoulder joint**

     ✓7th **S43.002** **Unspecified subluxation of left shoulder joint**

     ✓7th **S43.003** **Unspecified subluxation of unspecified shoulder joint**

     ✓7th **S43.004** **Unspecified dislocation of right shoulder joint**

     ✓7th **S43.005** **Unspecified dislocation of left shoulder joint**

     ✓7th **S43.006** **Unspecified dislocation of unspecified shoulder joint**

✓6th **S43.01** **Anterior subluxation and dislocation of humerus**

     ✓7th **S43.011** **Anterior subluxation of right humerus**

     ✓7th **S43.012** **Anterior subluxation of left humerus**

     ✓7th **S43.013** **Anterior subluxation of unspecified humerus**

     ✓7th **S43.014** **Anterior dislocation of right humerus**

     ✓7th **S43.015** **Anterior dislocation of left humerus**

     ✓7th **S43.016** **Anterior dislocation of unspecified humerus**

✓6th **S43.02** **Posterior subluxation and dislocation of humerus**

     ✓7th **S43.021** **Posterior subluxation of right humerus**

     ✓7th **S43.022** **Posterior subluxation of left humerus**

     ✓7th **S43.023** **Posterior subluxation of unspecified humerus**

     ✓7th **S43.024** **Posterior dislocation of right humerus**

     ✓7th **S43.025** **Posterior dislocation of left humerus**

     ✓7th **S43.026** **Posterior dislocation of unspecified humerus**

✓6th **S43.03** **Inferior subluxation and dislocation of humerus**

     ✓7th **S43.031** **Inferior subluxation of right humerus**

     ✓7th **S43.032** **Inferior subluxation of left humerus**

     ✓7th **S43.033** **Inferior subluxation of unspecified humerus**

     ✓7th **S43.034** **Inferior dislocation of right humerus**

     ✓7th **S43.035** **Inferior dislocation of left humerus**

     ✓7th **S43.036** **Inferior dislocation of unspecified humerus**

✓6th **S43.08** **Other subluxation and dislocation of shoulder joint**

     ✓7th **S43.081** **Other subluxation of right shoulder joint**

     ✓7th **S43.082** **Other subluxation of left shoulder joint**

     ✓7th **S43.083** **Other subluxation of unspecified shoulder joint**

     ✓7th **S43.084** **Other dislocation of right shoulder joint**

     ✓7th **S43.085** **Other dislocation of left shoulder joint**

     ✓7th **S43.086** **Other dislocation of unspecified shoulder joint**

---

**6** MCC when reported as an open fracture (7th character B or C – specific to category).
**7** CC when reported as an initial encounter (7th character A, B, or C – specific to category) OR a subsequent encounter for nonunion or malunion (7th character K, M, N, P, Q, or R – specific to category).

`N` Newborn: 0   `P` Pediatric: 0-17   `M` Maternity: 12-55   `A` Adult: 15-124   `MCC` Major CC Condition   `PDx MCC` PDx acts as own MCC   `CC` CC Condition   `PDx CC` PDx acts as own CC

**990**      ICD-10-CM 2018

Chapter 19. Injury, Poisoning and Certain Other Consequences of External Causes

S42.465–S43.086

✓5ᵗʰ **S43.1 Subluxation and dislocation of** acromioclavicular joint

  ✓6ᵗʰ **S43.10 Unspecified dislocation** of acromioclavicular joint

    ✓7ᵗʰ **S43.101 Unspecified dislocation of** right acromioclavicular joint

    ✓7ᵗʰ **S43.102 Unspecified dislocation of** left acromioclavicular joint

    ✓7ᵗʰ **S43.109 Unspecified dislocation of** unspecified acromioclavicular joint

  ✓6ᵗʰ **S43.11 Subluxation** of acromioclavicular joint

    ✓7ᵗʰ **S43.111 Subluxation of** right acromioclavicular joint

    ✓7ᵗʰ **S43.112 Subluxation of** left acromioclavicular joint

    ✓7ᵗʰ **S43.119 Subluxation of** unspecified acromioclavicular joint

  ✓6ᵗʰ **S43.12 Dislocation of acromioclavicular joint,** 100%-200% displacement

    ✓7ᵗʰ **S43.121 Dislocation of** right acromioclavicular joint, 100%-200% displacement

    ✓7ᵗʰ **S43.122 Dislocation of** left acromioclavicular joint, 100%-200% displacement

    ✓7ᵗʰ **S43.129 Dislocation of** unspecified acromioclavicular joint, 100%-200% displacement

  ✓6ᵗʰ **S43.13 Dislocation of acromioclavicular joint,** greater than 200% displacement

    ✓7ᵗʰ **S43.131 Dislocation of** right acromioclavicular joint, greater than 200% displacement

    ✓7ᵗʰ **S43.132 Dislocation of** left acromioclavicular joint, greater than 200% displacement

    ✓7ᵗʰ **S43.139 Dislocation of** unspecified acromioclavicular joint, greater than 200% displacement

  ✓6ᵗʰ **S43.14 Inferior dislocation of** acromioclavicular joint

    ✓7ᵗʰ **S43.141 Inferior dislocation of** right acromioclavicular joint

    ✓7ᵗʰ **S43.142 Inferior dislocation of** left acromioclavicular joint

    ✓7ᵗʰ **S43.149 Inferior dislocation of** unspecified acromioclavicular joint

  ✓6ᵗʰ **S43.15 Posterior dislocation of** acromioclavicular joint

    ✓7ᵗʰ **S43.151 Posterior dislocation of** right acromioclavicular joint

    ✓7ᵗʰ **S43.152 Posterior dislocation of** left acromioclavicular joint

    ✓7ᵗʰ **S43.159 Posterior dislocation of** unspecified acromioclavicular joint

✓5ᵗʰ **S43.2 Subluxation and dislocation of** sternoclavicular joint

> **CC Excl:** For CC codes in subcategory S43.2:
> **Right side:** PDX collection 1252
> **Left side:** PDX collection 1253
> **Unspecified side:** PDX collection 914

  ✓6ᵗʰ **S43.20 Unspecified subluxation and dislocation of** sternoclavicular joint

    ✓7ᵗʰ **S43.201 Unspecified subluxation of** right sternoclavicular joint   `CC` `H5`

    ✓7ᵗʰ **S43.202 Unspecified subluxation of** left sternoclavicular joint   `CC` `H5`

    ✓7ᵗʰ **S43.203 Unspecified subluxation of** unspecified sternoclavicular joint   `CC` `H5`

    ✓7ᵗʰ **S43.204 Unspecified dislocation of** right sternoclavicular joint   `CC` `H5`

    ✓7ᵗʰ **S43.205 Unspecified dislocation of** left sternoclavicular joint   `CC` `H5`

    ✓7ᵗʰ **S43.206 Unspecified dislocation of** unspecified sternoclavicular joint   `CC` `H5`

  ✓6ᵗʰ **S43.21 Anterior subluxation and dislocation of** sternoclavicular joint

    ✓7ᵗʰ **S43.211 Anterior subluxation of** right sternoclavicular joint   `CC` `H5`

    ✓7ᵗʰ **S43.212 Anterior subluxation of** left sternoclavicular joint   `CC` `H5`

    ✓7ᵗʰ **S43.213 Anterior subluxation of** unspecified sternoclavicular joint   `CC` `H5`

    ✓7ᵗʰ **S43.214 Anterior dislocation of** right sternoclavicular joint   `CC` `H5`

    ✓7ᵗʰ **S43.215 Anterior dislocation of** left sternoclavicular joint   `CC` `H5`

    ✓7ᵗʰ **S43.216 Anterior dislocation of** unspecified sternoclavicular joint   `CC` `H5`

  ✓6ᵗʰ **S43.22 Posterior subluxation and dislocation of** sternoclavicular joint

    ✓7ᵗʰ **S43.221 Posterior subluxation of** right sternoclavicular joint   `CC` `H5`

    ✓7ᵗʰ **S43.222 Posterior subluxation of** left sternoclavicular joint   `CC` `H5`

    ✓7ᵗʰ **S43.223 Posterior subluxation of** unspecified sternoclavicular joint   `CC` `H5`

    ✓7ᵗʰ **S43.224 Posterior dislocation of** right sternoclavicular joint   `CC` `H5`

    ✓7ᵗʰ **S43.225 Posterior dislocation of** left sternoclavicular joint   `CC` `H5`

    ✓7ᵗʰ **S43.226 Posterior dislocation of** unspecified sternoclavicular joint   `CC` `H5`

✓5ᵗʰ **S43.3 Subluxation and dislocation of other and unspecified parts of** shoulder girdle

  ✓6ᵗʰ **S43.30 Subluxation and dislocation of** unspecified parts of shoulder girdle
    Dislocation of shoulder girdle NOS
    Subluxation of shoulder girdle NOS

    ✓7ᵗʰ **S43.301 Subluxation of unspecified parts of** right shoulder girdle

    ✓7ᵗʰ **S43.302 Subluxation of unspecified parts of** left shoulder girdle

    ✓7ᵗʰ **S43.303 Subluxation of unspecified parts of** unspecified shoulder girdle

    ✓7ᵗʰ **S43.304 Dislocation of unspecified parts of** right shoulder girdle

    ✓7ᵗʰ **S43.305 Dislocation of unspecified parts of** left shoulder girdle

    ✓7ᵗʰ **S43.306 Dislocation of unspecified parts of** unspecified shoulder girdle

  ✓6ᵗʰ **S43.31 Subluxation and dislocation of** scapula

    ✓7ᵗʰ **S43.311 Subluxation of right** scapula

    ✓7ᵗʰ **S43.312 Subluxation of left** scapula

    ✓7ᵗʰ **S43.313 Subluxation of unspecified** scapula

    ✓7ᵗʰ **S43.314 Dislocation of right** scapula

    ✓7ᵗʰ **S43.315 Dislocation of left** scapula

    ✓7ᵗʰ **S43.316 Dislocation of unspecified** scapula

  ✓6ᵗʰ **S43.39 Subluxation and dislocation of other parts of** shoulder girdle

    ✓7ᵗʰ **S43.391 Subluxation of other parts of** right shoulder girdle

    ✓7ᵗʰ **S43.392 Subluxation of other parts of** left shoulder girdle

    ✓7ᵗʰ **S43.393 Subluxation of other parts of** unspecified shoulder girdle

    ✓7ᵗʰ **S43.394 Dislocation of other parts of** right shoulder girdle

    ✓7ᵗʰ **S43.395 Dislocation of other parts of** left shoulder girdle

    ✓7ᵗʰ **S43.396 Dislocation of other parts of** unspecified shoulder girdle

✓5ᵗʰ **S43.4 Sprain of** shoulder joint

  ✓6ᵗʰ **S43.40 Unspecified sprain of shoulder joint**

    ✓7ᵗʰ **S43.401 Unspecified sprain of** right shoulder joint

    ✓7ᵗʰ **S43.402 Unspecified sprain of** left shoulder joint

    ✓7ᵗʰ **S43.409 Unspecified sprain of** unspecified shoulder joint

  ✓6ᵗʰ **S43.41 Sprain of** coracohumeral (ligament)

    ✓7ᵗʰ **S43.411 Sprain of** right coracohumeral (ligament)

    ✓7ᵗʰ **S43.412 Sprain of** left coracohumeral (ligament)

    ✓7ᵗʰ **S43.419 Sprain of** unspecified coracohumeral (ligament)

✓ Additional Character Req   ✓×7ᵗʰ Placeholder Alert   Unacceptable PDx   Manifestation   `H1`-`H14` HAC   `HCC` CMS-HCC Condition   *EXCLUDES 1* Not Coded Here   *EXCLUDES 2* Not Included Here

ICD-10-CM 2018      991

S43.1–S43.419

✓6ᵗʰ **S43.42　Sprain of rotator cuff capsule**
> EXCLUDES 1　rotator cuff syndrome (complete)
> (incomplete), not specified as traumatic
> (M75.1-)
> EXCLUDES 2　injury of tendon of rotator cuff (S46.Ø-)

　　✓7ᵗʰ **S43.421　Sprain of right rotator cuff capsule**
　　✓7ᵗʰ **S43.422　Sprain of left rotator cuff capsule**
　　✓7ᵗʰ **S43.429　Sprain of unspecified rotator cuff capsule**

✓6ᵗʰ **S43.43　Superior glenoid labrum lesion**
　　SLAP lesion
> **DEF:** Detachment injury of the superior aspect of the
> glenoid labrum, which is the ring of fibrocartilage
> attached to the rim of the glenoid cavity of the scapula.

　　✓7ᵗʰ **S43.431　Superior glenoid labrum lesion of right shoulder**
　　✓7ᵗʰ **S43.432　Superior glenoid labrum lesion of left shoulder**
　　✓7ᵗʰ **S43.439　Superior glenoid labrum lesion of unspecified shoulder**

✓6ᵗʰ **S43.49　Other sprain of shoulder joint**
　　✓7ᵗʰ **S43.491　Other sprain of right shoulder joint**
　　✓7ᵗʰ **S43.492　Other sprain of left shoulder joint**
　　✓7ᵗʰ **S43.499　Other sprain of unspecified shoulder joint**

✓5ᵗʰ **S43.5　Sprain of acromioclavicular joint**
　　Sprain of acromioclavicular ligament
　　✓x7ᵗʰ **S43.5Ø　Sprain of unspecified acromioclavicular joint**
　　✓x7ᵗʰ **S43.51　Sprain of right acromioclavicular joint**
　　✓x7ᵗʰ **S43.52　Sprain of left acromioclavicular joint**

✓5ᵗʰ **S43.6　Sprain of sternoclavicular joint**
　　✓x7ᵗʰ **S43.6Ø　Sprain of unspecified sternoclavicular joint**
　　✓x7ᵗʰ **S43.61　Sprain of right sternoclavicular joint**
　　✓x7ᵗʰ **S43.62　Sprain of left sternoclavicular joint**

✓5ᵗʰ **S43.8　Sprain of other specified parts of shoulder girdle**
　　✓x7ᵗʰ **S43.8Ø　Sprain of other specified parts of unspecified shoulder girdle**
　　✓x7ᵗʰ **S43.81　Sprain of other specified parts of right shoulder girdle**
　　✓x7ᵗʰ **S43.82　Sprain of other specified parts of left shoulder girdle**

✓5ᵗʰ **S43.9　Sprain of unspecified parts of shoulder girdle**
　　✓x7ᵗʰ **S43.9Ø　Sprain of unspecified parts of unspecified shoulder girdle**
　　　　Sprain of shoulder girdle NOS
　　✓x7ᵗʰ **S43.91　Sprain of unspecified parts of right shoulder girdle**
　　✓x7ᵗʰ **S43.92　Sprain of unspecified parts of left shoulder girdle**

✓4ᵗʰ **S44　Injury of nerves at shoulder and upper arm level**
> Code also any associated open wound (S41.-)
> EXCLUDES 2　injury of brachial plexus (S14.3-)

> The appropriate 7th character is to be added to each code from
> category S44.
> A　initial encounter
> D　subsequent encounter
> S　sequela

✓5ᵗʰ **S44.Ø　Injury of ulnar nerve at upper arm level**
> EXCLUDES 1　ulnar nerve NOS (S54.Ø)

　　✓x7ᵗʰ **S44.ØØ　Injury of ulnar nerve at upper arm level, unspecified arm**
　　✓x7ᵗʰ **S44.Ø1　Injury of ulnar nerve at upper arm level, right arm**
　　✓x7ᵗʰ **S44.Ø2　Injury of ulnar nerve at upper arm level, left arm**

✓5ᵗʰ **S44.1　Injury of median nerve at upper arm level**
> EXCLUDES 1　median nerve NOS (S54.1)

　　✓x7ᵗʰ **S44.1Ø　Injury of median nerve at upper arm level, unspecified arm**
　　✓x7ᵗʰ **S44.11　Injury of median nerve at upper arm level, right arm**
　　✓x7ᵗʰ **S44.12　Injury of median nerve at upper arm level, left arm**

✓5ᵗʰ **S44.2　Injury of radial nerve at upper arm level**
> EXCLUDES 1　radial nerve NOS (S54.2)

　　✓x7ᵗʰ **S44.2Ø　Injury of radial nerve at upper arm level, unspecified arm**
　　✓x7ᵗʰ **S44.21　Injury of radial nerve at upper arm level, right arm**
　　✓x7ᵗʰ **S44.22　Injury of radial nerve at upper arm level, left arm**

✓5ᵗʰ **S44.3　Injury of axillary nerve**
　　✓x7ᵗʰ **S44.3Ø　Injury of axillary nerve, unspecified arm**
　　✓x7ᵗʰ **S44.31　Injury of axillary nerve, right arm**
　　✓x7ᵗʰ **S44.32　Injury of axillary nerve, left arm**

✓5ᵗʰ **S44.4　Injury of musculocutaneous nerve**
　　✓x7ᵗʰ **S44.4Ø　Injury of musculocutaneous nerve, unspecified arm**
　　✓x7ᵗʰ **S44.41　Injury of musculocutaneous nerve, right arm**
　　✓x7ᵗʰ **S44.42　Injury of musculocutaneous nerve, left arm**

✓5ᵗʰ **S44.5　Injury of cutaneous sensory nerve at shoulder and upper arm level**
　　✓x7ᵗʰ **S44.5Ø　Injury of cutaneous sensory nerve at shoulder and upper arm level, unspecified arm**
　　✓x7ᵗʰ **S44.51　Injury of cutaneous sensory nerve at shoulder and upper arm level, right arm**
　　✓x7ᵗʰ **S44.52　Injury of cutaneous sensory nerve at shoulder and upper arm level, left arm**

✓5ᵗʰ **S44.8　Injury of other nerves at shoulder and upper arm level**
　　✓6ᵗʰ **S44.8X　Injury of other nerves at shoulder and upper arm level**
　　　　✓7ᵗʰ **S44.8X1　Injury of other nerves at shoulder and upper arm level, right arm**
　　　　✓7ᵗʰ **S44.8X2　Injury of other nerves at shoulder and upper arm level, left arm**
　　　　✓7ᵗʰ **S44.8X9　Injury of other nerves at shoulder and upper arm level, unspecified arm**

✓5ᵗʰ **S44.9　Injury of unspecified nerve at shoulder and upper arm level**
　　✓x7ᵗʰ **S44.9Ø　Injury of unspecified nerve at shoulder and upper arm level, unspecified arm**
　　✓x7ᵗʰ **S44.91　Injury of unspecified nerve at shoulder and upper arm level, right arm**
　　✓x7ᵗʰ **S44.92　Injury of unspecified nerve at shoulder and upper arm level, left arm**

✓4ᵗʰ **S45　Injury of blood vessels at shoulder and upper arm level**
> Code also any associated open wound (S41.-)
> EXCLUDES 2　injury of subclavian artery (S25.1)
> injury of subclavian vein (S25.3)

> The appropriate 7th character is to be added to each code from
> category S45.
> A　initial encounter
> D　subsequent encounter
> S　sequela

✓5ᵗʰ **S45.Ø　Injury of axillary artery**

> **CC Excl: For MCC codes in subcategory S45.Ø:**
> **Right side:** PDX collection 1254
> **Left side:** PDX collection 1255
> **Unspecified side:** PDX collection 1256

　　✓6ᵗʰ **S45.ØØ　Unspecified injury of axillary artery**
　　　　✓7ᵗʰ **S45.ØØ1　Unspecified injury of axillary artery, right side**　MCC
　　　　✓7ᵗʰ **S45.ØØ2　Unspecified injury of axillary artery, left side**　MCC
　　　　✓7ᵗʰ **S45.ØØ9　Unspecified injury of axillary artery, unspecified side**　MCC

　　✓6ᵗʰ **S45.Ø1　Laceration of axillary artery**
　　　　✓7ᵗʰ **S45.Ø11　Laceration of axillary artery, right side**　MCC
　　　　✓7ᵗʰ **S45.Ø12　Laceration of axillary artery, left side**　MCC
　　　　✓7ᵗʰ **S45.Ø19　Laceration of axillary artery, unspecified side**　MCC

　　✓6ᵗʰ **S45.Ø9　Other specified injury of axillary artery**
　　　　✓7ᵗʰ **S45.Ø91　Other specified injury of axillary artery, right side**　MCC
　　　　✓7ᵗʰ **S45.Ø92　Other specified injury of axillary artery, left side**　MCC
　　　　✓7ᵗʰ **S45.Ø99　Other specified injury of axillary artery, unspecified side**　MCC

✓5ᵗʰ **S45.1**   **Injury of** brachial artery

> **CC Excl: For CC codes in subcategory S45.1:**
> **Right side:** PDX collection 1257
> **Left side:** PDX collection 1258
> **Unspecified side:** PDX collection 1259

   ✓6ᵗʰ **S45.10**   **Unspecified injury of brachial artery**

     ✓7ᵗʰ **S45.101**   Unspecified injury of brachial artery, right side   `CC`

     ✓7ᵗʰ **S45.102**   Unspecified injury of brachial artery, left side   `CC`

     ✓7ᵗʰ **S45.109**   Unspecified injury of brachial artery, unspecified side   `CC`

   ✓6ᵗʰ **S45.11**   **Laceration of brachial artery**

     ✓7ᵗʰ **S45.111**   Laceration of brachial artery, right side   `CC`

     ✓7ᵗʰ **S45.112**   Laceration of brachial artery, left side   `CC`

     ✓7ᵗʰ **S45.119**   Laceration of brachial artery, unspecified side   `CC`

   ✓6ᵗʰ **S45.19**   **Other specified injury of brachial artery**

     ✓7ᵗʰ **S45.191**   Other specified injury of brachial artery, right side   `CC`

     ✓7ᵗʰ **S45.192**   Other specified injury of brachial artery, left side   `CC`

     ✓7ᵗʰ **S45.199**   Other specified injury of brachial artery, unspecified side   `CC`

✓5ᵗʰ **S45.2**   **Injury of** axillary or brachial vein

> **CC Excl: For CC codes in subcategory S45.2:**
> **Right side:** PDX collection 1257
> **Left side:** PDX collection 1258
> **Unspecified side:** PDX collection 1259

   ✓6ᵗʰ **S45.20**   **Unspecified injury of axillary or brachial vein**

     ✓7ᵗʰ **S45.201**   Unspecified injury of axillary or brachial vein, right side   `CC`

     ✓7ᵗʰ **S45.202**   Unspecified injury of axillary or brachial vein, left side   `CC`

     ✓7ᵗʰ **S45.209**   Unspecified injury of axillary or brachial vein, unspecified side   `CC`

   ✓6ᵗʰ **S45.21**   **Laceration of axillary or brachial vein**

     ✓7ᵗʰ **S45.211**   Laceration of axillary or brachial vein, right side   `CC`

     ✓7ᵗʰ **S45.212**   Laceration of axillary or brachial vein, left side   `CC`

     ✓7ᵗʰ **S45.219**   Laceration of axillary or brachial vein, unspecified side   `CC`

   ✓6ᵗʰ **S45.29**   **Other specified injury of axillary or brachial vein**

     ✓7ᵗʰ **S45.291**   Other specified injury of axillary or brachial vein, right side   `CC`

     ✓7ᵗʰ **S45.292**   Other specified injury of axillary or brachial vein, left side   `CC`

     ✓7ᵗʰ **S45.299**   Other specified injury of axillary or brachial vein, unspecified side   `CC`

✓5ᵗʰ **S45.3**   **Injury of** superficial vein at shoulder and upper arm level

> **CC Excl: For CC codes in subcategory S45.3:**
> **Right side:** PDX collection 1260
> **Left side:** PDX collection 1261
> **Unspecified side:** PDX collection 1262

   ✓6ᵗʰ **S45.30**   **Unspecified injury of superficial vein at shoulder and upper arm level**

     ✓7ᵗʰ **S45.301**   Unspecified injury of superficial vein at shoulder and upper arm level, right arm   `CC`

     ✓7ᵗʰ **S45.302**   Unspecified injury of superficial vein at shoulder and upper arm level, left arm   `CC`

     ✓7ᵗʰ **S45.309**   Unspecified injury of superficial vein at shoulder and upper arm level, unspecified arm   `CC`

   ✓6ᵗʰ **S45.31**   **Laceration of superficial vein at shoulder and upper arm level**

     ✓7ᵗʰ **S45.311**   Laceration of superficial vein at shoulder and upper arm level, right arm   `CC`

     ✓7ᵗʰ **S45.312**   Laceration of superficial vein at shoulder and upper arm level, left arm   `CC`

     ✓7ᵗʰ **S45.319**   Laceration of superficial vein at shoulder and upper arm level, unspecified arm   `CC`

   ✓6ᵗʰ **S45.39**   **Other specified injury of superficial vein at shoulder and upper arm level**

     ✓7ᵗʰ **S45.391**   Other specified injury of superficial vein at shoulder and upper arm level, right arm   `CC`

     ✓7ᵗʰ **S45.392**   Other specified injury of superficial vein at shoulder and upper arm level, left arm   `CC`

     ✓7ᵗʰ **S45.399**   Other specified injury of superficial vein at shoulder and upper arm level, unspecified arm   `CC`

✓5ᵗʰ **S45.8**   **Injury of** other specified blood vessels at shoulder and upper arm level

> **CC Excl: For CC codes in subcategory S45.8:**
> **Right side:** PDX collection 1260
> **Left side:** PDX collection 1261
> **Unspecified side:** PDX collection 1262

   ✓6ᵗʰ **S45.80**   **Unspecified injury of other specified blood vessels at shoulder and upper arm level**

     ✓7ᵗʰ **S45.801**   Unspecified injury of other specified blood vessels at shoulder and upper arm level, right arm   `CC`

     ✓7ᵗʰ **S45.802**   Unspecified injury of other specified blood vessels at shoulder and upper arm level, left arm   `CC`

     ✓7ᵗʰ **S45.809**   Unspecified injury of other specified blood vessels at shoulder and upper arm level, unspecified arm   `CC`

   ✓6ᵗʰ **S45.81**   **Laceration of other specified blood vessels at shoulder and upper arm level**

     ✓7ᵗʰ **S45.811**   Laceration of other specified blood vessels at shoulder and upper arm level, right arm   `CC`

     ✓7ᵗʰ **S45.812**   Laceration of other specified blood vessels at shoulder and upper arm level, left arm   `CC`

     ✓7ᵗʰ **S45.819**   Laceration of other specified blood vessels at shoulder and upper arm level, unspecified arm   `CC`

   ✓6ᵗʰ **S45.89**   **Other specified injury of other specified blood vessels at shoulder and upper arm level**

     ✓7ᵗʰ **S45.891**   Other specified injury of other specified blood vessels at shoulder and upper arm level, right arm   `CC`

     ✓7ᵗʰ **S45.892**   Other specified injury of other specified blood vessels at shoulder and upper arm level, left arm   `CC`

     ✓7ᵗʰ **S45.899**   Other specified injury of other specified blood vessels at shoulder and upper arm level, unspecified arm   `CC`

✓5ᵗʰ **S45.9**   **Injury of** unspecified blood vessel at shoulder and upper arm level

> **CC Excl: For CC codes in subcategory S45.9:**
> **Right side:** PDX collection 1260
> **Left side:** PDX collection 1261
> **Unspecified side:** PDX collection 1262

   ✓6ᵗʰ **S45.90**   **Unspecified injury of unspecified blood vessel at shoulder and upper arm level**

     ✓7ᵗʰ **S45.901**   Unspecified injury of unspecified blood vessel at shoulder and upper arm level, right arm   `CC`

     ✓7ᵗʰ **S45.902**   Unspecified injury of unspecified blood vessel at shoulder and upper arm level, left arm   `CC`

     ✓7ᵗʰ **S45.909**   Unspecified injury of unspecified blood vessel at shoulder and upper arm level, unspecified arm   `CC`

   ✓6ᵗʰ **S45.91**   **Laceration of unspecified blood vessel at shoulder and upper arm level**

     ✓7ᵗʰ **S45.911**   Laceration of unspecified blood vessel at shoulder and upper arm level, right arm   `CC`

---

✓ Additional Character Req   ✓x7ᵗʰ Placeholder Alert   Unacceptable PDx   Manifestation   **H1**-**H14** HAC   **HCC** CMS-HCC Condition   *EXCLUDES1* Not Coded Here   *EXCLUDES2* Not Included Here

√7th **S45.912** **Laceration of unspecified blood vessel at shoulder and upper arm level, left arm** `CC`

√7th **S45.919** **Laceration of unspecified blood vessel at shoulder and upper arm level, unspecified arm** `CC`

√6th **S45.99** **Other specified injury of unspecified blood vessel at shoulder and upper arm level**

√7th **S45.991** **Other specified injury of unspecified blood vessel at shoulder and upper arm level, right arm** `CC`

√7th **S45.992** **Other specified injury of unspecified blood vessel at shoulder and upper arm level, left arm** `CC`

√7th **S45.999** **Other specified injury of unspecified blood vessel at shoulder and upper arm level, unspecified arm** `CC`

√4th **S46** **Injury of muscle, fascia and tendon at shoulder and upper arm level**

Code also any associated open wound (S41.-)

EXCLUDES 2 *injury of muscle, fascia and tendon at elbow (S56.-)*
*sprain of joints and ligaments of shoulder girdle (S43.9)*

**TIP:** Refer to the Muscle/Tendon table at the beginning of this chapter.

The appropriate 7th character is to be added to each code from category S46.
A    initial encounter
D    subsequent encounter
S    sequela

**CC Excl: For CC codes in category S46:**
**Right side:** PDX collection 1263
**Left side:** PDX collection 1264
**Unspecified side:** PDX collection 1265

√5th **S46.0** **Injury of muscle(s) and tendon(s) of the rotator cuff of shoulder**

√6th **S46.00** **Unspecified injury of muscle(s) and tendon(s) of the rotator cuff of shoulder**

√7th **S46.001** **Unspecified injury of muscle(s) and tendon(s) of the rotator cuff of right shoulder**

√7th **S46.002** **Unspecified injury of muscle(s) and tendon(s) of the rotator cuff of left shoulder**

√7th **S46.009** **Unspecified injury of muscle(s) and tendon(s) of the rotator cuff of unspecified shoulder**

√6th **S46.01** **Strain of muscle(s) and tendon(s) of the rotator cuff of shoulder**

√7th **S46.011** **Strain of muscle(s) and tendon(s) of the rotator cuff of right shoulder**

√7th **S46.012** **Strain of muscle(s) and tendon(s) of the rotator cuff of left shoulder**

√7th **S46.019** **Strain of muscle(s) and tendon(s) of the rotator cuff of unspecified shoulder**

√6th **S46.02** **Laceration of muscle(s) and tendon(s) of the rotator cuff of shoulder**

√7th **S46.021** **Laceration of muscle(s) and tendon(s) of the rotator cuff of right shoulder** `CC`

√7th **S46.022** **Laceration of muscle(s) and tendon(s) of the rotator cuff of left shoulder** `CC`

√7th **S46.029** **Laceration of muscle(s) and tendon(s) of the rotator cuff of unspecified shoulder** `CC`

√6th **S46.09** **Other injury of muscle(s) and tendon(s) of the rotator cuff of shoulder**

√7th **S46.091** **Other injury of muscle(s) and tendon(s) of the rotator cuff of right shoulder**

√7th **S46.092** **Other injury of muscle(s) and tendon(s) of the rotator cuff of left shoulder**

√7th **S46.099** **Other injury of muscle(s) and tendon(s) of the rotator cuff of unspecified shoulder**

√5th **S46.1** **Injury of muscle, fascia and tendon of long head of biceps**

√6th **S46.10** **Unspecified injury of muscle, fascia and tendon of long head of biceps**

√7th **S46.101** **Unspecified injury of muscle, fascia and tendon of long head of biceps, right arm**

√7th **S46.102** **Unspecified injury of muscle, fascia and tendon of long head of biceps, left arm**

√7th **S46.109** **Unspecified injury of muscle, fascia and tendon of long head of biceps, unspecified arm**

√6th **S46.11** **Strain of muscle, fascia and tendon of long head of biceps**

√7th **S46.111** **Strain of muscle, fascia and tendon of long head of biceps, right arm**

√7th **S46.112** **Strain of muscle, fascia and tendon of long head of biceps, left arm**

√7th **S46.119** **Strain of muscle, fascia and tendon of long head of biceps, unspecified arm**

√6th **S46.12** **Laceration of muscle, fascia and tendon of long head of biceps**

√7th **S46.121** **Laceration of muscle, fascia and tendon of long head of biceps, right arm** `CC`

√7th **S46.122** **Laceration of muscle, fascia and tendon of long head of biceps, left arm** `CC`

√7th **S46.129** **Laceration of muscle, fascia and tendon of long head of biceps, unspecified arm** `CC`

√6th **S46.19** **Other injury of muscle, fascia and tendon of long head of biceps**

√7th **S46.191** **Other injury of muscle, fascia and tendon of long head of biceps, right arm**

√7th **S46.192** **Other injury of muscle, fascia and tendon of long head of biceps, left arm**

√7th **S46.199** **Other injury of muscle, fascia and tendon of long head of biceps, unspecified arm**

√5th **S46.2** **Injury of muscle, fascia and tendon of other parts of biceps**

√6th **S46.20** **Unspecified injury of muscle, fascia and tendon of other parts of biceps**

√7th **S46.201** **Unspecified injury of muscle, fascia and tendon of other parts of biceps, right arm**

√7th **S46.202** **Unspecified injury of muscle, fascia and tendon of other parts of biceps, left arm**

√7th **S46.209** **Unspecified injury of muscle, fascia and tendon of other parts of biceps, unspecified arm**

√6th **S46.21** **Strain of muscle, fascia and tendon of other parts of biceps**

√7th **S46.211** **Strain of muscle, fascia and tendon of other parts of biceps, right arm**

√7th **S46.212** **Strain of muscle, fascia and tendon of other parts of biceps, left arm**

√7th **S46.219** **Strain of muscle, fascia and tendon of other parts of biceps, unspecified arm**

√6th **S46.22** **Laceration of muscle, fascia and tendon of other parts of biceps**

√7th **S46.221** **Laceration of muscle, fascia and tendon of other parts of biceps, right arm** `CC`

√7th **S46.222** **Laceration of muscle, fascia and tendon of other parts of biceps, left arm** `CC`

√7th **S46.229** **Laceration of muscle, fascia and tendon of other parts of biceps, unspecified arm** `CC`

√6th **S46.29** **Other injury of muscle, fascia and tendon of other parts of biceps**

√7th **S46.291** **Other injury of muscle, fascia and tendon of other parts of biceps, right arm**

√7th **S46.292** **Other injury of muscle, fascia and tendon of other parts of biceps, left arm**

√7th **S46.299** **Other injury of muscle, fascia and tendon of other parts of biceps, unspecified arm**

√5th **S46.3** **Injury of muscle, fascia and tendon of triceps**

√6th **S46.30** **Unspecified injury of muscle, fascia and tendon of triceps**

√7th **S46.301** **Unspecified injury of muscle, fascia and tendon of triceps, right arm**

√7th **S46.302** **Unspecified injury of muscle, fascia and tendon of triceps, left arm**

√7th **S46.309** **Unspecified injury of muscle, fascia and tendon of triceps, unspecified arm**

N Newborn: 0   P Pediatric: 0-17   M Maternity: 12-55   A Adult: 15-124   MCC Major CC Condition   PDxMCC PDx acts as own MCC   CC CC Condition   PDxCC PDx acts as own CC

**994**      ICD-10-CM 2018

✓6ᵗʰ **S46.31** Strain of muscle, fascia and tendon of triceps

✓7ᵗʰ **S46.311** Strain of muscle, fascia and tendon of triceps, right arm

✓7ᵗʰ **S46.312** Strain of muscle, fascia and tendon of triceps, left arm

✓7ᵗʰ **S46.319** Strain of muscle, fascia and tendon of triceps, unspecified arm

✓6ᵗʰ **S46.32** Laceration of muscle, fascia and tendon of triceps

✓7ᵗʰ **S46.321** Laceration of muscle, fascia and tendon of triceps, right arm ▫CC

✓7ᵗʰ **S46.322** Laceration of muscle, fascia and tendon of triceps, left arm ▫CC

✓7ᵗʰ **S46.329** Laceration of muscle, fascia and tendon of triceps, unspecified arm ▫CC

✓6ᵗʰ **S46.39** Other injury of muscle, fascia and tendon of triceps

✓7ᵗʰ **S46.391** Other injury of muscle, fascia and tendon of triceps, right arm

✓7ᵗʰ **S46.392** Other injury of muscle, fascia and tendon of triceps, left arm

✓7ᵗʰ **S46.399** Other injury of muscle, fascia and tendon of triceps, unspecified arm

✓5ᵗʰ **S46.8** Injury of other muscles, fascia and tendons at shoulder and upper arm level

✓6ᵗʰ **S46.80** Unspecified injury of other muscles, fascia and tendons at shoulder and upper arm level

✓7ᵗʰ **S46.801** Unspecified injury of other muscles, fascia and tendons at shoulder and upper arm level, right arm

✓7ᵗʰ **S46.802** Unspecified injury of other muscles, fascia and tendons at shoulder and upper arm level, left arm

✓7ᵗʰ **S46.809** Unspecified injury of other muscles, fascia and tendons at shoulder and upper arm level, unspecified arm

✓6ᵗʰ **S46.81** Strain of other muscles, fascia and tendons at shoulder and upper arm level

✓7ᵗʰ **S46.811** Strain of other muscles, fascia and tendons at shoulder and upper arm level, right arm

✓7ᵗʰ **S46.812** Strain of other muscles, fascia and tendons at shoulder and upper arm level, left arm

✓7ᵗʰ **S46.819** Strain of other muscles, fascia and tendons at shoulder and upper arm level, unspecified arm

✓6ᵗʰ **S46.82** Laceration of other muscles, fascia and tendons at shoulder and upper arm level

✓7ᵗʰ **S46.821** Laceration of other muscles, fascia and tendons at shoulder and upper arm level, right arm ▫CC

✓7ᵗʰ **S46.822** Laceration of other muscles, fascia and tendons at shoulder and upper arm level, left arm ▫CC

✓7ᵗʰ **S46.829** Laceration of other muscles, fascia and tendons at shoulder and upper arm level, unspecified arm ▫CC

✓6ᵗʰ **S46.89** Other injury of other muscles, fascia and tendons at shoulder and upper arm level

✓7ᵗʰ **S46.891** Other injury of other muscles, fascia and tendons at shoulder and upper arm level, right arm

✓7ᵗʰ **S46.892** Other injury of other muscles, fascia and tendons at shoulder and upper arm level, left arm

✓7ᵗʰ **S46.899** Other injury of other muscles, fascia and tendons at shoulder and upper arm level, unspecified arm

✓5ᵗʰ **S46.9** Injury of unspecified muscle, fascia and tendon at shoulder and upper arm level

✓6ᵗʰ **S46.90** Unspecified injury of unspecified muscle, fascia and tendon at shoulder and upper arm level

✓7ᵗʰ **S46.901** Unspecified injury of unspecified muscle, fascia and tendon at shoulder and upper arm level, right arm

✓7ᵗʰ **S46.902** Unspecified injury of unspecified muscle, fascia and tendon at shoulder and upper arm level, left arm

✓7ᵗʰ **S46.909** Unspecified injury of unspecified muscle, fascia and tendon at shoulder and upper arm level, unspecified arm

✓6ᵗʰ **S46.91** Strain of unspecified muscle, fascia and tendon at shoulder and upper arm level

✓7ᵗʰ **S46.911** Strain of unspecified muscle, fascia and tendon at shoulder and upper arm level, right arm

✓7ᵗʰ **S46.912** Strain of unspecified muscle, fascia and tendon at shoulder and upper arm level, left arm

✓7ᵗʰ **S46.919** Strain of unspecified muscle, fascia and tendon at shoulder and upper arm level, unspecified arm

✓6ᵗʰ **S46.92** Laceration of unspecified muscle, fascia and tendon at shoulder and upper arm level

✓7ᵗʰ **S46.921** Laceration of unspecified muscle, fascia and tendon at shoulder and upper arm level, right arm ▫CC

✓7ᵗʰ **S46.922** Laceration of unspecified muscle, fascia and tendon at shoulder and upper arm level, left arm ▫CC

✓7ᵗʰ **S46.929** Laceration of unspecified muscle, fascia and tendon at shoulder and upper arm level, unspecified arm ▫CC

✓6ᵗʰ **S46.99** Other injury of unspecified muscle, fascia and tendon at shoulder and upper arm level

✓7ᵗʰ **S46.991** Other injury of unspecified muscle, fascia and tendon at shoulder and upper arm level, right arm

✓7ᵗʰ **S46.992** Other injury of unspecified muscle, fascia and tendon at shoulder and upper arm level, left arm

✓7ᵗʰ **S46.999** Other injury of unspecified muscle, fascia and tendon at shoulder and upper arm level, unspecified arm

✓4ᵗʰ **S47** **Crushing injury of shoulder and upper arm**

Use additional code for all associated injuries

*EXCLUDES 2*   crushing injury of elbow (S57.0-)

> The appropriate 7th character is to be added to each code from category S47.
> A    initial encounter
> D    subsequent encounter
> S    sequela

✓x7ᵗʰ **S47.1** Crushing injury of right shoulder and upper arm

✓x7ᵗʰ **S47.2** Crushing injury of left shoulder and upper arm

✓x7ᵗʰ **S47.9** Crushing injury of shoulder and upper arm, unspecified arm

✓4ᵗʰ **S48** **Traumatic amputation of shoulder and upper arm**

An amputation not identified as partial or complete should be coded to complete.

*EXCLUDES 1*   traumatic amputation at elbow level (S58.0)

> The appropriate 7th character is to be added to each code from category S48.
> A    initial encounter
> D    subsequent encounter
> S    sequela

**CC Excl: For CC codes in category S48:**
**Right side:** PDX collection 1266
**Left side:** PDX collection 1267
**Unspecified side:** PDX collection 1268

✓5ᵗʰ **S48.0** Traumatic amputation at shoulder joint

✓6ᵗʰ **S48.01** Complete traumatic amputation at shoulder joint

11 ✓7ᵗʰ **S48.011** Complete traumatic amputation at right shoulder joint ▫CC ▫HCC

11 ✓7ᵗʰ **S48.012** Complete traumatic amputation at left shoulder joint ▫CC ▫HCC

11 ✓7ᵗʰ **S48.019** Complete traumatic amputation at unspecified shoulder joint ▫CC ▫HCC

---

11 HCC with 7th character indicating initial encounter (A or B - specific to category) OR sequela.

✓ Additional Character Req   ✓x7ᵗʰ Placeholder Alert   Unacceptable PDx   Manifestation   H1-H14 HAC   HCC CMS-HCC Condition   *EXCLUDES 1* Not Coded Here   *EXCLUDES 2* Not Included Here

√6ᵗʰ **S48.02** **Partial** traumatic amputation at shoulder joint

11 √7ᵗʰ **S48.021** **Partial traumatic amputation at right** shoulder joint   `CC` `HCC`

11 √7ᵗʰ **S48.022** **Partial traumatic amputation at left** shoulder joint   `CC` `HCC`

11 √7ᵗʰ **S48.029** **Partial traumatic amputation at unspecified** shoulder joint   `CC` `HCC`

√5ᵗʰ **S48.1** **Traumatic amputation at** level between shoulder and elbow

√6ᵗʰ **S48.11** **Complete** traumatic amputation at level between shoulder and elbow

11 √7ᵗʰ **S48.111** **Complete traumatic amputation at level between right** shoulder and elbow   `CC` `HCC`

11 √7ᵗʰ **S48.112** **Complete traumatic amputation at level between left** shoulder and elbow   `CC` `HCC`

11 √7ᵗʰ **S48.119** **Complete traumatic amputation at level between unspecified** shoulder and elbow   `CC` `HCC`

√6ᵗʰ **S48.12** **Partial** traumatic amputation at level between shoulder and elbow

11 √7ᵗʰ **S48.121** **Partial traumatic amputation at level between right** shoulder and elbow   `CC` `HCC`

11 √7ᵗʰ **S48.122** **Partial traumatic amputation at level between left** shoulder and elbow   `CC` `HCC`

11 √7ᵗʰ **S48.129** **Partial traumatic amputation at level between unspecified** shoulder and elbow   `CC` `HCC`

√5ᵗʰ **S48.9** **Traumatic amputation of shoulder and upper arm,** level unspecified

√6ᵗʰ **S48.91** **Complete** traumatic amputation of shoulder and upper arm, level unspecified

11 √7ᵗʰ **S48.911** **Complete traumatic amputation of right** shoulder and upper arm, level unspecified   `CC` `HCC`

11 √7ᵗʰ **S48.912** **Complete traumatic amputation of left** shoulder and upper arm, level unspecified   `CC` `HCC`

11 √7ᵗʰ **S48.919** **Complete traumatic amputation of unspecified** shoulder and upper arm, level unspecified   `CC` `HCC`

√6ᵗʰ **S48.92** **Partial** traumatic amputation of shoulder and upper arm, level unspecified

11 √7ᵗʰ **S48.921** **Partial traumatic amputation of right** shoulder and upper arm, level unspecified   `CC` `HCC`

11 √7ᵗʰ **S48.922** **Partial traumatic amputation of left** shoulder and upper arm, level unspecified   `CC` `HCC`

11 √7ᵗʰ **S48.929** **Partial traumatic amputation of unspecified** shoulder and upper arm, level unspecified   `CC` `HCC`

√4ᵗʰ **S49** **Other and unspecified injuries of shoulder and upper arm**

> The appropriate 7th character is to be added to each code from subcategories S49.0 and S49.1.
> A   initial encounter for closed fracture
> D   subsequent encounter for fracture with routine healing
> G   subsequent encounter for fracture with delayed healing
> K   subsequent encounter for fracture with nonunion
> P   subsequent encounter for fracture with malunion
> S   sequela
>
> **CC Excl: For CC codes in category S49:**
> **Right side:** See code S49.001
> **Left side:** See code S49.002
> **Unspecified side:** See code S49.009

√5ᵗʰ **S49.0** **Physeal fracture of** upper end of humerus

√6ᵗʰ **S49.00** **Unspecified** physeal fracture of upper end of humerus

7 √7ᵗʰ **S49.001** **Unspecified physeal fracture of upper end of humerus, right arm**   `CC` `H5`
CC Excl: CC with 7th character A:
PDX collection 1245
**CC with 7th character K or P:**
PDX collection 897

√7ᵗʰ **S49.002** **Unspecified physeal fracture of upper end of humerus, left arm**   `CC` `H5`
**CC Excl: CC with 7th character A:**
PDX collection 1247
**CC with 7th character K or P:**
PDX collection 897

7 √7ᵗʰ **S49.009** **Unspecified physeal fracture of upper end of humerus, unspecified arm**   `CC` `H5`
**CC Excl: CC with 7th character A:**
PDX collection 1248
**CC with 7th character K or P:**
PDX collection 897

√6ᵗʰ **S49.01** **Salter-Harris Type I physeal fracture of upper end of humerus**

7 √7ᵗʰ **S49.011** **Salter-Harris Type I physeal fracture of upper end of humerus, right arm**   `CC` `H5`

7 √7ᵗʰ **S49.012** **Salter-Harris Type I physeal fracture of upper end of humerus, left arm**   `CC` `H5`

7 √7ᵗʰ **S49.019** **Salter-Harris Type I physeal fracture of upper end of humerus, unspecified arm**   `CC` `H5`

√6ᵗʰ **S49.02** **Salter-Harris Type II physeal fracture of upper end of humerus**

7 √7ᵗʰ **S49.021** **Salter-Harris Type II physeal fracture of upper end of humerus, right arm**   `CC` `H5`

7 √7ᵗʰ **S49.022** **Salter-Harris Type II physeal fracture of upper end of humerus, left arm**   `CC` `H5`

7 √7ᵗʰ **S49.029** **Salter-Harris Type II physeal fracture of upper end of humerus, unspecified arm**   `CC` `H5`

√6ᵗʰ **S49.03** **Salter-Harris Type III physeal fracture of upper end of humerus**

√7ᵗʰ **S49.031** **Salter-Harris Type III physeal fracture of upper end of humerus, right arm**   `CC` `H5`

√7ᵗʰ **S49.032** **Salter-Harris Type III physeal fracture of upper end of humerus, left arm**   `CC` `H5`

√7ᵗʰ **S49.039** **Salter-Harris Type III physeal fracture of upper end of humerus, unspecified arm**   `CC` `H5`

√6ᵗʰ **S49.04** **Salter-Harris Type IV physeal fracture of upper end of humerus**

7 √7ᵗʰ **S49.041** **Salter-Harris Type IV physeal fracture of upper end of humerus, right arm**   `CC` `H5`

7 √7ᵗʰ **S49.042** **Salter-Harris Type IV physeal fracture of upper end of humerus, left arm**   `CC` `H5`

7 √7ᵗʰ **S49.049** **Salter-Harris Type IV physeal fracture of upper end of humerus, unspecified arm**   `CC` `H5`

√6ᵗʰ **S49.09** **Other physeal fracture of upper end of humerus**

7 √7ᵗʰ **S49.091** **Other physeal fracture of upper end of humerus, right arm**   `CC` `H5`

7 √7ᵗʰ **S49.092** **Other physeal fracture of upper end of humerus, left arm**   `CC` `H5`

7 √7ᵗʰ **S49.099** **Other physeal fracture of upper end of humerus, unspecified arm**   `CC` `H5`

√5ᵗʰ **S49.1** **Physeal fracture of** lower end of humerus

√6ᵗʰ **S49.10** **Unspecified** physeal fracture of lower end of humerus

7 √7ᵗʰ **S49.101** **Unspecified physeal fracture of lower end of humerus, right arm**   `CC` `H5`

7 √7ᵗʰ **S49.102** **Unspecified physeal fracture of lower end of humerus, left arm**   `CC` `H5`

7 √7ᵗʰ **S49.109** **Unspecified physeal fracture of lower end of humerus, unspecified arm**   `CC` `H5`

---

7   CC when reported as an initial encounter (7th character A, B, or C – specific to category) OR a subsequent encounter for nonunion or malunion (7th character K, M, N, P, Q, or R – specific to category).

11   HCC with 7th character indicating initial encounter (A or B - specific to category) OR sequela.

---

N Newborn: 0   P Pediatric: 0-17   M Maternity: 12-55   A Adult: 15-124   MCC Major CC Condition   PDxMCC PDx acts as own MCC   CC CC Condition   PDxCC PDx acts as own CC

996     ICD-10-CM 2018

☑6ᵗʰ **S49.11** **Salter-Harris Type I physeal fracture of lower end of humerus**

7 ☑7ᵗʰ **S49.111** **Salter-Harris Type I physeal fracture of lower end of humerus, right arm** `CC` `H5`

7 ☑7ᵗʰ **S49.112** **Salter-Harris Type I physeal fracture of lower end of humerus, left arm** `CC` `H5`

7 ☑7ᵗʰ **S49.119** **Salter-Harris Type I physeal fracture of lower end of humerus, unspecified arm** `CC` `H5`

☑6ᵗʰ **S49.12** **Salter-Harris Type II physeal fracture of lower end of humerus**

7 ☑7ᵗʰ **S49.121** **Salter-Harris Type II physeal fracture of lower end of humerus, right arm** `CC` `H5`

7 ☑7ᵗʰ **S49.122** **Salter-Harris Type II physeal fracture of lower end of humerus, left arm** `CC` `H5`

7 ☑7ᵗʰ **S49.129** **Salter-Harris Type II physeal fracture of lower end of humerus, unspecified arm** `CC` `H5`

☑6ᵗʰ **S49.13** **Salter-Harris Type III physeal fracture of lower end of humerus**

7 ☑7ᵗʰ **S49.131** **Salter-Harris Type III physeal fracture of lower end of humerus, right arm** `CC` `H5`

7 ☑7ᵗʰ **S49.132** **Salter-Harris Type III physeal fracture of lower end of humerus, left arm** `CC` `H5`

7 ☑7ᵗʰ **S49.139** **Salter-Harris Type III physeal fracture of lower end of humerus, unspecified arm** `CC` `H5`

☑6ᵗʰ **S49.14** **Salter-Harris Type IV physeal fracture of lower end of humerus**

7 ☑7ᵗʰ **S49.141** **Salter-Harris Type IV physeal fracture of lower end of humerus, right arm** `CC` `H5`

7 ☑7ᵗʰ **S49.142** **Salter-Harris Type IV physeal fracture of lower end of humerus, left arm** `CC` `H5`

7 ☑7ᵗʰ **S49.149** **Salter-Harris Type IV physeal fracture of lower end of humerus, unspecified arm** `CC` `H5`

☑6ᵗʰ **S49.19** **Other physeal fracture of lower end of humerus**

7 ☑7ᵗʰ **S49.191** **Other physeal fracture of lower end of humerus, right arm** `CC` `H5`

7 ☑7ᵗʰ **S49.192** **Other physeal fracture of lower end of humerus, left arm** `CC` `H5`

7 ☑7ᵗʰ **S49.199** **Other physeal fracture of lower end of humerus, unspecified arm** `CC` `H5`

☑5ᵗʰ **S49.8** **Other specified injuries of shoulder and upper arm**

The appropriate 7th character is to be added to each code in subcategory S49.8.
A   initial encounter
D   subsequent encounter
S   sequela

☑x7ᵗʰ **S49.80** **Other specified injuries of shoulder and upper arm, unspecified arm**

☑x7ᵗʰ **S49.81** **Other specified injuries of right shoulder and upper arm**

☑x7ᵗʰ **S49.82** **Other specified injuries of left shoulder and upper arm**

☑5ᵗʰ **S49.9** **Unspecified injury of shoulder and upper arm**

The appropriate 7th character is to be added to each code in subcategory S49.9.
A   initial encounter
D   subsequent encounter
S   sequela

☑x7ᵗʰ **S49.90** **Unspecified injury of shoulder and upper arm, unspecified arm**

☑x7ᵗʰ **S49.91** **Unspecified injury of right shoulder and upper arm**

☑x7ᵗʰ **S49.92** **Unspecified injury of left shoulder and upper arm**

## Injuries to the elbow and forearm (S50-S59)

EXCLUDES 2   burns and corrosions (T20-T32)
   frostbite (T33-T34)
   injuries of wrist and hand (S60-S69)
   insect bite or sting, venomous (T63.4)

☑4ᵗʰ **S50** **Superficial injury of elbow and forearm**

EXCLUDES 2   superficial injury of wrist and hand (S60.-)

The appropriate 7th character is to be added to each code from category S50.
A   initial encounter
D   subsequent encounter
S   sequela

☑5ᵗʰ **S50.0** **Contusion of elbow**

☑x7ᵗʰ **S50.00** **Contusion of unspecified elbow**

☑x7ᵗʰ **S50.01** **Contusion of right elbow**

☑x7ᵗʰ **S50.02** **Contusion of left elbow**

☑5ᵗʰ **S50.1** **Contusion of forearm**

☑x7ᵗʰ **S50.10** **Contusion of unspecified forearm**

☑x7ᵗʰ **S50.11** **Contusion of right forearm**

☑x7ᵗʰ **S50.12** **Contusion of left forearm**

☑5ᵗʰ **S50.3** **Other superficial injuries of elbow**

☑6ᵗʰ **S50.31** **Abrasion of elbow**

☑7ᵗʰ **S50.311** **Abrasion of right elbow**

☑7ᵗʰ **S50.312** **Abrasion of left elbow**

☑7ᵗʰ **S50.319** **Abrasion of unspecified elbow**

☑6ᵗʰ **S50.32** **Blister (nonthermal) of elbow**

☑7ᵗʰ **S50.321** **Blister (nonthermal) of right elbow**

☑7ᵗʰ **S50.322** **Blister (nonthermal) of left elbow**

☑7ᵗʰ **S50.329** **Blister (nonthermal) of unspecified elbow**

☑6ᵗʰ **S50.34** **External constriction of elbow**

☑7ᵗʰ **S50.341** **External constriction of right elbow**

☑7ᵗʰ **S50.342** **External constriction of left elbow**

☑7ᵗʰ **S50.349** **External constriction of unspecified elbow**

☑6ᵗʰ **S50.35** **Superficial foreign body of elbow**
Splinter in the elbow

☑7ᵗʰ **S50.351** **Superficial foreign body of right elbow**

☑7ᵗʰ **S50.352** **Superficial foreign body of left elbow**

☑7ᵗʰ **S50.359** **Superficial foreign body of unspecified elbow**

☑6ᵗʰ **S50.36** **Insect bite (nonvenomous) of elbow**

☑7ᵗʰ **S50.361** **Insect bite (nonvenomous) of right elbow**

☑7ᵗʰ **S50.362** **Insect bite (nonvenomous) of left elbow**

☑7ᵗʰ **S50.369** **Insect bite (nonvenomous) of unspecified elbow**

☑6ᵗʰ **S50.37** **Other superficial bite of elbow**
EXCLUDES 1   open bite of elbow (S51.04)

☑7ᵗʰ **S50.371** **Other superficial bite of right elbow**

☑7ᵗʰ **S50.372** **Other superficial bite of left elbow**

☑7ᵗʰ **S50.379** **Other superficial bite of unspecified elbow**

☑5ᵗʰ **S50.8** **Other superficial injuries of forearm**

☑6ᵗʰ **S50.81** **Abrasion of forearm**

☑7ᵗʰ **S50.811** **Abrasion of right forearm**

☑7ᵗʰ **S50.812** **Abrasion of left forearm**

☑7ᵗʰ **S50.819** **Abrasion of unspecified forearm**

☑6ᵗʰ **S50.82** **Blister (nonthermal) of forearm**

☑7ᵗʰ **S50.821** **Blister (nonthermal) of right forearm**

☑7ᵗʰ **S50.822** **Blister (nonthermal) of left forearm**

☑7ᵗʰ **S50.829** **Blister (nonthermal) of unspecified forearm**

☑6ᵗʰ **S50.84** **External constriction of forearm**

☑7ᵗʰ **S50.841** **External constriction of right forearm**

☑7ᵗʰ **S50.842** **External constriction of left forearm**

☑7ᵗʰ **S50.849** **External constriction of unspecified forearm**

☑6ᵗʰ **S50.85** **Superficial foreign body of forearm**
Splinter in the forearm

☑7ᵗʰ **S50.851** **Superficial foreign body of right forearm**

---

7   CC when reported as an initial encounter (7th character A, B, or C – specific to category) OR a subsequent encounter for nonunion or malunion (7th character K, M, N, P, Q, or R – specific to category).

☑ Additional Character Req    ☑x7ᵗʰ Placeholder Alert    Unacceptable PDx    Manifestation    `H1`-`H14` HAC    `HCC` CMS-HCC Condition    EXCLUDES 1 Not Coded Here    EXCLUDES 2 Not Included Here

√7ᵗʰ **S50.852** **Superficial foreign body of left forearm**

√7ᵗʰ **S50.859** **Superficial foreign body of unspecified forearm**

√6ᵗʰ **S50.86** **Insect bite (nonvenomous) of forearm**

√7ᵗʰ **S50.861** **Insect bite (nonvenomous) of right forearm**

√7ᵗʰ **S50.862** **Insect bite (nonvenomous) of left forearm**

√7ᵗʰ **S50.869** **Insect bite (nonvenomous) of unspecified forearm**

√6ᵗʰ **S50.87** **Other superficial bite of forearm**
> EXCLUDES 1   *open bite of forearm (S51.84)*

√7ᵗʰ **S50.871** **Other superficial bite of right forearm**

√7ᵗʰ **S50.872** **Other superficial bite of left forearm**

√7ᵗʰ **S50.879** **Other superficial bite of unspecified forearm**

√5ᵗʰ **S50.9** **Unspecified superficial injury of elbow and forearm**

√6ᵗʰ **S50.90** **Unspecified superficial injury of elbow**

√7ᵗʰ **S50.901** **Unspecified superficial injury of right elbow**

√7ᵗʰ **S50.902** **Unspecified superficial injury of left elbow**

√7ᵗʰ **S50.909** **Unspecified superficial injury of unspecified elbow**

√6ᵗʰ **S50.91** **Unspecified superficial injury of forearm**

√7ᵗʰ **S50.911** **Unspecified superficial injury of right forearm**

√7ᵗʰ **S50.912** **Unspecified superficial injury of left forearm**

√7ᵗʰ **S50.919** **Unspecified superficial injury of unspecified forearm**

√4ᵗʰ **S51** **Open wound of elbow and forearm**
Code also any associated wound infection
> EXCLUDES 1   *open fracture of elbow and forearm (S52- with open fracture 7th character)*
> *traumatic amputation of elbow and forearm (S58.-)*
> EXCLUDES 2   *open wound of wrist and hand (S61.-)*

The appropriate 7th character is to be added to each code from category S51.
A   initial encounter
D   subsequent encounter
S   sequela

√5ᵗʰ **S51.0** **Open wound of elbow**

√6ᵗʰ **S51.00** **Unspecified open wound of elbow**

√7ᵗʰ **S51.001** **Unspecified open wound of right elbow**
**AHA:** 2012, 4Q, 108

√7ᵗʰ **S51.002** **Unspecified open wound of left elbow**

√7ᵗʰ **S51.009** **Unspecified open wound of unspecified elbow**
Open wound of elbow NOS

√6ᵗʰ **S51.01** **Laceration without foreign body of elbow**

√7ᵗʰ **S51.011** **Laceration without foreign body of right elbow**

√7ᵗʰ **S51.012** **Laceration without foreign body of left elbow**

√7ᵗʰ **S51.019** **Laceration without foreign body of unspecified elbow**

√6ᵗʰ **S51.02** **Laceration with foreign body of elbow**

√7ᵗʰ **S51.021** **Laceration with foreign body of right elbow**

√7ᵗʰ **S51.022** **Laceration with foreign body of left elbow**

√7ᵗʰ **S51.029** **Laceration with foreign body of unspecified elbow**

√6ᵗʰ **S51.03** **Puncture wound without foreign body of elbow**

√7ᵗʰ **S51.031** **Puncture wound without foreign body of right elbow**

√7ᵗʰ **S51.032** **Puncture wound without foreign body of left elbow**

√7ᵗʰ **S51.039** **Puncture wound without foreign body of unspecified elbow**

√6ᵗʰ **S51.04** **Puncture wound with foreign body of elbow**

√7ᵗʰ **S51.041** **Puncture wound with foreign body of right elbow**

√7ᵗʰ **S51.042** **Puncture wound with foreign body of left elbow**

√7ᵗʰ **S51.049** **Puncture wound with foreign body of unspecified elbow**

√6ᵗʰ **S51.05** **Open bite of elbow**
Bite of elbow NOS
> EXCLUDES 1   *superficial bite of elbow (S50.36, S50.37)*

√7ᵗʰ **S51.051** **Open bite, right elbow**

√7ᵗʰ **S51.052** **Open bite, left elbow**

√7ᵗʰ **S51.059** **Open bite, unspecified elbow**

√5ᵗʰ **S51.8** **Open wound of forearm**
> EXCLUDES 2   *open wound of elbow (S51.0-)*

√6ᵗʰ **S51.80** **Unspecified open wound of forearm**
**AHA:** 2016, 3Q, 24

√7ᵗʰ **S51.801** **Unspecified open wound of right forearm**

√7ᵗʰ **S51.802** **Unspecified open wound of left forearm**

√7ᵗʰ **S51.809** **Unspecified open wound of unspecified forearm**
Open wound of forearm NOS

√6ᵗʰ **S51.81** **Laceration without foreign body of forearm**

√7ᵗʰ **S51.811** **Laceration without foreign body of right forearm**

√7ᵗʰ **S51.812** **Laceration without foreign body of left forearm**

√7ᵗʰ **S51.819** **Laceration without foreign body of unspecified forearm**

√6ᵗʰ **S51.82** **Laceration with foreign body of forearm**

√7ᵗʰ **S51.821** **Laceration with foreign body of right forearm**

√7ᵗʰ **S51.822** **Laceration with foreign body of left forearm**

√7ᵗʰ **S51.829** **Laceration with foreign body of unspecified forearm**

√6ᵗʰ **S51.83** **Puncture wound without foreign body of forearm**
**AHA:** 2016, 3Q, 24

√7ᵗʰ **S51.831** **Puncture wound without foreign body of right forearm**

√7ᵗʰ **S51.832** **Puncture wound without foreign body of left forearm**

√7ᵗʰ **S51.839** **Puncture wound without foreign body of unspecified forearm**

√6ᵗʰ **S51.84** **Puncture wound with foreign body of forearm**
**AHA:** 2016, 3Q, 24

√7ᵗʰ **S51.841** **Puncture wound with foreign body of right forearm**

√7ᵗʰ **S51.842** **Puncture wound with foreign body of left forearm**

√7ᵗʰ **S51.849** **Puncture wound with foreign body of unspecified forearm**

√6ᵗʰ **S51.85** **Open bite of forearm**
Bite of forearm NOS
> EXCLUDES 1   *superficial bite of forearm (S50.86, S50.87)*

√7ᵗʰ **S51.851** **Open bite of right forearm**

√7ᵗʰ **S51.852** **Open bite of left forearm**

√7ᵗʰ **S51.859** **Open bite of unspecified forearm**

## ✓4ᵗʰ S52 Fracture of forearm

**NOTE** A fracture not indicated as displaced or nondisplaced should be coded to displaced.
A fracture not indicated as open or closed should be coded to closed.
The open fracture designations are based on the Gustilo open fracture classification.

**EXCLUDES 1** traumatic amputation of forearm (S58.-)
**EXCLUDES 2** fracture at wrist and hand level (S62.-)
**AHA:** 2016, 1Q, 33; 2015, 3Q, 37-39

The appropriate 7th character is to be added to all codes from category S52 [unless otherwise indicated].
A   initial encounter for closed fracture
B   initial encounter for open fracture type I or II
    initial encounter for open fracture NOS
C   initial encounter for open fracture type IIIA, IIIB, or IIIC
D   subsequent encounter for closed fracture with routine healing
E   subsequent encounter for open fracture type I or II with routine healing
F   subsequent encounter for open fracture type IIIA, IIIB, or IIIC with routine healing
G   subsequent encounter for closed fracture with delayed healing
H   subsequent encounter for open fracture type I or II with delayed healing
J   subsequent encounter for open fracture type IIIA, IIIB, or IIIC with delayed healing
K   subsequent encounter for closed fracture with nonunion
M   subsequent encounter for open fracture type I or II with nonunion
N   subsequent encounter for open fracture type IIIA, IIIB, or IIIC with nonunion
P   subsequent encounter for closed fracture with malunion
Q   subsequent encounter for open fracture type I or II with malunion
R   subsequent encounter for open fracture type IIIA, IIIB, or IIIC with malunion
S   sequela

### ✓5ᵗʰ S52.0 Fracture of upper end of ulna
Fracture of proximal end of ulna
**EXCLUDES 2** fracture of elbow NOS (S42.40-)
fractures of shaft of ulna (S52.2-)

#### ✓6ᵗʰ S52.00 Unspecified fracture of upper end of ulna

CC Excl: For codes in subcatagory S52.00: MCC with 7th character B or C: PDX collection 1269
CC with 7th character K, M, N, P, Q, or R: PDX collection 897

6, 8   ✓7ᵗʰ **S52.001 Unspecified fracture of upper end of right ulna** MCC CC H5

6, 8   ✓7ᵗʰ **S52.002 Unspecified fracture of upper end of left ulna** MCC CC H5

6, 8   ✓7ᵗʰ **S52.009 Unspecified fracture of upper end of unspecified ulna** MCC CC H5

#### ✓6ᵗʰ S52.01 Torus fracture of upper end of ulna

The appropriate 7th character is to be added to all codes in subcategory S52.01.
A   initial encounter for closed fracture
D   subsequent encounter for fracture with routine healing
G   subsequent encounter for fracture with delayed healing
K   subsequent encounter for fracture with nonunion
P   subsequent encounter for fracture with malunion
S   sequela

7   ✓7ᵗʰ **S52.011 Torus fracture of upper end of right ulna** CC H5
CC Excl: CC with 7th character A: PDX collection 1270
CC with 7th character K or P: PDX collection 897

7   ✓7ᵗʰ **S52.012 Torus fracture of upper end of left ulna** CC H5
CC Excl: CC with 7th character A: PDX collection 1271
CC with 7th character K or P: PDX collection 897

7   ✓7ᵗʰ **S52.019 Torus fracture of upper end of unspecified ulna** CC H5
CC Excl: CC with 7th character A: PDX collection 1272
CC with 7th character K or P: PDX collection 897

### ✓6ᵗʰ S52.02 Fracture of olecranon process without intraarticular extension of ulna

CC Excl: For codes in subcatagory S52.02: MCC with 7th character B or C: PDX collection 1273
CC with 7th character K, M, N, P, Q, or R: PDX collection 897

6, 8   ✓7ᵗʰ **S52.021 Displaced fracture of olecranon process without intraarticular extension of right ulna** MCC CC H5

6, 8   ✓7ᵗʰ **S52.022 Displaced fracture of olecranon process without intraarticular extension of left ulna** MCC CC H5

6, 8   ✓7ᵗʰ **S52.023 Displaced fracture of olecranon process without intraarticular extension of unspecified ulna** MCC CC H5

6, 8   ✓7ᵗʰ **S52.024 Nondisplaced fracture of olecranon process without intraarticular extension of right ulna** MCC CC H5

6, 8   ✓7ᵗʰ **S52.025 Nondisplaced fracture of olecranon process without intraarticular extension of left ulna** MCC CC H5

6, 8   ✓7ᵗʰ **S52.026 Nondisplaced fracture of olecranon process without intraarticular extension of unspecified ulna** MCC CC H5

### ✓6ᵗʰ S52.03 Fracture of olecranon process with intraarticular extension of ulna

CC Excl: For codes in subcatagory S52.03: MCC with 7th character B or C: PDX collection 1273
CC with 7th character K, M, N, P, Q, or R: PDX collection 897

6, 8   ✓7ᵗʰ **S52.031 Displaced fracture of olecranon process with intraarticular extension of right ulna** MCC CC H5

6, 8   ✓7ᵗʰ **S52.032 Displaced fracture of olecranon process with intraarticular extension of left ulna** MCC CC H5

6, 8   ✓7ᵗʰ **S52.033 Displaced fracture of olecranon process with intraarticular extension of unspecified ulna** MCC CC H5

6, 8   ✓7ᵗʰ **S52.034 Nondisplaced fracture of olecranon process with intraarticular extension of right ulna** MCC CC H5

6, 8   ✓7ᵗʰ **S52.035 Nondisplaced fracture of olecranon process with intraarticular extension of left ulna** MCC CC H5

6, 8   ✓7ᵗʰ **S52.036 Nondisplaced fracture of olecranon process with intraarticular extension of unspecified ulna** MCC CC H5

### ✓6ᵗʰ S52.04 Fracture of coronoid process of ulna

CC Excl: For codes in subcatagory S52.04: MCC with 7th character B or C: PDX collection 1269
CC with 7th character K, M, N, P, Q, or R: PDX collection 897

6, 8   ✓7ᵗʰ **S52.041 Displaced fracture of coronoid process of right ulna** MCC CC H5

6, 8   ✓7ᵗʰ **S52.042 Displaced fracture of coronoid process of left ulna** MCC CC H5

6, 8   ✓7ᵗʰ **S52.043 Displaced fracture of coronoid process of unspecified ulna** MCC CC H5

---

6   MCC when reported as an open fracture (7th character B or C – specific to category).
7   CC when reported as an initial encounter (7th character A, B, or C – specific to category) OR a subsequent encounter for nonunion or malunion (7th character K, M, N, P, Q, or R – specific to category).
8   CC when reported as a subsequent encounter for nonunion or malunion (7th character K, M, N, P, Q, or R – specific to category).

✓Additional Character Req   ✓x7ᵗʰ Placeholder Alert   Unacceptable PDx   Manifestation   H1-H14 HAC   HCC CMS-HCC Condition   EXCLUDES 1 Not Coded Here   EXCLUDES 2 Not Included Here

6, 8 √7th **S52.044 Nondisplaced fracture of coronoid process of right ulna** MCC CC H5

6, 8 √7th **S52.045 Nondisplaced fracture of coronoid process of left ulna** MCC CC H5

6, 8 √7th **S52.046 Nondisplaced fracture of coronoid process of unspecified ulna** MCC CC H5

√6th **S52.09 Other fracture of upper end of ulna**

> **CC Excl: For codes in subcatagory S52.09:**
> **MCC with 7th character B or C:**
> PDX collection 1269
> **CC with 7th character K, M, N, P, Q, or R:**
> PDX collection 897

6, 8 √7th **S52.091 Other fracture of upper end of right ulna** MCC CC H5

6, 8 √7th **S52.092 Other fracture of upper end of left ulna** MCC CC H5

6, 8 √7th **S52.099 Other fracture of upper end of unspecified ulna** MCC CC H5

√5th **S52.1 Fracture of upper end of radius**
Fracture of proximal end of radius

EXCLUDES 2 *physeal fractures of upper end of radius (S59.2-)*
*fracture of shaft of radius (S52.3-)*

> **CC Excl: For CC/MCC codes in subcategory S52.1,**
> **unless otherwise noted:**
> **MCC with 7th character B or C:** PDX collection 1269
> **CC with 7th character K, M, N, P, Q, or R:**
> PDX collection 897

√6th **S52.10 Unspecified fracture of upper end of radius**

6, 8 √7th **S52.101 Unspecified fracture of upper end of right radius** MCC CC H5

6, 8 √7th **S52.102 Unspecified fracture of upper end of left radius** MCC CC H5

6, 8 √7th **S52.109 Unspecified fracture of upper end of unspecified radius** MCC CC H5

√6th **S52.11 Torus fracture of upper end of radius**

> The appropriate 7th character is to be added to all codes in subcategory S52.11.
> A initial encounter for closed fracture
> D subsequent encounter for fracture with routine healing
> G subsequent encounter for fracture with delayed healing
> K subsequent encounter for fracture with nonunion
> P subsequent encounter for fracture with malunion
> S sequela

7 √7th **S52.111 Torus fracture of upper end of right radius** CC H5
> **CC Excl: CC with 7th character A:**
> PDX collection 1270
> **CC with 7th character K, P:**
> PDX collection 897

7 √7th **S52.112 Torus fracture of upper end of left radius** CC H5
> **CC Excl: CC with 7th character A:**
> PDX collection 1271
> **CC with 7th character K or P:**
> PDX collection 897

7 √7th **S52.119 Torus fracture of upper end of unspecified radius** CC H5
> **CC Excl: CC with 7th character A:**
> PDX collection 1272
> **CC Excl: CC with 7th character K or P:**
> PDX collection 897

√6th **S52.12 Fracture of head of radius**

6, 8 √7th **S52.121 Displaced fracture of head of right radius** MCC CC H5

6, 8 √7th **S52.122 Displaced fracture of head of left radius** MCC CC H5

6, 8 √7th **S52.123 Displaced fracture of head of unspecified radius** MCC CC H5

6, 8 √7th **S52.124 Nondisplaced fracture of head of right radius** MCC CC H5

6, 8 √7th **S52.125 Nondisplaced fracture of head of left radius** MCC CC H5

6, 8 √7th **S52.126 Nondisplaced fracture of head of unspecified radius** MCC CC H5

√6th **S52.13 Fracture of neck of radius**

6, 8 √7th **S52.131 Displaced fracture of neck of right radius** MCC CC H5

6, 8 √7th **S52.132 Displaced fracture of neck of left radius** MCC CC H5

6, 8 √7th **S52.133 Displaced fracture of neck of unspecified radius** MCC CC H5

6, 8 √7th **S52.134 Nondisplaced fracture of neck of right radius** MCC CC H5

6, 8 √7th **S52.135 Nondisplaced fracture of neck of left radius** MCC CC H5

6, 8 √7th **S52.136 Nondisplaced fracture of neck of unspecified radius** MCC CC H5

√6th **S52.18 Other fracture of upper end of radius**

6, 8 √7th **S52.181 Other fracture of upper end of right radius** MCC CC H5

6, 8 √7th **S52.182 Other fracture of upper end of left radius** MCC CC H5

6, 8 √7th **S52.189 Other fracture of upper end of unspecified radius** MCC CC H5

√5th **S52.2 Fracture of shaft of ulna**

> **CC Excl: For CC/MCC codes in subcategory S52.2,**
> **unless otherwise noted:**
> **Right side:** See code S52.201
> **Left side:** See code S52.202
> **Unspecified side:** See code S52.209

√6th **S52.20 Unspecified fracture of shaft of ulna**
Fracture of ulna NOS

6, 7 √7th **S52.201 Unspecified fracture of shaft of right ulna** MCC CC H5
> **CC Excl: CC with 7th character A:**
> PDX collection 1270
> **MCC with 7th character B or C:**
> PDX collection 1269
> **CC with 7th character K, M, N, P, Q or R:**
> PDX collection 897

6, 7 √7th **S52.202 Unspecified fracture of shaft of left ulna** MCC CC H5
> **CC Excl: CC with 7th character A:**
> PDX collection 1271
> **MCC with 7th character B or C:**
> PDX collection 1269
> **CC with 7th character K, M, N, P, Q or R:**
> PDX collection 897

6, 7 √7th **S52.209 Unspecified fracture of shaft of unspecified ulna** MCC CC H5
> **CC Excl: CC with 7th character A:**
> PDX collection 1272
> **MCC with 7th character B or C:**
> PDX collection 1269
> **CC with 7th character K, M, N, P, Q or R:**
> PDX collection 897

---

6 MCC when reported as an open fracture (7th character B or C – specific to category).

7 CC when reported as an initial encounter (7th character A, B, or C – specific to category) OR a subsequent encounter for nonunion or malunion (7th character K, M, N, P, Q, or R – specific to category).

8 CC when reported as a subsequent encounter for nonunion or malunion (7th character K, M, N, P, Q, or R – specific to category).

N Newborn: 0 P Pediatric: 0-17 M Maternity: 12-55 A Adult: 15-124 MCC Major CC Condition PDxMCC PDx acts as own MCC CC CC Condition PDxCC PDx acts as own CC

**1000** ICD-10-CM 2018

**✓6ᵗʰ S52.21**   **Greenstick fracture of shaft of ulna**

The appropriate 7th character is to be added to all codes in subcategory S52.21.
- A   initial encounter for closed fracture
- D   subsequent encounter for fracture with routine healing
- G   subsequent encounter for fracture with delayed healing
- K   subsequent encounter for fracture with nonunion
- P   subsequent encounter for fracture with malunion
- S   sequela

**7**   **✓7ᵗʰ S52.211**   **Greenstick fracture of shaft of right ulna**   `CC` `H5`
CC Excl: CC with 7th character A: PDX collection 1270
CC with 7th character K or P: PDX collection 897

**7**   **✓7ᵗʰ S52.212**   **Greenstick fracture of shaft of left ulna**   `CC` `H5`
CC Excl: CC with 7th character A: PDX collection 1271
CC with 7th character K or P: PDX collection 897

**7**   **✓7ᵗʰ S52.219**   **Greenstick fracture of shaft of unspecified ulna**   `CC` `H5`
CC Excl: CC with 7th character A: PDX collection 1272
CC with 7th character K or P: PDX collection 897

**✓6ᵗʰ S52.22**   **Transverse fracture of shaft of ulna**

**6, 7**   **✓7ᵗʰ S52.221**   **Displaced transverse fracture of shaft of right ulna**   `MCC` `CC` `H5`

**6, 7**   **✓7ᵗʰ S52.222**   **Displaced transverse fracture of shaft of left ulna**   `MCC` `CC` `H5`

**6, 7**   **✓7ᵗʰ S52.223**   **Displaced transverse fracture of shaft of unspecified ulna**   `MCC` `CC` `H5`

**6, 7**   **✓7ᵗʰ S52.224**   **Nondisplaced transverse fracture of shaft of right ulna**   `MCC` `CC` `H5`

**6, 7**   **✓7ᵗʰ S52.225**   **Nondisplaced transverse fracture of shaft of left ulna**   `MCC` `CC` `H5`

**6, 7**   **✓7ᵗʰ S52.226**   **Nondisplaced transverse fracture of shaft of unspecified ulna**   `MCC` `CC` `H5`

**✓6ᵗʰ S52.23**   **Oblique fracture of shaft of ulna**

**6, 7**   **✓7ᵗʰ S52.231**   **Displaced oblique fracture of shaft of right ulna**   `MCC` `CC` `H5`

**6, 7**   **✓7ᵗʰ S52.232**   **Displaced oblique fracture of shaft of left ulna**   `MCC` `CC` `H5`

**6, 7**   **✓7ᵗʰ S52.233**   **Displaced oblique fracture of shaft of unspecified ulna**   `MCC` `CC` `H5`

**6, 7**   **✓7ᵗʰ S52.234**   **Nondisplaced oblique fracture of shaft of right ulna**   `MCC` `CC` `H5`

**6, 7**   **✓7ᵗʰ S52.235**   **Nondisplaced oblique fracture of shaft of left ulna**   `MCC` `CC` `H5`

**6, 7**   **✓7ᵗʰ S52.236**   **Nondisplaced oblique fracture of shaft of unspecified ulna**   `MCC` `CC` `H5`

**✓6ᵗʰ S52.24**   **Spiral fracture of shaft of ulna**

**6, 7**   **✓7ᵗʰ S52.241**   **Displaced spiral fracture of shaft of ulna, right arm**   `MCC` `CC` `H5`

**6, 7**   **✓7ᵗʰ S52.242**   **Displaced spiral fracture of shaft of ulna, left arm**   `MCC` `CC` `H5`

**6, 7**   **✓7ᵗʰ S52.243**   **Displaced spiral fracture of shaft of ulna, unspecified arm**   `MCC` `CC` `H5`

**6, 7**   **✓7ᵗʰ S52.244**   **Nondisplaced spiral fracture of shaft of ulna, right arm**   `MCC` `CC` `H5`

**6, 7**   **✓7ᵗʰ S52.245**   **Nondisplaced spiral fracture of shaft of ulna, left arm**   `MCC` `CC` `H5`

**6, 7**   **✓7ᵗʰ S52.246**   **Nondisplaced spiral fracture of shaft of ulna, unspecified arm**   `MCC` `CC` `H5`

**✓6ᵗʰ S52.25**   **Comminuted fracture of shaft of ulna**

**6, 7**   **✓7ᵗʰ S52.251**   **Displaced comminuted fracture of shaft of ulna, right arm**   `MCC` `CC` `H5`

**6, 7**   **✓7ᵗʰ S52.252**   **Displaced comminuted fracture of shaft of ulna, left arm**   `MCC` `CC` `H5`

**6, 7**   **✓7ᵗʰ S52.253**   **Displaced comminuted fracture of shaft of ulna, unspecified arm**   `MCC` `CC` `H5`

**6, 7**   **✓7ᵗʰ S52.254**   **Nondisplaced comminuted fracture of shaft of ulna, right arm**   `MCC` `CC` `H5`

**6, 7**   **✓7ᵗʰ S52.255**   **Nondisplaced comminuted fracture of shaft of ulna, left arm**   `MCC` `CC` `H5`

**6, 7**   **✓7ᵗʰ S52.256**   **Nondisplaced comminuted fracture of shaft of ulna, unspecified arm**   `MCC` `CC` `H5`

**✓6ᵗʰ S52.26**   **Segmental fracture of shaft of ulna**

**6, 7**   **✓7ᵗʰ S52.261**   **Displaced segmental fracture of shaft of ulna, right arm**   `MCC` `CC` `H5`

**6, 7**   **✓7ᵗʰ S52.262**   **Displaced segmental fracture of shaft of ulna, left arm**   `MCC` `CC` `H5`

**6, 7**   **✓7ᵗʰ S52.263**   **Displaced segmental fracture of shaft of ulna, unspecified arm**   `MCC` `CC` `H5`

**6, 7**   **✓7ᵗʰ S52.264**   **Nondisplaced segmental fracture of shaft of ulna, right arm**   `MCC` `CC` `H5`

**6, 7**   **✓7ᵗʰ S52.265**   **Nondisplaced segmental fracture of shaft of ulna, left arm**   `MCC` `CC` `H5`

**6, 7**   **✓7ᵗʰ S52.266**   **Nondisplaced segmental fracture of shaft of ulna, unspecified arm**   `MCC` `CC` `H5`

**✓6ᵗʰ S52.27**   **Monteggia's fracture of ulna**
Fracture of upper shaft of ulna with dislocation of radial head

CC Excl: For codes in subcategory S52.27:
MCC with 7th character B or C: PDX collection 1269
CC with 7th character K, M, N, P Q or R: PDX collection 897

**6, 8**   **✓7ᵗʰ S52.271**   **Monteggia's fracture of right ulna**   `MCC` `CC` `H5`

**6, 8**   **✓7ᵗʰ S52.272**   **Monteggia's fracture of left ulna**   `MCC` `CC` `H5`

**6, 8**   **✓7ᵗʰ S52.279**   **Monteggia's fracture of unspecified ulna**   `MCC` `CC` `H5`

**✓6ᵗʰ S52.28**   **Bent bone of ulna**

**6, 7**   **✓7ᵗʰ S52.281**   **Bent bone of right ulna**   `MCC` `CC` `H5`

**6, 7**   **✓7ᵗʰ S52.282**   **Bent bone of left ulna**   `MCC` `CC` `H5`

**6, 7**   **✓7ᵗʰ S52.283**   **Bent bone of unspecified ulna**   `MCC` `CC` `H5`

**✓6ᵗʰ S52.29**   **Other fracture of shaft of ulna**

**6, 7**   **✓7ᵗʰ S52.291**   **Other fracture of shaft of right ulna**   `MCC` `CC` `H5`

**6, 7**   **✓7ᵗʰ S52.292**   **Other fracture of shaft of left ulna**   `MCC` `CC` `H5`

**6, 7**   **✓7ᵗʰ S52.299**   **Other fracture of shaft of unspecified ulna**   `MCC` `CC` `H5`

**✓5ᵗʰ S52.3**   **Fracture of shaft of radius**

CC Excl: For CC/MCC codes in subcategory S52.3, unless otherwise noted:
**Right side:** See code S52.201
**Left side:** See code S52.202
**Unspecified side:** See code S52.209

**✓6ᵗʰ S52.30**   **Unspecified fracture of shaft of radius**

**6, 7**   **✓7ᵗʰ S52.301**   **Unspecified fracture of shaft of right radius**   `MCC` `CC` `H5`

**6, 7**   **✓7ᵗʰ S52.302**   **Unspecified fracture of shaft of left radius**   `MCC` `CC` `H5`

**6, 7**   **✓7ᵗʰ S52.309**   **Unspecified fracture of shaft of unspecified radius**   `MCC` `CC` `H5`

---

**6**   MCC when reported as an open fracture (7th character B or C – specific to category).
**7**   CC when reported as an initial encounter (7th character A, B, or C – specific to category) OR a subsequent encounter for nonunion or malunion (7th character K, M, N, P, Q, or R – specific to category).
**8**   CC when reported as a subsequent encounter for nonunion or malunion (7th character K, M, N, P, Q, or R – specific to category).

---

☑ Additional Character Req   ✓ₓ7ᵗʰ Placeholder Alert   Unacceptable PDx   Manifestation   `H1`-`H14` HAC   `HCC` CMS-HCC Condition   *EXCLUDES 1* Not Coded Here   *EXCLUDES 2* Not Included Here

✓6th **S52.31** Greenstick **fracture of shaft of radius**

The appropriate 7th character is to be added to all codes in subcategory S52.31.
A    initial encounter for closed fracture
D    subsequent encounter for fracture with routine healing
G    subsequent encounter for fracture with delayed healing
K    subsequent encounter for fracture with nonunion
P    subsequent encounter for fracture with malunion
S    sequela

7 ✓7th **S52.311** Greenstick **fracture of shaft of radius, right arm** `CC` `H5`
    **CC Excl:** See code: S52.211

7 ✓7th **S52.312** Greenstick **fracture of shaft of radius, left arm** `CC` `H5`
    **CC Excl:** See code: S52.212

7 ✓7th **S52.319** Greenstick **fracture of shaft of radius, unspecified arm** `CC` `H5`
    **CC Excl:** See code: S52.219

✓6th **S52.32** Transverse **fracture of shaft of radius**

6, 7 ✓7th **S52.321** Displaced transverse fracture **of shaft of right radius** `MCC` `CC` `H5`

6, 7 ✓7th **S52.322** Displaced transverse fracture **of shaft of left radius** `MCC` `CC` `H5`

6, 7 ✓7th **S52.323** Displaced transverse fracture **of shaft of unspecified radius** `MCC` `CC` `H5`

6, 7 ✓7th **S52.324** Nondisplaced transverse **fracture of shaft of right radius** `MCC` `CC` `H5`

6, 7 ✓7th **S52.325** Nondisplaced transverse **fracture of shaft of left radius** `MCC` `CC` `H5`

6, 7 ✓7th **S52.326** Nondisplaced transverse **fracture of shaft of unspecified radius** `MCC` `CC` `H5`

✓6th **S52.33** Oblique **fracture of shaft of radius**

6, 7 ✓7th **S52.331** Displaced oblique fracture of **shaft of right radius** `MCC` `CC` `H5`

6, 7 ✓7th **S52.332** Displaced oblique fracture of **shaft of left radius** `MCC` `CC` `H5`

6, 7 ✓7th **S52.333** Displaced oblique fracture of **shaft of unspecified radius** `MCC` `CC` `H5`

6, 7 ✓7th **S52.334** Nondisplaced oblique fracture **of shaft of right radius** `MCC` `CC` `H5`

6, 7 ✓7th **S52.335** Nondisplaced oblique fracture **of shaft of left radius** `MCC` `CC` `H5`

6, 7 ✓7th **S52.336** Nondisplaced oblique fracture **of shaft of unspecified radius** `MCC` `CC` `H5`

✓6th **S52.34** Spiral **fracture of shaft of radius**

6, 7 ✓7th **S52.341** Displaced spiral fracture of **shaft of radius, right arm** `MCC` `CC` `H5`

6, 7 ✓7th **S52.342** Displaced spiral fracture of **shaft of radius, left arm** `MCC` `CC` `H5`

6, 7 ✓7th **S52.343** Displaced spiral fracture of **shaft of radius, unspecified arm** `MCC` `CC` `H5`

6, 7 ✓7th **S52.344** Nondisplaced spiral fracture **of shaft of radius, right arm** `MCC` `CC` `H5`

6, 7 ✓7th **S52.345** Nondisplaced spiral fracture **of shaft of radius, left arm** `MCC` `CC` `H5`

6, 7 ✓7th **S52.346** Nondisplaced spiral fracture **of shaft of radius, unspecified arm** `MCC` `CC` `H5`

✓6th **S52.35** Comminuted **fracture of shaft of radius**

6, 7 ✓7th **S52.351** Displaced comminuted **fracture of shaft of radius, right arm** `MCC` `CC` `H5`

6, 7 ✓7th **S52.352** Displaced comminuted **fracture of shaft of radius, left arm** `MCC` `CC` `H5`

6, 7 ✓7th **S52.353** Displaced comminuted **fracture of shaft of radius, unspecified arm** `MCC` `CC` `H5`

6, 7 ✓7th **S52.354** Nondisplaced comminuted **fracture of shaft of radius, right arm** `MCC` `CC` `H5`

6, 7 ✓7th **S52.355** Nondisplaced comminuted **fracture of shaft of radius, left arm** `MCC` `CC` `H5`

6, 7 ✓7th **S52.356** Nondisplaced comminuted **fracture of shaft of radius, unspecified arm** `MCC` `CC` `H5`

✓6th **S52.36** Segmental **fracture of shaft of radius**

6, 7 ✓7th **S52.361** Displaced segmental fracture **of shaft of radius, right arm** `MCC` `CC` `H5`

6, 7 ✓7th **S52.362** Displaced segmental fracture **of shaft of radius, left arm** `MCC` `CC` `H5`

6, 7 ✓7th **S52.363** Displaced segmental fracture **of shaft of radius, unspecified arm** `MCC` `CC` `H5`

6, 7 ✓7th **S52.364** Nondisplaced segmental **fracture of shaft of radius, right arm** `MCC` `CC` `H5`

6, 7 ✓7th **S52.365** Nondisplaced segmental **fracture of shaft of radius, left arm** `MCC` `CC` `H5`

6, 7 ✓7th **S52.366** Nondisplaced segmental **fracture of shaft of radius, unspecified arm** `MCC` `CC` `H5`

✓6th **S52.37** Galeazzi's **fracture**
    Fracture of lower shaft of radius with radioulnar joint dislocation

6, 7 ✓7th **S52.371** Galeazzi's **fracture of right radius** `MCC` `CC` `H5`

6, 7 ✓7th **S52.372** Galeazzi's **fracture of left radius** `MCC` `CC` `H5`

6, 7 ✓7th **S52.379** Galeazzi's **fracture of unspecified radius** `MCC` `CC` `H5`

✓6th **S52.38** Bent bone **of radius**

6, 7 ✓7th **S52.381** Bent bone of **right radius** `MCC` `CC` `H5`

6, 7 ✓7th **S52.382** Bent bone of **left radius** `MCC` `CC` `H5`

6, 7 ✓7th **S52.389** Bent bone of **unspecified radius** `MCC` `CC` `H5`

✓6th **S52.39** Other **fracture of shaft of radius**

6, 7 ✓7th **S52.391** Other fracture of shaft of **radius, right arm** `MCC` `CC` `H5`

6, 7 ✓7th **S52.392** Other fracture of shaft of **radius, left arm** `MCC` `CC` `H5`

6, 7 ✓7th **S52.399** Other fracture of shaft of **radius, unspecified arm** `MCC` `CC` `H5`

✓5th **S52.5** **Fracture of lower end of radius**
    Fracture of distal end of radius
    *EXCLUDES 2*   *physeal fractures of lower end of radius (S59.2-)*
    **DEF:** Fracture of distal end of radius above the wrist; most commonly caused by fall onto an outstretched hand.

**CC Excl:** For CC/MCC codes in subcategory S52.5, unless otherwise noted:
**Right side:** See code S52.201
**Left side:** See code S52.202
**Unspecified side:** See code S52.209

✓6th **S52.50** **Unspecified fracture of the lower end of radius**

6, 7 ✓7th **S52.501** Unspecified fracture of the **lower end of right radius** `MCC` `CC` `H5`

6, 7 ✓7th **S52.502** Unspecified fracture of the **lower end of left radius** `MCC` `CC` `H5`

6, 7 ✓7th **S52.509** Unspecified fracture of the **lower nd of unspecified radius** `MCC` `CC` `H5`

✓6th **S52.51** **Fracture of radial styloid process**

6, 7 ✓7th **S52.511** Displaced fracture of **right radial styloid process** `MCC` `CC` `H5`

6, 7 ✓7th **S52.512** Displaced fracture of **left radial styloid process** `MCC` `CC` `H5`

6, 7 ✓7th **S52.513** Displaced fracture of **unspecified radial styloid process** `MCC` `CC` `H5`

6, 7 ✓7th **S52.514** Nondisplaced fracture of **right radial styloid process** `MCC` `CC` `H5`

6, 7 ✓7th **S52.515** Nondisplaced fracture of **left radial styloid process** `MCC` `CC` `H5`

6, 7 ✓7th **S52.516** Nondisplaced fracture of **unspecified radial styloid process** `MCC` `CC` `H5`

---

6   MCC when reported as an open fracture (7th character B or C – specific to category).
7   CC when reported as an initial encounter (7th character A, B, or C – specific to category) OR a subsequent encounter for nonunion or malunion (7th character K, M, N, P, Q, or R – specific to category).

√6ᵗʰ **S52.52**   **Torus fracture of lower end of radius**

> The appropriate 7th character is to be added to all codes in subcategory S52.52.
> A   initial encounter for closed fracture
> D   subsequent encounter for fracture with routine healing
> G   subsequent encounter for fracture with delayed healing
> K   subsequent encounter for fracture with nonunion
> P   subsequent encounter for fracture with malunion
> S   sequela

7   √7ᵗʰ   **S52.521**   **Torus fracture of lower end of right radius** `CC` `H5`
> CC Excl: See code: S52.211

7   √7ᵗʰ   **S52.522**   **Torus fracture of lower end of left radius** `CC` `H5`
> CC Excl: See code: S52.212

7   √7ᵗʰ   **S52.529**   **Torus fracture of lower end of unspecified radius** `CC` `H5`
> CC Excl: See code: S52.219

√6ᵗʰ **S52.53**   **Colles' fracture**

6, 7   √7ᵗʰ   **S52.531**   **Colles' fracture of right radius** `MCC` `CC` `H5`
> AHA: 2016, 2Q, 4

6, 7   √7ᵗʰ   **S52.532**   **Colles' fracture of left radius** `MCC` `CC` `H5`

6, 7   √7ᵗʰ   **S52.539**   **Colles' fracture of unspecified radius** `MCC` `CC` `H5`

√6ᵗʰ **S52.54**   **Smith's fracture**

6, 7   √7ᵗʰ   **S52.541**   **Smith's fracture of right radius** `MCC` `CC` `H5`

6, 7   √7ᵗʰ   **S52.542**   **Smith's fracture of left radius** `MCC` `CC` `H5`

6, 7   √7ᵗʰ   **S52.549**   **Smith's fracture of unspecified radius** `MCC` `CC` `H5`

√6ᵗʰ **S52.55**   **Other extraarticular fracture of lower end of radius**

6, 7   √7ᵗʰ   **S52.551**   **Other extraarticular fracture of lower end of right radius** `MCC` `CC` `H5`

6, 7   √7ᵗʰ   **S52.552**   **Other extraarticular fracture of lower end of left radius** `MCC` `CC` `H5`

6, 7   √7ᵗʰ   **S52.559**   **Other extraarticular fracture of lower end of unspecified radius** `MCC` `CC` `H5`

√6ᵗʰ **S52.56**   **Barton's fracture**

6, 7   √7ᵗʰ   **S52.561**   **Barton's fracture of right radius** `MCC` `CC` `H5`

6, 7   √7ᵗʰ   **S52.562**   **Barton's fracture of left radius** `MCC` `CC` `H5`

6, 7   √7ᵗʰ   **S52.569**   **Barton's fracture of unspecified radius** `MCC` `CC` `H5`

√6ᵗʰ **S52.57**   **Other intraarticular fracture of lower end of radius**

6, 7   √7ᵗʰ   **S52.571**   **Other intraarticular fracture of lower end of right radius** `MCC` `CC` `H5`

6, 7   √7ᵗʰ   **S52.572**   **Other intraarticular fracture of lower end of left radius** `MCC` `CC` `H5`

6, 7   √7ᵗʰ   **S52.579**   **Other intraarticular fracture of lower end of unspecified radius** `MCC` `CC` `H5`

√6ᵗʰ **S52.59**   **Other fractures of lower end of radius**

6, 7   √7ᵗʰ   **S52.591**   **Other fractures of lower end of right radius** `MCC` `CC` `H5`

6, 7   √7ᵗʰ   **S52.592**   **Other fractures of lower end of left radius** `MCC` `CC` `H5`

6, 7   √7ᵗʰ   **S52.599**   **Other fractures of lower end of unspecified radius** `MCC` `CC` `H5`

√5ᵗʰ **S52.6**   **Fracture of lower end of ulna**

> CC Excl: For CC/MCC codes in subcategory S52.6, unless otherwise noted:
> **Right side:** See code S52.201
> **Left side:** See code S52.202
> **Unspecified side:** See code S52.209

√6ᵗʰ **S52.60**   **Unspecified fracture of lower end of ulna**

6, 7   √7ᵗʰ   **S52.601**   **Unspecified fracture of lower end of right ulna** `MCC` `CC` `H5`

6, 7   √7ᵗʰ   **S52.602**   **Unspecified fracture of lower end of left ulna** `MCC` `CC` `H5`

6, 7   √7ᵗʰ   **S52.609**   **Unspecified fracture of lower end of unspecified ulna** `MCC` `CC` `H5`

√6ᵗʰ **S52.61**   **Fracture of ulna styloid process**

6, 7   √7ᵗʰ   **S52.611**   **Displaced fracture of right ulna styloid process** `MCC` `CC` `H5`

6, 7   √7ᵗʰ   **S52.612**   **Displaced fracture of left ulna styloid process** `MCC` `CC` `H5`

6, 7   √7ᵗʰ   **S52.613**   **Displaced fracture of unspecified ulna styloid process** `MCC` `CC` `H5`

6, 7   √7ᵗʰ   **S52.614**   **Nondisplaced fracture of right ulna styloid process** `MCC` `CC` `H5`

6, 7   √7ᵗʰ   **S52.615**   **Nondisplaced fracture of left ulna styloid process** `MCC` `CC` `H5`

6, 7   √7ᵗʰ   **S52.616**   **Nondisplaced fracture of unspecified ulna styloid process** `MCC` `CC` `H5`

√6ᵗʰ **S52.62**   **Torus fracture of lower end of ulna**

> The appropriate 7th character is to be added to all codes in subcategory S52.62.
> A   initial encounter for closed fracture
> D   subsequent encounter for fracture with routine healing
> G   subsequent encounter for fracture with delayed healing
> K   subsequent encounter for fracture with nonunion
> P   subsequent encounter for fracture with malunion
> S   sequela

7   √7ᵗʰ   **S52.621**   **Torus fracture of lower end of right ulna** `CC` `H5`
> CC Excl: See code: S52.211

7   √7ᵗʰ   **S52.622**   **Torus fracture of lower end of left ulna** `CC` `H5`
> CC Excl: See code: S52.212

7   √7ᵗʰ   **S52.629**   **Torus fracture of lower end of unspecified ulna** `CC` `H5`
> CC Excl: See code: S52.219

√6ᵗʰ **S52.69**   **Other fracture of lower end of ulna**

6, 7   √7ᵗʰ   **S52.691**   **Other fracture of lower end of right ulna** `MCC` `CC` `H5`

6, 7   √7ᵗʰ   **S52.692**   **Other fracture of lower end of left ulna** `MCC` `CC` `H5`

6, 7   √7ᵗʰ   **S52.699**   **Other fracture of lower end of unspecified ulna** `MCC` `CC` `H5`

√5ᵗʰ **S52.9**   **Unspecified fracture of forearm**

> CC Excl: For CC/MCC codes in subcategory S52.9:
> See code S52.209

6, 7   √x7ᵗʰ   **S52.90**   **Unspecified fracture of unspecified forearm** `MCC` `CC` `H5`

6, 7   √x7ᵗʰ   **S52.91**   **Unspecified fracture of right forearm** `MCC` `CC` `H5`

6, 7   √x7ᵗʰ   **S52.92**   **Unspecified fracture of left forearm** `MCC` `CC` `H5`

---

⁶   MCC when reported as an open fracture (7th character B or C – specific to category).

⁷   CC when reported as an initial encounter (7th character A, B, or C – specific to category) OR a subsequent encounter for nonunion or malunion (7th character K, M, N, P, Q, or R – specific to category).

---

✓ Additional Character Req   √x7ᵗʰ Placeholder Alert   Unacceptable PDx   ■ Manifestation   `H1`-`H14` HAC   `HCC` CMS-HCC Condition   *EXCLUDES 1* Not Coded Here   *EXCLUDES 2* Not Included Here

## ✓4ᵗʰ S53  Dislocation and sprain of joints and ligaments of elbow

INCLUDES  avulsion of joint or ligament of elbow
laceration of cartilage, joint or ligament of elbow
sprain of cartilage, joint or ligament of elbow
traumatic hemarthrosis of joint or ligament of elbow
traumatic rupture of joint or ligament of elbow
traumatic subluxation of joint or ligament of elbow
traumatic tear of joint or ligament of elbow

Code also any associated open wound

EXCLUDES 2  *strain of muscle, fascia and tendon at forearm level (S56.-)*

The appropriate 7th character is to be added to each code from category S53.
A    initial encounter
D    subsequent encounter
S    sequela

### ✓5ᵗʰ S53.0  Subluxation and dislocation of radial head
Dislocation of radiohumeral joint
Subluxation of radiohumeral joint
EXCLUDES 1  *Monteggia's fracture-dislocation (S52.27-)*

#### ✓6ᵗʰ S53.00  Unspecified subluxation and dislocation of radial head
- ✓7ᵗʰ **S53.001**  Unspecified subluxation of right radial head
- ✓7ᵗʰ **S53.002**  Unspecified subluxation of left radial head
- ✓7ᵗʰ **S53.003**  Unspecified subluxation of unspecified radial head
- ✓7ᵗʰ **S53.004**  Unspecified dislocation of right radial head
- ✓7ᵗʰ **S53.005**  Unspecified dislocation of left radial head
- ✓7ᵗʰ **S53.006**  Unspecified dislocation of unspecified radial head

#### ✓6ᵗʰ S53.01  Anterior subluxation and dislocation of radial head
Anteriomedial subluxation and dislocation of radial head
- ✓7ᵗʰ **S53.011**  Anterior subluxation of right radial head
- ✓7ᵗʰ **S53.012**  Anterior subluxation of left radial head
- ✓7ᵗʰ **S53.013**  Anterior subluxation of unspecified radial head
- ✓7ᵗʰ **S53.014**  Anterior dislocation of right radial head
- ✓7ᵗʰ **S53.015**  Anterior dislocation of left radial head
- ✓7ᵗʰ **S53.016**  Anterior dislocation of unspecified radial head

#### ✓6ᵗʰ S53.02  Posterior subluxation and dislocation of radial head
Posteriolateral subluxation and dislocation of radial head
- ✓7ᵗʰ **S53.021**  Posterior subluxation of right radial head
- ✓7ᵗʰ **S53.022**  Posterior subluxation of left radial head
- ✓7ᵗʰ **S53.023**  Posterior subluxation of unspecified radial head
- ✓7ᵗʰ **S53.024**  Posterior dislocation of right radial head
- ✓7ᵗʰ **S53.025**  Posterior dislocation of left radial head
- ✓7ᵗʰ **S53.026**  Posterior dislocation of unspecified radial head

#### ✓6ᵗʰ S53.03  Nursemaid's elbow
- ✓7ᵗʰ **S53.031**  Nursemaid's elbow, right elbow
- ✓7ᵗʰ **S53.032**  Nursemaid's elbow, left elbow
- ✓7ᵗʰ **S53.033**  Nursemaid's elbow, unspecified elbow

#### ✓6ᵗʰ S53.09  Other subluxation and dislocation of radial head
- ✓7ᵗʰ **S53.091**  Other subluxation of right radial head
- ✓7ᵗʰ **S53.092**  Other subluxation of left radial head
- ✓7ᵗʰ **S53.093**  Other subluxation of unspecified radial head
- ✓7ᵗʰ **S53.094**  Other dislocation of right radial head
- ✓7ᵗʰ **S53.095**  Other dislocation of left radial head
- ✓7ᵗʰ **S53.096**  Other dislocation of unspecified radial head

### ✓5ᵗʰ S53.1  Subluxation and dislocation of ulnohumeral joint
Subluxation and dislocation of elbow NOS
EXCLUDES 1  *dislocation of radial head alone (S53.0-)*

#### ✓6ᵗʰ S53.10  Unspecified subluxation and dislocation of ulnohumeral joint
- ✓7ᵗʰ **S53.101**  Unspecified subluxation of right ulnohumeral joint

- ✓7ᵗʰ **S53.102**  Unspecified subluxation of left ulnohumeral joint
- ✓7ᵗʰ **S53.103**  Unspecified subluxation of unspecified ulnohumeral joint
- ✓7ᵗʰ **S53.104**  Unspecified dislocation of right ulnohumeral joint
- ✓7ᵗʰ **S53.105**  Unspecified dislocation of left ulnohumeral joint
- ✓7ᵗʰ **S53.106**  Unspecified dislocation of unspecified ulnohumeral joint

#### ✓6ᵗʰ S53.11  Anterior subluxation and dislocation of ulnohumeral joint
- ✓7ᵗʰ **S53.111**  Anterior subluxation of right ulnohumeral joint
- ✓7ᵗʰ **S53.112**  Anterior subluxation of left ulnohumeral joint
- ✓7ᵗʰ **S53.113**  Anterior subluxation of unspecified ulnohumeral joint
- ✓7ᵗʰ **S53.114**  Anterior dislocation of right ulnohumeral joint
  AHA: 2012, 4Q, 108
- ✓7ᵗʰ **S53.115**  Anterior dislocation of left ulnohumeral joint
- ✓7ᵗʰ **S53.116**  Anterior dislocation of unspecified ulnohumeral joint

#### ✓6ᵗʰ S53.12  Posterior subluxation and dislocation of ulnohumeral joint
- ✓7ᵗʰ **S53.121**  Posterior subluxation of right ulnohumeral joint
- ✓7ᵗʰ **S53.122**  Posterior subluxation of left ulnohumeral joint
- ✓7ᵗʰ **S53.123**  Posterior subluxation of unspecified ulnohumeral joint
- ✓7ᵗʰ **S53.124**  Posterior dislocation of right ulnohumeral joint
- ✓7ᵗʰ **S53.125**  Posterior dislocation of left ulnohumeral joint
- ✓7ᵗʰ **S53.126**  Posterior dislocation of unspecified ulnohumeral joint

#### ✓6ᵗʰ S53.13  Medial subluxation and dislocation of ulnohumeral joint
- ✓7ᵗʰ **S53.131**  Medial subluxation of right ulnohumeral joint
- ✓7ᵗʰ **S53.132**  Medial subluxation of left ulnohumeral joint
- ✓7ᵗʰ **S53.133**  Medial subluxation of unspecified ulnohumeral joint
- ✓7ᵗʰ **S53.134**  Medial dislocation of right ulnohumeral joint
- ✓7ᵗʰ **S53.135**  Medial dislocation of left ulnohumeral joint
- ✓7ᵗʰ **S53.136**  Medial dislocation of unspecified ulnohumeral joint

#### ✓6ᵗʰ S53.14  Lateral subluxation and dislocation of ulnohumeral joint
- ✓7ᵗʰ **S53.141**  Lateral subluxation of right ulnohumeral joint
- ✓7ᵗʰ **S53.142**  Lateral subluxation of left ulnohumeral joint
- ✓7ᵗʰ **S53.143**  Lateral subluxation of unspecified ulnohumeral joint
- ✓7ᵗʰ **S53.144**  Lateral dislocation of right ulnohumeral joint
- ✓7ᵗʰ **S53.145**  Lateral dislocation of left ulnohumeral joint
- ✓7ᵗʰ **S53.146**  Lateral dislocation of unspecified ulnohumeral joint

#### ✓6ᵗʰ S53.19  Other subluxation and dislocation of ulnohumeral joint
- ✓7ᵗʰ **S53.191**  Other subluxation of right ulnohumeral joint
- ✓7ᵗʰ **S53.192**  Other subluxation of left ulnohumeral joint
- ✓7ᵗʰ **S53.193**  Other subluxation of unspecified ulnohumeral joint

Ⓝ Newborn: 0  Ⓟ Pediatric: 0-17  Ⓜ Maternity: 12-55  Ⓐ Adult: 15-124  MCC Major CC Condition  PDx MCC PDx acts as own MCC  CC CC Condition  PDx CC PDx acts as own CC

1004
ICD-10-CM 2018

✓7ᵗʰ **S53.194** Other dislocation of right ulnohumeral joint

✓7ᵗʰ **S53.195** Other dislocation of left ulnohumeral joint

✓7ᵗʰ **S53.196** Other dislocation of unspecified ulnohumeral joint

✓5ᵗʰ **S53.2 Traumatic rupture of radial collateral ligament**
 **EXCLUDES 1** *sprain of radial collateral ligament NOS (S53.43-)*

✓x7ᵗʰ **S53.20** Traumatic rupture of unspecified radial collateral ligament

✓x7ᵗʰ **S53.21** Traumatic rupture of right radial collateral ligament

✓x7ᵗʰ **S53.22** Traumatic rupture of left radial collateral ligament

✓5ᵗʰ **S53.3 Traumatic rupture of ulnar collateral ligament**
 **EXCLUDES 1** *sprain of ulnar collateral ligament (S53.44-)*

✓x7ᵗʰ **S53.30** Traumatic rupture of unspecified ulnar collateral ligament

✓x7ᵗʰ **S53.31** Traumatic rupture of right ulnar collateral ligament

✓x7ᵗʰ **S53.32** Traumatic rupture of left ulnar collateral ligament

✓5ᵗʰ **S53.4 Sprain of elbow**
 **EXCLUDES 2** *traumatic rupture of radial collateral ligament (S53.2-)*
 *traumatic rupture of ulnar collateral ligament (S53.3-)*

✓6ᵗʰ **S53.40** Unspecified sprain of elbow

 ✓7ᵗʰ **S53.401** Unspecified sprain of right elbow

 ✓7ᵗʰ **S53.402** Unspecified sprain of left elbow

 ✓7ᵗʰ **S53.409** Unspecified sprain of unspecified elbow
  Sprain of elbow NOS

✓6ᵗʰ **S53.41** Radiohumeral (joint) sprain

 ✓7ᵗʰ **S53.411** Radiohumeral (joint) sprain of right elbow

 ✓7ᵗʰ **S53.412** Radiohumeral (joint) sprain of left elbow

 ✓7ᵗʰ **S53.419** Radiohumeral (joint) sprain of unspecified elbow

✓6ᵗʰ **S53.42** Ulnohumeral (joint) sprain

 ✓7ᵗʰ **S53.421** Ulnohumeral (joint) sprain of right elbow

 ✓7ᵗʰ **S53.422** Ulnohumeral (joint) sprain of left elbow

 ✓7ᵗʰ **S53.429** Ulnohumeral (joint) sprain of unspecified elbow

✓6ᵗʰ **S53.43** Radial collateral ligament sprain

 ✓7ᵗʰ **S53.431** Radial collateral ligament sprain of right elbow

 ✓7ᵗʰ **S53.432** Radial collateral ligament sprain of left elbow

 ✓7ᵗʰ **S53.439** Radial collateral ligament sprain of unspecified elbow

✓6ᵗʰ **S53.44** Ulnar collateral ligament sprain

 ✓7ᵗʰ **S53.441** Ulnar collateral ligament sprain of right elbow

 ✓7ᵗʰ **S53.442** Ulnar collateral ligament sprain of left elbow

 ✓7ᵗʰ **S53.449** Ulnar collateral ligament sprain of unspecified elbow

✓6ᵗʰ **S53.49** Other sprain of elbow

 ✓7ᵗʰ **S53.491** Other sprain of right elbow

 ✓7ᵗʰ **S53.492** Other sprain of left elbow

 ✓7ᵗʰ **S53.499** Other sprain of unspecified elbow

✓4ᵗʰ **S54 Injury of nerves at forearm level**
 Code also any associated open wound (S51.-)
 **EXCLUDES 2** *injury of nerves at wrist and hand level (S64.-)*

 The appropriate 7th character is to be added to each code from category S54.
 A  initial encounter
 D  subsequent encounter
 S  sequela

✓5ᵗʰ **S54.0 Injury of ulnar nerve at forearm level**
 Injury of ulnar nerve NOS

✓x7ᵗʰ **S54.00** Injury of ulnar nerve at forearm level, unspecified arm

✓x7ᵗʰ **S54.01** Injury of ulnar nerve at forearm level, right arm

✓x7ᵗʰ **S54.02** Injury of ulnar nerve at forearm level, left arm

✓5ᵗʰ **S54.1 Injury of median nerve at forearm level**
 Injury of median nerve NOS

✓x7ᵗʰ **S54.10** Injury of median nerve at forearm level, unspecified arm

✓x7ᵗʰ **S54.11** Injury of median nerve at forearm level, right arm

✓x7ᵗʰ **S54.12** Injury of median nerve at forearm level, left arm

✓5ᵗʰ **S54.2 Injury of radial nerve at forearm level**
 Injury of radial nerve NOS

✓x7ᵗʰ **S54.20** Injury of radial nerve at forearm level, unspecified arm

✓x7ᵗʰ **S54.21** Injury of radial nerve at forearm level, right arm

✓x7ᵗʰ **S54.22** Injury of radial nerve at forearm level, left arm

✓5ᵗʰ **S54.3 Injury of cutaneous sensory nerve at forearm level**

✓x7ᵗʰ **S54.30** Injury of cutaneous sensory nerve at forearm level, unspecified arm

✓x7ᵗʰ **S54.31** Injury of cutaneous sensory nerve at forearm level, right arm

✓x7ᵗʰ **S54.32** Injury of cutaneous sensory nerve at forearm level, left arm

✓5ᵗʰ **S54.8 Injury of other nerves at forearm level**

✓6ᵗʰ **S54.8X** Injury of other nerves at forearm level

 ✓7ᵗʰ **S54.8X1** Injury of other nerves at forearm level, right arm

 ✓7ᵗʰ **S54.8X2** Injury of other nerves at forearm level, left arm

 ✓7ᵗʰ **S54.8X9** Injury of other nerves at forearm level, unspecified arm

✓5ᵗʰ **S54.9 Injury of unspecified nerve at forearm level**

✓x7ᵗʰ **S54.90** Injury of unspecified nerve at forearm level, unspecified arm

✓x7ᵗʰ **S54.91** Injury of unspecified nerve at forearm level, right arm

✓x7ᵗʰ **S54.92** Injury of unspecified nerve at forearm level, left arm

✓4ᵗʰ **S55 Injury of blood vessels at forearm level**
 Code also any associated open wound (S51.-)
 **EXCLUDES 2** *injury of blood vessels at wrist and hand level (S65.-)*
 *injury of brachial vessels (S45.1-S45.2)*

 The appropriate 7th character is to be added to each code from category S55.
 A  initial encounter
 D  subsequent encounter
 S  sequela

✓5ᵗʰ **S55.0 Injury of ulnar artery at forearm level**

 **CC Excl:** For CC codes in subcategory S55.0:
 **Right side:** PDX collection 1274
 **Left side:** PDX collection 1275
 **Unspecified side:** PDX collection 1276

✓6ᵗʰ **S55.00** Unspecified injury of ulnar artery at forearm level

 ✓7ᵗʰ **S55.001** Unspecified injury of ulnar artery at forearm level, right arm  CC

 ✓7ᵗʰ **S55.002** Unspecified injury of ulnar artery at forearm level, left arm  CC

 ✓7ᵗʰ **S55.009** Unspecified injury of ulnar artery at forearm level, unspecified arm  CC

✓6ᵗʰ **S55.01** Laceration of ulnar artery at forearm level

 ✓7ᵗʰ **S55.011** Laceration of ulnar artery at forearm level, right arm  CC

 ✓7ᵗʰ **S55.012** Laceration of ulnar artery at forearm level, left arm  CC

 ✓7ᵗʰ **S55.019** Laceration of ulnar artery at forearm level, unspecified arm  CC

✓6ᵗʰ **S55.09** Other specified injury of ulnar artery at forearm level

 ✓7ᵗʰ **S55.091** Other specified injury of ulnar artery at forearm level, right arm  CC

 ✓7ᵗʰ **S55.092** Other specified injury of ulnar artery at forearm level, left arm  CC

 ✓7ᵗʰ **S55.099** Other specified injury of ulnar artery at forearm level, unspecified arm  CC

✓ Additional Character Req   ✓x7ᵗʰ Placeholder Alert   Unacceptable PDx   ▬ Manifestation   H1-H14 HAC   HCC CMS-HCC Condition   **EXCLUDES 1** Not Coded Here   **EXCLUDES 2** Not Included Here

ICD-10-CM 2018     1005

√5ᵗʰ **S55.1 Injury of radial artery at forearm level**

> **CC Excl: For CC codes in subcategory S55.1:**
> **Right side:** PDX collection 1277
> **Left side:** PDX collection 1278
> **Unspecified side:** PDX collection 1279

√6ᵗʰ **S55.10 Unspecified injury of radial artery at forearm level**

√7ᵗʰ **S55.101 Unspecified injury of radial artery at forearm level, right arm** `CC`

√7ᵗʰ **S55.102 Unspecified injury of radial artery at forearm level, left arm** `CC`

√7ᵗʰ **S55.109 Unspecified injury of radial artery at forearm level, unspecified arm** `CC`

√6ᵗʰ **S55.11 Laceration of radial artery at forearm level**

√7ᵗʰ **S55.111 Laceration of radial artery at forearm level, right arm** `CC`

√7ᵗʰ **S55.112 Laceration of radial artery at forearm level, left arm** `CC`

√7ᵗʰ **S55.119 Laceration of radial artery at forearm level, unspecified arm** `CC`

√6ᵗʰ **S55.19 Other specified injury of radial artery at forearm level**

√7ᵗʰ **S55.191 Other specified injury of radial artery at forearm level, right arm** `CC`

√7ᵗʰ **S55.192 Other specified injury of radial artery at forearm level, left arm** `CC`

√7ᵗʰ **S55.199 Other specified injury of radial artery at forearm level, unspecified arm** `CC`

√5ᵗʰ **S55.2 Injury of vein at forearm level**

> **CC Excl: For CC codes in subcategory S55.2:**
> **Right side:** PDX collection 1260
> **Left side:** PDX collection 1261
> **Unspecified side:** PDX collection 1262

√6ᵗʰ **S55.20 Unspecified injury of vein at forearm level**

√7ᵗʰ **S55.201 Unspecified injury of vein at forearm level, right arm** `CC`

√7ᵗʰ **S55.202 Unspecified injury of vein at forearm level, left arm** `CC`

√7ᵗʰ **S55.209 Unspecified injury of vein at forearm level, unspecified arm** `CC`

√6ᵗʰ **S55.21 Laceration of vein at forearm level**

√7ᵗʰ **S55.211 Laceration of vein at forearm level, right arm** `CC`

√7ᵗʰ **S55.212 Laceration of vein at forearm level, left arm** `CC`

√7ᵗʰ **S55.219 Laceration of vein at forearm level, unspecified arm** `CC`

√6ᵗʰ **S55.29 Other specified injury of vein at forearm level**

√7ᵗʰ **S55.291 Other specified injury of vein at forearm level, right arm** `CC`

√7ᵗʰ **S55.292 Other specified injury of vein at forearm level, left arm** `CC`

√7ᵗʰ **S55.299 Other specified injury of vein at forearm level, unspecified arm** `CC`

√5ᵗʰ **S55.8 Injury of other blood vessels at forearm level**

> **CC Excl: For CC codes in subcategory S55.8:**
> **Right side:** PDX collection 1260
> **Left side:** PDX collection 1261
> **Unspecified side:** PDX collection 1262

√6ᵗʰ **S55.80 Unspecified injury of other blood vessels at forearm level**

√7ᵗʰ **S55.801 Unspecified injury of other blood vessels at forearm level, right arm** `CC`

√7ᵗʰ **S55.802 Unspecified injury of other blood vessels at forearm level, left arm** `CC`

√7ᵗʰ **S55.809 Unspecified injury of other blood vessels at forearm level, unspecified arm** `CC`

√6ᵗʰ **S55.81 Laceration of other blood vessels at forearm level**

√7ᵗʰ **S55.811 Laceration of other blood vessels at forearm level, right arm** `CC`

√7ᵗʰ **S55.812 Laceration of other blood vessels at forearm level, left arm** `CC`

√7ᵗʰ **S55.819 Laceration of other blood vessels at forearm level, unspecified arm** `CC`

√6ᵗʰ **S55.89 Other specified injury of other blood vessels at forearm level**

√7ᵗʰ **S55.891 Other specified injury of other blood vessels at forearm level, right arm** `CC`

√7ᵗʰ **S55.892 Other specified injury of other blood vessels at forearm level, left arm** `CC`

√7ᵗʰ **S55.899 Other specified injury of other blood vessels at forearm level, unspecified arm** `CC`

√5ᵗʰ **S55.9 Injury of unspecified blood vessel at forearm level**

> **CC Excl: For CC codes in subcategory S55.9:**
> **Right side:** PDX collection 1260
> **Left side:** PDX collection 1261
> **Unspecified side:** PDX collection 1262

√6ᵗʰ **S55.90 Unspecified injury of unspecified blood vessel at forearm level**

√7ᵗʰ **S55.901 Unspecified injury of unspecified blood vessel at forearm level, right arm** `CC`

√7ᵗʰ **S55.902 Unspecified injury of unspecified blood vessel at forearm level, left arm** `CC`

√7ᵗʰ **S55.909 Unspecified injury of unspecified blood vessel at forearm level, unspecified arm** `CC`

√6ᵗʰ **S55.91 Laceration of unspecified blood vessel at forearm level**

√7ᵗʰ **S55.911 Laceration of unspecified blood vessel at forearm level, right arm** `CC`

√7ᵗʰ **S55.912 Laceration of unspecified blood vessel at forearm level, left arm** `CC`

√7ᵗʰ **S55.919 Laceration of unspecified blood vessel at forearm level, unspecified arm** `CC`

√6ᵗʰ **S55.99 Other specified injury of unspecified blood vessel at forearm level**

√7ᵗʰ **S55.991 Other specified injury of unspecified blood vessel at forearm level, right arm** `CC`

√7ᵗʰ **S55.992 Other specified injury of unspecified blood vessel at forearm level, left arm** `CC`

√7ᵗʰ **S55.999 Other specified injury of unspecified blood vessel at forearm level, unspecified arm** `CC`

√4ᵗʰ **S56 Injury of muscle, fascia and tendon at forearm level**

Code also any associated open wound (S51.-)

**EXCLUDES 2** injury of muscle, fascia and tendon at or below wrist (S66.-)
sprain of joints and ligaments of elbow (S53.4-)

**TIP:** Refer to the Muscle/Tendon table at the beginning of this chapter.

> The appropriate 7th character is to be added to each code from category S56.
> A    initial encounter
> D    subsequent encounter
> S    sequela

> **CC Excl: For CC codes in category S56:**
> **Right side:** PDX collection 1280
> **Left side:** PDX collection 1281
> **Unspecified side:** PDX collection 1282

√5ᵗʰ **S56.0 Injury of flexor muscle, fascia and tendon of thumb at forearm level**

√6ᵗʰ **S56.00 Unspecified injury of flexor muscle, fascia and tendon of thumb at forearm level**

√7ᵗʰ **S56.001 Unspecified injury of flexor muscle, fascia and tendon of right thumb at forearm level**

√7ᵗʰ **S56.002 Unspecified injury of flexor muscle, fascia and tendon of left thumb at forearm level**

√7ᵗʰ **S56.009 Unspecified injury of flexor muscle, fascia and tendon of unspecified thumb at forearm level**

√6ᵗʰ **S56.01 Strain of flexor muscle, fascia and tendon of thumb at forearm level**

√7ᵗʰ **S56.011 Strain of flexor muscle, fascia and tendon of right thumb at forearm level**

√7ᵗʰ **S56.012 Strain of flexor muscle, fascia and tendon of left thumb at forearm level**

√7ᵗʰ **S56.019 Strain of flexor muscle, fascia and tendon of unspecified thumb at forearm level**

Ⓝ Newborn: 0   Ⓟ Pediatric: 0-17   Ⓜ Maternity: 12-55   Ⓐ Adult: 15-124   **MCC** Major CC Condition   **PDxMCC** PDx acts as own MCC   **CC** CC Condition   **PDxCC** PDx acts as own CC

1006       ICD-10-CM 2018

✓6ᵗʰ **S56.02** Laceration of flexor muscle, fascia and tendon of thumb at forearm level

  ✓7ᵗʰ **S56.021** Laceration of flexor muscle, fascia and ᴄᴄ tendon of right thumb at forearm level

  ✓7ᵗʰ **S56.022** Laceration of flexor muscle, fascia and ᴄᴄ tendon of left thumb at forearm level

  ✓7ᵗʰ **S56.029** Laceration of flexor muscle, fascia and ᴄᴄ tendon of unspecified thumb at forearm level

✓6ᵗʰ **S56.09** Other injury of flexor muscle, fascia and tendon of thumb at forearm level

  ✓7ᵗʰ **S56.091** Other injury of flexor muscle, fascia and tendon of right thumb at forearm level

  ✓7ᵗʰ **S56.092** Other injury of flexor muscle, fascia and tendon of left thumb at forearm level

  ✓7ᵗʰ **S56.099** Other injury of flexor muscle, fascia and tendon of unspecified thumb at forearm level

✓5ᵗʰ **S56.1** Injury of flexor muscle, fascia and tendon of other and unspecified finger at forearm level

  ✓6ᵗʰ **S56.10** Unspecified injury of flexor muscle, fascia and tendon of other and unspecified finger at forearm level

    ✓7ᵗʰ **S56.101** Unspecified injury of flexor muscle, fascia and tendon of right index finger at forearm level

    ✓7ᵗʰ **S56.102** Unspecified injury of flexor muscle, fascia and tendon of left index finger at forearm level

    ✓7ᵗʰ **S56.103** Unspecified injury of flexor muscle, fascia and tendon of right middle finger at forearm level

    ✓7ᵗʰ **S56.104** Unspecified injury of flexor muscle, fascia and tendon of left middle finger at forearm level

    ✓7ᵗʰ **S56.105** Unspecified injury of flexor muscle, fascia and tendon of right ring finger at forearm level

    ✓7ᵗʰ **S56.106** Unspecified injury of flexor muscle, fascia and tendon of left ring finger at forearm level

    ✓7ᵗʰ **S56.107** Unspecified injury of flexor muscle, fascia and tendon of right little finger at forearm level

    ✓7ᵗʰ **S56.108** Unspecified injury of flexor muscle, fascia and tendon of left little finger at forearm level

    ✓7ᵗʰ **S56.109** Unspecified injury of flexor muscle, fascia and tendon of unspecified finger at forearm level

  ✓6ᵗʰ **S56.11** Strain of flexor muscle, fascia and tendon of other and unspecified finger at forearm level

    ✓7ᵗʰ **S56.111** Strain of flexor muscle, fascia and tendon of right index finger at forearm level

    ✓7ᵗʰ **S56.112** Strain of flexor muscle, fascia and tendon of left index finger at forearm level

    ✓7ᵗʰ **S56.113** Strain of flexor muscle, fascia and tendon of right middle finger at forearm level

    ✓7ᵗʰ **S56.114** Strain of flexor muscle, fascia and tendon of left middle finger at forearm level

    ✓7ᵗʰ **S56.115** Strain of flexor muscle, fascia and tendon of right ring finger at forearm level

    ✓7ᵗʰ **S56.116** Strain of flexor muscle, fascia and tendon of left ring finger at forearm level

    ✓7ᵗʰ **S56.117** Strain of flexor muscle, fascia and tendon of right little finger at forearm level

    ✓7ᵗʰ **S56.118** Strain of flexor muscle, fascia and tendon of left little finger at forearm level

    ✓7ᵗʰ **S56.119** Strain of flexor muscle, fascia and tendon of finger of unspecified finger at forearm level

  ✓6ᵗʰ **S56.12** Laceration of flexor muscle, fascia and tendon of other and unspecified finger at forearm level

    ✓7ᵗʰ **S56.121** Laceration of flexor muscle, fascia and ᴄᴄ tendon of right index finger at forearm level

  ✓7ᵗʰ **S56.122** Laceration of flexor muscle, fascia and ᴄᴄ tendon of left index finger at forearm level

  ✓7ᵗʰ **S56.123** Laceration of flexor muscle, fascia and ᴄᴄ tendon of right middle finger at forearm level

  ✓7ᵗʰ **S56.124** Laceration of flexor muscle, fascia and ᴄᴄ tendon of left middle finger at forearm level

  ✓7ᵗʰ **S56.125** Laceration of flexor muscle, fascia and ᴄᴄ tendon of right ring finger at forearm level

  ✓7ᵗʰ **S56.126** Laceration of flexor muscle, fascia and ᴄᴄ tendon of left ring finger at forearm level

  ✓7ᵗʰ **S56.127** Laceration of flexor muscle, fascia and ᴄᴄ tendon of right little finger at forearm level

  ✓7ᵗʰ **S56.128** Laceration of flexor muscle, fascia and ᴄᴄ tendon of left little finger at forearm level

  ✓7ᵗʰ **S56.129** Laceration of flexor muscle, fascia and ᴄᴄ tendon of unspecified finger at forearm level

✓6ᵗʰ **S56.19** Other injury of flexor muscle, fascia and tendon of other and unspecified finger at forearm level

  ✓7ᵗʰ **S56.191** Other injury of flexor muscle, fascia and tendon of right index finger at forearm level

  ✓7ᵗʰ **S56.192** Other injury of flexor muscle, fascia and tendon of left index finger at forearm level

  ✓7ᵗʰ **S56.193** Other injury of flexor muscle, fascia and tendon of right middle finger at forearm level

  ✓7ᵗʰ **S56.194** Other injury of flexor muscle, fascia and tendon of left middle finger at forearm level

  ✓7ᵗʰ **S56.195** Other injury of flexor muscle, fascia and tendon of right ring finger at forearm level

  ✓7ᵗʰ **S56.196** Other injury of flexor muscle, fascia and tendon of left ring finger at forearm level

  ✓7ᵗʰ **S56.197** Other injury of flexor muscle, fascia and tendon of right little finger at forearm level

  ✓7ᵗʰ **S56.198** Other injury of flexor muscle, fascia and tendon of left little finger at forearm level

  ✓7ᵗʰ **S56.199** Other injury of flexor muscle, fascia and tendon of unspecified finger at forearm level

✓5ᵗʰ **S56.2** Injury of other flexor muscle, fascia and tendon at forearm level

  ✓6ᵗʰ **S56.20** Unspecified injury of other flexor muscle, fascia and tendon at forearm level

    ✓7ᵗʰ **S56.201** Unspecified injury of other flexor muscle, fascia and tendon at forearm level, right arm

    ✓7ᵗʰ **S56.202** Unspecified injury of other flexor muscle, fascia and tendon at forearm level, left arm

    ✓7ᵗʰ **S56.209** Unspecified injury of other flexor muscle, fascia and tendon at forearm level, unspecified arm

  ✓6ᵗʰ **S56.21** Strain of other flexor muscle, fascia and tendon at forearm level

    ✓7ᵗʰ **S56.211** Strain of other flexor muscle, fascia and tendon at forearm level, right arm

    ✓7ᵗʰ **S56.212** Strain of other flexor muscle, fascia and tendon at forearm level, left arm

    ✓7ᵗʰ **S56.219** Strain of other flexor muscle, fascia and tendon at forearm level, unspecified arm

  ✓6ᵗʰ **S56.22** Laceration of other flexor muscle, fascia and tendon at forearm level

    ✓7ᵗʰ **S56.221** Laceration of other flexor muscle, ᴄᴄ fascia and tendon at forearm level, right arm

☑ Additional Character Req   ✓x7ᵗʰ Placeholder Alert   Unacceptable PDx   **Manifestation**   **H1**–**H14** HAC   **HCC** CMS-HCC Condition   *EXCLUDES 1* Not Coded Here   *EXCLUDES 2* Not Included Here

ICD-10-CM 2018     1007

√7ᵗʰ **S56.222** **Laceration of other flexor muscle, fascia and tendon at forearm level, left arm** `CC`

√7ᵗʰ **S56.229** **Laceration of other flexor muscle, fascia and tendon at forearm level, unspecified arm** `CC`

√6ᵗʰ **S56.29** **Other injury** of other flexor muscle, fascia and tendon at forearm level

√7ᵗʰ **S56.291** **Other injury of other flexor muscle, fascia and tendon at forearm level, right arm**

√7ᵗʰ **S56.292** **Other injury of other flexor muscle, fascia and tendon at forearm level, left arm**

√7ᵗʰ **S56.299** **Other injury of other flexor muscle, fascia and tendon at forearm level, unspecified arm**

√5ᵗʰ **S56.3** **Injury of** extensor or abductor **muscles, fascia and tendons of thumb at forearm level**

√6ᵗʰ **S56.30** **Unspecified** injury of extensor or abductor muscles, fascia and tendons of thumb at forearm level

√7ᵗʰ **S56.301** **Unspecified injury of extensor or abductor muscles, fascia and tendons of right thumb at forearm level**

√7ᵗʰ **S56.302** **Unspecified injury of extensor or abductor muscles, fascia and tendons of left thumb at forearm level**

√7ᵗʰ **S56.309** **Unspecified injury of extensor or abductor muscles, fascia and tendons of unspecified thumb at forearm level**

√6ᵗʰ **S56.31** **Strain** of extensor or abductor muscles, fascia and tendons of thumb at forearm level

√7ᵗʰ **S56.311** **Strain of extensor or abductor muscles, fascia and tendons of right thumb at forearm level**

√7ᵗʰ **S56.312** **Strain of extensor or abductor muscles, fascia and tendons of left thumb at forearm level**

√7ᵗʰ **S56.319** **Strain of extensor or abductor muscles, fascia and tendons of unspecified thumb at forearm level**

√6ᵗʰ **S56.32** **Laceration** of extensor or abductor muscles, fascia and tendons of thumb at forearm level

√7ᵗʰ **S56.321** **Laceration of extensor or abductor muscles, fascia and tendons of right thumb at forearm level** `CC`

√7ᵗʰ **S56.322** **Laceration of extensor or abductor muscles, fascia and tendons of left thumb at forearm level** `CC`

√7ᵗʰ **S56.329** **Laceration of extensor or abductor muscles, fascia and tendons of unspecified thumb at forearm level** `CC`

√6ᵗʰ **S56.39** **Other injury** of extensor or abductor muscles, fascia and tendons of thumb at forearm level

√7ᵗʰ **S56.391** **Other injury of extensor or abductor muscles, fascia and tendons of right thumb at forearm level**

√7ᵗʰ **S56.392** **Other injury of extensor or abductor muscles, fascia and tendons of left thumb at forearm level**

√7ᵗʰ **S56.399** **Other injury of extensor or abductor muscles, fascia and tendons of unspecified thumb at forearm level**

√5ᵗʰ **S56.4** **Injury of** extensor **muscle, fascia and tendon of other and unspecified** finger **at forearm level**

√6ᵗʰ **S56.40** **Unspecified** injury of extensor muscle, fascia and tendon of other and unspecified finger at forearm level

√7ᵗʰ **S56.401** **Unspecified injury of extensor muscle, fascia and tendon of right index finger at forearm level**

√7ᵗʰ **S56.402** **Unspecified injury of extensor muscle, fascia and tendon of left index finger at forearm level**

√7ᵗʰ **S56.403** **Unspecified injury of extensor muscle, fascia and tendon of right middle finger at forearm level**

√7ᵗʰ **S56.404** **Unspecified injury of extensor muscle, fascia and tendon of left middle finger at forearm level**

√7ᵗʰ **S56.405** **Unspecified injury of extensor muscle, fascia and tendon of right ring finger at forearm level**

√7ᵗʰ **S56.406** **Unspecified injury of extensor muscle, fascia and tendon of left ring finger at forearm level**

√7ᵗʰ **S56.407** **Unspecified injury of extensor muscle, fascia and tendon of right little finger at forearm level**

√7ᵗʰ **S56.408** **Unspecified injury of extensor muscle, fascia and tendon of left little finger at forearm level**

√7ᵗʰ **S56.409** **Unspecified injury of extensor muscle, fascia and tendon of unspecified finger at forearm level**

√6ᵗʰ **S56.41** **Strain of** extensor muscle, fascia and tendon of other and unspecified finger at forearm level

√7ᵗʰ **S56.411** **Strain of extensor muscle, fascia and tendon of right index finger at forearm level**

√7ᵗʰ **S56.412** **Strain of extensor muscle, fascia and tendon of left index finger at forearm level**

√7ᵗʰ **S56.413** **Strain of extensor muscle, fascia and tendon of right middle finger at forearm level**

√7ᵗʰ **S56.414** **Strain of extensor muscle, fascia and tendon of left middle finger at forearm level**

√7ᵗʰ **S56.415** **Strain of extensor muscle, fascia and tendon of right ring finger at forearm level**

√7ᵗʰ **S56.416** **Strain of extensor muscle, fascia and tendon of left ring finger at forearm level**

√7ᵗʰ **S56.417** **Strain of extensor muscle, fascia and tendon of right little finger at forearm level**

√7ᵗʰ **S56.418** **Strain of extensor muscle, fascia and tendon of left little finger at forearm level**

√7ᵗʰ **S56.419** **Strain of extensor muscle, fascia and tendon of finger, unspecified finger at forearm level**

√6ᵗʰ **S56.42** **Laceration of** extensor muscle, fascia and tendon of other and unspecified finger at forearm level

√7ᵗʰ **S56.421** **Laceration of extensor muscle, fascia and tendon of right index finger at forearm level** `CC`

√7ᵗʰ **S56.422** **Laceration of extensor muscle, fascia and tendon of left index finger at forearm level** `CC`

√7ᵗʰ **S56.423** **Laceration of extensor muscle, fascia and tendon of right middle finger at forearm level** `CC`

√7ᵗʰ **S56.424** **Laceration of extensor muscle, fascia and tendon of left middle finger at forearm level** `CC`

√7ᵗʰ **S56.425** **Laceration of extensor muscle, fascia and tendon of right ring finger at forearm level** `CC`

√7ᵗʰ **S56.426** **Laceration of extensor muscle, fascia and tendon of left ring finger at forearm level** `CC`

√7ᵗʰ **S56.427** **Laceration of extensor muscle, fascia and tendon of right little finger at forearm level** `CC`

√7ᵗʰ **S56.428** **Laceration of extensor muscle, fascia and tendon of left little finger at forearm level** `CC`

√7ᵗʰ **S56.429** **Laceration of extensor muscle, fascia and tendon of unspecified finger at forearm level** `CC`

√6ᵗʰ **S56.49** **Other injury** of extensor muscle, fascia and tendon of other and unspecified finger at forearm level

√7ᵗʰ **S56.491** **Other injury of extensor muscle, fascia and tendon of right index finger at forearm level**

√7ᵗʰ **S56.492** **Other injury of extensor muscle, fascia and tendon of left index finger at forearm level**

☑7ᵗʰ **S56.493** Other injury of extensor muscle, fascia and tendon of right middle finger at forearm level

☑7ᵗʰ **S56.494** Other injury of extensor muscle, fascia and tendon of left middle finger at forearm level

☑7ᵗʰ **S56.495** Other injury of extensor muscle, fascia and tendon of right ring finger at forearm level

☑7ᵗʰ **S56.496** Other injury of extensor muscle, fascia and tendon of left ring finger at forearm level

☑7ᵗʰ **S56.497** Other injury of extensor muscle, fascia and tendon of right little finger at forearm level

☑7ᵗʰ **S56.498** Other injury of extensor muscle, fascia and tendon of left little finger at forearm level

☑7ᵗʰ **S56.499** Other injury of extensor muscle, fascia and tendon of unspecified finger at forearm level

☑5ᵗʰ **S56.5** Injury of other extensor muscle, fascia and tendon at forearm level

☑6ᵗʰ **S56.50** Unspecified injury of other extensor muscle, fascia and tendon at forearm level

☑7ᵗʰ **S56.501** Unspecified injury of other extensor muscle, fascia and tendon at forearm level, right arm

☑7ᵗʰ **S56.502** Unspecified injury of other extensor muscle, fascia and tendon at forearm level, left arm

☑7ᵗʰ **S56.509** Unspecified injury of other extensor muscle, fascia and tendon at forearm level, unspecified arm

☑6ᵗʰ **S56.51** Strain of other extensor muscle, fascia and tendon at forearm level

☑7ᵗʰ **S56.511** Strain of other extensor muscle, fascia and tendon at forearm level, right arm

☑7ᵗʰ **S56.512** Strain of other extensor muscle, fascia and tendon at forearm level, left arm

☑7ᵗʰ **S56.519** Strain of other extensor muscle, fascia and tendon at forearm level, unspecified arm

☑6ᵗʰ **S56.52** Laceration of other extensor muscle, fascia and tendon at forearm level

☑7ᵗʰ **S56.521** Laceration of other extensor muscle, fascia and tendon at forearm level, right arm   `CC`

☑7ᵗʰ **S56.522** Laceration of other extensor muscle, fascia and tendon at forearm level, left arm   `CC`

☑7ᵗʰ **S56.529** Laceration of other extensor muscle, fascia and tendon at forearm level, unspecified arm   `CC`

☑6ᵗʰ **S56.59** Other injury of other extensor muscle, fascia and tendon at forearm level

☑7ᵗʰ **S56.591** Other injury of other extensor muscle, fascia and tendon at forearm level, right arm

☑7ᵗʰ **S56.592** Other injury of other extensor muscle, fascia and tendon at forearm level, left arm

☑7ᵗʰ **S56.599** Other injury of other extensor muscle, fascia and tendon at forearm level, unspecified arm

☑5ᵗʰ **S56.8** Injury of other muscles, fascia and tendons at forearm level

☑6ᵗʰ **S56.80** Unspecified injury of other muscles, fascia and tendons at forearm level

☑7ᵗʰ **S56.801** Unspecified injury of other muscles, fascia and tendons at forearm level, right arm

☑7ᵗʰ **S56.802** Unspecified injury of other muscles, fascia and tendons at forearm level, left arm

☑7ᵗʰ **S56.809** Unspecified injury of other muscles, fascia and tendons at forearm level, unspecified arm

☑6ᵗʰ **S56.81** Strain of other muscles, fascia and tendons at forearm level

☑7ᵗʰ **S56.811** Strain of other muscles, fascia and tendons at forearm level, right arm

☑7ᵗʰ **S56.812** Strain of other muscles, fascia and tendons at forearm level, left arm

☑7ᵗʰ **S56.819** Strain of other muscles, fascia and tendons at forearm level, unspecified arm

☑6ᵗʰ **S56.82** Laceration of other muscles, fascia and tendons at forearm level

☑7ᵗʰ **S56.821** Laceration of other muscles, fascia and tendons at forearm level, right arm   `CC`

☑7ᵗʰ **S56.822** Laceration of other muscles, fascia and tendons at forearm level, left arm   `CC`

☑7ᵗʰ **S56.829** Laceration of other muscles, fascia and tendons at forearm level, unspecified arm   `CC`

☑6ᵗʰ **S56.89** Other injury of other muscles, fascia and tendons at forearm level

☑7ᵗʰ **S56.891** Other injury of other muscles, fascia and tendons at forearm level, right arm

☑7ᵗʰ **S56.892** Other injury of other muscles, fascia and tendons at forearm level, left arm

☑7ᵗʰ **S56.899** Other injury of other muscles, fascia and tendons at forearm level, unspecified arm

☑5ᵗʰ **S56.9** Injury of unspecified muscles, fascia and tendons at forearm level

☑6ᵗʰ **S56.90** Unspecified injury of unspecified muscles, fascia and tendons at forearm level

☑7ᵗʰ **S56.901** Unspecified injury of unspecified muscles, fascia and tendons at forearm level, right arm

☑7ᵗʰ **S56.902** Unspecified injury of unspecified muscles, fascia and tendons at forearm level, left arm

☑7ᵗʰ **S56.909** Unspecified injury of unspecified muscles, fascia and tendons at forearm level, unspecified arm

☑6ᵗʰ **S56.91** Strain of unspecified muscles, fascia and tendons at forearm level

☑7ᵗʰ **S56.911** Strain of unspecified muscles, fascia and tendons at forearm level, right arm

☑7ᵗʰ **S56.912** Strain of unspecified muscles, fascia and tendons at forearm level, left arm

☑7ᵗʰ **S56.919** Strain of unspecified muscles, fascia and tendons at forearm level, unspecified arm

☑6ᵗʰ **S56.92** Laceration of unspecified muscles, fascia and tendons at forearm level

☑7ᵗʰ **S56.921** Laceration of unspecified muscles, fascia and tendons at forearm level, right arm   `CC`

☑7ᵗʰ **S56.922** Laceration of unspecified muscles, fascia and tendons at forearm level, left arm   `CC`

☑7ᵗʰ **S56.929** Laceration of unspecified muscles, fascia and tendons at forearm level, unspecified arm   `CC`

☑6ᵗʰ **S56.99** Other injury of unspecified muscles, fascia and tendons at forearm level

☑7ᵗʰ **S56.991** Other injury of unspecified muscles, fascia and tendons at forearm level, right arm

☑7ᵗʰ **S56.992** Other injury of unspecified muscles, fascia and tendons at forearm level, left arm

☑7ᵗʰ **S56.999** Other injury of unspecified muscles, fascia and tendons at forearm level, unspecified arm

☑4ᵗʰ **S57** **Crushing injury of elbow and forearm**

Use additional code(s) for all associated injuries
*EXCLUDES 2*   crushing injury of wrist and hand (S67.-)

The appropriate 7th character is to be added to each code from category S57.
A   initial encounter
D   subsequent encounter
S   sequela

☑5ᵗʰ **S57.0** **Crushing injury of elbow**

☑×7ᵗʰ **S57.00** Crushing injury of unspecified elbow

☑×7ᵗʰ **S57.01** Crushing injury of right elbow

☑×7ᵗʰ **S57.02** Crushing injury of left elbow

☑5ᵗʰ **S57.8** **Crushing injury of forearm**

☑×7ᵗʰ **S57.80** Crushing injury of unspecified forearm

☑ Additional Character Req   ☑×7ᵗʰ Placeholder Alert   Unacceptable PDx   **Manifestation**   `H1`-`H14` HAC   `HCC` CMS-HCC Condition   *EXCLUDES 1* Not Coded Here   *EXCLUDES 2* Not Included Here

ICD-10-CM 2018      **1009**

**✓x7ᵗʰ S57.81 Crushing injury of right forearm**

**✓x7ᵗʰ S57.82 Crushing injury of left forearm**

**✓4ᵗʰ S58 Traumatic amputation of elbow and forearm**

An amputation not identified as partial or complete should be coded to complete.

**EXCLUDES 1** *traumatic amputation of wrist and hand (S68.-)*

The appropriate 7th character is to be added to each code from category S58.
A   initial encounter
D   subsequent encounter
S   sequela

**CC Excl: For CC codes in category S58:**
**Right side:** PDX collection 1266
**Left side:** PDX collection 1267
**Unspecified side:** PDX collection 1268

**✓5ᵗʰ S58.0 Traumatic amputation at elbow level**

**✓6ᵗʰ S58.01 Complete traumatic amputation at elbow level**

11 ✓7ᵗʰ **S58.011 Complete traumatic amputation at elbow level, right arm** `CC` `HCC`

11 ✓7ᵗʰ **S58.012 Complete traumatic amputation at elbow level, left arm** `CC` `HCC`

11 ✓7ᵗʰ **S58.019 Complete traumatic amputation at elbow level, unspecified arm** `CC` `HCC`

**✓6ᵗʰ S58.02 Partial traumatic amputation at elbow level**

11 ✓7ᵗʰ **S58.021 Partial traumatic amputation at elbow level, right arm** `CC` `HCC`

11 ✓7ᵗʰ **S58.022 Partial traumatic amputation at elbow level, left arm** `CC` `HCC`

11 ✓7ᵗʰ **S58.029 Partial traumatic amputation at elbow level, unspecified arm** `CC` `HCC`

**✓5ᵗʰ S58.1 Traumatic amputation at level between elbow and wrist**

**✓6ᵗʰ S58.11 Complete traumatic amputation at level between elbow and wrist**

11 ✓7ᵗʰ **S58.111 Complete traumatic amputation at level between elbow and wrist, right arm** `CC` `HCC`

11 ✓7ᵗʰ **S58.112 Complete traumatic amputation at level between elbow and wrist, left arm** `CC` `HCC`

11 ✓7ᵗʰ **S58.119 Complete traumatic amputation at level between elbow and wrist, unspecified arm** `CC` `HCC`

**✓6ᵗʰ S58.12 Partial traumatic amputation at level between elbow and wrist**

11 ✓7ᵗʰ **S58.121 Partial traumatic amputation at level between elbow and wrist, right arm** `CC` `HCC`

11 ✓7ᵗʰ **S58.122 Partial traumatic amputation at level between elbow and wrist, left arm** `CC` `HCC`

11 ✓7ᵗʰ **S58.129 Partial traumatic amputation at level between elbow and wrist, unspecified arm** `CC` `HCC`

**✓5ᵗʰ S58.9 Traumatic amputation of forearm, level unspecified**

**EXCLUDES 1** *traumatic amputation of wrist (S68.-)*

**✓6ᵗʰ S58.91 Complete traumatic amputation of forearm, level unspecified**

11 ✓7ᵗʰ **S58.911 Complete traumatic amputation of right forearm, level unspecified** `CC` `HCC`

11 ✓7ᵗʰ **S58.912 Complete traumatic amputation of left forearm, level unspecified** `CC` `HCC`

11 ✓7ᵗʰ **S58.919 Complete traumatic amputation of unspecified forearm, level unspecified** `CC` `HCC`

**✓6ᵗʰ S58.92 Partial traumatic amputation of forearm, level unspecified**

11 ✓7ᵗʰ **S58.921 Partial traumatic amputation of right forearm, level unspecified** `CC` `HCC`

11 ✓7ᵗʰ **S58.922 Partial traumatic amputation of left forearm, level unspecified** `CC` `HCC`

11 ✓7ᵗʰ **S58.929 Partial traumatic amputation of unspecified forearm, level unspecified** `CC` `HCC`

**✓4ᵗʰ S59 Other and unspecified injuries of elbow and forearm**

**EXCLUDES 2** *other and unspecified injuries of wrist and hand (S69.-)*
**AHA:** 2015, 3Q, 37-39

The appropriate 7th character is to be added to each code from subcategories S59.0, S59.1, and S59.2.
A   initial encounter for closed fracture
D   subsequent encounter for fracture with routine healing
G   subsequent encounter for fracture with delayed healing
K   subsequent encounter for fracture with nonunion
P   subsequent encounter for fracture with malunion
S   sequela

**✓5ᵗʰ S59.0 Physeal fracture of lower end of ulna**

**CC Excl: For CC codes in subcategory S59.0:**
**Right side:** See code S59.001
**Left side:** See code S59.002
**Unspecified side:** See code S59.009

**✓6ᵗʰ S59.00 Unspecified physeal fracture of lower end of ulna**

7 ✓7ᵗʰ **S59.001 Unspecified physeal fracture of lower end of ulna, right arm** `CC` `H5`
**CC Excl: CC with 7th character A:** PDX collection 1270
**CC with 7th character K or P:** PDX collection 897

7 ✓7ᵗʰ **S59.002 Unspecified physeal fracture of lower end of ulna, left arm** `CC` `H5`
**CC Excl: CC with 7th character A:** PDX collection 1271
**CC with 7th character K or P:** PDX collection 897

7 ✓7ᵗʰ **S59.009 Unspecified physeal fracture of lower end of ulna, unspecified arm** `CC` `H5`
**CC Excl: CC with 7th character A:** PDX collection 1272
**CC with 7th character K or P:** PDX collection 897

**✓6ᵗʰ S59.01 Salter-Harris Type I physeal fracture of lower end of ulna**

7 ✓7ᵗʰ **S59.011 Salter-Harris Type I physeal fracture of lower end of ulna, right arm** `CC` `H5`

7 ✓7ᵗʰ **S59.012 Salter-Harris Type I physeal fracture of lower end of ulna, left arm** `CC` `H5`

7 ✓7ᵗʰ **S59.019 Salter-Harris Type I physeal fracture of lower end of ulna, unspecified arm** `CC` `H5`

**✓6ᵗʰ S59.02 Salter-Harris Type II physeal fracture of lower end of ulna**

7 ✓7ᵗʰ **S59.021 Salter-Harris Type II physeal fracture of lower end of ulna, right arm** `CC` `H5`

7 ✓7ᵗʰ **S59.022 Salter-Harris Type II physeal fracture of lower end of ulna, left arm** `CC` `H5`

7 ✓7ᵗʰ **S59.029 Salter-Harris Type II physeal fracture of lower end of ulna, unspecified arm** `CC` `H5`

**✓6ᵗʰ S59.03 Salter-Harris Type III physeal fracture of lower end of ulna**

7 ✓7ᵗʰ **S59.031 Salter-Harris Type III physeal fracture of lower end of ulna, right arm** `CC` `H5`

7 ✓7ᵗʰ **S59.032 Salter-Harris Type III physeal fracture of lower end of ulna, left arm** `CC` `H5`

7 ✓7ᵗʰ **S59.039 Salter-Harris Type III physeal fracture of lower end of ulna, unspecified arm** `CC` `H5`

**✓6ᵗʰ S59.04 Salter-Harris Type IV physeal fracture of lower end of ulna**

7 ✓7ᵗʰ **S59.041 Salter-Harris Type IV physeal fracture of lower end of ulna, right arm** `CC` `H5`

7 ✓7ᵗʰ **S59.042 Salter-Harris Type IV physeal fracture of lower end of ulna, left arm** `CC` `H5`

7 ✓7ᵗʰ **S59.049 Salter-Harris Type IV physeal fracture of lower end of ulna, unspecified arm** `CC` `H5`

**✓6ᵗʰ S59.09 Other physeal fracture of lower end of ulna**

7 ✓7ᵗʰ **S59.091 Other physeal fracture of lower end of ulna, right arm** `CC` `H5`

7 ✓7ᵗʰ **S59.092 Other physeal fracture of lower end of ulna, left arm** `CC` `H5`

---

7   CC when reported as an initial encounter (7th character A, B or C - specific to category) OR a subsequent encounter for nonunion or malunion (7th character K, M, N, P, Q or R - specific to category).

11   HCC with 7th character indicating initial encounter (A or B - specific to category) OR sequela.

7 ✓7ᵗʰ **S59.099** Other physeal fracture of lower end **CC H5**
     of ulna, unspecified arm

✓5ᵗʰ **S59.1** Physeal fracture of upper end of radius

> **CC Excl:** For codes in subcategory S59.1:
> CC with 7th character K or P: PDX collection 897

✓6ᵗʰ **S59.10** Unspecified physeal fracture of upper end of radius

8 ✓7ᵗʰ **S59.101** Unspecified physeal fracture of upper **CC**
     end of radius, right arm

8 ✓7ᵗʰ **S59.102** Unspecified physeal fracture of upper **CC**
     end of radius, left arm

8 ✓7ᵗʰ **S59.109** Unspecified physeal fracture of upper **CC**
     end of radius, unspecified arm

✓6ᵗʰ **S59.11** Salter-Harris Type I physeal fracture of upper end of radius

8 ✓7ᵗʰ **S59.111** Salter-Harris Type I physeal fracture **CC**
     of upper end of radius, right arm

8 ✓7ᵗʰ **S59.112** Salter-Harris Type I physeal fracture **CC**
     of upper end of radius, left arm

8 ✓7ᵗʰ **S59.119** Salter-Harris Type I physeal fracture **CC**
     of upper end of radius, unspecified arm

✓6ᵗʰ **S59.12** Salter-Harris Type II physeal fracture of upper end of radius

8 ✓7ᵗʰ **S59.121** Salter-Harris Type II physeal fracture **CC**
     of upper end of radius, right arm

8 ✓7ᵗʰ **S59.122** Salter-Harris Type II physeal fracture **CC**
     of upper end of radius, left arm

8 ✓7ᵗʰ **S59.129** Salter-Harris Type II physeal fracture **CC**
     of upper end of radius, unspecified arm

✓6ᵗʰ **S59.13** Salter-Harris Type III physeal fracture of upper end of radius

8 ✓7ᵗʰ **S59.131** Salter-Harris Type III physeal fracture **CC**
     of upper end of radius, right arm

8 ✓7ᵗʰ **S59.132** Salter-Harris Type III physeal fracture **CC**
     of upper end of radius, left arm

8 ✓7ᵗʰ **S59.139** Salter-Harris Type III physeal fracture **CC**
     of upper end of radius, unspecified arm

✓6ᵗʰ **S59.14** Salter-Harris Type IV physeal fracture of upper end of radius

8 ✓7ᵗʰ **S59.141** Salter-Harris Type IV physeal fracture **CC**
     of upper end of radius, right arm

8 ✓7ᵗʰ **S59.142** Salter-Harris Type IV physeal fracture **CC**
     of upper end of radius, left arm

8 ✓7ᵗʰ **S59.149** Salter-Harris Type IV physeal fracture **CC**
     of upper end of radius, unspecified arm

✓6ᵗʰ **S59.19** Other physeal fracture of upper end of radius

8 ✓7ᵗʰ **S59.191** Other physeal fracture of upper end **CC**
     of radius, right arm

8 ✓7ᵗʰ **S59.192** Other physeal fracture of upper end **CC**
     of radius, left arm

8 ✓7ᵗʰ **S59.199** Other physeal fracture of upper end **CC**
     of radius, unspecified arm

✓5ᵗʰ **S59.2** Physeal fracture of lower end of radius

> **CC Excl:** For CC codes in subcategory S59.2:
> **Right side:** See code S59.201
> **Left side:** See code S59.202
> **Unspecified side:** See code S59.209

✓6ᵗʰ **S59.20** Unspecified physeal fracture of lower end of radius

7 ✓7ᵗʰ **S59.201** Unspecified physeal fracture of **CC H5**
     lower end of radius, right arm
     **CC Excl:** CC with 7th character A:
     PDX collection 1270
     **CC with 7th character K or P:**
     PDX collection 897

7 ✓7ᵗʰ **S59.202** Unspecified physeal fracture of **CC H5**
     lower end of radius, left arm
     **CC Excl:** CC with 7th character A:
     PDX collection 1271
     **CC with 7th character K or P:**
     PDX collection 897

7 ✓7ᵗʰ **S59.209** Unspecified physeal fracture of **CC H5**
     lower end of radius, unspecified arm
     **CC Excl:** CC with 7th character A:
     PDX collection 1272
     **CC with 7th character K or P:**
     PDX collection 897

✓6ᵗʰ **S59.21** Salter-Harris Type I physeal fracture of lower end of radius

7 ✓7ᵗʰ **S59.211** Salter-Harris Type I physeal **CC H5**
     fracture of lower end of radius, right arm

7 ✓7ᵗʰ **S59.212** Salter-Harris Type I physeal **CC H5**
     fracture of lower end of radius, left arm

7 ✓7ᵗʰ **S59.219** Salter-Harris Type I physeal **CC H5**
     fracture of lower end of radius,
     unspecified arm

✓6ᵗʰ **S59.22** Salter-Harris Type II physeal fracture of lower end of radius

7 ✓7ᵗʰ **S59.221** Salter-Harris Type II physeal **CC H5**
     fracture of lower end of radius, right arm

7 ✓7ᵗʰ **S59.222** Salter-Harris Type II physeal **CC H5**
     fracture of lower end of radius, left arm

7 ✓7ᵗʰ **S59.229** Salter-Harris Type II physeal **CC H5**
     fracture of lower end of radius,
     unspecified arm

✓6ᵗʰ **S59.23** Salter-Harris Type III physeal fracture of lower end of radius

7 ✓7ᵗʰ **S59.231** Salter-Harris Type III physeal **CC H5**
     fracture of lower end of radius, right arm

7 ✓7ᵗʰ **S59.232** Salter-Harris Type III physeal **CC H5**
     fracture of lower end of radius, left arm

7 ✓7ᵗʰ **S59.239** Salter-Harris Type III physeal **CC H5**
     fracture of lower end of radius,
     unspecified arm

✓6ᵗʰ **S59.24** Salter-Harris Type IV physeal fracture of lower end of radius

7 ✓7ᵗʰ **S59.241** Salter-Harris Type IV physeal **CC H5**
     fracture of lower end of radius, right arm

7 ✓7ᵗʰ **S59.242** Salter-Harris Type IV physeal **CC H5**
     fracture of lower end of radius, left arm

7 ✓7ᵗʰ **S59.249** Salter-Harris Type IV physeal **CC H5**
     fracture of lower end of radius,
     unspecified arm

✓6ᵗʰ **S59.29** Other physeal fracture of lower end of radius

7 ✓7ᵗʰ **S59.291** Other physeal fracture of lower **CC H5**
     end of radius, right arm

7 ✓7ᵗʰ **S59.292** Other physeal fracture of lower **CC H5**
     end of radius, left arm

7 ✓7ᵗʰ **S59.299** Other physeal fracture of lower **CC H5**
     end of radius, unspecified arm

✓5ᵗʰ **S59.8** Other specified injuries of elbow and forearm

> The appropriate 7th character is to be added to each code in subcategory S59.8.
> A    initial encounter
> D    subsequent encounter
> S    sequela

✓6ᵗʰ **S59.80** Other specified injuries of elbow

✓7ᵗʰ **S59.801** Other specified injuries of right elbow

✓7ᵗʰ **S59.802** Other specified injuries of left elbow

✓7ᵗʰ **S59.809** Other specified injuries of unspecified elbow

✓6ᵗʰ **S59.81** Other specified injuries of forearm

✓7ᵗʰ **S59.811** Other specified injuries right forearm

✓7ᵗʰ **S59.812** Other specified injuries left forearm

✓7ᵗʰ **S59.819** Other specified injuries unspecified forearm

---

7   CC when reported as an initial encounter (7th character A, B, or C – specific to category) OR a subsequent encounter for nonunion or malunion (7th character K, M, N, P, Q, or R – specific to category).

8   CC when reported as a subsequent encounter for nonunion or malunion (7th character K, M, N, P, Q, or R – specific to category).

---

✓ Additional Character Req    ✓x7ᵗʰ Placeholder Alert    Unacceptable PDx    Manifestation    **H1–H14** HAC    **HCC** CMS-HCC Condition    *EXCLUDES 1* Not Coded Here    *EXCLUDES 2* Not Included Here

ICD-10-CM 2018          **1011**

**✓5ᵗʰ S59.9   Unspecified injury of elbow and forearm**

> The appropriate 7th character is to be added to each code in subcategory S59.9.
> A    initial encounter
> D    subsequent encounter
> S    sequela

     ✓6ᵗʰ **S59.90   Unspecified injury of elbow**
         ✓7ᵗʰ **S59.901   Unspecified injury of right elbow**
         ✓7ᵗʰ **S59.902   Unspecified injury of left elbow**
         ✓7ᵗʰ **S59.909   Unspecified injury of unspecified elbow**

     ✓6ᵗʰ **S59.91   Unspecified injury of forearm**
         ✓7ᵗʰ **S59.911   Unspecified injury of right forearm**
         ✓7ᵗʰ **S59.912   Unspecified injury of left forearm**
         ✓7ᵗʰ **S59.919   Unspecified injury of unspecified forearm**

## Injuries to the wrist, hand and fingers (S60-S69)

**EXCLUDES 2**   burns and corrosions (T20-T32)
                frostbite (T33-T34)
                insect bite or sting, venomous (T63.4)

**✓4ᵗʰ S60   Superficial injury of wrist, hand and fingers**

> The appropriate 7th character is to be added to each code from category S60.
> A    initial encounter
> D    subsequent encounter
> S    sequela

     ✓5ᵗʰ **S60.0   Contusion of finger without damage to nail**
         **EXCLUDES 1**   contusion involving nail (matrix) (S60.1)

     ✓x7ᵗʰ **S60.00   Contusion of unspecified finger without damage to nail**
         Contusion of finger(s) NOS

     ✓6ᵗʰ **S60.01   Contusion of thumb without damage to nail**
         ✓7ᵗʰ **S60.011   Contusion of right thumb without damage to nail**
         ✓7ᵗʰ **S60.012   Contusion of left thumb without damage to nail**
         ✓7ᵗʰ **S60.019   Contusion of unspecified thumb without damage to nail**

     ✓6ᵗʰ **S60.02   Contusion of index finger without damage to nail**
         ✓7ᵗʰ **S60.021   Contusion of right index finger without damage to nail**
         ✓7ᵗʰ **S60.022   Contusion of left index finger without damage to nail**
         ✓7ᵗʰ **S60.029   Contusion of unspecified index finger without damage to nail**

     ✓6ᵗʰ **S60.03   Contusion of middle finger without damage to nail**
         ✓7ᵗʰ **S60.031   Contusion of right middle finger without damage to nail**
         ✓7ᵗʰ **S60.032   Contusion of left middle finger without damage to nail**
         ✓7ᵗʰ **S60.039   Contusion of unspecified middle finger without damage to nail**

     ✓6ᵗʰ **S60.04   Contusion of ring finger without damage to nail**
         ✓7ᵗʰ **S60.041   Contusion of right ring finger without damage to nail**
         ✓7ᵗʰ **S60.042   Contusion of left ring finger without damage to nail**
         ✓7ᵗʰ **S60.049   Contusion of unspecified ring finger without damage to nail**

     ✓6ᵗʰ **S60.05   Contusion of little finger without damage to nail**
         ✓7ᵗʰ **S60.051   Contusion of right little finger without damage to nail**
         ✓7ᵗʰ **S60.052   Contusion of left little finger without damage to nail**
         ✓7ᵗʰ **S60.059   Contusion of unspecified little finger without damage to nail**

     ✓5ᵗʰ **S60.1   Contusion of finger with damage to nail**
     ✓x7ᵗʰ **S60.10   Contusion of unspecified finger with damage to nail**
     ✓6ᵗʰ **S60.11   Contusion of thumb with damage to nail**
         ✓7ᵗʰ **S60.111   Contusion of right thumb with damage to nail**
         ✓7ᵗʰ **S60.112   Contusion of left thumb with damage to nail**

---

         ✓7ᵗʰ **S60.119   Contusion of unspecified thumb with damage to nail**

     ✓6ᵗʰ **S60.12   Contusion of index finger with damage to nail**
         ✓7ᵗʰ **S60.121   Contusion of right index finger with damage to nail**
         ✓7ᵗʰ **S60.122   Contusion of left index finger with damage to nail**
         ✓7ᵗʰ **S60.129   Contusion of unspecified index finger with damage to nail**

     ✓6ᵗʰ **S60.13   Contusion of middle finger with damage to nail**
         ✓7ᵗʰ **S60.131   Contusion of right middle finger with damage to nail**
         ✓7ᵗʰ **S60.132   Contusion of left middle finger with damage to nail**
         ✓7ᵗʰ **S60.139   Contusion of unspecified middle finger with damage to nail**

     ✓6ᵗʰ **S60.14   Contusion of ring finger with damage to nail**
         ✓7ᵗʰ **S60.141   Contusion of right ring finger with damage to nail**
         ✓7ᵗʰ **S60.142   Contusion of left ring finger with damage to nail**
         ✓7ᵗʰ **S60.149   Contusion of unspecified ring finger with damage to nail**

     ✓6ᵗʰ **S60.15   Contusion of little finger with damage to nail**
         ✓7ᵗʰ **S60.151   Contusion of right little finger with damage to nail**
         ✓7ᵗʰ **S60.152   Contusion of left little finger with damage to nail**
         ✓7ᵗʰ **S60.159   Contusion of unspecified little finger with damage to nail**

     ✓5ᵗʰ **S60.2   Contusion of wrist and hand**
         **EXCLUDES 2**   contusion of fingers (S60.0-, S60.1-)

     ✓6ᵗʰ **S60.21   Contusion of wrist**
         ✓7ᵗʰ **S60.211   Contusion of right wrist**
         ✓7ᵗʰ **S60.212   Contusion of left wrist**
         ✓7ᵗʰ **S60.219   Contusion of unspecified wrist**

     ✓6ᵗʰ **S60.22   Contusion of hand**
         ✓7ᵗʰ **S60.221   Contusion of right hand**
         ✓7ᵗʰ **S60.222   Contusion of left hand**
         ✓7ᵗʰ **S60.229   Contusion of unspecified hand**

     ✓5ᵗʰ **S60.3   Other superficial injuries of thumb**
     ✓6ᵗʰ **S60.31   Abrasion of thumb**
         ✓7ᵗʰ **S60.311   Abrasion of right thumb**
         ✓7ᵗʰ **S60.312   Abrasion of left thumb**
         ✓7ᵗʰ **S60.319   Abrasion of unspecified thumb**

     ✓6ᵗʰ **S60.32   Blister (nonthermal) of thumb**
         ✓7ᵗʰ **S60.321   Blister (nonthermal) of right thumb**
         ✓7ᵗʰ **S60.322   Blister (nonthermal) of left thumb**
         ✓7ᵗʰ **S60.329   Blister (nonthermal) of unspecified thumb**

     ✓6ᵗʰ **S60.34   External constriction of thumb**
         Hair tourniquet syndrome of thumb
         Use additional cause code to identify the constricting item (W49.0-)
         ✓7ᵗʰ **S60.341   External constriction of right thumb**
         ✓7ᵗʰ **S60.342   External constriction of left thumb**
         ✓7ᵗʰ **S60.349   External constriction of unspecified thumb**

     ✓6ᵗʰ **S60.35   Superficial foreign body of thumb**
         Splinter in the thumb
         ✓7ᵗʰ **S60.351   Superficial foreign body of right thumb**
         ✓7ᵗʰ **S60.352   Superficial foreign body of left thumb**
         ✓7ᵗʰ **S60.359   Superficial foreign body of unspecified thumb**

     ✓6ᵗʰ **S60.36   Insect bite (nonvenomous) of thumb**
         ✓7ᵗʰ **S60.361   Insect bite (nonvenomous) of right thumb**
         ✓7ᵗʰ **S60.362   Insect bite (nonvenomous) of left thumb**
         ✓7ᵗʰ **S60.369   Insect bite (nonvenomous) of unspecified thumb**

     ✓6ᵗʰ **S60.37   Other superficial bite of thumb**
         **EXCLUDES 1**   open bite of thumb (S61.05-, S61.15-)
         ✓7ᵗʰ **S60.371   Other superficial bite of right thumb**

N Newborn: 0    P Pediatric: 0-17    M Maternity: 12-55    A Adult: 15-124    MCC Major CC Condition    PDx MCC PDx acts as own MCC    CC CC Condition    PDx CC PDx acts as own CC

1012                                                    ICD-10-CM 2018

✓7ᵗʰ **S60.372**  Other superficial bite of left thumb
✓7ᵗʰ **S60.379**  Other superficial bite of unspecified thumb
✓6ᵗʰ **S60.39**  Other superficial injuries of thumb
✓7ᵗʰ **S60.391**  Other superficial injuries of right thumb
✓7ᵗʰ **S60.392**  Other superficial injuries of left thumb
✓7ᵗʰ **S60.399**  Other superficial injuries of unspecified thumb

✓5ᵗʰ **S60.4**  Other superficial injuries of other fingers
✓6ᵗʰ **S60.41**  Abrasion of fingers
✓7ᵗʰ **S60.410**  Abrasion of right index finger
✓7ᵗʰ **S60.411**  Abrasion of left index finger
✓7ᵗʰ **S60.412**  Abrasion of right middle finger
✓7ᵗʰ **S60.413**  Abrasion of left middle finger
✓7ᵗʰ **S60.414**  Abrasion of right ring finger
✓7ᵗʰ **S60.415**  Abrasion of left ring finger
✓7ᵗʰ **S60.416**  Abrasion of right little finger
✓7ᵗʰ **S60.417**  Abrasion of left little finger
✓7ᵗʰ **S60.418**  Abrasion of other finger
Abrasion of specified finger with unspecified laterality
✓7ᵗʰ **S60.419**  Abrasion of unspecified finger
✓6ᵗʰ **S60.42**  Blister (nonthermal) of fingers
✓7ᵗʰ **S60.420**  Blister (nonthermal) of right index finger
✓7ᵗʰ **S60.421**  Blister (nonthermal) of left index finger
✓7ᵗʰ **S60.422**  Blister (nonthermal) of right middle finger
✓7ᵗʰ **S60.423**  Blister (nonthermal) of left middle finger
✓7ᵗʰ **S60.424**  Blister (nonthermal) of right ring finger
✓7ᵗʰ **S60.425**  Blister (nonthermal) of left ring finger
✓7ᵗʰ **S60.426**  Blister (nonthermal) of right little finger
✓7ᵗʰ **S60.427**  Blister (nonthermal) of left little finger
✓7ᵗʰ **S60.428**  Blister (nonthermal) of other finger
Blister (nonthermal) of specified finger with unspecified laterality
✓7ᵗʰ **S60.429**  Blister (nonthermal) of unspecified finger
✓6ᵗʰ **S60.44**  External constriction of fingers
Hair tourniquet syndrome of finger
Use additional cause code to identify the constricting item (W49.0-)
✓7ᵗʰ **S60.440**  External constriction of right index finger
✓7ᵗʰ **S60.441**  External constriction of left index finger
✓7ᵗʰ **S60.442**  External constriction of right middle finger
✓7ᵗʰ **S60.443**  External constriction of left middle finger
✓7ᵗʰ **S60.444**  External constriction of right ring finger
✓7ᵗʰ **S60.445**  External constriction of left ring finger
✓7ᵗʰ **S60.446**  External constriction of right little finger
✓7ᵗʰ **S60.447**  External constriction of left little finger
✓7ᵗʰ **S60.448**  External constriction of other finger
External constriction of specified finger with unspecified laterality
✓7ᵗʰ **S60.449**  External constriction of unspecified finger
✓6ᵗʰ **S60.45**  Superficial foreign body of fingers
Splinter in the finger(s)
✓7ᵗʰ **S60.450**  Superficial foreign body of right index finger
✓7ᵗʰ **S60.451**  Superficial foreign body of left index finger
✓7ᵗʰ **S60.452**  Superficial foreign body of right middle finger
✓7ᵗʰ **S60.453**  Superficial foreign body of left middle finger
✓7ᵗʰ **S60.454**  Superficial foreign body of right ring finger
✓7ᵗʰ **S60.455**  Superficial foreign body of left ring finger
✓7ᵗʰ **S60.456**  Superficial foreign body of right little finger
✓7ᵗʰ **S60.457**  Superficial foreign body of left little finger
✓7ᵗʰ **S60.458**  Superficial foreign body of other finger
Superficial foreign body of specified finger with unspecified laterality

✓7ᵗʰ **S60.459**  Superficial foreign body of unspecified finger
✓6ᵗʰ **S60.46**  Insect bite (nonvenomous) of fingers
✓7ᵗʰ **S60.460**  Insect bite (nonvenomous) of right index finger
✓7ᵗʰ **S60.461**  Insect bite (nonvenomous) of left index finger
✓7ᵗʰ **S60.462**  Insect bite (nonvenomous) of right middle finger
✓7ᵗʰ **S60.463**  Insect bite (nonvenomous) of left middle finger
✓7ᵗʰ **S60.464**  Insect bite (nonvenomous) of right ring finger
✓7ᵗʰ **S60.465**  Insect bite (nonvenomous) of left ring finger
✓7ᵗʰ **S60.466**  Insect bite (nonvenomous) of right little finger
✓7ᵗʰ **S60.467**  Insect bite (nonvenomous) of left little finger
✓7ᵗʰ **S60.468**  Insect bite (nonvenomous) of other finger
Insect bite (nonvenomous) of specified finger with unspecified laterality
✓7ᵗʰ **S60.469**  Insect bite (nonvenomous) of unspecified finger
✓6ᵗʰ **S60.47**  Other superficial bite of fingers
*EXCLUDES 1*  open bite of fingers (S61.25-, S61.35-)
✓7ᵗʰ **S60.470**  Other superficial bite of right index finger
✓7ᵗʰ **S60.471**  Other superficial bite of left index finger
✓7ᵗʰ **S60.472**  Other superficial bite of right middle finger
✓7ᵗʰ **S60.473**  Other superficial bite of left middle finger
✓7ᵗʰ **S60.474**  Other superficial bite of right ring finger
✓7ᵗʰ **S60.475**  Other superficial bite of left ring finger
✓7ᵗʰ **S60.476**  Other superficial bite of right little finger
✓7ᵗʰ **S60.477**  Other superficial bite of left little finger
✓7ᵗʰ **S60.478**  Other superficial bite of other finger
Other superficial bite of specified finger with unspecified laterality
✓7ᵗʰ **S60.479**  Other superficial bite of unspecified finger
✓5ᵗʰ **S60.5**  Other superficial injuries of hand
*EXCLUDES 2*  superficial injuries of fingers (S60.3-, S60.4-)
✓6ᵗʰ **S60.51**  Abrasion of hand
✓7ᵗʰ **S60.511**  Abrasion of right hand
✓7ᵗʰ **S60.512**  Abrasion of left hand
✓7ᵗʰ **S60.519**  Abrasion of unspecified hand
✓6ᵗʰ **S60.52**  Blister (nonthermal) of hand
✓7ᵗʰ **S60.521**  Blister (nonthermal) of right hand
✓7ᵗʰ **S60.522**  Blister (nonthermal) of left hand
✓7ᵗʰ **S60.529**  Blister (nonthermal) of unspecified hand
✓6ᵗʰ **S60.54**  External constriction of hand
✓7ᵗʰ **S60.541**  External constriction of right hand
✓7ᵗʰ **S60.542**  External constriction of left hand
✓7ᵗʰ **S60.549**  External constriction of unspecified hand
✓6ᵗʰ **S60.55**  Superficial foreign body of hand
Splinter in the hand
✓7ᵗʰ **S60.551**  Superficial foreign body of right hand
✓7ᵗʰ **S60.552**  Superficial foreign body of left hand
✓7ᵗʰ **S60.559**  Superficial foreign body of unspecified hand
✓6ᵗʰ **S60.56**  Insect bite (nonvenomous) of hand
✓7ᵗʰ **S60.561**  Insect bite (nonvenomous) of right hand
✓7ᵗʰ **S60.562**  Insect bite (nonvenomous) of left hand
✓7ᵗʰ **S60.569**  Insect bite (nonvenomous) of unspecified hand
✓6ᵗʰ **S60.57**  Other superficial bite of hand
*EXCLUDES 1*  open bite of hand (S61.45-)
✓7ᵗʰ **S60.571**  Other superficial bite of hand of right hand
✓7ᵗʰ **S60.572**  Other superficial bite of hand of left hand
✓7ᵗʰ **S60.579**  Other superficial bite of hand of unspecified hand

**Chapter 19. Injury, Poisoning and Certain Other Consequences of External Causes**

**S60.8–S61.109**

✓5ᵗʰ **S60.8**   **Other superficial injuries of** wrist

   ✓6ᵗʰ **S60.81**   **Abrasion of** wrist

     ✓7ᵗʰ **S60.811**   **Abrasion of** right **wrist**

     ✓7ᵗʰ **S60.812**   **Abrasion of** left **wrist**

     ✓7ᵗʰ **S60.819**   **Abrasion of** unspecified **wrist**

   ✓6ᵗʰ **S60.82**   **Blister (nonthermal) of** wrist

     ✓7ᵗʰ **S60.821**   **Blister (nonthermal) of** right **wrist**

     ✓7ᵗʰ **S60.822**   **Blister (nonthermal) of** left **wrist**

     ✓7ᵗʰ **S60.829**   **Blister (nonthermal) of** unspecified **wrist**

   ✓6ᵗʰ **S60.84**   **External constriction of** wrist

     ✓7ᵗʰ **S60.841**   **External constriction of** right **wrist**

     ✓7ᵗʰ **S60.842**   **External constriction of** left **wrist**

     ✓7ᵗʰ **S60.849**   **External constriction of** unspecified **wrist**

   ✓6ᵗʰ **S60.85**   **Superficial** foreign body **of wrist**
     Splinter in the wrist

     ✓7ᵗʰ **S60.851**   **Superficial foreign body of** right **wrist**

     ✓7ᵗʰ **S60.852**   **Superficial foreign body of** left **wrist**

     ✓7ᵗʰ **S60.859**   **Superficial foreign body of** unspecified **wrist**

   ✓6ᵗʰ **S60.86**   **Insect bite (nonvenomous) of** wrist

     ✓7ᵗʰ **S60.861**   **Insect bite (nonvenomous) of** right **wrist**

     ✓7ᵗʰ **S60.862**   **Insect bite (nonvenomous) of** left **wrist**

     ✓7ᵗʰ **S60.869**   **Insect bite (nonvenomous) of** unspecified **wrist**

   ✓6ᵗʰ **S60.87**   **Other superficial** bite **of wrist**
     **EXCLUDES 1**   *open bite of wrist (S61.55)*

     ✓7ᵗʰ **S60.871**   **Other superficial bite of** right **wrist**

     ✓7ᵗʰ **S60.872**   **Other superficial bite of** left **wrist**

     ✓7ᵗʰ **S60.879**   **Other superficial bite of** unspecified **wrist**

✓5ᵗʰ **S60.9**   **Unspecified superficial injury of wrist, hand and fingers**

   ✓6ᵗʰ **S60.91**   **Unspecified superficial injury of** wrist

     ✓7ᵗʰ **S60.911**   **Unspecified superficial injury of** right **wrist**

     ✓7ᵗʰ **S60.912**   **Unspecified superficial injury of** left **wrist**

     ✓7ᵗʰ **S60.919**   **Unspecified superficial injury of** unspecified **wrist**

   ✓6ᵗʰ **S60.92**   **Unspecified superficial injury of** hand

     ✓7ᵗʰ **S60.921**   **Unspecified superficial injury of** right **hand**

     ✓7ᵗʰ **S60.922**   **Unspecified superficial injury of** left **hand**

     ✓7ᵗʰ **S60.929**   **Unspecified superficial injury of** unspecified **hand**

   ✓6ᵗʰ **S60.93**   **Unspecified superficial injury of** thumb

     ✓7ᵗʰ **S60.931**   **Unspecified superficial injury of** right **thumb**

     ✓7ᵗʰ **S60.932**   **Unspecified superficial injury of** left **thumb**

     ✓7ᵗʰ **S60.939**   **Unspecified superficial injury of** unspecified **thumb**

   ✓6ᵗʰ **S60.94**   **Unspecified superficial injury of other** fingers

     ✓7ᵗʰ **S60.940**   **Unspecified superficial injury of** right **index** finger

     ✓7ᵗʰ **S60.941**   **Unspecified superficial injury of** left index **finger**

     ✓7ᵗʰ **S60.942**   **Unspecified superficial injury of** right **middle** finger

     ✓7ᵗʰ **S60.943**   **Unspecified superficial injury of** left **middle** finger

     ✓7ᵗʰ **S60.944**   **Unspecified superficial injury of** right ring **finger**

     ✓7ᵗʰ **S60.945**   **Unspecified superficial injury of** left ring **finger**

     ✓7ᵗʰ **S60.946**   **Unspecified superficial injury of** right little **finger**

     ✓7ᵗʰ **S60.947**   **Unspecified superficial injury of** left little **finger**

     ✓7ᵗʰ **S60.948**   **Unspecified superficial injury of** other **finger**
       Unspecified superficial injury of specified finger with unspecified laterality

     ✓7ᵗʰ **S60.949**   **Unspecified superficial injury of** unspecified **finger**

---

✓4ᵗʰ **S61**   **Open wound of wrist, hand and fingers**
   Code also any associated wound infection
   **EXCLUDES 1**   *open fracture of wrist, hand and finger (S62- with 7th character B)*
       *traumatic amputation of wrist and hand (S68.-)*

   The appropriate 7th character is to be added to each code from category S61.
   A    initial encounter
   D    subsequent encounter
   S    sequela

✓5ᵗʰ **S61.0**   **Open wound of** thumb without damage to nail
   **EXCLUDES 1**   *open wound of thumb with damage to nail (S61.1-)*

   ✓6ᵗʰ **S61.00**   **Unspecified open wound of thumb without damage to nail**

     ✓7ᵗʰ **S61.001**   **Unspecified open wound of** right **thumb without damage to nail**

     ✓7ᵗʰ **S61.002**   **Unspecified open wound of** left **thumb without damage to nail**

     ✓7ᵗʰ **S61.009**   **Unspecified open wound of** unspecified **thumb without damage to nail**

   ✓6ᵗʰ **S61.01**   **Laceration without foreign body** of thumb without damage to nail

     ✓7ᵗʰ **S61.011**   **Laceration without foreign body of** right **thumb without damage to nail**

     ✓7ᵗʰ **S61.012**   **Laceration without foreign body of** left **thumb without damage to nail**

     ✓7ᵗʰ **S61.019**   **Laceration without foreign body of** unspecified **thumb without damage to nail**

   ✓6ᵗʰ **S61.02**   **Laceration with foreign body** of thumb without damage to nail

     ✓7ᵗʰ **S61.021**   **Laceration with foreign body of** right **thumb without damage to nail**

     ✓7ᵗʰ **S61.022**   **Laceration with foreign body of** left **thumb without damage to nail**

     ✓7ᵗʰ **S61.029**   **Laceration with foreign body of** unspecified **thumb without damage to nail**

   ✓6ᵗʰ **S61.03**   **Puncture wound without foreign body** of thumb without damage to nail

     ✓7ᵗʰ **S61.031**   **Puncture wound without foreign body of** right **thumb without damage to nail**

     ✓7ᵗʰ **S61.032**   **Puncture wound without foreign body of** left **thumb without damage to nail**

     ✓7ᵗʰ **S61.039**   **Puncture wound without foreign body of** unspecified **thumb without damage to nail**

   ✓6ᵗʰ **S61.04**   **Puncture wound with foreign body** of thumb without damage to nail

     ✓7ᵗʰ **S61.041**   **Puncture wound with foreign body of** right **thumb without damage to nail**

     ✓7ᵗʰ **S61.042**   **Puncture wound with foreign body of** left **thumb without damage to nail**

     ✓7ᵗʰ **S61.049**   **Puncture wound with foreign body of** unspecified **thumb without damage to nail**

   ✓6ᵗʰ **S61.05**   **Open bite of thumb without damage to nail**
     Bite of thumb NOS
     **EXCLUDES 1**   *superficial bite of thumb (S60.36-, S60.37-)*

     ✓7ᵗʰ **S61.051**   **Open bite of** right **thumb without damage to nail**

     ✓7ᵗʰ **S61.052**   **Open bite of** left **thumb without damage to nail**

     ✓7ᵗʰ **S61.059**   **Open bite of** unspecified **thumb without damage to nail**

✓5ᵗʰ **S61.1**   **Open wound of** thumb with damage to nail

   ✓6ᵗʰ **S61.10**   **Unspecified open wound of thumb with damage to nail**

     ✓7ᵗʰ **S61.101**   **Unspecified open wound of** right **thumb with damage to nail**

     ✓7ᵗʰ **S61.102**   **Unspecified open wound of** left **thumb with damage to nail**

     ✓7ᵗʰ **S61.109**   **Unspecified open wound of** unspecified **thumb with damage to nail**

N Newborn: 0   P Pediatric: 0-17   M Maternity: 12-55   A Adult: 15-124   MCC Major CC Condition   PDxMCC PDx acts as own MCC   CC CC Condition   PDxCC PDx acts as own CC

**1014**      ICD-10-CM 2018

✓6ᵗʰ **S61.11** Laceration without foreign body of thumb with damage to nail

✓7ᵗʰ **S61.111** Laceration without foreign body of right thumb with damage to nail

✓7ᵗʰ **S61.112** Laceration without foreign body of left thumb with damage to nail

✓7ᵗʰ **S61.119** Laceration without foreign body of unspecified thumb with damage to nail

✓6ᵗʰ **S61.12** Laceration with foreign body of thumb with damage to nail

✓7ᵗʰ **S61.121** Laceration with foreign body of right thumb with damage to nail

✓7ᵗʰ **S61.122** Laceration with foreign body of left thumb with damage to nail

✓7ᵗʰ **S61.129** Laceration with foreign body of unspecified thumb with damage to nail

✓6ᵗʰ **S61.13** Puncture wound without foreign body of thumb with damage to nail

✓7ᵗʰ **S61.131** Puncture wound without foreign body of right thumb with damage to nail

✓7ᵗʰ **S61.132** Puncture wound without foreign body of left thumb with damage to nail

✓7ᵗʰ **S61.139** Puncture wound without foreign body of unspecified thumb with damage to nail

✓6ᵗʰ **S61.14** Puncture wound with foreign body of thumb with damage to nail

✓7ᵗʰ **S61.141** Puncture wound with foreign body of right thumb with damage to nail

✓7ᵗʰ **S61.142** Puncture wound with foreign body of left thumb with damage to nail

✓7ᵗʰ **S61.149** Puncture wound with foreign body of unspecified thumb with damage to nail

✓6ᵗʰ **S61.15** Open bite with damage to nail
Bite of thumb with damage to nail NOS
*EXCLUDES 1* superficial bite of thumb (S60.36-, S60.37-)

✓7ᵗʰ **S61.151** Open bite of right thumb with damage to nail

✓7ᵗʰ **S61.152** Open bite of left thumb with damage to nail

✓7ᵗʰ **S61.159** Open bite of unspecified thumb with damage to nail

✓5ᵗʰ **S61.2** Open wound of other finger without damage to nail
*EXCLUDES 1* open wound of finger involving nail (matrix) (S61.3-)
*EXCLUDES 2* open wound of thumb without damage to nail (S61.0-)

✓6ᵗʰ **S61.20** Unspecified open wound of other finger without damage to nail

✓7ᵗʰ **S61.200** Unspecified open wound of right index finger without damage to nail

✓7ᵗʰ **S61.201** Unspecified open wound of left index finger without damage to nail

✓7ᵗʰ **S61.202** Unspecified open wound of right middle finger without damage to nail

✓7ᵗʰ **S61.203** Unspecified open wound of left middle finger without damage to nail

✓7ᵗʰ **S61.204** Unspecified open wound of right ring finger without damage to nail

✓7ᵗʰ **S61.205** Unspecified open wound of left ring finger without damage to nail

✓7ᵗʰ **S61.206** Unspecified open wound of right little finger without damage to nail

✓7ᵗʰ **S61.207** Unspecified open wound of left little finger without damage to nail

✓7ᵗʰ **S61.208** Unspecified open wound of other finger without damage to nail
Unspecified open wound of specified finger with unspecified laterality without damage to nail

✓7ᵗʰ **S61.209** Unspecified open wound of unspecified finger without damage to nail

✓6ᵗʰ **S61.21** Laceration without foreign body of finger without damage to nail

✓7ᵗʰ **S61.210** Laceration without foreign body of right index finger without damage to nail

✓7ᵗʰ **S61.211** Laceration without foreign body of left index finger without damage to nail

✓7ᵗʰ **S61.212** Laceration without foreign body of right middle finger without damage to nail

✓7ᵗʰ **S61.213** Laceration without foreign body of left middle finger without damage to nail

✓7ᵗʰ **S61.214** Laceration without foreign body of right ring finger without damage to nail

✓7ᵗʰ **S61.215** Laceration without foreign body of left ring finger without damage to nail

✓7ᵗʰ **S61.216** Laceration without foreign body of right little finger without damage to nail

✓7ᵗʰ **S61.217** Laceration without foreign body of left little finger without damage to nail

✓7ᵗʰ **S61.218** Laceration without foreign body of other finger without damage to nail
Laceration without foreign body of specified finger with unspecified laterality without damage to nail

✓7ᵗʰ **S61.219** Laceration without foreign body of unspecified finger without damage to nail

✓6ᵗʰ **S61.22** Laceration with foreign body of finger without damage to nail

✓7ᵗʰ **S61.220** Laceration with foreign body of right index finger without damage to nail

✓7ᵗʰ **S61.221** Laceration with foreign body of left index finger without damage to nail

✓7ᵗʰ **S61.222** Laceration with foreign body of right middle finger without damage to nail

✓7ᵗʰ **S61.223** Laceration with foreign body of left middle finger without damage to nail

✓7ᵗʰ **S61.224** Laceration with foreign body of right ring finger without damage to nail

✓7ᵗʰ **S61.225** Laceration with foreign body of left ring finger without damage to nail

✓7ᵗʰ **S61.226** Laceration with foreign body of right little finger without damage to nail

✓7ᵗʰ **S61.227** Laceration with foreign body of left little finger without damage to nail

✓7ᵗʰ **S61.228** Laceration with foreign body of other finger without damage to nail
Laceration with foreign body of specified finger with unspecified laterality without damage to nail

✓7ᵗʰ **S61.229** Laceration with foreign body of unspecified finger without damage to nail

✓6ᵗʰ **S61.23** Puncture wound without foreign body of finger without damage to nail

✓7ᵗʰ **S61.230** Puncture wound without foreign body of right index finger without damage to nail

✓7ᵗʰ **S61.231** Puncture wound without foreign body of left index finger without damage to nail

✓7ᵗʰ **S61.232** Puncture wound without foreign body of right middle finger without damage to nail

✓7ᵗʰ **S61.233** Puncture wound without foreign body of left middle finger without damage to nail

✓7ᵗʰ **S61.234** Puncture wound without foreign body of right ring finger without damage to nail

✓7ᵗʰ **S61.235** Puncture wound without foreign body of left ring finger without damage to nail

✓7ᵗʰ **S61.236** Puncture wound without foreign body of right little finger without damage to nail

✓7ᵗʰ **S61.237** Puncture wound without foreign body of left little finger without damage to nail

✓7ᵗʰ **S61.238** Puncture wound without foreign body of other finger without damage to nail
Puncture wound without foreign body of specified finger with unspecified laterality without damage to nail

✓7ᵗʰ **S61.239** Puncture wound without foreign body of unspecified finger without damage to nail

✓6ᵗʰ **S61.24** Puncture wound with foreign body of finger without damage to nail

✓7ᵗʰ **S61.240** Puncture wound with foreign body of right index finger without damage to nail

✓7ᵗʰ **S61.241** Puncture wound with foreign body of left index finger without damage to nail

✔ Additional Character Req  ✓ₓ7ᵗʰ Placeholder Alert  Unacceptable PDx  Manifestation  **H1-H14** HAC  **HCC** CMS-HCC Condition  *EXCLUDES 1* Not Coded Here  *EXCLUDES 2* Not Included Here

ICD-10-CM 2018  **1015**

√7ᵗʰ **S61.242 Puncture wound with foreign body of right middle finger without damage to nail**

√7ᵗʰ **S61.243 Puncture wound with foreign body of left middle finger without damage to nail**

√7ᵗʰ **S61.244 Puncture wound with foreign body of right ring finger without damage to nail**

√7ᵗʰ **S61.245 Puncture wound with foreign body of left ring finger without damage to nail**

√7ᵗʰ **S61.246 Puncture wound with foreign body of right little finger without damage to nail**

√7ᵗʰ **S61.247 Puncture wound with foreign body of left little finger without damage to nail**

√7ᵗʰ **S61.248 Puncture wound with foreign body of other finger without damage to nail**
     Puncture wound with foreign body of specified finger with unspecified laterality without damage to nail

√7ᵗʰ **S61.249 Puncture wound with foreign body of unspecified finger without damage to nail**

√6ᵗʰ **S61.25 Open bite of finger without damage to nail**
     Bite of finger without damage to nail NOS
     **EXCLUDES 1**   superficial bite of finger (S60.46-, S60.47-)

√7ᵗʰ **S61.250 Open bite of right index finger without damage to nail**

√7ᵗʰ **S61.251 Open bite of left index finger without damage to nail**

√7ᵗʰ **S61.252 Open bite of right middle finger without damage to nail**

√7ᵗʰ **S61.253 Open bite of left middle finger without damage to nail**

√7ᵗʰ **S61.254 Open bite of right ring finger without damage to nail**

√7ᵗʰ **S61.255 Open bite of left ring finger without damage to nail**

√7ᵗʰ **S61.256 Open bite of right little finger without damage to nail**

√7ᵗʰ **S61.257 Open bite of left little finger without damage to nail**

√7ᵗʰ **S61.258 Open bite of other finger without damage to nail**
     Open bite of specified finger with unspecified laterality without damage to nail

√7ᵗʰ **S61.259 Open bite of unspecified finger without damage to nail**

√5ᵗʰ **S61.3 Open wound of other finger with damage to nail**

√6ᵗʰ **S61.30 Unspecified open wound of finger with damage to nail**

√7ᵗʰ **S61.300 Unspecified open wound of right index finger with damage to nail**

√7ᵗʰ **S61.301 Unspecified open wound of left index finger with damage to nail**

√7ᵗʰ **S61.302 Unspecified open wound of right middle finger with damage to nail**

√7ᵗʰ **S61.303 Unspecified open wound of left middle finger with damage to nail**

√7ᵗʰ **S61.304 Unspecified open wound of right ring finger with damage to nail**

√7ᵗʰ **S61.305 Unspecified open wound of left ring finger with damage to nail**

√7ᵗʰ **S61.306 Unspecified open wound of right little finger with damage to nail**

√7ᵗʰ **S61.307 Unspecified open wound of left little finger with damage to nail**

√7ᵗʰ **S61.308 Unspecified open wound of other finger with damage to nail**
     Unspecified open wound of specified finger with unspecified laterality with damage to nail

√7ᵗʰ **S61.309 Unspecified open wound of unspecified finger with damage to nail**

√6ᵗʰ **S61.31 Laceration without foreign body of finger with damage to nail**

√7ᵗʰ **S61.310 Laceration without foreign body of right index finger with damage to nail**

√7ᵗʰ **S61.311 Laceration without foreign body of left index finger with damage to nail**

√7ᵗʰ **S61.312 Laceration without foreign body of right middle finger with damage to nail**

√7ᵗʰ **S61.313 Laceration without foreign body of left middle finger with damage to nail**

√7ᵗʰ **S61.314 Laceration without foreign body of right ring finger with damage to nail**

√7ᵗʰ **S61.315 Laceration without foreign body of left ring finger with damage to nail**

√7ᵗʰ **S61.316 Laceration without foreign body of right little finger with damage to nail**

√7ᵗʰ **S61.317 Laceration without foreign body of left little finger with damage to nail**

√7ᵗʰ **S61.318 Laceration without foreign body of other finger with damage to nail**
     Laceration without foreign body of specified finger with unspecified laterality with damage to nail

√7ᵗʰ **S61.319 Laceration without foreign body of unspecified finger with damage to nail**

√6ᵗʰ **S61.32 Laceration with foreign body of finger with damage to nail**

√7ᵗʰ **S61.320 Laceration with foreign body of right index finger with damage to nail**

√7ᵗʰ **S61.321 Laceration with foreign body of left index finger with damage to nail**

√7ᵗʰ **S61.322 Laceration with foreign body of right middle finger with damage to nail**

√7ᵗʰ **S61.323 Laceration with foreign body of left middle finger with damage to nail**

√7ᵗʰ **S61.324 Laceration with foreign body of right ring finger with damage to nail**

√7ᵗʰ **S61.325 Laceration with foreign body of left ring finger with damage to nail**

√7ᵗʰ **S61.326 Laceration with foreign body of right little finger with damage to nail**

√7ᵗʰ **S61.327 Laceration with foreign body of left little finger with damage to nail**

√7ᵗʰ **S61.328 Laceration with foreign body of other finger with damage to nail**
     Laceration with foreign body of specified finger with unspecified laterality with damage to nail

√7ᵗʰ **S61.329 Laceration with foreign body of unspecified finger with damage to nail**

√6ᵗʰ **S61.33 Puncture wound without foreign body of finger with damage to nail**

√7ᵗʰ **S61.330 Puncture wound without foreign body of right index finger with damage to nail**

√7ᵗʰ **S61.331 Puncture wound without foreign body of left index finger with damage to nail**

√7ᵗʰ **S61.332 Puncture wound without foreign body of right middle finger with damage to nail**

√7ᵗʰ **S61.333 Puncture wound without foreign body of left middle finger with damage to nail**

√7ᵗʰ **S61.334 Puncture wound without foreign body of right ring finger with damage to nail**

√7ᵗʰ **S61.335 Puncture wound without foreign body of left ring finger with damage to nail**

√7ᵗʰ **S61.336 Puncture wound without foreign body of right little finger with damage to nail**

√7ᵗʰ **S61.337 Puncture wound without foreign body of left little finger with damage to nail**

√7ᵗʰ **S61.338 Puncture wound without foreign body of other finger with damage to nail**
     Puncture wound without foreign body of specified finger with unspecified laterality with damage to nail

√7ᵗʰ **S61.339 Puncture wound without foreign body of unspecified finger with damage to nail**

N Newborn: 0   P Pediatric: 0-17   M Maternity: 12-55   A Adult: 15-124   MCC Major CC Condition   PDxMCC PDx acts as own MCC   CC CC Condition   PDxCC PDx acts as own CC

**1016**      ICD-10-CM 2018

√6ᵗʰ **S61.34** **Puncture wound with foreign body of finger with damage to nail**

√7ᵗʰ **S61.340** **Puncture wound with foreign body of right index finger with damage to nail**

√7ᵗʰ **S61.341** **Puncture wound with foreign body of left index finger with damage to nail**

√7ᵗʰ **S61.342** **Puncture wound with foreign body of right middle finger with damage to nail**

√7ᵗʰ **S61.343** **Puncture wound with foreign body of left middle finger with damage to nail**

√7ᵗʰ **S61.344** **Puncture wound with foreign body of right ring finger with damage to nail**

√7ᵗʰ **S61.345** **Puncture wound with foreign body of left ring finger with damage to nail**

√7ᵗʰ **S61.346** **Puncture wound with foreign body of right little finger with damage to nail**

√7ᵗʰ **S61.347** **Puncture wound with foreign body of left little finger with damage to nail**

√7ᵗʰ **S61.348** **Puncture wound with foreign body of other finger with damage to nail**
Puncture wound with foreign body of specified finger with unspecified laterality with damage to nail

√7ᵗʰ **S61.349** **Puncture wound with foreign body of unspecified finger with damage to nail**

√6ᵗʰ **S61.35** **Open bite of finger with damage to nail**
Bite of finger with damage to nail NOS
*EXCLUDES 1*   superficial bite of finger (S60.46-, S60.47-)

√7ᵗʰ **S61.350** **Open bite of right index finger with damage to nail**

√7ᵗʰ **S61.351** **Open bite of left index finger with damage to nail**

√7ᵗʰ **S61.352** **Open bite of right middle finger with damage to nail**

√7ᵗʰ **S61.353** **Open bite of left middle finger with damage to nail**

√7ᵗʰ **S61.354** **Open bite of right ring finger with damage to nail**

√7ᵗʰ **S61.355** **Open bite of left ring finger with damage to nail**

√7ᵗʰ **S61.356** **Open bite of right little finger with damage to nail**

√7ᵗʰ **S61.357** **Open bite of left little finger with damage to nail**

√7ᵗʰ **S61.358** **Open bite of other finger with damage to nail**
Open bite of specified finger with unspecified laterality with damage to nail

√7ᵗʰ **S61.359** **Open bite of unspecified finger with damage to nail**

√5ᵗʰ **S61.4** **Open wound of hand**

√6ᵗʰ **S61.40** **Unspecified open wound of hand**

√7ᵗʰ **S61.401** **Unspecified open wound of right hand**

√7ᵗʰ **S61.402** **Unspecified open wound of left hand**

√7ᵗʰ **S61.409** **Unspecified open wound of unspecified hand**

√6ᵗʰ **S61.41** **Laceration without foreign body of hand**

√7ᵗʰ **S61.411** **Laceration without foreign body of right hand**

√7ᵗʰ **S61.412** **Laceration without foreign body of left hand**

√7ᵗʰ **S61.419** **Laceration without foreign body of unspecified hand**

√6ᵗʰ **S61.42** **Laceration with foreign body of hand**

√7ᵗʰ **S61.421** **Laceration with foreign body of right hand**

√7ᵗʰ **S61.422** **Laceration with foreign body of left hand**

√7ᵗʰ **S61.429** **Laceration with foreign body of unspecified hand**

√6ᵗʰ **S61.43** **Puncture wound without foreign body of hand**

√7ᵗʰ **S61.431** **Puncture wound without foreign body of right hand**

√7ᵗʰ **S61.432** **Puncture wound without foreign body of left hand**

√7ᵗʰ **S61.439** **Puncture wound without foreign body of unspecified hand**

√6ᵗʰ **S61.44** **Puncture wound with foreign body of hand**

√7ᵗʰ **S61.441** **Puncture wound with foreign body of right hand**

√7ᵗʰ **S61.442** **Puncture wound with foreign body of left hand**

√7ᵗʰ **S61.449** **Puncture wound with foreign body of unspecified hand**

√6ᵗʰ **S61.45** **Open bite of hand**
Bite of hand NOS
*EXCLUDES 1*   superficial bite of hand (S60.56-, S60.57-)

√7ᵗʰ **S61.451** **Open bite of right hand**

√7ᵗʰ **S61.452** **Open bite of left hand**

√7ᵗʰ **S61.459** **Open bite of unspecified hand**

√5ᵗʰ **S61.5** **Open wound of wrist**

√6ᵗʰ **S61.50** **Unspecified open wound of wrist**

√7ᵗʰ **S61.501** **Unspecified open wound of right wrist**

√7ᵗʰ **S61.502** **Unspecified open wound of left wrist**

√7ᵗʰ **S61.509** **Unspecified open wound of unspecified wrist**

√6ᵗʰ **S61.51** **Laceration without foreign body of wrist**

√7ᵗʰ **S61.511** **Laceration without foreign body of right wrist**

√7ᵗʰ **S61.512** **Laceration without foreign body of left wrist**

√7ᵗʰ **S61.519** **Laceration without foreign body of unspecified wrist**

√6ᵗʰ **S61.52** **Laceration with foreign body of wrist**

√7ᵗʰ **S61.521** **Laceration with foreign body of right wrist**

√7ᵗʰ **S61.522** **Laceration with foreign body of left wrist**

√7ᵗʰ **S61.529** **Laceration with foreign body of unspecified wrist**

√6ᵗʰ **S61.53** **Puncture wound without foreign body of wrist**

√7ᵗʰ **S61.531** **Puncture wound without foreign body of right wrist**

√7ᵗʰ **S61.532** **Puncture wound without foreign body of left wrist**

√7ᵗʰ **S61.539** **Puncture wound without foreign body of unspecified wrist**

√6ᵗʰ **S61.54** **Puncture wound with foreign body of wrist**

√7ᵗʰ **S61.541** **Puncture wound with foreign body of right wrist**

√7ᵗʰ **S61.542** **Puncture wound with foreign body of left wrist**

√7ᵗʰ **S61.549** **Puncture wound with foreign body of unspecified wrist**

√6ᵗʰ **S61.55** **Open bite of wrist**
Bite of wrist NOS
*EXCLUDES 1*   superficial bite of wrist (S60.86-, S60.87-)

√7ᵗʰ **S61.551** **Open bite of right wrist**

√7ᵗʰ **S61.552** **Open bite of left wrist**

√7ᵗʰ **S61.559** **Open bite of unspecified wrist**

---

√ Additional Character Req    √×7ᵗʰ Placeholder Alert    Unacceptable PDx    Manifestation    **H1**-**H14** HAC    **HCC** CMS-HCC Condition    *EXCLUDES 1* Not Coded Here    *EXCLUDES 2* Not Included Here

ICD-10-CM 2018        **1017**

**✓4th S62 Fracture at wrist and hand level**

> **NOTE**    A fracture not indicated as displaced or nondisplaced should be coded to displaced.
> A fracture not indicated as open or closed should be coded to closed.
>
> **EXCLUDES 1**   *traumatic amputation of wrist and hand (S68.-)*
> **EXCLUDES 2**   *fracture of distal parts of ulna and radius (S52.-)*
> **AHA:** 2015, 3Q, 37-39

> The appropriate 7th character is to be added to each code from category S62.
> A    initial encounter for closed fracture
> B    initial encounter for open fracture
> D    subsequent encounter for fracture with routine healing
> G    subsequent encounter for fracture with delayed healing
> K    subsequent encounter for fracture with nonunion
> P    subsequent encounter for fracture with malunion
> S    sequela

**✓5th S62.0 Fracture of navicular [scaphoid] bone of wrist**

> **CC Excl: For codes in subcategory S62.0:**
> **CC with 7th character B:** PDX collection 1283
> **CC with 7th character K or P:** PDX collection 897

   **✓6th S62.00 Unspecified fracture of navicular [scaphoid] bone of wrist**

     7   **✓7th S62.001 Unspecified fracture of navicular [scaphoid] bone of right wrist**   CC H5

     7   **✓7th S62.002 Unspecified fracture of navicular [scaphoid] bone of left wrist**   CC H5
                 **AHA:** 2012, 4Q, 106

     7   **✓7th S62.009 Unspecified fracture of navicular [scaphoid] bone of unspecified wrist**   CC H5

   **✓6th S62.01 Fracture of distal pole of navicular [scaphoid] bone of wrist**
           Fracture of volar tuberosity of navicular [scaphoid] bone of wrist

     7   **✓7th S62.011 Displaced fracture of distal pole of navicular [scaphoid] bone of right wrist**   CC H5

     7   **✓7th S62.012 Displaced fracture of distal pole of navicular [scaphoid] bone of left wrist**   CC H5

     7   **✓7th S62.013 Displaced fracture of distal pole of navicular [scaphoid] bone of unspecified wrist**   CC H5

     7   **✓7th S62.014 Nondisplaced fracture of distal pole of navicular [scaphoid] bone of right wrist**   CC H5

     7   **✓7th S62.015 Nondisplaced fracture of distal pole of navicular [scaphoid] bone of left wrist**   CC H5

     7   **✓7th S62.016 Nondisplaced fracture of distal pole of navicular [scaphoid] bone of unspecified wrist**   CC H5

   **✓6th S62.02 Fracture of middle third of navicular [scaphoid] bone of wrist**

     7   **✓7th S62.021 Displaced fracture of middle third of navicular [scaphoid] bone of right wrist**   CC H5

     7   **✓7th S62.022 Displaced fracture of middle third of navicular [scaphoid] bone of left wrist**   CC H5

     7   **✓7th S62.023 Displaced fracture of middle third of navicular [scaphoid] bone of unspecified wrist**   CC H5

     7   **✓7th S62.024 Nondisplaced fracture of middle third of navicular [scaphoid] bone of right wrist**   CC H5

     7   **✓7th S62.025 Nondisplaced fracture of middle third of navicular [scaphoid] bone of left wrist**   CC H5

     7   **✓7th S62.026 Nondisplaced fracture of middle third of navicular [scaphoid] bone of unspecified wrist**   CC H5

   **✓6th S62.03 Fracture of proximal third of navicular [scaphoid] bone of wrist**

     7   **✓7th S62.031 Displaced fracture of proximal third of navicular [scaphoid] bone of right wrist**   CC H5

---

     7   **✓7th S62.032 Displaced fracture of proximal third of navicular [scaphoid] bone of left wrist**   CC H5

     7   **✓7th S62.033 Displaced fracture of proximal third of navicular [scaphoid] bone of unspecified wrist**   CC H5

     7   **✓7th S62.034 Nondisplaced fracture of proximal third of navicular [scaphoid] bone of right wrist**   CC H5

     7   **✓7th S62.035 Nondisplaced fracture of proximal third of navicular [scaphoid] bone of left wrist**   CC H5

     7   **✓7th S62.036 Nondisplaced fracture of proximal third of navicular [scaphoid] bone of unspecified wrist**   CC H5

**✓5th S62.1 Fracture of other and unspecified carpal bone(s)**

> **EXCLUDES 2**   *fracture of scaphoid of wrist (S62.0-)*

> **CC Excl: For codes in subcategory S62.1:**
> **CC with 7th character B:** PDX collection 1283
> **CC with 7th character K or P:** PDX collection 897

   **✓6th S62.10 Fracture of unspecified carpal bone**
           Fracture of wrist NOS

     7   **✓7th S62.101 Fracture of unspecified carpal bone, right wrist**   CC H5

     7   **✓7th S62.102 Fracture of unspecified carpal bone, left wrist**   CC H5
                 **AHA:** 2012, 4Q, 95

     7   **✓7th S62.109 Fracture of unspecified carpal bone, unspecified wrist**   CC H5

   **✓6th S62.11 Fracture of triquetrum [cuneiform] bone of wrist**

     7   **✓7th S62.111 Displaced fracture of triquetrum [cuneiform] bone, right wrist**   CC H5

     7   **✓7th S62.112 Displaced fracture of triquetrum [cuneiform] bone, left wrist**   CC H5

     7   **✓7th S62.113 Displaced fracture of triquetrum [cuneiform] bone, unspecified wrist**   CC H5

     7   **✓7th S62.114 Nondisplaced fracture of triquetrum [cuneiform] bone, right wrist**   CC H5

     7   **✓7th S62.115 Nondisplaced fracture of triquetrum [cuneiform] bone, left wrist**   CC H5

     7   **✓7th S62.116 Nondisplaced fracture of triquetrum [cuneiform] bone, unspecified wrist**   CC H5

   **✓6th S62.12 Fracture of lunate [semilunar]**

     7   **✓7th S62.121 Displaced fracture of lunate [semilunar], right wrist**   CC H5

     7   **✓7th S62.122 Displaced fracture of lunate [semilunar], left wrist**   CC H5

     7   **✓7th S62.123 Displaced fracture of lunate [semilunar], unspecified wrist**   CC H5

     7   **✓7th S62.124 Nondisplaced fracture of lunate [semilunar], right wrist**   CC H5

     7   **✓7th S62.125 Nondisplaced fracture of lunate [semilunar], left wrist**   CC H5

     7   **✓7th S62.126 Nondisplaced fracture of lunate [semilunar], unspecified wrist**   CC H5

   **✓6th S62.13 Fracture of capitate [os magnum] bone**

     7   **✓7th S62.131 Displaced fracture of capitate [os magnum] bone, right wrist**   CC H5

     7   **✓7th S62.132 Displaced fracture of capitate [os magnum] bone, left wrist**   CC H5

     7   **✓7th S62.133 Displaced fracture of capitate [os magnum] bone, unspecified wrist**   CC H5

     7   **✓7th S62.134 Nondisplaced fracture of capitate [os magnum] bone, right wrist**   CC H5

     7   **✓7th S62.135 Nondisplaced fracture of capitate [os magnum] bone, left wrist**   CC H5

     7   **✓7th S62.136 Nondisplaced fracture of capitate [os magnum] bone, unspecified wrist**   CC H5

   **✓6th S62.14 Fracture of body of hamate [unciform] bone**
           Fracture of hamate [unciform] bone NOS

     7   **✓7th S62.141 Displaced fracture of body of hamate [unciform] bone, right wrist**   CC H5

---

**7**   CC when reported as an initial encounter (7th character A, B, or C – specific to category) OR a subsequent encounter for nonunion or malunion (7th character K, M, N, P, Q, or R – specific to category).

Ⓝ Newborn: 0    Ⓟ Pediatric: 0-17    Ⓜ Maternity: 12-55    Ⓐ Adult: 15-124    **MCC** Major CC Condition    **PDxMCC** PDx acts as own MCC    **CC** CC Condition    **PDxCC** PDx acts as own CC

**1018**                                        ICD-10-CM 2018

**7** ✓7th **S62.142** Displaced **fracture of body of hamate [unciform] bone, left wrist** `CC` `H5`

**7** ✓7th **S62.143** Displaced **fracture of body of hamate [unciform] bone, unspecified wrist** `CC` `H5`

**7** ✓7th **S62.144** Nondisplaced **fracture of body of hamate [unciform] bone, right wrist** `CC` `H5`

**7** ✓7th **S62.145** Nondisplaced **fracture of body of hamate [unciform] bone, left wrist** `CC` `H5`

**7** ✓7th **S62.146** Nondisplaced **fracture of body of hamate [unciform] bone, unspecified wrist** `CC` `H5`

✓6th **S62.15** Fracture of **hook process of hamate [unciform] bone**
Fracture of unciform process of hamate [unciform] bone

**7** ✓7th **S62.151** Displaced **fracture of hook process of hamate [unciform] bone, right wrist** `CC` `H5`

**7** ✓7th **S62.152** Displaced **fracture of hook process of hamate [unciform] bone, left wrist** `CC` `H5`

**7** ✓7th **S62.153** Displaced **fracture of hook process of hamate [unciform] bone, unspecified wrist** `CC` `H5`

**7** ✓7th **S62.154** Nondisplaced **fracture of hook process of hamate [unciform] bone, right wrist** `CC` `H5`

**7** ✓7th **S62.155** Nondisplaced **fracture of hook process of hamate [unciform] bone, left wrist** `CC` `H5`

**7** ✓7th **S62.156** Nondisplaced **fracture of hook process of hamate [unciform] bone, unspecified wrist** `CC` `H5`

✓6th **S62.16** Fracture of **pisiform**

**7** ✓7th **S62.161** Displaced **fracture of pisiform, right wrist** `CC` `H5`

**7** ✓7th **S62.162** Displaced **fracture of pisiform, left wrist** `CC` `H5`

**7** ✓7th **S62.163** Displaced **fracture of pisiform, unspecified wrist** `CC` `H5`

**7** ✓7th **S62.164** Nondisplaced **fracture of pisiform, right wrist** `CC` `H5`

**7** ✓7th **S62.165** Nondisplaced **fracture of pisiform, left wrist** `CC` `H5`

**7** ✓7th **S62.166** Nondisplaced **fracture of pisiform, unspecified wrist** `CC` `H5`

✓6th **S62.17** Fracture of **trapezium [larger multangular]**

**7** ✓7th **S62.171** Displaced **fracture of trapezium [larger multangular], right wrist** `CC` `H5`

**7** ✓7th **S62.172** Displaced **fracture of trapezium [larger multangular], left wrist** `CC` `H5`

**7** ✓7th **S62.173** Displaced **fracture of trapezium [larger multangular], unspecified wrist** `CC` `H5`

**7** ✓7th **S62.174** Nondisplaced **fracture of trapezium [larger multangular], right wrist** `CC` `H5`

**7** ✓7th **S62.175** Nondisplaced **fracture of trapezium [larger multangular], left wrist** `CC` `H5`

**7** ✓7th **S62.176** Nondisplaced **fracture of trapezium [larger multangular], unspecified wrist** `CC` `H5`

✓6th **S62.18** Fracture of **trapezoid [smaller multangular]**

**7** ✓7th **S62.181** Displaced **fracture of trapezoid [smaller multangular], right wrist** `CC` `H5`

**7** ✓7th **S62.182** Displaced **fracture of trapezoid [smaller multangular], left wrist** `CC` `H5`

**7** ✓7th **S62.183** Displaced **fracture of trapezoid [smaller multangular], unspecified wrist** `CC` `H5`

**7** ✓7th **S62.184** Nondisplaced **fracture of trapezoid [smaller multangular], right wrist** `CC` `H5`

**7** ✓7th **S62.185** Nondisplaced **fracture of trapezoid [smaller multangular], left wrist** `CC` `H5`

**7** ✓7th **S62.186** Nondisplaced **fracture of trapezoid [smaller multangular], unspecified wrist** `CC` `H5`

✓5th **S62.2** Fracture of **first metacarpal bone**

> **CC Excl: For codes in subcategory S62.2:**
> **CC with 7th character B:** PDX collection 1284
> **CC with 7th character K or P:** PDX collection 897

✓6th **S62.20** Unspecified **fracture of first metacarpal bone**

**7** ✓7th **S62.201** Unspecified **fracture of first metacarpal bone, right hand** `CC` `H5`

**7** ✓7th **S62.202** Unspecified **fracture of first metacarpal bone, left hand** `CC` `H5`

**7** ✓7th **S62.209** Unspecified **fracture of first metacarpal bone, unspecified hand** `CC` `H5`

✓6th **S62.21** Bennett's **fracture**

**7** ✓7th **S62.211** Bennett's **fracture, right hand** `CC` `H5`

**7** ✓7th **S62.212** Bennett's **fracture, left hand** `CC` `H5`

**7** ✓7th **S62.213** Bennett's **fracture, unspecified hand** `CC` `H5`

✓6th **S62.22** Rolando's **fracture**

**7** ✓7th **S62.221** Displaced **Rolando's fracture, right hand** `CC` `H5`

**7** ✓7th **S62.222** Displaced **Rolando's fracture, left hand** `CC` `H5`

**7** ✓7th **S62.223** Displaced **Rolando's fracture, unspecified hand** `CC` `H5`

**7** ✓7th **S62.224** Nondisplaced **Rolando's fracture, right hand** `CC` `H5`

**7** ✓7th **S62.225** Nondisplaced **Rolando's fracture, left hand** `CC` `H5`

**7** ✓7th **S62.226** Nondisplaced **Rolando's fracture, unspecified hand** `CC` `H5`

✓6th **S62.23** Other fracture of **base of first metacarpal bone**

**7** ✓7th **S62.231** Other displaced **fracture of base of first metacarpal bone, right hand** `CC` `H5`

**7** ✓7th **S62.232** Other displaced **fracture of base of first metacarpal bone, left hand** `CC` `H5`

**7** ✓7th **S62.233** Other displaced **fracture of base of first metacarpal bone, unspecified hand** `CC` `H5`

**7** ✓7th **S62.234** Other nondisplaced **fracture of base of first metacarpal bone, right hand** `CC` `H5`

**7** ✓7th **S62.235** Other nondisplaced **fracture of base of first metacarpal bone, left hand** `CC` `H5`

**7** ✓7th **S62.236** Other nondisplaced **fracture of base of first metacarpal bone, unspecified hand** `CC` `H5`

✓6th **S62.24** Fracture of **shaft of first metacarpal bone**

**7** ✓7th **S62.241** Displaced **fracture of shaft of first metacarpal bone, right hand** `CC` `H5`

**7** ✓7th **S62.242** Displaced **fracture of shaft of first metacarpal bone, left hand** `CC` `H5`

**7** ✓7th **S62.243** Displaced **fracture of shaft of first metacarpal bone, unspecified hand** `CC` `H5`

**7** ✓7th **S62.244** Nondisplaced **fracture of shaft of first metacarpal bone, right hand** `CC` `H5`

**7** ✓7th **S62.245** Nondisplaced **fracture of shaft of first metacarpal bone, left hand** `CC` `H5`

**7** ✓7th **S62.246** Nondisplaced **fracture of shaft of first metacarpal bone, unspecified hand** `CC` `H5`

✓6th **S62.25** Fracture of **neck of first metacarpal bone**

**7** ✓7th **S62.251** Displaced **fracture of neck of first metacarpal bone, right hand** `CC` `H5`

**7** ✓7th **S62.252** Displaced **fracture of neck of first metacarpal bone, left hand** `CC` `H5`

**7** ✓7th **S62.253** Displaced **fracture of neck of first metacarpal bone, unspecified hand** `CC` `H5`

**7** ✓7th **S62.254** Nondisplaced **fracture of neck of first metacarpal bone, right hand** `CC` `H5`

**7** ✓7th **S62.255** Nondisplaced **fracture of neck of first metacarpal bone, left hand** `CC` `H5`

**7** ✓7th **S62.256** Nondisplaced **fracture of neck of first metacarpal bone, unspecified hand** `CC` `H5`

---

**7** CC when reported as an initial encounter (7th character A, B, or C – specific to category) OR a subsequent encounter for nonunion or malunion (7th character K, M, N, P, Q, or R – specific to category).

✓ Additional Character Req  ✓x7th Placeholder Alert  Unacceptable PDx  Manifestation  `H1`-`H14` HAC  `HCC` CMS-HCC Condition  *EXCLUDES 1* Not Coded Here  *EXCLUDES 2* Not Included Here

ICD-10-CM 2018                  **1019**

**✓6th S62.29 Other fracture of first metacarpal bone**

7   ✓7th **S62.291 Other fracture of first metacarpal bone, right hand** `CC` `H5`

7   ✓7th **S62.292 Other fracture of first metacarpal bone, left hand** `CC` `H5`

7   ✓7th **S62.299 Other fracture of first metacarpal bone, unspecified hand** `CC` `H5`

**✓5th S62.3 Fracture of other and unspecified metacarpal bone**

EXCLUDES 2   *fracture of first metacarpal bone (S62.2-)*

CC Excl: For codes in subcategory S62.3:
CC with 7th character B: PDX collection 1284
CC with 7th character K or P: PDX collection 897

**✓6th S62.30 Unspecified fracture of other metacarpal bone**

7   ✓7th **S62.300 Unspecified fracture of second metacarpal bone, right hand** `CC` `H5`

7   ✓7th **S62.301 Unspecified fracture of second metacarpal bone, left hand** `CC` `H5`

7   ✓7th **S62.302 Unspecified fracture of third metacarpal bone, right hand** `CC` `H5`

7   ✓7th **S62.303 Unspecified fracture of third metacarpal bone, left hand** `CC` `H5`

7   ✓7th **S62.304 Unspecified fracture of fourth metacarpal bone, right hand** `CC` `H5`

7   ✓7th **S62.305 Unspecified fracture of fourth metacarpal bone, left hand** `CC` `H5`

7   ✓7th **S62.306 Unspecified fracture of fifth metacarpal bone, right hand** `CC` `H5`

7   ✓7th **S62.307 Unspecified fracture of fifth metacarpal bone, left hand** `CC` `H5`

7   ✓7th **S62.308 Unspecified fracture of other metacarpal bone** `CC` `H5`

Unspecified fracture of specified metacarpal bone with unspecified laterality

7   ✓7th **S62.309 Unspecified fracture of unspecified metacarpal bone** `CC` `H5`

**✓6th S62.31 Displaced fracture of base of other metacarpal bone**

7   ✓7th **S62.37 Displaced fracture of base of second metacarpal bone, right hand** `CC` `H5`

▲ 7   ✓7th **S62.311 Displaced fracture of base of second metacarpal bone, left hand** `CC` `H5`

7   ✓7th **S62.312 Displaced fracture of base of third metacarpal bone, right hand** `CC` `H5`

7   ✓7th **S62.313 Displaced fracture of base of third metacarpal bone, left hand** `CC` `H5`

7   ✓7th **S62.314 Displaced fracture of base of fourth metacarpal bone, right hand** `CC` `H5`

7   ✓7th **S62.315 Displaced fracture of base of fourth metacarpal bone, left hand** `CC` `H5`

7   ✓7th **S62.316 Displaced fracture of base of fifth metacarpal bone, right hand** `CC` `H5`

▲ 7   ✓7th **S62.317 Displaced fracture of base of fifth metacarpal bone, left hand** `CC` `H5`

7   ✓7th **S62.318 Displaced fracture of base of other metacarpal bone** `CC` `H5`

Displaced fracture of base of specified metacarpal bone with unspecified laterality

7   ✓7th **S62.319 Displaced fracture of base of unspecified metacarpal bone** `CC` `H5`

**✓6th S62.32 Displaced fracture of shaft of other metacarpal bone**

7   ✓7th **S62.320 Displaced fracture of shaft of second metacarpal bone, right hand** `CC` `H5`

7   ✓7th **S62.321 Displaced fracture of shaft of second metacarpal bone, left hand** `CC` `H5`

7   ✓7th **S62.322 Displaced fracture of shaft of third metacarpal bone, right hand** `CC` `H5`

7   ✓7th **S62.323 Displaced fracture of shaft of third metacarpal bone, left hand** `CC` `H5`

7   ✓7th **S62.324 Displaced fracture of shaft of fourth metacarpal bone, right hand** `CC` `H5`

7   ✓7th **S62.325 Displaced fracture of shaft of fourth metacarpal bone, left hand** `CC` `H5`

7   ✓7th **S62.326 Displaced fracture of shaft of fifth metacarpal bone, right hand** `CC` `H5`

7   ✓7th **S62.327 Displaced fracture of shaft of fifth metacarpal bone, left hand** `CC` `H5`

7   ✓7th **S62.328 Displaced fracture of shaft of other metacarpal bone** `CC` `H5`

Displaced fracture of shaft of specified metacarpal bone with unspecified laterality

7   ✓7th **S62.329 Displaced fracture of shaft of unspecified metacarpal bone** `CC` `H5`

**✓6th S62.33 Displaced fracture of neck of other metacarpal bone**

7   ✓7th **S62.330 Displaced fracture of neck of second metacarpal bone, right hand** `CC` `H5`

7   ✓7th **S62.331 Displaced fracture of neck of second metacarpal bone, left hand** `CC` `H5`

7   ✓7th **S62.332 Displaced fracture of neck of third metacarpal bone, right hand** `CC` `H5`

7   ✓7th **S62.333 Displaced fracture of neck of third metacarpal bone, left hand** `CC` `H5`

7   ✓7th **S62.334 Displaced fracture of neck of fourth metacarpal bone, right hand** `CC` `H5`

7   ✓7th **S62.335 Displaced fracture of neck of fourth metacarpal bone, left hand** `CC` `H5`

7   ✓7th **S62.336 Displaced fracture of neck of fifth metacarpal bone, right hand** `CC` `H5`

7   ✓7th **S62.337 Displaced fracture of neck of fifth metacarpal bone, left hand** `CC` `H5`

7   ✓7th **S62.338 Displaced fracture of neck of other metacarpal bone** `CC` `H5`

Displaced fracture of neck of specified metacarpal bone with unspecified laterality

7   ✓7th **S62.339 Displaced fracture of neck of unspecified metacarpal bone** `CC` `H5`

**✓6th S62.34 Nondisplaced fracture of base of other metacarpal bone**

7   ✓7th **S62.340 Nondisplaced fracture of base of second metacarpal bone, right hand** `CC` `H5`

▲ 7   ✓7th **S62.341 Nondisplaced fracture of base of second metacarpal bone, left hand** `CC` `H5`

7   ✓7th **S62.342 Nondisplaced fracture of base of third metacarpal bone, right hand** `CC` `H5`

7   ✓7th **S62.343 Nondisplaced fracture of base of third metacarpal bone, left hand** `CC` `H5`

7   ✓7th **S62.344 Nondisplaced fracture of base of fourth metacarpal bone, right hand** `CC` `H5`

7   ✓7th **S62.345 Nondisplaced fracture of base of fourth metacarpal bone, left hand** `CC` `H5`

7   ✓7th **S62.346 Nondisplaced fracture of base of fifth metacarpal bone, right hand** `CC` `H5`

▲ 7   ✓7th **S62.347 Nondisplaced fracture of base of fifth metacarpal bone, left hand** `CC` `H5`

7   ✓7th **S62.348 Nondisplaced fracture of base of other metacarpal bone** `CC` `H5`

Nondisplaced fracture of base of specified metacarpal bone with unspecified laterality

7   ✓7th **S62.349 Nondisplaced fracture of base of unspecified metacarpal bone** `CC` `H5`

**✓6th S62.35 Nondisplaced fracture of shaft of other metacarpal bone**

7   ✓7th **S62.350 Nondisplaced fracture of shaft of second metacarpal bone, right hand** `CC` `H5`

7   ✓7th **S62.351 Nondisplaced fracture of shaft of second metacarpal bone, left hand** `CC` `H5`

7   ✓7th **S62.352 Nondisplaced fracture of shaft of third metacarpal bone, right hand** `CC` `H5`

7   ✓7th **S62.353 Nondisplaced fracture of shaft of third metacarpal bone, left hand** `CC` `H5`

7   ✓7th **S62.354 Nondisplaced fracture of shaft of fourth metacarpal bone, right hand** `CC` `H5`

7   ✓7th **S62.355 Nondisplaced fracture of shaft of fourth metacarpal bone, left hand** `CC` `H5`

---

7   CC when reported as an initial encounter (7th character A, B, or C – specific to category) OR a subsequent encounter for nonunion or malunion (7th character K, M, N, P, Q, or R – specific to category).

`N` Newborn: 0   `P` Pediatric: 0-17   `M` Maternity: 12-55   `A` Adult: 15-124   `MCC` Major CC Condition   `PDxMCC` PDx acts as own MCC   `CC` CC Condition   `PDxCC` PDx acts as own CC

7  √7ᵗʰ  **S62.356**  **Nondisplaced fracture of shaft of fifth metacarpal bone, right hand**  `CC` `H5`

7  √7ᵗʰ  **S62.357**  **Nondisplaced fracture of shaft of fifth metacarpal bone, left hand**  `CC` `H5`

7  √7ᵗʰ  **S62.358**  **Nondisplaced fracture of shaft of other metacarpal bone**  `CC` `H5`
Nondisplaced fracture of shaft of specified metacarpal bone with unspecified laterality

7  √7ᵗʰ  **S62.359**  **Nondisplaced fracture of shaft of unspecified metacarpal bone**  `CC` `H5`

√6ᵗʰ  **S62.36**  **Nondisplaced fracture of neck of other metacarpal bone**

7  √7ᵗʰ  **S62.360**  **Nondisplaced fracture of neck of second metacarpal bone, right hand**  `CC` `H5`

7  √7ᵗʰ  **S62.361**  **Nondisplaced fracture of neck of second metacarpal bone, left hand**  `CC` `H5`

7  √7ᵗʰ  **S62.362**  **Nondisplaced fracture of neck of third metacarpal bone, right hand**  `CC` `H5`

7  √7ᵗʰ  **S62.363**  **Nondisplaced fracture of neck of third metacarpal bone, left hand**  `CC` `H5`

7  √7ᵗʰ  **S62.364**  **Nondisplaced fracture of neck of fourth metacarpal bone, right hand**  `CC` `H5`

7  √7ᵗʰ  **S62.365**  **Nondisplaced fracture of neck of fourth metacarpal bone, left hand**  `CC` `H5`

7  √7ᵗʰ  **S62.366**  **Nondisplaced fracture of neck of fifth metacarpal bone, right hand**  `CC` `H5`

7  √7ᵗʰ  **S62.367**  **Nondisplaced fracture of neck of fifth metacarpal bone, left hand**  `CC` `H5`

7  √7ᵗʰ  **S62.368**  **Nondisplaced fracture of neck of other metacarpal bone**  `CC` `H5`
Nondisplaced fracture of neck of specified metacarpal bone with unspecified laterality

7  √7ᵗʰ  **S62.369**  **Nondisplaced fracture of neck of unspecified metacarpal bone**  `CC` `H5`

√6ᵗʰ  **S62.39**  **Other fracture of other metacarpal bone**

7  √7ᵗʰ  **S62.390**  **Other fracture of second metacarpal bone, right hand**  `CC` `H5`

7  √7ᵗʰ  **S62.391**  **Other fracture of second metacarpal bone, left hand**  `CC` `H5`

7  √7ᵗʰ  **S62.392**  **Other fracture of third metacarpal bone, right hand**  `CC` `H5`

7  √7ᵗʰ  **S62.393**  **Other fracture of third metacarpal bone, left hand**  `CC` `H5`

7  √7ᵗʰ  **S62.394**  **Other fracture of fourth metacarpal bone, right hand**  `CC` `H5`

7  √7ᵗʰ  **S62.395**  **Other fracture of fourth metacarpal bone, left hand**  `CC` `H5`

7  √7ᵗʰ  **S62.396**  **Other fracture of fifth metacarpal bone, right hand**  `CC` `H5`

7  √7ᵗʰ  **S62.397**  **Other fracture of fifth metacarpal bone, left hand**  `CC` `H5`

7  √7ᵗʰ  **S62.398**  **Other fracture of other metacarpal bone**  `CC` `H5`
Other fracture of specified metacarpal bone with unspecified laterality

7  √7ᵗʰ  **S62.399**  **Other fracture of unspecified metacarpal bone**  `CC` `H5`

√5ᵗʰ  **S62.5**  **Fracture of thumb**

**CC Excl: For codes in subcategory S62.5:**
**CC with 7th character B:** PDX collection 1285
**CC with 7th character K or P:** PDX collection 897

√6ᵗʰ  **S62.50**  **Fracture of unspecified phalanx of thumb**

7  √7ᵗʰ  **S62.501**  **Fracture of unspecified phalanx of right thumb**  `CC` `H5`

7  √7ᵗʰ  **S62.502**  **Fracture of unspecified phalanx of left thumb**  `CC` `H5`

7  √7ᵗʰ  **S62.509**  **Fracture of unspecified phalanx of unspecified thumb**  `CC` `H5`

√6ᵗʰ  **S62.51**  **Fracture of proximal phalanx of thumb**

7  √7ᵗʰ  **S62.511**  **Displaced fracture of proximal phalanx of right thumb**  `CC` `H5`

7  √7ᵗʰ  **S62.512**  **Displaced fracture of proximal phalanx of left thumb**  `CC` `H5`

7  √7ᵗʰ  **S62.513**  **Displaced fracture of proximal phalanx of unspecified thumb**  `CC` `H5`

7  √7ᵗʰ  **S62.514**  **Nondisplaced fracture of proximal phalanx of right thumb**  `CC` `H5`

7  √7ᵗʰ  **S62.515**  **Nondisplaced fracture of proximal phalanx of left thumb**  `CC` `H5`

7  √7ᵗʰ  **S62.516**  **Nondisplaced fracture of proximal phalanx of unspecified thumb**  `CC` `H5`

√6ᵗʰ  **S62.52**  **Fracture of distal phalanx of thumb**

7  √7ᵗʰ  **S62.521**  **Displaced fracture of distal phalanx of right thumb**  `CC` `H5`

7  √7ᵗʰ  **S62.522**  **Displaced fracture of distal phalanx of left thumb**  `CC` `H5`

7  √7ᵗʰ  **S62.523**  **Displaced fracture of distal phalanx of unspecified thumb**  `CC` `H5`

7  √7ᵗʰ  **S62.524**  **Nondisplaced fracture of distal phalanx of right thumb**  `CC` `H5`

7  √7ᵗʰ  **S62.525**  **Nondisplaced fracture of distal phalanx of left thumb**  `CC` `H5`

7  √7ᵗʰ  **S62.526**  **Nondisplaced fracture of distal phalanx of unspecified thumb**  `CC` `H5`

√5ᵗʰ  **S62.6**  **Fracture of other and unspecified finger(s)**
*EXCLUDES 2*  fracture of thumb (S62.5-)

**CC Excl: For codes in subcategory S62.6:**
**CC with 7th character B:** PDX collection 1285
**CC with 7th character K or P:** PDX collection 897

√6ᵗʰ  **S62.60**  **Fracture of unspecified phalanx of finger**

7  √7ᵗʰ  **S62.600**  **Fracture of unspecified phalanx of right index finger**  `CC` `H5`

7  √7ᵗʰ  **S62.601**  **Fracture of unspecified phalanx of left index finger**  `CC` `H5`

7  √7ᵗʰ  **S62.602**  **Fracture of unspecified phalanx of right middle finger**  `CC` `H5`

7  √7ᵗʰ  **S62.603**  **Fracture of unspecified phalanx of left middle finger**  `CC` `H5`

7  √7ᵗʰ  **S62.604**  **Fracture of unspecified phalanx of right ring finger**  `CC` `H5`

7  √7ᵗʰ  **S62.605**  **Fracture of unspecified phalanx of left ring finger**  `CC` `H5`

7  √7ᵗʰ  **S62.606**  **Fracture of unspecified phalanx of right little finger**  `CC` `H5`

7  √7ᵗʰ  **S62.607**  **Fracture of unspecified phalanx of left little finger**  `CC` `H5`

7  √7ᵗʰ  **S62.608**  **Fracture of unspecified phalanx of other finger**  `CC` `H5`
Fracture of unspecified phalanx of specified finger with unspecified laterality

7  √7ᵗʰ  **S62.609**  **Fracture of unspecified phalanx of unspecified finger**  `CC` `H5`

√6ᵗʰ  **S62.61**  **Displaced fracture of proximal phalanx of finger**

7  √7ᵗʰ  **S62.610**  **Displaced fracture of proximal phalanx of right index finger**  `CC` `H5`

7  √7ᵗʰ  **S62.611**  **Displaced fracture of proximal phalanx of left index finger**  `CC` `H5`

7  √7ᵗʰ  **S62.612**  **Displaced fracture of proximal phalanx of right middle finger**  `CC` `H5`

7  √7ᵗʰ  **S62.613**  **Displaced fracture of proximal phalanx of left middle finger**  `CC` `H5`

7  √7ᵗʰ  **S62.614**  **Displaced fracture of proximal phalanx of right ring finger**  `CC` `H5`

7  √7ᵗʰ  **S62.615**  **Displaced fracture of proximal phalanx of left ring finger**  `CC` `H5`

7  √7ᵗʰ  **S62.616**  **Displaced fracture of proximal phalanx of right little finger**  `CC` `H5`

7  √7ᵗʰ  **S62.617**  **Displaced fracture of proximal phalanx of left little finger**  `CC` `H5`

7  √7ᵗʰ  **S62.618**  **Displaced fracture of proximal phalanx of other finger**  `CC` `H5`
Displaced fracture of proximal phalanx of specified finger with unspecified laterality

---

7  CC when reported as an initial encounter (7th character A, B, or C – specific to category) OR a subsequent encounter for nonunion or malunion (7th character K, M, N, P, Q, or R – specific to category).

**Chapter 19. Injury, Poisoning and Certain Other Consequences of External Causes**

7 ✓7ᵗʰ **S62.619 Displaced fracture of proximal phalanx of unspecified finger** `CC` `H5`

▲ ✓6ᵗʰ **S62.62 Displaced fracture of middle phalanx of finger**

▲ 7 ✓7ᵗʰ **S62.620 Displaced fracture of middle phalanx of right index finger** `CC` `H5`

▲ 7 ✓7ᵗʰ **S62.621 Displaced fracture of middle phalanx of left index finger** `CC` `H5`

▲ 7 ✓7ᵗʰ **S62.622 Displaced fracture of middle phalanx of right middle finger** `CC` `H5`

▲ 7 ✓7ᵗʰ **S62.623 Displaced fracture of middle phalanx of left middle finger** `CC` `H5`

▲ 7 ✓7ᵗʰ **S62.624 Displaced fracture of middle phalanx of right ring finger** `CC` `H5`

▲ 7 ✓7ᵗʰ **S62.625 Displaced fracture of middle phalanx of left ring finger** `CC` `H5`

7 ✓7ᵗʰ **S62.626 Displaced fracture of medial phalanx of right little finger** `CC` `H5`

7 ✓7ᵗʰ **S62.627 Displaced fracture of medial phalanx of left little finger** `CC` `H5`

7 ✓7ᵗʰ **S62.628 Displaced fracture of medial phalanx of other finger** `CC` `H5`
  Displaced fracture of medial phalanx of specified finger with unspecified laterality

7 ✓7ᵗʰ **S62.629 Displaced fracture of medial phalanx of unspecified finger** `CC` `H5`

✓6ᵗʰ **S62.63 Displaced fracture of distal phalanx of finger**

7 ✓7ᵗʰ **S62.630 Displaced fracture of distal phalanx of right index finger** `CC` `H5`

7 ✓7ᵗʰ **S62.631 Displaced fracture of distal phalanx of left index finger** `CC` `H5`

7 ✓7ᵗʰ **S62.632 Displaced fracture of distal phalanx of right middle finger** `CC` `H5`

7 ✓7ᵗʰ **S62.633 Displaced fracture of distal phalanx of left middle finger** `CC` `H5`

7 ✓7ᵗʰ **S62.634 Displaced fracture of distal phalanx of right ring finger** `CC` `H5`

7 ✓7ᵗʰ **S62.635 Displaced fracture of distal phalanx of left ring finger** `CC` `H5`

7 ✓7ᵗʰ **S62.636 Displaced fracture of distal phalanx of right little finger** `CC` `H5`

7 ✓7ᵗʰ **S62.637 Displaced fracture of distal phalanx of left little finger** `CC` `H5`

7 ✓7ᵗʰ **S62.638 Displaced fracture of distal phalanx of other finger** `CC` `H5`
  Displaced fracture of distal phalanx of specified finger with unspecified laterality

7 ✓7ᵗʰ **S62.639 Displaced fracture of distal phalanx of unspecified finger** `CC` `H5`

✓6ᵗʰ **S62.64 Nondisplaced fracture of proximal phalanx of finger**

7 ✓7ᵗʰ **S62.640 Nondisplaced fracture of proximal phalanx of right index finger** `CC` `H5`

7 ✓7ᵗʰ **S62.641 Nondisplaced fracture of proximal phalanx of left index finger** `CC` `H5`

7 ✓7ᵗʰ **S62.642 Nondisplaced fracture of proximal phalanx of right middle finger** `CC` `H5`

7 ✓7ᵗʰ **S62.643 Nondisplaced fracture of proximal phalanx of left middle finger** `CC` `H5`

7 ✓7ᵗʰ **S62.644 Nondisplaced fracture of proximal phalanx of right ring finger** `CC` `H5`

7 ✓7ᵗʰ **S62.645 Nondisplaced fracture of proximal phalanx of left ring finger** `CC` `H5`

7 ✓7ᵗʰ **S62.646 Nondisplaced fracture of proximal phalanx of right little finger** `CC` `H5`

7 ✓7ᵗʰ **S62.647 Nondisplaced fracture of proximal phalanx of left little finger** `CC` `H5`

7 ✓7ᵗʰ **S62.648 Nondisplaced fracture of proximal phalanx of other finger** `CC` `H5`
  Nondisplaced fracture of proximal phalanx of specified finger with unspecified laterality

7 ✓7ᵗʰ **S62.649 Nondisplaced fracture of proximal phalanx of unspecified finger** `CC` `H5`

▲ ✓6ᵗʰ **S62.65 Nondisplaced fracture of middle phalanx of finger**

▲ 7 ✓7ᵗʰ **S62.650 Nondisplaced fracture of middle phalanx of right index finger** `CC` `H5`

▲ 7 ✓7ᵗʰ **S62.651 Nondisplaced fracture of middle phalanx of left index finger** `CC` `H5`

7 ✓7ᵗʰ **S62.652 Nondisplaced fracture of middle phalanx of right middle finger** `CC` `H5`

▲ 7 ✓7ᵗʰ **S62.653 Nondisplaced fracture of middle phalanx of left middle finger** `CC` `H5`

7 ✓7ᵗʰ **S62.654 Nondisplaced fracture of medial phalanx of right ring finger** `CC` `H5`

7 ✓7ᵗʰ **S62.655 Nondisplaced fracture of medial phalanx of left ring finger** `CC` `H5`

7 ✓7ᵗʰ **S62.656 Nondisplaced fracture of medial phalanx of right little finger** `CC` `H5`

7 ✓7ᵗʰ **S62.657 Nondisplaced fracture of medial phalanx of left little finger** `CC` `H5`

7 ✓7ᵗʰ **S62.658 Nondisplaced fracture of medial phalanx of other finger** `CC` `H5`
  Nondisplaced fracture of medial phalanx of specified finger with unspecified laterality

7 ✓7ᵗʰ **S62.659 Nondisplaced fracture of medial phalanx of unspecified finger** `CC` `H5`

✓6ᵗʰ **S62.66 Nondisplaced fracture of distal phalanx of finger**

7 ✓7ᵗʰ **S62.660 Nondisplaced fracture of distal phalanx of right index finger** `CC` `H5`

7 ✓7ᵗʰ **S62.661 Nondisplaced fracture of distal phalanx of left index finger** `CC` `H5`

7 ✓7ᵗʰ **S62.662 Nondisplaced fracture of distal phalanx of right middle finger** `CC` `H5`

7 ✓7ᵗʰ **S62.663 Nondisplaced fracture of distal phalanx of left middle finger** `CC` `H5`

7 ✓7ᵗʰ **S62.664 Nondisplaced fracture of distal phalanx of right ring finger** `CC` `H5`

7 ✓7ᵗʰ **S62.665 Nondisplaced fracture of distal phalanx of left ring finger** `CC` `H5`

7 ✓7ᵗʰ **S62.666 Nondisplaced fracture of distal phalanx of right little finger** `CC` `H5`

7 ✓7ᵗʰ **S62.667 Nondisplaced fracture of distal phalanx of left little finger** `CC` `H5`

7 ✓7ᵗʰ **S62.668 Nondisplaced fracture of distal phalanx of other finger** `CC` `H5`
  Nondisplaced fracture of distal phalanx of specified finger with unspecified laterality

7 ✓7ᵗʰ **S62.669 Nondisplaced fracture of distal phalanx of unspecified finger** `CC` `H5`

✓5ᵗʰ **S62.9 Unspecified fracture of wrist and hand**

7 ✓x7ᵗʰ **S62.90 Unspecified fracture of unspecified wrist and hand** `CC` `H5`
  **CC Excl: CC with 7th character B:** PDX collection 1286
  **CC with 7th character K or P:** PDX collection 897

7 ✓x7ᵗʰ **S62.91 Unspecified fracture of right wrist and hand** `CC` `H5`
  **CC Excl: CC with 7th character B:** PDX collection 1287
  **CC with 7th character K or P:** PDX collection 897

7 ✓x7ᵗʰ **S62.92 Unspecified fracture of left wrist and hand** `CC` `H5`
  **CC Excl: CC with 7th character B:** PDX collection 1287
  **CC with 7th character K or P:** PDX collection 897

---

**7** CC when reported as an initial encounter (7th character A, B, or C – specific to category) OR a subsequent encounter for nonunion or malunion (7th character K, M, N, P, Q, or R – specific to category).

`N` Newborn: 0   `P` Pediatric: 0-17   `M` Maternity: 12-55   `A` Adult: 15-124   `MCC` Major CC Condition   `PDxMCC` PDx acts as own MCC   `CC` CC Condition   `PDxCC` PDx acts as own CC

**1022**          ICD-10-CM 2018

✓4ᵗʰ **S63** **Dislocation and sprain of joints and ligaments at wrist and hand level**

     INCLUDES    avulsion of joint or ligament at wrist and hand level
         laceration of cartilage, joint or ligament at wrist and hand level
         sprain of cartilage, joint or ligament at wrist and hand level
         traumatic hemarthrosis of joint or ligament at wrist and hand level
         traumatic rupture of joint or ligament at wrist and hand level
         traumatic subluxation of joint or ligament at wrist and hand level
         traumatic tear of joint or ligament at wrist and hand level

     Code also any associated open wound

     EXCLUDES 2   *strain of muscle, fascia and tendon of wrist and hand (S66.-)*

     The appropriate 7th character is to be added to each code from category S63.
     A     initial encounter
     D     subsequent encounter
     S     sequela

✓5ᵗʰ **S63.0** **Subluxation and dislocation of** wrist and hand joints

     ✓6ᵗʰ **S63.00** **Unspecified subluxation and dislocation of wrist and hand**
         Dislocation of carpal bone NOS
         Dislocation of distal end of radius NOS
         Subluxation of carpal bone NOS
         Subluxation of distal end of radius NOS

         ✓7ᵗʰ **S63.001** **Unspecified subluxation of right wrist and hand**

         ✓7ᵗʰ **S63.002** **Unspecified subluxation of left wrist and hand**

         ✓7ᵗʰ **S63.003** **Unspecified subluxation of unspecified wrist and hand**

         ✓7ᵗʰ **S63.004** **Unspecified dislocation of right wrist and hand**

         ✓7ᵗʰ **S63.005** **Unspecified dislocation of left wrist and hand**

         ✓7ᵗʰ **S63.006** **Unspecified dislocation of unspecified wrist and hand**

     ✓6ᵗʰ **S63.01** **Subluxation and dislocation of distal radioulnar joint**

         ✓7ᵗʰ **S63.011** **Subluxation of distal radioulnar joint of right wrist**

         ✓7ᵗʰ **S63.012** **Subluxation of distal radioulnar joint of left wrist**

         ✓7ᵗʰ **S63.013** **Subluxation of distal radioulnar joint of unspecified wrist**

         ✓7ᵗʰ **S63.014** **Dislocation of distal radioulnar joint of right wrist**

         ✓7ᵗʰ **S63.015** **Dislocation of distal radioulnar joint of left wrist**

         ✓7ᵗʰ **S63.016** **Dislocation of distal radioulnar joint of unspecified wrist**

     ✓6ᵗʰ **S63.02** **Subluxation and dislocation of radiocarpal joint**

         ✓7ᵗʰ **S63.021** **Subluxation of radiocarpal joint of right wrist**

         ✓7ᵗʰ **S63.022** **Subluxation of radiocarpal joint of left wrist**

         ✓7ᵗʰ **S63.023** **Subluxation of radiocarpal joint of unspecified wrist**

         ✓7ᵗʰ **S63.024** **Dislocation of radiocarpal joint of right wrist**

         ✓7ᵗʰ **S63.025** **Dislocation of radiocarpal joint of left wrist**

         ✓7ᵗʰ **S63.026** **Dislocation of radiocarpal joint of unspecified wrist**

     ✓6ᵗʰ **S63.03** **Subluxation and dislocation of midcarpal joint**

         ✓7ᵗʰ **S63.031** **Subluxation of midcarpal joint of right wrist**

         ✓7ᵗʰ **S63.032** **Subluxation of midcarpal joint of left wrist**

         ✓7ᵗʰ **S63.033** **Subluxation of midcarpal joint of unspecified wrist**

         ✓7ᵗʰ **S63.034** **Dislocation of midcarpal joint of right wrist**

         ✓7ᵗʰ **S63.035** **Dislocation of midcarpal joint of left wrist**

         ✓7ᵗʰ **S63.036** **Dislocation of midcarpal joint of unspecified wrist**

     ✓6ᵗʰ **S63.04** **Subluxation and dislocation of** carpometacarpal joint of thumb

         EXCLUDES 2   *interphalangeal subluxation and dislocation of thumb (S63.1-)*

         ✓7ᵗʰ **S63.041** **Subluxation of carpometacarpal joint of right thumb**

         ✓7ᵗʰ **S63.042** **Subluxation of carpometacarpal joint of left thumb**

         ✓7ᵗʰ **S63.043** **Subluxation of carpometacarpal joint of unspecified thumb**

         ✓7ᵗʰ **S63.044** **Dislocation of carpometacarpal joint of right thumb**

         ✓7ᵗʰ **S63.045** **Dislocation of carpometacarpal joint of left thumb**

         ✓7ᵗʰ **S63.046** **Dislocation of carpometacarpal joint of unspecified thumb**

     ✓6ᵗʰ **S63.05** **Subluxation and dislocation of** other carpometacarpal joint

         EXCLUDES 2   *subluxation and dislocation of carpometacarpal joint of thumb (S63.04-)*

         ✓7ᵗʰ **S63.051** **Subluxation of other carpometacarpal joint of right hand**

         ✓7ᵗʰ **S63.052** **Subluxation of other carpometacarpal joint of left hand**

         ✓7ᵗʰ **S63.053** **Subluxation of other carpometacarpal joint of unspecified hand**

         ✓7ᵗʰ **S63.054** **Dislocation of other carpometacarpal joint of right hand**

         ✓7ᵗʰ **S63.055** **Dislocation of other carpometacarpal joint of left hand**

         ✓7ᵗʰ **S63.056** **Dislocation of other carpometacarpal joint of unspecified hand**

     ✓6ᵗʰ **S63.06** **Subluxation and dislocation of** metacarpal (bone), proximal end

         ✓7ᵗʰ **S63.061** **Subluxation of metacarpal (bone), proximal end of right hand**

         ✓7ᵗʰ **S63.062** **Subluxation of metacarpal (bone), proximal end of left hand**

         ✓7ᵗʰ **S63.063** **Subluxation of metacarpal (bone), proximal end of unspecified hand**

         ✓7ᵗʰ **S63.064** **Dislocation of metacarpal (bone), proximal end of right hand**

         ✓7ᵗʰ **S63.065** **Dislocation of metacarpal (bone), proximal end of left hand**

         ✓7ᵗʰ **S63.066** **Dislocation of metacarpal (bone), proximal end of unspecified hand**

     ✓6ᵗʰ **S63.07** **Subluxation and dislocation of** distal end of ulna

         ✓7ᵗʰ **S63.071** **Subluxation of distal end of right ulna**

         ✓7ᵗʰ **S63.072** **Subluxation of distal end of left ulna**

         ✓7ᵗʰ **S63.073** **Subluxation of distal end of unspecified ulna**

         ✓7ᵗʰ **S63.074** **Dislocation of distal end of right ulna**

         ✓7ᵗʰ **S63.075** **Dislocation of distal end of left ulna**

         ✓7ᵗʰ **S63.076** **Dislocation of distal end of unspecified ulna**

     ✓6ᵗʰ **S63.09** **Other subluxation and dislocation of** wrist and hand

         ✓7ᵗʰ **S63.091** **Other subluxation of right wrist and hand**

         ✓7ᵗʰ **S63.092** **Other subluxation of left wrist and hand**

         ✓7ᵗʰ **S63.093** **Other subluxation of unspecified wrist and hand**

         ✓7ᵗʰ **S63.094** **Other dislocation of right wrist and hand**

         ✓7ᵗʰ **S63.095** **Other dislocation of left wrist and hand**

         ✓7ᵗʰ **S63.096** **Other dislocation of unspecified wrist and hand**

✓5ᵗʰ **S63.1** **Subluxation and dislocation of** thumb

     ✓6ᵗʰ **S63.10** **Unspecified subluxation and dislocation of thumb**

         ✓7ᵗʰ **S63.101** **Unspecified subluxation of right thumb**

         ✓7ᵗʰ **S63.102** **Unspecified subluxation of left thumb**

         ✓7ᵗʰ **S63.103** **Unspecified subluxation of unspecified thumb**

         ✓7ᵗʰ **S63.104** **Unspecified dislocation of right thumb**

         ✓7ᵗʰ **S63.105** **Unspecified dislocation of left thumb**

✓ Additional Character Req    ✓x7ᵗʰ Placeholder Alert    Unacceptable PDx    Manifestation    H1 - H14 HAC    HCC CMS-HCC Condition    EXCLUDES 1 Not Coded Here    EXCLUDES 2 Not Included Here

ICD-10-CM 2018                                                    **1023**

√7ᵗʰ **S63.106** Unspecified dislocation of unspecified thumb

√6ᵗʰ **S63.11** Subluxation and dislocation of metacarpophalangeal joint of thumb

√7ᵗʰ **S63.111** Subluxation of metacarpophalangeal joint of right thumb

√7ᵗʰ **S63.112** Subluxation of metacarpophalangeal joint of left thumb

√7ᵗʰ **S63.113** Subluxation of metacarpophalangeal joint of unspecified thumb

√7ᵗʰ **S63.114** Dislocation of metacarpophalangeal joint of right thumb

√7ᵗʰ **S63.115** Dislocation of metacarpophalangeal joint of left thumb

√7ᵗʰ **S63.116** Dislocation of metacarpophalangeal joint of unspecified thumb

▲ √6ᵗʰ **S63.12** Subluxation and dislocation of interphalangeal joint of thumb

▲ √7ᵗʰ **S63.121** Subluxation of interphalangeal joint of right thumb

▲ √7ᵗʰ **S63.122** Subluxation of interphalangeal joint of left thumb

▲ √7ᵗʰ **S63.123** Subluxation of interphalangeal joint of unspecified thumb

▲ √7ᵗʰ **S63.124** Dislocation of interphalangeal joint of right thumb

▲ √7ᵗʰ **S63.125** Dislocation of interphalangeal joint of left thumb

▲ √7ᵗʰ **S63.126** Dislocation of interphalangeal joint of unspecified thumb

√6ᵗʰ **S63.13** ~~Subluxation and dislocation of proximal interphalangeal joint of thumb~~

√7ᵗʰ **S63.131** ~~Subluxation of proximal interphalangeal joint of right thumb~~

√7ᵗʰ **S63.132** ~~Subluxation of proximal interphalangeal joint of left thumb~~

√7ᵗʰ **S63.133** ~~Subluxation of proximal interphalangeal joint of unspecified thumb~~

√7ᵗʰ **S63.134** ~~Dislocation of proximal interphalangeal joint of right thumb~~

√7ᵗʰ **S63.135** ~~Dislocation of proximal interphalangeal joint of left thumb~~

√7ᵗʰ **S63.136** ~~Dislocation of proximal interphalangeal joint of unspecified thumb~~

√6ᵗʰ **S63.14** ~~Subluxation and dislocation of distal interphalangeal joint of thumb~~

√7ᵗʰ **S63.141** ~~Subluxation of distal interphalangeal joint of right thumb~~

√7ᵗʰ **S63.142** ~~Subluxation of distal interphalangeal joint of left thumb~~

√7ᵗʰ **S63.143** ~~Subluxation of distal interphalangeal joint of unspecified thumb~~

√7ᵗʰ **S63.144** ~~Dislocation of distal interphalangeal joint of right thumb~~

√7ᵗʰ **S63.145** ~~Dislocation of distal interphalangeal joint of left thumb~~

√7ᵗʰ **S63.146** ~~Dislocation of distal interphalangeal joint of unspecified thumb~~

√5ᵗʰ **S63.2** Subluxation and dislocation of other finger(s)

     **EXCLUDES 2**   subluxation and dislocation of thumb (S63.1-)

√6ᵗʰ **S63.20** Unspecified subluxation of other finger

√7ᵗʰ **S63.200** Unspecified subluxation of right index finger

√7ᵗʰ **S63.201** Unspecified subluxation of left index finger

√7ᵗʰ **S63.202** Unspecified subluxation of right middle finger

√7ᵗʰ **S63.203** Unspecified subluxation of left middle finger

√7ᵗʰ **S63.204** Unspecified subluxation of right ring finger

√7ᵗʰ **S63.205** Unspecified subluxation of left ring finger

√7ᵗʰ **S63.206** Unspecified subluxation of right little finger

√7ᵗʰ **S63.207** Unspecified subluxation of left little finger

√7ᵗʰ **S63.208** Unspecified subluxation of other finger

Unspecified subluxation of specified finger with unspecified laterality

√7ᵗʰ **S63.209** Unspecified subluxation of unspecified finger

√6ᵗʰ **S63.21** Subluxation of metacarpophalangeal joint of finger

√7ᵗʰ **S63.210** Subluxation of metacarpophalangeal joint of right index finger

√7ᵗʰ **S63.211** Subluxation of metacarpophalangeal joint of left index finger

√7ᵗʰ **S63.212** Subluxation of metacarpophalangeal joint of right middle finger

√7ᵗʰ **S63.213** Subluxation of metacarpophalangeal joint of left middle finger

√7ᵗʰ **S63.214** Subluxation of metacarpophalangeal joint of right ring finger

√7ᵗʰ **S63.215** Subluxation of metacarpophalangeal joint of left ring finger

√7ᵗʰ **S63.216** Subluxation of metacarpophalangeal joint of right little finger

√7ᵗʰ **S63.217** Subluxation of metacarpophalangeal joint of left little finger

√7ᵗʰ **S63.218** Subluxation of metacarpophalangeal joint of other finger

Subluxation of metacarpophalangeal joint of specified finger with unspecified laterality

√7ᵗʰ **S63.219** Subluxation of metacarpophalangeal joint of unspecified finger

√6ᵗʰ **S63.22** Subluxation of unspecified interphalangeal joint of finger

√7ᵗʰ **S63.220** Subluxation of unspecified interphalangeal joint of right index finger

√7ᵗʰ **S63.221** Subluxation of unspecified interphalangeal joint of left index finger

√7ᵗʰ **S63.222** Subluxation of unspecified interphalangeal joint of right middle finger

√7ᵗʰ **S63.223** Subluxation of unspecified interphalangeal joint of left middle finger

√7ᵗʰ **S63.224** Subluxation of unspecified interphalangeal joint of right ring finger

√7ᵗʰ **S63.225** Subluxation of unspecified interphalangeal joint of left ring finger

√7ᵗʰ **S63.226** Subluxation of unspecified interphalangeal joint of right little finger

√7ᵗʰ **S63.227** Subluxation of unspecified interphalangeal joint of left little finger

√7ᵗʰ **S63.228** Subluxation of unspecified interphalangeal joint of other finger

Subluxation of unspecified interphalangeal joint of specified finger with unspecified laterality

√7ᵗʰ **S63.229** Subluxation of unspecified interphalangeal joint of unspecified finger

√6ᵗʰ **S63.23** Subluxation of proximal interphalangeal joint of finger

√7ᵗʰ **S63.230** Subluxation of proximal interphalangeal joint of right index finger

√7ᵗʰ **S63.231** Subluxation of proximal interphalangeal joint of left index finger

√7ᵗʰ **S63.232** Subluxation of proximal interphalangeal joint of right middle finger

√7ᵗʰ **S63.233** Subluxation of proximal interphalangeal joint of left middle finger

√7ᵗʰ **S63.234** Subluxation of proximal interphalangeal joint of right ring finger

√7ᵗʰ **S63.235** Subluxation of proximal interphalangeal joint of left ring finger

√7ᵗʰ **S63.236** Subluxation of proximal interphalangeal joint of right little finger

√7ᵗʰ **S63.237** Subluxation of proximal interphalangeal joint of left little finger

ℕ Newborn: 0   ℙ Pediatric: 0-17   Ⓜ Maternity: 12-55   Ⓐ Adult: 15-124   **MCC** Major CC Condition   **PDxMCC** PDx acts as own MCC   **CC** CC Condition   **PDxCC** PDx acts as own CC

**1024**

ICD-10-CM 2018

√7ᵗʰ **S63.238** **Subluxation of proximal interphalangeal joint of** other **finger**
Subluxation of proximal interphalangeal joint of specified finger with unspecified laterality

√7ᵗʰ **S63.239** **Subluxation of proximal interphalangeal joint of** unspecified **finger**

√6ᵗʰ **S63.24** **Subluxation of** distal interphalangeal **joint of finger**

√7ᵗʰ **S63.240** **Subluxation of distal interphalangeal joint of** right index **finger**

√7ᵗʰ **S63.241** **Subluxation of distal interphalangeal joint of** left index **finger**

√7ᵗʰ **S63.242** **Subluxation of distal interphalangeal joint of** right middle **finger**

√7ᵗʰ **S63.243** **Subluxation of distal interphalangeal joint of** left middle **finger**

√7ᵗʰ **S63.244** **Subluxation of distal interphalangeal joint of** right ring **finger**

√7ᵗʰ **S63.245** **Subluxation of distal interphalangeal joint of** left ring **finger**

√7ᵗʰ **S63.246** **Subluxation of distal interphalangeal joint of** right little **finger**

√7ᵗʰ **S63.247** **Subluxation of distal interphalangeal joint of** left little **finger**

√7ᵗʰ **S63.248** **Subluxation of distal interphalangeal joint of** other **finger**
Subluxation of distal interphalangeal joint of specified finger with unspecified laterality

√7ᵗʰ **S63.249** **Subluxation of distal interphalangeal joint of** unspecified **finger**

√6ᵗʰ **S63.25** **Unspecified dislocation of** other **finger**

√7ᵗʰ **S63.250** **Unspecified dislocation of** right index **finger**

√7ᵗʰ **S63.251** **Unspecified dislocation of** left index **finger**

√7ᵗʰ **S63.252** **Unspecified dislocation of** right middle **finger**

√7ᵗʰ **S63.253** **Unspecified dislocation of** left middle **finger**

√7ᵗʰ **S63.254** **Unspecified dislocation of** right ring **finger**

√7ᵗʰ **S63.255** **Unspecified dislocation of** left ring **finger**

√7ᵗʰ **S63.256** **Unspecified dislocation of** right little **finger**

√7ᵗʰ **S63.257** **Unspecified dislocation of** left little **finger**

√7ᵗʰ **S63.258** **Unspecified dislocation of** other **finger**
Unspecified dislocation of specified finger with unspecified laterality

√7ᵗʰ **S63.259** **Unspecified dislocation of** unspecified **finger**
▶Unspecified dislocation of unspecified finger with unspecified laterality◀

√6ᵗʰ **S63.26** **Dislocation of** metacarpophalangeal **joint of finger**

√7ᵗʰ **S63.260** **Dislocation of metacarpophalangeal joint of** right index **finger**

√7ᵗʰ **S63.261** **Dislocation of metacarpophalangeal joint of** left index **finger**

√7ᵗʰ **S63.262** **Dislocation of metacarpophalangeal joint of** right middle **finger**

√7ᵗʰ **S63.263** **Dislocation of metacarpophalangeal joint of** left middle **finger**

√7ᵗʰ **S63.264** **Dislocation of metacarpophalangeal joint of** right ring **finger**

√7ᵗʰ **S63.265** **Dislocation of metacarpophalangeal joint of** left ring **finger**

√7ᵗʰ **S63.266** **Dislocation of metacarpophalangeal joint of** right little **finger**

√7ᵗʰ **S63.267** **Dislocation of metacarpophalangeal joint of** left little **finger**

√7ᵗʰ **S63.268** **Dislocation of metacarpophalangeal joint of** other **finger**
Dislocation of metacarpophalangeal joint of specified finger with unspecified laterality

√7ᵗʰ **S63.269** **Dislocation of metacarpophalangeal joint of** unspecified **finger**

√6ᵗʰ **S63.27** **Dislocation of unspecified** interphalangeal **joint of finger**

√7ᵗʰ **S63.270** **Dislocation of unspecified interphalangeal joint of** right index **finger**

√7ᵗʰ **S63.271** **Dislocation of unspecified interphalangeal joint of** left index **finger**

√7ᵗʰ **S63.272** **Dislocation of unspecified interphalangeal joint of** right middle **finger**

√7ᵗʰ **S63.273** **Dislocation of unspecified interphalangeal joint of** left middle **finger**

√7ᵗʰ **S63.274** **Dislocation of unspecified interphalangeal joint of** right ring **finger**

√7ᵗʰ **S63.275** **Dislocation of unspecified interphalangeal joint of** left ring **finger**

√7ᵗʰ **S63.276** **Dislocation of unspecified interphalangeal joint of** right little **finger**

√7ᵗʰ **S63.277** **Dislocation of unspecified interphalangeal joint of** left little **finger**

√7ᵗʰ **S63.278** **Dislocation of unspecified interphalangeal joint of** other **finger**
Dislocation of unspecified interphalangeal joint of specified finger with unspecified laterality

√7ᵗʰ **S63.279** **Dislocation of unspecified interphalangeal joint of** unspecified **finger**
▶Dislocation of unspecified interphalangeal joint of unspecified finger without specified laterality◀

√6ᵗʰ **S63.28** **Dislocation of** proximal interphalangeal joint **of finger**

√7ᵗʰ **S63.280** **Dislocation of proximal interphalangeal joint of** right index **finger**

√7ᵗʰ **S63.281** **Dislocation of proximal interphalangeal joint of** left index **finger**

√7ᵗʰ **S63.282** **Dislocation of proximal interphalangeal joint of** right middle **finger**

√7ᵗʰ **S63.283** **Dislocation of proximal interphalangeal joint of** left middle **finger**

√7ᵗʰ **S63.284** **Dislocation of proximal interphalangeal joint of** right ring **finger**

√7ᵗʰ **S63.285** **Dislocation of proximal interphalangeal joint of** left ring **finger**

√7ᵗʰ **S63.286** **Dislocation of proximal interphalangeal joint of** right little **finger**

√7ᵗʰ **S63.287** **Dislocation of proximal interphalangeal joint of** left little **finger**

√7ᵗʰ **S63.288** **Dislocation of proximal interphalangeal joint of** other **finger**
Dislocation of proximal interphalangeal joint of specified finger with unspecified laterality

√7ᵗʰ **S63.289** **Dislocation of proximal interphalangeal joint of** unspecified **finger**

√6ᵗʰ **S63.29** **Dislocation of** distal interphalangeal **joint of finger**

√7ᵗʰ **S63.290** **Dislocation of distal interphalangeal joint of** right index **finger**

√7ᵗʰ **S63.291** **Dislocation of distal interphalangeal joint of** left index **finger**

√7ᵗʰ **S63.292** **Dislocation of distal interphalangeal joint of** right middle **finger**

√7ᵗʰ **S63.293** **Dislocation of distal interphalangeal joint of** left middle **finger**

√7ᵗʰ **S63.294** **Dislocation of distal interphalangeal joint of** right ring **finger**

√7ᵗʰ **S63.295** **Dislocation of distal interphalangeal joint of** left ring **finger**

√7ᵗʰ **S63.296** **Dislocation of distal interphalangeal joint of** right little **finger**

√7ᵗʰ **S63.297** **Dislocation of distal interphalangeal joint of** left little **finger**

√7ᵗʰ **S63.298** **Dislocation of distal interphalangeal joint of** other **finger**
Dislocation of distal interphalangeal joint of specified finger with unspecified laterality

✓ Additional Character Req   ✓×7ᵗʰ Placeholder Alert   Unacceptable PDx   Manifestation   **H1**-**H14** HAC   **HCC** CMS-HCC Condition   *EXCLUDES 1* Not Coded Here   *EXCLUDES 2* Not Included Here

ICD-10-CM 2018      **1025**

S63.238–S63.298

√7ᵗʰ **S63.299**   **Dislocation of distal interphalangeal joint of unspecified finger**

√5ᵗʰ **S63.3**   **Traumatic rupture of ligament of wrist**

  √6ᵗʰ **S63.30**   **Traumatic rupture of unspecified ligament of wrist**

    √7ᵗʰ **S63.301**   **Traumatic rupture of unspecified ligament of right wrist**

    √7ᵗʰ **S63.302**   **Traumatic rupture of unspecified ligament of left wrist**

    √7ᵗʰ **S63.309**   **Traumatic rupture of unspecified ligament of unspecified wrist**

  √6ᵗʰ **S63.31**   **Traumatic rupture of collateral ligament of wrist**

    √7ᵗʰ **S63.311**   **Traumatic rupture of collateral ligament of right wrist**

    √7ᵗʰ **S63.312**   **Traumatic rupture of collateral ligament of left wrist**

    √7ᵗʰ **S63.319**   **Traumatic rupture of collateral ligament of unspecified wrist**

  √6ᵗʰ **S63.32**   **Traumatic rupture of radiocarpal ligament**

    √7ᵗʰ **S63.321**   **Traumatic rupture of right radiocarpal ligament**

    √7ᵗʰ **S63.322**   **Traumatic rupture of left radiocarpal ligament**

    √7ᵗʰ **S63.329**   **Traumatic rupture of unspecified radiocarpal ligament**

  √6ᵗʰ **S63.33**   **Traumatic rupture of ulnocarpal (palmar) ligament**

    √7ᵗʰ **S63.331**   **Traumatic rupture of right ulnocarpal (palmar) ligament**

    √7ᵗʰ **S63.332**   **Traumatic rupture of left ulnocarpal (palmar) ligament**

    √7ᵗʰ **S63.339**   **Traumatic rupture of unspecified ulnocarpal (palmar) ligament**

  √6ᵗʰ **S63.39**   **Traumatic rupture of other ligament of wrist**

    √7ᵗʰ **S63.391**   **Traumatic rupture of other ligament of right wrist**

    √7ᵗʰ **S63.392**   **Traumatic rupture of other ligament of left wrist**

    √7ᵗʰ **S63.399**   **Traumatic rupture of other ligament of unspecified wrist**

√5ᵗʰ **S63.4**   **Traumatic rupture of ligament of finger at metacarpophalangeal and interphalangeal joint(s)**

  √6ᵗʰ **S63.40**   **Traumatic rupture of unspecified ligament of finger at metacarpophalangeal and interphalangeal joint**

    √7ᵗʰ **S63.400**   **Traumatic rupture of unspecified ligament of right index finger at metacarpophalangeal and interphalangeal joint**

    √7ᵗʰ **S63.401**   **Traumatic rupture of unspecified ligament of left index finger at metacarpophalangeal and interphalangeal joint**

    √7ᵗʰ **S63.402**   **Traumatic rupture of unspecified ligament of right middle finger at metacarpophalangeal and interphalangeal joint**

    √7ᵗʰ **S63.403**   **Traumatic rupture of unspecified ligament of left middle finger at metacarpophalangeal and interphalangeal joint**

    √7ᵗʰ **S63.404**   **Traumatic rupture of unspecified ligament of right ring finger at metacarpophalangeal and interphalangeal joint**

    √7ᵗʰ **S63.405**   **Traumatic rupture of unspecified ligament of left ring finger at metacarpophalangeal and interphalangeal joint**

    √7ᵗʰ **S63.406**   **Traumatic rupture of unspecified ligament of right little finger at metacarpophalangeal and interphalangeal joint**

    √7ᵗʰ **S63.407**   **Traumatic rupture of unspecified ligament of left little finger at metacarpophalangeal and interphalangeal joint**

    √7ᵗʰ **S63.408**   **Traumatic rupture of unspecified ligament of other finger at metacarpophalangeal and interphalangeal joint**

      Traumatic rupture of unspecified ligament of specified finger with unspecified laterality at metacarpophalangeal and interphalangeal joint

    √7ᵗʰ **S63.409**   **Traumatic rupture of unspecified ligament of unspecified finger at metacarpophalangeal and interphalangeal joint**

  √6ᵗʰ **S63.41**   **Traumatic rupture of collateral ligament of finger at metacarpophalangeal and interphalangeal joint**

    √7ᵗʰ **S63.410**   **Traumatic rupture of collateral ligament of right index finger at metacarpophalangeal and interphalangeal joint**

    √7ᵗʰ **S63.411**   **Traumatic rupture of collateral ligament of left index finger at metacarpophalangeal and interphalangeal joint**

    √7ᵗʰ **S63.412**   **Traumatic rupture of collateral ligament of right middle finger at metacarpophalangeal and interphalangeal joint**

    √7ᵗʰ **S63.413**   **Traumatic rupture of collateral ligament of left middle finger at metacarpophalangeal and interphalangeal joint**

    √7ᵗʰ **S63.414**   **Traumatic rupture of collateral ligament of right ring finger at metacarpophalangeal and interphalangeal joint**

    √7ᵗʰ **S63.415**   **Traumatic rupture of collateral ligament of left ring finger at metacarpophalangeal and interphalangeal joint**

    √7ᵗʰ **S63.416**   **Traumatic rupture of collateral ligament of right little finger at metacarpophalangeal and interphalangeal joint**

    √7ᵗʰ **S63.417**   **Traumatic rupture of collateral ligament of left little finger at metacarpophalangeal and interphalangeal joint**

    √7ᵗʰ **S63.418**   **Traumatic rupture of collateral ligament of other finger at metacarpophalangeal and interphalangeal joint**

      Traumatic rupture of collateral ligament of specified finger with unspecified laterality at metacarpophalangeal and interphalangeal joint

    √7ᵗʰ **S63.419**   **Traumatic rupture of collateral ligament of unspecified finger at metacarpophalangeal and interphalangeal joint**

  √6ᵗʰ **S63.42**   **Traumatic rupture of palmar ligament of finger at metacarpophalangeal and interphalangeal joint**

    √7ᵗʰ **S63.420**   **Traumatic rupture of palmar ligament of right index finger at metacarpophalangeal and interphalangeal joint**

    √7ᵗʰ **S63.421**   **Traumatic rupture of palmar ligament of left index finger at metacarpophalangeal and interphalangeal joint**

    √7ᵗʰ **S63.422**   **Traumatic rupture of palmar ligament of right middle finger at metacarpophalangeal and interphalangeal joint**

    √7ᵗʰ **S63.423**   **Traumatic rupture of palmar ligament of left middle finger at metacarpophalangeal and interphalangeal joint**

    √7ᵗʰ **S63.424**   **Traumatic rupture of palmar ligament of right ring finger at metacarpophalangeal and interphalangeal joint**

    √7ᵗʰ **S63.425**   **Traumatic rupture of palmar ligament of left ring finger at metacarpophalangeal and interphalangeal joint**

    √7ᵗʰ **S63.426**   **Traumatic rupture of palmar ligament of right little finger at metacarpophalangeal and interphalangeal joint**

Ⓝ Newborn: 0   Ⓟ Pediatric: 0-17   Ⓜ Maternity: 12-55   Ⓐ Adult: 15-124   **MCC** Major CC Condition   **PDxMCC** PDx acts as own MCC   **CC** CC Condition   **PDxCC** PDx acts as own CC

**1026**      ICD-10-CM 2018

√7ᵗʰ **S63.427** **Traumatic rupture of palmar ligament of left little finger at metacarpophalangeal and interphalangeal joint**

√7ᵗʰ **S63.428** **Traumatic rupture of palmar ligament of other finger at metacarpophalangeal and interphalangeal joint**
Traumatic rupture of palmar ligament of specified finger with unspecified laterality at metacarpophalangeal and interphalangeal joint

√7ᵗʰ **S63.429** **Traumatic rupture of palmar ligament of unspecified finger at metacarpophalangeal and interphalangeal joint**

√6ᵗʰ **S63.43** **Traumatic rupture of** volar plate **of finger at metacarpophalangeal and interphalangeal joint**

√7ᵗʰ **S63.430** **Traumatic rupture of volar plate of** right **index finger at metacarpophalangeal and interphalangeal joint**

√7ᵗʰ **S63.431** **Traumatic rupture of volar plate of** left **index finger at metacarpophalangeal and interphalangeal joint**

√7ᵗʰ **S63.432** **Traumatic rupture of volar plate of** right **middle finger at metacarpophalangeal and interphalangeal joint**

√7ᵗʰ **S63.433** **Traumatic rupture of volar plate of** left **middle finger at metacarpophalangeal and interphalangeal joint**

√7ᵗʰ **S63.434** **Traumatic rupture of volar plate of** right **ring finger at metacarpophalangeal and interphalangeal joint**

√7ᵗʰ **S63.435** **Traumatic rupture of volar plate of** left **ring finger at metacarpophalangeal and interphalangeal joint**

√7ᵗʰ **S63.436** **Traumatic rupture of volar plate of** right **little finger at metacarpophalangeal and interphalangeal joint**

√7ᵗʰ **S63.437** **Traumatic rupture of volar plate of** left **little finger at metacarpophalangeal and interphalangeal joint**

√7ᵗʰ **S63.438** **Traumatic rupture of volar plate of** other **finger at metacarpophalangeal and interphalangeal joint**
Traumatic rupture of volar plate of specified finger with unspecified laterality at metacarpophalangeal and interphalangeal joint

√7ᵗʰ **S63.439** **Traumatic rupture of volar plate of** unspecified **finger at metacarpophalangeal and interphalangeal joint**

√6ᵗʰ **S63.49** **Traumatic rupture of** other ligament **of finger at metacarpophalangeal and interphalangeal joint**

√7ᵗʰ **S63.490** **Traumatic rupture of other ligament of** right index **finger at metacarpophalangeal and interphalangeal joint**

√7ᵗʰ **S63.491** **Traumatic rupture of other ligament of** left index **finger at metacarpophalangeal and interphalangeal joint**

√7ᵗʰ **S63.492** **Traumatic rupture of other ligament of** right middle **finger at metacarpophalangeal and interphalangeal joint**

√7ᵗʰ **S63.493** **Traumatic rupture of other ligament of** left middle **finger at metacarpophalangeal and interphalangeal joint**

√7ᵗʰ **S63.494** **Traumatic rupture of other ligament of** right ring **finger at metacarpophalangeal and interphalangeal joint**

√7ᵗʰ **S63.495** **Traumatic rupture of other ligament of** left ring **finger at metacarpophalangeal and interphalangeal joint**

√7ᵗʰ **S63.496** **Traumatic rupture of other ligament of** right little **finger at metacarpophalangeal and interphalangeal joint**

√7ᵗʰ **S63.497** **Traumatic rupture of other ligament of** left little **finger at metacarpophalangeal and interphalangeal joint**

√7ᵗʰ **S63.498** **Traumatic rupture of other ligament of** other **finger at metacarpophalangeal and interphalangeal joint**
Traumatic rupture of ligament of specified finger with unspecified laterality at metacarpophalangeal and interphalangeal joint

√7ᵗʰ **S63.499** **Traumatic rupture of other ligament of** unspecified **finger at metacarpophalangeal and interphalangeal joint**

√5ᵗʰ **S63.5** **Other and unspecified** sprain of wrist

√6ᵗʰ **S63.50** **Unspecified sprain of wrist**

√7ᵗʰ **S63.501** **Unspecified sprain of** right wrist

√7ᵗʰ **S63.502** **Unspecified sprain of** left wrist

√7ᵗʰ **S63.509** **Unspecified sprain of** unspecified wrist

√6ᵗʰ **S63.51** **Sprain of carpal (joint)**

√7ᵗʰ **S63.511** **Sprain of carpal joint of** right wrist

√7ᵗʰ **S63.512** **Sprain of carpal joint of** left wrist

√7ᵗʰ **S63.519** **Sprain of carpal joint of** unspecified wrist

√6ᵗʰ **S63.52** **Sprain of** radiocarpal **joint**
*EXCLUDES 1* traumatic rupture of radiocarpal ligament (S63.32-)

√7ᵗʰ **S63.521** **Sprain of radiocarpal joint of** right wrist

√7ᵗʰ **S63.522** **Sprain of radiocarpal joint of** left wrist

√7ᵗʰ **S63.529** **Sprain of radiocarpal joint of** unspecified wrist

√6ᵗʰ **S63.59** **Other** specified sprain of wrist

√7ᵗʰ **S63.591** **Other specified sprain of** right wrist

√7ᵗʰ **S63.592** **Other specified sprain of** left wrist

√7ᵗʰ **S63.599** **Other specified sprain of** unspecified wrist

√5ᵗʰ **S63.6** **Other and unspecified sprain of finger(s)**
*EXCLUDES 1* traumatic rupture of ligament of finger at metacarpophalangeal and interphalangeal joint(s) (S63.4-)

√6ᵗʰ **S63.60** **Unspecified sprain of thumb**

√7ᵗʰ **S63.601** **Unspecified sprain of** right thumb

√7ᵗʰ **S63.602** **Unspecified sprain of** left thumb

√7ᵗʰ **S63.609** **Unspecified sprain of** unspecified thumb

√6ᵗʰ **S63.61** **Unspecified sprain of other and unspecified finger(s)**

√7ᵗʰ **S63.610** **Unspecified sprain of** right index finger

√7ᵗʰ **S63.611** **Unspecified sprain of** left index finger

√7ᵗʰ **S63.612** **Unspecified sprain of** right middle finger

√7ᵗʰ **S63.613** **Unspecified sprain of** left middle finger

√7ᵗʰ **S63.614** **Unspecified sprain of** right ring finger

√7ᵗʰ **S63.615** **Unspecified sprain of** left ring finger

√7ᵗʰ **S63.616** **Unspecified sprain of** right little finger

√7ᵗʰ **S63.617** **Unspecified sprain of** left little finger

√7ᵗʰ **S63.618** **Unspecified sprain of** other finger
Unspecified sprain of specified finger with unspecified laterality

√7ᵗʰ **S63.619** **Unspecified sprain of** unspecified finger

√6ᵗʰ **S63.62** **Sprain of** interphalangeal joint of thumb

√7ᵗʰ **S63.621** **Sprain of interphalangeal joint of** right thumb

√7ᵗʰ **S63.622** **Sprain of interphalangeal joint of** left thumb

√7ᵗʰ **S63.629** **Sprain of interphalangeal joint of** unspecified thumb

√6ᵗʰ **S63.63** **Sprain of** interphalangeal joint of other and unspecified finger(s)

√7ᵗʰ **S63.630** **Sprain of interphalangeal joint of** right index finger

√7ᵗʰ **S63.631** **Sprain of interphalangeal joint of** left index finger

√7ᵗʰ **S63.632** **Sprain of interphalangeal joint of** right middle finger

√7ᵗʰ **S63.633** **Sprain of interphalangeal joint of** left middle finger

√7ᵗʰ **S63.634** **Sprain of interphalangeal joint of** right ring finger

√7ᵗʰ **S63.635** **Sprain of interphalangeal joint of** left ring finger

✔Additional Character Req   √ₓ7ᵗʰ Placeholder Alert   Unacceptable PDx   Manifestation   **H1**-**H14** HAC   **HCC** CMS-HCC Condition   *EXCLUDES 1* Not Coded Here   *EXCLUDES 2* Not Included Here

ICD-10-CM 2018     **1027**

**Chapter 19. Injury, Poisoning and Certain Other Consequences of External Causes**

☑6ᵗʰ **S63.636** Sprain of interphalangeal joint of right little **finger**

☑7ᵗʰ **S63.636** Sprain of interphalangeal joint of right little **finger**

☑7ᵗʰ **S63.637** Sprain of interphalangeal joint of left little **finger**

☑7ᵗʰ **S63.638** Sprain of interphalangeal joint of other **finger**

☑7ᵗʰ **S63.639** Sprain of interphalangeal joint of unspecified **finger**

☑6ᵗʰ **S63.64** Sprain of metacarpophalangeal joint of thumb

☑7ᵗʰ **S63.641** Sprain of metacarpophalangeal joint of right **thumb**

☑7ᵗʰ **S63.642** Sprain of metacarpophalangeal joint of left **thumb**

☑7ᵗʰ **S63.649** Sprain of metacarpophalangeal joint of unspecified **thumb**

☑6ᵗʰ **S63.65** Sprain of metacarpophalangeal joint of other and unspecified finger(s)

☑7ᵗʰ **S63.650** Sprain of metacarpophalangeal joint of right index **finger**

☑7ᵗʰ **S63.651** Sprain of metacarpophalangeal joint of left index **finger**

☑7ᵗʰ **S63.652** Sprain of metacarpophalangeal joint of right middle **finger**

☑7ᵗʰ **S63.653** Sprain of metacarpophalangeal joint of left middle **finger**

☑7ᵗʰ **S63.654** Sprain of metacarpophalangeal joint of right ring **finger**

☑7ᵗʰ **S63.655** Sprain of metacarpophalangeal joint of left ring **finger**

☑7ᵗʰ **S63.656** Sprain of metacarpophalangeal joint of right little **finger**

☑7ᵗʰ **S63.657** Sprain of metacarpophalangeal joint of left little **finger**

☑7ᵗʰ **S63.658** Sprain of metacarpophalangeal joint of other **finger**
Sprain of metacarpophalangeal joint of specified finger with unspecified laterality

☑7ᵗʰ **S63.659** Sprain of metacarpophalangeal joint of unspecified **finger**

☑6ᵗʰ **S63.68** Other sprain of thumb

☑7ᵗʰ **S63.681** Other sprain of right **thumb**

☑7ᵗʰ **S63.682** Other sprain of left **thumb**

☑7ᵗʰ **S63.689** Other sprain of unspecified **thumb**

☑6ᵗʰ **S63.69** Other sprain of other and unspecified finger(s)

☑7ᵗʰ **S63.690** Other sprain of right index **finger**

☑7ᵗʰ **S63.691** Other sprain of left index **finger**

☑7ᵗʰ **S63.692** Other sprain of right middle **finger**

☑7ᵗʰ **S63.693** Other sprain of left middle **finger**

☑7ᵗʰ **S63.694** Other sprain of right ring **finger**

☑7ᵗʰ **S63.695** Other sprain of left ring **finger**

☑7ᵗʰ **S63.696** Other sprain of right little **finger**

☑7ᵗʰ **S63.697** Other sprain of left little **finger**

☑7ᵗʰ **S63.698** Other sprain of other **finger**
Other sprain of specified finger with unspecified laterality

☑7ᵗʰ **S63.699** Other sprain of unspecified **finger**

☑5ᵗʰ **S63.8** Sprain of other part of wrist and hand

☑6ᵗʰ **S63.8X** Sprain of other part of wrist and hand

☑7ᵗʰ **S63.8X1** Sprain of other part of right wrist and hand

☑7ᵗʰ **S63.8X2** Sprain of other part of left wrist and hand

☑7ᵗʰ **S63.8X9** Sprain of other part of unspecified wrist and hand

☑5ᵗʰ **S63.9** Sprain of unspecified part of wrist and hand

☑x7ᵗʰ **S63.90** Sprain of unspecified part of unspecified wrist and hand

☑x7ᵗʰ **S63.91** Sprain of unspecified part of right wrist and hand

☑x7ᵗʰ **S63.92** Sprain of unspecified part of left wrist and hand

☑4ᵗʰ **S64** **Injury of nerves at wrist and hand level**
Code also any associated open wound (S61.-)

The appropriate 7th character is to be added to each code from category S64.
A   initial encounter
D   subsequent encounter
S   sequela

☑5ᵗʰ **S64.0** Injury of ulnar nerve at wrist and hand level

☑x7ᵗʰ **S64.00** Injury of ulnar nerve at wrist and hand level of unspecified **arm**

☑x7ᵗʰ **S64.01** Injury of ulnar nerve at wrist and hand level of right **arm**

☑x7ᵗʰ **S64.02** Injury of ulnar nerve at wrist and hand level of left **arm**

☑5ᵗʰ **S64.1** Injury of median nerve at wrist and hand level

☑x7ᵗʰ **S64.10** Injury of median nerve at wrist and hand level of unspecified **arm**

☑x7ᵗʰ **S64.11** Injury of median nerve at wrist and hand level of right **arm**

☑x7ᵗʰ **S64.12** Injury of median nerve at wrist and hand level of left **arm**

☑5ᵗʰ **S64.2** Injury of radial nerve at wrist and hand level

☑x7ᵗʰ **S64.20** Injury of radial nerve at wrist and hand level of unspecified **arm**

☑x7ᵗʰ **S64.21** Injury of radial nerve at wrist and hand level of right **arm**

☑x7ᵗʰ **S64.22** Injury of radial nerve at wrist and hand level of left **arm**

☑5ᵗʰ **S64.3** Injury of digital nerve of thumb

☑x7ᵗʰ **S64.30** Injury of digital nerve of unspecified **thumb**

☑x7ᵗʰ **S64.31** Injury of digital nerve of right **thumb**

☑x7ᵗʰ **S64.32** Injury of digital nerve of left **thumb**

☑5ᵗʰ **S64.4** Injury of digital nerve of other and unspecified finger

☑x7ᵗʰ **S64.40** Injury of digital nerve of unspecified **finger**

☑6ᵗʰ **S64.49** Injury of digital nerve of other **finger**

☑7ᵗʰ **S64.490** Injury of digital nerve of right index **finger**

☑7ᵗʰ **S64.491** Injury of digital nerve of left index **finger**

☑7ᵗʰ **S64.492** Injury of digital nerve of right middle **finger**

☑7ᵗʰ **S64.493** Injury of digital nerve of left middle **finger**

☑7ᵗʰ **S64.494** Injury of digital nerve of right ring **finger**

☑7ᵗʰ **S64.495** Injury of digital nerve of left ring **finger**

☑7ᵗʰ **S64.496** Injury of digital nerve of right little **finger**

☑7ᵗʰ **S64.497** Injury of digital nerve of left little **finger**

☑7ᵗʰ **S64.498** Injury of digital nerve of other **finger**
Injury of digital nerve of specified finger with unspecified laterality

☑5ᵗʰ **S64.8** Injury of other nerves at wrist and hand level

☑6ᵗʰ **S64.8X** Injury of other nerves at wrist and hand level

☑7ᵗʰ **S64.8X1** Injury of other nerves at wrist and hand level of right **arm**

☑7ᵗʰ **S64.8X2** Injury of other nerves at wrist and hand level of left **arm**

☑7ᵗʰ **S64.8X9** Injury of other nerves at wrist and hand level of unspecified **arm**

☑5ᵗʰ **S64.9** Injury of unspecified nerve at wrist and hand level

☑x7ᵗʰ **S64.90** Injury of unspecified nerve at wrist and hand level of unspecified **arm**

☑x7ᵗʰ **S64.91** Injury of unspecified nerve at wrist and hand level of right **arm**

☑x7ᵗʰ **S64.92** Injury of unspecified nerve at wrist and hand level of left **arm**

Ⓝ Newborn: 0   Ⓟ Pediatric: 0-17   Ⓜ Maternity: 12-55   Ⓐ Adult: 15-124   **MCC** Major CC Condition   **PDxMCC** PDx acts as own MCC   **CC** CC Condition   **PDxCC** PDx acts as own CC

**1028**
ICD-10-CM 2018

☑4ᵗʰ **S65 Injury of blood vessels at wrist and hand level**
Code also any associated open wound (S61.-)

The appropriate 7th character is to be added to each code from category S65.
A    initial encounter
D    subsequent encounter
S    sequela

☑5ᵗʰ **S65.0 Injury of ulnar artery at wrist and hand level**

**CC Excl: For CC codes in subcategory S65.0:**
**Right side:** PDX collection 1274
**Left side:** PDX collection 1275
**Unspecified side:** PDX collection 1276

☑6ᵗʰ **S65.00 Unspecified injury of ulnar artery at wrist and hand level**
   ☑7ᵗʰ **S65.001 Unspecified injury of ulnar artery at wrist and hand level of right arm** CC
   ☑7ᵗʰ **S65.002 Unspecified injury of ulnar artery at wrist and hand level of left arm** CC
   ☑7ᵗʰ **S65.009 Unspecified injury of ulnar artery at wrist and hand level of unspecified arm** CC

☑6ᵗʰ **S65.01 Laceration of ulnar artery at wrist and hand level**
   ☑7ᵗʰ **S65.011 Laceration of ulnar artery at wrist and hand level of right arm** CC
   ☑7ᵗʰ **S65.012 Laceration of ulnar artery at wrist and hand level of left arm** CC
   ☑7ᵗʰ **S65.019 Laceration of ulnar artery at wrist and hand level of unspecified arm** CC

☑6ᵗʰ **S65.09 Other specified injury of ulnar artery at wrist and hand level**
   ☑7ᵗʰ **S65.091 Other specified injury of ulnar artery at wrist and hand level of right arm** CC
   ☑7ᵗʰ **S65.092 Other specified injury of ulnar artery at wrist and hand level of left arm** CC
   ☑7ᵗʰ **S65.099 Other specified injury of ulnar artery at wrist and hand level of unspecified arm** CC

☑5ᵗʰ **S65.1 Injury of radial artery at wrist and hand level**

**CC Excl: For CC codes in subcategory S65.1:**
**Right side:** PDX collection 1277
**Left side:** PDX collection 1278
**Unspecified side:** PDX collection 1279

☑6ᵗʰ **S65.10 Unspecified injury of radial artery at wrist and hand level**
   ☑7ᵗʰ **S65.101 Unspecified injury of radial artery at wrist and hand level of right arm** CC
   ☑7ᵗʰ **S65.102 Unspecified injury of radial artery at wrist and hand level of left arm** CC
   ☑7ᵗʰ **S65.109 Unspecified injury of radial artery at wrist and hand level of unspecified arm** CC

☑6ᵗʰ **S65.11 Laceration of radial artery at wrist and hand level**
   ☑7ᵗʰ **S65.111 Laceration of radial artery at wrist and hand level of right arm** CC
   ☑7ᵗʰ **S65.112 Laceration of radial artery at wrist and hand level of left arm** CC
   ☑7ᵗʰ **S65.119 Laceration of radial artery at wrist and hand level of unspecified arm** CC

☑6ᵗʰ **S65.19 Other specified injury of radial artery at wrist and hand level**
   ☑7ᵗʰ **S65.191 Other specified injury of radial artery at wrist and hand level of right arm** CC
   ☑7ᵗʰ **S65.192 Other specified injury of radial artery at wrist and hand level of left arm** CC
   ☑7ᵗʰ **S65.199 Other specified injury of radial artery at wrist and hand level of unspecified arm** CC

☑5ᵗʰ **S65.2 Injury of superficial palmar arch**

**CC Excl: For CC codes in subcategory S65.2:**
**Right side:** PDX collection 1288
**Left side:** PDX collection 1289
**Unspecified side:** PDX collection 1290

☑6ᵗʰ **S65.20 Unspecified injury of superficial palmar arch**
   ☑7ᵗʰ **S65.201 Unspecified injury of superficial palmar arch of right hand** CC

---

   ☑7ᵗʰ **S65.202 Unspecified injury of superficial palmar arch of left hand** CC
   ☑7ᵗʰ **S65.209 Unspecified injury of superficial palmar arch of unspecified hand** CC

☑6ᵗʰ **S65.21 Laceration of superficial palmar arch**
   ☑7ᵗʰ **S65.211 Laceration of superficial palmar arch of right hand** CC
   ☑7ᵗʰ **S65.212 Laceration of superficial palmar arch of left hand** CC
   ☑7ᵗʰ **S65.219 Laceration of superficial palmar arch of unspecified hand** CC

☑6ᵗʰ **S65.29 Other specified injury of superficial palmar arch**
   ☑7ᵗʰ **S65.291 Other specified injury of superficial palmar arch of right hand** CC
   ☑7ᵗʰ **S65.292 Other specified injury of superficial palmar arch of left hand** CC
   ☑7ᵗʰ **S65.299 Other specified injury of superficial palmar arch of unspecified hand** CC

☑5ᵗʰ **S65.3 Injury of deep palmar arch**

**CC Excl: For CC codes in subcategory S65.3:**
**Right side:** PDX collection 1288
**Left side:** PDX collection 1289
**Unspecified side:** PDX collection 1290

☑6ᵗʰ **S65.30 Unspecified injury of deep palmar arch**
   ☑7ᵗʰ **S65.301 Unspecified injury of deep palmar arch of right hand** CC
   ☑7ᵗʰ **S65.302 Unspecified injury of deep palmar arch of left hand** CC
   ☑7ᵗʰ **S65.309 Unspecified injury of deep palmar arch of unspecified hand** CC

☑6ᵗʰ **S65.31 Laceration of deep palmar arch**
   ☑7ᵗʰ **S65.311 Laceration of deep palmar arch of right hand** CC
   ☑7ᵗʰ **S65.312 Laceration of deep palmar arch of left hand** CC
   ☑7ᵗʰ **S65.319 Laceration of deep palmar arch of unspecified hand** CC

☑6ᵗʰ **S65.39 Other specified injury of deep palmar arch**
   ☑7ᵗʰ **S65.391 Other specified injury of deep palmar arch of right hand** CC
   ☑7ᵗʰ **S65.392 Other specified injury of deep palmar arch of left hand** CC
   ☑7ᵗʰ **S65.399 Other specified injury of deep palmar arch of unspecified hand** CC

☑5ᵗʰ **S65.4 Injury of blood vessel of thumb**

**CC Excl: For CC codes in subcategory S65.4:**
**Right side:** PDX collection 1291
**Left side:** PDX collection 1292
**Unspecified side:** PDX collection 1293

☑6ᵗʰ **S65.40 Unspecified injury of blood vessel of thumb**
   ☑7ᵗʰ **S65.401 Unspecified injury of blood vessel of right thumb** CC
   ☑7ᵗʰ **S65.402 Unspecified injury of blood vessel of left thumb** CC
   ☑7ᵗʰ **S65.409 Unspecified injury of blood vessel of unspecified thumb** CC

☑6ᵗʰ **S65.41 Laceration of blood vessel of thumb**
   ☑7ᵗʰ **S65.411 Laceration of blood vessel of right thumb** CC
   ☑7ᵗʰ **S65.412 Laceration of blood vessel of left thumb** CC
   ☑7ᵗʰ **S65.419 Laceration of blood vessel of unspecified thumb** CC

☑6ᵗʰ **S65.49 Other specified injury of blood vessel of thumb**
   ☑7ᵗʰ **S65.491 Other specified injury of blood vessel of right thumb** CC
   ☑7ᵗʰ **S65.492 Other specified injury of blood vessel of left thumb** CC
   ☑7ᵗʰ **S65.499 Other specified injury of blood vessel of unspecified thumb** CC

---

☑ Additional Character Req    ☑x7ᵗʰ Placeholder Alert    Unacceptable PDx    Manifestation    **H1**-**H14** HAC    ᴴᶜᶜ CMS-HCC Condition    *EXCLUDES 1* Not Coded Here    *EXCLUDES 2* Not Included Here

✓5ᵗʰ **S65.5**   **Injury of blood vessel of** other and unspecified finger

> **CC Excl: For CC codes in subcategory S65.5:**
> **Right side:** PDX collection 1291
> **Left side:** PDX collection 1292
> **Other or unspecified side:** PDX collection 1293

✓6ᵗʰ **S65.50**   Unspecified **injury of blood vessel of other and unspecified finger**

    ✓7ᵗʰ **S65.500**   Unspecified **injury of blood vessel of** right index **finger**   **CC**

    ✓7ᵗʰ **S65.501**   Unspecified **injury of blood vessel of** left index **finger**   **CC**

    ✓7ᵗʰ **S65.502**   Unspecified **injury of blood vessel of** right middle **finger**   **CC**

    ✓7ᵗʰ **S65.503**   Unspecified **injury of blood vessel of** left middle **finger**   **CC**

    ✓7ᵗʰ **S65.504**   Unspecified **injury of blood vessel of** right ring **finger**   **CC**

    ✓7ᵗʰ **S65.505**   Unspecified **injury of blood vessel of** left ring **finger**   **CC**

    ✓7ᵗʰ **S65.506**   Unspecified **injury of blood vessel of** right little **finger**   **CC**

    ✓7ᵗʰ **S65.507**   Unspecified **injury of blood vessel of** left little **finger**   **CC**

    ✓7ᵗʰ **S65.508**   Unspecified **injury of blood vessel of** other **finger**   **CC**
       Unspecified injury of blood vessel of specified finger with unspecified laterality

    ✓7ᵗʰ **S65.509**   Unspecified **injury of blood vessel of** unspecified **finger**   **CC**

✓6ᵗʰ **S65.51**   Laceration **of blood vessel of other and unspecified finger**

    ✓7ᵗʰ **S65.510**   **Laceration of blood vessel of** right index **finger**   **CC**

    ✓7ᵗʰ **S65.511**   **Laceration of blood vessel of** left index **finger**   **CC**

    ✓7ᵗʰ **S65.512**   **Laceration of blood vessel of** right middle **finger**   **CC**

    ✓7ᵗʰ **S65.513**   **Laceration of blood vessel of** left middle **finger**   **CC**

    ✓7ᵗʰ **S65.514**   **Laceration of blood vessel of** right ring **finger**   **CC**

    ✓7ᵗʰ **S65.515**   **Laceration of blood vessel of** left ring **finger**   **CC**

    ✓7ᵗʰ **S65.516**   **Laceration of blood vessel of** right little **finger**   **CC**

    ✓7ᵗʰ **S65.517**   **Laceration of blood vessel of** left little **finger**   **CC**

    ✓7ᵗʰ **S65.518**   **Laceration of blood vessel of** other **finger**   **CC**
       Laceration of blood vessel of specified finger with unspecified laterality

    ✓7ᵗʰ **S65.519**   **Laceration of blood vessel of** unspecified **finger**   **CC**

✓6ᵗʰ **S65.59**   Other specified **injury of blood vessel of other and unspecified finger**

    ✓7ᵗʰ **S65.590**   **Other specified injury of blood vessel of** right index **finger**   **CC**

    ✓7ᵗʰ **S65.591**   **Other specified injury of blood vessel of** left index **finger**   **CC**

    ✓7ᵗʰ **S65.592**   **Other specified injury of blood vessel of** right middle **finger**   **CC**

    ✓7ᵗʰ **S65.593**   **Other specified injury of blood vessel of** left middle **finger**   **CC**

    ✓7ᵗʰ **S65.594**   **Other specified injury of blood vessel of** right ring **finger**   **CC**

    ✓7ᵗʰ **S65.595**   **Other specified injury of blood vessel of** left ring **finger**   **CC**

    ✓7ᵗʰ **S65.596**   **Other specified injury of blood vessel of** right little **finger**   **CC**

    ✓7ᵗʰ **S65.597**   **Other specified injury of blood vessel of** left little **finger**   **CC**

    ✓7ᵗʰ **S65.598**   **Other specified injury of blood vessel of** other **finger**   **CC**
       Other specified injury of blood vessel of specified finger with unspecified laterality

    ✓7ᵗʰ **S65.599**   **Other specified injury of blood vessel of** unspecified **finger**   **CC**

✓5ᵗʰ **S65.8**   **Injury of other blood vessels at** wrist and hand level

> **CC Excl: For CC codes in subcategory S65.8:**
> **Right side:** PDX collection 1260
> **Left side:** PDX collection 1261
> **Unspecified side:** PDX collection 1262

✓6ᵗʰ **S65.80**   Unspecified **injury of other blood vessels at wrist and hand level**

    ✓7ᵗʰ **S65.801**   **Unspecified injury of other blood vessels at wrist and hand level of** right **arm**   **CC**

    ✓7ᵗʰ **S65.802**   **Unspecified injury of other blood vessels at wrist and hand level of** left **arm**   **CC**

    ✓7ᵗʰ **S65.809**   **Unspecified injury of other blood vessels at wrist and hand level of** unspecified **arm**   **CC**

✓6ᵗʰ **S65.81**   Laceration **of other blood vessels at wrist and hand level**

    ✓7ᵗʰ **S65.811**   **Laceration of other blood vessels at wrist and hand level of** right **arm**   **CC**

    ✓7ᵗʰ **S65.812**   **Laceration of other blood vessels at wrist and hand level of** left **arm**   **CC**

    ✓7ᵗʰ **S65.819**   **Laceration of other blood vessels at wrist and hand level of** unspecified **arm**   **CC**

✓6ᵗʰ **S65.89**   Other specified **injury of other blood vessels at wrist and hand level**

    ✓7ᵗʰ **S65.891**   **Other specified injury of other blood vessels at wrist and hand level of** right **arm**   **CC**

    ✓7ᵗʰ **S65.892**   **Other specified injury of other blood vessels at wrist and hand level of** left **arm**   **CC**

    ✓7ᵗʰ **S65.899**   **Other specified injury of other blood vessels at wrist and hand level of** unspecified **arm**   **CC**

✓5ᵗʰ **S65.9**   **Injury of unspecified blood vessel at** wrist and hand level

> **CC Excl: For CC codes in subcategory S65.9:**
> **Right side:** PDX collection 1260
> **Left side:** PDX collection 1261
> **Unspecified side:** PDX collection 1262

✓6ᵗʰ **S65.90**   Unspecified **injury of unspecified blood vessel at wrist and hand level**

    ✓7ᵗʰ **S65.901**   **Unspecified injury of unspecified blood vessel at wrist and hand level of** right **arm**   **CC**

    ✓7ᵗʰ **S65.902**   **Unspecified injury of unspecified blood vessel at wrist and hand level of** left **arm**   **CC**

    ✓7ᵗʰ **S65.909**   **Unspecified injury of unspecified blood vessel at wrist and hand level of** unspecified **arm**   **CC**

✓6ᵗʰ **S65.91**   Laceration **of unspecified blood vessel at wrist and hand level**

    ✓7ᵗʰ **S65.911**   **Laceration of unspecified blood vessel at wrist and hand level of** right **arm**   **CC**

    ✓7ᵗʰ **S65.912**   **Laceration of unspecified blood vessel at wrist and hand level of** left **arm**   **CC**

    ✓7ᵗʰ **S65.919**   **Laceration of unspecified blood vessel at wrist and hand level of** unspecified **arm**   **CC**

✓6ᵗʰ **S65.99**   Other specified **injury of unspecified blood vessel at wrist and hand level**

    ✓7ᵗʰ **S65.991**   **Other specified injury of unspecified blood vessel at wrist and hand of** right **arm**   **CC**

**N** Newborn: 0   **P** Pediatric: 0-17   **M** Maternity: 12-55   **A** Adult: 15-124   **MCC** Major CC Condition   **PDxMCC** PDx acts as own MCC   **CC** CC Condition   **PDxCC** PDx acts as own CC

**1030**          ICD-10-CM 2018

√7ᵗʰ **S65.992** Other specified injury of unspecified blood vessel at wrist and hand of left arm `CC`

√7ᵗʰ **S65.999** Other specified injury of unspecified blood vessel at wrist and hand of unspecified arm `CC`

√4ᵗʰ **S66 Injury of muscle, fascia and tendon at wrist and hand level**
Code also any associated open wound (S61.-)
*EXCLUDES 2* *sprain of joints and ligaments of wrist and hand (S63.-)*
**TIP:** Refer to the Muscle/Tendon table at the beginning of this chapter.

The appropriate 7th character is to be added to each code from category S66.
A   initial encounter
D   subsequent encounter
S   sequela

**CC Excl: For CC codes in category S66:**
**Right side:** PDX collection 1294
**Left side:** PDX collection 1295
**Other or unspecified side:** PDX collection 1296

√5ᵗʰ **S66.0 Injury of long flexor muscle, fascia and tendon of thumb at wrist and hand level**

√6ᵗʰ **S66.00** Unspecified injury of long flexor muscle, fascia and tendon of thumb at wrist and hand level

√7ᵗʰ **S66.001** Unspecified injury of long flexor muscle, fascia and tendon of right thumb at wrist and hand level

√7ᵗʰ **S66.002** Unspecified injury of long flexor muscle, fascia and tendon of left thumb at wrist and hand level

√7ᵗʰ **S66.009** Unspecified injury of long flexor muscle, fascia and tendon of unspecified thumb at wrist and hand level

√6ᵗʰ **S66.01** Strain of long flexor muscle, fascia and tendon of thumb at wrist and hand level

√7ᵗʰ **S66.011** Strain of long flexor muscle, fascia and tendon of right thumb at wrist and hand level

√7ᵗʰ **S66.012** Strain of long flexor muscle, fascia and tendon of left thumb at wrist and hand level

√7ᵗʰ **S66.019** Strain of long flexor muscle, fascia and tendon of unspecified thumb at wrist and hand level

√6ᵗʰ **S66.02** Laceration of long flexor muscle, fascia and tendon of thumb at wrist and hand level

√7ᵗʰ **S66.021** Laceration of long flexor muscle, fascia and tendon of right thumb at wrist and hand level `CC`

√7ᵗʰ **S66.022** Laceration of long flexor muscle, fascia and tendon of left thumb at wrist and hand level `CC`

√7ᵗʰ **S66.029** Laceration of long flexor muscle, fascia and tendon of unspecified thumb at wrist and hand level `CC`

√6ᵗʰ **S66.09** Other specified injury of long flexor muscle, fascia and tendon of thumb at wrist and hand level

√7ᵗʰ **S66.091** Other specified injury of long flexor muscle, fascia and tendon of right thumb at wrist and hand level

√7ᵗʰ **S66.092** Other specified injury of long flexor muscle, fascia and tendon of left thumb at wrist and hand level

√7ᵗʰ **S66.099** Other specified injury of long flexor muscle, fascia and tendon of unspecified thumb at wrist and hand level

√5ᵗʰ **S66.1 Injury of flexor muscle, fascia and tendon of other and unspecified finger at wrist and hand level**
*EXCLUDES 2* *Injury of long flexor muscle, fascia and tendon of thumb at wrist and hand level (S66.0-)*

√6ᵗʰ **S66.10** Unspecified injury of flexor muscle, fascia and tendon of other and unspecified finger at wrist and hand level

√7ᵗʰ **S66.100** Unspecified injury of flexor muscle, fascia and tendon of right index finger at wrist and hand level

√7ᵗʰ **S66.101** Unspecified injury of flexor muscle, fascia and tendon of left index finger at wrist and hand level

√7ᵗʰ **S66.102** Unspecified injury of flexor muscle, fascia and tendon of right middle finger at wrist and hand level

√7ᵗʰ **S66.103** Unspecified injury of flexor muscle, fascia and tendon of left middle finger at wrist and hand level

√7ᵗʰ **S66.104** Unspecified injury of flexor muscle, fascia and tendon of right ring finger at wrist and hand level

√7ᵗʰ **S66.105** Unspecified injury of flexor muscle, fascia and tendon of left ring finger at wrist and hand level

√7ᵗʰ **S66.106** Unspecified injury of flexor muscle, fascia and tendon of right little finger at wrist and hand level

√7ᵗʰ **S66.107** Unspecified injury of flexor muscle, fascia and tendon of left little finger at wrist and hand level

√7ᵗʰ **S66.108** Unspecified injury of flexor muscle, fascia and tendon of other finger at wrist and hand level
Unspecified injury of flexor muscle, fascia and tendon of specified finger with unspecified laterality at wrist and hand level

√7ᵗʰ **S66.109** Unspecified injury of flexor muscle, fascia and tendon of unspecified finger at wrist and hand level

√6ᵗʰ **S66.11** Strain of flexor muscle, fascia and tendon of other and unspecified finger at wrist and hand level

√7ᵗʰ **S66.110** Strain of flexor muscle, fascia and tendon of right index finger at wrist and hand level

√7ᵗʰ **S66.111** Strain of flexor muscle, fascia and tendon of left index finger at wrist and hand level

√7ᵗʰ **S66.112** Strain of flexor muscle, fascia and tendon of right middle finger at wrist and hand level

√7ᵗʰ **S66.113** Strain of flexor muscle, fascia and tendon of left middle finger at wrist and hand level

√7ᵗʰ **S66.114** Strain of flexor muscle, fascia and tendon of right ring finger at wrist and hand level

√7ᵗʰ **S66.115** Strain of flexor muscle, fascia and tendon of left ring finger at wrist and hand level

√7ᵗʰ **S66.116** Strain of flexor muscle, fascia and tendon of right little finger at wrist and hand level

√7ᵗʰ **S66.117** Strain of flexor muscle, fascia and tendon of left little finger at wrist and hand level

√7ᵗʰ **S66.118** Strain of flexor muscle, fascia and tendon of other finger at wrist and hand level
Strain of flexor muscle, fascia and tendon of specified finger with unspecified laterality at wrist and hand level

√7ᵗʰ **S66.119** Strain of flexor muscle, fascia and tendon of unspecified finger at wrist and hand level

√6ᵗʰ **S66.12** Laceration of flexor muscle, fascia and tendon of other and unspecified finger at wrist and hand level

√7ᵗʰ **S66.120** Laceration of flexor muscle, fascia and tendon of right index finger at wrist and hand level `CC`

√7ᵗʰ **S66.121** Laceration of flexor muscle, fascia and tendon of left index finger at wrist and hand level `CC`

√7ᵗʰ **S66.122** Laceration of flexor muscle, fascia and tendon of right middle finger at wrist and hand level `CC`

√7ᵗʰ **S66.123** Laceration of flexor muscle, fascia and tendon of left middle finger at wrist and hand level `CC`

√7ᵗʰ **S66.124** Laceration of flexor muscle, fascia and tendon of right ring finger at wrist and hand level `CC`

√7ᵗʰ **S66.125** **Laceration of flexor muscle, fascia and tendon of left ring finger at wrist and hand level** CC

√7ᵗʰ **S66.126** **Laceration of flexor muscle, fascia and tendon of right little finger at wrist and hand level** CC

√7ᵗʰ **S66.127** **Laceration of flexor muscle, fascia and tendon of left little finger at wrist and hand level** CC

√7ᵗʰ **S66.128** **Laceration of flexor muscle, fascia and tendon of other finger at wrist and hand level** CC

Laceration of flexor muscle, fascia and tendon of specified finger with unspecified laterality at wrist and hand level

√7ᵗʰ **S66.129** **Laceration of flexor muscle, fascia and tendon of unspecified finger at wrist and hand level** CC

√6ᵗʰ **S66.19** **Other injury of flexor muscle, fascia and tendon of other and unspecified finger at wrist and hand level**

√7ᵗʰ **S66.190** **Other injury of flexor muscle, fascia and tendon of right index finger at wrist and hand level**

√7ᵗʰ **S66.191** **Other injury of flexor muscle, fascia and tendon of left index finger at wrist and hand level**

√7ᵗʰ **S66.192** **Other injury of flexor muscle, fascia and tendon of right middle finger at wrist and hand level**

√7ᵗʰ **S66.193** **Other injury of flexor muscle, fascia and tendon of left middle finger at wrist and hand level**

√7ᵗʰ **S66.194** **Other injury of flexor muscle, fascia and tendon of right ring finger at wrist and hand level**

√7ᵗʰ **S66.195** **Other injury of flexor muscle, fascia and tendon of left ring finger at wrist and hand level**

√7ᵗʰ **S66.196** **Other injury of flexor muscle, fascia and tendon of right little finger at wrist and hand level**

√7ᵗʰ **S66.197** **Other injury of flexor muscle, fascia and tendon of left little finger at wrist and hand level**

√7ᵗʰ **S66.198** **Other injury of flexor muscle, fascia and tendon of other finger at wrist and hand level**

Other injury of flexor muscle, fascia and tendon of specified finger with unspecified laterality at wrist and hand level

√7ᵗʰ **S66.199** **Other injury of flexor muscle, fascia and tendon of unspecified finger at wrist and hand level**

√5ᵗʰ **S66.2** **Injury of extensor muscle, fascia and tendon of thumb at wrist and hand level**

√6ᵗʰ **S66.20** **Unspecified injury of extensor muscle, fascia and tendon of thumb at wrist and hand level**

√7ᵗʰ **S66.201** **Unspecified injury of extensor muscle, fascia and tendon of right thumb at wrist and hand level**

√7ᵗʰ **S66.202** **Unspecified injury of extensor muscle, fascia and tendon of left thumb at wrist and hand level**

√7ᵗʰ **S66.209** **Unspecified injury of extensor muscle, fascia and tendon of unspecified thumb at wrist and hand level**

√6ᵗʰ **S66.21** **Strain of extensor muscle, fascia and tendon of thumb at wrist and hand level**

√7ᵗʰ **S66.211** **Strain of extensor muscle, fascia and tendon of right thumb at wrist and hand level**

√7ᵗʰ **S66.212** **Strain of extensor muscle, fascia and tendon of left thumb at wrist and hand level**

√7ᵗʰ **S66.219** **Strain of extensor muscle, fascia and tendon of unspecified thumb at wrist and hand level**

√6ᵗʰ **S66.22** **Laceration of extensor muscle, fascia and tendon of thumb at wrist and hand level**

√7ᵗʰ **S66.221** **Laceration of extensor muscle, fascia and tendon of right thumb at wrist and hand level** CC

√7ᵗʰ **S66.222** **Laceration of extensor muscle, fascia and tendon of left thumb at wrist and hand level** CC

√7ᵗʰ **S66.229** **Laceration of extensor muscle, fascia and tendon of unspecified thumb at wrist and hand level** CC

√6ᵗʰ **S66.29** **Other specified injury of extensor muscle, fascia and tendon of thumb at wrist and hand level**

√7ᵗʰ **S66.291** **Other specified injury of extensor muscle, fascia and tendon of right thumb at wrist and hand level**

√7ᵗʰ **S66.292** **Other specified injury of extensor muscle, fascia and tendon of left thumb at wrist and hand level**

√7ᵗʰ **S66.299** **Other specified injury of extensor muscle, fascia and tendon of unspecified thumb at wrist and hand level**

√5ᵗʰ **S66.3** **Injury of extensor muscle, fascia and tendon of other and unspecified finger at wrist and hand level**

EXCLUDES 2    *Injury of extensor muscle, fascia and tendon of thumb at wrist and hand level (S66.2-)*

√6ᵗʰ **S66.30** **Unspecified injury of extensor muscle, fascia and tendon of other and unspecified finger at wrist and hand level**

√7ᵗʰ **S66.300** **Unspecified injury of extensor muscle, fascia and tendon of right index finger at wrist and hand level**

√7ᵗʰ **S66.301** **Unspecified injury of extensor muscle, fascia and tendon of left index finger at wrist and hand level**

√7ᵗʰ **S66.302** **Unspecified injury of extensor muscle, fascia and tendon of right middle finger at wrist and hand level**

√7ᵗʰ **S66.303** **Unspecified injury of extensor muscle, fascia and tendon of left middle finger at wrist and hand level**

√7ᵗʰ **S66.304** **Unspecified injury of extensor muscle, fascia and tendon of right ring finger at wrist and hand level**

√7ᵗʰ **S66.305** **Unspecified injury of extensor muscle, fascia and tendon of left ring finger at wrist and hand level**

√7ᵗʰ **S66.306** **Unspecified injury of extensor muscle, fascia and tendon of right little finger at wrist and hand level**

√7ᵗʰ **S66.307** **Unspecified injury of extensor muscle, fascia and tendon of left little finger at wrist and hand level**

√7ᵗʰ **S66.308** **Unspecified injury of extensor muscle, fascia and tendon of other finger at wrist and hand level**

Unspecified injury of extensor muscle, fascia and tendon of specified finger with unspecified laterality at wrist and hand level

√7ᵗʰ **S66.309** **Unspecified injury of extensor muscle, fascia and tendon of unspecified finger at wrist and hand level**

√6ᵗʰ **S66.31** **Strain of extensor muscle, fascia and tendon of other and unspecified finger at wrist and hand level**

√7ᵗʰ **S66.310** **Strain of extensor muscle, fascia and tendon of right index finger at wrist and hand level**

√7ᵗʰ **S66.311** **Strain of extensor muscle, fascia and tendon of left index finger at wrist and hand level**

√7ᵗʰ **S66.312** **Strain of extensor muscle, fascia and tendon of right middle finger at wrist and hand level**

√7ᵗʰ **S66.313** **Strain of extensor muscle, fascia and tendon of left middle finger at wrist and hand level**

N Newborn: 0    P Pediatric: 0-17    M Maternity: 12-55    A Adult: 15-124    MCC Major CC Condition    PDx MCC PDx acts as own MCC    CC CC Condition    PDx CC PDx acts as own CC

**1032**      ICD-10-CM 2018

✓7ᵗʰ **S66.314** Strain of extensor muscle, fascia and tendon of right ring finger at wrist and hand level

✓7ᵗʰ **S66.315** Strain of extensor muscle, fascia and tendon of left ring finger at wrist and hand level

✓7ᵗʰ **S66.316** Strain of extensor muscle, fascia and tendon of right little finger at wrist and hand level

✓7ᵗʰ **S66.317** Strain of extensor muscle, fascia and tendon of left little finger at wrist and hand level

✓7ᵗʰ **S66.318** Strain of extensor muscle, fascia and tendon of other finger at wrist and hand level

     Strain of extensor muscle, fascia and tendon of specified finger with unspecified laterality at wrist and hand level

✓7ᵗʰ **S66.319** Strain of extensor muscle, fascia and tendon of unspecified finger at wrist and hand level

✓6ᵗʰ **S66.32** Laceration of extensor muscle, fascia and tendon of other and unspecified finger at wrist and hand level

✓7ᵗʰ **S66.320** Laceration of extensor muscle, fascia and tendon of right index finger at wrist and hand level   CC

✓7ᵗʰ **S66.321** Laceration of extensor muscle, fascia and tendon of left index finger at wrist and hand level   CC

✓7ᵗʰ **S66.322** Laceration of extensor muscle, fascia and tendon of right middle finger at wrist and hand level   CC

✓7ᵗʰ **S66.323** Laceration of extensor muscle, fascia and tendon of left middle finger at wrist and hand level   CC

✓7ᵗʰ **S66.324** Laceration of extensor muscle, fascia and tendon of right ring finger at wrist and hand level   CC

✓7ᵗʰ **S66.325** Laceration of extensor muscle, fascia and tendon of left ring finger at wrist and hand level   CC

✓7ᵗʰ **S66.326** Laceration of extensor muscle, fascia and tendon of right little finger at wrist and hand level   CC

✓7ᵗʰ **S66.327** Laceration of extensor muscle, fascia and tendon of left little finger at wrist and hand level   CC

✓7ᵗʰ **S66.328** Laceration of extensor muscle, fascia and tendon of other finger at wrist and hand level   CC

     Laceration of extensor muscle, fascia and tendon of specified finger with unspecified laterality at wrist and hand level

✓7ᵗʰ **S66.329** Laceration of extensor muscle, fascia and tendon of unspecified finger at wrist and hand level   CC

✓6ᵗʰ **S66.39** Other injury of extensor muscle, fascia and tendon of other and unspecified finger at wrist and hand level

✓7ᵗʰ **S66.390** Other injury of extensor muscle, fascia and tendon of right index finger at wrist and hand level

✓7ᵗʰ **S66.391** Other injury of extensor muscle, fascia and tendon of left index finger at wrist and hand level

✓7ᵗʰ **S66.392** Other injury of extensor muscle, fascia and tendon of right middle finger at wrist and hand level

✓7ᵗʰ **S66.393** Other injury of extensor muscle, fascia and tendon of left middle finger at wrist and hand level

✓7ᵗʰ **S66.394** Other injury of extensor muscle, fascia and tendon of right ring finger at wrist and hand level

✓7ᵗʰ **S66.395** Other injury of extensor muscle, fascia and tendon of left ring finger at wrist and hand level

✓7ᵗʰ **S66.396** Other injury of extensor muscle, fascia and tendon of right little finger at wrist and hand level

✓7ᵗʰ **S66.397** Other injury of extensor muscle, fascia and tendon of left little finger at wrist and hand level

✓7ᵗʰ **S66.398** Other injury of extensor muscle, fascia and tendon of other finger at wrist and hand level

     Other injury of extensor muscle, fascia and tendon of specified finger with unspecified laterality at wrist and hand level

✓7ᵗʰ **S66.399** Other injury of extensor muscle, fascia and tendon of unspecified finger at wrist and hand level

✓5ᵗʰ **S66.4 Injury of intrinsic muscle, fascia and tendon of thumb at wrist and hand level**

✓6ᵗʰ **S66.40** Unspecified injury of intrinsic muscle, fascia and tendon of thumb at wrist and hand level

✓7ᵗʰ **S66.401** Unspecified injury of intrinsic muscle, fascia and tendon of right thumb at wrist and hand level

✓7ᵗʰ **S66.402** Unspecified injury of intrinsic muscle, fascia and tendon of left thumb at wrist and hand level

✓7ᵗʰ **S66.409** Unspecified injury of intrinsic muscle, fascia and tendon of unspecified thumb at wrist and hand level

✓6ᵗʰ **S66.41** Strain of intrinsic muscle, fascia and tendon of thumb at wrist and hand level

✓7ᵗʰ **S66.411** Strain of intrinsic muscle, fascia and tendon of right thumb at wrist and hand level

✓7ᵗʰ **S66.412** Strain of intrinsic muscle, fascia and tendon of left thumb at wrist and hand level

✓7ᵗʰ **S66.419** Strain of intrinsic muscle, fascia and tendon of unspecified thumb at wrist and hand level

✓6ᵗʰ **S66.42** Laceration of intrinsic muscle, fascia and tendon of thumb at wrist and hand level

✓7ᵗʰ **S66.421** Laceration of intrinsic muscle, fascia and tendon of right thumb at wrist and hand level   CC

✓7ᵗʰ **S66.422** Laceration of intrinsic muscle, fascia and tendon of left thumb at wrist and hand level   CC

✓7ᵗʰ **S66.429** Laceration of intrinsic muscle, fascia and tendon of unspecified thumb at wrist and hand level   CC

✓6ᵗʰ **S66.49** Other specified injury of intrinsic muscle, fascia and tendon of thumb at wrist and hand level

✓7ᵗʰ **S66.491** Other specified injury of intrinsic muscle, fascia and tendon of right thumb at wrist and hand level

✓7ᵗʰ **S66.492** Other specified injury of intrinsic muscle, fascia and tendon of left thumb at wrist and hand level

✓7ᵗʰ **S66.499** Other specified injury of intrinsic muscle, fascia and tendon of unspecified thumb at wrist and hand level

✓5ᵗʰ **S66.5 Injury of intrinsic muscle, fascia and tendon of other and unspecified finger at wrist and hand level**

     *EXCLUDES 2*   *injury of intrinsic muscle, fascia and tendon of thumb at wrist and hand level (S66.4-)*

✓6ᵗʰ **S66.50** Unspecified injury of intrinsic muscle, fascia and tendon of other and unspecified finger at wrist and hand level

✓7ᵗʰ **S66.500** Unspecified injury of intrinsic muscle, fascia and tendon of right index finger at wrist and hand level

✓7ᵗʰ **S66.501** Unspecified injury of intrinsic muscle, fascia and tendon of left index finger at wrist and hand level

✓7ᵗʰ **S66.502** Unspecified injury of intrinsic muscle, fascia and tendon of right middle finger at wrist and hand level

☑Additional Character Req   ✓7ᵗʰ Placeholder Alert   Unacceptable PDx   Manifestation   **H1**-**H14** HAC   **HCC** CMS-HCC Condition   *EXCLUDES 1* Not Coded Here   *EXCLUDES 2* Not Included Here

ICD-10-CM 2018      1033

√7ᵗʰ **S66.503** **Unspecified injury of intrinsic muscle, fascia and tendon of left middle finger at wrist and hand level**

√7ᵗʰ **S66.504** **Unspecified injury of intrinsic muscle, fascia and tendon of right ring finger at wrist and hand level**

√7ᵗʰ **S66.505** **Unspecified injury of intrinsic muscle, fascia and tendon of left ring finger at wrist and hand level**

√7ᵗʰ **S66.506** **Unspecified injury of intrinsic muscle, fascia and tendon of right little finger at wrist and hand level**

√7ᵗʰ **S66.507** **Unspecified injury of intrinsic muscle, fascia and tendon of left little finger at wrist and hand level**

√7ᵗʰ **S66.508** **Unspecified injury of intrinsic muscle, fascia and tendon of other finger at wrist and hand level**

Unspecified injury of intrinsic muscle, fascia and tendon of specified finger with unspecified laterality at wrist and hand level

√7ᵗʰ **S66.509** **Unspecified injury of intrinsic muscle, fascia and tendon of unspecified finger at wrist and hand level**

√6ᵗʰ **S66.51** **Strain of intrinsic muscle, fascia and tendon of other and unspecified finger at wrist and hand level**

√7ᵗʰ **S66.510** **Strain of intrinsic muscle, fascia and tendon of right index finger at wrist and hand level**

√7ᵗʰ **S66.511** **Strain of intrinsic muscle, fascia and tendon of left index finger at wrist and hand level**

√7ᵗʰ **S66.512** **Strain of intrinsic muscle, fascia and tendon of right middle finger at wrist and hand level**

√7ᵗʰ **S66.513** **Strain of intrinsic muscle, fascia and tendon of left middle finger at wrist and hand level**

√7ᵗʰ **S66.514** **Strain of intrinsic muscle, fascia and tendon of right ring finger at wrist and hand level**

√7ᵗʰ **S66.515** **Strain of intrinsic muscle, fascia and tendon of left ring finger at wrist and hand level**

√7ᵗʰ **S66.516** **Strain of intrinsic muscle, fascia and tendon of right little finger at wrist and hand level**

√7ᵗʰ **S66.517** **Strain of intrinsic muscle, fascia and tendon of left little finger at wrist and hand level**

√7ᵗʰ **S66.518** **Strain of intrinsic muscle, fascia and tendon of other finger at wrist and hand level**

Strain of intrinsic muscle, fascia and tendon of specified finger with unspecified laterality at wrist and hand level

√7ᵗʰ **S66.519** **Strain of intrinsic muscle, fascia and tendon of unspecified finger at wrist and hand level**

√6ᵗʰ **S66.52** **Laceration of intrinsic muscle, fascia and tendon of other and unspecified finger at wrist and hand level**

√7ᵗʰ **S66.520** **Laceration of intrinsic muscle, fascia and tendon of right index finger at wrist and hand level** `CC`

√7ᵗʰ **S66.521** **Laceration of intrinsic muscle, fascia and tendon of left index finger at wrist and hand level** `CC`

√7ᵗʰ **S66.522** **Laceration of intrinsic muscle, fascia and tendon of right middle finger at wrist and hand level** `CC`

√7ᵗʰ **S66.523** **Laceration of intrinsic muscle, fascia and tendon of left middle finger at wrist and hand level** `CC`

√7ᵗʰ **S66.524** **Laceration of intrinsic muscle, fascia and tendon of right ring finger at wrist and hand level** `CC`

√7ᵗʰ **S66.525** **Laceration of intrinsic muscle, fascia and tendon of left ring finger at wrist and hand level** `CC`

√7ᵗʰ **S66.526** **Laceration of intrinsic muscle, fascia and tendon of right little finger at wrist and hand level** `CC`

√7ᵗʰ **S66.527** **Laceration of intrinsic muscle, fascia and tendon of left little finger at wrist and hand level** `CC`

√7ᵗʰ **S66.528** **Laceration of intrinsic muscle, fascia and tendon of other finger at wrist and hand level** `CC`

Laceration of intrinsic muscle, fascia and tendon of specified finger with unspecified laterality at wrist and hand level

√7ᵗʰ **S66.529** **Laceration of intrinsic muscle, fascia and tendon of unspecified finger at wrist and hand level** `CC`

√6ᵗʰ **S66.59** **Other injury of intrinsic muscle, fascia and tendon of other and unspecified finger at wrist and hand level**

√7ᵗʰ **S66.590** **Other injury of intrinsic muscle, fascia and tendon of right index finger at wrist and hand level**

√7ᵗʰ **S66.591** **Other injury of intrinsic muscle, fascia and tendon of left index finger at wrist and hand level**

√7ᵗʰ **S66.592** **Other injury of intrinsic muscle, fascia and tendon of right middle finger at wrist and hand level**

√7ᵗʰ **S66.593** **Other injury of intrinsic muscle, fascia and tendon of left middle finger at wrist and hand level**

√7ᵗʰ **S66.594** **Other injury of intrinsic muscle, fascia and tendon of right ring finger at wrist and hand level**

√7ᵗʰ **S66.595** **Other injury of intrinsic muscle, fascia and tendon of left ring finger at wrist and hand level**

√7ᵗʰ **S66.596** **Other injury of intrinsic muscle, fascia and tendon of right little finger at wrist and hand level**

√7ᵗʰ **S66.597** **Other injury of intrinsic muscle, fascia and tendon of left little finger at wrist and hand level**

√7ᵗʰ **S66.598** **Other injury of intrinsic muscle, fascia and tendon of other finger at wrist and hand level**

Other injury of intrinsic muscle, fascia and tendon of specified finger with unspecified laterality at wrist and hand level

√7ᵗʰ **S66.599** **Other injury of intrinsic muscle, fascia and tendon of unspecified finger at wrist and hand level**

√5ᵗʰ **S66.8** **Injury of other specified muscles, fascia and tendons at wrist and hand level**

√6ᵗʰ **S66.80** **Unspecified injury of other specified muscles, fascia and tendons at wrist and hand level**

√7ᵗʰ **S66.801** **Unspecified injury of other specified muscles, fascia and tendons at wrist and hand level, right hand**

√7ᵗʰ **S66.802** **Unspecified injury of other specified muscles, fascia and tendons at wrist and hand level, left hand**

√7ᵗʰ **S66.809** **Unspecified injury of other specified muscles, fascia and tendons at wrist and hand level, unspecified hand**

√6ᵗʰ **S66.81** **Strain of other specified muscles, fascia and tendons at wrist and hand level**

√7ᵗʰ **S66.811** **Strain of other specified muscles, fascia and tendons at wrist and hand level, right hand**

√7ᵗʰ **S66.812** **Strain of other specified muscles, fascia and tendons at wrist and hand level, left hand**

√7ᵗʰ **S66.819** **Strain of other specified muscles, fascia and tendons at wrist and hand level, unspecified hand**

Ⓝ Newborn: 0   Ⓟ Pediatric: 0-17   Ⓜ Maternity: 12-55   Ⓐ Adult: 15-124   `MCC` Major CC Condition   `PDxMCC` PDx acts as own MCC   `CC` CC Condition   `PDxCC` PDx acts as own CC

**1034**      ICD-10-CM 2018

☑6ᵗʰ **S66.82** Laceration of other specified muscles, fascia and tendons at wrist and hand level

  ☑7ᵗʰ **S66.821** Laceration of other specified muscles, `CC` fascia and tendons at wrist and hand level, **right** hand

  ☑7ᵗʰ **S66.822** Laceration of other specified muscles, `CC` fascia and tendons at wrist and hand level, **left** hand

  ☑7ᵗʰ **S66.829** Laceration of other specified muscles, `CC` fascia and tendons at wrist and hand level, **unspecified** hand

☑6ᵗʰ **S66.89** Other injury of other specified muscles, fascia and tendons at wrist and hand level

  ☑7ᵗʰ **S66.891** Other injury of other specified muscles, fascia and tendons at wrist and hand level, **right** hand

  ☑7ᵗʰ **S66.892** Other injury of other specified muscles, fascia and tendons at wrist and hand level, **left** hand

  ☑7ᵗʰ **S66.899** Other injury of other specified muscles, fascia and tendons at wrist and hand level, **unspecified** hand

☑5ᵗʰ **S66.9** Injury of **unspecified** muscle, fascia and tendon at wrist and hand level

 ☑6ᵗʰ **S66.90** Unspecified injury of unspecified muscle, fascia and tendon at wrist and hand level

  ☑7ᵗʰ **S66.901** Unspecified injury of unspecified muscle, fascia and tendon at wrist and hand level, **right** hand

  ☑7ᵗʰ **S66.902** Unspecified injury of unspecified muscle, fascia and tendon at wrist and hand level, **left** hand

  ☑7ᵗʰ **S66.909** Unspecified injury of unspecified muscle, fascia and tendon at wrist and hand level, **unspecified** hand

 ☑6ᵗʰ **S66.91** Strain of unspecified muscle, fascia and tendon at wrist and hand level

  ☑7ᵗʰ **S66.911** Strain of unspecified muscle, fascia and tendon at wrist and hand level, **right** hand

  ☑7ᵗʰ **S66.912** Strain of unspecified muscle, fascia and tendon at wrist and hand level, **left** hand

  ☑7ᵗʰ **S66.919** Strain of unspecified muscle, fascia and tendon at wrist and hand level, **unspecified** hand

 ☑6ᵗʰ **S66.92** Laceration of unspecified muscle, fascia and tendon at wrist and hand level

  ☑7ᵗʰ **S66.921** Laceration of unspecified muscle, `CC` fascia and tendon at wrist and hand level, **right** hand

  ☑7ᵗʰ **S66.922** Laceration of unspecified muscle, `CC` fascia and tendon at wrist and hand level, **left** hand

  ☑7ᵗʰ **S66.929** Laceration of unspecified muscle, `CC` fascia and tendon at wrist and hand level, **unspecified** hand

 ☑6ᵗʰ **S66.99** Other injury of unspecified muscle, fascia and tendon at wrist and hand level

  ☑7ᵗʰ **S66.991** Other injury of unspecified muscle, fascia and tendon at wrist and hand level, **right** hand

  ☑7ᵗʰ **S66.992** Other injury of unspecified muscle, fascia and tendon at wrist and hand level, **left** hand

  ☑7ᵗʰ **S66.999** Other injury of unspecified muscle, fascia and tendon at wrist and hand level, **unspecified** hand

☑4ᵗʰ **S67** **Crushing injury of wrist, hand and fingers**
Use additional code for all associated injuries, such as:
 fracture of wrist and hand (S62.-)
 open wound of wrist and hand (S61.-)

> The appropriate 7th character is to be added to each code from category S67.
> A initial encounter
> D subsequent encounter
> S sequela

☑5ᵗʰ **S67.0** Crushing injury of **thumb**

 ☑×7ᵗʰ **S67.00** Crushing injury of **unspecified** thumb

 ☑×7ᵗʰ **S67.01** Crushing injury of **right** thumb

 ☑×7ᵗʰ **S67.02** Crushing injury of **left** thumb

☑5ᵗʰ **S67.1** Crushing injury of **other and unspecified finger(s)**
 *EXCLUDES 2* *crushing injury of thumb (S67.0-)*

 ☑×7ᵗʰ **S67.10** Crushing injury of **unspecified** finger(s)

 ☑6ᵗʰ **S67.19** Crushing injury of **other** finger(s)

  ☑7ᵗʰ **S67.190** Crushing injury of **right index** finger

  ☑7ᵗʰ **S67.191** Crushing injury of **left index** finger

  ☑7ᵗʰ **S67.192** Crushing injury of **right middle** finger

  ☑7ᵗʰ **S67.193** Crushing injury of **left middle** finger

  ☑7ᵗʰ **S67.194** Crushing injury of **right ring** finger

  ☑7ᵗʰ **S67.195** Crushing injury of **left ring** finger

  ☑7ᵗʰ **S67.196** Crushing injury of **right little** finger

  ☑7ᵗʰ **S67.197** Crushing injury of **left little** finger

  ☑7ᵗʰ **S67.198** Crushing injury of **other** finger
   Crushing injury of specified finger with unspecified laterality

☑5ᵗʰ **S67.2** Crushing injury of **hand**
 *EXCLUDES 2* *crushing injury of fingers (S67.1-)*
    *crushing injury of thumb (S67.0-)*

 ☑×7ᵗʰ **S67.20** Crushing injury of **unspecified** hand

 ☑×7ᵗʰ **S67.21** Crushing injury of **right** hand

 ☑×7ᵗʰ **S67.22** Crushing injury of **left** hand

☑5ᵗʰ **S67.3** Crushing injury of **wrist**

 ☑×7ᵗʰ **S67.30** Crushing injury of **unspecified** wrist

 ☑×7ᵗʰ **S67.31** Crushing injury of **right** wrist

 ☑×7ᵗʰ **S67.32** Crushing injury of **left** wrist

☑5ᵗʰ **S67.4** Crushing injury of **wrist and hand**
 *EXCLUDES 1* *crushing injury of hand alone (S67.2-)*
    *crushing injury of wrist alone (S67.3-)*
 *EXCLUDES 2* *crushing injury of fingers (S67.1-)*
    *crushing injury of thumb (S67.0-)*

 ☑×7ᵗʰ **S67.40** Crushing injury of **unspecified** wrist and hand

 ☑×7ᵗʰ **S67.41** Crushing injury of **right** wrist and hand

 ☑×7ᵗʰ **S67.42** Crushing injury of **left** wrist and hand

☑5ᵗʰ **S67.9** Crushing injury of **unspecified part(s)** of wrist, hand and fingers

 ☑×7ᵗʰ **S67.90** Crushing injury of unspecified part(s) of **unspecified** wrist, hand and fingers

 ☑×7ᵗʰ **S67.91** Crushing injury of unspecified part(s) of **right** wrist, hand and fingers

 ☑×7ᵗʰ **S67.92** Crushing injury of unspecified part(s) of **left** wrist, hand and fingers

☑ Additional Character Req ☑×7ᵗʰ Placeholder Alert Unacceptable PDx Manifestation **H1**-**H14** HAC **HCC** CMS-HCC Condition *EXCLUDES 1* Not Coded Here *EXCLUDES 2* Not Included Here

ICD-10-CM 2018                             **1035**

Chapter 19. Injury, Poisoning and Certain Other Consequences of External Causes

✓4th **S68 Traumatic amputation of wrist, hand and fingers**
An amputation not identified as partial or complete should be coded to complete.

The appropriate 7th character is to be added to each code from category S68.
A    initial encounter
D    subsequent encounter
S    sequela

CC Excl: For CC codes in category S68:
**Right side:** PDX collection 1266
**Left side:** PDX collection 1267
**Unspecified side:** PDX collection 1268

✓5th **S68.0 Traumatic metacarpophalangeal amputation of thumb**
Traumatic amputation of thumb NOS

✓6th **S68.01 Complete traumatic metacarpophalangeal amputation of thumb**
12 ✓7th **S68.011 Complete traumatic metacarpophalangeal amputation of right thumb** HCC
12 ✓7th **S68.012 Complete traumatic metacarpophalangeal amputation of left thumb** HCC
12 ✓7th **S68.019 Complete traumatic metacarpophalangeal amputation of unspecified thumb** HCC

✓6th **S68.02 Partial traumatic metacarpophalangeal amputation of thumb**
12 ✓7th **S68.021 Partial traumatic metacarpophalangeal amputation of right thumb** HCC
12 ✓7th **S68.022 Partial traumatic metacarpophalangeal amputation of left thumb** HCC
12 ✓7th **S68.029 Partial traumatic metacarpophalangeal amputation of unspecified thumb** HCC

✓5th **S68.1 Traumatic metacarpophalangeal amputation of other and unspecified finger**
Traumatic amputation of finger NOS
EXCLUDES 2    *traumatic metacarpophalangeal amputation of thumb (S68.0-)*

✓6th **S68.11 Complete traumatic metacarpophalangeal amputation of other and unspecified finger**
12 ✓7th **S68.110 Complete traumatic metacarpophalangeal amputation of right index finger** HCC
12 ✓7th **S68.111 Complete traumatic metacarpophalangeal amputation of left index finger** HCC
12 ✓7th **S68.112 Complete traumatic metacarpophalangeal amputation of right middle finger** HCC
12 ✓7th **S68.113 Complete traumatic metacarpophalangeal amputation of left middle finger** HCC
12 ✓7th **S68.114 Complete traumatic metacarpophalangeal amputation of right ring finger** HCC
12 ✓7th **S68.115 Complete traumatic metacarpophalangeal amputation of left ring finger** HCC
12 ✓7th **S68.116 Complete traumatic metacarpophalangeal amputation of right little finger** HCC
12 ✓7th **S68.117 Complete traumatic metacarpophalangeal amputation of left little finger** HCC
12 ✓7th **S68.118 Complete traumatic metacarpophalangeal amputation of other finger** HCC
Complete traumatic metacarpophalangeal amputation of specified finger with unspecified laterality
12 ✓7th **S68.119 Complete traumatic metacarpophalangeal amputation of unspecified finger** HCC

✓6th **S68.12 Partial traumatic metacarpophalangeal amputation of other and unspecified finger**
12 ✓7th **S68.120 Partial traumatic metacarpophalangeal amputation of right index finger** HCC
12 ✓7th **S68.121 Partial traumatic metacarpophalangeal amputation of left index finger** HCC
12 ✓7th **S68.122 Partial traumatic metacarpophalangeal amputation of right middle finger** HCC
12 ✓7th **S68.123 Partial traumatic metacarpophalangeal amputation of left middle finger** HCC
12 ✓7th **S68.124 Partial traumatic metacarpophalangeal amputation of right ring finger** HCC
12 ✓7th **S68.125 Partial traumatic metacarpophalangeal amputation of left ring finger** HCC
12 ✓7th **S68.126 Partial traumatic metacarpophalangeal amputation of right little finger** HCC
12 ✓7th **S68.127 Partial traumatic metacarpophalangeal amputation of left little finger** HCC
12 ✓7th **S68.128 Partial traumatic metacarpophalangeal amputation of other finger** HCC
Partial traumatic metacarpophalangeal amputation of specified finger with unspecified laterality
12 ✓7th **S68.129 Partial traumatic metacarpophalangeal amputation of unspecified finger** HCC

✓5th **S68.4 Traumatic amputation of hand at wrist level**
Traumatic amputation of hand NOS
Traumatic amputation of wrist

✓6th **S68.41 Complete traumatic amputation of hand at wrist level**
11 ✓7th **S68.411 Complete traumatic amputation of right hand at wrist level** CC HCC
11 ✓7th **S68.412 Complete traumatic amputation of left hand at wrist level** CC HCC
11 ✓7th **S68.419 Complete traumatic amputation of unspecified hand at wrist level** CC HCC

✓6th **S68.42 Partial traumatic amputation of hand at wrist level**
11 ✓7th **S68.421 Partial traumatic amputation of right hand at wrist level** CC HCC
11 ✓7th **S68.422 Partial traumatic amputation of left hand at wrist level** CC HCC
11 ✓7th **S68.429 Partial traumatic amputation of unspecified hand at wrist level** CC HCC

✓5th **S68.5 Traumatic transphalangeal amputation of thumb**
Traumatic interphalangeal joint amputation of thumb

✓6th **S68.51 Complete traumatic transphalangeal amputation of thumb**
12 ✓7th **S68.511 Complete traumatic transphalangeal amputation of right thumb** HCC
12 ✓7th **S68.512 Complete traumatic transphalangeal amputation of left thumb** HCC
12 ✓7th **S68.519 Complete traumatic transphalangeal amputation of unspecified thumb** HCC

✓6th **S68.52 Partial traumatic transphalangeal amputation of thumb**
12 ✓7th **S68.521 Partial traumatic transphalangeal amputation of right thumb** HCC
12 ✓7th **S68.522 Partial traumatic transphalangeal amputation of left thumb** HCC
12 ✓7th **S68.529 Partial traumatic transphalangeal amputation of unspecified thumb** HCC

---

[11] HCC with 7th character indicating initial encounter (A or B - specific to category) OR sequela.
[12] HCC with 7th character indicating sequela.

✓5th **S68.6** **Traumatic** transphalangeal **amputation of** other and unspecified finger

　✓6th **S68.61** Complete **traumatic transphalangeal amputation of** other and unspecified finger(s)

　　12 ✓7th **S68.610** **Complete traumatic transphalangeal** HCC **amputation of** right index **finger**

　　12 ✓7th **S68.611** **Complete traumatic transphalangeal** HCC **amputation of** left index **finger**

　　12 ✓7th **S68.612** **Complete traumatic transphalangeal** HCC **amputation of** right middle **finger**

　　12 ✓7th **S68.613** **Complete traumatic transphalangeal** HCC **amputation of** left middle **finger**

　　12 ✓7th **S68.614** **Complete traumatic transphalangeal** HCC **amputation of** right ring **finger**

　　12 ✓7th **S68.615** **Complete traumatic transphalangeal** HCC **amputation of** left ring **finger**

　　12 ✓7th **S68.616** **Complete traumatic transphalangeal** HCC **amputation of** right little **finger**

　　12 ✓7th **S68.617** **Complete traumatic transphalangeal** HCC **amputation of** left little **finger**

　　12 ✓7th **S68.618** **Complete traumatic transphalangeal** HCC **amputation of** other **finger**
　　　　　Complete traumatic transphalangeal amputation of specified finger with unspecified laterality

　　12 ✓7th **S68.619** **Complete traumatic transphalangeal** HCC **amputation of** unspecified **finger**

　✓6th **S68.62** Partial **traumatic transphalangeal amputation of** other and unspecified finger

　　12 ✓7th **S68.620** **Partial traumatic transphalangeal** HCC **amputation of** right index **finger**

　　12 ✓7th **S68.621** **Partial traumatic transphalangeal** HCC **amputation of** left index **finger**

　　12 ✓7th **S68.622** **Partial traumatic transphalangeal** HCC **amputation of** right middle **finger**

　　12 ✓7th **S68.623** **Partial traumatic transphalangeal** HCC **amputation of** left middle **finger**

　　12 ✓7th **S68.624** **Partial traumatic transphalangeal** HCC **amputation of** right ring **finger**

　　12 ✓7th **S68.625** **Partial traumatic transphalangeal** HCC **amputation of** left ring **finger**

　　12 ✓7th **S68.626** **Partial traumatic transphalangeal** HCC **amputation of** right little **finger**

　　12 ✓7th **S68.627** **Partial traumatic transphalangeal** HCC **amputation of** left little **finger**

　　12 ✓7th **S68.628** **Partial traumatic transphalangeal** HCC **amputation of** other **finger**
　　　　　Partial traumatic transphalangeal amputation of specified finger with unspecified laterality

　　12 ✓7th **S68.629** **Partial traumatic transphalangeal** HCC **amputation of** unspecified **finger**

✓5th **S68.7** **Traumatic** transmetacarpal **amputation of** hand

　✓6th **S68.71** Complete **traumatic transmetacarpal amputation of** hand

　　11 ✓7th **S68.711** **Complete traumatic** CC HCC **transmetacarpal amputation of** right **hand**

　　11 ✓7th **S68.712** **Complete traumatic** CC HCC **transmetacarpal amputation of** left **hand**

　　11 ✓7th **S68.719** **Complete traumatic** CC HCC **transmetacarpal amputation of** unspecified **hand**

　✓6th **S68.72** Partial **traumatic transmetacarpal amputation of** hand

　　11 ✓7th **S68.721** **Partial traumatic transmetacarpal** CC HCC **amputation of** right **hand**

　　11 ✓7th **S68.722** **Partial traumatic transmetacarpal** CC HCC **amputation of** left **hand**

　　11 ✓7th **S68.729** **Partial traumatic transmetacarpal** CC HCC **amputation of** unspecified **hand**

✓4th **S69** **Other and unspecified injuries of wrist, hand and finger(s)**

　　The appropriate 7th character is to be added to each code from category S69.
　　A　　initial encounter
　　D　　subsequent encounter
　　S　　sequela

　✓5th **S69.8** **Other specified injuries of wrist, hand and finger(s)**

　　✓x7th **S69.80** **Other specified injuries of** unspecified **wrist, hand and finger(s)**

　　✓x7th **S69.81** **Other specified injuries of** right **wrist, hand and finger(s)**

　　✓x7th **S69.82** **Other specified injuries of** left **wrist, hand and finger(s)**

　✓5th **S69.9** **Unspecified injury of wrist, hand and finger(s)**

　　✓x7th **S69.90** **Unspecified injury of** unspecified **wrist, hand and finger(s)**

　　✓x7th **S69.91** **Unspecified injury of** right **wrist, hand and finger(s)**

　　✓x7th **S69.92** **Unspecified injury of** left **wrist, hand and finger(s)**

### Injuries to the hip and thigh (S70-S79)

EXCLUDES 2　burns and corrosions (T20-T32)
　　　　　frostbite (T33-T34)
　　　　　snake bite (T63.0-)
　　　　　venomous insect bite or sting (T63.4-)

✓4th **S70** **Superficial injury of hip and thigh**

　　The appropriate 7th character is to be added to each code from category S70.
　　A　　initial encounter
　　D　　subsequent encounter
　　S　　sequela

　✓5th **S70.0** **Contusion of hip**

　　✓x7th **S70.00** **Contusion of** unspecified **hip**

　　✓x7th **S70.01** **Contusion of** right **hip**

　　✓x7th **S70.02** **Contusion of** left **hip**

　✓5th **S70.1** **Contusion of thigh**

　　✓x7th **S70.10** **Contusion of** unspecified **thigh**

　　✓x7th **S70.11** **Contusion of** right **thigh**

　　✓x7th **S70.12** **Contusion of** left **thigh**

　✓5th **S70.2** **Other superficial injuries of hip**

　　✓6th **S70.21** Abrasion **of hip**

　　　✓7th **S70.211** **Abrasion,** right **hip**

　　　✓7th **S70.212** **Abrasion,** left **hip**

　　　✓7th **S70.219** **Abrasion,** unspecified **hip**

　　✓6th **S70.22** Blister (nonthermal) **of hip**

　　　✓7th **S70.221** **Blister (nonthermal),** right **hip**

　　　✓7th **S70.222** **Blister (nonthermal),** left **hip**

　　　✓7th **S70.229** **Blister (nonthermal),** unspecified **hip**

　　✓6th **S70.24** External constriction **of hip**

　　　✓7th **S70.241** **External constriction,** right **hip**

　　　✓7th **S70.242** **External constriction,** left **hip**

　　　✓7th **S70.249** **External constriction,** unspecified **hip**

　　✓6th **S70.25** Superficial foreign body **of hip**
　　　　　Splinter in the hip

　　　✓7th **S70.251** **Superficial foreign body,** right **hip**

　　　✓7th **S70.252** **Superficial foreign body,** left **hip**

　　　✓7th **S70.259** **Superficial foreign body,** unspecified **hip**

　　✓6th **S70.26** Insect bite (nonvenomous) **of hip**

　　　✓7th **S70.261** **Insect bite (nonvenomous),** right **hip**

　　　✓7th **S70.262** **Insect bite (nonvenomous),** left **hip**

　　　✓7th **S70.269** **Insect bite (nonvenomous),** unspecified **hip**

　　✓6th **S70.27** Other superficial bite **of hip**
　　　　　EXCLUDES 1　open bite of hip (S71.05-)

　　　✓7th **S70.271** **Other superficial bite of hip,** right **hip**

　　　✓7th **S70.272** **Other superficial bite of hip,** left **hip**

　　　✓7th **S70.279** **Other superficial bite of hip,** unspecified **hip**

---

**11** HCC with 7th character indicating initial encounter (A or B - specific to category) OR sequela.

**12** HCC with 7th character indicating sequela.

---

☑ Additional Character Req　✓x7th Placeholder Alert　Unacceptable PDx　Manifestation　H1-H4 HAC　HCC CMS-HCC Condition　EXCLUDES 1 Not Coded Here　EXCLUDES 2 Not Included Here

✓5ᵗʰ **S70.3** Other superficial injuries of thigh
- ✓6ᵗʰ **S70.31** Abrasion of thigh
  - ✓7ᵗʰ **S70.311** Abrasion, right thigh
  - ✓7ᵗʰ **S70.312** Abrasion, left thigh
  - ✓7ᵗʰ **S70.319** Abrasion, unspecified thigh
- ✓6ᵗʰ **S70.32** Blister (nonthermal) of thigh
  - ✓7ᵗʰ **S70.321** Blister (nonthermal), right thigh
  - ✓7ᵗʰ **S70.322** Blister (nonthermal), left thigh
  - ✓7ᵗʰ **S70.329** Blister (nonthermal), unspecified thigh
- ✓6ᵗʰ **S70.34** External constriction of thigh
  - ✓7ᵗʰ **S70.341** External constriction, right thigh
  - ✓7ᵗʰ **S70.342** External constriction, left thigh
  - ✓7ᵗʰ **S70.349** External constriction, unspecified thigh
- ✓6ᵗʰ **S70.35** Superficial foreign body of thigh
  Splinter in the thigh
  - ✓7ᵗʰ **S70.351** Superficial foreign body, right thigh
  - ✓7ᵗʰ **S70.352** Superficial foreign body, left thigh
  - ✓7ᵗʰ **S70.359** Superficial foreign body, unspecified thigh
- ✓6ᵗʰ **S70.36** Insect bite (nonvenomous) of thigh
  - ✓7ᵗʰ **S70.361** Insect bite (nonvenomous), right thigh
  - ✓7ᵗʰ **S70.362** Insect bite (nonvenomous), left thigh
  - ✓7ᵗʰ **S70.369** Insect bite (nonvenomous), unspecified thigh
- ✓6ᵗʰ **S70.37** Other superficial bite of thigh
  EXCLUDES 1 open bite of thigh (S71.15)
  - ✓7ᵗʰ **S70.371** Other superficial bite of right thigh
  - ✓7ᵗʰ **S70.372** Other superficial bite of left thigh
  - ✓7ᵗʰ **S70.379** Other superficial bite of unspecified thigh

✓5ᵗʰ **S70.9** Unspecified superficial injury of hip and thigh
- ✓6ᵗʰ **S70.91** Unspecified superficial injury of hip
  - ✓7ᵗʰ **S70.911** Unspecified superficial injury of right hip
  - ✓7ᵗʰ **S70.912** Unspecified superficial injury of left hip
  - ✓7ᵗʰ **S70.919** Unspecified superficial injury of unspecified hip
- ✓6ᵗʰ **S70.92** Unspecified superficial injury of thigh
  - ✓7ᵗʰ **S70.921** Unspecified superficial injury of right thigh
  - ✓7ᵗʰ **S70.922** Unspecified superficial injury of left thigh
  - ✓7ᵗʰ **S70.929** Unspecified superficial injury of unspecified thigh

✓4ᵗʰ **S71** Open wound of hip and thigh
Code also any associated wound infection
EXCLUDES 1 open fracture of hip and thigh (S72.-)
traumatic amputation of hip and thigh (S78.-)
EXCLUDES 2 bite of venomous animal (T63.-)
open wound of ankle, foot and toes (S91.-)
open wound of knee and lower leg (S81.-)

> The appropriate 7th character is to be added to each code from category S71.
> A    initial encounter
> D    subsequent encounter
> S    sequela

✓5ᵗʰ **S71.0** Open wound of hip
- ✓6ᵗʰ **S71.00** Unspecified open wound of hip
  - ✓7ᵗʰ **S71.001** Unspecified open wound, right hip
  - ✓7ᵗʰ **S71.002** Unspecified open wound, left hip
  - ✓7ᵗʰ **S71.009** Unspecified open wound, unspecified hip
- ✓6ᵗʰ **S71.01** Laceration without foreign body of hip
  - ✓7ᵗʰ **S71.011** Laceration without foreign body, right hip
  - ✓7ᵗʰ **S71.012** Laceration without foreign body, left hip
  - ✓7ᵗʰ **S71.019** Laceration without foreign body, unspecified hip
- ✓6ᵗʰ **S71.02** Laceration with foreign body of hip
  - ✓7ᵗʰ **S71.021** Laceration with foreign body, right hip
  - ✓7ᵗʰ **S71.022** Laceration with foreign body, left hip
  - ✓7ᵗʰ **S71.029** Laceration with foreign body, unspecified hip

- ✓6ᵗʰ **S71.03** Puncture wound without foreign body of hip
  - ✓7ᵗʰ **S71.031** Puncture wound without foreign body, right hip
  - ✓7ᵗʰ **S71.032** Puncture wound without foreign body, left hip
  - ✓7ᵗʰ **S71.039** Puncture wound without foreign body, unspecified hip
- ✓6ᵗʰ **S71.04** Puncture wound with foreign body of hip
  - ✓7ᵗʰ **S71.041** Puncture wound with foreign body, right hip
  - ✓7ᵗʰ **S71.042** Puncture wound with foreign body, left hip
  - ✓7ᵗʰ **S71.049** Puncture wound with foreign body, unspecified hip
- ✓6ᵗʰ **S71.05** Open bite of hip
  Bite of hip NOS
  EXCLUDES 1 superficial bite of hip (S70.26, S70.27)
  - ✓7ᵗʰ **S71.051** Open bite, right hip
  - ✓7ᵗʰ **S71.052** Open bite, left hip
  - ✓7ᵗʰ **S71.059** Open bite, unspecified hip

✓5ᵗʰ **S71.1** Open wound of thigh
- ✓6ᵗʰ **S71.10** Unspecified open wound of thigh
  AHA: 2016, 3Q, 24
  - ✓7ᵗʰ **S71.101** Unspecified open wound, right thigh
  - ✓7ᵗʰ **S71.102** Unspecified open wound, left thigh
  - ✓7ᵗʰ **S71.109** Unspecified open wound, unspecified thigh
- ✓6ᵗʰ **S71.11** Laceration without foreign body of thigh
  - ✓7ᵗʰ **S71.111** Laceration without foreign body, right thigh
  - ✓7ᵗʰ **S71.112** Laceration without foreign body, left thigh
  - ✓7ᵗʰ **S71.119** Laceration without foreign body, unspecified thigh
- ✓6ᵗʰ **S71.12** Laceration with foreign body of thigh
  - ✓7ᵗʰ **S71.121** Laceration with foreign body, right thigh
  - ✓7ᵗʰ **S71.122** Laceration with foreign body, left thigh
  - ✓7ᵗʰ **S71.129** Laceration with foreign body, unspecified thigh
- ✓6ᵗʰ **S71.13** Puncture wound without foreign body of thigh
  AHA: 2016, 3Q, 24
  - ✓7ᵗʰ **S71.131** Puncture wound without foreign body, right thigh
  - ✓7ᵗʰ **S71.132** Puncture wound without foreign body, left thigh
  - ✓7ᵗʰ **S71.139** Puncture wound without foreign body, unspecified thigh
- ✓6ᵗʰ **S71.14** Puncture wound with foreign body of thigh
  AHA: 2016, 3Q, 24
  - ✓7ᵗʰ **S71.141** Puncture wound with foreign body, right thigh
  - ✓7ᵗʰ **S71.142** Puncture wound with foreign body, left thigh
  - ✓7ᵗʰ **S71.149** Puncture wound with foreign body, unspecified thigh
- ✓6ᵗʰ **S71.15** Open bite of thigh
  Bite of thigh NOS
  EXCLUDES 1 superficial bite of thigh (S70.37-)
  - ✓7ᵗʰ **S71.151** Open bite, right thigh
  - ✓7ᵗʰ **S71.152** Open bite, left thigh
  - ✓7ᵗʰ **S71.159** Open bite, unspecified thigh

N Newborn: 0    P Pediatric: 0-17    M Maternity: 12-55    A Adult: 15-124    MCC Major CC Condition    PDx MCC PDx acts as own MCC    CC CC Condition    PDx CC PDx acts as own CC

1038    ICD-10-CM 2018

### ✓4ᵗʰ S72   Fracture of femur

NOTE   A fracture not indicated as displaced or nondisplaced should be coded to displaced.

The open fracture designations are based on the Gustilo open fracture classification A fracture not indicated as open or closed should be coded to closed.

EXCLUDES 1   *traumatic amputation of hip and thigh (S78.-)*
EXCLUDES 2   *fracture of lower leg and ankle (S82.-)*
         *fracture of foot (S92.-)*
         *periprosthetic fracture of prosthetic implant of hip ▶(M97.0-)◀*

AHA: 2016, 1Q, 33; 2015, 3Q, 37-39; 2015, 1Q, 17; 2013, 4Q, 128

The appropriate 7th character is to be added to all codes from category S72 [unless otherwise indicated].

| | |
|---|---|
| A | initial encounter for closed fracture |
| B | initial encounter for open fracture type I or II<br>initial encounter for open fracture NOS |
| C | initial encounter for open fracture type IIIA, IIIB, or IIIC |
| D | subsequent encounter for closed fracture with routine healing |
| E | subsequent encounter for open fracture type I or II with routine healing |
| F | subsequent encounter for open fracture type IIIA, IIIB, or IIIC with routine healing |
| G | subsequent encounter for closed fracture with delayed healing |
| H | subsequent encounter for open fracture type I or II with delayed healing |
| J | subsequent encounter for open fracture type IIIA, IIIB, or IIIC with delayed healing |
| K | subsequent encounter for closed fracture with nonunion |
| M | subsequent encounter for open fracture type I or II with nonunion |
| N | subsequent encounter for open fracture type IIIA, IIIB, or IIIC with nonunion |
| P | subsequent encounter for closed fracture with malunion |
| Q | subsequent encounter for open fracture type I or II with malunion |
| R | subsequent encounter for open fracture type IIIA, IIIB, or IIIC with malunion |
| S | sequela |

### ✓5ᵗʰ S72.0   Fracture of head and neck of femur

EXCLUDES 2   *physeal fracture of upper end of femur (S79.0-)*
AHA: 2016, 3Q, 16

**CC Excl: For CC/MCC codes in subcategory S72.0:**
**Right side:** See code S72.001
**Left side:** See code S72.002
**Unspecified side:** See code S72.009

✓6ᵗʰ **S72.00   Fracture of unspecified part of neck of femur**
Fracture of hip NOS
Fracture of neck of femur NOS

8,10   ✓7ᵗʰ   **S72.001   Fracture of unspecified part** MCC CC H5 HCC **of neck of right femur**
**CC Excl: MCC with 7th character A:**
PDX collection 1297
**MCC with 7th character B or C:**
PDX collection 1298
**CC with 7th character K, M, N, P, Q or R:**
PDX collection 897

8,10   ✓7ᵗʰ   **S72.002   Fracture of unspecified part** MCC CC H5 HCC **of neck of left femur**
**CC Excl: MCC with 7th character A:**
PDX collection 1299
**MCC with 7th character B or C:**
PDX collection 1298
**CC with 7th character K, M, N, P, Q or R:**
PDX collection 897

8,10   ✓7ᵗʰ   **S72.009   Fracture of unspecified part** MCC CC H5 HCC **of neck of unspecified femur**
**CC Excl: MCC with 7th character A, B or C:**
PDX collection 1298
**CC with 7th character K, M, N, P, Q or R:**
PDX collection 897

✓6ᵗʰ **S72.01   Unspecified intracapsular fracture of femur**
Subcapital fracture of femur

8,10   ✓7ᵗʰ   **S72.011   Unspecified intracapsular** MCC CC H5 HCC **fracture of right femur**

8,10   ✓7ᵗʰ   **S72.012   Unspecified intracapsular** MCC CC H5 HCC **fracture of left femur**

8,10   ✓7ᵗʰ   **S72.019   Unspecified intracapsular** MCC CC H5 HCC **fracture of unspecified femur**

✓6ᵗʰ **S72.02   Fracture of epiphysis (separation) (upper) of femur**
Transepiphyseal fracture of femur
EXCLUDES 1   *capital femoral epiphyseal fracture (pediatric) of femur (S79.01-)*
     *Salter-Harris Type I physeal fracture of upper end of femur (S79.01-)*

8,10   ✓7ᵗʰ   **S72.021   Displaced fracture of** MCC CC H5 HCC **epiphysis (separation) (upper) of right femur**

8,10   ✓7ᵗʰ   **S72.022   Displaced fracture of** MCC CC H5 HCC **epiphysis (separation) (upper) of left femur**

8,10   ✓7ᵗʰ   **S72.023   Displaced fracture of** MCC CC H5 HCC **epiphysis (separation) (upper) of unspecified femur**

8,10   ✓7ᵗʰ   **S72.024   Nondisplaced fracture of** MCC CC H5 HCC **epiphysis (separation) (upper) of right femur**

8,10   ✓7ᵗʰ   **S72.025   Nondisplaced fracture of** MCC CC H5 HCC **epiphysis (separation) (upper) of left femur**

8,10   ✓7ᵗʰ   **S72.026   Nondisplaced fracture of** MCC CC H5 HCC **epiphysis (separation) (upper) of unspecified femur**

✓6ᵗʰ **S72.03   Midcervical fracture of femur**
Transcervical fracture of femur NOS

8,10   ✓7ᵗʰ   **S72.031   Displaced midcervical** MCC CC H5 HCC **fracture of right femur**

8,10   ✓7ᵗʰ   **S72.032   Displaced midcervical** MCC CC H5 HCC **fracture of left femur**

8,10   ✓7ᵗʰ   **S72.033   Displaced midcervical** MCC CC H5 HCC **fracture of unspecified femur**

8,10   ✓7ᵗʰ   **S72.034   Nondisplaced midcervical** MCC CC H5 HCC **fracture of right femur**

8,10   ✓7ᵗʰ   **S72.035   Nondisplaced midcervical** MCC CC H5 HCC **fracture of left femur**

8,10   ✓7ᵗʰ   **S72.036   Nondisplaced midcervical** MCC CC H5 HCC **fracture of unspecified femur**

✓6ᵗʰ **S72.04   Fracture of base of neck of femur**
Cervicotrochanteric fracture of femur

8,10   ✓7ᵗʰ   **S72.041   Displaced fracture of base** MCC CC H5 HCC **of neck of right femur**

8,10   ✓7ᵗʰ   **S72.042   Displaced fracture of base** MCC CC H5 HCC **of neck of left femur**

8,10   ✓7ᵗʰ   **S72.043   Displaced fracture of base** MCC CC H5 HCC **of neck of unspecified femur**

8,10   ✓7ᵗʰ   **S72.044   Nondisplaced fracture of** MCC CC H5 HCC **base of neck of right femur**

8,10   ✓7ᵗʰ   **S72.045   Nondisplaced fracture of** MCC CC H5 HCC **base of neck of left femur**

8,10   ✓7ᵗʰ   **S72.046   Nondisplaced fracture of** MCC CC H5 HCC **base of neck of unspecified femur**

✓6ᵗʰ **S72.05   Unspecified fracture of head of femur**
Fracture of head of femur NOS

8,10   ✓7ᵗʰ   **S72.051   Unspecified fracture of** MCC CC H5 HCC **head of right femur**

8,10   ✓7ᵗʰ   **S72.052   Unspecified fracture of** MCC CC H5 HCC **head of left femur**

8,10   ✓7ᵗʰ   **S72.059   Unspecified fracture of** MCC CC H5 HCC **head of unspecified femur**

✓6ᵗʰ **S72.06   Articular fracture of head of femur**

8,10   ✓7ᵗʰ   **S72.061   Displaced articular fracture** MCC CC H5 HCC **of head of right femur**

8,10   ✓7ᵗʰ   **S72.062   Displaced articular fracture** MCC CC H5 HCC **of head of left femur**

8,10   ✓7ᵗʰ   **S72.063   Displaced articular** MCC CC H5 HCC **fracture of head of unspecified femur**

8,10   ✓7ᵗʰ   **S72.064   Nondisplaced articular** MCC CC H5 HCC **fracture of head of right femur**

8,10   ✓7ᵗʰ   **S72.065   Nondisplaced articular** MCC CC H5 HCC **fracture of head of left femur**

8,10   ✓7ᵗʰ   **S72.066   Nondisplaced articular** MCC CC H5 HCC **fracture of head of unspecified femur**

---

**8**   CC when reported as a subsequent encounter for nonunion or malunion (7th character K, M, N, P, Q, or R).
**10**   HCC with 7th character indicating initial encounter (A, B or C - specific to category).

---

✓Additional Character Req   ✓x7ᵗʰ Placeholder Alert   Unacceptable PDx   Manifestation   H1 - H14 HAC   HCC CMS-HCC Condition   EXCLUDES 1 Not Coded Here   EXCLUDES 2 Not Included Here

✓6th **S72.09**   Other fracture of head and neck of femur

   8,10   ✓7th **S72.091**   Other fracture of head and neck of right femur   `MCC` `CC` `H5` `HCC`

   8,10   ✓7th **S72.092**   Other fracture of head and neck of left femur   `MCC` `CC` `H5` `HCC`

   8,10   ✓7th **S72.099**   Other fracture of head and neck of unspecified femur   `MCC` `CC` `H5` `HCC`

✓5th **S72.1**   Pertrochanteric **fracture**
     **AHA:** 2016, 3Q, 16

> **CC Excl: For CC/MCC codes in subcategory S72.1:**
> **Right side:** See code S72.001
> **Left side:** See code S72.002
> **Unspecified side:** See code S72.009

✓6th **S72.10**   Unspecified trochanteric **fracture of femur**
     Fracture of trochanter NOS

   8,10   ✓7th **S72.101**   Unspecified trochanteric fracture of right femur   `MCC` `CC` `H5` `HCC`

   8,10   ✓7th **S72.102**   Unspecified trochanteric fracture of left femur   `MCC` `CC` `H5` `HCC`

   8,10   ✓7th **S72.109**   Unspecified trochanteric fracture of unspecified femur   `MCC` `CC` `H5` `HCC`

✓6th **S72.11**   Fracture of greater trochanter of femur

   8,10   ✓7th **S72.111**   Displaced fracture of greater trochanter of right femur   `MCC` `CC` `H5` `HCC`

   8,10   ✓7th **S72.112**   Displaced fracture of greater trochanter of left femur   `MCC` `CC` `H5` `HCC`

   8,10   ✓7th **S72.113**   Displaced fracture of greatertrochanter of unspecified femur   `MCC` `CC` `H5` `HCC`

   8,10   ✓7th **S72.114**   Nondisplaced fracture of greater trochanter of right femur   `MCC` `CC` `H5` `HCC`

   8,10   ✓7th **S72.115**   Nondisplaced fracture of greater trochanter of left femur   `MCC` `CC` `H5` `HCC`

   8,10   ✓7th **S72.116**   Nondisplaced fracture of greater trochanter of unspecified femur   `MCC` `CC` `H5` `HCC`

✓6th **S72.12**   Fracture of lesser trochanter of femur

   8,10   ✓7th **S72.121**   Displaced fracture of lesser trochanter of right femur   `MCC` `CC` `H5` `HCC`

   8,10   ✓7th **S72.122**   Displaced fracture of lesser trochanter of left femur   `MCC` `CC` `H5` `HCC`

   8,10   ✓7th **S72.123**   Displaced fracture of lesser trochanter of unspecified femur   `MCC` `CC` `H5` `HCC`

   8,10   ✓7th **S72.124**   Nondisplaced fracture of lesser trochanter of right femur   `MCC` `CC` `H5` `HCC`

   8,10   ✓7th **S72.125**   Nondisplaced fracture of lesser trochanter of left femur   `MCC` `CC` `H5` `HCC`

   8,10   ✓7th **S72.126**   Nondisplaced fracture of lesser trochanter of unspecified femur   `MCC` `CC` `H5` `HCC`

✓6th **S72.13**   Apophyseal **fracture of femur**
     `EXCLUDES 1`   *chronic (nontraumatic) slipped upper femoral epiphysis (M93.0-)*

   8,10   ✓7th **S72.131**   Displaced apophyseal fracture of right femur   `MCC` `CC` `H5` `HCC`

   8,10   ✓7th **S72.132**   Displaced apophyseal fracture of left femur   `MCC` `CC` `H5` `HCC`

   8,10   ✓7th **S72.133**   Displaced apophyseal fracture of unspecified femur   `MCC` `CC` `H5` `HCC`

   8,10   ✓7th **S72.134**   Nondisplaced apophyseal fracture of right femur   `MCC` `CC` `H5` `HCC`

   8,10   ✓7th **S72.135**   Nondisplaced apophyseal fractureof left femur   `MCC` `CC` `H5` `HCC`

   8,10   ✓7th **S72.136**   Nondisplaced apophyseal fracture of unspecified femur   `MCC` `CC` `H5` `HCC`

✓6th **S72.14**   Intertrochanteric fracture of femur

   8,10   ✓7th **S72.141**   Displaced intertrochanteric fracture of right femur   `MCC` `CC` `H5` `HCC`

   8,10   ✓7th **S72.142**   Displaced intertrochanteric fracture of left femur   `MCC` `CC` `H5` `HCC`

   8,10   ✓7th **S72.143**   Displaced intertrochanteric fracture of unspecified femur   `MCC` `CC` `H5` `HCC`

   8,10   ✓7th **S72.144**   Nondisplaced intertrochanteric fracture of right femur   `MCC` `CC` `H5` `HCC`

   8,10   ✓7th **S72.145**   Nondisplaced intertrochanteric fracture of left femur   `MCC` `CC` `H5` `HCC`

   8,10   ✓7th **S72.146**   Nondisplaced intertrochanteric fracture of unspecified femur   `MCC` `CC` `H5` `HCC`

✓5th **S72.2**   Subtrochanteric **fracture of femur**

> **CC Excl: For CC/MCC codes in subcategory S72.2:**
> **Right side:** See code S72.009
> **Left side:** See code S72.009
> **Unspecified side:** See code S72.009

   8,10   ✓x7th **S72.21**   Displaced subtrochanteric fracture of right femur   `MCC` `CC` `H5` `HCC`

   8,10   ✓x7th **S72.22**   Displaced subtrochanteric fracture of left femur   `MCC` `CC` `H5` `HCC`

   8,10   ✓x7th **S72.23**   Displaced subtrochanteric fracture of unspecified femur   `MCC` `CC` `H5` `HCC`

   8,10   ✓x7th **S72.24**   Nondisplaced subtrochanteric fracture of right femur   `MCC` `CC` `H5` `HCC`

   8,10   ✓x7th **S72.25**   Nondisplaced subtrochanteric fracture of left femur   `MCC` `CC` `H5` `HCC`

   8,10   ✓x7th **S72.26**   Nondisplaced subtrochanteric fracture of unspecified femur   `MCC` `CC` `H5` `HCC`

✓5th **S72.3**   Fracture of shaft of femur

> **CC Excl: For CC/MCC codes in subcategory S72.3:**
> **Right side:** See code S72.001
> **Left side:** See code S72.002
> **Unspecified side:** See code S72.009

✓6th **S72.30**   Unspecified fracture of shaft of femur

   8,10   ✓7th **S72.301**   Unspecified fracture of shaft of right femur   `MCC` `CC` `H5` `HCC`

   8,10   ✓7th **S72.302**   Unspecified fracture of shaft of left femur   `MCC` `CC` `H5` `HCC`

   8,10   ✓7th **S72.309**   Unspecified fracture of shaft of unspecified femur   `MCC` `CC` `H5` `HCC`

✓6th **S72.32**   Transverse fracture of shaft of femur

   8,10   ✓7th **S72.321**   Displaced transverse fracture of shaft of right femur   `MCC` `CC` `H5` `HCC`

   8,10   ✓7th **S72.322**   Displaced transverse fracture of shaft of left femur   `MCC` `CC` `H5` `HCC`

   8,10   ✓7th **S72.323**   Displaced transverse fracture of shaft of unspecified femur   `MCC` `CC` `H5` `HCC`

   8,10   ✓7th **S72.324**   Nondisplaced transverse fracture of shaft of right femur   `MCC` `CC` `H5` `HCC`

   8,10   ✓7th **S72.325**   Nondisplaced transverse fracture of shaft of left femur   `MCC` `CC` `H5` `HCC`

   8,10   ✓7th **S72.326**   Nondisplaced transverse fracture of shaft of unspecified femur   `MCC` `CC` `H5` `HCC`

✓6th **S72.33**   Oblique fracture of shaft of femur

   8,10   ✓7th **S72.331**   Displaced oblique fracture of shaft of right femur   `MCC` `CC` `H5` `HCC`

   8,10   ✓7th **S72.332**   Displaced oblique fracture of shaft of left femur   `MCC` `CC` `H5` `HCC`

   8,10   ✓7th **S72.333**   Displaced oblique fracture of shaft of unspecified femur   `MCC` `CC` `H5` `HCC`

   8,10   ✓7th **S72.334**   Nondisplaced oblique fracture of shaft of right femur   `MCC` `CC` `H5` `HCC`

   8,10   ✓7th **S72.335**   Nondisplaced oblique fracture of shaft of left femur   `MCC` `CC` `H5` `HCC`

   8,10   ✓7th **S72.336**   Nondisplaced oblique fracture of shaft of unspecified femur   `MCC` `CC` `H5` `HCC`

✓6th **S72.34**   Spiral fracture of shaft of femur

   8,10   ✓7th **S72.341**   Displaced spiral fracture of shaft of right femur   `MCC` `CC` `H5` `HCC`

   8,10   ✓7th **S72.342**   Displaced spiral fracture of shaft of left femur   `MCC` `CC` `H5` `HCC`

   8,10   ✓7th **S72.343**   Displaced spiral fracture of shaft of unspecified femur   `MCC` `CC` `H5` `HCC`

   8,10   ✓7th **S72.344**   Nondisplaced spiral fracture of shaft of right femur   `MCC` `CC` `H5` `HCC`

---

8   CC when reported as a subsequent encounter for nonunion or malunion (7th character K, M, N, P, Q, or R).

10   HCC with 7th character indicating initial encounter (A, B or C - specific to category).

N Newborn: 0   P Pediatric: 0-17   M Maternity: 12-55   A Adult: 15-124   `MCC` Major CC Condition   `PDxMCC` PDx acts as own MCC   `CC` CC Condition   `PDxCC` PDx acts as own CC

**1040**          ICD-10-CM 2018

8,10 ✓7ᵗʰ **S72.345** Nondisplaced spiral fracture of shaft of **left femur** `MCC` `CC` `H5` `HCC`

8,10 ✓7ᵗʰ **S72.346** Nondisplaced spiral fracture of shaft of **unspecified femur** `MCC` `CC` `H5` `HCC`

✓6ᵗʰ **S72.35** Comminuted fracture of shaft of femur

8,10 ✓7ᵗʰ **S72.351** Displaced comminuted fracture of shaft of **right femur** `MCC` `CC` `H5` `HCC`

8,10 ✓7ᵗʰ **S72.352** Displaced comminuted fracture of shaft of **left femur** `MCC` `CC` `H5` `HCC`

8,10 ✓7ᵗʰ **S72.353** Displaced comminuted fracture of shaft of **unspecified femur** `MCC` `CC` `H5` `HCC`

8,10 ✓7ᵗʰ **S72.354** Nondisplaced comminuted fracture of shaft of **right femur** `MCC` `CC` `H5` `HCC`

8,10 ✓7ᵗʰ **S72.355** Nondisplaced comminuted fracture of shaft of **left femur** `MCC` `CC` `H5` `HCC`

8,10 ✓7ᵗʰ **S72.356** Nondisplaced comminuted fracture of shaft of **unspecified femur** `MCC` `CC` `H5` `HCC`

✓6ᵗʰ **S72.36** Segmental fracture of shaft of femur

8,10 ✓7ᵗʰ **S72.361** Displaced segmental fracture of shaft of **right femur** `MCC` `CC` `H5` `HCC`

8,10 ✓7ᵗʰ **S72.362** Displaced segmental fracture of shaft of **left femur** `MCC` `CC` `H5` `HCC`

8,10 ✓7ᵗʰ **S72.363** Displaced segmental fracture of shaft of **unspecified femur** `MCC` `CC` `H5` `HCC`

8,10 ✓7ᵗʰ **S72.364** Nondisplaced segmental fracture of shaft of **right femur** `MCC` `CC` `H5` `HCC`

8,10 ✓7ᵗʰ **S72.365** Nondisplaced segmental fracture of shaft of **left femur** `MCC` `CC` `H5` `HCC`

8,10 ✓7ᵗʰ **S72.366** Nondisplaced segmental fracture of shaft of **unspecified femur** `MCC` `CC` `H5` `HCC`

✓6ᵗʰ **S72.39** Other fracture of shaft of femur

8,10 ✓7ᵗʰ **S72.391** Other fracture of shaft of **right femur** `MCC` `CC` `H5` `HCC`

8,10 ✓7ᵗʰ **S72.392** Other fracture of shaft of **left femur** `MCC` `CC` `H5` `HCC`

8,10 ✓7ᵗʰ **S72.399** Other fracture of shaft of **unspecified femur** `MCC` `CC` `H5` `HCC`

✓5ᵗʰ **S72.4** Fracture of lower end of femur
Fracture of distal end of femur
> **EXCLUDES 2**   fracture of shaft of femur (S72.3-)
>       physeal fracture of lower end of femur (S79.1-)

> **CC Excl: For CC/MCC codes in subcategory S72.4, unless otherwise noted:**
> **Right side:** See code S72.401
> **Left side:** See code S72.402
> **Unspecified side:** See code S72.409

✓6ᵗʰ **S72.40** Unspecified fracture of lower end of femur

6,7,10 ✓7ᵗʰ **S72.401** Unspecified fracture of lower end of **right femur** `MCC` `CC` `H5` `HCC`
> **CC Excl: MCC with 7th character A:**
> PDX collection 1300
> **MCC with 7th character B or C:**
> PDX collection 1301
> **CC with 7th character K, M, N, P, Q or R:**
> PDX collection 897

6,7,10 ✓7ᵗʰ **S72.402** Unspecified fracture of lower end of **left femur** `MCC` `CC` `H5` `HCC`
> **CC Excl: MCC with 7th character A:**
> PDX collection 1302
> **MCC with 7th character B or C:**
> PDX collection 1301
> **CC with 7th character K, M, N, P, Q or R:**
> PDX collection 897

6,7,10 ✓7ᵗʰ **S72.409** Unspecified fracture of lower end of **unspecified femur** `MCC` `CC` `H5` `HCC`
> **CC Excl: MCC with 7th character A, B or C:**
> PDX collection 1301
> **CC with 7th character K, M, N, P, Q or R:**
> PDX collection 897

✓6ᵗʰ **S72.41** Unspecified condyle fracture of lower end of femur
Condyle fracture of femur NOS

6,7,10 ✓7ᵗʰ **S72.411** Displaced unspecified condyle fracture of lower end of **right femur** `MCC` `CC` `H5` `HCC`

6,7,10 ✓7ᵗʰ **S72.412** Displaced unspecified condyle fracture of lower end of **left femur** `MCC` `CC` `H5` `HCC`

6,7,10 ✓7ᵗʰ **S72.413** Displaced unspecified condyle fracture of lower end of **unspecified femur** `MCC` `CC` `H5` `HCC`

6,7,10 ✓7ᵗʰ **S72.414** Nondisplaced unspecified condyle fracture of lower end of **right femur** `MCC` `CC` `H5` `HCC`

6,7,10 ✓7ᵗʰ **S72.415** Nondisplaced unspecified condyle fracture of lower end of **left femur** `MCC` `CC` `H5` `HCC`

6,7,10 ✓7ᵗʰ **S72.416** Nondisplaced unspecified condyle fracture of lower end of **unspecified femur** `MCC` `CC` `H5` `HCC`

✓6ᵗʰ **S72.42** Fracture of lateral condyle of femur

6,7,10 ✓7ᵗʰ **S72.421** Displaced fracture of lateral condyle of **right femur** `MCC` `CC` `H5` `HCC`

6,7,10 ✓7ᵗʰ **S72.422** Displaced fracture of lateral condyle of **left femur** `MCC` `CC` `H5` `HCC`

6,7,10 ✓7ᵗʰ **S72.423** Displaced fracture of lateral condyle of **unspecified femur** `MCC` `CC` `H5` `HCC`

6,7,10 ✓7ᵗʰ **S72.424** Nondisplaced fracture of lateral condyle of **right femur** `MCC` `CC` `H5` `HCC`

6,7,10 ✓7ᵗʰ **S72.425** Nondisplaced fracture of lateral condyle of **left femur** `MCC` `CC` `H5` `HCC`

6,7,10 ✓7ᵗʰ **S72.426** Nondisplaced fracture of lateral condyle of **unspecified femur** `MCC` `CC` `H5` `HCC`

✓6ᵗʰ **S72.43** Fracture of medial condyle of femur

6,7,10 ✓7ᵗʰ **S72.431** Displaced fracture of medial condyle of **right femur** `MCC` `CC` `H5` `HCC`

6,7,10 ✓7ᵗʰ **S72.432** Displaced fracture of medial condyle of **left femur** `MCC` `CC` `H5` `HCC`

6,7,10 ✓7ᵗʰ **S72.433** Displaced fracture of medial condyle of **unspecified femur** `MCC` `CC` `H5` `HCC`

6,7,10 ✓7ᵗʰ **S72.434** Nondisplaced fracture of medial condyle of **right femur** `MCC` `CC` `H5` `HCC`

6,7,10 ✓7ᵗʰ **S72.435** Nondisplaced fracture of medial condyle of **left femur** `MCC` `CC` `H5` `HCC`

6,7,10 ✓7ᵗʰ **S72.436** Nondisplaced fracture of medial condyle of **unspecified femur** `MCC` `CC` `H5` `HCC`

✓6ᵗʰ **S72.44** Fracture of lower epiphysis (separation) of femur
> **EXCLUDES 1**   Salter-Harris Type I physeal fracture of lower end of femur (S79.11-)

6,7,10 ✓7ᵗʰ **S72.441** Displaced fracture of lower epiphysis (separation) of **right femur** `MCC` `CC` `H5` `HCC`

6,7,10 ✓7ᵗʰ **S72.442** Displaced fracture of lower epiphysis (separation) of **left femur** `MCC` `CC` `H5` `HCC`

6,7,10 ✓7ᵗʰ **S72.443** Displaced fracture of lower epiphysis (separation) of **unspecified femur** `MCC` `CC` `H5` `HCC`

6,7,10 ✓7ᵗʰ **S72.444** Nondisplaced fracture of lower epiphysis (separation) of **right femur** `MCC` `CC` `H5` `HCC`

6,7,10 ✓7ᵗʰ **S72.445** Nondisplaced fracture of lower epiphysis (separation) of **left femur** `MCC` `CC` `H5` `HCC`

6,7,10 ✓7ᵗʰ **S72.446** Nondisplaced fracture of lower epiphysis (separation) of **unspecified femur** `MCC` `CC` `H5` `HCC`

---

**6**   MCC when reported as an open fracture (7th character B or C).

**7**   CC when reported as an initial encounter (7th character A, B, or C – specific to category) OR a subsequent encounter for nonunion or malunion (7th character K, M, N, P, Q, or R – specific to category).

**8**   CC when reported as a subsequent encounter for nonunion or malunion (7th character K, M, N, P, Q, or R).

**10**   HCC with 7th character indicating initial encounter (A, B or C - specific to category).

---

✓ Additional Character Req    ✓x7ᵗʰ Placeholder Alert    Unacceptable PDx    Manifestation    `H1`-`H14` HAC    `HCC` CMS-HCC Condition    **EXCLUDES 1** Not Coded Here    **EXCLUDES 2** Not Included Here

✓6ᵗʰ **S72.45  Supracondylar fracture without intracondylar extension of lower end of femur**
Supracondylar fracture of lower end of femur NOS
**EXCLUDES 1**  *supracondylar fracture with intracondylar extension of lower end of femur (S72.46-)*

6,7,10  ✓7ᵗʰ **S72.451  Displaced supracondylar**  MCC CC H5 HCC
**fracture without intracondylar extension of lower end of right femur**

6,7,10  ✓7ᵗʰ **S72.452  Displaced supracondylar**  MCC CC H5 HCC
**fracture without intracondylar extension of lower end of left femur**

6,7,10  ✓7ᵗʰ **S72.453  Displaced supracondylar**  MCC CC H5 HCC
**fracture without intracondylar extension of lower end of unspecified femur**

6,7,10  ✓7ᵗʰ **S72.454  Nondisplaced**  MCC CC H5 HCC
**supracondylar fracture without intracondylar extension of lower end of right femur**

6,7,10  ✓7ᵗʰ **S72.455  Nondisplaced**  MCC CC H5 HCC
**supracondylar fracture without intracondylar extension of lower end of left femur**

6,7,10  ✓7ᵗʰ **S72.456  Nondisplaced**  MCC CC H5 HCC
**supracondylar fracture without intracondylar extension of lower end of unspecified femur**

✓6ᵗʰ **S72.46  Supracondylar fracture with intracondylar extension of lower end of femur**
**EXCLUDES 1**  *supracondylar fracture without intracondylar extension of lower end of femur (S72.45-)*

6,7,10  ✓7ᵗʰ **S72.461  Displaced supracondylar**  MCC CC H5 HCC
**fracture with intracondylar extension of lower end of right femur**

6,7,10  ✓7ᵗʰ **S72.462  Displaced supracondylar**  MCC CC H5 HCC
**fracture with intracondylar extension of lower end of left femur**

6,7,10  ✓7ᵗʰ **S72.463  Displaced supracondylar**  MCC CC H5 HCC
**fracture with intracondylar extension of lower end of unspecified femur**

6,7,10  ✓7ᵗʰ **S72.464  Nondisplaced**  MCC CC H5 HCC
**supracondylar fracture with intracondylar extension of lower end of right femur**

6,7,10  ✓7ᵗʰ **S72.465  Nondisplaced**  MCC CC H5 HCC
**supracondylar fracture with intracondylar extension of lower end of left femur**

6,7,10  ✓7ᵗʰ **S72.466  Nondisplaced**  MCC CC H5 HCC
**supracondylar fracture with intracondylar extension of lower end of unspecified femur**

✓6ᵗʰ **S72.47  Torus fracture of lower end of femur**

The appropriate 7th character is to be added to all codes in subcategory S72.47.
A    initial encounter for closed fracture
D    subsequent encounter for fracture with routine healing
G    subsequent encounter for fracture with delayed healing
K    subsequent encounter for fracture with nonunion
P    subsequent encounter for fracture with malunion
S    sequela

7,10  ✓7ᵗʰ **S72.471  Torus fracture of lower end of**  CC H5 HCC
**right femur**
**CC Excl: CC with 7th character A:**
PDX collection 1300
**CC Excl: CC with 7th character K or P:**
PDX collection 897

7,10  ✓7ᵗʰ **S72.472  Torus fracture of lower end of**  CC H5 HCC
**left femur**
**CC Excl: CC with 7th character A:**
PDX collection 1302
**CC Excl: CC with 7th character K or P:**
PDX collection 897

7,10  ✓7ᵗʰ **S72.479  Torus fracture of lower end of**  CC H5 HCC
**unspecified femur**
**CC Excl: CC with 7th character A:**
PDX collection 1301
**CC Excl: CC with 7th character K or P:**
PDX collection 897

✓6ᵗʰ **S72.49  Other fracture of lower end of femur**

6,7,10  ✓7ᵗʰ **S72.491  Other fracture of lower end**  MCC CC H5 HCC
**of right femur**
**CC Excl: MCC with 7th character A:**
PDX collection 1300
**MCC with 7th character B or C:**
PDX collection 1303
**CC with 7th character K, M, N, P, Q or R:**
PDX collection 897

6,7,10  ✓7ᵗʰ **S72.492  Other fracture of lower end**  MCC CC H5 HCC
**of left femur**
**CC Excl: MCC with 7th character A:**
PDX collection 1302
**MCC with 7th character B or C:**
PDX collection 1303
**CC with 7th character K, M, N, P, Q or R:**
PDX collection 897

6,7,10  ✓7ᵗʰ **S72.499  Other fracture of lower end**  MCC CC H5 HCC
**of unspecified femur**
**CC Excl: MCC with 7th character A:**
PDX collection 1301
**MCC with 7th character B or C:**
PDX collection 1303
**CC with 7th character K, M, N, P, Q or R:**
PDX collection 897

✓5ᵗʰ **S72.8  Other fracture of femur**

✓6ᵗʰ **S72.8X  Other fracture of femur**

**CC Excl: For codes in subcategory S72.8X:**
**MCC with 7th character A, B or C:**
PDX collection 1298
**CC with 7th character K, M, N, P, Q or R:**
PDX collection 897

8,10  ✓7ᵗʰ **S72.8X1  Other fracture of right**  MCC CC H5 HCC
**femur**

8,10  ✓7ᵗʰ **S72.8X2  Other fracture of left femur**  MCC CC H5 HCC

8,10  ✓7ᵗʰ **S72.8X9  Other fracture of**  MCC CC H5 HCC
**unspecified femur**

✓5ᵗʰ **S72.9  Unspecified fracture of femur**
Fracture of thigh NOS
Fracture of upper leg NOS
**EXCLUDES 1**  *fracture of hip NOS (S72.00-, S72.01-)*

**CC Excl: For codes in subcategory S72.9:**
**MCC with 7th character A, B or C:**
PDX collection 1298
**CC with 7th character K, M, N, P, Q or R:**
PDX collection 897

8,10  ✓x7ᵗʰ **S72.90  Unspecified fracture of unspecified**  MCC CC H5 HCC
**femur**
**AHA:** 2012, 4Q, 93

8,10  ✓x7ᵗʰ **S72.91  Unspecified fracture of right femur**  MCC CC H5 HCC

8,10  ✓x7ᵗʰ **S72.92  Unspecified fracture of left femur**  MCC CC H5 HCC

---

6    MCC when reported as an open fracture (7th character B or C).
7    CC when reported as an initial encounter (7th character A, B, or C – specific to category) OR a subsequent encounter for nonunion or malunion (7th character K, M, N, P, Q, or R – specific to category).
8    CC when reported as a subsequent encounter for nonunion or malunion (7th character K, M, N, P, Q, or R).
10   HCC with 7th character indicating initial encounter (A, B or C - specific to category).

✓4ᵗʰ **S73**   **Dislocation and sprain of joint and ligaments of hip**
INCLUDES   avulsion of joint or ligament of hip
     laceration of cartilage, joint or ligament of hip
     sprain of cartilage, joint or ligament of hip
     traumatic hemarthrosis of joint or ligament of hip
     traumatic rupture of joint or ligament of hip
     traumatic subluxation of joint or ligament of hip
     traumatic tear of joint or ligament of hip
Code also any associated open wound
EXCLUDES 2   *strain of muscle, fascia and tendon of hip and thigh (S76.-)*

The appropriate 7th character is to be added to each code from category S73.
A    initial encounter
D    subsequent encounter
S    sequela

✓5ᵗʰ **S73.0**   **Subluxation and dislocation of** hip
   EXCLUDES 2   *dislocation and subluxation of hip prosthesis (T84.020, T84.021)*

   ✓6ᵗʰ **S73.00**   **Unspecified subluxation and dislocation of hip**
     Dislocation of hip NOS
     Subluxation of hip NOS
     10 ✓7ᵗʰ **S73.001**   **Unspecified subluxation of right hip**   CC H5 HCC
      CC Excl: CC with 7th character A:
      PDX collection 1304
     10 ✓7ᵗʰ **S73.002**   **Unspecified subluxation of left hip**   CC H5 HCC
      CC Excl: CC with 7th character A:
      PDX collection 1305
     10 ✓7ᵗʰ **S73.003**   **Unspecified subluxation of unspecified hip**   CC H5 HCC
      CC Excl: CC with 7th character A:
      PDX collection 1306
     10 ✓7ᵗʰ **S73.004**   **Unspecified dislocation of right hip**   CC H5 HCC
      CC Excl: CC with 7th character A:
      PDX collection 1304
     10 ✓7ᵗʰ **S73.005**   **Unspecified dislocation of left hip**   CC H5 HCC
      CC Excl: CC with 7th character A:
      PDX collection 1305
     10 ✓7ᵗʰ **S73.006**   **Unspecified dislocation of unspecified hip**   CC H5 HCC
      CC Excl: CC with 7th character A:
      PDX collection 1306

   ✓6ᵗʰ **S73.01**   **Posterior subluxation and dislocation of hip**
     10 ✓7ᵗʰ **S73.011**   **Posterior subluxation of right hip**   CC H5 HCC
      CC Excl: CC with 7th character A:
      PDX collection 1307
     10 ✓7ᵗʰ **S73.012**   **Posterior subluxation of left hip** CC H5 HCC
      CC Excl: CC with 7th character A:
      PDX collection 1308
     10 ✓7ᵗʰ **S73.013**   **Posterior subluxation of unspecified hip**   CC H5 HCC
      CC Excl: CC with 7th character A:
      PDX collection 1309
     10 ✓7ᵗʰ **S73.014**   **Posterior dislocation of right hip** CC H5 HCC
      CC Excl: CC with 7th character A:
      PDX collection 1307
     10 ✓7ᵗʰ **S73.015**   **Posterior dislocation of left hip**   CC H5 HCC
      CC Excl: CC with 7th character A:
      PDX collection 1308
     10 ✓7ᵗʰ **S73.016**   **Posterior dislocation of unspecified hip**   CC H5 HCC
      CC Excl: CC with 7th character A:
      PDX collection 1309

   ✓6ᵗʰ **S73.02**   **Obturator subluxation and dislocation of hip**
     10 ✓7ᵗʰ **S73.021**   **Obturator subluxation of right hip**   CC H5 HCC
      CC Excl: CC with 7th character A:
      PDX collection 1310
     10 ✓7ᵗʰ **S73.022**   **Obturator subluxation of left hip**   CC H5 HCC
      CC Excl: CC with 7th character A:
      PDX collection 1311
     10 ✓7ᵗʰ **S73.023**   **Obturator subluxation of unspecified hip**   CC H5 HCC
      CC Excl: CC with 7th character A:
      PDX collection 1312

     10 ✓7ᵗʰ **S73.024**   **Obturator dislocation of right hip**   CC H5 HCC
      CC Excl: CC with 7th character A:
      PDX collection 1310
     10 ✓7ᵗʰ **S73.025**   **Obturator dislocation of left hip** CC H5 HCC
      CC Excl: CC with 7th character A:
      PDX collection 1311
     10 ✓7ᵗʰ **S73.026**   **Obturator dislocation of unspecified hip**   CC H5 HCC
      CC Excl: CC with 7th character A:
      PDX collection 1312

   ▲ ✓6ᵗʰ **S73.03**   **Other anterior subluxation and dislocation of hip**
     10 ✓7ᵗʰ **S73.031**   **Other anterior subluxation of right hip**   CC H5 HCC
      CC Excl: CC with 7th character A:
      PDX collection 1313
     10 ✓7ᵗʰ **S73.032**   **Other anterior subluxation of left hip**   CC H5 HCC
      CC Excl: CC with 7th character A:
      PDX collection 1314
     10 ✓7ᵗʰ **S73.033**   **Other anterior subluxation of unspecified hip**   CC H5 HCC
      CC Excl: CC with 7th character A:
      PDX collection 1315
     10 ✓7ᵗʰ **S73.034**   **Other anterior dislocation of right hip**   CC H5 HCC
      CC Excl: CC with 7th character A:
      PDX collection 1313
     10 ✓7ᵗʰ **S73.035**   **Other anterior dislocation of left hip**   CC H5 HCC
      CC Excl: CC with 7th character A:
      PDX collection 1314
     10 ✓7ᵗʰ **S73.036**   **Other anterior dislocation of unspecified hip**   CC H5 HCC
      CC Excl: CC with 7th character A:
      PDX collection 1315

   ▲ ✓6ᵗʰ **S73.04**   **Central subluxation and dislocation of hip**
     10 ✓7ᵗʰ **S73.041**   **Central subluxation of right hip** CC H5 HCC
      CC Excl: CC with 7th character A:
      PDX collection 1304
     10 ✓7ᵗʰ **S73.042**   **Central subluxation of left hip** CC H5 HCC
      CC Excl: CC with 7th character A:
      PDX collection 1305
     10 ✓7ᵗʰ **S73.043**   **Central subluxation of unspecified hip**   CC H5 HCC
      CC Excl: CC with 7th character A:
      PDX collection 1306
     10 ✓7ᵗʰ **S73.044**   **Central dislocation of right hip**   CC H5 HCC
      CC Excl: CC with 7th character A:
      PDX collection 1304
     10 ✓7ᵗʰ **S73.045**   **Central dislocation of left hip**   CC H5 HCC
      CC Excl: CC with 7th character A:
      PDX collection 1305
     10 ✓7ᵗʰ **S73.046**   **Central dislocation of unspecified hip**   CC H5 HCC
      CC Excl: CC with 7th character A:
      PDX collection 1306

✓5ᵗʰ **S73.1**   **Sprain of hip**
   **AHA:** 2014, 4Q, 25
   ✓6ᵗʰ **S73.10**   **Unspecified sprain of hip**
     ✓7ᵗʰ **S73.101**   **Unspecified sprain of right hip**
     ✓7ᵗʰ **S73.102**   **Unspecified sprain of left hip**
     ✓7ᵗʰ **S73.109**   **Unspecified sprain of unspecified hip**
   ✓6ᵗʰ **S73.11**   **Iliofemoral ligament sprain of hip**
     ✓7ᵗʰ **S73.111**   **Iliofemoral ligament sprain of right hip**
     ✓7ᵗʰ **S73.112**   **Iliofemoral ligament sprain of left hip**
     ✓7ᵗʰ **S73.119**   **Iliofemoral ligament sprain of unspecified hip**
   ✓6ᵗʰ **S73.12**   **Ischiocapsular (ligament) sprain of hip**
     ✓7ᵗʰ **S73.121**   **Ischiocapsular ligament sprain of right hip**
     ✓7ᵗʰ **S73.122**   **Ischiocapsular ligament sprain of left hip**
     ✓7ᵗʰ **S73.129**   **Ischiocapsular ligament sprain of unspecified hip**
   ✓6ᵗʰ **S73.19**   **Other sprain of hip**
     ✓7ᵗʰ **S73.191**   **Other sprain of right hip**
     ✓7ᵗʰ **S73.192**   **Other sprain of left hip**
     ✓7ᵗʰ **S73.199**   **Other sprain of unspecified hip**

---

10 HCC with 7th character indicating initial encounter (A, B or C - specific to category).

✓ Additional Character Req    ✓x7ᵗʰ Placeholder Alert    Unacceptable PDx    Manifestation    H1-H14 HAC    HCC CMS-HCC Condition    EXCLUDES 1 Not Coded Here    EXCLUDES 2 Not Included Here

✓4ᵗʰ **S74** **Injury of nerves at hip and thigh level**
Code also any associated open wound (S71.-)
*EXCLUDES 2*   *injury of nerves at ankle and foot level (S94.-)*
*injury of nerves at lower leg level (S84.-)*

The appropriate 7th character is to be added to each code from category S74.
A   initial encounter
D   subsequent encounter
S   sequela

✓5ᵗʰ **S74.0** **Injury of sciatic nerve at hip and thigh level**

✓x7ᵗʰ **S74.00** **Injury of sciatic nerve at hip and thigh level, unspecified leg**

✓x7ᵗʰ **S74.01** **Injury of sciatic nerve at hip and thigh level, right leg**

✓x7ᵗʰ **S74.02** **Injury of sciatic nerve at hip and thigh level, left leg**

✓5ᵗʰ **S74.1** **Injury of femoral nerve at hip and thigh level**

✓x7ᵗʰ **S74.10** **Injury of femoral nerve at hip and thigh level, unspecified leg**

✓x7ᵗʰ **S74.11** **Injury of femoral nerve at hip and thigh level, right leg**

✓x7ᵗʰ **S74.12** **Injury of femoral nerve at hip and thigh level, left leg**

✓5ᵗʰ **S74.2** **Injury of cutaneous sensory nerve at hip and thigh level**

✓x7ᵗʰ **S74.20** **Injury of cutaneous sensory nerve at hip and thigh level, unspecified leg**

✓x7ᵗʰ **S74.21** **Injury of cutaneous sensory nerve at hip and high level, right leg**

✓x7ᵗʰ **S74.22** **Injury of cutaneous sensory nerve at hip and thigh level, left leg**

✓5ᵗʰ **S74.8** **Injury of other nerves at hip and thigh level**

✓6ᵗʰ **S74.8X** **Injury of other nerves at hip and thigh level**

✓7ᵗʰ **S74.8X1** **Injury of other nerves at hip and thigh level, right leg**

✓7ᵗʰ **S74.8X2** **Injury of other nerves at hip and thigh level, left leg**

✓7ᵗʰ **S74.8X9** **Injury of other nerves at hip and thigh level, unspecified leg**

✓5ᵗʰ **S74.9** **Injury of unspecified nerve at hip and thigh level**

✓x7ᵗʰ **S74.90** **Injury of unspecified nerve at hip and thigh level, unspecified leg**

✓x7ᵗʰ **S74.91** **Injury of unspecified nerve at hip and thigh level, right leg**

✓x7ᵗʰ **S74.92** **Injury of unspecified nerve at hip and thigh level, left leg**

✓4ᵗʰ **S75** **Injury of blood vessels at hip and thigh level**
Code also any associated open wound (S71.-)
*EXCLUDES 2*   *injury of blood vessels at lower leg level (S85.-)*
*injury of popliteal artery (S85.0)*

The appropriate 7th character is to be added to each code from category S75.
A   initial encounter
D   subsequent encounter
S   sequela

✓5ᵗʰ **S75.0** **Injury of femoral artery**

**CC Excl: For CC codes in subcategory S75.0:**
**Right side:** PDX collection 1316
**Left side:** PDX collection 1317
**Unspecified side:** PDX collection 1318

✓6ᵗʰ **S75.00** **Unspecified injury of femoral artery**

✓7ᵗʰ **S75.001** **Unspecified injury of femoral artery, right leg**   MCC

✓7ᵗʰ **S75.002** **Unspecified injury of femoral artery, left leg**   MCC

✓7ᵗʰ **S75.009** **Unspecified injury of femoral artery, unspecified leg**   MCC

✓6ᵗʰ **S75.01** **Minor laceration of femoral artery**
Incomplete transection of femoral artery
Laceration of femoral artery NOS
Superficial laceration of femoral artery

✓7ᵗʰ **S75.011** **Minor laceration of femoral artery, right leg**   MCC

✓7ᵗʰ **S75.012** **Minor laceration of femoral artery, left leg**   MCC

✓7ᵗʰ **S75.019** **Minor laceration of femoral artery, unspecified leg**   MCC

✓6ᵗʰ **S75.02** **Major laceration of femoral artery**
Complete transection of femoral artery
Traumatic rupture of femoral artery

✓7ᵗʰ **S75.021** **Major laceration of femoral artery, right leg**   MCC

✓7ᵗʰ **S75.022** **Major laceration of femoral artery, left leg**   MCC

✓7ᵗʰ **S75.029** **Major laceration of femoral artery, unspecified leg**   MCC

✓6ᵗʰ **S75.09** **Other specified injury of femoral artery**

✓7ᵗʰ **S75.091** **Other specified injury of femoral artery, right leg**   MCC

✓7ᵗʰ **S75.092** **Other specified injury of femoral artery, left leg**   MCC

✓7ᵗʰ **S75.099** **Other specified injury of femoral artery, unspecified leg**   MCC

✓5ᵗʰ **S75.1** **Injury of femoral vein at hip and thigh level**

**CC Excl: For CC codes in subcategory S75.1:**
**Right side:** PDX collection 1319
**Left side:** PDX collection 1320
**Unspecified side:** PDX collection 1321

✓6ᵗʰ **S75.10** **Unspecified injury of femoral vein at hip and thigh level**

✓7ᵗʰ **S75.101** **Unspecified injury of femoral vein at hip and thigh level, right leg**   MCC

✓7ᵗʰ **S75.102** **Unspecified injury of femoral vein at hip and thigh level, left leg**   MCC

✓7ᵗʰ **S75.109** **Unspecified injury of femoral vein at hip and thigh level, unspecified leg**   MCC

✓6ᵗʰ **S75.11** **Minor laceration of femoral vein at hip and thigh level**
Incomplete transection of femoral vein at hip and thigh level
Laceration of femoral vein at hip and thigh level NOS
Superficial laceration of femoral vein at hip and thigh level

✓7ᵗʰ **S75.111** **Minor laceration of femoral vein at hip and thigh level, right leg**   MCC

✓7ᵗʰ **S75.112** **Minor laceration of femoral vein at hip and thigh level, left leg**   MCC

✓7ᵗʰ **S75.119** **Minor laceration of femoral vein at hip and thigh level, unspecified leg**   MCC

✓6ᵗʰ **S75.12** **Major laceration of femoral vein at hip and thigh level**
Complete transection of femoral vein at hip and thigh level
Traumatic rupture of femoral vein at hip and thigh level

✓7ᵗʰ **S75.121** **Major laceration of femoral vein at hip and thigh level, right leg**   MCC

✓7ᵗʰ **S75.122** **Major laceration of femoral vein at hip and thigh level, left leg**   MCC

✓7ᵗʰ **S75.129** **Major laceration of femoral vein at hip and thigh level, unspecified leg**   MCC

✓6ᵗʰ **S75.19** **Other specified injury of femoral vein at hip and thigh level**

✓7ᵗʰ **S75.191** **Other specified injury of femoral vein at hip and thigh level, right leg**   MCC

✓7ᵗʰ **S75.192** **Other specified injury of femoral vein at hip and thigh level, left leg**   MCC

✓7ᵗʰ **S75.199** **Other specified injury of femoral vein at hip and thigh level, unspecified leg**   MCC

✓5ᵗʰ **S75.2** **Injury of greater saphenous vein at hip and thigh level**
*EXCLUDES 1*   *greater saphenous vein NOS (S85.3)*

**CC Excl: For CC codes in subcategory S75.2:**
**Right side:** PDX collection 1322
**Left side:** PDX collection 1323
**Unspecified side:** PDX collection 1324

✓6ᵗʰ **S75.20** **Unspecified injury of greater saphenous vein at hip and thigh level**

✓7ᵗʰ **S75.201** **Unspecified injury of greater saphenous vein at hip and thigh level, right leg**   CC

√7ᵗʰ **S75.202** **Unspecified injury of greater saphenous vein at hip and thigh level, left leg**   `CC`

√7ᵗʰ **S75.209** **Unspecified injury of greater saphenous vein at hip and thigh level, unspecified leg**   `CC`

√6ᵗʰ **S75.21** **Minor laceration of greater saphenous vein at hip and thigh level**
    Incomplete transection of greater saphenous vein at hip and thigh level
    Laceration of greater saphenous vein at hip and thigh level NOS
    Superficial laceration of greater saphenous vein at hip and thigh level

√7ᵗʰ **S75.211** **Minor laceration of greater saphenous vein at hip and thigh level, right leg**   `CC`

√7ᵗʰ **S75.212** **Minor laceration of greater saphenous vein at hip and thigh level, left leg**   `CC`

√7ᵗʰ **S75.219** **Minor laceration of greater saphenous vein at hip and thigh level, unspecified leg**   `CC`

√6ᵗʰ **S75.22** **Major laceration of greater saphenous vein at hip and thigh level**
    Complete transection of greater saphenous vein at hip and thigh level
    Traumatic rupture of greater saphenous vein at hip and thigh level

√7ᵗʰ **S75.221** **Major laceration of greater saphenous vein at hip and thigh level, right leg**   `CC`

√7ᵗʰ **S75.222** **Major laceration of greater saphenous vein at hip and thigh level, left leg**   `CC`

√7ᵗʰ **S75.229** **Major laceration of greater saphenous vein at hip and thigh level, unspecified leg**   `CC`

√6ᵗʰ **S75.29** **Other specified injury of greater saphenous vein at hip and thigh level**

√7ᵗʰ **S75.291** **Other specified injury of greater saphenous vein at hip and thigh level, right leg**   `CC`

√7ᵗʰ **S75.292** **Other specified injury of greater saphenous vein at hip and thigh level, left leg**   `CC`

√7ᵗʰ **S75.299** **Other specified injury of greater saphenous vein at hip and thigh level, unspecified leg**   `CC`

√5ᵗʰ **S75.8** **Injury of other blood vessels at hip and thigh level**

> **CC Excl: For CC codes in subcategory S75.8:**
> **Right side:** PDX collection 1325
> **Left side:** PDX collection 1326
> **Unspecified side:** PDX collection 1327

√6ᵗʰ **S75.80** **Unspecified injury of other blood vessels at hip and thigh level**

√7ᵗʰ **S75.801** **Unspecified injury of other blood vessels at hip and thigh level, right leg**   `CC`

√7ᵗʰ **S75.802** **Unspecified injury of other blood vessels at hip and thigh level, left leg**   `CC`

√7ᵗʰ **S75.809** **Unspecified injury of other blood vessels at hip and thigh level, unspecified leg**   `CC`

√6ᵗʰ **S75.81** **Laceration of other blood vessels at hip and thigh level**

√7ᵗʰ **S75.811** **Laceration of other blood vessels at hip and thigh level, right leg**   `CC`

√7ᵗʰ **S75.812** **Laceration of other blood vessels at hip and thigh level, left leg**   `CC`

√7ᵗʰ **S75.819** **Laceration of other blood vessels' at hip and thigh level, unspecified leg**   `CC`

√6ᵗʰ **S75.89** **Other specified injury of other blood vessels at hip and thigh level**

√7ᵗʰ **S75.891** **Other specified injury of other blood vessels at hip and thigh level, right leg**   `CC`

√7ᵗʰ **S75.892** **Other specified injury of other blood vessels at hip and thigh level, left leg**   `CC`

√7ᵗʰ **S75.899** **Other specified injury of other blood vessels at hip and thigh level, unspecified leg**   `CC`

√5ᵗʰ **S75.9** **Injury of unspecified blood vessel at hip and thigh level**

> **CC Excl: For CC codes in subcategory S75.9:**
> **Right side:** PDX collection 1325
> **Left side:** PDX collection 1326
> **Unspecified side:** PDX collection 1327

√6ᵗʰ **S75.90** **Unspecified injury of unspecified blood vessel at hip and thigh level**

√7ᵗʰ **S75.901** **Unspecified injury of unspecified blood vessel at hip and thigh level, right leg**   `CC`

√7ᵗʰ **S75.902** **Unspecified injury of unspecified blood vessel at hip and thigh level, left leg**   `CC`

√7ᵗʰ **S75.909** **Unspecified injury of unspecified blood vessel at hip and thigh level, unspecified leg**   `CC`

√6ᵗʰ **S75.91** **Laceration of unspecified blood vessel at hip and thigh level**

√7ᵗʰ **S75.911** **Laceration of unspecified blood vessel at hip and thigh level, right leg**   `CC`

√7ᵗʰ **S75.912** **Laceration of unspecified blood vessel at hip and thigh level, left leg**   `CC`

√7ᵗʰ **S75.919** **Laceration of unspecified blood vessel at hip and thigh level, unspecified leg**   `CC`

√6ᵗʰ **S75.99** **Other specified injury of unspecified blood vessel at hip and thigh level**

√7ᵗʰ **S75.991** **Other specified injury of unspecified blood vessel at hip and thigh level, right leg**   `CC`

√7ᵗʰ **S75.992** **Other specified injury of unspecified blood vessel at hip and thigh level, left leg**   `CC`

√7ᵗʰ **S75.999** **Other specified injury of unspecified blood vessel at hip and thigh level, unspecified leg**   `CC`

√4ᵗʰ **S76** **Injury of muscle, fascia and tendon at hip and thigh level**
    Code also any associated open wound (S71.-)
    *EXCLUDES 2*   injury of muscle, fascia and tendon at lower leg level (S86)
       sprain of joint and ligament of hip (S73.1)
    **TIP:** Refer to the Muscle/Tendon table at the beginning of this chapter.

> The appropriate 7th character is to be added to each code from category S76.
> A    initial encounter
> D    subsequent encounter
> S    sequela

> **CC Excl: For CC codes in category S76:**
> **Right side:** PDX collection 1328
> **Left side:** PDX collection 1329
> **Unspecified side:** PDX collection 1330

√5ᵗʰ **S76.0** **Injury of muscle, fascia and tendon of hip**

√6ᵗʰ **S76.00** **Unspecified injury of muscle, fascia and tendon of hip**

√7ᵗʰ **S76.001** **Unspecified injury of muscle, fascia and tendon of right hip**

√7ᵗʰ **S76.002** **Unspecified injury of muscle, fascia and tendon of left hip**

√7ᵗʰ **S76.009** **Unspecified injury of muscle, fascia and tendon of unspecified hip**

√6ᵗʰ **S76.01** **Strain of muscle, fascia and tendon of hip**

√7ᵗʰ **S76.011** **Strain of muscle, fascia and tendon of right hip**

√7ᵗʰ **S76.012** **Strain of muscle, fascia and tendon of left hip**

√7ᵗʰ **S76.019** **Strain of muscle, fascia and tendon of unspecified hip**

√6ᵗʰ **S76.02** **Laceration of muscle, fascia and tendon of hip**

√7ᵗʰ **S76.021** **Laceration of muscle, fascia and tendon of right hip**   `CC`

√7ᵗʰ **S76.022** **Laceration of muscle, fascia and tendon of left hip**   `CC`

√7ᵗʰ **S76.029** **Laceration of muscle, fascia and tendon of unspecified hip**   `CC`

✓ Additional Character Req   √x7ᵗʰ Placeholder Alert   Unacceptable PDx   Manifestation   `H1`-`H14` HAC   `HCC` CMS-HCC Condition   *EXCLUDES 1* Not Coded Here   *EXCLUDES 2* Not Included Here

ICD-10-CM 2018      1045

✓6ᵗʰ **S76.09** Other specified injury of muscle, fascia and tendon of hip

    ✓7ᵗʰ **S76.091** Other specified injury of muscle, fascia and tendon of right hip

    ✓7ᵗʰ **S76.092** Other specified injury of muscle, fascia and tendon of left hip

    ✓7ᵗʰ **S76.099** Other specified injury of muscle, fascia and tendon of unspecified hip

✓5ᵗʰ **S76.1** Injury of quadriceps muscle, fascia and tendon
    Injury of patellar ligament (tendon)

   ✓6ᵗʰ **S76.10** Unspecified injury of quadriceps muscle, fascia and tendon

    ✓7ᵗʰ **S76.101** Unspecified injury of right quadriceps muscle, fascia and tendon

    ✓7ᵗʰ **S76.102** Unspecified injury of left quadriceps muscle, fascia and tendon

    ✓7ᵗʰ **S76.109** Unspecified injury of unspecified quadriceps muscle, fascia and tendon

   ✓6ᵗʰ **S76.11** Strain of quadriceps muscle, fascia and tendon

    ✓7ᵗʰ **S76.111** Strain of right quadriceps muscle, fascia and tendon

    ✓7ᵗʰ **S76.112** Strain of left quadriceps muscle, fascia and tendon

    ✓7ᵗʰ **S76.119** Strain of unspecified quadriceps muscle, fascia and tendon

   ✓6ᵗʰ **S76.12** Laceration of quadriceps muscle, fascia and tendon

    ✓7ᵗʰ **S76.121** Laceration of right quadriceps muscle, fascia and tendon **CC**

    ✓7ᵗʰ **S76.122** Laceration of left quadriceps muscle, fascia and tendon **CC**

    ✓7ᵗʰ **S76.129** Laceration of unspecified quadriceps muscle, fascia and tendon **CC**

   ✓6ᵗʰ **S76.19** Other specified injury of quadriceps muscle, fascia and tendon

    ✓7ᵗʰ **S76.191** Other specified injury of right quadriceps muscle, fascia and tendon

    ✓7ᵗʰ **S76.192** Other specified injury of left quadriceps muscle, fascia and tendon

    ✓7ᵗʰ **S76.199** Other specified injury of unspecified quadriceps muscle, fascia and tendon

✓5ᵗʰ **S76.2** Injury of adductor muscle, fascia and tendon of thigh

   ✓6ᵗʰ **S76.20** Unspecified injury of adductor muscle, fascia and tendon of thigh

    ✓7ᵗʰ **S76.201** Unspecified injury of adductor muscle, fascia and tendon of right thigh

    ✓7ᵗʰ **S76.202** Unspecified injury of adductor muscle, fascia and tendon of left thigh

    ✓7ᵗʰ **S76.209** Unspecified injury of adductor muscle, fascia and tendon of unspecified thigh

   ✓6ᵗʰ **S76.21** Strain of adductor muscle, fascia and tendon of thigh

    ✓7ᵗʰ **S76.211** Strain of adductor muscle, fascia and tendon of right thigh

    ✓7ᵗʰ **S76.212** Strain of adductor muscle, fascia and tendon of left thigh

    ✓7ᵗʰ **S76.219** Strain of adductor muscle, fascia and tendon of unspecified thigh

   ✓6ᵗʰ **S76.22** Laceration of adductor muscle, fascia and tendon of thigh

    ✓7ᵗʰ **S76.221** Laceration of adductor muscle, fascia and tendon of right thigh **CC**

    ✓7ᵗʰ **S76.222** Laceration of adductor muscle, fascia and tendon of left thigh **CC**

    ✓7ᵗʰ **S76.229** Laceration of adductor muscle, fascia and tendon of unspecified thigh **CC**

   ✓6ᵗʰ **S76.29** Other injury of adductor muscle, fascia and tendon of thigh

    ✓7ᵗʰ **S76.291** Other injury of adductor muscle, fascia and tendon of right thigh

    ✓7ᵗʰ **S76.292** Other injury of adductor muscle, fascia and tendon of left thigh

    ✓7ᵗʰ **S76.299** Other injury of adductor muscle, fascia and tendon of unspecified thigh

✓5ᵗʰ **S76.3** Injury of muscle, fascia and tendon of the posterior muscle group at thigh level

   ✓6ᵗʰ **S76.30** Unspecified injury of muscle, fascia and tendon of the posterior muscle group at thigh level

    ✓7ᵗʰ **S76.301** Unspecified injury of muscle, fascia and tendon of the posterior muscle group at thigh level, right thigh

    ✓7ᵗʰ **S76.302** Unspecified injury of muscle, fascia and tendon of the posterior muscle group at thigh level, left thigh

    ✓7ᵗʰ **S76.309** Unspecified injury of muscle, fascia and tendon of the posterior muscle group at thigh level, unspecified thigh

   ✓6ᵗʰ **S76.31** Strain of muscle, fascia and tendon of the posterior muscle group at thigh level

    ✓7ᵗʰ **S76.311** Strain of muscle, fascia and tendon of the posterior muscle group at thigh level, right thigh

    ✓7ᵗʰ **S76.312** Strain of muscle, fascia and tendon of the posterior muscle group at thigh level, left thigh

    ✓7ᵗʰ **S76.319** Strain of muscle, fascia and tendon of the posterior muscle group at thigh level, unspecified thigh

   ✓6ᵗʰ **S76.32** Laceration of muscle, fascia and tendon of the posterior muscle group at thigh level

    ✓7ᵗʰ **S76.321** Laceration of muscle, fascia and tendon of the posterior muscle group at thigh level, right thigh **CC**

    ✓7ᵗʰ **S76.322** Laceration of muscle, fascia and tendon of the posterior muscle group at thigh level, left thigh **CC**

    ✓7ᵗʰ **S76.329** Laceration of muscle, fascia and tendon of the posterior muscle group at thigh level, unspecified thigh **CC**

   ✓6ᵗʰ **S76.39** Other specified injury of muscle, fascia and tendon of the posterior muscle group at thigh level

    ✓7ᵗʰ **S76.391** Other specified injury of muscle, fascia and tendon of the posterior muscle group at thigh level, right thigh

    ✓7ᵗʰ **S76.392** Other specified injury of muscle, fascia and tendon of the posterior muscle group at thigh level, left thigh

    ✓7ᵗʰ **S76.399** Other specified injury of muscle, fascia and tendon of the posterior muscle group at thigh level, unspecified thigh

✓5ᵗʰ **S76.8** Injury of other specified muscles, fascia and tendons at thigh level

   ✓6ᵗʰ **S76.80** Unspecified injury of other specified muscles, fascia and tendons at thigh level

    ✓7ᵗʰ **S76.801** Unspecified injury of other specified muscles, fascia and tendons at thigh level, right thigh

    ✓7ᵗʰ **S76.802** Unspecified injury of other specified muscles, fascia and tendons at thigh level, left thigh

    ✓7ᵗʰ **S76.809** Unspecified injury of other specified muscles, fascia and tendons at thigh level, unspecified thigh

   ✓6ᵗʰ **S76.81** Strain of other specified muscles, fascia and tendons at thigh level

    ✓7ᵗʰ **S76.811** Strain of other specified muscles, fascia and tendons at thigh level, right thigh

    ✓7ᵗʰ **S76.812** Strain of other specified muscles, fascia and tendons at thigh level, left thigh

    ✓7ᵗʰ **S76.819** Strain of other specified muscles, fascia and tendons at thigh level, unspecified thigh

   ✓6ᵗʰ **S76.82** Laceration of other specified muscles, fascia and tendons at thigh level

    ✓7ᵗʰ **S76.821** Laceration of other specified muscles, fascia and tendons at thigh level, right thigh **CC**

    ✓7ᵗʰ **S76.822** Laceration of other specified muscles, fascia and tendons at thigh level, left thigh **CC**

**N** Newborn: 0   **P** Pediatric: 0-17   **M** Maternity: 12-55   **A** Adult: 15-124   **MCC** Major CC Condition   **PDxMCC** PDx acts as own MCC   **CC** CC Condition   **PDxCC** PDx acts as own CC

1046                ICD-10-CM 2018

✓7th **S76.829** Laceration of other specified muscles, `CC` fascia and tendons at thigh level, unspecified thigh

✓6th **S76.89** Other injury of other specified muscles, fascia and tendons at thigh level

    ✓7th **S76.891** Other injury of other specified muscles, fascia and tendons at thigh level, right thigh

    ✓7th **S76.892** Other injury of other specified muscles, fascia and tendons at thigh level, left thigh

    ✓7th **S76.899** Other injury of other specified muscles, fascia and tendons at thigh level, unspecified thigh

✓5th **S76.9** Injury of unspecified muscles, fascia and tendons at thigh level

✓6th **S76.90** Unspecified injury of unspecified muscles and tendons at thigh level

    ✓7th **S76.901** Unspecified injury of unspecified muscles, fascia and tendons at thigh level, right thigh

    ✓7th **S76.902** Unspecified injury of unspecified muscles, fascia and tendons at thigh level, left thigh

    ✓7th **S76.909** Unspecified injury of unspecified muscles, fascia and tendons at thigh level, unspecified thigh

✓6th **S76.91** Strain of unspecified muscles, fascia and tendons at thigh level

    ✓7th **S76.911** Strain of unspecified muscles, fascia and tendons at thigh level, right thigh

    ✓7th **S76.912** Strain of unspecified muscles, fascia and tendons at thigh level, left thigh

    ✓7th **S76.919** Strain of unspecified muscles, fascia and tendons at thigh level, unspecified thigh

✓6th **S76.92** Laceration of unspecified muscles, fascia and tendons at thigh level

    ✓7th **S76.921** Laceration of unspecified muscles, `CC` fascia and tendons at thigh level, right thigh

    ✓7th **S76.922** Laceration of unspecified muscles, `CC` fascia and tendons at thigh level, left thigh

    ✓7th **S76.929** Laceration of unspecified muscles, `CC` fascia and tendons at thigh level, unspecified thigh

✓6th **S76.99** Other specified injury of unspecified muscles, fascia and tendons at thigh level

    ✓7th **S76.991** Other specified injury of unspecified muscles, fascia and tendons at thigh level, right thigh

    ✓7th **S76.992** Other specified injury of unspecified muscles, fascia and tendons at thigh level, left thigh

    ✓7th **S76.999** Other specified injury of unspecified muscles, fascia and tendons at thigh level, unspecified thigh

✓4th **S77** **Crushing injury of hip and thigh**

    Use additional code(s) for all associated injuries

    *EXCLUDES 2*   crushing injury of ankle and foot (S97.-)
                 crushing injury of lower leg (S87.-)

    The appropriate 7th character is to be added to each code from category S77.
    A     initial encounter
    D     subsequent encounter
    S     sequela

✓5th **S77.0** Crushing injury of hip

    **CC Excl: For CC codes in subcategory S77.0:**
    PDX collection 1331

    ✓x7th **S77.00** Crushing injury of unspecified hip   `CC` `H5`
    ✓x7th **S77.01** Crushing injury of right hip   `CC` `H5`
    ✓x7th **S77.02** Crushing injury of left hip   `CC` `H5`

✓5th **S77.1** Crushing injury of thigh

    **CC Excl: For CC codes in subcategory S77.1:**
    PDX collection 1332

    ✓x7th **S77.10** Crushing injury of unspecified thigh   `CC` `H5`
    ✓x7th **S77.11** Crushing injury of right thigh   `CC` `H5`
    ✓x7th **S77.12** Crushing injury of left thigh   `CC` `H5`

✓5th **S77.2** Crushing injury of hip with thigh

    ✓x7th **S77.20** Crushing injury of unspecified hip with thigh
    ✓x7th **S77.21** Crushing injury of right hip with thigh
    ✓x7th **S77.22** Crushing injury of left hip with thigh

✓4th **S78** **Traumatic amputation of hip and thigh**

    An amputation not identified as partial or complete should be coded to complete.

    *EXCLUDES 1*   traumatic amputation of knee (S88.0-)

    The appropriate 7th character is to be added to each code from category S78.
    A     initial encounter
    D     subsequent encounter
    S     sequela

    **CC Excl: For CC codes in category S78:**
    **Right side:** PDX collection 1333
    **Left side:** PDX collection 1334
    **Unspecified side:** PDX collection 1335

✓5th **S78.0** Traumatic amputation at hip joint

    ✓6th **S78.01** Complete traumatic amputation at hip joint

       ✓7th **S78.011** Complete traumatic amputation at `CC` `HCC` right hip joint

       ✓7th **S78.012** Complete traumatic amputation at `CC` `HCC` left hip joint

       ✓7th **S78.019** Complete traumatic amputation at unspecified hip joint

    ✓6th **S78.02** Partial traumatic amputation at hip joint

       ✓7th **S78.021** Partial traumatic amputation at `CC` `HCC` right hip joint

       ✓7th **S78.022** Partial traumatic amputation at `CC` `HCC` left hip joint

       ✓7th **S78.029** Partial traumatic amputation at unspecified hip joint

✓5th **S78.1** Traumatic amputation at level between hip and knee

    *EXCLUDES 1*   traumatic amputation of knee (S88.0-)

    ✓6th **S78.11** Complete traumatic amputation at level between hip and knee

       ✓7th **S78.111** Complete traumatic amputation at `CC` `HCC` level between right hip and knee

       ✓7th **S78.112** Complete traumatic amputation at `CC` `HCC` level between left hip and knee

       ✓7th **S78.119** Complete traumatic amputation at `CC` `HCC` level between unspecified hip and knee

    ✓6th **S78.12** Partial traumatic amputation at level between hip and knee

       ✓7th **S78.121** Partial traumatic amputation at `CC` `HCC` level between right hip and knee

       ✓7th **S78.122** Partial traumatic amputation at `CC` `HCC` level between left hip and knee

       ✓7th **S78.129** Partial traumatic amputation at `CC` `HCC` level between unspecified hip and knee

✓5th **S78.9** Traumatic amputation of hip and thigh, level unspecified

    ✓6th **S78.91** Complete traumatic amputation of hip and thigh, level unspecified

       ✓7th **S78.911** Complete traumatic amputation `CC` `HCC` of right hip and thigh, level unspecified

       ✓7th **S78.912** Complete traumatic amputation `CC` `HCC` of left hip and thigh, level unspecified

       ✓7th **S78.919** Complete traumatic amputation `CC` `HCC` of unspecified hip and thigh, level unspecified

    ✓6th **S78.92** Partial traumatic amputation of hip and thigh, level unspecified

       ✓7th **S78.921** Partial traumatic amputation of `CC` `HCC` right hip and thigh, level unspecified

       ✓7th **S78.922** Partial traumatic amputation of `CC` `HCC` left hip and thigh, level unspecified

✓ Additional Character Req   ✓x7th Placeholder Alert   Unacceptable PDx   Manifestation   `H1`-`H14` HAC   `HCC` CMS-HCC Condition   *EXCLUDES 1* Not Coded Here   *EXCLUDES 2* Not Included Here

ICD-10-CM 2018                                                         **1047**

√7ᵗʰ **S78.929** **Partial traumatic amputation of** CC HCC
**unspecified hip and thigh, level**
**unspecified**

√4ᵗʰ **S79** **Other and unspecified injuries of hip and thigh**

NOTE   A fracture not indicated as open or closed should
be coded to closed.

**AHA:** 2015, 3Q, 37-39

The appropriate 7th character is to be added to each code from
subcategory S79.0 and S79.1
- A   initial encounter for closed fracture
- D   subsequent encounter for fracture with routine healing
- G   subsequent encounter for fracture with delayed healing
- K   subsequent encounter for fracture with nonunion
- P   subsequent encounter for fracture with malunion
- S   sequela

√5ᵗʰ **S79.0** **Physeal fracture of upper end of femur**

EXCLUDES 1   *apophyseal fracture of upper end of femur (S72.13-)*
*nontraumatic slipped upper femoral epiphysis*
*(M93.0-)*

**CC Excl: For CC/MCC codes in subcategory S79.0:**
**Right side:** See code S79.001
**Left side:** See code S79.002
**Unspecified side:** See code S79.009

√6ᵗʰ **S79.00** **Unspecified physeal fracture of upper end of femur**

8,10 √7ᵗʰ **S79.001** **Unspecified physeal** MCC CC H5 HCC
**fracture of upper end**
**of right femur**
**CC Excl: MCC with 7th character A:**
PDX collection 1297
**CC with 7th character K or P:**
PDX collection 897

8,10 √7ᵗʰ **S79.002** **Unspecified physeal** MCC CC H5 HCC
**fracture of upper end**
**of left femur**
**CC Excl: MCC with 7th character A:**
PDX collection 1299
**CC with 7th character K or P:**
PDX collection 897

8,10 √7ᵗʰ **S79.009** **Unspecified physeal** MCC CC H5 HCC
**fracture of upper end of**
**unspecified femur**
**CC Excl: MCC with 7th character A:**
PDX collection 1298
**CC with 7th character K or P:**
PDX collection 897

√6ᵗʰ **S79.01** **Salter-Harris Type I physeal fracture of upper end of**
**femur**
Acute on chronic slipped capital femoral epiphysis
(traumatic)
Acute slipped capital femoral epiphysis (traumatic)
Capital femoral epiphyseal fracture
EXCLUDES 1   *chronic slipped upper femoral epiphysis*
*(nontraumatic) (M93.02-)*

8,10 √7ᵗʰ **S79.011** **Salter-Harris Type I physeal** MCC CC H5 HCC
**fracture of upper end of**
**right femur**

8,10 √7ᵗʰ **S79.012** **Salter-Harris Type I physeal** MCC CC H5 HCC
**fracture of upper end of**
**left femur**

8,10 √7ᵗʰ **S79.019** **Salter-Harris Type I physeal** MCC CC H5 HCC
**fracture of upper end of**
**unspecified femur**

√6ᵗʰ **S79.09** **Other physeal fracture of upper end of femur**

8,10 √7ᵗʰ **S79.091** **Other physeal fracture of** MCC CC H5 HCC
**upper end of right femur**

8,10 √7ᵗʰ **S79.092** **Other physeal fracture of** MCC CC H5 HCC
**upper end of left femur**

8,10 √7ᵗʰ **S79.099** **Other physeal fracture of** MCC CC H5 HCC
**upper end of unspecified femur**

√5ᵗʰ **S79.1** **Physeal fracture of lower end of femur**

**CC Excl: For CC/MCC codes in subcategory S79.1:**
**Right side:** See code S79.101
**Left side:** See code S79.102
**Unspecified side:** See code S79.109

√6ᵗʰ **S79.10** **Unspecified physeal fracture of lower end of femur**

7,10 √7ᵗʰ **S79.101** **Unspecified physeal fracture of** CC H5 HCC
**lower end of right femur**
**CC Excl: CC with 7th character A:**
PDX collection 1300
**CC with 7th character K or P:**
PDX collection 897

7,10 √7ᵗʰ **S79.102** **Unspecified physeal fracture of** CC H5 HCC
**lower end of left femur**
**CC Excl: CC with 7th character A:**
PDX collection 1302
**CC with 7th character K or P:**
PDX collection 897

7,10 √7ᵗʰ **S79.109** **Unspecified physeal fracture of** CC H5 HCC
**lower end of unspecified femur**
**CC Excl: CC with 7th character A:**
PDX collection 1301
**CC with 7th character K or P:**
PDX collection 897

√6ᵗʰ **S79.11** **Salter-Harris Type I physeal fracture of lower end of**
**femur**

7,10 √7ᵗʰ **S79.111** **Salter-Harris Type I physeal** CC H5 HCC
**fracture of lower end of right femur**

7,10 √7ᵗʰ **S79.112** **Salter-Harris Type I physeal** CC H5 HCC
**fracture of lower end of left femur**

7,10 √7ᵗʰ **S79.119** **Salter-Harris Type I physeal** CC H5 HCC
**fracture of lower end of unspecified femur**

√6ᵗʰ **S79.12** **Salter-Harris Type II physeal fracture of lower end of**
**femur**

7,10 √7ᵗʰ **S79.121** **Salter-Harris Type II physeal** CC H5 HCC
**fracture of lower end of right femur**

7,10 √7ᵗʰ **S79.122** **Salter-Harris Type II physeal** CC H5 HCC
**fracture of lower end of left femur**

7,10 √7ᵗʰ **S79.129** **Salter-Harris Type II physeal** CC H5 HCC
**fracture of lower end of unspecified femur**

√6ᵗʰ **S79.13** **Salter-Harris Type III physeal fracture of lower end of**
**femur**

7,10 √7ᵗʰ **S79.131** **Salter-Harris Type III physeal** CC H5 HCC
**fracture of lower end of right femur**

7,10 √7ᵗʰ **S79.132** **Salter-Harris Type III physeal** CC H5 HCC
**fracture of lower end of left femur**

7,10 √7ᵗʰ **S79.139** **Salter-Harris Type III physeal** CC H5 HCC
**fracture of lower end of unspecified femur**

√6ᵗʰ **S79.14** **Salter-Harris Type IV physeal fracture of lower end of**
**femur**

7,10 √7ᵗʰ **S79.141** **Salter-Harris Type IV physeal** CC H5 HCC
**fracture of lower end of right femur**

7,10 √7ᵗʰ **S79.142** **Salter-Harris Type IV physeal** CC H5 HCC
**fracture of lower end of left femur**

7,10 √7ᵗʰ **S79.149** **Salter-Harris Type IV physeal** CC H5 HCC
**fracture of lower end of unspecified femur**

√6ᵗʰ **S79.19** **Other physeal fracture of lower end of femur**

7,10 √7ᵗʰ **S79.191** **Other physeal fracture of lower** CC H5 HCC
**end of right femur**

7,10 √7ᵗʰ **S79.192** **Other physeal fracture of lower** CC H5 HCC
**end of left femur**

7,10 √7ᵗʰ **S79.199** **Other physeal fracture of lower** CC H5 HCC
**end of unspecified femur**

√5ᵗʰ **S79.8** **Other specified injuries of hip and thigh**

The appropriate 7th character is to be added to each code
in subcategory S79.8.
- A   initial encounter
- D   subsequent encounter
- S   sequela

√6ᵗʰ **S79.81** **Other specified injuries of hip**

√7ᵗʰ **S79.811** **Other specified injuries of right hip**

√7ᵗʰ **S79.812** **Other specified injuries of left hip**

---

7   CC when reported as an initial encounter (7th character A, B, or C – specific to category) OR a subsequent encounter for nonunion or malunion
(7th character K, M, N, P, Q, or R – specific to category).

8   CC when reported as a subsequent encounter for nonunion or malunion (7th character K, M, N, P, Q, or R – specific to category).

10   HCC with 7th character indicating initial encounter (A, B or C - specific to category).

---

Ⓝ Newborn: 0   Ⓟ Pediatric: 0-17   Ⓜ Maternity: 12-55   Ⓐ Adult: 15-124   **MCC** Major CC Condition   **PDxMCC** PDx acts as own MCC   **CC** CC Condition   **PDxCC** PDx acts as own CC

**1048**      ICD-10-CM 2018

√7ᵗʰ **S79.819**   Other specified injuries of unspecified hip

√6ᵗʰ **S79.82**   **Other specified injuries of thigh**
  √7ᵗʰ **S79.821**   Other specified injuries of right thigh
  √7ᵗʰ **S79.822**   Other specified injuries of left thigh
  √7ᵗʰ **S79.829**   Other specified injuries of unspecified thigh

√5ᵗʰ **S79.9**   **Unspecified injury of hip and thigh**

The appropriate 7th character is to be added to each code in subcategory S79.9.
A     initial encounter
D     subsequent encounter
S     sequela

√6ᵗʰ **S79.91**   **Unspecified injury of hip**
  √7ᵗʰ **S79.911**   Unspecified injury of right hip
  √7ᵗʰ **S79.912**   Unspecified injury of left hip
  √7ᵗʰ **S79.919**   Unspecified injury of unspecified hip

√6ᵗʰ **S79.92**   **Unspecified injury of thigh**
  √7ᵗʰ **S79.921**   Unspecified injury of right thigh
  √7ᵗʰ **S79.922**   Unspecified injury of left thigh
  √7ᵗʰ **S79.929**   Unspecified injury of unspecified thigh

## Injuries to the knee and lower leg (S80-S89)

EXCLUDES 2   *burns and corrosions (T20-T32)*
  *frostbite (T33-T34)*
  *injuries of ankle and foot, except fracture of ankle and malleolus (S90-S99)*
  *insect bite or sting, venomous (T63.4)*

√4ᵗʰ **S80**   **Superficial injury of knee and lower leg**
  EXCLUDES 2   *superficial injury of ankle and foot (S90.-)*

The appropriate 7th character is to be added to each code from category S80.
A     initial encounter
D     subsequent encounter
S     sequela

√5ᵗʰ **S80.0**   **Contusion of knee**
  √x7ᵗʰ **S80.00**   Contusion of unspecified knee
  √x7ᵗʰ **S80.01**   Contusion of right knee
  √x7ᵗʰ **S80.02**   Contusion of left knee

√5ᵗʰ **S80.1**   **Contusion of lower leg**
  √x7ᵗʰ **S80.10**   Contusion of unspecified lower leg
  √x7ᵗʰ **S80.11**   Contusion of right lower leg
  √x7ᵗʰ **S80.12**   Contusion of left lower leg

√5ᵗʰ **S80.2**   **Other superficial injuries of knee**
  √6ᵗʰ **S80.21**   **Abrasion of knee**
    √7ᵗʰ **S80.211**   Abrasion, right knee
    √7ᵗʰ **S80.212**   Abrasion, left knee
    √7ᵗʰ **S80.219**   Abrasion, unspecified knee
  √6ᵗʰ **S80.22**   **Blister (nonthermal) of knee**
    √7ᵗʰ **S80.221**   Blister (nonthermal), right knee
    √7ᵗʰ **S80.222**   Blister (nonthermal), left knee
    √7ᵗʰ **S80.229**   Blister (nonthermal), unspecified knee
  √6ᵗʰ **S80.24**   **External constriction of knee**
    √7ᵗʰ **S80.241**   External constriction, right knee
    √7ᵗʰ **S80.242**   External constriction, left knee
    √7ᵗʰ **S80.249**   External constriction, unspecified knee
  √6ᵗʰ **S80.25**   **Superficial foreign body of knee**
    Splinter in the knee
    √7ᵗʰ **S80.251**   Superficial foreign body, right knee
    √7ᵗʰ **S80.252**   Superficial foreign body, left knee
    √7ᵗʰ **S80.259**   Superficial foreign body, unspecified knee
  √6ᵗʰ **S80.26**   **Insect bite (nonvenomous) of knee**
    √7ᵗʰ **S80.261**   Insect bite (nonvenomous), right knee
    √7ᵗʰ **S80.262**   Insect bite (nonvenomous), left knee
    √7ᵗʰ **S80.269**   Insect bite (nonvenomous), unspecified knee
  √6ᵗʰ **S80.27**   **Other superficial bite of knee**
    EXCLUDES 1   *open bite of knee (S81.05-)*
    √7ᵗʰ **S80.271**   Other superficial bite of right knee
    √7ᵗʰ **S80.272**   Other superficial bite of left knee

√7ᵗʰ **S80.279**   Other superficial bite of unspecified knee

√5ᵗʰ **S80.8**   **Other superficial injuries of lower leg**
  √6ᵗʰ **S80.81**   **Abrasion of lower leg**
    √7ᵗʰ **S80.811**   Abrasion, right lower leg
    √7ᵗʰ **S80.812**   Abrasion, left lower leg
    √7ᵗʰ **S80.819**   Abrasion, unspecified lower leg
  √6ᵗʰ **S80.82**   **Blister (nonthermal) of lower leg**
    √7ᵗʰ **S80.821**   Blister (nonthermal), right lower leg
    √7ᵗʰ **S80.822**   Blister (nonthermal), left lower leg
    √7ᵗʰ **S80.829**   Blister (nonthermal), unspecified lower leg
  √6ᵗʰ **S80.84**   **External constriction of lower leg**
    √7ᵗʰ **S80.841**   External constriction, right lower leg
    √7ᵗʰ **S80.842**   External constriction, left lower leg
    √7ᵗʰ **S80.849**   External constriction, unspecified lower leg
  √6ᵗʰ **S80.85**   **Superficial foreign body of lower leg**
    Splinter in the lower leg
    √7ᵗʰ **S80.851**   Superficial foreign body, right lower leg
    √7ᵗʰ **S80.852**   Superficial foreign body, left lower leg
    √7ᵗʰ **S80.859**   Superficial foreign body, unspecified lower leg
  √6ᵗʰ **S80.86**   **Insect bite (nonvenomous) of lower leg**
    √7ᵗʰ **S80.861**   Insect bite (nonvenomous), right lower leg
    √7ᵗʰ **S80.862**   Insect bite (nonvenomous), left lower leg
    √7ᵗʰ **S80.869**   Insect bite (nonvenomous), unspecified lower leg
  √6ᵗʰ **S80.87**   **Other superficial bite of lower leg**
    EXCLUDES 1   *open bite of lower leg (S81.85-)*
    √7ᵗʰ **S80.871**   Other superficial bite, right lower leg
    √7ᵗʰ **S80.872**   Other superficial bite, left lower leg
    √7ᵗʰ **S80.879**   Other superficial bite, unspecified lower leg

√5ᵗʰ **S80.9**   **Unspecified superficial injury of knee and lower leg**
  √6ᵗʰ **S80.91**   **Unspecified superficial injury of knee**
    √7ᵗʰ **S80.911**   Unspecified superficial injury of right knee
    √7ᵗʰ **S80.912**   Unspecified superficial injury of left knee
    √7ᵗʰ **S80.919**   Unspecified superficial injury of unspecified knee
  √6ᵗʰ **S80.92**   **Unspecified superficial injury of lower leg**
    √7ᵗʰ **S80.921**   Unspecified superficial injury of right lower leg
    √7ᵗʰ **S80.922**   Unspecified superficial injury of left lower leg
    √7ᵗʰ **S80.929**   Unspecified superficial injury of unspecified lower leg

√4ᵗʰ **S81**   **Open wound of knee and lower leg**
  Code also any associated wound infection
  EXCLUDES 1   *open fracture of knee and lower leg (S82.-)*
    *traumatic amputation of lower leg (S88.-)*
  EXCLUDES 2   *open wound of ankle and foot (S91.-)*

The appropriate 7th character is to be added to each code from category S81.
A     initial encounter
D     subsequent encounter
S     sequela

√5ᵗʰ **S81.0**   **Open wound of knee**
  √6ᵗʰ **S81.00**   **Unspecified open wound of knee**
    √7ᵗʰ **S81.001**   Unspecified open wound, right knee
    √7ᵗʰ **S81.002**   Unspecified open wound, left knee
    √7ᵗʰ **S81.009**   Unspecified open wound, unspecified knee
  √6ᵗʰ **S81.01**   **Laceration without foreign body of knee**
    √7ᵗʰ **S81.011**   Laceration without foreign body, right knee
    √7ᵗʰ **S81.012**   Laceration without foreign body, left knee
    √7ᵗʰ **S81.019**   Laceration without foreign body, unspecified knee
  √6ᵗʰ **S81.02**   **Laceration with foreign body of knee**
    √7ᵗʰ **S81.021**   Laceration with foreign body, right knee

√ Additional Character Req   √x7ᵗʰ Placeholder Alert   Unacceptable PDx   Manifestation   H1–H14 HAC   HCC CMS-HCC Condition   EXCLUDES 1 Not Coded Here   EXCLUDES 2 Not Included Here

ICD-10-CM 2018   **1049**

✓7th **S81.022** Laceration with foreign body, left knee

✓7th **S81.029** Laceration with foreign body, unspecified knee

✓6th **S81.03** Puncture wound without foreign body of knee

    ✓7th **S81.031** Puncture wound without foreign body, right knee

    ✓7th **S81.032** Puncture wound without foreign body, left knee

    ✓7th **S81.039** Puncture wound without foreign body, unspecified knee

✓6th **S81.04** Puncture wound with foreign body of knee

    ✓7th **S81.041** Puncture wound with foreign body, right knee

    ✓7th **S81.042** Puncture wound with foreign body, left knee

    ✓7th **S81.049** Puncture wound with foreign body, unspecified knee

✓6th **S81.05** Open bite of knee
    Bite of knee NOS
    *EXCLUDES 1*   *superficial bite of knee (S80.27-)*

    ✓7th **S81.051** Open bite, right knee

    ✓7th **S81.052** Open bite, left knee

    ✓7th **S81.059** Open bite, unspecified knee

✓5th **S81.8** Open wound of lower leg

✓6th **S81.80** Unspecified open wound of lower leg
    AHA: 2016, 3Q, 24

    ✓7th **S81.801** Unspecified open wound, right lower leg

    ✓7th **S81.802** Unspecified open wound, left lower leg

    ✓7th **S81.809** Unspecified open wound, unspecified lower leg

✓6th **S81.81** Laceration without foreign body of lower leg

    ✓7th **S81.811** Laceration without foreign body, right lower leg

    ✓7th **S81.812** Laceration without foreign body, left lower leg

    ✓7th **S81.819** Laceration without foreign body, unspecified lower leg

✓6th **S81.82** Laceration with foreign body of lower leg

    ✓7th **S81.821** Laceration with foreign body, right lower leg

    ✓7th **S81.822** Laceration with foreign body, left lower leg

    ✓7th **S81.829** Laceration with foreign body, unspecified lower leg

✓6th **S81.83** Puncture wound without foreign body of lower leg
    AHA: 2016, 3Q, 24

    ✓7th **S81.831** Puncture wound without foreign body, right lower leg

    ✓7th **S81.832** Puncture wound without foreign body, left lower leg

    ✓7th **S81.839** Puncture wound without foreign body, unspecified lower leg

✓6th **S81.84** Puncture wound with foreign body of lower leg
    AHA: 2016, 3Q, 24

    ✓7th **S81.841** Puncture wound with foreign body, right lower leg

    ✓7th **S81.842** Puncture wound with foreign body, left lower leg

    ✓7th **S81.849** Puncture wound with foreign body, unspecified lower leg

✓6th **S81.85** Open bite of lower leg
    Bite of lower leg NOS
    *EXCLUDES 1*   *superficial bite of lower leg (S80.86-, S80.87-)*

    ✓7th **S81.851** Open bite, right lower leg

    ✓7th **S81.852** Open bite, left lower leg

    ✓7th **S81.859** Open bite, unspecified lower leg

---

✓4th **S82** Fracture of lower leg, including ankle

    **NOTE**   A fracture not indicated as displaced or nondisplaced should be coded to displaced.
    A fracture not designated as open or closed should be coded to closed.
    The open fracture designations are based on the Gustilo open fracture classification.

    **INCLUDES**   fracture of malleolus
    *EXCLUDES 1*   *traumatic amputation of lower leg (S88.-)*
    *EXCLUDES 2*   *fracture of foot, except ankle (S92.-)*
    *periprosthetic fracture of prosthetic implant of knee ▶(M97.0-)◀*

    **AHA:** 2016, 1Q, 33; 2015, 3Q, 37-39; 2015, 3Q, 37-39

The appropriate 7th character is to be added to all codes from category S82 [unless otherwise indicated].
A   initial encounter for closed fracture
B   initial encounter for open fracture type I or II
    initial encounter for open fracture NOS
C   initial encounter for open fracture type IIIA, IIIB, or IIIC
D   subsequent encounter for closed fracture with routine healing
E   subsequent encounter for open fracture type I or II with routine healing
F   subsequent encounter for open fracture type IIIA, IIIB, or IIIC with routine healing
G   subsequent encounter for closed fracture with delayed healing
H   subsequent encounter for open fracture type I or II with delayed healing
J   subsequent encounter for open fracture type IIIA, IIIB or IIIC with delayed healing
K   subsequent encounter for closed fracture with nonunion
M   subsequent encounter for open fracture type I or II with nonunion
N   subsequent encounter for open fracture type IIIA, IIIB or IIIC with nonunion
P   subsequent encounter for closed fracture with malunion
Q   subsequent encounter for open fracture type I or II with malunion
R   subsequent encounter for open fracture type IIIA, IIIB or IIIC with malunion
S   sequela

✓5th **S82.0** Fracture of patella
    Knee cap

    **CC Excl: For CC codes in subcategory S82.0:**
    **Right side:** See code S82.001
    **Left side:** See code S82.002
    **Unspecified side:** See code S82.009

✓6th **S82.00** Unspecified fracture of patella

    7   ✓7th **S82.001** Unspecified fracture of right patella **CC H5**
    **CC Excl: CC with 7th character A:**
    PDX collection 1336
    **CC with 7th character B or C:**
    PDX collection 1337
    **CC with 7th character K, M, N, P, Q or R:**
    PDX collection 897

    7   ✓7th **S82.002** Unspecified fracture of left patella **CC H5**
    **CC Excl: CC with 7th character A:**
    PDX collection 1338
    **CC with 7th character B or C:**
    PDX collection 1337
    **CC with 7th character K, M, N, P, Q or R:**
    PDX collection 897

    7   ✓7th **S82.009** Unspecified fracture of unspecified patella **CC H5**
    **CC Excl: CC with 7th character A:**
    PDX collection 1339
    **CC with 7th character B or C:**
    PDX collection 1337
    **CC with 7th character K, M, N, P, Q or R:**
    PDX collection 897

✓6th **S82.01** Osteochondral fracture of patella

    7   ✓7th **S82.011** Displaced osteochondral fracture of right patella **CC H5**

    7   ✓7th **S82.012** Displaced osteochondral fracture of left patella **CC H5**

    7   ✓7th **S82.013** Displaced osteochondral fracture of unspecified patella **CC H5**

    7   ✓7th **S82.014** Nondisplaced osteochondral fracture of right patella **CC H5**

---

**7**   CC when reported as an initial encounter (7th character A, B, or C – specific to category) OR a subsequent encounter for nonunion or malunion (7th character K, M, N, P, Q, or R – specific to category).

**N** Newborn: 0   **P** Pediatric: 0-17   **M** Maternity: 12-55   **A** Adult: 15-124   **MCC** Major CC Condition   **PDx MCC** PDx acts as own MCC   **CC** CC Condition   **PDx CC** PDx acts as own CC

1050     ICD-10-CM 2018

7  ✓7ᵗʰ **S82.015** Nondisplaced **osteochondral** `CC` `H5`
fracture of **left patella**

7  ✓7ᵗʰ **S82.016** Nondisplaced **osteochondral** `CC` `H5`
fracture of **unspecified patella**

✓6ᵗʰ **S82.02** Longitudinal **fracture of patella**

7  ✓7ᵗʰ **S82.021** Displaced **longitudinal fracture of** `CC` `H5`
**right patella**

7  ✓7ᵗʰ **S82.022** Displaced **longitudinal fracture of** `CC` `H5`
**left patella**

7  ✓7ᵗʰ **S82.023** Displaced **longitudinal fracture of** `CC` `H5`
**unspecified patella**

7  ✓7ᵗʰ **S82.024** Nondisplaced **longitudinal fracture** `CC` `H5`
**of right patella**

7  ✓7ᵗʰ **S82.025** Nondisplaced **longitudinal fracture** `CC` `H5`
**of left patella**

7  ✓7ᵗʰ **S82.026** Nondisplaced **longitudinal fracture** `CC` `H5`
**of unspecified patella**

✓6ᵗʰ **S82.03** Transverse **fracture of patella**

7  ✓7ᵗʰ **S82.031** Displaced **transverse fracture of** `CC` `H5`
**right patella**

7  ✓7ᵗʰ **S82.032** Displaced **transverse fracture of** `CC` `H5`
**left patella**

7  ✓7ᵗʰ **S82.033** Displaced **transverse fracture of** `CC` `H5`
**unspecified patella**

7  ✓7ᵗʰ **S82.034** Nondisplaced **transverse fracture** `CC` `H5`
**of right patella**

7  ✓7ᵗʰ **S82.035** Nondisplaced **transverse fracture** `CC` `H5`
**of left patella**

7  ✓7ᵗʰ **S82.036** Nondisplaced **transverse fracture** `CC` `H5`
**of unspecified patella**

✓6ᵗʰ **S82.04** Comminuted **fracture of patella**

7  ✓7ᵗʰ **S82.041** Displaced **comminuted fracture** `CC` `H5`
**of right patella**

7  ✓7ᵗʰ **S82.042** Displaced **comminuted fracture of** `CC` `H5`
**left patella**

7  ✓7ᵗʰ **S82.043** Displaced **comminuted fracture of** `CC` `H5`
**unspecified patella**

7  ✓7ᵗʰ **S82.044** Nondisplaced **comminuted fracture** `CC` `H5`
**of right patella**

7  ✓7ᵗʰ **S82.045** Nondisplaced **comminuted fracture** `CC` `H5`
**of left patella**

7  ✓7ᵗʰ **S82.046** Nondisplaced **comminuted fracture** `CC` `H5`
**of unspecified patella**

✓6ᵗʰ **S82.09** Other **fracture of patella**

7  ✓7ᵗʰ **S82.091** Other **fracture of right patella** `CC` `H5`

7  ✓7ᵗʰ **S82.092** Other **fracture of left patella** `CC` `H5`

7  ✓7ᵗʰ **S82.099** Other **fracture of unspecified** `CC` `H5`
**patella**

✓5ᵗʰ **S82.1** Fracture of **upper end of tibia**
Fracture of proximal end of tibia

*EXCLUDES 2* *fracture of shaft of tibia (S82.2-)*
*physeal fracture of upper end of tibia (S89.0-)*

**CC Excl: For CC/MCC codes in subcategory S82.1,**
**unless otherwise noted:**
**Right side:** See code S82.101
**Left side:** See code S82.102
**Unspecified side:** See code S82.109

✓6ᵗʰ **S82.10** Unspecified **fracture of upper end of tibia**

6, 7  ✓7ᵗʰ **S82.101** Unspecified **fracture of upper** `MCC` `CC` `H5`
**end of right tibia**
**CC Excl: CC with 7th character A:**
PDX collection 1340
**MCC with 7th character B or C:**
PDX collection 1341
**CC with 7th character K, M, N, P, Q or R:**
PDX collection 897

6, 7  ✓7ᵗʰ **S82.102** Unspecified **fracture of upper** `MCC` `CC` `H5`
**end of left tibia**
**CC Excl: CC with 7th character A:**
PDX collection 1342
**MCC with 7th character B or C:**
PDX collection 1341
**CC with 7th character K, M, N, P, Q or R:**
PDX collection 897

6, 7  ✓7ᵗʰ **S82.109** Unspecified **fracture of upper** `MCC` `CC` `H5`
**end of unspecified tibia**
**CC Excl:**
**CC or MCC with 7th character A, B or C:**
PDX collection 1341
**CC with 7th character K, M, N, P, Q or R:**
PDX collection 897

✓6ᵗʰ **S82.11** Fracture of **tibial spine**

6, 7  ✓7ᵗʰ **S82.111** Displaced **fracture of right** `MCC` `CC` `H5`
**tibial spine**

6, 7  ✓7ᵗʰ **S82.112** Displaced **fracture of left** `MCC` `CC` `H5`
**tibial spine**

6, 7  ✓7ᵗʰ **S82.113** Displaced **fracture of** `MCC` `CC` `H5`
**unspecified tibial spine**

6, 7  ✓7ᵗʰ **S82.114** Nondisplaced **fracture of** `MCC` `CC` `H5`
**right tibial spine**

6, 7  ✓7ᵗʰ **S82.115** Nondisplaced **fracture of left** `MCC` `CC` `H5`
**tibial spine**

6, 7  ✓7ᵗʰ **S82.116** Nondisplaced **fracture of** `MCC` `CC` `H5`
**unspecified tibial spine**

✓6ᵗʰ **S82.12** Fracture of **lateral condyle of tibia**

6, 7  ✓7ᵗʰ **S82.121** Displaced **fracture of lateral** `MCC` `CC` `H5`
**condyle of right tibia**

6, 7  ✓7ᵗʰ **S82.122** Displaced **fracture of lateral** `MCC` `CC` `H5`
**condyle of left tibia**

6, 7  ✓7ᵗʰ **S82.123** Displaced **fracture of lateral** `MCC` `CC` `H5`
**condyle of unspecified tibia**

6, 7  ✓7ᵗʰ **S82.124** Nondisplaced **fracture of** `MCC` `CC` `H5`
**lateral condyle of right tibia**

6, 7  ✓7ᵗʰ **S82.125** Nondisplaced **fracture of** `MCC` `CC` `H5`
**lateral condyle of left tibia**

6, 7  ✓7ᵗʰ **S82.126** Nondisplaced **fracture of** `MCC` `CC` `H5`
**lateral condyle of unspecified tibia**

✓6ᵗʰ **S82.13** Fracture of **medial condyle of tibia**

6, 7  ✓7ᵗʰ **S82.131** Displaced **fracture of medial** `MCC` `CC` `H5`
**condyle of right tibia**

6, 7  ✓7ᵗʰ **S82.132** Displaced **fracture of medial** `MCC` `CC` `H5`
**condyle of left tibia**

6, 7  ✓7ᵗʰ **S82.133** Displaced **fracture of medial** `MCC` `CC` `H5`
**condyle of unspecified tibia**

6, 7  ✓7ᵗʰ **S82.134** Nondisplaced **fracture of** `MCC` `CC` `H5`
**medial condyle of right tibia**

6, 7  ✓7ᵗʰ **S82.135** Nondisplaced **fracture of** `MCC` `CC` `H5`
**medial condyle of left tibia**

6, 7  ✓7ᵗʰ **S82.136** Nondisplaced **fracture of** `MCC` `CC` `H5`
**medial condyle of unspecified tibia**

✓6ᵗʰ **S82.14** Bicondylar **fracture of tibia**
Fracture of tibial plateau NOS

6, 7  ✓7ᵗʰ **S82.141** Displaced **bicondylar fracture** `MCC` `CC` `H5`
**of right tibia**

6, 7  ✓7ᵗʰ **S82.142** Displaced **bicondylar fracture** `MCC` `CC` `H5`
**of left tibia**

6, 7  ✓7ᵗʰ **S82.143** Displaced **bicondylar fracture** `MCC` `CC` `H5`
**of unspecified tibia**

6, 7  ✓7ᵗʰ **S82.144** Nondisplaced **bicondylar** `MCC` `CC` `H5`
**fracture of right tibia**

6, 7  ✓7ᵗʰ **S82.145** Nondisplaced **bicondylar** `MCC` `CC` `H5`
**fracture of left tibia**

6, 7  ✓7ᵗʰ **S82.146** Nondisplaced **bicondylar** `MCC` `CC` `H5`
**fracture of unspecified tibia**

✓6ᵗʰ **S82.15** Fracture of **tibial tuberosity**

6, 7  ✓7ᵗʰ **S82.151** Displaced **fracture of right** `MCC` `CC` `H5`
**tibial tuberosity**

6, 7  ✓7ᵗʰ **S82.152** Displaced **fracture of left** `MCC` `CC` `H5`
**tibial tuberosity**

6, 7  ✓7ᵗʰ **S82.153** Displaced **fracture of** `MCC` `CC` `H5`
**unspecified tibial tuberosity**

6, 7  ✓7ᵗʰ **S82.154** Nondisplaced **fracture of** `MCC` `CC` `H5`
**right tibial tuberosity**

6, 7  ✓7ᵗʰ **S82.155** Nondisplaced **fracture of left** `MCC` `CC` `H5`
**tibial tuberosity**

6, 7  ✓7ᵗʰ **S82.156** Nondisplaced **fracture of** `MCC` `CC` `H5`
**unspecified tibial tuberosity**

---

6  MCC when reported as an open fracture (7th character B or C).
7  CC when reported as an initial encounter (7th character A, B, or C – specific to category) OR a subsequent encounter for nonunion or malunion
(7th character K, M, N, P, Q, or R – specific to category).

---

✓ Additional Character Req  ✓x7ᵗʰ Placeholder Alert  Unacceptable PDx  **Manifestation**  `H1`-`H14` HAC  `HCC` CMS-HCC Condition  *EXCLUDES 1* Not Coded Here  *EXCLUDES 2* Not Included Here

✓6ᵗʰ **S82.16**   Torus **fracture of upper end of tibia**

> The appropriate 7th character is to be added to all codes in subcategory S82.16.
> A   initial encounter for closed fracture
> D   subsequent encounter for fracture with routine healing
> G   subsequent encounter for fracture with delayed healing
> K   subsequent encounter for fracture with nonunion
> P   subsequent encounter for fracture with malunion
> S   sequela

7   ✓7ᵗʰ **S82.161**   **Torus fracture of upper end of right tibia**   `CC` `H5`
> **CC Excl: CC with 7th character A:**
> PDX collection 1343
> **CC with 7th character K or P:**
> PDX collection 897

7   ✓7ᵗʰ **S82.162**   **Torus fracture of upper end of left tibia**   `CC` `H5`
> **CC Excl: CC with 7th character A:**
> PDX collection 1344
> **CC with 7th character K or P:**
> PDX collection 897

7   ✓7ᵗʰ **S82.169**   **Torus fracture of upper end of unspecified tibia**   `CC` `H5`
> **CC Excl: CC with 7th character A:**
> PDX collection 1345
> **CC with 7th character K or P:**
> PDX collection 897

✓6ᵗʰ **S82.19**   Other **fracture of upper end of tibia**

6, 7   ✓7ᵗʰ **S82.191**   **Other fracture of upper end of right tibia**   `MCC` `CC` `H5`

6, 7   ✓7ᵗʰ **S82.192**   **Other fracture of upper end of left tibia**   `MCC` `CC` `H5`

6, 7   ✓7ᵗʰ **S82.199**   **Other fracture of upper end of unspecified tibia**   `MCC` `CC` `H5`

✓5ᵗʰ **S82.2**   **Fracture of shaft of tibia**

> **CC Excl: For CC/MCC codes in subcategory S82.2, unless otherwise noted:**
> **Right side:** See code S82.101
> **Left side:** See code S82.102
> **Unspecified side:** See code S82.109

✓6ᵗʰ **S82.20**   **Unspecified fracture of shaft of tibia**
Fracture of tibia NOS

6, 7   ✓7ᵗʰ **S82.201**   **Unspecified fracture of shaft of right tibia**   `MCC` `CC` `H5`
> **CC Excl: CC with 7th character A:**
> PDX collection 1346
> **MCC with 7th character B or C:**
> PDX collection 1341
> **CC with 7th character K, M, N, P, Q or R:**
> PDX collection 897

6, 7   ✓7ᵗʰ **S82.202**   **Unspecified fracture of shaft of left tibia**   `MCC` `CC` `H5`
> **CC Excl: CC with 7th character A:**
> PDX collection 1342
> **MCC with 7th character B or C:**
> PDX collection 1341
> **CC with 7th character K, M, N, P, Q or R:**
> PDX collection 897

6, 7   ✓7ᵗʰ **S82.209**   **Unspecified fracture of shaft of unspecified tibia**   `MCC` `CC` `H5`
> **CC Excl:**
> **CC or MCC with 7th character A, B or C:**
> PDX collection 1341
> **CC with 7th character K, M, N, P, Q or R:**
> PDX collection 897

✓6ᵗʰ **S82.22**   Transverse **fracture of shaft of tibia**

6, 7   ✓7ᵗʰ **S82.221**   **Displaced transverse fracture of shaft of right tibia**   `MCC` `CC` `H5`

6, 7   ✓7ᵗʰ **S82.222**   **Displaced transverse fracture of shaft of left tibia**   `MCC` `CC` `H5`

6, 7   ✓7ᵗʰ **S82.223**   **Displaced transverse fracture of shaft of unspecified tibia**   `MCC` `CC` `H5`

6, 7   ✓7ᵗʰ **S82.224**   **Nondisplaced transverse fracture of shaft of right tibia**   `MCC` `CC` `H5`

6, 7   ✓7ᵗʰ **S82.225**   **Nondisplaced transverse fracture of shaft of left tibia**   `MCC` `CC` `H5`

6, 7   ✓7ᵗʰ **S82.226**   **Nondisplaced transverse fracture of shaft of unspecified tibia**   `MCC` `CC` `H5`

✓6ᵗʰ **S82.23**   Oblique **fracture of shaft of tibia**

6, 7   ✓7ᵗʰ **S82.231**   **Displaced oblique fracture of shaft of right tibia**   `MCC` `CC` `H5`

6, 7   ✓7ᵗʰ **S82.232**   **Displaced oblique fracture of shaft of left tibia**   `MCC` `CC` `H5`

6, 7   ✓7ᵗʰ **S82.233**   **Displaced oblique fracture of shaft of unspecified tibia**   `MCC` `CC` `H5`

6, 7   ✓7ᵗʰ **S82.234**   **Nondisplaced oblique fracture of shaft of right tibia**   `MCC` `CC` `H5`

6, 7   ✓7ᵗʰ **S82.235**   **Nondisplaced oblique fracture of shaft of left tibia**   `MCC` `CC` `H5`

6, 7   ✓7ᵗʰ **S82.236**   **Nondisplaced oblique fracture of shaft of unspecified tibia**   `MCC` `CC` `H5`

✓6ᵗʰ **S82.24**   Spiral **fracture of shaft of tibia**
Toddler fracture

6, 7   ✓7ᵗʰ **S82.241**   **Displaced spiral fracture of shaft of right tibia**   `MCC` `CC` `H5`

6, 7   ✓7ᵗʰ **S82.242**   **Displaced spiral fracture of shaft of left tibia**   `MCC` `CC` `H5`

6, 7   ✓7ᵗʰ **S82.243**   **Displaced spiral fracture of shaft of unspecified tibia**   `MCC` `CC` `H5`

6, 7   ✓7ᵗʰ **S82.244**   **Nondisplaced spiral fracture of shaft of right tibia**   `MCC` `CC` `H5`

6, 7   ✓7ᵗʰ **S82.245**   **Nondisplaced spiral fracture of shaft of left tibia**   `MCC` `CC` `H5`

6, 7   ✓7ᵗʰ **S82.246**   **Nondisplaced spiral fracture of shaft of unspecified tibia**   `MCC` `CC` `H5`

✓6ᵗʰ **S82.25**   Comminuted **fracture of shaft of tibia**

6, 7   ✓7ᵗʰ **S82.251**   **Displaced comminuted fracture of shaft of right tibia**   `MCC` `CC` `H5`

6, 7   ✓7ᵗʰ **S82.252**   **Displaced comminuted fracture of shaft of left tibia**   `MCC` `CC` `H5`

6, 7   ✓7ᵗʰ **S82.253**   **Displaced comminuted fracture of shaft of unspecified tibia**   `MCC` `CC` `H5`

6, 7   ✓7ᵗʰ **S82.254**   **Nondisplaced comminuted fracture of shaft of right tibia**   `MCC` `CC` `H5`

6, 7   ✓7ᵗʰ **S82.255**   **Nondisplaced comminuted fracture of shaft of left tibia**   `MCC` `CC` `H5`

6, 7   ✓7ᵗʰ **S82.256**   **Nondisplaced comminuted fracture of shaft of unspecified tibia**   `MCC` `CC` `H5`

✓6ᵗʰ **S82.26**   Segmental **fracture of shaft of tibia**

6, 7   ✓7ᵗʰ **S82.261**   **Displaced segmental fracture of shaft of right tibia**   `MCC` `CC` `H5`

6, 7   ✓7ᵗʰ **S82.262**   **Displaced segmental fracture of shaft of left tibia**   `MCC` `CC` `H5`

6, 7   ✓7ᵗʰ **S82.263**   **Displaced segmental fracture of shaft of unspecified tibia**   `MCC` `CC` `H5`

6, 7   ✓7ᵗʰ **S82.264**   **Nondisplaced segmental fracture of shaft of right tibia**   `MCC` `CC` `H5`

6, 7   ✓7ᵗʰ **S82.265**   **Nondisplaced segmental fracture of shaft of left tibia**   `MCC` `CC` `H5`

6, 7   ✓7ᵗʰ **S82.266**   **Nondisplaced segmental fracture of shaft of unspecified tibia**   `MCC` `CC` `H5`

✓6ᵗʰ **S82.29**   Other **fracture of shaft of tibia**

6, 7   ✓7ᵗʰ **S82.291**   **Other fracture of shaft of right tibia**   `MCC` `CC` `H5`

6, 7   ✓7ᵗʰ **S82.292**   **Other fracture of shaft of left tibia**   `MCC` `CC` `H5`

6, 7   ✓7ᵗʰ **S82.299**   **Other fracture of shaft of unspecified tibia**   `MCC` `CC` `H5`

---

**6**   MCC when reported as an open fracture (7th character B or C).

**7**   CC when reported as an initial encounter (7th character A, B, or C – specific to category) OR a subsequent encounter for nonunion or malunion (7th character K, M, N, P, Q, or R – specific to category).

---

Ⓝ Newborn: 0   Ⓟ Pediatric: 0-17   Ⓜ Maternity: 12-55   Ⓐ Adult: 15-124   `MCC` Major CC Condition   `PDxMCC` PDx acts as own MCC   `CC` CC Condition   `PDxCC` PDx acts as own CC

**☑5ᵗʰ S82.3　Fracture of lower end of tibia**

> EXCLUDES 1　bimalleolar fracture of lower leg (S82.84-)
> fracture of medial malleolus alone (S82.5-)
> Maisonneuve's fracture (S82.86-)
> pilon fracture of distal tibia (S82.87-)
> trimalleolar fractures of lower leg (S82.85-)

**☑6ᵗʰ S82.30　Unspecified fracture of lower end of tibia**

> **CC Excl: For codes in subcategory S82.30:**
> **CC with 7th character B or C:** PDX collection 1347
> **CC with 7th character K, M, N, P, Q or R:**
> PDX collection 897

7　☑7ᵗʰ **S82.301　Unspecified fracture of lower end of right tibia**　CC H5

7　☑7ᵗʰ **S82.302　Unspecified fracture of lower end of left tibia**　CC H5

7　☑7ᵗʰ **S82.309　Unspecified fracture of lower end of unspecified tibia**　CC H5

**☑6ᵗʰ S82.31　Torus fracture of lower end of tibia**

> The appropriate 7th character is to be added to all codes in subcategory S82.31.
> A　initial encounter for closed fracture
> D　subsequent encounter for fracture with routine healing
> G　subsequent encounter for fracture with delayed healing
> K　subsequent encounter for fracture with nonunion
> P　subsequent encounter for fracture with malunion
> S　sequela

7　☑7ᵗʰ **S82.311　Torus fracture of lower end of right tibia**　CC H5
> **CC Excl: CC with 7th character A:**
> PDX collection 1343
> **CC with 7th character K or P:**
> PDX collection 897

7　☑7ᵗʰ **S82.312　Torus fracture of lower end of left tibia**　CC H5
> **CC Excl: CC with 7th character A:**
> PDX collection 1344
> **CC with 7th character K or P:**
> PDX collection 897

7　☑7ᵗʰ **S82.319　Torus fracture of lower end of unspecified tibia**　CC H5
> **CC Excl: CC with 7th character A:**
> PDX collection 1345
> **CC with 7th character K or P:**
> PDX collection 897

**☑6ᵗʰ S82.39　Other fracture of lower end of tibia**

> AHA: 2015, 1Q, 25

> **CC Excl: For codes in subcategory S82.39:**
> **CC for codes with 7th character B or C:**
> PDX collection 1347
> **CC with 7th character K, M, N, P, Q or R:**
> PDX collection 897

7　☑7ᵗʰ **S82.391　Other fracture of lower end of right tibia**　CC H5

7　☑7ᵗʰ **S82.392　Other fracture of lower end of left tibia**　CC H5

7　☑7ᵗʰ **S82.399　Other fracture of lower end of unspecified tibia**　CC H5

**☑5ᵗʰ S82.4　Fracture of shaft of fibula**

> EXCLUDES 2　fracture of lateral malleolus alone (S82.6-)

> **CC Excl: For codes in subcategory S82.4:**
> **MCC for codes with 7th character B or C:**
> PDX collection 1341
> **CC with 7th character K, M, N, P, Q or R:** PDX collection 897

**☑6ᵗʰ S82.40　Unspecified fracture of shaft of fibula**

6, 8　☑7ᵗʰ **S82.401　Unspecified fracture of shaft of right fibula**　MCC CC H5

6, 8　☑7ᵗʰ **S82.402　Unspecified fracture of shaft of left fibula**　MCC CC H5

6, 8　☑7ᵗʰ **S82.409　Unspecified fracture of shaft of unspecified fibula**　MCC CC H5

**☑6ᵗʰ S82.42　Transverse fracture of shaft of fibula**

6, 8　☑7ᵗʰ **S82.421　Displaced transverse fracture of shaft of right fibula**　MCC CC H5

6, 8　☑7ᵗʰ **S82.422　Displaced transverse fracture of shaft of left fibula**　MCC CC H5

6, 8　☑7ᵗʰ **S82.423　Displaced transverse fracture of shaft of unspecified fibula**　MCC CC H5

6, 8　☑7ᵗʰ **S82.424　Nondisplaced transverse fracture of shaft of right fibula**　MCC CC H5

6, 8　☑7ᵗʰ **S82.425　Nondisplaced transverse fracture of shaft of left fibula**　MCC CC H5

6, 8　☑7ᵗʰ **S82.426　Nondisplaced transverse fracture of shaft of unspecified fibula**　MCC CC H5

**☑6ᵗʰ S82.43　Oblique fracture of shaft of fibula**

6, 8　☑7ᵗʰ **S82.431　Displaced oblique fracture of shaft of right fibula**　MCC CC H5

6, 8　☑7ᵗʰ **S82.432　Displaced oblique fracture of shaft of left fibula**　MCC CC H5

6, 8　☑7ᵗʰ **S82.433　Displaced oblique fracture of shaft of unspecified fibula**　MCC CC H5

6, 8　☑7ᵗʰ **S82.434　Nondisplaced oblique fracture of shaft of right fibula**　MCC CC H5

6, 8　☑7ᵗʰ **S82.435　Nondisplaced oblique fracture of shaft of left fibula**　MCC CC H5

6, 8　☑7ᵗʰ **S82.436　Nondisplaced oblique fracture of shaft of unspecified fibula**　MCC CC H5

**☑6ᵗʰ S82.44　Spiral fracture of shaft of fibula**

6, 8　☑7ᵗʰ **S82.441　Displaced spiral fracture of shaft of right fibula**　MCC CC H5

6, 8　☑7ᵗʰ **S82.442　Displaced spiral fracture of shaft of left fibula**　MCC CC H5

6, 8　☑7ᵗʰ **S82.443　Displaced spiral fracture of shaft of unspecified fibula**　MCC CC H5

6, 8　☑7ᵗʰ **S82.444　Nondisplaced spiral fracture of shaft of right fibula**　MCC CC H5

6, 8　☑7ᵗʰ **S82.445　Nondisplaced spiral fracture of shaft of left fibula**　MCC CC H5

6, 8　☑7ᵗʰ **S82.446　Nondisplaced spiral fracture of sahft of unspecified fibula**　MCC CC H5

**☑6ᵗʰ S82.45　Comminuted fracture of shaft of fibula**

6, 8　☑7ᵗʰ **S82.451　Displaced comminuted fracture of shaft of right fibula**　MCC CC H5

6, 8　☑7ᵗʰ **S82.452　Displaced comminuted fracture of shaft of left fibula**　MCC CC H5

6, 8　☑7ᵗʰ **S82.453　Displaced comminuted fracture of shaft of unspecified fibula**　MCC CC H5

6, 8　☑7ᵗʰ **S82.454　Nondisplaced comminuted fracture of shaft of right fibula**　MCC CC H5

6, 8　☑7ᵗʰ **S82.455　Nondisplaced comminuted fracture of shaft of left fibula**　MCC CC H5

6, 8　☑7ᵗʰ **S82.456　Nondisplaced comminuted fracture of shaft of unspecified fibula**　MCC CC H5

**☑6ᵗʰ S82.46　Segmental fracture of shaft of fibula**

6, 8　☑7ᵗʰ **S82.461　Displaced segmental fracture of shaft of right fibula**　MCC CC H5

6, 8　☑7ᵗʰ **S82.462　Displaced segmental fracture of shaft of left fibula**　MCC CC H5

6, 8　☑7ᵗʰ **S82.463　Displaced segmental fracture of shaft of unspecified fibula**　MCC CC H5

6, 8　☑7ᵗʰ **S82.464　Nondisplaced segmental fracture of shaft of right fibula**　MCC CC

6, 8　☑7ᵗʰ **S82.465　Nondisplaced segmental fracture of shaft of left fibula**　MCC CC H5

6, 8　☑7ᵗʰ **S82.466　Nondisplaced segmental fracture of shaft of unspecified fibula**　MCC CC H5

---

6　MCC when reported as an open fracture (7th character B or C).

7　CC when reported as an initial encounter (7th character A, B, or C – specific to category) OR a subsequent encounter for nonunion or malunion (7th character K, M, N, P, Q, or R – specific to category).

8　CC when reported as a subsequent encounter for nonunion or malunion (7th character K, M, N, P, Q, or R).

---

☑ Additional Character Req　✓ₓ7ᵗʰ Placeholder Alert　Unacceptable PDx　Manifestation　H1-H14 HAC　HCC CMS-HCC Condition　EXCLUDES 1 Not Coded Here　EXCLUDES 2 Not Included Here

ICD-10-CM 2018　　　　　　　　　　　　　　　　　　　　　　　　　　　　　　　　　　　　　　　　　　　　1053

√6ᵗʰ **S82.49**   **Other fracture of shaft of fibula**

6, 8   √7ᵗʰ   **S82.491**   **Other fracture of shaft of right fibula**   `MCC` `CC` `H5`

6, 8   √7ᵗʰ   **S82.492**   **Other fracture of shaft of left fibula**   `MCC` `CC` `H5`

6, 8   √7ᵗʰ   **S82.499**   **Other fracture of shaft of unspecified fibula**   `MCC` `CC` `H5`

√5ᵗʰ **S82.5**   **Fracture of medial malleolus**

    **EXCLUDES 1**   *pilon fracture of distal tibia (S82.87-)*
                *Salter-Harris type III of lower end of tibia (S89.13-)*
                *Salter-Harris type IV of lower end of tibia (S89.14-)*

> **CC Excl: For codes in subcategory S82.5:**
> **CC with 7th character B or C:** PDX collection 1347
> **CC with 7th character K, M, N, P, Q or R:** PDX collection 897

7   √x7ᵗʰ   **S82.51**   **Displaced fracture of medial malleolus of right tibia**   `CC` `H5`

7   √x7ᵗʰ   **S82.52**   **Displaced fracture of medial malleolus of left tibia**   `CC` `H5`

7   √x7ᵗʰ   **S82.53**   **Displaced fracture of medial malleolus of unspecified tibia**   `CC` `H5`

7   √x7ᵗʰ   **S82.54**   **Nondisplaced fracture of medial malleolus of right tibia**   `CC` `H5`

7   √x7ᵗʰ   **S82.55**   **Nondisplaced fracture of medial malleolus of left tibia**   `CC` `H5`

7   √x7ᵗʰ   **S82.56**   **Nondisplaced fracture of medial malleolus of unspecified tibia**   `CC` `H5`

√5ᵗʰ **S82.6**   **Fracture of lateral malleolus**

    **EXCLUDES 1**   *pilon fracture of distal tibia (S82.87-)*

> **CC Excl: For codes in subcategory S82.6:**
> **CC with 7th character B or C:** PDX collection 1347
> **CC with 7th character K, M, N, P, Q or R:** PDX collection 897

7   √x7ᵗʰ   **S82.61**   **Displaced fracture of lateral malleolus of right fibula**   `CC` `H5`

7   √x7ᵗʰ   **S82.62**   **Displaced fracture of lateral malleolus of left fibula**   `CC` `H5`

7   √x7ᵗʰ   **S82.63**   **Displaced fracture of lateral malleolus of unspecified fibula**   `CC` `H5`

7   √x7ᵗʰ   **S82.64**   **Nondisplaced fracture of lateral malleolus of right fibula**   `CC` `H5`

7   √x7ᵗʰ   **S82.65**   **Nondisplaced fracture of lateral malleolus of left fibula**   `CC` `H5`

7   √x7ᵗʰ   **S82.66**   **Nondisplaced fracture of lateral malleolus of unspecified fibula**   `CC` `H5`

√5ᵗʰ **S82.8**   **Other fractures of lower leg**

√6ᵗʰ **S82.81**   **Torus fracture of upper end of fibula**

> The appropriate 7th character is to be added to all codes in subcategory S82.81.
> A   initial encounter for closed fracture
> D   subsequent encounter for fracture with routine healing
> G   subsequent encounter for fracture with delayed healing
> K   subsequent encounter for fracture wit nonunion
> P   subsequent encounter for fracture with malunion
> S   sequela

> **CC Excl: For codes in subcatgory S82.81:**
> **CC with 7th character K or P:** PDX collection 897

8   √7ᵗʰ   **S82.811**   **Torus fracture of upper end of right fibula**   `CC`

8   √7ᵗʰ   **S82.812**   **Torus fracture of upper end of left fibula**   `CC`

8   √7ᵗʰ   **S82.819**   **Torus fracture of upper end of unspecified fibula**   `CC`

---

√6ᵗʰ **S82.82**   **Torus fracture of lower end of fibula**

> The appropriate 7th character is to be added to all codes in subcategory S82.82.
> A   initial encounter for closed fracture
> D   subsequent encounter for fracture with routine healing
> G   subsequent encounter for fracture with delayed healing
> K   subsequent encounter for fracture with nonunion
> P   subsequent encounter for fracture with malunion
> S   sequela

> **CC Excl: For codes in subcatgory S82.82:**
> **CC with 7th character K or P:** PDX collection 897

8   √7ᵗʰ   **S82.821**   **Torus fracture of lower end of right fibula**   `CC`

8   √7ᵗʰ   **S82.822**   **Torus fracture of lower end of left fibula**   `CC`

8   √7ᵗʰ   **S82.829**   **Torus fracture of lower end of unspecified fibula**   `CC`

√6ᵗʰ **S82.83**   **Other fracture of upper and lower end of fibula**

    **AHA:** 2015, 1Q, 25

> **CC Excl: For codes in subcatgory S82.83:**
> **MCC with 7th B or C:** PDX collection 1341
> **CC with 7th character K, M, N, P, Q or R:** PDX collection 897

6, 8   √7ᵗʰ   **S82.831**   **Other fracture of upper and lower end of right fibula**   `MCC` `CC` `H5`

6, 8   √7ᵗʰ   **S82.832**   **Other fracture of upper and lower end of left fibula**   `MCC` `CC` `H5`

6, 8   √7ᵗʰ   **S82.839**   **Other fracture of upper and lower end of unspecified fibula**   `MCC` `CC` `H5`

√6ᵗʰ **S82.84**   **Bimalleolar fracture of lower leg**

> **CC Excl: For codes in subcatgory S82.84:**
> **CC with 7th character B or C:** PDX collection 1347
> **CC with 7th character K, M, N, P, Q or R:** PDX collection 897

7   √7ᵗʰ   **S82.841**   **Displaced bimalleolar fracture of right lower leg**   `CC` `H5`

7   √7ᵗʰ   **S82.842**   **Displaced bimalleolar fracture of left lower leg**   `CC` `H5`

7   √7ᵗʰ   **S82.843**   **Displaced bimalleolar fracture of unspecified lower leg**   `CC` `H5`

### Right Bimalleolar Fracture

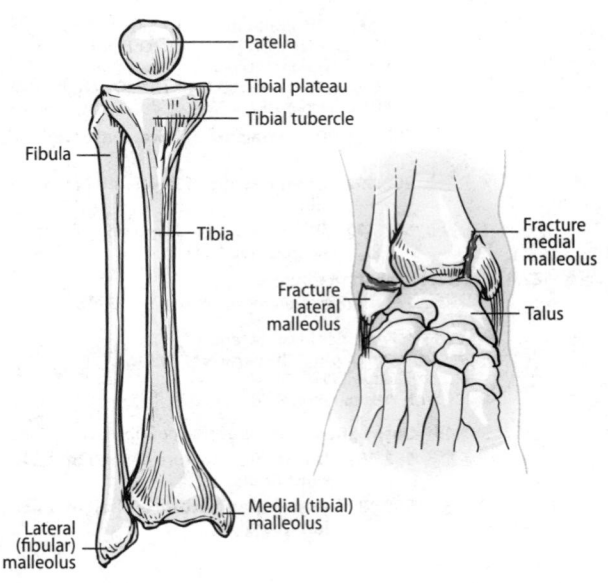

---

6   MCC when reported as an open fracture (7th character B or C).

7   CC when reported as an initial encounter (7th character A, B, or C – specific to category) OR a subsequent encounter for nonunion or malunion (7th character K, M, N, P, Q, or R – specific to category).

8   CC when reported as a subsequent encounter for nonunion or malunion (7th character K, M, N, P, Q, or R).

---

`N` Newborn: 0    `P` Pediatric: 0-17    `M` Maternity: 12-55    `A` Adult: 15-124    `MCC` Major CC Condition    `PDxMCC` PDx acts as own MCC    `CC` CC Condition    `PDxCC` PDx acts as own CC

7   ✓7th   **S82.844**   Nondisplaced **bimalleolar** fracture of **right lower leg**   CC H5

7   ✓7th   **S82.845**   Nondisplaced **bimalleolar** fracture of **left lower leg**   CC H5

7   ✓7th   **S82.846**   Nondisplaced **bimalleolar** fracture of **unspecified lower leg**   CC H5

✓6th   **S82.85**   **Trimalleolar** fracture of **lower leg**

> **CC Excl: For codes in subcatgory S82.85:**
> **CC with 7th character B or C:** PDX collection 1347
> **CC with 7th character K, M, N, P, Q or R:**
> PDX collection 897

7   ✓7th   **S82.851**   Displaced **trimalleolar** fracture of **right lower leg**   CC H5

7   ✓7th   **S82.852**   Displaced **trimalleolar** fracture of **left lower leg**   CC H5

7   ✓7th   **S82.853**   Displaced **trimalleolar** fracture of **unspecified lower leg**   CC H5

7   ✓7th   **S82.854**   Nondisplaced **trimalleolar** fracture of **right lower leg**   CC H5

7   ✓7th   **S82.855**   Nondisplaced **trimalleolar** fracture of **left lower leg**   CC H5

7   ✓7th   **S82.856**   Nondisplaced **trimalleolar** fracture of **unspecified lower leg**   CC H5

✓6th   **S82.86**   **Maisonneuve's fracture**

> **CC Excl: For codes in subcatgory S82.86:**
> **MCC with 7th character B or C:** PDX collection 1341
> **CC with 7th character K, M, N, P, Q or R:**
> PDX collection 897

6, 8   ✓7th   **S82.861**   Displaced **Maisonneuve's** fracture of **right leg**   MCC CC H5

6, 8   ✓7th   **S82.862**   Displaced **Maisonneuve's** fracture of **left leg**   MCC CC H5

6, 8   ✓7th   **S82.863**   Displaced **Maisonneuve's** fracture of **unspecified leg**   MCC CC H5

6, 8   ✓7th   **S82.864**   Nondisplaced **Maisonneuve's** fracture of **right leg**   MCC CC H5

6, 8   ✓7th   **S82.865**   Nondisplaced **Maisonneuve's** fracture of **left leg**   MCC CC H5

6, 8   ✓7th   **S82.866**   Nondisplaced **Maisonneuve's** fracture of **unspecified leg**   MCC CC H5

✓6th   **S82.87**   **Pilon** fracture of **tibia**

> **CC Excl: For codes in subcatgory S82.87:**
> **CC with 7th character B or C:** PDX collection 1347
> **CC with 7th character K, M, N, P, Q or R:**
> PDX collection 897

7   ✓7th   **S82.871**   Displaced **pilon** fracture of **right tibia**   CC H5

7   ✓7th   **S82.872**   Displaced **pilon** fracture of **left tibia**   CC H5

7   ✓7th   **S82.873**   Displaced **pilon** fracture of **unspecified tibia**   CC H5

7   ✓7th   **S82.874**   Nondisplaced **pilon** fracture of **right tibia**   CC H5

7   ✓7th   **S82.875**   Nondisplaced **pilon** fracture of **left tibia**   CC H5

7   ✓7th   **S82.876**   Nondisplaced **pilon** fracture of **unspecified tibia**   CC H5

✓6th   **S82.89**   **Other** fractures of **lower leg**
Fracture of ankle NOS

> **CC Excl: For codes in subcatgory S82.89:**
> **CC with 7th character B or C:** PDX collection 1347
> **CC with 7th character K, M, N, P, Q or R:**
> PDX collection 897

7   ✓7th   **S82.891**   Other fracture of **right lower leg**   CC H5

7   ✓7th   **S82.892**   Other fracture of **left lower leg**   CC H5

7   ✓7th   **S82.899**   Other fracture of **unspecified lower leg**   CC H5

✓5th   **S82.9**   **Unspecified** fracture of **lower leg**

> **CC Excl: For codes in subcatgory S82.9:**
> **CC with 7th character B or C:** PDX collection 1348
> **CC with 7th character K, M, N, P, Q or R:**
> PDX collection 897

7   ✓x7th   **S82.90**   Unspecified fracture of **unspecified lower leg**   CC H5

7   ✓x7th   **S82.91**   Unspecified fracture of **right lower leg**   CC H5

7   ✓x7th   **S82.92**   Unspecified fracture of **left lower leg**   CC H5

✓4th   **S83**   **Dislocation and sprain of joints and ligaments of knee**
   INCLUDES   avulsion of joint or ligament of knee
           laceration of cartilage, joint or ligament of knee
           sprain of cartilage, joint or ligament of knee
           traumatic hemarthrosis of joint or ligament of knee
           traumatic rupture of joint or ligament of knee
           traumatic subluxation of joint or ligament of knee
           traumatic tear of joint or ligament of knee
Code also any associated open wound
   EXCLUDES 1   *derangement of patella (M22.0-M22.3)*
           *injury of patellar ligament (tendon) (S76.1-)*
           *internal derangement of knee (M23.-)*
           *old dislocation of knee (M24.36)*
           *pathological dislocation of knee (M24.36)*
           *recurrent dislocation of knee (M22.0)*
   EXCLUDES 2   *strain of muscle, fascia and tendon of lower leg (S86.-)*

> The appropriate 7th character is to be added to each code from
> category S83.
> A     initial encounter
> D     subsequent encounter
> S     sequela

✓5th   **S83.0**   **Subluxation and dislocation of patella**

✓6th   **S83.00**   **Unspecified** subluxation and dislocation of **patella**

   ✓7th   **S83.001**   **Unspecified subluxation** of **right patella**

   ✓7th   **S83.002**   **Unspecified subluxation** of **left patella**

   ✓7th   **S83.003**   **Unspecified subluxation** of **unspecified patella**

   ✓7th   **S83.004**   **Unspecified dislocation** of **right patella**

   ✓7th   **S83.005**   **Unspecified dislocation** of **left patella**

   ✓7th   **S83.006**   **Unspecified dislocation** of **unspecified patella**

✓6th   **S83.01**   **Lateral** subluxation and dislocation of **patella**

   ✓7th   **S83.011**   **Lateral subluxation** of **right patella**

   ✓7th   **S83.012**   **Lateral subluxation** of **left patella**

   ✓7th   **S83.013**   **Lateral subluxation** of **unspecified patella**

   ✓7th   **S83.014**   **Lateral dislocation** of **right patella**

   ✓7th   **S83.015**   **Lateral dislocation** of **left patella**

   ✓7th   **S83.016**   **Lateral dislocation** of **unspecified patella**

✓6th   **S83.09**   **Other** subluxation and dislocation of **patella**

   ✓7th   **S83.091**   **Other subluxation** of **right patella**

   ✓7th   **S83.092**   **Other subluxation** of **left patella**

   ✓7th   **S83.093**   **Other subluxation** of **unspecified patella**

   ✓7th   **S83.094**   **Other dislocation** of **right patella**

   ✓7th   **S83.095**   **Other dislocation** of **left patella**

   ✓7th   **S83.096**   **Other dislocation** of **unspecified patella**

✓5th   **S83.1**   **Subluxation and dislocation of knee**
   EXCLUDES 2   *instability of knee prosthesis (T84.022, T84.023)*

✓6th   **S83.10**   **Unspecified** subluxation and dislocation of **knee**

   ✓7th   **S83.101**   **Unspecified subluxation** of **right knee**

   ✓7th   **S83.102**   **Unspecified subluxation** of **left knee**

   ✓7th   **S83.103**   **Unspecified subluxation** of **unspecified knee**

   ✓7th   **S83.104**   **Unspecified dislocation** of **right knee**

   ✓7th   **S83.105**   **Unspecified dislocation** of **left knee**

   ✓7th   **S83.106**   **Unspecified dislocation** of **unspecified knee**

---

6   MCC when reported as an open fracture (7th character B or C).
7   CC when reported as an initial encounter (7th character A, B, or C – specific to category) OR a subsequent encounter for nonunion or malunion
   (7th character K, M, N, P, Q, or R – specific to category).
8   CC when reported as a subsequent encounter for nonunion or malunion (7th character K, M, N, P, Q, or R).

✓Additional Character Req    ✓x7th Placeholder Alert    Unacceptable PDx    Manifestation    H1–H14 HAC    HCC CMS-HCC Condition    EXCLUDES 1 Not Coded Here    EXCLUDES 2 Not Included Here

✓6ᵗʰ **S83.11 Anterior subluxation and dislocation of proximal end of tibia**
Posterior subluxation and dislocation of distal end of femur

     ✓7ᵗʰ **S83.111 Anterior subluxation of proximal end of tibia, right knee**

     ✓7ᵗʰ **S83.112 Anterior subluxation of proximal end of tibia, left knee**

     ✓7ᵗʰ **S83.113 Anterior subluxation of proximal end of tibia, unspecified knee**

     ✓7ᵗʰ **S83.114 Anterior dislocation of proximal end of tibia, right knee**

     ✓7ᵗʰ **S83.115 Anterior dislocation of proximal end of tibia, left knee**

     ✓7ᵗʰ **S83.116 Anterior dislocation of proximal end of tibia, unspecified knee**

✓6ᵗʰ **S83.12 Posterior subluxation and dislocation of proximal end of tibia**
Anterior dislocation of distal end of femur

     ✓7ᵗʰ **S83.121 Posterior subluxation of proximal end of tibia, right knee**

     ✓7ᵗʰ **S83.122 Posterior subluxation of proximal end of tibia, left knee**

     ✓7ᵗʰ **S83.123 Posterior subluxation of proximal end of tibia, unspecified knee**

     ✓7ᵗʰ **S83.124 Posterior dislocation of proximal end of tibia, right knee**

     ✓7ᵗʰ **S83.125 Posterior dislocation of proximal end of tibia, left knee**

     ✓7ᵗʰ **S83.126 Posterior dislocation of proximal end of tibia, unspecified knee**

✓6ᵗʰ **S83.13 Medial subluxation and dislocation of proximal end of tibia**

     ✓7ᵗʰ **S83.131 Medial subluxation of proximal end of tibia, right knee**

     ✓7ᵗʰ **S83.132 Medial subluxation of proximal end of tibia, left knee**

     ✓7ᵗʰ **S83.133 Medial subluxation of proximal end of tibia, unspecified knee**

     ✓7ᵗʰ **S83.134 Medial dislocation of proximal end of tibia, right knee**

     ✓7ᵗʰ **S83.135 Medial dislocation of proximal end of tibia, left knee**

     ✓7ᵗʰ **S83.136 Medial dislocation of proximal end of tibia, unspecified knee**

✓6ᵗʰ **S83.14 Lateral subluxation and dislocation of proximal end of tibia**

     ✓7ᵗʰ **S83.141 Lateral subluxation of proximal end of tibia, right knee**

     ✓7ᵗʰ **S83.142 Lateral subluxation of proximal end of tibia, left knee**

     ✓7ᵗʰ **S83.143 Lateral subluxation of proximal end of tibia, unspecified knee**

     ✓7ᵗʰ **S83.144 Lateral dislocation of proximal end of tibia, right knee**

     ✓7ᵗʰ **S83.145 Lateral dislocation of proximal end of tibia, left knee**

     ✓7ᵗʰ **S83.146 Lateral dislocation of proximal end of tibia, unspecified knee**

✓6ᵗʰ **S83.19 Other subluxation and dislocation of knee**

     ✓7ᵗʰ **S83.191 Other subluxation of right knee**

     ✓7ᵗʰ **S83.192 Other subluxation of left knee**

     ✓7ᵗʰ **S83.193 Other subluxation of unspecified knee**

     ✓7ᵗʰ **S83.194 Other dislocation of right knee**

     ✓7ᵗʰ **S83.195 Other dislocation of left knee**

     ✓7ᵗʰ **S83.196 Other dislocation of unspecified knee**

✓5ᵗʰ **S83.2 Tear of meniscus, current injury**
     **EXCLUDES 1**   old bucket-handle tear (M23.2)

✓6ᵗʰ **S83.20 Tear of unspecified meniscus, current injury**
Tear of meniscus of knee NOS

     ✓7ᵗʰ **S83.200 Bucket-handle tear of unspecified meniscus, current injury, right knee**

     ✓7ᵗʰ **S83.201 Bucket-handle tear of unspecified meniscus, current injury, left knee**

     ✓7ᵗʰ **S83.202 Bucket-handle tear of unspecified meniscus, current injury, unspecified knee**

     ✓7ᵗʰ **S83.203 Other tear of unspecified meniscus, current injury, right knee**

     ✓7ᵗʰ **S83.204 Other tear of unspecified meniscus, current injury, left knee**

     ✓7ᵗʰ **S83.205 Other tear of unspecified meniscus, current injury, unspecified knee**

     ✓7ᵗʰ **S83.206 Unspecified tear of unspecified meniscus, current injury, right knee**

     ✓7ᵗʰ **S83.207 Unspecified tear of unspecified meniscus, current injury, left knee**

     ✓7ᵗʰ **S83.209 Unspecified tear of unspecified meniscus, current injury, unspecified knee**

✓6ᵗʰ **S83.21 Bucket-handle tear of medial meniscus, current injury**

     ✓7ᵗʰ **S83.211 Bucket-handle tear of medial meniscus, current injury, right knee**

     ✓7ᵗʰ **S83.212 Bucket-handle tear of medial meniscus, current injury, left knee**

     ✓7ᵗʰ **S83.219 Bucket-handle tear of medial meniscus, current injury, unspecified knee**

✓6ᵗʰ **S83.22 Peripheral tear of medial meniscus, current injury**

     ✓7ᵗʰ **S83.221 Peripheral tear of medial meniscus, current injury, right knee**

     ✓7ᵗʰ **S83.222 Peripheral tear of medial meniscus, current injury, left knee**

     ✓7ᵗʰ **S83.229 Peripheral tear of medial meniscus, current injury, unspecified knee**

✓6ᵗʰ **S83.23 Complex tear of medial meniscus, current injury**

     ✓7ᵗʰ **S83.231 Complex tear of medial meniscus, current injury, right knee**

     ✓7ᵗʰ **S83.232 Complex tear of medial meniscus, current injury, left knee**

     ✓7ᵗʰ **S83.239 Complex tear of medial meniscus, current injury, unspecified knee**

✓6ᵗʰ **S83.24 Other tear of medial meniscus, current injury**

     ✓7ᵗʰ **S83.241 Other tear of medial meniscus, current injury, right knee**

     ✓7ᵗʰ **S83.242 Other tear of medial meniscus, current injury, left knee**

     ✓7ᵗʰ **S83.249 Other tear of medial meniscus, current injury, unspecified knee**

✓6ᵗʰ **S83.25 Bucket-handle tear of lateral meniscus, current injury**

     ✓7ᵗʰ **S83.251 Bucket-handle tear of lateral meniscus, current injury, right knee**

     ✓7ᵗʰ **S83.252 Bucket-handle tear of lateral meniscus, current injury, left knee**

     ✓7ᵗʰ **S83.259 Bucket-handle tear of lateral meniscus, current injury, unspecified knee**

✓6ᵗʰ **S83.26 Peripheral tear of lateral meniscus, current injury**

     ✓7ᵗʰ **S83.261 Peripheral tear of lateral meniscus, current injury, right knee**

     ✓7ᵗʰ **S83.262 Peripheral tear of lateral meniscus, current injury, left knee**

     ✓7ᵗʰ **S83.269 Peripheral tear of lateral meniscus, current injury, unspecified knee**

✓6ᵗʰ **S83.27 Complex tear of lateral meniscus, current injury**

     ✓7ᵗʰ **S83.271 Complex tear of lateral meniscus, current injury, right knee**

     ✓7ᵗʰ **S83.272 Complex tear of lateral meniscus, current injury, left knee**

     ✓7ᵗʰ **S83.279 Complex tear of lateral meniscus, current injury, unspecified knee**

✓6ᵗʰ **S83.28 Other tear of lateral meniscus, current injury**

     ✓7ᵗʰ **S83.281 Other tear of lateral meniscus, current injury, right knee**

     ✓7ᵗʰ **S83.282 Other tear of lateral meniscus, current injury, left knee**

     ✓7ᵗʰ **S83.289 Other tear of lateral meniscus, current injury, unspecified knee**

Ⓝ Newborn: 0    Ⓟ Pediatric: 0-17    Ⓜ Maternity: 12-55    Ⓐ Adult: 15-124    **MCC** Major CC Condition    **PDxMCC** PDx acts as own MCC    **CC** CC Condition    **PDxCC** PDx acts as own CC

**1056**          ICD-10-CM 2018

✓5th **S83.3** Tear of articular cartilage of knee, current

   ✓x7th **S83.30** Tear of articular cartilage of unspecified knee, current

   ✓x7th **S83.31** Tear of articular cartilage of right knee, current

   ✓x7th **S83.32** Tear of articular cartilage of left knee, current

✓5th **S83.4** Sprain of collateral ligament of knee

   ✓6th **S83.40** Sprain of unspecified collateral ligament of knee

      ✓7th **S83.401** Sprain of unspecified collateral ligament of right knee

      ✓7th **S83.402** Sprain of unspecified collateral ligament of left knee

      ✓7th **S83.409** Sprain of unspecified collateral ligament of unspecified knee

   ✓6th **S83.41** Sprain of medial collateral ligament of knee
         Sprain of tibial collateral ligament

      ✓7th **S83.411** Sprain of medial collateral ligament of right knee

      ✓7th **S83.412** Sprain of medial collateral ligament of left knee

      ✓7th **S83.419** Sprain of medial collateral ligament of unspecified knee

   ✓6th **S83.42** Sprain of lateral collateral ligament of knee
         Sprain of fibular collateral ligament

      ✓7th **S83.421** Sprain of lateral collateral ligament of right knee

      ✓7th **S83.422** Sprain of lateral collateral ligament of left knee

      ✓7th **S83.429** Sprain of lateral collateral ligament of unspecified knee

✓5th **S83.5** Sprain of cruciate ligament of knee
      AHA: 2016, 2Q, 3

   ✓6th **S83.50** Sprain of unspecified cruciate ligament of knee

      ✓7th **S83.501** Sprain of unspecified cruciate ligament of right knee

      ✓7th **S83.502** Sprain of unspecified cruciate ligament of left knee

      ✓7th **S83.509** Sprain of unspecified cruciate ligament of unspecified knee

   ✓6th **S83.51** Sprain of anterior cruciate ligament of knee

      ✓7th **S83.511** Sprain of anterior cruciate ligament of right knee

      ✓7th **S83.512** Sprain of anterior cruciate ligament of left knee

      ✓7th **S83.519** Sprain of anterior cruciate ligament of unspecified knee

   ✓6th **S83.52** Sprain of posterior cruciate ligament of knee

      ✓7th **S83.521** Sprain of posterior cruciate ligament of right knee

      ✓7th **S83.522** Sprain of posterior cruciate ligament of left knee

      ✓7th **S83.529** Sprain of posterior cruciate ligament of unspecified knee

✓5th **S83.6** Sprain of the superior tibiofibular joint and ligament

   ✓x7th **S83.60** Sprain of the superior tibiofibular joint and ligament, unspecified knee

   ✓x7th **S83.61** Sprain of the superior tibiofibular joint and ligament, right knee

   ✓x7th **S83.62** Sprain of the superior tibiofibular joint and ligament, left knee

✓5th **S83.8** Sprain of other specified parts of knee

   ✓6th **S83.8X** Sprain of other specified parts of knee

      ✓7th **S83.8X1** Sprain of other specified parts of right knee

      ✓7th **S83.8X2** Sprain of other specified parts of left knee

      ✓7th **S83.8X9** Sprain of other specified parts of unspecified knee

✓5th **S83.9** Sprain of unspecified site of knee

   ✓x7th **S83.90** Sprain of unspecified site of unspecified knee

   ✓x7th **S83.91** Sprain of unspecified site of right knee

   ✓x7th **S83.92** Sprain of unspecified site of left knee

✓4th **S84** **Injury of nerves at lower leg level**

   Code also any associated open wound (S81.-)
   *EXCLUDES 2* injury of nerves at ankle and foot level (S94.-)

   The appropriate 7th character is to be added to each code from category S84.
   A   initial encounter
   D   subsequent encounter
   S   sequela

   ✓5th **S84.0** Injury of tibial nerve at lower leg level

      ✓x7th **S84.00** Injury of tibial nerve at lower leg level, unspecified leg

      ✓x7th **S84.01** Injury of tibial nerve at lower leg level, right leg

      ✓x7th **S84.02** Injury of tibial nerve at lower leg level, left leg

   ✓5th **S84.1** Injury of peroneal nerve at lower leg level

      ✓x7th **S84.10** Injury of peroneal nerve at lower leg level, unspecified leg

      ✓x7th **S84.11** Injury of peroneal nerve at lower leg level, right leg

      ✓x7th **S84.12** Injury of peroneal nerve at lower leg level, left leg

   ✓5th **S84.2** Injury of cutaneous sensory nerve at lower leg level

      ✓x7th **S84.20** Injury of cutaneous sensory nerve at lower leg level, unspecified leg

      ✓x7th **S84.21** Injury of cutaneous sensory nerve at lower leg level, right leg

      ✓x7th **S84.22** Injury of cutaneous sensory nerve at lower leg level, left leg

   ✓5th **S84.8** Injury of other nerves at lower leg level

      ✓6th **S84.80** Injury of other nerves at lower leg level

         ✓7th **S84.801** Injury of other nerves at lower leg level, right leg

         ✓7th **S84.802** Injury of other nerves at lower leg level, left leg

         ✓7th **S84.809** Injury of other nerves at lower leg level, unspecified leg

   ✓5th **S84.9** Injury of unspecified nerve at lower leg level

      ✓x7th **S84.90** Injury of unspecified nerve at lower leg level, unspecified leg

      ✓x7th **S84.91** Injury of unspecified nerve at lower leg level, right leg

      ✓x7th **S84.92** Injury of unspecified nerve at lower leg level, left leg

✓4th **S85** **Injury of blood vessels at lower leg level**

   Code also any associated open wound (S81.-)
   *EXCLUDES 2* injury of blood vessels at ankle and foot level (S95.-)

   The appropriate 7th character is to be added to each code from category S85.
   A   initial encounter
   D   subsequent encounter
   S   sequela

   ✓5th **S85.0** Injury of popliteal artery

      **CC Excl: For MCC codes in subcategory S85.0:**
      **Right side:** PDX collection 1349
      **Left side:** PDX collection 1350
      **Unspecified side:** PDX collection 1351

      ✓6th **S85.00** Unspecified injury of popliteal artery

         ✓7th **S85.001** Unspecified injury of popliteal artery, right leg `MCC`

         ✓7th **S85.002** Unspecified injury of popliteal artery, left leg `MCC`

         ✓7th **S85.009** Unspecified injury of popliteal artery, unspecified leg `MCC`

      ✓6th **S85.01** Laceration of popliteal artery

         ✓7th **S85.011** Laceration of popliteal artery, right leg `MCC`

         ✓7th **S85.012** Laceration of popliteal artery, left leg `MCC`

         ✓7th **S85.019** Laceration of popliteal artery, unspecified leg `MCC`

      ✓6th **S85.09** Other specified injury of popliteal artery

         ✓7th **S85.091** Other specified injury of popliteal artery, right leg `MCC`

         ✓7th **S85.092** Other specified injury of popliteal artery, left leg `MCC`

✓ Additional Character Req    ✓x7th Placeholder Alert    Unacceptable PDx    Manifestation    H1-H14 HAC    HCC CMS-HCC Condition    *EXCLUDES 1* Not Coded Here    *EXCLUDES 2* Not Included Here

ICD-10-CM 2018                                                       1057

✓7ᵗʰ **S85.099** Other specified injury of popliteal artery, unspecified **leg**   `MCC`

✓5ᵗʰ **S85.1** Injury of tibial artery

     ✓6ᵗʰ **S85.10** Unspecified injury of unspecified tibial artery
         Injury of tibial artery NOS

         ✓7ᵗʰ **S85.101** Unspecified injury of unspecified tibial artery, right **leg**   `CC`

         ✓7ᵗʰ **S85.102** Unspecified injury of unspecified tibial artery, left **leg**   `CC`

         ✓7ᵗʰ **S85.109** Unspecified injury of unspecified tibial artery, unspecified **leg**   `CC`

     ✓6ᵗʰ **S85.11** Laceration of unspecified tibial artery

         ✓7ᵗʰ **S85.111** Laceration of unspecified tibial artery, right **leg**   `CC`
             **CC Excl:** PDX collection 1352

         ✓7ᵗʰ **S85.112** Laceration of unspecified tibial artery, left **leg**   `CC`
             **CC Excl:** PDX collection 1353

         ✓7ᵗʰ **S85.119** Laceration of unspecified tibial artery, unspecified **leg**   `CC`
             **CC Excl:** PDX collection 1354

     ✓6ᵗʰ **S85.12** Other specified injury of unspecified tibial artery

         ✓7ᵗʰ **S85.121** Other specified injury of unspecified tibial artery, right **leg**   `CC`
             **CC Excl:** PDX collection 1352

         ✓7ᵗʰ **S85.122** Other specified injury of unspecified tibial artery, left **leg**   `CC`
             **CC Excl:** PDX collection 1353

         ✓7ᵗʰ **S85.129** Other specified injury of unspecified tibial artery, unspecified **leg**   `CC`
             **CC Excl:** PDX collection 1354

     ✓6ᵗʰ **S85.13** Unspecified injury of anterior tibial artery

         ✓7ᵗʰ **S85.131** Unspecified injury of anterior tibial artery, right **leg**   `CC`
             **CC Excl:** PDX collection 1355

         ✓7ᵗʰ **S85.132** Unspecified injury of anterior tibial artery, left **leg**   `CC`
             **CC Excl:** PDX collection 1356

         ✓7ᵗʰ **S85.139** Unspecified injury of anterior tibial artery, unspecified **leg**   `CC`
             **CC Excl:** PDX collection 1357

     ✓6ᵗʰ **S85.14** Laceration of anterior tibial artery

         ✓7ᵗʰ **S85.141** Laceration of anterior tibial artery, right **leg**   `CC`
             **CC Excl:** PDX collection 1355

         ✓7ᵗʰ **S85.142** Laceration of anterior tibial artery, left **leg**   `CC`
             **CC Excl:** PDX collection 1356

         ✓7ᵗʰ **S85.149** Laceration of anterior tibial artery, unspecified **leg**   `CC`
             **CC Excl:** PDX collection 1357

     ✓6ᵗʰ **S85.15** Other specified injury of anterior tibial artery

         ✓7ᵗʰ **S85.151** Other specified injury of anterior tibial artery, right **leg**   `CC`
             **CC Excl:** PDX collection 1355

         ✓7ᵗʰ **S85.152** Other specified injury of anterior tibial artery, left **leg**   `CC`
             **CC Excl:** PDX collection 1356

         ✓7ᵗʰ **S85.159** Other specified injury of anterior tibial artery, unspecified **leg**   `CC`
             **CC Excl:** PDX collection 1357

     ✓6ᵗʰ **S85.16** Unspecified injury of posterior tibial artery

         ✓7ᵗʰ **S85.161** Unspecified injury of posterior tibial artery, right **leg**   `CC`
             **CC Excl:** PDX collection 1358

         ✓7ᵗʰ **S85.162** Unspecified injury of posterior tibial artery, left **leg**   `CC`
             **CC Excl:** PDX collection 1359

         ✓7ᵗʰ **S85.169** Unspecified injury of posterior tibial artery, unspecified **leg**   `CC`
             **CC Excl:** PDX collection 1360

     ✓6ᵗʰ **S85.17** Laceration of posterior tibial artery

         ✓7ᵗʰ **S85.171** Laceration of posterior tibial artery, right **leg**   `CC`
             **CC Excl:** PDX collection 1358

         ✓7ᵗʰ **S85.172** Laceration of posterior tibial artery, left **leg**   `CC`
             **CC Excl:** PDX collection 1359

         ✓7ᵗʰ **S85.179** Laceration of posterior tibial artery, unspecified **leg**   `CC`
             **CC Excl:** PDX collection 1360

     ✓6ᵗʰ **S85.18** Other specified injury of posterior tibial artery

         ✓7ᵗʰ **S85.181** Other specified injury of posterior tibial artery, right **leg**   `CC`
             **CC Excl:** PDX collection 1358

         ✓7ᵗʰ **S85.182** Other specified injury of posterior tibial artery, left **leg**   `CC`
             **CC Excl:** PDX collection 1359

         ✓7ᵗʰ **S85.189** Other specified injury of posterior tibial artery, unspecified **leg**   `CC`
             **CC Excl:** PDX collection 1360

✓5ᵗʰ **S85.2** Injury of peroneal artery

     **CC Excl: For CC codes in subcategory S85.2:**
     **Right side:** PDX collection 1325
     **Left side:** PDX collection 1326
     **Unspecified side:** PDX collection 1327

     ✓6ᵗʰ **S85.20** Unspecified injury of peroneal artery

         ✓7ᵗʰ **S85.201** Unspecified injury of peroneal artery, right **leg**   `CC`

         ✓7ᵗʰ **S85.202** Unspecified injury of peroneal artery, left **leg**   `CC`

         ✓7ᵗʰ **S85.209** Unspecified injury of peroneal artery, unspecified **leg**   `CC`

     ✓6ᵗʰ **S85.21** Laceration of peroneal artery

         ✓7ᵗʰ **S85.211** Laceration of peroneal artery, right **leg**   `CC`

         ✓7ᵗʰ **S85.212** Laceration of peroneal artery, left **leg**   `CC`

         ✓7ᵗʰ **S85.219** Laceration of peroneal artery, unspecified **leg**   `CC`

     ✓6ᵗʰ **S85.29** Other specified injury of peroneal artery

         ✓7ᵗʰ **S85.291** Other specified injury of peroneal artery, right **leg**   `CC`

         ✓7ᵗʰ **S85.292** Other specified injury of peroneal artery, left **leg**   `CC`

         ✓7ᵗʰ **S85.299** Other specified injury of peroneal artery, unspecified **leg**   `CC`

✓5ᵗʰ **S85.3** Injury of greater saphenous vein at lower leg level
     Injury of greater saphenous vein NOS
     Injury of saphenous vein NOS

     **CC Excl: For CC codes in subcategory S85.3:**
     **Right side:** PDX collection 1322
     **Left side:** PDX collection 1323
     **Unspecified side:** PDX collection 1324

     ✓6ᵗʰ **S85.30** Unspecified injury of greater saphenous vein at lower leg level

         ✓7ᵗʰ **S85.301** Unspecified injury of greater saphenous vein at lower leg level, right **leg**   `CC`

         ✓7ᵗʰ **S85.302** Unspecified injury of greater saphenous vein at lower leg level, left **leg**   `CC`

         ✓7ᵗʰ **S85.309** Unspecified injury of greater saphenous vein at lower leg level, unspecified **leg**   `CC`

     ✓6ᵗʰ **S85.31** Laceration of greater saphenous vein at lower leg level

         ✓7ᵗʰ **S85.311** Laceration of greater saphenous vein at lower leg level, right **leg**   `CC`

         ✓7ᵗʰ **S85.312** Laceration of greater saphenous vein at lower leg level, left **leg**   `CC`

         ✓7ᵗʰ **S85.319** Laceration of greater saphenous vein at lower leg level, unspecified **leg**   `CC`

     ✓6ᵗʰ **S85.39** Other specified injury of greater saphenous vein at lower leg level

         ✓7ᵗʰ **S85.391** Other specified injury of greater saphenous vein at lower leg level, right **leg**   `CC`

         ✓7ᵗʰ **S85.392** Other specified injury of greater saphenous vein at lower leg level, left **leg**   `CC`

**N** Newborn: 0   **P** Pediatric: 0-17   **M** Maternity: 12-55   **A** Adult: 15-124   `MCC` Major CC Condition   `PDxMCC` PDx acts as own MCC   `CC` CC Condition   `PDxCC` PDx acts as own CC

**1058**          ICD-10-CM 2018

√7ᵗʰ **S85.399** Other specified injury of greater saphenous vein at lower leg level, unspecified leg   CC

√5ᵗʰ **S85.4** Injury of lesser saphenous vein at lower leg level

> **CC Excl: For CC codes in subcategory S85.4:**
> **Right side:** PDX collection 1322
> **Left side:** PDX collection 1323
> **Unspecified side:** PDX collection 1324

√6ᵗʰ **S85.40** Unspecified injury of lesser saphenous vein at lower leg level

√7ᵗʰ **S85.401** Unspecified injury of lesser saphenous vein at lower leg level, right leg   CC

√7ᵗʰ **S85.402** Unspecified injury of lesser saphenous vein at lower leg level, left leg   CC

√7ᵗʰ **S85.409** Unspecified injury of lesser saphenous vein at lower leg level, unspecified leg   CC

√6ᵗʰ **S85.41** Laceration of lesser saphenous vein at lower leg level

√7ᵗʰ **S85.411** Laceration of lesser saphenous vein at lower leg level, right leg   CC

√7ᵗʰ **S85.412** Laceration of lesser saphenous vein at lower leg level, left leg   CC

√7ᵗʰ **S85.419** Laceration of lesser saphenous vein at lower leg level, unspecified leg   CC

√6ᵗʰ **S85.49** Other specified injury of lesser saphenous vein at lower leg level

√7ᵗʰ **S85.491** Other specified injury of lesser saphenous vein at lower leg level, right leg   CC

√7ᵗʰ **S85.492** Other specified injury of lesser saphenous vein at lower leg level, left leg   CC

√7ᵗʰ **S85.499** Other specified injury of lesser saphenous vein at lower leg level, unspecified leg   CC

√5ᵗʰ **S85.5** Injury of popliteal vein

> **CC Excl: For MCC codes in subcategory S85.5:**
> **Right side:** PDX collection 1361
> **Left side:** PDX collection 1362
> **Unspecified side:** PDX collection 1363

√6ᵗʰ **S85.50** Unspecified injury of popliteal vein

√7ᵗʰ **S85.501** Unspecified injury of popliteal vein, right leg   MCC

√7ᵗʰ **S85.502** Unspecified injury of popliteal vein, left leg   MCC

√7ᵗʰ **S85.509** Unspecified injury of popliteal vein, unspecified leg   MCC

√6ᵗʰ **S85.51** Laceration of popliteal vein

√7ᵗʰ **S85.511** Laceration of popliteal vein, right leg   MCC

√7ᵗʰ **S85.512** Laceration of popliteal vein, left leg   MCC

√7ᵗʰ **S85.519** Laceration of popliteal vein, unspecified leg   MCC

√6ᵗʰ **S85.59** Other specified injury of popliteal vein

√7ᵗʰ **S85.591** Other specified injury of popliteal vein, right leg   MCC

√7ᵗʰ **S85.592** Other specified injury of popliteal vein, left leg   MCC

√7ᵗʰ **S85.599** Other specified injury of popliteal vein, unspecified leg   MCC

√5ᵗʰ **S85.8** Injury of other blood vessels at lower leg level

> **CC Excl: For CC codes in subcategory S85.8:**
> **Right side:** PDX collection 1325
> **Left side:** PDX collection 1326
> **Unspecified side:** PDX collection 1327

√6ᵗʰ **S85.80** Unspecified injury of other blood vessels at lower leg level

√7ᵗʰ **S85.801** Unspecified injury of other blood vessels at lower leg level, right leg   CC

√7ᵗʰ **S85.802** Unspecified injury of other blood vessels at lower leg level, left leg   CC

√7ᵗʰ **S85.809** Unspecified injury of other blood vessels at lower leg level, unspecified leg   CC

√6ᵗʰ **S85.81** Laceration of other blood vessels at lower leg level

√7ᵗʰ **S85.811** Laceration of other blood vessels at lower leg level, right leg   CC

√7ᵗʰ **S85.812** Laceration of other blood vessels at lower leg level, left leg   CC

√7ᵗʰ **S85.819** Laceration of other blood vessels at lower leg level, unspecified leg   CC

√6ᵗʰ **S85.89** Other specified injury of other blood vessels at lower leg level

√7ᵗʰ **S85.891** Other specified injury of other blood vessels at lower leg level, right leg   CC

√7ᵗʰ **S85.892** Other specified injury of other blood vessels at lower leg level, left leg   CC

√7ᵗʰ **S85.899** Other specified injury of other blood vessels at lower leg level, unspecified leg   CC

√5ᵗʰ **S85.9** Injury of unspecified blood vessel at lower leg level

> **CC Excl: For CC codes in subcategory S85.9:**
> **Right side:** PDX collection 1325
> **Left side:** PDX collection 1326
> **Unspecified side:** PDX collection 1327

√6ᵗʰ **S85.90** Unspecified injury of unspecified blood vessel at lower leg level

√7ᵗʰ **S85.901** Unspecified injury of unspecified blood vessel at lower leg level, right leg   CC

√7ᵗʰ **S85.902** Unspecified injury of unspecified blood vessel at lower leg level, left leg   CC

√7ᵗʰ **S85.909** Unspecified injury of unspecified blood vessel at lower leg level, unspecified leg   CC

√6ᵗʰ **S85.91** Laceration of unspecified blood vessel at lower leg level

√7ᵗʰ **S85.911** Laceration of unspecified blood vessel at lower leg level, right leg   CC

√7ᵗʰ **S85.912** Laceration of unspecified blood vessel at lower leg level, left leg   CC

√7ᵗʰ **S85.919** Laceration of unspecified blood vessel at lower leg level, unspecified leg   CC

√6ᵗʰ **S85.99** Other specified injury of unspecified blood vessel at lower leg level

√7ᵗʰ **S85.991** Other specified injury of unspecified blood vessel at lower leg level, right leg   CC

√7ᵗʰ **S85.992** Other specified injury of unspecified blood vessel at lower leg level, left leg   CC

√7ᵗʰ **S85.999** Other specified injury of unspecified blood vessel at lower leg level, unspecified leg   CC

√4ᵗʰ **S86 Injury of muscle, fascia and tendon at lower leg level**

Code also any associated open wound (S81.-)

*EXCLUDES 2* injury of muscle, fascia and tendon at ankle (S96.-)
injury of patellar ligament (tendon) (S76.1-)
sprain of joints and ligaments of knee (S83.-)

**TIP:** Refer to the Muscle/Tendon table at the beginning of this chapter

> The appropriate 7th character is to be added to each code from category S86.
> A    initial encounter
> D    subsequent encounter
> S    sequela

> **CC Excl: For CC codes in category S86:**
> **Right side:** PDX collection 1364
> **Left side:** PDX collection 1365
> **Unspecified side:** PDX collection 1366

√5ᵗʰ **S86.0** Injury of Achilles tendon

√6ᵗʰ **S86.00** Unspecified injury of Achilles tendon

√7ᵗʰ **S86.001** Unspecified injury of right Achilles tendon

√7ᵗʰ **S86.002** Unspecified injury of left Achilles tendon

✓ Additional Character Req   √x7ᵗʰ Placeholder Alert   Unacceptable PDx   Manifestation   H1-H14 HAC   HCC CMS-HCC Condition   *EXCLUDES 1* Not Coded Here   *EXCLUDES 2* Not Included Here

ICD-10-CM 2018     1059

√7ᵗʰ **S86.009** Unspecified injury of **unspecified** Achilles tendon

√6ᵗʰ **S86.01** **Strain** of Achilles tendon

    √7ᵗʰ **S86.011** **Strain** of **right** Achilles tendon

    √7ᵗʰ **S86.012** **Strain** of **left** Achilles tendon

    √7ᵗʰ **S86.019** **Strain** of **unspecified** Achilles tendon

√6ᵗʰ **S86.02** **Laceration** of Achilles tendon

    √7ᵗʰ **S86.021** **Laceration** of **right** Achilles tendon   CC

    √7ᵗʰ **S86.022** **Laceration** of **left** Achilles tendon   CC

    √7ᵗʰ **S86.029** **Laceration** of **unspecified** Achilles tendon   CC

√6ᵗʰ **S86.09** **Other specified** injury of Achilles tendon

    √7ᵗʰ **S86.091** **Other specified** injury of **right** Achilles tendon

    √7ᵗʰ **S86.092** **Other specified** injury of **left** Achilles tendon

    √7ᵗʰ **S86.099** **Other specified** injury of **unspecified** Achilles tendon

√5ᵗʰ **S86.1** **Injury of other muscle(s) and tendon(s) of posterior muscle group at lower leg level**

√6ᵗʰ **S86.10** **Unspecified** injury of other muscle(s) and tendon(s) of posterior muscle group at lower leg level

    √7ᵗʰ **S86.101** Unspecified injury of other muscle(s) and tendon(s) of posterior muscle group at lower leg level, **right leg**

    √7ᵗʰ **S86.102** Unspecified injury of other muscle(s) and tendon(s) of posterior muscle group at lower leg level, **left leg**

    √7ᵗʰ **S86.109** Unspecified injury of other muscle(s) and tendon(s) of posterior muscle group at lower leg level, **unspecified leg**

√6ᵗʰ **S86.11** **Strain** of other muscle(s) and tendon(s) of posterior muscle group at lower leg level

    √7ᵗʰ **S86.111** Strain of other muscle(s) and tendon(s) of posterior muscle group at lower leg level, **right leg**

    √7ᵗʰ **S86.112** Strain of other muscle(s) and tendon(s) of posterior muscle group at lower leg level, **left leg**

    √7ᵗʰ **S86.119** Strain of other muscle(s) and tendon(s) of posterior muscle group at lower leg level, **unspecified leg**

√6ᵗʰ **S86.12** **Laceration** of other muscle(s) and tendon(s) of posterior muscle group at lower leg level

    √7ᵗʰ **S86.121** Laceration of other muscle(s) and tendon(s) of posterior muscle group at lower leg level, **right leg**   CC

    √7ᵗʰ **S86.122** Laceration of other muscle(s) and tendon(s) of posterior muscle group at lower leg level, **left leg**   CC

    √7ᵗʰ **S86.129** Laceration of other muscle(s) and tendon(s) of posterior muscle group at lower leg level, **unspecified leg**   CC

√6ᵗʰ **S86.19** **Other** injury of other muscle(s) and tendon(s) of posterior muscle group at lower leg level

    √7ᵗʰ **S86.191** Other injury of other muscle(s) and tendon(s) of posterior muscle group at lower leg level, **right leg**

    √7ᵗʰ **S86.192** Other injury of other muscle(s) and tendon(s) of posterior muscle group at lower leg level, **left leg**

    √7ᵗʰ **S86.199** Other injury of other muscle(s) and tendon(s) of posterior muscle group at lower leg level, **unspecified leg**

√5ᵗʰ **S86.2** **Injury of muscle(s) and tendon(s) of anterior muscle group at lower leg level**

√6ᵗʰ **S86.20** **Unspecified** injury of muscle(s) and tendon(s) of anterior muscle group at lower leg level

    √7ᵗʰ **S86.201** Unspecified injury of muscle(s) and tendon(s) of anterior muscle group at lower leg level, **right leg**

    √7ᵗʰ **S86.202** Unspecified injury of muscle(s) and tendon(s) of anterior muscle group at lower leg level, **left leg**

√7ᵗʰ **S86.209** Unspecified injury of muscle(s) and tendon(s) of anterior muscle group at lower leg level, **unspecified leg**

√6ᵗʰ **S86.21** **Strain** of muscle(s) and tendon(s) of anterior muscle group at lower leg level

    √7ᵗʰ **S86.211** Strain of muscle(s) and tendon(s) of anterior muscle group at lower leg level, **right leg**

    √7ᵗʰ **S86.212** Strain of muscle(s) and tendon(s) of anterior muscle group at lower leg level, **left leg**

    √7ᵗʰ **S86.219** Strain of muscle(s) and tendon(s) of anterior muscle group at lower leg level, **unspecified leg**

√6ᵗʰ **S86.22** **Laceration** of muscle(s) and tendon(s) of anterior muscle group at lower leg level

    √7ᵗʰ **S86.221** Laceration of muscle(s) and tendon(s) of anterior muscle group at lower leg level, **right leg**   CC

    √7ᵗʰ **S86.222** Laceration of muscle(s) and tendon(s) of anterior muscle group at lower leg level, **left leg**   CC

    √7ᵗʰ **S86.229** Laceration of muscle(s) and tendon(s) of anterior muscle group at lower leg level, **unspecified leg**   CC

√6ᵗʰ **S86.29** **Other** injury of muscle(s) and tendon(s) of anterior muscle group at lower leg level

    √7ᵗʰ **S86.291** Other injury of muscle(s) and tendon(s) of anterior muscle group at lower leg level, **right leg**

    √7ᵗʰ **S86.292** Other injury of muscle(s) and tendon(s) of anterior muscle group at lower leg level, **left leg**

    √7ᵗʰ **S86.299** Other injury of muscle(s) and tendon(s) of anterior muscle group at lower leg level, **unspecified leg**

√5ᵗʰ **S86.3** **Injury of muscle(s) and tendon(s) of peroneal muscle group at lower leg level**

√6ᵗʰ **S86.30** **Unspecified** injury of muscle(s) and tendon(s) of peroneal muscle group at lower leg level

    √7ᵗʰ **S86.301** Unspecified injury of muscle(s) and tendon(s) of peroneal muscle group at lower leg level, **right leg**

    √7ᵗʰ **S86.302** Unspecified injury of muscle(s) and tendon(s) of peroneal muscle group at lower leg level, **left leg**

    √7ᵗʰ **S86.309** Unspecified injury of muscle(s) and tendon(s) of peroneal muscle group at lower leg level, **unspecified leg**

√6ᵗʰ **S86.31** **Strain** of muscle(s) and tendon(s) of peroneal muscle group at lower leg level

    √7ᵗʰ **S86.311** Strain of muscle(s) and tendon(s) of peroneal muscle group at lower leg level, **right leg**

    √7ᵗʰ **S86.312** Strain of muscle(s) and tendon(s) of peroneal muscle group at lower leg level, **left leg**

    √7ᵗʰ **S86.319** Strain of muscle(s) and tendon(s) of peroneal muscle group at lower leg level, **unspecified leg**

√6ᵗʰ **S86.32** **Laceration** of muscle(s) and tendon(s) of peroneal muscle group at lower leg level

    √7ᵗʰ **S86.321** Laceration of muscle(s) and tendon(s) of peroneal muscle group at lower leg level, **right leg**   CC

    √7ᵗʰ **S86.322** Laceration of muscle(s) and tendon(s) of peroneal muscle group at lower leg level, **left leg**   CC

    √7ᵗʰ **S86.329** Laceration of muscle(s) and tendon(s) of peroneal muscle group at lower leg level, **unspecified leg**   CC

√6ᵗʰ **S86.39** **Other** injury of muscle(s) and tendon(s) of peroneal muscle group at lower leg level

    √7ᵗʰ **S86.391** Other injury of muscle(s) and tendon(s) of peroneal muscle group at lower leg level, **right leg**

N Newborn: 0   P Pediatric: 0-17   M Maternity: 12-55   A Adult: 15-124   **MCC** Major CC Condition   **PDx MCC** PDx acts as own MCC   **CC** CC Condition   **PDx CC** PDx acts as own CC

**1060**      ICD-10-CM 2018

√7ᵗʰ **S86.392** **Other injury of muscle(s) and tendon(s) of peroneal muscle group at lower leg level, left leg**

√7ᵗʰ **S86.399** **Other injury of muscle(s) and tendon(s) of peroneal muscle group at lower leg level, unspecified leg**

√5ᵗʰ **S86.8** **Injury of other muscles and tendons at lower leg level**

√6ᵗʰ **S86.80** **Unspecified injury of other muscles and tendons at lower leg level**

√7ᵗʰ **S86.801** **Unspecified injury of other muscle(s) and tendon(s) at lower leg level, right leg**

√7ᵗʰ **S86.802** **Unspecified injury of other muscle(s) and tendon(s) at lower leg level, left leg**

√7ᵗʰ **S86.809** **Unspecified injury of other muscle(s) and tendon(s) at lower leg level, unspecified leg**

√6ᵗʰ **S86.81** **Strain of other muscles and tendons at lower leg level**

√7ᵗʰ **S86.811** **Strain of other muscle(s) and tendon(s) at lower leg level, right leg**

√7ᵗʰ **S86.812** **Strain of other muscle(s) and tendon(s) at lower leg level, left leg**

√7ᵗʰ **S86.819** **Strain of other muscle(s) and tendon(s) at lower leg level, unspecified leg**

√6ᵗʰ **S86.82** **Laceration of other muscles and tendons at lower leg level**

√7ᵗʰ **S86.821** **Laceration of other muscle(s) and tendon(s) at lower leg level, right leg** `CC`

√7ᵗʰ **S86.822** **Laceration of other muscle(s) and tendon(s) at lower leg level, left leg** `CC`

√7ᵗʰ **S86.829** **Laceration of other muscle(s) and tendon(s) at lower leg level, unspecified leg** `CC`

√6ᵗʰ **S86.89** **Other injury of other muscles and tendons at lower leg level**

√7ᵗʰ **S86.891** **Other injury of other muscle(s) and tendon(s) at lower leg level, right leg**

√7ᵗʰ **S86.892** **Other injury of other muscle(s) and tendon(s) at lower leg level, left leg**

√7ᵗʰ **S86.899** **Other injury of other muscle(s) and tendon(s) at lower leg level, unspecified leg**

√5ᵗʰ **S86.9** **Injury of unspecified muscle and tendon at lower leg level**

√6ᵗʰ **S86.90** **Unspecified injury of unspecified muscle and tendon at lower leg level**

√7ᵗʰ **S86.901** **Unspecified injury of unspecified muscle(s) and tendon(s) at lower leg level, right leg**

√7ᵗʰ **S86.902** **Unspecified injury of unspecified muscle(s) and tendon(s) at lower leg level, left leg**

√7ᵗʰ **S86.909** **Unspecified injury of unspecified muscle(s) and tendon(s) at lower leg level, unspecified leg**

√6ᵗʰ **S86.91** **Strain of unspecified muscle and tendon at lower leg level**

√7ᵗʰ **S86.911** **Strain of unspecified muscle(s) and tendon(s) at lower leg level, right leg**

√7ᵗʰ **S86.912** **Strain of unspecified muscle(s) and tendon(s) at lower leg level, left leg**

√7ᵗʰ **S86.919** **Strain of unspecified muscle(s) and tendon(s) at lower leg level, unspecified leg**

√6ᵗʰ **S86.92** **Laceration of unspecified muscle and tendon at lower leg level**

√7ᵗʰ **S86.921** **Laceration of unspecified muscle(s) and tendon(s) at lower leg level, right leg** `CC`

√7ᵗʰ **S86.922** **Laceration of unspecified muscle(s) and tendon(s) at lower leg level, left leg** `CC`

√7ᵗʰ **S86.929** **Laceration of unspecified muscle(s) and tendon(s) at lower leg level, unspecified leg** `CC`

√6ᵗʰ **S86.99** **Other injury of unspecified muscle and tendon at lower leg level**

√7ᵗʰ **S86.991** **Other injury of unspecified muscle(s) and tendon(s) at lower leg level, right leg**

√7ᵗʰ **S86.992** **Other injury of unspecified muscle(s) and tendon(s) at lower leg level, left leg**

√7ᵗʰ **S86.999** **Other injury of unspecified muscle(s) and tendon(s) at lower leg level, unspecified leg**

√4ᵗʰ **S87** **Crushing injury of lower leg**
Use additional code(s) for all associated injuries
*EXCLUDES 2*   crushing injury of ankle and foot (S97.-)

The appropriate 7th character is to be added to each code from category S87.
A   initial encounter
D   subsequent encounter
S   sequela

√5ᵗʰ **S87.0** **Crushing injury of knee**

√x7ᵗʰ **S87.00** **Crushing injury of unspecified knee**

√x7ᵗʰ **S87.01** **Crushing injury of right knee**

√x7ᵗʰ **S87.02** **Crushing injury of left knee**

√5ᵗʰ **S87.8** **Crushing injury of lower leg**

√x7ᵗʰ **S87.80** **Crushing injury of unspecified lower leg**

√x7ᵗʰ **S87.81** **Crushing injury of right lower leg**

√x7ᵗʰ **S87.82** **Crushing injury of left lower leg**

√4ᵗʰ **S88** **Traumatic amputation of lower leg**
An amputation not identified as partial or complete should be coded to complete.
*EXCLUDES 1*   traumatic amputation of ankle and foot (S98.-)

The appropriate 7th character is to be added to each code from category S88.
A   initial encounter
D   subsequent encounter
S   sequela

**CC Excl: For CC codes in category S88:**
**Right side:** PDX collection 1333
**Left side:** PDX collection 1334
**Unspecified side:** PDX collection 1335

√5ᵗʰ **S88.0** **Traumatic amputation at knee level**

√6ᵗʰ **S88.01** **Complete traumatic amputation at knee level**

√7ᵗʰ **S88.011** **Complete traumatic amputation at knee level, right lower leg** `CC` `HCC`

√7ᵗʰ **S88.012** **Complete traumatic amputation at knee level, left lower leg** `CC` `HCC`

√7ᵗʰ **S88.019** **Complete traumatic amputation at knee level, unspecified lower leg** `CC` `HCC`

√6ᵗʰ **S88.02** **Partial traumatic amputation at knee level**

√7ᵗʰ **S88.021** **Partial traumatic amputation at knee level, right lower leg** `CC` `HCC`

√7ᵗʰ **S88.022** **Partial traumatic amputation at knee level, left lower leg** `CC` `HCC`

√7ᵗʰ **S88.029** **Partial traumatic amputation at knee level, unspecified lower leg** `CC` `HCC`

√5ᵗʰ **S88.1** **Traumatic amputation at level between knee and ankle**

√6ᵗʰ **S88.11** **Complete traumatic amputation at level between knee and ankle**

√7ᵗʰ **S88.111** **Complete traumatic amputation at level between knee and ankle, right lower leg** `CC` `HCC`

√7ᵗʰ **S88.112** **Complete traumatic amputation at level between knee and ankle, left lower leg** `CC` `HCC`

√7ᵗʰ **S88.119** **Complete traumatic amputation at level between knee and ankle, unspecified lower leg** `CC` `HCC`

√6ᵗʰ **S88.12** **Partial traumatic amputation at level between knee and ankle**

√7ᵗʰ **S88.121** **Partial traumatic amputation at level between knee and ankle, right lower leg** `CC` `HCC`

√7ᵗʰ **S88.122** **Partial traumatic amputation at levelbetween knee and ankle, left lower leg** `CC` `HCC`

---

☑ Additional Character Req   √x7ᵗʰ Placeholder Alert   <u>Unacceptable PDx</u>   ▪ Manifestation   **H1**-**H14** HAC   `HCC` CMS-HCC Condition   *EXCLUDES 1* Not Coded Here   *EXCLUDES 2* Not Included Here

√7ᵗʰ **S88.129** **Partial traumatic amputation at** CC HCC
**level between knee and ankle,**
**unspecified lower leg**

√5ᵗʰ **S88.9** **Traumatic amputation of lower leg, level unspecified**

√6ᵗʰ **S88.91** **Complete traumatic amputation of lower leg, level unspecified**

√7ᵗʰ **S88.911** **Complete traumatic amputation** CC HCC
**of right lower leg, level unspecified**

√7ᵗʰ **S88.912** **Complete traumatic amputation** CC HCC
**of left lower leg, level unspecified**

√7ᵗʰ **S88.919** **Complete traumatic amputation** CC HCC
**of unspecified lower leg, level**
**unspecified**

√6ᵗʰ **S88.92** **Partial traumatic amputation of lower leg, level unspecified**

√7ᵗʰ **S88.921** **Partial traumatic amputation of** CC HCC
**right lower leg, level unspecified**

√7ᵗʰ **S88.922** **Partial traumatic amputation of** CC HCC
**left lower leg, level unspecified**

√7ᵗʰ **S88.929** **Partial traumatic amputation of** CC HCC
**unspecified lower leg, level unspecified**

√4ᵗʰ **S89** **Other and unspecified injuries of lower leg**

**NOTE** A fracture not indicated as open or closed should be coded to closed.

**EXCLUDES 2** *other and unspecified injuries of ankle and foot (S99.-)*
**AHA:** 2015, 3Q, 37-39

The appropriate 7th character is to be added to each code from subcategories S89.0, S89.1, S89.2, and S89.3.
A    initial encounter for closed fracture
D    subsequent encounter for fracture with routine healing
G    subsequent encounter for fracture with delayed healing
K    subsequent encounter for fracture with nonunion
P    subsequent encounter for fracture with malunion
S    sequela

√5ᵗʰ **S89.0** **Physeal fracture of upper end of tibia**

**CC Excl: For CC codes in subcategory S89.0:**
**Right side:** See code S89.001
**Left side:** See code S89.002
**Unspecified side:** See code S89.009

√6ᵗʰ **S89.00** **Unspecified physeal fracture of upper end of tibia**

7 √7ᵗʰ **S89.001** **Unspecified physeal fracture of** CC H5
**upper end of right tibia**
**CC Excl: CC with 7th character A:**
PDX collection 1340
**CC with 7th character K or P:**
PDX collection 897

7 √7ᵗʰ **S89.002** **Unspecified physeal fracture of** CC H5
**upper end of left tibia**
**CC Excl: CC with 7th character A:**
PDX collection 1342
**CC with 7th character K or P:**
PDX collection 897

7 √7ᵗʰ **S89.009** **Unspecified physeal fracture of** CC H5
**upper end of unspecified tibia**
**CC Excl: CC with 7th character A:**
PDX collection 1341
**CC with 7th character K or P:**
PDX collection 897

√6ᵗʰ **S89.01** **Salter-Harris Type I physeal fracture of upper end of tibia**

7 √7ᵗʰ **S89.011** **Salter-Harris Type I physeal** CC H5
**fracture of upper end of right tibia**

7 √7ᵗʰ **S89.012** **Salter-Harris Type I physeal** CC H5
**fracture of upper end of left tibia**

7 √7ᵗʰ **S89.019** **Salter-Harris Type I physeal** CC H5
**fracture of upper end of unspecified tibia**

√6ᵗʰ **S89.02** **Salter-Harris Type II physeal fracture of upper end of tibia**

7 √7ᵗʰ **S89.021** **Salter-Harris Type II physeal** CC H5
**fracture of upper end of right tibia**

7 √7ᵗʰ **S89.022** **Salter-Harris Type II physeal** CC H5
**fracture of upper end of left tibia**

7 √7ᵗʰ **S89.029** **Salter-Harris Type II physeal** CC H5
**fracture of upper end of unspecified tibia**

√6ᵗʰ **S89.03** **Salter-Harris Type III physeal fracture of upper end of tibia**

7 √7ᵗʰ **S89.031** **Salter-Harris Type III physeal** CC H5
**fracture of upper end of right tibia**

7 √7ᵗʰ **S89.032** **Salter-Harris Type III physeal** CC H5
**fracture of upper end of left tibia**

7 √7ᵗʰ **S89.039** **Salter-Harris Type III physeal** CC H5
**fracture of upper end of unspecified tibia**

√6ᵗʰ **S89.04** **Salter-Harris Type IV physeal fracture of upper end of tibia**

7 √7ᵗʰ **S89.041** **Salter-Harris Type IV physeal** CC H5
**fracture of upper end of right tibia**

7 √7ᵗʰ **S89.042** **Salter-Harris Type IV physeal** CC H5
**fracture of upper end of left tibia**

7 √7ᵗʰ **S89.049** **Salter-Harris Type IV physeal** CC H5
**fracture of upper end of unspecified tibia**

√6ᵗʰ **S89.09** **Other physeal fracture of upper end of tibia**

7 √7ᵗʰ **S89.091** **Other physeal fracture of upper** CC H5
**end of right tibia**

7 √7ᵗʰ **S89.092** **Other physeal fracture of upper** CC H5
**end of left tibia**

7 √7ᵗʰ **S89.099** **Other physeal fracture of upper** CC H5
**end of unspecified tibia**

√5ᵗʰ **S89.1** **Physeal fracture of lower end of tibia**

**CC Excl: For codes in subcategory S89.1:**
**CC with 7th character K or P:** PDX collection 897

√6ᵗʰ **S89.10** **Unspecified physeal fracture of lower end of tibia**

8 √7ᵗʰ **S89.101** **Unspecified physeal fracture of lower** CC
**end of right tibia**

8 √7ᵗʰ **S89.102** **Unspecified physeal fracture of lower** CC
**end of left tibia**

8 √7ᵗʰ **S89.109** **Unspecified physeal fracture of lower** CC
**end of unspecified tibia**

√6ᵗʰ **S89.11** **Salter-Harris Type I physeal fracture of ower end of tibia**

8 √7ᵗʰ **S89.111** **Salter-Harris Type I physeal fracture of** CC
**lower end of right tibia**

8 √7ᵗʰ **S89.112** **Salter-Harris Type I physeal fracture** CC
**oflower end of left tibia**

8 √7ᵗʰ **S89.119** **Salter-Harris Type I physeal fracture** CC
**of lower end of unspecified tibia**

√6ᵗʰ **S89.12** **Salter-Harris Type II physeal fracture of lower end of tibia**

8 √7ᵗʰ **S89.121** **Salter-Harris Type II physeal fracture** CC
**of lower end of right tibia**

8 √7ᵗʰ **S89.122** **Salter-Harris Type II physeal fracture** CC
**of lower end of left tibia**

8 √7ᵗʰ **S89.129** **Salter-Harris Type II physeal fracture** CC
**of lower end of unspecified tibia**

√6ᵗʰ **S89.13** **Salter-Harris Type III physeal fracture of lower end of tibia**

**EXCLUDES 1** *fracture of medial malleolus (adult) (S82.5-)*

8 √7ᵗʰ **S89.131** **Salter-Harris Type III physeal fracture** CC
**of lower end of right tibia**

8 √7ᵗʰ **S89.132** **Salter-Harris Type III physeal fracture** CC
**of lower end of left tibia**

8 √7ᵗʰ **S89.139** **Salter-Harris Type III physeal fracture** CC
**of lower end of unspecified tibia**

√6ᵗʰ **S89.14** **Salter-Harris Type IV physeal fracture of lower end of tibia**

**EXCLUDES 1** *fracture of medial malleolus (adult) (S82.5-)*

8 √7ᵗʰ **S89.141** **Salter-Harris Type IV physeal fracture** CC
**oflower end of right tibia**

8 √7ᵗʰ **S89.142** **Salter-Harris Type IV physeal fracture** CC
**of lower end of left tibia**

8 √7ᵗʰ **S89.149** **Salter-Harris Type IV physeal fracture** CC
**of lower end of unspecified tibia**

√6ᵗʰ **S89.19** **Other physeal fracture of lower end of tibia**

8 √7ᵗʰ **S89.191** **Other physeal fracture of lower end** CC
**of right tibia**

8 √7ᵗʰ **S89.192** **Other physeal fracture of lower end** CC
**of left tibia**

---

7   CC when reported as an initial encounter (7th character A, B, or C – specific to category) OR a subsequent encounter for nonunion or malunion (7th character K, M, N, P, Q, or R – specific to category).

8   CC when reported as a subsequent encounter for nonunion or malunion (7th character K, M, N, P, Q, or R – specific to category).

N Newborn: 0   P Pediatric: 0-17   M Maternity: 12-55   A Adult: 15-124   MCC Major CC Condition   PDxMCC PDx acts as own MCC   CC CC Condition   PDxCC PDx acts as own CC

**1062**     ICD-10-CM 2018

8 ✓7ᵗʰ **S89.199 Other physeal fracture of lower end** CC
of **unspecified** tibia

✓5ᵗʰ **S89.2 Physeal fracture of upper end of fibula**

**CC Excl: For codes in subcategory S89.2:**
**CC with 7th character K or P:** PDX collection 897

✓6ᵗʰ **S89.20 Unspecified physeal fracture of upper end of fibula**
8 ✓7ᵗʰ **S89.201 Unspecified physeal fracture of upper** CC
end of **right** fibula
8 ✓7ᵗʰ **S89.202 Unspecified physeal fracture of upper** CC
end of **left** fibula
8 ✓7ᵗʰ **S89.209 Unspecified physeal fracture of upper** CC
end of **unspecified** fibula

✓6ᵗʰ **S89.21 Salter-Harris Type I physeal fracture of upper end of**
**fibula**
8 ✓7ᵗʰ **S89.211 Salter-Harris Type I physeal fracture** CC
of upper end of **right** fibula
8 ✓7ᵗʰ **S89.212 Salter-Harris Type I physeal fracture** CC
of upper end of **left** fibula
8 ✓7ᵗʰ **S89.219 Salter-Harris Type I physeal fracture** CC
of upper end of **unspecified** fibula

✓6ᵗʰ **S89.22 Salter-Harris Type II physeal fracture of upper end of**
**fibula**
8 ✓7ᵗʰ **S89.221 Salter-Harris Type II physeal fracture** CC
of upper end of **right** fibula
8 ✓7ᵗʰ **S89.222 Salter-Harris Type II physeal fracture** CC
of upper end of **left** fibula
8 ✓7ᵗʰ **S89.229 Salter-Harris Type II physeal fracture** CC
of upper end of **unspecified** fibula

✓6ᵗʰ **S89.29 Other physeal fracture of upper end of fibula**
8 ✓7ᵗʰ **S89.291 Other physeal fracture of upper end** CC
of **right** fibula
8 ✓7ᵗʰ **S89.292 Other physeal fracture of upper end** CC
of **left** fibula
8 ✓7ᵗʰ **S89.299 Other physeal fracture of upper end** CC
of **unspecified** fibula

✓5ᵗʰ **S89.3 Physeal fracture of lower end of fibula**

**CC Excl: For codes in subcategory S89.3:**
**CC with 7th character K or P:** PDX collection 897

✓6ᵗʰ **S89.30 Unspecified physeal fracture of lower end of fibula**
8 ✓7ᵗʰ **S89.301 Unspecified physeal fracture of lower** CC
end of **right** fibula
8 ✓7ᵗʰ **S89.302 Unspecified physeal fracture of lower** CC
end of **left** fibula
8 ✓7ᵗʰ **S89.309 Unspecified physeal fracture of lower** CC
end of **unspecified** fibula

✓6ᵗʰ **S89.31 Salter-Harris Type I physeal fracture of lower end of**
**fibula**
8 ✓7ᵗʰ **S89.311 Salter-Harris Type I physeal fracture** CC
of lower end of **right** fibula
8 ✓7ᵗʰ **S89.312 Salter-Harris Type I physeal fracture** CC
of lower end of **left** fibula
8 ✓7ᵗʰ **S89.319 Salter-Harris Type I physeal fracture** CC
of lower end of **unspecified** fibula

✓6ᵗʰ **S89.32 Salter-Harris Type II physeal fracture of lower end of**
**fibula**
8 ✓7ᵗʰ **S89.321 Salter-Harris Type II physeal fracture** CC
of lower end of **right** fibula
8 ✓7ᵗʰ **S89.322 Salter-Harris Type II physeal fracture** CC
of lower end of **left** fibula
8 ✓7ᵗʰ **S89.329 Salter-Harris Type II physeal fracture** CC
of lower end of **unspecified** fibula

✓6ᵗʰ **S89.39 Other physeal fracture of lower end of fibula**
8 ✓7ᵗʰ **S89.391 Other physeal fracture of lower end of** CC
**right** fibula
8 ✓7ᵗʰ **S89.392 Other physeal fracture of lower end of** CC
**left** fibula
8 ✓7ᵗʰ **S89.399 Other physeal fracture of lower end of** CC
**unspecified** fibula

✓5ᵗʰ **S89.8 Other specified injuries of lower leg**

The appropriate 7th character is to be added to each code
in subcategory S89.8.
A    initial encounter
D    subsequent encounter
S    sequela

✓x7ᵗʰ **S89.80 Other specified injuries of unspecified lower leg**
✓x7ᵗʰ **S89.81 Other specified injuries of right lower leg**
✓x7ᵗʰ **S89.82 Other specified injuries of left lower leg**

✓5ᵗʰ **S89.9 Unspecified injury of lower leg**

The appropriate 7th character is to be added to each code
in subcategory S89.9.
A    initial encounter
D    subsequent encounter
S    sequela

✓x7ᵗʰ **S89.90 Unspecified injury of unspecified lower leg**
✓x7ᵗʰ **S89.91 Unspecified injury of right lower leg**
✓x7ᵗʰ **S89.92 Unspecified injury of left lower leg**

## Injuries to the ankle and foot (S90-S99)

EXCLUDES 2 *burns and corrosions (T20-T32)*
*fracture of ankle and malleolus (S82.-)*
*frostbite (T33-T34)*
*insect bite or sting, venomous (T63.4)*

✓4ᵗʰ **S90 Superficial injury of ankle, foot and toes**

The appropriate 7th character is to be added to each code from
category S90.
A    initial encounter
D    subsequent encounter
S    sequela

✓5ᵗʰ **S90.0 Contusion of ankle**
✓x7ᵗʰ **S90.00 Contusion of unspecified ankle**
✓x7ᵗʰ **S90.01 Contusion of right ankle**
✓x7ᵗʰ **S90.02 Contusion of left ankle**

✓5ᵗʰ **S90.1 Contusion of toe without damage to nail**
✓6ᵗʰ **S90.11 Contusion of great toe without damage to nail**
✓7ᵗʰ **S90.111 Contusion of right great toe without**
**damage to nail**
✓7ᵗʰ **S90.112 Contusion of left great toe without**
**damage to nail**
✓7ᵗʰ **S90.119 Contusion of unspecified great toe**
**without damage to nail**

✓6ᵗʰ **S90.12 Contusion of lesser toe without damage to nail**
✓7ᵗʰ **S90.121 Contusion of right lesser toe(s) without**
**damage to nail**
✓7ᵗʰ **S90.122 Contusion of left lesser toe(s) without**
**damage to nail**
✓7ᵗʰ **S90.129 Contusion of unspecified lesser toe(s)**
**without damage to nail**
Contusion of toe NOS

✓5ᵗʰ **S90.2 Contusion of toe with damage to nail**
✓6ᵗʰ **S90.21 Contusion of great toe with damage to nail**
✓7ᵗʰ **S90.211 Contusion of right great toe with damage**
**to nail**
✓7ᵗʰ **S90.212 Contusion of left great toe with damage**
**to nail**
✓7ᵗʰ **S90.219 Contusion of unspecified great toe with**
**damage to nail**

✓6ᵗʰ **S90.22 Contusion of lesser toe with damage to nail**
✓7ᵗʰ **S90.221 Contusion of right lesser toe(s) with**
**damage to nail**
✓7ᵗʰ **S90.222 Contusion of left lesser toe(s) with**
**damage to nail**
✓7ᵗʰ **S90.229 Contusion of unspecified lesser toe(s) with**
**damage to nail**

✓5ᵗʰ **S90.3 Contusion of foot**
EXCLUDES 2 *contusion of toes (S90.1-, S90.2-)*
✓x7ᵗʰ **S90.30 Contusion of unspecified foot**
Contusion of foot NOS
✓x7ᵗʰ **S90.31 Contusion of right foot**

---

8    CC when reported as a subsequent encounter for nonunion or malunion (7th character K, M, N, P, Q, or R – specific to category).

---

✓Additional Character Req | ✓x7ᵗʰ Placeholder Alert | Unacceptable PDx | Manifestation | **H1**-**H14** HAC | **HCC** CMS-HCC Condition | EXCLUDES 1 Not Coded Here | EXCLUDES 2 Not Included Here

**Chapter 19. Injury, Poisoning and Certain Other Consequences of External Causes**

√x7th **S90.32**   **Contusion of** left **foot**

√5th **S90.4**   **Other superficial injuries of toe**

√6th   **S90.41**   **Abrasion of toe**

√7th   **S90.411**   **Abrasion,** right great **toe**

√7th   **S90.412**   **Abrasion,** left great **toe**

√7th   **S90.413**   **Abrasion,** unspecified great **toe**

√7th   **S90.414**   **Abrasion,** right lesser **toe(s)**

√7th   **S90.415**   **Abrasion,** left lesser **toe(s)**

√7th   **S90.416**   **Abrasion,** unspecified lesser **toe(s)**

√6th   **S90.42**   **Blister (nonthermal) of toe**

√7th   **S90.421**   **Blister (nonthermal),** right great **toe**

√7th   **S90.422**   **Blister (nonthermal),** left great **toe**

√7th   **S90.423**   **Blister (nonthermal),** unspecified great **toe**

√7th   **S90.424**   **Blister (nonthermal),** right lesser **toe(s)**

√7th   **S90.425**   **Blister (nonthermal),** left lesser **toe(s)**

√7th   **S90.426**   **Blister (nonthermal),** unspecified lesser **toe(s)**

√6th   **S90.44**   **External constriction of toe**
Hair tourniquet syndrome of toe

√7th   **S90.441**   **External constriction,** right great **toe**

√7th   **S90.442**   **External constriction,** left great **toe**

√7th   **S90.443**   **External constriction,** unspecified great **toe**

√7th   **S90.444**   **External constriction,** right lesser **toe(s)**

√7th   **S90.445**   **External constriction,** left lesser **toe(s)**

√7th   **S90.446**   **External constriction,** unspecified lesser **toe(s)**

√6th   **S90.45**   **Superficial** foreign body **of toe**
Splinter in the toe

√7th   **S90.451**   **Superficial foreign body,** right great **toe**

√7th   **S90.452**   **Superficial foreign body,** left great **toe**

√7th   **S90.453**   **Superficial foreign body,** unspecified great **toe**

√7th   **S90.454**   **Superficial foreign body,** right lesser **toe(s)**

√7th   **S90.455**   **Superficial foreign body,** left lesser **toe(s)**

√7th   **S90.456**   **Superficial foreign body,** unspecified lesser **toe(s)**

√6th   **S90.46**   **Insect bite (nonvenomous) of toe**

√7th   **S90.461**   **Insect bite (nonvenomous),** right great **toe**

√7th   **S90.462**   **Insect bite (nonvenomous),** left great **toe**

√7th   **S90.463**   **Insect bite (nonvenomous),** unspecified great **toe**

√7th   **S90.464**   **Insect bite (nonvenomous),** right lesser **toe(s)**

√7th   **S90.465**   **Insect bite (nonvenomous),** left lesser **toe(s)**

√7th   **S90.466**   **Insect bite (nonvenomous),** unspecified lesser **toe(s)**

√6th   **S90.47**   **Other superficial** bite **of toe**
**EXCLUDES 1**   *open bite of toe (S91.15-, S91.25-)*

√7th   **S90.471**   **Other superficial bite of** right great **toe**

√7th   **S90.472**   **Other superficial bite of** left great **toe**

√7th   **S90.473**   **Other superficial bite of** unspecified great **toe**

√7th   **S90.474**   **Other superficial bite of** right lesser **toe(s)**

√7th   **S90.475**   **Other superficial bite of** left lesser **toe(s)**

√7th   **S90.476**   **Other superficial bite of** unspecified lesser **toe(s)**

√5th **S90.5**   **Other superficial injuries of ankle**

√6th   **S90.51**   **Abrasion of ankle**

√7th   **S90.511**   **Abrasion,** right ankle

√7th   **S90.512**   **Abrasion,** left ankle

√7th   **S90.519**   **Abrasion,** unspecified ankle

√6th   **S90.52**   **Blister (nonthermal) of ankle**

√7th   **S90.521**   **Blister (nonthermal),** right ankle

√7th   **S90.522**   **Blister (nonthermal),** left ankle

√7th   **S90.529**   **Blister (nonthermal),** unspecified ankle

√6th   **S90.54**   **External constriction of ankle**

√7th   **S90.541**   **External constriction,** right ankle

√7th   **S90.542**   **External constriction,** left ankle

√7th   **S90.549**   **External constriction,** unspecified ankle

√6th   **S90.55**   **Superficial** foreign body **of ankle**
Splinter in the ankle

√7th   **S90.551**   **Superficial foreign body,** right ankle

√7th   **S90.552**   **Superficial foreign body,** left ankle

√7th   **S90.559**   **Superficial foreign body,** unspecified ankle

√6th   **S90.56**   **Insect bite (nonvenomous) of ankle**

√7th   **S90.561**   **Insect bite (nonvenomous),** right ankle

√7th   **S90.562**   **Insect bite (nonvenomous),** left ankle

√7th   **S90.569**   **Insect bite (nonvenomous),** unspecified ankle

√6th   **S90.57**   **Other** superficial bite **of ankle**
**EXCLUDES 1**   *open bite of ankle (S91.05-)*

√7th   **S90.571**   **Other superficial bite of ankle,** right ankle

√7th   **S90.572**   **Other superficial bite of ankle,** left ankle

√7th   **S90.579**   **Other superficial bite of ankle,** unspecified ankle

√5th **S90.8**   **Other superficial injuries of** foot

√6th   **S90.81**   **Abrasion of foot**

√7th   **S90.811**   **Abrasion,** right **foot**

√7th   **S90.812**   **Abrasion,** left **foot**

√7th   **S90.819**   **Abrasion,** unspecified **foot**

√6th   **S90.82**   **Blister (nonthermal) of foot**

√7th   **S90.821**   **Blister (nonthermal),** right **foot**

√7th   **S90.822**   **Blister (nonthermal),** left **foot**

√7th   **S90.829**   **Blister (nonthermal),** unspecified **foot**

√6th   **S90.84**   **External constriction of foot**

√7th   **S90.841**   **External constriction,** right **foot**

√7th   **S90.842**   **External constriction,** left **foot**

√7th   **S90.849**   **External constriction,** unspecified **foot**

√6th   **S90.85**   **Superficial** foreign body **of foot**
Splinter in the foot

√7th   **S90.851**   **Superficial foreign body,** right **foot**

√7th   **S90.852**   **Superficial foreign body,** left **foot**

√7th   **S90.859**   **Superficial foreign body,** unspecified **foot**

√6th   **S90.86**   **Insect bite (nonvenomous) of foot**

√7th   **S90.861**   **Insect bite (nonvenomous),** right **foot**

√7th   **S90.862**   **Insect bite (nonvenomous),** left **foot**

√7th   **S90.869**   **Insect bite (nonvenomous),** unspecified **foot**

√6th   **S90.87**   **Other** superficial bite **of foot**
**EXCLUDES 1**   *open bite of foot (S91.35-)*

√7th   **S90.871**   **Other superficial bite of** right **foot**

√7th   **S90.872**   **Other superficial bite of** left **foot**

√7th   **S90.879**   **Other superficial bite of** unspecified **foot**

√5th **S90.9**   **Unspecified superficial injury of** ankle, foot and toe

√6th   **S90.91**   **Unspecified superficial injury of** ankle

√7th   **S90.911**   **Unspecified superficial injury of** right ankle

√7th   **S90.912**   **Unspecified superficial injury of** left ankle

√7th   **S90.919**   **Unspecified superficial injury of** unspecified ankle

√6th   **S90.92**   **Unspecified superficial injury of** foot

√7th   **S90.921**   **Unspecified superficial injury of** right foot

√7th   **S90.922**   **Unspecified superficial injury of** left foot

√7th   **S90.929**   **Unspecified superficial injury of** unspecified **foot**

√6th   **S90.93**   **Unspecified superficial injury of** toes

√7th   **S90.931**   **Unspecified superficial injury of** right great **toe**

√7th   **S90.932**   **Unspecified superficial injury of** left great **toe**

√7th   **S90.933**   **Unspecified superficial injury of** unspecified great **toe**

√7th   **S90.934**   **Unspecified superficial injury of** right lesser **toe(s)**

√7th   **S90.935**   **Unspecified superficial injury of** left lesser **toe(s)**

N Newborn: 0   P Pediatric: 0-17   M Maternity: 12-55   A Adult: 15-124   MCC Major CC Condition   PDx MCC PDx acts as own MCC   CC CC Condition   PDx CC PDx acts as own CC

**1064**

ICD-10-CM 2018

√7ᵗʰ **S90.936** Unspecified superficial injury of unspecified lesser **toe(s)**

√4ᵗʰ **S91** **Open wound of ankle, foot and toes**

Code also any associated wound infection

EXCLUDES 1 open fracture of ankle, foot and toes (S92-with 7th B)
traumatic amputation of ankle and foot (S98.-)

The appropriate 7th character is to be added to each code from category S91.
A    initial encounter
D    subsequent encounter
S    sequela

√5ᵗʰ **S91.0** **Open wound of ankle**

√6ᵗʰ **S91.00** Unspecified **open wound of ankle**

√7ᵗʰ **S91.001** Unspecified open wound, **right** ankle

√7ᵗʰ **S91.002** Unspecified open wound, **left** ankle

√7ᵗʰ **S91.009** Unspecified open wound, **unspecified** ankle

√6ᵗʰ **S91.01** Laceration without foreign body **of ankle**

√7ᵗʰ **S91.011** Laceration without foreign body, **right** ankle

√7ᵗʰ **S91.012** Laceration without foreign body, **left** ankle

√7ᵗʰ **S91.019** Laceration without foreign body, **unspecified** ankle

√6ᵗʰ **S91.02** Laceration with foreign body **of ankle**

√7ᵗʰ **S91.021** Laceration with foreign body, **right** ankle

√7ᵗʰ **S91.022** Laceration with foreign body, **left** ankle

√7ᵗʰ **S91.029** Laceration with foreign body, **unspecified** ankle

√6ᵗʰ **S91.03** Puncture wound without foreign body **of ankle**

√7ᵗʰ **S91.031** Puncture wound without foreign body, **right** ankle

√7ᵗʰ **S91.032** Puncture wound without foreign body, **left** ankle

√7ᵗʰ **S91.039** Puncture wound without foreign body, **unspecified** ankle

√6ᵗʰ **S91.04** Puncture wound with foreign body **of ankle**

√7ᵗʰ **S91.041** Puncture wound with foreign body, **right** ankle

√7ᵗʰ **S91.042** Puncture wound with foreign body, **left** ankle

√7ᵗʰ **S91.049** Puncture wound with foreign body, **unspecified** ankle

√6ᵗʰ **S91.05** Open bite **of ankle**

EXCLUDES 1 superficial bite of ankle (S90.56-, S90.57-)

√7ᵗʰ **S91.051** Open bite, **right** ankle

√7ᵗʰ **S91.052** Open bite, **left** ankle

√7ᵗʰ **S91.059** Open bite, **unspecified** ankle

√5ᵗʰ **S91.1** **Open wound of toe without damage to nail**

√6ᵗʰ **S91.10** Unspecified **open wound of toe without damage to nail**

√7ᵗʰ **S91.101** Unspecified open wound of **right great** **toe** without damage to nail

√7ᵗʰ **S91.102** Unspecified open wound of **left great** **toe** without damage to nail

√7ᵗʰ **S91.103** Unspecified open wound of **unspecified great** toe without damage to nail

√7ᵗʰ **S91.104** Unspecified open wound of **right lesser** toe(s) without damage to nail

√7ᵗʰ **S91.105** Unspecified open wound of **left lesser** toe(s) without damage to nail

√7ᵗʰ **S91.106** Unspecified open wound of **unspecified lesser** toe(s) without damage to nail

√7ᵗʰ **S91.109** Unspecified open wound of **unspecified** toe(s) without damage to nail

√6ᵗʰ **S91.11** Laceration without foreign body **of toe without damage to nail**

√7ᵗʰ **S91.111** Laceration without foreign body of **right great** toe without damage to nail

√7ᵗʰ **S91.112** Laceration without foreign body of **left great** toe without damage to nail

√7ᵗʰ **S91.113** Laceration without foreign body of **unspecified great** toe without damage to nail

√7ᵗʰ **S91.114** Laceration without foreign body of **right lesser** toe(s) without damage to nail

√7ᵗʰ **S91.115** Laceration without foreign body of **left lesser** toe(s) without damage to nail

√7ᵗʰ **S91.116** Laceration without foreign body of **unspecified lesser** toe(s) without damage to nail

√7ᵗʰ **S91.119** Laceration without foreign body of **unspecified** toe without damage to nail

√6ᵗʰ **S91.12** Laceration with foreign body **of toe without damage to nail**

√7ᵗʰ **S91.121** Laceration with foreign body of **right great** toe without damage to nail

√7ᵗʰ **S91.122** Laceration with foreign body of **left great** toe without damage to nail

√7ᵗʰ **S91.123** Laceration with foreign body of **unspecified great** toe without damage to nail

√7ᵗʰ **S91.124** Laceration with foreign body of **right lesser** toe(s) without damage to nail

√7ᵗʰ **S91.125** Laceration with foreign body of **left lesser** toe(s) without damage to nail

√7ᵗʰ **S91.126** Laceration with foreign body of **unspecified lesser** toe(s) without damage to nail

√7ᵗʰ **S91.129** Laceration with foreign body of **unspecified** toe(s) without damage to nail

√6ᵗʰ **S91.13** Puncture wound without foreign body **of toe without damage to nail**

√7ᵗʰ **S91.131** Puncture wound without foreign body of **right great** toe without damage to nail

√7ᵗʰ **S91.132** Puncture wound without foreign body of **left great** toe without damage to nail

√7ᵗʰ **S91.133** Puncture wound without foreign body of **unspecified great** toe without damage to nail

√7ᵗʰ **S91.134** Puncture wound without foreign body of **right lesser** toe(s) without damage to nail

√7ᵗʰ **S91.135** Puncture wound without foreign body of **left lesser** toe(s) without damage to nail

√7ᵗʰ **S91.136** Puncture wound without foreign body of **unspecified lesser** toe(s) without damage to nail

√7ᵗʰ **S91.139** Puncture wound without foreign body of **unspecified** toe(s) without damage to nail

√6ᵗʰ **S91.14** Puncture wound with foreign body **of toe without damage to nail**

√7ᵗʰ **S91.141** Puncture wound with foreign body of **right great** toe without damage to nail

√7ᵗʰ **S91.142** Puncture wound with foreign body of **left great** toe without damage to nail

√7ᵗʰ **S91.143** Puncture wound with foreign body of **unspecified great** toe without damage to nail

√7ᵗʰ **S91.144** Puncture wound with foreign body of **right lesser** toe(s) without damage to nail

√7ᵗʰ **S91.145** Puncture wound with foreign body of **left lesser** toe(s) without damage to nail

√7ᵗʰ **S91.146** Puncture wound with foreign body of **unspecified lesser** toe(s) without damage to nail

√7ᵗʰ **S91.149** Puncture wound with foreign body of **unspecified** toe(s) without damage to nail

√6ᵗʰ **S91.15** Open bite **of toe without damage to nail**

Bite of toe NOS

EXCLUDES 1 superficial bite of toe (S90.46-, S90.47-)

√7ᵗʰ **S91.151** Open bite of **right great** toe without damage to nail

√7ᵗʰ **S91.152** Open bite of **left great** toe without damage to nail

√7ᵗʰ **S91.153** Open bite of **unspecified great** toe without damage to nail

√7ᵗʰ **S91.154** Open bite of **right lesser** toe(s) without damage to nail

☑ Additional Character Req    √x7ᵗʰ Placeholder Alert    Unacceptable PDx    Manifestation    H1 - H14 HAC    HCC CMS-HCC Condition    EXCLUDES 1 Not Coded Here    EXCLUDES 2 Not Included Here

ICD-10-CM 2018    1065

☑7ᵗʰ **S91.155** Open bite of left lesser toe(s) without damage to nail

☑7ᵗʰ **S91.156** Open bite of unspecified lesser toe(s) without damage to nail

☑7ᵗʰ **S91.159** Open bite of unspecified toe(s) without damage to nail

☑5ᵗʰ **S91.2** Open wound of toe with damage to nail

☑6ᵗʰ **S91.20** Unspecified open wound of toe with damage to nail

☑7ᵗʰ **S91.201** Unspecified open wound of right great toe with damage to nail

☑7ᵗʰ **S91.202** Unspecified open wound of left great toe with damage to nail

☑7ᵗʰ **S91.203** Unspecified open wound of unspecified great toe with damage to nail

☑7ᵗʰ **S91.204** Unspecified open wound of right lesser toe(s) with damage to nail

☑7ᵗʰ **S91.205** Unspecified open wound of left lesser toe(s) with damage to nail

☑7ᵗʰ **S91.206** Unspecified open wound of unspecified lesser toe(s) with damage to nail

☑7ᵗʰ **S91.209** Unspecified open wound of unspecified toe(s) with damage to nail

☑6ᵗʰ **S91.21** Laceration without foreign body of toe with damage to nail

☑7ᵗʰ **S91.211** Laceration without foreign body of right great toe with damage to nail

☑7ᵗʰ **S91.212** Laceration without foreign body of left great toe with damage to nail

☑7ᵗʰ **S91.213** Laceration without foreign body of unspecified great toe with damage to nail

☑7ᵗʰ **S91.214** Laceration without foreign body of right lesser toe(s) with damage to nail

☑7ᵗʰ **S91.215** Laceration without foreign body of left lesser toe(s) with damage to nail

☑7ᵗʰ **S91.216** Laceration without foreign body of unspecified lesser toe(s) with damage to nail

☑7ᵗʰ **S91.219** Laceration without foreign body of unspecified toe(s) with damage to nail

☑6ᵗʰ **S91.22** Laceration with foreign body of toe with damage to nail

☑7ᵗʰ **S91.221** Laceration with foreign body of right great toe with damage to nail

☑7ᵗʰ **S91.222** Laceration with foreign body of left great toe with damage to nail

☑7ᵗʰ **S91.223** Laceration with foreign body of unspecified great toe with damage to nail

☑7ᵗʰ **S91.224** Laceration with foreign body of right lesser toe(s) with damage to nail

☑7ᵗʰ **S91.225** Laceration with foreign body of left lesser toe(s) with damage to nail

☑7ᵗʰ **S91.226** Laceration with foreign body of unspecified lesser toe(s) with damage to nail

☑7ᵗʰ **S91.229** Laceration with foreign body of unspecified toe(s) with damage to nail

☑6ᵗʰ **S91.23** Puncture wound without foreign body of toe with damage to nail

☑7ᵗʰ **S91.231** Puncture wound without foreign body of right great toe with damage to nail

☑7ᵗʰ **S91.232** Puncture wound without foreign body of left great toe with damage to nail

☑7ᵗʰ **S91.233** Puncture wound without foreign body of unspecified great toe with damage to nail

☑7ᵗʰ **S91.234** Puncture wound without foreign body of right lesser toe(s) with damage to nail

☑7ᵗʰ **S91.235** Puncture wound without foreign body of left lesser toe(s) with damage to nail

☑7ᵗʰ **S91.236** Puncture wound without foreign body of unspecified lesser toe(s) with damage to nail

☑7ᵗʰ **S91.239** Puncture wound without foreign body of unspecified toe(s) with damage to nail

☑6ᵗʰ **S91.24** Puncture wound with foreign body of toe with damage to nail

☑7ᵗʰ **S91.241** Puncture wound with foreign body of right great toe with damage to nail

☑7ᵗʰ **S91.242** Puncture wound with foreign body of left great toe with damage to nail

☑7ᵗʰ **S91.243** Puncture wound with foreign body of unspecified great toe with damage to nail

☑7ᵗʰ **S91.244** Puncture wound with foreign body of right lesser toe(s) with damage to nail

☑7ᵗʰ **S91.245** Puncture wound with foreign body of left lesser toe(s) with damage to nail

☑7ᵗʰ **S91.246** Puncture wound with foreign body of unspecified lesser toe(s) with damage to nail

☑7ᵗʰ **S91.249** Puncture wound with foreign body of unspecified toe(s) with damage to nail

☑6ᵗʰ **S91.25** Open bite of toe with damage to nail
Bite of toe with damage to nail NOS
**EXCLUDES 1** superficial bite of toe (S90.46-, S90.47-)

☑7ᵗʰ **S91.251** Open bite of right great toe with damage to nail

☑7ᵗʰ **S91.252** Open bite of left great toe with damage to nail

☑7ᵗʰ **S91.253** Open bite of unspecified great toe with damage to nail

☑7ᵗʰ **S91.254** Open bite of right lesser toe(s) with damage to nail

☑7ᵗʰ **S91.255** Open bite of left lesser toe(s) with damage to nail

☑7ᵗʰ **S91.256** Open bite of unspecified lesser toe(s) with damage to nail

☑7ᵗʰ **S91.259** Open bite of unspecified toe(s) with damage to nail

☑5ᵗʰ **S91.3** Open wound of foot

☑6ᵗʰ **S91.30** Unspecified open wound of foot

☑7ᵗʰ **S91.301** Unspecified open wound, right foot

☑7ᵗʰ **S91.302** Unspecified open wound, left foot

☑7ᵗʰ **S91.309** Unspecified open wound, unspecified foot

☑6ᵗʰ **S91.31** Laceration without foreign body of foot

☑7ᵗʰ **S91.311** Laceration without foreign body, right foot

☑7ᵗʰ **S91.312** Laceration without foreign body, left foot

☑7ᵗʰ **S91.319** Laceration without foreign body, unspecified foot

☑6ᵗʰ **S91.32** Laceration with foreign body of foot

☑7ᵗʰ **S91.321** Laceration with foreign body, right foot

☑7ᵗʰ **S91.322** Laceration with foreign body, left foot

☑7ᵗʰ **S91.329** Laceration with foreign body, unspecified foot

☑6ᵗʰ **S91.33** Puncture wound without foreign body of foot

☑7ᵗʰ **S91.331** Puncture wound without foreign body, right foot

☑7ᵗʰ **S91.332** Puncture wound without foreign body, left foot

☑7ᵗʰ **S91.339** Puncture wound without foreign body, unspecified foot

☑6ᵗʰ **S91.34** Puncture wound with foreign body of foot

☑7ᵗʰ **S91.341** Puncture wound with foreign body, right foot

☑7ᵗʰ **S91.342** Puncture wound with foreign body, left foot

☑7ᵗʰ **S91.349** Puncture wound with foreign body, unspecified foot

☑6ᵗʰ **S91.35** Open bite of foot
**EXCLUDES 1** superficial bite of foot (S90.86-, S90.87-)

☑7ᵗʰ **S91.351** Open bite, right foot

☑7ᵗʰ **S91.352** Open bite, left foot

☑7ᵗʰ **S91.359** Open bite, unspecified foot

N Newborn: 0   P Pediatric: 0-17   M Maternity: 12-55   A Adult: 15-124   **MCC** Major CC Condition   **PDxMCC** PDx acts as own MCC   **CC** CC Condition   **PDxCC** PDx acts as own CC

**1066**      ICD-10-CM 2018

## ✓4th S92 Fracture of foot and toe, except ankle

**NOTE**    A fracture not indicated as displaced or nondisplaced should be coded to displaced.

A fracture not indicated as open or closed should be coded to closed.

**EXCLUDES 1**   traumatic amputation of ankle and foot (S98.-)

**EXCLUDES 2**   fracture of ankle (S82.-)
fracture of malleolus (S82.-)

**AHA:** 2015, 3Q, 37-39

The appropriate 7th character is to be added to each code from category S92.
A    initial encounter for closed fracture
B    initial encounter for open fracture
D    subsequent encounter for fracture with routine healing
G    subsequent encounter for fracture with delayed healing
K    subsequent encounter for fracture with nonunion
P    subsequent encounter for fracture with malunion
S    sequela

### ✓5th S92.0 Fracture of calcaneus

Heel bone
Os calcis

**EXCLUDES 2**   physeal fracture of calcaneus (S99.0-)

**CC Excl: For codes in subcategory S92.0:**
**CC with 7th character B:** PDX collection 1367
**CC with 7th character K or P:** PDX collection 897

#### ✓6th S92.00 Unspecified fracture of calcaneus

- 7   ✓7th **S92.001** Unspecified fracture of right calcaneus   CC H5
- 7   ✓7th **S92.002** Unspecified fracture of left calcaneus   CC H5
- 7   ✓7th **S92.009** Unspecified fracture of unspecified calcaneus   CC H5

#### ✓6th S92.01 Fracture of body of calcaneus

- 7   ✓7th **S92.011** Displaced fracture of body of right calcaneus   CC H5
- 7   ✓7th **S92.012** Displaced fracture of body of left calcaneus   CC H5
- 7   ✓7th **S92.013** Displaced fracture of body of unspecified calcaneus   CC H5
- 7   ✓7th **S92.014** Nondisplaced fracture of body of right calcaneus   CC H5
- 7   ✓7th **S92.015** Nondisplaced fracture of body of left calcaneus   CC H5
- 7   ✓7th **S92.016** Nondisplaced fracture of body of unspecified calcaneus   CC H5

#### ✓6th S92.02 Fracture of anterior process of calcaneus

- 7   ✓7th **S92.021** Displaced fracture of anterior process of right calcaneus   CC H5
- 7   ✓7th **S92.022** Displaced fracture of anterior process of left calcaneus   CC H5
- 7   ✓7th **S92.023** Displaced fracture of anterior process of unspecified calcaneus   CC H5
- 7   ✓7th **S92.024** Nondisplaced fracture of anterior process of right calcaneus   CC H5
- 7   ✓7th **S92.025** Nondisplaced fracture of anterior process of left calcaneus   CC H5
- 7   ✓7th **S92.026** Nondisplaced fracture of anterior process of unspecified calcaneus   CC H5

#### ✓6th S92.03 Avulsion fracture of tuberosity of calcaneus

- 7   ✓7th **S92.031** Displaced avulsion fracture of tuberosity of right calcaneus   CC H5
- 7   ✓7th **S92.032** Displaced avulsion fracture of tuberosity of left calcaneus   CC H5
- 7   ✓7th **S92.033** Displaced avulsion fracture of tuberosity of unspecified calcaneus   CC H5
- 7   ✓7th **S92.034** Nondisplaced avulsion fracture of tuberosity of right calcaneus   CC H5
- 7   ✓7th **S92.035** Nondisplaced avulsion fracture of tuberosity of left calcaneus   CC H5
- 7   ✓7th **S92.036** Nondisplaced avulsion fracture of tuberosity of unspecified calcaneus   CC H5

#### ✓6th S92.04 Other fracture of tuberosity of calcaneus

- 7   ✓7th **S92.041** Displaced other fracture of tuberosity of right calcaneus   CC H5

- 7   ✓7th **S92.042** Displaced other fracture of tuberosity of left calcaneus   CC H5
- 7   ✓7th **S92.043** Displaced other fracture of tuberosity of unspecified calcaneus   CC H5
- 7   ✓7th **S92.044** Nondisplaced other fracture of tuberosity of right calcaneus   CC H5
- 7   ✓7th **S92.045** Nondisplaced other fracture of tuberosity of left calcaneus   CC H5
- 7   ✓7th **S92.046** Nondisplaced other fracture of tuberosity of unspecified calcaneus   CC H5

#### ✓6th S92.05 Other extraarticular fracture of calcaneus

- 7   ✓7th **S92.051** Displaced other extraarticular fracture of right calcaneus   CC H5
- 7   ✓7th **S92.052** Displaced other extraarticular fracture of left calcaneus   CC H5
- 7   ✓7th **S92.053** Displaced other extraarticular fracture of unspecified calcaneus   CC H5
- 7   ✓7th **S92.054** Nondisplaced other extraarticular fracture of right calcaneus   CC H5
- 7   ✓7th **S92.055** Nondisplaced other extraarticular fracture of left calcaneus   CC H5
- 7   ✓7th **S92.056** Nondisplaced other extraarticular fracture of unspecified calcaneus   CC H5

#### ✓6th S92.06 Intraarticular fracture of calcaneus

- 7   ✓7th **S92.061** Displaced intraarticular fracture of right calcaneus   CC H5
- 7   ✓7th **S92.062** Displaced intraarticular fracture of left calcaneus   CC H5
- 7   ✓7th **S92.063** Displaced intraarticular fracture of unspecified calcaneus   CC H5
- 7   ✓7th **S92.064** Nondisplaced intraarticular fracture of right calcaneus   CC H5
- 7   ✓7th **S92.065** Nondisplaced intraarticular fracture of left calcaneus   CC H5
- 7   ✓7th **S92.066** Nondisplaced intraarticular fracture of unspecified calcaneus   CC H5

### ✓5th S92.1 Fracture of talus

Astragalus

**CC Excl: For codes in subcategory S92.1:**
**CC with 7th character B:** PDX collection 1368
**CC with 7th character K or P:** PDX collection 897

#### ✓6th S92.10 Unspecified fracture of talus

- 7   ✓7th **S92.101** Unspecified fracture of right talus   CC H5
- 7   ✓7th **S92.102** Unspecified fracture of left talus   CC H5
- 7   ✓7th **S92.109** Unspecified fracture of unspecified talus   CC H5

#### ✓6th S92.11 Fracture of neck of talus

- 7   ✓7th **S92.111** Displaced fracture of neck of right talus   CC H5
- 7   ✓7th **S92.112** Displaced fracture of neck of left talus   CC H5
- 7   ✓7th **S92.113** Displaced fracture of neck of unspecified talus   CC H5
- 7   ✓7th **S92.114** Nondisplaced fracture of neck of right talus   CC H5
- 7   ✓7th **S92.115** Nondisplaced fracture of neck of left talus   CC H5
- 7   ✓7th **S92.116** Nondisplaced fracture of neck of unspecified talus   CC H5

#### ✓6th S92.12 Fracture of body of talus

- 7   ✓7th **S92.121** Displaced fracture of body of right talus   CC H5
- 7   ✓7th **S92.122** Displaced fracture of body of left talus   CC H5
- 7   ✓7th **S92.123** Displaced fracture of body of unspecified talus   CC H5
- 7   ✓7th **S92.124** Nondisplaced fracture of body of right talus   CC H5
- 7   ✓7th **S92.125** Nondisplaced fracture of body of left talus   CC H5
- 7   ✓7th **S92.126** Nondisplaced fracture of body of unspecified talus   CC H5

---

**7**   CC when reported as an initial encounter (7th character A, B, or C – specific to category) OR a subsequent encounter for nonunion or malunion (7th character K, M, N, P, Q, or R – specific to category).

✓ Additional Character Req    ✓x7th Placeholder Alert    Unacceptable PDx    Manifestation    H1-H14 HAC    HCC CMS-HCC Condition    EXCLUDES 1 Not Coded Here    EXCLUDES 2 Not Included Here

ICD-10-CM 2018      **1067**

√6ᵗʰ **S92.13** Fracture of posterior process of talus

7 √7ᵗʰ **S92.131** Displaced fracture of posterior process of right talus `CC` `H5`

7 √7ᵗʰ **S92.132** Displaced fracture of posterior process of left talus `CC` `H5`

7 √7ᵗʰ **S92.133** Displaced fracture of posterior process of unspecified talus `CC` `H5`

7 √7ᵗʰ **S92.134** Nondisplaced fracture of posterior process of right talus `CC` `H5`

7 √7ᵗʰ **S92.135** Nondisplaced fracture of posterior process of left talus `CC` `H5`

7 √7ᵗʰ **S92.136** Nondisplaced fracture of posterior process of unspecified talus `CC` `H5`

√6ᵗʰ **S92.14** Dome fracture of talus

**EXCLUDES 1** osteochondritis dissecans (M93.2)

7 √7ᵗʰ **S92.141** Displaced dome fracture of right talus `CC` `H5`

7 √7ᵗʰ **S92.142** Displaced dome fracture of left talus `CC` `H5`

7 √7ᵗʰ **S92.143** Displaced dome fracture of unspecified talus `CC` `H5`

7 √7ᵗʰ **S92.144** Nondisplaced dome fracture of right talus `CC` `H5`

7 √7ᵗʰ **S92.145** Nondisplaced dome fracture of left talus `CC` `H5`

7 √7ᵗʰ **S92.146** Nondisplaced dome fracture of unspecified talus `CC` `H5`

√6ᵗʰ **S92.15** Avulsion fracture (chip fracture) of talus

7 √7ᵗʰ **S92.151** Displaced avulsion fracture (chip fracture) of right talus `CC` `H5`

7 √7ᵗʰ **S92.152** Displaced avulsion fracture (chip fracture) of left talus `CC` `H5`

7 √7ᵗʰ **S92.153** Displaced avulsion fracture (chip fracture) of unspecified talus `CC` `H5`

7 √7ᵗʰ **S92.154** Nondisplaced avulsion fracture (chip fracture) of right talus `CC` `H5`

7 √7ᵗʰ **S92.155** Nondisplaced avulsion fracture (chip fracture) of left talus `CC` `H5`

7 √7ᵗʰ **S92.156** Nondisplaced avulsion fracture (chip fracture) of unspecified talus `CC` `H5`

√6ᵗʰ **S92.19** Other fracture of talus

7 √7ᵗʰ **S92.191** Other fracture of right talus `CC` `H5`

7 √7ᵗʰ **S92.192** Other fracture of left talus `CC` `H5`

7 √7ᵗʰ **S92.199** Other fracture of unspecified talus `CC` `H5`

√5ᵗʰ **S92.2** Fracture of other and unspecified tarsal bone(s)

> **CC Excl: For codes in subcategory S92.2, unless otherwise noted:**
> **CC with 7th character B:** PDX collection 1368
> **CC with 7th character K or P:** PDX collection 897

√6ᵗʰ **S92.20** Fracture of unspecified tarsal bone(s)

> **CC Excl: For codes in subcategory S92.20:**
> **CC with 7th character B:** PDX collection 1369
> **CC with 7th character K or P:** PDX collection 897

7 √7ᵗʰ **S92.201** Fracture of unspecified tarsal bone(s) of right foot `CC` `H5`

7 √7ᵗʰ **S92.202** Fracture of unspecified tarsal bone(s) of left foot `CC` `H5`

7 √7ᵗʰ **S92.209** Fracture of unspecified tarsal bone(s) of unspecified foot `CC` `H5`

√6ᵗʰ **S92.21** Fracture of cuboid bone

7 √7ᵗʰ **S92.211** Displaced fracture of cuboid bone of right foot `CC` `H5`

7 √7ᵗʰ **S92.212** Displaced fracture of cuboid bone of left foot `CC` `H5`

7 √7ᵗʰ **S92.213** Displaced fracture of cuboid bone of unspecified foot `CC` `H5`

7 √7ᵗʰ **S92.214** Nondisplaced fracture of cuboid bone of right foot `CC` `H5`

7 √7ᵗʰ **S92.215** Nondisplaced fracture of cuboid bone of left foot `CC` `H5`

7 √7ᵗʰ **S92.216** Nondisplaced fracture of cuboid bone of unspecified foot `CC` `H5`

√6ᵗʰ **S92.22** Fracture of lateral cuneiform

7 √7ᵗʰ **S92.221** Displaced fracture of lateral cuneiform of right foot `CC` `H5`

7 √7ᵗʰ **S92.222** Displaced fracture of lateral cuneiform of left foot `CC` `H5`

7 √7ᵗʰ **S92.223** Displaced fracture of lateral cuneiform of unspecified foot `CC` `H5`

7 √7ᵗʰ **S92.224** Nondisplaced fracture of lateral cuneiform of right foot `CC` `H5`

7 √7ᵗʰ **S92.225** Nondisplaced fracture of lateral cuneiform of left foot `CC` `H5`

7 √7ᵗʰ **S92.226** Nondisplaced fracture of lateral cuneiform of unspecified foot `CC` `H5`

√6ᵗʰ **S92.23** Fracture of intermediate cuneiform

7 √7ᵗʰ **S92.231** Displaced fracture of intermediate cuneiform of right foot `CC` `H5`

7 √7ᵗʰ **S92.232** Displaced fracture of intermediate cuneiform of left foot `CC` `H5`

7 √7ᵗʰ **S92.233** Displaced fracture of intermediate cuneiform of unspecified foot `CC` `H5`

7 √7ᵗʰ **S92.234** Nondisplaced fracture of intermediate cuneiform of right foot `CC` `H5`

7 √7ᵗʰ **S92.235** Nondisplaced fracture of intermediate cuneiform of left foot `CC` `H5`

7 √7ᵗʰ **S92.236** Nondisplaced fracture of intermediate cuneiform of unspecified foot `CC` `H5`

√6ᵗʰ **S92.24** Fracture of medial cuneiform

7 √7ᵗʰ **S92.241** Displaced fracture of medial cuneiform of right foot `CC` `H5`

7 √7ᵗʰ **S92.242** Displaced fracture of medial cuneiform of left foot `CC` `H5`

7 √7ᵗʰ **S92.243** Displaced fracture of medial cuneiform of unspecified foot `CC` `H5`

7 √7ᵗʰ **S92.244** Nondisplaced fracture of medial cuneiform of right foot `CC` `H5`

7 √7ᵗʰ **S92.245** Nondisplaced fracture of medial cuneiform of left foot `CC` `H5`

7 √7ᵗʰ **S92.246** Nondisplaced fracture of medial cuneiform of unspecified foot `CC` `H5`

√6ᵗʰ **S92.25** Fracture of navicular [scaphoid] of foot

7 √7ᵗʰ **S92.251** Displaced fracture of navicular [scaphoid] of right foot `CC` `H5`

7 √7ᵗʰ **S92.252** Displaced fracture of navicular [scaphoid] of left foot `CC` `H5`

7 √7ᵗʰ **S92.253** Displaced fracture of navicular [scaphoid] of unspecified foot `CC` `H5`

7 √7ᵗʰ **S92.254** Nondisplaced fracture of navicular [scaphoid] of right foot `CC` `H5`

7 √7ᵗʰ **S92.255** Nondisplaced fracture of navicular [scaphoid] of left foot `CC` `H5`

7 √7ᵗʰ **S92.256** Nondisplaced fracture of navicular [scaphoid] of unspecified foot `CC` `H5`

√5ᵗʰ **S92.3** Fracture of metatarsal bone(s)

**EXCLUDES 2** physeal fracture of metatarsal (S99.1-)

> **CC Excl: For codes in subcategory S92.3:**
> **CC with 7th character B:** PDX collection 1368
> **CC with 7th character K or P:** PDX collection 897

√6ᵗʰ **S92.30** Fracture of unspecified metatarsal bone(s)

7 √7ᵗʰ **S92.301** Fracture of unspecified metatarsal bone(s), right foot `CC` `H5`

7 √7ᵗʰ **S92.302** Fracture of unspecified metatarsal bone(s), left foot `CC` `H5`

7 √7ᵗʰ **S92.309** Fracture of unspecified metatarsal bone(s), unspecified foot `CC` `H5`

√6ᵗʰ **S92.31** Fracture of first metatarsal bone

7 √7ᵗʰ **S92.311** Displaced fracture of first metatarsal bone, right foot `CC` `H5`

7 √7ᵗʰ **S92.312** Displaced fracture of first metatarsal bone, left foot `CC` `H5`

7 √7ᵗʰ **S92.313** Displaced fracture of first metatarsal bone, unspecified foot `CC` `H5`

---

7 CC when reported as an initial encounter (7th character A, B, or C – specific to category) OR a subsequent encounter for nonunion or malunion (7th character K, M, N, P, Q, or R – specific to category).

`N` Newborn: 0 `P` Pediatric: 0-17 `M` Maternity: 12-55 `A` Adult: 15-124 `MCC` Major CC Condition `PDxMCC` PDx acts as own MCC `CC` CC Condition `PDxCC` PDx acts as own CC

**1068** ICD-10-CM 2018

**7** ✓7th **S92.314** Nondisplaced **fracture of first metatarsal bone, right foot** `CC` `H5`

**7** ✓7th **S92.315** Nondisplaced **fracture of first metatarsal bone, left foot** `CC` `H5`

**7** ✓7th **S92.316** Nondisplaced **fracture of first metatarsal bone, unspecified foot** `CC` `H5`

✓6th **S92.32** Fracture of second metatarsal bone

**7** ✓7th **S92.321** Displaced **fracture of second metatarsal bone, right foot** `CC` `H5`

**7** ✓7th **S92.322** Displaced **fracture of second metatarsal bone, left foot** `CC` `H5`

**7** ✓7th **S92.323** Displaced **fracture of second metatarsal bone, unspecified foot** `CC` `H5`

**7** ✓7th **S92.324** Nondisplaced **fracture of second metatarsal bone, right foot** `CC` `H5`

**7** ✓7th **S92.325** Nondisplaced **fracture of second metatarsal bone, left foot** `CC` `H5`

**7** ✓7th **S92.326** Nondisplaced **fracture of second metatarsal bone, unspecified foot** `CC` `H5`

✓6th **S92.33** Fracture of third metatarsal bone

**7** ✓7th **S92.331** Displaced **fracture of third metatarsal bone, right foot** `CC` `H5`

**7** ✓7th **S92.332** Displaced **fracture of third metatarsal bone, left foot** `CC` `H5`

**7** ✓7th **S92.333** Displaced **fracture of third metatarsal bone, unspecified foot** `CC` `H5`

**7** ✓7th **S92.334** Nondisplaced **fracture of third metatarsal bone, right foot** `CC` `H5`

**7** ✓7th **S92.335** Nondisplaced **fracture of third metatarsal bone, left foot** `CC` `H5`

**7** ✓7th **S92.336** Nondisplaced **fracture of third metatarsal bone, unspecified foot** `CC` `H5`

✓6th **S92.34** Fracture of fourth metatarsal bone

**7** ✓7th **S92.341** Displaced **fracture of fourth metatarsal bone, right foot** `CC` `H5`

**7** ✓7th **S92.342** Displaced **fracture of fourth metatarsal bone, left foot** `CC` `H5`

**7** ✓7th **S92.343** Displaced **fracture of fourth metatarsal bone, unspecified foot** `CC` `H5`

**7** ✓7th **S92.344** Nondisplaced **fracture of fourth metatarsal bone, right foot** `CC` `H5`

**7** ✓7th **S92.345** Nondisplaced **fracture of fourth metatarsal bone, left foot** `CC` `H5`

**7** ✓7th **S92.346** Nondisplaced **fracture of fourth metatarsal bone, unspecified foot** `CC` `H5`

✓6th **S92.35** Fracture of fifth metatarsal bone

**7** ✓7th **S92.351** Displaced **fracture of fifth metatarsal bone, right foot** `CC` `H5`

**7** ✓7th **S92.352** Displaced **fracture of fifth metatarsal bone, left foot** `CC` `H5`

**7** ✓7th **S92.353** Displaced **fracture of fifth metatarsal bone, unspecified foot** `CC` `H5`

**7** ✓7th **S92.354** Nondisplaced **fracture of fifth metatarsal bone, right foot** `CC` `H5`

**7** ✓7th **S92.355** Nondisplaced **fracture of fifth metatarsal bone, left foot** `CC` `H5`

**7** ✓7th **S92.356** Nondisplaced **fracture of fifth metatarsal bone, unspecified foot** `CC` `H5`

✓5th **S92.4** Fracture of great toe

> **EXCLUDES 2**    *physeal fracture of phalanx of toe (S99.2-)*

> **CC Excl: For codes in subcategory S92.4:**
> **CC with 7th character K or P:** PDX collection 897

✓6th **S92.40** Unspecified **fracture of great toe**

**8** ✓7th **S92.401** Displaced **unspecified fracture of right great toe** `CC`

**8** ✓7th **S92.402** Displaced **unspecified fracture of left great toe** `CC`

**8** ✓7th **S92.403** Displaced **unspecified fracture of unspecified great toe** `CC`

**8** ✓7th **S92.404** Nondisplaced **unspecified fracture of right great toe** `CC`

**8** ✓7th **S92.405** Nondisplaced **unspecified fracture of left great toe** `CC`

**8** ✓7th **S92.406** Nondisplaced **unspecified fracture of unspecified great toe** `CC`

✓6th **S92.41** Fracture of proximal phalanx of great toe

**8** ✓7th **S92.411** Displaced **fracture of proximal phalanx of right great toe** `CC`

**8** ✓7th **S92.412** Displaced **fracture of proximal phalanx of left great toe** `CC`

**8** ✓7th **S92.413** Displaced **fracture of proximal phalanx of unspecified great toe** `CC`

**8** ✓7th **S92.414** Nondisplaced **fracture of proximal phalanx of right great toe** `CC`

**8** ✓7th **S92.415** Nondisplaced **fracture of proximal phalanx of left great toe** `CC`

**8** ✓7th **S92.416** Nondisplaced **fracture of proximal phalanx of unspecified great toe** `CC`

✓6th **S92.42** Fracture of distal phalanx of great toe

**8** ✓7th **S92.421** Displaced **fracture of distal phalanx of right great toe** `CC`

**8** ✓7th **S92.422** Displaced **fracture of distal phalanx of left great toe** `CC`

**8** ✓7th **S92.423** Displaced **fracture of distal phalanx of unspecified great toe** `CC`

**8** ✓7th **S92.424** Nondisplaced **fracture of distal phalanx of right great toe** `CC`

**8** ✓7th **S92.425** Nondisplaced **fracture of distal phalanx of left great toe** `CC`

**8** ✓7th **S92.426** Nondisplaced **fracture of distal phalanx of unspecified great toe** `CC`

✓6th **S92.49** Other fracture of great toe

**8** ✓7th **S92.491** Other **fracture of right great toe** `CC`

**8** ✓7th **S92.492** Other **fracture of left great toe** `CC`

**8** ✓7th **S92.499** Other **fracture of unspecified great toe** `CC`

✓5th **S92.5** Fracture of lesser toe(s)

> **EXCLUDES 2**    *physeal fracture of phalanx of toe (S99.2-)*

> **CC Excl: For codes in subcategory S92.5:**
> **CC with 7th character K or P:** PDX collection 897

✓6th **S92.50** Unspecified **fracture of lesser toe(s)**

**8** ✓7th **S92.501** Displaced **unspecified fracture of right lesser toe(s)** `CC`

**8** ✓7th **S92.502** Displaced **unspecified fracture of left lesser toe(s)** `CC`

**8** ✓7th **S92.503** Displaced **unspecified fracture of unspecified lesser toe(s)** `CC`

**8** ✓7th **S92.504** Nondisplaced **unspecified fracture of right lesser toe(s)** `CC`

**8** ✓7th **S92.505** Nondisplaced **unspecified fracture of left lesser toe(s)** `CC`

**8** ✓7th **S92.506** Nondisplaced **unspecified fracture of unspecified lesser toe(s)** `CC`

✓6th **S92.51** Fracture of proximal phalanx of lesser toe(s)

**8** ✓7th **S92.511** Displaced **fracture of proximal phalanx of right lesser toe(s)** `CC`

**8** ✓7th **S92.512** Displaced **fracture of proximal phalanx of left lesser toe(s)** `CC`

**8** ✓7th **S92.513** Displaced **fracture of proximal phalanx of unspecified lesser toe(s)** `CC`

**8** ✓7th **S92.514** Nondisplaced **fracture of proximal phalanx of right lesser toe(s)** `CC`

**8** ✓7th **S92.515** Nondisplaced **fracture of proximal phalanx of left lesser toe(s)** `CC`

**8** ✓7th **S92.516** Nondisplaced **fracture of proximal phalanx of unspecified lesser toe(s)** `CC`

▲ ✓6th **S92.52** Fracture of middle phalanx of lesser toe(s)

▲ **8** ✓7th **S92.521** Displaced **fracture of middle phalanx of right lesser toe(s)** `CC`

▲ **8** ✓7th **S92.522** Displaced **fracture of middle phalanx of left lesser toe(s)** `CC`

▲ **8** ✓7th **S92.523** Displaced **fracture of middle phalanx of unspecified lesser toe(s)** `CC`

---

**7** CC when reported as an initial encounter (7th character A, B, or C – specific to category) OR a subsequent encounter for nonunion or malunion (7th character K, M, N, P, Q, or R – specific to category).

**8** CC when reported as a subsequent encounter for nonunion or malunion (7th character K, M, N, P, Q, or R – specific to category).

✓ Additional Character Req   ✓7th Placeholder Alert   Unacceptable PDx   Manifestation   `H1`-`H14` HAC   `HCC` CMS-HCC Condition   **EXCLUDES 1** Not Coded Here   **EXCLUDES 2** Not Included Here

ICD-10-CM 2018      **1069**

▲   8   √7ᵗʰ   **S92.524**   **Nondisplaced fracture of middle phalanx of right lesser toe(s)**   CC

▲   8   √7ᵗʰ   **S92.525**   **Nondisplaced fracture of middle phalanx of left lesser toe(s)**   CC

▲   8   √7ᵗʰ   **S92.526**   **Nondisplaced fracture of middle phalanx of unspecified lesser toe(s)**   CC

√6ᵗʰ   **S92.53**   **Fracture of distal phalanx of lesser toe(s)**

8   √7ᵗʰ   **S92.531**   **Displaced fracture of distal phalanx of right lesser toe(s)**   CC

8   √7ᵗʰ   **S92.532**   **Displaced fracture of distal phalanx of left lesser toe(s)**   CC

8   √7ᵗʰ   **S92.533**   **Displaced fracture of distal phalanx of unspecified lesser toe(s)**   CC

8   √7ᵗʰ   **S92.534**   **Nondisplaced fracture of distal phalanx of right lesser toe(s)**   CC

8   √7ᵗʰ   **S92.535**   **Nondisplaced fracture of distal phalanx of left lesser toe(s)**   CC

8   √7ᵗʰ   **S92.536**   **Nondisplaced fracture of distal phalanx of unspecified lesser toe(s)**   CC

√6ᵗʰ   **S92.59**   **Other fracture of lesser toe(s)**

8   √7ᵗʰ   **S92.591**   **Other fracture of right lesser toe(s)**   CC

8   √7ᵗʰ   **S92.592**   **Other fracture of left lesser toe(s)**   CC

8   √7ᵗʰ   **S92.599**   **Other fracture of unspecified lesser toe(s)**   CC

√5ᵗʰ   **S92.8**   **Other fracture of foot, except ankle**

√6ᵗʰ   **S92.81**   **Other fracture of foot**
    Sesamoid fracture of foot

> **CC Excl: For codes in subcategory S92.81:**
> **CC with 7th character B:** PDX collection 1369
> **CC with 7th character K or P:** PDX collection 897

7   √7ᵗʰ   **S92.811**   **Other fracture of right foot**   CC   H5

7   √7ᵗʰ   **S92.812**   **Other fracture of left foot**   CC   H5

7   √7ᵗʰ   **S92.819**   **Other fracture of unspecified foot**   CC   H5

√5ᵗʰ   **S92.9**   **Unspecified fracture of foot and toe**

√6ᵗʰ   **S92.90**   **Unspecified fracture of foot**

> **CC Excl: For codes in subcategory S92.90:**
> **CC with 7th character B:** PDX collection 1369
> **CC with 7th character K or P:** PDX collection 897

7   √7ᵗʰ   **S92.901**   **Unspecified fracture of right foot**   CC   H5

7   √7ᵗʰ   **S92.902**   **Unspecified fracture of left foot**   CC   H5

7   √7ᵗʰ   **S92.909**   **Unspecified fracture of unspecified foot**   CC   H5

√6ᵗʰ   **S92.91**   **Unspecified fracture of toe**

> **CC Excl: For codes in subcategory S92.91:**
> **CC with 7th character K or P:** PDX collection 897

8   √7ᵗʰ   **S92.911**   **Unspecified fracture of right toe(s)**   CC

8   √7ᵗʰ   **S92.912**   **Unspecified fracture of left toe(s)**   CC

8   √7ᵗʰ   **S92.919**   **Unspecified fracture of unspecified toe(s)**   CC

√4ᵗʰ   **S93**   **Dislocation and sprain of joints and ligaments at ankle, foot and toe level**

INCLUDES   avulsion of joint or ligament of ankle, foot and toe
laceration of cartilage, joint or ligament of ankle, foot and toe
sprain of cartilage, joint or ligament of ankle, foot and toe
traumatic hemarthrosis of joint or ligament of ankle, foot and toe
traumatic rupture of joint or ligament of ankle, foot and toe
traumatic subluxation of joint or ligament of ankle, foot and toe
traumatic tear of joint or ligament of ankle, foot and toe

Code also any associated open wound

EXCLUDES 2   *strain of muscle and tendon of ankle and foot (S96.-)*

> The appropriate 7th character is to be added to each code from category S93.
> A   initial encounter
> D   subsequent encounter
> S   sequela

√5ᵗʰ   **S93.0**   **Subluxation and dislocation of ankle joint**
    Subluxation and dislocation of astragalus
    Subluxation and dislocation of fibula, lower end
    Subluxation and dislocation of talus
    Subluxation and dislocation of tibia, lower end

√x7ᵗʰ   **S93.01**   **Subluxation of right ankle joint**

√x7ᵗʰ   **S93.02**   **Subluxation of left ankle joint**

√x7ᵗʰ   **S93.03**   **Subluxation of unspecified ankle joint**

√x7ᵗʰ   **S93.04**   **Dislocation of right ankle joint**

√x7ᵗʰ   **S93.05**   **Dislocation of left ankle joint**

√x7ᵗʰ   **S93.06**   **Dislocation of unspecified ankle joint**

√5ᵗʰ   **S93.1**   **Subluxation and dislocation of toe**

√6ᵗʰ   **S93.10**   **Unspecified subluxation and dislocation of toe**
    Dislocation of toe NOS
    Subluxation of toe NOS

√7ᵗʰ   **S93.101**   **Unspecified subluxation of right toe(s)**

√7ᵗʰ   **S93.102**   **Unspecified subluxation of left toe(s)**

√7ᵗʰ   **S93.103**   **Unspecified subluxation of unspecified toe(s)**

√7ᵗʰ   **S93.104**   **Unspecified dislocation of right toe(s)**

√7ᵗʰ   **S93.105**   **Unspecified dislocation of left toe(s)**

√7ᵗʰ   **S93.106**   **Unspecified dislocation of unspecified toe(s)**

√6ᵗʰ   **S93.11**   **Dislocation of interphalangeal joint**

√7ᵗʰ   **S93.111**   **Dislocation of interphalangeal joint of right great toe**

√7ᵗʰ   **S93.112**   **Dislocation of interphalangeal joint of left great toe**

√7ᵗʰ   **S93.113**   **Dislocation of interphalangeal joint of unspecified great toe**

√7ᵗʰ   **S93.114**   **Dislocation of interphalangeal joint of right lesser toe(s)**

√7ᵗʰ   **S93.115**   **Dislocation of interphalangeal joint of left lesser toe(s)**

√7ᵗʰ   **S93.116**   **Dislocation of interphalangeal joint of unspecified lesser toe(s)**

√7ᵗʰ   **S93.119**   **Dislocation of interphalangeal joint of unspecified toe(s)**

√6ᵗʰ   **S93.12**   **Dislocation of metatarsophalangeal joint**

√7ᵗʰ   **S93.121**   **Dislocation of metatarsophalangeal joint of right great toe**

√7ᵗʰ   **S93.122**   **Dislocation of metatarsophalangeal joint of left great toe**

√7ᵗʰ   **S93.123**   **Dislocation of metatarsophalangeal joint of unspecified great toe**

√7ᵗʰ   **S93.124**   **Dislocation of metatarsophalangeal joint of right lesser toe(s)**

√7ᵗʰ   **S93.125**   **Dislocation of metatarsophalangeal joint of left lesser toe(s)**

√7ᵗʰ   **S93.126**   **Dislocation of metatarsophalangeal joint of unspecified lesser toe(s)**

√7ᵗʰ   **S93.129**   **Dislocation of metatarsophalangeal joint of unspecified toe(s)**

√6ᵗʰ   **S93.13**   **Subluxation of interphalangeal joint**

√7ᵗʰ   **S93.131**   **Subluxation of interphalangeal joint of right great toe**

√7ᵗʰ   **S93.132**   **Subluxation of interphalangeal joint of left great toe**

√7ᵗʰ   **S93.133**   **Subluxation of interphalangeal joint of unspecified great toe**

√7ᵗʰ   **S93.134**   **Subluxation of interphalangeal joint of right lesser toe(s)**

√7ᵗʰ   **S93.135**   **Subluxation of interphalangeal joint of left lesser toe(s)**

√7ᵗʰ   **S93.136**   **Subluxation of interphalangeal joint of unspecified lesser toe(s)**

√7ᵗʰ   **S93.139**   **Subluxation of interphalangeal joint of unspecified toe(s)**

---

7   CC when reported as an initial encounter (7th character A, B, or C – specific to category) OR a subsequent encounter for nonunion or malunion (7th character K, M, N, P, Q, or R – specific to category).

8   CC when reported as a subsequent encounter for nonunion or malunion (7th character K, M, N, P, Q, or R – specific to category).

N Newborn: 0   P Pediatric: 0-17   M Maternity: 12-55   A Adult: 15-124   MCC Major CC Condition   PDx MCC PDx acts as own MCC   CC CC Condition   PDx CC PDx acts as own CC

**1070**      ICD-10-CM 2018

✓6ᵗʰ **S93.14** **Subluxation of** metatarsophalangeal joint

     ✓7ᵗʰ **S93.141** **Subluxation of metatarsophalangeal joint of** right great **toe**

     ✓7ᵗʰ **S93.142** **Subluxation of metatarsophalangeal joint of** left great **toe**

     ✓7ᵗʰ **S93.143** **Subluxation of metatarsophalangeal joint of** unspecified great **toe**

     ✓7ᵗʰ **S93.144** **Subluxation of metatarsophalangeal joint of** right lesser **toe(s)**

     ✓7ᵗʰ **S93.145** **Subluxation of metatarsophalangeal joint of** left lesser **toe(s)**

     ✓7ᵗʰ **S93.146** **Subluxation of metatarsophalangeal joint of** unspecified lesser **toe(s)**

     ✓7ᵗʰ **S93.149** **Subluxation of metatarsophalangeal joint of** unspecified **toe(s)**

✓5ᵗʰ **S93.3** **Subluxation and dislocation of** foot

     EXCLUDES 2   *dislocation of toe (S93.1-)*

     ✓6ᵗʰ **S93.30** **Unspecified subluxation and dislocation of foot**
         Dislocation of foot NOS
         Subluxation of foot NOS

         ✓7ᵗʰ **S93.301** **Unspecified** subluxation **of** right **foot**

         ✓7ᵗʰ **S93.302** **Unspecified** subluxation **of** left **foot**

         ✓7ᵗʰ **S93.303** **Unspecified** subluxation **of** unspecified **foot**

         ✓7ᵗʰ **S93.304** **Unspecified** dislocation **of** right **foot**

         ✓7ᵗʰ **S93.305** **Unspecified** dislocation **of** left **foot**

         ✓7ᵗʰ **S93.306** **Unspecified** dislocation **of** unspecified **foot**

     ✓6ᵗʰ **S93.31** **Subluxation and dislocation of** tarsal joint

         ✓7ᵗʰ **S93.311** **Subluxation of tarsal joint of** right **foot**

         ✓7ᵗʰ **S93.312** **Subluxation of tarsal joint of** left **foot**

         ✓7ᵗʰ **S93.313** **Subluxation of tarsal joint of** unspecified **foot**

         ✓7ᵗʰ **S93.314** **Dislocation of tarsal joint of** right **foot**

         ✓7ᵗʰ **S93.315** **Dislocation of tarsal joint of** left **foot**

         ✓7ᵗʰ **S93.316** **Dislocation of tarsal joint of** unspecified **foot**

     ✓6ᵗʰ **S93.32** **Subluxation and dislocation of** tarsometatarsal **joint**

         ✓7ᵗʰ **S93.321** **Subluxation of tarsometatarsal joint of** right **foot**

         ✓7ᵗʰ **S93.322** **Subluxation of tarsometatarsal joint of** left **foot**

         ✓7ᵗʰ **S93.323** **Subluxation of tarsometatarsal joint of** unspecified **foot**

         ✓7ᵗʰ **S93.324** **Dislocation of tarsometatarsal joint of** right **foot**

         ✓7ᵗʰ **S93.325** **Dislocation of tarsometatarsal joint of** left **foot**

         ✓7ᵗʰ **S93.326** **Dislocation of tarsometatarsal joint of** unspecified **foot**

     ✓6ᵗʰ **S93.33** **Other subluxation and dislocation of** foot

         ✓7ᵗʰ **S93.331** **Other** subluxation **of** right **foot**

         ✓7ᵗʰ **S93.332** **Other** subluxation **of** left **foot**

         ✓7ᵗʰ **S93.333** **Other** subluxation **of** unspecified **foot**

         ✓7ᵗʰ **S93.334** **Other** dislocation **of** right **foot**

         ✓7ᵗʰ **S93.335** **Other** dislocation **of** left **foot**

         ✓7ᵗʰ **S93.336** **Other** dislocation **of** unspecified **foot**

✓5ᵗʰ **S93.4** **Sprain of** ankle

     EXCLUDES 2   *injury of Achilles tendon (S86.0-)*

     ✓6ᵗʰ **S93.40** **Sprain of** unspecified **ligament of ankle**
         Sprain of ankle NOS
         Sprained ankle NOS

         ✓7ᵗʰ **S93.401** **Sprain of unspecified ligament of** right **ankle**

         ✓7ᵗʰ **S93.402** **Sprain of unspecified ligament of** left **ankle**

         ✓7ᵗʰ **S93.409** **Sprain of unspecified ligament of** unspecified **ankle**

     ✓6ᵗʰ **S93.41** **Sprain of** calcaneofibular **ligament**

         ✓7ᵗʰ **S93.411** **Sprain of calcaneofibular ligament of** right **ankle**

         ✓7ᵗʰ **S93.412** **Sprain of calcaneofibular ligament of** left **ankle**

         ✓7ᵗʰ **S93.419** **Sprain of calcaneofibular ligament of** unspecified **ankle**

     ✓6ᵗʰ **S93.42** **Sprain of** deltoid **ligament**

         ✓7ᵗʰ **S93.421** **Sprain of deltoid ligament of** right **ankle**

         ✓7ᵗʰ **S93.422** **Sprain of deltoid ligament of** left **ankle**

         ✓7ᵗʰ **S93.429** **Sprain of deltoid ligament of** unspecified **ankle**

     ✓6ᵗʰ **S93.43** **Sprain of** tibiofibular **ligament**

         ✓7ᵗʰ **S93.431** **Sprain of tibiofibular ligament of** right **ankle**

         ✓7ᵗʰ **S93.432** **Sprain of tibiofibular ligament of** left **ankle**

         ✓7ᵗʰ **S93.439** **Sprain of tibiofibular ligament of** unspecified **ankle**

     ✓6ᵗʰ **S93.49** **Sprain of** other **ligament of ankle**
         Sprain of internal collateral ligament
         Sprain of talofibular ligament

         ✓7ᵗʰ **S93.491** **Sprain of other ligament of** right **ankle**

         ✓7ᵗʰ **S93.492** **Sprain of other ligament of** left **ankle**

         ✓7ᵗʰ **S93.499** **Sprain of other ligament of** unspecified **ankle**

✓5ᵗʰ **S93.5** **Sprain of** toe

     ✓6ᵗʰ **S93.50** **Unspecified** sprain of toe

         ✓7ᵗʰ **S93.501** **Unspecified sprain of** right great **toe**

         ✓7ᵗʰ **S93.502** **Unspecified sprain of** left great **toe**

         ✓7ᵗʰ **S93.503** **Unspecified sprain of** unspecified great **toe**

         ✓7ᵗʰ **S93.504** **Unspecified sprain of** right lesser **toe(s)**

         ✓7ᵗʰ **S93.505** **Unspecified sprain of** left lesser **toe(s)**

         ✓7ᵗʰ **S93.506** **Unspecified sprain of** unspecified lesser **toe(s)**

         ✓7ᵗʰ **S93.509** **Unspecified sprain of** unspecified **toe(s)**

     ✓6ᵗʰ **S93.51** **Sprain of** interphalangeal joint **of toe**

         ✓7ᵗʰ **S93.511** **Sprain of interphalangeal joint of** right great **toe**

         ✓7ᵗʰ **S93.512** **Sprain of interphalangeal joint of** left great **toe**

         ✓7ᵗʰ **S93.513** **Sprain of interphalangeal joint of** unspecified great **toe**

         ✓7ᵗʰ **S93.514** **Sprain of interphalangeal joint of** right lesser **toe(s)**

         ✓7ᵗʰ **S93.515** **Sprain of interphalangeal joint of** left lesser **toe(s)**

         ✓7ᵗʰ **S93.516** **Sprain of interphalangeal joint of** unspecified lesser **toe(s)**

         ✓7ᵗʰ **S93.519** **Sprain of interphalangeal joint of** unspecified **toe(s)**

     ✓6ᵗʰ **S93.52** **Sprain of** metatarsophalangeal joint **of toe**

         ✓7ᵗʰ **S93.521** **Sprain of metatarsophalangeal joint of** right great **toe**

         ✓7ᵗʰ **S93.522** **Sprain of metatarsophalangeal joint of** left great **toe**

         ✓7ᵗʰ **S93.523** **Sprain of metatarsophalangeal joint of** unspecified great **toe**

         ✓7ᵗʰ **S93.524** **Sprain of metatarsophalangeal joint of** right lesser **toe(s)**

         ✓7ᵗʰ **S93.525** **Sprain of metatarsophalangeal joint of** left lesser **toe(s)**

         ✓7ᵗʰ **S93.526** **Sprain of metatarsophalangeal joint of** unspecified lesser **toe(s)**

         ✓7ᵗʰ **S93.529** **Sprain of metatarsophalangeal joint of** unspecified **toe(s)**

✓5ᵗʰ **S93.6** **Sprain of** foot

     EXCLUDES 2   *sprain of metatarsophalangeal joint of toe (S93.52-)*
                   *sprain of toe (S93.5-)*

     ✓6ᵗʰ **S93.60** **Unspecified** sprain of foot

         ✓7ᵗʰ **S93.601** **Unspecified sprain of** right **foot**

         ✓7ᵗʰ **S93.602** **Unspecified sprain of** left **foot**

         ✓7ᵗʰ **S93.609** **Unspecified sprain of** unspecified **foot**

     ✓6ᵗʰ **S93.61** **Sprain of** tarsal ligament **of foot**

         ✓7ᵗʰ **S93.611** **Sprain of tarsal ligament of** right **foot**

         ✓7ᵗʰ **S93.612** **Sprain of tarsal ligament of** left **foot**

---

✓ Additional Character Req    ✓ₓ7ᵗʰ Placeholder Alert    Unacceptable PDx    Manifestation    **H1**-**H14** HAC    **HCC** CMS-HCC Condition    *EXCLUDES 1* Not Coded Here    *EXCLUDES 2* Not Included Here

☑7ᵗʰ **S93.619**   **Sprain of tarsal ligament of** unspecified **foot**

☑6ᵗʰ **S93.62**   **Sprain of** tarsometatarsal ligament **of foot**

     ☑7ᵗʰ **S93.621**   **Sprain of tarsometatarsal ligament of** right **foot**

     ☑7ᵗʰ **S93.622**   **Sprain of tarsometatarsal ligament of** left **foot**

     ☑7ᵗʰ **S93.629**   **Sprain of tarsometatarsal ligament of** unspecified **foot**

☑6ᵗʰ **S93.69**   **Other sprain of foot**

     ☑7ᵗʰ **S93.691**   **Other sprain of** right **foot**

     ☑7ᵗʰ **S93.692**   **Other sprain of** left **foot**

     ☑7ᵗʰ **S93.699**   **Other sprain of** unspecified **foot**

☑4ᵗʰ **S94**   **Injury of nerves at ankle and foot level**

Code also any associated open wound (S91.-)

The appropriate 7th character is to be added to each code from category S94.
A   initial encounter
D   subsequent encounter
S   sequela

☑5ᵗʰ **S94.0**   **Injury of** lateral plantar **nerve**

     ☑ₓ7ᵗʰ **S94.00**   **Injury of lateral plantar nerve,** unspecified **leg**

     ☑ₓ7ᵗʰ **S94.01**   **Injury of lateral plantar nerve,** right **leg**

     ☑ₓ7ᵗʰ **S94.02**   **Injury of lateral plantar nerve,** left **leg**

☑5ᵗʰ **S94.1**   **Injury of** medial plantar **nerve**

     ☑ₓ7ᵗʰ **S94.10**   **Injury of medial plantar nerve,** unspecified **leg**

     ☑ₓ7ᵗʰ **S94.11**   **Injury of medial plantar nerve,** right **leg**

     ☑ₓ7ᵗʰ **S94.12**   **Injury of medial plantar nerve,** left **leg**

☑5ᵗʰ **S94.2**   **Injury of deep** peroneal **nerve at ankle and foot level**

Injury of terminal, lateral branch of deep peroneal nerve

     ☑ₓ7ᵗʰ **S94.20**   **Injury of deep peroneal nerve at ankle and foot level,** unspecified **leg**

     ☑ₓ7ᵗʰ **S94.21**   **Injury of deep peroneal nerve at ankle and foot level,** right **leg**

     ☑ₓ7ᵗʰ **S94.22**   **Injury of deep peroneal nerve at ankle and foot level,** left **leg**

☑5ᵗʰ **S94.3**   **Injury of** cutaneous sensory **nerve at ankle and foot level**

     ☑ₓ7ᵗʰ **S94.30**   **Injury of cutaneous sensory nerve at ankle and foot level,** unspecified **leg**

     ☑ₓ7ᵗʰ **S94.31**   **Injury of cutaneous sensory nerve at ankle and foot level,** right **leg**

     ☑ₓ7ᵗʰ **S94.32**   **Injury of cutaneous sensory nerve at ankle and foot level,** left **leg**

☑5ᵗʰ **S94.8**   **Injury of** other **nerves at ankle and foot level**

     ☑6ᵗʰ **S94.8X**   **Injury of other nerves at ankle and foot level**

         ☑7ᵗʰ **S94.8X1**   **Injury of other nerves at ankle and foot level,** right **leg**

         ☑7ᵗʰ **S94.8X2**   **Injury of other nerves at ankle and foot level,** left **leg**

         ☑7ᵗʰ **S94.8X9**   **Injury of other nerves at ankle and foot level,** unspecified **leg**

☑5ᵗʰ **S94.9**   **Injury of** unspecified **nerve at ankle and foot level**

     ☑ₓ7ᵗʰ **S94.90**   **Injury of unspecified nerve at ankle and foot level,** unspecified **leg**

     ☑ₓ7ᵗʰ **S94.91**   **Injury of unspecified nerve at ankle and foot level,** right **leg**

     ☑ₓ7ᵗʰ **S94.92**   **Injury of unspecified nerve at ankle and foot level,** left **leg**

☑4ᵗʰ **S95**   **Injury of blood vessels at ankle and foot level**

Code also any associated open wound (S91.-)

EXCLUDES 2   *injury of posterior tibial artery and vein (S85.1-, S85.8-)*

The appropriate 7th character is to be added to each code from category S95.
A   initial encounter
D   subsequent encounter
S   sequela

**CC Excl: For CC codes in category S95, unless otherwise noted:**
**Right side:** PDX collection 1325
**Left side:** PDX collection 1326
**Unspecified side:** PDX collection 1327

☑5ᵗʰ **S95.0**   **Injury of** dorsal artery **of foot**

     ☑6ᵗʰ **S95.00**   **Unspecified injury of dorsal artery of foot**

         ☑7ᵗʰ **S95.001**   **Unspecified injury of dorsal artery of** right **foot**   CC

         ☑7ᵗʰ **S95.002**   **Unspecified injury of dorsal artery of** left **foot**   CC

         ☑7ᵗʰ **S95.009**   **Unspecified injury of dorsal artery of** unspecified **foot**   CC

     ☑6ᵗʰ **S95.01**   **Laceration of dorsal artery of foot**

         ☑7ᵗʰ **S95.011**   **Laceration of dorsal artery of** left **foot**   CC

         ☑7ᵗʰ **S95.012**   **Laceration of dorsal artery of** left **foot**   CC

         ☑7ᵗʰ **S95.019**   **Laceration of dorsal artery of** unspecified **foot**   CC

     ☑6ᵗʰ **S95.09**   **Other specified injury of dorsal artery of foot**

         ☑7ᵗʰ **S95.091**   **Other specified injury of dorsal artery of** right **foot**   CC

         ☑7ᵗʰ **S95.092**   **Other specified injury of dorsal artery of** left **foot**   CC

         ☑7ᵗʰ **S95.099**   **Other specified injury of dorsal artery of** unspecified **foot**   CC

☑5ᵗʰ **S95.1**   **Injury of** plantar artery **of foot**

**CC Excl: For CC codes in subcategory S95.1:**
**Right side:** PDX collection 1370
**Left side:** PDX collection 1371
**Unspecified side:** PDX collection 1372

     ☑6ᵗʰ **S95.10**   **Unspecified injury of plantar artery of foot**

         ☑7ᵗʰ **S95.101**   **Unspecified injury of plantar artery of** right **foot**   CC

         ☑7ᵗʰ **S95.102**   **Unspecified injury of plantar artery of** left **foot**   CC

         ☑7ᵗʰ **S95.109**   **Unspecified injury of plantar artery of** unspecified **foot**   CC

     ☑6ᵗʰ **S95.11**   **Laceration of plantar artery of foot**

         ☑7ᵗʰ **S95.111**   **Laceration of plantar artery of** right **foot**   CC

         ☑7ᵗʰ **S95.112**   **Laceration of plantar artery of** left **foot**   CC

         ☑7ᵗʰ **S95.119**   **Laceration of plantar artery of** unspecified **foot**   CC

     ☑6ᵗʰ **S95.19**   **Other specified injury of plantar artery of foot**

         ☑7ᵗʰ **S95.191**   **Other specified injury of plantar artery of** right **foot**   CC

         ☑7ᵗʰ **S95.192**   **Other specified injury of plantar artery of** left **foot**   CC

         ☑7ᵗʰ **S95.199**   **Other specified injury of plantar artery of** unspecified **foot**   CC

☑5ᵗʰ **S95.2**   **Injury of** dorsal vein **of foot**

     ☑6ᵗʰ **S95.20**   **Unspecified injury of dorsal vein of foot**

         ☑7ᵗʰ **S95.201**   **Unspecified injury of dorsal vein of** right **foot**   CC

         ☑7ᵗʰ **S95.202**   **Unspecified injury of dorsal vein of** left **foot**   CC

         ☑7ᵗʰ **S95.209**   **Unspecified injury of dorsal vein of** unspecified **foot**   CC

     ☑6ᵗʰ **S95.21**   **Laceration of dorsal vein of foot**

         ☑7ᵗʰ **S95.211**   **Laceration of dorsal vein of** right **foot**   CC

         ☑7ᵗʰ **S95.212**   **Laceration of dorsal vein of** left **foot**   CC

         ☑7ᵗʰ **S95.219**   **Laceration of dorsal vein of** unspecified **foot**   CC

Ⓝ Newborn: 0   Ⓟ Pediatric: 0-17   Ⓜ Maternity: 12-55   Ⓐ Adult: 15-124   MCC Major CC Condition   PDx MCC PDx acts as own MCC   CC CC Condition   PDx CC PDx acts as own CC

**1072**

ICD-10-CM 2018

✓6ᵗʰ **S95.29** Other specified injury of dorsal vein of foot

     ✓7ᵗʰ **S95.291** Other specified injury of dorsal vein of **right** foot   **CC**

     ✓7ᵗʰ **S95.292** Other specified injury of dorsal vein of **left** foot   **CC**

     ✓7ᵗʰ **S95.299** Other specified injury of dorsal vein of **unspecified** foot   **CC**

✓5ᵗʰ **S95.8** Injury of other blood vessels at ankle and foot level

   ✓6ᵗʰ **S95.80** Unspecified injury of other blood vessels at ankle and foot level

     ✓7ᵗʰ **S95.801** Unspecified injury of other blood vessels at ankle and foot level, **right leg**   **CC**

     ✓7ᵗʰ **S95.802** Unspecified injury of other blood vessels at ankle and foot level, **left leg**   **CC**

     ✓7ᵗʰ **S95.809** Unspecified injury of other blood vessels at ankle and foot level, **unspecified leg**   **CC**

   ✓6ᵗʰ **S95.81** Laceration of other blood vessels at ankle and foot level

     ✓7ᵗʰ **S95.811** Laceration of other blood vessels at ankle and foot level, **right leg**   **CC**

     ✓7ᵗʰ **S95.812** Laceration of other blood vessels at ankle and foot level, **left leg**   **CC**

     ✓7ᵗʰ **S95.819** Laceration of other blood vessels at ankle and foot level, **unspecified leg**   **CC**

   ✓6ᵗʰ **S95.89** Other specified injury of other blood vessels at ankle and foot level

     ✓7ᵗʰ **S95.891** Other specified injury of other blood vessels at ankle and foot level, **right leg**   **CC**

     ✓7ᵗʰ **S95.892** Other specified injury of other blood vessels at ankle and foot level, **left leg**   **CC**

     ✓7ᵗʰ **S95.899** Other specified injury of other blood vessels at ankle and foot level, **unspecified leg**   **CC**

✓5ᵗʰ **S95.9** Injury of unspecified blood vessel at ankle and foot level

   ✓6ᵗʰ **S95.90** Unspecified injury of unspecified blood vessel at ankle and foot level

     ✓7ᵗʰ **S95.901** Unspecified injury of unspecified blood vessel at ankle and foot level, **right leg**   **CC**

     ✓7ᵗʰ **S95.902** Unspecified injury of unspecified blood vessel at ankle and foot level, **left leg**   **CC**

     ✓7ᵗʰ **S95.909** Unspecified injury of unspecified blood vessel at ankle and foot level, **unspecified leg**   **CC**

   ✓6ᵗʰ **S95.91** Laceration of unspecified blood vessel at ankle and foot level

     ✓7ᵗʰ **S95.911** Laceration of unspecified blood vessel at ankle and foot level, **right leg**   **CC**

     ✓7ᵗʰ **S95.912** Laceration of unspecified blood vessel at ankle and foot level, **left leg**   **CC**

     ✓7ᵗʰ **S95.919** Laceration of unspecified blood vessel at ankle and foot level, **unspecified leg**   **CC**

   ✓6ᵗʰ **S95.99** Other specified injury of unspecified blood vessel at ankle and foot level

     ✓7ᵗʰ **S95.991** Other specified injury of unspecified blood vessel at ankle and foot level, **right leg**   **CC**

     ✓7ᵗʰ **S95.992** Other specified injury of unspecified blood vessel at ankle and foot level, **left leg**   **CC**

     ✓7ᵗʰ **S95.999** Other specified injury of unspecified blood vessel at ankle and foot level, **unspecified leg**   **CC**

✓4ᵗʰ **S96** **Injury of muscle and tendon at ankle and foot level**

   Code also any associated open wound (S91.-)

   *EXCLUDES 2*   injury of Achilles tendon (S86.0-)
            sprain of joints and ligaments of ankle and foot (S93.-)

   **TIP:** Refer to the Muscle/Tendon table at the beginning of this chapter

The appropriate 7th character is to be added to each code from category S96.
A    initial encounter
D    subsequent encounter
S    sequela

**CC Excl: For CC codes in category S96:**
**Right side:** PDX collection 1364
**Left side:** PDX collection 1365
**Unspecified side:** PDX collection 1366

✓5ᵗʰ **S96.0** Injury of muscle and tendon of long flexor muscle of toe at ankle and foot level

   ✓6ᵗʰ **S96.00** Unspecified injury of muscle and tendon of long flexor muscle of toe at ankle and foot level

     ✓7ᵗʰ **S96.001** Unspecified injury of muscle and tendon of long flexor muscle of toe at ankle and foot level, **right** foot

     ✓7ᵗʰ **S96.002** Unspecified injury of muscle and tendon of long flexor muscle of toe at ankle and foot level, **left** foot

     ✓7ᵗʰ **S96.009** Unspecified injury of muscle and tendon of long flexor muscle of toe at ankle and foot level, **unspecified** foot

   ✓6ᵗʰ **S96.01** Strain of muscle and tendon of long flexor muscle of toe at ankle and foot level

     ✓7ᵗʰ **S96.011** Strain of muscle and tendon of long flexor muscle of toe at ankle and foot level, **right** foot

     ✓7ᵗʰ **S96.012** Strain of muscle and tendon of long flexor muscle of toe at ankle and foot level, **left** foot

     ✓7ᵗʰ **S96.019** Strain of muscle and tendon of long flexor muscle of toe at ankle and foot level, **unspecified** foot

   ✓6ᵗʰ **S96.02** Laceration of muscle and tendon of long flexor muscle of toe at ankle and foot level

     ✓7ᵗʰ **S96.021** Laceration of muscle and tendon of long flexor muscle of toe at ankle and foot level, **right** foot   **CC**

     ✓7ᵗʰ **S96.022** Laceration of muscle and tendon of long flexor muscle of toe at ankle and foot level, **left** foot   **CC**

     ✓7ᵗʰ **S96.029** Laceration of muscle and tendon of long flexor muscle of toe at ankle and foot level, **unspecified** foot   **CC**

   ✓6ᵗʰ **S96.09** Other injury of muscle and tendon of long flexor muscle of toe at ankle and foot level

     ✓7ᵗʰ **S96.091** Other injury of muscle and tendon of long flexor muscle of toe at ankle and foot level, **right** foot

     ✓7ᵗʰ **S96.092** Other injury of muscle and tendon of long flexor muscle of toe at ankle and foot level, **left** foot

     ✓7ᵗʰ **S96.099** Other injury of muscle and tendon of long flexor muscle of toe at ankle and foot level, **unspecified** foot

✓5ᵗʰ **S96.1** Injury of muscle and tendon of long extensor muscle of toe at ankle and foot level

   ✓6ᵗʰ **S96.10** Unspecified injury of muscle and tendon of long extensor muscle of toe at ankle and foot level

     ✓7ᵗʰ **S96.101** Unspecified injury of muscle and tendon of long extensor muscle of toe at ankle and foot level, **right** foot

     ✓7ᵗʰ **S96.102** Unspecified injury of muscle and tendon of long extensor muscle of toe at ankle and foot level, **left** foot

     ✓7ᵗʰ **S96.109** Unspecified injury of muscle and tendon of long extensor muscle of toe at ankle and foot level, **unspecified** foot

✓ Additional Character Req   ✓x7ᵗʰ Placeholder Alert   Unacceptable PDx   Manifestation   **H1 - H14** HAC   **HCC** CMS-HCC Condition   *EXCLUDES 1* Not Coded Here   *EXCLUDES 2* Not Included Here

ICD-10-CM 2018          1073

**√6th S96.11 Strain of muscle and tendon of long extensor muscle of toe at ankle and foot level**

√7th **S96.111** Strain of muscle and tendon of long extensor muscle of toe at ankle and foot level, **right** foot

√7th **S96.112** Strain of muscle and tendon of long extensor muscle of toe at ankle and foot level, **left** foot

√7th **S96.119** Strain of muscle and tendon of long extensor muscle of toe at ankle and foot level, **unspecified** foot

**√6th S96.12 Laceration of muscle and tendon of long extensor muscle of toe at ankle and foot level**

√7th **S96.121** Laceration of muscle and tendon of long extensor muscle of toe at ankle and foot level, **right** foot   **CC**

√7th **S96.122** Laceration of muscle and tendon of long extensor muscle of toe at ankle and foot level, **left** foot   **CC**

√7th **S96.129** Laceration of muscle and tendon of long extensor muscle of toe at ankle and foot level, **unspecified** foot   **CC**

**√6th S96.19 Other specified injury of muscle and tendon of long extensor muscle of toe at ankle and foot level**

√7th **S96.191** Other specified injury of muscle and tendon of long extensor muscle of toe at ankle and foot level, **right** foot

√7th **S96.192** Other specified injury of muscle and tendon of long extensor muscle of toe at ankle and foot level, **left** foot

√7th **S96.199** Other specified injury of muscle and tendon of long extensor muscle of toe at ankle and foot level, **unspecified** foot

**√5th S96.2 Injury of intrinsic muscle and tendon at ankle and foot level**

**√6th S96.20 Unspecified injury of intrinsic muscle and tendon at ankle and foot level**

√7th **S96.201** Unspecified injury of intrinsic muscle and tendon at ankle and foot level, **right** foot

√7th **S96.202** Unspecified injury of intrinsic muscle and tendon at ankle and foot level, **left** foot

√7th **S96.209** Unspecified injury of intrinsic muscle and tendon at ankle and foot level, **unspecified** foot

**√6th S96.21 Strain of intrinsic muscle and tendon at ankle and foot level**

√7th **S96.211** Strain of intrinsic muscle and tendon at ankle and foot level, **right** foot

√7th **S96.212** Strain of intrinsic muscle and tendon at ankle and foot level, **left** foot

√7th **S96.219** Strain of intrinsic muscle and tendon at ankle and foot level, **unspecified** foot

**√6th S96.22 Laceration of intrinsic muscle and tendon at ankle and foot level**

√7th **S96.221** Laceration of intrinsic muscle and tendon at ankle and foot level, **right** foot   **CC**

√7th **S96.222** Laceration of intrinsic muscle and tendon at ankle and foot level, **left** foot   **CC**

√7th **S96.229** Laceration of intrinsic muscle and tendon at ankle and foot level, **unspecified** foot   **CC**

**√6th S96.29 Other specified injury of intrinsic muscle and tendon at ankle and foot level**

√7th **S96.291** Other specified injury of intrinsic muscle and tendon at ankle and foot level, **right** foot

√7th **S96.292** Other specified injury of intrinsic muscle and tendon at ankle and foot level, **left** foot

√7th **S96.299** Other specified injury of intrinsic muscle and tendon at ankle and foot level, **unspecified** foot

**√5th S96.8 Injury of other specified muscles and tendons at ankle and foot level**

**√6th S96.80 Unspecified injury of other specified muscles and tendons at ankle and foot level**

√7th **S96.801** Unspecified injury of other specified muscles and tendons at ankle and foot level, **right** foot

√7th **S96.802** Unspecified injury of other specified muscles and tendons at ankle and foot level, **left** foot

√7th **S96.809** Unspecified injury of other specified muscles and tendons at ankle and foot level, **unspecified** foot

**√6th S96.81 Strain of other specified muscles and tendons at ankle and foot level**

√7th **S96.811** Strain of other specified muscles and tendons at ankle and foot level, **right** foot

√7th **S96.812** Strain of other specified muscles and tendons at ankle and foot level, **left** foot

√7th **S96.819** Strain of other specified muscles and tendons at ankle and foot level, **unspecified** foot

**√6th S96.82 Laceration of other specified muscles and tendons at ankle and foot level**

√7th **S96.821** Laceration of other specified muscles and tendons at ankle and foot level, **right** foot   **CC**

√7th **S96.822** Laceration of other specified muscles and tendons at ankle and foot level, **left** foot   **CC**

√7th **S96.829** Laceration of other specified muscles and tendons at ankle and foot level, **unspecified** foot   **CC**

**√6th S96.89 Other specified injury of other specified muscles and tendons at ankle and foot level**

√7th **S96.891** Other specified injury of other specified muscles and tendons at ankle and foot level, **right** foot

√7th **S96.892** Other specified injury of other specified muscles and tendons at ankle and foot level, **left** foot

√7th **S96.899** Other specified injury of other specified muscles and tendons at ankle and foot level, **unspecified** foot

**√5th S96.9 Injury of unspecified muscle and tendon at ankle and foot level**

**√6th S96.90 Unspecified injury of unspecified muscle and tendon at ankle and foot level**

√7th **S96.901** Unspecified injury of unspecified muscle and tendon at ankle and foot level, **right** foot

√7th **S96.902** Unspecified injury of unspecified muscle and tendon at ankle and foot level, **left** foot

√7th **S96.909** Unspecified injury of unspecified muscle and tendon at ankle and foot level, **unspecified** foot

**√6th S96.91 Strain of unspecified muscle and tendon at ankle and foot level**

√7th **S96.911** Strain of unspecified muscle and tendon at ankle and foot level, **right** foot

√7th **S96.912** Strain of unspecified muscle and tendon at ankle and foot level, **left** foot

√7th **S96.919** Strain of unspecified muscle and tendon at ankle and foot level, **unspecified** foot

**√6th S96.92 Laceration of unspecified muscle and tendon at ankle and foot level**

√7th **S96.921** Laceration of unspecified muscle and tendon at ankle and foot level, **right** foot   **CC**

√7th **S96.922** Laceration of unspecified muscle and tendon at ankle and foot level, **left** foot   **CC**

√7th **S96.929** Laceration of unspecified muscle and tendon at ankle and foot level, **unspecified** foot   **CC**

✓6th **S96.99** Other **specified injury of unspecified muscle and tendon at ankle and foot level**

    ✓7th **S96.991** Other specified injury of unspecified muscle and tendon at ankle and foot level, right **foot**

    ✓7th **S96.992** Other specified injury of unspecified muscle and tendon at ankle and foot level, left **foot**

    ✓7th **S96.999** Other specified injury of unspecified muscle and tendon at ankle and foot level, unspecified **foot**

✓4th **S97** **Crushing injury** of ankle and foot
    Use additional code(s) for all associated injuries

    The appropriate 7th character is to be added to each code from category S97.
    A   initial encounter
    D   subsequent encounter
    S   sequela

✓5th **S97.0** **Crushing injury of** ankle

    ✓x7th **S97.00** **Crushing injury of** unspecified **ankle**

    ✓x7th **S97.01** **Crushing injury of** right **ankle**

    ✓x7th **S97.02** **Crushing injury of** left **ankle**

✓5th **S97.1** **Crushing injury of** toe

    ✓6th **S97.10** **Crushing injury of** unspecified **toe(s)**

        ✓7th **S97.101** **Crushing injury of unspecified** right **toe(s)**

        ✓7th **S97.102** **Crushing injury of unspecified** left **toe(s)**

        ✓7th **S97.109** **Crushing injury of** unspecified **toe(s)**
        Crushing injury of toe NOS

    ✓6th **S97.11** **Crushing injury of** great toe

        ✓7th **S97.111** **Crushing injury of** right **great toe**

        ✓7th **S97.112** **Crushing injury of** left **great toe**

        ✓7th **S97.119** **Crushing injury of** unspecified **great toe**

    ✓6th **S97.12** **Crushing injury of** lesser **toe(s)**

        ✓7th **S97.121** **Crushing injury of** right **lesser toe(s)**

        ✓7th **S97.122** **Crushing injury of** left **lesser toe(s)**

        ✓7th **S97.129** **Crushing injury of** unspecified **lesser toe(s)**

✓5th **S97.8** **Crushing injury of** foot

    ✓x7th **S97.80** **Crushing injury of** unspecified **foot**
    Crushing injury of foot NOS

    ✓x7th **S97.81** **Crushing injury of** right **foot**

    ✓x7th **S97.82** **Crushing injury of** left **foot**

✓4th **S98** **Traumatic amputation of ankle and foot**
    An amputation not identified as partial or complete should be coded to complete

    The appropriate 7th character is to be added to each code from category S98.
    A   initial encounter
    D   subsequent encounter
    S   sequela

    **CC Excl: For CC codes in category S98:**
    **Right side:** PDX collection 1333
    **Left side:** PDX collection 1334
    **Unspecified side:** PDX collection 1335

✓5th **S98.0** **Traumatic amputation of** foot at ankle level

    ✓6th **S98.01** **Complete** traumatic amputation of foot at ankle level

        ✓7th **S98.011** **Complete traumatic amputation of** right **foot at ankle level** CC HCC

        ✓7th **S98.012** **Complete traumatic amputation of** left **foot at ankle level** CC HCC

        ✓7th **S98.019** **Complete traumatic amputation of** unspecified **foot at ankle level** CC HCC

    ✓6th **S98.02** **Partial** traumatic amputation of foot at ankle level

        ✓7th **S98.021** **Partial traumatic amputation of** right **foot at ankle level** CC HCC

        ✓7th **S98.022** **Partial traumatic amputation of** left **foot at ankle level** CC HCC

        ✓7th **S98.029** **Partial traumatic amputation of** unspecified **foot at ankle level** CC HCC

✓5th **S98.1** **Traumatic amputation of** one toe

    ✓6th **S98.11** **Complete** traumatic amputation of great toe

        ✓7th **S98.111** **Complete traumatic amputation of** right **great toe** HCC

        ✓7th **S98.112** **Complete traumatic amputation of** left **great toe** HCC

        ✓7th **S98.119** **Complete traumatic amputation of** unspecified **great toe** HCC

    ✓6th **S98.12** **Partial** traumatic amputation of great toe

        ✓7th **S98.121** **Partial traumatic amputation of** right **great toe** HCC

        ✓7th **S98.122** **Partial traumatic amputation of** left **great toe** HCC

        ✓7th **S98.129** **Partial traumatic amputation of** unspecified **great toe** HCC

    ✓6th **S98.13** **Complete** traumatic amputation of one lesser toe
    Traumatic amputation of toe NOS

        ✓7th **S98.131** **Complete traumatic amputation of** one right **lesser toe** HCC

        ✓7th **S98.132** **Complete traumatic amputation of** one left **lesser toe** HCC

        ✓7th **S98.139** **Complete traumatic amputation of** one unspecified **lesser toe** HCC

    ✓6th **S98.14** **Partial** traumatic amputation of one lesser toe

        ✓7th **S98.141** **Partial traumatic amputation of** one right **lesser toe** HCC

        ✓7th **S98.142** **Partial traumatic amputation of** one left **lesser toe** HCC

        ✓7th **S98.149** **Partial traumatic amputation of** one unspecified **lesser toe** HCC

✓5th **S98.2** **Traumatic amputation of** two or more lesser toes

    ✓6th **S98.21** **Complete** traumatic amputation of two or more lesser toes

        ✓7th **S98.211** **Complete traumatic amputation of** two or more right **lesser toes** HCC

        ✓7th **S98.212** **Complete traumatic amputation of** two or more left **lesser toes** HCC

        ✓7th **S98.219** **Complete traumatic amputation of** two or more unspecified **lesser toes** HCC

    ✓6th **S98.22** **Partial** traumatic amputation of two or more lesser toes

        ✓7th **S98.221** **Partial traumatic amputation of** two or more right **lesser toes** HCC

        ✓7th **S98.222** **Partial traumatic amputation of** two or more left **lesser toes** HCC

        ✓7th **S98.229** **Partial traumatic amputation of** two or more unspecified **lesser toes** HCC

✓5th **S98.3** **Traumatic amputation of** midfoot

    ✓6th **S98.31** **Complete** traumatic amputation of midfoot

        ✓7th **S98.311** **Complete traumatic amputation of** right **midfoot** CC HCC

        ✓7th **S98.312** **Complete traumatic amputation of** left **midfoot** CC HCC

        ✓7th **S98.319** **Complete traumatic amputation of** unspecified **midfoot** CC HCC

    ✓6th **S98.32** **Partial** traumatic amputation of midfoot

        ✓7th **S98.321** **Partial traumatic amputation of** right **midfoot** CC HCC

        ✓7th **S98.322** **Partial traumatic amputation of** left **midfoot** CC HCC

        ✓7th **S98.329** **Partial traumatic amputation of** unspecified **midfoot** CC HCC

✓5th **S98.9** **Traumatic amputation of** foot, level unspecified

    ✓6th **S98.91** **Complete** traumatic amputation of foot, level unspecified

        ✓7th **S98.911** **Complete traumatic amputation of** right **foot, level unspecified** CC HCC

        ✓7th **S98.912** **Complete traumatic amputation of** left **foot, level unspecified** CC HCC

        ✓7th **S98.919** **Complete traumatic amputation of** unspecified **foot, level** unspecified CC HCC

✓6th **S98.92** **Partial** traumatic amputation of foot, level unspecified

    ✓7th **S98.921** **Partial traumatic amputation of** right foot, level unspecified `CC` `HCC`

    ✓7th **S98.922** **Partial traumatic amputation of** left foot, level unspecified `CC` `HCC`

    ✓7th **S98.929** **Partial traumatic amputation of** unspecified foot, level unspecified `CC` `HCC`

✓4th **S99** **Other and unspecified injuries of ankle and foot**

  ✓5th **S99.0** **Physeal fracture of** calcaneus

> The appropriate 7th character is to be added to each code from subcategories S99.0.
> A　initial encounter for closed fracture
> B　initial encounter for open fracture
> D　subsequent encounter for fracture with routine healing
> G　subsequent encounter for fracture with delayed healing
> K　subsequent encounter for fracture with nonunion
> P　subsequent encounter for fracture with malunion
> S　sequela

    ✓6th **S99.00** **Unspecified** physeal fracture of calcaneus

      ✓7th **S99.001** **Unspecified physeal fracture of** right calcaneus

      ✓7th **S99.002** **Unspecified physeal fracture of** left calcaneus

      ✓7th **S99.009** **Unspecified physeal fracture of** unspecified calcaneus

    ✓6th **S99.01** Salter-Harris Type I physeal fracture of calcaneus

      ✓7th **S99.011** **Salter-Harris Type I physeal fracture of** right calcaneus

      ✓7th **S99.012** **Salter-Harris Type I physeal fracture of** left calcaneus

      ✓7th **S99.019** **Salter-Harris Type I physeal fracture of** unspecified calcaneus

    ✓6th **S99.02** Salter-Harris Type II physeal fracture of calcaneus

      ✓7th **S99.021** **Salter-Harris Type II physeal fracture of** right calcaneus

      ✓7th **S99.022** **Salter-Harris Type II physeal fracture of** left calcaneus

      ✓7th **S99.029** **Salter-Harris Type II physeal fracture of** unspecified calcaneus

    ✓6th **S99.03** Salter-Harris Type III physeal fracture of calcaneus

      ✓7th **S99.031** **Salter-Harris Type III physeal fracture of** right calcaneus

      ✓7th **S99.032** **Salter-Harris Type III physeal fracture of** left calcaneus

      ✓7th **S99.039** **Salter-Harris Type III physeal fracture of** unspecified calcaneus

    ✓6th **S99.04** Salter-Harris Type IV physeal fracture of calcaneus

      ✓7th **S99.041** **Salter-Harris Type IV physeal fracture of** right calcaneus

      ✓7th **S99.042** **Salter-Harris Type IV physeal fracture of** left calcaneus

      ✓7th **S99.049** **Salter-Harris Type IV physeal fracture of** unspecified calcaneus

    ✓6th **S99.09** Other physeal fracture of calcaneus

      ✓7th **S99.091** **Other physeal fracture of** right calcaneus

      ✓7th **S99.092** **Other physeal fracture of** left calcaneus

      ✓7th **S99.099** **Other physeal fracture of** unspecified calcaneus

  ✓5th **S99.1** **Physeal fracture of** metatarsal

> The appropriate 7th character is to be added to each code from subcategories S99.1.
> A　initial encounter for closed fracture
> B　initial encounter for open fracture
> D　subsequent encounter for fracture with routine healing
> G　subsequent encounter for fracture with delayed healing
> K　subsequent encounter for fracture with nonunion
> P　subsequent encounter for fracture with malunion
> S　sequela

    ✓6th **S99.10** **Unspecified** physeal fracture of metatarsal

      ✓7th **S99.101** **Unspecified physeal fracture of** right metatarsal

      ✓7th **S99.102** **Unspecified physeal fracture of** left metatarsal

      ✓7th **S99.109** **Unspecified physeal fracture of** unspecified metatarsal

    ✓6th **S99.11** Salter-Harris Type I physeal fracture of metatarsal

      ✓7th **S99.111** **Salter-Harris Type I physeal fracture of** right metatarsal

      ✓7th **S99.112** **Salter-Harris Type I physeal fracture of** left metatarsal

      ✓7th **S99.119** **Salter-Harris Type I physeal fracture of** unspecified metatarsal

    ✓6th **S99.12** Salter-Harris Type II physeal fracture of metatarsal

      ✓7th **S99.121** **Salter-Harris Type II physeal fracture of** right metatarsal

      ✓7th **S99.122** **Salter-Harris Type II physeal fracture of** left metatarsal

      ✓7th **S99.129** **Salter-Harris Type II physeal fracture of** unspecified metatarsal

    ✓6th **S99.13** Salter-Harris Type III physeal fracture of metatarsal

      ✓7th **S99.131** **Salter-Harris Type III physeal fracture of** right metatarsal

      ✓7th **S99.132** **Salter-Harris Type III physeal fracture of** left metatarsal

      ✓7th **S99.139** **Salter-Harris Type III physeal fracture of** unspecified metatarsal

    ✓6th **S99.14** Salter-Harris Type IV physeal fracture of metatarsal

      ✓7th **S99.141** **Salter-Harris Type IV physeal fracture of** right metatarsal

      ✓7th **S99.142** **Salter-Harris Type IV physeal fracture of** left metatarsal

      ✓7th **S99.149** **Salter-Harris Type IV physeal fracture of** unspecified metatarsal

    ✓6th **S99.19** Other physeal fracture of metatarsal

      ✓7th **S99.191** **Other physeal fracture of** right metatarsal

      ✓7th **S99.192** **Other physeal fracture of** left metatarsal

      ✓7th **S99.199** **Other physeal fracture of** unspecified metatarsal

  ✓5th **S99.2** **Physeal fracture of** phalanx of toe

> The appropriate 7th character is to be added to each code from subcategories S99.2.
> A　initial encounter for closed fracture
> B　initial encounter for open fracture
> D　subsequent encounter for fracture with routine healing
> G　subsequent encounter for fracture with delayed healing
> K　subsequent encounter for fracture with nonunion
> P　subsequent encounter for fracture with malunion
> S　sequela

    ✓6th **S99.20** **Unspecified** physeal fracture of phalanx of toe

      ✓7th **S99.201** **Unspecified physeal fracture of** phalanx of right toe

      ✓7th **S99.202** **Unspecified physeal fracture of** phalanx of left toe

      ✓7th **S99.209** **Unspecified physeal fracture of** phalanx of unspecified toe

    ✓6th **S99.21** Salter-Harris Type I physeal fracture of phalanx of toe

      ✓7th **S99.211** **Salter-Harris Type I physeal fracture of** phalanx of right toe

      ✓7th **S99.212** **Salter-Harris Type I physeal fracture of** phalanx of left toe

      ✓7th **S99.219** **Salter-Harris Type I physeal fracture of** phalanx of unspecified toe

    ✓6th **S99.22** Salter-Harris Type II physeal fracture of phalanx of toe

      ✓7th **S99.221** **Salter-Harris Type II physeal fracture of** phalanx of right toe

      ✓7th **S99.222** **Salter-Harris Type II physeal fracture of** phalanx of left toe

      ✓7th **S99.229** **Salter-Harris Type II physeal fracture of** phalanx of unspecified toe

    ✓6th **S99.23** Salter-Harris Type III physeal fracture of phalanx of toe

      ✓7th **S99.231** **Salter-Harris Type III physeal fracture of** phalanx of right toe

      ✓7th **S99.232** **Salter-Harris Type III physeal fracture of** phalanx of left toe

N Newborn: 0　P Pediatric: 0-17　M Maternity: 12-55　A Adult: 15-124　MCC Major CC Condition　PDxMCC PDx acts as own MCC　CC CC Condition　PDxCC PDx acts as own CC

**1076**　　　　ICD-10-CM 2018

✓7ᵗʰ **S99.239**   Salter-Harris Type III physeal fracture of phalanx of unspecified toe

✓6ᵗʰ **S99.24**   Salter-Harris Type IV physeal fracture of phalanx of toe

    ✓7ᵗʰ **S99.241**   Salter-Harris Type IV physeal fracture of phalanx of right toe

    ✓7ᵗʰ **S99.242**   Salter-Harris Type IV physeal fracture of phalanx of left toe

    ✓7ᵗʰ **S99.249**   Salter-Harris Type IV physeal fracture of phalanx of unspecified toe

✓6ᵗʰ **S99.29**   Other physeal fracture of phalanx of toe

    ✓7ᵗʰ **S99.291**   Other physeal fracture of phalanx of right toe

    ✓7ᵗʰ **S99.292**   Other physeal fracture of phalanx of left toe

    ✓7ᵗʰ **S99.299**   Other physeal fracture of phalanx of unspecified toe

✓5ᵗʰ **S99.8**   Other specified injuries of ankle and foot

The appropriate 7th character is to be added to each code from subcategory S99.8.
A   initial encounter
D   subsequent encounter
S   sequela

✓6ᵗʰ **S99.81**   Other specified injuries of ankle

    ✓7ᵗʰ **S99.811**   Other specified injuries of right ankle

    ✓7ᵗʰ **S99.812**   Other specified injuries of left ankle

    ✓7ᵗʰ **S99.819**   Other specified injuries of unspecified ankle

✓6ᵗʰ **S99.82**   Other specified injuries of foot

    ✓7ᵗʰ **S99.821**   Other specified injuries of right foot

    ✓7ᵗʰ **S99.822**   Other specified injuries of left foot

    ✓7ᵗʰ **S99.829**   Other specified injuries of unspecified foot

✓5ᵗʰ **S99.9**   Unspecified injury of ankle and foot

The appropriate 7th character is to be added to each code from subcategory S99.9.
A   initial encounter
D   subsequent encounter
S   sequela

✓6ᵗʰ **S99.91**   Unspecified injury of ankle

    ✓7ᵗʰ **S99.911**   Unspecified injury of right ankle

    ✓7ᵗʰ **S99.912**   Unspecified injury of left ankle

    ✓7ᵗʰ **S99.919**   Unspecified injury of unspecified ankle

✓6ᵗʰ **S99.92**   Unspecified injury of foot

    ✓7ᵗʰ **S99.921**   Unspecified injury of right foot

    ✓7ᵗʰ **S99.922**   Unspecified injury of left foot

    ✓7ᵗʰ **S99.929**   Unspecified injury of unspecified foot

## Injury, Poisoning And Certain Other Consequences Of External Causes (T07-T88)

### Injuries involving multiple body regions (T07)

EXCLUDES 1   burns and corrosions (T20-T32)
frostbite (T33-T34)
insect bite or sting, venomous (T63.4)
sunburn (L55.-)

✓x7ᵗʰ **T07**   **Unspecified multiple injuries**
    EXCLUDES 1   injury NOS ▶(T14.90)◀

The appropriate 7th character is to be added to code T07.
A   initial encounter
D   subsequent encounter
S   sequela

### Injury of unspecified body region (T14)

✓4ᵗʰ **T14**   **Injury of unspecified body region**
    EXCLUDES 1   multiple unspecified injuries (T07)

The appropriate 7th character is to be added to each code from category T14.
A   initial encounter
D   subsequent encounter
S   sequela

✓x7ᵗʰ **T14.8**   **Other injury of unspecified body region**
Abrasion NOS
Contusion NOS
Crush injury NOS
Fracture NOS
Skin injury NOS
Vascular injury NOS
▶Wound NOS◀

✓5ᵗʰ **T14.9**   **Unspecified injury**

    ✓x7ᵗʰ **T14.90**   Injury, unspecified
Injury NOS

    ✓x7ᵗʰ **T14.91**   Suicide attempt     **HCC**
Attempted suicide NOS

### Effects of foreign body entering through natural orifice (T15-T19)

EXCLUDES 2   foreign body accidentally left in operation wound (T81.5-)
foreign body in penetrating wound—See open wound by body region
residual foreign body in soft tissue (M79.5)
splinter, without open wound—See superficial injury by body region

✓4ᵗʰ **T15**   **Foreign body on external eye**
    EXCLUDES 2   foreign body in penetrating wound of orbit and eye ball (S05.4-, S05.5-)
open wound of eyelid and periocular area (S01.1-)
retained foreign body in eyelid (H02.8-)
retained (old) foreign body in penetrating wound of orbit and eye ball (H05.5-, H44.6-, H44.7-)
superficial foreign body of eyelid and periocular area (S00.25-)

The appropriate 7th character is to be added to each code from category T15.
A   initial encounter
D   subsequent encounter
S   sequela

✓5ᵗʰ **T15.0**   **Foreign body in cornea**

    ✓x7ᵗʰ **T15.00**   Foreign body in cornea, unspecified eye

    ✓x7ᵗʰ **T15.01**   Foreign body in cornea, right eye

    ✓x7ᵗʰ **T15.02**   Foreign body in cornea, left eye

✓5ᵗʰ **T15.1**   **Foreign body in conjunctival sac**

    ✓x7ᵗʰ **T15.10**   Foreign body in conjunctival sac, unspecified eye

    ✓x7ᵗʰ **T15.11**   Foreign body in conjunctival sac, right eye

    ✓x7ᵗʰ **T15.12**   Foreign body in conjunctival sac, left eye

✓5ᵗʰ **T15.8**   **Foreign body in other and multiple parts of external eye**
Foreign body in lacrimal punctum

    ✓x7ᵗʰ **T15.80**   Foreign body in other and multiple parts of external eye, unspecified eye

    ✓x7ᵗʰ **T15.81**   Foreign body in other and multiple parts of external eye, right eye

    ✓x7ᵗʰ **T15.82**   Foreign body in other and multiple parts of external eye, left eye

✓5ᵗʰ **T15.9**   **Foreign body on external eye, part unspecified**

    ✓x7ᵗʰ **T15.90**   Foreign body on external eye, part unspecified, unspecified eye

    ✓x7ᵗʰ **T15.91**   Foreign body on external eye, part unspecified, right eye

    ✓x7ᵗʰ **T15.92**   Foreign body on external eye, part unspecified, left eye

✓4ᵗʰ **T16**   **Foreign body in ear**
    INCLUDES   foreign body in auditory canal

The appropriate 7th character is to be added to each code from category T16.
A   initial encounter
D   subsequent encounter
S   sequela

    ✓x7ᵗʰ **T16.1**   Foreign body in right ear

    ✓x7ᵗʰ **T16.2**   Foreign body in left ear

    ✓x7ᵗʰ **T16.9**   Foreign body in ear, unspecified ear

√4ᵗʰ **T17**   **Foreign body in respiratory tract**

> The appropriate 7th character is to be added to each code from category T17.
> A    initial encounter
> D    subsequent encounter
> S    sequela

√x7ᵗʰ **T17.0**   **Foreign body in** nasal sinus

√x7ᵗʰ **T17.1**   **Foreign body in** nostril
Foreign body in nose NOS

√5ᵗʰ **T17.2**   **Foreign body in** pharynx
Foreign body in nasopharynx
Foreign body in throat NOS

   √6ᵗʰ **T17.20**   **Unspecified foreign body in** pharynx

     √7ᵗʰ **T17.200**   **Unspecified foreign body in pharynx** causing asphyxiation

     √7ᵗʰ **T17.208**   **Unspecified foreign body in pharynx** causing other injury

   √6ᵗʰ **T17.21**   **Gastric contents in** pharynx
Aspiration of gastric contents into pharynx
Vomitus in pharynx

     √7ᵗʰ **T17.210**   **Gastric contents in pharynx** causing asphyxiation

     √7ᵗʰ **T17.218**   **Gastric contents in pharynx** causing other injury

   √6ᵗʰ **T17.22**   **Food in** pharynx
Bones in pharynx
Seeds in pharynx

     √7ᵗʰ **T17.220**   **Food in pharynx** causing asphyxiation

     √7ᵗʰ **T17.228**   **Food in pharynx** causing other injury

   √6ᵗʰ **T17.29**   **Other** foreign object in pharynx

     √7ᵗʰ **T17.290**   **Other foreign object in pharynx** causing asphyxiation

     √7ᵗʰ **T17.298**   **Other foreign object in pharynx** causing other injury

√5ᵗʰ **T17.3**   **Foreign body in** larynx

   √6ᵗʰ **T17.30**   **Unspecified foreign body in** larynx

     √7ᵗʰ **T17.300**   **Unspecified foreign body in larynx** causing asphyxiation

     √7ᵗʰ **T17.308**   **Unspecified foreign body in larynx** causing other injury

   √6ᵗʰ **T17.31**   **Gastric contents in** larynx
Aspiration of gastric contents into larynx
Vomitus in larynx

     √7ᵗʰ **T17.310**   **Gastric contents in larynx** causing asphyxiation

     √7ᵗʰ **T17.318**   **Gastric contents in larynx** causing other injury

   √6ᵗʰ **T17.32**   **Food in** larynx
Bones in larynx
Seeds in larynx

     √7ᵗʰ **T17.320**   **Food in larynx** causing asphyxiation

     √7ᵗʰ **T17.328**   **Food in larynx** causing other injury

   √6ᵗʰ **T17.39**   **Other** foreign object in larynx

     √7ᵗʰ **T17.390**   **Other foreign object in larynx** causing asphyxiation

     √7ᵗʰ **T17.398**   **Other foreign object in larynx** causing other injury

√5ᵗʰ **T17.4**   **Foreign body in** trachea

> **CC Excl: For codes in subcategory T17.4:**
> PDX collection 1373

   √6ᵗʰ **T17.40**   **Unspecified foreign body in** trachea

     √7ᵗʰ **T17.400**   **Unspecified foreign body in trachea** causing asphyxiation   `CC`

     √7ᵗʰ **T17.408**   **Unspecified foreign body in trachea** causing other injury   `CC`

   √6ᵗʰ **T17.41**   **Gastric contents in** trachea
Aspiration of gastric contents into trachea
Vomitus in trachea

     √7ᵗʰ **T17.410**   **Gastric contents in trachea** causing asphyxiation   `CC`

     √7ᵗʰ **T17.418**   **Gastric contents in trachea** causing other injury   `CC`

   √6ᵗʰ **T17.42**   **Food in** trachea
Bones in trachea      Seeds in trachea

     √7ᵗʰ **T17.420**   **Food in trachea** causing asphyxiation   `CC`

     √7ᵗʰ **T17.428**   **Food in trachea** causing other injury   `CC`

   √6ᵗʰ **T17.49**   **Other** foreign object in trachea

     √7ᵗʰ **T17.490**   **Other foreign object in trachea** causing asphyxiation   `CC`

     √7ᵗʰ **T17.498**   **Other foreign object in trachea** causing other injury   `CC`

√5ᵗʰ **T17.5**   **Foreign body in** bronchus

> **CC Excl: For codes in subcategory T17.5:**
> PDX collection 1374

   √6ᵗʰ **T17.50**   **Unspecified foreign body in** bronchus

     √7ᵗʰ **T17.500**   **Unspecified foreign body in bronchus** causing asphyxiation   `CC`

     √7ᵗʰ **T17.508**   **Unspecified foreign body in bronchus** causing other injury   `CC`

   √6ᵗʰ **T17.51**   **Gastric contents in** bronchus
Aspiration of gastric contents into bronchus
Vomitus in bronchus

     √7ᵗʰ **T17.510**   **Gastric contents in bronchus** causing asphyxiation   `CC`

     √7ᵗʰ **T17.518**   **Gastric contents in bronchus** causing other injury   `CC`

   √6ᵗʰ **T17.52**   **Food in** bronchus
Bones in bronchus
Seeds in bronchus

     √7ᵗʰ **T17.520**   **Food in bronchus** causing asphyxiation   `CC`

     √7ᵗʰ **T17.528**   **Food in bronchus** causing other injury   `CC`

   √6ᵗʰ **T17.59**   **Other** foreign object in bronchus

     √7ᵗʰ **T17.590**   **Other foreign object in bronchus** causing asphyxiation   `CC`

     √7ᵗʰ **T17.598**   **Other foreign object in bronchus** causing other injury   `CC`

√5ᵗʰ **T17.8**   **Foreign body in** other parts of respiratory tract
Foreign body in bronchioles
Foreign body in lung

> **CC Excl: For codes in subcategory T17.8, unless otherwise noted:** PDX collection 1374

   √6ᵗʰ **T17.80**   **Unspecified foreign body in other parts of** respiratory tract

     √7ᵗʰ **T17.800**   **Unspecified foreign body in other parts of respiratory tract** causing asphyxiation   `CC`

     √7ᵗʰ **T17.808**   **Unspecified foreign body in other parts of respiratory tract** causing other injury   `CC`

   √6ᵗʰ **T17.81**   **Gastric contents in** other parts of respiratory tract
Aspiration of gastric contents into other parts of respiratory tract
Vomitus in other parts of respiratory tract

     √7ᵗʰ **T17.810**   **Gastric contents in other parts of respiratory tract** causing asphyxiation   `CC`

     √7ᵗʰ **T17.818**   **Gastric contents in other parts of respiratory tract** causing other injury   `CC`

   √6ᵗʰ **T17.82**   **Food in** other parts of respiratory tract
Bones in other parts of respiratory tract
Seeds in other parts of respiratory tract

     √7ᵗʰ **T17.820**   **Food in other parts of respiratory tract** causing asphyxiation   `CC`

     √7ᵗʰ **T17.828**   **Food in other parts of respiratory tract** causing other injury   `CC`

   √6ᵗʰ **T17.89**   **Other** foreign object in other parts of respiratory tract

     √7ᵗʰ **T17.890**   **Other foreign object in other parts of respiratory tract** causing asphyxiation   `CC`

     √7ᵗʰ **T17.898**   **Other foreign object in other parts of respiratory tract** causing other injury   `CC`

√5ᵗʰ **T17.9**   **Foreign body in respiratory tract**, part unspecified

   √6ᵗʰ **T17.90**   **Unspecified** foreign body in respiratory tract, part unspecified

N Newborn: 0   P Pediatric: 0-17   M Maternity: 12-55   A Adult: 15-124   MCC Major CC Condition   PDxMCC PDx acts as own MCC   CC CC Condition   PDxCC PDx acts as own CC

**1078**

ICD-10-CM 2018

✓7ᵗʰ **T17.900** **Unspecified foreign body in respiratory tract, part unspecified** causing **asphyxiation**

✓7ᵗʰ **T17.908** **Unspecified foreign body in respiratory tract, part unspecified** causing other injury

✓6ᵗʰ **T17.91** Gastric contents **in respiratory tract, part unspecified**
　　Aspiration of gastric contents into respiratory tract, part unspecified
　　Vomitus in trachea respiratory tract, part unspecified

✓7ᵗʰ **T17.910** **Gastric contents in respiratory tract, part unspecified** causing asphyxiation

✓7ᵗʰ **T17.918** **Gastric contents in respiratory tract, part unspecified** causing other injury

✓6ᵗʰ **T17.92** Food **in respiratory tract, part unspecified**
　　Bones in respiratory tract, part unspecified
　　Seeds in respiratory tract, part unspecified

✓7ᵗʰ **T17.920** **Food in respiratory tract, part unspecified** causing **asphyxiation**

✓7ᵗʰ **T17.928** **Food in respiratory tract, part unspecified** causing other injury

✓6ᵗʰ **T17.99** Other **foreign object in respiratory tract, part unspecified**

✓7ᵗʰ **T17.990** **Other foreign object in respiratory tract, part unspecified in** causing **asphyxiation**

✓7ᵗʰ **T17.998** **Other foreign object in respiratory tract, part unspecified** causing other injury

✓4ᵗʰ **T18** **Foreign body in alimentary tract**
　　*EXCLUDES 2*　foreign body in pharynx (T17.2-)

The appropriate 7th character is to be added to each code from category T18.
A　initial encounter
D　subsequent encounter
S　sequela

✓x7ᵗʰ **T18.0** **Foreign body in** mouth

✓5ᵗʰ **T18.1** **Foreign body in** esophagus
　　*EXCLUDES 2*　foreign body in respiratory tract (T17.-)

✓6ᵗʰ **T18.10** Unspecified **foreign body in esophagus**

✓7ᵗʰ **T18.100** **Unspecified foreign body in esophagus** causing compression of trachea
　　Unspecified foreign body in esophagus causing obstruction of respiration

✓7ᵗʰ **T18.108** **Unspecified foreign body in esophagus** causing other injury

✓6ᵗʰ **T18.11** Gastric contents **in esophagus**
　　Vomitus in esophagus

✓7ᵗʰ **T18.110** **Gastric contents in esophagus** causing compression of trachea
　　Gastric contents in esophagus causing obstruction of respiration

✓7ᵗʰ **T18.118** **Gastric contents in esophagus** causing other injury

✓6ᵗʰ **T18.12** Food **in esophagus**
　　Bones in esophagus
　　Seeds in esophagus

✓7ᵗʰ **T18.120** **Food in esophagus** causing compression of trachea
　　Food in esophagus causing obstruction of respiration

✓7ᵗʰ **T18.128** **Food in esophagus** causing other injury

✓6ᵗʰ **T18.19** Other **foreign object in esophagus**
　　AHA: 2015, 1Q, 23

✓7ᵗʰ **T18.190** **Other foreign object in esophagus** causing compression of trachea
　　Other foreign body in esophagus causing obstruction of respiration

✓7ᵗʰ **T18.198** **Other foreign object in esophagus** causing other injury

✓x7ᵗʰ **T18.2** **Foreign body in** stomach

✓x7ᵗʰ **T18.3** **Foreign body in** small intestine

✓x7ᵗʰ **T18.4** **Foreign body in** colon

✓x7ᵗʰ **T18.5** **Foreign body in** anus and rectum
　　Foreign body in rectosigmoid (junction)

✓x7ᵗʰ **T18.8** **Foreign body in** other parts **of alimentary tract**

✓x7ᵗʰ **T18.9** **Foreign body of alimentary tract,** part unspecified
　　Foreign body in digestive system NOS
　　Swallowed foreign body NOS

✓4ᵗʰ **T19** **Foreign body in genitourinary tract**
　　*EXCLUDES 2*　complications due to implanted mesh (T83.7-)
　　　mechanical complications of contraceptive device (intrauterine) (vaginal) (T83.3-)
　　　presence of contraceptive device (intrauterine) (vaginal) (Z97.5)

The appropriate 7th character is to be added to each code from category T19.
A　initial encounter
D　subsequent encounter
S　sequela

✓x7ᵗʰ **T19.0** **Foreign body in** urethra

✓x7ᵗʰ **T19.1** **Foreign body in** bladder

✓x7ᵗʰ **T19.2** **Foreign body in** vulva and vagina　　♀

✓x7ᵗʰ **T19.3** **Foreign body in** uterus　　♀

✓x7ᵗʰ **T19.4** **Foreign body in** penis　　♂

✓x7ᵗʰ **T19.8** **Foreign body in** other parts **of genitourinary tract**

✓x7ᵗʰ **T19.9** **Foreign body in genitourinary tract,** part unspecified

## Burns and corrosions (T20-T32)

**INCLUDES**　burns (thermal) from electrical heating appliances
　　burns (thermal) from electricity
　　burns (thermal) from flame
　　burns (thermal) from friction
　　burns (thermal) from hot air and hot gases
　　burns (thermal) from hot objects
　　burns (thermal) from lightning
　　burns (thermal) from radiation
　　chemical burn [corrosion] (external) (internal)
　　scalds
*EXCLUDES 2*　erythema [dermatitis] ab igne (L59.0)
　　radiation-related disorders of the skin and subcutaneous tissue (L55-L59)
　　sunburn (L55.-)
**AHA:** 2016, 2Q, 4

## Burns and corrosions of external body surface, specified by site (T20-T25)

**INCLUDES**　burns and corrosions of first degree [erythema]
　　burns and corrosions of second degree [blisters] [epidermal loss]
　　burns and corrosions of third degree [deep necrosis of underlying tissue] [full-thickness skin loss]
Use additional code from category T31 or T32 to identify extent of body surface involved

✓4ᵗʰ **T20** **Burn and corrosion of head, face, and neck**
　　*EXCLUDES 2*　burn and corrosion of ear drum (T28.41, T28.91)
　　　burn and corrosion of eye and adnexa (T26.-)
　　　burn and corrosion of mouth and pharynx (T28.0)
　　AHA: 2015, 1Q, 18-19

The appropriate 7th character is to be added to each code from category T20.
A　initial encounter
D　subsequent encounter
S　sequela

✓5ᵗʰ **T20.0** **Burn of** unspecified degree **of head, face, and neck**
　　Use additional external cause code to identify the source, place and intent of the burn (X00-X19, X75-X77, X96-X98, Y92)

✓x7ᵗʰ **T20.00** **Burn of unspecified degree of head, face, and neck,** unspecified site

✓6ᵗʰ **T20.01** **Burn of unspecified degree of** ear [any part, except ear drum]
　　*EXCLUDES 2*　burn of ear drum (T28.41-)

✓7ᵗʰ **T20.011** **Burn of unspecified degree of** right ear **[any part, except ear drum]**

✓7ᵗʰ **T20.012** **Burn of unspecified degree of** left ear **[any part, except ear drum]**

✓7ᵗʰ **T20.019** **Burn of unspecified degree of** unspecified ear **[any part, except ear drum]**

✓x7ᵗʰ **T20.02** **Burn of unspecified degree of** lip(s)

✓x7ᵗʰ **T20.03** **Burn of unspecified degree of** chin

✓x7ᵗʰ **T20.04** **Burn of unspecified degree of** nose (septum)

✓x7ᵗʰ **T20.05** **Burn of unspecified degree of** scalp [any part]

✓x7ᵗʰ **T20.06** **Burn of unspecified degree of** forehead and cheek

✓Additional Character Req　✓x7ᵗʰ Placeholder Alert　Unacceptable PDx　Manifestation　**H1**-**H14** HAC　**HCC** CMS-HCC Condition　*EXCLUDES 1* Not Coded Here　*EXCLUDES 2* Not Included Here

ICD-10-CM 2018　　　　1079

## Rule of Nines Estimation of Total Body Surface Burned

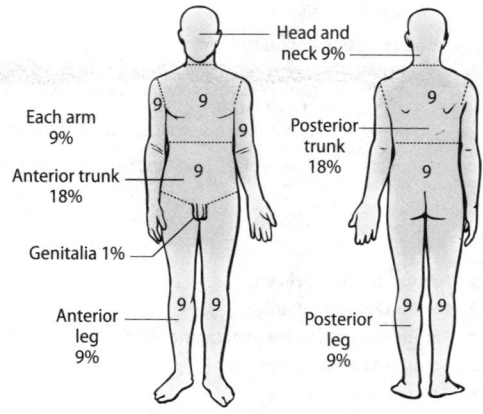

- Head and neck 9%
- Each arm 9%
- Anterior trunk 18%
- Genitalia 1%
- Anterior leg 9%
- Posterior trunk 18%
- Posterior leg 9%

## Degree of Burns

Epidermis
Dermis
Subcutaneous

Normal      First Degree Burn

Second Degree Burn      Third Degree Burn

---

√7ᵗʰ **T20.07** Burn of unspecified degree of neck

√7ᵗʰ **T20.09** Burn of unspecified degree of multiple sites of head, face, and neck

√5ᵗʰ **T20.1** Burn of first degree of head, face, and neck
      Use additional external cause code to identify the source, place and intent of the burn (X00-X19, X75-X77, X96-X98, Y92)

√7ᵗʰ **T20.10** Burn of first degree of head, face, and neck, unspecified site

√6ᵗʰ **T20.11** Burn of first degree of ear [any part, except ear drum]
      **EXCLUDES 2** burn of ear drum (T28.41-)

 √7ᵗʰ **T20.111** Burn of first degree of right ear [any part, except ear drum]

 √7ᵗʰ **T20.112** Burn of first degree of left ear [any part, except ear drum]

 √7ᵗʰ **T20.119** Burn of first degree of unspecified ear [any part, except ear drum]

√x7ᵗʰ **T20.12** Burn of first degree of lip(s)

√x7ᵗʰ **T20.13** Burn of first degree of chin

√x7ᵗʰ **T20.14** Burn of first degree of nose (septum)

√x7ᵗʰ **T20.15** Burn of first degree of scalp [any part]

√x7ᵗʰ **T20.16** Burn of first degree of forehead and cheek

√x7ᵗʰ **T20.17** Burn of first degree of neck

√x7ᵗʰ **T20.19** Burn of first degree of multiple sites of head, face, and neck

√5ᵗʰ **T20.2** Burn of second degree of head, face, and neck
      Use additional external cause code to identify the source, place and intent of the burn (X00-X19, X75-X77, X96-X98, Y92)

√x7ᵗʰ **T20.20** Burn of second degree of head, face, and neck, unspecified site

√6ᵗʰ **T20.21** Burn of second degree of ear [any part, except ear drum]
      **EXCLUDES 2** burn of ear drum (T28.41-)

 √7ᵗʰ **T20.211** Burn of second degree of right ear [any part, except ear drum]

 √7ᵗʰ **T20.212** Burn of second degree of left ear [any part, except ear drum]

 √7ᵗʰ **T20.219** Burn of second degree of unspecified ear [any part, except ear drum]

√x7ᵗʰ **T20.22** Burn of second degree of lip(s)

√x7ᵗʰ **T20.23** Burn of second degree of chin

√x7ᵗʰ **T20.24** Burn of second degree of nose (septum)

√x7ᵗʰ **T20.25** Burn of second degree of scalp [any part]

√x7ᵗʰ **T20.26** Burn of second degree of forehead and cheek

√x7ᵗʰ **T20.27** Burn of second degree of neck

√x7ᵗʰ **T20.29** Burn of second degree of multiple sites of head, face, and neck

---

√5ᵗʰ **T20.3** Burn of third degree of head, face, and neck
      Use additional external cause code to identify the source, place and intent of the burn (X00-X19, X75-X77, X96-X98, Y92)

√x7ᵗʰ **T20.30** Burn of third degree of head, face, and neck, unspecified site   **CC H5**
      CC Excl: PDX collection 1375

√6ᵗʰ **T20.31** Burn of third degree of ear [any part, except ear drum]
      **EXCLUDES 2** burn of ear drum (T28.41-)
      **AHA:** 2015, 1Q, 18

      **CC Excl: For codes in subcategory T20.31:**
      PDX collection 1376

 √7ᵗʰ **T20.311** Burn of third degree of right ear [any part, except ear drum]   **CC H5**

 √7ᵗʰ **T20.312** Burn of third degree of left ear [any part, except ear drum]   **CC H5**

 √7ᵗʰ **T20.319** Burn of third degree of unspecified ear [any part, except ear drum]   **CC H5**

√x7ᵗʰ **T20.32** Burn of third degree of lip(s)   **CC H5**
      CC Excl: PDX collection 1377

√x7ᵗʰ **T20.33** Burn of third degree of chin   **CC H5**
      CC Excl: PDX collection 1378

√x7ᵗʰ **T20.34** Burn of third degree of nose (septum)   **CC H5**
      CC Excl: PDX collection 1379

√x7ᵗʰ **T20.35** Burn of third degree of scalp [any part]   **CC H5**
      CC Excl: PDX collection 1380

√x7ᵗʰ **T20.36** Burn of third degree of forehead and cheek   **CC H5**
      CC Excl: PDX collection 1381

√x7ᵗʰ **T20.37** Burn of third degree of neck   **CC H5**
      CC Excl: PDX collection 1382

√x7ᵗʰ **T20.39** Burn of third degree of multiple sites of head, face, and neck   **CC H5**
      CC Excl: PDX collection 1383

√5ᵗʰ **T20.4** Corrosion of unspecified degree of head, face, and neck
      Code first (T51-T65) to identify chemical and intent
      Use additional external cause code to identify place (Y92)

√x7ᵗʰ **T20.40** Corrosion of unspecified degree of head, face, and neck, unspecified site

√6ᵗʰ **T20.41** Corrosion of unspecified degree of ear [any part, except ear drum]
      **EXCLUDES 2** corrosion of ear drum (T28.91-)

 √7ᵗʰ **T20.411** Corrosion of unspecified degree of right ear [any part, except ear drum]

 √7ᵗʰ **T20.412** Corrosion of unspecified degree of left ear [any part, except ear drum]

 √7ᵗʰ **T20.419** Corrosion of unspecified degree of unspecified ear [any part, except ear drum]

√x7ᵗʰ **T20.42** Corrosion of unspecified degree of lip(s)

√x7ᵗʰ **T20.43** Corrosion of unspecified degree of chin

---

**N** Newborn: 0   **P** Pediatric: 0-17   **M** Maternity: 12-55   **A** Adult: 15-124   **MCC** Major CC Condition   **PDxMCC** PDx acts as own MCC   **CC** CC Condition   **PDxCC** PDx acts as own CC

**1080**      ICD-10-CM 2018

√x 7ᵗʰ **T20.44** **Corrosion of unspecified degree of nose (septum)**

√x 7ᵗʰ **T20.45** **Corrosion of unspecified degree of scalp [any part]**

√x 7ᵗʰ **T20.46** **Corrosion of unspecified degree of forehead and cheek**

√x 7ᵗʰ **T20.47** **Corrosion of unspecified degree of neck**

√x 7ᵗʰ **T20.49** **Corrosion of unspecified degree of multiple sites of head, face, and neck**

√ 5ᵗʰ **T20.5** **Corrosion of first degree of head, face, and neck**
Code first (T51-T65) to identify chemical and intent
Use additional external cause code to identify place (Y92)

√x 7ᵗʰ **T20.50** **Corrosion of first degree of head, face, and neck, unspecified site**

√ 6ᵗʰ **T20.51** **Corrosion of first degree of ear [any part, except ear drum]**
*EXCLUDES 2*   corrosion of ear drum (T28.91-)

√ 7ᵗʰ **T20.511** **Corrosion of first degree of right ear [any part, except ear drum]**

√ 7ᵗʰ **T20.512** **Corrosion of first degree of left ear [any part, except ear drum]**

√ 7ᵗʰ **T20.519** **Corrosion of first degree of unspecified ear [any part, except ear drum]**

√x 7ᵗʰ **T20.52** **Corrosion of first degree of lip(s)**

√x 7ᵗʰ **T20.53** **Corrosion of first degree of chin**

√x 7ᵗʰ **T20.54** **Corrosion of first degree of nose (septum)**

√x 7ᵗʰ **T20.55** **Corrosion of first degree of scalp [any part]**

√x 7ᵗʰ **T20.56** **Corrosion of first degree of forehead and cheek**

√x 7ᵗʰ **T20.57** **Corrosion of first degree of neck**

√x 7ᵗʰ **T20.59** **Corrosion of first degree of multiple sites of head, face, and neck**

√ 5ᵗʰ **T20.6** **Corrosion of second degree of head, face, and neck**
Code first (T51-T65) to identify chemical and intent
Use additional external cause code to identify place (Y92)

√x 7ᵗʰ **T20.60** **Corrosion of second degree of head, face, and neck, unspecified site**

√ 6ᵗʰ **T20.61** **Corrosion of second degree of ear [any part, except ear drum]**
*EXCLUDES 2*   corrosion of ear drum (T28.91-)

√ 7ᵗʰ **T20.611** **Corrosion of second degree of right ear [any part, except ear drum]**

√ 7ᵗʰ **T20.612** **Corrosion of second degree of left ear [any part, except ear drum]**

√ 7ᵗʰ **T20.619** **Corrosion of second degree of unspecified ear [any part, except ear drum]**

√x 7ᵗʰ **T20.62** **Corrosion of second degree of lip(s)**

√x 7ᵗʰ **T20.63** **Corrosion of second degree of chin**

√x 7ᵗʰ **T20.64** **Corrosion of second degree of nose (septum)**

√x 7ᵗʰ **T20.65** **Corrosion of second degree of scalp [any part]**

√x 7ᵗʰ **T20.66** **Corrosion of second degree of forehead and cheek**

√x 7ᵗʰ **T20.67** **Corrosion of second degree of neck**

√x 7ᵗʰ **T20.69** **Corrosion of second degree of multiple sites of head, face, and neck**

√ 5ᵗʰ **T20.7** **Corrosion of third degree of head, face, and neck**
Code first (T51-T65) to identify chemical and intent
Use additional external cause code to identify place (Y92)

√x 7ᵗʰ **T20.70** **Corrosion of third degree of head, face, and neck, unspecified site**   CC H5
**CC Excl:** PDX collection 1375

√ 6ᵗʰ **T20.71** **Corrosion of third degree of ear [any part, except ear drum]**
*EXCLUDES 2*   corrosion of ear drum (T28.91-)

**CC Excl: For codes in subcategory T20.71:**
PDX collection 1376

√ 7ᵗʰ **T20.711** **Corrosion of third degree of right ear [any part, except ear drum]**   CC H5

√ 7ᵗʰ **T20.712** **Corrosion of third degree of left ear [any part, except ear drum]**   CC H5

√ 7ᵗʰ **T20.719** **Corrosion of third degree of unspecified ear [any part, except ear drum]**   CC H5

√x 7ᵗʰ **T20.72** **Corrosion of third degree of lip(s)**   CC H5
**CC Excl:** PDX collection 1377

√x 7ᵗʰ **T20.73** **Corrosion of third degree of chin**   CC H5
**CC Excl:** PDX collection 1378

√x 7ᵗʰ **T20.74** **Corrosion of third degree of nose (septum)**   CC H5
**CC Excl:** PDX collection 1379

√x 7ᵗʰ **T20.75** **Corrosion of third degree of scalp [any part]**   CC H5
**CC Excl:** PDX collection 1380

√x 7ᵗʰ **T20.76** **Corrosion of third degree of forehead and cheek**   CC H5
**CC Excl:** PDX collection 1381

√x 7ᵗʰ **T20.77** **Corrosion of third degree of neck**   CC H5
**CC Excl:** PDX collection 1382

√x 7ᵗʰ **T20.79** **Corrosion of third degree of multiple sites of head, face, and neck**   CC H5
**CC Excl:** PDX collection 1383

√ 4ᵗʰ **T21** **Burn and corrosion of trunk**
*INCLUDES*   burns and corrosion of hip region
*EXCLUDES 2*   burns and corrosion of axilla (T22.- with fifth character 4)
    burns and corrosion of scapular region (T22.- with fifth character 6)
    burns and corrosion of shoulder (T22.- with fifth character 5)

The appropriate 7th character is to be added to each code from category T21.
A   initial encounter
D   subsequent encounter
S   sequela

√ 5ᵗʰ **T21.0** **Burn of unspecified degree of trunk**
Use additional external cause code to identify the source, place and intent of the burn (X00-X19, X75-X77, X96-X98, Y92)

√x 7ᵗʰ **T21.00** **Burn of unspecified degree of trunk, unspecified site**

√x 7ᵗʰ **T21.01** **Burn of unspecified degree of chest wall**
Burn of of unspecified degree of breast

√x 7ᵗʰ **T21.02** **Burn of unspecified degree of abdominal wall**
Burn of unspecified degree of flank
Burn of unspecified degree of groin

√x 7ᵗʰ **T21.03** **Burn of unspecified degree of upper back**
Burn of unspecified degree of interscapular region

√x 7ᵗʰ **T21.04** **Burn of unspecified degree of lower back**

√x 7ᵗʰ **T21.05** **Burn of unspecified degree of buttock**
Burn of unspecified degree of anus

√x 7ᵗʰ **T21.06** **Burn of unspecified degree of male genital region** ♂
Burn of unspecified degree of penis
Burn of unspecified degree of scrotum
Burn of unspecified degree of testis

√x 7ᵗʰ **T21.07** **Burn of unspecified degree of female genital region** ♀
Burn of unspecified degree of labium (majus) (minus)
Burn of unspecified degree of perineum
Burn of unspecified degree of vulva
*EXCLUDES 2*   burn of vagina (T28.3)

√x 7ᵗʰ **T21.09** **Burn of unspecified degree of other site of trunk**

√ 5ᵗʰ **T21.1** **Burn of first degree of trunk**
Use additional external cause code to identify the source, place and intent of the burn (X00-X19, X75-X77, X96-X98, Y92)

√x 7ᵗʰ **T21.10** **Burn of first degree of trunk, unspecified site**

√x 7ᵗʰ **T21.11** **Burn of first degree of chest wall**
Burn of first degree of breast

√x 7ᵗʰ **T21.12** **Burn of first degree of abdominal wall**
Burn of first degree of flank
Burn of first degree of groin

√x 7ᵗʰ **T21.13** **Burn of first degree of upper back**
Burn of first degree of interscapular region

√x 7ᵗʰ **T21.14** **Burn of first degree of lower back**

√x 7ᵗʰ **T21.15** **Burn of first degree of buttock**
Burn of first degree of anus

√x 7ᵗʰ **T21.16** **Burn of first degree of male genital region** ♂
Burn of first degree of penis
Burn of first degree of scrotum
Burn of first degree of testis

√x 7ᵗʰ **T21.17** **Burn of first degree of female genital region** ♀
Burn of first degree of labium (majus) (minus)
Burn of first degree of perineum
Burn of first degree of vulva
*EXCLUDES 2*   burn of vagina (T28.3)

√x 7ᵗʰ **T21.19** **Burn of first degree of other site of trunk**

---

**Chapter 19. Injury, Poisoning and Certain Other Consequences of External Causes**

√5ᵗʰ **T21.2** **Burn of** second degree **of trunk**
> Use additional external cause code to identify the source, place and intent of the burn (X00-X19, X75-X77, X96-X98, Y92)

√x7ᵗʰ **T21.20** **Burn of second degree of trunk, unspecified site**

√x7ᵗʰ **T21.21** **Burn of second degree of** chest wall
> Burn of second degree of breast

√x7ᵗʰ **T21.22** **Burn of second degree of** abdominal wall
> Burn of second degree of flank
> Burn of second degree of groin

√x7ᵗʰ **T21.23** **Burn of second degree of** upper back
> Burn of second degree of interscapular region

√x7ᵗʰ **T21.24** **Burn of second degree of** lower back

√x7ᵗʰ **T21.25** **Burn of second degree of** buttock
> Burn of second degree of anus

√x7ᵗʰ **T21.26** **Burn of second degree of** male genital region ♂
> Burn of second degree of penis
> Burn of second degree of scrotum
> Burn of second degree of testis

√x7ᵗʰ **T21.27** **Burn of second degree of** female genital region ♀
> Burn of second degree of labium (majus) (minus)
> Burn of second degree of perineum
> Burn of second degree of vulva
> **EXCLUDES 2** *burn of vagina (T28.3)*

√x7ᵗʰ **T21.29** **Burn of second degree of** other site **of trunk**

√5ᵗʰ **T21.3** **Burn of** third degree **of trunk**
> Use additional external cause code to identify the source, place and intent of the burn (X00-X19, X75-X77, X96-X98, Y92)

√x7ᵗʰ **T21.30** **Burn of third degree of trunk, unspecified site** CC H5
> **CC Excl:** PDX collection 1384

√x7ᵗʰ **T21.31** **Burn of third degree of** chest wall CC H5
> Burn of third degree of breast
> **AHA:** 2016, 2Q, 5
> **CC Excl:** PDX collection 1385

√x7ᵗʰ **T21.32** **Burn of third degree of** abdominal wall CC H5
> Burn of third degree of flank
> Burn of third degree of groin
> **CC Excl:** PDX collection 1386

√x7ᵗʰ **T21.33** **Burn of third degree of** upper back CC H5
> Burn of third degree of interscapular region
> **CC Excl:** PDX collection 1387

√x7ᵗʰ **T21.34** **Burn of third degree of** lower back CC H5
> **CC Excl:** PDX collection 1387

√x7ᵗʰ **T21.35** **Burn of third degree of** buttock CC H5
> Burn of third degree of anus
> **CC Excl:** PDX collection 1387

√x7ᵗʰ **T21.36** **Burn of third degree of** male genital region CC H5 ♂
> Burn of third degree of penis
> Burn of third degree of scrotum
> Burn of third degree of testis
> **CC Excl:** PDX collection 1388

√x7ᵗʰ **T21.37** **Burn of third degree of** female genital region CC H5 ♀
> Burn of third degree of labium (majus) (minus)
> Burn of third degree of perineum
> Burn of third degree of vulva
> **EXCLUDES 2** *burn of vagina (T28.3)*
> **CC Excl:** PDX collection 1388

√x7ᵗʰ **T21.39** **Burn of third degree of** other site **of trunk** CC H5
> **CC Excl:** PDX collection 1384

√5ᵗʰ **T21.4** **Corrosion of** unspecified degree **of trunk**
> Code first (T51-T65) to identify chemical and intent
> Use additional external cause code to identify place (Y92)

√x7ᵗʰ **T21.40** **Corrosion of unspecified degree of trunk, unspecified site**

√x7ᵗʰ **T21.41** **Corrosion of unspecified degree of** chest wall
> Corrosion of unspecified degree of breast

√x7ᵗʰ **T21.42** **Corrosion of unspecified degree of** abdominal wall
> Corrosion of unspecified degree of flank
> Corrosion of unspecified degree of groin

√x7ᵗʰ **T21.43** **Corrosion of unspecified degree of** upper back
> Corrosion of unspecified degree of interscapular region

√x7ᵗʰ **T21.44** **Corrosion of unspecified degree of** lower back

√x7ᵗʰ **T21.45** **Corrosion of unspecified degree of** buttock
> Corrosion of unspecified degree of anus

√x7ᵗʰ **T21.46** **Corrosion of unspecified degree of** male genital region ♂
> Corrosion of unspecified degree of penis
> Corrosion of unspecified degree of scrotum
> Corrosion of unspecified degree of testis

√x7ᵗʰ **T21.47** **Corrosion of unspecified degree of** female genital region ♀
> Corrosion of unspecified degree of labium (majus) (minus)
> Corrosion of unspecified degree of perineum
> Corrosion of unspecified degree of vulva
> **EXCLUDES 2** *corrosion of vagina (T28.8)*

√x7ᵗʰ **T21.49** **Corrosion of unspecified degree of** other site **of trunk**

√5ᵗʰ **T21.5** **Corrosion of** first degree **of trunk**
> Code first (T51-T65) to identify chemical and intent
> Use additional external cause code to identify place (Y92)

√x7ᵗʰ **T21.50** **Corrosion of first degree of trunk, unspecified site**

√x7ᵗʰ **T21.51** **Corrosion of first degree of** chest wall
> Corrosion of first degree of breast

√x7ᵗʰ **T21.52** **Corrosion of first degree of** abdominal wall
> Corrosion of first degree of flank
> Corrosion of first degree of groin

√x7ᵗʰ **T21.53** **Corrosion of first degree of** upper back
> Corrosion of first degree of interscapular region

√x7ᵗʰ **T21.54** **Corrosion of first degree of** lower back

√x7ᵗʰ **T21.55** **Corrosion of first degree of** buttock
> Corrosion of first degree of anus

√x7ᵗʰ **T21.56** **Corrosion of first degree of** male genital region ♂
> Corrosion of first degree of penis
> Corrosion of first degree of scrotum
> Corrosion of first degree of testis

√x7ᵗʰ **T21.57** **Corrosion of first degree of** female genital region ♀
> Corrosion of first degree of labium (majus) (minus)
> Corrosion of first degree of perineum
> Corrosion of first degree of vulva
> **EXCLUDES 2** *corrosion of vagina (T28.8)*

√x7ᵗʰ **T21.59** **Corrosion of first degree of** other site **of trunk**

√5ᵗʰ **T21.6** **Corrosion of** second degree **of trunk**
> Code first (T51-T65) to identify chemical and intent
> Use additional external cause code to identify place (Y92)

√x7ᵗʰ **T21.60** **Corrosion of second degree of trunk, unspecified site**

√x7ᵗʰ **T21.61** **Corrosion of second degree of** chest wall
> Corrosion of second degree of breast

√x7ᵗʰ **T21.62** **Corrosion of second degree of** abdominal wall
> Corrosion of second degree of flank
> Corrosion of second degree of groin

√x7ᵗʰ **T21.63** **Corrosion of second degree of** upper back
> Corrosion of second degree of interscapular region

√x7ᵗʰ **T21.64** **Corrosion of second degree of** lower back

√x7ᵗʰ **T21.65** **Corrosion of second degree of** buttock
> Corrosion of second degree of anus

√x7ᵗʰ **T21.66** **Corrosion of second degree of** male genital region ♂
> Corrosion of second degree of penis
> Corrosion of second degree of scrotum
> Corrosion of second degree of testis

√x7ᵗʰ **T21.67** **Corrosion of second degree of** female genital region ♀
> Corrosion of second degree of labium (majus) (minus)
> Corrosion of second degree of perineum
> Corrosion of second degree of vulva
> **EXCLUDES 2** *corrosion of vagina (T28.8)*

√x7ᵗʰ **T21.69** **Corrosion of second degree of** other site **of trunk**

√5ᵗʰ **T21.7** **Corrosion of** third degree **of trunk**
> Code first (T51-T65) to identify chemical and intent
> Use additional external cause code to identify place (Y92)

√x7ᵗʰ **T21.70** **Corrosion of third degree of trunk, unspecified site** CC H5
> **CC Excl:** PDX collection 1384

√x7ᵗʰ **T21.71** **Corrosion of third degree of** chest wall CC H5
> Corrosion of third degree of breast
> **CC Excl:** PDX collection 1385

√x7ᵗʰ **T21.72** **Corrosion of third degree of** abdominal wall CC H5
> Corrosion of third degree of flank
> Corrosion of third degree of groin
> **CC Excl:** PDX collection 1386

N Newborn: 0    P Pediatric: 0-17    M Maternity: 12-55    A Adult: 15-124    MCC Major CC Condition    PDxMCC PDx acts as own MCC    CC CC Condition    PDxCC PDx acts as own CC

**1082**            ICD-10-CM 2018

✓x7ᵗʰ **T21.73** **Corrosion of third degree of** upper back  CC H5
　Corrosion of third degree of interscapular region
　**CC Excl:** PDX collection 1387

✓x7ᵗʰ **T21.74** **Corrosion of third degree of** lower back  CC H5
　**CC Excl:** PDX collection 1387

✓x7ᵗʰ **T21.75** **Corrosion of third degree of** buttock  CC H5
　Corrosion of third degree of anus
　**CC Excl:** PDX collection 1387

✓x7ᵗʰ **T21.76** **Corrosion of third degree of** male genital region  CC H5 ♂
　Corrosion of third degree of penis
　Corrosion of third degree of scrotum
　Corrosion of third degree of testis
　**CC Excl:** PDX collection 1388

✓x7ᵗʰ **T21.77** **Corrosion of third degree of** female genital region  CC H5 ♀
　Corrosion of third degree of labium (majus) (minus)
　Corrosion of third degree of perineum
　Corrosion of third degree of vulva
　*EXCLUDES 2*　corrosion of vagina (T28.8)
　**CC Excl:** PDX collection 1388

✓x7ᵗʰ **T21.79** **Corrosion of third degree of** other site **of trunk**  CC H5
　**CC Excl:** PDX collection 1384

✓4ᵗʰ **T22** **Burn and corrosion of shoulder and upper limb, except wrist and hand**
　*EXCLUDES 2*　burn and corrosion of interscapular region (T21.-)
　　　　burn and corrosion of wrist and hand (T23.-)

> The appropriate 7th character is to be added to each code from category T22.
> A　initial encounter
> D　subsequent encounter
> S　sequela

✓5ᵗʰ **T22.0** **Burn of** unspecified degree **of shoulder and upper limb, except wrist and hand**
　Use additional external cause code to identify the source, place and intent of the burn (X00-X19, X75-X77, X96-X98, Y92)

✓x7ᵗʰ **T22.00** **Burn of unspecified degree of shoulder and upper limb, except wrist and hand,** unspecified site

✓6ᵗʰ **T22.01** **Burn of unspecified degree of** forearm
　✓7ᵗʰ **T22.011** **Burn of unspecified degree of** right forearm
　✓7ᵗʰ **T22.012** **Burn of unspecified degree of** left forearm
　✓7ᵗʰ **T22.019** **Burn of unspecified degree of** unspecified forearm

✓6ᵗʰ **T22.02** **Burn of unspecified degree of** elbow
　✓7ᵗʰ **T22.021** **Burn of unspecified degree of** right elbow
　✓7ᵗʰ **T22.022** **Burn of unspecified degree of** left elbow
　✓7ᵗʰ **T22.029** **Burn of unspecified degree of** unspecified elbow

✓6ᵗʰ **T22.03** **Burn of unspecified degree of** upper arm
　✓7ᵗʰ **T22.031** **Burn of unspecified degree of** right upper arm
　✓7ᵗʰ **T22.032** **Burn of unspecified degree of** left upper arm
　✓7ᵗʰ **T22.039** **Burn of unspecified degree of** unspecified upper arm

✓6ᵗʰ **T22.04** **Burn of unspecified degree of** axilla
　✓7ᵗʰ **T22.041** **Burn of unspecified degree of** right axilla
　✓7ᵗʰ **T22.042** **Burn of unspecified degree of** left axilla
　✓7ᵗʰ **T22.049** **Burn of unspecified degree of** unspecified axilla

✓6ᵗʰ **T22.05** **Burn of unspecified degree of** shoulder
　✓7ᵗʰ **T22.051** **Burn of unspecified degree of** right shoulder
　✓7ᵗʰ **T22.052** **Burn of unspecified degree of** left shoulder
　✓7ᵗʰ **T22.059** **Burn of unspecified degree of** unspecified shoulder

✓6ᵗʰ **T22.06** **Burn of unspecified degree of** scapular region
　✓7ᵗʰ **T22.061** **Burn of unspecified degree of** right scapular region
　✓7ᵗʰ **T22.062** **Burn of unspecified degree of** left scapular region

✓7ᵗʰ **T22.069** **Burn of unspecified degree of** unspecified scapular region

✓6ᵗʰ **T22.09** **Burn of unspecified degree of** multiple sites of shoulder and upper limb, except wrist and hand
　✓7ᵗʰ **T22.091** **Burn of unspecified degree of multiple sites of** right shoulder and upper limb, except wrist and hand
　✓7ᵗʰ **T22.092** **Burn of unspecified degree of multiple sites of** left shoulder and upper limb, except wrist and hand
　✓7ᵗʰ **T22.099** **Burn of unspecified degree of multiple sites of** unspecified shoulder and upper limb, except wrist and hand

✓5ᵗʰ **T22.1** **Burn of** first degree **of shoulder and upper limb, except wrist and hand**
　Use additional external cause code to identify the source, place and intent of the burn (X00-X19, X75-X77, X96-X98, Y92)

✓x7ᵗʰ **T22.10** **Burn of first degree of shoulder and upper limb, except wrist and hand,** unspecified site

✓6ᵗʰ **T22.11** **Burn of first degree of** forearm
　✓7ᵗʰ **T22.111** **Burn of first degree of** right forearm
　✓7ᵗʰ **T22.112** **Burn of first degree of** left forearm
　✓7ᵗʰ **T22.119** **Burn of first degree of** unspecified forearm

✓6ᵗʰ **T22.12** **Burn of first degree of** elbow
　✓7ᵗʰ **T22.121** **Burn of first degree of** right elbow
　✓7ᵗʰ **T22.122** **Burn of first degree of** left elbow
　✓7ᵗʰ **T22.129** **Burn of first degree of** unspecified elbow

✓6ᵗʰ **T22.13** **Burn of first degree of** upper arm
　✓7ᵗʰ **T22.131** **Burn of first degree of** right upper arm
　✓7ᵗʰ **T22.132** **Burn of first degree of** left upper arm
　✓7ᵗʰ **T22.139** **Burn of first degree of** unspecified upper arm

✓6ᵗʰ **T22.14** **Burn of first degree of** axilla
　✓7ᵗʰ **T22.141** **Burn of first degree of** right axilla
　✓7ᵗʰ **T22.142** **Burn of first degree of** left axilla
　✓7ᵗʰ **T22.149** **Burn of first degree of** unspecified axilla

✓6ᵗʰ **T22.15** **Burn of first degree of** shoulder
　✓7ᵗʰ **T22.151** **Burn of first degree of** right shoulder
　✓7ᵗʰ **T22.152** **Burn of first degree of** left shoulder
　✓7ᵗʰ **T22.159** **Burn of first degree of** unspecified shoulder

✓6ᵗʰ **T22.16** **Burn of first degree of** scapular region
　✓7ᵗʰ **T22.161** **Burn of first degree of** right scapular region
　✓7ᵗʰ **T22.162** **Burn of first degree of** left scapular region
　✓7ᵗʰ **T22.169** **Burn of first degree of** unspecified scapular region

✓6ᵗʰ **T22.19** **Burn of first degree of** multiple sites of shoulder and upper limb, except wrist and hand
　✓7ᵗʰ **T22.191** **Burn of first degree of multiple sites of** right shoulder and upper limb, except wrist and hand
　✓7ᵗʰ **T22.192** **Burn of first degree of multiple sites of** left shoulder and upper limb, except wrist and hand
　✓7ᵗʰ **T22.199** **Burn of first degree of multiple sites of** unspecified shoulder and upper limb, except wrist and hand

✓5ᵗʰ **T22.2** **Burn of** second degree **of shoulder and upper limb, except wrist and hand**
　Use additional external cause code to identify the source, place and intent of the burn (X00-X19, X75-X77, X96-X98, Y92)

✓x7ᵗʰ **T22.20** **Burn of second degree of shoulder and upper limb, except wrist and hand,** unspecified site

✓6ᵗʰ **T22.21** **Burn of second degree of** forearm
　✓7ᵗʰ **T22.211** **Burn of second degree of** right forearm
　✓7ᵗʰ **T22.212** **Burn of second degree of** left forearm
　✓7ᵗʰ **T22.219** **Burn of second degree of** unspecified forearm

✓6ᵗʰ **T22.22** **Burn of second degree of** elbow
　✓7ᵗʰ **T22.221** **Burn of second degree of** right elbow
　✓7ᵗʰ **T22.222** **Burn of second degree of** left elbow

**Chapter 19. Injury, Poisoning and Certain Other Consequences of External Causes**

✓7ᵗʰ **T22.229** Burn of second degree of unspecified elbow

✓6ᵗʰ **T22.23** **Burn of second degree of upper arm**
     ✓7ᵗʰ **T22.231** Burn of second degree of right upper arm
     ✓7ᵗʰ **T22.232** Burn of second degree of left upper arm
     ✓7ᵗʰ **T22.239** Burn of second degree of unspecified upper arm

✓6ᵗʰ **T22.24** **Burn of second degree of axilla**
     ✓7ᵗʰ **T22.241** Burn of second degree of right axilla
     ✓7ᵗʰ **T22.242** Burn of second degree of left axilla
     ✓7ᵗʰ **T22.249** Burn of second degree of unspecified axilla

✓6ᵗʰ **T22.25** **Burn of second degree of shoulder**
     ✓7ᵗʰ **T22.251** Burn of second degree of right shoulder
     ✓7ᵗʰ **T22.252** Burn of second degree of left shoulder
     ✓7ᵗʰ **T22.259** Burn of second degree of unspecified shoulder

✓6ᵗʰ **T22.26** **Burn of second degree of scapular region**
     ✓7ᵗʰ **T22.261** Burn of second degree of right scapular region
     ✓7ᵗʰ **T22.262** Burn of second degree of left scapular region
     ✓7ᵗʰ **T22.269** Burn of second degree of unspecified scapular region

✓6ᵗʰ **T22.29** **Burn of second degree of multiple sites of shoulder and upper limb, except wrist and hand**
     ✓7ᵗʰ **T22.291** Burn of second degree of multiple sites of right shoulder and upper limb, except wrist and hand
     ✓7ᵗʰ **T22.292** Burn of second degree of multiple sites of left shoulder and upper limb, except wrist and hand
     ✓7ᵗʰ **T22.299** Burn of second degree of multiple sites of unspecified shoulder and upper limb, except wrist and hand

✓5ᵗʰ **T22.3** **Burn of third degree of shoulder and upper limb, except wrist and hand**
     Use additional external cause code to identify the source, place and intent of the burn (X00-X19, X75-X77, X96-X98, Y92)

✓x7ᵗʰ **T22.30** **Burn of third degree of shoulder and upper limb, except wrist and hand, unspecified site** CC H5
     **CC Excl:** PDX collection 1389

✓6ᵗʰ **T22.31** **Burn of third degree of forearm**

     **CC Excl: For codes in subcategory T22.31:** PDX collection 1390

     ✓7ᵗʰ **T22.311** Burn of third degree of right forearm CC H5
     ✓7ᵗʰ **T22.312** Burn of third degree of left forearm CC H5
     ✓7ᵗʰ **T22.319** Burn of third degree of unspecified forearm CC H5

✓6ᵗʰ **T22.32** **Burn of third degree of elbow**

     **CC Excl: For codes in subcategory T22.32:** PDX collection 1391

     ✓7ᵗʰ **T22.321** Burn of third degree of right elbow CC H5
     ✓7ᵗʰ **T22.322** Burn of third degree of left elbow CC H5
     ✓7ᵗʰ **T22.329** Burn of third degree of unspecified elbow CC H5

✓6ᵗʰ **T22.33** **Burn of third degree of upper arm**

     **CC Excl: For codes in subcategory T22.33:** PDX collection 1392

     ✓7ᵗʰ **T22.331** Burn of third degree of right upper arm CC H5
     ✓7ᵗʰ **T22.332** Burn of third degree of left upper arm CC H5
     ✓7ᵗʰ **T22.339** Burn of third degree of unspecified upper arm CC H5

✓6ᵗʰ **T22.34** **Burn of third degree of axilla**

     **CC Excl: For codes in subcategory T22.34:** PDX collection 1393

     ✓7ᵗʰ **T22.341** Burn of third degree of right axilla CC H5
     ✓7ᵗʰ **T22.342** Burn of third degree of left axilla CC H5

✓7ᵗʰ **T22.349** Burn of third degree of unspecified axilla CC H5

✓6ᵗʰ **T22.35** **Burn of third degree of shoulder**

     **CC Excl: For codes in subcategory T22.35:** PDX collection 1394

     ✓7ᵗʰ **T22.351** Burn of third degree of right shoulder CC H5
     ✓7ᵗʰ **T22.352** Burn of third degree of left shoulder CC H5
     ✓7ᵗʰ **T22.359** Burn of third degree of unspecified shoulder CC H5

✓6ᵗʰ **T22.36** **Burn of third degree of scapular region**

     **CC Excl: For codes in subcategory T22.36:** PDX collection 1395

     ✓7ᵗʰ **T22.361** Burn of third degree of right scapular region CC H5
     ✓7ᵗʰ **T22.362** Burn of third degree of left scapular region CC H5
     ✓7ᵗʰ **T22.369** Burn of third degree of unspecified scapular region CC H5

✓6ᵗʰ **T22.39** **Burn of third degree of multiple sites of shoulder and upper limb, except wrist and hand**

     **CC Excl: For codes in subcategory T22.39:** PDX collection 1389

     ✓7ᵗʰ **T22.391** Burn of third degree of multiple sites of right shoulder and upper limb, except wrist and hand CC H5
     ✓7ᵗʰ **T22.392** Burn of third degree of multiple sites of left shoulder and upper limb, except wrist and hand CC H5
     ✓7ᵗʰ **T22.399** Burn of third degree of multiple sites of unspecified shoulder and upper limb, except wrist and hand CC H5

✓5ᵗʰ **T22.4** **Corrosion of unspecified degree of shoulder and upper limb, except wrist and hand**
     Code first (T51-T65) to identify chemical and intent
     Use additional external cause code to identify place (Y92)

✓x7ᵗʰ **T22.40** **Corrosion of unspecified degree of shoulder and upper limb, except wrist and hand, unspecified site**

✓6ᵗʰ **T22.41** **Corrosion of unspecified degree of forearm**
     ✓7ᵗʰ **T22.411** Corrosion of unspecified degree of right forearm
     ✓7ᵗʰ **T22.412** Corrosion of unspecified degree of left forearm
     ✓7ᵗʰ **T22.419** Corrosion of unspecified degree of unspecified forearm

✓6ᵗʰ **T22.42** **Corrosion of unspecified degree of elbow**
     ✓7ᵗʰ **T22.421** Corrosion of unspecified degree of right elbow
     ✓7ᵗʰ **T22.422** Corrosion of unspecified degree of left elbow
     ✓7ᵗʰ **T22.429** Corrosion of unspecified degree of unspecified elbow

✓6ᵗʰ **T22.43** **Corrosion of unspecified degree of upper arm**
     ✓7ᵗʰ **T22.431** Corrosion of unspecified degree of right upper arm
     ✓7ᵗʰ **T22.432** Corrosion of unspecified degree of left upper arm
     ✓7ᵗʰ **T22.439** Corrosion of unspecified degree of unspecified upper arm

✓6ᵗʰ **T22.44** **Corrosion of unspecified degree of axilla**
     ✓7ᵗʰ **T22.441** Corrosion of unspecified degree of right axilla
     ✓7ᵗʰ **T22.442** Corrosion of unspecified degree of left axilla
     ✓7ᵗʰ **T22.449** Corrosion of unspecified degree of unspecified axilla

✓6ᵗʰ **T22.45** **Corrosion of unspecified degree of shoulder**
     ✓7ᵗʰ **T22.451** Corrosion of unspecified degree of right shoulder
     ✓7ᵗʰ **T22.452** Corrosion of unspecified degree of left shoulder
     ✓7ᵗʰ **T22.459** Corrosion of unspecified degree of unspecified shoulder

Ⓝ Newborn: 0   Ⓟ Pediatric: 0-17   Ⓜ Maternity: 12-55   Ⓐ Adult: 15-124   **MCC** Major CC Condition   **PDxMCC** PDx acts as own MCC   **CC** CC Condition   **PDxCC** PDx acts as own CC

**1084**      ICD-10-CM 2018

√6ᵗʰ **T22.46** Corrosion of unspecified degree of scapular region

√7ᵗʰ **T22.461** Corrosion of unspecified degree of right scapular region

√7ᵗʰ **T22.462** Corrosion of unspecified degree of left scapular region

√7ᵗʰ **T22.469** Corrosion of unspecified degree of unspecified scapular region

√6ᵗʰ **T22.49** Corrosion of unspecified degree of multiple sites of shoulder and upper limb, except wrist and hand

√7ᵗʰ **T22.491** Corrosion of unspecified degree of multiple sites of right shoulder and upper limb, except wrist and hand

√7ᵗʰ **T22.492** Corrosion of unspecified degree of multiple sites of left shoulder and upper limb, except wrist and hand

√7ᵗʰ **T22.499** Corrosion of unspecified degree of multiple sites of unspecified shoulder and upper limb, except wrist and hand

√5ᵗʰ **T22.5** Corrosion of first degree of shoulder and upper limb, except wrist and hand

Code first (T51-T65) to identify chemical and intent
Use additional external cause code to identify place (Y92)

√x7ᵗʰ **T22.50** Corrosion of first degree of shoulder and upper limb, except wrist and hand unspecified site

√6ᵗʰ **T22.51** Corrosion of first degree of forearm

√7ᵗʰ **T22.511** Corrosion of first degree of right forearm

√7ᵗʰ **T22.512** Corrosion of first degree of left forearm

√7ᵗʰ **T22.519** Corrosion of first degree of unspecified forearm

√6ᵗʰ **T22.52** Corrosion of first degree of elbow

√7ᵗʰ **T22.521** Corrosion of first degree of right elbow

√7ᵗʰ **T22.522** Corrosion of first degree of left elbow

√7ᵗʰ **T22.529** Corrosion of first degree of unspecified elbow

√6ᵗʰ **T22.53** Corrosion of first degree of upper arm

√7ᵗʰ **T22.531** Corrosion of first degree of right upper arm

√7ᵗʰ **T22.532** Corrosion of first degree of left upper arm

√7ᵗʰ **T22.539** Corrosion of first degree of unspecified upper arm

√6ᵗʰ **T22.54** Corrosion of first degree of axilla

√7ᵗʰ **T22.541** Corrosion of first degree of right axilla

√7ᵗʰ **T22.542** Corrosion of first degree of left axilla

√7ᵗʰ **T22.549** Corrosion of first degree of unspecified axilla

√6ᵗʰ **T22.55** Corrosion of first degree of shoulder

√7ᵗʰ **T22.551** Corrosion of first degree of right shoulder

√7ᵗʰ **T22.552** Corrosion of first degree of left shoulder

√7ᵗʰ **T22.559** Corrosion of first degree of unspecified shoulder

√6ᵗʰ **T22.56** Corrosion of first degree of scapular region

√7ᵗʰ **T22.561** Corrosion of first degree of right scapular region

√7ᵗʰ **T22.562** Corrosion of first degree of left scapular region

√7ᵗʰ **T22.569** Corrosion of first degree of unspecified scapular region

√6ᵗʰ **T22.59** Corrosion of first degree of multiple sites of shoulder and upper limb, except wrist and hand

√7ᵗʰ **T22.591** Corrosion of first degree of multiple sites of right shoulder and upper limb, except wrist and hand

√7ᵗʰ **T22.592** Corrosion of first degree of multiple sites of left shoulder and upper limb, except wrist and hand

√7ᵗʰ **T22.599** Corrosion of first degree of multiple sites of unspecified shoulder and upper limb, except wrist and hand

√5ᵗʰ **T22.6** Corrosion of second degree of shoulder and upper limb, except wrist and hand

Code first (T51-T65) to identify chemical and intent
Use additional external cause code to identify place (Y92)

√x7ᵗʰ **T22.60** Corrosion of second degree of shoulder and upper limb, except wrist and hand, unspecified site

√6ᵗʰ **T22.61** Corrosion of second degree of forearm

√7ᵗʰ **T22.611** Corrosion of second degree of right forearm

√7ᵗʰ **T22.612** Corrosion of second degree of left forearm

√7ᵗʰ **T22.619** Corrosion of second degree of unspecified forearm

√6ᵗʰ **T22.62** Corrosion of second degree of elbow

√7ᵗʰ **T22.621** Corrosion of second degree of right elbow

√7ᵗʰ **T22.622** Corrosion of second degree of left elbow

√7ᵗʰ **T22.629** Corrosion of second degree of unspecified elbow

√6ᵗʰ **T22.63** Corrosion of second degree of upper arm

√7ᵗʰ **T22.631** Corrosion of second degree of right upper arm

√7ᵗʰ **T22.632** Corrosion of second degree of left upper arm

√7ᵗʰ **T22.639** Corrosion of second degree of unspecified upper arm

√6ᵗʰ **T22.64** Corrosion of second degree of axilla

√7ᵗʰ **T22.641** Corrosion of second degree of right axilla

√7ᵗʰ **T22.642** Corrosion of second degree of left axilla

√7ᵗʰ **T22.649** Corrosion of second degree of unspecified axilla

√6ᵗʰ **T22.65** Corrosion of second degree of shoulder

√7ᵗʰ **T22.651** Corrosion of second degree of right shoulder

√7ᵗʰ **T22.652** Corrosion of second degree of left shoulder

√7ᵗʰ **T22.659** Corrosion of second degree of unspecified shoulder

√6ᵗʰ **T22.66** Corrosion of second degree of scapular region

√7ᵗʰ **T22.661** Corrosion of second degree of right scapular region

√7ᵗʰ **T22.662** Corrosion of second degree of left scapular region

√7ᵗʰ **T22.669** Corrosion of second degree of unspecified scapular region

√6ᵗʰ **T22.69** Corrosion of second degree of multiple sites of shoulder and upper limb, except wrist and hand

√7ᵗʰ **T22.691** Corrosion of second degree of multiple sites of right shoulder and upper limb, except wrist and hand

√7ᵗʰ **T22.692** Corrosion of second degree of multiple sites of left shoulder and upper limb, except wrist and hand

√7ᵗʰ **T22.699** Corrosion of second degree of multiple sites of unspecified shoulder and upper limb, except wrist and hand

√5ᵗʰ **T22.7** Corrosion of third degree of shoulder and upper limb, except wrist and hand

Code first (T51-T65) to identify chemical and intent
Use additional external cause code to identify place (Y92)

√x7ᵗʰ **T22.70** Corrosion of third degree of shoulder and upper limb, except wrist and hand, unspecified site   CC H5
CC Excl: PDX collection 1389

√6ᵗʰ **T22.71** Corrosion of third degree of forearm

CC Excl: For codes in subcategory T22.71: PDX collection 1390

√7ᵗʰ **T22.711** Corrosion of third degree of right forearm   CC H5

√7ᵗʰ **T22.712** Corrosion of third degree of left forearm   CC H5

√7ᵗʰ **T22.719** Corrosion of third degree of unspecified forearm   CC H5

√6ᵗʰ **T22.72** Corrosion of third degree of elbow

CC Excl: For codes in subcategory T22.72: PDX collection 1391

√7ᵗʰ **T22.721** Corrosion of third degree of right elbow   CC H5

√7ᵗʰ **T22.722** Corrosion of third degree of left elbow   CC H5

√7ᵗʰ **T22.729** Corrosion of third degree of unspecified elbow   CC H5

✔ Additional Character Req   √x7ᵗʰ Placeholder Alert   Unacceptable PDx   Manifestation   H1-H14 HAC   HCC CMS-HCC Condition   EXCLUDES 1 Not Coded Here   EXCLUDES 2 Not Included Here

ICD-10-CM 2018     T22.46–T22.729     1085

✓6ᵗʰ **T22.73** Corrosion of third degree of upper arm

> **CC Excl:** For codes in subcategory T22.73: PDX collection 1392

> ✓7ᵗʰ **T22.731** Corrosion of third degree of right upper arm `CC` `H5`

> ✓7ᵗʰ **T22.732** Corrosion of third degree of left upper arm `CC` `H5`

> ✓7ᵗʰ **T22.739** Corrosion of third degree of unspecified upper arm `CC` `H5`

✓6ᵗʰ **T22.74** Corrosion of third degree of axilla

> **CC Excl:** For codes in subcategory T22.74: PDX collection 1393

> ✓7ᵗʰ **T22.741** Corrosion of third degree of right axilla `CC` `H5`

> ✓7ᵗʰ **T22.742** Corrosion of third degree of left axilla `CC` `H5`

> ✓7ᵗʰ **T22.749** Corrosion of third degree of unspecified axilla `CC` `H5`

✓6ᵗʰ **T22.75** Corrosion of third degree of shoulder

> **CC Excl:** For codes in subcategory T22.75: PDX collection 1394

> ✓7ᵗʰ **T22.751** Corrosion of third degree of right shoulder `CC` `H5`

> ✓7ᵗʰ **T22.752** Corrosion of third degree of left shoulder `CC` `H5`

> ✓7ᵗʰ **T22.759** Corrosion of third degree of unspecified shoulder `CC` `H5`

✓6ᵗʰ **T22.76** Corrosion of third degree of scapular region

> **CC Excl:** For codes in subcategory T22.76: PDX collection 1395

> ✓7ᵗʰ **T22.761** Corrosion of third degree of right scapular region `CC` `H5`

> ✓7ᵗʰ **T22.762** Corrosion of third degree of left scapular region `CC` `H5`

> ✓7ᵗʰ **T22.769** Corrosion of third degree of unspecified scapular region `CC` `H5`

✓6ᵗʰ **T22.79** Corrosion of third degree of multiple sites of shoulder and upper limb, except wrist and hand

> **CC Excl:** For codes in subcategory T22.79: PDX collection 1389

> ✓7ᵗʰ **T22.791** Corrosion of third degree of multiple sites of right shoulder and upper limb, except wrist and hand `CC` `H5`

> ✓7ᵗʰ **T22.792** Corrosion of third degree of multiple sites of left shoulder and upper limb, except wrist and hand `CC` `H5`

> ✓7ᵗʰ **T22.799** Corrosion of third degree of multiple sites of unspecified shoulder and upper limb, except wrist and hand `CC` `H5`

✓4ᵗʰ **T23** **Burn and corrosion of wrist and hand**
**AHA:** 2015, 1Q, 19

> The appropriate 7th character is to be added to each code from category T23.
> A  initial encounter
> D  subsequent encounter
> S  sequela

✓5ᵗʰ **T23.0** Burn of unspecified degree of wrist and hand

> Use additional external cause code to identify the source, place and intent of the burn (X00-X19, X75-X77, X96-X98, Y92)

✓6ᵗʰ **T23.00** Burn of unspecified degree of hand, unspecified site

> ✓7ᵗʰ **T23.001** Burn of unspecified degree of right hand, unspecified site

> ✓7ᵗʰ **T23.002** Burn of unspecified degree of left hand, unspecified site

> ✓7ᵗʰ **T23.009** Burn of unspecified degree of unspecified hand, unspecified site

✓6ᵗʰ **T23.01** Burn of unspecified degree of thumb (nail)

> ✓7ᵗʰ **T23.011** Burn of unspecified degree of right thumb (nail)

> ✓7ᵗʰ **T23.012** Burn of unspecified degree of left thumb (nail)

> ✓7ᵗʰ **T23.019** Burn of unspecified degree of unspecified thumb (nail)

✓6ᵗʰ **T23.02** Burn of unspecified degree of single finger (nail) except thumb

> ✓7ᵗʰ **T23.021** Burn of unspecified degree of single right finger (nail) except thumb

> ✓7ᵗʰ **T23.022** Burn of unspecified degree of single left finger (nail) except thumb

> ✓7ᵗʰ **T23.029** Burn of unspecified degree of unspecified single finger (nail) except thumb

✓6ᵗʰ **T23.03** Burn of unspecified degree of multiple fingers (nail), not including thumb

> ✓7ᵗʰ **T23.031** Burn of unspecified degree of multiple right fingers (nail), not including thumb

> ✓7ᵗʰ **T23.032** Burn of unspecified degree of multiple left fingers (nail), not including thumb

> ✓7ᵗʰ **T23.039** Burn of unspecified degree of unspecified multiple fingers (nail), not including thumb

✓6ᵗʰ **T23.04** Burn of unspecified degree of multiple fingers (nail), including thumb

> ✓7ᵗʰ **T23.041** Burn of unspecified degree of multiple right fingers (nail), including thumb

> ✓7ᵗʰ **T23.042** Burn of unspecified degree of multiple left fingers (nail), including thumb

> ✓7ᵗʰ **T23.049** Burn of unspecified degree of unspecified multiple fingers (nail), including thumb

✓6ᵗʰ **T23.05** Burn of unspecified degree of palm

> ✓7ᵗʰ **T23.051** Burn of unspecified degree of right palm

> ✓7ᵗʰ **T23.052** Burn of unspecified degree of left palm

> ✓7ᵗʰ **T23.059** Burn of unspecified degree of unspecified palm

✓6ᵗʰ **T23.06** Burn of unspecified degree of back of hand

> ✓7ᵗʰ **T23.061** Burn of unspecified degree of back of right hand

> ✓7ᵗʰ **T23.062** Burn of unspecified degree of back of left hand

> ✓7ᵗʰ **T23.069** Burn of unspecified degree of back of unspecified hand

✓6ᵗʰ **T23.07** Burn of unspecified degree of wrist

> ✓7ᵗʰ **T23.071** Burn of unspecified degree of right wrist

> ✓7ᵗʰ **T23.072** Burn of unspecified degree of left wrist

> ✓7ᵗʰ **T23.079** Burn of unspecified degree of unspecified wrist

✓6ᵗʰ **T23.09** Burn of unspecified degree of multiple sites of wrist and hand

> ✓7ᵗʰ **T23.091** Burn of unspecified degree of multiple sites of right wrist and hand

> ✓7ᵗʰ **T23.092** Burn of unspecified degree of multiple sites of left wrist and hand

> ✓7ᵗʰ **T23.099** Burn of unspecified degree of multiple sites of unspecified wrist and hand

✓5ᵗʰ **T23.1** Burn of first degree of wrist and hand

> Use additional external cause code to identify the source, place and intent of the burn (X00-X19, X75-X77, X96-X98, Y92)

✓6ᵗʰ **T23.10** Burn of first degree of hand, unspecified site

> ✓7ᵗʰ **T23.101** Burn of first degree of right hand, unspecified site

> ✓7ᵗʰ **T23.102** Burn of first degree of left hand, unspecified site

> ✓7ᵗʰ **T23.109** Burn of first degree of unspecified hand, unspecified site

✓6ᵗʰ **T23.11** Burn of first degree of thumb (nail)

> ✓7ᵗʰ **T23.111** Burn of first degree of right thumb (nail)

> ✓7ᵗʰ **T23.112** Burn of first degree of left thumb (nail)

> ✓7ᵗʰ **T23.119** Burn of first degree of unspecified thumb (nail)

✓6ᵗʰ **T23.12** Burn of first degree of single finger (nail) except thumb

> ✓7ᵗʰ **T23.121** Burn of first degree of single right finger (nail) except thumb

> ✓7ᵗʰ **T23.122** Burn of first degree of single left finger (nail) except thumb

√7ᵗʰ **T23.129** **Burn of first degree of** unspecified single finger (nail) except thumb

√6ᵗʰ **T23.13** **Burn of first degree of** multiple fingers (nail), not including thumb

  √7ᵗʰ **T23.131** **Burn of first degree of multiple** right fingers (nail), not including thumb

  √7ᵗʰ **T23.132** **Burn of first degree of multiple** left fingers (nail), not including thumb

  √7ᵗʰ **T23.139** **Burn of first degree of** unspecified multiple fingers (nail), not including thumb

√6ᵗʰ **T23.14** **Burn of first degree of** multiple fingers (nail), including thumb

  √7ᵗʰ **T23.141** **Burn of first degree of multiple** right fingers (nail), including thumb

  √7ᵗʰ **T23.142** **Burn of first degree of multiple** left fingers (nail), including thumb

  √7ᵗʰ **T23.149** **Burn of first degree of** unspecified multiple fingers (nail), including thumb

√6ᵗʰ **T23.15** **Burn of first degree of** palm

  √7ᵗʰ **T23.151** **Burn of first degree of** right palm

  √7ᵗʰ **T23.152** **Burn of first degree of** left palm

  √7ᵗʰ **T23.159** **Burn of first degree of** unspecified palm

√6ᵗʰ **T23.16** **Burn of first degree of** back of hand

  √7ᵗʰ **T23.161** **Burn of first degree of back of** right hand

  √7ᵗʰ **T23.162** **Burn of first degree of back of** left hand

  √7ᵗʰ **T23.169** **Burn of first degree of back of** unspecified hand

√6ᵗʰ **T23.17** **Burn of first degree of** wrist

  √7ᵗʰ **T23.171** **Burn of first degree of** right wrist

  √7ᵗʰ **T23.172** **Burn of first degree of** left wrist

  √7ᵗʰ **T23.179** **Burn of first degree of** unspecified wrist

√6ᵗʰ **T23.19** **Burn of first degree of** multiple sites of wrist and hand

  √7ᵗʰ **T23.191** **Burn of first degree of multiple sites of** right wrist and hand

  √7ᵗʰ **T23.192** **Burn of first degree of multiple sites of** left wrist and hand

  √7ᵗʰ **T23.199** **Burn of first degree of multiple sites of** unspecified wrist and hand

√5ᵗʰ **T23.2** **Burn of** second degree **of wrist and hand**

Use additional external cause code to identify the source, place and intent of the burn (X00-X19, X75-X77, X96-X98, Y92)

√6ᵗʰ **T23.20** **Burn of second degree of hand,** unspecified site

  √7ᵗʰ **T23.201** **Burn of second degree of** right hand, unspecified site

  √7ᵗʰ **T23.202** **Burn of second degree of** left hand, unspecified site

  √7ᵗʰ **T23.209** **Burn of second degree of** unspecified hand, unspecified site

√6ᵗʰ **T23.21** **Burn of second degree of** thumb (nail)

  √7ᵗʰ **T23.211** **Burn of second degree of** right thumb (nail)

  √7ᵗʰ **T23.212** **Burn of second degree of** left thumb (nail)

  √7ᵗʰ **T23.219** **Burn of second degree of** unspecified thumb (nail)

√6ᵗʰ **T23.22** **Burn of second degree of** single finger (nail) except thumb

  √7ᵗʰ **T23.221** **Burn of second degree of single** right finger (nail) except thumb

  √7ᵗʰ **T23.222** **Burn of second degree of single** left finger (nail) except thumb

  √7ᵗʰ **T23.229** **Burn of second degree of** unspecified single finger (nail) except thumb

√6ᵗʰ **T23.23** **Burn of second degree of** multiple fingers (nail), not including thumb

  √7ᵗʰ **T23.231** **Burn of second degree of multiple** right fingers (nail), not including thumb

  √7ᵗʰ **T23.232** **Burn of second degree of multiple** left fingers (nail), not including thumb

  √7ᵗʰ **T23.239** **Burn of second degree of** unspecified multiple fingers (nail), not including thumb

√6ᵗʰ **T23.24** **Burn of second degree of** multiple fingers (nail), including thumb

  √7ᵗʰ **T23.241** **Burn of second degree of multiple** right fingers (nail), including thumb

  √7ᵗʰ **T23.242** **Burn of second degree of multiple** left fingers (nail), including thumb

  √7ᵗʰ **T23.249** **Burn of second degree of** unspecified multiple fingers (nail), including thumb

√6ᵗʰ **T23.25** **Burn of second degree of** palm

  √7ᵗʰ **T23.251** **Burn of second degree of** right palm

  √7ᵗʰ **T23.252** **Burn of second degree of** left palm

  √7ᵗʰ **T23.259** **Burn of second degree of** unspecified palm

√6ᵗʰ **T23.26** **Burn of second degree of** back of hand

  √7ᵗʰ **T23.261** **Burn of second degree of** back of right hand

  √7ᵗʰ **T23.262** **Burn of second degree of** back of left hand

  √7ᵗʰ **T23.269** **Burn of second degree of** back of unspecified hand

√6ᵗʰ **T23.27** **Burn of second degree of** wrist

  √7ᵗʰ **T23.271** **Burn of second degree of** right wrist

  √7ᵗʰ **T23.272** **Burn of second degree of** left wrist

  √7ᵗʰ **T23.279** **Burn of second degree of** unspecified wrist

√6ᵗʰ **T23.29** **Burn of second degree of** multiple sites of wrist and hand

  √7ᵗʰ **T23.291** **Burn of second degree of multiple sites of** right wrist and hand

  √7ᵗʰ **T23.292** **Burn of second degree of multiple sites of** left wrist and hand

  √7ᵗʰ **T23.299** **Burn of second degree of multiple sites of** unspecified wrist and hand

√5ᵗʰ **T23.3** **Burn of** third degree **of wrist and hand**

Use additional external cause code to identify the source, place and intent of the burn (X00-X19, X75-X77, X96-X98, Y92)

√6ᵗʰ **T23.30** **Burn of third degree of hand,** unspecified site
**AHA:** 2016, 2Q, 5

> **CC Excl: For codes in subcategory T23.30:**
> PDX collection 1396

  √7ᵗʰ **T23.301** **Burn of third degree of** right hand, unspecified site   **CC H5**

  √7ᵗʰ **T23.302** **Burn of third degree of** left hand, unspecified site   **CC H5**

  √7ᵗʰ **T23.309** **Burn of third degree of** unspecified hand, unspecified site   **CC H5**

√6ᵗʰ **T23.31** **Burn of third degree of** thumb (nail)

> **CC Excl: For codes in subcategory T23.31:**
> PDX collection 1397

  √7ᵗʰ **T23.311** **Burn of third degree of** right thumb (nail)   **CC H5**

  √7ᵗʰ **T23.312** **Burn of third degree of** left thumb (nail)   **CC H5**

  √7ᵗʰ **T23.319** **Burn of third degree of** unspecified thumb (nail)   **CC H5**

√6ᵗʰ **T23.32** **Burn of third degree of** single finger (nail) except thumb

> **CC Excl: For codes in subcategory T23.32:**
> PDX collection 1398

  √7ᵗʰ **T23.321** **Burn of third degree of single** right finger (nail) except thumb   **CC H5**

  √7ᵗʰ **T23.322** **Burn of third degree of single** left finger (nail) except thumb   **CC H5**

  √7ᵗʰ **T23.329** **Burn of third degree of** unspecified single finger (nail) except thumb   **CC H5**

√6ᵗʰ **T23.33** **Burn of third degree of** multiple fingers (nail), not including thumb

> **CC Excl: For codes in subcategory T23.33:**
> PDX collection 1399

  √7ᵗʰ **T23.331** **Burn of third degree of multiple** right fingers (nail), not including thumb   **CC H5**

  √7ᵗʰ **T23.332** **Burn of third degree of multiple** left fingers (nail), not including thumb   **CC H5**

☑ Additional Character Req   √x7ᵗʰ Placeholder Alert   Unacceptable PDx   Manifestation   **H1-H14** HAC   **HCC** CMS-HCC Condition   *EXCLUDES 1* Not Coded Here   *EXCLUDES 2* Not Included Here

ICD-10-CM 2018      **1087**

**T23.339** ✓7th Burn of third degree of unspecified **CC H5** multiple fingers (nail), not including thumb

✓6th **T23.34** Burn of third degree of multiple fingers (nail), including thumb

> **CC Excl: For codes in subcategory T23.34:**
> PDX collection 1400

✓7th **T23.341** Burn of third degree of multiple **CC H5** right fingers (nail), including thumb

✓7th **T23.342** Burn of third degree of multiple **CC H5** left fingers (nail), including thumb

✓7th **T23.349** Burn of third degree of unspecified **CC H5** multiple fingers (nail), including thumb

✓6th **T23.35** Burn of third degree of palm

> **CC Excl: For codes in subcategory T23.35:**
> PDX collection 1401

✓7th **T23.351** Burn of third degree of right palm **CC H5**

✓7th **T23.352** Burn of third degree of left palm **CC H5**

✓7th **T23.359** Burn of third degree of unspecified **CC H5** palm

✓6th **T23.36** Burn of third degree of back of hand

> **CC Excl: For codes in subcategory T23.36:**
> PDX collection 1402

✓7th **T23.361** Burn of third degree of back of **CC H5** right hand

✓7th **T23.362** Burn of third degree of back of left **CC H5** hand

✓7th **T23.369** Burn of third degree of back of **CC H5** unspecified hand

✓6th **T23.37** Burn of third degree of wrist

> **CC Excl: For codes in subcategory T23.37:**
> PDX collection 1403

✓7th **T23.371** Burn of third degree of right wrist **CC H5**

✓7th **T23.372** Burn of third degree of left wrist **CC H5**

✓7th **T23.379** Burn of third degree of unspecified **CC H5** wrist

✓6th **T23.39** Burn of third degree of multiple sites of wrist and hand

> **CC Excl: For codes in subcategory T23.39:**
> PDX collection 1396

✓7th **T23.391** Burn of third degree of multiple **CC H5** sites of right wrist and hand

✓7th **T23.392** Burn of third degree of multiple **CC H5** sites of left wrist and hand

✓7th **T23.399** Burn of third degree of multiple **CC H5** sites of unspecified wrist and hand

✓5th **T23.4** Corrosion of unspecified degree of wrist and hand
Code first (T51-T65) to identify chemical and intent
Use additional external cause code to identify place (Y92)

✓6th **T23.40** Corrosion of unspecified degree of hand, unspecified site

✓7th **T23.401** Corrosion of unspecified degree of right hand, unspecified site

✓7th **T23.402** Corrosion of unspecified degree of left hand, unspecified site

✓7th **T23.409** Corrosion of unspecified degree of unspecified hand, unspecified site

✓6th **T23.41** Corrosion of unspecified degree of thumb (nail)

✓7th **T23.411** Corrosion of unspecified degree of right thumb (nail)

✓7th **T23.412** Corrosion of unspecified degree of left thumb (nail)

✓7th **T23.419** Corrosion of unspecified degree of unspecified thumb (nail)

✓6th **T23.42** Corrosion of unspecified degree of single finger (nail) except thumb

✓7th **T23.421** Corrosion of unspecified degree of single right finger (nail) except thumb

✓7th **T23.422** Corrosion of unspecified degree of single left finger (nail) except thumb

✓7th **T23.429** Corrosion of unspecified degree of unspecified single finger (nail) except thumb

✓6th **T23.43** Corrosion of unspecified degree of multiple fingers (nail), not including thumb

✓7th **T23.431** Corrosion of unspecified degree of multiple right fingers (nail), not including thumb

✓7th **T23.432** Corrosion of unspecified degree of multiple left fingers (nail), not including thumb

✓7th **T23.439** Corrosion of unspecified degree of unspecified multiple fingers (nail), not including thumb

✓6th **T23.44** Corrosion of unspecified degree of multiple fingers (nail), including thumb

✓7th **T23.441** Corrosion of unspecified degree of multiple right fingers (nail), including thumb

✓7th **T23.442** Corrosion of unspecified degree of multiple left fingers (nail), including thumb

✓7th **T23.449** Corrosion of unspecified degree of unspecified multiple fingers (nail), including thumb

✓6th **T23.45** Corrosion of unspecified degree of palm

✓7th **T23.451** Corrosion of unspecified degree of right palm

✓7th **T23.452** Corrosion of unspecified degree of left palm

✓7th **T23.459** Corrosion of unspecified degree of unspecified palm

✓6th **T23.46** Corrosion of unspecified degree of back of hand

✓7th **T23.461** Corrosion of unspecified degree of back of right hand

✓7th **T23.462** Corrosion of unspecified degree of back of left hand

✓7th **T23.469** Corrosion of unspecified degree of back of unspecified hand

✓6th **T23.47** Corrosion of unspecified degree of wrist

✓7th **T23.471** Corrosion of unspecified degree of right wrist

✓7th **T23.472** Corrosion of unspecified degree of left wrist

✓7th **T23.479** Corrosion of unspecified degree of unspecified wrist

✓6th **T23.49** Corrosion of unspecified degree of multiple sites of wrist and hand

✓7th **T23.491** Corrosion of unspecified degree of multiple sites of right wrist and hand

✓7th **T23.492** Corrosion of unspecified degree of multiple sites of left wrist and hand

✓7th **T23.499** Corrosion of unspecified degree of multiple sites of unspecified wrist and hand

✓5th **T23.5** Corrosion of first degree of wrist and hand
Code first (T51-T65) to identify chemical and intent
Use additional external cause code to identify place (Y92)

✓6th **T23.50** Corrosion of first degree of hand, unspecified site

✓7th **T23.501** Corrosion of first degree of right hand, unspecified site

✓7th **T23.502** Corrosion of first degree of left hand, unspecified site

✓7th **T23.509** Corrosion of first degree of unspecified hand, unspecified site

✓6th **T23.51** Corrosion of first degree of thumb (nail)

✓7th **T23.511** Corrosion of first degree of right thumb (nail)

✓7th **T23.512** Corrosion of first degree of left thumb (nail)

✓7th **T23.519** Corrosion of first degree of unspecified thumb (nail)

✓6th **T23.52** Corrosion of first degree of single finger (nail) except thumb

✓7th **T23.521** Corrosion of first degree of single right finger (nail) except thumb

√7ᵗʰ **T23.522** **Corrosion of first degree of single left finger (nail) except thumb**

√7ᵗʰ **T23.529** **Corrosion of first degree of unspecified single finger (nail) except thumb**

√6ᵗʰ **T23.53** **Corrosion of first degree of** multiple fingers (nail), not including thumb

√7ᵗʰ **T23.531** **Corrosion of first degree of multiple right fingers (nail), not including thumb**

√7ᵗʰ **T23.532** **Corrosion of first degree of multiple left fingers (nail), not including thumb**

√7ᵗʰ **T23.539** **Corrosion of first degree of unspecified multiple fingers (nail), not including thumb**

√6ᵗʰ **T23.54** **Corrosion of first degree of** multiple fingers (nail), including thumb

√7ᵗʰ **T23.541** **Corrosion of first degree of multiple right fingers (nail), including thumb**

√7ᵗʰ **T23.542** **Corrosion of first degree of multiple left fingers (nail), including thumb**

√7ᵗʰ **T23.549** **Corrosion of first degree of unspecified multiple fingers (nail), including thumb**

√6ᵗʰ **T23.55** **Corrosion of first degree of** palm

√7ᵗʰ **T23.551** **Corrosion of first degree of right palm**

√7ᵗʰ **T23.552** **Corrosion of first degree of left palm**

√7ᵗʰ **T23.559** **Corrosion of first degree of unspecified palm**

√6ᵗʰ **T23.56** **Corrosion of first degree of** back of hand

√7ᵗʰ **T23.561** **Corrosion of first degree of back of right hand**

√7ᵗʰ **T23.562** **Corrosion of first degree of back of left hand**

√7ᵗʰ **T23.569** **Corrosion of first degree of back of unspecified hand**

√6ᵗʰ **T23.57** **Corrosion of first degree of** wrist

√7ᵗʰ **T23.571** **Corrosion of first degree of right wrist**

√7ᵗʰ **T23.572** **Corrosion of first degree of left wrist**

√7ᵗʰ **T23.579** **Corrosion of first degree of unspecified wrist**

√6ᵗʰ **T23.59** **Corrosion of first degree of** multiple sites of wrist and hand

√7ᵗʰ **T23.591** **Corrosion of first degree of multiple sites of right wrist and hand**

√7ᵗʰ **T23.592** **Corrosion of first degree of multiple sites of left wrist and hand**

√7ᵗʰ **T23.599** **Corrosion of first degree of multiple sites of unspecified wrist and hand**

√5ᵗʰ **T23.6** **Corrosion of** second degree of wrist and hand

Code first (T51-T65) to identify chemical and intent
Use additional external cause code to identify place (Y92)

√6ᵗʰ **T23.60** **Corrosion of second degree of hand, unspecified site**

√7ᵗʰ **T23.601** **Corrosion of second degree of right hand, unspecified site**

√7ᵗʰ **T23.602** **Corrosion of second degree of left hand, unspecified site**

√7ᵗʰ **T23.609** **Corrosion of second degree of unspecified hand, unspecified site**

√6ᵗʰ **T23.61** **Corrosion of second degree of** thumb (nail)

√7ᵗʰ **T23.611** **Corrosion of second degree of right thumb (nail)**

√7ᵗʰ **T23.612** **Corrosion of second degree of left thumb (nail)**

√7ᵗʰ **T23.619** **Corrosion of second degree of unspecified thumb (nail)**

√6ᵗʰ **T23.62** **Corrosion of second degree of** single finger (nail) except thumb

√7ᵗʰ **T23.621** **Corrosion of second degree of single right finger (nail) except thumb**

√7ᵗʰ **T23.622** **Corrosion of second degree of single left finger (nail) except thumb**

√7ᵗʰ **T23.629** **Corrosion of second degree of unspecified single finger (nail) except thumb**

√6ᵗʰ **T23.63** **Corrosion of second degree of** multiple fingers (nail), not including thumb

√7ᵗʰ **T23.631** **Corrosion of second degree of multiple right fingers (nail), not including thumb**

√7ᵗʰ **T23.632** **Corrosion of second degree of multiple left fingers (nail), not including thumb**

√7ᵗʰ **T23.639** **Corrosion of second degree of unspecified multiple fingers (nail), not including thumb**

√6ᵗʰ **T23.64** **Corrosion of second degree of** multiple fingers (nail), including thumb

√7ᵗʰ **T23.641** **Corrosion of second degree of multiple right fingers (nail), including thumb**

√7ᵗʰ **T23.642** **Corrosion of second degree of multiple left fingers (nail), including thumb**

√7ᵗʰ **T23.649** **Corrosion of second degree of unspecified multiple fingers (nail), including thumb**

√6ᵗʰ **T23.65** **Corrosion of second degree of** palm

√7ᵗʰ **T23.651** **Corrosion of second degree of right palm**

√7ᵗʰ **T23.652** **Corrosion of second degree of left palm**

√7ᵗʰ **T23.659** **Corrosion of second degree of unspecified palm**

√6ᵗʰ **T23.66** **Corrosion of second degree of** back of hand

√7ᵗʰ **T23.661** **Corrosion of second degree back of right hand**

√7ᵗʰ **T23.662** **Corrosion of second degree back of left hand**

√7ᵗʰ **T23.669** **Corrosion of second degree back of unspecified hand**

√6ᵗʰ **T23.67** **Corrosion of second degree of** wrist

√7ᵗʰ **T23.671** **Corrosion of second degree of right wrist**

√7ᵗʰ **T23.672** **Corrosion of second degree of left wrist**

√7ᵗʰ **T23.679** **Corrosion of second degree of unspecified wrist**

√6ᵗʰ **T23.69** **Corrosion of second degree of** multiple sites of wrist and hand

√7ᵗʰ **T23.691** **Corrosion of second degree of multiple sites of right wrist and hand**

√7ᵗʰ **T23.692** **Corrosion of second degree of multiple sites of left wrist and hand**

√7ᵗʰ **T23.699** **Corrosion of second degree of multiple sites of unspecified wrist and hand**

√5ᵗʰ **T23.7** **Corrosion of** third degree of wrist and hand

Code first (T51-T65) to identify chemical and intent
Use additional external cause code to identify place (Y92)

√6ᵗʰ **T23.70** **Corrosion of third degree of hand, unspecified site**

> **CC Excl: For codes in subcategory T23.70:**
> PDX collection 1396

√7ᵗʰ **T23.701** **Corrosion of third degree of right hand, unspecified site** `CC` `H5`

√7ᵗʰ **T23.702** **Corrosion of third degree of left hand, unspecified site** `CC` `H5`

√7ᵗʰ **T23.709** **Corrosion of third degree of unspecified hand, unspecified site** `CC` `H5`

√6ᵗʰ **T23.71** **Corrosion of third degree of** thumb (nail)

> **CC Excl: For codes in subcategory T23.71:**
> PDX collection 1397

√7ᵗʰ **T23.711** **Corrosion of third degree of right thumb (nail)** `CC` `H5`

√7ᵗʰ **T23.712** **Corrosion of third degree of left thumb (nail)** `CC` `H5`

√7ᵗʰ **T23.719** **Corrosion of third degree of unspecified thumb (nail)** `CC` `H5`

√6ᵗʰ **T23.72** **Corrosion of third degree of** single finger (nail) except thumb

> **CC Excl: For codes in subcategory T23.72:**
> PDX collection 1398

√7ᵗʰ **T23.721** **Corrosion of third degree of single right finger (nail) except thumb** `CC` `H5`

√7ᵗʰ **T23.722** **Corrosion of third degree of single left finger (nail) except thumb** `CC` `H5`

✓ Additional Character Req   √ₓ7ᵗʰ Placeholder Alert   Unacceptable PDx   Manifestation   **H1**-**H14** HAC   **HCC** CMS-HCC Condition   **EXCLUDES 1** Not Coded Here   **EXCLUDES 2** Not Included Here

ICD-10-CM 2018        **1089**

☑7ᵗʰ **T23.729**   **Corrosion of third degree of unspecified single finger (nail) except thumb**   CC H5

☑6ᵗʰ **T23.73**   **Corrosion of third degree of multiple fingers (nail), not including thumb**

> **CC Excl: For codes in subcategory T23.73:** PDX collection 1399

☑7ᵗʰ **T23.731**   **Corrosion of third degree of multiple right fingers (nail), not including thumb**   CC H5

☑7ᵗʰ **T23.732**   **Corrosion of third degree of multiple left fingers (nail), not including thumb**   CC H5

☑7ᵗʰ **T23.739**   **Corrosion of third degree of unspecified multiple fingers (nail), not including thumb**   CC H5

☑6ᵗʰ **T23.74**   **Corrosion of third degree of multiple fingers (nail), including thumb**

> **CC Excl: For codes in subcategory T23.74:** PDX collection 1400

☑7ᵗʰ **T23.741**   **Corrosion of third degree of multiple right fingers (nail), including thumb**   CC H5

☑7ᵗʰ **T23.742**   **Corrosion of third degree of multiple left fingers (nail), including thumb**   CC H5

☑7ᵗʰ **T23.749**   **Corrosion of third degree of unspecified multiple fingers (nail), including thumb**   CC H5

☑6ᵗʰ **T23.75**   **Corrosion of third degree of palm**

> **CC Excl: For codes in subcategory T23.75:** PDX collection 1401

☑7ᵗʰ **T23.751**   **Corrosion of third degree of right palm**   CC H5

☑7ᵗʰ **T23.752**   **Corrosion of third degree of left palm**   CC H5

☑7ᵗʰ **T23.759**   **Corrosion of third degree of unspecified palm**   CC H5

☑6ᵗʰ **T23.76**   **Corrosion of third degree of back of hand**

> **CC Excl: For codes in subcategory T23.76:** PDX collection 1402

☑7ᵗʰ **T23.761**   **Corrosion of third degree of back of right hand**   CC H5

☑7ᵗʰ **T23.762**   **Corrosion of third degree of back of left hand**   CC H5

☑7ᵗʰ **T23.769**   **Corrosion of third degree back of unspecified hand**   CC H5

☑6ᵗʰ **T23.77**   **Corrosion of third degree of wrist**

> **CC Excl: For codes in subcategory T23.77:** PDX collection 1403

☑7ᵗʰ **T23.771**   **Corrosion of third degree of right wrist**   CC H5

☑7ᵗʰ **T23.772**   **Corrosion of third degree of left wrist**   CC H5

☑7ᵗʰ **T23.779**   **Corrosion of third degree of unspecified wrist**   CC H5

☑6ᵗʰ **T23.79**   **Corrosion of third degree of multiple sites of wrist and hand**

> **CC Excl: For codes in subcategory T23.79:** PDX collection 1396

☑7ᵗʰ **T23.791**   **Corrosion of third degree of multiple sites of right wrist and hand**   CC H5

☑7ᵗʰ **T23.792**   **Corrosion of third degree of multiple sites of left wrist and hand**   CC H5

☑7ᵗʰ **T23.799**   **Corrosion of third degree of multiple sites of unspecified wrist and hand**

---

☑4ᵗʰ **T24**   **Burn and corrosion of lower limb, except ankle and foot**

> **EXCLUDES 2**   *burn and corrosion of ankle and foot (T25.-)*
> *burn and corrosion of hip region (T21.-)*

> The appropriate 7th character is to be added to each code from category T24.
> A   initial encounter
> D   subsequent encounter
> S   sequela

☑5ᵗʰ **T24.0**   **Burn of unspecified degree of lower limb, except ankle and foot**

> Use additional external cause code to identify the source, place and intent of the burn (X00-X19, X75-X77, X96-X98, Y92)

☑6ᵗʰ **T24.00**   **Burn of unspecified degree of unspecified site of lower limb, except ankle and foot**

☑7ᵗʰ **T24.001**   **Burn of unspecified degree of unspecified site of right lower limb, except ankle and foot**

☑7ᵗʰ **T24.002**   **Burn of unspecified degree of unspecified site of left lower limb, except ankle and foot**

☑7ᵗʰ **T24.009**   **Burn of unspecified degree of unspecified site of unspecified lower limb, except ankle and foot**

☑6ᵗʰ **T24.01**   **Burn of unspecified degree of thigh**

☑7ᵗʰ **T24.011**   **Burn of unspecified degree of right thigh**

☑7ᵗʰ **T24.012**   **Burn of unspecified degree of left thigh**

☑7ᵗʰ **T24.019**   **Burn of unspecified degree of unspecified thigh**

☑6ᵗʰ **T24.02**   **Burn of unspecified degree of knee**

☑7ᵗʰ **T24.021**   **Burn of unspecified degree of right knee**

☑7ᵗʰ **T24.022**   **Burn of unspecified degree of left knee**

☑7ᵗʰ **T24.029**   **Burn of unspecified degree of unspecified knee**

☑6ᵗʰ **T24.03**   **Burn of unspecified degree of lower leg**

☑7ᵗʰ **T24.031**   **Burn of unspecified degree of right lower leg**

☑7ᵗʰ **T24.032**   **Burn of unspecified degree of left lower leg**

☑7ᵗʰ **T24.039**   **Burn of unspecified degree of unspecified lower leg**

☑6ᵗʰ **T24.09**   **Burn of unspecified degree of multiple sites of lower limb, except ankle and foot**

☑7ᵗʰ **T24.091**   **Burn of unspecified degree of multiple sites of right lower limb, except ankle and foot**

☑7ᵗʰ **T24.092**   **Burn of unspecified degree of multiple sites of left lower limb, except ankle and foot**

☑7ᵗʰ **T24.099**   **Burn of unspecified degree of multiple sites of unspecified lower limb, except ankle and foot**

☑5ᵗʰ **T24.1**   **Burn of first degree of lower limb, except ankle and foot**

> Use additional external cause code to identify the source, and intent of the burn (X00-X19, X75-X77, X96-X98, Y92)

☑6ᵗʰ **T24.10**   **Burn of first degree of unspecified site of lower limb, except ankle and foot**

☑7ᵗʰ **T24.101**   **Burn of first degree of unspecified site of right lower limb, except ankle and foot**

☑7ᵗʰ **T24.102**   **Burn of first degree of unspecified site of left lower limb, except ankle and foot**

☑7ᵗʰ **T24.109**   **Burn of first degree of unspecified site of unspecified lower limb, except ankle and foot**

☑6ᵗʰ **T24.11**   **Burn of first degree of thigh**

☑7ᵗʰ **T24.111**   **Burn of first degree of right thigh**

☑7ᵗʰ **T24.112**   **Burn of first degree of left thigh**

☑7ᵗʰ **T24.119**   **Burn of first degree of unspecified thigh**

☑6ᵗʰ **T24.12**   **Burn of first degree of knee**

☑7ᵗʰ **T24.121**   **Burn of first degree of right knee**

☑7ᵗʰ **T24.122**   **Burn of first degree of left knee**

☑7ᵗʰ **T24.129**   **Burn of first degree of unspecified knee**

☑6ᵗʰ **T24.13**   **Burn of first degree of lower leg**

☑7ᵗʰ **T24.131**   **Burn of first degree of right lower leg**

☑7ᵗʰ **T24.132**   **Burn of first degree of left lower leg**

N Newborn: 0   P Pediatric: 0-17   M Maternity: 12-55   A Adult: 15-124   MCC Major CC Condition   PDxMCC PDx acts as own MCC   CC CC Condition   PDxCC PDx acts as own CC

1090      ICD-10-CM 2018

√7ᵗʰ **T24.139** **Burn of first degree of** unspecified **lower leg**

√6ᵗʰ **T24.19** **Burn of first degree of** multiple sites **of lower limb, except ankle and foot**

   √7ᵗʰ **T24.191** **Burn of first degree of multiple sites of** right **lower limb, except ankle and foot**

   √7ᵗʰ **T24.192** **Burn of first degree of multiple sites of** left **lower limb, except ankle and foot**

   √7ᵗʰ **T24.199** **Burn of first degree of multiple sites of** unspecified **lower limb, except ankle and foot**

√5ᵗʰ **T24.2** **Burn of** second degree **of lower limb, except ankle and foot**

Use additional external cause code to identify the source, place and intent of the burn (X00-X19, X75-X77, X96-X98, Y92)

√6ᵗʰ **T24.20** **Burn of second degree of** unspecified site **of lower limb, except ankle and foot**

   √7ᵗʰ **T24.201** **Burn of second degree of unspecified site of** right **lower limb, except ankle and foot**

   √7ᵗʰ **T24.202** **Burn of second degree of unspecified site of** left **lower limb, except ankle and foot**

   √7ᵗʰ **T24.209** **Burn of second degree of unspecified site of** unspecified **lower limb, except ankle and foot**

√6ᵗʰ **T24.21** **Burn of second degree of** thigh

   √7ᵗʰ **T24.211** **Burn of second degree of** right **thigh**

   √7ᵗʰ **T24.212** **Burn of second degree of** left **thigh**

   √7ᵗʰ **T24.219** **Burn of second degree of** unspecified **thigh**

√6ᵗʰ **T24.22** **Burn of second degree of** knee

   √7ᵗʰ **T24.221** **Burn of second degree of** right **knee**

   √7ᵗʰ **T24.222** **Burn of second degree of** left **knee**

   √7ᵗʰ **T24.229** **Burn of second degree of** unspecified **knee**

√6ᵗʰ **T24.23** **Burn of second degree of** lower leg

   √7ᵗʰ **T24.231** **Burn of second degree of** right **lower leg**

   √7ᵗʰ **T24.232** **Burn of second degree of** left **lower leg**

   √7ᵗʰ **T24.239** **Burn of second degree of** unspecified **lower leg**

√6ᵗʰ **T24.29** **Burn of second degree of** multiple sites **of lower limb, except ankle and foot**

   √7ᵗʰ **T24.291** **Burn of second degree of multiple sites of** right **lower limb, except ankle and foot**

   √7ᵗʰ **T24.292** **Burn of second degree of multiple sites of** left **lower limb, except ankle and foot**

   √7ᵗʰ **T24.299** **Burn of second degree of multiple sites of** unspecified **lower limb, except ankle and foot**

√5ᵗʰ **T24.3** **Burn of** third degree **of lower limb, except ankle and foot**

Use additional external cause code to identify the source, place and intent of the burn (X00-X19, X75-X77, X96-X98, Y92)

√6ᵗʰ **T24.30** **Burn of third degree of** unspecified site **of lower limb, except ankle and foot**

**CC Excl: For codes in subcategory T24.30:**
PDX collection 1404

   √7ᵗʰ **T24.301** **Burn of third degree of unspecified site of** right **lower limb, except ankle and foot** `CC` `H5`

   √7ᵗʰ **T24.302** **Burn of third degree of unspecified site of** left **lower limb, except ankle and foot** `CC` `H5`

   √7ᵗʰ **T24.309** **Burn of third degree of unspecified site of** unspecified **lower limb, except ankle and foot** `CC` `H5`

√6ᵗʰ **T24.31** **Burn of third degree of** thigh

**CC Excl: For codes in subcategory T24.31:**
PDX collection 1405

   √7ᵗʰ **T24.311** **Burn of third degree of** right **thigh** `CC` `H5`

   √7ᵗʰ **T24.312** **Burn of third degree of** left **thigh** `CC` `H5`

   √7ᵗʰ **T24.319** **Burn of third degree of** unspecified **thigh** `CC` `H5`

√6ᵗʰ **T24.32** **Burn of third degree of** knee

**CC Excl: For codes in subcategory T24.32:**
PDX collection 1406

   √7ᵗʰ **T24.321** **Burn of third degree of** right **knee** `CC` `H5`

   √7ᵗʰ **T24.322** **Burn of third degree of** left **knee** `CC` `H5`

   √7ᵗʰ **T24.329** **Burn of third degree of** unspecified **knee** `CC` `H5`

√6ᵗʰ **T24.33** **Burn of third degree of** lower leg

**CC Excl: For codes in subcategory T24.33:**
PDX collection 1407

   √7ᵗʰ **T24.331** **Burn of third degree of** right **lower leg** `CC` `H5`

   √7ᵗʰ **T24.332** **Burn of third degree of** left **lower leg** `CC` `H5`

   √7ᵗʰ **T24.339** **Burn of third degree of** unspecified **lower leg** `CC` `H5`

√6ᵗʰ **T24.39** **Burn of third degree of** multiple sites **of lower limb, except ankle and foot**
**AHA:** 2016, 2Q, 4

**CC Excl: For codes in subcategory T24.39:**
PDX collection 1404

   √7ᵗʰ **T24.391** **Burn of third degree of multiple sites of** right **lower limb, except ankle and foot** `CC` `H5`

   √7ᵗʰ **T24.392** **Burn of third degree of multiple sites of** left **lower limb, except ankle and foot** `CC` `H5`

   √7ᵗʰ **T24.399** **Burn of third degree of multiple sites of** unspecified **lower limb, except ankle and foot** `CC` `H5`

√5ᵗʰ **T24.4** **Corrosion of** unspecified degree **of lower limb, except ankle and foot**

Code first (T51-T65) to identify chemical and intent
Use additional external cause code to identify place (Y92)

√6ᵗʰ **T24.40** **Corrosion of unspecified degree of** unspecified site **of lower limb, except ankle and foot**

   √7ᵗʰ **T24.401** **Corrosion of unspecified degree of unspecified site of** right **lower limb, except ankle and foot**

   √7ᵗʰ **T24.402** **Corrosion of unspecified degree of unspecified site of** left **lower limb, except ankle and foot**

   √7ᵗʰ **T24.409** **Corrosion of unspecified degree of unspecified site of** unspecified **lower limb, except ankle and foot**

√6ᵗʰ **T24.41** **Corrosion of unspecified degree of** thigh

   √7ᵗʰ **T24.411** **Corrosion of unspecified degree of** right **thigh**

   √7ᵗʰ **T24.412** **Corrosion of unspecified degree of** left **thigh**

   √7ᵗʰ **T24.419** **Corrosion of unspecified degree of** unspecified **thigh**

√6ᵗʰ **T24.42** **Corrosion of unspecified degree of** knee

   √7ᵗʰ **T24.421** **Corrosion of unspecified degree of** right **knee**

   √7ᵗʰ **T24.422** **Corrosion of unspecified degree of** left **knee**

   √7ᵗʰ **T24.429** **Corrosion of unspecified degree of** unspecified **knee**

√6ᵗʰ **T24.43** **Corrosion of unspecified degree of** lower leg

   √7ᵗʰ **T24.431** **Corrosion of unspecified degree of** right **lower leg**

   √7ᵗʰ **T24.432** **Corrosion of unspecified degree of** left **lower leg**

   √7ᵗʰ **T24.439** **Corrosion of unspecified degree of** unspecified **lower leg**

√6ᵗʰ **T24.49** **Corrosion of unspecified degree of** multiple sites **of lower limb, except ankle and foot**

   √7ᵗʰ **T24.491** **Corrosion of unspecified degree of multiple sites of** right **lower limb, except ankle and foot**

   √7ᵗʰ **T24.492** **Corrosion of unspecified degree of multiple sites of** left **lower limb, except ankle and foot**

☑ Additional Character Req   √ₓ7ᵗʰ Placeholder Alert   Unacceptable PDx   Manifestation   `H1`-`H14` HAC   `HCC` CMS-HCC Condition   *EXCLUDES 1* Not Coded Here   *EXCLUDES 2* Not Included Here

ICD-10-CM 2018     1091

Chapter 19. Injury, Poisoning and Certain Other Consequences of External Causes

T24.139-T24.492

√7ᵗʰ **T24.499** Corrosion of unspecified degree of multiple sites of unspecified lower limb, except ankle and foot

√5ᵗʰ **T24.5** Corrosion of first degree of lower limb, except ankle and foot
Code first (T51-T65) to identify chemical and intent
Use additional external cause code to identify place (Y92)

√6ᵗʰ **T24.50** Corrosion of first degree of unspecified site of lower limb, except ankle and foot

√7ᵗʰ **T24.501** Corrosion of first degree of unspecified site of right lower limb, except ankle and foot

√7ᵗʰ **T24.502** Corrosion of first degree of unspecified site of left lower limb, except ankle and foot

√7ᵗʰ **T24.509** Corrosion of first degree of unspecified site of unspecified lower limb, except ankle and foot

√6ᵗʰ **T24.51** Corrosion of first degree of thigh

√7ᵗʰ **T24.511** Corrosion of first degree of right thigh

√7ᵗʰ **T24.512** Corrosion of first degree of left thigh

√7ᵗʰ **T24.519** Corrosion of first degree of unspecified thigh

√6ᵗʰ **T24.52** Corrosion of first degree of knee

√7ᵗʰ **T24.521** Corrosion of first degree of right knee

√7ᵗʰ **T24.522** Corrosion of first degree of left knee

√7ᵗʰ **T24.529** Corrosion of first degree of unspecified knee

√6ᵗʰ **T24.53** Corrosion of first degree of lower leg

√7ᵗʰ **T24.531** Corrosion of first degree of right lower leg

√7ᵗʰ **T24.532** Corrosion of first degree of left lower leg

√7ᵗʰ **T24.539** Corrosion of first degree of unspecified lower leg

√6ᵗʰ **T24.59** Corrosion of first degree of multiple sites of lower limb, except ankle and foot

√7ᵗʰ **T24.591** Corrosion of first degree of multiple sites of right lower limb, except ankle and foot

√7ᵗʰ **T24.592** Corrosion of first degree of multiple sites of left lower limb, except ankle and foot

√7ᵗʰ **T24.599** Corrosion of first degree of multiple sites of unspecified lower limb, except ankle and foot

√5ᵗʰ **T24.6** Corrosion of second degree of lower limb, except ankle and foot
Code first (T51-T65) to identify chemical and intent
Use additional external cause code to identify place (Y92)

√6ᵗʰ **T24.60** Corrosion of second degree of unspecified site of lower limb, except ankle and foot

√7ᵗʰ **T24.601** Corrosion of second degree of unspecified site of right lower limb, except ankle and foot

√7ᵗʰ **T24.602** Corrosion of second degree of unspecified site of left lower limb, except ankle and foot

√7ᵗʰ **T24.609** Corrosion of second degree of unspecified site of unspecified lower limb, except ankle and foot

√6ᵗʰ **T24.61** Corrosion of second degree of thigh

√7ᵗʰ **T24.611** Corrosion of second degree of right thigh

√7ᵗʰ **T24.612** Corrosion of second degree of left thigh

√7ᵗʰ **T24.619** Corrosion of second degree of unspecified thigh

√6ᵗʰ **T24.62** Corrosion of second degree of knee

√7ᵗʰ **T24.621** Corrosion of second degree of right knee

√7ᵗʰ **T24.622** Corrosion of second degree of left knee

√7ᵗʰ **T24.629** Corrosion of second degree of unspecified knee

√6ᵗʰ **T24.63** Corrosion of second degree of lower leg

√7ᵗʰ **T24.631** Corrosion of second degree of right lower leg

√7ᵗʰ **T24.632** Corrosion of second degree of left lower leg

√7ᵗʰ **T24.639** Corrosion of second degree of unspecified lower leg

√6ᵗʰ **T24.69** Corrosion of second degree of multiple sites of lower limb, except ankle and foot

√7ᵗʰ **T24.691** Corrosion of second degree of multiple sites of right lower limb, except ankle and foot

√7ᵗʰ **T24.692** Corrosion of second degree of multiple sites of left lower limb, except ankle and foot

√7ᵗʰ **T24.699** Corrosion of second degree of multiple sites of unspecified lower limb, except ankle and foot

√5ᵗʰ **T24.7** Corrosion of third degree of lower limb, except ankle and foot
Code first (T51-T65) to identify chemical and intent
Use additional external cause code to identify place (Y92)

√6ᵗʰ **T24.70** Corrosion of third degree of unspecified site of lower limb, except ankle and foot

**CC Excl:** For codes in subcategory T24.70:
PDX collection 1404

√7ᵗʰ **T24.701** Corrosion of third degree of unspecified site of right lower limb, except ankle and foot `CC` `H5`

√7ᵗʰ **T24.702** Corrosion of third degree of unspecified site of left lower limb, except ankle and foot `CC` `H5`

√7ᵗʰ **T24.709** Corrosion of third degree of unspecified site of unspecified lower limb, except ankle and foot `CC` `H5`

√6ᵗʰ **T24.71** Corrosion of third degree of thigh

**CC Excl:** For codes in subcategory T24.71:
PDX collection 1405

√7ᵗʰ **T24.711** Corrosion of third degree of right thigh `CC` `H5`

√7ᵗʰ **T24.712** Corrosion of third degree of left thigh `CC` `H5`

√7ᵗʰ **T24.719** Corrosion of third degree of unspecified thigh `CC` `H5`

√6ᵗʰ **T24.72** Corrosion of third degree of knee

**CC Excl:** For codes in subcategory T24.72:
PDX collection 1406

√7ᵗʰ **T24.721** Corrosion of third degree of right knee `CC` `H5`

√7ᵗʰ **T24.722** Corrosion of third degree of left knee `CC` `H5`

√7ᵗʰ **T24.729** Corrosion of third degree of unspecified knee `CC` `H5`

√6ᵗʰ **T24.73** Corrosion of third degree of lower leg

**CC Excl:** For codes in subcategory T24.73:
PDX collection 1407

√7ᵗʰ **T24.731** Corrosion of third degree of right lower leg `CC` `H5`

√7ᵗʰ **T24.732** Corrosion of third degree of left lower leg `CC` `H5`

√7ᵗʰ **T24.739** Corrosion of third degree of unspecified lower leg `CC` `H5`

√6ᵗʰ **T24.79** Corrosion of third degree of multiple sites of lower limb, except ankle and foot

**CC Excl:** For codes in subcategory T24.79:
PDX collection 1404

√7ᵗʰ **T24.791** Corrosion of third degree of multiple sites of right lower limb, except ankle and foot `CC` `H5`

√7ᵗʰ **T24.792** Corrosion of third degree of multiple sites of left lower limb, except ankle and foot `CC` `H5`

√7ᵗʰ **T24.799** Corrosion of third degree of multiple sites of unspecified lower limb, except ankle and foot `CC` `H5`

Ⓝ Newborn: 0　Ⓟ Pediatric: 0-17　Ⓜ Maternity: 12-55　Ⓐ Adult: 15-124　`MCC` Major CC Condition　`PDxMCC` PDx acts as own MCC　`CC` CC Condition　`PDxCC` PDx acts as own CC

**1092**　ICD-10-CM 2018

✓4ᵗʰ **T25　Burn and corrosion of ankle and foot**

> The appropriate 7th character is to be added to each code from category T25.
> A　initial encounter
> D　subsequent encounter
> S　sequela

✓5ᵗʰ **T25.0　Burn of unspecified degree of ankle and foot**
> Use additional external cause code to identify the source, place and intent of the burn (X00-X19, X75-X77, X96-X98, Y92)

✓6ᵗʰ **T25.01　Burn of unspecified degree of ankle**
- ✓7ᵗʰ **T25.011　Burn of unspecified degree of right ankle**
- ✓7ᵗʰ **T25.012　Burn of unspecified degree of left ankle**
- ✓7ᵗʰ **T25.019　Burn of unspecified degree of unspecified ankle**

✓6ᵗʰ **T25.02　Burn of unspecified degree of foot**
> EXCLUDES 2　burn of unspecified degree of toe(s) (nail) (T25.03-)
- ✓7ᵗʰ **T25.021　Burn of unspecified degree of right foot**
- ✓7ᵗʰ **T25.022　Burn of unspecified degree of left foot**
- ✓7ᵗʰ **T25.029　Burn of unspecified degree of unspecified foot**

✓6ᵗʰ **T25.03　Burn of unspecified degree of toe(s) (nail)**
- ✓7ᵗʰ **T25.031　Burn of unspecified degree of right toe(s) (nail)**
- ✓7ᵗʰ **T25.032　Burn of unspecified degree of left toe(s) (nail)**
- ✓7ᵗʰ **T25.039　Burn of unspecified degree of unspecified toe(s) (nail)**

✓6ᵗʰ **T25.09　Burn of unspecified degree of multiple sites of ankle and foot**
- ✓7ᵗʰ **T25.091　Burn of unspecified degree of multiple sites of right ankle and foot**
- ✓7ᵗʰ **T25.092　Burn of unspecified degree of multiple sites of left ankle and foot**
- ✓7ᵗʰ **T25.099　Burn of unspecified degree of multiple sites of unspecified ankle and foot**

✓5ᵗʰ **T25.1　Burn of first degree of ankle and foot**
> Use additional external cause code to identify the source, place and intent of the burn (X00-X19, X75-X77, X96-X98, Y92)

✓6ᵗʰ **T25.11　Burn of first degree of ankle**
- ✓7ᵗʰ **T25.111　Burn of first degree of right ankle**
- ✓7ᵗʰ **T25.112　Burn of first degree of left ankle**
- ✓7ᵗʰ **T25.119　Burn of first degree of unspecified ankle**

✓6ᵗʰ **T25.12　Burn of first degree of foot**
> EXCLUDES 2　burn of first degree of toe(s) (nail) (T25.13-)
- ✓7ᵗʰ **T25.121　Burn of first degree of right foot**
- ✓7ᵗʰ **T25.122　Burn of first degree of left foot**
- ✓7ᵗʰ **T25.129　Burn of first degree of unspecified foot**

✓6ᵗʰ **T25.13　Burn of first degree of toe(s) (nail)**
- ✓7ᵗʰ **T25.131　Burn of first degree of right toe(s) (nail)**
- ✓7ᵗʰ **T25.132　Burn of first degree of left toe(s) (nail)**
- ✓7ᵗʰ **T25.139　Burn of first degree of unspecified toe(s) (nail)**

✓6ᵗʰ **T25.19　Burn of first degree of multiple sites of ankle and foot**
- ✓7ᵗʰ **T25.191　Burn of first degree of multiple sites of right ankle and foot**
- ✓7ᵗʰ **T25.192　Burn of first degree of multiple sites of left ankle and foot**
- ✓7ᵗʰ **T25.199　Burn of first degree of multiple sites of unspecified ankle and foot**

✓5ᵗʰ **T25.2　Burn of second degree of ankle and foot**
> Use additional external cause code to identify the source, place and intent of the burn (X00-X19, X75-X77, X96-X98, Y92)

✓6ᵗʰ **T25.21　Burn of second degree of ankle**
- ✓7ᵗʰ **T25.211　Burn of second degree of right ankle**
- ✓7ᵗʰ **T25.212　Burn of second degree of left ankle**
- ✓7ᵗʰ **T25.219　Burn of second degree of unspecified ankle**

✓6ᵗʰ **T25.22　Burn of second degree of foot**
> EXCLUDES 2　burn of second degree of toe(s) (nail) (T25.23-)
- ✓7ᵗʰ **T25.221　Burn of second degree of right foot**

- ✓7ᵗʰ **T25.222　Burn of second degree of left foot**
- ✓7ᵗʰ **T25.229　Burn of second degree of unspecified foot**

✓6ᵗʰ **T25.23　Burn of second degree of toe(s) (nail)**
- ✓7ᵗʰ **T25.231　Burn of second degree of right toe(s) (nail)**
- ✓7ᵗʰ **T25.232　Burn of second degree of left toe(s) (nail)**
- ✓7ᵗʰ **T25.239　Burn of second degree of unspecified toe(s) (nail)**

✓6ᵗʰ **T25.29　Burn of second degree of multiple sites of ankle and foot**
- ✓7ᵗʰ **T25.291　Burn of second degree of multiple sites of right ankle and foot**
- ✓7ᵗʰ **T25.292　Burn of second degree of multiple sites of left ankle and foot**
- ✓7ᵗʰ **T25.299　Burn of second degree of multiple sites of unspecified ankle and foot**

✓5ᵗʰ **T25.3　Burn of third degree of ankle and foot**
> Use additional external cause code to identify the source, place and intent of the burn (X00-X19, X75-X77, X96-X98, Y92)

✓6ᵗʰ **T25.31　Burn of third degree of ankle**
> **CC Excl: For codes in subcategory T25.31:** PDX collection 1408
- ✓7ᵗʰ **T25.311　Burn of third degree of right ankle** CC H5
- ✓7ᵗʰ **T25.312　Burn of third degree of left ankle** CC H5
- ✓7ᵗʰ **T25.319　Burn of third degree of unspecified ankle** CC H5

✓6ᵗʰ **T25.32　Burn of third degree of foot**
> EXCLUDES 2　burn of third degree of toe(s) (nail) (T25.33-)
> **CC Excl: For codes in subcategory T25.32:** PDX collection 1409
- ✓7ᵗʰ **T25.321　Burn of third degree of right foot** CC H5
- ✓7ᵗʰ **T25.322　Burn of third degree of left foot** CC H5
- ✓7ᵗʰ **T25.329　Burn of third degree of unspecified foot** CC H5

✓6ᵗʰ **T25.33　Burn of third degree of toe(s) (nail)**
> **CC Excl: For codes in subcategory T25.33:** PDX collection 1410
- ✓7ᵗʰ **T25.331　Burn of third degree of right toe(s) (nail)** CC H5
- ✓7ᵗʰ **T25.332　Burn of third degree of left toe(s) (nail)** CC H5
- ✓7ᵗʰ **T25.339　Burn of third degree of unspecified toe(s) (nail)** CC H5

✓6ᵗʰ **T25.39　Burn of third degree of multiple sites of ankle and foot**
> **CC Excl: For codes in subcategory T25.39:** PDX collection 1404
- ✓7ᵗʰ **T25.391　Burn of third degree of multiple sites of right ankle and foot** CC H5
- ✓7ᵗʰ **T25.392　Burn of third degree of multiple sites of left ankle and foot** CC H5
- ✓7ᵗʰ **T25.399　Burn of third degree of multiple sites of unspecified ankle and foot** CC H5

✓5ᵗʰ **T25.4　Corrosion of unspecified degree of ankle and foot**
> Code first (T51-T65) to identify chemical and intent
> Use additional external cause code to identify place (Y92)

✓6ᵗʰ **T25.41　Corrosion of unspecified degree of ankle**
- ✓7ᵗʰ **T25.411　Corrosion of unspecified degree of right ankle**
- ✓7ᵗʰ **T25.412　Corrosion of unspecified degree of left ankle**
- ✓7ᵗʰ **T25.419　Corrosion of unspecified degree of unspecified ankle**

✓6ᵗʰ **T25.42　Corrosion of unspecified degree of foot**
> EXCLUDES 2　corrosion of unspecified degree of toe(s) (nail) (T25.43-)
- ✓7ᵗʰ **T25.421　Corrosion of unspecified degree of right foot**
- ✓7ᵗʰ **T25.422　Corrosion of unspecified degree of left foot**
- ✓7ᵗʰ **T25.429　Corrosion of unspecified degree of unspecified foot**

---

✓ Additional Character Req　✓x7ᵗʰ Placeholder Alert　Unacceptable PDx　■ Manifestation　H1-H14 HAC　HCC CMS-HCC Condition　EXCLUDES 1 Not Coded Here　EXCLUDES 2 Not Included Here

✓6ᵗʰ **T25.43** **Corrosion of unspecified degree of** toe(s) (nail)

     ✓7ᵗʰ **T25.431** **Corrosion of unspecified degree of** right toe(s) (nail)

     ✓7ᵗʰ **T25.432** **Corrosion of unspecified degree of** left toe(s) (nail)

     ✓7ᵗʰ **T25.439** **Corrosion of unspecified degree of** unspecified toe(s) (nail)

✓6ᵗʰ **T25.49** **Corrosion of unspecified degree of** multiple sites **of ankle and foot**

     ✓7ᵗʰ **T25.491** **Corrosion of unspecified degree of multiple sites of** right **ankle and foot**

     ✓7ᵗʰ **T25.492** **Corrosion of unspecified degree of multiple sites of** left **ankle and foot**

     ✓7ᵗʰ **T25.499** **Corrosion of unspecified degree of multiple sites of** unspecified **ankle and foot**

✓5ᵗʰ **T25.5** **Corrosion of** first degree **of ankle and foot**

     Code first (T51-T65) to identify chemical and intent
     Use additional external cause code to identify place (Y92)

✓6ᵗʰ **T25.51** **Corrosion of first degree of** ankle

     ✓7ᵗʰ **T25.511** **Corrosion of first degree of** right ankle

     ✓7ᵗʰ **T25.512** **Corrosion of first degree of** left ankle

     ✓7ᵗʰ **T25.519** **Corrosion of first degree of** unspecified ankle

✓6ᵗʰ **T25.52** **Corrosion of first degree of** foot

     EXCLUDES 2   corrosion of first degree of toe(s) (nail) (T25.53-)

     ✓7ᵗʰ **T25.521** **Corrosion of first degree of** right foot

     ✓7ᵗʰ **T25.522** **Corrosion of first degree of** left foot

     ✓7ᵗʰ **T25.529** **Corrosion of first degree of** unspecified foot

✓6ᵗʰ **T25.53** **Corrosion of first degree of** toe(s) (nail)

     ✓7ᵗʰ **T25.531** **Corrosion of first degree of** right toe(s) (nail)

     ✓7ᵗʰ **T25.532** **Corrosion of first degree of** left toe(s) (nail)

     ✓7ᵗʰ **T25.539** **Corrosion of first degree of** unspecified toe(s) (nail)

✓6ᵗʰ **T25.59** **Corrosion of first degree of** multiple sites **of ankle and foot**

     ✓7ᵗʰ **T25.591** **Corrosion of first degree of multiple sites of** right **ankle and foot**

     ✓7ᵗʰ **T25.592** **Corrosion of first degree of multiple sites of** left **ankle and foot**

     ✓7ᵗʰ **T25.599** **Corrosion of first degree of multiple sites of** unspecified **ankle and foot**

✓5ᵗʰ **T25.6** **Corrosion of** second degree **of ankle and foot**

     Code first (T51-T65) to identify chemical and intent
     Use additional external cause code to identify place (Y92)

✓6ᵗʰ **T25.61** **Corrosion of second degree of** ankle

     ✓7ᵗʰ **T25.611** **Corrosion of second degree of** right ankle

     ✓7ᵗʰ **T25.612** **Corrosion of second degree of** left ankle

     ✓7ᵗʰ **T25.619** **Corrosion of second degree of** unspecified ankle

✓6ᵗʰ **T25.62** **Corrosion of second degree of** foot

     EXCLUDES 2   corrosion of second degree of toe(s) (nail) (T25.63-)

     ✓7ᵗʰ **T25.621** **Corrosion of second degree of** right foot

     ✓7ᵗʰ **T25.622** **Corrosion of second degree of** left foot

     ✓7ᵗʰ **T25.629** **Corrosion of second degree of** unspecified foot

✓6ᵗʰ **T25.63** **Corrosion of second degree of** toe(s) (nail)

     ✓7ᵗʰ **T25.631** **Corrosion of second degree of** right toe(s) (nail)

     ✓7ᵗʰ **T25.632** **Corrosion of second degree of** left toe(s) (nail)

     ✓7ᵗʰ **T25.639** **Corrosion of second degree of** unspecified toe(s) (nail)

✓6ᵗʰ **T25.69** **Corrosion of second degree of** multiple sites **of ankle and foot**

     ✓7ᵗʰ **T25.691** **Corrosion of second degree of** right **ankle and foot**

     ✓7ᵗʰ **T25.692** **Corrosion of second degree of** left **ankle and foot**

---

     ✓7ᵗʰ **T25.699** **Corrosion of second degree of** unspecified **ankle and foot**

✓5ᵗʰ **T25.7** **Corrosion of** third degree **of ankle and foot**

     Code first (T51-T65) to identify chemical and intent
     Use additional external cause code to identify place (Y92)

✓6ᵗʰ **T25.71** **Corrosion of third degree of** ankle

> **CC Excl: For codes in subcategory T25.71:**
> PDX collection 1408

     ✓7ᵗʰ **T25.711** **Corrosion of third degree of** right ankle   CC H5

     ✓7ᵗʰ **T25.712** **Corrosion of third degree of** left ankle   CC H5

     ✓7ᵗʰ **T25.719** **Corrosion of third degree of** unspecified **ankle**   CC H5

✓6ᵗʰ **T25.72** **Corrosion of third degree of** foot

     EXCLUDES 2   corrosion of third degree of toe(s) (nail) (T25.73-)

> **CC Excl: For codes in subcategory T25.72:**
> PDX collection 1409

     ✓7ᵗʰ **T25.721** **Corrosion of third degree of** right foot   CC H5

     ✓7ᵗʰ **T25.722** **Corrosion of third degree of** left foot   CC H5

     ✓7ᵗʰ **T25.729** **Corrosion of third degree of** unspecified **foot**   CC H5

✓6ᵗʰ **T25.73** **Corrosion of third degree of** toe(s) (nail)

> **CC Excl: For codes in subcategory T25.73:**
> PDX collection 1410

     ✓7ᵗʰ **T25.731** **Corrosion of third degree of** right toe(s) (nail)   CC H5

     ✓7ᵗʰ **T25.732** **Corrosion of third degree of** left toe(s) (nail)   CC H5

     ✓7ᵗʰ **T25.739** **Corrosion of third degree of** unspecified **toe(s) (nail)**   CC H5

✓6ᵗʰ **T25.79** **Corrosion of third degree of** multiple sites **of ankle and foot**

> **CC Excl: For codes in subcategory T25.79:**
> PDX collection 1404

     ✓7ᵗʰ **T25.791** **Corrosion of third degree of multiple sites of** right **ankle and foot**   CC H5

     ✓7ᵗʰ **T25.792** **Corrosion of third degree of multiple sites of** left **ankle and foot**   CC H5

     ✓7ᵗʰ **T25.799** **Corrosion of third degree of multiple sites of** unspecified **ankle and foot**   CC H5

## Burns and corrosions confined to eye and internal organs (T26-T28)

✓4ᵗʰ **T26** **Burn and corrosion confined to eye and adnexa**

> The appropriate 7th character is to be added to each code from category T26.
> A   initial encounter
> D   subsequent encounter
> S   sequela

✓5ᵗʰ **T26.0** **Burn of** eyelid and periocular area

     Use additional external cause code to identify the source, place and intent of the burn (X00-X19, X75-X77, X96-X98, Y92)

     ✓x7ᵗʰ **T26.00** **Burn of** unspecified eyelid and periocular area

     ✓x7ᵗʰ **T26.01** **Burn of** right eyelid and periocular area

     ✓x7ᵗʰ **T26.02** **Burn of** left eyelid and periocular area

✓5ᵗʰ **T26.1** **Burn of** cornea and conjunctival sac

     Use additional external cause code to identify the source, place and intent of the burn (X00-X19, X75-X77, X96-X98, Y92)

     ✓x7ᵗʰ **T26.10** **Burn of cornea and conjunctival sac,** unspecified **eye**

     ✓x7ᵗʰ **T26.11** **Burn of cornea and conjunctival sac,** right **eye**

     ✓x7ᵗʰ **T26.12** **Burn of cornea and conjunctival sac,** left **eye**

---

N Newborn: 0   P Pediatric: 0-17   M Maternity: 12-55   A Adult: 15-124   MCC Major CC Condition   PDxMCC PDx acts as own MCC   CC CC Condition   PDxCC PDx acts as own CC

1094      ICD-10-CM 2018

☑5ᵗʰ **T26.2 Burn with resulting rupture and destruction of eyeball**
Use additional external cause code to identify the source, place and intent of the burn (X00-X19, X75-X77, X96-X98, Y92)

  √x7ᵗʰ **T26.20 Burn with resulting rupture and destruction of unspecified eyeball** ᴄᴄ ʜ5
    CC Excl: No Excl

  √x7ᵗʰ **T26.21 Burn with resulting rupture and destruction of right eyeball** ᴄᴄ ʜ5
    CC Excl: No Excl

  √x7ᵗʰ **T26.22 Burn with resulting rupture and destruction of left eyeball** ᴄᴄ ʜ5
    CC Excl: No Excl

☑5ᵗʰ **T26.3 Burns of other specified parts of eye and adnexa**
Use additional external cause code to identify the source, place and intent of the burn (X00-X19, X75-X77, X96-X98, Y92)

  √x7ᵗʰ **T26.30 Burns of other specified parts of unspecified eye and adnexa**

  √x7ᵗʰ **T26.31 Burns of other specified parts of right eye and adnexa**

  √x7ᵗʰ **T26.32 Burns of other specified parts of left eye and adnexa**

☑5ᵗʰ **T26.4 Burn of eye and adnexa, part unspecified**
Use additional external cause code to identify the source, place and intent of the burn (X00-X19, X75-X77, X96-X98, Y92)

  √x7ᵗʰ **T26.40 Burn of unspecified eye and adnexa, part unspecified**

  √x7ᵗʰ **T26.41 Burn of right eye and adnexa, part unspecified**

  √x7ᵗʰ **T26.42 Burn of left eye and adnexa, part unspecified**

☑5ᵗʰ **T26.5 Corrosion of eyelid and periocular area**
Code first (T51-T65) to identify chemical and intent
Use additional external cause code to identify place (Y92)

  √x7ᵗʰ **T26.50 Corrosion of unspecified eyelid and periocular area**

  √x7ᵗʰ **T26.51 Corrosion of right eyelid and periocular area**

  √x7ᵗʰ **T26.52 Corrosion of left eyelid and periocular area**

☑5ᵗʰ **T26.6 Corrosion of cornea and conjunctival sac**
Code first (T51-T65) to identify chemical and intent
Use additional external cause code to identify place (Y92)

  √x7ᵗʰ **T26.60 Corrosion of cornea and conjunctival sac, unspecified eye**

  √x7ᵗʰ **T26.61 Corrosion of cornea and conjunctival sac, right eye**

  √x7ᵗʰ **T26.62 Corrosion of cornea and conjunctival sac, left eye**

☑5ᵗʰ **T26.7 Corrosion with resulting rupture and destruction of eyeball**
Code first (T51-T65) to identify chemical and intent
Use additional external cause code to identify place (Y92)

  √x7ᵗʰ **T26.70 Corrosion with resulting rupture and destruction of unspecified eyeball** ᴄᴄ ʜ5
    CC Excl: No Excl

  √x7ᵗʰ **T26.71 Corrosion with resulting rupture and destruction of right eyeball** ᴄᴄ ʜ5
    CC Excl: No Excl

  √x7ᵗʰ **T26.72 Corrosion with resulting rupture and destruction of left eyeball** ᴄᴄ ʜ5
    CC Excl: No Excl

☑5ᵗʰ **T26.8 Corrosions of other specified parts of eye and adnexa**
Code first (T51-T65) to identify chemical and intent
Use additional external cause code to identify place (Y92)

  √x7ᵗʰ **T26.80 Corrosions of other specified parts of unspecified eye and adnexa**

  √x7ᵗʰ **T26.81 Corrosions of other specified parts of right eye and adnexa**

  √x7ᵗʰ **T26.82 Corrosions of other specified parts of left eye and adnexa**

☑5ᵗʰ **T26.9 Corrosion of eye and adnexa, part unspecified**
Code first (T51-T65) to identify chemical and intent
Use additional external cause code to identify place (Y92)

  √x7ᵗʰ **T26.90 Corrosion of unspecified eye and adnexa, part unspecified**

  √x7ᵗʰ **T26.91 Corrosion of right eye and adnexa, part unspecified**

  √x7ᵗʰ **T26.92 Corrosion of left eye and adnexa, part unspecified**

☑4ᵗʰ **T27 Burn and corrosion of respiratory tract**
Use additional external cause code to identify the source and intent of the burn (X00-X19, X75-X77, X96-X98)
Use additional external cause code to identify place (Y92)

The appropriate 7th character is to be added to each code from category T27.
A   initial encounter
D   subsequent encounter
S   sequela

**CC Excl: For codes in subcategory T27:** PDX collection 1411

√x7ᵗʰ **T27.0 Burn of larynx and trachea** ᴄᴄ ʜ5

√x7ᵗʰ **T27.1 Burn involving larynx and trachea with lung** ᴄᴄ ʜ5

√x7ᵗʰ **T27.2 Burn of other parts of respiratory tract** ᴄᴄ ʜ5
  Burn of thoracic cavity

√x7ᵗʰ **T27.3 Burn of respiratory tract, part unspecified** ᴄᴄ ʜ5
  ~~Code first (T51-T65) to identify chemical and intent for codes T27.4-T27.7~~

√x7ᵗʰ **T27.4 Corrosion of larynx and trachea** ᴄᴄ ʜ5
  ►Code first (T51-T65) to identify chemical and intent◄

√x7ᵗʰ **T27.5 Corrosion involving larynx and trachea with lung** ᴄᴄ ʜ5

√x7ᵗʰ **T27.6 Corrosion of other parts of respiratory tract** ᴄᴄ ʜ5
  ►Code first (T51-T65) to identify chemical and intent◄

√x7ᵗʰ **T27.7 Corrosion of respiratory tract, part unspecified** ᴄᴄ ʜ5
  ►Code first (T51-T65) to identify chemical and intent◄

☑4ᵗʰ **T28 Burn and corrosion of other internal organs**
Use additional external cause code to identify the source and intent of the burn (X00- X19, X75-X77, X96-X98)
Use additional external cause code to identify place (Y92)

The appropriate 7th character is to be added to each code from category T28.
A   initial encounter
D   subsequent encounter
S   sequela

√x7ᵗʰ **T28.0 Burn of mouth and pharynx**

√x7ᵗʰ **T28.1 Burn of esophagus** ᴄᴄ ʜ5
  **CC Excl: CC with 7th character A:** PDX collection 1412

√x7ᵗʰ **T28.2 Burn of other parts of alimentary tract** ᴄᴄ ʜ5
  **CC Excl: CC with 7th character A:** PDX collection 1413

√x7ᵗʰ **T28.3 Burn of internal genitourinary organs**

☑5ᵗʰ **T28.4 Burns of other and unspecified internal organs**
  ►Code first (T51-T65) to identify chemical and intent◄

  √x7ᵗʰ **T28.40 Burn of unspecified internal organ**

  ☑6ᵗʰ **T28.41 Burn of ear drum**

    √7ᵗʰ **T28.411 Burn of right ear drum**

    √7ᵗʰ **T28.412 Burn of left ear drum**

    √7ᵗʰ **T28.419 Burn of unspecified ear drum**

  √x7ᵗʰ **T28.49 Burn of other internal organ**
    ~~Code first (T51-T65) to identify chemical and intent for T28.5-T28.9~~

√x7ᵗʰ **T28.5 Corrosion of mouth and pharynx**
  ►Code first (T51-T65) to identify chemical and intent◄

√x7ᵗʰ **T28.6 Corrosion of esophagus** ᴄᴄ ʜ5
  ►Code first (T51-T65) to identify chemical and intent◄
  **CC Excl: CC with 7th character A:** PDX collection 1412

√x7ᵗʰ **T28.7 Corrosion of other parts of alimentary tract** ᴄᴄ ʜ5
  ►Code first (T51-T65) to identify chemical and intent◄
  **CC Excl: CC with 7th character A:** PDX collection 1413

√x7ᵗʰ **T28.8 Corrosion of internal genitourinary organs**
  ►Code first (T51-T65) to identify chemical and intent◄

☑5ᵗʰ **T28.9 Corrosions of other and unspecified internal organs**
  ►Code first (T51-T65) to identify chemical and intent◄

  √x7ᵗʰ **T28.90 Corrosions of unspecified internal organs**

  ☑6ᵗʰ **T28.91 Corrosions of ear drum**

    √7ᵗʰ **T28.911 Corrosions of right ear drum**

    √7ᵗʰ **T28.912 Corrosions of left ear drum**

    √7ᵗʰ **T28.919 Corrosions of unspecified ear drum**

  √x7ᵗʰ **T28.99 Corrosions of other internal organs**

Chapter 19. Injury, Poisoning and Certain Other Consequences of External Causes

T26.2–T28.99

☑ Additional Character Req   √x7ᵗʰ Placeholder Alert   Unacceptable PDx   Manifestation   H1 - H14 HAC   ʜᴄᴄ CMS-HCC Condition   *EXCLUDES 1* Not Coded Here   *EXCLUDES 2* Not Included Here

ICD-10-CM 2018      1095

## Burns and corrosions of multiple and unspecified body regions (T30-T32)

**✓4ᵗʰ T30   Burn and corrosion, body region unspecified**

**T30.0   Burn of unspecified body region, unspecified degree**
This code is not for inpatient use. Code to specified site and degree of burns.
Burn NOS
Multiple burns NOS

**T30.4   Corrosion of unspecified body region, unspecified degree**
This code is not for inpatient use. Code to specified site and degree of corrosion.
Corrosion NOS
Multiple corrosion NOS

**✓4ᵗʰ T31   Burns classified according to extent of body surface involved**
**NOTE**   This category is to be used as the primary code only when the site of the burn is unspecified. It should be used as a supplementary code with categories T20-T25 when the site is specified.

**CC Excl: For CC/MCC codes in category T31:** PDX collection 1414

**T31.0   Burns involving less than 10% of body surface**

**✓5ᵗʰ T31.1   Burns involving 10-19% of body surface**

**T31.10   Burns involving 10-19% of body surface** `CC` `H5`
**with 0% to 9% third degree burns**
Burns involving 10-19% of body surface NOS

**T31.11   Burns involving 10-19% of body surface** `CC` `H5` `HCC`
**with 10-19% third degree burns**

**✓5ᵗʰ T31.2   Burns involving 20-29% of body surface**

**T31.20   Burns involving 20-29% of body surface** `CC` `H5`
**with 0% to 9% third degree burns**
Burns involving 20-29% of body surface NOS

**T31.21   Burns involving 20-29% of body surface** `MCC` `H5` `HCC`
**with 10-19% third degree burns**

**T31.22   Burns involving 20-29% of body surface** `MCC` `H5` `HCC`
**with 20-29% third degree burns**

**✓5ᵗʰ T31.3   Burns involving 30-39% of body surface**

**T31.30   Burns involving 30-39% of body surface** `CC` `H5`
**with 0% to 9% third degree burns**
Burns involving 30-39% of body surface NOS

**T31.31   Burns involving 30-39% of body surface** `MCC` `H5` `HCC`
**with 10-19% third degree burns**

**T31.32   Burns involving 30-39% of body surface** `MCC` `H5` `HCC`
**with 20-29% third degree burns**

**T31.33   Burns involving 30-39% of body surface** `MCC` `H5` `HCC`
**30-39% third degree burns**

**✓5ᵗʰ T31.4   Burns involving 40-49% of body surface**

**T31.40   Burns involving 40-49% of body surface** `CC` `H5`
**with 0% to 9% third degree burns**
Burns involving 40-49% of body surface NOS

**T31.41   Burns involving 40-49% of body surface** `MCC` `H5` `HCC`
**with 10-19% third degree burns**

**T31.42   Burns involving 40-49% of body surface** `MCC` `H5` `HCC`
**with 20-29% third degree burns**

**T31.43   Burns involving 40-49% of body surface** `MCC` `H5` `HCC`
**with 30-39% third degree burns**

**T31.44   Burns involving 40-49% of body surface** `MCC` `H5` `HCC`
**with 40-49% third degree burns**

**✓5ᵗʰ T31.5   Burns involving 50-59% of body surface**

**T31.50   Burns involving 50-59% of body surface with** `CC` `H5`
**0% to 9% third degree burns**
Burns involving 50-59% of body surface NOS

**T31.51   Burns involving 50-59% of body surface** `MCC` `H5` `HCC`
**with 10-19% third degree burns**

**T31.52   Burns involving 50-59% of body surface** `MCC` `H5` `HCC`
**with 20-29% third degree burns**

**T31.53   Burns involving 50-59% of body surface** `MCC` `H5` `HCC`
**with 30-39% third degree burns**

**T31.54   Burns involving 50-59% of body surface** `MCC` `H5` `HCC`
**with 40-49% third degree burns**

**T31.55   Burns involving 50-59% of body surface** `MCC` `H5` `HCC`
**with 50-59% third degree burns**

**✓5ᵗʰ T31.6   Burns involving 60-69% of body surface**

**T31.60   Burns involving 60-69% of body surface** `CC` `H5`
**with 0% to 9% third degree burns**
Burns involving 60-69% of body surface NOS

**T31.61   Burns involving 60-69% of body surface** `MCC` `H5` `HCC`
**with 10-19% third degree burns**

**T31.62   Burns involving 60-69% of body surface** `MCC` `H5` `HCC`
**with 20-29% third degree burns**

**T31.63   Burns involving 60-69% of body surface** `MCC` `H5` `HCC`
**with 30-39% third degree burns**

**T31.64   Burns involving 60-69% of body surface** `MCC` `H5` `HCC`
**with 40-49% third degree burns**

**T31.65   Burns involving 60-69% of body surface** `MCC` `H5` `HCC`
**with 50-59% third degree burns**

**T31.66   Burns involving 60-69% of body surface** `MCC` `H5` `HCC`
**with 60-69% third degree burns**

**✓5ᵗʰ T31.7   Burns involving 70-79% of body surface**

**T31.70   Burns involving 70-79% of body surface** `CC` `H5`
**with 0% to 9% third degree burns**
Burns involving 70-79% of body surface NOS

**T31.71   Burns involving 70-79% of body surface** `MCC` `H5` `HCC`
**with 10-19% third degree burns**

**T31.72   Burns involving 70-79% of body surface** `MCC` `H5` `HCC`
**with 20-29% third degree burns**

**T31.73   Burns involving 70-79% of body surface** `MCC` `H5` `HCC`
**with 30-39% third degree burns**

**T31.74   Burns involving 70-79% of body surface** `MCC` `H5` `HCC`
**with 40-49% third degree burns**

**T31.75   Burns involving 70-79% of body surface** `MCC` `H5` `HCC`
**with 50-59% third degree burns**

**T31.76   Burns involving 70-79% of body surface** `MCC` `H5` `HCC`
**with 60-69% third degree burns**

**T31.77   Burns involving 70-79% of body surface** `MCC` `H5` `HCC`
**with 70-79% third degree burns**

**✓5ᵗʰ T31.8   Burns involving 80-89% of body surface**

**T31.80   Burns involving 80-89% of body surface** `CC` `H5`
**with 0% to 9% third degree burns**
Burns involving 80-89% of body surface NOS

**T31.81   Burns involving 80-89% of body surface** `MCC` `H5` `HCC`
**with 10-19% third degree burns**

**T31.82   Burns involving 80-89% of body surface** `MCC` `H5` `HCC`
**with 20-29% third degree burns**

**T31.83   Burns involving 80-89% of body surface** `MCC` `H5` `HCC`
**with 30-39% third degree burns**

**T31.84   Burns involving 80-89% of body surface** `MCC` `H5` `HCC`
**with 40-49% third degree burns**

**T31.85   Burns involving 80-89% of body surface** `MCC` `H5` `HCC`
**with 50-59% third degree burns**

**T31.86   Burns involving 80-89% of body surface** `MCC` `H5` `HCC`
**with 60-69% third degree burns**

**T31.87   Burns involving 80-89% of body surface** `MCC` `H5` `HCC`
**with 70-79% third degree burns**

**T31.88   Burns involving 80-89% of body surface** `MCC` `H5` `HCC`
**with 80-89% third degree burns**

**✓5ᵗʰ T31.9   Burns involving 90% or more of body surface**

**T31.90   Burns involving 90% or more of body surface** `CC` `H5`
**with 0% to 9% third degree burns**
Burns involving 90% or more of body surface NOS

**T31.91   Burns involving 90% or more of body** `MCC` `H5` `HCC`
**surface with 10-19% third degree burns**

**T31.92   Burns involving 90% or more of body** `MCC` `H5` `HCC`
**surface with 20-29% third degree burns**

**T31.93   Burns involving 90% or more of body** `MCC` `H5` `HCC`
**surface with 30-39% third degree burns**

**T31.94   Burns involving 90% or more of body** `MCC` `H5` `HCC`
**surface with 40-49% third degree burns**

**T31.95   Burns involving 90% or more of body** `MCC` `H5` `HCC`
**surface with 50-59% third degree burns**

**T31.96   Burns involving 90% or more of body** `MCC` `H5` `HCC`
**surface with 60-69% third degree burns**

**T31.97   Burns involving 90% or more of body** `MCC` `H5` `HCC`
**surface with 70-79% third degree burns**

**T31.98   Burns involving 90% or more of body** `MCC` `H5` `HCC`
**surface with 80-89% third degree burns**

**T31.99   Burns involving 90% or more of body** `MCC` `H5` `HCC`
**surface with 90% or more third degree burns**

☑4th **T32** **Corrosions** **classified** according to extent of body surface involved

NOTE　This category is to be used as the primary code only when the site of the corrosion is unspecified. It may be used as a supplementary code with categories T20-T25 when the site is specified.

CC Excl: For CC/MCC codes in category T32: PDX collection 1414

**T32.0** **Corrosions involving** less than 10% of body surface

☑5th **T32.1** **Corrosions involving** 10-19% of body surface

　　**T32.10** **Corrosions involving** 10-19% of body surface with 0% to 9% third degree **corrosion** `CC` `H5`
　　　　Corrosions involving 10-19% of body surface NOS

　　**T32.11** **Corrosions involving** 10-19% of body surface with 10-19% third degree **corrosion** `CC` `H5` `HCC`

☑5th **T32.2** **Corrosions involving** 20-29% of body surface

　　**T32.20** **Corrosions involving** 20-29% of body surface with 0% to 9% third degree **corrosion** `CC` `H5`

　　**T32.21** **Corrosions involving** 20-29% of body surface with 10-19% third degree **corrosion** `MCC` `H5` `HCC`

　　**T32.22** **Corrosions involving** 20-29% of body surface with 20-29% third degree **corrosion** `MCC` `H5` `HCC`

☑5th **T32.3** **Corrosions involving** 30-39% of body surface

　　**T32.30** **Corrosions involving** 30-39% of body surface with 0% to 9% third degree **corrosion** `CC` `H5`

　　**T32.31** **Corrosions involving** 30-39% of body surface with 10-19% third degree **corrosion** `MCC` `H5` `HCC`

　　**T32.32** **Corrosions involving** 30-39% of body surface with 20-29% third degree **corrosion** `MCC` `H5` `HCC`

　　**T32.33** **Corrosions involving** 30-39% of body surface with 30-39% third degree **corrosion** `MCC` `H5` `HCC`

☑5th **T32.4** **Corrosions involving** 40-49% of body surface

　　**T32.40** **Corrosions involving** 40-49% of body surface with 0% to 9% third degree **corrosion** `CC` `H5`

　　**T32.41** **Corrosions involving** 40-49% of body surface with 10-19% third degree **corrosion** `MCC` `H5` `HCC`

　　**T32.42** **Corrosions involving** 40-49% of body surface with 20-29% third degree **corrosion** `MCC` `H5` `HCC`

　　**T32.43** **Corrosions involving** 40-49% of body surface with 30-39% third degree **corrosion** `MCC` `H5` `HCC`

　　**T32.44** **Corrosions involving** 40-49% of body surface with 40-49% third degree **corrosion** `MCC` `H5` `HCC`

☑5th **T32.5** **Corrosions involving** 50-59% of body surface

　　**T32.50** **Corrosions involving** 50-59% of body surface with 0% to 9% third degree **corrosion** `CC` `H5`

　　**T32.51** **Corrosions involving** 50-59% of body surface with 10-19% third degree **corrosion** `MCC` `H5` `HCC`

　　**T32.52** **Corrosions involving** 50-59% of body surface with 20-29% third degree **corrosion** `MCC` `H5` `HCC`

　　**T32.53** **Corrosions involving** 50-59% of body surface with 30-39% third degree **corrosion** `MCC` `H5` `HCC`

　　**T32.54** **Corrosions involving** 50-59% of body surface with 40-49% third degree **corrosion** `MCC` `H5` `HCC`

　　**T32.55** **Corrosions involving** 50-59% of body surface with 50-59% third degree **corrosion** `MCC` `H5` `HCC`

☑5th **T32.6** **Corrosions involving** 60-69% of body surface

　　**T32.60** **Corrosions involving** 60-69% of body surface with 0% to 9% third degree **corrosion** `CC` `H5`

　　**T32.61** **Corrosions involving** 60-69% of body surface with 10-19% third degree **corrosion** `MCC` `H5` `HCC`

　　**T32.62** **Corrosions involving** 60-69% of body surface with 20-29% third degree **corrosion** `MCC` `H5` `HCC`

　　**T32.63** **Corrosions involving** 60-69% of body surface with 30-39% third degree **corrosion** `MCC` `H5` `HCC`

　　**T32.64** **Corrosions involving** 60-69% of body surface with 40-49% third degree **corrosion** `MCC` `H5` `HCC`

　　**T32.65** **Corrosions involving** 60-69% of body surface with 50-59% third degree **corrosion** `MCC` `H5` `HCC`

　　**T32.66** **Corrosions involving** 60-69% of body surface with 60-69% third degree **corrosion** `MCC` `H5` `HCC`

☑5th **T32.7** **Corrosions involving** 70-79% of body surface

　　**T32.70** **Corrosions involving** 70-79% of body surface with 0% to 9% third degree **corrosion** `CC` `H5`

　　**T32.71** **Corrosions involving** 70-79% of body surface with 10-19% third degree **corrosion** `MCC` `H5` `HCC`

　　**T32.72** **Corrosions involving** 70-79% of body surface with 20-29% third degree **corrosion** `MCC` `H5` `HCC`

　　**T32.73** **Corrosions involving** 70-79% of body surface with 30-39% third degree **corrosion** `MCC` `H5` `HCC`

　　**T32.74** **Corrosions involving** 70-79% of body surface with 40-49% third degree **corrosion** `MCC` `H5` `HCC`

　　**T32.75** **Corrosions involving** 70-79% of body surface with 50-59% third degree **corrosion** `MCC` `H5` `HCC`

　　**T32.76** **Corrosions involving** 70-79% of body surface with 60-69% third degree **corrosion** `MCC` `H5` `HCC`

　　**T32.77** **Corrosions involving** 70-79% of body surface with 70-79% third degree **corrosion** `MCC` `H5` `HCC`

☑5th **T32.8** **Corrosions involving** 80-89% of body surface

　　**T32.80** **Corrosions involving** 80-89% of body surface with 0% to 9% third degree **corrosion** `CC` `H5`

　　**T32.81** **Corrosions involving** 80-89% of body surface with 10-19% third degree **corrosion** `MCC` `H5` `HCC`

　　**T32.82** **Corrosions involving** 80-89% of body surface with 20-29% third degree **corrosion** `MCC` `H5` `HCC`

　　**T32.83** **Corrosions involving** 80-89% of body surface with 30-39% third degree **corrosion** `MCC` `H5` `HCC`

　　**T32.84** **Corrosions involving** 80-89% of body surface with 40-49% third degree **corrosion** `MCC` `H5` `HCC`

　　**T32.85** **Corrosions involving** 80-89% of body surface with 50-59% third degree **corrosion** `MCC` `H5` `HCC`

　　**T32.86** **Corrosions involving** 80-89% of body surface with 60-69% third degree **corrosion** `MCC` `H5` `HCC`

　　**T32.87** **Corrosions involving** 80-89% of body surface with 70-79% third degree **corrosion** `MCC` `H5` `HCC`

　　**T32.88** **Corrosions involving** 80-89% of body surface with 80-89% third degree **corrosion** `MCC` `H5` `HCC`

☑5th **T32.9** **Corrosions involving** 90% or more of body surface

　　**T32.90** **Corrosions involving** 90% or more of body surface with 0% to 9% third degree **corrosion** `CC` `H5`

　　**T32.91** **Corrosions involving** 90% or more of body surface with 10-19% third degree **corrosion** `MCC` `H5` `HCC`

　　**T32.92** **Corrosions involving** 90% or more of body surface with 20-29% third degree **corrosion** `MCC` `H5` `HCC`

　　**T32.93** **Corrosions involving** 90% or more of body surface with 30-39% third degree **corrosion** `MCC` `H5` `HCC`

　　**T32.94** **Corrosions involving** 90% or more of body surface with 40-49% third degree **corrosion** `MCC` `H5` `HCC`

　　**T32.95** **Corrosions involving** 90% or more of body surface with 50-59% third degree **corrosion** `MCC` `H5` `HCC`

　　**T32.96** **Corrosions involving** 90% or more of body surface with 60-69% third degree **corrosion** `MCC` `H5` `HCC`

　　**T32.97** **Corrosions involving** 90% or more of body surface with 70-79% third degree **corrosion** `MCC` `H5` `HCC`

　　**T32.98** **Corrosions involving** 90% or more of body surface with 80-89% third degree **corrosion** `MCC` `H5` `HCC`

　　**T32.99** **Corrosions involving** 90% or more of body surface with 90% or more third degree **corrosion** `MCC` `H5` `HCC`

## Frostbite (T33-T34)

EXCLUDES 2　hypothermia and other effects of reduced temperature (T68, T69-)

☑4th **T33** **Superficial** **frostbite**

INCLUDES　frostbite with partial thickness skin loss

The appropriate 7th character is to be added to each code from category T33.
A　initial encounter
D　subsequent encounter
S　sequela

CC Excl: For CC codes in category T33, unless otherwise noted: PDX collection 1416

☑5th **T33.0** **Superficial frostbite of** head

CC Excl: For CC codes in subcategory T33.0: PDX collection 1415

☑6th **T33.01** **Superficial frostbite of** ear

　☑7th **T33.011** **Superficial frostbite of** right ear `CC` `H5`

　☑7th **T33.012** **Superficial frostbite of** left ear `CC` `H5`

　☑7th **T33.019** **Superficial frostbite of** unspecified ear `CC` `H5`

☑x7th **T33.02** **Superficial frostbite of** nose `CC` `H5`

☑x7th **T33.09** **Superficial frostbite of** other part of head `CC` `H5`

**√x7th T33.1 Superficial frostbite of neck** `CC` `H5`
     CC Excl: CC with 7th character A: PDX collection 1415

**√x7th T33.2 Superficial frostbite of thorax** `CC` `H5`

**√x7th T33.3 Superficial frostbite of abdominal wall, lower back and pelvis** `CC` `H5`

**√5th T33.4 Superficial frostbite of arm**
     *EXCLUDES 2*   superficial frostbite of wrist and hand (T33.5-)

     **√x7th T33.40 Superficial frostbite of unspecified arm** `CC` `H5`

     **√x7th T33.41 Superficial frostbite of right arm** `CC` `H5`

     **√x7th T33.42 Superficial frostbite of left arm** `CC` `H5`

**√5th T33.5 Superficial frostbite of wrist, hand, and fingers**

     **CC Excl: For codes in subcategory T33.5:**
     PDX collection 1417

     **√6th T33.51 Superficial frostbite of wrist**

       **√7th T33.511 Superficial frostbite of right wrist** `CC` `H5`

       **√7th T33.512 Superficial frostbite of left wrist** `CC` `H5`

       **√7th T33.519 Superficial frostbite of unspecified wrist** `CC` `H5`

     **√6th T33.52 Superficial frostbite of hand**
       *EXCLUDES 2*   superficial frostbite of fingers (T33.53-)

       **√7th T33.521 Superficial frostbite of right hand** `CC` `H5`

       **√7th T33.522 Superficial frostbite of left hand** `CC` `H5`

       **√7th T33.529 Superficial frostbite of unspecified hand** `CC` `H5`

     **√6th T33.53 Superficial frostbite of finger(s)**

       **√7th T33.531 Superficial frostbite of right finger(s)** `CC` `H5`

       **√7th T33.532 Superficial frostbite of left finger(s)** `CC` `H5`

       **√7th T33.539 Superficial frostbite of unspecified finger(s)** `CC` `H5`

**√5th T33.6 Superficial frostbite of hip and thigh**

     **√x7th T33.60 Superficial frostbite of unspecified hip and thigh** `CC` `H5`

     **√x7th T33.61 Superficial frostbite of right hip and thigh** `CC` `H5`

     **√x7th T33.62 Superficial frostbite of left hip and thigh** `CC` `H5`

**√5th T33.7 Superficial frostbite of knee and lower leg**
     *EXCLUDES 2*   superficial frostbite of ankle and foot (T33.8-)

     **√x7th T33.70 Superficial frostbite of unspecified knee and lower leg** `CC` `H5`

     **√x7th T33.71 Superficial frostbite of right knee and lower leg** `CC` `H5`

     **√x7th T33.72 Superficial frostbite of left knee and lower leg** `CC` `H5`

**√5th T33.8 Superficial frostbite of ankle, foot, and toe(s)**

     **CC Excl: For codes in subcategory T33.8:**
     PDX collection 1418

     **√6th T33.81 Superficial frostbite of ankle**

       **√7th T33.811 Superficial frostbite of right ankle** `CC` `H5`

       **√7th T33.812 Superficial frostbite of left ankle** `CC` `H5`

       **√7th T33.819 Superficial frostbite of unspecified ankle** `CC` `H5`

     **√6th T33.82 Superficial frostbite of foot**

       **√7th T33.821 Superficial frostbite of right foot** `CC` `H5`

       **√7th T33.822 Superficial frostbite of left foot** `CC` `H5`

       **√7th T33.829 Superficial frostbite of unspecified foot** `CC` `H5`

     **√6th T33.83 Superficial frostbite of toe(s)**

       **√7th T33.831 Superficial frostbite of right toe(s)** `CC` `H5`

       **√7th T33.832 Superficial frostbite of left toe(s)** `CC` `H5`

       **√7th T33.839 Superficial frostbite of unspecified toe(s)** `CC` `H5`

**√5th T33.9 Superficial frostbite of other and unspecified sites**

     **√x7th T33.90 Superficial frostbite of unspecified sites** `CC` `H5`
     Superficial frostbite NOS

     **√x7th T33.99 Superficial frostbite of other sites** `CC` `H5`
     Superficial frostbite of leg NOS
     Superficial frostbite of trunk NOS

**√4th T34 Frostbite with tissue necrosis**

The appropriate 7th character is to be added to each code from category T34.
A   initial encounter
D   subsequent encounter
S   sequela

**CC Excl: For CC codes in category T34, unless otherwise noted:**
PDX collection 1416

**√5th T34.0 Frostbite with tissue necrosis of head**

     **CC Excl: For CC codes in subcategory T34.0:**
     PDX collection 1415

     **√6th T34.01 Frostbite with tissue necrosis of ear**

       **√7th T34.011 Frostbite with tissue necrosis of right ear** `CC` `H5`

       **√7th T34.012 Frostbite with tissue necrosis of left ear** `CC` `H5`

       **√7th T34.019 Frostbite with tissue necrosis of unspecified ear** `CC` `H5`

     **√x7th T34.02 Frostbite with tissue necrosis of nose** `CC` `H5`

     **√x7th T34.09 Frostbite with tissue necrosis of other part of head** `CC` `H5`

**√x7th T34.1 Frostbite with tissue necrosis of neck** `CC` `H5`
     CC Excl: PDX collection 1415

**√x7th T34.2 Frostbite with tissue necrosis of thorax** `CC` `H5`

**√x7th T34.3 Frostbite with tissue necrosis of abdominal wall, lower back and pelvis** `CC` `H5`

**√5th T34.4 Frostbite with tissue necrosis of arm**
     *EXCLUDES 2*   frostbite with tissue necrosis of wrist and hand (T34.5-)

     **√x7th T34.40 Frostbite with tissue necrosis of unspecified arm** `CC` `H5`

     **√x7th T34.41 Frostbite with tissue necrosis of right arm** `CC` `H5`

     **√x7th T34.42 Frostbite with tissue necrosis of left arm** `CC` `H5`

**√5th T34.5 Frostbite with tissue necrosis of wrist, hand, and finger(s)**

     **CC Excl: For CC codes in subcategory T34.5:** PDX collection 1417

     **√6th T34.51 Frostbite with tissue necrosis of wrist**

       **√7th T34.511 Frostbite with tissue necrosis of right wrist** `CC` `H5`

       **√7th T34.512 Frostbite with tissue necrosis of left wrist** `CC` `H5`

       **√7th T34.519 Frostbite with tissue necrosis of unspecified wrist** `CC` `H5`

     **√6th T34.52 Frostbite with tissue necrosis of hand**
       *EXCLUDES 2*   frostbite with tissue necrosis of finger(s) (T34.53-)

       **√7th T34.521 Frostbite with tissue necrosis of right hand** `CC` `H5`

       **√7th T34.522 Frostbite with tissue necrosis of left hand** `CC` `H5`

       **√7th T34.529 Frostbite with tissue necrosis of unspecified hand** `CC` `H5`

     **√6th T34.53 Frostbite with tissue necrosis of finger(s)**

       **√7th T34.531 Frostbite with tissue necrosis of right finger(s)** `CC` `H5`

       **√7th T34.532 Frostbite with tissue necrosis of left finger(s)** `CC` `H5`

       **√7th T34.539 Frostbite with tissue necrosis of unspecified finger(s)** `CC` `H5`

**√5th T34.6 Frostbite with tissue necrosis of hip and thigh**

     **√x7th T34.60 Frostbite with tissue necrosis of unspecified hip and thigh** `CC` `H5`

     **√x7th T34.61 Frostbite with tissue necrosis of right hip and thigh** `CC` `H5`

     **√x7th T34.62 Frostbite with tissue necrosis of left hip and thigh** `CC` `H5`

**√5th T34.7 Frostbite with tissue necrosis of knee and lower leg**
     *EXCLUDES 2*   frostbite with tissue necrosis of ankle and foot (T34.8-)

     **√x7th T34.70 Frostbite with tissue necrosis of unspecified knee and lower leg** `CC` `H5`

     **√x7th T34.71 Frostbite with tissue necrosis of right knee and lower leg** `CC` `H5`

N Newborn: 0   P Pediatric: 0-17   M Maternity: 12-55   A Adult: 15-124   **MCC** Major CC Condition   **PDxMCC** PDx acts as own MCC   **CC** CC Condition   **PDxCC** PDx acts as own CC

**1098**      ICD-10-CM 2018

√x7ᵗʰ **T34.72** **Frostbite with tissue necrosis of** left knee and lower leg   CC H5

√5ᵗʰ **T34.8** **Frostbite with tissue necrosis of** ankle, foot, and toe(s)

> **CC Excl:** For CC codes in subcategory T34.8: PDX collection 1418

√6ᵗʰ **T34.81** **Frostbite with tissue necrosis of** ankle

√7ᵗʰ **T34.811** **Frostbite with tissue necrosis of** right **ankle**   CC H5

√7ᵗʰ **T34.812** **Frostbite with tissue necrosis of** left **ankle**   CC H5

√7ᵗʰ **T34.819** **Frostbite with tissue necrosis of** unspecified **ankle**   CC H5

√6ᵗʰ **T34.82** **Frostbite with tissue necrosis of** foot

√7ᵗʰ **T34.821** **Frostbite with tissue necrosis of** right **foot**   CC H5

√7ᵗʰ **T34.822** **Frostbite with tissue necrosis of** left **foot**   CC H5

√7ᵗʰ **T34.829** **Frostbite with tissue necrosis of** unspecified **foot**   CC H5

√6ᵗʰ **T34.83** **Frostbite with tissue necrosis of** toe(s)

√7ᵗʰ **T34.831** **Frostbite with tissue necrosis of** right **toe(s)**   CC H5

√7ᵗʰ **T34.832** **Frostbite with tissue necrosis of** left **toe(s)**   CC H5

√7ᵗʰ **T34.839** **Frostbite with tissue necrosis of** unspecified **toe(s)**   CC H5

√5ᵗʰ **T34.9** **Frostbite with tissue necrosis of** other and unspecified sites

√x7ᵗʰ **T34.90** **Frostbite with tissue necrosis of** unspecified sites   CC H5
Frostbite with tissue necrosis NOS

√x7ᵗʰ **T34.99** **Frostbite with tissue necrosis of** other sites   CC H5
Frostbite with tissue necrosis of leg NOS
Frostbite with tissue necrosis of trunk NOS

## Poisoning by, adverse effects of and underdosing of drugs, medicaments and biological substances (T36-T50)

INCLUDES   adverse effect of correct substance properly administered
poisoning by overdose of substance
poisoning by wrong substance given or taken in error
underdosing by (inadvertently) (deliberately) taking less substance than prescribed or instructed

Code first, for adverse effects, the nature of the adverse effect, such as:
adverse effect NOS (T88.7)
aspirin gastritis (K29.-)
blood disorders (D56-D76)
contact dermatitis (L23-L25)
dermatitis due to substances taken internally (L27.-)
nephropathy (N14.0-N14.2)

NOTE   The drug giving rise to the adverse effect should be identified by use of codes from categories T36-T50 with fifth or sixth character 5.

Use additional code(s) to specify:
manifestations of poisoning
underdosing or failure in dosage during medical and surgical care (Y63.6, Y63.8-Y63.9)
underdosing of medication regimen (Z91.12-, Z91.13-)

EXCLUDES 1   toxic reaction to local anesthesia in pregnancy (O29.3-)
EXCLUDES 2   abuse and dependence of psychoactive substances (F10-F19)
abuse of non-dependence-producing substances (F55.-)
drug reaction and poisoning affecting newborn (P00-P96)
pathological drug intoxication (inebriation) (F10-F19)

AHA: 2016, 2Q, 8; 2015, 3Q, 22

√4ᵗʰ **T36** **Poisoning by, adverse effect of and underdosing of systemic antibiotics**

EXCLUDES 1   antineoplastic antibiotics (T45.1-)
locally applied antibiotic NEC (T49.0)
topically used antibiotic for ear, nose and throat (T49.6)
topically used antibiotic for eye (T49.5)

> The appropriate 7th character is to be added to each code from category T36.
> A   initial encounter
> D   subsequent encounter
> S   sequela

√5ᵗʰ **T36.0** **Poisoning by, adverse effect of and underdosing of** penicillins

√6ᵗʰ **T36.0X** **Poisoning by, adverse effect of and underdosing of** penicillins

√7ᵗʰ **T36.0X1** **Poisoning by penicillins,** accidental **(unintentional)**
Poisoning by penicillins NOS

11 √7ᵗʰ **T36.0X2** **Poisoning by penicillins,** intentional self-harm   HCC

√7ᵗʰ **T36.0X3** **Poisoning by penicillins,** assault

√7ᵗʰ **T36.0X4** **Poisoning by penicillins,** undetermined

√7ᵗʰ **T36.0X5** **Adverse effect** of penicillins

√7ᵗʰ **T36.0X6** **Underdosing** of penicillins

√5ᵗʰ **T36.1** **Poisoning by, adverse effect of and underdosing of** cephalosporins and other beta-lactam antibiotics

√6ᵗʰ **T36.1X** **Poisoning by, adverse effect of and underdosing of** cephalosporins and other beta-lactam antibiotics

√7ᵗʰ **T36.1X1** **Poisoning by cephalosporins and other beta-lactam antibiotics,** accidental **(unintentional)**
Poisoning by cephalosporins and other beta-lactam antibiotics NOS

11 √7ᵗʰ **T36.1X2** **Poisoning by cephalosporins and other beta-lactam antibiotics,** intentional self-harm   HCC

√7ᵗʰ **T36.1X3** **Poisoning by cephalosporins and other beta-lactam antibiotics,** assault

√7ᵗʰ **T36.1X4** **Poisoning by cephalosporins and other beta-lactam antibiotics,** undetermined

√7ᵗʰ **T36.1X5** **Adverse effect** of cephalosporins and other beta-lactam antibiotics

√7ᵗʰ **T36.1X6** **Underdosing** of cephalosporins and other beta-lactam antibiotics

√5ᵗʰ **T36.2** **Poisoning by, adverse effect of and underdosing of** chloramphenicol group

√6ᵗʰ **T36.2X** **Poisoning by, adverse effect of and underdosing of** chloramphenicol group

√7ᵗʰ **T36.2X1** **Poisoning by chloramphenicol group,** accidental **(unintentional)**
Poisoning by chloramphenicol group NOS

11 √7ᵗʰ **T36.2X2** **Poisoning by chloramphenicol group,** intentional self-harm   HCC

√7ᵗʰ **T36.2X3** **Poisoning by chloramphenicol group,** assault

√7ᵗʰ **T36.2X4** **Poisoning by chloramphenicol group,** undetermined

√7ᵗʰ **T36.2X5** **Adverse effect** of chloramphenicol group

√7ᵗʰ **T36.2X6** **Underdosing** of chloramphenicol group

√5ᵗʰ **T36.3** **Poisoning by, adverse effect of and underdosing of** macrolides

√6ᵗʰ **T36.3X** **Poisoning by, adverse effect of and underdosing of** macrolides

√7ᵗʰ **T36.3X1** **Poisoning by macrolides,** accidental **(unintentional)**
Poisoning by macrolides NOS

11 √7ᵗʰ **T36.3X2** **Poisoning by macrolides,** intentional self-harm   HCC

√7ᵗʰ **T36.3X3** **Poisoning by macrolides,** assault

√7ᵗʰ **T36.3X4** **Poisoning by macrolides,** undetermined

√7ᵗʰ **T36.3X5** **Adverse effect** of macrolides

√7ᵗʰ **T36.3X6** **Underdosing** of macrolides

√5ᵗʰ **T36.4** **Poisoning by, adverse effect of and underdosing of** tetracyclines

√6ᵗʰ **T36.4X** **Poisoning by, adverse effect of and underdosing of** tetracyclines

√7ᵗʰ **T36.4X1** **Poisoning by tetracyclines,** accidental **(unintentional)**
Poisoning by tetracyclines NOS

11 √7ᵗʰ **T36.4X2** **Poisoning by tetracyclines,** intentional self-harm   HCC

√7ᵗʰ **T36.4X3** **Poisoning by tetracyclines,** assault

√7ᵗʰ **T36.4X4** **Poisoning by tetracyclines,** undetermined

√7ᵗʰ **T36.4X5** **Adverse effect** of tetracyclines

√7ᵗʰ **T36.4X6** **Underdosing** of tetracyclines

---

11 HCC with 7th character indicating initial encounter (A or B - specific to category) OR sequela.

☑ Additional Character Req   √x7ᵗʰ Placeholder Alert   Unacceptable PDx   Manifestation   H1-H14 HAC   HCC CMS-HCC Condition   EXCLUDES 1 Not Coded Here   EXCLUDES 2 Not Included Here

ICD-10-CM 2018     1099

✓5ᵗʰ **T36.5** **Poisoning by, adverse effect of and underdosing of aminoglycosides**
Poisoning by, adverse effect of and underdosing of streptomycin

    ✓6ᵗʰ **T36.5X** **Poisoning by, adverse effect of and underdosing of aminoglycosides**

       ✓7ᵗʰ **T36.5X1** **Poisoning by aminoglycosides,** accidental **(unintentional)**
Poisoning by aminoglycosides NOS

       [11] ✓7ᵗʰ **T36.5X2** **Poisoning by aminoglycosides, intentional self-harm** `HCC`

       ✓7ᵗʰ **T36.5X3** **Poisoning by aminoglycosides,** assault

       ✓7ᵗʰ **T36.5X4** **Poisoning by aminoglycosides, undetermined**

       ✓7ᵗʰ **T36.5X5** Adverse effect **of aminoglycosides**

       ✓7ᵗʰ **T36.5X6** Underdosing **of aminoglycosides**

✓5ᵗʰ **T36.6** **Poisoning by, adverse effect of and underdosing of rifampicins**

    ✓6ᵗʰ **T36.6X** **Poisoning by, adverse effect of and underdosing of rifampicins**

       ✓7ᵗʰ **T36.6X1** **Poisoning by rifampicins,** accidental **(unintentional)**
Poisoning by rifampicins NOS

       [11] ✓7ᵗʰ **T36.6X2** **Poisoning by rifampicins, intentional self-harm** `HCC`

       ✓7ᵗʰ **T36.6X3** **Poisoning by rifampicins,** assault

       ✓7ᵗʰ **T36.6X4** **Poisoning by rifampicins,** undetermined

       ✓7ᵗʰ **T36.6X5** Adverse effect **of rifampicins**

       ✓7ᵗʰ **T36.6X6** Underdosing **of rifampicins**

✓5ᵗʰ **T36.7** **Poisoning by, adverse effect of and underdosing of antifungal antibiotics, systemically used**

    ✓6ᵗʰ **T36.7X** **Poisoning by, adverse effect of and underdosing of antifungal antibiotics, systemically used**

       ✓7ᵗʰ **T36.7X1** **Poisoning by antifungal antibiotics, systemically used,** accidental **(unintentional)**
Poisoning by antifungal antibiotics, systemically used NOS

       [11] ✓7ᵗʰ **T36.7X2** **Poisoning by antifungal antibiotics, systemically used, intentional self-harm** `HCC`

       ✓7ᵗʰ **T36.7X3** **Poisoning by antifungal antibiotics, systemically used,** assault

       ✓7ᵗʰ **T36.7X4** **Poisoning by antifungal antibiotics, systemically used,** undetermined

       ✓7ᵗʰ **T36.7X5** Adverse effect **of antifungal antibiotics, systemically used**

       ✓7ᵗʰ **T36.7X6** Underdosing **of antifungal antibiotics, systemically used**

✓5ᵗʰ **T36.8** **Poisoning by, adverse effect of and underdosing of other systemic antibiotics**

    ✓6ᵗʰ **T36.8X** **Poisoning by, adverse effect of and underdosing of other systemic antibiotics**
**AHA:** 2017, 1Q, 39

       ✓7ᵗʰ **T36.8X1** **Poisoning by other systemic antibiotics,** accidental **(unintentional)**
Poisoning by other systemic antibiotics NOS

       [11] ✓7ᵗʰ **T36.8X2** **Poisoning by other systemic antibiotics, intentional self-harm** `HCC`

       ✓7ᵗʰ **T36.8X3** **Poisoning by other systemic antibiotics,** assault

       ✓7ᵗʰ **T36.8X4** **Poisoning by other systemic antibiotics,** undetermined

       ✓7ᵗʰ **T36.8X5** Adverse effect **of other systemic antibiotics**

       ✓7ᵗʰ **T36.8X6** Underdosing **of other systemic antibiotics**

✓5ᵗʰ **T36.9** **Poisoning by, adverse effect of and underdosing of unspecified systemic antibiotic**

    ✓x7ᵗʰ **T36.91** **Poisoning by unspecified systemic antibiotic,** accidental **(unintentional)**
Poisoning by systemic antibiotic NOS

    [11] ✓x7ᵗʰ **T36.92** **Poisoning by unspecified systemic antibiotic, intentional self-harm** `HCC`

    ✓x7ᵗʰ **T36.93** **Poisoning by unspecified systemic antibiotic,** assault

    ✓x7ᵗʰ **T36.94** **Poisoning by unspecified systemic antibiotic, undetermined**

    ✓x7ᵗʰ **T36.95** Adverse effect **of unspecified systemic antibiotic**

    ✓x7ᵗʰ **T36.96** Underdosing **of unspecified systemic antibiotic**

✓4ᵗʰ **T37** **Poisoning by, adverse effect of and underdosing of other systemic anti- infectives and antiparasitics**
**EXCLUDES 1** *anti-infectives topically used for ear, nose and throat (T49.6-)*
*anti-infectives topically used for eye (T49.5-)*
*locally applied anti-infectives NEC (T49.0-)*

The appropriate 7th character is to be added to each code from category T37.
A    initial encounter
D    subsequent encounter
S    sequela

✓5ᵗʰ **T37.0** **Poisoning by, adverse effect of and underdosing of sulfonamides**

    ✓6ᵗʰ **T37.0X** **Poisoning by, adverse effect of and underdosing of sulfonamides**

       ✓7ᵗʰ **T37.0X1** **Poisoning by sulfonamides,** accidental **(unintentional)**
Poisoning by sulfonamides NOS

       [11] ✓7ᵗʰ **T37.0X2** **Poisoning by sulfonamides, intentional self-harm** `HCC`

       ✓7ᵗʰ **T37.0X3** **Poisoning by sulfonamides,** assault

       ✓7ᵗʰ **T37.0X4** **Poisoning by sulfonamides, undetermined**

       ✓7ᵗʰ **T37.0X5** Adverse effect **of sulfonamides**

       ✓7ᵗʰ **T37.0X6** Underdosing **of sulfonamides**

✓5ᵗʰ **T37.1** **Poisoning by, adverse effect of and underdosing of antimycobacterial drugs**
**EXCLUDES 1** *rifampicins (T36.6-)*
*streptomycin (T36.5-)*

    ✓6ᵗʰ **T37.1X** **Poisoning by, adverse effect of and underdosing of antimycobacterial drugs**

       ✓7ᵗʰ **T37.1X1** **Poisoning by antimycobacterial drugs,** accidental **(unintentional)**
Poisoning by antimycobacterial drugs NOS

       [11] ✓7ᵗʰ **T37.1X2** **Poisoning by antimycobacterial drugs, intentional self-harm** `HCC`

       ✓7ᵗʰ **T37.1X3** **Poisoning by antimycobacterial drugs,** assault

       ✓7ᵗʰ **T37.1X4** **Poisoning by antimycobacterial drugs,** undetermined

       ✓7ᵗʰ **T37.1X5** Adverse effect **of antimycobacterial drugs**

       ✓7ᵗʰ **T37.1X6** Underdosing **of antimycobacterial drugs**

✓5ᵗʰ **T37.2** **Poisoning by, adverse effect of and underdosing of antimalarials and drugs acting on other blood protozoa**
**EXCLUDES 1** *hydroxyquinoline derivatives (T37.8-)*

    ✓6ᵗʰ **T37.2X** **Poisoning by, adverse effect of and underdosing of antimalarials and drugs acting on other blood protozoa**

       ✓7ᵗʰ **T37.2X1** **Poisoning by antimalarials and drugs acting on other blood protozoa,** accidental **(unintentional)**
Poisoning by antimalarials and drugs acting on other blood protozoa NOS

       [11] ✓7ᵗʰ **T37.2X2** **Poisoning by antimalarials and drugs acting on other blood protozoa, intentional self-harm** `HCC`

       ✓7ᵗʰ **T37.2X3** **Poisoning by antimalarials and drugs acting on other blood protozoa,** assault

       ✓7ᵗʰ **T37.2X4** **Poisoning by antimalarials and drugs acting on other blood protozoa, undetermined**

       ✓7ᵗʰ **T37.2X5** Adverse effect **of antimalarials and drugs acting on other blood protozoa**

       ✓7ᵗʰ **T37.2X6** Underdosing **of antimalarials and drugs acting on other blood protozoa**

---

[11] HCC with 7th character indicating initial encounter (A or B - specific to category) OR sequela.

√5th **T37.3** **Poisoning by, adverse effect of and underdosing of other antiprotozoal drugs**

  √6th **T37.3X** Poisoning by, adverse effect of and underdosing of other antiprotozoal drugs

    √7th **T37.3X1** **Poisoning by other antiprotozoal drugs, accidental (unintentional)**
         Poisoning by other antiprotozoal drugs NOS

    11 √7th **T37.3X2** **Poisoning by other antiprotozoal drugs, intentional self-harm** HCC

    √7th **T37.3X3** **Poisoning by other antiprotozoal drugs, assault**

    √7th **T37.3X4** **Poisoning by other antiprotozoal drugs, undetermined**

    √7th **T37.3X5** Adverse effect of other antiprotozoal drugs

    √7th **T37.3X6** Underdosing of other antiprotozoal drugs

√5th **T37.4** **Poisoning by, adverse effect of and underdosing of anthelminthics**

  √6th **T37.4X** Poisoning by, adverse effect of and underdosing of anthelminthics

    √7th **T37.4X1** **Poisoning by anthelminthics, accidental (unintentional)**
         Poisoning by anthelminthics NOS

    11 √7th **T37.4X2** **Poisoning by anthelminthics, intentional self-harm** HCC

    √7th **T37.4X3** **Poisoning by anthelminthics, assault**

    √7th **T37.4X4** **Poisoning by anthelminthics, undetermined**

    √7th **T37.4X5** Adverse effect of anthelminthics

    √7th **T37.4X6** Underdosing of anthelminthics

√5th **T37.5** **Poisoning by, adverse effect of and underdosing of antiviral drugs**
    EXCLUDES 1   amantadine (T42.8-)
               cytarabine (T45.1-)

  √6th **T37.5X** **Poisoning by, adverse effect of and underdosing of antiviral drugs**

    √7th **T37.5X1** **Poisoning by antiviral drugs, accidental (unintentional)**
         Poisoning by antiviral drugs NOS

    11 √7th **T37.5X2** **Poisoning by antiviral drugs, intentional self-harm** HCC

    √7th **T37.5X3** **Poisoning by antiviral drugs, assault**

    √7th **T37.5X4** **Poisoning by antiviral drugs, undetermined**

    √7th **T37.5X5** Adverse effect of antiviral drugs

    √7th **T37.5X6** Underdosing of antiviral drugs

√5th **T37.8** **Poisoning by, adverse effect of and underdosing of other specified systemic anti-infectives and antiparasitics**
     Poisoning by, adverse effect of and underdosing of hydroxyquinoline derivatives
    EXCLUDES 1   antimalarial drugs (T37.2-)

  √6th **T37.8X** **Poisoning by, adverse effect of and underdosing of other specified systemic anti-infectives and antiparasitics**

    √7th **T37.8X1** **Poisoning by other specified systemic anti-infectives and antiparasitics, accidental (unintentional)**
         Poisoning by other specified systemic anti-infectives and antiparasitics NOS

    11 √7th **T37.8X2** **Poisoning by other specified systemic anti-infectives and antiparasitics, intentional self-harm** HCC

    √7th **T37.8X3** **Poisoning by other specified systemic anti-infectives and antiparasitics, assault**

    √7th **T37.8X4** **Poisoning by other specified systemic anti-infectives and antiparasitics, undetermined**

    √7th **T37.8X5** Adverse effect of other specified systemic anti-infectives and antiparasitics

    √7th **T37.8X6** Underdosing of other specified systemic anti-infectives and antiparasitics

√5th **T37.9** **Poisoning by, adverse effect of and underdosing of unspecified systemic anti-infective and antiparasitics**

  √x7th **T37.91** **Poisoning by unspecified systemic anti-infective and antiparasitics, accidental (unintentional)**
     Poisoning by, adverse effect of and underdosing of systemic anti-infective and antiparasitics NOS

  11 √x7th **T37.92** **Poisoning by unspecified systemic anti-infective and antiparasitics, intentional self-harm** HCC

  √x7th **T37.93** **Poisoning by unspecified systemic anti-infective and antiparasitics, assault**

  √x7th **T37.94** **Poisoning by unspecified systemic anti-infective and antiparasitics, undetermined**

  √x7th **T37.95** Adverse effect of unspecified systemic anti-infective and antiparasitic

  √x7th **T37.96** Underdosing of unspecified systemic anti-infectives and antiparasitics

√4th **T38** **Poisoning by, adverse effect of and underdosing of hormones and their synthetic substitutes and antagonists, not elsewhere classified**
    EXCLUDES 1   mineralocorticoids and their antagonists (T50.0-)
               oxytocic hormones (T48.0-)
               parathyroid hormones and derivatives (T50.9-)

     The appropriate 7th character is to be added to each code from category T38.
     A     initial encounter
     D     subsequent encounter
     S     sequela

√5th **T38.0** **Poisoning by, adverse effect of and underdosing of glucocorticoids and synthetic analogues**
    EXCLUDES 1   glucocorticoids, topically used (T49.-)

  √6th **T38.0X** **Poisoning by, adverse effect of and underdosing of glucocorticoids and synthetic analogues**

    √7th **T38.0X1** **Poisoning by glucocorticoids and synthetic analogues, accidental (unintentional)**
         Poisoning by glucocorticoids and synthetic analogues NOS

    11 √7th **T38.0X2** **Poisoning by glucocorticoids and synthetic analogues, intentional self-harm** HCC

    √7th **T38.0X3** **Poisoning by glucocorticoids and synthetic analogues, assault**

    √7th **T38.0X4** **Poisoning by glucocorticoids and synthetic analogues, undetermined**

    √7th **T38.0X5** Adverse effect of glucocorticoids and synthetic analogues

    √7th **T38.0X6** Underdosing of glucocorticoids and synthetic analogues

√5th **T38.1** **Poisoning by, adverse effect of and underdosing of thyroid hormones and substitutes**

  √6th **T38.1X** **Poisoning by, adverse effect of and underdosing of thyroid hormones and substitutes**

    √7th **T38.1X1** **Poisoning by thyroid hormones and substitutes, accidental (unintentional)**
         Poisoning by thyroid hormones and substitutes NOS

    11 √7th **T38.1X2** **Poisoning by thyroid hormones and substitutes, intentional self-harm** HCC

    √7th **T38.1X3** **Poisoning by thyroid hormones and substitutes, assault**

    √7th **T38.1X4** **Poisoning by thyroid hormones and substitutes, undetermined**

    √7th **T38.1X5** Adverse effect of thyroid hormones and substitutes

    √7th **T38.1X6** Underdosing of thyroid hormones and substitutes

√5th **T38.2** **Poisoning by, adverse effect of and underdosing of antithyroid drugs**

  √6th **T38.2X** **Poisoning by, adverse effect of and underdosing of antithyroid drugs**

    √7th **T38.2X1** **Poisoning by antithyroid drugs, accidental (unintentional)**
         Poisoning by antithyroid drugs NOS

    11 √7th **T38.2X2** **Poisoning by antithyroid drugs, intentional self-harm** HCC

---

11 HCC with 7th character indicating initial encounter (A or B - specific to category) OR sequela.

✓ Additional Character Req    √x7th Placeholder Alert    Unacceptable PDx    Manifestation    H1 - H14 HAC    HCC CMS-HCC Condition    EXCLUDES 1 Not Coded Here    EXCLUDES 2 Not Included Here

ICD-10-CM 2018          **1101**

√7ᵗʰ **T38.2X3** **Poisoning by antithyroid drugs,** assault

√7ᵗʰ **T38.2X4** **Poisoning by antithyroid drugs, undetermined**

√7ᵗʰ **T38.2X5** **Adverse effect of antithyroid drugs**

√7ᵗʰ **T38.2X6** **Underdosing of antithyroid drugs**

✓5ᵗʰ **T38.3** **Poisoning by, adverse effect of and underdosing of insulin and oral hypoglycemic [antidiabetic] drugs**

✓6ᵗʰ **T38.3X** **Poisoning by, adverse effect of and underdosing of insulin and oral hypoglycemic [antidiabetic] drugs**

√7ᵗʰ **T38.3X1** **Poisoning by insulin and oral hypoglycemic [antidiabetic] drugs, accidental (unintentional)**
Poisoning by insulin and oral hypoglycemic [antidiabetic] drugs NOS

11 √7ᵗʰ **T38.3X2** **Poisoning by insulin and oral** HCC **hypoglycemic [antidiabetic] drugs, intentional self-harm**

√7ᵗʰ **T38.3X3** **Poisoning by insulin and oral hypoglycemic [antidiabetic] drugs,** assault

√7ᵗʰ **T38.3X4** **Poisoning by insulin and oral hypoglycemic [antidiabetic] drugs, undetermined**

√7ᵗʰ **T38.3X5** **Adverse effect of insulin and oral hypoglycemic [antidiabetic] drugs**

√7ᵗʰ **T38.3X6** **Underdosing of insulin and oral hypoglycemic [antidiabetic] drugs**

✓5ᵗʰ **T38.4** **Poisoning by, adverse effect of and underdosing of oral contraceptives**
Poisoning by, adverse effect of and underdosing of multiple- and single-ingredient oral contraceptive preparations

✓6ᵗʰ **T38.4X** **Poisoning by, adverse effect of and underdosing of oral contraceptives**

√7ᵗʰ **T38.4X1** **Poisoning by oral contraceptives, accidental (unintentional)**
Poisoning by oral contraceptives NOS

11 √7ᵗʰ **T38.4X2** **Poisoning by oral contraceptives,** HCC **intentional self-harm**

√7ᵗʰ **T38.4X3** **Poisoning by oral contraceptives,** assault

√7ᵗʰ **T38.4X4** **Poisoning by oral contraceptives, undetermined**

√7ᵗʰ **T38.4X5** **Adverse effect of oral contraceptives**

√7ᵗʰ **T38.4X6** **Underdosing of oral contraceptives**

✓5ᵗʰ **T38.5** **Poisoning by, adverse effect of and underdosing of other estrogens and progestogens**
Poisoning by, adverse effect of and underdosing of estrogens and progestogens mixtures and substitutes

✓6ᵗʰ **T38.5X** **Poisoning by, adverse effect of and underdosing of other estrogens and progestogens**

√7ᵗʰ **T38.5X1** **Poisoning by other estrogens and progestogens, accidental (unintentional)**
Poisoning by other estrogens and progestogens NOS

11 √7ᵗʰ **T38.5X2** **Poisoning by other estrogens and** HCC **progestogens, intentional self-harm**

√7ᵗʰ **T38.5X3** **Poisoning by other estrogens and progestogens,** assault

√7ᵗʰ **T38.5X4** **Poisoning by other estrogens and progestogens, undetermined**

√7ᵗʰ **T38.5X5** **Adverse effect of other estrogens and progestogens**

√7ᵗʰ **T38.5X6** **Underdosing of other estrogens and progestogens**

✓5ᵗʰ **T38.6** **Poisoning by, adverse effect of and underdosing of antigonadotrophins, antiestrogens, antiandrogens, not elsewhere classified**
Poisoning by, adverse effect of and underdosing of tamoxifen

✓6ᵗʰ **T38.6X** **Poisoning by, adverse effect of and underdosing of antigonadotrophins, antiestrogens, antiandrogens, not elsewhere classified**

√7ᵗʰ **T38.6X1** **Poisoning by antigonadotrophins, antiestrogens, antiandrogens, not elsewhere classified, accidental (unintentional)**
Poisoning by antigonadotrophins, antiestrogens, antiandrogens, not elsewhere classified NOS

11 √7ᵗʰ **T38.6X2** **Poisoning by antigonadotrophins,** HCC **antiestrogens, antiandrogens, not elsewhere classified, intentional self-harm**

√7ᵗʰ **T38.6X3** **Poisoning by antigonadotrophins, antiestrogens, antiandrogens, not elsewhere classified,** assault

√7ᵗʰ **T38.6X4** **Poisoning by antigonadotrophins, antiestrogens, antiandrogens, not elsewhere classified, undetermined**

√7ᵗʰ **T38.6X5** **Adverse effect of antigonadotrophins, antiestrogens, antiandrogens, not elsewhere classified**

√7ᵗʰ **T38.6X6** **Underdosing of antigonadotrophins, antiestrogens, antiandrogens, not elsewhere classified**

✓5ᵗʰ **T38.7** **Poisoning by, adverse effect of and underdosing of androgens and anabolic congeners**

✓6ᵗʰ **T38.7X** **Poisoning by, adverse effect of and underdosing of androgens and anabolic congeners**

√7ᵗʰ **T38.7X1** **Poisoning by androgens and anabolic congeners, accidental (unintentional)**
Poisoning by androgens and anabolic congeners NOS

11 √7ᵗʰ **T38.7X2** **Poisoning by androgens and anabolic** HCC **congeners, intentional self-harm**

√7ᵗʰ **T38.7X3** **Poisoning by androgens and anabolic congeners,** assault

√7ᵗʰ **T38.7X4** **Poisoning by androgens and anabolic congeners, undetermined**

√7ᵗʰ **T38.7X5** **Adverse effect of androgens and anabolic congeners**

√7ᵗʰ **T38.7X6** **Underdosing of androgens and anabolic congeners**

✓5ᵗʰ **T38.8** **Poisoning by, adverse effect of and underdosing of other and unspecified hormones and synthetic substitutes**

✓6ᵗʰ **T38.80** **Poisoning by, adverse effect of and underdosing of unspecified hormones and synthetic substitutes**

√7ᵗʰ **T38.801** **Poisoning by unspecified hormones and synthetic substitutes, accidental (unintentional)**
Poisoning by unspecified hormones and synthetic substitutes NOS

11 √7ᵗʰ **T38.802** **Poisoning by unspecified hormones** HCC **and synthetic substitutes, intentional self-harm**

√7ᵗʰ **T38.803** **Poisoning by unspecified hormones and synthetic substitutes,** assault

√7ᵗʰ **T38.804** **Poisoning by unspecified hormones and synthetic substitutes, undetermined**

√7ᵗʰ **T38.805** **Adverse effect of unspecified hormones and synthetic substitutes**

√7ᵗʰ **T38.806** **Underdosing of unspecified hormones and synthetic substitutes**

✓6ᵗʰ **T38.81** **Poisoning by, adverse effect of and underdosing of anterior pituitary [adenohypophyseal] hormones**

√7ᵗʰ **T38.811** **Poisoning by anterior pituitary [adenohypophyseal] hormones, accidental (unintentional)**
Poisoning by anterior pituitary [adenohypophyseal] hormones NOS

11 √7ᵗʰ **T38.812** **Poisoning by anterior pituitary** HCC **[adenohypophyseal] hormones, intentional self-harm**

√7ᵗʰ **T38.813** **Poisoning by anterior pituitary [adenohypophyseal] hormones,** assault

√7ᵗʰ **T38.814** **Poisoning by anterior pituitary [adenohypophyseal] hormones, undetermined**

√7ᵗʰ **T38.815** **Adverse effect of anterior pituitary [adenohypophyseal] hormones**

√7ᵗʰ **T38.816** **Underdosing of anterior pituitary [adenohypophyseal] hormones**

---

11 HCC with 7th character indicating initial encounter (A or B - specific to category) OR sequela.

Ⓝ Newborn: 0   Ⓟ Pediatric: 0-17   Ⓜ Maternity: 12-55   Ⓐ Adult: 15-124   **MCC** Major CC Condition   **PDxMCC** PDx acts as own MCC   **CC** CC Condition   **PDxCC** PDx acts as own CC

**1102**      ICD-10-CM 2018

**Chapter 19. Injury, Poisoning and Certain Other Consequences of External Causes**

✓6ᵗʰ **T38.89** **Poisoning by, adverse effect of and underdosing of** other hormones and synthetic substitutes

    ✓7ᵗʰ **T38.891** **Poisoning by other hormones and synthetic substitutes,** accidental (unintentional)
      Poisoning by other hormones and synthetic substitutes NOS

    11 ✓7ᵗʰ **T38.892** **Poisoning by other hormones and synthetic substitutes,** intentional self-harm   HCC

    ✓7ᵗʰ **T38.893** **Poisoning by other hormones and synthetic substitutes,** assault

    ✓7ᵗʰ **T38.894** **Poisoning by other hormones and synthetic substitutes,** undetermined

    ✓7ᵗʰ **T38.895** Adverse effect of other hormones and synthetic substitutes

    ✓7ᵗʰ **T38.896** Underdosing of other hormones and synthetic substitutes

✓5ᵗʰ **T38.9** **Poisoning by, adverse effect of and underdosing of other and unspecified hormone antagonists**

    ✓6ᵗʰ **T38.90** **Poisoning by, adverse effect of and underdosing of** unspecified hormone antagonists

      ✓7ᵗʰ **T38.901** **Poisoning by unspecified hormone antagonists,** accidental (unintentional)
        Poisoning by unspecified hormone antagonists NOS

      11 ✓7ᵗʰ **T38.902** **Poisoning by unspecified hormone antagonists,** intentional self-harm   HCC

      ✓7ᵗʰ **T38.903** **Poisoning by unspecified hormone antagonists,** assault

      ✓7ᵗʰ **T38.904** **Poisoning by unspecified hormone antagonists,** undetermined

      ✓7ᵗʰ **T38.905** Adverse effect of unspecified hormone antagonists

      ✓7ᵗʰ **T38.906** Underdosing of unspecified hormone antagonists

    ✓6ᵗʰ **T38.99** **Poisoning by, adverse effect of and underdosing of** other hormone antagonists

      ✓7ᵗʰ **T38.991** **Poisoning by other hormone antagonists,** accidental (unintentional)
        Poisoning by other hormone antagonists NOS

      11 ✓7ᵗʰ **T38.992** **Poisoning by other hormone antagonists,** intentional self-harm   HCC

      ✓7ᵗʰ **T38.993** **Poisoning by other hormone antagonists,** assault

      ✓7ᵗʰ **T38.994** **Poisoning by other hormone antagonists,** undetermined

      ✓7ᵗʰ **T38.995** Adverse effect of other hormone antagonists

      ✓7ᵗʰ **T38.996** Underdosing of other hormone antagonists

✓4ᵗʰ **T39** **Poisoning by, adverse effect of and underdosing of nonopioid analgesics, antipyretics and antirheumatics**

    The appropriate 7th character is to be added to each code from category T39.
    A    initial encounter
    D    subsequent encounter
    S    sequela

✓5ᵗʰ **T39.0** **Poisoning by, adverse effect of and underdosing of** salicylates

    ✓6ᵗʰ **T39.01** **Poisoning by, adverse effect of and underdosing of** aspirin
      Poisoning by, adverse effect of and underdosing of acetylsalicylic acid

      ✓7ᵗʰ **T39.011** **Poisoning by aspirin,** accidental (unintentional)

      11 ✓7ᵗʰ **T39.012** **Poisoning by aspirin,** intentional self-harm   HCC

      ✓7ᵗʰ **T39.013** **Poisoning by aspirin,** assault

      ✓7ᵗʰ **T39.014** **Poisoning by aspirin,** undetermined

      ✓7ᵗʰ **T39.015** Adverse effect of aspirin
        **AHA:** 2016, 1Q, 15

      ✓7ᵗʰ **T39.016** Underdosing of aspirin

✓6ᵗʰ **T39.09** **Poisoning by, adverse effect of and underdosing of** other salicylates

    ✓7ᵗʰ **T39.091** **Poisoning by salicylates,** accidental (unintentional)
      Poisoning by salicylates NOS

    11 ✓7ᵗʰ **T39.092** **Poisoning by salicylates,** intentional self-harm   HCC

    ✓7ᵗʰ **T39.093** **Poisoning by salicylates,** assault

    ✓7ᵗʰ **T39.094** **Poisoning by salicylates,** undetermined

    ✓7ᵗʰ **T39.095** Adverse effect of salicylates

    ✓7ᵗʰ **T39.096** Underdosing of salicylates

✓5ᵗʰ **T39.1** **Poisoning by, adverse effect of and underdosing of 4-Aminophenol derivatives**

    ✓6ᵗʰ **T39.1X** **Poisoning by, adverse effect of and underdosing of** 4-Aminophenol derivatives

      ✓7ᵗʰ **T39.1X1** **Poisoning by 4-Aminophenol derivatives,** accidental (unintentional)
        Poisoning by 4-Aminophenol derivatives NOS

      11 ✓7ᵗʰ **T39.1X2** **Poisoning by 4-Aminophenol derivatives,** intentional self-harm   HCC

      ✓7ᵗʰ **T39.1X3** **Poisoning by 4-Aminophenol derivatives,** assault

      ✓7ᵗʰ **T39.1X4** **Poisoning by 4-Aminophenol derivatives,** undetermined

      ✓7ᵗʰ **T39.1X5** Adverse effect of 4-Aminophenol derivatives

      ✓7ᵗʰ **T39.1X6** Underdosing of 4-Aminophenol derivatives

✓5ᵗʰ **T39.2** **Poisoning by, adverse effect of and underdosing of pyrazolone derivatives**

    ✓6ᵗʰ **T39.2X** **Poisoning by, adverse effect of and underdosing of** pyrazolone derivatives

      ✓7ᵗʰ **T39.2X1** **Poisoning by pyrazolone derivatives,** accidental (unintentional)
        Poisoning by pyrazolone derivatives NOS

      11 ✓7ᵗʰ **T39.2X2** **Poisoning by pyrazolone derivatives,** intentional self-harm   HCC

      ✓7ᵗʰ **T39.2X3** **Poisoning by pyrazolone derivatives,** assault

      ✓7ᵗʰ **T39.2X4** **Poisoning by pyrazolone derivatives,** undetermined

      ✓7ᵗʰ **T39.2X5** Adverse effect of pyrazolone derivatives

      ✓7ᵗʰ **T39.2X6** Underdosing of pyrazolone derivatives

✓5ᵗʰ **T39.3** **Poisoning by, adverse effect of and underdosing of other nonsteroidal anti-inflammatory drugs [NSAID]**

    ✓6ᵗʰ **T39.31** **Poisoning by, adverse effect of and underdosing of** propionic acid derivatives
      Poisoning by, adverse effect of and underdosing of fenoprofen
      Poisoning by, adverse effect of and underdosing of flurbiprofen
      Poisoning by, adverse effect of and underdosing of ibuprofen
      Poisoning by, adverse effect of and underdosing of ketoprofen
      Poisoning by, adverse effect of and underdosing of naproxen
      Poisoning by, adverse effect of and underdosing of oxaprozin

      ✓7ᵗʰ **T39.311** **Poisoning by propionic acid derivatives,** accidental (unintentional)

      11 ✓7ᵗʰ **T39.312** **Poisoning by propionic acid derivatives,** intentional self-harm   HCC

      ✓7ᵗʰ **T39.313** **Poisoning by propionic acid derivatives,** assault

      ✓7ᵗʰ **T39.314** **Poisoning by propionic acid derivatives,** undetermined

      ✓7ᵗʰ **T39.315** Adverse effect of propionic acid derivatives

      ✓7ᵗʰ **T39.316** Underdosing of propionic acid derivatives

---

11 HCC with 7th character indicating initial encounter (A or B - specific to category) OR sequela.

---

✓ Additional Character Req    ✓x7ᵗʰ Placeholder Alert    Unacceptable PDx    Manifestation    H1 - H14 HAC    HCC CMS-HCC Condition    *EXCLUDES 1* Not Coded Here    *EXCLUDES 2* Not Included Here

**✓6ᵗʰ T39.39 Poisoning by, adverse effect of and underdosing of other nonsteroidal anti-inflammatory drugs [NSAID]**

    **✓7ᵗʰ T39.391 Poisoning by other nonsteroidal anti-inflammatory drugs [NSAID], accidental (unintentional)**
        Poisoning by other nonsteroidal anti-inflammatory drugs NOS

    ¹¹ **✓7ᵗʰ T39.392 Poisoning by other nonsteroidal anti-inflammatory drugs [NSAID], intentional self-harm**    HCC

    **✓7ᵗʰ T39.393 Poisoning by other nonsteroidal anti-inflammatory drugs [NSAID], assault**

    **✓7ᵗʰ T39.394 Poisoning by other nonsteroidal anti-inflammatory drugs [NSAID], undetermined**

    **✓7ᵗʰ T39.395 Adverse effect of other nonsteroidal anti-inflammatory drugs [NSAID]**

    **✓7ᵗʰ T39.396 Underdosing of other nonsteroidal anti-inflammatory drugs [NSAID]**

**✓5ᵗʰ T39.4 Poisoning by, adverse effect of and underdosing of antirheumatics, not elsewhere classified**
    **EXCLUDES 1**   poisoning by, adverse effect of and underdosing of glucocorticoids (T38.0-)
           poisoning by, adverse effect of and underdosing of salicylates (T39.0-)

    **✓6ᵗʰ T39.4X Poisoning by, adverse effect of and underdosing of antirheumatics, not elsewhere classified**

        **✓7ᵗʰ T39.4X1 Poisoning by antirheumatics, not elsewhere classified, accidental (unintentional)**
           Poisoning by antirheumatics, not elsewhere classified NOS

        ¹¹ **✓7ᵗʰ T39.4X2 Poisoning by antirheumatics, not elsewhere classified, intentional self-harm**   HCC

        **✓7ᵗʰ T39.4X3 Poisoning by antirheumatics, not elsewhere classified, assault**

        **✓7ᵗʰ T39.4X4 Poisoning by antirheumatics, not elsewhere classified, undetermined**

        **✓7ᵗʰ T39.4X5 Adverse effect of antirheumatics, not elsewhere classified**

        **✓7ᵗʰ T39.4X6 Underdosing of antirheumatics, not elsewhere classified**

**✓5ᵗʰ T39.8 Poisoning by, adverse effect of and underdosing of other nonopioid analgesics and antipyretics, not elsewhere classified**

    **✓6ᵗʰ T39.8X Poisoning by, adverse effect of and underdosing of other nonopioid analgesics and antipyretics, not elsewhere classified**

        **✓7ᵗʰ T39.8X1 Poisoning by other nonopioid analgesics and antipyretics, not elsewhere classified, accidental (unintentional)**
           Poisoning by other nonopioid analgesics and antipyretics, not elsewhere classified NOS

        ¹¹ **✓7ᵗʰ T39.8X2 Poisoning by other nonopioid analgesics and antipyretics, not elsewhere classified, intentional self-harm**   HCC

        **✓7ᵗʰ T39.8X3 Poisoning by other nonopioid analgesics and antipyretics, not elsewhere classified, assault**

        **✓7ᵗʰ T39.8X4 Poisoning by other nonopioid analgesics and antipyretics, not elsewhere classified, undetermined**

        **✓7ᵗʰ T39.8X5 Adverse effect of other nonopioid analgesics and antipyretics, not elsewhere classified**

        **✓7ᵗʰ T39.8X6 Underdosing of other nonopioid analgesics and antipyretics, not elsewhere classified**

**✓5ᵗʰ T39.9 Poisoning by, adverse effect of and underdosing of unspecified nonopioid analgesic, antipyretic and antirheumatic**

    **✓x7ᵗʰ T39.91 Poisoning by unspecified nonopioid analgesic, antipyretic and antirheumatic, accidental (unintentional)**
        Poisoning by nonopioid analgesic, antipyretic and antirheumatic NOS

---

    ¹¹ **✓x7ᵗʰ T39.92 Poisoning by unspecified nonopioid analgesic, antipyretic and antirheumatic, intentional self-harm**   HCC

    **✓x7ᵗʰ T39.93 Poisoning by unspecified nonopioid analgesic, antipyretic and antirheumatic, assault**

    **✓x7ᵗʰ T39.94 Poisoning by unspecified nonopioid analgesic, antipyretic and antirheumatic, undetermined**

    **✓x7ᵗʰ T39.95 Adverse effect of unspecified nonopioid analgesic, antipyretic and antirheumatic**

    **✓x7ᵗʰ T39.96 Underdosing of unspecified nonopioid analgesic, antipyretic and antirheumatic**

**✓4ᵗʰ T40 Poisoning by, adverse effect of and underdosing of narcotics and psychodysleptics [hallucinogens]**
    **EXCLUDES 2**   drug dependence and related mental and behavioral disorders due to psychoactive substance use (F10-F19-)

    The appropriate 7th character is to be added to each code from category T40.
    A    initial encounter
    D    subsequent encounter
    S    sequela

**✓5ᵗʰ T40.0 Poisoning by, adverse effect of and underdosing of opium**

    **✓6ᵗʰ T40.0X Poisoning by, adverse effect of and underdosing of opium**

        **✓7ᵗʰ T40.0X1 Poisoning by opium, accidental (unintentional)**
           Poisoning by opium NOS

        ¹¹ **✓7ᵗʰ T40.0X2 Poisoning by opium, intentional self-harm**   HCC

        **✓7ᵗʰ T40.0X3 Poisoning by opium, assault**

        **✓7ᵗʰ T40.0X4 Poisoning by opium, undetermined**

        **✓7ᵗʰ T40.0X5 Adverse effect of opium**

        **✓7ᵗʰ T40.0X6 Underdosing of opium**

**✓5ᵗʰ T40.1 Poisoning by and adverse effect of heroin**

    **✓6ᵗʰ T40.1X Poisoning by and adverse effect of heroin**

        **✓7ᵗʰ T40.1X1 Poisoning by heroin, accidental (unintentional)**
           Poisoning by heroin NOS

        ¹¹ **✓7ᵗʰ T40.1X2 Poisoning by heroin, intentional self-harm**   HCC

        **✓7ᵗʰ T40.1X3 Poisoning by heroin, assault**

        **✓7ᵗʰ T40.1X4 Poisoning by heroin, undetermined**

**✓5ᵗʰ T40.2 Poisoning by, adverse effect of and underdosing of other opioids**

    **✓6ᵗʰ T40.2X Poisoning by, adverse effect of and underdosing of other opioids**

        **✓7ᵗʰ T40.2X1 Poisoning by other opioids, accidental (unintentional)**
           Poisoning by other opioids NOS

        ¹¹ **✓7ᵗʰ T40.2X2 Poisoning by other opioids, intentional self-harm**   HCC

        **✓7ᵗʰ T40.2X3 Poisoning by other opioids, assault**

        **✓7ᵗʰ T40.2X4 Poisoning by other opioids, undetermined**

        **✓7ᵗʰ T40.2X5 Adverse effect of other opioids**

        **✓7ᵗʰ T40.2X6 Underdosing of other opioids**

**✓5ᵗʰ T40.3 Poisoning by, adverse effect of and underdosing of methadone**

    **✓6ᵗʰ T40.3X Poisoning by, adverse effect of and underdosing of methadone**

        **✓7ᵗʰ T40.3X1 Poisoning by methadone, accidental (unintentional)**
           Poisoning by methadone NOS

        ¹¹ **✓7ᵗʰ T40.3X2 Poisoning by methadone, intentional self-harm**   HCC

        **✓7ᵗʰ T40.3X3 Poisoning by methadone, assault**

        **✓7ᵗʰ T40.3X4 Poisoning by methadone, undetermined**

        **✓7ᵗʰ T40.3X5 Adverse effect of methadone**

        **✓7ᵗʰ T40.3X6 Underdosing of methadone**

---

¹¹ HCC with 7th character indicating initial encounter (A or B - specific to category) OR sequela.

Ⓝ Newborn: 0    Ⓟ Pediatric: 0-17    Ⓜ Maternity: 12-55    Ⓐ Adult: 15-124    **MCC** Major CC Condition    **PDxMCC** PDx acts as own MCC    **CC** CC Condition    **PDxCC** PDx acts as own CC

**1104**      ICD-10-CM 2018

√5th **T40.4** **Poisoning by, adverse effect of and underdosing of other synthetic narcotics**

  √6th **T40.4X** **Poisoning by, adverse effect of and underdosing of other synthetic narcotics**

    √7th **T40.4X1** **Poisoning by other synthetic narcotics, accidental (unintentional)**
        Poisoning by other synthetic narcotics NOS

    11 √7th **T40.4X2** **Poisoning by other synthetic narcotics, intentional self-harm** `HCC`

    √7th **T40.4X3** **Poisoning by other synthetic narcotics, assault**

    √7th **T40.4X4** **Poisoning by other synthetic narcotics, undetermined**

    √7th **T40.4X5** **Adverse effect** of other synthetic narcotics

    √7th **T40.4X6** **Underdosing** of other synthetic narcotics

√5th **T40.5** **Poisoning by, adverse effect of and underdosing of cocaine**

  √6th **T40.5X** **Poisoning by, adverse effect of and underdosing of cocaine**

    √7th **T40.5X1** **Poisoning by cocaine, accidental (unintentional)**
        Poisoning by cocaine NOS
        **AHA:** 2016, 2Q, 8

    11 √7th **T40.5X2** **Poisoning by cocaine, intentional self-harm** `HCC`

    √7th **T40.5X3** **Poisoning by cocaine, assault**

    √7th **T40.5X4** **Poisoning by cocaine, undetermined**

    √7th **T40.5X5** **Adverse effect** of cocaine

    √7th **T40.5X6** **Underdosing** of cocaine

√5th **T40.6** **Poisoning by, adverse effect of and underdosing of other and unspecified narcotics**

  √6th **T40.60** **Poisoning by, adverse effect of and underdosing of unspecified narcotics**

    √7th **T40.601** **Poisoning by unspecified narcotics, accidental (unintentional)**
        Poisoning by narcotics NOS

    11 √7th **T40.602** **Poisoning by unspecified narcotics, intentional self-harm** `HCC`

    √7th **T40.603** **Poisoning by unspecified narcotics, assault**

    √7th **T40.604** **Poisoning by unspecified narcotics, undetermined**

    √7th **T40.605** **Adverse effect** of unspecified narcotics

    √7th **T40.606** **Underdosing** of unspecified narcotics

  √6th **T40.69** **Poisoning by, adverse effect of and underdosing of other narcotics**

    √7th **T40.691** **Poisoning by other narcotics, accidental (unintentional)**
        Poisoning by other narcotics NOS

    11 √7th **T40.692** **Poisoning by other narcotics, intentional self-harm** `HCC`

    √7th **T40.693** **Poisoning by other narcotics, assault**

    √7th **T40.694** **Poisoning by other narcotics, undetermined**

    √7th **T40.695** **Adverse effect** of other narcotics

    √7th **T40.696** **Underdosing** of other narcotics

√5th **T40.7** **Poisoning by, adverse effect of and underdosing of cannabis (derivatives)**

  √6th **T40.7X** **Poisoning by, adverse effect of and underdosing of cannabis (derivatives)**

    √7th **T40.7X1** **Poisoning by cannabis (derivatives), accidental (unintentional)**
        Poisoning by cannabis NOS

    11 √7th **T40.7X2** **Poisoning by cannabis (derivatives), intentional self-harm** `HCC`

    √7th **T40.7X3** **Poisoning by cannabis (derivatives), assault**

    √7th **T40.7X4** **Poisoning by cannabis (derivatives), undetermined**

    √7th **T40.7X5** **Adverse effect** of cannabis (derivatives)

    √7th **T40.7X6** **Underdosing** of cannabis (derivatives)

√5th **T40.8** **Poisoning by and adverse effect of lysergide [LSD]**

  √6th **T40.8X** **Poisoning by and adverse effect of lysergide [LSD]**

    √7th **T40.8X1** **Poisoning by lysergide [LSD], accidental (unintentional)**
        Poisoning by lysergide [LSD]NOS

    11 √7th **T40.8X2** **Poisoning by lysergide [LSD], intentional self-harm** `HCC`

    √7th **T40.8X3** **Poisoning by lysergide [LSD], assault**

    √7th **T40.8X4** **Poisoning by lysergide [LSD], undetermined**

√5th **T40.9** **Poisoning by, adverse effect of and underdosing of other and unspecified psychodysleptics [hallucinogens]**

  √6th **T40.90** **Poisoning by, adverse effect of and underdosing of unspecified psychodysleptics [hallucinogens]**

    √7th **T40.901** **Poisoning by unspecified psychodysleptics [hallucinogens], accidental (unintentional)**

    11 √7th **T40.902** **Poisoning by unspecified psychodysleptics [hallucinogens], intentional self-harm** `HCC`

    √7th **T40.903** **Poisoning by unspecified psychodysleptics [hallucinogens], assault**

    √7th **T40.904** **Poisoning by unspecified psychodysleptics [hallucinogens], undetermined**

    √7th **T40.905** **Adverse effect** of unspecified psychodysleptics [hallucinogens]

    √7th **T40.906** **Underdosing** of unspecified psychodysleptics

  √6th **T40.99** **Poisoning by, adverse effect of and underdosing of other psychodysleptics [hallucinogens]**

    √7th **T40.991** **Poisoning by other psychodysleptics [hallucinogens], accidental (unintentional)**
        Poisoning by other psychodysleptics [hallucinogens] NOS

    11 √7th **T40.992** **Poisoning by other psychodysleptics [hallucinogens], intentional self-harm** `HCC`

    √7th **T40.993** **Poisoning by other psychodysleptics [hallucinogens], assault**

    √7th **T40.994** **Poisoning by other psychodysleptics [hallucinogens], undetermined**

    √7th **T40.995** **Adverse effect** of other psychodysleptics [hallucinogens]

    √7th **T40.996** **Underdosing** of other psychodysleptics

√4th **T41** **Poisoning by, adverse effect of and underdosing of anesthetics and therapeutic gases**

  `EXCLUDES 1`  *benzodiazepines (T42.4-)*
           *cocaine (T40.5-)*
           *complications of anesthesia during labor and delivery (O74.-)*
           *complications of anesthesia during pregnancy (O29.-)*
           *complications of anesthesia during the puerperium (O89.-)*
           *opioids (T40.0-T40.2-)*

  The appropriate 7th character is to be added to each code from category T41.
  A    initial encounter
  D    subsequent encounter
  S    sequela

√5th **T41.0** **Poisoning by, adverse effect of and underdosing of inhaled anesthetics**
  `EXCLUDES 1`  *oxygen (T41.5-)*

  √6th **T41.0X** **Poisoning by, adverse effect of and underdosing of inhaled anesthetics**

    √7th **T41.0X1** **Poisoning by inhaled anesthetics, accidental (unintentional)**
        Poisoning by inhaled anesthetics NOS

    11 √7th **T41.0X2** **Poisoning by inhaled anesthetics, intentional self-harm** `HCC`

    √7th **T41.0X3** **Poisoning by inhaled anesthetics, assault**

    √7th **T41.0X4** **Poisoning by inhaled anesthetics, undetermined**

    √7th **T41.0X5** **Adverse effect** of inhaled anesthetics

    √7th **T41.0X6** **Underdosing** of inhaled anesthetics

---

11 HCC with 7th character indicating initial encounter (A or B - specific to category) OR sequela.

☑ Additional Character Req  √x7th Placeholder Alert  Unacceptable PDx  Manifestation  `H1`-`H14` HAC  `HCC` CMS-HCC Condition  `EXCLUDES 1` Not Coded Here  `EXCLUDES 2` Not Included Here

ICD-10-CM 2018          **1105**

Chapter 19. Injury, Poisoning and Certain Other Consequences of External Causes

T41.1–T42.2X5

✓5th **T41.1** **Poisoning by, adverse effect of and underdosing of intravenous anesthetics**
Poisoning by, adverse effect of and underdosing of thiobarbiturates

    ✓6th **T41.1X** **Poisoning by, adverse effect of and underdosing of intravenous anesthetics**

        ✓7th **T41.1X1** **Poisoning by intravenous anesthetics, accidental (unintentional)**
Poisoning by intravenous anesthetics NOS

        11 ✓7th **T41.1X2** **Poisoning by intravenous anesthetics,** HCC **intentional self-harm**

        ✓7th **T41.1X3** **Poisoning by intravenous anesthetics, assault**

        ✓7th **T41.1X4** **Poisoning by intravenous anesthetics, undetermined**

        ✓7th **T41.1X5** Adverse effect **of intravenous anesthetics**

        ✓7th **T41.1X6** Underdosing **of intravenous anesthetics**

✓5th **T41.2** **Poisoning by, adverse effect of and underdosing of other and unspecified general anesthetics**

    ✓6th **T41.20** **Poisoning by, adverse effect of and underdosing of unspecified general anesthetics**

        ✓7th **T41.201** **Poisoning by unspecified general anesthetics, accidental (unintentional)**
Poisoning by general anesthetics NOS

        11 ✓7th **T41.202** **Poisoning by unspecified general** HCC **anesthetics, intentional self-harm**

        ✓7th **T41.203** **Poisoning by unspecified general anesthetics, assault**

        ✓7th **T41.204** **Poisoning by unspecified general anesthetics, undetermined**

        ✓7th **T41.205** Adverse effect **of unspecified general anesthetics**

        ✓7th **T41.206** Underdosing **of unspecified general anesthetics**

    ✓6th **T41.29** **Poisoning by, adverse effect of and underdosing of other general anesthetics**

        ✓7th **T41.291** **Poisoning by other general anesthetics, accidental (unintentional)**
Poisoning by other general anesthetics NOS

        11 ✓7th **T41.292** **Poisoning by other general** HCC **anesthetics, intentional self-harm**

        ✓7th **T41.293** **Poisoning by other general anesthetics, assault**

        ✓7th **T41.294** **Poisoning by other general anesthetics, undetermined**

        ✓7th **T41.295** Adverse effect **of other general anesthetics**

        ✓7th **T41.296** Underdosing **of other general anesthetics**

✓5th **T41.3** **Poisoning by, adverse effect of and underdosing of local anesthetics**
Cocaine (topical)
EXCLUDES 2 *poisoning by cocaine used as a central nervous system stimulant (T40.5X1-T40.5X4)*

    ✓6th **T41.3X** **Poisoning by, adverse effect of and underdosing of local anesthetics**

        ✓7th **T41.3X1** **Poisoning by local anesthetics, accidental (unintentional)**
Poisoning by local anesthetics NOS

        11 ✓7th **T41.3X2** **Poisoning by local anesthetics,** HCC **intentional self-harm**

        ✓7th **T41.3X3** **Poisoning by local anesthetics, assault**

        ✓7th **T41.3X4** **Poisoning by local anesthetics, undetermined**

        ✓7th **T41.3X5** Adverse effect **of local anesthetics**

        ✓7th **T41.3X6** Underdosing **of local anesthetics**

✓5th **T41.4** **Poisoning by, adverse effect of and underdosing of unspecified anesthetic**

    ✓x7th **T41.41** **Poisoning by unspecified anesthetic, accidental (unintentional)**
Poisoning by anesthetic NOS

    11 ✓x7th **T41.42** **Poisoning by unspecified anesthetic,** HCC **intentional self-harm**

    ✓x7th **T41.43** **Poisoning by unspecified anesthetic, assault**

    ✓x7th **T41.44** **Poisoning by unspecified anesthetic, undetermined**

    ✓x7th **T41.45** Adverse effect **of unspecified anesthetic**

    ✓x7th **T41.46** Underdosing **of unspecified anesthetics**

✓5th **T41.5** **Poisoning by, adverse effect of and underdosing of therapeutic gases**

    ✓6th **T41.5X** **Poisoning by, adverse effect of and underdosing of therapeutic gases**

        ✓7th **T41.5X1** **Poisoning by therapeutic gases, accidental (unintentional)**
Poisoning by therapeutic gases NOS

        11 ✓7th **T41.5X2** **Poisoning by therapeutic gases,** HCC **intentional self-harm**

        ✓7th **T41.5X3** **Poisoning by therapeutic gases, assault**

        ✓7th **T41.5X4** **Poisoning by therapeutic gases, undetermined**

        ✓7th **T41.5X5** Adverse effect **of therapeutic gases**

        ✓7th **T41.5X6** Underdosing **of therapeutic gases**

✓4th **T42** **Poisoning by, adverse effect of and underdosing of antiepileptic, sedative- hypnotic and antiparkinsonism drugs**
EXCLUDES 2 *drug dependence and related mental and behavioral disorders due to psychoactive substance use (F10- – F19-)*

> The appropriate 7th character is to be added to each code from category T42.
> A    initial encounter
> D    subsequent encounter
> S    sequela

✓5th **T42.0** **Poisoning by, adverse effect of and underdosing of hydantoin derivatives**

    ✓6th **T42.0X** **Poisoning by, adverse effect of and underdosing of hydantoin derivatives**

        ✓7th **T42.0X1** **Poisoning by hydantoin derivatives, accidental (unintentional)**
Poisoning by hydantoin derivatives NOS

        11 ✓7th **T42.0X2** **Poisoning by hydantoin derivatives,** HCC **intentional self-harm**

        ✓7th **T42.0X3** **Poisoning by hydantoin derivatives, assault**

        ✓7th **T42.0X4** **Poisoning by hydantoin derivatives, undetermined**

        ✓7th **T42.0X5** Adverse effect **of hydantoin derivatives**

        ✓7th **T42.0X6** Underdosing **of hydantoin derivatives**

✓5th **T42.1** **Poisoning by, adverse effect of and underdosing of iminostilbenes**
Poisoning by, adverse effect of and underdosing of carbamazepine

    ✓6th **T42.1X** **Poisoning by, adverse effect of and underdosing of iminostilbenes**

        ✓7th **T42.1X1** **Poisoning by iminostilbenes, accidental (unintentional)**
Poisoning by iminostilbenes NOS

        11 ✓7th **T42.1X2** **Poisoning by iminostilbenes,** HCC **intentional self-harm**

        ✓7th **T42.1X3** **Poisoning by iminostilbenes, assault**

        ✓7th **T42.1X4** **Poisoning by iminostilbenes, undetermined**

        ✓7th **T42.1X5** Adverse effect **of iminostilbenes**

        ✓7th **T42.1X6** Underdosing **of iminostilbenes**

✓5th **T42.2** **Poisoning by, adverse effect of and underdosing of succinimides and oxazolidinediones**

    ✓6th **T42.2X** **Poisoning by, adverse effect of and underdosing of succinimides and oxazolidinediones**

        ✓7th **T42.2X1** **Poisoning by succinimides and oxazolidinediones, accidental (unintentional)**
Poisoning by succinimides and oxazolidinediones NOS

        11 ✓7th **T42.2X2** **Poisoning by succinimides and** HCC **oxazolidinediones, intentional self-harm**

        ✓7th **T42.2X3** **Poisoning by succinimides and oxazolidinediones, assault**

        ✓7th **T42.2X4** **Poisoning by succinimides and oxazolidinediones, undetermined**

        ✓7th **T42.2X5** Adverse effect **of succinimides and oxazolidinediones**

---

11 HCC with 7th character indicating initial encounter (A or B - specific to category) OR sequela.

Ⓝ Newborn: 0   Ⓟ Pediatric: 0-17   Ⓜ Maternity: 12-55   Ⓐ Adult: 15-124   MCC Major CC Condition   PDxMCC PDx acts as own MCC   CC CC Condition   PDxCC PDx acts as own CC

**1106**                                                                                                                 ICD-10-CM 2018

☑7ᵗʰ **T42.2X6**  Underdosing of succinimides and oxazolidinediones

☑5ᵗʰ **T42.3**  **Poisoning by, adverse effect of and underdosing of barbiturates**
  *EXCLUDES 1*  poisoning by, adverse effect of and underdosing of thiobarbiturates (T41.1-)

  ☑6ᵗʰ **T42.3X**  **Poisoning by, adverse effect of and underdosing of barbiturates**

    ☑7ᵗʰ **T42.3X1**  **Poisoning by barbiturates, accidental (unintentional)**
        Poisoning by barbiturates NOS

    11  ☑7ᵗʰ **T42.3X2**  **Poisoning by barbiturates, intentional self-harm**  ᴴᶜᶜ

    ☑7ᵗʰ **T42.3X3**  **Poisoning by barbiturates, assault**

    ☑7ᵗʰ **T42.3X4**  **Poisoning by barbiturates, undetermined**

    ☑7ᵗʰ **T42.3X5**  Adverse effect of barbiturates

    ☑7ᵗʰ **T42.3X6**  Underdosing of barbiturates

☑5ᵗʰ **T42.4**  **Poisoning by, adverse effect of and underdosing of benzodiazepines**

  ☑6ᵗʰ **T42.4X**  **Poisoning by, adverse effect of and underdosing of benzodiazepines**

    ☑7ᵗʰ **T42.4X1**  **Poisoning by benzodiazepines, accidental (unintentional)**
        Poisoning by benzodiazepines NOS

    11  ☑7ᵗʰ **T42.4X2**  **Poisoning by benzodiazepines, intentional self-harm**  ᴴᶜᶜ

    ☑7ᵗʰ **T42.4X3**  **Poisoning by benzodiazepines, assault**

    ☑7ᵗʰ **T42.4X4**  **Poisoning by benzodiazepines, undetermined**

    ☑7ᵗʰ **T42.4X5**  Adverse effect of benzodiazepines

    ☑7ᵗʰ **T42.4X6**  Underdosing of benzodiazepines

☑5ᵗʰ **T42.5**  **Poisoning by, adverse effect of and underdosing of mixed antiepileptics**

  ☑6ᵗʰ **T42.5X**  **Poisoning by, adverse effect of and underdosing of antiepileptics**

    ☑7ᵗʰ **T42.5X1**  **Poisoning by mixed antiepileptics, accidental (unintentional)**
        Poisoning by mixed antiepileptics NOS

    11  ☑7ᵗʰ **T42.5X2**  **Poisoning by mixed antiepileptics, intentional self-harm**  ᴴᶜᶜ

    ☑7ᵗʰ **T42.5X3**  **Poisoning by mixed antiepileptics, assault**

    ☑7ᵗʰ **T42.5X4**  **Poisoning by mixed antiepileptics, undetermined**

    ☑7ᵗʰ **T42.5X5**  Adverse effect of mixed antiepileptics

    ☑7ᵗʰ **T42.5X6**  Underdosing of mixed antiepileptics

☑5ᵗʰ **T42.6**  **Poisoning by, adverse effect of and underdosing of other antiepileptic and sedative-hypnotic drugs**
    Poisoning by, adverse effect of and underdosing of methaqualone
    Poisoning by, adverse effect of and underdosing of valproic acid
  *EXCLUDES 1*  poisoning by, adverse effect of and underdosing of carbamazepine (T42.1-)

  ☑6ᵗʰ **T42.6X**  **Poisoning by, adverse effect of and underdosing of other antiepileptic and sedative-hypnotic drugs**

    ☑7ᵗʰ **T42.6X1**  **Poisoning by other antiepileptic and sedative-hypnotic drugs, accidental (unintentional)**
        Poisoning by other antiepileptic and sedative-hypnotic drugs NOS

    11  ☑7ᵗʰ **T42.6X2**  **Poisoning by other antiepileptic and sedative-hypnotic drugs, intentional self-harm**  ᴴᶜᶜ

    ☑7ᵗʰ **T42.6X3**  **Poisoning by other antiepileptic and sedative-hypnotic drugs, assault**

    ☑7ᵗʰ **T42.6X4**  **Poisoning by other antiepileptic and sedative-hypnotic drugs, undetermined**

    ☑7ᵗʰ **T42.6X5**  Adverse effect of other antiepileptic and sedative-hypnotic drugs

    ☑7ᵗʰ **T42.6X6**  Underdosing of other antiepileptic and sedative-hypnotic drugs

☑5ᵗʰ **T42.7**  **Poisoning by, adverse effect of and underdosing of unspecified antiepileptic and sedative-hypnotic drugs**

  ☑ₓ7ᵗʰ **T42.71**  **Poisoning by unspecified antiepileptic and sedative-hypnotic drugs, accidental (unintentional)**
        Poisoning by antiepileptic and sedative-hypnotic drugs NOS

  11  ☑ₓ7ᵗʰ **T42.72**  **Poisoning by unspecified antiepileptic and sedative-hypnotic drugs, intentional self-harm**  ᴴᶜᶜ

  ☑ₓ7ᵗʰ **T42.73**  **Poisoning by unspecified antiepileptic and sedative-hypnotic drugs, assault**

  ☑ₓ7ᵗʰ **T42.74**  **Poisoning by unspecified antiepileptic and sedative-hypnotic drugs, undetermined**

  ☑ₓ7ᵗʰ **T42.75**  Adverse effect of unspecified antiepileptic and sedative-hypnotic drugs

  ☑ₓ7ᵗʰ **T42.76**  Underdosing of unspecified antiepileptic and sedative-hypnotic drugs

☑5ᵗʰ **T42.8**  **Poisoning by, adverse effect of and underdosing of antiparkinsonism drugs and other central muscle-tone depressants**
    Poisoning by, adverse effect of and underdosing of amantadine

  ☑6ᵗʰ **T42.8X**  **Poisoning by, adverse effect of and underdosing of antiparkinsonism drugs and other central muscle-tone depressants**

    ☑7ᵗʰ **T42.8X1**  **Poisoning by antiparkinsonism drugs and other central muscle-tone depressants, accidental (unintentional)**
        Poisoning by antiparkinsonism drugs and other central muscle-tone depressants NOS

    11  ☑7ᵗʰ **T42.8X2**  **Poisoning by antiparkinsonism drugs and other central muscle-tone depressants, intentional self-harm**  ᴴᶜᶜ

    ☑7ᵗʰ **T42.8X3**  **Poisoning by antiparkinsonism drugs and other central muscle-tone depressants, assault**

    ☑7ᵗʰ **T42.8X4**  **Poisoning by antiparkinsonism drugs and other central muscle-tone depressants, undetermined**

    ☑7ᵗʰ **T42.8X5**  Adverse effect of antiparkinsonism drugs and other central muscle-tone depressants

    ☑7ᵗʰ **T42.8X6**  Underdosing of antiparkinsonism drugs and other central muscle-tone depressants

☑4ᵗʰ **T43**  **Poisoning by, adverse effect of and underdosing of psychotropic drugs, not elsewhere classified**
  *EXCLUDES 1*  appetite depressants (T50.5-)
        barbiturates (T42.3-)
        benzodiazepines (T42.4-)
        methaqualone (T42.6-)
        psychodysleptics [hallucinogens] (T40.7-T40.9-)
  *EXCLUDES 2*  drug dependence and related mental and behavioral disorders due to psychoactive substance use (F10.- – F19.-)

  The appropriate 7th character is to be added to each code from category T43.
  A    initial encounter
  D    subsequent encounter
  S    sequela

☑5ᵗʰ **T43.0**  **Poisoning by, adverse effect of and underdosing of tricyclic and tetracyclic antidepressants**

  ☑6ᵗʰ **T43.01**  **Poisoning by, adverse effect of and underdosing of tricyclic antidepressants**

    ☑7ᵗʰ **T43.011**  **Poisoning by tricyclic antidepressants, accidental (unintentional)**
        Poisoning by tricyclic antidepressants NOS

    11  ☑7ᵗʰ **T43.012**  **Poisoning by tricyclic antidepressants, intentional self-harm**  ᴴᶜᶜ

    ☑7ᵗʰ **T43.013**  **Poisoning by tricyclic antidepressants, assault**

    ☑7ᵗʰ **T43.014**  **Poisoning by tricyclic antidepressants, undetermined**

    ☑7ᵗʰ **T43.015**  Adverse effect of tricyclic antidepressants

    ☑7ᵗʰ **T43.016**  Underdosing of tricyclic antidepressants

---

¹¹ HCC with 7th character indicating initial encounter (A or B - specific to category) OR sequela.

**Chapter 19. Injury, Poisoning and Certain Other Consequences of External Causes**

  ✓6ᵗʰ **T43.02** **Poisoning by, adverse effect of and underdosing of tetracyclic antidepressants**

    ✓7ᵗʰ **T43.021** **Poisoning by tetracyclic antidepressants, accidental (unintentional)**
      Poisoning by tetracyclic antidepressants NOS

    11 ✓7ᵗʰ **T43.022** **Poisoning by tetracyclic antidepressants, intentional self-harm** `HCC`

    ✓7ᵗʰ **T43.023** **Poisoning by tetracyclic antidepressants, assault**

    ✓7ᵗʰ **T43.024** **Poisoning by tetracyclic antidepressants, undetermined**

    ✓7ᵗʰ **T43.025** **Adverse effect of tetracyclic antidepressants**

    ✓7ᵗʰ **T43.026** **Underdosing of tetracyclic antidepressants**

 ✓5ᵗʰ **T43.1** **Poisoning by, adverse effect of and underdosing of monoamine-oxidase-inhibitor antidepressants**

  ✓6ᵗʰ **T43.1X** **Poisoning by, adverse effect of and underdosing of monoamine-oxidase-inhibitor antidepressants**

    ✓7ᵗʰ **T43.1X1** **Poisoning by monoamine-oxidase-inhibitor antidepressants, accidental (unintentional)**
      Poisoning by monoamine-oxidase-inhibitor antidepressants NOS

    11 ✓7ᵗʰ **T43.1X2** **Poisoning by monoamine-oxidase-inhibitor antidepressants, intentional self-harm** `HCC`

    ✓7ᵗʰ **T43.1X3** **Poisoning by monoamine-oxidase-inhibitor antidepressants, assault**

    ✓7ᵗʰ **T43.1X4** **Poisoning by monoamine-oxidase-inhibitor antidepressants, undetermined**

    ✓7ᵗʰ **T43.1X5** **Adverse effect of monoamine-oxidase-inhibitor antidepressants**

    ✓7ᵗʰ **T43.1X6** **Underdosing of monoamine-oxidase-inhibitor antidepressants**

 ✓5ᵗʰ **T43.2** **Poisoning by, adverse effect of and underdosing of other and unspecified antidepressants**

  ✓6ᵗʰ **T43.20** **Poisoning by, adverse effect of and underdosing of unspecified antidepressants**

    ✓7ᵗʰ **T43.201** **Poisoning by unspecified antidepressants, accidental (unintentional)**
      Poisoning by antidepressants NOS

    11 ✓7ᵗʰ **T43.202** **Poisoning by unspecified antidepressants, intentional self-harm** `HCC`

    ✓7ᵗʰ **T43.203** **Poisoning by unspecified antidepressants, assault**

    ✓7ᵗʰ **T43.204** **Poisoning by unspecified antidepressants, undetermined**

    ✓7ᵗʰ **T43.205** **Adverse effect of unspecified antidepressants**
      ▶Antidepressant discontinuation syndrome◄

    ✓7ᵗʰ **T43.206** **Underdosing of unspecified antidepressants**

  ✓6ᵗʰ **T43.21** **Poisoning by, adverse effect of and underdosing of selective serotonin and norepinephrine reuptake inhibitors**
    Poisoning by, adverse effect of and underdosing of SSNRI antidepressants

    ✓7ᵗʰ **T43.211** **Poisoning by selective serotonin and norepinephrine reuptake inhibitors, accidental (unintentional)**

    11 ✓7ᵗʰ **T43.212** **Poisoning by selective serotonin and norepinephrine reuptake inhibitors, intentional self-harm** `HCC`

    ✓7ᵗʰ **T43.213** **Poisoning by selective serotonin and norepinephrine reuptake inhibitors, assault**

    ✓7ᵗʰ **T43.214** **Poisoning by selective serotonin and norepinephrine reuptake inhibitors, undetermined**

    ✓7ᵗʰ **T43.215** **Adverse effect of selective serotonin and norepinephrine reuptake inhibitors**

    ✓7ᵗʰ **T43.216** **Underdosing of selective serotonin and norepinephrine reuptake inhibitors**

  ✓6ᵗʰ **T43.22** **Poisoning by, adverse effect of and underdosing of selective serotonin reuptake inhibitors**
    Poisoning by, adverse effect of and underdosing of SSRI antidepressants

    ✓7ᵗʰ **T43.221** **Poisoning by selective serotonin reuptake inhibitors, accidental (unintentional)**

    11 ✓7ᵗʰ **T43.222** **Poisoning by selective serotonin reuptake inhibitors, intentional self-harm** `HCC`

    ✓7ᵗʰ **T43.223** **Poisoning by selective serotonin reuptake inhibitors, assault**

    ✓7ᵗʰ **T43.224** **Poisoning by selective serotonin reuptake inhibitors, undetermined**

    ✓7ᵗʰ **T43.225** **Adverse effect of selective serotonin reuptake inhibitors**

    ✓7ᵗʰ **T43.226** **Underdosing of selective serotonin reuptake inhibitors**

  ✓6ᵗʰ **T43.29** **Poisoning by, adverse effect of and underdosing of other antidepressants**

    ✓7ᵗʰ **T43.291** **Poisoning by other antidepressants, accidental (unintentional)**
      Poisoning by other antidepressants NOS

    11 ✓7ᵗʰ **T43.292** **Poisoning by other antidepressants, intentional self-harm** `HCC`

    ✓7ᵗʰ **T43.293** **Poisoning by other antidepressants, assault**

    ✓7ᵗʰ **T43.294** **Poisoning by other antidepressants, undetermined**

    ✓7ᵗʰ **T43.295** **Adverse effect of other antidepressants**

    ✓7ᵗʰ **T43.296** **Underdosing of other antidepressants**

 ✓5ᵗʰ **T43.3** **Poisoning by, adverse effect of and underdosing of phenothiazine antipsychotics and neuroleptics**

  ✓6ᵗʰ **T43.3X** **Poisoning by, adverse effect of and underdosing of phenothiazine antipsychotics and neuroleptics**

    ✓7ᵗʰ **T43.3X1** **Poisoning by phenothiazine antipsychotics and neuroleptics, accidental (unintentional)**
      Poisoning by phenothiazine antipsychotics and neuroleptics NOS

    11 ✓7ᵗʰ **T43.3X2** **Poisoning by phenothiazine antipsychotics and neuroleptics, intentional self-harm** `HCC`

    ✓7ᵗʰ **T43.3X3** **Poisoning by phenothiazine antipsychotics and neuroleptics, assault**

    ✓7ᵗʰ **T43.3X4** **Poisoning by phenothiazine antipsychotics and neuroleptics, undetermined**

    ✓7ᵗʰ **T43.3X5** **Adverse effect of phenothiazine antipsychotics and neuroleptics**

    ✓7ᵗʰ **T43.3X6** **Underdosing of phenothiazine antipsychotics and neuroleptics**

 ✓5ᵗʰ **T43.4** **Poisoning by, adverse effect of and underdosing of butyrophenone and thiothixene neuroleptics**

  ✓6ᵗʰ **T43.4X** **Poisoning by, adverse effect of and underdosing of butyrophenone and thiothixene neuroleptics**

    ✓7ᵗʰ **T43.4X1** **Poisoning by butyrophenone and thiothixene neuroleptics, accidental (unintentional)**
      Poisoning by butyrophenone and thiothixene neuroleptics NOS

    11 ✓7ᵗʰ **T43.4X2** **Poisoning by butyrophenone and thiothixene neuroleptics, intentional self-harm** `HCC`

    ✓7ᵗʰ **T43.4X3** **Poisoning by butyrophenone and thiothixene neuroleptics, assault**

    ✓7ᵗʰ **T43.4X4** **Poisoning by butyrophenone and thiothixene neuroleptics, undetermined**

    ✓7ᵗʰ **T43.4X5** **Adverse effect of butyrophenone and thiothixene neuroleptics**

    ✓7ᵗʰ **T43.4X6** **Underdosing of butyrophenone and thiothixene neuroleptics**

---

[11] HCC with 7th character indicating initial encounter (A or B - specific to category) OR sequela.

N Newborn: 0    P Pediatric: 0-17    M Maternity: 12-55    A Adult: 15-124    `MCC` Major CC Condition    `PDxMCC` PDx acts as own MCC    `CC` CC Condition    `PDxCC` PDx acts as own CC

1108            ICD-10-CM 2018

√5ᵗʰ **T43.5**  **Poisoning by, adverse effect of and underdosing of other and unspecified antipsychotics and neuroleptics**
> EXCLUDES 1  *poisoning by, adverse effect of and underdosing of rauwolfia (T46.5-)*

√6ᵗʰ **T43.50**  **Poisoning by, adverse effect of and underdosing of unspecified antipsychotics and neuroleptics**

√7ᵗʰ **T43.501**  **Poisoning by unspecified antipsychotics and neuroleptics, accidental (unintentional)**
> Poisoning by antipsychotics and neuroleptics NOS

11  √7ᵗʰ **T43.502**  **Poisoning by unspecified antipsychotics and neuroleptics, intentional self-harm**  HCC

√7ᵗʰ **T43.503**  **Poisoning by unspecified antipsychotics and neuroleptics, assault**

√7ᵗʰ **T43.504**  **Poisoning by unspecified antipsychotics and neuroleptics, undetermined**

√7ᵗʰ **T43.505**  **Adverse effect of unspecified antipsychotics and neuroleptics**

√7ᵗʰ **T43.506**  **Underdosing of unspecified antipsychotics and neuroleptics**

√6ᵗʰ **T43.59**  **Poisoning by, adverse effect of and underdosing of other antipsychotics and neuroleptics**
> **AHA:** 2017, 1Q, 40

√7ᵗʰ **T43.591**  **Poisoning by other antipsychotics and neuroleptics, accidental (unintentional)**
> Poisoning by other antipsychotics and neuroleptics NOS

11  √7ᵗʰ **T43.592**  **Poisoning by other antipsychotics and neuroleptics, intentional self-harm**  HCC

√7ᵗʰ **T43.593**  **Poisoning by other antipsychotics and neuroleptics, assault**

√7ᵗʰ **T43.594**  **Poisoning by other antipsychotics and neuroleptics, undetermined**

√7ᵗʰ **T43.595**  **Adverse effect of other antipsychotics and neuroleptics**

√7ᵗʰ **T43.596**  **Underdosing of other antipsychotics and neuroleptics**

√5ᵗʰ **T43.6**  **Poisoning by, adverse effect of and underdosing of psychostimulants**
> EXCLUDES 1  *poisoning by, adverse effect of and underdosing of cocaine (T40.5-)*

√6ᵗʰ **T43.60**  **Poisoning by, adverse effect of and underdosing of unspecified psychostimulant**

√7ᵗʰ **T43.601**  **Poisoning by unspecified psychostimulants, accidental (unintentional)**
> Poisoning by psychostimulants NOS

11  √7ᵗʰ **T43.602**  **Poisoning by unspecified psychostimulants, intentional self-harm**  HCC

√7ᵗʰ **T43.603**  **Poisoning by unspecified psychostimulants, assault**

√7ᵗʰ **T43.604**  **Poisoning by unspecified psychostimulants, undetermined**

√7ᵗʰ **T43.605**  **Adverse effect of unspecified psychostimulants**

√7ᵗʰ **T43.606**  **Underdosing of unspecified psychostimulants**

√6ᵗʰ **T43.61**  **Poisoning by, adverse effect of and underdosing of caffeine**

√7ᵗʰ **T43.611**  **Poisoning by caffeine, accidental (unintentional)**
> Poisoning by caffeine NOS

11  √7ᵗʰ **T43.612**  **Poisoning by caffeine, intentional self-harm**  HCC

√7ᵗʰ **T43.613**  **Poisoning by caffeine, assault**

√7ᵗʰ **T43.614**  **Poisoning by caffeine, undetermined**

√7ᵗʰ **T43.615**  **Adverse effect of caffeine**

√7ᵗʰ **T43.616**  **Underdosing of caffeine**

√6ᵗʰ **T43.62**  **Poisoning by, adverse effect of and underdosing of amphetamines**
> Poisoning by, adverse effect of and underdosing of methamphetamines

√7ᵗʰ **T43.621**  **Poisoning by amphetamines, accidental (unintentional)**
> Poisoning by amphetamines NOS

11  √7ᵗʰ **T43.622**  **Poisoning by amphetamines, intentional self-harm**  HCC

√7ᵗʰ **T43.623**  **Poisoning by amphetamines, assault**

√7ᵗʰ **T43.624**  **Poisoning by amphetamines, undetermined**

√7ᵗʰ **T43.625**  **Adverse effect of amphetamines**

√7ᵗʰ **T43.626**  **Underdosing of amphetamines**

√6ᵗʰ **T43.63**  **Poisoning by, adverse effect of and underdosing of methylphenidate**

√7ᵗʰ **T43.631**  **Poisoning by methylphenidate, accidental (unintentional)**
> Poisoning by methylphenidate NOS

11  √7ᵗʰ **T43.632**  **Poisoning by methylphenidate, intentional self-harm**  HCC

√7ᵗʰ **T43.633**  **Poisoning by methylphenidate, assault**

√7ᵗʰ **T43.634**  **Poisoning by methylphenidate, undetermined**

√7ᵗʰ **T43.635**  **Adverse effect of methylphenidate**

√7ᵗʰ **T43.636**  **Underdosing of methylphenidate**

√6ᵗʰ **T43.69**  **Poisoning by, adverse effect of and underdosing of other psychostimulants**

√7ᵗʰ **T43.691**  **Poisoning by other psychostimulants, accidental (unintentional)**
> Poisoning by other psychostimulants NOS

11  √7ᵗʰ **T43.692**  **Poisoning by other psychostimulants, intentional self-harm**  HCC

√7ᵗʰ **T43.693**  **Poisoning by other psychostimulants, assault**

√7ᵗʰ **T43.694**  **Poisoning by other psychostimulants, undetermined**

√7ᵗʰ **T43.695**  **Adverse effect of other psychostimulants**

√7ᵗʰ **T43.696**  **Underdosing of other psychostimulants**

√5ᵗʰ **T43.8**  **Poisoning by, adverse effect of and underdosing of other psychotropic drugs**

√6ᵗʰ **T43.8X**  **Poisoning by, adverse effect of and underdosing of other psychotropic drugs**

√7ᵗʰ **T43.8X1**  **Poisoning by other psychotropic drugs, accidental (unintentional)**
> Poisoning by other psychotropic drugs NOS

11  √7ᵗʰ **T43.8X2**  **Poisoning by other psychotropic drugs, intentional self-harm**  HCC

√7ᵗʰ **T43.8X3**  **Poisoning by other psychotropic drugs, assault**

√7ᵗʰ **T43.8X4**  **Poisoning by other psychotropic drugs, undetermined**

√7ᵗʰ **T43.8X5**  **Adverse effect of other psychotropic drugs**

√7ᵗʰ **T43.8X6**  **Underdosing of other psychotropic drugs**

√5ᵗʰ **T43.9**  **Poisoning by, adverse effect of and underdosing of unspecified psychotropic drug**

√x7ᵗʰ **T43.91**  **Poisoning by unspecified psychotropic drug, accidental (unintentional)**
> Poisoning by psychotropic drug NOS

11  √x7ᵗʰ **T43.92**  **Poisoning by unspecified psychotropic drug, intentional self-harm**  HCC

√x7ᵗʰ **T43.93**  **Poisoning by unspecified psychotropic drug, assault**

√x7ᵗʰ **T43.94**  **Poisoning by unspecified psychotropic drug, undetermined**

√x7ᵗʰ **T43.95**  **Adverse effect of unspecified psychotropic drug**

√x7ᵗʰ **T43.96**  **Underdosing of unspecified psychotropic drug**

---

**11** HCC with 7th character indicating initial encounter (A or B - specific to category) OR sequela.

✓4ᵗʰ **T44    Poisoning by, adverse effect of and underdosing of drugs primarily affecting the autonomic nervous system**

> The appropriate 7th character is to be added to each code from category T44.
> A    initial encounter
> D    subsequent encounter
> S    sequela

✓5ᵗʰ **T44.Ø    Poisoning by, adverse effect of and underdosing of anticholinesterase agents**

  ✓6ᵗʰ **T44.ØX    Poisoning by, adverse effect of and underdosing of anticholinesterase agents**

    ✓7ᵗʰ **T44.ØX1    Poisoning by anticholinesterase agents, accidental (unintentional)**
      Poisoning by anticholinesterase agents NOS

    [11] ✓7ᵗʰ **T44.ØX2    Poisoning by anticholinesterase agents, intentional self-harm**    HCC

    ✓7ᵗʰ **T44.ØX3    Poisoning by anticholinesterase agents, assault**

    ✓7ᵗʰ **T44.ØX4    Poisoning by anticholinesterase agents, undetermined**

    ✓7ᵗʰ **T44.ØX5    Adverse effect of anticholinesterase agents**

    ✓7ᵗʰ **T44.ØX6    Underdosing of anticholinesterase agents**

✓5ᵗʰ **T44.1    Poisoning by, adverse effect of and underdosing of other parasympathomimetics [cholinergics]**

  ✓6ᵗʰ **T44.1X    Poisoning by, adverse effect of and underdosing of other parasympathomimetics [cholinergics]**

    ✓7ᵗʰ **T44.1X1    Poisoning by other parasympathomimetics [cholinergics], accidental (unintentional)**
      Poisoning by other parasympathomimetics [cholinergics] NOS

    [11] ✓7ᵗʰ **T44.1X2    Poisoning by other parasympathomimetics [cholinergics], intentional self-harm**    HCC

    ✓7ᵗʰ **T44.1X3    Poisoning by other parasympathomimetics [cholinergics], assault**

    ✓7ᵗʰ **T44.1X4    Poisoning by other parasympathomimetics [cholinergics], undetermined**

    ✓7ᵗʰ **T44.1X5    Adverse effect of other parasympathomimetics [cholinergics]**

    ✓7ᵗʰ **T44.1X6    Underdosing of other parasympathomimetics**

✓5ᵗʰ **T44.2    Poisoning by, adverse effect of and underdosing of ganglionic blocking drugs**

  ✓6ᵗʰ **T44.2X    Poisoning by, adverse effect of and underdosing of ganglionic blocking drugs**

    ✓7ᵗʰ **T44.2X1    Poisoning by ganglionic blocking drugs, accidental (unintentional)**
      Poisoning by ganglionic blocking drugs NOS

    [11] ✓7ᵗʰ **T44.2X2    Poisoning by ganglionic blocking drugs, intentional self-harm**    HCC

    ✓7ᵗʰ **T44.2X3    Poisoning by ganglionic blocking drugs, assault**

    ✓7ᵗʰ **T44.2X4    Poisoning by ganglionic blocking drugs, undetermined**

    ✓7ᵗʰ **T44.2X5    Adverse effect of ganglionic blocking drugs**

    ✓7ᵗʰ **T44.2X6    Underdosing of ganglionic blocking drugs**

✓5ᵗʰ **T44.3    Poisoning by, adverse effect of and underdosing of other parasympatholytics [anticholinergics and antimuscarinics] and spasmolytics**
  Poisoning by, adverse effect of and underdosing of papaverine

  ✓6ᵗʰ **T44.3X    Poisoning by, adverse effect of and underdosing of other parasympatholytics [anticholinergics and antimuscarinics] and spasmolytics**

    ✓7ᵗʰ **T44.3X1    Poisoning by other parasympatholytics [anticholinergics and antimuscarinics] and spasmolytics, accidental (unintentional)**
      Poisoning by other parasympatholytics [anticholinergics and antimuscarinics] and spasmolytics NOS

    [11] ✓7ᵗʰ **T44.3X2    Poisoning by other parasympatholytics [anticholinergics and antimuscarinics] and spasmolytics, intentional self-harm**    HCC

    ✓7ᵗʰ **T44.3X3    Poisoning by other parasympatholytics [anticholinergics and antimuscarinics] and spasmolytics, assault**

    ✓7ᵗʰ **T44.3X4    Poisoning by other parasympatholytics [anticholinergics and antimuscarinics] and spasmolytics, undetermined**

    ✓7ᵗʰ **T44.3X5    Adverse effect of other parasympatholytics [anticholinergics and antimuscarinics] and spasmolytics**

    ✓7ᵗʰ **T44.3X6    Underdosing of other parasympatholytics [anticholinergics and antimuscarinics] and spasmolytics**

✓5ᵗʰ **T44.4    Poisoning by, adverse effect of and underdosing of predominantly alpha-adrenoreceptor agonists**
  Poisoning by, adverse effect of and underdosing of metaraminol

  ✓6ᵗʰ **T44.4X    Poisoning by, adverse effect of and underdosing of predominantly alpha-adrenoreceptor agonists**

    ✓7ᵗʰ **T44.4X1    Poisoning by predominantly alpha-adrenoreceptor agonists, accidental (unintentional)**
      Poisoning by predominantly alpha-adrenoreceptor agonists NOS

    [11] ✓7ᵗʰ **T44.4X2    Poisoning by predominantly alpha-adrenoreceptor agonists, intentional self-harm**    HCC

    ✓7ᵗʰ **T44.4X3    Poisoning by predominantly alpha-adrenoreceptor agonists, assault**

    ✓7ᵗʰ **T44.4X4    Poisoning by predominantly alpha-adrenoreceptor agonists, undetermined**

    ✓7ᵗʰ **T44.4X5    Adverse effect of predominantly alpha-adrenoreceptor agonists**

    ✓7ᵗʰ **T44.4X6    Underdosing of predominantly alpha-adrenoreceptor agonists**

✓5ᵗʰ **T44.5    Poisoning by, adverse effect of and underdosing of predominantly beta-adrenoreceptor agonists**
  **EXCLUDES 1**    *poisoning by, adverse effect of and underdosing of beta-adrenoreceptor agonists used in asthma therapy (T48.6-)*

  ✓6ᵗʰ **T44.5X    Poisoning by, adverse effect of and underdosing of predominantly beta-adrenoreceptor agonists**

    ✓7ᵗʰ **T44.5X1    Poisoning by predominantly beta-adrenoreceptor agonists, accidental (unintentional)**
      Poisoning by predominantly beta-adrenoreceptor agonists NOS

    [11] ✓7ᵗʰ **T44.5X2    Poisoning by predominantly beta-adrenoreceptor agonists, intentional self-harm**    HCC

    ✓7ᵗʰ **T44.5X3    Poisoning by predominantly beta-adrenoreceptor agonists, assault**

    ✓7ᵗʰ **T44.5X4    Poisoning by predominantly beta-adrenoreceptor agonists, undetermined**

    ✓7ᵗʰ **T44.5X5    Adverse effect of predominantly beta-adrenoreceptor agonists**

    ✓7ᵗʰ **T44.5X6    Underdosing of predominantly beta-adrenoreceptor agonists**

✓5ᵗʰ **T44.6    Poisoning by, adverse effect of and underdosing of alpha-adrenoreceptor antagonists**
  **EXCLUDES 1**    *poisoning by, adverse effect of and underdosing of ergot alkaloids (T48.Ø)*

  ✓6ᵗʰ **T44.6X    Poisoning by, adverse effect of and underdosing of alpha-adrenoreceptor antagonists**

    ✓7ᵗʰ **T44.6X1    Poisoning by alpha-adrenoreceptor antagonists, accidental (unintentional)**
      Poisoning by alpha-adrenoreceptor antagonists NOS

    [11] ✓7ᵗʰ **T44.6X2    Poisoning by alpha-adrenoreceptor antagonists, intentional self-harm**    HCC

    ✓7ᵗʰ **T44.6X3    Poisoning by alpha-adrenoreceptor antagonists, assault**

    ✓7ᵗʰ **T44.6X4    Poisoning by alpha-adrenoreceptor antagonists, undetermined**

---

[11] HCC with 7th character indicating initial encounter (A or B - specific to category) OR sequela.

N Newborn: 0    P Pediatric: 0-17    M Maternity: 12-55    A Adult: 15-124    MCC Major CC Condition    PDxMCC PDx acts as own MCC    CC CC Condition    PDxCC PDx acts as own CC

**1110**    ICD-10-CM 2018

√7th **T44.6X5** Adverse effect of alpha-adrenoreceptor antagonists

√7th **T44.6X6** Underdosing of alpha-adrenoreceptor antagonists

√5th **T44.7** Poisoning by, adverse effect of and underdosing of beta-adrenoreceptor antagonists

  √6th **T44.7X** Poisoning by, adverse effect of and underdosing of beta-adrenoreceptor antagonists

    √7th **T44.7X1** Poisoning by beta-adrenoreceptor antagonists, accidental (unintentional)
        Poisoning by beta-adrenoreceptor antagonists NOS

    11 √7th **T44.7X2** Poisoning by beta-adrenoreceptor antagonists, intentional self-harm   HCC

    √7th **T44.7X3** Poisoning by beta-adrenoreceptor antagonists, assault

    √7th **T44.7X4** Poisoning by beta-adrenoreceptor antagonists, undetermined

    √7th **T44.7X5** Adverse effect of beta-adrenoreceptor antagonists

    √7th **T44.7X6** Underdosing of beta-adrenoreceptor antagonists

√5th **T44.8** Poisoning by, adverse effect of and underdosing of centrally-acting and adrenergic-neuron- blocking agents

    **EXCLUDES 1**   poisoning by, adverse effect of and underdosing of clonidine (T46.5)
        poisoning by, adverse effect of and underdosing of guanethidine (T46.5)

  √6th **T44.8X** Poisoning by, adverse effect of and underdosing of centrally-acting and adrenergic-neuron-blocking agents

    √7th **T44.8X1** Poisoning by centrally-acting and adrenergic-neuron-blocking agents, accidental (unintentional)
        Poisoning by centrally-acting and adrenergic-neuron-blocking agents NOS

    11 √7th **T44.8X2** Poisoning by centrally-acting and adrenergic-neuron-blocking agents, intentional self-harm   HCC

    √7th **T44.8X3** Poisoning by centrally-acting and adrenergic-neuron-blocking agents, assault

    √7th **T44.8X4** Poisoning by centrally-acting and adrenergic-neuron-blocking agents, undetermined

    √7th **T44.8X5** Adverse effect of centrally-acting and adrenergic-neuron-blocking agents

    √7th **T44.8X6** Underdosing of centrally-acting and adrenergic-neuron-blocking agents

√5th **T44.9** Poisoning by, adverse effect of and underdosing of other and unspecified drugs primarily affecting the autonomic nervous system
    Poisoning by, adverse effect of and underdosing of drug stimulating both alpha and beta-adrenoreceptors

  √6th **T44.90** Poisoning by, adverse effect of and underdosing of unspecified drugs primarily affecting the autonomic nervous system

    √7th **T44.901** Poisoning by unspecified drugs primarily affecting the autonomic nervous system, accidental (unintentional)
        Poisoning by unspecified drugs primarily affecting the autonomic nervous system NOS

    11 √7th **T44.902** Poisoning by unspecified drugs primarily affecting the autonomic nervous system, intentional self-harm   HCC

    √7th **T44.903** Poisoning by unspecified drugs primarily affecting the autonomic nervous system, assault

    √7th **T44.904** Poisoning by unspecified drugs primarily affecting the autonomic nervous system, undetermined

    √7th **T44.905** Adverse effect of unspecified drugs primarily affecting the autonomic nervous system

    √7th **T44.906** Underdosing of unspecified drugs primarily affecting the autonomic nervous system

  √6th **T44.99** Poisoning by, adverse effect of and underdosing of other drugs primarily affecting the autonomic nervous system

    √7th **T44.991** Poisoning by other drug primarily affecting the autonomic nervous system, accidental (unintentional)
        Poisoning by other drugs primarily affecting the autonomic nervous system NOS

    11 √7th **T44.992** Poisoning by other drug primarily affecting the autonomic nervous system, intentional self-harm   HCC

    √7th **T44.993** Poisoning by other drug primarily affecting the autonomic nervous system, assault

    √7th **T44.994** Poisoning by other drug primarily affecting the autonomic nervous system, undetermined

    √7th **T44.995** Adverse effect of other drug primarily affecting the autonomic nervous system

    √7th **T44.996** Underdosing of other drug primarily affecting the autonomic nervous system

√4th **T45** Poisoning by, adverse effect of and underdosing of primarily systemic and hematological agents, not elsewhere classified

    The appropriate 7th character is to be added to each code from category T45.
    A     initial encounter
    D     subsequent encounter
    S     sequela

√5th **T45.0** Poisoning by, adverse effect of and underdosing of antiallergic and antiemetic drugs

    **EXCLUDES 1**   poisoning by, adverse effect of and underdosing of phenothiazine-based neuroleptics (T43.3)

  √6th **T45.0X** Poisoning by, adverse effect of and underdosing of antiallergic and antiemetic drugs

    √7th **T45.0X1** Poisoning by antiallergic and antiemetic drugs, accidental (unintentional)
        Poisoning by antiallergic and antiemetic drugs NOS

    11 √7th **T45.0X2** Poisoning by antiallergic and antiemetic drugs, intentional self-harm   HCC

    √7th **T45.0X3** Poisoning by antiallergic and antiemetic drugs, assault

    √7th **T45.0X4** Poisoning by antiallergic and antiemetic drugs, undetermined

    √7th **T45.0X5** Adverse effect of antiallergic and antiemetic drugs

    √7th **T45.0X6** Underdosing of antiallergic and antiemetic drugs

√5th **T45.1** Poisoning by, adverse effect of and underdosing of antineoplastic and immunosuppressive drugs

    **EXCLUDES 1**   poisoning by, adverse effect of and underdosing of tamoxifen (T38.6)

    **AHA:** 2014, 4Q, 22

  √6th **T45.1X** Poisoning by, adverse effect of and underdosing of antineoplastic and immunosuppressive drugs

    √7th **T45.1X1** Poisoning by antineoplastic and immunosuppressive drugs, accidental (unintentional)
        Poisoning by antineoplastic and immunosuppressive drugs NOS

    11 √7th **T45.1X2** Poisoning by antineoplastic and immunosuppressive drugs, intentional self-harm   HCC

    √7th **T45.1X3** Poisoning by antineoplastic and immunosuppressive drugs, assault

    √7th **T45.1X4** Poisoning by antineoplastic and immunosuppressive drugs, undetermined

    √7th **T45.1X5** Adverse effect of antineoplastic and immunosuppressive drugs

    √7th **T45.1X6** Underdosing of antineoplastic and immunosuppressive drugs

---

11 HCC with 7th character indicating initial encounter (A or B - specific to category) OR sequela.

✔ Additional Character Req   √x7th Placeholder Alert   Unacceptable PDx   Manifestation   H1 - H14 HAC   HCC CMS-HCC Condition   EXCLUDES 1 Not Coded Here   EXCLUDES 2 Not Included Here

ICD-10-CM 2018        1111

**√5ᵗʰ T45.2 Poisoning by, adverse effect of and underdosing of vitamins**

EXCLUDES 2   poisoning by, adverse effect of and underdosing of iron (T45.4)

poisoning by, adverse effect of and underdosing of nicotinic acid (derivatives) (T46.7)

poisoning by, adverse effect of and underdosing of vitamin K (T45.7)

**√6ᵗʰ T45.2X Poisoning by, adverse effect of and underdosing of vitamins**

√7ᵗʰ **T45.2X1 Poisoning by vitamins, accidental (unintentional)**
Poisoning by vitamins NOS

11 √7ᵗʰ **T45.2X2 Poisoning by vitamins, intentional**   HCC
**self-harm**

√7ᵗʰ **T45.2X3 Poisoning by vitamins, assault**

√7ᵗʰ **T45.2X4 Poisoning by vitamins, undetermined**

√7ᵗʰ **T45.2X5 Adverse effect of vitamins**

√7ᵗʰ **T45.2X6 Underdosing of vitamins**
EXCLUDES 1   vitamin deficiencies (E50-E56)

**√5ᵗʰ T45.3 Poisoning by, adverse effect of and underdosing of enzymes**

**√6ᵗʰ T45.3X Poisoning by, adverse effect of and underdosing of enzymes**

√7ᵗʰ **T45.3X1 Poisoning by enzymes, accidental (unintentional)**
Poisoning by enzymes NOS

11 √7ᵗʰ **T45.3X2 Poisoning by enzymes, intentional**   HCC
**self-harm**

√7ᵗʰ **T45.3X3 Poisoning by enzymes, assault**

√7ᵗʰ **T45.3X4 Poisoning by enzymes, undetermined**

√7ᵗʰ **T45.3X5 Adverse effect of enzymes**

√7ᵗʰ **T45.3X6 Underdosing of enzymes**

**√5ᵗʰ T45.4 Poisoning by, adverse effect of and underdosing of iron and its compounds**

**√6ᵗʰ T45.4X Poisoning by, adverse effect of and underdosing of iron and its compounds**

√7ᵗʰ **T45.4X1 Poisoning by iron and its compounds, accidental (unintentional)**
Poisoning by iron and its compounds NOS

11 √7ᵗʰ **T45.4X2 Poisoning by iron and its compounds,**   HCC
**intentional self-harm**

√7ᵗʰ **T45.4X3 Poisoning by iron and its compounds, assault**

√7ᵗʰ **T45.4X4 Poisoning by iron and its compounds, undetermined**

√7ᵗʰ **T45.4X5 Adverse effect of iron and its compounds**

√7ᵗʰ **T45.4X6 Underdosing of iron and its compounds**
EXCLUDES 1   iron deficiency (E61.1)

**√5ᵗʰ T45.5 Poisoning by, adverse effect of and underdosing of anticoagulants and antithrombotic drugs**

**√6ᵗʰ T45.51 Poisoning by, adverse effect of and underdosing of anticoagulants**

√7ᵗʰ **T45.511 Poisoning by anticoagulants, accidental (unintentional)**
Poisoning by anticoagulants NOS

11 √7ᵗʰ **T45.512 Poisoning by anticoagulants,**   HCC
**intentional self-harm**

√7ᵗʰ **T45.513 Poisoning by anticoagulants, assault**

√7ᵗʰ **T45.514 Poisoning by anticoagulants, undetermined**

√7ᵗʰ **T45.515 Adverse effect of anticoagulants**
AHA: 2016, 1Q, 14; 2013, 2Q, 34

√7ᵗʰ **T45.516 Underdosing of anticoagulants**

**√6ᵗʰ T45.52 Poisoning by, adverse effect of and underdosing of antithrombotic drugs**
Poisoning by, adverse effect of and underdosing of antiplatelet drugs
EXCLUDES 2   poisoning by, adverse effect of and underdosing of aspirin (T39.01-)
poisoning by, adverse effect of and underdosing of acetylsalicylic acid (T39.01-)

√7ᵗʰ **T45.521 Poisoning by antithrombotic drugs, accidental (unintentional)**
Poisoning by antithrombotic drug NOS

11 √7ᵗʰ **T45.522 Poisoning by antithrombotic drugs,**   HCC
**intentional self-harm**

√7ᵗʰ **T45.523 Poisoning by antithrombotic drugs, assault**

√7ᵗʰ **T45.524 Poisoning by antithrombotic drugs, undetermined**

√7ᵗʰ **T45.525 Adverse effect of antithrombotic drugs**
AHA: 2016, 1Q, 15

√7ᵗʰ **T45.526 Underdosing of antithrombotic drugs**

**√5ᵗʰ T45.6 Poisoning by, adverse effect of and underdosing of fibrinolysis-affecting drugs**

**√6ᵗʰ T45.60 Poisoning by, adverse effect of and underdosing of unspecified fibrinolysis-affecting drugs**

√7ᵗʰ **T45.601 Poisoning by unspecified fibrinolysis-affecting drugs, accidental (unintentional)**
Poisoning by fibrinolysis-affecting drug NOS

11 √7ᵗʰ **T45.602 Poisoning by unspecified fibrinolysis-**   HCC
**affecting drugs, intentional self-harm**

√7ᵗʰ **T45.603 Poisoning by unspecified fibrinolysis-affecting drugs, assault**

√7ᵗʰ **T45.604 Poisoning by unspecified fibrinolysis-affecting drugs, undetermined**

√7ᵗʰ **T45.605 Adverse effect of unspecified fibrinolysis-affecting drugs**

√7ᵗʰ **T45.606 Underdosing of unspecified fibrinolysis-affecting drugs**

**√6ᵗʰ T45.61 Poisoning by, adverse effect of and underdosing of thrombolytic drugs**

√7ᵗʰ **T45.611 Poisoning by thrombolytic drug, accidental (unintentional)**
Poisoning by thrombolytic drug NOS

11 √7ᵗʰ **T45.612 Poisoning by thrombolytic drug,**   HCC
**intentional self-harm**

√7ᵗʰ **T45.613 Poisoning by thrombolytic drug, assault**

√7ᵗʰ **T45.614 Poisoning by thrombolytic drug, undetermined**

√7ᵗʰ **T45.615 Adverse effect of thrombolytic drugs**
AHA: 2017, 2Q, 9

√7ᵗʰ **T45.616 Underdosing of thrombolytic drugs**

**√6ᵗʰ T45.62 Poisoning by, adverse effect of and underdosing of hemostatic drugs**

√7ᵗʰ **T45.621 Poisoning by hemostatic drug, accidental (unintentional)**
Poisoning by hemostatic drug NOS

11 √7ᵗʰ **T45.622 Poisoning by hemostatic drug,**   HCC
**intentional self-harm**

√7ᵗʰ **T45.623 Poisoning by hemostatic drug, assault**

√7ᵗʰ **T45.624 Poisoning by hemostatic drug, undetermined**

√7ᵗʰ **T45.625 Adverse effect of hemostatic drug**

√7ᵗʰ **T45.626 Underdosing of hemostatic drugs**

**√6ᵗʰ T45.69 Poisoning by, adverse effect of and underdosing of other fibrinolysis-affecting drugs**

√7ᵗʰ **T45.691 Poisoning by other fibrinolysis-affecting drugs, accidental (unintentional)**
Poisoning by other fibrinolysis-affecting drug NOS

11 √7ᵗʰ **T45.692 Poisoning by other fibrinolysis-**   HCC
**affecting drugs, intentional self-harm**

√7ᵗʰ **T45.693 Poisoning by other fibrinolysis-affecting drugs, assault**

√7ᵗʰ **T45.694 Poisoning by other fibrinolysis-affecting drugs, undetermined**

√7ᵗʰ **T45.695 Adverse effect of other fibrinolysis-affecting drugs**

√7ᵗʰ **T45.696 Underdosing of other fibrinolysis-affecting drugs**

---

11 HCC with 7th character indicating initial encounter (A or B - specific to category) OR sequela.

N Newborn: 0   P Pediatric: 0-17   M Maternity: 12-55   A Adult: 15-124   MCC Major CC Condition   PDxMCC PDx acts as own MCC   CC CC Condition   PDxCC PDx acts as own CC

**1112**      ICD-10-CM 2018

✓5ᵗʰ **T45.7**  **Poisoning by, adverse effect of and underdosing of anticoagulant antagonists, vitamin K and other coagulants**

  ✓6ᵗʰ **T45.7X**  **Poisoning by, adverse effect of and underdosing of anticoagulant antagonists, vitamin K and other coagulants**

    ✓7ᵗʰ **T45.7X1**  **Poisoning by anticoagulant antagonists, vitamin K and other coagulants, accidental (unintentional)**
      Poisoning by anticoagulant antagonists, vitamin K and other coagulants NOS

    11 ✓7ᵗʰ **T45.7X2**  **Poisoning by anticoagulant antagonists, vitamin K and other coagulants, intentional self-harm**  `HCC`

    ✓7ᵗʰ **T45.7X3**  **Poisoning by anticoagulant antagonists, vitamin K and other coagulants, assault**

    ✓7ᵗʰ **T45.7X4**  **Poisoning by anticoagulant antagonists, vitamin K and other coagulants, undetermined**

    ✓7ᵗʰ **T45.7X5**  **Adverse effect of anticoagulant antagonists, vitamin K and other coagulants**

    ✓7ᵗʰ **T45.7X6**  **Underdosing of anticoagulant antagonist, vitamin K and other coagulants**
      *EXCLUDES 1*  *vitamin K deficiency (E56.1)*

✓5ᵗʰ **T45.8**  **Poisoning by, adverse effect of and underdosing of other primarily systemic and hematological agents**
  Poisoning by, adverse effect of and underdosing of liver preparations and other antianemic agents
  Poisoning by, adverse effect of and underdosing of natural blood and blood products
  Poisoning by, adverse effect of and underdosing of plasma substitute
  *EXCLUDES 2*  *poisoning by, adverse effect of and underdosing of immunoglobulin (T50.Z1)*
    *poisoning by, adverse effect of and underdosing of iron (T45.4)*
    *transfusion reactions (T80.-)*

  ✓6ᵗʰ **T45.8X**  **Poisoning by, adverse effect of and underdosing of other primarily systemic and hematological agents**

    ✓7ᵗʰ **T45.8X1**  **Poisoning by other primarily systemic and hematological agents, accidental (unintentional)**
      Poisoning by other primarily systemic and hematological agents NOS

    11 ✓7ᵗʰ **T45.8X2**  **Poisoning by other primarily systemic and hematological agents, intentional self-harm**  `HCC`

    ✓7ᵗʰ **T45.8X3**  **Poisoning by other primarily systemic and hematological agents, assault**

    ✓7ᵗʰ **T45.8X4**  **Poisoning by other primarily systemic and hematological agents, undetermined**

    ✓7ᵗʰ **T45.8X5**  **Adverse effect of other primarily systemic and hematological agents**

    ✓7ᵗʰ **T45.8X6**  **Underdosing of other primarily systemic and hematological agents**

✓5ᵗʰ **T45.9**  **Poisoning by, adverse effect of and underdosing of unspecified primarily systemic and hematological agent**

  ✓x7ᵗʰ **T45.91**  **Poisoning by unspecified primarily systemic and hematological agent, accidental (unintentional)**
    Poisoning by primarily systemic and hematological agent NOS

  11 ✓x7ᵗʰ **T45.92**  **Poisoning by unspecified primarily systemic and hematological agent, intentional self-harm**  `HCC`

  ✓x7ᵗʰ **T45.93**  **Poisoning by unspecified primarily systemic and hematological agent, assault**

  ✓x7ᵗʰ **T45.94**  **Poisoning by unspecified primarily systemic and hematological agent, undetermined**

  ✓x7ᵗʰ **T45.95**  **Adverse effect of unspecified primarily systemic and hematological agent**

  ✓x7ᵗʰ **T45.96**  **Underdosing of unspecified primarily systemic and hematological agent**

✓4ᵗʰ **T46**  **Poisoning by, adverse effect of and underdosing of agents primarily affecting the cardiovascular system**
  *EXCLUDES 1*  *poisoning by, adverse effect of and underdosing of metaraminol (T44.4)*

  The appropriate 7th character is to be added to each code from category T46.
  A   initial encounter
  D   subsequent encounter
  S   sequela

✓5ᵗʰ **T46.0**  **Poisoning by, adverse effect of and underdosing of cardiac-stimulant glycosides and drugs of similar action**

  ✓6ᵗʰ **T46.0X**  **Poisoning by, adverse effect of and underdosing of cardiac-stimulant glycosides and drugs of similar action**

    ✓7ᵗʰ **T46.0X1**  **Poisoning by cardiac-stimulant glycosides and drugs of similar action, accidental (unintentional)**
      Poisoning by cardiac-stimulant glycosides and drugs of similar action NOS

    11 ✓7ᵗʰ **T46.0X2**  **Poisoning by cardiac-stimulant glycosides and drugs of similar action, intentional self-harm**  `HCC`

    ✓7ᵗʰ **T46.0X3**  **Poisoning by cardiac-stimulant glycosides and drugs of similar action, assault**

    ✓7ᵗʰ **T46.0X4**  **Poisoning by cardiac-stimulant glycosides and drugs of similar action, undetermined**

    ✓7ᵗʰ **T46.0X5**  **Adverse effect of cardiac-stimulant glycosides and drugs of similar action**

    ✓7ᵗʰ **T46.0X6**  **Underdosing of cardiac-stimulant glycosides and drugs of similar action**

✓5ᵗʰ **T46.1**  **Poisoning by, adverse effect of and underdosing of calcium-channel blockers**

  ✓6ᵗʰ **T46.1X**  **Poisoning by, adverse effect of and underdosing of calcium-channel blockers**

    ✓7ᵗʰ **T46.1X1**  **Poisoning by calcium-channel blockers, accidental (unintentional)**
      Poisoning by calcium-channel blockers NOS

    11 ✓7ᵗʰ **T46.1X2**  **Poisoning by calcium-channel blockers, intentional self-harm**  `HCC`

    ✓7ᵗʰ **T46.1X3**  **Poisoning by calcium-channel blockers, assault**

    ✓7ᵗʰ **T46.1X4**  **Poisoning by calcium-channel blockers, undetermined**

    ✓7ᵗʰ **T46.1X5**  **Adverse effect of calcium-channel blockers**

    ✓7ᵗʰ **T46.1X6**  **Underdosing of calcium-channel blockers**

✓5ᵗʰ **T46.2**  **Poisoning by, adverse effect of and underdosing of other antidysrhythmic drugs, not elsewhere classified**
  *EXCLUDES 1*  *poisoning by, adverse effect of and underdosing of beta-adrenoreceptor antagonists (T44.7-)*

  ✓6ᵗʰ **T46.2X**  **Poisoning by, adverse effect of and underdosing of other antidysrhythmic drugs**

    ✓7ᵗʰ **T46.2X1**  **Poisoning by other antidysrhythmic drugs, accidental (unintentional)**
      Poisoning by other antidysrhythmic drugs NOS

    11 ✓7ᵗʰ **T46.2X2**  **Poisoning by other antidysrhythmic drugs, intentional self-harm**  `HCC`

    ✓7ᵗʰ **T46.2X3**  **Poisoning by other antidysrhythmic drugs, assault**

    ✓7ᵗʰ **T46.2X4**  **Poisoning by other antidysrhythmic drugs, undetermined**

    ✓7ᵗʰ **T46.2X5**  **Adverse effect of other antidysrhythmic drugs**

    ✓7ᵗʰ **T46.2X6**  **Underdosing of other antidysrhythmic drugs**

---

[11] HCC with 7th character indicating initial encounter (A or B - specific to category) OR sequela.

✓ Additional Character Req  ✓x7ᵗʰ Placeholder Alert  Unacceptable PDx  Manifestation  `H1`-`H14` HAC  `HCC` CMS-HCC Condition  *EXCLUDES 1* Not Coded Here  *EXCLUDES 2* Not Included Here

ICD-10-CM 2018      1113

√5th **T46.3** **Poisoning by, adverse effect of and underdosing of coronary vasodilators**

Poisoning by, adverse effect of and underdosing of dipyridamole

> EXCLUDES 1   poisoning by, adverse effect of and underdosing of calcium-channel blockers (T46.1)

√6th **T46.3X** **Poisoning by, adverse effect of and underdosing of coronary vasodilators**

√7th **T46.3X1** **Poisoning by coronary vasodilators, accidental (unintentional)**

Poisoning by coronary vasodilators NOS

11 √7th **T46.3X2** **Poisoning by coronary vasodilators, intentional self-harm**   HCC

√7th **T46.3X3** **Poisoning by coronary vasodilators, assault**

√7th **T46.3X4** **Poisoning by coronary vasodilators, undetermined**

√7th **T46.3X5** **Adverse effect of coronary vasodilators**

√7th **T46.3X6** **Underdosing of coronary vasodilators**

√5th **T46.4** **Poisoning by, adverse effect of and underdosing of angiotensin-converting-enzyme inhibitors**

√6th **T46.4X** **Poisoning by, adverse effect of and underdosing of angiotensin-converting-enzyme inhibitors**

√7th **T46.4X1** **Poisoning by angiotensin-converting-enzyme inhibitors, accidental (unintentional)**

Poisoning by angiotensin-converting-enzyme inhibitors NOS

11 √7th **T46.4X2** **Poisoning by angiotensin-converting-enzyme inhibitors, intentional self-harm**   HCC

√7th **T46.4X3** **Poisoning by angiotensin-converting-enzyme inhibitors, assault**

√7th **T46.4X4** **Poisoning by angiotensin-converting-enzyme inhibitors, undetermined**

√7th **T46.4X5** **Adverse effect of angiotensin-converting-enzyme inhibitors**

√7th **T46.4X6** **Underdosing of angiotensin-converting-enzyme inhibitors**

√5th **T46.5** **Poisoning by, adverse effect of and underdosing of other antihypertensive drugs**

> EXCLUDES 2   poisoning by, adverse effect of and underdosing of beta-adrenoreceptor antagonists (T44.7)
> poisoning by, adverse effect of and underdosing of calcium-channel blockers (T46.1)
> poisoning by, adverse effect of and underdosing of diuretics (T50.0-T50.2)

√6th **T46.5X** **Poisoning by, adverse effect of and underdosing of other antihypertensive drugs**

√7th **T46.5X1** **Poisoning by other antihypertensive drugs, accidental (unintentional)**

Poisoning by other antihypertensive drugs NOS

11 √7th **T46.5X2** **Poisoning by other antihypertensive drugs, intentional self-harm**   HCC

√7th **T46.5X3** **Poisoning by other antihypertensive drugs, assault**

√7th **T46.5X4** **Poisoning by other antihypertensive drugs, undetermined**

√7th **T46.5X5** **Adverse effect of other antihypertensive drugs**

√7th **T46.5X6** **Underdosing of other antihypertensive drugs**

√5th **T46.6** **Poisoning by, adverse effect of and underdosing of antihyperlipidemic and antiarteriosclerotic drugs**

√6th **T46.6X** **Poisoning by, adverse effect of and underdosing of antihyperlipidemic and antiarteriosclerotic drugs**

√7th **T46.6X1** **Poisoning by antihyperlipidemic and antiarteriosclerotic drugs, accidental (unintentional)**

Poisoning by antihyperlipidemic and antiarteriosclerotic drugs NOS

11 √7th **T46.6X2** **Poisoning by antihyperlipidemic and antiarteriosclerotic drugs, intentional self-harm**   HCC

√7th **T46.6X3** **Poisoning by antihyperlipidemic and antiarteriosclerotic drugs, assault**

√7th **T46.6X4** **Poisoning by antihyperlipidemic and antiarteriosclerotic drugs, undetermined**

√7th **T46.6X5** **Adverse effect of antihyperlipidemic and antiarteriosclerotic drugs**

√7th **T46.6X6** **Underdosing of antihyperlipidemic and antiarteriosclerotic drugs**

√5th **T46.7** **Poisoning by, adverse effect of and underdosing of peripheral vasodilators**

Poisoning by, adverse effect of and underdosing of nicotinic acid (derivatives)

> EXCLUDES 1   poisoning by, adverse effect of and underdosing of papaverine (T44.3)

√6th **T46.7X** **Poisoning by, adverse effect of and underdosing of peripheral vasodilators**

√7th **T46.7X1** **Poisoning by peripheral vasodilators, accidental (unintentional)**

Poisoning by peripheral vasodilators NOS

11 √7th **T46.7X2** **Poisoning by peripheral vasodilators, intentional self-harm**   HCC

√7th **T46.7X3** **Poisoning by peripheral vasodilators, assault**

√7th **T46.7X4** **Poisoning by peripheral vasodilators, undetermined**

√7th **T46.7X5** **Adverse effect of peripheral vasodilators**

√7th **T46.7X6** **Underdosing of peripheral vasodilators**

√5th **T46.8** **Poisoning by, adverse effect of and underdosing of antivaricose drugs, including sclerosing agents**

√6th **T46.8X** **Poisoning by, adverse effect of and underdosing of antivaricose drugs, including sclerosing agents**

√7th **T46.8X1** **Poisoning by antivaricose drugs, including sclerosing agents, accidental (unintentional)**

Poisoning by antivaricose drugs, including sclerosing agents NOS

11 √7th **T46.8X2** **Poisoning by antivaricose drugs, including sclerosing agents, intentional self-harm**   HCC

√7th **T46.8X3** **Poisoning by antivaricose drugs, including sclerosing agents, assault**

√7th **T46.8X4** **Poisoning by antivaricose drugs, including sclerosing agents, undetermined**

√7th **T46.8X5** **Adverse effect of antivaricose drugs, including sclerosing agents**

√7th **T46.8X6** **Underdosing of antivaricose drugs, including sclerosing agents**

√5th **T46.9** **Poisoning by, adverse effect of and underdosing of other and unspecified agents primarily affecting the cardiovascular system**

√6th **T46.90** **Poisoning by, adverse effect of and underdosing of unspecified agents primarily affecting the cardiovascular system**

√7th **T46.901** **Poisoning by unspecified agents primarily affecting the cardiovascular system, accidental (unintentional)**

11 √7th **T46.902** **Poisoning by unspecified agents primarily affecting the cardiovascular system, intentional self-harm**   HCC

√7th **T46.903** **Poisoning by unspecified agents primarily affecting the cardiovascular system, assault**

√7th **T46.904** **Poisoning by unspecified agents primarily affecting the cardiovascular system, undetermined**

√7th **T46.905** **Adverse effect of unspecified agents primarily affecting the cardiovascular system**

√7th **T46.906** **Underdosing of unspecified agents primarily affecting the cardiovascular system**

√6th **T46.99** **Poisoning by, adverse effect of and underdosing of other agents primarily affecting the cardiovascular system**

√7th **T46.991** **Poisoning by other agents primarily affecting the cardiovascular system, accidental (unintentional)**

---

11 HCC with 7th character indicating initial encounter (A or B - specific to category) OR sequela.

N Newborn: 0   P Pediatric: 0-17   M Maternity: 12-55   A Adult: 15-124   MCC Major CC Condition   PDxMCC PDx acts as own MCC   CC CC Condition   PDxCC PDx acts as own CC

**1114**     ICD-10-CM 2018

**11** ✓7th **T46.992** **Poisoning by other agents primarily affecting the cardiovascular system, intentional self-harm** `HCC`

✓7th **T46.993** **Poisoning by other agents primarily affecting the cardiovascular system, assault**

✓7th **T46.994** **Poisoning by other agents primarily affecting the cardiovascular system, undetermined**

✓7th **T46.995** **Adverse effect of other agents primarily affecting the cardiovascular system**

✓7th **T46.996** **Underdosing of other agents primarily affecting the cardiovascular system**

✓4th **T47** **Poisoning by, adverse effect of and underdosing of agents primarily affecting the gastrointestinal system**

> The appropriate 7th character is to be added to each code from category T47.
> A    initial encounter
> D    subsequent encounter
> S    sequela

✓5th **T47.0** **Poisoning by, adverse effect of and underdosing of histamine H2-receptor blockers**

✓6th **T47.0X** **Poisoning by, adverse effect of and underdosing of histamine H2-receptor blockers**

✓7th **T47.0X1** **Poisoning by histamine H2-receptor blockers, accidental (unintentional)**
Poisoning by histamine H2-receptor blockers NOS

**11** ✓7th **T47.0X2** **Poisoning by histamine H2-receptor blockers, intentional self-harm** `HCC`

✓7th **T47.0X3** **Poisoning by histamine H2-receptor blockers, assault**

✓7th **T47.0X4** **Poisoning by histamine H2-receptor blockers, undetermined**

✓7th **T47.0X5** **Adverse effect of histamine H2-receptor blockers**

✓7th **T47.0X6** **Underdosing of histamine H2-receptor blockers**

✓5th **T47.1** **Poisoning by, adverse effect of and underdosing of other antacids and anti-gastric-secretion drugs**

✓6th **T47.1X** **Poisoning by, adverse effect of and underdosing of other antacids and anti-gastric-secretion drugs**

✓7th **T47.1X1** **Poisoning by other antacids and anti-gastric-secretion drugs, accidental (unintentional)**
Poisoning by other antacids and anti-gastric-secretion drugs NOS

**11** ✓7th **T47.1X2** **Poisoning by other antacids and anti-gastric-secretion drugs, intentional self-harm** `HCC`

✓7th **T47.1X3** **Poisoning by other antacids and anti-gastric-secretion drugs, assault**

✓7th **T47.1X4** **Poisoning by other antacids and anti-gastric-secretion drugs, undetermined**

✓7th **T47.1X5** **Adverse effect of other antacids and anti-gastric-secretion drugs**

✓7th **T47.1X6** **Underdosing of other antacids and anti-gastric-secretion drugs**

✓5th **T47.2** **Poisoning by, adverse effect of and underdosing of stimulant laxatives**

✓6th **T47.2X** **Poisoning by, adverse effect of and underdosing of stimulant laxatives**

✓7th **T47.2X1** **Poisoning by stimulant laxatives, accidental (unintentional)**
Poisoning by stimulant laxatives NOS

**11** ✓7th **T47.2X2** **Poisoning by stimulant laxatives, intentional self-harm** `HCC`

✓7th **T47.2X3** **Poisoning by stimulant laxatives, assault**

✓7th **T47.2X4** **Poisoning by stimulant laxatives, undetermined**

✓7th **T47.2X5** **Adverse effect of stimulant laxatives**

✓7th **T47.2X6** **Underdosing of stimulant laxatives**

✓5th **T47.3** **Poisoning by, adverse effect of and underdosing of saline and osmotic laxatives**

✓6th **T47.3X** **Poisoning by and adverse effect of saline and osmotic laxatives**

✓7th **T47.3X1** **Poisoning by saline and osmotic laxatives, accidental (unintentional)**
Poisoning by saline and osmotic laxatives NOS

**11** ✓7th **T47.3X2** **Poisoning by saline and osmotic laxatives, intentional self-harm** `HCC`

✓7th **T47.3X3** **Poisoning by saline and osmotic laxatives, assault**

✓7th **T47.3X4** **Poisoning by saline and osmotic laxatives, undetermined**

✓7th **T47.3X5** **Adverse effect of saline and osmotic laxatives**

✓7th **T47.3X6** **Underdosing of saline and osmotic laxatives**

✓5th **T47.4** **Poisoning by, adverse effect of and underdosing of other laxatives**

✓6th **T47.4X** **Poisoning by, adverse effect of and underdosing of other laxatives**

✓7th **T47.4X1** **Poisoning by other laxatives, accidental (unintentional)**
Poisoning by other laxatives NOS

**11** ✓7th **T47.4X2** **Poisoning by other laxatives, intentional self-harm** `HCC`

✓7th **T47.4X3** **Poisoning by other laxatives, assault**

✓7th **T47.4X4** **Poisoning by other laxatives, undetermined**

✓7th **T47.4X5** **Adverse effect of other laxatives**

✓7th **T47.4X6** **Underdosing of other laxatives**

✓5th **T47.5** **Poisoning by, adverse effect of and underdosing of digestants**

✓6th **T47.5X** **Poisoning by, adverse effect of and underdosing of digestants**

✓7th **T47.5X1** **Poisoning by digestants, accidental (unintentional)**
Poisoning by digestants NOS

**11** ✓7th **T47.5X2** **Poisoning by digestants, intentional self-harm** `HCC`

✓7th **T47.5X3** **Poisoning by digestants, assault**

✓7th **T47.5X4** **Poisoning by digestants, undetermined**

✓7th **T47.5X5** **Adverse effect of digestants**

✓7th **T47.5X6** **Underdosing of digestants**

✓5th **T47.6** **Poisoning by, adverse effect of and underdosing of antidiarrheal drugs**

> *EXCLUDES 2*    poisoning by, adverse effect of and underdosing of systemic antibiotics and other anti-infectives (T36-T37)

✓6th **T47.6X** **Poisoning by, adverse effect of and underdosing of antidiarrheal drugs**

✓7th **T47.6X1** **Poisoning by antidiarrheal drugs, accidental (unintentional)**
Poisoning by antidiarrheal drugs NOS

**11** ✓7th **T47.6X2** **Poisoning by antidiarrheal drugs, intentional self-harm** `HCC`

✓7th **T47.6X3** **Poisoning by antidiarrheal drugs, assault**

✓7th **T47.6X4** **Poisoning by antidiarrheal drugs, undetermined**

✓7th **T47.6X5** **Adverse effect of antidiarrheal drugs**

✓7th **T47.6X6** **Underdosing of antidiarrheal drugs**

✓5th **T47.7** **Poisoning by, adverse effect of and underdosing of emetics**

✓6th **T47.7X** **Poisoning by, adverse effect of and underdosing of emetics**

✓7th **T47.7X1** **Poisoning by emetics, accidental (unintentional)**
Poisoning by emetics NOS

**11** ✓7th **T47.7X2** **Poisoning by emetics, intentional self-harm** `HCC`

✓7th **T47.7X3** **Poisoning by emetics, assault**

✓7th **T47.7X4** **Poisoning by emetics, undetermined**

✓7th **T47.7X5** **Adverse effect of emetics**

---

**11** HCC with 7th character indicating initial encounter (A or B - specific to category) OR sequela.

☑7ᵗʰ **T47.7X6** Underdosing of emetics

☑5ᵗʰ **T47.8** Poisoning by, adverse effect of and underdosing of other agents primarily affecting gastrointestinal system

   ☑6ᵗʰ **T47.8X** Poisoning by, adverse effect of and underdosing of other agents primarily affecting gastrointestinal system

      ☑7ᵗʰ **T47.8X1** Poisoning by other agents primarily affecting gastrointestinal system, accidental (unintentional)
         Poisoning by other agents primarily affecting gastrointestinal system NOS

     11 ☑7ᵗʰ **T47.8X2** Poisoning by other agents primarily affecting gastrointestinal system, intentional self-harm   HCC

      ☑7ᵗʰ **T47.8X3** Poisoning by other agents primarily affecting gastrointestinal system, assault

      ☑7ᵗʰ **T47.8X4** Poisoning by other agents primarily affecting gastrointestinal system, undetermined

      ☑7ᵗʰ **T47.8X5** Adverse effect of other agents primarily affecting gastrointestinal system

      ☑7ᵗʰ **T47.8X6** Underdosing of other agents primarily affecting gastrointestinal system

☑5ᵗʰ **T47.9** Poisoning by, adverse effect of and underdosing of unspecified agents primarily affecting the gastrointestinal system

   ☑x7ᵗʰ **T47.91** Poisoning by unspecified agents primarily affecting the gastrointestinal system, accidental (unintentional)
      Poisoning by agents primarily affecting the gastrointestinal system NOS

  11 ☑x7ᵗʰ **T47.92** Poisoning by unspecified agents primarily affecting the gastrointestinal system, intentional self-harm   HCC

   ☑x7ᵗʰ **T47.93** Poisoning by unspecified agents primarily affecting the gastrointestinal system, assault

   ☑x7ᵗʰ **T47.94** Poisoning by unspecified agents primarily affecting the gastrointestinal system, undetermined

   ☑x7ᵗʰ **T47.95** Adverse effect of unspecified agents primarily affecting the gastrointestinal system

   ☑x7ᵗʰ **T47.96** Underdosing of unspecified agents primarily affecting the gastrointestinal system

☑4ᵗʰ **T48** Poisoning by, adverse effect of and underdosing of agents primarily acting on smooth and skeletal muscles and the respiratory system

   The appropriate 7th character is to be added to each code from category T48.
   A   initial encounter
   D   subsequent encounter
   S   sequela

☑5ᵗʰ **T48.0** Poisoning by, adverse effect of and underdosing of oxytocic drugs

      *EXCLUDES 1*  *poisoning by, adverse effect of and underdosing of estrogens, progestogens and antagonists (T38.4-T38.6)*

   ☑6ᵗʰ **T48.0X** Poisoning by, adverse effect of and underdosing of oxytocic drugs

      ☑7ᵗʰ **T48.0X1** Poisoning by oxytocic drugs, accidental (unintentional)
         Poisoning by oxytocic drugs NOS

     11 ☑7ᵗʰ **T48.0X2** Poisoning by oxytocic drugs, intentional self-harm   HCC

      ☑7ᵗʰ **T48.0X3** Poisoning by oxytocic drugs, assault

      ☑7ᵗʰ **T48.0X4** Poisoning by oxytocic drugs, undetermined

      ☑7ᵗʰ **T48.0X5** Adverse effect of oxytocic drugs

      ☑7ᵗʰ **T48.0X6** Underdosing of oxytocic drugs

☑5ᵗʰ **T48.1** Poisoning by, adverse effect of and underdosing of skeletal muscle relaxants [neuromuscular blocking agents]

   ☑6ᵗʰ **T48.1X** Poisoning by, adverse effect of and underdosing of skeletal muscle relaxants [neuromuscular blocking agents]

      ☑7ᵗʰ **T48.1X1** Poisoning by skeletal muscle relaxants [neuromuscular blocking agents], accidental (unintentional)
         Poisoning by skeletal muscle relaxants [neuromuscular blocking agents] NOS

     11 ☑7ᵗʰ **T48.1X2** Poisoning by skeletal muscle relaxants [neuromuscular blocking agents], intentional self-harm   HCC

      ☑7ᵗʰ **T48.1X3** Poisoning by skeletal muscle relaxants [neuromuscular blocking agents], assault

      ☑7ᵗʰ **T48.1X4** Poisoning by skeletal muscle relaxants [neuromuscular blocking agents], undetermined

      ☑7ᵗʰ **T48.1X5** Adverse effect of skeletal muscle relaxants [neuromuscular blocking agents]

      ☑7ᵗʰ **T48.1X6** Underdosing of skeletal muscle relaxants [neuromuscular blocking agents]

☑5ᵗʰ **T48.2** Poisoning by, adverse effect of and underdosing of other and unspecified drugs acting on muscles

   ☑6ᵗʰ **T48.20** Poisoning by, adverse effect of and underdosing of unspecified drugs acting on muscles

      ☑7ᵗʰ **T48.201** Poisoning by unspecified drugs acting on muscles, accidental (unintentional)
         Poisoning by unspecified drugs acting on muscles NOS

     11 ☑7ᵗʰ **T48.202** Poisoning by unspecified drugs acting on muscles, intentional self-harm   HCC

      ☑7ᵗʰ **T48.203** Poisoning by unspecified drugs acting on muscles, assault

      ☑7ᵗʰ **T48.204** Poisoning by unspecified drugs acting on muscles, undetermined

      ☑7ᵗʰ **T48.205** Adverse effect of unspecified drugs acting on muscles

      ☑7ᵗʰ **T48.206** Underdosing of unspecified drugs acting on muscles

   ☑6ᵗʰ **T48.29** Poisoning by, adverse effect of and underdosing of other drugs acting on muscles

      ☑7ᵗʰ **T48.291** Poisoning by other drugs acting on muscles, accidental (unintentional)
         Poisoning by other drugs acting on muscles NOS

     11 ☑7ᵗʰ **T48.292** Poisoning by other drugs acting on muscles, intentional self-harm   HCC

      ☑7ᵗʰ **T48.293** Poisoning by other drugs acting on muscles, assault

      ☑7ᵗʰ **T48.294** Poisoning by other drugs acting on muscles, undetermined

      ☑7ᵗʰ **T48.295** Adverse effect of other drugs acting on muscles

      ☑7ᵗʰ **T48.296** Underdosing of other drugs acting on muscles

☑5ᵗʰ **T48.3** Poisoning by, adverse effect of and underdosing of antitussives

   ☑6ᵗʰ **T48.3X** Poisoning by, adverse effect of and underdosing of antitussives

      ☑7ᵗʰ **T48.3X1** Poisoning by antitussives, accidental (unintentional)
         Poisoning by antitussives NOS

     11 ☑7ᵗʰ **T48.3X2** Poisoning by antitussives, intentional self-harm   HCC

      ☑7ᵗʰ **T48.3X3** Poisoning by antitussives, assault

      ☑7ᵗʰ **T48.3X4** Poisoning by antitussives, undetermined

      ☑7ᵗʰ **T48.3X5** Adverse effect of antitussives

      ☑7ᵗʰ **T48.3X6** Underdosing of antitussives

---

¹¹ HCC with 7th character indicating initial encounter (A or B - specific to category) OR sequela.

Ⓝ Newborn: 0  Ⓟ Pediatric: 0-17  Ⓜ Maternity: 12-55  Ⓐ Adult: 15-124  **MCC** Major CC Condition  **PDxMCC** PDx acts as own MCC  **CC** CC Condition  **PDxCC** PDx acts as own CC

**1116** ICD-10-CM 2018

✓5ᵗʰ **T48.4** **Poisoning by, adverse effect of and underdosing of expectorants**

  ✓6ᵗʰ **T48.4X** **Poisoning by, adverse effect of and underdosing of expectorants**

    ✓7ᵗʰ **T48.4X1** **Poisoning by expectorants, accidental (unintentional)**
Poisoning by expectorants NOS

    11 ✓7ᵗʰ **T48.4X2** **Poisoning by expectorants, intentional self-harm** `HCC`

    ✓7ᵗʰ **T48.4X3** **Poisoning by expectorants, assault**

    ✓7ᵗʰ **T48.4X4** **Poisoning by expectorants, undetermined**

    ✓7ᵗʰ **T48.4X5** **Adverse effect of expectorants**

    ✓7ᵗʰ **T48.4X6** **Underdosing of expectorants**

✓5ᵗʰ **T48.5** **Poisoning by, adverse effect of and underdosing of other anti-common-cold drugs**
Poisoning by, adverse effect of and underdosing of decongestants

  EXCLUDES 2   poisoning by, adverse effect of and underdosing of antipyretics, NEC (T39.9-)
poisoning by, adverse effect of and underdosing of non-steroidal antiinflammatory drugs (T39.3-)
poisoning by, adverse effect of and underdosing of salicylates (T39.0-)

  ✓6ᵗʰ **T48.5X** **Poisoning by, adverse effect of and underdosing of other anti-common-cold drugs**

    ✓7ᵗʰ **T48.5X1** **Poisoning by other anti-common-cold drugs, accidental (unintentional)**
Poisoning by other anti-common-cold drugs NOS

    11 ✓7ᵗʰ **T48.5X2** **Poisoning by other anti-common-cold drugs, intentional self-harm** `HCC`

    ✓7ᵗʰ **T48.5X3** **Poisoning by other anti-common-cold drugs, assault**

    ✓7ᵗʰ **T48.5X4** **Poisoning by other anti-common-cold drugs, undetermined**

    ✓7ᵗʰ **T48.5X5** **Adverse effect of other anti-common-cold drugs**

    ✓7ᵗʰ **T48.5X6** **Underdosing of other anti-common-cold drugs**

✓5ᵗʰ **T48.6** **Poisoning by, adverse effect of and underdosing of antiasthmatics, not elsewhere classified**
Poisoning by, adverse effect of and underdosing of beta-adrenoreceptor agonists used in asthma therapy

  EXCLUDES 1   poisoning by, adverse effect of and underdosing of anterior pituitary [adenohypophyseal] hormones (T38.8)
poisoning by, adverse effect of and underdosing of beta-adrenoreceptor agonists not used in asthma therapy (T44.5)

  ✓6ᵗʰ **T48.6X** **Poisoning by, adverse effect of and underdosing of antiasthmatics**

    ✓7ᵗʰ **T48.6X1** **Poisoning by antiasthmatics, accidental (unintentional)**
Poisoning by antiasthmatics NOS

    11 ✓7ᵗʰ **T48.6X2** **Poisoning by antiasthmatics, intentional self-harm** `HCC`

    ✓7ᵗʰ **T48.6X3** **Poisoning by antiasthmatics, assault**

    ✓7ᵗʰ **T48.6X4** **Poisoning by antiasthmatics, undetermined**

    ✓7ᵗʰ **T48.6X5** **Adverse effect of antiasthmatics**

    ✓7ᵗʰ **T48.6X6** **Underdosing of antiasthmatics**

✓5ᵗʰ **T48.9** **Poisoning by, adverse effect of and underdosing of other and unspecified agents primarily acting on the respiratory system**

  ✓6ᵗʰ **T48.90** **Poisoning by, adverse effect of and underdosing of unspecified agents primarily acting on the respiratory system**

    ✓7ᵗʰ **T48.901** **Poisoning by unspecified agents primarily acting on the respiratory system, accidental (unintentional)**

    11 ✓7ᵗʰ **T48.902** **Poisoning by unspecified agents primarily acting on the respiratory system, intentional self-harm** `HCC`

    ✓7ᵗʰ **T48.903** **Poisoning by unspecified agents primarily acting on the respiratory system, assault**

    ✓7ᵗʰ **T48.904** **Poisoning by unspecified agents primarily acting on the respiratory system, undetermined**

    ✓7ᵗʰ **T48.905** **Adverse effect of unspecified agents primarily acting on the respiratory system**

    ✓7ᵗʰ **T48.906** **Underdosing of unspecified agents primarily acting on the respiratory system**

  ✓6ᵗʰ **T48.99** **Poisoning by, adverse effect of and underdosing of other agents primarily acting on the respiratory system**

    ✓7ᵗʰ **T48.991** **Poisoning by other agents primarily acting on the respiratory system, accidental (unintentional)**

    11 ✓7ᵗʰ **T48.992** **Poisoning by other agents primarily acting on the respiratory system, intentional self-harm** `HCC`

    ✓7ᵗʰ **T48.993** **Poisoning by other agents primarily acting on the respiratory system, assault**

    ✓7ᵗʰ **T48.994** **Poisoning by other agents primarily acting on the respiratory system, undetermined**

    ✓7ᵗʰ **T48.995** **Adverse effect of other agents primarily acting on the respiratory system**

    ✓7ᵗʰ **T48.996** **Underdosing of other agents primarily acting on the respiratory system**

✓4ᵗʰ **T49** **Poisoning by, adverse effect of and underdosing of topical agents primarily affecting skin and mucous membrane and by ophthalmological, otorhinolaryngological and dental drugs**
  INCLUDES   poisoning by, adverse effect of and underdosing of glucocorticoids, topically used

  The appropriate 7th character is to be added to each code from category T49.
  A   initial encounter
  D   subsequent encounter
  S   sequela

✓5ᵗʰ **T49.0** **Poisoning by, adverse effect of and underdosing of local antifungal, anti-infective and anti-inflammatory drugs**

  ✓6ᵗʰ **T49.0X** **Poisoning by, adverse effect of and underdosing of local antifungal, anti-infective and anti-inflammatory drugs**

    ✓7ᵗʰ **T49.0X1** **Poisoning by local antifungal, anti-infective and anti-inflammatory drugs, accidental (unintentional)**
Poisoning by local antifungal, anti-infective and anti-inflammatory drugs NOS

    11 ✓7ᵗʰ **T49.0X2** **Poisoning by local antifungal, anti-infective and anti-inflammatory drugs, intentional self-harm** `HCC`

    ✓7ᵗʰ **T49.0X3** **Poisoning by local antifungal, anti-infective and anti-inflammatory drugs, assault**

    ✓7ᵗʰ **T49.0X4** **Poisoning by local antifungal, anti-infective and anti-inflammatory drugs, undetermined**

    ✓7ᵗʰ **T49.0X5** **Adverse effect of local antifungal, anti-infective and anti-inflammatory drugs**

    ✓7ᵗʰ **T49.0X6** **Underdosing of local antifungal, anti-infective and anti-inflammatory drugs**

✓5ᵗʰ **T49.1** **Poisoning by, adverse effect of and underdosing of antipruritics**

  ✓6ᵗʰ **T49.1X** **Poisoning by, adverse effect of and underdosing of antipruritics**

    ✓7ᵗʰ **T49.1X1** **Poisoning by antipruritics, accidental (unintentional)**
Poisoning by antipruritics NOS

    11 ✓7ᵗʰ **T49.1X2** **Poisoning by antipruritics, intentional self-harm** `HCC`

    ✓7ᵗʰ **T49.1X3** **Poisoning by antipruritics, assault**

    ✓7ᵗʰ **T49.1X4** **Poisoning by antipruritics, undetermined**

    ✓7ᵗʰ **T49.1X5** **Adverse effect of antipruritics**

    ✓7ᵗʰ **T49.1X6** **Underdosing of antipruritics**

---

[11] HCC with 7th character indicating initial encounter (A or B - specific to category) OR sequela.

✓ Additional Character Req    ✓x7ᵗʰ Placeholder Alert    Unacceptable PDx    Manifestation    H1 - H14 HAC    HCC CMS-HCC Condition    EXCLUDES 1 Not Coded Here    EXCLUDES 2 Not Included Here

ICD-10-CM 2018      **1117**

√5ᵗʰ **T49.2** Poisoning by, adverse effect of and underdosing of local astringents and local detergents

> √6ᵗʰ **T49.2X** Poisoning by, adverse effect of and underdosing of local astringents and local detergents

>> √7ᵗʰ **T49.2X1** Poisoning by local astringents and local detergents, accidental (unintentional)
>> Poisoning by local astringents and local detergents NOS

>> 11 √7ᵗʰ **T49.2X2** Poisoning by local astringents and local detergents, intentional self-harm   HCC

>> √7ᵗʰ **T49.2X3** Poisoning by local astringents and local detergents, assault

>> √7ᵗʰ **T49.2X4** Poisoning by local astringents and local detergents, undetermined

>> √7ᵗʰ **T49.2X5** Adverse effect of local astringents and local detergents

>> √7ᵗʰ **T49.2X6** Underdosing of local astringents and local detergents

√5ᵗʰ **T49.3** Poisoning by, adverse effect of and underdosing of emollients, demulcents and protectants

> √6ᵗʰ **T49.3X** Poisoning by, adverse effect of and underdosing of emollients, demulcents and protectants

>> √7ᵗʰ **T49.3X1** Poisoning by emollients, demulcents and protectants, accidental (unintentional)
>> Poisoning by emollients, demulcents and protectants NOS

>> 11 √7ᵗʰ **T49.3X2** Poisoning by emollients, demulcents and protectants, intentional self-harm   HCC

>> √7ᵗʰ **T49.3X3** Poisoning by emollients, demulcents and protectants, assault

>> √7ᵗʰ **T49.3X4** Poisoning by emollients, demulcents and protectants, undetermined

>> √7ᵗʰ **T49.3X5** Adverse effect of emollients, demulcents and protectants

>> √7ᵗʰ **T49.3X6** Underdosing of emollients, demulcents and protectants

√5ᵗʰ **T49.4** Poisoning by, adverse effect of and underdosing of keratolytics, keratoplastics, and other hair treatment drugs and preparations

> √6ᵗʰ **T49.4X** Poisoning by, adverse effect of and underdosing of keratolytics, keratoplastics, and other hair treatment drugs and preparations

>> √7ᵗʰ **T49.4X1** Poisoning by keratolytics, keratoplastics, and other hair treatment drugs and preparations, accidental (unintentional)
>> Poisoning by keratolytics, keratoplastics, and other hair treatment drugs and preparations NOS

>> 11 √7ᵗʰ **T49.4X2** Poisoning by keratolytics, keratoplastics, and other hair treatment drugs and preparations, intentional self-harm   HCC

>> √7ᵗʰ **T49.4X3** Poisoning by keratolytics, keratoplastics, and other hair treatment drugs and preparations, assault

>> √7ᵗʰ **T49.4X4** Poisoning by keratolytics, keratoplastics, and other hair treatment drugs and preparations, undetermined

>> √7ᵗʰ **T49.4X5** Adverse effect of keratolytics, keratoplastics, and other hair treatment drugs and preparations

>> √7ᵗʰ **T49.4X6** Underdosing of keratolytics, keratoplastics, and other hair treatment drugs and preparations

√5ᵗʰ **T49.5** Poisoning by, adverse effect of and underdosing of ophthalmological drugs and preparations

> √6ᵗʰ **T49.5X** Poisoning by, adverse effect of and underdosing of ophthalmological drugs and preparations

>> √7ᵗʰ **T49.5X1** Poisoning by ophthalmological drugs and preparations, accidental (unintentional)
>> Poisoning by ophthalmological drugs and preparations NOS

>> 11 √7ᵗʰ **T49.5X2** Poisoning by ophthalmological drugs and preparations, intentional self-harm   HCC

>> √7ᵗʰ **T49.5X3** Poisoning by ophthalmological drugs and preparations, assault

>> √7ᵗʰ **T49.5X4** Poisoning by ophthalmological drugs and preparations, undetermined

>> √7ᵗʰ **T49.5X5** Adverse effect of ophthalmological drugs and preparations

>> √7ᵗʰ **T49.5X6** Underdosing of ophthalmological drugs and preparations

√5ᵗʰ **T49.6** Poisoning by, adverse effect of and underdosing of otorhinolaryngological drugs and preparations

> √6ᵗʰ **T49.6X** Poisoning by, adverse effect of and underdosing of otorhinolaryngological drugs and preparations

>> √7ᵗʰ **T49.6X1** Poisoning by otorhinolaryngological drugs and preparations, accidental (unintentional)
>> Poisoning by otorhinolaryngological drugs and preparations NOS

>> 11 √7ᵗʰ **T49.6X2** Poisoning by otorhinolaryngological drugs and preparations, intentional self-harm   HCC

>> √7ᵗʰ **T49.6X3** Poisoning by otorhinolaryngological drugs and preparations, assault

>> √7ᵗʰ **T49.6X4** Poisoning by otorhinolaryngological drugs and preparations, undetermined

>> √7ᵗʰ **T49.6X5** Adverse effect of otorhinolaryngological drugs and preparations

>> √7ᵗʰ **T49.6X6** Underdosing of otorhinolaryngological drugs and preparations

√5ᵗʰ **T49.7** Poisoning by, adverse effect of and underdosing of dental drugs, topically applied

> √6ᵗʰ **T49.7X** Poisoning by, adverse effect of and underdosing of dental drugs, topically applied

>> √7ᵗʰ **T49.7X1** Poisoning by dental drugs, topically applied, accidental (unintentional)
>> Poisoning by dental drugs, topically applied NOS

>> 11 √7ᵗʰ **T49.7X2** Poisoning by dental drugs, topically applied, intentional self-harm   HCC

>> √7ᵗʰ **T49.7X3** Poisoning by dental drugs, topically applied, assault

>> √7ᵗʰ **T49.7X4** Poisoning by dental drugs, topically applied, undetermined

>> √7ᵗʰ **T49.7X5** Adverse effect of dental drugs, topically applied

>> √7ᵗʰ **T49.7X6** Underdosing of dental drugs, topically applied

√5ᵗʰ **T49.8** Poisoning by, adverse effect of and underdosing of other topical agents
Poisoning by, adverse effect of and underdosing of spermicides

> √6ᵗʰ **T49.8X** Poisoning by, adverse effect of and underdosing of other topical agents

>> √7ᵗʰ **T49.8X1** Poisoning by other topical agents, accidental (unintentional)
>> Poisoning by other topical agents NOS

>> 11 √7ᵗʰ **T49.8X2** Poisoning by other topical agents, intentional self-harm   HCC

>> √7ᵗʰ **T49.8X3** Poisoning by other topical agents, assault

>> √7ᵗʰ **T49.8X4** Poisoning by other topical agents, undetermined

>> √7ᵗʰ **T49.8X5** Adverse effect of other topical agents

>> √7ᵗʰ **T49.8X6** Underdosing of other topical agents

√5ᵗʰ **T49.9** Poisoning by, adverse effect of and underdosing of unspecified topical agent

> √x7ᵗʰ **T49.91** Poisoning by unspecified topical agent, accidental (unintentional)

> 11 √x7ᵗʰ **T49.92** Poisoning by unspecified topical agent, intentional self-harm   HCC

> √x7ᵗʰ **T49.93** Poisoning by unspecified topical agent, assault

> √x7ᵗʰ **T49.94** Poisoning by unspecified topical agent, undetermined

> √x7ᵗʰ **T49.95** Adverse effect of unspecified topical agent

> √x7ᵗʰ **T49.96** Underdosing of unspecified topical agent

---

11 HCC with 7th character indicating initial encounter (A or B - specific to category) OR sequela.

N Newborn: 0   P Pediatric: 0-17   M Maternity: 12-55   A Adult: 15-124   **MCC** Major CC Condition   **PDxMCC** PDx acts as own MCC   **CC** CC Condition   **PDxCC** PDx acts as own CC

**1118**

ICD-10-CM 2018

✓4th **T50 Poisoning by, adverse effect of and underdosing of diuretics and other and unspecified drugs, medicaments and biological substances**

> The appropriate 7th character is to be added to each code from category T50.
> A    initial encounter
> D    subsequent encounter
> S    sequela

✓5th **T50.0 Poisoning by, adverse effect of and underdosing of mineralocorticoids and their antagonists**

✓6th **T50.0X Poisoning by, adverse effect of and underdosing of mineralocorticoids and their antagonists**

✓7th **T50.0X1 Poisoning by mineralocorticoids and their antagonists, accidental (unintentional)**
> Poisoning by mineralocorticoids and their antagonists NOS

11 ✓7th **T50.0X2 Poisoning by mineralocorticoids and their antagonists, intentional self-harm** HCC

✓7th **T50.0X3 Poisoning by mineralocorticoids and their antagonists, assault**

✓7th **T50.0X4 Poisoning by mineralocorticoids and their antagonists, undetermined**

✓7th **T50.0X5 Adverse effect of mineralocorticoids and their antagonists**

✓7th **T50.0X6 Underdosing of mineralocorticoids and their antagonists**

✓5th **T50.1 Poisoning by, adverse effect of and underdosing of loop [high-ceiling] diuretics**

✓6th **T50.1X Poisoning by, adverse effect of and underdosing of loop [high-ceiling] diuretics**

✓7th **T50.1X1 Poisoning by loop [high-ceiling] diuretics, accidental (unintentional)**
> Poisoning by loop [high-ceiling] diuretics NOS

11 ✓7th **T50.1X2 Poisoning by loop [high-ceiling] diuretics, intentional self-harm** HCC

✓7th **T50.1X3 Poisoning by loop [high-ceiling] diuretics, assault**

✓7th **T50.1X4 Poisoning by loop [high-ceiling] diuretics, undetermined**

✓7th **T50.1X5 Adverse effect of loop [high-ceiling] diuretics**

✓7th **T50.1X6 Underdosing of loop [high-ceiling] diuretics**

✓5th **T50.2 Poisoning by, adverse effect of and underdosing of carbonic-anhydrase inhibitors, benzothiadiazides and other diuretics**
> Poisoning by, adverse effect of and underdosing of acetazolamide

✓6th **T50.2X Poisoning by, adverse effect of and underdosing of carbonic-anhydrase inhibitors, benzothiadiazides and other diuretics**

✓7th **T50.2X1 Poisoning by carbonic-anhydrase inhibitors, benzothiadiazides and other diuretics, accidental (unintentional)**
> Poisoning by carbonic-anhydrase inhibitors, benzothiadiazides and other diuretics NOS

11 ✓7th **T50.2X2 Poisoning by carbonic-anhydrase inhibitors, benzothiadiazides and other diuretics, intentional self-harm** HCC

✓7th **T50.2X3 Poisoning by carbonic-anhydrase inhibitors, benzothiadiazides and other diuretics, assault**

✓7th **T50.2X4 Poisoning by carbonic-anhydrase inhibitors, benzothiadiazides and other diuretics, undetermined**

✓7th **T50.2X5 Adverse effect of carbonic-anhydrase inhibitors, benzothiadiazides and other diuretics**

✓7th **T50.2X6 Underdosing of carbonic-anhydrase inhibitors, benzothiadiazides and other diuretics**

✓5th **T50.3 Poisoning by, adverse effect of and underdosing of electrolytic, caloric and water-balance agents**
> Poisoning by, adverse effect of and underdosing of oral rehydration salts

✓6th **T50.3X Poisoning by, adverse effect of and underdosing of electrolytic, caloric and water-balance agents**

✓7th **T50.3X1 Poisoning by electrolytic, caloric and water-balance agents, accidental (unintentional)**
> Poisoning by electrolytic, caloric and water-balance agents NOS

11 ✓7th **T50.3X2 Poisoning by electrolytic, caloric and water-balance agents, intentional self-harm** HCC

✓7th **T50.3X3 Poisoning by electrolytic, caloric and water-balance agents, assault**

✓7th **T50.3X4 Poisoning by electrolytic, caloric and water-balance agents, undetermined**

✓7th **T50.3X5 Adverse effect of electrolytic, caloric and water-balance agents**

✓7th **T50.3X6 Underdosing of electrolytic, caloric and water-balance agents**

✓5th **T50.4 Poisoning by, adverse effect of and underdosing of drugs affecting uric acid metabolism**

✓6th **T50.4X Poisoning by, adverse effect of and underdosing of drugs affecting uric acid metabolism**

✓7th **T50.4X1 Poisoning by drugs affecting uric acid metabolism, accidental (unintentional)**
> Poisoning by drugs affecting uric acid metabolism NOS

11 ✓7th **T50.4X2 Poisoning by drugs affecting uric acid metabolism, intentional self-harm** HCC

✓7th **T50.4X3 Poisoning by drugs affecting uric acid metabolism, assault**

✓7th **T50.4X4 Poisoning by drugs affecting uric acid metabolism, undetermined**

✓7th **T50.4X5 Adverse effect of drugs affecting uric acid metabolism**

✓7th **T50.4X6 Underdosing of drugs affecting uric acid metabolism**

✓5th **T50.5 Poisoning by, adverse effect of and underdosing of appetite depressants**

✓6th **T50.5X Poisoning by, adverse effect of and underdosing of appetite depressants**

✓7th **T50.5X1 Poisoning by appetite depressants, accidental (unintentional)**
> Poisoning by appetite depressants NOS

11 ✓7th **T50.5X2 Poisoning by appetite depressants, intentional self-harm** HCC

✓7th **T50.5X3 Poisoning by appetite depressants, assault**

✓7th **T50.5X4 Poisoning by appetite depressants, undetermined**

✓7th **T50.5X5 Adverse effect of appetite depressants**

✓7th **T50.5X6 Underdosing of appetite depressants**

✓5th **T50.6 Poisoning by, adverse effect of and underdosing of antidotes and chelating agents**
> Poisoning by, adverse effect of and underdosing of alcohol deterrents

✓6th **T50.6X Poisoning by, adverse effect of and underdosing of antidotes and chelating agents**

✓7th **T50.6X1 Poisoning by antidotes and chelating agents, accidental (unintentional)**
> Poisoning by antidotes and chelating agents NOS

11 ✓7th **T50.6X2 Poisoning by antidotes and chelating agents, intentional self-harm** HCC

✓7th **T50.6X3 Poisoning by antidotes and chelating agents, assault**

✓7th **T50.6X4 Poisoning by antidotes and chelating agents, undetermined**

✓7th **T50.6X5 Adverse effect of antidotes and chelating agents**

✓7th **T50.6X6 Underdosing of antidotes and chelating agents**

---

11 HCC with 7th character indicating initial encounter (A or B - specific to category) OR sequela.

✓ Additional Character Req   ✓x7th Placeholder Alert   Unacceptable PDx   Manifestation   H1 - H14 HAC   HCC CMS-HCC Condition   EXCLUDES 1 Not Coded Here   EXCLUDES 2 Not Included Here

☑5ᵗʰ **T50.7** **Poisoning by, adverse effect of and underdosing of analeptics and opioid receptor antagonists**

   ☑6ᵗʰ **T50.7X** **Poisoning by, adverse effect of and underdosing of analeptics and opioid receptor antagonists**

     ☑7ᵗʰ **T50.7X1** **Poisoning by analeptics and opioid receptor antagonists, accidental (unintentional)**
        Poisoning by analeptics and opioid receptor antagonists NOS

     11 ☑7ᵗʰ **T50.7X2** **Poisoning by analeptics and opioid** HCC **receptor antagonists, intentional self-harm**

     ☑7ᵗʰ **T50.7X3** **Poisoning by analeptics and opioid receptor antagonists, assault**

     ☑7ᵗʰ **T50.7X4** **Poisoning by analeptics and opioid receptor antagonists, undetermined**

     ☑7ᵗʰ **T50.7X5** **Adverse effect of analeptics and opioid receptor antagonists**

     ☑7ᵗʰ **T50.7X6** **Underdosing of analeptics and opioid receptor antagonists**

☑5ᵗʰ **T50.8** **Poisoning by, adverse effect of and underdosing of diagnostic agents**

   ☑6ᵗʰ **T50.8X** **Poisoning by, adverse effect of and underdosing of diagnostic agents**

     ☑7ᵗʰ **T50.8X1** **Poisoning by diagnostic agents, accidental (unintentional)**
        Poisoning by diagnostic agents NOS

     11 ☑7ᵗʰ **T50.8X2** **Poisoning by diagnostic agents,** HCC **intentional self-harm**

     ☑7ᵗʰ **T50.8X3** **Poisoning by diagnostic agents, assault**

     ☑7ᵗʰ **T50.8X4** **Poisoning by diagnostic agents, undetermined**

     ☑7ᵗʰ **T50.8X5** **Adverse effect of diagnostic agents**

     ☑7ᵗʰ **T50.8X6** **Underdosing of diagnostic agents**

☑5ᵗʰ **T50.A** **Poisoning by, adverse effect of and underdosing of bacterial vaccines**

   ☑6ᵗʰ **T50.A1** **Poisoning by, adverse effect of and underdosing of pertussis vaccine, including combinations with a pertussis component**

     ☑7ᵗʰ **T50.A11** **Poisoning by pertussis vaccine, including combinations with a pertussis component, accidental (unintentional)**

     11 ☑7ᵗʰ **T50.A12** **Poisoning by pertussis vaccine,** HCC **including combinations with a pertussis component, intentional self-harm**

     ☑7ᵗʰ **T50.A13** **Poisoning by pertussis vaccine, including combinations with a pertussis component, assault**

     ☑7ᵗʰ **T50.A14** **Poisoning by pertussis vaccine, including combinations with a pertussis component, undetermined**

     ☑7ᵗʰ **T50.A15** **Adverse effect of pertussis vaccine, including combinations with a pertussis component**

     ☑7ᵗʰ **T50.A16** **Underdosing of pertussis vaccine, including combinations with a pertussis component**

   ☑6ᵗʰ **T50.A2** **Poisoning by, adverse effect of and underdosing of mixed bacterial vaccines without a pertussis component**

     ☑7ᵗʰ **T50.A21** **Poisoning by mixed bacterial vaccines without a pertussis component, accidental (unintentional)**

     11 ☑7ᵗʰ **T50.A22** **Poisoning by mixed bacterial vaccines** HCC **without a pertussis component, intentional self-harm**

     ☑7ᵗʰ **T50.A23** **Poisoning by mixed bacterial vaccines without a pertussis component, assault**

     ☑7ᵗʰ **T50.A24** **Poisoning by mixed bacterial vaccines without a pertussis component, undetermined**

     ☑7ᵗʰ **T50.A25** **Adverse effect of mixed bacterial vaccines without a pertussis component**

     ☑7ᵗʰ **T50.A26** **Underdosing of mixed bacterial vaccines without a pertussis component**

   ☑6ᵗʰ **T50.A9** **Poisoning by, adverse effect of and underdosing of other bacterial vaccines**

     ☑7ᵗʰ **T50.A91** **Poisoning by other bacterial vaccines, accidental (unintentional)**

     11 ☑7ᵗʰ **T50.A92** **Poisoning by other bacterial vaccines,** HCC **intentional self-harm**

     ☑7ᵗʰ **T50.A93** **Poisoning by other bacterial vaccines, assault**

     ☑7ᵗʰ **T50.A94** **Poisoning by other bacterial vaccines, undetermined**

     ☑7ᵗʰ **T50.A95** **Adverse effect of other bacterial vaccines**

     ☑7ᵗʰ **T50.A96** **Underdosing of other bacterial vaccines**

☑5ᵗʰ **T50.B** **Poisoning by, adverse effect of and underdosing of viral vaccines**

   ☑6ᵗʰ **T50.B1** **Poisoning by, adverse effect of and underdosing of smallpox vaccines**

     ☑7ᵗʰ **T50.B11** **Poisoning by smallpox vaccines, accidental (unintentional)**

     11 ☑7ᵗʰ **T50.B12** **Poisoning by smallpox vaccines,** HCC **intentional self-harm**

     ☑7ᵗʰ **T50.B13** **Poisoning by smallpox vaccines, assault**

     ☑7ᵗʰ **T50.B14** **Poisoning by smallpox vaccines, undetermined**

     ☑7ᵗʰ **T50.B15** **Adverse effect of smallpox vaccines**

     ☑7ᵗʰ **T50.B16** **Underdosing of smallpox vaccines**

   ☑6ᵗʰ **T50.B9** **Poisoning by, adverse effect of and underdosing of other viral vaccines**

     ☑7ᵗʰ **T50.B91** **Poisoning by other viral vaccines, accidental (unintentional)**

     11 ☑7ᵗʰ **T50.B92** **Poisoning by other viral vaccines,** HCC **intentional self-harm**

     ☑7ᵗʰ **T50.B93** **Poisoning by other viral vaccines, assault**

     ☑7ᵗʰ **T50.B94** **Poisoning by other viral vaccines, undetermined**

     ☑7ᵗʰ **T50.B95** **Adverse effect of other viral vaccines**

     ☑7ᵗʰ **T50.B96** **Underdosing of other viral vaccines**

☑5ᵗʰ **T50.Z** **Poisoning by, adverse effect of and underdosing of other vaccines and biological substances**

   ☑6ᵗʰ **T50.Z1** **Poisoning by, adverse effect of and underdosing of immunoglobulin**

     ☑7ᵗʰ **T50.Z11** **Poisoning by immunoglobulin, accidental (unintentional)**

     11 ☑7ᵗʰ **T50.Z12** **Poisoning by immunoglobulin,** HCC **intentional self-harm**

     ☑7ᵗʰ **T50.Z13** **Poisoning by immunoglobulin, assault**

     ☑7ᵗʰ **T50.Z14** **Poisoning by immunoglobulin, undetermined**

     ☑7ᵗʰ **T50.Z15** **Adverse effect of immunoglobulin**

     ☑7ᵗʰ **T50.Z16** **Underdosing of immunoglobulin**

   ☑6ᵗʰ **T50.Z9** **Poisoning by, adverse effect of and underdosing of other vaccines and biological substances**

     ☑7ᵗʰ **T50.Z91** **Poisoning by other vaccines and biological substances, accidental (unintentional)**

     11 ☑7ᵗʰ **T50.Z92** **Poisoning by other vaccines and** HCC **biological substances, intentional self-harm**

     ☑7ᵗʰ **T50.Z93** **Poisoning by other vaccines and biological substances, assault**

     ☑7ᵗʰ **T50.Z94** **Poisoning by other vaccines and biological substances, undetermined**

     ☑7ᵗʰ **T50.Z95** **Adverse effect of other vaccines and biological substances**

     ☑7ᵗʰ **T50.Z96** **Underdosing of other vaccines and biological substances**

☑5ᵗʰ **T50.9** **Poisoning by, adverse effect of and underdosing of other and unspecified drugs, medicaments and biological substances**
     AHA: 2016, 1Q, 38; 2015, 1Q, 21

   ☑6ᵗʰ **T50.90** **Poisoning by, adverse effect of and underdosing of unspecified drugs, medicaments and biological substances**

     ☑7ᵗʰ **T50.901** **Poisoning by unspecified drugs, medicaments and biological substances, accidental (unintentional)**

---

**11** HCC with 7th character indicating initial encounter (A or B - specific to category) OR sequela.

Ⓝ Newborn: 0   Ⓟ Pediatric: 0-17   Ⓜ Maternity: 12-55   Ⓐ Adult: 15-124   **MCC** Major CC Condition   **PDxMCC** PDx acts as own MCC   **CC** CC Condition   **PDxCC** PDx acts as own CC

**1120**                                                ICD-10-CM 2018

**11** ✓7ᵗʰ **T50.902 Poisoning by unspecified drugs,** HCC
**medicaments and biological substances,**
**intentional self-harm**

✓7ᵗʰ **T50.903 Poisoning by unspecified drugs,**
**medicaments and biological substances,**
**assault**

✓7ᵗʰ **T50.904 Poisoning by unspecified drugs,**
**medicaments and biological substances,**
**undetermined**

✓7ᵗʰ **T50.905 Adverse effect of unspecified drugs,**
**medicaments and biological substances**

✓7ᵗʰ **T50.906 Underdosing of unspecified drugs,**
**medicaments and biological substances**

✓6ᵗʰ **T50.99 Poisoning by, adverse effect of and underdosing of**
**other drugs, medicaments and biological substances**

✓7ᵗʰ **T50.991 Poisoning by other drugs, medicaments**
**and biological substances, accidental**
**(unintentional)**

**11** ✓7ᵗʰ **T50.992 Poisoning by other drugs,** HCC
**medicaments and biological substances,**
**intentional self-harm**

✓7ᵗʰ **T50.993 Poisoning by other drugs, medicaments**
**and biological substances, assault**

✓7ᵗʰ **T50.994 Poisoning by other drugs, medicaments**
**and biological substances, undetermined**

✓7ᵗʰ **T50.995 Adverse effect of other drugs,**
**medicaments and biological substances**

✓7ᵗʰ **T50.996 Underdosing of other drugs, medicaments**
**and biological substances**

## Toxic effects of substances chiefly nonmedicinal as to source
## (T51-T65)

NOTE    When no intent is indicated code to accidental. Undetermined intent
is only for use when there is specific documentation in the record
that the intent of the toxic effect cannot be determined.

Use additional code(s) for all associated manifestations of toxic effect, such as:
personal history of foreign body fully removed (Z87.821)
respiratory conditions due to external agents (J60-J70)
to identify any retained foreign body, if applicable (Z18.-)

EXCLUDES 1   contact with and (suspected) exposure to toxic substances (Z77.-)
**AHA:** 2017, 1Q, 39-40

✓4ᵗʰ **T51 Toxic effect of alcohol**

The appropriate 7th character is to be added to each code from
category T51.
A    initial encounter
D    subsequent encounter
S    sequela

✓5ᵗʰ **T51.0 Toxic effect of ethanol**
Toxic effect of ethyl alcohol
EXCLUDES 2   acute alcohol intoxication or 'hangover' effects
(F10.129, F10.229, F10.929)
drunkenness (F10.129, F10.229, F10.929)
pathological alcohol intoxication (F10.129, F10.229,
F10.929)

✓6ᵗʰ **T51.0X Toxic effect of ethanol**

✓7ᵗʰ **T51.0X1 Toxic effect of ethanol, accidental**
**(unintentional)**
Toxic effect of ethanol NOS

**11** ✓7ᵗʰ **T51.0X2 Toxic effect of ethanol, intentional** HCC
**self-harm**

✓7ᵗʰ **T51.0X3 Toxic effect of ethanol, assault**

✓7ᵗʰ **T51.0X4 Toxic effect of ethanol, undetermined**

✓5ᵗʰ **T51.1 Toxic effect of methanol**
Toxic effect of methyl alcohol

✓6ᵗʰ **T51.1X Toxic effect of methanol**

✓7ᵗʰ **T51.1X1 Toxic effect of methanol, accidental**
**(unintentional)**
Toxic effect of methanol NOS

**11** ✓7ᵗʰ **T51.1X2 Toxic effect of methanol, intentional** HCC
**self-harm**

✓7ᵗʰ **T51.1X3 Toxic effect of methanol, assault**

✓7ᵗʰ **T51.1X4 Toxic effect of methanol, undetermined**

✓5ᵗʰ **T51.2 Toxic effect of 2-Propanol**
Toxic effect of isopropyl alcohol

✓6ᵗʰ **T51.2X Toxic effect of 2-Propanol**

✓7ᵗʰ **T51.2X1 Toxic effect of 2-Propanol, accidental**
**(unintentional)**
Toxic effect of 2-Propanol NOS

**11** ✓7ᵗʰ **T51.2X2 Toxic effect of 2-Propanol,** HCC
**intentional self-harm**

✓7ᵗʰ **T51.2X3 Toxic effect of 2-Propanol, assault**

✓7ᵗʰ **T51.2X4 Toxic effect of 2-Propanol, undetermined**

✓5ᵗʰ **T51.3 Toxic effect of fusel oil**
Toxic effect of amyl alcohol
Toxic effect of butyl [1-butanol] alcohol
Toxic effect of propyl [1-propanol] alcohol

✓6ᵗʰ **T51.3X Toxic effect of fusel oil**

✓7ᵗʰ **T51.3X1 Toxic effect of fusel oil, accidental**
**(unintentional)**
Toxic effect of fusel oil NOS

**11** ✓7ᵗʰ **T51.3X2 Toxic effect of fusel oil, intentional** HCC
**self-harm**

✓7ᵗʰ **T51.3X3 Toxic effect of fusel oil, assault**

✓7ᵗʰ **T51.3X4 Toxic effect of fusel oil, undetermined**

✓5ᵗʰ **T51.8 Toxic effect of other alcohols**

✓6ᵗʰ **T51.8X Toxic effect of other alcohols**

✓7ᵗʰ **T51.8X1 Toxic effect of other alcohols, accidental**
**(unintentional)**
Toxic effect of other alcohols NOS

**11** ✓7ᵗʰ **T51.8X2 Toxic effect of other alcohols,** HCC
**intentional self-harm**

✓7ᵗʰ **T51.8X3 Toxic effect of other alcohols, assault**

✓7ᵗʰ **T51.8X4 Toxic effect of other alcohols,**
**undetermined**

✓5ᵗʰ **T51.9 Toxic effect of unspecified alcohol**

✓ₓ7ᵗʰ **T51.91 Toxic effect of unspecified alcohol, accidental**
**(unintentional)**

**11** ✓ₓ7ᵗʰ **T51.92 Toxic effect of unspecified alcohol, intentional** HCC
**self-harm**

✓ₓ7ᵗʰ **T51.93 Toxic effect of unspecified alcohol, assault**

✓ₓ7ᵗʰ **T51.94 Toxic effect of unspecified alcohol, undetermined**

✓4ᵗʰ **T52 Toxic effect of organic solvents**
EXCLUDES 1   halogen derivatives of aliphatic and aromatic hydrocarbons
(T53.-)

The appropriate 7th character is to be added to each code from
category T52.
A    initial encounter
D    subsequent encounter
S    sequela

✓5ᵗʰ **T52.0 Toxic effects of petroleum products**
Toxic effects of ether petroleum
Toxic effects of gasoline [petrol]
Toxic effects of kerosene [paraffin oil]
Toxic effects of naphtha petroleum
Toxic effects of paraffin wax
Toxic effects of spirit petroleum

✓6ᵗʰ **T52.0X Toxic effects of petroleum products**

✓7ᵗʰ **T52.0X1 Toxic effect of petroleum products,**
**accidental (unintentional)**
Toxic effects of petroleum products NOS

**11** ✓7ᵗʰ **T52.0X2 Toxic effect of petroleum products,** HCC
**intentional self-harm**

✓7ᵗʰ **T52.0X3 Toxic effect of petroleum products,**
**assault**

✓7ᵗʰ **T52.0X4 Toxic effect of petroleum products,**
**undetermined**

✓5ᵗʰ **T52.1 Toxic effects of benzene**
EXCLUDES 1   homologues of benzene (T52.2)
nitroderivatives and aminoderivatives of benzene and
its homologues (T65.3)

✓6ᵗʰ **T52.1X Toxic effects of benzene**

✓7ᵗʰ **T52.1X1 Toxic effect of benzene, accidental**
**(unintentional)**
Toxic effects of benzene NOS

---

**11** HCC with 7th character indicating initial encounter (A or B - specific to category) OR sequela.

✓ Additional Character Req    ✓ₓ7ᵗʰ Placeholder Alert    Unacceptable PDx    Manifestation    H1-H14 HAC    HCC CMS-HCC Condition    EXCLUDES 1 Not Coded Here    EXCLUDES 2 Not Included Here

**11** ✓7ᵗʰ **T52.1X2** **Toxic effect of benzene,** intentional **self-harm** `HCC`

✓7ᵗʰ **T52.1X3** **Toxic effect of benzene,** assault

✓7ᵗʰ **T52.1X4** **Toxic effect of benzene,** undetermined

✓5ᵗʰ **T52.2** **Toxic effects of homologues of benzene**
Toxic effects of toluene [methylbenzene]
Toxic effects of xylene [dimethylbenzene]

✓6ᵗʰ **T52.2X** **Toxic effects of** homologues of benzene

✓7ᵗʰ **T52.2X1** **Toxic effect of homologues of benzene,** accidental **(unintentional)**
Toxic effects of homologues of benzene NOS

**11** ✓7ᵗʰ **T52.2X2** **Toxic effect of homologues of benzene,** intentional self-harm `HCC`

✓7ᵗʰ **T52.2X3** **Toxic effect of homologues of benzene,** assault

✓7ᵗʰ **T52.2X4** **Toxic effect of homologues of benzene,** undetermined

✓5ᵗʰ **T52.3** **Toxic effects of glycols**

✓6ᵗʰ **T52.3X** **Toxic effects of** glycols

✓7ᵗʰ **T52.3X1** **Toxic effect of glycols,** accidental **(unintentional)**
Toxic effects of glycols NOS

**11** ✓7ᵗʰ **T52.3X2** **Toxic effect of glycols,** intentional **self-harm** `HCC`

✓7ᵗʰ **T52.3X3** **Toxic effect of glycols,** assault

✓7ᵗʰ **T52.3X4** **Toxic effect of glycols,** undetermined

✓5ᵗʰ **T52.4** **Toxic effects of ketones**

✓6ᵗʰ **T52.4X** **Toxic effects of** ketones

✓7ᵗʰ **T52.4X1** **Toxic effect of ketones,** accidental **(unintentional)**
Toxic effects of ketones NOS

**11** ✓7ᵗʰ **T52.4X2** **Toxic effect of ketones,** intentional **self-harm** `HCC`

✓7ᵗʰ **T52.4X3** **Toxic effect of ketones,** assault

✓7ᵗʰ **T52.4X4** **Toxic effect of ketones,** undetermined

✓5ᵗʰ **T52.8** **Toxic effects of other organic solvents**

✓6ᵗʰ **T52.8X** **Toxic effects of** other organic solvents

✓7ᵗʰ **T52.8X1** **Toxic effect of other organic solvents,** accidental **(unintentional)**
Toxic effects of other organic solvents NOS

**11** ✓7ᵗʰ **T52.8X2** **Toxic effect of other organic solvents,** `HCC` intentional self-harm

✓7ᵗʰ **T52.8X3** **Toxic effect of other organic solvents,** assault

✓7ᵗʰ **T52.8X4** **Toxic effect of other organic solvents,** undetermined

✓5ᵗʰ **T52.9** **Toxic effects of** unspecified **organic solvent**

✓x7ᵗʰ **T52.91** **Toxic effect of unspecified organic solvent,** accidental **(unintentional)**

**11** ✓x7ᵗʰ **T52.92** **Toxic effect of unspecified organic solvent,** intentional self-harm `HCC`

✓x7ᵗʰ **T52.93** **Toxic effect of unspecified organic solvent,** assault

✓x7ᵗʰ **T52.94** **Toxic effect of unspecified organic solvent,** undetermined

✓4ᵗʰ **T53** **Toxic effect of halogen derivatives of aliphatic and aromatic hydrocarbons**

> The appropriate 7th character is to be added to each code from category T53.
> A    initial encounter
> D    subsequent encounter
> S    sequela

✓5ᵗʰ **T53.0** **Toxic effects of** carbon tetrachloride
Toxic effects of tetrachloromethane

✓6ᵗʰ **T53.0X** **Toxic effects of carbon tetrachloride**

✓7ᵗʰ **T53.0X1** **Toxic effect of carbon tetrachloride,** accidental **(unintentional)**
Toxic effects of carbon tetrachloride NOS

**11** ✓7ᵗʰ **T53.0X2** **Toxic effect of carbon tetrachloride,** intentional self-harm `HCC`

✓7ᵗʰ **T53.0X3** **Toxic effect of carbon tetrachloride,** assault

✓7ᵗʰ **T53.0X4** **Toxic effect of carbon tetrachloride,** undetermined

✓5ᵗʰ **T53.1** **Toxic effects of chloroform**
Toxic effects of trichloromethane

✓6ᵗʰ **T53.1X** **Toxic effects of** chloroform

✓7ᵗʰ **T53.1X1** **Toxic effect of chloroform,** accidental **(unintentional)**
Toxic effects of chloroform NOS

**11** ✓7ᵗʰ **T53.1X2** **Toxic effect of chloroform,** `HCC` intentional self-harm

✓7ᵗʰ **T53.1X3** **Toxic effect of chloroform,** assault

✓7ᵗʰ **T53.1X4** **Toxic effect of chloroform,** undetermined

✓5ᵗʰ **T53.2** **Toxic effects of trichloroethylene**
Toxic effects of trichloroethene

✓6ᵗʰ **T53.2X** **Toxic effects of** trichloroethylene

✓7ᵗʰ **T53.2X1** **Toxic effect of trichloroethylene,** accidental **(unintentional)**
Toxic effects of trichloroethylene NOS

**11** ✓7ᵗʰ **T53.2X2** **Toxic effect of trichloroethylene,** intentional self-harm `HCC`

✓7ᵗʰ **T53.2X3** **Toxic effect of trichloroethylene,** assault

✓7ᵗʰ **T53.2X4** **Toxic effect of trichloroethylene,** undetermined

✓5ᵗʰ **T53.3** **Toxic effects of tetrachloroethylene**
Toxic effects of perchloroethylene
Toxic effect of tetrachloroethene

✓6ᵗʰ **T53.3X** **Toxic effects of** tetrachloroethylene

✓7ᵗʰ **T53.3X1** **Toxic effect of tetrachloroethylene,** accidental **(unintentional)**
Toxic effects of tetrachloroethylene NOS

**11** ✓7ᵗʰ **T53.3X2** **Toxic effect of tetrachloroethylene,** intentional self-harm `HCC`

✓7ᵗʰ **T53.3X3** **Toxic effect of tetrachloroethylene,** assault

✓7ᵗʰ **T53.3X4** **Toxic effect of tetrachloroethylene,** undetermined

✓5ᵗʰ **T53.4** **Toxic effects of dichloromethane**
Toxic effects of methylene chloride

✓6ᵗʰ **T53.4X** **Toxic effects of** dichloromethane

✓7ᵗʰ **T53.4X1** **Toxic effect of dichloromethane,** accidental **(unintentional)**
Toxic effects of dichloromethane NOS

**11** ✓7ᵗʰ **T53.4X2** **Toxic effect of dichloromethane,** `HCC` intentional self-harm

✓7ᵗʰ **T53.4X3** **Toxic effect of dichloromethane,** assault

✓7ᵗʰ **T53.4X4** **Toxic effect of dichloromethane,** undetermined

✓5ᵗʰ **T53.5** **Toxic effects of chlorofluorocarbons**

✓6ᵗʰ **T53.5X** **Toxic effects of** chlorofluorocarbons

✓7ᵗʰ **T53.5X1** **Toxic effect of chlorofluorocarbons,** accidental **(unintentional)**
Toxic effects of chlorofluorocarbons NOS

**11** ✓7ᵗʰ **T53.5X2** **Toxic effect of chlorofluorocarbons,** `HCC` intentional self-harm

✓7ᵗʰ **T53.5X3** **Toxic effect of chlorofluorocarbons,** assault

✓7ᵗʰ **T53.5X4** **Toxic effect of chlorofluorocarbons,** undetermined

✓5ᵗʰ **T53.6** **Toxic effects of other halogen derivatives of aliphatic hydrocarbons**

✓6ᵗʰ **T53.6X** **Toxic effects of other** halogen derivatives of aliphatic hydrocarbons

✓7ᵗʰ **T53.6X1** **Toxic effect of other halogen derivatives of aliphatic hydrocarbons,** accidental **(unintentional)**
Toxic effects of other halogen derivatives of aliphatic hydrocarbons NOS

**11** ✓7ᵗʰ **T53.6X2** **Toxic effect of other halogen derivatives of aliphatic hydrocarbons,** intentional self-harm `HCC`

✓7ᵗʰ **T53.6X3** **Toxic effect of other halogen derivatives of aliphatic hydrocarbons,** assault

✓7ᵗʰ **T53.6X4** **Toxic effect of other halogen derivatives of aliphatic hydrocarbons,** undetermined

---

**11** HCC with 7th character indicating initial encounter (A or B - specific to category) OR sequela.

Ⓝ Newborn: 0   Ⓟ Pediatric: 0-17   Ⓜ Maternity: 12-55   Ⓐ Adult: 15-124   `MCC` Major CC Condition   `PDxMCC` PDx acts as own MCC   `CC` CC Condition   `PDxCC` PDx acts as own CC

**1122**        ICD-10-CM 2018

✓5ᵗʰ **T53.7** **Toxic effects of other halogen derivatives of aromatic hydrocarbons**

   ✓6ᵗʰ **T53.7X** **Toxic effects of other** halogen derivatives of aromatic hydrocarbons

     ✓7ᵗʰ **T53.7X1** **Toxic effect of other halogen derivatives of aromatic hydrocarbons,** accidental (unintentional)
        Toxic effects of other halogen derivatives of aromatic hydrocarbons NOS

     [11] ✓7ᵗʰ **T53.7X2** **Toxic effect of other halogen**    `HCC` **derivatives of aromatic hydrocarbons,** intentional self-harm

     ✓7ᵗʰ **T53.7X3** **Toxic effect of other halogen derivatives of aromatic hydrocarbons,** assault

     ✓7ᵗʰ **T53.7X4** **Toxic effect of other halogen derivatives of aromatic hydrocarbons,** undetermined

✓5ᵗʰ **T53.9** **Toxic effects of** unspecified halogen derivatives of aliphatic and aromatic hydrocarbons

   ✓x7ᵗʰ **T53.91** **Toxic effect of unspecified halogen derivatives of aliphatic and aromatic hydrocarbons,** accidental (unintentional)

   [11] ✓x7ᵗʰ **T53.92** **Toxic effect of unspecified halogen derivatives**    `HCC` **of aliphatic and aromatic hydrocarbons,** intentional self-harm

   ✓x7ᵗʰ **T53.93** **Toxic effect of unspecified halogen derivatives of aliphatic and aromatic hydrocarbons,** assault

   ✓x7ᵗʰ **T53.94** **Toxic effect of unspecified halogen derivatives of aliphatic and aromatic hydrocarbons,** undetermined

✓4ᵗʰ **T54** **Toxic effect of corrosive substances**

> The appropriate 7th character is to be added to each code from category T54.
> A     initial encounter
> D     subsequent encounter
> S     sequela

✓5ᵗʰ **T54.0** **Toxic effects of phenol and phenol homologues**

   ✓6ᵗʰ **T54.0X** **Toxic effects of** phenol and phenol homologues

     ✓7ᵗʰ **T54.0X1** **Toxic effect of phenol and phenol homologues,** accidental (unintentional)
        Toxic effects of phenol and phenol homologues NOS

     [11] ✓7ᵗʰ **T54.0X2** **Toxic effect of phenol and phenol**    `HCC` **homologues,** intentional self-harm

     ✓7ᵗʰ **T54.0X3** **Toxic effect of phenol and phenol homologues,** assault

     ✓7ᵗʰ **T54.0X4** **Toxic effect of phenol and phenol homologues,** undetermined

✓5ᵗʰ **T54.1** **Toxic effects of other corrosive organic compounds**

   ✓6ᵗʰ **T54.1X** **Toxic effects of** other corrosive organic compounds

     ✓7ᵗʰ **T54.1X1** **Toxic effect of other corrosive organic compounds,** accidental (unintentional)
        Toxic effects of other corrosive organic compounds NOS

     [11] ✓7ᵗʰ **T54.1X2** **Toxic effect of other corrosive organic** `HCC` **compounds,** intentional self-harm

     ✓7ᵗʰ **T54.1X3** **Toxic effect of other corrosive organic compounds,** assault

     ✓7ᵗʰ **T54.1X4** **Toxic effect of other corrosive organic compounds,** undetermined

✓5ᵗʰ **T54.2** **Toxic effects of corrosive acids and acid-like substances**
   Toxic effects of hydrochloric acid
   Toxic effects of sulfuric acid

   ✓6ᵗʰ **T54.2X** **Toxic effects of corrosive** acids and acid-like substances

     ✓7ᵗʰ **T54.2X1** **Toxic effect of corrosive acids and acid-like substances,** accidental (unintentional)
        Toxic effects of corrosive acids and acid-like substances NOS

     [11] ✓7ᵗʰ **T54.2X2** **Toxic effect of corrosive acids and**    `HCC` **acid-like substances,** intentional self-harm

     ✓7ᵗʰ **T54.2X3** **Toxic effect of corrosive acids and acid-like substances,** assault

     ✓7ᵗʰ **T54.2X4** **Toxic effect of corrosive acids and acid-like substances,** undetermined

✓5ᵗʰ **T54.3** **Toxic effects of corrosive alkalis and alkali-like substances**
   Toxic effects of potassium hydroxide
   Toxic effects of sodium hydroxide

   ✓6ᵗʰ **T54.3X** **Toxic effects of corrosive** alkalis and alkali-like substances

     ✓7ᵗʰ **T54.3X1** **Toxic effect of corrosive alkalis and alkali-like substances,** accidental (unintentional)
        Toxic effects of corrosive alkalis and alkali-like substances NOS

     [11] ✓7ᵗʰ **T54.3X2** **Toxic effect of corrosive alkalis and**    `HCC` **alkali-like substances,** intentional self-harm

     ✓7ᵗʰ **T54.3X3** **Toxic effect of corrosive alkalis and alkali-like substances,** assault

     ✓7ᵗʰ **T54.3X4** **Toxic effect of corrosive alkalis and alkali-like substances,** undetermined

✓5ᵗʰ **T54.9** **Toxic effects of** unspecified corrosive substance

   ✓x7ᵗʰ **T54.91** **Toxic effect of unspecified corrosive substance,** accidental (unintentional)

   [11] ✓x7ᵗʰ **T54.92** **Toxic effect of unspecified corrosive substance,**    `HCC` intentional self-harm

   ✓x7ᵗʰ **T54.93** **Toxic effect of unspecified corrosive substance,** assault

   ✓x7ᵗʰ **T54.94** **Toxic effect of unspecified corrosive substance,** undetermined

✓4ᵗʰ **T55** **Toxic effect of soaps and detergents**

> The appropriate 7th character is to be added to each code from category T55.
> A     initial encounter
> D     subsequent encounter
> S     sequela

✓5ᵗʰ **T55.0** **Toxic effect of soaps**

   ✓6ᵗʰ **T55.0X** **Toxic effect of** soaps

     ✓7ᵗʰ **T55.0X1** **Toxic effect of soaps,** accidental (unintentional)
        Toxic effect of soaps NOS

     [11] ✓7ᵗʰ **T55.0X2** **Toxic effect of soaps,** intentional    `HCC` self-harm

     ✓7ᵗʰ **T55.0X3** **Toxic effect of soaps,** assault

     ✓7ᵗʰ **T55.0X4** **Toxic effect of soaps,** undetermined

✓5ᵗʰ **T55.1** **Toxic effect of detergents**

   ✓6ᵗʰ **T55.1X** **Toxic effect of** detergents

     ✓7ᵗʰ **T55.1X1** **Toxic effect of detergents,** accidental (unintentional)
        Toxic effect of detergents NOS

     [11] ✓7ᵗʰ **T55.1X2** **Toxic effect of detergents,** intentional `HCC` self-harm

     ✓7ᵗʰ **T55.1X3** **Toxic effect of detergents,** assault

     ✓7ᵗʰ **T55.1X4** **Toxic effect of detergents,** undetermined

✓4ᵗʰ **T56** **Toxic effect of metals**
   `INCLUDES`   toxic effects of fumes and vapors of metals
          toxic effects of metals from all sources, except medicinal substances
   Use additional code to identify any retained metal foreign body, if applicable (Z18.0-, T18.1-)
   `EXCLUDES 1`   arsenic and its compounds (T57.0)
          manganese and its compounds (T57.2)

> The appropriate 7th character is to be added to each code from category T56.
> A     initial encounter
> D     subsequent encounter
> S     sequela

✓5ᵗʰ **T56.0** **Toxic effects of lead and its compounds**

   ✓6ᵗʰ **T56.0X** **Toxic effects of** lead and its compounds

     ✓7ᵗʰ **T56.0X1** **Toxic effect of lead and its compounds,** accidental (unintentional)
        Toxic effects of lead and its compounds NOS

     [11] ✓7ᵗʰ **T56.0X2** **Toxic effect of lead and its**    `HCC` **compounds,** intentional self-harm

     ✓7ᵗʰ **T56.0X3** **Toxic effect of lead and its compounds,** assault

---

[11] HCC with 7th character indicating initial encounter (A or B - specific to category) OR sequela.

---

✓ Additional Character Req    ✓x7ᵗʰ Placeholder Alert    Unacceptable PDx    Manifestation    `H1`-`H14` HAC    `HCC` CMS-HCC Condition    `EXCLUDES 1` Not Coded Here    `EXCLUDES 2` Not Included Here

√7ᵗʰ **T56.0X4 Toxic effect of lead and its compounds, undetermined**

√5ᵗʰ **T56.1 Toxic effects of mercury and its compounds**

√6ᵗʰ **T56.1X Toxic effects of mercury and its compounds**

√7ᵗʰ **T56.1X1 Toxic effect of mercury and its compounds, accidental (unintentional)**
Toxic effects of mercury and its compounds NOS

11 √7ᵗʰ **T56.1X2 Toxic effect of mercury and its compounds, intentional self-harm** HCC

√7ᵗʰ **T56.1X3 Toxic effect of mercury and its compounds, assault**

√7ᵗʰ **T56.1X4 Toxic effect of mercury and its compounds, undetermined**

√5ᵗʰ **T56.2 Toxic effects of chromium and its compounds**

√6ᵗʰ **T56.2X Toxic effects of chromium and its compounds**

√7ᵗʰ **T56.2X1 Toxic effect of chromium and its compounds, accidental (unintentional)**
Toxic effects of chromium and its compounds NOS

11 √7ᵗʰ **T56.2X2 Toxic effect of chromium and its compounds, intentional self-harm** HCC

√7ᵗʰ **T56.2X3 Toxic effect of chromium and its compounds, assault**

√7ᵗʰ **T56.2X4 Toxic effect of chromium and its compounds, undetermined**

√5ᵗʰ **T56.3 Toxic effects of cadmium and its compounds**

√6ᵗʰ **T56.3X Toxic effects of cadmium and its compounds**

√7ᵗʰ **T56.3X1 Toxic effect of cadmium and its compounds, accidental (unintentional)**
Toxic effects of cadmium and its compounds NOS

11 √7ᵗʰ **T56.3X2 Toxic effect of cadmium and its compounds, intentional self-harm** HCC

√7ᵗʰ **T56.3X3 Toxic effect of cadmium and its compounds, assault**

√7ᵗʰ **T56.3X4 Toxic effect of cadmium and its compounds, undetermined**

√5ᵗʰ **T56.4 Toxic effects of copper and its compounds**

√6ᵗʰ **T56.4X Toxic effects of copper and its compounds**

√7ᵗʰ **T56.4X1 Toxic effect of copper and its compounds, accidental (unintentional)**
Toxic effects of copper and its compounds NOS

11 √7ᵗʰ **T56.4X2 Toxic effect of copper and its compounds, intentional self-harm** HCC

√7ᵗʰ **T56.4X3 Toxic effect of copper and its compounds, assault**

√7ᵗʰ **T56.4X4 Toxic effect of copper and its compounds, undetermined**

√5ᵗʰ **T56.5 Toxic effects of zinc and its compounds**

√6ᵗʰ **T56.5X Toxic effects of zinc and its compounds**

√7ᵗʰ **T56.5X1 Toxic effect of zinc and its compounds, accidental (unintentional)**
Toxic effects of zinc and its compounds NOS

11 √7ᵗʰ **T56.5X2 Toxic effect of zinc and its compounds, intentional self-harm** HCC

√7ᵗʰ **T56.5X3 Toxic effect of zinc and its compounds, assault**

√7ᵗʰ **T56.5X4 Toxic effect of zinc and its compounds, undetermined**

√5ᵗʰ **T56.6 Toxic effects of tin and its compounds**

√6ᵗʰ **T56.6X Toxic effects of tin and its compounds**

√7ᵗʰ **T56.6X1 Toxic effect of tin and its compounds, accidental (unintentional)**
Toxic effects of tin and its compounds NOS

11 √7ᵗʰ **T56.6X2 Toxic effect of tin and its compounds, intentional self-harm** HCC

√7ᵗʰ **T56.6X3 Toxic effect of tin and its compounds, assault**

√7ᵗʰ **T56.6X4 Toxic effect of tin and its compounds, undetermined**

√5ᵗʰ **T56.7 Toxic effects of beryllium and its compounds**

√6ᵗʰ **T56.7X Toxic effects of beryllium and its compounds**

√7ᵗʰ **T56.7X1 Toxic effect of beryllium and its compounds, accidental (unintentional)**
Toxic effects of beryllium and its compounds NOS

11 √7ᵗʰ **T56.7X2 Toxic effect of beryllium and its compounds, intentional self-harm** HCC

√7ᵗʰ **T56.7X3 Toxic effect of beryllium and its compounds, assault**

√7ᵗʰ **T56.7X4 Toxic effect of beryllium and its compounds, undetermined**

√5ᵗʰ **T56.8 Toxic effects of other metals**

√6ᵗʰ **T56.81 Toxic effect of thallium**

√7ᵗʰ **T56.811 Toxic effect of thallium, accidental (unintentional)**
Toxic effect of thallium NOS

11 √7ᵗʰ **T56.812 Toxic effect of thallium, intentional self-harm** HCC

√7ᵗʰ **T56.813 Toxic effect of thallium, assault**

√7ᵗʰ **T56.814 Toxic effect of thallium, undetermined**

√6ᵗʰ **T56.89 Toxic effects of other metals**

√7ᵗʰ **T56.891 Toxic effect of other metals, accidental (unintentional)**
Toxic effects of other metals NOS

11 √7ᵗʰ **T56.892 Toxic effect of other metals, intentional self-harm** HCC

√7ᵗʰ **T56.893 Toxic effect of other metals, assault**

√7ᵗʰ **T56.894 Toxic effect of other metals, undetermined**

√5ᵗʰ **T56.9 Toxic effects of unspecified metal**

√x7ᵗʰ **T56.91 Toxic effect of unspecified metal, accidental (unintentional)**

11 √x7ᵗʰ **T56.92 Toxic effect of unspecified metal, intentional self-harm** HCC

√x7ᵗʰ **T56.93 Toxic effect of unspecified metal, assault**

√x7ᵗʰ **T56.94 Toxic effect of unspecified metal, undetermined**

√4ᵗʰ **T57 Toxic effect of other inorganic substances**

The appropriate 7th character is to be added to each code from category T57.
A initial encounter
D subsequent encounter
S sequela

√5ᵗʰ **T57.0 Toxic effect of arsenic and its compounds**

√6ᵗʰ **T57.0X Toxic effect of arsenic and its compounds**

√7ᵗʰ **T57.0X1 Toxic effect of arsenic and its compounds, accidental (unintentional)**
Toxic effect of arsenic and its compounds NOS

11 √7ᵗʰ **T57.0X2 Toxic effect of arsenic and its compounds, intentional self-harm** HCC

√7ᵗʰ **T57.0X3 Toxic effect of arsenic and its compounds, assault**

√7ᵗʰ **T57.0X4 Toxic effect of arsenic and its compounds, undetermined**

√5ᵗʰ **T57.1 Toxic effect of phosphorus and its compounds**
EXCLUDES 1 organophosphate insecticides (T60.0)

√6ᵗʰ **T57.1X Toxic effect of phosphorus and its compounds**

√7ᵗʰ **T57.1X1 Toxic effect of phosphorus and its compounds, accidental (unintentional)**
Toxic effect of phosphorus and its compounds NOS

11 √7ᵗʰ **T57.1X2 Toxic effect of phosphorus and its compounds, intentional self-harm** HCC

√7ᵗʰ **T57.1X3 Toxic effect of phosphorus and its compounds, assault**

√7ᵗʰ **T57.1X4 Toxic effect of phosphorus and its compounds, undetermined**

---

11 HCC with 7th character indicating initial encounter (A or B - specific to category) OR sequela.

Ⓝ Newborn: 0 Ⓟ Pediatric: 0-17 Ⓜ Maternity: 12-55 Ⓐ Adult: 15-124 **MCC** Major CC Condition **PDxMCC** PDx acts as own MCC **CC** CC Condition **PDxCC** PDx acts as own CC

**1124**

**ICD-10-CM 2018**

✓5ᵗʰ **T57.2** **Toxic effect of manganese and its compounds**

   ✓6ᵗʰ **T57.2X** **Toxic effect of** manganese and its compounds

      ✓7ᵗʰ **T57.2X1** **Toxic effect of** manganese and its compounds, accidental (unintentional)
Toxic effect of manganese and its compounds NOS

      [11] ✓7ᵗʰ **T57.2X2** **Toxic effect of** manganese and its compounds, intentional self-harm   HCC

      ✓7ᵗʰ **T57.2X3** **Toxic effect of** manganese and its compounds, assault

      ✓7ᵗʰ **T57.2X4** **Toxic effect of** manganese and its compounds, undetermined

✓5ᵗʰ **T57.3** **Toxic effect of hydrogen cyanide**

   ✓6ᵗʰ **T57.3X** **Toxic effect of** hydrogen cyanide

      ✓7ᵗʰ **T57.3X1** **Toxic effect of** hydrogen cyanide, accidental (unintentional)
Toxic effect of hydrogen cyanide NOS

      [11] ✓7ᵗʰ **T57.3X2** **Toxic effect of** hydrogen cyanide, intentional self-harm   HCC

      ✓7ᵗʰ **T57.3X3** **Toxic effect of** hydrogen cyanide, assault

      ✓7ᵗʰ **T57.3X4** **Toxic effect of** hydrogen cyanide, undetermined

✓5ᵗʰ **T57.8** **Toxic effect of other specified inorganic substances**

   ✓6ᵗʰ **T57.8X** **Toxic effect of** other specified inorganic substances

      ✓7ᵗʰ **T57.8X1** **Toxic effect of other specified inorganic substances**, accidental (unintentional)
Toxic effect of other specified inorganic substances NOS

      [11] ✓7ᵗʰ **T57.8X2** **Toxic effect of other specified inorganic substances**, intentional self-harm   HCC

      ✓7ᵗʰ **T57.8X3** **Toxic effect of other specified inorganic substances**, assault

      ✓7ᵗʰ **T57.8X4** **Toxic effect of other specified inorganic substances**, undetermined

✓5ᵗʰ **T57.9** **Toxic effect of** unspecified inorganic substance

   ✓x7ᵗʰ **T57.91** **Toxic effect of unspecified inorganic substance, accidental (unintentional)**

   [11] ✓x7ᵗʰ **T57.92** **Toxic effect of unspecified inorganic substance, intentional self-harm**   HCC

   ✓x7ᵗʰ **T57.93** **Toxic effect of unspecified inorganic substance, assault**

   ✓x7ᵗʰ **T57.94** **Toxic effect of unspecified inorganic substance, undetermined**

✓4ᵗʰ **T58** **Toxic effect of carbon monoxide**

   **INCLUDES** asphyxiation from carbon monoxide
toxic effect of carbon monoxide from all sources

> The appropriate 7th character is to be added to each code from category T58.
> A    initial encounter
> D    subsequent encounter
> S    sequela

✓5ᵗʰ **T58.0** **Toxic effect of carbon monoxide** from motor vehicle exhaust
Toxic effect of exhaust gas from gas engine
Toxic effect of exhaust gas from motor pump

   ✓x7ᵗʰ **T58.01** **Toxic effect of carbon monoxide from motor vehicle exhaust**, accidental (unintentional)

   [11] ✓x7ᵗʰ **T58.02** **Toxic effect of carbon monoxide from motor vehicle exhaust**, intentional self-harm   HCC

   ✓x7ᵗʰ **T58.03** **Toxic effect of carbon monoxide from motor vehicle exhaust**, assault

   ✓x7ᵗʰ **T58.04** **Toxic effect of carbon monoxide from motor vehicle exhaust**, undetermined

✓5ᵗʰ **T58.1** **Toxic effect of carbon monoxide** from utility gas
Toxic effect of acetylene
Toxic effect of gas NOS used for lighting, heating, cooking
Toxic effect of water gas

   ✓x7ᵗʰ **T58.11** **Toxic effect of carbon monoxide from utility gas, accidental (unintentional)**

   [11] ✓x7ᵗʰ **T58.12** **Toxic effect of carbon monoxide from utility gas, intentional self-harm**   HCC

   ✓x7ᵗʰ **T58.13** **Toxic effect of carbon monoxide from utility gas, assault**

   ✓x7ᵗʰ **T58.14** **Toxic effect of carbon monoxide from utility gas, undetermined**

✓5ᵗʰ **T58.2** **Toxic effect of carbon monoxide** from incomplete combustion of other domestic fuels
Toxic effect of carbon monoxide from incomplete combustion of coal, coke, kerosene, wood

   ✓6ᵗʰ **T58.2X** **Toxic effect of carbon monoxide from incomplete combustion of other domestic fuels**

      ✓7ᵗʰ **T58.2X1** **Toxic effect of carbon monoxide from incomplete combustion of other domestic fuels**, accidental (unintentional)

      [11] ✓7ᵗʰ **T58.2X2** **Toxic effect of carbon monoxide from incomplete combustion of other domestic fuels**, intentional self-harm   HCC

      ✓7ᵗʰ **T58.2X3** **Toxic effect of carbon monoxide from incomplete combustion of other domestic fuels**, assault

      ✓7ᵗʰ **T58.2X4** **Toxic effect of carbon monoxide from incomplete combustion of other domestic fuels**, undetermined

✓5ᵗʰ **T58.8** **Toxic effect of carbon monoxide** from other source
Toxic effect of carbon monoxide from blast furnace gas
Toxic effect of carbon monoxide from fuels in industrial use
Toxic effect of carbon monoxide from kiln vapor

   ✓6ᵗʰ **T58.8X** **Toxic effect of carbon monoxide from other source**

      ✓7ᵗʰ **T58.8X1** **Toxic effect of carbon monoxide from other source**, accidental (unintentional)

      [11] ✓7ᵗʰ **T58.8X2** **Toxic effect of carbon monoxide from other source**, intentional self-harm   HCC

      ✓7ᵗʰ **T58.8X3** **Toxic effect of carbon monoxide from other source**, assault

      ✓7ᵗʰ **T58.8X4** **Toxic effect of carbon monoxide from other source**, undetermined

✓5ᵗʰ **T58.9** **Toxic effect of carbon monoxide** from unspecified source

   ✓x7ᵗʰ **T58.91** **Toxic effect of carbon monoxide from unspecified source**, accidental (unintentional)

   [11] ✓x7ᵗʰ **T58.92** **Toxic effect of carbon monoxide from unspecified source**, intentional self-harm   HCC

   ✓x7ᵗʰ **T58.93** **Toxic effect of carbon monoxide from unspecified source**, assault

   ✓x7ᵗʰ **T58.94** **Toxic effect of carbon monoxide from unspecified source**, undetermined

✓4ᵗʰ **T59** **Toxic effect of other gases, fumes and vapors**

   **INCLUDES** aerosol propellants
   **EXCLUDES 1** chlorofluorocarbons (T53.5)

> The appropriate 7th character is to be added to each code from category T59.
> A    initial encounter
> D    subsequent encounter
> S    sequela

✓5ᵗʰ **T59.0** **Toxic effect of nitrogen oxides**

   ✓6ᵗʰ **T59.0X** **Toxic effect of** nitrogen oxides

      ✓7ᵗʰ **T59.0X1** **Toxic effect of nitrogen oxides**, accidental (unintentional)
Toxic effect of nitrogen oxides NOS

      [11] ✓7ᵗʰ **T59.0X2** **Toxic effect of nitrogen oxides**, intentional self-harm   HCC

      ✓7ᵗʰ **T59.0X3** **Toxic effect of nitrogen oxides**, assault

      ✓7ᵗʰ **T59.0X4** **Toxic effect of nitrogen oxides**, undetermined

✓5ᵗʰ **T59.1** **Toxic effect of sulfur dioxide**

   ✓6ᵗʰ **T59.1X** **Toxic effect of** sulfur dioxide

      ✓7ᵗʰ **T59.1X1** **Toxic effect of sulfur dioxide**, accidental (unintentional)
Toxic effect of sulfur dioxide NOS

      [11] ✓7ᵗʰ **T59.1X2** **Toxic effect of sulfur dioxide**, intentional self-harm   HCC

      ✓7ᵗʰ **T59.1X3** **Toxic effect of sulfur dioxide**, assault

      ✓7ᵗʰ **T59.1X4** **Toxic effect of sulfur dioxide**, undetermined

---

[11] HCC with 7th character indicating initial encounter (A or B - specific to category) OR sequela.

✓ Additional Character Req   ✓x7ᵗʰ Placeholder Alert   Unacceptable PDx   ■ Manifestation   H1-H14 HAC   HCC CMS-HCC Condition   EXCLUDES 1 Not Coded Here   EXCLUDES 2 Not Included Here

ICD-10-CM 2018                            **1125**

✓5th **T59.2** **Toxic effect of formaldehyde**

    ✓6th **T59.2X** **Toxic effect of** formaldehyde

        ✓7th **T59.2X1** **Toxic effect of formaldehyde,** accidental **(unintentional)**
                Toxic effect of formaldehyde NOS

      11 ✓7th **T59.2X2** **Toxic effect of formaldehyde,** HCC **intentional self-harm**

        ✓7th **T59.2X3** **Toxic effect of formaldehyde,** assault

        ✓7th **T59.2X4** **Toxic effect of formaldehyde, undetermined**

✓5th **T59.3** **Toxic effect of lacrimogenic gas**
    Toxic effect of tear gas

    ✓6th **T59.3X** **Toxic effect of** lacrimogenic gas

        ✓7th **T59.3X1** **Toxic effect of lacrimogenic gas, accidental (unintentional)**
                Toxic effect of lacrimogenic gas NOS

      11 ✓7th **T59.3X2** **Toxic effect of lacrimogenic gas,** HCC **intentional self-harm**

        ✓7th **T59.3X3** **Toxic effect of lacrimogenic gas,** assault

        ✓7th **T59.3X4** **Toxic effect of lacrimogenic gas, undetermined**

✓5th **T59.4** **Toxic effect of chlorine gas**

    ✓6th **T59.4X** **Toxic effect of** chlorine gas

        ✓7th **T59.4X1** **Toxic effect of chlorine gas, accidental (unintentional)**
                Toxic effect of chlorine gas NOS

      11 ✓7th **T59.4X2** **Toxic effect of chlorine gas,** HCC **intentional self-harm**

        ✓7th **T59.4X3** **Toxic effect of chlorine gas,** assault

        ✓7th **T59.4X4** **Toxic effect of chlorine gas,** undetermined

✓5th **T59.5** **Toxic effect of fluorine gas and hydrogen fluoride**

    ✓6th **T59.5X** **Toxic effect of** fluorine gas and hydrogen fluoride

        ✓7th **T59.5X1** **Toxic effect of fluorine gas and hydrogen fluoride, accidental (unintentional)**
                Toxic effect of fluorine gas and hydrogen fluoride NOS

      11 ✓7th **T59.5X2** **Toxic effect of fluorine gas and hydrogen fluoride, intentional self-harm** HCC

        ✓7th **T59.5X3** **Toxic effect of fluorine gas and hydrogen fluoride, assault**

        ✓7th **T59.5X4** **Toxic effect of fluorine gas and hydrogen fluoride, undetermined**

✓5th **T59.6** **Toxic effect of hydrogen sulfide**

    ✓6th **T59.6X** **Toxic effect of** hydrogen sulfide

        ✓7th **T59.6X1** **Toxic effect of hydrogen sulfide, accidental (unintentional)**
                Toxic effect of hydrogen sulfide NOS

      11 ✓7th **T59.6X2** **Toxic effect of hydrogen sulfide,** HCC **intentional self-harm**

        ✓7th **T59.6X3** **Toxic effect of hydrogen sulfide,** assault

        ✓7th **T59.6X4** **Toxic effect of hydrogen sulfide, undetermined**

✓5th **T59.7** **Toxic effect of carbon dioxide**

    ✓6th **T59.7X** **Toxic effect of** carbon dioxide

        ✓7th **T59.7X1** **Toxic effect of carbon dioxide,** accidental **(unintentional)**
                Toxic effect of carbon dioxide NOS

      11 ✓7th **T59.7X2** **Toxic effect of carbon dioxide,** HCC **intentional self-harm**

        ✓7th **T59.7X3** **Toxic effect of carbon dioxide,** assault

        ✓7th **T59.7X4** **Toxic effect of carbon dioxide, undetermined**

✓5th **T59.8** **Toxic effect of** other specified gases, fumes and vapors

    ✓6th **T59.81** **Toxic effect of** smoke
        Smoke inhalation
        EXCLUDES 2 toxic effect of cigarette (tobacco) smoke (T65.22-)

        ✓7th **T59.811** **Toxic effect of smoke,** accidental **(unintentional)**
                Toxic effect of smoke NOS
                **AHA:** 2013, 4Q, 121

      11 ✓7th **T59.812** **Toxic effect of smoke,** intentional **self-harm** HCC

        ✓7th **T59.813** **Toxic effect of smoke,** assault

        ✓7th **T59.814** **Toxic effect of smoke,** undetermined

    ✓6th **T59.89** **Toxic effect of** other specified gases, fumes and vapors

        ✓7th **T59.891** **Toxic effect of other specified gases, fumes and vapors,** accidental **(unintentional)**

      11 ✓7th **T59.892** **Toxic effect of other specified gases,** HCC **fumes and vapors,** intentional self-harm

        ✓7th **T59.893** **Toxic effect of other specified gases, fumes and vapors,** assault

        ✓7th **T59.894** **Toxic effect of other specified gases, fumes and vapors,** undetermined

✓5th **T59.9** **Toxic effect of** unspecified gases, fumes and vapors

    ✓x7th **T59.91** **Toxic effect of unspecified gases, fumes and vapors,** accidental **(unintentional)**

    11 ✓x7th **T59.92** **Toxic effect of unspecified gases, fumes and** HCC **vapors,** intentional self-harm

    ✓x7th **T59.93** **Toxic effect of unspecified gases, fumes and vapors,** assault

    ✓x7th **T59.94** **Toxic effect of unspecified gases, fumes and vapors,** undetermined

✓4th **T60** **Toxic effect of pesticides**
    INCLUDES toxic effect of wood preservatives

    The appropriate 7th character is to be added to each code from category T60.
    A    initial encounter
    D    subsequent encounter
    S    sequela

✓5th **T60.0** **Toxic effect of organophosphate and carbamate insecticides**

    ✓6th **T60.0X** **Toxic effect of** organophosphate and carbamate insecticides

        ✓7th **T60.0X1** **Toxic effect of organophosphate and carbamate insecticides, accidental (unintentional)**
                Toxic effect of organophosphate and carbamate insecticides NOS

      11 ✓7th **T60.0X2** **Toxic effect of organophosphate and** HCC **carbamate insecticides,** intentional self-harm

        ✓7th **T60.0X3** **Toxic effect of organophosphate and carbamate insecticides,** assault

        ✓7th **T60.0X4** **Toxic effect of organophosphate and carbamate insecticides,** undetermined

✓5th **T60.1** **Toxic effect of halogenated insecticides**
    EXCLUDES 1 chlorinated hydrocarbon (T53.-)

    ✓6th **T60.1X** **Toxic effect of** halogenated insecticides

        ✓7th **T60.1X1** **Toxic effect of halogenated insecticides, accidental (unintentional)**
                Toxic effect of halogenated insecticides NOS

      11 ✓7th **T60.1X2** **Toxic effect of halogenated** HCC **insecticides,** intentional self-harm

        ✓7th **T60.1X3** **Toxic effect of halogenated insecticides,** assault

        ✓7th **T60.1X4** **Toxic effect of halogenated insecticides, undetermined**

✓5th **T60.2** **Toxic effect of other insecticides**

    ✓6th **T60.2X** **Toxic effect of** other insecticides

        ✓7th **T60.2X1** **Toxic effect of other insecticides, accidental (unintentional)**
                Toxic effect of other insecticides NOS

      11 ✓7th **T60.2X2** **Toxic effect of other insecticides,** HCC **intentional self-harm**

        ✓7th **T60.2X3** **Toxic effect of other insecticides,** assault

        ✓7th **T60.2X4** **Toxic effect of other insecticides, undetermined**

✓5th **T60.3** **Toxic effect of herbicides and fungicides**

    ✓6th **T60.3X** **Toxic effect of** herbicides and fungicides

        ✓7th **T60.3X1** **Toxic effect of herbicides and fungicides, accidental (unintentional)**
                Toxic effect of herbicides and fungicides NOS

---

11 HCC with 7th character indicating initial encounter (A or B - specific to category) OR sequela.

N Newborn: 0   P Pediatric: 0-17   M Maternity: 12-55   A Adult: 15-124   MCC Major CC Condition   PDx MCC PDx acts as own MCC   CC CC Condition   PDx CC PDx acts as own CC

1126
ICD-10-CM 2018

11 ✓7ᵗʰ **T60.3X2** **Toxic effect of herbicides and fungicides, intentional self-harm** HCC

✓7ᵗʰ **T60.3X3** **Toxic effect of herbicides and fungicides, assault**

✓7ᵗʰ **T60.3X4** **Toxic effect of herbicides and fungicides, undetermined**

✓5ᵗʰ **T60.4** **Toxic effect of rodenticides**

EXCLUDES 1   strychnine and its salts (T65.1)
thallium (T56.81-)

✓6ᵗʰ **T60.4X** **Toxic effect of rodenticides**

✓7ᵗʰ **T60.4X1** **Toxic effect of rodenticides, accidental (unintentional)**
Toxic effect of rodenticides NOS

11 ✓7ᵗʰ **T60.4X2** **Toxic effect of rodenticides, intentional self-harm** HCC

✓7ᵗʰ **T60.4X3** **Toxic effect of rodenticides, assault**

✓7ᵗʰ **T60.4X4** **Toxic effect of rodenticides, undetermined**

✓5ᵗʰ **T60.8** **Toxic effect of other pesticides**

✓6ᵗʰ **T60.8X** **Toxic effect of other pesticides**

✓7ᵗʰ **T60.8X1** **Toxic effect of other pesticides, accidental (unintentional)**
Toxic effect of other pesticides NOS

11 ✓7ᵗʰ **T60.8X2** **Toxic effect of other pesticides, intentional self-harm** HCC

✓7ᵗʰ **T60.8X3** **Toxic effect of other pesticides, assault**

✓7ᵗʰ **T60.8X4** **Toxic effect of other pesticides, undetermined**

✓5ᵗʰ **T60.9** **Toxic effect of unspecified pesticide**

✓ₓ7ᵗʰ **T60.91** **Toxic effect of unspecified pesticide, accidental (unintentional)**

11 ✓ₓ7ᵗʰ **T60.92** **Toxic effect of unspecified pesticide, intentional self-harm** HCC

✓ₓ7ᵗʰ **T60.93** **Toxic effect of unspecified pesticide, assault**

✓ₓ7ᵗʰ **T60.94** **Toxic effect of unspecified pesticide, undetermined**

✓4ᵗʰ **T61** **Toxic effect of noxious substances eaten as seafood**

EXCLUDES 1   allergic reaction to food, such as:
anaphylactic reaction or shock due to adverse food reaction (T78.0-)
bacterial foodborne intoxications (A05.-)
dermatitis (L23.6, L25.4, L27.2)
food protein-induced enterocolitis syndrome (K52.21)
food protein-induced enteropathy (K52.22)
gastroenteritis (noninfective) (K52.29)
toxic effect of aflatoxin and other mycotoxins (T64)
toxic effect of cyanides (T65.0-)
toxic effect of harmful algae bloom (T65.82-)
toxic effect of hydrogen cyanide (T57.3-)
toxic effect of mercury (T56.1-)
toxic effect of red tide (T65.82-)

The appropriate 7th character is to be added to each code from category T61.
A   initial encounter
D   subsequent encounter
S   sequela

✓5ᵗʰ **T61.0** **Ciguatera fish poisoning**

✓ₓ7ᵗʰ **T61.01** **Ciguatera fish poisoning, accidental (unintentional)**

11 ✓ₓ7ᵗʰ **T61.02** **Ciguatera fish poisoning, intentional self-harm** HCC

✓ₓ7ᵗʰ **T61.03** **Ciguatera fish poisoning, assault**

✓ₓ7ᵗʰ **T61.04** **Ciguatera fish poisoning, undetermined**

✓5ᵗʰ **T61.1** **Scombroid fish poisoning**
Histamine-like syndrome

✓ₓ7ᵗʰ **T61.11** **Scombroid fish poisoning, accidental (unintentional)**

11 ✓ₓ7ᵗʰ **T61.12** **Scombroid fish poisoning, intentional self-harm** HCC

✓ₓ7ᵗʰ **T61.13** **Scombroid fish poisoning, assault**

✓ₓ7ᵗʰ **T61.14** **Scombroid fish poisoning, undetermined**

✓5ᵗʰ **T61.7** **Other fish and shellfish poisoning**

✓6ᵗʰ **T61.77** **Other fish poisoning**

✓7ᵗʰ **T61.771** **Other fish poisoning, accidental (unintentional)**

11 ✓7ᵗʰ **T61.772** **Other fish poisoning, intentional self-harm** HCC

✓7ᵗʰ **T61.773** **Other fish poisoning, assault**

✓7ᵗʰ **T61.774** **Other fish poisoning, undetermined**

✓6ᵗʰ **T61.78** **Other shellfish poisoning**

✓7ᵗʰ **T61.781** **Other shellfish poisoning, accidental (unintentional)**

11 ✓7ᵗʰ **T61.782** **Other shellfish poisoning, intentional self-harm** HCC

✓7ᵗʰ **T61.783** **Other shellfish poisoning, assault**

✓7ᵗʰ **T61.784** **Other shellfish poisoning, undetermined**

✓5ᵗʰ **T61.8** **Toxic effect of other seafood**

✓6ᵗʰ **T61.8X** **Toxic effect of other seafood**

✓7ᵗʰ **T61.8X1** **Toxic effect of other seafood, accidental (unintentional)**

11 ✓7ᵗʰ **T61.8X2** **Toxic effect of other seafood, intentional self-harm** HCC

✓7ᵗʰ **T61.8X3** **Toxic effect of other seafood, assault**

✓7ᵗʰ **T61.8X4** **Toxic effect of other seafood, undetermined**

✓5ᵗʰ **T61.9** **Toxic effect of unspecified seafood**

✓ₓ7ᵗʰ **T61.91** **Toxic effect of unspecified seafood, accidental (unintentional)**

11 ✓ₓ7ᵗʰ **T61.92** **Toxic effect of unspecified seafood, intentional self-harm** HCC

✓ₓ7ᵗʰ **T61.93** **Toxic effect of unspecified seafood, assault**

✓ₓ7ᵗʰ **T61.94** **Toxic effect of unspecified seafood, undetermined**

✓4ᵗʰ **T62** **Toxic effect of other noxious substances eaten as food**

EXCLUDES 1   allergic reaction to food, such as:
anaphylactic shock (reaction) due to adverse food reaction (T78.0-)
bacterial food borne intoxications (A05.-)
dermatitis (L23.6, L25.4, L27.2)
food protein-induced enterocolitis syndrome (K52.21)
food protein-induced enteropathy (K52.22)
gastroenteritis (noninfective) (K52.29)
toxic effect of aflatoxin and other mycotoxins (T64)
toxic effect of cyanides (T65.0-)
toxic effect of hydrogen cyanide (T57.3-)
toxic effect of mercury (T56.1-)

The appropriate 7th character is to be added to each code from category T62.
A   initial encounter
D   subsequent encounter
S   sequela

✓5ᵗʰ **T62.0** **Toxic effect of ingested mushrooms**

✓6ᵗʰ **T62.0X** **Toxic effect of ingested mushrooms**

✓7ᵗʰ **T62.0X1** **Toxic effect of ingested mushrooms, accidental (unintentional)**
Toxic effect of ingested mushrooms NOS

11 ✓7ᵗʰ **T62.0X2** **Toxic effect of ingested mushrooms, intentional self-harm** HCC

✓7ᵗʰ **T62.0X3** **Toxic effect of ingested mushrooms, assault**

✓7ᵗʰ **T62.0X4** **Toxic effect of ingested mushrooms, undetermined**

✓5ᵗʰ **T62.1** **Toxic effect of ingested berries**

✓6ᵗʰ **T62.1X** **Toxic effect of ingested berries**

✓7ᵗʰ **T62.1X1** **Toxic effect of ingested berries, accidental (unintentional)**
Toxic effect of ingested berries NOS

11 ✓7ᵗʰ **T62.1X2** **Toxic effect of ingested berries, intentional self-harm** HCC

✓7ᵗʰ **T62.1X3** **Toxic effect of ingested berries, assault**

✓7ᵗʰ **T62.1X4** **Toxic effect of ingested berries, undetermined**

✓5ᵗʰ **T62.2** **Toxic effect of other ingested (parts of) plant(s)**

✓6ᵗʰ **T62.2X** **Toxic effect of other ingested (parts of) plant(s)**

✓7ᵗʰ **T62.2X1** **Toxic effect of other ingested (parts of) plant(s), accidental (unintentional)**
Toxic effect of other ingested (parts of) plant(s) NOS

11 ✓7ᵗʰ **T62.2X2** **Toxic effect of other ingested (parts of) plant(s), intentional self-harm** HCC

---

11 HCC with 7th character indicating initial encounter (A or B - specific to category) OR sequela.

✓ Additional Character Req   ✓ₓ7ᵗʰ Placeholder Alert   Unacceptable PDx   Manifestation   H1 -H14 HAC   HCC CMS-HCC Condition   EXCLUDES 1 Not Coded Here   EXCLUDES 2 Not Included Here

ICD-10-CM 2018      **1127**

✓7th **T62.2X3** **Toxic effect of other ingested (parts of) plant(s)**, assault

✓7th **T62.2X4** **Toxic effect of other ingested (parts of) plant(s)**, undetermined

✓5th **T62.8** **Toxic effect of other specified** noxious substances eaten as food

  ✓6th **T62.8X** **Toxic effect of** other specified noxious substances eaten as food

    ✓7th **T62.8X1** **Toxic effect of other specified noxious substances eaten as food, accidental (unintentional)**
      Toxic effect of other specified noxious substances eaten as food NOS

    11 ✓7th **T62.8X2** **Toxic effect of other specified noxious substances eaten as food, intentional self-harm** `HCC`

    ✓7th **T62.8X3** **Toxic effect of other specified noxious substances eaten as food, assault**

    ✓7th **T62.8X4** **Toxic effect of other specified noxious substances eaten as food, undetermined**

✓5th **T62.9** **Toxic effect of** unspecified noxious substance eaten as food

  ✓x7th **T62.91** **Toxic effect of unspecified noxious substance eaten as food, accidental (unintentional)**
    Toxic effect of unspecified noxious substance eaten as food NOS

  11 ✓x7th **T62.92** **Toxic effect of unspecified noxious substance eaten as food, intentional self-harm** `HCC`

  ✓x7th **T62.93** **Toxic effect of unspecified noxious substance eaten as food, assault**

  ✓x7th **T62.94** **Toxic effect of unspecified noxious substance eaten as food, undetermined**

✓4th **T63** **Toxic effect of contact with venomous animals and plants**
  **INCLUDES**   bite or touch of venomous animal
      pricked or stuck by thorn or leaf
  **EXCLUDES 2**   *ingestion of toxic animal or plant (T61.-, T62.-)*

> The appropriate 7th character is to be added to each code from category T63.
> A     initial encounter
> D     subsequent encounter
> S     sequela

✓5th **T63.0** **Toxic effect of** snake venom

  ✓6th **T63.00** **Toxic effect of** unspecified snake venom

    ✓7th **T63.001** **Toxic effect of unspecified snake venom, accidental (unintentional)**
      Toxic effect of unspecified snake venom NOS

    11 ✓7th **T63.002** **Toxic effect of unspecified snake venom, intentional self-harm** `HCC`

    ✓7th **T63.003** **Toxic effect of unspecified snake venom, assault**

    ✓7th **T63.004** **Toxic effect of unspecified snake venom, undetermined**

  ✓6th **T63.01** **Toxic effect of** rattlesnake venom

    ✓7th **T63.011** **Toxic effect of rattlesnake venom, accidental (unintentional)**
      Toxic effect of rattlesnake venom NOS

    11 ✓7th **T63.012** **Toxic effect of rattlesnake venom, intentional self-harm** `HCC`

    ✓7th **T63.013** **Toxic effect of rattlesnake venom,** assault

    ✓7th **T63.014** **Toxic effect of rattlesnake venom, undetermined**

  ✓6th **T63.02** **Toxic effect of** coral snake venom

    ✓7th **T63.021** **Toxic effect of coral snake venom, accidental (unintentional)**
      Toxic effect of coral snake venom NOS

    11 ✓7th **T63.022** **Toxic effect of coral snake venom, intentional self-harm** `HCC`

    ✓7th **T63.023** **Toxic effect of coral snake venom,** assault

    ✓7th **T63.024** **Toxic effect of coral snake venom, undetermined**

  ✓6th **T63.03** **Toxic effect of** taipan venom

    ✓7th **T63.031** **Toxic effect of taipan venom,** accidental **(unintentional)**
      Toxic effect of taipan venom NOS

  11 ✓7th **T63.032** **Toxic effect of taipan venom, intentional self-harm** `HCC`

  ✓7th **T63.033** **Toxic effect of taipan venom,** assault

  ✓7th **T63.034** **Toxic effect of taipan venom, undetermined**

  ✓6th **T63.04** **Toxic effect of** cobra venom

    ✓7th **T63.041** **Toxic effect of cobra venom, accidental (unintentional)**
      Toxic effect of cobra venom NOS

    11 ✓7th **T63.042** **Toxic effect of cobra venom, intentional self-harm** `HCC`

    ✓7th **T63.043** **Toxic effect of cobra venom,** assault

    ✓7th **T63.044** **Toxic effect of cobra venom, undetermined**

  ✓6th **T63.06** **Toxic effect of venom of** other North and South American snake

    ✓7th **T63.061** **Toxic effect of venom of other North and South American snake, accidental (unintentional)**
      Toxic effect of venom of other North and South American snake NOS

    11 ✓7th **T63.062** **Toxic effect of venom of other North and South American snake, intentional self-harm** `HCC`

    ✓7th **T63.063** **Toxic effect of venom of other North and South American snake,** assault

    ✓7th **T63.064** **Toxic effect of venom of other North and South American snake, undetermined**

  ✓6th **T63.07** **Toxic effect of venom of** other Australian snake

    ✓7th **T63.071** **Toxic effect of venom of other Australian snake, accidental (unintentional)**
      Toxic effect of venom of other Australian snake NOS

    11 ✓7th **T63.072** **Toxic effect of venom of other Australian snake, intentional self-harm** `HCC`

    ✓7th **T63.073** **Toxic effect of venom of other Australian snake,** assault

    ✓7th **T63.074** **Toxic effect of venom of other Australian snake, undetermined**

  ✓6th **T63.08** **Toxic effect of venom of** other African and Asian snake

    ✓7th **T63.081** **Toxic effect of venom of other African and Asian snake, accidental (unintentional)**
      Toxic effect of venom of other African and Asian snake NOS

    11 ✓7th **T63.082** **Toxic effect of venom of other African and Asian snake, intentional self-harm** `HCC`

    ✓7th **T63.083** **Toxic effect of venom of other African and Asian snake,** assault

    ✓7th **T63.084** **Toxic effect of venom of other African and Asian snake, undetermined**

  ✓6th **T63.09** **Toxic effect of venom of** other snake

    ✓7th **T63.091** **Toxic effect of venom of other snake, accidental (unintentional)**
      Toxic effect of venom of other snake NOS

    11 ✓7th **T63.092** **Toxic effect of venom of other snake, intentional self-harm** `HCC`

    ✓7th **T63.093** **Toxic effect of venom of other snake, assault**

    ✓7th **T63.094** **Toxic effect of venom of other snake, undetermined**

✓5th **T63.1** **Toxic effect of venom of** other reptiles

  ✓6th **T63.11** **Toxic effect of venom of** gila monster

    ✓7th **T63.111** **Toxic effect of venom of gila monster, accidental (unintentional)**
      Toxic effect of venom of gila monster NOS

    11 ✓7th **T63.112** **Toxic effect of venom of gila monster, intentional self-harm** `HCC`

    ✓7th **T63.113** **Toxic effect of venom of gila monster, assault**

    ✓7th **T63.114** **Toxic effect of venom of gila monster, undetermined**

---

11 HCC with 7th character indicating initial encounter (A or B - specific to category) OR sequela.

N Newborn: 0   P Pediatric: 0-17   M Maternity: 12-55   A Adult: 15-124   **MCC** Major CC Condition   **PDxMCC** PDx acts as own MCC   **CC** CC Condition   **PDxCC** PDx acts as own CC

1128      ICD-10-CM 2018

✓6th **T63.12** **Toxic effect of venom of** other venomous lizard

  ✓7th **T63.121** **Toxic effect of venom of other venomous lizard,** accidental (unintentional)
      Toxic effect of venom of other venomous lizard NOS

  11 ✓7th **T63.122** **Toxic effect of venom of other venomous lizard,** intentional self-harm  HCC

  ✓7th **T63.123** **Toxic effect of venom of other venomous lizard,** assault

  ✓7th **T63.124** **Toxic effect of venom of other venomous lizard,** undetermined

✓6th **T63.19** **Toxic effect of venom of** other reptiles

  ✓7th **T63.191** **Toxic effect of venom of other reptiles,** accidental (unintentional)
      Toxic effect of venom of other reptiles NOS

  11 ✓7th **T63.192** **Toxic effect of venom of other reptiles,** intentional self-harm  HCC

  ✓7th **T63.193** **Toxic effect of venom of other reptiles,** assault

  ✓7th **T63.194** **Toxic effect of venom of other reptiles,** undetermined

✓5th **T63.2** **Toxic effect of venom of** scorpion

  ✓6th **T63.2X** **Toxic effect of venom of scorpion**

    ✓7th **T63.2X1** **Toxic effect of venom of scorpion,** accidental (unintentional)
        Toxic effect of venom of scorpion NOS

    11 ✓7th **T63.2X2** **Toxic effect of venom of scorpion,** intentional self-harm  HCC

    ✓7th **T63.2X3** **Toxic effect of venom of scorpion,** assault

    ✓7th **T63.2X4** **Toxic effect of venom of scorpion,** undetermined

✓5th **T63.3** **Toxic effect of venom of** spider

  ✓6th **T63.30** **Toxic effect of** unspecified **spider venom**

    ✓7th **T63.301** **Toxic effect of unspecified spider venom,** accidental (unintentional)

    11 ✓7th **T63.302** **Toxic effect of unspecified spider venom,** intentional self-harm  HCC

    ✓7th **T63.303** **Toxic effect of unspecified spider venom,** assault

    ✓7th **T63.304** **Toxic effect of unspecified spider venom,** undetermined

  ✓6th **T63.31** **Toxic effect of venom of** black widow **spider**

    ✓7th **T63.311** **Toxic effect of venom of black widow spider,** accidental (unintentional)

    11 ✓7th **T63.312** **Toxic effect of venom of black widow spider,** intentional self-harm  HCC

    ✓7th **T63.313** **Toxic effect of venom of black widow spider,** assault

    ✓7th **T63.314** **Toxic effect of venom of black widow spider,** undetermined

  ✓6th **T63.32** **Toxic effect of venom of** tarantula

    ✓7th **T63.321** **Toxic effect of venom of tarantula,** accidental (unintentional)

    11 ✓7th **T63.322** **Toxic effect of venom of tarantula,** intentional self-harm  HCC

    ✓7th **T63.323** **Toxic effect of venom of tarantula,** assault

    ✓7th **T63.324** **Toxic effect of venom of tarantula,** undetermined

  ✓6th **T63.33** **Toxic effect of venom of** brown recluse **spider**

    ✓7th **T63.331** **Toxic effect of venom of brown recluse spider,** accidental (unintentional)

    11 ✓7th **T63.332** **Toxic effect of venom of brown recluse spider,** intentional self-harm  HCC

    ✓7th **T63.333** **Toxic effect of venom of brown recluse spider,** assault

    ✓7th **T63.334** **Toxic effect of venom of brown recluse spider,** undetermined

  ✓6th **T63.39** **Toxic effect of venom of** other spider

    ✓7th **T63.391** **Toxic effect of venom of other spider,** accidental (unintentional)

    11 ✓7th **T63.392** **Toxic effect of venom of other spider,** intentional self-harm  HCC

    ✓7th **T63.393** **Toxic effect of venom of other spider,** assault

    ✓7th **T63.394** **Toxic effect of venom of other spider,** undetermined

✓5th **T63.4** **Toxic effect of venom of** other arthropods

  ✓6th **T63.41** **Toxic effect of venom of** centipedes and venomous millipedes

    ✓7th **T63.411** **Toxic effect of venom of centipedes and venomous millipedes,** accidental (unintentional)

    11 ✓7th **T63.412** **Toxic effect of venom of centipedes and venomous millipedes,** intentional self-harm  HCC

    ✓7th **T63.413** **Toxic effect of venom of centipedes and venomous millipedes,** assault

    ✓7th **T63.414** **Toxic effect of venom of centipedes and venomous millipedes,** undetermined

  ✓6th **T63.42** **Toxic effect of venom of** ants

    ✓7th **T63.421** **Toxic effect of venom of ants,** accidental (unintentional)

    11 ✓7th **T63.422** **Toxic effect of venom of ants,** intentional self-harm  HCC

    ✓7th **T63.423** **Toxic effect of venom of ants,** assault

    ✓7th **T63.424** **Toxic effect of venom of ants,** undetermined

  ✓6th **T63.43** **Toxic effect of venom of** caterpillars

    ✓7th **T63.431** **Toxic effect of venom of caterpillars,** accidental (unintentional)

    11 ✓7th **T63.432** **Toxic effect of venom of caterpillars,** intentional self-harm  HCC

    ✓7th **T63.433** **Toxic effect of venom of caterpillars,** assault

    ✓7th **T63.434** **Toxic effect of venom of caterpillars,** undetermined

  ✓6th **T63.44** **Toxic effect of venom of** bees

    ✓7th **T63.441** **Toxic effect of venom of bees,** accidental (unintentional)

    11 ✓7th **T63.442** **Toxic effect of venom of bees,** intentional self-harm  HCC

    ✓7th **T63.443** **Toxic effect of venom of bees,** assault

    ✓7th **T63.444** **Toxic effect of venom of bees,** undetermined

  ✓6th **T63.45** **Toxic effect of venom of** hornets

    ✓7th **T63.451** **Toxic effect of venom of hornets,** accidental (unintentional)

    11 ✓7th **T63.452** **Toxic effect of venom of hornets,** intentional self-harm  HCC

    ✓7th **T63.453** **Toxic effect of venom of hornets,** assault

    ✓7th **T63.454** **Toxic effect of venom of hornets,** undetermined

  ✓6th **T63.46** **Toxic effect of venom of** wasps
    Toxic effect of yellow jacket

    ✓7th **T63.461** **Toxic effect of venom of wasps,** accidental (unintentional)

    11 ✓7th **T63.462** **Toxic effect of venom of wasps,** intentional self-harm  HCC

    ✓7th **T63.463** **Toxic effect of venom of wasps,** assault

    ✓7th **T63.464** **Toxic effect of venom of wasps,** undetermined

  ✓6th **T63.48** **Toxic effect of venom of** other arthropod

    ✓7th **T63.481** **Toxic effect of venom of other arthropod,** accidental (unintentional)

    11 ✓7th **T63.482** **Toxic effect of venom of other arthropod,** intentional self-harm  HCC

    ✓7th **T63.483** **Toxic effect of venom of other arthropod,** assault

    ✓7th **T63.484** **Toxic effect of venom of other arthropod,** undetermined

✓5th **T63.5** **Toxic effect of contact with** venomous fish
    EXCLUDES 2    poisoning by ingestion of fish (T61.-)

  ✓6th **T63.51** **Toxic effect of contact with** stingray

    ✓7th **T63.511** **Toxic effect of contact with stingray,** accidental (unintentional)

---

11 HCC with 7th character indicating initial encounter (A or B - specific to category) OR sequela.

✓ Additional Character Req    ✓x7th Placeholder Alert    Unacceptable PDx    Manifestation    H1-H14 HAC    HCC CMS-HCC Condition    EXCLUDES 1 Not Coded Here    EXCLUDES 2 Not Included Here

**11** ✓7th **T63.512 Toxic effect of contact with stingray, intentional self-harm** HCC

✓7th **T63.513 Toxic effect of contact with stingray, assault**

✓7th **T63.514 Toxic effect of contact with stingray, undetermined**

✓6th **T63.59 Toxic effect of contact with** other venomous fish

✓7th **T63.591 Toxic effect of contact with other venomous fish,** accidental (unintentional)

**11** ✓7th **T63.592 Toxic effect of contact with other venomous fish,** intentional self-harm HCC

✓7th **T63.593 Toxic effect of contact with other venomous fish,** assault

✓7th **T63.594 Toxic effect of contact with other venomous fish,** undetermined

✓5th **T63.6 Toxic effect of contact with other** venomous marine animals

     EXCLUDES 1   *sea-snake venom (T63.09)*

     EXCLUDES 2   *poisoning by ingestion of shellfish (T61.78-)*

✓6th **T63.61 Toxic effect of contact with** Portugese Man-o-war
     Toxic effect of contact with bluebottle

✓7th **T63.611 Toxic effect of contact with Portugese Man-o-war,** accidental (unintentional)

**11** ✓7th **T63.612 Toxic effect of contact with Portugese Man-o-war,** intentional self-harm HCC

✓7th **T63.613 Toxic effect of contact with Portugese Man-o-war,** assault

✓7th **T63.614 Toxic effect of contact with Portugese Man-o-war,** undetermined

✓6th **T63.62 Toxic effect of contact with** other jellyfish

✓7th **T63.621 Toxic effect of contact with other jellyfish,** accidental (unintentional)

**11** ✓7th **T63.622 Toxic effect of contact with other jellyfish,** intentional self-harm HCC

✓7th **T63.623 Toxic effect of contact with other jellyfish,** assault

✓7th **T63.624 Toxic effect of contact with other jellyfish,** undetermined

✓6th **T63.63 Toxic effect of contact with** sea anemone

✓7th **T63.631 Toxic effect of contact with sea anemone,** accidental (unintentional)

**11** ✓7th **T63.632 Toxic effect of contact with sea anemone,** intentional self-harm HCC

✓7th **T63.633 Toxic effect of contact with sea anemone,** assault

✓7th **T63.634 Toxic effect of contact with sea anemone,** undetermined

✓6th **T63.69 Toxic effect of contact with** other venomous marine animals

✓7th **T63.691 Toxic effect of contact with other venomous marine animals,** accidental (unintentional)

**11** ✓7th **T63.692 Toxic effect of contact with other venomous marine animals,** intentional self-harm HCC

✓7th **T63.693 Toxic effect of contact with other venomous marine animals,** assault

✓7th **T63.694 Toxic effect of contact with other venomous marine animals,** undetermined

✓5th **T63.7 Toxic effect of contact with** venomous plant

✓6th **T63.71 Toxic effect of contact with venomous** marine plant

✓7th **T63.711 Toxic effect of contact with venomous marine plant,** accidental (unintentional)

**11** ✓7th **T63.712 Toxic effect of contact with venomous marine plant,** intentional self-harm HCC

✓7th **T63.713 Toxic effect of contact with venomous marine plant,** assault

✓7th **T63.714 Toxic effect of contact with venomous marine plant,** undetermined

✓6th **T63.79 Toxic effect of contact with** other venomous plant

✓7th **T63.791 Toxic effect of contact with other venomous plant,** accidental (unintentional)

**11** ✓7th **T63.792 Toxic effect of contact with other venomous plant,** intentional self-harm HCC

✓7th **T63.793 Toxic effect of contact with other venomous plant,** assault

✓7th **T63.794 Toxic effect of contact with other venomous plant,** undetermined

✓5th **T63.8 Toxic effect of contact with** other venomous animals

✓6th **T63.81 Toxic effect of contact with venomous** frog

     EXCLUDES 1   *contact with nonvenomous frog (W62.0)*

✓7th **T63.811 Toxic effect of contact with venomous frog,** accidental (unintentional)

**11** ✓7th **T63.812 Toxic effect of contact with venomous frog,** intentional self-harm HCC

✓7th **T63.813 Toxic effect of contact with venomous frog,** assault

✓7th **T63.814 Toxic effect of contact with venomous frog,** undetermined

✓6th **T63.82 Toxic effect of contact with venomous** toad

     EXCLUDES 1   *contact with nonvenomous toad (W62.1)*

✓7th **T63.821 Toxic effect of contact with venomous toad,** accidental (unintentional)

**11** ✓7th **T63.822 Toxic effect of contact with venomous toad,** intentional self-harm HCC

✓7th **T63.823 Toxic effect of contact with venomous toad,** assault

✓7th **T63.824 Toxic effect of contact with venomous toad,** undetermined

✓6th **T63.83 Toxic effect of contact with** other venomous amphibian

     EXCLUDES 1   *contact with nonvenomous amphibian (W62.9)*

✓7th **T63.831 Toxic effect of contact with other venomous amphibian,** accidental (unintentional)

**11** ✓7th **T63.832 Toxic effect of contact with other venomous amphibian,** intentional self-harm HCC

✓7th **T63.833 Toxic effect of contact with other venomous amphibian,** assault

✓7th **T63.834 Toxic effect of contact with other venomous amphibian,** undetermined

✓6th **T63.89 Toxic effect of contact with** other venomous animals

✓7th **T63.891 Toxic effect of contact with other venomous animals,** accidental (unintentional)

**11** ✓7th **T63.892 Toxic effect of contact with other venomous animals,** intentional self-harm HCC

✓7th **T63.893 Toxic effect of contact with other venomous animals,** assault

✓7th **T63.894 Toxic effect of contact with other venomous animals,** undetermined

✓5th **T63.9 Toxic effect of contact with** unspecified venomous animal

✓x7th **T63.91 Toxic effect of contact with unspecified venomous animal,** accidental (unintentional)

**11** ✓x7th **T63.92 Toxic effect of contact with unspecified venomous animal,** intentional self-harm HCC

✓x7th **T63.93 Toxic effect of contact with unspecified venomous animal,** assault

✓x7th **T63.94 Toxic effect of contact with unspecified venomous animal,** undetermined

✓4th **T64 Toxic effect of aflatoxin and other mycotoxin food contaminants**

     The appropriate 7th character is to be added to each code from category T64.
     A   initial encounter
     D   subsequent encounter
     S   sequela

✓5th **T64.0 Toxic effect of** aflatoxin

✓x7th **T64.01 Toxic effect of aflatoxin,** accidental (unintentional)

**11** ✓x7th **T64.02 Toxic effect of aflatoxin,** intentional self-harm HCC

✓x7th **T64.03 Toxic effect of aflatoxin,** assault

✓x7th **T64.04 Toxic effect of aflatoxin,** undetermined

---

**11** HCC with 7th character indicating initial encounter (A or B - specific to category) OR sequela.

N Newborn: 0   P Pediatric: 0-17   M Maternity: 12-55   A Adult: 15-124   MCC Major CC Condition   PDxMCC PDx acts as own MCC   CC CC Condition   PDxCC PDx acts as own CC

**1130**              ICD-10-CM 2018

√5ᵗʰ **T64.8   Toxic effect of** other mycotoxin food contaminants

√x7ᵗʰ **T64.81   Toxic effect of other mycotoxin food contaminants, accidental (unintentional)**

11  √x7ᵗʰ **T64.82   Toxic effect of other mycotoxin food contaminants, intentional self-harm**   HCC

√x7ᵗʰ **T64.83   Toxic effect of other mycotoxin food contaminants, assault**

√x7ᵗʰ **T64.84   Toxic effect of other mycotoxin food contaminants, undetermined**

√4ᵗʰ **T65   Toxic effect of other and unspecified substances**

The appropriate 7th character is to be added to each code from category T65.
A    initial encounter
D    subsequent encounter
S    sequela

√5ᵗʰ **T65.0   Toxic effect of** cyanides

EXCLUDES 1    hydrogen cyanide (T57.3-)

√6ᵗʰ **T65.0X   Toxic effect of cyanides**

√7ᵗʰ **T65.0X1   Toxic effect of cyanides, accidental (unintentional)**
Toxic effect of cyanides NOS

11  √7ᵗʰ **T65.0X2   Toxic effect of cyanides, intentional self-harm**   HCC

√7ᵗʰ **T65.0X3   Toxic effect of cyanides, assault**

√7ᵗʰ **T65.0X4   Toxic effect of cyanides, undetermined**

√5ᵗʰ **T65.1   Toxic effect of** strychnine and its salts

√6ᵗʰ **T65.1X   Toxic effect of strychnine and its salts**

√7ᵗʰ **T65.1X1   Toxic effect of strychnine and its salts, accidental (unintentional)**
Toxic effect of strychnine and its salts NOS

11  √7ᵗʰ **T65.1X2   Toxic effect of strychnine and its salts, intentional self-harm**   HCC

√7ᵗʰ **T65.1X3   Toxic effect of strychnine and its salts, assault**

√7ᵗʰ **T65.1X4   Toxic effect of strychnine and its salts, undetermined**

√5ᵗʰ **T65.2   Toxic effect of** tobacco and nicotine

EXCLUDES 2    nicotine dependence (F17.-)

√6ᵗʰ **T65.21   Toxic effect of** chewing tobacco

√7ᵗʰ **T65.211   Toxic effect of chewing tobacco, accidental (unintentional)**
Toxic effect of chewing tobacco NOS

11  √7ᵗʰ **T65.212   Toxic effect of chewing tobacco, intentional self-harm**   HCC

√7ᵗʰ **T65.213   Toxic effect of chewing tobacco, assault**

√7ᵗʰ **T65.214   Toxic effect of chewing tobacco, undetermined**

√6ᵗʰ **T65.22   Toxic effect of** tobacco cigarettes
Toxic effect of tobacco smoke
Use additional code for exposure to second hand tobacco smoke (Z57.31, Z77.22)

√7ᵗʰ **T65.221   Toxic effect of tobacco cigarettes, accidental (unintentional)**
Toxic effect of tobacco cigarettes NOS

11  √7ᵗʰ **T65.222   Toxic effect of tobacco cigarettes, intentional self-harm**   HCC

√7ᵗʰ **T65.223   Toxic effect of tobacco cigarettes, assault**

√7ᵗʰ **T65.224   Toxic effect of tobacco cigarettes, undetermined**

√6ᵗʰ **T65.29   Toxic effect of** other tobacco and nicotine

√7ᵗʰ **T65.291   Toxic effect of other tobacco and nicotine, accidental (unintentional)**
Toxic effect of other tobacco and nicotine NOS

11  √7ᵗʰ **T65.292   Toxic effect of other tobacco and nicotine, intentional self-harm**   HCC

√7ᵗʰ **T65.293   Toxic effect of other tobacco and nicotine, assault**

√7ᵗʰ **T65.294   Toxic effect of other tobacco and nicotine, undetermined**

√5ᵗʰ **T65.3   Toxic effect of** nitroderivatives and aminoderivatives of benzene and its homologues
Toxic effect of anilin [benzenamine]
Toxic effect of nitrobenzene
Toxic effect of trinitrotoluene

√6ᵗʰ **T65.3X   Toxic effect of nitroderivatives and aminoderivatives of benzene and its homologues**

√7ᵗʰ **T65.3X1   Toxic effect of nitroderivatives and aminoderivatives of benzene and its homologues, accidental (unintentional)**
Toxic effect of nitroderivatives and aminoderivatives of benzene and its homologues NOS

11  √7ᵗʰ **T65.3X2   Toxic effect of nitroderivatives and aminoderivatives of benzene and its homologues, intentional self-harm**   HCC

√7ᵗʰ **T65.3X3   Toxic effect of nitroderivatives and aminoderivatives of benzene and its homologues, assault**

√7ᵗʰ **T65.3X4   Toxic effect of nitroderivatives and aminoderivatives of benzene and its homologues, undetermined**

√5ᵗʰ **T65.4   Toxic effect of** carbon disulfide

√6ᵗʰ **T65.4X   Toxic effect of carbon disulfide**

√7ᵗʰ **T65.4X1   Toxic effect of carbon disulfide, accidental (unintentional)**
Toxic effect of carbon disulfide NOS

11  √7ᵗʰ **T65.4X2   Toxic effect of carbon disulfide, intentional self-harm**   HCC

√7ᵗʰ **T65.4X3   Toxic effect of carbon disulfide, assault**

√7ᵗʰ **T65.4X4   Toxic effect of carbon disulfide, undetermined**

√5ᵗʰ **T65.5   Toxic effect of** nitroglycerin and other nitric acids and esters
Toxic effect of 1,2,3-Propanetriol trinitrate

√6ᵗʰ **T65.5X   Toxic effect of nitroglycerin and other nitric acids and esters**

√7ᵗʰ **T65.5X1   Toxic effect of nitroglycerin and other nitric acids and esters, accidental (unintentional)**
Toxic effect of nitroglycerin and other nitric acids and esters NOS

11  √7ᵗʰ **T65.5X2   Toxic effect of nitroglycerin and other nitric acids and esters, intentional self-harm**   HCC

√7ᵗʰ **T65.5X3   Toxic effect of nitroglycerin and other nitric acids and esters, assault**

√7ᵗʰ **T65.5X4   Toxic effect of nitroglycerin and other nitric acids and esters, undetermined**

√5ᵗʰ **T65.6   Toxic effect of** paints and dyes, not elsewhere classified

√6ᵗʰ **T65.6X   Toxic effect of paints and dyes, not elsewhere classified**

√7ᵗʰ **T65.6X1   Toxic effect of paints and dyes, not elsewhere classified, accidental (unintentional)**
Toxic effect of paints and dyes NOS

11  √7ᵗʰ **T65.6X2   Toxic effect of paints and dyes, not elsewhere classified, intentional self-harm**   HCC

√7ᵗʰ **T65.6X3   Toxic effect of paints and dyes, not elsewhere classified, assault**

√7ᵗʰ **T65.6X4   Toxic effect of paints and dyes, not elsewhere classified, undetermined**

√5ᵗʰ **T65.8   Toxic effect of** other specified substances

√6ᵗʰ **T65.81   Toxic effect of** latex

√7ᵗʰ **T65.811   Toxic effect of latex, accidental (unintentional)**
Toxic effect of latex NOS

11  √7ᵗʰ **T65.812   Toxic effect of latex, intentional self-harm**   HCC

√7ᵗʰ **T65.813   Toxic effect of latex, assault**

√7ᵗʰ **T65.814   Toxic effect of latex, undetermined**

---

11 HCC with 7th character indicating initial encounter (A or B - specific to category) OR sequela.

---

√ Additional Character Req   √x7ᵗʰ Placeholder Alert   Unacceptable PDx   Manifestation   H1-H14 HAC   HCC CMS-HCC Condition   EXCLUDES 1 Not Coded Here   EXCLUDES 2 Not Included Here

**√6th T65.82 Toxic effect of harmful algae and algae toxins**
Toxic effect of (harmful) algae bloom NOS
Toxic effect of blue-green algae bloom
Toxic effect of brown tide
Toxic effect of cyanobacteria bloom
Toxic effect of Florida red tide
Toxic effect of pfiesteria piscicida
Toxic effect of red tide

√7th **T65.821 Toxic effect of harmful algae and algae toxins, accidental (unintentional)**
Toxic effect of harmful algae and algae toxins NOS

11 √7th **T65.822 Toxic effect of harmful algae and algae toxins, intentional self-harm** HCC

√7th **T65.823 Toxic effect of harmful algae and algae toxins, assault**

√7th **T65.824 Toxic effect of harmful algae and algae toxins, undetermined**

**√6th T65.83 Toxic effect of fiberglass**

√7th **T65.831 Toxic effect of fiberglass, accidental (unintentional)**
Toxic effect of fiberglass NOS

11 √7th **T65.832 Toxic effect of fiberglass, intentional self-harm** HCC

√7th **T65.833 Toxic effect of fiberglass, assault**

√7th **T65.834 Toxic effect of fiberglass, undetermined**

**√6th T65.89 Toxic effect of other specified substances**

√7th **T65.891 Toxic effect of other specified substances, accidental (unintentional)**
Toxic effect of other specified substances NOS

11 √7th **T65.892 Toxic effect of other specified substances, intentional self-harm** HCC

√7th **T65.893 Toxic effect of other specified substances, assault**

√7th **T65.894 Toxic effect of other specified substances, undetermined**

**√5th T65.9 Toxic effect of unspecified substance**

√x7th **T65.91 Toxic effect of unspecified substance, accidental (unintentional)**
Poisoning NOS

11 √x7th **T65.92 Toxic effect of unspecified substance, intentional self-harm** HCC

√x7th **T65.93 Toxic effect of unspecified substance, assault**

√x7th **T65.94 Toxic effect of unspecified substance, undetermined**

## Other and unspecified effects of external causes (T66-T78)

√x7th **T66 Radiation sickness, unspecified**
EXCLUDES 1    specified adverse effects of radiation, such as:
  burns (T20-T31)
  leukemia (C91-C95)
  radiation gastroenteritis and colitis (K52.0)
  radiation pneumonitis (J70.0)
  radiation related disorders of the skin and subcutaneous tissue
    (L55-L59)
  radiation sunburn (L55.-)

The appropriate 7th character is to be added to code T66.
A    initial encounter
D    subsequent encounter
S    sequela

√4th **T67 Effects of heat and light**
EXCLUDES 1    erythema [dermatitis] ab igne (L59.0)
  malignant hyperpyrexia due to anesthesia (T88.3)
  radiation-related disorders of the skin and subcutaneous tissue
    (L55-L59)
EXCLUDES 2    burns (T20-T31)
  sunburn (L55.-)
  sweat disorder due to heat (L74-L75)

The appropriate 7th character is to be added to each code from
category T67.
A    initial encounter
D    subsequent encounter
S    sequela

√x7th **T67.0 Heatstroke and sunstroke** CC H5
Heat apoplexy          Siriasis
Heat pyrexia           Thermoplegia
Use additional code(s) to identify any associated complications
  of heatstroke, such as:
  coma and stupor (R40.-)
  systemic inflammatory response syndrome (R65.1-)
**DEF:** Headache, vertigo, cramps, and elevated body temperature
due to prolonged exposure to high environmental temperatures;
requires emergency intervention.
**CC Excl:** PDX collection 1419

√x7th **T67.1 Heat syncope**
Heat collapse

√x7th **T67.2 Heat cramp**

√x7th **T67.3 Heat exhaustion, anhydrotic**
Heat prostration due to water depletion
EXCLUDES 1    heat exhaustion due to salt depletion (T67.4)

√x7th **T67.4 Heat exhaustion due to salt depletion**
Heat prostration due to salt (and water) depletion

√x7th **T67.5 Heat exhaustion, unspecified**
Heat prostration NOS

√x7th **T67.6 Heat fatigue, transient**

√x7th **T67.7 Heat edema**

√x7th **T67.8 Other effects of heat and light**

√x7th **T67.9 Effect of heat and light, unspecified**

√x7th **T68 Hypothermia**
Accidental hypothermia
Hypothermia NOS
Use additional code to identify source of exposure:
  exposure to excessive cold of man-made origin (W93)
  exposure to excessive cold of natural origin (X31)
EXCLUDES 1    hypothermia following anesthesia (T88.51)
  hypothermia not associated with low environmental
    temperature (R68.0)
  hypothermia of newborn (P80.-)
EXCLUDES 2    frostbite (T33-T34)

The appropriate 7th character is to be added to code T68.
A    initial encounter
D    subsequent encounter
S    sequela

√4th **T69 Other effects of reduced temperature**
Use additional code to identify source of exposure:
  exposure to excessive cold of man-made origin (W93)
  exposure to excessive cold of natural origin (X31)
EXCLUDES 2    frostbite (T33-T34)

The appropriate 7th character is to be added to each code from
category T69.
A    initial encounter
D    subsequent encounter
S    sequela

√5th **T69.0 Immersion hand and foot**

√6th **T69.01 Immersion hand**

√7th **T69.011 Immersion hand, right hand**

√7th **T69.012 Immersion hand, left hand**

√7th **T69.019 Immersion hand, unspecified hand**

√6th **T69.02 Immersion foot**
Trench foot

**CC Excl:** For codes in subcategory T69.02:
PDX collection 1420

√7th **T69.021 Immersion foot, right foot** CC H5

√7th **T69.022 Immersion foot, left foot** CC H5

√7th **T69.029 Immersion foot, unspecified foot** CC H5

√x7th **T69.1 Chilblains**
**DEF:** Red, swollen, itchy skin primarily affecting the fingers and
toes, nose and ears, and legs; follows damp-cold exposure; can
also be associated with pruritus and a burning feeling.

√x7th **T69.8 Other specified effects of reduced temperature**

√x7th **T69.9 Effect of reduced temperature, unspecified**

---

11 HCC with 7th character indicating initial encounter (A or B - specific to category) OR sequela.

☑4ᵗʰ **T70   Effects of air pressure and water pressure**

> The appropriate 7th character is to be added to each code from category T70.
> A    initial encounter
> D    subsequent encounter
> S    sequela

☑x7ᵗʰ **T70.0   Otitic barotrauma**
> Aero-otitis media
> Effects of change in ambient atmospheric pressure or water pressure on ears

☑x7ᵗʰ **T70.1   Sinus barotrauma**
> Aerosinusitis
> Effects of change in ambient atmospheric pressure on sinuses

☑5ᵗʰ **T70.2   Other and unspecified effects of high altitude**
> EXCLUDES 2   *polycythemia due to high altitude (D75.1)*

> ☑x7ᵗʰ **T70.20   Unspecified effects of high altitude**

> ☑x7ᵗʰ **T70.29   Other effects of high altitude**
> > Alpine sickness       Hypobaropathy
> > Anoxia due to high altitude    Mountain sickness
> > Barotrauma NOS

☑x7ᵗʰ **T70.3   Caisson disease [decompression sickness]**   `CC` `H5`
> Compressed-air disease
> Diver's palsy or paralysis
> **DEF:** Rapid reduction in air pressure while breathing compressed air; symptoms include skin lesions, joint pains, and respiratory and neurological problems.
> **CC Excl:** PDX collection 1421

☑x7ᵗʰ **T70.4   Effects of high-pressure fluids**
> Hydraulic jet injection (industrial)
> Pneumatic jet injection (industrial)
> Traumatic jet injection (industrial)

☑x7ᵗʰ **T70.8   Other effects of air pressure and water pressure**

☑x7ᵗʰ **T70.9   Effect of air pressure and water pressure, unspecified**

☑4ᵗʰ **T71   Asphyxiation**
> Mechanical suffocation
> Traumatic suffocation
> EXCLUDES 1   *acute respiratory distress (syndrome) (J80)*
> > *anoxia due to high altitude (T70.2)*
> > *asphyxia NOS (R09.01)*
> > *asphyxia from carbon monoxide (T58.-)*
> > *asphyxia from inhalation of food or foreign body (T17.-)*
> > *asphyxia from other gases, fumes and vapors (T59.-)*
> > *respiratory distress (syndrome) in newborn (P22.-)*

> The appropriate 7th character is to be added to each code from category T71.
> A    initial encounter
> D    subsequent encounter
> S    sequela

> **CC Excl: For codes in category T71:** PDX collection 1422

☑5ᵗʰ **T71.1   Asphyxiation due to mechanical threat to breathing**
> Suffocation due to mechanical threat to breathing

> ☑6ᵗʰ **T71.11   Asphyxiation due to smothering under pillow**

> > ☑7ᵗʰ **T71.111   Asphyxiation due to smothering under pillow, accidental**   `CC` `H5`
> > > Asphyxiation due to smothering under pillow NOS

> > 11   ☑7ᵗʰ **T71.112   Asphyxiation due to smothering under pillow, intentional self-harm**   `CC` `H5` `HCC`

> > ☑7ᵗʰ **T71.113   Asphyxiation due to smothering under pillow, assault**   `CC` `H5`

> > ☑7ᵗʰ **T71.114   Asphyxiation due to smothering under pillow, undetermined**   `CC` `H5`

> ☑6ᵗʰ **T71.12   Asphyxiation due to plastic bag**

> > ☑7ᵗʰ **T71.121   Asphyxiation due to plastic bag, accidental**   `CC` `H5`
> > > Asphyxiation due to plastic bag NOS

> > 11   ☑7ᵗʰ **T71.122   Asphyxiation due to plastic bag, intentional self-harm**   `CC` `H5` `HCC`

> > ☑7ᵗʰ **T71.123   Asphyxiation due to plastic bag, assault**   `CC` `H5`

> > ☑7ᵗʰ **T71.124   Asphyxiation due to plastic bag, undetermined**   `CC` `H5`

☑6ᵗʰ **T71.13   Asphyxiation due to being trapped in bed linens**

> ☑7ᵗʰ **T71.131   Asphyxiation due to being trapped in bed linens, accidental**   `CC` `H5`
> > Asphyxiation due to being trapped in bed linens NOS

> 11   ☑7ᵗʰ **T71.132   Asphyxiation due to being trapped in bed linens, intentional self-harm**   `CC` `H5` `HCC`

> ☑7ᵗʰ **T71.133   Asphyxiation due to being trapped in bed linens, assault**   `CC` `H5`

> ☑7ᵗʰ **T71.134   Asphyxiation due to being trapped in bed linens, undetermined**   `CC` `H5`

☑6ᵗʰ **T71.14   Asphyxiation due to smothering under another person's body (in bed)**

> ☑7ᵗʰ **T71.141   Asphyxiation due to smothering under another person's body (in bed), accidental**   `CC` `H5`
> > Asphyxiation due to smothering under another person's body (in bed) NOS

> ☑7ᵗʰ **T71.143   Asphyxiation due to smothering under another person's body (in bed), assault**   `CC` `H5`

> ☑7ᵗʰ **T71.144   Asphyxiation due to smothering under another person's body (in bed), undetermined**   `CC` `H5`

☑6ᵗʰ **T71.15   Asphyxiation due to smothering in furniture**

> ☑7ᵗʰ **T71.151   Asphyxiation due to smothering in furniture, accidental**   `CC` `H5`
> > Asphyxiation due to smothering in furniture NOS

> 11   ☑7ᵗʰ **T71.152   Asphyxiation due to smothering in furniture, intentional self-harm**   `CC` `H5` `HCC`

> ☑7ᵗʰ **T71.153   Asphyxiation due to smothering in furniture, assault**   `CC` `H5`

> ☑7ᵗʰ **T71.154   Asphyxiation due to smothering in furniture, undetermined**   `CC` `H5`

☑6ᵗʰ **T71.16   Asphyxiation due to hanging**
> Hanging by window shade cord
> Use additional code for any associated injuries, such as:
> crushing injury of neck (S17.-)
> fracture of cervical vertebrae (S12.0-S12.2-)
> open wound of neck (S11.-)

> ☑7ᵗʰ **T71.161   Asphyxiation due to hanging, accidental**   `CC` `H5`
> > Asphyxiation due to hanging NOS
> > Hanging NOS

> 11   ☑7ᵗʰ **T71.162   Asphyxiation due to hanging, intentional self-harm**   `CC` `H5` `HCC`

> ☑7ᵗʰ **T71.163   Asphyxiation due to hanging, assault**   `CC` `H5`

> ☑7ᵗʰ **T71.164   Asphyxiation due to hanging, undetermined**   `CC` `H5`

☑6ᵗʰ **T71.19   Asphyxiation due to mechanical threat to breathing due to other causes**

> ☑7ᵗʰ **T71.191   Asphyxiation due to mechanical threat to breathing due to other causes, accidental**   `CC` `H5`
> > Asphyxiation due to other causes NOS

> 11   ☑7ᵗʰ **T71.192   Asphyxiation due to mechanical threat to breathing due to other causes, intentional self-harm**   `CC` `H5` `HCC`

> ☑7ᵗʰ **T71.193   Asphyxiation due to mechanical threat to breathing due to other causes, assault**   `CC` `H5`

> ☑7ᵗʰ **T71.194   Asphyxiation due to mechanical threat to breathing due to other causes, undetermined**   `CC` `H5`

☑5ᵗʰ **T71.2   Asphyxiation due to systemic oxygen deficiency due to low oxygen content in ambient air**
> Suffocation due to systemic oxygen deficiency due to low oxygen content in ambient air

> ☑x7ᵗʰ **T71.20   Asphyxiation due to systemic oxygen deficiency due to low oxygen content in ambient air due to unspecified cause**   `CC` `H5`

---

11   HCC with 7th character indicating initial encounter (A or B - specific to category) OR sequela.

---

☑ Additional Character Req    ☑x7ᵗʰ Placeholder Alert    Unacceptable PDx    Manifestation    `H1`-`H14` HAC    `HCC` CMS-HCC Condition    EXCLUDES 1 Not Coded Here    EXCLUDES 2 Not Included Here

√x7th **T71.21** **Asphyxiation due to cave-in or falling earth** CC H5
Use additional code for any associated cataclysm (X34-X38)

√6th **T71.22** **Asphyxiation due to being trapped in a car trunk**

√7th **T71.221** **Asphyxiation due to being trapped in a car trunk, accidental** CC

11 √7th **T71.222** **Asphyxiation due to being trapped in a car trunk, intentional self-harm** CC HCC

√7th **T71.223** **Asphyxiation due to being trapped in a car trunk, assault** CC

√7th **T71.224** **Asphyxiation due to being trapped in a car trunk, undetermined** CC

√6th **T71.23** **Asphyxiation due to being trapped in a (discarded) refrigerator**

√7th **T71.231** **Asphyxiation due to being trapped in a (discarded) refrigerator, accidental** CC

11 √7th **T71.232** **Asphyxiation due to being trapped in a (discarded) refrigerator, intentional self-harm** CC HCC

√7th **T71.233** **Asphyxiation due to being trapped in a (discarded) refrigerator, assault** CC

√7th **T71.234** **Asphyxiation due to being trapped in a (discarded) refrigerator, undetermined** CC

√x7th **T71.29** **Asphyxiation due to being trapped in other low oxygen environment** CC H5

√x7th **T71.9** **Asphyxiation due to unspecified cause** CC H5
Suffocation (by strangulation) due to unspecified cause
Suffocation NOS
Systemic oxygen deficiency due to low oxygen content in ambient air due to unspecified cause
Systemic oxygen deficiency due to mechanical threat to breathing due to unspecified cause
Traumatic asphyxia NOS

√4th **T73** **Effects of other deprivation**

The appropriate 7th character is to be added to each code from category T73.
A   initial encounter
D   subsequent encounter
S   sequela

√x7th **T73.0** **Starvation**
Deprivation of food

√x7th **T73.1** **Deprivation of water**

√x7th **T73.2** **Exhaustion due to exposure**

√x7th **T73.3** **Exhaustion due to excessive exertion**
Exhaustion due to overexertion

√x7th **T73.8** **Other effects of deprivation**

√x7th **T73.9** **Effect of deprivation, unspecified**

√4th **T74** **Adult and child abuse, neglect and other maltreatment, confirmed**
Use additional code, if applicable, to identify any associated current injury
Use additional external cause code to identify perpetrator, if known (Y07.-)
EXCLUDES 1   abuse and maltreatment in pregnancy (O9A.3-, O9A.4-, O9A.5-)
adult and child maltreatment, suspected (T76.-)

The appropriate 7th character is to be added to each code from category T74.
A   initial encounter
D   subsequent encounter
S   sequela

CC Excl: For codes in category T74, unless otherwise noted: PDX collection 1423

√5th **T74.0** **Neglect or abandonment, confirmed**

√x7th **T74.01** **Adult neglect or abandonment, confirmed** CC A

√x7th **T74.02** **Child neglect or abandonment, confirmed** CC P

√5th **T74.1** **Physical abuse, confirmed**
EXCLUDES 2   sexual abuse (T74.2-)

√x7th **T74.11** **Adult physical abuse, confirmed** CC A

√x7th **T74.12** **Child physical abuse, confirmed** CC P
EXCLUDES 2   shaken infant syndrome (T74.4)

√5th **T74.2** **Sexual abuse, confirmed**
Rape, confirmed
Sexual assault, confirmed

√x7th **T74.21** **Adult sexual abuse, confirmed** CC A

√x7th **T74.22** **Child sexual abuse, confirmed** CC P

√5th **T74.3** **Psychological abuse, confirmed**

√x7th **T74.31** **Adult psychological abuse, confirmed** A

√x7th **T74.32** **Child psychological abuse, confirmed** CC P

√x7th **T74.4** **Shaken infant syndrome** CC P

√5th **T74.9** **Unspecified maltreatment, confirmed**

√x7th **T74.91** **Unspecified adult maltreatment, confirmed** CC A
CC Excl: CC with 7th character A: PDX collection 1424

√x7th **T74.92** **Unspecified child maltreatment, confirmed** CC P

√4th **T75** **Other and unspecified effects of other external causes**
EXCLUDES 1   adverse effects NEC (T78.-)
EXCLUDES 2   burns (electric) (T20-T31)

The appropriate 7th character is to be added to each code from category T75.
A   initial encounter
D   subsequent encounter
S   sequela

√5th **T75.0** **Effects of lightning**
Struck by lightning

√x7th **T75.00** **Unspecified effects of lightning**
Struck by lightning NOS

√x7th **T75.01** **Shock due to being struck by lightning**

√x7th **T75.09** **Other effects of lightning**
Use additional code for other effects of lightning

√x7th **T75.1** **Unspecified effects of drowning and nonfatal submersion** CC H5
Immersion
EXCLUDES 1   specified effects of drowning—code to effects
CC Excl: PDX collection 1425

√5th **T75.2** **Effects of vibration**

√x7th **T75.20** **Unspecified effects of vibration**

√x7th **T75.21** **Pneumatic hammer syndrome**

√x7th **T75.22** **Traumatic vasospastic syndrome**

√x7th **T75.23** **Vertigo from infrasound**
EXCLUDES 1   vertigo NOS (R42)

**T75.29** **Other effects of vibration**

√x7th **T75.3** **Motion sickness**
Airsickness
Seasickness
Travel sickness
Use additional external cause code to identify vehicle or type of motion (Y92.81-, Y93.5-)

√x7th **T75.4** **Electrocution**
Shock from electric current
Shock from electroshock gun (taser)

√5th **T75.8** **Other specified effects of external causes**

√x7th **T75.81** **Effects of abnormal gravitation [G] forces**

√x7th **T75.82** **Effects of weightlessness**

√x7th **T75.89** **Other specified effects of external causes**

---

11 HCC with 7th character indicating initial encounter (A or B - specific to category) OR sequela.

N Newborn: 0   P Pediatric: 0-17   M Maternity: 12-55   A Adult: 15-124   MCC Major CC Condition   PDxMCC PDx acts as own MCC   CC CC Condition   PDxCC PDx acts as own CC

✓4th **T76 Adult and child abuse, neglect and other maltreatment, suspected**

Use additional code, if applicable, to identify any associated current injury

EXCLUDES 1   adult and child maltreatment, confirmed (T74.-)
suspected abuse and maltreatment in pregnancy (O9A.3-, O9A.4-, O9A.5-)
suspected adult physical and sexual abuse, ruled out (Z04.71)
suspected adult sexual abused, ruled out (Z04.41)
suspected child physical abuse, ruled out (Z04.72)
suspected child sexual abuse, ruled out (Z04.42)

The appropriate 7th character is to be added to each code from category T76.
A   initial encounter
D   subsequent encounter
S   sequela

**CC Excl: For codes in category T76, unless otherwise noted:** PDX collection 1423

✓5th **T76.0 Neglect or abandonment, suspected**
✓x7th **T76.01 Adult neglect or abandonment, suspected** CC A
✓x7th **T76.02 Child neglect or abandonment, suspected** CC P

✓5th **T76.1 Physical abuse, suspected**
✓x7th **T76.11 Adult physical abuse, suspected** CC A
✓x7th **T76.12 Child physical abuse, suspected** CC P

✓5th **T76.2 Sexual abuse, suspected**
Rape, suspected
~~Sexual abuse, suspected~~
EXCLUDES 1   alleged abuse, ruled out (Z04.7)
✓x7th **T76.21 Adult sexual abuse, suspected** CC A
✓x7th **T76.22 Child sexual abuse, suspected** CC P

✓5th **T76.3 Psychological abuse, suspected**
✓x7th **T76.31 Adult psychological abuse, suspected** A
✓x7th **T76.32 Child psychological abuse, suspected** CC P

✓5th **T76.9 Unspecified maltreatment, suspected**
✓x7th **T76.91 Unspecified adult maltreatment, suspected** CC A
**CC Excl: CC with 7th character A:** PDX collection 1424
✓x7th **T76.92 Unspecified child maltreatment, suspected** CC P

✓4th **T78 Adverse effects, not elsewhere classified**
EXCLUDES 2   complications of surgical and medical care NEC (T80-T88)

The appropriate 7th character is to be added to each code from category T78.
A   initial encounter
D   subsequent encounter
S   sequela

**CC Excl: For CC codes in category T78:** PDX collection 1426

✓5th **T78.0 Anaphylactic reaction due to food**
Anaphylactic reaction due to adverse food reaction
Anaphylactic shock or reaction due to nonpoisonous foods
Anaphylactoid reaction due to food

✓x7th **T78.00 Anaphylactic reaction due to unspecified food** CC
✓x7th **T78.01 Anaphylactic reaction due to peanuts** CC
✓x7th **T78.02 Anaphylactic reaction due to shellfish (crustaceans)** CC
✓x7th **T78.03 Anaphylactic reaction due to other fish** CC
✓x7th **T78.04 Anaphylactic reaction due to fruits and vegetables** CC
✓x7th **T78.05 Anaphylactic reaction due to tree nuts and seeds** CC
EXCLUDES 2   anaphylactic reaction due to peanuts (T78.01)
✓x7th **T78.06 Anaphylactic reaction due to food additives** CC
✓x7th **T78.07 Anaphylactic reaction due to milk and dairy products** CC
✓x7th **T78.08 Anaphylactic reaction due to eggs** CC
✓x7th **T78.09 Anaphylactic reaction due to other food products** CC

✓x7th **T78.1 Other adverse food reactions, not elsewhere classified**
Use additional code to identify the type of reaction, if applicable
EXCLUDES 1   anaphylactic reaction or shock due to adverse food reaction (T78.0-)
anaphylactic reaction due to food (T78.0-)
bacterial food borne intoxications (A05.-)
EXCLUDES 2   allergic and dietetic gastroenteritis and colitis (K52.29)
allergic rhinitis due to food (J30.5)
dermatitis due to food in contact with skin (L23.6, L24.6, L25.4)
dermatitis due to ingested food (L27.2)
food protein-induced enterocolitis syndrome (K52.21)
food protein-induced enteropathy (K52.22)

✓x7th **T78.2 Anaphylactic shock, unspecified** CC
Allergic shock               Anaphylaxis
Anaphylactic reaction
EXCLUDES 1   anaphylactic reaction or shock due to adverse effect of correct medicinal substance properly administered (T88.6)
anaphylactic reaction or shock due to adverse food reaction (T78.0-)
anaphylactic reaction or shock due to serum (T80.5-)

✓x7th **T78.3 Angioneurotic edema**
Allergic angioedema
Giant urticaria
Quincke's edema
EXCLUDES 1   serum urticaria (T80.6-)
urticaria (L50.-)

✓5th **T78.4 Other and unspecified allergy**
EXCLUDES 1   specified types of allergic reaction such as:
allergic diarrhea (K52.29)
allergic gastroenteritis and colitis (K52.29)
dermatitis (L23-L25, L27-)
food protein-induced enterocolitis syndrome (K52.21)
food protein-induced enteropathy (K52.22)
hay fever (J30.1)

✓x7th **T78.40 Allergy, unspecified**
Allergic reaction NOS
Hypersensitivity NOS
✓x7th **T78.41 Arthus phenomenon**
Arthus reaction
✓x7th **T78.49 Other allergy**
✓x7th **T78.8 Other adverse effects, not elsewhere classified**

## Certain early complications of trauma (T79)

✓4th **T79 Certain early complications of trauma, not elsewhere classified**
EXCLUDES 2   acute respiratory distress syndrome (J80)
complications occurring during or following medical procedures (T80-T88)
complications of surgical and medical care NEC (T80-T88)
newborn respiratory distress syndrome (P22.0)

The appropriate 7th character is to be added to each code from category T79.
A   initial encounter
D   subsequent encounter
S   sequela

10 ✓x7th **T79.0 Air embolism (traumatic)** MCC HCC
EXCLUDES 1   air embolism complicating abortion or ectopic or molar pregnancy (O00-O07, O08.2)
air embolism complicating pregnancy, childbirth and the puerperium (O88.0)
air embolism following infusion, transfusion, and therapeutic injection (T80.0)
air embolism following procedure NEC (T81.7-)
**DEF:** Arterial or venous obstruction due to introduction of air bubbles into the blood vessels following surgery or trauma.
**CC Excl:** PDX collection 1427

10 ✓x7th **T79.1 Fat embolism (traumatic)** MCC HCC
EXCLUDES 1   fat embolism complicating:
abortion or ectopic or molar pregnancy (O00-O07, O08.2)
pregnancy, childbirth and the puerperium (O88.8)
**DEF:** Arterial blockage due to the entrance of fat into the circulatory system after fracture of large bones or administration of corticosteroids.
**CC Excl:** PDX collection 1428

10 ✓x7th **T79.2 Traumatic secondary and recurrent hemorrhage and seroma** CC HCC
**CC Excl:** PDX collection 1429

---

10 HCC with 7th character indicating initial encounter (A, B or C - specific to category).

**10** ✓x7ᵗʰ **T79.4 Traumatic shock**    MCC HCC

Shock (immediate) (delayed) following injury

EXCLUDES 1    *anaphylactic shock due to adverse food reaction (T78.0-)*
*anaphylactic shock due to correct medicinal substance properly administered (T88.6)*
*anaphylactic shock due to serum (T80.5-)*
*anaphylactic shock NOS (T78.2)*
*anesthetic shock (T88.2)*
*electric shock (T75.4)*
*nontraumatic shock NEC (R57.-)*
*obstetric shock (O75.1)*
*postprocedural shock (T81.1-)*
*septic shock (R65.21)*
*shock complicating abortion or ectopic or molar pregnancy (O00-O07, O08.3)*
*shock due to lightning (T75.01)*
*shock NOS (R57.9)*

**CC Excl:** PDX collection 1430

**10** ✓x7ᵗʰ **T79.5 Traumatic anuria**    MCC HCC

Crush syndrome
Renal failure following crushing
**CC Excl:** PDX collection 1431

**10** ✓x7ᵗʰ **T79.6 Traumatic ischemia of muscle**    HCC

Traumatic rhabdomyolysis
Volkmann's ischemic contracture

EXCLUDES 2    *anterior tibial syndrome (M76.8)*
*compartment syndrome (traumatic) (T79.A-)*
*nontraumatic ischemia of muscle (M62.2-)*

**10** ✓x7ᵗʰ **T79.7 Traumatic subcutaneous emphysema**    CC HCC

EXCLUDES 1    *emphysema NOS (J43)*
*emphysema (subcutaneous) resulting from a procedure (T81.82)*

**CC Excl:** PDX collection 1432

✓5ᵗʰ **T79.A Traumatic compartment syndrome**

EXCLUDES 1    *fibromyalgia (M79.7)*
*nontraumatic compartment syndrome (M79.A-)*
*traumatic ischemic infarction of muscle (T79.6)*

**DEF:** Compression of nerves and blood vessels within an enclosed muscle space due to previous trauma, which leads to impaired blood flow and muscle and nerve damage.

**10** ✓x7ᵗʰ **T79.A0 Compartment syndrome, unspecified**    CC HCC

Compartment syndrome NOS
**CC Excl:** PDX collection 896

✓6ᵗʰ **T79.A1 Traumatic compartment syndrome of upper extremity**

Traumatic compartment syndrome of shoulder, arm, forearm, wrist, hand, and fingers

**CC Excl: For codes in category T79.A1:** PDX collection 1433

**10** ✓7ᵗʰ **T79.A11 Traumatic compartment syndrome** CC HCC **of right upper extremity**

**10** ✓7ᵗʰ **T79.A12 Traumatic compartment syndrome** CC HCC **of left upper extremity**

**10** ✓7ᵗʰ **T79.A19 Traumatic compartment syndrome** CC HCC **of unspecified upper extremity**

✓6ᵗʰ **T79.A2 Traumatic compartment syndrome of lower extremity**

Traumatic compartment syndrome of hip, buttock, thigh, leg, foot, and toes

**CC Excl: For codes in category T79.A2:** PDX collection 1433

**10** ✓7ᵗʰ **T79.A21 Traumatic compartment syndrome** CC HCC **of right lower extremity**

**10** ✓7ᵗʰ **T79.A22 Traumatic compartment syndrome** CC HCC **of left lower extremity**

**10** ✓7ᵗʰ **T79.A29 Traumatic compartment syndrome** CC HCC **of unspecified lower extremity**

**10** ✓x7ᵗʰ **T79.A3 Traumatic compartment syndrome of** CC HCC **abdomen**

**CC Excl:** PDX collection 1434

**10** ✓x7ᵗʰ **T79.A9 Traumatic compartment syndrome of other** CC HCC **sites**

**CC Excl:** PDX collection 896

**10** ✓x7ᵗʰ **T79.8 Other early complications of trauma**    HCC

**10** ✓x7ᵗʰ **T79.9 Unspecified early complication of trauma**    HCC

---

## Complications of surgical and medical care, not elsewhere classified (T80-T88)

Use additional code for adverse effect, if applicable, to identify drug (T36-T50 with fifth or sixth character 5)

Use additional code(s) to identify the specified condition resulting from the complication

Use additional code to identify devices involved and details of circumstances (Y62-Y82)

EXCLUDES 2    *any encounters with medical care for postprocedural conditions in which no complications are present, such as:*
     *artificial opening status (Z93.-)*
     *closure of external stoma (Z43.-)*
     *fitting and adjustment of external prosthetic device (Z44.-)*
*burns and corrosions from local applications and irradiation (T20-T32)*
*complications of surgical procedures during pregnancy, childbirth and the puerperium (O00-O9A)*
*mechanical complication of respirator [ventilator] (J95.850)*
*poisoning and toxic effects of drugs and chemicals (T36-T65 with fifth or sixth character 1-4 or 6)*
*postprocedural fever (R50.82)*
*specified complications classified elsewhere, such as:*
     *cerebrospinal fluid leak from spinal puncture (G97.0)*
     *colostomy malfunction (K94.0-)*
     *disorders of fluid and electrolyte imbalance (E86-E87)*
     *functional disturbances following cardiac surgery (I97.0-I97.1)*
     *intraoperative and postprocedural complications of specified body systems (D78.-, E36.-, E89.-, G97.3-, G97.4, H59.3-, H59.-, H95.2-, H95.3, I97.4-, I97.5, J95.6-, J95.7, K91.6-, L76.-, M96.-, N99.-)*
*ostomy complications (J95.0-, K94-, N99.5-)*
*postgastric surgery syndromes (K91.1)*
*postlaminectomy syndrome NEC (M96.1)*
*postmastectomy lymphedema syndrome (I97.2)*
*postsurgical blind-loop syndrome (K91.2)*
*ventilator associated pneumonia (J95.851)*

**AHA:** 2015, 1Q, 15

✓4ᵗʰ **T80 Complications following infusion, transfusion and therapeutic injection**

INCLUDES    complications following perfusion

EXCLUDES 2    *bone marrow transplant rejection (T86.01)*
*febrile nonhemolytic transfusion reaction (R50.84)*
*fluid overload due to transfusion (E87.71)*
*posttransfusion purpura (D69.51)*
*transfusion associated circulatory overload (TACO) (E87.71)*
*transfusion (red blood cell) associated hemochromatosis (E83.111)*
*transfusion related acute lung injury (TRALI) (J95.84)*

The appropriate 7th character is to be added to each code from category T80.
A    initial encounter
D    subsequent encounter
S    sequela

✓x7ᵗʰ **T80.0 Air embolism following infusion, transfusion and** MCC H2 **therapeutic injection**

**CC Excl:** PDX collection 1435

✓x7ᵗʰ **T80.1 Vascular complications following infusion, transfusion** CC **and therapeutic injection**

Use additional code to identify the vascular complication

EXCLUDES 2    *extravasation of vesicant agent (T80.81-)*
*infiltration of vesicant agent (T80.81-)*
*postprocedural vascular complications (T81.7-)*
*vascular complications specified as due to prosthetic devices, implants and grafts (T82.8-, T83.8-, T84.8-, T85.8-)*

**CC Excl:** PDX collection 1436

✓5ᵗʰ **T80.2 Infections following infusion, transfusion and therapeutic injection**

Use additional code to identify the specific infection, such as: sepsis (A41.9)

Use additional code (R65.2-) to identify severe sepsis, if applicable

EXCLUDES 2    *infections specified as due to prosthetic devices, implants and grafts (T82.6-T82.7, T83.5-T83.6, T84.5-T84.7, T85.7)*
*postprocedural infections (T81.4-)*

**CC Excl: For codes in subcategory T80.2:** PDX collection 948

---

**10** HCC with 7th character indicating initial encounter (A, B or C - specific to category).

Ⓝ Newborn: 0    Ⓟ Pediatric: 0-17    Ⓜ Maternity: 12-55    Ⓐ Adult: 15-124    MCC Major CC Condition    PDx MCC PDx acts as own MCC    CC CC Condition    PDx CC PDx acts as own CC

**1136**      ICD-10-CM 2018

√6ᵗʰ **T80.21**   **Infection due to central venous catheter**
Infection due to pulmonary artery catheter (Swan-Ganz catheter)

√7ᵗʰ **T80.211**   **Bloodstream infection due to central venous catheter**   `CC` `H7`
Catheter-related bloodstream infection (CRBSI) NOS
Central line-associated bloodstream infection (CLABSI)
Bloodstream infection due to Hickman catheter
Bloodstream infection due to peripherally inserted central catheter (PICC)
Bloodstream infection due to portacath (port-a-cath)
Bloodstream infection due to pulmonary artery catheter
Bloodstream infection due to triple lumen catheter
Bloodstream infection due to umbilical venous catheter

√7ᵗʰ **T80.212**   **Local infection due to central venous catheter**   `CC` `H7`
Exit or insertion site infection
Local infection due to Hickman catheter
Local infection due to peripherally inserted central catheter (PICC)
Local infection due to portacath (port-a-cath)
Local infection due to pulmonary artery catheter
Local infection due to triple lumen catheter
Local infection due to umbilical venous catheter
Port or reservoir infection
Tunnel infection

√7ᵗʰ **T80.218**   **Other infection due to central venous catheter**   `CC` `H7`
Other central line-associated infection
Other infection due to Hickman catheter
Other infection due to peripherally inserted central catheter (PICC)
Other infection due to portacath (port-a-cath)
Other infection due to pulmonary artery catheter
Other infection due to triple lumen catheter
Other infection due to umbilical venous catheter

√7ᵗʰ **T80.219**   **Unspecified infection due to central venous catheter**   `CC` `H7`
Central line-associated infection NOS
Unspecified infection due to Hickman catheter
Unspecified infection due to peripherally inserted central catheter (PICC)
Unspecified infection due to portacath (port-a-cath)
Unspecified infection due to pulmonary artery catheter
Unspecified infection due to triple lumen catheter
Unspecified infection due to umbilical venous catheter

√x7ᵗʰ **T80.22**   **Acute infection following transfusion, infusion, or injection of blood and blood products**   `CC`

√x7ᵗʰ **T80.29**   **Infection following other infusion, transfusion and therapeutic injection**   `CC`

√5ᵗʰ **T80.3**   **ABO incompatibility reaction due to transfusion of blood or blood products**
*EXCLUDES 1*   *minor blood group antigens reactions (Duffy) (E) (K(ell)) (Kidd) (Lewis) (M) (N) (P) (S) (T80.A)*

**CC Excl: For codes in subcategory T80.3:**
**PDX collection 1437**

√x7ᵗʰ **T80.30**   **ABO incompatibility reaction due to transfusion of blood or blood products, unspecified**   `CC` `H3`
ABO incompatibility blood transfusion NOS
Reaction to ABO incompatibility from transfusion NOS

√6ᵗʰ **T80.31**   **ABO incompatibility with hemolytic transfusion reaction**

√7ᵗʰ **T80.310**   **ABO incompatibility with acute hemolytic transfusion reaction**   `CC` `H3`
ABO incompatibility with hemolytic transfusion reaction less than 24 hours after transfusion
Acute hemolytic transfusion reaction (AHTR) due to ABO incompatibility

√7ᵗʰ **T80.311**   **ABO incompatibility with delayed hemolytic transfusion reaction**   `CC` `H3`
ABO incompatibility with hemolytic transfusion reaction 24 hours or more after transfusion
Delayed hemolytic transfusion reaction (DHTR) due to ABO incompatibility

√7ᵗʰ **T80.319**   **ABO incompatibility with hemolytic transfusion reaction, unspecified**   `CC` `H3`
ABO incompatibility with hemolytic transfusion reaction at unspecified time after transfusion
Hemolytic transfusion reaction (HTR) due to ABO incompatibility NOS

√x7ᵗʰ **T80.39**   **Other ABO incompatibility reaction due to transfusion of blood or blood products**   `CC` `H3`
Delayed serologic transfusion reaction (DSTR) from ABO incompatibility
Other ABO incompatible blood transfusion
Other reaction to ABO incompatible blood transfusion

√5ᵗʰ **T80.4**   **Rh incompatibility reaction due to transfusion of blood or blood products**
Reaction due to incompatibility of Rh antigens (C) (c) (D) (E) (e)

**CC Excl: For codes in subcategory T80.4, unless otherwise noted:** PDX collection 1437

√x7ᵗʰ **T80.40**   **Rh incompatibility reaction due to transfusion of blood or blood products, unspecified**   `CC`
Reaction due to Rh factor in transfusion NOS
Rh incompatible blood transfusion NOS

√6ᵗʰ **T80.41**   **Rh incompatibility with hemolytic transfusion reaction**

√7ᵗʰ **T80.410**   **Rh incompatibility with acute hemolytic transfusion reaction**   `CC`
Acute hemolytic transfusion reaction (AHTR) due to Rh incompatibility
Rh incompatibility with hemolytic transfusion reaction less than 24 hours after transfusion

√7ᵗʰ **T80.411**   **Rh incompatibility with delayed hemolytic transfusion reaction**   `CC`
Delayed hemolytic transfusion reaction (DHTR) due to Rh incompatibility
Rh incompatibility with hemolytic transfusion reaction 24 hours or more after transfusion

√7ᵗʰ **T80.419**   **Rh incompatibility with hemolytic transfusion reaction, unspecified**   `CC`
Hemolytic transfusion reaction (HTR) due to Rh incompatibility NOS
Rh incompatibility with hemolytic transfusion reaction at unspecified time after transfusion

√x7ᵗʰ **T80.49**   **Other Rh incompatibility reaction due to transfusion of blood or blood products**   `CC`
Delayed serologic transfusion reaction (DSTR) from Rh incompatibility
Other reaction to Rh incompatible blood transfusion
**CC Excl:** PDX collection 1438

√5ᵗʰ **T80.A**   **Non-ABO incompatibility reaction due to transfusion of blood or blood products**
Reaction due to incompatibility of minor antigens (Duffy) (Kell) (Kidd) (Lewis) (M) (N) (P) (S)

**CC Excl: For codes in subcategory T80.A, unless otherwise noted:** PDX collection 1438

√x7ᵗʰ **T80.A0**   **Non-ABO incompatibility reaction due to transfusion of blood or blood products, unspecified**   `CC`
Non-ABO antigen incompatibility reaction from transfusion NOS

---

√6ᵗʰ **T80.A1** **Non-ABO incompatibility** with hemolytic transfusion reaction

    √7ᵗʰ **T80.A10** **Non-ABO incompatibility with acute** `CC` **hemolytic transfusion reaction**

        Acute hemolytic transfusion reaction (AHTR) due to non-ABO incompatibility

        Non-ABO incompatibility with hemolytic transfusion reaction less than 24 hours after transfusion

    √7ᵗʰ **T80.A11** **Non-ABO incompatibility with** `CC` **delayed hemolytic transfusion reaction**

        Delayed hemolytic transfusion reaction (DHTR) due to non-ABO incompatibility

        Non-ABO incompatibility with hemolytic transfusion reaction 24 or more hours after transfusion

    √7ᵗʰ **T80.A19** **Non-ABO incompatibility with** `CC` **hemolytic transfusion reaction, unspecified**

        Hemolytic transfusion reaction (HTR) due to non-ABO incompatibility NOS

        Non-ABO incompatibility with hemolytic transfusion reaction at unspecified time after transfusion

√x7ᵗʰ **T80.A9** **Other non-ABO incompatibility reaction due to** `CC` **transfusion of blood or blood products**

    Delayed serologic transfusion reaction (DSTR) from non-ABO incompatibility

    Other reaction to non-ABO incompatible blood transfusion

    **CC Excl:** PDX collection 1437

√5ᵗʰ **T80.5** **Anaphylactic reaction due to serum**

    Allergic shock due to serum
    Anaphylactic shock due to serum
    Anaphylactoid reaction due to serum
    Anaphylaxis due to serum

    *EXCLUDES 1*   ABO incompatibility reaction due to transfusion of blood or blood products (T80.3-)
        allergic reaction or shock NOS (T78.2)
        anaphylactic reaction or shock NOS (T78.2)
        anaphylactic reaction or shock due to adverse effect of correct medicinal substance properly administered (T88.6)
        other serum reaction (T80.6-)

    **DEF:** Life-threatening hypersensitivity to foreign serum; causes respiratory distress, vascular collapse, and shock.

    **CC Excl: For codes in subcategory T80.5:**
    PDX collection 1439

  √x7ᵗʰ **T80.51** **Anaphylactic reaction due to administration of** `CC` **blood and blood products**

  √x7ᵗʰ **T80.52** **Anaphylactic reaction due to vaccination** `CC`

  √x7ᵗʰ **T80.59** **Anaphylactic reaction due to other serum** `CC`

√5ᵗʰ **T80.6** **Other serum reactions**

    Intoxication by serum       Serum sickness
    Protein sickness           Serum urticaria
    Serum rash

    *EXCLUDES 2*   serum hepatitis (B16-B19)

    **DEF:** Serum sickness: Hypersensitivity to foreign serum; causes fever, hives, swelling, and lymphadenopathy.

    **CC Excl: For codes in subcategory T80.6, unless otherwise noted: CC with 7th character A:**
    PDX collection 1439

  √x7ᵗʰ **T80.61** **Other serum reaction due to administration of** `CC` **blood and blood products**

  √x7ᵗʰ **T80.62** **Other serum reaction due to vaccination** `CC`

  √x7ᵗʰ **T80.69** **Other serum reaction due to other serum** `CC`

    ►Code also, if applicable, arthropathy in hypersensitivity reactions classified elsewhere (M36.4)◄

    **CC Excl:** PDX collection 1440

√5ᵗʰ **T80.8** **Other complications following infusion, transfusion and therapeutic injection**

  √6ᵗʰ **T80.81** **Extravasation of vesicant agent**
    Infiltration of vesicant agent

    √7ᵗʰ **T80.810** **Extravasation of vesicant** `CC` **antineoplastic chemotherapy**

        Infiltration of vesicant antineoplastic chemotherapy
        **CC Excl:** PDX collection 1436

    √7ᵗʰ **T80.818** **Extravasation of other vesicant agent** `CC`
        Infiltration of other vesicant agent
        **CC Excl:** PDX collection 1436

  √x7ᵗʰ **T80.89** **Other complications following infusion, transfusion and therapeutic injection**

    Delayed serologic transfusion reaction (DSTR), unspecified incompatibility

    Use additional code to identify graft-versus-host reaction, if applicable, (D89.81-)

√5ᵗʰ **T80.9** **Unspecified complication following infusion, transfusion and therapeutic injection**

  √x7ᵗʰ **T80.90** **Unspecified complication** following infusion and therapeutic injection

  √6ᵗʰ **T80.91** **Hemolytic transfusion reaction, unspecified incompatibility**

    *EXCLUDES 1*   ABO incompatibility with hemolytic transfusion reaction (T80.31-)
        Non-ABO incompatibility with hemolytic transfusion reaction (T80.A1-)
        Rh incompatibility with hemolytic transfusion reaction (T80.41-)

    **CC Excl: For codes in subcategory T80.91:**
    PDX collection 1437

    √7ᵗʰ **T80.910** **Acute hemolytic transfusion reaction,** `CC` **unspecified incompatibility**

    √7ᵗʰ **T80.911** **Delayed hemolytic transfusion** `CC` **reaction, unspecified incompatibility**

    √7ᵗʰ **T80.919** **Hemolytic transfusion reaction,** `CC` **unspecified incompatibility, unspecified as acute or delayed**
        Hemolytic transfusion reaction NOS

  √x7ᵗʰ **T80.92** **Unspecified transfusion reaction**
    Transfusion reaction NOS

√4ᵗʰ **T81** **Complications of procedures, not elsewhere classified**

    Use additional code for adverse effect, if applicable, to identify drug (T36-T50 with fifth or sixth character 5)

    *EXCLUDES 2*   complications following immunization (T88.0-T88.1)
        complications following infusion, transfusion and therapeutic injection (T80.-)
        complications of transplanted organs and tissue (T86.-)
        specified complications classified elsewhere, such as:
            complication of prosthetic devices, implants and grafts (T82-T85)
            dermatitis due to drugs and medicaments (L23.3, L24.4, L25.1, L27.0-L27.1)
            endosseous dental implant failure (M27.6-)
            floppy iris syndrome (IFIS) (intraoperative) (H21.81)
            intraoperative and postprocedural complications of specific body system (D78.-, E36.-, E89.-, G97.3-, G97.4, H59.3-, H59.-, H95.2-, H95.3, I97.4-, I97.5, J95.-, K91.-, L76.-, M96.-, N99.-)
            ostomy complications (J95.0-, K94.-, N99.5-)
            plateau iris syndrome (post-iridectomy) (postprocedural) (H21.82)
            poisoning and toxic effects of drugs and chemicals (T36-T65 with fifth or sixth character 1-4 or 6)

    The appropriate 7th character is to be added to each code from category T81.
    A    initial encounter
    D    subsequent encounter
    S    sequela

N Newborn: 0    P Pediatric: 0-17    M Maternity: 12-55    A Adult: 15-124    MCC Major CC Condition    PDxMCC PDx acts as own MCC    CC CC Condition    PDxCC PDx acts as own CC

1138

ICD-10-CM 2018

✓5ᵗʰ **T81.1 Postprocedural shock**
Shock during or resulting from a procedure, not elsewhere classified

*EXCLUDES 1* *anaphylactic shock due to correct substance properly administered (T88.6)*
*anaphylactic shock due to serum (T80.5-)*
*anaphylactic shock NOS (T78.2)*
*anesthetic shock (T88.2)*
*electric shock (T75.4)*
*obstetric shock (O75.1)*
*septic shock (R65.21)*
*shock following abortion or ectopic or molar pregnancy (O00-O07, O08.3)*
*traumatic shock (T79.4)*

**CC Excl: For codes in subcategory T81.1:**
PDX collection 1441

✓x7ᵗʰ **T81.10 Postprocedural shock unspecified** `CC`
Collapse NOS during or resulting from a procedure, not elsewhere classified
Postprocedural failure of peripheral circulation
Postprocedural shock NOS

10 ✓x7ᵗʰ **T81.11 Postprocedural cardiogenic shock** `MCC` `HCC`

3,10 ✓x7ᵗʰ **T81.12 Postprocedural septic shock** `MCC` `HCC`
Postprocedural endotoxic shock resulting from a procedure, not elsewhere classified
Postprocedural gram-negative shock resulting from a procedure, not elsewhere classified
Code first underlying infection
Use additional code, to identify any associated acute organ dysfunction, if applicable

✓x7ᵗʰ **T81.19 Other postprocedural shock** `MCC`
Postprocedural hypovolemic shock

✓5ᵗʰ **T81.3 Disruption of wound, not elsewhere classified**
Disruption of any suture materials or other closure methods

*EXCLUDES 1* *breakdown (mechanical) of permanent sutures (T85.612)*
*displacement of permanent sutures (T85.622)*
*disruption of cesarean delivery wound (O90.0)*
*disruption of perineal obstetric wound (O90.1)*
*mechanical complication of permanent sutures NEC (T85.692)*

**AHA:** 2014, 1Q, 23

**CC Excl: For codes in subcategory T81.3:**
PDX collection 1442

✓x7ᵗʰ **T81.30 Disruption of wound, unspecified** `CC`
Disruption of wound NOS

✓x7ᵗʰ **T81.31 Disruption of external operation (surgical) wound, not elsewhere classified** `CC`
Dehiscence of operation wound NOS
Disruption of operation wound NOS
Disruption or dehiscence of closure of cornea
Disruption or dehiscence of closure of mucosa
Disruption or dehiscence of closure of skin and subcutaneous tissue
Full-thickness skin disruption or dehiscence
Superficial disruption or dehiscence of operation wound

*EXCLUDES 1* *dehiscence of amputation stump (T87.81)*

✓x7ᵗʰ **T81.32 Disruption of internal operation (surgical) wound, not elsewhere classified** `CC`
Deep disruption or dehiscence of operation wound NOS
Disruption or dehiscence of closure of internal organ or other internal tissue
Disruption or dehiscence of closure of muscle or muscle flap
Disruption or dehiscence of closure of ribs or rib cage
Disruption or dehiscence of closure of skull or craniotomy
Disruption or dehiscence of closure of sternum or sternotomy
Disruption or dehiscence of closure of tendon or ligament
Disruption or dehiscence of closure of superficial or muscular fascia

✓x7ᵗʰ **T81.33 Disruption of traumatic injury wound repair** `CC`
Disruption or dehiscence of closure of traumatic laceration (external) (internal)

✓x7ᵗʰ **T81.4 Infection following a procedure** `CC` `H11` `H12` `H13`
Intra-abdominal abscess following a procedure
Postprocedural infection, not elsewhere classified
Sepsis following a procedure
Stitch abscess following a procedure
Subphrenic abscess following a procedure
Wound abscess following a procedure
Use additional code to identify infection
Use additional code (R65.2-) to identify severe sepsis, if applicable

*EXCLUDES 1* *obstetric surgical wound infection (O86.0)*
*postprocedural fever NOS (R50.82)*
*postprocedural retroperitoneal abscess (K68.11)*

*EXCLUDES 2* *bleb associated endophthalmitis (H59.4-)*
*infection due to infusion, transfusion and therapeutic injection (T80.2-)*
*infection due to prosthetic devices, implants and grafts (T82.6-T82.7, T83.5-T83.6, T84.5-T84.7, T85.7)*

**AHA:** 2014, 1Q, 23
**CC Excl:** PDX collection 805

✓5ᵗʰ **T81.5 Complications of foreign body accidentally left in body following procedure**
**AHA:** 2014, 4Q, 24

**CC Excl: For codes in subcategory T81.5:**
PDX collection 1443

✓6ᵗʰ **T81.50 Unspecified complication of foreign body accidentally left in body following procedure**

✓7ᵗʰ **T81.500 Unspecified complication of foreign body accidentally left in body following surgical operation** `CC` `H1`

✓7ᵗʰ **T81.501 Unspecified complication of foreign body accidentally left in body following infusion or transfusion** `CC` `H1`

✓7ᵗʰ **T81.502 Unspecified complication of foreign body accidentally left in body following kidney dialysis** `CC` `H1` `HCC`

✓7ᵗʰ **T81.503 Unspecified complication of foreign body accidentally left in body following injection or immunization** `CC` `H1`

✓7ᵗʰ **T81.504 Unspecified complication of foreign body accidentally left in body following endoscopic examination** `CC` `H1`

✓7ᵗʰ **T81.505 Unspecified complication of foreign body accidentally left in body following heart catheterization** `CC` `H1`

✓7ᵗʰ **T81.506 Unspecified complication of foreign body accidentally left in body following aspiration, puncture or other catheterization** `CC` `H1`

✓7ᵗʰ **T81.507 Unspecified complication of foreign body accidentally left in body following removal of catheter or packing** `CC` `H1`

✓7ᵗʰ **T81.508 Unspecified complication of foreign body accidentally left in body following other procedure** `CC` `H1`

✓7ᵗʰ **T81.509 Unspecified complication of foreign body accidentally left in body following unspecified procedure** `CC` `H1`

✓6ᵗʰ **T81.51 Adhesions due to foreign body accidentally left in body following procedure**

✓7ᵗʰ **T81.510 Adhesions due to foreign body accidentally left in body following surgical operation** `CC` `H1`

✓7ᵗʰ **T81.511 Adhesions due to foreign body accidentally left in body following infusion or transfusion** `CC` `H1`

✓7ᵗʰ **T81.512 Adhesions due to foreign body accidentally left in body following kidney dialysis** `CC` `H1` `HCC`

✓7ᵗʰ **T81.513 Adhesions due to foreign body accidentally left in body following injection or immunization** `CC` `H1`

✓7ᵗʰ **T81.514 Adhesions due to foreign body accidentally left in body following endoscopic examination** `CC` `H1`

---

3 Unacceptable PDx for all encounters (7th character A, D, OR S).
10 HCC with 7th character indicating initial encounter (A, B or C - specific to category).

✓ Additional Character Req ✓x7ᵗʰ Placeholder Alert Unacceptable PDx Manifestation `H1`-`H14` HAC `HCC` CMS-HCC Condition *EXCLUDES 1* Not Coded Here *EXCLUDES 2* Not Included Here

√7th **T81.515** Adhesions due to foreign body accidentally left in body following **heart catheterization** `CC` `H1`

√7th **T81.516** Adhesions due to foreign body accidentally left in body following **aspiration, puncture or other catheterization** `CC` `H1`

√7th **T81.517** Adhesions due to foreign body accidentally left in body following **removal of catheter or packing** `CC` `H1`

√7th **T81.518** Adhesions due to foreign body accidentally left in body following **other procedure** `CC` `H1`

√7th **T81.519** Adhesions due to foreign body accidentally left in body following **unspecified procedure** `CC` `H1`

√6th **T81.52** Obstruction due to foreign body accidentally left in body following procedure

√7th **T81.520** Obstruction due to foreign body accidentally left in body following **surgical operation** `CC` `H1`

√7th **T81.521** Obstruction due to foreign body accidentally left in body following **infusion or transfusion** `CC` `H1`

√7th **T81.522** Obstruction due to foreign body accidentally left in body following **kidney dialysis** `CC` `H1` `HCC`

√7th **T81.523** Obstruction due to foreign body accidentally left in body following **injection or immunization** `CC` `H1`

√7th **T81.524** Obstruction due to foreign body accidentally left in body following **endoscopic examination** `CC` `H1`

√7th **T81.525** Obstruction due to foreign body accidentally left in body following **heart catheterization** `CC` `H1`

√7th **T81.526** Obstruction due to foreign body accidentally left in body following **aspiration, puncture or other catheterization** `CC` `H1`

√7th **T81.527** Obstruction due to foreign body accidentally left in body following **removal of catheter or packing** `CC` `H1`

√7th **T81.528** Obstruction due to foreign body accidentally left in body following **other procedure** `CC` `H1`

√7th **T81.529** Obstruction due to foreign body accidentally left in body following **unspecified procedure** `CC` `H1`

√6th **T81.53** Perforation due to foreign body accidentally left in body following procedure

√7th **T81.530** Perforation due to foreign body accidentally left in body following **surgical operation** `CC` `H1`

√7th **T81.531** Perforation due to foreign body accidentally left in body following **infusion or transfusion** `CC` `H1`

√7th **T81.532** Perforation due to foreign body accidentally left in body following **kidney dialysis** `CC` `H1` `HCC`

√7th **T81.533** Perforation due to foreign body accidentally left in body following **injection or immunization** `CC` `H1`

√7th **T81.534** Perforation due to foreign body accidentally left in body following **endoscopic examination** `CC` `H1`

√7th **T81.535** Perforation due to foreign body accidentally left in body following **heart catheterization** `CC` `H1`

√7th **T81.536** Perforation due to foreign body accidentally left in body following **aspiration, puncture or other catheterization** `CC` `H1`

√7th **T81.537** Perforation due to foreign body accidentally left in body following **removal of catheter or packing** `CC` `H1`

√7th **T81.538** Perforation due to foreign body accidentally left in body following **other procedure** `CC` `H1`

√7th **T81.539** Perforation due to foreign body accidentally left in body following **unspecified procedure** `CC` `H1`

√6th **T81.59** Other complications of foreign body accidentally left in body following procedure

EXCLUDES 2 obstruction or perforation due to prosthetic devices and implants intentionally left in body (T82.0-T82.5, T83.0-T83.4, T83.7, T84.0-T84.4, T85.0-T85.6)

√7th **T81.590** Other complications of foreign body accidentally left in body following **surgical operation** `CC` `H1`

√7th **T81.591** Other complications of foreign body accidentally left in body following **infusion or transfusion** `CC` `H1`

√7th **T81.592** Other complications of foreign body accidentally left in body following **kidney dialysis** `CC` `H1` `HCC`

√7th **T81.593** Other complications of foreign body accidentally left in body following **injection or immunization** `CC` `H1`

√7th **T81.594** Other complications of foreign body accidentally left in body following **endoscopic examination** `CC` `H1`

√7th **T81.595** Other complications of foreign body accidentally left in body following **heart catheterization** `CC` `H1`

√7th **T81.596** Other complications of foreign body accidentally left in body following **aspiration, puncture or other catheterization** `CC` `H1`

√7th **T81.597** Other complications of foreign body accidentally left in body following **removal of catheter or packing** `CC` `H1`

√7th **T81.598** Other complications of foreign body accidentally left in body following **other procedure** `CC` `H1`

√7th **T81.599** Other complications of foreign body accidentally left in body following **unspecified procedure** `CC` `H1`

√5th **T81.6** Acute reaction to foreign substance accidentally left during a procedure

EXCLUDES 2 complications of foreign body accidentally left in body cavity or operation wound following procedure (T81.5-)

**CC Excl: For codes in subcategory T81.6:**
PDX collection 1444

√x7th **T81.60** Unspecified acute reaction to foreign substance accidentally left during a procedure `CC` `H1`

√x7th **T81.61** Aseptic peritonitis due to foreign substance accidentally left during a procedure `CC` `H1`
Chemical peritonitis

√x7th **T81.69** Other acute reaction to foreign substance accidentally left during a procedure `CC` `H1`

√5th **T81.7** Vascular complications following a procedure, not elsewhere classified
Air embolism following procedure NEC
Phlebitis or thrombophlebitis resulting from a procedure

EXCLUDES 1 embolism complicating abortion or ectopic or molar pregnancy (O00-O07, O08.2)
embolism complicating pregnancy, childbirth and the puerperium (O88.-)
traumatic embolism (T79.0)

EXCLUDES 2 embolism due to prosthetic devices, implants and grafts (T82.8-, T83.81, T84.8-, T85.81-)
embolism following infusion, transfusion and therapeutic injection (T80.0)

√6th **T81.71** Complication of artery following a procedure, not elsewhere classified

√7th **T81.710** Complication of mesenteric artery following a procedure, not elsewhere classified `CC`
**CC Excl:** PDX collection 1445

√7th **T81.711** Complication of renal artery following a procedure, not elsewhere classified `CC`
**CC Excl:** PDX collection 1445

N Newborn: 0   P Pediatric: 0-17   M Maternity: 12-55   A Adult: 15-124   MCC Major CC Condition   PDxMCC PDx acts as own MCC   CC CC Condition   PDxCC PDx acts as own CC

1140

ICD-10-CM 2018

√7ᵗʰ **T81.718** **Complication of** other **artery following a procedure, not elsewhere classified**   CC
     CC Excl: PDX collection 1446

√7ᵗʰ **T81.719** **Complication of** unspecified **artery following a procedure, not elsewhere classified**   CC
     CC Excl: PDX collection 1446

√x7ᵗʰ **T81.72** **Complication of** vein **following a procedure, not elsewhere classified**
     CC Excl: PDX collection 1446

√5ᵗʰ **T81.8** **Other complications of procedures, not elsewhere classified**
     EXCLUDES 2   *hypothermia following anesthesia (T88.51)*
            *malignant hyperpyrexia due to anesthesia (T88.3)*

√x7ᵗʰ **T81.81** **Complication of inhalation therapy**

√x7ᵗʰ **T81.82** **Emphysema (subcutaneous) resulting from a procedure**

√x7ᵗʰ **T81.83** **Persistent postprocedural fistula**   CC
     CC Excl: PDX collection 1447

√x7ᵗʰ **T81.89** **Other complications of procedures, not elsewhere classified**
     Use additional code to specify complication, such as:
       postprocedural delirium (F05)
     **AHA:** 2014, 1Q, 23

√x7ᵗʰ **T81.9** **Unspecified complication of procedure**

√4ᵗʰ **T82** **Complications of cardiac and vascular prosthetic devices, implants and grafts**
     EXCLUDES 2   *failure and rejection of transplanted organs and tissue (T86.-)*

     The appropriate 7th character is to be added to each code from category T82.
     A     initial encounter
     D     subsequent encounter
     S     sequela

√5ᵗʰ **T82.0** **Mechanical complication of** heart valve prosthesis
     Mechanical complication of artificial heart valve
     EXCLUDES 1   *mechanical complication of biological heart valve graft (T82.22-)*

     **CC Excl: For codes in subcategory T82.0:** PDX collection 1448

√x7ᵗʰ **T82.01** **Breakdown (mechanical) of heart valve prosthesis**   CC

√x7ᵗʰ **T82.02** **Displacement of heart valve prosthesis**   CC
     Malposition of heart valve prosthesis

√x7ᵗʰ **T82.03** **Leakage of heart valve prosthesis**   CC

√x7ᵗʰ **T82.09** **Other mechanical complication of heart valve prosthesis**   CC
     Obstruction (mechanical) of heart valve prosthesis
     Perforation of heart valve prosthesis
     Protrusion of heart valve prosthesis

√5ᵗʰ **T82.1** **Mechanical complication of** cardiac electronic device

     **CC Excl: For codes in subcategory T82.1, unless otherwise noted:** PDX collection 1449

√6ᵗʰ **T82.11** **Breakdown (mechanical) of cardiac electronic device**

√7ᵗʰ **T82.110** **Breakdown (mechanical) of cardiac electrode**   CC

√7ᵗʰ **T82.111** **Breakdown (mechanical) of cardiac pulse generator (battery)**

√7ᵗʰ **T82.118** **Breakdown (mechanical) of other cardiac electronic device**   CC
     CC Excl: PDX collection 1450

√7ᵗʰ **T82.119** **Breakdown (mechanical) of** unspecified **cardiac electronic device**   CC
     CC Excl: No Excl

√6ᵗʰ **T82.12** **Displacement of cardiac electronic device**
     Malposition of cardiac electronic device

√7ᵗʰ **T82.120** **Displacement of** cardiac electrode   CC

√7ᵗʰ **T82.121** **Displacement of cardiac** pulse generator (battery)   CC

√7ᵗʰ **T82.128** **Displacement of other cardiac electronic device**   CC
     CC Excl: PDX collection 1450

√7ᵗʰ **T82.129** **Displacement of** unspecified cardiac electronic device   CC
     CC Excl: No Excl

√6ᵗʰ **T82.19** **Other mechanical complication of cardiac electronic device**
     Leakage of cardiac electronic device
     Obstruction of cardiac electronic device
     Perforation of cardiac electronic device
     Protrusion of cardiac electronic device

√7ᵗʰ **T82.190** **Other mechanical complication of cardiac electrode**   CC

√7ᵗʰ **T82.191** **Other mechanical complication of cardiac** pulse generator (battery)   CC

√7ᵗʰ **T82.198** **Other mechanical complication of** other cardiac electronic device   CC
     CC Excl: PDX collection 1450

√7ᵗʰ **T82.199** **Other mechanical complication of** unspecified **cardiac device**   CC
     CC Excl: No Excl

√5ᵗʰ **T82.2** **Mechanical complication of** coronary artery bypass graft and biological heart valve graft
     EXCLUDES 1   *mechanical complication of artificial heart valve prosthesis (T82.0-)*

√6ᵗʰ **T82.21** **Mechanical complication of** coronary artery bypass graft

     **CC Excl: For codes in subcategory T82.21:** PDX collection 1451

√7ᵗʰ **T82.211** **Breakdown (mechanical) of coronary artery bypass graft**   CC

√7ᵗʰ **T82.212** **Displacement of coronary artery bypass graft**   CC
     Malposition of coronary artery bypass graft

√7ᵗʰ **T82.213** **Leakage of coronary artery bypass graft**   CC

√7ᵗʰ **T82.218** **Other mechanical complication of coronary artery bypass graft**   CC
     Obstruction, mechanical of coronary artery bypass graft
     Perforation of coronary artery bypass graft
     Protrusion of coronary artery bypass graft

√6ᵗʰ **T82.22** **Mechanical complication of** biological heart valve graft

     **CC Excl: For codes in subcategory T82.22:** PDX collection 1450

√7ᵗʰ **T82.221** **Breakdown (mechanical) of biological heart valve graft**   CC

√7ᵗʰ **T82.222** **Displacement of biological heart valve graft**   CC
     Malposition of biological heart valve graft

√7ᵗʰ **T82.223** **Leakage of biological heart valve graft**   CC

√7ᵗʰ **T82.228** **Other mechanical complication of biological heart valve graft**   CC
     Obstruction of biological heart valve graft
     Perforation of biological heart valve graft
     Protrusion of biological heart valve graft

√5ᵗʰ **T82.3** **Mechanical complication of** other vascular grafts

     **CC Excl: For codes in subcategory T82.3:** PDX collection 1452

√6ᵗʰ **T82.31** **Breakdown (mechanical) of other vascular grafts**

10 √7ᵗʰ **T82.310** **Breakdown (mechanical) of** aortic **(bifurcation) graft (replacement)**   CC HCC

10 √7ᵗʰ **T82.311** **Breakdown (mechanical) of** carotid **arterial graft (bypass)**   CC HCC

10 √7ᵗʰ **T82.312** **Breakdown (mechanical) of** femoral **arterial graft (bypass)**   CC HCC

10 √7ᵗʰ **T82.318** **Breakdown (mechanical) of** other **vascular grafts**   CC HCC

10 √7ᵗʰ **T82.319** **Breakdown (mechanical) of** unspecified **vascular grafts**   CC HCC

√6ᵗʰ **T82.32** **Displacement of other vascular grafts**
     Malposition of other vascular grafts

10 √7ᵗʰ **T82.320** **Displacement of** aortic **(bifurcation) graft (replacement)**   CC HCC

10 √7ᵗʰ **T82.321** **Displacement of** carotid arterial **graft (bypass)**   CC HCC

10 √7ᵗʰ **T82.322** **Displacement of** femoral arterial **graft (bypass)**   CC HCC

---

10   HCC with 7th character indicating initial encounter (A, B or C - specific to category).

√ Additional Character Req    √x7ᵗʰ Placeholder Alert    Unacceptable PDx    Manifestation    H1-H14 HAC    HCC CMS-HCC Condition    EXCLUDES 1 Not Coded Here    EXCLUDES 2 Not Included Here

**Chapter 19. Injury, Poisoning and Certain Other Consequences of External Causes** *(side margin)*

10 ✓7ᵗʰ **T82.328** **Displacement of** other **vascular grafts** `CC` `HCC`

10 ✓7ᵗʰ **T82.329** **Displacement of** unspecified **vascular grafts** `CC` `HCC`

✓6ᵗʰ **T82.33** **Leakage of other vascular grafts**

10 ✓7ᵗʰ **T82.330** **Leakage of** aortic (bifurcation) **graft (replacement)** `CC` `HCC`

10 ✓7ᵗʰ **T82.331** **Leakage of** carotid arterial graft (bypass) `CC` `HCC`

10 ✓7ᵗʰ **T82.332** **Leakage of** femoral arterial graft (bypass) `CC` `HCC`

10 ✓7ᵗʰ **T82.338** **Leakage of** other **vascular grafts** `CC` `HCC`

10 ✓7ᵗʰ **T82.339** **Leakage of** unspecified **vascular graft** `CC` `HCC`

✓6ᵗʰ **T82.39** **Other** mechanical complication of other **vascular grafts**

    Obstruction (mechanical) of other vascular grafts
    Perforation of other vascular grafts
    Protrusion of other vascular grafts

10 ✓7ᵗʰ **T82.390** **Other mechanical complication of** aortic (bifurcation) graft (replacement) `CC` `HCC`

10 ✓7ᵗʰ **T82.391** **Other mechanical complication of** carotid arterial graft (bypass) `CC` `HCC`

10 ✓7ᵗʰ **T82.392** **Other mechanical complication of** femoral arterial graft (bypass) `CC` `HCC`

10 ✓7ᵗʰ **T82.398** **Other mechanical complication of** other **vascular grafts** `CC` `HCC`

10 ✓7ᵗʰ **T82.399** **Other mechanical complication of** unspecified **vascular grafts** `CC` `HCC`

✓5ᵗʰ **T82.4** **Mechanical complication of** vascular dialysis catheter

    Mechanical complication of hemodialysis catheter

    **EXCLUDES 1**   *mechanical complication of intraperitoneal dialysis catheter (T85.62)*

    **CC Excl: For codes in subcategory T82.4:**
    PDX collection 1452

✓x7ᵗʰ **T82.41** **Breakdown (mechanical) of vascular dialysis catheter** `CC` `HCC`

✓x7ᵗʰ **T82.42** **Displacement of vascular dialysis catheter** `CC` `HCC`

    Malposition of vascular dialysis catheter

✓x7ᵗʰ **T82.43** **Leakage of vascular dialysis catheter** `CC` `HCC`

✓x7ᵗʰ **T82.49** **Other complication of vascular dialysis catheter** `CC` `HCC`

    Obstruction (mechanical) of vascular dialysis catheter
    Perforation of vascular dialysis catheter
    Protrusion of vascular dialysis catheter

✓5ᵗʰ **T82.5** **Mechanical complication of** other cardiac and vascular devices and implants

    **EXCLUDES 2**   *mechanical complication of epidural and subdural infusion catheter (T85.61)*

    **CC Excl: For codes in subcategory T82.5, unless otherwise noted:** PDX collection 1452

✓6ᵗʰ **T82.51** **Breakdown (mechanical) of other cardiac and vascular devices and implants**

10 ✓7ᵗʰ **T82.510** **Breakdown (mechanical) of** surgically created arteriovenous fistula `CC` `HCC`

10 ✓7ᵗʰ **T82.511** **Breakdown (mechanical) of** surgically created arteriovenous shunt `CC` `HCC`

✓7ᵗʰ **T82.512** **Breakdown (mechanical) of artificial heart** `CC`
    **CC Excl:** PDX collection 1450

10 ✓7ᵗʰ **T82.513** **Breakdown (mechanical) of** balloon (counterpulsation) device `CC` `HCC`

10 ✓7ᵗʰ **T82.514** **Breakdown (mechanical) of infusion catheter** `CC` `HCC`

10 ✓7ᵗʰ **T82.515** **Breakdown (mechanical) of umbrella device** `CC` `HCC`

10 ✓7ᵗʰ **T82.518** **Breakdown (mechanical) of** other **cardiac and vascular devices and implants** `CC` `HCC`

✓7ᵗʰ **T82.519** **Breakdown (mechanical) of** unspecified **cardiac and vascular devices and implants** `CC`
    **CC Excl:** PDX collection 1453

✓6ᵗʰ **T82.52** **Displacement** of other cardiac and vascular devices and implants

    Malposition of other cardiac and vascular devices and implants

10 ✓7ᵗʰ **T82.520** **Displacement of** surgically created arteriovenous fistula `CC` `HCC`

10 ✓7ᵗʰ **T82.521** **Displacement of** surgically created arteriovenous shunt `CC` `HCC`

✓7ᵗʰ **T82.522** **Displacement of** artificial heart `CC`
    **CC Excl:** PDX collection 1450

10 ✓7ᵗʰ **T82.523** **Displacement of** balloon (counterpulsation) device `CC` `HCC`

10 ✓7ᵗʰ **T82.524** **Displacement of** infusion catheter `CC` `HCC`

10 ✓7ᵗʰ **T82.525** **Displacement of** umbrella device `CC` `HCC`

10 ✓7ᵗʰ **T82.528** **Displacement of** other **cardiac and vascular devices and implants** `CC` `HCC`

✓7ᵗʰ **T82.529** **Displacement of** unspecified **cardiac and vascular devices and implants** `CC`

✓6ᵗʰ **T82.53** **Leakage** of other cardiac and vascular devices and implants

10 ✓7ᵗʰ **T82.530** **Leakage of** surgically created arteriovenous fistula `CC` `HCC`

10 ✓7ᵗʰ **T82.531** **Leakage of** surgically created arteriovenous shunt `CC` `HCC`

✓7ᵗʰ **T82.532** **Leakage of** artificial heart `CC`
    **CC Excl:** PDX collection 1450

10 ✓7ᵗʰ **T82.533** **Leakage of** balloon (counterpulsation) device `CC` `HCC`

10 ✓7ᵗʰ **T82.534** **Leakage of** infusion catheter `CC` `HCC`

10 ✓7ᵗʰ **T82.535** **Leakage of** umbrella device `CC` `HCC`

10 ✓7ᵗʰ **T82.538** **Leakage of** other **cardiac and vascular devices and implants** `CC` `HCC`

✓7ᵗʰ **T82.539** **Leakage of** unspecified **cardiac and vascular devices and implants** `CC`
    **CC Excl:** PDX collection 1453

✓6ᵗʰ **T82.59** **Other** mechanical complication of other cardiac and vascular devices and implants

    Obstruction (mechanical) of other cardiac and vascular devices and implants
    Perforation of other cardiac and vascular devices and implants
    Protrusion of other cardiac and vascular devices and implants

10 ✓7ᵗʰ **T82.590** **Other mechanical complication of** surgically created arteriovenous fistula `CC` `HCC`

10 ✓7ᵗʰ **T82.591** **Other mechanical complication of** surgically created arteriovenous shunt `CC` `HCC`

✓7ᵗʰ **T82.592** **Other mechanical complication of** artificial heart `CC`
    **CC Excl:** PDX collection 1450

10 ✓7ᵗʰ **T82.593** **Other mechanical complication of** balloon (counterpulsation) device `CC` `HCC`

10 ✓7ᵗʰ **T82.594** **Other mechanical complication of** infusion catheter `CC` `HCC`
    **CC Excl:** PDX collection 1450

10 ✓7ᵗʰ **T82.595** **Other mechanical complication of** umbrella device `CC` `HCC`

10 ✓7ᵗʰ **T82.598** **Other mechanical complication of** other **cardiac and vascular devices and implants** `CC` `HCC`
    **CC Excl:** PDX collection 1450

✓7ᵗʰ **T82.599** **Other mechanical complication of** unspecified **cardiac and vascular devices and implants** `CC`
    **CC Excl:** PDX collection 1453

10 ✓x7ᵗʰ **T82.6** **Infection and inflammatory reaction due to** cardiac valve prosthesis `CC` `H13` `HCC`
    Use additional code to identify infection
    **CC Excl:** PDX collection 1454

10 ✓x7ᵗʰ **T82.7** **Infection and inflammatory reaction due to** other **cardiac and vascular devices, implants and grafts** `CC` `H13` `HCC`
    Use additional code to identify infection
    **CC Excl:** PDX collection 1454

---

10 HCC with 7th character indicating initial encounter (A, B or C - specific to category).

Ⓝ Newborn: 0   Ⓟ Pediatric: 0-17   Ⓜ Maternity: 12-55   Ⓐ Adult: 15-124   `MCC` Major CC Condition   `PDxMCC` PDx acts as own MCC   `CC` CC Condition   `PDxCC` PDx acts as own CC

1142      ICD-10-CM 2018

✓5ᵗʰ **T82.8** **Other specified complications of cardiac and vascular prosthetic devices, implants and grafts**

✓6ᵗʰ   **T82.81** **Embolism due to cardiac and vascular prosthetic devices, implants and grafts**

✓7ᵗʰ   **T82.817** **Embolism due to cardiac prosthetic** `CC` **devices, implants and grafts**
CC Excl: PDX collection 1455

10 ✓7ᵗʰ   **T82.818** **Embolism due to vascular** `CC` `HCC` **prosthetic devices, implants and grafts**
CC Excl: PDX collection 1454

✓6ᵗʰ   **T82.82** **Fibrosis due to cardiac and vascular prosthetic devices, implants and grafts**

✓7ᵗʰ   **T82.827** **Fibrosis due to cardiac prosthetic** `CC` **devices, implants and grafts**
CC Excl: PDX collection 1455

10 ✓7ᵗʰ   **T82.828** **Fibrosis due to vascular prosthetic** `CC` `HCC` **devices, implants and grafts**
CC Excl: PDX collection 1454

✓6ᵗʰ   **T82.83** **Hemorrhage due to cardiac and vascular prosthetic devices, implants and grafts**

✓7ᵗʰ   **T82.837** **Hemorrhage due to cardiac prosthetic** `CC` **devices, implants and grafts**
CC Excl: PDX collection 1455

10 ✓7ᵗʰ   **T82.838** **Hemorrhage due to vascular** `CC` `HCC` **prosthetic devices, implants and grafts**
CC Excl: PDX collection 1454

✓6ᵗʰ   **T82.84** **Pain due to cardiac and vascular prosthetic devices, implants and grafts**

✓7ᵗʰ   **T82.847** **Pain due to cardiac prosthetic devices,** `CC` **implants and grafts**
CC Excl: PDX collection 1455

10 ✓7ᵗʰ   **T82.848** **Pain due to vascular prosthetic** `CC` `HCC` **devices, implants and grafts**
CC Excl: PDX collection 1454

✓6ᵗʰ   **T82.85** **Stenosis due to cardiac and vascular prosthetic devices, implants and grafts**

✓7ᵗʰ   **T82.855** **Stenosis of coronary artery stent** `CC`
In-stent stenosis (restenosis) of coronary artery stent
Restenosis of coronary artery stent
CC Excl: PDX collection 1455

10 ✓7ᵗʰ   **T82.856** **Stenosis of peripheral vascular** `CC` `HCC` **stent**
In-stent stenosis (restenosis) of peripheral vascular stent
Restenosis of peripheral vascular stent
CC Excl: PDX collection 1454

✓7ᵗʰ   **T82.857** **Stenosis of other cardiac prosthetic** `CC` **devices, implants and grafts**
CC Excl: PDX collection 1455

10 ✓7ᵗʰ   **T82.858** **Stenosis of other vascular** `CC` `HCC` **prostheticdevices, implants and grafts**
CC Excl: PDX collection 1454

✓6ᵗʰ   **T82.86** **Thrombosis of cardiac and vascular prosthetic devices, implants and grafts**

✓7ᵗʰ   **T82.867** **Thrombosis due to cardiac prosthetic** `CC` **devices, implants and grafts**
CC Excl: PDX collection 1455

10 ✓7ᵗʰ   **T82.868** **Thrombosis due to vascular** `CC` `HCC` **prosthetic devices, implants and grafts**
CC Excl: PDX collection 1454

✓6ᵗʰ   **T82.89** **Other specified complication of cardiac and vascular prosthetic devices, implants and grafts**

✓7ᵗʰ   **T82.897** **Other specified complication of** `CC` **cardiac prosthetic devices, implants and grafts**
CC Excl: PDX collection 1455

10 ✓7ᵗʰ   **T82.898** **Other specified complication of** `CC` `HCC` **vascular prosthetic devices, implants and grafts**
CC Excl: PDX collection 1454

✓ˣ7ᵗʰ **T82.9** **Unspecified complication of cardiac and vascular** `CC` **prosthetic device, implant and graft**
CC Excl: PDX collection 1455

✓4ᵗʰ **T83** **Complications of genitourinary prosthetic devices, implants and grafts**

*EXCLUDES 2*   *failure and rejection of transplanted organs and tissue (T86.-)*

The appropriate 7th character is to be added to each code from category T83.
A   initial encounter
D   subsequent encounter
S   sequela

**CC Excl: For CC codes in category T83, unless otherwise noted:**
PDX collection 1456

✓5ᵗʰ **T83.0** **Mechanical complication of urinary catheter**

*EXCLUDES 2*   *complications of stoma of urinary tract (N99.5-)*

✓6ᵗʰ   **T83.01** **Breakdown (mechanical) of urinary catheter**

10 ✓7ᵗʰ   **T83.010** **Breakdown (mechanical) of** `CC` `HCC` **cystostomy catheter**

10 ✓7ᵗʰ   **T83.011** **Breakdown (mechanical) of** `HCC` **indwelling urethral catheter**

10 ✓7ᵗʰ   **T83.012** **Breakdown (mechanical) of** `HCC` **nephrostomy catheter**

10 ✓7ᵗʰ   **T83.018** **Breakdown (mechanical) of other** `HCC` **urinary catheter**
Breakdown (mechanical) of Hopkins catheter
Breakdown (mechanical) of ileostomy catheter
Breakdown (mechanical) urostomy catheter

✓6ᵗʰ   **T83.02** **Displacement of urinary catheter**
Malposition of urinary catheter

10 ✓7ᵗʰ   **T83.020** **Displacement of cystostomy** `CC` `HCC` **catheter**

10 ✓7ᵗʰ   **T83.021** **Displacement of indwelling urethral** `HCC` **catheter**

10 ✓7ᵗʰ   **T83.022** **Displacement of nephrostomy** `HCC` **catheter**

10 ✓7ᵗʰ   **T83.028** **Displacement of other urinary** `HCC` **catheter**
Displacement of Hopkins catheter
Displacement of ileostomy catheter
Displacement of urostomy catheter

✓6ᵗʰ   **T83.03** **Leakage of urinary catheter**

10 ✓7ᵗʰ   **T83.030** **Leakage of cystostomy catheter** `CC` `HCC`

10 ✓7ᵗʰ   **T83.031** **Leakage of indwelling urethral** `HCC` **catheter**

10 ✓7ᵗʰ   **T83.032** **Leakage of nephrostomy catheter** `HCC`

10 ✓7ᵗʰ   **T83.038** **Leakage of other urinary catheter** `HCC`
Leakage of Hopkins catheter
Leakage of ileostomy catheter
Leakage of urostomy catheter

✓6ᵗʰ   **T83.09** **Other mechanical complication of urinary catheter**
Obstruction (mechanical) of urinary catheter
Perforation of urinary catheter
Protrusion of urinary catheter

10 ✓7ᵗʰ   **T83.090** **Other mechanical complication of** `CC` `HCC` **cystostomy catheter**

10 ✓7ᵗʰ   **T83.091** **Other mechanical complication of** `HCC` **indwelling urethral catheter**

10 ✓7ᵗʰ   **T83.092** **Other mechanical complication of** `HCC` **nephrostomy catheter**

10 ✓7ᵗʰ   **T83.098** **Other mechanical complication of** `HCC` **other urinary catheter**
Other mechanical complication of Hopkins catheter
Other mechanical complication of ileostomy catheter
Other mechanical complication of urostomy catheter

---

[10] HCC with 7th character indicating initial encounter (A, B or C - specific to category).

✓ Additional Character Req   ✓ˣ7ᵗʰ Placeholder Alert   Unacceptable PDx   Manifestation   `H1`-`H14` HAC   `HCC` CMS-HCC Condition   *EXCLUDES 1* Not Coded Here   *EXCLUDES 2* Not Included Here

✓5ᵗʰ **T83.1** Mechanical complication of other urinary devices and implants

✓6ᵗʰ **T83.11** Breakdown (mechanical) of other urinary devices and implants

10 ✓7ᵗʰ **T83.110** Breakdown (mechanical) of urinary **CC HCC** electronic stimulator device

EXCLUDES 2 breakdown (mechanical) of electrode (lead) for sacral nerve neurostimulator (T85.111)
breakdown (mechanical) of implanted electronic sacral neurostimulator, pulse generator or receiver (T85.113)

10 ✓7ᵗʰ **T83.111** Breakdown (mechanical) of **CC HCC** implanted urinary sphincter

10 ✓7ᵗʰ **T83.112** Breakdown (mechanical) of **CC HCC** indwelling ureteral stent

10 ✓7ᵗʰ **T83.113** Breakdown (mechanical) of other **CC HCC** urinary stents

Breakdown (mechanical) of ileal conduit stent
Breakdown (mechanical) of nephroureteral stent

10 ✓7ᵗʰ **T83.118** Breakdown (mechanical) of other **CC HCC** urinary devices and implants

✓6ᵗʰ **T83.12** Displacement of other urinary devices and implants

Malposition of other urinary devices and implants

10 ✓7ᵗʰ **T83.120** Displacement of urinary electronic **CC HCC** stimulator device

EXCLUDES 2 displacement of electrode (lead) for sacral nerve neurostimulator (T85.121)
displacement of implanted electronic sacral neurostimulator, pulse generator or receiver (T85.123)

10 ✓7ᵗʰ **T83.121** Displacement of implanted **CC HCC** urinary sphincter

10 ✓7ᵗʰ **T83.122** Displacement of indwelling **CC HCC** ureteral stent

10 ✓7ᵗʰ **T83.123** Displacement of other urinary **CC HCC** stents

Displacement of ileal conduit stent
Displacement of nephroureteral stent

10 ✓7ᵗʰ **T83.128** Displacement of other urinary **CC HCC** devices and implants

✓6ᵗʰ **T83.19** Other mechanical complication of other urinary devices and implants

Leakage of other urinary devices and implants
Obstruction (mechanical) of other urinary devices and implants
Perforation of other urinary devices and implants
Protrusion of other urinary devices and implants

10 ✓7ᵗʰ **T83.190** Other mechanical complication of **CC HCC** urinary electronic stimulator device

EXCLUDES 2 other mechanical complication of electrode (lead) for sacral nerve neurostimulator (T85.191)
other mechanical complication of implanted electronic sacral neurostimulator, pulse generator or receiver (T85.193)

10 ✓7ᵗʰ **T83.191** Other mechanical complication of **CC HCC** implanted urinary sphincter

10 ✓7ᵗʰ **T83.192** Other mechanical complication of **CC HCC** indwelling ureteral stent

10 ✓7ᵗʰ **T83.193** Other mechanical complication of **CC HCC** other urinary stent

Other mechanical complication of ileal conduit stent
Other mechanical complication of nephroureteral stent

10 ✓7ᵗʰ **T83.198** Other mechanical complication of **CC HCC** other urinary devices and implants

✓5ᵗʰ **T83.2** Mechanical complication of graft of urinary organ

10 ✓x7ᵗʰ **T83.21** Breakdown (mechanical) of graft of urinary **CC HCC** organ

10 ✓x7ᵗʰ **T83.22** Displacement of graft of urinary organ **CC HCC**

Malposition of graft of urinary organ

10 ✓x7ᵗʰ **T83.23** Leakage of graft of urinary organ **CC HCC**

10 ✓x7ᵗʰ **T83.24** Erosion of graft of urinary organ **CC HCC**

10 ✓x7ᵗʰ **T83.25** Exposure of graft of urinary organ **CC HCC**

10 ✓x7ᵗʰ **T83.29** Other mechanical complication of graft of **CC HCC** urinary organ

Obstruction (mechanical) of graft of urinary organ
Perforation of graft of urinary organ
Protrusion of graft of urinary organ

✓5ᵗʰ **T83.3** Mechanical complication of intrauterine contraceptive device

✓x7ᵗʰ **T83.31** Breakdown (mechanical) of intrauterine ♀ contraceptive device

✓x7ᵗʰ **T83.32** Displacement of intrauterine contraceptive ♀ device

Malposition of intrauterine contraceptive device
Missing string of intrauterine contraceptive device

✓x7ᵗʰ **T83.39** Other mechanical complication of intrauterine ♀ contraceptive device

Leakage of intrauterine contraceptive device
Obstruction (mechanical) of intrauterine contraceptive device
Perforation of intrauterine contraceptive device
Protrusion of intrauterine contraceptive device

✓5ᵗʰ **T83.4** Mechanical complication of other prosthetic devices, implants and grafts of genital tract

✓6ᵗʰ **T83.41** Breakdown (mechanical) of other prosthetic devices, implants and grafts of genital tract

10 ✓7ᵗʰ **T83.410** Breakdown (mechanical) of **CC HCC** ♂ implanted penile prosthesis

Breakdown (mechanical) of penile prosthesis cylinder
Breakdown (mechanical) of penile prosthesis pump
Breakdown (mechanical) of penile prosthesis reservoir

10 ✓7ᵗʰ **T83.411** Breakdown (mechanical) of **CC HCC** implanted testicular prosthesis

10 ✓7ᵗʰ **T83.418** Breakdown (mechanical) of other **CC HCC** prosthetic devices, implants and grafts of genital tract

✓6ᵗʰ **T83.42** Displacement of other prosthetic devices, implants and grafts of genital tract

Malposition of other prosthetic devices, implants and grafts of genital tract

10 ✓7ᵗʰ **T83.420** Displacement of implanted penile **CC HCC** ♂ prosthesis

Displacement of penile prosthesis cylinder
Displacement of penile prosthesis pump
Displacement of penile prosthesis reservoir

10 ✓7ᵗʰ **T83.421** Displacement of implanted **CC HCC** testicular prosthesis

10 ✓7ᵗʰ **T83.428** Displacement of other prosthetic **CC HCC** devices, implants and grafts of genital tract

✓6ᵗʰ **T83.49** Other mechanical complication of other prosthetic devices, implants and grafts of genital tract

Leakage of other prosthetic devices, implants and grafts of genital tract
Obstruction, mechanical of other prosthetic devices, implants and grafts of genital tract
Perforation of other prosthetic devices, implants and grafts of genital tract
Protrusion of other prosthetic devices, implants and grafts of genital tract

10 ✓7ᵗʰ **T83.490** Other mechanical complication **CC HCC** ♂ of implanted penile prosthesis

Other mechanical complication of penile prosthesis cylinder
Other mechanical complication of penile prosthesis pump
Other mechanical complication of penile prosthesis reservoir

---

10 HCC with 7th character indicating initial encounter (A, B or C - specific to category).

**10** ☑7ᵗʰ **T83.491** **Other mechanical complication of** CC HCC
**implanted testicular prosthesis**

**10** ☑7ᵗʰ **T83.498** **Other mechanical complication of** CC HCC
**other prosthetic devices, implants and grafts of genital tract**

☑5ᵗʰ **T83.5** **Infection and inflammatory reaction due to prosthetic device, implant and graft in urinary system**
Use additional code to identify infection

CC Excl: For codes in subcategory T83.5, unless otherwise noted: PDX collection 1458

☑6ᵗʰ **T83.51** **Infection and inflammatory reaction due to urinary catheter**
EXCLUDES 2   complications of stoma of urinary tract (N99.5-)

**10** ☑7ᵗʰ **T83.510** **Infection and inflammatory** CC HCC
**reaction due to cystostomy catheter**

**10** ☑7ᵗʰ **T83.511** **Infection and inflammatory** CC H5 HCC
**reaction due to indwelling urethral catheter**
CC Excl: PDX collection 1457

**10** ☑7ᵗʰ **T83.512** **Infection and inflammatory** CC HCC
**reaction due to nephrostomy catheter**

**10** ☑7ᵗʰ **T83.518** **Infection and inflammatory** CC H5 HCC
**reaction due to other urinary catheter**
Infection and inflammatory reaction due to Hopkins catheter
Infection and inflammatory reaction due to ileostomy catheter
Infection and inflammatory reaction due to urostomy catheter

☑6ᵗʰ **T83.59** **Infection and inflammatory reaction due to prosthetic device, implant and graft in urinary system**

**10** ☑7ᵗʰ **T83.590** **Infection and inflammatory** CC HCC
**reaction due to implanted urinary neurostimulation device**
EXCLUDES 2   infection and inflammatory reaction due to electrode lead of sacral nerve neurostimulator (T85.732)
infection and inflammatory reaction due to pulse generator or receiver of sacral nerve neurostimulator (T85.734)

**10** ☑7ᵗʰ **T83.591** **Infection and inflammatory** CC HCC
**reaction due to implanted urinary sphincter**

**10** ☑7ᵗʰ **T83.592** **Infection and inflammatory** CC HCC
**reaction due to indwelling ureteral stent**

**10** ☑7ᵗʰ **T83.593** **Infection and inflammatory** CC HCC
**reaction due to other urinary stents**
Infection and inflammatory reaction due to ileal conduit stents
Infection and inflammatory reaction due to nephroureteral stent

**10** ☑7ᵗʰ **T83.598** **Infection and inflammatory** CC HCC
**reaction due to other prosthetic device, implant and graft in urinary system**

☑5ᵗʰ **T83.6** **Infection and inflammatory reaction due to prosthetic device, implant and graft in genital tract**
Use additional code to identify infection

CC Excl: For codes in subcategory T83.6: PDX collection 1458

**10** ☑ₓ7ᵗʰ **T83.61** **Infection and inflammatory reaction due to** CC HCC
**implanted penile prosthesis**
Infection and inflammatory reaction due to penile prosthesis cylinder
Infection and inflammatory reaction due to penile prosthesis pump
Infection and inflammatory reaction due to penile prosthesis reservoir

**10** ☑ₓ7ᵗʰ **T83.62** **Infection and inflammatory reaction due to** CC HCC
**implanted testicular prosthesis**

**10** ☑ₓ7ᵗʰ **T83.69** **Infection and inflammatory reaction due to** CC HCC
**other prosthetic device, implant and graft in genital tract**

☑5ᵗʰ **T83.7** **Complications due to implanted mesh and other prosthetic materials**

☑6ᵗʰ **T83.71** **Erosion of implanted mesh and other prosthetic materials to surrounding organ or tissue**

**10** ☑7ᵗʰ **T83.711** **Erosion of implanted vaginal mesh** HCC ♀
**to surrounding organ or tissue**
Erosion of implanted vaginal mesh into pelvic floor muscles

**10** ☑7ᵗʰ **T83.712** **Erosion of implanted urethral** CC HCC
**mesh to surrounding organ or tissue**
Erosion of implanted female urethral sling
Erosion of implanted male urethral sling
Erosion of implanted urethral mesh into pelvic floor muscles

**10** ☑7ᵗʰ **T83.713** **Erosion of implanted urethral** CC HCC
**bulking agent to surrounding organ or tissue**

**10** ☑7ᵗʰ **T83.714** **Erosion of implanted ureteral** CC HCC
**bulking agent to surrounding organ or tissue**

**10** ☑7ᵗʰ **T83.718** **Erosion of other implanted mesh** CC HCC
**to organ or tissue**

**10** ☑7ᵗʰ **T83.719** **Erosion of other prosthetic** CC HCC
**materials to surrounding organ or tissue**

☑6ᵗʰ **T83.72** **Exposure of implanted mesh and other prosthetic materials into surrounding organ or tissue**
Extrusion of implanted mesh

**10** ☑7ᵗʰ **T83.721** **Exposure of implanted vaginal mesh** HCC ♀
**into vagina**
Exposure of implanted vaginal mesh through vaginal wall

**10** ☑7ᵗʰ **T83.722** **Exposure of implanted urethral** CC HCC
**mesh into urethra**
Exposure of implanted female urethral sling
Exposure of implanted male urethral sling
Exposure of implanted urethral mesh through urethral wall

**10** ☑7ᵗʰ **T83.723** **Exposure of implanted urethral** CC HCC
**bulking agent into urethra**

**10** ☑7ᵗʰ **T83.724** **Exposure of implanted ureteral** CC HCC
**bulking agent into ureter**

**10** ☑7ᵗʰ **T83.728** **Exposure of other implanted mesh** CC HCC
**into organ or tissue**

**10** ☑7ᵗʰ **T83.729** **Exposure of other prosthetic** CC HCC
**materials into organ or tissue**

**10** ☑ₓ7ᵗʰ **T83.79** **Other specified complications due to other** CC HCC
**genitourinary prosthetic materials**
CC Excl: PDX collection 1458

☑5ᵗʰ **T83.8** **Other specified complications of genitourinary prosthetic devices, implants and grafts**

CC Excl: For codes in subcategory T83.8: PDX collection 1458

**10** ☑ₓ7ᵗʰ **T83.81** **Embolism due to genitourinary prosthetic** CC HCC
**devices, implants and grafts**

**10** ☑ₓ7ᵗʰ **T83.82** **Fibrosis due to genitourinary prosthetic** CC HCC
**devices, implants and grafts**

**10** ☑ₓ7ᵗʰ **T83.83** **Hemorrhage due to genitourinary prosthetic** CC HCC
**devices, implants and grafts**

**10** ☑ₓ7ᵗʰ **T83.84** **Pain due to genitourinary prosthetic devices,** CC HCC
**implants and grafts**

**10** ☑ₓ7ᵗʰ **T83.85** **Stenosis due to genitourinary prosthetic** CC HCC
**devices, implants and grafts**

**10** ☑ₓ7ᵗʰ **T83.86** **Thrombosis due to genitourinary prosthetic** CC HCC
**devices, implants and grafts**

**10** ☑ₓ7ᵗʰ **T83.89** **Other specified complication of genitourinary** CC HCC
**prosthetic devices, implants and grafts**

**10** ☑ₓ7ᵗʰ **T83.9** **Unspecified complication of genitourinary prosthetic** CC HCC
**device, implant and graft**
CC Excl: PDX collection 1458

---

**10** HCC with 7th character indicating initial encounter (A, B or C - specific to category).

**Chapter 19. Injury, Poisoning and Certain Other Consequences of External Causes**

**T84.119**

✓4th **T84  Complications of internal orthopedic prosthetic devices, implants and grafts**

> EXCLUDES 2  *failure and rejection of transplanted organs and tissues (T86.-)*
> *fracture of bone following insertion of orthopedic implant, joint prosthesis or bone plate (M96.6)*

> The appropriate 7th character is to be added to each code from category T84.
> A     initial encounter
> D     subsequent encounter
> S     sequela

> **CC Excl: For codes in category T84, unless otherwise noted:**
> PDX collection 911

✓5th **T84.0  Mechanical complication of internal joint prosthesis**

✓6th **T84.01  Broken internal joint prosthesis**
Breakage (fracture) of prosthetic joint
Broken prosthetic joint implant
> EXCLUDES 1  *periprosthetic joint implant fracture ►(M97-)◄*

10 ✓7th **T84.010  Broken internal right hip prosthesis** CC HCC
10 ✓7th **T84.011  Broken internal left hip prosthesis** CC HCC
10 ✓7th **T84.012  Broken internal right knee prosthesis** CC HCC
10 ✓7th **T84.013  Broken internal left knee prosthesis** CC HCC
10 ✓7th **T84.018  Broken internal joint prosthesis, other site** CC HCC
Use additional code to identify the joint (Z96.6-)
10 ✓7th **T84.019  Broken internal joint prosthesis, unspecified site** CC HCC

✓6th **T84.02  Dislocation of internal joint prosthesis**
Instability of internal joint prosthesis
Subluxation of internal joint prosthesis

10 ✓7th **T84.020  Dislocation of internal right hip prosthesis** CC HCC
10 ✓7th **T84.021  Dislocation of internal left hip prosthesis** CC HCC
10 ✓7th **T84.022  Instability of internal right knee prosthesis** CC HCC
10 ✓7th **T84.023  Instability of internal left knee prosthesis** CC HCC
10 ✓7th **T84.028  Dislocation of other internal joint prosthesis** CC HCC
Use additional code to identify the joint (Z96.6-)
10 ✓7th **T84.029  Dislocation of unspecified internal joint prosthesis** CC HCC

✓6th **T84.03  Mechanical loosening of internal prosthetic joint**
Aseptic loosening of prosthetic joint

10 ✓7th **T84.030  Mechanical loosening of internal right hip prosthetic joint** CC HCC
10 ✓7th **T84.031  Mechanical loosening of internal left hip prosthetic joint** CC HCC
10 ✓7th **T84.032  Mechanical loosening of internal right knee prosthetic joint** CC HCC
10 ✓7th **T84.033  Mechanical loosening of internal left knee prosthetic joint** CC HCC
10 ✓7th **T84.038  Mechanical loosening of other internal prosthetic joint** CC HCC
Use additional code to identify the joint (Z96.6-)
10 ✓7th **T84.039  Mechanical loosening of unspecified internal prosthetic joint** CC HCC

✓6th **T84.05  Periprosthetic osteolysis of internal prosthetic joint**
Use additional code to identify major osseous defect, if applicable (M89.7-)

10 ✓7th **T84.050  Periprosthetic osteolysis of internal prosthetic right hip joint** CC HCC
10 ✓7th **T84.051  Periprosthetic osteolysis of internal prosthetic left hip joint** CC HCC
10 ✓7th **T84.052  Periprosthetic osteolysis of internal prosthetic right knee joint** CC HCC
10 ✓7th **T84.053  Periprosthetic osteolysis of internal prosthetic left knee joint** CC HCC

10 ✓7th **T84.058  Periprosthetic osteolysis of other internal prosthetic joint** CC HCC
Use additional code to identify the joint (Z96.6-)
10 ✓7th **T84.059  Periprosthetic osteolysis of unspecified internal prosthetic joint** CC HCC

✓6th **T84.06  Wear of articular bearing surface of internal prosthetic joint**

10 ✓7th **T84.060  Wear of articular bearing surface of internal prosthetic right hip joint** CC HCC
10 ✓7th **T84.061  Wear of articular bearing surface of internal prosthetic left hip joint** CC HCC
10 ✓7th **T84.062  Wear of articular bearing surface of internal prosthetic right knee joint** CC HCC
10 ✓7th **T84.063  Wear of articular bearing surface of internal prosthetic left knee joint** CC HCC
10 ✓7th **T84.068  Wear of articular bearing surface of other internal prosthetic joint** CC HCC
Use additional code to identify the joint (Z96.6-)
10 ✓7th **T84.069  Wear of articular bearing surface of unspecified internal prosthetic joint** CC HCC

✓6th **T84.09  Other mechanical complication of internal joint prosthesis**
Prosthetic joint implant failure NOS

10 ✓7th **T84.090  Other mechanical complication of internal right hip prosthesis** CC HCC
10 ✓7th **T84.091  Other mechanical complication of internal left hip prosthesis** CC HCC
10 ✓7th **T84.092  Other mechanical complication of internal right knee prosthesis** CC HCC
10 ✓7th **T84.093  Other mechanical complication of internal left knee prosthesis** CC HCC
10 ✓7th **T84.098  Other mechanical complication of other internal joint prosthesis** CC HCC
Use additional code to identify the joint (Z96.6-)
10 ✓7th **T84.099  Other mechanical complication of unspecified internal joint prosthesis** CC HCC

✓5th **T84.1  Mechanical complication of internal fixation device of bones of limb**

> EXCLUDES 2  *mechanical complication of internal fixation device of bones of feet (T84.2-)*
> *mechanical complication of internal fixation device of bones of fingers (T84.2-)*
> *mechanical complication of internal fixation device of bones of hands (T84.2-)*
> *mechanical complication of internal fixation device of bones of toes (T84.2-)*

✓6th **T84.11  Breakdown (mechanical) of internal fixation device of bones of limb**

10 ✓7th **T84.110  Breakdown (mechanical) of internal fixation device of right humerus** CC HCC
10 ✓7th **T84.111  Breakdown (mechanical) of internal fixation device of left humerus** CC HCC
10 ✓7th **T84.112  Breakdown (mechanical) of internal fixation device of bone of right forearm** CC HCC
10 ✓7th **T84.113  Breakdown (mechanical) of internal fixation device of bone of left forearm** CC HCC
10 ✓7th **T84.114  Breakdown (mechanical) of internal fixation device of right femur** CC HCC
10 ✓7th **T84.115  Breakdown (mechanical) of internal fixation device of left femur** CC HCC
10 ✓7th **T84.116  Breakdown (mechanical) of internal fixation device of bone of right lower leg** CC HCC
10 ✓7th **T84.117  Breakdown (mechanical) of internal fixation device of bone of left lower leg** CC HCC
10 ✓7th **T84.119  Breakdown (mechanical) of internal fixation device of unspecified bone of limb** CC HCC

---
10  HCC with 7th character indicating initial encounter (A, B or C - specific to category).

√6th **T84.12** **Displacement** of internal fixation device of bones of limb
Malposition of internal fixation device of bones of limb

10 √7th **T84.120** **Displacement of internal fixation device of right humerus** `CC` `HCC`

10 √7th **T84.121** **Displacement of internal fixation device of left humerus** `CC` `HCC`

10 √7th **T84.122** **Displacement of internal fixation device of bone of right forearm** `CC` `HCC`

10 √7th **T84.123** **Displacement of internal fixation device of bone of left forearm** `CC` `HCC`

10 √7th **T84.124** **Displacement of internal fixation device of right femur** `CC` `HCC`

10 √7th **T84.125** **Displacement of internal fixation device of left femur** `CC` `HCC`

10 √7th **T84.126** **Displacement of internal fixation device of bone of right lower leg** `CC` `HCC`

10 √7th **T84.127** **Displacement of internal fixation device of bone of left lower leg** `CC` `HCC`

10 √7th **T84.129** **Displacement of internal fixation device of unspecified bone of limb** `CC` `HCC`

√6th **T84.19** **Other mechanical complication of internal fixation device of bones of limb**
Obstruction (mechanical) of internal fixation device of bones of limb
Perforation of internal fixation device of bones of limb
Protrusion of internal fixation device of bones of limb

10 √7th **T84.190** **Other mechanical complication of internal fixation device of right humerus** `CC` `HCC`

10 √7th **T84.191** **Other mechanical complication of internal fixation device of left humerus** `CC` `HCC`

10 √7th **T84.192** **Other mechanical complication of internal fixation device of bone of right forearm** `CC` `HCC`

10 √7th **T84.193** **Other mechanical complication of internal fixation device of bone of left forearm** `CC` `HCC`

10 √7th **T84.194** **Other mechanical complication of internal fixation device of right femur** `CC` `HCC`

10 √7th **T84.195** **Other mechanical complication of internal fixation device of left femur** `CC` `HCC`

10 √7th **T84.196** **Other mechanical complication of internal fixation device of bone of right lower leg** `CC` `HCC`

10 √7th **T84.197** **Other mechanical complication of internal fixation device of bone of left lower leg** `CC` `HCC`

10 √7th **T84.199** **Other mechanical complication of internal fixation device of unspecified bone of limb** `CC` `HCC`

√5th **T84.2** **Mechanical complication of internal fixation device of other bones**

√6th **T84.21** **Breakdown (mechanical) of internal fixation device of other bones**

10 √7th **T84.210** **Breakdown (mechanical) of internal fixation device of bones of hand and fingers** `CC` `HCC`

10 √7th **T84.213** **Breakdown (mechanical) of internal fixation device of bones of foot and toes** `CC` `HCC`

10 √7th **T84.216** **Breakdown (mechanical) of internal fixation device of vertebrae** `CC` `HCC`

10 √7th **T84.218** **Breakdown (mechanical) of internal fixation device of other bones** `CC` `HCC`

√6th **T84.22** **Displacement of internal fixation device of other bones**
Malposition of internal fixation device of other bones

10 √7th **T84.220** **Displacement of internal fixation device of bones of hand and fingers** `CC` `HCC`

10 √7th **T84.223** **Displacement of internal fixation device of bones of foot and toes** `CC` `HCC`

10 √7th **T84.226** **Displacement of internal fixation device of vertebrae** `CC` `HCC`

10 √7th **T84.228** **Displacement of internal fixation device of other bones** `CC` `HCC`

√6th **T84.29** **Other mechanical complication of internal fixation device of other bones**
Obstruction (mechanical) of internal fixation device of other bones
Perforation of internal fixation device of other bones
Protrusion of internal fixation device of other bones

10 √7th **T84.290** **Other mechanical complication of internal fixation device of bones of hand and fingers** `CC` `HCC`

10 √7th **T84.293** **Other mechanical complication of internal fixation device of bones of foot and toes** `CC` `HCC`

10 √7th **T84.296** **Other mechanical complication of internal fixation device of vertebrae** `CC` `HCC`

10 √7th **T84.298** **Other mechanical complication of internal fixation device of other bones** `CC` `HCC`

√5th **T84.3** **Mechanical complication of other bone devices, implants and grafts**
EXCLUDES 2   other complications of bone graft (T86.83-)

√6th **T84.31** **Breakdown (mechanical) of other bone devices, implants and grafts**

10 √7th **T84.310** **Breakdown (mechanical) of electronic bone stimulator** `CC` `HCC`

10 √7th **T84.318** **Breakdown (mechanical) of other bone devices, implants and grafts** `CC` `HCC`

√6th **T84.32** **Displacement of other bone devices, implants and grafts**
Malposition of other bone devices, implants and grafts

10 √7th **T84.320** **Displacement of electronic bone stimulator** `CC` `HCC`

10 √7th **T84.328** **Displacement of other bone devices, implants and grafts** `CC` `HCC`
**AHA:** 2014, 4Q, 28

√6th **T84.39** **Other mechanical complication of other bone devices, implants and grafts**
Obstruction (mechanical) of other bone devices, implants and grafts
Perforation of other bone devices, implants and grafts
Protrusion of other bone devices, implants and grafts

10 √7th **T84.390** **Other mechanical complication of electronic bone stimulator** `CC` `HCC`

10 √7th **T84.398** **Other mechanical complication of other bone devices, implants and grafts** `CC` `HCC`

√5th **T84.4** **Mechanical complication of other internal orthopedic devices, implants and grafts**

√6th **T84.41** **Breakdown (mechanical) of other internal orthopedic devices, implants and grafts**

10 √7th **T84.410** **Breakdown (mechanical) of muscle and tendon graft** `CC` `HCC`

10 √7th **T84.418** **Breakdown (mechanical) of other internal orthopedic devices, implants and grafts** `CC` `HCC`

√6th **T84.42** **Displacement of other internal orthopedic devices, implants and grafts**
Malposition of other internal orthopedic devices, implants and grafts

10 √7th **T84.420** **Displacement of muscle and tendon graft** `CC` `HCC`

10 √7th **T84.428** **Displacement of other internal orthopedic devices, implants and grafts** `CC` `HCC`

√6th **T84.49** **Other mechanical complication of other internal orthopedic devices, implants and grafts**
Mechanical complication of other internal orthopedic devices, implants and grafts NOS
Obstruction (mechanical) of other internal orthopedic devices, implants and grafts
Perforation of other internal orthopedic devices, implants and grafts
Protrusion of other internal orthopedic devices, implants and grafts

10 √7th **T84.490** **Other mechanical complication of muscle and tendon graft** `CC` `HCC`

10 √7th **T84.498** **Other mechanical complication of other internal orthopedic devices, implants and grafts** `CC` `HCC`

---

**10** HCC with 7th character indicating initial encounter (A, B or C - specific to category).

✔ Additional Character Req   √x7th Placeholder Alert   Unacceptable PDx   Manifestation   H1 - H14 HAC   HCC CMS-HCC Condition   EXCLUDES 1 Not Coded Here   EXCLUDES 2 Not Included Here

ICD-10-CM 2018       1147

T84.12–T84.498

√5ᵗʰ **T84.5** **Infection and inflammatory reaction due to** internal joint prosthesis

Use additional code to identify infection

AHA: 2015, 1Q, 16

> **CC Excl: For codes in subcategory T84.5:**
> PDX collection 1459

10 √x7ᵗʰ **T84.50** **Infection and inflammatory reaction due to** unspecified **internal joint prosthesis**   CC HCC

10 √x7ᵗʰ **T84.51** **Infection and inflammatory reaction due to internal** right hip **prosthesis**   CC HCC

10 √x7ᵗʰ **T84.52** **Infection and inflammatory reaction due to internal** left hip **prosthesis**   CC HCC

10 √x7ᵗʰ **T84.53** **Infection and inflammatory reaction due to internal** right knee **prosthesis**   CC HCC

10 √x7ᵗʰ **T84.54** **Infection and inflammatory reaction due to internal** left knee **prosthesis**   CC HCC

10 √x7ᵗʰ **T84.59** **Infection and inflammatory reaction due to** other **internal joint prosthesis**   CC HCC

√5ᵗʰ **T84.6** **Infection and inflammatory reaction due to** internal fixation device

Use additional code to identify infection

> **CC Excl: For codes in subcategory T84.6:**
> PDX collection 1459

10 √x7ᵗʰ **T84.60** **Infection and inflammatory reaction due to internal fixation device of** unspecified **site**   CC H12 HCC

√6ᵗʰ **T84.61** **Infection and inflammatory reaction due to internal fixation device of** arm

   10 √7ᵗʰ **T84.610** **Infection and inflammatory reaction due to internal fixation device of** right humerus   CC H12 HCC

   10 √7ᵗʰ **T84.611** **Infection and inflammatory reaction due to internal fixation device of** left humerus   CC H12 HCC

   10 √7ᵗʰ **T84.612** **Infection and inflammatory reaction due to internal fixation device of** right radius   CC H12 HCC

   10 √7ᵗʰ **T84.613** **Infection and inflammatory reaction due to internal fixation device of** left radius   CC H12 HCC

   10 √7ᵗʰ **T84.614** **Infection and inflammatory reaction due to internal fixation device of** right ulna   CC H12 HCC

   10 √7ᵗʰ **T84.615** **Infection and inflammatory reaction due to internal fixation device of** left ulna   CC H12 HCC

   10 √7ᵗʰ **T84.619** **Infection and inflammatory reaction due to internal fixation device of** unspecified bone **of arm**   CC H12 HCC

√6ᵗʰ **T84.62** **Infection and inflammatory reaction due to internal fixation device of** leg

   10 √7ᵗʰ **T84.620** **Infection and inflammatory reaction due to internal fixation device of** right femur   CC HCC

   10 √7ᵗʰ **T84.621** **Infection and inflammatory reaction due to internal fixation device of** left femur   CC HCC

   10 √7ᵗʰ **T84.622** **Infection and inflammatory reaction due to internal fixation device of** right tibia   CC HCC

   10 √7ᵗʰ **T84.623** **Infection and inflammatory reaction due to internal fixation device of** left tibia   CC HCC

   10 √7ᵗʰ **T84.624** **Infection and inflammatory reaction due to internal fixation device of** right fibula   CC HCC

   10 √7ᵗʰ **T84.625** **Infection and inflammatory reaction due to internal fixation device of** left fibula   CC HCC

   10 √7ᵗʰ **T84.629** **Infection and inflammatory reaction due to internal fixation device of** unspecified bone **of leg**   CC HCC

10 √x7ᵗʰ **T84.63** **Infection and inflammatory reaction due to internal fixation device of** spine   CC H12 HCC

10 √x7ᵗʰ **T84.69** **Infection and inflammatory reaction due to internal fixation device of** other **site**   CC H12 HCC

10 √x7ᵗʰ **T84.7** **Infection and inflammatory reaction due to** other internal orthopedic prosthetic devices, implants and grafts   CC H12 HCC

Use additional code to identify infection

**CC Excl:** PDX collection 1459

√5ᵗʰ **T84.8** **Other specified complications of internal orthopedic prosthetic devices, implants and grafts**

> **CC Excl: For codes in subcategory T84.8:**
> PDX collection 1459

10 √x7ᵗʰ **T84.81** Embolism **due to internal orthopedic prosthetic devices, implants and grafts**   CC HCC

10 √x7ᵗʰ **T84.82** Fibrosis **due to internal orthopedic prosthetic devices, implants and grafts**   CC HCC

10 √x7ᵗʰ **T84.83** Hemorrhage **due to internal orthopedic prosthetic devices, implants and grafts**   CC HCC

10 √x7ᵗʰ **T84.84** Pain **due to internal orthopedic prosthetic devices, implants and grafts**   CC HCC

10 √x7ᵗʰ **T84.85** Stenosis **due to internal orthopedic prosthetic devices, implants and grafts**   CC HCC

10 √x7ᵗʰ **T84.86** Thrombosis **due to internal orthopedic prosthetic devices, implants and grafts**   CC HCC

10 √x7ᵗʰ **T84.89** Other **specified complication of internal orthopedic prosthetic devices, implants and grafts**   CC HCC

10 √x7ᵗʰ **T84.9** **Unspecified complication of internal orthopedic prosthetic device, implant and graft**   CC HCC

**CC Excl:** PDX collection 1459

√4ᵗʰ **T85** **Complications of other internal prosthetic devices, implants and grafts**

EXCLUDES 2   *failure and rejection of transplanted organs and tissue (T86.-)*

> The appropriate 7th character is to be added to each code from category T85.
> A   initial encounter
> D   subsequent encounter
> S   sequela

√5ᵗʰ **T85.0** **Mechanical complication of** ventricular intracranial (communicating) shunt

> **CC Excl: For codes in subcategory T85.0:**
> PDX collection 1460

10 √x7ᵗʰ **T85.01** Breakdown **(mechanical) of ventricular intracranial (communicating) shunt**   CC HCC

10 √x7ᵗʰ **T85.02** Displacement **of ventricular intracranial (communicating) shunt**   CC HCC

Malposition of ventricular intracranial (communicating) shunt

10 √x7ᵗʰ **T85.03** Leakage **of ventricular intracranial (communicating) shunt**   CC HCC

10 √x7ᵗʰ **T85.09** Other **mechanical complication of ventricular intracranial (communicating) shunt**   CC HCC

Obstruction (mechanical) of ventricular intracranial (communicating) shunt

Perforation of ventricular intracranial (communicating) shunt

Protrusion of ventricular intracranial (communicating) shunt

√5ᵗʰ **T85.1** **Mechanical complication of** implanted electronic stimulator of nervous system

> **CC Excl: For codes in subcategory T85.1:**
> PDX collection 1460

√6ᵗʰ **T85.11** Breakdown **(mechanical) of implanted electronic stimulator of nervous system**

   10 √7ᵗʰ **T85.110** Breakdown (mechanical) of implanted electronic neurostimulator of brain electrode (lead)   CC HCC

   10 √7ᵗʰ **T85.111** Breakdown (mechanical) of implanted electronic neurostimulator of peripheral nerve electrode (lead)   CC HCC

Breakdown of electrode (lead) for cranial nerve neurostimulators

Breakdown of electrode (lead) for gastric neurostimulator

Breakdown of electrode (lead) for sacral nerve neurostimulator

Breakdown of electrode (lead) for vagal nerve neurostimulators

---

10 HCC with 7th character indicating initial encounter (A, B or C - specific to category).

Ⓝ Newborn: 0   Ⓟ Pediatric: 0-17   Ⓜ Maternity: 12-55   Ⓐ Adult: 15-124   MCC Major CC Condition   PDxMCC PDx acts as own MCC   CC CC Condition   PDxCC PDx acts as own CC

**1148**        ICD-10-CM 2018

**10** ☑7ᵗʰ **T85.112** **Breakdown (mechanical) of** ᴄᴄ ʜᴄᴄ
**implanted electronic neurostimulator**
**of spinal cord electrode (lead)**

**10** ☑7ᵗʰ **T85.113** **Breakdown (mechanical) of** ᴄᴄ ʜᴄᴄ
**implanted electronic neurostimulator,**
**generator**
Breakdown (mechanical) of implanted
electronic neurostimuator generator,
brain, peripheral, gastric, spinal
Breakdown (mechanical) of implanted
electronic sacral neurostimulator,
pulse generator or receiver

**10** ☑7ᵗʰ **T85.118** **Breakdown (mechanical) of other** ᴄᴄ ʜᴄᴄ
**implanted electronic stimulator**
**of nervous system**

☑6ᵗʰ **T85.12** **Displacement of implanted electronic stimulator of**
**nervous system**
Malposition of implanted electronic stimulator of
nervous system

**10** ☑7ᵗʰ **T85.120** **Displacement of implanted** ᴄᴄ ʜᴄᴄ
**electronic neurostimulator**
**of brain electrode (lead)**

**10** ☑7ᵗʰ **T85.121** **Displacement of implanted** ᴄᴄ ʜᴄᴄ
**electronic neurostimulator of**
**peripheral nerve electrode (lead)**
Displacement of electrode (lead) for cranial
nerve neurostimulators
Displacement of electrode (lead) for gastric
neurostimulator
Displacement of electrode (lead) for sacral
nerve neurostimulator
Displacement of electrode (lead) for vagal
nerve neurostimulators

**10** ☑7ᵗʰ **T85.122** **Displacement of implanted** ᴄᴄ ʜᴄᴄ
**electronic neurostimulator of**
**spinal cord electrode (lead)**

**10** ☑7ᵗʰ **T85.123** **Displacement of implanted** ᴄᴄ ʜᴄᴄ
**electronic neurostimulator,**
**generator**
Displacement of implanted electronic
neurostimulator generator, brain,
peripheral, gastric, spinal
Displacement of implanted electronic
sacral neurostimulator, pulse
generator or receiver

**10** ☑7ᵗʰ **T85.128** **Displacement of other implanted** ᴄᴄ ʜᴄᴄ
**electronic stimulator of nervous system**

☑6ᵗʰ **T85.19** **Other mechanical complication of implanted**
**electronic stimulator of nervous system**
Leakage of implanted electronic stimulator of nervous
system
Obstruction (mechanical) of implanted electronic
stimulator of nervous system
Perforation of implanted electronic stimulator of
nervous system
Protrusion of implanted electronic stimulator of
nervous system

**10** ☑7ᵗʰ **T85.190** **Other mechanical complication of** ᴄᴄ ʜᴄᴄ
**implanted electronic neurostimulator**
**of brain electrode (lead)**

**10** ☑7ᵗʰ **T85.191** **Other mechanical complication of** ᴄᴄ ʜᴄᴄ
**implanted electronic neurostimulator**
**of peripheral nerve electrode (lead)**
Other mechanical complication of
electrode (lead) for cranial nerve
neurostimulators
Other mechanical complication of
electrode (lead) for gastric
neurostimulator
Other mechanical complication of
electrode (lead) for sacral nerve
neurostimulator
Other mechanical complication of
electrode (lead) for vagal nerve
neurostimulators

**10** ☑7ᵗʰ **T85.192** **Other mechanical complication of** ᴄᴄ ʜᴄᴄ
**implanted electronic neurostimulator**
**of spinal cord electrode (lead)**

**10** ☑7ᵗʰ **T85.193** **Other mechanical complication of** ᴄᴄ ʜᴄᴄ
**implanted electronic neurostimulator,**
**generator**
Other mechanical complication of
implanted electronic neurostimulator
generator, brain, peripheral, gastric,
spinal
Other mechanical complication of
implanted electronic sacral
neurostimulator, pulse generator or
receiver

**10** ☑7ᵗʰ **T85.199** **Other mechanical complication of** ᴄᴄ ʜᴄᴄ
**other implanted electronic stimulator**
**of nervous system**

☑5ᵗʰ **T85.2** **Mechanical complication of intraocular lens**

**CC Excl: For codes in subcategory T85.2:**
PDX collection 1461

☑x7ᵗʰ **T85.21** **Breakdown (mechanical) of intraocular lens** ᴄᴄ

☑x7ᵗʰ **T85.22** **Displacement of intraocular lens** ᴄᴄ
Malposition of intraocular lens

☑x7ᵗʰ **T85.29** **Other mechanical complication of intraocular** ᴄᴄ
**lens**
Obstruction (mechanical) of intraocular lens
Perforation of intraocular lens
Protrusion of intraocular lens

☑5ᵗʰ **T85.3** **Mechanical complication of other ocular prosthetic devices,**
**implants and grafts**
*EXCLUDES 2*   other complications of corneal graft (T86.84-)

**CC Excl: For codes in subcategory T85.3:**
PDX collection 1462

☑6ᵗʰ **T85.31** **Breakdown (mechanical) of other ocular prosthetic**
**devices, implants and grafts**

☑7ᵗʰ **T85.310** **Breakdown (mechanical) of prosthetic** ᴄᴄ
**orbit of right eye**

☑7ᵗʰ **T85.311** **Breakdown (mechanical) of prosthetic** ᴄᴄ
**orbit of left eye**

☑7ᵗʰ **T85.318** **Breakdown (mechanical) of other ocular**
**prosthetic devices, implants and grafts**

☑6ᵗʰ **T85.32** **Displacement of other ocular prosthetic devices,**
**implants and grafts**
Malposition of other ocular prosthetic devices,
implants and grafts

☑7ᵗʰ **T85.320** **Displacement of prosthetic orbit of** ᴄᴄ
**right eye**

☑7ᵗʰ **T85.321** **Displacement of prosthetic orbit of** ᴄᴄ
**left eye**

☑7ᵗʰ **T85.328** **Displacement of other ocular prosthetic**
**devices, implants and grafts**

☑6ᵗʰ **T85.39** **Other mechanical complication of other ocular**
**prosthetic devices, implants and grafts**
Obstruction (mechanical) of other ocular
devices, implants and grafts
Perforation of other ocular prosthetic devices,
implants and grafts
Protrusion of other ocular prosthetic devices, implants
and grafts

☑7ᵗʰ **T85.390** **Other mechanical complication of** ᴄᴄ
**prosthetic orbit of right eye**

☑7ᵗʰ **T85.391** **Other mechanical complication of** ᴄᴄ
**prosthetic orbit of left eye**

☑7ᵗʰ **T85.398** **Other mechanical complication of other**
**ocular prosthetic devices, implants and**
**grafts**

☑5ᵗʰ **T85.4** **Mechanical complication of breast prosthesis and implant**

**CC Excl: For codes in subcategory T85.4:**
PDX collection 1463

☑x7ᵗʰ **T85.41** **Breakdown (mechanical) of breast prosthesis** ᴄᴄ
**and implant**

☑x7ᵗʰ **T85.42** **Displacement of breast prosthesis and implant** ᴄᴄ
Malposition of breast prosthesis and implant

☑x7ᵗʰ **T85.43** **Leakage of breast prosthesis and implant** ᴄᴄ

☑x7ᵗʰ **T85.44** **Capsular contracture of breast implant** ᴄᴄ

---

**10** HCC with 7th character indicating initial encounter (A, B or C - specific to category).

☑Additional Character Req   ☑x7ᵗʰ Placeholder Alert   Unacceptable PDx   Manifestation   H1-H14 HAC   ʜᴄᴄ CMS-HCC Condition   *EXCLUDES 1* Not Coded Here   *EXCLUDES 2* Not Included Here

√x7ᵗʰ **T85.49** Other **mechanical complication of breast prosthesis and implant** `CC`
- Obstruction (mechanical) of breast prosthesis and implant
- Perforation of breast prosthesis and implant
- Protrusion of breast prosthesis and implant

√5ᵗʰ **T85.5** **Mechanical complication of** gastrointestinal prosthetic devices, implants and grafts

> **CC Excl:** For codes in subcategory T85.5:
> PDX collection 1464

√6ᵗʰ **T85.51** Breakdown (mechanical) of gastrointestinal prosthetic devices, implants and grafts
- √7ᵗʰ **T85.510** Breakdown (mechanical) of bile duct prosthesis `CC`
- √7ᵗʰ **T85.511** Breakdown (mechanical) of esophageal anti-reflux device `CC`
- √7ᵗʰ **T85.518** Breakdown (mechanical) of other gastrointestinal prosthetic devices, implants and grafts `CC`

√6ᵗʰ **T85.52** Displacement of gastrointestinal prosthetic devices, implants and grafts
- Malposition of gastrointestinal prosthetic devices, implants and grafts
- √7ᵗʰ **T85.520** Displacement of bile duct prosthesis `CC`
- √7ᵗʰ **T85.521** Displacement of esophageal anti-reflux device `CC`
- √7ᵗʰ **T85.528** Displacement of other gastrointestinal prosthetic devices, implants and grafts `CC`

√6ᵗʰ **T85.59** Other **mechanical complication of** gastrointestinal prosthetic devices, implants and grafts
- Obstruction, mechanical of gastrointestinal prosthetic devices, implants and grafts
- Perforation of gastrointestinal prosthetic devices, implants and grafts
- Protrusion of gastrointestinal prosthetic devices, implants and grafts
- √7ᵗʰ **T85.590** Other mechanical complication of bile duct prosthesis `CC`
- √7ᵗʰ **T85.591** Other mechanical complication of esophageal anti-reflux device `CC`
- √7ᵗʰ **T85.598** Other mechanical complication of other gastrointestinal prosthetic devices, implants and grafts `CC`

√5ᵗʰ **T85.6** **Mechanical complication of** other specified internal and external prosthetic devices, implants and grafts

√6ᵗʰ **T85.61** Breakdown (mechanical) of other specified internal prosthetic devices, implants and grafts
- √7ᵗʰ **T85.610** Breakdown (mechanical) of cranial or spinal infusion catheter `CC`
  - Breakdown (mechanical) of epidural infusion catheter
  - Breakdown (mechanical) of intrathecal infusion catheter
  - Breakdown (mechanical) of subarachnoid infusion catheter
  - Breakdown (mechanical) of subdural infusion catheter
  - **CC Excl:** PDX collection 1465
- √7ᵗʰ **T85.611** Breakdown (mechanical) of intraperitoneal dialysis catheter `CC` `HCC`
  - **EXCLUDES 1** *mechanical complication of vascular dialysis catheter (T82.4-)*
  - **CC Excl:** PDX collection 1466
- √7ᵗʰ **T85.612** Breakdown (mechanical) of permanent sutures `CC`
  - **EXCLUDES 1** *mechanical complication of permanent (wire) suture used in bone repair (T84.1-T84.2)*
  - **CC Excl:** PDX collection 1467

√7ᵗʰ **T85.613** Breakdown (mechanical) of artificial skin graft and decellularized allodermis `CC`
- Failure of artificial skin graft and decellularized allodermis
- Non-adherence of artificial skin graft and decellularized allodermis
- Poor incorporation of artificial skin graft and decellularized allodermis
- Shearing of artificial skin graft and decellularized allodermis
- **CC Excl:** PDX collection 1468

√7ᵗʰ **T85.614** Breakdown (mechanical) of insulin pump `CC`
- **CC Excl:** PDX collection 1469

10 √7ᵗʰ **T85.615** Breakdown (mechanical) of other nervous system device, implant or graft `CC` `HCC`
- Breakdown (mechanical) of intrathecal infusion pump
- **CC Excl:** PDX collection 1467

√7ᵗʰ **T85.618** Breakdown (mechanical) of other specified internal prosthetic devices, implants and grafts `CC`
- **CC Excl:** PDX collection 1467

√6ᵗʰ **T85.62** Displacement of other specified internal prosthetic devices, implants and grafts
- Malposition of other specified internal prosthetic devices, implants and grafts
- √7ᵗʰ **T85.620** Displacement of cranial or spinal infusion catheter `CC`
  - Displacement of epidural infusion catheter
  - Displacement of intrathecal infusion catheter
  - Displacement of subarachnoid infusion catheter
  - Displacement of subdural infusion catheter
  - **CC Excl:** PDX collection 1465
- √7ᵗʰ **T85.621** Displacement of intraperitoneal dialysis catheter `CC` `HCC`
  - **EXCLUDES 1** *mechanical complication of vascular dialysis catheter (T82.4-)*
  - **CC Excl:** PDX collection 1466
- √7ᵗʰ **T85.622** Displacement of permanent sutures `CC`
  - **EXCLUDES 1** *mechanical complication of permanent (wire) suture used in bone repair (T84.1-T84.2)*
  - **CC Excl:** PDX collection 1467
- √7ᵗʰ **T85.623** Displacement of artificial skin graft and decellularized allodermis `CC`
  - Dislodgement of artificial skin graft and decellularized allodermis
  - Displacement of artificial skin graft and decellularized allodermis
  - **CC Excl:** PDX collection 1468
- √7ᵗʰ **T85.624** Displacement of insulin pump `CC`
  - **CC Excl:** PDX collection 1469
- 10 √7ᵗʰ **T85.625** Displacement of other nervous system device, implant or graft `CC` `HCC`
  - Displacement of intrathecal infusion pump
  - **CC Excl:** PDX collection 1467
- √7ᵗʰ **T85.628** Displacement of other specified internal prosthetic devices, implants and grafts `CC`
  - **CC Excl:** PDX collection 1467

√6ᵗʰ **T85.63** Leakage of other specified internal prosthetic devices, implants and grafts
- √7ᵗʰ **T85.630** Leakage of cranial or spinal infusion catheter `CC`
  - Leakage of epidural infusion catheter
  - Leakage of intrathecal infusion catheter infusion catheter
  - Leakage of subdural infusion catheter
  - Leakage of subarachnoid infusion catheter
  - **CC Excl:** PDX collection 1465
- √7ᵗʰ **T85.631** Leakage of intraperitoneal dialysis catheter `CC` `HCC`
  - **EXCLUDES 1** *mechanical complication of vascular dialysis catheter (T82.4)*
  - **CC Excl:** PDX collection 1466

---

[10] HCC with 7th character indicating initial encounter (A, B or C - specific to category).

---

N Newborn: 0   P Pediatric: 0-17   M Maternity: 12-55   A Adult: 15-124   **MCC** Major CC Condition   **PDxMCC** PDx acts as own MCC   **CC** CC Condition   **PDxCC** PDx acts as own CC

**1150**        ICD-10-CM 2018

✓7ᵗʰ **T85.633** **Leakage of** insulin pump    CC
     CC Excl: PDX collection 1469

10 ✓7ᵗʰ **T85.635** **Leakage of** other nervous system CC HCC
     **device, implant or graft**
       Leakage of intrathecal infusion pump
     CC Excl: PDX collection 1467

✓7ᵗʰ **T85.638** **Leakage of** other specified internal CC
     **prosthetic devices, implants and grafts**
     CC Excl: PDX collection 1467

✓6ᵗʰ **T85.69** **Other** mechanical **complication of** other specified
     **internal prosthetic** devices, implants and grafts
       Obstruction, mechanical of other specified internal
         prosthetic devices, implants and grafts
       Perforation of other specified internal prosthetic
         devices, implants and grafts
       Protrusion of other specified internal prosthetic
         devices, implants and grafts

✓7ᵗʰ **T85.690** **Other mechanical complication of** CC
     **cranial or spinal infusion catheter**
       Other mechanical complication of epidural
         infusion catheter
       Other mechanical complication of
         intrathecal infusion catheter
       Other mechanical complication of
         subarachnoid infusion catheter
       Other mechanical complication of subdural
         infusion catheter
     CC Excl: PDX collection 1465

✓7ᵗʰ **T85.691** **Other mechanical complication of** CC HCC
     **intraperitoneal dialysis catheter**
       EXCLUDES 1   mechanical complication of
          vascular dialysis catheter
          (T82.4)
     CC Excl: PDX collection 1466

✓7ᵗʰ **T85.692** **Other mechanical complication of** CC
     **permanent sutures**
       EXCLUDES 1   mechanical complication of
          permanent (wire) suture
          used in bone repair
          (T84.1-T84.2)
     CC Excl: PDX collection 1467

✓7ᵗʰ **T85.693** **Other mechanical complication of** CC
     **artificial skin graft and decellularized**
     **allodermis**
     CC Excl: PDX collection 1468

✓7ᵗʰ **T85.694** **Other mechanical complication of** CC
     **insulin pump**
     CC Excl: PDX collection 1469

10 ✓7ᵗʰ **T85.695** **Other mechanical complication of** CC HCC
     other **nervous system device, implant**
     **or graft**
       Other mechanical complication of
         intrathecal infusion pump
     CC Excl: PDX collection 1467

✓7ᵗʰ **T85.698** **Other mechanical complication of** CC
     other **specified internal prosthetic**
     **devices, implants and grafts**
       Mechanical complication of nonabsorbable
         surgical material NOS
     CC Excl: PDX collection 1467

✓5ᵗʰ **T85.7** **Infection and inflammatory reaction due to other internal**
     **prosthetic devices, implants and grafts**
     Use additional code to identify infection

     CC Excl: For codes in subcategory T85.7, unless
     otherwise noted: PDX collection 1470

✓x7ᵗʰ **T85.71** **Infection and inflammatory reaction due to** CC HCC
     **peritoneal dialysis catheter**
     CC Excl: PDX collection 1467

10 ✓x7ᵗʰ **T85.72** **Infection and inflammatory reaction due to** CC HCC
     **insulin pump**
     CC Excl: PDX collection 1470

✓6ᵗʰ **T85.73** **Infection and inflammatory reaction due to** nervous
     system **devices, implants and graft**

10 ✓7ᵗʰ **T85.730** **Infection and inflammatory** CC HCC
     **reaction due to** ventricular intracranial
     **(communicating)** shunt

10 ✓7ᵗʰ **T85.731** **Infection and inflammatory** CC HCC
     **reaction due to implanted electronic**
     **neurostimulator of** brain, electrode (lead)

10 ✓7ᵗʰ **T85.732** **Infection and inflammatory** CC HCC
     **reaction due to implanted electronic**
     **neurostimulator of** peripheral nerve,
     **electrode (lead)**
       Infection and inflammatory reaction due to
         electrode (lead) for cranial nerve
         neurostimulators
       Infection and inflammatory reaction due to
         electrode (lead) for gastric
         neurostimulator
       Infection and inflammatory reaction due to
         electrode (lead) for sacral nerve
         neurostimulator
       Infection and inflammatory reaction due to
         electrode (lead) for vagal nerve
         neurostimulators

10 ✓7ᵗʰ **T85.733** **Infection and inflammatory** CC HCC
     **reaction due to implanted electronic**
     **neurostimulator of** spinal cord, electrode
     **(lead)**

10 ✓7ᵗʰ **T85.734** **Infection and inflammatory** CC HCC
     **reaction due to implanted electronic**
     **neurostimulator,** generator
       Generator pocket infection

10 ✓7ᵗʰ **T85.735** **Infection and inflammatory** CC HCC
     **reaction due to** cranial or spinal infusion
     catheter
       Infection and inflammatory reaction due to
         epidural catheter
       Infection and inflammatory reaction due to
         intrathecal infusion catheter
       Infection and inflammatory reaction due to
         subarachnoid catheter
       Infection and inflammatory reaction due to
         subdural catheter

10 ✓7ᵗʰ **T85.738** **Infection and inflammatory** CC HCC
     **reaction due to** other nervous system
     **device, implant or graft**
       Infection and inflammatory reaction due to
         intrathecal infusion pump

10 ✓x7ᵗʰ **T85.79** **Infection and inflammatory reaction due to** CC HCC
     other **internal prosthetic devices, implants and**
     **grafts**
     CC Excl: PDX collection 1470

✓5ᵗʰ **T85.8** **Other specified complications of internal prosthetic devices,**
     **implants and grafts, not elsewhere classified**

     CC Excl: For CC codes in subcategory T85.8:
     CC with 7th character A or D: PDX collection 1470

✓6ᵗʰ **T85.81** **Embolism due to internal prosthetic devices,**
     **implants and grafts, not elsewhere classified**

9,10 ✓7ᵗʰ **T85.810** **Embolism due to** nervous system CC HCC
     **prosthetic devices, implants and grafts**

✓7ᵗʰ **T85.818** **Embolism due to** other internal prosthetic
     **devices, implants and grafts**

✓6ᵗʰ **T85.82** **Fibrosis due to internal prosthetic devices, implants**
     **and grafts, not elsewhere classified**

9,10 ✓7ᵗʰ **T85.820** **Fibrosis due to** nervous system CC HCC
     **prosthetic devices, implants and grafts**

✓7ᵗʰ **T85.828** **Fibrosis due to** other internal prosthetic
     **devices, implants and grafts**

✓6ᵗʰ **T85.83** **Hemorrhage due to internal prosthetic devices,**
     **implants and grafts, not elsewhere classified**

9,10 ✓7ᵗʰ **T85.830** **Hemorrhage due to** nervous CC HCC
     system **prosthetic devices, implants and**
     **grafts**

✓7ᵗʰ **T85.838** **Hemorrhage due to** other internal
     **prosthetic devices, implants and grafts**

✓6ᵗʰ **T85.84** **Pain due to internal prosthetic devices, implants and**
     **grafts, not elsewhere classified**

9,10 ✓7ᵗʰ **T85.840** **Pain due to** nervous system CC HCC
     **prosthetic devices, implants and grafts**

✓7ᵗʰ **T85.848** **Pain due to** other internal prosthetic
     **devices, implants and grafts**

✓6ᵗʰ **T85.85** **Stenosis due to internal prosthetic devices, implants**
     **and grafts, not elsewhere classified**

9,10 ✓7ᵗʰ **T85.850** **Stenosis due to** nervous system CC HCC
     **prosthetic devices, implants and grafts**

---

9   CC when reported as an initial or subsequent encounter (7th character A or D).
10   HCC with 7th character indicating initial encounter (A, B or C - specific to category).

✓ Additional Character Req   ✓x7ᵗʰ Placeholder Alert   Unacceptable PDx   Manifestation   H1-H14 HAC   HCC CMS-HCC Condition   EXCLUDES 1 Not Coded Here   EXCLUDES 2 Not Included Here

ICD-10-CM 2018      1151

**√7ᵗʰ** **T85.858** **Stenosis due to** other **internal prosthetic devices, implants and grafts**

**√6ᵗʰ** **T85.86** **Thrombosis due to internal prosthetic devices, implants and grafts, not elsewhere classified**

9,10 **√7ᵗʰ** **T85.860** **Thrombosis due to** nervous system **CC HCC** **prosthetic devices, implants and grafts**

**√7ᵗʰ** **T85.868** **Thrombosis due to** other **internal prosthetic devices, implants and grafts**

**√6ᵗʰ** **T85.89** **Other** specified complication of internal prosthetic **devices, implants and grafts, not elsewhere classified**
Erosion or breakdown of subcutaneous device pocket

9,10 **√7ᵗʰ** **T85.890** **Other specified complication of** **CC HCC** nervous system **prosthetic devices, implants and grafts**

**√7ᵗʰ** **T85.898** **Other specified complication of** other **internal prosthetic devices, implants and grafts**

**√x7ᵗʰ** **T85.9** **Unspecified complication of internal prosthetic device, implant and graft**
Complication of internal prosthetic device, implant and graft NOS

**√4ᵗʰ** **T86** **Complications of transplanted organs and tissue**
Use additional code to identify other transplant complications, such as:
graft-versus-host disease (D89.81-)
malignancy associated with organ transplant (C80.2)
post-transplant lymphoproliferative disorders (PTLD) (D47.Z1)

**√5ᵗʰ** **T86.0** **Complications of** bone marrow **transplant**

**CC Excl: For codes in subcategory T86.0:**
PDX collection 514

**T86.00** **Unspecified complication of bone marrow** **CC HCC** **transplant**

**T86.01** **Bone marrow transplant** rejection **CC HCC**

**T86.02** **Bone marrow transplant** failure **CC HCC**

**T86.03** **Bone marrow transplant** infection **CC HCC**

**T86.09** **Other** complications of bone marrow **CC HCC** **transplant**

**√5ᵗʰ** **T86.1** **Complications of** kidney **transplant**

**CC Excl: For codes in subcategory T86.1:**
PDX collection 1471

**T86.10** **Unspecified complication of kidney transplant** **CC**

**T86.11** **Kidney transplant** rejection **CC**

**T86.12** **Kidney transplant** failure **CC**
**AHA:** 2013, 1Q, 24

**T86.13** **Kidney transplant** infection **CC**
Use additional code to specify infection

**T86.19** **Other complication of kidney transplant** **CC**

**√5ᵗʰ** **T86.2** **Complications of** heart **transplant**
**EXCLUDES 1** complication of:
artificial heart device (T82.5)
heart-lung transplant (T86.3)

**CC Excl: For codes in subcategory T86.2:**
PDX collection 1472

**T86.20** **Unspecified complication of heart transplant** **CC HCC**

**T86.21** **Heart transplant** rejection **CC HCC**

**T86.22** **Heart transplant** failure **CC HCC**

**T86.23** **Heart transplant** infection **CC HCC**
Use additional code to specify infection

**√6ᵗʰ** **T86.29** **Other** complications of heart transplant

**T86.290** **Cardiac allograft vasculopathy** **CC HCC**
**EXCLUDES 1** atherosclerosis of coronary arteries (I25.75-, I25.76-, I25.81-)

**T86.298** **Other complications of heart** **CC HCC** **transplant**

**√5ᵗʰ** **T86.3** **Complications of** heart-lung **transplant**

**CC Excl: For codes in subcategory T86.3:**
PDX collection 1472

**T86.30** **Unspecified complication of heart-lung** **PDxCC CC HCC** **transplant**

**T86.31** **Heart-lung transplant** rejection **PDxCC CC HCC**

**T86.32** **Heart-lung transplant** failure **PDxCC CC HCC**

**T86.33** **Heart-lung transplant** infection **PDxCC CC HCC**
Use additional code to specify infection

**T86.39** **Other** complications of heart-lung **PDxCC CC HCC** **transplant**

**√5ᵗʰ** **T86.4** **Complications of** liver **transplant**

**CC Excl: For codes in subcategory T86.4:**
PDX collection 1473

**T86.40** **Unspecified complication of liver transplant** **CC HCC**

**T86.41** **Liver transplant** rejection **CC HCC**

**T86.42** **Liver transplant** failure **CC HCC**

**T86.43** **Liver transplant** infection **CC HCC**
Use additional code to identify infection, such as:
cytomegalovirus (CMV) infection (B25.-)

**T86.49** **Other complications of liver transplant** **CC HCC**

**T86.5** **Complications of** stem cell **transplant** **CC HCC**
Complications from stem cells from peripheral blood
Complications from stem cells from umbilical cord
**CC Excl:** PDX collection 1474

**√5ᵗʰ** **T86.8** **Complications of other transplanted organs and tissues**

**√6ᵗʰ** **T86.81** **Complications of** lung **transplant**
**EXCLUDES 1** complication of heart-lung transplant (T86.3-)

**CC Excl: For codes in subcategory T86.81:**
PDX collection 1475

**T86.810** **Lung transplant** rejection **CC HCC**

**T86.811** **Lung transplant** failure **CC HCC**

**T86.812** **Lung transplant** infection **CC HCC**
Use additional code to specify infection

**T86.818** **Other** complications of lung **CC HCC** **transplant**

**T86.819** **Unspecified complication of lung** **CC HCC** **transplant**

**√6ᵗʰ** **T86.82** **Complications of** skin graft (allograft) (autograft)
**EXCLUDES 2** complication of artificial skin graft (T85.693)

**CC Excl: For codes in subcategory T86.82:**
PDX collection 1476

**T86.820** **Skin graft (allograft)** rejection **CC**

**T86.821** **Skin graft (allograft) (autograft)** **CC** **failure**

**T86.822** **Skin graft (allograft) (autograft)** **CC** **infection**
Use additional code to specify infection

**T86.828** **Other** complications of skin graft **CC** **(allograft) (autograft)**

**T86.829** **Unspecified complication of skin graft** **CC** **(allograft) (autograft)**

**√6ᵗʰ** **T86.83** **Complications of** bone graft
**EXCLUDES 2** mechanical complications of bone graft (T84.3-)

**CC Excl: For codes in subcategory T86.83:**
PDX collection 1477

**T86.830** **Bone graft** rejection **CC**

**T86.831** **Bone graft** failure **CC**

**T86.832** **Bone graft** infection **CC**
Use additional code to specify infection

**T86.838** **Other complications of bone graft** **CC**

**T86.839** **Unspecified complication of bone** **CC** **graft**

**√6ᵗʰ** **T86.84** **Complications of** corneal **transplant**
**EXCLUDES 2** mechanical complications of corneal graft (T85.3-)

**T86.840** **Corneal transplant** rejection **CC**
**CC Excl:** PDX collection 1478

**T86.841** **Corneal transplant** failure **CC**
**CC Excl:** PDX collection 1478

**T86.842** **Corneal transplant** infection **CC HCC**
Use additional code to specify infection
**CC Excl:** PDX collection 1479

**T86.848** **Other** complications of corneal **CC** **transplant**
**CC Excl:** PDX collection 1479

---

**9** CC when reported as an initial or subsequent encounter (7th character A or D).
**10** HCC with 7th character indicating initial encounter (A, B or C - specific to category).

**N** Newborn: 0 **P** Pediatric: 0-17 **M** Maternity: 12-55 **A** Adult: 15-124 **MCC** Major CC Condition **PDxMCC** PDx acts as own MCC **CC** CC Condition **PDxCC** PDx acts as own CC

**T86.849** Unspecified complication of corneal transplant
    **CC Excl:** PDX collection 1479

✓6ᵗʰ **T86.85** Complication of intestine transplant

    **CC Excl: For codes in subcategory T86.85:** PDX collection 495

    **T86.850** Intestine transplant rejection    CC HCC
    **T86.851** Intestine transplant failure    CC HCC
    **T86.852** Intestine transplant infection    CC HCC
        Use additional code to specify infection
    **T86.858** Other complications of intestine transplant    CC HCC
    **T86.859** Unspecified complication of intestine transplant    CC HCC

✓6ᵗʰ **T86.89** Complications of other transplanted tissue
    Transplant failure or rejection of pancreas

    **CC Excl: For codes in subcategory T86.89:** PDX collection 1480

    **T86.890** Other transplanted tissue rejection    CC
    **T86.891** Other transplanted tissue failure    CC
    **T86.892** Other transplanted tissue infection    CC
        Use additional code to specify infection
    **T86.898** Other complications of other transplanted tissue    CC
    **T86.899** Unspecified complication of other transplanted tissue    CC

✓5ᵗʰ **T86.9** Complication of unspecified transplanted organ and tissue

    **CC Excl: For codes in subcategory T86.9:** PDX collection 495

    **T86.90** Unspecified complication of unspecified transplanted organ and tissue    CC
    **T86.91** Unspecified transplanted organ and tissue rejection    CC
    **T86.92** Unspecified transplanted organ and tissue failure    CC
    **T86.93** Unspecified transplanted organ and tissue infection    CC
        Use additional code to specify infection
    **T86.99** Other complications of unspecified transplanted organ and tissue    CC

✓4ᵗʰ **T87** Complications peculiar to reattachment and amputation

✓5ᵗʰ **T87.0** Complications of reattached (part of) upper extremity

    ✓6ᵗʰ **T87.0X** Complications of reattached (part of) upper extremity

        **CC Excl: For codes in subcategory T87.0X:** PDX collection 1481

        **T87.0X1** Complications of reattached (part of) right upper extremity    CC HCC
        **T87.0X2** Complications of reattached (part of) left upper extremity    CC HCC
        **T87.0X9** Complications of reattached (part of) unspecified upper extremity    CC HCC

✓5ᵗʰ **T87.1** Complications of reattached (part of) lower extremity

    ✓6ᵗʰ **T87.1X** Complications of reattached (part of) lower extremity

        **CC Excl: For codes in subcategory T87.1X:** PDX collection 1482

        **T87.1X1** Complications of reattached (part of) right lower extremity    CC HCC
        **T87.1X2** Complications of reattached (part of) left lower extremity    CC HCC
        **T87.1X9** Complications of reattached (part of) unspecified lower extremity    CC HCC

**T87.2** Complications of other reattached body part    CC HCC
    **CC Excl:** PDX collection 1483

✓5ᵗʰ **T87.3** Neuroma of amputation stump
    **DEF:** Non-neoplastic tumor generated at the proximal end of severed, partially transected, or injured nerve following amputation.

    **T87.30** Neuroma of amputation stump, unspecified extremity    HCC
    **T87.31** Neuroma of amputation stump, right upper extremity    HCC
    **T87.32** Neuroma of amputation stump, left upper extremity    HCC
    **T87.33** Neuroma of amputation stump, right lower extremity    HCC
    **T87.34** Neuroma of amputation stump, left lower extremity    HCC

✓5ᵗʰ **T87.4** Infection of amputation stump

    **CC Excl: For codes in subcategory T87.4:** PDX collection 1484

    **T87.40** Infection of amputation stump, unspecified extremity    CC HCC
    **T87.41** Infection of amputation stump, right upper extremity    CC HCC
    **T87.42** Infection of amputation stump, left upper extremity    CC HCC
    **T87.43** Infection of amputation stump, right lower extremity    CC HCC
    **T87.44** Infection of amputation stump, left lower extremity    CC HCC

✓5ᵗʰ **T87.5** Necrosis of amputation stump
    **T87.50** Necrosis of amputation stump, unspecified extremity    HCC
    **T87.51** Necrosis of amputation stump, right upper extremity    HCC
    **T87.52** Necrosis of amputation stump, left upper extremity    HCC
    **T87.53** Necrosis of amputation stump, right lower extremity    HCC
    **T87.54** Necrosis of amputation stump, left lower extremity    HCC

✓5ᵗʰ **T87.8** Other complications of amputation stump
    **T87.81** Dehiscence of amputation stump    HCC
    **T87.89** Other complications of amputation stump    HCC
        Amputation stump contracture
        Amputation stump contracture of next proximal joint
        Amputation stump flexion
        Amputation stump edema
        Amputation stump hematoma
        *EXCLUDES 2*   *phantom limb syndrome (G54.6-G54.7)*

**T87.9** Unspecified complications of amputation stump    HCC

✓4ᵗʰ **T88** Other complications of surgical and medical care, not elsewhere classified
    *EXCLUDES 2*   *complication following infusion, transfusion and therapeutic injection (T80.-)*
        *complication following procedure NEC (T81.-)*
        *complications of anesthesia in labor and delivery (O74.-)*
        *complications of anesthesia in pregnancy (O29.-)*
        *complications of anesthesia in puerperium (O89.-)*
        *complications of devices, implants and grafts (T82-T85)*
        *complications of obstetric surgery and procedure (O75.4)*
        *dermatitis due to drugs and medicaments (L23.3, L24.4, L25.1, L27.0-L27.1)*
        *poisoning and toxic effects of drugs and chemicals (T36-T65 with fifth or sixth character 1-4 or 6)*
        *specified complications classified elsewhere*

    The appropriate 7th character is to be added to each code from category T88.
    A    initial encounter
    D    subsequent encounter
    S    sequela

✓x7ᵗʰ **T88.0** Infection following immunization    CC
    Sepsis following immunization
    **CC Excl:** PDX collection 948

✓x7ᵗʰ **T88.1** Other complications following immunization, not elsewhere classified    CC
    Generalized vaccinia
    Rash following immunization
    *EXCLUDES 1*   *vaccinia not from vaccine (B08.011)*
    *EXCLUDES 2*   *anaphylactic shock due to serum (T80.5-)*
        *other serum reactions (T80.6-)*
        *postimmunization arthropathy (M02.2)*
        *postimmunization encephalitis (G04.02)*
        *postimmunization fever (R50.83)*
    **CC Excl:** PDX collection 1485

√x7ᵗʰ **T88.2   Shock due to anesthesia**        `CC`

Use additional code for adverse effect, if applicable, to identify drug (T41.- with fifth or sixth character 5)

> EXCLUDES 1    complications of anesthesia (in):
> labor and delivery (O74.-)
> postprocedural shock NOS (T81.1-)
> pregnancy (O29.-)
> puerperium (O89.-)

**CC Excl:** PDX collection 1441

√x7ᵗʰ **T88.3   Malignant hyperthermia due to anesthesia**        `CC`

Use additional code for adverse effect, if applicable, to identify drug (T41.- with fifth or sixth character 5)

**CC Excl:** PDX collection 1486

√x7ᵗʰ **T88.4   Failed or difficult intubation**

√5ᵗʰ **T88.5   Other complications of anesthesia**

Use additional code for adverse effect, if applicable, to identify drug (T41.- with fifth or sixth character 5)

√x7ᵗʰ **T88.51   Hypothermia following anesthesia**

√x7ᵗʰ **T88.52   Failed moderate sedation during procedure**

Failed conscious sedation during procedure

> EXCLUDES 2    personal history of failed moderate sedation (Z92.83)

√x7ᵗʰ **T88.53   Unintended awareness under general anesthesia during procedure**

> EXCLUDES 2    personal history of unintended awareness under general anesthesia (Z92.84)

√x7ᵗʰ **T88.59   Other complications of anesthesia**

√x7ᵗʰ **T88.6   Anaphylactic reaction due to adverse effect of correct drug or medicament properly administered**        `CC`

Anaphylactic shock due to adverse effect of correct drug or medicament properly administered

Anaphylactoid reaction NOS

Use additional code for adverse effect, if applicable, to identify drug (T41.- with fifth or sixth character 5)

> EXCLUDES 1    anaphylactic reaction due to serum (T80.5-)
> anaphylactic shock or reaction due to adverse food reaction (T78.0-)

**CC Excl:** PDX collection 1426

√x7ᵗʰ **T88.7   Unspecified adverse effect of drug or medicament**

Drug hypersensitivity NOS

Drug reaction NOS

Use additional code for adverse effect, if applicable, to identify drug (T41.- with fifth or sixth character 5)

> EXCLUDES 1    specified adverse effects of drugs and medicaments (A00-R94 and T80-T88.6, T88.8)

√x7ᵗʰ **T88.8   Other specified complications of surgical and medical care, not elsewhere classified**

Use additional code to identify the complication

√x7ᵗʰ **T88.9   Complication of surgical and medical care, unspecified**

N Newborn: 0    P Pediatric: 0-17    M Maternity: 12-55    A Adult: 15-124    MCC Major CC Condition    PDxMCC PDx acts as own MCC    CC CC Condition    PDxCC PDx acts as own CC

**1154**        ICD-10-CM 2018

# Chapter 20. External Causes of Morbidity (VØØ–Y99)

## Chapter Specific Guidelines with Coding Examples

The chapter specific guidelines from the ICD-10-CM Official Guidelines for Coding and Reporting have been provided below. Along with these guidelines are coding examples, contained in the shaded boxes, that have been developed to help illustrate the coding and/or sequencing guidance found in these guidelines.

The external causes of morbidity codes should never be sequenced as the first-listed or principal diagnosis.

External cause codes are intended to provide data for injury research and evaluation of injury prevention strategies. These codes capture how the injury or health condition happened (cause), the intent (unintentional or accidental; or intentional, such as suicide or assault), the place where the event occurred the activity of the patient at the time of the event, and the person's status (e.g., civilian, military).

There is no national requirement for mandatory ICD-10-CM external cause code reporting. Unless a provider is subject to a state-based external cause code reporting mandate or these codes are required by a particular payer, reporting of ICD-10-CM codes in Chapter 20, External Causes of Morbidity, is not required. In the absence of a mandatory reporting requirement, providers are encouraged to voluntarily report external cause codes, as they provide valuable data for injury research and evaluation of injury prevention strategies.

### a. General external cause coding guidelines

#### 1) Used with any code in the range of AØØ.Ø–T88.9, ZØØ–Z99

An external cause code may be used with any code in the range of AØØ.Ø-T88.9, ZØØ-Z99, classification that is a health condition due to an external cause. Though they are most applicable to injuries, they are also valid for use with such things as infections or diseases due to an external source, and other health conditions, such as a heart attack that occurs during strenuous physical activity.

> Actinic reticuloid due to tanning bed use
>
> | **L57.1** | **Actinic reticuloid** |
> |---|---|
> | **W89.1XXA** | **Exposure to tanning bed, initial encounter** |
>
> *Explanation:* An external cause code may be used with any code in the range of AØØ.Ø–T88.9, ZØØ–Z99, classifications that describe health conditions due to an external cause. Code W89.1 Exposure to tanning bed requires a seventh character of A to report this initial encounter, with a placeholder X for the fifth and sixth characters.

#### 2) External cause code used for length of treatment

Assign the external cause code, with the appropriate 7th character (initial encounter, subsequent encounter or sequela) for each encounter for which the injury or condition is being treated.

Most categories in chapter 20 have a 7th character requirement for each applicable code. Most categories in this chapter have three 7th character values: A, initial encounter, D, subsequent encounter and S, sequela. While the patient may be seen by a new or different provider over the course of treatment for an injury or condition, assignment of the 7th character for external cause should match the 7th character of the code assigned for the associated injury or condition for the encounter.

#### 3) Use the full range of external cause codes

Use the full range of external cause codes to completely describe the cause, the intent, the place of occurrence, and if applicable, the activity of the patient at the time of the event, and the patient's status, for all injuries, and other health conditions due to an external cause.

#### 4) Assign as many external cause codes as necessary

Assign as many external cause codes as necessary to fully explain each cause. If only one external code can be recorded, assign the code most related to the principal diagnosis.

#### 5) The selection of the appropriate external cause code

The selection of the appropriate external cause code is guided by the Alphabetic Index of External Causes and by Inclusion and Exclusion notes in the Tabular List.

#### 6) External cause code can never be a principal diagnosis

An external cause code can never be a principal (first-listed) diagnosis.

#### 7) Combination external cause codes

Certain of the external cause codes are combination codes that identify sequential events that result in an injury, such as a fall which results in striking against an object. The injury may be due to either event or both.

The combination external cause code used should correspond to the sequence of events regardless of which caused the most serious injury.

> Toddler tripped and fell while walking and struck his head on an end table, sustaining a scalp contusion
>
> | **SØØ.Ø3XA** | **Contusion of scalp, initial encounter** |
> |---|---|
> | **WØ1.19ØA** | **Fall on same level from slipping, tripping and stumbling with subsequent striking against furniture, initial encounter** |
>
> *Explanation:* Combination external cause codes identify sequential events that result in an injury, such as a fall resulting in striking against an object. The injury may be due to either or both events.

#### 8) No external cause code needed in certain circumstances

No external cause code from Chapter 20 is needed if the external cause and intent are included in a code from another chapter (e.g. T36.ØX1-Poisoning by penicillins, accidental (unintentional)).

### b. Place of occurrence guideline

Codes from category Y92, Place of occurrence of the external cause, are secondary codes for use after other external cause codes to identify the location of the patient at the time of injury or other condition.

Generally, a place of occurrence code is assigned only once, at the initial encounter for treatment. However, in the rare instance that a new injury occurs during hospitalization, an additional place of occurrence code may be assigned. No 7th characters are used for Y92.

Do not use place of occurrence code Y92.9 if the place is not stated or is not applicable.

> A farmer was working in his barn and sustained a foot contusion when the horse stepped on his left foot
>
> | **S9Ø.32XA** | **Contusion of left foot, initial encounter** |
> |---|---|
> | **W55.19XA** | **Other contact with horse, initial encounter** |
> | **Y92.71** | **Barn as the place of occurrence of the external cause** |
>
> *Explanation:* A place-of-occurrence code from category Y92 is assigned at the initial encounter to identify the location of the patient at the time the injury occurred.

### c. Activity code

Assign a code from category Y93, Activity code, to describe the activity of the patient at the time the injury or other health condition occurred.

An activity code is used only once, at the initial encounter for treatment. Only one code from Y93 should be recorded on a medical record.

The activity codes are not applicable to poisonings, adverse effects, misadventures or sequela.

Do not assign Y93.9, Unspecified activity, if the activity is not stated.

A code from category Y93 is appropriate for use with external cause and intent codes if identifying the activity provides additional information about the event.

> Ranch hand who was grooming a horse sustained a foot contusion when the horse stepped on his left foot
>
> | **S9Ø.32XA** | **Contusion of left foot, initial encounter** |
> |---|---|
> | **W55.19XA** | **Other contact with horse, initial encounter** |
> | **Y93.K3** | **Activity, grooming and shearing an animal** |
>
> *Explanation:* One activity code from category Y93 is assigned at the initial encounter only to describe the activity of the patient at the time the injury occurred.

### d. Place of occurrence, activity, and status codes used with other external cause code

When applicable, place of occurrence, activity, and external cause status codes are sequenced after the main external cause code(s). Regardless of the number of external cause codes assigned, generally there should be only one place of occurrence code, one activity code, and one external cause status code assigned to an encounter. However, in the rare instance that a new injury occurs during hospitalization, an additional place of occurrence code may be assigned.

### e. If the reporting format limits the number of external cause codes

If the reporting format limits the number of external cause codes that can be used in reporting clinical data, report the code for the cause/intent most related to the principal diagnosis. If the format permits capture of additional external cause codes, the cause/intent, including medical misadventures, of the additional events should be reported rather than the codes for place, activity, or external status.

### f. Multiple external cause coding guidelines

More than one external cause code is required to fully describe the external cause of an illness or injury. The assignment of external cause codes should be sequenced in the following priority:

If two or more events cause separate injuries, an external cause code should be assigned for each cause. The first-listed external cause code will be selected in the following order:

External codes for child and adult abuse take priority over all other external cause codes.

*See Section I.C.19., Child and Adult abuse guidelines.*

External cause codes for terrorism events take priority over all other external cause codes except child and adult abuse.

External cause codes for cataclysmic events take priority over all other external cause codes except child and adult abuse and terrorism.

External cause codes for transport accidents take priority over all other external cause codes except cataclysmic events, child and adult abuse and terrorism.

Activity and external cause status codes are assigned following all causal (intent) external cause codes.

The first-listed external cause code should correspond to the cause of the most serious diagnosis due to an assault, accident, or self-harm, following the order of hierarchy listed above..

30-year-old man accidentally discharged his hunting rifle, sustaining an open gunshot wound to the right thigh, which caused him to fall down the stairs, resulting in closed displaced comminuted fracture of his left radial shaft

| | |
|---|---|
| **S71.101A** | **Unspecified open wound, right thigh, initial encounter** |
| **W33.02XA** | **Accidental discharge of hunting rifle, initial encounter** |
| **S52.352A** | **Displaced comminuted fracture of shaft of radius, left arm, initial encounter for closed fracture** |
| **W10.9XXA** | **Fall (on) (from) unspecified stairs and steps, initial encounter** |

*Explanation:* If two or more events cause separate injuries, an external cause code should be assigned for each cause.

### g. Child and adult abuse guideline

Adult and child abuse, neglect and maltreatment are classified as assault. Any of the assault codes may be used to indicate the external cause of any injury resulting from the confirmed abuse.

For confirmed cases of abuse, neglect and maltreatment, when the perpetrator is known, a code from Y07, Perpetrator of maltreatment and neglect, should accompany any other assault codes.

*See Section I.C.19. Adult and child abuse, neglect and other maltreatment*

### h. Unknown or undetermined intent guideline

If the intent (accident, self-harm, assault) of the cause of an injury or other condition is unknown or unspecified, code the intent as accidental intent. All transport accident categories assume accidental intent.

#### 1) Use of undetermined intent

External cause codes for events of undetermined intent are only for use if the documentation in the record specifies that the intent cannot be determined.

### i. Sequelae (late effects) of external cause guidelines

#### 1) Sequelae external cause codes

Sequela are reported using the external cause code with the 7th character "S" for sequela. These codes should be used with any report of a late effect or sequela resulting from a previous injury.

*See Section I.B.10 Sequela (Late Effects)*

#### 2) Sequela external cause code with a related current injury

A sequela external cause code should never be used with a related current nature of injury code.

#### 3) Use of sequela external cause codes for subsequent visits

Use a late effect external cause code for subsequent visits when a late effect of the initial injury is being treated. Do not use a late effect external cause code for subsequent visits for follow-up care (e.g., to assess healing, to receive rehabilitative therapy) of the injury when no late effect of the injury has been documented.

### j. Terrorism guidelines

#### 1) Cause of injury identified by the Federal Government (FBI) as terrorism

When the cause of an injury is identified by the Federal Government (FBI) as terrorism, the first-listed external cause code should be a code from category Y38, Terrorism. The definition of terrorism employed by the FBI is found at the inclusion note at the beginning of category Y38. Use additional code for place of occurrence (Y92.-). More than one Y38 code may be assigned if the injury is the result of more than one mechanism of terrorism.

#### 2) Cause of an injury is suspected to be the result of terrorism

When the cause of an injury is suspected to be the result of terrorism a code from category Y38 should not be assigned. Suspected cases should be classified as assault.

#### 3) Code Y38.9, Terrorism, secondary effects

Assign code Y38.9, Terrorism, secondary effects, for conditions occurring subsequent to the terrorist event. This code should not be assigned for conditions that are due to the initial terrorist act.

It is acceptable to assign code Y38.9 with another code from Y38 if there is an injury due to the initial terrorist event and an injury that is a subsequent result of the terrorist event.

### k. External cause status

A code from category Y99, External cause status, should be assigned whenever any other external cause code is assigned for an encounter, including an Activity code, except for the events noted below. Assign a code from category Y99, External cause status, to indicate the work status of the person at the time the event occurred. The status code indicates whether the event occurred during military activity, whether a non-military person was at work, whether an individual including a student or volunteer was involved in a non-work activity at the time of the causal event.

A code from Y99, External cause status, should be assigned, when applicable, with other external cause codes, such as transport accidents and falls. The external cause status codes are not applicable to poisonings, adverse effects, misadventures or late effects.

Do not assign a code from category Y99 if no other external cause codes (cause, activity) are applicable for the encounter.

An external cause status code is used only once, at the initial encounter for treatment. Only one code from Y99 should be recorded on a medical record.

Do not assign code Y99.9, Unspecified external cause status, if the status is not stated.

# Chapter 20. External Causes of Morbidity (V00-Y99)

**NOTE** This chapter permits the classification of environmental events and circumstances as the cause of injury, and other adverse effects. Where a code from this section is applicable, it is intended that it shall be used secondary to a code from another chapter of the Classification indicating the nature of the condition. Most often, the condition will be classifiable to Chapter 19, Injury, poisoning and certain other consequences of external causes (S00-T88). Other conditions that may be stated to be due to external causes are classified in Chapters I to XVIII. For these conditions, codes from Chapter 20 should be used to provide additional information as to the cause of the condition.

This chapter contains the following blocks:

| | |
|---|---|
| V00-X58 | Accidents |
| V00-V99 | Transport accidents |
| V00-V09 | Pedestrian injured in transport accident |
| V10-V19 | Pedal cycle rider injured in transport accident |
| V20-V29 | Motorcycle rider injured in transport accident |
| V30-V39 | Occupant of three-wheeled motor vehicle injured in transport accident |
| V40-V49 | Car occupant injured in transport accident |
| V50-V59 | Occupant of pick-up truck or van injured in transport accident |
| V60-V69 | Occupant of heavy transport vehicle injured in transport accident |
| V70-V79 | Bus occupant injured in transport accident |
| V80-V89 | Other land transport accidents |
| V90-V94 | Water transport accidents |
| V95-V97 | Air and space transport accidents |
| V98-V99 | Other and unspecified transport accidents |
| W00-X58 | Other external causes of accidental injury |
| W00-W19 | Slipping, tripping, stumbling and falls |
| W20-W49 | Exposure to inanimate mechanical forces |
| W50-W64 | Exposure to animate mechanical forces |
| W65-W74 | Accidental non-transport drowning and submersion |
| W85-W99 | Exposure to electric current, radiation and extreme ambient air temperature and pressure |
| X00-X08 | Exposure to smoke, fire and flames |
| X10-X19 | Contact with heat and hot substances |
| X30-X39 | Exposure to forces of nature |
| X50 | ~~Overexertion and strenuous or repetitive movements~~ |
| X52-X58 | Accidental exposure to other specified factors |
| X71-X83 | Intentional self-harm |
| X92-Y09 | Assault |
| Y21-Y33 | Event of undetermined intent |
| Y35-Y38 | Legal intervention, operations of war, military operations, and terrorism |
| Y62-Y84 | Complications of medical and surgical care |
| Y62-Y69 | Misadventures to patients during surgical and medical care |
| Y70-Y82 | Medical devices associated with adverse incidents in diagnostic and therapeutic use |
| Y83-Y84 | Surgical and other medical procedures as the cause of abnormal reaction of the patient, or of later complication, without mention of misadventure at the time of the procedure |
| Y90-Y99 | Supplementary factors related to causes of morbidity classified elsewhere |

### Accidents (V00-X58)

### Transport accidents (V00-V99)

**NOTE** This section is structured in 12 groups. Those relating to land transport accidents (V00-V89) reflect the victim's mode of transport and are subdivided to identify the victim's 'counterpart' or the type of event. The vehicle of which the injured person is an occupant is identified in the first two characters since it is seen as the most important factor to identify for prevention purposes. A transport accident is one in which the vehicle involved must be moving or running or in use for transport purposes at the time of the accident.

Use additional code to identify:
  airbag injury (W22.1)
  type of street or road (Y92.4-)
  use of cellular telephone and other electronic equipment at the time of the transport accident (Y93.C-)

**EXCLUDES 1** *agricultural vehicles in stationary use or maintenance (W31.-)*
*assault by crashing of motor vehicle (Y03.-)*
*automobile or motor cycle in stationary use or maintenance—code to type of accident*
*crashing of motor vehicle, undetermined intent (Y32)*
*intentional self-harm by crashing of motor vehicle (X82)*

**EXCLUDES 2** *transport accidents due to cataclysm (X34-X38)*

**NOTE** Definitions related to transport accidents:

(a) A transport accident (V00-V99) is any accident involving a device designed primarily for, or used at the time primarily for, conveying persons or good from one place to another.

(b) A public highway [trafficway] or street is the entire width between property lines (or other boundary lines) of land open to the public as a matter of right or custom for purposes of moving persons or property from one place to another. A roadway is that part of the public highway designed, improved and customarily used for vehicular traffic.

(c) A traffic accident is any vehicle accident occurring on the public highway [i.e. originating on, terminating on, or involving a vehicle partially on the highway]. A vehicle accident is assumed to have occurred on the public highway unless another place is specified, except in the case of accidents involving only off-road motor vehicles, which are classified as nontraffic accidents unless the contrary is stated.

(d) A nontraffic accident is any vehicle accident that occurs entirely in any place other than a public highway.

(e) A pedestrian is any person involved in an accident who was not at the time of the accident riding in or on a motor vehicle, railway train, streetcar or animal-drawn or other vehicle, or on a pedal cycle or animal. This includes, a person changing a tire, working on a parked car, or a person on foot. It also includes the user of a pedestrian conveyance such as a babystroller, ice-skates, skis, sled, roller skates, a skateboard, nonmotorized or motorized wheelchair, motorized mobility scooter, or nonmotorized scooter.

(f) A driver is an occupant of a transport vehicle who is operating or intending to operate it.

(g) A passenger is any occupant of a transport vehicle other than the driver, except a person traveling on the outside of the vehicle.

(h) A person on the outside of a vehicle is any person being transported by a vehicle but not occupying the space normally reserved for the driver or passengers, or the space intended for the transport of property. This includes a person travelling on the bodywork, bumper, fender, roof, running board or step of a vehicle, as well as, hanging on the outside of the vehicle.

(i) A pedal cycle is any land transport vehicle operated solely by nonmotorized pedals including a bicycle or tricycle.

(j) A pedal cyclist is any person riding a pedal cycle or in a sidecar or trailer attached to a pedal cycle.

(k) A motorcycle is a two-wheeled motor vehicle with one or two riding saddles and sometimes with a third wheel for the support of a sidecar. The sidecar is considered part of the motorcycle. This includes a moped, motor scooter, or motorized bicycle.

(l) A motorcycle rider is any person riding a motorcycle or in a sidecar or trailer attached to the motorcycle.

(m) A three-wheeled motor vehicle is a motorized tricycle designed primarily for on-road use. This includes a motor-driven tricycle, a motorized rickshaw, or a three-wheeled motor car.

(n) A car [automobile] is a four-wheeled motor vehicle designed primarily for carrying up to 7 persons. A trailer being towed by the car is considered part of the car. It does not include a van or minivan - see definition (o).

(o) A pick-up truck or van is a four or six-wheeled motor vehicle designed for carrying passengers as well as property or cargo weighing less than the local limit for classification as a heavy goods vehicle, and not requiring a special driver's license. This includes a minivan and a sport-utility vehicle (SUV).

(p) A heavy transport vehicle is a motor vehicle designed primarily for carrying property, meeting local criteria for classification as a heavy goods vehicle in terms of weight and requiring a special driver's license.

(q) A bus (coach) is a motor vehicle designed or adapted primarily for carrying more than 10 passengers, and requiring a special driver's license.

(r) A railway train or railway vehicle is any device, with or without freight or passenger cars couple to it, designed for traffic on a railway track. This includes subterranean (subways) or elevated trains.

(s) A streetcar, is a device designed and used primarily for transporting passengers within a municipality, running on rails, usually subject to normal traffic control signals, and operated principally on a right-of-way that forms part of the roadway. This includes a tram or trolley that runs on rails. A trailer being towed by a streetcar is considered part of the streetcar.

(t) A special vehicle mainly used on industrial premises is a motor vehicle designed primarily for use within the buildings and premises of industrial or commercial establishments. This includes battery-powered airport passenger vehicles or baggage/mail trucks, forklifts, coal-cars in a coal mine, logging cars and trucks used in mines or quarries.

✓ Additional Character Req    ✓x7ᵗʰ Placeholder Alert    Unacceptable PDx    Manifestation    **H1** - **H14** HAC    **HCC** CMS-HCC Condition    **EXCLUDES 1** Not Coded Here    **EXCLUDES 2** Not Included Here

ICD-10-CM 2018      1157

(u) A special vehicle mainly used in agriculture is a motor vehicle designed specifically for use in farming and agriculture (horticulture), to work the land, tend and harvest crops and transport materials on the farm. This includes harvesters, farm machinery and tractor and trailers.

(v) A special construction vehicle is a motor vehicle designed specifically for use on construction and demolition sites. This includes bulldozers, diggers, earth levellers, dump trucks, backhoes, front-end loaders, pavers, and mechanical shovels.

(w) A special all-terrain vehicle is a motor vehicle of special design to enable it to negotiate over rough or soft terrain, snow or sand. Examples of special design are high construction, special wheels and tires, tracks, and support on a cushion of air. This includes snow mobiles, All-terrain vehicles (ATV), and dune buggies. It does not include passenger vehicle designated as Sport Utility Vehicles. (SUV)

(x) A watercraft is any device designed for transporting passengers or goods on water. This includes motor or sailboats, ships, and hovercraft.

(y) An aircraft is any device for transporting passengers or goods in the air. This includes hot-air balloons, gliders, helicopters and airplanes.

(z) A military vehicle is any motorized vehicle operating on a public roadway owned by the military and being operated by a member of the military

## Pedestrian injured in transport accident (V00-V09)

**INCLUDES** person changing tire on transport vehicle
person examining engine of vehicle broken down in (on side of) road

**EXCLUDES 1** *fall due to non-transport collision with other person (W03)*
*pedestrian on foot falling (slipping) on ice and snow (W00.-)*
*struck or bumped by another person (W51)*

The appropriate 7th character is to be added to each code from categories V00-V09.
A   initial encounter
D   subsequent encounter
S   sequela

✓4ᵗʰ **V00   Pedestrian conveyance accident**
Use additional place of occurrence and activity external cause codes, if known (Y92-, Y93-)

**EXCLUDES 1** *collision with another person without fall (W51)*
*fall due to person on foot colliding with another person on foot (W03)*
*fall from non-moving wheelchair, nonmotorized scooter and motorized mobility scooter without collision (W05.-)*
*pedestrian (conveyance) collision with other land transport vehicle (V01-V09)*
*pedestrian on foot falling (slipping) on ice and snow (W00.-)*

✓5ᵗʰ **V00.0   Pedestrian on foot injured in collision with pedestrian conveyance**

✓x7ᵗʰ **V00.01   Pedestrian on foot injured in collision with roller-skater**

✓x7ᵗʰ **V00.02   Pedestrian on foot injured in collision with skateboarder**

✓x7ᵗʰ **V00.09   Pedestrian on foot injured in collision with other pedestrian conveyance**

✓5ᵗʰ **V00.1   Rolling-type pedestrian conveyance accident**
**EXCLUDES 1** *accident with babystroller (V00.82-)*
*accident with motorized mobility scooter (V00.83-)*
*accident with wheelchair (powered) (V00.81-)*

✓6ᵗʰ **V00.11   In-line roller-skate accident**

✓7ᵗʰ **V00.111   Fall from in-line roller-skates**

✓7ᵗʰ **V00.112   In-line roller-skater colliding with stationary object**

✓7ᵗʰ **V00.118   Other in-line roller-skate accident**
**EXCLUDES 1** *roller-skater collision with other land transport vehicle (V01-V09 with 5th character 1)*

✓6ᵗʰ **V00.12   Non-in- line roller-skate accident**

✓7ᵗʰ **V00.121   Fall from non-in-line roller-skates**

✓7ᵗʰ **V00.122   Non-in-line roller-skater colliding with stationary object**

✓7ᵗʰ **V00.128   Other non-in-line roller-skating accident**
**EXCLUDES 1** *roller-skater collision with other land transport vehicle (V01-V09 with 5th character 1)*

✓6ᵗʰ **V00.13   Skateboard accident**

✓7ᵗʰ **V00.131   Fall from skateboard**

✓7ᵗʰ **V00.132   Skateboarder colliding with stationary object**

✓7ᵗʰ **V00.138   Other skateboard accident**
**EXCLUDES 1** *skateboarder collision with other land transport vehicle (V01-V09 with 5th character 2)*

✓6ᵗʰ **V00.14   Scooter (nonmotorized) accident**
**EXCLUDES 1** *motorscooter accident (V20-V29)*

✓7ᵗʰ **V00.141   Fall from scooter (nonmotorized)**

✓7ᵗʰ **V00.142   Scooter (nonmotorized) colliding with stationary object**

✓7ᵗʰ **V00.148   Other scooter (nonmotorized) accident**
**EXCLUDES 1** *scooter (nonmotorized) collision with other land transport vehicle (V01-V09 with fifth character 9)*

✓6ᵗʰ **V00.15   Heelies accident**
Rolling shoe
Wheeled shoe
Wheelies accident

✓7ᵗʰ **V00.151   Fall from heelies**

✓7ᵗʰ **V00.152   Heelies colliding with stationary object**

✓7ᵗʰ **V00.158   Other heelies accident**

✓6ᵗʰ **V00.18   Accident on other rolling-type pedestrian conveyance**

✓7ᵗʰ **V00.181   Fall from other rolling-type pedestrian conveyance**

✓7ᵗʰ **V00.182   Pedestrian on other rolling-type pedestrian conveyance colliding with stationary object**

✓7ᵗʰ **V00.188   Other accident on other rolling-type pedestrian conveyance**

✓5ᵗʰ **V00.2   Gliding-type pedestrian conveyance accident**

✓6ᵗʰ **V00.21   Ice-skates accident**

✓7ᵗʰ **V00.211   Fall from ice-skates**

✓7ᵗʰ **V00.212   Ice-skater colliding with stationary object**

✓7ᵗʰ **V00.218   Other ice-skates accident**
**EXCLUDES 1** *ice-skater collision with other land transport vehicle (V01-V09 with 5th digit 9)*

✓6ᵗʰ **V00.22   Sled accident**

✓7ᵗʰ **V00.221   Fall from sled**

✓7ᵗʰ **V00.222   Sledder colliding with stationary object**

✓7ᵗʰ **V00.228   Other sled accident**
**EXCLUDES 1** *sled collision with other land transport vehicle (V01-V09 with 5th digit 9)*

✓6ᵗʰ **V00.28   Other gliding-type pedestrian conveyance accident**

✓7ᵗʰ **V00.281   Fall from other gliding-type pedestrian conveyance**

✓7ᵗʰ **V00.282   Pedestrian on other gliding-type pedestrian conveyance colliding with stationary object**

✓7ᵗʰ **V00.288   Other accident on other gliding-type pedestrian conveyance**
**EXCLUDES 1** *gliding-type pedestrian conveyance collision with other land transport vehicle (V01-V09 with 5th digit 9)*

✓5ᵗʰ **V00.3   Flat-bottomed pedestrian conveyance accident**

✓6ᵗʰ **V00.31   Snowboard accident**

✓7ᵗʰ **V00.311   Fall from snowboard**

✓7ᵗʰ **V00.312   Snowboarder colliding with stationary object**

✓7ᵗʰ **V00.318   Other snowboard accident**
**EXCLUDES 1** *snowboarder collision with other land transport vehicle (V01-V09 with 5th digit 9)*

✓6ᵗʰ **V00.32   Snow-ski accident**

✓7ᵗʰ **V00.321   Fall from snow-skis**

✓7ᵗʰ **V00.322   Snow-skier colliding with stationary object**

✓7ᵗʰ **V00.328   Other snow-ski accident**
**EXCLUDES 1** *snow-skier collision with other land transport vehicle (V01-V09 with 5th digit 9)*

✓6ᵗʰ **V00.38** Other flat-bottomed **pedestrian conveyance accident**

    ✓7ᵗʰ **V00.381** Fall from other flat-bottomed **conveyance**

    ✓7ᵗʰ **V00.382** Pedestrian on other flat-bottomed **pedestrian conveyance** colliding with stationary object

    ✓7ᵗʰ **V00.388** Other **accident on other flat-bottomed pedestrian conveyance**

✓5ᵗʰ **V00.8** **Accident on other pedestrian conveyance**

  ✓6ᵗʰ **V00.81** **Accident with** wheelchair **(powered)**

    ✓7ᵗʰ **V00.811** Fall from **moving wheelchair (powered)**
       **EXCLUDES 1** *fall from non-moving wheelchair (W05.0)*

    ✓7ᵗʰ **V00.812** **Wheelchair (powered)** colliding with stationary object

    ✓7ᵗʰ **V00.818** Other **accident with wheelchair (powered)**

  ✓6ᵗʰ **V00.82** **Accident with** babystroller

    ✓7ᵗʰ **V00.821** Fall from **babystroller**

    ✓7ᵗʰ **V00.822** **Babystroller** colliding with stationary object

    ✓7ᵗʰ **V00.828** Other **accident with babystroller**

  ✓6ᵗʰ **V00.83** **Accident with motorized** mobility scooter

    ✓7ᵗʰ **V00.831** Fall from **motorized mobility scooter**
       **EXCLUDES 1** *fall from non-moving motorized mobility scooter (W05.2)*

    ✓7ᵗʰ **V00.832** **Motorized mobility scooter** colliding with stationary object

    ✓7ᵗʰ **V00.838** Other **accident with motorized mobility scooter**

  ✓6ᵗʰ **V00.89** **Accident on** other pedestrian conveyance

    ✓7ᵗʰ **V00.891** Fall from **other pedestrian conveyance**

    ✓7ᵗʰ **V00.892** Pedestrian on other pedestrian **conveyance** colliding with stationary object

    ✓7ᵗʰ **V00.898** Other **accident on other pedestrian conveyance**
       **EXCLUDES 1** *other pedestrian (conveyance) collision with other land transport vehicle (V01-V09 with 5th digit 9)*

✓4ᵗʰ **V01** **Pedestrian injured in collision with pedal cycle**

  ✓5ᵗʰ **V01.0** **Pedestrian injured in collision with pedal cycle in** nontraffic accident

    ✓x7ᵗʰ **V01.00** **Pedestrian** on foot **injured in collision with pedal cycle in nontraffic accident**
       Pedestrian NOS injured in collision with pedal cycle in nontraffic accident

    ✓x7ᵗʰ **V01.01** **Pedestrian** on roller-skates **injured in collision with pedal cycle in nontraffic accident**

    ✓x7ᵗʰ **V01.02** **Pedestrian** on skateboard **injured in collision with pedal cycle in nontraffic accident**

    ✓x7ᵗʰ **V01.09** **Pedestrian** with other conveyance **injured in collision with pedal cycle in nontraffic accident**
       Pedestrian with babystroller injured in collision with pedal cycle in nontraffic accident
       Pedestrian on ice-skates injured in collision with pedal cycle in nontraffic accident
       Pedestrian on nonmotorized scooter injured in collision with pedal cycle in nontraffic accident
       Pedestrian on sled injured in collision with pedal cycle in nontraffic accident
       Pedestrian on snowboard injured in collision with pedal cycle in nontraffic accident
       Pedestrian on snow-skis injured in collision with pedal cycle in nontraffic accident
       Pedestrian in wheelchair (powered) injured in collision with pedal cycle in nontraffic accident
       Pedestrian in motorized mobility scooter injured in collision with pedal cycle in nontraffic accident

  ✓5ᵗʰ **V01.1** **Pedestrian injured in collision with pedal cycle in** traffic accident

    ✓x7ᵗʰ **V01.10** **Pedestrian** on foot **injured in collision with pedal cycle in traffic accident**
       Pedestrian NOS injured in collision with pedal cycle in traffic accident

    ✓x7ᵗʰ **V01.11** **Pedestrian** on roller-skates **injured in collision with pedal cycle in traffic accident**

    ✓x7ᵗʰ **V01.12** **Pedestrian** on skateboard **injured in collision with pedal cycle in traffic accident**

    ✓x7ᵗʰ **V01.19** **Pedestrian** with other conveyance **injured in collision with pedal cycle in traffic accident**
       Pedestrian with babystroller injured in collision with pedal cycle in traffic accident
       Pedestrian on ice-skates injured in collision with pedal cycle in traffic accident
       Pedestrian on nonmotorized scooter injured in collision with pedal cycle in traffic accident
       Pedestrian on sled injured in collision with pedal cycle in traffic accident
       Pedestrian on snowboard injured in collision with pedal cycle in traffic accident
       Pedestrian on snow-skis injured in collision with pedal cycle in traffic accident
       Pedestrian in wheelchair (powered) injured in collision with pedal cycle in traffic accident
       Pedestrian in motorized mobility scooter injured in collision with pedal cycle in traffic accident

  ✓5ᵗʰ **V01.9** **Pedestrian injured in collision with pedal cycle,** unspecified whether traffic or nontraffic accident

    ✓x7ᵗʰ **V01.90** **Pedestrian** on foot **injured in collision with pedal cycle, unspecified whether traffic or nontraffic accident**
       Pedestrian NOS injured in collision with pedal cycle, unspecified whether traffic or nontraffic accident

    ✓x7ᵗʰ **V01.91** **Pedestrian** on roller-skates **injured in collision with pedal cycle, unspecified whether traffic or nontraffic accident**

    ✓x7ᵗʰ **V01.92** **Pedestrian** on skateboard **injured in collision with pedal cycle, unspecified whether traffic or nontraffic accident**

    ✓x7ᵗʰ **V01.99** **Pedestrian** with other conveyance **injured in collision with pedal cycle, unspecified whether traffic or nontraffic accident**
       Pedestrian with babystroller injured in collision with pedal cycle, unspecified whether traffic or nontraffic accident
       Pedestrian on ice-skates injured in collision with pedal cycle unspecified, whether traffic or nontraffic accident
       Pedestrian on nonmotorized scooter injured in collision with pedal cycle, unspecified whether traffic or nontraffic accident
       Pedestrian on sled injured in collision with pedal cycle unspecified, whether traffic or nontraffic accident
       Pedestrian on snowboard injured in collision with pedal cycle, unspecified whether traffic or nontraffic accident
       Pedestrian on snow-skis injured in collision with pedal cycle, unspecified whether traffic or nontraffic accident
       Pedestrian in wheelchair (powered) injured in collision with pedal cycle, unspecified whether traffic or nontraffic accident
       Pedestrian in motorized mobility scooter injured in collision with pedal cycle, unspecified whether traffic or nontraffic accident

✓4ᵗʰ **V02** **Pedestrian injured in collision with two- or three-wheeled motor vehicle**

  ✓5ᵗʰ **V02.0** **Pedestrian injured in collision with two- or three-wheeled motor vehicle in** nontraffic accident

    ✓x7ᵗʰ **V02.00** **Pedestrian** on foot **injured in collision with two- or three-wheeled motor vehicle in nontraffic accident**
       Pedestrian NOS injured in collision with two- or three-wheeled motor vehicle in nontraffic accident

    ✓x7ᵗʰ **V02.01** **Pedestrian** on roller-skates **injured in collision with two- or three-wheeled motor vehicle in nontraffic accident**

    ✓x7ᵗʰ **V02.02** **Pedestrian** on skateboard **injured in collision with two- or three-wheeled motor vehicle in nontraffic accident**

---

√x7ᵗʰ **V02.09** **Pedestrian** with other conveyance **injured in collision with two- or three-wheeled motor vehicle in nontraffic accident**

    Pedestrian with babystroller injured in collision with two- or three-wheeled motor vehicle in nontraffic accident

    Pedestrian on ice-skates injured in collision with two- or three-wheeled motor vehicle in nontraffic accident

    Pedestrian on nonmotorized scooter injured in collision with two- or three-wheeled motor vehicle in nontraffic accident

    Pedestrian on sled injured in collision with two- or three-wheeled motor vehicle in nontraffic accident

    Pedestrian on snowboard injured in collision with two- or three-wheeled motor vehicle in nontraffic accident

    Pedestrian on snow-skis injured in collision with two- or three-wheeled motor vehicle in nontraffic accident

    Pedestrian in wheelchair (powered) injured in collision with two- or three-wheeled motor vehicle in nontraffic accident

    Pedestrian in motorized mobility scooter injured in collision with two- or three-wheeled motor vehicle in nontraffic accident

√5ᵗʰ **V02.1** **Pedestrian injured in collision with two- or three-wheeled motor vehicle in** traffic accident

√x7ᵗʰ **V02.10** **Pedestrian** on foot **injured in collision with two- or three-wheeled motor vehicle in traffic accident**

    Pedestrian NOS injured in collision with two- or three-wheeled motor vehicle in traffic accident

√x7ᵗʰ **V02.11** **Pedestrian** on roller-skates **injured in collision with two- or three-wheeled motor vehicle in traffic accident**

√x7ᵗʰ **V02.12** **Pedestrian** on skateboard **injured in collision with two- or three-wheeled motor vehicle in traffic accident**

√x7ᵗʰ **V02.19** **Pedestrian** with other conveyance **injured in collision with two- or three-wheeled motor vehicle in traffic accident**

    Pedestrian with babystroller injured in collision with two- or three-wheeled motor vehicle in traffic accident

    Pedestrian on ice-skates injured in collision with two- or three-wheeled motor vehicle in traffic accident

    Pedestrian on nonmotorized scooter injured in collision with two- or three-wheeled motor vehicle in traffic accident

    Pedestrian on sled injured in collision with two- or three-wheeled motor vehicle in traffic accident

    Pedestrian on snowboard injured in collision with two- or three-wheeled motor vehicle in traffic accident

    Pedestrian on snow-skis injured in collision with two- or three-wheeled motor vehicle in traffic accident

    Pedestrian in wheelchair (powered) injured in collision with two- or three-wheeled motor vehicle in traffic accident

    Pedestrian in motorized mobility scooter injured in collision with two- or three-wheeled motor vehicle in traffic accident

√5ᵗʰ **V02.9** **Pedestrian injured in collision with two- or three-wheeled motor vehicle,** unspecified whether traffic or nontraffic accident

√x7ᵗʰ **V02.90** **Pedestrian** on foot **injured in collision with two- or three-wheeled motor vehicle, unspecified whether traffic or nontraffic accident**

    Pedestrian NOS injured in collision with two- or three-wheeled motor vehicle, unspecified whether traffic or nontraffic accident

√x7ᵗʰ **V02.91** **Pedestrian** on roller-skates **injured in collision with two- or three-wheeled motor vehicle, unspecified whether traffic or nontraffic accident**

√x7ᵗʰ **V02.92** **Pedestrian** on skateboard **injured in collision with two- or three-wheeled motor vehicle, unspecified whether traffic or nontraffic accident**

√x7ᵗʰ **V02.99** **Pedestrian** with other conveyance **injured in collision with two- or three-wheeled motor vehicle, unspecified whether traffic or nontraffic accident**

    Pedestrian with babystroller injured in collision with two- or three-wheeled motor vehicle, unspecified whether traffic or nontraffic accident

    Pedestrian on ice-skates injured in collision with two- or three-wheeled motor vehicle, unspecified whether traffic or nontraffic accident

    Pedestrian on nonmotorized scooter injured in collision with two- or three-wheeled motor vehicle, unspecified whether traffic or nontraffic accident

    Pedestrian on sled injured in collision with two- or three-wheeled motor vehicle, unspecified whether traffic or nontraffic accident

    Pedestrian on snowboard injured in collision with two- or three-wheeled motor vehicle, unspecified whether traffic or nontraffic accident

    Pedestrian on snow-skis injured in collision with two- or three-wheeled motor vehicle, unspecified whether traffic or nontraffic accident

    Pedestrian in wheelchair (powered) injured in collision with two- or three-wheeled motor vehicle, unspecified whether traffic or nontraffic accident

    Pedestrian in motorized mobility scooter injured in collision with two- or three-wheeled motor vehicle, unspecified whether traffic or nontraffic accident

√4ᵗʰ **V03** **Pedestrian injured in collision with car, pick-up truck or van**

√5ᵗʰ **V03.0** **Pedestrian injured in collision with car, pick-up truck or van in** nontraffic accident

√x7ᵗʰ **V03.00** **Pedestrian** on foot **injured in collision with car, pick-up truck or van in nontraffic accident**

    Pedestrian NOS injured in collision with car, pick-up truck or van in nontraffic accident

√x7ᵗʰ **V03.01** **Pedestrian** on roller-skates **injured in collision with car, pick-up truck or van in nontraffic accident**

√x7ᵗʰ **V03.02** **Pedestrian** on skateboard **injured in collision with car, pick-up truck or van in nontraffic accident**

√x7ᵗʰ **V03.09** **Pedestrian** with other conveyance **injured in collision with car, pick-up truck or van in nontraffic accident**

    Pedestrian with babystroller injured in collision with car, pick-up truck or van in nontraffic accident

    Pedestrian on ice-skates injured in collision with car, pick-up truck or van in nontraffic accident

    Pedestrian on nonmotorized scooter injured in collision with car, pick-up truck or van in nontraffic accident

    Pedestrian on sled injured in collision with car, pick-up truck or van in nontraffic accident

    Pedestrian on snowboard injured in collision with car, pick-up truck or van in nontraffic accident

    Pedestrian on snow-skis injured in collision with car, pick-up truck or van in nontraffic accident

    Pedestrian in wheelchair (powered) injured in collision with car, pick-up truck or van in nontraffic accident

    Pedestrian in motorized mobility scooter injured in collision with car, pick-up truck or van in nontraffic accident

√5ᵗʰ **V03.1** **Pedestrian injured in collision with car, pick-up truck or van in** traffic accident

√x7ᵗʰ **V03.10** **Pedestrian** on foot **injured in collision with car, pick-up truck or van in traffic accident**

    Pedestrian NOS injured in collision with car, pick-up truck or van in traffic accident

√x7ᵗʰ **V03.11** **Pedestrian** on roller-skates **injured in collision with car, pick-up truck or van in traffic accident**

√x7ᵗʰ **V03.12** **Pedestrian** on skateboard **injured in collision with car, pick-up truck or van in traffic accident**

Ⓝ Newborn: 0    Ⓟ Pediatric: 0-17    Ⓜ Maternity: 12-55    Ⓐ Adult: 15-124    **MCC** Major CC Condition    **PDxMCC** PDx acts as own MCC    **CC** CC Condition    **PDxCC** PDx acts as own CC

1160      ICD-10-CM 2018

√x7ᵗʰ **V03.19** **Pedestrian with other conveyance injured in collision with car, pick-up truck or van in traffic accident**
Pedestrian with babystroller injured in collision with car, pick-up truck or van in traffic accident
Pedestrian on ice-skates injured in collision with car, pick-up truck or van in traffic accident
Pedestrian on nonmotorized scooter injured in collision with car, pick-up truck or van in traffic accident
Pedestrian on sled injured in collision with car, pick-up truck or van in traffic accident
Pedestrian on snowboard injured in collision with car, pick-up truck or van in traffic accident
Pedestrian on snow-skis injured in collision with car, pick-up truck or van in traffic accident
Pedestrian in wheelchair (powered) injured in collision with car, pick-up truck or van in traffic accident
Pedestrian in motorized mobility scooter injured in collision with car, pick-up truck or van in traffic accident

√5ᵗʰ **V03.9** **Pedestrian injured in collision with car, pick-up truck or van, unspecified whether traffic or nontraffic accident**

√x7ᵗʰ **V03.90** **Pedestrian on foot injured in collision with car, pick-up truck or van, unspecified whether traffic or nontraffic accident**
Pedestrian NOS injured in collision with car, pick-up truck or van, unspecified whether traffic or nontraffic accident

√x7ᵗʰ **V03.91** **Pedestrian on roller-skates injured in collision with car, pick-up truck or van, unspecified whether traffic or nontraffic accident**

√x7ᵗʰ **V03.92** **Pedestrian on skateboard injured in collision with car, pick-up truck or van, unspecified whether traffic or nontraffic accident**

√x7ᵗʰ **V03.99** **Pedestrian with other conveyance injured in collision with car, pick-up truck or van, unspecified whether traffic or nontraffic accident**
Pedestrian with babystroller injured in collision with car, pick-up truck or van, unspecified whether traffic or nontraffic accident
Pedestrian on ice-skates injured in collision with car, pick-up truck or van, unspecified whether traffic or nontraffic accident
Pedestrian on nonmotorized scooter injured in collision with car, pick-up truck or van, unspecified whether traffic or nontraffic accident
Pedestrian on sled injured in collision with car, pick-up truck or van in nontraffic accident
Pedestrian on snowboard injured in collision with car, pick-up truck or van, unspecified whether traffic or nontraffic accident
Pedestrian on snow-skis injured in collision with car, pick-up truck or van, unspecified whether traffic or nontraffic accident
Pedestrian in wheelchair (powered) injured in collision with car, pick-up truck or van, unspecified whether traffic or nontraffic accident
Pedestrian in motorized mobility scooter injured in collision with car, pick-up truck or van, unspecified whether traffic or nontraffic accident

√4ᵗʰ **V04** **Pedestrian injured in collision with heavy transport vehicle or bus**
EXCLUDES1 *pedestrian injured in collision with military vehicle (V09.01, V09.21)*

√5ᵗʰ **V04.0** **Pedestrian injured in collision with heavy transport vehicle or bus in nontraffic accident**

√x7ᵗʰ **V04.00** **Pedestrian on foot injured in collision with heavy transport vehicle or bus in nontraffic accident**
Pedestrian NOS injured in collision with heavy transport vehicle or bus in nontraffic accident

√x7ᵗʰ **V04.01** **Pedestrian on roller-skates injured in collision with heavy transport vehicle or bus in nontraffic accident**

√x7ᵗʰ **V04.02** **Pedestrian on skateboard injured in collision with heavy transport vehicle or bus in nontraffic accident**

√x7ᵗʰ **V04.09** **Pedestrian with other conveyance injured in collision with heavy transport vehicle or bus in nontraffic accident**
Pedestrian with babystroller injured in collision with heavy transport vehicle or bus in nontraffic accident
Pedestrian on ice-skates injured in collision with heavy transport vehicle or bus in nontraffic accident
Pedestrian on nonmotorized scooter injured in collision with heavy transport vehicle or bus in nontraffic accident
Pedestrian on sled injured in collision with heavy transport vehicle or bus in nontraffic accident
Pedestrian on snowboard injured in collision with heavy transport vehicle or bus in nontraffic accident
Pedestrian on snow-skis injured in collision with heavy transport vehicle or bus in nontraffic accident
Pedestrian in wheelchair (powered) injured in collision with heavy transport vehicle or bus in nontraffic accident
Pedestrian in motorized mobility scooter injured in collision with heavy transport vehicle or bus in nontraffic accident

√5ᵗʰ **V04.1** **Pedestrian injured in collision with heavy transport vehicle or bus in traffic accident**

√x7ᵗʰ **V04.10** **Pedestrian on foot injured in collision with heavy transport vehicle or bus in traffic accident**
Pedestrian NOS injured in collision with heavy transport vehicle or bus in traffic accident

√x7ᵗʰ **V04.11** **Pedestrian on roller-skates injured in collision with heavy transport vehicle or bus in traffic accident**

√x7ᵗʰ **V04.12** **Pedestrian on skateboard injured in collision with heavy transport vehicle or bus in traffic accident**

√x7ᵗʰ **V04.19** **Pedestrian with other conveyance injured in collision with heavy transport vehicle or bus in traffic accident**
Pedestrian with babystroller injured in collision with heavy transport vehicle or bus in traffic accident
Pedestrian on ice-skates injured in collision with heavy transport vehicle or bus in traffic accident
Pedestrian on nonmotorized scooter injured in collision with heavy transport vehicle or bus in traffic accident
Pedestrian on sled injured in collision with heavy transport vehicle or bus in traffic accident
Pedestrian on snowboard injured in collision with heavy transport vehicle or bus in traffic accident
Pedestrian on snow-skis injured in collision with heavy transport vehicle or bus in traffic accident
Pedestrian in wheelchair (powered) injured in collision with heavy transport vehicle or bus in traffic accident
Pedestrian in motorized mobility scooter injured in collision with heavy transport vehicle or bus in traffic accident

√5ᵗʰ **V04.9** **Pedestrian injured in collision with heavy transport vehicle or bus, unspecified whether traffic or nontraffic accident**

√x7ᵗʰ **V04.90** **Pedestrian on foot injured in collision with heavy transport vehicle or bus, unspecified whether traffic or nontraffic accident**
Pedestrian NOS injured in collision with heavy transport vehicle or bus, unspecified whether traffic or nontraffic accident

√x7ᵗʰ **V04.91** **Pedestrian on roller-skates injured in collision with heavy transport vehicle or bus, unspecified whether traffic or nontraffic accident**

√x7ᵗʰ **V04.92** **Pedestrian on skateboard injured in collision with heavy transport vehicle or bus, unspecified whether traffic or nontraffic accident**

√ Additional Character Req   √x7ᵗʰ Placeholder Alert   Unacceptable PDx   Manifestation   H1-H14 HAC   HCC CMS-HCC Condition   EXCLUDES1 Not Coded Here   EXCLUDES2 Not Included Here

ICD-10-CM 2018      1161

V03.19–V04.92

**Chapter 20. External Causes of Morbidity**

**V04.99–V06.02**

  ✓x7th **V04.99 Pedestrian with other conveyance injured in collision with heavy transport vehicle or bus, unspecified whether traffic or nontraffic accident**

Pedestrian with babystroller injured in collision with heavy transport vehicle or bus, unspecified whether traffic or nontraffic accident

Pedestrian on ice-skates injured in collision with heavy transport vehicle or bus, unspecified whether traffic or nontraffic accident

Pedestrian on nonmotorized scooter injured in collision with heavy transport vehicle or bus, unspecified whether traffic or nontraffic accident

Pedestrian on sled injured in collision with heavy transport vehicle or bus, unspecified whether traffic or nontraffic accident

Pedestrian on snowboard injured in collision with heavy transport vehicle or bus, unspecified whether traffic or nontraffic accident

Pedestrian on snow-skis injured in collision with heavy transport vehicle or bus, unspecified whether traffic or nontraffic accident

Pedestrian in wheelchair (powered) injured in collision with heavy transport vehicle or bus, unspecified whether traffic or nontraffic accident

Pedestrian in motorized mobility scooter injured in collision with heavy transport vehicle or bus, unspecified whether traffic or nontraffic accident

✓4th **V05 Pedestrian injured in collision with railway train or railway vehicle**

  ✓5th **V05.0 Pedestrian injured in collision with railway train or railway vehicle in nontraffic accident**

    ✓x7th **V05.00 Pedestrian on foot injured in collision with railway train or railway vehicle in nontraffic accident**

Pedestrian NOS injured in collision with railway train or railway vehicle in nontraffic accident

    ✓x7th **V05.01 Pedestrian on roller-skates injured in collision with railway train or railway vehicle in nontraffic accident**

    ✓x7th **V05.02 Pedestrian on skateboard injured in collision with railway train or railway vehicle in nontraffic accident**

    ✓x7th **V05.09 Pedestrian with other conveyance injured in collision with railway train or railway vehicle in nontraffic accident**

Pedestrian with babystroller injured in collision with railway train or railway vehicle in nontraffic accident

Pedestrian on ice-skates injured in collision with railway train or railway vehicle in nontraffic accident

Pedestrian on nonmotorized scooter injured in collision with railway train or railway vehicle in nontraffic accident

Pedestrian on sled injured in collision with railway train or railway vehicle in nontraffic accident

Pedestrian on snowboard injured in collision with railway train or railway vehicle in nontraffic accident

Pedestrian on snow-skis injured in collision with railway train or railway vehicle in nontraffic accident

Pedestrian in wheelchair (powered) injured in collision with railway train or railway vehicle in nontraffic accident

Pedestrian in motorized mobility scooter injured in collision with railway train or railway vehicle in nontraffic accident

  ✓5th **V05.1 Pedestrian injured in collision with railway train or railway vehicle in traffic accident**

    ✓x7th **V05.10 Pedestrian on foot injured in collision with railway train or railway vehicle in traffic accident**

Pedestrian NOS injured in collision with railway train or railway vehicle in traffic accident

    ✓x7th **V05.11 Pedestrian on roller-skates injured in collision with railway train or railway vehicle in traffic accident**

    ✓x7th **V05.12 Pedestrian on skateboard injured in collision with railway train or railway vehicle in traffic accident**

  ✓x7th **V05.19 Pedestrian with other conveyance injured in collision with railway train or railway vehicle in traffic accident**

Pedestrian with babystroller injured in collision with railway train or railway vehicle in traffic accident

Pedestrian on ice-skates injured in collision with railway train or railway vehicle in traffic accident

Pedestrian on nonmotorized scooter injured in collision with railway train or railway vehicle in traffic accident

Pedestrian on sled injured in collision with railway train or railway vehicle in traffic accident

Pedestrian on snowboard injured in collision with railway train or railway vehicle in traffic accident

Pedestrian on snow-skis injured in collision with railway train or railway vehicle in traffic accident

Pedestrian in wheelchair (powered) injured in collision with railway train or railway vehicle in traffic accident

Pedestrian in motorized mobility scooter injured in collision with railway train or railway vehicle in traffic accident

  ✓5th **V05.9 Pedestrian injured in collision with railway train or railway vehicle, unspecified whether traffic or nontraffic accident**

    ✓x7th **V05.90 Pedestrian on foot injured in collision with railway train or railway vehicle, unspecified whether traffic or nontraffic accident**

Pedestrian NOS injured in collision with railway train or railway vehicle, unspecified whether traffic or nontraffic accident

    ✓x7th **V05.91 Pedestrian on roller-skates injured in collision with railway train or railway vehicle, unspecified whether traffic or nontraffic accident**

    ✓x7th **V05.92 Pedestrian on skateboard injured in collision with railway train or railway vehicle, unspecified whether traffic or nontraffic accident**

    ✓x7th **V05.99 Pedestrian with other conveyance injured in collision with railway train or railway vehicle, unspecified whether traffic or nontraffic accident**

Pedestrian with babystroller injured in collision with railway train or railway vehicle, unspecified whether traffic or nontraffic

Pedestrian on ice-skates injured in collision with railway train or railway vehicle, unspecified whether traffic or nontraffic

Pedestrian on nonmotorized scooter injured in collision with railway train or railway vehicle, unspecified whether traffic or nontraffic

Pedestrian on sled injured in collision with railway train or railway vehicle, unspecified whether traffic or nontraffic

Pedestrian on snowboard injured in collision with railway train or railway vehicle, unspecified whether traffic or nontraffic

Pedestrian on snow-skis injured in collision with railway train or railway vehicle, unspecified whether traffic or nontraffic

Pedestrian in wheelchair (powered) injured in collision with railway train or railway vehicle, unspecified whether traffic or nontraffic

Pedestrian in motorized mobility scooter injured in collision with railway train or railway vehicle, unspecified whether traffic or nontraffic

✓4th **V06 Pedestrian injured in collision with other nonmotor vehicle**

  **INCLUDES** collision with animal-drawn vehicle, animal being ridden, nonpowered streetcar

  **EXCLUDES 1** pedestrian injured in collision with pedestrian conveyance (V00.0-)

  ✓5th **V06.0 Pedestrian injured in collision with other nonmotor vehicle in nontraffic accident**

    ✓x7th **V06.00 Pedestrian on foot injured in collision with other nonmotor vehicle in nontraffic accident**

Pedestrian NOS injured in collision with other nonmotor vehicle in nontraffic accident

    ✓x7th **V06.01 Pedestrian on roller-skates injured in collision with other nonmotor vehicle in nontraffic accident**

    ✓x7th **V06.02 Pedestrian on skateboard injured in collision with other nonmotor vehicle in nontraffic accident**

N Newborn: 0   P Pediatric: 0-17   M Maternity: 12-55   A Adult: 15-124   **MCC** Major CC Condition   **PDxMCC** PDx acts as own MCC   **CC** CC Condition   **PDxCC** PDx acts as own CC

1162                ICD-10-CM 2018

√x7ᵗʰ **V06.09 Pedestrian** with other conveyance **injured in collision with other nonmotor vehicle in nontraffic accident**

> Pedestrian with babystroller injured in collision with other nonmotor vehicle in nontraffic accident
> Pedestrian on ice-skates injured in collision with other nonmotor vehicle in nontraffic accident
> Pedestrian on nonmotorized scooter injured in collision with other nonmotor vehicle in nontraffic accident
> Pedestrian on sled injured in collision with other nonmotor vehicle in nontraffic accident
> Pedestrian on snowboard injured in collision with other nonmotor vehicle in nontraffic accident
> Pedestrian on snow-skis injured in collision with other nonmotor vehicle in nontraffic accident
> Pedestrian in wheelchair (powered) injured in collision with other nonmotor vehicle in nontraffic accident
> Pedestrian in motorized mobility scooter injured in collision with other nonmotor vehicle in nontraffic accident

√5ᵗʰ **V06.1 Pedestrian injured in collision with other nonmotor vehicle** in traffic accident

√x7ᵗʰ **V06.10 Pedestrian** on foot **injured in collision with other nonmotor vehicle in traffic accident**

> Pedestrian NOS injured in collision with other nonmotor vehicle in traffic accident

√x7ᵗʰ **V06.11 Pedestrian** on roller-skates **injured in collision with other nonmotor vehicle in traffic accident**

√x7ᵗʰ **V06.12 Pedestrian** on skateboard **injured in collision with other nonmotor vehicle in traffic accident**

√x7ᵗʰ **V06.19 Pedestrian** with other conveyance **injured in collision with other nonmotor vehicle in traffic accident**

> Pedestrian with babystroller injured in collision with other nonmotor vehicle in nontraffic accident
> Pedestrian on ice-skates injured in collision with other nonmotor vehicle in traffic accident
> Pedestrian on nonmotorized scooter injured in collision with other nonmotor vehicle in traffic accident
> Pedestrian on sled injured in collision with other nonmotor vehicle in traffic accident
> Pedestrian on snowboard injured in collision with other nonmotor vehicle in traffic  accident
> Pedestrian on snow-skis injured in collision with other nonmotor vehicle in traffic accident
> Pedestrian in wheelchair (powered) injured in collision with other nonmotor vehicle in traffic accident
> Pedestrian in motorized mobility scooter injured in collision with other nonmotor vehicle in traffic accident

√5ᵗʰ **V06.9 Pedestrian injured in collision with other nonmotor vehicle,** unspecified whether traffic or nontraffic accident

√x7ᵗʰ **V06.90 Pedestrian** on foot **injured in collision with other nonmotor vehicle, unspecified whether traffic or nontraffic accident**

> Pedestrian NOS injured in collision with other nonmotor vehicle, unspecified whether traffic or nontraffic accident

√x7ᵗʰ **V06.91 Pedestrian** on roller-skates **injured in collision with other nonmotor vehicle, unspecified whether traffic or nontraffic accident**

√x7ᵗʰ **V06.92 Pedestrian** on skateboard **injured in collision with other nonmotor vehicle, unspecified whether traffic or nontraffic accident**

√x7ᵗʰ **V06.99 Pedestrian** with other conveyance **injured in collision with other nonmotor vehicle, unspecified whether traffic or nontraffic accident**

> Pedestrian with babystroller injured in collision with other nonmotor vehicle, unspecified whether traffic or nontraffic accident
> Pedestrian on ice-skates injured in collision with other nonmotor vehicle, unspecified whether traffic or nontraffic accident
> Pedestrian on nonmotorized scooter injured in collision with other nonmotor vehicle, unspecified whether traffic or nontraffic accident
> Pedestrian on sled injured in collision with other nonmotor vehicle, unspecified whether traffic or nontraffic accident
> Pedestrian on snowboard injured in collision with other nonmotor vehicle, unspecified whether traffic or nontraffic accident
> Pedestrian on snow-skis injured in collision with other nonmotor vehicle, unspecified whether traffic or nontraffic accident
> Pedestrian in wheelchair (powered) injured in collision with other nonmotor vehicle, unspecified whether traffic or nontraffic accident
> Pedestrian in motorized mobility scooter injured in collision with other nonmotor vehicle, unspecified whether traffic or nontraffic accident

√4ᵗʰ **V09 Pedestrian injured in other and unspecified transport accidents**

√5ᵗʰ **V09.0 Pedestrian injured in** nontraffic **accident involving** other and unspecified motor vehicles

√x7ᵗʰ **V09.00 Pedestrian injured in nontraffic accident involving** unspecified **motor vehicles**

√x7ᵗʰ **V09.01 Pedestrian injured in nontraffic accident involving** military **vehicle**

√x7ᵗʰ **V09.09 Pedestrian injured in nontraffic accident involving** other **motor vehicles**

> Pedestrian injured in nontraffic accident by special vehicle

√x7ᵗʰ **V09.1 Pedestrian injured in** unspecified nontraffic **accident**

√5ᵗʰ **V09.2 Pedestrian injured in** traffic accident **involving other and unspecified motor vehicles**

√x7ᵗʰ **V09.20 Pedestrian injured in traffic accident involving** unspecified **motor vehicles**

√x7ᵗʰ **V09.21 Pedestrian injured in traffic accident involving** military **vehicle**

√x7ᵗʰ **V09.29 Pedestrian injured in traffic accident involving** other **motor vehicles**

√x7ᵗʰ **V09.3 Pedestrian injured in** unspecified traffic **accident**

√x7ᵗʰ **V09.9 Pedestrian injured in** unspecified transport **accident**

## Pedal cycle rider injured in transport accident (V10-V19)

**INCLUDES**   any non-motorized vehicle, excluding an animal-drawn vehicle, or a sidecar or trailer attached to the pedal cycle

**EXCLUDES 2**   *rupture of pedal cycle tire (W37.0)*

> The appropriate 7th character is to be added to each code from categories V10-V19.
> A   initial encounter
> D   subsequent encounter
> S   sequela

√4ᵗʰ **V10 Pedal cycle rider injured in collision with pedestrian or animal**

> **EXCLUDES 1**   *pedal cycle rider collision with animal-drawn vehicle or animal being ridden (V16.-)*

√x7ᵗʰ **V10.0 Pedal cycle** driver **injured in collision with pedestrian or animal in** nontraffic **accident**

√x7ᵗʰ **V10.1 Pedal cycle** passenger **injured in collision with pedestrian or animal in** nontraffic **accident**

√x7ᵗʰ **V10.2** Unspecified **pedal cyclist injured in collision with pedestrian or animal in** nontraffic **accident**

√x7ᵗʰ **V10.3** Person boarding or alighting **a pedal cycle injured in collision with pedestrian or animal**

√x7ᵗʰ **V10.4 Pedal cycle** driver **injured in collision with pedestrian or animal in** traffic **accident**

√x7ᵗʰ **V10.5 Pedal cycle** passenger **injured in collision with pedestrian or animal in** traffic **accident**

√x7ᵗʰ **V10.9** Unspecified **pedal cyclist injured in collision with pedestrian or animal in** traffic **accident**

✓ Additional Character Req   √x7ᵗʰ Placeholder Alert   Unacceptable PDx   **Manifestation**   **H1**-**H14** HAC   **HCC** CMS-HCC Condition   **EXCLUDES 1** Not Coded Here   **EXCLUDES 2** Not Included Here

ICD-10-CM 2018      1163

✓4th **V11 Pedal cycle rider injured in collision with other pedal cycle**

✓x7th **V11.0** Pedal cycle driver injured in collision with other pedal cycle in nontraffic accident

✓x7th **V11.1** Pedal cycle passenger injured in collision with other pedal cycle in nontraffic accident

✓x7th **V11.2** Unspecified pedal cyclist injured in collision with other pedal cycle in nontraffic accident

✓x7th **V11.3** Person boarding or alighting a pedal cycle injured in collision with other pedal cycle

✓x7th **V11.4** Pedal cycle driver injured in collision with other pedal cycle in traffic accident

✓x7th **V11.5** Pedal cycle passenger injured in collision with other pedal cycle in traffic accident

✓x7th **V11.9** Unspecified pedal cyclist injured in collision with other pedal cycle in traffic accident

✓4th **V12 Pedal cycle rider injured in collision with two- or three-wheeled motor vehicle**

✓x7th **V12.0** Pedal cycle driver injured in collision with two- or three-wheeled motor vehicle in nontraffic accident

✓x7th **V12.1** Pedal cycle passenger injured in collision with two- or three-wheeled motor vehicle in nontraffic accident

✓x7th **V12.2** Unspecified pedal cyclist injured in collision with two- or three-wheeled motor vehicle in nontraffic accident

✓x7th **V12.3** Person boarding or alighting a pedal cycle injured in collision with two- or three-wheeled motor vehicle

✓x7th **V12.4** Pedal cycle driver injured in collision with two- or three-wheeled motor vehicle in traffic accident

✓x7th **V12.5** Pedal cycle passenger injured in collision with two- or three-wheeled motor vehicle in traffic accident

✓x7th **V12.9** Unspecified pedal cyclist injured in collision with two- or three-wheeled motor vehicle in traffic accident

✓4th **V13 Pedal cycle rider injured in collision with car, pick-up truck or van**

✓x7th **V13.0** Pedal cycle driver injured in collision with car, pick-up truck or van in nontraffic accident

✓x7th **V13.1** Pedal cycle passenger injured in collision with car, pick-up truck or van in nontraffic accident

✓x7th **V13.2** Unspecified pedal cyclist injured in collision with car, pick-up truck or van in nontraffic accident

✓x7th **V13.3** Person boarding or alighting a pedal cycle injured in collision with car, pick-up truck or van

✓x7th **V13.4** Pedal cycle driver injured in collision with car, pick-up truck or van in traffic accident

✓x7th **V13.5** Pedal cycle passenger injured in collision with car, pick-up truck or van in traffic accident

✓x7th **V13.9** Unspecified pedal cyclist injured in collision with car, pick-up truck or van in traffic accident

✓4th **V14 Pedal cycle rider injured in collision with heavy transport vehicle or bus**

> EXCLUDES 1 *pedal cycle rider injured in collision with military vehicle (V19.81)*

✓x7th **V14.0** Pedal cycle driver injured in collision with heavy transport vehicle or bus in nontraffic accident

✓x7th **V14.1** Pedal cycle passenger injured in collision with heavy transport vehicle or bus in nontraffic accident

✓x7th **V14.2** Unspecified pedal cyclist injured in collision with heavy transport vehicle or bus in nontraffic accident

✓x7th **V14.3** Person boarding or alighting a pedal cycle injured in collision with heavy transport vehicle or bus

✓x7th **V14.4** Pedal cycle driver injured in collision with heavy transport vehicle or bus in traffic accident

✓x7th **V14.5** Pedal cycle passenger injured in collision with heavy transport vehicle or bus in traffic accident

✓x7th **V14.9** Unspecified pedal cyclist injured in collision with heavy transport vehicle or bus in traffic accident

✓4th **V15 Pedal cycle rider injured in collision with railway train or railway vehicle**

✓x7th **V15.0** Pedal cycle driver injured in collision with railway train or railway vehicle in nontraffic accident

✓x7th **V15.1** Pedal cycle passenger injured in collision with railway train or railway vehicle in nontraffic accident

✓x7th **V15.2** Unspecified pedal cyclist injured in collision with railway train or railway vehicle in nontraffic accident

✓x7th **V15.3** Person boarding or alighting a pedal cycle injured in collision with railway train or railway vehicle

✓x7th **V15.4** Pedal cycle driver injured in collision with railway train or railway vehicle in traffic accident

✓x7th **V15.5** Pedal cycle passenger injured in collision with railway train or railway vehicle in traffic accident

✓x7th **V15.9** Unspecified pedal cyclist injured in collision with railway train or railway vehicle in traffic accident

✓4th **V16 Pedal cycle rider injured in collision with other nonmotor vehicle**

> INCLUDES collision with animal-drawn vehicle, animal being ridden, streetcar

✓x7th **V16.0** Pedal cycle driver injured in collision with other nonmotor vehicle in nontraffic accident

✓x7th **V16.1** Pedal cycle passenger injured in collision with other nonmotor vehicle in nontraffic accident

✓x7th **V16.2** Unspecified pedal cyclist injured in collision with other nonmotor vehicle in nontraffic accident

✓x7th **V16.3** Person boarding or alighting a pedal cycle injured in collision with other nonmotor vehicle in nontraffic accident

✓x7th **V16.4** Pedal cycle driver injured in collision with other nonmotor vehicle in traffic accident

✓x7th **V16.5** Pedal cycle passenger injured in collision with other nonmotor vehicle in traffic accident

✓x7th **V16.9** Unspecified pedal cyclist injured in collision with other nonmotor vehicle in traffic accident

✓4th **V17 Pedal cycle rider injured in collision with fixed or stationary object**

✓x7th **V17.0** Pedal cycle driver injured in collision with fixed or stationary object in nontraffic accident

✓x7th **V17.1** Pedal cycle passenger injured in collision with fixed or stationary object in nontraffic accident

✓x7th **V17.2** Unspecified pedal cyclist injured in collision with fixed or stationary object in nontraffic accident

✓x7th **V17.3** Person boarding or alighting a pedal cycle injured in collision with fixed or stationary object

✓x7th **V17.4** Pedal cycle driver injured in collision with fixed or stationary object in traffic accident

✓x7th **V17.5** Pedal cycle passenger injured in collision with fixed or stationary object in traffic accident

✓x7th **V17.9** Unspecified pedal cyclist injured in collision with fixed or stationary object in traffic accident

✓4th **V18 Pedal cycle rider injured in noncollision transport accident**

> INCLUDES fall or thrown from pedal cycle (without antecedent collision)
> overturning pedal cycle NOS
> overturning pedal cycle without collision

✓x7th **V18.0** Pedal cycle driver injured in noncollision transport accident in nontraffic accident

✓x7th **V18.1** Pedal cycle passenger injured in noncollision transport accident in nontraffic accident

✓x7th **V18.2** Unspecified pedal cyclist injured in noncollision transport accident in nontraffic accident

✓x7th **V18.3** Person boarding or alighting a pedal cycle injured in noncollision transport accident

✓x7th **V18.4** Pedal cycle driver injured in noncollision transport accident in traffic accident

✓x7th **V18.5** Pedal cycle passenger injured in noncollision transport accident in traffic accident

✓x7th **V18.9** Unspecified pedal cyclist injured in noncollision transport accident in traffic accident

✓4th **V19 Pedal cycle rider injured in other and unspecified transport accidents**

✓5th **V19.0** Pedal cycle driver injured in collision with other and unspecified motor vehicles in nontraffic accident

✓x7th **V19.00** Pedal cycle driver injured in collision with unspecified motor vehicles in nontraffic accident

✓x7th **V19.09** Pedal cycle driver injured in collision with other motor vehicles in nontraffic accident

✓5th **V19.1** Pedal cycle passenger injured in collision with other and unspecified motor vehicles in nontraffic accident

✓x7th **V19.10** Pedal cycle passenger injured in collision with unspecified motor vehicles in nontraffic accident

✓x7th **V19.19** Pedal cycle passenger injured in collision with other motor vehicles in nontraffic accident

N Newborn: 0 | P Pediatric: 0-17 | M Maternity: 12-55 | A Adult: 15-124 | MCC Major CC Condition | PDxMCC PDx acts as own MCC | CC CC Condition | PDxCC PDx acts as own CC

1164 | ICD-10-CM 2018

✓5ᵗʰ **V19.2** **Unspecified pedal cyclist injured in collision with** other and unspecified motor vehicles in nontraffic accident

     ✓x7ᵗʰ **V19.20** **Unspecified pedal cyclist injured in collision with** unspecified **motor vehicles in nontraffic accident**
         Pedal cycle collision NOS, nontraffic

     ✓x7ᵗʰ **V19.29** **Unspecified pedal cyclist injured in collision with** other **motor vehicles in nontraffic accident**

✓x7ᵗʰ **V19.3** **Pedal cyclist (driver) (passenger) injured in unspecified nontraffic accident**
     Pedal cycle accident NOS, nontraffic
     Pedal cyclist injured in nontraffic accident NOS

✓5ᵗʰ **V19.4** **Pedal cycle** driver **injured in collision with other and unspecified motor vehicles in traffic accident**

     ✓x7ᵗʰ **V19.40** **Pedal cycle driver injured in collision with** unspecified **motor vehicles in traffic accident**

     ✓x7ᵗʰ **V19.49** **Pedal cycle driver injured in collision with** other **motor vehicles in traffic accident**

✓5ᵗʰ **V19.5** **Pedal cycle** passenger **injured in collision with other and unspecified motor vehicles in traffic accident**

     ✓x7ᵗʰ **V19.50** **Pedal cycle passenger injured in collision with** unspecified **motor vehicles in traffic accident**

     ✓x7ᵗʰ **V19.59** **Pedal cycle passenger injured in collision with** other **motor vehicles in traffic accident**

✓5ᵗʰ **V19.6** **Unspecified** pedal cyclist injured in collision with other and unspecified motor vehicles in traffic accident

     ✓x7ᵗʰ **V19.60** **Unspecified pedal cyclist injured in collision with** unspecified **motor vehicles in traffic accident**
         Pedal cycle collision NOS (traffic)

     ✓x7ᵗʰ **V19.69** **Unspecified pedal cyclist injured in collision with** other **motor vehicles in traffic accident**

✓5ᵗʰ **V19.8** **Pedal cyclist (driver) (passenger) injured in** other specified transport accidents

     ✓x7ᵗʰ **V19.81** **Pedal cyclist (driver) (passenger) injured in transport accident with** military vehicle

     ✓x7ᵗʰ **V19.88** **Pedal cyclist (driver) (passenger) injured in** other **specified transport accidents**

✓x7ᵗʰ **V19.9** **Pedal cyclist (driver) (passenger) injured in unspecified traffic accident**
     Pedal cycle accident NOS

## Motorcycle rider injured in transport accident (V20-V29)

**INCLUDES**   moped
          motorcycle with sidecar
          motorized bicycle
          motor scooter

**EXCLUDES 1**   *three-wheeled motor vehicle (V30-V39)*

> The appropriate 7th character is to be added to each code from categories V20-V29.
> A    initial encounter
> D    subsequent encounter
> S    sequela

✓4ᵗʰ **V20** **Motorcycle rider injured in collision with pedestrian or animal**
     **EXCLUDES 1**   *motorcycle rider collision with animal-drawn vehicle or animal being ridden (V26.-)*

✓x7ᵗʰ **V20.0** **Motorcycle** driver **injured in collision with pedestrian or animal** in nontraffic accident

✓x7ᵗʰ **V20.1** **Motorcycle** passenger **injured in collision with pedestrian or animal** in nontraffic accident

✓x7ᵗʰ **V20.2** **Unspecified** motorcycle rider injured in collision with pedestrian or animal in nontraffic accident

✓x7ᵗʰ **V20.3** **Person boarding or alighting** a motorcycle injured in collision **with pedestrian or animal**

✓x7ᵗʰ **V20.4** **Motorcycle** driver **injured in collision with pedestrian or animal** in traffic accident

✓x7ᵗʰ **V20.5** **Motorcycle** passenger **injured in collision with pedestrian or animal** in traffic accident

✓x7ᵗʰ **V20.9** **Unspecified** motorcycle rider injured in collision with pedestrian or animal in traffic accident

✓4ᵗʰ **V21** **Motorcycle rider injured in collision with pedal cycle**

✓x7ᵗʰ **V21.0** **Motorcycle** driver **injured in collision with pedal cycle in** nontraffic accident

✓x7ᵗʰ **V21.1** **Motorcycle** passenger **injured in collision with pedal cycle in** nontraffic accident

✓x7ᵗʰ **V21.2** **Unspecified** motorcycle rider injured in collision with pedal cycle in nontraffic accident

✓x7ᵗʰ **V21.3** **Person boarding or alighting** a motorcycle injured in collision **with pedal cycle**

✓x7ᵗʰ **V21.4** **Motorcycle** driver **injured in collision with pedal cycle in** traffic accident

✓x7ᵗʰ **V21.5** **Motorcycle** passenger **injured in collision with pedal cycle in** traffic accident

✓x7ᵗʰ **V21.9** **Unspecified** motorcycle rider injured in collision with pedal cycle in traffic accident

✓4ᵗʰ **V22** **Motorcycle rider injured in collision with two- or three-wheeled motor vehicle**

✓x7ᵗʰ **V22.0** **Motorcycle** driver **injured in collision with two- or three-wheeled motor vehicle** in nontraffic accident

✓x7ᵗʰ **V22.1** **Motorcycle** passenger **injured in collision with two- or three-wheeled motor vehicle** in nontraffic accident

✓x7ᵗʰ **V22.2** **Unspecified** motorcycle rider injured in collision with two- or three-wheeled motor vehicle in nontraffic accident

✓x7ᵗʰ **V22.3** **Person boarding or alighting** a motorcycle injured in collision **with two- or three-wheeled motor vehicle**

✓x7ᵗʰ **V22.4** **Motorcycle** driver **injured in collision with two- or three-wheeled motor vehicle** in traffic accident

✓x7ᵗʰ **V22.5** **Motorcycle** passenger **injured in collision with two- or three-wheeled motor vehicle** in traffic accident

✓x7ᵗʰ **V22.9** **Unspecified** motorcycle rider injured in collision with two- or three-wheeled motor vehicle in traffic accident

✓4ᵗʰ **V23** **Motorcycle rider injured in collision with car, pick-up truck or van**

✓x7ᵗʰ **V23.0** **Motorcycle** driver **injured in collision with car, pick-up truck or van** in nontraffic accident

✓x7ᵗʰ **V23.1** **Motorcycle** passenger **injured in collision with car, pick-up truck or van** in nontraffic accident

✓x7ᵗʰ **V23.2** **Unspecified** motorcycle rider injured in collision with car, pick-up truck or van in nontraffic accident

✓x7ᵗʰ **V23.3** **Person boarding or alighting** a motorcycle injured in collision **with car, pick-up truck or van**

✓x7ᵗʰ **V23.4** **Motorcycle** driver **injured in collision with car, pick-up truck or van** in traffic accident

✓x7ᵗʰ **V23.5** **Motorcycle** passenger **injured in collision with car, pick-up truck or van** in traffic accident

✓x7ᵗʰ **V23.9** **Unspecified** motorcycle rider injured in collision with car, pick-up truck or van in traffic accident

✓4ᵗʰ **V24** **Motorcycle rider injured in collision with heavy transport vehicle or bus**
     **EXCLUDES 1**   *motorcycle rider injured in collision with military vehicle (V29.81)*

✓x7ᵗʰ **V24.0** **Motorcycle** driver **injured in collision with heavy transport vehicle or bus** in nontraffic accident

✓x7ᵗʰ **V24.1** **Motorcycle** passenger **injured in collision with heavy transport vehicle or bus** in nontraffic accident

✓x7ᵗʰ **V24.2** **Unspecified** motorcycle rider injured in collision with heavy transport vehicle or bus in nontraffic accident

✓x7ᵗʰ **V24.3** **Person boarding or alighting** a motorcycle injured in collision **with heavy transport vehicle or bus**

✓x7ᵗʰ **V24.4** **Motorcycle** driver **injured in collision with heavy transport vehicle or bus** in traffic accident

✓x7ᵗʰ **V24.5** **Motorcycle** passenger **injured in collision with heavy transport vehicle or bus** in traffic accident

✓x7ᵗʰ **V24.9** **Unspecified** motorcycle rider injured in collision with heavy transport vehicle or bus in traffic accident

✓4ᵗʰ **V25** **Motorcycle rider injured in collision with railway train or railway vehicle**

✓x7ᵗʰ **V25.0** **Motorcycle** driver **injured in collision with railway train or railway vehicle** in nontraffic accident

✓x7ᵗʰ **V25.1** **Motorcycle** passenger **injured in collision with railway train or railway vehicle** in nontraffic accident

✓x7ᵗʰ **V25.2** **Unspecified** motorcycle rider injured in collision with railway train or railway vehicle in nontraffic accident

✓x7ᵗʰ **V25.3** **Person boarding or alighting** a motorcycle injured in collision **with railway train or railway vehicle**

✓x7ᵗʰ **V25.4** **Motorcycle** driver **injured in collision with railway train or railway vehicle** in traffic accident

✓x7ᵗʰ **V25.5** **Motorcycle** passenger **injured in collision with railway train or railway vehicle** in traffic accident

☑ Additional Character Req   ✓x7ᵗʰ Placeholder Alert   Unacceptable PDx   Manifestation   **H1**-**H14** HAC   **HCC** CMS-HCC Condition   **EXCLUDES1** Not Coded Here   **EXCLUDES2** Not Included Here

ICD-10-CM 2018          1165

✓x7ᵗʰ **V25.9** Unspecified motorcycle rider injured in collision with railway train or railway vehicle in traffic accident

✓4ᵗʰ **V26** **Motorcycle rider injured in collision with other nonmotor vehicle**
    INCLUDES   collision with animal-drawn vehicle, animal being ridden, streetcar

✓x7ᵗʰ **V26.0** Motorcycle driver injured in collision with other nonmotor vehicle in nontraffic accident

✓x7ᵗʰ **V26.1** Motorcycle passenger injured in collision with other nonmotor vehicle in nontraffic accident

✓x7ᵗʰ **V26.2** Unspecified motorcycle rider injured in collision with other nonmotor vehicle in nontraffic accident

✓x7ᵗʰ **V26.3** Person boarding or alighting a motorcycle injured in collision with other nonmotor vehicle

✓x7ᵗʰ **V26.4** Motorcycle driver injured in collision with other nonmotor vehicle in traffic accident

✓x7ᵗʰ **V26.5** Motorcycle passenger injured in collision with other nonmotor vehicle in traffic accident

✓x7ᵗʰ **V26.9** Unspecified motorcycle rider injured in collision with other nonmotor vehicle in traffic accident

✓4ᵗʰ **V27** **Motorcycle rider injured in collision with fixed or stationary object**

✓x7ᵗʰ **V27.0** Motorcycle driver injured in collision with fixed or stationary object in nontraffic accident

✓x7ᵗʰ **V27.1** Motorcycle passenger injured in collision with fixed or stationary object in nontraffic accident

✓x7ᵗʰ **V27.2** Unspecified motorcycle rider injured in collision with fixed or stationary object in nontraffic accident

✓x7ᵗʰ **V27.3** Person boarding or alighting a motorcycle injured in collision with fixed or stationary object

✓x7ᵗʰ **V27.4** Motorcycle driver injured in collision with fixed or stationary object in traffic accident

✓x7ᵗʰ **V27.5** Motorcycle passenger injured in collision with fixed or stationary object in traffic accident

✓x7ᵗʰ **V27.9** Unspecified motorcycle rider injured in collision with fixed or stationary object in traffic accident

✓4ᵗʰ **V28** **Motorcycle rider injured in noncollision transport accident**
    INCLUDES   fall or thrown from motorcycle (without antecedent collision)
       overturning motorcycle NOS
       overturning motorcycle without collision

✓x7ᵗʰ **V28.0** Motorcycle driver injured in noncollision transport accident in nontraffic accident

✓x7ᵗʰ **V28.1** Motorcycle passenger injured in noncollision transport accident in nontraffic accident

✓x7ᵗʰ **V28.2** Unspecified motorcycle rider injured in noncollision transport accident in nontraffic accident

✓x7ᵗʰ **V28.3** Person boarding or alighting a motorcycle injured in noncollision transport accident

✓x7ᵗʰ **V28.4** Motorcycle driver injured in noncollision transport accident in traffic accident

✓x7ᵗʰ **V28.5** Motorcycle passenger injured in noncollision transport accident in traffic accident

✓x7ᵗʰ **V28.9** Unspecified motorcycle rider injured in noncollision transport accident in traffic accident

✓4ᵗʰ **V29** **Motorcycle rider injured in other and unspecified transport accidents**

✓5ᵗʰ **V29.0** Motorcycle driver injured in collision with other and unspecified motor vehicles in nontraffic accident

   ✓x7ᵗʰ **V29.00** Motorcycle driver injured in collision with unspecified motor vehicles in nontraffic accident

   ✓x7ᵗʰ **V29.09** Motorcycle driver injured in collision with other motor vehicles in nontraffic accident

✓5ᵗʰ **V29.1** Motorcycle passenger injured in collision with other and unspecified motor vehicles in nontraffic accident

   ✓x7ᵗʰ **V29.10** Motorcycle passenger injured in collision with unspecified motor vehicles in nontraffic accident

   ✓x7ᵗʰ **V29.19** Motorcycle passenger injured in collision with other motor vehicles in nontraffic accident

✓5ᵗʰ **V29.2** Unspecified motorcycle rider injured in collision with other and unspecified motor vehicles in nontraffic accident

   ✓x7ᵗʰ **V29.20** Unspecified motorcycle rider injured in collision with unspecified motor vehicles in nontraffic accident
         Motorcycle collision NOS, nontraffic

✓x7ᵗʰ **V29.29** Unspecified motorcycle rider injured in collision with other motor vehicles in nontraffic accident

✓x7ᵗʰ **V29.3** Motorcycle rider (driver) (passenger) injured in unspecified nontraffic accident
    Motorcycle accident NOS, nontraffic
    Motorcycle rider injured in nontraffic accident NOS

✓5ᵗʰ **V29.4** Motorcycle driver injured in collision with other and unspecified motor vehicles in traffic accident

   ✓x7ᵗʰ **V29.40** Motorcycle driver injured in collision with unspecified motor vehicles in traffic accident

   ✓x7ᵗʰ **V29.49** Motorcycle driver injured in collision with other motor vehicles in traffic accident

✓5ᵗʰ **V29.5** Motorcycle passenger injured in collision with other and unspecified motor vehicles in traffic accident

   ✓x7ᵗʰ **V29.50** Motorcycle passenger injured in collision with unspecified motor vehicles in traffic accident

   ✓x7ᵗʰ **V29.59** Motorcycle passenger injured in collision with other motor vehicles in traffic accident

✓5ᵗʰ **V29.6** Unspecified motorcycle rider injured in collision with other and unspecified motor vehicles in traffic accident

   ✓x7ᵗʰ **V29.60** Unspecified motorcycle rider injured in collision with unspecified motor vehicles in traffic accident
         Motorcycle collision NOS (traffic)

   ✓x7ᵗʰ **V29.69** Unspecified motorcycle rider injured in collision with other motor vehicles in traffic accident

✓5ᵗʰ **V29.8** Motorcycle rider (driver) (passenger) injured in other specified transport accidents

   ✓x7ᵗʰ **V29.81** Motorcycle rider (driver) (passenger) injured in transport accident with military vehicle

   ✓x7ᵗʰ **V29.88** Motorcycle rider (driver) (passenger) injured in other specified transport accidents

✓x7ᵗʰ **V29.9** Motorcycle rider (driver) (passenger) injured in unspecified traffic accident
    Motorcycle accident NOS

## Occupant of three-wheeled motor vehicle injured in transport accident (V30-V39)

    INCLUDES   motorized tricycle
       motorized rickshaw
       three-wheeled motor car
    EXCLUDES 1   all-terrain vehicles (V86.-)
       motorcycle with sidecar (V20-V29)
       vehicle designed primarily for off-road use (V86.-)

The appropriate 7th character is to be added to each code from categories V30-V39.
A   initial encounter
D   subsequent encounter
S   sequela

✓4ᵗʰ **V30** **Occupant of three-wheeled motor vehicle injured in collision with pedestrian or animal**
    EXCLUDES 1   three-wheeled motor vehicle collision with animal-drawn vehicle or animal being ridden (V36.-)

✓x7ᵗʰ **V30.0** Driver of three-wheeled motor vehicle injured in collision with pedestrian or animal in nontraffic accident

✓x7ᵗʰ **V30.1** Passenger in three-wheeled motor vehicle injured in collision with pedestrian or animal in nontraffic accident

✓x7ᵗʰ **V30.2** Person on outside of three-wheeled motor vehicle injured in collision with pedestrian or animal in nontraffic accident

✓x7ᵗʰ **V30.3** Unspecified occupant of three-wheeled motor vehicle injured in collision with pedestrian or animal in nontraffic accident

✓x7ᵗʰ **V30.4** Person boarding or alighting a three-wheeled motor vehicle injured in collision with pedestrian or animal

✓x7ᵗʰ **V30.5** Driver of three-wheeled motor vehicle injured in collision with pedestrian or animal in traffic accident

✓x7ᵗʰ **V30.6** Passenger in three-wheeled motor vehicle injured in collision with pedestrian or animal in traffic accident

✓x7ᵗʰ **V30.7** Person on outside of three-wheeled motor vehicle injured in collision with pedestrian or animal in traffic accident

✓x7ᵗʰ **V30.9** Unspecified occupant of three-wheeled motor vehicle injured in collision with pedestrian or animal in traffic accident

✓4ᵗʰ **V31** **Occupant of three-wheeled motor vehicle injured in collision with pedal cycle**

✓x7ᵗʰ **V31.0** Driver of three-wheeled motor vehicle injured in collision with pedal cycle in nontraffic accident

√x7ᵗʰ **V31.1** Passenger in three-wheeled motor vehicle injured in collision with pedal cycle in nontraffic accident

√x7ᵗʰ **V31.2** Person on outside of three-wheeled motor vehicle injured in collision with pedal cycle in nontraffic accident

√x7ᵗʰ **V31.3** Unspecified occupant of three-wheeled motor vehicle injured in collision with pedal cycle in nontraffic accident

√x7ᵗʰ **V31.4** Person boarding or alighting a three-wheeled motor vehicle injured in collision with pedal cycle

√x7ᵗʰ **V31.5** Driver of three-wheeled motor vehicle injured in collision with pedal cycle in traffic accident

√x7ᵗʰ **V31.6** Passenger in three-wheeled motor vehicle injured in collision with pedal cycle in traffic accident

√x7ᵗʰ **V31.7** Person on outside of three-wheeled motor vehicle injured in collision with pedal cycle in traffic accident

√x7ᵗʰ **V31.9** Unspecified occupant of three-wheeled motor vehicle injured in collision with pedal cycle in traffic accident

√4ᵗʰ **V32** **Occupant of three-wheeled motor vehicle injured in collision with two- or three-wheeled motor vehicle**

√x7ᵗʰ **V32.0** Driver of three-wheeled motor vehicle injured in collision with two- or three-wheeled motor vehicle in nontraffic accident

√x7ᵗʰ **V32.1** Passenger in three-wheeled motor vehicle injured in collision with two- or three-wheeled motor vehicle in nontraffic accident

√x7ᵗʰ **V32.2** Person on outside of three-wheeled motor vehicle injured in collision with two- or three-wheeled motor vehicle in nontraffic accident

√x7ᵗʰ **V32.3** Unspecified occupant of three-wheeled motor vehicle injured in collision with two- or three-wheeled motor vehicle in nontraffic accident

√x7ᵗʰ **V32.4** Person boarding or alighting a three-wheeled motor vehicle injured in collision with two- or three-wheeled motor vehicle

√x7ᵗʰ **V32.5** Driver of three-wheeled motor vehicle injured in collision with two- or three-wheeled motor vehicle in traffic accident

√x7ᵗʰ **V32.6** Passenger in three-wheeled motor vehicle injured in collision with two- or three-wheeled motor vehicle in traffic accident

√x7ᵗʰ **V32.7** Person on outside of three-wheeled motor vehicle injured in collision with two- or three-wheeled motor vehicle in traffic accident

√x7ᵗʰ **V32.9** Unspecified occupant of three-wheeled motor vehicle injured in collision with two- or three-wheeled motor vehicle in traffic accident

√4ᵗʰ **V33** **Occupant of three-wheeled motor vehicle injured in collision with car, pick-up truck or van**

√x7ᵗʰ **V33.0** Driver of three-wheeled motor vehicle injured in collision with car, pick-up truck or van in nontraffic accident

√x7ᵗʰ **V33.1** Passenger in three-wheeled motor vehicle injured in collision with car, pick-up truck or van in nontraffic accident

√x7ᵗʰ **V33.2** Person on outside of three-wheeled motor vehicle injured in collision with car, pick-up truck or van in nontraffic accident

√x7ᵗʰ **V33.3** Unspecified occupant of three-wheeled motor vehicle injured in collision with car, pick-up truck or van in nontraffic accident

√x7ᵗʰ **V33.4** Person boarding or alighting a three-wheeled motor vehicle injured in collision with car, pick-up truck or van

√x7ᵗʰ **V33.5** Driver of three-wheeled motor vehicle injured in collision with car, pick-up truck or van in traffic accident

√x7ᵗʰ **V33.6** Passenger in three-wheeled motor vehicle injured in collision with car, pick-up truck or van in traffic accident

√x7ᵗʰ **V33.7** Person on outside of three-wheeled motor vehicle injured in collision with car, pick-up truck or van in traffic accident

√x7ᵗʰ **V33.9** Unspecified occupant of three-wheeled motor vehicle injured in collision with car, pick-up truck or van in traffic accident

√4ᵗʰ **V34** **Occupant of three-wheeled motor vehicle injured in collision with heavy transport vehicle or bus**

     **EXCLUDES 1** occupant of three-wheeled motor vehicle injured in collision with military vehicle (V39.81)

√x7ᵗʰ **V34.0** Driver of three-wheeled motor vehicle injured in collision with heavy transport vehicle or bus in nontraffic accident

√x7ᵗʰ **V34.1** Passenger in three-wheeled motor vehicle injured in collision with heavy transport vehicle or bus in nontraffic accident

√x7ᵗʰ **V34.2** Person on outside of three-wheeled motor vehicle injured in collision with heavy transport vehicle or bus in nontraffic accident

√x7ᵗʰ **V34.3** Unspecified occupant of three-wheeled motor vehicle injured in collision with heavy transport vehicle or bus in nontraffic accident

√x7ᵗʰ **V34.4** Person boarding or alighting a three-wheeled motor vehicle injured in collision with heavy transport vehicle or bus

√x7ᵗʰ **V34.5** Driver of three-wheeled motor vehicle injured in collision with heavy transport vehicle or bus in traffic accident

√x7ᵗʰ **V34.6** Passenger in three-wheeled motor vehicle injured in collision with heavy transport vehicle or bus in traffic accident

√x7ᵗʰ **V34.7** Person on outside of three-wheeled motor vehicle injured in collision with heavy transport vehicle or bus in traffic accident

√x7ᵗʰ **V34.9** Unspecified occupant of three-wheeled motor vehicle injured in collision with heavy transport vehicle or bus in traffic accident

√4ᵗʰ **V35** **Occupant of three-wheeled motor vehicle injured in collision with railway train or railway vehicle**

√x7ᵗʰ **V35.0** Driver of three-wheeled motor vehicle injured in collision with railway train or railway vehicle in nontraffic accident

√x7ᵗʰ **V35.1** Passenger in three-wheeled motor vehicle injured in collision with railway train or railway vehicle in nontraffic accident

√x7ᵗʰ **V35.2** Person on outside of three-wheeled motor vehicle injured in collision with railway train or railway vehicle in nontraffic accident

√x7ᵗʰ **V35.3** Unspecified occupant of three-wheeled motor vehicle injured in collision with railway train or railway vehicle in nontraffic accident

√x7ᵗʰ **V35.4** Person boarding or alighting a three-wheeled motor vehicle injured in collision with railway train or railway vehicle

√x7ᵗʰ **V35.5** Driver of three-wheeled motor vehicle injured in collision with railway train or railway vehicle in traffic accident

√x7ᵗʰ **V35.6** Passenger in three-wheeled motor vehicle injured in collision with railway train or railway vehicle in traffic accident

√x7ᵗʰ **V35.7** Person on outside of three-wheeled motor vehicle injured in collision with railway train or railway vehicle in traffic accident

√x7ᵗʰ **V35.9** Unspecified occupant of three-wheeled motor vehicle injured in collision with railway train or railway vehicle in traffic accident

√4ᵗʰ **V36** **Occupant of three-wheeled motor vehicle injured in collision with other nonmotor vehicle**

     **INCLUDES** collision with animal-drawn vehicle, animal being ridden, streetcar

√x7ᵗʰ **V36.0** Driver of three-wheeled motor vehicle injured in collision with other nonmotor vehicle in nontraffic accident

√x7ᵗʰ **V36.1** Passenger in three-wheeled motor vehicle injured in collision with other nonmotor vehicle in nontraffic accident

√x7ᵗʰ **V36.2** Person on outside of three-wheeled motor vehicle injured in collision with other nonmotor vehicle in nontraffic accident

√x7ᵗʰ **V36.3** Unspecified occupant of three-wheeled motor vehicle injured in collision with other nonmotor vehicle in nontraffic accident

√x7ᵗʰ **V36.4** Person boarding or alighting a three-wheeled motor vehicle injured in collision with other nonmotor vehicle

√x7ᵗʰ **V36.5** Driver of three-wheeled motor vehicle injured in collision with other nonmotor vehicle in traffic accident

√x7ᵗʰ **V36.6** Passenger in three-wheeled motor vehicle injured in collision with other nonmotor vehicle in traffic accident

√x7ᵗʰ **V36.7** Person on outside of three-wheeled motor vehicle injured in collision with other nonmotor vehicle in traffic accident

√x7ᵗʰ **V36.9** Unspecified occupant of three-wheeled motor vehicle injured in collision with other nonmotor vehicle in traffic accident

√4ᵗʰ **V37** **Occupant of three-wheeled motor vehicle injured in collision with fixed or stationary object**

√x7ᵗʰ **V37.0** Driver of three-wheeled motor vehicle injured in collision with fixed or stationary object in nontraffic accident

√x7ᵗʰ **V37.1** Passenger in three-wheeled motor vehicle injured in collision with fixed or stationary object in nontraffic accident

√x7ᵗʰ **V37.2** Person on outside of three-wheeled motor vehicle injured in collision with fixed or stationary object in nontraffic accident

√x7ᵗʰ **V37.3** Unspecified occupant of three-wheeled motor vehicle injured in collision with fixed or stationary object in nontraffic accident

√x7ᵗʰ **V37.4** Person boarding or alighting a three-wheeled motor vehicle injured in collision with fixed or stationary object

---

☑ Additional Character Req    √x7ᵗʰ Placeholder Alert    Unacceptable PDx    Manifestation    **H1**-**H14** HAC    **HCC** CMS-HCC Condition    **EXCLUDES 1** Not Coded Here    **EXCLUDES 2** Not Included Here

**✓x7ᵗʰ V37.5** Driver of three-wheeled motor vehicle injured in collision with fixed or stationary object in traffic accident

**✓x7ᵗʰ V37.6** Passenger in three-wheeled motor vehicle injured in collision with fixed or stationary object in traffic accident

**✓x7ᵗʰ V37.7** Person on outside of three-wheeled motor vehicle injured in collision with fixed or stationary object in traffic accident

**✓x7ᵗʰ V37.9** Unspecified occupant of three-wheeled motor vehicle injured in collision with fixed or stationary object in traffic accident

**✓4ᵗʰ V38 Occupant of three-wheeled motor vehicle injured in noncollision transport accident**
> INCLUDES fall or thrown from three-wheeled motor vehicle
> overturning of three-wheeled motor vehicle NOS
> overturning of three-wheeled motor vehicle without collision

**✓x7ᵗʰ V38.0** Driver of three-wheeled motor vehicle injured in noncollision transport accident in nontraffic accident

**✓x7ᵗʰ V38.1** Passenger in three-wheeled motor vehicle injured in noncollision transport accident in nontraffic accident

**✓x7ᵗʰ V38.2** Person on outside of three-wheeled motor vehicle injured in noncollision transport accident in nontraffic accident

**✓x7ᵗʰ V38.3** Unspecified occupant of three-wheeled motor vehicle injured in noncollision transport accident in nontraffic accident

**✓x7ᵗʰ V38.4** Person boarding or alighting a three-wheeled motor vehicle injured in noncollision transport accident

**✓x7ᵗʰ V38.5** Driver of three-wheeled motor vehicle injured in noncollision transport accident in traffic accident

**✓x7ᵗʰ V38.6** Passenger in three-wheeled motor vehicle injured in noncollision transport accident in traffic accident

**✓x7ᵗʰ V38.7** Person on outside of three-wheeled motor vehicle injured in noncollision transport accident in traffic accident

**✓x7ᵗʰ V38.9** Unspecified occupant of three-wheeled motor vehicle injured in noncollision transport accident in traffic accident

**✓4ᵗʰ V39 Occupant of three-wheeled motor vehicle injured in other and unspecified transport accidents**

**✓5ᵗʰ V39.0** Driver of three-wheeled motor vehicle injured in collision with other and unspecified motor vehicles in nontraffic accident

**✓x7ᵗʰ V39.00** Driver of three-wheeled motor vehicle injured in collision with unspecified motor vehicles in nontraffic accident

**✓x7ᵗʰ V39.09** Driver of three-wheeled motor vehicle injured in collision with other motor vehicles in nontraffic accident

**✓5ᵗʰ V39.1** Passenger in three-wheeled motor vehicle injured in collision with other and unspecified motor vehicles in nontraffic accident

**✓x7ᵗʰ V39.10** Passenger in three-wheeled motor vehicle injured in collision with unspecified motor vehicles in nontraffic accident

**✓x7ᵗʰ V39.19** Passenger in three-wheeled motor vehicle injured in collision with other motor vehicles in nontraffic accident

**✓5ᵗʰ V39.2** Unspecified occupant of three-wheeled motor vehicle injured in collision with other and unspecified motor vehicles in nontraffic accident

**✓x7ᵗʰ V39.20** Unspecified occupant of three-wheeled motor vehicle injured in collision with unspecified motor vehicles in nontraffic accident
> Collision NOS involving three-wheeled motor vehicle, nontraffic

**✓x7ᵗʰ V39.29** Unspecified occupant of three-wheeled motor vehicle injured in collision with other motor vehicles in nontraffic accident

**✓x7ᵗʰ V39.3** Occupant (driver) (passenger) of three-wheeled motor vehicle injured in unspecified nontraffic accident
> Accident NOS involving three-wheeled motor vehicle, nontraffic
> Occupant of three-wheeled motor vehicle injured in nontraffic accident NOS

**✓5ᵗʰ V39.4** Driver of three-wheeled motor vehicle injured in collision with other and unspecified motor vehicles in traffic accident

**✓x7ᵗʰ V39.40** Driver of three-wheeled motor vehicle injured in collision with unspecified motor vehicles in traffic accident

**✓x7ᵗʰ V39.49** Driver of three-wheeled motor vehicle injured in collision with other motor vehicles in traffic accident

**✓5ᵗʰ V39.5** Passenger in three-wheeled motor vehicle injured in collision with other and unspecified motor vehicles in traffic accident

**✓x7ᵗʰ V39.50** Passenger in three-wheeled motor vehicle injured in collision with unspecified motor vehicles in traffic accident

**✓x7ᵗʰ V39.59** Passenger in three-wheeled motor vehicle injured in collision with other motor vehicles in traffic accident

**✓5ᵗʰ V39.6** Unspecified occupant of three-wheeled motor vehicle injured in collision with other and unspecified motor vehicles in traffic accident

**✓x7ᵗʰ V39.60** Unspecified occupant of three-wheeled motor vehicle injured in collision with unspecified motor vehicles in traffic accident
> Collision NOS involving three-wheeled motor vehicle (traffic)

**✓x7ᵗʰ V39.69** Unspecified occupant of three-wheeled motor vehicle injured in collision with other motor vehicles in traffic accident

**✓5ᵗʰ V39.8** Occupant (driver) (passenger) of three-wheeled motor vehicle injured in other specified transport accidents

**✓x7ᵗʰ V39.81** Occupant (driver) (passenger) of three-wheeled motor vehicle injured in transport accident with military vehicle

**✓x7ᵗʰ V39.89** Occupant (driver) (passenger) of three-wheeled motor vehicle injured in other specified transport accidents

**✓x7ᵗʰ V39.9** Occupant (driver) (passenger) of three-wheeled motor vehicle injured in unspecified traffic accident
> Accident NOS involving three-wheeled motor vehicle

### Car occupant injured in transport accident (V40-V49)
> INCLUDES a four-wheeled motor vehicle designed primarily for carrying passengers
> automobile (pulling a trailer or camper)
> EXCLUDES 1 bus (V50-V59)
> minibus (V50-V59)
> minivan (V50-V59)
> motorcoach (V70-V79)
> pick-up truck (V50-V59)
> sport utility vehicle (SUV) (V50-V59)

The appropriate 7th character is to be added to each code from categories V40-V49.
A   initial encounter
D   subsequent encounter
S   sequela

**✓4ᵗʰ V40 Car occupant injured in collision with pedestrian or animal**
> EXCLUDES 1 car collision with animal-drawn vehicle or animal being ridden (V46.-)

**✓x7ᵗʰ V40.0** Car driver injured in collision with pedestrian or animal in nontraffic accident

**✓x7ᵗʰ V40.1** Car passenger injured in collision with pedestrian or animal in nontraffic accident

**✓x7ᵗʰ V40.2** Person on outside of car injured in collision with pedestrian or animal in nontraffic accident

**✓x7ᵗʰ V40.3** Unspecified car occupant injured in collision with pedestrian or animal in nontraffic accident

**✓x7ᵗʰ V40.4** Person boarding or alighting a car injured in collision with pedestrian or animal

**✓x7ᵗʰ V40.5** Car driver injured in collision with pedestrian or animal in traffic accident

**✓x7ᵗʰ V40.6** Car passenger injured in collision with pedestrian or animal in traffic accident

**✓x7ᵗʰ V40.7** Person on outside of car injured in collision with pedestrian or animal in traffic accident

**✓x7ᵗʰ V40.9** Unspecified car occupant injured in collision with pedestrian or animal in traffic accident

**✓4ᵗʰ V41 Car occupant injured in collision with pedal cycle**

**✓x7ᵗʰ V41.0** Car driver injured in collision with pedal cycle in nontraffic accident

**✓x7ᵗʰ V41.1** Car passenger injured in collision with pedal cycle in nontraffic accident

**✓x7ᵗʰ V41.2** Person on outside of car injured in collision with pedal cycle in nontraffic accident

**✓x7ᵗʰ V41.3** Unspecified car occupant injured in collision with pedal cycle in nontraffic accident

Ⓝ Newborn: 0   Ⓟ Pediatric: 0-17   Ⓜ Maternity: 12-55   Ⓐ Adult: 15-124   **MCC** Major CC Condition   **PDx MCC** PDx acts as own MCC   **CC** CC Condition   **PDx CC** PDx acts as own CC

1168     ICD-10-CM 2018

✓x 7ᵗʰ **V41.4** Person boarding or alighting a car injured in collision with pedal cycle

✓x 7ᵗʰ **V41.5** Car driver injured in collision with pedal cycle in traffic accident

✓x 7ᵗʰ **V41.6** Car passenger injured in collision with pedal cycle in traffic accident

✓x 7ᵗʰ **V41.7** Person on outside of car injured in collision with pedal cycle in traffic accident

✓x 7ᵗʰ **V41.9** Unspecified car occupant injured in collision with pedal cycle in traffic accident

✓4ᵗʰ **V42 Car occupant injured in collision with two- or three-wheeled motor vehicle**

✓x 7ᵗʰ **V42.0** Car driver injured in collision with two- or three-wheeled motor vehicle in nontraffic accident

✓x 7ᵗʰ **V42.1** Car passenger injured in collision with two- or three-wheeled motor vehicle in nontraffic accident

✓x 7ᵗʰ **V42.2** Person on outside of car injured in collision with two- or three-wheeled motor vehicle in nontraffic accident

✓x 7ᵗʰ **V42.3** Unspecified car occupant injured in collision with two- or three-wheeled motor vehicle in nontraffic accident

✓x 7ᵗʰ **V42.4** Person boarding or alighting a car injured in collision with two- or three-wheeled motor vehicle

✓x 7ᵗʰ **V42.5** Car driver injured in collision with two- or three-wheeled motor vehicle in traffic accident

✓x 7ᵗʰ **V42.6** Car passenger injured in collision with two- or three-wheeled motor vehicle in traffic accident

✓x 7ᵗʰ **V42.7** Person on outside of car injured in collision with two- or three-wheeled motor vehicle in traffic accident

✓x 7ᵗʰ **V42.9** Unspecified car occupant injured in collision with two- or three-wheeled motor vehicle in traffic accident

✓4ᵗʰ **V43 Car occupant injured in collision with car, pick-up truck or van**

✓5ᵗʰ **V43.0** Car driver injured in collision with car, pick-up truck or van in nontraffic accident

✓x 7ᵗʰ **V43.01** Car driver injured in collision with sport utility vehicle in nontraffic accident

✓x 7ᵗʰ **V43.02** Car driver injured in collision with other type car in nontraffic accident

✓x 7ᵗʰ **V43.03** Car driver injured in collision with pick-up truck in nontraffic accident

✓x 7ᵗʰ **V43.04** Car driver injured in collision with van in nontraffic accident

✓5ᵗʰ **V43.1** Car passenger injured in collision with car, pick-up truck or van in nontraffic accident

✓x 7ᵗʰ **V43.11** Car passenger injured in collision with sport utility vehicle in nontraffic accident

✓x 7ᵗʰ **V43.12** Car passenger injured in collision with other type car in nontraffic accident

✓x 7ᵗʰ **V43.13** Car passenger injured in collision with pick-up in nontraffic accident

✓x 7ᵗʰ **V43.14** Car passenger injured in collision with van in nontraffic accident

✓5ᵗʰ **V43.2** Person on outside of car injured in collision with car, pick-up truck or van in nontraffic accident

✓x 7ᵗʰ **V43.21** Person on outside of car injured in collision with sport utility vehicle in nontraffic accident

✓x 7ᵗʰ **V43.22** Person on outside of car injured in collision with other type car in nontraffic accident

✓x 7ᵗʰ **V43.23** Person on outside of car injured in collision with pick-up truck in nontraffic accident

✓x 7ᵗʰ **V43.24** Person on outside of car injured in collision with van in nontraffic accident

✓5ᵗʰ **V43.3** Unspecified car occupant injured in collision with car, pick-up truck or van in nontraffic accident

✓x 7ᵗʰ **V43.31** Unspecified car occupant injured in collision with sport utility vehicle in nontraffic accident

✓x 7ᵗʰ **V43.32** Unspecified car occupant injured in collision with other type car in nontraffic accident

✓x 7ᵗʰ **V43.33** Unspecified car occupant injured in collision with pick-up truck in nontraffic accident

✓x 7ᵗʰ **V43.34** Unspecified car occupant injured in collision with van in nontraffic accident

✓5ᵗʰ **V43.4** Person boarding or alighting a car injured in collision with car, pick-up truck or van

✓x 7ᵗʰ **V43.41** Person boarding or alighting a car injured in collision with sport utility vehicle

✓x 7ᵗʰ **V43.42** Person boarding or alighting a car injured in collision with other type car

✓x 7ᵗʰ **V43.43** Person boarding or alighting a car injured in collision with pick-up truck

✓x 7ᵗʰ **V43.44** Person boarding or alighting a car injured in collision with van

✓5ᵗʰ **V43.5** Car driver injured in collision with car, pick-up truck or van in traffic accident

✓x 7ᵗʰ **V43.51** Car driver injured in collision with sport utility vehicle in traffic accident

✓x 7ᵗʰ **V43.52** Car driver injured in collision with other type car in traffic accident

✓x 7ᵗʰ **V43.53** Car driver injured in collision with pick-up truck in traffic accident

✓x 7ᵗʰ **V43.54** Car driver injured in collision with van in traffic accident

✓5ᵗʰ **V43.6** Car passenger injured in collision with car, pick-up truck or van in traffic accident

✓x 7ᵗʰ **V43.61** Car passenger injured in collision with sport utility vehicle in traffic accident

✓x 7ᵗʰ **V43.62** Car passenger injured in collision with other type car in traffic accident

✓x 7ᵗʰ **V43.63** Car passenger injured in collision with pick-up truck in traffic accident

✓x 7ᵗʰ **V43.64** Car passenger injured in collision with van in traffic accident

✓5ᵗʰ **V43.7** Person on outside of car injured in collision with car, pick-up truck or van in traffic accident

✓x 7ᵗʰ **V43.71** Person on outside of car injured in collision with sport utility vehicle in traffic accident

✓x 7ᵗʰ **V43.72** Person on outside of car injured in collision with other type car in traffic accident

✓x 7ᵗʰ **V43.73** Person on outside of car injured in collision with pick-up truck in traffic accident

✓x 7ᵗʰ **V43.74** Person on outside of car injured in collision with van in traffic accident

✓5ᵗʰ **V43.9** Unspecified car occupant injured in collision with car, pick-up truck or van in traffic accident

✓x 7ᵗʰ **V43.91** Unspecified car occupant injured in collision with sport utility vehicle in traffic accident

✓x 7ᵗʰ **V43.92** Unspecified car occupant injured in collision with other type car in traffic accident

✓x 7ᵗʰ **V43.93** Unspecified car occupant injured in collision with pick-up truck in traffic accident

✓x 7ᵗʰ **V43.94** Unspecified car occupant injured in collision with van in traffic accident

✓4ᵗʰ **V44 Car occupant injured in collision with heavy transport vehicle or bus**

     *EXCLUDES 1*    car occupant injured in collision with military vehicle (V49.81)

✓x 7ᵗʰ **V44.0** Car driver injured in collision with heavy transport vehicle or bus in nontraffic accident

✓x 7ᵗʰ **V44.1** Car passenger injured in collision with heavy transport vehicle or bus in nontraffic accident

✓x 7ᵗʰ **V44.2** Person on outside of car injured in collision with heavy transport vehicle or bus in nontraffic accident

✓x 7ᵗʰ **V44.3** Unspecified car occupant injured in collision with heavy transport vehicle or bus in nontraffic accident

✓x 7ᵗʰ **V44.4** Person boarding or alighting a car injured in collision with heavy transport vehicle or bus

✓x 7ᵗʰ **V44.5** Car driver injured in collision with heavy transport vehicle or bus in traffic accident

✓x 7ᵗʰ **V44.6** Car passenger injured in collision with heavy transport vehicle or bus in traffic accident

✓x 7ᵗʰ **V44.7** Person on outside of car injured in collision with heavy transport vehicle or bus in traffic accident

✓x 7ᵗʰ **V44.9** Unspecified car occupant injured in collision with heavy transport vehicle or bus in traffic accident

---

✓ Additional Character Req   ✓x7ᵗʰ Placeholder Alert   Unacceptable PDx   Manifestation   **H1 - H14** HAC   **HCC** CMS-HCC Condition   *EXCLUDES 1* Not Coded Here   *EXCLUDES 2* Not Included Here

ICD-10-CM 2018                            **1169**

V41.4–V44.9

√4ᵗʰ **V45 Car occupant injured in collision with railway train or railway vehicle**

√7ᵗʰ **V45.0** Car driver injured in collision with railway train or railway vehicle in nontraffic accident

√7ᵗʰ **V45.1** Car passenger injured in collision with railway train or railway vehicle in nontraffic accident

√7ᵗʰ **V45.2** Person on outside of car injured in collision with railway train or railway vehicle in nontraffic accident

√7ᵗʰ **V45.3** Unspecified car occupant injured in collision with railway train or railway vehicle in nontraffic accident

√7ᵗʰ **V45.4** Person boarding or alighting a car injured in collision with railway train or railway vehicle

√7ᵗʰ **V45.5** Car driver injured in collision with railway train or railway vehicle in traffic accident

√7ᵗʰ **V45.6** Car passenger injured in collision with railway train or railway vehicle in traffic accident

√7ᵗʰ **V45.7** Person on outside of car injured in collision with railway train or railway vehicle in traffic accident

√7ᵗʰ **V45.9** Unspecified car occupant injured in collision with railway train or railway vehicle in traffic accident

√4ᵗʰ **V46 Car occupant injured in collision with other nonmotor vehicle**

     INCLUDES   collision with animal-drawn vehicle, animal being ridden, streetcar

√7ᵗʰ **V46.0** Car driver injured in collision with other nonmotor vehicle in nontraffic accident

√7ᵗʰ **V46.1** Car passenger injured in collision with other nonmotor vehicle in nontraffic accident

√7ᵗʰ **V46.2** Person on outside of car injured in collision with other nonmotor vehicle in nontraffic accident

√7ᵗʰ **V46.3** Unspecified car occupant injured in collision with other nonmotor vehicle in nontraffic accident

√7ᵗʰ **V46.4** Person boarding or alighting a car injured in collision with other nonmotor vehicle

√7ᵗʰ **V46.5** Car driver injured in collision with other nonmotor vehicle in traffic accident

√7ᵗʰ **V46.6** Car passenger injured in collision with other nonmotor vehicle in traffic accident

√7ᵗʰ **V46.7** Person on outside of car injured in collision with other nonmotor vehicle in traffic accident

√7ᵗʰ **V46.9** Unspecified car occupant injured in collision with other nonmotor vehicle in traffic accident

√4ᵗʰ **V47 Car occupant injured in collision with fixed or stationary object**

√7ᵗʰ **V47.0** Car driver injured in collision with fixed or stationary object in nontraffic accident

√7ᵗʰ **V47.1** Car passenger injured in collision with fixed or stationary object in nontraffic accident

√7ᵗʰ **V47.2** Person on outside of car injured in collision with fixed or stationary object in nontraffic accident

√7ᵗʰ **V47.3** Unspecified car occupant injured in collision with fixed or stationary object in nontraffic accident

√7ᵗʰ **V47.4** Person boarding or alighting a car injured in collision with fixed or stationary object

√7ᵗʰ **V47.5** Car driver injured in collision with fixed or stationary object in traffic accident

√7ᵗʰ **V47.6** Car passenger injured in collision with fixed or stationary object in traffic accident

√7ᵗʰ **V47.7** Person on outside of car injured in collision with fixed or stationary object in traffic accident

√7ᵗʰ **V47.9** Unspecified car occupant injured in collision with fixed or stationary object in traffic accident

√4ᵗʰ **V48 Car occupant injured in noncollision transport accident**

     INCLUDES   overturning car NOS
                 overturning car without collision

√7ᵗʰ **V48.0** Car driver injured in noncollision transport accident in nontraffic accident

√7ᵗʰ **V48.1** Car passenger injured in noncollision transport accident in nontraffic accident

√7ᵗʰ **V48.2** Person on outside of car injured in noncollision transport accident in nontraffic accident

√7ᵗʰ **V48.3** Unspecified car occupant injured in noncollision transport accident in nontraffic accident

√7ᵗʰ **V48.4** Person boarding or alighting a car injured in noncollision transport accident

√7ᵗʰ **V48.5** Car driver injured in noncollision transport accident in traffic accident

√7ᵗʰ **V48.6** Car passenger injured in noncollision transport accident in traffic accident

√7ᵗʰ **V48.7** Person on outside of car injured in noncollision transport accident in traffic accident

√7ᵗʰ **V48.9** Unspecified car occupant injured in noncollision transport accident in traffic accident

√4ᵗʰ **V49 Car occupant injured in other and unspecified transport accidents**

√5ᵗʰ **V49.0** Driver injured in collision with other and unspecified motor vehicles in nontraffic accident

√7ᵗʰ **V49.00** Driver injured in collision with unspecified motor vehicles in nontraffic accident

√7ᵗʰ **V49.09** Driver injured in collision with other motor vehicles in nontraffic accident

√5ᵗʰ **V49.1** Passenger injured in collision with other and unspecified motor vehicles in nontraffic accident

√7ᵗʰ **V49.10** Passenger injured in collision with unspecified motor vehicles in nontraffic accident

√7ᵗʰ **V49.19** Passenger injured in collision with other motor vehicles in nontraffic accident

√5ᵗʰ **V49.2** Unspecified car occupant injured in collision with other and unspecified motor vehicles in nontraffic accident

√7ᵗʰ **V49.20** Unspecified car occupant injured in collision with unspecified motor vehicles in nontraffic accident
     Car collision NOS, nontraffic

√7ᵗʰ **V49.29** Unspecified car occupant injured in collision with other motor vehicles in nontraffic accident

√7ᵗʰ **V49.3** Car occupant (driver) (passenger) injured in unspecified nontraffic accident
     Car accident NOS, nontraffic
     Car occupant injured in nontraffic accident NOS

√5ᵗʰ **V49.4** Driver injured in collision with other and unspecified motor vehicles in traffic accident

√7ᵗʰ **V49.40** Driver injured in collision with unspecified motor vehicles in traffic accident

√7ᵗʰ **V49.49** Driver injured in collision with other motor vehicles in traffic accident

√5ᵗʰ **V49.5** Passenger injured in collision with other and unspecified motor vehicles in traffic accident

√7ᵗʰ **V49.50** Passenger injured in collision with unspecified motor vehicles in traffic accident

√7ᵗʰ **V49.59** Passenger injured in collision with other motor vehicles in traffic accident

√5ᵗʰ **V49.6** Unspecified car occupant injured in collision with other and unspecified motor vehicles in traffic accident

√7ᵗʰ **V49.60** Unspecified car occupant injured in collision with unspecified motor vehicles in traffic accident
     Car collision NOS (traffic)

√7ᵗʰ **V49.69** Unspecified car occupant injured in collision with other motor vehicles in traffic accident

√5ᵗʰ **V49.8** Car occupant (driver) (passenger) injured in other specified transport accidents

√7ᵗʰ **V49.81** Car occupant (driver) (passenger) injured in transport accident with military vehicle

√7ᵗʰ **V49.88** Car occupant (driver) (passenger) injured in other specified transport accidents

√7ᵗʰ **V49.9** Car occupant (driver) (passenger) injured in unspecified traffic accident
     Car accident NOS

---

## Occupant of pick-up truck or van injured in transport accident (V50-V59)

| INCLUDES | a four or six wheel motor vehicle designed primarily for carrying passengers and property but weighing less than the local limit for classification as a heavy goods vehicle |

  minibus
  minivan
  sport utility vehicle (SUV)
  truck
  van

**EXCLUDES 1** *heavy transport vehicle (V60-V69)*

The appropriate 7th character is to be added to each code from categories V50-V59.
  A    initial encounter
  D    subsequent encounter
  S    sequela

✓4ᵗʰ **V50  Occupant of pick-up truck or van injured in collision with pedestrian or animal**
  **EXCLUDES 1** *pick-up truck or van collision with animal-drawn vehicle or animal being ridden (V56.-)*

✓x7ᵗʰ **V50.0  Driver** of pick-up truck or van injured in collision with pedestrian or animal in nontraffic accident

✓x7ᵗʰ **V50.1  Passenger** in pick-up truck or van injured in collision with pedestrian or animal in nontraffic accident

✓x7ᵗʰ **V50.2  Person on outside** of pick-up truck or van injured in collision with pedestrian or animal in nontraffic accident

✓x7ᵗʰ **V50.3  Unspecified** occupant of pick-up truck or van injured in collision with pedestrian or animal in nontraffic accident

✓x7ᵗʰ **V50.4  Person boarding or alighting** a pick-up truck or van injured in collision with pedestrian or animal

✓x7ᵗʰ **V50.5  Driver** of pick-up truck or van injured in collision with pedestrian or animal in traffic accident

✓x7ᵗʰ **V50.6  Passenger** in pick-up truck or van injured in collision with pedestrian or animal in traffic accident

✓x7ᵗʰ **V50.7  Person on outside** of pick-up truck or van injured in collision with pedestrian or animal in traffic accident

✓x7ᵗʰ **V50.9  Unspecified** occupant of pick-up truck or van injured in collision with pedestrian or animal in traffic accident

✓4ᵗʰ **V51  Occupant of pick-up truck or van injured in collision with pedal cycle**

✓x7ᵗʰ **V51.0  Driver** of pick-up truck or van injured in collision with pedal cycle in nontraffic accident

✓x7ᵗʰ **V51.1  Passenger** in pick-up truck or van injured in collision with pedal cycle in nontraffic accident

✓x7ᵗʰ **V51.2  Person on outside** of pick-up truck or van injured in collision with pedal cycle in nontraffic accident

✓x7ᵗʰ **V51.3  Unspecified** occupant of pick-up truck or van injured in collision with pedal cycle in nontraffic accident

✓x7ᵗʰ **V51.4  Person boarding or alighting** a pick-up truck or van injured in collision with pedal cycle

✓x7ᵗʰ **V51.5  Driver** of pick-up truck or van injured in collision with pedal cycle in traffic accident

✓x7ᵗʰ **V51.6  Passenger** in pick-up truck or van injured in collision with pedal cycle in traffic accident

✓x7ᵗʰ **V51.7  Person on outside** of pick-up truck or van injured in collision with pedal cycle in traffic accident

✓x7ᵗʰ **V51.9  Unspecified** occupant of pick-up truck or van injured in collision with pedal cycle in traffic accident

✓4ᵗʰ **V52  Occupant of pick-up truck or van injured in collision with two- or three-wheeled motor vehicle**

✓x7ᵗʰ **V52.0  Driver** of pick-up truck or van injured in collision with two- or three-wheeled motor vehicle in nontraffic accident

✓x7ᵗʰ **V52.1  Passenger** in pick-up truck or van injured in collision with two- or three-wheeled motor vehicle in nontraffic accident

✓x7ᵗʰ **V52.2  Person on outside** of pick-up truck or van injured in collision with two- or three-wheeled motor vehicle in nontraffic accident

✓x7ᵗʰ **V52.3  Unspecified** occupant of pick-up truck or van injured in collision with two- or three-wheeled motor vehicle in nontraffic accident

✓x7ᵗʰ **V52.4  Person boarding or alighting** a pick-up truck or van injured in collision with two- or three-wheeled motor vehicle

✓x7ᵗʰ **V52.5  Driver** of pick-up truck or van injured in collision with two- or three-wheeled motor vehicle in traffic accident

✓x7ᵗʰ **V52.6  Passenger** in pick-up truck or van injured in collision with two- or three-wheeled motor vehicle in traffic accident

✓x7ᵗʰ **V52.7  Person on outside** of pick-up truck or van injured in collision with two- or three-wheeled motor vehicle in traffic accident

✓x7ᵗʰ **V52.9  Unspecified** occupant of pick-up truck or van injured in collision with two- or three-wheeled motor vehicle in traffic accident

✓4ᵗʰ **V53  Occupant of pick-up truck or van injured in collision with car, pick-up truck or van**

✓x7ᵗʰ **V53.0  Driver** of pick-up truck or van injured in collision with car, pick-up truck or van in nontraffic accident

✓x7ᵗʰ **V53.1  Passenger** in pick-up truck or van injured in collision with car, pick-up truck or van in nontraffic accident

✓x7ᵗʰ **V53.2  Person on outside** of pick-up truck or van injured in collision with car, pick-up truck or van in nontraffic accident

✓x7ᵗʰ **V53.3  Unspecified** occupant of pick-up truck or van injured in collision with car, pick-up truck or van in nontraffic accident

✓x7ᵗʰ **V53.4  Person boarding or alighting** a pick-up truck or van injured in collision with car, pick-up truck or van

✓x7ᵗʰ **V53.5  Driver** of pick-up truck or van injured in collision with car, pick-up truck or van in traffic accident

✓x7ᵗʰ **V53.6  Passenger** in pick-up truck or van injured in collision with car, pick-up truck or van in traffic accident

✓x7ᵗʰ **V53.7  Person on outside** of pick-up truck or van injured in collision with car, pick-up truck or van in traffic accident

✓x7ᵗʰ **V53.9  Unspecified** occupant of pick-up truck or van injured in collision with car, pick-up truck or van in traffic accident

✓4ᵗʰ **V54  Occupant of pick-up truck or van injured in collision with heavy transport vehicle or bus**
  **EXCLUDES 1** *occupant of pick-up truck or van injured in collision with military vehicle (V59.81)*

✓x7ᵗʰ **V54.0  Driver** of pick-up truck or van injured in collision with heavy transport vehicle or bus in nontraffic accident

✓x7ᵗʰ **V54.1  Passenger** in pick-up truck or van injured in collision with heavy transport vehicle or bus in nontraffic accident

✓x7ᵗʰ **V54.2  Person on outside** of pick-up truck or van injured in collision with heavy transport vehicle or bus in nontraffic accident

✓x7ᵗʰ **V54.3  Unspecified** occupant of pick-up truck or van injured in collision with heavy transport vehicle or bus in nontraffic accident

✓x7ᵗʰ **V54.4  Person boarding or alighting** a pick-up truck or van injured in collision with heavy transport vehicle or bus

✓x7ᵗʰ **V54.5  Driver** of pick-up truck or van injured in collision with heavy transport vehicle or bus in traffic accident

✓x7ᵗʰ **V54.6  Passenger** in pick-up truck or van injured in collision with heavy transport vehicle or bus in traffic accident

✓x7ᵗʰ **V54.7  Person on outside** of pick-up truck or van injured in collision with heavy transport vehicle or bus in traffic accident

✓x7ᵗʰ **V54.9  Unspecified** occupant of pick-up truck or van injured in collision with heavy transport vehicle or bus in traffic accident

✓4ᵗʰ **V55  Occupant of pick-up truck or van injured in collision with railway train or railway vehicle**

✓x7ᵗʰ **V55.0  Driver** of pick-up truck or van injured in collision with railway train or railway vehicle in nontraffic accident

✓x7ᵗʰ **V55.1  Passenger** in pick-up truck or van injured in collision with railway train or railway vehicle in nontraffic accident

✓x7ᵗʰ **V55.2  Person on outside** of pick-up truck or van injured in collision with railway train or railway vehicle in nontraffic accident

✓x7ᵗʰ **V55.3  Unspecified** occupant of pick-up truck or van injured in collision with railway train or railway vehicle in nontraffic accident

✓x7ᵗʰ **V55.4  Person boarding or alighting** a pick-up truck or van injured in collision with railway train or railway vehicle

✓x7ᵗʰ **V55.5  Driver** of pick-up truck or van injured in collision with railway train or railway vehicle in traffic accident

✓x7ᵗʰ **V55.6  Passenger** in pick-up truck or van injured in collision with railway train or railway vehicle in traffic accident

✓x7ᵗʰ **V55.7  Person on outside** of pick-up truck or van injured in collision with railway train or railway vehicle in traffic accident

✓x7ᵗʰ **V55.9  Unspecified** occupant of pick-up truck or van injured in collision with railway train or railway vehicle in traffic accident

---

✓ Additional Character Req   ✓x7ᵗʰ Placeholder Alert   Unacceptable PDx   Manifestation   ■ H1 - H14 HAC   HCC CMS-HCC Condition   EXCLUDES 1 Not Coded Here   EXCLUDES 2 Not Included Here

ICD-10-CM 2018                                                                1171

**✓4ᵗʰ V56 Occupant of pick-up truck or van injured in collision with other nonmotor vehicle**
- **INCLUDES** collision with animal-drawn vehicle, animal being ridden, streetcar

**✓x7ᵗʰ V56.0 Driver** of pick-up truck or van injured in collision with other nonmotor vehicle in nontraffic accident

**✓x7ᵗʰ V56.1 Passenger** in pick-up truck or van injured in collision with other nonmotor vehicle in nontraffic accident

**✓x7ᵗʰ V56.2 Person on outside** of pick-up truck or van injured in collision with other nonmotor vehicle in nontraffic accident

**✓x7ᵗʰ V56.3 Unspecified** occupant of pick-up truck or van injured in collision with other nonmotor vehicle in nontraffic accident

**✓x7ᵗʰ V56.4 Person boarding or alighting** a pick-up truck or van injured in collision with other nonmotor vehicle

**✓x7ᵗʰ V56.5 Driver** of pick-up truck or van injured in collision with other nonmotor vehicle in traffic accident

**✓x7ᵗʰ V56.6 Passenger** in pick-up truck or van injured in collision with other nonmotor vehicle in traffic accident

**✓x7ᵗʰ V56.7 Person on outside** of pick-up truck or van injured in collision with other nonmotor vehicle in traffic accident

**✓x7ᵗʰ V56.9 Unspecified** occupant of pick-up truck or van injured in collision with other nonmotor vehicle in traffic accident

**✓4ᵗʰ V57 Occupant of pick-up truck or van injured in collision with fixed or stationary object**

**✓x7ᵗʰ V57.0 Driver** of pick-up truck or van injured in collision with fixed or stationary object in nontraffic accident

**✓x7ᵗʰ V57.1 Passenger** in pick-up truck or van injured in collision with fixed or stationary object in nontraffic accident

**✓x7ᵗʰ V57.2 Person on outside** of pick-up truck or van injured in collision with fixed or stationary object in nontraffic accident

**✓x7ᵗʰ V57.3 Unspecified** occupant of pick-up truck or van injured in collision with fixed or stationary object in nontraffic accident

**✓x7ᵗʰ V57.4 Person boarding or alighting** a pick-up truck or van injured in collision with fixed or stationary object

**✓x7ᵗʰ V57.5 Driver** of pick-up truck or van injured in collision with fixed or stationary object in traffic accident

**✓x7ᵗʰ V57.6 Passenger** in pick-up truck or van injured in collision with fixed or stationary object in traffic accident

**✓x7ᵗʰ V57.7 Person on outside** of pick-up truck or van injured in collision with fixed or stationary object in traffic accident

**✓x7ᵗʰ V57.9 Unspecified** occupant of pick-up truck or van injured in collision with fixed or stationary object in traffic accident

**✓4ᵗʰ V58 Occupant of pick-up truck or van injured in noncollision transport accident**
- **INCLUDES** overturning pick-up truck or van NOS
  overturning pick-up truck or van without collision

**✓x7ᵗʰ V58.0 Driver** of pick-up truck or van injured in noncollision transport accident in nontraffic accident

**✓x7ᵗʰ V58.1 Passenger** in pick-up truck or van injured in noncollision transport accident in nontraffic accident

**✓x7ᵗʰ V58.2 Person on outside** of pick-up truck or van injured in noncollision transport accident in nontraffic accident

**✓x7ᵗʰ V58.3 Unspecified** occupant of pick-up truck or van injured in noncollision transport accident in nontraffic accident

**✓x7ᵗʰ V58.4 Person boarding or alighting** a pick-up truck or van injured in noncollision transport accident

**✓x7ᵗʰ V58.5 Driver** of pick-up truck or van injured in noncollision transport accident in traffic accident

**✓x7ᵗʰ V58.6 Passenger** in pick-up truck or van injured in noncollision transport accident in traffic accident

**✓x7ᵗʰ V58.7 Person on outside** of pick-up truck or van injured in noncollision transport accident in traffic accident

**✓x7ᵗʰ V58.9 Unspecified** occupant of pick-up truck or van injured in noncollision transport accident in traffic accident

**✓4ᵗʰ V59 Occupant of pick-up truck or van injured in other and unspecified transport accidents**

**✓5ᵗʰ V59.0 Driver** of pick-up truck or van injured in collision with other and unspecified motor vehicles in nontraffic accident

**✓x7ᵗʰ V59.00 Driver** of pick-up truck or van injured in collision with unspecified motor vehicles in nontraffic accident

**✓x7ᵗʰ V59.09 Driver** of pick-up truck or van injured in collision with other motor vehicles in nontraffic accident

**✓5ᵗʰ V59.1 Passenger** in pick-up truck or van injured in collision with other and unspecified motor vehicles in nontraffic accident

**✓x7ᵗʰ V59.10 Passenger** in pick-up truck or van injured in collision with unspecified motor vehicles in nontraffic accident

**✓x7ᵗʰ V59.19 Passenger** in pick-up truck or van injured in collision with other motor vehicles in nontraffic accident

**✓5ᵗʰ V59.2 Unspecified** occupant of pick-up truck or van injured in collision with other and unspecified motor vehicles in nontraffic accident

**✓x7ᵗʰ V59.20 Unspecified** occupant of pick-up truck or van injured in collision with unspecified motor vehicles in nontraffic accident
  Collision NOS involving pick-up truck or van, nontraffic

**✓x7ᵗʰ V59.29 Unspecified** occupant of pick-up truck or van injured in collision with other motor vehicles in nontraffic accident

**✓x7ᵗʰ V59.3 Occupant (driver) (passenger)** of pick-up truck or van injured in unspecified nontraffic accident
  Accident NOS involving pick-up truck or van, nontraffic
  Occupant of pick-up truck or van injured in nontraffic accident NOS

**✓5ᵗʰ V59.4 Driver** of pick-up truck or van injured in collision with other and unspecified motor vehicles in traffic accident

**✓x7ᵗʰ V59.40 Driver** of pick-up truck or van injured in collision with unspecified motor vehicles in traffic accident

**✓x7ᵗʰ V59.49 Driver** of pick-up truck or van injured in collision with other motor vehicles in traffic accident

**✓5ᵗʰ V59.5 Passenger** in pick-up truck or van injured in collision with other and unspecified motor vehicles in traffic accident

**✓x7ᵗʰ V59.50 Passenger** in pick-up truck or van injured in collision with unspecified motor vehicles in traffic accident

**✓x7ᵗʰ V59.59 Passenger** in pick-up truck or van injured in collision with other motor vehicles in traffic accident

**✓5ᵗʰ V59.6 Unspecified** occupant of pick-up truck or van injured in collision with other and unspecified motor vehicles in traffic accident

**✓x7ᵗʰ V59.60 Unspecified** occupant of pick-up truck or van injured in collision with unspecified motor vehicles in traffic accident
  Collision NOS involving pick-up truck or van (traffic)

**✓x7ᵗʰ V59.69 Unspecified** occupant of pick-up truck or van injured in collision with other motor vehicles in traffic accident

**✓5ᵗʰ V59.8 Occupant (driver) (passenger)** of pick-up truck or van injured in other specified transport accidents

**✓x7ᵗʰ V59.81 Occupant (driver) (passenger)** of pick-up truck or van injured in transport accident with military vehicle

**✓x7ᵗʰ V59.88 Occupant (driver) (passenger)** of pick-up truck or van injured in other specified transport accidents

**✓x7ᵗʰ V59.9 Occupant (driver) (passenger)** of pick-up truck or van injured in unspecified traffic accident
  Accident NOS involving pick-up truck or van

## Occupant of heavy transport vehicle injured in transport accident (V60-V69)

- **INCLUDES** 18 wheeler
  armored car
  panel truck
- **EXCLUDES 1** bus
  motorcoach

> The appropriate 7th character is to be added to each code from categories V60-V69.
> A    initial encounter
> D    subsequent encounter
> S    sequela

**✓4ᵗʰ V60 Occupant of heavy transport vehicle injured in collision with pedestrian or animal**
- **EXCLUDES 1** heavy transport vehicle collision with animal-drawn vehicle or animal being ridden (V66.-)

**✓x7ᵗʰ V60.0 Driver** of heavy transport vehicle injured in collision with pedestrian or animal in nontraffic accident

**✓x7ᵗʰ V60.1 Passenger** in heavy transport vehicle injured in collision with pedestrian or animal in nontraffic accident

**✓x7ᵗʰ V60.2 Person on outside** of heavy transport vehicle injured in collision with pedestrian or animal in nontraffic accident

---

Ⓝ Newborn: 0   Ⓟ Pediatric: 0-17   Ⓜ Maternity: 12-55   Ⓐ Adult: 15-124   **MCC** Major CC Condition   **PDxMCC** PDx acts as own MCC   **CC** CC Condition   **PDxCC** PDx acts as own CC

**1172**
ICD-10-CM 2018

√x7ᵗʰ **V60.3** Unspecified **occupant of heavy transport vehicle injured in collision with pedestrian or animal** in nontraffic accident

√x7ᵗʰ **V60.4** Person boarding or alighting **a heavy transport vehicle injured in collision with pedestrian or animal**

√x7ᵗʰ **V60.5** Driver **of heavy transport vehicle injured in collision with pedestrian or animal** in traffic accident

√x7ᵗʰ **V60.6** Passenger **in heavy transport vehicle injured in collision with pedestrian or animal** in traffic accident

√x7ᵗʰ **V60.7** Person on outside **of heavy transport vehicle injured in collision with pedestrian or animal** in traffic accident

√x7ᵗʰ **V60.9** Unspecified **occupant of heavy transport vehicle injured in collision with pedestrian or animal** in traffic accident

√4ᵗʰ **V61** **Occupant of heavy transport vehicle injured in collision with pedal cycle**

√x7ᵗʰ **V61.0** Driver **of heavy transport vehicle injured in collision with pedal cycle** in nontraffic accident

√x7ᵗʰ **V61.1** Passenger **in heavy transport vehicle injured in collision with pedal cycle** in nontraffic accident

√x7ᵗʰ **V61.2** Person on outside **of heavy transport vehicle injured in collision with pedal cycle** in nontraffic accident

√x7ᵗʰ **V61.3** Unspecified **occupant of heavy transport vehicle injured in collision with pedal cycle** in nontraffic accident

√x7ᵗʰ **V61.4** Person boarding or alighting **a heavy transport vehicle injured in collision with pedal cycle while boarding or alighting**

√x7ᵗʰ **V61.5** Driver **of heavy transport vehicle injured in collision with pedal cycle** in traffic accident

√x7ᵗʰ **V61.6** Passenger **in heavy transport vehicle injured in collision with pedal cycle** in traffic accident

√x7ᵗʰ **V61.7** Person on outside **of heavy transport vehicle injured in collision with pedal cycle** in traffic accident

√x7ᵗʰ **V61.9** Unspecified **occupant of heavy transport vehicle injured in collision with pedal cycle** in traffic accident

√4ᵗʰ **V62** **Occupant of heavy transport vehicle injured in collision with two- or three-wheeled motor vehicle**

√x7ᵗʰ **V62.0** Driver **of heavy transport vehicle injured in collision with two- or three-wheeled motor vehicle** in nontraffic accident

√x7ᵗʰ **V62.1** Passenger **in heavy transport vehicle injured in collision with two- or three-wheeled motor vehicle** in nontraffic accident

√x7ᵗʰ **V62.2** Person on outside **of heavy transport vehicle injured in collision with two- or three-wheeled motor vehicle** in nontraffic accident

√x7ᵗʰ **V62.3** Unspecified **occupant of heavy transport vehicle injured in collision with two- or three-wheeled motor vehicle** in nontraffic accident

√x7ᵗʰ **V62.4** Person **boarding or alighting a heavy transport vehicle injured in collision with two- or three-wheeled motor vehicle**

√x7ᵗʰ **V62.5** Driver **of heavy transport vehicle injured in collision with two- or three-wheeled motor vehicle** in traffic accident

√x7ᵗʰ **V62.6** Passenger **in heavy transport vehicle injured in collision with two- or three-wheeled motor vehicle** in traffic accident

√x7ᵗʰ **V62.7** Person on outside **of heavy transport vehicle injured in collision with two- or three-wheeled motor vehicle** in traffic accident

√x7ᵗʰ **V62.9** Unspecified **occupant of heavy transport vehicle injured in collision with two- or three-wheeled motor vehicle** in traffic accident

√4ᵗʰ **V63** **Occupant of heavy transport vehicle injured in collision with car, pick-up truck or van**

√x7ᵗʰ **V63.0** Driver **of heavy transport vehicle injured in collision with car, pick-up truck or van** in nontraffic accident

√x7ᵗʰ **V63.1** Passenger **in heavy transport vehicle injured in collision with car, pick-up truck or van** in nontraffic accident

√x7ᵗʰ **V63.2** Person on outside **of heavy transport vehicle injured in collision with car, pick-up truck or van** in nontraffic accident

√x7ᵗʰ **V63.3** Unspecified **occupant of heavy transport vehicle injured in collision with car, pick-up truck or van** in nontraffic accident

√x7ᵗʰ **V63.4** Person boarding or alighting **a heavy transport vehicle injured in collision with car, pick-up truck or van**

√x7ᵗʰ **V63.5** Driver **of heavy transport vehicle injured in collision with car, pick-up truck or van** in traffic accident

√x7ᵗʰ **V63.6** Passenger **in heavy transport vehicle injured in collision with car, pick-up truck or van** in traffic accident

√x7ᵗʰ **V63.7** Person on outside **of heavy transport vehicle injured in collision with car, pick-up truck or van** in traffic accident

√x7ᵗʰ **V63.9** Unspecified **occupant of heavy transport vehicle injured in collision with car, pick-up truck or van** in traffic accident

√4ᵗʰ **V64** **Occupant of heavy transport vehicle injured in collision with heavy transport vehicle or bus**

> EXCLUDES 1   *occupant of heavy transport vehicle injured in collision with military vehicle (V69.81)*

√x7ᵗʰ **V64.0** Driver **of heavy transport vehicle injured in collision with heavy transport vehicle or bus** in nontraffic accident

√x7ᵗʰ **V64.1** Passenger **in heavy transport vehicle injured in collision with heavy transport vehicle or bus** in nontraffic accident

√x7ᵗʰ **V64.2** Person on outside **of heavy transport vehicle injured in collision with heavy transport vehicle or bus** in nontraffic accident

√x7ᵗʰ **V64.3** Unspecified **occupant of heavy transport vehicle injured in collision with heavy transport vehicle or bus** in nontraffic accident

√x7ᵗʰ **V64.4** Person boarding or alighting **a heavy transport vehicle injured in collision with heavy transport vehicle or bus while boarding or alighting**

√x7ᵗʰ **V64.5** Driver **of heavy transport vehicle injured in collision with heavy transport vehicle or bus** in traffic accident

√x7ᵗʰ **V64.6** Passenger **in heavy transport vehicle injured in collision with heavy transport vehicle or bus** in traffic accident

√x7ᵗʰ **V64.7** Person on outside **of heavy transport vehicle injured in collision with heavy transport vehicle or bus** in traffic accident

√x7ᵗʰ **V64.9** Unspecified **occupant of heavy transport vehicle injured in collision with heavy transport vehicle or bus** in traffic accident

√4ᵗʰ **V65** **Occupant of heavy transport vehicle injured in collision with railway train or railway vehicle**

√x7ᵗʰ **V65.0** Driver **of heavy transport vehicle injured in collision with railway train or railway vehicle** in nontraffic accident

√x7ᵗʰ **V65.1** Passenger **in heavy transport vehicle injured in collision with railway train or railway vehicle** in nontraffic accident

√x7ᵗʰ **V65.2** Person on outside **of heavy transport vehicle injured in collision with railway train or railway vehicle** in nontraffic accident

√x7ᵗʰ **V65.3** Unspecified **occupant of heavy transport vehicle injured in collision with railway train or railway vehicle** in nontraffic accident

√x7ᵗʰ **V65.4** Person boarding or alighting **a heavy transport vehicle injured in collision with railway train or railway vehicle**

√x7ᵗʰ **V65.5** Driver **of heavy transport vehicle injured in collision with railway train or railway vehicle** in traffic accident

√x7ᵗʰ **V65.6** Passenger **in heavy transport vehicle injured in collision with railway train or railway vehicle** in traffic accident

√x7ᵗʰ **V65.7** Person on outside **of heavy transport vehicle injured in collision with railway train or railway vehicle** in traffic accident

√x7ᵗʰ **V65.9** Unspecified **occupant of heavy transport vehicle injured in collision with railway train or railway vehicle** in traffic accident

√4ᵗʰ **V66** **Occupant of heavy transport vehicle injured in collision with other nonmotor vehicle**

> INCLUDES   collision with animal-drawn vehicle, animal being ridden, streetcar

√x7ᵗʰ **V66.0** Driver **of heavy transport vehicle injured in collision with other nonmotor vehicle** in nontraffic accident

√x7ᵗʰ **V66.1** Passenger **in heavy transport vehicle injured in collision with other nonmotor vehicle** in nontraffic accident

√x7ᵗʰ **V66.2** Person on outside **of heavy transport vehicle injured in collision with other nonmotor vehicle** in nontraffic accident

√x7ᵗʰ **V66.3** Unspecified **occupant of heavy transport vehicle injured in collision with other nonmotor vehicle** in nontraffic accident

√x7ᵗʰ **V66.4** Person boarding or alighting **a heavy transport vehicle injured in collision with other nonmotor vehicle**

√x7ᵗʰ **V66.5** Driver **of heavy transport vehicle injured in collision with other nonmotor vehicle** in traffic accident

√x7ᵗʰ **V66.6** Passenger **in heavy transport vehicle injured in collision with other nonmotor vehicle** in traffic accident

√x7ᵗʰ **V66.7** Person on outside **of heavy transport vehicle injured in collision with other nonmotor vehicle** in traffic accident

---

✓ Additional Character Req   √x7ᵗʰ Placeholder Alert   Unacceptable PDx   Manifestation   H1-H14 HAC   HCC CMS-HCC Condition   EXCLUDES 1 Not Coded Here   EXCLUDES 2 Not Included Here

√x7ᵗʰ **V66.9** Unspecified occupant of heavy transport vehicle injured in collision with other nonmotor vehicle in traffic accident

√4ᵗʰ **V67** Occupant of heavy transport vehicle injured in collision with fixed or stationary object

√x7ᵗʰ **V67.0** Driver of heavy transport vehicle injured in collision with fixed or stationary object in nontraffic accident

√x7ᵗʰ **V67.1** Passenger in heavy transport vehicle injured in collision with fixed or stationary object in nontraffic accident

√x7ᵗʰ **V67.2** Person on outside of heavy transport vehicle injured in collision with fixed or stationary object in nontraffic accident

√x7ᵗʰ **V67.3** Unspecified occupant of heavy transport vehicle injured in collision with fixed or stationary object in nontraffic accident

√x7ᵗʰ **V67.4** Person boarding or alighting a heavy transport vehicle injured in collision with fixed or stationary object

√x7ᵗʰ **V67.5** Driver of heavy transport vehicle injured in collision with fixed or stationary object in traffic accident

√x7ᵗʰ **V67.6** Passenger in heavy transport vehicle injured in collision with fixed or stationary object in traffic accident

√x7ᵗʰ **V67.7** Person on outside of heavy transport vehicle injured in collision with fixed or stationary object in traffic accident

√x7ᵗʰ **V67.9** Unspecified occupant of heavy transport vehicle injured in collision with fixed or stationary object in traffic accident

√4ᵗʰ **V68** Occupant of heavy transport vehicle injured in noncollision transport accident

    **INCLUDES** overturning heavy transport vehicle NOS
           overturning heavy transport vehicle without collision

√x7ᵗʰ **V68.0** Driver of heavy transport vehicle injured in noncollision transport accident in nontraffic accident

√x7ᵗʰ **V68.1** Passenger in heavy transport vehicle injured in noncollision transport accident in nontraffic accident

√x7ᵗʰ **V68.2** Person on outside of heavy transport vehicle injured in noncollision transport accident in nontraffic accident

√x7ᵗʰ **V68.3** Unspecified occupant of heavy transport vehicle injured in noncollision transport accident in nontraffic accident

√x7ᵗʰ **V68.4** Person boarding or alighting a heavy transport vehicle injured in noncollision transport accident

√x7ᵗʰ **V68.5** Driver of heavy transport vehicle injured in noncollision transport accident in traffic accident

√x7ᵗʰ **V68.6** Passenger in heavy transport vehicle injured in noncollision transport accident in traffic accident

√x7ᵗʰ **V68.7** Person on outside of heavy transport vehicle injured in noncollision transport accident in traffic accident

√x7ᵗʰ **V68.9** Unspecified occupant of heavy transport vehicle injured in noncollision transport accident in traffic accident

√4ᵗʰ **V69** Occupant of heavy transport vehicle injured in other and unspecified transport accidents

√5ᵗʰ **V69.0** Driver of heavy transport vehicle injured in collision with other and unspecified motor vehicles in nontraffic accident

√x7ᵗʰ **V69.00** Driver of heavy transport vehicle injured in collision with unspecified motor vehicles in nontraffic accident

√x7ᵗʰ **V69.09** Driver of heavy transport vehicle injured in collision with other motor vehicles in nontraffic accident

√5ᵗʰ **V69.1** Passenger in heavy transport vehicle injured in collision with other and unspecified motor vehicles in nontraffic accident

√x7ᵗʰ **V69.10** Passenger in heavy transport vehicle injured in collision with unspecified motor vehicles in nontraffic accident

√x7ᵗʰ **V69.19** Passenger in heavy transport vehicle injured in collision with other motor vehicles in nontraffic accident

√5ᵗʰ **V69.2** Unspecified occupant of heavy transport vehicle injured in collision with other and unspecified motor vehicles in nontraffic accident

√x7ᵗʰ **V69.20** Unspecified occupant of heavy transport vehicle injured in collision with unspecified motor vehicles in nontraffic accident
    Collision NOS involving heavy transport vehicle, nontraffic

√x7ᵗʰ **V69.29** Unspecified occupant of heavy transport vehicle injured in collision with other motor vehicles in nontraffic accident

√x7ᵗʰ **V69.3** Occupant (driver) (passenger) of heavy transport vehicle injured in unspecified nontraffic accident
    Accident NOS involving heavy transport vehicle, nontraffic
    Occupant of heavy transport vehicle injured in nontraffic accident NOS

√5ᵗʰ **V69.4** Driver of heavy transport vehicle injured in collision with other and unspecified motor vehicles in traffic accident

√x7ᵗʰ **V69.40** Driver of heavy transport vehicle injured in collision with unspecified motor vehicles in traffic accident

√x7ᵗʰ **V69.49** Driver of heavy transport vehicle injured in collision with other motor vehicles in traffic accident

√5ᵗʰ **V69.5** Passenger in heavy transport vehicle injured in collision with other and unspecified motor vehicles in traffic accident

√x7ᵗʰ **V69.50** Passenger in heavy transport vehicle injured in collision with unspecified motor vehicles in traffic accident

√x7ᵗʰ **V69.59** Passenger in heavy transport vehicle injured in collision with other motor vehicles in traffic accident

√5ᵗʰ **V69.6** Unspecified occupant of heavy transport vehicle injured in collision with other and unspecified motor vehicles in traffic accident

√x7ᵗʰ **V69.60** Unspecified occupant of heavy transport vehicle injured in collision with unspecified motor vehicles in traffic accident
    Collision NOS involving heavy transport vehicle (traffic)

√x7ᵗʰ **V69.69** Unspecified occupant of heavy transport vehicle injured in collision with other motor vehicles in traffic accident

√5ᵗʰ **V69.8** Occupant (driver) (passenger) of heavy transport vehicle injured in other specified transport accidents

√x7ᵗʰ **V69.81** Occupant (driver) (passenger) of heavy transport vehicle injured in transport accidents with military vehicle

√x7ᵗʰ **V69.88** Occupant (driver) (passenger) of heavy transport vehicle injured in other specified transport accidents

√x7ᵗʰ **V69.9** Occupant (driver) (passenger) of heavy transport vehicle injured in unspecified traffic accident
    Accident NOS involving heavy transport vehicle

### Bus occupant injured in transport accident (V70-V79)

    **INCLUDES** motorcoach
    **EXCLUDES 1** minibus (V50-V59)

> The appropriate 7th character is to be added to each code from categories V70-V79.
> A    initial encounter
> D    subsequent encounter
> S    sequela

√4ᵗʰ **V70** Bus occupant injured in collision with pedestrian or animal
    **EXCLUDES 1** bus collision with animal-drawn vehicle or animal being ridden (V76.-)

√x7ᵗʰ **V70.0** Driver of bus injured in collision with pedestrian or animal in nontraffic accident

√x7ᵗʰ **V70.1** Passenger on bus injured in collision with pedestrian or animal in nontraffic accident

√x7ᵗʰ **V70.2** Person on outside of bus injured in collision with pedestrian or animal in nontraffic accident

√x7ᵗʰ **V70.3** Unspecified occupant of bus injured in collision with pedestrian or animal in nontraffic accident

√x7ᵗʰ **V70.4** Person boarding or alighting from bus injured in collision with pedestrian or animal

√x7ᵗʰ **V70.5** Driver of bus injured in collision with pedestrian or animal in traffic accident

√x7ᵗʰ **V70.6** Passenger on bus injured in collision with pedestrian or animal in traffic accident

√x7ᵗʰ **V70.7** Person on outside of bus injured in collision with pedestrian or animal in traffic accident

√x7ᵗʰ **V70.9** Unspecified occupant of bus injured in collision with pedestrian or animal in traffic accident

√4ᵗʰ **V71** Bus occupant injured in collision with pedal cycle

√x7ᵗʰ **V71.0** Driver of bus injured in collision with pedal cycle in nontraffic accident

√x7ᵗʰ **V71.1** Passenger on bus injured in collision with pedal cycle in nontraffic accident

---

**N** Newborn: 0   **P** Pediatric: 0-17   **M** Maternity: 12-55   **A** Adult: 15-124   **MCC** Major CC Condition   **PDx MCC** PDx acts as own MCC   **CC** CC Condition   **PDx CC** PDx acts as own CC

**1174**

ICD-10-CM 2018

√x7th **V71.2** Person on outside of bus injured in collision with pedal cycle in nontraffic accident

√x7th **V71.3** Unspecified occupant of bus injured in collision with pedal cycle in nontraffic accident

√x7th **V71.4** Person boarding or alighting from bus injured in collision with pedal cycle

√x7th **V71.5** Driver of bus injured in collision with pedal cycle in traffic accident

√x7th **V71.6** Passenger on bus injured in collision with pedal cycle in traffic accident

√x7th **V71.7** Person on outside of bus injured in collision with pedal cycle in traffic accident

√x7th **V71.9** Unspecified occupant of bus injured in collision with pedal cycle in traffic accident

√4th **V72** Bus occupant injured in collision with two- or three-wheeled motor vehicle

√x7th **V72.0** Driver of bus injured in collision with two- or three-wheeled motor vehicle in nontraffic accident

√x7th **V72.1** Passenger on bus injured in collision with two- or three-wheeled motor vehicle in nontraffic accident

√x7th **V72.2** Person on outside of bus injured in collision with two- or three-wheeled motor vehicle in nontraffic accident

√x7th **V72.3** Unspecified occupant of bus injured in collision with two- or three-wheeled motor vehicle in nontraffic accident

√x7th **V72.4** Person boarding or alighting from bus injured in collision with two- or three-wheeled motor vehicle

√x7th **V72.5** Driver of bus injured in collision with two- or three-wheeled motor vehicle in traffic accident

√x7th **V72.6** Passenger on bus injured in collision with two- or three-wheeled motor vehicle in traffic accident

√x7th **V72.7** Person on outside of bus injured in collision with two- or three-wheeled motor vehicle in traffic accident

√x7th **V72.9** Unspecified occupant of bus injured in collision with two- or three-wheeled motor vehicle in traffic accident

√4th **V73** Bus occupant injured in collision with car, pick-up truck or van

√x7th **V73.0** Driver of bus injured in collision with car, pick-up truck or van in nontraffic accident

√x7th **V73.1** Passenger on bus injured in collision with car, pick-up truck or van in nontraffic accident

√x7th **V73.2** Person on outside of bus injured in collision with car, pick-up truck or van in nontraffic accident

√x7th **V73.3** Unspecified occupant of bus injured in collision with car, pick-up truck or van in nontraffic accident

√x7th **V73.4** Person boarding or alighting from bus injured in collision with car, pick-up truck or van

√x7th **V73.5** Driver of bus injured in collision with car, pick-up truck or van in traffic accident

√x7th **V73.6** Passenger on bus injured in collision with car, pick-up truck or van in traffic accident

√x7th **V73.7** Person on outside of bus injured in collision with car, pick-up truck or van in traffic accident

√x7th **V73.9** Unspecified occupant of bus injured in collision with car, pick-up truck or van in traffic accident

√4th **V74** Bus occupant injured in collision with heavy transport vehicle or bus

  *EXCLUDES 1*   *bus occupant injured in collision with military vehicle (V79.81)*

√x7th **V74.0** Driver of bus injured in collision with heavy transport vehicle or bus in nontraffic accident

√x7th **V74.1** Passenger on bus injured in collision with heavy transport vehicle or bus in nontraffic accident

√x7th **V74.2** Person on outside of bus injured in collision with heavy transport vehicle or bus in nontraffic accident

√x7th **V74.3** Unspecified occupant of bus injured in collision with heavy transport vehicle or bus in nontraffic accident

√x7th **V74.4** Person boarding or alighting from bus injured in collision with heavy transport vehicle or bus

√x7th **V74.5** Driver of bus injured in collision with heavy transport vehicle or bus in traffic accident

√x7th **V74.6** Passenger on bus injured in collision with heavy transport vehicle or bus in traffic accident

√x7th **V74.7** Person on outside of bus injured in collision with heavy transport vehicle or bus in traffic accident

√x7th **V74.9** Unspecified occupant of bus injured in collision with heavy transport vehicle or bus in traffic accident

√4th **V75** Bus occupant injured in collision with railway train or railway vehicle

√x7th **V75.0** Driver of bus injured in collision with railway train or railway vehicle in nontraffic accident

√x7th **V75.1** Passenger on bus injured in collision with railway train or railway vehicle in nontraffic accident

√x7th **V75.2** Person on outside of bus injured in collision with railway train or railway vehicle in nontraffic accident

√x7th **V75.3** Unspecified occupant of bus injured in collision with railway train or railway vehicle in nontraffic accident

√x7th **V75.4** Person boarding or alighting from bus injured in collision with railway train or railway vehicle

√x7th **V75.5** Driver of bus injured in collision with railway train or railway vehicle in traffic accident

√x7th **V75.6** Passenger on bus injured in collision with railway train or railway vehicle in traffic accident

√x7th **V75.7** Person on outside of bus injured in collision with railway train or railway vehicle in traffic accident

√x7th **V75.9** Unspecified occupant of bus injured in collision with railway train or railway vehicle in traffic accident

√4th **V76** Bus occupant injured in collision with other nonmotor vehicle

  *INCLUDES*   collision with animal-drawn vehicle, animal being ridden, streetcar

√x7th **V76.0** Driver of bus injured in collision with other nonmotor vehicle in nontraffic accident

√x7th **V76.1** Passenger on bus injured in collision with other nonmotor vehicle in nontraffic accident

√x7th **V76.2** Person on outside of bus injured in collision with other nonmotor vehicle in nontraffic accident

√x7th **V76.3** Unspecified occupant of bus injured in collision with other nonmotor vehicle in nontraffic accident

√x7th **V76.4** Person boarding or alighting from bus injured in collision with other nonmotor vehicle

√x7th **V76.5** Driver of bus injured in collision with other nonmotor vehicle in traffic accident

√x7th **V76.6** Passenger on bus injured in collision with other nonmotor vehicle in traffic accident

√x7th **V76.7** Person on outside of bus injured in collision with other nonmotor vehicle in traffic accident

√x7th **V76.9** Unspecified occupant of bus injured in collision with other nonmotor vehicle in traffic accident

√4th **V77** Bus occupant injured in collision with fixed or stationary object

√x7th **V77.0** Driver of bus injured in collision with fixed or stationary object in nontraffic accident

√x7th **V77.1** Passenger on bus injured in collision with fixed or stationary object in nontraffic accident

√x7th **V77.2** Person on outside of bus injured in collision with fixed or stationary object in nontraffic accident

√x7th **V77.3** Unspecified occupant of bus injured in collision with fixed or stationary object in nontraffic accident

√x7th **V77.4** Person boarding or alighting from bus injured in collision with fixed or stationary object

√x7th **V77.5** Driver of bus injured in collision with fixed or stationary object in traffic accident

√x7th **V77.6** Passenger on bus injured in collision with fixed or stationary object in traffic accident

√x7th **V77.7** Person on outside of bus injured in collision with fixed or stationary object in traffic accident

√x7th **V77.9** Unspecified occupant of bus injured in collision with fixed or stationary object in traffic accident

√4th **V78** Bus occupant injured in noncollision transport accident

  *INCLUDES*   overturning bus NOS
      overturning bus without collision

√x7th **V78.0** Driver of bus injured in noncollision transport accident in nontraffic accident

√x7th **V78.1** Passenger on bus injured in noncollision transport accident in nontraffic accident

√x7th **V78.2** Person on outside of bus injured in noncollision transport accident in nontraffic accident

√x7th **V78.3** Unspecified occupant of bus injured in noncollision transport accident in nontraffic accident

---

✔ Additional Character Req   √x7th Placeholder Alert   Unacceptable PDx   Manifestation   H1-H14 HAC   HCC CMS-HCC Condition   *EXCLUDES 1* Not Coded Here   *EXCLUDES 2* Not Included Here

ICD-10-CM 2018                                                                        **1175**

**Chapter 20. External Causes of Morbidity**

✓x7ᵗʰ **V78.4** Person boarding or alighting from bus injured in noncollision transport accident

✓x7ᵗʰ **V78.5** Driver of bus injured in noncollision transport accident in traffic accident

✓x7ᵗʰ **V78.6** Passenger on bus injured in noncollision transport accident in traffic accident

✓x7ᵗʰ **V78.7** Person on outside of bus injured in noncollision transport accident in traffic accident

✓x7ᵗʰ **V78.9** Unspecified occupant of bus injured in noncollision transport accident in traffic accident

✓4ᵗʰ **V79 Bus occupant injured in other and unspecified transport accidents**

✓5ᵗʰ **V79.0** Driver of bus injured in collision with other and unspecified motor vehicles in nontraffic accident

  ✓x7ᵗʰ **V79.00** Driver of bus injured in collision with unspecified motor vehicles in nontraffic accident

  ✓x7ᵗʰ **V79.09** Driver of bus injured in collision with other motor vehicles in nontraffic accident

✓5ᵗʰ **V79.1** Passenger on bus injured in collision with other and unspecified motor vehicles in nontraffic accident

  ✓x7ᵗʰ **V79.10** Passenger on bus injured in collision with unspecified motor vehicles in nontraffic accident

  ✓x7ᵗʰ **V79.19** Passenger on bus injured in collision with other motor vehicles in nontraffic accident

✓5ᵗʰ **V79.2** Unspecified bus occupant injured in collision with other and unspecified motor vehicles in nontraffic accident

  ✓x7ᵗʰ **V79.20** Unspecified bus occupant injured in collision with unspecified motor vehicles in nontraffic accident
      Bus collision NOS, nontraffic

  ✓x7ᵗʰ **V79.29** Unspecified bus occupant injured in collision with other motor vehicles in nontraffic accident

✓x7ᵗʰ **V79.3** Bus occupant (driver) (passenger) injured in unspecified nontraffic accident
      Bus accident NOS, nontraffic
      Bus occupant injured in nontraffic accident NOS

✓5ᵗʰ **V79.4** Driver of bus injured in collision with other and unspecified motor vehicles in traffic accident

  ✓x7ᵗʰ **V79.40** Driver of bus injured in collision with unspecified motor vehicles in traffic accident

  ✓x7ᵗʰ **V79.49** Driver of bus injured in collision with other motor vehicles in traffic accident

✓5ᵗʰ **V79.5** Passenger on bus injured in collision with other and unspecified motor vehicles in traffic accident

  ✓x7ᵗʰ **V79.50** Passenger on bus injured in collision with unspecified motor vehicles in traffic accident

  ✓x7ᵗʰ **V79.59** Passenger on bus injured in collision with other motor vehicles in traffic accident

✓5ᵗʰ **V79.6** Unspecified bus occupant injured in collision with other and unspecified motor vehicles in traffic accident

  ✓x7ᵗʰ **V79.60** Unspecified bus occupant injured in collision with unspecified motor vehicles in traffic accident
      Bus collision NOS (traffic)

  ✓x7ᵗʰ **V79.69** Unspecified bus occupant injured in collision with other motor vehicles in traffic accident

✓5ᵗʰ **V79.8** Bus occupant (driver) (passenger) injured in other specified transport accidents

  ✓x7ᵗʰ **V79.81** Bus occupant (driver) (passenger) injured in transport accidents with military vehicle

  ✓x7ᵗʰ **V79.88** Bus occupant (driver) (passenger) injured in other specified transport accidents

✓x7ᵗʰ **V79.9** Bus occupant (driver) (passenger) injured in unspecified traffic accident
      Bus accident NOS

## Other land transport accidents (V80-V89)

The appropriate 7th character is to be added to each code from categories V80-V89.
A    initial encounter
D    subsequent encounter
S    sequela

✓4ᵗʰ **V80 Animal-rider or occupant of animal-drawn vehicle injured in transport accident**

✓5ᵗʰ **V80.0** Animal-rider or occupant of animal drawn vehicle injured by fall from or being thrown from animal or animal-drawn vehicle in noncollision accident

  ✓6ᵗʰ **V80.01** Animal-rider injured by fall from or being thrown from animal in noncollision accident

    ✓7ᵗʰ **V80.010** Animal-rider injured by fall from or being thrown from horse in noncollision accident

    ✓7ᵗʰ **V80.018** Animal-rider injured by fall from or being thrown from other animal in noncollision accident

  ✓x7ᵗʰ **V80.02** Occupant of animal-drawn vehicle injured by fall from or being thrown from animal-drawn vehicle in noncollision accident
      Overturning animal-drawn vehicle NOS
      Overturning animal-drawn vehicle without collision

✓5ᵗʰ **V80.1** Animal-rider or occupant of animal-drawn vehicle injured in collision with pedestrian or animal
    **EXCLUDES 1**   *animal-rider or animal-drawn vehicle collision with animal-drawn vehicle or animal being ridden (V80.7)*

  ✓x7ᵗʰ **V80.11** Animal-rider injured in collision with pedestrian or animal

  ✓x7ᵗʰ **V80.12** Occupant of animal-drawn vehicle injured in collision with pedestrian or animal

✓5ᵗʰ **V80.2** Animal-rider or occupant of animal-drawn vehicle injured in collision with pedal cycle

  ✓x7ᵗʰ **V80.21** Animal-rider injured in collision with pedal cycle

  ✓x7ᵗʰ **V80.22** Occupant of animal-drawn vehicle injured in collision with pedal cycle

✓5ᵗʰ **V80.3** Animal-rider or occupant of animal-drawn vehicle injured in collision with two- or three-wheeled motor vehicle

  ✓x7ᵗʰ **V80.31** Animal-rider injured in collision with two- or three-wheeled motor vehicle

  ✓x7ᵗʰ **V80.32** Occupant of animal-drawn vehicle injured in collision with two- or three-wheeled motor vehicle

✓5ᵗʰ **V80.4** Animal-rider or occupant of animal-drawn vehicle injured in collision with car, pick-up truck, van, heavy transport vehicle or bus
    **EXCLUDES 1**   *animal-rider injured in collision with military vehicle (V80.910)*
          *occupant of animal-drawn vehicle injured in collision with military vehicle (V80.920)*

  ✓x7ᵗʰ **V80.41** Animal-rider injured in collision with car, pick-up truck, van, heavy transport vehicle or bus

  ✓x7ᵗʰ **V80.42** Occupant of animal-drawn vehicle injured in collision with car, pick-up truck, van, heavy transport vehicle or bus

✓5ᵗʰ **V80.5** Animal-rider or occupant of animal-drawn vehicle injured in collision with other specified motor vehicle

  ✓x7ᵗʰ **V80.51** Animal-rider injured in collision with other specified motor vehicle

  ✓x7ᵗʰ **V80.52** Occupant of animal-drawn vehicle injured in collision with other specified motor vehicle

✓5ᵗʰ **V80.6** Animal-rider or occupant of animal-drawn vehicle injured in collision with railway train or railway vehicle

  ✓x7ᵗʰ **V80.61** Animal-rider injured in collision with railway train or railway vehicle

  ✓x7ᵗʰ **V80.62** Occupant of animal-drawn vehicle injured in collision with railway train or railway vehicle

✓5ᵗʰ **V80.7** Animal-rider or occupant of animal-drawn vehicle injured in collision with other nonmotor vehicles

  ✓6ᵗʰ **V80.71** Animal-rider or occupant of animal-drawn vehicle injured in collision with animal being ridden

    ✓7ᵗʰ **V80.710** Animal-rider injured in collision with other animal being ridden

N Newborn: 0    P Pediatric: 0-17    M Maternity: 12-55    A Adult: 15-124    **MCC** Major CC Condition    **PDx MCC** PDx acts as own MCC    **CC** CC Condition    **PDx CC** PDx acts as own CC

**1176**        ICD-10-CM 2018

✓7ᵗʰ **V80.711** Occupant of animal-drawn vehicle injured in collision with animal being ridden

✓6ᵗʰ **V80.72** Animal-rider or occupant of animal-drawn vehicle injured in collision with other animal-drawn vehicle

    ✓7ᵗʰ **V80.720** Animal-rider injured in collision with animal-drawn vehicle

    ✓7ᵗʰ **V80.721** Occupant of animal-drawn vehicle injured in collision with other animal-drawn vehicle

✓6ᵗʰ **V80.73** Animal-rider or occupant of animal-drawn vehicle injured in collision with streetcar

    ✓7ᵗʰ **V80.730** Animal-rider injured in collision with streetcar

    ✓7ᵗʰ **V80.731** Occupant of animal-drawn vehicle injured in collision with streetcar

✓6ᵗʰ **V80.79** Animal-rider or occupant of animal-drawn vehicle injured in collision with other nonmotor vehicles

    ✓7ᵗʰ **V80.790** Animal-rider injured in collision with other nonmotor vehicles

    ✓7ᵗʰ **V80.791** Occupant of animal-drawn vehicle injured in collision with other nonmotor vehicles

✓5ᵗʰ **V80.8** Animal-rider or occupant of animal-drawn vehicle injured in collision with fixed or stationary object

    ✓x7ᵗʰ **V80.81** Animal-rider injured in collision with fixed or stationary object

    ✓x7ᵗʰ **V80.82** Occupant of animal-drawn vehicle injured in collision with fixed or stationary object

✓5ᵗʰ **V80.9** Animal-rider or occupant of animal-drawn vehicle injured in other and unspecified transport accidents

    ✓6ᵗʰ **V80.91** Animal-rider injured in other and unspecified transport accidents

        ✓7ᵗʰ **V80.910** Animal-rider injured in transport accident with military vehicle

        ✓7ᵗʰ **V80.918** Animal-rider injured in other transport accident

        ✓7ᵗʰ **V80.919** Animal-rider injured in unspecified transport accident
            Animal rider accident NOS

    ✓6ᵗʰ **V80.92** Occupant of animal-drawn vehicle injured in other and unspecified transport accidents

        ✓7ᵗʰ **V80.920** Occupant of animal-drawn vehicle injured in transport accident with military vehicle

        ✓7ᵗʰ **V80.928** Occupant of animal-drawn vehicle injured in other transport accident

        ✓7ᵗʰ **V80.929** Occupant of animal-drawn vehicle injured in unspecified transport accident
            Animal-drawn vehicle accident NOS

✓4ᵗʰ **V81** Occupant of railway train or railway vehicle injured in transport accident
    **INCLUDES** derailment of railway train or railway vehicle
                person on outside of train
    **EXCLUDES 1** *streetcar (V82.-)*

✓x7ᵗʰ **V81.0** Occupant of railway train or railway vehicle injured in collision with motor vehicle in nontraffic accident
    **EXCLUDES 1** *occupant of railway train or railway vehicle injured due to collision with military vehicle (V81.83)*

✓x7ᵗʰ **V81.1** Occupant of railway train or railway vehicle injured in collision with motor vehicle in traffic accident
    **EXCLUDES 1** *occupant of railway train or railway vehicle injured due to collision with military vehicle (V81.83)*

✓x7ᵗʰ **V81.2** Occupant of railway train or railway vehicle injured in collision with or hit by rolling stock

✓x7ᵗʰ **V81.3** Occupant of railway train or railway vehicle injured in collision with other object
    Railway collision NOS

✓x7ᵗʰ **V81.4** Person injured while boarding or alighting from railway train or railway vehicle

✓x7ᵗʰ **V81.5** Occupant of railway train or railway vehicle injured by fall in railway train or railway vehicle

✓x7ᵗʰ **V81.6** Occupant of railway train or railway vehicle injured by fall from railway train or railway vehicle

✓x7ᵗʰ **V81.7** Occupant of railway train or railway vehicle injured in derailment without antecedent collision

✓5ᵗʰ **V81.8** Occupant of railway train or railway vehicle injured in other specified railway accidents

    ✓x7ᵗʰ **V81.81** Occupant of railway train or railway vehicle injured due to explosion or fire on train

    ✓x7ᵗʰ **V81.82** Occupant of railway train or railway vehicle injured due to object falling onto train
        Occupant of railway train or railway vehicle injured due to falling earth onto train
        Occupant of railway train or railway vehicle injured due to falling rocks onto train
        Occupant of railway train or railway vehicle injured due to falling snow onto train
        Occupant of railway train or railway vehicle injured due to falling trees onto train

    ✓x7ᵗʰ **V81.83** Occupant of railway train or railway vehicle injured due to collision with military vehicle

    ✓x7ᵗʰ **V81.89** Occupant of railway train or railway vehicle injured due to other specified railway accident

✓x7ᵗʰ **V81.9** Occupant of railway train or railway vehicle injured in unspecified railway accident
    Railway accident NOS

✓4ᵗʰ **V82** Occupant of powered streetcar injured in transport accident
    **INCLUDES** interurban electric car
                person on outside of streetcar
                tram (car)
                trolley (car)
    **EXCLUDES 1** *bus (V70-V79)*
                *motorcoach (V70-V79)*
                *nonpowered streetcar (V76.-)*
                *train (V81.-)*

✓x7ᵗʰ **V82.0** Occupant of streetcar injured in collision with motor vehicle in nontraffic accident

✓x7ᵗʰ **V82.1** Occupant of streetcar injured in collision with motor vehicle in traffic accident

✓x7ᵗʰ **V82.2** Occupant of streetcar injured in collision with or hit by rolling stock

✓x7ᵗʰ **V82.3** Occupant of streetcar injured in collision with other object
    **EXCLUDES 1** *collision with animal-drawn vehicle or animal being ridden (V82.8)*

✓x7ᵗʰ **V82.4** Person injured while boarding or alighting from streetcar

✓x7ᵗʰ **V82.5** Occupant of streetcar injured by fall in streetcar
    **EXCLUDES 1** *fall in streetcar:*
        *while boarding or alighting (V82.4)*
        *with antecedent collision (V82.0-V82.3)*

✓x7ᵗʰ **V82.6** Occupant of streetcar injured by fall from streetcar
    **EXCLUDES 1** *fall from streetcar:*
        *while boarding or alighting (V82.4)*
        *with antecedent collision (V82.0-V82.3)*

✓x7ᵗʰ **V82.7** Occupant of streetcar injured in derailment without antecedent collision
    **EXCLUDES 1** *occupant of streetcar injured in derailment with antecedent collision (V82.0-V82.3)*

✓x7ᵗʰ **V82.8** Occupant of streetcar injured in other specified transport accidents
    Streetcar collision with military vehicle
    Streetcar collision with train or nonmotor vehicles

✓x7ᵗʰ **V82.9** Occupant of streetcar injured in unspecified traffic accident
    Streetcar accident NOS

✓4ᵗʰ **V83** Occupant of special vehicle mainly used on industrial premises injured in transport accident
    **INCLUDES** battery-powered airport passenger vehicle
                battery-powered truck (baggage) (mail)
                coal-car in mine
                forklift (truck)
                logging car
                self-propelled industrial truck
                station baggage truck (powered)
                tram, truck, or tub (powered) in mine or quarry
    **EXCLUDES 1** *special construction vehicles (V85.-)*
                *special industrial vehicle in stationary use or maintenance (W31.-)*

✓x7ᵗʰ **V83.0** Driver of special industrial vehicle injured in traffic accident

✓x7ᵗʰ **V83.1** Passenger of special industrial vehicle injured in traffic accident

✓x7ᵗʰ **V83.2** Person on outside of special industrial vehicle injured in traffic accident

✓x7ᵗʰ **V83.3** Unspecified occupant of special industrial vehicle injured in traffic accident

---

✓ Additional Character Req    ✓x7ᵗʰ Placeholder Alert    Unacceptable PDx    Manifestation    H1 - H14 HAC    HCC CMS-HCC Condition    EXCLUDES 1 Not Coded Here    EXCLUDES 2 Not Included Here

**Chapter 20. External Causes of Morbidity**

**V83.4–V86.36**

√x7ᵗʰ **V83.4** **Person injured while** boarding or alighting **from special industrial vehicle**

√x7ᵗʰ **V83.5** **Driver of special industrial vehicle injured** in nontraffic accident

√x7ᵗʰ **V83.6** **Passenger of special industrial vehicle injured** in nontraffic accident

√x7ᵗʰ **V83.7** **Person on outside of special industrial vehicle injured** in nontraffic accident

√x7ᵗʰ **V83.9** **Unspecified occupant of special industrial vehicle injured** in nontraffic accident
Special-industrial-vehicle accident NOS

√4ᵗʰ **V84** **Occupant of special vehicle mainly used in agriculture injured in transport accident**
INCLUDES   self-propelled farm machinery
tractor (and trailer)
EXCLUDES 1   animal-powered farm machinery accident (W30.8-)
contact with combine harvester (W30.0)
special agricultural vehicle in stationary use or maintenance (W30.-)

√x7ᵗʰ **V84.0** **Driver of special agricultural vehicle injured** in traffic accident

√x7ᵗʰ **V84.1** **Passenger of special agricultural vehicle injured** in traffic accident

√x7ᵗʰ **V84.2** **Person on outside of special agricultural vehicle injured** in traffic accident

√x7ᵗʰ **V84.3** **Unspecified occupant of special agricultural vehicle injured** in traffic accident

√x7ᵗʰ **V84.4** **Person injured while** boarding or alighting **from special agricultural vehicle**

√x7ᵗʰ **V84.5** **Driver of special agricultural vehicle injured** in nontraffic accident

√x7ᵗʰ **V84.6** **Passenger of special agricultural vehicle injured** in nontraffic accident

√x7ᵗʰ **V84.7** **Person on outside of special agricultural vehicle injured** in nontraffic accident

√x7ᵗʰ **V84.9** **Unspecified occupant of special agricultural vehicle injured** in nontraffic accident
Special-agricultural vehicle accident NOS

√4ᵗʰ **V85** **Occupant of special construction vehicle injured in transport accident**
INCLUDES   bulldozer
digger
dump truck
earth-leveller
mechanical shovel
road-roller
EXCLUDES 1   special industrial vehicle (V83.-)
special construction vehicle in stationary use or maintenance (W31.-)

√x7ᵗʰ **V85.0** **Driver of special construction vehicle injured** in traffic accident

√x7ᵗʰ **V85.1** **Passenger of special construction vehicle injured** in traffic accident

√x7ᵗʰ **V85.2** **Person on outside of special construction vehicle injured** in traffic accident

√x7ᵗʰ **V85.3** **Unspecified occupant of special construction vehicle injured** in traffic accident

√x7ᵗʰ **V85.4** **Person injured while** boarding or alighting **from special construction vehicle**

√x7ᵗʰ **V85.5** **Driver of special construction vehicle injured** in nontraffic accident

√x7ᵗʰ **V85.6** **Passenger of special construction vehicle injured** in nontraffic accident

√x7ᵗʰ **V85.7** **Person on outside of special construction vehicle injured** in nontraffic accident

√x7ᵗʰ **V85.9** **Unspecified occupant of special construction vehicle injured** in nontraffic accident
Special-construction-vehicle accident NOS

√4ᵗʰ **V86** **Occupant of special all-terrain or other off-road motor vehicle, injured in transport accident**
EXCLUDES 1   special all-terrain vehicle in stationary use or maintenance (W31.-)
sport-utility vehicle (V50-V59)
three-wheeled motor vehicle designed for on-road use (V30-V39)

√5ᵗʰ **V86.0** **Driver of special all-terrain or other off-road motor vehicle injured** in traffic accident

√x7ᵗʰ **V86.01** **Driver of** ambulance **or** fire engine **injured in traffic accident**

√x7ᵗʰ **V86.02** **Driver of** snowmobile **injured in traffic accident**

√x7ᵗʰ **V86.03** **Driver of** dune buggy **injured in traffic accident**

√x7ᵗʰ **V86.04** **Driver of** military vehicle **injured in traffic accident**

● √x7ᵗʰ **V86.05** **Driver of** 3- or 4- wheeled all-terrain vehicle (ATV) **injured in traffic accident**

● √x7ᵗʰ **V86.06** **Driver of** dirt bike or motor/cross bike **injured in traffic accident**

√x7ᵗʰ **V86.09** **Driver of** other **special all-terrain or other off-road motor vehicle injured in traffic accident**
Driver of dirt bike injured in traffic accident
Driver of go cart injured in traffic accident
Driver of golf cart injured in traffic accident

√5ᵗʰ **V86.1** **Passenger of special all-terrain or other off-road motor vehicle injured** in traffic accident

√x7ᵗʰ **V86.11** **Passenger of** ambulance **or** fire engine **injured in traffic accident**

√x7ᵗʰ **V86.12** **Passenger of** snowmobile **injured in traffic accident**

√x7ᵗʰ **V86.13** **Passenger of** dune buggy **injured in traffic accident**

√x7ᵗʰ **V86.14** **Passenger of** military vehicle **injured in traffic accident**

● √x7ᵗʰ **V86.15** **Passenger of** 3- or 4- wheeled all-terrain vehicle (ATV) **injured in traffic accident**

● √x7ᵗʰ **V86.16** **Passenger of** dirt bike or motor/cross bike **injured in traffic accident**

√x7ᵗʰ **V86.19** **Passenger of** other **special all-terrain or other off-road motor vehicle injured in traffic accident**
Passenger of dirt bike injured in traffic accident
Passenger of go cart injured in traffic accident
Passenger of golf cart injured in traffic accident

√5ᵗʰ **V86.2** **Person on outside of special all-terrain or other off-road motor vehicle injured** in traffic accident

√x7ᵗʰ **V86.21** **Person on outside of** ambulance **or** fire engine **injured in traffic accident**

√x7ᵗʰ **V86.22** **Person on outside of** snowmobile **injured in traffic accident**

√x7ᵗʰ **V86.23** **Person on outside of** dune buggy **injured in traffic accident**

√x7ᵗʰ **V86.24** **Person on outside of** military vehicle **injured in traffic accident**

● √x7ᵗʰ **V86.25** **Person on outside of** 3- or 4- wheeled all-terrain vehicle (ATV) **injured in traffic accident**

● √x7ᵗʰ **V86.26** **Person on outside of** dirt bike or motor/cross bike **injured in traffic accident**

√x7ᵗʰ **V86.29** **Person on outside of** other **special all-terrain or other off-road motor vehicle injured in traffic accident**
Person on outside of dirt bike injured in traffic accident
Person on outside of go cart in traffic accident
Person on outside of golf cart injured in traffic accident

√5ᵗʰ **V86.3** **Unspecified occupant of special all-terrain or other off-road motor vehicle injured** in traffic accident

√x7ᵗʰ **V86.31** **Unspecified occupant of** ambulance **or** fire engine **injured in traffic accident**

√x7ᵗʰ **V86.32** **Unspecified occupant of** snowmobile **injured in traffic accident**

√x7ᵗʰ **V86.33** **Unspecified occupant of** dune buggy **injured in traffic accident**

√x7ᵗʰ **V86.34** **Unspecified occupant of** military vehicle **injured in traffic accident**

● √x7ᵗʰ **V86.35** **Unspecified occupant of** 3- or 4- wheeled all-terrain vehicle (ATV) **injured in traffic accident**

● √x7ᵗʰ **V86.36** **Unspecified occupant of** dirt bike or motor/cross bike **injured in traffic accident**

√x7ᵗʰ **V86.39** **Unspecified occupant of other special all-terrain or other off-road motor vehicle injured in traffic accident**
> Unspecified occupant of dirt bike injured in traffic accident
> Unspecified occupant of go cart injured in traffic accident
> Unspecified occupant of golf cart injured in traffic accident

√5ᵗʰ **V86.4** **Person injured while boarding or alighting from special all-terrain or other off-road motor vehicle**

√x7ᵗʰ **V86.41** **Person injured while boarding or alighting from ambulance or fire engine**

√x7ᵗʰ **V86.42** **Person injured while boarding or alighting from snowmobile**

√x7ᵗʰ **V86.43** **Person injured while boarding or alighting from dune buggy**

√x7ᵗʰ **V86.44** **Person injured while boarding or alighting from military vehicle**

● √x7ᵗʰ **V86.45** **Person injured while boarding or alighting from a 3- or 4- wheeled all-terrain vehicle (ATV)**

● √x7ᵗʰ **V86.46** **Person injured while boarding or alighting from a dirt bike or motor/cross bike**

√x7ᵗʰ **V86.49** **Person injured while boarding or alighting from other special all-terrain or other off-road motor vehicle**
> Person injured while boarding or alighting from dirt bike
> Person injured while boarding or alighting from go cart
> Person injured while boarding or alighting from golf cart

√5ᵗʰ **V86.5** **Driver of special all-terrain or other off-road motor vehicle injured in nontraffic accident**

√x7ᵗʰ **V86.51** **Driver of ambulance or fire engine injured in nontraffic accident**

√x7ᵗʰ **V86.52** **Driver of snowmobile injured in nontraffic accident**

√x7ᵗʰ **V86.53** **Driver of dune buggy injured in nontraffic accident**

√x7ᵗʰ **V86.54** **Driver of military vehicle injured in nontraffic accident**

● √x7ᵗʰ **V86.55** **Driver of 3- or 4- wheeled all-terrain vehicle (ATV) injured in nontraffic accident**

● √x7ᵗʰ **V86.56** **Driver of dirt bike or motor/cross bike injured in nontraffic accident**

√x7ᵗʰ **V86.59** **Driver of other special all-terrain or other off-road motor vehicle injured in nontraffic accident**
> Driver of dirt bike injured in nontraffic accident
> Driver of go cart injured in nontraffic accident
> Driver of golf cart injured in nontraffic accident

√5ᵗʰ **V86.6** **Passenger of special all-terrain or other off-road motor vehicle injured in nontraffic accident**

√x7ᵗʰ **V86.61** **Passenger of ambulance or fire engine injured in nontraffic accident**

√x7ᵗʰ **V86.62** **Passenger of snowmobile injured in nontraffic accident**

√x7ᵗʰ **V86.63** **Passenger of dune buggy injured in nontraffic accident**

√x7ᵗʰ **V86.64** **Passenger of military vehicle injured in nontraffic accident**

● √x7ᵗʰ **V86.65** **Passenger of 3- or 4- wheeled all-terrain vehicle (ATV) injured in nontraffic accident**

● √x7ᵗʰ **V86.66** **Passenger of dirt bike or motor/cross bike injured in nontraffic accident**

√x7ᵗʰ **V86.69** **Passenger of other special all-terrain or other off-road motor vehicle injured in nontraffic accident**
> Passenger of dirt bike injured in nontraffic accident
> Passenger of go cart injured in nontraffic accident
> Passenger of golf cart injured in nontraffic accident

√5ᵗʰ **V86.7** **Person on outside of special all-terrain or other off-road motor vehicle injured in nontraffic accident**

√x7ᵗʰ **V86.71** **Person on outside of ambulance or fire engine injured in nontraffic accident**

√x7ᵗʰ **V86.72** **Person on outside of snowmobile injured in nontraffic accident**

√x7ᵗʰ **V86.73** **Person on outside of dune buggy injured in nontraffic accident**

√x7ᵗʰ **V86.74** **Person on outside of military vehicle injured in nontraffic accident**

● √x7ᵗʰ **V86.75** **Person on outside of 3- or 4- wheeled all-terrain vehicle (ATV) injured in nontraffic accident**

● √x7ᵗʰ **V86.76** **Person on outside of dirt bike or motor/cross bike injured in nontraffic accident**

√x7ᵗʰ **V86.79** **Person on outside of other special all-terrain or other off-road motor vehicles injured in nontraffic accident**
> Person on outside of dirt bike injured in nontraffic accident
> Person on outside of go cart injured in nontraffic accident
> Person on outside of golf cart injured in nontraffic accident

√5ᵗʰ **V86.9** **Unspecified occupant of special all-terrain or other off-road motor vehicle injured in nontraffic accident**

√x7ᵗʰ **V86.91** **Unspecified occupant of ambulance or fire engine injured in nontraffic accident**

√x7ᵗʰ **V86.92** **Unspecified occupant of snowmobile injured in nontraffic accident**

√x7ᵗʰ **V86.93** **Unspecified occupant of dune buggy injured in nontraffic accident**

√x7ᵗʰ **V86.94** **Unspecified occupant of military vehicle injured in nontraffic accident**

● √x7ᵗʰ **V86.95** **Unspecified occupant of 3- or 4- wheeled all-terrain vehicle (ATV) injured in nontraffic accident**

● √x7ᵗʰ **V86.96** **Unspecified occupant of dirt bike or motor/cross bike injured in nontraffic accident**

√x7ᵗʰ **V86.99** **Unspecified occupant of other special all-terrain or other off-road motor vehicle injured in nontraffic accident**
> All-terrain motor-vehicle accident NOS
> Off-road motor-vehicle accident NOS
> Other motor-vehicle accident NOS
> ~~Unspecified occupant of dirt bike injured in nontraffic accident~~
> Unspecified occupant of go cart injured in nontraffic accident
> Unspecified occupant of golf cart injured in nontraffic accident

√4ᵗʰ **V87** **Traffic accident of specified type but victim's mode of transport unknown**
> *EXCLUDES 1*   collision involving:
> > pedal cycle (V10-V19)
> > pedestrian (V01-V09)

√x7ᵗʰ **V87.0** **Person injured in collision between car and two- or three-wheeled powered vehicle (traffic)**

√x7ᵗʰ **V87.1** **Person injured in collision between other motor vehicle and two- or three-wheeled motor vehicle (traffic)**

√x7ᵗʰ **V87.2** **Person injured in collision between car and pick-up truck or van (traffic)**

√x7ᵗʰ **V87.3** **Person injured in collision between car and bus (traffic)**

√x7ᵗʰ **V87.4** **Person injured in collision between car and heavy transport vehicle (traffic)**

√x7ᵗʰ **V87.5** **Person injured in collision between heavy transport vehicle and bus (traffic)**

√x7ᵗʰ **V87.6** **Person injured in collision between railway train or railway vehicle and car (traffic)**

√x7ᵗʰ **V87.7** **Person injured in collision between other specified motor vehicles (traffic)**

√x7ᵗʰ **V87.8** **Person injured in other specified noncollision transport accidents involving motor vehicle (traffic)**

√x7ᵗʰ **V87.9** **Person injured in other specified (collision)(noncollision) transport accidents involving nonmotor vehicle (traffic)**

√4ᵗʰ **V88** **Nontraffic accident of specified type but victim's mode of transport unknown**
> *EXCLUDES 1*   collision involving:
> > pedal cycle (V10-V19)
> > pedestrian (V01-V09)

√x7ᵗʰ **V88.0** **Person injured in collision between car and two- or three-wheeled motor vehicle, nontraffic**

√x7ᵗʰ **V88.1** **Person injured in collision between other motor vehicle and two- or three-wheeled motor vehicle, nontraffic**

√x7ᵗʰ **V88.2** **Person injured in collision between car and pick-up truck or van, nontraffic**

√x7ᵗʰ **V88.3** **Person injured in collision between car and bus, nontraffic**

√ Additional Character Req   √x7ᵗʰ Placeholder Alert   Unacceptable PDx   Manifestation   H1 - H14 HAC   HCC CMS-HCC Condition   *EXCLUDES 1* Not Coded Here   *EXCLUDES 2* Not Included Here

ICD-10-CM 2018      1179

√x7ᵗʰ **V88.4** **Person injured in collision between** car and heavy transport vehicle, **nontraffic**

√x7ᵗʰ **V88.5** **Person injured in collision between** heavy transport vehicle and bus, **nontraffic**

√x7ᵗʰ **V88.6** **Person injured in collision between** railway train or railway vehicle and car, **nontraffic**

√x7ᵗʰ **V88.7** **Person injured in collision between** other specified motor vehicle, **nontraffic**

√x7ᵗʰ **V88.8** **Person injured in** other specified noncollision transport accidents **involving** motor vehicle, **nontraffic**

√x7ᵗʰ **V88.9** **Person injured in** other specified (collision)(noncollision) transport accidents **involving** nonmotor vehicle, **nontraffic**

√4ᵗʰ **V89** **Motor- or nonmotor-vehicle accident, type of vehicle unspecified**

√x7ᵗʰ **V89.0** **Person injured in unspecified** motor-vehicle **accident, nontraffic**
Motor-vehicle accident NOS, nontraffic

√x7ᵗʰ **V89.1** **Person injured in unspecified** nonmotor-vehicle **accident, nontraffic**
Nonmotor-vehicle accident NOS (nontraffic)

√x7ᵗʰ **V89.2** **Person injured in** unspecified motor-vehicle **accident, traffic**
Motor-vehicle accident [MVA] NOS
Road (traffic) accident [RTA] NOS

√x7ᵗʰ **V89.3** **Person injured in** unspecified nonmotor-vehicle **accident, traffic**
Nonmotor-vehicle traffic accident NOS

√x7ᵗʰ **V89.9** **Person injured in** unspecified vehicle accident
Collision NOS

### Water transport accidents (V90-V94)

The appropriate 7th character is to be added to each code from categories V90-V94.
A    initial encounter
D    subsequent encounter
S    sequela

√4ᵗʰ **V90** **Drowning and submersion due to accident to watercraft**
**EXCLUDES 1** *civilian water transport accident involving military watercraft (V94.81-)*
*fall into water not from watercraft (W16.-)*
*military watercraft accident in military or war operations (Y36.0-, Y37.0-)*
*water-transport-related drowning or submersion without accident to watercraft (V92.-)*

√5ᵗʰ **V90.0** **Drowning and submersion due to** watercraft overturning

√x7ᵗʰ **V90.00** **Drowning and submersion due to** merchant ship **overturning**

√x7ᵗʰ **V90.01** **Drowning and submersion due to** passenger ship **overturning**
Drowning and submersion due to Ferry-boat overturning
Drowning and submersion due to Liner overturning

√x7ᵗʰ **V90.02** **Drowning and submersion due to** fishing boat **overturning**

√x7ᵗʰ **V90.03** **Drowning and submersion due to** other powered watercraft **overturning**
Drowning and submersion due to Hovercraft (on open water) overturning
Drowning and submersion due to Jet ski overturning

√x7ᵗʰ **V90.04** **Drowning and submersion due to** sailboat **overturning**

√x7ᵗʰ **V90.05** **Drowning and submersion due to** canoe or kayak **overturning**

√x7ᵗʰ **V90.06** **Drowning and submersion due to** (nonpowered) inflatable craft **overturning**

√x7ᵗʰ **V90.08** **Drowning and submersion due to** other unpowered watercraft **overturning**
Drowning and submersion due to windsurfer overturning

√x7ᵗʰ **V90.09** **Drowning and submersion due to** unspecified watercraft **overturning**
Drowning and submersion due to boat NOS overturning
Drowning and submersion due to ship NOS overturning
Drowning and submersion due to watercraft NOS overturning

√5ᵗʰ **V90.1** **Drowning and submersion due to** watercraft sinking

√x7ᵗʰ **V90.10** **Drowning and submersion due to** merchant ship **sinking**

√x7ᵗʰ **V90.11** **Drowning and submersion due to** passenger ship **sinking**
Drowning and submersion due to Ferry-boat sinking
Drowning and submersion due to Liner sinking

√x7ᵗʰ **V90.12** **Drowning and submersion due to** fishing boat **sinking**

√x7ᵗʰ **V90.13** **Drowning and submersion due to** other powered watercraft **sinking**
Drowning and submersion due to Hovercraft (on open water) sinking
Drowning and submersion due to Jet ski sinking

√x7ᵗʰ **V90.14** **Drowning and submersion due to** sailboat **sinking**

√x7ᵗʰ **V90.15** **Drowning and submersion due to** canoe or kayak **sinking**

√x7ᵗʰ **V90.16** **Drowning and submersion due to** (nonpowered) inflatable craft **sinking**

√x7ᵗʰ **V90.18** **Drowning and submersion due to** other unpowered watercraft sinking

√x7ᵗʰ **V90.19** **Drowning and submersion due to** unspecified watercraft **sinking**
Drowning and submersion due to boat NOS sinking
Drowning and submersion due to ship NOS sinking
Drowning and submersion due to watercraft NOS sinking

√5ᵗʰ **V90.2** **Drowning and submersion due to** falling or jumping from burning watercraft

√x7ᵗʰ **V90.20** **Drowning and submersion due to falling or jumping from burning** merchant ship

√x7ᵗʰ **V90.21** **Drowning and submersion due to falling or jumping from burning** passenger ship
Drowning and submersion due to falling or jumping from burning Ferry-boat
Drowning and submersion due to falling or jumping from burning Liner

√x7ᵗʰ **V90.22** **Drowning and submersion due to falling or jumping from burning** fishing boat

√x7ᵗʰ **V90.23** **Drowning and submersion due to falling or jumping from** other burning powered **watercraft**
Drowning and submersion due to falling and jumping from burning Hovercraft (on open water)
Drowning and submersion due to falling and jumping from burning Jet ski

√x7ᵗʰ **V90.24** **Drowning and submersion due to falling or jumping from burning** sailboat

√x7ᵗʰ **V90.25** **Drowning and submersion due to falling or jumping from burning** canoe or kayak

√x7ᵗʰ **V90.26** **Drowning and submersion due to falling or jumping from burning** (nonpowered) inflatable craft

√x7ᵗʰ **V90.27** **Drowning and submersion due to falling or jumping from burning** water-skis

√x7ᵗʰ **V90.28** **Drowning and submersion due to falling or jumping from** other burning unpowered **watercraft**
Drowning and submersion due to falling and jumping from burning surf-board
Drowning and submersion due to falling and jumping from burning windsurfer

√x7ᵗʰ **V90.29** **Drowning and submersion due to falling or jumping from** unspecified burning watercraft
Drowning and submersion due to falling or jumping from burning boat NOS
Drowning and submersion due to falling or jumping from burning ship NOS
Drowning and submersion due to falling or jumping from burning watercraft NOS

√5ᵗʰ **V90.3** **Drowning and submersion due to** falling or jumping from crushed watercraft

√x7ᵗʰ **V90.30** **Drowning and submersion due to falling or jumping from crushed** merchant ship

√x7ᵗʰ **V90.31** **Drowning and submersion due to falling or jumping from crushed** passenger ship
Drowning and submersion due to falling and jumping from crushed Ferry boat
Drowning and submersion due to falling and jumping from crushed Liner

**✓x7ᵗʰ V90.32 Drowning and submersion due to falling or jumping from crushed** fishing boat

**✓x7ᵗʰ V90.33 Drowning and submersion due to falling or jumping from** other crushed powered **watercraft**
    Drowning and submersion due to falling and jumping from crushed Hovercraft
    Drowning and submersion due to falling and jumping from crushed Jet ski

**✓x7ᵗʰ V90.34 Drowning and submersion due to falling or jumping from crushed** sailboat

**✓x7ᵗʰ V90.35 Drowning and submersion due to falling or jumping from crushed** canoe or kayak

**✓x7ᵗʰ V90.36 Drowning and submersion due to falling or jumping from crushed (nonpowered)** inflatable craft

**✓x7ᵗʰ V90.37 Drowning and submersion due to falling or jumping from crushed** water-skis

**✓x7ᵗʰ V90.38 Drowning and submersion due to falling or jumping from** other crushed unpowered **watercraft**
    Drowning and submersion due to falling and jumping from crushed surf-board
    Drowning and submersion due to falling and jumping from crushed windsurfer

**✓x7ᵗʰ V90.39 Drowning and submersion due to falling or jumping from crushed** unspecified **watercraft**
    Drowning and submersion due to falling and jumping from crushed boat NOS
    Drowning and submersion due to falling and jumping from crushed ship NOS
    Drowning and submersion due to falling and jumping from crushed watercraft NOS

**✓5ᵗʰ V90.8 Drowning and submersion due to** other accident to watercraft

**✓x7ᵗʰ V90.80 Drowning and submersion due to other accident to** merchant ship

**✓x7ᵗʰ V90.81 Drowning and submersion due to other accident to** passenger ship
    Drowning and submersion due to other accident to Ferry-boat
    Drowning and submersion due to other accident to Liner

**✓x7ᵗʰ V90.82 Drowning and submersion due to other accident to** fishing boat

**✓x7ᵗʰ V90.83 Drowning and submersion due to other accident to** other powered **watercraft**
    Drowning and submersion due to other accident to Hovercraft (on open water)
    Drowning and submersion due to other accident to Jet ski

**✓x7ᵗʰ V90.84 Drowning and submersion due to other accident to** sailboat

**✓x7ᵗʰ V90.85 Drowning and submersion due to other accident to** canoe or kayak

**✓x7ᵗʰ V90.86 Drowning and submersion due to other accident to (nonpowered)** inflatable craft

**✓x7ᵗʰ V90.87 Drowning and submersion due to other accident to** water-skis

**✓x7ᵗʰ V90.88 Drowning and submersion due to other accident to** other unpowered **watercraft**
    Drowning and submersion due to other accident to surf-board
    Drowning and submersion due to other accident to windsurfer

**✓x7ᵗʰ V90.89 Drowning and submersion due to other accident to** unspecified **watercraft**
    Drowning and submersion due to other accident to boat NOS
    Drowning and submersion due to other accident to ship NOS
    Drowning and submersion due to other accident to watercraft NOS

**✓4ᵗʰ V91 Other injury due to accident to watercraft**
    **INCLUDES** any injury except drowning and submersion as a result of an accident to watercraft
    **EXCLUDES 1** civilian water transport accident involving military watercraft (V94.81-)
        military watercraft accident in military or war operations (Y36, Y37.-)
    **EXCLUDES 2** drowning and submersion due to accident to watercraft (V90.-)

**✓5ᵗʰ V91.0 Burn due to watercraft on fire**
    **EXCLUDES 1** burn from localized fire or explosion on board ship without accident to watercraft (V93.-)

**✓x7ᵗʰ V91.00 Burn due to** merchant ship **on fire**

**✓x7ᵗʰ V91.01 Burn due to** passenger ship **on fire**
    Burn due to Ferry-boat on fire
    Burn due to Liner on fire

**✓x7ᵗʰ V91.02 Burn due to** fishing boat **on fire**

**✓x7ᵗʰ V91.03 Burn due to** other powered **watercraft on fire**
    Burn due to Hovercraft (on open water) on fire
    Burn due to Jet ski on fire

**✓x7ᵗʰ V91.04 Burn due to** sailboat **on fire**

**✓x7ᵗʰ V91.05 Burn due to** canoe or kayak **on fire**

**✓x7ᵗʰ V91.06 Burn due to (nonpowered)** inflatable craft **on fire**

**✓x7ᵗʰ V91.07 Burn due to** water-skis **on fire**

**✓x7ᵗʰ V91.08 Burn due to** other unpowered **watercraft on fire**

**✓x7ᵗʰ V91.09 Burn due to** unspecified **watercraft on fire**
    Burn due to boat NOS on fire
    Burn due to ship NOS on fire
    Burn due to watercraft NOS on fire

**✓5ᵗʰ V91.1 Crushed between watercraft and other watercraft or other object due to collision**
    Crushed by lifeboat after abandoning ship in a collision
    **NOTE** Select the specified type of watercraft that the victim was on at the time of the collision

**✓x7ᵗʰ V91.10 Crushed between** merchant ship **and other watercraft or other object due to collision**

**✓x7ᵗʰ V91.11 Crushed between** passenger ship **and other watercraft or other object due to collision**
    Crushed between Ferry-boat and other watercraft or other object due to collision
    Crushed between Liner and other watercraft or other object due to collision

**✓x7ᵗʰ V91.12 Crushed between** fishing boat **and other watercraft or other object due to collision**

**✓x7ᵗʰ V91.13 Crushed between** other powered **watercraft and other watercraft or other object due to collision**
    Crushed between Hovercraft (on open water) and other watercraft or other object due to collision
    Crushed between Jet ski and other watercraft or other object due to collision

**✓x7ᵗʰ V91.14 Crushed between** sailboat **and other watercraft or other object due to collision**

**✓x7ᵗʰ V91.15 Crushed between** canoe or kayak **and other watercraft or other object due to collision**

**✓x7ᵗʰ V91.16 Crushed between (nonpowered)** inflatable craft **and other watercraft or other object due to collision**

**✓x7ᵗʰ V91.18 Crushed between other** unpowered **watercraft and other watercraft or other object due to collision**
    Crushed between surfboard and other watercraft or other object due to collision
    Crushed between windsurfer and other watercraft or other object due to collision

**✓x7ᵗʰ V91.19 Crushed between** unspecified **watercraft and other watercraft or other object due to collision**
    Crushed between boat NOS and other watercraft or other object due to collision
    Crushed between ship NOS and other watercraft or other object due to collision
    Crushed between watercraft NOS and other watercraft or other object due to collision

✓ Additional Character Req    ✓x7ᵗʰ Placeholder Alert    Unacceptable PDx    Manifestation    **H1**-**H14** HAC    **HCC** CMS-HCC Condition    **EXCLUDES 1** Not Coded Here    **EXCLUDES 2** Not Included Here

ICD-10-CM 2018          1181

☑5ᵗʰ **V91.2** **Fall due to collision between watercraft and other watercraft or other object**
Fall while remaining on watercraft after collision

> **NOTE**   Select the specified type of watercraft that the victim was on at the time of the collision.
>
> **EXCLUDES 1**   *crushed between watercraft and other watercraft and other object due to collision (V91.1-)*
> *drowning and submersion due to falling from crushed watercraft (V90.3-)*

√x 7ᵗʰ **V91.20** **Fall due to collision between merchant ship and other watercraft or other object**

√x 7ᵗʰ **V91.21** **Fall due to collision between passenger ship and other watercraft or other object**
Fall due to collision between Ferry-boat and other watercraft or other object
Fall due to collision between Liner and other watercraft or other object

√x 7ᵗʰ **V91.22** **Fall due to collision between fishing boat and other watercraft or other object**

√x 7ᵗʰ **V91.23** **Fall due to collision between other powered watercraft and other watercraft or other object**
Fall due to collision between Hovercraft (on open water) and other watercraft or other object
Fall due to collision between Jet ski and other watercraft or other object

√x 7ᵗʰ **V91.24** **Fall due to collision between sailboat and other watercraft or other object**

√x 7ᵗʰ **V91.25** **Fall due to collision between canoe or kayak and other watercraft or other object**

√x 7ᵗʰ **V91.26** **Fall due to collision between (nonpowered) inflatable craft and other watercraft or other object**

√x 7ᵗʰ **V91.29** **Fall due to collision between unspecified watercraft and other watercraft or other object**
Fall due to collision between boat NOS and other watercraft or other object
Fall due to collision between ship NOS and other watercraft or other object
Fall due to collision between watercraft NOS and other watercraft or other object

☑5ᵗʰ **V91.3** **Hit or struck by falling object due to accident to watercraft**
Hit or struck by falling object (part of damaged watercraft or other object) after falling or jumping from damaged watercraft

> **EXCLUDES 2**   *drowning or submersion due to fall or jumping from damaged watercraft (V90.2-, V90.3-)*

√x 7ᵗʰ **V91.30** **Hit or struck by falling object due to accident to merchant ship**

√x 7ᵗʰ **V91.31** **Hit or struck by falling object due to accident to passenger ship**
Hit or struck by falling object due to accident to Ferry-boat
Hit or struck by falling object due to accident to Liner

√x 7ᵗʰ **V91.32** **Hit or struck by falling object due to accident to fishing boat**

√x 7ᵗʰ **V91.33** **Hit or struck by falling object due to accident to other powered watercraft**
Hit or struck by falling object due to accident to Hovercraft (on open water)
Hit or struck by falling object due to accident to Jet ski

√x 7ᵗʰ **V91.34** **Hit or struck by falling object due to accident to sailboat**

√x 7ᵗʰ **V91.35** **Hit or struck by falling object due to accident to canoe or kayak**

√x 7ᵗʰ **V91.36** **Hit or struck by falling object due to accident to (nonpowered) inflatable craft**

√x 7ᵗʰ **V91.37** **Hit or struck by falling object due to accident to water-skis**
Hit by water-skis after jumping off of waterskis

√x 7ᵗʰ **V91.38** **Hit or struck by falling object due to accident to other unpowered watercraft**
Hit or struck by surf-board after falling off damaged surf-board
Hit or struck by object after falling off damaged windsurfer

√x 7ᵗʰ **V91.39** **Hit or struck by falling object due to accident to unspecified watercraft**
Hit or struck by falling object due to accident to boat NOS
Hit or struck by falling object due to accident to ship NOS
Hit or struck by falling object due to accident to watercraft NOS

☑5ᵗʰ **V91.8** **Other injury due to other accident to watercraft**

√x 7ᵗʰ **V91.80** **Other injury due to other accident to merchant ship**

√x 7ᵗʰ **V91.81** **Other injury due to other accident to passenger ship**
Other injury due to other accident to Ferry-boat
Other injury due to other accident to Liner

√x 7ᵗʰ **V91.82** **Other injury due to other accident to fishing boat**

√x 7ᵗʰ **V91.83** **Other injury due to other accident to other powered watercraft**
Other injury due to other accident to Hovercraft (on open water)
Other injury due to other accident to Jet ski

√x 7ᵗʰ **V91.84** **Other injury due to other accident to sailboat**

√x 7ᵗʰ **V91.85** **Other injury due to other accident to canoe or kayak**

√x 7ᵗʰ **V91.86** **Other injury due to other accident to (nonpowered) inflatable craft**

√x 7ᵗʰ **V91.87** **Other injury due to other accident to water-skis**

√x 7ᵗʰ **V91.88** **Other injury due to other accident to other unpowered watercraft**
Other injury due to other accident to surf-board
Other injury due to other accident to windsurfer

√x 7ᵗʰ **V91.89** **Other injury due to other accident to unspecified watercraft**
Other injury due to other accident to boat NOS
Other injury due to other accident to ship NOS
Other injury due to other accident to watercraft NOS

☑4ᵗʰ **V92** **Drowning and submersion due to accident on board watercraft, without accident to watercraft**

> **EXCLUDES 1**   *civilian water transport accident involving military watercraft (V94.81-)*
> *drowning or submersion due to accident to watercraft (V90-V91)*
> *drowning or submersion of diver who voluntarily jumps from boat not involved in an accident (W16.711, W16.721)*
> *fall into water without watercraft (W16.-)*
> *military watercraft accident in military or war operations (Y36, Y37)*

☑5ᵗʰ **V92.0** **Drowning and submersion due to fall off watercraft**
Drowning and submersion due to fall from gangplank of watercraft
Drowning and submersion due to fall overboard watercraft

> **EXCLUDES 2**   *hitting head on object or bottom of body of water due to fall from watercraft (V94.0-)*

√x 7ᵗʰ **V92.00** **Drowning and submersion due to fall off merchant ship**

√x 7ᵗʰ **V92.01** **Drowning and submersion due to fall off passenger ship**
Drowning and submersion due to fall off Ferry-boat
Drowning and submersion due to fall off Liner

√x 7ᵗʰ **V92.02** **Drowning and submersion due to fall off fishing boat**

√x 7ᵗʰ **V92.03** **Drowning and submersion due to fall off other powered watercraft**
Drowning and submersion due to fall off Hovercraft (on open water)
Drowning and submersion due to fall off Jet ski

√x 7ᵗʰ **V92.04** **Drowning and submersion due to fall off sailboat**

√x 7ᵗʰ **V92.05** **Drowning and submersion due to fall off canoe or kayak**

√x 7ᵗʰ **V92.06** **Drowning and submersion due to fall off (nonpowered) inflatable craft**

√x 7ᵗʰ **V92.07** **Drowning and submersion due to fall off water-skis**

> **EXCLUDES 1**   *drowning and submersion due to falling off burning water-skis (V90.27)*
> *drowning and submersion due to falling off crushed water-skis (V90.37)*
> *hit by boat while water-skiing NOS (V94.X)*

---

N Newborn: 0   P Pediatric: 0-17   M Maternity: 12-55   A Adult: 15-124   **MCC** Major CC Condition   **PDx MCC** PDx acts as own MCC   **CC** CC Condition   **PDx CC** PDx acts as own CC

**1182**      ICD-10-CM 2018

√x7ᵗʰ **V92.08  Drowning and submersion due to fall off** other unpowered **watercraft**

Drowning and submersion due to fall off surf-board
Drowning and submersion due to fall off windsurfer

EXCLUDES 1  *drowning and submersion due to fall off burning unpowered watercraft (V90.28)*
*drowning and submersion due to fall off crushed unpowered watercraft (V90.38)*
*drowning and submersion due to fall off damaged unpowered watercraft (V90.88)*
*drowning and submersion due to rider of nonpowered watercraft being hit by other watercraft (V94.-)*
*other injury due to rider of nonpowered watercraft being hit by other watercraft (V94.-)*

√x7ᵗʰ **V92.09  Drowning and submersion due to fall off** unspecified **watercraft**

Drowning and submersion due to fall off boat NOS
Drowning and submersion due to fall off ship
Drowning and submersion due to fall off watercraft NOS

√5ᵗʰ **V92.1  Drowning and submersion due to being** thrown overboard **by motion of watercraft**

EXCLUDES 1  *drowning and submersion due to fall off surf-board (V92.08)*
*drowning and submersion due to fall off water-skis (V92.07)*
*drowning and submersion due to fall off windsurfer (V92.08)*

√x7ᵗʰ **V92.10  Drowning and submersion due to being thrown overboard by motion of** merchant ship

√x7ᵗʰ **V92.11  Drowning and submersion due to being thrown overboard by motion of** passenger ship

Drowning and submersion due to being thrown overboard by motion of Ferry-boat
Drowning and submersion due to being thrown overboard by motion of Liner

√x7ᵗʰ **V92.12  Drowning and submersion due to being thrown overboard by motion of** fishing boat

√x7ᵗʰ **V92.13  Drowning and submersion due to being thrown overboard by motion of** other powered **watercraft**

Drowning and submersion due to being thrown overboard by motion of Hovercraft

√x7ᵗʰ **V92.14  Drowning and submersion due to being thrown overboard by motion of** sailboat

√x7ᵗʰ **V92.15  Drowning and submersion due to being thrown overboard by motion of** canoe or kayak

√x7ᵗʰ **V92.16  Drowning and submersion due to being thrown overboard by motion of (nonpowered)** inflatable craft

√x7ᵗʰ **V92.19  Drowning and submersion due to being thrown overboard by motion of** unspecified **watercraft**

Drowning and submersion due to being thrown overboard by motion of boat NOS
Drowning and submersion due to being thrown overboard by motion of ship NOS
Drowning and submersion due to being thrown overboard by motion of watercraft NOS

√5ᵗʰ **V92.2  Drowning and submersion due to being** washed overboard **from watercraft**

Code first any associated cataclysm (X37.0-)

√x7ᵗʰ **V92.20  Drowning and submersion due to being washed overboard from** merchant ship

√x7ᵗʰ **V92.21  Drowning and submersion due to being washed overboard from** passenger ship

Drowning and submersion due to being washed overboard from Ferry-boat
Drowning and submersion due to being washed overboard from Liner

√x7ᵗʰ **V92.22  Drowning and submersion due to being washed overboard from** fishing boat

√x7ᵗʰ **V92.23  Drowning and submersion due to being washed overboard from** other powered **watercraft**

Drowning and submersion due to being washed overboard from Hovercraft (on open water)
Drowning and submersion due to being washed overboard from Jet ski

√x7ᵗʰ **V92.24  Drowning and submersion due to being washed overboard from** sailboat

√x7ᵗʰ **V92.25  Drowning and submersion due to being washed overboard from** canoe or kayak

√x7ᵗʰ **V92.26  Drowning and submersion due to being washed overboard from (nonpowered)** inflatable craft

√x7ᵗʰ **V92.27  Drowning and submersion due to being washed overboard from** water-skis

EXCLUDES 1  *drowning and submersion due to fall off water-skis (V92.07)*

√x7ᵗʰ **V92.28  Drowning and submersion due to being washed overboard from** other unpowered **watercraft**

Drowning and submersion due to being washed overboard from surf-board
Drowning and submersion due to being washed overboard from windsurfer

√x7ᵗʰ **V92.29  Drowning and submersion due to being washed overboard from** unspecified **watercraft**

Drowning and submersion due to being washed overboard from boat NOS
Drowning and submersion due to being washed overboard from ship NOS
Drowning and submersion due to being washed overboard from watercraft NOS

√4ᵗʰ **V93  Other injury due to accident on board watercraft, without accident to watercraft**

EXCLUDES 1  *civilian water transport accident involving military watercraft (V94.81-)*
*other injury due to accident to watercraft (V91.-)*
*military watercraft accident in military or war operations (Y36, Y37.-)*

EXCLUDES 2  *drowning and submersion due to accident on board watercraft, without accident to watercraft (V92.-)*

√5ᵗʰ **V93.0  Burn due to localized fire on board watercraft**

EXCLUDES 1  *burn due to watercraft on fire (V91.0-)*

√x7ᵗʰ **V93.00  Burn due to localized fire on board** merchant vessel

√x7ᵗʰ **V93.01  Burn due to localized fire on board** passenger vessel

Burn due to localized fire on board Ferry-boat
Burn due to localized fire on board Liner

√x7ᵗʰ **V93.02  Burn due to localized fire on board** fishing boat

√x7ᵗʰ **V93.03  Burn due to localized fire on board** other powered **watercraft**

Burn due to localized fire on board Hovercraft
Burn due to localized fire on board Jet ski

√x7ᵗʰ **V93.04  Burn due to localized fire on board** sailboat

√x7ᵗʰ **V93.09  Burn due to localized fire on board** unspecified **watercraft**

Burn due to localized fire on board boat NOS
Burn due to localized fire on board ship NOS
Burn due to localized fire on board watercraft NOS

√5ᵗʰ **V93.1  Other burn on board watercraft**

Burn due to source other than fire on board watercraft

EXCLUDES 1  *burn due to watercraft on fire (V91.0-)*

√x7ᵗʰ **V93.10  Other burn on board** merchant vessel

√x7ᵗʰ **V93.11  Other burn on board** passenger vessel

Other burn on board Ferry-boat
Other burn on board Liner

√x7ᵗʰ **V93.12  Other burn on board** fishing boat

√x7ᵗʰ **V93.13  Other burn on board** other powered **watercraft**

Other burn on board Hovercraft
Other burn on board Jet ski

√x7ᵗʰ **V93.14  Other burn on board** sailboat

√x7ᵗʰ **V93.19  Other burn on board** unspecified **watercraft**

Other burn on board boat NOS
Other burn on board ship NOS
Other burn on board watercraft NOS

√5ᵗʰ **V93.2  Heat exposure on board watercraft**

EXCLUDES 1  *exposure to man-made heat not aboard watercraft (W92)*
*exposure to natural heat while on board watercraft (X30)*
*exposure to sunlight while on board watercraft (X32)*

EXCLUDES 2  *burn due to fire on board watercraft (V93.0-)*

√x7ᵗʰ **V93.20  Heat exposure on board** merchant ship

√x7ᵗʰ **V93.21  Heat exposure on board** passenger ship

Heat exposure on board Ferry-boat
Heat exposure on board Liner

√x7ᵗʰ **V93.22  Heat exposure on board** fishing boat

---

✓Additional Character Req  √x7ᵗʰ Placeholder Alert  Unacceptable PDx  Manifestation  H1 - H14 HAC  HCC CMS-HCC Condition  EXCLUDES 1 Not Coded Here  EXCLUDES 2 Not Included Here

ICD-10-CM 2018     1183

✓x7th **V93.23 Heat exposure on board** other powered **watercraft**
Heat exposure on board hovercraft

✓x7th **V93.24 Heat exposure on board** sailboat

✓x7th **V93.29 Heat exposure on board** unspecified **watercraft**
Heat exposure on board boat NOS
Heat exposure on board ship NOS
Heat exposure on board watercraft NOS

✓5th **V93.3 Fall on board watercraft**
EXCLUDES 1 *fall due to collision of watercraft (V91.2-)*

✓x7th **V93.30 Fall on board** merchant ship

✓x7th **V93.31 Fall on board** passenger ship
Fall on board Ferry-boat
Fall on board Liner

✓x7th **V93.32 Fall on board** fishing boat

✓x7th **V93.33 Fall on board** other powered **watercraft**
Fall on board Hovercraft (on open water)
Fall on board Jet ski

✓x7th **V93.34 Fall on board** sailboat

✓x7th **V93.35 Fall on board** canoe or kayak

✓x7th **V93.36 Fall on board (nonpowered)** inflatable craft

✓x7th **V93.38 Fall on board** other unpowered **watercraft**

✓x7th **V93.39 Fall on board** unspecified **watercraft**
Fall on board boat NOS
Fall on board ship NOS
Fall on board watercraft NOS

✓5th **V93.4 Struck by falling object on board watercraft**
Hit by falling object on board watercraft
EXCLUDES 1 *struck by falling object due to accident to watercraft (V91.3)*

✓x7th **V93.40 Struck by falling object on** merchant ship

✓x7th **V93.41 Struck by falling object on** passenger ship
Struck by falling object on Ferry-boat
Struck by falling object on Liner

✓x7th **V93.42 Struck by falling object on** fishing boat

✓x7th **V93.43 Struck by falling object on** other powered **watercraft**
Struck by falling object on Hovercraft

✓x7th **V93.44 Struck by falling object on** sailboat

✓x7th **V93.48 Struck by falling object on** other unpowered **watercraft**

✓x7th **V93.49 Struck by falling object on** unspecified **watercraft**

✓5th **V93.5 Explosion on board watercraft**
Boiler explosion on steamship
EXCLUDES 2 *fire on board watercraft (V93.0-)*

✓x7th **V93.50 Explosion on board** merchant ship

✓x7th **V93.51 Explosion on board** passenger ship
Explosion on board Ferry-boat
Explosion on board Liner

✓x7th **V93.52 Explosion on board** fishing boat

✓x7th **V93.53 Explosion on board** other powered **watercraft**
Explosion on board Hovercraft
Explosion on board Jet ski

✓x7th **V93.54 Explosion on board** sailboat

✓x7th **V93.59 Explosion on board** unspecified **watercraft**
Explosion on board boat NOS
Explosion on board ship NOS
Explosion on board watercraft NOS

✓5th **V93.6 Machinery accident on board watercraft**
EXCLUDES 1 *machinery explosion on board watercraft (V93.4-)*
*machinery fire on board watercraft (V93.0-)*

✓x7th **V93.60 Machinery accident on board** merchant ship

✓x7th **V93.61 Machinery accident on board** passenger ship
Machinery accident on board Ferry-boat
Machinery accident on board Liner

✓x7th **V93.62 Machinery accident on board** fishing boat

✓x7th **V93.63 Machinery accident on board** other powered **watercraft**
Machinery accident on board Hovercraft

✓x7th **V93.64 Machinery accident on board** sailboat

✓x7th **V93.69 Machinery accident on board** unspecified **watercraft**
Machinery accident on board boat NOS
Machinery accident on board ship NOS
Machinery accident on board watercraft NOS

✓5th **V93.8 Other injury due to other accident on board watercraft**
Accidental poisoning by gases or fumes on watercraft

✓x7th **V93.80 Other injury due to other accident on board** merchant ship

✓x7th **V93.81 Other injury due to other accident on board** passenger ship
Other injury due to other accident on board Ferry-boat
Other injury due to other accident on board Liner

✓x7th **V93.82 Other injury due to other accident on board** fishing boat

✓x7th **V93.83 Other injury due to other accident on board** other powered **watercraft**
Other injury due to other accident on board Hovercraft
Other injury due to other accident on board Jet ski

✓x7th **V93.84 Other injury due to other accident on board** sailboat

✓x7th **V93.85 Other injury due to other accident on board** canoe or kayak

✓x7th **V93.86 Other injury due to other accident on board (nonpowered)** inflatable craft

✓x7th **V93.87 Other injury due to other accident on board** water-skis
Hit or struck by object while waterskiing

✓x7th **V93.88 Other injury due to other accident on board** other unpowered **watercraft**
Hit or struck by object while surfing
Hit or struck by object while on board windsurfer

✓x7th **V93.89 Other injury due to other accident on board** unspecified **watercraft**
Other injury due to other accident on board boat NOS
Other injury due to other accident on board ship NOS
Other injury due to other accident on board watercraft NOS

✓4th **V94 Other and unspecified water transport accidents**
EXCLUDES 1 *military watercraft accidents in military or war operations (Y36, Y37)*

✓x7th **V94.0 Hitting object or bottom of body of water due to fall from watercraft**
EXCLUDES 2 *drowning and submersion due to fall from watercraft (V92.0-)*

✓5th **V94.1 Bather struck by watercraft**
Swimmer hit by watercraft

✓x7th **V94.11 Bather struck by** powered **watercraft**

✓x7th **V94.12 Bather struck by** nonpowered **watercraft**

✓5th **V94.2 Rider of nonpowered watercraft struck by other watercraft**

✓x7th **V94.21 Rider of nonpowered watercraft struck by** other nonpowered **watercraft**
Canoer hit by other nonpowered watercraft
Surfer hit by other nonpowered watercraft
Windsurfer hit by other nonpowered watercraft

✓x7th **V94.22 Rider of nonpowered watercraft struck by** powered **watercraft**
Canoer hit by motorboat
Surfer hit by motorboat
Windsurfer hit by motorboat

✓5th **V94.3 Injury to rider of (inflatable) watercraft being pulled behind other watercraft**

✓x7th **V94.31 Injury to rider of (inflatable)** recreational **watercraft being pulled behind other watercraft**
Injury to rider of inner-tube pulled behind motor boat

✓x7th **V94.32 Injury to rider of** non-recreational **watercraft being pulled behind other watercraft**
Injury to occupant of dingy being pulled behind boat or ship
Injury to occupant of life-raft being pulled behind boat or ship

✓x7th **V94.4 Injury to barefoot water-skier**
Injury to person being pulled behind boat or ship

✓5th **V94.8 Other water transport accident**

✓6th **V94.81 Water transport accident involving military watercraft**

✓7th **V94.810 Civilian watercraft involved in water transport accident with military watercraft**
Passenger on civilian watercraft injured due to accident with military watercraft

☑7ᵗʰ **V94.811**   Civilian in water injured by military watercraft

☑7ᵗʰ **V94.818**   Other water transport accident involving military watercraft

✓x7ᵗʰ **V94.89**   Other water transport accident

✓x7ᵗʰ **V94.9**   Unspecified water transport accident
Water transport accident NOS

### Air and space transport accidents (V95-V97)

EXCLUDES 1   *military aircraft accidents in military or war operations (Y36, Y37)*

The appropriate 7th character is to be added to each code from categories V95-V97.
A   initial encounter
D   subsequent encounter
S   sequela

✓4ᵗʰ **V95**   Accident to powered aircraft causing injury to occupant

✓5ᵗʰ **V95.0**   Helicopter accident injuring occupant

✓x7ᵗʰ **V95.00**   Unspecified helicopter accident injuring occupant

✓x7ᵗʰ **V95.01**   Helicopter crash injuring occupant

✓x7ᵗʰ **V95.02**   Forced landing of helicopter injuring occupant

✓x7ᵗʰ **V95.03**   Helicopter collision injuring occupant
Helicopter collision with any object, fixed, movable or moving

✓x7ᵗʰ **V95.04**   Helicopter fire injuring occupant

✓x7ᵗʰ **V95.05**   Helicopter explosion injuring occupant

✓x7ᵗʰ **V95.09**   Other helicopter accident injuring occupant

✓5ᵗʰ **V95.1**   Ultralight, microlight or powered-glider accident injuring occupant

✓x7ᵗʰ **V95.10**   Unspecified ultralight, microlight or powered-glider accident injuring occupant

✓x7ᵗʰ **V95.11**   Ultralight, microlight or powered-glider crash injuring occupant

✓x7ᵗʰ **V95.12**   Forced landing of ultralight, microlight or powered-glider injuring occupant

✓x7ᵗʰ **V95.13**   Ultralight, microlight or powered-glider collision injuring occupant
Ultralight, microlight or powered-glider collision with any object, fixed, movable or moving

✓x7ᵗʰ **V95.14**   Ultralight, microlight or powered-glider fire injuring occupant

✓x7ᵗʰ **V95.15**   Ultralight, microlight or powered-glider explosion injuring occupant

✓x7ᵗʰ **V95.19**   Other ultralight, microlight or powered-glider accident injuring occupant

✓5ᵗʰ **V95.2**   Other private fixed-wing aircraft accident injuring occupant

✓x7ᵗʰ **V95.20**   Unspecified accident to other private fixed-wing aircraft, injuring occupant

✓x7ᵗʰ **V95.21**   Other private fixed-wing aircraft crash injuring occupant

✓x7ᵗʰ **V95.22**   Forced landing of other private fixed-wing aircraft injuring occupant

✓x7ᵗʰ **V95.23**   Other private fixed-wing aircraft collision injuring occupant
Other private fixed-wing aircraft collision with any object, fixed, movable or moving

✓x7ᵗʰ **V95.24**   Other private fixed-wing aircraft fire injuring occupant

✓x7ᵗʰ **V95.25**   Other private fixed-wing aircraft explosion injuring occupant

✓x7ᵗʰ **V95.29**   Other accident to other private fixed-wing aircraft injuring occupant

✓5ᵗʰ **V95.3**   Commercial fixed-wing aircraft accident injuring occupant

✓x7ᵗʰ **V95.30**   Unspecified accident to commercial fixed-wing aircraft injuring occupant

✓x7ᵗʰ **V95.31**   Commercial fixed-wing aircraft crash injuring occupant

✓x7ᵗʰ **V95.32**   Forced landing of commercial fixed-wing aircraft injuring occupant

✓x7ᵗʰ **V95.33**   Commercial fixed-wing aircraft collision injuring occupant
Commercial fixed-wing aircraft collision with any object, fixed, movable or moving

✓x7ᵗʰ **V95.34**   Commercial fixed-wing aircraft fire injuring occupant

✓x7ᵗʰ **V95.35**   Commercial fixed-wing aircraft explosion injuring occupant

✓x7ᵗʰ **V95.39**   Other accident to commercial fixed-wing aircraft injuring occupant

✓5ᵗʰ **V95.4**   Spacecraft accident injuring occupant

✓x7ᵗʰ **V95.40**   Unspecified spacecraft accident injuring occupant

✓x7ᵗʰ **V95.41**   Spacecraft crash injuring occupant

✓x7ᵗʰ **V95.42**   Forced landing of spacecraft injuring occupant

✓x7ᵗʰ **V95.43**   Spacecraft collision injuring occupant
Spacecraft collision with any object, fixed, moveable or moving

✓x7ᵗʰ **V95.44**   Spacecraft fire injuring occupant

✓x7ᵗʰ **V95.45**   Spacecraft explosion injuring occupant

✓x7ᵗʰ **V95.49**   Other spacecraft accident injuring occupant

✓x7ᵗʰ **V95.8**   Other powered aircraft accidents injuring occupant

✓x7ᵗʰ **V95.9**   Unspecified aircraft accident injuring occupant
Aircraft accident NOS
Air transport accident NOS

✓4ᵗʰ **V96**   Accident to nonpowered aircraft causing injury to occupant

✓5ᵗʰ **V96.0**   Balloon accident injuring occupant

✓x7ᵗʰ **V96.00**   Unspecified balloon accident injuring occupant

✓x7ᵗʰ **V96.01**   Balloon crash injuring occupant

✓x7ᵗʰ **V96.02**   Forced landing of balloon injuring occupant

✓x7ᵗʰ **V96.03**   Balloon collision injuring occupant
Balloon collision with any object, fixed, moveable or moving

✓x7ᵗʰ **V96.04**   Balloon fire injuring occupant

✓x7ᵗʰ **V96.05**   Balloon explosion injuring occupant

✓x7ᵗʰ **V96.09**   Other balloon accident injuring occupant

✓5ᵗʰ **V96.1**   Hang-glider accident injuring occupant

✓x7ᵗʰ **V96.10**   Unspecified hang-glider accident injuring occupant

✓x7ᵗʰ **V96.11**   Hang-glider crash injuring occupant

✓x7ᵗʰ **V96.12**   Forced landing of hang-glider injuring occupant

✓x7ᵗʰ **V96.13**   Hang-glider collision injuring occupant
Hang-glider collision with any object, fixed, moveable or moving

✓x7ᵗʰ **V96.14**   Hang-glider fire injuring occupant

✓x7ᵗʰ **V96.15**   Hang-glider explosion injuring occupant

✓x7ᵗʰ **V96.19**   Other hang-glider accident injuring occupant

✓5ᵗʰ **V96.2**   Glider (nonpowered) accident injuring occupant

✓x7ᵗʰ **V96.20**   Unspecified glider (nonpowered) accident injuring occupant

✓x7ᵗʰ **V96.21**   Glider (nonpowered) crash injuring occupant

✓x7ᵗʰ **V96.22**   Forced landing of glider (nonpowered) injuring occupant

✓x7ᵗʰ **V96.23**   Glider (nonpowered) collision injuring occupant
Glider (nonpowered) collision with any object, fixed, moveable or moving

✓x7ᵗʰ **V96.24**   Glider (nonpowered) fire injuring occupant

✓x7ᵗʰ **V96.25**   Glider (nonpowered) explosion injuring occupant

✓x7ᵗʰ **V96.29**   Other glider (nonpowered) accident injuring occupant

✓x7ᵗʰ **V96.8**   Other nonpowered-aircraft accidents injuring occupant
Kite carrying a person accident injuring occupant

✓x7ᵗʰ **V96.9**   Unspecified nonpowered-aircraft accident injuring occupant
Nonpowered-aircraft accident NOS

✓4ᵗʰ **V97**   Other specified air transport accidents

✓x7ᵗʰ **V97.0**   Occupant of aircraft injured in other specified air transport accidents
Fall in, on or from aircraft in air transport accident
EXCLUDES 1   *accident while boarding or alighting aircraft (V97.1)*

✓x7ᵗʰ **V97.1**   Person injured while boarding or alighting from aircraft

✓5ᵗʰ **V97.2**   Parachutist accident

✓x7ᵗʰ **V97.21**   Parachutist entangled in object
Parachutist landing in tree

✓x7ᵗʰ **V97.22**   Parachutist injured on landing

✓x7ᵗʰ **V97.29**   Other parachutist accident

☑ Additional Character Req    ✓x7ᵗʰ Placeholder Alert    Unacceptable PDx    Manifestation    **H1**-**H14** HAC    **HCC** CMS-HCC Condition    EXCLUDES 1 Not Coded Here    EXCLUDES 2 Not Included Here

ICD-10-CM 2018        1185

√5ᵗʰ **V97.3 Person on ground injured in air transport accident**

√x7ᵗʰ **V97.31 Hit by object falling from aircraft**
Hit by crashing aircraft
Injured by aircraft hitting house
Injured by aircraft hitting car

√x7ᵗʰ **V97.32 Injured by rotating propeller**

√x7ᵗʰ **V97.33 Sucked into jet engine**

√x7ᵗʰ **V97.39 Other injury to person on ground due to air transport accident**

√5ᵗʰ **V97.8 Other air transport accidents, not elsewhere classified**
EXCLUDES 1 *aircraft accident NOS (V95.9)*
*exposure to changes in air pressure during ascent or descent (W94.-)*

√6ᵗʰ **V97.81 Air transport accident involving military aircraft**

√7ᵗʰ **V97.810 Civilian aircraft involved in air transport accident with military aircraft**
Passenger in civilian aircraft injured due to accident with military aircraft

√7ᵗʰ **V97.811 Civilian injured by military aircraft**

√7ᵗʰ **V97.818 Other air transport accident involving military aircraft**

√x7ᵗʰ **V97.89 Other air transport accidents, not elsewhere classified**
Injury from machinery on aircraft

### Other and unspecified transport accidents (V98-V99)
EXCLUDES 1 *vehicle accident, type of vehicle unspecified (V89.-)*

The appropriate 7th character is to be added to each code from categories V98-V99.
A    initial encounter
D    subsequent encounter
S    sequela

√4ᵗʰ **V98 Other specified transport accidents**

√x7ᵗʰ **V98.0 Accident to, on or involving cable-car, not on rails**
Caught or dragged by cable-car, not on rails
Fall or jump from cable-car, not on rails
Object thrown from or in cable-car, not on rails

√x7ᵗʰ **V98.1 Accident to, on or involving land-yacht**

√x7ᵗʰ **V98.2 Accident to, on or involving ice yacht**

√x7ᵗʰ **V98.3 Accident to, on or involving ski lift**
Accident to, on or involving ski chair-lift
Accident to, on or involving ski-lift with gondola

√x7ᵗʰ **V98.8 Other specified transport accidents**

√x7ᵗʰ **V99 Unspecified transport accident**

## OTHER EXTERNAL CAUSES OF ACCIDENTAL INJURY (W00-X58)

### Slipping, tripping, stumbling and falls (W00-W19)
EXCLUDES 1 *assault involving a fall (Y01-Y02)*
*fall from animal (V80.-)*
*fall (in) (from) machinery (in operation) (W28-W31)*
*fall (in) (from) transport vehicle (V01-V99)*
*intentional self-harm involving a fall (X80-X81)*
EXCLUDES 2 *at risk for fall (history of fall) (Z91.81)*
*fall (in) (from) burning building (X00.-)*
*fall into fire ▶(X00-X04, X08)◄*

The appropriate 7th character is to be added to each code from category W00-W19.
A    initial encounter
D    subsequent encounter
S    sequela

√4ᵗʰ **W00 Fall due to ice and snow**
INCLUDES    pedestrian on foot falling (slipping) on ice and snow
EXCLUDES 1 *fall on (from) ice and snow involving pedestrian conveyance (V00.-)*
*fall from stairs and steps not due to ice and snow (W10.-)*
AHA: 2016, 2Q, 4

√x7ᵗʰ **W00.0 Fall on same level due to ice and snow**

√x7ᵗʰ **W00.1 Fall from stairs and steps due to ice and snow**

√x7ᵗʰ **W00.2 Other fall from one level to another due to ice and snow**

√x7ᵗʰ **W00.9 Unspecified fall due to ice and snow**

√4ᵗʰ **W01 Fall on same level from slipping, tripping and stumbling**
INCLUDES    fall on moving sidewalk
EXCLUDES 1 *fall due to bumping (striking) against object (W18.0-)*
*fall in shower or bathtub (W18.2-)*
*fall on same level NOS (W18.30)*
*fall on same level from slipping, tripping and stumbling due to ice or snow (W00.0)*
*fall off or from toilet (W18.1-)*
*slipping, tripping and stumbling NOS (W18.40)*
*slipping, tripping and stumbling without falling (W18.4-)*

√x7ᵗʰ **W01.0 Fall on same level from slipping, tripping and stumbling without subsequent striking against object**
Falling over animal

√5ᵗʰ **W01.1 Fall on same level from slipping, tripping and stumbling with subsequent striking against object**

√x7ᵗʰ **W01.10 Fall on same level from slipping, tripping and stumbling with subsequent striking against unspecified object**

√6ᵗʰ **W01.11 Fall on same level from slipping, tripping and stumbling with subsequent striking against sharp object**

√7ᵗʰ **W01.110 Fall on same level from slipping, tripping and stumbling with subsequent striking against sharp glass**

√7ᵗʰ **W01.111 Fall on same level from slipping, tripping and stumbling with subsequent striking against power tool or machine**

√7ᵗʰ **W01.118 Fall on same level from slipping, tripping and stumbling with subsequent striking against other sharp object**

√7ᵗʰ **W01.119 Fall on same level from slipping, tripping and stumbling with subsequent striking against unspecified sharp object**

√6ᵗʰ **W01.19 Fall on same level from slipping, tripping and stumbling with subsequent striking against other object**

√7ᵗʰ **W01.190 Fall on same level from slipping, tripping and stumbling with subsequent striking against furniture**

√7ᵗʰ **W01.198 Fall on same level from slipping, tripping and stumbling with subsequent striking against other object**

√x7ᵗʰ **W03 Other fall on same level due to collision with another person**
Fall due to non-transport collision with other person
EXCLUDES 1 *collision with another person without fall (W51)*
*crushed or pushed by a crowd or human stampede (W52)*
*fall involving pedestrian conveyance (V00-V09)*
*fall due to ice or snow (W00)*
*fall on same level NOS (W18.30)*
AHA: 2012, 4Q, 108

√x7ᵗʰ **W04 Fall while being carried or supported by other persons**
Accidentally dropped while being carried

√4ᵗʰ **W05 Fall from non-moving wheelchair, nonmotorized scooter and motorized mobility scooter**
EXCLUDES 1 *fall from moving motorized mobility scooter (V00.831)*
*fall from moving wheelchair (powered) (V00.811)*
*fall from nonmotorized scooter (V00.141)*

√x7ᵗʰ **W05.0 Fall from non-moving wheelchair**

√x7ᵗʰ **W05.1 Fall from non-moving nonmotorized scooter**

√x7ᵗʰ **W05.2 Fall from non-moving motorized mobility scooter**

√x7ᵗʰ **W06 Fall from bed**

√x7ᵗʰ **W07 Fall from chair**

√x7ᵗʰ **W08 Fall from other furniture**

√4ᵗʰ **W09 Fall on and from playground equipment**
EXCLUDES 1 *fall involving recreational machinery (W31)*

√x7ᵗʰ **W09.0 Fall on or from playground slide**

√x7ᵗʰ **W09.1 Fall from playground swing**

√x7ᵗʰ **W09.2 Fall on or from jungle gym**

√x7ᵗʰ **W09.8 Fall on or from other playground equipment**

√4ᵗʰ **W10 Fall on and from stairs and steps**
EXCLUDES 1 *Fall from stairs and steps due to ice and snow (W00.1)*

√x7ᵗʰ **W10.0 Fall (on)(from) escalator**

√x7ᵗʰ **W10.1 Fall (on)(from) sidewalk curb**

√x7ᵗʰ **W10.2 Fall (on)(from) incline**
Fall (on) (from) ramp

√x7ᵗʰ **W10.8 Fall (on) (from) other stairs and steps**

√x7ᵗʰ **W10.9 Fall (on) (from) unspecified stairs and steps**

√x7ᵗʰ **W11 Fall on and from ladder**

√x7ᵗʰ **W12 Fall on and from scaffolding**

√4ᵗʰ **W13 Fall from, out of or through building or structure**

√x7ᵗʰ **W13.0 Fall from, out of or through balcony**
Fall from, out of or through railing

√x7ᵗʰ **W13.1 Fall from, out of or through bridge**

√x7ᵗʰ **W13.2 Fall from, out of or through roof**

√x7ᵗʰ **W13.3 Fall through floor**

√x7ᵗʰ **W13.4 Fall from, out of or through window**
> *EXCLUDES 2*   *fall with subsequent striking against sharp glass (W01.110)*

√x7ᵗʰ **W13.8 Fall from, out of or through other building or structure**
Fall from, out of or through viaduct
Fall from, out of or through wall
Fall from, out of or through flag-pole

√x7ᵗʰ **W13.9 Fall from, out of or through building, not otherwise specified**
> *EXCLUDES 1*   *collapse of a building or structure (W20.-)*
> *fall or jump from burning building or structure (X00.-)*

√x7ᵗʰ **W14 Fall from tree**

√x7ᵗʰ **W15 Fall from cliff**

√4ᵗʰ **W16 Fall, jump or diving into water**
> *EXCLUDES 1*   *accidental non-watercraft drowning and submersion not involving fall (W65-W74)*
> *effects of air pressure from diving (W94.-)*
> *fall into water from watercraft (V90-V94)*
> *hitting an object or against bottom when falling from watercraft (V94.0)*
> *EXCLUDES 2*   *striking or hitting diving board (W21.4)*

√5ᵗʰ **W16.0 Fall into swimming pool**
Fall into swimming pool NOS
> *EXCLUDES 1*   *fall into empty swimming pool (W17.3)*

√6ᵗʰ **W16.01 Fall into swimming pool striking water surface**

√7ᵗʰ **W16.011 Fall into swimming pool striking water surface causing drowning and submersion**
> *EXCLUDES 1*   *drowning and submersion while in swimming pool without fall (W67)*

√7ᵗʰ **W16.012 Fall into swimming pool striking water surface causing other injury**

√6ᵗʰ **W16.02 Fall into swimming pool striking bottom**

√7ᵗʰ **W16.021 Fall into swimming pool striking bottom causing drowning and submersion**
> *EXCLUDES 1*   *drowning and submersion while in swimming pool without fall (W67)*

√7ᵗʰ **W16.022 Fall into swimming pool striking bottom causing other injury**

√6ᵗʰ **W16.03 Fall into swimming pool striking wall**

√7ᵗʰ **W16.031 Fall into swimming pool striking wall causing drowning and submersion**
> *EXCLUDES 1*   *drowning and submersion while in swimming pool without fall (W67)*

√7ᵗʰ **W16.032 Fall into swimming pool striking wall causing other injury**

√5ᵗʰ **W16.1 Fall into natural body of water**
Fall into laker
Fall into open sea
Fall into river
Fall into stream

√6ᵗʰ **W16.11 Fall into natural body of water striking water surface**

√7ᵗʰ **W16.111 Fall into natural body of water striking water surface causing drowning and submersion**
> *EXCLUDES 1*   *drowning and submersion while in natural body of water without fall (W69)*

√7ᵗʰ **W16.112 Fall into natural body of water striking water surface causing other injury**

√6ᵗʰ **W16.12 Fall into natural body of water striking bottom**

√7ᵗʰ **W16.121 Fall into natural body of water striking bottom causing drowning and submersion**
> *EXCLUDES 1*   *drowning and submersion while in natural body of water without fall (W69)*

√7ᵗʰ **W16.122 Fall into natural body of water striking bottom causing other injury**

√6ᵗʰ **W16.13 Fall into natural body of water striking side**

√7ᵗʰ **W16.131 Fall into natural body of water striking side causing drowning and submersion**
> *EXCLUDES 1*   *drowning and submersion while in natural body of water without fall (W69)*

√7ᵗʰ **W16.132 Fall into natural body of water striking side causing other injury**

√5ᵗʰ **W16.2 Fall in (into) filled bathtub or bucket of water**

√6ᵗʰ **W16.21 Fall in (into) filled bathtub**
> *EXCLUDES 1*   *fall into empty bathtub (W18.2)*

√7ᵗʰ **W16.211 Fall in (into) filled bathtub causing drowning and submersion**
> *EXCLUDES 1*   *drowning and submersion while in filled bathtub without fall (W65)*

√7ᵗʰ **W16.212 Fall in (into) filled bathtub causing other injury**

√6ᵗʰ **W16.22 Fall in (into) bucket of water**

√7ᵗʰ **W16.221 Fall in (into) bucket of water causing drowning and submersion**

√7ᵗʰ **W16.222 Fall in (into) bucket of water causing other injury**

√5ᵗʰ **W16.3 Fall into other water**
Fall into fountain
Fall into reservoir

√6ᵗʰ **W16.31 Fall into other water striking water surface**

√7ᵗʰ **W16.311 Fall into other water striking water surface causing drowning and submersion**
> *EXCLUDES 1*   *drowning and submersion while in other water without fall (W73)*

√7ᵗʰ **W16.312 Fall into other water striking water surface causing other injury**

√6ᵗʰ **W16.32 Fall into other water striking bottom**

√7ᵗʰ **W16.321 Fall into other water striking bottom causing drowning and submersion**
> *EXCLUDES 1*   *drowning and submersion while in other water without fall (W73)*

√7ᵗʰ **W16.322 Fall into other water striking bottom causing other injury**

√6ᵗʰ **W16.33 Fall into other water striking wall**

√7ᵗʰ **W16.331 Fall into other water striking wall causing drowning and submersion**
> *EXCLUDES 1*   *drowning and submersion while in other water without fall (W73)*

√7ᵗʰ **W16.332 Fall into other water striking wall causing other injury**

√5ᵗʰ **W16.4 Fall into unspecified water**

√x7ᵗʰ **W16.41 Fall into unspecified water causing drowning and submersion**

√x7ᵗʰ **W16.42 Fall into unspecified water causing other injury**

√5ᵗʰ **W16.5 Jumping or diving into swimming pool**

√6ᵗʰ **W16.51 Jumping or diving into swimming pool striking water surface**

√7ᵗʰ **W16.511 Jumping or diving into swimming pool striking water surface causing drowning and submersion**
> *EXCLUDES 1*   *drowning and submersion while in swimming pool without jumping or diving (W67)*

√7ᵗʰ **W16.512 Jumping or diving into swimming pool striking water surface causing other injury**

✓ Additional Character Req   √x7ᵗʰ Placeholder Alert   Unacceptable PDx   Manifestation   **H1**–**H14** HAC   **HCC** CMS-HCC Condition   *EXCLUDES 1* Not Coded Here   *EXCLUDES 2* Not Included Here

ICD-10-CM 2018      1187

Chapter 20. External Causes of Morbidity

W10.8–W16.512

✓6ᵗʰ **W16.52 Jumping or diving into swimming pool striking bottom**

     ✓7ᵗʰ **W16.521 Jumping or diving into swimming pool striking bottom causing drowning and submersion**

         **EXCLUDES 1** *drowning and submersion while in swimming pool without jumping or diving (W67)*

     ✓7ᵗʰ **W16.522 Jumping or diving into swimming pool striking bottom causing other injury**

✓6ᵗʰ **W16.53 Jumping or diving into swimming pool striking wall**

     ✓7ᵗʰ **W16.531 Jumping or diving into swimming pool striking wall causing drowning and submersion**

         **EXCLUDES 1** *drowning and submersion while in swimming pool without jumping or diving (W67)*

     ✓7ᵗʰ **W16.532 Jumping or diving into swimming pool striking wall causing other injury**

✓5ᵗʰ **W16.6 Jumping or diving into natural body of water**

     Jumping or diving into lake
     Jumping or diving into open sea
     Jumping or diving into river
     Jumping or diving into stream

     ✓6ᵗʰ **W16.61 Jumping or diving into natural body of water striking water surface**

         ✓7ᵗʰ **W16.611 Jumping or diving into natural body of water striking water surface causing drowning and submersion**

             **EXCLUDES 1** *drowning and submersion while in natural body of water without jumping or diving (W69)*

         ✓7ᵗʰ **W16.612 Jumping or diving into natural body of water striking water surface causing other injury**

     ✓6ᵗʰ **W16.62 Jumping or diving into natural body of water striking bottom**

         ✓7ᵗʰ **W16.621 Jumping or diving into natural body of water striking bottom causing drowning and submersion**

             **EXCLUDES 1** *drowning and submersion while in natural body of water without jumping or diving (W69)*

         ✓7ᵗʰ **W16.622 Jumping or diving into natural body of water striking bottom causing other injury**

✓5ᵗʰ **W16.7 Jumping or diving from boat**

     **EXCLUDES 1** *fall from boat into water—see watercraft accident (V90-V94)*

     ✓6ᵗʰ **W16.71 Jumping or diving from boat striking water surface**

         ✓7ᵗʰ **W16.711 Jumping or diving from boat striking water surface causing drowning and submersion**

         ✓7ᵗʰ **W16.712 Jumping or diving from boat striking water surface causing other injury**

     ✓6ᵗʰ **W16.72 Jumping or diving from boat striking bottom**

         ✓7ᵗʰ **W16.721 Jumping or diving from boat striking bottom causing drowning and submersion**

         ✓7ᵗʰ **W16.722 Jumping or diving from boat striking bottom causing other injury**

✓5ᵗʰ **W16.8 Jumping or diving into other water**

     Jumping or diving into fountain
     Jumping or diving into reservoir

     ✓6ᵗʰ **W16.81 Jumping or diving into other water striking water surface**

         ✓7ᵗʰ **W16.811 Jumping or diving into other water striking water surface causing drowning and submersion**

             **EXCLUDES 1** *drowning and submersion while in other water without jumping or diving (W73)*

         ✓7ᵗʰ **W16.812 Jumping or diving into other water striking water surface causing other injury**

✓6ᵗʰ **W16.82 Jumping or diving into other water striking bottom**

     ✓7ᵗʰ **W16.821 Jumping or diving into other water striking bottom causing drowning and submersion**

         **EXCLUDES 1** *drowning and submersion while in other water without jumping or diving (W73)*

     ✓7ᵗʰ **W16.822 Jumping or diving into other water striking bottom causing other injury**

✓6ᵗʰ **W16.83 Jumping or diving into other water striking wall**

     ✓7ᵗʰ **W16.831 Jumping or diving into other water striking wall causing drowning and submersion**

         **EXCLUDES 1** *drowning and submersion while in other water without jumping or diving (W73)*

     ✓7ᵗʰ **W16.832 Jumping or diving into other water striking wall causing other injury**

✓5ᵗʰ **W16.9 Jumping or diving into unspecified water**

     ✓x7ᵗʰ **W16.91 Jumping or diving into unspecified water causing drowning and submersion**

     ✓x7ᵗʰ **W16.92 Jumping or diving into unspecified water causing other injury**

✓4ᵗʰ **W17 Other fall from one level to another**

     ✓x7ᵗʰ **W17.0 Fall into well**

     ✓x7ᵗʰ **W17.1 Fall into storm drain or manhole**

     ✓x7ᵗʰ **W17.2 Fall into hole**

         Fall into pit

     ✓x7ᵗʰ **W17.3 Fall into empty swimming pool**

         **EXCLUDES 1** *fall into filled swimming pool (W16.0-)*

     ✓x7ᵗʰ **W17.4 Fall from dock**

     ✓5ᵗʰ **W17.8 Other fall from one level to another**

         ✓x7ᵗʰ **W17.81 Fall down embankment (hill)**

         ✓x7ᵗʰ **W17.82 Fall from (out of) grocery cart**

             Fall due to grocery cart tipping over

         ✓x7ᵗʰ **W17.89 Other fall from one level to another**

             Fall from cherry picker
             Fall from lifting device
             Fall from mobile elevated work platform [MEWP]
             Fall from sky lift
             **AHA:** 2015, 2Q, 6

✓4ᵗʰ **W18 Other slipping, tripping and stumbling and falls**

     ✓5ᵗʰ **W18.0 Fall due to bumping against object**

         Striking against object with subsequent fall

         **EXCLUDES 1** *fall on same level due to slipping, tripping, or stumbling with subsequent striking against object (W01.1-)*

         ✓x7ᵗʰ **W18.00 Striking against unspecified object with subsequent fall**

         ✓x7ᵗʰ **W18.01 Striking against sports equipment with subsequent fall**

         ✓x7ᵗʰ **W18.02 Striking against glass with subsequent fall**

         ✓x7ᵗʰ **W18.09 Striking against other object with subsequent fall**

     ✓5ᵗʰ **W18.1 Fall from or off toilet**

         ✓x7ᵗʰ **W18.11 Fall from or off toilet without subsequent striking against object**

             Fall from (off) toilet NOS

         ✓x7ᵗʰ **W18.12 Fall from or off toilet with subsequent striking against object**

     ✓x7ᵗʰ **W18.2 Fall in (into) shower or empty bathtub**

         **EXCLUDES 1** *fall in full bathtub causing drowning or submersion (W16.21-)*

     ✓5ᵗʰ **W18.3 Other and unspecified fall on same level**

         ✓x7ᵗʰ **W18.30 Fall on same level, unspecified**

         ✓x7ᵗʰ **W18.31 Fall on same level due to stepping on an object**

             Fall on same level due to stepping on an animal

             **EXCLUDES 1** *slipping, tripping and stumbling without fall due to stepping on animal (W18.41)*

         ✓x7ᵗʰ **W18.39 Other fall on same level**

     ✓5ᵗʰ **W18.4 Slipping, tripping and stumbling without falling**

         **EXCLUDES 1** *collision with another person without fall (W51)*

         ✓x7ᵗʰ **W18.40 Slipping, tripping and stumbling without falling, unspecified**

---

N Newborn: 0    P Pediatric: 0-17    M Maternity: 12-55    A Adult: 15-124    **MCC** Major CC Condition    **PDxMCC** PDx acts as own MCC    **CC** CC Condition    **PDxCC** PDx acts as own CC

**1188**          ICD-10-CM 2018

✓x7ᵗʰ **W18.41** **Slipping, tripping and stumbling without falling due to stepping on object**
Slipping, tripping and stumbling without falling due to stepping on animal
*EXCLUDES 1*   *slipping, tripping and stumbling with fall due to stepping on animal (W18.31)*

✓x7ᵗʰ **W18.42** **Slipping, tripping and stumbling without falling due to stepping into hole or opening**

✓x7ᵗʰ **W18.43** **Slipping, tripping and stumbling without falling due to stepping from one level to another**

✓x7ᵗʰ **W18.49** **Other slipping, tripping and stumbling without falling**

✓x7ᵗʰ **W19 Unspecified fall**
Accidental fall NOS
**AHA:** 2012, 4Q, 95

### Exposure to inanimate mechanical forces (W20-W49)

*EXCLUDES 1*   *assault (X92-Y09)*
*contact or collision with animals or persons (W50-W64)*
*exposure to inanimate mechanical forces involving military or war operations (Y36.-, Y37.-)*
*intentional self-harm (X71-X83)*

The appropriate 7th character is to be added to each code from categories W20-W49.
A    initial encounter
D    subsequent encounter
S    sequela

✓4ᵗʰ **W20 Struck by thrown, projected or falling object**
Code first any associated:
   cataclysm (X34-X39)
   lightning strike (T75.00)
*EXCLUDES 1*   *falling object in machinery accident (W24, W28-W31)*
*falling object in transport accident (V01-V99)*
*object set in motion by explosion (W35-W40)*
*object set in motion by firearm (W32-W34)*
*struck by thrown sports equipment (W21.-)*

✓x7ᵗʰ **W20.0** **Struck by falling object in cave-in**
*EXCLUDES 2*   *asphyxiation due to cave-in (T71.21)*

✓x7ᵗʰ **W20.1** **Struck by object due to collapse of building**
*EXCLUDES 1*   *struck by object due to collapse of burning building (X00.2, X02.2)*

✓x7ᵗʰ **W20.8** **Other cause of strike by thrown, projected or falling object**
*EXCLUDES 1*   *struck by thrown sports equipment (W21.-)*

✓4ᵗʰ **W21 Striking against or struck by sports equipment**
*EXCLUDES 1*   *assault with sports equipment (Y08.0-)*
*striking against or struck by sports equipment with subsequent fall (W18.01)*

✓5ᵗʰ **W21.0** **Struck by hit or thrown ball**
   ✓x7ᵗʰ **W21.00** **Struck by hit or thrown ball, unspecified type**
   ✓x7ᵗʰ **W21.01** **Struck by football**
   ✓x7ᵗʰ **W21.02** **Struck by soccer ball**
   ✓x7ᵗʰ **W21.03** **Struck by baseball**
   ✓x7ᵗʰ **W21.04** **Struck by golf ball**
   ✓x7ᵗʰ **W21.05** **Struck by basketball**
   ✓x7ᵗʰ **W21.06** **Struck by volleyball**
   ✓x7ᵗʰ **W21.07** **Struck by softball**
   ✓x7ᵗʰ **W21.09** **Struck by other hit or thrown ball**

✓5ᵗʰ **W21.1** **Struck by bat, racquet or club**
   ✓x7ᵗʰ **W21.11** **Struck by baseball bat**
   ✓x7ᵗʰ **W21.12** **Struck by tennis racquet**
   ✓x7ᵗʰ **W21.13** **Struck by golf club**
   ✓x7ᵗʰ **W21.19** **Struck by other bat, racquet or club**

✓5ᵗʰ **W21.2** **Struck by hockey stick or puck**
   ✓6ᵗʰ **W21.21** **Struck by hockey stick**
     ✓7ᵗʰ **W21.210** **Struck by ice hockey stick**
     ✓7ᵗʰ **W21.211** **Struck by field hockey stick**
   ✓6ᵗʰ **W21.22** **Struck by hockey puck**
     ✓7ᵗʰ **W21.220** **Struck by ice hockey puck**
     ✓7ᵗʰ **W21.221** **Struck by field hockey puck**

✓5ᵗʰ **W21.3** **Struck by sports foot wear**
   ✓x7ᵗʰ **W21.31** **Struck by shoe cleats**
     Stepped on by shoe cleats

✓x7ᵗʰ **W21.32** **Struck by skate blades**
     Skated over by skate blades

✓x7ᵗʰ **W21.39** **Struck by other sports foot wear**

✓x7ᵗʰ **W21.4** **Striking against diving board**
Use additional code for subsequent falling into water, if applicable (W16.-)

✓5ᵗʰ **W21.8** **Striking against or struck by other sports equipment**
   ✓x7ᵗʰ **W21.81** **Striking against or struck by football helmet**
   ✓x7ᵗʰ **W21.89** **Striking against or struck by other sports equipment**

✓x7ᵗʰ **W21.9** **Striking against or struck by unspecified sports equipment**

✓4ᵗʰ **W22 Striking against or struck by other objects**
*EXCLUDES 1*   *striking against or struck by object with subsequent fall (W18.09)*

✓5ᵗʰ **W22.0** **Striking against stationary object**
*EXCLUDES 1*   *striking against stationary sports equipment (W21.8)*
   ✓x7ᵗʰ **W22.01** **Walked into wall**
   ✓x7ᵗʰ **W22.02** **Walked into lamppost**
   ✓x7ᵗʰ **W22.03** **Walked into furniture**
   ✓6ᵗʰ **W22.04** **Striking against wall of swimming pool**
     ✓7ᵗʰ **W22.041** **Striking against wall of swimming pool causing drowning and submersion**
       *EXCLUDES 1*   *drowning and submersion while swimming without striking against wall (W67)*
     ✓7ᵗʰ **W22.042** **Striking against wall of swimming pool causing other injury**
   ✓x7ᵗʰ **W22.09** **Striking against other stationary object**

✓5ᵗʰ **W22.1** **Striking against or struck by automobile airbag**
   ✓x7ᵗʰ **W22.10** **Striking against or struck by unspecified automobile airbag**
   ✓x7ᵗʰ **W22.11** **Striking against or struck by driver side automobile airbag**
   ✓x7ᵗʰ **W22.12** **Striking against or struck by front passenger side automobile airbag**
   ✓x7ᵗʰ **W22.19** **Striking against or struck by other automobile airbag**

✓x7ᵗʰ **W22.8** **Striking against or struck by other objects**
Striking against or struck by object NOS
*EXCLUDES 1*   *struck by thrown, projected or falling object (W20.-)*

✓4ᵗʰ **W23 Caught, crushed, jammed or pinched in or between objects**
*EXCLUDES 1*   *injury caused by cutting or piercing instruments (W25-W27)*
*injury caused by firearms malfunction (W32.1, W33.1-, W34.1-)*
*injury caused by lifting and transmission devices (W24.-)*
*injury caused by machinery (W28-W31)*
*injury caused by nonpowered hand tools (W27.-)*
*injury caused by transport vehicle being used as a means of transportation (V01-V99)*
*injury caused by struck by thrown, projected or falling object (W20.-)*

✓x7ᵗʰ **W23.0** **Caught, crushed, jammed, or pinched between moving objects**

✓x7ᵗʰ **W23.1** **Caught, crushed, jammed, or pinched between stationary objects**

✓4ᵗʰ **W24 Contact with lifting and transmission devices, not elsewhere classified**
*EXCLUDES 1*   *transport accidents (V01-V99)*

✓x7ᵗʰ **W24.0** **Contact with lifting devices, not elsewhere classified**
Contact with chain hoist
Contact with drive belt
Contact with pulley (block)

✓x7ᵗʰ **W24.1** **Contact with transmission devices, not elsewhere classified**
Contact with transmission belt or cable

✓x7ᵗʰ **W25 Contact with sharp glass**
Code first any associated:
   injury due to flying glass from explosion or firearm discharge (W32-W40)
   transport accident (V00-V99)
*EXCLUDES 1*   *fall on same level due to slipping, tripping and stumbling with subsequent striking against sharp glass (W01.10)*
*striking against sharp glass with subsequent fall (W18.02)*
*EXCLUDES 2*   *glass embedded in skin (W45)*

**Chapter 20. External Causes of Morbidity**

**W26–W31.9**

✓4th **W26 Contact with other sharp objects**
> EXCLUDES 2   sharp object(s) embedded in skin (W45)

✓x7th **W26.0 Contact with knife**
> EXCLUDES 1   contact with electric knife (W29.1)

✓x7th **W26.1 Contact with sword or dagger**

✓x7th **W26.2 Contact with edge of stiff paper**
> Paper cut

✓x7th **W26.8 Contact with other sharp object(s), not elsewhere classified**
> Contact with tin can lid

✓x7th **W26.9 Contact with unspecified sharp object(s)**

✓4th **W27 Contact with nonpowered hand tool**

✓x7th **W27.0 Contact with workbench tool**
> Contact with auger       Contact with handsaw
> Contact with axe       Contact with screwdriver
> Contact with chisel

✓x7th **W27.1 Contact with garden tool**
> Contact with hoe
> Contact with nonpowered lawn mower
> Contact with pitchfork
> Contact with rake

✓x7th **W27.2 Contact with scissors**

✓x7th **W27.3 Contact with needle (sewing)**
> EXCLUDES 1   contact with hypodermic needle (W46.-)

✓x7th **W27.4 Contact with kitchen utensil**
> Contact with fork
> Contact with ice-pick
> Contact with can-opener NOS

✓x7th **W27.5 Contact with paper-cutter**

✓x7th **W27.8 Contact with other nonpowered hand tool**
> Contact with nonpowered sewing machine
> Contact with shovel

✓x7th **W28 Contact with powered lawn mower**
> Powered lawn mower (commercial) (residential)
> EXCLUDES 1   contact with nonpowered lawn mower (W27.1)
> EXCLUDES 2   exposure to electric current (W86.-)

✓4th **W29 Contact with other powered hand tools and household machinery**
> EXCLUDES 1   contact with commercial machinery (W31.82)
> contact with hot household appliance (X15)
> contact with nonpowered hand tool (W27.-)
> exposure to electric current (W86)

✓x7th **W29.0 Contact with powered kitchen appliance**
> Contact with blender       Contact with garbage disposal
> Contact with can-opener       Contact with mixer

✓x7th **W29.1 Contact with electric knife**

✓x7th **W29.2 Contact with other powered household machinery**
> Contact with electric fan
> Contact with powered dryer (clothes) (powered) (spin)
> Contact with washing-machine
> Contact with sewing machine

✓x7th **W29.3 Contact with powered garden and outdoor hand tools and machinery**
> Contact with chainsaw
> Contact with edger
> Contact with garden cultivator (tiller)
> Contact with hedge trimmer
> Contact with other powered garden tool
> EXCLUDES 1   contact with powered lawn mower (W28)

✓x7th **W29.4 Contact with nail gun**

▲ ✓x7th **W29.8 Contact with other powered hand tools and household machinery**
> Contact with do-it-yourself tool NOS

✓4th **W30 Contact with agricultural machinery**
> INCLUDES   animal-powered farm machine
> EXCLUDES 1   agricultural transport vehicle accident (V01-V99)
> explosion of grain store (W40.8)
> exposure to electric current (W86.-)

✓x7th **W30.0 Contact with combine harvester**
> Contact with reaper       Contact with thresher

✓x7th **W30.1 Contact with power take-off devices (PTO)**

✓x7th **W30.2 Contact with hay derrick**

✓x7th **W30.3 Contact with grain storage elevator**
> EXCLUDES 1   explosion of grain store (W40.8)

✓5th **W30.8 Contact with other specified agricultural machinery**

✓x7th **W30.81 Contact with agricultural transport vehicle in stationary use**
> Contact with agricultural transport vehicle under repair, not on public roadway
> EXCLUDES 1   agricultural transport vehicle accident (V01-V99)

✓x7th **W30.89 Contact with other specified agricultural machinery**

✓x7th **W30.9 Contact with unspecified agricultural machinery**
> Contact with farm machinery NOS

✓4th **W31 Contact with other and unspecified machinery**
> EXCLUDES 1   contact with agricultural machinery (W30.-)
> contact with machinery in transport under own power or being towed by a vehicle (V01-V99)
> exposure to electric current (W86)

✓x7th **W31.0 Contact with mining and earth-drilling machinery**
> Contact with bore or drill (land) (seabed)
> Contact with shaft hoist
> Contact with shaft lift
> Contact with undercutter

✓x7th **W31.1 Contact with metalworking machines**
> Contact with abrasive wheel
> Contact with forging machine
> Contact with lathe
> Contact with mechanical shears
> Contact with metal drilling machine
> Contact with milling machine
> Contact with power press
> Contact with rolling-mill
> Contact with metal sawing machine

✓x7th **W31.2 Contact with powered woodworking and forming machines**
> Contact with band saw       Contact with overhead plane
> Contact with bench saw       Contact with powered saw
> Contact with circular saw       Contact with radial saw
> Contact with molding machine     Contact with sander
> EXCLUDES 1   nonpowered woodworking tools (W27.0)

✓x7th **W31.3 Contact with prime movers**
> Contact with gas turbine
> Contact with internal combustion engine
> Contact with steam engine
> Contact with water driven turbine

✓5th **W31.8 Contact with other specified machinery**

✓x7th **W31.81 Contact with recreational machinery**
> Contact with roller coaster

✓x7th **W31.82 Contact with other commercial machinery**
> Contact with commercial electric fan
> Contact with commercial kitchen appliances
> Contact with commercial powered dryer (clothes) (powered) (spin)
> Contact with commercial washing-machine
> Contact with commercial sewing machine
> EXCLUDES 1   contact with household machinery (W29.-)
> contact with powered lawn mower (W28)

✓x7th **W31.83 Contact with special construction vehicle in stationary use**
> Contact with special construction vehicle under repair, not on public roadway
> EXCLUDES 1   special construction vehicle accident (V01-V99)

✓x7th **W31.89 Contact with other specified machinery**

✓x7th **W31.9 Contact with unspecified machinery**
> Contact with machinery NOS

N Newborn: 0   P Pediatric: 0-17   M Maternity: 12-55   A Adult: 15-124   MCC Major CC Condition   PDxMCC PDx acts as own MCC   CC CC Condition   PDxCC PDx acts as own CC

1190                                                            ICD-10-CM 2018

☑4ᵗʰ **W32　Accidental handgun discharge and malfunction**
　　INCLUDES　accidental discharge and malfunction of gun for single hand use
　　　　　　accidental discharge and malfunction of pistol
　　　　　　accidental discharge and malfunction of revolver
　　　　　　handgun discharge and malfunction NOS
　　EXCLUDES 1　*accidental airgun discharge and malfunction (W34.010, W34.110)*
　　　　　　*accidental BB gun discharge and malfunction (W34.010, W34.110)*
　　　　　　*accidental pellet gun discharge and malfunction (W34.010, W34.110)*
　　　　　　*accidental shotgun discharge and malfunction (W33.01, W33.11)*
　　　　　　*assault by handgun discharge (X93)*
　　　　　　*handgun discharge involving legal intervention (Y35.0-)*
　　　　　　*handgun discharge involving military or war operations (Y36.4-)*
　　　　　　*intentional self-harm by handgun discharge (X72)*
　　　　　　*Very pistol discharge and malfunction (W34.09, W34.19)*

☑x7ᵗʰ **W32.0　Accidental handgun discharge**

☑x7ᵗʰ **W32.1　Accidental handgun malfunction**
　　　　Injury due to explosion of handgun (parts)
　　　　Injury due to malfunction of mechanism or component of handgun
　　　　Injury due to recoil of handgun
　　　　Powder burn from handgun

☑4ᵗʰ **W33　Accidental rifle, shotgun and larger firearm discharge and malfunction**
　　INCLUDES　rifle, shotgun and larger firearm discharge and malfunction NOS
　　EXCLUDES 1　*accidental airgun discharge and malfunction (W34.010, W34.110)*
　　　　　　*accidental BB gun discharge and malfunction (W34.010, W34.110)*
　　　　　　*accidental handgun discharge and malfunction (W32.-)*
　　　　　　*accidental pellet gun discharge and malfunction (W34.010, W34.110)*
　　　　　　*assault by rifle, shotgun and larger firearm discharge (X94)*
　　　　　　*firearm discharge involving legal intervention (Y35.0-)*
　　　　　　*firearm discharge involving military or war operations (Y36.4-)*
　　　　　　*intentional self-harm by rifle, shotgun and larger firearm discharge (X73)*

☑5ᵗʰ **W33.0　Accidental rifle, shotgun and larger firearm discharge**

☑x7ᵗʰ **W33.00　Accidental discharge of unspecified larger firearm**
　　　　Discharge of unspecified larger firearm NOS

☑x7ᵗʰ **W33.01　Accidental discharge of shotgun**
　　　　Discharge of shotgun NOS

☑x7ᵗʰ **W33.02　Accidental discharge of hunting rifle**
　　　　Discharge of hunting rifle NOS

☑x7ᵗʰ **W33.03　Accidental discharge of machine gun**
　　　　Discharge of machine gun NOS

☑x7ᵗʰ **W33.09　Accidental discharge of other larger firearm**
　　　　Discharge of other larger firearm NOS

☑5ᵗʰ **W33.1　Accidental rifle, shotgun and larger firearm malfunction**
　　　　Injury due to explosion of rifle, shotgun and larger firearm (parts)
　　　　Injury due to malfunction of mechanism or component of rifle, shotgun and larger firearm
　　　　Injury due to piercing, cutting, crushing or pinching due to (by) slide trigger mechanism, scope or other gun part
　　　　Injury due to recoil of rifle, shotgun and larger firearm
　　　　Powder burn from rifle, shotgun and larger firearm

☑x7ᵗʰ **W33.10　Accidental malfunction of unspecified larger firearm**
　　　　Malfunction of unspecified larger firearm NOS

☑x7ᵗʰ **W33.11　Accidental malfunction of shotgun**
　　　　Malfunction of shotgun NOS

☑x7ᵗʰ **W33.12　Accidental malfunction of hunting rifle**
　　　　Malfunction of hunting rifle NOS

☑x7ᵗʰ **W33.13　Accidental malfunction of machine gun**
　　　　Malfunction of machine gun NOS

☑x7ᵗʰ **W33.19　Accidental malfunction of other larger firearm**
　　　　Malfunction of other larger firearm NOS

☑4ᵗʰ **W34　Accidental discharge and malfunction from other and unspecified firearms and guns**

☑5ᵗʰ **W34.0　Accidental discharge from other and unspecified firearms and guns**

☑x7ᵗʰ **W34.00　Accidental discharge from unspecified firearms or gun**
　　　　Discharge from firearm NOS
　　　　Gunshot wound NOS
　　　　Shot NOS

☑6ᵗʰ **W34.01　Accidental discharge of gas, air or spring-operated guns**

☑7ᵗʰ **W34.010　Accidental discharge of airgun**
　　　　Accidental discharge of BB gun
　　　　Accidental discharge of pellet gun

☑7ᵗʰ **W34.011　Accidental discharge of paintball gun**
　　　　Accidental injury due to paintball discharge

☑7ᵗʰ **W34.018　Accidental discharge of other gas, air or spring-operated gun**

☑x7ᵗʰ **W34.09　Accidental discharge from other specified firearms**
　　　　Accidental discharge from Very pistol [flare]

☑5ᵗʰ **W34.1　Accidental malfunction from other and unspecified firearms and guns**

☑x7ᵗʰ **W34.10　Accidental malfunction from unspecified firearms or gun**
　　　　Firearm malfunction NOS

☑6ᵗʰ **W34.11　Accidental malfunction of gas, air or spring-operated guns**

☑7ᵗʰ **W34.110　Accidental malfunction of airgun**
　　　　Accidental malfunction of BB gun
　　　　Accidental malfunction of pellet gun

☑7ᵗʰ **W34.111　Accidental malfunction of paintball gun**
　　　　Accidental injury due to paintball gun malfunction

☑7ᵗʰ **W34.118　Accidental malfunction of other gas, air or spring-operated gun**

☑x7ᵗʰ **W34.19　Accidental malfunction from other specified firearms**
　　　　Accidental malfunction from Very pistol [flare]

☑x7ᵗʰ **W35　Explosion and rupture of boiler**
　　EXCLUDES 1　*explosion and rupture of boiler on watercraft (V93.4)*

☑4ᵗʰ **W36　Explosion and rupture of gas cylinder**

☑x7ᵗʰ **W36.1　Explosion and rupture of aerosol can**

☑x7ᵗʰ **W36.2　Explosion and rupture of air tank**

☑x7ᵗʰ **W36.3　Explosion and rupture of pressurized-gas tank**

☑x7ᵗʰ **W36.8　Explosion and rupture of other gas cylinder**

☑x7ᵗʰ **W36.9　Explosion and rupture of unspecified gas cylinder**

☑4ᵗʰ **W37　Explosion and rupture of pressurized tire, pipe or hose**

☑x7ᵗʰ **W37.0　Explosion of bicycle tire**

☑x7ᵗʰ **W37.8　Explosion and rupture of other pressurized tire, pipe or hose**

☑x7ᵗʰ **W38　Explosion and rupture of other specified pressurized devices**

☑x7ᵗʰ **W39　Discharge of firework**

☑4ᵗʰ **W40　Explosion of other materials**
　　EXCLUDES 1　*assault by explosive material (X96)*
　　　　　　*explosion involving legal intervention (Y35.1-)*
　　　　　　*explosion involving military or war operations (Y36.0-, Y36.2-)*
　　　　　　*intentional self-harm by explosive material (X75)*

☑x7ᵗʰ **W40.0　Explosion of blasting material**
　　　　Explosion of blasting cap
　　　　Explosion of detonator
　　　　Explosion of dynamite
　　　　Explosion of explosive (any) used in blasting operations

☑x7ᵗʰ **W40.1　Explosion of explosive gases**
　　　　Explosion of acetylene　　　　Explosion of fire damp
　　　　Explosion of butane　　　　Explosion of gasoline fumes
　　　　Explosion of coal gas　　　　Explosion of methane
　　　　Explosion in mine NOS　　　　Explosion of propane
　　　　Explosion of explosive gas

☑x7ᵗʰ **W40.8　Explosion of other specified explosive materials**
　　　　Explosion in dump NOS　　　　Explosion in grain store
　　　　Explosion in factory NOS　　　　Explosion in munitions
　　EXCLUDES 1　*explosion involving legal intervention (Y35.1-)*
　　　　　　*explosion involving military or war operations (Y36.0-, Y36.2-)*

☑ Additional Character Req　　☑x7ᵗʰ Placeholder Alert　　Unacceptable PDx　　Manifestation　　H1–H14 HAC　　HCC CMS-HCC Condition　　EXCLUDES 1 Not Coded Here　　EXCLUDES 2 Not Included Here

ICD-10-CM 2018　　　　　　　　　　　　　　　　　　　　　　　　　　　　　　　　　　　　　　1191

✓x7ᵗʰ **W40.9 Explosion of unspecified explosive materials**
Explosion NOS

✓4ᵗʰ **W42 Exposure to noise**

✓x7ᵗʰ **W42.0 Exposure to supersonic waves**

✓x7ᵗʰ **W42.9 Exposure to other noise**
Exposure to sound waves NOS

✓4ᵗʰ **W45 Foreign body or object entering through skin**
INCLUDES  foreign body or object embedded in skin
nail embedded in skin
EXCLUDES 2  *contact with hand tools (nonpowered) (powered) (W27-W29)*
*contact with other sharp object(s) (W26.-)*
*contact with sharp glass (W25.-)*
*struck by objects (W20-W22)*

✓x7ᵗʰ **W45.0 Nail entering through skin**

✓x7ᵗʰ **W45.8 Other foreign body or object entering through skin**
Splinter in skin NOS

✓4ᵗʰ **W46 Contact with hypodermic needle**

✓x7ᵗʰ **W46.0 Contact with hypodermic needle**
Hypodermic needle stick NOS

✓x7ᵗʰ **W46.1 Contact with contaminated hypodermic needle**

✓4ᵗʰ **W49 Exposure to other inanimate mechanical forces**
INCLUDES  exposure to abnormal gravitational [G] forces
exposure to inanimate mechanical forces NEC
EXCLUDES 1  *exposure to inanimate mechanical forces involving military or*
*war operations (Y36.-, Y37.-)*

✓5ᵗʰ **W49.0 Item causing external constriction**

✓x7ᵗʰ **W49.01 Hair causing external constriction**

✓x7ᵗʰ **W49.02 String or thread causing external constriction**

✓x7ᵗʰ **W49.03 Rubber band causing external constriction**

✓x7ᵗʰ **W49.04 Ring or other jewelry causing external constriction**

✓x7ᵗʰ **W49.09 Other specified item causing external constriction**

✓x7ᵗʰ **W49.9 Exposure to other inanimate mechanical forces**

## Exposure to animate mechanical forces (W50-W64)

EXCLUDES 1  *Toxic effect of contact with venomous animals and plants (T63.-)*

The appropriate 7th character is to be added to each code from
categories W50-W64.
A    initial encounter
D    subsequent encounter
S    sequela

✓4ᵗʰ **W50 Accidental hit, strike, kick, twist, bite or scratch by another
person**
INCLUDES  hit, strike, kick, twist, bite, or scratch by another person NOS
EXCLUDES 1  *assault by bodily force (Y04)*
*struck by objects (W20-W22)*

✓x7ᵗʰ **W50.0 Accidental hit or strike by another person**
Hit or strike by another person NOS

✓x7ᵗʰ **W50.1 Accidental kick by another person**
Kick by another person NOS

✓x7ᵗʰ **W50.2 Accidental twist by another person**
Twist by another person NOS

✓x7ᵗʰ **W50.3 Accidental bite by another person**
Human bite                    Bite by another person NOS

✓x7ᵗʰ **W50.4 Accidental scratch by another person**
Scratch by another person NOS

✓x7ᵗʰ **W51 Accidental striking against or bumped into by another person**
EXCLUDES 1  *assault by striking against or bumping into by another person*
*(Y04.2)*
*fall due to collision with another person (W03)*

✓x7ᵗʰ **W52 Crushed, pushed or stepped on by crowd or human stampede**
Crushed, pushed or stepped on by crowd or human stampede with or
without fall

✓4ᵗʰ **W53 Contact with rodent**
INCLUDES  contact with saliva, feces or urine of rodent

✓5ᵗʰ **W53.0 Contact with mouse**

✓x7ᵗʰ **W53.01 Bitten by mouse**

✓x7ᵗʰ **W53.09 Other contact with mouse**

✓5ᵗʰ **W53.1 Contact with rat**

✓x7ᵗʰ **W53.11 Bitten by rat**

✓x7ᵗʰ **W53.19 Other contact with rat**

✓5ᵗʰ **W53.2 Contact with squirrel**

✓x7ᵗʰ **W53.21 Bitten by squirrel**

✓x7ᵗʰ **W53.29 Other contact with squirrel**

✓5ᵗʰ **W53.8 Contact with other rodent**

✓x7ᵗʰ **W53.81 Bitten by other rodent**

✓x7ᵗʰ **W53.89 Other contact with other rodent**

✓4ᵗʰ **W54 Contact with dog**
INCLUDES  contact with saliva, feces or urine of dog

✓x7ᵗʰ **W54.0 Bitten by dog**

✓x7ᵗʰ **W54.1 Struck by dog**
Knocked over by dog

✓x7ᵗʰ **W54.8 Other contact with dog**

✓4ᵗʰ **W55 Contact with other mammals**
INCLUDES  contact with saliva, feces or urine of mammal
EXCLUDES 1  *animal being ridden—see transport accidents*
*bitten or struck by dog (W54)*
*bitten or struck by rodent (W53.-)*
*contact with marine mammals (W56.-)*

✓5ᵗʰ **W55.0 Contact with cat**

✓x7ᵗʰ **W55.01 Bitten by cat**

✓x7ᵗʰ **W55.03 Scratched by cat**

✓x7ᵗʰ **W55.09 Other contact with cat**

✓5ᵗʰ **W55.1 Contact with horse**

✓x7ᵗʰ **W55.11 Bitten by horse**

✓x7ᵗʰ **W55.12 Struck by horse**

✓x7ᵗʰ **W55.19 Other contact with horse**

✓5ᵗʰ **W55.2 Contact with cow**
Contact with bull

✓x7ᵗʰ **W55.21 Bitten by cow**

✓x7ᵗʰ **W55.22 Struck by cow**
Gored by bull

✓x7ᵗʰ **W55.29 Other contact with cow**

✓5ᵗʰ **W55.3 Contact with other hoof stock**
Contact with goats
Contact with sheep

✓x7ᵗʰ **W55.31 Bitten by other hoof stock**

✓x7ᵗʰ **W55.32 Struck by other hoof stock**
Gored by goat
Gored by ram

✓x7ᵗʰ **W55.39 Other contact with other hoof stock**

✓5ᵗʰ **W55.4 Contact with pig**

✓x7ᵗʰ **W55.41 Bitten by pig**

✓x7ᵗʰ **W55.42 Struck by pig**

✓x7ᵗʰ **W55.49 Other contact with pig**

✓5ᵗʰ **W55.5 Contact with raccoon**

✓x7ᵗʰ **W55.51 Bitten by raccoon**

✓x7ᵗʰ **W55.52 Struck by raccoon**

✓x7ᵗʰ **W55.59 Other contact with raccoon**

✓5ᵗʰ **W55.8 Contact with other mammals**

✓x7ᵗʰ **W55.81 Bitten by other mammals**

✓x7ᵗʰ **W55.82 Struck by other mammals**

✓x7ᵗʰ **W55.89 Other contact with other mammals**

✓4ᵗʰ **W56 Contact with nonvenomous marine animal**
EXCLUDES 1  *contact with venomous marine animal (T63.-)*

✓5ᵗʰ **W56.0 Contact with dolphin**

✓x7ᵗʰ **W56.01 Bitten by dolphin**

✓x7ᵗʰ **W56.02 Struck by dolphin**

✓x7ᵗʰ **W56.09 Other contact with dolphin**

✓5ᵗʰ **W56.1 Contact with sea lion**

✓x7ᵗʰ **W56.11 Bitten by sea lion**

✓x7ᵗʰ **W56.12 Struck by sea lion**

✓x7ᵗʰ **W56.19 Other contact with sea lion**

✓5ᵗʰ **W56.2 Contact with orca**
Contact with killer whale

✓x7ᵗʰ **W56.21 Bitten by orca**

✓x7ᵗʰ **W56.22 Struck by orca**

✓x7ᵗʰ **W56.29 Other contact with orca**

✓5ᵗʰ **W56.3 Contact with** other marine mammals
    ✓x7ᵗʰ **W56.31 Bitten by other marine mammals**
    ✓x7ᵗʰ **W56.32 Struck by other marine mammals**
    ✓x7ᵗʰ **W56.39 Other contact with other marine mammals**

✓5ᵗʰ **W56.4 Contact with** shark
    ✓x7ᵗʰ **W56.41 Bitten by shark**
    ✓x7ᵗʰ **W56.42 Struck by shark**
    ✓x7ᵗʰ **W56.49 Other contact with shark**

✓5ᵗʰ **W56.5 Contact with other** fish
    ✓x7ᵗʰ **W56.51 Bitten by other fish**
    ✓x7ᵗʰ **W56.52 Struck by other fish**
    ✓x7ᵗʰ **W56.59 Other contact with other fish**

✓5ᵗʰ **W56.8 Contact with** other nonvenomous marine animals
    ✓x7ᵗʰ **W56.81 Bitten by other nonvenomous marine animals**
    ✓x7ᵗʰ **W56.82 Struck by other nonvenomous marine animals**
    ✓x7ᵗʰ **W56.89 Other contact with other nonvenomous marine animals**

✓x7ᵗʰ **W57 Bitten or stung by nonvenomous insect and other nonvenomous arthropods**
    **EXCLUDES 1** *contact with venomous insects and arthropods (T63.2-, T63.3-, T63.4-)*

✓4ᵗʰ **W58 Contact with crocodile or alligator**
✓5ᵗʰ **W58.0 Contact with** alligator
    ✓x7ᵗʰ **W58.01 Bitten by alligator**
    ✓x7ᵗʰ **W58.02 Struck by alligator**
    ✓x7ᵗʰ **W58.03 Crushed by alligator**
    ✓x7ᵗʰ **W58.09 Other contact with alligator**

✓5ᵗʰ **W58.1 Contact with** crocodile
    ✓x7ᵗʰ **W58.11 Bitten by crocodile**
    ✓x7ᵗʰ **W58.12 Struck by crocodile**
    ✓x7ᵗʰ **W58.13 Crushed by crocodile**
    ✓x7ᵗʰ **W58.19 Other contact with crocodile**

✓4ᵗʰ **W59 Contact with other nonvenomous reptiles**
    **EXCLUDES 1** *contact with venomous reptile (T63.0-, T63.1-)*

✓5ᵗʰ **W59.0 Contact with nonvenomous** lizards
    ✓x7ᵗʰ **W59.01 Bitten by nonvenomous lizards**
    ✓x7ᵗʰ **W59.02 Struck by nonvenomous lizards**
    ✓x7ᵗʰ **W59.09 Other contact with nonvenomous lizards**
      Exposure to nonvenomous lizards

✓5ᵗʰ **W59.1 Contact with nonvenomous** snakes
    ✓x7ᵗʰ **W59.11 Bitten by nonvenomous snake**
    ✓x7ᵗʰ **W59.12 Struck by nonvenomous snake**
    ✓x7ᵗʰ **W59.13 Crushed by nonvenomous snake**
    ✓x7ᵗʰ **W59.19 Other contact with nonvenomous snake**

✓5ᵗʰ **W59.2 Contact with** turtles
    **EXCLUDES 1** *contact with tortoises (W59.8-)*
    ✓x7ᵗʰ **W59.21 Bitten by turtle**
    ✓x7ᵗʰ **W59.22 Struck by turtle**
    ✓x7ᵗʰ **W59.29 Other contact with turtle**
      Exposure to turtles

✓5ᵗʰ **W59.8 Contact with** other nonvenomous reptiles
    ✓x7ᵗʰ **W59.81 Bitten by other nonvenomous reptiles**
    ✓x7ᵗʰ **W59.82 Struck by other nonvenomous reptiles**
    ✓x7ᵗʰ **W59.83 Crushed by other nonvenomous reptiles**
    ✓x7ᵗʰ **W59.89 Other contact with other nonvenomous reptiles**

✓x7ᵗʰ **W60 Contact with nonvenomous plant thorns and spines and sharp leaves**
    **EXCLUDES 1** *contact with venomous plants (T63.7-)*

✓4ᵗʰ **W61 Contact with birds (domestic) (wild)**
    **INCLUDES** contact with excreta of birds
✓5ᵗʰ **W61.0 Contact with** parrot
    ✓x7ᵗʰ **W61.01 Bitten by parrot**
    ✓x7ᵗʰ **W61.02 Struck by parrot**
    ✓x7ᵗʰ **W61.09 Other contact with parrot**
      Exposure to parrots

✓5ᵗʰ **W61.1 Contact with** macaw
    ✓x7ᵗʰ **W61.11 Bitten by macaw**
    ✓x7ᵗʰ **W61.12 Struck by macaw**
    ✓x7ᵗʰ **W61.19 Other contact with macaw**
      Exposure to macaws

✓5ᵗʰ **W61.2 Contact with other** psittacines
    ✓x7ᵗʰ **W61.21 Bitten by other psittacines**
    ✓x7ᵗʰ **W61.22 Struck by other psittacines**
    ✓x7ᵗʰ **W61.29 Other contact with other psittacines**
      Exposure to other psittacines

✓5ᵗʰ **W61.3 Contact with** chicken
    ✓x7ᵗʰ **W61.32 Struck by chicken**
    ✓x7ᵗʰ **W61.33 Pecked by chicken**
    ✓x7ᵗʰ **W61.39 Other contact with chicken**
      Exposure to chickens

✓5ᵗʰ **W61.4 Contact with** turkey
    ✓x7ᵗʰ **W61.42 Struck by turkey**
    ✓x7ᵗʰ **W61.43 Pecked by turkey**
    ✓x7ᵗʰ **W61.49 Other contact with turkey**

✓5ᵗʰ **W61.5 Contact with** goose
    ✓x7ᵗʰ **W61.51 Bitten by goose**
    ✓x7ᵗʰ **W61.52 Struck by goose**
    ✓x7ᵗʰ **W61.59 Other contact with goose**

✓5ᵗʰ **W61.6 Contact with** duck
    ✓x7ᵗʰ **W61.61 Bitten by duck**
    ✓x7ᵗʰ **W61.62 Struck by duck**
    ✓x7ᵗʰ **W61.69 Other contact with duck**

✓5ᵗʰ **W61.9 Contact with** other birds
    ✓x7ᵗʰ **W61.91 Bitten by other birds**
    ✓x7ᵗʰ **W61.92 Struck by other birds**
    ✓x7ᵗʰ **W61.99 Other contact with other birds**
      Contact with bird NOS

✓4ᵗʰ **W62 Contact with nonvenomous amphibians**
    **EXCLUDES 1** *contact with venomous amphibians (T63.81-R63.83)*
    ✓x7ᵗʰ **W62.0 Contact with nonvenomous** frogs
    ✓x7ᵗʰ **W62.1 Contact with nonvenomous** toads
    ✓x7ᵗʰ **W62.9 Contact with other nonvenomous** amphibians

✓x7ᵗʰ **W64 Exposure to other animate mechanical forces**
    **INCLUDES** exposure to nonvenomous animal NOS
    **EXCLUDES 1** *contact with venomous animal (T63.-)*

## Accidental non-transport drowning and submersion (W65-W74)
    **EXCLUDES 1** *accidental drowning and submersion due to fall into water (W16.-)*
      *accidental drowning and submersion due to water transport accident (V90.-, V92.-)*
    **EXCLUDES 2** *accidental drowning and submersion due to cataclysm (X34-X39)*

    The appropriate 7th character is to be added to each code from categories W65-W74.
    A    initial encounter
    D    subsequent encounter
    S    sequela

✓x7ᵗʰ **W65 Accidental drowning and submersion while in** bath-tub
    **EXCLUDES 1** *accidental drowning and submersion due to fall in (into) bathtub (W16.211)*

✓x7ᵗʰ **W67 Accidental drowning and submersion while in** swimming-pool
    **EXCLUDES 1** *accidental drowning and submersion due to fall into swimming pool (W16.011, W16.021, W16.031)*
      *accidental drowning and submersion due to striking into wall of swimming pool (W22.041)*

✓x7ᵗʰ **W69 Accidental drowning and submersion while in** natural water
    Accidental drowning and submersion while in lake
    Accidental drowning and submersion while in open sea
    Accidental drowning and submersion while in river
    Accidental drowning and submersion while in stream
    **EXCLUDES 1** *accidental drowning and submersion due to fall into natural body of water (W16.111, W16.121, W16.131)*

✓ Additional Character Req   ✓x7ᵗʰ Placeholder Alert   Unacceptable PDx   Manifestation   **H1**-**H14** HAC   **HCC** CMS-HCC Condition   **EXCLUDES 1** Not Coded Here   **EXCLUDES 2** Not Included Here

ICD-10-CM 2018      1193

√x7ᵗʰ **W73 Other specified cause of accidental non-transport drowning and submersion**
Accidental drowning and submersion while in quenching tank
Accidental drowning and submersion while in reservoir
**EXCLUDES 1**   *accidental drowning and submersion due to fall into other water (W16.311, W16.321, W16.331)*

√x7ᵗʰ **W74 Unspecified cause of accidental drowning and submersion**
Drowning NOS

## Exposure to electric current, radiation and extreme ambient air temperature and pressure (W85-W99)

**EXCLUDES 1**   *exposure to:*
    *failure in dosage of radiation or temperature during surgical and medical care (Y63.2-Y63.5)*
    *lightning (T75.0-)*
    *natural cold (X31)*
    *natural heat (X30)*
    *natural radiation NOS (X39)*
    *radiological procedure and radiotherapy (Y84.2)*
    *sunlight (X32)*

The appropriate 7th character is to be added to each code from categories W85-W99.
A    initial encounter
D    subsequent encounter
S    sequela

√x7ᵗʰ **W85 Exposure to electric transmission lines**
Broken power line

√4ᵗʰ **W86 Exposure to other specified electric current**
   √x7ᵗʰ **W86.0 Exposure to domestic wiring and appliances**
   √x7ᵗʰ **W86.1 Exposure to industrial wiring, appliances and electrical machinery**
       Exposure to conductors
       Exposure to control apparatus
       Exposure to electrical equipment and machinery
       Exposure to transformers
   √x7ᵗʰ **W86.8 Exposure to other electric current**
       Exposure to wiring and appliances in or on farm (not farmhouse)
       Exposure to wiring and appliances outdoors
       Exposure to wiring and appliances in or on public building
       Exposure to wiring and appliances in or on residential institutions
       Exposure to wiring and appliances in or on schools

√4ᵗʰ **W88 Exposure to ionizing radiation**
   **EXCLUDES 1**   *exposure to sunlight (X32)*
   √x7ᵗʰ **W88.0 Exposure to X-rays**
   √x7ᵗʰ **W88.1 Exposure to radioactive isotopes**
   √x7ᵗʰ **W88.8 Exposure to other ionizing radiation**

√4ᵗʰ **W89 Exposure to man-made visible and ultraviolet light**
   **INCLUDES**   exposure to welding light (arc)
   **EXCLUDES 1**   *exposure to sunlight (X32)*
   √x7ᵗʰ **W89.0 Exposure to welding light (arc)**
   √x7ᵗʰ **W89.1 Exposure to tanning bed**
   √x7ᵗʰ **W89.8 Exposure to other man-made visible and ultraviolet light**
   √x7ᵗʰ **W89.9 Exposure to unspecified man-made visible and ultraviolet light**

√4ᵗʰ **W90 Exposure to other nonionizing radiation**
   **EXCLUDES 1**   *exposure to sunlight (X32)*
   √x7ᵗʰ **W90.0 Exposure to radiofrequency**
   √x7ᵗʰ **W90.1 Exposure to infrared radiation**
   √x7ᵗʰ **W90.2 Exposure to laser radiation**
   √x7ᵗʰ **W90.8 Exposure to other nonionizing radiation**

√x7ᵗʰ **W92 Exposure to excessive heat of man-made origin**

√4ᵗʰ **W93 Exposure to excessive cold of man-made origin**
   √5ᵗʰ **W93.0 Contact with or inhalation of dry ice**
     √x7ᵗʰ **W93.01 Contact with dry ice**
     √x7ᵗʰ **W93.02 Inhalation of dry ice**
   √5ᵗʰ **W93.1 Contact with or inhalation of liquid air**
     √x7ᵗʰ **W93.11 Contact with liquid air**
       Contact with liquid hydrogen
       Contact with liquid nitrogen
     √x7ᵗʰ **W93.12 Inhalation of liquid air**
       Inhalation of liquid hydrogen
       Inhalation of liquid nitrogen

√x7ᵗʰ **W93.2 Prolonged exposure in deep freeze unit or refrigerator**
√x7ᵗʰ **W93.8 Exposure to other excessive cold of man-made origin**

√4ᵗʰ **W94 Exposure to high and low air pressure and changes in air pressure**
   √x7ᵗʰ **W94.0 Exposure to prolonged high air pressure**
   √5ᵗʰ **W94.1 Exposure to prolonged low air pressure**
     √x7ᵗʰ **W94.11 Exposure to residence or prolonged visit at high altitude**
     √x7ᵗʰ **W94.12 Exposure to other prolonged low air pressure**
   √5ᵗʰ **W94.2 Exposure to rapid changes in air pressure during ascent**
     √x7ᵗʰ **W94.21 Exposure to reduction in atmospheric pressure while surfacing from deep-water diving**
     √x7ᵗʰ **W94.22 Exposure to reduction in atmospheric pressure while surfacing from underground**
     √x7ᵗʰ **W94.23 Exposure to sudden change in air pressure in aircraft during ascent**
     √x7ᵗʰ **W94.29 Exposure to other rapid changes in air pressure during ascent**
   √5ᵗʰ **W94.3 Exposure to rapid changes in air pressure during descent**
     √x7ᵗʰ **W94.31 Exposure to sudden change in air pressure in aircraft during descent**
     √x7ᵗʰ **W94.32 Exposure to high air pressure from rapid descent in water**
     √x7ᵗʰ **W94.39 Exposure to other rapid changes in air pressure during descent**

√x7ᵗʰ **W99 Exposure to other man-made environmental factors**

## Exposure to smoke, fire and flames (X00-X08)

**EXCLUDES 1**   *arson (X97)*
**EXCLUDES 2**   *explosions (W35-W40)*
    *lightning (T75.0-)*
    *transport accident (V01-V99)*

The appropriate 7th character is to be added to each code from categories X00-X08.
A    initial encounter
D    subsequent encounter
S    sequela

√4ᵗʰ **X00 Exposure to uncontrolled fire in building or structure**
   **INCLUDES**   conflagration in building or structure
   Code first any associated cataclysm
   **EXCLUDES 2**   *exposure to ignition or melting of nightwear (X05)*
    *exposure to ignition or melting of other clothing and apparel (X06.-)*
    *exposure to other specified smoke, fire and flames (X08.-)*
   **AHA:** 2016, 2Q, 5
   √x7ᵗʰ **X00.0 Exposure to flames in uncontrolled fire in building or structure**
   √x7ᵗʰ **X00.1 Exposure to smoke in uncontrolled fire in building or structure**
   √x7ᵗʰ **X00.2 Injury due to collapse of burning building or structure in uncontrolled fire**
     **EXCLUDES 1**   *injury due to collapse of building not on fire (W20.1)*
   √x7ᵗʰ **X00.3 Fall from burning building or structure in uncontrolled fire**
   √x7ᵗʰ **X00.4 Hit by object from burning building or structure in uncontrolled fire**
     **AHA:** 2016, 2Q, 4
   √x7ᵗʰ **X00.5 Jump from burning building or structure in uncontrolled fire**
   √x7ᵗʰ **X00.8 Other exposure to uncontrolled fire in building or structure**

√4ᵗʰ **X01 Exposure to uncontrolled fire, not in building or structure**
   **INCLUDES**   exposure to forest fire
   √x7ᵗʰ **X01.0 Exposure to flames in uncontrolled fire, not in building or structure**
   √x7ᵗʰ **X01.1 Exposure to smoke in uncontrolled fire, not in building or structure**
   √x7ᵗʰ **X01.3 Fall due to uncontrolled fire, not in building or structure**
   √x7ᵗʰ **X01.4 Hit by object due to uncontrolled fire, not in building or structure**
   √x7ᵗʰ **X01.8 Other exposure to uncontrolled fire, not in building or structure**

☑4th **X02**   **Exposure to controlled fire in building or structure**
    INCLUDES   exposure to fire in fireplace
            exposure to fire in stove

   ✓x7th **X02.0**   **Exposure to flames in controlled fire in building or structure**

   ✓x7th **X02.1**   **Exposure to smoke in controlled fire in building or structure**

   ✓x7th **X02.2**   **Injury due to collapse of burning building or structure in controlled fire**
          EXCLUDES 1   injury due to collapse of building not on fire (W20.1)

   ✓x7th **X02.3**   **Fall from burning building or structure in controlled fire**

   ✓x7th **X02.4**   **Hit by object from burning building or structure in controlled fire**

   ✓x7th **X02.5**   **Jump from burning building or structure in controlled fire**

   ✓x7th **X02.8**   **Other exposure to controlled fire in building or structure**

☑4th **X03**   **Exposure to controlled fire, not in building or structure**
    INCLUDES   exposure to bon fire
            exposure to camp-fire
            exposure to trash fire

   ✓x7th **X03.0**   **Exposure to flames in controlled fire, not in building or structure**

   ✓x7th **X03.1**   **Exposure to smoke in controlled fire, not in building or structure**

   ✓x7th **X03.3**   **Fall due to controlled fire, not in building or structure**

   ✓x7th **X03.4**   **Hit by object due to controlled fire, not in building or structure**

   ✓x7th **X03.8**   **Other exposure to controlled fire, not in building or structure**

✓x7th **X04**   **Exposure to ignition of highly flammable material**
    Exposure to ignition of gasoline
    Exposure to ignition of kerosene
    Exposure to ignition of petrol
    EXCLUDES 2   exposure to ignition or melting of nightwear (X05)
           exposure to ignition or melting of other clothing and apparel (X06)
    AHA: 2016, 2Q, 4

✓x7th **X05**   **Exposure to ignition or melting of nightwear**
    EXCLUDES 2   exposure to uncontrolled fire in building or structure (X00.-)
           exposure to uncontrolled fire, not in building or structure (X01.-)
           exposure to controlled fire in building or structure (X02.-)
           exposure to controlled fire, not in building or structure (X03.-)
           exposure to ignition of highly flammable materials (X04.-)

☑4th **X06**   **Exposure to ignition or melting of other clothing and apparel**
    EXCLUDES 2   exposure to uncontrolled fire in building or structure (X00.-)
           exposure to uncontrolled fire, not in building or structure (X01.-)
           exposure to controlled fire in building or structure (X02.-)
           exposure to controlled fire, not in building or structure (X03.-)
           exposure to ignition of highly flammable materials (X04.-)

   ✓x7th **X06.0**   **Exposure to ignition of plastic jewelry**

   ✓x7th **X06.1**   **Exposure to melting of plastic jewelry**

   ✓x7th **X06.2**   **Exposure to ignition of other clothing and apparel**

   ✓x7th **X06.3**   **Exposure to melting of other clothing and apparel**

☑4th **X08**   **Exposure to other specified smoke, fire and flames**

   ✓5th **X08.0**   **Exposure to bed fire**
         Exposure to mattress fire

     ✓x7th **X08.00**   **Exposure to bed fire due to unspecified burning material**

     ✓x7th **X08.01**   **Exposure to bed fire due to burning cigarette**

     ✓x7th **X08.09**   **Exposure to bed fire due to other burning material**

   ✓5th **X08.1**   **Exposure to sofa fire**

     ✓x7th **X08.10**   **Exposure to sofa fire due to unspecified burning material**

     ✓x7th **X08.11**   **Exposure to sofa fire due to burning cigarette**

     ✓x7th **X08.19**   **Exposure to sofa fire due to other burning material**

   ✓5th **X08.2**   **Exposure to other furniture fire**

     ✓x7th **X08.20**   **Exposure to other furniture fire due to unspecified burning material**

     ✓x7th **X08.21**   **Exposure to other furniture fire due to burning cigarette**

     ✓x7th **X08.29**   **Exposure to other furniture fire due to other burning material**

   ✓x7th **X08.8**   **Exposure to other specified smoke, fire and flames**

## Contact with heat and hot substances (X10-X19)

   EXCLUDES 1   exposure to excessive natural heat (X30)
           exposure to fire and flames ▶(X00-X08)◀

The appropriate 7th character is to be added to each code from categories X10-X19.
A    initial encounter
D    subsequent encounter
S    sequela

☑4th **X10**   **Contact with hot drinks, food, fats and cooking oils**

   ✓x7th **X10.0**   **Contact with hot drinks**

   ✓x7th **X10.1**   **Contact with hot food**

   ✓x7th **X10.2**   **Contact with fats and cooking oils**

☑4th **X11**   **Contact with hot tap-water**
    INCLUDES   contact with boiling tap-water
            contact with boiling water NOS
    EXCLUDES 1   contact with water heated on stove (X12)

   ✓x7th **X11.0**   **Contact with hot water in bath or tub**
          EXCLUDES 1   contact with running hot water in bath or tub (X11.1)

   ✓x7th **X11.1**   **Contact with running hot water**
         Contact with hot water running out of hose
         Contact with hot water running out of tap

   ✓x7th **X11.8**   **Contact with other hot tap-water**
         Contact with hot water in bucket
         Contact with hot tap-water NOS

✓x7th **X12**   **Contact with other hot fluids**
    Contact with water heated on stove
    EXCLUDES 1   hot (liquid) metals (X18)

☑4th **X13**   **Contact with steam and other hot vapors**

   ✓x7th **X13.0**   **Inhalation of steam and other hot vapors**

   ✓x7th **X13.1**   **Other contact with steam and other hot vapors**

☑4th **X14**   **Contact with hot air and other hot gases**

   ✓x7th **X14.0**   **Inhalation of hot air and gases**

   ✓x7th **X14.1**   **Other contact with hot air and other hot gases**

☑4th **X15**   **Contact with hot household appliances**
    EXCLUDES 1   contact with heating appliances (X16)
           contact with powered household appliances (W29.-)
           exposure to controlled fire in building or structure due to household appliance (X02.8)
           exposure to household appliances electrical current (W86.0)

   ✓x7th **X15.0**   **Contact with hot stove (kitchen)**

   ✓x7th **X15.1**   **Contact with hot toaster**

   ✓x7th **X15.2**   **Contact with hotplate**

   ✓x7th **X15.3**   **Contact with hot saucepan or skillet**

   ✓x7th **X15.8**   **Contact with other hot household appliances**
         Contact with cooker
         Contact with kettle
         Contact with light bulbs

✓x7th **X16**   **Contact with hot heating appliances, radiators and pipes**
    EXCLUDES 1   contact with powered appliances (W29.-)
           exposure to controlled fire in building or structure due to appliance (X02.8)
           exposure to industrial appliances electrical current (W86.1)

✓x7th **X17**   **Contact with hot engines, machinery and tools**
    EXCLUDES 1   contact with hot heating appliances, radiators and pipes (X16)
           contact with hot household appliances (X15)

✓x7th **X18**   **Contact with other hot metals**
    Contact with liquid metal

✓x7th **X19**   **Contact with other heat and hot substances**
    EXCLUDES 1   objects that are not normally hot, e.g., an object made hot by a house fire ▶(X00-X08)◀

✓ Additional Character Req    ✓x7th Placeholder Alert    Unacceptable PDx    Manifestation    H1 - H14 HAC    HCC CMS-HCC Condition    EXCLUDES 1 Not Coded Here    EXCLUDES 2 Not Included Here

ICD-10-CM 2018                                                            1195

**Chapter 20. External Causes of Morbidity**

## Exposure to forces of nature (X30-X39)

The appropriate 7th character is to be added to each code from categories X30-X39.
A    initial encounter
D    subsequent encounter
S    sequela

✓x7th **X30** **Exposure to excessive natural heat**
Exposure to excessive heat as the cause of sunstroke
Exposure to heat NOS
  EXCLUDES 1   excessive heat of man-made origin (W92)
        exposure to man-made radiation (W89)
        exposure to sunlight (X32)
        exposure to tanning bed (W89)

✓x7th **X31** **Exposure to excessive natural cold**
Excessive cold as the cause of chilblains NOS
Excessive cold as the cause of immersion foot or hand
Exposure to cold NOS
Exposure to weather conditions
  EXCLUDES 1   cold of man-made origin (W93.-)
        contact with or inhalation of dry ice (W93.-)
        contact with or inhalation of liquefied gas (W93.-)

✓x7th **X32** **Exposure to sunlight**
  EXCLUDES 1   man-made radiation (tanning bed) (W89)
  EXCLUDES 2 ▶radiation-related disorders of the skin and subcutaneous tissue (L55-L59)◀

✓x7th **X34** **Earthquake**
  EXCLUDES 2   tidal wave (tsunami) due to earthquake (X37.41)

✓x7th **X35** **Volcanic eruption**
  EXCLUDES 2   tidal wave (tsunami) due to volcanic eruption (X37.41)

✓4th **X36** **Avalanche, landslide and other earth movements**
  INCLUDES   victim of mudslide of cataclysmic nature
  EXCLUDES 1   earthquake (X34)
  EXCLUDES 2   transport accident involving collision with avalanche or landslide not in motion (V01-V99)

  ✓x7th **X36.0** **Collapse of dam or man-made structure causing earth movement**

  ✓x7th **X36.1** **Avalanche, landslide, or mudslide**

✓4th **X37** **Cataclysmic storm**

  ✓x7th **X37.0** **Hurricane**
       Storm surge
       Typhoon

  ✓x7th **X37.1** **Tornado**
       Cyclone
       Twister

  ✓x7th **X37.2** **Blizzard (snow)(ice)**

  ✓x7th **X37.3** **Dust storm**

  ✓5th **X37.4** **Tidalwave**

    ✓x7th **X37.41** **Tidal wave due to earthquake or volcanic eruption**
         Tidal wave NOS
         Tsunami

    ✓x7th **X37.42** **Tidal wave due to storm**

    ✓x7th **X37.43** **Tidal wave due to landslide**

  ✓x7th **X37.8** **Other cataclysmic storms**
       Cloudburst
       Torrential rain
      EXCLUDES 2   flood (X38)

  ✓x7th **X37.9** **Unspecified cataclysmic storm**
       Storm NOS
      EXCLUDES 1   collapse of dam or man-made structure causing earth movement (X39.0)

✓x7th **X38** **Flood**
Flood arising from remote storm
Flood of cataclysmic nature arising from melting snow
Flood resulting directly from storm
  EXCLUDES 1   collapse of dam or man-made structure causing earth movement (X39.0)
        tidal wave NOS (X37.41)
        tidal wave caused by storm (X37.2)

✓4th **X39** **Exposure to other forces of nature**

  ✓5th **X39.0** **Exposure to natural radiation**
      EXCLUDES 1   contact with and (suspected) exposure to radon and other naturally occuring radiation (Z77.123)
           exposure to man-made radiation (W88-W90)
           exposure to sunlight (X32)

    ✓x7th **X39.01** **Exposure to radon**

    ✓x7th **X39.08** **Exposure to other natural radiation**

  ✓x7th **X39.8** **Other exposure to forces of nature**

## Overexertion and strenuous or repetitive movements (X50)

✓4th **X50** **Overexertion and strenuous or repetitive movements**

The appropriate 7th character is to be added to each code from category X50.
A    initial encounter
D    subsequent encounter
S    sequela

  ✓x7th **X50.0** **Overexertion from strenuous movement or load**
       Lifting heavy objects
       Lifting weights

  ✓x7th **X50.1** **Overexertion from prolonged static or awkward postures**
       Prolonged bending
       Prolonged kneeling
       Prolonged reaching
       Prolonged sitting
       Prolonged standing
       Prolonged twisting
       Static bending
       Static kneeling
       Static reaching
       Static sitting
       Static standing
       Static twisting

  ✓x7th **X50.3** **Overexertion from repetitive movements**
       Use of hand as hammer
      EXCLUDES 2   overuse from prolonged static or awkward postures (X50.1)

  ✓x7th **X50.9** **Other and unspecified overexertion or strenuous movements or postures**
       Contact pressure
       Contact stress

## Accidental exposure to other specified factors (X52-X58)

The appropriate 7th character is to be added to each code from categories X52 and X58.
A    initial encounter
D    subsequent encounter
S    sequela

✓x7th **X52** **Prolonged stay in weightless environment**
Weightlessness in spacecraft (simulator)

✓x7th **X58** **Exposure to other specified factors**
Accident NOS                Exposure NOS

## Intentional self-harm (X71-X83)

Purposely self-inflicted injury
Suicide (attempted)

The appropriate 7th character is to be added to each code from categories X71-X83.
A    initial encounter
D    subsequent encounter
S    sequela

✓4th **X71** **Intentional self-harm by drowning and submersion**

  ✓x7th **X71.0** **Intentional self-harm by drowning and submersion while in bathtub**    HCC

  ✓x7th **X71.1** **Intentional self-harm by drowning and submersion while in swimming pool**    HCC

  ✓x7th **X71.2** **Intentional self-harm by drowning and submersion after jump into swimming pool**    HCC

  ✓x7th **X71.3** **Intentional self-harm by drowning and submersion in natural water**    HCC

  ✓x7th **X71.8** **Other intentional self-harm by drowning and submersion**    HCC

  ✓x7th **X71.9** **Intentional self-harm by drowning and submersion, unspecified**    HCC

√x7th **X72  Intentional self-harm by** handgun **discharge**     HCC
  Intentional self-harm by gun for single hand use
  Intentional self-harm by pistol
  Intentional self-harm by revolver
  *EXCLUDES 1*     *Very pistol (X74.8)*

√4th **X73  Intentional self-harm by** rifle, shotgun and larger firearm **discharge**
  *EXCLUDES 1*     *airgun (X74.Ø1)*

  √x7th  **X73.Ø  Intentional self-harm by** shotgun **discharge**     HCC
  √x7th  **X73.1  Intentional self-harm by** hunting rifle **discharge**     HCC
  √x7th  **X73.2  Intentional self-harm by** machine gun **discharge**     HCC
  √x7th  **X73.8  Intentional self-harm by** other **larger firearm discharge**     HCC
  √x7th  **X73.9  Intentional self-harm by** unspecified **larger firearm discharge**     HCC

√4th **X74  Intentional self-harm by other and unspecified firearm and gun discharge**

  √5th  **X74.Ø  Intentional self-harm by** gas, air or spring-operated guns
    √x7th  **X74.Ø1  Intentional self-harm by** airgun     HCC
      Intentional self-harm by BB gun discharge
      Intentional self-harm by pellet gun discharge
    √x7th  **X74.Ø2  Intentional self-harm by** paintball gun     HCC
    √x7th  **X74.Ø9  Intentional self-harm by** other **gas, air or spring-operated gun**     HCC
  √x7th  **X74.8  Intentional self-harm by** other **firearm discharge**     HCC
    Intentional self-harm by Very pistol [flare] discharge
  √x7th  **X74.9  Intentional self-harm by** unspecified **firearm discharge**     HCC

√x7th **X75  Intentional self-harm by explosive material**     HCC

√x7th **X76  Intentional self-harm by smoke, fire and flames**     HCC

√4th **X77  Intentional self-harm by steam, hot vapors and hot objects**
  √x7th  **X77.Ø  Intentional self-harm by** steam **or hot** vapors     HCC
  √x7th  **X77.1  Intentional self-harm by** hot **tap water**     HCC
  √x7th  **X77.2  Intentional self-harm by** other **hot fluids**     HCC
  √x7th  **X77.3  Intentional self-harm by** hot **household appliances**     HCC
  √x7th  **X77.8  Intentional self-harm by** other **hot objects**     HCC
  √x7th  **X77.9  Intentional self-harm by** unspecified **hot objects**     HCC

√4th **X78  Intentional self-harm by sharp object**
  √x7th  **X78.Ø  Intentional self-harm by** sharp glass     HCC
  √x7th  **X78.1  Intentional self-harm by** knife     HCC
  √x7th  **X78.2  Intentional self-harm by** sword or dagger     HCC
  √x7th  **X78.8  Intentional self-harm by** other **sharp object**     HCC
  √x7th  **X78.9  Intentional self-harm by** unspecified **sharp object**     HCC

√x7th **X79  Intentional self-harm by blunt object**     HCC

√x7th **X80  Intentional self-harm by jumping from a high place**     HCC
  Intentional fall from one level to another

√4th **X81  Intentional self-harm by jumping or lying in front of moving object**
  √x7th  **X81.Ø  Intentional self-harm by jumping or lying in front of** motor vehicle     HCC
  √x7th  **X81.1  Intentional self-harm by jumping or lying in front of** (subway) train     HCC
  √x7th  **X81.8  Intentional self-harm by jumping or lying in front of** other **moving object**     HCC

√4th **X82  Intentional self-harm by crashing of motor vehicle**
  √x7th  **X82.Ø  Intentional collision of motor vehicle with** other motor vehicle     HCC
  √x7th  **X82.1  Intentional collision of motor vehicle with** train     HCC
  √x7th  **X82.2  Intentional collision of motor vehicle with** tree     HCC
  √x7th  **X82.8  Other intentional self-harm by crashing of motor vehicle**     HCC

√4th **X83  Intentional self-harm by other specified means**
  *EXCLUDES 1*     *intentional self-harm by poisoning or contact with toxic substance—see Table of Drugs and Chemicals*
  √x7th  **X83.Ø  Intentional self-harm by** crashing of aircraft     HCC
  √x7th  **X83.1  Intentional self-harm by** electrocution     HCC
  √x7th  **X83.2  Intentional self-harm by** exposure to extremes of cold     HCC
  √x7th  **X83.8  Intentional self-harm by** other specified means     HCC

## Assault (X92-Y09)

*INCLUDES*  homicide
  injuries inflicted by another person with intent to injure or kill, by any means
*EXCLUDES 1*  *injuries due to legal intervention (Y35.-)*
  *injuries due to operations of war (Y36.-)*
  *injuries due to terrorism (Y38.-)*

The appropriate 7th character is to be added to each code from categories X92-YØ4 and YØ8.
A     initial encounter
D     subsequent encounter
S     sequela

√4th **X92  Assault by drowning and submersion**
  √x7th  **X92.Ø  Assault by drowning and submersion while in** bathtub
  √x7th  **X92.1  Assault by drowning and submersion while in** swimming pool
  √x7th  **X92.2  Assault by drowning and submersion** after push into **swimming pool**
  √x7th  **X92.3  Assault by drowning and submersion** in natural water
  √x7th  **X92.8  Other assault by drowning and submersion**
  √x7th  **X92.9  Assault by drowning and submersion,** unspecified

√x7th **X93  Assault by** handgun **discharge**
  Assault by discharge of gun for single hand use
  Assault by discharge of pistol
  Assault by discharge of revolver
  *EXCLUDES 1*     *Very pistol (X95.8)*

√4th **X94  Assault by** rifle, shotgun and larger firearm **discharge**
  *EXCLUDES 1*     *airgun (X95.Ø1)*
  √x7th  **X94.Ø  Assault by** shotgun
  √x7th  **X94.1  Assault by** hunting rifle
  √x7th  **X94.2  Assault by** machine gun
  √x7th  **X94.8  Assault by** other **larger firearm discharge**
  √x7th  **X94.9  Assault by** unspecified **larger firearm discharge**

√4th **X95  Assault by other and unspecified firearm and gun discharge**
  √5th  **X95.Ø  Assault by** gas, air or spring-operated guns
    √x7th  **X95.Ø1  Assault by** airgun **discharge**
      Assault by BB gun discharge
      Assault by pellet gun discharge
    √x7th  **X95.Ø2  Assault by** paintball gun **discharge**
    √x7th  **X95.Ø9  Assault by** other **gas, air or spring-operated gun**
  √x7th  **X95.8  Assault by** other **firearm discharge**
    Assault by Very pistol [flare] discharge
  √x7th  **X95.9  Assault by** unspecified **firearm discharge**

√4th **X96  Assault by explosive material**
  *EXCLUDES 1*     *incendiary device (X97)*
    *terrorism involving explosive material (Y38.2-)*
  √x7th  **X96.Ø  Assault by** antipersonnel **bomb**
    *EXCLUDES 1*     *antipersonnel bomb use in military or war (Y36.2-)*
  √x7th  **X96.1  Assault by** gasoline **bomb**
  √x7th  **X96.2  Assault by** letter **bomb**
  √x7th  **X96.3  Assault by** fertilizer **bomb**
  √x7th  **X96.4  Assault by** pipe **bomb**
  √x7th  **X96.8  Assault by** other **specified explosive**
  √x7th  **X96.9  Assault by** unspecified **explosive**

√x7th **X97  Assault by smoke, fire and flames**
  Assault by arson
  Assault by cigarettes
  Assault by incendiary device

√4th **X98  Assault by steam, hot vapors and hot objects**
  √x7th  **X98.Ø  Assault by** steam or hot **vapors**
  √x7th  **X98.1  Assault by** hot **tap water**
  √x7th  **X98.2  Assault by** hot **fluids**
  √x7th  **X98.3  Assault by** hot household **appliances**
  √x7th  **X98.8  Assault by** other **hot objects**
  √x7th  **X98.9  Assault by** unspecified **hot objects**

√4th **X99  Assault by sharp object**
  *EXCLUDES 1*     *assault by strike by sports equipment (YØ8.Ø-)*
  √x7th  **X99.Ø  Assault by** sharp **glass**
  √x7th  **X99.1  Assault by** knife
  √x7th  **X99.2  Assault by** sword **or** dagger

---

✓Additional Character Req     √x7th Placeholder Alert     Unacceptable PDx     Manifestation     **H1**-**H14** HAC     **HCC** CMS-HCC Condition     *EXCLUDES 1* Not Coded Here     *EXCLUDES 2* Not Included Here

√x 7th **X99.8**    **Assault by other sharp object**

√x 7th **X99.9**    **Assault by unspecified sharp object**
      Assault by stabbing NOS

√x 7th **Y00**    **Assault by blunt object**
     EXCLUDES 1   *assault by strike by sports equipment (Y08.0-)*

√x 7th **Y01**    **Assault by pushing from high place**

√4th **Y02**    **Assault by pushing or placing victim in front of moving object**

√x 7th **Y02.0**    **Assault by pushing or placing victim in front of motor vehicle**

√x 7th **Y02.1**    **Assault by pushing or placing victim in front of (subway) train**

√x 7th **Y02.8**    **Assault by pushing or placing victim in front of other moving object**

√4th **Y03**    **Assault by crashing of motor vehicle**

√x 7th **Y03.0**    **Assault by being hit or run over by motor vehicle**

√x 7th **Y03.8**    **Other assault by crashing of motor vehicle**

√4th **Y04**    **Assault by bodily force**
     EXCLUDES 1   *assault by:*
        *submersion (X92.-)*
        *use of weapon (X93-X95, X99, Y00)*

√x 7th **Y04.0**    **Assault by unarmed brawl or fight**

√x 7th **Y04.1**    **Assault by human bite**

√x 7th **Y04.2**    **Assault by strike against or bumped into by another person**

√x 7th **Y04.8**    **Assault by other bodily force**
      Assault by bodily force NOS

√4th **Y07**    **Perpetrator of assault, maltreatment and neglect**
     NOTE   Codes from this category are for use only in cases of confirmed abuse (T74.-)
        Selection of the correct perpetrator code is based on the relationship between the perpetrator and the victim
     INCLUDES   perpetrator of abandonment
        perpetrator of emotional neglect
        perpetrator of mental cruelty
        perpetrator of physical abuse
        perpetrator of physical neglect
        perpetrator of sexual abuse
        perpetrator of torture

√5th **Y07.0**    **Spouse or partner, perpetrator of maltreatment and neglect**
      Spouse or partner, perpetrator of maltreatment and neglect against spouse or partner

**Y07.01**    **Husband, perpetrator of maltreatment and neglect**

**Y07.02**    **Wife, perpetrator of maltreatment and neglect**

**Y07.03**    **Male partner, perpetrator of maltreatment and neglect**

**Y07.04**    **Female partner, perpetrator of maltreatment and neglect**

√5th **Y07.1**    **Parent (adoptive) (biological), perpetrator of maltreatment and neglect**

**Y07.11**    **Biological father, perpetrator of maltreatment and neglect**

**Y07.12**    **Biological mother, perpetrator of maltreatment and neglect**

**Y07.13**    **Adoptive father, perpetrator of maltreatment and neglect**

**Y07.14**    **Adoptive mother, perpetrator of maltreatment and neglect**

√5th **Y07.4**    **Other family member, perpetrator of maltreatment and neglect**

√6th **Y07.41**    **Sibling, perpetrator of maltreatment and neglect**
      EXCLUDES 1   *stepsibling, perpetrator of maltreatment and neglect (Y07.435, Y07.436)*

**Y07.410**    **Brother, perpetrator of maltreatment and neglect**

**Y07.411**    **Sister, perpetrator of maltreatment and neglect**

√6th **Y07.42**    **Foster parent, perpetrator of maltreatment and neglect**

**Y07.420**    **Foster father, perpetrator of maltreatment and neglect**

**Y07.421**    **Foster mother, perpetrator of maltreatment and neglect**

√6th **Y07.43**    **Stepparent or stepsibling, perpetrator of maltreatment and neglect**

**Y07.430**    **Stepfather, perpetrator of maltreatment and neglect**

**Y07.432**    **Male friend of parent (co-residing in household), perpetrator of maltreatment and neglect**

**Y07.433**    **Stepmother, perpetrator of maltreatment and neglect**

**Y07.434**    **Female friend of parent (co-residing in household), perpetrator of maltreatment and neglect**

**Y07.435**    **Stepbrother, perpetrator or maltreatment and neglect**

**Y07.436**    **Stepsister, perpetrator of maltreatment and neglect**

√6th **Y07.49**    **Other family member, perpetrator of maltreatment and neglect**

**Y07.490**    **Male cousin, perpetrator of maltreatment and neglect**

**Y07.491**    **Female cousin, perpetrator of maltreatment and neglect**

**Y07.499**    **Other family member, perpetrator of maltreatment and neglect**

√5th **Y07.5**    **Non-family member, perpetrator of maltreatment and neglect**

**Y07.50**    **Unspecified non-family member, perpetrator of maltreatment and neglect**

√6th **Y07.51**    **Daycare provider, perpetrator of maltreatment and neglect**

**Y07.510**    **At-home childcare provider, perpetrator of maltreatment and neglect**

**Y07.511**    **Daycare center childcare provider, perpetrator of maltreatment and neglect**

**Y07.512**    **At-home adultcare provider, perpetrator of maltreatment and neglect**

**Y07.513**    **Adultcare center provider, perpetrator of maltreatment and neglect**

**Y07.519**    **Unspecified daycare provider, perpetrator of maltreatment and neglect**

√6th **Y07.52**    **Healthcare provider, perpetrator of maltreatment and neglect**

**Y07.521**    **Mental health provider, perpetrator of maltreatment and neglect**

**Y07.528**    **Other therapist or healthcare provider, perpetrator of maltreatment and neglect**
      Nurse, perpetrator of maltreatment and neglect
      Occupational therapist, perpetrator of maltreatment and neglect
      Physical therapist, perpetrator of maltreatment and neglect
      Speech therapist, perpetrator of maltreatment and neglect

**Y07.529**    **Unspecified healthcare provider, perpetrator of maltreatment and neglect**

**Y07.53**    **Teacher or instructor, perpetrator of maltreatment and neglect**
      Coach, perpetrator of maltreatment and neglect

**Y07.59**    **Other non-family member, perpetrator of maltreatment and neglect**

**Y07.9**    **Unspecified perpetrator of maltreatment and neglect**

√4th **Y08**    **Assault by other specified means**

√5th **Y08.0**    **Assault by strike by sport equipment**

√x 7th **Y08.01**    **Assault by strike by hockey stick**

√x 7th **Y08.02**    **Assault by strike by baseball bat**

√x 7th **Y08.09**    **Assault by strike by other specified type of sport equipment**

√5th **Y08.8**    **Assault by other specified means**

√x 7th **Y08.81**    **Assault by crashing of aircraft**

√x 7th **Y08.89**    **Assault by other specified means**

**Y09**    **Assault by unspecified means**
      Assassination (attempted) NOS
      Homicide (attempted) NOS
      Manslaughter (attempted) NOS
      Murder (attempted) NOS

---

N Newborn: 0    P Pediatric: 0-17    M Maternity: 12-55    A Adult: 15-124    MCC Major CC Condition    PDxMCC PDx acts as own MCC    CC CC Condition    PDxCC PDx acts as own CC

### Event of undetermined intent (Y21-Y33)

Undetermined intent is only for use when there is specific documentation in the record that the intent of the injury cannot be determined. If no such documentation is present, code to accidental (unintentional)

☑4ᵗʰ **Y21 Drowning and submersion, undetermined intent**

> The appropriate 7th character is to be added to each code from categories Y21-Y33.
> A    initial encounter
> D    subsequent encounter
> S    sequela

☑x7ᵗʰ **Y21.Ø Drowning and submersion** while in bathtub, **undetermined intent**

☑x7ᵗʰ **Y21.1 Drowning and submersion** after fall into bathtub, **undetermined intent**

☑x7ᵗʰ **Y21.2 Drowning and submersion** while in swimming pool, **undetermined intent**

☑x7ᵗʰ **Y21.3 Drowning and submersion** after fall into swimming pool, **undetermined intent**

☑x7ᵗʰ **Y21.4 Drowning and submersion** in natural water, **undetermined intent**

☑x7ᵗʰ **Y21.8** Other drowning and submersion, undetermined intent

☑x7ᵗʰ **Y21.9** Unspecified drowning and submersion, undetermined intent

☑x7ᵗʰ **Y22 Handgun discharge, undetermined intent**
> Discharge of gun for single hand use, undetermined intent
> Discharge of pistol, undetermined intent
> Discharge of revolver, undetermined intent
> *EXCLUDES 2*   Very pistol (Y24.8)

☑4ᵗʰ **Y23 Rifle, shotgun and larger firearm discharge, undetermined intent**
> *EXCLUDES 2*   airgun (Y24.Ø)

☑x7ᵗʰ **Y23.Ø Shotgun** discharge, undetermined intent

☑x7ᵗʰ **Y23.1** Hunting rifle discharge, undetermined intent

☑x7ᵗʰ **Y23.2** Military firearm discharge, undetermined intent

☑x7ᵗʰ **Y23.3** Machine gun discharge, undetermined intent

☑x7ᵗʰ **Y23.8** Other larger firearm discharge, undetermined intent

☑x7ᵗʰ **Y23.9** Unspecified larger firearm discharge, undetermined intent

☑4ᵗʰ **Y24 Other and unspecified firearm discharge, undetermined intent**

☑x7ᵗʰ **Y24.Ø Airgun** discharge, undetermined intent
> BB gun discharge, undetermined intent
> Pellet gun discharge, undetermined intent

☑x7ᵗʰ **Y24.8** Other firearm discharge, undetermined intent
> Paintball gun discharge, undetermined intent
> Very pistol [flare] discharge, undetermined intent

☑x7ᵗʰ **Y24.9** Unspecified firearm discharge, undetermined intent

☑x7ᵗʰ **Y25 Contact with explosive material, undetermined intent**

☑x7ᵗʰ **Y26 Exposure to smoke, fire and flames, undetermined intent**

☑4ᵗʰ **Y27 Contact with steam, hot vapors and hot objects, undetermined intent**

☑x7ᵗʰ **Y27.Ø Contact with steam and hot** vapors, **undetermined intent**

☑x7ᵗʰ **Y27.1 Contact with hot** tap water, **undetermined intent**

☑x7ᵗʰ **Y27.2 Contact with hot** fluids, **undetermined intent**

☑x7ᵗʰ **Y27.3 Contact with hot household** appliance, **undetermined intent**

☑x7ᵗʰ **Y27.8 Contact with** other **hot objects, undetermined intent**

☑x7ᵗʰ **Y27.9 Contact with** unspecified **hot objects, undetermined intent**

☑4ᵗʰ **Y28 Contact with sharp object, undetermined intent**

☑x7ᵗʰ **Y28.Ø Contact with sharp** glass, **undetermined intent**

☑x7ᵗʰ **Y28.1 Contact with** knife, **undetermined intent**

☑x7ᵗʰ **Y28.2 Contact with** sword or dagger, **undetermined intent**

☑x7ᵗʰ **Y28.8 Contact with** other **sharp object, undetermined intent**

☑x7ᵗʰ **Y28.9 Contact with** unspecified **sharp object, undetermined intent**

☑x7ᵗʰ **Y29 Contact with blunt object, undetermined intent**

☑x7ᵗʰ **Y3Ø Falling, jumping or pushed from a high place, undetermined intent**
> Victim falling from one level to another, undetermined intent

☑x7ᵗʰ **Y31 Falling, lying or running before or into moving object, undetermined intent**

☑x7ᵗʰ **Y32 Crashing of motor vehicle, undetermined intent**

☑x7ᵗʰ **Y33 Other specified events, undetermined intent**

### Legal intervention, operations of war, military operations, and terrorism (Y35-Y38)

> The appropriate 7th character is to be added to each code from categories Y35-Y38.
> A    initial encounter
> D    subsequent encounter
> S    sequela

☑4ᵗʰ **Y35 Legal intervention**
> **INCLUDES**   any injury sustained as a result of an encounter with any law enforcement official, serving in any capacity at the time of the encounter, whether on-duty or off-duty.
> Includes: injury to law enforcement official, suspect and bystander

☑5ᵗʰ **Y35.Ø Legal intervention involving** firearm discharge

☑6ᵗʰ **Y35.ØØ Legal intervention involving** unspecified firearm discharge
> Legal intervention involving gunshot wound
> Legal intervention involving shot NOS

☑7ᵗʰ **Y35.ØØ1 Legal intervention involving unspecified firearm discharge,** law enforcement official injured

☑7ᵗʰ **Y35.ØØ2 Legal intervention involving unspecified firearm discharge,** bystander injured

☑7ᵗʰ **Y35.ØØ3 Legal intervention involving unspecified firearm discharge,** suspect injured

☑6ᵗʰ **Y35.Ø1 Legal intervention involving injury by** machine gun

☑7ᵗʰ **Y35.Ø11 Legal intervention involving injury by machine gun,** law enforcement official injured

☑7ᵗʰ **Y35.Ø12 Legal intervention involving injury by machine gun,** bystander injured

☑7ᵗʰ **Y35.Ø13 Legal intervention involving injury by machine gun,** suspect injured

☑6ᵗʰ **Y35.Ø2 Legal intervention involving injury by** handgun

☑7ᵗʰ **Y35.Ø21 Legal intervention involving injury by handgun,** law enforcement official injured

☑7ᵗʰ **Y35.Ø22 Legal intervention involving injury by handgun,** bystander injured

☑7ᵗʰ **Y35.Ø23 Legal intervention involving injury by handgun,** suspect injured

☑6ᵗʰ **Y35.Ø3 Legal intervention involving injury by** rifle pellet

☑7ᵗʰ **Y35.Ø31 Legal intervention involving injury by rifle pellet,** law enforcement official injured

☑7ᵗʰ **Y35.Ø32 Legal intervention involving injury by rifle pellet,** bystander injured

☑7ᵗʰ **Y35.Ø33 Legal intervention involving injury by rifle pellet,** suspect injured

☑6ᵗʰ **Y35.Ø4 Legal intervention involving injury by** rubber bullet

☑7ᵗʰ **Y35.Ø41 Legal intervention involving injury by rubber bullet,** law enforcement official injured

☑7ᵗʰ **Y35.Ø42 Legal intervention involving injury by rubber bullet,** bystander injured

☑7ᵗʰ **Y35.Ø43 Legal intervention involving injury by rubber bullet,** suspect injured

☑6ᵗʰ **Y35.Ø9 Legal intervention involving** other firearm discharge

☑7ᵗʰ **Y35.Ø91 Legal intervention involving other firearm discharge,** law enforcement official injured

☑7ᵗʰ **Y35.Ø92 Legal intervention involving other firearm discharge,** bystander injured

☑7ᵗʰ **Y35.Ø93 Legal intervention involving other firearm discharge,** suspect injured

☑Additional Character Req   ☑x7ᵗʰ Placeholder Alert   Unacceptable PDx   Manifestation   **H1**-**H14** HAC   **HCC** CMS-HCC Condition   *EXCLUDES 1* Not Coded Here   *EXCLUDES 2* Not Included Here

ICD-10-CM 2018                1199

✓5ᵗʰ **Y35.1 Legal intervention involving** explosives

    ✓6ᵗʰ **Y35.10 Legal intervention involving** unspecified explosives

       ✓7ᵗʰ **Y35.101 Legal intervention involving unspecified explosives,** law enforcement **official injured**

       ✓7ᵗʰ **Y35.102 Legal intervention involving unspecified explosives,** bystander **injured**

       ✓7ᵗʰ **Y35.103 Legal intervention involving unspecified explosives,** suspect **injured**

    ✓6ᵗʰ **Y35.11 Legal intervention involving injury by** dynamite

       ✓7ᵗʰ **Y35.111 Legal intervention involving injury by dynamite,** law enforcement **official injured**

       ✓7ᵗʰ **Y35.112 Legal intervention involving injury by dynamite,** bystander **injured**

       ✓7ᵗʰ **Y35.113 Legal intervention involving injury by dynamite,** suspect **injured**

    ✓6ᵗʰ **Y35.12 Legal intervention involving injury by** explosive shell

       ✓7ᵗʰ **Y35.121 Legal intervention involving injury by explosive shell,** law enforcement **official injured**

       ✓7ᵗʰ **Y35.122 Legal intervention involving injury by explosive shell,** bystander **injured**

       ✓7ᵗʰ **Y35.123 Legal intervention involving injury by explosive shell,** suspect **injured**

    ✓6ᵗʰ **Y35.19 Legal intervention involving** other explosives

       Legal intervention involving injury by grenade

       Legal intervention involving injury by mortar bomb

       ✓7ᵗʰ **Y35.191 Legal intervention involving other explosives,** law enforcement **official injured**

       ✓7ᵗʰ **Y35.192 Legal intervention involving other explosives,** bystander **injured**

       ✓7ᵗʰ **Y35.193 Legal intervention involving other explosives,** suspect **injured**

✓5ᵗʰ **Y35.2 Legal intervention involving** gas

    Legal intervention involving asphyxiation by gas

    Legal intervention involving poisoning by gas

    ✓6ᵗʰ **Y35.20 Legal intervention involving** unspecified gas

       ✓7ᵗʰ **Y35.201 Legal intervention involving unspecified gas,** law enforcement **official injured**

       ✓7ᵗʰ **Y35.202 Legal intervention involving unspecified gas,** bystander **injured**

       ✓7ᵗʰ **Y35.203 Legal intervention involving unspecified gas,** suspect **injured**

    ✓6ᵗʰ **Y35.21 Legal intervention involving injury by** tear gas

       ✓7ᵗʰ **Y35.211 Legal intervention involving injury by tear gas,** law enforcement **official injured**

       ✓7ᵗʰ **Y35.212 Legal intervention involving injury by tear gas,** bystander **injured**

       ✓7ᵗʰ **Y35.213 Legal intervention involving injury by tear gas,** suspect **injured**

    ✓6ᵗʰ **Y35.29 Legal intervention involving** other gas

       ✓7ᵗʰ **Y35.291 Legal intervention involving other gas,** law enforcement **official injured**

       ✓7ᵗʰ **Y35.292 Legal intervention involving other gas,** bystander **injured**

       ✓7ᵗʰ **Y35.293 Legal intervention involving other gas,** suspect **injured**

✓5ᵗʰ **Y35.3 Legal intervention involving** blunt objects

    Legal intervention involving being hit or struck by blunt object

    ✓6ᵗʰ **Y35.30 Legal intervention involving** unspecified blunt objects

       ✓7ᵗʰ **Y35.301 Legal intervention involving unspecified blunt objects,** law enforcement **official injured**

       ✓7ᵗʰ **Y35.302 Legal intervention involving unspecified blunt objects,** bystander **injured**

       ✓7ᵗʰ **Y35.303 Legal intervention involving unspecified blunt objects,** suspect **injured**

    ✓6ᵗʰ **Y35.31 Legal intervention involving** baton

       ✓7ᵗʰ **Y35.311 Legal intervention involving baton,** law enforcement **official injured**

       ✓7ᵗʰ **Y35.312 Legal intervention involving baton,** bystander **injured**

       ✓7ᵗʰ **Y35.313 Legal intervention involving baton,** suspect **injured**

    ✓6ᵗʰ **Y35.39 Legal intervention involving** other **blunt objects**

       ✓7ᵗʰ **Y35.391 Legal intervention involving other blunt objects,** law enforcement **official injured**

       ✓7ᵗʰ **Y35.392 Legal intervention involving other blunt objects,** bystander **injured**

       ✓7ᵗʰ **Y35.393 Legal intervention involving other blunt objects,** suspect **injured**

✓5ᵗʰ **Y35.4 Legal intervention involving** sharp objects

    Legal intervention involving being cut by sharp objects

    Legal intervention involving being stabbed by sharp objects

    ✓6ᵗʰ **Y35.40 Legal intervention involving** unspecified **sharp objects**

       ✓7ᵗʰ **Y35.401 Legal intervention involving unspecified sharp objects,** law enforcement **official injured**

       ✓7ᵗʰ **Y35.402 Legal intervention involving unspecified sharp objects,** bystander **injured**

       ✓7ᵗʰ **Y35.403 Legal intervention involving unspecified sharp objects,** suspect **injured**

    ✓6ᵗʰ **Y35.41 Legal intervention involving** bayonet

       ✓7ᵗʰ **Y35.411 Legal intervention involving bayonet,** law enforcement **official injured**

       ✓7ᵗʰ **Y35.412 Legal intervention involving bayonet,** bystander **injured**

       ✓7ᵗʰ **Y35.413 Legal intervention involving bayonet,** suspect **injured**

    ✓6ᵗʰ **Y35.49 Legal intervention involving** other **sharp objects**

       ✓7ᵗʰ **Y35.491 Legal intervention involving other sharp objects,** law enforcement **official injured**

       ✓7ᵗʰ **Y35.492 Legal intervention involving other sharp objects,** bystander **injured**

       ✓7ᵗʰ **Y35.493 Legal intervention involving other sharp objects,** suspect **injured**

✓5ᵗʰ **Y35.8 Legal intervention involving** other **specified** means

    ✓6ᵗʰ **Y35.81 Legal intervention involving** manhandling

       ✓7ᵗʰ **Y35.811 Legal intervention involving manhandling,** law enforcement **official injured**

       ✓7ᵗʰ **Y35.812 Legal intervention involving manhandling,** bystander **injured**

       ✓7ᵗʰ **Y35.813 Legal intervention involving manhandling,** suspect **injured**

    ✓6ᵗʰ **Y35.89 Legal intervention involving** other specified means

       ✓7ᵗʰ **Y35.891 Legal intervention involving other specified means,** law enforcement **official injured**

       ✓7ᵗʰ **Y35.892 Legal intervention involving other specified means,** bystander **injured**

       ✓7ᵗʰ **Y35.893 Legal intervention involving other specified means,** suspect **injured**

✓5ᵗʰ **Y35.9 Legal intervention, means** unspecified

    ✓x7ᵗʰ **Y35.91 Legal intervention, means unspecified,** law enforcement **official injured**

    ✓x7ᵗʰ **Y35.92 Legal intervention, means unspecified,** bystander **injured**

    ✓x7ᵗʰ **Y35.93 Legal intervention, means unspecified,** suspect **injured**

---

Ⓝ Newborn: 0   Ⓟ Pediatric: 0-17   Ⓜ Maternity: 12-55   Ⓐ Adult: 15-124   **MCC** Major CC Condition   **PDxMCC** PDx acts as own MCC   **CC** CC Condition   **PDxCC** PDx acts as own CC

☑️4ᵗʰ **Y36**   **Operations of war**

> **INCLUDES**   injuries to military personnel and civilians caused by war, civil insurrection, and peacekeeping missions
>
> **EXCLUDES 1**   *injury to military personnel occurring during peacetime military operations (Y37.-)*
> *military vehicles involved in transport accidents with non-military vehicle during peacetime (V09.01, V09.21, V19.81, V29.81, V39.81, V49.81, V59.81, V69.81, V79.81)*
>
> **AHA:** 2014, 3Q, 4

☑️5ᵗʰ **Y36.0**   **War operations involving** explosion of marine weapons

☑️6ᵗʰ   **Y36.00**   **War operations involving explosion of** unspecified marine weapon
> War operations involving underwater blast NOS

☑️7ᵗʰ   **Y36.000**   **War operations involving explosion of unspecified marine weapon, military personnel**

☑️7ᵗʰ   **Y36.001**   **War operations involving explosion of unspecified marine weapon, civilian**

☑️6ᵗʰ   **Y36.01**   **War operations involving explosion of** depth-charge

☑️7ᵗʰ   **Y36.010**   **War operations involving explosion of depth-charge, military personnel**

☑️7ᵗʰ   **Y36.011**   **War operations involving explosion of depth-charge, civilian**

☑️6ᵗʰ   **Y36.02**   **War operations involving explosion of** marine mine
> War operations involving explosion of marine mine, at sea or in harbor

☑️7ᵗʰ   **Y36.020**   **War operations involving explosion of marine mine, military personnel**

☑️7ᵗʰ   **Y36.021**   **War operations involving explosion of marine mine, civilian**

☑️6ᵗʰ   **Y36.03**   **War operations involving explosion of** sea-based artillery shell

☑️7ᵗʰ   **Y36.030**   **War operations involving explosion of sea-based artillery shell, military personnel**

☑️7ᵗʰ   **Y36.031**   **War operations involving explosion of sea-based artillery shell, civilian**

☑️6ᵗʰ   **Y36.04**   **War operations involving explosion of** torpedo

☑️7ᵗʰ   **Y36.040**   **War operations involving explosion of torpedo, military personnel**

☑️7ᵗʰ   **Y36.041**   **War operations involving explosion of torpedo, civilian**

☑️6ᵗʰ   **Y36.05**   **War operations involving** accidental detonation of onboard marine weapons

☑️7ᵗʰ   **Y36.050**   **War operations involving accidental detonation of onboard marine weapons, military personnel**

☑️7ᵗʰ   **Y36.051**   **War operations involving accidental detonation of onboard marine weapons, civilian**

☑️6ᵗʰ   **Y36.09**   **War operations involving explosion of** other marine weapons

☑️7ᵗʰ   **Y36.090**   **War operations involving explosion of other marine weapons, military personnel**

☑️7ᵗʰ   **Y36.091**   **War operations involving explosion of other marine weapons, civilian**

☑️5ᵗʰ **Y36.1**   **War operations involving** destruction of aircraft

☑️6ᵗʰ   **Y36.10**   **War operations involving** unspecified **destruction of aircraft**

☑️7ᵗʰ   **Y36.100**   **War operations involving unspecified destruction of aircraft, military personnel**

☑️7ᵗʰ   **Y36.101**   **War operations involving unspecified destruction of aircraft, civilian**

☑️6ᵗʰ   **Y36.11**   **War operations involving destruction of aircraft due to** enemy fire or explosives
> War operations involving destruction of aircraft due to air to air missile
> War operations involving destruction of aircraft due to explosive placed on aircraft
> War operations involving destruction of aircraft due to rocket propelled grenade [RPG]
> War operations involving destruction of aircraft due to small arms fire
> War operations involving destruction of aircraft due to surface to air missile

☑️7ᵗʰ   **Y36.110**   **War operations involving destruction of aircraft due to enemy fire or explosives, military personnel**

☑️7ᵗʰ   **Y36.111**   **War operations involving destruction of aircraft due to enemy fire or explosives, civilian**

☑️6ᵗʰ   **Y36.12**   **War operations involving destruction of aircraft due to** collision with other aircraft

☑️7ᵗʰ   **Y36.120**   **War operations involving destruction of aircraft due to collision with other aircraft, military personnel**

☑️7ᵗʰ   **Y36.121**   **War operations involving destruction of aircraft due to collision with other aircraft, civilian**

☑️6ᵗʰ   **Y36.13**   **War operations involving destruction of aircraft due to** onboard fire

☑️7ᵗʰ   **Y36.130**   **War operations involving destruction of aircraft due to onboard fire, military personnel**

☑️7ᵗʰ   **Y36.131**   **War operations involving destruction of aircraft due to onboard fire, civilian**

☑️6ᵗʰ   **Y36.14**   **War operations involving destruction of aircraft due to** accidental detonation of onboard munitions and explosives

☑️7ᵗʰ   **Y36.140**   **War operations involving destruction of aircraft due to accidental detonation of onboard munitions and explosives, military personnel**

☑️7ᵗʰ   **Y36.141**   **War operations involving destruction of aircraft due to accidental detonation of onboard munitions and explosives, civilian**

☑️6ᵗʰ   **Y36.19**   **War operations involving** other destruction of aircraft

☑️7ᵗʰ   **Y36.190**   **War operations involving other destruction of aircraft, military personnel**

☑️7ᵗʰ   **Y36.191**   **War operations involving other destruction of aircraft, civilian**

☑️5ᵗʰ **Y36.2**   **War operations involving** other explosions and fragments

> **EXCLUDES 1**   *war operations involving explosion of aircraft (Y36.1-)*
> *war operations involving explosion of marine weapons (Y36.0-)*
> *war operations involving explosion of nuclear weapons (Y36.5-)*
> *war operations involving explosion occurring after cessation of hostilities (Y36.8-)*

☑️6ᵗʰ   **Y36.20**   **War operations involving** unspecified **explosion and fragments**
> War operations involving air blast NOS
> War operations involving blast NOS
> War operations involving blast fragments NOS
> War operations involving blast wave NOS
> War operations involving blast wind NOS
> War operations involving explosion NOS
> War operations involving explosion of bomb NOS

☑️7ᵗʰ   **Y36.200**   **War operations involving unspecified explosion and fragments, military personnel**

☑️7ᵗʰ   **Y36.201**   **War operations involving unspecified explosion and fragments, civilian**

☑️6ᵗʰ   **Y36.21**   **War operations involving explosion of** aerial bomb

☑️7ᵗʰ   **Y36.210**   **War operations involving explosion of aerial bomb, military personnel**

☑️7ᵗʰ   **Y36.211**   **War operations involving explosion of aerial bomb, civilian**

☑️6ᵗʰ   **Y36.22**   **War operations involving explosion of** guided missile

☑️7ᵗʰ   **Y36.220**   **War operations involving explosion of guided missile, military personnel**

☑️7ᵗʰ   **Y36.221**   **War operations involving explosion of guided missile, civilian**

☑️ Additional Character Req   ☑️x7ᵗʰ Placeholder Alert   Unacceptable PDx   Manifestation   **H1**-**H14** HAC   **HCC** CMS-HCC Condition   **EXCLUDES 1** Not Coded Here   **EXCLUDES 2** Not Included Here

ICD-10-CM 2018                                                           **1201**

**Chapter 20. External Causes of Morbidity**

✓6ᵗʰ **Y36.23** **War operations involving explosion of** improvised explosive device [IED]
War operations involving explosion of person-borne improvised explosive device [IED]
War operations involving explosion of vehicle-borne improvised explosive device [IED]
War operations involving explosion of roadside improvised explosive device [IED]

    ✓7ᵗʰ **Y36.230** **War operations involving explosion of improvised explosive device [IED],** military personnel

    ✓7ᵗʰ **Y36.231** **War operations involving explosion of improvised explosive device [IED],** civilian

✓6ᵗʰ **Y36.24** **War operations involving explosion due to** accidental detonation and discharge of own munitions or munitions launch device

    ✓7ᵗʰ **Y36.240** **War operations involving explosion due to accidental detonation and discharge of own munitions or munitions launch device,** military personnel

    ✓7ᵗʰ **Y36.241** **War operations involving explosion due to accidental detonation and discharge of own munitions or munitions launch device,** civilian

✓6ᵗʰ **Y36.25** **War operations involving** fragments from munitions

    ✓7ᵗʰ **Y36.250** **War operations involving fragments from munitions,** military personnel

    ✓7ᵗʰ **Y36.251** **War operations involving fragments from munitions,** civilian

✓6ᵗʰ **Y36.26** **War operations involving fragments of** improvised explosive device [IED]
War operations involving fragments of person-borne improvised explosive device [IED]
War operations involving fragments of vehicle-borne improvised explosive device [IED]
War operations involving fragments of roadside improvised explosive device [IED]

    ✓7ᵗʰ **Y36.260** **War operations involving fragments of improvised explosive device [IED],** military personnel

    ✓7ᵗʰ **Y36.261** **War operations involving fragments of improvised explosive device [IED],** civilian

✓6ᵗʰ **Y36.27** **War operations involving** fragments from weapons

    ✓7ᵗʰ **Y36.270** **War operations involving fragments from weapons,** military personnel

    ✓7ᵗʰ **Y36.271** **War operations involving fragments from weapons,** civilian

✓6ᵗʰ **Y36.29** **War operations involving** other explosions and fragments
War operations involving explosion of grenade
War operations involving explosions of land mine
War operations involving shrapnel NOS

    ✓7ᵗʰ **Y36.290** **War operations involving other explosions and fragments,** military personnel

    ✓7ᵗʰ **Y36.291** **War operations involving other explosions and fragments,** civilian

✓5ᵗʰ **Y36.3** **War operations involving** fires, conflagrations and hot substances
War operations involving smoke, fumes, and heat from fires, conflagrations and hot substances

    **EXCLUDES 1**   *war operations involving fires and conflagrations aboard military aircraft (Y36.1-)*
*war operations involving fires and conflagrations aboard military watercraft (Y36.0-)*
*war operations involving fires and conflagrations caused indirectly by conventional weapons (Y36.2-)*
*war operations involving fires and thermal effects of nuclear weapons (Y36.53-)*

✓6ᵗʰ **Y36.30** **War operations involving** unspecified fire, conflagration and hot substance

    ✓7ᵗʰ **Y36.300** **War operations involving unspecified fire, conflagration and hot substance,** military personnel

    ✓7ᵗʰ **Y36.301** **War operations involving unspecified fire, conflagration and hot substance,** civilian

✓6ᵗʰ **Y36.31** **War operations involving** gasoline bomb
War operations involving incendiary bomb
War operations involving petrol bomb

    ✓7ᵗʰ **Y36.310** **War operations involving gasoline bomb,** military personnel

    ✓7ᵗʰ **Y36.311** **War operations involving gasoline bomb,** civilian

✓6ᵗʰ **Y36.32** **War operations involving** incendiary bullet

    ✓7ᵗʰ **Y36.320** **War operations involving incendiary bullet,** military personnel

    ✓7ᵗʰ **Y36.321** **War operations involving incendiary bullet,** civilian

✓6ᵗʰ **Y36.33** **War operations involving** flamethrower

    ✓7ᵗʰ **Y36.330** **War operations involving flamethrower,** military personnel

    ✓7ᵗʰ **Y36.331** **War operations involving flamethrower,** civilian

✓6ᵗʰ **Y36.39** **War operations involving other fires,** conflagrations and hot substances

    ✓7ᵗʰ **Y36.390** **War operations involving other fires, conflagrations and hot substances,** military personnel

    ✓7ᵗʰ **Y36.391** **War operations involving other fires, conflagrations and hot substances,** civilian

✓5ᵗʰ **Y36.4** **War operations involving firearm discharge and other forms of conventional warfare**

✓6ᵗʰ **Y36.41** **War operations involving** rubber bullets

    ✓7ᵗʰ **Y36.410** **War operations involving rubber bullets,** military personnel

    ✓7ᵗʰ **Y36.411** **War operations involving rubber bullets,** civilian

✓6ᵗʰ **Y36.42** **War operations involving** firearms pellets

    ✓7ᵗʰ **Y36.420** **War operations involving firearms pellets,** military personnel

    ✓7ᵗʰ **Y36.421** **War operations involving firearms pellets,** civilian

✓6ᵗʰ **Y36.43** **War operations involving** other firearms discharge
War operations involving bullets NOS

    **EXCLUDES 1**   *war operations involving munitions fragments (Y36.25-)*
*war operations involving incendiary bullets (Y36.32-)*

    ✓7ᵗʰ **Y36.430** **War operations involving other firearms discharge,** military personnel

    ✓7ᵗʰ **Y36.431** **War operations involving other firearms discharge,** civilian

✓6ᵗʰ **Y36.44** **War operations involving** unarmed hand to hand combat

    **EXCLUDES 1**   *war operations involving combat using blunt or piercing object (Y36.45-)*
*war operations involving intentional restriction of air and airway (Y36.46-)*
*war operations involving unintentional restriction of air and airway (Y36.47-)*

    ✓7ᵗʰ **Y36.440** **War operations involving unarmed hand to hand combat,** military personnel

    ✓7ᵗʰ **Y36.441** **War operations involving unarmed hand to hand combat,** civilian

✓6ᵗʰ **Y36.45** **War operations involving combat using blunt or piercing object**

    ✓7ᵗʰ **Y36.450** **War operations involving combat using blunt or piercing object,** military personnel

    ✓7ᵗʰ **Y36.451** **War operations involving combat using blunt or piercing object,** civilian

✓6ᵗʰ **Y36.46** **War operations involving** intentional restriction of air and airway

    ✓7ᵗʰ **Y36.460** **War operations involving intentional restriction of air and airway,** military personnel

    ✓7ᵗʰ **Y36.461** **War operations involving intentional restriction of air and airway,** civilian

N Newborn: 0   P Pediatric: 0-17   M Maternity: 12-55   A Adult: 15-124   MCC Major CC Condition   PDx MCC PDx acts as own MCC   CC CC Condition   PDx CC PDx acts as own CC

**1202**      ICD-10-CM 2018

√6th **Y36.47** **War operations involving** unintentional restriction of air and airway

√7th **Y36.470** **War operations involving unintentional restriction of air and airway,** military personnel

√7th **Y36.471** **War operations involving unintentional restriction of air and airway,** civilian

√6th **Y36.49** **War operations involving** other forms of conventional warfare

√7th **Y36.490** **War operations involving other forms of conventional warfare,** military personnel

√7th **Y36.491** **War operations involving other forms of conventional warfare,** civilian

√5th **Y36.5** **War operations involving** nuclear weapons
War operations involving dirty bomb NOS

√6th **Y36.50** **War operations involving** unspecified effect of nuclear weapon

√7th **Y36.500** **War operations involving unspecified effect of nuclear weapon,** military personnel

√7th **Y36.501** **War operations involving unspecified effect of nuclear weapon,** civilian

√6th **Y36.51** **War operations involving** direct blast effect of nuclear weapon
War operations involving blast pressure of nuclear weapon

√7th **Y36.510** **War operations involving direct blast effect of nuclear weapon,** military personnel

√7th **Y36.511** **War operations involving direct blast effect of nuclear weapon,** civilian

√6th **Y36.52** **War operations involving** indirect blast effect of nuclear weapon
War operations involving being thrown by blast of nuclear weapon
War operations involving being struck or crushed by blast debris of nuclear weapon

√7th **Y36.520** **War operations involving indirect blast effect of nuclear weapon,** military personnel

√7th **Y36.521** **War operations involving indirect blast effect of nuclear weapon,** civilian

√6th **Y36.53** **War operations involving** thermal radiation effect of nuclear weapon
War operations involving direct heat from nuclear weapon
War operation involving fireball effects from nuclear weapon

√7th **Y36.530** **War operations involving thermal radiation effect of nuclear weapon,** military personnel

√7th **Y36.531** **War operations involving thermal radiation effect of nuclear weapon,** civilian

√6th **Y36.54** **War operation involving** nuclear radiation effects of nuclear weapon
War operation involving acute radiation exposure from nuclear weapon
War operation involving exposure to immediate ionizing radiation from nuclear weapon
War operation involving fallout exposure from nuclear weapon
War operation involving secondary effects of nuclear weapons

√7th **Y36.540** **War operation involving nuclear radiation effects of nuclear weapon,** military personnel

√7th **Y36.541** **War operation involving nuclear radiation effects of nuclear weapon,** civilian

√6th **Y36.59** **War operation involving** other effects of nuclear weapons

√7th **Y36.590** **War operation involving other effects of nuclear weapons,** military personnel

√7th **Y36.591** **War operation involving other effects of nuclear weapons,** civilian

√5th **Y36.6** **War operations involving** biological weapons

√6th **Y36.6X** **War operations involving** biological weapons

√7th **Y36.6X0** **War operations involving biological weapons,** military personnel

√7th **Y36.6X1** **War operations involving biological weapons,** civilian

√5th **Y36.7** **War operations involving** chemical weapons and other forms of unconventional warfare

EXCLUDES 1    *war operations involving incendiary devices (Y36.3-, Y36.5-)*

√6th **Y36.7X** **War operations involving** chemical weapons and other forms of unconventional warfare

√7th **Y36.7X0** **War operations involving chemical weapons and other forms of unconventional warfare,** military personnel

√7th **Y36.7X1** **War operations involving chemical weapons and other forms of unconventional warfare,** civilian

√5th **Y36.8** **War operations occurring** after cessation of hostilities
War operations classifiable to categories Y36.0-Y36.8 but occurring after cessation of hostilities

√6th **Y36.81** **Explosion of** mine placed during war operations but exploding after cessation of hostilities

√7th **Y36.810** **Explosion of mine placed during war operations but exploding after cessation of hostilities,** military personnel

√7th **Y36.811** **Explosion of mine placed during war operations but exploding after cessation of hostilities,** civilian

√6th **Y36.82** **Explosion of** bomb placed during war operations but exploding after cessation of hostilities

√7th **Y36.820** **Explosion of bomb placed during war operations but exploding after cessation of hostilities,** military personnel

√7th **Y36.821** **Explosion of bomb placed during war operations but exploding after cessation of hostilities,** civilian

√6th **Y36.88** **Other** war operations occurring after cessation of hostilities

√7th **Y36.880** **Other war operations occurring after cessation of hostilities,** military personnel

√7th **Y36.881** **Other war operations occurring after cessation of hostilities,** civilian

√6th **Y36.89** **Unspecified** war operations occurring after cessation of hostilities

√7th **Y36.890** **Unspecified war operations occurring after cessation of hostilities,** military personnel

√7th **Y36.891** **Unspecified war operations occurring after cessation of hostilities,** civilian

√5th **Y36.9** **Other and unspecified war operations**

√x7th **Y36.90** **War operations,** unspecified

√x7th **Y36.91** **War operations** involving unspecified weapon of mass destruction [WMD]

√x7th **Y36.92** **War operations** involving friendly fire

√4th **Y37** **Military operations**
INCLUDES    injuries to military personnel and civilians occurring during peacetime on military property and during routine military exercises and operations

EXCLUDES 1    *military aircraft involved in aircraft accident with civilian aircraft (V97.81-)*
*military vehicles involved in transport accident with civilian vehicle (V09.01, V09.21, V19.81, V29.81, V39.81, V49.81, V59.81, V69.81, V79.81)*
*military watercraft involved in water transport accident with civilian watercraft (V94.81-)*
*war operations (Y36.-)*

√5th **Y37.0** **Military operations involving** explosion of marine weapons

√6th **Y37.00** **Military operations involving explosion of** unspecified marine weapon
Military operations involving underwater blast NOS

√7th **Y37.000** **Military operations involving explosion of unspecified marine weapon,** military personnel

√7th **Y37.001** **Military operations involving explosion of unspecified marine weapon,** civilian

---

√ Additional Character Req    √x7th Placeholder Alert    Unacceptable PDx    Manifestation    H1-H14 HAC    HCC CMS-HCC Condition    EXCLUDES 1 Not Coded Here    EXCLUDES 2 Not Included Here

✓6th   **Y37.01**   **Military operations involving explosion of** depth-charge

    ✓7th   **Y37.010**   **Military operations involving explosion of depth-charge, military personnel**

    ✓7th   **Y37.011**   **Military operations involving explosion of depth-charge, civilian**

✓6th   **Y37.02**   **Military operations involving explosion of** marine mine

      Military operations involving explosion of marine mine, at sea or in harbor

    ✓7th   **Y37.020**   **Military operations involving explosion of marine mine, military personnel**

    ✓7th   **Y37.021**   **Military operations involving explosion of marine mine, civilian**

✓6th   **Y37.03**   **Military operations involving explosion of** sea-based artillery shell

    ✓7th   **Y37.030**   **Military operations involving explosion of sea-based artillery shell, military personnel**

    ✓7th   **Y37.031**   **Military operations involving explosion of sea-based artillery shell, civilian**

✓6th   **Y37.04**   **Military operations involving explosion of** torpedo

    ✓7th   **Y37.040**   **Military operations involving explosion of torpedo, military personnel**

    ✓7th   **Y37.041**   **Military operations involving explosion of torpedo, civilian**

✓6th   **Y37.05**   **Military operations involving accidental detonation of** onboard marine weapons

    ✓7th   **Y37.050**   **Military operations involving accidental detonation of onboard marine weapons, military personnel**

    ✓7th   **Y37.051**   **Military operations involving accidental detonation of onboard marine weapons, civilian**

✓6th   **Y37.09**   **Military operations involving explosion of** other marine weapons

    ✓7th   **Y37.090**   **Military operations involving explosion of other marine weapons, military personnel**

    ✓7th   **Y37.091**   **Military operations involving explosion of other marine weapons, civilian**

✓5th   **Y37.1**   **Military operations involving** destruction of aircraft

   ✓6th   **Y37.10**   **Military operations involving** unspecified **destruction of aircraft**

    ✓7th   **Y37.100**   **Military operations involving unspecified destruction of aircraft, military personnel**

    ✓7th   **Y37.101**   **Military operations involving unspecified destruction of aircraft, civilian**

   ✓6th   **Y37.11**   **Military operations involving destruction of aircraft** due to enemy fire or explosives

      Military operations involving destruction of aircraft due to air to air missile

      Military operations involving destruction of aircraft due to explosive placed on aircraft

      Military operations involving destruction of aircraft due to rocket propelled grenade [RPG]

      Military operations involving destruction of aircraft due to small arms fire

      Military operations involving destruction of aircraft due to surface to air missile

    ✓7th   **Y37.110**   **Military operations involving destruction of aircraft due to enemy fire or explosives, military personnel**

    ✓7th   **Y37.111**   **Military operations involving destruction of aircraft due to enemy fire or explosives, civilian**

   ✓6th   **Y37.12**   **Military operations involving destruction of aircraft** due to collision with other aircraft

    ✓7th   **Y37.120**   **Military operations involving destruction of aircraft due to collision with other aircraft, military personnel**

    ✓7th   **Y37.121**   **Military operations involving destruction of aircraft due to collision with other aircraft, civilian**

   ✓6th   **Y37.13**   **Military operations involving destruction of aircraft** due to onboard fire

    ✓7th   **Y37.130**   **Military operations involving destruction of aircraft due to onboard fire, military personnel**

    ✓7th   **Y37.131**   **Military operations involving destruction of aircraft due to onboard fire, civilian**

   ✓6th   **Y37.14**   **Military operations involving destruction of aircraft due to** accidental detonation of onboard munitions and explosives

    ✓7th   **Y37.140**   **Military operations involving destruction of aircraft due to accidental detonation of onboard munitions and explosives, military personnel**

    ✓7th   **Y37.141**   **Military operations involving destruction of aircraft due to accidental detonation of onboard munitions and explosives, civilian**

   ✓6th   **Y37.19**   **Military operations involving other** destruction of aircraft

    ✓7th   **Y37.190**   **Military operations involving other destruction of aircraft, military personnel**

    ✓7th   **Y37.191**   **Military operations involving other destruction of aircraft, civilian**

✓5th   **Y37.2**   **Military operations involving** other explosions and fragments

     **EXCLUDES 1**   *military operations involving explosion of aircraft (Y37.1-)*

       *military operations involving explosion of marine weapons (Y37.0-)*

       *military operations involving explosion of nuclear weapons (Y37.5-)*

   ✓6th   **Y37.20**   **Military operations involving** unspecified **explosion and fragments**

      Military operations involving air blast NOS

      Military operations involving blast NOS

      Military operations involving blast fragments NOS

      Military operations involving blast wave NOS

      Military operations involving blast wind NOS

      Military operations involving explosion NOS

      Military operations involving explosion of bomb NOS

    ✓7th   **Y37.200**   **Military operations involving unspecified explosion and fragments, military personnel**

    ✓7th   **Y37.201**   **Military operations involving unspecified explosion and fragments, civilian**

   ✓6th   **Y37.21**   **Military operations involving explosion of** aerial bomb

    ✓7th   **Y37.210**   **Military operations involving explosion of aerial bomb, military personnel**

    ✓7th   **Y37.211**   **Military operations involving explosion of aerial bomb, civilian**

   ✓6th   **Y37.22**   **Military operations involving explosion of** guided missile

    ✓7th   **Y37.220**   **Military operations involving explosion of guided missile, military personnel**

    ✓7th   **Y37.221**   **Military operations involving explosion of guided missile, civilian**

   ✓6th   **Y37.23**   **Military operations involving explosion of** improvised explosive device [IED]

      Military operations involving explosion of person-borne improvised explosive device [IED]

      Military operations involving explosion of vehicle-borne improvised explosive device [IED]

      Military operations involving explosion of roadside improvised explosive device [IED]

    ✓7th   **Y37.230**   **Military operations involving explosion of improvised explosive device [IED], military personnel**

    ✓7th   **Y37.231**   **Military operations involving explosion of improvised explosive device [IED], civilian**

   ✓6th   **Y37.24**   **Military operations involving explosion** due to accidental detonation and discharge of own munitions or munitions launch device

    ✓7th   **Y37.240**   **Military operations involving explosion due to accidental detonation and discharge of own munitions or munitions launch device, military personnel**

    ✓7th   **Y37.241**   **Military operations involving explosion due to accidental detonation and discharge of own munitions or munitions launch device, civilian**

N Newborn: 0    P Pediatric: 0-17    M Maternity: 12-55    A Adult: 15-124    **MCC** Major CC Condition    **PDx MCC** PDx acts as own MCC    **CC** CC Condition    **PDx CC** PDx acts as own CC

1204        ICD-10-CM 2018

☑6ᵗʰ **Y37.25** **Military operations involving** fragments from munitions

     ☑7ᵗʰ **Y37.250** **Military operations involving fragments from munitions,** military personnel

     ☑7ᵗʰ **Y37.251** **Military operations involving fragments from munitions,** civilian

☑6ᵗʰ **Y37.26** **Military operations involving fragments of** improvised explosive device [IED]

     Military operations involving fragments of person-borne improvised explosive device [IED]

     Military operations involving fragments of vehicle-borne improvised explosive device [IED]

     Military operations involving fragments of roadside improvised explosive device [IED]

     ☑7ᵗʰ **Y37.260** **Military operations involving fragments of improvised explosive device [IED],** military personnel

     ☑7ᵗʰ **Y37.261** **Military operations involving fragments of improvised explosive device [IED],** civilian

☑6ᵗʰ **Y37.27** **Military operations involving fragments from** weapons

     ☑7ᵗʰ **Y37.270** **Military operations involving fragments from weapons,** military personnel

     ☑7ᵗʰ **Y37.271** **Military operations involving fragments from weapons,** civilian

☑6ᵗʰ **Y37.29** **Military operations involving** other explosions and fragments

     Military operations involving explosion of grenade

     Military operations involving explosions of land mine

     Military operations involving shrapnel NOS

     ☑7ᵗʰ **Y37.290** **Military operations involving other explosions and fragments,** military personnel

     ☑7ᵗʰ **Y37.291** **Military operations involving other explosions and fragments,** civilian

☑5ᵗʰ **Y37.3** **Military operations involving** fires, conflagrations and hot substances

     Military operations involving smoke, fumes, and heat from fires, conflagrations and hot substances

     *EXCLUDES 1*   *military operations involving fires and conflagrations aboard military aircraft (Y37.1-)*

     *military operations involving fires and conflagrations aboard military watercraft (Y37.0-)*

     *military operations involving fires and conflagrations caused indirectly by conventional weapons (Y37.2-)*

     *military operations involving fires and thermal effects of nuclear weapons (Y36.53-)*

☑6ᵗʰ **Y37.30** **Military operations involving** unspecified fire, conflagration and hot substance

     ☑7ᵗʰ **Y37.300** **Military operations involving unspecified fire, conflagration and hot substance,** military personnel

     ☑7ᵗʰ **Y37.301** **Military operations involving unspecified fire, conflagration and hot substance,** civilian

☑6ᵗʰ **Y37.31** **Military operations involving** gasoline bomb

     Military operations involving incendiary bomb

     Military operations involving petrol bomb

     ☑7ᵗʰ **Y37.310** **Military operations involving gasoline bomb,** military personnel

     ☑7ᵗʰ **Y37.311** **Military operations involving gasoline bomb,** civilian

☑6ᵗʰ **Y37.32** **Military operations involving** incendiary bullet

     ☑7ᵗʰ **Y37.320** **Military operations involving incendiary bullet,** military personnel

     ☑7ᵗʰ **Y37.321** **Military operations involving incendiary bullet,** civilian

☑6ᵗʰ **Y37.33** **Military operations involving** flamethrower

     ☑7ᵗʰ **Y37.330** **Military operations involving flamethrower,** military personnel

     ☑7ᵗʰ **Y37.331** **Military operations involving flamethrower,** civilian

☑6ᵗʰ **Y37.39** **Military operations involving** other fires, conflagrations and hot substances

     ☑7ᵗʰ **Y37.390** **Military operations involving other fires, conflagrations and hot substances,** military personnel

     ☑7ᵗʰ **Y37.391** **Military operations involving other fires, conflagrations and hot substances,** civilian

☑5ᵗʰ **Y37.4** **Military operations involving firearm discharge and other forms of conventional warfare**

☑6ᵗʰ **Y37.41** **Military operations involving** rubber bullets

     ☑7ᵗʰ **Y37.410** **Military operations involving rubber bullets,** military personnel

     ☑7ᵗʰ **Y37.411** **Military operations involving rubber bullets,** civilian

☑6ᵗʰ **Y37.42** **Military operations involving** firearms pellets

     ☑7ᵗʰ **Y37.420** **Military operations involving firearms pellets,** military personnel

     ☑7ᵗʰ **Y37.421** **Military operations involving firearms pellets,** civilian

☑6ᵗʰ **Y37.43** **Military operations involving** other firearms discharge

     Military operations involving bullets NOS

     *EXCLUDES 1*   *military operations involving munitions fragments (Y37.25-)*

     *military operations involving incendiary bullets (Y37.32-)*

     ☑7ᵗʰ **Y37.430** **Military operations involving other firearms discharge,** military personnel

     ☑7ᵗʰ **Y37.431** **Military operations involving other firearms discharge,** civilian

☑6ᵗʰ **Y37.44** **Military operations involving** unarmed hand to hand combat

     *EXCLUDES 1*   *military operations involving combat using blunt or piercing object (Y37.45-)*

     *military operations involving intentional restriction of air and airway (Y37.46-)*

     *military operations involving unintentional restriction of air and airway (Y37.47-)*

     ☑7ᵗʰ **Y37.440** **Military operations involving unarmed hand to hand combat,** military personnel

     ☑7ᵗʰ **Y37.441** **Military operations involving unarmed hand to hand combat,** civilian

☑6ᵗʰ **Y37.45** **Military operations involving** combat using blunt or piercing object

     ☑7ᵗʰ **Y37.450** **Military operations involving combat using blunt or piercing object,** military personnel

     ☑7ᵗʰ **Y37.451** **Military operations involving combat using blunt or piercing object,** civilian

☑6ᵗʰ **Y37.46** **Military operations involving** intentional restriction of air and airway

     ☑7ᵗʰ **Y37.460** **Military operations involving intentional restriction of air and airway,** military personnel

     ☑7ᵗʰ **Y37.461** **Military operations involving intentional restriction of air and airway,** civilian

☑6ᵗʰ **Y37.47** **Military operations involving** unintentional restriction of air and airway

     ☑7ᵗʰ **Y37.470** **Military operations involving unintentional restriction of air and airway,** military personnel

     ☑7ᵗʰ **Y37.471** **Military operations involving unintentional restriction of air and airway,** civilian

☑6ᵗʰ **Y37.49** **Military operations involving** other forms of conventional warfare

     ☑7ᵗʰ **Y37.490** **Military operations involving other forms of conventional warfare,** military personnel

     ☑7ᵗʰ **Y37.491** **Military operations involving other forms of conventional warfare,** civilian

---

☑ Additional Character Req   ☑7ᵗʰ Placeholder Alert   Unacceptable PDx   Manifestation   **H1**-**H14** HAC   **HCC** CMS-HCC Condition   *EXCLUDES 1* Not Coded Here   *EXCLUDES 2* Not Included Here

**Chapter 20. External Causes of Morbidity**

**Y37.5–Y38.2X3**

✓5ᵗʰ **Y37.5 Military operations involving nuclear weapons**
Military operation involving dirty bomb NOS

  ✓6ᵗʰ **Y37.50 Military operations involving unspecified effect of nuclear weapon**

    ✓7ᵗʰ **Y37.500 Military operations involving unspecified effect of nuclear weapon, military personnel**

    ✓7ᵗʰ **Y37.501 Military operations involving unspecified effect of nuclear weapon, civilian**

  ✓6ᵗʰ **Y37.51 Military operations involving direct blast effect of nuclear weapon**
Military operations involving blast pressure of nuclear weapon

    ✓7ᵗʰ **Y37.510 Military operations involving direct blast effect of nuclear weapon, military personnel**

    ✓7ᵗʰ **Y37.511 Military operations involving direct blast effect of nuclear weapon, civilian**

  ✓6ᵗʰ **Y37.52 Military operations involving indirect blast effect of nuclear weapon**
Military operations involving being thrown by blast of nuclear weapon
Military operations involving being struck or crushed by blast debris of nuclear weapon

    ✓7ᵗʰ **Y37.520 Military operations involving indirect blast effect of nuclear weapon, military personnel**

    ✓7ᵗʰ **Y37.521 Military operations involving indirect blast effect of nuclear weapon, civilian**

  ✓6ᵗʰ **Y37.53 Military operations involving thermal radiation effect of nuclear weapon**
Military operations involving direct heat from nuclear weapon
Military operation involving fireball effects from nuclear weapon

    ✓7ᵗʰ **Y37.530 Military operations involving thermal radiation effect of nuclear weapon, military personnel**

    ✓7ᵗʰ **Y37.531 Military operations involving thermal radiation effect of nuclear weapon, civilian**

  ✓6ᵗʰ **Y37.54 Military operation involving nuclear radiation effects of nuclear weapon**
Military operation involving acute radiation exposure from nuclear weapon
Military operation involving exposure to immediate ionizing radiation from nuclear weapon
Military operation involving fallout exposure from nuclear weapon
Military operation involving secondary effects of nuclear weapons

    ✓7ᵗʰ **Y37.540 Military operation involving nuclear radiation effects of nuclear weapon, military personnel**

    ✓7ᵗʰ **Y37.541 Military operation involving nuclear radiation effects of nuclear weapon, civilian**

  ✓6ᵗʰ **Y37.59 Military operation involving other effects of nuclear weapons**

    ✓7ᵗʰ **Y37.590 Military operation involving other effects of nuclear weapons, military personnel**

    ✓7ᵗʰ **Y37.591 Military operation involving other effects of nuclear weapons, civilian**

✓5ᵗʰ **Y37.6 Military operations involving biological weapons**

  ✓6ᵗʰ **Y37.6X Military operations involving biological weapons**

    ✓7ᵗʰ **Y37.6X0 Military operations involving biological weapons, military personnel**

    ✓7ᵗʰ **Y37.6X1 Military operations involving biological weapons, civilian**

✓5ᵗʰ **Y37.7 Military operations involving chemical weapons and other forms of unconventional warfare**

    **EXCLUDES 1** *military operations involving incendiary devices (Y36.3-, Y36.5-)*

  ✓6ᵗʰ **Y37.7X Military operations involving chemical weapons and other forms of unconventional warfare**

    ✓7ᵗʰ **Y37.7X0 Military operations involving chemical weapons and other forms of unconventional warfare, military personnel**

    ✓7ᵗʰ **Y37.7X1 Military operations involving chemical weapons and other forms of unconventional warfare, civilian**

✓5ᵗʰ **Y37.9 Other and unspecified military operations**

  ✓x7ᵗʰ **Y37.90 Military operations, unspecified**

  ✓x7ᵗʰ **Y37.91 Military operations involving unspecified weapon of mass destruction [WMD]**

  ✓x7ᵗʰ **Y37.92 Military operations involving friendly fire**

✓4ᵗʰ **Y38 Terrorism**

  **NOTE** These codes are for use to identify injuries resulting from the unlawful use of force or violence against persons or property to intimidate or coerce a Government, the civilian population, or any segment thereof, in furtherance of political or social objective.
Use additional code for place of occurrence (Y92.-)

✓5ᵗʰ **Y38.0 Terrorism involving explosion of marine weapons**
Terrorism involving depth-charge
Terrorism involving marine mine
Terrorism involving mine NOS, at sea or in harbor
Terrorism involving sea-based artillery shell
Terrorism involving torpedo
Terrorism involving underwater blast

  ✓6ᵗʰ **Y38.0X Terrorism involving explosion of marine weapons**

    ✓7ᵗʰ **Y38.0X1 Terrorism involving explosion of marine weapons, public safety official injured**

    ✓7ᵗʰ **Y38.0X2 Terrorism involving explosion of marine weapons, civilian injured**

    ✓7ᵗʰ **Y38.0X3 Terrorism involving explosion of marine weapons, terrorist injured**

✓5ᵗʰ **Y38.1 Terrorism involving destruction of aircraft**
Terrorism involving aircraft burned
Terrorism involving aircraft exploded
Terrorism involving aircraft being shot down
Terrorism involving aircraft used as a weapon

  ✓6ᵗʰ **Y38.1X Terrorism involving destruction of aircraft**

    ✓7ᵗʰ **Y38.1X1 Terrorism involving destruction of aircraft, public safety official injured**

    ✓7ᵗʰ **Y38.1X2 Terrorism involving destruction of aircraft, civilian injured**

    ✓7ᵗʰ **Y38.1X3 Terrorism involving destruction of aircraft, terrorist injured**

✓5ᵗʰ **Y38.2 Terrorism involving other explosions and fragments**
Terrorism involving antipersonnel (fragments) bomb
Terrorism involving blast NOS
Terrorism involving explosion NOS
Terrorism involving explosion of breech block
Terrorism involving explosion of cannon block
Terrorism involving explosion (fragments) of artillery shell
Terrorism involving explosion (fragments) of bomb
Terrorism involving explosion (fragments) of grenade
Terrorism involving explosion (fragments) of guided missile
Terrorism involving explosion (fragments) of land mine
Terrorism involving explosion of mortar bomb
Terrorism involving explosion of munitions
Terrorism involving explosion (fragments) of rocket
Terrorism involving explosion (fragments) of shell
Terrorism involving shrapnel
Terrorism involving mine NOS, on land

    **EXCLUDES 1** *terrorism involving explosion of nuclear weapon (Y38.5)*
*terrorism involving suicide bomber (Y38.81)*

  ✓6ᵗʰ **Y38.2X Terrorism involving other explosions and fragments**

    ✓7ᵗʰ **Y38.2X1 Terrorism involving other explosions and fragments, public safety official injured**

    ✓7ᵗʰ **Y38.2X2 Terrorism involving other explosions and fragments, civilian injured**

    ✓7ᵗʰ **Y38.2X3 Terrorism involving other explosions and fragments, terrorist injured**

**N** Newborn: 0    **P** Pediatric: 0-17    **M** Maternity: 12-55    **A** Adult: 15-124    **MCC** Major CC Condition    **PDxMCC** PDx acts as own MCC    **CC** CC Condition    **PDxCC** PDx acts as own CC

1206          ICD-10-CM 2018

✓5ᵗʰ **Y38.3** **Terrorism involving fires, conflagration and hot substances**
Terrorism involving conflagration NOS
Terrorism involving fire NOS
Terrorism involving petrol bomb
> *EXCLUDES 1*   *terrorism involving fire or heat of nuclear weapon (Y38.5)*

✓6ᵗʰ **Y38.3X** **Terrorism involving** fires, conflagration and hot substances

✓7ᵗʰ **Y38.3X1** **Terrorism involving fires, conflagration and hot substances, public safety official injured**

✓7ᵗʰ **Y38.3X2** **Terrorism involving fires, conflagration and hot substances, civilian injured**

✓7ᵗʰ **Y38.3X3** **Terrorism involving fires, conflagration and hot substances, terrorist injured**

✓5ᵗʰ **Y38.4** **Terrorism involving firearms**
Terrorism involving carbine bullet
Terrorism involving machine gun bullet
Terrorism involving pellets (shotgun)
Terrorism involving pistol bullet
Terrorism involving rifle bullet
Terrorism involving rubber (rifle) bullet

✓6ᵗʰ **Y38.4X** **Terrorism involving** firearms

✓7ᵗʰ **Y38.4X1** **Terrorism involving firearms, public safety official injured**

✓7ᵗʰ **Y38.4X2** **Terrorism involving firearms, civilian injured**

✓7ᵗʰ **Y38.4X3** **Terrorism involving firearms, terrorist injured**

✓5ᵗʰ **Y38.5** **Terrorism involving nuclear weapons**
Terrorism involving blast effects of nuclear weapon
Terrorism involving exposure to ionizing radiation from nuclear weapon
Terrorism involving fireball effect of nuclear weapon
Terrorism involving heat from nuclear weapon

✓6ᵗʰ **Y38.5X** **Terrorism involving** nuclear weapons

✓7ᵗʰ **Y38.5X1** **Terrorism involving nuclear weapons, public safety official injured**

✓7ᵗʰ **Y38.5X2** **Terrorism involving nuclear weapons, civilian injured**

✓7ᵗʰ **Y38.5X3** **Terrorism involving nuclear weapons, terrorist injured**

✓5ᵗʰ **Y38.6** **Terrorism involving biological weapons**
Terrorism involving anthrax
Terrorism involving cholera
Terrorism involving smallpox

✓6ᵗʰ **Y38.6X** **Terrorism involving** biological weapons

✓7ᵗʰ **Y38.6X1** **Terrorism involving biological weapons, public safety official injured**

✓7ᵗʰ **Y38.6X2** **Terrorism involving biological weapons, civilian injured**

✓7ᵗʰ **Y38.6X3** **Terrorism involving biological weapons, terrorist injured**

✓5ᵗʰ **Y38.7** **Terrorism involving chemical weapons**
Terrorism involving gases, fumes, chemicals
Terrorism involving hydrogen cyanide
Terrorism involving phosgene
Terrorism involving sarin

✓6ᵗʰ **Y38.7X** **Terrorism involving** chemical weapons

✓7ᵗʰ **Y38.7X1** **Terrorism involving chemical weapons, public safety official injured**

✓7ᵗʰ **Y38.7X2** **Terrorism involving chemical weapons, civilian injured**

✓7ᵗʰ **Y38.7X3** **Terrorism involving chemical weapons, terrorist injured**

✓5ᵗʰ **Y38.8** **Terrorism involving other and unspecified means**

✓x7ᵗʰ **Y38.80** **Terrorism involving unspecified means**
Terrorism NOS

✓6ᵗʰ **Y38.81** **Terrorism involving** suicide bomber

✓7ᵗʰ **Y38.811** **Terrorism involving suicide bomber, public safety official injured**

✓7ᵗʰ **Y38.812** **Terrorism involving suicide bomber, civilian injured**

✓6ᵗʰ **Y38.89** **Terrorism involving** other **means**
Terrorism involving drowning and submersion
Terrorism involving lasers
Terrorism involving piercing or stabbing instruments

✓7ᵗʰ **Y38.891** **Terrorism involving other means, public safety official injured**

✓7ᵗʰ **Y38.892** **Terrorism involving other means, civilian injured**

✓7ᵗʰ **Y38.893** **Terrorism involving other means, terrorist injured**

✓5ᵗʰ **Y38.9** **Terrorism, secondary effects**
> *NOTE*   This code is for use to identify injuries occurring subsequent to a terrorist attack, not those that are due to the initial terrorist attack.

✓6ᵗʰ **Y38.9X** **Terrorism,** secondary effects

✓7ᵗʰ **Y38.9X1** **Terrorism, secondary effects, public safety official injured**

✓7ᵗʰ **Y38.9X2** **Terrorism, secondary effects, civilian injured**

## Complications of medical and surgical care (Y62-Y84)

> *INCLUDES*   complications of medical devices
> surgical and medical procedures as the cause of abnormal reaction of the patient, or of later complication, without mention of misadventure at the time of the procedure

## Misadventures to patients during surgical and medical care (Y62-Y69)

> *EXCLUDES 1*   *surgical and medical procedures as the cause of abnormal reaction of the patient, without mention of misadventure at the time of the procedure (Y83-Y84)*
> *EXCLUDES 2*   *breakdown or malfunctioning of medical device (during procedure) (after implantation) (ongoing use) (Y70-Y82)*

✓4ᵗʰ **Y62** **Failure of** sterile precautions **during surgical and medical care**

**Y62.0** **Failure of sterile precautions during** surgical operation

**Y62.1** **Failure of sterile precautions during** infusion or transfusion

**Y62.2** **Failure of sterile precautions during** kidney dialysis and other perfusion    `HCC`

**Y62.3** **Failure of sterile precautions during** injection or immunization

**Y62.4** **Failure of sterile precautions during** endoscopic examination

**Y62.5** **Failure of sterile precautions during** heart catheterization

**Y62.6** **Failure of sterile precautions during** aspiration, puncture and other catheterization

**Y62.8** **Failure of sterile precautions during** other **surgical and medical care**

**Y62.9** **Failure of sterile precautions during** unspecified **surgical and medical care**

✓4ᵗʰ **Y63** **Failure in** dosage **during surgical and medical care**
> *EXCLUDES 2*   *accidental overdose of drug or wrong drug given in error (T36-T50)*

**Y63.0** **Excessive amount of blood or other fluid given during transfusion or infusion**

**Y63.1** **Incorrect dilution of fluid used during infusion**

**Y63.2** **Overdose of radiation given during therapy**

**Y63.3** **Inadvertent exposure of patient to radiation during medical care**

**Y63.4** **Failure in dosage in electroshock or insulin-shock therapy**

**Y63.5** **Inappropriate temperature in local application and packing**

**Y63.6** **Underdosing and nonadministration of necessary drug, medicament or biological substance**

**Y63.8** **Failure in dosage during other surgical and medical care**

**Y63.9** **Failure in dosage during unspecified surgical and medical care**

✓4ᵗʰ **Y64** **Contaminated** medical or biological **substances**

**Y64.0** **Contaminated medical or biological substance,** transfused or infused

**Y64.1** **Contaminated medical or biological substance,** injected or used for immunization

**Y64.8** **Contaminated medical or biological substance administered by** other means

**Y64.9** **Contaminated medical or biological substance administered by** unspecified means
Administered contaminated medical or biological substance NOS

---

✓ Additional Character Req    ✓x7ᵗʰ Placeholder Alert    Unacceptable PDx    **Manifestation**    H1 - H14 HAC    HCC CMS-HCC Condition    *EXCLUDES 1* Not Coded Here    *EXCLUDES 2* Not Included Here

ICD-10-CM 2018          1207

Y38.3–Y64.9

✓4ᵗʰ **Y65** **Other misadventures during surgical and medical care**

**Y65.0** **Mismatched blood in transfusion**

**Y65.1** **Wrong fluid used in infusion**

**Y65.2** **Failure in suture or ligature during surgical operation**

**Y65.3** **Endotracheal tube wrongly placed during anesthetic procedure**

**Y65.4** **Failure to introduce or to remove other tube or instrument**

✓5ᵗʰ **Y65.5** **Performance of wrong procedure (operation)**

² **Y65.51** **Performance of wrong procedure (operation) on correct patient**
Wrong device implanted into correct surgical site
EXCLUDES 1 *performance of correct procedure (operation) on wrong side or body part (Y65.53)*

² **Y65.52** **Performance of procedure (operation) on patient not scheduled for surgery**
Performance of procedure (operation) intended for another patient
Performance of procedure (operation) on wrong patient

² **Y65.53** **Performance of correct procedure (operation) on wrong side or body part**
Performance of correct procedure (operation) on wrong side
Performance of correct procedure (operation) on wrong site

**Y65.8** **Other specified misadventures during surgical and medical care**

**Y66** **Nonadministration of surgical and medical care**
Premature cessation of surgical and medical care
EXCLUDES 1 *DNR status (Z66)*
*palliative care (Z51.5)*

**Y69** **Unspecified misadventure during surgical and medical care**

## Medical devices associated with adverse incidents in diagnostic and therapeutic use (Y70-Y82)

INCLUDES breakdown or malfunction of medical devices (during use) (after implantation) (ongoing use)
EXCLUDES 2 *breakdown or malfunctioning of medical device (after implantation) (during procedure) (ongoing use) (Y70-Y82)*
*later complications following use of medical devices without breakdown or malfunctioning of device (Y83-Y84)*
*misadventure to patients during surgical and medical care, classifiable to (Y62-Y69)*
*surgical and other medical procedures as the cause of abnormal reaction of the patient, or of later complication, without mention of misadventure at the time of the procedure (Y83-Y84)*

✓4ᵗʰ **Y70** **Anesthesiology devices associated with adverse incidents**

**Y70.0** **Diagnostic and monitoring anesthesiology devices associated with adverse incidents**

**Y70.1** **Therapeutic (nonsurgical) and rehabilitative anesthesiology devices associated with adverse incidents**

**Y70.2** **Prosthetic and other implants, materials and accessory anesthesiology devices associated with adverse incidents**

**Y70.3** **Surgical instruments, materials and anesthesiology devices (including sutures) associated with adverse incidents**

**Y70.8** **Miscellaneous anesthesiology devices associated with adverse incidents, not elsewhere classified**

✓4ᵗʰ **Y71** **Cardiovascular devices associated with adverse incidents**

**Y71.0** **Diagnostic and monitoring cardiovascular devices associated with adverse incidents**

**Y71.1** **Therapeutic (nonsurgical) and rehabilitative cardiovascular devices associated with adverse incidents**

**Y71.2** **Prosthetic and other implants, materials and accessory cardiovascular devices associated with adverse incidents**

**Y71.3** **Surgical instruments, materials and cardiovascular devices (including sutures) associated with adverse incidents**

**Y71.8** **Miscellaneous cardiovascular devices associated with adverse incidents, not elsewhere classified**

✓4ᵗʰ **Y72** **Otorhinolaryngological devices associated with adverse incidents**

**Y72.0** **Diagnostic and monitoring otorhinolaryngological devices associated with adverse incidents**

**Y72.1** **Therapeutic (nonsurgical) and rehabilitative otorhinolaryngological devices associated with adverse incidents**

**Y72.2** **Prosthetic and other implants, materials and accessory otorhinolaryngological devices associated with adverse incidents**

**Y72.3** **Surgical instruments, materials and otorhinolaryngological devices (including sutures) associated with adverse incidents**

**Y72.8** **Miscellaneous otorhinolaryngological devices associated with adverse incidents, not elsewhere classified**

✓4ᵗʰ **Y73** **Gastroenterology and urology devices associated with adverse incidents**

**Y73.0** **Diagnostic and monitoring gastroenterology and urology devices associated with adverse incidents**

**Y73.1** **Therapeutic (nonsurgical) and rehabilitative gastroenterology and urology devices associated with adverse incidents**

**Y73.2** **Prosthetic and other implants, materials and accessory gastroenterology and urology devices associated with adverse incidents**

**Y73.3** **Surgical instruments, materials and gastroenterology and urology devices (including sutures) associated with adverse incidents**

**Y73.8** **Miscellaneous gastroenterology and urology devices associated with adverse incidents, not elsewhere classified**

✓4ᵗʰ **Y74** **General hospital and personal-use devices associated with adverse incidents**

**Y74.0** **Diagnostic and monitoring general hospital and personal-use devices associated with adverse incidents**

**Y74.1** **Therapeutic (nonsurgical) and rehabilitative general hospital and personal-use devices associated with adverse incidents**

**Y74.2** **Prosthetic and other implants, materials and accessory general hospital and personal-use devices associated with adverse incidents**

**Y74.3** **Surgical instruments, materials and general hospital and personal-use devices (including sutures) associated with adverse incidents**

**Y74.8** **Miscellaneous general hospital and personal-use devices associated with adverse incidents, not elsewhere classified**

✓4ᵗʰ **Y75** **Neurological devices associated with adverse incidents**

**Y75.0** **Diagnostic and monitoring neurological devices associated with adverse incidents**

**Y75.1** **Therapeutic (nonsurgical) and rehabilitative neurological devices associated with adverse incidents**

**Y75.2** **Prosthetic and other implants, materials and neurological devices associated with adverse incidents**

**Y75.3** **Surgical instruments, materials and neurological devices (including sutures) associated with adverse incidents**

**Y75.8** **Miscellaneous neurological devices associated with adverse incidents, not elsewhere classified**

✓4ᵗʰ **Y76** **Obstetric and gynecological devices associated with adverse incidents**

**Y76.0** **Diagnostic and monitoring obstetric and gynecological devices associated with adverse incidents** ♀

**Y76.1** **Therapeutic (nonsurgical) and rehabilitative obstetric and gynecological devices associated with adverse incidents** ♀

**Y76.2** **Prosthetic and other implants, materials and accessory obstetric and gynecological devices associated with adverse incidents** ♀

**Y76.3** **Surgical instruments, materials and obstetric and gynecological devices (including sutures) associated with adverse incidents** ♀

**Y76.8** **Miscellaneous obstetric and gynecological devices associated with adverse incidents, not elsewhere classified** ♀

✓4ᵗʰ **Y77** **Ophthalmic devices associated with adverse incidents**

**Y77.0** **Diagnostic and monitoring ophthalmic devices associated with adverse incidents**

**Y77.1** **Therapeutic (nonsurgical) and rehabilitative ophthalmic devices associated with adverse incidents**

**Y77.2** **Prosthetic and other implants, materials and accessory ophthalmic devices associated with adverse incidents**

**Y77.3** **Surgical instruments, materials and ophthalmic devices (including sutures) associated with adverse incidents**

**Y77.8** **Miscellaneous ophthalmic devices associated with adverse incidents, not elsewhere classified**

---

² Wrong procedure performed edit applies.

Ⓝ Newborn: 0 | Ⓟ Pediatric: 0-17 | Ⓜ Maternity: 12-55 | Ⓐ Adult: 15-124 | MCC Major CC Condition | PDxMCC PDx acts as own MCC | CC CC Condition | PDxCC PDx acts as own CC

☑4ᵗʰ **Y78  Radiological devices associated with adverse incidents**

   **Y78.0  Diagnostic and monitoring radiological devices associated with adverse incidents**

   **Y78.1  Therapeutic (nonsurgical) and rehabilitative radiological devices associated with adverse incidents**

   **Y78.2  Prosthetic and other implants, materials and accessory radiological devices associated with adverse incidents**

   **Y78.3  Surgical instruments, materials and radiological devices (including sutures) associated with adverse incidents**

   **Y78.8  Miscellaneous radiological devices associated with adverse incidents, not elsewhere classified**

☑4ᵗʰ **Y79  Orthopedic devices associated with adverse incidents**

   **Y79.0  Diagnostic and monitoring orthopedic devices associated with adverse incidents**

   **Y79.1  Therapeutic (nonsurgical) and rehabilitative orthopedic devices associated with adverse incidents**

   **Y79.2  Prosthetic and other implants, materials and accessory orthopedic devices associated with adverse incidents**

   **Y79.3  Surgical instruments, materials and orthopedic devices (including sutures) associated with adverse incidents**

   **Y79.8  Miscellaneous orthopedic devices associated with adverse incidents, not elsewhere classified**

☑4ᵗʰ **Y80  Physical medicine devices associated with adverse incidents**

   **Y80.0  Diagnostic and monitoring physical medicine devices associated with adverse incidents**

   **Y80.1  Therapeutic (nonsurgical) and rehabilitative physical medicine devices associated with adverse incidents**

   **Y80.2  Prosthetic and other implants, materials and accessory physical medicine devices associated with adverse incidents**

   **Y80.3  Surgical instruments, materials and physical medicine devices (including sutures) associated with adverse incidents**

   **Y80.8  Miscellaneous physical medicine devices associated with adverse incidents, not elsewhere classified**

☑4ᵗʰ **Y81  General- and plastic-surgery devices associated with adverse incidents**

   **Y81.0  Diagnostic and monitoring general- and plastic-surgery devices associated with adverse incidents**

   **Y81.1  Therapeutic (nonsurgical) and rehabilitative general- and plastic-surgery devices associated with adverse incidents**

   **Y81.2  Prosthetic and other implants, materials and accessory general- and plastic-surgery devices associated with adverse incidents**

   **Y81.3  Surgical instruments, materials and general- and plastic-surgery devices (including sutures) associated with adverse incidents**

   **Y81.8  Miscellaneous general- and plastic-surgery devices associated with adverse incidents, not elsewhere classified**

☑4ᵗʰ **Y82  Other and unspecified medical devices associated with adverse incidents**

   **Y82.8  Other medical devices associated with adverse incidents**

   **Y82.9  Unspecified medical devices associated with adverse incidents**

**Surgical and other medical procedures as the cause of abnormal reaction of the patient, or of later complication, without mention of misadventure at the time of the procedure (Y83-Y84)**

   EXCLUDES 1  *misadventures to patients during surgical and medical care, classifiable to (Y62-Y69)*

   EXCLUDES 2  *breakdown or malfunctioning of medical device (after implantation) (during procedure) (ongoing use) (Y70-Y82)*

☑4ᵗʰ **Y83  Surgical operation and other surgical procedures as the cause of abnormal reaction of the patient, or of later complication, without mention of misadventure at the time of the procedure**

   **Y83.0  Surgical operation with transplant of whole organ as the cause of abnormal reaction of the patient, or of later complication, without mention of misadventure at the time of the procedure**

   **Y83.1  Surgical operation with implant of artificial internal device as the cause of abnormal reaction of the patient, or of later complication, without mention of misadventure at the time of the procedure**

   **Y83.2  Surgical operation with anastomosis, bypass or graft as the cause of abnormal reaction of the patient, or of later complication, without mention of misadventure at the time of the procedure**

   **Y83.3  Surgical operation with formation of external stoma as the cause of abnormal reaction of the patient, or of later complication, without mention of misadventure at the time of the procedure**

   **Y83.4  Other reconstructive surgery as the cause of abnormal reaction of the patient, or of later complication, without mention of misadventure at the time of the procedure**

   **Y83.5  Amputation of limb(s) as the cause of abnormal reaction of the patient, or of later complication, without mention of misadventure at the time of the procedure**

   **Y83.6  Removal of other organ (partial) (total) as the cause of abnormal reaction of the patient, or of later complication, without mention of misadventure at the time of the procedure**

   **Y83.8  Other surgical procedures as the cause of abnormal reaction of the patient, or of later complication, without mention of misadventure at the time of the procedure**

   **Y83.9  Surgical procedure, unspecified as the cause of abnormal reaction of the patient, or of later complication, without mention of misadventure at the time of the procedure**

☑4ᵗʰ **Y84  Other medical procedures as the cause of abnormal reaction of the patient, or of later complication, without misadventure at the time of the procedure**

   **Y84.0  Cardiac catheterization as the cause of abnormal reaction of the patient, or of later complication, without mention of misadventure at the time of the procedure**

   **Y84.1  Kidney dialysis as the cause of abnormal reaction of the patient, or of later complication, without mention of misadventure at the time of the procedure**

   **Y84.2  Radiological procedure and radiotherapy as the cause of abnormal reaction of the patient, or of later complication, without mention of misadventure at the time of the procedure**
     AHA: 2017, 1Q, 33

   **Y84.3  Shock therapy as the cause of abnormal reaction of the patient, or of later complication, without mention of misadventure at the time of the procedure**

   **Y84.4  Aspiration of fluid as the cause of abnormal reaction of the patient, or of later complication, without mention of misadventure at the time of the procedure**

   **Y84.5  Insertion of gastric or duodenal sound as the cause of abnormal reaction of the patient, or of later complication, without mention of misadventure at the time of the procedure**

   **Y84.6  Urinary catheterization as the cause of abnormal reaction of the patient, or of later complication, without mention of misadventure at the time of the procedure**

   **Y84.7  Blood-sampling as the cause of abnormal reaction of the patient, or of later complication, without mention of misadventure at the time of the procedure**

   **Y84.8  Other medical procedures as the cause of abnormal reaction of the patient, or of later complication, without mention of misadventure at the time of the procedure**
     AHA: 2014, 4Q, 24

   **Y84.9  Medical procedure, unspecified as the cause of abnormal reaction of the patient, or of later complication, without mention of misadventure at the time of the procedure**

**Supplementary factors related to causes of morbidity classified elsewhere (Y90-Y99)**

   NOTE  These categories may be used to provide supplementary information concerning causes of morbidity. They are not to be used for single-condition coding.

☑4ᵗʰ **Y90  Evidence of alcohol involvement determined by blood alcohol level**

   Code first any associated alcohol related disorders (F10)

   **Y90.0  Blood alcohol level of less than 20 mg/100 ml**

   **Y90.1  Blood alcohol level of 20-39 mg/100 ml**

   **Y90.2  Blood alcohol level of 40-59 mg/100 ml**

   **Y90.3  Blood alcohol level of 60-79 mg/100 ml**

   **Y90.4  Blood alcohol level of 80-99 mg/100 ml**

   **Y90.5  Blood alcohol level of 100-119 mg/100 ml**

   **Y90.6  Blood alcohol level of 120-199 mg/100 ml**

   **Y90.7  Blood alcohol level of 200-239 mg/100 ml**

   **Y90.8  Blood alcohol level of 240 mg/100 ml or more**

   **Y90.9  Presence of alcohol in blood, level not specified**

☑ Additional Character Req  ✓7ᵗʰ Placeholder Alert  Unacceptable PDx  **Manifestation**  H1 - H14 HAC  HCC CMS-HCC Condition  EXCLUDES 1 Not Coded Here  EXCLUDES 2 Not Included Here

**ICD-10-CM 2018**             **1209**

**Chapter 20. External Causes of Morbidity**

**☑4ᵗʰ Y92 Place of occurrence of the external cause**

The following category is for use, when relevant, to identify the place of occurrence of the external cause. Use in conjunction with an activity code.

Place of occurrence should be recorded only at the initial encounter for treatment

**☑5ᵗʰ Y92.0 Non-institutional (private) residence as the place of occurrence of the external cause**

EXCLUDES 1  *abandoned or derelict house (Y92.89)*
*home under construction but not yet occupied (Y92.6-)*
*institutional place of residence (Y92.1-)*

**☑6ᵗʰ Y92.00 Unspecified non-institutional (private) residence as the place of occurrence of the external cause**

**Y92.000 Kitchen of unspecified non-institutional (private) residence as the place of occurrence of the external cause**

**Y92.001 Dining room of unspecified non-institutional (private) residence as the place of occurrence of the external cause**

**Y92.002 Bathroom of unspecified non-institutional (private) residence single-family (private) house as the place of occurrence of the external cause**

**Y92.003 Bedroom of unspecified non-institutional (private) residence as the place of occurrence of the external cause**

**Y92.007 Garden or yard of unspecified non-institutional (private) residence as the place of occurrence of the external cause**

**Y92.008 Other place in unspecified non-institutional (private) residence as the place of occurrence of the external cause**

**Y92.009 Unspecified place in unspecified non-institutional (private) residence as the place of occurrence of the external cause**
Home (NOS) as the place of occurrence of the external cause

**☑6ᵗʰ Y92.01 Single-family non-institutional (private) house as the place of occurrence of the external cause**
Farmhouse as the place of occurrence of the external cause

EXCLUDES 1  *barn (Y92.71)*
*chicken coop or hen house (Y92.72)*
*farm field (Y92.73)*
*orchard (Y92.74)*
*single family mobile home or trailer (Y92.02-)*
*slaughter house (Y92.86)*

**Y92.010 Kitchen of single-family (private) house as the place of occurrence of the external cause**

**Y92.011 Dining room of single-family (private) house as the place of occurrence of the external cause**

**Y92.012 Bathroom of single-family (private) house as the place of occurrence of the external cause**

**Y92.013 Bedroom of single-family (private) house as the place of occurrence of the external cause**

**Y92.014 Private driveway to single-family (private) house as the place of occurrence of the external cause**

**Y92.015 Private garage of single-family (private) house as the place of occurrence of the external cause**

**Y92.016 Swimming-pool in single-family (private) house or garden as the place of occurrence of the external cause**

**Y92.017 Garden or yard in single-family (private) house as the place of occurrence of the external cause**

**Y92.018 Other place in single-family (private) house as the place of occurrence of the external cause**

**Y92.019 Unspecified place in single-family (private) house as the place of occurrence of the external cause**

**☑6ᵗʰ Y92.02 Mobile home as the place of occurrence of the external cause**

**Y92.020 Kitchen in mobile home as the place of occurrence of the external cause**

**Y92.021 Dining room in mobile home as the place of occurrence of the external cause**

**Y92.022 Bathroom in mobile home as the place of occurrence of the external cause**

**Y92.023 Bedroom in mobile home as the place of occurrence of the external cause**

**Y92.024 Driveway of mobile home as the place of occurrence of the external cause**

**Y92.025 Garage of mobile home as the place of occurrence of the external cause**

**Y92.026 Swimming-pool of mobile home as the place of occurrence of the external cause**

**Y92.027 Garden or yard of mobile home as the place of occurrence of the external cause**

**Y92.028 Other place in mobile home as the place of occurrence of the external cause**

**Y92.029 Unspecified place in mobile home as the place of occurrence of the external cause**

**☑6ᵗʰ Y92.03 Apartment as the place of occurrence of the external cause**
Condominium as the place of occurrence of the external cause
Co-op apartment as the place of occurrence of the external cause

**Y92.030 Kitchen in apartment as the place of occurrence of the external cause**

**Y92.031 Bathroom in apartment as the place of occurrence of the external cause**

**Y92.032 Bedroom in apartment as the place of occurrence of the external cause**

**Y92.038 Other place in apartment as the place of occurrence of the external cause**

**Y92.039 Unspecified place in apartment as the place of occurrence of the external cause**

**☑6ᵗʰ Y92.04 Boarding-house as the place of occurrence of the external cause**

**Y92.040 Kitchen in boarding-house as the place of occurrence of the external cause**

**Y92.041 Bathroom in boarding-house as the place of occurrence of the external cause**

**Y92.042 Bedroom in boarding-house as the place of occurrence of the external cause**

**Y92.043 Driveway of boarding-house as the place of occurrence of the external cause**

**Y92.044 Garage of boarding-house as the place of occurrence of the external cause**

**Y92.045 Swimming-pool of boarding-house as the place of occurrence of the external cause**

**Y92.046 Garden or yard of boarding-house as the place of occurrence of the external cause**

**Y92.048 Other place in boarding-house as the place of occurrence of the external cause**

**Y92.049 Unspecified place in boarding-house as the place of occurrence of the external cause**

**☑6ᵗʰ Y92.09 Other non-institutional residence as the place of occurrence of the external cause**
AHA: 2017, 2Q, 10

**Y92.090 Kitchen in other non-institutional residence as the place of occurrence of the external cause**

**Y92.091 Bathroom in other non-institutional residence as the place of occurrence of the external cause**

**Y92.092 Bedroom in other non-institutional residence as the place of occurrence of the external cause**

**Y92.093 Driveway of other non-institutional residence as the place of occurrence of the external cause**

**Y92.094 Garage of other non-institutional residence as the place of occurrence of the external cause**

**Y92.095 Swimming-pool of other non-institutional residence as the place of occurrence of the external cause**

**Y92.096 Garden or yard of other non-institutional residence as the place of occurrence of the external cause**

Ⓝ Newborn: 0   Ⓟ Pediatric: 0-17   Ⓜ Maternity: 12-55   Ⓐ Adult: 15-124   MCC Major CC Condition   PDxMCC PDx acts as own MCC   CC CC Condition   PDxCC PDx acts as own CC

1210

ICD-10-CM 2018

**Y92.098**  Other place in other non-institutional residence as the place of occurrence of the external cause

**Y92.099**  Unspecified place in other non-institutional residence as the place of occurrence of the external cause

✓5ᵗʰ  **Y92.1**  Institutional (nonprivate) residence as the place of occurrence of the external cause

**Y92.10**  Unspecified residential institution as the place of occurrence of the external cause

✓6ᵗʰ  **Y92.11**  Children's home and orphanage as the place of occurrence of the external cause

**Y92.110**  Kitchen in children's home and orphanage as the place of occurrence of the external cause

**Y92.111**  Bathroom in children's home and orphanage as the place of occurrence of the external cause

**Y92.112**  Bedroom in children's home and orphanage as the place of occurrence of the external cause

**Y92.113**  Driveway of children's home and orphanage as the place of occurrence of the external cause

**Y92.114**  Garage of children's home and orphanage as the place of occurrence of the external cause

**Y92.115**  Swimming-pool of children's home and orphanage as the place of occurrence of the external cause

**Y92.116**  Garden or yard of children's home and orphanage as the place of occurrence of the external cause

**Y92.118**  Other place in children's home and orphanage as the place of occurrence of the external cause

**Y92.119**  Unspecified place in children's home and orphanage as the place of occurrence of the external cause

✓6ᵗʰ  **Y92.12**  Nursing home as the place of occurrence of the external cause
Home for the sick as the place of occurrence of the external cause
Hospice as the place of occurrence of the external cause
**AHA:** 2017, 2Q, 10

**Y92.120**  Kitchen in nursing home as the place of occurrence of the external cause

**Y92.121**  Bathroom in nursing home as the place of occurrence of the external cause

**Y92.122**  Bedroom in nursing home as the place of occurrence of the external cause

**Y92.123**  Driveway of nursing home as the place of occurrence of the external cause

**Y92.124**  Garage of nursing home as the place of occurrence of the external cause

**Y92.125**  Swimming-pool of nursing home as the place of occurrence of the external cause

**Y92.126**  Garden or yard of nursing home as the place of occurrence of the external cause

**Y92.128**  Other place in nursing home as the place of occurrence of the external cause

**Y92.129**  Unspecified place in nursing home as the place of occurrence of the external cause

✓6ᵗʰ  **Y92.13**  Military base as the place of occurrence of the external cause
*EXCLUDES 1*  military training grounds (Y92.83)

**Y92.130**  Kitchen on military base as the place of occurrence of the external cause

**Y92.131**  Mess hall on military base as the place of occurrence of the external cause

**Y92.133**  Barracks on military base as the place of occurrence of the external cause

**Y92.135**  Garage on military base as the place of occurrence of the external cause

**Y92.136**  Swimming-pool on military base as the place of occurrence of the external cause

**Y92.137**  Garden or yard on military base as the place of occurrence of the external cause

**Y92.138**  Other place on military base as the place of occurrence of the external cause

**Y92.139**  Unspecified place military base as the place of occurrence of the external cause

✓6ᵗʰ  **Y92.14**  Prison as the place of occurrence of the external cause

**Y92.140**  Kitchen in prison as the place of occurrence of the external cause

**Y92.141**  Dining room in prison as the place of occurrence of the external cause

**Y92.142**  Bathroom in prison as the place of occurrence of the external cause

**Y92.143**  Cell of prison as the place of occurrence of the external cause

**Y92.146**  Swimming-pool of prison as the place of occurrence of the external cause

**Y92.147**  Courtyard of prison as the place of occurrence of the external cause

**Y92.148**  Other place in prison as the place of occurrence of the external cause

**Y92.149**  Unspecified place in prison as the place of occurrence of the external cause

✓6ᵗʰ  **Y92.15**  Reform school as the place of occurrence of the external cause

**Y92.150**  Kitchen in reform school as the place of occurrence of the external cause

**Y92.151**  Dining room in reform school as the place of occurrence of the external cause

**Y92.152**  Bathroom in reform school as the place of occurrence of the external cause

**Y92.153**  Bedroom in reform school as the place of occurrence of the external cause

**Y92.154**  Driveway of reform school as the place of occurrence of the external cause

**Y92.155**  Garage of reform school as the place of occurrence of the external cause

**Y92.156**  Swimming-pool of reform school as the place of occurrence of the external cause

**Y92.157**  Garden or yard of reform school as the place of occurrence of the external cause

**Y92.158**  Other place in reform school as the place of occurrence of the external cause

**Y92.159**  Unspecified place in reform school as the place of occurrence of the external cause

✓6ᵗʰ  **Y92.16**  School dormitory as the place of occurrence of the external cause
*EXCLUDES 1*  reform school as the place of occurrence of the external cause (Y92.15-)
school buildings and grounds as the place of occurrence of the external cause (Y92.2-)
school sports and athletic areas as the place of occurrence of the external cause (Y92.3-)

**Y92.160**  Kitchen in school dormitory as the place of occurrence of the external cause

**Y92.161**  Dining room in school dormitory as the place of occurrence of the external cause

**Y92.162**  Bathroom in school dormitory as the place of occurrence of the external cause

**Y92.163**  Bedroom in school dormitory as the place of occurrence of the external cause

**Y92.168**  Other place in school dormitory as the place of occurrence of the external cause

**Y92.169**  Unspecified place in school dormitory as the place of occurrence of the external cause

✓6ᵗʰ  **Y92.19**  Other specified residential institution as the place of occurrence of the external cause
**AHA:** 2017, 2Q, 10

**Y92.190**  Kitchen in other specified residential institution as the place of occurrence of the external cause

**Y92.191**  Dining room in other specified residential institution as the place of occurrence of the external cause

**Y92.192**  Bathroom in other specified residential institution as the place of occurrence of the external cause

---

**Y92.193**   **Bedroom** in other specified residential institution as the place of occurrence of the external cause

**Y92.194**   **Driveway** of other specified residential institution as the place of occurrence of the external cause

**Y92.195**   **Garage** of other specified residential institution as the place of occurrence of the external cause

**Y92.196**   **Pool** of other specified residential institution as the place of occurrence of the external cause

**Y92.197**   **Garden or yard** of other specified residential institution as the place of occurrence of the external cause

**Y92.198**   **Other place** in other specified residential institution as the place of occurrence of the external cause

**Y92.199**   **Unspecified place** in other specified residential institution as the place of occurrence of the external cause

√5ᵗʰ **Y92.2**   **School, other institution and public administrative area as the place of occurrence of the external cause**

Building and adjacent grounds used by the general public or by a particular group of the public

> **EXCLUDES 1**   *building under construction as the place of occurrence of the external cause (Y92.6)*
> *residential institution as the place of occurrence of the external cause (Y92.1)*
> *school dormitory as the place of occurrence of the external cause (Y92.16-)*
> *sports and athletics area of schools as the place of occurrence of the external cause (Y92.3-)*

√6ᵗʰ **Y92.21**   **School (private) (public) (state) as the place of occurrence of the external cause**

**Y92.210**   **Daycare center** as the place of occurrence of the external cause

**Y92.211**   **Elementary school** as the place of occurrence of the external cause

Kindergarten as the place of occurrence of the external cause

**Y92.212**   **Middle school** as the place of occurrence of the external cause

**Y92.213**   **High school** as the place of occurrence of the external cause

**AHA:** 2012, 4Q, 108

**Y92.214**   **College** as the place of occurrence of the external cause

University as the place of occurrence of the external cause

**Y92.215**   **Trade school** as the place of occurrence of the external cause

**Y92.218**   **Other school** as the place of occurrence of the external cause

**Y92.219**   **Unspecified school** as the place of occurrence of the external cause

**Y92.22**   **Religious institution** as the place of occurrence of the external cause

Church as the place of occurrence of the external cause

Mosque as the place of occurrence of the external cause

Synagogue as the place of occurrence of the external cause

√6ᵗʰ **Y92.23**   **Hospital as the place of occurrence of the external cause**

> **EXCLUDES 1**   *ambulatory (outpatient) health services establishments (Y92.53-)*
> *home for the sick as the place of occurrence of the external cause (Y92.12-)*
> *hospice as the place of occurrence of the external cause (Y92.12-)*
> *nursing home as the place of occurrence of the external cause (Y92.12-)*

**Y92.230**   **Patient room** in hospital as the place of occurrence of the external cause

**Y92.231**   **Patient bathroom** in hospital as the place of occurrence of the external cause

**Y92.232**   **Corridor** of hospital as the place of occurrence of the external cause

**Y92.233**   **Cafeteria** of hospital as the place of occurrence of the external cause

**Y92.234**   **Operating room** of hospital as the place of occurrence of the external cause

**Y92.238**   **Other place** in hospital as the place of occurrence of the external cause

**Y92.239**   **Unspecified place** in hospital as the place of occurrence of the external cause

√6ᵗʰ **Y92.24**   **Public administrative building as the place of occurrence of the external cause**

**Y92.240**   **Courthouse** as the place of occurrence of the external cause

**Y92.241**   **Library** as the place of occurrence of the external cause

**Y92.242**   **Post office** as the place of occurrence of the external cause

**Y92.243**   **City hall** as the place of occurrence of the external cause

**Y92.248**   **Other public administrative building** as the place of occurrence of the external cause

√6ᵗʰ **Y92.25**   **Cultural building as the place of occurrence of the external cause**

**Y92.250**   **Art Gallery** as the place of occurrence of the external cause

**Y92.251**   **Museum** as the place of occurrence of the external cause

**Y92.252**   **Music hall** as the place of occurrence of the external cause

**Y92.253**   **Opera house** as the place of occurrence of the external cause

**Y92.254**   **Theater (live)** as the place of occurrence of the external cause

**Y92.258**   **Other cultural public building** as the place of occurrence of the external cause

**Y92.26**   **Movie house or cinema** as the place of occurrence of the external cause

**Y92.29**   **Other specified public building** as the place of occurrence of the external cause

Assembly hall as the place of occurrence of the external cause

Clubhouse as the place of occurrence of the external cause

√5ᵗʰ **Y92.3**   **Sports and athletics area as the place of occurrence of the external cause**

√6ᵗʰ **Y92.31**   **Athletic court as the place of occurrence of the external cause**

> **EXCLUDES 1**   *tennis court in private home or garden (Y92.09)*

**Y92.310**   **Basketball court** as the place of occurrence of the external cause

**Y92.311**   **Squash court** as the place of occurrence of the external cause

**Y92.312**   **Tennis court** as the place of occurrence of the external cause

**Y92.318**   **Other athletic court** as the place of occurrence of the external cause

√6ᵗʰ **Y92.32**   **Athletic field as the place of occurrence of the external cause**

**Y92.320**   **Baseball field** as the place of occurrence of the external cause

**Y92.321**   **Football field** as the place of occurrence of the external cause

**Y92.322**   **Soccer field** as the place of occurrence of the external cause

**Y92.328**   **Other athletic field** as the place of occurrence of the external cause

Cricket field as the place of occurrence of the external cause

Hockey field as the place of occurrence of the external cause

√6ᵗʰ **Y92.33**   **Skating rink as the place of occurrence of the external cause**

**Y92.330**   **Ice skating rink (indoor) (outdoor)** as the place of occurrence of the external cause

**Y92.331**   **Roller skating rink** as the place of occurrence of the external cause

**Y92.34**   **Swimming pool (public)** as the place of occurrence of the external cause

> **EXCLUDES 1**   *swimming pool in private home or garden (Y92.016)*

N Newborn: 0   P Pediatric: 0-17   M Maternity: 12-55   A Adult: 15-124   MCC Major CC Condition   PDxMCC PDx acts as own MCC   CC CC Condition   PDxCC PDx acts as own CC

**1212**                                                    ICD-10-CM 2018

**Y92.39**   **Other** specified **sports and athletic area as the place of occurrence of the external cause**

Golf-course as the place of occurrence of the external cause

Gymnasium as the place of occurrence of the external cause

Riding-school as the place of occurrence of the external cause

Stadium as the place of occurrence of the external cause

✓5th **Y92.4**   **Street, highway and other paved roadways as the place of occurrence of the external cause**

> EXCLUDES 1   *private driveway of residence (Y92.014, Y92.024, Y92.043, Y92.093, Y92.113, Y92.123, Y92.154, Y92.194)*

✓6th **Y92.41**   **Street and highway as the place of occurrence of the external cause**

**Y92.410**   **Unspecified** street and highway **as the place of occurrence of the external cause**

Road NOS as the place of occurrence of the external cause

**Y92.411**   **Interstate** highway **as the place of occurrence of the external cause**

Freeway as the place of occurrence of the external cause

Motorway as the place of occurrence of the external cause

**Y92.412**   **Parkway as the place of occurrence of the external cause**

**Y92.413**   **State road as the place of occurrence of the external cause**

**Y92.414**   **Local residential or business street as the place of occurrence of the external cause**

**Y92.415**   **Exit ramp or entrance ramp** of street or **highway as the place of occurrence of the external cause**

✓6th **Y92.48**   **Other paved roadways as the place of occurrence of the external cause**

**Y92.480**   **Sidewalk as the place of occurrence of the external cause**

**Y92.481**   **Parking lot as the place of occurrence of the external cause**

**Y92.482**   **Bike path as the place of occurrence of the external cause**

**Y92.488**   **Other** paved roadways as the place of occurrence of the external cause

✓5th **Y92.5**   **Trade and service area as the place of occurrence of the external cause**

> EXCLUDES 1   *garage in private home (Y92.015)*
> *schools and other public administration buildings (Y92.2-)*

✓6th **Y92.51**   **Private commercial establishments as the place of occurrence of the external cause**

**Y92.510**   **Bank as the place of occurrence of the external cause**

**Y92.511**   **Restaurant** or **café as the place of occurrence of the external cause**

**Y92.512**   **Supermarket, store** or **market as the place of occurrence of the external cause**

**Y92.513**   **Shop** (commercial) **as the place of occurrence of the external cause**

✓6th **Y92.52**   **Service areas as the place of occurrence of the external cause**

**Y92.520**   **Airport as the place of occurrence of the external cause**

**Y92.521**   **Bus station as the place of occurrence of the external cause**

**Y92.522**   **Railway station as the place of occurrence of the external cause**

**Y92.523**   **Highway rest stop as the place of occurrence of the external cause**

**Y92.524**   **Gas station as the place of occurrence of the external cause**

Petroleum station as the place of occurrence of the external cause

Service station as the place of occurrence of the external cause

✓6th **Y92.53**   **Ambulatory health services establishments as the place of occurrence of the external cause**

**Y92.530**   **Ambulatory surgery center as the place of occurrence of the external cause**

Outpatient surgery center, including that connected with a hospital as the place of occurrence of the external cause

Same day surgery center, including that connected with a hospital as the place of occurrence of the external cause

**Y92.531**   **Health care provider office as the place of occurrence of the external cause**

Physician office as the place of occurrence of the external cause

**Y92.532**   **Urgent care center as the place of occurrence of the external cause**

**Y92.538**   **Other ambulatory** health services **establishments as the place of occurrence of the external cause**

**Y92.59**   **Other trade areas as the place of occurrence of the external cause**

Office building as the place of occurrence of the external cause

Casino as the place of occurrence of the external cause

Garage (commercial) as the place of occurrence of the external cause

Hotel as the place of occurrence of the external cause

Radio or television station as the place of occurrence of the external cause

Shopping mall as the place of occurrence of the external cause

Warehouse as the place of occurrence of the external cause

✓5th **Y92.6**   **Industrial and construction area as the place of occurrence of the external cause**

**Y92.61**   **Building [any] under construction as the place of occurrence of the external cause**

**Y92.62**   **Dock or shipyard as the place of occurrence of the external cause**

Dockyard as the place of occurrence of the external cause

Dry dock as the place of occurrence of the external cause

Shipyard as the place of occurrence of the external cause

**Y92.63**   **Factory as the place of occurrence of the external cause**

Factory building as the place of occurrence of the external cause

Factory premises as the place of occurrence of the external cause

Industrial yard as the place of occurrence of the external cause

**Y92.64**   **Mine or pit as the place of occurrence of the external cause**

Mine as the place of occurrence of the external cause

**Y92.65**   **Oil rig as the place of occurrence of the external cause**

Pit (coal) (gravel) (sand) as the place of occurrence of the external cause

**Y92.69**   **Other** specified **industrial and construction area as the place of occurrence of the external cause**

Gasworks as the place of occurrence of the external cause

Power-station (coal) (nuclear) (oil) as the place of occurrence of the external cause

Tunnel under construction as the place of occurrence of the external cause

Workshop as the place of occurrence of the external cause

✓5th **Y92.7**   **Farm as the place of occurrence of the external cause**

Ranch as the place of occurrence of the external cause

> EXCLUDES 1   *farmhouse and home premises of farm (Y92.01-)*

**Y92.71**   **Barn as the place of occurrence of the external cause**

**Y92.72**   **Chicken coop as the place of occurrence of the external cause**

Hen house as the place of occurrence of the external cause

**Y92.73**   **Farm field as the place of occurrence of the external cause**

**Y92.74**   **Orchard as the place of occurrence of the external cause**

✓ Additional Character Req   ✓x7th Placeholder Alert   Unacceptable PDx   Manifestation   H1 - H14 HAC   HCC CMS-HCC Condition   EXCLUDES 1 Not Coded Here   EXCLUDES 2 Not Included Here

ICD-10-CM 2018      1213

Y92.39–Y92.74

**Y92.79** Other **farm location as the place of occurrence of the external cause**

✓5ᵗʰ **Y92.8** Other **places as the place of occurrence of the external cause**

✓6ᵗʰ **Y92.81** Transport **vehicle as the place of occurrence of the external cause**

**EXCLUDES 1** *transport accidents (V00-V99)*

**Y92.810** Car **as the place of occurrence of the external cause**

**Y92.811** Bus **as the place of occurrence of the external cause**

**Y92.812** Truck **as the place of occurrence of the external cause**

**Y92.813** Airplane **as the place of occurrence of the external cause**

**Y92.814** Boat **as the place of occurrence of the external cause**

**Y92.815** Train **as the place of occurrence of the external cause**

**Y92.816** Subway **car as the place of occurrence of the external cause**

**Y92.818** Other **transport vehicle as the place of occurrence of the external cause**

✓6ᵗʰ **Y92.82** Wilderness **area**

**Y92.820** Desert **as the place of occurrence of the external cause**

**Y92.821** Forest **as the place of occurrence of the external cause**

**Y92.828** Other **wilderness area as the place of occurrence of the external cause**
Swamp as the place of occurrence of the external cause
Mountain as the place of occurrence of the external cause
Marsh as the place of occurrence of the external cause
Prairie as the place of occurrence of the external cause

✓6ᵗʰ **Y92.83** Recreation **area as the place of occurrence of the external cause**

**Y92.830** Public **park as the place of occurrence of the external cause**

**Y92.831** Amusement **park as the place of occurrence of the external cause**

**Y92.832** Beach **as the place of occurrence of the external cause**
Seashore as the place of occurrence of the external cause

**Y92.833** Campsite **as the place of occurrence of the external cause**

**Y92.834** Zoological **garden (Zoo) as the place of occurrence of the external cause**

**Y92.838** Other **recreation area as the place of occurrence of the external cause**

**Y92.84** Military **training ground as the place of occurrence of the external cause**

**Y92.85** Railroad **track as the place of occurrence of the external cause**

**Y92.86** Slaughter **house as the place of occurrence of the external cause**

**Y92.89** Other **specified places as the place of occurrence of the external cause**
Derelict house as the place of occurrence of the external cause

**Y92.9** Unspecified **place or not applicable**

✓4ᵗʰ **Y93** **Activity codes**

**NOTE** Category Y93 is provided for use to indicate the activity of the person seeking healthcare for an injury or health condition, such as a heart attack while shoveling snow, which resulted from, or was contributed to, by the activity. These codes are appropriate for use for both acute injuries, such as those from chapter 19, and conditions that are due to the long-term, cumulative effects of an activity, such as those from chapter 13. They are also appropriate for use with external cause codes for cause and intent if identifying the activity provides additional information on the event. These codes should be used in conjunction with codes for external cause status (Y99) and place of occurrence (Y92).

This section contains the following broad activity categories:

Y93.0 Activities involving walking and running
Y93.1 Activities involving water and water craft
Y93.2 Activities involving ice and snow
Y93.3 Activities involving climbing, rappelling, and jumping off
Y93.4 Activities involving dancing and other rhythmic movement
Y93.5 Activities involving other sports and athletics played individually
Y93.6 Activities involving other sports and athletics played as a team or group
Y93.7 Activities involving other specified sports and athletics
Y93.A Activities involving other cardiorespiratory exercise
Y93.B Activities involving other muscle strengthening exercises
Y93.C Activities involving computer technology and electronic devices
Y93.D Activities involving arts and handcrafts
Y93.E Activities involving personal hygiene and interior property and clothing maintenance
Y93.F Activities involving caregiving
Y93.G Activities involving food preparation, cooking and grilling
Y93.H Activities involving exterior property and land maintenance, building and construction
Y93.I Activities involving roller coasters and other types of external motion
Y93.J Activities involving playing musical instrument
Y93.K Activities involving animal care
Y93.8 Activities, other specified
Y93.9 Activity, unspecified

✓5ᵗʰ **Y93.0** **Activities involving walking and running**

**EXCLUDES 1** *activity, walking an animal (Y93.K1)*
*activity, walking or running on a treadmill (Y93.A1)*

**Y93.01** **Activity,** walking, marching and hiking
Activity, walking, marching and hiking on level or elevated terrain
**EXCLUDES 1** *activity, mountain climbing (Y93.31)*

**Y93.02** **Activity,** running

✓5ᵗʰ **Y93.1** **Activities involving water and water craft**

**EXCLUDES 1** *activities involving ice (Y93.2-)*

**Y93.11** **Activity,** swimming

**Y93.12** **Activity,** springboard and platform diving

**Y93.13** **Activity,** water polo

**Y93.14** **Activity,** water aerobics and water exercise

**Y93.15** **Activity,** underwater diving and snorkeling
Activity, SCUBA diving

**Y93.16** **Activity,** rowing, canoeing, kayaking, rafting and tubing
Activity, canoeing, kayaking, rafting and tubing in calm and turbulent water

**Y93.17** **Activity,** water skiing and wake boarding

**Y93.18** **Activity,** surfing, windsurfing and boogie boarding
Activity, water sliding

**Y93.19** **Activity,** other involving water and watercraft
Activity involving water NOS
Activity, parasailing
Activity, water survival training and testing

✓5ᵗʰ **Y93.2** **Activities involving ice and snow**

**EXCLUDES 1** *activity, shoveling ice and snow (Y93.H1)*

**Y93.21** **Activity,** ice skating
Activity, figure skating (singles) (pairs)
Activity, ice dancing
**EXCLUDES 1** *activity, ice hockey (Y93.22)*

**Y93.22** **Activity,** ice hockey

**Y93.23** **Activity,** snow (alpine) (downhill) skiing, snow boarding, sledding, tobogganing and snow tubing
**EXCLUDES 1** *activity, cross country skiing (Y93.24)*

**Y93.24** **Activity,** cross country skiing
Activity, nordic skiing

**Y93.29** **Activity,** other involving ice and snow
Activity involving ice and snow NOS

✓5ᵗʰ **Y93.3** **Activities involving climbing, rappelling and jumping off**
*EXCLUDES 1* *activity, hiking on level or elevated terrain (Y93.01)*
*activity, jumping rope (Y93.56)*
*activity, trampoline jumping (Y93.44)*

**Y93.31** **Activity,** mountain climbing, rock climbing and wall climbing

**Y93.32** **Activity,** rappelling

**Y93.33** **Activity,** BASE jumping
Activity, Building, Antenna, Span, Earth jumping

**Y93.34** **Activity,** bungee jumping

**Y93.35** **Activity,** hang gliding

**Y93.39** **Activity,** other involving climbing, rappelling and jumping off

✓5ᵗʰ **Y93.4** **Activities involving dancing and other rhythmic movement**
*EXCLUDES 1* *activity, martial arts (Y93.75)*

**Y93.41** **Activity,** dancing
**AHA:** 2012, 4Q, 108

**Y93.42** **Activity,** yoga

**Y93.43** **Activity,** gymnastics
Activity, rhythmic gymnastics
*EXCLUDES 1* *activity, trampolining (Y93.44)*

**Y93.44** **Activity,** trampolining

**Y93.45** **Activity,** cheerleading

**Y93.49** **Activity,** other involving dancing and other rhythmic movements

✓5ᵗʰ **Y93.5** **Activities involving other sports and athletics played individually**
*EXCLUDES 1* *activity, dancing (Y93.41)*
*activity, gymnastic (Y93.43)*
*activity, trampolining (Y93.44)*
*activity, yoga (Y93.42)*

**Y93.51** **Activity,** roller skating (inline) and skateboarding

**Y93.52** **Activity,** horseback riding

**Y93.53** **Activity,** golf

**Y93.54** **Activity,** bowling

**Y93.55** **Activity,** bike riding

**Y93.56** **Activity,** jumping rope

**Y93.57** **Activity,** non-running track and field events
*EXCLUDES 1* *activity, running (any form) (Y93.02)*

**Y93.59** **Activity,** other involving other sports and athletics played individually
*EXCLUDES 1* *activities involving climbing, rappelling, and jumping (Y93.3-)*
*activities involving ice and snow (Y93.2-)*
*activities involving walking and running (Y93.0-)*
*activities involving water and watercraft (Y93.1-)*

✓5ᵗʰ **Y93.6** **Activities involving other sports and athletics played as a team or group**
*EXCLUDES 1* *activity, ice hockey (Y93.22)*
*activity, water polo (Y93.13)*

**Y93.61** **Activity,** American tackle football
Activity, football NOS

**Y93.62** **Activity,** American flag or touch football

**Y93.63** **Activity,** rugby

**Y93.64** **Activity,** baseball
Activity, softball

**Y93.65** **Activity,** lacrosse and field hockey

**Y93.66** **Activity,** soccer

**Y93.67** **Activity,** basketball

**Y93.68** **Activity,** volleyball (beach) (court)

**Y93.6A** **Activity,** physical games generally associated with school recess, summer camp and children
Activity, capture the flag     Activity, four square
Activity, dodge ball     Activity, kickball

**Y93.69** **Activity,** other involving other sports and athletics played as a team or group
Activity, cricket

✓5ᵗʰ **Y93.7** **Activities involving other specified sports and athletics**

**Y93.71** **Activity,** boxing

**Y93.72** **Activity,** wrestling

**Y93.73** **Activity,** racquet and hand sports
Activity, handball     Activity, squash
Activity, racquetball     Activity, tennis

**Y93.74** **Activity,** frisbee
Activity, ultimate frisbee

**Y93.75** **Activity,** martial arts
Activity, combatives

**Y93.79** **Activity,** other specified sports and athletics
*EXCLUDES 1* *sports and athletics activities specified in categories Y93.0-Y93.6*

✓5ᵗʰ **Y93.A** **Activities involving other cardiorespiratory exercise**
Activities involving physical training

**Y93.A1** **Activity,** exercise machines primarily for cardiorespiratory conditioning
Activity, elliptical and stepper machines
Activity, stationary bike
Activity, treadmill

**Y93.A2** **Activity,** calisthenics
Activity, jumping jacks
Activity, warm up and cool down

**Y93.A3** **Activity,** aerobic and step exercise

**Y93.A4** **Activity,** circuit training

**Y93.A5** **Activity,** obstacle course
Activity, challenge course
Activity, confidence course

**Y93.A6** **Activity,** grass drills
Activity, guerilla drills

**Y93.A9** **Activity,** other involving cardiorespiratory exercise
*EXCLUDES 1* *activities involving cardiorespiratory exercise specified in categories Y93.0-Y93.7*

✓5ᵗʰ **Y93.B** **Activities involving other muscle strengthening exercises**

**Y93.B1** **Activity,** exercise machines primarily for muscle strengthening

**Y93.B2** **Activity,** push-ups, pull-ups, sit-ups

**Y93.B3** **Activity,** free weights
Activity, barbells     Activity, dumbbells

**Y93.B4** **Activity,** pilates

**Y93.B9** **Activity,** other involving muscle strengthening exercises
*EXCLUDES 1* *activities involving muscle strengthening specified in categories Y93.0-Y93.A*

✓5ᵗʰ **Y93.C** **Activities involving computer technology and electronic devices**
*EXCLUDES 1* *activity, electronic musical keyboard or instruments (Y93.J-)*

**Y93.C1** **Activity,** computer keyboarding
Activity, electronic game playing using keyboard or other stationary device

**Y93.C2** **Activity,** hand held interactive electronic device
Activity, cellular telephone and communication device
Activity, electronic game playing using interactive device
*EXCLUDES 1* *activity, electronic game playing using keyboard or other stationary device (Y93.C1)*

**Y93.C9** **Activity,** other involving computer technology and electronic devices

✓5ᵗʰ **Y93.D** **Activities involving arts and handcrafts**
*EXCLUDES 1* *activities involving playing musical instrument (Y93.J-)*

**Y93.D1** **Activity,** knitting and crocheting

**Y93.D2** **Activity,** sewing

**Y93.D3** **Activity,** furniture building and finishing
Activity, furniture repair

**Y93.D9** **Activity,** other involving arts and handcrafts

✓5ᵗʰ **Y93.E** **Activities involving personal hygiene and interior property and clothing maintenance**
*EXCLUDES 1* *activities involving cooking and grilling (Y93.G-)*
*activities involving exterior property and land maintenance, building and construction (Y93.H-)*
*activities involving caregiving (Y93.F-)*
*activity, dishwashing (Y93.G1)*
*activity, food preparation (Y93.G1)*
*activity, gardening (Y93.H2)*

**Y93.E1** **Activity,** personal bathing and showering

**Y93.E2** **Activity,** laundry

**Y93.E3** **Activity,** vacuuming

**Y93.E4** **Activity,** ironing

✓Additional Character Req   ✓7ᵗʰ Placeholder Alert   Unacceptable PDx   Manifestation   **H1**-**H14** HAC   **HCC** CMS-HCC Condition   *EXCLUDES 1* Not Coded Here   *EXCLUDES 2* Not Included Here

ICD-10-CM 2018     **1215**

Y93.E5    **Activity,** floor mopping and cleaning

Y93.E6    **Activity,** residential relocation
Activity, packing up and unpacking involved in moving to a new residence

Y93.E8    **Activity,** other personal hygiene

Y93.E9    **Activity,** other interior property and clothing maintenance

✓5ᵗʰ Y93.F    **Activities involving** caregiving
Activity involving the provider of caregiving

Y93.F1    **Activity, caregiving,** bathing

Y93.F2    **Activity, caregiving,** lifting

Y93.F9    **Activity,** other **caregiving**

✓5ᵗʰ Y93.G    **Activities involving food preparation, cooking and grilling**

Y93.G1    **Activity, food** preparation and clean up
Activity, dishwashing

Y93.G2    **Activity,** grilling and smoking food

Y93.G3    **Activity,** cooking and baking
Activity, use of stove, oven and microwave oven

Y93.G9    **Activity,** other **involving cooking and grilling**

✓5ᵗʰ Y93.H    **Activities involving exterior property and land maintenance, building and construction**

Y93.H1    **Activity,** digging, shoveling and raking
Activity, dirt digging
Activity, raking leaves
Activity, snow shoveling

Y93.H2    **Activity,** gardening and landscaping
Activity, pruning, trimming shrubs, weeding

Y93.H3    **Activity,** building and construction

Y93.H9    **Activity,** other **involving exterior property and land maintenance, building and construction**

✓5ᵗʰ Y93.I    **Activities involving roller coasters and other types of external motion**

Y93.I1    **Activity,** rollercoaster riding

Y93.I9    **Activity,** other **involving external motion**

✓5ᵗʰ Y93.J    **Activities involving playing musical instrument**
Activity involving playing electric musical instrument

Y93.J1    **Activity,** piano **playing**
Activity, musical keyboard (electronic) playing

Y93.J2    **Activity,** drum and other percussion instrument **playing**

Y93.J3    **Activity,** string instrument **playing**

Y93.J4    **Activity,** winds and brass instrument **playing**

✓5ᵗʰ Y93.K    **Activities involving** animal care
EXCLUDES 1    *activity, horseback riding (Y93.52)*

Y93.K1    **Activity,** walking **an animal**

Y93.K2    **Activity,** milking **an animal**

Y93.K3    **Activity,** grooming and shearing **an animal**

Y93.K9    **Activity,** other **involving animal care**

✓5ᵗʰ Y93.8    **Activities, other specified**

Y93.81    **Activity,** refereeing a sports activity

Y93.82    **Activity,** spectator at an event

Y93.83    **Activity,** rough housing and horseplay

Y93.84    **Activity,** sleeping

Y93.85    **Activity,** choking game
Activity, blackout game
Activity, fainting game
Activity, pass out game

Y93.89    **Activity,** other **specified**

Y93.9    **Activity,** unspecified

**Y95    Nosocomial condition**
**AHA:** 2013, 4Q, 119

✓4ᵗʰ **Y99    External cause status**
NOTE    A single code from category Y99 should be used in conjunction with the external cause code(s) assigned to a record to indicate the status of the person at the time the event occurred.

**Y99.0    Civilian activity done for income or pay**
Civilian activity done for financial or other compensation
EXCLUDES 1    *military activity (Y99.1)*
*volunteer activity (Y99.2)*

**Y99.1    Military activity**
EXCLUDES 1    *activity of off duty military personnel (Y99.8)*

**Y99.2    Volunteer activity**
EXCLUDES 1    *activity of child or other family member assisting in compensated work of other family member (Y99.8)*

**Y99.8    Other external cause status**
Activity NEC
Activity of child or other family member assisting in compensated work of other family member
Hobby not done for income
Leisure activity
Off-duty activity of military personnel
Recreation or sport not for income or while a student
Student activity
EXCLUDES 1    *civilian activity done for income or compensation (Y99.0)*
*military activity (Y99.1)*
**AHA:** 2012, 4Q, 108

**Y99.9    Unspecified external cause status**

N Newborn: 0    P Pediatric: 0-17    M Maternity: 12-55    A Adult: 15-124    MCC Major CC Condition    PDxMCC PDx acts as own MCC    CC CC Condition    PDxCC PDx acts as own CC

1216    ICD-10-CM 2018

# Chapter 21. Factors Influencing Health Status and Contact with Health Services (ZØØ–Z99)

## Chapter Specific Guidelines with Coding Examples

The chapter specific guidelines from the ICD-10-CM Official Guidelines for Coding and Reporting have been provided below. Along with these guidelines are coding examples, contained in the shaded boxes, that have been developed to help illustrate the coding and/or sequencing guidance found in these guidelines.

**Note:** The chapter specific guidelines provide additional information about the use of Z codes for specified encounters.

### a. Use of Z codes in any healthcare setting

Z codes are for use in any healthcare setting. Z codes may be used as either a first-listed (principal diagnosis code in the inpatient setting) or secondary code, depending on the circumstances of the encounter. Certain Z codes may only be used as first-listed or principal diagnosis.

| | |
|---|---|
| Patient with middle lobe lung cancer admitted for initiation of chemotherapy | |
| **Z51.11** | **Encounter for antineoplastic chemotherapy** |
| **C34.2** | **Malignant neoplasm of middle lobe, bronchus or lung** |

*Explanation:* A Z code can be used as first-listed in this situation based on guidelines in this chapter as well as chapter 2, "Neoplasms."

| | |
|---|---|
| Patient has chronic lymphocytic leukemia for which the patient had previous chemotherapy and is now in remission | |
| **C91.11** | **Chronic lymphocytic leukemia of B-cell type in remission** |
| **Z92.21** | **Personal history of antineoplastic chemotherapy** |

*Explanation:*The personal history Z code is used to describe a secondary (supplementary) diagnosis to identify that this patient has had chemotherapy in the past.

### b. Z codes indicate a reason for an encounter

Z codes are not procedure codes. A corresponding procedure code must accompany a Z code to describe any procedure performed.

### c. Categories of Z codes

#### 1) Contact/exposure

Category Z2Ø indicates contact with, and suspected exposure to, communicable diseases. These codes are for patients who do not show any sign or symptom of a disease but are suspected to have been exposed to it by close personal contact with an infected individual or are in an area where a disease is epidemic.

Category Z77, Other contact with and (suspected) exposures hazardous to health, indicates contact with and suspected exposures hazardous to health.

Contact/exposure codes may be used as a first-listed code to explain an encounter for testing, or, more commonly, as a secondary code to identify a potential risk.

#### 2) Inoculations and vaccinations

Code Z23 is for encounters for inoculations and vaccinations. It indicates that a patient is being seen to receive a prophylactic inoculation against a disease. Procedure codes are required to identify the actual administration of the injection and the type(s) of immunizations given. Code Z23 may be used as a secondary code if the inoculation is given as a routine part of preventive health care, such as a well-baby visit.

#### 3) Status

Status codes indicate that a patient is either a carrier of a disease or has the sequelae or residual of a past disease or condition. This includes such things as the presence of prosthetic or mechanical devices resulting from past treatment. A status code is informative, because the status may affect the course of treatment and its outcome. A status code is distinct from a history code. The history code indicates that the patient no longer has the condition.

A status code should not be used with a diagnosis code from one of the body system chapters, if the diagnosis code includes the information provided by the status code. For example, code Z94.1, Heart transplant status, should not be used with a code from subcategory T86.2, Complications of heart transplant. The status code does not provide

additional information. The complication code indicates that the patient is a heart transplant patient.

For encounters for weaning from a mechanical ventilator, assign a code from subcategory J96.1, Chronic respiratory failure, followed by code Z99.11, Dependence on respirator [ventilator] status.

The status Z codes/categories are:

| | |
|---|---|
| Z14 | Genetic carrier |

Genetic carrier status indicates that a person carries a gene, associated with a particular disease, which may be passed to offspring who may develop that disease. The person does not have the disease and is not at risk of developing the disease.

| | |
|---|---|
| Z15 | Genetic susceptibility to disease |

Genetic susceptibility indicates that a person has a gene that increases the risk of that person developing the disease.

Codes from category Z15 should not be used as principal or first-listed codes. If the patient has the condition to which he/she is susceptible, and that condition is the reason for the encounter, the code for the current condition should be sequenced first. If the patient is being seen for follow-up after completed treatment for this condition, and the condition no longer exists, a follow-up code should be sequenced first, followed by the appropriate personal history and genetic susceptibility codes. If the purpose of the encounter is genetic counseling associated with procreative management, code Z31.5, Encounter for genetic counseling, should be assigned as the first-listed code, followed by a code from category Z15. Additional codes should be assigned for any applicable family or personal history.

| | |
|---|---|
| Z16 | Resistance to antimicrobial drugs |

This code indicates that a patient has a condition that is resistant to antimicrobial drug treatment. Sequence the infection code first.

| | |
|---|---|
| Z17 | Estrogen receptor status |
| Z18 | Retained foreign body fragments |
| Z19 | Hormone sensitivity malignancy status |
| Z21 | Asymptomatic HIV infection status |

This code indicates that a patient has tested positive for HIV but has manifested no signs or symptoms of the disease.

| | |
|---|---|
| Z22 | Carrier of infectious disease |

Carrier status indicates that a person harbors the specific organisms of a disease without manifest symptoms and is capable of transmitting the infection.

| | |
|---|---|
| Z28.3 | Underimmunization status |
| Z33.1 | Pregnant state, incidental |

This code is a secondary code only for use when the pregnancy is in no way complicating the reason for visit. Otherwise, a code from the obstetric chapter is required.

| | |
|---|---|
| Z66 | Do not resuscitate |

This code may be used when it is documented by the provider that a patient is on do not resuscitate status at any time during the stay.

| | |
|---|---|
| Z67 | Blood type |
| Z68 | Body mass index (BMI) |

As with all other secondary diagnosis codes, the BMI codes should only be assigned when they meet the definition of a reportable diagnosis (see Section III, Reporting Additional Diagnoses).

| | |
|---|---|
| Z74.Ø1 | Bed confinement status |
| Z76.82 | Awaiting organ transplant status |
| Z78 | Other specified health status |

Code Z78.1, Physical restraint status, may be used when it is documented by the provider that a patient has been put in restraints during the current encounter. Please note that this code should not be reported when it is documented by the provider that a patient is temporarily restrained during a procedure.

| | |
|---|---|
| Z79 | Long-term (current) drug therapy |

Codes from this category indicate a patient's continuous use of a prescribed drug (including such things as aspirin therapy) for the long-term treatment of a condition or for prophylactic use. It is not for use for patients who have addictions to drugs. This subcategory is not for use of medications for detoxification or maintenance programs to prevent withdrawal symptoms in patients with drug dependence (e.g., methadone maintenance for opiate dependence). Assign the appropriate code for the drug dependence instead.

Assign a code from Z79 if the patient is receiving a medication for an extended period as a prophylactic measure (such as for the prevention of deep vein thrombosis) or as treatment of a chronic condition (such as arthritis) or a disease requiring a lengthy course of treatment (such as cancer). Do not assign a code from category Z79 for medication being administered for a brief period of time to treat an acute illness or injury (such as a course of antibiotics to treat acute bronchitis).

| | |
|---|---|
| Z88 | Allergy status to drugs, medicaments and biological substances |

Except: Z88.9, Allergy status to unspecified drugs, medicaments and biological substances status

| | |
|---|---|
| Z89 | Acquired absence of limb |
| Z90 | Acquired absence of organs, not elsewhere classified |
| Z91.0- | Allergy status, other than to drugs and biological substances |
| Z92.82 | Status post administration of tPA (rtPA) in a different facility within the last 24 hours prior to admission to a current facility |

Assign code Z92.82, Status post administration of tPA (rtPA) in a different facility within the last 24 hours prior to admission to current facility, as a secondary diagnosis when a patient is received by transfer into a facility and documentation indicates they were administered tissue plasminogen activator (tPA) within the last 24 hours prior to admission to the current facility.

This guideline applies even if the patient is still receiving the tPA at the time they are received into the current facility.

The appropriate code for the condition for which the tPA was administered (such as cerebrovascular disease or myocardial infarction) should be assigned first.

Code Z92.82 is only applicable to the receiving facility record and not to the transferring facility record.

| | |
|---|---|
| Z93 | Artificial opening status |
| Z94 | Transplanted organ and tissue status |
| Z95 | Presence of cardiac and vascular implants and grafts |
| Z96 | Presence of other functional implants |
| Z97 | Presence of other devices |
| Z98 | Other postprocedural states |

Assign code Z98.85, Transplanted organ removal status, to indicate that a transplanted organ has been previously removed. This code should not be assigned for the encounter in which the transplanted organ is removed. The complication necessitating removal of the transplant organ should be assigned for that encounter.

*See section I.C19. for information on the coding of organ transplant complications.*

| | |
|---|---|
| Z99 | Dependence on enabling machines and devices, not elsewhere classified |

**Note:** Categories Z89-Z90 and Z93-Z99 are for use only if there are no complications or malfunctions of the organ or tissue replaced, the amputation site or the equipment on which the patient is dependent.

### 4) History (of)

There are two types of history Z codes, personal and family. Personal history codes explain a patient's past medical condition that no longer exists and is not receiving any treatment, but that has the potential for recurrence, and therefore may require continued monitoring.

Family history codes are for use when a patient has a family member(s) who has had a particular disease that causes the patient to be at higher risk of also contracting the disease.

Personal history codes may be used in conjunction with follow-up codes and family history codes may be used in conjunction with screening codes to explain the need for a test or procedure. History codes are also acceptable on any medical record regardless of the reason for visit. A history of an illness, even if no longer present, is important information that may alter the type of treatment ordered.

The history Z code categories are:

| | |
|---|---|
| Z80 | Family history of primary malignant neoplasm |
| Z81 | Family history of mental and behavioral disorders |
| Z82 | Family history of certain disabilities and chronic diseases (leading to disablement) |
| Z83 | Family history of other specific disorders |
| Z84 | Family history of other conditions |
| Z85 | Personal history of malignant neoplasm |
| Z86 | Personal history of certain other diseases |
| Z87 | Personal history of other diseases and conditions |
| Z91.4- | Personal history of psychological trauma, not elsewhere classified |
| Z91.5 | Personal history of self-harm |
| Z91.8- | Other specified personal risk factors, not elsewhere classified |

Exception: Z91.83, Wandering in diseases classified elsewhere

| | |
|---|---|
| Z92 | Personal history of medical treatment |

Except: Z92.0, Personal history of contraception

Except: Z92.82, Status post administration of tPA (rtPA) in a different facility within the last 24 hours prior to admission to a current facility

### 5) Screening

Screening is the testing for disease or disease precursors in seemingly well individuals so that early detection and treatment can be provided for those who test positive for the disease (e.g., screening mammogram).

The testing of a person to rule out or confirm a suspected diagnosis because the patient has some sign or symptom is a diagnostic examination, not a screening. In these cases, the sign or symptom is used to explain the reason for the test.

A screening code may be a first-listed code if the reason for the visit is specifically the screening exam. It may also be used as an additional code if the screening is done during an office visit for other health problems. A screening code is not necessary if the screening is inherent to a routine examination, such as a pap smear done during a routine pelvic examination.

Should a condition be discovered during the screening then the code for the condition may be assigned as an additional diagnosis.

The Z code indicates that a screening exam is planned. A procedure code is required to confirm that the screening was performed.

The screening Z codes/categories:

| | |
|---|---|
| Z11 | Encounter for screening for infectious and parasitic diseases |
| Z12 | Encounter for screening for malignant neoplasms |
| Z13 | Encounter for screening for other diseases and disorders |

Except: Z13.9, Encounter for screening, unspecified

| | |
|---|---|
| Z36 | Encounter for antenatal screening for mother |

### 6) Observation

There are three observation Z code categories. They are for use in very limited circumstances when a person is being observed for a suspected condition that is ruled out. The observation codes are not for use if an injury or illness or any signs or symptoms related to the suspected condition are present. In such cases the diagnosis/symptom code is used with the corresponding external cause code.

The observation codes are to be used as principal diagnosis only. The only exception to this is when the principal diagnosis is required to be a code from category Z38, Liveborn infants according to place of birth and type of delivery. Then a code from category Z05, Encounter for observation and evaluation of newborn for suspected diseases and conditions ruled out, is sequenced after the Z38 code. Additional codes may be used in addition to the observation code but only if they are unrelated to the suspected condition being observed.

Codes from subcategory Z03.7, Encounter for suspected maternal and fetal conditions ruled out, may either be used as a first-listed or as an additional code assignment depending on the case. They are for use in very limited circumstances on a maternal record when an encounter is for a suspected maternal or fetal condition that is ruled out during that encounter (for example, a maternal or fetal condition may be suspected due to an abnormal test result). These codes should not be used when the condition is confirmed. In those cases, the confirmed condition should be coded. In addition, these codes are not for use if an illness or any signs or symptoms related to the suspected condition or problem are present. In such cases the diagnosis/symptom code is used.

Additional codes may be used in addition to the code from subcategory Z03.7, but only if they are unrelated to the suspected condition being evaluated.

Codes from subcategory Z03.7 may not be used for encounters for antenatal screening of mother. *See Section I.C.21. Screening.*

For encounters for suspected fetal condition that are inconclusive following testing and evaluation, assign the appropriate code from category O35, O36, O40 or O41.

The observation Z code categories:

Z03     Encounter for medical observation for suspected diseases and conditions ruled out

Z04     Encounter for examination and observation for other reasons

Except: Z04.9, Encounter for examination and observation for unspecified reason

Z05     Encounter for observation and evaluation of newborn for suspected diseases and conditions ruled out

---

Upon initial examination, a heart murmur was heard in a newborn infant delivered vaginally in the hospital; however, after further observation, any serious cardiac conditions were ruled out.

**Z38.00     Single liveborn infant, delivered vaginally**

**Z05.0     Observation and evaluation of newborn for suspected cardiac condition ruled out**

*Explanation:* Normally an observation code is used as the principal diagnosis except when the patient is a newborn. A code from category Z38 Liveborn infants according to place of birth and type of delivery code would be sequenced first, followed by the encounter for observation and evaluation of newborn for suspected diseases and conditions ruled out.

---

### 7) Aftercare

Aftercare visit codes cover situations when the initial treatment of a disease has been performed and the patient requires continued care during the healing or recovery phase, or for the long-term consequences of the disease. The aftercare Z code should not be used if treatment is directed at a current, acute disease. The diagnosis code is to be used in these cases. Exceptions to this rule are codes Z51.0, Encounter for antineoplastic radiation therapy, and codes from subcategory Z51.1, Encounter for antineoplastic chemotherapy and immunotherapy. These codes are to be first-listed, followed by the diagnosis code when a patient's encounter is solely to receive radiation therapy, chemotherapy, or immunotherapy for the treatment of a neoplasm. If the reason for the encounter is more than one type of antineoplastic therapy, code Z51.0 and a code from subcategory Z51.1 may be assigned together, in which case one of these codes would be reported as a secondary diagnosis.

The aftercare Z codes should also not be used for aftercare for injuries. For aftercare of an injury, assign the acute injury code with the appropriate 7th character (for subsequent encounter).

The aftercare codes are generally first-listed to explain the specific reason for the encounter. An aftercare code may be used as an additional code when some type of aftercare is provided in addition to the reason for admission and no diagnosis code is applicable. An example of this would be the closure of a colostomy during an encounter for treatment of another condition.

Aftercare codes should be used in conjunction with other aftercare codes or diagnosis codes to provide better detail on the specifics of an aftercare encounter visit, unless otherwise directed by the classification. Should a patient receive multiple types of antineoplastic therapy during the same encounter, code Z51.0, Encounter for antineoplastic radiation therapy, and codes from subcategory Z51.1, Encounter for antineoplastic chemotherapy and immunotherapy, may be used together on a record. The sequencing of multiple aftercare codes depends on the circumstances of the encounter.

Certain aftercare Z code categories need a secondary diagnosis code to describe the resolving condition or sequelae. For others, the condition is included in the code title.

Additional Z code aftercare category terms include fitting and adjustment, and attention to artificial openings.

Status Z codes may be used with aftercare Z codes to indicate the nature of the aftercare. For example code Z95.1, Presence of aortocoronary bypass graft, may be used with code Z48.812, Encounter for surgical aftercare following surgery on the circulatory system, to indicate the surgery for which the aftercare is being performed. A status code should not be used when the aftercare code indicates the type of status, such as using Z43.0, Encounter for attention to tracheostomy, with Z93.0, Tracheostomy status.

The aftercare Z category/codes:

Z42     Encounter for plastic and reconstructive surgery following medical procedure or healed injury

Z43     Encounter for attention to artificial openings

Z44     Encounter for fitting and adjustment of external prosthetic device

Z45     Encounter for adjustment and management of implanted device

Z46     Encounter for fitting and adjustment of other devices

Z47     Orthopedic aftercare

Z48     Encounter for other postprocedural aftercare

Z49     Encounter for care involving renal dialysis

Z51     Encounter for other aftercare and medical care

### 8) Follow-up

The follow-up codes are used to explain continuing surveillance following completed treatment of a disease, condition, or injury. They imply that the condition has been fully treated and no longer exists. They should not be confused with aftercare codes, or injury codes with a 7th character for subsequent encounter, that explain ongoing care of a healing condition or its sequelae. Follow-up codes may be used in conjunction with history codes to provide the full picture of the healed condition and its treatment. The follow-up code is sequenced first, followed by the history code.

A follow-up code may be used to explain multiple visits. Should a condition be found to have recurred on the follow-up visit, then the diagnosis code for the condition should be assigned in place of the follow-up code.

The follow-up Z code categories:

Z08     Encounter for follow-up examination after completed treatment for malignant neoplasm

Z09     Encounter for follow-up examination after completed treatment for conditions other than malignant neoplasm

Z39     Encounter for maternal postpartum care and examination

### 9) Donor

Codes in category Z52, Donors of organs and tissues, are used for living individuals who are donating blood or other body tissue. These codes are only for individuals donating for others, not for self-donations. They are not used to identify cadaveric donations.

### 10) Counseling

Counseling Z codes are used when a patient or family member receives assistance in the aftermath of an illness or injury, or when support is required in coping with family or social problems. They are not used in conjunction with a diagnosis code when the counseling component of care is considered integral to standard treatment.

The counseling Z codes/categories:

Z30.0-     Encounter for general counseling and advice on contraception

Z31.5     Encounter for genetic counseling

Z31.6-     Encounter for general counseling and advice on procreation

Z32.2     Encounter for childbirth instruction

Z32.3     Encounter for childcare instruction

Z69     Encounter for mental health services for victim and perpetrator of abuse

Z70     Counseling related to sexual attitude, behavior and orientation

Z71     Persons encountering health services for other counseling and medical advice, not elsewhere classified

Z76.81     Expectant mother prebirth pediatrician visit

### 11) Encounters for obstetrical and reproductive services

*See Section I.C.15. Pregnancy, Childbirth, and the Puerperium, for further instruction on the use of these codes.*

Z codes for pregnancy are for use in those circumstances when none of the problems or complications included in the codes from the Obstetrics chapter exist (a routine prenatal visit or postpartum care). Codes in category Z34, Encounter for supervision of normal pregnancy, are always first-listed and are not to be used with any other code from the OB chapter.

Codes in category Z3A, Weeks of gestation, may be assigned to provide additional information about the pregnancy. Category Z3A codes should not be assigned for pregnancies with abortive outcomes (categories O00-O08), elective termination of pregnancy (code Z33.32), nor for postpartum conditions, as category Z3A is not applicable to these conditions. The date of the admission should be used to determine weeks of gestation for inpatient admissions that encompass more than one gestational week.

The outcome of delivery, category Z37, should be included on all maternal delivery records. It is always a secondary code. Codes in category Z37 should not be used on the newborn record.

Z codes for family planning (contraceptive) or procreative management and counseling should be included on an obstetric record either during the pregnancy or the postpartum stage, if applicable.

Z codes/categories for obstetrical and reproductive services:

| | |
|---|---|
| Z30 | Encounter for contraceptive management |
| Z31 | Encounter for procreative management |
| Z32.2 | Encounter for childbirth instruction |
| Z32.3 | Encounter for childcare instruction |
| Z33 | Pregnant state |
| Z34 | Encounter for supervision of normal pregnancy |
| Z36 | Encounter for antenatal screening of mother |
| Z3A | Weeks of gestation |
| Z37 | Outcome of delivery |
| Z39 | Encounter for maternal postpartum care and examination |
| Z76.81 | Expectant mother prebirth pediatrician visit |

### 12) Newborns and infants

*See Section I.C.16. Newborn (Perinatal) Guidelines, for further instruction on the use of these codes.*

Newborn Z codes/categories:

| | |
|---|---|
| Z76.1 | Encounter for health supervision and care of foundling |
| Z00.1- | Encounter for routine child health examination |
| Z38 | Liveborn infants according to place of birth and type of delivery |

### 13) Routine and administrative examinations

The Z codes allow for the description of encounters for routine examinations, such as, a general check-up, or, examinations for administrative purposes, such as, a pre-employment physical. The codes are not to be used if the examination is for diagnosis of a suspected condition or for treatment purposes. In such cases the diagnosis code is used. During a routine exam, should a diagnosis or condition be discovered, it should be coded as an additional code. Pre-existing and chronic conditions and history codes may also be included as additional codes as long as the examination is for administrative purposes and not focused on any particular condition.

Some of the codes for routine health examinations distinguish between "with" and "without" abnormal findings. Code assignment depends on the information that is known at the time the encounter is being coded. For example, if no abnormal findings were found during the examination, but the encounter is being coded before test results are back, it is acceptable to assign the code for "without abnormal findings." When assigning a code for "with abnormal findings," additional code(s) should be assigned to identify the specific abnormal finding(s).

Pre-operative examination and pre-procedural laboratory examination Z codes are for use only in those situations when a patient is being cleared for a procedure or surgery and no treatment is given.

The Z codes/categories for routine and administrative examinations:

| | |
|---|---|
| Z00 | Encounter for general examination without complaint, suspected or reported diagnosis |
| Z01 | Encounter for other special examination without complaint, suspected or reported diagnosis |
| Z02 | Encounter for administrative examination |
| | Except: Z02.9, Encounter for administrative examinations, unspecified |
| Z32.0- | Encounter for pregnancy test |

### 14) Miscellaneous Z codes

The miscellaneous Z codes capture a number of other health care encounters that do not fall into one of the other categories. Certain of these codes identify the reason for the encounter; others are for use as additional codes that provide useful information on circumstances that may affect a patient's care and treatment.

**Prophylactic organ removal**

For encounters specifically for prophylactic removal of an organ (such as prophylactic removal of breasts due to a genetic susceptibility to cancer or a family history of cancer), the principal or first-listed code should be a code from category Z40, Encounter for prophylactic surgery, followed by the appropriate codes to identify the associated risk factor (such as genetic susceptibility or family history).

If the patient has a malignancy of one site and is having prophylactic removal at another site to prevent either a new primary malignancy or metastatic disease, a code for the malignancy should also be assigned in addition to a code from subcategory Z40.0, Encounter for prophylactic surgery for risk factors related to malignant neoplasms. A Z40.0 code should not be assigned if the patient is having organ removal for treatment of a malignancy, such as the removal of the testes for the treatment of prostate cancer.

Miscellaneous Z codes/categories:

| | |
|---|---|
| Z28 | Immunization not carried out |
| | Except: Z28.3, Underimmunization status |

| | |
|---|---|
| Z29 | Encounter for other prophylactic measures |
| Z40 | Encounter for prophylactic surgery |
| Z41 | Encounter for procedures for purposes other than remedying health state |
| | Except: Z41.9, Encounter for procedure for purposes other than remedying health state, unspecified |
| Z53 | Persons encountering health services for specific procedures and treatment, not carried out |
| Z55 | Problems related to education and literacy |
| Z56 | Problems related to employment and unemployment |
| Z57 | Occupational exposure to risk factors |
| Z58 | Problems related to physical environment |
| Z59 | Problems related to housing and economic circumstances |
| Z60 | Problems related to social environment |
| Z62 | Problems related to upbringing |
| Z63 | Other problems related to primary support group, including family circumstances |
| Z64 | Problems related to certain psychosocial circumstances |
| Z65 | Problems related to other psychosocial circumstances |
| Z72 | Problems related to lifestyle |
| | **Note:** These codes should be assigned only when the documentation specifies that the patient has an associated problem |
| Z73 | Problems related to life management difficulty |
| Z74 | Problems related to care provider dependency |
| | Except: Z74.01, Bed confinement status |
| Z75 | Problems related to medical facilities and other health care |
| Z76.0 | Encounter for issue of repeat prescription |
| Z76.3 | Healthy person accompanying sick person |
| Z76.4 | Other boarder to healthcare facility |
| Z76.5 | Malingerer [conscious simulation] |
| Z91.1- | Patient's noncompliance with medical treatment and regimen |
| Z91.83 | Wandering in diseases classified elsewhere |
| Z91.89 | Other specified personal risk factors, not elsewhere classified |

### 15) Nonspecific Z codes

Certain Z codes are so non-specific, or potentially redundant with other codes in the classification, that there can be little justification for their use in the inpatient setting. Their use in the outpatient setting should be limited to those instances when there is no further documentation to permit more precise coding. Otherwise, any sign or symptom or any other reason for visit that is captured in another code should be used.

Nonspecific Z codes/categories:

| | |
|---|---|
| Z02.9 | Encounter for administrative examinations, unspecified |
| Z04.9 | Encounter for examination and observation for unspecified reason |
| Z13.9 | Encounter for screening, unspecified |
| Z41.9 | Encounter for procedure for purposes other than remedying health state, unspecified |
| Z52.9 | Donor of unspecified organ or tissue |
| Z86.59 | Personal history of other mental and behavioral disorders |
| Z88.9 | Allergy status to unspecified drugs, medicaments and biological substances status |
| Z92.0 | Personal history of contraception |

### 16) Z codes that may only be principal/first-listed diagnosis

The following Z codes/categories may only be reported as the principal/first-listed diagnosis, except when there are multiple encounters on the same day and the medical records for the encounters are combined:

| | |
|---|---|
| Z00 | Encounter for general examination without complaint, suspected or reported diagnosis |
| | Except: Z00.6 |
| Z01 | Encounter for other special examination without complaint, suspected or reported diagnosis |
| Z02 | Encounter for administrative examination |
| Z03 | Encounter for medical observation for suspected diseases and conditions ruled out |
| Z04 | Encounter for examination and observation for other reasons |
| Z33.2 | Encounter for elective termination of pregnancy |
| Z31.81 | Encounter for male factor infertility in female patient |
| Z31.83 | Encounter for assisted reproductive fertility procedure cycle |

Z31.84   Encounter for fertility preservation procedure

Z34       Encounter for supervision of normal pregnancy

Z39       Encounter for maternal postpartum care and examination

Z38       Liveborn infants according to place of birth and type of delivery

Z42       Encounter for plastic and reconstructive surgery following medical procedure or healed injury

Z51.Ø    Encounter for antineoplastic radiation therapy

Z51.1-   Encounter for antineoplastic chemotherapy and immunotherapy

Z52       Donors of organs and tissues
          Except: Z52.9, Donor of unspecified organ or tissue

Z76.1    Encounter for health supervision and care of foundling

Z76.2    Encounter for health supervision and care of other healthy infant and child

Z99.12   Encounter for respirator [ventilator] dependence during power failure

# Chapter 21. Factors Influencing Health Status and Contact With Health Services (Z00-Z99)

**NOTE**   Z codes represent reasons for encounters. A corresponding procedure code must accompany a Z code if a procedure is performed. Categories Z00-Z99 are provided for occasions when circumstances other than a disease, injury or external cause classifiable to categories A00-Y89 are recorded as "diagnoses" or "problems". This can arise in two main ways:

(a) When a person who may or may not be sick encounters the health services for some specific purpose, such as to receive limited care or service for a current condition, to donate an organ or tissue, to receive prophylactic vaccination (immunization), or to discuss a problem which is in itself not a disease or injury.

(b) When some circumstance or problem is present which influences the person's health status but is not in itself a current illness or injury.

This chapter contains the following blocks:

| | |
|---|---|
| Z00-Z13 | Persons encountering health services for examinations |
| Z14-Z15 | Genetic carrier and genetic susceptibility to disease |
| Z16 | Resistance to antimicrobial drugs |
| Z17 | Estrogen receptor status |
| Z18 | Retained foreign body fragments |
| ~~Z19~~ | ~~Hormone sensitivity malignancy status~~ |
| Z20-Z29 | Persons with potential health hazards related to communicable diseases |
| Z30-Z39 | Persons encountering health services in circumstances related to reproduction |
| Z40-Z53 | Encounters for other specific health care |
| Z55-Z65 | Persons with potential health hazards related to socioeconomic and psychosocial circumstances |
| Z66 | Do not resuscitate status |
| Z67 | Blood type |
| Z68 | Body mass index (BMI) |
| Z69-Z76 | Persons encountering health services in other circumstances |
| Z77-Z99 | Persons with potential health hazards related to family and personal history and certain conditions influencing health status |

## Persons encountering health services for examinations (Z00-Z13)

**NOTE**   Nonspecific abnormal findings disclosed at the time of these examinations are classified to categories R70-R94.

**EXCLUDES 1**   *examinations related to pregnancy and reproduction (Z30-Z36, Z39-)*

√4ᵗʰ **Z00**   **Encounter for general examination without complaint, suspected or reported diagnosis**

**EXCLUDES 1**   *encounter for examination for administrative purposes (Z02.-)*

**EXCLUDES 2**   *encounter for pre-procedural examinations (Z01.81-)*
*special screening examinations (Z11-Z13)*

√5ᵗʰ **Z00.0**   **Encounter for general adult medical examination**
Encounter for adult periodic examination (annual) (physical) and any associated laboratory and radiologic examinations

**EXCLUDES 1**   *encounter for examination of sign or symptom—code to sign or symptom*
*general health check-up of infant or child (Z00.12-)*

**Z00.00**   **Encounter for general adult medical examination without abnormal findings**   Ⓐ
Encounter for adult health check-up NOS
**AHA:** 2016, 1Q, 36

**Z00.01**   **Encounter for general adult medical examination with abnormal findings**   Ⓐ
Use additional code to identify abnormal findings
**AHA:** 2016, 1Q, 35-36

√5ᵗʰ **Z00.1**   **Encounter for newborn, infant and child health examinations**

√6ᵗʰ **Z00.11**   **Newborn health examination**
Health check for child under 29 days old
Use additional code to identify any abnormal findings
**EXCLUDES 1**   *health check for child over 28 days old (Z00.12-)*

**Z00.110**   **Health examination for newborn under 8 days old**   Ⓝ
Health check for newborn under 8 days old

**Z00.111**   **Health examination for newborn 8 to 28 days old**   Ⓝ
Health check for newborn 8 to 28 days old
Newborn weight check

√6ᵗʰ **Z00.12**   **Encounter for routine child health examination**
Encounter for development testing of infant or child
Health check (routine) for child over 28 days old
**EXCLUDES 1**   *health check for child under 29 days old (Z00.11-)*
*health supervision of foundling or other healthy infant or child (Z76.1-Z76.2)*
*newborn health examination (Z00.11-)*

**Z00.121**   **Encounter for routine child health examination with abnormal findings**   Ⓟ
Use additional code to identify abnormal findings
**AHA:** 2016, 1Q, 34-35

**Z00.129**   **Encounter for routine child health examination without abnormal findings**   Ⓟ
Encounter for routine child health examination NOS
**AHA:** 2016, 1Q, 34

**Z00.2**   **Encounter for examination for period of rapid growth in childhood**   Ⓟ

**Z00.3**   **Encounter for examination for adolescent development state**   Ⓟ
Encounter for puberty development state

**Z00.5**   **Encounter for examination of potential donor of organ and tissue**   Ⓟ

**Z00.6**   **Encounter for examination for normal comparison and control in clinical research program**
Examination of participant or control in clinical research program

√5ᵗʰ **Z00.7**   **Encounter for examination for period of delayed growth in childhood**

**Z00.70**   **Encounter for examination for period of delayed growth in childhood without abnormal findings**   Ⓟ

**Z00.71**   **Encounter for examination for period of delayed growth in childhood with abnormal findings**   Ⓟ
Use additional code to identify abnormal findings

**Z00.8**   **Encounter for other general examination**
Encounter for health examination in population surveys

√4ᵗʰ **Z01**   **Encounter for other special examination without complaint, suspected or reported diagnosis**

**INCLUDES**   routine examination of specific system

**NOTE**   Codes from category Z01 represent the reason for the encounter. A separate procedure code is required to identify any examinations or procedures performed.

**EXCLUDES 1**   *encounter for examination for administrative purposes (Z02.-)*
*encounter for examination for suspected conditions, proven not to exist (Z03.-)*
*encounter for laboratory and radiologic examinations as a component of general medical examinations (Z00.0-)*
*encounter for laboratory, radiologic and imaging examinations for sign(s) and symptom(s)—code to the sign(s) or symptom(s)*

**EXCLUDES 2**   *screening examinations (Z11-Z13)*

√5ᵗʰ **Z01.0**   **Encounter for examination of eyes and vision**
**EXCLUDES 1**   *examination for driving license (Z02.4)*

**Z01.00**   **Encounter for examination of eyes and vision without abnormal findings**
Encounter for examination of eyes and vision NOS

**Z01.01**   **Encounter for examination of eyes and vision with abnormal findings**
Use additional code to identify abnormal findings

√5ᵗʰ **Z01.1**   **Encounter for examination of ears and hearing**

**Z01.10**   **Encounter for examination of ears and hearing without abnormal findings**
Encounter for examination of ears and hearing NOS
**AHA:** 2016, 4Q, 24

√6ᵗʰ **Z01.11**   **Encounter for examination of ears and hearing with abnormal findings**
**AHA:** 2016, 3Q, 17-18

**Z01.110**   **Encounter for hearing examination following failed hearing screening**

**Z01.118**   **Encounter for examination of ears and hearing with other abnormal findings**
Use additional code to identify abnormal findings

**Z01.12**   **Encounter for hearing conservation and treatment**

√5ᵗʰ **Z01.2**   **Encounter for dental examination and cleaning**

**Z01.20**   **Encounter for dental examination and cleaning without abnormal findings**
Encounter for dental examination and cleaning NOS

Ⓝ Newborn: 0   Ⓟ Pediatric: 0-17   Ⓜ Maternity: 12-55   Ⓐ Adult: 15-124   **MCC** Major CC Condition   **PDxMCC** PDx acts as own MCC   **CC** CC Condition   **PDxCC** PDx acts as own CC

**1222**      ICD-10-CM 2018

**Z01.21** **Encounter for dental examination and cleaning with abnormal findings**
Use additional code to identify abnormal findings

√5th **Z01.3** **Encounter for examination of blood pressure**

**Z01.30** **Encounter for examination of blood pressure without abnormal findings**
Encounter for examination of blood pressure NOS

**Z01.31** **Encounter for examination of blood pressure with abnormal findings**
Use additional code to identify abnormal findings

√5th **Z01.4** **Encounter for gynecological examination**
*EXCLUDES 2*  *pregnancy examination or test (Z32.0-)*
*routine examination for contraceptive maintenance (Z30.4-)*

√6th **Z01.41** **Encounter for routine gynecological examination**
Encounter for general gynecological examination with or without cervical smear
Encounter for gynecological examination (general) (routine) NOS
Encounter for pelvic examination (annual) (periodic)
Use additional code:
for screening for human papillomavirus, if applicable, (Z11.51)
for screening vaginal pap smear, if applicable (Z12.72)
to identify acquired absence of uterus, if applicable (Z90.71-)
*EXCLUDES 1*  *gynecologic examination status-post hysterectomy for malignant condition (Z08)*
*screening cervical pap smear not a part of a routine gynecological examination (Z12.4)*

**Z01.411** **Encounter for gynecological examination (general) (routine) with abnormal findings**   ♀
Use additional code to identify abnormal findings

**Z01.419** **Encounter for gynecological examination (general) (routine) without abnormal findings**   ♀

**Z01.42** **Encounter for cervical smear to confirm findings of recent normal smear following initial abnormal smear**   ♀

√5th **Z01.8** **Encounter for other specified special examinations**

√6th **Z01.81** **Encounter for preprocedural examinations**
Encounter for preoperative examinations
Encounter for radiological and imaging examinations as part of preprocedural examination

**Z01.810** **Encounter for preprocedural cardiovascular examination**

**Z01.811** **Encounter for preprocedural respiratory examination**

**Z01.812** **Encounter for preprocedural laboratory examination**
Blood and urine tests prior to treatment or procedure

**Z01.818** **Encounter for other preprocedural examination**
Encounter for preprocedural examination NOS
Encounter for examinations prior to antineoplastic chemotherapy

**Z01.82** **Encounter for allergy testing**
*EXCLUDES 1*  *encounter for antibody response examination (Z01.84)*

**Z01.83** **Encounter for blood typing**
Encounter for Rh typing

**Z01.84** **Encounter for antibody response examination**
Encounter for immunity status testing
*EXCLUDES 1*  *encounter for allergy testing (Z01.82)*

**Z01.89** **Encounter for other specified special examinations**

√4th **Z02** **Encounter for administrative examination**

**Z02.0** **Encounter for examination for admission to educational institution**
Encounter for examination for admission to preschool (education)
Encounter for examination for re-admission to school following illness or medical treatment

**Z02.1** **Encounter for pre-employment examination**

**Z02.2** **Encounter for examination for admission to residential institution**
*EXCLUDES 1*  *examination for admission to prison (Z02.89)*

**Z02.3** **Encounter for examination for recruitment to armed forces**

**Z02.4** **Encounter for examination for driving license**

**Z02.5** **Encounter for examination for participation in sport**
*EXCLUDES 1*  *blood-alcohol and blood-drug test (Z02.83)*

**Z02.6** **Encounter for examination for insurance purposes**

√5th **Z02.7** **Encounter for issue of medical certificate**
*EXCLUDES 1*  *encounter for general medical examination (Z00-Z01, Z02.0-Z02.6, Z02.8-Z02.9)*

**Z02.71** **Encounter for disability determination**
Encounter for issue of medical certificate of incapacity
Encounter for issue of medical certificate of invalidity

**Z02.79** **Encounter for issue of other medical certificate**

√5th **Z02.8** **Encounter for other administrative examinations**

**Z02.81** **Encounter for paternity testing**

**Z02.82** **Encounter for adoption services**

**Z02.83** **Encounter for blood-alcohol and blood-drug test**
Use additional code for findings of alcohol or drugs in blood (R78.-)

**Z02.89** **Encounter for other administrative examinations**
Encounter for examination for admission to prison
Encounter for examination for admission to summer camp
Encounter for immigration examination
Encounter for naturalization examination
Encounter for premarital examination
*EXCLUDES 1*  *health supervision of foundling or other healthy infant or child (Z76.1-Z76.2)*

**Z02.9** **Encounter for administrative examinations, unspecified**

√4th **Z03** **Encounter for medical observation for suspected diseases and conditions ruled out**
*NOTE*  This category is to be used when a person without a diagnosis is suspected of having an abnormal condition, without signs or symptoms, which requires study, but after examination and observation, is ruled out. This category is also for use for administrative and legal observation status.
*EXCLUDES 1*  *contact with and (suspected) exposures hazardous to health (Z77.-)*
▶*encounter for observation and evaluation of newborn for suspected diseases and conditions ruled out (Z05.0-)*◀
*newborn observation for suspected condition, ruled out (P00-P04)*
*person with feared complaint in whom no diagnosis is made (Z71.1)*
*signs or symptoms under study—code to signs or symptoms*

**Z03.6** **Encounter for observation for suspected toxic effect from ingested substance ruled out**
Encounter for observation for suspected adverse effect from drug
Encounter for observation for suspected poisoning

√5th **Z03.7** **Encounter for suspected maternal and fetal conditions ruled out**
Encounter for suspected maternal and fetal conditions not found
*EXCLUDES 1*  *known or suspected fetal anomalies affecting management of mother, not ruled out (O26-, O35-, O36-, O40-, O41-)*

**Z03.71** **Encounter for suspected problem with amniotic cavity and membrane ruled out**   M♀
Encounter for suspected oligohydramnios ruled out
Encounter for suspected polyhydramnios ruled out

**Z03.72** **Encounter for suspected placental problem ruled out**   M♀

**Z03.73** **Encounter for suspected fetal anomaly ruled out**   M♀

**Z03.74** **Encounter for suspected problem with fetal growth ruled out**   M♀

**Z03.75** **Encounter for suspected cervical shortening ruled out**   M♀

**Z03.79** **Encounter for other suspected maternal and fetal conditions ruled out**   M♀

√5th **Z03.8** **Encounter for observation for other suspected diseases and conditions ruled out**

√6th **Z03.81** **Encounter for observation for suspected exposure to biological agents ruled out**

**Z03.810** **Encounter for observation for suspected exposure to anthrax ruled out**

---

√ Additional Character Req   √x7th Placeholder Alert   Unacceptable PDx   Manifestation   H1 - H14 HAC   HCC CMS-HCC Condition   *EXCLUDES 1* Not Coded Here   *EXCLUDES 2* Not Included Here

**Z03.818**   **Encounter for observation for suspected exposure to** other **biological agents ruled out**

**Z03.89**   **Encounter for observation for** other **suspected diseases and conditions ruled out**

√4ᵗʰ **Z04**   **Encounter for examination and observation for other reasons**

INCLUDES   encounter for examination for medicolegal reasons

This category is to be used when a person without a diagnosis is suspected of having an abnormal condition, without signs or symptoms, which requires study, but after examination and observation, is ruled-out. This category is also for use for administrative and legal observation status.

**Z04.1**   **Encounter for examination and observation following** transport accident

EXCLUDES 1   *encounter for examination and observation following work accident (Z04.2)*

**Z04.2**   **Encounter for examination and observation following** work accident

**Z04.3**   **Encounter for examination and observation following** other accident

√5ᵗʰ **Z04.4**   **Encounter for examination and observation following** alleged rape

Encounter for examination and observation of victim following alleged rape

Encounter for examination and observation of victim following alleged sexual abuse

**Z04.41**   **Encounter for examination and observation following alleged** adult **rape**    A

Suspected adult rape, ruled out

Suspected adult sexual abuse, ruled out

**Z04.42**   **Encounter for examination and observation following alleged** child **rape**    P

Suspected child rape, ruled out

Suspected child sexual abuse, ruled out

**Z04.6**   **Encounter for** general psychiatric examination, requested by authority

√5ᵗʰ **Z04.7**   **Encounter for examination and observation following** alleged physical abuse

**Z04.71**   **Encounter for examination and observation following alleged** adult **physical abuse**    A

Suspected adult physical abuse, ruled out

EXCLUDES 1   *confirmed case of adult physical abuse (T74.-)*

*encounter for examination and observation following alleged adult sexual abuse (Z04.41)*

*suspected case of adult physical abuse, not ruled out (T76.-)*

**Z04.72**   **Encounter for examination and observation following alleged** child **physical abuse**    P

Suspected child physical abuse, ruled out

EXCLUDES 1   *confirmed case of child physical abuse (T74.-)*

*encounter for examination and observation following alleged child sexual abuse (Z04.42)*

*suspected case of child physical abuse, not ruled out (T76.-)*

**Z04.8**   **Encounter for examination and observation for** other **specified reasons**

Encounter for examination and observation for request for expert evidence

**Z04.9**   **Encounter for examination and observation for** unspecified **reason**

Encounter for observation NOS

√4ᵗʰ **Z05**   **Encounter for observation of newborn for suspected diseases and conditions ruled out**

▶This category is to be used for newborns, within the neonatal period (the first 28 days of life), who are suspected of having an abnormal condition, but without signs or symptoms, and which, after examination and observation, is ruled out.◀

EXCLUDES 2   *newborn observation for suspected condition, related to exposure from the mother or birth process (P00-P04)*

**Z05.0**   **Observation and evaluation of newborn for suspected** cardiac **condition ruled out**

**Z05.1**   **Observation and evaluation of newborn for suspected** infectious **condition ruled out**

**Z05.2**   **Observation and evaluation of newborn for suspected** neurological **condition ruled out**

**Z05.3**   **Observation and evaluation of newborn for suspected** respiratory **condition ruled out**

√5ᵗʰ **Z05.4**   **Observation and evaluation of newborn for suspected** genetic, metabolic or immunologic **condition ruled out**

**Z05.41**   **Observation and evaluation of newborn for suspected** genetic **condition ruled out**

**Z05.42**   **Observation and evaluation of newborn for suspected** metabolic **condition ruled out**

**Z05.43**   **Observation and evaluation of newborn for suspected** immunologic **condition ruled out**

**Z05.5**   **Observation and evaluation of newborn for suspected** gastrointestinal **condition ruled out**

**Z05.6**   **Observation and evaluation of newborn for suspected** genitourinary **condition ruled out**

√5ᵗʰ **Z05.7**   **Observation and evaluation of newborn for suspected** skin, subcutaneous, musculoskeletal and connective tissue **condition ruled out**

**Z05.71**   **Observation and evaluation of newborn for suspected** skin and subcutaneous **tissue condition ruled out**

**Z05.72**   **Observation and evaluation of newborn for suspected** musculoskeletal **condition ruled out**

**Z05.73**   **Observation and evaluation of newborn for suspected** connective tissue **condition ruled out**

**Z05.8**   **Observation and evaluation of newborn for** other **specified suspected condition ruled out**

**Z05.9**   **Observation and evaluation of newborn for** unspecified **suspected condition ruled out**

**Z08**   **Encounter for** follow-up **examination** after completed treatment **for malignant neoplasm**

Medical surveillance following completed treatment

Use additional code to identify any acquired absence of organs (Z90.-)

Use additional code to identify the personal history of malignant neoplasm (Z85.-)

EXCLUDES 1   *aftercare following medical care (Z43-Z49, Z51)*

**Z09**   **Encounter for** follow-up **examination** after completed treatment **for conditions** other **than malignant neoplasm**

Medical surveillance following completed treatment

Use additional code to identify any applicable history of disease code (Z86-. Z87-)

EXCLUDES 1   *aftercare following medical care (Z43-Z49, Z51)*

*surveillance of contraception (Z30.4-)*

*surveillance of prosthetic and other medical devices (Z44-Z46)*

**AHA:** 2017, 1Q, 9; 2015, 1Q, 8

√4ᵗʰ **Z11**   **Encounter for** screening for infectious and parasitic diseases

Screening is the testing for disease or disease precursors in asymptomatic individuals so that early detection and treatment can be provided for those who test positive for the disease.

EXCLUDES 1   *encounter for diagnostic examination—code to sign or symptom*

**Z11.0**   **Encounter for screening for** intestinal infectious diseases

**Z11.1**   **Encounter for screening for** respiratory tuberculosis

**Z11.2**   **Encounter for screening for** other bacterial diseases

**Z11.3**   **Encounter for screening for infections with a** predominantly sexual mode of transmission

EXCLUDES 2   *encounter for screening for human immunodeficiency virus [HIV] (Z11.4)*

*encounter for screening for human papillomavirus (Z11.51)*

**Z11.4**   **Encounter for screening for** human immunodeficiency virus [HIV]

√5ᵗʰ **Z11.5**   **Encounter for screening for** other viral diseases

EXCLUDES 2   *encounter for screening for viral intestinal disease (Z11.0)*

**Z11.51**   **Encounter for screening for** human papillomavirus (HPV)

**Z11.59**   **Encounter for screening for** other viral diseases

**Z11.6**   **Encounter for screening for** other protozoal diseases and helminthiases

EXCLUDES 2   *encounter for screening for protozoal intestinal disease (Z11.0)*

**Z11.8**   **Encounter for screening for** other infectious and parasitic diseases

Encounter for screening for chlamydia

Encounter for screening for rickettsial

Encounter for screening for spirochetal

Encounter for screening for mycoses

**Z11.9**   **Encounter for screening for infectious and parasitic diseases, unspecified**

N Newborn: 0   P Pediatric: 0-17   M Maternity: 12-55   A Adult: 15-124   MCC Major CC Condition   PDxMCC PDx acts as own MCC   CC CC Condition   PDxCC PDx acts as own CC

1224

ICD-10-CM 2018

**✓4ᵗʰ Z12   Encounter for screening for malignant neoplasms**

Screening is the testing for disease or disease precursors in asymptomatic individuals so that early detection and treatment can be provided for those who test positive for the disease.

Use additional code to identify any family history of malignant neoplasm (Z80.-)

*EXCLUDES 1*   *encounter for diagnostic examination—code to sign or symptom*

**Z12.0   Encounter for screening for malignant neoplasm of stomach**

**✓5ᵗʰ Z12.1   Encounter for screening for malignant neoplasm of intestinal tract**

AHA: 2017, 1Q, 8, 9

**Z12.10   Encounter for screening for malignant neoplasm of intestinal tract, unspecified**

**Z12.11   Encounter for screening for malignant neoplasm of colon**

Encounter for screening colonoscopy NOS

**Z12.12   Encounter for screening for malignant neoplasm of rectum**

**Z12.13   Encounter for screening for malignant neoplasm of small intestine**

**Z12.2   Encounter for screening for malignant neoplasm of respiratory organs**

**✓5ᵗʰ Z12.3   Encounter for screening for malignant neoplasm of breast**

**Z12.31   Encounter for screening mammogram for malignant neoplasm of breast**

*EXCLUDES 1*   *inconclusive mammogram (R92.2)*

AHA: 2015, 1Q, 24

**Z12.39   Encounter for other screening for malignant neoplasm of breast**

**Z12.4   Encounter for screening for malignant neoplasm of cervix ♀**

Encounter for screening pap smear for malignant neoplasm of cervix

*EXCLUDES 1*   *when screening is part of general gynecological examination (Z01.4-)*

*EXCLUDES 2*   *encounter for screening for human papillomavirus (Z11.51)*

**Z12.5   Encounter for screening for malignant neoplasm of prostate ♂**

**Z12.6   Encounter for screening for malignant neoplasm of bladder**

**✓5ᵗʰ Z12.7   Encounter for screening for malignant neoplasm of other genitourinary organs**

**Z12.71   Encounter for screening for malignant neoplasm of testis ♂**

**Z12.72   Encounter for screening for malignant neoplasm of vagina ♀**

Vaginal pap smear status-post hysterectomy for non-malignant condition

Use additional code to identify acquired absence of uterus (Z90.71-)

*EXCLUDES 1*   *vaginal pap smear status-post hysterectomy for malignant conditions (Z08)*

**Z12.73   Encounter for screening for malignant neoplasm of ovary ♀**

**Z12.79   Encounter for screening for malignant neoplasm of other genitourinary organs**

**✓5ᵗʰ Z12.8   Encounter for screening for malignant neoplasm of other sites**

**Z12.81   Encounter for screening for malignant neoplasm of oral cavity**

**Z12.82   Encounter for screening for malignant neoplasm of nervous system**

**Z12.83   Encounter for screening for malignant neoplasm of skin**

**Z12.89   Encounter for screening for malignant neoplasm of other sites**

**Z12.9   Encounter for screening for malignant neoplasm, site unspecified**

**✓4ᵗʰ Z13   Encounter for screening for other diseases and disorders**

Screening is the testing for disease or disease precursors in asymptomatic individuals so that early detection and treatment can be provided for those who test positive for the disease.

*EXCLUDES 1*   *encounter for diagnostic examination—code to sign or symptom*

**Z13.0   Encounter for screening for diseases of the blood and blood-forming organs and certain disorders involving the immune mechanism**

**Z13.1   Encounter for screening for diabetes mellitus**

**✓5ᵗʰ Z13.2   Encounter for screening for nutritional, metabolic and other endocrine disorders**

**Z13.21   Encounter for screening for nutritional disorder**

**✓6ᵗʰ Z13.22   Encounter for screening for metabolic disorder**

**Z13.220   Encounter for screening for lipoid disorders**

Encounter for screening for cholesterol level

Encounter for screening for hypercholesterolemia

Encounter for screening for hyperlipidemia

**Z13.228   Encounter for screening for other metabolic disorders**

**Z13.29   Encounter for screening for other suspected endocrine disorder**

*EXCLUDES 1*   *encounter for screening for diabetes mellitus (Z13.1)*

**Z13.4   Encounter for screening for certain developmental disorders in childhood**   P

Encounter for screening for developmental handicaps in early childhood

*EXCLUDES 1*   *routine development testing of infant or child (Z00.1-)*

**Z13.5   Encounter for screening for eye and ear disorders**

*EXCLUDES 2*   *encounter for general hearing examination (Z01.1-)*

*encounter for general vision examination (Z01.0-)*

AHA: 2016, 3Q, 17

**Z13.6   Encounter for screening for cardiovascular disorders**

**✓5ᵗʰ Z13.7   Encounter for screening for genetic and chromosomal anomalies**

*EXCLUDES 1*   *genetic testing for procreative management (Z31.4-)*

**Z13.71   Encounter for nonprocreative screening for genetic disease carrier status**

**Z13.79   Encounter for other screening for genetic and chromosomal anomalies**

**✓5ᵗʰ Z13.8   Encounter for screening for other specified diseases and disorders**

*EXCLUDES 2*   *screening for malignant neoplasms (Z12.-)*

**✓6ᵗʰ Z13.81   Encounter for screening for digestive system disorders**

**Z13.810   Encounter for screening for upper gastrointestinal disorder**

**Z13.811   Encounter for screening for lower gastrointestinal disorder**

*EXCLUDES 1*   *encounter for screening for intestinal infectious disease (Z11.0)*

**Z13.818   Encounter for screening for other digestive system disorders**

**✓6ᵗʰ Z13.82   Encounter for screening for musculoskeletal disorder**

**Z13.820   Encounter for screening for osteoporosis**

**Z13.828   Encounter for screening for other musculoskeletal disorder**

**Z13.83   Encounter for screening for respiratory disorder NEC**

*EXCLUDES 1*   *encounter for screening for respiratory tuberculosis (Z11.1)*

**Z13.84   Encounter for screening for dental disorders**

**✓6ᵗʰ Z13.85   Encounter for screening for nervous system disorders**

**Z13.850   Encounter for screening for traumatic brain injury**

**Z13.858   Encounter for screening for other nervous system disorders**

**Z13.88   Encounter for screening for disorder due to exposure to contaminants**

*EXCLUDES 1*   *those exposed to contaminants without suspected disorders (Z57-Z77-)*

**Z13.89   Encounter for screening for other disorder**

Encounter for screening for genitourinary disorders

**Z13.9   Encounter for screening, unspecified**

**✓** Additional Character Req   **✓x7ᵗʰ** Placeholder Alert   Unacceptable PDx   Manifestation   **H1**-**H14** HAC   **HCC** CMS-HCC Condition   *EXCLUDES 1* Not Coded Here   *EXCLUDES 2* Not Included Here

ICD-10-CM 2018          **1225**

**Chapter 21. Factors Influencing Health Status and Contact with Health Services**

## Genetic carrier and genetic susceptibility to disease (Z14-Z15)

√4th **Z14 Genetic carrier**
**DEF:** Individuals carrying a gene mutation associated with a certain disease who typically do not develop the disease but are able to pass mutated gene to offspring.

√5th **Z14.0 Hemophilia A carrier**
**Z14.01 Asymptomatic hemophilia A carrier**
**Z14.02 Symptomatic hemophilia A carrier**

**Z14.1 Cystic fibrosis carrier**

**Z14.8 Genetic carrier of other disease**

√4th **Z15 Genetic susceptibility to disease**
INCLUDES confirmed abnormal gene
Use additional code, if applicable, for any associated family history of the disease (Z80-Z84)
EXCLUDES 1 chromosomal anomalies (Q90-Q99)

√5th **Z15.0 Genetic susceptibility to malignant neoplasm**
Code first, if applicable, any current malignant neoplasm (C00-C75, C81-C96)
Use additional code, if applicable, for any personal history of malignant neoplasm (Z85.-)

**Z15.01 Genetic susceptibility to malignant neoplasm of breast**

**Z15.02 Genetic susceptibility to malignant neoplasm of ovary** ♀

**Z15.03 Genetic susceptibility to malignant neoplasm of prostate** ♂

**Z15.04 Genetic susceptibility to malignant neoplasm of endometrium** ♀

**Z15.09 Genetic susceptibility to other malignant neoplasm**

√5th **Z15.8 Genetic susceptibility to other disease**
**Z15.81 Genetic susceptibility to multiple endocrine neoplasia [MEN]**
EXCLUDES 1 multiple endocrine neoplasia [MEN] syndromes (E31.2-)

**Z15.89 Genetic susceptibility to other disease**

## Resistance to antimicrobial drugs (Z16)

√4th **Z16 Resistance to antimicrobial drugs**
NOTE The codes in this category are provided for use as additional codes to identify the resistance and non-responsiveness of a condition to antimicrobial drugs.
Code first the infection
EXCLUDES 1 Methicillin resistant Staphylococcus aureus infection (A49.02)
~~Methicillin resistant Staphylococcus aureus infection in diseases classified elsewhere (B95.62)~~
Methicillin resistant Staphylococcus aureus pneumonia (J15.212)
sepsis due to Methicillin resistant Staphylococcus aureus (A41.02)

√5th **Z16.1 Resistance to beta lactam antibiotics**
**Z16.10 Resistance to unspecified beta lactam antibiotics**
**Z16.11 Resistance to penicillins**
Resistance to amoxicillin
Resistance to ampicillin
**Z16.12 Extended spectrum beta lactamase (ESBL) resistance**
EXCLUDES 2 ►Methicillin resistant Staphylococcus aureus infection in diseases classified elsewhere (B95.62)◄
**Z16.19 Resistance to other specified beta lactam antibiotics**
Resistance to cephalosporins

√5th **Z16.2 Resistance to other antibiotics**
**Z16.20 Resistance to unspecified antibiotic**
Resistance to antibiotics NOS
**Z16.21 Resistance to vancomycin**
**Z16.22 Resistance to vancomycin related antibiotics**
**Z16.23 Resistance to quinolones and fluoroquinolones**
**Z16.24 Resistance to multiple antibiotics**
**Z16.29 Resistance to other single specified antibiotic**
Resistance to aminoglycosides
Resistance to macrolides
Resistance to sulfonamides
Resistance to tetracyclines

√5th **Z16.3 Resistance to other antimicrobial drugs**
EXCLUDES 1 resistance to antibiotics (Z16.1-, Z16.2-)
**Z16.30 Resistance to unspecified antimicrobial drugs**
Drug resistance NOS
**Z16.31 Resistance to antiparasitic drug(s)**
Resistance to quinine and related compounds
**Z16.32 Resistance to antifungal drug(s)**
**Z16.33 Resistance to antiviral drug(s)**
√6th **Z16.34 Resistance to antimycobacterial drug(s)**
Resistance to tuberculostatics
**Z16.341 Resistance to single antimycobacterial drug**
Resistance to antimycobacterial drug NOS
**Z16.342 Resistance to multiple antimycobacterial drugs**
**Z16.35 Resistance to multiple antimicrobial drugs**
EXCLUDES 1 Resistance to multiple antibiotics only (Z16.24)
**Z16.39 Resistance to other specified antimicrobial drug**

## Estrogen receptor status (Z17)

√4th **Z17 Estrogen receptor status**
Code first malignant neoplasm of breast (C50.-)
**Z17.0 Estrogen receptor positive status [ER+]**
**Z17.1 Estrogen receptor negative status [ER-]**

## Retained foreign body fragment (Z18)

√4th **Z18 Retained foreign body fragments**
INCLUDES embedded fragment (status)
embedded splinter (status)
retained foreign body status
EXCLUDES 1 artificial joint prosthesis status (Z96.6-)
foreign body accidentally left during a procedure (T81.5-)
foreign body entering through orifice (T15-T19)
in situ cardiac device (Z95.-)
organ or tissue replaced by means other than transplant (Z96.-, Z97.-)
organ or tissue replaced by transplant (Z94.-)
personal history of retained foreign body fully removed (Z87.821)
superficial foreign body (non-embedded splinter)—code to superficial foreign body, by site
**DEF:** Embedded or retained fragment, splinter, or foreign body; natural or synthetic; can cause infection.

√5th **Z18.0 Retained radioactive fragments**
**Z18.01 Retained depleted uranium fragments**
**Z18.09 Other retained radioactive fragments**
Other retained depleted isotope fragments
Retained nontherapeutic radioactive fragments

√5th **Z18.1 Retained metal fragments**
EXCLUDES 1 retained radioactive metal fragments (Z18.01-Z18.09)
**Z18.10 Retained metal fragments, unspecified**
Retained metal fragment NOS
**Z18.11 Retained magnetic metal fragments**
**Z18.12 Retained nonmagnetic metal fragments**

**Z18.2 Retained plastic fragments**
Acrylics fragments
Diethylhexylphthalates fragments
Isocyanate fragments

√5th **Z18.3 Retained organic fragments**
**Z18.31 Retained animal quills or spines**
**Z18.32 Retained tooth**
**Z18.33 Retained wood fragments**
**Z18.39 Other retained organic fragments**

√5th **Z18.8 Other specified retained foreign body**
**Z18.81 Retained glass fragments**
**Z18.83 Retained stone or crystalline fragments**
Retained concrete or cement fragments
**Z18.89 Other specified retained foreign body fragments**
**Z18.9 Retained foreign body fragments, unspecified material**

N Newborn: 0   P Pediatric: 0-17   M Maternity: 12-55   A Adult: 15-124   MCC Major CC Condition   PDxMCC PDx acts as own MCC   CC CC Condition   PDxCC PDx acts as own CC

**1226**      ICD-10-CM 2018

## Hormone sensitivity malignancy status (Z19)

**☑4ᵗʰ Z19 Hormone sensitivity malignancy status**
> Code first malignant neoplasm — see Table of Neoplasms, by site, malignant

**Z19.1 Hormone sensitive malignancy status**

**Z19.2 Hormone resistant malignancy status**
> Castrate resistant prostate malignancy status

## Persons with potential health hazards related to communicable diseases (Z20-Z29)

**☑4ᵗʰ Z20 Contact with and (suspected) exposure to communicable diseases**
> *EXCLUDES 1*   carrier of infectious disease (Z22.-)
> diagnosed current infectious or parasitic disease—see Alphabetic Index
> *EXCLUDES 2*   personal history of infectious and parasitic diseases (Z86.1-)

**☑5ᵗʰ Z20.0 Contact with and (suspected) exposure to intestinal infectious diseases**

**Z20.01 Contact with and (suspected) exposure to intestinal infectious diseases due to Escherichia coli (E. coli)**

**Z20.09 Contact with and (suspected) exposure to other intestinal infectious diseases**

**Z20.1 Contact with and (suspected) exposure to tuberculosis**

**Z20.2 Contact with and (suspected) exposure to infections with a predominantly sexual mode of transmission**

**Z20.3 Contact with and (suspected) exposure to rabies**

**Z20.4 Contact with and (suspected) exposure to rubella**

**Z20.5 Contact with and (suspected) exposure to viral hepatitis**

**Z20.6 Contact with and (suspected) exposure to human immunodeficiency virus [HIV]**
> *EXCLUDES 1*   asymptomatic human immunodeficiency virus [HIV] HIV infection status (Z21)

**Z20.7 Contact with and (suspected) exposure to pediculosis, acariasis and other infestations**

**☑5ᵗʰ Z20.8 Contact with and (suspected) exposure to other communicable diseases**

**☑6ᵗʰ Z20.81 Contact with and (suspected) exposure to other bacterial communicable diseases**

**Z20.810 Contact with and (suspected) exposure to anthrax**

**Z20.811 Contact with and (suspected) exposure to meningococcus**

**Z20.818 Contact with and (suspected) exposure to other bacterial communicable diseases**

**☑6ᵗʰ Z20.82 Contact with and (suspected) exposure to other viral communicable diseases**

**Z20.820 Contact with and (suspected) exposure to varicella**

**Z20.828 Contact with and (suspected) exposure to other viral communicable diseases**

**Z20.89 Contact with and (suspected) exposure to other communicable diseases**

**Z20.9 Contact with and (suspected) exposure to unspecified communicable disease**

**⁴ Z21 Asymptomatic human immunodeficiency virus [HIV] infection status**   HCC
> HIV positive NOS
> Code first human immunodeficiency virus [HIV] disease complicating pregnancy, childbirth and the puerperium, if applicable (O98.7-)
> *EXCLUDES 1*   acquired immunodeficiency syndrome (B20)
> contact with human immunodeficiency virus [HIV] (Z20.6)
> exposure to human immunodeficiency virus [HIV] (Z20.6)
> human immunodeficiency virus [HIV] disease (B20)
> inconclusive laboratory evidence of human immunodeficiency virus [HIV] (R75)
>
> **DEF:** Phase of human immunodeficiency virus (HIV) infection with no clinical symptoms; may last for 10 years or more.

**☑4ᵗʰ Z22 Carrier of infectious disease**
> *INCLUDES*   colonization status
> suspected carrier
> *EXCLUDES 2*   carrier of viral hepatitis (B18.-)

**Z22.0 Carrier of typhoid**

**Z22.1 Carrier of other intestinal infectious diseases**

**Z22.2 Carrier of diphtheria**

**☑5ᵗʰ Z22.3 Carrier of other specified bacterial diseases**

**Z22.31 Carrier of bacterial disease due to meningococci**

**☑6ᵗʰ Z22.32 Carrier of bacterial disease due to staphylococci**

**Z22.321 Carrier or suspected carrier of Methicillin susceptible Staphylococcus aureus**
> MSSA colonization

**Z22.322 Carrier or suspected carrier of Methicillin resistant Staphylococcus aureus**
> MRSA colonization

**☑6ᵗʰ Z22.33 Carrier of bacterial disease due to streptococci**

**Z22.330 Carrier of Group B streptococcus**
> *EXCLUDES 1*   carrier of streptococcus group B (GBS) complicating pregnancy, childbirth and the puerperium (O99.82-)

**Z22.338 Carrier of other streptococcus**

**Z22.39 Carrier of other specified bacterial diseases**

**Z22.4 Carrier of infections with a predominantly sexual mode of transmission**

**Z22.6 Carrier of human T-lymphotropic virus type-1 [HTLV-1] infection**

**Z22.8 Carrier of other infectious diseases**

**Z22.9 Carrier of infectious disease, unspecified**

**Z23 Encounter for immunization**
> Code first any routine childhood examination
> *NOTE*   Procedure codes are required to identify the types of immunizations given

**☑4ᵗʰ Z28 Immunization not carried out and underimmunization status**
> *INCLUDES*   vaccination not carried out

**☑5ᵗʰ Z28.0 Immunization not carried out because of contraindication**

**Z28.01 Immunization not carried out because of acute illness of patient**

**Z28.02 Immunization not carried out because of chronic illness or condition of patient**

**Z28.03 Immunization not carried out because of immune compromised state of patient**

**Z28.04 Immunization not carried out because of patient allergy to vaccine or component**

**Z28.09 Immunization not carried out because of other contraindication**

**Z28.1 Immunization not carried out because of patient decision for reasons of belief or group pressure**
> Immunization not carried out because of religious belief

**☑5ᵗʰ Z28.2 Immunization not carried out because of patient decision for other and unspecified reason**

**Z28.20 Immunization not carried out because of patient decision for unspecified reason**

**Z28.21 Immunization not carried out because of patient refusal**

**Z28.29 Immunization not carried out because of patient decision for other reason**

**Z28.3 Underimmunization status**
> Delinquent immunization status
> Lapsed immunization schedule status

**☑5ᵗʰ Z28.8 Immunization not carried out for other reason**

**Z28.81 Immunization not carried out due to patient having had the disease**

**Z28.82 Immunization not carried out because of caregiver refusal**
> Immunization not carried out because of guardian refusal
> Immunization not carried out because of parent refusal
> *EXCLUDES 1*   immunization not carried out because of caregiver refusal because of religious belief (Z28.1)

**Z28.89 Immunization not carried out for other reason**

**Z28.9 Immunization not carried out for unspecified reason**

**☑4ᵗʰ Z29 Encounter for other prophylactic measures**
> *EXCLUDES 1*   desensitization to allergens (Z51.6)
> prophylactic surgery (Z40.-)

**☑5ᵗʰ Z29.1 Encounter for prophylactic immunotherapy**
> Encounter for administration of immunoglobulin

**Z29.11 Encounter for prophylactic immunotherapy for respiratory syncytial virus (RSV)**

---

⁴   Questionable admission when used as PDx.

Chapter 21. Factors Influencing Health Status and Contact with Health Services

Z19–Z29.11

**Z29.12**   **Encounter for** prophylactic antivenin

**Z29.13**   **Encounter for** prophylactic Rho(D) immune globulin

**Z29.14**   **Encounter for** prophylactic rabies immune globin

**Z29.3**   **Encounter for** prophylactic fluoride administration

**Z29.8**   **Encounter for** other specified prophylactic measures

**Z29.9**   **Encounter for** prophylactic measures, unspecified

## Persons encountering health services in circumstances related to reproduction (Z30-Z39)

✓4ᵗʰ **Z30**   **Encounter for contraceptive management**

DEF: Contraceptive management to prevent pregnancy; methods include oral medications, intrauterine devices, and surgical procedures for males and females (sterilization).

✓5ᵗʰ **Z30.0**   **Encounter for general counseling and advice on contraception**

✓6ᵗʰ **Z30.01**   **Encounter for** initial prescription of contraceptives

EXCLUDES 1   *encounter for surveillance of contraceptives (Z30.4-)*

**Z30.011**   **Encounter for** initial prescription of contraceptive pills   ♀

**Z30.012**   **Encounter for** prescription of emergency contraception   ♀
Encounter for postcoital contraception

**Z30.013**   **Encounter for** initial prescription of injectable contraceptive   ♀

**Z30.014**   **Encounter for** initial prescription of intrauterine contraceptive device   ♀
EXCLUDES 1   *encounter for insertion of intrauterine contraceptive device (Z30.430, Z30.432)*

**Z30.015**   **Encounter for** initial prescription of vaginal ring hormonal contraceptive   ♀

**Z30.016**   **Encounter for** initial prescription of transdermal patch hormonal contraceptive device   ♀

**Z30.017**   **Encounter for** initial prescription of implantable subdermal contraceptive   ♀

**Z30.018**   **Encounter for** initial prescription of other contraceptives   ♀
Encounter for initial prescription of barrier contraception
Encounter for initial prescription of diaphragm

**Z30.019**   **Encounter for** initial prescription of contraceptives, unspecified   ♀

**Z30.02**   **Counseling and instruction in** natural family planning to avoid pregnancy

**Z30.09**   **Encounter for** other general counseling and advice on contraception
Encounter for family planning advice NOS

**Z30.2**   **Encounter for sterilization**

✓5ᵗʰ **Z30.4**   **Encounter for surveillance of contraceptives**

**Z30.40**   **Encounter for surveillance of contraceptives, unspecified**

**Z30.41**   **Encounter for surveillance of** contraceptive pills   ♀
Encounter for repeat prescription for contraceptive pill

**Z30.42**   **Encounter for surveillance of** injectable contraceptive   ♀

✓6ᵗʰ **Z30.43**   **Encounter for surveillance of** intrauterine contraceptive device

**Z30.430**   **Encounter for** insertion of intrauterine contraceptive device   ♀

**Z30.431**   **Encounter for** routine checking of intrauterine contraceptive device   ♀

**Z30.432**   **Encounter for** removal of intrauterine contraceptive device   ♀

**Z30.433**   **Encounter for** removal and reinsertion of intrauterine contraceptive device   ♀
Encounter for replacement of intrauterine contraceptive device

**Z30.44**   **Encounter for surveillance of** vaginal ring hormonal contraceptive device   ♀

**Z30.45**   **Encounter for surveillance of** transdermal patch hormonal contraceptive device   ♀

**Z30.46**   **Encounter for surveillance of** implantable subdermal contraceptive   ♀
Encounter for checking, reinsertion or removal of implantable subdermal contraceptive

**Z30.49**   **Encounter for** surveillance of other contraceptives   ♀
Encounter for surveillance of barrier contraception
Encounter for surveillance of diaphragm

**Z30.8**   **Encounter for** other contraceptive management
Encounter for postvasectomy sperm count
Encounter for routine examination for contraceptive maintenance
EXCLUDES 1   *sperm count following sterilization reversal (Z31.42)*
*sperm count for fertility testing (Z31.41)*

**Z30.9**   **Encounter for contraceptive management, unspecified**

✓4ᵗʰ **Z31**   **Encounter for procreative management**
EXCLUDES 1   *complications associated with artificial fertilization (N98.-)*
*female infertility (N97.-)*
*male infertility (N46.-)*

**Z31.0**   **Encounter for reversal of previous sterilization**

✓5ᵗʰ **Z31.4**   **Encounter for** procreative investigation and testing
EXCLUDES 1   *postvasectomy sperm count (Z30.8)*

**Z31.41**   **Encounter for** fertility testing
Encounter for fallopian tube patency testing
Encounter for sperm count for fertility testing

**Z31.42**   **Aftercare following** sterilization reversal
Sperm count following sterilization reversal

✓6ᵗʰ **Z31.43**   **Encounter for genetic testing of** female for procreative management
Use additional code for recurrent pregnancy loss, if applicable (N96, O26.2-)
EXCLUDES 1   *nonprocreative genetic testing (Z13.7-)*

**Z31.430**   **Encounter of female for testing for genetic** disease carrier status for procreative management   ♀

**Z31.438**   **Encounter for** other genetic testing of female for procreative management   ♀

✓6ᵗʰ **Z31.44**   **Encounter for genetic testing of** male for procreative management
EXCLUDES 1   *nonprocreative genetic testing (Z13.7-)*

**Z31.440**   **Encounter of male for testing for genetic** disease carrier status for procreative management   ♂

**Z31.441**   **Encounter for testing of male partner** 🅰 ♂ of patient with recurrent pregnancy loss

**Z31.448**   **Encounter for** other genetic testing of 🅰 ♂ male for procreative management

**Z31.49**   **Encounter for** other procreative investigation and testing

▲   **Z31.5**   **Encounter for procreative genetic counseling**

✓5ᵗʰ **Z31.6**   **Encounter for general counseling and advice on procreation**

**Z31.61**   **Procreative counseling and advice using** natural family planning

**Z31.62**   **Encounter for** fertility preservation counseling
Encounter for fertility preservation counseling prior to cancer therapy
Encounter for fertility preservation counseling prior to surgical removal of gonads

**Z31.69**   **Encounter for** other general counseling and advice on procreation

**Z31.7**   **Encounter for procreative management and counseling for gestational carrier**
EXCLUDES 1   *pregnant state, gestational carrier (Z33.3)*

✓5ᵗʰ **Z31.8**   **Encounter for** other procreative management

**Z31.81**   **Encounter for** male factor infertility in female patient   ♀

**Z31.82**   **Encounter for** Rh incompatibility status   ♀
AHA: 2015, 3Q, 40; 2014, 4Q, 17

**Z31.83**   **Encounter for** assisted reproductive fertility procedure cycle   ♀
Patient undergoing in vitro fertilization cycle
Use additional code to identify the type of infertility
EXCLUDES 1   *pre-cycle diagnosis and testing—code to reason for encounter*

**Z31.84**   **Encounter for** fertility preservation procedure
Encounter for fertility preservation procedure prior to cancer therapy
Encounter for fertility preservation procedure prior to surgical removal of gonads

**Z31.89**   **Encounter for** other procreative management

**Z31.9**   **Encounter for procreative management, unspecified**

---

🅽 Newborn: 0   🅿 Pediatric: 0-17   🅼 Maternity: 12-55   🅰 Adult: 15-124   **MCC** Major CC Condition   **PDxMCC** PDx acts as own MCC   **CC** CC Condition   **PDxCC** PDx acts as own CC

**1228**      ICD-10-CM 2018

✅4ᵗʰ **Z32** **Encounter for pregnancy test and childbirth and childcare instruction**

  ✅5ᵗʰ **Z32.0** **Encounter for pregnancy test**

    **Z32.00** **Encounter for pregnancy test, result unknown** ♀
      Encounter for pregnancy test NOS

    **Z32.01** **Encounter for pregnancy test, result positive** Ⓜ♀

    **Z32.02** **Encounter for pregnancy test, result negative** ♀

  **Z32.2** **Encounter for childbirth instruction**

  **Z32.3** **Encounter for childcare instruction**
    Encounter for prenatal or postpartum childcare instruction

✅4ᵗʰ **Z33** **Pregnant state**

  **Z33.1** **Pregnant state, incidental** Ⓜ♀
    Pregnant state NOS
    *EXCLUDES 1*   complications of pregnancy (O00–O9A)
          pregnant state, gestational carrier (Z33.3)

  **Z33.2** **Encounter for elective termination of pregnancy** Ⓜ♀
    *EXCLUDES 1*   early fetal death with retention of dead fetus (O02.1)
          late fetal death (O36.4)
          spontaneous abortion (O03)

  **Z33.3** **Pregnant state, gestational carrier** Ⓜ♀
    *EXCLUDES 1*   encounter for procreative management and
          counseling for gestational carrier (Z31.7)

✅4ᵗʰ **Z34** **Encounter for supervision of normal pregnancy**
  *EXCLUDES 1*   any complication of pregnancy (O00–O9A)
        encounter for pregnancy test (Z32.0-)
        encounter for supervision of high risk pregnancy (O09.-)
  AHA: 2014, 4Q, 17

  ✅5ᵗʰ **Z34.0** **Encounter for supervision of normal first pregnancy**

    **Z34.00** **Encounter for supervision of normal first pregnancy, unspecified trimester** Ⓜ♀

    **Z34.01** **Encounter for supervision of normal first pregnancy, first trimester** Ⓜ♀

    **Z34.02** **Encounter for supervision of normal first pregnancy, second trimester** Ⓜ♀

    **Z34.03** **Encounter for supervision of normal first pregnancy, third trimester** Ⓜ♀

  ✅5ᵗʰ **Z34.8** **Encounter for supervision of other normal pregnancy**

    **Z34.80** **Encounter for supervision of other normal pregnancy, unspecified trimester** Ⓜ♀

    **Z34.81** **Encounter for supervision of other normal pregnancy, first trimester** Ⓜ♀

    **Z34.82** **Encounter for supervision of other normal pregnancy, second trimester** Ⓜ♀

    **Z34.83** **Encounter for supervision of other normal pregnancy, third trimester** Ⓜ♀

  ✅5ᵗʰ **Z34.9** **Encounter for supervision of normal pregnancy, unspecified**

    **Z34.90** **Encounter for supervision of normal pregnancy, unspecified, unspecified trimester** Ⓜ♀

    **Z34.91** **Encounter for supervision of normal pregnancy, unspecified, first trimester** Ⓜ♀

    **Z34.92** **Encounter for supervision of normal pregnancy, unspecified, second trimester** Ⓜ♀

    **Z34.93** **Encounter for supervision of normal pregnancy, unspecified, third trimester** Ⓜ♀

✅4ᵗʰ **Z36** **Encounter for antenatal screening of mother**
  *INCLUDES* ▶encounter for placental sample (taken vaginally)
    screening is the testing for disease or disease precursors in
    asymptomatic individuals so that early detection and
    treatment can be provided for those who test positive
    for the disease◀
  *EXCLUDES 1* ~~abnormal findings on antenatal screening of mother (O28.-)~~
    diagnostic examination—code to sign or symptom
    encounter for suspected maternal and fetal conditions ruled out
    (Z03.7-)
    suspected fetal condition affecting management of
    pregnancy—code to condition in Chapter 15
  *EXCLUDES 2* ▶abnormal findings on antenatal screening of mother (O28.-)◀
    genetic counseling and testing (Z31.43-, Z31.5)
    routine prenatal care (Z34)

●   **Z36.0** **Encounter for antenatal screening for chromosomal anomalies**

●   **Z36.1** **Encounter for antenatal screening for raised alphafetoprotein level**
    Encounter for antenatal screening for elevated maternal serum
    alphafetoprotein level

●   **Z36.2** **Encounter for other antenatal screening follow-up**
    Non-visualized anatomy on a previous scan

●   **Z36.3** **Encounter for antenatal screening for malformations**
    Screening for a suspected anomaly

●   **Z36.4** **Encounter for antenatal screening for fetal growth retardation**
    Intrauterine growth restriction (IUGR)/small-for-dates

●   **Z36.5** **Encounter for antenatal screening for isoimmunization**

● ✅5ᵗʰ **Z36.8** **Encounter for other antenatal screening**

    **Z36.81** **Encounter for antenatal screening for hydrops fetalis**

    **Z36.82** **Encounter for antenatal screening for nuchal translucency**

    **Z36.83** **Encounter for fetal screening for congenital cardiac abnormalities**

    **Z36.84** **Encounter for antenatal screening for fetal lung maturity**

    **Z36.85** **Encounter for antenatal screening for Streptococcus B**

    **Z36.86** **Encounter for antenatal screening for cervical length**
      Screening for risk of pre-term labor

    **Z36.87** **Encounter for antenatal screening for uncertain dates**

    **Z36.88** **Encounter for antenatal screening for fetal macrosomia**
      Screening for large-for-dates

    **Z36.89** **Encounter for other specified antenatal screening**

    **Z36.8A** **Encounter for antenatal screening for other genetic defects**

●   **Z36.9** **Encounter for antenatal screening, unspecified**

✅4ᵗʰ **Z3A** **Weeks of gestation**
  *NOTE*   Codes from category Z3A are for use, only on the maternal
    record, to indicate the weeks of gestation of the pregnancy, if
    known.
  Code first complications of pregnancy, childbirth and the puerperium
    ▶(O09-O9A)◀
  AHA: 2016, 2Q, 34; 2014, 3Q, 17; 2014, 2Q, 9; 2013, 2Q, 33

  ✅5ᵗʰ **Z3A.0** **Weeks of gestation of pregnancy, unspecified or less than 10 weeks**

    **Z3A.00** **Weeks of gestation of pregnancy not specified** Ⓜ♀
    **Z3A.01** **Less than 8 weeks gestation of pregnancy** Ⓜ♀
    **Z3A.08** **8 weeks gestation of pregnancy** Ⓜ♀
    **Z3A.09** **9 weeks gestation of pregnancy** Ⓜ♀

  ✅5ᵗʰ **Z3A.1** **Weeks of gestation of pregnancy, weeks 10-19**

    **Z3A.10** **10 weeks gestation of pregnancy** Ⓜ♀
    **Z3A.11** **11 weeks gestation of pregnancy** Ⓜ♀
    **Z3A.12** **12 weeks gestation of pregnancy** Ⓜ♀
    **Z3A.13** **13 weeks gestation of pregnancy** Ⓜ♀
    **Z3A.14** **14 weeks gestation of pregnancy** Ⓜ♀
    **Z3A.15** **15 weeks gestation of pregnancy** Ⓜ♀
    **Z3A.16** **16 weeks gestation of pregnancy** Ⓜ♀
    **Z3A.17** **17 weeks gestation of pregnancy** Ⓜ♀
    **Z3A.18** **18 weeks gestation of pregnancy** Ⓜ♀
    **Z3A.19** **19 weeks gestation of pregnancy** Ⓜ♀

  ✅5ᵗʰ **Z3A.2** **Weeks of gestation of pregnancy, weeks 20-29**

    **Z3A.20** **20 weeks gestation of pregnancy** Ⓜ♀
    **Z3A.21** **21 weeks gestation of pregnancy** Ⓜ♀
    **Z3A.22** **22 weeks gestation of pregnancy** Ⓜ♀
    **Z3A.23** **23 weeks gestation of pregnancy** Ⓜ♀
    **Z3A.24** **24 weeks gestation of pregnancy** Ⓜ♀
    **Z3A.25** **25 weeks gestation of pregnancy** Ⓜ♀
    **Z3A.26** **26 weeks gestation of pregnancy** Ⓜ♀
    **Z3A.27** **27 weeks gestation of pregnancy** Ⓜ♀
    **Z3A.28** **28 weeks gestation of pregnancy** Ⓜ♀
    **Z3A.29** **29 weeks gestation of pregnancy** Ⓜ♀

  ✅5ᵗʰ **Z3A.3** **Weeks of gestation of pregnancy, weeks 30-39**

    **Z3A.30** **30 weeks gestation of pregnancy** Ⓜ♀
    **Z3A.31** **31 weeks gestation of pregnancy** Ⓜ♀
    **Z3A.32** **32 weeks gestation of pregnancy** Ⓜ♀
    **Z3A.33** **33 weeks gestation of pregnancy** Ⓜ♀
    **Z3A.34** **34 weeks gestation of pregnancy** Ⓜ♀
    **Z3A.35** **35 weeks gestation of pregnancy** Ⓜ♀
    **Z3A.36** **36 weeks gestation of pregnancy** Ⓜ♀
    **Z3A.37** **37 weeks gestation of pregnancy** Ⓜ♀

✅ Additional Character Req   ✅x7ᵗʰ Placeholder Alert   Unacceptable PDx   Manifestation   H1 - H14 HAC   HCC CMS-HCC Condition   *EXCLUDES 1* Not Coded Here   *EXCLUDES 2* Not Included Here

ICD-10-CM 2018      1229

    Z3A.38   **38 weeks** gestation of pregnancy   Ⓜ♀

    Z3A.39   **39 weeks** gestation of pregnancy   Ⓜ♀

✓5ᵗʰ **Z3A.4**   **Weeks of gestation of pregnancy, weeks 4Ø or greater**
       AHA: 2014, 4Q, 23

    Z3A.4Ø   **4Ø weeks** gestation of pregnancy   Ⓜ♀

    Z3A.41   **41 weeks** gestation of pregnancy   Ⓜ♀

    Z3A.42   **42 weeks** gestation of pregnancy   Ⓜ♀

    Z3A.49   **Greater than 42 weeks** gestation of pregnancy   Ⓜ♀

✓4ᵗʰ **Z37**   **Outcome of delivery**
    This category is intended for use as an additional code to identify the outcome of delivery on the mother's record. It is not for use on the newborn record.
    *EXCLUDES 1*   *stillbirth (P95)*

    **Z37.Ø**   **Single live birth**   Ⓜ♀
       AHA: 2016, 2Q, 34; 2014, 2Q, 9

    **Z37.1**   **Single stillbirth**   Ⓜ♀

    **Z37.2**   **Twins, both liveborn**   Ⓜ♀

    **Z37.3**   **Twins, one liveborn and one stillborn**   Ⓜ♀

    **Z37.4**   **Twins, both stillborn**   Ⓜ♀

✓5ᵗʰ   **Z37.5**   **Other multiple births, all liveborn**

    **Z37.5Ø**   **Multiple births, unspecified, all liveborn**   Ⓜ♀

    **Z37.51**   **Triplets, all liveborn**   Ⓜ♀

    **Z37.52**   **Quadruplets, all liveborn**   Ⓜ♀

    **Z37.53**   **Quintuplets, all liveborn**   Ⓜ♀

    **Z37.54**   **Sextuplets, all liveborn**   Ⓜ♀

    **Z37.59**   **Other multiple births, all liveborn**   Ⓜ♀

✓5ᵗʰ   **Z37.6**   **Other multiple births, some liveborn**

    **Z37.6Ø**   **Multiple births, unspecified, some liveborn**   Ⓜ♀

    **Z37.61**   **Triplets, some liveborn**   Ⓜ♀

    **Z37.62**   **Quadruplets, some liveborn**   Ⓜ♀

    **Z37.63**   **Quintuplets, some liveborn**   Ⓜ♀

    **Z37.64**   **Sextuplets, some liveborn**   Ⓜ♀

    **Z37.69**   **Other multiple births, some liveborn**   Ⓜ♀

    **Z37.7**   **Other multiple births, all stillborn**   Ⓜ♀

    **Z37.9**   **Outcome of delivery, unspecified**   Ⓜ♀
       Multiple birth NOS
       Single birth NOS

✓4ᵗʰ **Z38**   **Liveborn infants according to place of birth and type of delivery**
    This category is for use as the principal code on the initial record of a newborn baby. It is to be used for the initial birth record only. It is not to be used on the mother's record.
    AHA: 2017, 2Q, 5-7; 2016, 3Q, 18; 2015, 2Q, 15

✓5ᵗʰ   **Z38.Ø**   **Single liveborn infant, born in hospital**
       Single liveborn infant, born in birthing center or other health care facility

    **Z38.ØØ**   **Single liveborn infant, delivered vaginally**   Ⓝ

    **Z38.Ø1**   **Single liveborn infant, delivered by cesarean**   Ⓝ

    **Z38.1**   **Single liveborn infant, born outside hospital**   Ⓝ

    **Z38.2**   **Single liveborn infant, unspecified as to place of birth**   Ⓝ
       Single liveborn infant NOS

✓5ᵗʰ   **Z38.3**   **Twin liveborn infant, born in hospital**

    **Z38.3Ø**   **Twin liveborn infant, delivered vaginally**   Ⓝ

    **Z38.31**   **Twin liveborn infant, delivered by cesarean**   Ⓝ

    **Z38.4**   **Twin liveborn infant, born outside hospital**   Ⓝ

    **Z38.5**   **Twin liveborn infant, unspecified as to place of birth**   Ⓝ

✓5ᵗʰ   **Z38.6**   **Other multiple liveborn infant, born in hospital**

    **Z38.61**   **Triplet liveborn infant, delivered vaginally**   Ⓝ

    **Z38.62**   **Triplet liveborn infant, delivered by cesarean**   Ⓝ

    **Z38.63**   **Quadruplet liveborn infant, delivered vaginally**   Ⓝ

    **Z38.64**   **Quadruplet liveborn infant, delivered by cesarean**   Ⓝ

    **Z38.65**   **Quintuplet liveborn infant, delivered vaginally**   Ⓝ

    **Z38.66**   **Quintuplet liveborn infant, delivered by cesarean**   Ⓝ

    **Z38.68**   **Other multiple liveborn infant, delivered vaginally**   Ⓝ

    **Z38.69**   **Other multiple liveborn infant, delivered by cesarean**   Ⓝ

    **Z38.7**   **Other multiple liveborn infant, born outside hospital**   Ⓝ

    **Z38.8**   **Other multiple liveborn infant, unspecified as to place of birth**   Ⓝ

✓4ᵗʰ **Z39**   **Encounter for maternal postpartum care and examination**

    **Z39.Ø**   **Encounter for care and examination of mother immediately after delivery**   Ⓜ♀
       Care and observation in uncomplicated cases when the delivery occurs outside a healthcare facility
       *EXCLUDES 1*   *care for postpartum complication—see Alphabetic index*

    **Z39.1**   **Encounter for care and examination of lactating mother**   Ⓜ♀
       Encounter for supervision of lactation
       *EXCLUDES 1*   *disorders of lactation (O92.-)*

    **Z39.2**   **Encounter for routine postpartum follow-up**   Ⓜ♀

### Encounters for other specific health care (Z4Ø-Z53)

Categories Z4Ø-Z53 are intended for use to indicate a reason for care. They may be used for patients who have already been treated for a disease or injury, but who are receiving aftercare or prophylactic care, or care to consolidate the treatment, or to deal with a residual state.

*EXCLUDES 2*   *follow-up examination for medical surveillance after treatment (ZØ8-ZØ9)*

✓4ᵗʰ **Z4Ø**   **Encounter for prophylactic surgery**
    *EXCLUDES 1*   *organ donations (Z52.-)*
       *therapeutic organ removal—code to condition*

✓5ᵗʰ   **Z4Ø.Ø**   **Encounter for prophylactic surgery for risk factors related to malignant neoplasms**
       Admission for prophylactic organ removal
       Use additional code to identify risk factor

    **Z4Ø.ØØ**   **Encounter for prophylactic removal of unspecified organ**

    **Z4Ø.Ø1**   **Encounter for prophylactic removal of breast**

▲     **Z4Ø.Ø2**   **Encounter for prophylactic removal of ovary(s)**   ♀
       ▶Encounter for prophylactic removal of ovary(s) and fallopian tube(s)◀

●     **Z4Ø.Ø3**   **Encounter for prophylactic removal of fallopian tube(s)**   ♀

    **Z4Ø.Ø9**   **Encounter for prophylactic removal of other organ**

    **Z4Ø.8**   **Encounter for other prophylactic surgery**

    **Z4Ø.9**   **Encounter for prophylactic surgery, unspecified**

✓4ᵗʰ **Z41**   **Encounter for procedures for purposes other than remedying health state**

    **Z41.1**   **Encounter for cosmetic surgery**
       Encounter for cosmetic breast implant
       Encounter for cosmetic procedure
       *EXCLUDES 1*   *encounter for plastic and reconstructive surgery following medical procedure or healed injury (Z42.-)*
       *encounter for post-mastectomy breast implantation (Z42.1)*

    **Z41.2**   **Encounter for routine and ritual male circumcision**   ♂

    **Z41.3**   **Encounter for ear piercing**

    **Z41.8**   **Encounter for other procedures for purposes other than remedying health state**

    **Z41.9**   **Encounter for procedure for purposes other than remedying health state, unspecified**

✓4ᵗʰ **Z42**   **Encounter for plastic and reconstructive surgery following medical procedure or healed injury**
    *EXCLUDES 1*   *encounter for cosmetic plastic surgery (Z41.1)*
       *encounter for plastic surgery for treatment of current injury—code to relevant injury*

    **Z42.1**   **Encounter for breast reconstruction following mastectomy**   Ⓐ
       *EXCLUDES 1*   *deformity and disproportion of reconstructed breast (N65.1-)*

    **Z42.8**   **Encounter for other plastic and reconstructive surgery following medical procedure or healed injury**
       AHA: 2017, 1Q, 42

✓4ᵗʰ **Z43**   **Encounter for attention to artificial openings**
    **INCLUDES**   closure of artificial openings
       passage of sounds or bougies through artificial openings
       reforming artificial openings
       removal of catheter from artificial openings
       toilet or cleansing of artificial openings
    *EXCLUDES 1*   *artificial opening status only, without need for care (Z93.-)*
       *complications of external stoma (J95.Ø-, K94.-, N99.5-)*
    *EXCLUDES 2*   *fitting and adjustment of prosthetic and other devices (Z44-Z46)*

    **Z43.Ø**   **Encounter for attention to tracheostomy**   HCC

Ⓝ Newborn: 0   Ⓟ Pediatric: 0-17   Ⓜ Maternity: 12-55   Ⓐ Adult: 15-124   **MCC** Major CC Condition   **PDxMCC** PDx acts as own MCC   **CC** CC Condition   **PDxCC** PDx acts as own CC

1230              ICD-10-CM 2018

**Z43.1** Encounter for attention to gastrostomy `CC` `HCC`
  EXCLUDES 2 ▶artificial opening status only, without need for care (Z93.-)◄
  **CC Excl:** PDX collection 1487

**Z43.2** Encounter for attention to ileostomy `HCC`

**Z43.3** Encounter for attention to colostomy `HCC`

**Z43.4** Encounter for attention to other artificial openings of digestive tract `HCC`

**Z43.5** Encounter for attention to cystostomy `HCC`

**Z43.6** Encounter for attention to other artificial openings of urinary tract `HCC`
  Encounter for attention to nephrostomy
  Encounter for attention to ureterostomy
  Encounter for attention to urethrostomy

**Z43.7** Encounter for attention to artificial vagina

**Z43.8** Encounter for attention to other artificial openings `HCC`

**Z43.9** Encounter for attention to unspecified artificial opening `HCC`

✓4th **Z44** Encounter for fitting and adjustment of external prosthetic device
  INCLUDES   removal or replacement of external prosthetic device
  EXCLUDES 1 malfunction or other complications of device—see Alphabetical Index
    presence of prosthetic device (Z97.-)

✓5th **Z44.0** Encounter for fitting and adjustment of artificial arm

  ✓6th **Z44.00** Encounter for fitting and adjustment of unspecified artificial arm

    **Z44.001** Encounter for fitting and adjustment of unspecified right artificial arm

    **Z44.002** Encounter for fitting and adjustment of unspecified left artificial arm

    **Z44.009** Encounter for fitting and adjustment of unspecified artificial arm, unspecified arm

  ✓6th **Z44.01** Encounter for fitting and adjustment of complete artificial arm

    **Z44.011** Encounter for fitting and adjustment of complete right artificial arm

    **Z44.012** Encounter for fitting and adjustment of complete left artificial arm

    **Z44.019** Encounter for fitting and adjustment of complete artificial arm, unspecified arm

  ✓6th **Z44.02** Encounter for fitting and adjustment of partial artificial arm

    **Z44.021** Encounter for fitting and adjustment of partial artificial right arm

    **Z44.022** Encounter for fitting and adjustment of partial artificial left arm

    **Z44.029** Encounter for fitting and adjustment of partial artificial arm, unspecified arm

✓5th **Z44.1** Encounter for fitting and adjustment of artificial leg

  ✓6th **Z44.10** Encounter for fitting and adjustment of unspecified artificial leg

    **Z44.101** Encounter for fitting and adjustment of unspecified right artificial leg `HCC`

    **Z44.102** Encounter for fitting and adjustment of unspecified left artificial leg `HCC`

    **Z44.109** Encounter for fitting and adjustment of unspecified artificial leg, unspecified leg `HCC`

  ✓6th **Z44.11** Encounter for fitting and adjustment of complete artificial leg

    **Z44.111** Encounter for fitting and adjustment of complete right artificial leg `HCC`

    **Z44.112** Encounter for fitting and adjustment of complete left artificial leg `HCC`

    **Z44.119** Encounter for fitting and adjustment of complete artificial leg, unspecified leg `HCC`

  ✓6th **Z44.12** Encounter for fitting and adjustment of partial artificial leg

    **Z44.121** Encounter for fitting and adjustment of partial artificial right leg `HCC`

    **Z44.122** Encounter for fitting and adjustment of partial artificial left leg `HCC`

    **Z44.129** Encounter for fitting and adjustment of partial artificial leg, unspecified leg `HCC`

✓5th **Z44.2** Encounter for fitting and adjustment of artificial eye
  EXCLUDES 1 mechanical complication of ocular prosthesis (T85.3)

  **Z44.20** Encounter for fitting and adjustment of artificial eye, unspecified

  **Z44.21** Encounter for fitting and adjustment of artificial right eye

  **Z44.22** Encounter for fitting and adjustment of artificial left eye

✓5th **Z44.3** Encounter for fitting and adjustment of external breast prosthesis
  EXCLUDES 1 complications of breast implant (T85.4-)
    encounter for adjustment or removal of breast implant (Z45.81-)
    encounter for initial breast implant insertion for cosmetic breast augmentation (Z41.1)
    encounter for breast reconstruction following mastectomy (Z42.1)

  **Z44.30** Encounter for fitting and adjustment of external breast prosthesis, unspecified breast

  **Z44.31** Encounter for fitting and adjustment of external right breast prosthesis

  **Z44.32** Encounter for fitting and adjustment of external left breast prosthesis

  **Z44.8** Encounter for fitting and adjustment of other external prosthetic devices

  **Z44.9** Encounter for fitting and adjustment of unspecified external prosthetic device

✓4th **Z45** Encounter for adjustment and management of implanted device
  INCLUDES   removal or replacement of implanted device
  EXCLUDES 1 malfunction or other complications of device – see Alphabetical Index
    presence of prosthetic and other devices (Z95-Z97)
  EXCLUDES 2 encounter for fitting and adjustment of non-implanted device (Z46.-)

✓5th **Z45.0** Encounter for adjustment and management of cardiac device

  ✓6th **Z45.01** Encounter for adjustment and management of cardiac pacemaker
    Encounter for adjustment and management of cardiac resynchronization therapy pacemaker (CRT-P)
    EXCLUDES 1 encounter for adjustment and management of automatic implantable cardiac defibrillator with synchronous cardiac pacemaker (Z45.02)

    4 **Z45.010** Encounter for checking and testing of cardiac pacemaker pulse generator [battery]
      Encounter for replacing cardiac pacemaker pulse generator [battery]

    4 **Z45.018** Encounter for adjustment and management of other part of cardiac pacemaker
      EXCLUDES 2 ▶presence of prosthetic and other devices (Z95-Z97)◄

  4 **Z45.02** Encounter for adjustment and management of automatic implantable cardiac defibrillator
    Encounter for adjustment and management of automatic implantable cardiac defibrillator with synchronous cardiac pacemaker
    Encounter for adjustment and management of cardiac resynchronization therapy defibrillator (CRT-D)

  4 **Z45.09** Encounter for adjustment and management of other cardiac device

  **Z45.1** Encounter for adjustment and management of infusion pump

  **Z45.2** Encounter for adjustment and management of vascular access device
    Encounter for adjustment and management of vascular catheters
    EXCLUDES 1 encounter for adjustment and management of renal dialysis catheter (Z49.01)

✓5th **Z45.3** Encounter for adjustment and management of implanted devices of the special senses

  **Z45.31** Encounter for adjustment and management of implanted visual substitution device

---

⁴ Questionable admission when used as PDx.

☑6ᵗʰ **Z45.32** **Encounter for adjustment and management of implanted hearing device**

> EXCLUDES 1 *encounter for fitting and adjustment of hearing aide (Z46.1)*

**Z45.320** **Encounter for adjustment and management of bone conduction device**

**Z45.321** **Encounter for adjustment and management of cochlear device**

**Z45.328** **Encounter for adjustment and management of other implanted hearing device**

☑5ᵗʰ **Z45.4** **Encounter for adjustment and management of implanted nervous system device**

**Z45.41** **Encounter for adjustment and management of cerebrospinal fluid drainage device**

> Encounter for adjustment and management of cerebral ventricular (communicating) shunt

**Z45.42** **Encounter for adjustment and management of neuropacemaker (brain) (peripheral nerve) (spinal cord)**

**Z45.49** **Encounter for adjustment and management of other implanted nervous system device**

> AHA: 2014, 3Q, 19

☑5ᵗʰ **Z45.8** **Encounter for adjustment and management of other implanted devices**

☑6ᵗʰ **Z45.81** **Encounter for adjustment or removal of breast implant**

> Encounter for elective implant exchange (different material) (different size)
> Encounter removal of tissue expander without synchronous insertion of permanent implant
>
> EXCLUDES 1 *complications of breast implant (T85.4-)*
> *encounter for initial breast implant insertion for cosmetic breast augmentation (Z41.1)*
> *encounter for breast reconstruction following mastectomy (Z42.1)*

**Z45.811** **Encounter for adjustment or removal of right breast implant**

**Z45.812** **Encounter for adjustment or removal of left breast implant**

**Z45.819** **Encounter for adjustment or removal of unspecified breast implant**

**Z45.82** **Encounter for adjustment or removal of myringotomy device (stent) (tube)**

**Z45.89** **Encounter for adjustment and management of other implanted devices**

> AHA: 2014, 4Q, 26-28

**Z45.9** **Encounter for adjustment and management of unspecified implanted device**

☑4ᵗʰ **Z46** **Encounter for fitting and adjustment of other devices**

> INCLUDES removal or replacement of other device
>
> EXCLUDES 1 *malfunction or other complications of device—see Alphabetical Index*
>
> EXCLUDES 2 *encounter for fitting and management of implanted devices (Z45.-)*
> *issue of repeat prescription only (Z76.0)*
> *presence of prosthetic and other devices (Z95-Z97)*

**Z46.0** **Encounter for fitting and adjustment of spectacles and contact lenses**

**Z46.1** **Encounter for fitting and adjustment of hearing aid**

> EXCLUDES 1 *encounter for adjustment and management of implanted hearing device (Z45.32-)*

**Z46.2** **Encounter for fitting and adjustment of other devices related to nervous system and special senses**

> EXCLUDES 2 *encounter for adjustment and management of implanted nervous system device (Z45.4-)*
> *encounter for adjustment and management of implanted visual substitution device (Z45.31)*

**Z46.3** **Encounter for fitting and adjustment of dental prosthetic device**

> Encounter for fitting and adjustment of dentures

**Z46.4** **Encounter for fitting and adjustment of orthodontic device**

☑5ᵗʰ **Z46.5** **Encounter for fitting and adjustment of other gastrointestinal appliance and device**

> EXCLUDES 1 *encounter for attention to artificial openings of digestive tract (Z43.1-Z43.4)*

**Z46.51** **Encounter for fitting and adjustment of gastric lap band**

**Z46.59** **Encounter for fitting and adjustment of other gastrointestinal appliance and device**

**Z46.6** **Encounter for fitting and adjustment of urinary device**

> EXCLUDES 2 *attention to artificial openings of urinary tract (Z43.5, Z43.6)*

☑5ᵗʰ **Z46.8** **Encounter for fitting and adjustment of other specified devices**

**Z46.81** **Encounter for fitting and adjustment of insulin pump**

> Encounter for insulin pump instruction and training
> Encounter for insulin pump titration

**Z46.82** **Encounter for fitting and adjustment of non-vascular catheter**

**Z46.89** **Encounter for fitting and adjustment of other specified devices**

> Encounter for fitting and adjustment of wheelchair
> AHA: 2014, 4Q, 26-28

**Z46.9** **Encounter for fitting and adjustment of unspecified device**

☑4ᵗʰ **Z47** **Orthopedic aftercare**

> EXCLUDES 1 *aftercare for healing fracture—code to fracture with 7th character D*

**Z47.1** **Aftercare following joint replacement surgery**

> Use additional code to identify the joint (Z96.6-)

**Z47.2** **Encounter for removal of internal fixation device**

> EXCLUDES 1 *encounter for adjustment of internal fixation device for fracture treatment—code to fracture with appropriate 7th character*
> *encounter for removal of external fixation device—code to fracture with 7th character D*
> *infection or inflammatory reaction to internal fixation device (T84.6-)*
> *mechanical complication of internal fixation device (T84.1-)*

☑5ᵗʰ **Z47.3** **Aftercare following explantation of joint prosthesis**

> Aftercare following explantation of joint prosthesis, staged procedure
> Encounter for joint prosthesis insertion following prior explantation of joint prosthesis
> AHA: 2015, 1Q, 16

**Z47.31** **Aftercare following explantation of shoulder joint prosthesis**

> EXCLUDES 1 *acquired absence of shoulder joint following prior explantation of shoulder joint prosthesis (Z89.23-)*
> *shoulder joint prosthesis explantation status (Z89.23-)*

**Z47.32** **Aftercare following explantation of hip joint prosthesis**

> EXCLUDES 1 *acquired absence of hip joint following prior explantation of hip joint prosthesis (Z89.62-)*
> *hip joint prosthesis explantation status (Z89.62-)*

**Z47.33** **Aftercare following explantation of knee joint prosthesis**

> EXCLUDES 1 *acquired absence of knee joint following prior explantation of knee prosthesis (Z89.52-)*
> *knee joint prosthesis explantation status (Z89.52-)*

☑5ᵗʰ **Z47.8** **Encounter for other orthopedic aftercare**

**Z47.81** **Encounter for orthopedic aftercare following surgical amputation**

> Use additional code to identify the limb amputated (Z89.-)

**Z47.82** **Encounter for orthopedic aftercare following scoliosis surgery**

**Z47.89** **Encounter for other orthopedic aftercare**

> AHA: 2015, 1Q, 8

---

✓4th **Z48 Encounter for other postprocedural aftercare**

> *EXCLUDES 1* ▶encounter for aftercare following injury – code to Injury, by site, with appropriate 7th character for subsequent encounter◀
> encounter for follow-up examination after completed treatment (Z08-Z09)
>
> *EXCLUDES 2* encounter for attention to artificial openings (Z43.-)
> encounter for fitting and adjustment of prosthetic and other devices (Z44-Z46)
>
> **AHA:** 2015, 4Q, 38; 2015, 1Q, 6-7

✓5th **Z48.0 Encounter for attention to dressings, sutures and drains**

> *EXCLUDES 1* encounter for planned postprocedural wound closure (Z48.1)

     **Z48.00 Encounter for change or removal of nonsurgical wound dressing**
         Encounter for change or removal of wound dressing NOS

     **Z48.01 Encounter for change or removal of surgical wound dressing**

     **Z48.02 Encounter for removal of sutures**
         Encounter for removal of staples

     **Z48.03 Encounter for change or removal of drains**

**Z48.1 Encounter for planned postprocedural wound closure**

> *EXCLUDES 1* encounter for attention to dressings and sutures (Z48.0-)

✓5th **Z48.2 Encounter for aftercare following organ transplant**

     **Z48.21 Encounter for aftercare following heart transplant** `PDxCC` `CC` `HCC`
         **CC Excl:** PDX collection 1488

     **Z48.22 Encounter for aftercare following kidney transplant** `PDxCC` `CC`
         **CC Excl:** PDX collection 1489

     **Z48.23 Encounter for aftercare following liver transplant** `PDxCC` `CC` `HCC`
         **CC Excl:** PDX collection 1490

     **Z48.24 Encounter for aftercare following lung transplant** `PDxCC` `CC` `HCC`
         **CC Excl:** PDX collection 1491

✓6th **Z48.28 Encounter for aftercare following multiple organ transplant**

     **Z48.280 Encounter for aftercare following heart-lung transplant** `PDxCC` `CC` `HCC`
         **CC Excl:** PDX collection 1488

     **Z48.288 Encounter for aftercare following multiple organ transplant**

✓6th **Z48.29 Encounter for aftercare following other organ transplant**

     **Z48.290 Encounter for aftercare following bone marrow transplant** `PDxCC` `CC` `HCC`
         **CC Excl:** PDX collection 1492

     **Z48.298 Encounter for aftercare following other organ transplant**

**Z48.3 Aftercare following surgery for neoplasm**
     Use additional code to identify the neoplasm

✓5th **Z48.8 Encounter for other specified postprocedural aftercare**

✓6th **Z48.81 Encounter for surgical aftercare following surgery on specified body systems**

> **NOTE** These codes identify the body system requiring aftercare. They are for use in conjunction with other aftercare codes to fully explain the aftercare encounter. The condition treated should also be coded if still present.
>
> *EXCLUDES 1* aftercare for injury—code the injury with 7th character D
> aftercare following surgery for neoplasm (Z48.3)
>
> *EXCLUDES 2* aftercare following organ transplant (Z48.2-)
> orthopedic aftercare (Z47.-)
>
> **AHA:** 2015, 4Q, 38

     **Z48.810 Encounter for surgical aftercare following surgery on the sense organs**

     **Z48.811 Encounter for surgical aftercare following surgery on the nervous system**

> *EXCLUDES 2* encounter for surgical aftercare following surgery on the sense organs (Z48.810)

     **Z48.812 Encounter for surgical aftercare following surgery on the circulatory system**
         **AHA:** 2012, 4Q, 96

     **Z48.813 Encounter for surgical aftercare following surgery on the respiratory system**

     **Z48.814 Encounter for surgical aftercare following surgery on the teeth or oral cavity**

     **Z48.815 Encounter for surgical aftercare following surgery on the digestive system**

     **Z48.816 Encounter for surgical aftercare following surgery on the genitourinary system**

> *EXCLUDES 1* encounter for aftercare following sterilization reversal (Z31.42)

     **Z48.817 Encounter for surgical aftercare following surgery on the skin and subcutaneous tissue**

     **Z48.89 Encounter for other specified surgical aftercare**

✓4th **Z49 Encounter for care involving renal dialysis**

> Code also associated end stage renal disease (N18.6)

✓5th **Z49.0 Preparatory care for renal dialysis**
     Encounter for dialysis instruction and training

     **Z49.01 Encounter for fitting and adjustment of extracorporeal dialysis catheter** `HCC`
         Removal or replacement of renal dialysis catheter
         Toilet or cleansing of renal dialysis catheter

     **Z49.02 Encounter for fitting and adjustment of peritoneal dialysis catheter** `HCC`

✓5th **Z49.3 Encounter for adequacy testing for dialysis**

     **Z49.31 Encounter for adequacy testing for hemodialysis** `HCC`

     **Z49.32 Encounter for adequacy testing for peritoneal dialysis** `HCC`
         Encounter for peritoneal equilibration test

✓4th **Z51 Encounter for other aftercare and medical care**

> Code also condition requiring care
>
> *EXCLUDES 1* follow-up examination after treatment (Z08-Z09)

**Z51.0 Encounter for antineoplastic radiation therapy**

✓5th **Z51.1 Encounter for antineoplastic chemotherapy and immunotherapy**

> *EXCLUDES 2* encounter for chemotherapy and immunotherapy for nonneoplastic condition—code to condition

     **Z51.11 Encounter for antineoplastic chemotherapy**
         **AHA:** 2015, 3Q, 19

     **Z51.12 Encounter for antineoplastic immunotherapy**

**Z51.5 Encounter for palliative care**
     **AHA:** 2017, 1Q, 48

**Z51.6 Encounter for desensitization to allergens**

✓5th **Z51.8 Encounter for other specified aftercare**

> *EXCLUDES 1* holiday relief care (Z75.5)

     **Z51.81 Encounter for therapeutic drug level monitoring**
         Code also any long-term (current) drug therapy (Z79.-)

> *EXCLUDES 1* encounter for blood-drug test for administrative or medicolegal reasons (Z02.83)

         **DEF:** Drug monitoring: Measurement of the level of a specific drug in the body or measurement of a specific function to assess effectiveness of a drug.

     5 **Z51.89 Encounter for other specified aftercare**
         **AHA:** 2012, 4Q, 95-97

✓4th **Z52 Donors of organs and tissues**

> **INCLUDES** autologous and other living donors
>
> *EXCLUDES 1* cadaveric donor—omit code
> examination of potential donor (Z00.5)
>
> **AHA:** 2012, 4Q, 99

✓5th **Z52.0 Blood donor**

✓6th **Z52.00 Unspecified blood donor**

     **Z52.000 Unspecified donor, whole blood**
     **Z52.001 Unspecified donor, stem cells**
     **Z52.008 Unspecified donor, other blood**

✓6th **Z52.01 Autologous blood donor**

     **Z52.010 Autologous donor, whole blood**
     **Z52.011 Autologous donor, stem cells**
     **Z52.018 Autologous donor, other blood**

✓6th **Z52.09 Other blood donor**
     Volunteer donor

     **Z52.090 Other blood donor, whole blood**
     **Z52.091 Other blood donor, stem cells**
     **Z52.098 Other blood donor, other blood**

---

5 Unacceptable PDx unless a secondary diagnosis is present.

✓ Additional Character Req   ✓x7th Placeholder Alert   Unacceptable PDx   Manifestation   **H1**-**H14** HAC   `HCC` CMS-HCC Condition   *EXCLUDES 1* Not Coded Here   *EXCLUDES 2* Not Included Here

**Z52.1**    Skin **donor**

     **Z52.10**    **Skin donor,** unspecified

     **Z52.11**    **Skin donor,** autologous

     **Z52.19**    **Skin donor,** other

**Z52.2**    Bone **donor**

     **Z52.20**    **Bone donor,** unspecified

     **Z52.21**    **Bone donor,** autologous

     **Z52.29**    **Bone donor,** other

**Z52.3**    Bone marrow **donor**

**Z52.4**    Kidney **donor**

**Z52.5**    Cornea **donor**

**Z52.6**    Liver **donor**

**Z52.8**    Donor of other specified organs or tissues

     **Z52.81**    Egg (Oocyte) **donor**

         **Z52.810**    **Egg (Oocyte) donor** under age 35, **anonymous** recipient ♀

             Egg donor under age 35 NOS

         **Z52.811**    **Egg (Oocyte) donor** under age 35, **designated** recipient ♀

         **Z52.812**    **Egg (Oocyte) donor** age 35 and over, **anonymous** recipient ♀

             Egg donor age 35 and over NOS

         **Z52.813**    **Egg (Oocyte) donor** age 35 and over, **designated** recipient ♀

         **Z52.819**    **Egg (Oocyte) donor,** unspecified ♀

     **Z52.89**    Donor of other specified organs or tissues

**Z52.9**    Donor of unspecified organ or tissue

     Donor NOS

**Z53**    **Persons encountering health services for specific procedures and treatment, not carried out**

**Z53.0**    **Procedure and treatment not carried out because of contraindication**

     **Z53.01**    **Procedure and treatment not carried out due to patient smoking**

     **Z53.09**    **Procedure and treatment not carried out because of other contraindication**

**Z53.1**    **Procedure and treatment not carried out because of patient's decision for reasons of belief and group pressure**

**Z53.2**    **Procedure and treatment not carried out because of patient's decision for other and unspecified reasons**

     **Z53.20**    **Procedure and treatment not carried out because of patient's decision for unspecified reasons**

     **Z53.21**    **Procedure and treatment not carried out due to patient leaving prior to being seen by health care provider**

     **Z53.29**    **Procedure and treatment not carried out because of patient's decision for other reasons**

**Z53.3**    **Procedure converted to open procedure**

     **Z53.31**    **Laparoscopic surgical procedure converted to open procedure**

     **Z53.32**    **Thoracoscopic surgical procedure converted to open procedure**

     **Z53.33**    **Arthroscopic surgical procedure converted to open procedure**

     **Z53.39**    **Other specified procedure converted to open procedure**

**Z53.8**    **Procedure and treatment not carried out for other reasons**

**Z53.9**    **Procedure and treatment not carried out, unspecified reason**

## Persons with potential health hazards related to socioeconomic and psychosocial circumstances (Z55-Z65)

**Z55**    **Problems related to education and literacy**

     EXCLUDES 1    disorders of psychological development (F80-F89)

**Z55.0**    **Illiteracy and low-level literacy**

**Z55.1**    **Schooling unavailable and unattainable**

**Z55.2**    **Failed school examinations**

**Z55.3**    **Underachievement in school**

**Z55.4**    **Educational maladjustment and discord with teachers and classmates**

**Z55.8**    **Other problems related to education and literacy**

     Problems related to inadequate teaching

**Z55.9**    **Problems related to education and literacy, unspecified**

     Academic problems NOS

**Z56**    **Problems related to employment and unemployment**

     EXCLUDES 2    occupational exposure to risk factors (Z57.-)

            problems related to housing and economic circumstances (Z59.-)

**Z56.0**    **Unemployment, unspecified**

**Z56.1**    **Change of job**    A

**Z56.2**    **Threat of job loss**

**Z56.3**    **Stressful work schedule**

**Z56.4**    **Discord with boss and workmates**

**Z56.5**    **Uncongenial work environment**

     Difficult conditions at work

**Z56.6**    **Other physical and mental strain related to work**

**Z56.8**    **Other problems related to employment**

     **Z56.81**    **Sexual harassment on the job**

     **Z56.82**    **Military deployment status**

         Individual (civilian or military) currently deployed in theater or in support of military war, peacekeeping and humanitarian operations

     **Z56.89**    **Other problems related to employment**

**Z56.9**    **Unspecified problems related to employment**

     Occupational problems NOS

**Z57**    **Occupational exposure to risk factors**

**Z57.0**    **Occupational exposure to noise**

**Z57.1**    **Occupational exposure to radiation**

**Z57.2**    **Occupational exposure to dust**

**Z57.3**    **Occupational exposure to other air contaminants**

     **Z57.31**    **Occupational exposure to environmental tobacco smoke**

         EXCLUDES 2    exposure to environmental tobacco smoke (Z77.22)

     **Z57.39**    **Occupational exposure to other air contaminants**

**Z57.4**    **Occupational exposure to toxic agents in agriculture**

     Occupational exposure to solids, liquids, gases or vapors in agriculture

**Z57.5**    **Occupational exposure to toxic agents in other industries**

     Occupational exposure to solids, liquids, gases or vapors in other industries

**Z57.6**    **Occupational exposure to extreme temperature**

**Z57.7**    **Occupational exposure to vibration**

**Z57.8**    **Occupational exposure to other risk factors**

**Z57.9**    **Occupational exposure to unspecified risk factor**

**Z59**    **Problems related to housing and economic circumstances**

     EXCLUDES 2    problems related to upbringing (Z62.-)

**Z59.0**    **Homelessness**

**Z59.1**    **Inadequate housing**

     Lack of heating

     Restriction of space

     Technical defects in home preventing adequate care

     Unsatisfactory surroundings

     EXCLUDES 1    problems related to the natural and physical environment (Z77.1-)

**Z59.2**    **Discord with neighbors, lodgers and landlord**

**Z59.3**    **Problems related to living in residential institution**

     Boarding-school resident

     EXCLUDES 1    institutional upbringing (Z62.2)

**Z59.4**    **Lack of adequate food and safe drinking water**

     Inadequate drinking water supply

     EXCLUDES 1    effects of hunger (T73.0)

            inappropriate diet or eating habits (Z72.4)

            malnutrition (E40-E46)

**Z59.5**    **Extreme poverty**

**Z59.6**    **Low income**

**Z59.7**    **Insufficient social insurance and welfare support**

**Z59.8**    **Other problems related to housing and economic circumstances**

     Foreclosure on loan      Problems with creditors

     Isolated dwelling

**Z59.9**    **Problem related to housing and economic circumstances, unspecified**

**Z60**    **Problems related to social environment**

**Z60.0**    **Problems of adjustment to life-cycle transitions**

     Empty nest syndrome      Problem with adjustment

     Phase of life problem      to retirement [pension]

**Z60.2**    **Problems related to living alone**

N Newborn: 0    P Pediatric: 0-17    M Maternity: 12-55    A Adult: 15-124    MCC Major CC Condition    PDxMCC PDx acts as own MCC    CC CC Condition    PDxCC PDx acts as own CC

1234      ICD-10-CM 2018

**Z60.3** **Acculturation difficulty**
Problem with migration
Problem with social transplantation
**DEF:** A problem in adapting to a different culture or environment not based on any coexisting mental disorder.

**Z60.4** **Social exclusion and rejection**
Exclusion and rejection on the basis of personal characteristics, such as unusual physical appearance, illness or behavior.
*EXCLUDES 1* *target of adverse discrimination such as for racial or religious reasons (Z60.5)*

**Z60.5** **Target of (perceived) adverse discrimination and persecution**
*EXCLUDES 1* *social exclusion and rejection (Z60.4)*

**Z60.8** **Other problems related to social environment**

**Z60.9** **Problem related to social environment, unspecified**

✓4th **Z62** **Problems related to upbringing**
*INCLUDES* current and past negative life events in childhood
current and past problems of a child related to upbringing
*EXCLUDES 2* *maltreatment syndrome (T74.-)*
*problems related to housing and economic circumstances (Z59.-)*

**Z62.0** **Inadequate parental supervision and control**

**Z62.1** **Parental overprotection**

✓5th **Z62.2** **Upbringing away from parents**
*EXCLUDES 1* *problems with boarding school (Z59.3)*

**Z62.21** **Child in welfare custody** ℗
Child in care of non-parental family member
Child in foster care
*EXCLUDES 2* *problem for parent due to child in welfare custody (Z63.5)*

**Z62.22** **Institutional upbringing**
Child living in orphanage or group home

**Z62.29** **Other upbringing away from parents**

**Z62.3** **Hostility towards and scapegoating of child** ℗

**Z62.6** **Inappropriate (excessive) parental pressure**

✓5th **Z62.8** **Other specified problems related to upbringing**

✓6th **Z62.81** **Personal history of abuse in childhood**

**Z62.810** **Personal history of physical and sexual abuse in childhood**
*EXCLUDES 1* *current child physical abuse (T74.12, T76.12)*
*current child sexual abuse (T74.22, T76.22)*

**Z62.811** **Personal history of psychological abuse in childhood**
*EXCLUDES 1* *current child psychological abuse (T74.32, T76.32)*

**Z62.812** **Personal history of neglect in childhood**
*EXCLUDES 1* *current child neglect (T74.02, T76.02)*

**Z62.819** **Personal history of unspecified abuse in childhood**
*EXCLUDES 1* *current child abuse NOS (T74.92, T76.92)*

✓6th **Z62.82** **Parent-child conflict**

**Z62.820** **Parent-biological child conflict**
Parent-child problem NOS

**Z62.821** **Parent-adopted child conflict**

**Z62.822** **Parent-foster child conflict**

✓6th **Z62.89** **Other specified problems related to upbringing**

**Z62.890** **Parent-child estrangement NEC**

**Z62.891** **Sibling rivalry**

**Z62.898** **Other specified problems related to upbringing**

**Z62.9** **Problem related to upbringing, unspecified**

✓4th **Z63** **Other problems related to primary support group, including family circumstances**
*EXCLUDES 2* *maltreatment syndrome (T74-, T76)*
*parent-child problems (Z62.-)*
*problems related to negative life events in childhood (Z62.-)*
*problems related to upbringing (Z62.-)*

**Z63.0** **Problems in relationship with spouse or partner**
▶Relationship distress with spouse or intimate partner◀
*EXCLUDES 1* *counseling for spousal or partner abuse problems (Z69.1)*
*counseling related to sexual attitude, behavior, and orientation (Z70.-)*

**Z63.1** **Problems in relationship with in-laws**

✓5th **Z63.3** **Absence of family member**
*EXCLUDES 1* *absence of family member due to disappearance and death (Z63.4)*
*absence of family member due to separation and divorce (Z63.5)*

**Z63.31** **Absence of family member due to military deployment**
Individual or family affected by other family member being on military deployment
*EXCLUDES 1* *family disruption due to return of family member from military deployment (Z63.71)*

**Z63.32** **Other absence of family member**

**Z63.4** **Disappearance and death of family member**
Assumed death of family member
Bereavement
**AHA:** 2014, 1Q, 25

**Z63.5** **Disruption of family by separation and divorce**
Marital estrangement

**Z63.6** **Dependent relative needing care at home**

✓5th **Z63.7** **Other stressful life events affecting family and household**

**Z63.71** **Stress on family due to return of family member from military deployment**
Individual or family affected by family member having returned from military deployment (current or past conflict)

**Z63.72** **Alcoholism and drug addiction in family**

**Z63.79** **Other stressful life events affecting family and household**
Anxiety (normal) about sick person in family
Health problems within family
Ill or disturbed family member
Isolated family

**Z63.8** **Other specified problems related to primary support group**
Family discord NOS
Family estrangement NOS
High expressed emotional level within family
Inadequate family support NOS
Inadequate or distorted communication within family

**Z63.9** **Problem related to primary support group, unspecified**
Relationship disorder NOS

✓4th **Z64** **Problems related to certain psychosocial circumstances**

**Z64.0** **Problems related to unwanted pregnancy** ♀

**Z64.1** **Problems related to multiparity** ♀

**Z64.4** **Discord with counselors**
Discord with probation officer
Discord with social worker

✓4th **Z65** **Problems related to other psychosocial circumstances**

**Z65.0** **Conviction in civil and criminal proceedings without imprisonment**

**Z65.1** **Imprisonment and other incarceration**

**Z65.2** **Problems related to release from prison**

**Z65.3** **Problems related to other legal circumstances**
Arrest
Child custody or support proceedings
Litigation
Prosecution

**Z65.4** **Victim of crime and terrorism**
Victim of torture

**Z65.5** **Exposure to disaster, war and other hostilities**
*EXCLUDES 1* *target of perceived discrimination or persecution (Z60.5)*

**Z65.8** **Other specified problems related to psychosocial circumstances**
▶Religious or spiritual problem◀

**Z65.9** **Problem related to unspecified psychosocial circumstances**

### Do not resuscitate status (Z66)

**Z66** **Do not resuscitate**
DNR status
**DEF:** Medical order written by a physician that instructs others not to perform cardiopulmonary resuscitation (CPR), intubation, or advanced life support (ACLS); prevents unnecessary invasive treatment to prolong life should breathing stop or cardiac arrest occur.

---

☑Additional Character Req  ✓x7th Placeholder Alert  Unacceptable PDx  Manifestation  **H1**-**H14** HAC  **HCC** CMS-HCC Condition  *EXCLUDES 1* Not Coded Here  *EXCLUDES 2* Not Included Here

**Chapter 21. Factors Influencing Health Status and Contact with Health Services**

**Blood Types**

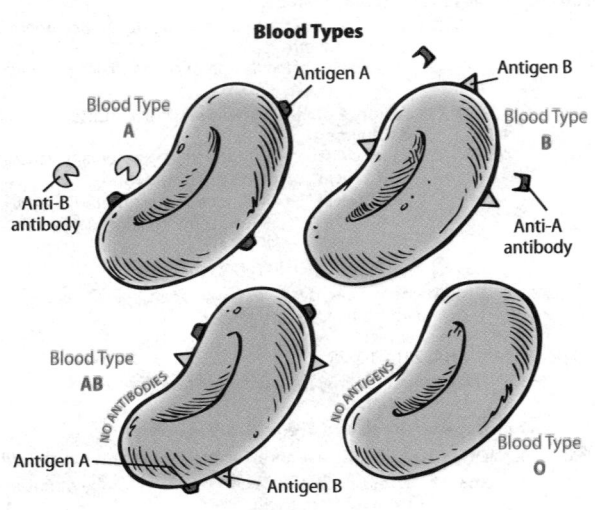

Antigen A   Antigen B

Blood Type A

Blood Type B

Anti-B antibody

Anti-A antibody

Blood Type AB

NO ANTIBODIES

NO ANTIGENS

Antigen A

Antigen B

Blood Type O

### Blood type (Z67)

✓4ᵗʰ **Z67** **Blood type**
AHA: 2015, 3Q, 40

✓5ᵗʰ **Z67.1** **Type A blood**
- Z67.10   Type A blood, Rh positive
- Z67.11   Type A blood, Rh negative

✓5ᵗʰ **Z67.2** **Type B blood**
- Z67.20   Type B blood, Rh positive
- Z67.21   Type B blood, Rh negative

✓5ᵗʰ **Z67.3** **Type AB blood**
- Z67.30   Type AB blood, Rh positive
- Z67.31   Type AB blood, Rh negative

✓5ᵗʰ **Z67.4** **Type O blood**
- Z67.40   Type O blood, Rh positive
- Z67.41   Type O blood, Rh negative

✓5ᵗʰ **Z67.9** **Unspecified blood type**
- Z67.90   Unspecified blood type, Rh positive
- Z67.91   Unspecified blood type, Rh negative

### Body mass index [BMI] (Z68)

✓4ᵗʰ **Z68** **Body mass index [BMI]**
Kilograms per meters squared
**NOTE**   BMI adult codes are for use for persons 21 years of age or older.
BMI pediatric codes are for use for persons 2-20 years of age. These percentiles are based on the growth charts published by the Centers for Disease Control and Prevention (CDC)
AHA: 2017, 1Q, 39
DEF: Index used to help determine whether an individual is underweight, a healthy weight, overweight, or obese.

▲ **Z68.1**   Body mass index [BMI] 19.9 or less, adult    CC A
CC Excl: PDX collection 1493

✓5ᵗʰ **Z68.2** **Body mass index [BMI] 20-29, adult**
- Z68.20   Body mass index [BMI] 20.0-20.9, adult   A
- Z68.21   Body mass index [BMI] 21.0-21.9, adult   A
- Z68.22   Body mass index [BMI] 22.0-22.9, adult   A
- Z68.23   Body mass index [BMI] 23.0-23.9, adult   A
- Z68.24   Body mass index [BMI] 24.0-24.9, adult   A
- Z68.25   Body mass index [BMI] 25.0-25.9, adult   A
- Z68.26   Body mass index [BMI] 26.0-26.9, adult   A
- Z68.27   Body mass index [BMI] 27.0-27.9, adult   A
- Z68.28   Body mass index [BMI] 28.0-28.9, adult   A
- Z68.29   Body mass index [BMI] 29.0-29.9, adult   A

✓5ᵗʰ **Z68.3** **Body mass index [BMI] 30-39, adult**
- Z68.30   Body mass index [BMI] 30.0-30.9, adult   A
- Z68.31   Body mass index [BMI] 31.0-31.9, adult   A
- Z68.32   Body mass index [BMI] 32.0-32.9, adult   A
- Z68.33   Body mass index [BMI] 33.0-33.9, adult   A
- Z68.34   Body mass index [BMI] 34.0-34.9, adult   A

- Z68.35   Body mass index [BMI] 35.0-35.9, adult   A
- Z68.36   Body mass index [BMI] 36.0-36.9, adult   A
- Z68.37   Body mass index [BMI] 37.0-37.9, adult   A
- Z68.38   Body mass index [BMI] 38.0-38.9, adult   A
- Z68.39   Body mass index [BMI] 39.0-39.9, adult   A

✓5ᵗʰ **Z68.4** **Body mass index [BMI] 40 or greater, adult**

> **CC Excl:** For CC codes in subcategory Z68.4, unless otherwise noted: PDX collection 1494

- Z68.41   Body mass index [BMI] 40.0-44.9, adult   CC MCC A
- Z68.42   Body mass index [BMI] 45.0-49.9, adult   CC MCC A
- Z68.43   Body mass index [BMI] 50-59.9, adult   CC MCC A
- Z68.44   Body mass index [BMI] 60.0-69.9, adult   CC MCC A
- Z68.45   Body mass index [BMI] 70 or greater, adult   CC MCC A

✓5ᵗʰ **Z68.5** **Body mass index [BMI] pediatric**
- Z68.51   Body mass index [BMI] pediatric, less than 5th percentile for age
- Z68.52   Body mass index [BMI] pediatric, 5th percentile to less than 85th percentile for age
- Z68.53   Body mass index [BMI] pediatric, 85th percentile to less than 95th percentile for age
- Z68.54   Body mass index [BMI] pediatric, greater than or equal to 95th percentile for age

### Persons encountering health services in other circumstances (Z69-Z76)

✓4ᵗʰ **Z69** **Encounter for mental health services for victim and perpetrator of abuse**
**INCLUDES**   counseling for victims and perpetrators of abuse

✓5ᵗʰ **Z69.0** **Encounter for mental health services for child abuse problems**

✓6ᵗʰ **Z69.01** **Encounter for mental health services for parental child abuse**
- Z69.010   **Encounter for mental health services for victim of parental child abuse**   P
  ▶Encounter for mental health services for victim of child abuse by parent
  Encounter for mental health services for victim of child neglect by parent
  Encounter for mental health services for victim of child psychological abuse by parent
  Encounter for mental health services for victim of child sexual abuse by parent◀
- Z69.011   **Encounter for mental health services for perpetrator of parental child abuse**
  ▶Encounter for mental health services for perpetrator of parental child neglect
  Encounter for mental health services for perpetrator of parental child psychological abuse
  Encounter for mental health services for perpetrator of parental child sexual abuse◀
  **EXCLUDES 1**   encounter for mental health services for non-parental child abuse (Z69.02-)

✓6ᵗʰ **Z69.02** **Encounter for mental health services for non-parental child abuse**
- Z69.020   **Encounter for mental health services for victim of non-parental child abuse**   P
  ▶Encounter for mental health services for victim of non-parental child neglect
  Encounter for mental health services for victim of non-parental child psychological abuse
  Encounter for mental health services for victim of non-parental child sexual abuse◀

---

N Newborn: 0   P Pediatric: 0-17   M Maternity: 12-55   A Adult: 15-124   MCC Major CC Condition   PDxMCC PDx acts as own MCC   CC CC Condition   PDxCC PDx acts as own CC

1236            ICD-10-CM 2018

Z69.021 **Encounter for mental health services for perpetrator of** non-parental child abuse
▶Encounter for mental health services for perpetrator of non-parental child neglect
Encounter for mental health services for perpetrator of non-parental child psychological abuse
Encounter for mental health services for perpetrator of non-parental child sexual abuse◀

√5ᵗʰ **Z69.1** **Encounter for mental health services for** spousal or partner abuse problems

Z69.11 **Encounter for mental health services for** victim of spousal or partner abuse
▶Encounter for mental health services for victim of spouse or partner neglect
Encounter for mental health services for victim of spouse or partner psychological abuse
Encounter for mental health services for victim of spouse or partner violence, physical◀

Z69.12 **Encounter for mental health services for** perpetrator of spousal or partner abuse
▶Encounter for mental health services for perpetrator of spouse or partner neglect
Encounter for mental health services for perpetrator of spouse or partner psychological abuse
Encounter for mental health services for perpetrator of spouse or partner violence, physical
Encounter for mental health services for perpetrator of spouse or partner violence, sexual◀

√5ᵗʰ **Z69.8** **Encounter for mental health services for** victim or perpetrator of other abuse

Z69.81 **Encounter for mental health services for** victim of other abuse
▶Encounter for mental health services for perpetrator of non-spousal adult abuse
Encounter for mental health services for victim of non-spousal adult abuse
Encounter for mental health services for victim of spouse or partner violence, sexual◀
Encounter for rape victim counseling

Z69.82 **Encounter for mental health services for** perpetrator of other abuse

√4ᵗʰ **Z70** **Counseling related to sexual attitude, behavior and orientation**
INCLUDES encounter for mental health services for sexual attitude, behavior and orientation
EXCLUDES 2 contraceptive or procreative counseling (Z30-Z31)

Z70.0 **Counseling related to sexual attitude**

Z70.1 **Counseling related to patient's sexual behavior and orientation**
Patient concerned regarding impotence
Patient concerned regarding non-responsiveness
Patient concerned regarding promiscuity
Patient concerned regarding sexual orientation

Z70.2 **Counseling related to sexual behavior and orientation of third party**
Advice sought regarding sexual behavior and orientation of child
Advice sought regarding sexual behavior and orientation of partner
Advice sought regarding sexual behavior and orientation of spouse

Z70.3 **Counseling related to combined concerns regarding sexual attitude, behavior and orientation**

Z70.8 **Other sex counseling**
Encounter for sex education

Z70.9 **Sex counseling, unspecified**

√4ᵗʰ **Z71** **Persons encountering health services for other counseling and medical advice, not elsewhere classified**
EXCLUDES 2 contraceptive or procreation counseling (Z30-Z31)
sex counseling (Z70.-)

Z71.0 **Person encountering health services to consult on behalf of another person**
Person encountering health services to seek advice or treatment for non-attending third party
EXCLUDES 2 anxiety (normal) about sick person in family (Z63.7)
expectant (adoptive) parent(s) pre-birth pediatrician visit (Z76.81)

Z71.1 **Person with feared health complaint in whom no diagnosis is made**
Person encountering health services with feared condition which was not demonstrated
Person encountering health services in which problem was normal state
"Worried well"
EXCLUDES 1 medical observation for suspected diseases and conditions proven not to exist (Z03.-)

Z71.2 **Person consulting for explanation of examination or test findings**

Z71.3 **Dietary counseling and surveillance**
Use additional code for any associated underlying medical condition
Use additional code to identify body mass index (BMI), if known (Z68.-)

√5ᵗʰ **Z71.4** **Alcohol abuse counseling and surveillance**
Use additional code for alcohol abuse or dependence (F10.-)

Z71.41 **Alcohol abuse counseling and surveillance of alcoholic**

Z71.42 **Counseling for** family member of alcoholic
Counseling for significant other, partner, or friend of alcoholic

√5ᵗʰ **Z71.5** **Drug abuse counseling and surveillance**
Use additional code for drug abuse or dependence (F11-F16, F18-F19)

Z71.51 **Drug abuse counseling and surveillance of** drug abuser

Z71.52 **Counseling for** family member of drug abuser
Counseling for significant other, partner, or friend of drug abuser

Z71.6 **Tobacco** abuse counseling
Use additional code for nicotine dependence (F17.-)

Z71.7 **Human immunodeficiency virus [HIV] counseling**

√5ᵗʰ **Z71.8** **Other specified counseling**
EXCLUDES 2 counseling for contraception (Z30.0-)
counseling for genetics (Z31.5)
counseling for procreative management (Z31.6-)

Z71.81 **Spiritual or religious** counseling

● Z71.82 **Exercise** counseling

● Z71.83 **Encounter for nonprocreative genetic counseling**
EXCLUDES 1 counseling for procreative genetics (Z31.5)
counseling for procreative management (Z31.6)

Z71.89 **Other specified counseling**

Z71.9 **Counseling, unspecified**
Encounter for medical advice NOS

√4ᵗʰ **Z72** **Problems related to lifestyle**
EXCLUDES 2 problems related to life-management difficulty (Z73.-)
problems related to socioeconomic and psychosocial circumstances (Z55-Z65)

Z72.0 **Tobacco use**
Tobacco use NOS
EXCLUDES 1 history of tobacco dependence (Z87.891)
nicotine dependence (F17.2-)
tobacco dependence (F17.2-)
tobacco use during pregnancy (O99.33-)

Z72.3 **Lack of physical exercise**

Z72.4 **Inappropriate diet and eating habits**
EXCLUDES 1 behavioral eating disorders of infancy or childhood (F98.2- F98.3)
eating disorders (F50.-)
lack of adequate food (Z59.4)
malnutrition and other nutritional deficiencies (E40-E64)

√5ᵗʰ **Z72.5** **High risk sexual behavior**
Promiscuity
EXCLUDES 1 paraphilias (F65)

Z72.51 **High risk** heterosexual **behavior**

Z72.52 **High risk** homosexual **behavior**

Z72.53 **High risk** bisexual **behavior**

Z72.6 **Gambling and betting**
EXCLUDES 1 compulsive or pathological gambling (F63.0)

**Z72.8 Other problems related to lifestyle**

☑6ᵗʰ **Z72.81 Antisocial behavior**
: EXCLUDES 1   conduct disorders (F91.-)

**Z72.810 Child and adolescent antisocial behavior**  P
: Antisocial behavior (child) (adolescent) without manifest psychiatric disorder
: Delinquency NOS
: Group delinquency
: Offenses in the context of gang membership
: Stealing in company with others
: Truancy from school

**Z72.811 Adult antisocial behavior**  A
: Adult antisocial behavior without manifest psychiatric disorder

☑6ᵗʰ **Z72.82 Problems related to sleep**

**Z72.820 Sleep deprivation**
: Lack of adequate sleep
: EXCLUDES 1   insomnia (G47.0-)

**Z72.821 Inadequate sleep hygiene**
: Bad sleep habits
: Irregular sleep habits
: Unhealthy sleep wake schedule
: EXCLUDES 1   insomnia (F51.0-, G47.0-)

**Z72.89 Other problems related to lifestyle**
: Self-damaging behavior

**Z72.9 Problem related to lifestyle, unspecified**

☑4ᵗʰ **Z73 Problems related to life management difficulty**
: EXCLUDES 2   problems related to socioeconomic and psychosocial circumstances (Z55-Z65)
: **DEF:** State of emotional, mental, and physical exhaustion; causing difficulties in managing personal, school, or work circumstances; usually due to prolonged stress; poor interpersonal relationship skills, or parenting skills.

**Z73.0 Burn-out**

**Z73.1 Type A behavior pattern**

**Z73.2 Lack of relaxation and leisure**

**Z73.3 Stress, not elsewhere classified**
: Physical and mental strain NOS
: EXCLUDES 1   stress related to employment or unemployment (Z56.-)

**Z73.4 Inadequate social skills, not elsewhere classified**

**Z73.5 Social role conflict, not elsewhere classified**

**Z73.6 Limitation of activities due to disability**
: EXCLUDES 1   care-provider dependency (Z74.-)

☑5ᵗʰ **Z73.8 Other problems related to life management difficulty**

☑6ᵗʰ **Z73.81 Behavioral insomnia of childhood**
: **DEF:** Behaviors on the part of the child or caregivers that cause negative compliance with a child's sleep schedule; results in lack of adequate sleep.

**Z73.810 Behavioral insomnia of childhood, sleep-onset association type**  P

**Z73.811 Behavioral insomnia of childhood, limit setting type**  P

**Z73.812 Behavioral insomnia of childhood, combined type**  P

**Z73.819 Behavioral insomnia of childhood, unspecified type**  P

**Z73.82 Dual sensory impairment**

**Z73.89 Other problems related to life management difficulty**

**Z73.9 Problem related to life management difficulty, unspecified**

☑4ᵗʰ **Z74 Problems related to care provider dependency**
: EXCLUDES 2   dependence on enabling machines or devices NEC (Z99.-)

☑5ᵗʰ **Z74.0 Reduced mobility**

**Z74.01 Bed confinement status**
: Bedridden

**Z74.09 Other reduced mobility**
: Chair ridden
: Reduced mobility NOS
: EXCLUDES 2   wheelchair dependence (Z99.3)

**Z74.1 Need for assistance with personal care**

**Z74.2 Need for assistance at home and no other household member able to render care**

**Z74.3 Need for continuous supervision**

**Z74.8 Other problems related to care provider dependency**

**Z74.9 Problem related to care provider dependency, unspecified**

☑4ᵗʰ **Z75 Problems related to medical facilities and other health care**

**Z75.0 Medical services not available in home**
: EXCLUDES 1   no other household member able to render care (Z74.2)

**Z75.1 Person awaiting admission to adequate facility elsewhere**

**Z75.2 Other waiting period for investigation and treatment**

**Z75.3 Unavailability and inaccessibility of health-care facilities**
: EXCLUDES 1   bed unavailable (Z75.1)

**Z75.4 Unavailability and inaccessibility of other helping agencies**

**Z75.5 Holiday relief care**

**Z75.8 Other problems related to medical facilities and other health care**

**Z75.9 Unspecified problem related to medical facilities and other health care**

☑4ᵗʰ **Z76 Persons encountering health services in other circumstances**

**Z76.0 Encounter for issue of repeat prescription**
: Encounter for issue of repeat prescription for appliance
: Encounter for issue of repeat prescription for medicaments
: Encounter for issue of repeat prescription for spectacles
: EXCLUDES 2   issue of medical certificate (Z02.7)
:      repeat prescription for contraceptive (Z30.4-)

**Z76.1 Encounter for health supervision and care of foundling**

**Z76.2 Encounter for health supervision and care of other healthy infant and child**  P
: Encounter for medical or nursing care or supervision of healthy infant under circumstances such as adverse socioeconomic conditions at home
: Encounter for medical or nursing care or supervision of healthy infant under circumstances such as awaiting foster or adoptive placement
: Encounter for medical or nursing care or supervision of healthy infant under circumstances such as maternal illness
: Encounter for medical or nursing care or supervision of healthy infant under circumstances such as number of children at home preventing or interfering with normal care

**Z76.3 Healthy person accompanying sick person**

**Z76.4 Other boarder to healthcare facility**
: EXCLUDES 1   homelessness (Z59.0)

**Z76.5 Malingerer [conscious simulation]**
: Person feigning illness (with obvious motivation)
: EXCLUDES 1   factitious disorder (F68.1-)
:      peregrinating patient (F68.1-)
: **DEF:** Act of intentionally exaggerating an illness or disability in order to receive personal gain; or to avoid punishment or responsibility.

☑5ᵗʰ **Z76.8 Persons encountering health services in other specified circumstances**

**Z76.81 Expectant parent(s) prebirth pediatrician visit**
: Pre-adoption pediatrician visit for adoptive parent(s)

**Z76.82 Awaiting organ transplant status**
: Patient waiting for organ availability

**Z76.89 Persons encountering health services in other specified circumstances**
: Persons encountering health services NOS
: **AHA:** 2014, 2Q, 10

N Newborn: 0    P Pediatric: 0-17    M Maternity: 12-55    A Adult: 15-124    MCC Major CC Condition    PDxMCC PDx acts as own MCC    CC CC Condition    PDxCC PDx acts as own CC

**1238**      ICD-10-CM 2018

## Persons with potential health hazards related to family and personal history and certain conditions influencing health status (Z77-Z99)

Code also any follow-up examination (Z08-Z09)

**✓4ᵗʰ Z77 Other contact with and (suspected) exposures hazardous to health**

INCLUDES contact with and (suspected) exposures to potential hazards to health

EXCLUDES 2 contact with and (suspected) exposure to communicable diseases (Z20.-)

exposure to (parental) (environmental) tobacco smoke in the perinatal period (P96.81)

newborn affected by noxious substances transmitted via placenta or breast milk (P04.-)

occupational exposure to risk factors (Z57.-)

retained foreign body (Z18.-)

retained foreign body fully removed (Z87.821)

toxic effects of substances chiefly nonmedicinal as to source (T51-T65)

**✓5ᵗʰ Z77.0 Contact with and (suspected) exposure to hazardous, chiefly nonmedicinal, chemicals**

**✓6ᵗʰ Z77.01 Contact with and (suspected) exposure to hazardous metals**

**Z77.010 Contact with and (suspected) exposure to arsenic**

**Z77.011 Contact with and (suspected) exposure to lead**

**Z77.012 Contact with and (suspected) exposure to uranium**

EXCLUDES 1 retained depleted uranium fragments (Z18.01)

**Z77.018 Contact with and (suspected) exposure to other hazardous metals**

Contact with and (suspected) exposure to chromium compounds

Contact with and (suspected) exposure to nickel dust

**✓6ᵗʰ Z77.02 Contact with and (suspected) exposure to hazardous aromatic compounds**

**Z77.020 Contact with and (suspected) exposure to aromatic amines**

**Z77.021 Contact with and (suspected) exposure to benzene**

**Z77.028 Contact with and (suspected) exposure to other hazardous aromatic compounds**

Aromatic dyes NOS

Polycyclic aromatic hydrocarbons

**✓6ᵗʰ Z77.09 Contact with and (suspected) exposure to other hazardous, chiefly nonmedicinal, chemicals**

**Z77.090 Contact with and (suspected) exposure to asbestos**

**Z77.098 Contact with and (suspected) exposure to other hazardous, chiefly nonmedicinal, chemicals**

Dyes NOS

**✓5ᵗʰ Z77.1 Contact with and (suspected) exposure to environmental pollution and hazards in the physical environment**

**✓6ᵗʰ Z77.11 Contact with and (suspected) exposure to environmental pollution**

**Z77.110 Contact with and (suspected) exposure to air pollution**

**Z77.111 Contact with and (suspected) exposure to water pollution**

**Z77.112 Contact with and (suspected) exposure to soil pollution**

**Z77.118 Contact with and (suspected) exposure to other environmental pollution**

**✓6ᵗʰ Z77.12 Contact with and (suspected) exposure to hazards in the physical environment**

**Z77.120 Contact with and (suspected) exposure to mold (toxic)**

**Z77.121 Contact with and (suspected) exposure to harmful algae and algae toxins**

Contact with and (suspected) exposure to (harmful) algae bloom NOS

Contact with and (suspected) exposure to blue-green algae bloom

Contact with and (suspected) exposure to brown tide

Contact with and (suspected) exposure to cyanobacteria bloom

Contact with and (suspected) exposure to Florida red tide

Contact with and (suspected) exposure to pfiesteria piscicida

Contact with and (suspected) exposure to red tide

**Z77.122 Contact with and (suspected) exposure to noise**

**Z77.123 Contact with and (suspected) exposure to radon and other naturally occuring radiation**

EXCLUDES 2 radiation exposure as the cause of a confirmed condition (W88-W90, X39.0-)

radiation sickness NOS (T66)

**Z77.128 Contact with and (suspected) exposure to other hazards in the physical environment**

**✓5ᵗʰ Z77.2 Contact with and (suspected ) exposure to other hazardous substances**

**Z77.21 Contact with and (suspected) exposure to potentially hazardous body fluids**

**Z77.22 Contact with and (suspected) exposure to environmental tobacco smoke (acute) (chronic)**

Exposure to second hand tobacco smoke (acute) (chronic)

Passive smoking (acute) (chronic)

EXCLUDES 1 nicotine dependence (F17.-)

tobacco use (Z72.0)

EXCLUDES 2 occupational exposure to environmental tobacco smoke (Z57.31)

**Z77.29 Contact with and (suspected ) exposure to other hazardous substances**

AHA: 2016, 2Q, 33

**Z77.9 Other contact with and (suspected) exposures hazardous to health**

**✓4ᵗʰ Z78 Other specified health status**

EXCLUDES 2 asymptomatic human immunodeficiency virus [HIV] infection status (Z21)

postprocedural status (Z93- Z99)

sex reassignment status (Z87.890)

**Z78.0 Asymptomatic menopausal state**    Ⓐ ♀

Menopausal state NOS

Postmenopausal status NOS

EXCLUDES 2 symptomatic menopausal state (N95.1)

**Z78.1 Physical restraint status**

EXCLUDES 1 physical restraint due to a procedure - omit code

DEF: Application of mechanical restraining devices or manual restraints; used to limit physical mobility of a patient.

**Z78.9 Other specified health status**

**✓4ᵗʰ Z79 Long term (current) drug therapy**

INCLUDES long term (current) drug use for prophylactic purposes

Code also any therapeutic drug level monitoring (Z51.81)

EXCLUDES 2 drug abuse and dependence (F11-F19)

drug use complicating pregnancy, childbirth, and the puerperium (O99.32-)

long term (current) use of oral antidiabetic drugs (Z79.84)

long term (current) use of oral hypoglycemic drugs (Z79.84)

**✓5ᵗʰ Z79.0 Long term (current) use of anticoagulants and antithrombotics/antiplatelets**

EXCLUDES 2 long term (current) use of aspirin (Z79.82)

**Z79.01 Long term (current) use of anticoagulants**

**Z79.02 Long term (current) use of antithrombotics/antiplatelets**

**Z79.1 Long term (current) use of non-steroidal anti-inflammatories (NSAID)**

EXCLUDES 2 long term (current) use of aspirin (Z79.82)

**Z79.2 Long term (current) use of antibiotics**

**Z79.3 Long term (current) use of hormonal contraceptives**

Long term (current) use of birth control pill or patch

**Z79.4 Long term (current) use of insulin**    HCC

---

✓ Additional Character Req   ✓x7ᵗʰ Placeholder Alert   Unacceptable PDx   Manifestation   H1-H14 HAC   HCC CMS-HCC Condition   EXCLUDES 1 Not Coded Here   EXCLUDES 2 Not Included Here

ICD-10-CM 2018          1239

**Chapter 21. Factors Influencing Health Status and Contact with Health Services**

✓5ᵗʰ **Z79.5** **Long term (current) use of steroids**

    **Z79.51** Long term (current) use of inhaled steroids

    **Z79.52** Long term (current) use of systemic steroids

✓5ᵗʰ **Z79.8** **Other long term (current) drug therapy**

  ✓6ᵗʰ **Z79.81** **Long term (current) use of agents affecting estrogen receptors and estrogen levels**

    Code first, if applicable:
      malignant neoplasm of breast (C50.-)
      malignant neoplasm of prostate (C61)
    Use additional code, if applicable, to identify:
      estrogen receptor positive status (Z17.0)
      family history of breast cancer (Z80.3)
      genetic susceptibility to malignant neoplasm (cancer) (Z15.0-)
      personal history of breast cancer (Z85.3)
      personal history of prostate cancer (Z85.46)
      postmenopausal status (Z78.0)
    **EXCLUDES 1** ▶hormone replacement therapy◀ (Z79.890)

    **Z79.810** **Long term (current) use of selective estrogen receptor modulators (SERMs)**
      Long term (current) use of raloxifene (Evista)
      Long term (current) use of tamoxifen (Nolvadex)
      Long term (current) use of toremifene (Fareston)

    **Z79.811** **Long term (current) use of aromatase inhibitors**
      Long term (current) use of anastrozole (Arimidex)
      Long term (current) use of exemestane (Aromasin)
      Long term (current) use of letrozole (Femara)

    **Z79.818** **Long term (current) use of other agents affecting estrogen receptors and estrogen levels**
      Long term (current) use of estrogen receptor downregulators
      Long term (current) use of fulvestrant (Faslodex)
      Long term (current) use of gonadotropin-releasing hormone (GnRH) agonist
      Long term (current) use of goserelin acetate (Zoladex)
      Long term (current) use of leuprolide acetate (leuprorelin) (Lupron)
      Long term (current) use of megestrol acetate (Megace)

    **Z79.82** Long term (current) use of aspirin

    **Z79.83** Long term (current) use of bisphosphonates

    **Z79.84** **Long term (current) use of oral hypoglycemic drugs**
      Long term (current) use of oral antidiabetic drugs
      **EXCLUDES 2** long term (current) use of insulin (Z79.4)

  ✓6ᵗʰ **Z79.89** **Other long term (current) drug therapy**

    **Z79.890** Hormone replacement therapy

    **Z79.891** **Long term (current) use of opiate analgesic**
      Long term (current) use of methadone for pain management
      **EXCLUDES 1** methodone use NOS (F11.9-)
      use of methodone for treatment of heroin addiction (F11.2-)

    **Z79.899** **Other long term (current) drug therapy**
      AHA: 2015, 4Q, 34; 2015, 3Q, 21

✓4ᵗʰ **Z80** **Family history of primary malignant neoplasm**

  **Z80.0** **Family history of malignant neoplasm of digestive organs**
    Conditions classifiable to C15-C26

  **Z80.1** **Family history of malignant neoplasm of trachea, bronchus and lung**
    Conditions classifiable to C33-C34

  **Z80.2** **Family history of malignant neoplasm of other respiratory and intrathoracic organs**
    Conditions classifiable to C30-C32, C37-C39

  **Z80.3** **Family history of malignant neoplasm of breast**
    Conditions classifiable to C50-

✓5ᵗʰ **Z80.4** **Family history of malignant neoplasm of genital organs**
    Conditions classifiable to C51-C63

    **Z80.41** Family history of malignant neoplasm of ovary

    **Z80.42** Family history of malignant neoplasm of prostate

    **Z80.43** Family history of malignant neoplasm of testis

    **Z80.49** Family history of malignant neoplasm of other genital organs

✓5ᵗʰ **Z80.5** **Family history of malignant neoplasm of urinary tract**
    Conditions classifiable to C64-C68

    **Z80.51** Family history of malignant neoplasm of kidney

    **Z80.52** Family history of malignant neoplasm of bladder

    **Z80.59** Family history of malignant neoplasm of other urinary tract organ

  **Z80.6** **Family history of leukemia**
    Conditions classifiable to C91-C95

  **Z80.7** **Family history of other malignant neoplasms of lymphoid, hematopoietic and related tissues**
    Conditions classifiable to C81-C90, C96-

  **Z80.8** **Family history of malignant neoplasm of other organs or systems**
    Conditions classifiable to C00-C14, C40-C49, C69-C79

  **Z80.9** **Family history of malignant neoplasm, unspecified**
    Conditions classifiable to C80.1

✓4ᵗʰ **Z81** **Family history of mental and behavioral disorders**

  **Z81.0** **Family history of intellectual disabilities**
    Conditions classifiable to F70-F79

  **Z81.1** **Family history of alcohol abuse and dependence**
    Conditions classifiable to F10-

  **Z81.2** **Family history of tobacco abuse and dependence**
    Conditions classifiable to F17-

  **Z81.3** **Family history of other psychoactive substance abuse and dependence**
    Conditions classifiable to F11-F16, F18-F19

  **Z81.4** **Family history of other substance abuse and dependence**
    Conditions classifiable to F55

  **Z81.8** **Family history of other mental and behavioral disorders**
    Conditions classifiable elsewhere in F01-F99

✓4ᵗʰ **Z82** **Family history of certain disabilities and chronic diseases (leading to disablement)**

  **Z82.0** **Family history of epilepsy and other diseases of the nervous system**
    Conditions classifiable to G00-G99

  **Z82.1** **Family history of blindness and visual loss**
    Conditions classifiable to H54-

  **Z82.2** **Family history of deafness and hearing loss**
    Conditions classifiable to H90-H91

  **Z82.3** **Family history of stroke**
    Conditions classifiable to I60-I64

✓5ᵗʰ **Z82.4** **Family history of ischemic heart disease and other diseases of the circulatory system**
    Conditions classifiable to I00-I52, I65-I99

    **Z82.41** Family history of sudden cardiac death

    **Z82.49** Family history of ischemic heart disease and other diseases of the circulatory system

  **Z82.5** **Family history of asthma and other chronic lower respiratory diseases**
    Conditions classifiable to J40-J47
    **EXCLUDES 2** family history of other diseases of the respiratory system (Z83.6)

✓5ᵗʰ **Z82.6** **Family history of arthritis and other diseases of the musculoskeletal system and connective tissue**
    Conditions classifiable to M00-M99

    **Z82.61** Family history of arthritis

    **Z82.62** Family history of osteoporosis

    **Z82.69** Family history of other diseases of the musculoskeletal system and connective tissue

✓5ᵗʰ **Z82.7** **Family history of congenital malformations, deformations and chromosomal abnormalities**
    Conditions classifiable to Q00-Q99

    **Z82.71** Family history of polycystic kidney

    **Z82.79** Family history of other congenital malformations, deformations and chromosomal abnormalities

  **Z82.8** **Family history of other disabilities and chronic diseases leading to disablement, not elsewhere classified**

N Newborn: 0   P Pediatric: 0-17   M Maternity: 12-55   A Adult: 15-124   **MCC** Major CC Condition   **PDxMCC** PDx acts as own MCC   **CC** CC Condition   **PDxCC** PDx acts as own CC

**1240**     ICD-10-CM 2018

✓4th **Z83** **Family history of other specific disorders**

     EXCLUDES 2   *contact with and (suspected) exposure to communicable disease in the family (Z20.-)*

**Z83.0** **Family history of human immunodeficiency virus [HIV] disease**
     Conditions classifiable to B20

**Z83.1** **Family history of other infectious and parasitic diseases**
     Conditions classifiable to A00-B19, B25-B94, B99

**Z83.2** **Family history of diseases of the blood and blood-forming organs and certain disorders involving the immune mechanism**
     Conditions classifiable to D50-D89

**Z83.3** **Family history of diabetes mellitus**
     Conditions classifiable to E08-E13

✓5th **Z83.4** **Family history of other endocrine, nutritional and metabolic diseases**
     Conditions classifiable to E00-E07, E15-E88

     **Z83.41** **Family history of multiple endocrine neoplasia [MEN] syndrome**

     **Z83.42** **Family history of familial hypercholesterolemia**

     **Z83.49** **Family history of other endocrine, nutritional and metabolic diseases**

✓5th **Z83.5** **Family history of eye and ear disorders**

     ✓6th **Z83.51** **Family history of eye disorders**
       Conditions classifiable to H00-H53, H55-H59
       EXCLUDES 2   *family history of blindness and visual loss (Z82.1)*

       **Z83.511** **Family history of glaucoma**
       **Z83.518** **Family history of other specified eye disorder**

     **Z83.52** **Family history of ear disorders**
       Conditions classifiable to H60-H83, H92-H95
       EXCLUDES 2   *family history of deafness and hearing loss (Z82.2)*

**Z83.6** **Family history of other diseases of the respiratory system**
     Conditions classifiable to J00-J39, J60-J99
     EXCLUDES 2   *family history of asthma and other chronic lower respiratory diseases (Z82.5)*

✓5th **Z83.7** **Family history of diseases of the digestive system**
     Conditions classifiable to K00-K93

     **Z83.71** **Family history of colonic polyps**
       EXCLUDES 1   *family history of malignant neoplasm of digestive organs (Z80.0)*
       EXCLUDES 2   ▶*family history of malignant neoplasm of digestive organs (Z80.0)*◄

     **Z83.79** **Family history of other diseases of the digestive system**

✓4th **Z84** **Family history of other conditions**

**Z84.0** **Family history of diseases of the skin and subcutaneous tissue**
     Conditions classifiable to L00-L99

**Z84.1** **Family history of disorders of kidney and ureter**
     Conditions classifiable to N00-N29

**Z84.2** **Family history of other diseases of the genitourinary system**
     Conditions classifiable to N30-N99

**Z84.3** **Family history of consanguinity**

✓5th **Z84.8** **Family history of other specified conditions**

     **Z84.81** **Family history of carrier of genetic disease**

     **Z84.82** **Family history of sudden infant death syndrome**
       Family history of SIDS

     **Z84.89** **Family history of other specified conditions**

✓4th **Z85** **Personal history of malignant neoplasm**
     Code first any follow-up examination after treatment of malignant neoplasm (Z08)
     Use additional code to identify:
       alcohol use and dependence (F10.-)
       exposure to environmental tobacco smoke (Z77.22)
       history of tobacco dependence (Z87.891)
       occupational exposure to environmental tobacco smoke (Z57.31)
       tobacco dependence (F17.-)
       tobacco use (Z72.0)
     EXCLUDES 2   *personal history of benign neoplasm (Z86.01-)*
          *personal history of carcinoma-in-situ (Z86.00-)*

✓5th **Z85.0** **Personal history of malignant neoplasm of digestive organs**
     AHA: 2017, 1Q, 9

     **Z85.00** **Personal history of malignant neoplasm of unspecified digestive organ**

     **Z85.01** **Personal history of malignant neoplasm of esophagus**
       Conditions classifiable to C15

     ✓6th **Z85.02** **Personal history of malignant neoplasm of stomach**

       **Z85.020** **Personal history of malignant carcinoid tumor of stomach**
         Conditions classifiable to C7A.092

       **Z85.028** **Personal history of other malignant neoplasm of stomach**
         Conditions classifiable to C16

     ✓6th **Z85.03** **Personal history of malignant neoplasm of large intestine**

       **Z85.030** **Personal history of malignant carcinoid tumor of large intestine**
         Conditions classifiable to C7A.022-C7A.025, C7A.029

       **Z85.038** **Personal history of other malignant neoplasm of large intestine**
         Conditions classifiable to C18

     ✓6th **Z85.04** **Personal history of malignant neoplasm of rectum, rectosigmoid junction, and anus**

       **Z85.040** **Personal history of malignant carcinoid tumor of rectum**
         Conditions classifiable to C7A.026

       **Z85.048** **Personal history of other malignant neoplasm of rectum, rectosigmoid junction, and anus**
         Conditions classifiable to C19-C21

     **Z85.05** **Personal history of malignant neoplasm of liver**
       Conditions classifiable to C22

     ✓6th **Z85.06** **Personal history of malignant neoplasm of small intestine**

       **Z85.060** **Personal history of malignant carcinoid tumor of small intestine**
         Conditions classifiable to C7A.01-

       **Z85.068** **Personal history of other malignant neoplasm of small intestine**
         Conditions classifiable to C17

     **Z85.07** **Personal history of malignant neoplasm of pancreas**
       Conditions classifiable to C25

     **Z85.09** **Personal history of malignant neoplasm of other digestive organs**

✓5th **Z85.1** **Personal history of malignant neoplasm of trachea, bronchus and lung**

     ✓6th **Z85.11** **Personal history of malignant neoplasm of bronchus and lung**

       **Z85.110** **Personal history of malignant carcinoid tumor of bronchus and lung**
         Conditions classifiable to C7A.090

       **Z85.118** **Personal history of other malignant neoplasm of bronchus and lung**
         Conditions classifiable to C34

     **Z85.12** **Personal history of malignant neoplasm of trachea**
       Conditions classifiable to C33

✓5th **Z85.2** **Personal history of malignant neoplasm of other respiratory and intrathoracic organs**

     **Z85.20** **Personal history of malignant neoplasm of unspecified respiratory organ**

     **Z85.21** **Personal history of malignant neoplasm of larynx**
       Conditions classifiable to C32

     **Z85.22** **Personal history of malignant neoplasm of nasal cavities, middle ear, and accessory sinuses**
       Conditions classifiable to C30-C31

     ✓6th **Z85.23** **Personal history of malignant neoplasm of thymus**

       **Z85.230** **Personal history of malignant carcinoid tumor of thymus**
         Conditions classifiable to C7A.091

       **Z85.238** **Personal history of other malignant neoplasm of thymus**
         Conditions classifiable to C37

     **Z85.29** **Personal history of malignant neoplasm of other respiratory and intrathoracic organs**

**Z85.3** **Personal history of malignant neoplasm of breast**
     Conditions classifiable to C50.-

✓5th **Z85.4** **Personal history of malignant neoplasm of genital organs**
     Conditions classifiable to C51-C63

     **Z85.40** **Personal history of malignant neoplasm of unspecified female genital organ** ♀

✓ Additional Character Req   ✓x7th Placeholder Alert   Unacceptable PDx   Manifestation   H1 - H14 HAC   HCC CMS-HCC Condition   EXCLUDES 1 Not Coded Here   EXCLUDES 2 Not Included Here

ICD-10-CM 2018

1241

**Z85.41** Personal history of malignant neoplasm of cervix uteri ♀

**Z85.42** Personal history of malignant neoplasm of other parts of uterus ♀

**Z85.43** Personal history of malignant neoplasm of ovary ♀

**Z85.44** Personal history of malignant neoplasm of other female genital organs ♀

**Z85.45** Personal history of malignant neoplasm of unspecified male genital organ ♂

**Z85.46** Personal history of malignant neoplasm of prostate ♂

**Z85.47** Personal history of malignant neoplasm of testis ♂

**Z85.48** Personal history of malignant neoplasm of epididymis ♂

**Z85.49** Personal history of malignant neoplasm of other male genital organs ♂

✓5ᵗʰ **Z85.5** Personal history of malignant neoplasm of urinary tract
Conditions classifiable to C64–C68

**Z85.50** Personal history of malignant neoplasm of unspecified urinary tract organ

**Z85.51** Personal history of malignant neoplasm of bladder

✓6ᵗʰ **Z85.52** Personal history of malignant neoplasm of kidney
EXCLUDES 1   personal history of malignant neoplasm of renal pelvis (Z85.53)

**Z85.520** Personal history of malignant carcinoid tumor of kidney
Conditions classifiable to C7A.093

**Z85.528** Personal history of other malignant neoplasm of kidney
Conditions classifiable to C64

**Z85.53** Personal history of malignant neoplasm of renal pelvis

**Z85.54** Personal history of malignant neoplasm of ureter

**Z85.59** Personal history of malignant neoplasm of other urinary tract organ

**Z85.6** Personal history of leukemia
Conditions classifiable to C91–C95
EXCLUDES 1   leukemia in remission C91.0–C95.9 with 5th character 1

✓5ᵗʰ **Z85.7** Personal history of other malignant neoplasms of lymphoid, hematopoietic and related tissues

**Z85.71** Personal history of Hodgkin lymphoma
Conditions classifiable to C81

**Z85.72** Personal history of non-Hodgkin lymphomas
Conditions classifiable to C82–C85

**Z85.79** Personal history of other malignant neoplasms of lymphoid, hematopoietic and related tissues
Conditions classifiable to C88–C90, C96
EXCLUDES 1   multiple myeloma in remission (C90.01)
plasma cell leukemia in remission (C90.11)
plasmacytoma in remission (C90.21)

✓5ᵗʰ **Z85.8** Personal history of malignant neoplasms of other organs and systems
Conditions classifiable to C00–C14, C40–C49, C69–C75, C7A.098, C76–C79

✓6ᵗʰ **Z85.81** Personal history of malignant neoplasm of lip, oral cavity, and pharynx

**Z85.810** Personal history of malignant neoplasm of tongue

**Z85.818** Personal history of malignant neoplasm of other sites of lip, oral cavity, and pharynx

**Z85.819** Personal history of malignant neoplasm of unspecified site of lip, oral cavity, and pharynx

✓6ᵗʰ **Z85.82** Personal history of malignant neoplasm of skin

**Z85.820** Personal history of malignant melanoma of skin
Conditions classifiable to C43

**Z85.821** Personal history of Merkel cell carcinoma
Conditions classifiable to C4A

**Z85.828** Personal history of other malignant neoplasm of skin
Conditions classifiable to C44

✓6ᵗʰ **Z85.83** Personal history of malignant neoplasm of bone and soft tissue

**Z85.830** Personal history of malignant neoplasm of bone

**Z85.831** Personal history of malignant neoplasm of soft tissue
EXCLUDES 2   personal history of malignant neoplasm of skin (Z85.82-)

✓6ᵗʰ **Z85.84** Personal history of malignant neoplasm of eye and nervous tissue

**Z85.840** Personal history of malignant neoplasm of eye

**Z85.841** Personal history of malignant neoplasm of brain

**Z85.848** Personal history of malignant neoplasm of other parts of nervous tissue

✓6ᵗʰ **Z85.85** Personal history of malignant neoplasm of endocrine glands

**Z85.850** Personal history of malignant neoplasm of thyroid

**Z85.858** Personal history of malignant neoplasm of other endocrine glands

**Z85.89** Personal history of malignant neoplasm of other organs and systems

**Z85.9** Personal history of malignant neoplasm, unspecified
Conditions classifiable to C7A.00, C80.1

✓4ᵗʰ **Z86** Personal history of certain other diseases
Code first any follow-up examination after treatment (Z09)

✓5ᵗʰ **Z86.0** Personal history of in-situ and benign neoplasms and neoplasms of uncertain behavior
EXCLUDES 2   personal history of malignant neoplasms (Z85.-)
AHA: 2017, 1Q, 9

✓6ᵗʰ **Z86.00** Personal history of in-situ neoplasm
Conditions classifiable to D00–D09

**Z86.000** Personal history of in-situ neoplasm of breast

**Z86.001** Personal history of in-situ neoplasm of cervix uteri ♀
Personal history of cervical intraepithelial neoplasia III [CIN III]

**Z86.008** Personal history of in-situ neoplasm of other site
Personal history of vaginal intraepithelial neoplasia III [VAIN III]
Personal history of vulvar intraepithelial neoplasia III [VIN III]

✓6ᵗʰ **Z86.01** Personal history of benign neoplasm

**Z86.010** Personal history of colonic polyps
AHA: 2017, 1Q, 14

**Z86.011** Personal history of benign neoplasm of the brain

**Z86.012** Personal history of benign carcinoid tumor

**Z86.018** Personal history of other benign neoplasm
AHA: 2017, 1Q, 14

**Z86.03** Personal history of neoplasm of uncertain behavior

✓5ᵗʰ **Z86.1** Personal history of infectious and parasitic diseases
Conditions classifiable to A00–B89, B99
EXCLUDES 1   personal history of infectious diseases specific to a body system
sequelae of infectious and parasitic diseases (B90–B94)

**Z86.11** Personal history of tuberculosis

**Z86.12** Personal history of poliomyelitis

**Z86.13** Personal history of malaria

**Z86.14** Personal history of Methicillin resistant Staphylococcus aureus infection
Personal history of MRSA infection

**Z86.19** Personal history of other infectious and parasitic diseases

**Z86.2** Personal history of diseases of the blood and blood-forming organs and certain disorders involving the immune mechanism
Conditions classifiable to D50–D89

✓5ᵗʰ **Z86.3** Personal history of endocrine, nutritional and metabolic diseases
Conditions classifiable to E00–E88

**Z86.31** Personal history of diabetic foot ulcer
EXCLUDES 2   current diabetic foot ulcer (E08.621, E09.621, E10.621, E11.621, E13.621)

---

N Newborn: 0   P Pediatric: 0-17   M Maternity: 12-55   A Adult: 15-124   MCC Major CC Condition   PDxMCC PDx acts as own MCC   CC CC Condition   PDxCC PDx acts as own CC

1242   ICD-10-CM 2018

**Z86.32**  **Personal history of gestational diabetes**  ♀
Personal history of conditions classifiable to O24.4-
EXCLUDES 1  *gestational diabetes mellitus in current pregnancy (O24.4-)*

**Z86.39**  **Personal history of other endocrine, nutritional and metabolic disease**

√5th **Z86.5**  **Personal history of mental and behavioral disorders**
Conditions classifiable to F40-F59

**Z86.51**  **Personal history of combat and operational stress reaction**  A

**Z86.59**  **Personal history of other mental and behavioral disorders**

√5th **Z86.6**  **Personal history of diseases of the nervous system and sense organs**
Conditions classifiable to G00-G99, H00-H95
EXCLUDES 2  *personal history of anaphylactic shock (Z87.892)*

**Z86.61**  **Personal history of infections of the central nervous system**
Personal history of encephalitis
Personal history of meningitis

**Z86.69**  **Personal history of other diseases of the nervous system and sense organs**

√5th **Z86.7**  **Personal history of diseases of the circulatory system**
Conditions classifiable to I00-I99
EXCLUDES 2  *old myocardial infarction (I25.2)*
*personal history of anaphylactic shock (Z87.892)*
*postmyocardial infarction syndrome (I24.1)*

√6th **Z86.71**  **Personal history of venous thrombosis and embolism**

**Z86.711**  **Personal history of pulmonary embolism**

**Z86.718**  **Personal history of other venous thrombosis and embolism**

**Z86.72**  **Personal history of thrombophlebitis**

**Z86.73**  **Personal history of transient ischemic attack (TIA), and cerebral infarction without residual deficits**
Personal history of prolonged reversible ischemic neurological deficit (PRIND)
Personal history of stroke NOS without residual deficits
EXCLUDES 1  *personal history of traumatic brain injury (Z87.820)*
*sequelae of cerebrovascular disease (I69.-)*
**AHA:** 2012, 4Q, 92

**Z86.74**  **Personal history of sudden cardiac arrest**
Personal history of sudden cardiac death successfully resuscitated

**Z86.79**  **Personal history of other diseases of the circulatory system**

√4th **Z87**  **Personal history of other diseases and conditions**
Code first any follow-up examination after treatment (Z09)

√5th **Z87.0**  **Personal history of diseases of the respiratory system**
Conditions classifiable to J00-J99

**Z87.01**  **Personal history of pneumonia (recurrent)**

**Z87.09**  **Personal history of other diseases of the respiratory system**

√5th **Z87.1**  **Personal history of diseases of the digestive system**
Conditions classifiable to K00-K93

**Z87.11**  **Personal history of peptic ulcer disease**

**Z87.19**  **Personal history of other diseases of the digestive system**
**AHA:** 2017, 1Q, 14

**Z87.2**  **Personal history of diseases of the skin and subcutaneous tissue**
Conditions classifiable to L00-L99
EXCLUDES 2  *personal history of diabetic foot ulcer (Z86.31)*

√5th **Z87.3**  **Personal history of diseases of the musculoskeletal system and connective tissue**
Conditions classifiable to M00-M99
EXCLUDES 2  *personal history of (healed) traumatic fracture (Z87.81)*

√6th **Z87.31**  **Personal history of (healed) nontraumatic fracture**

**Z87.310**  **Personal history of (healed) osteoporosis fracture**
Personal history of (healed) fragility fracture
Personal history of (healed) collapsed vertebra due to osteoporosis

**Z87.311**  **Personal history of (healed) other pathological fracture**
Personal history of (healed) collapsed vertebra NOS
EXCLUDES 2  *personal history of osteoporosis fracture (Z87.310)*

**Z87.312**  **Personal history of (healed) stress fracture**
Personal history of (healed) fatigue fracture

**Z87.39**  **Personal history of other diseases of the musculoskeletal system and connective tissue**

√5th **Z87.4**  **Personal history of diseases of genitourinary system**
Conditions classifiable to N00-N99

√6th **Z87.41**  **Personal history of dysplasia of the female genital tract**
EXCLUDES 1  *personal history of intraepithelial neoplasia III of female genital tract ▶(Z86.001, Z86.008)◀*
*personal history of malignant neoplasm of female genital tract (Z85.40-Z85.44)*

**Z87.410**  **Personal history of cervical dysplasia**  ♀

**Z87.411**  **Personal history of vaginal dysplasia**  ♀

**Z87.412**  **Personal history of vulvar dysplasia**  ♀

**Z87.42**  **Personal history of other diseases of the female genital tract**  ♀

√6th **Z87.43**  **Personal history of diseases of the male genital organs**

**Z87.430**  **Personal history of prostatic dysplasia**  ♂
EXCLUDES 1  *personal history of malignant neoplasm of prostate (Z85.46)*

**Z87.438**  **Personal history of other diseases of male genital organs**  ♂

√6th **Z87.44**  **Personal history of diseases of the urinary system**
EXCLUDES 1  *personal history of malignant neoplasm of cervix uteri (Z85.41)*

**Z87.440**  **Personal history of urinary (tract) infections**

**Z87.441**  **Personal history of nephrotic syndrome**

**Z87.442**  **Personal history of urinary calculi**
Personal history of kidney stones

**Z87.448**  **Personal history of other diseases of urinary system**

√5th **Z87.5**  **Personal history of complications of pregnancy, ~~childbirth~~ and the puerperium**
Conditions classifiable to O00-O9A
EXCLUDES 2  *recurrent pregnancy loss (N96)*

**Z87.51**  **Personal history of pre-term labor**  ♀
EXCLUDES 1  *current pregnancy with history of pre-term labor (O09.21-)*

**Z87.59**  **Personal history of other complications of pregnancy, childbirth and the puerperium**  ♀
Personal history of trophoblastic disease

**✓5ᵗʰ Z87.7 Personal history of (corrected) congenital malformations**
Conditions classifiable to Q00-Q89 that have been repaired or corrected
> **EXCLUDES 1** *congenital malformations that have been partially corrected or repaired but which still require medical treatment—code to condition*
> **EXCLUDES 2** *other postprocedural states (Z98.-)*
> *personal history of medical treatment (Z92.-)*
> *presence of cardiac and vascular implants and grafts (Z95.-)*
> *presence of other devices (Z97.-)*
> *presence of other functional implants (Z96.-)*
> *transplanted organ and tissue status (Z94.-)*

   **✓6ᵗʰ Z87.71 Personal history of (corrected) congenital malformations of genitourinary system**
      **Z87.710 Personal history of (corrected) hypospadias** ♂
      **Z87.718 Personal history of other specified (corrected) congenital malformations of genitourinary system**

   **✓6ᵗʰ Z87.72 Personal history of (corrected) congenital malformations of nervous system and sense organs**
      **Z87.720 Personal history of (corrected) congenital malformations of eye**
      **Z87.721 Personal history of (corrected) congenital malformations of ear**
      **Z87.728 Personal history of other specified (corrected) congenital malformations of nervous system and sense organs**

   **✓6ᵗʰ Z87.73 Personal history of (corrected) congenital malformations of digestive system**
      **Z87.730 Personal history of (corrected) cleft lip and palate**
      **Z87.738 Personal history of other specified (corrected) congenital malformations of digestive system**

   **Z87.74 Personal history of (corrected) congenital malformations of heart and circulatory system**

   **Z87.75 Personal history of (corrected) congenital malformations of respiratory system**

   **Z87.76 Personal history of (corrected) congenital malformations of integument, limbs and musculoskeletal system**

   **✓6ᵗʰ Z87.79 Personal history of other (corrected) congenital malformations**
      **Z87.790 Personal history of (corrected) congenital malformations of face and neck**
      **Z87.798 Personal history of other (corrected) congenital malformations**

**✓5ᵗʰ Z87.8 Personal history of other specified conditions**
> **EXCLUDES 2** *personal history of self harm (Z91.5)*

   **Z87.81 Personal history of (healed) traumatic fracture**
> **EXCLUDES 2** *personal history of (healed) nontraumatic fracture (Z87.31-)*

   **✓6ᵗʰ Z87.82 Personal history of other (healed) physical injury and trauma**
Conditions classifiable to S00-T88, except traumatic fractures
      **Z87.820 Personal history of traumatic brain injury**
> **EXCLUDES 1** *personal history of transient ischemic attack (TIA), and cerebral infarction without residual deficits (Z86.73)*
      **Z87.821 Personal history of retained foreign body fully removed**
      **Z87.828 Personal history of other (healed) physical injury and trauma**

   **✓6ᵗʰ Z87.89 Personal history of other specified conditions**
      **Z87.890 Personal history of sex reassignment**
      **Z87.891 Personal history of nicotine dependence**
> **EXCLUDES 1** *current nicotine dependence (F17.2-)*
> **AHA:** 2017, 2Q, 27
      **Z87.892 Personal history of anaphylaxis**
Code also allergy status such as:
allergy status to drugs, medicaments and biological substances (Z88.-)
allergy status, other than to drugs and biological substances (Z91.0-)

      **Z87.898 Personal history of other specified conditions**
> **AHA:** 2013, 1Q, 21

**✓4ᵗʰ Z88 Allergy status to drugs, medicaments and biological substances**
> **EXCLUDES 2** *allergy status, other than to drugs and biological substances (Z91.0-)*
> **AHA:** 2015, 3Q, 23

   **Z88.0 Allergy status to penicillin**
   **Z88.1 Allergy status to other antibiotic agents status**
   **Z88.2 Allergy status to sulfonamides status**
   **Z88.3 Allergy status to other anti-infective agents status**
   **Z88.4 Allergy status to anesthetic agent status**
   **Z88.5 Allergy status to narcotic agent status**
   **Z88.6 Allergy status to analgesic agent status**
   **Z88.7 Allergy status to serum and vaccine status**
   **Z88.8 Allergy status to other drugs, medicaments and biological substances status**
   **Z88.9 Allergy status to unspecified drugs, medicaments and biological substances status**

**✓4ᵗʰ Z89 Acquired absence of limb**
> **INCLUDES** amputation status
> postprocedural loss of limb
> post-traumatic loss of limb
> **EXCLUDES 1** *acquired deformities of limbs (M20-M21)*
> *congenital absence of limbs (Q71-Q73)*

   **✓5ᵗʰ Z89.0 Acquired absence of thumb and other finger(s)**
     **✓6ᵗʰ Z89.01 Acquired absence of thumb**
      **Z89.011 Acquired absence of right thumb**
      **Z89.012 Acquired absence of left thumb**
      **Z89.019 Acquired absence of unspecified thumb**
     **✓6ᵗʰ Z89.02 Acquired absence of other finger(s)**
> **EXCLUDES 2** *acquired absence of thumb (Z89.01-)*
      **Z89.021 Acquired absence of right finger(s)**
      **Z89.022 Acquired absence of left finger(s)**
      **Z89.029 Acquired absence of unspecified finger(s)**

   **✓5ᵗʰ Z89.1 Acquired absence of hand and wrist**
     **✓6ᵗʰ Z89.11 Acquired absence of hand**
      **Z89.111 Acquired absence of right hand**
      **Z89.112 Acquired absence of left hand**
      **Z89.119 Acquired absence of unspecified hand**
     **✓6ᵗʰ Z89.12 Acquired absence of wrist**
Disarticulation at wrist
      **Z89.121 Acquired absence of right wrist**
      **Z89.122 Acquired absence of left wrist**
      **Z89.129 Acquired absence of unspecified wrist**

   **✓5ᵗʰ Z89.2 Acquired absence of upper limb above wrist**
     **✓6ᵗʰ Z89.20 Acquired absence of upper limb, unspecified level**
      **Z89.201 Acquired absence of right upper limb, unspecified level**
      **Z89.202 Acquired absence of left upper limb, unspecified level**
      **Z89.209 Acquired absence of unspecified upper limb, unspecified level**
Acquired absence of arm NOS
     **✓6ᵗʰ Z89.21 Acquired absence of upper limb below elbow**
      **Z89.211 Acquired absence of right upper limb below elbow**
      **Z89.212 Acquired absence of left upper limb below elbow**
      **Z89.219 Acquired absence of unspecified upper limb below elbow**
     **✓6ᵗʰ Z89.22 Acquired absence of upper limb above elbow**
Disarticulation at elbow
      **Z89.221 Acquired absence of right upper limb above elbow**
      **Z89.222 Acquired absence of left upper limb above elbow**
      **Z89.229 Acquired absence of unspecified upper limb above elbow**
     **✓6ᵗʰ Z89.23 Acquired absence of shoulder**
Acquired absence of shoulder joint following explantation of shoulder joint prosthesis, with or without presence of antibiotic-impregnated cement spacer
      **Z89.231 Acquired absence of right shoulder**

**N** Newborn: 0   **P** Pediatric: 0-17   **M** Maternity: 12-55   **A** Adult: 15-124   **MCC** Major CC Condition   **PDxMCC** PDx acts as own MCC   **CC** CC Condition   **PDxCC** PDx acts as own CC

1244                                                        ICD-10-CM 2018

Z89.232   Acquired absence of left shoulder
Z89.239   Acquired absence of unspecified shoulder

√5th **Z89.4**   **Acquired absence of toe(s), foot, and ankle**

√6th **Z89.41**   **Acquired absence of great toe**
Z89.411   Acquired absence of right great toe   `HCC`
Z89.412   Acquired absence of left great toe   `HCC`
Z89.419   Acquired absence of unspecified great toe   `HCC`

√6th **Z89.42**   **Acquired absence of other toe(s)**
*EXCLUDES 2*   acquired absence of great toe (Z89.41-)
Z89.421   Acquired absence of other right toe(s)   `HCC`
Z89.422   Acquired absence of other left toe(s)   `HCC`
Z89.429   Acquired absence of other toe(s), unspecified side   `HCC`

√6th **Z89.43**   **Acquired absence of foot**
Z89.431   Acquired absence of right foot   `HCC`
Z89.432   Acquired absence of left foot   `HCC`
Z89.439   Acquired absence of unspecified foot   `HCC`

√6th **Z89.44**   **Acquired absence of ankle**
Disarticulation of ankle
Z89.441   Acquired absence of right ankle   `HCC`
Z89.442   Acquired absence of left ankle   `HCC`
Z89.449   Acquired absence of unspecified ankle   `HCC`

√5th **Z89.5**   **Acquired absence of leg below knee**

√6th **Z89.51**   **Acquired absence of leg below knee**
Z89.511   Acquired absence of right leg below knee   `HCC`
Z89.512   Acquired absence of left leg below knee   `HCC`
Z89.519   Acquired absence of unspecified leg below knee   `HCC`

√6th **Z89.52**   **Acquired absence of knee**
Acquired absence of knee joint following explantation of knee joint prosthesis, with or without presence of antibiotic-impregnated cement spacer
Z89.521   Acquired absence of right knee
Z89.522   Acquired absence of left knee
Z89.529   Acquired absence of unspecified knee

√5th **Z89.6**   **Acquired absence of leg above knee**

√6th **Z89.61**   **Acquired absence of leg above knee**
Acquired absence of leg NOS
Disarticulation at knee
Z89.611   Acquired absence of right leg above knee   `HCC`
Z89.612   Acquired absence of left leg above knee   `HCC`
Z89.619   Acquired absence of unspecified leg above knee   `HCC`

√6th **Z89.62**   **Acquired absence of hip**
Acquired absence of hip joint following explantation of hip joint prosthesis, with or without presence of antibiotic-impregnated cement spacer
Disarticulation at hip
Z89.621   Acquired absence of right hip joint
Z89.622   Acquired absence of left hip joint
Z89.629   Acquired absence of unspecified hip joint

**Z89.9**   **Acquired absence of limb, unspecified**

√4th **Z90**   **Acquired absence of organs, not elsewhere classified**
*INCLUDES*   postprocedural or post-traumatic loss of body part NEC
*EXCLUDES 1*   congenital absence—see Alphabetical Index
*EXCLUDES 2*   postprocedural absence of endocrine glands (E89.-)

√5th **Z90.0**   **Acquired absence of part of head and neck**
Z90.01   Acquired absence of eye
Z90.02   Acquired absence of larynx
Z90.09   Acquired absence of other part of head and neck
Acquired absence of nose
*EXCLUDES 2*   teeth (K08.1)

√5th **Z90.1**   **Acquired absence of breast and nipple**
Z90.10   Acquired absence of unspecified breast and nipple
Z90.11   Acquired absence of right breast and nipple
Z90.12   Acquired absence of left breast and nipple
Z90.13   Acquired absence of bilateral breasts and nipples

**Z90.2**   **Acquired absence of lung [part of]**
**Z90.3**   **Acquired absence of stomach [part of]**

√5th **Z90.4**   **Acquired absence of other specified parts of digestive tract**

√6th **Z90.41**   **Acquired absence of pancreas**
Code also exocrine pancreatic insufficiency (K86.81)
Use additional code to identify any associated:
insulin use (Z79.4)
diabetes mellitus, postpancreatectomy (E13.-)
Z90.410   Acquired total absence of pancreas
Acquired absence of pancreas NOS
Z90.411   Acquired partial absence of pancreas
Z90.49   Acquired absence of other specified parts of digestive tract

**Z90.5**   **Acquired absence of kidney**
**Z90.6**   **Acquired absence of other parts of urinary tract**
Acquired absence of bladder

√5th **Z90.7**   **Acquired absence of genital organ(s)**
*EXCLUDES 1*   personal history of sex reassignment (Z87.890)
*EXCLUDES 2*   female genital mutilation status (N90.81-)

√6th **Z90.71**   **Acquired absence of cervix and uterus**
Z90.710   Acquired absence of both cervix and uterus   ♀
Acquired absence of uterus NOS
Status post total hysterectomy
Z90.711   Acquired absence of uterus with remaining cervical stump   ♀
Status post partial hysterectomy with remaining cervical stump
Z90.712   Acquired absence of cervix with remaining uterus   ♀

√6th **Z90.72**   **Acquired absence of ovaries**
Z90.721   Acquired absence of ovaries, unilateral   ♀
Z90.722   Acquired absence of ovaries, bilateral   ♀
Z90.79   Acquired absence of other genital organ(s)

√5th **Z90.8**   **Acquired absence of other organs**
Z90.81   Acquired absence of spleen
Z90.89   Acquired absence of other organs

√4th **Z91**   **Personal risk factors, not elsewhere classified**
*EXCLUDES 2*   contact with and (suspected) exposures hazardous to health (Z77.-)
exposure to pollution and other problems related to physical environment (Z77.1-)
►female genital mutilation status (N90.81-)◄
personal history of physical injury and trauma (Z87.81, Z87.82-)
occupational exposure to risk factors (Z57.-)

√5th **Z91.0**   **Allergy status, other than to drugs and biological substances**
*EXCLUDES 2*   allergy status to drugs, medicaments, and biological substances (Z88.-)

√6th **Z91.01**   **Food allergy status**
*EXCLUDES 2*   food additives allergy status (Z91.02)
Z91.010   Allergy to peanuts
Z91.011   Allergy to milk products
*EXCLUDES 1*   lactose intolerance (E73.-)
Z91.012   Allergy to eggs
Z91.013   Allergy to seafood
Allergy to shellfish
Allergy to octopus or squid ink
Z91.018   Allergy to other foods
Allergy to nuts other than peanuts

**Z91.02**   **Food additives allergy status**

√6th **Z91.03**   **Insect allergy status**
Z91.030   Bee allergy status
Z91.038   Other insect allergy status

√6th **Z91.04**   **Nonmedicinal substance allergy status**
Z91.040   Latex allergy status
Latex sensitivity status
Z91.041   Radiographic dye allergy status
Allergy status to contrast media used for diagnostic X-ray procedure
Z91.048   Other nonmedicinal substance allergy status
Z91.09   Other allergy status, other than to drugs and biological substances

√5th **Z91.1**   **Patient's noncompliance with medical treatment and regimen**
Z91.11   Patient's noncompliance with dietary regimen

---

√ Additional Character Req    √x7th Placeholder Alert    Unacceptable PDx    Manifestation    H1 - H14 HAC    `HCC` CMS-HCC Condition    *EXCLUDES 1* Not Coded Here    *EXCLUDES 2* Not Included Here

ICD-10-CM 2018        1245

**✓6ᵗʰ Z91.12 Patient's intentional underdosing of medication regimen**
Code first underdosing of medication (T36-T5Ø) with fifth or sixth character 6
> **EXCLUDES 1** adverse effect of prescribed drug taken as directed—code to adverse effect
> poisoning (overdose)—code to poisoning

**Z91.12Ø Patient's intentional underdosing of medication regimen due to financial hardship**

**Z91.128 Patient's intentional underdosing of medication regimen for other reason**

**✓6ᵗʰ Z91.13 Patient's unintentional underdosing of medication regimen**
Code first underdosing of medication (T36-T5Ø) with fifth or sixth character 6
> **EXCLUDES 1** adverse effect of prescribed drug taken as directed—code to adverse effect
> poisoning (overdose)—code to poisoning

**Z91.13Ø Patient's unintentional underdosing of medication regimen due to age-related debility**

**Z91.138 Patient's unintentional underdosing of medication regimen for other reason**

**Z91.14 Patient's other noncompliance with medication regimen**
Patient's underdosing of medication NOS

**Z91.15 Patient's noncompliance with renal dialysis** HCC

**Z91.19 Patient's noncompliance with other medical treatment and regimen**
▶Nonadherence to medical treatment◀

**✓5ᵗʰ Z91.4 Personal history of psychological trauma, not elsewhere classified**

**✓6ᵗʰ Z91.41 Personal history of adult abuse**
> **EXCLUDES 2** personal history of abuse in childhood (Z62.81-)

**Z91.41Ø Personal history of adult physical and sexual abuse** A
> **EXCLUDES 1** current adult physical abuse (T74.11, T76.11)
> current adult sexual abuse (T74.21, T76.11)

**Z91.411 Personal history of adult psychological abuse** A

**Z91.412 Personal history of adult neglect** A
> **EXCLUDES 1** current adult neglect (T74.Ø1, T76.Ø1)

**Z91.419 Personal history of unspecified adult abuse** A

**Z91.49 Other personal history of psychological trauma, not elsewhere classified**

**Z91.5 Personal history of self-harm**
Personal history of parasuicide
Personal history of self-poisoning
Personal history of suicide attempt

**✓5ᵗʰ Z91.8 Other specified personal risk factors, not elsewhere classified**

**Z91.81 History of falling**
At risk for falling

**Z91.82 Personal history of military deployment** A
Individual (civilian or military) with past history of military war, peacekeeping and humanitarian deployment (current or past conflict)
Returned from military deployment

**Z91.83 Wandering in diseases classified elsewhere**
Code first underlying disorder such as:
Alzheimer's disease (G3Ø.-)
autism or pervasive developmental disorder (F84.-)
intellectual disabilities (F7Ø-F79)
unspecified dementia with behavioral disturbance (FØ3.9-)

**✓6ᵗʰ Z91.84 Oral health risk factors**

**Z91.841 Risk for dental caries, low**

**Z91.842 Risk for dental caries, moderate**

**Z91.843 Risk for dental caries, high**

**Z91.849 Unspecified risk for dental caries**

**Z91.89 Other specified personal risk factors, not elsewhere classified**
AHA: 2017, 1Q, 45

**✓4ᵗʰ Z92 Personal history of medical treatment**
> **EXCLUDES 2** postprocedural states (Z98.-)

**Z92.Ø Personal history of contraception**
> **EXCLUDES 1** counseling or management of current contraceptive practices (Z3Ø.-)
> long term (current) use of contraception (Z79.3)
> presence of (intrauterine) contraceptive device (Z97.5)

**✓5ᵗʰ Z92.2 Personal history of drug therapy**
> **EXCLUDES 2** long term (current) drug therapy (Z79.-)

**Z92.21 Personal history of antineoplastic chemotherapy**

**Z92.22 Personal history of monoclonal drug therapy**

**Z92.23 Personal history of estrogen therapy**

**✓6ᵗʰ Z92.24 Personal history of steroid therapy**

**Z92.24Ø Personal history of inhaled steroid therapy**

**Z92.241 Personal history of systemic steroid therapy**
Personal history of steroid therapy NOS

**Z92.25 Personal history of immunosupression therapy**
> **EXCLUDES 2** personal history of steroid therapy (Z92.24)

**Z92.29 Personal history of other drug therapy**

**Z92.3 Personal history of irradiation**
Personal history of exposure to therapeutic radiation
> **EXCLUDES 1** exposure to radiation in the physical environment (Z77.12)
> occupational exposure to radiation (Z57.1)

**✓5ᵗʰ Z92.8 Personal history of other medical treatment**

**Z92.81 Personal history of extracorporeal membrane oxygenation (ECMO)**

**Z92.82 Status post administration of tPA (rtPA) in a different facility within the last 24 hours prior to admission to current facility**
Code first condition requiring tPA administration, such as:
acute cerebral infarction (I63.-)
acute myocardial infarction (I21-, I22-)
AHA: 2013, 4Q, 124

**Z92.83 Personal history of failed moderate sedation**
Personal history of failed conscious sedation
> **EXCLUDES 2** failed moderate sedation during procedure (T88.52)

**Z92.84 Personal history of unintended awareness under general anesthesia**
> **EXCLUDES 2** unintended awareness under general anesthesia during procedure (T88.53)

**Z92.89 Personal history of other medical treatment**

**✓4ᵗʰ Z93 Artificial opening status**
> **EXCLUDES 1** artificial openings requiring attention or management (Z43.-)
> complications of external stoma (J95.Ø-, K94.-, N99.5-)

**Z93.Ø Tracheostomy status** HCC
AHA: 2013, 4Q, 129

**Z93.1 Gastrostomy status** HCC

**Z93.2 Ileostomy status** HCC

**Z93.3 Colostomy status** HCC

**Z93.4 Other artificial openings of gastrointestinal tract status** HCC

**✓5ᵗʰ Z93.5 Cystostomy status**

**Z93.5Ø Unspecified cystostomy status** HCC

**Z93.51 Cutaneous-vesicostomy status** HCC

**Z93.52 Appendico-vesicostomy status** HCC

**Z93.59 Other cystostomy status** HCC

**Z93.6 Other artificial openings of urinary tract status** HCC
Nephrostomy status
Ureterostomy status
Urethrostomy status

**Z93.8 Other artificial opening status** HCC

**Z93.9 Artificial opening status, unspecified** HCC

**✓4ᵗʰ Z94 Transplanted organ and tissue status**
> **INCLUDES** organ or tissue replaced by heterogenous or homogenous transplant
> **EXCLUDES 1** complications of transplanted organ or tissue—see Alphabetical Index
> **EXCLUDES 2** presence of vascular grafts (Z95.-)

**Z94.Ø Kidney transplant status** CC
CC Excl: PDX collection 1489

**Z94.1** **Heart** transplant status `CC` `HCC`
　　EXCLUDES 1　*artificial heart status (Z95.812)*
　　　　　　　*heart-valve replacement status (Z95.2-Z95.4)*
　　**CC Excl:** PDX collection 1488

**Z94.2** **Lung** transplant status `CC` `HCC`
　　**CC Excl:** PDX collection 1491

**Z94.3** **Heart and lungs** transplant status `PDxCC` `CC` `HCC`
　　**CC Excl:** PDX collection 1488

**Z94.4** **Liver** transplant status `CC` `HCC`
　　**CC Excl:** PDX collection 1490

**Z94.5** **Skin** transplant status
　　Autogenous skin transplant status

**Z94.6** **Bone** transplant status

**Z94.7** **Corneal** transplant status

✓5ᵗʰ **Z94.8** **Other transplanted organ and tissue status**
　　**Z94.81** **Bone marrow** transplant status `CC` `HCC`
　　　　**CC Excl:** PDX collection 1492
　　**Z94.82** **Intestine** transplant status `CC` `HCC`
　　　　**CC Excl:** PDX collection 1495
　　**Z94.83** **Pancreas** transplant status `CC` `HCC`
　　　　**CC Excl:** PDX collection 1496
　　**Z94.84** **Stem cells** transplant status `CC` `HCC`
　　　　**CC Excl:** PDX collection 1497
　　**Z94.89** Other transplanted organ and tissue status

**Z94.9** **Transplanted organ and tissue status, unspecified**

✓4ᵗʰ **Z95** **Presence of cardiac and vascular implants and grafts**
　　EXCLUDES 1　*complications of cardiac and vascular devices, implants and grafts (T82.-)*
　　EXCLUDES 2　▶*complications of cardiac and vascular devices, implants and grafts (T82.-)*◄

**Z95.0** **Presence of cardiac pacemaker**
　　Presence of cardiac resynchronization therapy (CRT-P) pacemaker
　　EXCLUDES 1　*adjustment or management of cardiac device (Z45.0-)*
　　　　　　　*adjustment or management of cardiac pacemaker (Z45.0)*
　　　　　　　*presence of automatic (implantable) cardiac defibrillator with synchronous cardiac pacemaker (Z95.810)*

**Z95.1** **Presence of aortocoronary bypass graft**
　　Presence of coronary artery bypass graft

**Z95.2** **Presence of prosthetic heart valve**
　　Presence of heart valve NOS

**Z95.3** **Presence of xenogenic heart valve**

**Z95.4** **Presence of other heart-valve replacement**

**Z95.5** **Presence of coronary angioplasty implant and graft**
　　EXCLUDES 1　*coronary angioplasty status without implant and graft (Z98.61)*

✓5ᵗʰ **Z95.8** **Presence of other cardiac and vascular implants and grafts**
　　✓6ᵗʰ **Z95.81** **Presence of other cardiac implants and grafts**
　　　　**Z95.810** **Presence of automatic (implantable) cardiac defibrillator**
　　　　　　Presence of automatic (implantable) cardiac defibrillator with synchronous cardiac pacemaker
　　　　　　Presence of cardiac resynchronization therapy defibrillator (CRT-D)
　　　　　　Presence of cardioverter-defibrillator (ICD)
　　　　**Z95.811** **Presence of heart assist device** `CC` `HCC`
　　　　　　**CC Excl:** PDX collection 1498
　　　　**Z95.812** **Presence of fully implantable artificial heart** `CC` `HCC`
　　　　　　**CC Excl:** PDX collection 1498
　　　　**Z95.818** **Presence of other cardiac implants and grafts**
　　✓6ᵗʰ **Z95.82** **Presence of other vascular implants and grafts**
　　　　**Z95.820** **Peripheral vascular angioplasty status with implants and grafts**
　　　　　　EXCLUDES 1　*peripheral vascular angioplasty without implant and graft (Z98.62)*
　　　　**Z95.828** **Presence of other vascular implants and grafts**
　　　　　　Presence of intravascular prosthesis NEC

**Z95.9** **Presence of cardiac and vascular implant and graft, unspecified**

✓4ᵗʰ **Z96** **Presence of other functional implants**
　　EXCLUDES 2　*complications of internal prosthetic devices, implants and grafts (T82-T85)*
　　　　　　　*fitting and adjustment of prosthetic and other devices (Z44-Z46)*

**Z96.0** **Presence of urogenital implants**

**Z96.1** **Presence of intraocular lens**
　　Presence of pseudophakia

✓5ᵗʰ **Z96.2** **Presence of otological and audiological implants**
　　**Z96.20** **Presence of otological and audiological implant, unspecified**
　　**Z96.21** **Cochlear implant status**
　　**Z96.22** **Myringotomy tube(s) status**
　　**Z96.29** **Presence of other otological and audiological implants**
　　　　Presence of bone-conduction hearing device
　　　　Presence of eustachian tube stent
　　　　Stapes replacement

**Z96.3** **Presence of artificial larynx**

✓5ᵗʰ **Z96.4** **Presence of endocrine implants**
　　**Z96.41** **Presence of insulin pump (external) (internal)**
　　**Z96.49** **Presence of other endocrine implants**

**Z96.5** **Presence of tooth-root and mandibular implants**

✓5ᵗʰ **Z96.6** **Presence of orthopedic joint implants**
　　**Z96.60** **Presence of unspecified orthopedic joint implant**
　　✓6ᵗʰ **Z96.61** **Presence of artificial shoulder joint**
　　　　**Z96.611** **Presence of right artificial shoulder joint**
　　　　**Z96.612** **Presence of left artificial shoulder joint**
　　　　**Z96.619** **Presence of unspecified artificial shoulder joint**
　　✓6ᵗʰ **Z96.62** **Presence of artificial elbow joint**
　　　　**Z96.621** **Presence of right artificial elbow joint**
　　　　**Z96.622** **Presence of left artificial elbow joint**
　　　　**Z96.629** **Presence of unspecified artificial elbow joint**
　　✓6ᵗʰ **Z96.63** **Presence of artificial wrist joint**
　　　　**Z96.631** **Presence of right artificial wrist joint**
　　　　**Z96.632** **Presence of left artificial wrist joint**
　　　　**Z96.639** **Presence of unspecified artificial wrist joint**
　　✓6ᵗʰ **Z96.64** **Presence of artificial hip joint**
　　　　Hip-joint replacement (partial) (total)
　　　　**Z96.641** **Presence of right artificial hip joint**
　　　　**Z96.642** **Presence of left artificial hip joint**
　　　　**Z96.643** **Presence of artificial hip joint, bilateral**
　　　　**Z96.649** **Presence of unspecified artificial hip joint**
　　✓6ᵗʰ **Z96.65** **Presence of artificial knee joint**
　　　　**Z96.651** **Presence of right artificial knee joint**
　　　　**Z96.652** **Presence of left artificial knee joint**
　　　　**Z96.653** **Presence of artificial knee joint, bilateral**
　　　　**Z96.659** **Presence of unspecified artificial knee joint**
　　✓6ᵗʰ **Z96.66** **Presence of artificial ankle joint**
　　　　**Z96.661** **Presence of right artificial ankle joint**
　　　　**Z96.662** **Presence of left artificial ankle joint**
　　　　**Z96.669** **Presence of unspecified artificial ankle joint**
　　✓6ᵗʰ **Z96.69** **Presence of other orthopedic joint implants**
　　　　**Z96.691** **Finger-joint replacement of right hand**
　　　　**Z96.692** **Finger-joint replacement of left hand**
　　　　**Z96.693** **Finger-joint replacement, bilateral**
　　　　**Z96.698** **Presence of other orthopedic joint implants**

**Z96.7** **Presence of other bone and tendon implants**
　　Presence of skull plate

✓5ᵗʰ **Z96.8** **Presence of other specified functional implants**
　　**Z96.81** **Presence of artificial skin**
　　**Z96.89** **Presence of other specified functional implants**

**Z96.9** **Presence of functional implant, unspecified**

☑4ᵗʰ **Z97 Presence of other devices**

> EXCLUDES 1   *complications of internal prosthetic devices, implants and grafts (T82-T85)*
> *fitting and adjustment of prosthetic and other devices (Z44-Z46)*
>
> EXCLUDES 2   *presence of cerebrospinal fluid drainage device (Z98.2)*

**Z97.0 Presence of artificial eye**

✓5ᵗʰ **Z97.1 Presence of artificial limb (complete) (partial)**

    **Z97.10 Presence of artificial limb (complete) (partial), unspecified**

    **Z97.11 Presence of artificial right arm (complete) (partial)**

    **Z97.12 Presence of artificial left arm (complete) (partial)**

    **Z97.13 Presence of artificial right leg (complete) (partial)**

    **Z97.14 Presence of artificial left leg (complete) (partial)**

    **Z97.15 Presence of artificial arms, bilateral (complete) (partial)**

    **Z97.16 Presence of artificial legs, bilateral (complete) (partial)**

**Z97.2 Presence of dental prosthetic device (complete) (partial)**
    Presence of dentures (complete) (partial)

**Z97.3 Presence of spectacles and contact lenses**

**Z97.4 Presence of external hearing-aid**

**Z97.5 Presence of (intrauterine) contraceptive device** ♀

> EXCLUDES 1   *checking, reinsertion or removal of implantable subdermal contraceptive (Z30.46)*
> *checking, reinsertion or removal of intrauterine contraceptive device (Z30.43-)*

**Z97.8 Presence of other specified devices**

☑4ᵗʰ **Z98 Other postprocedural states**

> EXCLUDES 2   *aftercare (Z43-Z49, Z51)*
> *follow-up medical care (Z08- Z09)*
> *postprocedural complication—see Alphabetical Index*

**Z98.0 Intestinal bypass and anastomosis status**

> EXCLUDES 2   *bariatric surgery status (Z98.84)*
> *gastric bypass status (Z98.84)*
> *obesity surgery status (Z98.84)*

**Z98.1 Arthrodesis status**

**Z98.2 Presence of cerebrospinal fluid drainage device**
    Presence of CSF shunt

**Z98.3 Post therapeutic collapse of lung status**
    Code first underlying disease

✓5ᵗʰ **Z98.4 Cataract extraction status**
    Use additional code to identify intraocular lens implant status (Z96.1)

> EXCLUDES 1   *aphakia (H27.0)*

    **Z98.41 Cataract extraction status, right eye**

    **Z98.42 Cataract extraction status, left eye**

    **Z98.49 Cataract extraction status, unspecified eye**

✓5ᵗʰ **Z98.5 Sterilization status**

> EXCLUDES 1   *female infertility (N97.-)*
> *male infertility (N46.-)*

    **Z98.51 Tubal ligation status** ♀

    **Z98.52 Vasectomy status** Ⓐ♂

✓5ᵗʰ **Z98.6 Angioplasty status**

    **Z98.61 Coronary angioplasty status**

> EXCLUDES 1   *coronary angioplasty status with implant and graft (Z95.5)*

    **Z98.62 Peripheral vascular angioplasty status**

> EXCLUDES 1   *peripheral vascular angioplasty status with implant and graft (Z95.820)*

✓5ᵗʰ **Z98.8 Other specified postprocedural states**

    ✓6ᵗʰ **Z98.81 Dental procedure status**

      **Z98.810 Dental sealant status**

      **Z98.811 Dental restoration status**
       Dental crown status
       Dental fillings status

      **Z98.818 Other dental procedure status**

    **Z98.82 Breast implant status**

> EXCLUDES 1   *breast implant removal status (Z98.86)*

    **Z98.83 Filtering (vitreous) bleb after glaucoma surgery status**

> EXCLUDES 1   *inflammation (infection) of postprocedural bleb (H59.4-)*

**Z98.84 Bariatric surgery status**
    Gastric banding status
    Gastric bypass status for obesity
    Obesity surgery status

> EXCLUDES 1   *bariatric surgery status complicating pregnancy, childbirth, or the puerperium (O99.84)*
>
> EXCLUDES 2   *intestinal bypass and anastomosis status (Z98.0)*

**Z98.85 Transplanted organ removal status**
    Transplanted organ previously removed due to complication, failure, rejection or infection

> EXCLUDES 1   *encounter for removal of transplanted organ—code to complication of transplanted organ (T86.-)*

**Z98.86 Personal history of breast implant removal**

✓6ᵗʰ **Z98.87 Personal history of in utero procedure**

    **Z98.870 Personal history of in utero procedure during pregnancy** ♀

> EXCLUDES 2   *complications from in utero procedure for current pregnancy (O35.7)*
> *supervision of current pregnancy with history of in utero procedure during previous pregnancy (O09.82-)*

    **Z98.871 Personal history of in utero procedure while a fetus**

✓6ᵗʰ **Z98.89 Other specified postprocedural states**

    **Z98.890 Other specified postprocedural states**
      Personal history of surgery, not elsewhere classified

    **Z98.891 History of uterine scar from previous surgery**

> EXCLUDES 1   *maternal care due to uterine scar from previous surgery (O34.2-)*

✓4ᵗʰ **Z99 Dependence on enabling machines and devices, not elsewhere classified**

> EXCLUDES 1   *cardiac pacemaker status (Z95.0)*

**Z99.0 Dependence on aspirator**

✓5ᵗʰ **Z99.1 Dependence on respirator**
    Dependence on ventilator

> **CC Excl: For CC codes in subcategory Z99.1, unless otherwise noted:** PDX collection 759

    **Z99.11 Dependence on respirator [ventilator] status** CC HCC
      **AHA:** 2015, 1Q, 21

    **Z99.12 Encounter for respirator [ventilator] dependence during power failure** CC HCC

> EXCLUDES 1   *mechanical complication of respirator [ventilator] (J95.850)*

**Z99.2 Dependence on renal dialysis** HCC
    Hemodialysis status
    Peritoneal dialysis status
    Presence of arteriovenous shunt for dialysis
    Renal dialysis status NOS

> EXCLUDES 1   *encounter for fitting and adjustment of dialysis catheter (Z49.0-)*
>
> EXCLUDES 2   *noncompliance with renal dialysis (Z91.15)*

    **AHA:** 2016, 1Q, 12; 2013, 4Q, 125

**Z99.3 Dependence on wheelchair**
    Wheelchair confinement status
    Code first cause of dependence, such as:
      muscular dystrophy (G71.0)
      obesity (E66.-)

✓5ᵗʰ **Z99.8 Dependence on other enabling machines and devices**

    **Z99.81 Dependence on supplemental oxygen**
      Dependence on long-term oxygen
      **AHA:** 2013, 4Q, 129

    **Z99.89 Dependence on other enabling machines and devices**
      Dependence on machine or device NOS

Ⓝ Newborn: 0   Ⓟ Pediatric: 0-17   Ⓜ Maternity: 12-55   Ⓐ Adult: 15-124   MCC Major CC Condition   PDxMCC PDx acts as own MCC   CC CC Condition   PDxCC PDx acts as own CC

1248       ICD-10-CM 2018

# Appendixes

## Appendix A: 10 Steps to Correct Coding

Follow the 10 steps below to correctly code encounters for health care services.

### Step 1: Identify the reason for the visit or encounter (i.e., a sign, symptom, diagnosis and/or condition).
The medical record documentation should accurately reflect the patient's condition, using terminology that includes specific diagnoses and symptoms or clearly states the reasons for the encounter.

Choosing the main term that best describes the reason chiefly responsible for the service provided is the most important step in coding. If symptoms are present and documented but a definitive diagnosis has not yet been determined, code the symptoms. **For outpatient cases, do not code conditions that are referred to as "rule out," "suspected," "probable," or "questionable."** Diagnoses often are not established at the time of the initial encounter/visit and may require two or more visits to be established. Code only what is documented in the available records and only to the highest degree of certainty known at the time of the patient's visit, unless it is an inpatient medical record, in which case uncertain diagnoses may be reported if documented at the time of discharge.

### Step 2: After selecting the reason for the encounter, always consult the alphabetic index before verifying code selection in the tabular section.
The most critical rule is to begin code selection in the *alphabetic index.* Never turn first to the tabular list. The index provides cross-references, essential and nonessential modifiers, and inclusion terms not found in the tabular list. To prevent coding errors, always use both the alphabetic index (to identify a code) and the tabular list (to verify a code), as the index does not include the important instructional notes found in the tabular list. An added benefit of using the tabular list, which groups like things together, is that while looking at one code in the list, a coder might see a more specific one that would have been missed had the coder relied solely on the alphabetic index. Additionally, many of the codes require a fourth, fifth, sixth, or seventh, character to be valid, and many of these characters can be found only in the tabular list.

### Step 3: Locate the main term entry.
The alphabetic index is a listing of conditions, which may be expressed as nouns or eponyms, with critical use of adjectives. Some conditions known by several names have multiple main entries. Reasons for encounters may be located under general terms such as admission, encounter, and examination. Other general terms such as history of, status post, or presence (of) are used to locate factors influencing health.

### Step 4: Read cross-references listed with the main term or the subterm.
Cross-references such as *"see"* and *"see also"* are identified by italicized type and should always be checked to ensure that all alternative terms are researched.

### Step 5: Review entries for modifiers.
Nonessential modifiers are the terms in parentheses following the main term entry. These parenthetical terms are supplementary words or explanatory information that may or may not appear in the diagnostic statement and do not affect code selection. The subterms listed under the main term are essential modifiers that do affect coding assignment. Each line of indent represents a more specific code entry. The nonessential modifiers apply to the subterms following a main term except when they are mutually exclusive, in which case the subterm takes precedence. For example, if "acute" is listed as a nonessential modifier but there is a subentry for "chronic," then the nonessential modifier of "acute" does not apply.

### Step 6: Interpret abbreviations, cross-references, default codes, additional characters, and brackets.
The abbreviation NEC (not elsewhere classified) that follows some main terms or subterms indicates that there is no specific code for the condition even though the medical documentation may be very specific. The code next to the main term is called the default code. It represents the condition most commonly associated with the main term or the unspecified code for the main term. Additional characters may be required to construct the code; the tabular list must be referenced to determine what those specific characters should be. The alphabetic index uses brackets [ ] to enclose manifestation codes that can be

used only as secondary codes to the underlying condition code immediately preceding it. Both codes must be reported in this multiple-coding situation.

### Step 7: Choose a potential code and locate it in the tabular list.
The coder must follow any Includes, Excludes 1 and Excludes 2 notes, and other instructional notes, such as "Code first" and "Use additional code," listed in the tabular list for the chapter, category, subcategory, and subclassification level of code selection that direct the coder to use a different or additional code. Any codes in the tabular range, A00.0- through T88.9-, may be used to identify the diagnostic reason for the encounter. The tabular list encompasses many codes describing disease and injury classifications (e.g., infectious and parasitic diseases, neoplasms, symptoms, nervous and circulatory system etc.).

Codes that describe symptoms and signs, as opposed to definitive diagnoses, should be reported when an established diagnosis has not been made (confirmed) by the physician. Chapter 18 of the ICD-10-CM code book, "Symptoms, Signs, and Abnormal Clinical and Laboratory Findings, Not Elsewhere Classified" (codes R00.--R99), contains many, but not all, codes for symptoms.

ICD-10-CM classifies encounters with health care providers for circumstances other than a disease or injury using codes in chapter 21, "Factors Influencing Health Status and Contact with Health Services" (codes Z00–Z99). Circumstances other than a disease or injury often are recorded as chiefly responsible for the encounter.

### Step 8: Determine whether the code is at the highest level of specificity.
A code is invalid if it has not been coded to the full number of characters (greatest level of specificity) required. Codes in ICD-10-CM can contain from three up to seven alphanumeric characters. A three-character code is to be used only if the category is not further subdivided into four-, five-, six-, or seven-character codes. Placeholder character X is used both to allow for future expansion and as a placeholder for empty characters in a code that requires a seventh character but has no fourth, fifth, or sixth character. Certain categories require seventh characters that apply to all codes in that category. Always check the category level for applicable seventh characters for that category.

### Step 9: Assign the code.
Having reviewed all relevant information concerning the possible code choices, assign the code that most completely describes the condition.

Repeat steps one through nine for all additional documented conditions that meet the following criteria:

- Conditions that currently exist at the time of the visit
- Conditions that require or affect patient care, treatment, or management

### Step 10: Sequence codes correctly.
Sequencing is the order in which the codes are listed on the claim. List first the ICD-10-CM code for the diagnosis, condition, problem, or other reason for the encounter/visit, which is shown in the medical record to be chiefly responsible for the services provided. List additional codes that describe any coexisting conditions. Follow the official coding guidelines (see section II, "Selection of Principal Diagnosis"; section III, "Reporting Additional Diagnoses"; and section IV, "Diagnostic Coding and Reporting Guidelines for Outpatient Services") on proper sequencing of codes.

## Coding Examples

### Diagnosis: Anorexia
**Step 1:** The reason for the encounter was the condition, anorexia.

**Step 2:** Consult the alphabetic index.

**Step 3:** Locate the main term "Anorexia."

**Step 4:** There are no cross-references to check.

**Step 5:** Note that there are two possible subterms (essential modifiers), "hysterical" and "nervosa," neither of which is documented in this instance and therefore cannot be used in code selection. The code listed next to the main term is called the default code selection.

**Step 6:** There are no abbreviations, cross-references, additional character icons, or brackets.

**Step 7:** Turn to code R63.0 in the tabular list and read the instructional notes. In this case the Excludes 1 note indicates that anorexia nervosa and loss of appetite determined to be of nonorganic origin should be coded to a code from chapter 5. The diagnostic statement does not indicate nonorganic origin.

**Step 8:** There is no further division of the category past the fourth character subcategory. Therefore, the subcategory code level is the highest level of specificity.

**Step 9:** The default code, R63.0 Anorexia, is the correct code selection.

**Step 10:** Since anorexia is listed as the chief reason for the health care encounter, the first-listed, or principal, diagnosis is R63.0. Note that this is a chapter 18 symptom code but can be assigned since the provider did not establish a more definitive diagnosis.

## Diagnosis: Acute bronchitis

**Step 1:** The reason for the encounter was the condition, acute bronchitis.

**Step 2:** Consult the alphabetic index.

**Step 3:** Locate the main term "Bronchitis."

**Step 4:** There are cross-references to interpret.

**Step 5:** Review entries for modifiers. Since "acute" is not listed as a nonessential modifier, read past the "with" modifier until you find the subterm "acute or subacute" with a nonessential modifier of "with bronchospasm or obstruction," code J20.9.

**Step 6:** There are no abbreviations, cross-references, additional character icons, or brackets.

**Step 7:** Since there are no more appropriate subterms, turn to code J20.9 in the tabular list. The Includes note under category J20 does refer to other alternative terms for acute bronchitis. Note that the inclusion term list is not exhaustive but is only a representative selection of diagnoses that are included in the subcategory. The Excludes 1 note refers bronchitis and tracheobronchitis NOS to category J40. There are several Excludes 2 notes that, if applicable, can be coded in addition to this code.

**Step 8:** Note that the subcategories included in J20 represent acute bronchitis due to various infectious organisms that would be selected if identified in the documentation. In this case, the organism was not identified and there is no further division of the category past the fourth character subcategory. Therefore, the subcategory code level is the highest level of specificity.

**Step 9:** Assign code J20.9 Acute bronchitis, unspecified.

**Step 10:** Repeat steps 1-9 for any additional code assignments.

## Diagnosis: Infectious diarrhea

**Step 1:** The reason for the encounter was the condition, infectious diarrhea.

**Step 2:** Consult the alphabetic index.

**Step 3:** Locate the main term "Diarrhea" in the alphabetic index.

**Step 4:** There are no cross-references to check.

**Step 5:** Review entries for modifiers. Note that the nonessential modifiers (in parentheses) after the main term do not include the term "infectious," which means that the coder should search the subterms for the term "infectious." The subterm "infectious" refers to code A09.

**Step 6:** There are no abbreviations, cross-references, additional character icons, or brackets.

**Step 7:** Locate code A09 in the tabular list, and read all instructional notes under the main category and subcategories. The Includes notes does not list the term "infectious diarrhea" under code A09; however, as instructed by the alphabetic index, you should code the condition to A09. The ICD-10-CM code book implies that infectious diarrhea is the same as infectious gastroenteritis, enteritis, and colitis.

**Step 8:** There is no further division of the category past the third-character category level. Therefore, the category code level is the highest level of specificity. The final code assignment would be A09.

**Step 9:** Assign code A09 Infectious gastroenteritis and colitis, unspecified.

**Step 10:** Since infectious diarrhea is listed as the chief reason for the health care encounter, the first-listed, or principal, diagnosis is A09.

## Diagnosis: Decubitus ulcer of right elbow with skin loss and necrosis of subcutaneous tissue

**Step 1:** The reason for the encounter was the condition, decubitus ulcer.

**Step 2:** Consult the alphabetic index.

**Step 3:** Locate the main term "Ulcer" in the alphabetic index.

**Step 4:** There are no cross-references to check.

**Step 5:** This entry does not have any important nonessential modifiers; however, there are other terms such as ulcerated, ulcerating, etc., that are included as main terms. Locate the subterm "decubitus" and note that there is an italicized cross-reference to "*see* Ulcer, pressure, by site." Go to the subterm "pressure" and locate "elbow," which refers to code L89.0-.

**Step 6:** Note that the code L89.0 is followed by a dash and an additional character icon, which indicate that more characters are required. From here, the tabular list can be consulted at code L89.0-.

**Step 7:** Locate code L89.0 in the tabular list, and check the category level L89 for any instructional, Includes, and Excludes 1 and 2 notes. Note that "decubitus" is an Includes note under L89 Pressure ulcer. Excludes 2 notes indicate that if this were documented as a diabetic pressure ulcer, it would be necessary to use a code from chapter 4.

**Step 8:** Read through the subcategory codes under L89.0 and note that the fifth character describes laterality. Locate the right elbow at subcategory L89.01. See that an additional sixth character is now needed to complete the code. The sixth character specifies the stage of the ulcer, which can be determined either by the specific documentation of the stage (e.g., stage 1, stage 2) or in this case, a description that matches one of the Includes notes that follow each stage code. For example, the description in this case of "skin loss and necrosis of the subcutaneous tissue" matches the Includes notes under L89.013 Pressure ulcer of right elbow, stage 3.

**Step 9:** Assign code L89.013 Pressure ulcer of right elbow, stage 3

**Step 10:** Since the decubitus ulcer is listed as the chief reason for the health care encounter, the first-listed, or principal, diagnosis is L89.013. However, according to the Code first instructional note at the L89 category level, gangrene would be sequenced before the pressure ulcer if it were documented.

## Diagnosis: First visit for bimalleolar fracture of the right ankle due to trauma

**Step 1:** The reason for the encounter was the condition, bimalleolar fracture of the right ankle.

**Step 2:** Consult the alphabetic index.

**Step 3:** Locate the main term "Fracture" in the alphabetic index.

**Step 4:** Note that the first main term for Fracture is pathological with cross-reference to "*see also* Fracture, traumatic." Locate the main term "Fracture, traumatic."

**Step 5:** Review entries for nonessential modifiers. Locate the subterms "ankle," "bimalleolar." Note that "displaced" is a nonessential modifier following "bimalleolar," indicating that S82.84- is the default code unless the fracture is specified as nondisplaced.

**Step 6:** Note that code S82.84- is followed by a dash and an additional character icon, both of which indicate that more characters are required. From here, the tabular list can be consulted at code S82.84.

**Step 7:** Locate code S82.84 Bimalleolar fracture of lower leg, in the tabular list and check the category level S82 for any instructional, Includes, and Excludes 1 and 2 notes. See the instructional notes indicating that fractures not specified as displaced or nondisplaced default to displaced, and fractures not designated as open or closed default to closed. See also the list of appropriate seventh characters to be added to all codes from category S82.

**Step 8:** Read through the subcategory codes under S82.84, and note that the sixth character specifies displaced or nondisplaced and laterality. Locate the displaced bimalleolar fracture of the right lower leg at code S82.841. See that an additional seventh character is still needed to complete the code. The seventh character specifies the type of encounter and whether the fracture is open or closed. Use character A listed in the box at the category level to describe initial encounter, closed fracture.

**Step 9:** Assign code S82.841A Displaced bimalleolar fracture of right lower leg, initial encounter for closed fracture.

**Step 10:** Since this is an injury code, code additionally any external cause, place of occurrence, and activity codes, with the injury (fracture) sequenced first.

# Appendix B: Valid 3-character ICD-10-CM Codes

| | | | |
|---|---|---|---|
| A09 | Infectious gastroenteritis and colitis, unspecified | E46 | Unspecified protein-calorie malnutrition |
| A33 | Tetanus neonatorum | E52 | Niacin deficiency [pellagra] |
| A34 | Obstetrical tetanus | E54 | Ascorbic acid deficiency |
| A35 | Other tetanus | E58 | Dietary calcium deficiency |
| A46 | Erysipelas | E59 | Dietary selenium deficiency |
| A55 | Chlamydial lymphogranuloma (venereum) | E60 | Dietary zinc deficiency |
| A57 | Chancroid | E65 | Localized adiposity |
| A58 | Granuloma inguinale | E68 | Sequelae of hyperalimentation |
| A64 | Unspecified sexually transmitted disease | F04 | Amnestic disorder due to known physiological condition |
| A65 | Nonvenereal syphilis | F05 | Delirium due to known physiological condition |
| A70 | Chlamydia psittaci infections | F09 | Unspecified mental disorder due to known physiological condition |
| A78 | Q fever | F21 | Schizotypal disorder |
| A86 | Unspecified viral encephalitis | F22 | Delusional disorders |
| A89 | Unspecified viral infection of central nervous system | F23 | Brief psychotic disorder |
| A90 | Dengue fever [classical dengue] | F24 | Shared psychotic disorder |
| A91 | Dengue hemorrhagic fever | F28 | Other psychotic disorder not due to a substance or known physiological condition |
| A94 | Unspecified arthropod-borne viral fever | F29 | Unspecified psychosis not due to a substance or known physiological condition |
| A99 | Unspecified viral hemorrhagic fever | F39 | Unspecified mood [affective] disorder |
| B03 | Smallpox | F53 | Puerperal psychosis |
| B04 | Monkeypox | F54 | Psychological and behavioral factors associated with disorders or diseases classified elsewhere |
| B09 | Unspecified viral infection characterized by skin and mucous membrane lesions | F59 | Unspecified behavioral syndromes associated with physiological disturbances and physical factors |
| B20 | Human immunodeficiency virus [HIV] disease | F66 | Other sexual disorders |
| B49 | Unspecified mycosis | F69 | Unspecified disorder of adult personality and behavior |
| B54 | Unspecified malaria | F70 | Mild intellectual disabilities |
| B59 | Pneumocystosis | F71 | Moderate intellectual disabilities |
| B64 | Unspecified protozoal disease | F72 | Severe intellectual disabilities |
| B72 | Dracunculiasis | F73 | Profound intellectual disabilities |
| B75 | Trichinellosis | F78 | Other intellectual disabilities |
| B79 | Trichuriasis | F79 | Unspecified intellectual disabilities |
| B80 | Enterobiasis | F82 | Specific developmental disorder of motor function |
| B86 | Scabies | F88 | Other disorders of psychological development |
| B89 | Unspecified parasitic disease | F89 | Unspecified disorder of psychological development |
| B91 | Sequelae of poliomyelitis | F99 | Mental disorder, not otherwise specified |
| B92 | Sequelae of leprosy | G01 | Meningitis in bacterial diseases classified elsewhere |
| C01 | Malignant neoplasm of base of tongue | G02 | Meningitis in other infectious and parasitic diseases classified elsewhere |
| C07 | Malignant neoplasm of parotid gland | G07 | Intracranial and intraspinal abscess and granuloma in diseases classified elsewhere |
| C12 | Malignant neoplasm of pyriform sinus | | |
| C19 | Malignant neoplasm of rectosigmoid junction | G08 | Intracranial and intraspinal phlebitis and thrombophlebitis |
| C20 | Malignant neoplasm of rectum | G09 | Sequelae of inflammatory diseases of central nervous system |
| C23 | Malignant neoplasm of gallbladder | G10 | Huntington's disease |
| C33 | Malignant neoplasm of trachea | G14 | Postpolio syndrome |
| C37 | Malignant neoplasm of thymus | G20 | Parkinson's disease |
| C52 | Malignant neoplasm of vagina | G26 | Extrapyramidal and movement disorders in diseases classified elsewhere |
| C55 | Malignant neoplasm of uterus, part unspecified | | |
| C58 | Malignant neoplasm of placenta | G35 | Multiple sclerosis |
| C61 | Malignant neoplasm of prostate | G53 | Cranial nerve disorders in diseases classified elsewhere |
| C73 | Malignant neoplasm of thyroid gland | G55 | Nerve root and plexus compressions in diseases classified elsewhere |
| D34 | Benign neoplasm of thyroid gland | G59 | Mononeuropathy in diseases classified elsewhere |
| D45 | Polycythemia vera | G63 | Polyneuropathy in diseases classified elsewhere |
| D62 | Acute posthemorrhagic anemia | G64 | Other disorders of peripheral nervous system |
| D65 | Disseminated intravascular coagulation [defibrination A syndrome] | G92 | Toxic encephalopathy |
| D66 | Hereditary factor VIII deficiency | G94 | Other disorders of brain in diseases classified elsewhere |
| D67 | Hereditary factor IX deficiency | H22 | Disorders of iris and ciliary body in diseases classified elsewhere |
| D71 | Functional disorders of polymorphonuclear neutrophils | H28 | Cataract in diseases classified elsewhere |
| D77 | Other disorders of blood and blood-forming organs in diseases classified elsewhere | H32 | Chorioretinal disorders in diseases classified elsewhere |
| | | H36 | Retinal disorders in diseases classified elsewhere |
| E02 | Subclinical iodine-deficiency hypothyroidism | H42 | Glaucoma in diseases classified elsewhere |
| E15 | Nondiabetic hypoglycemic coma | I00 | Rheumatic fever without heart involvement |
| E35 | Disorders of endocrine glands in diseases classified elsewhere | I10 | Essential (primary) hypertension |
| E40 | Kwashiorkor | I32 | Pericarditis in diseases classified elsewhere |
| E41 | Nutritional marasmus | I38 | Endocarditis, valve unspecified |
| E42 | Marasmic kwashiorkor | | |
| E43 | Unspecified severe protein-calorie malnutrition | | |
| E45 | Retarded development following protein-calorie malnutrition | | |

| | |
|---|---|
| I39 | Endocarditis and heart valve disorders in diseases classified elsewhere |
| I41 | Myocarditis in diseases classified elsewhere |
| I43 | Cardiomyopathy in diseases classified elsewhere |
| I52 | Other heart disorders in diseases classified elsewhere |
| I76 | Septic arterial embolism |
| I81 | Portal vein thrombosis |
| I96 | Gangrene, not elsewhere classified |
| J00 | Acute nasopharyngitis (common cold) |
| J13 | Pneumonia due to Streptococcus pneumoniae |
| J14 | Pneumonia due to Hemophilus influenzae |
| J17 | Pneumonia in diseases classified elsewhere |
| J22 | Unspecified acute lower respiratory infection |
| J36 | Peritonsillar abscess |
| J40 | Bronchitis, not specified as acute or chronic |
| J42 | Unspecified chronic bronchitis |
| J60 | Coalworker's pneumoconiosis |
| J61 | Pneumoconiosis due to asbestos and other mineral fibers |
| J64 | Unspecified pneumoconiosis |
| J65 | Pneumoconiosis associated with tuberculosis |
| J80 | Acute respiratory distress syndrome |
| J82 | Pulmonary eosinophilia, not elsewhere classified |
| J90 | Pleural effusion, not elsewhere classified |
| J99 | Respiratory disorders in diseases classified elsewhere |
| K23 | Disorders of esophagus in diseases classified elsewhere |
| K30 | Functional dyspepsia |
| K36 | Other appendicitis |
| K37 | Unspecified appendicitis |
| K67 | Disorders of peritoneum in infectious diseases classified elsewhere |
| K77 | Liver disorders in diseases classified elsewhere |
| K87 | Disorders of gallbladder, biliary tract and pancreas in diseases classified elsewhere |
| L00 | Staphylococcal scalded skin syndrome |
| L14 | Bullous disorders in diseases classified elsewhere |
| L22 | Diaper dermatitis |
| L26 | Exfoliative dermatitis |
| L42 | Pityriasis rosea |
| L45 | Papulosquamous disorders in diseases classified elsewhere |
| L52 | Erythema nodosum |
| L54 | Erythema in diseases classified elsewhere |
| L62 | Nail disorders in diseases classified elsewhere |
| L80 | Vitiligo |
| L83 | Acanthosis nigricans |
| L84 | Corns and callosities |
| L86 | Keratoderma in diseases classified elsewhere |
| L88 | Pyoderma gangrenosum |
| L99 | Other disorders of skin and subcutaneous tissue in diseases classified elsewhere |
| N08 | Glomerular disorders in diseases classified elsewhere |
| N10 | Acute tubulo-interstitial nephritis |
| N12 | Tubulo-interstitial nephritis, not specified as acute or chronic |
| N16 | Renal tubulo-interstitial disorders in diseases classified elsewhere |
| N19 | Unspecified kidney failure |
| N22 | Calculus of urinary tract in diseases classified elsewhere |
| N23 | Unspecified renal colic |
| N29 | Other disorders of kidney and ureter in diseases classified elsewhere |
| N33 | Bladder disorders in diseases classified elsewhere |
| N37 | Urethral disorders in diseases classified elsewhere |
| N51 | Disorders of male genital organs in diseases classified elsewhere |
| N62 | Hypertrophy of breast |
| N72 | Inflammatory disease of cervix uteri |
| N74 | Female pelvic inflammatory disorders in diseases classified elsewhere |
| N86 | Erosion and ectropion of cervix uteri |
| N96 | Recurrent pregnancy loss |
| O68 | Labor and delivery complicated by abnormality of fetal acid-base balance |
| O76 | Abnormality in fetal heart rate and rhythm complicating labor and delivery |
| O80 | Encounter for full-term uncomplicated delivery |
| O82 | Encounter for cesarean delivery without indication |
| O85 | Puerperal sepsis |
| O94 | Sequelae of complication of pregnancy, childbirth, and the puerperium |
| P09 | Abnormal findings on neonatal screening |
| P53 | Hemorrhagic disease of newborn |
| P60 | Disseminated intravascular coagulation of newborn |
| P84 | Other problems with newborn |
| P90 | Convulsions of newborn |
| P95 | Stillbirth |
| Q02 | Microcephaly |
| R05 | Cough |
| R12 | Heartburn |
| R17 | Unspecified jaundice |
| R21 | Rash and other nonspecific skin eruption |
| R32 | Unspecified urinary incontinence |
| R34 | Anuria and oliguria |
| R37 | Sexual dysfunction, unspecified |
| R42 | Dizziness and giddiness |
| R51 | Headache |
| R52 | Pain, unspecified |
| R54 | Age-related physical debility |
| R55 | Syncope and collapse |
| R58 | Hemorrhage, not elsewhere classified |
| R61 | Generalized hyperhidrosis |
| R64 | Cachexia |
| R69 | Illness, unspecified |
| R75 | Inconclusive laboratory evidence of human immunodeficiency virus [HIV] |
| R81 | Glycosuria |
| R99 | Ill-defined and unknown cause of mortality |
| Y09 | Assault by unspecified means |
| Y66 | Nonadministration of surgical and medical care |
| Y69 | Unspecified misadventure during surgical and medical care |
| Y95 | Nosocomial condition |
| Z08 | Encounter for follow-up examination after completed treatment for malignant neoplasm |
| Z09 | Encounter for follow-up examination after completed treatment for conditions other than malignant neoplasm |
| Z21 | Asymptomatic human immunodeficiency virus [HIV] infection status |
| Z23 | Encounter for immunization |
| Z66 | Do not resuscitate |

Appendix B: Valid 3-character ICD-10-CM Codes

# Appendix C: Pharmacology List 2018

This section enables the coder to quickly review drugs, drug actions, and indications that are often associated with overlooked or undocumented diagnoses. The coder should review the patient's medication record and know what condition the physician is treating with the prescribed medication based on documentation in the medical record. When documentation is lacking, the coder can reference this section to locate the drug, determine the drug action, confirm drug indications, and when necessary query the physician.

| Drug | Z Code | Drug Action | Indications |
|---|---|---|---|
| Abilify [aripiprazole] | | Antipsychotic | Depression, bipolar disorder, schizophrenia, autism symptoms |
| Acarbose [acarbose] | Z79.84 | Blood glucose regulator | Diabetes mellitus |
| Accupril [quinapril hydrochloride] | | ACE inhibitor; antihypertensive | Congestive heart failure; essential hypertension |
| Acetaminophen with codeine [acetominophen/codeine phosphate] | Z79.891 | Analgesic, general; analgesic-narcotic | Pain, moderate to severe |
| Actemra [tocilizumab] | | Antirheumatic | Rheumatoid arthritis |
| Actimmune [interferon gamma-1b] | Z79.899 | Antineoplastic interferons; antiviral interferons | Chronic granulomatous disease; malignant osteopetrosis |
| Activella [estradiol/norethindrone acetate] | Z79.890 | Estrogen therapy | Menopause symptoms; vaginal and vulvar atrophy; osteoporosis prevention |
| Actonel [risedronate sodium] | Z79.83 | Electrolytic and renal agent; bone resorption inhibitor | Decrease in bone loss in multiple myeloma patients; Paget's disease; hyperparathyroidism; osteoporosis |
| Actoplus Met [metformin hydrochloride/pioglitazone hydrochloride] | Z79.84 | Blood glucose regulator | Diabetes mellitus |
| Actos [pioglitazone hydrochloride] | Z79.84 | Blood glucose regulator | Diabetes mellitus |
| Adalat CC [nifedipine] | | Calcium channel blocker | Vasospastic angina; chronic stable angina; essential hypertension |
| Advair [fluticasone propionate/salmeterol xinafoate] | Z79.51 | Corticosteroids--inhaled; antiasthmatic | Prophylaxis and treatment of asthma and COPD |
| Advil [ibuprofen] | Z79.1 | Nonsteroidal anti-inflammatory drug (NSAID) | Pain or fever relief |
| Aerospan [flunisolide] | Z79.51 | Corticosteroids--inhaled; antiasthmatic | Prophylaxis and treatment of asthma |
| Afrezza [human insulin recombinant] | Z79.4 | Blood glucose regulator | Diabetes mellitus |
| Aggrastat [tirofiban hydrochloride] | Z79.02 | Antithrombotic platelet aggregation inhibitor | Unstable angina or heart attacks |
| Aggrenox [aspirin/dipyridamole] | Z79.02 | Antithrombotic platelet aggregation inhibitor | Lessening of the chance of heart attack or stroke |
| Akne-Mycin [erythromycin] | Z79.2 | Antibacterial | Severe acne treatment |
| Aldactone [spironolactone] | | Cardiovascular agent; antihypertensive agent; diuretic; electrolytic and renal agent | Severe heart failure; ascites associated with cirrhosis; hypokalemia |
| Aleve [naproxen sodium] | Z79.1 | Nonsteroidal anti-inflammatory drug (NSAID) | Reduction of temporary aches and pains |
| Allegra [fexofenadine hydrochloride] | | Antihistamine | Seasonal allergic rhinitis |
| Allopurinol [allopurinol] | | Antigout | Gouty arthritis, renal calculus, hyperuricemia, hyperuricemia secondary to leukemia, hyperuricemia secondary to lymphoma |
| Alora [estradiol] | Z79.890 | Estrogen therapy | Menopause symptoms |
| Alphagan P [brimonidine tartrate] | | Antiglaucoma agent (ophthalmic) antihypertensive, ocular | Open angle glaucoma or another condition in which pressure in the eye is too high (ocular hypertension) |
| Alprazolam [alprazolam] | | Antianxiety; sedative/hypnotic | |
| Altabax [retapamulin] | Z79.2 | Antibacterial | Skin infections |
| Altace [ramipril] | | ACE inhibitor; antihypertensive | Congestive heart failure, essential hypertension |
| Altavera [ethinyl estradiol/levonorgestrel] | Z79.3 | Contraceptive | Contraception |
| Alvesco [ciclesonide] | Z79.51 | Corticosteroids--inhaled; antiasthmatic | Prophylaxis and treatment of asthma |
| Alyacen [ethinyl estradiol/norethindrone] | Z79.3 | Contraceptive | Contraception |
| Amaryl [glimepiride] | Z79.84 | Blood glucose regulator | Diabetes mellitus |
| Ambien [zolpidem tartrate] | | Sedative/hypnotic | Insomnia |
| A-Methapred [methylprednisolone sodium succinate] | Z79.52 | Corticosteroids | Severe inflammation |
| Amikacin [amikacin sulfate] | | Aminoglycoside antibiotic | Active in treatment of gram-negative bacterial infections such as *Pseudomonas, Escherichia coli (E. coli), Proteus, Klebsiella-Enterobacter-Serratia* |

| Drug | Z Code | Drug Action | Indications |
|------|--------|-------------|-------------|
| Aminophylline [aminophylline] | | Bronchodilator, pulmonary vasodilator, smooth muscle relaxant | Relief and/or prevention of symptoms from asthma and reversible bronchospasms in bronchitis and emphysema |
| Amitriptyline hydrochloride [amitriptyline hydrochloride] | | Anorexiant/CNS stimulant; antidepressant | Depression |
| Amoxicillin [amoxicillin] | Z79.2 | Penicillin | Effective for infections with a broad spectrum of bactericidal activity against many gram-positive and gram-negative micro-organisms; otitis media, gonorrhea, skin, respiratory, gastrointestinal, and genitourinary infections |
| Ampicillin [ampicillin sodium] | Z79.2 | Antibacterial | Bacterial infections |
| Amrix [cyclobenzaprine hydrochloride] | | Muscle relaxant | Adjunct to rest and physical therapy for muscle spasms |
| Anaprox [naproxen sodium] | Z79.1 | Nonsteroidal anti-inflammatory drug (NSAID) | Pain, inflammation, or fever relief |
| Anastrozole [anastrozole] | Z79.811 | Aromatase inhibitor | Postmenopausal breast cancer |
| Ancef [cefazolin sodium] | Z79.2 | Semisynthetic cephalosporin antibiotic | Respiratory tract infections due to *Streptococcus pneumoniae*, *Klebsiella species*, *Haemophilus influenzae (H. influenzae)*, *Staphylococcus aureus*, and group A betahemolytic streptococci; urinary tract infections due to *E. coli*, *Proteus mirabilis*, *Klebsiella* species and some strains of *Enterobacter* and enterococci; skin and skin structure infections, biliary tract infections, bone and joint infections, genital infections, septicemia, and endocarditis |
| Angeliq [drospirenone/estradiol] | Z79.89 | Estrogen therapy | Menopause symptoms |
| Angiomax [bivalirudin] | Z79.02 | Antithrombotic platelet aggregation inhibitor | Prevention of blood clots |
| Antabuse [disulfiram] | | Alcohol treatment | Alcoholism |
| Antineoplastic/chemotherapy | Z79.899 | Antineoplastic | Cancer |
| Anzemet [dolasetron mesylate] | | Antiemetic/antinauseant | Management of nausea/vomiting following surgery or from effects of chemotherapy or cancer |
| Apidra [insulin glulisine recombinant] | Z79.4 | Blood glucose regulator | Diabetes mellitus |
| Aranelle [ethinyl estradiol/norethindrone] | Z79.3 | Contraceptive | Contraception; acne |
| Aranesp [darbepoetin alfa] | | Erythropoiesis-stimulating agent (ESA) | Lower than normal blood cell count (anemia) from disorders such as CKD and neoplasms |
| Argatroban [argatroban] | Z79.2 | Antithrombotic platelet aggregation inhibitor | Prophylaxis and treatment of venous thrombosis in thrombocytopenia patients |
| Aricept [donepezil hydrochloride] | | Acetylcholine sterase inhibitor | Symptoms of mild to moderate Alzheimer's disease; can improve thinking ability in some patients |
| Arimidex [anastrozole] | Z79.811 | Aromatase inhibitor | Postmenopausal breast cancer |
| Aristospan [triamcinolone hexacetonide] | Z79.52 | Corticosteroids | Severe inflammation |
| Arixtra [fondaparinux sodium] | Z79.01 | Anticoagulant | Venous thrombosis and pulmonary embolism |
| Arnuity Ellipta [fluticasone furoate] | Z79.51 | Corticosteroids--inhaled; antiasthmatic | Prophylaxis and treatment of asthma |
| Aromasin [exemestane] | Z79.811 | Aromatase inhibitor | Postmenopausal breast cancer |
| Arthrotec [diclofenac sodium/misoprostol] | Z79.1 | Analgesic | Arthritis in patients who may develop stomach ulcers from taking nonsteroidal anti-inflammatory drugs (NSAIDs) alone; used to help relieve some symptoms of arthritis, such as inflammation, swelling, stiffness, and joint pain |
| Ashlyna [ethinyl estradiol/levonorgestrel] | Z79.3 | Contraceptive | Contraception |
| Asmanex [mometasone furoate] | Z79.51 | Corticosteroids--inhaled; antiasthmatic | Prophylaxis and treatment of asthma |
| Astagraf XL [tacrolimus] | Z79.899 | Immunosuppressant | Prophylaxis of organ transplant rejection |
| Astramorph [morphine sulfate] | Z79.891 | Narcotic analgesic | Pain |
| Atelvia [risedronate sodium] | Z79.83 | Bisphosphonates | Prevention of thinning of the bones (osteoporosis) |
| Atenolol [atenolol] | | Antianginal; antihypertensive; beta blocker | Chronic stable angina pectoris; essential hypertension; reduces cardiovascular mortality in those with definite or suspected acute myocardial infarction |
| Ativan [lorazepam] | | Antianxiety; sedative/hypnotic | Anxiety disorder associated with depressive symptoms; controls tension, agitation, irritability, and insomnia |
| Atrovent [ipratropium bromide] | | Antiasthmatic/bronchodilator | Chronic bronchitis, emphysema; bronchial asthma |
| Augmentin [amoxicillin/clavulanate potassium] | Z79.2 | Antibacterial | Middle ear, lower respiratory, sinus, skin and skin structures, and urinary tract infections |
| Avandia [rosiglitazone maleate] | Z79.84 | Blood glucose regulator | Diabetes mellitus |

| Drug | Z Code | Drug Action | Indications |
|---|---|---|---|
| Avapro [irbesartan] | | Antihypertensive | Hypertension |
| Aviane [ethinyl estradiol/levonorgestrel] | Z79.3 | Contraceptive | Contraception |
| Avonex [interferon beta-1a] | Z79.899 | Antiviral interferon | Relapsing multiple sclerosis |
| Axid AR [nizatidine] | | Histamine H2-receptor antagonist | Acid/peptic disorder; gastroesophageal reflux; duodenal, gastric, and peptic ulcers |
| Aygestin [norethindrone acetate] | Z79.3 | Contraceptive | Contraception; menstrual disorders |
| Azactam [aztreonam] | Z79.2 | Antibacterial | Severe or life-threatening bacterial infections |
| Azithromycin [azithromycin] | Z79.2 | Antibacterial | Treatment of bacterial infections |
| Bactrim [sulfamethoxazole/trimethoprim] | Z79.2 | Antibacterial | Urinary tract infections, acute otitis media, acute exacerbation of chronic bronchitis, shigellosis, and *Pneumocystis carinii* |
| Bactroban [mupirocin] | Z79.2 | Dermatologic; topical anti-infective | Topical treatment of impetigo |
| Balziva [ethinyl estradiol/norethindrone] | Z79.3 | Contraceptive | Contraception |
| Basaglar [insulin glargine] | Z79.4 | Blood glucose regulator | Diabetes mellitus |
| Bayer [acetylsalicylic acid] | Z79.82 | Aspirin | Prophylaxis and treatment of heart attacks, angina, or strokes; reduction of fever, pain, and inflammation |
| Beconase AQ [beclomethasone dipropionate monohydrate] | | Corticosteroids; antiasthmatic | Bronchial asthma, prevention of nasal polyps, perennial allergies, seasonal allergies, and vasomotor rhinitis |
| Bekyree [desogestrel/ethinyl estradiol] | Z79.3 | Contraceptive | Contraception |
| Betoptic [betaxolol hydrochloride] | | Cardioselective beta-adrenergic receptor blocking agent | Lowering of intraocular pressure; also used for treatment of ocular hypertension and chronic open-angle glaucoma |
| Beyaz [drospirenone/ethinyl estradiol/levomefolate calcium] | Z79.3 | Contraceptive | Contraception; acne |
| Biaxin [clarithromycin] | | Macrolide | Acid/peptic disorder or ulcer, acute exacerbation chronic bronchitis, HIV, lower and upper respiratory tract infections, sinus infection, prophylaxis mycobacterium avium complex, pharyngitis, pneumonia, tonsillitis |
| Binosto [alendronate sodium] | Z79.83 | Bisphosphonates | Prevention of thinning of the bones (osteoporosis) |
| Boniva [ibandronate sodium] | Z79.83 | Bisphosphonates | Prevention of thinning of the bones (osteoporosis) |
| Brevicon [ethinyl estradiol/norethindrone] | Z79.3 | Contraceptive | Contraception; acne |
| Briellyn [ethinyl estradiol/norethindrone] | Z79.3 | Contraceptive | Contraception |
| Brilinta [ticagrelor] | Z79.02 | Antithrombotic platelet aggregation inhibitor | Unstable angina or heart attacks and prevention of blood clots |
| Bufferin [acetylsalicylic acid] | Z79.82 | Aspirin | Prophylaxis and treatment of heart attacks, angina or strokes; reduction of fever, pain, and inflammation |
| Buprenex [buprenorphine hydrochloride] | Z79.891 | Narcotic analgesic | Moderate to severe pain |
| Buprenorphine HCl [buprenorphine hydrochloride] | Z79.891 | Narcotic analgesic | Moderate to severe pain |
| Buspirone [buspirone hydrochloride] | | Antianxiety agent | Generalized anxiety disorder |
| Butorphanol Tartrate [butorphanol tartrate] | | Narcotic analgesic | Moderate to severe postsurgical pain |
| Butrans [buprenorphine] | Z79.891 | Narcotic analgesic | Chronic pain |
| Calan [verapamil hydrochloride] | | Antianginal; antiarrhythmic, antiarthritic, antihypertensive, calcium channel blocker | Angina pectoris at rest and chronic stable, arrhythmia, atrial fibrillation, atrial flutter, paroxysmal supraventricular tachycardia, ventricular arrhythmia, essential hypertension |
| Caldolor [ibuprofen] | Z79.1 | Nonsteroidal anti-inflammatory drug (NSAID) | Pain or fever relief |
| Cambia [diclofenac potassium] | Z79.1 | Nonsteroidal anti-inflammatory drug (NSAID) | Migraine headaches |
| Camila [norethindrone] | Z79.3 | Contraceptive | Contraception; menstrual disorders |
| Cardizem CD [diltiazem hydrochloride] | | Antianginal, antiarrhythmic, antihypertensive, channel blocker, coronary vasodilator | Chronic stable angina, atrial fibrillation, atrial flutter, essential hypertension, paroxysmal supraventricular tachycardia |
| Cardura [doxazosin mesylate] | | Antihypertensive | Benign prostatic hyperplasia, essential hypertension |
| Catapres [clonidine hydrochloride] | | Antihypertensive | Hypertension |
| Cefprozil [cefprozil] | | Antibiotic: second generation cephalosporins | Acute exacerbation and chronic bronchitis, lower and upper respiratory tract infections, pharyngitis, tonsillitis |

| Drug | Z Code | Drug Action | Indications |
|---|---|---|---|
| Ceftin [cefuroxime axetil] | | Antibiotic: second generation cephalosporins | Acute exacerbation and chronic bronchitis, middle ear infection, sexually transmitted gonorrhea infection, upper respiratory tract infection, urinary tract infection, pharyngitis, tonsillitis |
| Ceftriaxone [ceftriaxone sodium] | Z79.2 | Antibacterial | Bacterial infections |
| Celebrex [celecoxib] | Z79.1 | Antirheumatic, nonsteroidal anti-inflammatory | Relief of some symptoms caused by arthritis, such as inflammation, swelling, stiffness, and joint pain |
| Celestone Soluspan [betamethasone acetate/ betamethasone sodium phosphate] | Z79.52 | Corticosteroids; antiasthmatic | Asthma; severe inflammation |
| Celexa [citalopram hydrobromide] | | Antidepressant | Depression |
| Cellcept [mycophenolate mofetil] | Z79.899 | Immunosuppressant | Prophylaxis of organ transplant rejection |
| Centany [mupirocin] | Z79.2 | Antibacterial | Topical treatment of skin infections |
| Cephalexin [cephalexin] | Z79.2 | Antibacterial | Bacterial infections |
| Chantix [varenicline tartrate] | | Smoking cessation aid | Nicotine addiction, smoking |
| Cipro [ciprofloxacin hydrochloride] | Z79.2 | Anti-infective; quinolone | Cystitis, infectious diarrhea, gonorrhea, bone and joint infection, gastrointestinal tract infection, lower and upper respiratory tract infections, sinus infection, urinary tract infection, nosocomial pneumonia, chronic prostatitis |
| Ciprofloxacin [ciprofloxacin] | Z79.2 | Antibacterial | Bacterial infections |
| Clarithromycin [clarithromycin] | Z79.2 | Antibacterial | Skin and respiratory bacterial infections |
| Claritin [loratadine] | | Antihistamine | Seasonal allergic rhinitis, chronic idiopathic urticaria |
| Cleocin [clindamycin phosphate] | Z79.2 | Antibacterial | Bacterial infections |
| Climara [estradiol] | Z79.890 | Estrogen therapy | Osteoporosis prevention and menopausal symptoms; vaginal and vulvar atrophy; hypoestrogenism; ovarian failure |
| Clindamycin [clindamycin phosphate] | Z79.2 | Antibacterial | Bacterial infections |
| Clonazepam [clonazepam] | | Anticonvulsant | Absence, akinetic, and myoclonic epilepsy, Lennox-Gastaut syndrome |
| Clonidine [clonidine hydrochloride] | | Antihypertensive | Hypertension |
| Clopidogrel bisulfate [clopidogrel bisulfate] | Z79.02 | Antithrombotic platelet aggregation inhibitor | Treatment of unstable angina or heart attacks and prevention of blood clots |
| Codeine [codeine sulfate] | Z79.891 | Narcotic analgesic | Mild to moderate pain |
| Cogentin [benztropine mesylate] | | Antiparkinsonism | Parkinson's disease |
| Colace [docusate sodium] | | Gastrointestinal agent; laxative, stool softener | Constipation |
| Colocort [hydrocortisone] | Z79.52 | Corticosteroids | Inflammation of the colon |
| CombiPatch [ethinyl estradiol/norethindrone acetate] | Z79.890 | Estrogen therapy | Menopause symptoms; vaginal and vulvar atrophy; osteoporosis prevention |
| Combivent [ipratropium bromide/albuterol sulfate] | | Antiasthmatic/bronchodilator | Chronic bronchitis, emphysema; bronchial asthma |
| Compro [prochlorperazine] | | Antiemetic, antipsychotic | Nausea, vomiting, and manic phase of bipolar syndrome or schizophrenia |
| Cortef [hydrocortisone] | Z79.52 | Corticosteroids | Severe inflammation |
| Cortenema [hydrocortisone] | Z79.52 | Corticosteroids | Inflammation of the colon |
| Cortifoam [hydrocortisone acetate] | Z79.52 | Corticosteroids | Colon and rectum inflammation |
| Cortisone acetate [cortisone acetate] | Z79.52 | Corticosteroids | Inflammation |
| Cortisporin [hydrocortisone acetate/neomycin sulfate/polymyxin B sulfate] | | Topical anti-infective, topical steroid | Dermatosis |
| Coumadin [warfarin sodium] | Z79.01 | Anticoagulant | Prophylaxis and treatment of venous thrombosis, treatment of atrial fibrillation with embolization (pulmonary embolism), arrhythmias, myocardial infarction, and stroke prevention |
| Cozaar [losartan potassium] | | Antihypertensive | Essential hypertension |
| Crestor [rosuvastatin calcium] | | HMG-CoA reductase inhibitor (statin) | Hypercholesterolemia, hyperlipidemia, hyperproteinemia |
| Crixivan [indinavir sulfate] | | HIV inhibitor | HIV, asymptomatic HIV |
| Cryselle [ethinyl estradiol/norgestrel] | Z79.3 | Contraceptive | Contraception |
| Cyclafem [ethinyl estradiol/norethindrone] | Z79.3 | Contraceptive | Contraception |
| Cyclessa [desogestrel/ethinyl estradiol] | Z79.3 | Contraceptive | Contraception |

| Drug | Z Code | Drug Action | Indications |
|------|--------|-------------|-------------|
| Cyclosporine [cyclosporine] | Z79.899 | Immunosuppressant | Prophylaxis of organ transplant rejection |
| Cytomel [liothyronine sodium] | | Thyroid hormone | Treatment of hypothyroidism or prevention of euthyroid goiters |
| Daptomycin [daptomycin] | Z79.2 | Antibacterial | Skin and underlying tissue bacterial infections |
| Dasetta [ethinyl estradiol/norethindrone] | Z79.3 | Contraceptive | Contraception |
| Daypro [oxaprozin] | Z79.1 | Nonsteroidal anti-inflammatory drug (NSAID) | Osteoarthritis and rheumatoid arthritis |
| Daysee [ethinyl estradiol/levonorgestrel] | Z79.3 | Contraceptive | Contraception |
| Delestrogen [estradiol valerate] | Z79.890 | Estrogen therapy | Menopause symptoms |
| Demerol [meperidine hydrochloride] | Z79.891 | Narcotic analgesic | Moderate to severe pain |
| Depakote [divalproex sodium] | | Anticonvulsant | Bipolar affective disorder; complex absence, complex partial, and mixed pattern epilepsy; migraine headache |
| Depo-Medrol [methylprednisolone acetate] | Z79.52 | Corticosteroids | Arthritis and joint disorders |
| Depo-Provera [medroxyprogesterone acetate] | Z79.3, Z79.890 | Antineoplastic; contraceptive; progestin | Amenorrhea; carcinoma, endometrium, adjunct; carcinoma, renal; contraception; hemorrhage |
| Depo-SubQ Provera [medroxyprogesterone acetate] | Z79.3 | Contraceptive | Contraception; menstrual disorder pain |
| Desogen [desogestrel/ethinyl estradiol] | Z79.3 | Contraceptive; estrogen/progestin | Contraception |
| Detrol [tolterodine tartrate] | | Muscarinic receptor antagonist | Overactive bladders in patients with urinary frequency, urgency, or urge incontinence |
| Dexamethasone Intensol [dexamethasone] | Z79.52 | Corticosteroids | Arthritis; allergic disorders; breathing disorders; lupus |
| Didronel [etidronate disodium] | Z79.83 | Bisphosphonates | Paget's disease and irregular bone growth |
| Dificid [fidaxomicin] | Z79.2 | Antibacterial | *Clostridium difficile* |
| Diflucan [fluconazole] | | Antifungal agent | Oropharyngeal and esophageal candidiasis and cryptococcal meningitis in AIDS patients |
| Digoxin [digoxin] | | Cardiotonic glycoside | Heart failure, atrial flutter, atrial fibrillation, and supraventricular tachycardia |
| Dilantin [phenytoin sodium] | | Anticonvulsant | Control of grand mal and psychomotor seizures |
| Dilaudid [hydromorphone hydrochloride] | Z79.891 | Narcotic analgesic | Moderate to severe pain |
| Diovan [valsartan] | | ACE inhibitor | Essential hypertension |
| Divigel [estradiol] | Z79.890 | Estrogen therapy | Menopause symptoms |
| Dolophine HCl [methadone hydrochloride] | Z79.891 | Narcotic analgesic | Pain; treatment of opioid addiction |
| Doxycycline [doxycycline] | Z79.2 | Antibacterial | Treatment of bacterial infections; acne |
| Duavee [bazedoxifene acetate/conjugated estrogens] | Z79.890 | Estrogen therapy | Treatment of menopause symptoms; osteoporosis prevention |
| Duetact [glimepiride/pioglitazone hydrochloride] | Z79.84 | Blood glucose regulator | Diabetes mellitus |
| Duexis [famotidine/ibuprofen] | Z79.1 | Nonsteroidal anti-inflammatory drug (NSAID) | Symptomatic treatment of osteoarthritis and rheumatoid arthritis; reduction of risk of ulcers |
| Dulera [formoterol fumarate/mometasone furoate] | Z79.51 | Corticosteroids -inhaled; antiasthmatic | Prophylaxis and treatment of asthma |
| Duragesic [fentanyl] | Z79.891 | Narcotic analgesic | Chronic pain |
| Duramorph [morphine sulfate] | Z79.891 | Narcotic analgesic | Moderate to severe pain |
| Dyloject [diclofenac sodium] | Z79.1 | Nonsteroidal anti-inflammatory drug (NSAID) | Pain relief |
| Dynacin [minocycline hydrochloride] | Z79.2 | Antibacterial | Severe acne treatment |
| E.E.S. [erythromycin ethylsuccinate] | Z79.2 | Antibacterial | Bacterial infections |
| Ecotrin [acetylsalicylic acid] | Z79.82 | Aspirin | Prophylaxis and treatment of heart attacks, angina or strokes; reduction of fever, pain and inflammation |
| Effexor XR [venlafaxine hydrochloride] | | Antidepressant | Depression |
| Effient [prasugrel hydrochloride] | Z79.02 | Antithrombotic platelet aggregation inhibitor | Lessening of the chance of heart attack or stroke |
| Elestrin [estradiol] | Z79.890 | Estrogen therapy | Menopause symptoms |
| Eligard [leuprolide acetate] | Z79.818 | Agents affecting estrogen receptors and estrogen levels | Endometriosis; uterine fibroids; symptoms of prostate cancer |

| Drug | Z Code | Drug Action | Indications |
|------|--------|-------------|-------------|
| Elinest [norgestrel/ethinyl estradiol] | Z79.3 | Contraceptive | Contraception |
| Eliquis [apixaban] | Z79.01 | Anticoagulant | Venous thrombosis |
| Embeda [morphine sulfate/naltrexone hydrochloride] | Z79.891 | Narcotic analgesic | Moderate to severe pain |
| Emoquette [ethinyl estradiol/desogestrel] | Z79.3 | Contraceptive | Contraception |
| Enjuvia [conjugated synthetic b estrogens] | Z79.890 | Estrogen therapy | Osteoporosis prevention and to treat menopausal symptoms; vaginal and vulvar atrophy; hypoestrogenism; ovarian failure |
| Enpresse [ethinyl estradiol/levonorgestrel] | Z79.3 | Contraceptive | Contraception |
| Enskyce [desogestrel/ethinyl estradiol] | Z79.3 | Contraceptive | Contraception |
| Entocort EC [budesonide] | Z79.52 | Corticosteroids | Crohn's disease; ulcerative colitis |
| Envarsus XR [tacrolimus] | Z79.899 | Immunosuppressant | Prophylaxis of organ transplant rejection |
| Epinephrine [epinephrine] | | Bronchodilator, cardiotonic | Most commonly, relief of respiratory distress due to bronchospasm and restoration of cardiac rhythm in cardiac arrest |
| Epivir, Epivir-HBV [lamivudine] | | HIV and HBV inhibitor | HIV, hepatitis B (HBV), asymptomatic HIV |
| Errin [norethindrone] | Z79.3 | Contraceptive | Contraception |
| Ertapenem [ertapenem sodium] | Z79.2 | Antibacterial | Stomach, urinary tract, pelvis, skin and lung infections |
| ERYC [erythromycin] | Z79.2 | Antibacterial | Lower respiratory tract infections |
| Erygel [erythromycin] | Z79.2 | Antibacterial | Treatment of bacterial infections; rheumatic fever attacks |
| EryPed [erythromycin ethylsuccinate] | Z79.2 | Antibacterial | Treatment of bacterial infections; rheumatic fever attacks |
| Ery-Tab [erythromycin] | Z79.2 | Acne product; macrolide; ocular anti-infective; topical anti-infective | Acne vulgaris, intestinal amebiasis, infectious conjunctivitis, diphtheria, endocarditis, prevention, treatment of erythrasma infections: endocervical, gynecologic, lower and upper respiratory tract, ophthalmic, and rectal; skin and skin structures, and urethral; Legionnaires' disease, pelvic inflammatory disease, pertussis, pneumonia, rheumatic fever, prophylaxis, syphilis |
| Erythrocin [erythromycin lactobionate] | Z79.2 | Antibacterial | Bacterial infections |
| Erythromycin [erythromycin] | Z79.2 | Antibacterial | Respiratory tract infections |
| Estarylla [ethinyl estradiol/norgestimate] | Z79.3 | Contraceptive | Contraception |
| Estrace [estradiol] | Z79.890 | Estrogen therapy | Vaginal cream used to treat vaginal and vulvar atrophy |
| Estraderm [estradiol] | Z79.890 | Estrogen therapy | Osteoporosis prevention and to treat menopausal symptoms, vaginal and vulvar atrophy, hypoestrogenism, ovarian failure |
| Estrasorb [estradiol hemihydrate] | Z79.890 | Estrogen therapy | Menopause symptoms |
| EstroGel [estradiol] | Z79.890 | Estrogen therapy | Menopause symptoms |
| Estrostep Fe [ethinyl estradiol/norethindrone acetate] | Z79.3 | Contraceptive | Contraception |
| Evista [raloxifene hydrochloride] | Z79.810 | Estrogen receptor modulator, selective osteoporosis prophylactic | Prevention of thinning of the bones (osteoporosis) only in postmenopausal women |
| Exalgo [hydromorphone hydrochloride] | Z79.891 | Narcotic analgesic | Moderate to severe pain |
| Exemestane [exemestane] | Z79.811 | Aromatase inhibitor | Postmenopausal breast cancer |
| Factive [gemifloxacin mesylate] | Z79.2 | Antibacterial | Bacterial lung infections |
| Falmina [ethinyl estradiol/levonorgestrel] | Z79.3 | Contraceptive | Contraception |
| Fareston [toremifene citrate] | Z79.810 | Selective estrogen receptor modulator (SERM) | Metastatic breast cancer in postmenopausal women |
| Faslodex [fulvestrant] | Z79.818 | Agents affecting estrogen receptors and estrogen levels | Metastatic breast cancer in postmenopausal women |
| Feldene [piroxicam] | Z79.1 | Nonsteroidal anti-inflammatory drug (NSAID) | Treatment of pain and inflammation due to arthritis |
| Femara [letrozole] | Z79.811 | Aromatase inhibitor | Postmenopausal breast cancer |
| Femcon Fe [ethinyl estradiol/norethindrone] | Z79.3 | Contraceptive | Contraception; acne |
| Femhrt [ethinyl estradiol/norethindrone acetate] | Z79.3, Z79.890 | Contraceptive; estrogen therapy | Contraception; menopause symptoms; osteoporosis prevention |
| Femring [estradiol acetate] | Z79.890 | Estrogen therapy | Osteoporosis prevention and to treat menopausal symptoms; hypoestrogenism; ovarian failure |
| Femtrace [estradiol acetate] | Z79.890 | Estrogen therapy | Menopause symptoms |

| Drug | Z Code | Drug Action | Indications |
|------|--------|-------------|-------------|
| Fentanyl [fentanyl] | Z79.891 | Narcotic analgesic | Postprocedural or chronic pain |
| Fentora [fentanyl citrate] | Z79.891 | Narcotic analgesic | Breakthrough cancer pain |
| Fioricet with codeine [acetaminophen/butalbital/caffeine/codeine phosphate] | Z79.891 | Narcotic analgesic | Tension headaches |
| Flagyl [metronidazole] | Z79.2 | Antibacterial | Treatment of bacterial infections |
| Flavoxate hydrochloride [flavoxate hydrochloride] | | Urinary tract spasmolytic | Relief of dysuria, urgency, nocturia, suprapubic pain, frequency, and incontinence associated with cystitis, prostatitis, urethritis, and urethrocystitis/urethrotrigonitis |
| Flomax [tamsulosin hydrochloride] | | Alpha-adrenergic blocker, benign prostatic hypertrophy therapy agent | Signs and symptoms of benign enlargement of the prostate (benign prostatic hyperplasia, or BPH) |
| Flonase [fluticasone propionate] | | Corticosteroid-inhalation/nasal; topical steroid | Corticosteroid-responsive dermatosis; perennial allergic and seasonal allergic rhinitis |
| Flovent HFA [fluticasone propionate] | Z79.51 | Corticosteroid-inhaled/nasal; topical steroid | Corticosteroid-responsive dermatosis, perennial allergic and seasonal allergic rhinitis |
| Fortamet [metformin hydrochloride] | Z79.84 | Blood glucose regulator | Diabetes mellitus |
| Fortaz [ceftazidime] | Z79.2 | Antibacterial | Pneumonia and lower respiratory infections |
| Fosamax [alendronate sodium] | Z79.83 | Calcium metabolism | Osteoporosis; Paget's disease |
| Fosinopril sodium [fosinopril sodium] | | ACE inhibitor; antihypertensive | Essential hypertension |
| Fragmin [dalteparin sodium] | Z79.01 | Anticoagulant | Prophylaxis and treatment of blood clots |
| Fulvestrant [fulvestrant] | Z79.818 | Agents affecting estrogen receptors and estrogen levels | Treatment of metastatic breast cancer in postmenopausal women |
| Gengraf [cyclosporine] | Z79.899 | Immunosuppressant | Prophylaxis of organ transplant rejection |
| Gentamicin sulfate [gentamicin sulfate] | Z79.2 | Antibacterial | Severe bacterial infections |
| Gildagia [ethinyl estradiol/norethindrone] | Z79.3 | Contraceptive | Contraception |
| Gildess [ethinyl estradiol/norethindrone acetate] | Z79.3 | Contraceptive | Contraception |
| Glimepiride [glimepiride] | Z79.84 | Blood glucose regulator | Diabetes mellitus |
| Glucophage [metformin hydrochloride] | Z79.84 | Blood glucose regulator | Diabetes mellitus |
| Glucotrol [glipizide] | Z79.84 | Oral blood-glucose-lowering agent | Diabetes mellitus |
| Glucovance [glyburide/metformin hydrochloride] | Z79.84 | Blood glucose regulator | Diabetes mellitus |
| Glumetza [metformin hydrochloride] | Z79.84 | Blood glucose regulator | Diabetes mellitus |
| Glyburide (micronized) [glyburide] | Z79.84 | Blood glucose regulator | Diabetes mellitus |
| Heparin sodium [heparin sodium] | Z79.01 | Anticoagulant | Prophylaxis and treatment of venous thrombosis, pulmonary embolism; prevention of cerebral thrombosis, and treatment of consumptive coagulopathies |
| Humalog [insulin lispro recombinant] | Z79.4 | Blood glucose regulator | Diabetes mellitus |
| Humulin [insulin recombinant] | Z79.4 | Blood glucose regulator | Diabetes mellitus |
| Hydrochlorothiazide [hydrochlorothiazide] | | Diuretic, antihypertensive | Management of hypertension and in adjunctive therapy for edema associated with congestive heart failure, hepatic cirrhosis, corticosteroid, and estrogen therapy |
| Hydrocodone [acetaminophen/hydrocodone bitartrate] | Z79.891 | Narcotic analgesic | Moderate to severe pain |
| Hydrocodone bitartrate and acetaminophen [acetaminophen/ hydrocodone bitartrate] | Z79.891 | Analgesic, general; analgesic-narcotic; antitussive/expectorant | Pain, moderate to severe |
| Hydrocortisone [hydrocortisone] | Z79.52 | Corticosteroids | Addison's disease; arthritis; immune disorders; allergies; breathing problems |
| Hydromorphone HCl [hydromorphone hydrochloride] | Z79.891 | Narcotic analgesic | Moderate to severe pain |
| Hyzaar [hydrochlorothiazide/ losartan potassium] | | Antihypertensive | Hypertension |
| Ibuprofen [ibuprofen] | Z79.1 | Nonsteroidal anti-inflammatory drug (NSAID) | Pain or fever relief |
| Imitrex [sumatriptan succinate] | | Antimigraine | Migraine headache |
| Imuran [azathioprine] | Z79.899 | Immunosuppressant | Rheumatoid arthritis |

| Drug | Z Code | Drug Action | Indications |
|------|--------|-------------|-------------|
| Inderal [propranolol hydrochloride] | | Beta-adrenergic blocking agent | Management of hypertension, long-term management of angina pectoris due to coronary atherosclerosis, cardiac arrhythmias |
| Indocin [indomethacin] | Z79.1 | Nonsteroidal anti-inflammatory drug (NSAID) | Treatment of pain and inflammation |
| Integrilin [eptifibatide] | Z79.02 | Antithrombotic platelet aggregation inhibitor | Treatment of unstable angina or heart attacks and prevention of blood clots |
| Intron [interferon alfa 2-b] | Z79.899 | Antineoplastic interferons; antiviral interferons | Cancer; hepatitis |
| Introvale [levonorgestrel/ethinyl estradiol] | Z79.3 | Contraceptive | Contraception |
| Invanz [ertapeneum sodium] | Z79.2 | Antibacterial | Stomach, urinary tract, pelvis, skin and lung infections |
| Invokamet [canagliflozin/metformin hydrochloride] | Z79.84 | Blood glucose regulator | Diabetes mellitus |
| Iprivask [desirudin recombinant] | Z79.02 | Antithrombotic platelet aggregation inhibitor | Prophylaxis and treatment of venous thrombosis and pulmonary embolism |
| Isoniazid [isoniazid] | Z79.2 | Antibacterial | Prophylaxis and treatment of tuberculosis |
| Isordil [isosorbide dinitrate] | | Smooth muscle relaxant | Acute anginal attacks |
| Isuprel [isoproterenol hydrochloride] | | Adrenergic agent | Bronchodilator for asthma, chronic pulmonary emphysema, bronchitis, and other conditions accompanied by bronchospasm; can be used in cardiogenic shock cases |
| Jantoven [warfarin sodium] | Z79.01 | Anticoagulant | Prophylaxis and treatment of venous thrombosis, pulmonary embolism; prevention of cerebral thrombosis, and treatment of consumptive coagulopathies |
| Janumet [metformin hydrochloride/sitagliptin phosphate] | Z79.84 | Blood glucose regulator | Diabetes mellitus |
| Januvia [sitagliptin phosphate] | Z79.84 | Blood glucose regulator | Diabetes mellitus |
| Jencycla [norethindrone] | Z79.3 | Contraceptive | Contraception |
| Jentadueto [linagliptin/metformin hydrochloride] | Z79.84 | Blood glucose regulator | Diabetes mellitus |
| Junel [ethinyl estradiol/norethindrone acetate] | Z79.3 | Contraceptive | Contraception |
| Kadian [morphine sulfate] | Z79.891 | Narcotic analgesic | Moderate to severe pain |
| Kariva [desogestrel/ethinyl estradiol] | Z79.3 | Contraceptive | Contraception |
| Kazano [alogliptin benzoate/metformin hydrochloride] | Z79.84 | Blood glucose regulator | Diabetes mellitus |
| Keflex [cephalexin] | Z79.2 | Antibacterial | Bone, middle ear, skin and skin structures, upper respiratory tract and urinary tract infections; acute prostatitis |
| Kefzol [cefazolin sodium] | Z79.2 | Antibacterial | Skin, ear, urinary tract, and upper respiratory bacterial infections |
| Kelnor [ethynodiol diacetate/ethinyl estradiol] | Z79.3 | Contraceptive | Contraception |
| Kenalog [triamcinolone acetonide] | Z79.52 | Corticosteroids | Eczema; allergic reactions; psoriasis |
| Kimidess [ethinyl estradiol/desogestrel] | Z79.3 | Contraceptive | Contraception |
| Klaron [sulfacetamide sodium] | Z79.2 | Antibacterial | Acne |
| Klonopin [clonazepam] | | Anticonvulsant, anxiolytic - benzodiazepine | Epilepsy, seizures, panic disorder |
| Klor-Con [potassium chloride] | | Replaces potassium and maintains potassium level | Hypokalemia |
| Kombiglyze [metformin hydrochloride/saxagliptin hydrochloride] | Z79.84 | Blood glucose regulator | Diabetes mellitus |
| K-Tab [potassium chloride] | | Replaces potassium and maintains potassium level | Hypokalemia |
| Kurvelo [ethinyl estradiol/levonorgestrel] | Z79.3 | Contraceptive | Contraception; menstrual disorders |
| Lamisil [terbinafine hydrochloride] | | Antifungal | *Tinea cruris* (jock itch), *T. pedis* (athlete's foot), *T. corporis* (ringworm) |
| Lanoxin [digoxin] | | Cardiotonic glycoside | Congestive heart failure |
| Lantus [insulin glargine recombinant] | Z79.4 | Blood glucose regulator | Diabetes mellitus |
| Larin [ethinyl estradiol/norethindrone acetate] | Z79.3 | Contraceptive | Contraception |
| Lasix [furosemide] | | Antihypertensive; diuretic | Management of edema associated with congestive heart failure, renal disease, including nephrotic syndrome and hypertension |

| Drug | Z Code | Drug Action | Indications |
|---|---|---|---|
| Lescol [fluvastatin sodium] | | HMG-CoA reductase inhibitor (statin) | Hypercholesterolemia; hyperlipidemia; hyperlipoproteinemia |
| Lessina [ethinyl estradiol/levonorgestrel] | Z79.3 | Contraceptive | Contraception |
| Letrozole [letrozole] | Z79.811 | Aromatase inhibitor | Postmenopausal breast cancer |
| Levaquin [levofloxacin] | Z79.2 | Fluoroquinolone antibacterial | Acute exacerbation chronic bronchitis; cellulitis; furuncle; impetigo; infections of the lower and upper respiratory tracts, sinus, skin and skin structures, and urinary tract; pneumonia, community-acquired; pyoderma |
| Levemir [insulin detemir recombinant] | Z79.4 | Blood glucose regulator | Diabetes mellitus |
| Levonest [levonorgestrel/ethinyl estradiol] | Z79.3 | Contraceptive | Contraception; menstrual disorders; acne |
| Levora [levonorgestrel/ethinyl estradiol] | Z79.3 | Contraceptive | Contraception |
| Levothroid [levothyroxine sodium] | | Thyroid hormone | Treatment of hypothyroidism |
| Levoxyl [levothyroxine sodium] | | Synthetic thyroid hormone | Euthyroid goiter; hypothyroidism |
| Lexapro [escitalopram oxalate] | | Antidepressant—selective serotonin reuptake inhibitor (SSRI) | Depression, anxiety |
| Librium [chlordiazepoxide hydrochloride] | | Antianxiety agent | Acute withdrawal symptoms, especially from alcohol, or for other anxiety-producing conditions |
| Lidocaine hydrochloride [lidocaine hydrochloride] | | Antiarrhythmic | Management of ventricular arrhythmias or during cardiac manipulation, such as cardiac surgery |
| Liletta [levonorgestrel] | Z79.3 | Contraceptive | Intrauterine device for contraception |
| Lincocin [lincocin hydrochloride] | Z79.2 | Antibacterial | Serious bacterial infections |
| Lipitor [atorvastatin calcium] | | HMG-CoA reductase inhibitor (statin) | Hypercholesterolemia, hyperlipidemia, hyperproteinemia |
| Lithium [lithium carbonate] | | Antimanic | Control of manic episodes in bipolar disorders |
| Lo Loestrin Fe [ethinyl estradiol/norethindrone acetate] | Z79.3 | Contraceptive | Contraception |
| Lo Minastrin Fe [ethinyl estradiol/norethindrone acetate] | Z79.3 | Contraceptive | Contraception |
| Loestrin [ethinyl estradiol/norethindrone acetate] | Z79.3 | Contraceptive | Contraception |
| Lomotil [diphenoxylate hydrochloride/atropine sulfate] | | Antidiarrheal | Treatment of symptoms of chronic and functional diarrhea |
| Lopid [gemfibrozil] | | Lipid regulating agent | Hypercholesterolemia, hyperlipidemia, hyperlipoproteinemia, hypertriglyceridemia |
| Lopressor [metoprolol tartrate] | | Antihypertensive, betablocker antianginal; antihypertensive; betablocker | Essential hypertension therapy, angina pectoris, and myocardial infarction |
| Lorazepam [lorazepam] | | Antianxiety; sedative/hypnotic | Anxiety disorder associated with depressive symptoms; controls tension, agitation, irritability, and insomnia |
| Loryna [drospirenone/ethinyl estradiol] | Z79.3 | Contraceptive | Contraception |
| LoSeasonique [ethinyl estradiol/levonorgestrel] | Z79.3 | Contraceptive | Contraception |
| Lotensin [benazepril hydrochloride] | | ACE inhibitor; antihypertensive | Essential hypertension |
| Lotrel [amlodipine besylate/benazepril hydrochloride] | | Antihypertensive | Hypertension |
| Lotrisone [clotrimazole/ betamethasone dipropionate] | | Antifungal-corticosteroid | Relief of redness, swelling, itching, and other discomfort of fungus infections |
| Lovastatin [lovastatin] | | HMG-CoA reductase inhibitor (statin) | Hypercholesterolemia; hyperlipidemia, hyperlipoproteinemia |
| Lovenox [enoxaparin sodium ] | Z79.Ø1 | Anticoagulant | Prophylaxis and treatment of venous thrombosis and pulmonary embolism |
| Low-Ogestrel [norgestrel/ethinyl estradiol] | Z79.3 | Contraceptive | Contraception |
| Lupron [leuprolide acetate] | Z79.818 | Agents affecting estrogen receptors and estrogen levels | Treatment of metastatic breast cancer in postmenopausal women; prostate cancer symptoms |
| Macrobid [nitrofuantoin] | Z79.2 | Antibacterial | Bacterial urinary tract infections |
| Macrodantin [nitrofurantoin] | | Antibacterial | Urinary tract infection; prophylaxis |
| Marlissa [ethinyl estradiol/levonorgestrel] | Z79.3 | Contraceptive | Contraception |
| Maxipime [cefepime hydrochloride] | Z79.2 | Antibacterial | Treatment of bacterial infections |
| Meclizine hydrochloride [meclizine hydrochloride] | | Antihistamine | Management of nausea and vomiting, and dizziness associated with motion sickness |

| Drug | Z Code | Drug Action | Indications |
|---|---|---|---|
| Medrol [methylprednisolone] | Z79.52 | Glucocorticoid; anti-inflammatory | Acute/chronic adrenal insufficiency, congenital adrenal hyperplasia, adrenal insufficiency secondary to pituitary insufficiency; nonendocrine disorders, including arthritis, rheumatic carditis, bronchial asthma, cerebral edema, and allergic, collagen, intestinal tract, liver, ocular, renal, and skin diseases |
| Mefoxin [cefoxitin sodium] | Z79.2 | Antibacterial | Bacterial infections |
| Megace ES [megestrol acetate] | Z79.818 | Agents affecting estrogen receptors and estrogen levels | Endometrial or advanced breast cancers; weight loss due to AIDS |
| Menest [esteriefied estrogens] | Z79.890 | Estrogen therapy | Menopause symptoms; ovarian failure |
| Menostar [estradiol] | Z79.890 | Estrogen therapy | Menopause symptoms; osteoporosis prevention |
| Mepron [atovaquone] | Z79.2 | Antibacterial | Pneumonia |
| Merrem [meropenem] | Z79.2 | Antibacterial | Bacterial infections of skin or stomach; bacterial meningitis |
| Metformin [metformin hydrochloride] | Z79.84 | Blood glucose regulator | Diabetes mellitus |
| Methadone HCl [methadone hydrochloride] | Z79.891 | Narcotic analgesic | Pain; treatment of opoid addiction |
| Methadose [methadone hydrochloride] | Z79.891 | Narcotic analgesic | Acute and chronic pain |
| Methergine [methylergonovine maleate] | | Oxytocic agent | Routine management of postpartum hemorrhage after delivery of placenta |
| Methylprednisolone [methylprednisolone] | Z79.52 | Corticosteroids | Inflammatory disorders |
| Metro [metronidazole] | Z79.2 | Antibacterial | Bacterial infections |
| Metronidazole [metronidazole] | Z79.2 | Antibacterial | Bacterial infections |
| Miacalcin [calcitonin salmon] | | Calcitonin; a peptide hormone | Hypercalcemia, osteoporosis, postmenopausal symptoms, Paget's disease |
| Microgestin [ethinyl estradiol/norethindrone acetate] | Z79.3 | Contraceptive | Contraception |
| Micronor [norethindrone] | Z79.3 | Contraceptive | Contraception |
| Minastrin [ethinyl estradiol/norethindrone acetate] | Z79.3 | Contraceptive | Contraception |
| Minivelle [estradiol] | Z79.890 | Estrogen therapy | Menopause symptoms; osteoporosis prevention |
| Minocin [minocycline hydrochloride] | Z79.2 | Antibacterial | Bacterial infections; acne |
| Mirena [levonorgestrel] | Z79.3 | Contraceptive | Intrauterine device for contraception; menstrual disorders |
| Mobic [meloxicam] | Z79.1 | Nonsteroidal anti-inflammatory drug (NSAID) | Pain and inflammation due to osteoarthritis and rheumatoid arthritis |
| Modicon [ethinyl estradiol/norethindrone] | Z79.3 | Contraceptive | Contraception |
| Monoclonal antibodies | Z79.899 | Monoclonal antibodies | Cancer; prophylaxis of organ transplant rejection |
| Monodox [doxycycline] | Z79.2 | Antibacterial | Bacterial infections; acne |
| Monoket [isosorbide mononitrate] | | Antianginal; coronary vasodilator, nitrate | Angina pectoris |
| Mono-Linyah [norgestimate/ethinyl estradiol] | Z79.3 | Contraceptive | Contraception; menstrual disorders; acne |
| Monurol [fosfomycin tromethamine] | Z79.2 | Antibacterial | Bacterial bladder infections |
| Morphine [morphine sulfate] | Z79.891 | Narcotic analgesic | Moderate to severe pain |
| Motrin [ibuprofen] | Z79.1 | Analgesic, general; analgesic, non-narcotic; antiarthritic; antigout; antipyretic; NSAID | Osteoarthritis and rheumatoid arthritis, dysmenorrhea, fever; pain, mild to moderate |
| Moxatag [amoxicillin] | Z79.2 | Antibacterial | Bacterial tonsillitis and pharyngitis |
| MS Contin [morphine sulfate] | Z79.891 | Narcotic analgesic | Moderate to severe pain |
| Multaq [dronedarone hydrochloride] | | Cardiac rhythm regulator | Treatment of patients with recent episodes of atrial fibrillation or atrial flutter |
| Mycobutin [rifabutin] | Z79.2 | Antibacterial | Mycobacterium avium complex (MAC) prophylactic |
| Myzilra [ethinyl estradiol/levonorgestrel] | Z79.3 | Contraceptive | Contraception |
| Nabumetone [nabumetone] | Z79.1 | Non-steroidal anti-inflammatory drug (NSAID) | Osteoarthritis and rheumatoid arthritis |
| Nalfon [fenoprofen calcium] | Z79.1 | Nonsteroidal anti-inflammatory drug (NSAID) | Pain or inflammation relief |
| Naprelan [naproxen sodium] | Z79.1 | Nonsteroidal anti-inflammatory drug (NSAID) | Pain or inflammation relief |

| Drug | Z Code | Drug Action | Indications |
|---|---|---|---|
| Naprosyn [naproxen] | Z79.1 | Anti-inflammatory analgesic, general; analgesic, non-narcotic; antiarthritic; antigout; NSAID | Rheumatoid, gouty arthritis and osteoarthritis; ankylosing spondylitis; bursitis; dysmenorrhea; pain, mild to moderate; tendonitis |
| Natazia [estradiol valerate/dienogest] | Z79.3 | Contraceptive | Contraception; menstrual disorders |
| Nebupent [pentamidine isethionate] | Z79.2 | Antibacterial | Serious bacterial lung infection in high-risk patients with HIV |
| Nefazodone hydrochloride [nefazodone hydrochloride] | | Antidepressant | Depression |
| Nembutal sodium [pentobarbital sodium] | | Sedative; hypnotic | Adjunct medication in diagnostic procedures or for emergency use with convulsive disorders |
| NeoProfen [ibuprofen lysine] | Z79.1 | Nonsteroidal anti-inflammatory drug (NSAID) | Pain or fever relief |
| Neoral [cyclosporine] | Z79.899 | Immunosuppressant | Prophylaxis of organ transplant rejection |
| Neurontin [gabapentin] | | Anticonvulsant | Epilepsy, partial |
| Nexium [esomeprazole magnesium] | | Proton pump inhibitor | Gastroesophageal reflux disease (GERD), erosive esophagitis |
| Nexplanon [etonogestrel] | Z79.3 | Contraceptive | Implantable contraception |
| Nitrofurantoin [nitrofurantoin] | Z79.2 | Antibacterial | Bacterial urinary tract infections |
| Nitropress [sodium nitroprusside] | | Vasodilator | Potent, rapid action in reducing blood pressure in hypertensive crisis or for controlling bleeding during anesthesia by producing controlled hypotension |
| Nitrostat [nitroglycerin] | | Muscle relaxant antianginal; antihypertensive; coronary vasodilator | Prophylaxis and treatment of angina pectoris; heart failure associated with myocardial infarction; hypertension, perioperative; surgery, adjunct |
| Norco [acetaminophen/hydrocodone bitartrate] | Z79.891 | Narcotic analgesic | Moderate to severe pain |
| Norinyl [mestranol/norethisterone] | Z79.3 | Contraceptive | Contraception |
| Norpace [disopyramide phosphate] | | Antiarrhythmic | Coronary artery disease, for prevention, recurrence, and control of unifocal, multifocal, and paired PVCs |
| Nor-QD [norethindrone] | Z79.3 | Contraceptive | Contraception |
| Nortrel [ethinyl estradiol/norethindrone] | Z79.3 | Contraceptive | Contraception |
| Norvasc [amlodipine besylate] | | Calcium channel blocker | Hypertension, chronic stable angina, and vasospastic angina |
| Novolin [insulin recombinant] | Z79.4 | Blood glucose regulator | Diabetes mellitus |
| NovoLog [insulin recombinant] | Z79.4 | Blood glucose regulator | Diabetes mellitus |
| Nucynta [tapentadol hydrochloride] | Z79.891 | Narcotic analgesic | Moderate to severe pain |
| NuvaRing [etonogestrel/ethinyl estradiol] | Z79.3 | Contraceptive | Vaginal ring for contraception |
| Ogestrel [norgestrel/ethinyl estradiol] | Z79.3 | Contraceptive | Contraception |
| Onglyza [saxagliptin hydrochloride] | Z79.84 | Blood glucose regulator | Diabetes mellitus |
| Opana [oxymorphone hydrochloride] | Z79.891 | Narcotic analgesic | Moderate to severe pain |
| Oracea [doxycycline] | Z79.2 | Antibacterial | Rosacea |
| Orapred ODT [prednisolone sodium phosphate] | Z79.52 | Corticosteroids | Inflammatory disorders |
| Orbactiv [oritavancin diphosphate] | Z79.2 | Antibacterial | Bacterial skin infections |
| Orphenadrine citrate [orphenadrine citrate] | | Muscle relaxant | Acute spasms, tension, and post-trauma cases |
| Orsythia [ethinyl estradiol/levonorgestrel] | Z79.3 | Contraceptive | Contraception |
| Ortho Cyclen [ethinyl estradiol/norgestimate] | Z79.3 | Contraceptive | Contraception |
| Ortho-Novum [norethindrone/ethinyl estradiol] | Z79.3 | Contraceptive | Contraception |
| Ortho-Tri-Cyclen [ethinyl estradiol/norgestimate] | Z79.3 | Contraceptive | Contraception |
| Oseni [alogliptin benzoate/pioglitazone hydrochloride] | Z79.84 | Blood glucose regulator | Diabetes mellitus |
| Osphena [ospemifene] | Z79.810, Z79.890 | Selective estrogen receptor modulator (SERM) | Postmenopausal dyspareunia due to vaginal atrophy; osteoporosis prevention and treatment of menopause symptoms |
| Oxazepam [oxazepam] | | Antianxiety agent | Anxiety, tension, and alcohol withdrawal |
| Oxycodone HCl [oxycodone hydrochloride] | Z79.891 | Narcotic analgesic | Moderate to severe pain |

| Drug | Z Code | Drug Action | Indications |
|---|---|---|---|
| OxyContin [oxycodone hydrochloride] | Z79.891 | Narcotic analgesic | Moderate to severe pain |
| Pavabid [papaverine hydrochloride] | | Vasodilator | Relief of cerebral and peripheral ischemia |
| Paxil [paroxetine hydrochloride] | | Antidepressant | Anxiety with panic disorder and depression; obsessive-compulsive disorder |
| PCE [erythromycin] | Z79.2 | Antibacterial | Bacterial infections |
| PediaPred [prednisolone sodium phosphate] | Z79.52 | Corticosteroids | Inflammatory disorders |
| Pegintron [peginterferon alfa-2b] | Z79.899 | Antiviral interferon | Hepatitis C |
| Penicillin-VK [penicillin V potassium] | Z79.2 | Natural penicillin | Chorea prevention; endocarditis prevention, secondary to tooth extraction; erysipelas; infections of the skin and skin structures, upper respiratory tract; rheumatic fever, prophylaxis; scarlet fever; Vincent's gingivitis; Vincent's pharyngitis |
| Pentam [pentamidine isethionate] | Z79.2 | Antibacterial | Serious bacterial lung infections |
| Pepcid [famotidine] | | Histamine H2-receptor inhibitor | Acid/peptic disorder; adenoma, secretory; gastroesophageal reflux; duodenal and gastric ulcer; Zollinger-Ellison syndrome |
| Percocet [oxycodone hydrochloride/acetaminophen] | Z79.891 | Analgesic, general; analgesic-narcotic | Pain, moderate to severe |
| Persantine [dipyridamole] | Z79.02 | Platelet inhibitor | Therapy for chronic angina pectoris, preventing clots post heart valve surgery |
| Pfizerpen [penicillin g potassium] | Z79.2 | Antibacterial | Severe bacterial infections |
| Phenobarbital [phenobarbital sodium] | | Barbiturate | Grand mal epilepsy |
| Philith [ethinyl estradiol/norethindrone] | Z79.3 | Contraceptive | Contraception |
| Pimtrea [desogestrel/ethinyl estradiol] | Z79.3 | Contraceptive | Contraception |
| Pirmella [ethinyl estradiol/norethindrone] | Z79.3 | Contraceptive | Contraception |
| Pitocin [oxytocin] | | Synthetic oxytocin | Induction or stimulation of labor at term |
| Plan B One-Step [levonorgestrel] | Z79.3 | Contraceptive | Contraception |
| Plasmanate [plasma, plasma protein fraction] | | Blood volume expander | Hypovolemic shock, burn patients, and hemorrhages when whole blood is unavailable |
| Plavix [clopidogrel bisulfate] | Z79.02 | Antithrombotic platelet aggregation inhibitor | Lessening of the chance of heart attack or stroke |
| Ponstel [mefenamic acid] | Z79.1 | Nonsteroidal anti-inflammatory drug (NSAID) | Pain |
| Portia [ethinyl estradiol/levonorgestrel] | Z79.3 | Contraceptive | Contraception |
| Pradaxa [dabigatran etexilate mesylate] | Z79.01 | Anticoagulant | Prophylaxis and treatment of blood clots in patients with atrial fibrillation |
| Prandimet [metformin hydrochloride/repaglinide] | Z79.84 | Blood glucose regulator | Diabetes mellitus |
| Prandin [repaglinide] | Z79.84 | Blood glucose regulator | Diabetes mellitus |
| Pravachol [pravastatin sodium] | | HMG-CoA reductase inhibitor (statin) | Hypercholesterolemia, hyperlipidemia, hyperlipoproteinemia |
| Precose [acarbose] | Z79.84 | Blood glucose regulator | Diabetes mellitus |
| Prednisolone [prednisolone] | Z79.52 | Corticosteroids | Inflammatory disorders |
| Prednisone [prednisone] | Z79.52 | Adrenocorticoid, corticosteroid | Used for its immunosuppressant effects and for relief of inflammations; used in arthritis, polymyositis and other systemic diseases |
| Pregnyl [chorionic gonadotropin] | | Gonadotropic hormone | Prepubertal cryptorchidism, hypogonadism, corpus luteum insufficiency and infertility |
| Prelone [prednisolone] | Z79.52 | Corticosteroids; antiasthmatic | Inflammatory disorders |
| Premarin [conjugated estrogens] | Z79.890 | Antineoplastic; estrogen | Vasomotor symptoms associated with menopause; atrophic vaginitis; kraurosis vulvae, female hypogonadism; primary ovarian failure |
| Prempro [conjugated estrogens/medroxyprogesterone acetate] | Z79.890 | Estrogen/progestin | Menopause, osteoporosis, atrophic vaginitis |
| Prevacid [lansoprazole] | | Proton pump inhibitor (PPI) | Acid/peptic disorder, erosive esophagitis, duodenal ulcer, Zollinger-Ellison syndrome |
| Previfem [ethinyl estradiol/norgestimate] | Z79.3 | Contraceptive | Contraception |
| Priftin [rifapentine] | Z79.2 | Antibacterial | Prophylaxis and treatment of tuberculosis |

| Drug | Z Code | Drug Action | Indications |
|------|--------|-------------|-------------|
| Prilosec [omeprazole magnesium] | | Proton pump inhibitor | Acid/peptic disorder; endocrine adenoma; erosive esophagitis; systemic mastocytosis; gastroesophageal reflux; duodenal, peptic and gastric ulcer; Zollinger-Ellison syndrome |
| Primaxin [cilastatin sodium/imipenem] | Z79.2 | Antibacterial | Skin, stomach, female reproductive organs or lower respiratory tract infections |
| Prinivil [lisinopril] | | Synthetic peptide derivative, long-acting angiotensin converting enzyme inhibitor | Congestive heart failure, essential hypertension |
| Procardia [nifedipine] | | Antianginal agent; calcium channel blocker | Management of vasospastic angina and chronic stable angina, essential hypertension |
| Prograf [tacrolimus] | Z79.899 | Immunosuppressant | Prophylaxis of organ transplant rejection |
| Promethazine hydrochloride [promethazine hydrochloride] | | Anesthesia, adjunct to; antiemetic; antihistamine; antitussive/expectorant; sedative/hypnotic; vertigo/motion sickness/vomiting | Anesthesia; adjunct; angioedema; conjunctivitis; dermographism; hypersensitivity, motion sickness; pain; perennial, seasonal, and allergic rhinitis; sedation, obstetrical; urticaria |
| Protonix [pantoprazole] | | Proton pump inhibitor (PPI) | Short-term treatment and maintenance therapy of erosive esophagitis associated with gastroesophageal reflux disease (GERD) |
| Protopic [tacrolimus] | Z79.899 | Immunosuppressant | Atomic dermatitis (eczema) |
| Proventil-HFA [albuterol sulfate] | | Antiasthmatic/bronchodilator | Asthma |
| Provera [medroxyprogesterone acetate] | Z79.3, Z79.890 | Antineoplastic; contraceptive; progestin | Amenorrhea; carcinoma, endometrium, adjunct; carcinoma, renal; contraception; hemorrhage |
| Prozac [fluoxetine hydrochloride] | | Serotonin reuptake inhibitor | Bulimia nervosa; depression; obsessive-compulsive disorder |
| Pulmicort [budesonide] | Z79.51 | Corticosteroids -inhaled; antiasthmatic | Prophylaxis and treatment of asthma |
| Qnasl [beclomethasone dipropionate] | | Corticosteroid | Perennial allergies, seasonal allergies, and vasomotor rhinitis |
| Qtern [dapagliflozin propanediol/saxagliptin hydrochloride] | Z79.84 | Blood glucose regulator | Diabetes mellitus |
| Quartette [levonorgestrel/ethinyl estradiol] | Z79.3 | Contraceptive | Contraception |
| Quasense [ethinyl estradiol/levonorgestrel] | Z79.3 | Contraceptive | Contraception |
| Quinidine gluconate [quinidine gluconate] | | Antiarrhythmic | Management of cardiac arrhythmias |
| Qvar [beclomethasone dipropionate] | Z79.51 | Corticosteroids -inhaled; antiasthmatic | Prevention and control of symptoms related to asthma |
| Raloxifene [raloxifene hydrochloride] | Z79.810 | Selective estrogen receptor modulator (SERM) | Prevention of thinning of the bones (osteoporosis) only in postmenopausal women |
| Rapamune [sirolimus] | Z79.899 | Immunosuppressant | Prophylaxis of organ transplant rejection |
| Rayos [prednisone] | Z79.52 | Corticosteroids; antiasthmatic | Arthritis, blood disorders, allergies, asthma |
| Rebif [interferon beta-1a] | Z79.899 | Antiviral interferon | Relapsing multiple sclerosis |
| Reclast [zoledronic acid] | Z79.83 | Bisphosphonates | Prevention of thinning of the bones (osteoporosis); Paget's disease; bone cancer |
| Repaglinide [repaglinide] | Z79.84 | Blood glucose regulator | Diabetes mellitus |
| Reprexain [hydrocodone bitartrate/ibuprofen] | Z79.891 | Opioid analgesic/Nonsteroidal anti-inflammatory drug (NSAID) | Pain, inflammation, or fever relief |
| Restoril [temazepam] | | Sedative/hypnotic | Insomnia |
| Retrovir [zidovudine] | | Antiretroviral agent | Indicated in symptomatic HIV infection |
| Rifadin [rifampin] | Z79.2 | Antibacterial | Prophylaxis and treatment of tuberculosis |
| Rimactane [rifampin] | Z79.2 | Antibacterial | Prophylaxis and treatment of tuberculosis |
| Riomet [metformin hydrochloride] | Z79.84 | Blood glucose regulator | Diabetes mellitus |
| Risperdal [risperidone] | | Antipsychotic/antimanic | Schizophrenia; bipolar I disorder |
| Ritalin [methylphenidate hydrochloride] | | Central nervous system (CNS) stimulant | Treatment of depression and hyperkinetic activity in children |
| Roxicet [oxycodone hydrochloride/acetaminophen] | Z79.891 | Analgesic, general; analgesic-narcotic | Pain, moderate to severe |
| Roxicodone [oxycodone hydrochloride] | Z79.891 | Narcotic analgesic | Pain relief |
| Ryzodeg [insulin aspart/insulin degludec] | Z79.4 | Blood glucose regulator | Diabetes mellitus |
| Sabril [vigabatrin] | | Anticonvulsant | Refractory complex partial seizures |
| Safyral [drospirenone/ethinyl estradiol/levomefolate calcium] | Z79.3 | Contraceptive | Contraception |
| Sandimmune [cyclosporine] | Z79.899 | Immunosuppressant | Prophylaxis of organ transplant rejection |

| Drug | Z Code | Drug Action | Indications |
|------|--------|-------------|-------------|
| Savaysa [edoxaban tosylate] | Z79.Ø1 | Anticoagulant | Prophylaxis and treatment of venous thrombosis, pulmonary embolism; prevention of blood clots due to atrial fibrillation |
| Seasonale [levonorgestrel/ethinyl estradiol] | Z79.3 | Contraceptive | Contraception |
| Seasonique [ethinyl estradiol/levonorgestrel] | Z79.3 | Contraceptive | Contraception |
| Septra [sulfamethoxazole trimethoprim] | Z79.2 | Antibacterial | Treatment of urinary tract infections, acute otitis media, acute exacerbations of chronic bronchitis, and shigellosis |
| Serevent [salmeterol xinafoate] | | Bronchodilator | Asthma |
| Seromycin [cycloserine] | Z79.2 | Antibacterial | Tuberculosis; urinary tract infections |
| Setlakin [ethinyl estradiol/levonorgestrel] | Z79.3 | Contraceptive | Contraception |
| Simulect [basiliximab] | Z79.899 | Immunosuppressant | Prophylaxis of organ transplant rejection |
| Sinemet [carbidopa/levodopa] | | Antiparkinsonian | Parkinson's disease |
| Singulair [montelukast sodium] | | Antiasthmatic, leukotriene receptor antagonist | Treatment of mild to moderate asthma to decrease the symptoms of asthma and the number of acute asthma attacks |
| Sirolimus [sirolimus] | Z79.899 | Immunosuppressant | Prophylaxis of organ transplant rejection |
| Sitagliptin [sitagliptin/metformin hydrochloride] | Z79.84 | Blood glucose regulator | Diabetes mellitus |
| Sivextro [tedizolid phosphate] | Z79.2 | Antibacterial | Skin infections including MRSA |
| Skyla [levonorgestrel] | Z79.3 | Contraceptive | Intrauterine device for contraception |
| Solodyn [minocycline hydrochloride] | Z79.2 | Antibacterial | Bacterial infections |
| Soltamox [tamoxifen citrate] | Z79.81Ø | Selective estrogen receptor modulator (SERM) | Breast cancer |
| Solu-Cortef [hydrocortisone sodium succinate] | Z79.52 | Corticosteroids; antiasthmatic | Asthma; severe inflammation; allergic reactions |
| Solu-Medrol [methylprednisolone sodium succinate] | Z79.52 | Adrenocorticosteroid | Anti-inflammatory and antiallergenic for shock and ulcerative colitis |
| Sprintec [norgestimate/ethinyl estradiol] | Z79.3 | Contraceptive | Contraception |
| Streptomycin sulfate [streptomycin sulfate] | Z79.2 | Antibacterial | Severe bacterial infections |
| Sublimaze [fentanyl citrate] | Z79.891 | Narcotic analgesic | Pain relief |
| Supprelin LA [histrelin acetate] | Z79.818 | Agents affecting estrogen receptors and estrogen levels | Precocious puberty; prostate cancer symptoms |
| Suprax [cefixime] | Z79.2 | Antibacterial | Bacterial infections |
| Syeda [drospirenone/ethinyl estradiol] | Z79.3 | Contraceptive | Contraception |
| Sylatron [peginterferon alfa-2b] | Z79.899 | Antineoplastic interferons; antiviral interferons | Prevention of recurrent malignant melanoma |
| Symbicort [budesonide/formoterol fumarate dihydrate] | Z79.51 | Corticosteroids -inhaled; antiasthmatic | Prophylaxis and treatment of asthma and COPD |
| Synarel [nafarelin acetate] | Z79.818 | Agents affecting estrogen receptors and estrogen levels | Endometriosis symptoms; precocious puberty |
| Synercid [dalfopristin/quinupristin] | Z79.2 | Antibacterial | Severe blood infections |
| Synjardy [empagliflozin/metformin hydrochloride] | Z79.84 | Blood glucose regulator | Diabetes mellitus |
| Synthroid [levothyroxine sodium] | | Thyroid hormone | Treatment of hypothyroidism |
| Tacrolimus [tacrolimus] | Z79.899 | Immunosuppressant | Prophylaxis of organ transplant rejection |
| Tagamet HB [cimetidine] | | Acid reducer | Treatment of active duodenal ulcer, short-term treatment of active, benign gastric ulcer, and treatment of pathological hypersecretory conditions |
| Tamoxifen [tamoxifen citrate] | Z79.81Ø | Selective estrogen receptor modulator (SERM) | Metastatic breast cancer in postmenopausal women |
| Tazicef [ceftazidime] | Z79.2 | Antibacterial | Confirmed or suspected bacterial infections |
| Teflaro [ceftaroline fosamil] | Z79.2 | Antibacterial | Bacterial skin infections; pneumonia |
| Tegretol [carbamazepine] | | Anticonvulsant; analgesic | Epilepsy, especially with complex symptomatology; specific analgesic for trigeminal neuralgia |
| Tenormin [atenolol] | | Antianginal; antihypertensive; beta blocker | Treatment of hypertension; lowering blood pressure lowers the risk of fatal and nonfatal cardiovascular events, primarily strokes and myocardial infarctions |

| Drug | Z Code | Drug Action | Indications |
|------|--------|-------------|-------------|
| Terazosin hydrochloride [terazosin hydrochloride] | | Alpha-blocker; antihypertensive; diuretic | Benign prostatic hypertrophy; essential hypertension |
| Tetracycline HCl [tetracycline hydrochloride] | Z79.2 | Antibacterial | Bacterial infections |
| Tiazac [diltiazem hydrochloride] | | Antianginal, antiarrhythmic, antihypertensive, channel blocker, coronary vasodilator | Chronic stable angina, atrial fibrillation, atrial flutter, essential hypertension, paroxysmal supraventricular tachycardia |
| Tivorbex [indomethacin] | Z79.1 | Nonsteroidal anti-inflammatory drug (NSAID) | Pain, inflammation and joint stiffness |
| Tobradex [tobramycin/dexamethasone] | | Aminoglycoside ocular anti-infective; anti-inflammatory | Infectious conjunctivitis; dermatosis, corticosteroid-responsive with secondary infection; foreign body in eye; corneal inflammation; uveitis |
| Tobramycin [dexamethasone/tobramycin] | Z79.2 | Antibacterial | Bacterial eye infections |
| Toprol-XL [metoprolol succinate] | | Antianginal antihypertensive beta blocker | Angina pectoris, essential hypertension |
| Toremifene [toremifene citrate] | Z79.810 | Selective estrogen receptor modulator (SERM) | Metastatic breast cancer in postmenopausal women |
| Torisel [temsirolimus] | Z79.899 | Antineoplastic | Renal cell carcinoma |
| Toujeo Solostar [insulin glargine recombinant] | Z79.4 | Blood glucose regulator | Diabetes mellitus |
| Trazodone hydrochloride [trazodone hydrochloride] | | Antidepressant | Depression |
| Trelstar [triptorelin pamoate] | Z79.818 | Agents affecting estrogen receptors and estrogen levels | Prophylaxis of chemo-induced menopause; prostate cancer symptoms |
| Tresiba [insulin degludec] | Z79.4 | Blood glucose regulator | Diabetes mellitus |
| Triamterene and hydrochlorothiazide [triamterene/ hydrochlorothiazide] | | Antihypertensive, diuretic | Edema; essential hypertension |
| Tri-Estarylla [ethinyl estradiol/norgestimate] | Z79.3 | Contraceptive | Contraception; acne |
| Tri-Legest [ethinyl estradiol/norethindrone acetate] | Z79.3 | Contraceptive | Contraception |
| Tri-Linyah [ethinyl estradiol/norgestimate] | Z79.3 | Contraceptive | Contraception |
| Tri-Lo-Estarylla [ethinyl estradiol/norgestimate] | Z79.3 | Contraceptive | Contraception |
| Tri-Lo-Sprintec [ethinyl estradiol/norgestimate] | Z79.3 | Contraceptive | Contraception |
| Trimethoprim [trimethoprim] | Z79.2 | Antibacterial | Acute exacerbation chronic bronchitis; travelers' diarrhea; infections of the middle and lower respiratory tracts, and urinary tract; pneumonia, pneumocystis; shigellosis |
| Tri-Norinyl [ethinyl estradiol/norethindrone] | Z79.3 | Contraceptive | Contraception |
| Tri-Previfem [ethinyl estradiol/norgestimate] | Z79.3 | Contraceptive | Contraception |
| Tri-Sprintec [ethinyl estradiol/norgestimate] | Z79.3 | Contraceptive | Contraception; acne |
| Trivora [ethinyl estradiol/ levonorgestrel] | Z79.3 | Contraceptive | Contraception |
| Tygacil [tigecycline] | Z79.2 | Antibacterial | Bacterial skin or digestive system infections; pneumonia |
| Tylenol with codeine [acetaminophen/codeine phosphate] | Z79.891 | Narcotic analgesic | Pain and cough |
| Ultram [tramadol hydrochloride] | Z79.891 | Analgesic, non-narcotic (opiate, narcotic-like) | Pain, moderate to moderately severe |
| Unasyn [ampicillin sodium/sulbactam sodium] | Z79.2 | Antibacterial | Bacterial infections |
| Vagifem [estradiol] | Z79.890 | Estrogen therapy | Menopause symptoms |
| Valium [diazepam] | | Antianxiety, muscle relaxant, anticonvulsant | Anxiety, tension, withdrawal from alcohol, muscle spasms and anticonvulsant therapy; epilepsy, generalized tonic-clonic; status epilepticus; stiff-man syndrome; tetanus |
| Vancocin HCl [vancomycin hydrochloride] | Z79.2 | Antibacterial | Serious bacterial infections |
| Vancomycin HCl [vancomycin hydrochloride] | Z79.2 | Antibacterial | Serious bacterial infections |

| Drug | Z Code | Drug Action | Indications |
|---|---|---|---|
| Vantas [histrelin acetate] | Z79.818 | Agents affecting estrogen receptors and estrogen levels | Prostate cancer symptoms; breast cancer; endometriosis |
| Vasotec [enalaprilat maleate] | | ACE inhibitor; antihypertensive | Congestive heart failure; essential hypertension |
| Velivet [desogestrel/ethinyl estradiol] | Z79.3 | Contraceptive | Contraception |
| Ventolin HFA [albuterol sulfate] | | Antiasthmatic/bronchodilator | Asthma |
| Verapamil HCL [verapamil hydrochloride] | | Antianginal, antiarrhythmic, antiarthritic, antihypertensive, calcium channel blocker | Angina pectoris, chronic stable angina, atrial fibrillation, atrial flutter, paroxysmal supraventricular tachycardia, ventricular arrhythmia, essential hypertension |
| Viagra [sildenafil citrate] | | Phosphodiesterase-5 (PDE5) inhibitor | Erectile dysfunction |
| Vibativ [telavancin hydrochloride] | Z79.2 | Antibacterial | Pneumonia; severe bacterial skin infections |
| Vibramycin [doxycycline calcium] | Z79.2 | Antibacterial | Bacterial infections |
| Vicoprofen [hydrocodone bitartrate/ibuprofen] | Z79.891 | Opioid analgesic/ Nonsteroidal anti-inflammatory drug (NSAID) | Pain, inflammation, or fever relief |
| Victoza [liraglutide (rDNA) injection] | | Glucagon-like peptide-1 (GLP-1) receptor agonist | Diabetes mellitus |
| Vienva [ethinyl estradiol/levonorgestrel] | Z79.3 | Contraceptive | Contraception |
| Viorele [desogestrel/ethinyl estradiol] | Z79.3 | Contraceptive | Contraception |
| Virazole [ribavirin] | | Antiviral | Respiratory syncytial virus (RSV) |
| Vistaril [hydroxyzine pamoate] | | Antianxiety agent, antiemetic | Treatment of nausea and vomiting, for reducing narcotic requirement in surgery and as tranquilizer for tension, anxiety, or agitation states |
| Vivelle [estradiol] | Z79.890 | Estrogen therapy | Menopause symptoms; osteoporosis prevention |
| Voltaren [diclofenac sodium] | Z79.1 | Nonsteroidal anti-inflammatory drug (NSAID) | Treatment of pain, inflammation, and joint stiffness due to arthritis |
| Warfarin [warfarin sodium] | Z79.01 | Anticoagulant | Prophylaxis and treatment of venous thrombosis, treatment of atrial fibrillation with embolization (pulmonary embolism), arrhythmias, myocardial infarction, and stroke prevention |
| Wellbutrin SR, Wellbutrin XL [bupropion hydrochloride] | | Antidepressant; CNS | Depression; smoking cessation |
| Wera [ethinyl estradiol/norethindrone] | Z79.3 | Contraceptive | Contraception |
| Xalatan [latanoprost] | | Prostaglandin F2α analogue | Glaucoma, open-angle; ocular hypertension |
| Xanax, Xanax XR [alprazolam] | | Antianxiety; sedative/hypnotic | Anxiety disorders with panic disorder and depression |
| Xarelto [rivaraxaban] | Z79.01 | Anticoagulant | Prophylaxis and treatment of venous thrombosis, pulmonary embolism; prevention of blood clots due to atrial fibrillation |
| Xifaxan [rifaximin] | Z79.2 | Antibacterial | E. coli diarrhea |
| Xigduo [dapagliflozin propanediol/metformin hydrochloride] | Z79.84 | Blood glucose regulator | Diabetes mellitus |
| Xigris [drotrecogin alfa] | | Biologic response modifier | Severe sepsis |
| Yasmin [drospirenone/ethinyl estradiol] | Z79.3 | Contraceptive | Contraception |
| Yaz [drospirenone/ethinyl estradiol] | Z79.3 | Contraceptive | Contraception; menstrual disorders |
| Zantac [ranitidine hydrochloride] | | Histamine H2-receptors inhibitor | Acid/peptic disorder, erosive esophagitis, gastrointestinal hypersecretion, mastocytosis, gastroesophageal reflux, peptic ulcer, Zollinger-Ellison syndrome |
| Zerbaxa [ceftolozane sulfate/tazobactam sodium] | Z79.2 | Antibacterial | Complicated urinary tract and intra-abdominal infections |
| Zestoretic [lisinopril/hydrochlorothiazide] | | ACE inhibitor; antihypertensive | Congestive heart failure; essential hypertension |
| Zestril [lisinopril] | | ACE inhibitor; antihypertensive | Congestive heart failure; essential hypertension |
| Ziac [bisoprolol fumarate/ hydrochlorothiazide] | | Antihypertensive | Essential hypertension |
| Zinacef [cefuroxime sodium] | Z79.2 | Antibacterial | Bacterial infections |
| Zipsor [diclofenac potassium] | Z79.1 | Nonsteroidal anti-inflammatory drug (NSAID) | Pain and inflammation relief |
| Zithromax [azithromycin] | Z79.2 | Macrolide | Infections of the cervix, lower respiratory tract, skin and skin structures, urethra, nongonococcal; mycobacterium avium complex; pharyngitis, streptococcal pneumonia; tonsillitis |
| Zmax [azithromycin] | Z79.2 | Antibacterial | Pneumonia; sinusitis |
| Zocor [simvastatin] | | HMG-CoA reductase inhibitor (statin) | Hypercholesterolemia, hyperlipidemia, hyperlipoproteinemia, hypertriglyceridemia |

| Drug | Z Code | Drug Action | Indications |
|------|--------|-------------|-------------|
| Zoladex [goserelin acetate] | Z79.818 | Agents affecting estrogen receptors and estrogen levels | Prostate cancer symptoms and advanced breast cancer |
| Zoloft [sertraline hydrochloride] | | Antidepressant | Anxiety with panic disorder and depression; obsessive-compulsive disorder |
| Zometa [zoledronic acid] | Z79.83 | Bisphosphonates | Multiple myeloma; Paget's disease |
| Zorvolex [diclofenac] | Z79.1 | Nonsteroidal anti-inflammatory drug (NSAID) | Pain, inflammation or fever relief |
| Zosyn [piperacillin sodium/tazobactam sodium] | Z79.2 | Antibacterial | Bacterial infections |
| Zovia [ethynodiol diacetate/ethinyl estradiol] | Z79.3 | Contraceptive | Contraception |
| Zovirax [acyclovir] | | Antiviral | Genital herpes and herpes zoster infections |
| Zyloprim [allopurinol] | | Antigout | Gouty arthritis, renal calculus, hyperuricemia, hyperuricemia secondary to leukemia, hyperuricemia secondary to lymphoma |
| Zyprexa [olanzapine] | | Antipsychotic/antimanic | Psychotic disorders; schizophrenia |
| Zyrtec [cetirizine hydrochloride] | | Antihistamine | Perennial allergic and seasonal allergic rhinitis; chronic urticaria |
| Zyvox [linezolid] | Z79.2 | Antibacterial | Serious bacterial infections |

**Z79.Ø1**  **Long term (current) use of anticoagulants**
Arixtra
Coumadin
Eliquis
Fragmin
Heparin
Jantoven
Lovenox
Pradaxa
Savaysa
Warfarin
Xarelto

**Z79.Ø2**  **Long term (current) use of antithrombotics/antiplatelets**
Aggrastat
Aggrenox
Angiomax
Argatroban
Brilinta
Clopidogrel bisulfate
Effient
Integrilin
Iprivask
Persantine
Plavix

**Z79.1**  **Long term (current) use of non-steroidal anti-inflammatories (NSAID)**
Advil
Aleve
Anaprox
Arthrotec
Caldolor
Cambia
Celebrex
Daypro
Duexis
Dyloject
Feldene
Ibuprofen
Indocin
Mobic
Motrin
Nabumetone
Nalfon
Naprelan
Naprosyn
NeoProfen
Ponstel
Tivorbex
Voltaren
Zipsor
Zorvolex

**Z79.2**  **Long term (current) use of antibiotics**
Akne-Mycin
Altabax
Amoxicillin
Ampicillin
Ancef
Augmentin
Azactam
Azithromycin
Bactrim
Bactroban
Ceftriaxone
Centany
Cephalexin
Cipro
Ciprofloxacin
Clarithromycin
Cleocin
Clindamycin
Daptomycin
Dificid

Doxycycline
Dynacin
E.E.S.
Ertapenem
ERYC
Erygel
EryPed
Ery-Tab
Erythrocin
Erythromycin
Factive
Flagyl
Fortaz
Gentamicin sulfate
Invanz
Isoniazid
Keflex
Kefzol
Klaron
Levaquin
Lincocin
Macrobid
Maxipime
Mefoxin
Mepron
Merrem
Metro
Metronidazole
Minocin
Monodox
Monurol
Moxatag
Mycobutin
Nebupent
Nitrofurantoin
Oracea
Orbactiv
PCE
Penicillin-VK
Pentam
Pfizerpen
Priftin
Primaxin
Rifadin
Rimactane
Septra
Seromycin
Sivextro
Solodyn
Streptomycin sulfate
Suprax
Synercid
Tazicef
Teflaro
Tetracycline HCl
Tobramycin
Trimethoprim
Tygacil
Unasyn
Vancocin HCl
Vancomycin HCl
Vibativ
Vibramycin
Xifaxan
Zerbaxa
Zinacef
Zithromax
Zmax
Zosyn
Zyvox

**Z79.3**  **Long term (current) use of hormonal contraceptives**
Altavera
Alyacen
Aranelle

Ashlyna
Aviane
Aygestin
Balziva
Bekyree
Beyaz
Brevicon
Briellyn
Camila
Cryselle
Cyclafem
Cyclessa
Dasetta
Daysee
Depo-Provera
Depo-SubQ Provera
Desogen
Elinest
Emoquette
Enpresse
Enskyce
Errin
Estarylla
Estrostep Fe
Falmina
Femcon Fe
Femhrt
Gildagia
Gildess
Introvale
Jencycla
Junel
Kariva
Kelnor
Kimidess
Kurvelo
Larin
Lessina
Levonest
Levora
Liletta
Lo Loestrin Fe
Lo Minastrin Fe
Loestrin
Loryna
LoSeasonique
Low-Ogestrel
Marlissa
Microgestin
Micronor
Minastrin
Mirena
Modicon
Mono-Linyah
Myzilra
Natazia
Nexplanon
Norinyl
Nor-QD
Nortrel
NuvaRing
Ogestrel
Orsythia
Ortho Cyclen
Ortho-Novum
Ortho-Tri-Cyclen
Philith
Pimtrea
Pirmella
Plan B One-Step
Portia
Previfem
Provera
Quartette
Quasense

Safyral
Seasonale
Seasonique
Setlakin
Skyla
Sprintec
Syeda
Tri-Estarylla
Tri-Legest
Tri-Linyah
Tri-Lo-Estarylla
Tri-Lo-Sprintec
Tri-Norinyl
Tri-Previfem
Tri-Sprintec
Trivora
Velivet
Vienva
Viorele
Wera
Yasmin
Yaz
Zovia

**Z79.4    Long term (current) use of insulin**
Afrezza
Apidra
Basaglar
Humalog
Humulin
Lantus
Levemir
Novolin
NovoLog
Ryzodeg
Toujeo Solostar
Tresiba

**Z79.51   Long term (current) use of inhaled steroids**
Advair
Aerospan
Alvesco
Arnuity Ellipta
Asmanex
Dulera
Flovent
Pulmicort
Qvar
Symbicort

**Z79.52   Long term (current) use of systemic steroids**
A-Methapred
Aristospan
Celestone Soluspan
Colocort
Cortef
Cortenema
Cortifoam
Cortisone acetate
Depo-Medrol
Dexamethasone Intensol
Entocort EC
Hydrocortisone
Kenalog
Medrol
Methylprednisolone
Orapred ODT
PediaPred
Prednisolone
Prednisone
Prelone
Rayos
Solu-Cortef
Solu-Medrol

**Z79.810  Long term (current) use of selective estrogen receptor modulators (SERMs)**
Evista
Fareston
Osphena
Raloxifene
Soltamox
Tamoxifen
Toremifene

**Z79.811  Long term (current) use of aromatase inhibitors**
Anastrozole
Arimidex
Aromasin
Exemestane
Femara
Letrozole

**Z79.818  Long term (current) use of other agents affecting estrogen receptors and estrogen levels**
Eligard
Faslodex
Fulvestrant
Lupron
Megace ES
Supprelin LA
Synarel
Trelstar
Vantas
Zoladex

**Z79.82   Long term (current) use of aspirin**
Bayer
Bufferin
Ecotrin

**Z79.83   Long term (current) use of bisphosphonates**
Actonel
Atelvia
Binosto
Boniva
Didronel
Fosamax
Reclast
Zometa

**Z79.84   Long term (current) use of oral hypoglycemic drugs**
Acarbose
Actoplus Met
Actos
Amaryl
Avandia
Duetact
Fortamet
Glimepiride
Glucophage
Glucotrol
Glucovance
Glumetza
Glyburide
Invokamet
Janumet
Januvia
Jentadueto
Kazano
Kombiglyze
Metformin
Onglyza
Oseni
PrandiMet
Prandin
Precose
Qtern
Repaglinide
Riomet
Sitagliptin

Synjardy
Xigduo

**Z79.890  Hormone replacement therapy**
Activella
Alora
Angeliq
Climara
CombiPatch
Delestrogen
Divigel
Duavee
Elestrin
Enjuvia
Estrace
Estraderm
Estrasorb
EstroGel
Femhrt
Femring
Femtrace
Menest
Menostar
Minivelle
Osphena
Premarin
Prempro
Provera
Vagifem
Vivelle

**Z79.891  Long term (current) use of opiate analgesic**
Acetaminophen with codeine
Astramorph
Buprenex
Buprenorphine HCl
Butrans
Codeine
Demerol
Dilaudid
Dolophine HCl
Duragesic
Duramorph
Embeda
Exalgo
Fentanyl
Fentora
Fioricet with codeine
Hydrocodone
Hydrocodone bitartrate and acetaminophen
Hydromorphone HCl
Kadian
Methadone HCl
Methadose
Morphine
MS Contin
Norco
Nucynta
Opana
Oxycodone HCl
OxyContin
Percocet
Reprexain
Roxicet
Roxicodone
Sublimaze
Tylenol with codeine
Ultram
Vicoprofen

**Z79.899** **Other long term (current) drug therapy**
    Actimmune
    Antineoplastic/chemotherapy
    Astagraf XL
    Avonex
    Cellcept
    Cyclosporine
    Envarsus XR
    Gengraf
    Imuran
    Intron
    Monoclonal antibodies
    Neoral
    Pegintron
    Prograf
    Protopic
    Rapamune
    Rebif
    Sandimmune
    Simulect
    Sirolimus
    Sylatron
    Tacrolimus
    Torisel

# Appendix E: Major Complication and Comorbidity (MCC) Code List

**Note:** The following list of MCCs are based on the *Federal Register,* volume 82, number 81, April 28, 2017 ("Hospital Inpatient Prospective Payment Systems for Acute Care Hospitals and the Long-Term Care Hospital Prospective Payment System and Proposed Policy Changes and Fiscal Year 2018 Rates; Proposed Rule"). The most current version, v35, of the ICD-10 MS-DRG Definitions Manual was not available at the time this book was printed. For the most current files related to IPPS please refer to the following:
https://www.cms.gov/Medicare/Medicare-Fee-for-Service-Payment/AcuteInpatientPPS/IPPS-Regulations-and-Notices.html.

| | | | | | | | |
|---|---|---|---|---|---|---|---|
| A02.1 | A48.1 | B45.1 | E13.00 | I21.09 | I61.9 | I63.432 | J12.3 | K25.5 |
| A02.21 | A48.3 | B46.0 | E13.01 | I21.11 | I62.00 | I63.433 | J12.81 | K25.6 |
| A02.22 | A50.41 | B46.1 | E13.10 | I21.19 | I62.01 | I63.439 | J12.89 | K26.0 |
| A06.4 | A50.42 | B46.2 | E13.11 | I21.21 | I62.02 | I63.441 | J12.9 | K26.1 |
| A06.5 | A51.41 | B46.3 | E13.641 | I21.29 | I62.03 | I63.442 | J13 | K26.2 |
| A06.6 | A52.13 | B46.4 | E40 | I21.3 | I62.1 | I63.443 | J14 | K26.4 |
| A17.0 | A52.14 | B46.5 | E41 | I21.4 | I63.00 | I63.449 | J15.0 | K26.5 |
| A17.1 | A54.81 | B46.8 | E42 | I22.0 | I63.011 | I63.49 | J15.1 | K26.6 |
| A17.81 | A54.86 | B46.9 | E43 | I22.1 | I63.012 | I63.50 | J15.20 | K27.0 |
| A17.82 | A80.0 | B50.9 | E84.0 | I22.2 | I63.013 | I63.511 | J15.211 | K27.1 |
| A17.83 | A80.1 | B58.2 | E84.11 | I22.8 | I63.019 | I63.512 | J15.212 | K27.2 |
| A17.89 | A80.2 | B58.3 | E88.3 | I22.9 | I63.02 | I63.513 | J15.29 | K27.4 |
| A18.31 | A80.30 | B58.81 | G00.0 | I23.4 | I63.031 | I63.519 | J15.3 | K27.5 |
| A19.0 | A80.39 | B59 | G00.1 | I23.5 | I63.032 | I63.521 | J15.4 | K27.6 |
| A19.1 | A83.0 | B77.81 | G00.2 | I25.42 | I63.033 | I63.522 | J15.5 | K28.0 |
| A19.2 | A83.1 | D57.00 | G00.3 | I26.01 | I63.039 | I63.523 | J15.6 | K28.1 |
| A19.8 | A83.2 | D57.01 | G00.8 | I26.02 | I63.09 | I63.529 | J15.7 | K28.2 |
| A19.9 | A83.3 | D57.02 | G00.9 | I26.09 | I63.10 | I63.531 | J15.8 | K28.4 |
| A20.0 | A83.4 | D57.211 | G01 | I26.90 | I63.111 | I63.532 | J15.9 | K28.5 |
| A20.1 | A83.5 | D57.212 | G02 | I26.92 | I63.112 | I63.533 | J16.0 | K28.6 |
| A20.2 | A83.6 | D57.219 | G03.0 | I26.99 | I63.113 | I63.539 | J16.8 | K29.01 |
| A20.3 | A83.8 | D57.411 | G03.8 | I33.0 | I63.119 | I63.541 | J17 | K29.21 |
| A20.7 | A83.9 | D57.412 | G03.9 | I33.9 | I63.12 | I63.542 | J18.0 | K29.31 |
| A20.8 | A84.0 | D57.419 | G04.00 | I40.0 | I63.131 | I63.543 | J18.1 | K29.41 |
| A20.9 | A84.1 | D57.811 | G04.01 | I40.1 | I63.132 | I63.549 | J18.8 | K29.51 |
| A22.1 | A84.8 | D57.812 | G04.02 | I40.8 | I63.133 | I63.59 | J18.9 | K29.61 |
| A22.7 | A84.9 | D57.819 | G04.2 | I40.9 | I63.139 | I63.6 | J68.1 | K29.71 |
| A26.7 | A85.2 | D59.3 | G04.30 | I41 | I63.19 | I63.8 | J69.0 | K29.81 |
| A27.81 | A92.30 | D60.0 | G04.31 | I46.2 | I63.20 | I63.9 | J69.1 | K29.91 |
| A32.7 | A92.31 | D60.1 | G04.32 | I46.8 | I63.211 | I67.0 | J69.8 | K31.811 |
| A33 | A92.32 | D60.8 | G04.39 | I46.9 | I63.212 | I67.83 | J81.0 | K31.82 |
| A35 | A92.39 | D60.9 | G04.81 | I49.01 | I63.213 | I71.00 | J84.81 | K35.2 |
| A37.01 | B00.3 | D61.1 | G04.89 | I49.02 | I63.219 | I71.01 | J84.83 | K35.3 |
| A37.11 | B00.4 | D61.2 | G04.90 | I50.21 | I63.22 | I71.02 | J84.841 | K40.10 |
| A37.81 | B00.7 | D61.3 | G04.91 | I50.23 | I63.231 | I71.03 | J84.842 | K40.11 |
| A37.91 | B00.82 | D61.810 | G05.3 | I50.31 | I63.232 | I71.1 | J84.843 | K40.40 |
| A39.0 | B01.11 | D61.811 | G05.4 | I50.33 | I63.233 | I71.3 | J84.848 | K40.41 |
| A39.1 | B01.12 | D61.89 | G06.0 | I50.41 | I63.239 | I71.5 | J85.0 | K41.10 |
| A39.2 | B01.2 | D65 | G06.1 | I50.43 | I63.29 | I71.8 | J85.1 | K41.11 |
| A39.3 | B02.1 | D66 | G06.2 | I51.1 | I63.30 | I74.01 | J85.2 | K41.40 |
| A39.4 | B02.24 | D67 | G07 | I51.2 | I63.311 | I77.70 | J85.3 | K41.41 |
| A39.50 | B05.0 | E03.5 | G08 | I60.00 | I63.312 | I77.71 | J86.0 | K42.1 |
| A39.51 | B05.2 | E05.01 | G21.0 | I60.01 | I63.313 | I77.72 | J86.9 | K43.1 |
| A39.52 | B06.01 | E05.11 | G37.4 | I60.02 | I63.319 | I77.73 | J93.0 | K43.4 |
| A39.53 | B10.01 | E05.21 | G40.301 | I60.10 | I63.321 | I77.74 | J95.1 | K43.7 |
| A39.81 | B10.09 | E05.31 | G40.311 | I60.11 | I63.322 | I77.75 | J95.2 | K44.1 |
| A40.0 | B15.0 | E05.41 | G40.319 | I60.12 | I63.323 | I77.76 | J95.3 | K45.1 |
| A40.1 | B16.0 | E05.81 | G70.01 | I60.2 | I63.329 | I77.77 | J95.821 | K46.1 |
| A40.3 | B16.2 | E05.91 | G80.0 | I60.30 | I63.331 | I77.79 | J95.822 | K55.011 |
| A40.8 | B17.11 | E08.00 | G82.50 | I60.31 | I63.332 | I81 | J96.00 | K55.012 |
| A40.9 | B19.0 | E08.01 | G82.51 | I60.32 | I63.333 | I82.0 | J96.01 | K55.019 |
| A41.01 | B19.11 | E08.10 | G82.52 | I60.4 | I63.339 | I82.220 | J96.02 | K55.021 |
| A41.02 | B19.21 | E08.11 | G82.53 | I60.50 | I63.341 | I82.221 | J96.20 | K55.022 |
| A41.1 | B20 | E08.641 | G82.54 | I60.51 | I63.342 | I85.01 | J96.21 | K55.029 |
| A41.2 | B25.0 | E09.00 | G83.5 | I60.52 | I63.343 | I85.11 | J96.22 | K55.031 |
| A41.3 | B25.2 | E09.01 | G92 | I60.6 | I63.349 | J04.11 | J96.90 | K55.032 |
| A41.4 | B26.1 | E09.10 | G93.40 | I60.7 | I63.39 | J04.31 | J96.91 | K55.039 |
| A41.50 | B26.2 | E09.11 | G93.41 | I60.8 | I63.40 | J05.11 | J96.92 | K55.041 |
| A41.51 | B37.1 | E09.641 | G93.49 | I60.9 | I63.411 | J09.X1 | J98.51 | K55.042 |
| A41.52 | B37.5 | E10.10 | G93.5 | I61.0 | I63.412 | J10.00 | J98.59 | K55.049 |
| A41.53 | B37.6 | E10.11 | G93.6 | I61.1 | I63.413 | J10.01 | K22.11 | K55.051 |
| A41.59 | B37.7 | E10.641 | G93.7 | I61.2 | I63.419 | J10.08 | K22.3 | K55.052 |
| A41.81 | B38.4 | E11.00 | G93.82 | I61.3 | I63.421 | J11.00 | K22.6 | K55.059 |
| A41.89 | B39.0 | E11.01 | G95.11 | I61.4 | I63.422 | J11.08 | K25.0 | K55.061 |
| A41.9 | B39.1 | E11.10 | G95.19 | I61.5 | I63.423 | J12.0 | K25.1 | K55.062 |
| A42.7 | B39.2 | E11.11 | I21.01 | I61.6 | I63.429 | J12.1 | K25.2 | K55.069 |
| A48.0 | B44.0 | E11.641 | I21.02 | I61.8 | I63.431 | J12.2 | K25.4 | K55.21 |

Appendix E: Major Complication and Comorbidity (MCC) Code List

| | | | | | | | | |
|---|---|---|---|---|---|---|---|---|
| K55.30 | L89.143 | O08.4 | O41.1425 | O60.22X9 | P26.8 | Q04.3 | R40.2342 | S06.341A |
| K55.31 | L89.144 | O10.42 | O41.1429 | O60.23X0 | P26.9 | Q20.0 | R40.2343 | S06.342A |
| K55.32 | L89.153 | O11.1 | O41.1430 | O60.23X1 | P27.0 | Q20.1 | R40.2344 | S06.343A |
| K55.33 | L89.154 | O11.2 | O41.1431 | O60.23X2 | P27.1 | Q20.2 | R53.2 | S06.344A |
| K56.2 | L89.203 | O11.3 | O41.1432 | O60.23X3 | P27.8 | Q20.3 | R57.0 | S06.345A |
| K57.01 | L89.204 | O14.12 | O41.1433 | O60.23X4 | P27.9 | Q20.4 | R57.1 | S06.346A |
| K57.11 | L89.213 | O14.13 | O41.1434 | O60.23X5 | P28.5 | Q21.3 | R57.8 | S06.347A |
| K57.13 | L89.214 | O14.22 | O41.1435 | O60.23X9 | P28.81 | Q22.0 | R65.11 | S06.348A |
| K57.21 | L89.223 | O14.23 | O41.1439 | O67.0 | P29.30 | Q22.4 | R65.20 | S06.349A |
| K57.31 | L89.224 | O15.02 | O44.11 | O71.02 | P29.38 | Q22.5 | R65.21 | S06.350A |
| K57.33 | L89.303 | O15.03 | O44.12 | O71.03 | P29.81 | Q22.6 | S02.0XXB | S06.351A |
| K57.41 | L89.304 | O15.1 | O44.13 | O71.1 | P35.1 | Q22.8 | S02.101B | S06.352A |
| K57.51 | L89.313 | O15.2 | O44.31 | O75.1 | P35.2 | Q22.9 | S02.102B | S06.353A |
| K57.53 | L89.314 | O22.31 | O44.32 | O75.3 | P35.3 | Q23.4 | S02.109B | S06.354A |
| K57.81 | L89.323 | O22.32 | O44.33 | O85 | P35.8 | Q24.2 | S02.110B | S06.355A |
| K57.91 | L89.324 | O22.33 | O44.51 | O86.81 | P35.9 | Q24.4 | S02.111B | S06.356A |
| K57.93 | L89.43 | O24.02 | O44.52 | O86.89 | P36.0 | Q24.6 | S02.112B | S06.357A |
| K63.1 | L89.44 | O24.12 | O44.53 | O87.1 | P36.10 | Q25.5 | S02.113B | S06.358A |
| K63.81 | L89.503 | O24.32 | O45.001 | O88.011 | P36.19 | Q25.6 | S02.118B | S06.359A |
| K65.0 | L89.504 | O24.82 | O45.002 | O88.012 | P36.2 | Q25.71 | S02.119B | S06.360A |
| K65.1 | L89.513 | O34.31 | O45.003 | O88.013 | P36.30 | Q25.72 | S02.11AB | S06.361A |
| K65.2 | L89.514 | O34.32 | O45.011 | O88.02 | P36.39 | Q25.79 | S02.11BB | S06.362A |
| K65.3 | L89.523 | O34.33 | O45.012 | O88.03 | P36.4 | Q28.2 | S02.11CB | S06.363A |
| K65.8 | L89.524 | O41.1010 | O45.013 | O88.111 | P36.5 | Q28.3 | S02.11DB | S06.364A |
| K65.9 | L89.603 | O41.1011 | O45.021 | O88.112 | P36.8 | Q33.2 | S02.11EB | S06.365A |
| K66.1 | L89.604 | O41.1012 | O45.022 | O88.113 | P36.9 | Q33.3 | S02.11FB | S06.366A |
| K67 | L89.613 | O41.1013 | O45.023 | O88.12 | P37.0 | Q33.6 | S02.11GB | S06.367A |
| K68.12 | L89.614 | O41.1014 | O45.091 | O88.13 | P37.1 | Q39.0 | S02.11HB | S06.368A |
| K68.19 | L89.623 | O41.1015 | O45.092 | O88.211 | P37.2 | Q39.1 | S02.19XB | S06.369A |
| K68.9 | L89.624 | O41.1019 | O45.093 | O88.212 | P37.3 | Q39.3 | S02.91XB | S06.370A |
| K70.41 | L89.813 | O41.1020 | O45.8X1 | O88.213 | P37.4 | Q39.4 | S06.1X0A | S06.376A |
| K71.11 | L89.814 | O41.1021 | O45.8X2 | O88.22 | P37.8 | Q44.2 | S06.1X1A | S06.377A |
| K72.00 | L89.893 | O41.1022 | O45.8X3 | O88.23 | P37.9 | Q44.3 | S06.1X2A | S06.378A |
| K72.01 | L89.894 | O41.1023 | O45.91 | O88.311 | P52.21 | Q79.0 | S06.1X3A | S06.380A |
| K72.11 | L89.93 | O41.1024 | O45.92 | O88.312 | P52.22 | Q79.1 | S06.1X4A | S06.386A |
| K72.91 | L89.94 | O41.1025 | O45.93 | O88.313 | P52.4 | Q79.2 | S06.1X5A | S06.387A |
| K75.0 | M31.1 | O41.1029 | O46.001 | O88.32 | P52.5 | Q79.3 | S06.1X6A | S06.388A |
| K75.1 | M72.6 | O41.1030 | O46.002 | O88.33 | P52.6 | Q79.4 | S06.1X7A | S06.4X0A |
| K76.2 | N00.0 | O41.1031 | O46.003 | O88.811 | P52.8 | Q79.51 | S06.1X8A | S06.4X1A |
| K76.3 | N00.1 | O41.1032 | O46.011 | O88.812 | P52.9 | Q79.59 | S06.1X9A | S06.4X2A |
| K76.7 | N00.2 | O41.1033 | O46.012 | O88.813 | P54.1 | Q89.4 | S06.2X6A | S06.4X3A |
| K80.67 | N00.3 | O41.1034 | O46.013 | O88.82 | P54.2 | Q93.81 | S06.2X7A | S06.4X4A |
| K82.2 | N00.4 | O41.1035 | O46.021 | O88.83 | P54.3 | R09.2 | S06.2X8A | S06.4X5A |
| K83.1 | N00.5 | O41.1039 | O46.022 | O90.3 | P56.0 | R40.20 | S06.306A | S06.4X6A |
| K83.2 | N00.6 | O41.1210 | O46.023 | O90.4 | P56.90 | R40.2110 | S06.307A | S06.4X7A |
| K85.00 | N00.7 | O41.1211 | O46.091 | O99.42 | P56.99 | R40.2111 | S06.308A | S06.4X8A |
| K85.01 | N00.8 | O41.1212 | O46.092 | P10.0 | P57.0 | R40.2112 | S06.310A | S06.4X9A |
| K85.02 | N00.9 | O41.1213 | O46.093 | P10.1 | P57.8 | R40.2113 | S06.311A | S06.5X0A |
| K85.10 | N01.0 | O41.1214 | O60.02 | P10.3 | P57.9 | R40.2114 | S06.312A | S06.5X1A |
| K85.11 | N01.1 | O41.1215 | O60.03 | P10.4 | P59.1 | R40.2120 | S06.313A | S06.5X2A |
| K85.12 | N01.2 | O41.1219 | O60.12X0 | P10.8 | P59.20 | R40.2121 | S06.314A | S06.5X3A |
| K85.20 | N01.3 | O41.1220 | O60.12X1 | P10.9 | P59.29 | R40.2122 | S06.315A | S06.5X4A |
| K85.21 | N01.4 | O41.1221 | O60.12X2 | P11.0 | P60 | R40.2123 | S06.316A | S06.5X5A |
| K85.22 | N01.5 | O41.1222 | O60.12X3 | P11.2 | P61.0 | R40.2124 | S06.317A | S06.5X6A |
| K85.30 | N01.6 | O41.1223 | O60.12X4 | P11.9 | P61.5 | R40.2210 | S06.318A | S06.5X7A |
| K85.31 | N01.7 | O41.1224 | O60.12X5 | P22.0 | P74.0 | R40.2211 | S06.319A | S06.5X8A |
| K85.32 | N01.8 | O41.1225 | O60.12X9 | P23.0 | P77.1 | R40.2212 | S06.320A | S06.5X9A |
| K85.80 | N01.9 | O41.1229 | O60.13X0 | P23.1 | P77.2 | R40.2213 | S06.321A | S06.6X0A |
| K85.81 | N15.1 | O41.1230 | O60.13X1 | P23.2 | P77.3 | R40.2214 | S06.322A | S06.6X1A |
| K85.82 | N17.0 | O41.1231 | O60.13X2 | P23.3 | P77.9 | R40.2220 | S06.323A | S06.6X2A |
| K85.90 | N17.1 | O41.1232 | O60.13X3 | P23.4 | P78.0 | R40.2221 | S06.324A | S06.6X3A |
| K85.91 | N17.2 | O41.1233 | O60.13X4 | P23.5 | P83.2 | R40.2222 | S06.325A | S06.6X4A |
| K85.92 | N18.6 | O41.1234 | O60.13X5 | P23.6 | P90 | R40.2223 | S06.326A | S06.6X5A |
| L89.003 | N73.3 | O41.1235 | O60.13X9 | P23.8 | P91.0 | R40.2224 | S06.327A | S06.6X6A |
| L89.004 | O03.2 | O41.1239 | O60.14X0 | P23.9 | P91.1 | R40.2310 | S06.328A | S06.6X7A |
| L89.013 | O03.31 | O41.1410 | O60.14X1 | P24.01 | P91.2 | R40.2311 | S06.329A | S06.6X8A |
| L89.014 | O03.32 | O41.1411 | O60.14X2 | P24.11 | P91.3 | R40.2312 | S06.330A | S06.6X9A |
| L89.023 | O03.81 | O41.1412 | O60.14X3 | P24.21 | P91.4 | R40.2313 | S06.331A | S06.816A |
| L89.024 | O03.82 | O41.1413 | O60.14X4 | P24.31 | P91.5 | R40.2314 | S06.332A | S06.817A |
| L89.103 | O04.7 | O41.1414 | O60.14X5 | P24.81 | P91.63 | R40.2320 | S06.333A | S06.818A |
| L89.104 | O04.81 | O41.1415 | O60.14X9 | P25.0 | P92.01 | R40.2321 | S06.334A | S06.826A |
| L89.113 | O04.82 | O41.1419 | O60.22X0 | P25.1 | Q00.0 | R40.2322 | S06.335A | S06.827A |
| L89.114 | O07.2 | O41.1420 | O60.22X1 | P25.2 | Q00.1 | R40.2323 | S06.336A | S06.828A |
| L89.123 | O07.31 | O41.1421 | O60.22X2 | P25.3 | Q00.2 | R40.2324 | S06.337A | S06.896A |
| L89.124 | O07.32 | O41.1422 | O60.22X3 | P25.8 | Q04.0 | R40.2340 | S06.338A | S06.897A |
| L89.133 | O08.2 | O41.1423 | O60.22X4 | P26.0 | Q04.1 | R40.2341 | S06.339A | S06.898A |
| L89.134 | O08.3 | O41.1424 | O60.22X5 | P26.1 | Q04.2 | | S06.340A | S06.9X6A |

Appendix E: Major Complication and Comorbidity (MCC) Code List

| | | | | | | | | |
|---|---|---|---|---|---|---|---|---|
| S06.9X7A | S12.551B | S21.351A | S22.49XB | S27.332A | S32.018B | S32.424A | S32.486B | S35.291A |
| S06.9X8A | S12.590B | S21.352A | S22.5XXA | S27.339A | S32.019B | S32.424B | S32.491A | S35.292A |
| S11.011A | S12.591B | S21.359A | S22.5XXB | S27.401A | S32.020B | S32.425A | S32.491B | S35.298A |
| S11.012A | S12.600B | S21.401A | S22.9XXB | S27.402A | S32.021B | S32.425B | S32.492A | S35.299A |
| S11.013A | S12.601B | S21.402A | S24.0XXA | S27.409A | S32.022B | S32.426A | S32.492B | S35.311A |
| S11.014A | S12.630B | S21.409A | S24.101A | S27.411A | S32.028B | S32.426B | S32.499A | S35.318A |
| S11.015A | S12.631B | S21.411A | S24.102A | S27.412A | S32.029B | S32.431A | S32.499B | S35.319A |
| S11.019A | S12.64XB | S21.412A | S24.103A | S27.419A | S32.030B | S32.431B | S32.501B | S35.321A |
| S11.021A | S12.650B | S21.419A | S24.104A | S27.421A | S32.031B | S32.432A | S32.502B | S35.328A |
| S11.022A | S12.651B | S21.421A | S24.111A | S27.422A | S32.032B | S32.432B | S32.509B | S35.329A |
| S11.023A | S12.690B | S21.422A | S24.112A | S27.429A | S32.038B | S32.433A | S32.511B | S35.331A |
| S11.024A | S12.691B | S21.429A | S24.113A | S27.431A | S32.039B | S32.433B | S32.512B | S35.338A |
| S11.025A | S12.8XXA | S21.431A | S24.114A | S27.432A | S32.040B | S32.434A | S32.519B | S35.339A |
| S11.029A | S14.0XXA | S21.432A | S24.131A | S27.439A | S32.041B | S32.434B | S32.591B | S35.341A |
| S11.031A | S14.101A | S21.439A | S24.132A | S27.491A | S32.042B | S32.435A | S32.592B | S35.348A |
| S11.032A | S14.102A | S21.441A | S24.133A | S27.492A | S32.048B | S32.435B | S32.599B | S35.349A |
| S11.033A | S14.103A | S21.442A | S24.134A | S27.499A | S32.049B | S32.436A | S32.601B | S35.401A |
| S11.034A | S14.104A | S21.449A | S24.141A | S27.812A | S32.050B | S32.436B | S32.602B | S35.402A |
| S11.035A | S14.105A | S21.451A | S24.142A | S27.813A | S32.051B | S32.441A | S32.609B | S35.403A |
| S11.039A | S14.106A | S21.452A | S24.143A | S27.818A | S32.052B | S32.441B | S32.611B | S35.404A |
| S12.000B | S14.107A | S21.459A | S24.144A | S27.819A | S32.058B | S32.442A | S32.612B | S35.405A |
| S12.001B | S14.108A | S22.000B | S24.151A | S31.001A | S32.059B | S32.442B | S32.613B | S35.406A |
| S12.01XB | S14.111A | S22.001B | S24.152A | S31.011A | S32.10XB | S32.443A | S32.614B | S35.411A |
| S12.02XB | S14.112A | S22.002B | S24.153A | S31.021A | S32.110B | S32.443B | S32.615B | S35.412A |
| S12.030B | S14.113A | S22.008B | S24.154A | S31.031A | S32.111B | S32.444A | S32.616B | S35.413A |
| S12.031B | S14.114A | S22.009B | S25.00XA | S31.041A | S32.112B | S32.444B | S32.691B | S35.414A |
| S12.040B | S14.115A | S22.010B | S25.01XA | S31.051A | S32.119B | S32.445A | S32.692B | S35.415A |
| S12.041B | S14.116A | S22.011B | S25.02XA | S31.600A | S32.120B | S32.445B | S32.699B | S35.416A |
| S12.090B | S14.117A | S22.012B | S25.09XA | S31.601A | S32.121B | S32.446A | S32.810B | S35.491A |
| S12.091B | S14.118A | S22.018B | S25.101A | S31.602A | S32.122B | S32.446B | S32.82XB | S35.492A |
| S12.100B | S14.121A | S22.019B | S25.102A | S31.603A | S32.129B | S32.451A | S32.89XB | S35.493A |
| S12.101B | S14.122A | S22.020B | S25.109A | S31.604A | S32.130B | S32.451B | S32.9XXB | S35.494A |
| S12.110B | S14.123A | S22.021B | S25.111A | S31.605A | S32.131B | S32.452A | S34.01XA | S35.495A |
| S12.111B | S14.124A | S22.022B | S25.112A | S31.609A | S32.132B | S32.452B | S34.02XA | S35.496A |
| S12.112B | S14.125A | S22.028B | S25.119A | S31.610A | S32.139B | S32.453A | S34.101A | S35.50XA |
| S12.120B | S14.126A | S22.029B | S25.121A | S31.611A | S32.14XB | S32.453B | S34.102A | S35.511A |
| S12.121B | S14.127A | S22.030B | S25.122A | S31.612A | S32.15XB | S32.454A | S34.103A | S35.512A |
| S12.130B | S14.128A | S22.031B | S25.129A | S31.613A | S32.16XB | S32.454B | S34.104A | S35.513A |
| S12.131B | S14.131A | S22.032B | S25.191A | S31.614A | S32.17XB | S32.455A | S34.105A | S35.514A |
| S12.14XB | S14.132A | S22.038B | S25.192A | S31.615A | S32.19XB | S32.455B | S34.109A | S35.515A |
| S12.150B | S14.133A | S22.039B | S25.199A | S31.619A | S32.2XXB | S32.456A | S34.111A | S35.516A |
| S12.151B | S14.134A | S22.040B | S25.20XA | S31.620A | S32.301B | S32.456B | S34.112A | S35.59XA |
| S12.190B | S14.135A | S22.041B | S25.21XA | S31.621A | S32.302B | S32.461A | S34.113A | S36.031A |
| S12.191B | S14.136A | S22.042B | S25.22XA | S31.622A | S32.309B | S32.461B | S34.114A | S36.032A |
| S12.200B | S14.137A | S22.048B | S25.29XA | S31.623A | S32.311B | S32.462A | S34.115A | S36.115A |
| S12.201B | S14.138A | S22.049B | S25.301A | S31.624A | S32.312B | S32.462B | S34.119A | S36.116A |
| S12.230B | S14.141A | S22.050B | S25.302A | S31.625A | S32.313B | S32.463A | S34.121A | S37.061A |
| S12.231B | S14.142A | S22.051B | S25.309A | S31.629A | S32.314B | S32.463B | S34.122A | S37.062A |
| S12.24XB | S14.143A | S22.052B | S25.311A | S31.630A | S32.315B | S32.464A | S34.123A | S37.069A |
| S12.250B | S14.144A | S22.058B | S25.312A | S31.631A | S32.316B | S32.464B | S34.124A | S37.091A |
| S12.251B | S14.145A | S22.059B | S25.319A | S31.632A | S32.391B | S32.465A | S34.125A | S37.092A |
| S12.290B | S14.146A | S22.060B | S25.321A | S31.633A | S32.392B | S32.465B | S34.129A | S37.099A |
| S12.291B | S14.147A | S22.061B | S25.322A | S31.634A | S32.399B | S32.466A | S34.131A | S42.201A |
| S12.300B | S14.148A | S22.062B | S25.329A | S31.635A | S32.401A | S32.466B | S34.132A | S42.202B |
| S12.301B | S14.151A | S22.068B | S25.391A | S31.639A | S32.401B | S32.471A | S34.139A | S42.209B |
| S12.330B | S14.152A | S22.069B | S25.392A | S31.640A | S32.402A | S32.471B | S34.3XXA | S42.211B |
| S12.331B | S14.153A | S22.070B | S25.399A | S31.641A | S32.402B | S32.472A | S35.00XA | S42.212B |
| S12.34XB | S14.154A | S22.071B | S25.401A | S31.642A | S32.409A | S32.472B | S35.01XA | S42.213B |
| S12.350B | S14.155A | S22.072B | S25.402A | S31.643A | S32.409B | S32.473A | S35.02XA | S42.214B |
| S12.351B | S14.156A | S22.078B | S25.409A | S31.644A | S32.411A | S32.473B | S35.09XA | S42.215B |
| S12.390B | S14.157A | S22.079B | S25.411A | S31.645A | S32.411B | S32.474A | S35.10XA | S42.216B |
| S12.391B | S14.158A | S22.080B | S25.412A | S31.649A | S32.412A | S32.474B | S35.11XA | S42.221B |
| S12.400B | S21.301A | S22.081B | S25.419A | S31.650A | S32.412B | S32.475A | S35.12XA | S42.222B |
| S12.401B | S21.302A | S22.082B | S25.421A | S31.651A | S32.413A | S32.475B | S35.19XA | S42.223B |
| S12.430B | S21.309A | S22.088B | S25.422A | S31.652A | S32.413B | S32.476A | S35.211A | S42.224B |
| S12.431B | S21.311A | S22.089B | S25.429A | S31.653A | S32.414A | S32.476B | S35.212A | S42.225B |
| S12.44XB | S21.312A | S22.20XB | S25.491A | S31.654A | S32.414B | S32.481A | S35.218A | S42.226B |
| S12.450B | S21.319A | S22.21XB | S25.492A | S31.655A | S32.415A | S32.481B | S35.219A | S42.231B |
| S12.451B | S21.321A | S22.22XB | S25.499A | S31.659A | S32.415B | S32.482A | S35.221A | S42.232B |
| S12.490B | S21.322A | S22.23XB | S26.020A | S32.000A | S32.416A | S32.482B | S35.222A | S42.239B |
| S12.491B | S21.329A | S22.24XB | S26.021A | S32.001B | S32.416B | S32.483A | S35.228A | S42.241B |
| S12.500B | S21.331A | S22.31XB | S26.022A | S32.002B | S32.421A | S32.483B | S35.229A | S42.242B |
| S12.501B | S21.332A | S22.32XB | S26.12XA | S32.008B | S32.421B | S32.484A | S35.231A | S42.249B |
| S12.530B | S21.339A | S22.39XB | S26.92XA | S32.009B | S32.422A | S32.484B | S35.232A | S42.251B |
| S12.531B | S21.341A | S22.41XB | S27.1XXA | S32.010B | S32.422B | S32.485A | S35.238A | S42.252B |
| S12.54XB | S21.342A | S22.42XB | S27.2XXA | S32.011B | S32.423A | S32.485B | S35.239A | S42.253B |
| S12.550B | S21.349A | S22.43XB | S27.331A | S32.012B | S32.423B | S32.486A | | S42.254B |

| | | | | | | | | |
|---|---|---|---|---|---|---|---|---|
| S42.255B | S42.447B | S52.045B | S52.241C | S52.334B | S52.516C | S72.011B | S72.063A | S72.134C |
| S42.256B | S42.448B | S52.045C | S52.242B | S52.334C | S52.531B | S72.011C | S72.063B | S72.135A |
| S42.261B | S42.449B | S52.046B | S52.242C | S52.335B | S52.531C | S72.012A | S72.063C | S72.135B |
| S42.262B | S42.451B | S52.046C | S52.243B | S52.335C | S52.532B | S72.012B | S72.064A | S72.135C |
| S42.263B | S42.452B | S52.091B | S52.243C | S52.336B | S52.532C | S72.012C | S72.064B | S72.136A |
| S42.264B | S42.453B | S52.091C | S52.244B | S52.336C | S52.539B | S72.019A | S72.064C | S72.136B |
| S42.265B | S42.454B | S52.092B | S52.244C | S52.341B | S52.539C | S72.019B | S72.065A | S72.136C |
| S42.266B | S42.455B | S52.092C | S52.245B | S52.341C | S52.541B | S72.019C | S72.065B | S72.141A |
| S42.291B | S42.456B | S52.099B | S52.245C | S52.342B | S52.541C | S72.021A | S72.065C | S72.141B |
| S42.292B | S42.461B | S52.099C | S52.246B | S52.342C | S52.542B | S72.021B | S72.066A | S72.141C |
| S42.293B | S42.462B | S52.101B | S52.246C | S52.343B | S52.542C | S72.021C | S72.066B | S72.142A |
| S42.294B | S42.463B | S52.101C | S52.251B | S52.343C | S52.549B | S72.022A | S72.066C | S72.142B |
| S42.295B | S42.464B | S52.102B | S52.251C | S52.344B | S52.549C | S72.022B | S72.091A | S72.142C |
| S42.296B | S42.465B | S52.102C | S52.252B | S52.344C | S52.551B | S72.022C | S72.091B | S72.143A |
| S42.301B | S42.466B | S52.109B | S52.252C | S52.345B | S52.551C | S72.023A | S72.091C | S72.143B |
| S42.302B | S42.471B | S52.109C | S52.253B | S52.345C | S52.552B | S72.023B | S72.092A | S72.143C |
| S42.309B | S42.472B | S52.121B | S52.253C | S52.346B | S52.552C | S72.023C | S72.092B | S72.144A |
| S42.321B | S42.473B | S52.121C | S52.254B | S52.346C | S52.559B | S72.024A | S72.092C | S72.144B |
| S42.322B | S42.474B | S52.122B | S52.254C | S52.351B | S52.559C | S72.024B | S72.099A | S72.144C |
| S42.323B | S42.475B | S52.122C | S52.255B | S52.351C | S52.561B | S72.024C | S72.099B | S72.145A |
| S42.324B | S42.476B | S52.123B | S52.255C | S52.352B | S52.561C | S72.025A | S72.099C | S72.145B |
| S42.325B | S42.491B | S52.123C | S52.256B | S52.352C | S52.562B | S72.025B | S72.101A | S72.145C |
| S42.326B | S42.492B | S52.124B | S52.256C | S52.353B | S52.562C | S72.025C | S72.101B | S72.146A |
| S42.331B | S42.493B | S52.124C | S52.261B | S52.353C | S52.569B | S72.026A | S72.101C | S72.146B |
| S42.332B | S42.494B | S52.125B | S52.261C | S52.354B | S52.569C | S72.026B | S72.102A | S72.146C |
| S42.333B | S42.495B | S52.125C | S52.262B | S52.354C | S52.571B | S72.026C | S72.102B | S72.21XA |
| S42.334B | S42.496B | S52.126B | S52.262C | S52.355B | S52.571C | S72.031A | S72.102C | S72.21XB |
| S42.335B | S42.90XB | S52.126C | S52.263B | S52.355C | S52.572B | S72.031B | S72.109A | S72.21XC |
| S42.336B | S42.91XB | S52.131B | S52.263C | S52.356B | S52.572C | S72.031C | S72.109B | S72.22XA |
| S42.341B | S42.92XB | S52.131C | S52.264B | S52.356C | S52.579B | S72.032A | S72.109C | S72.22XB |
| S42.342B | S45.001A | S52.132B | S52.264C | S52.361B | S52.579C | S72.032B | S72.111A | S72.22XC |
| S42.343B | S45.002A | S52.132C | S52.265B | S52.361C | S52.591B | S72.032C | S72.111B | S72.23XA |
| S42.344B | S45.009A | S52.133B | S52.265C | S52.362B | S52.591C | S72.033A | S72.111C | S72.23XB |
| S42.345B | S45.011A | S52.133C | S52.266B | S52.362C | S52.592B | S72.033B | S72.112A | S72.23XC |
| S42.346B | S45.012A | S52.134B | S52.266C | S52.363B | S52.592C | S72.033C | S72.112B | S72.24XA |
| S42.351B | S45.019A | S52.134C | S52.271B | S52.363C | S52.599B | S72.034A | S72.112C | S72.24XB |
| S42.352B | S45.091A | S52.135B | S52.271C | S52.364B | S52.599C | S72.034B | S72.113A | S72.24XC |
| S42.353B | S45.092A | S52.135C | S52.272B | S52.364C | S52.601B | S72.034C | S72.113B | S72.25XA |
| S42.354B | S45.099A | S52.136B | S52.272C | S52.365B | S52.601C | S72.035A | S72.113C | S72.25XB |
| S42.355B | S52.001B | S52.136C | S52.279B | S52.365C | S52.602B | S72.035B | S72.114A | S72.25XC |
| S42.356B | S52.001C | S52.181B | S52.279C | S52.366B | S52.602C | S72.035C | S72.114B | S72.26XA |
| S42.361B | S52.002B | S52.181C | S52.281B | S52.366C | S52.609B | S72.036A | S72.114C | S72.26XB |
| S42.362B | S52.002C | S52.182B | S52.281C | S52.371B | S52.609C | S72.036B | S72.115A | S72.26XC |
| S42.363B | S52.009B | S52.182C | S52.282B | S52.371C | S52.611B | S72.036C | S72.115B | S72.301A |
| S42.364B | S52.009C | S52.189B | S52.282C | S52.372B | S52.611C | S72.041A | S72.115C | S72.301B |
| S42.365B | S52.021B | S52.189C | S52.283B | S52.372C | S52.612B | S72.041B | S72.116A | S72.301C |
| S42.366B | S52.021C | S52.201B | S52.283C | S52.379B | S52.612C | S72.041C | S72.116B | S72.302A |
| S42.391B | S52.022B | S52.201C | S52.291B | S52.379C | S52.613B | S72.042A | S72.116C | S72.302B |
| S42.392B | S52.022C | S52.202B | S52.291C | S52.381B | S52.613C | S72.042B | S72.121A | S72.302C |
| S42.399B | S52.023B | S52.202C | S52.292B | S52.381C | S52.614B | S72.042C | S72.121B | S72.309A |
| S42.401B | S52.023C | S52.209B | S52.292C | S52.382B | S52.614C | S72.043A | S72.121C | S72.309B |
| S42.402B | S52.024B | S52.209C | S52.299B | S52.382C | S52.615B | S72.043B | S72.122A | S72.309C |
| S42.409B | S52.024C | S52.221B | S52.299C | S52.389B | S52.615C | S72.043C | S72.122B | S72.321A |
| S42.411B | S52.025B | S52.221C | S52.301B | S52.389C | S52.616B | S72.044A | S72.122C | S72.321B |
| S42.412B | S52.025C | S52.222B | S52.301C | S52.391B | S52.616C | S72.044B | S72.123A | S72.321C |
| S42.413B | S52.026B | S52.222C | S52.302B | S52.391C | S52.691B | S72.044C | S72.123B | S72.322A |
| S42.414B | S52.026C | S52.223B | S52.302C | S52.392B | S52.691C | S72.045A | S72.123C | S72.322B |
| S42.415B | S52.031B | S52.223C | S52.309B | S52.392C | S52.692B | S72.045B | S72.124A | S72.322C |
| S42.416B | S52.031C | S52.224B | S52.309C | S52.399B | S52.692C | S72.045C | S72.124B | S72.323A |
| S42.421B | S52.032B | S52.224C | S52.321B | S52.399C | S52.699B | S72.046A | S72.124C | S72.323B |
| S42.422B | S52.032C | S52.225B | S52.321C | S52.501B | S52.699C | S72.046B | S72.125A | S72.323C |
| S42.423B | S52.033B | S52.225C | S52.322B | S52.501C | S52.90XB | S72.046C | S72.125B | S72.324A |
| S42.424B | S52.033C | S52.226B | S52.322C | S52.502B | S52.90XC | S72.051A | S72.125C | S72.324B |
| S42.425B | S52.034B | S52.226C | S52.323B | S52.502C | S52.91XB | S72.051B | S72.126A | S72.324C |
| S42.426B | S52.034C | S52.231B | S52.323C | S52.509B | S52.91XC | S72.051C | S72.126B | S72.325A |
| S42.431B | S52.035B | S52.231C | S52.324B | S52.509C | S52.92XB | S72.052A | S72.126C | S72.325B |
| S42.432B | S52.035C | S52.232B | S52.324C | S52.511B | S52.92XC | S72.052B | S72.131A | S72.325C |
| S42.433B | S52.036B | S52.232C | S52.325B | S52.511C | S72.001A | S72.052C | S72.131B | S72.326A |
| S42.434B | S52.036C | S52.233B | S52.325C | S52.512B | S72.001B | S72.059A | S72.131C | S72.326B |
| S42.435B | S52.041B | S52.233C | S52.326B | S52.512C | S72.001C | S72.059B | S72.132A | S72.326C |
| S42.436B | S52.041C | S52.234B | S52.326C | S52.513B | S72.002A | S72.059C | S72.132B | S72.331A |
| S42.441B | S52.042B | S52.234C | S52.331B | S52.513C | S72.002B | S72.061A | S72.132C | S72.331B |
| S42.442B | S52.042C | S52.235B | S52.331C | S52.514B | S72.002C | S72.061B | S72.133A | S72.331C |
| S42.443B | S52.043B | S52.235C | S52.332B | S52.514C | S72.009A | S72.061C | S72.133B | S72.332A |
| S42.444B | S52.043C | S52.236B | S52.332C | S52.515B | S72.009B | S72.062A | S72.133C | S72.332B |
| S42.445B | S52.044B | S52.236C | S52.333B | S52.515C | S72.009C | S72.062B | S72.134A | S72.332C |
| S42.446B | S52.044C | S52.241B | S52.333C | S52.516B | S72.011A | S72.062C | S72.134B | S72.333A |

| | | | | | | | | |
|---|---|---|---|---|---|---|---|---|
| S72.333B | S72.366A | S72.445B | S75.092A | S82.135C | S82.236C | S82.431C | S82.862C | T31.91 |
| S72.333C | S72.366B | S72.445C | S75.099A | S82.136B | S82.241B | S82.432B | S82.863B | T31.92 |
| S72.334A | S72.366C | S72.446B | S75.101A | S82.136C | S82.241C | S82.432C | S82.863C | T31.93 |
| S72.334B | S72.391A | S72.446C | S75.102A | S82.141B | S82.242B | S82.433B | S82.864B | T31.94 |
| S72.334C | S72.391B | S72.451B | S75.109A | S82.141C | S82.242C | S82.433C | S82.864C | T31.95 |
| S72.335A | S72.391C | S72.451C | S75.111A | S82.142B | S82.243B | S82.434B | S82.865B | T31.96 |
| S72.335B | S72.392A | S72.452B | S75.112A | S82.142C | S82.243C | S82.434C | S82.865C | T31.97 |
| S72.335C | S72.392B | S72.452C | S75.119A | S82.143B | S82.244B | S82.435B | S82.866B | T31.98 |
| S72.336A | S72.392C | S72.453B | S75.121A | S82.143C | S82.244C | S82.435C | S82.866C | T31.99 |
| S72.336B | S72.399A | S72.453C | S75.122A | S82.144B | S82.245B | S82.436B | S85.001A | T32.21 |
| S72.336C | S72.399B | S72.454B | S75.129A | S82.144C | S82.245C | S82.436C | S85.002A | T32.22 |
| S72.341A | S72.399C | S72.454C | S75.191A | S82.145B | S82.246B | S82.441B | S85.009A | T32.31 |
| S72.341B | S72.401B | S72.455B | S75.192A | S82.145C | S82.246C | S82.441C | S85.011A | T32.32 |
| S72.341C | S72.401C | S72.455C | S75.199A | S82.146B | S82.251B | S82.442B | S85.012A | T32.33 |
| S72.342A | S72.402B | S72.456B | S79.001A | S82.146C | S82.251C | S82.442C | S85.019A | T32.41 |
| S72.342B | S72.402C | S72.456C | S79.002A | S82.151B | S82.252B | S82.443B | S85.091A | T32.42 |
| S72.342C | S72.409B | S72.461B | S79.009A | S82.151C | S82.252C | S82.443C | S85.092A | T32.43 |
| S72.343A | S72.409C | S72.461C | S79.011A | S82.152B | S82.253B | S82.444B | S85.099A | T32.44 |
| S72.343B | S72.411B | S72.462B | S79.012A | S82.152C | S82.253C | S82.444C | S85.501A | T32.51 |
| S72.343C | S72.411C | S72.462C | S79.019A | S82.153B | S82.254B | S82.445B | S85.502A | T32.52 |
| S72.344A | S72.412B | S72.463B | S79.091A | S82.153C | S82.254C | S82.445C | S85.509A | T32.53 |
| S72.344B | S72.412C | S72.463C | S79.092A | S82.154B | S82.255B | S82.446B | S85.511A | T32.54 |
| S72.344C | S72.413B | S72.464B | S79.099A | S82.154C | S82.255C | S82.446C | S85.512A | T32.55 |
| S72.345A | S72.413C | S72.464C | S82.101B | S82.155B | S82.256B | S82.451B | S85.519A | T32.61 |
| S72.345B | S72.414B | S72.465B | S82.101C | S82.155C | S82.256C | S82.451C | S85.591A | T32.62 |
| S72.345C | S72.414C | S72.465C | S82.102B | S82.156B | S82.261B | S82.452B | S85.592A | T32.63 |
| S72.346A | S72.415B | S72.466B | S82.102C | S82.156C | S82.261C | S82.452C | S85.599A | T32.64 |
| S72.346B | S72.415C | S72.466C | S82.109B | S82.191B | S82.262B | S82.453B | T31.21 | T32.65 |
| S72.346C | S72.416B | S72.491B | S82.109C | S82.191C | S82.262C | S82.453C | T31.22 | T32.66 |
| S72.351A | S72.416C | S72.491C | S82.111B | S82.192B | S82.263B | S82.454B | T31.31 | T32.71 |
| S72.351B | S72.421B | S72.492B | S82.111C | S82.192C | S82.263C | S82.454C | T31.32 | T32.72 |
| S72.351C | S72.421C | S72.492C | S82.112B | S82.199B | S82.264B | S82.455B | T31.33 | T32.73 |
| S72.352A | S72.422B | S72.499B | S82.112C | S82.199C | S82.264C | S82.455C | T31.41 | T32.74 |
| S72.352B | S72.422C | S72.499C | S82.113B | S82.201B | S82.265B | S82.456B | T31.42 | T32.75 |
| S72.352C | S72.423B | S72.8X1A | S82.113C | S82.201C | S82.265C | S82.456C | T31.43 | T32.76 |
| S72.353A | S72.423C | S72.8X1B | S82.114B | S82.202B | S82.266B | S82.461B | T31.44 | T32.77 |
| S72.353B | S72.424B | S72.8X1C | S82.114C | S82.202C | S82.266C | S82.461C | T31.51 | T32.81 |
| S72.353C | S72.424C | S72.8X2A | S82.115B | S82.209B | S82.291B | S82.462B | T31.52 | T32.82 |
| S72.354A | S72.425B | S72.8X2B | S82.115C | S82.209C | S82.291C | S82.462C | T31.53 | T32.83 |
| S72.354B | S72.425C | S72.8X2C | S82.116B | S82.221B | S82.292B | S82.463B | T31.54 | T32.84 |
| S72.354C | S72.426B | S72.8X9A | S82.116C | S82.221C | S82.292C | S82.463C | T31.55 | T32.85 |
| S72.355A | S72.426C | S72.8X9B | S82.121B | S82.222B | S82.299B | S82.464B | T31.61 | T32.86 |
| S72.355B | S72.431B | S72.8X9C | S82.121C | S82.222C | S82.299C | S82.464C | T31.62 | T32.87 |
| S72.355C | S72.431C | S72.90XA | S82.122B | S82.223B | S82.401B | S82.465B | T31.63 | T32.88 |
| S72.356A | S72.432B | S72.90XB | S82.122C | S82.223C | S82.401C | S82.465C | T31.64 | T32.91 |
| S72.356B | S72.432C | S72.90XC | S82.123B | S82.224B | S82.402B | S82.466B | T31.65 | T32.92 |
| S72.356C | S72.433B | S72.91XA | S82.123C | S82.224C | S82.402C | S82.466C | T31.66 | T32.93 |
| S72.361A | S72.433C | S72.91XB | S82.124B | S82.225B | S82.409B | S82.491B | T31.71 | T32.94 |
| S72.361B | S72.434B | S72.91XC | S82.124C | S82.225C | S82.409C | S82.491C | T31.72 | T32.95 |
| S72.361C | S72.434C | S72.92XA | S82.125B | S82.226B | S82.421B | S82.492B | T31.73 | T32.96 |
| S72.362A | S72.435B | S72.92XB | S82.125C | S82.226C | S82.421C | S82.492C | T31.74 | T32.97 |
| S72.362B | S72.435C | S72.92XC | S82.126B | S82.231B | S82.422B | S82.499B | T31.75 | T32.98 |
| S72.362C | S72.436B | S75.001A | S82.126C | S82.231C | S82.422C | S82.499C | T31.76 | T32.99 |
| S72.363A | S72.436C | S75.002A | S82.131B | S82.232B | S82.423B | S82.831B | T31.77 | T79.0XXA |
| S72.363B | S72.441B | S75.009A | S82.131C | S82.232C | S82.423C | S82.831C | T31.81 | T79.1XXA |
| S72.363C | S72.441C | S75.011A | S82.132B | S82.233B | S82.424B | S82.832B | T31.82 | T79.4XXA |
| S72.364A | S72.442B | S75.012A | S82.132C | S82.233C | S82.424C | S82.832C | T31.83 | T79.5XXA |
| S72.364B | S72.442C | S75.019A | S82.133B | S82.234B | S82.425B | S82.839B | T31.84 | T80.0XXA |
| S72.364C | S72.443B | S75.021A | S82.133C | S82.234C | S82.425C | S82.839C | T31.85 | T81.11XA |
| S72.365A | S72.443C | S75.022A | S82.134B | S82.235B | S82.426B | S82.861B | T31.86 | T81.12XA |
| S72.365B | S72.444B | S75.029A | S82.134C | S82.235C | S82.426C | S82.861C | T31.87 | T81.19XA |
| S72.365C | S72.444C | S75.091A | S82.135B | S82.236B | S82.431B | S82.862B | T31.88 | |

# Appendix F: Complication and Comorbidity (CC) Code List

**Note:** The following list of CCs are based on the *Federal Register,* volume 82, number 81, April 28, 2017 ("Hospital Inpatient Prospective Payment Systems for Acute Care Hospitals and the Long-Term Care Hospital Prospective Payment System and Proposed Policy Changes and Fiscal Year 2018 Rates; Proposed Rule"). The most current version, v35, of the ICD-10 MS-DRG Definitions Manual was not available at the time this book was printed. For the most current files related to IPPS please refer to the following:
https://www.cms.gov/Medicare/Medicare-Fee-for-Service-Payment/AcuteInpatientPPS/IPPS-Regulations-and-Notices.html.

| | | | | | | | | |
|---|---|---|---|---|---|---|---|---|
| A00.0 | A15.9 | A30.5 | A50.2 | A54.33 | A89 | B15.9 | B45.0 | B66.4 |
| A00.1 | A17.9 | A30.8 | A50.30 | A54.39 | A90 | B16.1 | B45.2 | B66.5 |
| A00.9 | A18.01 | A30.9 | A50.31 | A54.40 | A91 | B16.9 | B45.3 | B66.8 |
| A01.00 | A18.02 | A31.0 | A50.32 | A54.41 | A92.0 | B17.0 | B45.7 | B67.0 |
| A01.01 | A18.03 | A31.1 | A50.39 | A54.42 | A92.1 | B17.10 | B45.8 | B67.1 |
| A01.02 | A18.09 | A31.2 | A50.40 | A54.43 | A92.2 | B17.2 | B45.9 | B67.2 |
| A01.03 | A18.10 | A31.8 | A50.43 | A54.49 | A92.4 | B17.8 | B47.0 | B67.31 |
| A01.04 | A18.11 | A31.9 | A50.44 | A54.82 | A92.5 | B17.9 | B47.1 | B67.32 |
| A01.05 | A18.12 | A32.0 | A50.45 | A54.83 | A92.8 | B18.0 | B47.9 | B67.39 |
| A01.09 | A18.13 | A32.11 | A50.49 | A54.84 | A92.9 | B18.1 | B48.2 | B67.4 |
| A01.1 | A18.14 | A32.12 | A50.51 | A54.85 | A93.0 | B18.8 | B48.3 | B67.5 |
| A01.2 | A18.15 | A32.81 | A50.52 | A54.89 | A93.1 | B18.9 | B48.4 | B67.61 |
| A01.3 | A18.16 | A32.82 | A50.53 | A54.9 | A93.2 | B19.10 | B48.8 | B67.69 |
| A01.4 | A18.17 | A32.89 | A50.54 | A68.0 | A93.8 | B19.9 | B49 | B67.7 |
| A02.0 | A18.18 | A32.9 | A50.55 | A68.1 | A94 | B25.1 | B50.0 | B67.8 |
| A02.23 | A18.2 | A34 | A50.56 | A68.9 | A95.0 | B25.8 | B50.8 | B67.90 |
| A02.24 | A18.32 | A36.0 | A50.57 | A69.1 | A95.1 | B25.9 | B51.0 | B67.99 |
| A02.25 | A18.39 | A36.1 | A50.59 | A69.20 | A95.9 | B26.0 | B51.8 | B68.0 |
| A02.29 | A18.4 | A36.2 | A51.31 | A69.21 | A96.0 | B26.3 | B51.9 | B68.1 |
| A02.8 | A18.50 | A36.3 | A51.32 | A69.22 | A96.1 | B26.81 | B52.0 | B68.9 |
| A02.9 | A18.51 | A36.81 | A51.39 | A69.23 | A96.8 | B26.82 | B52.8 | B69.0 |
| A03.0 | A18.52 | A36.82 | A51.42 | A69.29 | A96.9 | B26.83 | B52.9 | B69.1 |
| A04.0 | A18.53 | A36.83 | A51.43 | A70 | A98.0 | B26.84 | B53.0 | B69.81 |
| A04.1 | A18.54 | A36.84 | A51.44 | A75.0 | A98.1 | B26.85 | B53.1 | B69.89 |
| A04.2 | A18.59 | A36.85 | A51.45 | A75.1 | A98.2 | B26.89 | B53.8 | B69.9 |
| A04.3 | A18.6 | A36.86 | A51.46 | A75.2 | A98.5 | B33.1 | B54 | B70.0 |
| A04.4 | A18.7 | A36.89 | A51.49 | A75.3 | A98.8 | B33.20 | B55.0 | B70.1 |
| A04.5 | A18.81 | A36.9 | A52.00 | A75.9 | A99 | B33.21 | B55.1 | B71.0 |
| A04.6 | A18.82 | A37.00 | A52.01 | A77.0 | B00.2 | B33.22 | B55.2 | B71.1 |
| A04.71 | A18.83 | A37.10 | A52.02 | A77.1 | B00.50 | B33.23 | B55.9 | B71.8 |
| A04.72 | A18.84 | A37.80 | A52.03 | A77.2 | B00.51 | B33.4 | B56.0 | B72 |
| A04.8 | A18.85 | A37.90 | A52.04 | A77.3 | B00.52 | B34.2 | B56.1 | B73.00 |
| A04.9 | A18.89 | A38.0 | A52.05 | A77.40 | B00.53 | B37.0 | B56.9 | B73.01 |
| A05.0 | A21.0 | A38.1 | A52.06 | A77.41 | B00.59 | B37.41 | B57.0 | B73.02 |
| A05.1 | A21.1 | A38.8 | A52.09 | A77.49 | B00.81 | B37.49 | B57.1 | B73.09 |
| A05.2 | A21.2 | A38.9 | A52.10 | A77.8 | B00.89 | B37.81 | B57.2 | B73.1 |
| A05.3 | A21.3 | A39.82 | A52.11 | A77.9 | B01.0 | B37.82 | B57.30 | B74.0 |
| A05.4 | A21.7 | A39.83 | A52.12 | A78 | B01.81 | B37.83 | B57.31 | B74.1 |
| A05.5 | A21.8 | A39.84 | A52.15 | A79.0 | B01.89 | B37.84 | B57.32 | B74.2 |
| A05.8 | A21.9 | A39.89 | A52.16 | A79.1 | B01.9 | B37.89 | B57.39 | B74.3 |
| A06.0 | A22.0 | A39.9 | A52.17 | A79.81 | B02.0 | B38.0 | B57.40 | B74.4 |
| A06.1 | A22.2 | A42.0 | A52.19 | A79.89 | B02.21 | B38.1 | B57.41 | B74.8 |
| A06.2 | A22.8 | A42.1 | A52.2 | A79.9 | B02.22 | B38.2 | B57.42 | B74.9 |
| A06.3 | A22.9 | A42.2 | A52.3 | A81.00 | B02.23 | B38.3 | B57.49 | B75 |
| A06.81 | A23.8 | A42.81 | A52.71 | A81.01 | B02.29 | B38.7 | B57.5 | B76.0 |
| A06.82 | A23.9 | A42.82 | A52.72 | A81.09 | B02.30 | B38.81 | B58.00 | B76.1 |
| A06.89 | A24.0 | A42.89 | A52.73 | A81.1 | B02.31 | B38.89 | B58.01 | B76.8 |
| A07.1 | A24.1 | A42.9 | A52.74 | A81.2 | B02.32 | B38.9 | B58.09 | B76.9 |
| A07.2 | A24.2 | A43.0 | A52.75 | A81.81 | B02.33 | B39.3 | B58.1 | B77.0 |
| A07.3 | A24.3 | A43.1 | A52.76 | A81.82 | B02.34 | B40.0 | B58.82 | B77.89 |
| A07.4 | A24.9 | A43.8 | A52.77 | A81.83 | B02.39 | B40.1 | B58.83 | B77.9 |
| A07.8 | A25.0 | A43.9 | A52.78 | A81.89 | B02.7 | B40.2 | B58.89 | B78.0 |
| A07.9 | A25.1 | A44.0 | A52.79 | A81.9 | B02.8 | B40.3 | B58.9 | B78.7 |
| A08.0 | A25.9 | A44.1 | A54.00 | A82.0 | B03 | B40.7 | B60.0 | B78.9 |
| A08.11 | A27.0 | A44.8 | A54.01 | A82.1 | B04 | B40.81 | B60.10 | B79 |
| A08.19 | A27.89 | A44.9 | A54.02 | A82.9 | B05.1 | B40.89 | B60.19 | B80 |
| A08.2 | A27.9 | A48.51 | A54.03 | A85.0 | B05.4 | B40.9 | B60.2 | B81.0 |
| A08.31 | A28.0 | A48.52 | A54.09 | A85.1 | B05.81 | B41.0 | B65.0 | B81.1 |
| A08.32 | A28.1 | A50.01 | A54.1 | A85.8 | B05.89 | B41.7 | B65.1 | B81.2 |
| A08.39 | A28.2 | A50.02 | A54.21 | A86 | B06.00 | B41.8 | B65.2 | B81.3 |
| A09 | A28.8 | A50.03 | A54.22 | A87.0 | B06.02 | B41.9 | B65.3 | B81.4 |
| A15.0 | A28.9 | A50.04 | A54.23 | A87.1 | B06.09 | B44.1 | B65.8 | B81.8 |
| A15.4 | A30.0 | A50.05 | A54.24 | A87.2 | B06.81 | B44.2 | B65.9 | B82.0 |
| A15.5 | A30.1 | A50.06 | A54.29 | A87.8 | B06.82 | B44.7 | B66.0 | B97.21 |
| A15.6 | A30.2 | A50.07 | A54.30 | A87.9 | B06.89 | B44.81 | B66.1 | B97.33 |
| A15.7 | A30.3 | A50.08 | A54.31 | A88.0 | B08.3 | B44.89 | B66.2 | B97.34 |
| A15.8 | A30.4 | A50.09 | A54.32 | A88.8 | B08.71 | B44.9 | B66.3 | B97.35 |

Appendix F: Complication and Comorbidity (CC) Code List

| | | | | | | | | |
|---|---|---|---|---|---|---|---|---|
| C15.3 | C38.2 | C49.A9 | C78.5 | C81.18 | C82.25 | C83.12 | C84.19 | C85.26 |
| C15.4 | C38.3 | C56.1 | C78.6 | C81.19 | C82.26 | C83.13 | C84.40 | C85.27 |
| C15.5 | C38.4 | C56.2 | C78.7 | C81.20 | C82.27 | C83.14 | C84.41 | C85.28 |
| C15.8 | C38.8 | C56.9 | C78.80 | C81.21 | C82.28 | C83.15 | C84.42 | C85.29 |
| C15.9 | C40.00 | C64.1 | C78.89 | C81.22 | C82.29 | C83.16 | C84.43 | C85.80 |
| C16.0 | C40.01 | C64.2 | C79.00 | C81.23 | C82.30 | C83.17 | C84.44 | C85.81 |
| C16.1 | C40.02 | C64.9 | C79.01 | C81.24 | C82.31 | C83.18 | C84.45 | C85.82 |
| C16.2 | C40.10 | C65.1 | C79.02 | C81.25 | C82.32 | C83.19 | C84.46 | C85.83 |
| C16.3 | C40.11 | C65.2 | C79.10 | C81.26 | C82.33 | C83.30 | C84.47 | C85.84 |
| C16.4 | C40.12 | C65.9 | C79.11 | C81.27 | C82.34 | C83.31 | C84.48 | C85.85 |
| C16.5 | C40.20 | C66.1 | C79.19 | C81.28 | C82.35 | C83.32 | C84.49 | C85.86 |
| C16.6 | C40.21 | C66.2 | C79.2 | C81.29 | C82.36 | C83.33 | C84.60 | C85.87 |
| C16.8 | C40.22 | C66.9 | C79.31 | C81.30 | C82.37 | C83.34 | C84.61 | C85.88 |
| C16.9 | C40.30 | C68.0 | C79.32 | C81.31 | C82.38 | C83.35 | C84.62 | C85.89 |
| C17.0 | C40.31 | C68.1 | C79.40 | C81.32 | C82.39 | C83.36 | C84.63 | C85.90 |
| C17.1 | C40.32 | C68.8 | C79.49 | C81.33 | C82.40 | C83.37 | C84.64 | C85.91 |
| C17.2 | C40.80 | C68.9 | C79.51 | C81.34 | C82.41 | C83.38 | C84.65 | C85.92 |
| C17.3 | C40.81 | C70.0 | C79.52 | C81.35 | C82.42 | C83.39 | C84.66 | C85.93 |
| C17.8 | C40.82 | C70.1 | C79.60 | C81.36 | C82.43 | C83.50 | C84.67 | C85.94 |
| C17.9 | C40.90 | C70.9 | C79.61 | C81.37 | C82.44` | C83.51 | C84.68 | C85.95 |
| C18.0 | C40.91 | C71.0 | C79.62 | C81.38 | C82.45 | C83.52 | C84.69 | C85.96 |
| C18.1 | C40.92 | C71.1 | C79.70 | C81.39 | C82.46 | C83.53 | C84.70 | C85.97 |
| C18.2 | C41.0 | C71.2 | C79.71 | C81.40 | C82.47 | C83.54 | C84.71 | C85.98 |
| C18.3 | C41.1 | C71.3 | C79.72 | C81.41 | C82.48 | C83.55 | C84.72 | C85.99 |
| C18.4 | C41.2 | C71.4 | C79.81 | C81.42 | C82.49 | C83.56 | C84.73 | C86.0 |
| C18.5 | C41.3 | C71.5 | C79.82 | C81.43 | C82.50 | C83.57 | C84.74 | C86.1 |
| C18.6 | C41.4 | C71.6 | C79.89 | C81.44 | C82.51 | C83.58 | C84.75 | C86.2 |
| C18.7 | C41.9 | C71.7 | C79.9 | C81.45 | C82.52 | C83.59 | C84.76 | C86.3 |
| C18.8 | C45.0 | C71.8 | C7A.00 | C81.46 | C82.53 | C83.70 | C84.77 | C86.4 |
| C18.9 | C45.1 | C71.9 | C7A.010 | C81.47 | C82.54 | C83.71 | C84.78 | C86.5 |
| C19 | C45.2 | C72.0 | C7A.011 | C81.48 | C82.55 | C83.72 | C84.79 | C86.6 |
| C20 | C46.0 | C72.1 | C7A.012 | C81.49 | C82.56 | C83.73 | C84.90 | C88.2 |
| C21.0 | C46.1 | C72.20 | C7A.019 | C81.70 | C82.57 | C83.74 | C84.91 | C88.3 |
| C21.1 | C46.2 | C72.21 | C7A.020 | C81.71 | C82.58 | C83.75 | C84.92 | C88.4 |
| C21.2 | C46.3 | C72.22 | C7A.021 | C81.72 | C82.59 | C83.76 | C84.93 | C88.8 |
| C21.8 | C46.4 | C72.30 | C7A.022 | C81.73 | C82.60 | C83.77 | C84.94 | C88.9 |
| C22.0 | C46.50 | C72.31 | C7A.023 | C81.74 | C82.61 | C83.78 | C84.95 | C90.00 |
| C22.1 | C46.51 | C72.32 | C7A.024 | C81.75 | C82.62 | C83.79 | C84.96 | C90.01 |
| C22.2 | C46.52 | C72.40 | C7A.025 | C81.76 | C82.63 | C83.80 | C84.97 | C90.02 |
| C22.3 | C46.7 | C72.41 | C7A.026 | C81.77 | C82.64 | C83.81 | C84.98 | C90.10 |
| C22.4 | C46.9 | C72.42 | C7A.029 | C81.78 | C82.65 | C83.82 | C84.99 | C90.11 |
| C22.7 | C47.0 | C72.50 | C7A.090 | C81.79 | C82.66 | C83.83 | C84.A0 | C90.12 |
| C22.8 | C47.10 | C72.59 | C7A.091 | C81.90 | C82.67 | C83.84 | C84.A1 | C90.20 |
| C22.9 | C47.11 | C72.9 | C7A.092 | C81.91 | C82.68 | C83.85 | C84.A2 | C90.21 |
| C23 | C47.12 | C74.00 | C7A.093 | C81.92 | C82.69 | C83.86 | C84.A3 | C90.22 |
| C24.0 | C47.20 | C74.01 | C7A.094 | C81.93 | C82.80 | C83.87 | C84.A4 | C90.30 |
| C24.1 | C47.21 | C74.02 | C7A.095 | C81.94 | C82.81 | C83.88 | C84.A5 | C90.31 |
| C24.8 | C47.22 | C74.10 | C7A.096 | C81.95 | C82.82 | C83.89 | C84.A6 | C90.32 |
| C24.9 | C47.3 | C74.11 | C7A.098 | C81.96 | C82.83 | C83.90 | C84.A7 | C91.00 |
| C25.0 | C47.4 | C74.12 | C7A.1 | C81.97 | C82.84 | C83.91 | C84.A8 | C91.01 |
| C25.1 | C47.5 | C74.90 | C7A.8 | C81.98 | C82.85 | C83.92 | C84.A9 | C91.02 |
| C25.2 | C47.6 | C74.91 | C7B.01 | C81.99 | C82.86 | C83.93 | C84.Z0 | C91.10 |
| C25.3 | C47.8 | C74.92 | C7B.02 | C82.00 | C82.87 | C83.94 | C84.Z1 | C91.11 |
| C25.4 | C47.9 | C75.0 | C7B.03 | C82.01 | C82.88 | C83.95 | C84.Z2 | C91.12 |
| C25.7 | C48.0 | C75.1 | C7B.04 | C82.02 | C82.89 | C83.96 | C84.Z3 | C91.30 |
| C25.8 | C48.1 | C75.2 | C7B.09 | C82.03 | C82.90 | C83.97 | C84.Z4 | C91.31 |
| C25.9 | C48.2 | C75.3 | C7B.8 | C82.04 | C82.91 | C83.98 | C84.Z5 | C91.32 |
| C33 | C48.8 | C75.4 | C80.0 | C82.05 | C82.92 | C83.99 | C84.Z6 | C91.40 |
| C34.00 | C49.0 | C75.5 | C80.2 | C82.06 | C82.93 | C84.00 | C84.Z7 | C91.41 |
| C34.01 | C49.10 | C75.8 | C81.00 | C82.07 | C82.94 | C84.01 | C84.Z8 | C91.42 |
| C34.02 | C49.11 | C75.9 | C81.01 | C82.08 | C82.95 | C84.02 | C84.Z9 | C91.50 |
| C34.10 | C49.12 | C77.0 | C81.02 | C82.09 | C82.96 | C84.03 | C85.10 | C91.51 |
| C34.11 | C49.20 | C77.1 | C81.03 | C82.10 | C82.97 | C84.04 | C85.11 | C91.52 |
| C34.12 | C49.21 | C77.2 | C81.04 | C82.11 | C82.98 | C84.05 | C85.12 | C91.60 |
| C34.2 | C49.22 | C77.3 | C81.05 | C82.12 | C82.99 | C84.06 | C85.13 | C91.61 |
| C34.30 | C49.3 | C77.4 | C81.06 | C82.13 | C83.00 | C84.07 | C85.14 | C91.62 |
| C34.31 | C49.4 | C77.5 | C81.07 | C82.14 | C83.01 | C84.08 | C85.15 | C91.90 |
| C34.32 | C49.5 | C77.8 | C81.08 | C82.15 | C83.02 | C84.09 | C85.16 | C91.91 |
| C34.80 | C49.6 | C77.9 | C81.09 | C82.16 | C83.03 | C84.10 | C85.17 | C91.92 |
| C34.81 | C49.8 | C78.00 | C81.10 | C82.17 | C83.04 | C84.11 | C85.18 | C91.A0 |
| C34.82 | C49.9 | C78.01 | C81.11 | C82.18 | C83.05 | C84.12 | C85.19 | C91.A1 |
| C34.90 | C49.A0 | C78.02 | C81.12 | C82.19 | C83.06 | C84.13 | C85.20 | C91.A2 |
| C34.91 | C49.A1 | C78.1 | C81.13 | C82.20 | C83.07 | C84.14 | C85.21 | C91.Z0 |
| C34.92 | C49.A2 | C78.2 | C81.14 | C82.21 | C83.08 | C84.15 | C85.22 | C91.Z1 |
| C37 | C49.A3 | C78.30 | C81.15 | C82.22 | C83.09 | C84.16 | C85.23 | C91.Z2 |
| C38.0 | C49.A4 | C78.39 | C81.16 | C82.23 | C83.10 | C84.17 | C85.24 | C92.00 |
| C38.1 | C49.A5 | C78.4 | C81.17 | C82.24 | C83.11 | C84.18 | C85.25 | C92.01 |

| | | | | | | | | |
|---|---|---|---|---|---|---|---|---|
| C92.02 | C96.A | D81.3 | E70.328 | E74.4 | F10.180 | F14.121 | F19.230 | F84.5 |
| C92.10 | C96.Z | D81.4 | E70.329 | E74.8 | F10.181 | F14.150 | F19.231 | F84.8 |
| C92.11 | D46.22 | D81.5 | E70.330 | E75.00 | F10.188 | F14.151 | F19.232 | F84.9 |
| C92.12 | D46.C | D81.6 | E70.331 | E75.01 | F10.19 | F14.20 | F19.239 | G03.1 |
| C92.20 | D47.01 | D81.7 | E70.338 | E75.02 | F10.221 | F14.221 | F19.250 | G03.2 |
| C92.21 | D47.02 | D81.89 | E70.339 | E75.09 | F10.230 | F14.222 | F19.251 | G04.1 |
| C92.22 | D47.09 | D81.9 | E70.39 | E75.10 | F10.231 | F14.229 | F19.259 | G10 |
| C92.30 | D47.1 | D82.0 | E70.40 | E75.11 | F10.232 | F14.23 | F19.26 | G11.0 |
| C92.31 | D47.9 | D82.1 | E70.41 | E75.19 | F10.239 | F14.250 | F19.27 | G11.1 |
| C92.32 | D47.Z1 | D83.0 | E70.49 | E75.23 | F10.24 | F14.251 | F19.280 | G11.2 |
| C92.40 | D47.Z2 | D83.1 | E70.5 | E75.25 | F10.251 | F14.259 | F19.281 | G11.3 |
| C92.41 | D47.Z9 | D83.2 | E70.8 | E75.29 | F10.259 | F14.280 | F19.282 | G11.4 |
| C92.42 | D58.8 | D83.8 | E70.9 | E75.4 | F10.27 | F14.281 | F19.288 | G11.8 |
| C92.50 | D58.9 | D83.9 | E71.0 | E76.01 | F10.280 | F14.282 | F19.921 | G11.9 |
| C92.51 | D59.0 | D84.8 | E71.110 | E76.02 | F10.281 | F14.288 | F19.930 | G12.0 |
| C92.52 | D59.1 | D84.9 | E71.111 | E76.03 | F10.288 | F14.921 | F19.931 | G12.1 |
| C92.60 | D59.2 | D89.810 | E71.118 | E76.1 | F10.29 | F14.950 | F19.932 | G12.20 |
| C92.61 | D59.4 | D89.811 | E71.120 | E76.210 | F10.921 | F14.951 | F19.939 | G12.21 |
| C92.62 | D59.9 | D89.812 | E71.121 | E76.211 | F10.94 | F15.121 | F19.950 | G12.22 |
| C92.90 | D61.01 | D89.813 | E71.128 | E76.219 | F10.951 | F15.150 | F19.951 | G12.23 |
| C92.91 | D61.09 | E06.0 | E71.19 | E76.22 | F10.959 | F15.151 | F19.97 | G12.24 |
| C92.92 | D61.818 | E08.52 | E71.2 | E76.29 | F10.980 | F15.20 | F20.0 | G12.25 |
| C92.A0 | D61.82 | E09.52 | E71.310 | E76.3 | F10.981 | F15.221 | F20.1 | G12.29 |
| C92.A1 | D61.9 | E10.52 | E71.311 | E76.8 | F10.988 | F15.222 | F20.2 | G12.8 |
| C92.A2 | D62 | E11.52 | E71.312 | E76.9 | F10.99 | F15.23 | F20.5 | G12.9 |
| C92.Z0 | D68.0 | E13.52 | E71.313 | E78.71 | F11.121 | F15.250 | F20.81 | G21.11 |
| C92.Z1 | D68.1 | E15 | E71.314 | E78.72 | F11.150 | F15.251 | F20.89 | G21.19 |
| C92.Z2 | D68.2 | E22.1 | E71.318 | E79.1 | F11.151 | F15.259 | F23 | G21.2 |
| C93.00 | D68.311 | E22.2 | E71.32 | E79.2 | F11.20 | F15.280 | F30.10 | G21.3 |
| C93.01 | D68.312 | E22.8 | E71.39 | E79.8 | F11.221 | F15.281 | F30.11 | G21.8 |
| C93.02 | D68.318 | E22.9 | E71.50 | E79.9 | F11.222 | F15.282 | F30.12 | G21.9 |
| C93.10 | D68.32 | E23.0 | E71.510 | E80.0 | F11.23 | F15.288 | F30.13 | G23.0 |
| C93.11 | D68.4 | E23.2 | E71.511 | E80.1 | F11.250 | F15.921 | F30.2 | G23.1 |
| C93.12 | D68.51 | E24.0 | E71.518 | E80.20 | F11.251 | F15.93 | F30.9 | G23.2 |
| C93.30 | D68.52 | E24.2 | E71.520 | E80.21 | F11.259 | F15.950 | F31.0 | G23.8 |
| C93.31 | D68.59 | E24.3 | E71.521 | E80.29 | F11.281 | F15.951 | F31.10 | G23.9 |
| C93.32 | D68.61 | E24.4 | E71.522 | E80.3 | F11.282 | F16.121 | F31.11 | G24.02 |
| C93.90 | D68.62 | E24.8 | E71.528 | E84.19 | F11.288 | F16.150 | F31.12 | G24.09 |
| C93.91 | D68.69 | E24.9 | E71.529 | E84.8 | F11.921 | F16.151 | F31.13 | G24.2 |
| C93.92 | D68.8 | E27.0 | E71.53 | E84.9 | F11.93 | F16.20 | F31.2 | G24.8 |
| C93.Z0 | D68.9 | E27.1 | E71.540 | E85.0 | F11.950 | F16.221 | F31.30 | G25.82 |
| C93.Z1 | D69.0 | E27.2 | E71.541 | E85.1 | F11.951 | F16.250 | F31.31 | G25.9 |
| C93.Z2 | D69.3 | E27.3 | E71.542 | E85.2 | F12.121 | F16.251 | F31.32 | G31.81 |
| C94.00 | D69.41 | E27.40 | E71.548 | E85.3 | F12.150 | F16.259 | F31.4 | G31.82 |
| C94.01 | D69.42 | E27.49 | E72.00 | E85.4 | F12.151 | F16.280 | F31.5 | G32.0 |
| C94.02 | D74.0 | E27.5 | E72.01 | E85.81 | F12.221 | F16.283 | F31.60 | G32.81 |
| C94.20 | D74.8 | E32.1 | E72.02 | E85.82 | F12.250 | F16.288 | F31.61 | G36.0 |
| C94.21 | D74.9 | E34.0 | E72.03 | E85.89 | F12.251 | F16.921 | F31.62 | G36.1 |
| C94.22 | D75.81 | E36.01 | E72.04 | E85.9 | F12.921 | F16.950 | F31.63 | G36.8 |
| C94.30 | D76.1 | E36.02 | E72.09 | E87.0 | F12.950 | F16.951 | F31.64 | G36.9 |
| C94.31 | D76.2 | E36.11 | E72.10 | E87.1 | F12.951 | F17.203 | F31.81 | G37.0 |
| C94.32 | D76.3 | E36.12 | E72.11 | E87.2 | F13.121 | F17.213 | F31.89 | G37.1 |
| C94.40 | D78.01 | E44.0 | E72.12 | E87.3 | F13.150 | F17.223 | F32.0 | G37.3 |
| C94.41 | D78.02 | E44.1 | E72.19 | E87.4 | F13.151 | F17.293 | F32.1 | G37.5 |
| C94.42 | D78.11 | E45 | E72.20 | E88.40 | F13.20 | F18.121 | F32.2 | G37.8 |
| C94.6 | D78.12 | E46 | E72.21 | E88.41 | F13.221 | F18.150 | F32.3 | G37.9 |
| C94.80 | D78.21 | E51.11 | E72.22 | E88.42 | F13.230 | F18.151 | F33.0 | G40.001 |
| C94.81 | D78.22 | E51.12 | E72.23 | E88.49 | F13.231 | F18.17 | F33.1 | G40.009 |
| C94.82 | D78.31 | E51.2 | E72.29 | E89.1 | F13.232 | F18.20 | F33.2 | G40.011 |
| C95.00 | D78.32 | E51.8 | E72.3 | E89.6 | F13.239 | F18.221 | F33.3 | G40.019 |
| C95.01 | D78.33 | E51.9 | E72.4 | E89.810 | F13.250 | F18.250 | F33.40 | G40.101 |
| C95.02 | D78.34 | E53.0 | E72.50 | E89.811 | F13.251 | F18.251 | F33.8 | G40.109 |
| C95.10 | D78.81 | E55.0 | E72.51 | E89.820 | F13.259 | F18.259 | F33.9 | G40.111 |
| C95.11 | D78.89 | E64.0 | E72.52 | E89.821 | F13.26 | F18.27 | F34.81 | G40.119 |
| C95.12 | D80.0 | E66.2 | E72.53 | E89.822 | F13.27 | F18.280 | F34.89 | G40.201 |
| C95.90 | D80.1 | E70.0 | E72.59 | E89.823 | F13.280 | F18.288 | F34.9 | G40.209 |
| C95.91 | D80.2 | E70.1 | E72.8 | E89.89 | F13.281 | F18.921 | F50.00 | G40.211 |
| C95.92 | D80.3 | E70.20 | E72.9 | F01.51 | F13.282 | F18.950 | F50.01 | G40.219 |
| C96.0 | D80.4 | E70.21 | E74.00 | F02.81 | F13.288 | F18.951 | F50.02 | G40.411 |
| C96.20 | D80.5 | E70.29 | E74.01 | F03.91 | F13.921 | F18.97 | F50.2 | G40.419 |
| C96.21 | D80.6 | E70.30 | E74.02 | F05 | F13.930 | F19.121 | F68.10 | G40.501 |
| C96.22 | D80.7 | E70.310 | E74.03 | F06.0 | F13.931 | F19.150 | F68.12 | G40.509 |
| C96.29 | D80.8 | E70.311 | E74.04 | F06.2 | F13.932 | F19.151 | F72 | G40.801 |
| C96.4 | D80.9 | E70.318 | E74.09 | F10.121 | F13.939 | F19.17 | F73 | G40.802 |
| C96.5 | D81.0 | E70.319 | E74.20 | F10.14 | F13.950 | F19.20 | F84.0 | G40.803 |
| C96.6 | D81.1 | E70.320 | E74.21 | F10.151 | F13.951 | F19.221 | F84.2 | G40.804 |
| C96.9 | D81.2 | E70.321 | E74.29 | F10.159 | F13.97 | F19.222 | F84.3 | |

| | | | | | | | | |
|---|---|---|---|---|---|---|---|---|
| G40.811 | G90.59 | H30.133 | H35.731 | H53.132 | H95.21 | I27.82 | I69.352 | I70.642 |
| G40.812 | G91.0 | H30.139 | H35.732 | H53.133 | H95.22 | I28.0 | I69.353 | I70.643 |
| G40.813 | G91.1 | H30.141 | H35.733 | H53.139 | H95.31 | I28.1 | I69.354 | I70.644 |
| G40.814 | G91.2 | H30.142 | H35.739 | H59.011 | H95.32 | I30.0 | I69.359 | I70.648 |
| G40.821 | G91.3 | H30.143 | H35.82 | H59.012 | H95.41 | I30.1 | I69.851 | I70.649 |
| G40.822 | G91.8 | H30.149 | H40.211 | H59.013 | H95.42 | I30.8 | I69.852 | I70.661 |
| G40.823 | G91.9 | H30.891 | H40.212 | H59.019 | H95.51 | I30.9 | I69.853 | I70.662 |
| G40.824 | G93.1 | H30.892 | H40.213 | H59.031 | H95.52 | I31.0 | I69.854 | I70.663 |
| G40.89 | G95.0 | H30.893 | H40.219 | H59.032 | H95.53 | I31.1 | I69.859 | I70.668 |
| G40.911 | G95.20 | H30.899 | H44.001 | H59.033 | H95.54 | I31.2 | I69.951 | I70.669 |
| G40.919 | G95.29 | H30.90 | H44.002 | H59.039 | H95.811 | I31.3 | I69.952 | I70.731 |
| G40.A11 | G95.81 | H30.91 | H44.003 | H59.091 | H95.812 | I31.4 | I69.953 | I70.732 |
| G40.A19 | G95.89 | H30.92 | H44.009 | H59.092 | H95.813 | I31.8 | I69.954 | I70.733 |
| G40.B01 | G95.9 | H30.93 | H44.011 | H59.093 | H95.819 | I31.9 | I69.959 | I70.734 |
| G40.B09 | G96.0 | H31.321 | H44.012 | H59.099 | H95.88 | I32 | I70.261 | I70.738 |
| G40.B11 | G96.11 | H31.322 | H44.013 | H59.111 | H95.89 | I38 | I70.262 | I70.739 |
| G40.B19 | G97.0 | H31.323 | H44.019 | H59.112 | I01.0 | I39 | I70.263 | I70.741 |
| G43.601 | G97.2 | H31.329 | H44.021 | H59.113 | I01.1 | I42.0 | I70.268 | I70.742 |
| G43.609 | G97.31 | H31.401 | H44.022 | H59.119 | I01.2 | I42.1 | I70.269 | I70.743 |
| G43.611 | G97.32 | H31.402 | H44.023 | H59.121 | I01.8 | I42.2 | I70.331 | I70.744 |
| G43.619 | G97.41 | H31.403 | H44.029 | H59.122 | I01.9 | I42.3 | I70.332 | I70.748 |
| G45.0 | G97.48 | H31.409 | H44.111 | H59.123 | I02.0 | I42.4 | I70.333 | I70.749 |
| G45.1 | G97.49 | H31.411 | H44.112 | H59.129 | I02.9 | I42.5 | I70.334 | I70.761 |
| G45.2 | G97.51 | H31.412 | H44.113 | H59.211 | I09.0 | I42.6 | I70.338 | I70.762 |
| G45.3 | G97.52 | H31.413 | H44.119 | H59.212 | I09.2 | I42.7 | I70.339 | I70.763 |
| G45.8 | G97.61 | H31.419 | H44.121 | H59.213 | I09.81 | I42.8 | I70.341 | I70.768 |
| G45.9 | G97.62 | H31.421 | H44.122 | H59.219 | I12.0 | I42.9 | I70.342 | I70.769 |
| G46.0 | G97.63 | H31.422 | H44.123 | H59.221 | I13.0 | I43 | I70.343 | I70.92 |
| G46.1 | G97.64 | H31.423 | H44.129 | H59.222 | I13.11 | I44.2 | I70.344 | I73.01 |
| G46.2 | G97.81 | H31.429 | H44.131 | H59.223 | I13.2 | I45.2 | I70.348 | I74.09 |
| G60.1 | G97.82 | H33.121 | H44.132 | H59.229 | I16.1 | I45.3 | I70.349 | I74.10 |
| G61.0 | G99.0 | H33.122 | H44.133 | H59.311 | I16.9 | I45.89 | I70.361 | I74.11 |
| G61.81 | G99.2 | H33.123 | H44.139 | H59.312 | I20.0 | I47.0 | I70.362 | I74.19 |
| G62.81 | H05.011 | H33.129 | H44.19 | H59.313 | I20.1 | I47.1 | I70.363 | I74.2 |
| G70.80 | H05.012 | H33.20 | H46.00 | H59.319 | I23.0 | I47.2 | I70.368 | I74.3 |
| G70.81 | H05.013 | H33.21 | H46.01 | H59.321 | I23.1 | I48.1 | I70.369 | I74.4 |
| G71.0 | H05.019 | H33.22 | H46.02 | H59.322 | I23.2 | I48.3 | I70.431 | I74.5 |
| G71.2 | H05.021 | H33.23 | H46.03 | H59.323 | I23.3 | I48.4 | I70.432 | I74.8 |
| G72.0 | H05.022 | H33.40 | H46.10 | H59.329 | I23.6 | I48.92 | I70.433 | I74.9 |
| G72.1 | H05.023 | H33.41 | H46.11 | H59.331 | I23.7 | I49.2 | I70.434 | I75.011 |
| G72.2 | H05.029 | H33.42 | H46.12 | H59.332 | I23.8 | I50.1 | I70.438 | I75.012 |
| G72.81 | H05.031 | H33.43 | H46.13 | H59.333 | I24.0 | I50.20 | I70.439 | I75.013 |
| G73.1 | H05.032 | H33.8 | H46.8 | H59.339 | I24.1 | I50.22 | I70.441 | I75.019 |
| G73.3 | H05.033 | H34.00 | H46.9 | H59.341 | I24.8 | I50.30 | I70.442 | I75.021 |
| G80.1 | H05.039 | H34.01 | H47.10 | H59.342 | I24.9 | I50.32 | I70.443 | I75.022 |
| G80.2 | H20.00 | H34.02 | H47.11 | H59.343 | I25.110 | I50.40 | I70.444 | I75.023 |
| G80.3 | H20.011 | H34.03 | H47.41 | H59.349 | I25.3 | I50.42 | I70.448 | I75.029 |
| G81.00 | H20.012 | H34.10 | H47.42 | H59.351 | I25.700 | I51.0 | I70.449 | I75.81 |
| G81.01 | H20.013 | H34.11 | H47.43 | H59.352 | I25.710 | I51.81 | I70.461 | I75.89 |
| G81.02 | H20.019 | H34.12 | H47.49 | H59.353 | I25.711 | I62.9 | I70.462 | I76 |
| G81.03 | H20.021 | H34.13 | H47.511 | H59.359 | I25.718 | I67.3 | I70.463 | I77.2 |
| G81.04 | H20.022 | H34.211 | H47.512 | H59.361 | I25.719 | I67.4 | I70.468 | I77.4 |
| G81.10 | H20.023 | H34.212 | H47.519 | H59.362 | I25.720 | I67.5 | I70.469 | I77.5 |
| G81.11 | H20.029 | H34.213 | H47.521 | H59.363 | I25.721 | I67.6 | I70.531 | I80.10 |
| G81.12 | H20.031 | H34.219 | H47.522 | H59.369 | I25.728 | I67.7 | I70.532 | I80.11 |
| G81.13 | H20.032 | H34.231 | H47.529 | H59.811 | I25.729 | I67.81 | I70.533 | I80.12 |
| G81.14 | H20.033 | H34.232 | H47.531 | H59.812 | I25.730 | I67.82 | I70.534 | I80.13 |
| G81.90 | H20.039 | H34.233 | H47.532 | H59.813 | I25.731 | I67.841 | I70.538 | I80.201 |
| G81.91 | H20.9 | H34.239 | H47.539 | H59.819 | I25.738 | I67.848 | I70.539 | I80.202 |
| G81.92 | H21.331 | H34.8110 | H47.621 | H59.88 | I25.739 | I67.89 | I70.541 | I80.203 |
| G81.93 | H21.332 | H34.8111 | H47.622 | H59.89 | I25.750 | I68.2 | I70.542 | I80.209 |
| G81.94 | H21.333 | H34.8112 | H47.629 | H60.20 | I25.751 | I69.051 | I70.543 | I80.211 |
| G82.20 | H21.339 | H34.8120 | H47.631 | H60.21 | I25.758 | I69.052 | I70.544 | I80.212 |
| G82.21 | H30.101 | H34.8121 | H47.632 | H60.22 | I25.759 | I69.053 | I70.548 | I80.213 |
| G82.22 | H30.102 | H34.8122 | H47.639 | H60.23 | I25.760 | I69.054 | I70.549 | I80.219 |
| G83.0 | H30.103 | H34.8130 | H47.641 | H70.001 | I25.761 | I69.059 | I70.561 | I80.221 |
| G83.4 | H30.109 | H34.8131 | H47.642 | H70.002 | I25.768 | I69.151 | I70.562 | I80.222 |
| G90.3 | H30.111 | H34.8132 | H47.649 | H70.003 | I25.769 | I69.152 | I70.563 | I80.223 |
| G90.50 | H30.112 | H34.8190 | H49.811 | H70.009 | I25.790 | I69.153 | I70.568 | I80.229 |
| G90.511 | H30.113 | H34.8191 | H49.812 | H70.011 | I25.791 | I69.154 | I70.569 | I80.231 |
| G90.512 | H30.119 | H34.8192 | H49.813 | H70.012 | I25.798 | I69.159 | I70.631 | I80.232 |
| G90.513 | H30.121 | H34.9 | H49.819 | H70.013 | I25.799 | I69.251 | I70.632 | I80.233 |
| G90.519 | H30.122 | H35.70 | H53.121 | H70.019 | I25.810 | I69.252 | I70.633 | I80.239 |
| G90.521 | H30.123 | H35.721 | H53.122 | H70.091 | I25.811 | I69.253 | I70.634 | I80.291 |
| G90.522 | H30.129 | H35.722 | H53.123 | H70.092 | I25.812 | I69.254 | I70.638 | I80.292 |
| G90.523 | H30.131 | H35.723 | H53.129 | H70.093 | I27.0 | I69.259 | I70.639 | I80.293 |
| G90.529 | H30.132 | H35.729 | H53.131 | H70.099 | I27.1 | I69.351 | I70.641 | I80.299 |

**Appendix F: Complication and Comorbidity (CC) Code List**

| | | | | | | | | |
|---|---|---|---|---|---|---|---|---|
| I82.1 | I82.619 | I87.032 | J70.1 | K40.31 | K51.812 | K80.44 | L02.01 | L10.89 |
| I82.210 | I82.621 | I87.033 | J80 | K41.00 | K51.813 | K80.45 | L02.11 | L10.9 |
| I82.211 | I82.622 | I87.039 | J81.1 | K41.01 | K51.814 | K80.46 | L02.211 | L12.0 |
| I82.290 | I82.623 | I87.1 | J82 | K41.30 | K51.818 | K80.47 | L02.212 | L12.30 |
| I82.291 | I82.629 | I87.311 | J84.01 | K41.31 | K51.819 | K80.51 | L02.213 | L12.31 |
| I82.3 | I82.701 | I87.312 | J84.02 | K42.0 | K51.90 | K80.60 | L02.214 | L12.35 |
| I82.401 | I82.702 | I87.313 | J84.03 | K43.0 | K51.911 | K80.61 | L02.215 | L12.8 |
| I82.402 | I82.703 | I87.319 | J84.09 | K43.3 | K51.912 | K80.62 | L02.216 | L12.9 |
| I82.403 | I82.709 | I87.331 | J84.114 | K43.6 | K51.913 | K80.63 | L02.219 | L49.3 |
| I82.409 | I82.711 | I87.332 | J84.116 | K44.0 | K51.914 | K80.64 | L02.31 | L49.4 |
| I82.411 | I82.712 | I87.333 | J84.117 | K45.0 | K51.918 | K80.65 | L02.411 | L49.5 |
| I82.412 | I82.713 | I87.339 | J84.2 | K46.0 | K51.919 | K80.66 | L02.412 | L49.6 |
| I82.413 | I82.719 | I96 | J84.82 | K50.00 | K52.0 | K80.71 | L02.413 | L49.7 |
| I82.419 | I82.721 | I97.110 | J84.9 | K50.011 | K52.1 | K80.81 | L02.414 | L49.8 |
| I82.421 | I82.722 | I97.111 | J90 | K50.012 | K55.1 | K81.0 | L02.415 | L49.9 |
| I82.422 | I82.723 | I97.120 | J91.0 | K50.013 | K55.8 | K81.2 | L02.416 | L51.1 |
| I82.423 | I82.729 | I97.121 | J91.8 | K50.014 | K55.9 | K82.0 | L02.419 | L51.2 |
| I82.429 | I82.811 | I97.130 | J93.11 | K50.018 | K56.0 | K82.1 | L02.511 | L51.3 |
| I82.431 | I82.812 | I97.131 | J93.12 | K50.019 | K56.1 | K82.3 | L02.512 | L53.0 |
| I82.432 | I82.813 | I97.190 | J93.81 | K50.10 | K56.3 | K83.0 | L02.519 | L53.1 |
| I82.433 | I82.819 | I97.191 | J93.82 | K50.111 | K56.49 | K83.3 | L02.611 | L53.2 |
| I82.439 | I82.890 | I97.410 | J93.83 | K50.112 | K56.50 | K86.0 | L02.612 | L53.3 |
| I82.441 | I82.891 | I97.411 | J93.9 | K50.113 | K56.51 | K86.1 | L02.619 | L76.01 |
| I82.442 | I82.90 | I97.418 | J94.0 | K50.114 | K56.52 | K86.2 | L02.811 | L76.02 |
| I82.443 | I82.91 | I97.42 | J94.2 | K50.118 | K56.600 | K86.3 | L02.818 | L76.11 |
| I82.449 | I82.A11 | I97.51 | J94.8 | K50.119 | K56.601 | K90.1 | L02.91 | L76.12 |
| I82.491 | I82.A12 | I97.52 | J95.00 | K50.80 | K56.609 | K90.2 | L03.111 | L76.21 |
| I82.492 | I82.A13 | I97.610 | J95.01 | K50.811 | K56.690 | K90.3 | L03.112 | L76.22 |
| I82.493 | I82.A19 | I97.611 | J95.02 | K50.812 | K56.691 | K90.41 | L03.113 | L76.31 |
| I82.499 | I82.A21 | I97.618 | J95.03 | K50.813 | K56.699 | K90.49 | L03.114 | L76.32 |
| I82.4Y1 | I82.A22 | I97.620 | J95.04 | K50.814 | K56.7 | K90.81 | L03.115 | L76.33 |
| I82.4Y2 | I82.A23 | I97.621 | J95.09 | K50.818 | K57.00 | K90.89 | L03.116 | L76.34 |
| I82.4Y3 | I82.A29 | I97.622 | J95.4 | K50.819 | K57.12 | K90.9 | L03.119 | L88 |
| I82.4Y9 | I82.B11 | I97.630 | J95.5 | K50.90 | K57.20 | K91.2 | L03.121 | L97.101 |
| I82.4Z1 | I82.B12 | I97.631 | J95.61 | K50.911 | K57.32 | K91.30 | L03.122 | L97.102 |
| I82.4Z2 | I82.B13 | I97.638 | J95.62 | K50.912 | K57.40 | K91.31 | L03.123 | L97.103 |
| I82.4Z3 | I82.B19 | I97.640 | J95.71 | K50.913 | K57.52 | K91.32 | L03.124 | L97.104 |
| I82.4Z9 | I82.B21 | I97.641 | J95.72 | K50.914 | K57.80 | K91.61 | L03.125 | L97.105 |
| I82.501 | I82.B22 | I97.648 | J95.811 | K50.918 | K57.92 | K91.62 | L03.126 | L97.106 |
| I82.502 | I82.B23 | I97.710 | J95.812 | K50.919 | K59.2 | K91.71 | L03.129 | L97.108 |
| I82.503 | I82.B29 | I97.711 | J95.830 | K51.00 | K59.31 | K91.72 | L03.211 | L97.109 |
| I82.509 | I82.C11 | I97.790 | J95.831 | K51.011 | K59.39 | K91.81 | L03.212 | L97.111 |
| I82.511 | I82.C12 | I97.791 | J95.84 | K51.012 | K61.0 | K91.82 | L03.213 | L97.112 |
| I82.512 | I82.C13 | I97.810 | J95.850 | K51.013 | K61.1 | K91.83 | L03.221 | L97.113 |
| I82.513 | I82.C19 | I97.811 | J95.851 | K51.014 | K61.2 | K91.840 | L03.222 | L97.114 |
| I82.519 | I82.C21 | I97.820 | J95.859 | K51.018 | K61.3 | K91.841 | L03.311 | L97.115 |
| I82.521 | I82.C22 | I97.821 | J95.860 | K51.019 | K61.4 | K91.850 | L03.312 | L97.116 |
| I82.522 | I82.C23 | I97.88 | J95.861 | K51.20 | K62.5 | K91.858 | L03.313 | L97.119 |
| I82.523 | I82.C29 | I97.89 | J95.862 | K51.211 | K62.6 | K91.86 | L03.314 | L97.121 |
| I82.529 | I83.201 | J05.10 | J95.863 | K51.212 | K63.0 | K91.870 | L03.315 | L97.122 |
| I82.531 | I83.202 | J18.2 | J95.88 | K51.213 | K63.2 | K91.871 | L03.316 | L97.123 |
| I82.532 | I83.203 | J21.0 | J95.89 | K51.214 | K63.3 | K91.872 | L03.317 | L97.124 |
| I82.533 | I83.204 | J21.1 | J96.10 | K51.218 | K65.4 | K91.873 | L03.319 | L97.125 |
| I82.539 | I83.205 | J21.8 | J96.11 | K51.219 | K68.11 | K91.89 | L03.321 | L97.126 |
| I82.541 | I83.208 | J21.9 | J96.12 | K51.30 | K76.6 | K92.0 | L03.322 | L97.128 |
| I82.542 | I83.209 | J36 | J98.11 | K51.311 | K77 | K92.1 | L03.323 | L97.129 |
| I82.543 | I83.211 | J39.0 | J98.19 | K51.312 | K80.00 | K92.2 | L03.324 | L97.201 |
| I82.549 | I83.212 | J39.1 | K04.01 | K51.313 | K80.01 | K92.81 | L03.325 | L97.202 |
| I82.591 | I83.213 | J44.0 | K04.02 | K51.314 | K80.10 | K94.01 | L03.326 | L97.203 |
| I82.592 | I83.214 | J44.1 | K04.4 | K51.318 | K80.11 | K94.02 | L03.327 | L97.204 |
| I82.593 | I83.215 | J45.21 | K11.3 | K51.319 | K80.12 | K94.03 | L03.329 | L97.205 |
| I82.599 | I83.218 | J45.22 | K11.4 | K51.40 | K80.13 | K94.09 | L03.811 | L97.206 |
| I82.5Y1 | I83.219 | J45.31 | K12.2 | K51.411 | K80.18 | K94.11 | L03.818 | L97.208 |
| I82.5Y2 | I83.221 | J45.32 | K22.10 | K51.412 | K80.19 | K94.12 | L03.891 | L97.209 |
| I82.5Y3 | I83.222 | J45.41 | K25.3 | K51.413 | K80.21 | K94.13 | L03.898 | L97.211 |
| I82.5Y9 | I83.223 | J45.42 | K26.3 | K51.414 | K80.30 | K94.19 | L03.90 | L97.212 |
| I82.5Z1 | I83.224 | J45.51 | K27.3 | K51.418 | K80.31 | K94.22 | L03.91 | L97.213 |
| I82.5Z2 | I83.225 | J45.52 | K28.3 | K51.419 | K80.32 | K94.23 | L05.01 | L97.214 |
| I82.5Z3 | I83.228 | J45.901 | K31.0 | K51.50 | K80.33 | K94.30 | L05.02 | L97.215 |
| I82.5Z9 | I83.229 | J45.902 | K31.1 | K51.511 | K80.34 | K94.31 | L08.1 | L97.216 |
| I82.601 | I85.00 | J47.0 | K31.5 | K51.512 | K80.35 | K94.32 | L10.0 | L97.218 |
| I82.602 | I85.10 | J47.1 | K31.6 | K51.513 | K80.36 | K94.33 | L10.1 | L97.219 |
| I82.603 | I87.011 | J67.7 | K35.80 | K51.514 | K80.37 | K94.39 | L10.2 | L97.221 |
| I82.609 | I87.012 | J67.8 | K35.89 | K51.518 | K80.40 | K95.01 | L10.3 | L97.222 |
| I82.611 | I87.013 | J67.9 | K40.00 | K51.519 | K80.41 | K95.09 | L10.4 | L97.223 |
| I82.612 | I87.019 | J68.0 | K40.01 | K51.80 | K80.42 | K95.81 | L10.5 | L97.224 |
| I82.613 | I87.031 | J70.0 | K40.30 | K51.811 | K80.43 | K95.89 | L10.81 | |

| | | | | | | | | |
|---|---|---|---|---|---|---|---|---|
| L97.225 | L97.821 | M00.142 | M01.X59 | M02.872 | M33.19 | M50.023 | M80.032A | M80.841P |
| L97.226 | L97.822 | M00.149 | M01.X61 | M02.879 | M33.20 | M50.03 | M80.032K | M80.842A |
| L97.228 | L97.823 | M00.151 | M01.X62 | M02.88 | M33.21 | M51.04 | M80.032P | M80.842K |
| L97.229 | L97.824 | M00.152 | M01.X69 | M02.89 | M33.22 | M51.05 | M80.039A | M80.842P |
| L97.301 | L97.825 | M00.159 | M01.X71 | M05.40 | M33.29 | M51.06 | M80.039K | M80.849A |
| L97.302 | L97.826 | M00.161 | M01.X72 | M05.411 | M33.90 | M60.000 | M80.039P | M80.849K |
| L97.303 | L97.828 | M00.162 | M01.X79 | M05.412 | M33.91 | M60.001 | M80.041A | M80.849P |
| L97.304 | L97.829 | M00.169 | M01.X8 | M05.419 | M33.92 | M60.002 | M80.041K | M80.851A |
| L97.305 | L97.901 | M00.171 | M01.X9 | M05.421 | M33.93 | M60.003 | M80.041P | M80.851K |
| L97.306 | L97.902 | M00.172 | M02.10 | M05.422 | M33.99 | M60.004 | M80.042A | M80.851P |
| L97.308 | L97.903 | M00.179 | M02.111 | M05.429 | M34.81 | M60.005 | M80.042K | M80.852A |
| L97.309 | L97.904 | M00.18 | M02.112 | M05.431 | M34.82 | M60.009 | M80.042P | M80.852K |
| L97.311 | L97.905 | M00.19 | M02.119 | M05.432 | M35.03 | M60.011 | M80.049A | M80.859A |
| L97.312 | L97.906 | M00.20 | M02.121 | M05.439 | M35.1 | M60.012 | M80.049K | M80.859K |
| L97.313 | L97.908 | M00.211 | M02.122 | M05.441 | M35.2 | M60.019 | M80.049P | M80.859P |
| L97.314 | L97.909 | M00.212 | M02.129 | M05.442 | M35.5 | M60.021 | M80.051A | M80.861A |
| L97.315 | L97.911 | M00.219 | M02.131 | M05.449 | M35.8 | M60.022 | M80.051K | M80.861K |
| L97.316 | L97.912 | M00.221 | M02.132 | M05.451 | M36.0 | M60.029 | M80.051P | M80.861P |
| L97.318 | L97.913 | M00.222 | M02.139 | M05.452 | M46.20 | M60.031 | M80.052A | M80.862A |
| L97.319 | L97.914 | M00.229 | M02.141 | M05.459 | M46.21 | M60.032 | M80.052K | M80.862K |
| L97.321 | L97.915 | M00.231 | M02.142 | M05.461 | M46.22 | M60.039 | M80.052P | M80.862P |
| L97.322 | L97.916 | M00.232 | M02.149 | M05.462 | M46.23 | M60.041 | M80.059A | M80.869A |
| L97.323 | L97.918 | M00.239 | M02.151 | M05.469 | M46.24 | M60.042 | M80.059K | M80.869K |
| L97.324 | L97.919 | M00.241 | M02.152 | M05.471 | M46.25 | M60.043 | M80.059P | M80.869P |
| L97.325 | L97.921 | M00.242 | M02.159 | M05.472 | M46.26 | M60.044 | M80.061A | M80.871A |
| L97.326 | L97.922 | M00.249 | M02.161 | M05.479 | M46.27 | M60.045 | M80.061K | M80.871K |
| L97.328 | L97.923 | M00.251 | M02.162 | M05.49 | M46.28 | M60.046 | M80.061P | M80.871P |
| L97.329 | L97.924 | M00.252 | M02.169 | M25.00 | M46.30 | M60.051 | M80.062A | M80.872A |
| L97.401 | L97.925 | M00.259 | M02.171 | M25.011 | M46.31 | M60.052 | M80.062K | M80.872K |
| L97.402 | L97.926 | M00.261 | M02.172 | M25.012 | M46.32 | M60.059 | M80.062P | M80.872P |
| L97.403 | L97.928 | M00.262 | M02.179 | M25.019 | M46.33 | M60.061 | M80.069A | M80.879A |
| L97.404 | L97.929 | M00.269 | M02.18 | M25.021 | M46.34 | M60.062 | M80.069K | M80.879K |
| L97.405 | L98.3 | M00.271 | M02.19 | M25.022 | M46.35 | M60.069 | M80.069P | M80.879P |
| L97.406 | L98.415 | M00.272 | M02.30 | M25.029 | M46.36 | M60.070 | M80.071A | M80.88XA |
| L97.408 | L98.416 | M00.279 | M02.311 | M25.031 | M46.37 | M60.071 | M80.071K | M80.88XK |
| L97.409 | L98.418 | M00.28 | M02.312 | M25.032 | M46.38 | M60.072 | M80.071P | M80.88XP |
| L97.411 | L98.425 | M00.29 | M02.319 | M25.039 | M46.39 | M60.073 | M80.072A | M84.30XK |
| L97.412 | L98.426 | M00.80 | M02.321 | M25.041 | M47.011 | M60.074 | M80.072K | M84.30XP |
| L97.413 | L98.428 | M00.811 | M02.322 | M25.042 | M47.012 | M60.075 | M80.072P | M84.311K |
| L97.414 | L98.495 | M00.812 | M02.329 | M25.049 | M47.013 | M60.076 | M80.079A | M84.311P |
| L97.415 | L98.496 | M00.819 | M02.331 | M25.051 | M47.014 | M60.077 | M80.079K | M84.312K |
| L97.416 | L98.498 | M00.821 | M02.332 | M25.052 | M47.015 | M60.078 | M80.079P | M84.312P |
| L97.418 | M00.00 | M00.822 | M02.339 | M25.059 | M47.016 | M60.08 | M80.08XA | M84.319K |
| L97.419 | M00.011 | M00.829 | M02.341 | M25.061 | M47.019 | M60.09 | M80.08XK | M84.319P |
| L97.421 | M00.012 | M00.831 | M02.342 | M25.062 | M47.021 | M62.82 | M80.08XP | M84.321K |
| L97.422 | M00.019 | M00.832 | M02.349 | M25.069 | M47.022 | M79.A11 | M80.80XA | M84.321P |
| L97.423 | M00.021 | M00.839 | M02.351 | M25.071 | M47.029 | M79.A12 | M80.80XK | M84.322K |
| L97.424 | M00.022 | M00.841 | M02.352 | M25.072 | M47.10 | M79.A19 | M80.80XP | M84.322P |
| L97.425 | M00.029 | M00.842 | M02.359 | M25.073 | M47.11 | M79.A21 | M80.811A | M84.329K |
| L97.426 | M00.031 | M00.849 | M02.361 | M25.074 | M47.12 | M79.A22 | M80.811K | M84.329P |
| L97.428 | M00.032 | M00.851 | M02.362 | M25.075 | M47.13 | M79.A29 | M80.811P | M84.331K |
| L97.429 | M00.039 | M00.852 | M02.369 | M25.076 | M47.14 | M79.A3 | M80.812A | M84.331P |
| L97.505 | M00.041 | M00.859 | M02.371 | M25.08 | M47.15 | M79.A9 | M80.812K | M84.332K |
| L97.506 | M00.042 | M00.861 | M02.372 | M30.0 | M47.16 | M80.00XA | M80.812P | M84.332P |
| L97.508 | M00.049 | M00.862 | M02.379 | M30.1 | M48.30 | M80.00XK | M80.819A | M84.333K |
| L97.515 | M00.051 | M00.869 | M02.38 | M30.2 | M48.31 | M80.00XP | M80.819K | M84.333P |
| L97.516 | M00.052 | M00.871 | M02.39 | M30.3 | M48.32 | M80.011A | M80.819P | M84.334K |
| L97.518 | M00.059 | M00.872 | M02.80 | M30.8 | M48.33 | M80.011K | M80.821A | M84.334P |
| L97.525 | M00.061 | M00.879 | M02.811 | M31.0 | M48.34 | M80.011P | M80.821K | M84.339K |
| L97.526 | M00.062 | M00.88 | M02.812 | M31.2 | M48.35 | M80.012A | M80.821P | M84.339P |
| L97.528 | M00.069 | M00.89 | M02.819 | M31.30 | M48.36 | M80.012K | M80.822A | M84.341K |
| L97.801 | M00.071 | M00.9 | M02.821 | M31.31 | M48.37 | M80.012P | M80.822K | M84.341P |
| L97.802 | M00.072 | M01.X0 | M02.822 | M31.4 | M48.38 | M80.019A | M80.822P | M84.342K |
| L97.803 | M00.079 | M01.X11 | M02.829 | M31.7 | M48.50XA | M80.019K | M80.829A | M84.342P |
| L97.804 | M00.08 | M01.X12 | M02.831 | M31.8 | M48.51XA | M80.019P | M80.829K | M84.343K |
| L97.805 | M00.09 | M01.X19 | M02.832 | M31.9 | M48.52XA | M80.021A | M80.829P | M84.343P |
| L97.806 | M00.10 | M01.X21 | M02.839 | M32.11 | M48.53XA | M80.021K | M80.831A | M84.344K |
| L97.808 | M00.111 | M01.X22 | M02.841 | M32.12 | M48.54XA | M80.021P | M80.831K | M84.344P |
| L97.809 | M00.112 | M01.X29 | M02.842 | M33.00 | M48.55XA | M80.022A | M80.831P | M84.345K |
| L97.811 | M00.119 | M01.X31 | M02.849 | M33.01 | M48.56XA | M80.022K | M80.832A | M84.345P |
| L97.812 | M00.121 | M01.X32 | M02.851 | M33.02 | M48.57XA | M80.022P | M80.832K | M84.346K |
| L97.813 | M00.122 | M01.X39 | M02.852 | M33.03 | M48.58XA | M80.029A | M80.832P | M84.346P |
| L97.814 | M00.129 | M01.X41 | M02.859 | M33.09 | M50.00 | M80.029K | M80.839A | M84.350K |
| L97.815 | M00.131 | M01.X42 | M02.861 | M33.10 | M50.01 | M80.029P | M80.839K | M84.350P |
| L97.816 | M00.132 | M01.X49 | M02.862 | M33.11 | M50.020 | M80.031A | M80.839P | M84.351K |
| L97.818 | M00.139 | M01.X51 | M02.869 | M33.12 | M50.021 | M80.031K | M80.841A | M84.351P |
| L97.819 | M00.141 | M01.X52 | M02.871 | M33.13 | M50.022 | M80.031P | M80.841K | |

| | | | | | | | | |
|---|---|---|---|---|---|---|---|---|
| M84.352K | M84.442P | M84.511K | M84.573A | M84.661P | M86.051 | M86.369 | M86.69 | M87.150 |
| M84.352P | M84.443A | M84.511P | M84.573K | M84.662A | M86.052 | M86.371 | M86.8X0 | M87.151 |
| M84.353K | M84.443K | M84.512A | M84.573P | M84.662K | M86.059 | M86.372 | M86.8X1 | M87.152 |
| M84.353P | M84.443P | M84.512K | M84.574A | M84.662P | M86.061 | M86.379 | M86.8X2 | M87.159 |
| M84.359K | M84.444A | M84.512P | M84.574K | M84.663A | M86.062 | M86.38 | M86.8X3 | M87.161 |
| M84.359P | M84.444K | M84.519A | M84.574P | M84.663K | M86.069 | M86.39 | M86.8X4 | M87.162 |
| M84.361K | M84.444P | M84.519K | M84.575A | M84.663P | M86.071 | M86.40 | M86.8X5 | M87.163 |
| M84.361P | M84.445A | M84.519P | M84.575K | M84.664A | M86.072 | M86.411 | M86.8X6 | M87.164 |
| M84.362K | M84.445K | M84.521A | M84.575P | M84.664K | M86.079 | M86.412 | M86.8X7 | M87.165 |
| M84.362P | M84.445P | M84.521K | M84.576A | M84.664P | M86.08 | M86.419 | M86.8X8 | M87.166 |
| M84.363K | M84.446A | M84.521P | M84.576K | M84.669A | M86.09 | M86.421 | M86.8X9 | M87.171 |
| M84.363P | M84.446K | M84.522A | M84.576P | M84.669K | M86.10 | M86.422 | M86.9 | M87.172 |
| M84.364K | M84.446P | M84.522K | M84.58XA | M84.669P | M86.111 | M86.429 | M87.00 | M87.173 |
| M84.364P | M84.451A | M84.522P | M84.58XK | M84.671A | M86.112 | M86.431 | M87.011 | M87.174 |
| M84.369K | M84.451K | M84.529A | M84.58XP | M84.671K | M86.119 | M86.432 | M87.012 | M87.175 |
| M84.369P | M84.451P | M84.529K | M84.60XA | M84.671P | M86.121 | M86.439 | M87.019 | M87.176 |
| M84.371K | M84.452A | M84.529P | M84.60XK | M84.672A | M86.122 | M86.441 | M87.021 | M87.177 |
| M84.371P | M84.452K | M84.531A | M84.60XP | M84.672K | M86.129 | M86.442 | M87.022 | M87.178 |
| M84.372K | M84.452P | M84.531K | M84.611A | M84.672P | M86.131 | M86.449 | M87.029 | M87.179 |
| M84.372P | M84.453A | M84.531P | M84.611K | M84.673A | M86.132 | M86.451 | M87.031 | M87.180 |
| M84.373K | M84.453K | M84.532A | M84.611P | M84.673K | M86.139 | M86.452 | M87.032 | M87.188 |
| M84.373P | M84.453P | M84.532K | M84.612A | M84.673P | M86.141 | M86.459 | M87.033 | M87.19 |
| M84.374K | M84.454A | M84.532P | M84.612K | M84.674A | M86.142 | M86.461 | M87.034 | M87.20 |
| M84.374P | M84.454K | M84.533A | M84.612P | M84.674K | M86.149 | M86.462 | M87.035 | M87.211 |
| M84.375K | M84.454P | M84.533K | M84.619A | M84.674P | M86.151 | M86.469 | M87.036 | M87.212 |
| M84.375P | M84.459A | M84.533P | M84.619K | M84.675A | M86.152 | M86.471 | M87.037 | M87.219 |
| M84.376K | M84.459K | M84.534A | M84.619P | M84.675K | M86.159 | M86.472 | M87.038 | M87.221 |
| M84.376P | M84.459P | M84.534K | M84.621A | M84.675P | M86.161 | M86.479 | M87.039 | M87.222 |
| M84.377K | M84.461A | M84.534P | M84.621K | M84.676A | M86.162 | M86.48 | M87.041 | M87.229 |
| M84.377P | M84.461K | M84.539A | M84.621P | M84.676K | M86.169 | M86.49 | M87.042 | M87.231 |
| M84.378K | M84.461P | M84.539K | M84.622A | M84.676P | M86.171 | M86.50 | M87.043 | M87.232 |
| M84.378P | M84.462A | M84.539P | M84.622K | M84.68XA | M86.172 | M86.511 | M87.044 | M87.233 |
| M84.379K | M84.462K | M84.541A | M84.622P | M84.68XK | M86.179 | M86.512 | M87.045 | M87.234 |
| M84.379P | M84.462P | M84.541K | M84.629A | M84.68XP | M86.18 | M86.519 | M87.046 | M87.235 |
| M84.38XK | M84.463A | M84.541P | M84.629K | M84.750A | M86.19 | M86.521 | M87.050 | M87.236 |
| M84.38XP | M84.463K | M84.542A | M84.629P | M84.750K | M86.20 | M86.522 | M87.051 | M87.237 |
| M84.40XA | M84.463P | M84.542K | M84.631A | M84.750P | M86.211 | M86.529 | M87.052 | M87.238 |
| M84.40XK | M84.464A | M84.542P | M84.631K | M84.751A | M86.212 | M86.531 | M87.059 | M87.239 |
| M84.40XP | M84.464K | M84.549A | M84.631P | M84.751K | M86.219 | M86.532 | M87.061 | M87.241 |
| M84.411A | M84.464P | M84.549K | M84.632A | M84.751P | M86.221 | M86.539 | M87.062 | M87.242 |
| M84.411K | M84.469A | M84.549P | M84.632K | M84.752A | M86.222 | M86.541 | M87.063 | M87.243 |
| M84.411P | M84.469K | M84.550A | M84.632P | M84.752K | M86.229 | M86.542 | M87.064 | M87.244 |
| M84.412A | M84.469P | M84.550K | M84.633A | M84.752P | M86.231 | M86.549 | M87.065 | M87.245 |
| M84.412K | M84.471A | M84.550P | M84.633K | M84.753A | M86.232 | M86.551 | M87.066 | M87.246 |
| M84.412P | M84.471K | M84.551A | M84.633P | M84.753K | M86.239 | M86.552 | M87.071 | M87.250 |
| M84.419A | M84.471P | M84.551K | M84.634A | M84.753P | M86.241 | M86.559 | M87.072 | M87.251 |
| M84.419K | M84.472A | M84.551P | M84.634K | M84.754A | M86.242 | M86.561 | M87.073 | M87.252 |
| M84.419P | M84.472K | M84.552A | M84.634P | M84.754K | M86.249 | M86.562 | M87.074 | M87.256 |
| M84.421A | M84.472P | M84.552K | M84.639A | M84.754P | M86.251 | M86.569 | M87.075 | M87.261 |
| M84.421K | M84.473A | M84.552P | M84.639K | M84.755A | M86.252 | M86.571 | M87.076 | M87.262 |
| M84.421P | M84.473K | M84.553A | M84.639P | M84.755K | M86.259 | M86.572 | M87.077 | M87.263 |
| M84.422A | M84.473P | M84.553K | M84.641A | M84.755P | M86.261 | M86.579 | M87.078 | M87.264 |
| M84.422K | M84.474A | M84.553P | M84.641K | M84.756A | M86.262 | M86.58 | M87.079 | M87.265 |
| M84.422P | M84.474K | M84.559A | M84.641P | M84.756K | M86.269 | M86.59 | M87.08 | M87.266 |
| M84.429A | M84.474P | M84.559K | M84.642A | M84.756P | M86.271 | M86.60 | M87.09 | M87.271 |
| M84.429K | M84.475A | M84.559P | M84.642K | M84.757A | M86.272 | M86.611 | M87.10 | M87.272 |
| M84.429P | M84.475K | M84.561A | M84.642P | M84.757K | M86.279 | M86.612 | M87.111 | M87.273 |
| M84.431A | M84.475P | M84.561K | M84.649A | M84.757P | M86.28 | M86.619 | M87.112 | M87.274 |
| M84.431K | M84.476A | M84.561P | M84.649K | M84.758A | M86.29 | M86.621 | M87.119 | M87.275 |
| M84.431P | M84.476K | M84.562A | M84.649P | M84.758K | M86.30 | M86.622 | M87.121 | M87.276 |
| M84.432A | M84.476P | M84.562K | M84.650A | M84.758P | M86.311 | M86.629 | M87.122 | M87.277 |
| M84.432K | M84.477A | M84.562P | M84.650K | M84.759A | M86.312 | M86.631 | M87.129 | M87.278 |
| M84.432P | M84.477K | M84.563A | M84.650P | M84.759K | M86.319 | M86.632 | M87.131 | M87.279 |
| M84.433A | M84.477P | M84.563K | M84.651A | M84.759P | M86.321 | M86.639 | M87.132 | M87.28 |
| M84.433K | M84.478A | M84.563P | M84.651K | M86.00 | M86.322 | M86.641 | M87.133 | M87.29 |
| M84.433P | M84.478K | M84.564A | M84.651P | M86.011 | M86.329 | M86.642 | M87.134 | M87.30 |
| M84.434A | M84.478P | M84.564K | M84.652A | M86.012 | M86.331 | M86.649 | M87.135 | M87.311 |
| M84.434K | M84.479A | M84.564P | M84.652K | M86.019 | M86.332 | M86.651 | M87.136 | M87.312 |
| M84.434P | M84.479K | M84.569A | M84.652P | M86.021 | M86.339 | M86.652 | M87.137 | M87.319 |
| M84.439A | M84.479P | M84.569K | M84.653A | M86.022 | M86.341 | M86.659 | M87.138 | M87.321 |
| M84.439K | M84.48XA | M84.569P | M84.653K | M86.029 | M86.342 | M86.661 | M87.139 | M87.322 |
| M84.439P | M84.48XK | M84.571A | M84.653P | M86.031 | M86.349 | M86.662 | M87.141 | M87.329 |
| M84.441A | M84.48XP | M84.571K | M84.659A | M86.032 | M86.351 | M86.669 | M87.142 | M87.331 |
| M84.441K | M84.50XA | M84.571P | M84.659K | M86.039 | M86.352 | M86.671 | M87.143 | M87.332 |
| M84.441P | M84.50XK | M84.572A | M84.659P | M86.041 | M86.359 | M86.672 | M87.144 | M87.333 |
| M84.442A | M84.50XP | M84.572K | M84.661A | M86.042 | M86.361 | M86.679 | M87.145 | M87.334 |
| M84.442K | M84.511A | M84.572P | M84.661K | M86.049 | M86.362 | M86.68 | M87.146 | M87.335 |

Appendix F: Complication and Comorbidity (CC) Code List

| | | | | | | | | |
|---|---|---|---|---|---|---|---|---|
| M87.336 | M90.512 | N03.4 | N70.02 | O03.87 | O23.01 | O30.211 | O36.0929 | O72.1 |
| M87.337 | M90.519 | N03.5 | N70.03 | O03.88 | O23.02 | O30.212 | O36.0930 | O72.2 |
| M87.338 | M90.521 | N03.6 | N71.0 | O03.89 | O23.03 | O30.213 | O36.0931 | O75.2 |
| M87.339 | M90.522 | N03.7 | N73.0 | O04.5 | O23.11 | O30.221 | O36.0932 | O86.11 |
| M87.341 | M90.529 | N03.8 | N73.4 | O04.80 | O23.12 | O30.222 | O36.0933 | O86.12 |
| M87.342 | M90.531 | N03.9 | N75.1 | O04.83 | O23.13 | O30.223 | O36.0934 | O86.13 |
| M87.343 | M90.532 | N04.0 | N76.4 | O04.84 | O23.21 | O30.291 | O36.0935 | O86.19 |
| M87.344 | M90.539 | N04.1 | N76.81 | O04.85 | O23.22 | O30.292 | O36.0939 | O86.20 |
| M87.345 | M90.541 | N04.2 | N82.0 | O04.86 | O23.23 | O30.293 | O36.4XX0 | O86.21 |
| M87.346 | M90.542 | N04.3 | N82.1 | O04.87 | O23.31 | O30.801 | O36.4XX1 | O86.22 |
| M87.350 | M90.549 | N04.4 | N82.2 | O04.88 | O23.32 | O30.802 | O36.4XX2 | O86.29 |
| M87.351 | M90.551 | N04.5 | N82.3 | O04.89 | O23.33 | O30.803 | O36.4XX3 | O86.4 |
| M87.352 | M90.552 | N04.6 | N82.4 | O07.0 | O23.41 | O30.811 | O36.4XX4 | O87.0 |
| M87.353 | M90.559 | N04.7 | N82.5 | O07.1 | O23.42 | O30.812 | O36.4XX5 | O87.2 |
| M87.361 | M90.561 | N04.8 | N82.8 | O07.30 | O23.43 | O30.813 | O36.4XX9 | O87.3 |
| M87.362 | M90.562 | N04.9 | N82.9 | O07.33 | O23.511 | O30.821 | O41.01X0 | O87.8 |
| M87.363 | M90.569 | N05.2 | N83.511 | O07.34 | O23.512 | O30.822 | O41.01X1 | O88.319 |
| M87.364 | M90.571 | N05.3 | N83.512 | O07.35 | O23.513 | O30.823 | O41.01X2 | O98.011 |
| M87.365 | M90.572 | N05.4 | N83.519 | O07.36 | O23.521 | O30.891 | O41.01X3 | O98.012 |
| M87.366 | M90.579 | N05.5 | N83.521 | O07.37 | O23.522 | O30.892 | O41.01X4 | O98.013 |
| M87.371 | M90.58 | N06.2 | N83.522 | O07.38 | O23.523 | O30.893 | O41.01X5 | O98.02 |
| M87.372 | M90.59 | N06.3 | N83.529 | O07.39 | O23.591 | O31.8X10 | O41.01X9 | O98.03 |
| M87.373 | M96.0 | N06.4 | N83.53 | O08.0 | O23.592 | O31.8X11 | O41.02X0 | O98.111 |
| M87.374 | M96.621 | N06.5 | N98.0 | O08.1 | O23.593 | O31.8X12 | O41.02X1 | O98.112 |
| M87.375 | M96.622 | N07.2 | N98.1 | O08.5 | O23.91 | O31.8X13 | O41.02X2 | O98.113 |
| M87.376 | M96.629 | N07.3 | N98.2 | O08.6 | O23.92 | O31.8X14 | O41.02X3 | O98.12 |
| M87.377 | M96.631 | N07.4 | N98.3 | O08.7 | O23.93 | O31.8X15 | O41.02X4 | O98.13 |
| M87.378 | M96.632 | N07.5 | N98.8 | O08.81 | O24.011 | O31.8X19 | O41.02X5 | O98.211 |
| M87.379 | M96.639 | N10 | N98.9 | O08.82 | O24.012 | O31.8X20 | O41.02X9 | O98.212 |
| M87.38 | M96.65 | N11.1 | N99.510 | O08.83 | O24.013 | O31.8X21 | O41.03X0 | O98.213 |
| M87.39 | M96.661 | N11.8 | N99.511 | O08.89 | O24.019 | O31.8X22 | O41.03X1 | O98.22 |
| M87.80 | M96.662 | N11.9 | N99.512 | O08.9 | O24.03 | O31.8X23 | O41.03X2 | O98.23 |
| M87.811 | M96.669 | N12 | N99.518 | O10.011 | O24.111 | O31.8X24 | O41.03X3 | O98.311 |
| M87.812 | M96.671 | N13.0 | N99.61 | O10.012 | O24.112 | O31.8X25 | O41.03X4 | O98.312 |
| M87.819 | M96.672 | N13.1 | N99.62 | O10.013 | O24.113 | O31.8X29 | O41.03X5 | O98.313 |
| M87.821 | M96.679 | N13.2 | N99.71 | O10.02 | O24.119 | O31.8X30 | O41.03X9 | O98.32 |
| M87.822 | M96.69 | N13.30 | N99.72 | O10.411 | O24.13 | O31.8X31 | O44.01 | O98.33 |
| M87.829 | M96.810 | N13.39 | N99.820 | O10.412 | O24.311 | O31.8X32 | O44.02 | O98.411 |
| M87.831 | M96.811 | N13.4 | N99.821 | O10.413 | O24.312 | O31.8X33 | O44.03 | O98.412 |
| M87.832 | M96.820 | N13.6 | N99.840 | O10.419 | O24.313 | O31.8X34 | O44.21 | O98.413 |
| M87.833 | M96.821 | N13.8 | N99.841 | O10.43 | O24.319 | O31.8X35 | O44.22 | O98.42 |
| M87.834 | M96.830 | N17.8 | N99.842 | O10.911 | O24.33 | O31.8X39 | O44.23 | O98.43 |
| M87.835 | M96.831 | N17.9 | N99.843 | O10.912 | O24.811 | O33.0 | O44.41 | O98.511 |
| M87.836 | M96.840 | N18.4 | O00.00 | O10.913 | O24.812 | O36.0110 | O44.42 | O98.512 |
| M87.837 | M96.841 | N18.5 | O00.01 | O10.92 | O24.813 | O36.0111 | O44.43 | O98.513 |
| M87.838 | M96.842 | N20.1 | O00.101 | O12.11 | O24.819 | O36.0112 | O47.02 | O98.52 |
| M87.839 | M96.843 | N20.2 | O00.102 | O12.12 | O24.83 | O36.0113 | O47.03 | O98.53 |
| M87.841 | M96.89 | N25.1 | O00.109 | O12.13 | O24.911 | O36.0114 | O47.1 | O98.611 |
| M87.842 | M97.01XA | N25.81 | O00.111 | O12.21 | O24.912 | O36.0115 | O60.10X0 | O98.612 |
| M87.843 | M97.02XA | N28.0 | O00.112 | O12.22 | O24.913 | O36.0119 | O60.10X1 | O98.613 |
| M87.844 | M97.11XA | N28.84 | O00.119 | O12.23 | O24.919 | O36.0120 | O60.10X2 | O98.62 |
| M87.845 | M97.12XA | N28.85 | O00.201 | O14.02 | O24.93 | O36.0121 | O60.10X3 | O98.63 |
| M87.849 | M97.21XA | N28.86 | O00.202 | O14.03 | O26.611 | O36.0122 | O60.10X4 | O98.711 |
| M87.850 | M97.22XA | N30.00 | O00.209 | O14.92 | O26.612 | O36.0123 | O60.10X5 | O98.712 |
| M87.851 | M97.31XA | N30.01 | O00.211 | O14.93 | O26.613 | O36.0124 | O60.10X9 | O98.713 |
| M87.852 | M97.32XA | N30.40 | O00.212 | O16.1 | O26.62 | O36.0125 | O60.20X0 | O98.72 |
| M87.859 | M97.41XA | N30.41 | O00.219 | O16.2 | O26.831 | O36.0129 | O60.20X1 | O98.73 |
| M87.861 | M97.42XA | N32.1 | O00.80 | O16.3 | O26.832 | O36.0130 | O60.20X2 | O98.811 |
| M87.862 | M97.8XXA | N32.2 | O00.81 | O20.0 | O26.833 | O36.0131 | O60.20X3 | O98.812 |
| M87.863 | M97.9XXA | N34.0 | O00.90 | O20.9 | O26.872 | O36.0132 | O60.20X4 | O98.813 |
| M87.864 | M99.10 | N36.0 | O00.91 | O22.20 | O26.873 | O36.0133 | O60.20X5 | O98.82 |
| M87.865 | M99.11 | N39.0 | O03.0 | O22.21 | O26.879 | O36.0134 | O60.20X9 | O98.83 |
| M87.869 | M99.18 | N41.0 | O03.30 | O22.22 | O30.101 | O36.0135 | O63.9 | O98.911 |
| M87.871 | N02.0 | N41.2 | O03.33 | O22.23 | O30.102 | O36.0139 | O68 | O98.912 |
| M87.872 | N02.1 | N43.1 | O03.34 | O22.30 | O30.103 | O36.0910 | O70.20 | O98.913 |
| M87.873 | N02.2 | N44.00 | O03.35 | O22.40 | O30.111 | O36.0911 | O70.21 | O98.92 |
| M87.874 | N02.3 | N44.01 | O03.36 | O22.41 | O30.112 | O36.0912 | O70.22 | O98.93 |
| M87.875 | N02.4 | N44.02 | O03.37 | O22.42 | O30.113 | O36.0913 | O70.23 | O99.111 |
| M87.876 | N02.5 | N44.03 | O03.38 | O22.43 | O30.121 | O36.0914 | O70.3 | O99.112 |
| M87.877 | N02.6 | N44.04 | O03.39 | O22.50 | O30.122 | O36.0915 | O70.4 | O99.113 |
| M87.878 | N02.7 | N45.4 | O03.5 | O22.51 | O30.123 | O36.0919 | O71.2 | O99.119 |
| M87.879 | N02.8 | N48.30 | O03.7 | O22.52 | O30.191 | O36.0920 | O71.3 | O99.12 |
| M87.88 | N02.9 | N48.31 | O03.80 | O22.53 | O30.192 | O36.0921 | O71.4 | O99.13 |
| M87.89 | N03.0 | N48.32 | O03.83 | O22.8X1 | O30.193 | O36.0922 | O71.5 | O99.321 |
| M87.9 | N03.1 | N48.33 | O03.84 | O22.8X2 | O30.201 | O36.0923 | O71.6 | O99.322 |
| M90.50 | N03.2 | N48.39 | O03.85 | O22.8X3 | O30.202 | O36.0924 | O71.7 | O99.323 |
| M90.511 | N03.3 | N70.01 | O03.86 | O22.8X9 | O30.203 | O36.0925 | O72.0 | O99.324 |
| | | | | O22.90 | | | | |

| | | | | | | | | |
|---|---|---|---|---|---|---|---|---|
| O99.325 | Q05.3 | Q43.1 | Q87.3 | S02.113A | S02.600K | S02.81XB | S06.302A | S12.02XA |
| O99.354 | Q05.4 | Q43.2 | Q87.40 | S02.113K | S02.601A | S02.81XK | S06.303A | S12.02XK |
| O99.355 | Q07.02 | Q43.3 | Q87.410 | S02.118A | S02.601B | S02.82XA | S06.304A | S12.030A |
| O99.411 | Q07.03 | Q43.4 | Q87.418 | S02.118K | S02.601K | S02.82XB | S06.305A | S12.030K |
| O99.412 | Q20.5 | Q43.5 | Q87.42 | S02.119A | S02.602A | S02.82XK | S06.309A | S12.031A |
| O99.413 | Q21.0 | Q43.6 | Q87.43 | S02.119K | S02.602B | S02.91XA | S06.371A | S12.031K |
| O99.43 | Q21.1 | Q43.7 | Q87.5 | S02.11AA | S02.602K | S02.91XK | S06.372A | S12.040A |
| O99.830 | Q21.2 | Q43.8 | Q87.81 | S02.11AK | S02.609A | S02.92XA | S06.373A | S12.040K |
| O99.834 | Q22.1 | Q43.9 | Q87.82 | S02.11BA | S02.609B | S02.92XB | S06.374A | S12.041A |
| O99.835 | Q22.2 | Q44.0 | Q87.89 | S02.11BK | S02.609K | S02.92XK | S06.375A | S12.041K |
| P10.2 | Q22.3 | Q44.1 | Q89.01 | S02.11CA | S02.610A | S04.011A | S06.379A | S12.090A |
| P12.2 | Q23.0 | Q44.4 | Q89.09 | S02.11CK | S02.610B | S04.012A | S06.381A | S12.090K |
| P28.0 | Q23.1 | Q44.5 | Q89.3 | S02.11DA | S02.610K | S04.019A | S06.382A | S12.091A |
| P28.10 | Q23.2 | Q44.6 | Q89.7 | S02.11DK | S02.611A | S04.02XA | S06.383A | S12.091K |
| P28.11 | Q23.3 | Q44.7 | Q89.8 | S02.11EA | S02.611B | S04.031A | S06.384A | S12.100A |
| P28.19 | Q24.0 | Q45.0 | Q91.0 | S02.11EK | S02.611K | S04.032A | S06.385A | S12.100K |
| P28.2 | Q24.1 | Q45.1 | Q91.1 | S02.11FA | S02.612A | S04.039A | S06.389A | S12.101A |
| P28.3 | Q24.3 | Q45.2 | Q91.2 | S02.11FK | S02.612B | S04.041A | S06.811A | S12.101K |
| P28.4 | Q24.5 | Q45.3 | Q91.3 | S02.11GA | S02.612K | S04.042A | S06.812A | S12.110A |
| P35.0 | Q25.0 | Q60.0 | Q91.4 | S02.11GK | S02.620A | S04.049A | S06.813A | S12.110K |
| P38.1 | Q25.1 | Q60.1 | Q91.5 | S02.11HA | S02.620B | S04.10XA | S06.814A | S12.111A |
| P38.9 | Q25.21 | Q60.2 | Q91.6 | S02.11HK | S02.620K | S04.11XA | S06.815A | S12.111K |
| P39.0 | Q25.29 | Q60.3 | Q91.7 | S02.19XA | S02.621A | S04.12XA | S06.819A | S12.112A |
| P39.2 | Q25.3 | Q60.4 | Q93.3 | S02.19XK | S02.621B | S04.20XA | S06.821A | S12.112K |
| P39.3 | Q25.40 | Q60.5 | Q93.4 | S02.2XXB | S02.621K | S04.21XA | S06.822A | S12.120A |
| P39.4 | Q25.41 | Q60.6 | Q93.5 | S02.2XXK | S02.622A | S04.22XA | S06.823A | S12.120K |
| P39.8 | Q25.42 | Q61.00 | Q93.7 | S02.30XA | S02.622B | S04.30XA | S06.824A | S12.121A |
| P39.9 | Q25.43 | Q61.01 | Q93.88 | S02.30XB | S02.622K | S04.31XA | S06.825A | S12.121K |
| P52.0 | Q25.44 | Q61.02 | Q93.89 | S02.30XK | S02.630A | S04.32XA | S06.829A | S12.130A |
| P52.1 | Q25.45 | Q61.11 | Q93.9 | S02.31XA | S02.630B | S04.40XA | S06.891A | S12.130K |
| P52.3 | Q25.46 | Q61.19 | R04.2 | S02.31XB | S02.630K | S04.41XA | S06.892A | S12.131A |
| P53 | Q25.47 | Q61.2 | R04.81 | S02.31XK | S02.631A | S04.42XA | S06.893A | S12.131K |
| P54.4 | Q25.48 | Q61.3 | R04.89 | S02.32XA | S02.631B | S04.50XA | S06.894A | S12.14XA |
| P61.2 | Q25.49 | Q61.4 | R04.9 | S02.32XB | S02.631K | S04.51XA | S06.895A | S12.14XK |
| P61.3 | Q25.8 | Q61.5 | R06.3 | S02.32XK | S02.632A | S04.52XA | S06.899A | S12.150A |
| P61.4 | Q25.9 | Q61.8 | R09.01 | S02.400A | S02.632B | S04.60XA | S06.9X1A | S12.150K |
| P61.6 | Q26.0 | Q61.9 | R17 | S02.400B | S02.632K | S04.61XA | S06.9X2A | S12.151A |
| P70.2 | Q26.1 | Q62.0 | R18.0 | S02.400K | S02.63XA | S04.62XA | S06.9X3A | S12.151K |
| P70.8 | Q26.2 | Q62.10 | R18.8 | S02.401A | S02.63XB | S04.70XA | S06.9X4A | S12.190A |
| P71.0 | Q26.3 | Q62.11 | R29.0 | S02.401B | S02.63XK | S04.71XA | S06.9X5A | S12.190K |
| P71.1 | Q26.4 | Q62.12 | R29.1 | S02.401K | S02.640A | S04.72XA | S06.9X9A | S12.191A |
| P71.2 | Q26.8 | Q62.2 | R29.5 | S02.402A | S02.640B | S04.811A | S07.0XXA | S12.191K |
| P71.3 | Q26.9 | Q62.31 | R39.0 | S02.402B | S02.640K | S04.812A | S07.1XXA | S12.200A |
| P71.4 | Q27.30 | Q62.32 | R40.3 | S02.402K | S02.641A | S04.819A | S07.8XXA | S12.200K |
| P71.8 | Q27.4 | Q62.39 | R41.4 | S02.40AA | S02.641B | S04.891A | S07.9XXA | S12.201A |
| P71.9 | Q28.0 | Q64.10 | R44.0 | S02.40AB | S02.641K | S04.892A | S09.0XXA | S12.201K |
| P72.0 | Q28.1 | Q64.11 | R44.2 | S02.40AK | S02.642A | S04.899A | S09.20XA | S12.230A |
| P72.1 | Q28.8 | Q64.12 | R44.3 | S02.40BA | S02.642B | S04.9XXA | S09.21XA | S12.230K |
| P72.2 | Q28.9 | Q64.19 | R45.851 | S02.40BB | S02.642K | S05.20XA | S09.22XA | S12.231A |
| P72.8 | Q31.1 | Q64.2 | R47.01 | S02.40BK | S02.650A | S05.21XA | S09.301A | S12.231K |
| P74.5 | Q31.2 | Q64.31 | R56.00 | S02.40CA | S02.650B | S05.22XA | S09.302A | S12.24XA |
| P74.6 | Q31.3 | Q64.32 | R56.01 | S02.40CB | S02.650K | S05.30XA | S09.309A | S12.24XK |
| P74.8 | Q31.5 | Q64.33 | R56.1 | S02.40CK | S02.651A | S05.31XA | S09.311A | S12.250A |
| P76.1 | Q31.8 | Q64.39 | R57.9 | S02.40DA | S02.651B | S05.32XA | S09.312A | S12.250K |
| P83.0 | Q31.9 | Q67.5 | R64 | S02.40DB | S02.651K | S05.40XA | S09.313A | S12.251A |
| P83.30 | Q32.0 | Q67.8 | R65.10 | S02.40DK | S02.652A | S05.41XA | S09.319A | S12.251K |
| P83.39 | Q32.1 | Q68.1 | R71.0 | S02.40EA | S02.652B | S05.42XA | S09.391A | S12.290A |
| P91.60 | Q32.2 | Q74.3 | R74.3 | S02.40EB | S02.652K | S05.50XA | S09.392A | S12.290K |
| P91.61 | Q32.3 | Q76.3 | R78.81 | S02.40EK | S02.66XA | S05.51XA | S09.399A | S12.291A |
| P91.62 | Q32.4 | Q76.425 | R82.0 | S02.40FA | S02.66XB | S05.52XA | S11.10XA | S12.291K |
| P93.0 | Q33.0 | Q76.426 | R82.1 | S02.40FB | S02.66XK | S05.70XA | S11.11XA | S12.300A |
| P93.8 | Q33.4 | Q76.427 | S01.101A | S02.40FK | S02.670A | S05.71XA | S11.12XA | S12.300K |
| P94.0 | Q39.5 | Q76.428 | S01.102A | S02.411A | S02.670B | S05.72XA | S11.13XA | S12.301A |
| P96.1 | Q39.6 | Q76.429 | S01.109A | S02.411B | S02.670K | S05.8X1A | S11.14XA | S12.301K |
| P96.2 | Q39.8 | Q76.6 | S02.0XXA | S02.411K | S02.671A | S05.8X2A | S11.15XA | S12.330A |
| Q01.0 | Q39.9 | Q76.7 | S02.0XXK | S02.412A | S02.671B | S05.8X9A | S11.20XA | S12.330K |
| Q01.1 | Q41.0 | Q76.8 | S02.101A | S02.412B | S02.671K | S05.91XA | S11.21XA | S12.331A |
| Q01.2 | Q41.1 | Q76.9 | S02.101K | S02.412K | S02.672A | S05.92XA | S11.22XA | S12.331K |
| Q01.8 | Q41.2 | Q77.2 | S02.102A | S02.413A | S02.672B | S06.0X1A | S11.23XA | S12.34XA |
| Q01.9 | Q41.8 | Q78.0 | S02.102K | S02.413B | S02.672K | S06.0X9A | S11.24XA | S12.34XK |
| Q04.4 | Q41.9 | Q78.2 | S02.109A | S02.413K | S02.69XA | S06.2X1A | S11.25XA | S12.350A |
| Q04.5 | Q42.0 | Q79.6 | S02.109K | S02.42XA | S02.69XB | S06.2X2A | S12.000A | S12.350K |
| Q04.6 | Q42.1 | Q85.1 | S02.110A | S02.42XB | S02.69XK | S06.2X3A | S12.000K | S12.351A |
| Q04.8 | Q42.2 | Q85.8 | S02.110K | S02.42XK | S02.80XA | S06.2X4A | S12.001A | S12.351K |
| Q05.0 | Q42.3 | Q85.9 | S02.111A | S02.5XXK | S02.80XB | S06.2X5A | S12.001K | S12.390A |
| Q05.1 | Q42.8 | Q87.1 | S02.111K | S02.600A | S02.80XK | S06.2X9A | S12.01XA | S12.390K |
| Q05.2 | Q42.9 | Q87.2 | S02.112A | S02.600B | S02.81XA | S06.301A | S12.01XK | S12.391A |
| | | | S02.112K | | | | | |

| | | | | | | | | | |
|---|---|---|---|---|---|---|---|---|---|
| S12.391K | S15.001A | S22.000A | S22.078K | S27.321A | S32.050K | S32.414K | S32.613K | S36.291A |
| S12.400A | S15.002A | S22.000K | S22.079A | S27.322A | S32.051A | S32.415K | S32.614A | S36.292A |
| S12.400K | S15.009A | S22.001A | S22.079K | S27.329A | S32.051K | S32.416K | S32.614K | S36.299A |
| S12.401A | S15.011A | S22.001K | S22.080A | S27.391A | S32.052A | S32.421K | S32.615A | S36.30XA |
| S12.401K | S15.012A | S22.002A | S22.080K | S27.392A | S32.052K | S32.422K | S32.615K | S36.32XA |
| S12.430A | S15.019A | S22.002K | S22.081A | S27.399A | S32.058A | S32.423K | S32.616A | S36.33XA |
| S12.430K | S15.021A | S22.008A | S22.081K | S27.50XA | S32.058K | S32.424K | S32.616K | S36.39XA |
| S12.431A | S15.022A | S22.008K | S22.082A | S27.51XA | S32.059A | S32.425K | S32.691A | S36.400A |
| S12.431K | S15.029A | S22.009A | S22.082K | S27.52XA | S32.059K | S32.426K | S32.691K | S36.408A |
| S12.44XA | S15.091A | S22.009K | S22.088A | S27.53XA | S32.10XA | S32.431K | S32.692A | S36.409A |
| S12.44XK | S15.092A | S22.010A | S22.088K | S27.59XA | S32.10XK | S32.432K | S32.692K | S36.410A |
| S12.450A | S15.099A | S22.010K | S22.089A | S27.60XA | S32.110A | S32.433K | S32.699A | S36.418A |
| S12.450K | S15.101A | S22.011A | S22.089K | S27.63XA | S32.110K | S32.434K | S32.699K | S36.419A |
| S12.451A | S15.102A | S22.011K | S22.20XA | S27.69XA | S32.111A | S32.435K | S32.810A | S36.420A |
| S12.451K | S15.109A | S22.012A | S22.20XK | S27.802A | S32.111K | S32.436K | S32.810K | S36.428A |
| S12.490A | S15.111A | S22.012K | S22.21XA | S27.803A | S32.112A | S32.441K | S32.811A | S36.429A |
| S12.490K | S15.112A | S22.018A | S22.21XK | S27.808A | S32.112K | S32.442K | S32.811K | S36.430A |
| S12.491A | S15.119A | S22.018K | S22.22XA | S27.809A | S32.119A | S32.443K | S32.82XA | S36.438A |
| S12.491K | S15.121A | S22.019A | S22.22XK | S27.892A | S32.119K | S32.444K | S32.82XK | S36.439A |
| S12.500A | S15.122A | S22.019K | S22.23XA | S27.893A | S32.120A | S32.445K | S32.89XA | S36.490A |
| S12.500K | S15.129A | S22.020A | S22.23XK | S27.898A | S32.120K | S32.446K | S32.89XK | S36.498A |
| S12.501A | S15.191A | S22.020K | S22.24XA | S27.899A | S32.121A | S32.451K | S32.9XXA | S36.499A |
| S12.501K | S15.192A | S22.021A | S22.24XK | S27.9XXA | S32.121K | S32.452K | S32.9XXK | S36.500A |
| S12.530A | S15.199A | S22.021K | S22.31XA | S28.1XXA | S32.122A | S32.453K | S35.531A | S36.501A |
| S12.530K | S15.201A | S22.022A | S22.31XK | S29.021A | S32.122K | S32.454K | S35.532A | S36.502A |
| S12.531A | S15.202A | S22.022K | S22.32XA | S29.029A | S32.129A | S32.455K | S35.533A | S36.503A |
| S12.531K | S15.209A | S22.028A | S22.32XK | S32.000A | S32.129K | S32.456K | S35.534A | S36.508A |
| S12.54XA | S15.211A | S22.028K | S22.39XA | S32.000K | S32.130A | S32.461K | S35.535A | S36.509A |
| S12.54XK | S15.212A | S22.029A | S22.39XK | S32.001A | S32.130K | S32.462K | S35.536A | S36.510A |
| S12.550A | S15.219A | S22.029K | S22.41XA | S32.001K | S32.131A | S32.463K | S35.8X1A | S36.511A |
| S12.550K | S15.221A | S22.030A | S22.41XK | S32.002A | S32.131K | S32.464K | S35.8X8A | S36.512A |
| S12.551A | S15.222A | S22.030K | S22.42XA | S32.002K | S32.132A | S32.465K | S35.8X9A | S36.513A |
| S12.551K | S15.229A | S22.031A | S22.42XK | S32.008A | S32.132K | S32.466K | S35.90XA | S36.518A |
| S12.590A | S15.291A | S22.031K | S22.43XA | S32.008K | S32.139A | S32.471K | S35.91XA | S36.519A |
| S12.590K | S15.292A | S22.032A | S22.43XK | S32.009A | S32.139K | S32.472K | S35.99XA | S36.520A |
| S12.591A | S15.299A | S22.032K | S22.49XA | S32.009K | S32.14XA | S32.473K | S36.00XA | S36.521A |
| S12.591K | S15.301A | S22.038A | S22.49XK | S32.010A | S32.14XK | S32.474K | S36.020A | S36.522A |
| S12.600A | S15.302A | S22.038K | S22.5XXK | S32.010K | S32.15XA | S32.475K | S36.021A | S36.523A |
| S12.600K | S15.309A | S22.039A | S22.9XXA | S32.011A | S32.15XK | S32.476K | S36.029A | S36.528A |
| S12.601A | S15.311A | S22.039K | S22.9XXK | S32.011K | S32.16XA | S32.481K | S36.030A | S36.529A |
| S12.601K | S15.312A | S22.040A | S25.501A | S32.012A | S32.16XK | S32.482K | S36.039A | S36.530A |
| S12.630A | S15.319A | S22.040K | S25.502A | S32.012K | S32.17XA | S32.483K | S36.09XA | S36.531A |
| S12.630K | S15.321A | S22.041A | S25.509A | S32.018A | S32.17XK | S32.484K | S36.112A | S36.532A |
| S12.631A | S15.322A | S22.041K | S25.511A | S32.018K | S32.19XA | S32.485K | S36.113A | S36.533A |
| S12.631K | S15.329A | S22.042A | S25.512A | S32.019A | S32.19XK | S32.486K | S36.114A | S36.538A |
| S12.64XA | S15.391A | S22.042K | S25.519A | S32.019K | S32.2XXA | S32.491K | S36.118A | S36.539A |
| S12.64XK | S15.392A | S22.048A | S25.591A | S32.020A | S32.2XXK | S32.492K | S36.119A | S36.590A |
| S12.650A | S15.399A | S22.048K | S25.592A | S32.020K | S32.301A | S32.499K | S36.122A | S36.591A |
| S12.650K | S15.8XXA | S22.049A | S25.599A | S32.021A | S32.301K | S32.501A | S36.123A | S36.592A |
| S12.651A | S15.9XXA | S22.049K | S25.801A | S32.021K | S32.302A | S32.501K | S36.128A | S36.593A |
| S12.651K | S17.0XXA | S22.050A | S25.802A | S32.022A | S32.302K | S32.502A | S36.129A | S36.598A |
| S12.690A | S17.8XXA | S22.050K | S25.809A | S32.022K | S32.309A | S32.502K | S36.13XA | S36.599A |
| S12.690K | S17.9XXA | S22.051A | S25.811A | S32.028A | S32.309K | S32.509A | S36.200A | S36.60XA |
| S12.691A | S21.101A | S22.051K | S25.812A | S32.028K | S32.311A | S32.509K | S36.201A | S36.61XA |
| S12.691K | S21.102A | S22.052A | S25.819A | S32.029A | S32.311K | S32.511A | S36.202A | S36.62XA |
| S12.9XXA | S21.109A | S22.052K | S25.891A | S32.029K | S32.312A | S32.511K | S36.209A | S36.63XA |
| S13.0XXA | S21.111A | S22.058A | S25.892A | S32.030A | S32.312K | S32.512A | S36.220A | S36.69XA |
| S13.100A | S21.112A | S22.058K | S25.899A | S32.030K | S32.313A | S32.512K | S36.221A | S36.81XA |
| S13.101A | S21.119A | S22.059A | S25.90XA | S32.031A | S32.313K | S32.519A | S36.222A | S36.892A |
| S13.110A | S21.121A | S22.059K | S25.91XA | S32.031K | S32.314A | S32.519K | S36.229A | S36.893A |
| S13.111A | S21.122A | S22.060A | S25.99XA | S32.032A | S32.314K | S32.591A | S36.230A | S36.898A |
| S13.120A | S21.129A | S22.060K | S26.00XA | S32.032K | S32.315A | S32.591K | S36.231A | S36.899A |
| S13.121A | S21.131A | S22.061A | S26.01XA | S32.038A | S32.315K | S32.592A | S36.232A | S36.90XA |
| S13.130A | S21.132A | S22.061K | S26.09XA | S32.038K | S32.316A | S32.592K | S36.239A | S36.92XA |
| S13.131A | S21.139A | S22.062A | S26.10XA | S32.039A | S32.316K | S32.599A | S36.240A | S36.93XA |
| S13.140A | S21.141A | S22.062K | S26.11XA | S32.039K | S32.391A | S32.599K | S36.241A | S36.99XA |
| S13.141A | S21.142A | S22.068A | S26.19XA | S32.040A | S32.391K | S32.601A | S36.242A | S37.001A |
| S13.150A | S21.149A | S22.068K | S26.90XA | S32.040K | S32.392A | S32.601K | S36.249A | S37.002A |
| S13.151A | S21.151A | S22.069A | S26.91XA | S32.041A | S32.392K | S32.602A | S36.250A | S37.009A |
| S13.160A | S21.152A | S22.069K | S26.99XA | S32.041K | S32.399A | S32.602K | S36.251A | S37.011A |
| S13.161A | S21.159A | S22.070A | S27.0XXA | S32.042A | S32.399K | S32.609A | S36.252A | S37.012A |
| S13.170A | S21.90XA | S22.070K | S27.301A | S32.042K | S32.401K | S32.609K | S36.259A | S37.019A |
| S13.171A | S21.91XA | S22.071A | S27.302A | S32.048A | S32.402K | S32.611A | S36.260A | S37.021A |
| S13.180A | S21.92XA | S22.071K | S27.309A | S32.048K | S32.409K | S32.611K | S36.261A | S37.022A |
| S13.181A | S21.93XA | S22.072A | S27.311A | S32.049A | S32.411K | S32.612A | S36.262A | S37.029A |
| S13.20XA | S21.94XA | S22.072K | S27.312A | S32.049K | S32.412K | S32.612K | S36.269A | S37.031A |
| S13.29XA | S21.95XA | S22.078A | S27.319A | S32.050A | S32.413K | S32.613A | S36.290A | S37.032A |

| | | | | | | | | |
|---|---|---|---|---|---|---|---|---|
| S37.039A | S42.023B | S42.131P | S42.213K | S42.265A | S42.333P | S42.402K | S42.447A | S42.492P |
| S37.041A | S42.023K | S42.132B | S42.213P | S42.265K | S42.334A | S42.402P | S42.447K | S42.493A |
| S37.042A | S42.023P | S42.132K | S42.214A | S42.265P | S42.334K | S42.409A | S42.447P | S42.493K |
| S37.049A | S42.024B | S42.132P | S42.214K | S42.266A | S42.335A | S42.409K | S42.448A | S42.493P |
| S37.051A | S42.024K | S42.133B | S42.214P | S42.266K | S42.335K | S42.409P | S42.448K | S42.494A |
| S37.052A | S42.024P | S42.133K | S42.215A | S42.266P | S42.335P | S42.411A | S42.448P | S42.494K |
| S37.059A | S42.025B | S42.133P | S42.215K | S42.271A | S42.336A | S42.411K | S42.449A | S42.494P |
| S37.10XA | S42.025K | S42.134B | S42.215P | S42.271K | S42.336K | S42.411P | S42.449K | S42.495A |
| S37.12XA | S42.025P | S42.134K | S42.216A | S42.271P | S42.336P | S42.412A | S42.449P | S42.495K |
| S37.13XA | S42.026B | S42.134P | S42.216K | S42.272A | S42.341A | S42.412K | S42.451A | S42.495P |
| S37.19XA | S42.026K | S42.135B | S42.216P | S42.272K | S42.341K | S42.412P | S42.451K | S42.496A |
| S37.20XA | S42.026P | S42.135K | S42.221A | S42.272P | S42.341P | S42.413A | S42.451P | S42.496K |
| S37.22XA | S42.031B | S42.135P | S42.221K | S42.279A | S42.342A | S42.413K | S42.452A | S42.496P |
| S37.23XA | S42.031K | S42.136B | S42.221P | S42.279K | S42.342K | S42.413P | S42.452K | S42.90XA |
| S37.29XA | S42.031P | S42.136K | S42.222A | S42.279P | S42.342P | S42.414A | S42.452P | S42.90XK |
| S37.30XA | S42.032B | S42.136P | S42.222K | S42.291A | S42.343A | S42.414K | S42.453A | S42.90XP |
| S37.32XA | S42.032K | S42.141B | S42.222P | S42.291K | S42.343K | S42.414P | S42.453K | S42.91XA |
| S37.33XA | S42.032P | S42.141K | S42.223A | S42.291P | S42.343P | S42.415A | S42.453P | S42.91XK |
| S37.39XA | S42.033B | S42.141P | S42.223K | S42.292A | S42.344A | S42.415K | S42.454A | S42.91XP |
| S37.60XA | S42.033K | S42.142B | S42.223P | S42.292K | S42.344K | S42.415P | S42.454K | S42.92XA |
| S37.62XA | S42.033P | S42.142K | S42.224A | S42.292P | S42.344P | S42.416A | S42.454P | S42.92XK |
| S37.63XA | S42.034B | S42.142P | S42.224K | S42.293A | S42.345A | S42.416K | S42.455A | S42.92XP |
| S37.69XA | S42.034K | S42.143B | S42.224P | S42.293K | S42.345K | S42.421A | S42.455K | S43.201A |
| S37.812A | S42.034P | S42.143K | S42.225A | S42.293P | S42.345P | S42.421K | S42.455P | S43.202A |
| S37.813A | S42.035B | S42.143P | S42.225K | S42.294A | S42.346A | S42.421P | S42.456A | S43.203A |
| S37.818A | S42.035K | S42.144B | S42.225P | S42.294K | S42.346K | S42.422A | S42.456K | S43.204A |
| S37.819A | S42.035P | S42.144K | S42.226A | S42.294P | S42.346P | S42.422K | S42.456P | S43.205A |
| S37.892A | S42.036B | S42.144P | S42.226K | S42.295A | S42.351A | S42.422P | S42.461A | S43.206A |
| S37.893A | S42.036K | S42.145B | S42.226P | S42.295K | S42.351K | S42.423A | S42.461K | S43.211A |
| S37.898A | S42.036P | S42.145K | S42.231A | S42.295P | S42.351P | S42.423K | S42.461P | S43.212A |
| S37.899A | S42.101B | S42.145P | S42.231K | S42.296A | S42.352A | S42.423P | S42.462A | S43.213A |
| S37.90XA | S42.101K | S42.146B | S42.231P | S42.296K | S42.352K | S42.424A | S42.462K | S43.214A |
| S37.92XA | S42.101P | S42.146K | S42.232A | S42.296P | S42.352P | S42.424K | S42.462P | S43.215A |
| S37.93XA | S42.102B | S42.146P | S42.232K | S42.301A | S42.353A | S42.424P | S42.463A | S43.216A |
| S37.99XA | S42.102K | S42.151B | S42.232P | S42.301K | S42.353K | S42.425A | S42.463K | S43.221A |
| S42.001B | S42.102P | S42.151K | S42.239A | S42.301P | S42.353P | S42.425K | S42.463P | S43.222A |
| S42.001K | S42.109B | S42.151P | S42.239K | S42.302A | S42.354A | S42.425P | S42.464A | S43.223A |
| S42.001P | S42.109K | S42.152B | S42.239P | S42.302K | S42.354K | S42.426A | S42.464K | S43.224A |
| S42.002B | S42.109P | S42.152K | S42.241A | S42.302P | S42.354P | S42.426K | S42.464P | S43.225A |
| S42.002K | S42.111B | S42.152P | S42.241K | S42.309A | S42.355A | S42.426P | S42.465A | S43.226A |
| S42.002P | S42.111K | S42.153B | S42.241P | S42.309K | S42.355K | S42.431A | S42.465K | S45.101A |
| S42.009B | S42.111P | S42.153K | S42.242A | S42.309P | S42.355P | S42.431K | S42.465P | S45.102A |
| S42.009K | S42.112B | S42.153P | S42.242K | S42.311A | S42.356A | S42.431P | S42.466A | S45.109A |
| S42.009P | S42.112K | S42.154B | S42.242P | S42.311K | S42.356K | S42.432A | S42.466K | S45.111A |
| S42.011B | S42.112P | S42.154K | S42.249A | S42.311P | S42.356P | S42.432K | S42.466P | S45.112A |
| S42.011K | S42.113B | S42.154P | S42.249K | S42.312A | S42.361A | S42.432P | S42.471A | S45.119A |
| S42.011P | S42.113K | S42.155B | S42.249P | S42.312K | S42.361K | S42.433A | S42.471K | S45.191A |
| S42.012B | S42.113P | S42.155K | S42.251A | S42.312P | S42.361P | S42.433K | S42.471P | S45.192A |
| S42.012K | S42.114B | S42.155P | S42.251K | S42.319A | S42.362A | S42.433P | S42.472A | S45.199A |
| S42.012P | S42.114K | S42.156B | S42.251P | S42.319K | S42.362K | S42.434A | S42.472K | S45.201A |
| S42.013B | S42.114P | S42.156K | S42.252A | S42.319P | S42.362P | S42.434K | S42.472P | S45.202A |
| S42.013K | S42.115B | S42.156P | S42.252K | S42.321A | S42.363A | S42.434P | S42.473A | S45.209A |
| S42.013P | S42.115K | S42.191B | S42.252P | S42.321K | S42.363K | S42.435A | S42.473K | S45.211A |
| S42.014B | S42.115P | S42.191K | S42.253A | S42.321P | S42.363P | S42.435K | S42.473P | S45.212A |
| S42.014K | S42.116B | S42.191P | S42.253K | S42.322A | S42.364A | S42.435P | S42.474A | S45.219A |
| S42.014P | S42.116K | S42.192B | S42.253P | S42.322K | S42.364K | S42.436A | S42.474K | S45.291A |
| S42.015B | S42.116P | S42.192K | S42.254A | S42.322P | S42.364P | S42.436K | S42.474P | S45.292A |
| S42.015K | S42.121B | S42.192P | S42.254K | S42.323A | S42.365A | S42.436P | S42.475A | S45.299A |
| S42.015P | S42.121K | S42.199B | S42.254P | S42.323K | S42.365K | S42.441A | S42.475K | S45.301A |
| S42.016B | S42.121P | S42.199K | S42.255A | S42.323P | S42.365P | S42.441K | S42.475P | S45.302A |
| S42.016K | S42.122B | S42.199P | S42.255K | S42.324A | S42.366A | S42.441P | S42.476A | S45.309A |
| S42.016P | S42.122K | S42.201A | S42.255P | S42.324K | S42.366K | S42.442A | S42.476K | S45.311A |
| S42.017B | S42.122P | S42.201K | S42.256A | S42.324P | S42.366P | S42.442K | S42.476P | S45.312A |
| S42.017K | S42.123B | S42.201P | S42.256K | S42.325A | S42.391A | S42.442P | S42.481A | S45.319A |
| S42.017P | S42.123K | S42.202A | S42.256P | S42.325K | S42.391K | S42.443A | S42.481K | S45.391A |
| S42.018B | S42.123P | S42.202K | S42.261A | S42.325P | S42.391P | S42.443K | S42.481P | S45.392A |
| S42.018K | S42.124B | S42.202P | S42.261K | S42.326A | S42.392A | S42.443P | S42.482A | S45.399A |
| S42.018P | S42.124K | S42.209A | S42.261P | S42.326K | S42.392K | S42.444A | S42.482K | S45.801A |
| S42.019B | S42.124P | S42.209K | S42.262A | S42.326P | S42.392P | S42.444K | S42.482P | S45.802A |
| S42.019K | S42.125B | S42.209P | S42.262K | S42.331A | S42.399A | S42.444P | S42.489A | S45.809A |
| S42.019P | S42.125K | S42.211A | S42.262P | S42.331K | S42.399K | S42.445A | S42.489K | S45.811A |
| S42.021B | S42.125P | S42.211K | S42.263A | S42.331P | S42.399P | S42.445K | S42.489P | S45.812A |
| S42.021K | S42.126B | S42.211P | S42.263K | S42.332A | S42.401A | S42.445P | S42.491A | S45.819A |
| S42.021P | S42.126K | S42.212A | S42.263P | S42.332K | S42.401K | S42.446A | S42.491K | S45.891A |
| S42.022B | S42.126P | S42.212K | S42.264A | S42.332P | S42.401P | S42.446K | S42.491P | S45.892A |
| S42.022K | S42.131B | S42.212P | S42.264K | S42.333A | S42.402A | S42.446P | S42.492A | S45.899A |
| S42.022P | S42.131K | S42.213A | S42.264P | S42.333K | | | S42.492K | S45.901A |

Appendix F: Complication and Comorbidity (CC) Code List

| | | | | | | | | |
|---|---|---|---|---|---|---|---|---|
| S45.902A | S49.039A | S52.001N | S52.033Q | S52.101P | S52.133R | S52.222N | S52.241N | S52.256N |
| S45.909A | S49.039K | S52.001P | S52.033R | S52.101Q | S52.134K | S52.222P | S52.241P | S52.256P |
| S45.911A | S49.039P | S52.001Q | S52.034K | S52.101R | S52.134M | S52.222Q | S52.241Q | S52.256Q |
| S45.912A | S49.041A | S52.001R | S52.034M | S52.102K | S52.134N | S52.222R | S52.241R | S52.256R |
| S45.919A | S49.041K | S52.002K | S52.034N | S52.102M | S52.134P | S52.223A | S52.242A | S52.261A |
| S45.991A | S49.041P | S52.002M | S52.034P | S52.102N | S52.134Q | S52.223K | S52.242K | S52.261K |
| S45.992A | S49.042A | S52.002N | S52.034Q | S52.102P | S52.134R | S52.223M | S52.242M | S52.261M |
| S45.999A | S49.042K | S52.002P | S52.034R | S52.102Q | S52.135K | S52.223N | S52.242N | S52.261N |
| S46.021A | S49.042P | S52.002Q | S52.035K | S52.102R | S52.135M | S52.223P | S52.242P | S52.261P |
| S46.022A | S49.049A | S52.002R | S52.035M | S52.109K | S52.135N | S52.223Q | S52.242Q | S52.261Q |
| S46.029A | S49.049K | S52.009K | S52.035N | S52.109M | S52.135P | S52.223R | S52.242R | S52.261R |
| S46.121A | S49.049P | S52.009M | S52.035P | S52.109N | S52.135Q | S52.224A | S52.243A | S52.262A |
| S46.122A | S49.091A | S52.009N | S52.035Q | S52.109P | S52.135R | S52.224K | S52.243K | S52.262K |
| S46.129A | S49.091K | S52.009P | S52.035R | S52.109Q | S52.136K | S52.224M | S52.243M | S52.262M |
| S46.221A | S49.091P | S52.009Q | S52.036K | S52.109R | S52.136M | S52.224N | S52.243N | S52.262N |
| S46.222A | S49.092A | S52.009R | S52.036M | S52.111A | S52.136N | S52.224P | S52.243P | S52.262P |
| S46.229A | S49.092K | S52.011A | S52.036N | S52.111K | S52.136P | S52.224Q | S52.243Q | S52.262Q |
| S46.321A | S49.092P | S52.011K | S52.036Q | S52.111P | S52.136Q | S52.224R | S52.243R | S52.263A |
| S46.322A | S49.099A | S52.011P | S52.036R | S52.112A | S52.136R | S52.225A | S52.244A | S52.263K |
| S46.329A | S49.099K | S52.012A | S52.041K | S52.112K | S52.181K | S52.225K | S52.244K | S52.263M |
| S46.821A | S49.099P | S52.012K | S52.041M | S52.112P | S52.181M | S52.225M | S52.244M | S52.263N |
| S46.822A | S49.101A | S52.012P | S52.041N | S52.119A | S52.181N | S52.225N | S52.244N | S52.263P |
| S46.829A | S49.101K | S52.019A | S52.041P | S52.119K | S52.181P | S52.225P | S52.244P | S52.263R |
| S46.921A | S49.101P | S52.019K | S52.041Q | S52.119P | S52.181Q | S52.225Q | S52.244Q | S52.264A |
| S46.922A | S49.102A | S52.019P | S52.041R | S52.121K | S52.181R | S52.225R | S52.244R | S52.264K |
| S46.929A | S49.102K | S52.021K | S52.042K | S52.121M | S52.182K | S52.226A | S52.245A | S52.264M |
| S48.011A | S49.102P | S52.021M | S52.042M | S52.121N | S52.182M | S52.226K | S52.245K | S52.264N |
| S48.012A | S49.109A | S52.021N | S52.042N | S52.121P | S52.182N | S52.226M | S52.245M | S52.264P |
| S48.019A | S49.109K | S52.021P | S52.042P | S52.121Q | S52.182P | S52.226N | S52.245N | S52.264Q |
| S48.021A | S49.109P | S52.021Q | S52.042Q | S52.121R | S52.182Q | S52.226P | S52.245P | S52.264R |
| S48.022A | S49.111A | S52.021R | S52.042R | S52.122K | S52.182R | S52.226Q | S52.245Q | S52.265A |
| S48.029A | S49.111K | S52.022K | S52.043K | S52.122M | S52.189K | S52.226R | S52.245R | S52.265K |
| S48.111A | S49.111P | S52.022M | S52.043M | S52.122N | S52.189M | S52.231A | S52.246A | S52.265M |
| S48.112A | S49.112A | S52.022N | S52.043N | S52.122P | S52.189N | S52.231K | S52.246K | S52.265P |
| S48.119A | S49.112K | S52.022P | S52.043P | S52.122Q | S52.189P | S52.231M | S52.246M | S52.265Q |
| S48.121A | S49.112P | S52.022Q | S52.043Q | S52.122R | S52.189Q | S52.231N | S52.246N | S52.265R |
| S48.122A | S49.119A | S52.022R | S52.043R | S52.123K | S52.189R | S52.231P | S52.246P | S52.266A |
| S48.129A | S49.119K | S52.023K | S52.044K | S52.123M | S52.201A | S52.231Q | S52.246Q | S52.266K |
| S48.911A | S49.119P | S52.023M | S52.044M | S52.123N | S52.201K | S52.231R | S52.246R | S52.266M |
| S48.912A | S49.121A | S52.023N | S52.044N | S52.123P | S52.201M | S52.232A | S52.251A | S52.266N |
| S48.919A | S49.121K | S52.023P | S52.044P | S52.123R | S52.201N | S52.232K | S52.251K | S52.266P |
| S48.921A | S49.121P | S52.023Q | S52.044Q | S52.124K | S52.201P | S52.232M | S52.251M | S52.266Q |
| S48.922A | S49.122A | S52.023R | S52.044R | S52.124M | S52.201Q | S52.232N | S52.251N | S52.266R |
| S48.929A | S49.122K | S52.024K | S52.045K | S52.124N | S52.201R | S52.232P | S52.251P | S52.271A |
| S49.001A | S49.122P | S52.024M | S52.045M | S52.124P | S52.202A | S52.232Q | S52.251Q | S52.271M |
| S49.001K | S49.129A | S52.024N | S52.045N | S52.124R | S52.202K | S52.232R | S52.251R | S52.271N |
| S49.001P | S49.129K | S52.024P | S52.045P | S52.125K | S52.202M | S52.233A | S52.252A | S52.271P |
| S49.002A | S49.129P | S52.024Q | S52.045Q | S52.125M | S52.202N | S52.233K | S52.252K | S52.271Q |
| S49.002K | S49.131A | S52.024R | S52.045R | S52.125N | S52.202P | S52.233M | S52.252M | S52.271R |
| S49.002P | S49.131K | S52.025K | S52.046K | S52.125P | S52.202Q | S52.233N | S52.252N | S52.272K |
| S49.009A | S49.131P | S52.025M | S52.046M | S52.125Q | S52.202R | S52.233P | S52.252P | S52.272M |
| S49.009K | S49.132A | S52.025N | S52.046N | S52.125R | S52.209A | S52.233Q | S52.252Q | S52.272N |
| S49.009P | S49.132K | S52.025P | S52.046P | S52.126K | S52.209K | S52.233R | S52.252R | S52.272P |
| S49.011A | S49.132P | S52.025Q | S52.046Q | S52.126M | S52.209M | S52.234A | S52.253A | S52.272Q |
| S49.011K | S49.139A | S52.025R | S52.046R | S52.126N | S52.209N | S52.234K | S52.253K | S52.272R |
| S49.011P | S49.139K | S52.026K | S52.091K | S52.126P | S52.209P | S52.234M | S52.253M | S52.279K |
| S49.012A | S49.139P | S52.026M | S52.091M | S52.126Q | S52.209Q | S52.234N | S52.253N | S52.279M |
| S49.012K | S49.141A | S52.026N | S52.091N | S52.126R | S52.209R | S52.234Q | S52.253P | S52.279N |
| S49.012P | S49.141K | S52.026P | S52.091P | S52.131K | S52.211A | S52.234R | S52.253Q | S52.279P |
| S49.019A | S49.141P | S52.026Q | S52.091Q | S52.131M | S52.211K | S52.235A | S52.253R | S52.279Q |
| S49.019K | S49.142A | S52.026R | S52.091R | S52.131N | S52.211P | S52.235K | S52.254A | S52.279R |
| S49.019P | S49.142K | S52.031K | S52.092K | S52.131P | S52.212A | S52.235M | S52.254K | S52.281A |
| S49.021A | S49.142P | S52.031M | S52.092M | S52.131Q | S52.212K | S52.235N | S52.254M | S52.281K |
| S49.021K | S49.149A | S52.031N | S52.092N | S52.131R | S52.212P | S52.235P | S52.254N | S52.281M |
| S49.021P | S49.149K | S52.031P | S52.092P | S52.132K | S52.219A | S52.235Q | S52.254P | S52.281N |
| S49.022A | S49.149P | S52.031Q | S52.092Q | S52.132M | S52.219K | S52.235R | S52.254Q | S52.281P |
| S49.022K | S49.191A | S52.031R | S52.092R | S52.132N | S52.219P | S52.236A | S52.254R | S52.281Q |
| S49.022P | S49.191K | S52.032K | S52.099K | S52.132P | S52.221A | S52.236K | S52.255A | S52.281R |
| S49.029A | S49.191P | S52.032M | S52.099M | S52.132Q | S52.221K | S52.236M | S52.255K | S52.282A |
| S49.029K | S49.192A | S52.032N | S52.099N | S52.132R | S52.221N | S52.236N | S52.255M | S52.282K |
| S49.029P | S49.192K | S52.032P | S52.099P | S52.133K | S52.221P | S52.236P | S52.255N | S52.282M |
| S49.031A | S49.192P | S52.032Q | S52.099Q | S52.133M | S52.221Q | S52.236Q | S52.255P | S52.282N |
| S49.031K | S49.199A | S52.032R | S52.099R | S52.133N | S52.221R | S52.236R | S52.255Q | S52.282P |
| S49.031P | S49.199K | S52.033K | S52.101K | S52.133P | S52.222A | S52.241A | S52.255R | S52.282Q |
| S49.032A | S49.199P | S52.033M | S52.101M | S52.133Q | S52.222K | S52.241K | S52.256K | |
| S49.032K | S52.001K | S52.033N | S52.101N | | S52.222M | S52.241M | S52.256M | |
| S49.032P | S52.001M | S52.033P | | | | | | |

| | | | | | | | | |
|---|---|---|---|---|---|---|---|---|
| S52.282R | S52.323P | S52.342P | S52.361P | S52.389P | S52.515P | S52.559M | S52.602M | S52.699A |
| S52.283A | S52.323Q | S52.342Q | S52.361Q | S52.389Q | S52.515Q | S52.559N | S52.602N | S52.699K |
| S52.283K | S52.323R | S52.342R | S52.361R | S52.389R | S52.515R | S52.559P | S52.602P | S52.699M |
| S52.283M | S52.324A | S52.343A | S52.362A | S52.391A | S52.516A | S52.559Q | S52.602Q | S52.699N |
| S52.283N | S52.324K | S52.343K | S52.362K | S52.391K | S52.516K | S52.559R | S52.602R | S52.699P |
| S52.283P | S52.324M | S52.343M | S52.362M | S52.391M | S52.516M | S52.561A | S52.609A | S52.699Q |
| S52.283Q | S52.324N | S52.343N | S52.362N | S52.391N | S52.516N | S52.561K | S52.609K | S52.699R |
| S52.283R | S52.324P | S52.343P | S52.362P | S52.391P | S52.516P | S52.561M | S52.609M | S52.90XA |
| S52.291A | S52.324Q | S52.343Q | S52.362Q | S52.391Q | S52.516Q | S52.561N | S52.609N | S52.90XK |
| S52.291K | S52.324R | S52.343R | S52.362R | S52.391R | S52.516R | S52.561P | S52.609P | S52.90XM |
| S52.291M | S52.325A | S52.344A | S52.363A | S52.392A | S52.521A | S52.561Q | S52.609Q | S52.90XN |
| S52.291N | S52.325K | S52.344K | S52.363K | S52.392K | S52.521K | S52.561R | S52.609R | S52.90XP |
| S52.291P | S52.325M | S52.344M | S52.363M | S52.392M | S52.521P | S52.562A | S52.611A | S52.90XQ |
| S52.291Q | S52.325N | S52.344N | S52.363N | S52.392N | S52.522A | S52.562K | S52.611K | S52.90XR |
| S52.291R | S52.325P | S52.344P | S52.363P | S52.392P | S52.522K | S52.562M | S52.611M | S52.91XA |
| S52.292A | S52.325Q | S52.344Q | S52.363Q | S52.392Q | S52.522P | S52.562N | S52.611N | S52.91XK |
| S52.292K | S52.325R | S52.344R | S52.363R | S52.392R | S52.529A | S52.562P | S52.611P | S52.91XM |
| S52.292M | S52.326A | S52.345A | S52.364A | S52.399A | S52.529K | S52.562Q | S52.611Q | S52.91XN |
| S52.292N | S52.326K | S52.345K | S52.364K | S52.399K | S52.529P | S52.562R | S52.611R | S52.91XP |
| S52.292P | S52.326M | S52.345M | S52.364M | S52.399M | S52.531A | S52.569A | S52.612A | S52.91XQ |
| S52.292Q | S52.326N | S52.345N | S52.364N | S52.399N | S52.531K | S52.569K | S52.612K | S52.91XR |
| S52.292R | S52.326P | S52.345P | S52.364P | S52.399P | S52.531M | S52.569M | S52.612M | S52.92XA |
| S52.299A | S52.326Q | S52.345Q | S52.364Q | S52.399Q | S52.531N | S52.569N | S52.612N | S52.92XK |
| S52.299K | S52.326R | S52.345R | S52.364R | S52.399R | S52.531P | S52.569P | S52.612P | S52.92XM |
| S52.299M | S52.331A | S52.346A | S52.365A | S52.501A | S52.531Q | S52.569Q | S52.612Q | S52.92XN |
| S52.299N | S52.331K | S52.346K | S52.365K | S52.501K | S52.531R | S52.569R | S52.612R | S52.92XP |
| S52.299P | S52.331M | S52.346M | S52.365M | S52.501M | S52.532A | S52.571A | S52.613A | S52.92XQ |
| S52.299Q | S52.331N | S52.346N | S52.365N | S52.501N | S52.532K | S52.571K | S52.613K | S52.92XR |
| S52.299R | S52.331P | S52.346P | S52.365P | S52.501P | S52.532M | S52.571M | S52.613M | S55.001A |
| S52.301A | S52.331Q | S52.346Q | S52.365Q | S52.501Q | S52.532N | S52.571N | S52.613N | S55.002A |
| S52.301K | S52.331R | S52.346R | S52.365R | S52.501R | S52.532P | S52.571P | S52.613P | S55.009A |
| S52.301M | S52.332A | S52.351A | S52.366A | S52.502A | S52.532Q | S52.571Q | S52.613Q | S55.011A |
| S52.301N | S52.332K | S52.351K | S52.366K | S52.502K | S52.532R | S52.571R | S52.613R | S55.012A |
| S52.301P | S52.332M | S52.351M | S52.366M | S52.502M | S52.539A | S52.572A | S52.614A | S55.019A |
| S52.301Q | S52.332N | S52.351N | S52.366N | S52.502N | S52.539K | S52.572K | S52.614K | S55.091A |
| S52.301R | S52.332P | S52.351P | S52.366P | S52.502P | S52.539M | S52.572M | S52.614M | S55.092A |
| S52.302A | S52.332Q | S52.351Q | S52.366Q | S52.502Q | S52.539N | S52.572N | S52.614N | S55.099A |
| S52.302K | S52.332R | S52.351R | S52.366R | S52.502R | S52.539P | S52.572P | S52.614P | S55.101A |
| S52.302M | S52.333A | S52.352A | S52.371A | S52.509A | S52.539Q | S52.572Q | S52.614Q | S55.102A |
| S52.302N | S52.333K | S52.352K | S52.371K | S52.509K | S52.539R | S52.572R | S52.614R | S55.109A |
| S52.302P | S52.333M | S52.352M | S52.371M | S52.509M | S52.541A | S52.579A | S52.615A | S55.111A |
| S52.302Q | S52.333N | S52.352N | S52.371N | S52.509N | S52.541K | S52.579K | S52.615K | S55.112A |
| S52.302R | S52.333P | S52.352P | S52.371P | S52.509P | S52.541M | S52.579M | S52.615M | S55.119A |
| S52.309A | S52.333Q | S52.352Q | S52.371Q | S52.509Q | S52.541N | S52.579N | S52.615N | S55.191A |
| S52.309K | S52.333R | S52.352R | S52.371R | S52.509R | S52.541P | S52.579P | S52.615P | S55.192A |
| S52.309M | S52.334A | S52.353A | S52.372A | S52.511A | S52.541Q | S52.579Q | S52.615Q | S55.199A |
| S52.309N | S52.334K | S52.353K | S52.372K | S52.511K | S52.541R | S52.579R | S52.615R | S55.201A |
| S52.309P | S52.334M | S52.353M | S52.372M | S52.511M | S52.542A | S52.591A | S52.616A | S55.202A |
| S52.309Q | S52.334N | S52.353N | S52.372N | S52.511N | S52.542K | S52.591K | S52.616K | S55.209A |
| S52.309R | S52.334P | S52.353P | S52.372P | S52.511P | S52.542M | S52.591M | S52.616M | S55.211A |
| S52.311A | S52.334Q | S52.353Q | S52.372Q | S52.511Q | S52.542N | S52.591N | S52.616P | S55.212A |
| S52.311K | S52.334R | S52.353R | S52.372R | S52.511R | S52.542P | S52.591P | S52.616Q | S55.219A |
| S52.311P | S52.335A | S52.354A | S52.379A | S52.512A | S52.542Q | S52.591Q | S52.616R | S55.291A |
| S52.312A | S52.335K | S52.354K | S52.379K | S52.512K | S52.542R | S52.591R | S52.621A | S55.292A |
| S52.312K | S52.335M | S52.354M | S52.379M | S52.512M | S52.549A | S52.592A | S52.621K | S55.299A |
| S52.312P | S52.335N | S52.354N | S52.379N | S52.512N | S52.549K | S52.592K | S52.621P | S55.801A |
| S52.319A | S52.335P | S52.354P | S52.379P | S52.512P | S52.549M | S52.592M | S52.622A | S55.802A |
| S52.319K | S52.335Q | S52.354Q | S52.379Q | S52.512Q | S52.549N | S52.592N | S52.622K | S55.809A |
| S52.319P | S52.335R | S52.354R | S52.379R | S52.512R | S52.549P | S52.592P | S52.622P | S55.811A |
| S52.321A | S52.336A | S52.355A | S52.381A | S52.513A | S52.549Q | S52.592Q | S52.629A | S55.812A |
| S52.321K | S52.336K | S52.355K | S52.381K | S52.513K | S52.549R | S52.592R | S52.629K | S55.819A |
| S52.321M | S52.336M | S52.355M | S52.381M | S52.513M | S52.551A | S52.599A | S52.629P | S55.891A |
| S52.321N | S52.336N | S52.355N | S52.381N | S52.513N | S52.551K | S52.599K | S52.691A | S55.892A |
| S52.321P | S52.336P | S52.355P | S52.381P | S52.513P | S52.551M | S52.599M | S52.691K | S55.899A |
| S52.321Q | S52.336Q | S52.355Q | S52.381Q | S52.513Q | S52.551N | S52.599N | S52.691M | S55.901A |
| S52.321R | S52.336R | S52.355R | S52.381R | S52.513R | S52.551P | S52.599P | S52.691N | S55.902A |
| S52.322A | S52.341A | S52.356A | S52.382A | S52.514A | S52.551Q | S52.599Q | S52.691P | S55.909A |
| S52.322K | S52.341K | S52.356K | S52.382K | S52.514K | S52.551R | S52.599R | S52.691Q | S55.911A |
| S52.322M | S52.341M | S52.356M | S52.382M | S52.514M | S52.552A | S52.601A | S52.691R | S55.912A |
| S52.322N | S52.341N | S52.356N | S52.382N | S52.514N | S52.552K | S52.601K | S52.692A | S55.919A |
| S52.322P | S52.341P | S52.356P | S52.382P | S52.514P | S52.552M | S52.601M | S52.692K | S55.991A |
| S52.322Q | S52.341Q | S52.356Q | S52.382Q | S52.514Q | S52.552N | S52.601N | S52.692M | S55.992A |
| S52.322R | S52.341R | S52.356R | S52.382R | S52.514R | S52.552P | S52.601P | S52.692N | S55.999A |
| S52.323A | S52.342A | S52.361A | S52.389A | S52.515A | S52.552Q | S52.601Q | S52.692P | S56.021A |
| S52.323K | S52.342K | S52.361K | S52.389K | S52.515K | S52.552R | S52.601R | S52.692Q | S56.022A |
| S52.323M | S52.342M | S52.361M | S52.389M | S52.515M | S52.559A | S52.602A | S52.692R | S56.029A |
| S52.323N | S52.342N | S52.361N | S52.389N | S52.515N | S52.559K | S52.602K | | S56.121A |

| | | | | | | | | |
|---|---|---|---|---|---|---|---|---|
| S56.122A | S59.031A | S59.212P | S62.024K | S62.133B | S62.174P | S62.236K | S62.310B | S62.335P |
| S56.123A | S59.031K | S59.219A | S62.024P | S62.133K | S62.175B | S62.236P | S62.310K | S62.336B |
| S56.124A | S59.031P | S59.219K | S62.025B | S62.133P | S62.175K | S62.241B | S62.310P | S62.336K |
| S56.125A | S59.032A | S59.219P | S62.025K | S62.134B | S62.175P | S62.241K | S62.311B | S62.336P |
| S56.126A | S59.032K | S59.221A | S62.025P | S62.134K | S62.176B | S62.241P | S62.311K | S62.337B |
| S56.127A | S59.032P | S59.221K | S62.026B | S62.134P | S62.176K | S62.242B | S62.311P | S62.337K |
| S56.128A | S59.039A | S59.221P | S62.026K | S62.135B | S62.176P | S62.242K | S62.312B | S62.337P |
| S56.129A | S59.039K | S59.222A | S62.026P | S62.135K | S62.181B | S62.242P | S62.312K | S62.338B |
| S56.221A | S59.039P | S59.222K | S62.031B | S62.135P | S62.181K | S62.243B | S62.312P | S62.338K |
| S56.222A | S59.041A | S59.222P | S62.031K | S62.136B | S62.181P | S62.243K | S62.313B | S62.338P |
| S56.229A | S59.041K | S59.229A | S62.031P | S62.136K | S62.182B | S62.243P | S62.313K | S62.339B |
| S56.321A | S59.041P | S59.229K | S62.032B | S62.136P | S62.182K | S62.244B | S62.313P | S62.339K |
| S56.322A | S59.042A | S59.229P | S62.032K | S62.141B | S62.182P | S62.244K | S62.314B | S62.339P |
| S56.329A | S59.042K | S59.231A | S62.032P | S62.141K | S62.183B | S62.244P | S62.314K | S62.340B |
| S56.421A | S59.042P | S59.231K | S62.033B | S62.141P | S62.183K | S62.245B | S62.314P | S62.340K |
| S56.422A | S59.049A | S59.231P | S62.033K | S62.142B | S62.183P | S62.245K | S62.315B | S62.340P |
| S56.423A | S59.049K | S59.232A | S62.033P | S62.142K | S62.184B | S62.245P | S62.315P | S62.341B |
| S56.424A | S59.049P | S59.232K | S62.034B | S62.142P | S62.184K | S62.246B | S62.316B | S62.341K |
| S56.425A | S59.091A | S59.232P | S62.034K | S62.143B | S62.184P | S62.246K | S62.316K | S62.341P |
| S56.426A | S59.091K | S59.239A | S62.034P | S62.143K | S62.185B | S62.246P | S62.316P | S62.342B |
| S56.427A | S59.091P | S59.239K | S62.035B | S62.143P | S62.185K | S62.251B | S62.317B | S62.342K |
| S56.428A | S59.092A | S59.239P | S62.035K | S62.144B | S62.185P | S62.251K | S62.317K | S62.342P |
| S56.429A | S59.092K | S59.241A | S62.035P | S62.144K | S62.186B | S62.251P | S62.317P | S62.343B |
| S56.521A | S59.092P | S59.241K | S62.036B | S62.144P | S62.186K | S62.252B | S62.318B | S62.343K |
| S56.522A | S59.099A | S59.241P | S62.036K | S62.145B | S62.186P | S62.252K | S62.318K | S62.343P |
| S56.529A | S59.099K | S59.242A | S62.036P | S62.145K | S62.201B | S62.252P | S62.318P | S62.344B |
| S56.821A | S59.099P | S59.242K | S62.101B | S62.145P | S62.201K | S62.253B | S62.319B | S62.344K |
| S56.822A | S59.101K | S59.242P | S62.101K | S62.146B | S62.201P | S62.253K | S62.319K | S62.344P |
| S56.829A | S59.101P | S59.249A | S62.101P | S62.146K | S62.202B | S62.253P | S62.319P | S62.345B |
| S56.921A | S59.102K | S59.249K | S62.102B | S62.146P | S62.202K | S62.254B | S62.320B | S62.345K |
| S56.922A | S59.102P | S59.249P | S62.102K | S62.151B | S62.202P | S62.254K | S62.320K | S62.345P |
| S56.929A | S59.109K | S59.291A | S62.102P | S62.151K | S62.209B | S62.254P | S62.320P | S62.346B |
| S58.011A | S59.109P | S59.291K | S62.109B | S62.151P | S62.209K | S62.255B | S62.321B | S62.346K |
| S58.012A | S59.111K | S59.291P | S62.109K | S62.152B | S62.209P | S62.255K | S62.321K | S62.346P |
| S58.019A | S59.111P | S59.292A | S62.109P | S62.152K | S62.211B | S62.255P | S62.321P | S62.347B |
| S58.021A | S59.112K | S59.292K | S62.111B | S62.152P | S62.211K | S62.256B | S62.322B | S62.347K |
| S58.022A | S59.112P | S59.292P | S62.111K | S62.153B | S62.211P | S62.256K | S62.322K | S62.347P |
| S58.029A | S59.119K | S59.299A | S62.111P | S62.153K | S62.212B | S62.256P | S62.322P | S62.348B |
| S58.111A | S59.119P | S59.299K | S62.112B | S62.153P | S62.212K | S62.291B | S62.323B | S62.348K |
| S58.112A | S59.121K | S59.299P | S62.112K | S62.154B | S62.212P | S62.291K | S62.323K | S62.348P |
| S58.119A | S59.121P | S62.001B | S62.112P | S62.154K | S62.213B | S62.291P | S62.323P | S62.349B |
| S58.121A | S59.122K | S62.001K | S62.113B | S62.154P | S62.213K | S62.292B | S62.324B | S62.349K |
| S58.122A | S59.122P | S62.001P | S62.113K | S62.155B | S62.213P | S62.292K | S62.324K | S62.349P |
| S58.129A | S59.129K | S62.002B | S62.113P | S62.155K | S62.221B | S62.292P | S62.324P | S62.350B |
| S58.911A | S59.129P | S62.002K | S62.114B | S62.155P | S62.221K | S62.299B | S62.325B | S62.350K |
| S58.912A | S59.131K | S62.002P | S62.114K | S62.156B | S62.221P | S62.299K | S62.325K | S62.350P |
| S58.919A | S59.131P | S62.009B | S62.114P | S62.156K | S62.222B | S62.299P | S62.325P | S62.351B |
| S58.921A | S59.132K | S62.009K | S62.115B | S62.156P | S62.222K | S62.300B | S62.326B | S62.351K |
| S58.922A | S59.132P | S62.009P | S62.115K | S62.161B | S62.222P | S62.300K | S62.326K | S62.351P |
| S58.929A | S59.139K | S62.011B | S62.115P | S62.161K | S62.223B | S62.300P | S62.326P | S62.352B |
| S59.001A | S59.139P | S62.011K | S62.116B | S62.161P | S62.223K | S62.301B | S62.327B | S62.352K |
| S59.001K | S59.141K | S62.011P | S62.116K | S62.162B | S62.223P | S62.301K | S62.327K | S62.352P |
| S59.001P | S59.141P | S62.012B | S62.116P | S62.162K | S62.224B | S62.301P | S62.327P | S62.353B |
| S59.002A | S59.142K | S62.012K | S62.121B | S62.162P | S62.224K | S62.302B | S62.328B | S62.353K |
| S59.002K | S59.142P | S62.012P | S62.121K | S62.163B | S62.224P | S62.302K | S62.328K | S62.353P |
| S59.002P | S59.149K | S62.013B | S62.121P | S62.163K | S62.225B | S62.302P | S62.328P | S62.354B |
| S59.009A | S59.149P | S62.013K | S62.122B | S62.163P | S62.225K | S62.303B | S62.329B | S62.354K |
| S59.009K | S59.191K | S62.013P | S62.122K | S62.164B | S62.225P | S62.303K | S62.329K | S62.354P |
| S59.009P | S59.191P | S62.014B | S62.122P | S62.164K | S62.226B | S62.303P | S62.329P | S62.355B |
| S59.011A | S59.192K | S62.014K | S62.123B | S62.164P | S62.226K | S62.304B | S62.330B | S62.355K |
| S59.011K | S59.192P | S62.014P | S62.123K | S62.165B | S62.226P | S62.304K | S62.330K | S62.355P |
| S59.011P | S59.199K | S62.015B | S62.123P | S62.165K | S62.231B | S62.304P | S62.330P | S62.356B |
| S59.012A | S59.199P | S62.015K | S62.124B | S62.165P | S62.231K | S62.305B | S62.331B | S62.356K |
| S59.012K | S59.201A | S62.015P | S62.124K | S62.166B | S62.231P | S62.305K | S62.331K | S62.356P |
| S59.012P | S59.201K | S62.016B | S62.124P | S62.166K | S62.232B | S62.305P | S62.331P | S62.357B |
| S59.019A | S59.201P | S62.016K | S62.125B | S62.166P | S62.232K | S62.306B | S62.332B | S62.357K |
| S59.019K | S59.202A | S62.016P | S62.125K | S62.171B | S62.232P | S62.306K | S62.332K | S62.357P |
| S59.019P | S59.202K | S62.021B | S62.125P | S62.171K | S62.233B | S62.306P | S62.332P | S62.358B |
| S59.021A | S59.202P | S62.021K | S62.126B | S62.171P | S62.233K | S62.307B | S62.333B | S62.358K |
| S59.021K | S59.209A | S62.021P | S62.126K | S62.172B | S62.233P | S62.307K | S62.333K | S62.358P |
| S59.021P | S59.209K | S62.022B | S62.126P | S62.172K | S62.234B | S62.307P | S62.333P | S62.359B |
| S59.022A | S59.209P | S62.022K | S62.131B | S62.172P | S62.234K | S62.308B | S62.334B | S62.359K |
| S59.022K | S59.211A | S62.022P | S62.131K | S62.173B | S62.234P | S62.308K | S62.334K | S62.359P |
| S59.022P | S59.211K | S62.023B | S62.131P | S62.173K | S62.235B | S62.308P | S62.334P | S62.360B |
| S59.029A | S59.211P | S62.023K | S62.132B | S62.173P | S62.235K | S62.309B | S62.335B | S62.360K |
| S59.029K | S59.212A | S62.023P | S62.132K | S62.174B | S62.235P | S62.309K | S62.335B | S62.360P |
| S59.029P | S59.212K | S62.024B | S62.132P | S62.174K | S62.236B | S62.309P | S62.335K | S62.361B |

| | | | | | | | | |
|---|---|---|---|---|---|---|---|---|
| S62.361K | S62.515B | S62.617P | S62.643K | S62.669B | S65.590A | S68.422A | S72.026P | S72.051N |
| S62.361P | S62.515K | S62.618B | S62.643P | S62.669K | S65.591A | S68.429A | S72.026Q | S72.051P |
| S62.362B | S62.515P | S62.618K | S62.644B | S62.669P | S65.592A | S68.711A | S72.026R | S72.051Q |
| S62.362K | S62.516B | S62.618P | S62.644K | S62.90XB | S65.593A | S68.712A | S72.031K | S72.051R |
| S62.362P | S62.516K | S62.619B | S62.644P | S62.90XK | S65.594A | S68.719A | S72.031M | S72.052K |
| S62.363B | S62.516P | S62.619K | S62.645B | S62.90XP | S65.595A | S68.721A | S72.031N | S72.052M |
| S62.363K | S62.521B | S62.619P | S62.645K | S62.91XB | S65.596A | S68.722A | S72.031P | S72.052N |
| S62.363P | S62.521K | S62.620B | S62.645P | S62.91XK | S65.597A | S68.729A | S72.031Q | S72.052P |
| S62.364B | S62.521P | S62.620K | S62.646B | S62.91XP | S65.598A | S72.001K | S72.031R | S72.052Q |
| S62.364K | S62.522B | S62.620P | S62.646K | S62.92XB | S65.599A | S72.001M | S72.032K | S72.052R |
| S62.364P | S62.522K | S62.621B | S62.646P | S62.92XK | S65.801A | S72.001N | S72.032M | S72.059K |
| S62.365B | S62.522P | S62.621K | S62.647B | S62.92XP | S65.802A | S72.001P | S72.032N | S72.059M |
| S62.365K | S62.523B | S62.621P | S62.647K | S65.001A | S65.809A | S72.001Q | S72.032P | S72.059N |
| S62.365P | S62.523K | S62.622B | S62.647P | S65.002A | S65.811A | S72.001R | S72.032Q | S72.059P |
| S62.366B | S62.523P | S62.622K | S62.648B | S65.009A | S65.812A | S72.002K | S72.032R | S72.059Q |
| S62.366K | S62.524B | S62.622P | S62.648K | S65.011A | S65.819A | S72.002M | S72.033K | S72.059R |
| S62.366P | S62.524K | S62.623B | S62.648P | S65.012A | S65.891A | S72.002N | S72.033M | S72.061K |
| S62.367B | S62.524P | S62.623K | S62.649B | S65.019A | S65.892A | S72.002P | S72.033N | S72.061M |
| S62.367K | S62.525B | S62.623P | S62.649K | S65.091A | S65.899A | S72.002Q | S72.033P | S72.061N |
| S62.367P | S62.525K | S62.624B | S62.649P | S65.092A | S65.901A | S72.002R | S72.033Q | S72.061P |
| S62.368B | S62.525P | S62.624K | S62.650B | S65.099A | S65.902A | S72.009K | S72.033R | S72.061Q |
| S62.368K | S62.526B | S62.624P | S62.650K | S65.101A | S65.909A | S72.009M | S72.034K | S72.061R |
| S62.368P | S62.526K | S62.625B | S62.650P | S65.102A | S65.911A | S72.009N | S72.034M | S72.062K |
| S62.369B | S62.526P | S62.625K | S62.651B | S65.109A | S65.912A | S72.009P | S72.034N | S72.062M |
| S62.369K | S62.600B | S62.625P | S62.651K | S65.111A | S65.919A | S72.009Q | S72.034P | S72.062N |
| S62.369P | S62.600K | S62.626B | S62.651P | S65.112A | S65.991A | S72.009R | S72.034Q | S72.062P |
| S62.390B | S62.600P | S62.626K | S62.652B | S65.119A | S65.992A | S72.011K | S72.034R | S72.062Q |
| S62.390K | S62.601B | S62.626P | S62.652K | S65.191A | S65.999A | S72.011M | S72.035K | S72.062R |
| S62.390P | S62.601K | S62.627B | S62.652P | S65.192A | S66.021A | S72.011N | S72.035M | S72.063K |
| S62.391B | S62.601P | S62.627K | S62.653B | S65.199A | S66.022A | S72.011P | S72.035N | S72.063M |
| S62.391K | S62.602B | S62.627P | S62.653K | S65.201A | S66.029A | S72.011Q | S72.035P | S72.063N |
| S62.391P | S62.602K | S62.628B | S62.653P | S65.202A | S66.120A | S72.011R | S72.035Q | S72.063P |
| S62.392B | S62.602P | S62.628K | S62.654B | S65.209A | S66.121A | S72.012K | S72.035R | S72.063Q |
| S62.392K | S62.603B | S62.628P | S62.654K | S65.211A | S66.122A | S72.012M | S72.036K | S72.063R |
| S62.392P | S62.603K | S62.629B | S62.654P | S65.212A | S66.123A | S72.012N | S72.036M | S72.064K |
| S62.393B | S62.603P | S62.629K | S62.655B | S65.219A | S66.124A | S72.012P | S72.036N | S72.064M |
| S62.393K | S62.604B | S62.629P | S62.655K | S65.291A | S66.125A | S72.012Q | S72.036P | S72.064N |
| S62.393P | S62.604K | S62.630B | S62.655P | S65.292A | S66.126A | S72.012R | S72.036Q | S72.064P |
| S62.394B | S62.604P | S62.630K | S62.656B | S65.299A | S66.127A | S72.019K | S72.036R | S72.064Q |
| S62.394K | S62.605B | S62.630P | S62.656K | S65.301A | S66.128A | S72.019M | S72.041K | S72.064R |
| S62.394P | S62.605K | S62.631B | S62.656P | S65.302A | S66.129A | S72.019N | S72.041M | S72.065K |
| S62.395B | S62.605P | S62.631K | S62.657B | S65.309A | S66.221A | S72.019P | S72.041N | S72.065M |
| S62.395K | S62.606B | S62.631P | S62.657K | S65.311A | S66.222A | S72.019Q | S72.041P | S72.065N |
| S62.395P | S62.606K | S62.632B | S62.657P | S65.312A | S66.229A | S72.019R | S72.041Q | S72.065P |
| S62.396B | S62.606P | S62.632K | S62.658B | S65.319A | S66.320A | S72.021K | S72.041R | S72.065Q |
| S62.396K | S62.607B | S62.632P | S62.658K | S65.391A | S66.321A | S72.021M | S72.042K | S72.065R |
| S62.396P | S62.607K | S62.633B | S62.658P | S65.392A | S66.322A | S72.021N | S72.042M | S72.066K |
| S62.397B | S62.607P | S62.633K | S62.659B | S65.399A | S66.323A | S72.021P | S72.042N | S72.066M |
| S62.397K | S62.608B | S62.633P | S62.659K | S65.401A | S66.324A | S72.021Q | S72.042P | S72.066N |
| S62.397P | S62.608K | S62.634B | S62.659P | S65.402A | S66.325A | S72.021R | S72.042Q | S72.066P |
| S62.398B | S62.608P | S62.634K | S62.660B | S65.409A | S66.326A | S72.022K | S72.042R | S72.066Q |
| S62.398K | S62.609B | S62.634P | S62.660K | S65.411A | S66.327A | S72.022M | S72.043K | S72.066R |
| S62.398P | S62.609K | S62.635B | S62.660P | S65.412A | S66.328A | S72.022N | S72.043M | S72.091K |
| S62.399B | S62.609P | S62.635K | S62.661B | S65.419A | S66.329A | S72.022P | S72.043N | S72.091M |
| S62.399K | S62.610B | S62.635P | S62.661K | S65.491A | S66.421A | S72.022Q | S72.043P | S72.091N |
| S62.399P | S62.610K | S62.636B | S62.661P | S65.492A | S66.422A | S72.022R | S72.043Q | S72.091P |
| S62.501B | S62.610P | S62.636K | S62.662B | S65.499A | S66.429A | S72.023K | S72.043R | S72.091Q |
| S62.501K | S62.611B | S62.636P | S62.662K | S65.500A | S66.520A | S72.023M | S72.044K | S72.091R |
| S62.501P | S62.611K | S62.637B | S62.662P | S65.501A | S66.521A | S72.023N | S72.044M | S72.092K |
| S62.502B | S62.611P | S62.637K | S62.663B | S65.502A | S66.522A | S72.023P | S72.044N | S72.092M |
| S62.502K | S62.612B | S62.637P | S62.663K | S65.503A | S66.523A | S72.023Q | S72.044P | S72.092N |
| S62.502P | S62.612K | S62.638B | S62.663P | S65.504A | S66.524A | S72.023R | S72.044Q | S72.092P |
| S62.509B | S62.612P | S62.638K | S62.664B | S65.505A | S66.525A | S72.024K | S72.044R | S72.092Q |
| S62.509K | S62.613B | S62.638P | S62.664K | S65.506A | S66.526A | S72.024M | S72.045K | S72.092R |
| S62.509P | S62.613K | S62.639B | S62.664P | S65.507A | S66.527A | S72.024N | S72.045M | S72.099K |
| S62.511B | S62.613P | S62.639K | S62.665B | S65.508A | S66.528A | S72.024P | S72.045N | S72.099M |
| S62.511K | S62.614B | S62.639P | S62.665K | S65.509A | S66.529A | S72.024Q | S72.045P | S72.099N |
| S62.511P | S62.614K | S62.640B | S62.665P | S65.510A | S66.821A | S72.024R | S72.045Q | S72.099P |
| S62.512B | S62.614P | S62.640K | S62.666B | S65.511A | S66.822A | S72.025K | S72.045R | S72.099Q |
| S62.512K | S62.615B | S62.640P | S62.666K | S65.512A | S66.829A | S72.025M | S72.046K | S72.099R |
| S62.512P | S62.615K | S62.641B | S62.666P | S65.513A | S66.921A | S72.025N | S72.046M | S72.101K |
| S62.513B | S62.615P | S62.641K | S62.667B | S65.514A | S66.922A | S72.025P | S72.046N | S72.101M |
| S62.513K | S62.616B | S62.641P | S62.667K | S65.515A | S66.929A | S72.025Q | S72.046P | S72.101N |
| S62.513P | S62.616K | S62.642B | S62.667P | S65.516A | S68.411A | S72.025R | S72.046Q | S72.101P |
| S62.514B | S62.616P | S62.642K | S62.668B | S65.517A | S68.412A | S72.026K | S72.046R | S72.101Q |
| S62.514K | S62.617B | S62.642P | S62.668K | S65.518A | S68.419A | S72.026M | S72.051K | S72.101R |
| S62.514P | S62.617K | S62.643B | S62.668P | S65.519A | S68.421A | S72.026N | S72.051M | S72.102K |

Appendix F: Complication and Comorbidity (CC) Code List

| | | | | | | | | | |
|---|---|---|---|---|---|---|---|---|---|
| S72.102M | S72.126K | S72.146R | S72.324Q | S72.345P | S72.366N | S72.415R | S72.434R | S72.453R |
| S72.102N | S72.126M | S72.21XK | S72.324R | S72.345Q | S72.366P | S72.416A | S72.435A | S72.454A |
| S72.102P | S72.126N | S72.21XM | S72.325K | S72.345R | S72.366Q | S72.416K | S72.435K | S72.454K |
| S72.102Q | S72.126P | S72.21XN | S72.325M | S72.346K | S72.366R | S72.416M | S72.435N | S72.454M |
| S72.102R | S72.126Q | S72.21XP | S72.325N | S72.346M | S72.391K | S72.416N | S72.435P | S72.454N |
| S72.109K | S72.126R | S72.21XQ | S72.325P | S72.346N | S72.391M | S72.416P | S72.435Q | S72.454P |
| S72.109M | S72.131K | S72.21XR | S72.325Q | S72.346P | S72.391N | S72.416Q | S72.435R | S72.454Q |
| S72.109N | S72.131M | S72.22XK | S72.325R | S72.346Q | S72.391P | S72.416R | S72.436A | S72.454R |
| S72.109P | S72.131N | S72.22XM | S72.326K | S72.346R | S72.391Q | S72.421A | S72.436K | S72.455A |
| S72.109Q | S72.131P | S72.22XN | S72.326M | S72.351K | S72.391R | S72.421K | S72.436M | S72.455K |
| S72.109R | S72.131Q | S72.22XP | S72.326N | S72.351M | S72.392K | S72.421M | S72.436N | S72.455M |
| S72.111K | S72.131R | S72.22XQ | S72.326P | S72.351N | S72.392M | S72.421N | S72.436P | S72.455N |
| S72.111M | S72.132K | S72.22XR | S72.326Q | S72.351P | S72.392N | S72.421P | S72.436Q | S72.455P |
| S72.111N | S72.132M | S72.23XK | S72.326R | S72.351Q | S72.392P | S72.421Q | S72.436R | S72.455Q |
| S72.111P | S72.132N | S72.23XM | S72.331K | S72.351R | S72.392Q | S72.421R | S72.441A | S72.455R |
| S72.111Q | S72.132P | S72.23XN | S72.331M | S72.352K | S72.392R | S72.422A | S72.441K | S72.456A |
| S72.111R | S72.132Q | S72.23XP | S72.331N | S72.352M | S72.399K | S72.422K | S72.441M | S72.456K |
| S72.112K | S72.132R | S72.23XQ | S72.331P | S72.352N | S72.399M | S72.422M | S72.441N | S72.456M |
| S72.112M | S72.133K | S72.23XR | S72.331Q | S72.352P | S72.399N | S72.422N | S72.441P | S72.456N |
| S72.112N | S72.133M | S72.24XK | S72.331R | S72.352Q | S72.399P | S72.422P | S72.441Q | S72.456P |
| S72.112P | S72.133N | S72.24XM | S72.332K | S72.352R | S72.399Q | S72.422Q | S72.441R | S72.456Q |
| S72.112Q | S72.133P | S72.24XN | S72.332M | S72.353K | S72.399R | S72.422R | S72.442A | S72.456R |
| S72.112R | S72.133Q | S72.24XP | S72.332N | S72.353M | S72.401A | S72.423A | S72.442K | S72.461A |
| S72.113K | S72.133R | S72.24XQ | S72.332P | S72.353N | S72.401K | S72.423K | S72.442M | S72.461K |
| S72.113M | S72.134K | S72.24XR | S72.332Q | S72.353P | S72.401M | S72.423M | S72.442N | S72.461M |
| S72.113N | S72.134M | S72.25XK | S72.332R | S72.353Q | S72.401N | S72.423N | S72.442P | S72.461N |
| S72.113P | S72.134N | S72.25XM | S72.333K | S72.353R | S72.401P | S72.423P | S72.442Q | S72.461P |
| S72.113Q | S72.134P | S72.25XN | S72.333M | S72.354K | S72.401Q | S72.423Q | S72.442R | S72.461Q |
| S72.113R | S72.134Q | S72.25XP | S72.333N | S72.354M | S72.401R | S72.423R | S72.443A | S72.461R |
| S72.114K | S72.134R | S72.25XQ | S72.333P | S72.354N | S72.402A | S72.424A | S72.443K | S72.462A |
| S72.114M | S72.135K | S72.25XR | S72.333Q | S72.354P | S72.402K | S72.424K | S72.443M | S72.462K |
| S72.114N | S72.135M | S72.26XK | S72.333R | S72.354Q | S72.402M | S72.424M | S72.443N | S72.462M |
| S72.114P | S72.135N | S72.26XM | S72.334K | S72.354R | S72.402N | S72.424N | S72.443P | S72.462N |
| S72.114Q | S72.135P | S72.26XN | S72.334M | S72.355K | S72.402P | S72.424P | S72.443Q | S72.462P |
| S72.114R | S72.135Q | S72.26XP | S72.334N | S72.355M | S72.402Q | S72.424Q | S72.443R | S72.462Q |
| S72.115K | S72.135R | S72.26XQ | S72.334P | S72.355N | S72.402R | S72.424R | S72.444A | S72.462R |
| S72.115M | S72.136K | S72.26XR | S72.334Q | S72.355P | S72.409A | S72.425A | S72.444K | S72.463A |
| S72.115N | S72.136M | S72.301K | S72.334R | S72.355Q | S72.409K | S72.425K | S72.444M | S72.463K |
| S72.115P | S72.136N | S72.301M | S72.335K | S72.355R | S72.409M | S72.425M | S72.444N | S72.463M |
| S72.115Q | S72.136P | S72.301N | S72.335M | S72.356K | S72.409N | S72.425N | S72.444P | S72.463N |
| S72.115R | S72.136Q | S72.301P | S72.335N | S72.356M | S72.409P | S72.425P | S72.444Q | S72.463P |
| S72.116K | S72.136R | S72.301Q | S72.335P | S72.356N | S72.409Q | S72.425Q | S72.444R | S72.463Q |
| S72.116M | S72.141K | S72.301R | S72.335Q | S72.356P | S72.409R | S72.425R | S72.445A | S72.463R |
| S72.116N | S72.141M | S72.302K | S72.335R | S72.356Q | S72.411A | S72.426A | S72.445K | S72.464A |
| S72.116P | S72.141N | S72.302M | S72.336K | S72.356R | S72.411K | S72.426K | S72.445M | S72.464K |
| S72.116Q | S72.141P | S72.302N | S72.336M | S72.361K | S72.411M | S72.426M | S72.445N | S72.464M |
| S72.116R | S72.141Q | S72.302P | S72.336N | S72.361M | S72.411N | S72.426N | S72.445P | S72.464N |
| S72.121K | S72.141R | S72.302Q | S72.336P | S72.361N | S72.411P | S72.426P | S72.445Q | S72.464P |
| S72.121M | S72.142K | S72.302R | S72.336Q | S72.361P | S72.411Q | S72.426Q | S72.445R | S72.464Q |
| S72.121N | S72.142M | S72.309K | S72.336R | S72.361Q | S72.411R | S72.426R | S72.446A | S72.464R |
| S72.121P | S72.142N | S72.309M | S72.341K | S72.361R | S72.412A | S72.431A | S72.446K | S72.465A |
| S72.121Q | S72.142P | S72.309N | S72.341M | S72.362K | S72.412K | S72.431K | S72.446M | S72.465K |
| S72.121R | S72.142Q | S72.309P | S72.341N | S72.362M | S72.412M | S72.431M | S72.446N | S72.465M |
| S72.122K | S72.142R | S72.309Q | S72.341P | S72.362N | S72.412N | S72.431N | S72.446P | S72.465N |
| S72.122M | S72.143K | S72.309R | S72.341Q | S72.362P | S72.412P | S72.431P | S72.446Q | S72.465P |
| S72.122N | S72.143M | S72.321K | S72.341R | S72.362Q | S72.412Q | S72.431Q | S72.446R | S72.465Q |
| S72.122P | S72.143N | S72.321M | S72.342K | S72.362R | S72.412R | S72.431R | S72.451A | S72.465R |
| S72.122Q | S72.143P | S72.321N | S72.342M | S72.363K | S72.413A | S72.432A | S72.451K | S72.466A |
| S72.122R | S72.143Q | S72.321P | S72.342N | S72.363M | S72.413K | S72.432K | S72.451M | S72.466K |
| S72.123K | S72.143R | S72.321Q | S72.342P | S72.363N | S72.413M | S72.432M | S72.451N | S72.466M |
| S72.123M | S72.144K | S72.321R | S72.342Q | S72.363P | S72.413N | S72.432N | S72.451P | S72.466N |
| S72.123N | S72.144M | S72.322K | S72.342R | S72.363Q | S72.413P | S72.432P | S72.451Q | S72.466P |
| S72.123P | S72.144N | S72.322M | S72.343K | S72.363R | S72.413Q | S72.432Q | S72.451R | S72.466Q |
| S72.123Q | S72.144P | S72.322N | S72.343M | S72.364K | S72.413R | S72.432R | S72.452A | S72.466R |
| S72.123R | S72.144Q | S72.322P | S72.343N | S72.364M | S72.414A | S72.433A | S72.452K | S72.471A |
| S72.124K | S72.144R | S72.322Q | S72.343P | S72.364N | S72.414K | S72.433K | S72.452M | S72.471K |
| S72.124M | S72.145K | S72.322R | S72.343Q | S72.364P | S72.414M | S72.433M | S72.452N | S72.471P |
| S72.124N | S72.145M | S72.323K | S72.343R | S72.364Q | S72.414N | S72.433N | S72.452P | S72.472A |
| S72.124P | S72.145N | S72.323M | S72.344K | S72.364R | S72.414P | S72.433P | S72.452Q | S72.472K |
| S72.124Q | S72.145P | S72.323N | S72.344M | S72.365K | S72.414Q | S72.433Q | S72.452R | S72.472P |
| S72.124R | S72.145Q | S72.323P | S72.344N | S72.365M | S72.414R | S72.433R | S72.453A | S72.479A |
| S72.125K | S72.145R | S72.323Q | S72.344P | S72.365N | S72.415A | S72.434A | S72.453K | S72.479K |
| S72.125M | S72.146K | S72.323R | S72.344Q | S72.365P | S72.415K | S72.434K | S72.453M | S72.479P |
| S72.125N | S72.146M | S72.324K | S72.344R | S72.365Q | S72.415M | S72.434M | S72.453N | S72.491A |
| S72.125P | S72.146N | S72.324M | S72.345K | S72.365R | S72.415N | S72.434N | S72.453P | S72.491K |
| S72.125Q | S72.146P | S72.324N | S72.345M | S72.366K | S72.415P | S72.434P | S72.453Q | S72.491M |
| S72.125R | S72.146Q | S72.324P | S72.345N | S72.366M | S72.415Q | S72.434Q | | S72.491N |

| | | | | | | | | |
|---|---|---|---|---|---|---|---|---|
| S72.491P | S73.041A | S78.929A | S82.001M | S82.021A | S82.033N | S82.046B | S82.114A | S82.133A |
| S72.491Q | S73.042A | S79.001K | S82.001N | S82.021B | S82.033P | S82.046C | S82.114K | S82.133K |
| S72.491R | S73.043A | S79.001P | S82.001P | S82.021C | S82.033Q | S82.046K | S82.114M | S82.133M |
| S72.492A | S73.044A | S79.002K | S82.001Q | S82.021K | S82.033R | S82.046M | S82.114N | S82.133N |
| S72.492K | S73.045A | S79.002P | S82.001R | S82.021M | S82.034B | S82.046N | S82.114P | S82.133P |
| S72.492M | S73.046A | S79.009K | S82.002A | S82.021N | S82.034C | S82.046P | S82.114Q | S82.133Q |
| S72.492N | S75.201A | S79.009P | S82.002B | S82.021P | S82.034K | S82.046Q | S82.114R | S82.133R |
| S72.492P | S75.202A | S79.011K | S82.002C | S82.021Q | S82.034M | S82.046R | S82.115A | S82.134A |
| S72.492Q | S75.209A | S79.011P | S82.002K | S82.021R | S82.034N | S82.091A | S82.115K | S82.134K |
| S72.499A | S75.211A | S79.012K | S82.002M | S82.022A | S82.034P | S82.091B | S82.115M | S82.134M |
| S72.499K | S75.212A | S79.012P | S82.002N | S82.022B | S82.034Q | S82.091C | S82.115N | S82.134N |
| S72.499M | S75.219A | S79.019K | S82.002P | S82.022C | S82.034R | S82.091K | S82.115P | S82.134P |
| S72.499N | S75.221A | S79.019P | S82.002Q | S82.022K | S82.035A | S82.091M | S82.115Q | S82.134Q |
| S72.499P | S75.222A | S79.091K | S82.002R | S82.022M | S82.035B | S82.091N | S82.115R | S82.134R |
| S72.499Q | S75.229A | S79.091P | S82.009A | S82.022N | S82.035C | S82.091P | S82.116A | S82.135A |
| S72.499R | S75.291A | S79.092K | S82.009B | S82.022P | S82.035K | S82.091Q | S82.116K | S82.135K |
| S72.8X1K | S75.292A | S79.092P | S82.009C | S82.022Q | S82.035M | S82.091R | S82.116M | S82.135M |
| S72.8X1M | S75.299A | S79.099K | S82.009K | S82.022R | S82.035N | S82.092A | S82.116N | S82.135N |
| S72.8X1N | S75.801A | S79.099P | S82.009M | S82.023A | S82.035P | S82.092B | S82.116P | S82.135P |
| S72.8X1P | S75.802A | S79.101A | S82.009N | S82.023B | S82.035Q | S82.092C | S82.116Q | S82.135Q |
| S72.8X1Q | S75.809A | S79.101K | S82.009P | S82.023C | S82.035R | S82.092K | S82.116R | S82.135R |
| S72.8X1R | S75.811A | S79.101P | S82.009Q | S82.023K | S82.036A | S82.092N | S82.121A | S82.136A |
| S72.8X2K | S75.812A | S79.102A | S82.009R | S82.023M | S82.036B | S82.092P | S82.121K | S82.136K |
| S72.8X2M | S75.819A | S79.102K | S82.011A | S82.023N | S82.036C | S82.092Q | S82.121M | S82.136M |
| S72.8X2N | S75.891A | S79.102P | S82.011B | S82.023P | S82.036K | S82.092R | S82.121N | S82.136N |
| S72.8X2P | S75.892A | S79.109A | S82.011C | S82.023Q | S82.036M | S82.099A | S82.121P | S82.136P |
| S72.8X2Q | S75.899A | S79.109K | S82.011K | S82.023R | S82.036N | S82.099B | S82.121Q | S82.136Q |
| S72.8X2R | S75.901A | S79.109P | S82.011M | S82.024A | S82.036P | S82.099C | S82.121R | S82.136R |
| S72.8X9K | S75.902A | S79.111A | S82.011N | S82.024B | S82.036Q | S82.099K | S82.122A | S82.141A |
| S72.8X9M | S75.909A | S79.111K | S82.011P | S82.024C | S82.036R | S82.099M | S82.122K | S82.141K |
| S72.8X9N | S75.911A | S79.111P | S82.011Q | S82.024K | S82.041A | S82.099N | S82.122M | S82.141M |
| S72.8X9P | S75.912A | S79.112A | S82.011R | S82.024M | S82.041B | S82.099P | S82.122N | S82.141N |
| S72.8X9Q | S75.919A | S79.112K | S82.012A | S82.024N | S82.041K | S82.099Q | S82.122P | S82.141P |
| S72.8X9R | S75.991A | S79.112P | S82.012B | S82.024P | S82.041M | S82.099R | S82.122Q | S82.141Q |
| S72.90XK | S75.992A | S79.119A | S82.012C | S82.024Q | S82.041N | S82.101A | S82.122R | S82.141R |
| S72.90XM | S75.999A | S79.119K | S82.012K | S82.024R | S82.041P | S82.101K | S82.123A | S82.142A |
| S72.90XN | S76.021A | S79.119P | S82.012M | S82.025A | S82.041Q | S82.101M | S82.123K | S82.142K |
| S72.90XP | S76.022A | S79.121A | S82.012N | S82.025B | S82.041R | S82.101N | S82.123M | S82.142M |
| S72.90XQ | S76.029A | S79.121K | S82.012P | S82.025K | S82.042A | S82.101P | S82.123N | S82.142N |
| S72.90XR | S76.121A | S79.121P | S82.012Q | S82.025M | S82.042B | S82.101Q | S82.123Q | S82.142P |
| S72.91XK | S76.122A | S79.122A | S82.012R | S82.025N | S82.042C | S82.101R | S82.123R | S82.142Q |
| S72.91XM | S76.129A | S79.122K | S82.013A | S82.025P | S82.042K | S82.102A | S82.124A | S82.142R |
| S72.91XN | S76.221A | S79.122P | S82.013B | S82.025Q | S82.042M | S82.102K | S82.124K | S82.143A |
| S72.91XP | S76.222A | S79.129A | S82.013C | S82.025R | S82.042N | S82.102M | S82.124M | S82.143K |
| S72.91XQ | S76.321A | S79.129K | S82.013K | S82.026A | S82.042P | S82.102N | S82.124N | S82.143N |
| S72.91XR | S76.322A | S79.129P | S82.013M | S82.026B | S82.042Q | S82.102P | S82.124P | S82.143P |
| S72.92XK | S76.329A | S79.131A | S82.013N | S82.026C | S82.042R | S82.102Q | S82.124Q | S82.143Q |
| S72.92XM | S76.821A | S79.131K | S82.013P | S82.026K | S82.043A | S82.102R | S82.124R | S82.143R |
| S72.92XN | S76.822A | S79.131P | S82.013Q | S82.026M | S82.043B | S82.109A | S82.125A | S82.144A |
| S72.92XP | S76.829A | S79.132A | S82.013R | S82.026N | S82.043C | S82.109K | S82.125K | S82.144K |
| S72.92XQ | S76.921A | S79.132K | S82.014A | S82.026P | S82.043K | S82.109M | S82.125M | S82.144M |
| S72.92XR | S76.922A | S79.132P | S82.014B | S82.026Q | S82.043M | S82.109N | S82.125N | S82.144N |
| S73.001A | S76.929A | S79.139A | S82.014C | S82.026R | S82.043N | S82.109P | S82.125P | S82.144P |
| S73.002A | S77.00XA | S79.139K | S82.014K | S82.031A | S82.043P | S82.109Q | S82.125Q | S82.144Q |
| S73.003A | S77.01XA | S79.139P | S82.014M | S82.031B | S82.043Q | S82.109R | S82.125R | S82.144R |
| S73.004A | S77.02XA | S79.141A | S82.014N | S82.031C | S82.043R | S82.111A | S82.126A | S82.145A |
| S73.005A | S77.10XA | S79.141K | S82.014P | S82.031K | S82.044A | S82.111K | S82.126K | S82.145K |
| S73.006A | S77.11XA | S79.141P | S82.014Q | S82.031M | S82.044B | S82.111M | S82.126M | S82.145M |
| S73.011A | S77.12XA | S79.142A | S82.014R | S82.031N | S82.044C | S82.111N | S82.126N | S82.145N |
| S73.012A | S78.011A | S79.142K | S82.015A | S82.031P | S82.044K | S82.111P | S82.126P | S82.145P |
| S73.013A | S78.012A | S79.142P | S82.015B | S82.031Q | S82.044M | S82.111Q | S82.126Q | S82.145Q |
| S73.014A | S78.019A | S79.149A | S82.015C | S82.031R | S82.044N | S82.111R | S82.126R | S82.145R |
| S73.015A | S78.021A | S79.149K | S82.015K | S82.032A | S82.044P | S82.112A | S82.131A | S82.146A |
| S73.016A | S78.022A | S79.149P | S82.015M | S82.032B | S82.044Q | S82.112K | S82.131K | S82.146K |
| S73.021A | S78.029A | S79.191A | S82.015N | S82.032C | S82.044R | S82.112M | S82.131M | S82.146M |
| S73.022A | S78.111A | S79.191K | S82.015P | S82.032K | S82.045A | S82.112N | S82.131N | S82.146N |
| S73.023A | S78.112A | S79.191P | S82.015Q | S82.032N | S82.045B | S82.112P | S82.131P | S82.146P |
| S73.024A | S78.119A | S79.192A | S82.015R | S82.032P | S82.045C | S82.112Q | S82.131Q | S82.146Q |
| S73.025A | S78.121A | S79.192K | S82.016A | S82.032Q | S82.045K | S82.112R | S82.131R | S82.146R |
| S73.026A | S78.122A | S79.192P | S82.016B | S82.032R | S82.045M | S82.113A | S82.132A | S82.151A |
| S73.031A | S78.129A | S79.199A | S82.016C | S82.033A | S82.045N | S82.113K | S82.132K | S82.151K |
| S73.032A | S78.911A | S79.199K | S82.016K | S82.033B | S82.045P | S82.113M | S82.132M | S82.151M |
| S73.033A | S78.912A | S79.199P | S82.016M | S82.033C | S82.045Q | S82.113N | S82.132N | S82.151N |
| S73.034A | S78.919A | S82.001A | S82.016N | S82.033K | S82.045R | S82.113P | S82.132P | S82.151P |
| S73.035A | S78.921A | S82.001B | S82.016P | S82.033M | S82.046A | S82.113Q | S82.132Q | S82.151Q |
| S73.036A | S78.922A | S82.001C | S82.016Q | S82.033M | S82.046A | S82.113R | S82.132R | S82.151R |

| | | | | | | | | |
|---|---|---|---|---|---|---|---|---|
| S82.152A | S82.202Q | S82.234Q | S82.253Q | S82.292Q | S82.402R | S82.436Q | S82.461P | S82.54XK |
| S82.152K | S82.202R | S82.234R | S82.253R | S82.292R | S82.409K | S82.436R | S82.461Q | S82.54XM |
| S82.152M | S82.209A | S82.235A | S82.254A | S82.299A | S82.409M | S82.441K | S82.461R | S82.54XN |
| S82.152N | S82.209K | S82.235K | S82.254K | S82.299K | S82.409P | S82.441M | S82.462K | S82.54XP |
| S82.152P | S82.209M | S82.235M | S82.254M | S82.299M | S82.409Q | S82.441N | S82.462M | S82.54XQ |
| S82.152Q | S82.209N | S82.235N | S82.254N | S82.299N | S82.409R | S82.441P | S82.462N | S82.54XR |
| S82.152R | S82.209P | S82.235P | S82.254P | S82.299P | S82.421K | S82.441Q | S82.462P | S82.55XB |
| S82.153A | S82.209Q | S82.235Q | S82.254Q | S82.299Q | S82.421M | S82.441R | S82.462Q | S82.55XC |
| S82.153K | S82.209R | S82.235R | S82.254R | S82.299R | S82.421N | S82.442K | S82.462R | S82.55XK |
| S82.153M | S82.221A | S82.236A | S82.255A | S82.301B | S82.421P | S82.442M | S82.463K | S82.55XM |
| S82.153N | S82.221K | S82.236K | S82.255K | S82.301C | S82.421Q | S82.442N | S82.463M | S82.55XN |
| S82.153P | S82.221M | S82.236M | S82.255M | S82.301K | S82.421R | S82.442P | S82.463N | S82.55XP |
| S82.153Q | S82.221N | S82.236N | S82.255N | S82.301M | S82.422K | S82.442Q | S82.463P | S82.55XQ |
| S82.153R | S82.221P | S82.236P | S82.255P | S82.301N | S82.422M | S82.442R | S82.463Q | S82.55XR |
| S82.154A | S82.221Q | S82.236Q | S82.255Q | S82.301P | S82.422N | S82.443K | S82.463R | S82.56XB |
| S82.154K | S82.221R | S82.236R | S82.255R | S82.301Q | S82.422P | S82.443M | S82.464K | S82.56XC |
| S82.154M | S82.222A | S82.241A | S82.256A | S82.301R | S82.422Q | S82.443N | S82.464M | S82.56XK |
| S82.154N | S82.222K | S82.241K | S82.256K | S82.302B | S82.422R | S82.443P | S82.464N | S82.56XM |
| S82.154P | S82.222M | S82.241M | S82.256M | S82.302C | S82.423K | S82.443Q | S82.464P | S82.56XN |
| S82.154Q | S82.222N | S82.241N | S82.256N | S82.302K | S82.423M | S82.443R | S82.464Q | S82.56XP |
| S82.154R | S82.222P | S82.241P | S82.256P | S82.302M | S82.423N | S82.444K | S82.464R | S82.56XQ |
| S82.155A | S82.222Q | S82.241Q | S82.256Q | S82.302N | S82.423P | S82.444M | S82.465K | S82.56XR |
| S82.155K | S82.222R | S82.241R | S82.256R | S82.302P | S82.423Q | S82.444N | S82.465M | S82.61XB |
| S82.155M | S82.223A | S82.242A | S82.261A | S82.302Q | S82.423R | S82.444P | S82.465N | S82.61XC |
| S82.155N | S82.223K | S82.242K | S82.261K | S82.302R | S82.424K | S82.444Q | S82.465P | S82.61XK |
| S82.155P | S82.223M | S82.242M | S82.261M | S82.309B | S82.424M | S82.444R | S82.465Q | S82.61XM |
| S82.155Q | S82.223N | S82.242N | S82.261N | S82.309C | S82.424N | S82.445K | S82.465R | S82.61XN |
| S82.155R | S82.223P | S82.242P | S82.261P | S82.309K | S82.424P | S82.445N | S82.466K | S82.61XP |
| S82.156A | S82.223Q | S82.242Q | S82.261Q | S82.309M | S82.424Q | S82.445P | S82.466M | S82.61XQ |
| S82.156K | S82.223R | S82.242R | S82.261R | S82.309N | S82.424R | S82.445Q | S82.466N | S82.61XR |
| S82.156M | S82.224A | S82.243A | S82.262A | S82.309P | S82.425K | S82.445R | S82.466P | S82.62XB |
| S82.156N | S82.224K | S82.243K | S82.262K | S82.309Q | S82.425M | S82.446K | S82.466Q | S82.62XC |
| S82.156P | S82.224M | S82.243M | S82.262M | S82.309R | S82.425N | S82.446M | S82.466R | S82.62XK |
| S82.156Q | S82.224N | S82.243N | S82.262N | S82.311A | S82.425P | S82.446N | S82.491K | S82.62XM |
| S82.156R | S82.224P | S82.243P | S82.262P | S82.311K | S82.425Q | S82.446P | S82.491M | S82.62XN |
| S82.161A | S82.224Q | S82.243Q | S82.262Q | S82.311P | S82.425R | S82.446Q | S82.491N | S82.62XP |
| S82.161K | S82.224R | S82.243R | S82.262R | S82.312A | S82.426K | S82.446R | S82.491P | S82.62XQ |
| S82.161P | S82.225A | S82.244A | S82.263A | S82.312K | S82.426M | S82.451K | S82.491Q | S82.62XR |
| S82.162A | S82.225K | S82.244K | S82.263K | S82.312P | S82.426N | S82.451M | S82.491R | S82.63XB |
| S82.162K | S82.225M | S82.244M | S82.263M | S82.319A | S82.426P | S82.451N | S82.492K | S82.63XC |
| S82.162P | S82.225N | S82.244N | S82.263N | S82.319K | S82.426Q | S82.451P | S82.492M | S82.63XK |
| S82.169A | S82.225P | S82.244P | S82.263P | S82.319P | S82.426R | S82.451Q | S82.492N | S82.63XM |
| S82.169K | S82.225Q | S82.244Q | S82.263Q | S82.391B | S82.431K | S82.451R | S82.492P | S82.63XN |
| S82.169P | S82.225R | S82.244R | S82.263R | S82.391C | S82.431M | S82.452K | S82.492Q | S82.63XP |
| S82.191A | S82.226A | S82.245A | S82.264A | S82.391K | S82.431N | S82.452M | S82.492R | S82.63XQ |
| S82.191K | S82.226K | S82.245K | S82.264K | S82.391M | S82.431P | S82.452N | S82.499K | S82.63XR |
| S82.191M | S82.226M | S82.245M | S82.264M | S82.391N | S82.431Q | S82.452P | S82.499M | S82.64XB |
| S82.191N | S82.226N | S82.245N | S82.264N | S82.391P | S82.431R | S82.452Q | S82.499N | S82.64XC |
| S82.191P | S82.226P | S82.245P | S82.264P | S82.391Q | S82.432K | S82.452R | S82.499P | S82.64XK |
| S82.191Q | S82.226Q | S82.245Q | S82.264Q | S82.391R | S82.432M | S82.453K | S82.499Q | S82.64XN |
| S82.191R | S82.226R | S82.245R | S82.264R | S82.392B | S82.432N | S82.453M | S82.499R | S82.64XM |
| S82.192A | S82.231A | S82.246A | S82.265A | S82.392C | S82.432P | S82.453N | S82.51XB | S82.64XP |
| S82.192K | S82.231K | S82.246K | S82.265K | S82.392K | S82.432Q | S82.453P | S82.51XC | S82.64XQ |
| S82.192M | S82.231M | S82.246M | S82.265M | S82.392M | S82.432R | S82.453Q | S82.51XK | S82.64XR |
| S82.192N | S82.231N | S82.246N | S82.265N | S82.392N | S82.433K | S82.453R | S82.51XM | S82.65XB |
| S82.192P | S82.231P | S82.246P | S82.265P | S82.392P | S82.433N | S82.454K | S82.51XN | S82.65XC |
| S82.192Q | S82.231Q | S82.246Q | S82.265Q | S82.392Q | S82.433P | S82.454M | S82.51XP | S82.65XK |
| S82.192R | S82.231R | S82.246R | S82.265R | S82.392R | S82.433Q | S82.454N | S82.51XQ | S82.65XM |
| S82.199A | S82.232A | S82.251A | S82.266A | S82.399B | S82.433R | S82.454P | S82.51XR | S82.65XN |
| S82.199K | S82.232K | S82.251K | S82.266K | S82.399C | S82.434K | S82.454Q | S82.52XB | S82.65XP |
| S82.199M | S82.232M | S82.251M | S82.266M | S82.399K | S82.434M | S82.454R | S82.52XC | S82.65XQ |
| S82.199N | S82.232N | S82.251N | S82.266N | S82.399M | S82.434N | S82.455K | S82.52XK | S82.65XR |
| S82.199P | S82.232P | S82.251P | S82.266P | S82.399N | S82.434P | S82.455M | S82.52XM | S82.66XB |
| S82.199Q | S82.232Q | S82.251Q | S82.266Q | S82.399P | S82.434Q | S82.455N | S82.52XN | S82.66XC |
| S82.199R | S82.232R | S82.251R | S82.266R | S82.399Q | S82.434R | S82.455P | S82.52XP | S82.66XK |
| S82.201A | S82.233A | S82.252A | S82.291A | S82.399R | S82.435K | S82.455Q | S82.52XQ | S82.66XM |
| S82.201K | S82.233K | S82.252K | S82.291K | S82.401K | S82.435M | S82.455R | S82.52XR | S82.66XN |
| S82.201M | S82.233M | S82.252M | S82.291M | S82.401M | S82.435N | S82.456K | S82.53XB | S82.66XP |
| S82.201N | S82.233N | S82.252N | S82.291N | S82.401N | S82.435P | S82.456M | S82.53XC | S82.66XQ |
| S82.201P | S82.233P | S82.252P | S82.291P | S82.401P | S82.435Q | S82.456N | S82.53XK | S82.66XR |
| S82.201Q | S82.233Q | S82.252Q | S82.291Q | S82.401Q | S82.435R | S82.456P | S82.53XM | S82.811K |
| S82.201R | S82.233R | S82.252R | S82.291R | S82.401R | S82.434R | S82.456Q | S82.53XN | S82.811P |
| S82.202A | S82.234A | S82.253A | S82.292A | S82.402K | S82.435K | S82.456R | S82.53XP | S82.812K |
| S82.202K | S82.234K | S82.253K | S82.292K | S82.402M | S82.436K | S82.461K | S82.53XQ | S82.812P |
| S82.202M | S82.234M | S82.253M | S82.292M | S82.402N | S82.436M | S82.461M | S82.53XR | S82.819K |
| S82.202N | S82.234N | S82.253N | S82.292N | S82.402P | S82.436N | S82.461N | S82.54XB | S82.819P |
| S82.202P | S82.234P | S82.253P | S82.292P | S82.402Q | S82.436P | | S82.54XC | S82.821K |

| | | | | | | | | |
|---|---|---|---|---|---|---|---|---|
| S82.821P | S82.851Q | S82.866R | S82.90XN | S85.811A | S89.029P | S89.221P | S92.026B | S92.101P |
| S82.822K | S82.851R | S82.871B | S82.90XP | S85.812A | S89.031A | S89.222K | S92.026K | S92.102B |
| S82.822P | S82.852B | S82.871C | S82.90XQ | S85.819A | S89.031K | S89.222P | S92.026P | S92.102K |
| S82.829K | S82.852C | S82.871K | S82.90XR | S85.891A | S89.031P | S89.229K | S92.031B | S92.102P |
| S82.829P | S82.852K | S82.871M | S82.91XB | S85.892A | S89.032A | S89.229P | S92.031K | S92.109B |
| S82.831K | S82.852M | S82.871N | S82.91XC | S85.899A | S89.032K | S89.291K | S92.031P | S92.109K |
| S82.831M | S82.852N | S82.871P | S82.91XK | S85.901A | S89.032P | S89.291P | S92.032B | S92.109P |
| S82.831N | S82.852P | S82.871Q | S82.91XM | S85.902A | S89.039A | S89.292K | S92.032K | S92.111B |
| S82.831P | S82.852Q | S82.871R | S82.91XN | S85.909A | S89.039K | S89.292P | S92.032P | S92.111K |
| S82.831Q | S82.852R | S82.872B | S82.91XP | S85.911A | S89.039P | S89.299K | S92.033B | S92.111P |
| S82.831R | S82.853B | S82.872C | S82.91XQ | S85.912A | S89.041A | S89.299P | S92.033K | S92.112B |
| S82.832K | S82.853C | S82.872K | S82.91XR | S85.919A | S89.041K | S89.301K | S92.033P | S92.112K |
| S82.832M | S82.853K | S82.872M | S82.92XB | S85.991A | S89.041P | S89.301P | S92.034B | S92.112P |
| S82.832N | S82.853M | S82.872N | S82.92XC | S85.992A | S89.042A | S89.302K | S92.034K | S92.113B |
| S82.832P | S82.853N | S82.872P | S82.92XK | S85.999A | S89.042K | S89.302P | S92.034P | S92.113K |
| S82.832Q | S82.853P | S82.872Q | S82.92XM | S86.021A | S89.042P | S89.309K | S92.035B | S92.113P |
| S82.832R | S82.853Q | S82.872R | S82.92XN | S86.022A | S89.049A | S89.309P | S92.035K | S92.114B |
| S82.839K | S82.853R | S82.873B | S82.92XP | S86.029A | S89.049K | S89.311K | S92.035P | S92.114K |
| S82.839M | S82.854B | S82.873C | S82.92XQ | S86.121A | S89.049P | S89.311P | S92.036B | S92.114P |
| S82.839N | S82.854C | S82.873K | S82.92XR | S86.122A | S89.091A | S89.312K | S92.036K | S92.115B |
| S82.839P | S82.854K | S82.873M | S85.101A | S86.129A | S89.091K | S89.312P | S92.036P | S92.115K |
| S82.839Q | S82.854M | S82.873N | S85.102A | S86.221A | S89.091P | S89.319K | S92.041B | S92.115P |
| S82.839R | S82.854N | S82.873P | S85.109A | S86.222A | S89.092A | S89.319P | S92.041K | S92.116B |
| S82.841B | S82.854P | S82.873Q | S85.111A | S86.229A | S89.092K | S89.321K | S92.041P | S92.116K |
| S82.841C | S82.854Q | S82.873R | S85.112A | S86.321A | S89.092P | S89.321P | S92.042B | S92.116P |
| S82.841K | S82.854R | S82.874B | S85.119A | S86.322A | S89.099A | S89.322K | S92.042K | S92.121B |
| S82.841M | S82.855B | S82.874C | S85.121A | S86.329A | S89.099K | S89.322P | S92.042P | S92.121K |
| S82.841N | S82.855C | S82.874K | S85.122A | S86.821A | S89.099P | S89.329K | S92.043B | S92.121P |
| S82.841P | S82.855K | S82.874M | S85.129A | S86.822A | S89.101K | S89.329P | S92.043P | S92.122B |
| S82.841Q | S82.855M | S82.874N | S85.131A | S86.829A | S89.101P | S89.391K | S92.044B | S92.122K |
| S82.841R | S82.855N | S82.874P | S85.132A | S86.921A | S89.102K | S89.391P | S92.044K | S92.122P |
| S82.842B | S82.855P | S82.874Q | S85.139A | S86.922A | S89.102P | S89.392K | S92.044P | S92.123B |
| S82.842C | S82.855Q | S82.874R | S85.141A | S86.929A | S89.109K | S89.392P | S92.045B | S92.123K |
| S82.842K | S82.855R | S82.875B | S85.142A | S88.011A | S89.109P | S89.399K | S92.045K | S92.123P |
| S82.842M | S82.856B | S82.875C | S85.149A | S88.012A | S89.111K | S89.399P | S92.045P | S92.124B |
| S82.842N | S82.856C | S82.875K | S85.151A | S88.019A | S89.111P | S92.001B | S92.046B | S92.124K |
| S82.842P | S82.856K | S82.875M | S85.152A | S88.021A | S89.112K | S92.001K | S92.046K | S92.124P |
| S82.842Q | S82.856M | S82.875N | S85.159A | S88.022A | S89.112P | S92.001P | S92.046P | S92.125B |
| S82.842R | S82.856N | S82.875P | S85.161A | S88.029A | S89.119K | S92.002B | S92.051B | S92.125K |
| S82.843B | S82.856P | S82.875Q | S85.162A | S88.111A | S89.119P | S92.002P | S92.051K | S92.125P |
| S82.843C | S82.856Q | S82.875R | S85.169A | S88.112A | S89.121K | S92.009B | S92.051P | S92.126B |
| S82.843K | S82.856R | S82.876B | S85.171A | S88.119A | S89.121P | S92.009K | S92.052B | S92.126K |
| S82.843M | S82.861K | S82.876C | S85.172A | S88.121A | S89.122K | S92.009P | S92.052K | S92.126P |
| S82.843N | S82.861M | S82.876K | S85.179A | S88.122A | S89.122P | S92.011B | S92.052P | S92.131B |
| S82.843P | S82.861N | S82.876M | S85.181A | S88.129A | S89.129K | S92.011K | S92.053B | S92.131K |
| S82.843Q | S82.861P | S82.876N | S85.182A | S88.911A | S89.129P | S92.011P | S92.053K | S92.131P |
| S82.843R | S82.861Q | S82.876P | S85.189A | S88.912A | S89.131K | S92.012B | S92.053P | S92.132B |
| S82.844B | S82.861R | S82.876Q | S85.201A | S88.919A | S89.131P | S92.012K | S92.054B | S92.132K |
| S82.844C | S82.862K | S82.876R | S85.202A | S88.921A | S89.132K | S92.012P | S92.054K | S92.132P |
| S82.844K | S82.862M | S82.891B | S85.209A | S88.922A | S89.132P | S92.013B | S92.054P | S92.133B |
| S82.844M | S82.862N | S82.891C | S85.211A | S88.929A | S89.139K | S92.013K | S92.055B | S92.133K |
| S82.844N | S82.862P | S82.891K | S85.212A | S89.001A | S89.139P | S92.013P | S92.055K | S92.133P |
| S82.844P | S82.862Q | S82.891M | S85.219A | S89.001K | S89.141K | S92.014B | S92.055P | S92.134B |
| S82.844Q | S82.862R | S82.891N | S85.291A | S89.001P | S89.141P | S92.014K | S92.056B | S92.134K |
| S82.844R | S82.863K | S82.891P | S85.292A | S89.002A | S89.142K | S92.014P | S92.056K | S92.134P |
| S82.845B | S82.863M | S82.891Q | S85.299A | S89.002K | S89.142P | S92.015B | S92.056P | S92.135B |
| S82.845C | S82.863N | S82.891R | S85.301A | S89.002P | S89.149K | S92.015K | S92.061B | S92.135K |
| S82.845K | S82.863P | S82.892B | S85.302A | S89.009A | S89.149P | S92.015P | S92.061K | S92.135P |
| S82.845M | S82.863Q | S82.892C | S85.309A | S89.009K | S89.191K | S92.016B | S92.061P | S92.136B |
| S82.845N | S82.863R | S82.892K | S85.311A | S89.009P | S89.191P | S92.016K | S92.062B | S92.136K |
| S82.845P | S82.864K | S82.892M | S85.312A | S89.011A | S89.192K | S92.016P | S92.062K | S92.136P |
| S82.845Q | S82.864M | S82.892N | S85.319A | S89.011K | S89.192P | S92.021B | S92.062P | S92.141B |
| S82.845R | S82.864N | S82.892P | S85.391A | S89.011P | S89.199K | S92.021K | S92.063B | S92.141K |
| S82.846B | S82.864P | S82.892Q | S85.392A | S89.012A | S89.199P | S92.021P | S92.063K | S92.141P |
| S82.846C | S82.864Q | S82.892R | S85.399A | S89.012K | S89.201K | S92.022B | S92.063P | S92.142B |
| S82.846K | S82.864R | S82.899B | S85.401A | S89.012P | S89.201P | S92.022K | S92.064B | S92.142K |
| S82.846M | S82.865K | S82.899C | S85.402A | S89.019A | S89.202K | S92.022P | S92.064K | S92.142P |
| S82.846N | S82.865M | S82.899K | S85.409A | S89.019K | S89.202P | S92.023B | S92.064P | S92.143B |
| S82.846P | S82.865N | S82.899M | S85.411A | S89.019P | S89.209K | S92.023K | S92.065B | S92.143K |
| S82.846Q | S82.865P | S82.899N | S85.412A | S89.021A | S89.209P | S92.023P | S92.065K | S92.143P |
| S82.846R | S82.865Q | S82.899P | S85.419A | S89.021K | S89.211K | S92.024B | S92.065P | S92.144B |
| S82.851B | S82.865R | S82.899Q | S85.491A | S89.021P | S89.211P | S92.024K | S92.066B | S92.144K |
| S82.851C | S82.866K | S82.899R | S85.492A | S89.022A | S89.212K | S92.024P | S92.066K | S92.144P |
| S82.851K | S82.866M | S82.90XB | S85.499A | S89.022K | S89.212P | S92.025B | S92.066P | S92.145B |
| S82.851M | S82.866N | S82.90XC | S85.801A | S89.022P | S89.219K | S92.025K | S92.101B | S92.145K |
| S82.851N | S82.866P | S82.90XK | S85.802A | S89.029A | S89.219P | S92.025P | S92.101K | S92.145P |
| S82.851P | S82.866Q | S82.90XM | S85.809A | S89.029K | S89.221K | | | S92.146B |

| | | | | | | | | |
|---|---|---|---|---|---|---|---|---|
| S92.146K | S92.232B | S92.316P | S92.403K | S92.532P | S95.909A | T20.712A | T23.321A | T24.799A |
| S92.146P | S92.232K | S92.321B | S92.403P | S92.533K | S95.911A | T20.719A | T23.322A | T25.311A |
| S92.151B | S92.232P | S92.321K | S92.404K | S92.533P | S95.912A | T20.72XA | T23.329A | T25.312A |
| S92.151K | S92.233B | S92.321P | S92.404P | S92.534K | S95.919A | T20.73XA | T23.331A | T25.319A |
| S92.151P | S92.233K | S92.322B | S92.405K | S92.534P | S95.991A | T20.74XA | T23.332A | T25.321A |
| S92.152B | S92.233P | S92.322K | S92.405P | S92.535K | S95.992A | T20.75XA | T23.339A | T25.322A |
| S92.152K | S92.234B | S92.322P | S92.406K | S92.535P | S95.999A | T20.76XA | T23.341A | T25.329A |
| S92.152P | S92.234K | S92.323B | S92.406P | S92.536K | S96.021A | T20.77XA | T23.342A | T25.331A |
| S92.153B | S92.234P | S92.323K | S92.411K | S92.536P | S96.022A | T20.79XA | T23.349A | T25.332A |
| S92.153K | S92.235B | S92.323P | S92.411P | S92.591K | S96.029A | T21.30XA | T23.351A | T25.339A |
| S92.153P | S92.235K | S92.324B | S92.412K | S92.591P | S96.121A | T21.31XA | T23.352A | T25.391A |
| S92.154B | S92.235P | S92.324K | S92.412P | S92.592K | S96.122A | T21.32XA | T23.359A | T25.392A |
| S92.154K | S92.236B | S92.324P | S92.413K | S92.592P | S96.129A | T21.33XA | T23.361A | T25.399A |
| S92.154P | S92.236K | S92.325B | S92.413P | S92.599K | S96.221A | T21.34XA | T23.362A | T25.711A |
| S92.155B | S92.236P | S92.325K | S92.414K | S92.599P | S96.222A | T21.35XA | T23.369A | T25.712A |
| S92.155K | S92.241B | S92.325P | S92.414P | S92.811B | S96.229A | T21.36XA | T23.371A | T25.719A |
| S92.155P | S92.241K | S92.326B | S92.415K | S92.811K | S96.821A | T21.37XA | T23.372A | T25.721A |
| S92.156B | S92.241P | S92.326K | S92.415P | S92.811P | S96.822A | T21.39XA | T23.379A | T25.722A |
| S92.156K | S92.242B | S92.326P | S92.416K | S92.812B | S96.829A | T21.70XA | T23.391A | T25.729A |
| S92.156P | S92.242K | S92.331B | S92.416P | S92.812K | S96.921A | T21.71XA | T23.392A | T25.731A |
| S92.191B | S92.242P | S92.331K | S92.421K | S92.812P | S96.922A | T21.72XA | T23.399A | T25.732A |
| S92.191K | S92.243B | S92.331P | S92.421P | S92.819K | S96.929A | T21.73XA | T23.701A | T25.739A |
| S92.191P | S92.243K | S92.332B | S92.422K | S92.819P | S98.011A | T21.74XA | T23.702A | T25.791A |
| S92.192B | S92.243P | S92.332K | S92.422P | S92.901B | S98.012A | T21.75XA | T23.709A | T25.792A |
| S92.192K | S92.244B | S92.332P | S92.423K | S92.901K | S98.019A | T21.76XA | T23.711A | T25.799A |
| S92.192P | S92.244K | S92.333B | S92.423P | S92.901P | S98.021A | T21.77XA | T23.712A | T26.20XA |
| S92.199B | S92.244P | S92.333K | S92.424K | S92.902B | S98.022A | T21.79XA | T23.719A | T26.21XA |
| S92.199K | S92.245B | S92.333P | S92.424P | S92.902K | S98.029A | T22.30XA | T23.721A | T26.22XA |
| S92.199P | S92.245K | S92.334B | S92.425K | S92.902P | S98.311A | T22.311A | T23.722A | T26.70XA |
| S92.201B | S92.245P | S92.334K | S92.425P | S92.909B | S98.312A | T22.312A | T23.729A | T26.71XA |
| S92.201K | S92.246B | S92.334P | S92.426K | S92.909K | S98.319A | T22.319A | T23.731A | T26.72XA |
| S92.201P | S92.246K | S92.335B | S92.426P | S92.909P | S98.321A | T22.321A | T23.732A | T27.0XXA |
| S92.202B | S92.246P | S92.335K | S92.491K | S92.911K | S98.322A | T22.322A | T23.739A | T27.1XXA |
| S92.202K | S92.251B | S92.335P | S92.491P | S92.911P | S98.329A | T22.329A | T23.741A | T27.2XXA |
| S92.202P | S92.251K | S92.336B | S92.492K | S92.912K | S98.911A | T22.331A | T23.742A | T27.3XXA |
| S92.209B | S92.251P | S92.336K | S92.492P | S92.912P | S98.912A | T22.332A | T23.749A | T27.4XXA |
| S92.209K | S92.252B | S92.336P | S92.499K | S92.919K | S98.919A | T22.339A | T23.751A | T27.5XXA |
| S92.209P | S92.252K | S92.341B | S92.499P | S92.919P | S98.921A | T22.341A | T23.752A | T27.6XXA |
| S92.211B | S92.252P | S92.341K | S92.501K | S95.001A | S98.922A | T22.342A | T23.759A | T27.7XXA |
| S92.211K | S92.253B | S92.341P | S92.501P | S95.002A | S98.929A | T22.349A | T23.761A | T28.1XXA |
| S92.211P | S92.253K | S92.342B | S92.502K | S95.009A | T17.400A | T22.351A | T23.762A | T28.2XXA |
| S92.212B | S92.253P | S92.342K | S92.502P | S95.011A | T17.408A | T22.352A | T23.769A | T28.6XXA |
| S92.212K | S92.254B | S92.342P | S92.503K | S95.012A | T17.410A | T22.359A | T23.771A | T28.7XXA |
| S92.212P | S92.254K | S92.343B | S92.503P | S95.019A | T17.418A | T22.361A | T23.772A | T31.10 |
| S92.213B | S92.254P | S92.343K | S92.504K | S95.091A | T17.420A | T22.362A | T23.779A | T31.11 |
| S92.213K | S92.255B | S92.343P | S92.504P | S95.092A | T17.428A | T22.369A | T23.791A | T31.20 |
| S92.213P | S92.255K | S92.344B | S92.505K | S95.099A | T17.490A | T22.391A | T23.792A | T31.30 |
| S92.214B | S92.255P | S92.344K | S92.505P | S95.101A | T17.498A | T22.392A | T23.799A | T31.40 |
| S92.214K | S92.256B | S92.344P | S92.506K | S95.102A | T17.500A | T22.399A | T24.301A | T31.50 |
| S92.214P | S92.256K | S92.345B | S92.506P | S95.109A | T17.508A | T22.70XA | T24.302A | T31.60 |
| S92.215B | S92.256P | S92.345K | S92.511K | S95.111A | T17.510A | T22.711A | T24.309A | T31.70 |
| S92.215K | S92.301B | S92.345P | S92.511P | S95.112A | T17.518A | T22.712A | T24.311A | T31.80 |
| S92.215P | S92.301K | S92.346B | S92.512K | S95.119A | T17.520A | T22.719A | T24.312A | T31.90 |
| S92.216B | S92.301P | S92.346K | S92.512P | S95.191A | T17.528A | T22.721A | T24.319A | T32.10 |
| S92.216K | S92.302B | S92.346P | S92.513K | S95.192A | T17.590A | T22.722A | T24.321A | T32.11 |
| S92.216P | S92.302K | S92.351B | S92.513P | S95.199A | T17.598A | T22.729A | T24.322A | T32.20 |
| S92.221B | S92.302P | S92.351K | S92.514K | S95.201A | T17.800A | T22.731A | T24.329A | T32.30 |
| S92.221K | S92.309B | S92.351P | S92.514P | S95.202A | T17.808A | T22.732A | T24.331A | T32.40 |
| S92.221P | S92.309K | S92.352B | S92.515K | S95.209A | T17.810A | T22.739A | T24.332A | T32.50 |
| S92.222B | S92.309P | S92.352K | S92.515P | S95.211A | T17.818A | T22.741A | T24.339A | T32.60 |
| S92.222K | S92.311B | S92.352P | S92.516K | S95.212A | T17.820A | T22.742A | T24.391A | T32.70 |
| S92.222P | S92.311K | S92.353B | S92.516P | S95.219A | T17.828A | T22.749A | T24.392A | T32.80 |
| S92.223B | S92.311P | S92.353K | S92.521K | S95.291A | T17.890A | T22.751A | T24.399A | T32.90 |
| S92.223K | S92.312B | S92.353P | S92.521P | S95.292A | T17.898A | T22.752A | T24.701A | T33.011A |
| S92.223P | S92.312K | S92.354B | S92.522K | S95.299A | T20.30XA | T22.759A | T24.702A | T33.012A |
| S92.224B | S92.312P | S92.354K | S92.522P | S95.801A | T20.311A | T22.761A | T24.709A | T33.019A |
| S92.224K | S92.313B | S92.354P | S92.523K | S95.802A | T20.312A | T22.762A | T24.711A | T33.02XA |
| S92.224P | S92.313K | S92.355B | S92.523P | S95.809A | T20.319A | T22.769A | T24.712A | T33.09XA |
| S92.225B | S92.313P | S92.355K | S92.524K | S95.811A | T20.32XA | T22.791A | T24.719A | T33.1XXA |
| S92.225K | S92.314B | S92.355P | S92.524P | S95.812A | T20.33XA | T22.792A | T24.721A | T33.2XXA |
| S92.225P | S92.314K | S92.356B | S92.525K | S95.819A | T20.34XA | T22.799A | T24.722A | T33.3XXA |
| S92.226B | S92.314P | S92.356K | S92.525P | S95.891A | T20.35XA | T23.301A | T24.729A | T33.40XA |
| S92.226K | S92.315B | S92.356P | S92.526K | S95.892A | T20.36XA | T23.302A | T24.731A | T33.41XA |
| S92.226P | S92.315K | S92.401K | S92.526P | S95.899A | T20.37XA | T23.309A | T24.732A | T33.42XA |
| S92.231B | S92.315P | S92.401P | S92.531K | S95.901A | T20.39XA | T23.311A | T24.739A | T33.511A |
| S92.231K | S92.316B | S92.402K | S92.531P | S95.902A | T20.70XA | T23.312A | T24.791A | T33.512A |
| S92.231P | S92.316K | S92.402P | S92.532K | S95.902A | T20.711A | T23.319A | T24.792A | T33.519A |

| | | | | | | | | |
|---|---|---|---|---|---|---|---|---|
| T33.521A | T71.141A | T80.310A | T81.596A | T82.530A | T83.598A | T84.190A | T85.123A | T85.860D |
| T33.522A | T71.143A | T80.311A | T81.597A | T82.531A | T83.61XA | T84.191A | T85.128A | T85.890A |
| T33.529A | T71.144A | T80.319A | T81.598A | T82.532A | T83.62XA | T84.192A | T85.190A | T85.890D |
| T33.531A | T71.151A | T80.39XA | T81.599A | T82.533A | T83.69XA | T84.193A | T85.191A | T86.00 |
| T33.532A | T71.152A | T80.40XA | T81.60XA | T82.534A | T83.712A | T84.194A | T85.192A | T86.01 |
| T33.539A | T71.153A | T80.410A | T81.61XA | T82.535A | T83.713A | T84.195A | T85.193A | T86.02 |
| T33.60XA | T71.154A | T80.411A | T81.69XA | T82.538A | T83.714A | T84.196A | T85.199A | T86.03 |
| T33.61XA | T71.161A | T80.419A | T81.710A | T82.539A | T83.718A | T84.197A | T85.21XA | T86.09 |
| T33.62XA | T71.162A | T80.49XA | T81.711A | T82.590A | T83.719A | T84.199A | T85.22XA | T86.10 |
| T33.70XA | T71.163A | T80.51XA | T81.718A | T82.591A | T83.722A | T84.210A | T85.29XA | T86.11 |
| T33.71XA | T71.164A | T80.52XA | T81.719A | T82.592A | T83.723A | T84.213A | T85.310A | T86.12 |
| T33.72XA | T71.191A | T80.59XA | T81.72XA | T82.593A | T83.724A | T84.216A | T85.311A | T86.13 |
| T33.811A | T71.192A | T80.61XA | T81.83XA | T82.594A | T83.728A | T84.218A | T85.320A | T86.19 |
| T33.812A | T71.193A | T80.62XA | T82.01XA | T82.595A | T83.729A | T84.220A | T85.321A | T86.20 |
| T33.819A | T71.194A | T80.69XA | T82.02XA | T82.598A | T83.79XA | T84.223A | T85.390A | T86.21 |
| T33.821A | T71.20XA | T80.810A | T82.03XA | T82.599A | T83.81XA | T84.226A | T85.391A | T86.22 |
| T33.822A | T71.21XA | T80.818A | T82.09XA | T82.6XXA | T83.82XA | T84.228A | T85.41XA | T86.23 |
| T33.829A | T71.221A | T80.910A | T82.110A | T82.7XXA | T83.83XA | T84.290A | T85.42XA | T86.290 |
| T33.831A | T71.222A | T80.911A | T82.111A | T82.817A | T83.84XA | T84.293A | T85.43XA | T86.298 |
| T33.832A | T71.223A | T80.919A | T82.118A | T82.818A | T83.85XA | T84.296A | T85.44XA | T86.30 |
| T33.839A | T71.224A | T80.A0XA | T82.119A | T82.827A | T83.86XA | T84.298A | T85.49XA | T86.31 |
| T33.90XA | T71.231A | T80.A1XA | T82.120A | T82.828A | T83.89XA | T84.310A | T85.510A | T86.32 |
| T33.99XA | T71.232A | T80.A11A | T82.121A | T82.837A | T83.9XXA | T84.318A | T85.511A | T86.33 |
| T34.011A | T71.233A | T80.A19A | T82.128A | T82.838A | T84.010A | T84.320A | T85.518A | T86.39 |
| T34.012A | T71.234A | T80.A9XA | T82.129A | T82.847A | T84.011A | T84.328A | T85.520A | T86.40 |
| T34.019A | T71.29XA | T81.10XA | T82.190A | T82.848A | T84.012A | T84.390A | T85.521A | T86.41 |
| T34.02XA | T71.9XXA | T81.30XA | T82.191A | T82.855A | T84.013A | T84.398A | T85.528A | T86.42 |
| T34.09XA | T74.01XA | T81.31XA | T82.198A | T82.856A | T84.018A | T84.410A | T85.590A | T86.43 |
| T34.1XXA | T74.02XA | T81.32XA | T82.199A | T82.857A | T84.019A | T84.418A | T85.591A | T86.49 |
| T34.2XXA | T74.11XA | T81.33XA | T82.211A | T82.858A | T84.020A | T84.420A | T85.598A | T86.5 |
| T34.3XXA | T74.12XA | T81.4XXA | T82.212A | T82.867A | T84.021A | T84.428A | T85.610A | T86.810 |
| T34.40XA | T74.21XA | T81.500A | T82.213A | T82.868A | T84.022A | T84.490A | T85.611A | T86.811 |
| T34.41XA | T74.22XA | T81.501A | T82.218A | T82.897A | T84.023A | T84.498A | T85.612A | T86.812 |
| T34.42XA | T74.32XA | T81.502A | T82.221A | T82.898A | T84.029A | T84.50XA | T85.613A | T86.818 |
| T34.511A | T74.4XXA | T81.503A | T82.222A | T82.9XXA | T84.030A | T84.51XA | T85.614A | T86.819 |
| T34.512A | T74.91XA | T81.504A | T82.223A | T83.010A | T84.031A | T84.52XA | T85.615A | T86.820 |
| T34.519A | T74.92XA | T81.505A | T82.228A | T83.020A | T84.032A | T84.53XA | T85.618A | T86.821 |
| T34.521A | T75.1XXA | T81.506A | T82.310A | T83.030A | T84.033A | T84.54XA | T85.620A | T86.822 |
| T34.522A | T76.01XA | T81.507A | T82.311A | T83.090A | T84.038A | T84.59XA | T85.621A | T86.828 |
| T34.529A | T76.02XA | T81.508A | T82.312A | T83.110A | T84.039A | T84.60XA | T85.622A | T86.829 |
| T34.531A | T76.11XA | T81.509A | T82.318A | T83.111A | T84.050A | T84.610A | T85.623A | T86.830 |
| T34.532A | T76.12XA | T81.510A | T82.319A | T83.112A | T84.051A | T84.611A | T85.624A | T86.831 |
| T34.539A | T76.21XA | T81.511A | T82.320A | T83.113A | T84.052A | T84.612A | T85.625A | T86.832 |
| T34.60XA | T76.22XA | T81.512A | T82.321A | T83.118A | T84.053A | T84.613A | T85.628A | T86.838 |
| T34.61XA | T76.32XA | T81.513A | T82.322A | T83.120A | T84.058A | T84.614A | T85.630A | T86.839 |
| T34.62XA | T76.91XA | T81.514A | T82.328A | T83.121A | T84.059A | T84.615A | T85.631A | T86.840 |
| T34.70XA | T76.92XA | T81.515A | T82.329A | T83.122A | T84.060A | T84.619A | T85.633A | T86.841 |
| T34.71XA | T78.00XA | T81.516A | T82.330A | T83.123A | T84.061A | T84.620A | T85.635A | T86.842 |
| T34.72XA | T78.01XA | T81.517A | T82.331A | T83.128A | T84.062A | T84.621A | T85.638A | T86.848 |
| T34.811A | T78.02XA | T81.518A | T82.332A | T83.190A | T84.063A | T84.622A | T85.690A | T86.849 |
| T34.812A | T78.03XA | T81.519A | T82.338A | T83.191A | T84.068A | T84.623A | T85.691A | T86.850 |
| T34.819A | T78.04XA | T81.520A | T82.339A | T83.192A | T84.069A | T84.624A | T85.692A | T86.851 |
| T34.821A | T78.05XA | T81.521A | T82.390A | T83.193A | T84.090A | T84.625A | T85.693A | T86.852 |
| T34.822A | T78.06XA | T81.522A | T82.391A | T83.198A | T84.091A | T84.629A | T85.694A | T86.858 |
| T34.829A | T78.07XA | T81.523A | T82.392A | T83.21XA | T84.092A | T84.63XA | T85.695A | T86.859 |
| T34.831A | T78.08XA | T81.524A | T82.398A | T83.22XA | T84.093A | T84.69XA | T85.698A | T86.890 |
| T34.832A | T78.09XA | T81.525A | T82.399A | T83.23XA | T84.098A | T84.7XXA | T85.71XA | T86.891 |
| T34.839A | T78.2XXA | T81.526A | T82.41XA | T83.24XA | T84.099A | T84.81XA | T85.72XA | T86.892 |
| T34.90XA | T79.2XXA | T81.527A | T82.42XA | T83.25XA | T84.110A | T84.82XA | T85.730A | T86.898 |
| T34.99XA | T79.7XXA | T81.528A | T82.43XA | T83.29XA | T84.111A | T84.83XA | T85.731A | T86.899 |
| T67.0XXA | T79.A0XA | T81.529A | T82.49XA | T83.410A | T84.112A | T84.84XA | T85.732A | T86.90 |
| T69.021A | T79.A11A | T81.530A | T82.510A | T83.411A | T84.113A | T84.85XA | T85.733A | T86.91 |
| T69.022A | T79.A12A | T81.531A | T82.511A | T83.418A | T84.114A | T84.86XA | T85.734A | T86.92 |
| T69.029A | T79.A19A | T81.532A | T82.512A | T83.420A | T84.115A | T84.89XA | T85.735A | T86.93 |
| T70.3XXA | T79.A21A | T81.533A | T82.513A | T83.421A | T84.116A | T84.9XXA | T85.738A | T86.99 |
| T71.111A | T79.A22A | T81.534A | T82.514A | T83.428A | T84.117A | T85.01XA | T85.79XA | T87.0X1 |
| T71.112A | T79.A29A | T81.535A | T82.515A | T83.490A | T84.119A | T85.02XA | T85.810A | T87.0X2 |
| T71.113A | T79.A3XA | T81.536A | T82.518A | T83.491A | T84.120A | T85.03XA | T85.810D | T87.0X9 |
| T71.114A | T79.A9XA | T81.537A | T82.519A | T83.498A | T84.121A | T85.09XA | T85.820A | T87.1X1 |
| T71.121A | T80.1XXA | T81.538A | T82.520A | T83.510A | T84.122A | T85.110A | T85.820D | T87.1X2 |
| T71.122A | T80.211A | T81.539A | T82.521A | T83.511A | T84.123A | T85.111A | T85.830A | T87.1X9 |
| T71.123A | T80.212A | T81.590A | T82.522A | T83.512A | T84.124A | T85.112A | T85.830D | T87.2 |
| T71.124A | T80.218A | T81.591A | T82.523A | T83.518A | T84.125A | T85.113A | T85.840A | T87.40 |
| T71.131A | T80.219A | T81.592A | T82.524A | T83.590A | T84.126A | T85.118A | T85.840D | T87.41 |
| T71.132A | T80.22XA | T81.593A | T82.525A | T83.591A | T84.127A | T85.120A | T85.850A | T87.42 |
| T71.133A | T80.29XA | T81.594A | T82.528A | T83.592A | T84.129A | T85.121A | T85.850D | T87.43 |
| T71.134A | T80.30XA | T81.595A | T82.529A | T83.593A | | T85.122A | T85.860A | T87.44 |

| | | | | | |
|---|---|---|---|---|---|
| T88.ØXXA | Z48.21 | Z68.1 | Z94.Ø | Z94.82 | Z99.12 |
| T88.1XXA | Z48.22 | Z68.41 | Z94.1 | Z94.83 | |
| T88.2XXA | Z48.23 | Z68.42 | Z94.2 | Z94.84 | |
| T88.3XXA | Z48.24 | Z68.43 | Z94.3 | Z95.811 | |
| T88.6XXA | Z48.28Ø | Z68.44 | Z94.4 | Z95.812 | |
| Z43.1 | Z48.29Ø | Z68.45 | Z94.81 | Z99.11 | |

# Appendix G: Lists of Principal Diagnoses That Are Their Own CC and Their Own MCC

**Note:** The following lists are based on the *Federal Register,* volume 82, number 81, April 28, 2017 ("Hospital Inpatient Prospective Payment Systems for Acute Care Hospitals and the Long-Term Care Hospital Prospective Payment System and Proposed Policy Changes and Fiscal Year 2018 Rates; Proposed Rule"). The most current version, v35, of the ICD-10 MS-DRG Definitions Manual was not available at the time this book was printed. For the most current files related to IPPS please refer to the following: https://www.cms.gov/Medicare/Medicare-Fee-for-Service-Payment/AcuteInpatientPPS/IPPS-Regulations-and-Notices.html.

## Principal Diagnoses That Are Their Own CC

| | | | | | | | |
|---|---|---|---|---|---|---|---|
| B25.1 | I70.368 | I70.562 | I70.749 | K51.513 | M02.331 | M05.459 | M90.559 |
| B52.0 | I70.369 | I70.563 | I70.761 | K51.514 | M02.332 | M05.461 | M90.561 |
| D57.211 | I70.431 | I70.568 | I70.762 | K51.812 | M02.339 | M05.462 | M90.562 |
| D57.411 | I70.432 | I70.569 | I70.763 | K51.813 | M02.341 | M05.469 | M90.569 |
| E08.52 | I70.433 | I70.631 | I70.768 | K51.814 | M02.342 | M05.471 | M90.571 |
| E09.52 | I70.434 | I70.632 | I70.769 | K51.912 | M02.349 | M05.472 | M90.572 |
| E10.52 | I70.438 | I70.633 | I73.01 | K51.913 | M02.351 | M05.479 | M90.579 |
| E11.52 | I70.439 | I70.634 | K50.012 | K51.914 | M02.352 | M05.49 | M90.58 |
| E13.52 | I70.441 | I70.638 | K50.013 | K57.00 | M02.359 | M32.11 | M90.59 |
| I25.110 | I70.442 | I70.639 | K50.014 | K57.01 | M02.361 | M32.12 | N11.1 |
| I25.700 | I70.443 | I70.641 | K50.112 | K57.20 | M02.362 | M33.02 | N13.0 |
| I25.710 | I70.444 | I70.642 | K50.113 | K57.21 | M02.369 | M33.12 | N13.1 |
| I25.720 | I70.448 | I70.643 | K50.114 | K57.40 | M02.371 | M33.22 | N13.2 |
| I25.730 | I70.449 | I70.644 | K50.812 | K57.41 | M02.372 | M33.92 | O12.21 |
| I25.750 | I70.461 | I70.648 | K50.813 | K57.52 | M02.379 | M34.81 | O12.22 |
| I25.760 | I70.462 | I70.649 | K50.814 | K57.80 | M02.38 | M34.82 | O12.23 |
| I25.790 | I70.463 | I70.661 | K50.912 | K57.81 | M02.39 | M35.03 | T86.30 |
| I70.331 | I70.468 | I70.662 | K50.913 | K80.30 | M05.40 | M90.50 | T86.31 |
| I70.332 | I70.469 | I70.663 | K50.914 | K80.31 | M05.411 | M90.511 | T86.32 |
| I70.333 | I70.531 | I70.668 | K51.012 | K80.32 | M05.412 | M90.512 | T86.33 |
| I70.334 | I70.532 | I70.669 | K51.013 | K80.33 | M05.419 | M90.519 | T86.39 |
| I70.338 | I70.533 | I70.731 | K51.014 | K80.34 | M05.421 | M90.521 | Z48.21 |
| I70.339 | I70.534 | I70.732 | K51.212 | K80.35 | M05.422 | M90.522 | Z48.22 |
| I70.341 | I70.538 | I70.733 | K51.213 | K80.36 | M05.429 | M90.529 | Z48.23 |
| I70.342 | I70.539 | I70.734 | K51.214 | K80.37 | M05.431 | M90.531 | Z48.24 |
| I70.343 | I70.541 | I70.738 | K51.312 | M02.30 | M05.432 | M90.532 | Z48.280 |
| I70.344 | I70.542 | I70.739 | K51.313 | M02.311 | M05.439 | M90.539 | Z48.290 |
| I70.348 | I70.543 | I70.741 | K51.314 | M02.312 | M05.441 | M90.541 | Z94.3 |
| I70.349 | I70.544 | I70.742 | K51.412 | M02.319 | M05.442 | M90.542 | |
| I70.361 | I70.548 | I70.743 | K51.413 | M02.321 | M05.449 | M90.549 | |
| I70.362 | I70.549 | I70.744 | K51.414 | M02.322 | M05.451 | M90.551 | |
| I70.363 | I70.561 | I70.748 | K51.512 | M02.329 | M05.452 | M90.552 | |

## Principal Diagnoses That Are Their Own MCC

| | | | | | | | |
|---|---|---|---|---|---|---|---|
| A22.7 | B44.0 | L89.004 | L89.133 | L89.224 | L89.513 | L89.814 | S06.1X5A |
| A26.7 | B45.1 | L89.013 | L89.134 | L89.303 | L89.514 | L89.893 | S06.1X6A |
| A32.7 | B77.81 | L89.014 | L89.143 | L89.304 | L89.523 | L89.894 | S06.1X7A |
| A37.01 | I26.01 | L89.023 | L89.144 | L89.313 | L89.524 | L89.93 | S06.1X8A |
| A37.11 | I26.02 | L89.024 | L89.153 | L89.314 | L89.603 | L89.94 | S06.1X9A |
| A37.81 | I26.09 | L89.103 | L89.154 | L89.323 | L89.604 | R65.21 | |
| A37.91 | K70.41 | L89.104 | L89.203 | L89.324 | L89.613 | S06.1X0A | |
| A54.86 | K71.11 | L89.113 | L89.204 | L89.43 | L89.614 | S06.1X1A | |
| B25.0 | K72.01 | L89.114 | L89.213 | L89.44 | L89.623 | S06.1X2A | |
| B25.2 | K72.11 | L89.123 | L89.214 | L89.503 | L89.624 | S06.1X3A | |
| B37.7 | L89.003 | L89.124 | L89.223 | L89.504 | L89.813 | S06.1X4A | |

Present-on-admission (POA) indicators are required on all diagnoses and external cause-of-injury codes for all inpatient acute care hospital discharges, according to the requirement outlined in the Deficit Reduction Act of 2005, section 5001(c). The only exception is for a select group of codes that have been designated as exempt from the POA regulations. Certain facilities are also exempt from this reporting requirement and include the following:

- Critical access hospitals
- Long-term care hospitals
- Cancer hospitals
- Inpatient psychiatric hospitals
- Inpatient rehabilitation facilities
- Veterans Administration/Department of Defense Hospitals
- Children's inpatient facilities

The POA indicator guidelines are not intended to replace the official *ICD-10-CM Official Guidelines for Coding and Reporting*. Nor will the POA guidelines supersede the Uniform Hospital Discharge Data Set (UHDDS) definition of principal diagnosis, defined as the condition established after study to be chiefly responsible for occasioning the admission of the patient to the hospital. The definition of "additional diagnoses" also remains the same. Coders must report all conditions that coexist at the time of admission, develop subsequently, or that affect the treatment received and/or the length of stay. This significantly affects assignment of the POA indicators. Because the POA indicator should accurately reflect the patient's conditions upon admission as well as POA guidelines, review of POA guidelines in the *ICD-10-CM Official Guidelines for Coding and Reporting* is required.

The following is a summary of the POA guidelines:

- A POA condition is defined not only as one that is clearly present at the time of admission, but also one that was clearly present but not diagnosed until after the time of admission.

- Present on admission is defined as present at the time the order for an inpatient admission is made, whether or not the patient's episode of care originated in the emergency department, ambulatory surgery area, or other outpatient area. Conditions that develop during an outpatient encounter are considered present on admission.

- A POA indicator is assigned to the principal diagnosis, secondary diagnoses, and the external cause-of-injury codes.

- The POA guidelines are not intended to replace any of the other *ICD-10-CM Official Guidelines for Coding and Reporting*.

- The intent of the POA guidelines is not to determine whether or not a condition should be coded, but rather how to apply the POA indicator.

The following reporting options, with definitions, should be used to indicate whether a condition was POA:

Y    *Yes: Present at the time of inpatient admission*

N    *No: Not present at the time of inpatient admission*

U    *Unknown: Documentation is insufficient to determine if condition is present at the time of inpatient admission*

W    *Clinically undetermined: Provider is unable to clinically determine whether condition was or was not present at the time of inpatient admission*

*Unreported/not used—(exempt from POA reporting)—Most ICD-10-CM codes require the assignment of a POA indicator. However, there are some diagnoses that are considered exempt from the POA reporting. For these exempt conditions the POA field should be left blank.*

**Note:** A data file of all POA exempt codes can be accessed at the following: http://www.optum360coding.com/ProdcutUpdates/ Title: "2018 ICD-10-CM for Hospitals POA Exemption Data File" Password: OptumPOAExempt18

## Timeframe for POA identification and documentation

There is no timeframe during the encounter in which a condition must be diagnosed to be considered present on admission. In many cases, it is not clinically possible for the provider to determine a definitive diagnosis until well into the admission, after labs, imaging, and other tests have been performed and results examined. In these cases the condition is still considered to be present on admission, indicated with Y.

*Examples*

- A patient was admitted for diagnostic work-up for cachexia. The final diagnosis was malignant neoplasm of lung with metastasis.

  *Assign Y in the POA field for the malignant neoplasm, which was clearly present on admission, although it was not diagnosed until after the admission occurred.*

- A patient with severe cough and difficulty breathing was diagnosed during his hospitalization to have lung cancer.

  *Assign Y in the POA field for the lung cancer. Even though the cancer was not diagnosed until after admission, it is a chronic condition that was clearly present before the patient's admission.*

- A urine culture was obtained on admission. The provider documented urinary tract infection when the culture results became available a few days later.

  *Assign Y to the urinary tract infection since the diagnosis is based on test results from a specimen obtained on admission. It may not be possible for a provider to make a definitive diagnosis for a period of time after admission. There is no required timeframe as to when a provider must identify or document a condition for it to be considered present on admission.*

## Condition is on the "Exempt from Reporting" list

Several codes are exempt from POA reporting. A detailed list of codes can be found as an official download at http://www.cms.gov/Medicare/Coding/ICD10/Downloads/2017-POA-Exempt-List.zip. The POA field is left blank for codes excluded from POA reporting.

*Examples*

- A patient was admitted for inpatient surgery on a burn contracture from scar tissue from a burn five years ago.

  *Assign Y for the principal condition of the scar; however, the secondary code for the specifics of the burn injury with a seventh character for sequela is left blank since it is excluded from POA reporting.*

- A patient was admitted to inpatient for a PEG tube insertion because of residual dysphagia due to a recent CVA.

  *No POA indicator is assigned for the dysphagia following a CVA. Codes under I69.- are defined as sequela of cerebrovascular disease and are exempt from POA reporting.*

- A patient was admitted to inpatient for corrective surgery for a malunion of a closed femur fracture.

  *No POA indicator is assigned for the malunion of a closed fracture because the seventh character for malunion of fractures is considered a subsequent encounter and is exempt from POA reporting.*

- A patient was admitted for breast reconstruction following mastectomy.

  *The POA indicator field is left blank as this Z code is exempt from POA reporting.*

- A patient was admitted for changing the battery in his AICD as it is at the end of its useful life.

  *The POA indicator field is left blank as this Z code is exempt from POA reporting.*

## POA explicitly documented

If the provider explicitly documents a condition as being present on admission or not present on admission, assign the appropriate Y or N POA indicator based on that documentation. If there is conflicting documentation by different providers, query the attending physician.

*Examples*

- Even though sepsis is not diagnosed in the ED, the discharge summary states that the patient presented with sepsis at the time of admission.

  *The provider explicitly stated that the sepsis was present on admission and therefore the Y POA indicator should be used.*

- The patient was admitted with chills and cough and two days later diagnosed with pneumonia. The discharge summary documents that the pneumonia was not present on admission.

  *Although the patient showed some symptoms of pneumonia on admission, the provider may have clinical evidence (e.g., chest x-rays, cultures) that indicates that pneumonia did not develop until after admission. Since this was explicitly stated in the discharge summary, the appropriate POA indicator is N.*

- A consult note states that a patient came in with renal failure while the discharge summary states that the renal failure was not present on admission.

*When in doubt and there is conflicting documentation, query the attending physician.*

## Conditions diagnosed prior to inpatient admission

Conditions that were diagnosed prior to admission—for example, chronic conditions such as hypertension, diabetes, and asthma—are assigned the POA indicator of Y. A tip to help establish that a condition was POA is to check the patient's medication history for drugs that are routinely prescribed for these types of chronic conditions.

### Examples

- The history and physical states that the patient has a history of hypertension and seizure disorder, and it is noted that the patient is currently on Atenolol and Dilantin.

  *The hypertension and seizure disorder existed prior to admission; therefore, the appropriate POA indicator is Y. Verification that the patient is on long-term use of Atenolol and Dilantin can help solidify that these conditions are currently being treated.*

- A 56-year-old male was admitted as an inpatient for multi-trauma wounds. Because the patient was unconscious on admission, his medical history was unknown. A progress note two days into the stay noted that the patient was on Metformin for history of type 2 diabetes.

  *The timeframe of the diagnosis is irrelevant to POA. Even though it was not discovered until two days into the encounter that the patient had a history of DM2, the DM2 was still present prior to this admission and would be identified as such with the Y POA indicator.*

- A patient was admitted to an inpatient facility from the ED. The admitting provider indicated that the patient had a current history of lung cancer and chronic kidney disease.

  *Both of these conditions are indicated with Y, present on admission.*

- During the course of an eight-day inpatient stay with surgery, a patient was diagnosed postoperatively with hypertension and discharged on Metoprolol.

  *The hypertension was not diagnosed prior to admission and would be reported with an N POA indicator.*

## Conditions diagnosed during the admission but clearly present before admission

The POA indicator Y is assigned for conditions that clearly presented with applicable signs and symptoms but may have not been definitively diagnosed until later on, or even at the end of the encounter. Even if the presenting diagnosis was documented on admission as suspected, possible, or rule out, or written as a differential diagnosis and later confirmed, it is still considered present on admission.

### Examples

- A patient was admitted with jaundice, fatigue, and mental confusion. Differential diagnosis on admission lists possible liver failure. The definitive diagnosis of liver failure is not made until two days after admission.

  *Assign Y to the liver failure since the symptoms were present on admission and the differential diagnosis listed "possible" liver failure on admission even though the final diagnosis was two days later.*

- An aid worker recently returned from Afghanistan presents to the ED with hematemesis, chest pain, and fever. Patient is put into inpatient isolation with suspected TB documented on the H & P. TB is confirmed the next day.

  *The POA indicator Y is assigned because, even though the TB was only "suspected" on admission, it was confirmed the next day.*

## Condition develops during outpatient encounter prior to inpatient admission

Assign Y for any condition that develops during an outpatient encounter such as same-day surgery, observation, or extended recovery prior to a written order for inpatient admission. This also pertains to conditions that develop in facilities such as transitional care units, skilled nursing homes, long-term care, hospice, or rehabilitation facilities with the patient transferring to inpatient hospital admission.

### Examples

- A patient underwent outpatient surgery. During the recovery period, the patient developed atrial fibrillation and was subsequently admitted to the hospital as an inpatient.

*Assign Y on the POA field for the atrial fibrillation since it developed prior to a written order for inpatient admission.*

- A patient was treated in observation and while in observation fell out of bed and broke a hip. The patient was subsequently admitted as an inpatient to treat the hip fracture.

  *Assign Y on the POA field for the hip fracture since it developed prior to a written order for inpatient admission.*

- An elderly patient underwent outpatient surgery with plans to go home after the surgery. In recovery, the patient developed shortness of breath, chest pain, and fever. A sputum sample was taken, and the surgeon decided to admit the patient to inpatient. The next day the patient was diagnosed with staphylococcal pneumonia based on sputum results and admitting chest x-ray.

  *Assign Y to the staphylococcal pneumonia even though it was not diagnosed until the day following the admission. Even though the patient had undergone outpatient surgery, the sputum sample, signs, and symptoms were evident prior to the inpatient admission.*

## Documentation does not indicate whether condition was present on admission

If the documentation in the medical record is unclear as to the presence of a condition on admission, assign a U for unknown. This should be used sparingly and, if possible, the physician should be queried for further clarification.

### Example

- A wheelchair-bound patient was admitted in respiratory failure from a long-term care facility to an inpatient hospital with severe aspiration pneumonia. A progress note three days into the admission listed a pressure ulcer stage 2 on the lower back.

  *Assign U for the stage 2 pressure ulcer if unknown whether it was present on admission. Since the patient was wheelchair-bound and critically ill on admission, it is possible that the ulcer was present and not immediately addressed. The admitting physician can be queried to clarify, or a U is assigned if that is not possible.*

## Documentation states it cannot be determined whether the condition was or was not present on admission

A W is assigned when the documentation states that it cannot be clinically determined whether the condition was POA or not.

### Examples

- An elderly patient was admitted with multi-trauma injuries from a motor vehicle accident. Two days into the admission, a urinary tract infection was diagnosed. No labs or urine cultures had been taken on admission as focus was stabilization from traumatic wounds. Documentation from the provider in a progress note stated that it was not clinically possible to determine whether the UTI was present on admission.

  *Assign W for the UTI as it was specifically stated that it was not clinically possible to determine whether it was present on admission.*

- A patient was admitted with high fever and pneumonia. The patient rapidly deteriorated and became septic. The discharge diagnosis listed sepsis and pneumonia. The documentation was unclear as to whether the sepsis was present on admission or developed shortly after admission.

  *Query the physician as to whether the sepsis was present on admission, developed shortly after admission, or it cannot be clinically determined as to whether it was or was not present on admission.*

## Chronic condition with acute exacerbation during the admission

If a single code identifies only the chronic condition and not the acute exacerbation, assign Y. For instance, when there is no code for the acute exacerbation of a chronic condition as in acute exacerbation of chronic leukemia, the Y is assigned for the chronic leukemia.

For a single combination code that identifies both the chronic and acute exacerbation, see the combination code instructions.

*Example*

- Documentation on admission stated that the patient had chronic myelomonocytic leukemia. A progress note three days into the stay stated that the patient had, since admission, developed an acute exacerbation of his myelomonocytic leukemia.

  *There is no code for an acute exacerbation of chronic myelomonocytic leukemia; therefore, assign Y since the chronic leukemia (either not specified as in remission, or in relapse) is represented by a single code and was present on admission.*

## Acute and chronic conditions

Assign Y to acute conditions present on admission and N to acute conditions not present at the time of admission.

Assign Y to conditions specified as chronic, even though they may not be diagnosed until after admission.

See the POA guideline "Codes that contain multiple clinical concepts" for a single code that identifies both the acute and chronic condition.

*Examples*

- A patient was admitted to the hospital for coronary artery bypass surgery. Postoperatively he developed a pulmonary embolism.

  *Assign N in the POA field for the pulmonary embolism. This is an acute condition that was not present on admission.*
- A patient admitted with sepsis due to pneumonia with acute respiratory failure, developed acute renal failure on day three.

  *Assign Y for the sepsis, pneumonia, and acute respiratory failure, which were all acute conditions, present on admission. Assign N for the acute renal failure; even though it is an acute condition, it was not present until after the patient was admitted.*
- A patient admitted with hypoglycemia, weakness, confusion, and slurred speech was diagnosed the next day with type 2 diabetes.

  *Assign Y to the type 2 diabetes since it is a chronic condition that was present on admission, even though it was not diagnosed until the next day.*

## Codes that contain multiple clinical concepts

If at least one of the clinical concepts included in a code was not present on admission, assign N. If all the clinical concepts included in a code are present on admission, assign Y.

*Examples*

- Patient has history of gastrojejunal ulcer which started bleeding two days into the encounter.

  *Assign a POA indicator of N to chronic gastrojejunal ulcer with bleeding; although the gastrojejunal ulcer is a chronic condition that was present at the time of admission, the bleeding did not occur until after the admission.*
- A patient with chronic diastolic heart failure decompensated after admission.

  *Assign N to the code for acute on chronic diastolic (congestive) heart failure. Although the heart failure was present on admission, the acute decompensation of the failure was not.*
- A patient with viral hepatitis B progressed to hepatic coma after admission.

  *Assign N for the viral hepatitis B with hepatic coma because a condition described by part of the code description did not develop until after admission.*
- A patient with known systolic congestive heart failure was admitted to the hospital with decompensated systolic heart failure.

  *Assign Y in the POA field for the acute on chronic systolic (congestive) heart failure as both the chronic and acute parts of the condition were present on admission.*

Assign Y for infection codes that include the organism if the infection was present on admission even though the culture results are not available until after admission.

*Example*

- A patient was septic on admission with blood, sputum, and urine cultures taken. Two days later, *E. coli* was determined to be the causal organism.

  *Assign Y even though the test results were not confirmed until after admission.*

## Conditions documented as possible, probable, suspected, or rule out at the time of discharge or conditions documented as impending or threatened at the time of discharge

If the final diagnosis contains language identifying a condition as possible, probable, suspected, or rule out, or as an impending or threatened diagnosis but the diagnosis is based on signs and symptoms that were present on admission, the POA indicator is Y. If those signs and symptoms were not present on admission, the appropriate POA indicator is N.

*Examples*

- A patient underwent inpatient surgery, after which the patient developed fever and was treated aggressively. The physician's final diagnosis documented "possible postoperative infection following surgery."

  *Assign N on the POA field for the postoperative infection since final diagnoses that contain the terms "possible," "probable," "suspected," or "rule out" and that are based on symptoms or clinical findings that were not present on admission should be reported as N.*
- A patient with prior cardiac intervention history was admitted with chest pain. After two days, the chest pain diminished with no underlying cause found. The discharge summary stated, "Suspected costochondritis or coronary artery spasm. Pain resolved. Follow up at regular cardiology office visit."

  *Since the chest pain was present on admission, both suspected conditions of costochondritis and coronary artery spasm are represented by the POA indicator of Y.*
- A patient was admitted with a known history of coronary atherosclerosis, status post myocardial infarction five years ago, and was then admitted for treatment of impending myocardial infarction. The patient was transferred to a larger facility with a cath lab. The final diagnosis was documented as "impending myocardial infarction."

  *Assign Y to the impending myocardial infarction because the condition is present on admission.*

## Same diagnosis code for two or more conditions

When two or more separate conditions are classified to the same diagnosis code in the same encounter, assign Y if all conditions represented by the single code were present on admission and N if any of the conditions were not present on admission.

*Examples*

- A patient was admitted with diabetes type 2 with ketoacidosis.

  *Assign Y since both the diabetes and ketoacidosis were present on admission.*
- A patient involved in a car accident was admitted with hemorrhage to the abdomen secondary to the trauma; shortly after being admitted the patient also developed a seroma as a result of the trauma.

  *The secondary traumatic hemorrhage was present on admission, and the traumatic seroma did not develop until after admission. Both of these conditions are classified to one code, but because both conditions were not present when the patient was admitted, a POA of N should be assigned.*

## Obstetrical conditions

The POA assignment for obstetrical conditions is not affected by whether the patient delivers during the encounter but rather by whether the pregnancy complication was or was not present at the time of admission. If two or more conditions are classified to a single code, all conditions represented by that single code must be present on admission to correctly assign a Y. If all conditions are not present at the time of admission, the appropriate POA indicator is N. Several obstetrics codes are listed in the POA exclusion list; for obstetrics codes that are not on the exclusion list, all applicable POA guidelines apply.

*Examples*

- A female patient was admitted to the hospital and underwent a normal delivery.

  *Leave the "present on admission" (POA) field blank. Code O80 Normal delivery, is on the "exempt from reporting" list.*
- A patient was admitted in late pregnancy due to excessive vomiting and dehydration. During admission, the patient went into premature labor.

  *Assign Y for the excessive vomiting and the dehydration. Assign N for the premature labor.*

- A patient was admitted in active labor. During the stay, a breast abscess was noted when the mother attempted to breastfeed. The provider was unable to clinically determine whether the abscess was present on admission.

  *Assign W for the breast abscess since the provider was unable to clinically determine whether the abscess was present on admission.*

- A patient was admitted in active labor. After 12 hours of labor, it was noted that the infant was in fetal distress, and a cesarean section was performed.

  *Assign N for the fetal distress even if it is used for the principal diagnosis, since it did not develop until later in the admission. In obstetrics cases, the principal diagnosis may have a POA indicator of N.*

## Perinatal and congenital conditions

Newborns are not considered admitted until after birth; therefore all conditions that develop in utero, occur during delivery, or are present at birth are represented by the POA indicator Y. Any conditions that develop after birth and admission are represented by N.

All congenital conditions and anomalies not found in chapter 17 should have a POA indicator of Y assigned. Chapter 17 codes in categories Q00–Q99 are exempt from POA reporting. All congenital conditions, regardless of the coding chapter to which they are assigned, are considered present on admission.

### Examples

- A single liveborn infant was delivered in the hospital via cesarean section. The physician documented fetal bradycardia during labor as the final diagnosis in the newborn record.

  *Assign Y because the bradycardia developed prior to the newborn admission (birth).*

- A newborn developed diarrhea, which was believed to be due to the hospital baby formula.

  *Assign N because the diarrhea developed after admission.*

- A newborn was diagnosed with cephalhematoma due to birth injury.

  *Assign Y because the injury occurred during delivery.*

- A newborn was diagnosed with congenital pneumonia.

  *Assign Y for the congenital pneumonia. Congenital conditions from chapter 16 are always considered present on admission and require the POA indicator.*

- A newborn was diagnosed with congenital hydrocephalus.

  *There should be no POA indicator assigned. This condition is coded in chapter 17 and is excluded from POA reporting.*

- A 10-year-old boy was admitted for complications of spina bifida with hydrocephalus.

  *No POA indicator is assigned. This condition is coded in chapter 17 and is excluded from POA reporting.*

## External cause and injury codes

If an injury or poisoning occurred prior to or at the time of admission and the seventh character indicates an initial encounter or active treatment, the code for the injury/poisoning is reported with POA indicator Y. Injury and poisoning codes S00–T88 with the seventh character indicating subsequent or sequela are exempt from POA indicators since, in order to be a subsequent or sequela encounter, the condition must have occurred before the admission. Many of the external causes of morbidity codes from chapters V, W, and X are also exempt from POA reporting when the seventh character of S or D, representing subsequent or sequela encounters, are used.

Coders should be extremely careful in assigning the appropriate POA indicator if a patient suffers an injury while an inpatient. For example, if a patient falls from the hospital bed and fractures a hip, the codes representing that injury (along with the appropriate initial-encounter seventh character) should be assigned N for the corresponding POA indicator.

### Examples

- A 12-year-old was admitted for treatment of fractured arm from falling out of a tree house.

  *The injury itself and the cause of the injury are both assigned a Y POA indicator.* **Note:** *The injury code and external cause code POA indicators should always match.*

- A patient admitted for pneumonia sustained a laceration of the right arm after falling and hitting his arm against a cart in the hospital room, requiring stitches.

  *Assign N for the laceration for the right arm because it was not present on admission. The external cause code POA indicator should also be N.*

- A patient was admitted for manipulation of a knee contracture due to a scar from a burn injury 10 years ago.

  *Assign Y for the code for the scar, but leave blank the POA indicator for the burn injury with the seventh character of S for sequela. Sequela and subsequent-encounter codes in chapter 19 are exempt from POA reporting.*

# Appendix I: Hospital Acquired Conditions

Hospital-acquired conditions (HACs) are conditions considered reasonably preventable through the application of evidence-based guidelines. These conditions, in and of themselves, are either a complication or comorbidity (CC) or major complication or comorbidity (MCC) that as a secondary diagnosis will move the MS-DRG assignment from a lower-paying MS-DRG to a higher-paying MS-DRG. However, if these conditions are not present on admission (meaning they developed during the hospital stay), the CC or MCC designation is nullified and the case will not group to the higher-paying MS-DRG based solely upon the reporting of the HAC code.

HACs are grouped into 14 categories. ICD-10-CM codes in the tabular section of this book that are grouped to one of these HAC categories are identified by an icon specific to that category. As many of these HACs are conditional, this resource provides any additional stipulations that may be required before the code can be considered a HAC. For example, code I26.02 has an **H10** indicating it falls in the HAC 10 category for Deep Vein Thrombosis (DVT) or Pulmonary Embolism (PE) with Total Knee or Hip Replacement. However I26.02 is not, by itself, a HAC there must also be a specific ICD-10-PCS code, such as ØSR9Ø19 Replacement of Right Hip Joint with Metal Synthetic Substitute, Cemented, Open Approach, applied in order for I26.02 to act as a HAC.

**Note:** The resource used to compile this list is the fiscal 2017 ICD-10 MS-DRG Definitions Manual Files v34. The most current version, v35, of ICD-10 MS-DRG Definitions Manual was not available at the time this book was printed. For the most current files related to IPPS please refer to the following: https://www.cms.gov/Medicare/Medicare-Fee-for-Service-Payment/AcuteInpatientPPS/IPPS-Regulations-and-Notices.html.

**HAC 01: Foreign Object Retained After Surgery**
Secondary diagnosis not POA:

T81.5ØØA
T81.5Ø1A
T81.5Ø2A
T81.5Ø3A
T81.5Ø4A
T81.5Ø5A
T81.5Ø6A
T81.5Ø7A
T81.5Ø8A
T81.5Ø9A
T81.51ØA
T81.511A
T81.512A
T81.513A
T81.514A
T81.515A
T81.516A
T81.517A
T81.518A
T81.519A
T81.52ØA
T81.521A
T81.522A
T81.523A
T81.524A
T81.525A
T81.526A
T81.527A
T81.528A
T81.529A
T81.53ØA
T81.531A
T81.532A
T81.533A
T81.534A
T81.535A
T81.536A
T81.537A
T81.538A
T81.539A
T81.59ØA
T81.591A
T81.592A
T81.593A
T81.594A
T81.595A
T81.596A
T81.597A
T81.598A
T81.599A
T81.6ØXA
T81.61XA
T81.69XA

**HAC 02: Air Embolism**
Secondary diagnosis not POA:

T8Ø.ØXXA

**HAC 03: Blood Incompatibility**
Secondary diagnosis not POA:

T8Ø.3ØXA
T8Ø.31ØA
T8Ø.311A
T8Ø.319A
T8Ø.39XA

**HAC 04: Stage III and IV Pressure Ulcers**
Secondary diagnosis not POA:

L89.ØØ3
L89.ØØ4
L89.Ø13
L89.Ø14
L89.Ø23
L89.Ø24
L89.1Ø3
L89.1Ø4
L89.113
L89.114
L89.123
L89.124
L89.133
L89.134
L89.143
L89.144
L89.153
L89.154
L89.2Ø3
L89.2Ø4
L89.213
L89.214
L89.223
L89.224
L89.3Ø3
L89.3Ø4
L89.313
L89.314
L89.323
L89.324
L89.43
L89.44
L89.5Ø3
L89.5Ø4
L89.513
L89.514
L89.523
L89.524
L89.6Ø3
L89.6Ø4
L89.613
L89.614
L89.623
L89.624
L89.813
L89.814
L89.893
L89.894
L89.93
L89.94

**HAC 05: Falls and Trauma**
Secondary diagnosis not POA:

M99.1Ø
M99.11
M99.18
SØ2.ØXXA
SØ2.ØXXB
SØ2.1Ø1A
SØ2.1Ø1B
SØ2.1Ø2A
SØ2.1Ø2B
SØ2.1Ø9A
SØ2.1Ø9B
SØ2.11ØA
SØ2.11ØB
SØ2.111A
SØ2.111B
SØ2.112A
SØ2.112B
SØ2.113A
SØ2.113B
SØ2.118A
SØ2.118B
SØ2.119A
SØ2.119B
SØ2.11AA
SØ2.11AB
SØ2.11BA
SØ2.11BB
SØ2.11CA
SØ2.11CB
SØ2.11DA
SØ2.11DB
SØ2.11EA
SØ2.11EB
SØ2.11FA
SØ2.11FB
SØ2.11GA
SØ2.11GB
SØ2.11HA
SØ2.11HB
SØ2.19XA
SØ2.19XB
SØ2.2XXB
SØ2.3ØXA
SØ2.3ØXB
SØ2.31XA
SØ2.31XB
SØ2.32XA
SØ2.32XB
SØ2.4ØØA
SØ2.4ØØB
SØ2.4Ø1A
SØ2.4Ø1B
SØ2.4Ø2A
SØ2.4Ø2B
SØ2.4ØAA
SØ2.4ØAB
SØ2.4ØBA
SØ2.4ØBB
SØ2.4ØCA
SØ2.4ØCB
SØ2.4ØDA
SØ2.4ØDB
SØ2.4ØEA
SØ2.4ØEB
SØ2.4ØFA
SØ2.4ØFB
SØ2.411A
SØ2.411B
SØ2.412A
SØ2.412B
SØ2.413A
SØ2.413B
SØ2.42XA
SØ2.42XB
SØ2.6ØØA
SØ2.6ØØB
SØ2.6Ø1A
SØ2.6Ø1B
SØ2.6Ø2A
SØ2.6Ø2B
SØ2.6Ø9A
SØ2.6Ø9B
SØ2.61ØA
SØ2.61ØB
SØ2.611A
SØ2.611B
SØ2.612A
SØ2.612B
SØ2.62ØA
SØ2.62ØB
SØ2.621A
SØ2.621B
SØ2.622A
SØ2.622B
SØ2.63ØA
SØ2.63ØB
SØ2.631A
SØ2.631B
SØ2.632A
SØ2.632B
SØ2.64ØA
SØ2.64ØB
SØ2.641A
SØ2.641B
SØ2.642A
SØ2.642B
SØ2.65ØA
SØ2.65ØB
SØ2.651A
SØ2.651B
SØ2.652A
SØ2.652B
SØ2.66XA
SØ2.66XB
SØ2.67ØA
SØ2.67ØB
SØ2.671A
SØ2.671B
SØ2.672A
SØ2.672B
SØ2.69XA
SØ2.69XB
SØ2.8ØXA
SØ2.8ØXB
SØ2.81XA
SØ2.81XB
SØ2.82XA
SØ2.82XB
SØ2.91XA
SØ2.91XB
SØ2.92XA
SØ2.92XB
SØ6.ØX1A
SØ6.ØX9A
SØ6.1X1A
SØ6.1X2A
SØ6.1X3A
SØ6.1X4A
SØ6.1X5A
SØ6.1X6A
SØ6.1X7A
SØ6.1X8A
SØ6.1X9A
SØ6.2X1A
SØ6.2X2A
SØ6.2X3A
SØ6.2X4A
SØ6.2X5A
SØ6.2X6A
SØ6.2X7A
SØ6.2X8A
SØ6.2X9A
SØ6.3Ø1A
SØ6.3Ø2A
SØ6.3Ø3A
SØ6.3Ø4A
SØ6.3Ø5A
SØ6.3Ø6A
SØ6.3Ø7A
SØ6.3Ø8A
SØ6.3Ø9A
SØ6.31ØA
SØ6.311A
SØ6.312A
SØ6.313A
SØ6.314A
SØ6.315A
SØ6.316A
SØ6.317A
SØ6.318A
SØ6.319A
SØ6.32ØA
SØ6.321A
SØ6.322A
SØ6.323A
SØ6.324A
SØ6.325A
SØ6.326A
SØ6.327A
SØ6.328A
SØ6.329A
SØ6.33ØA
SØ6.331A
SØ6.332A
SØ6.333A
SØ6.334A
SØ6.335A
SØ6.336A
SØ6.337A
SØ6.338A
SØ6.339A
SØ6.34ØA
SØ6.341A
SØ6.342A
SØ6.343A
SØ6.344A
SØ6.345A
SØ6.346A
SØ6.347A
SØ6.348A
SØ6.349A
SØ6.35ØA
SØ6.351A
SØ6.352A
SØ6.353A
SØ6.354A
SØ6.355A
SØ6.356A
SØ6.357A
SØ6.358A
SØ6.359A
SØ6.36ØA
SØ6.361A

**HAC 05: Falls and Trauma (continued)**

| | | | | | |
|---|---|---|---|---|---|
| S06.362A | S06.829A | S12.231A | S12.650B | S22.009A | S22.082B |
| S06.363A | S06.891A | S12.231B | S12.651A | S22.009B | S22.088A |
| S06.364A | S06.892A | S12.24XA | S12.651B | S22.010A | S22.088B |
| S06.365A | S06.893A | S12.24XB | S12.690A | S22.010B | S22.089A |
| S06.366A | S06.894A | S12.250A | S12.690B | S22.011A | S22.089B |
| S06.367A | S06.895A | S12.250B | S12.691A | S22.011B | S22.20XA |
| S06.368A | S06.896A | S12.251A | S12.691B | S22.012A | S22.20XB |
| S06.369A | S06.897A | S12.251B | S12.8XXA | S22.012B | S22.21XA |
| S06.370A | S06.898A | S12.290A | S12.9XXA | S22.018A | S22.21XB |
| S06.371A | S06.899A | S12.290B | S13.0XXA | S22.018B | S22.22XA |
| S06.372A | S06.9X1A | S12.291A | S13.100A | S22.019A | S22.22XB |
| S06.373A | S06.9X2A | S12.291B | S13.101A | S22.019B | S22.23XA |
| S06.374A | S06.9X3A | S12.300A | S13.110A | S22.020A | S22.23XB |
| S06.375A | S06.9X4A | S12.300B | S13.111A | S22.020B | S22.24XA |
| S06.376A | S06.9X5A | S12.301A | S13.120A | S22.021A | S22.24XB |
| S06.377A | S06.9X6A | S12.301B | S13.121A | S22.021B | S22.31XA |
| S06.378A | S06.9X7A | S12.330A | S13.130A | S22.022A | S22.31XB |
| S06.379A | S06.9X8A | S12.330B | S13.131A | S22.022B | S22.32XA |
| S06.380A | S06.9X9A | S12.331A | S13.140A | S22.028A | S22.32XB |
| S06.381A | S07.0XXA | S12.331B | S13.141A | S22.028B | S22.39XA |
| S06.382A | S07.1XXA | S12.34XA | S13.150A | S22.029A | S22.39XB |
| S06.383A | S07.8XXA | S12.34XB | S13.151A | S22.029B | S22.41XA |
| S06.384A | S07.9XXA | S12.350A | S13.160A | S22.030A | S22.41XB |
| S06.385A | S12.000A | S12.350B | S13.161A | S22.030B | S22.42XA |
| S06.386A | S12.000B | S12.351A | S13.170A | S22.031A | S22.42XB |
| S06.387A | S12.001A | S12.351B | S13.171A | S22.031B | S22.43XA |
| S06.388A | S12.001B | S12.390A | S13.180A | S22.032A | S22.43XB |
| S06.389A | S12.01XA | S12.390B | S13.181A | S22.032B | S22.49XA |
| S06.4X0A | S12.01XB | S12.391A | S13.20XA | S22.038A | S22.49XB |
| S06.4X1A | S12.02XA | S12.391B | S13.29XA | S22.038B | S22.5XXA |
| S06.4X2A | S12.02XB | S12.400A | S14.101A | S22.039A | S22.5XXB |
| S06.4X3A | S12.030A | S12.400B | S14.102A | S22.039B | S22.9XXA |
| S06.4X4A | S12.030B | S12.401A | S14.103A | S22.040A | S22.9XXB |
| S06.4X5A | S12.031A | S12.401B | S14.104A | S22.040B | S24.101A |
| S06.4X6A | S12.031B | S12.430A | S14.105A | S22.041A | S24.102A |
| S06.4X7A | S12.040A | S12.430B | S14.106A | S22.041B | S24.103A |
| S06.4X8A | S12.040B | S12.431A | S14.107A | S22.042A | S24.104A |
| S06.4X9A | S12.041A | S12.431B | S14.109A | S22.042B | S24.109A |
| S06.5X0A | S12.041B | S12.44XA | S14.111A | S22.048A | S24.111A |
| S06.5X1A | S12.090A | S12.44XB | S14.112A | S22.048B | S24.112A |
| S06.5X2A | S12.090B | S12.450A | S14.113A | S22.049A | S24.113A |
| S06.5X3A | S12.091A | S12.450B | S14.114A | S22.049B | S24.114A |
| S06.5X4A | S12.091B | S12.451A | S14.115A | S22.050A | S24.131A |
| S06.5X5A | S12.100A | S12.451B | S14.116A | S22.050B | S24.132A |
| S06.5X6A | S12.100B | S12.490A | S14.117A | S22.051A | S24.133A |
| S06.5X7A | S12.101A | S12.490B | S14.121A | S22.051B | S24.134A |
| S06.5X8A | S12.101B | S12.491A | S14.122A | S22.052A | S24.151A |
| S06.5X9A | S12.110A | S12.491B | S14.123A | S22.052B | S24.152A |
| S06.6X0A | S12.110B | S12.500A | S14.124A | S22.058A | S24.153A |
| S06.6X1A | S12.111A | S12.500B | S14.125A | S22.058B | S24.154A |
| S06.6X2A | S12.111B | S12.501A | S14.126A | S22.059A | S32.000A |
| S06.6X3A | S12.112A | S12.501B | S14.127A | S22.059B | S32.000B |
| S06.6X4A | S12.112B | S12.530A | S14.131A | S22.060A | S32.001A |
| S06.6X5A | S12.120A | S12.530B | S14.132A | S22.060B | S32.001B |
| S06.6X6A | S12.120B | S12.531A | S14.133A | S22.061A | S32.002A |
| S06.6X7A | S12.121A | S12.531B | S14.134A | S22.061B | S32.002B |
| S06.6X8A | S12.121B | S12.54XA | S14.135A | S22.062A | S32.008A |
| S06.6X9A | S12.130A | S12.54XB | S14.136A | S22.062B | S32.008B |
| S06.811A | S12.130B | S12.550A | S14.137A | S22.068A | S32.009A |
| S06.812A | S12.131A | S12.550B | S14.151A | S22.068B | S32.009B |
| S06.813A | S12.131B | S12.551A | S14.152A | S22.069A | S32.010A |
| S06.814A | S12.14XA | S12.551B | S14.153A | S22.069B | S32.010B |
| S06.815A | S12.14XB | S12.590A | S14.154A | S22.070A | S32.011A |
| S06.816A | S12.150A | S12.590B | S14.155A | S22.070B | S32.011B |
| S06.817A | S12.150B | S12.591A | S14.156A | S22.071A | S32.012A |
| S06.818A | S12.151A | S12.591B | S14.157A | S22.071B | S32.012B |
| S06.819A | S12.151B | S12.600A | S17.0XXA | S22.072A | S32.018A |
| S06.821A | S12.190A | S12.600B | S17.8XXA | S22.072B | S32.018B |
| S06.822A | S12.190B | S12.601A | S17.9XXA | S22.078A | S32.019A |
| S06.823A | S12.191A | S12.601B | S22.000A | S22.078B | S32.019B |
| S06.824A | S12.191B | S12.630A | S22.000B | S22.079A | S32.020A |
| S06.825A | S12.200A | S12.630B | S22.001A | S22.079B | S32.020B |
| S06.826A | S12.200B | S12.631A | S22.001B | S22.080A | S32.021A |
| S06.827A | S12.201A | S12.631B | S22.002A | S22.080B | S32.021B |
| S06.828A | S12.201B | S12.64XA | S22.002B | S22.081A | S32.022A |
| | S12.230A | S12.64XB | S22.008A | S22.081B | S32.022B |
| | S12.230B | S12.650A | S22.008B | S22.082A | S32.028A |

## HAC 05: Falls and Trauma (continued)

| | | | | |
|---|---|---|---|---|
| S32.028B | S32.309A | S32.452B | S32.612A | S42.113B | S42.253A |
| S32.029A | S32.309B | S32.453A | S32.612B | S42.114B | S42.253B |
| S32.029B | S32.311A | S32.453B | S32.613A | S42.115B | S42.254A |
| S32.030A | S32.311B | S32.454A | S32.613B | S42.116B | S42.254B |
| S32.030B | S32.312A | S32.454B | S32.614A | S42.121B | S42.255A |
| S32.031A | S32.312B | S32.455A | S32.614B | S42.122B | S42.255B |
| S32.031B | S32.313A | S32.455B | S32.615A | S42.123B | S42.256A |
| S32.032A | S32.313B | S32.456A | S32.615B | S42.124B | S42.256B |
| S32.032B | S32.314A | S32.456B | S32.616A | S42.125B | S42.261A |
| S32.038A | S32.314B | S32.461A | S32.616B | S42.126B | S42.261B |
| S32.038B | S32.315A | S32.461B | S32.691A | S42.131B | S42.262A |
| S32.039A | S32.315B | S32.462A | S32.691B | S42.132B | S42.262B |
| S32.039B | S32.316A | S32.462B | S32.692A | S42.133B | S42.263A |
| S32.040A | S32.316B | S32.463A | S32.692B | S42.134B | S42.263B |
| S32.040B | S32.391A | S32.463B | S32.699A | S42.135B | S42.264A |
| S32.041A | S32.391B | S32.464A | S32.699B | S42.136B | S42.264B |
| S32.041B | S32.392A | S32.464B | S32.810A | S42.141B | S42.265A |
| S32.042A | S32.392B | S32.465A | S32.810B | S42.142B | S42.265B |
| S32.042B | S32.399A | S32.465B | S32.811A | S42.143B | S42.266A |
| S32.048A | S32.399B | S32.466A | S32.811B | S42.144B | S42.266B |
| S32.048B | S32.401A | S32.466B | S32.82XA | S42.145B | S42.271A |
| S32.049A | S32.401B | S32.471A | S32.82XB | S42.146B | S42.272A |
| S32.049B | S32.402A | S32.471B | S32.89XA | S42.151B | S42.279A |
| S32.050A | S32.402B | S32.472A | S32.89XB | S42.152B | S42.291A |
| S32.050B | S32.409A | S32.472B | S32.9XXA | S42.153B | S42.291B |
| S32.051A | S32.409B | S32.473A | S32.9XXB | S42.154B | S42.292A |
| S32.051B | S32.411A | S32.473B | S34.101A | S42.155B | S42.292B |
| S32.052A | S32.411B | S32.474A | S34.102A | S42.156B | S42.293A |
| S32.052B | S32.412A | S32.474B | S34.103A | S42.191B | S42.293B |
| S32.058A | S32.412B | S32.475A | S34.104A | S42.192B | S42.294A |
| S32.058B | S32.413A | S32.475B | S34.105A | S42.199B | S42.294B |
| S32.059A | S32.413B | S32.476A | S34.109A | S42.201A | S42.295A |
| S32.059B | S32.414A | S32.476B | S34.111A | S42.201B | S42.295B |
| S32.10XA | S32.414B | S32.481A | S34.112A | S42.202A | S42.296A |
| S32.10XB | S32.415A | S32.481B | S34.113A | S42.202B | S42.296B |
| S32.110A | S32.415B | S32.482A | S34.114A | S42.209A | S42.301A |
| S32.110B | S32.416A | S32.482B | S34.115A | S42.209B | S42.301B |
| S32.111A | S32.416B | S32.483A | S34.119A | S42.211A | S42.302A |
| S32.111B | S32.421A | S32.483B | S34.121A | S42.211B | S42.302B |
| S32.112A | S32.421B | S32.484A | S34.122A | S42.212A | S42.309A |
| S32.112B | S32.422A | S32.484B | S34.123A | S42.212B | S42.309B |
| S32.119A | S32.422B | S32.485A | S34.124A | S42.213A | S42.311A |
| S32.119B | S32.423A | S32.485B | S34.125A | S42.213B | S42.312A |
| S32.120A | S32.423B | S32.486A | S34.129A | S42.214A | S42.319A |
| S32.120B | S32.424A | S32.486B | S34.131A | S42.214B | S42.321A |
| S32.121A | S32.424B | S32.491A | S34.132A | S42.215A | S42.321B |
| S32.121B | S32.425A | S32.491B | S34.139A | S42.215B | S42.322A |
| S32.122A | S32.425B | S32.492A | S34.3XXA | S42.216A | S42.322B |
| S32.122B | S32.426A | S32.492B | S42.001B | S42.216B | S42.323A |
| S32.129A | S32.426B | S32.499A | S42.002B | S42.221A | S42.323B |
| S32.129B | S32.431A | S32.499B | S42.009B | S42.221B | S42.324A |
| S32.130A | S32.431B | S32.501A | S42.011B | S42.222A | S42.324B |
| S32.130B | S32.432A | S32.501B | S42.012B | S42.222B | S42.325A |
| S32.131A | S32.432B | S32.502A | S42.013B | S42.223A | S42.325B |
| S32.131B | S32.433A | S32.502B | S42.014B | S42.223B | S42.326A |
| S32.132A | S32.433B | S32.509A | S42.015B | S42.224A | S42.326B |
| S32.132B | S32.434A | S32.509B | S42.016B | S42.224B | S42.331A |
| S32.139A | S32.434B | S32.511A | S42.017B | S42.225A | S42.331B |
| S32.139B | S32.435A | S32.511B | S42.018B | S42.225B | S42.332A |
| S32.14XA | S32.435B | S32.512A | S42.019B | S42.226A | S42.332B |
| S32.14XB | S32.436A | S32.512B | S42.021B | S42.226B | S42.333A |
| S32.15XA | S32.436B | S32.519A | S42.022B | S42.231A | S42.333B |
| S32.15XB | S32.441A | S32.519B | S42.023B | S42.231B | S42.334A |
| S32.16XA | S32.441B | S32.591A | S42.024B | S42.232A | S42.334B |
| S32.16XB | S32.442A | S32.591B | S42.025B | S42.232B | S42.335A |
| S32.17XA | S32.442B | S32.592A | S42.026B | S42.239A | S42.335B |
| S32.17XB | S32.443A | S32.592B | S42.031B | S42.239B | S42.336A |
| S32.19XA | S32.443B | S32.599A | S42.032B | S42.241A | S42.336B |
| S32.19XB | S32.444A | S32.599B | S42.033B | S42.241B | S42.341A |
| S32.2XXA | S32.444B | S32.601A | S42.034B | S42.242A | S42.341B |
| S32.2XXB | S32.445A | S32.601B | S42.035B | S42.242B | S42.342A |
| S32.301A | S32.445B | S32.602A | S42.036B | S42.249A | S42.342B |
| S32.301B | S32.446A | S32.602B | S42.101B | S42.249B | S42.343A |
| S32.302A | S32.446B | S32.609A | S42.102B | S42.251A | S42.343B |
| S32.302B | S32.451A | S32.609B | S42.109B | S42.251B | S42.344A |
| | S32.451B | S32.611A | S42.111B | S42.252A | S42.344B |
| | S32.452A | S32.611B | S42.112B | S42.252B | S42.345A |

**HAC 05: Falls and Trauma (continued)**

| | | | | |
|---|---|---|---|---|
| S42.345B | S42.441A | S43.203A | S52.033B | S52.221A | S52.262C |
| S42.346A | S42.441B | S43.204A | S52.033C | S52.221B | S52.263A |
| S42.346B | S42.442A | S43.205A | S52.034B | S52.221C | S52.263B |
| S42.351A | S42.442B | S43.206A | S52.034C | S52.222A | S52.263C |
| S42.351B | S42.443A | S43.211A | S52.035B | S52.222B | S52.264A |
| S42.352A | S42.443B | S43.212A | S52.035C | S52.222C | S52.264B |
| S42.352B | S42.444A | S43.213A | S52.036B | S52.223A | S52.264C |
| S42.353A | S42.444B | S43.214A | S52.036C | S52.223B | S52.265A |
| S42.353B | S42.445A | S43.215A | S52.041B | S52.223C | S52.265B |
| S42.354A | S42.445B | S43.216A | S52.041C | S52.224A | S52.265C |
| S42.354B | S42.446A | S43.221A | S52.042B | S52.224B | S52.266A |
| S42.355A | S42.446B | S43.222A | S52.042C | S52.224C | S52.266B |
| S42.355B | S42.447A | S43.223A | S52.043B | S52.225A | S52.266C |
| S42.356A | S42.447B | S43.224A | S52.043C | S52.225B | S52.271B |
| S42.356B | S42.448A | S43.225A | S52.044B | S52.225C | S52.271C |
| S42.361A | S42.448B | S43.226A | S52.044C | S52.226A | S52.272B |
| S42.361B | S42.449A | S49.001A | S52.045B | S52.226B | S52.272C |
| S42.362A | S42.449B | S49.002A | S52.045C | S52.226C | S52.279B |
| S42.362B | S42.451A | S49.009A | S52.046B | S52.231A | S52.279C |
| S42.363A | S42.451B | S49.011A | S52.046C | S52.231B | S52.281A |
| S42.363B | S42.452A | S49.012A | S52.091B | S52.231C | S52.281B |
| S42.364A | S42.452B | S49.019A | S52.091C | S52.232A | S52.281C |
| S42.364B | S42.453A | S49.021A | S52.092B | S52.232B | S52.282A |
| S42.365A | S42.453B | S49.022A | S52.092C | S52.232C | S52.282B |
| S42.365B | S42.454A | S49.029A | S52.099B | S52.233A | S52.282C |
| S42.366A | S42.454B | S49.031A | S52.099C | S52.233B | S52.283A |
| S42.366B | S42.455A | S49.032A | S52.101B | S52.233C | S52.283B |
| S42.391A | S42.455B | S49.039A | S52.101C | S52.234A | S52.283C |
| S42.391B | S42.456A | S49.041A | S52.102B | S52.234B | S52.291A |
| S42.392A | S42.456B | S49.042A | S52.102C | S52.234C | S52.291B |
| S42.392B | S42.461A | S49.049A | S52.109B | S52.235A | S52.291C |
| S42.399A | S42.461B | S49.091A | S52.109C | S52.235B | S52.292A |
| S42.399B | S42.462A | S49.092A | S52.111A | S52.235C | S52.292B |
| S42.401A | S42.462B | S49.099A | S52.112A | S52.236A | S52.292C |
| S42.401B | S42.463A | S49.101A | S52.119A | S52.236B | S52.299A |
| S42.402A | S42.463B | S49.102A | S52.121B | S52.236C | S52.299B |
| S42.402B | S42.464A | S49.109A | S52.121C | S52.241A | S52.299C |
| S42.409A | S42.464B | S49.111A | S52.122B | S52.241B | S52.301A |
| S42.409B | S42.465A | S49.112A | S52.122C | S52.241C | S52.301B |
| S42.411A | S42.465B | S49.119A | S52.123B | S52.242A | S52.301C |
| S42.411B | S42.466A | S49.121A | S52.123C | S52.242B | S52.302A |
| S42.412A | S42.466B | S49.122A | S52.124B | S52.242C | S52.302B |
| S42.412B | S42.471A | S49.129A | S52.124C | S52.243A | S52.302C |
| S42.413A | S42.471B | S49.131A | S52.125B | S52.243B | S52.309A |
| S42.413B | S42.472A | S49.132A | S52.125C | S52.243C | S52.309B |
| S42.414A | S42.472B | S49.139A | S52.126B | S52.244A | S52.309C |
| S42.414B | S42.473A | S49.141A | S52.126C | S52.244B | S52.311A |
| S42.415A | S42.473B | S49.142A | S52.131B | S52.244C | S52.312A |
| S42.415B | S42.474A | S49.149A | S52.131C | S52.245A | S52.319A |
| S42.416A | S42.474B | S49.191A | S52.132B | S52.245B | S52.321A |
| S42.416B | S42.475A | S49.192A | S52.132C | S52.245C | S52.321B |
| S42.421A | S42.475B | S49.199A | S52.133B | S52.246A | S52.321C |
| S42.421B | S42.476A | S52.001B | S52.133C | S52.246B | S52.322A |
| S42.422A | S42.476B | S52.001C | S52.134B | S52.246C | S52.322B |
| S42.422B | S42.481A | S52.002B | S52.134C | S52.251A | S52.322C |
| S42.423A | S42.482A | S52.002C | S52.135B | S52.251B | S52.323A |
| S42.423B | S42.489A | S52.009B | S52.135C | S52.251C | S52.323B |
| S42.424A | S42.491A | S52.009C | S52.136B | S52.252A | S52.323C |
| S42.424B | S42.491B | S52.011A | S52.136C | S52.252B | S52.324A |
| S42.425A | S42.492A | S52.012A | S52.181B | S52.252C | S52.324B |
| S42.425B | S42.492B | S52.019A | S52.181C | S52.253A | S52.324C |
| S42.426A | S42.493A | S52.021B | S52.182B | S52.253B | S52.325A |
| S42.426B | S42.493B | S52.021C | S52.182C | S52.253C | S52.325B |
| S42.431A | S42.494A | S52.022B | S52.189B | S52.254A | S52.325C |
| S42.431B | S42.494B | S52.022C | S52.189C | S52.254B | S52.326A |
| S42.432A | S42.495A | S52.023B | S52.201A | S52.254C | S52.326B |
| S42.432B | S42.495B | S52.023C | S52.201B | S52.255A | S52.326C |
| S42.433A | S42.496A | S52.024B | S52.201C | S52.255B | S52.331A |
| S42.433B | S42.496B | S52.024C | S52.202A | S52.255C | S52.331B |
| S42.434A | S42.90XA | S52.025B | S52.202B | S52.256A | S52.331C |
| S42.434B | S42.90XB | S52.025C | S52.202C | S52.256B | S52.332A |
| S42.435A | S42.91XA | S52.026B | S52.209A | S52.256C | S52.332B |
| S42.435B | S42.91XB | S52.026C | S52.209B | S52.261A | S52.332C |
| S42.436A | S42.92XA | S52.031B | S52.209C | S52.261B | S52.333A |
| S42.436B | S42.92XB | S52.031C | S52.211A | S52.261C | S52.333B |
| | S43.201A | S52.032B | S52.212A | S52.262A | S52.333C |
| | S43.202A | S52.032C | S52.219A | S52.262B | S52.334A |

## HAC 05: Falls and Trauma (continued)

| | | | | |
|---|---|---|---|---|
| S52.334B | S52.382B | S52.569A | S59.029A | S62.152B | S62.321B |
| S52.334C | S52.382C | S52.569B | S59.031A | S62.153B | S62.322B |
| S52.335A | S52.389A | S52.569C | S59.032A | S62.154B | S62.323B |
| S52.335B | S52.389B | S52.571A | S59.039A | S62.155B | S62.324B |
| S52.335C | S52.389C | S52.571B | S59.041A | S62.156B | S62.325B |
| S52.336A | S52.391A | S52.571C | S59.042A | S62.161B | S62.326B |
| S52.336B | S52.391B | S52.572A | S59.049A | S62.162B | S62.327B |
| S52.336C | S52.391C | S52.572B | S59.091A | S62.163B | S62.328B |
| S52.341A | S52.392A | S52.572C | S59.092A | S62.164B | S62.329B |
| S52.341B | S52.392B | S52.579A | S59.099A | S62.165B | S62.330B |
| S52.341C | S52.392C | S52.579B | S59.201A | S62.166B | S62.331B |
| S52.342A | S52.399A | S52.579C | S59.202A | S62.171B | S62.332B |
| S52.342B | S52.399B | S52.591A | S59.209A | S62.172B | S62.333B |
| S52.342C | S52.399C | S52.591B | S59.211A | S62.173B | S62.334B |
| S52.343A | S52.501A | S52.591C | S59.212A | S62.174B | S62.335B |
| S52.343B | S52.501B | S52.592A | S59.219A | S62.175B | S62.336B |
| S52.343C | S52.501C | S52.592B | S59.221A | S62.176B | S62.337B |
| S52.344A | S52.502A | S52.592C | S59.222A | S62.181B | S62.338B |
| S52.344B | S52.502B | S52.599A | S59.229A | S62.182B | S62.339B |
| S52.344C | S52.502C | S52.599B | S59.231A | S62.183B | S62.340B |
| S52.345A | S52.509A | S52.599C | S59.232A | S62.184B | S62.341B |
| S52.345B | S52.509B | S52.601A | S59.239A | S62.185B | S62.342B |
| S52.345C | S52.509C | S52.601B | S59.241A | S62.186B | S62.343B |
| S52.346A | S52.511A | S52.601C | S59.242A | S62.201B | S62.344B |
| S52.346B | S52.511B | S52.602A | S59.249A | S62.202B | S62.345B |
| S52.346C | S52.511C | S52.602B | S59.291A | S62.209B | S62.346B |
| S52.351A | S52.512A | S52.602C | S59.292A | S62.211B | S62.347B |
| S52.351B | S52.512B | S52.609A | S59.299A | S62.212B | S62.348B |
| S52.351C | S52.512C | S52.609B | S62.001B | S62.213B | S62.349B |
| S52.352A | S52.513A | S52.609C | S62.002B | S62.221B | S62.350B |
| S52.352B | S52.513B | S52.611A | S62.009B | S62.222B | S62.351B |
| S52.352C | S52.513C | S52.611B | S62.011B | S62.223B | S62.352B |
| S52.353A | S52.514A | S52.611C | S62.012B | S62.224B | S62.353B |
| S52.353B | S52.514B | S52.612A | S62.013B | S62.225B | S62.354B |
| S52.353C | S52.514C | S52.612B | S62.014B | S62.226B | S62.355B |
| S52.354A | S52.515A | S52.612C | S62.015B | S62.231B | S62.356B |
| S52.354B | S52.515B | S52.613A | S62.016B | S62.232B | S62.357B |
| S52.354C | S52.515C | S52.613B | S62.021B | S62.233B | S62.358B |
| S52.355A | S52.516A | S52.613C | S62.022B | S62.234B | S62.359B |
| S52.355B | S52.516B | S52.614A | S62.023B | S62.235B | S62.360B |
| S52.355C | S52.516C | S52.614B | S62.024B | S62.236B | S62.361B |
| S52.356A | S52.521A | S52.614C | S62.025B | S62.241B | S62.362B |
| S52.356B | S52.522A | S52.615A | S62.026B | S62.242B | S62.363B |
| S52.356C | S52.529A | S52.615B | S62.031B | S62.243B | S62.364B |
| S52.361A | S52.531A | S52.615C | S62.032B | S62.244B | S62.365B |
| S52.361B | S52.531B | S52.616A | S62.033B | S62.245B | S62.366B |
| S52.361C | S52.531C | S52.616B | S62.034B | S62.246B | S62.367B |
| S52.362A | S52.532A | S52.616C | S62.035B | S62.251B | S62.368B |
| S52.362B | S52.532B | S52.621A | S62.036B | S62.252B | S62.369B |
| S52.362C | S52.532C | S52.622A | S62.101B | S62.253B | S62.390B |
| S52.363A | S52.539A | S52.629A | S62.102B | S62.254B | S62.391B |
| S52.363B | S52.539B | S52.691A | S62.109B | S62.255B | S62.392B |
| S52.363C | S52.539C | S52.691B | S62.111B | S62.256B | S62.393B |
| S52.364A | S52.541A | S52.691C | S62.112B | S62.291B | S62.394B |
| S52.364B | S52.541B | S52.692A | S62.113B | S62.292B | S62.395B |
| S52.364C | S52.541C | S52.692B | S62.114B | S62.299B | S62.396B |
| S52.365A | S52.542A | S52.692C | S62.115B | S62.300B | S62.397B |
| S52.365B | S52.542B | S52.699A | S62.116B | S62.301B | S62.398B |
| S52.365C | S52.542C | S52.699B | S62.121B | S62.302B | S62.399B |
| S52.366A | S52.549A | S52.699C | S62.122B | S62.303B | S62.501B |
| S52.366B | S52.549B | S52.90XA | S62.123B | S62.304B | S62.502B |
| S52.366C | S52.549C | S52.90XB | S62.124B | S62.305B | S62.509B |
| S52.371A | S52.551A | S52.90XC | S62.125B | S62.306B | S62.511B |
| S52.371B | S52.551B | S52.91XA | S62.126B | S62.307B | S62.512B |
| S52.371C | S52.551C | S52.91XB | S62.131B | S62.308B | S62.513B |
| S52.372A | S52.552A | S52.91XC | S62.132B | S62.309B | S62.514B |
| S52.372B | S52.552B | S52.92XA | S62.133B | S62.310B | S62.515B |
| S52.372C | S52.552C | S52.92XB | S62.134B | S62.311B | S62.516B |
| S52.379A | S52.559A | S52.92XC | S62.135B | S62.312B | S62.521B |
| S52.379B | S52.559B | S59.001A | S62.136B | S62.313B | S62.522B |
| S52.379C | S52.559C | S59.002A | S62.141B | S62.314B | S62.523B |
| S52.381A | S52.561A | S59.009A | S62.142B | S62.315B | S62.524B |
| S52.381B | S52.561B | S59.011A | S62.143B | S62.316B | S62.525B |
| S52.381C | S52.561C | S59.012A | S62.144B | S62.317B | S62.526B |
| S52.382A | S52.562A | S59.019A | S62.145B | S62.318B | S62.600B |
| | S52.562B | S59.021A | S62.146B | S62.319B | S62.601B |
| | S52.562C | S59.022A | S62.151B | S62.320B | S62.602B |

**Appendix I: Hospital Acquired Conditions**

**HAC 05: Falls and Trauma (continued)**

| | | | | |
|---|---|---|---|---|
| S62.603B | S72.002C | S72.061B | S72.133A | S72.331C | S72.399B |
| S62.604B | S72.009A | S72.061C | S72.133B | S72.332A | S72.399C |
| S62.605B | S72.009B | S72.062A | S72.133C | S72.332B | S72.401A |
| S62.606B | S72.009C | S72.062B | S72.134A | S72.332C | S72.401B |
| S62.607B | S72.011A | S72.062C | S72.134B | S72.333A | S72.401C |
| S62.608B | S72.011B | S72.063A | S72.134C | S72.333B | S72.402A |
| S62.609B | S72.011C | S72.063B | S72.135A | S72.333C | S72.402B |
| S62.610B | S72.012A | S72.063C | S72.135B | S72.334A | S72.402C |
| S62.611B | S72.012B | S72.064A | S72.135C | S72.334B | S72.409A |
| S62.612B | S72.012C | S72.064B | S72.136A | S72.334C | S72.409B |
| S62.613B | S72.019A | S72.064C | S72.136B | S72.335A | S72.409C |
| S62.614B | S72.019B | S72.065A | S72.136C | S72.335B | S72.411A |
| S62.615B | S72.019C | S72.065B | S72.141A | S72.335C | S72.411B |
| S62.616B | S72.021A | S72.065C | S72.141B | S72.336A | S72.411C |
| S62.617B | S72.021B | S72.066A | S72.141C | S72.336B | S72.412A |
| S62.618B | S72.021C | S72.066B | S72.142A | S72.336C | S72.412B |
| S62.619B | S72.022A | S72.066C | S72.142B | S72.341A | S72.412C |
| S62.620B | S72.022B | S72.091A | S72.142C | S72.341B | S72.413A |
| S62.621B | S72.022C | S72.091B | S72.143A | S72.341C | S72.413B |
| S62.622B | S72.023A | S72.091C | S72.143B | S72.342A | S72.413C |
| S62.623B | S72.023B | S72.092A | S72.143C | S72.342B | S72.414A |
| S62.624B | S72.023C | S72.092B | S72.144A | S72.342C | S72.414B |
| S62.625B | S72.024A | S72.092C | S72.144B | S72.343A | S72.414C |
| S62.626B | S72.024B | S72.099A | S72.144C | S72.343B | S72.415A |
| S62.627B | S72.024C | S72.099B | S72.145A | S72.343C | S72.415B |
| S62.628B | S72.025A | S72.099C | S72.145B | S72.344A | S72.415C |
| S62.629B | S72.025B | S72.101A | S72.145C | S72.344B | S72.416A |
| S62.630B | S72.025C | S72.101B | S72.146A | S72.344C | S72.416B |
| S62.631B | S72.026A | S72.101C | S72.146B | S72.345A | S72.416C |
| S62.632B | S72.026B | S72.102A | S72.146C | S72.345B | S72.421A |
| S62.633B | S72.026C | S72.102B | S72.21XA | S72.345C | S72.421B |
| S62.634B | S72.031A | S72.102C | S72.21XB | S72.346A | S72.421C |
| S62.635B | S72.031B | S72.109A | S72.21XC | S72.346B | S72.422A |
| S62.636B | S72.031C | S72.109B | S72.22XA | S72.346C | S72.422B |
| S62.637B | S72.032A | S72.109C | S72.22XB | S72.351A | S72.422C |
| S62.638B | S72.032B | S72.111A | S72.22XC | S72.351B | S72.423A |
| S62.639B | S72.032C | S72.111B | S72.23XA | S72.351C | S72.423B |
| S62.640B | S72.033A | S72.111C | S72.23XB | S72.352A | S72.423C |
| S62.641B | S72.033B | S72.112A | S72.23XC | S72.352B | S72.424A |
| S62.642B | S72.033C | S72.112B | S72.24XA | S72.352C | S72.424B |
| S62.643B | S72.034A | S72.112C | S72.24XB | S72.353A | S72.424C |
| S62.644B | S72.034B | S72.113A | S72.24XC | S72.353B | S72.425A |
| S62.645B | S72.034C | S72.113B | S72.25XA | S72.353C | S72.425B |
| S62.646B | S72.035A | S72.113C | S72.25XB | S72.354A | S72.425C |
| S62.647B | S72.035B | S72.114A | S72.25XC | S72.354B | S72.426A |
| S62.648B | S72.035C | S72.114B | S72.26XA | S72.354C | S72.426B |
| S62.649B | S72.036A | S72.114C | S72.26XB | S72.355A | S72.426C |
| S62.650B | S72.036B | S72.115A | S72.26XC | S72.355B | S72.431A |
| S62.651B | S72.036C | S72.115B | S72.301A | S72.355C | S72.431B |
| S62.652B | S72.041A | S72.115C | S72.301B | S72.356A | S72.431C |
| S62.653B | S72.041B | S72.116A | S72.301C | S72.356B | S72.432A |
| S62.654B | S72.041C | S72.116B | S72.302A | S72.356C | S72.432B |
| S62.655B | S72.042A | S72.116C | S72.302B | S72.361A | S72.432C |
| S62.656B | S72.042B | S72.121A | S72.302C | S72.361B | S72.433A |
| S62.657B | S72.042C | S72.121B | S72.309A | S72.361C | S72.433B |
| S62.658B | S72.043A | S72.121C | S72.309B | S72.362A | S72.433C |
| S62.659B | S72.043B | S72.122A | S72.309C | S72.362B | S72.434A |
| S62.660B | S72.043C | S72.122B | S72.321A | S72.362C | S72.434B |
| S62.661B | S72.044A | S72.122C | S72.321B | S72.363A | S72.434C |
| S62.662B | S72.044B | S72.123A | S72.321C | S72.363B | S72.435A |
| S62.663B | S72.044C | S72.123B | S72.322A | S72.363C | S72.435B |
| S62.664B | S72.045A | S72.123C | S72.322B | S72.364A | S72.435C |
| S62.665B | S72.045B | S72.124A | S72.322C | S72.364B | S72.436A |
| S62.666B | S72.045C | S72.124B | S72.323A | S72.364C | S72.436B |
| S62.667B | S72.046A | S72.124C | S72.323B | S72.365A | S72.436C |
| S62.668B | S72.046B | S72.125A | S72.323C | S72.365B | S72.441A |
| S62.669B | S72.046C | S72.125B | S72.324A | S72.365C | S72.441B |
| S62.90XB | S72.051A | S72.125C | S72.324B | S72.366A | S72.441C |
| S62.91XB | S72.051B | S72.126A | S72.324C | S72.366B | S72.442A |
| S62.92XB | S72.051C | S72.126B | S72.325A | S72.366C | S72.442B |
| S72.001A | S72.052A | S72.126C | S72.325B | S72.391A | S72.442C |
| S72.001B | S72.052B | S72.131A | S72.325C | S72.391B | S72.443A |
| S72.001C | S72.052C | S72.131B | S72.326A | S72.391C | S72.443B |
| S72.002A | S72.059A | S72.131C | S72.326B | S72.392A | S72.443C |
| S72.002B | S72.059B | S72.132A | S72.326C | S72.392B | S72.444A |
| | S72.059C | S72.132B | S72.331A | S72.392C | S72.444B |
| | S72.061A | S72.132C | S72.331B | S72.399A | S72.444C |

**HAC 05: Falls and Trauma (continued)**

| | | | | | |
|---|---|---|---|---|---|
| S72.445A | S73.004A | S82.013C | S82.102B | S82.151A | S82.241C |
| S72.445B | S73.005A | S82.014A | S82.102C | S82.151B | S82.242A |
| S72.445C | S73.006A | S82.014B | S82.109A | S82.151C | S82.242B |
| S72.446A | S73.011A | S82.014C | S82.109B | S82.152A | S82.242C |
| S72.446B | S73.012A | S82.015A | S82.109C | S82.152B | S82.243A |
| S72.446C | S73.013A | S82.015B | S82.111A | S82.152C | S82.243B |
| S72.451A | S73.014A | S82.015C | S82.111B | S82.153A | S82.244A |
| S72.451B | S73.015A | S82.016A | S82.111C | S82.153B | S82.244B |
| S72.451C | S73.016A | S82.016B | S82.112A | S82.153C | S82.244C |
| S72.452A | S73.021A | S82.016C | S82.112B | S82.154A | S82.245A |
| S72.452B | S73.022A | S82.021A | S82.112C | S82.154B | S82.245B |
| S72.452C | S73.023A | S82.021B | S82.113A | S82.154C | S82.245C |
| S72.453A | S73.024A | S82.021C | S82.113B | S82.155A | S82.246A |
| S72.453B | S73.025A | S82.022A | S82.113C | S82.155B | S82.246B |
| S72.453C | S73.026A | S82.022B | S82.114A | S82.155C | S82.246C |
| S72.454A | S73.031A | S82.022C | S82.114B | S82.156A | S82.251A |
| S72.454B | S73.032A | S82.023A | S82.114C | S82.156B | S82.251B |
| S72.454C | S73.033A | S82.023B | S82.115A | S82.156C | S82.251C |
| S72.455A | S73.034A | S82.023C | S82.115B | S82.161A | S82.252A |
| S72.455B | S73.035A | S82.024A | S82.115C | S82.162A | S82.252B |
| S72.455C | S73.036A | S82.024B | S82.116A | S82.169A | S82.252C |
| S72.456A | S73.041A | S82.024C | S82.116B | S82.191A | S82.253A |
| S72.456B | S73.042A | S82.025A | S82.116C | S82.191B | S82.253B |
| S72.456C | S73.043A | S82.025B | S82.121A | S82.191C | S82.253C |
| S72.461A | S73.044A | S82.025C | S82.121B | S82.192A | S82.254A |
| S72.461B | S73.045A | S82.026A | S82.121C | S82.192B | S82.254B |
| S72.461C | S73.046A | S82.026B | S82.122A | S82.192C | S82.254C |
| S72.462A | S77.00XA | S82.026C | S82.122B | S82.199A | S82.255A |
| S72.462B | S77.01XA | S82.031A | S82.122C | S82.199B | S82.255B |
| S72.462C | S77.02XA | S82.031B | S82.123A | S82.199C | S82.255C |
| S72.463A | S77.10XA | S82.031C | S82.123B | S82.201A | S82.256A |
| S72.463B | S77.11XA | S82.032A | S82.123C | S82.201B | S82.256B |
| S72.463C | S77.12XA | S82.032B | S82.124A | S82.201C | S82.256C |
| S72.464A | S79.001A | S82.032C | S82.124B | S82.202A | S82.261A |
| S72.464B | S79.002A | S82.033A | S82.124C | S82.202B | S82.261B |
| S72.464C | S79.009A | S82.033B | S82.125A | S82.202C | S82.261C |
| S72.465A | S79.011A | S82.033C | S82.125B | S82.209A | S82.262A |
| S72.465B | S79.012A | S82.034A | S82.125C | S82.209B | S82.262B |
| S72.465C | S79.019A | S82.034B | S82.126A | S82.209C | S82.262C |
| S72.466A | S79.091A | S82.034C | S82.126B | S82.221A | S82.263A |
| S72.466B | S79.092A | S82.035A | S82.126C | S82.221B | S82.263B |
| S72.466C | S79.099A | S82.035B | S82.131A | S82.221C | S82.263C |
| S72.471A | S79.101A | S82.035C | S82.131B | S82.222A | S82.264A |
| S72.472A | S79.102A | S82.036A | S82.131C | S82.222B | S82.264B |
| S72.479A | S79.109A | S82.036B | S82.132A | S82.222C | S82.264C |
| S72.491A | S79.111A | S82.036C | S82.132B | S82.223A | S82.265A |
| S72.491B | S79.112A | S82.041A | S82.132C | S82.223B | S82.265B |
| S72.491C | S79.119A | S82.041B | S82.133A | S82.223C | S82.265C |
| S72.492A | S79.121A | S82.041C | S82.133B | S82.224A | S82.266A |
| S72.492B | S79.122A | S82.042A | S82.133C | S82.224B | S82.266B |
| S72.492C | S79.129A | S82.042B | S82.134A | S82.224C | S82.266C |
| S72.499A | S79.131A | S82.042C | S82.134B | S82.225A | S82.291A |
| S72.499B | S79.132A | S82.043A | S82.134C | S82.225B | S82.291B |
| S72.499C | S79.139A | S82.043B | S82.135A | S82.225C | S82.291C |
| S72.8X1A | S79.141A | S82.043C | S82.135B | S82.226A | S82.292A |
| S72.8X1B | S79.142A | S82.044A | S82.135C | S82.226B | S82.292B |
| S72.8X1C | S79.149A | S82.044B | S82.136A | S82.226C | S82.292C |
| S72.8X2A | S79.191A | S82.044C | S82.136B | S82.231A | S82.299A |
| S72.8X2B | S79.192A | S82.045A | S82.136C | S82.231B | S82.299B |
| S72.8X2C | S79.199A | S82.045B | S82.141A | S82.231C | S82.299C |
| S72.8X9A | S82.001A | S82.045C | S82.141B | S82.232A | S82.301B |
| S72.8X9B | S82.001B | S82.046A | S82.141C | S82.232B | S82.301C |
| S72.8X9C | S82.001C | S82.046B | S82.142A | S82.232C | S82.302B |
| S72.90XA | S82.002A | S82.046C | S82.142B | S82.233A | S82.302C |
| S72.90XB | S82.002B | S82.091A | S82.142C | S82.233B | S82.309B |
| S72.90XC | S82.002C | S82.091B | S82.143A | S82.233C | S82.309C |
| S72.91XA | S82.009A | S82.091C | S82.143B | S82.234A | S82.311A |
| S72.91XB | S82.009B | S82.092A | S82.143C | S82.234B | S82.312A |
| S72.91XC | S82.009C | S82.092B | S82.144A | S82.234C | S82.319A |
| S72.92XA | S82.011A | S82.092C | S82.144B | S82.235A | S82.391B |
| S72.92XB | S82.011B | S82.099A | S82.144C | S82.235B | S82.391C |
| S72.92XC | S82.011C | S82.099B | S82.145A | S82.235C | S82.392B |
| S73.001A | S82.012A | S82.099C | S82.145B | S82.236A | S82.392C |
| S73.002A | S82.012B | S82.101A | S82.145C | S82.236B | S82.399B |
| S73.003A | S82.012C | S82.101B | S82.146A | S82.236C | S82.399C |
| | S82.013A | S82.101C | S82.146B | S82.241A | S82.401B |
| | S82.013B | S82.102A | S82.146C | S82.241B | |

**Appendix I: Hospital Acquired Conditions**

**HAC 05: Falls and Trauma (continued)**

| | | | | |
|---|---|---|---|---|
| S82.401C | S82.53XB | S82.892C | S92.123B | S92.335B | T22.362A |
| S82.402B | S82.53XC | S82.899B | S92.124B | S92.336B | T22.369A |
| S82.402C | S82.54XB | S82.899C | S92.125B | S92.341B | T22.391A |
| S82.409B | S82.54XC | S82.90XB | S92.126B | S92.342B | T22.392A |
| S82.409C | S82.55XB | S82.90XC | S92.131B | S92.343B | T22.399A |
| S82.421B | S82.55XC | S82.91XB | S92.132B | S92.344B | T22.70XA |
| S82.421C | S82.56XB | S82.91XC | S92.133B | S92.345B | T22.711A |
| S82.422B | S82.56XC | S82.92XB | S92.134B | S92.346B | T22.712A |
| S82.422C | S82.61XB | S82.92XC | S92.135B | S92.351B | T22.719A |
| S82.423B | S82.61XC | S89.001A | S92.136B | S92.352B | T22.721A |
| S82.423C | S82.62XB | S89.002A | S92.141B | S92.353B | T22.722A |
| S82.424B | S82.62XC | S89.009A | S92.142B | S92.354B | T22.729A |
| S82.424C | S82.63XB | S89.011A | S92.143B | S92.355B | T22.731A |
| S82.425B | S82.63XC | S89.012A | S92.144B | S92.356B | T22.732A |
| S82.425C | S82.64XB | S89.019A | S92.145B | S92.811B | T22.739A |
| S82.426B | S82.64XC | S89.021A | S92.146B | S92.812B | T22.741A |
| S82.426C | S82.65XB | S89.022A | S92.151B | S92.819B | T22.742A |
| S82.431B | S82.65XC | S89.029A | S92.152B | S92.901B | T22.749A |
| S82.431C | S82.66XB | S89.031A | S92.153B | S92.902B | T22.751A |
| S82.432B | S82.66XC | S89.032A | S92.154B | S92.909B | T22.752A |
| S82.432C | S82.831B | S89.039A | S92.155B | T20.30XA | T22.759A |
| S82.433B | S82.831C | S89.041A | S92.156B | T20.311A | T22.761A |
| S82.433C | S82.832B | S89.042A | S92.191B | T20.312A | T22.762A |
| S82.434B | S82.832C | S89.049A | S92.192B | T20.319A | T22.769A |
| S82.434C | S82.839B | S89.091A | S92.199B | T20.32XA | T22.791A |
| S82.435B | S82.839C | S89.092A | S92.201B | T20.33XA | T22.792A |
| S82.435C | S82.841B | S89.099A | S92.202B | T20.34XA | T22.799A |
| S82.436B | S82.841C | S92.001B | S92.209B | T20.35XA | T23.301A |
| S82.436C | S82.842B | S92.002B | S92.211B | T20.36XA | T23.302A |
| S82.441B | S82.842C | S92.009B | S92.212B | T20.37XA | T23.309A |
| S82.441C | S82.843B | S92.011B | S92.213B | T20.39XA | T23.311A |
| S82.442B | S82.843C | S92.012B | S92.214B | T20.70XA | T23.312A |
| S82.442C | S82.844B | S92.013B | S92.215B | T20.711A | T23.319A |
| S82.443B | S82.844C | S92.014B | S92.216B | T20.712A | T23.321A |
| S82.443C | S82.845B | S92.015B | S92.221B | T20.719A | T23.322A |
| S82.444B | S82.845C | S92.016B | S92.222B | T20.72XA | T23.329A |
| S82.444C | S82.846B | S92.021B | S92.223B | T20.73XA | T23.331A |
| S82.445B | S82.846C | S92.022B | S92.224B | T20.74XA | T23.332A |
| S82.445C | S82.851B | S92.023B | S92.225B | T20.75XA | T23.339A |
| S82.446B | S82.851C | S92.024B | S92.226B | T20.76XA | T23.341A |
| S82.446C | S82.852B | S92.025B | S92.231B | T20.77XA | T23.342A |
| S82.451B | S82.852C | S92.026B | S92.232B | T20.79XA | T23.349A |
| S82.451C | S82.853B | S92.031B | S92.233B | T21.30XA | T23.351A |
| S82.452B | S82.853C | S92.032B | S92.234B | T21.31XA | T23.352A |
| S82.452C | S82.854B | S92.033B | S92.235B | T21.32XA | T23.359A |
| S82.453B | S82.854C | S92.034B | S92.236B | T21.33XA | T23.361A |
| S82.453C | S82.855B | S92.035B | S92.241B | T21.34XA | T23.362A |
| S82.454B | S82.855C | S92.036B | S92.242B | T21.35XA | T23.369A |
| S82.454C | S82.856B | S92.041B | S92.243B | T21.36XA | T23.371A |
| S82.455B | S82.856C | S92.042B | S92.244B | T21.37XA | T23.372A |
| S82.455C | S82.861B | S92.043B | S92.245B | T21.39XA | T23.379A |
| S82.456B | S82.861C | S92.044B | S92.246B | T21.70XA | T23.391A |
| S82.456C | S82.862B | S92.045B | S92.251B | T21.71XA | T23.392A |
| S82.461B | S82.862C | S92.046B | S92.252B | T21.72XA | T23.399A |
| S82.461C | S82.863B | S92.051B | S92.253B | T21.73XA | T23.701A |
| S82.462B | S82.863C | S92.052B | S92.254B | T21.74XA | T23.702A |
| S82.462C | S82.864B | S92.053B | S92.255B | T21.75XA | T23.709A |
| S82.463B | S82.864C | S92.054B | S92.256B | T21.76XA | T23.711A |
| S82.463C | S82.865B | S92.055B | S92.301B | T21.77XA | T23.712A |
| S82.464B | S82.865C | S92.056B | S92.302B | T21.79XA | T23.719A |
| S82.464C | S82.866B | S92.061B | S92.309B | T22.30XA | T23.721A |
| S82.465B | S82.866C | S92.062B | S92.311B | T22.311A | T23.722A |
| S82.465C | S82.871B | S92.063B | S92.312B | T22.312A | T23.729A |
| S82.466B | S82.871C | S92.064B | S92.313B | T22.319A | T23.731A |
| S82.466C | S82.872B | S92.065B | S92.314B | T22.321A | T23.732A |
| S82.491B | S82.872C | S92.066B | S92.315B | T22.322A | T23.739A |
| S82.491C | S82.873B | S92.101B | S92.316B | T22.329A | T23.741A |
| S82.492B | S82.873C | S92.102B | S92.321B | T22.331A | T23.742A |
| S82.492C | S82.874B | S92.109B | S92.322B | T22.332A | T23.749A |
| S82.499B | S82.874C | S92.111B | S92.323B | T22.339A | T23.751A |
| S82.499C | S82.875B | S92.112B | S92.324B | T22.341A | T23.752A |
| S82.51XB | S82.875C | S92.113B | S92.325B | T22.342A | T23.759A |
| S82.51XC | S82.876B | S92.114B | S92.326B | T22.349A | T23.761A |
| S82.52XB | S82.876C | S92.115B | S92.331B | T22.351A | T23.762A |
| S82.52XC | S82.891B | S92.116B | S92.332B | T22.352A | T23.769A |
| | S82.891C | S92.121B | S92.333B | T22.359A | T23.771A |
| | S82.892B | S92.122B | S92.334B | T22.361A | T23.772A |

**HAC 05: Falls and Trauma (continued)**

| | | | | | |
|---|---|---|---|---|---|
| T23.779A | T25.791A | T31.81 | T32.84 | T34.1XXA | T71.162A |
| T23.791A | T25.792A | T31.82 | T32.85 | T34.2XXA | T71.163A |
| T23.792A | T25.799A | T31.83 | T32.86 | T34.3XXA | T71.164A |
| T23.799A | T26.20XA | T31.84 | T32.87 | T34.40XA | T71.191A |
| T24.301A | T26.21XA | T31.85 | T32.88 | T34.41XA | T71.192A |
| T24.302A | T26.22XA | T31.86 | T32.90 | T34.42XA | T71.193A |
| T24.309A | T26.70XA | T31.87 | T32.91 | T34.511A | T71.194A |
| T24.311A | T26.71XA | T31.88 | T32.92 | T34.512A | T71.20XA |
| T24.312A | T26.72XA | T31.90 | T32.93 | T34.519A | T71.21XA |
| T24.319A | T27.0XXA | T31.91 | T32.94 | T34.521A | T71.29XA |
| T24.321A | T27.1XXA | T31.92 | T32.95 | T34.522A | T71.9XXA |
| T24.322A | T27.2XXA | T31.93 | T32.96 | T34.529A | T75.1XXA |
| T24.329A | T27.3XXA | T31.94 | T32.97 | T34.531A | |
| T24.331A | T27.4XXA | T31.95 | T32.98 | T34.532A | **HAC 06: Catheter** |
| T24.332A | T27.5XXA | T31.96 | T32.99 | T34.539A | **Associated Urinary** |
| T24.339A | T27.6XXA | T31.97 | T33.011A | T34.60XA | **Tract Infection (UTI)** |
| T24.391A | T27.7XXA | T31.98 | T33.012A | T34.61XA | Secondary diagnosis not |
| T24.392A | T28.1XXA | T31.99 | T33.019A | T34.62XA | POA: |
| T24.399A | T28.2XXA | T32.10 | T33.02XA | T34.70XA | T83.511A |
| T24.701A | T28.6XXA | T32.11 | T33.09XA | T34.71XA | T83.518A |
| T24.702A | T28.7XXA | T32.20 | T33.1XXA | T34.72XA | |
| T24.709A | T31.10 | T32.21 | T33.2XXA | T34.811A | **With or Without** |
| T24.711A | T31.11 | T32.22 | T33.3XXA | T34.812A | Secondary diagnosis (also |
| T24.712A | T31.20 | T32.30 | T33.40XA | T34.819A | not POA) of: |
| T24.719A | T31.21 | T32.31 | T33.41XA | T34.821A | B37.41 |
| T24.721A | T31.22 | T32.32 | T33.42XA | T34.822A | B37.49 |
| T24.722A | T31.30 | T32.33 | T33.511A | T34.829A | N10 |
| T24.729A | T31.31 | T32.40 | T33.512A | T34.831A | N11.9 |
| T24.731A | T31.32 | T32.41 | T33.519A | T34.832A | N12 |
| T24.732A | T31.33 | T32.42 | T33.521A | T34.839A | N13.6 |
| T24.739A | T31.40 | T32.43 | T33.522A | T34.90XA | N15.1 |
| T24.791A | T31.41 | T32.44 | T33.529A | T34.99XA | N28.84 |
| T24.792A | T31.42 | T32.50 | T33.531A | T67.0XXA | N28.85 |
| T24.799A | T31.43 | T32.51 | T33.532A | T69.021A | N28.86 |
| T25.311A | T31.44 | T32.52 | T33.539A | T69.022A | N30.00 |
| T25.312A | T31.50 | T32.53 | T33.60XA | T69.029A | N30.01 |
| T25.319A | T31.51 | T32.54 | T33.61XA | T70.3XXA | N34.0 |
| T25.321A | T31.52 | T32.55 | T33.62XA | T71.111A | N39.0 |
| T25.322A | T31.53 | T32.60 | T33.70XA | T71.112A | |
| T25.329A | T31.54 | T32.61 | T33.71XA | T71.113A | **HAC 07: Vascular** |
| T25.331A | T31.55 | T32.62 | T33.72XA | T71.114A | **Catheter Associated** |
| T25.332A | T31.60 | T32.63 | T33.811A | T71.121A | **Infection** |
| T25.339A | T31.61 | T32.64 | T33.812A | T71.122A | Secondary diagnosis not |
| T25.391A | T31.62 | T32.65 | T33.819A | T71.123A | POA: |
| T25.392A | T31.63 | T32.66 | T33.821A | T71.124A | T80.211A |
| T25.399A | T31.64 | T32.70 | T33.822A | T71.131A | T80.212A |
| T25.711A | T31.65 | T32.71 | T33.829A | T71.132A | T80.218A |
| T25.712A | T31.66 | T32.72 | T33.831A | T71.133A | T80.219A |
| T25.719A | T31.70 | T32.73 | T33.832A | T71.134A | |
| T25.721A | T31.71 | T32.74 | T33.839A | T71.141A | |
| T25.722A | T31.72 | T32.75 | T33.90XA | T71.143A | |
| T25.729A | T31.73 | T32.76 | T33.99XA | T71.144A | |
| T25.731A | T31.74 | T32.77 | T34.011A | T71.151A | |
| T25.732A | T31.75 | T32.80 | T34.012A | T71.152A | |
| T25.739A | T31.76 | T32.81 | T34.019A | T71.153A | |
| | T31.77 | T32.82 | T34.02XA | T71.154A | |
| | T31.80 | T32.83 | T34.09XA | T71.161A | |

## HAC 08: Surgical Site Infection of Mediastinitis Following Coronary Bypass Graft (CABG) Procedures

Secondary diagnosis not POA:

J98.51

J98.59

**AND**

Any of the following procedures:

0210083   Bypass Coronary Artery, One Artery from Coronary Artery with Zooplastic Tissue, Open Approach

0210088   Bypass Coronary Artery, One Artery from Right Internal Mammary with Zooplastic Tissue, Open Approach

0210089   Bypass Coronary Artery, One Artery from Left Internal Mammary with Zooplastic Tissue, Open Approach

021008C   Bypass Coronary Artery, One Artery from Thoracic Artery with Zooplastic Tissue, Open Approach

021008F   Bypass Coronary Artery, One Artery from Abdominal Artery with Zooplastic Tissue, Open Approach

021008W   Bypass Coronary Artery, One Artery from Aorta with Zooplastic Tissue, Open Approach

0210093   Bypass Coronary Artery, One Artery from Coronary Artery with Autologous Venous Tissue, Open Approach

0210098   Bypass Coronary Artery, One Artery from Right Internal Mammary with Autologous Venous Tissue, Open Approach

0210099   Bypass Coronary Artery, One Artery from Left Internal Mammary with Autologous Venous Tissue, Open Approach

021009C   Bypass Coronary Artery, One Artery from Thoracic Artery with Autologous Venous Tissue, Open Approach

021009F   Bypass Coronary Artery, One Artery from Abdominal Artery with Autologous Venous Tissue, Open Approach

021009W   Bypass Coronary Artery, One Artery from Aorta with Autologous Venous Tissue, Open Approach

02100A3   Bypass Coronary Artery, One Artery from Coronary Artery with Autologous Arterial Tissue, Open Approach

02100A8   Bypass Coronary Artery, One Artery from Right Internal Mammary with Autologous Arterial Tissue, Open Approach

02100A9   Bypass Coronary Artery, One Artery from Left Internal Mammary with Autologous Arterial Tissue, Open Approach

02100AC   Bypass Coronary Artery, One Artery from Thoracic Artery with Autologous Arterial Tissue, Open Approach

02100AF   Bypass Coronary Artery, One Artery from Abdominal Artery with Autologous Arterial Tissue, Open Approach

02100AW   Bypass Coronary Artery, One Artery from Aorta with Autologous Arterial Tissue, Open Approach

02100J3   Bypass Coronary Artery, One Artery from Coronary Artery with Synthetic Substitute, Open Approach

02100J8   Bypass Coronary Artery, One Artery from Right Internal Mammary with Synthetic Substitute, Open Approach

02100J9   Bypass Coronary Artery, One Artery from Left Internal Mammary with Synthetic Substitute, Open Approach

02100JC   Bypass Coronary Artery, One Artery from Thoracic Artery with Synthetic Substitute, Open Approach

02100JF   Bypass Coronary Artery, One Artery from Abdominal Artery with Synthetic Substitute, Open Approach

02100JW   Bypass Coronary Artery, One Artery from Aorta with Synthetic Substitute, Open Approach

02100K3   Bypass Coronary Artery, One Artery from Coronary Artery with Nonautologous Tissue Substitute, Open Approach

02100K8   Bypass Coronary Artery, One Artery from Right Internal Mammary with Nonautologous Tissue Substitute, Open Approach

02100K9   Bypass Coronary Artery, One Artery from Left Internal Mammary with Nonautologous Tissue Substitute, Open Approach

02100KC   Bypass Coronary Artery, One Artery from Thoracic Artery with Nonautologous Tissue Substitute, Open Approach

02100KF   Bypass Coronary Artery, One Artery from Abdominal Artery with Nonautologous Tissue Substitute, Open Approach

02100KW   Bypass Coronary Artery, One Artery from Aorta with Nonautologous Tissue Substitute, Open Approach

02100Z3   Bypass Coronary Artery, One Artery from Coronary Artery, Open Approach

02100Z8   Bypass Coronary Artery, One Artery from Right Internal Mammary, Open Approach

02100Z9   Bypass Coronary Artery, One Artery from Left Internal Mammary, Open Approach

02100ZC   Bypass Coronary Artery, One Artery from Thoracic Artery, Open Approach

02100ZF   Bypass Coronary Artery, One Artery from Abdominal Artery, Open Approach

0210483   Bypass Coronary Artery, One Artery from Coronary Artery with Zooplastic Tissue, Percutaneous Endoscopic Approach

0210488   Bypass Coronary Artery, One Artery from Right Internal Mammary with Zooplastic Tissue, Percutaneous Endoscopic Approach

0210489   Bypass Coronary Artery, One Artery from Left Internal Mammary with Zooplastic Tissue, Percutaneous Endoscopic Approach

021048C   Bypass Coronary Artery, One Artery from Thoracic Artery with Zooplastic Tissue, Percutaneous Endoscopic Approach

021048F   Bypass Coronary Artery, One Artery from Abdominal Artery with Zooplastic Tissue, Percutaneous Endoscopic Approach

021048W   Bypass Coronary Artery, One Artery from Aorta with Zooplastic Tissue, Percutaneous Endoscopic Approach

0210493   Bypass Coronary Artery, One Artery from Coronary Artery with Autologous Venous Tissue, Percutaneous Endoscopic Approach

0210498   Bypass Coronary Artery, One Artery from Right Internal Mammary with Autologous Venous Tissue, Percutaneous Endoscopic Approach

0210499   Bypass Coronary Artery, One Artery from Left Internal Mammary with Autologous Venous Tissue, Percutaneous Endoscopic Approach

021049C   Bypass Coronary Artery, One Artery from Thoracic Artery with Autologous Venous Tissue, Percutaneous Endoscopic Approach

021049F   Bypass Coronary Artery, One Artery from Abdominal Artery with Autologous Venous Tissue, Percutaneous Endoscopic Approach

021049W   Bypass Coronary Artery, One Artery from Aorta with Autologous Venous Tissue, Percutaneous Endoscopic Approach

02104A3   Bypass Coronary Artery, One Artery from Coronary Artery with Autologous Arterial Tissue, Percutaneous Endoscopic Approach

02104A8   Bypass Coronary Artery, One Artery from Right Internal Mammary with Autologous Arterial Tissue, Percutaneous Endoscopic Approach

02104A9   Bypass Coronary Artery, One Artery from Left Internal Mammary with Autologous Arterial Tissue, Percutaneous Endoscopic Approach

02104AC   Bypass Coronary Artery, One Artery from Thoracic Artery with Autologous Arterial Tissue, Percutaneous Endoscopic Approach

02104AF   Bypass Coronary Artery, One Artery from Abdominal Artery with Autologous Arterial Tissue, Percutaneous Endoscopic Approach

02104AW   Bypass Coronary Artery, One Artery from Aorta with Autologous Arterial Tissue, Percutaneous Endoscopic Approach

02104J3   Bypass Coronary Artery, One Artery from Coronary Artery with Synthetic Substitute, Percutaneous Endoscopic Approach

02104J8   Bypass Coronary Artery, One Artery from Right Internal Mammary with Synthetic Substitute, Percutaneous Endoscopic Approach

02104J9   Bypass Coronary Artery, One Artery from Left Internal Mammary with Synthetic Substitute, Percutaneous Endoscopic Approach

02104JC   Bypass Coronary Artery, One Artery from Thoracic Artery with Synthetic Substitute, Percutaneous Endoscopic Approach

02104JF   Bypass Coronary Artery, One Artery from Abdominal Artery with Synthetic Substitute, Percutaneous Endoscopic Approach

02104JW   Bypass Coronary Artery, One Artery from Aorta with Synthetic Substitute, Percutaneous Endoscopic Approach

02104K3   Bypass Coronary Artery, One Artery from Coronary Artery with Nonautologous Tissue Substitute, Percutaneous Endoscopic Approach

02104K8   Bypass Coronary Artery, One Artery from Right Internal Mammary with Nonautologous Tissue Substitute, Percutaneous Endoscopic Approach

02104K9   Bypass Coronary Artery, One Artery from Left Internal Mammary with Nonautologous Tissue Substitute, Percutaneous Endoscopic Approach

02104KC   Bypass Coronary Artery, One Artery from Thoracic Artery with Nonautologous Tissue Substitute, Percutaneous Endoscopic Approach

02104KF   Bypass Coronary Artery, One Artery from Abdominal Artery with Nonautologous Tissue Substitute, Percutaneous Endoscopic Approach

02104KW   Bypass Coronary Artery, One Artery from Aorta with Nonautologous Tissue Substitute, Percutaneous Endoscopic Approach

02104Z3   Bypass Coronary Artery, One Artery from Coronary Artery, Percutaneous Endoscopic Approach

**HAC 08: Surgical Artery Infection of Mediastinitis Following Coronary Bypass Graft (CABG) Procedures (continued)**

02104Z8    Bypass Coronary Artery, One Artery from Right Internal Mammary, Percutaneous Endoscopic Approach

02104Z9    Bypass Coronary Artery, One Artery from Left Internal Mammary, Percutaneous Endoscopic Approach

02104ZC    Bypass Coronary Artery, One Artery from Thoracic Artery, Percutaneous Endoscopic Approach

02104ZF    Bypass Coronary Artery, One Artery from Abdominal Artery, Percutaneous Endoscopic Approach

0211083    Bypass Coronary Artery, Two Arteries from Coronary Artery with Zooplastic Tissue, Open Approach

0211088    Bypass Coronary Artery, Two Arteries from Right Internal Mammary with Zooplastic Tissue, Open Approach

0211089    Bypass Coronary Artery, Two Arteries from Left Internal Mammary with Zooplastic Tissue, Open Approach

021108C    Bypass Coronary Artery, Two Arteries from Thoracic Artery with Zooplastic Tissue, Open Approach

021108F    Bypass Coronary Artery, Two Arteries from Abdominal Artery with Zooplastic Tissue, Open Approach

021108W    Bypass Coronary Artery, Two Arteries from Aorta with Zooplastic Tissue, Open Approach

0211093    Bypass Coronary Artery, Two Arteries from Coronary Artery with Autologous Venous Tissue, Open Approach

0211098    Bypass Coronary Artery, Two Arteries from Right Internal Mammary with Autologous Venous Tissue, Open Approach

0211099    Bypass Coronary Artery, Two Arteries from Left Internal Mammary with Autologous Venous Tissue, Open Approach

021109C    Bypass Coronary Artery, Two Arteries from Thoracic Artery with Autologous Venous Tissue, Open Approach

021109F    Bypass Coronary Artery, Two Arteries from Abdominal Artery with Autologous Venous Tissue, Open Approach

021109W    Bypass Coronary Artery, Two Arteries from Aorta with Autologous Venous Tissue, Open Approach

02110A3    Bypass Coronary Artery, Two Arteries from Coronary Artery with Autologous Arterial Tissue, Open Approach

02110A8    Bypass Coronary Artery, Two Arteries from Right Internal Mammary with Autologous Arterial Tissue, Open Approach

02110A9    Bypass Coronary Artery, Two Arteries from Left Internal Mammary with Autologous Arterial Tissue, Open Approach

02110AC    Bypass Coronary Artery, Two Arteries from Thoracic Artery with Autologous Arterial Tissue, Open Approach

02110AF    Bypass Coronary Artery, Two Arteries from Abdominal Artery with Autologous Arterial Tissue, Open Approach

02110AW    Bypass Coronary Artery, Two Arteries from Aorta with Autologous Arterial Tissue, Open Approach

02110J3    Bypass Coronary Artery, Two Arteries from Coronary Artery with Synthetic Substitute, Open Approach

02110J8    Bypass Coronary Artery, Two Arteries from Right Internal Mammary with Synthetic Substitute, Open Approach

02110J9    Bypass Coronary Artery, Two Arteries from Left Internal Mammary with Synthetic Substitute, Open Approach

02110JC    Bypass Coronary Artery, Two Arteries from Thoracic Artery with Synthetic Substitute, Open Approach

02110JF    Bypass Coronary Artery, Two Arteries from Abdominal Artery with Synthetic Substitute, Open Approach

02110JW    Bypass Coronary Artery, Two Arteries from Aorta with Synthetic Substitute, Open Approach

02110K3    Bypass Coronary Artery, Two Arteries from Coronary Artery with Nonautologous Tissue Substitute, Open Approach

02110K8    Bypass Coronary Artery, Two Arteries from Right Internal Mammary with Nonautologous Tissue Substitute, Open Approach

02110K9    Bypass Coronary Artery, Two Arteries from Left Internal Mammary with Nonautologous Tissue Substitute, Open Approach

02110KC    Bypass Coronary Artery, Two Arteries from Thoracic Artery with Nonautologous Tissue Substitute, Open Approach

02110KF    Bypass Coronary Artery, Two Arteries from Abdominal Artery with Nonautologous Tissue Substitute, Open Approach

02110KW    Bypass Coronary Artery, Two Arteries from Aorta with Nonautologous Tissue Substitute, Open Approach

02110Z3    Bypass Coronary Artery, Two Arteries from Coronary Artery, Open Approach

02110Z8    Bypass Coronary Artery, Two Arteries from Right Internal Mammary, Open Approach

02110Z9    Bypass Coronary Artery, Two Arteries from Left Internal Mammary, Open Approach

02110ZC    Bypass Coronary Artery, Two Arteries from Thoracic Artery, Open Approach

02110ZF    Bypass Coronary Artery, Two Arteries from Abdominal Artery, Open Approach

0211483    Bypass Coronary Artery, Two Arteries from Coronary Artery with Zooplastic Tissue, Percutaneous Endoscopic Approach

0211488    Bypass Coronary Artery, Two Arteries from Right Internal Mammary with Zooplastic Tissue, Percutaneous Endoscopic Approach

0211489    Bypass Coronary Artery, Two Arteries from Left Internal Mammary with Zooplastic Tissue, Percutaneous Endoscopic Approach

021148C    Bypass Coronary Artery, Two Arteries from Thoracic Artery with Zooplastic Tissue, Percutaneous Endoscopic Approach

021148F    Bypass Coronary Artery, Two Arteries from Abdominal Artery with Zooplastic Tissue, Percutaneous Endoscopic Approach

021148W    Bypass Coronary Artery, Two Arteries from Aorta with Zooplastic Tissue, Percutaneous Endoscopic Approach

0211493    Bypass Coronary Artery, Two Arteries from Coronary Artery with Autologous Venous Tissue, Percutaneous Endoscopic Approach

0211498    Bypass Coronary Artery, Two Arteries from Right Internal Mammary with Autologous Venous Tissue, Percutaneous Endoscopic Approach

0211499    Bypass Coronary Artery, Two Arteries from Left Internal Mammary with Autologous Venous Tissue, Percutaneous Endoscopic Approach

021149C    Bypass Coronary Artery, Two Arteries from Thoracic Artery with Autologous Venous Tissue, Percutaneous Endoscopic Approach

021149F    Bypass Coronary Artery, Two Arteries from Abdominal Artery with Autologous Venous Tissue, Percutaneous Endoscopic Approach

021149W    Bypass Coronary Artery, Two Arteries from Aorta with Autologous Venous Tissue, Percutaneous Endoscopic Approach

02114A3    Bypass Coronary Artery, Two Arteries from Coronary Artery with Autologous Arterial Tissue, Percutaneous Endoscopic Approach

02114A8    Bypass Coronary Artery, Two Arteries from Right Internal Mammary with Autologous Arterial Tissue, Percutaneous Endoscopic Approach

02114A9    Bypass Coronary Artery, Two Arteries from Left Internal Mammary with Autologous Arterial Tissue, Percutaneous Endoscopic Approach

02114AC    Bypass Coronary Artery, Two Arteries from Thoracic Artery with Autologous Arterial Tissue, Percutaneous Endoscopic Approach

02114AF    Bypass Coronary Artery, Two Arteries from Abdominal Artery with Autologous Arterial Tissue, Percutaneous Endoscopic Approach

02114AW    Bypass Coronary Artery, Two Arteries from Aorta with Autologous Arterial Tissue, Percutaneous Endoscopic Approach

02114J3    Bypass Coronary Artery, Two Arteries from Coronary Artery with Synthetic Substitute, Percutaneous Endoscopic Approach

02114J8    Bypass Coronary Artery, Two Arteries from Right Internal Mammary with Synthetic Substitute, Percutaneous Endoscopic Approach

02114J9    Bypass Coronary Artery, Two Arteries from Left Internal Mammary with Synthetic Substitute, Percutaneous Endoscopic Approach

02114JC    Bypass Coronary Artery, Two Arteries from Thoracic Artery with Synthetic Substitute, Percutaneous Endoscopic Approach

02114JF    Bypass Coronary Artery, Two Arteries from Abdominal Artery with Synthetic Substitute, Percutaneous Endoscopic Approach

02114JW    Bypass Coronary Artery, Two Arteries from Aorta with Synthetic Substitute, Percutaneous Endoscopic Approach

02114K3    Bypass Coronary Artery, Two Arteries from Coronary Artery with Nonautologous Tissue Substitute, Percutaneous Endoscopic Approach

02114K8    Bypass Coronary Artery, Two Arteries from Right Internal Mammary with Nonautologous Tissue Substitute, Percutaneous Endoscopic Approach

**HAC 08: Surgical Site Infection of Mediastinitis Following Coronary Bypass Graft (CABG) Procedures (continued)**

02114K9 Bypass Coronary Artery, Two Arteries from Left Internal Mammary with Nonautologous Tissue Substitute, Percutaneous Endoscopic Approach

02114KC Bypass Coronary Artery, Two Arteries from Thoracic Artery with Nonautologous Tissue Substitute, Percutaneous Endoscopic Approach

02114KF Bypass Coronary Artery, Two Arteries from Abdominal Artery with Nonautologous Tissue Substitute, Percutaneous Endoscopic Approach

02114KW Bypass Coronary Artery, Two Arteries from Aorta with Nonautologous Tissue Substitute, Percutaneous Endoscopic Approach

02114Z3 Bypass Coronary Artery, Two Arteries from Coronary Artery, Percutaneous Endoscopic Approach

02114Z8 Bypass Coronary Artery, Two Arteries from Right Internal Mammary, Percutaneous Endoscopic Approach

02114Z9 Bypass Coronary Artery, Two Arteries from Left Internal Mammary, Percutaneous Endoscopic Approach

02114ZC Bypass Coronary Artery, Two Arteries from Thoracic Artery, Percutaneous Endoscopic Approach

02114ZF Bypass Coronary Artery, Two Arteries from Abdominal Artery, Percutaneous Endoscopic Approach

0212083 Bypass Coronary Artery, Three Arteries from Coronary Artery with Zooplastic Tissue, Open Approach

0212088 Bypass Coronary Artery, Three Arteries from Right Internal Mammary with Zooplastic Tissue, Open Approach

0212089 Bypass Coronary Artery, Three Arteries from Left Internal Mammary with Zooplastic Tissue, Open Approach

021208C Bypass Coronary Artery, Three Arteries from Thoracic Artery with Zooplastic Tissue, Open Approach

021208F Bypass Coronary Artery, Three Arteries from Abdominal Artery with Zooplastic Tissue, Open Approach

021208W Bypass Coronary Artery, Three Arteries from Aorta with Zooplastic Tissue, Open Approach

0212093 Bypass Coronary Artery, Three Arteries from Coronary Artery with Autologous Venous Tissue, Open Approach

0212098 Bypass Coronary Artery, Three Arteries from Right Internal Mammary with Autologous Venous Tissue, Open Approach

0212099 Bypass Coronary Artery, Three Arteries from Left Internal Mammary with Autologous Venous Tissue, Open Approach

021209C Bypass Coronary Artery, Three Arteries from Thoracic Artery with Autologous Venous Tissue, Open Approach

021209F Bypass Coronary Artery, Three Arteries from Abdominal Artery with Autologous Venous Tissue, Open Approach

021209W Bypass Coronary Artery, Three Arteries from Aorta with Autologous Venous Tissue, Open Approach

02120A3 Bypass Coronary Artery, Three Arteries from Coronary Artery with Autologous Arterial Tissue, Open Approach

02120A8 Bypass Coronary Artery, Three Arteries from Right Internal Mammary with Autologous Arterial Tissue, Open Approach

02120A9 Bypass Coronary Artery, Three Arteries from Left Internal Mammary with Autologous Arterial Tissue, Open Approach

02120AC Bypass Coronary Artery, Three Arteries from Thoracic Artery with Autologous Arterial Tissue, Open Approach

02120AF Bypass Coronary Artery, Three Arteries from Abdominal Artery with Autologous Arterial Tissue, Open Approach

02120AW Bypass Coronary Artery, Three Arteries from Aorta with Autologous Arterial Tissue, Open Approach

02120J3 Bypass Coronary Artery, Three Arteries from Coronary Artery with Synthetic Substitute, Open Approach

02120J8 Bypass Coronary Artery, Three Arteries from Right Internal Mammary with Synthetic Substitute, Open Approach

02120J9 Bypass Coronary Artery, Three Arteries from Left Internal Mammary with Synthetic Substitute, Open Approach

02120JC Bypass Coronary Artery, Three Arteries from Thoracic Artery with Synthetic Substitute, Open Approach

02120JF Bypass Coronary Artery, Three Arteries from Abdominal Artery with Synthetic Substitute, Open Approach

02120JW Bypass Coronary Artery, Three Arteries from Aorta with Synthetic Substitute, Open Approach

02120K3 Bypass Coronary Artery, Three Arteries from Coronary Artery with Nonautologous Tissue Substitute, Open Approach

02120K8 Bypass Coronary Artery, Three Arteries from Right Internal Mammary with Nonautologous Tissue Substitute, Open Approach

02120K9 Bypass Coronary Artery, Three Arteries from Left Internal Mammary with Nonautologous Tissue Substitute, Open Approach

02120KC Bypass Coronary Artery, Three Arteries from Thoracic Artery with Nonautologous Tissue Substitute, Open Approach

02120KF Bypass Coronary Artery, Three Arteries from Abdominal Artery with Nonautologous Tissue Substitute, Open Approach

02120KW Bypass Coronary Artery, Three Arteries from Aorta with Nonautologous Tissue Substitute, Open Approach

02120Z3 Bypass Coronary Artery, Three Arteries from Coronary Artery, Open Approach

02120Z8 Bypass Coronary Artery, Three Arteries from Right Internal Mammary, Open Approach

02120Z9 Bypass Coronary Artery, Three Arteries from Left Internal Mammary, Open Approach

02120ZC Bypass Coronary Artery, Three Arteries from Thoracic Artery, Open Approach

02120ZF Bypass Coronary Artery, Three Arteries from Abdominal Artery, Open Approach

0212483 Bypass Coronary Artery, Three Arteries from Coronary Artery with Zooplastic Tissue, Percutaneous Endoscopic Approach

0212488 Bypass Coronary Artery, Three Arteries from Right Internal Mammary with Zooplastic Tissue, Percutaneous Endoscopic Approach

0212489 Bypass Coronary Artery, Three Arteries from Left Internal Mammary with Zooplastic Tissue, Percutaneous Endoscopic Approach

021248C Bypass Coronary Artery, Three Arteries from Thoracic Artery with Zooplastic Tissue, Percutaneous Endoscopic Approach

021248F Bypass Coronary Artery, Three Arteries from Abdominal Artery with Zooplastic Tissue, Percutaneous Endoscopic Approach

021248W Bypass Coronary Artery, Three Arteries from Aorta with Zooplastic Tissue, Percutaneous Endoscopic Approach

0212493 Bypass Coronary Artery, Three Arteries from Coronary Artery with Autologous Venous Tissue, Percutaneous Endoscopic Approach

0212498 Bypass Coronary Artery, Three Arteries from Right Internal Mammary with Autologous Venous Tissue, Percutaneous Endoscopic Approach

0212499 Bypass Coronary Artery, Three Arteries from Left Internal Mammary with Autologous Venous Tissue, Percutaneous Endoscopic Approach

021249C Bypass Coronary Artery, Three Arteries from Thoracic Artery with Autologous Venous Tissue, Percutaneous Endoscopic Approach

021249F Bypass Coronary Artery, Three Arteries from Abdominal Artery with Autologous Venous Tissue, Percutaneous Endoscopic Approach

021249W Bypass Coronary Artery, Three Arteries from Aorta with Autologous Venous Tissue, Percutaneous Endoscopic Approach

02124A3 Bypass Coronary Artery, Three Arteries from Coronary Artery with Autologous Arterial Tissue, Percutaneous Endoscopic Approach

02124A8 Bypass Coronary Artery, Three Arteries from Right Internal Mammary with Autologous Arterial Tissue, Percutaneous Endoscopic Approach

02124A9 Bypass Coronary Artery, Three Arteries from Left Internal Mammary with Autologous Arterial Tissue, Percutaneous Endoscopic Approach

02124AC Bypass Coronary Artery, Three Arteries from Thoracic Artery with Autologous Arterial Tissue, Percutaneous Endoscopic Approach

02124AF Bypass Coronary Artery, Three Arteries from Abdominal Artery with Autologous Arterial Tissue, Percutaneous Endoscopic Approach

02124AW Bypass Coronary Artery, Three Arteries from Aorta with Autologous Arterial Tissue, Percutaneous Endoscopic Approach

02124J3 Bypass Coronary Artery, Three Arteries from Coronary Artery with Synthetic Substitute, Percutaneous Endoscopic Approach

02124J8 Bypass Coronary Artery, Three Arteries from Right Internal Mammary with Synthetic Substitute, Percutaneous Endoscopic Approach

**HAC 08: Surgical Site Infection of Mediastinitis Following Coronary Bypass Graft (CABG) Procedures (continued)**

Ø2124J9  Bypass Coronary Artery, Three Arteries from Left Internal Mammary with Synthetic Substitute, Percutaneous Endoscopic Approach

Ø2124JC  Bypass Coronary Artery, Three Arteries from Thoracic Artery with Synthetic Substitute, Percutaneous Endoscopic Approach

Ø2124JF  Bypass Coronary Artery, Three Arteries from Abdominal Artery with Synthetic Substitute, Percutaneous Endoscopic Approach

Ø2124JW  Bypass Coronary Artery, Three Arteries from Aorta with Synthetic Substitute, Percutaneous Endoscopic Approach

Ø2124K3  Bypass Coronary Artery, Three Arteries from Coronary Artery with Nonautologous Tissue Substitute, Percutaneous Endoscopic Approach

Ø2124K8  Bypass Coronary Artery, Three Arteries from Right Internal Mammary with Nonautologous Tissue Substitute, Percutaneous Endoscopic Approach

Ø2124K9  Bypass Coronary Artery, Three Arteries from Left Internal Mammary with Nonautologous Tissue Substitute, Percutaneous Endoscopic Approach

Ø2124KC  Bypass Coronary Artery, Three Arteries from Thoracic Artery with Nonautologous Tissue Substitute, Percutaneous Endoscopic Approach

Ø2124KF  Bypass Coronary Artery, Three Arteries from Abdominal Artery with Nonautologous Tissue Substitute, Percutaneous Endoscopic Approach

Ø2124KW  Bypass Coronary Artery, Three Arteries from Aorta with Nonautologous Tissue Substitute, Percutaneous Endoscopic Approach

Ø2124Z3  Bypass Coronary Artery, Three Arteries from Coronary Artery, Percutaneous Endoscopic Approach

Ø2124Z8  Bypass Coronary Artery, Three Arteries from Right Internal Mammary, Percutaneous Endoscopic Approach

Ø2124Z9  Bypass Coronary Artery, Three Arteries from Left Internal Mammary, Percutaneous Endoscopic Approach

Ø2124ZC  Bypass Coronary Artery, Three Arteries from Thoracic Artery, Percutaneous Endoscopic Approach

Ø2124ZF  Bypass Coronary Artery, Three Arteries from Abdominal Artery, Percutaneous Endoscopic Approach

Ø213Ø83  Bypass Coronary Artery, Four or More Arteries from Coronary Artery with Zooplastic Tissue, Open Approach

Ø213Ø88  Bypass Coronary Artery, Four or More Arteries from Right Internal Mammary with Zooplastic Tissue, Open Approach

Ø213Ø89  Bypass Coronary Artery, Four or More Arteries from Left Internal Mammary with Zooplastic Tissue, Open Approach

Ø213Ø8C  Bypass Coronary Artery, Four or More Arteries from Thoracic Artery with Zooplastic Tissue, Open Approach

Ø213Ø8F  Bypass Coronary Artery, Four or More Arteries from Abdominal Artery with Zooplastic Tissue, Open Approach

Ø213Ø8W  Bypass Coronary Artery, Four or More Arteries from Aorta with Zooplastic Tissue, Open Approach

Ø213Ø93  Bypass Coronary Artery, Four or More Arteries from Coronary Artery with Autologous Venous Tissue, Open Approach

Ø213Ø98  Bypass Coronary Artery, Four or More Arteries from Right Internal Mammary with Autologous Venous Tissue, Open Approach

Ø213Ø99  Bypass Coronary Artery, Four or More Arteries from Left Internal Mammary with Autologous Venous Tissue, Open Approach

Ø213Ø9C  Bypass Coronary Artery, Four or More Arteries from Thoracic Artery with Autologous Venous Tissue, Open Approach

Ø213Ø9F  Bypass Coronary Artery, Four or More Arteries from Abdominal Artery with Autologous Venous Tissue, Open Approach

Ø213Ø9W  Bypass Coronary Artery, Four or More Arteries from Aorta with Autologous Venous Tissue, Open Approach

Ø213ØA3  Bypass Coronary Artery, Four or More Arteries from Coronary Artery with Autologous Arterial Tissue, Open Approach

Ø213ØA8  Bypass Coronary Artery, Four or More Arteries from Right Internal Mammary with Autologous Arterial Tissue, Open Approach

Ø213ØA9  Bypass Coronary Artery, Four or More Arteries from Left Internal Mammary with Autologous Arterial Tissue, Open Approach

Ø213ØAC  Bypass Coronary Artery, Four or More Arteries from Thoracic Artery with Autologous Arterial Tissue, Open Approach

Ø213ØAF  Bypass Coronary Artery, Four or More Arteries from Abdominal Artery with Autologous Arterial Tissue, Open Approach

Ø213ØAW  Bypass Coronary Artery, Four or More Arteries from Aorta with Autologous Arterial Tissue, Open Approach

Ø213ØJ3  Bypass Coronary Artery, Four or More Arteries from Coronary Artery with Synthetic Substitute, Open Approach

Ø213ØJ8  Bypass Coronary Artery, Four or More Arteries from Right Internal Mammary with Synthetic Substitute, Open Approach

Ø213ØJ9  Bypass Coronary Artery, Four or More Arteries from Left Internal Mammary with Synthetic Substitute, Open Approach

Ø213ØJC  Bypass Coronary Artery, Four or More Arteries from Thoracic Artery with Synthetic Substitute, Open Approach

Ø213ØJF  Bypass Coronary Artery, Four or More Arteries from Abdominal Artery with Synthetic Substitute, Open Approach

Ø213ØJW  Bypass Coronary Artery, Four or More Arteries from Aorta with Synthetic Substitute, Open Approach

Ø213ØK3  Bypass Coronary Artery, Four or More Arteries from Coronary Artery with Nonautologous Tissue Substitute, Open Approach

Ø213ØK8  Bypass Coronary Artery, Four or More Arteries from Right Internal Mammary with Nonautologous Tissue Substitute, Open Approach

Ø213ØK9  Bypass Coronary Artery, Four or More Arteries from Left Internal Mammary with Nonautologous Tissue Substitute, Open Approach

Ø213ØKC  Bypass Coronary Artery, Four or More Arteries from Thoracic Artery with Nonautologous Tissue Substitute, Open Approach

Ø213ØKF  Bypass Coronary Artery, Four or More Arteries from Abdominal Artery with Nonautologous Tissue Substitute, Open Approach

Ø213ØKW  Bypass Coronary Artery, Four or More Arteries from Aorta with Nonautologous Tissue Substitute, Open Approach

Ø213ØZ3  Bypass Coronary Artery, Four or More Arteries from Coronary Artery, Open Approach

Ø213ØZ8  Bypass Coronary Artery, Four or More Arteries from Right Internal Mammary, Open Approach

Ø213ØZ9  Bypass Coronary Artery, Four or More Arteries from Left Internal Mammary, Open Approach

Ø213ØZC  Bypass Coronary Artery, Four or More Arteries from Thoracic Artery, Open Approach

Ø213ØZF  Bypass Coronary Artery, Four or More Arteries from Abdominal Artery, Open Approach

Ø213483  Bypass Coronary Artery, Four or More Arteries from Coronary Artery with Zooplastic Tissue, Percutaneous Endoscopic Approach

Ø213488  Bypass Coronary Artery, Four or More Arteries from Right Internal Mammary with Zooplastic Tissue, Percutaneous Endoscopic Approach

Ø213489  Bypass Coronary Artery, Four or More Arteries from Left Internal Mammary with Zooplastic Tissue, Percutaneous Endoscopic Approach

Ø21348C  Bypass Coronary Artery, Four or More Arteries from Thoracic Artery with Zooplastic Tissue, Percutaneous Endoscopic Approach

Ø21348F  Bypass Coronary Artery, Four or More Arteries from Abdominal Artery with Zooplastic Tissue, Percutaneous Endoscopic Approach

Ø21348W  Bypass Coronary Artery, Four or More Arteries from Aorta with Zooplastic Tissue, Percutaneous Endoscopic Approach

Ø213493  Bypass Coronary Artery, Four or More Arteries from Coronary Artery with Autologous Venous Tissue, Percutaneous Endoscopic Approach

Ø213498  Bypass Coronary Artery, Four or More Arteries from Right Internal Mammary with Autologous Venous Tissue, Percutaneous Endoscopic Approach

Ø213499  Bypass Coronary Artery, Four or More Arteries from Left Internal Mammary with Autologous Venous Tissue, Percutaneous Endoscopic Approach

Ø21349C  Bypass Coronary Artery, Four or More Arteries from Thoracic Artery with Autologous Venous Tissue, Percutaneous Endoscopic Approach

Ø21349F  Bypass Coronary Artery, Four or More Arteries from Abdominal Artery with Autologous Venous Tissue, Percutaneous Endoscopic Approach

Ø21349W  Bypass Coronary Artery, Four or More Arteries from Aorta with Autologous Venous Tissue, Percutaneous Endoscopic Approach

## HAC 08: Surgical Site Infection of Mediastinitis Following Coronary Bypass Graft (CABG) Procedures (continued)

02134A3   Bypass Coronary Artery, Four or More Arteries from Coronary Artery with Autologous Arterial Tissue, Percutaneous Endoscopic Approach

02134A8   Bypass Coronary Artery, Four or More Arteries from Right Internal Mammary with Autologous Arterial Tissue, Percutaneous Endoscopic Approach

02134A9   Bypass Coronary Artery, Four or More Arteries from Left Internal Mammary with Autologous Arterial Tissue, Percutaneous Endoscopic Approach

02134AC   Bypass Coronary Artery, Four or More Arteries from Thoracic Artery with Autologous Arterial Tissue, Percutaneous Endoscopic Approach

02134AF   Bypass Coronary Artery, Four or More Arteries from Abdominal Artery with Autologous Arterial Tissue, Percutaneous Endoscopic Approach

02134AW   Bypass Coronary Artery, Four or More Arteries from Aorta with Autologous Arterial Tissue, Percutaneous Endoscopic Approach

02134J3   Bypass Coronary Artery, Four or More Arteries from Coronary Artery with Synthetic Substitute, Percutaneous Endoscopic Approach

02134J8   Bypass Coronary Artery, Four or More Arteries from Right Internal Mammary with Synthetic Substitute, Percutaneous Endoscopic Approach

02134J9   Bypass Coronary Artery, Four or More Arteries from Left Internal Mammary with Synthetic Substitute, Percutaneous Endoscopic Approach

02134JC   Bypass Coronary Artery, Four or More Arteries from Thoracic Artery with Synthetic Substitute, Percutaneous Endoscopic Approach

02134JF   Bypass Coronary Artery, Four or More Arteries from Abdominal Artery with Synthetic Substitute, Percutaneous Endoscopic Approach

02134JW   Bypass Coronary Artery, Four or More Arteries from Aorta with Synthetic Substitute, Percutaneous Endoscopic Approach

02134K3   Bypass Coronary Artery, Four or More Arteries from Coronary Artery with Nonautologous Tissue Substitute, Percutaneous Endoscopic Approach

02134K8   Bypass Coronary Artery, Four or More Arteries from Right Internal Mammary with Nonautologous Tissue Substitute, Percutaneous Endoscopic Approach

02134K9   Bypass Coronary Artery, Four or More Arteries from Left Internal Mammary with Nonautologous Tissue Substitute, Percutaneous Endoscopic Approach

02134KC   Bypass Coronary Artery, Four or More Arteries from Thoracic Artery with Nonautologous Tissue Substitute, Percutaneous Endoscopic Approach

02134KF   Bypass Coronary Artery, Four or More Arteries from Abdominal Artery with Nonautologous Tissue Substitute, Percutaneous Endoscopic Approach

02134KW   Bypass Coronary Artery, Four or More Arteries from Aorta with Nonautologous Tissue Substitute, Percutaneous Endoscopic Approach

02134Z3   Bypass Coronary Artery, Four or More Arteries from Coronary Artery, Percutaneous Endoscopic Approach

02134Z8   Bypass Coronary Artery, Four or More Arteries from Right Internal Mammary, Percutaneous Endoscopic Approach

02134Z9   Bypass Coronary Artery, Four or More Arteries from Left Internal Mammary, Percutaneous Endoscopic Approach

02134ZC   Bypass Coronary Artery, Four or More Arteries from Thoracic Artery, Percutaneous Endoscopic Approach

02134ZF   Bypass Coronary Artery, Four or More Arteries from Abdominal Artery, Percutaneous Endoscopic Approach

## HAC 09: Manifestations of Poor Glycemic Control

Secondary diagnosis not POA:

E08.00
E08.01
E08.10
E09.00
E09.01
E09.10
E10.10
E11.00
E11.01
E13.00
E13.01
E13.10
E15

## HAC 10: Deep Vein Thrombosis (DVT) or Pulmonary Embolism (PE) with Total Knee or Hip Replacement

Secondary diagnosis not POA:

I26.02
I26.09
I26.92
I26.99
I82.401
I82.402
I82.403
I82.409
I82.411
I82.412
I82.413
I82.419
I82.421
I82.422
I82.423
I82.429
I82.431
I82.432
I82.433
I82.439
I82.441
I82.442
I82.443
I82.449
I82.491
I82.492
I82.493
I82.499
I82.4Y1
I82.4Y2
I82.4Y3
I82.4Y9
I82.4Z1
I82.4Z2
I82.4Z3
I82.4Z9

**AND**

Any of the following procedures:

0SR9019   Replacement of Right Hip Joint with Metal Synthetic Substitute, Cemented, Open Approach

0SR901A   Replacement of Right Hip Joint with Metal Synthetic Substitute, Uncemented, Open Approach

0SR901Z   Replacement of Right Hip Joint with Metal Synthetic Substitute, Open Approach

0SR9029   Replacement of Right Hip Joint with Metal on Polyethylene Synthetic Substitute, Cemented, Open Approach

0SR902A   Replacement of Right Hip Joint with Metal on Polyethylene Synthetic Substitute, Uncemented, Open Approach

0SR902Z   Replacement of Right Hip Joint with Metal on Polyethylene Synthetic Substitute, Open Approach

0SR9039   Replacement of Right Hip Joint with Ceramic Synthetic Substitute, Cemented, Open Approach

0SR903A   Replacement of Right Hip Joint with Ceramic Synthetic Substitute, Uncemented, Open Approach

0SR903Z   Replacement of Right Hip Joint with Ceramic Synthetic Substitute, Open Approach

0SR9049   Replacement of Right Hip Joint with Ceramic on Polyethylene Synthetic Substitute, Cemented, Open Approach

0SR904A   Replacement of Right Hip Joint with Ceramic on Polyethylene Synthetic Substitute, Uncemented, Open Approach

0SR904Z   Replacement of Right Hip Joint with Ceramic on Polyethylene Synthetic Substitute, Open Approach

0SR907Z   Replacement of Right Hip Joint with Autologous Tissue Substitute, Open Approach

0SR90J9   Replacement of Right Hip Joint with Synthetic Substitute, Cemented, Open Approach

0SR90JA   Replacement of Right Hip Joint with Synthetic Substitute, Uncemented, Open Approach

0SR90JZ   Replacement of Right Hip Joint with Synthetic Substitute, Open Approach

0SR90KZ   Replacement of Right Hip Joint with Nonautologous Tissue Substitute, Open Approach

0SRA009   Replacement of Right Hip Joint, Acetabular Surface with Polyethylene Synthetic Substitute, Cemented, Open Approach

0SRA00A   Replacement of Right Hip Joint, Acetabular Surface with Polyethylene Synthetic Substitute, Uncemented, Open Approach

0SRA00Z   Replacement of Right Hip Joint, Acetabular Surface with Polyethylene Synthetic Substitute, Open Approach

0SRA019   Replacement of Right Hip Joint, Acetabular Surface with Metal Synthetic Substitute, Cemented, Open Approach

0SRA01A   Replacement of Right Hip Joint, Acetabular Surface with Metal Synthetic Substitute, Uncemented, Open Approach

0SRA01Z   Replacement of Right Hip Joint, Acetabular Surface with Metal Synthetic Substitute, Open Approach

0SRA039   Replacement of Right Hip Joint, Acetabular Surface with Ceramic Synthetic Substitute, Cemented, Open Approach

0SRA03A   Replacement of Right Hip Joint, Acetabular Surface with Ceramic Synthetic Substitute, Uncemented, Open Approach

## HAC 10: Deep Vein Thrombosis (DVT) or Pulmonary Embolism (PE) with Total Knee or Hip Replacement (continued)

ØSRAØ3Z   Replacement of Right Hip Joint, Acetabular Surface with Ceramic Synthetic Substitute, Open Approach

ØSRAØ7Z   Replacement of Right Hip Joint, Acetabular Surface with Autologous Tissue Substitute, Open Approach

ØSRAØJ9   Replacement of Right Hip Joint, Acetabular Surface with Synthetic Substitute, Cemented, Open Approach

ØSRAØJA   Replacement of Right Hip Joint, Acetabular Surface with Synthetic Substitute, Uncemented, Open Approach

ØSRAØJZ   Replacement of Right Hip Joint, Acetabular Surface with Synthetic Substitute, Open Approach

ØSRAØKZ   Replacement of Right Hip Joint, Acetabular Surface with Nonautologous Tissue Substitute, Open Approach

ØSRBØ19   Replacement of Left Hip Joint with Metal Synthetic Substitute, Cemented, Open Approach

ØSRBØ1A   Replacement of Left Hip Joint with Metal Synthetic Substitute, Uncemented, Open Approach

ØSRBØ1Z   Replacement of Left Hip Joint with Metal Synthetic Substitute, Open Approach

ØSRBØ29   Replacement of Left Hip Joint with Metal on Polyethylene Synthetic Substitute, Cemented, Open Approach

ØSRBØ2A   Replacement of Left Hip Joint with Metal on Polyethylene Synthetic Substitute, Uncemented, Open Approach

ØSRBØ2Z   Replacement of Left Hip Joint with Metal on Polyethylene Synthetic Substitute, Open Approach

ØSRBØ39   Replacement of Left Hip Joint with Ceramic Synthetic Substitute, Cemented, Open Approach

ØSRBØ3A   Replacement of Left Hip Joint with Ceramic Synthetic Substitute, Uncemented, Open Approach

ØSRBØ3Z   Replacement of Left Hip Joint with Ceramic Synthetic Substitute, Open Approach

ØSRBØ49   Replacement of Left Hip Joint with Ceramic on Polyethylene Synthetic Substitute, Cemented, Open Approach

ØSRBØ4A   Replacement of Left Hip Joint with Ceramic on Polyethylene Synthetic Substitute, Uncemented, Open Approach

ØSRBØ4Z   Replacement of Left Hip Joint with Ceramic on Polyethylene Synthetic Substitute, Open Approach

ØSRBØ7Z   Replacement of Left Hip Joint with Autologous Tissue Substitute, Open Approach

ØSRBØJ9   Replacement of Left Hip Joint with Synthetic Substitute, Cemented, Open Approach

ØSRBØJA   Replacement of Left Hip Joint with Synthetic Substitute, Uncemented, Open Approach

ØSRBØJZ   Replacement of Left Hip Joint with Synthetic Substitute, Open Approach

ØSRBØKZ   Replacement of Left Hip Joint with Nonautologous Tissue Substitute, Open Approach

ØSRCØ7Z   Replacement of Right Knee Joint with Autologous Tissue Substitute, Open Approach

ØSRCØJ9   Replacement of Right Knee Joint with Synthetic Substitute, Cemented, Open Approach

ØSRCØJA   Replacement of Right Knee Joint with Synthetic Substitute, Uncemented, Open Approach

ØSRCØJZ   Replacement of Right Knee Joint with Synthetic Substitute, Open Approach

ØSRCØKZ   Replacement of Right Knee Joint with Nonautologous Tissue Substitute, Open Approach

ØSRCØL9   Replacement of Right Knee Joint with Unicondylar Synthetic Substitute, Cemented, Open Approach

ØSRCØLA   Replacement of Right Knee Joint with Unicondylar Synthetic Substitute, Uncemented, Open Approach

ØSRCØLZ   Replacement of Right Knee Joint with Unicondylar Synthetic Substitute, Open Approach

ØSRDØ7Z   Replacement of Left Knee Joint with Autologous Tissue Substitute, Open Approach

ØSRDØJ9   Replacement of Left Knee Joint with Synthetic Substitute, Cemented, Open Approach

ØSRDØJA   Replacement of Left Knee Joint with Synthetic Substitute, Uncemented, Open Approach

ØSRDØJZ   Replacement of Left Knee Joint with Synthetic Substitute, Open Approach

ØSRDØKZ   Replacement of Left Knee Joint with Nonautologous Tissue Substitute, Open Approach

ØSRDØL9   Replacement of Left Knee Joint with Unicondylar Synthetic Substitute, Cemented, Open Approach

ØSRDØLA   Replacement of Left Knee Joint with Unicondylar Synthetic Substitute, Uncemented, Open Approach

ØSRDØLZ   Replacement of Left Knee Joint with Unicondylar Synthetic Substitute, Open Approach

ØSREØØ9   Replacement of Left Hip Joint, Acetabular Surface with Polyethylene Synthetic Substitute, Cemented, Open Approach

ØSREØØA   Replacement of Left Hip Joint, Acetabular Surface with Polyethylene Synthetic Substitute, Uncemented, Open Approach

ØSREØØZ   Replacement of Left Hip Joint, Acetabular Surface with Polyethylene Synthetic Substitute, Open Approach

ØSREØ19   Replacement of Left Hip Joint, Acetabular Surface with Metal Synthetic Substitute, Cemented, Open Approach

ØSREØ1A   Replacement of Left Hip Joint, Acetabular Surface with Metal Synthetic Substitute, Uncemented, Open Approach

ØSREØ1Z   Replacement of Left Hip Joint, Acetabular Surface with Metal Synthetic Substitute, Open Approach

ØSREØ39   Replacement of Left Hip Joint, Acetabular Surface with Ceramic Synthetic Substitute, Cemented, Open Approach

ØSREØ3A   Replacement of Left Hip Joint, Acetabular Surface with Ceramic Synthetic Substitute, Uncemented, Open Approach

ØSREØ3Z   Replacement of Left Hip Joint, Acetabular Surface with Ceramic Synthetic Substitute, Open Approach

ØSREØ7Z   Replacement of Left Hip Joint, Acetabular Surface with Autologous Tissue Substitute, Open Approach

ØSREØJ9   Replacement of Left Hip Joint, Acetabular Surface with Synthetic Substitute, Cemented, Open Approach

ØSREØJA   Replacement of Left Hip Joint, Acetabular Surface with Synthetic Substitute, Uncemented, Open Approach

ØSREØJZ   Replacement of Left Hip Joint, Acetabular Surface with Synthetic Substitute, Open Approach

ØSREØKZ   Replacement of Left Hip Joint, Acetabular Surface with Nonautologous Tissue Substitute, Open Approach

ØSRRØ19   Replacement of Right Hip Joint, Femoral Surface with Metal Synthetic Substitute, Cemented, Open Approach

ØSRRØ1A   Replacement of Right Hip Joint, Femoral Surface with Metal Synthetic Substitute, Uncemented, Open Approach

ØSRRØ1Z   Replacement of Right Hip Joint, Femoral Surface with Metal Synthetic Substitute, Open Approach

ØSRRØ39   Replacement of Right Hip Joint, Femoral Surface with Ceramic Synthetic Substitute, Cemented, Open Approach

ØSRRØ3A   Replacement of Right Hip Joint, Femoral Surface with Ceramic Synthetic Substitute, Uncemented, Open Approach

ØSRRØ3Z   Replacement of Right Hip Joint, Femoral Surface with Ceramic Synthetic Substitute, Open Approach

ØSRRØ7Z   Replacement of Right Hip Joint, Femoral Surface with Autologous Tissue Substitute, Open Approach

ØSRRØJ9   Replacement of Right Hip Joint, Femoral Surface with Synthetic Substitute, Cemented, Open Approach

ØSRRØJA   Replacement of Right Hip Joint, Femoral Surface with Synthetic Substitute, Uncemented, Open Approach

ØSRRØJZ   Replacement of Right Hip Joint, Femoral Surface with Synthetic Substitute, Open Approach

ØSRRØKZ   Replacement of Right Hip Joint, Femoral Surface with Nonautologous Tissue Substitute, Open Approach

ØSRSØ19   Replacement of Left Hip Joint, Femoral Surface with Metal Synthetic Substitute, Cemented, Open Approach

ØSRSØ1A   Replacement of Left Hip Joint, Femoral Surface with Metal Synthetic Substitute, Uncemented, Open Approach

ØSRSØ1Z   Replacement of Left Hip Joint, Femoral Surface with Metal Synthetic Substitute, Open Approach

ØSRSØ39   Replacement of Left Hip Joint, Femoral Surface with Ceramic Synthetic Substitute, Cemented, Open Approach

ØSRSØ3A   Replacement of Left Hip Joint, Femoral Surface with Ceramic Synthetic Substitute, Uncemented, Open Approach

ØSRSØ3Z   Replacement of Left Hip Joint, Femoral Surface with Ceramic Synthetic Substitute, Open Approach

ØSRSØ7Z   Replacement of Left Hip Joint, Femoral Surface with Autologous Tissue Substitute, Open Approach

ØSRSØJ9   Replacement of Left Hip Joint, Femoral Surface with Synthetic Substitute, Cemented, Open Approach

ØSRSØJA   Replacement of Left Hip Joint, Femoral Surface with Synthetic Substitute, Uncemented, Open Approach

ØSRSØJZ   Replacement of Left Hip Joint, Femoral Surface with Synthetic Substitute, Open Approach

ØSRSØKZ   Replacement of Left Hip Joint, Femoral Surface with Nonautologous Tissue Substitute, Open Approach

ØSRTØ7Z   Replacement of Right Knee Joint, Femoral Surface with Autologous Tissue Substitute, Open Approach

**HAC 10: Deep Vein Thrombosis (DVT) or Pulmonary Embolism (PE) with Total Knee or Hip Replacement (continued)**

ØSRTØJ9  Replacement of Right Knee Joint, Femoral Surface with Synthetic Substitute, Cemented, Open Approach

ØSRTØJA  Replacement of Right Knee Joint, Femoral Surface with Synthetic Substitute, Uncemented, Open Approach

ØSRTØJZ  Replacement of Right Knee Joint, Femoral Surface with Synthetic Substitute, Open Approach

ØSRTØKZ  Replacement of Right Knee Joint, Femoral Surface with Nonautologous Tissue Substitute, Open Approach

ØSRUØ7Z  Replacement of Left Knee Joint, Femoral Surface with Autologous Tissue Substitute, Open Approach

ØSRUØJ9  Replacement of Left Knee Joint, Femoral Surface with Synthetic Substitute, Cemented, Open Approach

ØSRUØJA  Replacement of Left Knee Joint, Femoral Surface with Synthetic Substitute, Uncemented, Open Approach

ØSRUØJZ  Replacement of Left Knee Joint, Femoral Surface with Synthetic Substitute, Open Approach

ØSRUØKZ  Replacement of Left Knee Joint, Femoral Surface with Nonautologous Tissue Substitute, Open Approach

ØSRVØ7Z  Replacement of Right Knee Joint, Tibial Surface with Autologous Tissue Substitute, Open Approach

ØSRVØJ9  Replacement of Right Knee Joint, Tibial Surface with Synthetic Substitute, Cemented, Open Approach

ØSRVØJA  Replacement of Right Knee Joint, Tibial Surface with Synthetic Substitute, Uncemented, Open Approach

ØSRVØJZ  Replacement of Right Knee Joint, Tibial Surface with Synthetic Substitute, Open Approach

ØSRVØKZ  Replacement of Right Knee Joint, Tibial Surface with Nonautologous Tissue Substitute, Open Approach

ØSRWØ7Z  Replacement of Left Knee Joint, Tibial Surface with Autologous Tissue Substitute, Open Approach

ØSRWØJ9  Replacement of Left Knee Joint, Tibial Surface with Synthetic Substitute, Cemented, Open Approach

ØSRWØJA  Replacement of Left Knee Joint, Tibial Surface with Synthetic Substitute, Uncemented, Open Approach

ØSRWØJZ  Replacement of Left Knee Joint, Tibial Surface with Synthetic Substitute, Open Approach

ØSRWØKZ  Replacement of Left Knee Joint, Tibial Surface with Nonautologous Tissue Substitute, Open Approach

ØSU9ØBZ  Supplement Right Hip Joint with Resurfacing Device, Open Approach

ØSUAØBZ  Supplement Right Hip Joint, Acetabular Surface with Resurfacing Device, Open Approach

ØSUBØBZ  Supplement Left Hip Joint with Resurfacing Device, Open Approach

ØSUEØBZ  Supplement Left Hip Joint, Acetabular Surface with Resurfacing Device, Open Approach

ØSURØBZ  Supplement Right Hip Joint, Femoral Surface with Resurfacing Device, Open Approach

ØSUSØBZ  Supplement Left Hip Joint, Femoral Surface with Resurfacing Device, Open Approach

**HAC 11: Surgical Site Infection Following Bariatric Surgery**

Principal diagnosis of:

E66.Ø1

**AND**

Secondary diagnosis not POA:

K68.11

K95.Ø1

K95.81

T81.4XXA

**AND**

Any of the following procedures:

ØD16Ø79  Bypass Stomach to Duodenum with Autologous Tissue Substitute, Open Approach

ØD16Ø7A  Bypass Stomach to Jejunum with Autologous Tissue Substitute, Open Approach

ØD16Ø7B  Bypass Stomach to Ileum with Autologous Tissue Substitute, Open Approach

ØD16Ø7L  Bypass Stomach to Transverse Colon with Autologous Tissue Substitute, Open Approach

ØD16ØJ9  Bypass Stomach to Duodenum with Synthetic Substitute, Open Approach

ØD16ØJA  Bypass Stomach to Jejunum with Synthetic Substitute, Open Approach

ØD16ØJB  Bypass Stomach to Ileum with Synthetic Substitute, Open Approach

ØD16ØJL  Bypass Stomach to Transverse Colon with Synthetic Substitute, Open Approach

ØD16ØK9  Bypass Stomach to Duodenum with Nonautologous Tissue Substitute, Open Approach

ØD16ØKA  Bypass Stomach to Jejunum with Nonautologous Tissue Substitute, Open Approach

ØD16ØKB  Bypass Stomach to Ileum with Nonautologous Tissue Substitute, Open Approach

ØD16ØKL  Bypass Stomach to Transverse Colon with Nonautologous Tissue Substitute, Open Approach

ØD16ØZ9  Bypass Stomach to Duodenum, Open Approach

ØD16ØZA  Bypass Stomach to Jejunum, Open Approach

ØD16ØZB  Bypass Stomach to Ileum, Open Approach

ØD16ØZL  Bypass Stomach to Transverse Colon, Open Approach

ØD16479  Bypass Stomach to Duodenum with Autologous Tissue Substitute, Percutaneous Endoscopic Approach

ØD1647A  Bypass Stomach to Jejunum with Autologous Tissue Substitute, Percutaneous Endoscopic Approach

ØD1647B  Bypass Stomach to Ileum with Autologous Tissue Substitute, Percutaneous Endoscopic Approach

ØD1647L  Bypass Stomach to Transverse Colon with Autologous Tissue Substitute, Percutaneous Endoscopic Approach

ØD164J9  Bypass Stomach to Duodenum with Synthetic Substitute, Percutaneous Endoscopic Approach

ØD164JA  Bypass Stomach to Jejunum with Synthetic Substitute, Percutaneous Endoscopic Approach

ØD164JB  Bypass Stomach to Ileum with Synthetic Substitute, Percutaneous Endoscopic Approach

ØD164JL  Bypass Stomach to Transverse Colon with Synthetic Substitute, Percutaneous Endoscopic Approach

ØD164K9  Bypass Stomach to Duodenum with Nonautologous Tissue Substitute, Percutaneous Endoscopic Approach

ØD164KA  Bypass Stomach to Jejunum with Nonautologous Tissue Substitute, Percutaneous Endoscopic Approach

ØD164KB  Bypass Stomach to Ileum with Nonautologous Tissue Substitute, Percutaneous Endoscopic Approach

ØD164KL  Bypass Stomach to Transverse Colon with Nonautologous Tissue Substitute, Percutaneous Endoscopic Approach

ØD164Z9  Bypass Stomach to Duodenum, Percutaneous Endoscopic Approach

ØD164ZA  Bypass Stomach to Jejunum, Percutaneous Endoscopic Approach

ØD164ZB  Bypass Stomach to Ileum, Percutaneous Endoscopic Approach

ØD164ZL  Bypass Stomach to Transverse Colon, Percutaneous Endoscopic Approach

ØD16879  Bypass Stomach to Duodenum with Autologous Tissue Substitute, Via Natural or Artificial Opening Endoscopic

ØD1687A  Bypass Stomach to Jejunum with Autologous Tissue Substitute, Via Natural or Artificial Opening Endoscopic

ØD1687B  Bypass Stomach to Ileum with Autologous Tissue Substitute, Via Natural or Artificial Opening Endoscopic

ØD1687L  Bypass Stomach to Transverse Colon with Autologous Tissue Substitute, Via Natural or Artificial Opening Endoscopic

ØD168J9  Bypass Stomach to Duodenum with Synthetic Substitute, Via Natural or Artificial Opening Endoscopic

ØD168JA  Bypass Stomach to Jejunum with Synthetic Substitute, Via Natural or Artificial Opening Endoscopic

ØD168JB  Bypass Stomach to Ileum with Synthetic Substitute, Via Natural or Artificial Opening Endoscopic

ØD168JL  Bypass Stomach to Transverse Colon with Synthetic Substitute, Via Natural or Artificial Opening Endoscopic

ØD168K9  Bypass Stomach to Duodenum with Nonautologous Tissue Substitute, Via Natural or Artificial Opening Endoscopic

ØD168KA  Bypass Stomach to Jejunum with Nonautologous Tissue Substitute, Via Natural or Artificial Opening Endoscopic

ØD168KB  Bypass Stomach to Ileum with Nonautologous Tissue Substitute, Via Natural or Artificial Opening Endoscopic

ØD168KL  Bypass Stomach to Transverse Colon with Nonautologous Tissue Substitute, Via Natural or Artificial Opening Endoscopic

ØD168Z9  Bypass Stomach to Duodenum, Via Natural or Artificial Opening Endoscopic

ØD168ZA  Bypass Stomach to Jejunum, Via Natural or Artificial Opening Endoscopic

ØD168ZB  Bypass Stomach to Ileum, Via Natural or Artificial Opening Endoscopic

ØD168ZL  Bypass Stomach to Transverse Colon, Via Natural or Artificial Opening Endoscopic

ØDV64CZ  Restriction of Stomach with Extraluminal Device, Percutaneous Endoscopic Approach

## HAC 12: Surgical Site Infection Following Certain Orthopedic Procedures of the Spine, Shoulder, and Elbow

Secondary diagnosis not POA:

K68.11
T81.4XXA
T84.60XA
T84.610A
T84.611A
T84.612A
T84.613A
T84.614A
T84.615A
T84.619A
T84.63XA
T84.69XA
T84.7XXA

### AND

Any of the following procedures:

ØRG0070   Fusion of Occipital-cervical Joint with Autologous Tissue Substitute, Anterior Approach, Anterior Column, Open Approach

ØRG0071   Fusion of Occipital-cervical Joint with Autologous Tissue Substitute, Posterior Approach, Posterior Column, Open Approach

ØRG007J   Fusion of Occipital-cervical Joint with Autologous Tissue Substitute, Posterior Approach, Anterior Column, Open Approach

ØRG00A0   Fusion of Occipital-cervical Joint with Interbody Fusion Device, Anterior Approach, Anterior Column, Open Approach

ØRG00A1   Fusion of Occipital-cervical Joint with Interbody Fusion Device, Posterior Approach, Posterior Column, Open Approach

ØRG00AJ   Fusion of Occipital-cervical Joint with Interbody Fusion Device, Posterior Approach, Anterior Column, Open Approach

ØRG00J0   Fusion of Occipital-cervical Joint with Synthetic Substitute, Anterior Approach, Anterior Column, Open Approach

ØRG00J1   Fusion of Occipital-cervical Joint with Synthetic Substitute, Posterior Approach, Posterior Column, Open Approach

ØRG00JJ   Fusion of Occipital-cervical Joint with Synthetic Substitute, Posterior Approach, Anterior Column, Open Approach

ØRG00K0   Fusion of Occipital-cervical Joint with Nonautologous Tissue Substitute, Anterior Approach, Anterior Column, Open Approach

ØRG00K1   Fusion of Occipital-cervical Joint with Nonautologous Tissue Substitute, Posterior Approach, Posterior Column, Open Approach

ØRG00KJ   Fusion of Occipital-cervical Joint with Nonautologous Tissue Substitute, Posterior Approach, Anterior Column, Open Approach

ØRG00Z0   Fusion of Occipital-cervical Joint, Anterior Approach, Anterior Column, Open Approach

ØRG00Z1   Fusion of Occipital-cervical Joint, Posterior Approach, Posterior Column, Open Approach

ØRG00ZJ   Fusion of Occipital-cervical Joint, Posterior Approach, Anterior Column, Open Approach

ØRG0370   Fusion of Occipital-cervical Joint with Autologous Tissue Substitute, Anterior Approach, Anterior Column, Percutaneous Approach

ØRG0371   Fusion of Occipital-cervical Joint with Autologous Tissue Substitute, Posterior Approach, Posterior Column, Percutaneous Approach

ØRG037J   Fusion of Occipital-cervical Joint with Autologous Tissue Substitute, Posterior Approach, Anterior Column, Percutaneous Approach

ØRG03A0   Fusion of Occipital-cervical Joint with Interbody Fusion Device, Anterior Approach, Anterior Column, Percutaneous Approach

ØRG03A1   Fusion of Occipital-cervical Joint with Interbody Fusion Device, Posterior Approach, Posterior Column, Percutaneous Approach

ØRG03AJ   Fusion of Occipital-cervical Joint with Interbody Fusion Device, Posterior Approach, Anterior Column, Percutaneous Approach

ØRG03J0   Fusion of Occipital-cervical Joint with Synthetic Substitute, Anterior Approach, Anterior Column, Percutaneous Approach

ØRG03J1   Fusion of Occipital-cervical Joint with Synthetic Substitute, Posterior Approach, Posterior Column, Percutaneous Approach

ØRG03JJ   Fusion of Occipital-cervical Joint with Synthetic Substitute, Posterior Approach, Anterior Column, Percutaneous Approach

ØRG03K0   Fusion of Occipital-cervical Joint with Nonautologous Tissue Substitute, Anterior Approach, Anterior Column, Percutaneous Approach

ØRG03K1   Fusion of Occipital-cervical Joint with Nonautologous Tissue Substitute, Posterior Approach, Posterior Column, Percutaneous Approach

ØRG03KJ   Fusion of Occipital-cervical Joint with Nonautologous Tissue Substitute, Posterior Approach, Anterior Column, Percutaneous Approach

ØRG03Z0   Fusion of Occipital-cervical Joint, Anterior Approach, Anterior Column, Percutaneous Approach

ØRG03Z1   Fusion of Occipital-cervical Joint, Posterior Approach, Posterior Column, Percutaneous Approach

ØRG03ZJ   Fusion of Occipital-cervical Joint, Posterior Approach, Anterior Column, Percutaneous Approach

ØRG0470   Fusion of Occipital-cervical Joint with Autologous Tissue Substitute, Anterior Approach, Anterior Column, Percutaneous Endoscopic Approach

ØRG0471   Fusion of Occipital-cervical Joint with Autologous Tissue Substitute, Posterior Approach, Posterior Column, Percutaneous Endoscopic Approach

ØRG047J   Fusion of Occipital-cervical Joint with Autologous Tissue Substitute, Posterior Approach, Anterior Column, Percutaneous Endoscopic Approach

ØRG04A0   Fusion of Occipital-cervical Joint with Interbody Fusion Device, Anterior Approach, Anterior Column, Percutaneous Endoscopic Approach

ØRG04A1   Fusion of Occipital-cervical Joint with Interbody Fusion Device, Posterior Approach, Posterior Column, Percutaneous Endoscopic Approach

ØRG04AJ   Fusion of Occipital-cervical Joint with Interbody Fusion Device, Posterior Approach, Anterior Column, Percutaneous Endoscopic Approach

ØRG04J0   Fusion of Occipital-cervical Joint with Synthetic Substitute, Anterior Approach, Anterior Column, Percutaneous Endoscopic Approach

ØRG04J1   Fusion of Occipital-cervical Joint with Synthetic Substitute, Posterior Approach, Posterior Column, Percutaneous Endoscopic Approach

ØRG04JJ   Fusion of Occipital-cervical Joint with Synthetic Substitute, Posterior Approach, Anterior Column, Percutaneous Endoscopic Approach

ØRG04K0   Fusion of Occipital-cervical Joint with Nonautologous Tissue Substitute, Anterior Approach, Anterior Column, Percutaneous Endoscopic Approach

ØRG04K1   Fusion of Occipital-cervical Joint with Nonautologous Tissue Substitute, Posterior Approach, Posterior Column, Percutaneous Endoscopic Approach

ØRG04KJ   Fusion of Occipital-cervical Joint with Nonautologous Tissue Substitute, Posterior Approach, Anterior Column, Percutaneous Endoscopic Approach

ØRG04Z0   Fusion of Occipital-cervical Joint, Anterior Approach, Anterior Column, Percutaneous Endoscopic Approach

ØRG04Z1   Fusion of Occipital-cervical Joint, Posterior Approach, Posterior Column, Percutaneous Endoscopic Approach

ØRG04ZJ   Fusion of Occipital-cervical Joint, Posterior Approach, Anterior Column, Percutaneous Endoscopic Approach

ØRG1070   Fusion of Cervical Vertebral Joint with Autologous Tissue Substitute, Anterior Approach, Anterior Column, Open Approach

ØRG1071   Fusion of Cervical Vertebral Joint with Autologous Tissue Substitute, Posterior Approach, Posterior Column, Open Approach

ØRG107J   Fusion of Cervical Vertebral Joint with Autologous Tissue Substitute, Posterior Approach, Anterior Column, Open Approach

ØRG10A0   Fusion of Cervical Vertebral Joint with Interbody Fusion Device, Anterior Approach, Anterior Column, Open Approach

ØRG10A1   Fusion of Cervical Vertebral Joint with Interbody Fusion Device, Posterior Approach, Posterior Column, Open Approach

ØRG10AJ   Fusion of Cervical Vertebral Joint with Interbody Fusion Device, Posterior Approach, Anterior Column, Open Approach

ØRG10J0   Fusion of Cervical Vertebral Joint with Synthetic Substitute, Anterior Approach, Anterior Column, Open Approach

ØRG10J1   Fusion of Cervical Vertebral Joint with Synthetic Substitute, Posterior Approach, Posterior Column, Open Approach

ØRG10JJ   Fusion of Cervical Vertebral Joint with Synthetic Substitute, Posterior Approach, Anterior Column, Open Approach

ØRG10K0   Fusion of Cervical Vertebral Joint with Nonautologous Tissue Substitute, Anterior Approach, Anterior Column, Open Approach

**HAC 12: Surgical Site Infection Following Certain Orthopedic Procedures of the Spine, Shoulder, and Elbow (continued)**

ØRG10K1 Fusion of Cervical Vertebral Joint with Nonautologous Tissue Substitute, Posterior Approach, Posterior Column, Open Approach

ØRG10KJ Fusion of Cervical Vertebral Joint with Nonautologous Tissue Substitute, Posterior Approach, Anterior Column, Open Approach

ØRG10ZØ Fusion of Cervical Vertebral Joint, Anterior Approach, Anterior Column, Open Approach

ØRG10Z1 Fusion of Cervical Vertebral Joint, Posterior Approach, Posterior Column, Open Approach

ØRG10ZJ Fusion of Cervical Vertebral Joint, Posterior Approach, Anterior Column, Open Approach

ØRG137Ø Fusion of Cervical Vertebral Joint with Autologous Tissue Substitute, Anterior Approach, Anterior Column, Percutaneous Approach

ØRG1371 Fusion of Cervical Vertebral Joint with Autologous Tissue Substitute, Posterior Approach, Posterior Column, Percutaneous Approach

ØRG137J Fusion of Cervical Vertebral Joint with Autologous Tissue Substitute, Posterior Approach, Anterior Column, Percutaneous Approach

ØRG13AØ Fusion of Cervical Vertebral Joint with Interbody Fusion Device, Anterior Approach, Anterior Column, Percutaneous Approach

ØRG13A1 Fusion of Cervical Vertebral Joint with Interbody Fusion Device, Posterior Approach, Posterior Column, Percutaneous Approach

ØRG13AJ Fusion of Cervical Vertebral Joint with Interbody Fusion Device, Posterior Approach, Anterior Column, Percutaneous Approach

ØRG13JØ Fusion of Cervical Vertebral Joint with Synthetic Substitute, Anterior Approach, Anterior Column, Percutaneous Approach

ØRG13J1 Fusion of Cervical Vertebral Joint with Synthetic Substitute, Posterior Approach, Posterior Column, Percutaneous Approach

ØRG13JJ Fusion of Cervical Vertebral Joint with Synthetic Substitute, Posterior Approach, Anterior Column, Percutaneous Approach

ØRG13KØ Fusion of Cervical Vertebral Joint with Nonautologous Tissue Substitute, Anterior Approach, Anterior Column, Percutaneous Approach

ØRG13K1 Fusion of Cervical Vertebral Joint with Nonautologous Tissue Substitute, Posterior Approach, Posterior Column, Percutaneous Approach

ØRG13KJ Fusion of Cervical Vertebral Joint with Nonautologous Tissue Substitute, Posterior Approach, Anterior Column, Percutaneous Approach

ØRG13ZØ Fusion of Cervical Vertebral Joint, Anterior Approach, Anterior Column, Percutaneous Approach

ØRG13Z1 Fusion of Cervical Vertebral Joint, Posterior Approach, Posterior Column, Percutaneous Approach

ØRG13ZJ Fusion of Cervical Vertebral Joint, Posterior Approach, Anterior Column, Percutaneous Approach

ØRG147Ø Fusion of Cervical Vertebral Joint with Autologous Tissue Substitute, Anterior Approach, Anterior Column, Percutaneous Endoscopic Approach

ØRG1471 Fusion of Cervical Vertebral Joint with Autologous Tissue Substitute, Posterior Approach, Posterior Column, Percutaneous Endoscopic Approach

ØRG147J Fusion of Cervical Vertebral Joint with Autologous Tissue Substitute, Posterior Approach, Anterior Column, Percutaneous Endoscopic Approach

ØRG14AØ Fusion of Cervical Vertebral Joint with Interbody Fusion Device, Anterior Approach, Anterior Column, Percutaneous Endoscopic Approach

ØRG14A1 Fusion of Cervical Vertebral Joint with Interbody Fusion Device, Posterior Approach, Posterior Column, Percutaneous Endoscopic Approach

ØRG14AJ Fusion of Cervical Vertebral Joint with Interbody Fusion Device, Posterior Approach, Anterior Column, Percutaneous Endoscopic Approach

ØRG14JØ Fusion of Cervical Vertebral Joint with Synthetic Substitute, Anterior Approach, Anterior Column, Percutaneous Endoscopic Approach

ØRG14J1 Fusion of Cervical Vertebral Joint with Synthetic Substitute, Posterior Approach, Posterior Column, Percutaneous Endoscopic Approach

ØRG14JJ Fusion of Cervical Vertebral Joint with Synthetic Substitute, Posterior Approach, Anterior Column, Percutaneous Endoscopic Approach

ØRG14KØ Fusion of Cervical Vertebral Joint with Nonautologous Tissue Substitute, Anterior Approach, Anterior Column, Percutaneous Endoscopic Approach

ØRG14K1 Fusion of Cervical Vertebral Joint with Nonautologous Tissue Substitute, Posterior Approach, Posterior Column, Percutaneous Endoscopic Approach

ØRG14KJ Fusion of Cervical Vertebral Joint with Nonautologous Tissue Substitute, Posterior Approach, Anterior Column, Percutaneous Endoscopic Approach

ØRG14ZØ Fusion of Cervical Vertebral Joint, Anterior Approach, Anterior Column, Percutaneous Endoscopic Approach

ØRG14Z1 Fusion of Cervical Vertebral Joint, Posterior Approach, Posterior Column, Percutaneous Endoscopic Approach

ØRG14ZJ Fusion of Cervical Vertebral Joint, Posterior Approach, Anterior Column, Percutaneous Endoscopic Approach

ØRG207Ø Fusion of 2 or more Cervical Vertebral Joints with Autologous Tissue Substitute, Anterior Approach, Anterior Column, Open Approach

ØRG2071 Fusion of 2 or more Cervical Vertebral Joints with Autologous Tissue Substitute, Posterior Approach, Posterior Column, Open Approach

ØRG207J Fusion of 2 or more Cervical Vertebral Joints with Autologous Tissue Substitute, Posterior Approach, Anterior Column, Open Approach

ØRG20AØ Fusion of 2 or more Cervical Vertebral Joints with Interbody Fusion Device, Anterior Approach, Anterior Column, Open Approach

ØRG20A1 Fusion of 2 or more Cervical Vertebral Joints with Interbody Fusion Device, Posterior Approach, Posterior Column, Open Approach

ØRG20AJ Fusion of 2 or more Cervical Vertebral Joints with Interbody Fusion Device, Posterior Approach, Anterior Column, Open Approach

ØRG20JØ Fusion of 2 or more Cervical Vertebral Joints with Synthetic Substitute, Anterior Approach, Anterior Column, Open Approach

ØRG20J1 Fusion of 2 or more Cervical Vertebral Joints with Synthetic Substitute, Posterior Approach, Posterior Column, Open Approach

ØRG20JJ Fusion of 2 or more Cervical Vertebral Joints with Synthetic Substitute, Posterior Approach, Anterior Column, Open Approach

ØRG20KØ Fusion of 2 or more Cervical Vertebral Joints with Nonautologous Tissue Substitute, Anterior Approach, Anterior Column, Open Approach

ØRG20K1 Fusion of 2 or more Cervical Vertebral Joints with Nonautologous Tissue Substitute, Posterior Approach, Posterior Column, Open Approach

ØRG20KJ Fusion of 2 or more Cervical Vertebral Joints with Nonautologous Tissue Substitute, Posterior Approach, Anterior Column, Open Approach

ØRG20ZØ Fusion of 2 or more Cervical Vertebral Joints, Anterior Approach, Anterior Column, Open Approach

ØRG20Z1 Fusion of 2 or more Cervical Vertebral Joints, Posterior Approach, Posterior Column, Open Approach

ØRG20ZJ Fusion of 2 or more Cervical Vertebral Joints, Posterior Approach, Anterior Column, Open Approach

ØRG237Ø Fusion of 2 or more Cervical Vertebral Joints with Autologous Tissue Substitute, Anterior Approach, Anterior Column, Percutaneous Approach

ØRG2371 Fusion of 2 or more Cervical Vertebral Joints with Autologous Tissue Substitute, Posterior Approach, Posterior Column, Percutaneous Approach

ØRG237J Fusion of 2 or more Cervical Vertebral Joints with Autologous Tissue Substitute, Posterior Approach, Anterior Column, Percutaneous Approach

ØRG23AØ Fusion of 2 or more Cervical Vertebral Joints with Interbody Fusion Device, Anterior Approach, Anterior Column, Percutaneous Approach

ØRG23A1 Fusion of 2 or more Cervical Vertebral Joints with Interbody Fusion Device, Posterior Approach, Posterior Column, Percutaneous Approach

ØRG23AJ Fusion of 2 or more Cervical Vertebral Joints with Interbody Fusion Device, Posterior Approach, Anterior Column, Percutaneous Approach

ØRG23JØ Fusion of 2 or more Cervical Vertebral Joints with Synthetic Substitute, Anterior Approach, Anterior Column, Percutaneous Approach

ØRG23J1 Fusion of 2 or more Cervical Vertebral Joints with Synthetic Substitute, Posterior Approach, Posterior Column, Percutaneous Approach

ØRG23JJ Fusion of 2 or more Cervical Vertebral Joints with Synthetic Substitute, Posterior Approach, Anterior Column, Percutaneous Approach

ØRG23KØ Fusion of 2 or more Cervical Vertebral Joints with Nonautologous Tissue Substitute, Anterior Approach, Anterior Column, Percutaneous Approach

**HAC 12: Surgical Site Infection Following Certain Orthopedic Procedures of the Spine, Shoulder, and Elbow (continued)**

ØRG23K1   Fusion of 2 or more Cervical Vertebral Joints with Nonautologous Tissue Substitute, Posterior Approach, Posterior Column, Percutaneous Approach

ØRG23KJ   Fusion of 2 or more Cervical Vertebral Joints with Nonautologous Tissue Substitute, Posterior Approach, Anterior Column, Percutaneous Approach

ØRG23Z0   Fusion of 2 or more Cervical Vertebral Joints, Anterior Approach, Anterior Column, Percutaneous Approach

ØRG23Z1   Fusion of 2 or more Cervical Vertebral Joints, Posterior Approach, Posterior Column, Percutaneous Approach

ØRG23ZJ   Fusion of 2 or more Cervical Vertebral Joints, Posterior Approach, Anterior Column, Percutaneous Approach

ØRG2470   Fusion of 2 or more Cervical Vertebral Joints with Autologous Tissue Substitute, Anterior Approach, Anterior Column, Percutaneous Endoscopic Approach

ØRG2471   Fusion of 2 or more Cervical Vertebral Joints with Autologous Tissue Substitute, Posterior Approach, Posterior Column, Percutaneous Endoscopic Approach

ØRG247J   Fusion of 2 or more Cervical Vertebral Joints with Autologous Tissue Substitute, Posterior Approach, Anterior Column, Percutaneous Endoscopic Approach

ØRG24A0   Fusion of 2 or more Cervical Vertebral Joints with Interbody Fusion Device, Anterior Approach, Anterior Column, Percutaneous Endoscopic Approach

ØRG24A1   Fusion of 2 or more Cervical Vertebral Joints with Interbody Fusion Device, Posterior Approach, Posterior Column, Percutaneous Endoscopic Approach

ØRG24AJ   Fusion of 2 or more Cervical Vertebral Joints with Interbody Fusion Device, Posterior Approach, Anterior Column, Percutaneous Endoscopic Approach

ØRG24J0   Fusion of 2 or more Cervical Vertebral Joints with Synthetic Substitute, Anterior Approach, Anterior Column, Percutaneous Endoscopic Approach

ØRG24J1   Fusion of 2 or more Cervical Vertebral Joints with Synthetic Substitute, Posterior Approach, Posterior Column, Percutaneous Endoscopic Approach

ØRG24JJ   Fusion of 2 or more Cervical Vertebral Joints with Synthetic Substitute, Posterior Approach, Anterior Column, Percutaneous Endoscopic Approach

ØRG24K0   Fusion of 2 or more Cervical Vertebral Joints with Nonautologous Tissue Substitute, Anterior Approach, Anterior Column, Percutaneous Endoscopic Approach

ØRG24K1   Fusion of 2 or more Cervical Vertebral Joints with Nonautologous Tissue Substitute, Posterior Approach, Posterior Column, Percutaneous Endoscopic Approach

ØRG24KJ   Fusion of 2 or more Cervical Vertebral Joints with Nonautologous Tissue Substitute, Posterior Approach, Anterior Column, Percutaneous Endoscopic Approach

ØRG24Z0   Fusion of 2 or more Cervical Vertebral Joints, Anterior Approach, Anterior Column, Percutaneous Endoscopic Approach

ØRG24Z1   Fusion of 2 or more Cervical Vertebral Joints, Posterior Approach, Posterior Column, Percutaneous Endoscopic Approach

ØRG24ZJ   Fusion of 2 or more Cervical Vertebral Joints, Posterior Approach, Anterior Column, Percutaneous Endoscopic Approach

ØRG4070   Fusion of Cervicothoracic Vertebral Joint with Autologous Tissue Substitute, Anterior Approach, Anterior Column, Open Approach

ØRG4071   Fusion of Cervicothoracic Vertebral Joint with Autologous Tissue Substitute, Posterior Approach, Posterior Column, Open Approach

ØRG407J   Fusion of Cervicothoracic Vertebral Joint with Autologous Tissue Substitute, Posterior Approach, Anterior Column, Open Approach

ØRG40A0   Fusion of Cervicothoracic Vertebral Joint with Interbody Fusion Device, Anterior Approach, Anterior Column, Open Approach

ØRG40A1   Fusion of Cervicothoracic Vertebral Joint with Interbody Fusion Device, Posterior Approach, Posterior Column, Open Approach

ØRG40AJ   Fusion of Cervicothoracic Vertebral Joint with Interbody Fusion Device, Posterior Approach, Anterior Column, Open Approach

ØRG40J0   Fusion of Cervicothoracic Vertebral Joint with Synthetic Substitute, Anterior Approach, Anterior Column, Open Approach

ØRG40J1   Fusion of Cervicothoracic Vertebral Joint with Synthetic Substitute, Posterior Approach, Posterior Column, Open Approach

ØRG40JJ   Fusion of Cervicothoracic Vertebral Joint with Synthetic Substitute, Posterior Approach, Anterior Column, Open Approach

ØRG40K0   Fusion of Cervicothoracic Vertebral Joint with Nonautologous Tissue Substitute, Anterior Approach, Anterior Column, Open Approach

ØRG40K1   Fusion of Cervicothoracic Vertebral Joint with Nonautologous Tissue Substitute, Posterior Approach, Posterior Column, Open Approach

ØRG40KJ   Fusion of Cervicothoracic Vertebral Joint with Nonautologous Tissue Substitute, Posterior Approach, Anterior Column, Open Approach

ØRG40Z0   Fusion of Cervicothoracic Vertebral Joint, Anterior Approach, Anterior Column, Open Approach

ØRG40Z1   Fusion of Cervicothoracic Vertebral Joint, Posterior Approach, Posterior Column, Open Approach

ØRG40ZJ   Fusion of Cervicothoracic Vertebral Joint, Posterior Approach, Anterior Column, Open Approach

ØRG4370   Fusion of Cervicothoracic Vertebral Joint with Autologous Tissue Substitute, Anterior Approach, Anterior Column, Percutaneous Approach

ØRG4371   Fusion of Cervicothoracic Vertebral Joint with Autologous Tissue Substitute, Posterior Approach, Posterior Column, Percutaneous Approach

ØRG437J   Fusion of Cervicothoracic Vertebral Joint with Autologous Tissue Substitute, Posterior Approach, Anterior Column, Percutaneous Approach

ØRG43A0   Fusion of Cervicothoracic Vertebral Joint with Interbody Fusion Device, Anterior Approach, Anterior Column, Percutaneous Approach

ØRG43A1   Fusion of Cervicothoracic Vertebral Joint with Interbody Fusion Device, Posterior Approach, Posterior Column, Percutaneous Approach

ØRG43AJ   Fusion of Cervicothoracic Vertebral Joint with Interbody Fusion Device, Posterior Approach, Anterior Column, Percutaneous Approach

ØRG43J0   Fusion of Cervicothoracic Vertebral Joint with Synthetic Substitute, Anterior Approach, Anterior Column, Percutaneous Approach

ØRG43J1   Fusion of Cervicothoracic Vertebral Joint with Synthetic Substitute, Posterior Approach, Posterior Column, Percutaneous Approach

ØRG43JJ   Fusion of Cervicothoracic Vertebral Joint with Synthetic Substitute, Posterior Approach, Anterior Column, Percutaneous Approach

ØRG43K0   Fusion of Cervicothoracic Vertebral Joint with Nonautologous Tissue Substitute, Anterior Approach, Anterior Column, Percutaneous Approach

ØRG43K1   Fusion of Cervicothoracic Vertebral Joint with Nonautologous Tissue Substitute, Posterior Approach, Posterior Column, Percutaneous Approach

ØRG43KJ   Fusion of Cervicothoracic Vertebral Joint with Nonautologous Tissue Substitute, Posterior Approach, Anterior Column, Percutaneous Approach

ØRG43Z0   Fusion of Cervicothoracic Vertebral Joint, Anterior Approach, Anterior Column, Percutaneous Approach

ØRG43Z1   Fusion of Cervicothoracic Vertebral Joint, Posterior Approach, Posterior Column, Percutaneous Approach

ØRG43ZJ   Fusion of Cervicothoracic Vertebral Joint, Posterior Approach, Anterior Column, Percutaneous Approach

ØRG4470   Fusion of Cervicothoracic Vertebral Joint with Autologous Tissue Substitute, Anterior Approach, Anterior Column, Percutaneous Endoscopic Approach

ØRG4471   Fusion of Cervicothoracic Vertebral Joint with Autologous Tissue Substitute, Posterior Approach, Posterior Column, Percutaneous Endoscopic Approach

ØRG447J   Fusion of Cervicothoracic Vertebral Joint with Autologous Tissue Substitute, Posterior Approach, Anterior Column, Percutaneous Endoscopic Approach

ØRG44A0   Fusion of Cervicothoracic Vertebral Joint with Interbody Fusion Device, Anterior Approach, Anterior Column, Percutaneous Endoscopic Approach

ØRG44A1   Fusion of Cervicothoracic Vertebral Joint with Interbody Fusion Device, Posterior Approach, Posterior Column, Percutaneous Endoscopic Approach

ØRG44AJ   Fusion of Cervicothoracic Vertebral Joint with Interbody Fusion Device, Posterior Approach, Anterior Column, Percutaneous Endoscopic Approach

ØRG44J0   Fusion of Cervicothoracic Vertebral Joint with Synthetic Substitute, Anterior Approach, Anterior Column, Percutaneous Endoscopic Approach

ØRG44J1   Fusion of Cervicothoracic Vertebral Joint with Synthetic Substitute, Posterior Approach, Posterior Column, Percutaneous Endoscopic Approach

**HAC 12: Surgical Site Infection Following Certain Orthopedic Procedures of the Spine, Shoulder, and Elbow (continued)**

ØRG44JJ  Fusion of Cervicothoracic Vertebral Joint with Synthetic Substitute, Posterior Approach, Anterior Column, Percutaneous Endoscopic Approach

ØRG44KØ  Fusion of Cervicothoracic Vertebral Joint with Nonautologous Tissue Substitute, Anterior Approach, Anterior Column, Percutaneous Endoscopic Approach

ØRG44K1  Fusion of Cervicothoracic Vertebral Joint with Nonautologous Tissue Substitute, Posterior Approach, Posterior Column, Percutaneous Endoscopic Approach

ØRG44KJ  Fusion of Cervicothoracic Vertebral Joint with Nonautologous Tissue Substitute, Posterior Approach, Anterior Column, Percutaneous Endoscopic Approach

ØRG44ZØ  Fusion of Cervicothoracic Vertebral Joint, Anterior Approach, Anterior Column, Percutaneous Endoscopic Approach

ØRG44Z1  Fusion of Cervicothoracic Vertebral Joint, Posterior Approach, Posterior Column, Percutaneous Endoscopic Approach

ØRG44ZJ  Fusion of Cervicothoracic Vertebral Joint, Posterior Approach, Anterior Column, Percutaneous Endoscopic Approach

ØRG6Ø7Ø  Fusion of Thoracic Vertebral Joint with Autologous Tissue Substitute, Anterior Approach, Anterior Column, Open Approach

ØRG6Ø71  Fusion of Thoracic Vertebral Joint with Autologous Tissue Substitute, Posterior Approach, Posterior Column, Open Approach

ØRG6Ø7J  Fusion of Thoracic Vertebral Joint with Autologous Tissue Substitute, Posterior Approach, Anterior Column, Open Approach

ØRG6ØAØ  Fusion of Thoracic Vertebral Joint with Interbody Fusion Device, Anterior Approach, Anterior Column, Open Approach

ØRG6ØA1  Fusion of Thoracic Vertebral Joint with Interbody Fusion Device, Posterior Approach, Posterior Column, Open Approach

ØRG6ØAJ  Fusion of Thoracic Vertebral Joint with Interbody Fusion Device, Posterior Approach, Anterior Column, Open Approach

ØRG6ØJØ  Fusion of Thoracic Vertebral Joint with Synthetic Substitute, Anterior Approach, Anterior Column, Open Approach

ØRG6ØJ1  Fusion of Thoracic Vertebral Joint with Synthetic Substitute, Posterior Approach, Posterior Column, Open Approach

ØRG6ØJJ  Fusion of Thoracic Vertebral Joint with Synthetic Substitute, Posterior Approach, Anterior Column, Open Approach

ØRG6ØKØ  Fusion of Thoracic Vertebral Joint with Nonautologous Tissue Substitute, Anterior Approach, Anterior Column, Open Approach

ØRG6ØK1  Fusion of Thoracic Vertebral Joint with Nonautologous Tissue Substitute, Posterior Approach, Posterior Column, Open Approach

ØRG6ØKJ  Fusion of Thoracic Vertebral Joint with Nonautologous Tissue Substitute, Posterior Approach, Anterior Column, Open Approach

ØRG6ØZØ  Fusion of Thoracic Vertebral Joint, Anterior Approach, Anterior Column, Open Approach

ØRG6ØZ1  Fusion of Thoracic Vertebral Joint, Posterior Approach, Posterior Column, Open Approach

ØRG6ØZJ  Fusion of Thoracic Vertebral Joint, Posterior Approach, Anterior Column, Open Approach

ØRG637Ø  Fusion of Thoracic Vertebral Joint with Autologous Tissue Substitute, Anterior Approach, Anterior Column, Percutaneous Approach

ØRG6371  Fusion of Thoracic Vertebral Joint with Autologous Tissue Substitute, Posterior Approach, Posterior Column, Percutaneous Approach

ØRG637J  Fusion of Thoracic Vertebral Joint with Autologous Tissue Substitute, Posterior Approach, Anterior Column, Percutaneous Approach

ØRG63AØ  Fusion of Thoracic Vertebral Joint with Interbody Fusion Device, Anterior Approach, Anterior Column, Percutaneous Approach

ØRG63A1  Fusion of Thoracic Vertebral Joint with Interbody Fusion Device, Posterior Approach, Posterior Column, Percutaneous Approach

ØRG63AJ  Fusion of Thoracic Vertebral Joint with Interbody Fusion Device, Posterior Approach, Anterior Column, Percutaneous Approach

ØRG63JØ  Fusion of Thoracic Vertebral Joint with Synthetic Substitute, Anterior Approach, Anterior Column, Percutaneous Approach

ØRG63J1  Fusion of Thoracic Vertebral Joint with Synthetic Substitute, Posterior Approach, Posterior Column, Percutaneous Approach

ØRG63JJ  Fusion of Thoracic Vertebral Joint with Synthetic Substitute, Posterior Approach, Anterior Column, Percutaneous Approach

ØRG63KØ  Fusion of Thoracic Vertebral Joint with Nonautologous Tissue Substitute, Anterior Approach, Anterior Column, Percutaneous Approach

ØRG63K1  Fusion of Thoracic Vertebral Joint with Nonautologous Tissue Substitute, Posterior Approach, Posterior Column, Percutaneous Approach

ØRG63KJ  Fusion of Thoracic Vertebral Joint with Nonautologous Tissue Substitute, Posterior Approach, Anterior Column, Percutaneous Approach

ØRG63ZØ  Fusion of Thoracic Vertebral Joint, Anterior Approach, Anterior Column, Percutaneous Approach

ØRG63Z1  Fusion of Thoracic Vertebral Joint, Posterior Approach, Posterior Column, Percutaneous Approach

ØRG63ZJ  Fusion of Thoracic Vertebral Joint, Posterior Approach, Anterior Column, Percutaneous Approach

ØRG647Ø  Fusion of Thoracic Vertebral Joint with Autologous Tissue Substitute, Anterior Approach, Anterior Column, Percutaneous Endoscopic Approach

ØRG6471  Fusion of Thoracic Vertebral Joint with Autologous Tissue Substitute, Posterior Approach, Posterior Column, Percutaneous Endoscopic Approach

ØRG647J  Fusion of Thoracic Vertebral Joint with Autologous Tissue Substitute, Posterior Approach, Anterior Column, Percutaneous Endoscopic Approach

ØRG64AØ  Fusion of Thoracic Vertebral Joint with Interbody Fusion Device, Anterior Approach, Anterior Column, Percutaneous Endoscopic Approach

ØRG64A1  Fusion of Thoracic Vertebral Joint with Interbody Fusion Device, Posterior Approach, Posterior Column, Percutaneous Endoscopic Approach

ØRG64AJ  Fusion of Thoracic Vertebral Joint with Interbody Fusion Device, Posterior Approach, Anterior Column, Percutaneous Endoscopic Approach

ØRG64JØ  Fusion of Thoracic Vertebral Joint with Synthetic Substitute, Anterior Approach, Anterior Column, Percutaneous Endoscopic Approach

ØRG64J1  Fusion of Thoracic Vertebral Joint with Synthetic Substitute, Posterior Approach, Posterior Column, Percutaneous Endoscopic Approach

ØRG64JJ  Fusion of Thoracic Vertebral Joint with Synthetic Substitute, Posterior Approach, Anterior Column, Percutaneous Endoscopic Approach

ØRG64KØ  Fusion of Thoracic Vertebral Joint with Nonautologous Tissue Substitute, Anterior Approach, Anterior Column, Percutaneous Endoscopic Approach

ØRG64K1  Fusion of Thoracic Vertebral Joint with Nonautologous Tissue Substitute, Posterior Approach, Posterior Column, Percutaneous Endoscopic Approach

ØRG64KJ  Fusion of Thoracic Vertebral Joint with Nonautologous Tissue Substitute, Posterior Approach, Anterior Column, Percutaneous Endoscopic Approach

ØRG64ZØ  Fusion of Thoracic Vertebral Joint, Anterior Approach, Anterior Column, Percutaneous Endoscopic Approach

ØRG64Z1  Fusion of Thoracic Vertebral Joint, Posterior Approach, Posterior Column, Percutaneous Endoscopic Approach

ØRG64ZJ  Fusion of Thoracic Vertebral Joint, Posterior Approach, Anterior Column, Percutaneous Endoscopic Approach

ØRG7Ø7Ø  Fusion of 2 to 7 Thoracic Vertebral Joints with Autologous Tissue Substitute, Anterior Approach, Anterior Column, Open Approach

ØRG7Ø71  Fusion of 2 to 7 Thoracic Vertebral Joints with Autologous Tissue Substitute, Posterior Approach, Posterior Column, Open Approach

ØRG7Ø7J  Fusion of 2 to 7 Thoracic Vertebral Joints with Autologous Tissue Substitute, Posterior Approach, Anterior Column, Open Approach

ØRG7ØAØ  Fusion of 2 to 7 Thoracic Vertebral Joints with Interbody Fusion Device, Anterior Approach, Anterior Column, Open Approach

ØRG7ØA1  Fusion of 2 to 7 Thoracic Vertebral Joints with Interbody Fusion Device, Posterior Approach, Posterior Column, Open Approach

ØRG7ØAJ  Fusion of 2 to 7 Thoracic Vertebral Joints with Interbody Fusion Device, Posterior Approach, Anterior Column, Open Approach

ØRG7ØJØ  Fusion of 2 to 7 Thoracic Vertebral Joints with Synthetic Substitute, Anterior Approach, Anterior Column, Open Approach

ØRG7ØJ1  Fusion of 2 to 7 Thoracic Vertebral Joints with Synthetic Substitute, Posterior Approach, Posterior Column, Open Approach

**HAC 12: Surgical Site Infection Following Certain Orthopedic Procedures of the Spine, Shoulder, and Elbow (continued)**

ØRG70JJ    Fusion of 2 to 7 Thoracic Vertebral Joints with Synthetic Substitute, Posterior Approach, Anterior Column, Open Approach

ØRG70KØ    Fusion of 2 to 7 Thoracic Vertebral Joints with Nonautologous Tissue Substitute, Anterior Approach, Anterior Column, Open Approach

ØRG70K1    Fusion of 2 to 7 Thoracic Vertebral Joints with Nonautologous Tissue Substitute, Posterior Approach, Posterior Column, Open Approach

ØRG70KJ    Fusion of 2 to 7 Thoracic Vertebral Joints with Nonautologous Tissue Substitute, Posterior Approach, Anterior Column, Open Approach

ØRG70ZØ    Fusion of 2 to 7 Thoracic Vertebral Joints, Anterior Approach, Anterior Column, Open Approach

ØRG70Z1    Fusion of 2 to 7 Thoracic Vertebral Joints, Posterior Approach, Posterior Column, Open Approach

ØRG70ZJ    Fusion of 2 to 7 Thoracic Vertebral Joints, Posterior Approach, Anterior Column, Open Approach

ØRG737Ø    Fusion of 2 to 7 Thoracic Vertebral Joints with Autologous Tissue Substitute, Anterior Approach, Anterior Column, Percutaneous Approach

ØRG7371    Fusion of 2 to 7 Thoracic Vertebral Joints with Autologous Tissue Substitute, Posterior Approach, Posterior Column, Percutaneous Approach

ØRG737J    Fusion of 2 to 7 Thoracic Vertebral Joints with Autologous Tissue Substitute, Posterior Approach, Anterior Column, Percutaneous Approach

ØRG73AØ    Fusion of 2 to 7 Thoracic Vertebral Joints with Interbody Fusion Device, Anterior Approach, Anterior Column, Percutaneous Approach

ØRG73A1    Fusion of 2 to 7 Thoracic Vertebral Joints with Interbody Fusion Device, Posterior Approach, Posterior Column, Percutaneous Approach

ØRG73AJ    Fusion of 2 to 7 Thoracic Vertebral Joints with Interbody Fusion Device, Posterior Approach, Anterior Column, Percutaneous Approach

ØRG73JØ    Fusion of 2 to 7 Thoracic Vertebral Joints with Synthetic Substitute, Anterior Approach, Anterior Column, Percutaneous Approach

ØRG73J1    Fusion of 2 to 7 Thoracic Vertebral Joints with Synthetic Substitute, Posterior Approach, Posterior Column, Percutaneous Approach

ØRG73JJ    Fusion of 2 to 7 Thoracic Vertebral Joints with Synthetic Substitute, Posterior Approach, Anterior Column, Percutaneous Approach

ØRG73KØ    Fusion of 2 to 7 Thoracic Vertebral Joints with Nonautologous Tissue Substitute, Anterior Approach, Anterior Column, Percutaneous Approach

ØRG73K1    Fusion of 2 to 7 Thoracic Vertebral Joints with Nonautologous Tissue Substitute, Posterior Approach, Posterior Column, Percutaneous Approach

ØRG73KJ    Fusion of 2 to 7 Thoracic Vertebral Joints with Nonautologous Tissue Substitute, Posterior Approach, Anterior Column, Percutaneous Approach

ØRG73ZØ    Fusion of 2 to 7 Thoracic Vertebral Joints, Anterior Approach, Anterior Column, Percutaneous Approach

ØRG73Z1    Fusion of 2 to 7 Thoracic Vertebral Joints, Posterior Approach, Posterior Column, Percutaneous Approach

ØRG73ZJ    Fusion of 2 to 7 Thoracic Vertebral Joints, Posterior Approach, Anterior Column, Percutaneous Approach

ØRG747Ø    Fusion of 2 to 7 Thoracic Vertebral Joints with Autologous Tissue Substitute, Anterior Approach, Anterior Column, Percutaneous Endoscopic Approach

ØRG7471    Fusion of 2 to 7 Thoracic Vertebral Joints with Autologous Tissue Substitute, Posterior Approach, Posterior Column, Percutaneous Endoscopic Approach

ØRG747J    Fusion of 2 to 7 Thoracic Vertebral Joints with Autologous Tissue Substitute, Posterior Approach, Anterior Column, Percutaneous Endoscopic Approach

ØRG74AØ    Fusion of 2 to 7 Thoracic Vertebral Joints with Interbody Fusion Device, Anterior Approach, Anterior Column, Percutaneous Endoscopic Approach

ØRG74A1    Fusion of 2 to 7 Thoracic Vertebral Joints with Interbody Fusion Device, Posterior Approach, Posterior Column, Percutaneous Endoscopic Approach

ØRG74AJ    Fusion of 2 to 7 Thoracic Vertebral Joints with Interbody Fusion Device, Posterior Approach, Anterior Column, Percutaneous Endoscopic Approach

ØRG74JØ    Fusion of 2 to 7 Thoracic Vertebral Joints with Synthetic Substitute, Anterior Approach, Anterior Column, Percutaneous Endoscopic Approach

ØRG74J1    Fusion of 2 to 7 Thoracic Vertebral Joints with Synthetic Substitute, Posterior Approach, Posterior Column, Percutaneous Endoscopic Approach

ØRG74JJ    Fusion of 2 to 7 Thoracic Vertebral Joints with Synthetic Substitute, Posterior Approach, Anterior Column, Percutaneous Endoscopic Approach

ØRG74KØ    Fusion of 2 to 7 Thoracic Vertebral Joints with Nonautologous Tissue Substitute, Anterior Approach, Anterior Column, Percutaneous Endoscopic Approach

ØRG74K1    Fusion of 2 to 7 Thoracic Vertebral Joints with Nonautologous Tissue Substitute, Posterior Approach, Posterior Column, Percutaneous Endoscopic Approach

ØRG74KJ    Fusion of 2 to 7 Thoracic Vertebral Joints with Nonautologous Tissue Substitute, Posterior Approach, Anterior Column, Percutaneous Endoscopic Approach

ØRG74ZØ    Fusion of 2 to 7 Thoracic Vertebral Joints, Anterior Approach, Anterior Column, Percutaneous Endoscopic Approach

ØRG74Z1    Fusion of 2 to 7 Thoracic Vertebral Joints, Posterior Approach, Posterior Column, Percutaneous Endoscopic Approach

ØRG74ZJ    Fusion of 2 to 7 Thoracic Vertebral Joints, Posterior Approach, Anterior Column, Percutaneous Endoscopic Approach

ØRG807Ø    Fusion of 8 or More Thoracic Vertebral Joints with Autologous Tissue Substitute, Anterior Approach, Anterior Column, Open Approach

ØRG8071    Fusion of 8 or More Thoracic Vertebral Joints with Autologous Tissue Substitute, Posterior Approach, Posterior Column, Open Approach

ØRG807J    Fusion of 8 or More Thoracic Vertebral Joints with Autologous Tissue Substitute, Posterior Approach, Anterior Column, Open Approach

ØRG80AØ    Fusion of 8 or More Thoracic Vertebral Joints with Interbody Fusion Device, Anterior Approach, Anterior Column, Open Approach

ØRG80A1    Fusion of 8 or More Thoracic Vertebral Joints with Interbody Fusion Device, Posterior Approach, Posterior Column, Open Approach

ØRG80AJ    Fusion of 8 or More Thoracic Vertebral Joints with Interbody Fusion Device, Posterior Approach, Anterior Column, Open Approach

ØRG80JØ    Fusion of 8 or More Thoracic Vertebral Joints with Synthetic Substitute, Anterior Approach, Anterior Column, Open Approach

ØRG80J1    Fusion of 8 or More Thoracic Vertebral Joints with Synthetic Substitute, Posterior Approach, Posterior Column, Open Approach

ØRG80JJ    Fusion of 8 or More Thoracic Vertebral Joints with Synthetic Substitute, Posterior Approach, Anterior Column, Open Approach

ØRG80KØ    Fusion of 8 or More Thoracic Vertebral Joints with Nonautologous Tissue Substitute, Anterior Approach, Anterior Column, Open Approach

ØRG80K1    Fusion of 8 or More Thoracic Vertebral Joints with Nonautologous Tissue Substitute, Posterior Approach, Posterior Column, Open Approach

ØRG80KJ    Fusion of 8 or More Thoracic Vertebral Joints with Nonautologous Tissue Substitute, Posterior Approach, Anterior Column, Open Approach

ØRG80ZØ    Fusion of 8 or More Thoracic Vertebral Joints, Anterior Approach, Anterior Column, Open Approach

ØRG80Z1    Fusion of 8 or More Thoracic Vertebral Joints, Posterior Approach, Posterior Column, Open Approach

ØRG80ZJ    Fusion of 8 or More Thoracic Vertebral Joints, Posterior Approach, Anterior Column, Open Approach

ØRG837Ø    Fusion of 8 or More Thoracic Vertebral Joints with Autologous Tissue Substitute, Anterior Approach, Anterior Column, Percutaneous Approach

ØRG8371    Fusion of 8 or More Thoracic Vertebral Joints with Autologous Tissue Substitute, Posterior Approach, Posterior Column, Percutaneous Approach

ØRG837J    Fusion of 8 or More Thoracic Vertebral Joints with Autologous Tissue Substitute, Posterior Approach, Anterior Column, Percutaneous Approach

ØRG83AØ    Fusion of 8 or More Thoracic Vertebral Joints with Interbody Fusion Device, Anterior Approach, Anterior Column, Percutaneous Approach

ØRG83A1    Fusion of 8 or More Thoracic Vertebral Joints with Interbody Fusion Device, Posterior Approach, Posterior Column, Percutaneous Approach

ØRG83AJ    Fusion of 8 or More Thoracic Vertebral Joints with Interbody Fusion Device, Posterior Approach, Anterior Column, Percutaneous Approach

ØRG83JØ    Fusion of 8 or More Thoracic Vertebral Joints with Synthetic Substitute, Anterior Approach, Anterior Column, Percutaneous Approach

**HAC 12: Surgical Site Infection Following Certain Orthopedic Procedures of the Spine, Shoulder, and Elbow (continued)**

ØRG83J1 Fusion of 8 or More Thoracic Vertebral Joints with Synthetic Substitute, Posterior Approach, Posterior Column, Percutaneous Approach

ØRG83JJ Fusion of 8 or More Thoracic Vertebral Joints with Synthetic Substitute, Posterior Approach, Anterior Column, Percutaneous Approach

ØRG83KØ Fusion of 8 or More Thoracic Vertebral Joints with Nonautologous Tissue Substitute, Anterior Approach, Anterior Column, Percutaneous Approach

ØRG83K1 Fusion of 8 or More Thoracic Vertebral Joints with Nonautologous Tissue Substitute, Posterior Approach, Posterior Column, Percutaneous Approach

ØRG83KJ Fusion of 8 or More Thoracic Vertebral Joints with Nonautologous Tissue Substitute, Posterior Approach, Anterior Column, Percutaneous Approach

ØRG83ZØ Fusion of 8 or More Thoracic Vertebral Joints, Anterior Approach, Anterior Column, Percutaneous Approach

ØRG83Z1 Fusion of 8 or More Thoracic Vertebral Joints, Posterior Approach, Posterior Column, Percutaneous Approach

ØRG83ZJ Fusion of 8 or More Thoracic Vertebral Joints, Posterior Approach, Anterior Column, Percutaneous Approach

ØRG847Ø Fusion of 8 or More Thoracic Vertebral Joints with Autologous Tissue Substitute, Anterior Approach, Anterior Column, Percutaneous Endoscopic Approach

ØRG8471 Fusion of 8 or More Thoracic Vertebral Joints with Autologous Tissue Substitute, Posterior Approach, Posterior Column, Percutaneous Endoscopic Approach

ØRG847J Fusion of 8 or More Thoracic Vertebral Joints with Autologous Tissue Substitute, Posterior Approach, Anterior Column, Percutaneous Endoscopic Approach

ØRG84AØ Fusion of 8 or More Thoracic Vertebral Joints with Interbody Fusion Device, Anterior Approach, Anterior Column, Percutaneous Endoscopic Approach

ØRG84A1 Fusion of 8 or More Thoracic Vertebral Joints with Interbody Fusion Device, Posterior Approach, Posterior Column, Percutaneous Endoscopic Approach

ØRG84AJ Fusion of 8 or More Thoracic Vertebral Joints with Interbody Fusion Device, Posterior Approach, Anterior Column, Percutaneous Endoscopic Approach

ØRG84JØ Fusion of 8 or More Thoracic Vertebral Joints with Synthetic Substitute, Anterior Approach, Anterior Column, Percutaneous Endoscopic Approach

ØRG84J1 Fusion of 8 or More Thoracic Vertebral Joints with Synthetic Substitute, Posterior Approach, Posterior Column, Percutaneous Endoscopic Approach

ØRG84JJ Fusion of 8 or More Thoracic Vertebral Joints with Synthetic Substitute, Posterior Approach, Anterior Column, Percutaneous Endoscopic Approach

ØRG84KØ Fusion of 8 or More Thoracic Vertebral Joints with Nonautologous Tissue Substitute, Anterior Approach, Anterior Column, Percutaneous Endoscopic Approach

ØRG84K1 Fusion of 8 or More Thoracic Vertebral Joints with Nonautologous Tissue Substitute, Posterior Approach, Posterior Column, Percutaneous Endoscopic Approach

ØRG84KJ Fusion of 8 or More Thoracic Vertebral Joints with Nonautologous Tissue Substitute, Posterior Approach, Anterior Column, Percutaneous Endoscopic Approach

ØRG84ZØ Fusion of 8 or More Thoracic Vertebral Joints, Anterior Approach, Anterior Column, Percutaneous Endoscopic Approach

ØRG84Z1 Fusion of 8 or More Thoracic Vertebral Joints, Posterior Approach, Posterior Column, Percutaneous Endoscopic Approach

ØRG84ZJ Fusion of 8 or More Thoracic Vertebral Joints, Posterior Approach, Anterior Column, Percutaneous Endoscopic Approach

ØRGAØ7Ø Fusion of Thoracolumbar Vertebral Joint with Autologous Tissue Substitute, Anterior Approach, Anterior Column, Open Approach

ØRGAØ71 Fusion of Thoracolumbar Vertebral Joint with Autologous Tissue Substitute, Posterior Approach, Posterior Column, Open Approach

ØRGAØ7J Fusion of Thoracolumbar Vertebral Joint with Autologous Tissue Substitute, Posterior Approach, Anterior Column, Open Approach

ØRGAØAØ Fusion of Thoracolumbar Vertebral Joint with Interbody Fusion Device, Anterior Approach, Anterior Column, Open Approach

ØRGAØA1 Fusion of Thoracolumbar Vertebral Joint with Interbody Fusion Device, Posterior Approach, Posterior Column, Open Approach

ØRGAØAJ Fusion of Thoracolumbar Vertebral Joint with Interbody Fusion Device, Posterior Approach, Anterior Column, Open Approach

ØRGAØJØ Fusion of Thoracolumbar Vertebral Joint with Synthetic Substitute, Anterior Approach, Anterior Column, Open Approach

ØRGAØJ1 Fusion of Thoracolumbar Vertebral Joint with Synthetic Substitute, Posterior Approach, Posterior Column, Open Approach

ØRGAØJJ Fusion of Thoracolumbar Vertebral Joint with Synthetic Substitute, Posterior Approach, Anterior Column, Open Approach

ØRGAØKØ Fusion of Thoracolumbar Vertebral Joint with Nonautologous Tissue Substitute, Anterior Approach, Anterior Column, Open Approach

ØRGAØK1 Fusion of Thoracolumbar Vertebral Joint with Nonautologous Tissue Substitute, Posterior Approach, Posterior Column, Open Approach

ØRGAØKJ Fusion of Thoracolumbar Vertebral Joint with Nonautologous Tissue Substitute, Posterior Approach, Anterior Column, Open Approach

ØRGAØZØ Fusion of Thoracolumbar Vertebral Joint, Anterior Approach, Anterior Column, Open Approach

ØRGAØZ1 Fusion of Thoracolumbar Vertebral Joint, Posterior Approach, Posterior Column, Open Approach

ØRGAØZJ Fusion of Thoracolumbar Vertebral Joint, Posterior Approach, Anterior Column, Open Approach

ØRGA37Ø Fusion of Thoracolumbar Vertebral Joint with Autologous Tissue Substitute, Anterior Approach, Anterior Column, Percutaneous Approach

ØRGA371 Fusion of Thoracolumbar Vertebral Joint with Autologous Tissue Substitute, Posterior Approach, Posterior Column, Percutaneous Approach

ØRGA37J Fusion of Thoracolumbar Vertebral Joint with Autologous Tissue Substitute, Posterior Approach, Anterior Column, Percutaneous Approach

ØRGA3AØ Fusion of Thoracolumbar Vertebral Joint with Interbody Fusion Device, Anterior Approach, Anterior Column, Percutaneous Approach

ØRGA3A1 Fusion of Thoracolumbar Vertebral Joint with Interbody Fusion Device, Posterior Approach, Posterior Column, Percutaneous Approach

ØRGA3AJ Fusion of Thoracolumbar Vertebral Joint with Interbody Fusion Device, Posterior Approach, Anterior Column, Percutaneous Approach

ØRGA3JØ Fusion of Thoracolumbar Vertebral Joint with Synthetic Substitute, Anterior Approach, Anterior Column, Percutaneous Approach

ØRGA3J1 Fusion of Thoracolumbar Vertebral Joint with Synthetic Substitute, Posterior Approach, Posterior Column, Percutaneous Approach

ØRGA3JJ Fusion of Thoracolumbar Vertebral Joint with Synthetic Substitute, Posterior Approach, Anterior Column, Percutaneous Approach

ØRGA3KØ Fusion of Thoracolumbar Vertebral Joint with Nonautologous Tissue Substitute, Anterior Approach, Anterior Column, Percutaneous Approach

ØRGA3K1 Fusion of Thoracolumbar Vertebral Joint with Nonautologous Tissue Substitute, Posterior Approach, Posterior Column, Percutaneous Approach

ØRGA3KJ Fusion of Thoracolumbar Vertebral Joint with Nonautologous Tissue Substitute, Posterior Approach, Anterior Column, Percutaneous Approach

ØRGA3ZØ Fusion of Thoracolumbar Vertebral Joint, Anterior Approach, Anterior Column, Percutaneous Approach

ØRGA3Z1 Fusion of Thoracolumbar Vertebral Joint, Posterior Approach, Posterior Column, Percutaneous Approach

ØRGA3ZJ Fusion of Thoracolumbar Vertebral Joint, Posterior Approach, Anterior Column, Percutaneous Approach

ØRGA47Ø Fusion of Thoracolumbar Vertebral Joint with Autologous Tissue Substitute, Anterior Approach, Anterior Column, Percutaneous Endoscopic Approach

ØRGA471 Fusion of Thoracolumbar Vertebral Joint with Autologous Tissue Substitute, Posterior Approach, Posterior Column, Percutaneous Endoscopic Approach

ØRGA47J Fusion of Thoracolumbar Vertebral Joint with Autologous Tissue Substitute, Posterior Approach, Anterior Column, Percutaneous Endoscopic Approach

ØRGA4AØ Fusion of Thoracolumbar Vertebral Joint with Interbody Fusion Device, Anterior Approach, Anterior Column, Percutaneous Endoscopic Approach

## HAC 12: Surgical Site Infection Following Certain Orthopedic Procedures of the Spine, Shoulder, and Elbow (continued)

ØRGA4A1   Fusion of Thoracolumbar Vertebral Joint with Interbody Fusion Device, Posterior Approach, Posterior Column, Percutaneous Endoscopic Approach

ØRGA4AJ   Fusion of Thoracolumbar Vertebral Joint with Interbody Fusion Device, Posterior Approach, Anterior Column, Percutaneous Endoscopic Approach

ØRGA4JØ   Fusion of Thoracolumbar Vertebral Joint with Synthetic Substitute, Anterior Approach, Anterior Column, Percutaneous Endoscopic Approach

ØRGA4J1   Fusion of Thoracolumbar Vertebral Joint with Synthetic Substitute, Posterior Approach, Posterior Column, Percutaneous Endoscopic Approach

ØRGA4JJ   Fusion of Thoracolumbar Vertebral Joint with Synthetic Substitute, Posterior Approach, Anterior Column, Percutaneous Endoscopic Approach

ØRGA4KØ   Fusion of Thoracolumbar Vertebral Joint with Nonautologous Tissue Substitute, Anterior Approach, Anterior Column, Percutaneous Endoscopic Approach

ØRGA4K1   Fusion of Thoracolumbar Vertebral Joint with Nonautologous Tissue Substitute, Posterior Approach, Posterior Column, Percutaneous Endoscopic Approach

ØRGA4KJ   Fusion of Thoracolumbar Vertebral Joint with Nonautologous Tissue Substitute, Posterior Approach, Anterior Column, Percutaneous Endoscopic Approach

ØRGA4ZØ   Fusion of Thoracolumbar Vertebral Joint, Anterior Approach, Anterior Column, Percutaneous Endoscopic Approach

ØRGA4Z1   Fusion of Thoracolumbar Vertebral Joint, Posterior Approach, Posterior Column, Percutaneous Endoscopic Approach

ØRGA4ZJ   Fusion of Thoracolumbar Vertebral Joint, Posterior Approach, Anterior Column, Percutaneous Endoscopic Approach

ØRGE04Z   Fusion of Right Sternoclavicular Joint with Internal Fixation Device, Open Approach

ØRGE07Z   Fusion of Right Sternoclavicular Joint with Autologous Tissue Substitute, Open Approach

ØRGE0JZ   Fusion of Right Sternoclavicular Joint with Synthetic Substitute, Open Approach

ØRGE0KZ   Fusion of Right Sternoclavicular Joint with Nonautologous Tissue Substitute, Open Approach

ØRGE0ZZ   Fusion of Right Sternoclavicular Joint, Open Approach

ØRGE34Z   Fusion of Right Sternoclavicular Joint with Internal Fixation Device, Percutaneous Approach

ØRGE37Z   Fusion of Right Sternoclavicular Joint with Autologous Tissue Substitute, Percutaneous Approach

ØRGE3JZ   Fusion of Right Sternoclavicular Joint with Synthetic Substitute, Percutaneous Approach

ØRGE3KZ   Fusion of Right Sternoclavicular Joint with Nonautologous Tissue Substitute, Percutaneous Approach

ØRGE3ZZ   Fusion of Right Sternoclavicular Joint, Percutaneous Approach

ØRGE44Z   Fusion of Right Sternoclavicular Joint with Internal Fixation Device, Percutaneous Endoscopic Approach

ØRGE47Z   Fusion of Right Sternoclavicular Joint with Autologous Tissue Substitute, Percutaneous Endoscopic Approach

ØRGE4JZ   Fusion of Right Sternoclavicular Joint with Synthetic Substitute, Percutaneous Endoscopic Approach

ØRGE4KZ   Fusion of Right Sternoclavicular Joint with Nonautologous Tissue Substitute, Percutaneous Endoscopic Approach

ØRGE4ZZ   Fusion of Right Sternoclavicular Joint, Percutaneous Endoscopic Approach

ØRGF04Z   Fusion of Left Sternoclavicular Joint with Internal Fixation Device, Open Approach

ØRGF07Z   Fusion of Left Sternoclavicular Joint with Autologous Tissue Substitute, Open Approach

ØRGF0JZ   Fusion of Left Sternoclavicular Joint with Synthetic Substitute, Open Approach

ØRGF0KZ   Fusion of Left Sternoclavicular Joint with Nonautologous Tissue Substitute, Open Approach

ØRGF0ZZ   Fusion of Left Sternoclavicular Joint, Open Approach

ØRGF34Z   Fusion of Left Sternoclavicular Joint with Internal Fixation Device, Percutaneous Approach

ØRGF37Z   Fusion of Left Sternoclavicular Joint with Autologous Tissue Substitute, Percutaneous Approach

ØRGF3JZ   Fusion of Left Sternoclavicular Joint with Synthetic Substitute, Percutaneous Approach

ØRGF3KZ   Fusion of Left Sternoclavicular Joint with Nonautologous Tissue Substitute, Percutaneous Approach

ØRGF3ZZ   Fusion of Left Sternoclavicular Joint, Percutaneous Approach

ØRGF44Z   Fusion of Left Sternoclavicular Joint with Internal Fixation Device, Percutaneous Endoscopic Approach

ØRGF47Z   Fusion of Left Sternoclavicular Joint with Autologous Tissue Substitute, Percutaneous Endoscopic Approach

ØRGF4JZ   Fusion of Left Sternoclavicular Joint with Synthetic Substitute, Percutaneous Endoscopic Approach

ØRGF4KZ   Fusion of Left Sternoclavicular Joint with Nonautologous Tissue Substitute, Percutaneous Endoscopic Approach

ØRGF4ZZ   Fusion of Left Sternoclavicular Joint, Percutaneous Endoscopic Approach

ØRGG04Z   Fusion of Right Acromioclavicular Joint with Internal Fixation Device, Open Approach

ØRGG07Z   Fusion of Right Acromioclavicular Joint with Autologous Tissue Substitute, Open Approach

ØRGG0JZ   Fusion of Right Acromioclavicular Joint with Synthetic Substitute, Open Approach

ØRGG0KZ   Fusion of Right Acromioclavicular Joint with Nonautologous Tissue Substitute, Open Approach

ØRGG0ZZ   Fusion of Right Acromioclavicular Joint, Open Approach

ØRGG34Z   Fusion of Right Acromioclavicular Joint with Internal Fixation Device, Percutaneous Approach

ØRGG37Z   Fusion of Right Acromioclavicular Joint with Autologous Tissue Substitute, Percutaneous Approach

ØRGG3JZ   Fusion of Right Acromioclavicular Joint with Synthetic Substitute, Percutaneous Approach

ØRGG3KZ   Fusion of Right Acromioclavicular Joint with Nonautologous Tissue Substitute, Percutaneous Approach

ØRGG3ZZ   Fusion of Right Acromioclavicular Joint, Percutaneous Approach

ØRGG44Z   Fusion of Right Acromioclavicular Joint with Internal Fixation Device, Percutaneous Endoscopic Approach

ØRGG47Z   Fusion of Right Acromioclavicular Joint with Autologous Tissue Substitute, Percutaneous Endoscopic Approach

ØRGG4JZ   Fusion of Right Acromioclavicular Joint with Synthetic Substitute, Percutaneous Endoscopic Approach

ØRGG4KZ   Fusion of Right Acromioclavicular Joint with Nonautologous Tissue Substitute, Percutaneous Endoscopic Approach

ØRGG4ZZ   Fusion of Right Acromioclavicular Joint, Percutaneous Endoscopic Approach

ØRGH04Z   Fusion of Left Acromioclavicular Joint with Internal Fixation Device, Open Approach

ØRGH07Z   Fusion of Left Acromioclavicular Joint with Autologous Tissue Substitute, Open Approach

ØRGH0JZ   Fusion of Left Acromioclavicular Joint with Synthetic Substitute, Open Approach

ØRGH0KZ   Fusion of Left Acromioclavicular Joint with Nonautologous Tissue Substitute, Open Approach

ØRGH0ZZ   Fusion of Left Acromioclavicular Joint, Open Approach

ØRGH34Z   Fusion of Left Acromioclavicular Joint with Internal Fixation Device, Percutaneous Approach

ØRGH37Z   Fusion of Left Acromioclavicular Joint with Autologous Tissue Substitute, Percutaneous Approach

ØRGH3JZ   Fusion of Left Acromioclavicular Joint with Synthetic Substitute, Percutaneous Approach

ØRGH3KZ   Fusion of Left Acromioclavicular Joint with Nonautologous Tissue Substitute, Percutaneous Approach

ØRGH3ZZ   Fusion of Left Acromioclavicular Joint, Percutaneous Approach

ØRGH44Z   Fusion of Left Acromioclavicular Joint with Internal Fixation Device, Percutaneous Endoscopic Approach

ØRGH47Z   Fusion of Left Acromioclavicular Joint with Autologous Tissue Substitute, Percutaneous Endoscopic Approach

ØRGH4JZ   Fusion of Left Acromioclavicular Joint with Synthetic Substitute, Percutaneous Endoscopic Approach

ØRGH4KZ   Fusion of Left Acromioclavicular Joint with Nonautologous Tissue Substitute, Percutaneous Endoscopic Approach

ØRGH4ZZ   Fusion of Left Acromioclavicular Joint, Percutaneous Endoscopic Approach

ØRGJ04Z   Fusion of Right Shoulder Joint with Internal Fixation Device, Open Approach

ØRGJ07Z   Fusion of Right Shoulder Joint with Autologous Tissue Substitute, Open Approach

ØRGJ0JZ   Fusion of Right Shoulder Joint with Synthetic Substitute, Open Approach

ØRGJ0KZ   Fusion of Right Shoulder Joint with Nonautologous Tissue Substitute, Open Approach

ØRGJ0ZZ   Fusion of Right Shoulder Joint, Open Approach

ØRGJ34Z   Fusion of Right Shoulder Joint with Internal Fixation Device, Percutaneous Approach

ØRGJ37Z   Fusion of Right Shoulder Joint with Autologous Tissue Substitute, Percutaneous Approach

**HAC 12: Surgical Site Infection Following Certain Orthopedic Procedures of the Spine, Shoulder, and Elbow (continued)**

ØRGJ3JZ  Fusion of Right Shoulder Joint with Synthetic Substitute, Percutaneous Approach

ØRGJ3KZ  Fusion of Right Shoulder Joint with Nonautologous Tissue Substitute, Percutaneous Approach

ØRGJ3ZZ  Fusion of Right Shoulder Joint, Percutaneous Approach

ØRGJ44Z  Fusion of Right Shoulder Joint with Internal Fixation Device, Percutaneous Endoscopic Approach

ØRGJ47Z  Fusion of Right Shoulder Joint with Autologous Tissue Substitute, Percutaneous Endoscopic Approach

ØRGJ4JZ  Fusion of Right Shoulder Joint with Synthetic Substitute, Percutaneous Endoscopic Approach

ØRGJ4KZ  Fusion of Right Shoulder Joint with Nonautologous Tissue Substitute, Percutaneous Endoscopic Approach

ØRGJ4ZZ  Fusion of Right Shoulder Joint, Percutaneous Endoscopic Approach

ØRGK04Z  Fusion of Left Shoulder Joint with Internal Fixation Device, Open Approach

ØRGK07Z  Fusion of Left Shoulder Joint with Autologous Tissue Substitute, Open Approach

ØRGKØJZ  Fusion of Left Shoulder Joint with Synthetic Substitute, Open Approach

ØRGKØKZ  Fusion of Left Shoulder Joint with Nonautologous Tissue Substitute, Open Approach

ØRGKØZZ  Fusion of Left Shoulder Joint, Open Approach

ØRGK34Z  Fusion of Left Shoulder Joint with Internal Fixation Device, Percutaneous Approach

ØRGK37Z  Fusion of Left Shoulder Joint with Autologous Tissue Substitute, Percutaneous Approach

ØRGK3JZ  Fusion of Left Shoulder Joint with Synthetic Substitute, Percutaneous Approach

ØRGK3KZ  Fusion of Left Shoulder Joint with Nonautologous Tissue Substitute, Percutaneous Approach

ØRGK3ZZ  Fusion of Left Shoulder Joint, Percutaneous Approach

ØRGK44Z  Fusion of Left Shoulder Joint with Internal Fixation Device, Percutaneous Endoscopic Approach

ØRGK47Z  Fusion of Left Shoulder Joint with Autologous Tissue Substitute, Percutaneous Endoscopic Approach

ØRGK4JZ  Fusion of Left Shoulder Joint with Synthetic Substitute, Percutaneous Endoscopic Approach

ØRGK4KZ  Fusion of Left Shoulder Joint with Nonautologous Tissue Substitute, Percutaneous Endoscopic Approach

ØRGK4ZZ  Fusion of Left Shoulder Joint, Percutaneous Endoscopic Approach

ØRGL04Z  Fusion of Right Elbow Joint with Internal Fixation Device, Open Approach

ØRGL05Z  Fusion of Right Elbow Joint with External Fixation Device, Open Approach

ØRGL07Z  Fusion of Right Elbow Joint with Autologous Tissue Substitute, Open Approach

ØRGLØJZ  Fusion of Right Elbow Joint with Synthetic Substitute, Open Approach

ØRGLØKZ  Fusion of Right Elbow Joint with Nonautologous Tissue Substitute, Open Approach

ØRGLØZZ  Fusion of Right Elbow Joint, Open Approach

ØRGL34Z  Fusion of Right Elbow Joint with Internal Fixation Device, Percutaneous Approach

ØRGL35Z  Fusion of Right Elbow Joint with External Fixation Device, Percutaneous Approach

ØRGL37Z  Fusion of Right Elbow Joint with Autologous Tissue Substitute, Percutaneous Approach

ØRGL3JZ  Fusion of Right Elbow Joint with Synthetic Substitute, Percutaneous Approach

ØRGL3KZ  Fusion of Right Elbow Joint with Nonautologous Tissue Substitute, Percutaneous Approach

ØRGL3ZZ  Fusion of Right Elbow Joint, Percutaneous Approach

ØRGL44Z  Fusion of Right Elbow Joint with Internal Fixation Device, Percutaneous Endoscopic Approach

ØRGL45Z  Fusion of Right Elbow Joint with External Fixation Device, Percutaneous Endoscopic Approach

ØRGL47Z  Fusion of Right Elbow Joint with Autologous Tissue Substitute, Percutaneous Endoscopic Approach

ØRGL4JZ  Fusion of Right Elbow Joint with Synthetic Substitute, Percutaneous Endoscopic Approach

ØRGL4KZ  Fusion of Right Elbow Joint with Nonautologous Tissue Substitute, Percutaneous Endoscopic Approach

ØRGL4ZZ  Fusion of Right Elbow Joint, Percutaneous Endoscopic Approach

ØRGM04Z  Fusion of Left Elbow Joint with Internal Fixation Device, Open Approach

ØRGM05Z  Fusion of Left Elbow Joint with External Fixation Device, Open Approach

ØRGM07Z  Fusion of Left Elbow Joint with Autologous Tissue Substitute, Open Approach

ØRGMØJZ  Fusion of Left Elbow Joint with Synthetic Substitute, Open Approach

ØRGMØKZ  Fusion of Left Elbow Joint with Nonautologous Tissue Substitute, Open Approach

ØRGMØZZ  Fusion of Left Elbow Joint, Open Approach

ØRGM34Z  Fusion of Left Elbow Joint with Internal Fixation Device, Percutaneous Approach

ØRGM35Z  Fusion of Left Elbow Joint with External Fixation Device, Percutaneous Approach

ØRGM37Z  Fusion of Left Elbow Joint with Autologous Tissue Substitute, Percutaneous Approach

ØRGM3JZ  Fusion of Left Elbow Joint with Synthetic Substitute, Percutaneous Approach

ØRGM3KZ  Fusion of Left Elbow Joint with Nonautologous Tissue Substitute, Percutaneous Approach

ØRGM3ZZ  Fusion of Left Elbow Joint, Percutaneous Approach

ØRGM44Z  Fusion of Left Elbow Joint with Internal Fixation Device, Percutaneous Endoscopic Approach

ØRGM45Z  Fusion of Left Elbow Joint with External Fixation Device, Percutaneous Endoscopic Approach

ØRGM47Z  Fusion of Left Elbow Joint with Autologous Tissue Substitute, Percutaneous Endoscopic Approach

ØRGM4JZ  Fusion of Left Elbow Joint with Synthetic Substitute, Percutaneous Endoscopic Approach

ØRGM4KZ  Fusion of Left Elbow Joint with Nonautologous Tissue Substitute, Percutaneous Endoscopic Approach

ØRGM4ZZ  Fusion of Left Elbow Joint, Percutaneous Endoscopic Approach

ØRQE0ZZ  Repair Right Sternoclavicular Joint, Open Approach

ØRQE3ZZ  Repair Right Sternoclavicular Joint, Percutaneous Approach

ØRQE4ZZ  Repair Right Sternoclavicular Joint, Percutaneous Endoscopic Approach

ØRQEXZZ  Repair Right Sternoclavicular Joint, External Approach

ØRQF0ZZ  Repair Left Sternoclavicular Joint, Open Approach

ØRQF3ZZ  Repair Left Sternoclavicular Joint, Percutaneous Approach

ØRQF4ZZ  Repair Left Sternoclavicular Joint, Percutaneous Endoscopic Approach

ØRQFXZZ  Repair Left Sternoclavicular Joint, External Approach

ØRQG0ZZ  Repair Right Acromioclavicular Joint, Open Approach

ØRQG3ZZ  Repair Right Acromioclavicular Joint, Percutaneous Approach

ØRQG4ZZ  Repair Right Acromioclavicular Joint, Percutaneous Endoscopic Approach

ØRQGXZZ  Repair Right Acromioclavicular Joint, External Approach

ØRQH0ZZ  Repair Left Acromioclavicular Joint, Open Approach

ØRQH3ZZ  Repair Left Acromioclavicular Joint, Percutaneous Approach

ØRQH4ZZ  Repair Left Acromioclavicular Joint, Percutaneous Endoscopic Approach

ØRQHXZZ  Repair Left Acromioclavicular Joint, External Approach

ØRQJ0ZZ  Repair Right Shoulder Joint, Open Approach

ØRQJ3ZZ  Repair Right Shoulder Joint, Percutaneous Approach

ØRQJ4ZZ  Repair Right Shoulder Joint, Percutaneous Endoscopic Approach

ØRQJXZZ  Repair Right Shoulder Joint, External Approach

ØRQK0ZZ  Repair Left Shoulder Joint, Open Approach

ØRQK3ZZ  Repair Left Shoulder Joint, Percutaneous Approach

ØRQK4ZZ  Repair Left Shoulder Joint, Percutaneous Endoscopic Approach

ØRQKXZZ  Repair Left Shoulder Joint, External Approach

ØRQL0ZZ  Repair Right Elbow Joint, Open Approach

ØRQL3ZZ  Repair Right Elbow Joint, Percutaneous Approach

ØRQL4ZZ  Repair Right Elbow Joint, Percutaneous Endoscopic Approach

ØRQLXZZ  Repair Right Elbow Joint, External Approach

ØRQM0ZZ  Repair Left Elbow Joint, Open Approach

ØRQM3ZZ  Repair Left Elbow Joint, Percutaneous Approach

ØRQM4ZZ  Repair Left Elbow Joint, Percutaneous Endoscopic Approach

ØRQMXZZ  Repair Left Elbow Joint, External Approach

ØRUE07Z  Supplement Right Sternoclavicular Joint with Autologous Tissue Substitute, Open Approach

ØRUE0JZ  Supplement Right Sternoclavicular Joint with Synthetic Substitute, Open Approach

ØRUE0KZ  Supplement Right Sternoclavicular Joint with Nonautologous Tissue Substitute, Open Approach

ØRUE37Z  Supplement Right Sternoclavicular Joint with Autologous Tissue Substitute, Percutaneous Approach

**HAC 12: Surgical Site Infection Following Certain Orthopedic Procedures of the Spine, Shoulder, and Elbow (continued)**

ØRUE3JZ  Supplement Right Sternoclavicular Joint with Synthetic Substitute, Percutaneous Approach

ØRUE3KZ  Supplement Right Sternoclavicular Joint with Nonautologous Tissue Substitute, Percutaneous Approach

ØRUE47Z  Supplement Right Sternoclavicular Joint with Autologous Tissue Substitute, Percutaneous Endoscopic Approach

ØRUE4JZ  Supplement Right Sternoclavicular Joint with Synthetic Substitute, Percutaneous Endoscopic Approach

ØRUE4KZ  Supplement Right Sternoclavicular Joint with Nonautologous Tissue Substitute, Percutaneous Endoscopic Approach

ØRUF07Z  Supplement Left Sternoclavicular Joint with Autologous Tissue Substitute, Open Approach

ØRUF0JZ  Supplement Left Sternoclavicular Joint with Synthetic Substitute, Open Approach

ØRUF0KZ  Supplement Left Sternoclavicular Joint with Nonautologous Tissue Substitute, Open Approach

ØRUF37Z  Supplement Left Sternoclavicular Joint with Autologous Tissue Substitute, Percutaneous Approach

ØRUF3JZ  Supplement Left Sternoclavicular Joint with Synthetic Substitute, Percutaneous Approach

ØRUF3KZ  Supplement Left Sternoclavicular Joint with Nonautologous Tissue Substitute, Percutaneous Approach

ØRUF47Z  Supplement Left Sternoclavicular Joint with Autologous Tissue Substitute, Percutaneous Endoscopic Approach

ØRUF4JZ  Supplement Left Sternoclavicular Joint with Synthetic Substitute, Percutaneous Endoscopic Approach

ØRUF4KZ  Supplement Left Sternoclavicular Joint with Nonautologous Tissue Substitute, Percutaneous Endoscopic Approach

ØRUG07Z  Supplement Right Acromioclavicular Joint with Autologous Tissue Substitute, Open Approach

ØRUG0JZ  Supplement Right Acromioclavicular Joint with Synthetic Substitute, Open Approach

ØRUG0KZ  Supplement Right Acromioclavicular Joint with Nonautologous Tissue Substitute, Open Approach

ØRUG37Z  Supplement Right Acromioclavicular Joint with Autologous Tissue Substitute, Percutaneous Approach

ØRUG3JZ  Supplement Right Acromioclavicular Joint with Synthetic Substitute, Percutaneous Approach

ØRUG3KZ  Supplement Right Acromioclavicular Joint with Nonautologous Tissue Substitute, Percutaneous Approach

ØRUG47Z  Supplement Right Acromioclavicular Joint with Autologous Tissue Substitute, Percutaneous Endoscopic Approach

ØRUG4JZ  Supplement Right Acromioclavicular Joint with Synthetic Substitute, Percutaneous Endoscopic Approach

ØRUG4KZ  Supplement Right Acromioclavicular Joint with Nonautologous Tissue Substitute, Percutaneous Endoscopic Approach

ØRUH07Z  Supplement Left Acromioclavicular Joint with Autologous Tissue Substitute, Open Approach

ØRUH0JZ  Supplement Left Acromioclavicular Joint with Synthetic Substitute, Open Approach

ØRUH0KZ  Supplement Left Acromioclavicular Joint with Nonautologous Tissue Substitute, Open Approach

ØRUH37Z  Supplement Left Acromioclavicular Joint with Autologous Tissue Substitute, Percutaneous Approach

ØRUH3JZ  Supplement Left Acromioclavicular Joint with Synthetic Substitute, Percutaneous Approach

ØRUH3KZ  Supplement Left Acromioclavicular Joint with Nonautologous Tissue Substitute, Percutaneous Approach

ØRUH47Z  Supplement Left Acromioclavicular Joint with Autologous Tissue Substitute, Percutaneous Endoscopic Approach

ØRUH4JZ  Supplement Left Acromioclavicular Joint with Synthetic Substitute, Percutaneous Endoscopic Approach

ØRUH4KZ  Supplement Left Acromioclavicular Joint with Nonautologous Tissue Substitute, Percutaneous Endoscopic Approach

ØRUJ07Z  Supplement Right Shoulder Joint with Autologous Tissue Substitute, Open Approach

ØRUJ0JZ  Supplement Right Shoulder Joint with Synthetic Substitute, Open Approach

ØRUJ0KZ  Supplement Right Shoulder Joint with Nonautologous Tissue Substitute, Open Approach

ØRUJ37Z  Supplement Right Shoulder Joint with Autologous Tissue Substitute, Percutaneous Approach

ØRUJ3JZ  Supplement Right Shoulder Joint with Synthetic Substitute, Percutaneous Approach

ØRUJ3KZ  Supplement Right Shoulder Joint with Nonautologous Tissue Substitute, Percutaneous Approach

ØRUJ47Z  Supplement Right Shoulder Joint with Autologous Tissue Substitute, Percutaneous Endoscopic Approach

ØRUJ4JZ  Supplement Right Shoulder Joint with Synthetic Substitute, Percutaneous Endoscopic Approach

ØRUJ4KZ  Supplement Right Shoulder Joint with Nonautologous Tissue Substitute, Percutaneous Endoscopic Approach

ØRUK07Z  Supplement Left Shoulder Joint with Autologous Tissue Substitute, Open Approach

ØRUK0JZ  Supplement Left Shoulder Joint with Synthetic Substitute, Open Approach

ØRUK0KZ  Supplement Left Shoulder Joint with Nonautologous Tissue Substitute, Open Approach

ØRUK37Z  Supplement Left Shoulder Joint with Autologous Tissue Substitute, Percutaneous Approach

ØRUK3JZ  Supplement Left Shoulder Joint with Synthetic Substitute, Percutaneous Approach

ØRUK3KZ  Supplement Left Shoulder Joint with Nonautologous Tissue Substitute, Percutaneous Approach

ØRUK47Z  Supplement Left Shoulder Joint with Autologous Tissue Substitute, Percutaneous Endoscopic Approach

ØRUK4JZ  Supplement Left Shoulder Joint with Synthetic Substitute, Percutaneous Endoscopic Approach

ØRUK4KZ  Supplement Left Shoulder Joint with Nonautologous Tissue Substitute, Percutaneous Endoscopic Approach

ØRUL07Z  Supplement Right Elbow Joint with Autologous Tissue Substitute, Open Approach

ØRUL0JZ  Supplement Right Elbow Joint with Synthetic Substitute, Open Approach

ØRUL0KZ  Supplement Right Elbow Joint with Nonautologous Tissue Substitute, Open Approach

ØRUL37Z  Supplement Right Elbow Joint with Autologous Tissue Substitute, Percutaneous Approach

ØRUL3JZ  Supplement Right Elbow Joint with Synthetic Substitute, Percutaneous Approach

ØRUL3KZ  Supplement Right Elbow Joint with Nonautologous Tissue Substitute, Percutaneous Approach

ØRUL47Z  Supplement Right Elbow Joint with Autologous Tissue Substitute, Percutaneous Endoscopic Approach

ØRUL4JZ  Supplement Right Elbow Joint with Synthetic Substitute, Percutaneous Endoscopic Approach

ØRUL4KZ  Supplement Right Elbow Joint with Nonautologous Tissue Substitute, Percutaneous Endoscopic Approach

ØRUM07Z  Supplement Left Elbow Joint with Autologous Tissue Substitute, Open Approach

ØRUM0JZ  Supplement Left Elbow Joint with Synthetic Substitute, Open Approach

ØRUM0KZ  Supplement Left Elbow Joint with Nonautologous Tissue Substitute, Open Approach

ØRUM37Z  Supplement Left Elbow Joint with Autologous Tissue Substitute, Percutaneous Approach

ØRUM3JZ  Supplement Left Elbow Joint with Synthetic Substitute, Percutaneous Approach

ØRUM3KZ  Supplement Left Elbow Joint with Nonautologous Tissue Substitute, Percutaneous Approach

ØRUM47Z  Supplement Left Elbow Joint with Autologous Tissue Substitute, Percutaneous Endoscopic Approach

ØRUM4JZ  Supplement Left Elbow Joint with Synthetic Substitute, Percutaneous Endoscopic Approach

ØRUM4KZ  Supplement Left Elbow Joint with Nonautologous Tissue Substitute, Percutaneous Endoscopic Approach

ØSG0070  Fusion of Lumbar Vertebral Joint with Autologous Tissue Substitute, Anterior Approach, Anterior Column, Open Approach

ØSG0071  Fusion of Lumbar Vertebral Joint with Autologous Tissue Substitute, Posterior Approach, Posterior Column, Open Approach

ØSG007J  Fusion of Lumbar Vertebral Joint with Autologous Tissue Substitute, Posterior Approach, Anterior Column, Open Approach

ØSG00A0  Fusion of Lumbar Vertebral Joint with Interbody Fusion Device, Anterior Approach, Anterior Column, Open Approach

ØSG00A1  Fusion of Lumbar Vertebral Joint with Interbody Fusion Device, Posterior Approach, Posterior Column, Open Approach

ØSG00AJ  Fusion of Lumbar Vertebral Joint with Interbody Fusion Device, Posterior Approach, Anterior Column, Open Approach

**Appendix I: Hospital Acquired Conditions**

**HAC 12: Surgical Site Infection Following Certain Orthopedic Procedures of the Spine, Shoulder, and Elbow (continued)**

ØSG00JØ Fusion of Lumbar Vertebral Joint with Synthetic Substitute, Anterior Approach, Anterior Column, Open Approach

ØSG00J1 Fusion of Lumbar Vertebral Joint with Synthetic Substitute, Posterior Approach, Posterior Column, Open Approach

ØSG00JJ Fusion of Lumbar Vertebral Joint with Synthetic Substitute, Posterior Approach, Anterior Column, Open Approach

ØSG00KØ Fusion of Lumbar Vertebral Joint with Nonautologous Tissue Substitute, Anterior Approach, Anterior Column, Open Approach

ØSG00K1 Fusion of Lumbar Vertebral Joint with Nonautologous Tissue Substitute, Posterior Approach, Posterior Column, Open Approach

ØSG00KJ Fusion of Lumbar Vertebral Joint with Nonautologous Tissue Substitute, Posterior Approach, Anterior Column, Open Approach

ØSG00ZØ Fusion of Lumbar Vertebral Joint, Anterior Approach, Anterior Column, Open Approach

ØSG00Z1 Fusion of Lumbar Vertebral Joint, Posterior Approach, Posterior Column, Open Approach

ØSG00ZJ Fusion of Lumbar Vertebral Joint, Posterior Approach, Anterior Column, Open Approach

ØSG037Ø Fusion of Lumbar Vertebral Joint with Autologous Tissue Substitute, Anterior Approach, Anterior Column, Percutaneous Approach

ØSG0371 Fusion of Lumbar Vertebral Joint with Autologous Tissue Substitute, Posterior Approach, Posterior Column, Percutaneous Approach

ØSG037J Fusion of Lumbar Vertebral Joint with Autologous Tissue Substitute, Posterior Approach, Anterior Column, Percutaneous Approach

ØSG03AØ Fusion of Lumbar Vertebral Joint with Interbody Fusion Device, Anterior Approach, Anterior Column, Percutaneous Approach

ØSG03A1 Fusion of Lumbar Vertebral Joint with Interbody Fusion Device, Posterior Approach, Posterior Column, Percutaneous Approach

ØSG03AJ Fusion of Lumbar Vertebral Joint with Interbody Fusion Device, Posterior Approach, Anterior Column, Percutaneous Approach

ØSG03JØ Fusion of Lumbar Vertebral Joint with Synthetic Substitute, Anterior Approach, Anterior Column, Percutaneous Approach

ØSG03J1 Fusion of Lumbar Vertebral Joint with Synthetic Substitute, Posterior Approach, Posterior Column, Percutaneous Approach

ØSG03JJ Fusion of Lumbar Vertebral Joint with Synthetic Substitute, Posterior Approach, Anterior Column, Percutaneous Approach

ØSG03KØ Fusion of Lumbar Vertebral Joint with Nonautologous Tissue Substitute, Anterior Approach, Anterior Column, Percutaneous Approach

ØSG03K1 Fusion of Lumbar Vertebral Joint with Nonautologous Tissue Substitute, Posterior Approach, Posterior Column, Percutaneous Approach

ØSG03KJ Fusion of Lumbar Vertebral Joint with Nonautologous Tissue Substitute, Posterior Approach, Anterior Column, Percutaneous Approach

ØSG03ZØ Fusion of Lumbar Vertebral Joint, Anterior Approach, Anterior Column, Percutaneous Approach

ØSG03Z1 Fusion of Lumbar Vertebral Joint, Posterior Approach, Posterior Column, Percutaneous Approach

ØSG03ZJ Fusion of Lumbar Vertebral Joint, Posterior Approach, Anterior Column, Percutaneous Approach

ØSG047Ø Fusion of Lumbar Vertebral Joint with Autologous Tissue Substitute, Anterior Approach, Anterior Column, Percutaneous Endoscopic Approach

ØSG0471 Fusion of Lumbar Vertebral Joint with Autologous Tissue Substitute, Posterior Approach, Posterior Column, Percutaneous Endoscopic Approach

ØSG047J Fusion of Lumbar Vertebral Joint with Autologous Tissue Substitute, Posterior Approach, Anterior Column, Percutaneous Endoscopic Approach

ØSG04AØ Fusion of Lumbar Vertebral Joint with Interbody Fusion Device, Anterior Approach, Anterior Column, Percutaneous Endoscopic Approach

ØSG04A1 Fusion of Lumbar Vertebral Joint with Interbody Fusion Device, Posterior Approach, Posterior Column, Percutaneous Endoscopic Approach

ØSG04AJ Fusion of Lumbar Vertebral Joint with Interbody Fusion Device, Posterior Approach, Anterior Column, Percutaneous Endoscopic Approach

ØSG04JØ Fusion of Lumbar Vertebral Joint with Synthetic Substitute, Anterior Approach, Anterior Column, Percutaneous Endoscopic Approach

ØSG04J1 Fusion of Lumbar Vertebral Joint with Synthetic Substitute, Posterior Approach, Posterior Column, Percutaneous Endoscopic Approach

ØSG04JJ Fusion of Lumbar Vertebral Joint with Synthetic Substitute, Posterior Approach, Anterior Column, Percutaneous Endoscopic Approach

ØSG04KØ Fusion of Lumbar Vertebral Joint with Nonautologous Tissue Substitute, Anterior Approach, Anterior Column, Percutaneous Endoscopic Approach

ØSG04K1 Fusion of Lumbar Vertebral Joint with Nonautologous Tissue Substitute, Posterior Approach, Posterior Column, Percutaneous Endoscopic Approach

ØSG04KJ Fusion of Lumbar Vertebral Joint with Nonautologous Tissue Substitute, Posterior Approach, Anterior Column, Percutaneous Endoscopic Approach

ØSG04ZØ Fusion of Lumbar Vertebral Joint, Anterior Approach, Anterior Column, Percutaneous Endoscopic Approach

ØSG04Z1 Fusion of Lumbar Vertebral Joint, Posterior Approach, Posterior Column, Percutaneous Endoscopic Approach

ØSG04ZJ Fusion of Lumbar Vertebral Joint, Posterior Approach, Anterior Column, Percutaneous Endoscopic Approach

ØSG1070 Fusion of 2 or More Lumbar Vertebral Joints with Autologous Tissue Substitute, Anterior Approach, Anterior Column, Open Approach

ØSG1071 Fusion of 2 or More Lumbar Vertebral Joints with Autologous Tissue Substitute, Posterior Approach, Posterior Column, Open Approach

ØSG107J Fusion of 2 or More Lumbar Vertebral Joints with Autologous Tissue Substitute, Posterior Approach, Anterior Column, Open Approach

ØSG10AØ Fusion of 2 or More Lumbar Vertebral Joints with Interbody Fusion Device, Anterior Approach, Anterior Column, Open Approach

ØSG10A1 Fusion of 2 or More Lumbar Vertebral Joints with Interbody Fusion Device, Posterior Approach, Posterior Column, Open Approach

ØSG10AJ Fusion of 2 or More Lumbar Vertebral Joints with Interbody Fusion Device, Posterior Approach, Anterior Column, Open Approach

ØSG10JØ Fusion of 2 or More Lumbar Vertebral Joints with Synthetic Substitute, Anterior Approach, Anterior Column, Open Approach

ØSG10J1 Fusion of 2 or More Lumbar Vertebral Joints with Synthetic Substitute, Posterior Approach, Posterior Column, Open Approach

ØSG10JJ Fusion of 2 or More Lumbar Vertebral Joints with Synthetic Substitute, Posterior Approach, Anterior Column, Open Approach

ØSG10KØ Fusion of 2 or More Lumbar Vertebral Joints with Nonautologous Tissue Substitute, Anterior Approach, Anterior Column, Open Approach

ØSG10K1 Fusion of 2 or More Lumbar Vertebral Joints with Nonautologous Tissue Substitute, Posterior Approach, Posterior Column, Open Approach

ØSG10KJ Fusion of 2 or More Lumbar Vertebral Joints with Nonautologous Tissue Substitute, Posterior Approach, Anterior Column, Open Approach

ØSG10ZØ Fusion of 2 or More Lumbar Vertebral Joints, Anterior Approach, Anterior Column, Open Approach

ØSG10Z1 Fusion of 2 or More Lumbar Vertebral Joints, Posterior Approach, Posterior Column, Open Approach

ØSG10ZJ Fusion of 2 or More Lumbar Vertebral Joints, Posterior Approach, Anterior Column, Open Approach

ØSG1370 Fusion of 2 or More Lumbar Vertebral Joints with Autologous Tissue Substitute, Anterior Approach, Anterior Column, Percutaneous Approach

ØSG1371 Fusion of 2 or More Lumbar Vertebral Joints with Autologous Tissue Substitute, Posterior Approach, Posterior Column, Percutaneous Approach

ØSG137J Fusion of 2 or More Lumbar Vertebral Joints with Autologous Tissue Substitute, Posterior Approach, Anterior Column, Percutaneous Approach

ØSG13AØ Fusion of 2 or More Lumbar Vertebral Joints with Interbody Fusion Device, Anterior Approach, Anterior Column, Percutaneous Approach

ØSG13A1 Fusion of 2 or More Lumbar Vertebral Joints with Interbody Fusion Device, Posterior Approach, Posterior Column, Percutaneous Approach

ØSG13AJ Fusion of 2 or More Lumbar Vertebral Joints with Interbody Fusion Device, Posterior Approach, Anterior Column, Percutaneous Approach

**HAC 12: Surgical Site Infection Following Certain Orthopedic Procedures of the Spine, Shoulder, and Elbow (continued)**

ØSG13JØ  Fusion of 2 or More Lumbar Vertebral Joints with Synthetic Substitute, Anterior Approach, Anterior Column, Percutaneous Approach

ØSG13J1  Fusion of 2 or More Lumbar Vertebral Joints with Synthetic Substitute, Posterior Approach, Posterior Column, Percutaneous Approach

ØSG13JJ  Fusion of 2 or More Lumbar Vertebral Joints with Synthetic Substitute, Posterior Approach, Anterior Column, Percutaneous Approach

ØSG13KØ  Fusion of 2 or More Lumbar Vertebral Joints with Nonautologous Tissue Substitute, Anterior Approach, Anterior Column, Percutaneous Approach

ØSG13K1  Fusion of 2 or More Lumbar Vertebral Joints with Nonautologous Tissue Substitute, Posterior Approach, Posterior Column, Percutaneous Approach

ØSG13KJ  Fusion of 2 or More Lumbar Vertebral Joints with Nonautologous Tissue Substitute, Posterior Approach, Anterior Column, Percutaneous Approach

ØSG13ZØ  Fusion of 2 or More Lumbar Vertebral Joints, Anterior Approach, Anterior Column, Percutaneous Approach

ØSG13Z1  Fusion of 2 or More Lumbar Vertebral Joints, Posterior Approach, Posterior Column, Percutaneous Approach

ØSG13ZJ  Fusion of 2 or More Lumbar Vertebral Joints, Posterior Approach, Anterior Column, Percutaneous Approach

ØSG147Ø  Fusion of 2 or More Lumbar Vertebral Joints with Autologous Tissue Substitute, Anterior Approach, Anterior Column, Percutaneous Endoscopic Approach

ØSG1471  Fusion of 2 or More Lumbar Vertebral Joints with Autologous Tissue Substitute, Posterior Approach, Posterior Column, Percutaneous Endoscopic Approach

ØSG147J  Fusion of 2 or More Lumbar Vertebral Joints with Autologous Tissue Substitute, Posterior Approach, Anterior Column, Percutaneous Endoscopic Approach

ØSG14AØ  Fusion of 2 or More Lumbar Vertebral Joints with Interbody Fusion Device, Anterior Approach, Anterior Column, Percutaneous Endoscopic Approach

ØSG14A1  Fusion of 2 or More Lumbar Vertebral Joints with Interbody Fusion Device, Posterior Approach, Posterior Column, Percutaneous Endoscopic Approach

ØSG14AJ  Fusion of 2 or More Lumbar Vertebral Joints with Interbody Fusion Device, Posterior Approach, Anterior Column, Percutaneous Endoscopic Approach

ØSG14JØ  Fusion of 2 or More Lumbar Vertebral Joints with Synthetic Substitute, Anterior Approach, Anterior Column, Percutaneous Endoscopic Approach

ØSG14J1  Fusion of 2 or More Lumbar Vertebral Joints with Synthetic Substitute, Posterior Approach, Posterior Column, Percutaneous Endoscopic Approach

ØSG14JJ  Fusion of 2 or More Lumbar Vertebral Joints with Synthetic Substitute, Posterior Approach, Anterior Column, Percutaneous Endoscopic Approach

ØSG14KØ  Fusion of 2 or More Lumbar Vertebral Joints with Nonautologous Tissue Substitute, Anterior Approach, Anterior Column, Percutaneous Endoscopic Approach

ØSG14K1  Fusion of 2 or More Lumbar Vertebral Joints with Nonautologous Tissue Substitute, Posterior Approach, Posterior Column, Percutaneous Endoscopic Approach

ØSG14KJ  Fusion of 2 or More Lumbar Vertebral Joints with Nonautologous Tissue Substitute, Posterior Approach, Anterior Column, Percutaneous Endoscopic Approach

ØSG14ZØ  Fusion of 2 or More Lumbar Vertebral Joints, Anterior Approach, Anterior Column, Percutaneous Endoscopic Approach

ØSG14Z1  Fusion of 2 or More Lumbar Vertebral Joints, Posterior Approach, Posterior Column, Percutaneous Endoscopic Approach

ØSG14ZJ  Fusion of 2 or More Lumbar Vertebral Joints, Posterior Approach, Anterior Column, Percutaneous Endoscopic Approach

ØSG3Ø7Ø  Fusion of Lumbosacral Joint with Autologous Tissue Substitute, Anterior Approach, Anterior Column, Open Approach

ØSG3Ø71  Fusion of Lumbosacral Joint with Autologous Tissue Substitute, Posterior Approach, Posterior Column, Open Approach

ØSG3Ø7J  Fusion of Lumbosacral Joint with Autologous Tissue Substitute, Posterior Approach, Anterior Column, Open Approach

ØSG3ØAØ  Fusion of Lumbosacral Joint with Interbody Fusion Device, Anterior Approach, Anterior Column, Open Approach

ØSG3ØA1  Fusion of Lumbosacral Joint with Interbody Fusion Device, Posterior Approach, Posterior Column, Open Approach

ØSG3ØAJ  Fusion of Lumbosacral Joint with Interbody Fusion Device, Posterior Approach, Anterior Column, Open Approach

ØSG3ØJØ  Fusion of Lumbosacral Joint with Synthetic Substitute, Anterior Approach, Anterior Column, Open Approach

ØSG3ØJ1  Fusion of Lumbosacral Joint with Synthetic Substitute, Posterior Approach, Posterior Column, Open Approach

ØSG3ØJJ  Fusion of Lumbosacral Joint with Synthetic Substitute, Posterior Approach, Anterior Column, Open Approach

ØSG3ØKØ  Fusion of Lumbosacral Joint with Nonautologous Tissue Substitute, Anterior Approach, Anterior Column, Open Approach

ØSG3ØK1  Fusion of Lumbosacral Joint with Nonautologous Tissue Substitute, Posterior Approach, Posterior Column, Open Approach

ØSG3ØKJ  Fusion of Lumbosacral Joint with Nonautologous Tissue Substitute, Posterior Approach, Anterior Column, Open Approach

ØSG3ØZØ  Fusion of Lumbosacral Joint, Anterior Approach, Anterior Column, Open Approach

ØSG3ØZ1  Fusion of Lumbosacral Joint, Posterior Approach, Posterior Column, Open Approach

ØSG3ØZJ  Fusion of Lumbosacral Joint, Posterior Approach, Anterior Column, Open Approach

ØSG337Ø  Fusion of Lumbosacral Joint with Autologous Tissue Substitute, Anterior Approach, Anterior Column, Percutaneous Approach

ØSG3371  Fusion of Lumbosacral Joint with Autologous Tissue Substitute, Posterior Approach, Posterior Column, Percutaneous Approach

ØSG337J  Fusion of Lumbosacral Joint with Autologous Tissue Substitute, Posterior Approach, Anterior Column, Percutaneous Approach

ØSG33AØ  Fusion of Lumbosacral Joint with Interbody Fusion Device, Anterior Approach, Anterior Column, Percutaneous Approach

ØSG33A1  Fusion of Lumbosacral Joint with Interbody Fusion Device, Posterior Approach, Posterior Column, Percutaneous Approach

ØSG33AJ  Fusion of Lumbosacral Joint with Interbody Fusion Device, Posterior Approach, Anterior Column, Percutaneous Approach

ØSG33JØ  Fusion of Lumbosacral Joint with Synthetic Substitute, Anterior Approach, Anterior Column, Percutaneous Approach

ØSG33J1  Fusion of Lumbosacral Joint with Synthetic Substitute, Posterior Approach, Posterior Column, Percutaneous Approach

ØSG33JJ  Fusion of Lumbosacral Joint with Synthetic Substitute, Posterior Approach, Anterior Column, Percutaneous Approach

ØSG33KØ  Fusion of Lumbosacral Joint with Nonautologous Tissue Substitute, Anterior Approach, Anterior Column, Percutaneous Approach

ØSG33K1  Fusion of Lumbosacral Joint with Nonautologous Tissue Substitute, Posterior Approach, Posterior Column, Percutaneous Approach

ØSG33KJ  Fusion of Lumbosacral Joint with Nonautologous Tissue Substitute, Posterior Approach, Anterior Column, Percutaneous Approach

ØSG33ZØ  Fusion of Lumbosacral Joint, Anterior Approach, Anterior Column, Percutaneous Approach

ØSG33Z1  Fusion of Lumbosacral Joint, Posterior Approach, Posterior Column, Percutaneous Approach

ØSG33ZJ  Fusion of Lumbosacral Joint, Posterior Approach, Anterior Column, Percutaneous Approach

ØSG347Ø  Fusion of Lumbosacral Joint with Autologous Tissue Substitute, Anterior Approach, Anterior Column, Percutaneous Endoscopic Approach

ØSG3471  Fusion of Lumbosacral Joint with Autologous Tissue Substitute, Posterior Approach, Posterior Column, Percutaneous Endoscopic Approach

ØSG347J  Fusion of Lumbosacral Joint with Autologous Tissue Substitute, Posterior Approach, Anterior Column, Percutaneous Endoscopic Approach

ØSG34AØ  Fusion of Lumbosacral Joint with Interbody Fusion Device, Anterior Approach, Anterior Column, Percutaneous Endoscopic Approach

ØSG34A1  Fusion of Lumbosacral Joint with Interbody Fusion Device, Posterior Approach, Posterior Column, Percutaneous Endoscopic Approach

**HAC 12: Surgical Site Infection Following Certain Orthopedic Procedures of the Spine, Shoulder, and Elbow (continued)**

ØSG34AJ Fusion of Lumbosacral Joint with Interbody Fusion Device, Posterior Approach, Anterior Column, Percutaneous Endoscopic Approach

ØSG34J0 Fusion of Lumbosacral Joint with Synthetic Substitute, Anterior Approach, Anterior Column, Percutaneous Endoscopic Approach

ØSG34J1 Fusion of Lumbosacral Joint with Synthetic Substitute, Posterior Approach, Posterior Column, Percutaneous Endoscopic Approach

ØSG34JJ Fusion of Lumbosacral Joint with Synthetic Substitute, Posterior Approach, Anterior Column, Percutaneous Endoscopic Approach

ØSG34K0 Fusion of Lumbosacral Joint with Nonautologous Tissue Substitute, Anterior Approach, Anterior Column, Percutaneous Endoscopic Approach

ØSG34K1 Fusion of Lumbosacral Joint with Nonautologous Tissue Substitute, Posterior Approach, Posterior Column, Percutaneous Endoscopic Approach

ØSG34KJ Fusion of Lumbosacral Joint with Nonautologous Tissue Substitute, Posterior Approach, Anterior Column, Percutaneous Endoscopic Approach

ØSG34Z0 Fusion of Lumbosacral Joint, Anterior Approach, Anterior Column, Percutaneous Endoscopic Approach

ØSG34Z1 Fusion of Lumbosacral Joint, Posterior Approach, Posterior Column, Percutaneous Endoscopic Approach

ØSG34ZJ Fusion of Lumbosacral Joint, Posterior Approach, Anterior Column, Percutaneous Endoscopic Approach

ØSG704Z Fusion of Right Sacroiliac Joint with Internal Fixation Device, Open Approach

ØSG707Z Fusion of Right Sacroiliac Joint with Autologous Tissue Substitute, Open Approach

ØSG70JZ Fusion of Right Sacroiliac Joint with Synthetic Substitute, Open Approach

ØSG70KZ Fusion of Right Sacroiliac Joint with Nonautologous Tissue Substitute, Open Approach

ØSG70ZZ Fusion of Right Sacroiliac Joint, Open Approach

ØSG734Z Fusion of Right Sacroiliac Joint with Internal Fixation Device, Percutaneous Approach

ØSG737Z Fusion of Right Sacroiliac Joint with Autologous Tissue Substitute, Percutaneous Approach

ØSG73JZ Fusion of Right Sacroiliac Joint with Synthetic Substitute, Percutaneous Approach

ØSG73KZ Fusion of Right Sacroiliac Joint with Nonautologous Tissue Substitute, Percutaneous Approach

ØSG73ZZ Fusion of Right Sacroiliac Joint, Percutaneous Approach

ØSG744Z Fusion of Right Sacroiliac Joint with Internal Fixation Device, Percutaneous Endoscopic Approach

ØSG747Z Fusion of Right Sacroiliac Joint with Autologous Tissue Substitute, Percutaneous Endoscopic Approach

ØSG74JZ Fusion of Right Sacroiliac Joint with Synthetic Substitute, Percutaneous Endoscopic Approach

ØSG74KZ Fusion of Right Sacroiliac Joint with Nonautologous Tissue Substitute, Percutaneous Endoscopic Approach

ØSG74ZZ Fusion of Right Sacroiliac Joint, Percutaneous Endoscopic Approach

ØSG804Z Fusion of Left Sacroiliac Joint with Internal Fixation Device, Open Approach

ØSG807Z Fusion of Left Sacroiliac Joint with Autologous Tissue Substitute, Open Approach

ØSG80JZ Fusion of Left Sacroiliac Joint with Synthetic Substitute, Open Approach

ØSG80KZ Fusion of Left Sacroiliac Joint with Nonautologous Tissue Substitute, Open Approach

ØSG80ZZ Fusion of Left Sacroiliac Joint, Open Approach

ØSG834Z Fusion of Left Sacroiliac Joint with Internal Fixation Device, Percutaneous Approach

ØSG837Z Fusion of Left Sacroiliac Joint with Autologous Tissue Substitute, Percutaneous Approach

ØSG83JZ Fusion of Left Sacroiliac Joint with Synthetic Substitute, Percutaneous Approach

ØSG83KZ Fusion of Left Sacroiliac Joint with Nonautologous Tissue Substitute, Percutaneous Approach

ØSG83ZZ Fusion of Left Sacroiliac Joint, Percutaneous Approach

ØSG844Z Fusion of Left Sacroiliac Joint with Internal Fixation Device, Percutaneous Endoscopic Approach

ØSG847Z Fusion of Left Sacroiliac Joint with Autologous Tissue Substitute, Percutaneous Endoscopic Approach

ØSG84JZ Fusion of Left Sacroiliac Joint with Synthetic Substitute, Percutaneous Endoscopic Approach

ØSG84KZ Fusion of Left Sacroiliac Joint with Nonautologous Tissue Substitute, Percutaneous Endoscopic Approach

ØSG84ZZ Fusion of Left Sacroiliac Joint, Percutaneous Endoscopic Approach

XRG0092 Fusion of Occipital-cervical Joint using Nanotextured Surface Interbody Fusion Device, Open Approach, New Technology Group 2

XRG1092 Fusion of Cervical Vertebral Joint using Nanotextured Surface Interbody Fusion Device, Open Approach, New Technology Group 2

XRG2092 Fusion of 2 or more Cervical Vertebral Joints using Nanotextured Surface Interbody Fusion Device, Open Approach, New Technology Group 2

XRG4092 Fusion of Cervicothoracic Vertebral Joint using Nanotextured Surface Interbody Fusion Device, Open Approach, New Technology Group 2

XRG6092 Fusion of Thoracic Vertebral Joint using Nanotextured Surface Interbody Fusion Device, Open Approach, New Technology Group 2

XRG7092 Fusion of 2 to 7 Thoracic Vertebral Joints using Nanotextured Surface Interbody Fusion Device, Open Approach, New Technology Group 2

XRG8092 Fusion of 8 or more Thoracic Vertebral Joints using Nanotextured Surface Interbody Fusion Device, Open Approach, New Technology Group 2

XRGA092 Fusion of Thoracolumbar Vertebral Joint using Nanotextured Surface Interbody Fusion Device, Open Approach, New Technology Group 2

XRGB092 Fusion of Lumbar Vertebral Joint using Nanotextured Surface Interbody Fusion Device, Open Approach, New Technology Group 2

XRGC092 Fusion of 2 or more Lumbar Vertebral Joints using Nanotextured Surface Interbody Fusion Device, Open Approach, New Technology Group 2

XRGD092 Fusion of Lumbosacral Joint using Nanotextured Surface Interbody Fusion Device, Open Approach, New Technology Group 2

**HAC 13: Surgical Site Infection (SSI) Following Cardiac Implantable Electronic Device (CIED) Procedures**

Secondary diagnosis not POA:

K68.11
T81.4XXA
T82.6XXA
T82.7XXA

**AND**

Any of the following procedures:

02H43JZ Insertion of Pacemaker Lead into Coronary Vein, Percutaneous Approach

02H43KZ Insertion of Defibrillator Lead into Coronary Vein, Percutaneous Approach

02H43MZ Insertion of Cardiac Lead into Coronary Vein, Percutaneous Approach

02H63JZ Insertion of Pacemaker Lead into Right Atrium, Percutaneous Approach

02H63MZ Insertion of Cardiac Lead into Right Atrium, Percutaneous Approach

02H73JZ Insertion of Pacemaker Lead into Left Atrium, Percutaneous Approach

02H73MZ Insertion of Cardiac Lead into Left Atrium, Percutaneous Approach

02HK3JZ Insertion of Pacemaker Lead into Right Ventricle, Percutaneous Approach

02HL3JZ Insertion of Pacemaker Lead into Left Ventricle, Percutaneous Approach

02HN0JZ Insertion of Pacemaker Lead into Pericardium, Open Approach

02HN0MZ Insertion of Cardiac Lead into Pericardium, Open Approach

02HN3JZ Insertion of Pacemaker Lead into Pericardium, Percutaneous Approach

02HN3MZ Insertion of Cardiac Lead into Pericardium, Percutaneous Approach

02HN4JZ Insertion of Pacemaker Lead into Pericardium, Percutaneous Endoscopic Approach

02HN4MZ Insertion of Cardiac Lead into Pericardium, Percutaneous Endoscopic Approach

02PA0MZ Removal of Cardiac Lead from Heart, Open Approach

02PA3MZ Removal of Cardiac Lead from Heart, Percutaneous Approach

02PA4MZ Removal of Cardiac Lead from Heart, Percutaneous Endoscopic Approach

02PAXMZ Removal of Cardiac Lead from Heart, External Approach

02WA0MZ Revision of Cardiac Lead in Heart, Open Approach

02WA3MZ Revision of Cardiac Lead in Heart, Percutaneous Approach

02WA4MZ Revision of Cardiac Lead in Heart, Percutaneous Endoscopic Approach

0JH604Z Insertion of Pacemaker, Single Chamber into Chest Subcutaneous Tissue and Fascia, Open Approach

0JH605Z Insertion of Pacemaker, Single Chamber Rate Responsive into Chest Subcutaneous Tissue and Fascia, Open Approach

**HAC 13: Surgical Site Infection (SSI) Following Cardiac Implantable Electronic Device (CIED) Procedures (continued)**

ØJH6Ø6Z    Insertion of Pacemaker, Dual Chamber into Chest Subcutaneous Tissue and Fascia, Open Approach

ØJH6Ø7Z    Insertion of Cardiac Resynchronization Pacemaker Pulse Generator into Chest Subcutaneous Tissue and Fascia, Open Approach

ØJH6Ø8Z    Insertion of Defibrillator Generator into Chest Subcutaneous Tissue and Fascia, Open Approach

ØJH6Ø9Z    Insertion of Cardiac Resynchronization Defibrillator Pulse Generator into Chest Subcutaneous Tissue and Fascia, Open Approach

ØJH6ØPZ    Insertion of Cardiac Rhythm Related Device into Chest Subcutaneous Tissue and Fascia, Open Approach

ØJH634Z    Insertion of Pacemaker, Single Chamber into Chest Subcutaneous Tissue and Fascia, Percutaneous Approach

ØJH635Z    Insertion of Pacemaker, Single Chamber Rate Responsive into Chest Subcutaneous Tissue and Fascia, Percutaneous Approach

ØJH636Z    Insertion of Pacemaker, Dual Chamber into Chest Subcutaneous Tissue and Fascia, Percutaneous Approach

ØJH637Z    Insertion of Cardiac Resynchronization Pacemaker Pulse Generator into Chest Subcutaneous Tissue and Fascia, Percutaneous Approach

ØJH638Z    Insertion of Defibrillator Generator into Chest Subcutaneous Tissue and Fascia, Percutaneous Approach

ØJH639Z    Insertion of Cardiac Resynchronization Defibrillator Pulse Generator into Chest Subcutaneous Tissue and Fascia, Percutaneous Approach

ØJH63PZ    Insertion of Cardiac Rhythm Related Device into Chest Subcutaneous Tissue and Fascia, Percutaneous Approach

ØJH8Ø4Z    Insertion of Pacemaker, Single Chamber into Abdomen Subcutaneous Tissue and Fascia, Open Approach

ØJH8Ø5Z    Insertion of Pacemaker, Single Chamber Rate Responsive into Abdomen Subcutaneous Tissue and Fascia, Open Approach

ØJH8Ø6Z    Insertion of Pacemaker, Dual Chamber into Abdomen Subcutaneous Tissue and Fascia, Open Approach

ØJH8Ø7Z    Insertion of Cardiac Resynchronization Pacemaker Pulse Generator into Abdomen Subcutaneous Tissue and Fascia, Open Approach

ØJH8Ø8Z    Insertion of Defibrillator Generator into Abdomen Subcutaneous Tissue and Fascia, Open Approach

ØJH8Ø9Z    Insertion of Cardiac Resynchronization Defibrillator Pulse Generator into Abdomen Subcutaneous Tissue and Fascia, Open Approach

ØJH8ØPZ    Insertion of Cardiac Rhythm Related Device into Abdomen Subcutaneous Tissue and Fascia, Open Approach

ØJH834Z    Insertion of Pacemaker, Single Chamber into Abdomen Subcutaneous Tissue and Fascia, Percutaneous Approach

ØJH835Z    Insertion of Pacemaker, Single Chamber Rate Responsive into Abdomen Subcutaneous Tissue and Fascia, Percutaneous Approach

ØJH836Z    Insertion of Pacemaker, Dual Chamber into Abdomen Subcutaneous Tissue and Fascia, Percutaneous Approach

ØJH837Z    Insertion of Cardiac Resynchronization Pacemaker Pulse Generator into Abdomen Subcutaneous Tissue and Fascia, Percutaneous Approach

ØJH838Z    Insertion of Defibrillator Generator into Abdomen Subcutaneous Tissue and Fascia, Percutaneous Approach

ØJH839Z    Insertion of Cardiac Resynchronization Defibrillator Pulse Generator into Abdomen Subcutaneous Tissue and Fascia, Percutaneous Approach

ØJH83PZ    Insertion of Cardiac Rhythm Related Device into Abdomen Subcutaneous Tissue and Fascia, Percutaneous Approach

ØJPTØPZ    Removal of Cardiac Rhythm Related Device from Trunk Subcutaneous Tissue and Fascia, Open Approach

ØJPT3PZ    Removal of Cardiac Rhythm Related Device from Trunk Subcutaneous Tissue and Fascia, Percutaneous Approach

ØJWTØPZ    Revision of Cardiac Rhythm Related Device in Trunk Subcutaneous Tissue and Fascia, Open Approach

ØJWT3PZ    Revision of Cardiac Rhythm Related Device in Trunk Subcutaneous Tissue and Fascia, Percutaneous Approach

**HAC 14: Iatrogenic Pneumothorax with Venous Catheterization**

Secondary diagnosis not POA:

J95.811

**AND**

Any of the following procedures:

02H633Z    Insertion of Infusion Device into Right Atrium, Percutaneous Approach

02HK33Z    Insertion of Infusion Device into Right Ventricle, Percutaneous Approach

02HS33Z    Insertion of Infusion Device into Right Pulmonary Vein, Percutaneous Approach

02HS43Z    Insertion of Infusion Device into Right Pulmonary Vein, Percutaneous Endoscopic Approach

02HT33Z    Insertion of Infusion Device into Left Pulmonary Vein, Percutaneous Approach

02HT43Z    Insertion of Infusion Device into Left Pulmonary Vein, Percutaneous Endoscopic Approach

02HV33Z    Insertion of Infusion Device into Superior Vena Cava, Percutaneous Approach

02HV43Z    Insertion of Infusion Device into Superior Vena Cava, Percutaneous Endoscopic Approach

05HØ33Z    Insertion of Infusion Device into Azygos Vein, Percutaneous Approach

05HØ43Z    Insertion of Infusion Device into Azygos Vein, Percutaneous Endoscopic Approach

05H133Z    Insertion of Infusion Device into Hemiazygos Vein, Percutaneous Approach

05H143Z    Insertion of Infusion Device into Hemiazygos Vein, Percutaneous Endoscopic Approach

05H333Z    Insertion of Infusion Device into Right Innominate Vein, Percutaneous Approach

05H343Z    Insertion of Infusion Device into Right Innominate Vein, Percutaneous Endoscopic Approach

05H433Z    Insertion of Infusion Device into Left Innominate Vein, Percutaneous Approach

05H443Z    Insertion of Infusion Device into Left Innominate Vein, Percutaneous Endoscopic Approach

05H533Z    Insertion of Infusion Device into Right Subclavian Vein, Percutaneous Approach

05H543Z    Insertion of Infusion Device into Right Subclavian Vein, Percutaneous Endoscopic Approach

05H633Z    Insertion of Infusion Device into Left Subclavian Vein, Percutaneous Approach

05H643Z    Insertion of Infusion Device into Left Subclavian Vein, Percutaneous Endoscopic Approach

05HM33Z    Insertion of Infusion Device into Right Internal Jugular Vein, Percutaneous Approach

05HN33Z    Insertion of Infusion Device into Left Internal Jugular Vein, Percutaneous Approach

05HP33Z    Insertion of Infusion Device into Right External Jugular Vein, Percutaneous Approach

05HQ33Z    Insertion of Infusion Device into Left External Jugular Vein, Percutaneous Approach

ØJH63XZ    Insertion of Vascular Access Device into Chest Subcutaneous Tissue and Fascia, Percutaneous Approach

In the 1970s, Medicare began demonstration projects that contracted with health maintenance organizations (HMO) to provide care for Medicare beneficiaries in exchange for prospective payments. In 1985, this project changed from demonstration status to a regular part of the Medicare program, Medicare Part C. The Balanced Budget Act (BBA) of 1997 named Medicare's Part C managed care program Medicare+Choice, and the Medicare Modernization Act (MMA) of 2003 again renamed it to Medicare Advantage (MA).

Medicare is one of the world's largest health insurance programs, and about one-fourth of the beneficiaries on Medicare are enrolled in a MA private health care plan. Due to the great variance in the health status of Medicare beneficiaries, risk adjustment provides a means of adequately compensating those plans with large numbers of seriously ill patients while not overburdening other plans that have healthier individuals. Medicare Advantage (MA) plans have been using the HCC/risk adjustment model since 2004.

## The Risk Adjustment Model

The primary purpose of a risk adjustment model is to predict (on average) the future health care costs for specific consortiums enrolled in Medicare Advantage (MA) health plans. CMS is then able to provide capitation payments to these private health plans. Capitation payments are an incentive for health plans to enroll not only healthier individuals but those with chronic conditions or who are more seriously ill by removing some of the financial burden.

The MA risk adjustment model uses hierarchical condition categories (HCC) to assess the disease burden of its enrollees. HCC diagnostic groupings were created after examining claims data so that enrollees with similar disease processes, and consequently similar health care expenditures, could be pooled into a larger data set in which an average expenditure rate could be determined. The medical conditions included in HCC categories are those that were determined to most predictably affect the health status and health care costs of any individual. Several important principles to the risk adjustment model and the development of the HCC categories include but are not limited to:

1. The HCC diagnostic categories should be clinically meaningful.
   - Diagnostic categories are well-defined.
   - Clinically specific diseases or medical conditions are grouped to each category.
2. The HCC diagnostic categories should predict medical expenditures.
   - The diagnoses grouped to a specific category should have as close to the same cost burden not only in the current year but also in the future.
3. The HCC diagnostic categories should have adequate sample sizes and discretionary categories excluded to be as accurate and stable in their estimate of costs as possible.
   - A diagnostic category that groups extremely rare diseases or conditions would not be reliably effective in determining current or future costs.
   - Codes that are not credible as cost predictors or may be subject to coding variation should be excluded, when possible.
4. The HCC diagnostic categories should be both hierarchical and accumulative.
   - Hierarchical measurement is used within a specific disease process.
   - Disease processes that are unrelated to each other are measured accumulatively.
5. The diagnostic classification should encourage specificity and should not reward coding proliferation.
   - More diagnosis codes and vague diagnosis codes do not equal greater disease burden.

More than 9,000 ICD-10-CM diagnosis codes map to 79 HCCs in the current risk adjustment model. Diagnoses are excluded from mapping when they do not predict future cost or are vague or variable in diagnosis, coding, or treatment, such as symptoms or osteoarthritis. Also excluded are diagnosis codes from laboratories, radiology, and home health claims.

## Risk Adjustment Factors

The CMS-HCC risk adjustment model uses "risk adjustment factors" to calculate a risk score for each member. This score summarizes that particular patient's expected cost of care relative to other members'. Each member's risk score is based on demographic and health status information and is calculated as the sum of these demographic and health factors weighted by their estimated marginal contributions to total risk. The model also takes into account where the patient resides (community or institutional), Medicaid eligibility (full or partial benefits), the patient's Medicare enrollment status (new or established), age, disability status, whether the patient is frail or has end-stage renal disease (ESRD), and even prescription drug use.

No procedure codes, ICD-10-PCS or CPT, are included in the MA risk adjustment model. The model relies solely on diagnostic and demographic data. Not all ICD-10-CM diagnoses map to an HCC, and there is no specific code sequencing involved. The CMS-HCC model is accumulative as well as hierarchical. The accumulative functionality allows a patient to have more than one HCC category assigned, providing a more complete clinical picture and prediction of resource consumption. The hierarchical aspect of the model provides a means of ranking diagnoses that are similar in disease process, by severity. The hierarchy of the condition categories ensures the patient's conditions are classified to the most severe condition within the related group. Less severe conditions within a particular hierarchy are superseded by more severe diagnoses within the same group. The hierarchy and accumulative relationship permits this model to characterize the person's illness level within each disease process, while still allowing the effects of unrelated disease processes to be counted in the patient's overall score.

Certain combinations of coexisting diagnoses for an individual can increase medical costs. The CMS-HCC model adjusts for these higher costs by the addition of "disease interaction" factors. For each patient, multiple HCCs assigned, along with demographic and disease interaction factors, are used to calculate a single, combined risk adjustment factor (RAF). The RAF score for an individual member represents all of the HCCs that have been submitted from all sources for that member to CMS during the course of an entire calendar year.

There are separate CMS-HCC models for new enrollees and continuing enrollees. The new enrollee model uses demographic factors only, such as age, sex, and disability status, and is used when the enrollee has less than 12 months of medical history. The community model accounts for age, sex, original reason for Medicare entitlement (age or disability), Medicaid eligibility, and clinical conditions as measured by HCCs. In the second step, expected costs are adjusted for outliers based on the member's risk score and whether the patient has ESRD.

Demographic data (age, sex, eligibility) as well as health status (diagnoses codes submitted on claims to CMS) of an MA population are used to determine the reimbursement to the health plan to care for their members.

RAF scores, which range from 0.118 to 2.4888, indicate patient health status. A RAF score of 1.0 or below is the benchmark CMS uses to indicate the average healthy patient with the same demographic and diagnostic factors. These patients are expected to use average or lower-than-average resources. When the RAF score is higher than 1.0, CMS considers the patient to be sicker than the average patient with the same criteria and expects greater-than-average resource utilization.

A low RAF score may accurately indicate a healthier patient, but it may also falsely indicate a healthier patient due to incomplete or inaccurate coding, incomplete or insufficient record documentation, or patients who fail to complete an annual assessment.

A high RAF score may accurately indicate a sicker patient, or it may be falsely inflated from overcoding due to diagnoses that are reported but not documented, or from copying and pasting from previous encounters or problem lists of resolved conditions.

## Documentation Requirements

Payment is made per HCC category (not per diagnosis code). No matter how many times in the year the diagnosis codes are reported, a single payment is made to the MA plan each year. Each year the list of HCCs and the RAF for each patient is "reset." This means the annual health assessment is extremely important, and adequate documentation is critical. Accurate risk adjustment payment relies on complete medical record documentation and diagnosis coding. CMS requires that all applicable diagnosis codes be reported and that all diagnoses be reported to the highest level of specificity and that these be substantiated by the medical record.

CMS's Guiding Principle:

The risk adjustment diagnosis must be based on clinical medical record documentation from a face-to-face encounter, coded according to the *ICD-10-CM Guidelines for Coding and Reporting*; assigned based on dates of service within the data collection period, submitted to the MA organization from an appropriate risk adjustment provider type and an appropriate risk adjustment physician data source.

A "face-to-face" health service encounter between a patient and healthcare provider describes an encounter between the patient and the provider (MD, DO), including qualified nonphysician practitioners (NPP) (e.g. nurse practitioner or physician's assistant), which is face-to-face with the patient. CMS provides a current listing of acceptable physician specialty types for risk adjustment data submission within the 2012 Regional Technical Assistance Participant Guide. The only exception to the face-to-face encounter requirement is pathology services (professional component only). Currently, CMS does not provide a listing of all services that are considered face-to-face visits for risk adjustment data, but does provide guidance on what types of services are not acceptable for risk adjustment in the Participant Guide. For example, diagnostic radiology does not qualify because diagnostic radiologists typically do not document confirmed diagnoses. Other examples of services that are not acceptable include diagnostic reports that have not been interpreted, such as laboratory reports.

It is essential that the medical record documentation show evidence by provider authentication that the direct face-to-face service was personally furnished by the physician or qualified NPP. Examples of these services include office visits, hospital visits, preoperative anesthesia assessment, and surgical and invasive procedures.

Risk adjustment relies on annual health information. Each enrollee is assigned an individual risk score based on the health status information obtained from the diagnosis codes on the claims. The CMS-HCC model relies on ICD-10-CM coding specificity for accurate risk adjustment by using the most specific code available that is substantiated by the documentation in the medical record. Providers should fully document and accurately code the evaluation and management of all severe and chronic conditions to ensure a full, complete, and accurate clinical record of the patient's condition and reflect the work involved in caring for the patient, particularly those with complex and challenging health issues. All conditions affecting the treatment or management of the patient's health should be documented at least once a year, as applicable to care provided, to accurately describe the true complexity and severity of the patient's health. If the diagnosis coding on the claim is not accurate or complete, the claim may indicate that the provider did much less medical decision-making, evaluation, and management than was actually performed.

Documentation for a valid reportable diagnosis must clearly indicate evidence of M.E.A.T., for each diagnosis:

| | |
|---|---|
| M | managed |
| E | evaluated |
| A | assessed |
| T | treated |

It is recommended that providers use the Subjective and Objective observation, Assessment and Plan (S.O.A.P.) format for progress notes to document evidence of M.E.A.T. A problem list, active condition list, past medical history list, etc., are not suitable examples of documentation of M.E.A.T. Diagnoses and documentation may not be captured from past encounters that have been copied and pasted. Each encounter must be unique and reflect only that visit as it occurred. Chronic conditions require long-term attention and management, and should be reported when treated but are often inadequately documented due to familiarity with the patient. Insufficient documentation influences the assignment of diagnosis codes and directly affects the patient's risk score.

Documentation should be concise, include the reason for the face-to-face visit, and support the need for the patient to be monitored, evaluated, assessed, and/or treated for the conditions listed through clinical rationale and/or plan of care described in clear (legible) notes. Each page of progress notes should be properly authenticated and include the patient's name and the date.

Providers should document each clinical diagnosis to the highest degree of specificity per encounter, including all complications and/or manifestations, including clear links to causal conditions. Only confirmed conditions should be documented—no rule-out conditions or abnormal findings without clinical significance. All known conditions, including chronic conditions, that affect the care and treatment of the patient at least once per year should be noted.

Providers should specifically document the condition and test or report results, and document the status of any changes to the condition, using terminology such as decreased, increased, worsening, improving, or unchanged. Documentation should include supporting evidence of the results or plan of care.

## Documentation Tips

- Document all cause-and-effect relationships.
- Report the most specific diagnosis code available that is supported by the documentation.
- Include all current diagnoses as part of the current medical decision-making, and document for every visit.
- Identify diagnoses that are current or chronic problems rather than a past medical history or previous resolved condition.
- Document history of heart attack, status codes, etc., that affect the patient's care as "history of" or "PMH" when they no longer exist or are not current conditions.
- Ensure each progress note has the date, signature, and credentials/specialty.
- Document the thought processes used to assess each condition.
- Know high revenue HCCs that are often undiagnosed or undercoded.
- Avoid "unspecified" codes.
- Ensure the codes reported are accurate.
- Ensure each encounter is billed.
- Review rejection reports, and audit reports to assess risks.

## Audits

Because reimbursement is by patient, rather than based on an average of the entire population, and is based upon documentation, there is the potential for upcoding. Audits are conducted by the MA plan and CMS recovery auditors.

### Initial Validation Audit (IVA)

CMS requires that the MA plan validate HCCs. This is usually performed by an independent auditor working with the plan or a contracted vendor to validate the MA plan's data submitted to CMS.

The MA plan submits the one best medical record that supports each HCC identified for the beneficiary.

### Risk Adjustment Data Validation Audit

Risk adjustment data validation (RADV) audits were introduced in 2011 and updated for 2015. They are performed by CMS to validate the integrity and accuracy of risk-adjusted payments by verifying that the diagnosis codes the MA plans submit are supported by the medical record documentation for a member.

MA plans can be selected by CMS for RADV audits annually and if chosen are required to submit their members' medical records to CMS. Providers are required to assist the MA plan by providing the medical record documentation included in the audit. Even though each diagnosis needs to be reported only once in a calendar year, during a RADV audit up to five dates of service may be submitted to support any one HCC.

To be validated, medical record documentation must meet certain criteria and standards. Even if the diagnosis is documented and coded correctly, any deficiency in the documentation can make the encounter and the HCC invalid. Diagnoses that cannot be validated are considered payment errors. The results of the audit are communicated to the MA plan, which then communicates these results to the provider. Under- and overpayments are subject to payment adjustment. The results of RADV audits can be extrapolated over the MA plan population to calculate potential payment errors and overpayments/recoupments. Regulations include a RADV appeal process, a document dispute process, and a procedure for obtaining physician-signature attestations.

The following items are reviewed during the validation process:

- The record is for the correct enrollee.
- The record is from the correct calendar year for the payment year being audited.
- The record is legible.
- The date of service is present on the records and is for a face-to-face visit.
- The record is from a valid provider type.

- Valid credentials and/or a valid physician specialty are documented on the record.

- The record contains a signature from an acceptable type of physician.

- There is a diagnosis on the record.

- The diagnosis supports an HCC.

- The diagnosis supports the submitted HCC.

Mitigate audit risk by coding each reportable diagnosis each time it meets reporting guidelines. Audit regularly to assess areas of risk and in need of improvement and to capture conditions documented but not coded. Check for additional qualifying HCCs. Ensure claims are submitted and that corrected claims are submitted when indicated. There are three claims submission deadlines: January, March, and September. CMS adjusts each member's risk score twice a year, with the final reconciliation in August of the year after the plan year.

If providers emphasize correct coding and documentation and perform internal audits to determine where the risks are and prepare for audits, incorrect payment is less likely.

## Chapter 3. Diseases of the Blood and Blood-forming Organs and Certain Disorders Involving the Immune Mechanism (D50–D89)

**Red Blood Cells**

**White Blood Cell**

## Platelet

## Coagulation

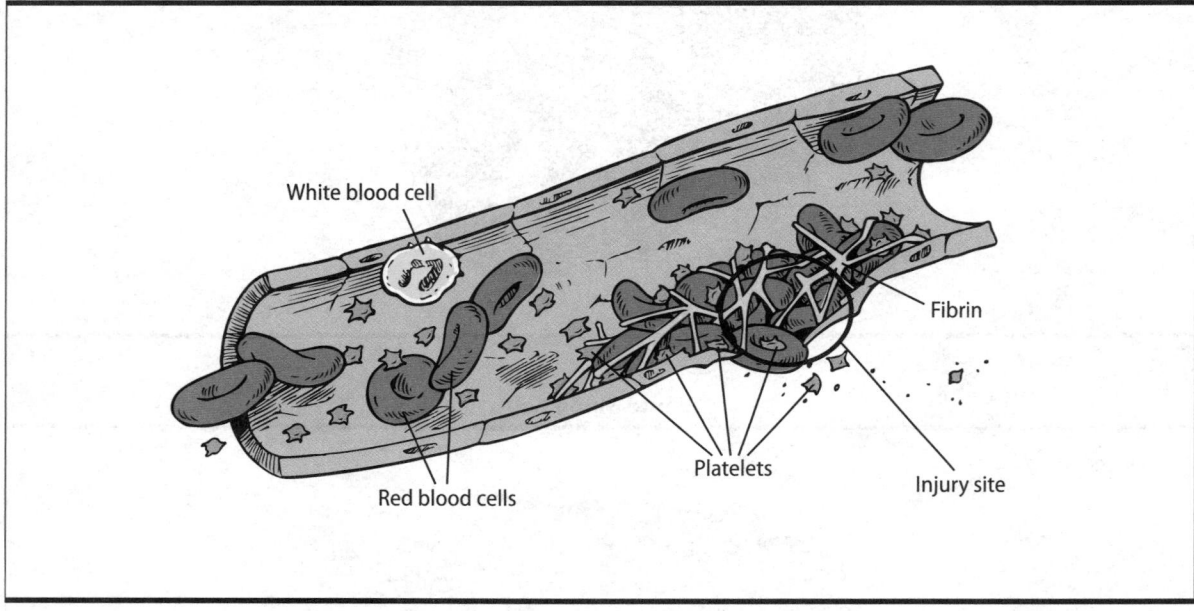

## Spleen Anatomical Location and External Structures

## Spleen Interior Structures

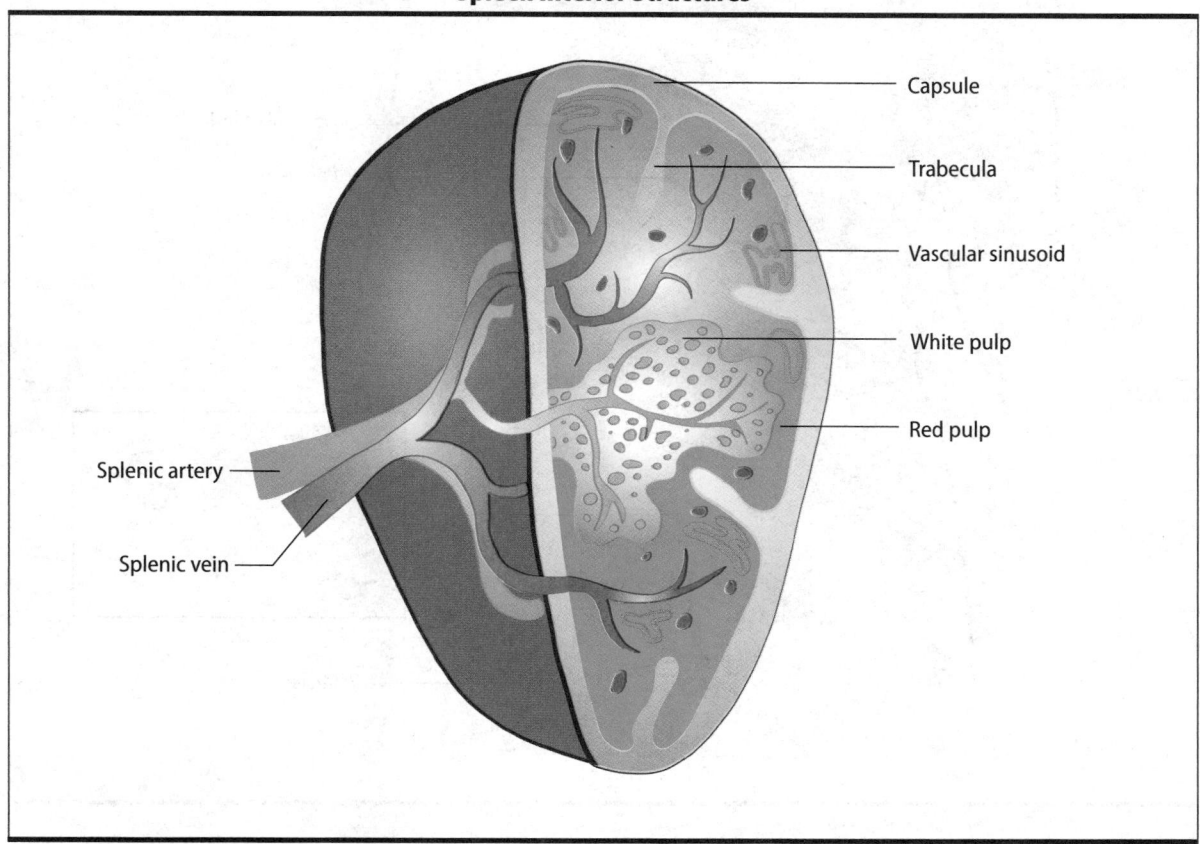

# Chapter 4. Endocrine, Nutritional and Metabolic Diseases (EØØ–E89)

## Endocrine System

## Thyroid

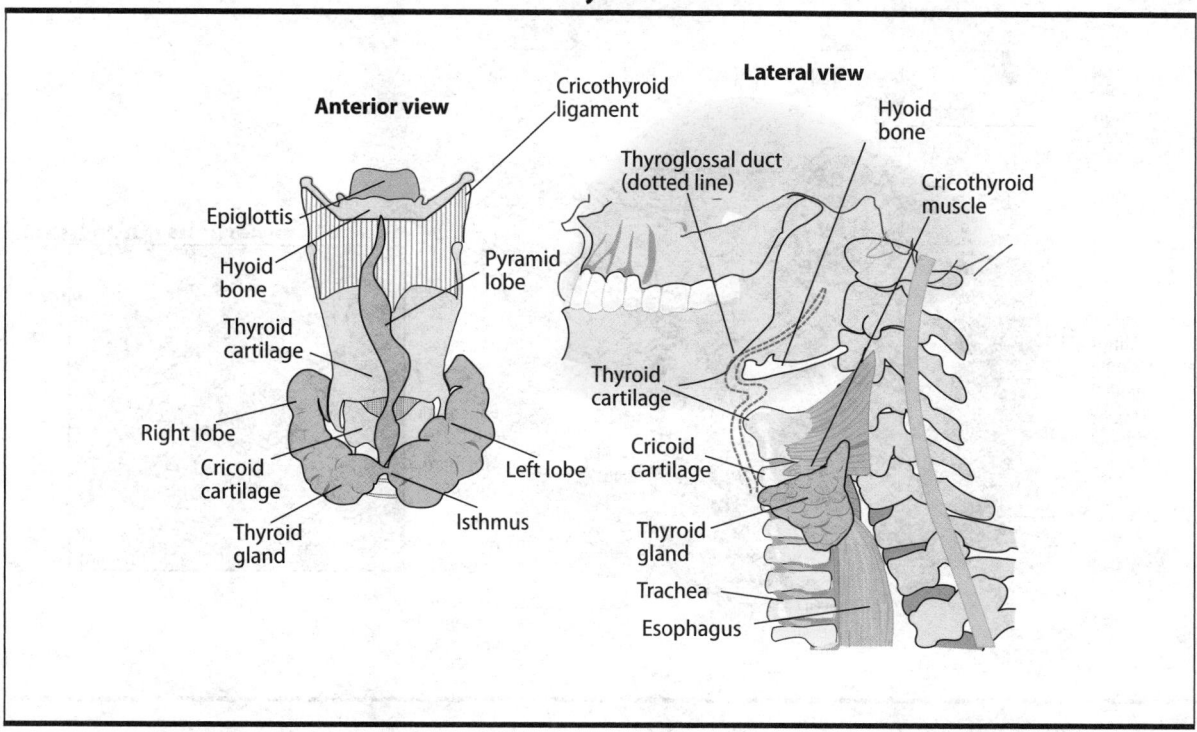

## Thyroid and Parathyroid Glands

# Pancreas

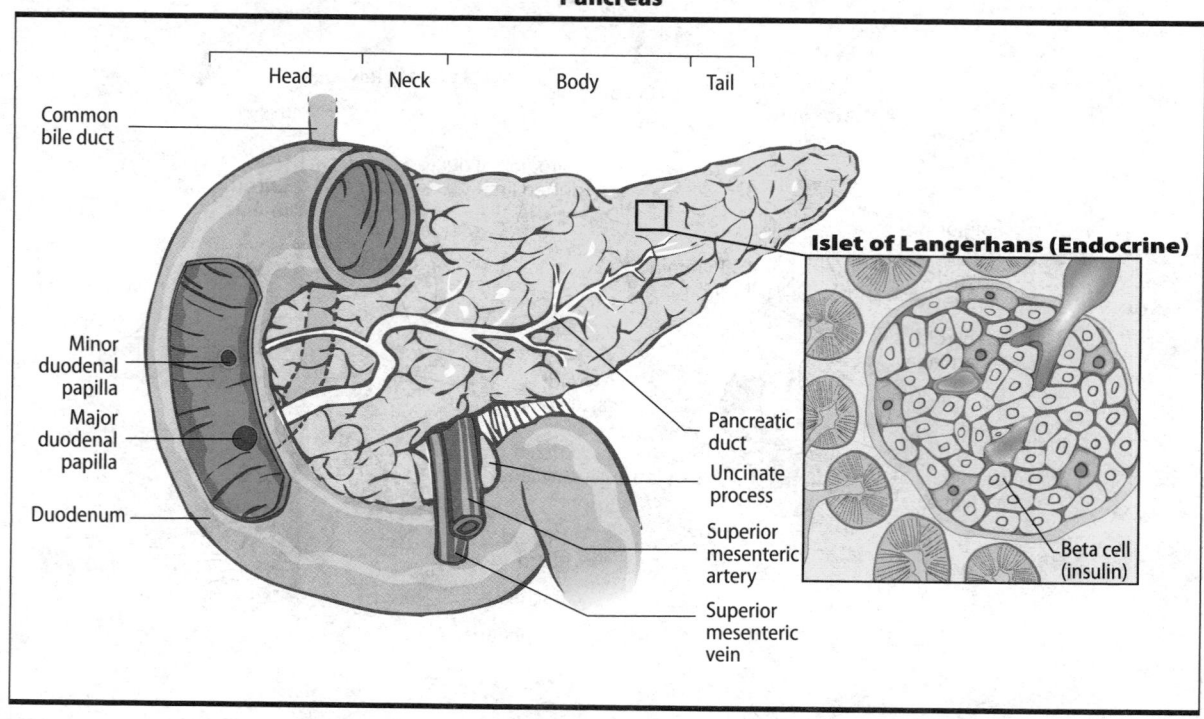

## Anatomy of the Adrenal Gland

## Structure of an Ovary

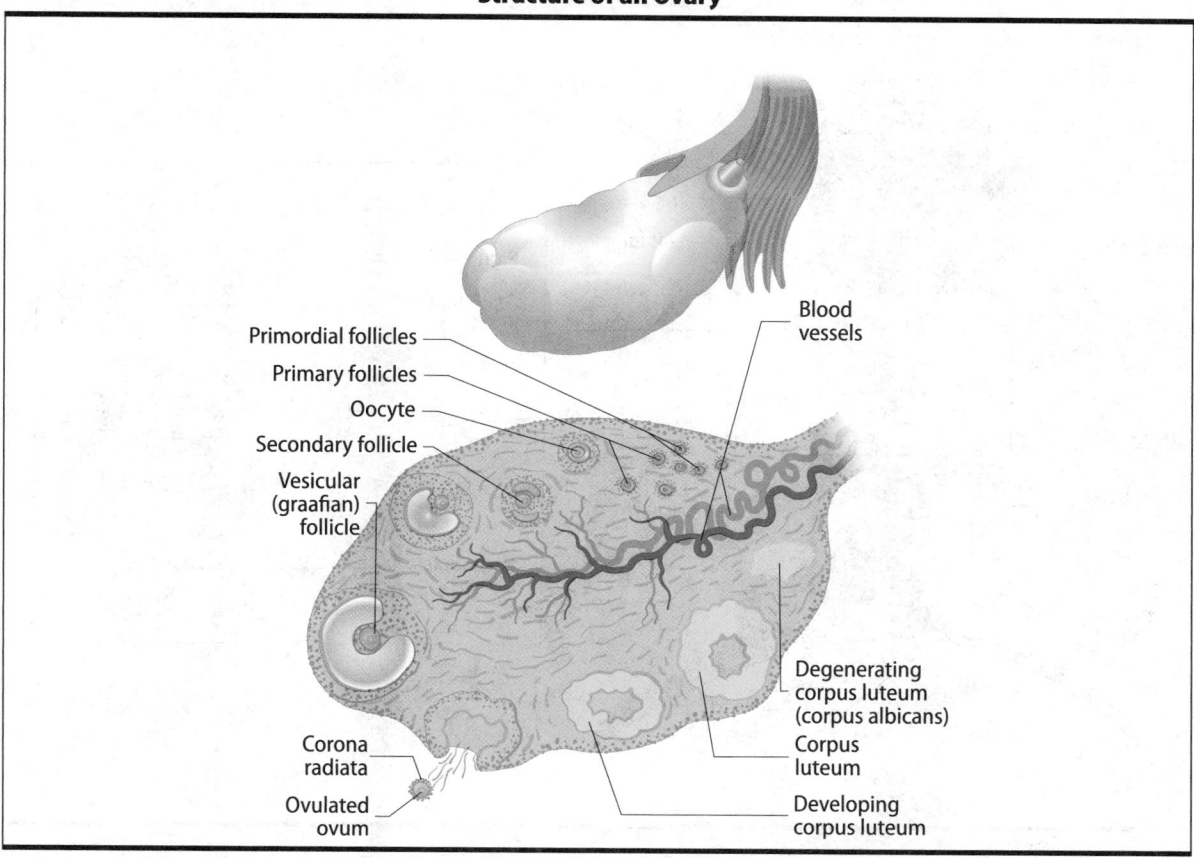

## Testis and Associated Structures

# Thymus

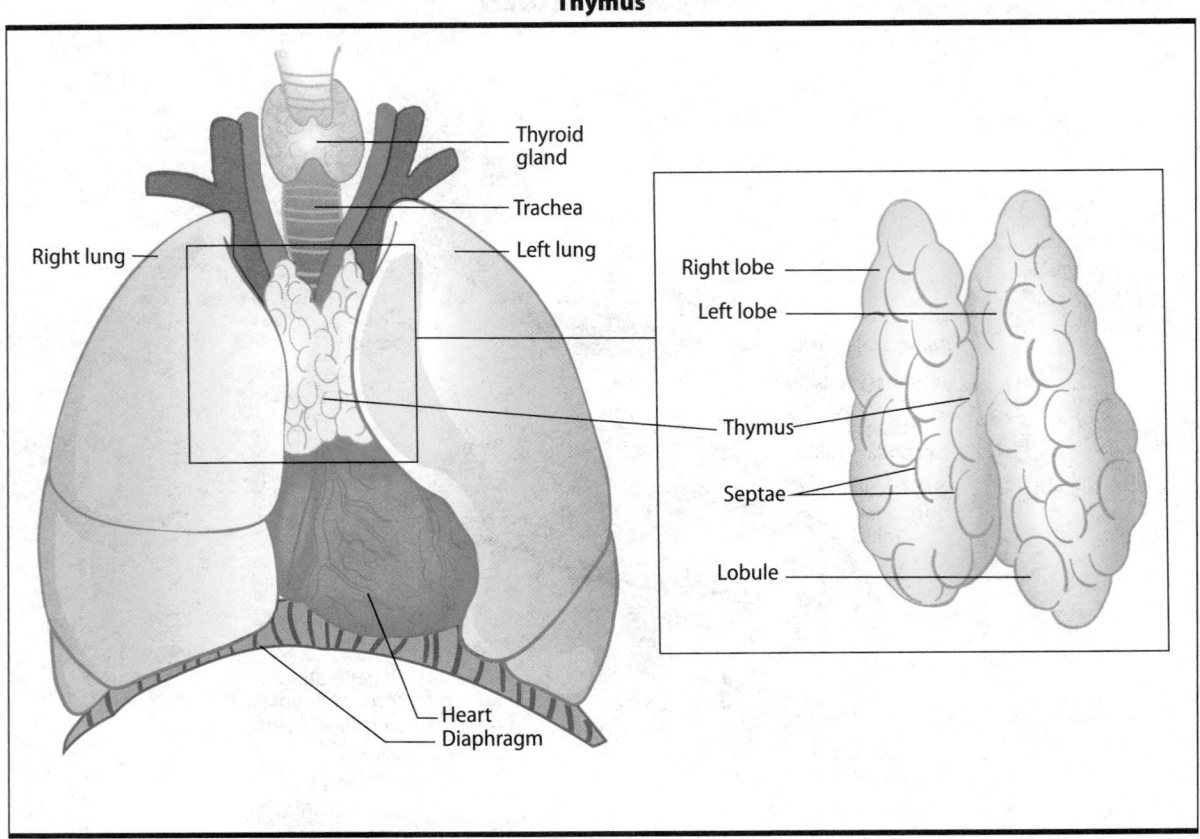

# Chapter 6. Diseases of the Nervous System (GØØ–G99)

**Brain**

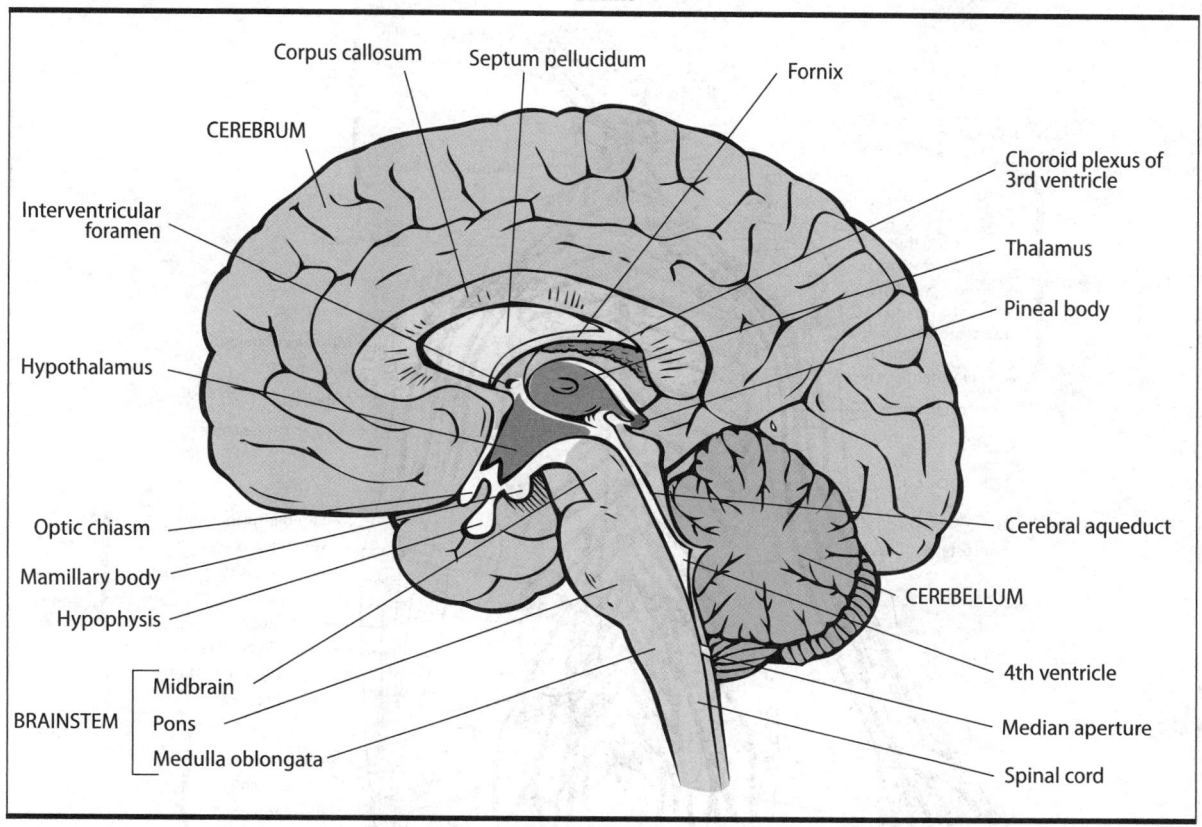

- Corpus callosum
- Septum pellucidum
- Fornix
- CEREBRUM
- Choroid plexus of 3rd ventricle
- Interventricular foramen
- Thalamus
- Pineal body
- Hypothalamus
- Optic chiasm
- Cerebral aqueduct
- Mamillary body
- CEREBELLUM
- Hypophysis
- 4th ventricle
- BRAINSTEM
  - Midbrain
  - Pons
  - Medulla oblongata
- Median aperture
- Spinal cord

**Cranial Nerves**

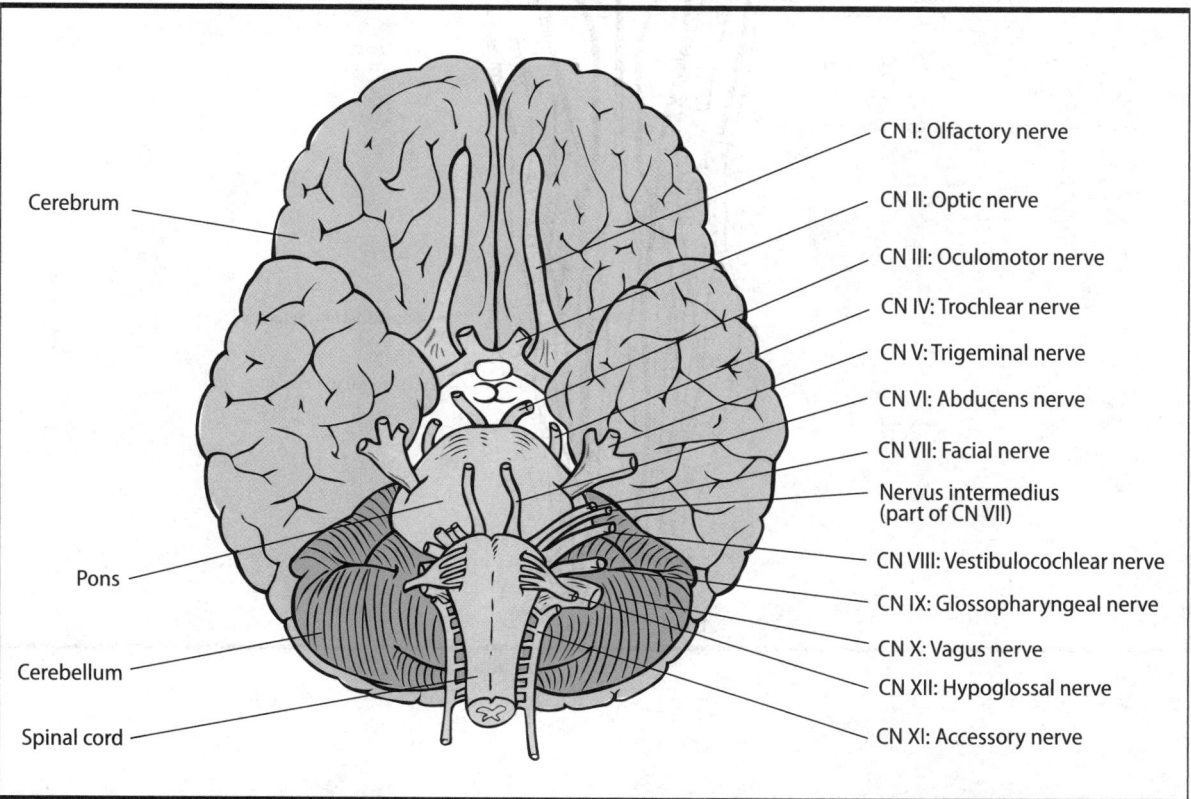

- Cerebrum
- CN I: Olfactory nerve
- CN II: Optic nerve
- CN III: Oculomotor nerve
- CN IV: Trochlear nerve
- CN V: Trigeminal nerve
- CN VI: Abducens nerve
- CN VII: Facial nerve
- Nervus intermedius (part of CN VII)
- CN VIII: Vestibulocochlear nerve
- CN IX: Glossopharyngeal nerve
- Pons
- CN X: Vagus nerve
- CN XII: Hypoglossal nerve
- Cerebellum
- CN XI: Accessory nerve
- Spinal cord

# Peripheral Nervous System

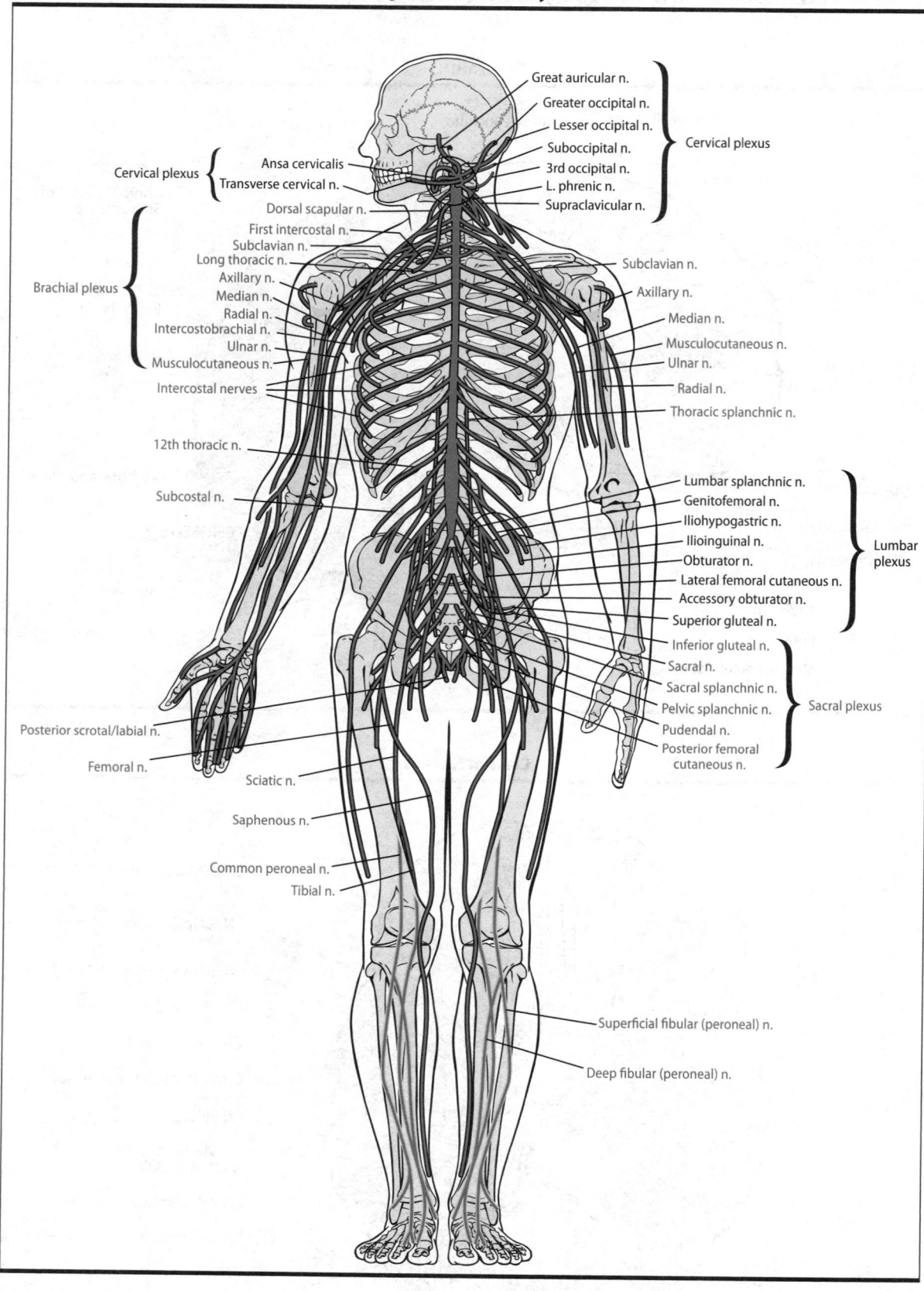

## Spinal Cord and Spinal Nerves

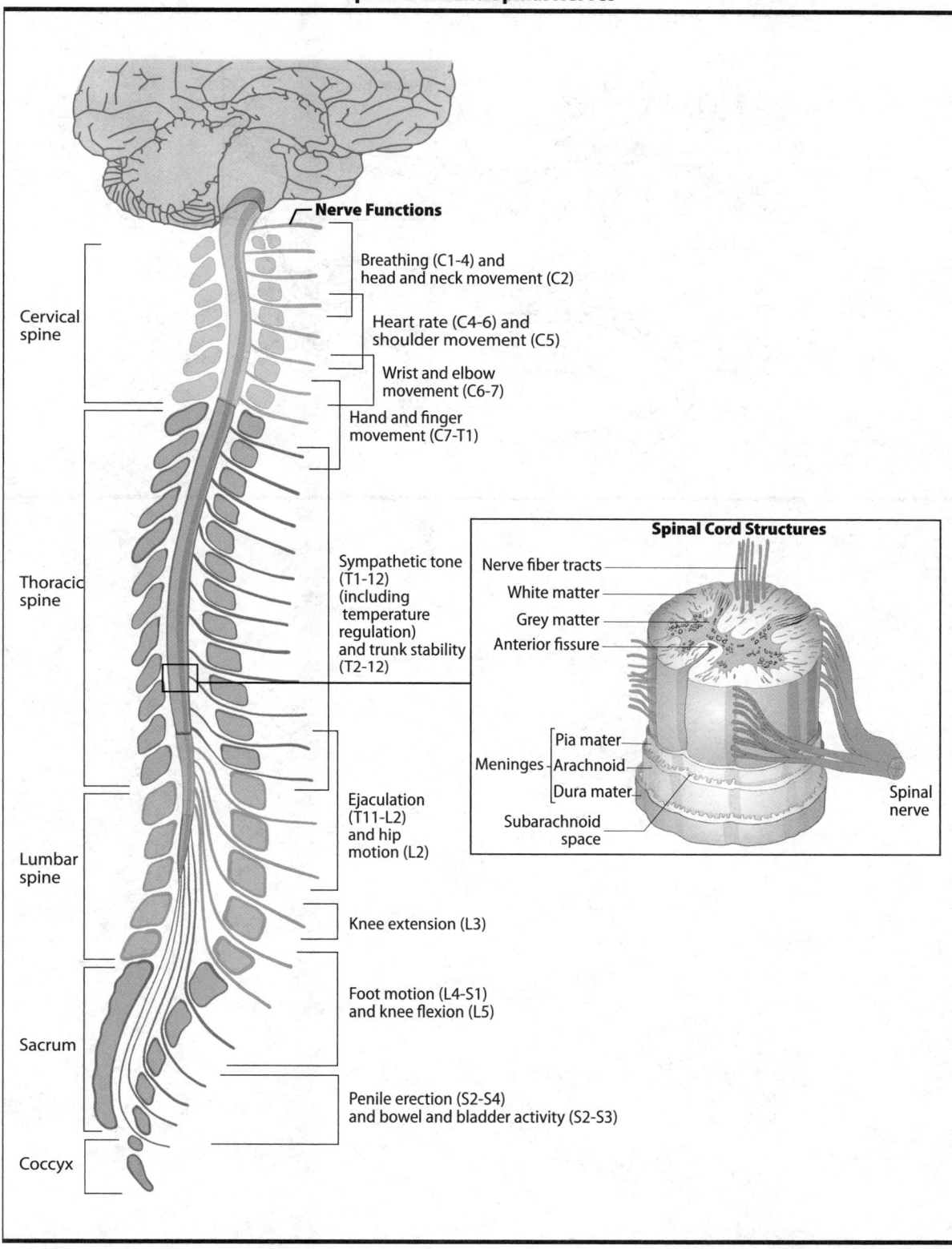

**Nerve Functions**

Breathing (C1-4) and head and neck movement (C2)

Heart rate (C4-6) and shoulder movement (C5)

Wrist and elbow movement (C6-7)

Hand and finger movement (C7-T1)

Cervical spine

Sympathetic tone (T1-12) (including temperature regulation) and trunk stability (T2-12)

Thoracic spine

Ejaculation (T11-L2) and hip motion (L2)

Knee extension (L3)

Lumbar spine

Foot motion (L4-S1) and knee flexion (L5)

Sacrum

Penile erection (S2-S4) and bowel and bladder activity (S2-S3)

Coccyx

**Spinal Cord Structures**

Nerve fiber tracts

White matter

Grey matter

Anterior fissure

Pia mater

Meninges — Arachnoid

Dura mater

Subarachnoid space

Spinal nerve

# Nerve Cell

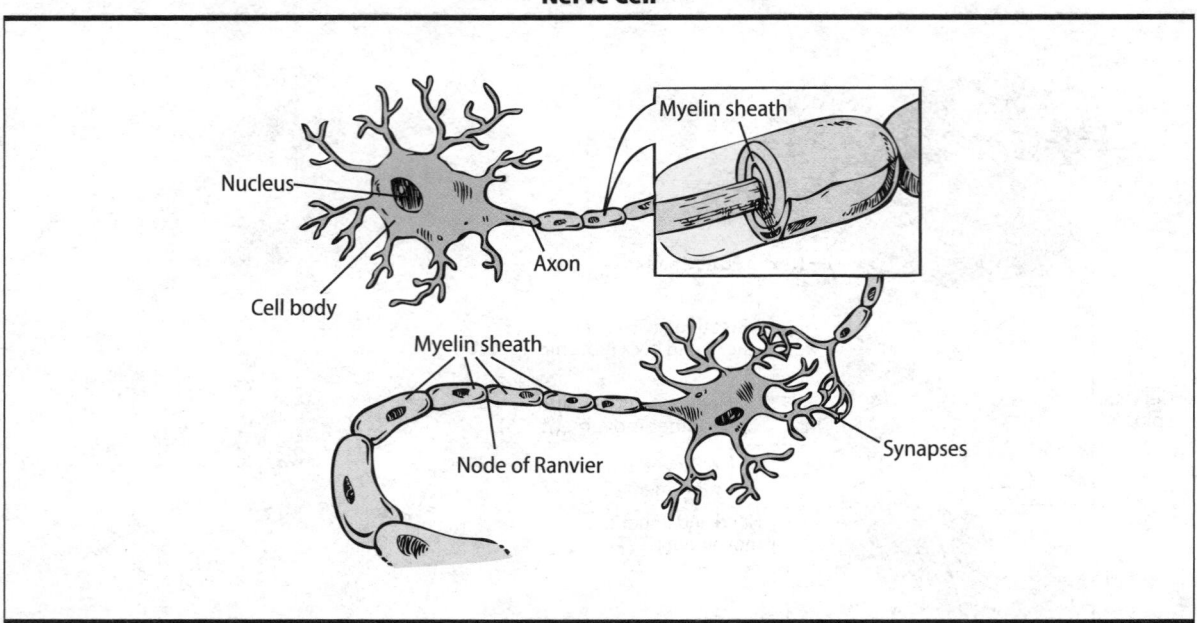

# Chapter 7. Diseases of the Eye and Adnexa (H00–H59)

**Eye**

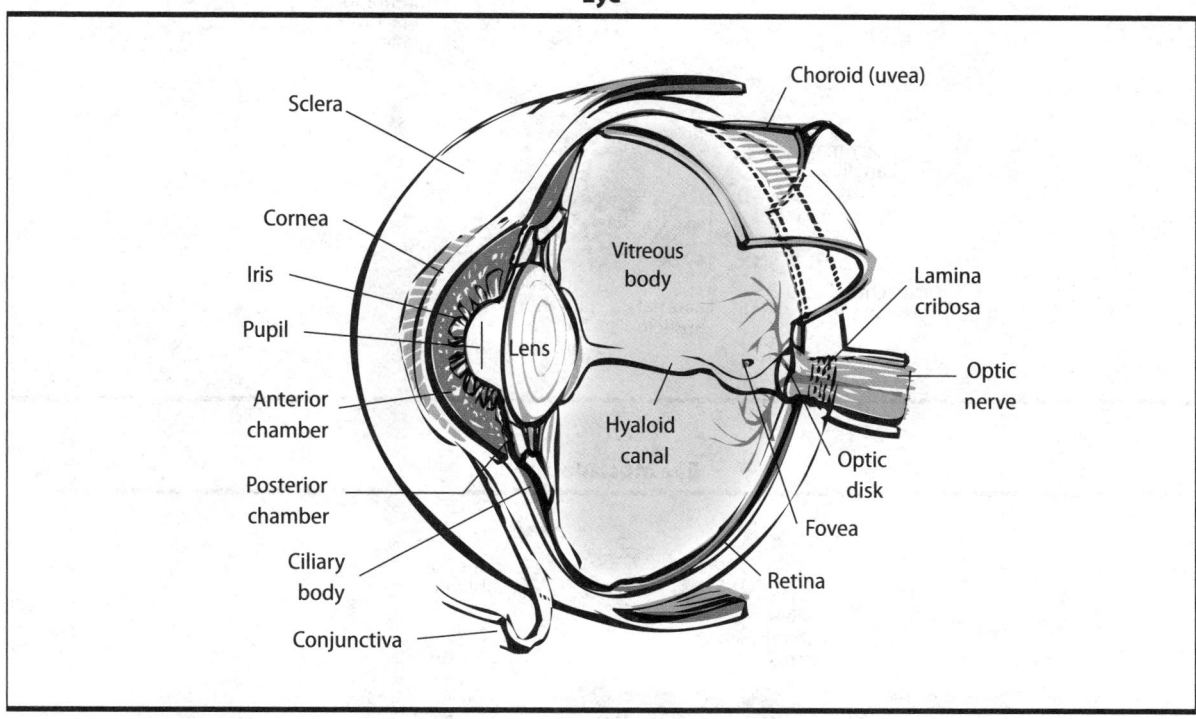

**Posterior Pole of Globe/Flow of Aqueous Humor**

## Lacrimal System

## Eye Musculature

## Eyelid Structures

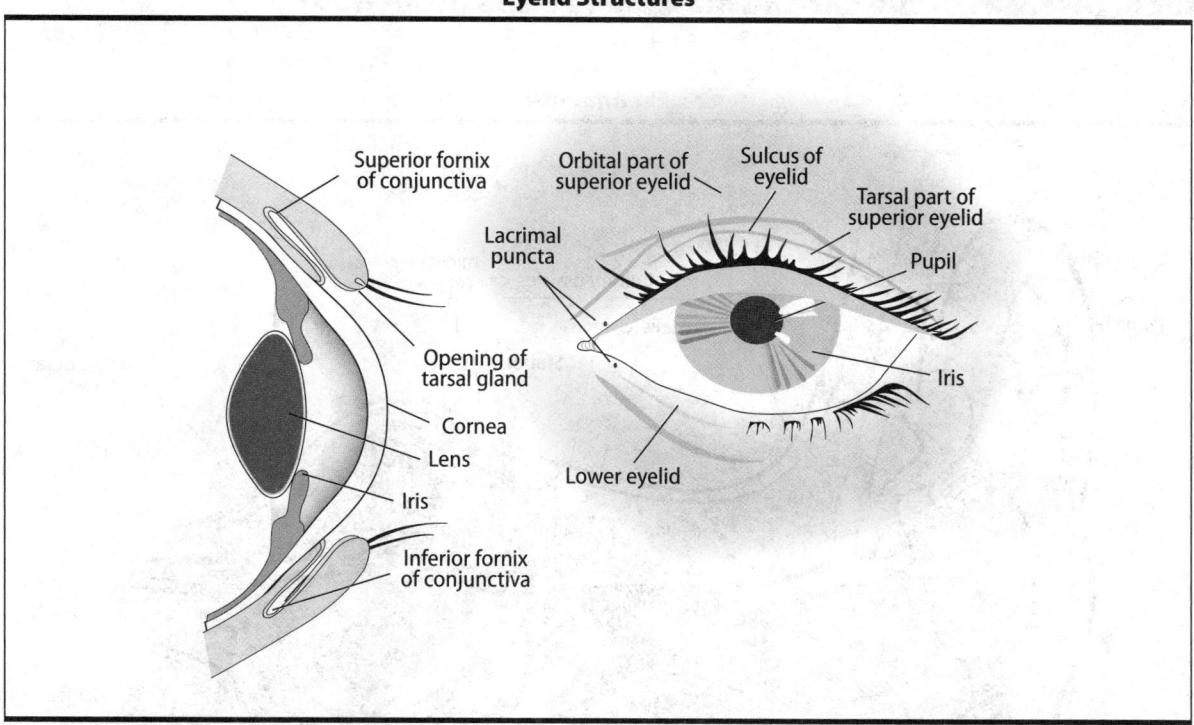

# Chapter 8. Diseases of the Ear and Mastoid Process (H60–H95)

**Ear Anatomy**

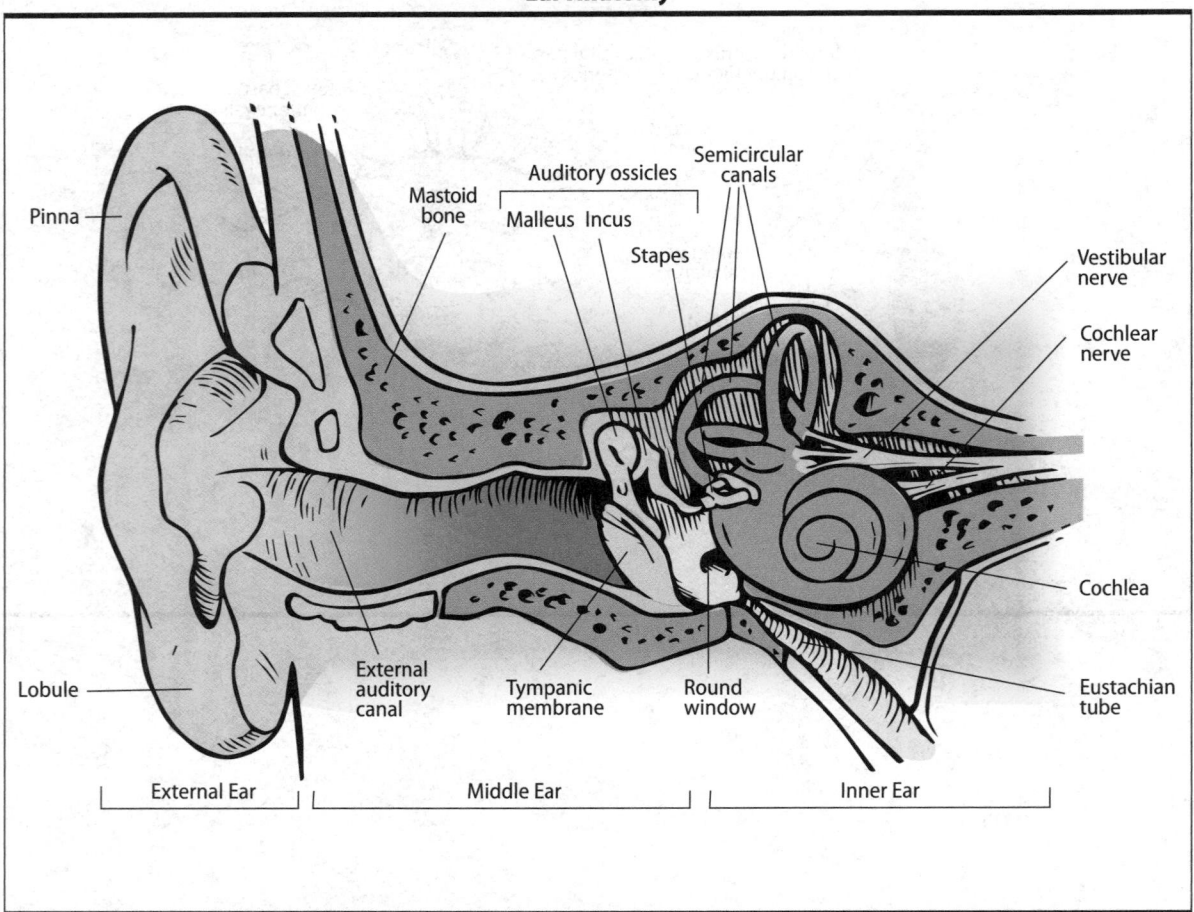

# Chapter 9. Diseases of the Circulatory System (I00–I99)

## Anatomy of the Heart

Aorta

Superior vena cava

Pulmonary artery

Pulmonary vein

Aortic valve

Pulmonary valve

Right atrium

Left atrium

Mitral valve

Tricuspid valve

Chorda tendinae

Right ventricle

Left ventricle

Inferior vena cava

## Heart Cross Section

Pericardial layers:

Sectional schematic

Pleura
Fibrous pleura
Parietal pleura
Epicardium
Serous (fluid)
Pericardial cavity
Endocardium
Myocardium (muscular)
Endocardial cavity
Septum

Pericardial sac

Pericardial reflection (layers fused)

Pericardial sinus

## Heart Valves

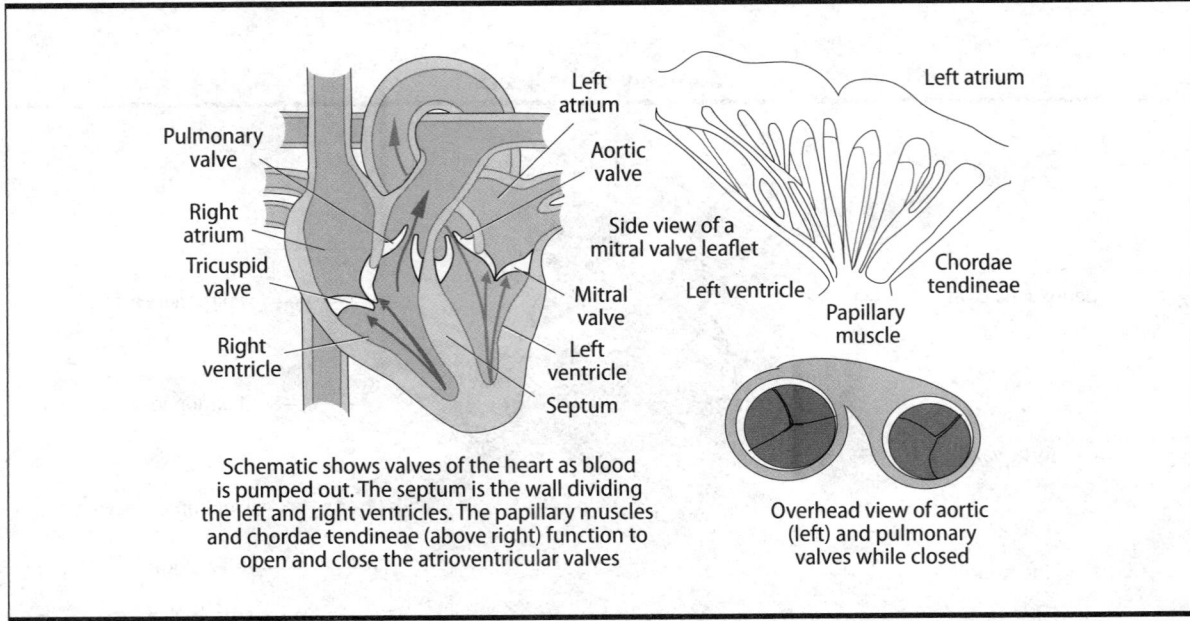

Schematic shows valves of the heart as blood is pumped out. The septum is the wall dividing the left and right ventricles. The papillary muscles and chordae tendineae (above right) function to open and close the atrioventricular valves

Overhead view of aortic (left) and pulmonary valves while closed

## Heart Conduction System

## Coronary Arteries

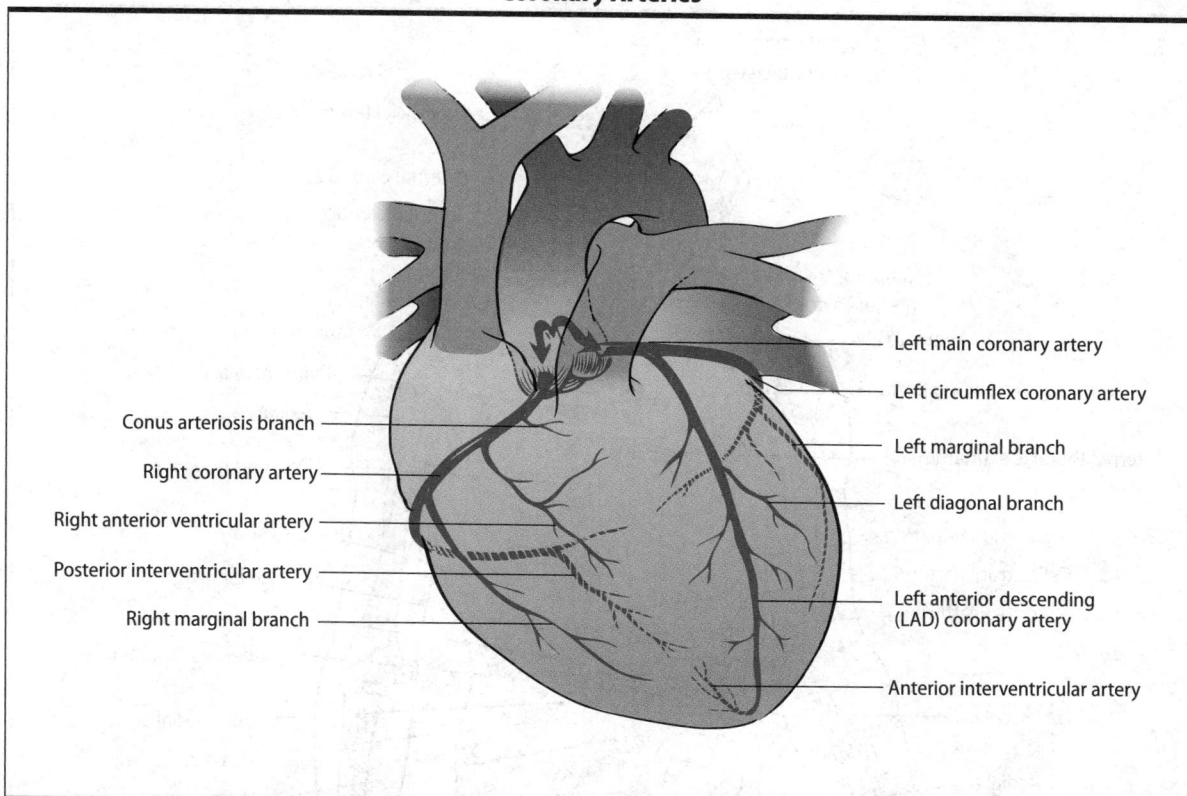

Left main coronary artery

Left circumflex coronary artery

Left marginal branch

Left diagonal branch

Conus arteriosis branch

Right coronary artery

Right anterior ventricular artery

Posterior interventricular artery

Left anterior descending (LAD) coronary artery

Right marginal branch

Anterior interventricular artery

# Arteries

# Veins

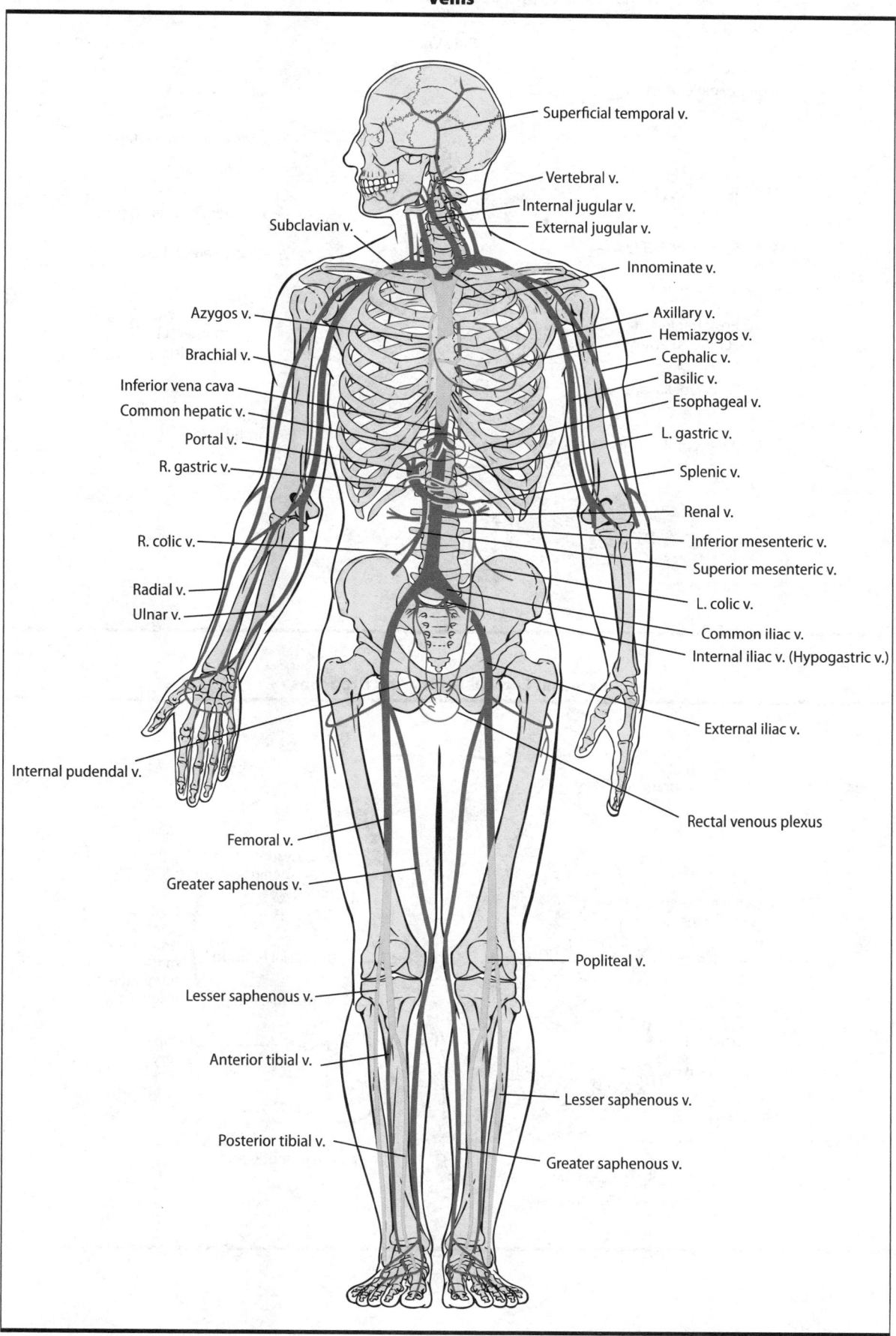

## Internal Carotid and Vertebral Arteries and Branches

### Side View

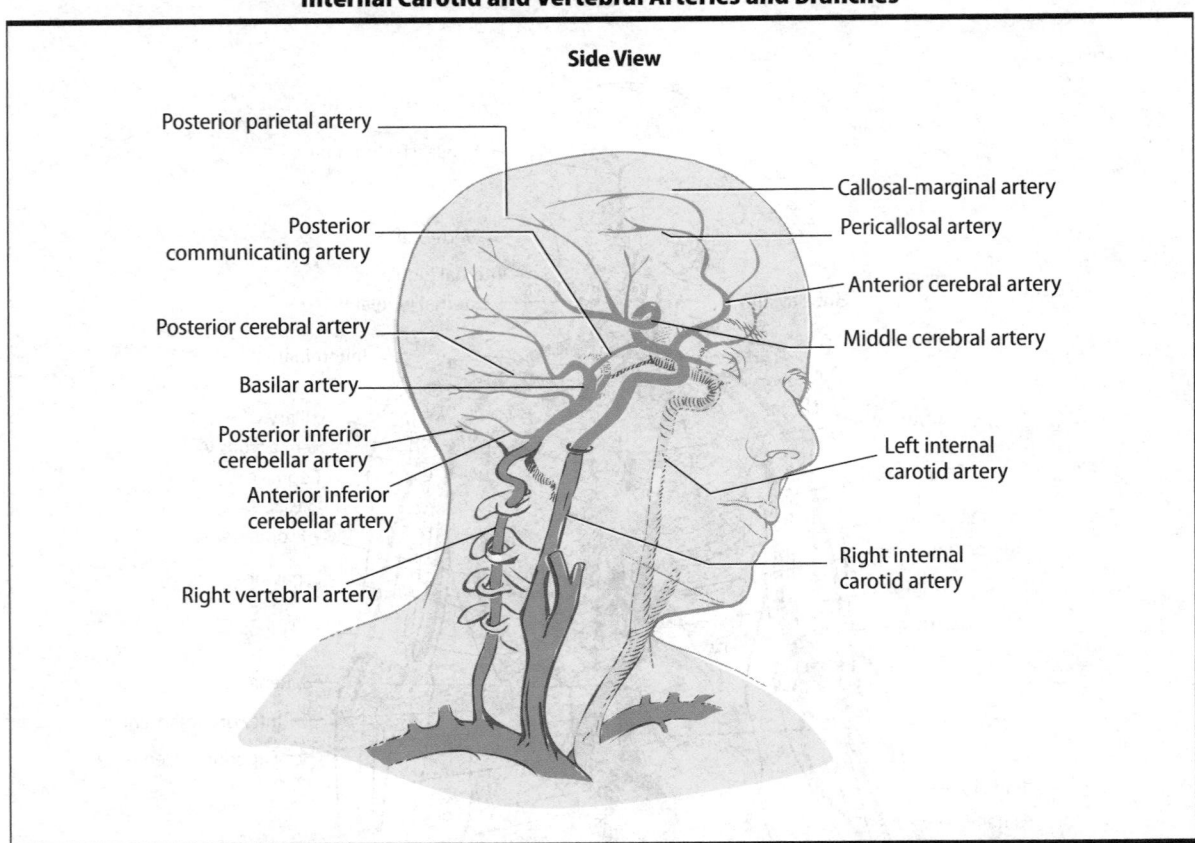

## External Carotid Artery and Branches

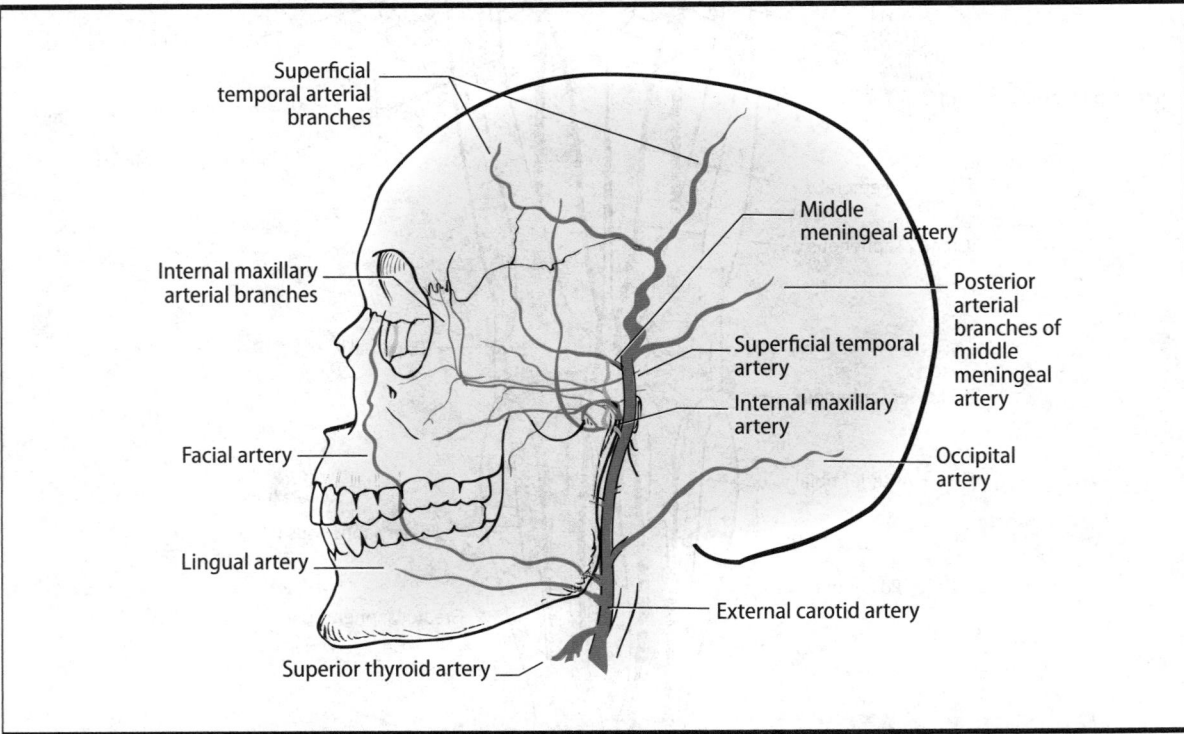

## Branches of Abdominal Aorta

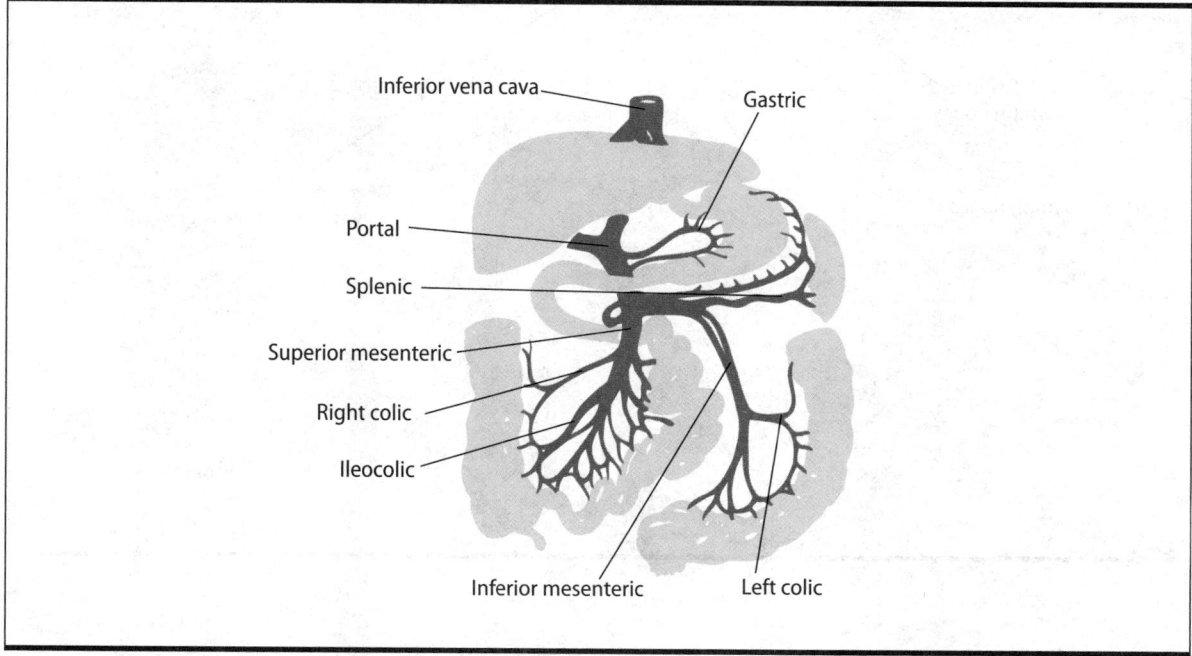

## Portal Venous Circulation

## Lymphatic System

## Axillary Lymph Nodes

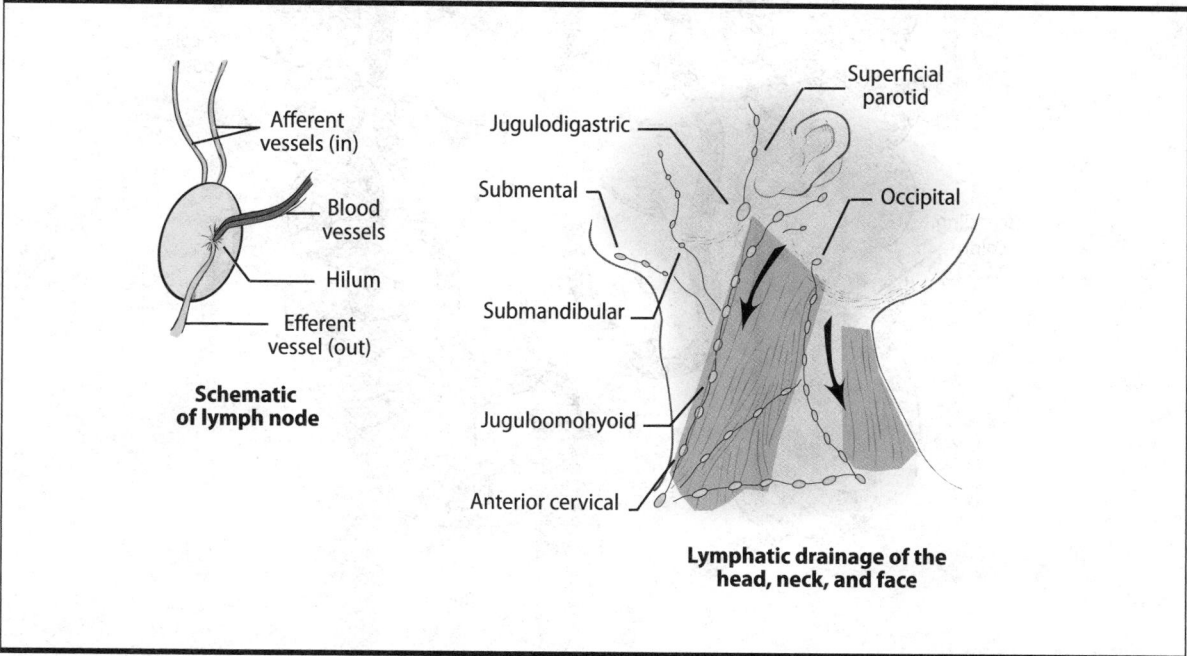

Parasternal nodes

Sternum

Clavicle

Deltoid muscle

Brachialis muscle

Lateral nodes

Subscapular nodes

Pectoral nodes

Axillary lymph nodes

Central nodes

Latissimus dorsi muscle

Rectus abdominis muscle

## Lymphatic System of Head and Neck

Afferent vessels (in)

Blood vessels

Hilum

Efferent vessel (out)

**Schematic of lymph node**

Jugulodigastric

Submental

Submandibular

Juguloomohyoid

Anterior cervical

Superficial parotid

Occipital

**Lymphatic drainage of the head, neck, and face**

## Lymphatic Capillaries

### Schematic of lymphatic capillaries

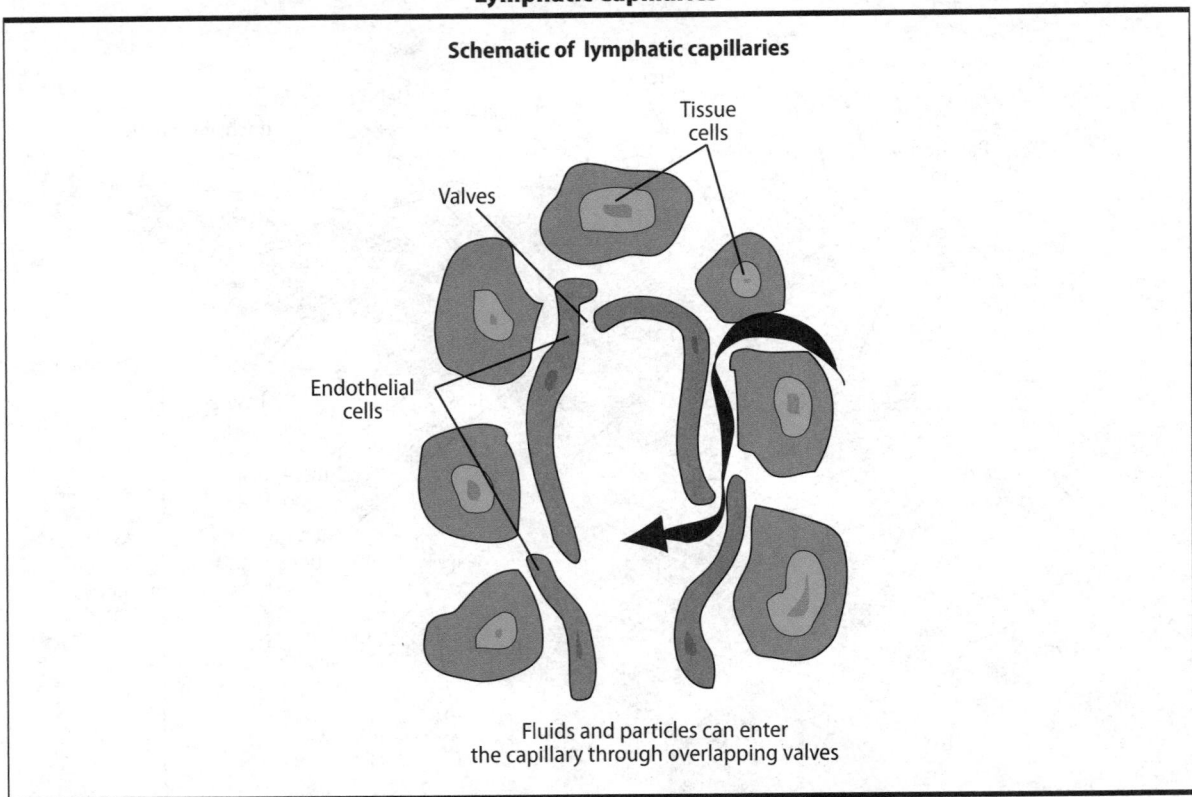

Fluids and particles can enter
the capillary through overlapping valves

## Lymphatic Drainage

### Lymphatic drainage of the colon follows blood supply

# Chapter 10. Diseases of the Respiratory System (J00–J99)

**Respiratory System**

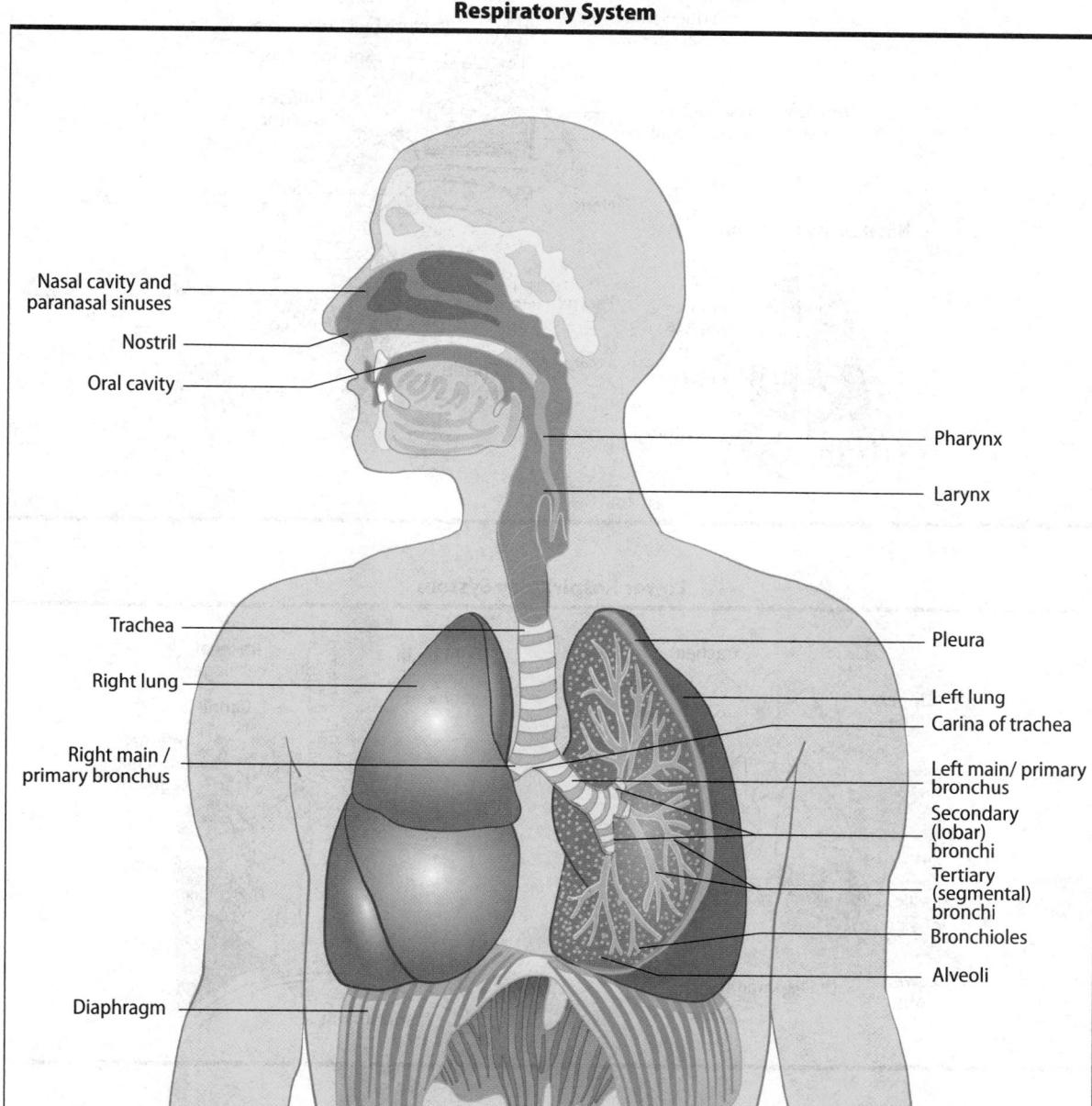

Nasal cavity and paranasal sinuses

Nostril

Oral cavity

Pharynx

Larynx

Trachea

Right lung

Right main / primary bronchus

Diaphragm

Pleura

Left lung

Carina of trachea

Left main/ primary bronchus

Secondary (lobar) bronchi

Tertiary (segmental) bronchi

Bronchioles

Alveoli

## Upper Respiratory System

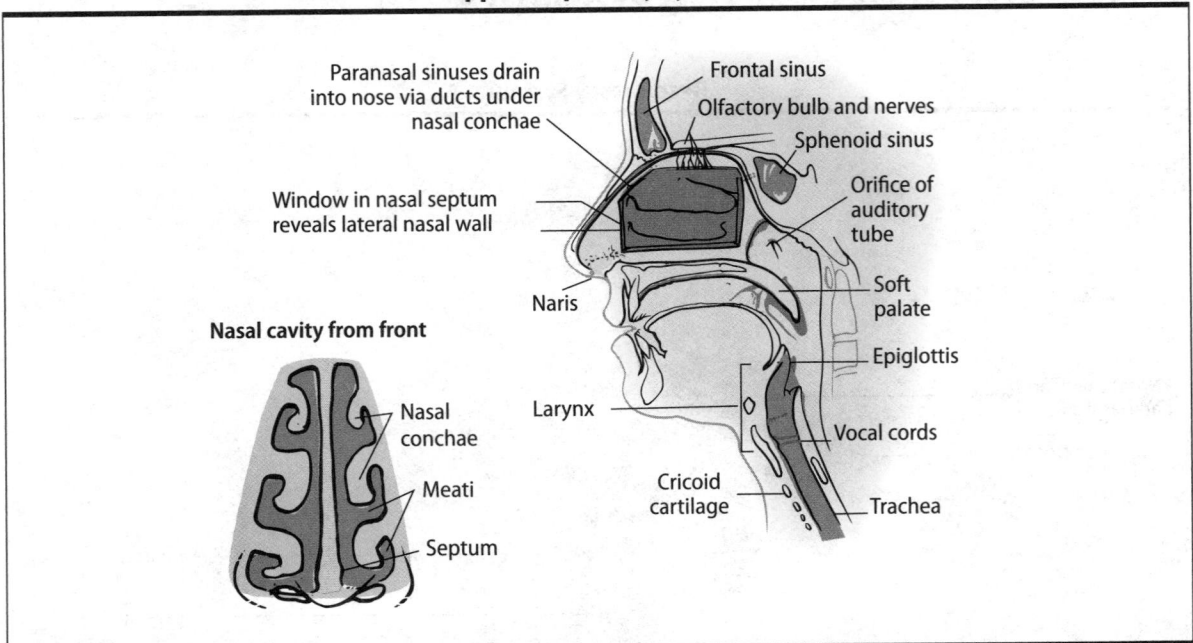

Paranasal sinuses drain into nose via ducts under nasal conchae

Frontal sinus

Olfactory bulb and nerves

Sphenoid sinus

Orifice of auditory tube

Window in nasal septum reveals lateral nasal wall

Naris

Soft palate

**Nasal cavity from front**

Nasal conchae

Meati

Septum

Larynx

Epiglottis

Vocal cords

Cricoid cartilage

Trachea

## Lower Respiratory System

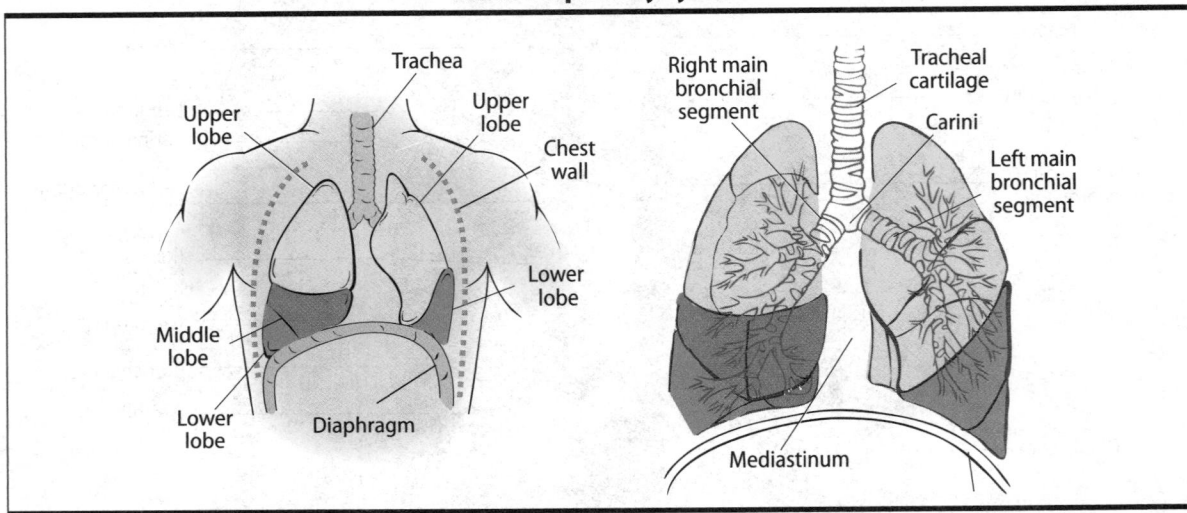

Trachea

Upper lobe

Upper lobe

Chest wall

Lower lobe

Middle lobe

Lower lobe

Diaphragm

Right main bronchial segment

Tracheal cartilage

Carini

Left main bronchial segment

Mediastinum

## Paranasal Sinuses

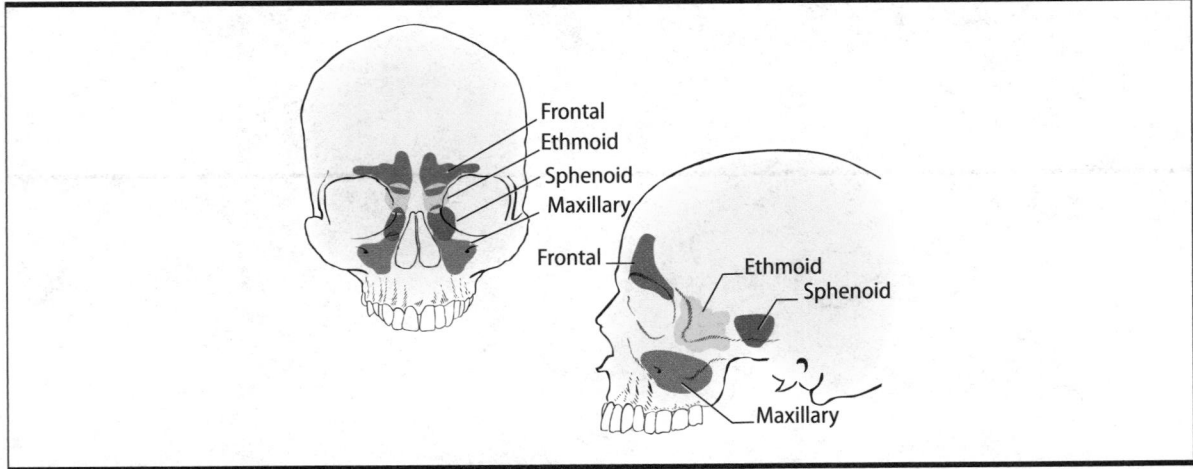

Frontal

Ethmoid

Sphenoid

Maxillary

Frontal

Ethmoid

Sphenoid

Maxillary

## Lung Segments

## Alveoli

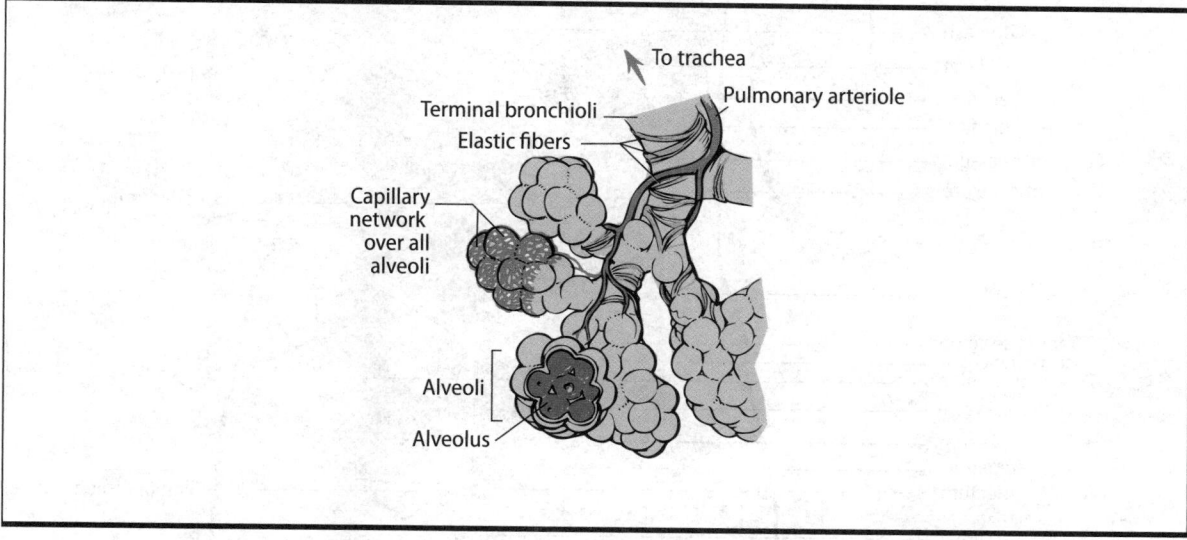

# Chapter 11. Diseases of the Digestive System (K00–K95)

**Digestive System**

## Omentum and Mesentery

## Peritoneum and Retroperitoneum

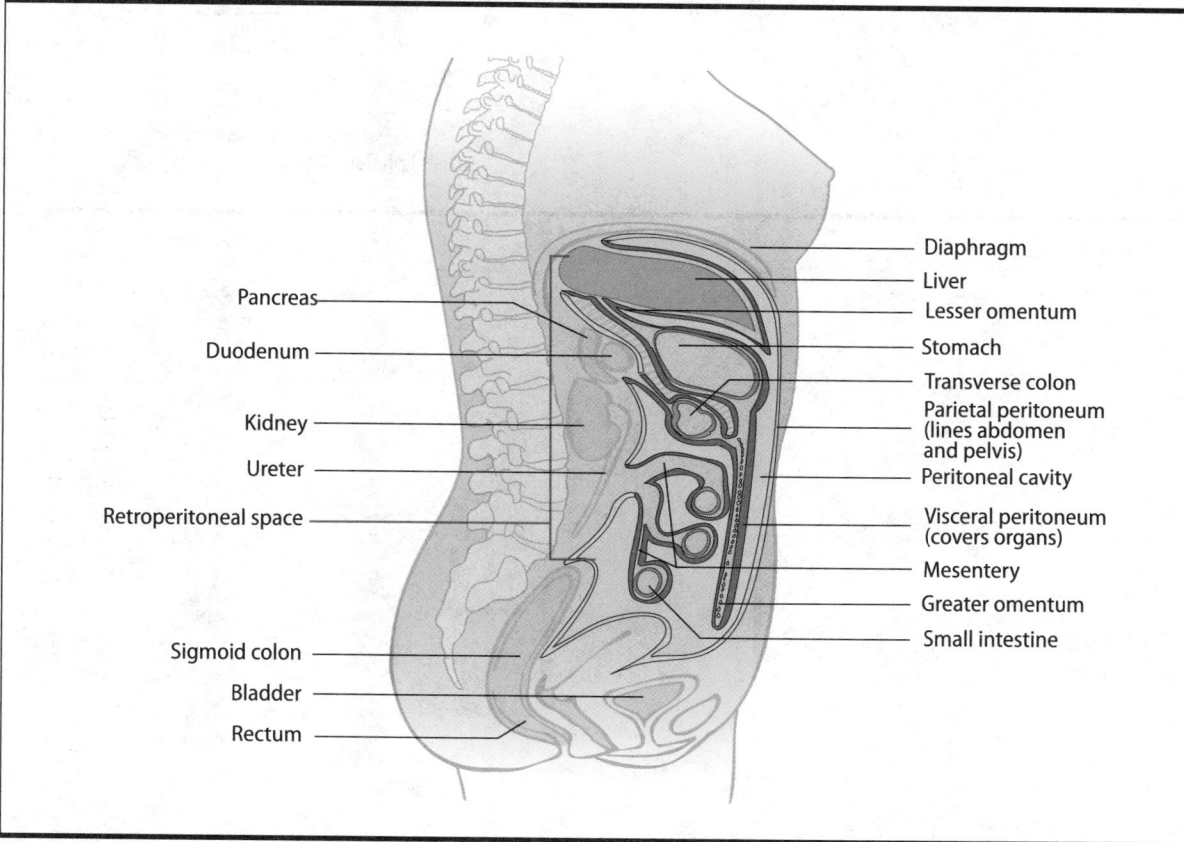

# Chapter 12. Diseases of the Skin and Subcutaneous Tissue (LØØ–L99)

**Nail Anatomy**

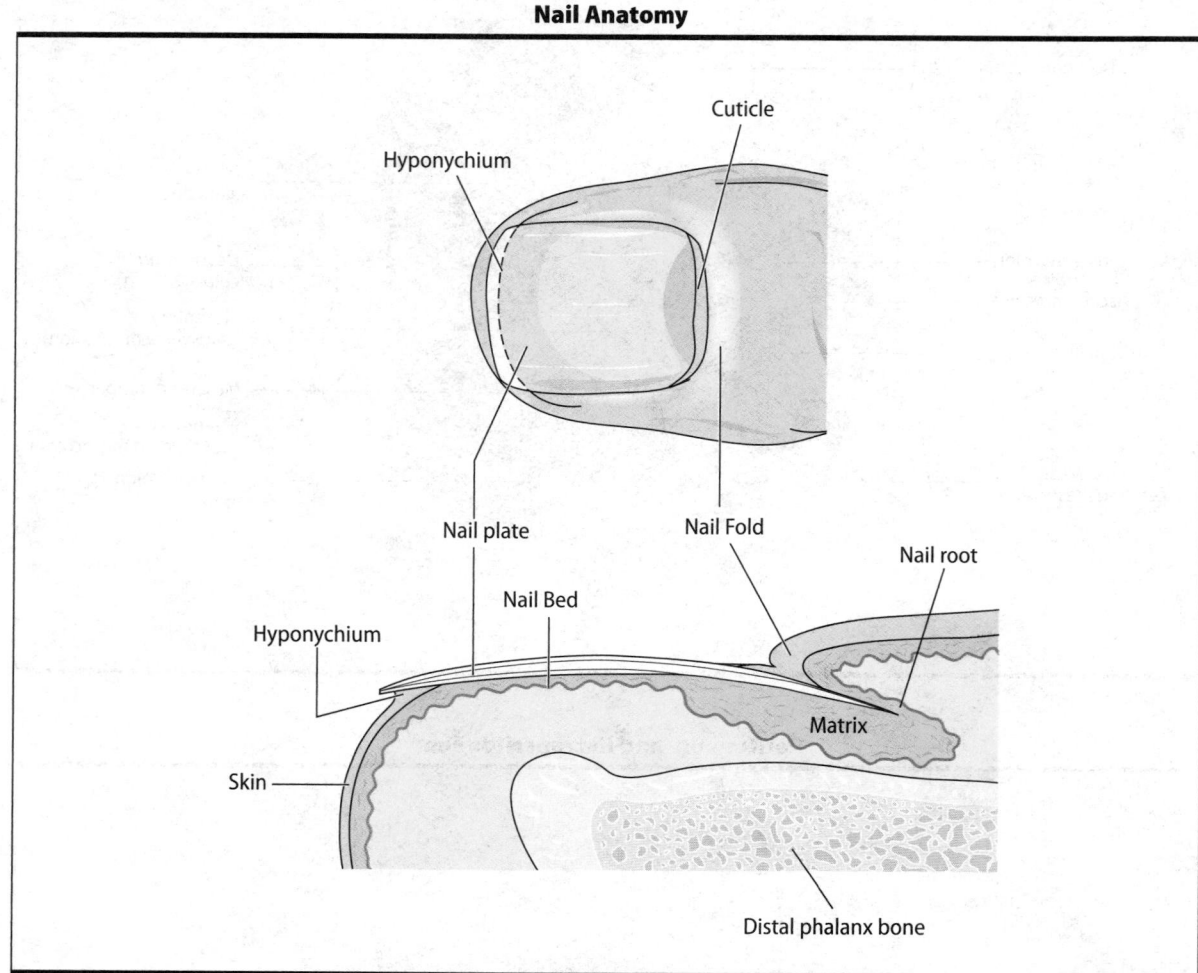

## Skin and Subcutaneous Tissue

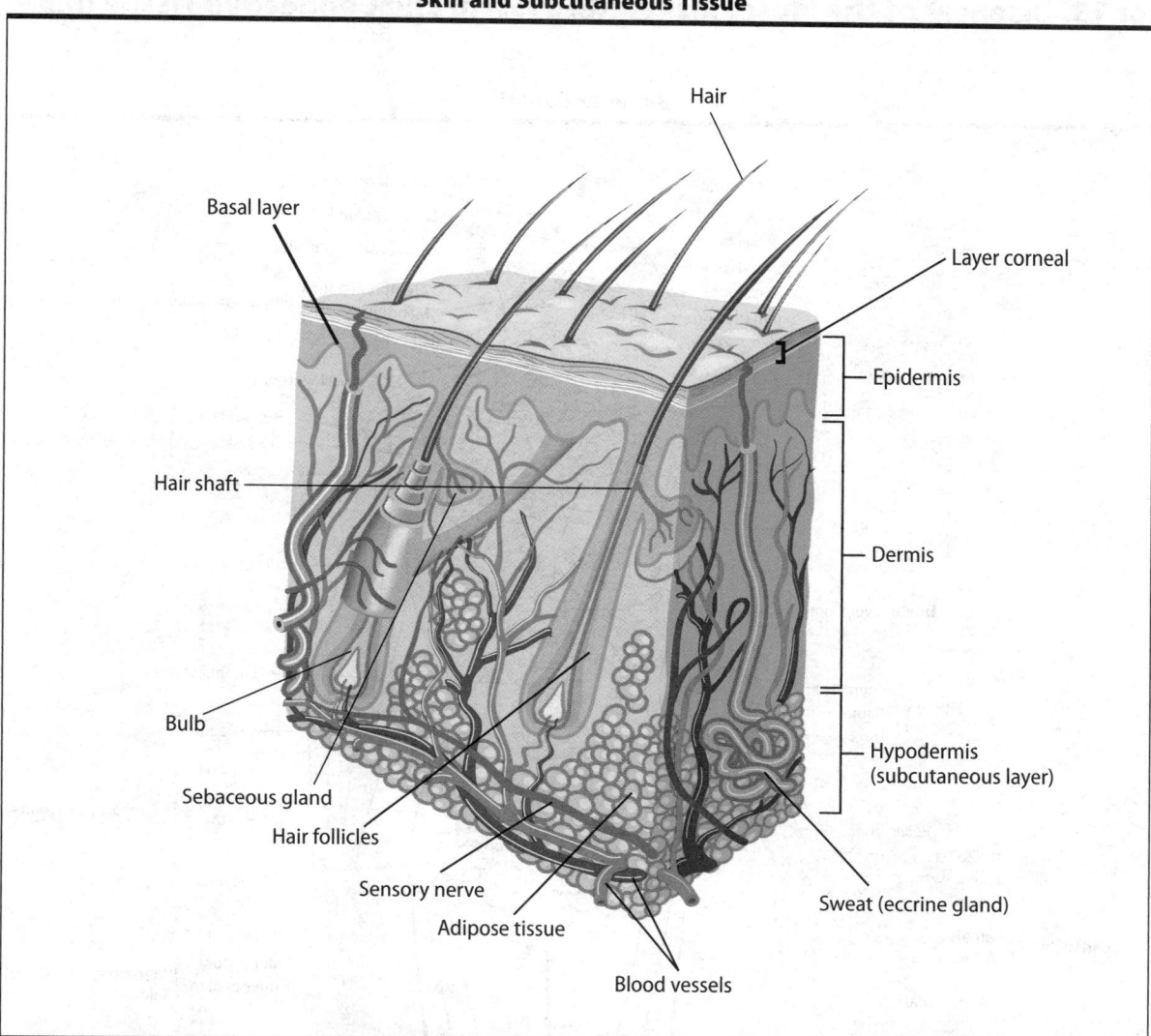

# Chapter 13. Diseases of the Musculoskeletal System and Connective Tissue (MØØ–M99)

## Bones and Joints

## Shoulder Anterior View

## Shoulder Posterior View

## Elbow Anterior View

## Elbow Posterior View

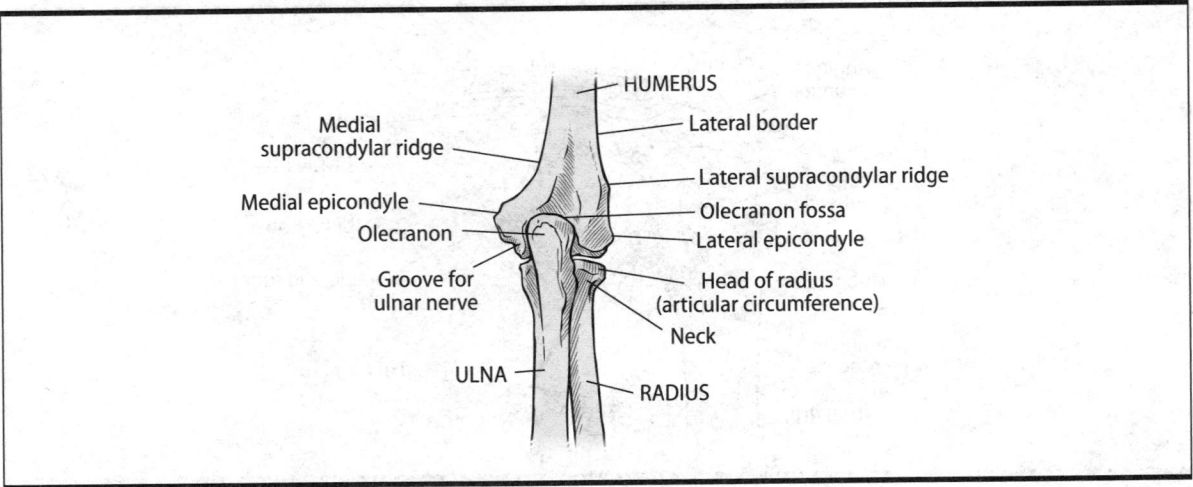

Medial supracondylar ridge

HUMERUS

Lateral border

Lateral supracondylar ridge

Medial epicondyle

Olecranon fossa

Olecranon

Lateral epicondyle

Groove for ulnar nerve

Head of radius (articular circumference)

Neck

ULNA

RADIUS

## Hand

Distal phalanx

Middle phalanx

Phalanges (digits)

Proximal phalanx

Interphalangeal joints

Distal phalanx (thumb)

Metacarpophalangeal joint

Proximal phalanx (thumb)

Metacarpals

5  4  3  2  1

Carpometacarpal joint

Hamate

Trapezium

Pisiform

Carpals

Trapezoid

Scaphoid

Triquetral   Lunate   Cuboid

## Hip Anterior View

## Hip Posterior View

## Knee Anterior View

## Knee Posterior View

## Foot

# Muscles

# Chapter 14. Diseases of the Genitourinary System (NØØ–N99)

**Urinary System**

## Male Genitourinary System

## Female Internal Genitalia

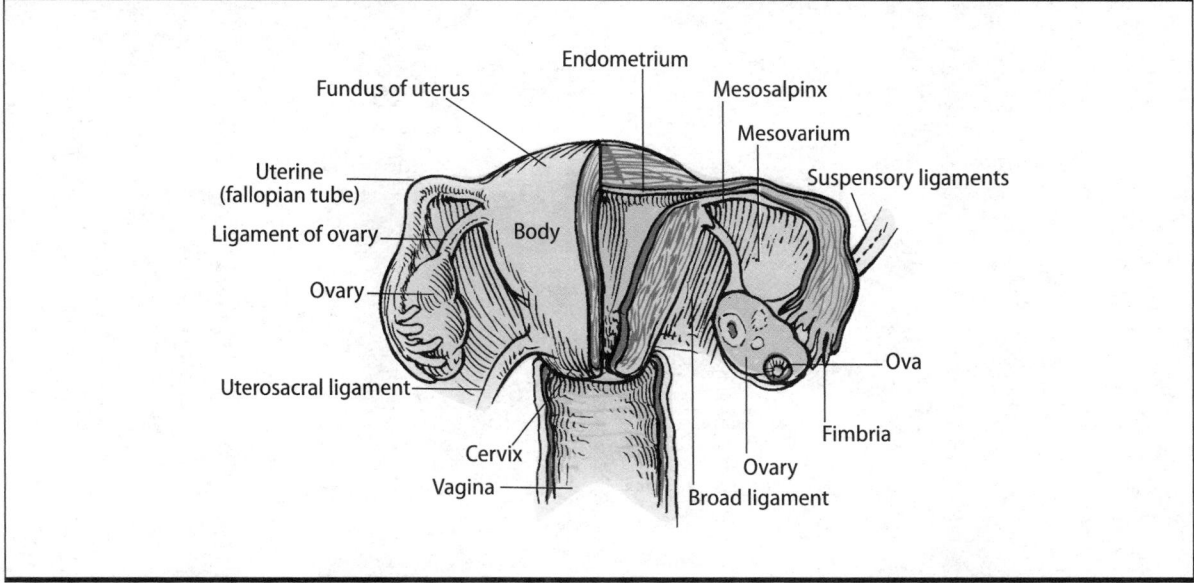

## Female Genitourinary Tract Lateral View

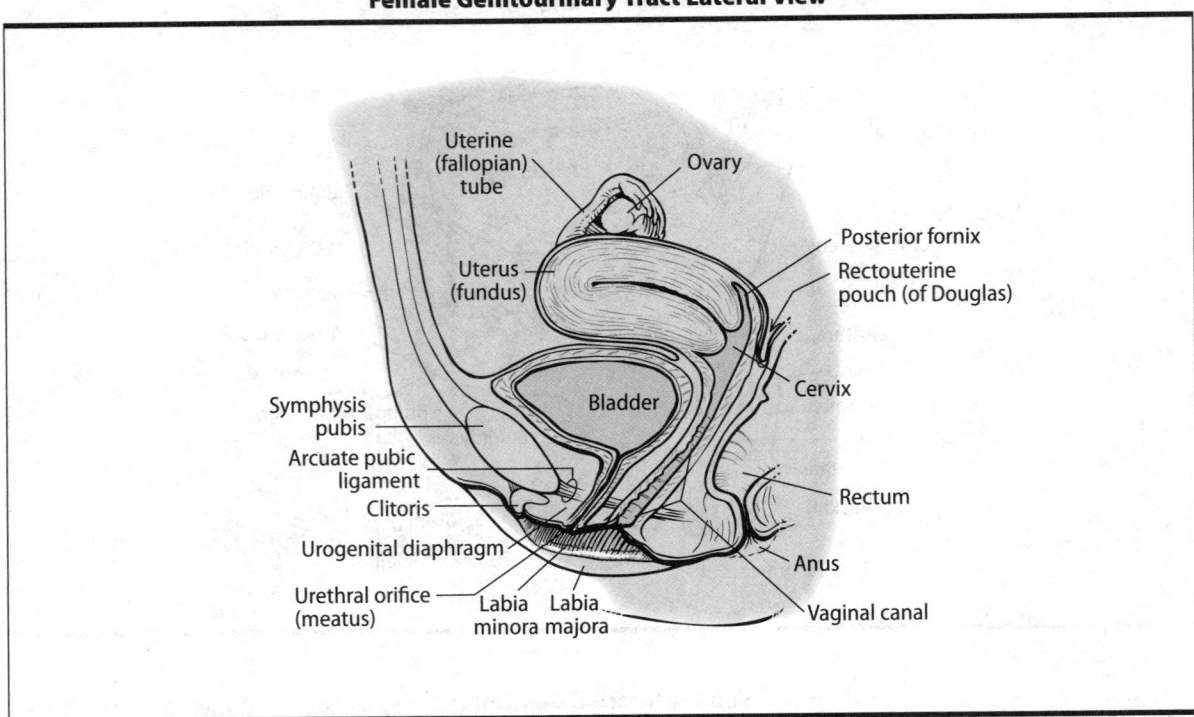

# Chapter 15. Pregnancy, Childbirth and the Puerperium (O00–O9A)

## Term Pregnancy – Single Gestation

## Twin Gestation–Dichorionic–Diamniotic (DI-DI)

## Twin Gestation–Monochorionic–Diamniotic (MO-DI)

1 Chorionic sac

2 Amniotic sacs

2 Fetuses

2 Umbilical cords

1 Placenta

## Twin Gestation–Monochorionic–Monoamniotic (MO-MO)

1 Chorionic sac

1 Amniotic sac

2 Fetuses

2 Umbilical cords

1 Placenta

# Chapter 19. Injury, Poisoning and Certain Other Consequences of External Causes (S00–T88)

## Types of Fractures

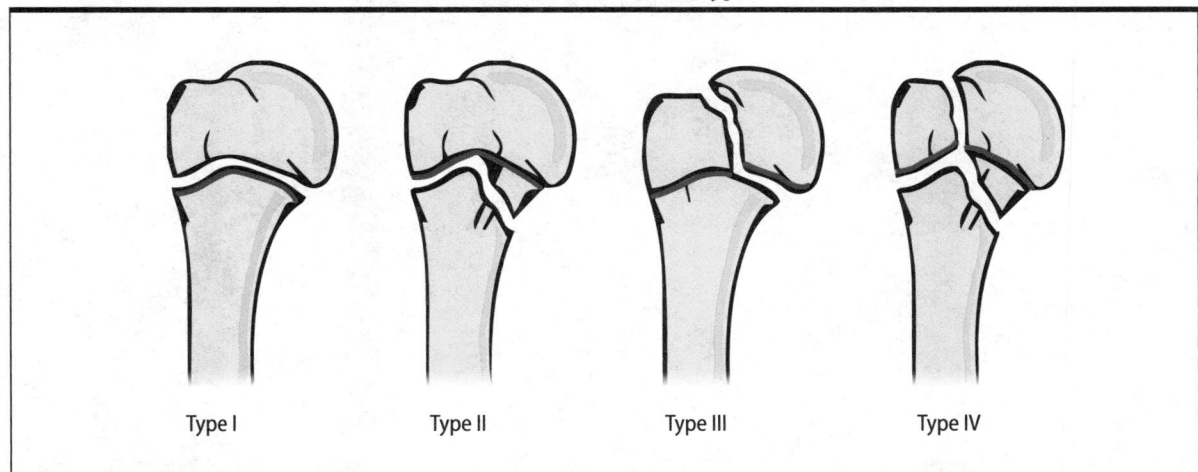

| Normal | Transverse | Open/Compound | Oblique | Oblique displaced |

| Comminuted | Segmental | Avulsed | Spiral | Greenstick |

## Salter-Harris Fracture Types

| Type I | Type II | Type III | Type IV |

# Notes

# Notes